2017 SoftCover
ICD-10-CM

The Educational Annotation of ICD-10-CM

DISEASES TABULAR LIST & INDEX

CRAIG D. PUCKETT

D1370758

Channel Publishing, Ltd.

Complete Official ICD-10-CM Text, FY2017 Version
Effective October 1, 2016
as standardized by
**U.S. DEPARTMENT OF HEALTH AND HUMAN SERVICES
CENTERS FOR DISEASE CONTROL AND PREVENTION
NATIONAL CENTER FOR HEALTH STATISTICS**

ISBN: 978-1-933053-79-0

9 781933 053790

DISCLAIMER

Every effort has been made to ensure the accuracy and reliability of the information contained in this publication. However, complete accuracy cannot be guaranteed. The editor and publisher will not be held responsible or liable for any errors.

Corrections Identification and Reporting

In an effort to provide our customers with the best code books possible, Channel Publishing has added a "Channel Errata Page" for each of its ICD-10 code books on its web site: www.channelpublishing.com. These Channel Errata Pages will be updated whenever an error is identified. Check the appropriate web page periodically for any changes to your Channel Publishing ICD-10 code book.

In addition, if at any time you identify a potential error, please copy the page and fax/mail/e-mail it to: Channel Publishing, Ltd., Attn: ICD-10 Book Production Department, 4750 Longley Lane, Suite 110, Reno, NV 89502. FAX (775) 825-5633. E-mail: info@channelpublishing.com

ICD-10-CM, FY2017 Version, Effective October 1, 2016

This edition contains the Complete, Official ICD-10-CM Text, FY2017 Version as standardized by the U.S. Department of Health and Human Services, Centers for Disease Control and Prevention, National Center for Health Statistics.

Published by CHANNEL PUBLISHING, Ltd., Reno, Nevada

Produced by Craig Puckett, Editor; Susan Dely, Assistant Editor;
Jo Ann Jones, RHIA, CCS, Editorial Assistant; Charisse Puckett, Editorial Assistant;
Trey Puckett, Editorial Assistant

Printed in the United States of America

Additional sets may be ordered from Channel Publishing, Ltd., 4750 Longley Lane, Suite 110, Reno, Nevada 89502, 1-800-248-2882, www.channelpublishing.com

ISBN: 978-1-933053-79-0

Errata #1
for
Channel Publishing's 2017 ICD-10-CM Code Books
2017 ICD-10-CM, The Educational Annotation of ICD-10-CM (All Versions)

Posting Date: October 10, 2016

Publication: 2017 ICD-10-CM, The Educational Annotation of ICD-10-CM (All Binding Versions)

Instructions: Make the Errata corrections below in your book, and keep this Errata page for your reference.

Coding Guidelines, pages: CG-11 and 721

Delete the lined-through words below:

9. Chapter 9: Diseases of Circulatory System (I00-I99)
   a. Hypertension
      1) Hypertension with Heart Disease
      Hypertension with heart conditions classified to I50.- or I51.4-I51.9, are assigned to, a code from category I11, Hypertensive heart disease, when a causal relationship is stated (due to hypertension) or implied (hypertensive).

Index to Diseases

Delete the lined-through 5th digits on the underlined codes as indicated. Although these 5th digit Index changes were included in the 2017 Official Addenda, the corresponding Tabular List codes were not added and therefore do not exist.

Abscess ... (p.6-7)
  intra-abdominal ...
    postprocedural T81.43
  intra-muscular, postprocedural T81.42
  operative wound T81.40
  peritoneum, peritoneal ...
    postoperative T81.43
  postoperative (any site) T81.40
  stitch T81.48
  subcutaneous ...
    postprocedural T81.44
  subphrenic ...
    postoperative T81.43
  wound T81.40

Cellulitis ... (p.61)
  drainage site (following operation) T81.48

Complication ... (p.80)
  surgical procedure ...
    stitch abscess T81.48
    wound infection T81.40

Fever ... (p.166)
  postoperative ...
    due to infection T81.40

Infection ... (p.215, 217)
  due to or resulting from
    surgery T81.40
  operation wound T81.40
  postoperative T81.40
  postoperative wound T81.40
  postprocedural T81.40
    deep incisional surgical site T81.42
    organ and space surgical site T81.43
    sepsis T81.49
    specified surgical site NEC T81.48
    superficial incisional surgical site T81.44

Sepsis ... (p.354-355)
  localized ...
    in operation wound T81.49
  postprocedural T81.49

Stitch (p.367)
  abscess T81.48

4750 Longley Lane, Suite 110 • Reno, NV 89502-5977 • 775-825-0880 • 800-248-2882 • FAX 775-825-5633
Web Site: www.channelpublishing.com • E-Mail: info@channelpublishing.com

Channel Publishing, Ltd.

Publishers of

"THE EDUCATIONAL ANNOTATION OF ICD-10-CM & ICD-10-PCS"

August 2016

Dear ICD-10 Colleague:

First, I would like to personally thank each and every Channel Publishing customer who has purchased and enjoyed our ICD-9-CM and ICD-10 coding products and services over these past 30 years.

Thank you for purchasing Channel Publishing's *2017Educational Annotation of ICD-10-CM* code book. I trust you will enjoy the design, layout, and all the new, coder-helpful features that we have created for you. I would also like to thank everyone who shared their ICD-10 comments and suggestions over the years from our "Preparing for ICD-10" seminars sixteen years ago, to those of you who called or wrote in, and those who stopped by our booth at AHIMA. We listened and made note of those comments and suggestions to bring you what we believe is an excellent ICD-10-CM code book, and at an incredibly low price.

In addition to this *2017 Educational Annotation of ICD-10-CM* code book, I'd like to remind you about all our ICD-10 products and services. Please visit our web site www.channelpublishing.com for details and sample content.

Once again, thank you for your purchase and I look forward to providing quality ICD-10 products and services to you in the years to come.

Sincerely,

Craig D. Puckett

Craig D. Puckett,
President, and Publisher

4750 Longley Lane, Suite 110 • Reno, NV 89502-5977 • (775) 825-0880 • Customer Service 1-800-248-2882 • FAX (775) 825-5633
WEB SITE: www.channelpublishing.com • E-MAIL: info@channelpublishing.com

1. CUSTOMER INFORMATION (Ship books to address below)

❑ Organization or ❑ Individual   ATTN: Name/Title/Dept.   Customer ID #   Order Date

Shipping Address (Street address required for FedEx delivery)   E-Mail Address

City   State   Zip   Telephone   Fax

2. ORDER INFORMATION

Product	See Web Site for Complete Product Descriptions and Sample Pages	Quantity	Regular Price	Fall Sale Price	Total(s)
CODE BOOKS	**2017 ICD-10-CM, The Educational Annotation of ICD-10-CM**			Exp. 12/31/16	
	Annual Version ICD-10-CM (Paperback) (ISBN: 9781933053-**76-9**)		$69⁹⁵ ea.	—	
	Spiral Version ICD-10-CM (Spiral coil) (ISBN: 9781933053-**77-6**)		$74⁹⁵ ea.	—	
	Spiral Version ICD-10-CM with Tabs (Spiral coil) (ISBN: 9781933053-**78-3**)		$89⁹⁵ ea.	—	
	SoftCover Version ICD-10-CM (Vinyl cover, updateable) (ISBN: 9781933053-**79-0**)		$79⁹⁵ ea.	—	
	2017 Update ICD-10-CM (Full text replacement) (ISBN: 9781933053-**80-6**)		$55⁹⁵ ea.	—	
	Tab Set for ICD-10-CM (SoftCover only, reusable) (ITEM: TABCM)		$17⁹⁵ ea.	—	
	2017 ICD-10-PCS, The Educational Annotation of ICD-10-PCS				
	Annual Version ICD-10-PCS (Paperback) (ISBN: 9781933053-**81-3**)		$59⁹⁵ ea.	—	
	Spiral Version ICD-10-PCS (Spiral coil) (ISBN: 9781933053-**82-0**)		$64⁹⁵ ea.	—	
	Spiral Version ICD-10-PCS with Tabs (Spiral coil) (ISBN: 9781933053-**83-7**)		$79⁹⁵ ea.	—	
	SoftCover Version ICD-10-PCS (Vinyl cover, updateable) (ISBN: 9781933053-**84-4**)		$69⁹⁵ ea.	—	
	2017 Update ICD-10-PCS (Full text replacement) (ISBN: 9781933053-**85-1**)		$48⁹⁵ ea.	—	
	Tab Set for ICD-10-PCS (SoftCover only, reusable) (ITEM: TABPCS)		$17⁹⁵ ea.	—	
TRAINING	(Professional Version – Includes: PowerPoint Slides, Instructor's Manual, DVD set, Workbook & Code Book) (Individual Version – Includes: DVD set, Workbook & Code Book - CM-12 CEUs, PCS-20 CEUs)				
	Professional Version – Learning ICD-10-CM (Step 1) (ITEM: SBCM-P)		$599⁹⁵ ea.	$559⁹⁵ ea.	
	Additional Learning ICD-10-CM Workbook & Book Packages (ITEM: ACM16W)		$65⁹⁵ ea.		
	Professional Version – Learning ICD-10-PCS (Step 1) (ITEM: SBPCS-P)		$699⁹⁵ ea.	$649⁹⁵ ea.	
	Additional Learning ICD-10-PCS Workbook & Book Packages (ITEM: APCS16W)		$55⁹⁵ ea.		
	Individual Version – Learning ICD-10-CM (Step 1) (12 CEUs) (ITEM: SBCM-I)		$299⁹⁵ ea.	$269⁹⁵ ea.	
	Individual Version – Learning ICD-10-PCS (Step 1) (20 CEUs) (ITEM: SBPCS-I)		$399⁹⁵ ea.	$359⁹⁵ ea.	
	2016 Mastering ICD-10-CM Exercise Book (Step 2) (ISBN: 9781933053-**88-2**)		$59⁹⁵ ea.	—	
	2016 Mastering ICD-10-PCS Exercise Book (Step 2) (ISBN: 9781933053-**89-9**)		$59⁹⁵ ea.	—	
	2016 Mastering ICD-10-CM Guidelines Exercise Book (Step 3) (ISBN: 9781933053-**90-5**)		$59⁹⁵ ea.	—	
	2016 Mastering ICD-10-PCS Guidelines Exercise Book (Step 3) (ISBN: 9781933053-**91-2**)		$59⁹⁵ ea.	—	
	The Last Word on ICD-10 (Step 4) (ISBN: 9781933053-**61-5**)		$69⁹⁵ ea.	—	
OTHER	**2017 Clinotes for ICD-10-CM** (ISBN: 9781933053-**87-5**)		$39⁹⁵ ea.	$29⁹⁵ ea.	
	2017 Expanded ICD-10-CM Table of Drugs & Chemicals (ISBN: 9781933053-**86-8**)		$39⁹⁵ ea.	$29⁹⁵ ea.	
	Acrylic Bookstand ❑ **One-piece** (ITEM: BSOP) ❑ **Two-piece** (ITEM: BSTP)		$34⁹⁵ ea.		
	CPT® 2017 Standard Edition (ISBN: 978162202-**398-1**)		$94⁹⁵ ea.		
	CPT® 2017 Professional Edition (ISBN: 978162202-**400-1**)		$119⁹⁵ ea.		

- OUTSIDE CONTINENTAL U.S.: Call for rates and shipping options. U.S. Dollars.
- EXPRESS SHIPPING: Call for delivery options and rates.

Fall Sale Prices Expire 12/31/16

Continental U.S. Shipping & Handling	
Less than $50	$7
$50-$99	$12
$100-$199	$19
$200-$299	$29
$300+	$39

Product Subtotal	
Shipping & Handling	
Nevada Res. Only Add Local Sales Tax	
Total Order Amount	

3. PAYMENT METHOD
❑ **Purchase Order** (Attach copy)   ❑ **Check Enclosed**
❑ **Credit Card: MC, VISA, DISC, AMEX** (Charged date order received)

_____

_____ / _____   _____   _____
Exp. Date   Sec. Code   Authorized Cardholder Signature

Billing Address (Street number or PO Box and Zip Code) ❑ Same as shipping

MAKE CHECKS PAYABLE AND MAIL TO:
Channel Publishing, Ltd.
4750 Longley Lane, Suite 110
Reno, NV 89502-5977
1-800-248-2882
(775) 825-0880
Fax (775) 825-5633
E-Mail: info@channelpublishing.com
Web Site: www.channelpublishing.com

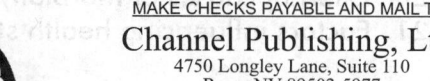

TABLE OF CONTENTS

Disease Index

Disease Tabular

ICD-10-CM PREFACE (FY 2017 Release)

Introduction

This FY 2017 update of the International Statistical Classification of Diseases and Related Health Problems, 10th revision, Clinical Modification (ICD-10-CM) is being published by the United States Government in recognition of its responsibility to promulgate this classification throughout the United States for morbidity coding. The International Statistical Classification of Diseases and Related Health Problems, 10th Revision (ICD-10), published by the World Health Organization (WHO), is the foundation of ICD-10-CM. ICD-10 continues to be the classification used in cause-of-death coding in the United States. The ICD-10-CM is comparable with the ICD-10. The WHO Collaborating Center for the Family of International Classifications in North America, housed at the Centers for Disease Control and Prevention's National Center for Health Statistics (NCHS), has responsibility for the implementation of ICD and other WHO-FIC classifications and serves as a liaison with the WHO, fulfilling international obligations for comparable classifications and the national health data needs of the United States.

Historical background

The historical background of ICD and ICD-10 can be found in the Introduction to the International Classification of Diseases and Related Health Problems (ICD-10), 2008, World Health Organization, Geneva, Switzerland.

Clinical modification

ICD-10-CM is the United States' clinical modification of the World Health Organization's ICD-10. The term "clinical" is used to emphasize the modification's intent: to serve as a useful tool in the area of classification of morbidity data for indexing of health records, medical care review, and ambulatory and other health care programs, as well as for basic health statistics. To describe the clinical picture of the patient the codes must be more precise than those needed only for statistical groupings and trend analysis.

Characteristics of ICD-10-CM

ICD-10-CM far exceeds its predecessors in the number of concepts and codes provided. The disease classification has been expanded to include health-related conditions and to provide greater specificity at the sixth and seventh character level. The sixth and seventh characters are not optional and are intended for use in recording the information documented in the clinical record.

ICD-10-CM extensions, interpretations, modifications, addenda, or errata other than those approved by the Centers for Disease Control and Prevention are not to be considered official and should not be utilized. Continuous maintenance of the ICD-10-CM is the responsibility of the aforementioned agencies. However, because the ICD-10-CM represents the best in contemporary thinking of clinicians, nosologists, epidemiologists, and statisticians from both public and private sectors, when future modifications are considered, advice will be sought from all stakeholders.

All official authorized addenda since the last update, October 1, 2015, have been included in this revision. For more information please see the complete official authorized addenda to ICD-10-CM, including the "ICD-10-CM Official Guidelines for Coding and Reporting," and a description of the ICD-10-CM updating and maintenance process.

The complete official authorized addenda to ICD-10-CM, including the "ICD-10-CM Official Guidelines for Coding and Reporting," can be accessed at the following website:
    http://www.cdc.gov/nchs/icd/icd10cm.htm#10update

A description of the ICD-10-CM updating and maintenance process can be found at the following website:
    http://www.cdc.gov/nchs/icd/icd9cm_maintenance.htm

INTRODUCTION TO ICD-10-CM (FY2017 Release)

The National Center for Health Statistics (NCHS), the Federal agency responsible for use of the International Statistical Classification of Diseases and Related Health Problems, 10th revision (ICD-10) in the United States, has developed a clinical modification of the classification for morbidity purposes. The ICD-10 is used to code and classify mortality data from death certificates, having replaced ICD-9 for this purpose as of January 1, 1999. ICD-10-CM is the replacement for ICD-9-CM, volumes 1 and 2.

The ICD-10 is copyrighted by the World Health Organization (WHO), which owns and publishes the classification. WHO has authorized the development of an adaptation of ICD-10 for use in the United States for U.S. government purposes. As agreed, all modifications to the ICD-10 must conform to WHO conventions for the ICD. ICD-10-CM was developed following a thorough evaluation by a Technical Advisory Panel and extensive additional consultation with physician groups, clinical coders, and others to assure clinical accuracy and utility.

The entire draft of the Tabular List of ICD-10-CM, and the preliminary crosswalk between ICD-9-CM and ICD-10-CM were made available on the NCHS website for public comment. The public comment period ran from December 1997 through February 1998. The American Hospital Association and the American Health Information Management Association conducted a field test for ICD-10-CM in the summer of 2003, with a subsequent report. All comments and suggestions from the open comment period and the field test were reviewed, and additional modifications to ICD-10-CM were made based on these comments and suggestions. Additionally, new concepts have been added to ICD-10-CM based on the established update process for ICD-9-CM (the ICD-9-CM Coordination and Maintenance Committee) and the World Health Organization's ICD-10 (the Update and Revision Committee). This represents ICD-9-CM modifications from 2003-2009 and ICD-10 modifications from 2002-2008.

The clinical modification represents a significant improvement over ICD-9-CM and ICD-10. Specific improvements include: the addition of information relevant to ambulatory and managed care encounters; expanded injury codes; the creation of combination diagnosis/symptom codes to reduce the number of codes needed to fully describe a condition; the addition of sixth and seventh characters; incorporation of common 4th and 5th digit subclassifications; laterality; and greater specificity in code assignment. The new structure will allow further expansion than was possible with ICD-9-CM.

On January 16, 2009 HHS published a Final Rule adopting ICD-10-CM (and ICD-10-PCS) to replace ICD-9-CM in HIPAA transactions, effective implementation date of October 1, 2013 (delayed two years to October 1, 2015).

ICD-10-CM Conventions (FY2017 Version)

The conventions for the ICD-10-CM are the general rules for use of the classification independent of the guidelines. These conventions are incorporated within the **Alphabetic Index** and **Tabular List** of the ICD-10-CM as instructional notes. The conventions and instructions of the classification take precedence over guidelines.

Organization of ICD-10-CM

The ICD-10-CM is divided into the Alphabetic Index, an alphabetical list of terms and their corresponding code, and the Tabular List, a chronological list of codes divided into chapters based on body system or condition.

Alphabetic Index

The Alphabetic Index consists of the following parts:
- Index of Diseases and Injury
- Table of Neoplasms
- Table of Drugs and Chemicals
- Index of External Causes of Injury

Tabular List

The Tabular List consists of the following chapters:
- Chapter 1 – Certain infectious and parasitic diseases (A00-B99)
- Chapter 2 – Neoplasms (C00-D49)
- Chapter 3 – Diseases of the blood and blood-forming organs and certain disorders involving the immune mechanism (D50-D89)
- Chapter 4 – Endocrine, nutritional and metabolic diseases (E00-E89)
- Chapter 5 – Mental, behavioral and neurodevelopmental disorders (F01-F99)
- Chapter 6 – Diseases of the nervous system (G00-G99)
- Chapter 7 – Diseases of the eye and adnexa (H00-H59)
- Chapter 8 – Diseases of the ear and mastoid process (H60-H95)
- Chapter 9 – Diseases of the circulatory system (I00-I99)
- Chapter 10 – Diseases of the respiratory system (J00-J99)
- Chapter 11 – Diseases of the digestive system (K00-K95)
- Chapter 12 – Diseases of the skin and subcutaneous tissue (L00-L99)
- Chapter 13 – Diseases of the musculoskeletal system and connective tissue (M00-M99)
- Chapter 14 – Diseases of the genitourinary system (N00-N99)
- Chapter 15 – Pregnancy, childbirth and the puerperium (O00-O99)
- Chapter 16 – Certain conditions originating in the perinatal period (P00-P96)
- Chapter 17 – Congenital malformations, deformations and chromosomal abnormalities (Q00-Q99)
- Chapter 18 – Symptoms, signs and abnormal clinical and laboratory findings, not elsewhere classified (R00-R99)
- Chapter 19 – Injury, poisoning and certain other consequences of external causes (S00-T88)
- Chapter 20 – External causes of morbidity (V00-Y99)
- Chapter 21 – Factors influencing health status and contact with health services (Z00-Z99)

Appendices

There are no appendices.

How to Use ICD-10-CM, General Coding Guidelines, and Chapter-Specific Coding Guidelines

See the 2017 ICD-10-CM Official Guidelines for Coding and Reporting following this Introduction.

Characteristics of ICD-10-CM

Format and Structure:

The ICD-10-CM Tabular List contains categories, subcategories and codes. Characters for categories, subcategories and codes may be either a letter or a number. All categories are 3 characters. A three-character category that has no further subdivision is equivalent to a code. Subcategories are either 4 or 5 characters. Codes may be 3, 4, 5, 6 or 7 characters. That is, each level of subdivision after a category is a subcategory. The final level of subdivision is a code. Codes that have applicable 7th characters are still referred to as codes, not subcategories. A code that has an applicable 7th character is considered invalid without the 7th character.

The ICD-10-CM uses an indented format for ease in reference.

Use of codes for reporting purposes

For reporting purposes only codes are permissible, not categories or subcategories, and any applicable 7th character is required.

Placeholder character

The ICD-10-CM utilizes a placeholder character "x". The "x" is used as a placeholder at certain codes to allow for future expansion. An example of this is at the poisoning, adverse effect and underdosing codes, categories T36-T50.

Where a placeholder "x" exists, the "x" must be used in order for the code to be considered a valid code.

7th Characters

Certain ICD-10-CM categories have applicable 7th characters. The applicable 7th character is required for all codes within the category, or as the notes in the Tabular List instruct. The 7th character must always be the 7th character in the data field. If a code that requires a 7th character is not 6 characters, a placeholder "x" must be used to fill in the empty characters.

Abbreviations

Alphabetic Index abbreviations

NEC "Not elsewhere classifiable"
This abbreviation in the Alphabetic Index represents "other specified." When a specific code is not available for a condition, the Alphabetic Index directs the coder to the "other specified" code in the Tabular List.

NOS "Not otherwise specified"
This abbreviation is the equivalent of unspecified.

Tabular List abbreviations

NEC "Not elsewhere classifiable"
This abbreviation in the Tabular List represents "other specified." When a specific code is not available for a condition the Tabular List includes an NEC entry under a code to identify the code as the "other specified" code.

NOS "Not otherwise specified"
This abbreviation is the equivalent of unspecified.

Punctuation

[ ] Brackets are used in the Tabular List to enclose synonyms, alternative wording or explanatory phrases. Brackets are used in the Alphabetic Index to identify manifestation codes.

( ) Parentheses are used in both the Alphabetic Index and Tabular List to enclose supplementary words that may be present or absent in the statement of a disease or procedure without affecting the code number to which it is assigned. The terms within the parentheses are referred to as nonessential modifiers.

: Colons are used in the Tabular List after an incomplete term which needs one or more of the modifiers following the colon to make it assignable to a given category.

Use of "and"

When the term "and" is used in a narrative statement it represents and/or.

Other and Unspecified codes

"Other" codes

Codes titled "other" or "other specified" are for use when the information in the medical record provides detail for which a specific code does not exist. Alphabetic Index entries with NEC in the line designate "other" codes in the Tabular List. These Alphabetic Index entries represent specific disease entities for which no specific code exists so the term is included within an "other" code.

"Unspecified" codes

Codes titled "unspecified" are for use when the information in the medical record is insufficient to assign a more specific code. For those categories for which an unspecified code is not provided, the "other specified" code may represent both other and unspecified.

Includes Notes

This note appears immediately under a three character code title to further define, or give examples of, the content of the category.

Inclusion terms

List of terms is included under some codes. These terms are the conditions for which that code is to be used. The terms may be synonyms of the code title, or, in the case of "other specified" codes, the terms are a list of the various conditions assigned to that code. The inclusion terms are not necessarily exhaustive. Additional terms found only in the Alphabetic Index may also be assigned to a code.

Excludes Notes

The ICD-10-CM has two types of excludes notes. Each type of note has a different definition for use but they are all similar in that they indicate that codes excluded from each other are independent of each other.

Excludes 1

A type 1 Excludes note is a pure excludes. It means "NOT CODED HERE!" An Excludes 1 note indicates that the code excluded should never be used at the same time as the code above the Excludes 1 note. An Excludes 1 is used when two conditions cannot occur together, such as a congenital form versus an acquired form of the same condition.

Excludes 2

A type 2 excludes note represents "Not included here". An Excludes 2 note indicates that the condition excluded is not part of the condition it is excluded from but a patient may have both conditions at the same time. When an Excludes 2 note appears under a code it is acceptable to use both the code and the excluded code together.

Etiology/manifestation convention ("code first", "use additional code" and "in diseases classified elsewhere" notes)

Certain conditions have both an underlying etiology and multiple body system manifestations due to the underlying etiology. For such conditions, the ICD-10-CM has a coding convention that requires the underlying condition be sequenced first followed by the manifestation. Wherever such a combination exists, there is a "use additional code" note at the etiology code, and a "code first" note at the manifestation code. These instructional notes indicate the proper sequencing order of the codes, etiology followed by manifestation.

In most cases the manifestation codes will have in the code title, "in diseases classified elsewhere." Codes with this title are a component of the etiology/manifestation convention. The code title indicates that it is a manifestation code. "In diseases classified elsewhere" codes are never permitted to be used as first-listed or principal diagnosis codes. They must be used in conjunction with an underlying condition code and they must be listed following the underlying condition. See category F02, Dementia in other diseases classified elsewhere, for an example of this convention.

There are manifestation codes that do not have "in diseases classified elsewhere" in the title. For such codes a "use additional code" note will still be present and the rules for sequencing apply.

In addition to the notes in the Tabular List, these conditions also have a specific Alphabetic Index entry structure. In the Alphabetic Index both conditions are listed together with the etiology code first followed by the manifestation codes in brackets. The code in brackets is always to be sequenced second.

An example of the etiology/manifestation convention is dementia in Parkinson's disease. In the Alphabetic Index, code G20 is listed first, followed by code F02.80 or F02.81 in brackets. Code G20 represents the underlying etiology, Parkinson's disease, and must be sequenced first, whereas codes F02.80 and F02.81 represent the manifestation of dementia in diseases classified elsewhere, with or without behavioral disturbance.

"Code first" and "Use additional code" notes are also used as sequencing rules in the classification for certain codes that are not part of an etiology/ manifestation combination.

"And"

The word "and" should be interpreted to mean either "and" or "or" when it appears in a title.

"With"

The word "with" should be interpreted to mean "associated with" or "due to" when it appears in a code title, the Alphabetic Index, or an instructional note in the Tabular List.

The word "with" in the Alphabetic Index is sequenced immediately following the main term, not in alphabetical order.

"See" and "See Also"

The "*see*" instruction following a main term in the Alphabetic Index indicates that another term should be referenced. It is necessary to go to the main term referenced with the "*see*" note to locate the correct code.

A "*see also*" instruction following a main term in the Alphabetic Index instructs that there is another main term that may also be referenced that may provide additional Alphabetic Index entries that may be useful. It is not necessary to follow the "*see also*" note when the original main term provides the necessary code.

"Code also note"

A "code also" note instructs that two codes may be required to fully describe a condition, but this note does not provide sequencing direction.

Default codes

A code listed next to a main term in the ICD-10-CM Alphabetic Index is referred to as a default code. The default code represents that condition that is most commonly associated with the main term, or is the unspecified code for the condition. If a condition is documented in a medical record (for example, appendicitis) without any additional information, such as acute or chronic, the default code should be assigned.

Syndromes

Follow the Alphabetic Index guidance when coding syndromes. In the absence of Alphabetic Index guidance, assign codes for the documented manifestations of the syndrome.

Typeface

Bold: Bold typeface is used for all codes and code titles in the Tabular List and for main terms in the Alphabetic Index.

Italics: Italicized typeface is used for all exclusion notes in the Tabular list and for *"see"* and *"see also"* instructions in the Alphabetic Index.

<u>Underscore:</u> See Channel Publishing Additional *Enhanced* Features.

DRG Pinciples and Medicare Code Editor Edits Key

DRG Principles

Identifies codes that are recognized and affected by the DRG Grouper.
- CC – Identifies codes that are defined as a complication or comorbidity when used as a secondary diagnosis.
- MCC – Identifies codes that are defined as a major complication or comorbidity when used as a secondary diagnosis.
- [Not Allowed as PDX] – Identifies codes that are not allowed as a principal diagnosis for an acute care hospital admission.
- [Questionable Admission] – Identifies some diagnoses that are usually not sufficient justification for admission to an acute care hospital.
- [Unacceptable PDX] – Identifies codes that are considered unacceptable as a principal diagnosis for an acute care hospital admission.
- [Wrong Procedure Performed] – Identifies codes that indicate that the wrong procedure was performed.

Medicare Code Editor Edits

Identifies codes that are edit-reviewed for age and sex-related discrepancies and principal diagnosis criteria.
- [♂] – Identifies diagnoses allowed for males.
- [♀] – Identifies diagnoses allowed for females.
- [Age/0] – Identifies perinatal/newborn diagnoses for patient's age of 0 years only.
- [Age/0-17] – Identifies pediatric diagnoses for patient's age range of 0-17 years inclusive.
- [Age/12-55] – Identifies maternity diagnoses for patient's age of 12-55 years inclusive.
- [Age/15-124] – Identifies adult diagnoses for patient's age of 15-124 years inclusive.

Channel Publishing Additional 2017 *Enhanced* Features

Definitions and Illustrations

Medical definitions of diseases written by a coder for coders. Anatomical illustrations with call outs of body parts.

Anatomy and Physiology Reviews

Anatomy and physiology reviews that help coders understand the anatomical structures and physiology of the various systems.

Color Highlighting

Color highlighting of key terms:
- Excludes 1 – Burgundy
- Excludes ❷ – Burgundy
- AHA Coding Clinic® Reference Notations – Burgundy
- Highlighted 7th Digit Subclassifications – Screened Burgundy
- Tab-Edge Printing – Screened Burgundy
- Index "continueds" – Burgundy
- Highlighted columns in Neoplasm Table – Screened Burgundy
- Highlighted columns in Drugs & Chemicals Table – Screened Burgundy

DRG Principles

Identifies codes that are recognized and affected by the DRG Grouper.

Medicare Code Editor Edits

Identifies codes that are edit-reviewed for age and sex-related discrepancies and principal diagnosis criteria.

AHA Coding Clinic® Reference Notations

Identifies AHA Coding Clinic® articles and Q&As (with descriptive title) that have relevant information for certain codes or code categories.

Highlighted Term <u>Differentiation</u>

Selected terms within code categories and code titles have been <u>underscored</u> to help coders more easily and accurately identify the correct code in the Tabular List.

Further use of dashes (-)

All code categories and codes requiring additional digits in the Tabular List have a dash (-) at the end of the last digit that helps coders be aware that additional characters are required for a complete code.

Further use of placeholder "x"

All codes requiring the coder to use the placeholder "x" to make a complete code have been placed in advance to help coders clearly identify when these "x" placeholders are required.

Excludes ❷:

All Excludes 2 listings have a graphic "❷" to help coders more clearly identify those unique excludes notations where a coder may code both conditions, if present.

Excludes 1 and Excludes ❷ key

The short descriptions of Excludes 1 and Excludes ❷ are listed on the bottom of each page throughout the Tabular List to help coders identify the difference between the two without referring back to the introduction.

Highlighted 7th digit subclassifications

Burgundy screen bars over the 7th digit subclassifications in the Tabular List help coders easily identify those code categories requiring a variable 7th digit.

Highlighted columns in the Neoplasm and Drugs & Chemical Tables

Burgundy screen bars over selected columns to help coders easily identify the appropriate column of codes.

Tab-Edge printing

Chapter-by-chapter, and section-by-section stair-stepped, tab-edge printing screen bars with code ranges for that page printed inside that helps coders locate the correct section quickly.

INTRODUCTION TO AHA CODING CLINIC® REFERENCE NOTATIONS

BACKGROUND
AHA Coding Clinic® is a registered trademark of the American Hospital Association. AHA Coding Clinic® Reference Notations is not a product of the American Hospital Association, and Channel Publishing, Ltd. is not affiliated with or endorsed by the American Hospital Association. The American Hospital coding website can be accessed at www.ahacentraloffice.org.

The AHA Coding Clinic® for ICD-10-CM/PCS is published quarterly by the American Hospital Association. The *Coding Clinic* is the official publication for *ICD-10-CM/PCS* coding guidelines and advice as designated by the four cooperating parties. The cooperating parties listed below have final approval of the coding advice provided in the *Coding Clinic*: American Hospital Association, American Health Information Management Association, Centers for Medicare and Medicaid Services, National Center for Health Statistics.

The *Coding Clinic* provides specific information and guidelines that are helpful for determining proper coding, and is used by CMS in reviewing claims. The goal of the *Coding Clinic* is to provide coding advice, official coding decisions, and news. It promotes accuracy and consistency in the use of ICD-10-CM/PCS. It offers coding guidelines and advice based on adherence to the statistical classification scheme of ICD-10-CM/PCS and the definitions specified in the Uniform Hospital Discharge Data Set (UHDDS).

INTRODUCTION
Channel Publishing has developed the AHA Coding Clinic® Reference Notations to help coders access the official coding advice found throughout all issues of the *Coding Clinic*. This information has been referenced in two ways: 1) direct code-by-code reference notations, 2) a categorical index of articles that are too broad in scope to be assigned to a particular code. Any comments regarding these reference notations should be directed to: *Coding Clinic* Reference Notations, c/o Channel Publishing, Ltd., 4750 Longley Lane, Suite 110, Reno, Nevada 89502.

GUIDANCE IN USE
Coders are encouraged to reference all relevant information contained in the *Coding Clinic* to promote the most accurate coding possible for their organization. It is important to understand the basic criteria for assigning the *Coding Clinic* Reference Notations. The basic criteria consists of: Assignment to codes with direct or indirect information concerning the proper use of each particular code, assignment to a code category when the information is relevant to all codes in that category, and assignment to codes where a coder might commonly attempt to use a code in error.

AHA CODING CLINIC® REFERENCE NOTATION INDEX

AHA CODING CLINIC® REFERENCE NOTATION INDEX – *continued*

2017 OFFICIAL CODING GUIDELINES

TABLE OF CONTENTS

**2017 ICD-10-CM Official Guidelines for Coding and Reporting
FY 2017 (October 1, 2016 – September 30, 2017)**

Channel Publishing Changes Highlighting
The Channel Publishing highlighting is designed to show what has changed in the Official Coding Guidelines from the 2016 to 2017 version including text that has been deleted or replaced.

- **Additions and revisions are in** burgundy-colored type
- **Deletions are in** burgundy-colored type with ~~strikethrough~~
- **Items/text moved within the guidelines since the 2016 version are** underlined **in** burgundy-colored type
- **Revisions to headings are in** burgundy-colored *italics* type

The Centers for Medicare and Medicaid Services (CMS) and the National Center for Health Statistics (NCHS), two departments within the U.S. Federal Government's Department of Health and Human Services (DHHS) provide the following guidelines for coding and reporting using the International Classification of Diseases, 10th Revision, Clinical Modification (ICD-10-CM). These guidelines should be used as a companion document to the official version of the ICD-10-CM as published on the NCHS website. The ICD-10-CM is a morbidity classification published by the United States for classifying diagnoses and reason for visits in all health care settings. The ICD-10-CM is based on the ICD-10, the statistical classification of disease published by the World Health Organization (WHO).

These guidelines have been approved by the four organizations that make up the Cooperating Parties for the ICD-10-CM: the American Hospital Association (AHA), the American Health Information Management Association (AHIMA), CMS, and NCHS.

These guidelines are a set of rules that have been developed to accompany and complement the official conventions and instructions provided within the ICD-10-CM itself. The instructions and conventions of the classification take precedence over guidelines. These guidelines are based on the coding and sequencing instructions in the Tabular List and Alphabetic Index of ICD-10-CM, but provide additional instruction. Adherence to these guidelines when assigning ICD-10-CM diagnosis codes is required under the Health Insurance Portability and Accountability Act (HIPAA). The diagnosis codes (Tabular List and Alphabetic Index) have been adopted under HIPAA for all healthcare settings. A joint effort between the healthcare provider and the coder is essential to achieve complete and accurate documentation, code assignment, and reporting of diagnoses and procedures. These guidelines have been developed to assist both the healthcare provider and the coder in identifying those diagnoses and procedures that are to be reported. The importance of consistent, complete documentation in the medical record cannot be overemphasized. Without such documentation accurate coding cannot be achieved. The entire record should be reviewed to determine the specific reason for the encounter and the conditions treated.

The term encounter is used for all settings, including hospital admissions. In the context of these guidelines, the term provider is used throughout the guidelines to mean physician or any qualified health care practitioner who is legally accountable for establishing the patient's diagnosis. Only this set of guidelines, approved by the Cooperating Parties, is official.

The guidelines are organized into sections. Section I includes the structure and conventions of the classification and general guidelines that apply to the entire classification, and chapter-specific guidelines that correspond to the chapters as they are arranged in the classification. Section II includes guidelines for selection of principal diagnosis for non-outpatient settings. Section III includes guidelines for reporting additional diagnoses in non-outpatient settings. Section IV is for outpatient coding and reporting. It is necessary to review all sections of the guidelines to fully understand all of the rules and instructions needed to code properly.

ICD-10-CM Official Guidelines Table of Contents

GUIDELINES

TABLE OF CONTENTS

SECTION I – CONVENTIONS
Section I. A. 1.

Section I. Conventions, general coding guidelines and chapter specific guidelines

The conventions, general guidelines and chapter-specific guidelines are applicable to all health care settings unless otherwise indicated. The conventions and instructions of the classification take precedence over guidelines.

A.   Conventions for the ICD-10-CM

The conventions for the ICD-10-CM are the general rules for use of the classification independent of the guidelines. These conventions are incorporated within the Alphabetic Index and Tabular List of the ICD-10-CM as instructional notes.

1.   The Alphabetic Index and Tabular List
The ICD-10-CM is divided into the Alphabetic Index, an alphabetical list of terms and their corresponding code, and the Tabular List, a structured list of codes divided into chapters based on body system or condition. The Alphabetic Index consists of the following parts: the Index of Diseases and Injury, the Index of External Causes of Injury, the Table of Neoplasms and the Table of Drugs and Chemicals.

See Section I.C2. General guidelines
See Section I.C.19. Adverse effects, poisoning, underdosing and toxic effects

2.   Format and Structure
The ICD-10-CM Tabular List contains categories, subcategories and codes. Characters for categories, subcategories and codes may be either a letter or a number. All categories are 3 characters. A three-character category that has no further subdivision is equivalent to a code. Subcategories are either 4 or 5 characters. Codes may be 3, 4, 5, 6 or 7 characters. That is, each level of subdivision after a category is a subcategory. The final level of subdivision is a code. Codes that have applicable 7th characters are still referred to as codes, not subcategories. A code that has an applicable 7th character is considered invalid without the 7th character.

The ICD-10-CM uses an indented format for ease in reference.

3.   Use of codes for reporting purposes
For reporting purposes only codes are permissible, not categories or subcategories, and any applicable 7th character is required.

4.   Placeholder character
The ICD-10-CM utilizes a placeholder character "X". The "X" is used as a placeholder at certain codes to allow for future expansion. An example of this is at the poisoning, adverse effect and underdosing codes, categories T36-T50.

Where a placeholder exists, the X must be used in order for the code to be considered a valid code.

5.   7th Characters
Certain ICD-10-CM categories have applicable 7th characters. The applicable 7th character is required for all codes within the category, or as the notes in the Tabular List instruct. The 7th character must always be the 7th character in the data field. If a code that requires a 7th character is not 6 characters, a placeholder X must be used to fill in the empty characters.

6.   Abbreviations

a.   Alphabetic Index abbreviations
NEC "Not elsewhere classifiable"
This abbreviation in the Alphabetic Index represents "other specified". When a specific code is not available for a condition, the Alphabetic Index directs the coder to the "other specified" code in the Tabular List.

NOS "Not otherwise specified"
This abbreviation is the equivalent of unspecified.

b.   Tabular List abbreviations
NEC "Not elsewhere classifiable"
This abbreviation in the Tabular List represents "other specified". When a specific code is not available for a condition, the Tabular List includes an NEC entry under a code to identify the code as the "other specified" code.

NOS "Not otherwise specified"
This abbreviation is the equivalent of unspecified.

7.   Punctuation
[ ] Brackets are used in the Tabular List to enclose synonyms, alternative wording or explanatory phrases. Brackets are used in the Alphabetic Index to identify manifestation codes.

SECTION I – CONVENTIONS
Section I. A. 8.

( ) Parentheses are used in both the Alphabetic Index and Tabular List to enclose supplementary words that may be present or absent in the statement of a disease or procedure without affecting the code number to which it is assigned. The terms within the parentheses are referred to as nonessential modifiers. The nonessential modifiers in the Alphabetic Index to Diseases apply to subterms following a main term except when a nonessential modifier and a subentry are mutually exclusive, the subentry takes precedence. For example, in the ICD-10-CM Alphabetic Index under the main term Enteritis, "acute" is a nonessential modifier and "chronic" is a subentry. In this case, the nonessential modifier "acute" does not apply to the subentry "chronic".

: Colons are used in the Tabular List after an incomplete term which needs one or more of the modifiers following the colon to make it assignable to a given category.

8.   Use of "and"
See Section I.A.14. Use of the term "And".

9.   Other and Unspecified codes

a.   "Other" codes
Codes titled "other" or "other specified" are for use when the information in the medical record provides detail for which a specific code does not exist. Alphabetic Index entries with NEC in the line designate "other" codes in the Tabular List. These Alphabetic Index entries represent specific disease entities for which no specific code exists so the term is included within an "other" code.

b.   "Unspecified" codes
Codes titled "unspecified" are for use when the information in the medical record is insufficient to assign a more specific code. For those categories for which an unspecified code is not provided, the "other specified" code may represent both other and unspecified.

See Section I.B.18 Use of Sign/Symptom/Unspecified Codes.

10.   Includes Notes
This note appears immediately under a three character code title to further define, or give examples of, the content of the category.

11.   Inclusion terms
List of terms is included under some codes. These terms are the conditions for which that code is to be used. The terms may be synonyms of the code title, or, in the case of "other specified" codes, the terms are a list of the various conditions assigned to that code. The inclusion terms are not necessarily exhaustive. Additional terms found only in the Alphabetic Index may also be assigned to a code.

12.   Excludes Notes
The ICD-10-CM has two types of excludes notes. Each type of note has a different definition for use but they are all similar in that they indicate that codes excluded from each other are independent of each other.

a.   Excludes 1
A type 1 Excludes note is a pure excludes note. It means "NOT CODED HERE!" An Excludes1 note indicates that the code excluded should never be used at the same time as the code above the Excludes1 note. An Excludes1 is used when two conditions cannot occur together, such as a congenital form versus an acquired form of the same condition.

b.   Excludes 2
A type 2 Excludes note represents "Not included here". An Excludes2 note indicates that the condition excluded is not part of the condition represented by the code, but a patient may have both conditions at the same time. When an Excludes2 note appears under a code, it is acceptable to use both the code and the excluded code together, when appropriate.

An exception to the Excludes1 definition is the circumstance when the two conditions are unrelated to each other. If it is not clear whether the two conditions involving an Excludes1 note are related or not, query the provider. For example, code F45.8, Other somatoform disorders, has an Excludes1 note for "sleep related teeth grinding (G47.63)," because "teeth grinding" is an inclusion term under F45.8. Only one of these two codes should be assigned for teeth grinding. However psychogenic dysmenorrhea is also an inclusion term under F45.8, and a patient could have both this condition and sleep related teeth grinding. In this case, the two conditions are clearly unrelated to each other, and so it would be appropriate to report F45.8 and G47.63 together.

13.   Etiology/manifestation convention ("code first", "use additional code" and "in diseases classified elsewhere" notes)
Certain conditions have both an underlying etiology and multiple body system manifestations due to the underlying etiology. For such conditions, the ICD-10-CM has a coding convention that requires the underlying condition be sequenced first, if applicable, followed by the manifestation. Wherever such a combination exists, there is a "use additional code" note at the etiology code, and a "code first" note at the manifestation code. These instructional notes indicate the proper sequencing order of the codes, etiology followed by manifestation.

SECTION I – CONVENTIONS
Section I. A. 14.

In most cases the manifestation codes will have in the code title, "in diseases classified elsewhere." Codes with this title are a component of the etiology/ manifestation convention. The code title indicates that it is a manifestation code. "In diseases classified elsewhere" codes are never permitted to be used as first-listed or principal diagnosis codes. They must be used in conjunction with an underlying condition code and they must be listed following the underlying condition. See category F02, Dementia in other diseases classified elsewhere, for an example of this convention.

There are manifestation codes that do not have "in diseases classified elsewhere" in the title. For such codes, there is a "use additional code" note at the etiology code and a "code first" note at the manifestation code and the rules for sequencing apply.

In addition to the notes in the Tabular List, these conditions also have a specific Alphabetic Index entry structure. In the Alphabetic Index both conditions are listed together with the etiology code first followed by the manifestation codes in brackets. The code in brackets is always to be sequenced second.

An example of the etiology/manifestation convention is dementia in Parkinson's disease. In the Alphabetic Index, code G20 is listed first, followed by code F02.80 or F02.81 in brackets. Code G20 represents the underlying etiology, Parkinson's disease, and must be sequenced first, whereas codes F02.80 and F02.81 represent the manifestation of dementia in diseases classified elsewhere, with or without behavioral disturbance.

"Code first" and "Use additional code" notes are also used as sequencing rules in the classification for certain codes that are not part of an etiology/ manifestation combination.

See Section I.B.7. Multiple coding for a single condition.

14. "And"
The word "and" should be interpreted to mean either "and" or "or" when it appears in a title.

For example, cases of "tuberculosis of bones", "tuberculosis of joints" and "tuberculosis of bones and joints" are classified to subcategory A18.0, Tuberculosis of bones and joints.

15. "With"
The word "with" should be interpreted to mean "associated with" or "due to" when it appears in a code title, the Alphabetic Index, or an instructional note in the Tabular List. The classification presumes a causal relationship between the two conditions linked by these terms in the Alphabetic Index or Tabular List. These conditions should be coded as related even in the absence of provider documentation explicitly linking them, unless the documentation clearly states the conditions are unrelated. For conditions not specifically linked by these relational terms in the classification, provider documentation must link the conditions in order to code them as related.

The word "with" in the Alphabetic Index is sequenced immediately following the main term, not in alphabetical order.

16. "See" and "See Also"
The "see" instruction following a main term in the Alphabetic Index indicates that another term should be referenced. It is necessary to go to the main term referenced with the "see" note to locate the correct code.

A "see also" instruction following a main term in the Alphabetic Index instructs that there is another main term that may also be referenced that may provide additional Alphabetic Index entries that may be useful. It is not necessary to follow the "see also" note when the original main term provides the necessary code.

17. "Code also note"
A "code also" note instructs that two codes may be required to fully describe a condition, but this note does not provide sequencing direction.

18. Default codes
A code listed next to a main term in the ICD-10-CM Alphabetic Index is referred to as a default code. The default code represents that condition that is most commonly associated with the main term, or is the unspecified code for the condition. If a condition is documented in a medical record (for example, appendicitis) without any additional information, such as acute or chronic, the default code should be assigned.

19. Code assignment and Clinical Criteria
The assignment of a diagnosis code is based on the provider's diagnostic statement that the condition exists. The provider's statement that the patient has a particular condition is sufficient. Code assignment is not based on clinical criteria used by the provider to establish the diagnosis.

SECTION I – CONVENTIONS
Section I. B. 1.

B. General Coding Guidelines

1. Locating a code in the ICD-10-CM
To select a code in the classification that corresponds to a diagnosis or reason for visit documented in a medical record, first locate the term in the Alphabetic Index, and then verify the code in the Tabular List. Read and be guided by instructional notations that appear in both the Alphabetic Index and the Tabular List.

It is essential to use both the Alphabetic Index and Tabular List when locating and assigning a code. The Alphabetic Index does not always provide the full code. Selection of the full code, including laterality and any applicable 7th character can only be done in the Tabular List. A dash (-) at the end of an Alphabetic Index entry indicates that additional characters are required. Even if a dash is not included at the Alphabetic Index entry, it is necessary to refer to the Tabular List to verify that no 7th character is required.

2. Level of Detail in Coding
Diagnosis codes are to be used and reported at their highest number of characters available.

ICD-10-CM diagnosis codes are composed of codes with 3, 4, 5, 6 or 7 characters. Codes with three characters are included in ICD-10-CM as the heading of a category of codes that may be further subdivided by the use of fourth and/or fifth characters and/or sixth characters, which provide greater detail.

A three-character code is to be used only if it is not further subdivided. A code is invalid if it has not been coded to the full number of characters required for that code, including the 7th character, if applicable.

3. Code or codes from A00.0 through T88.9, Z00-Z99.8
The appropriate code or codes from A00.0 through T88.9, Z00-Z99.8 must be used to identify diagnoses, symptoms, conditions, problems, complaints or other reason(s) for the encounter/visit.

4. Signs and symptoms
Codes that describe symptoms and signs, as opposed to diagnoses, are acceptable for reporting purposes when a related definitive diagnosis has not been established (confirmed) by the provider. Chapter 18 of ICD-10-CM, Symptoms, Signs, and Abnormal Clinical and Laboratory Findings, Not Elsewhere Classified (codes R00.0 - R99) contains many, but not all codes for symptoms.

See Section I.B.18 Use of Sign/Symptom/Unspecified Codes.

5. Conditions that are an integral part of a disease process
Signs and symptoms that are associated routinely with a disease process should not be assigned as additional codes, unless otherwise instructed by the classification.

6. Conditions that are not an integral part of a disease process
Additional signs and symptoms that may not be associated routinely with a disease process should be coded when present.

7. Multiple coding for a single condition
In addition to the etiology/manifestation convention that requires two codes to fully describe a single condition that affects multiple body systems, there are other single conditions that also require more than one code. "Use additional code" notes are found in the Tabular List at codes that are not part of an etiology/manifestation pair where a secondary code is useful to fully describe a condition. The sequencing rule is the same as the etiology/manifestation pair, "use additional code" indicates that a secondary code should be added.

For example, for bacterial infections that are not included in chapter 1, a secondary code from category B95, Streptococcus, Staphylococcus, and Enterococcus, as the cause of diseases classified elsewhere, or B96, Other bacterial agents as the cause of diseases classified elsewhere, may be required to identify the bacterial organism causing the infection. A "use additional code" note will normally be found at the infectious disease code, indicating a need for the organism code to be added as a secondary code.

"Code first" notes are also under certain codes that are not specifically manifestation codes but may be due to an underlying cause. When there is a "code first" note and an underlying condition is present, the underlying condition should be sequenced first.

"Code, if applicable, any causal condition first" notes indicate that this code may be assigned as a principal diagnosis when the causal condition is unknown or not applicable. If a causal condition is known, then the code for that condition should be sequenced as the principal or first-listed diagnosis.

Multiple codes may be needed for sequela, complication codes and obstetric codes to more fully describe a condition. See the specific guidelines for these conditions for further instruction.

8. Acute and Chronic Conditions
If the same condition is described as both acute (subacute) and chronic, and separate subentries exist in the Alphabetic Index at the same indentation level, code both and sequence the acute (subacute) code first.

9. Combination Code
A combination code is a single code used to classify:
    Two diagnoses, or
    A diagnosis with an associated secondary process (manifestation)
    A diagnosis with an associated complication

Combination codes are identified by referring to subterm entries in the Alphabetic Index and by reading the inclusion and exclusion notes in the Tabular List.

Assign only the combination code when that code fully identifies the diagnostic conditions involved or when the Alphabetic Index so directs. Multiple coding should not be used when the classification provides a combination code that clearly identifies all of the elements documented in the diagnosis. When the combination code lacks necessary specificity in describing the manifestation or complication, an additional code should be used as a secondary code.

10. Sequela (Late Effects)
A sequela is the residual effect (condition produced) after the acute phase of an illness or injury has terminated. There is no time limit on when a sequela code can be used. The residual may be apparent early, such as in cerebral infarction, or it may occur months or years later, such as that due to a previous injury. Examples of sequela include: scar formation resulting from a burn, deviated septum due to a nasal fracture, and infertility due to tubal occlusion from old tuberculosis. Coding of sequela generally requires two codes sequenced in the following order: The condition or nature of the sequela is sequenced first. The sequela code is sequenced second.

An exception to the above guidelines are those instances where the code for sequela is followed by a manifestation code identified in the Tabular List and title, or the sequela code has been expanded (at the fourth, fifth or sixth character levels) to include the manifestation(s). The code for the acute phase of an illness or injury that led to the sequela is never used with a code for the late effect.

See Section I.C.9. Sequelae of cerebrovascular disease.
See Section I.C.15. Sequelae of complication of pregnancy, childbirth and the puerperium.
See Section I.C.19. Application of 7th characters for Chapter 19.

11. Impending or Threatened Condition
Code any condition described at the time of discharge as "impending" or "threatened" as follows:
    If it did occur, code as confirmed diagnosis.
    If it did not occur, reference the Alphabetic Index to determine if the condition has a subentry term for "impending" or "threatened" and also reference main term entries for "Impending" and for "Threatened."
    If the subterms are listed, assign the given code.
    If the subterms are not listed, code the existing underlying condition(s) and not the condition described as impending or threatened.

12. Reporting Same Diagnosis Code More than Once
Each unique ICD-10-CM diagnosis code may be reported only once for an encounter. This applies to bilateral conditions when there are no distinct codes identifying laterality or two different conditions classified to the same ICD-10-CM diagnosis code.

13. Laterality
Some ICD-10-CM codes indicate laterality, specifying whether the condition occurs on the left, right or is bilateral. If no bilateral code is provided and the condition is bilateral, assign separate codes for both the left and right side. If the side is not identified in the medical record, assign the code for the unspecified side.

When a patient has a bilateral condition and each side is treated during separate encounters, assign the "bilateral" code (as the condition still exists on both sides), including for the encounter to treat the first side. For the second encounter for treatment after one side has previously been treated and the condition no longer exists on that side, assign the appropriate unilateral code for the side where the condition still exists (e.g., cataract surgery performed on each eye in separate encounters). The bilateral code would not be assigned for the subsequent encounter, as the patient no longer has the condition in the previously-treated site. If the treatment on the first side did not completely resolve the condition, then the bilateral code would still be appropriate.

14. Documentation for BMI, *Depth of* Non-pressure ulcers, Pressure Ulcer Stages, *Coma Scale, and NIH Stroke Scale*
For the Body Mass Index (BMI), depth of non-pressure chronic ulcers, pressure ulcer stage, coma scale, and NIH stroke scale (NIHSS) codes, code assignment may be based on medical record documentation from clinicians who are not the patient's provider (i.e., physician or other qualified healthcare practitioner legally accountable for establishing the patient's diagnosis), since this information is typically documented by other clinicians involved in the care of the patient (e.g., a dietitian often documents the BMI, a nurse often documents the pressure ulcer stages, and an emergency medical technician often documents the coma scale). However, the associated diagnosis (such as overweight, obesity, acute stroke, or pressure ulcer) must be documented by the patient's provider. If there is conflicting medical record documentation, either from the same clinician or different clinicians, the patient's attending provider should be queried for clarification.

The BMI, coma scale, and NIHSS codes should only be reported as secondary diagnoses. As with all other secondary diagnosis codes, the BMI codes should only be assigned when they meet the definition of a reportable additional diagnosis (see Section III, Reporting Additional Diagnoses).

15. Syndromes
Follow the Alphabetic Index guidance when coding syndromes. In the absence of Alphabetic Index guidance, assign codes for the documented manifestations of the syndrome. Additional codes for manifestations that are not an integral part of the disease process may also be assigned when the condition does not have a unique code.

16. Documentation of Complications of Care
Code assignment is based on the provider's documentaion of the relationship between the condition and the care or procedure, unless otherwise instructed by the classification. The guideline extends to any complications of care, regardless of the chapter the code is located in. It is important to note that not all conditions that occur during or following medical care or surgery are classified as complications. There must be a cause-and-effect relationship between the care provided and the condition, and an indication in the documentation that it is a complication. Query the provider for clarification, if the complication is not clearly documented.

17. Borderline diagnosis
If the provider documents a "borderline" diagnosis at the time of discharge, the diagnosis is coded as confirmed, unless the classification provides a specific entry (e.g., borderline diabetes). If a borderline condition has a specific index entry in ICD-10-CM, it should be coded as such. Since borderline conditions are not uncertain diagnoses, no distinction is made between the care setting (inpatient versus outpatient). Whenever the documentation is unclear regarding a borderline condition, coders are encouraged to query for clarification.

18. Use of Sign/Symptom/Unspecified Codes
Sign/symptom and "unspecified" codes have acceptable, even necessary, uses. While specific diagnosis codes should be reported when they are supported by the available medical record documentation and clinical knowledge of the patient's health condition, there are instances when signs/symptoms or unspecified codes are the best choices for accurately reflecting the healthcare encounter. Each healthcare encounter should be coded to the level of certainty known for that encounter.

If a definitive diagnosis has not been established by the end of the encounter, it is appropriate to report codes for sign(s) and/or symptoms(s) in lieu of a definitive diagnosis. When sufficient clinical information isn't known or available about a particular health condition to assign a more specific code, it is acceptable to report the appropriate "unspecified" code (e.g., a diagnosis of pneumonia has been determined, but not the specific type). Unspecified codes should be reported when they are the codes that most accurately reflects what is known about the patient's condition at the time of that particular encounter. It would be inappropriate to select a specific code that is not supported by the medical record documentation or conduct medically unnecessary diagnostic testing in order to determine a more specific code.

CHAPTER 1 – INFECTIOUS DISEASES
Section I. C. 1.

C. Chapter-Specific Coding Guidelines
In addition to general coding guidelines, there are guidelines for specific diagnoses and/or conditions in the classification. Unless otherwise indicated, these guidelines apply to all health care settings. Please refer to Section II for guidelines on the selection of principal diagnosis.

1. Chapter 1: Certain Infectious and Parasitic Diseases (A00-B99)

a. Human Immunodeficiency Virus (HIV) Infections

1) Code only confirmed cases
Code only confirmed cases of HIV infection/illness. This is an exception to the hospital inpatient guideline Section II, H.

In this context, "confirmation" does not require documentation of positive serology or culture for HIV; the provider's diagnostic statement that the patient is HIV positive, or has an HIV-related illness is sufficient.

2) Selection and sequencing of HIV codes

(a) Patient admitted for HIV-related condition
If a patient is admitted for an HIV-related condition, the principal diagnosis should be B20, Human immunodeficiency virus [HIV] disease followed by additional diagnosis codes for all reported HIV-related conditions.

(b) Patient with HIV disease admitted for unrelated condition
If a patient with HIV disease is admitted for an unrelated condition (such as a traumatic injury), the code for the unrelated condition (e.g., the nature of injury code) should be the principal diagnosis. Other diagnoses would be B20 followed by additional diagnosis codes for all reported HIV-related conditions.

(c) Whether the patient is newly diagnosed
Whether the patient is newly diagnosed or has had previous admissions/encounters for HIV conditions is irrelevant to the sequencing decision.

(d) Asymptomatic human immunodeficiency virus
Z21, Asymptomatic human immunodeficiency virus [HIV] infection status, is to be applied when the patient without any documentation of symptoms is listed as being "HIV positive," "known HIV," "HIV test positive," or similar terminology. Do not use this code if the term "AIDS" is used or if the patient is treated for any HIV-related illness or is described as having any condition(s) resulting from his/her HIV positive status; use B20 in these cases.

(e) Patients with inconclusive HIV serology
Patients with inconclusive HIV serology, but no definitive diagnosis or manifestations of the illness, may be assigned code R75, Inconclusive laboratory evidence of human immunodeficiency virus [HIV].

(f) Previously diagnosed HIV-related illness
Patients with any known prior diagnosis of an HIV-related illness should be coded to B20. Once a patient has developed an HIV-related illness, the patient should always be assigned code B20 on every subsequent admission/encounter. Patients previously diagnosed with any HIV illness (B20) should never be assigned to R75 or Z21, Asymptomatic human immunodeficiency virus [HIV] infection status.

(g) HIV Infection in Pregnancy, Childbirth and the Puerperium
During pregnancy, childbirth or the puerperium, a patient admitted (or presenting for a health care encounter) because of an HIV-related illness should receive a principal diagnosis code of O98.7-, Human immunodeficiency [HIV] disease complicating pregnancy, childbirth and the puerperium, followed by B20 and the code(s) for the HIV-related illness(es). Codes from Chapter 15 always take sequencing priority.

Patients with asymptomatic HIV infection status admitted (or presenting for a health care encounter) during pregnancy, childbirth, or the puerperium should receive codes of O98.7- and Z21.

(h) Encounters for testing for HIV
If a patient is being seen to determine his/her HIV status, use code Z11.4, Encounter for screening for human immunodeficiency virus [HIV]. Use additional codes for any associated high risk behavior.

If a patient with signs or symptoms is being seen for HIV testing, code the signs and symptoms. An additional counseling code Z71.7, Human immunodeficiency virus [HIV] counseling, may be used if counseling is provided during the encounter for the test.

When a patient returns to be informed of his/her HIV test results and the test result is negative, use code Z71.7, Human immunodeficiency virus [HIV] counseling.

If the results are positive, see previous guidelines and assign codes as appropriate.

CHAPTER 1 – INFECTIOUS DISEASES
Section I. C. 1. b.

b. Infectious agents as the cause of diseases classified to other chapters
Certain infections are classified in chapters other than Chapter 1 and no organism is identified as part of the infection code. In these instances, it is necessary to use an additional code from Chapter 1 to identify the organism. A code from category B95, Streptococcus, Staphylococcus, and Enterococcus as the cause of diseases classified to other chapters, B96, Other bacterial agents as the cause of diseases classified to other chapters, or B97, Viral agents as the cause of diseases classified to other chapters, is to be used as an additional code to identify the organism. An instructional note will be found at the infection code advising that an additional organism code is required.

c. Infections resistant to antibiotics
Many bacterial infections are resistant to current antibiotics. It is necessary to identify all infections documented as antibiotic resistant. Assign a code from category Z16, Resistance to antimicrobial drugs, following the infection code only if the infection code does not identify drug resistance.

d. Sepsis, Severe Sepsis, and Septic Shock

1) Coding of Sepsis and Severe Sepsis

(a) Sepsis
For a diagnosis of sepsis, assign the appropriate code for the underlying systemic infection. If the type of infection or causal organism is not further specified, assign code A41.9, Sepsis, unspecified organism.

A code from subcategory R65.2, Severe sepsis, should not be assigned unless severe sepsis or an associated acute organ dysfunction is documented.

(i) Negative or inconclusive blood cultures and sepsis
Negative or inconclusive blood cultures do not preclude a diagnosis of sepsis in patients with clinical evidence of the condition, however, the provider should be queried.

(ii) Urosepsis
The term urosepsis is a nonspecific term. It is not to be considered synonymous with sepsis. It has no default code in the Alphabetic Index. Should a provider use this term, he/she must be queried for clarification.

(iii) Sepsis with organ dysfunction
If a patient has sepsis and associated acute organ dysfunction or multiple organ dysfunction (MOD), follow the instructions for coding severe sepsis.

(iv) Acute organ dysfunction that is not clearly associated with the sepsis
If a patient has sepsis and an acute organ dysfunction, but the medical record documentation indicates that the acute organ dysfunction is related to a medical condition other than the sepsis, do not assign a code from subcategory R65.2, Severe sepsis. An acute organ dysfunction must be associated with the sepsis in order to assign the severe sepsis code. If the documentation is not clear as to whether an acute organ dysfunction is related to the sepsis or another medical condition, query the provider.

(b) Severe sepsis
The coding of severe sepsis requires a minimum of 2 codes: first a code for the underlying systemic infection, followed by a code from subcategory R65.2, Severe sepsis. If the causal organism is not documented, assign code A41.9, Sepsis, unspecified organism, for the infection. Additional code(s) for the associated acute organ dysfunction are also required.

Due to the complex nature of severe sepsis, some cases may require querying the provider prior to assignment of the codes.

2) Septic shock

(a) Septic shock
Septic shock generally refers to circulatory failure associated with severe sepsis, and therefore, it represents a type of acute organ dysfunction.

For cases of septic shock, the code for the systemic infection should be sequenced first, followed by code R65.21, Severe sepsis with septic shock or code T81.12, Postprocedural septic shock. Any additional codes for the other acute organ dysfunctions should also be assigned. As noted in the sequencing instructions in the Tabular List, the code for septic shock cannot be assigned as a principal diagnosis.

3) Sequencing of severe sepsis

If severe sepsis is present on admission, and meets the definition of principal diagnosis, the underlying systemic infection should be assigned as principal diagnosis followed by the appropriate code from subcategory R65.2 as required by the sequencing rules in the Tabular List. A code from subcategory R65.2 can never be assigned as a principal diagnosis.

When severe sepsis develops during an encounter (it was not present on admission) the underlying systemic infection and the appropriate code from subcategory R65.2 should be assigned as secondary diagnoses.

Severe sepsis may be present on admission but the diagnosis may not be confirmed until sometime after admission. If the documentation is not clear whether severe sepsis was present on admission, the provider should be queried.

4) Sepsis and severe sepsis with a localized infection

If the reason for admission is both sepsis or severe sepsis and a localized infection, such as pneumonia or cellulitis, a code(s) for the underlying systemic infection should be assigned first and the code for the localized infection should be assigned as a secondary diagnosis. If the patient has severe sepsis, a code from subcategory R65.2 should also be assigned as a secondary diagnosis. If the patient is admitted with a localized infection, such as pneumonia, and sepsis/severe sepsis doesn't develop until after admission, the localized infection should be assigned first, followed by the appropriate sepsis/severe sepsis codes.

5) Sepsis due to a postprocedural infection

(a) Documentation of causal relationship

As with all postprocedural complications, code assignment is based on the provider's documentation of the relationship between the infection and the procedure.

(b) Sepsis due to a postprocedural infection

For such cases, the postprocedural infection code, such as, T80.2, Infections following infusion, transfusion, and therapeutic injection, T81.4, Infection following a procedure, or T88.0, Infection following immunization, or O86.0, Infection of obstetric surgical wound, should be coded first, followed by the code for the specific infection. If the patient has severe sepsis the appropriate code from subcategory R65.2 should also be assigned with the additional code(s) for any acute organ dysfunction.

(c) Postprocedural infection and postprocedural septic shock

In cases where a postprocedural infection has occurred and has resulted in severe sepsis the code for the precipitating complication such as code T81.4, Infection following a procedure, or O86.0, Infection of obstetrical surgical wound should be coded first followed by code R65.20, Severe sepsis without septic shock and a code for the systemic infection. A code for the systemic infection should also be assigned.

If a postprocedural infection has resulted in postprocedural septic shock, the code for the precipitating complication such as T81.4, Infection following a procedure, or O86.0, Infection of obstetrical surgical wound should be coded first followed by code T81.12-, Postprocedural septic shock. A code for the systemic infection should also be assigned.

6) Sepsis and severe sepsis associated with a noninfectious process (condition)

In some cases a noninfectious process (condition), such as trauma, may lead to an infection which can result in sepsis or severe sepsis. If sepsis or severe sepsis is documented as associated with a noninfectious condition, such as a burn or serious injury, and this condition meets the definition for principal diagnosis, the code for the noninfectious condition should be sequenced first, followed by the code for the resulting infection. If severe sepsis, is present a code from subcategory R65.2 should also be assigned with any associated organ dysfunction(s) codes. It is not necessary to assign a code from subcategory R65.1, Systemic inflammatory response syndrome (SIRS) of non-infectious origin, for these cases.

If the infection meets the definition of principal diagnosis it should be sequenced before the non-infectious condition. When both the associated non-infectious condition and the infection meet the definition of principal diagnosis either may be assigned as principal diagnosis.

Only one code from category R65, Symptoms and signs specifically associated with systemic inflammation and infection, should be assigned. Therefore, when a non-infectious condition leads to an infection resulting in severe sepsis, assign the appropriate code from subcategory R65.2, Severe sepsis. Do not additionally assign a code from subcategory R65.1, Systemic inflammatory response syndrome (SIRS) of non-infectious origin.

See Section I.C.18. SIRS due to non-infectious process.

7) Sepsis and septic shock complicating abortion, pregnancy, childbirth, and the puerperium

See Section I.C.15. Sepsis and septic shock complicating abortion, pregnancy, childbirth and the puerperium.

8) Newborn sepsis

See Section I.C.16.f. Bacterial sepsis of Newborn.

e. Methicillin Resistant *Staphylococcus aureus* (MRSA) Conditions

1) Selection and sequencing of MRSA codes

(a) Combination codes for MRSA infection

When a patient is diagnosed with an infection that is due to methicillin resistant *Staphylococcus aureus* (MRSA), and that infection that has a combination code that includes the causal organism (e.g., sepsis, pneumonia) assign the appropriate combination code for the condition (e.g., code A41.02, Sepsis due to methicillin resistant Staphylococcus aureus or code J15.212, Pneumonia due to methicillin resistant Staphylococcus aureus). Do not assign code B95.62, Methicillin resistant Staphylococcus aureus infection as the cause of the diseases classified elsewhere, as an additional code because the combination code includes the type of infection and the MRSA organism. Do not assign a code from subcategory Z16.11, Resistance to penicillins, as an additional diagnosis.

See Section C.1. for instructions on coding and sequencing of sepsis and severe sepsis.

(b) Other codes for MRSA infection

When there is documentation of a current infection (e.g., wound infection, stitch abscess, urinary tract infection) due to MRSA, and that infection does not have a combination code that includes the causal organism, assign the appropriate code to identify the condition along with code B95.62, Methicillin resistant Staphylococcus aureus infection as the cause of diseases classified elsewhere for the MRSA infection. Do not assign a code from subcategory Z16.11, Resistance to penicillins.

(c) Methicillin susceptible Staphylococcus aureus (MSSA) and MRSA colonization

The condition or state of being colonized or carrying MSSA or MRSA is called colonization or carriage, while an individual person is described as being colonized or being a carrier. Colonization means that MSSA and MSRA is present on or in the body without necessarily causing illness. A positive MRSA colonization test might be documented by the provider as "MRSA screen positive" or "MRSA nasal swab positive".

Assign code Z22.322, Carrier or suspected carrier of methicillin resistant Staphylococcus aureus, for patients documented as having MRSA colonization. Assign code Z22.321, Carrier or suspected carrier of methicillin susceptible Staphylococcus aureus, for patient documented as having MSSA colonization. Colonization is not necessarily indicative of a disease process or as the cause of a specific condition the patient may have unless documented as such by the provider.

(d) MRSA colonization and infection

If a patient is documented as having both MRSA colonization and infection during a hospital admission, code Z22.322, Carrier or suspected carrier of methicillin resistant Staphylococcus aureus, and a code for the MRSA infection may both be assigned.

f. Zika virus infections

1) Code only confirmed cases

Code only a confirmed diagnosis of Zika virus (A92.5, Zika virus disease) as documented by the provider. This is an exception to the hospital inpatient guideline Section II, H. In this context, "confirmation" does not require documentation of the type of test performed; the physician's diagnostic statement that the condition is confirmed is sufficient. This code should be assigned regardless of the stated mode of transmission.

If the provider documents "suspected", "possible" or "probable" Zika, do not assign code A92.5. Assign a code(s) explaining the reason for the encounter (such as fever, rash, or joint pain) or Z20.828, Contact with and (suspected) exposure to other viral communicable diseases.

2. Chapter 2: Neoplasms (C00-D49)

General guidelines

Chapter 2 of the ICD-10-CM contains the codes for most benign and all malignant neoplasms. Certain benign neoplasms, such as prostatic adenomas, may be found in the specific body system chapters. To properly code a neoplasm it is necessary to determine from the record if the neoplasm is benign, in-situ, malignant, or of uncertain histologic behavior. If malignant, any secondary (metastatic) sites should also be determined.

Primary malignant neoplasms overlapping site boundaries

A primary malignant neoplasm that overlaps two or more contiguous (next to each other) sites should be classified to the subcategory/code .8 ('overlapping lesion'), unless the combination is specifically indexed elsewhere. For multiple neoplasms of the same site that are not contiguous such as tumors in different quadrants of the same breast, codes for each site should be assigned.

Malignant neoplasm of ectopic tissue

Malignant neoplasms of ectopic tissue are to be coded to the site of origin mentioned, e.g., ectopic pancreatic malignant neoplasms involving the stomach are coded to pancreas, unspecified (C25.9).
The neoplasm table in the Alphabetic Index should be referenced first. However, if the histological term is documented, that term should be referenced first, rather than going immediately to the Neoplasm Table, in order to determine which column in the Neoplasm Table is appropriate. For example, if the documentation indicates "adenoma," refer to the term in the Alphabetic Index to review the entries under this term and the instructional note to "see also neoplasm, by site, benign." The table provides the proper code based on the type of neoplasm and the site. It is important to select the proper column in the table that corresponds to the type of neoplasm. The Tabular List should then be referenced to verify that the correct code has been selected from the table and that a more specific site code does not exist.

See Section I.C.21. Factors influencing health status and contact with health services, Status, for information regarding Z15.0, codes for genetic susceptibility to cancer.

a. Treatment directed at the malignancy
If the treatment is directed at the malignancy, designate the malignancy as the principal diagnosis.

The only exception to this guideline is if a patient admission/encounter is solely for the administration of chemotherapy, immunotherapy or radiation therapy, assign the appropriate Z51.– code as the first-listed or principal diagnosis, and the diagnosis or problem for which the service is being performed as a secondary diagnosis.

b. Treatment of secondary site
When a patient is admitted because of a primary neoplasm with metastasis and treatment is directed toward the secondary site only, the secondary neoplasm is designated as the principal diagnosis even though the primary malignancy is still present.

c. Coding and sequencing of complications
Coding and sequencing of complications associated with the malignancies or with the therapy thereof are subject to the following guidelines:

1) Anemia associated with malignancy
When admission/encounter is for management of an anemia associated with the malignancy, and the treatment is only for anemia, the appropriate code for the malignancy is sequenced as the principal or first-listed diagnosis followed by the appropriate code for the anemia (such as code D63.0, Anemia in neoplastic disease).

2) Anemia associated with chemotherapy, immunotherapy and radiation therapy
When the admission/encounter is for management of an anemia associated with an adverse effect of the administration of chemotherapy or immunotherapy and the only treatment is for the anemia, the anemia code is sequenced first followed by the appropriate codes for the neoplasm and the adverse effect (T45.1X5, Adverse effect of antineoplastic and immunosuppressive drugs).

When the admission/encounter is for management of an anemia associated with an adverse effect of radiotherapy, the anemia code should be sequenced first, followed by the appropriate neoplasm code and code Y84.2, Radiological procedure and radiotherapy as the cause of abnormal reaction of the patient, or of later complication, without mention of misadventure at the time of the procedure.

3) Management of dehydration due to the malignancy
When the admission/encounter is for management of dehydration due to the malignancy and only the dehydration is being treated (intravenous rehydration), the dehydration is sequenced first, followed by the code(s) for the malignancy.

4) Treatment of a complication resulting from a surgical procedure
When the admission/encounter is for treatment of a complication resulting from a surgical procedure, designate the complication as the principal or first-listed diagnosis if treatment is directed at resolving the complication.

d. Primary malignancy previously excised
When a primary malignancy has been previously excised or eradicated from its site and there is no further treatment directed to that site and there is no evidence of any existing primary malignancy, a code from category Z85, Personal history of malignant neoplasm, should be used to indicate the former site of the malignancy. Any mention of extension, invasion, or metastasis to another site is coded as a secondary malignant neoplasm to that site. The secondary site may be the principal or first-listed with the Z85 code used as a secondary code.

e. Admissions/Encounters involving chemotherapy, immunotherapy and radiation therapy

1) Episode of care involves surgical removal of neoplasm
When an episode of care involves the surgical removal of a neoplasm, primary or secondary site, followed by adjunct chemotherapy or radiation treatment during the same episode of care, the code for the neoplasm should be assigned as principal or first-listed diagnosis.

2) Patient admission/encounter solely for administration of chemotherapy, immunotherapy and radiation therapy
If a patient admission/encounter is solely for the administration of chemotherapy, immunotherapy or radiation therapy assign code Z51.0, Encounter for antineoplastic radiation therapy, or Z51.11, Encounter for antineoplastic chemotherapy, or Z51.12, Encounter for antineoplastic immunotherapy as the first-listed or principal diagnosis. If a patient receives more than one of these therapies during the same admission more than one of these codes may be assigned, in any sequence.

The malignancy for which the therapy is being administered should be assigned as a secondary diagnosis.

3) Patient admitted for radiation therapy, chemotherapy or immunotherapy and develops complications
When a patient is admitted for the purpose of radiotherapy, immunotherapy or chemotherapy and develops complications such as uncontrolled nausea and vomiting or dehydration, the principal or first-listed diagnosis is Z51.0, Encounter for antineoplastic radiation therapy, or Z51.11, Encounter for antineoplastic chemotherapy, or Z51.12, Encounter for antineoplastic immunotherapy followed by any codes for the complications.

f. Admission/encounter to determine extent of malignancy
When the reason for admission/encounter is to determine the extent of the malignancy, or for a procedure such as paracentesis or thoracentesis, the primary malignancy or appropriate metastatic site is designated as the principal or first-listed diagnosis, even though chemotherapy or radiotherapy is administered.

g. Symptoms, signs, and abnormal findings listed in Chapter 18 associated with neoplasms
Symptoms, signs, and ill-defined conditions listed in Chapter 18 characteristic of, or associated with, an existing primary or secondary site malignancy cannot be used to replace the malignancy as principal or first-listed diagnosis, regardless of the number of admissions or encounters for treatment and care of the neoplasm.

See section I.C.21. Factors influencing health status and contact with health services, Encounter for prophylactic organ removal.

h. Admission/encounter for pain control/management
See Section I.C.6. for information on coding admission/encounter for pain control/management.

i. Malignancy in two or more noncontiguous sites
A patient may have more than one malignant tumor in the same organ. These tumors may represent different primaries or metastatic disease, depending on the site. Should the documentation be unclear, the provider should be queried as to the status of each tumor so that the correct codes can be assigned.

j. Disseminated malignant neoplasm, unspecified
Code C80.0, Disseminated malignant neoplasm, unspecified, is for use only in those cases where the patient has advanced metastatic disease and no known primary or secondary sites are specified. It should not be used in place of assigning codes for the primary site and all known secondary sites.

k. Malignant neoplasm without specification of site
Code C80.1, Malignant (primary) neoplasm, unspecified, equates to Cancer, unspecified. This code should only be used when no determination can be made as to the primary site of a malignancy. This code should rarely be used in the inpatient setting.

CHAPTER 2 – NEOPLASMS
Section I. C. 2. l. 1)

l.   Sequencing of neoplasm codes

1)   Encounter for treatment of primary malignancy
If the reason for the encounter is for treatment of a primary malignancy, assign the malignancy as the principal/first-listed diagnosis. The primary site is to be sequenced first, followed by any metastatic sites.

2)   Encounter for treatment of secondary malignancy
When an encounter is for a primary malignancy with metastasis and treatment is directed toward the metastatic (secondary) site(s) only, the metastatic site(s) is designated as the principal/first-listed diagnosis. The primary malignancy is coded as an additional code.

3)   Malignant neoplasm in a pregnant patient
When a pregnant woman has a malignant neoplasm, a code from subcategory O9A.1-, Malignant neoplasm complicating pregnancy, childbirth, and the puerperium, should be sequenced first, followed by the appropriate code from Chapter 2 to indicate the type of neoplasm.

4)   Encounter for complication associated with a neoplasm
When an encounter is for management of a complication associated with a neoplasm, such as dehydration, and the treatment is only for the complication, the complication is coded first, followed by the appropriate code(s) for the neoplasm.
The exception to this guideline is anemia. When the admission/encounter is for management of an anemia associated with the malignancy, and the treatment is only for anemia, the appropriate code for the malignancy is sequenced as the principal or first-listed diagnosis followed by code D63.0, Anemia in neoplastic disease.

5)   Complication from surgical procedure for treatment of a neoplasm
When an encounter is for treatment of a complication resulting from a surgical procedure performed for the treatment of the neoplasm, designate the complication as the principal/first-listed diagnosis. See guideline regarding the coding of a current malignancy versus personal history to determine if the code for the neoplasm should also be assigned.

6)   Pathologic fracture due to a neoplasm
When an encounter is for a pathological fracture due to a neoplasm, and the focus of treatment is the fracture, a code from subcategory M84.5, Pathological fracture in neoplastic disease, should be sequenced first, followed by the code for the neoplasm.

If the focus of treatment is the neoplasm with an associated pathological fracture, the neoplasm code should be sequenced first, followed by a code from M84.5 for the pathological fracture.

m.   Current malignancy versus personal history of malignancy
When a primary malignancy has been excised but further treatment, such as an additional surgery for the malignancy, radiation therapy or chemotherapy is directed to that site, the primary malignancy code should be used until treatment is completed.

When a primary malignancy has been previously excised or eradicated from its site, there is no further treatment (of the malignancy) directed to that site, and there is no evidence of any existing primary malignancy, a code from category Z85, Personal history of malignant neoplasm, should be used to indicate the former site of the malignancy.

See Section I.C.21. Factors influencing health status and contact with health services, History (of).

n.   Leukemia, Multiple Myeloma, and Malignant Plasma Cell Neoplasms in remission versus personal history
The categories for leukemia, and category C90, Multiple myeloma and malignant plasma cell neoplasms, have codes indicating whether or not the leukemia has achieved remission. There are also codes Z85.6, Personal history of leukemia, and Z85.79, Personal history of other malignant neoplasms of lymphoid, hematopoietic and related tissues. If the documentation is unclear, as to whether the leukemia has achieved remission, the provider should be queried.

See Section I.C.21. Factors influencing health status and contact with health services, History (of).

o.   Aftercare following surgery for neoplasm
See Section I.C.21. Factors influencing health status and contact with health services, Aftercare.

p.   Follow-up care for completed treatment of a malignancy
See Section I.C.21. Factors influencing health status and contact with health services, Follow-up.

CHAPTER 2 – NEOPLASMS
Section I. C. 2. q.

q.   Prophylactic organ removal for prevention of malignancy
See Section I.C.21. Factors influencing health status and contact with health services, Prophylactic organ removal.

r.   Malignant neoplasm associated with transplanted organ
A malignant neoplasm of a transplanted organ should be coded as a transplant complication. Assign first the appropriate code from category T86.-, Complications of transplanted organs and tissue, followed by code C80.2, Malignant neoplasm associated with transplanted organ. Use an additional code for the specific malignancy.

3.   Chapter 3: Disease of the Blood and Blood-forming Organs and Certain Disorders Involving the Immune Mechanism (D50-D89)

Reserved for future guideline expansion

4.   Chapter 4: Endocrine, Nutritional, and Metabolic Diseases (E00-E89)

a.   Diabetes mellitus
The diabetes mellitus codes are combination codes that include the type of diabetes mellitus, the body system affected, and the complications affecting that body system. As many codes within a particular category as are necessary to describe all of the complications of the disease may be used. They should be sequenced based on the reason for a particular encounter. Assign as many codes from categories E08 – E13 as needed to identify all of the associated conditions that the patient has.

1)   Type of diabetes
The age of a patient is not the sole determining factor, though most type 1 diabetics develop the condition before reaching puberty. For this reason type 1 diabetes mellitus is also referred to as juvenile diabetes.

2)   Type of diabetes mellitus not documented
If the type of diabetes mellitus is not documented in the medical record the default is E11.-, Type 2 diabetes mellitus.

3)   Diabetes mellitus and the use of insulin *and oral hypoglycemics*
If the documentation in a medical record does not indicate the type of diabetes but does indicate that the patient uses insulin, code E11, Type 2 diabetes mellitus, should be assigned. Code Z79.4, Long-term (current) use of insulin, or Z79.84, Long term (current) use of oral hypoglycemic drugs, should also be assigned to indicate that the patient uses insulin or hypoglycemic drugs. Code Z79.4 should not be assigned if insulin is given temporarily to bring a type 2 patient's blood sugar under control during an encounter.

4)   Diabetes mellitus in pregnancy and gestational diabetes
See Section I.C.15. Diabetes mellitus in pregnancy.
See Section I.C.15. Gestational (pregnancy induced) diabetes.

5)   Complications due to insulin pump malfunction

(a)   Underdose of insulin due to insulin pump failure
An underdose of insulin due to an insulin pump failure should be assigned to a code from subcategory T85.6, Mechanical complication of other specified internal and external prosthetic devices, implants and grafts, that specifies the type of pump malfunction, as the principal or first-listed code, followed by code T38.3x6-, Underdosing of insulin and oral hypoglycemic [antidiabetic] drugs. Additional codes for the type of diabetes mellitus and any associated complications due to the underdosing should also be assigned.

(b)   Overdose of insulin due to insulin pump failure
The principal or first-listed code for an encounter due to an insulin pump malfunction resulting in an overdose of insulin, should also be T85.6-, Mechanical complication of other specified internal and external prosthetic devices, implants and grafts, followed by code T38.3x1-, Poisoning by insulin and oral hypoglycemic [antidiabetic] drugs, accidental (unintentional).

GUIDELINES

6)   Secondary diabetes mellitus
Codes under categories E08, Diabetes mellitus due to underlying condition, and E09, Drug or chemical induced diabetes mellitus, and E13, Other specified diabetes mellitus, identify complications/manifestations associated with secondary diabetes mellitus. Secondary diabetes is always caused by another condition or event (e.g., cystic fibrosis, malignant neoplasm of pancreas, pancreatectomy, adverse effect of drug, or poisoning).

(a)   Secondary diabetes mellitus and the use of insulin *or oral hypoglycemic drugs*
For patients who routinely use insulin or hypoglycemic drugs, code Z79.4, Long-term (current) use of insulin, or Z79.84, Long term (current) use of oral hypoglycemic drugs, should also be assigned. Code Z79.4 should not be assigned if insulin is given temporarily to bring a patient's blood sugar under control during an encounter.

(b)   Assigning and sequencing secondary diabetes codes and its causes
The sequencing of the secondary diabetes codes in relationship to codes for the cause of the diabetes is based on the Tabular List instructions for categories E08, E09 and E13.

(i)   Secondary diabetes mellitus due to pancreatectomy
For postpancreatectomy diabetes mellitus (lack of insulin due to the surgical removal of all or part of the pancreas), assign code E89.1, Postprocedural hypoinsulinemia. Assign a code from category E13 and a code from subcategory Z90.41-, Acquired absence of pancreas, as additional codes.

(ii)   Secondary diabetes due to drugs
Secondary diabetes may be caused by an adverse effect of correctly administered medications, poisoning or sequela of poisoning.

See section I.C.19.e for coding of adverse effects and poisoning, and section I.C.20 for external cause code reporting.

5.   Chapter 5: Mental and Behavioral Disorders (F01 – F99)

a.   Pain disorders related to psychological factors
Assign code F45.41, for pain that is exclusively related to psychological disorders. As indicated by the Excludes1 note under category G89, a code from category G89 should not be assigned with code F45.41.

Code F45.42, Pain disorders with related psychological factors, should be used should be used with a code from category G89, Pain, not elsewhere classified, if there is documentation of a psychological component for a patient with acute or chronic pain.

See Section I.C.6. Pain.

b.   Mental and behavioral disorders due to psychoactive substance use

1)   In Remission
Selection of codes for "in remission" for categories F10-F19, Mental and behavioral disorders due to psychoactive substance use (categories F10-F19 with -.21) requires the provider's clinical judgment. The appropriate codes for "in remission" are assigned only on the basis of provider documentation (as defined in the Official Guidelines for Coding and Reporting).

2)   Psychoactive Substance Use, Abuse And Dependence
When the provider documentation refers to use, abuse and dependence of the same substance (e.g. alcohol, opioid, cannabis, etc.), only one code should be assigned to identify the pattern of use based on the following hierarchy:
• If both use and abuse are documented, assign only the code for abuse
• If both abuse and dependence are documented, assign only the code for dependence
• If use, abuse and dependence are all documented, assign only the code for dependence
• If both use and dependence are documented, assign only the code for dependence

3)   Psychoactive Substance Use
As with all other diagnoses, the codes for psychoactive substance use (F10.9-, F11.9-, F12.9-, F13.9-, F14.9-, F15.9-, F16.9-) should only be assigned based on provider documentation and when they meet the definition of a reportable diagnosis (see Section III, Reporting Additional Diagnoses). The codes are to be used only when the psychoactive substance use is associated with a mental or behavioral disorder, and such a relationship is documented by the provider.

6.   Chapter 6: Diseases of Nervous System and Sense Organs (G00-G99)

a.   Dominant/nondominant side
Codes from category G81, Hemiplegia and hemiparesis, and subcategories, G83.1, Monoplegia of lower limb, G83.2, Monoplegia of upper limb, and G83.3, Monoplegia, unspecified, identify whether the dominant or nondominant side is affected. Should the affected side be documented, but not specified as dominant or nondominant, and the classification system does not indicate a default, code selection is as follows:
• For ambidextrous patients, the default should be dominant.
• If the left side is affected, the default is non-dominant.
• If the right side is affected, the default is dominant.

b.   Pain - Category G89

1)   General coding information
Codes in category G89, Pain, not elsewhere classified, may be used in conjunction with codes from other categories and chapters to provide more detail about acute or chronic pain and neoplasm-related pain, unless otherwise indicated below.

If the pain is not specified as acute or chronic, post-thoracotomy, postprocedural, or neoplasm-related, do not assign codes from category G89.

A code from category G89 should not be assigned if the underlying (definitive) diagnosis is known, unless the reason for the encounter is pain control/management and not management of the underlying condition.

When an admission or encounter is for a procedure aimed at treating the underlying condition (e.g., spinal fusion, kyphoplasty), a code for the underlying condition (e.g., vertebral fracture, spinal stenosis) should be assigned as the principal diagnosis. No code from category G89 should be assigned.

(a)   Category G89 Codes as Principal or First-Listed Diagnosis
Category G89 codes are acceptable as principal diagnosis or the first-listed code:
• When pain control or pain management is the reason for the admission/encounter (e.g., a patient with displaced intervertebral disc, nerve impingement and severe back pain presents for injection of steroid into the spinal canal). The underlying cause of the pain should be reported as an additional diagnosis, if known.

• When a patient is admitted for the insertion of a neurostimulator for pain control, assign the appropriate pain code as the principal or first-listed diagnosis. When an admission or encounter is for a procedure aimed at treating the underlying condition and a neurostimulator is inserted for pain control during the same admission/encounter, a code for the underlying condition should be assigned as the principal diagnosis and the appropriate pain code should be assigned as a secondary diagnosis.

(b)   Use of Category G89 Codes in Conjunction with Site Specific Pain Codes

(i)   Assigning Category G89 and Site-Specific Pain Codes
Codes from category G89 may be used in conjunction with codes that identify the site of pain (including codes from chapter 18) if the category G89 code provides additional information. For example, if the code describes the site of the pain, but does not fully describe whether the pain is acute or chronic, then both codes should be assigned.

(ii)   Sequencing of Category G89 Codes with Site-Specific Pain Codes
The sequencing of category G89 codes with site-specific pain codes (including chapter 18 codes), is dependent on the circumstances of the encounter/admission as follows:
• If the encounter is for pain control or pain management, assign the code from category G89 followed by the code identifying the specific site of pain (e.g., a patient with displaced intervertebral disc, nerve impingement and severe back pain presents for injection of steroid into the spinal canal). The underlying cause of the pain should be reported as an additional diagnosis, if known.
Cervicalgia, to identify the site of pain).

• If the encounter is for any other reason except pain control or pain management, and a related definitive diagnosis has not been established (confirmed) by the provider, assign the code for the specific site of pain first, followed by the appropriate code from category G89.

2)   Pain due to devices, implants and grafts
See Section I.C.19. Pain due to medical devices.

CHAPTER 6 – NERVOUS SYSTEM
Section I. C. 6. b. 3)

3) Postoperative Pain

The provider's documentation should be used to guide the coding of postoperative pain, as well as *Section III. Reporting Additional Diagnoses and Section IV. Diagnostic Coding and Reporting in the Outpatient Setting.*

The default for post-thoracotomy and other postoperative pain not specified as acute or chronic is the code for the acute form.

Routine or expected postoperative pain immediately after surgery should not be coded.

(a) Postoperative pain not associated with specific postoperative complication

Postoperative pain not associated with a specific postoperative complication is assigned to the appropriate postoperative pain code in category G89.

(b) Postoperative pain associated with specific postoperative complication

Postoperative pain associated with a specific postoperative complication (such as painful wire sutures) is assigned to the appropriate code(s) found in Chapter 19, Injury, poisoning, and certain other consequences of external causes. If appropriate, use additional code(s) from category G89 to identify acute or chronic pain (G89.18 or G89.28).

4) Chronic pain

Chronic pain is classified to subcategory G89.2. There is no time frame defining when pain becomes chronic pain. The provider's documentation should be used to guide use of these codes.

5) Neoplasm Related Pain

Code G89.3 is assigned to pain documented as being related, associated or due to cancer, primary or secondary malignancy, or tumor. This code is assigned regardless of whether the pain is acute or chronic.

This code may be assigned as the principal or first-listed code when the stated reason for the admission/encounter is documented as pain control/pain management. The underlying neoplasm should be reported as an additional diagnosis. When the reason for the admission/encounter is management of the neoplasm and the pain associated with the neoplasm is also documented, code G89.3 may be assigned as an additional diagnosis. It is not necessary to assign an additional code for the site of the pain.

See Section I.C.2 for instructions on the sequencing of neoplasms for all other stated reasons for the admission/encounter (except for pain control/pain management).

6) Chronic pain syndrome

Central pain syndrome (G89.0) and chronic pain syndrome (G89.4) are different than the term "chronic pain," and therefore codes should only be used when the provider has specifically documented this condition.

See Section I.C.5. Pain disorders related to psychological factors.

7. Chapter 7: Diseases of Eye and Adnexa (H00-H59)

a. Glaucoma

1) Assigning Glaucoma Codes

Assign as many codes from category H40, Glaucoma, as needed to identify the type of glaucoma, the affected eye, and the glaucoma stage.

2) Bilateral glaucoma with same type and stage

When a patient has bilateral glaucoma and both eyes are documented as being the same type and stage, and there is a code for bilateral glaucoma, report only the code for the type of glaucoma, bilateral, with the seventh character for the stage.

When a patient has bilateral glaucoma and both eyes are documented as being the same type and stage, and the classification does not provide a code for bilateral glaucoma (i.e. subcategories H40.10, H40.11 and H40.20) report only one code for the type of glaucoma with the appropriate seventh character for the stage.

3) Bilateral glaucoma stage with different types or stages

When a patient has bilateral glaucoma and each eye is documented as having a different type or stage, and the classification distinguishes laterality, assign the appropriate code for each eye rather than the code for bilateral glaucoma.

When a patient has bilateral glaucoma and each eye is documented as having a different type, and the classification does not distinguish laterality (i.e. subcategories H40.10, H40.11 and H40.20), assign one code for each type of glaucoma with the appropriate seventh character for the stage.

CHAPTER 7 – EYE AND ADNEXA
Section I. C. 7. a. 3)

When a patient has bilateral glaucoma and each eye is documented as having the same type, but different stage, and the classification does not distinguish laterality (i.e. subcategories H40.10, H40.11 and H40.20), assign a code for the type of glaucoma for each eye with the seventh character for the specific glaucoma stage documented for each eye.

4) Patient admitted with glaucoma and stage evolves during the admission

If a patient is admitted with glaucoma and the stage progresses during the admission, assign the code for highest stage documented.

5) Indeterminate stage glaucoma

Assignment of the seventh character "4" for "indeterminate stage" should be based on the clinical documentation. The seventh character "4" is used for glaucomas whose stage cannot be clinically determined. This seventh character should not be confused with the seventh character "0", unspecified, which should be assigned when there is no documentation regarding the stage of the glaucoma.

8. Chapter 8: Diseases of Ear and Mastoid Process (H60-H95)

Reserved for future guideline expansion

9. Chapter 9: Diseases of Circulatory System (I00-I99)

a. Hypertension

The classification presumes a causal relationship between hypertension and heart involvement and between hypertension and kidney involvement, as the two conditions are linked by the term "with" in the Alphabetic Index. These conditions should be coded as related even in the absence of provider documentation explicitly linking them, unless the documentation clearly states the conditions are unrelated.

For hypertension and conditions not specifically linked by relational terms such as "with," "associated with" or "due to" in the classification, provider documentaton must link the conditions in order to code them as related.

1) Hypertension with Heart Disease

Hypertension with heart conditions classified to I50.- or I51.4-I51.9, are assigned to, a code from category I11, Hypertensive heart disease, when a causal relationship is stated (due to hypertension) or implied (hypertensive). Use an additional code from category I50, Heart failure, to identify the type of heart failure in those patients with heart failure.

The same heart conditions (I50.-, I51.4-I51.9) with hypertension, ~~but without a stated causal relationship~~, are coded separately if the provider has specifically documented a different cause. Sequence according to the circumstances of the admission/encounter.

2) Hypertensive Chronic Kidney Disease

Assign codes from category I12, Hypertensive chronic kidney disease, when both hypertension and a condition classifiable to category N18, Chronic kidney disease (CKD), are present. ~~Unlike hypertension with heart disease, ICD-10-CM presumes a cause-and-effect relationship and classifies chronic kidney disease with hypertension as hypertensive chronic kidney disease.~~ CKD should not be coded as hypertensive if the physician has specifically documented a different cause.

The appropriate code from category N18 should be used as a secondary code with a code from category I12 to identify the stage of chronic kidney disease.

See Section I.C.14. Chronic kidney disease.

If a patient has hypertensive chronic kidney disease and acute renal failure, an additional code for the acute renal failure is required.

3) Hypertensive Heart and Chronic Kidney Disease

Assign codes from combination category I13, Hypertensive heart and chronic kidney disease, when ~~both hypertensive kidney disease and hypertensive heart disease are stated in the diagnosis~~ there is hypertension with both heart and kidney involvement. ~~Assume a relationship between the hypertension and the chronic kidney disease, whether or not the condition is so designated.~~ If heart failure is present, assign an additional code from category I50 to identify the type of heart failure.

The appropriate code from category N18, Chronic kidney disease, should be used as a secondary code with a code from category I13 to identify the stage of chronic kidney disease.

See Section I.C.14. Chronic kidney disease.

GUIDELINES

CHAPTER 9 – CIRCULATORY SYSTEM
Section I. C. 9. a. 3)

The codes in category I13, Hypertensive heart and chronic kidney disease, are combination codes that include hypertension, heart disease and chronic kidney disease. The Includes note at I13 specifies that the conditions included at I11 and I12 are included together in I13. If apatient has hypertension, heart disease and chronic kidney disease then a code from I13 should be used, not individual codes for hypertension, heart disease and chronic kidney disease, or codes from I11 or I12.

For patients with both acute renal failure and chronic kidney disease, an additional code for acute renal failure is required.

4) Hypertensive Cerebrovascular Disease
For hypertensive cerebrovascular disease, first assign the appropriate code from categories I60-I69, followed by the appropriate hypertension code.

5) Hypertensive Retinopathy
Subcategory H35.0, Background retinopathy and retinal vascular changes, should be used with a code from category I10-I15, Hypertensive disease to include the systemic hypertension. The sequencing is based on the reason for the encounter.

6) Hypertension, Secondary
Secondary hypertension is due to an underlying condition. Two codes are required: one to identify the underlying etiology and one from category I15 to identify the hypertension. Sequencing of codes is determined by the reason for admission/encounter.

7) Hypertension, Transient
Assign code R03.0, Elevated blood pressure reading without diagnosis of hypertension, unless patient has an established diagnosis of hypertension. Assign code O13.-, Gestational [pregnancy-induced] hypertension without significant proteinuria, or O14.-, Pre-eclampsia, for transient hypertension of pregnancy.

8) Hypertension, Controlled
This diagnostic statement usually refers to an existing state of hypertension under control by therapy. Assign the appropriate code from categories I10-I15, Hypertensive diseases.

9) Hypertension, Uncontrolled
Uncontrolled hypertension may refer to untreated hypertension or hypertension not responding to current therapeutic regimen. In either case, assign the appropriate code from categories I10-I15, Hypertensive diseases.

10) Hypertensive Crisis
Assign a code from category I16, Hypertensive crisis, for documented hypertensive urgency, hypertensive emergency or unspecified hypertensive crisis. Code also any identified hypertensive disease (I10-I15). The sequencing is based on the reason for the encounter.

b. Atherosclerotic Coronary Artery Disease and Angina
ICD-10-CM has combination codes for atherosclerotic heart disease with angina pectoris. The subcategories for these codes are I25.11, Atherosclerotic heart disease of native coronary artery with angina pectoris and I25.7, Atherosclerosis of coronary artery bypass graft(s) and coronary artery of transplanted heart with angina pectoris.

When using one of these combination codes it is not necessary to use an additional code for angina pectoris. A causal relationship can be assumed in a patient with both atherosclerosis and angina pectoris, unless the documentation indicates the angina is due to something other than the atherosclerosis.

If a patient with coronary artery disease is admitted due to an acute myocardial infarction (AMI), the AMI should be sequenced before the coronary artery disease.

See Section I.C.9. Acute myocardial infarction (AMI).

c. Intraoperative and Postprocedural Cerebrovascular Accident
Medical record documentation should clearly specify the cause-and-effect relationship between the medical intervention and the cerebrovascular accident in order to assign a code for intraoperative or postprocedural cerebrovascular accident.

Proper code assignment depends on whether it was an infarction or hemorrhage and whether it occurred intraoperatively or postoperatively. If it was a cerebral hemorrhage, code assignment depends on the type of procedure performed.

CHAPTER 9 – CIRCULATORY SYSTEM
Section I. C. 9. d. 1)

d. Sequelae of Cerebrovascular Disease

1) Category I69, Sequelae of Cerebrovascular disease
Category I69 is used to indicate conditions classifiable to categories I60-I67 as the causes of sequela (neurologic deficits), themselves classified elsewhere. These "late effects" include neurologic deficits that persist after initial onset of conditions classifiable to categories I60-I67. The neurologic deficits caused by cerebrovascular disease may be present from the onset or may arise at any time after the onset of the condition classifiable to categories I60-I67.

Codes from category I69, Sequelae of cerebrovascular disease, that specify hemiplegia, hemiparesis and monoplegia identify whether the dominant or nondominant side is affected. Should the affected side be documented, but not specified as dominant or nondominant, and the classification system does not indicate a default, code selection is as follows:

- For ambidextrous patients, the default should be dominant.
- If the left side is affected, the default is nondominant.
- If the right side is affected, the default is dominant.

2) Codes from category I69 with codes from I60-I67
Codes from category I69 may be assigned on a health care record with codes from I60-I67, if the patient has a current cerebrovascular disease and deficits from an old cerebrovascular disease.

3) Codes from category I69 and Personal history of transient ischemic attack (TIA) and cerebral infarction (Z86.73)
Codes from category I69 should not be assigned if the patient does not have neurologic deficits.

See Section I.C.21.c4. History (of) for use of personal history codes.

e. Acute myocardial infarction (AMI)

1) ST elevation myocardial infarction (STEMI) and non ST elevation myocardial infarction (NSTEMI)
The ICD-10-CM codes for acute myocardial infarction (AMI) identify the site, such as anterolateral wall or true posterior wall. Subcategories I21.0-I21.2 and code I21.3 are used for ST elevation myocardial infarction (STEMI). Code I21.4, Non-ST elevation (NSTEMI) myocardial infarction, is used for non ST elevation myocardial infarction (NSTEMI) and nontransmural MIs.

If NSTEMI evolves to STEMI, assign the STEMI code. If STEMI converts to NSTEMI due to thrombolytic therapy, it is still coded as STEMI.

For encounters occurring while the myocardial infarction is equal to, or less than, four weeks old, including transfers to another acute setting or a postacute setting, and ~~the patient requires continued care for~~ the myocardial infarction meets the definition for "other diagnoses" (see Section III, Reporting Additional Diagnoses), codes from category I21 may continue to be reported. For encounters after the 4 week time frame and the patient is still receiving care related to the myocardial infarction, the appropriate aftercare code should be assigned, rather than a code from category I21. For old or healed myocardial infarctions not requiring further care, code I25.2, Old myocardial infarction, may be assigned.

2) Acute myocardial infarction, unspecified
Code I21.3, ST elevation (STEMI) myocardial infarction of unspecified site, is the default for the unspecified acute myocardial infarction. If only STEMI or transmural MI without the site is documented, assign code I21.3.

3) AMI documented as nontransmural or subendocardial but site provided
If an AMI is documented as nontransmural or subendocardial, but the site is provided, it is still coded as a subendocardial AMI.

See Section I.C.21.3 for information on coding status post administration of tPA in a different facility within the last 24 hours.

4) Subsequent acute myocardial infarction
A code from category I22, Subsequent ST elevation (STEMI) and non ST elevation (NSTEMI) myocardial infarction, is to be used when a patient who has suffered an AMI has a new AMI within the 4 week time frame of the initial AMI. A code from category I22 must be used in conjunction with a code from category I21. The sequencing of the I22 and I21 codes depends on the circumstances of the encounter.

CHAPTER 10 – RESPIRATORY SYSTEM
Section I. C. 10. a.

10. Chapter 10: Diseases of the Respiratory System (J00-J99)

a. Chronic Obstructive Pulmonary Disease [COPD] and Asthma

1) Acute exacerbation of chronic obstructive bronchitis and asthma
The codes in categories J44 and J45 distinguish between uncomplicated cases and those in acute exacerbation. An acute exacerbation is a worsening or a decompensation of a chronic condition. An acute exacerbation is not equivalent to an infection superimposed on a chronic condition, though an exacerbation may be triggered by an infection.

b. Acute Respiratory Failure

1) Acute respiratory failure as principal diagnosis
A code from subcategory J96.0, Acute respiratory failure, or subcategory J96.2, Acute and chronic respiratory failure, may be assigned as a principal diagnosis when it is the condition established after study to be chiefly responsible for occasioning the admission to the hospital, and the selection is supported by the Alphabetic Index and Tabular List. However, chapter-specific coding guidelines (such as obstetrics, poisoning, HIV, newborn) that provide sequencing direction take precedence.

2) Acute respiratory failure as secondary diagnosis
Respiratory failure may be listed as a secondary diagnosis if it occurs after admission, or if it is present on admission, but does not meet the definition of principal diagnosis.

3) Sequencing of acute respiratory failure and another acute condition
When a patient is admitted with respiratory failure and another acute condition, (e.g., myocardial infarction, cerebrovascular accident, aspiration pneumonia), the principal diagnosis will not be the same in every situation. This applies whether the other acute condition is a respiratory or nonrespiratory condition. Selection of the principal diagnosis will be dependent on the circumstances of admission. If both the respiratory failure and the other acute condition are equally responsible for occasioning the admission to the hospital, and there are no chapter-specific sequencing rules, the guideline regarding two or more diagnoses that equally meet the definition for principal diagnosis *(Section II, C.)* may be applied in these situations.

If the documentation is not clear as to whether acute respiratory failure and another condition are equally responsible for occasioning the admission, query the provider for clarification.

c. Influenza due to certain identified influenza viruses
Code only confirmed cases of influenza due to certain identified influenza viruses (category J09), and due to other identified influenza virus (category J10). This is an exception to the hospital inpatient guideline Section II, H. (Uncertain Diagnosis).

In this context, "confirmation" does not require documentation of positive laboratory testing specific for avian or other novel influenza A or other identified influenza virus. However, coding should be based on the provider's diagnostic statement that the patient has avian influenza, or other novel influenza A, for category J09, or has another particular identified strain of influenza, such as H1N1 or H3N2, but not identified as novel or variant, for category J10.

If the provider records "suspected" or "possible" or "probable" avian influenza, or novel influenza, or other identified influenza, then the appropriate influenza code from category J11, Influenza due to unidentified influenza virus, should be assigned. A code from category J09, Influenza due to certain identified influenza viruses, should not be assigned nor should a code from category J10, Influenza due to other identified influenza virus.

d. Ventilator associated Pneumonia

1) Documentation of Ventilator associated Pneumonia
As with all procedural or postprocedural complications, code assignment is based on the provider's documentation of the relationship between the condition and the procedure.

Code J95.851, Ventilator associated pneumonia, should be assigned only when the provider has documented ventilator associated pneumonia (VAP). An additional code to identify the organism (e.g., Pseudomonas aeruginosa, code B96.5) should also be assigned. Do not assign an additional code from categories J12-J18 to identify the type of pneumonia.

Code J95.851 should not be assigned for cases where the patient has pneumonia and is on a mechanical ventilator and the provider has not specifically stated that the pneumonia is ventilator-associated pneumonia. If the documentation is unclear as to whether the patient has a pneumonia that is a complication attributable to the mechanical ventilator, query the provider.

CHAPTER 10 – RESPIRATORY SYSTEM
Section I. C. 11. d. 2)

2) Ventilator associated Pneumonia Develops after Admission
A patient may be admitted with one type of pneumonia (e.g., code J13, Pneumonia due to Streptococcus pneumonia) and subsequently develop VAP. In this instance, the principal diagnosis would be the appropriate code from categories J12-J18 for the pneumonia diagnosed at the time of admission. Code J95.851, Ventilator associated pneumonia, would be assigned as an additional diagnosis when the provider has also documented the presence of ventilator associated pneumonia.

11. Chapter 11: Diseases of the Digestive System (K00-K94)

Reserved for future guideline expansion

12. Chapter 12: Diseases of the Skin and Subcutaneous Tissue (L00-L99)

a. Pressure ulcer stage codes

1) Pressure ulcer stages
Codes from category L89, Pressure ulcer, ~~are combination codes that~~ identify the site of the pressure ulcer as well as the stage of the ulcer.

The ICD-10-CM classifies pressure ulcer stages based on severity, which is designated by stages 1-4, unspecified stage and unstageable.

Assign as many codes from category L89 as needed to identify all the pressure ulcers the patient has, if applicable.

2) Unstageable pressure ulcers
Assignment of the code for unstageable pressure ulcer (L89.--0) should be based on the clinical documentation. These codes are used for pressure ulcers whose stage cannot be clinically determined (e.g., the ulcer is covered by eschar or has been treated with a skin or muscle graft) and pressure ulcers that are documented as deep tissue injury but not documented as due to trauma. This code should not be confused with the codes for unspecified stage (L89.--9). When there is no documentation regarding the stage of the pressure ulcer, assign the appropriate code for unspecified stage (L89.--9).

3) Documented pressure ulcer stage
Assignment of the pressure ulcer stage code should be guided by clinical documentation of the stage or documentation of the terms found in the Alphabetic Index. For clinical terms describing the stage that are not found in the Alphabetic Index, and there is no documentation of the stage, the provider should be queried.

4) Patients admitted with pressure ulcers documented as healed
No code is assigned if the documentation states that the pressure ulcer is completely healed.

5) Patients admitted with pressure ulcers documented as healing
Pressure ulcers described as healing should be assigned the appropriate pressure ulcer stage code based on the documentation in the medical record. If the documentation does not provide information about the stage of the healing pressure ulcer, assign the appropriate code for unspecified stage.

If the documentation is unclear as to whether the patient has a current (new) pressure ulcer or if the patient is being treated for a healing pressure ulcer, query the provider.

For ulcers that were present on admission but healed at the time of discharge, assign the code for the site and stage of the pressure ulcer at the time of admission.

6) Patient admitted with pressure ulcer evolving into another stage during the admission
If a patient is admitted with a pressure ulcer at one stage and it progresses to a higher stage, ~~assign the code for the highest stage reported for that site~~ two separate codes should be assigned: one code for the site and stage of the ulcer on admission and a second code for the same ulcer site and the highest stage reported during the stay.

CHAPTER 13 – MUSCULOSKELETAL SYSTEM
Section I. C. 13. a.

13. Chapter 13: Diseases of the Musculoskeletal System and Connective Tissue (M00-M99)

a. Site and laterality

Most of the codes within Chapter 13 have site and laterality designations. The site represents the bone, joint or the muscle involved. For some conditions where more than one bone, joint or muscle is usually involved, such as osteoarthritis, there is a "multiple sites" code available. For categories where no multiple site code is provided and more than one bone, joint or muscle is involved, multiple codes should be used to indicate the different sites involved.

1) Bone versus joint

For certain conditions, the bone may be affected at the upper or lower end, (e.g., avascular necrosis of bone, M87, Osteoporosis, M80, M81). Though the portion of the bone affected may be at the joint, the site designation will be the bone, not the joint.

b. Acute traumatic versus chronic or recurrent musculoskeletal conditions

Many musculoskeletal conditions are a result of previous injury or trauma to a site, or are recurrent conditions. Bone, joint or muscle conditions that are the result of a healed injury are usually found in chapter 13. Recurrent bone, joint or muscle conditions are also usually found in chapter 13. Any current, acute injury should be coded to the appropriate injury code from chapter 19. Chronic or recurrent conditions should generally be coded with a code from chapter 13. If it is difficult to determine from the documentation in the record which code is best to describe a condition, query the provider.

c. Coding of Pathologic Fractures

7th character A is for use as long as the patient is receiving active treatment for the fracture. ~~Examples of active treatment are: surgical treatment, emergency department encounter, evaluation and continuing treatment by the same or a different physician.~~ While the patient may be seen by a new or different provider over the course of treatment for a pathological fracture, assignment of the 7th character is based on whether the patient is undergoing active treatment and not whether the provider is seeing the patient for the first time.

7th character D is to be used for encounters after the patient has completed active treatment. The other 7th characters, listed under each subcategory in the Tabular List, are to be used for subsequent encounters for routine care of fractures during the healing and recovery phase as well as treatment of problems associated with the healing, such as malunions, nonunions, and sequelae.

Care for complications of surgical treatment for fracture repairs during the healing or recovery phase should be coded with the appropriate complication codes.

See Section I.C.19. Coding of traumatic fractures.

d. Osteoporosis

Osteoporosis is a systemic condition, meaning that all bones of the musculoskeletal system are affected. Therefore, site is not a component of the codes under category M81, Osteoporosis without current pathological fracture. The site codes under category M80, Osteoporosis with current pathological fracture, identify the site of the fracture, not the osteoporosis.

1) Osteoporosis without pathological fracture

Category M81, Osteoporosis without current pathological fracture, is for use for patients with osteoporosis who do not currently have a pathologic fracture due to the osteoporosis, even if they have had a fracture in the past. For patients with a history of osteoporosis fractures, status code Z87.310, Personal history of (healed) osteoporosis fracture, should follow the code from M81.

2) Osteoporosis with current pathological fracture

Category M80, Osteoporosis with current pathological fracture, is for patients who have a current pathologic fracture at the time of an encounter. The codes under M80 identify the site of the fracture. A code from category M80, not a traumatic fracture code, should be used for any patient with known osteoporosis who suffers a fracture, even if the patient had a minor fall or trauma, if that fall or trauma would not usually break a normal, healthy bone.

CHAPTER 14 – GENITOURINARY SYSTEM
Section I. C. 14. a.

14. Chapter 14: Diseases of Genitourinary System (N00-N99)

a. Chronic kidney disease

1) Stages of chronic kidney disease (CKD)

The ICD-10-CM classifies CKD based on severity. The severity of CKD is designated by stages 1-5. Stage 2, code N18.2, equates to mild CKD; stage 3, code N18.3, equates to moderate CKD; and stage 4, code N18.4, equates to severe CKD. Code N18.6, End stage renal disease (ESRD), is assigned when the provider has documented end-stage-renal disease (ESRD).

If both a stage of CKD and ESRD are documented, assign code N18.6 only.

2) Chronic kidney disease and kidney transplant status

Patients who have undergone kidney transplant may still have some form of chronic kidney disease (CKD) because the kidney transplant may not fully restore kidney function. Therefore, the presence of CKD alone does not constitute a transplant complication. Assign the appropriate N18 code for the patient's stage of CKD and code Z94.0, Kidney transplant status. If a transplant complication such as failure or rejection or other transplant complication is documented, see section I.C.19.g for information on coding complications of a kidney transplant. If the documentation is unclear as to whether the patient has a complication of the transplant, query the provider.

3) Chronic kidney disease with other conditions

Patients with CKD may also suffer from other serious conditions, most commonly diabetes mellitus and hypertension. The sequencing of the CKD code in relationship to codes for other contributing conditions is based on the conventions in the Tabular List.

See I.C.9. Hypertensive chronic kidney disease.
See I.C.19. Chronic kidney disease and kidney transplant complications.

15. Chapter 15: Pregnancy, Childbirth, and the Puerperium (O00-O9A)

a. General Rules for Obstetric Cases

1) Codes from chapter 15 and sequencing priority

Obstetric cases require codes from chapter 15, codes in the range O00-O9A, Pregnancy, Childbirth, and the Puerperium. Chapter 15 codes have sequencing priority over codes from other chapters. Additional codes from other chapters may be used in conjunction with chapter 15 codes to further specify conditions. Should the provider document that the pregnancy is incidental to the encounter, then code Z33.1, Pregnant state, incidental, should be used in place of any chapter 15 codes. It is the provider's responsibility to state that the condition being treated is not affecting the pregnancy.

2) Chapter 15 codes used only on the maternal record

Chapter 15 codes are to be used only on the maternal record, never on the record of the newborn.

3) Final character for trimester

The majority of codes in Chapter 15 have a final character indicating the trimester of pregnancy. The timeframes for the trimesters are indicated at the beginning of the chapter. If trimester is not a component of a code it is because the condition always occurs in a specific trimester, or the concept of trimester of pregnancy is not applicable. Certain codes have characters for only certain trimesters because the condition does not occur in all trimesters, but it may occur in more than just one.

Assignment of the final character for trimester should be based on the provider's documentation of the trimester (or number of weeks) for the current admission/encounter. This applies to the assignment of trimester for pre-existing conditions as well as those that develop during or are due to the pregnancy. The provider's documentation of the number of weeks may be used to assign the appropriate code identifying the trimester.

Whenever delivery occurs during the current admission, and there is an "in childbirth" option for the obstetric complication being coded, the "in childbirth" code should be assigned.

4) Selection of trimester for inpatient admissions that encompass more than one trimesters

In instances when a patient is admitted to a hospital for complications of pregnancy during one trimester and remains in the hospital into a subsequent trimester, the trimester character for the antepartum complication code should be assigned on the basis of the trimester when the complication developed, not the trimester of the discharge. If the condition developed prior to the current admission/encounter or represents a pre-existing condition, the trimester character for the trimester at the time of the admission/encounter should be assigned.

5) Unspecified trimester

Each category that includes codes for trimester has a code for "unspecified trimester." The "unspecified trimester" code should rarely be used, such as when the documentation in the record is insufficient to determine the trimester and it is not possible to obtain clarification.

6) 7th character for Fetus Identification

Where applicable, a 7th character is to be assigned for certain categories (O31, O32, O33.3 - O33.6, O35, O36, O40, O41, O60.1, O60.2, O64, and O69) to identify the fetus for which the complication code applies.

Assign 7th character "0":
- For single gestations
- When the documentation in the record is insufficient to determine the fetus affected and it is not possible to obtain clarification.
- When it is not possible to clinically determine which fetus is affected.

b. Selection of OB Principal or First-listed Diagnosis

1) Routine outpatient prenatal visits

For routine outpatient prenatal visits when no complications are present, a code from category Z34, Encounter for supervision of normal pregnancy, should be used as the first-listed diagnosis. These codes should not be used in conjunction with chapter 15 codes.

2) Supervision of High-Risk Pregnancy

Codes from category O09, Supervision of high-risk pregnancy, are intended for use only during the prenatal period. For complications during the labor or delivery episode as a result of a high-risk pregnancy, assign the applicable complication codes from Chapter 15. If there are no complications during the labor and delivery episode, assign code O80, Encounter for full-term uncomplicated delivery.

For routine prenatal outpatient visits for patients with high-risk pregnancies, a code from category O09, Supervision of high-risk pregnancy, should be used as the first-listed diagnosis. Secondary chapter 15 codes may be used in conjunction with these codes if appropriate.

3) Episodes when no delivery occurs

In episodes when no delivery occurs, the principal diagnosis should correspond to the principal complication of the pregnancy which necessitated the encounter. Should more than one complication exist, all of which are treated or monitored, any of the complications codes may be sequenced first.

4) When a delivery occurs

~~When a delivery occurs, the principal diagnosis should correspond to the main circumstances or complication of the delivery.~~ When an obstetric patient is admitted and delivers during that admission, the condition that prompted the admission should be sequenced as the principal diagnosis. If multiple conditions prompted the admission, sequence the one most related to the delivery as the principal diagnosis. A code for any complication of the delivery should be assigned as an additional diagnosis. In cases of cesarean delivery, ~~the selection of the principal diagnosis should be the condition established after study that was responsible for the patient's admission. If~~ if the patient was admitted with a condition that resulted in the performance of a cesarean procedure, that condition should be selected as the principal diagnosis. If the reason for the admission/~~encounter~~ was unrelated to the condition resulting in the cesarean delivery, the condition related to the reason for the admission/~~encounter~~ should be selected as the principal diagnosis.

5) Outcome of delivery

A code from category Z37, Outcome of delivery, should be included on every maternal record when a delivery has occurred. These codes are not to be used on subsequent records or on the newborn record.

c. Pre-existing conditions versus conditions due to the pregnancy

Certain categories in Chapter 15 distinguish between conditions of the mother that existed prior to pregnancy (pre-existing) and those that are a direct result of pregnancy. When assigning codes from Chapter 15, it is important to assess if a condition was pre-existing prior to pregnancy or developed during or due to the pregnancy in order to assign the correct code.

Categories that do not distinguish between pre-existing and pregnancy-related conditions may be used for either. It is acceptable to use codes specifically for the puerperium with codes complicating pregnancy and childbirth if a condition arises postpartum during the delivery encounter.

d. Pre-existing hypertension in pregnancy

Category O10, Pre-existing hypertension complicating pregnancy, childbirth and the puerperium, includes codes for hypertensive heart and hypertensive chronic kidney disease. When assigning one of the O10 codes that includes hypertensive heart disease or hypertensive chronic kidney disease, it is necessary to add a secondary code from the appropriate hypertension category to specify the type of heart failure or chronic kidney disease.

See Section I.C.9. Hypertension.

e. Fetal Conditions Affecting the Management of the Mother

1) Codes from categories O35 and O36

Codes from categories O35, Maternal care for known or suspected fetal abnormality and damage, and O36, Maternal care for other fetal problems, are assigned only when the fetal condition is actually responsible for modifying the management of the mother, i.e., by requiring diagnostic studies, additional observation, special care, or termination of pregnancy. The fact that the fetal condition exists does not justify assigning a code from this series to the mother's record.

2) In utero surgery

In cases when surgery is performed on the fetus, a diagnosis code from category O35, Maternal care for known or suspected fetal abnormality and damage, should be assigned identifying the fetal condition. Assign the appropriate procedure code for the procedure performed.

No code from Chapter 16, the perinatal codes, should be used on the mother's record to identify fetal conditions. Surgery performed in utero on a fetus is still to be coded as an obstetric encounter.

f. HIV Infection in Pregnancy, Childbirth and the Puerperium

During pregnancy, childbirth or the puerperium, a patient admitted because of an HIV-related illness should receive a principal diagnosis from subcategory O98.7-, Human immunodeficiency [HIV] disease complicating pregnancy, childbirth and the puerperium, followed by the code(s) for the HIV-related illness(es).

Patients with asymptomatic HIV infection status admitted during pregnancy, childbirth, or the puerperium should receive codes of O98.7- and Z21, Asymptomatic human immunodeficiency virus [HIV] infection status.

g. Diabetes mellitus in pregnancy

Diabetes mellitus is a significant complicating factor in pregnancy. Pregnant women who are diabetic should be assigned a code from category O24, Diabetes mellitus in pregnancy, childbirth, and the puerperium, first, followed by the appropriate diabetes code(s) (E08-E13) from Chapter 4.

h. Long-term use of insulin *and oral hypoglycemics*

Code Z79.4, Long-term (current) use of insulin, or code Z79.84, Long-term (current) use of oral hypoglycemic drugs, should also be assigned if the diabetes mellitus is being treated with insulin or oral medications. If the patient is treated with both oral medications and insulin, only the code for insulin-controlled should be assigned.

i. Gestational (pregnancy induced) diabetes

Gestational (pregnancy induced) diabetes can occur during the second and third trimester of pregnancy in women who were not diabetic prior to pregnancy. Gestational diabetes can cause complications in the pregnancy similar to those of pre-existing diabetes mellitus. It also puts the woman at greater risk of developing diabetes after the pregnancy. Codes for gestational diabetes are in subcategory O24.4, Gestational diabetes mellitus. No other code from category O24, Diabetes mellitus in pregnancy, childbirth, and the puerperium, should be used with a code from O24.4.

The codes under subcategory O24.4 include diet controlled, ~~and~~ insulin controlled, and controlled by oral hypoglycemic drugs. If a patient with gestational diabetes is treated with both diet and insulin, only the code for insulin-controlled is required. If a patient with gestational diabetes is treated with both diet and oral hypoglycemic medications, only the code for "controlled by oral hypoglycemic drugs" is required. Code Z79.4, Long-term (current) use of insulin or code Z79.84, Long-term (current) use of oral hypoglycemic drugs, should not be assigned with codes from subcategory O24.4.

An abnormal glucose tolerance in pregnancy is assigned a code from subcategory O99.81, Abnormal glucose complicating pregnancy, childbirth, and the puerperium.

j. Sepsis and septic shock complicating abortion, pregnancy, childbirth and the puerperium

When assigning a chapter 15 code for sepsis complicating abortion, pregnancy, childbirth, and the puerperium, a code for the specific type of infection should be assigned as an additional diagnosis. If severe sepsis is present, a code from subcategory R65.2, Severe sepsis, and code(s) for associated organ dysfunction(s) should also be assigned as additional diagnoses.

CHAPTER 15 – PREGNANCY
Section I. C. 15. k.

k.   Puerperal sepsis

Code O85, Puerperal sepsis, should be assigned with a secondary code to identify the causal organism (e.g., for a bacterial infection, assign a code from category B95-B96, Bacterial infections in conditions classified elsewhere). A code from category A40, Streptococcal sepsis, or A41, Other sepsis, should not be used for puerperal sepsis. If applicable, use additional codes to identify severe sepsis (R65.2-) and any associated acute organ dysfunction.

l.   Alcohol and tobacco use during pregnancy, childbirth and the puerperium

1)   Alcohol use during pregnancy, childbirth and the puerperium

Codes under subcategory O99.31, Alcohol use complicating pregnancy, childbirth, and the puerperium, should be assigned for any pregnancy case when a mother uses alcohol during the pregnancy or postpartum. A secondary code from category F10, Alcohol related disorders, should also be assigned to identify manifestations of the alcohol use.

2)   Tobacco use during pregnancy, childbirth and the puerperium

Codes under subcategory O99.33, Smoking (tobacco) complicating pregnancy, childbirth, and the puerperium, should be assigned for any pregnancy case when a mother uses any type of tobacco product during the pregnancy or postpartum. A secondary code from category F17, Nicotine dependence, Tobacco use, should also be assigned to identify the type of nicotine dependence.

m.   Poisoning, toxic effects, adverse effects and underdosing in a pregnant patient

A code from subcategory O9A.2, Injury, poisoning and certain other consequences of external causes complicating pregnancy, childbirth, and the puerperium, should be sequenced first, followed by the appropriate injury, poisoning, toxic effect, adverse effect or underdosing code, and then the additional code(s) that specifies the condition caused by the poisoning, toxic effect, adverse effect or underdosing.

See Section I.C.19. Adverse effects, poisoning, underdosing and toxic effects.

n.   Normal Delivery, Code O80

1)   Encounter for full term uncomplicated delivery

Code O80 should be assigned when a woman is admitted for a full-term normal delivery and delivers a single, healthy infant without any complications antepartum, during the delivery, or postpartum during the delivery episode. Code O80 is always a principal diagnosis. It is not to be used if any other code from chapter 15 is needed to describe a current complication of the antenatal, delivery, or perinatal period. Additional codes from other chapters may be used with code O80 if they are not related to or are in any way complicating the pregnancy.

2)   Uncomplicated delivery with resolved antepartum complication

Code O80 may be used if the patient had a complication at some point during the pregnancy, but the complication is not present at the time of the admission for delivery.

3)   Outcome of delivery for O80

Z37.0, Single live birth, is the only outcome of delivery code appropriate for use with O80.

o.   The Peripartum and Postpartum Periods

1)   Peripartum and Postpartum periods

The postpartum period begins immediately after delivery and continues for six weeks following delivery. The peripartum period is defined as the last month of pregnancy to five months postpartum.

2)   Peripartum and postpartum complication

A postpartum complication is any complication occurring within the six-week period.

3)   Pregnancy-related complications after 6 week period

Chapter 15 codes may also be used to describe pregnancy-related complications after the peripartum or postpartum period if the provider documents that a condition is pregnancy related.

4)   Admission for routine postpartum care following delivery outside hospital

When the mother delivers outside the hospital prior to admission and is admitted for routine postpartum care and no complications are noted, code Z39.0, Encounter for care and examination of mother immediately after delivery, should be assigned as the principal diagnosis.

5)   Pregnancy associated cardiomyopathy

Pregnancy associated cardiomyopathy, code O90.3, is unique in that it may be diagnosed in the third trimester of pregnancy but may continue to progress months after delivery. For this reason, it is referred to as peripartum cardiomyopathy. Code O90.3 is only for use when the cardiomyopathy develops as a result of pregnancy in a woman who did not have pre-existing heart disease.

CHAPTER 15 – PREGNANCY
Section I. C. 16. p. 1)

p.   Code O94, Sequelae of complication of pregnancy, childbirth, and the puerperium

1)   Code O94

Code O94, Sequelae of complication of pregnancy, childbirth, and the puerperium, is for use in those cases when an initial complication of a pregnancy develops a sequelae requiring care or treatment at a future date.

2)   After the initial postpartum period

This code may be used at any time after the initial postpartum period.

3)   Sequencing of Code O94

This code, like all sequela codes, is to be sequenced following the code describing the sequelae of the complication.

q.   Termination of Pregnancy and Spontaneous abortions

1)   Abortion with Liveborn Fetus

When an attempted termination of pregnancy results in a liveborn fetus, assign code Z33.2, Encounter for elective termination of pregnancy and a code from category Z37, Outcome of Delivery.

2)   Retained Products of Conception following an abortion

Subsequent encounters for retained products of conception following a spontaneous abortion or elective termination of pregnancy are assigned the appropriate code from category O03, Spontaneous abortion, or codes O07.4, Failed attempted termination of pregnancy without complication and Z33.2, Encounter for elective termination of pregnancy. This advice is appropriate even when the patient was discharged previously with a discharge diagnosis of complete abortion.

3)   Complications leading to abortion

Codes from Chapter 15 may be used as additional codes to identify any documented complications of the pregnancy in conjunction with codes in categories in O07 and O08.

r.   Abuse in a pregnant patient

For suspected or confirmed cases of abuse of a pregnant patient, a code(s) from subcategories O9A.3, Physical abuse complicating pregnancy, childbirth, and the puerperium, O9A.4, Sexual abuse complicating pregnancy, childbirth, and the puerperium, and O9A.5, Psychological abuse complicating pregnancy, childbirth, and the puerperium, should be sequenced first, followed by the appropriate codes (if applicable) to identify any associated current injury due to physical abuse, sexual abuse, and the perpetrator of abuse.

See Section I.C.19.f. Adult and child abuse, neglect and other maltreatment.

16.   Chapter 16: Certain Conditions Originating in the Perinatal Period (P00-P96)

For coding and reporting purposes the perinatal period is defined as before birth through the 28th day following birth. The following guidelines are provided for reporting purposes

a.   General Perinatal Rules

1)   Use of Chapter 16 Codes

Codes in this chapter are never for use on the maternal record.

Codes from Chapter 15, the obstetric chapter, are never permitted on the newborn record. Chapter 16 codes may be used throughout the life of the patient if the condition is still present.

2)   Principal Diagnosis for Birth Record

When coding the birth episode in a newborn record, assign a code from category Z38, Liveborn infants according to place of birth and type of delivery, as the principal diagnosis. A code from category Z38 is assigned only once, to a newborn at the time of birth. If a newborn is transferred to another institution, a code from category Z38 should not be used at the receiving hospital.

A code from category Z38 is used only on the newborn record, not on the mother's record.

3)   Use of Codes from other Chapters with Codes from Chapter 16

Codes from other chapters may be used with codes from chapter 16 if the codes from the other chapters provide more specific detail. Codes for signs and symptoms may be assigned when a definitive diagnosis has not been established. If the reason for the encounter is a perinatal condition, the code from chapter 16 should be sequenced first.

CHAPTER 16 – PERINATAL PERIOD
Section I. C. 16. a. 4)

4) Use of Chapter 16 Codes after the Perinatal Period
Should a condition originate in the perinatal period, and continue throughout the life of the patient, the perinatal code should continue to be used regardless of the patient's age.

5) Birth process or community acquired conditions
If a newborn has a condition that may be either due to the birth process or community acquired and the documentation does not indicate which it is, the default is due to the birth process and the code from Chapter 16 should be used. If the condition is community-acquired, a code from Chapter 16 should not be assigned.

6) Code all clinically significant conditions
All clinically significant conditions noted on routine newborn examination should be coded. A condition is clinically significant if it requires:
- clinical evaluation; or
- therapeutic treatment; or
- diagnostic procedures; or
- extended length of hospital stay; or
- increased nursing care and/or monitoring; or
- has implications for future health care needs

Note: The perinatal guidelines listed above are the same as the general coding guidelines for "additional diagnoses", except for the final point regarding implications for future health care needs. Codes should be assigned for conditions that have been specified by the provider as having implications for future health care needs.

b. Observation and Evaluation of Newborns for Suspected Conditions not Found
~~Reserved for future expansion~~

1) Assign a code from category Z05, Observation and evaluation of newborns and infants for suspected conditions ruled out, to identify those instances when a healthy newborn is evaluated for a suspected condition that is determined after study not to be present. Do not use a code from category Z05 when the patient has identified signs or symptoms of a suspected problem; in such cases code the sign or symptom.

2) A code from category Z05 may also be assigned as a principal or first-listed code for readmissions or encounters when the code from category Z38 code no longer applies. Codes from category Z05 are for use only for healthy newborns and infants for which no condition after study is found to be present.

3) Z05 on a birth record
A code from category Z05 is to be used as a secondary code after the code from category Z38, Liveborn infants according to place of birth and type of delivery.

c. Coding Additional Perinatal Diagnoses

1) Assigning codes for conditions that require treatment
Assign codes for conditions that require treatment or further investigation, prolong the length of stay, or require resource utilization.

2) Codes for conditions specified as having implications for future health care needs
Assign codes for conditions that have been specified by the provider as having implications for future health care needs.

Note: This guideline should not be used for adult patients.

d. Prematurity and Fetal Growth Retardation
Providers utilize different criteria in determining prematurity. A code for prematurity should not be assigned unless it is documented. Assignment of codes in categories P05, Disorders of newborn related to slow fetal growth and fetal malnutrition, and P07, Disorders of newborn related to short gestation and low birth weight, not elsewhere classified, should be based on the recorded birth weight and estimated gestational age. Codes from category P05 should not be assigned with codes from category P07.

When both birth weight and gestational age are available, two codes from category P07 should be assigned, with the code for birth weight sequenced before the code for gestational age.

e. Low birth weight and immaturity status
Codes from category P07, Disorders of newborn related to short gestation and low birth weight, not elsewhere classified, are for use for a child or adult who was premature or had a low birth weight as a newborn and this is affecting the patient's current health status.

See Section I.C.21. Factors influencing health status and contact with health services, Status.

CHAPTER 16 – PERINATAL PERIOD
Section I. C. 16. f.

f. Bacterial Sepsis of Newborn
Category P36, Bacterial sepsis of newborn, includes congenital sepsis. If a perinate is documented as having sepsis without documentation of congenital or community acquired, the default is congenital and a code from category P36 should be assigned. If the P36 code includes the causal organism, an additional code from category B95, Streptococcus, Staphylococcus, and Enterococcus as the cause of diseases classified elsewhere, or B96, Other bacterial agents as the cause of diseases classified elsewhere, should not be assigned. If the P36 code does not include the causal organism, assign an additional code from category B96. If applicable, use additional codes to identify severe sepsis (R65.2-) and any associated acute organ dysfunction.

g. Stillbirth
Code P95, Stillbirth, is only for use in institutions that maintain separate records for stillbirths. No other code should be used with P95. Code P95 should not be used on the mother's record.

17. Chapter 17: Congenital Malformations, Deformations, and Chromosomal Abnormalities (Q00-Q99)

Assign an appropriate code(s) from categories Q00-Q99, Congenital malformations, deformations, and chromosomal abnormalities when a malformation/deformation or chromosomal abnormality is documented. A malformation/deformation/or chromosomal abnormality may be the principal/first-listed diagnosis on a record or a secondary diagnosis.

When a malformation/deformation/or chromosomal abnormality does not have a unique code assignment, assign additional code(s) for any manifestations that may be present.

When the code assignment specifically identifies the malformation/deformation/or chromosomal abnormality, manifestations that are an inherent component of the anomaly should not be coded separately. Additional codes should be assigned for manifestations that are not an inherent component.

Codes from Chapter 17 may be used throughout the life of the patient. If a congenital malformation or deformity has been corrected, a personal history code should be used to identify the history of the malformation or deformity. Although present at birth, malformation/deformation/or chromosomal abnormality may not be identified until later in life. Whenever the condition is diagnosed by the physician, it is appropriate to assign a code from codes Q00-Q99.

For the birth admission, the appropriate code from category Z38, Liveborn infants, according to place of birth and type of delivery, should be sequenced as the principal diagnosis, followed by any congenital anomaly codes, Q00-Q99.

18. Chapter 18: Symptoms, Signs, and Abnormal Clinical and Laboratory Findings, Not Elsewhere Classified (R00-R99)

Chapter 18 includes symptoms, signs, abnormal results of clinical or other investigative procedures, and ill-defined conditions regarding which no diagnosis classifiable elsewhere is recorded. Signs and symptoms that point to a specific diagnosis have been assigned to a category in other chapters of the classification.

a. Use of symptom codes
Codes that describe symptoms and signs are acceptable for reporting purposes when a related definitive diagnosis has not been established (confirmed) by the provider.

b. Use of a symptom code with a definitive diagnosis code
Codes for signs and symptoms may be reported in addition to a related definitive diagnosis when the sign or symptom is not routinely associated with that diagnosis, such as the various signs and symptoms associated with complex syndromes. The definitive diagnosis code should be sequenced before the symptom code.

Signs or symptoms that are associated routinely with a disease process should not be assigned as additional codes, unless otherwise instructed by the classification.

c. Combination codes that include symptoms
ICD-10-CM contains a number of combination codes that identify both the definitive diagnosis and common symptoms of that diagnosis. When using one of these combination codes, an additional code should not be assigned for the symptom.

d. Repeated falls
Code R29.6, Repeated falls, is for use for encounters when a patient has recently fallen and the reason for the fall is being investigated.

Code Z91.81, History of falling, is for use when a patient has fallen in the past and is at risk for future falls. When appropriate, both codes R29.6 and Z91.81 may be assigned together.

CHAPTER 18 – SYMPTOMS & SIGNS
Section I. C. 18. e.

e.   Coma scale

The coma scale codes (R40.2-) can be used in conjunction with traumatic brain injury codes, acute cerebrovascular disease or sequelae of cerebrovascular disease codes. These codes are primarily for use by trauma registries, but they may be used in any setting where this information is collected. The coma scale may also be used to assess the status of the central nervous system for other non-trauma conditions, such as monitoring patients in the intensive care unit regardless of medical condition. The coma scale codes should be sequenced after the diagnosis code(s).

These codes, one from each subcategory, are needed to complete the scale. The 7th character indicates when the scale was recorded. The 7th character should match for all three codes.

At a minimum, report the initial score documented on presentation at your facility. This may be a score from the emergency medicine technician (EMT) or in the emergency department. If desired, a facility may choose to capture multiple coma scale scores.

Assign code R40.24, Glasgow coma scale, total score, when only the total score is documented in the medical record and not the individual score(s).

f.   Functional quadriplegia

Functional quadriplegia (code R53.2) is the lack of ability to use one's limbs or to ambulate due to extreme debility. It is not associated with neurologic deficit or injury, and code R53.2 should not be used for cases of neurologic quadriplegia. It should only be assigned if functional quadriplegia is specifically documented in the medical record.

g.   SIRS due to Non-Infectious Process

The systemic inflammatory response syndrome (SIRS) can develop as a result of certain non-infectious disease processes, such as trauma, malignant neoplasm, or pancreatitis. When SIRS is documented with a noninfectious condition, and no subsequent infection is documented, the code for the underlying condition, such as an injury, should be assigned, followed by code R65.10, Systemic inflammatory response syndrome (SIRS) of non-infectious origin without acute organ dysfunction, or code R65.11, Systemic inflammatory response syndrome (SIRS) of non-infectious origin with acute organ dysfunction. If an associated acute organ dysfunction is documented, the appropriate code(s) for the specific type of organ dysfunction(s) should be assigned in addition to code R65.11. If acute organ dysfunction is documented, but it cannot be determined if the acute organ dysfunction is associated with SIRS or due to another condition (e.g., directly due to the trauma), the provider should be queried.

h.   Death NOS

Code R99, Ill-defined and unknown cause of mortality, is only for use in the very limited circumstance when a patient who has already died is brought into an emergency department or other healthcare facility and is pronounced dead upon arrival. It does not represent the discharge disposition of death.

i.   NIHSS Stroke Scale

The NIH stroke scale (NIHSS) codes (R29.7- -) can be used in conjunction with acute stroke codes (I63) to identify the patient's neurological status and the severity of the stroke. The stroke scale codes should be sequenced after the acute stroke diagnosis code(s).

At a minimum, report the initial score documented. If desired, a facility may choose to capture multiple stroke scale scores.

See Section I.B.14. for information concerning the medical record documentation that may be used for assignment of the NIHSS codes.

19.   Chapter 19: Injury, Poisoning, and Certain Other Consequences of External Causes (S00-T88)

a.   Application of 7th Characters in Chapter 19

Most categories in chapter 19 have a 7th character requirement for each applicable code. Most categories in this chapter have three 7th character values (with the exception of fractures): A, initial encounter, D, subsequent encounter and S, sequela. Categories for traumatic fractures have additional 7th character values. While the patient may be seen by a new or different provider over the course of treatment for an injury, assignment of the 7th character is based on whether the patient is undergoing active treatment and not whether the provider is seeing the patient for the first time.

For complication codes, active treatment refers to treatment for the condition described by the code, even though it may be related to an earlier precipitating problem. For example, code T84.50xA, Infection and inflammatory reaction due to unspecified internal joint prosthesis, initial encounter, is used when active treatment is provided for the infection, even though the condition relates to the prosthetic device, implant or graft that was placed at a previous encounter.

CHAPTER 19 – INJURY & POISONING
Section I. C. 19. a.

7th character "A" initial encounter is used ~~while~~ for each encounter where the patient is receiving active treatment for the condition. ~~Examples of active treatment are: surgical treatment, emergency department encounter, and evaluation and continuing treatment by the same or a different physician.~~

7th character "D" subsequent encounter is used for encounters after the patient has ~~received~~ completed active treatment of the condition and is receiving routine care for the condition during the healing or recovery phase. ~~Examples of subsequent care are: cast change or removal, an x-ray to check healing status of fracture, removal of external or internal fixation device, medication adjustment, other aftercare and follow up visits following treatment of the injury or condition.~~

The aftercare Z codes should not be used for aftercare for conditions such as injuries or poisonings, where 7th characters are provided to identify subsequent care. For example, for aftercare of an injury, assign the acute injury code with the 7th character "D" (subsequent encounter).

7th character "S", sequela, is for use for complications or conditions that arise as a direct result of an condition, such as scar formation after a burn. The scars are sequelae of the burn. When using 7th character "S", it is necessary to use both the injury code that precipitated the sequela and the code for the sequela itself. The "S" is added only to the injury code, not the sequela code. The 7th character "S" identifies the injury responsible for the sequela. The specific type of sequela (e.g., scar) is sequenced first, followed by the injury code.

See Section I.B.10 Sequela (Late Effects).

b.   Coding of Injuries

When coding injuries, assign separate codes for each injury unless a combination code is provided, in which case the combination code is assigned. Code T07, Unspecified multiple injuries should not be assigned in the inpatient setting unless information for a more specific code is not available. Traumatic injury codes (S00-T14.9) are not to be used for normal, healing surgical wounds or to identify complications of surgical wounds.

The code for the most serious injury, as determined by the provider and the focus of treatment, is sequenced first.

1)   Superficial injuries

Superficial injuries such as abrasions or contusions are not coded when associated with more severe injuries of the same site.

2)   Primary injury with damage to nerves/blood vessels

When a primary injury results in minor damage to peripheral nerves or blood vessels, the primary injury is sequenced first with additional code(s) for injuries to nerves and spinal cord (such as category S04), and/or injury to blood vessels (such as category S15). When the primary injury is to the blood vessels or nerves, that injury should be sequenced first.

c.   Coding of Traumatic Fractures

The principles of multiple coding of injuries should be followed in coding fractures. Fractures of specified sites are coded individually by site in accordance with both the provisions within categories S02, S12, S22, S32, S42, S49, S52, S59, S62, S72, S79, S82, S89, S92 and the level of detail furnished by medical record content.

A fracture not indicated as open or closed should be coded to closed. A fracture not indicated whether displaced or not displaced should be coded to displaced.

More specific guidelines are as follows:

1)   Initial vs. Subsequent Encounter for Fractures

Traumatic fractures are coded using the appropriate 7th character for initial encounter (A, B, C) ~~while~~ for each encounter where the patient is receiving active treatment for the fracture. ~~Examples of active treatment are: surgical treatment, emergency department encounter, and evaluation and continuing (ongoing) treatment by the same or different physician.~~ The appropriate 7th character for initial encounter should also be assigned for a patient who delayed seeking treatment for the fracture or nonunion.

Fractures are coded using the appropriate 7th character for subsequent care for encounters after the patient has completed active treatment of the fracture and is receiving routine care for the fracture during the healing or recovery phase. ~~Examples of fracture aftercare are: cast change or removal, an x-ray to check healing status of fracture, removal of external or internal fixation device, medication adjustment, and follow-up visits following fracture treatment.~~

Care for complications of surgical treatment for fracture repairs during the healing or recovery phase should be coded with the appropriate complication codes.

CHAPTER 19 – INJURY & POISONING
Section I. C. 19. c. 1)

Care of complications of fractures, such as malunion and nonunion, should be reported with the appropriate 7th character for subsequent care with nonunion (K, M, N,) or subsequent care with malunion (P, Q, R).

Malunion/nonunion: The appropriate 7th character for initial encounter should also be assigned for a patient who delayed seeking treatment for the fracture or nonunion.

The open fracture designations in the assignment of the 7th character for fractures of the forearm, femur and lower leg, including ankle are based on the Gustilo open fracture classification. When the Gustilo classification type is not specified for an open fracture, the 7th character for open fracture type I or II should be assigned (B, E, H, M, Q).

A code from category M80, not a traumatic fracture code, should be used for any patient with known osteoporosis who suffers a fracture, even if the patient had a minor fall or trauma, if that fall or trauma would not usually break a normal, healthy bone.

See Section I.C.13. Osteoporosis.

The aftercare Z codes should not be used for aftercare for traumatic fractures. For aftercare of a traumatic fracture, assign the acute fracture code with the appropriate 7th character.

2)   Multiple fractures sequencing
Multiple fractures are sequenced in accordance with the severity of the fracture.

d.   Coding of Burns and Corrosions
The ICD-10-CM makes a distinction between burns and corrosions. The burn codes are for thermal burns, except sunburns, that come from a heat source, such as a fire or hot appliance. The burn codes are also for burns resulting from electricity and radiation. Corrosions are burns due to chemicals. The guidelines are the same for burns and corrosions.

Current burns (T20-T25) are classified by depth, extent and by agent (X code). Burns are classified by depth as first degree (erythema), second degree (blistering), and third degree (full-thickness involvement). Burns of the eye and internal organs (T26-T28) are classified by site, but not by degree.

1)   Sequencing of burn and related condition codes
Sequence first the code that reflects the highest degree of burn when more than one burn is present.

a. When the reason for the admission or encounter is for treatment of external multiple burns, sequence first the code that reflects the burn of the highest degree.

b. When a patient has both internal and external burns, the circumstances of admission govern the selection of the principal diagnosis or first-listed diagnosis.

c. When a patient is admitted for burn injuries and other related conditions such as smoke inhalation and/or respiratory failure, the circumstances of admission govern the selection of the principal or first-listed diagnosis.

2)   Burns of the same local site
Classify burns of the same local site (three-character category level, T20-T28) but of different degrees to the subcategory identifying the highest degree recorded in the diagnosis.

3)   Non-healing burns
Non-healing burns are coded as acute burns.

Necrosis of burned skin should be coded as a non-healed burn.

4)   Infected Burn
For any documented infected burn site, use an additional code for the infection.

5)   Assign separate codes for each burn site
When coding burns, assign separate codes for each burn site. Category T30, Burn and corrosion, body region unspecified is extremely vague and should rarely be used.

6)   Burns and Corrosions Classified According to Extent of Body Surface Involved
Assign codes from category T31, Burns classified according to extent of body surface involved, or T32, Corrosions classified according to extent of body surface involved, when the site of the burn is not specified or when there is a need for additional data. It is advisable to use category T31 as additional coding when needed to provide data for evaluating burn mortality, such as that needed by burn units. It is also advisable to use category T31 as an additional code for reporting purposes when there is mention of a third-degree burn involving 20 percent or more of the body surface.

CHAPTER 19 – INJURY & POISONING
Section I. C. 19. d. 6)

Categories T31 and T32 are based on the classic "rule of nines" in estimating body surface involved: head and neck are assigned nine percent, each arm nine percent, each leg 18 percent, the anterior trunk 18 percent, posterior trunk 18 percent, and genitalia one percent. Providers may change these percentage assignments where necessary to accommodate infants and children who have proportionately larger heads than adults, and patients who have large buttocks, thighs, or abdomen that involve burns.

7)   Encounters for treatment of sequela of burns
Encounters for the treatment of the late effects of burns or corrosions (i.e., scars or joint contractures) should be coded with a burn or corrosion code with the 7th character "S" for sequela.

8)   Sequelae with a late effect code and current burn
When appropriate, both a code for a current burn or corrosion with 7th character "A" or "D" and a burn or corrosion code with 7th character "S" may be assigned on the same record (when both a current burn and sequelae of an old burn exist). Burns and corrosions do not heal at the same rate and a current healing wound may still exist with sequela of a healed burn or corrosion.

See Section I.B.10 Sequela (Late Effects).

9)   Use of an external cause code with burns and corrosions
An external cause code should be used with burns and corrosions to identify the source and intent of the burn, as well as the place where it occurred.

e.   Adverse Effects, Poisoning, Underdosing and Toxic Effects
Codes in categories T36-T65 are combination codes that include the substance that was taken as well as the intent. No additional external cause code is required for poisonings, toxic effects, adverse effects and underdosing codes.

1)   Do not code directly from the Table of Drugs
Do not code directly from the Table of Drugs and Chemicals. Always refer back to the Tabular List.

2)   Use as many codes as necessary to describe
Use as many codes as necessary to describe completely all drugs, medicinal or biological substances.

3)   If the same code would describe the causative agent
If the same code would describe the causative agent for more than one adverse reaction, poisoning, toxic effect or underdosing, assign the code only once.

4)   If two or more drugs, medicinal or biological substances
If two or more drugs, medicinal or biological substances are reported, code each individually unless a combination code is listed in the Table of Drugs and Chemicals.

5)   The occurrence of drug toxicity is classified in ICD-10-CM as follows:

(a)   Adverse Effect
When coding an adverse effect of a drug that has been correctly prescribed and properly administered, assign the appropriate code for the nature of the adverse effect followed by the appropriate code for the adverse effect of the drug (T36-T50). The code for the drug should have a 5th or 6th character "5" (for example T36.0X5-). Examples of the nature of an adverse effect are tachycardia, delirium, gastrointestinal hemorrhaging, vomiting, hypokalemia, hepatitis, renal failure, or respiratory failure.

(b)   Poisoning
When coding a poisoning or reaction to the improper use of a medication (e.g., overdose, wrong substance given or taken in error, wrong route of administration), first assign the appropriate code from categories T36-T50. The poisoning codes have an associated intent as their 5th or 6th character accidental, intentional self-harm, assault and undetermined. If the intent of the poisoning is unknown or unspecified, code the intent as accidental intent. The undetermined intent is only for use if the documentation in the record specifies that the intent cannot be determined. Use additional code(s) for all manifestations of poisonings.

If there is also a diagnosis of abuse or dependence of the substance, the abuse or dependence is assigned as an additional code.

Examples of poisoning include:

(i)   Error was made in drug prescription
Errors made in drug prescription or in the administration of the drug by provider, nurse, patient, or other person.

(ii) **Overdose of a drug intentionally taken**
If an overdose of a drug was intentionally taken or administered and resulted in drug toxicity, it would be coded as a poisoning.

(iii) **Nonprescribed drug taken with correctly prescribed and properly administered drug**
If a nonprescribed drug or medicinal agent was taken in combination with a correctly prescribed and properly administered drug, any drug toxicity or other reaction resulting from the interaction of the two drugs would be classified as a poisoning.

(iv) **Interaction of drug(s) and alcohol**
When a reaction results from the interaction of a drug(s) and alcohol, this would be classified as poisoning.

See Section I.C.4. if poisoning is the result of insulin pump malfunctions.

(c) **Underdosing**
Underdosing refers to taking less of a medication than is prescribed by a provider or a manufacturer's instruction. For underdosing, assign the code from categories T36-T50 (fifth or sixth character "6").

Codes for underdosing should never be assigned as principal or first-listed codes. If a patient has a relapse or exacerbation of the medical condition for which the drug is prescribed because of the reduction in dose, then the medical condition itself should be coded.

Noncompliance (Z91.12-, Z91.13-) or complication of care (Y63.61, Y63.6-Y63.9) codes are to be used with an underdosing code to indicate intent, if known.

(d) **Toxic Effects**
When a harmful substance is ingested or comes in contact with a person, this is classified as a toxic effect. The toxic effect codes are in categories T51-T65.

Toxic effect codes have an associated intent: accidental, intentional self-harm, assault and undetermined.

f. **Adult and child abuse, neglect and other maltreatment**
Sequence first the appropriate code from categories T74.- (Adult and child abuse, neglect and other maltreatment, confirmed) or T76.- (Adult and child abuse, neglect and other maltreatment, suspected) for abuse, neglect and other maltreatment, followed by any accompanying mental health or injury code(s).

If the documentation in the medical record states abuse or neglect it is coded as confirmed (T74.-). It is coded as suspected if it is documented as suspected (T76.-).

For cases of confirmed abuse or neglect an external cause code from the assault section (X92-Y09) should be added to identify the cause of any physical injuries. A perpetrator code (Y07) should be added when the perpetrator of the abuse is known. For suspected cases of abuse or neglect, do not report external cause or perpetrator code.

If a suspected case of abuse, neglect or mistreatment is ruled out during an encounter code Z04.71, Encounter for examination and observation following alleged physical adult abuse, ruled out, or code Z04.72, Encounter for examination and observation following alleged physical child abuse, ruled out, should be used, not a code from T76.

If a suspected case of alleged rape or sexual abuse is ruled out during an encounter code Z04.41, Encounter for examination and observation following alleged ~~physical~~ adult rape ~~abuse, ruled out~~, or code Z04.42, Encounter for examination and observation following alleged child rape ~~or sexual abuse, ruled out~~, should be used, not a code from T76.

See Section I.C.15. Abuse in a pregnant patient.

g. **Complications of care**

1) **General guidelines for complications of care**

(a) **Documentation of complications of care**

See section I.B.16. for information on documentation of complications of care.

2) **Pain due to medical devices**
Pain associated with devices, implants or grafts left in a surgical site (for example painful hip prosthesis) is assigned to the appropriate code(s) found in Chapter 19, Injury, poisoning, and certain other consequences of external causes. Specific codes for pain due to medical devices are found in the T code section of the ICD-10-CM. Use additional code(s) from category G89 to identify acute or chronic pain due to presence of the device, implant or graft (G89.18 or G89.28).

3) **Transplant complications**

(a) **Transplant complications other than kidney**
Codes under category T86, Complications of transplanted organs and tissues, are for use for both complications and rejection of transplanted organs. A transplant complication code is only assigned if the complication affects the function of the transplanted organ. Two codes are required to fully describe a transplant complication: the appropriate code from category T86 and a secondary code that identifies the complication.

Pre-existing conditions or conditions that develop after the transplant are not coded as complications unless they affect the function of the transplanted organs.

See I.C.21. for transplant organ removal status.
See I.C.2. for malignant neoplasm associated with transplanted organ.

(b) **Kidney transplant complications**
Patients who have undergone kidney transplant may still have some form of chronic kidney disease (CKD) because the kidney transplant may not fully restore kidney function. Code T86.1- should be assigned for documented complications of a kidney transplant, such as transplant failure or rejection or other transplant complication. Code T86.1- should not be assigned for post kidney transplant patients who have chronic kidney (CKD) unless a transplant complication such as transplant failure or rejection is documented. If the documentation is unclear as to whether the patient has a complication of the transplant, query the provider.

Conditions that affect the function of the transplanted kidney, other than CKD, should be assigned a code from subcategory T86.1, Complications of transplanted organ, kidney, and a secondary code that identifies the complication.

For patients with CKD following a kidney transplant, but who do not have a complication such as failure or rejection, *see section I.C.14. Chronic kidney disease and kidney transplant status.*

4) **Complication codes that include the external cause**
As with certain other T codes, some of the complications of care codes have the external cause included in the code. The code includes the nature of the complication as well as the type of procedure that caused the complication. No external cause code indicating the type of procedure is necessary for these codes.

5) **Complications of care codes within the body system chapters**
Intraoperative and postprocedural complication codes are found within the body system chapters with codes specific to the organs and structures of that body system. These codes should be sequenced first, followed by a code(s) for the specific complication, if applicable.

20. **Chapter 20: External Causes of Morbidity (V00-Y99)**

The external causes of morbidity codes should never be sequenced as the first-listed or principal diagnosis.

External cause codes are intended to provide data for injury research and evaluation of injury prevention strategies. These codes capture how the injury or health condition happened (cause), the intent (unintentional or accidental; or intentional, such as suicide or assault), the place where the event occurred the activity of the patient at the time of the event, and the person's status (e.g., civilian, military).

There is no national requirement for mandatory ICD-10-CM external cause code reporting. Unless a provider is subject to a state-based external cause code reporting mandate or these codes are required by a particular payer, reporting of ICD-10-CM codes in Chapter 20, External Causes of Morbidity, is not required. In the absence of a mandatory reporting requirement, providers are encouraged to voluntarily report external cause codes, as they provide valuable data for injury research and evaluation of injury prevention strategies.

a. **General External Cause Coding Guidelines**

1) **Used with any code in the range of A00.0-T88.9, Z00-Z99**
An external cause code may be used with any code in the range of A00.0-T88.9, Z00-Z99, classification that is a health condition due to an external cause. Though they are most applicable to injuries, they are also valid for use with such things as infections or diseases due to an external source, and other health conditions, such as a heart attack that occurs during strenuous physical activity.

2) **External cause code used for length of treatment**
Assign the external cause code, with the appropriate 7th character (initial encounter, subsequent encounter or sequela) for each encounter for which the injury or condition is being treated.

CHAPTER 20 – EXTERNAL CAUSES
Section I. C. 20. a. 2)

Most categories in chapter 20 have a 7th character requirement for each applicable code. Most categories in this chapter have three 7th character values: A, initial encounter, D, subsequent encounter and S, sequela. While the patient may be seen by a new or different provider over the course of treatment for an injury or condition, assignment of the 7th character for external cause should match the 7th character of the code assigned for the associated injury or condition for the encounter.

3) Use the full range of external cause codes
Use the full range of external cause codes to completely describe the cause, the intent, the place of occurrence, and if applicable, the activity of the patient at the time of the event, and the patient's status, for all injuries, and other health conditions due to an external cause.

4) Assign as many external cause codes as necessary
Assign as many external cause codes as necessary to fully explain each cause. If only one external code can be recorded, assign the code most related to the principal diagnosis.

5) The selection of the appropriate external cause code
The selection of the appropriate external cause code is guided by the Alphabetic Index of External Causes and by Inclusion and Exclusion notes in the Tabular List.

6) External cause code can never be a principal diagnosis
An external cause code can never be a principal (first-listed) diagnosis.

7) Combination external cause codes
Certain of the external cause codes are combination codes that identify sequential events that result in an injury, such as a fall which results in striking against an object. The injury may be due to either event or both. The combination external cause code used should correspond to the sequence of events regardless of which caused the most serious injury.

8) No external cause code needed in certain circumstances
No external cause code from Chapter 20 is needed if the external cause and intent are included in a code from another chapter (e.g. T36.0x1- Poisoning by penicillins, accidental (unintentional)).

b. Place of Occurrence Guideline
Codes from category Y92, Place of occurrence of the external cause, are secondary codes for use after other external cause codes to identify the location of the patient at the time of injury or other condition.

Generally, a place of occurrence code is assigned only once, at the initial encounter for treatment. However, in the rare instance that a new injury occurs during hospitalization, an additional place of occurrence code may be assigned. No 7th characters are used for Y92.

Do not use place of occurrence code Y92.9 if the place is not stated or is not applicable.

c. Activity Code
Assign a code from category Y93, Activity code, to describe the activity of the patient at the time the injury or other health condition occurred.

An activity code is used only once, at the initial encounter for treatment. Only one code from Y93 should be recorded on a medical record.

The activity codes are not applicable to poisonings, adverse effects, misadventures or sequela.

Do not assign Y93.9, Unspecified activity, if the activity is not stated.

A code from category Y93 is appropriate for use with external cause and intent codes if identifying the activity provides additional information about the event.

d. Place of Occurrence, Activity, and Status Codes Used with other External Cause Code
When applicable, place of occurrence, activity, and external cause status codes are sequenced after the main external cause code(s). Regardless of the number of external cause codes assigned, there should be only one place of occurrence code, one activity code, and one external cause status code assigned to an encounter.

e. If the Reporting Format Limits the Number of External Cause Codes
If the reporting format limits the number of external cause codes that can be used in reporting clinical data, report the code for the cause/intent most related to the principal diagnosis. If the format permits capture of additional external cause codes, the cause/intent, including medical misadventures, of the additional events should be reported rather than the codes for place, activity, or external status.

CHAPTER 20 – EXTERNAL CAUSES
Section I. C. 20. f.

f. Multiple External Cause Coding Guidelines
More than one external cause code is required to fully describe the external cause of an illness or injury. The assignment of external cause codes should be sequenced in the following priority:
If two or more events cause separate injuries, an external cause code should be assigned for each cause. The first-listed external cause code will be selected in the following order:

External codes for child and adult abuse take priority over all other external cause codes.
See Section I.C.19. Child and Adult abuse guidelines.

External cause codes for terrorism events take priority over all other external cause codes except child and adult abuse.

External cause codes for cataclysmic events take priority over all other external cause codes except child and adult abuse and terrorism.

External cause codes for transport accidents take priority over all other external cause codes except cataclysmic events, child and adult abuse and terrorism.

Activity and external cause status codes are assigned following all causal (intent) external cause codes.

The first-listed external cause code should correspond to the cause of the most serious diagnosis due to an assault, accident, or self-harm, following the order of hierarchy listed above.

g. Child and Adult Abuse Guideline
Adult and child abuse, neglect and maltreatment are classified as assault. Any of the assault codes may be used to indicate the external cause of any injury resulting from the confirmed abuse.

For confirmed cases of abuse, neglect and maltreatment, when the perpetrator is known, a code from Y07, Perpetrator of maltreatment and neglect, should accompany any other assault codes.

See Section I.C.19. Adult and child abuse, neglect and other maltreatment.

h. Unknown or Undetermined Intent Guideline
If the intent (accident, self-harm, assault) of the cause of an injury or other condition is unknown or unspecified, code the intent as accidental intent. All transport accident categories assume accidental intent.

1) Use of undetermined intent
External cause codes for events of undetermined intent are only for use if the documentation in the record specifies that the intent cannot be determined.

i. Sequelae (Late Effects) of External Cause Guidelines

1) Sequelae external cause codes
Sequela are reported using the external cause code with the 7th character "S" for sequela. These codes should be used with any report of a late effect or sequela resulting from a previous injury.

See Section I.B.10 Sequela (Late Effects).

2) Sequela external cause code with a related current injury
A sequela external cause code should never be used with a related current nature of injury code.

3) Use of sequela external cause codes for subsequent visits
Use a late effect external cause code for subsequent visits when a late effect of the initial injury is being treated. Do not use a late effect external cause code for subsequent visits for follow-up care (e.g., to assess healing, to receive rehabilitative therapy) of the injury when no late effect of the injury has been documented.

j. Terrorism Guidelines

1) Cause of injury identified by the Federal Government (FBI) as terrorism
When the cause of an injury is identified by the Federal Government (FBI) as terrorism, the first-listed external cause code should be a code from category Y38, Terrorism. The definition of terrorism employed by the FBI is found at the inclusion note at the beginning of category Y38. Use additional code for place of occurrence (Y92.-). More than one Y38 code may be assigned if the injury is the result of more than one mechanism of terrorism.

2) Cause of an injury is suspected to be the result of terrorism
When the cause of an injury is suspected to be the result of terrorism a code from category Y38 should not be assigned. Suspected cases should be classified as assault.

GUIDELINES

3) Code Y38.9, Terrorism, secondary effects
Assign code Y38.9, Terrorism, secondary effects, for conditions occurring subsequent to the terrorist event. This code should not be assigned for conditions that are due to the initial terrorist act.

It is acceptable to assign code Y38.9 with another code from Y38 if there is an injury due to the initial terrorist event and an injury that is a subsequent result of the terrorist event.

k. External cause status
A code from category Y99, External cause status, should be assigned whenever any other external cause code is assigned for an encounter, including an Activity code, except for the events noted below. Assign a code from category Y99, External cause status, to indicate the work status of the person at the time the event occurred. The status code indicates whether the event occurred during military activity, whether a non-military person was at work, whether an individual including a student or volunteer was involved in a non-work activity at the time of the causal event.

A code from Y99, External cause status, should be assigned, when applicable, with other external cause codes, such as transport accidents and falls. The external cause status codes are not applicable to poisonings, adverse effects, misadventures or late effects.

Do not assign a code from category Y99 if no other external cause codes (cause, activity) are applicable for the encounter.

An external cause status code is used only once, at the initial encounter for treatment. Only one code from Y99 should be recorded on a medical record.

Do not assign code Y99.9, Unspecified external cause status, if the status is not stated.

21. Chapter 21: Factors Influencing Health Status and Contact with Health Services (Z00-Z99)

Note: The chapter specific guidelines provide additional information about the use of Z codes for specified encounters.

a. Use of Z codes in any healthcare setting
Z codes are for use in any healthcare setting. Z codes may be used as either a first-listed (principal diagnosis code in the inpatient setting) or secondary code, depending on the circumstances of the encounter.
Certain Z codes may only be used as first-listed or principal diagnosis.

b. Z Codes indicate a reason for an encounter
Z codes are not procedure codes. A corresponding procedure code must accompany a Z code to describe any procedure performed.

c. Categories of Z Codes

1) Contact/Exposure
Category Z20 indicates contact with, and suspected exposure to, communicable diseases. These codes are for patients who do not show any sign or symptom of a disease but are suspected to have been exposed to it by close personal contact with an infected individual or are in an area where a disease is epidemic.

Category Z77, Other contact with and (suspected) exposures hazardous to health, indicates contact with and suspected exposures hazardous to health.

Contact/exposure codes may be used as a first-listed code to explain an encounter for testing, or, more commonly, as a secondary code to identify a potential risk.

2) Inoculations and vaccinations
Code Z23 is for encounters for inoculations and vaccinations. It indicates that a patient is being seen to receive a prophylactic inoculation against a disease. Procedure codes are required to identify the actual administration of the injection and the type(s) of immunizations given. Code Z23 may be used as a secondary code if the inoculation is given as a routine part of preventive health care, such as a well-baby visit.

3) Status
Status codes indicate that a patient is either a carrier of a disease or has the sequelae or residual of a past disease or condition. This includes such things as the presence of prosthetic or mechanical devices resulting from past treatment. A status code is informative, because the status may affect the course of treatment and its outcome. A status code is distinct from a history code. The history code indicates that the patient no longer has the condition.

A status code should not be used with a diagnosis code from one of the body system chapters, if the diagnosis code includes the information provided by the status code. For example, code Z94.1, Heart transplant status, should not be used with a code from subcategory T86.2, Complications of heart transplant. The status code does not provide additional information. The complication code indicates that the patient is a heart transplant patient.

For encounters for weaning from a mechanical ventilator, assign a code from subcategory J96.1, Chronic respiratory failure, followed by code Z99.11, Dependence on respirator [ventilator] status.

The status Z codes/categories are:

Z14   Genetic carrier
Genetic carrier status indicates that a person carries a gene, associated with a particular disease, which may be passed to offspring who may develop that disease. The person does not have the disease and is not at risk of developing the disease.

Z15   Genetic susceptibility to disease
Genetic susceptibility indicates that a person has a gene that increases the risk of that person developing the disease.
Codes from category Z15 should not be used as principal or first-listed codes. If the patient has the condition to which he/she is susceptible, and that condition is the reason for the encounter, the code for the current condition should be sequenced first. If the patient is being seen for follow-up after completed treatment for this condition, and the condition no longer exists, a follow-up code should be sequenced first, followed by the appropriate personal history and genetic susceptibility codes. If the purpose of the encounter is genetic counseling associated with procreative management, code Z31.5, Encounter for genetic counseling, should be assigned as the first-listed code, followed by a code from category Z15. Additional codes should be assigned for any applicable family or personal history.

Z16   Resistance to antimicrobial drugs
This code indicates that a patient has a condition that is resistant to antimicrobial drug treatment. Sequence the infection code first.

Z17   Estrogen receptor status
Z18   Retained foreign body fragments
Z19   Hormone sensitivity malignancy status
Z21   Asymptomatic HIV infection status
This code indicates that a patient has tested positive for HIV but has manifested no signs or symptoms of the disease.

Z22   Carrier of infectious disease
Carrier status indicates that a person harbors the specific organisms of a disease without manifest symptoms and is capable of transmitting the infection.

Z28.3   Underimmunization status
Z33.1   Pregnant state, incidental
This code is a secondary code only for use when the pregnancy is in no way complicating the reason for visit. Otherwise, a code from the obstetric chapter is required.

Z66   Do not resuscitate
This code may be used when it is documented by the provider that a patient is on do not resuscitate status at any time during the stay.

Z67   Blood type
Z68   Body mass index (BMI)
As with all other secondary diagnosis codes, the BMI codes should only be assigned when they meet the definition of a reportable diagnosis (see Section III, Reporting Additional Diagnoses).

Z74.01   Bed confinement status
Z76.82   Awaiting organ transplant status
Z78   Other specified health status
Code Z78.1, Physical restraint status, may be used when it is documented by the provider that a patient has been put in restraints during the current encounter. Please note that this code should not be reported when it is documented by the provider that a patient is temporarily restrained during a procedure.

Z79   Long-term (current) drug therapy
Codes from this category indicate a patient's continuous use of a prescribed drug (including such things as aspirin therapy) for the long-term treatment of a condition or for prophylactic use. It is not for use for patients who have addictions to drugs. This subcategory is not for use of medications for detoxification or maintenance programs to prevent withdrawal symptoms in patients with drug dependence (e.g., methadone maintenance for opiate dependence). Assign the appropriate code for the drug dependence instead.

CHAPTER 21 – FACTORS INFLUENCING HEALTH
Section I. C. 21. c. 3)

Assign a code from Z79 if the patient is receiving a medication for an extended period as a prophylactic measure (such as for the prevention of deep vein thrombosis) or as treatment of a chronic condition (such as arthritis) or a disease requiring a lengthy course of treatment (such as cancer). Do not assign a code from category Z79 for medication being administered for a brief period of time to treat an acute illness or injury (such as a course of antibiotics to treat acute bronchitis).

Z88   Allergy status to drugs, medicaments and biological substances
       Except: Z88.9, Allergy status to unspecified drugs, medicaments and biological substances status
Z89   Acquired absence of limb
Z90   Acquired absence of organs, not elsewhere classified
Z91.0- Allergy status, other than to drugs and biological substances
Z92.82 Status post administration of tPA (rtPA) in a different facility within the last 24 hours prior to admission to a current facility.

       Assign code Z92.82, Status post administration of tPA (rtPA) in a different facility within the last 24 hours prior to admission to a current facility, as a secondary diagnosis when a patient is received by transfer into a facility and documentation indicates they were administered tissue plasminogen activator (tPA) within the last 24 hours prior to admission to the current facility.

       This guideline applies even if the patient is still receiving the tPA at the time they are received into the current facility.

       The appropriate code for the condition for which the tPA was administered (such as cerebrovascular disease or myocardial infarction) should be assigned first.

       Code Z92.82 is only applicable to the receiving facility record and not to the transferring facility record.

Z93   Artificial opening status
Z94   Transplanted organ and tissue status
Z95   Presence of cardiac and vascular implants and grafts
Z96   Presence of other functional implants
Z97   Presence of other devices
Z98   Other postprocedural states
       Assign code Z98.85, Transplanted organ removal status, to indicate that a transplanted organ has been previously removed. This code should not be assigned for the encounter in which the transplanted organ is removed. The complication necessitating removal of the transplant organ should be assigned for that encounter.

       See section I.C19. for information on the coding of organ transplant complications.

Z99   Dependence on enabling machines and devices, not elsewhere classified
       Note: Categories Z89-Z90 and Z93-Z99 are for use only if there are no complications or malfunctions of the organ or tissue replaced, the amputation site or the equipment on which the patient is dependent.

4)   **History (of)**
      There are two types of history Z codes, personal and family. Personal history codes explain a patient's past medical condition that no longer exists and is not receiving any treatment, but that has the potential for recurrence, and therefore may require continued monitoring.

      Family history codes are for use when a patient has a family member(s) who has had a particular disease that causes the patient to be at higher risk of also contracting the disease.

      Personal history codes may be used in conjunction with follow-up codes and family history codes may be used in conjunction with screening codes to explain the need for a test or procedure. History codes are also acceptable on any medical record regardless of the reason for visit. A history of an illness, even if no longer present, is important information that may alter the type of treatment ordered.

      The history Z code categories are:
Z80   Family history of primary malignant neoplasm
Z81   Family history of mental and behavioral disorders
Z82   Family history of certain disabilities and chronic diseases (leading to disablement)
Z83   Family history of other specific disorders
Z84   Family history of other conditions
Z85   Personal history of malignant neoplasm
Z86   Personal history of certain other diseases
Z87   Personal history of other diseases and conditions
Z91.4- Personal history of psychological trauma, not elsewhere classified
Z91.5 Personal history of self-harm

CHAPTER 21 – FACTORS INFLUENCING HEALTH
Section I. C. 21. c. 4)

Z91.8- Other specified personal risk factors, not elsewhere classified
       Exception: Z91.83, Wandering in diseases classified elsewhere
Z92   Personal history of medical treatment
       Except: Z92.0, Personal history of contraception
       Except: Z92.82, Status post administration of tPA (rtPA) in a different facility within the last 24 hours prior to admission to a current facility

5)   **Screening**
      Screening is the testing for disease or disease precursors in seemingly well individuals so that early detection and treatment can be provided for those who test positive for the disease (e.g., screening mammogram).

      The testing of a person to rule out or confirm a suspected diagnosis because the patient has some sign or symptom is a diagnostic examination, not a screening. In these cases, the sign or symptom is used to explain the reason for the test.

      A screening code may be a first-listed code if the reason for the visit is specifically the screening exam. It may also be used as an additional code if the screening is done during an office visit for other health problems. A screening code is not necessary if the screening is inherent to a routine examination, such as a pap smear done during a routine pelvic examination.

      Should a condition be discovered during the screening then the code for the condition may be assigned as an additional diagnosis.

      The Z code indicates that a screening exam is planned. A procedure code is required to confirm that the screening was performed.

      The screening Z codes/categories:
Z11   Encounter for screening for infectious and parasitic diseases
Z12   Encounter for screening for malignant neoplasms
Z13   Encounter for screening for other diseases and disorders
       Except: Z13.9, Encounter for screening, unspecified
Z36   Encounter for antenatal screening for mother

6)   **Observation**
      There are ~~two~~ three observation Z code categories. They are for use in very limited circumstances when a person is being observed for a suspected condition that is ruled out. The observation codes are not for use if an injury or illness or any signs or symptoms related to the suspected condition are present. In such cases the diagnosis/symptom code is used with the corresponding external cause code.

      The observation codes are to be used as principal diagnosis only. The only exception to this is when the principal diagnosis is required to be a code from category Z38, Live-born infants according to place of birth and type of delivery. Then a code from category Z05, Encounter for observation and evaluation of newborn for suspected diseases and conditions ruled out, is sequenced after the Z38 code. Additional codes may be used in addition to the observation code but only if they are unrelated to the suspected condition being observed.

      Codes from subcategory Z03.7, Encounter for suspected maternal and fetal conditions ruled out, may either be used as a first-listed or as an additional code assignment depending on the case. They are for use in very limited circumstances on a maternal record when an encounter is for a suspected maternal or fetal condition that is ruled out during that encounter (for example, a maternal or fetal condition may be suspected due to an abnormal test result). These codes should not be used when the condition is confirmed. In those cases, the confirmed condition should be coded. In addition, these codes are not for use if an illness or any signs or symptoms related to the suspected condition or problem are present. In such cases the diagnosis/symptom code is used.

      Additional codes may be used in addition to the code from subcategory Z03.7, but only if they are unrelated to the suspected condition being evaluated.

      Codes from subcategory Z03.7 may not be used for encounters for antenatal screening of mother. *See Section I.C.21. Screening.*

      For encounters for suspected fetal condition that are inconclusive following testing and evaluation, assign the appropriate code from category O35, O36, O40 or O41.

      The observation Z code categories:
Z03   Encounter for medical observation for suspected diseases and conditions ruled out
Z04   Encounter for examination and observation for other reasons
       Except: Z04.9, Encounter for examination and observation for unspecified reason
Z05   Encounter for observation and evaluation of newborn for suspected diseases and conditions ruled out

7) Aftercare

Aftercare visit codes cover situations when the initial treatment of a disease has been performed and the patient requires continued care during the healing or recovery phase, or for the long-term consequences of the disease. The aftercare Z code should not be used if treatment is directed at a current, acute disease. The diagnosis code is to be used in these cases. Exceptions to this rule are codes Z51.0, Encounter for antineoplastic radiation therapy, and codes from subcategory Z51.1, Encounter for antineoplastic chemotherapy and immunotherapy. These codes are to be first-listed, followed by the diagnosis code when a patient's encounter is solely to receive radiation therapy, chemotherapy, or immunotherapy for the treatment of a neoplasm. If the reason for the encounter is more than one type of antineoplastic therapy, code Z51.0 and a code from subcategory Z51.1 may be assigned together, in which case one of these codes would be reported as a secondary diagnosis.

The aftercare Z codes should also not be used for aftercare for injuries. For aftercare of an injury, assign the acute injury code with the appropriate 7th character (for subsequent encounter).

The aftercare codes are generally first-listed to explain the specific reason for the encounter. An aftercare code may be used as an additional code when some type of aftercare is provided in addition to the reason for admission and no diagnosis code is applicable. An example of this would be the closure of a colostomy during an encounter for treatment of another condition.

Aftercare codes should be used in conjunction with other aftercare codes or diagnosis codes to provide better detail on the specifics of an aftercare encounter visit, unless otherwise directed by the classification. Should a patient receive multiple types of antineoplastic therapy during the same encounter, code Z51.0, Encounter for antineoplastic radiation therapy, and codes from subcategory Z51.1, Encounter for antineoplastic chemotherapy and immunotherapy, may be used together on a record. The sequencing of multiple aftercare codes depends on the circumstances of the encounter.

Certain aftercare Z code categories need a secondary diagnosis code to describe the resolving condition or sequelae. For others, the condition is included in the code title.

Additional Z code aftercare category terms include fitting and adjustment, and attention to artificial openings.

Status Z codes may be used with aftercare Z codes to indicate the nature of the aftercare. For example code Z95.1, Presence of aortocoronary bypass graft, may be used with code Z48.812, Encounter for surgical aftercare following surgery on the circulatory system, to indicate the surgery for which the aftercare is being performed. A status code should not be used when the aftercare code indicates the type of status, such as using Z43.0, Encounter for attention to tracheostomy, with Z93.0, Tracheostomy status.

The aftercare Z category/codes:

Z42	Encounter for plastic and reconstructive surgery following medical procedure or healed injury
Z43	Encounter for attention to artificial openings
Z44	Encounter for fitting and adjustment of external prosthetic device
Z45	Encounter for adjustment and management of implanted device
Z46	Encounter for fitting and adjustment of other devices
Z47	Orthopedic aftercare
Z48	Encounter for other postprocedural aftercare
Z49	Encounter for care involving renal dialysis
Z51	Encounter for other aftercare and medical care

8) Follow-up

The follow-up codes are used to explain continuing surveillance following completed treatment of a disease, condition, or injury. They imply that the condition has been fully treated and no longer exists. They should not be confused with aftercare codes, or injury codes with a 7th character for subsequent encounter, that explain ongoing care of a healing condition or its sequelae. Follow-up codes may be used in conjunction with history codes to provide the full picture of the healed condition and its treatment. The follow-up code is sequenced first, followed by the history code.

A follow-up code may be used to explain multiple visits. Should a condition be found to have recurred on the follow-up visit, then the diagnosis code for the condition should be assigned in place of the follow-up code.

The follow-up Z code categories:

Z08	Encounter for follow-up examination after completed treatment for malignant neoplasm
Z09	Encounter for follow-up examination after completed treatment for conditions other than malignant neoplasm
Z39	Encounter for maternal postpartum care and examination

9) Donor

Codes in category Z52, Donors of organs and tissues, are used for living individuals who are donating blood or other body tissue. These codes are only for individuals donating for others, not for self-donations. They are not used to identify cadaveric donations.

10) Counseling

Counseling Z codes are used when a patient or family member receives assistance in the aftermath of an illness or injury, or when support is required in coping with family or social problems. They are not used in conjunction with a diagnosis code when the counseling component of care is considered integral to standard treatment.

The counseling Z codes/categories:

Z30.0-	Encounter for general counseling and advice on contraception
Z31.5	Encounter for genetic counseling
Z31.6	Encounter for general counseling and advice on procreation
Z32.2	Encounter for childbirth instruction
Z32.3	Encounter for childcare instruction
Z69	Encounter for mental health services for victim and perpetrator of abuse
Z70	Counseling related to sexual attitude, behavior and orientation
Z71	Persons encountering health services for other counseling and medical advice, not elsewhere classified
Z76.81	Expectant mother prebirth pediatrician visit

11) Encounters for Obstetrical and Reproductive Services

See Section I.C.15. Pregnancy, Childbirth, and the Puerperium, for further instruction on the use of these codes.

Z codes for pregnancy are for use in those circumstances when none of the problems or complications included in the codes from the Obstetrics chapter exist (a routine prenatal visit or postpartum care). Codes in category Z34, Encounter for supervision of normal pregnancy, are always first-listed and are not to be used with any other code from the OB chapter.

Codes in category Z3A, Weeks of gestation, may be assigned to provide additional information about the pregnancy. Category Z3A codes should not be assigned for pregnancies with abortive outcomes (categories O00-O08), elective termination of pregnancy (code Z33.32), nor for postpartum conditions, as category Z3A is not applicable to these conditions. The date of the admission should be used to determine weeks of gestation for inpatient admissions that encompass more than one gestational week.

The outcome of delivery, category Z37, should be included on all maternal delivery records. It is always a secondary code. Codes in category Z37 should not be used on the newborn record.

Z codes for family planning (contraceptive) or procreative management and counseling should be included on an obstetric record either during the pregnancy or the postpartum stage, if applicable.

Z codes/categories for obstetrical and reproductive services:

Z30	Encounter for contraceptive management
Z31	Encounter for procreative management
Z32.2	Encounter for childbirth instruction
Z32.3	Encounter for childcare instruction
Z33	Pregnant state
Z34	Encounter for supervision of normal pregnancy
Z36	Encounter for antenatal screening of mother
Z3A	Weeks of gestation
Z37	Outcome of delivery
Z39	Encounter for maternal postpartum care and examination
Z76.81	Expectant mother prebirth pediatrician visit

12) Newborns and Infants

See Section I.C.16. Newborn (Perinatal) Guidelines, for further instruction on the use of these codes.

Newborn Z codes/categories:

Z76.1	Encounter for health supervision and care of foundling
Z00.1-	Encounter for routine child health examination
Z38	Liveborn infants according to place of birth and type of delivery

13) Routine and administrative examinations

The Z codes allow for the description of encounters for routine examinations, such as, a general check-up, or, examinations for administrative purposes, such as, a pre-employment physical. The codes are not to be used if the examination is for diagnosis of a suspected condition or for treatment purposes. In such cases the diagnosis code is used. During a routine exam, should a diagnosis or condition be discovered, it should be coded as an additional code. Pre-existing and chronic conditions and history codes may also be included as additional codes as long as the examination is for administrative purposes and not focused on any particular condition.

Some of the codes for routine health examinations distinguish between "with" and "without" abnormal findings. Code assignment depends on the information that is known at the time the encounter is being coded. For example, if no abnormal findings were found during the examination, but the encounter is being coded before test results are back, it is acceptable to assign the code for "without abnormal findings." When assigning a code for "with abnormal findings," additional code(s) should be assigned to identify the specific abnormal finding(s).

Pre-operative examination and pre-procedural laboratory examination Z codes are for use only in those situations when a patient is being cleared for a procedure or surgery and no treatment is given.

The Z codes/categories for routine and administrative examinations:

Z00   Encounter for general examination without complaint, suspected or reported diagnosis
Z01   Encounter for other special examination without complaint, suspected or reported diagnosis
Z02   Encounter for administrative examination
       Except: Z02.9, Encounter for administrative examinations, unspecified
Z32.0- Encounter for pregnancy test

14) Miscellaneous Z codes

The miscellaneous Z codes capture a number of other health care encounters that do not fall into one of the other categories. Certain of these codes identify the reason for the encounter; others are for use as additional codes that provide useful information on circumstances that may affect a patient's care and treatment.

Prophylactic Organ Removal

For encounters specifically for prophylactic removal of an organ (such as prophylactic removal of breasts due to a genetic susceptibility to cancer or a family history of cancer), the principal or first-listed code should be a code from category Z40, Encounter for prophylactic surgery, followed by the appropriate codes to identify the associated risk factor (such as genetic susceptibility or family history).

If the patient has a malignancy of one site and is having prophylactic removal at another site to prevent either a new primary malignancy or metastatic disease, a code for the malignancy should also be assigned in addition to a code from subcategory Z40.0, Encounter for prophylactic surgery for risk factors related to malignant neoplasms. A Z40.0 code should not be assigned if the patient is having organ removal for treatment of a malignancy, such as the removal of the testes for the treatment of prostate cancer.

Miscellaneous Z codes/categories:

Z28   Immunization not carried out
       Except: Z28.3, Underimmunization status
Z29   Encounter for other prophylactic measures
Z40   Encounter for prophylactic surgery
Z41   Encounter for procedures for purposes other than remedying health state
       Except: Z41.9, Encounter for procedure for purposes other than remedying health state, unspecified
Z53   Persons encountering health services for specific procedures and treatment, not carried out
Z55   Problems related to education and literacy
Z56   Problems related to employment and unemployment
Z57   Occupational exposure to risk factors
Z58   Problems related to physical environment
Z59   Problems related to housing and economic circumstances
Z60   Problems related to social environment
Z62   Problems related to upbringing
Z63   Other problems related to primary support group, including family circumstances
Z64   Problems related to certain psychosocial circumstances
Z65   Problems related to other psychosocial circumstances
Z72   Problems related to lifestyle
       Note: These codes should be assigned only when the documentation specifies that the patient has an associated problem
Z73   Problems related to life management difficulty
Z74   Problems related to care provider dependency
       Except: Z74.01, Bed confinement status
Z75   Problems related to medical facilities and other health care
Z76.0 Encounter for issue of repeat prescription
Z76.3 Healthy person accompanying sick person
Z76.4 Other boarder to healthcare facility
Z76.5 Malingerer [conscious simulation]
Z91.1- Patient's noncompliance with medical treatment and regimen
Z91.83 Wandering in diseases classified elsewhere
Z91.89 Other specified personal risk factors, not elsewhere classified

15) Nonspecific Z codes

Certain Z codes are so non-specific, or potentially redundant with other codes in the classification, that there can be little justification for their use in the inpatient setting. Their use in the outpatient setting should be limited to those instances when there is no further documentation to permit more precise coding. Otherwise, any sign or symptom or any other reason for visit that is captured in another code should be used.

Nonspecific Z codes/categories:

Z02.9 Encounter for administrative examinations, unspecified
Z04.9 Encounter for examination and observation for unspecified reason
Z13.9 Encounter for screening, unspecified
Z41.9 Encounter for procedure for purposes other than remedying health state, unspecified
Z52.9 Donor of unspecified organ or tissue
Z86.59 Personal history of other mental and behavioral disorders
Z88.9 Allergy status to unspecified drugs, medicaments and biological substances status
Z92.0 Personal history of contraception

16) Z Codes That May Only be Principal/First-Listed Diagnosis

The following Z codes/categories may only be reported as the principal/first-listed diagnosis, except when there are multiple encounters on the same day and the medical records for the encounters are combined:

Z00   Encounter for general examination without complaint, suspected or reported diagnosis Except: Z00.6
Z01   Encounter for other special examination without complaint, suspected or reported diagnosis
Z02   Encounter for administrative examination
Z03   Encounter for medical observation for suspected diseases and conditions ruled out
Z04   Encounter for examination and observation for other reasons
Z31.81 Encounter for male factor infertility in female patient
Z31.82 Encounter for Rh incompatibility status
Z31.83 Encounter for assisted reproductive fertility procedure cycle
Z31.84 Encounter for fertility preservation procedure
Z34   Encounter for supervision of normal pregnancy
Z39   Encounter for maternal postpartum care and examination
Z38   Liveborn infants according to place of birth and type of delivery
Z42   Encounter for plastic and reconstructive surgery following medical procedure or healed injury
Z51.0 Encounter for antineoplastic radiation therapy
Z51.1- Encounter for antineoplastic chemotherapy and immunotherapy
Z52   Donors of organs and tissues
       Except: Z52.9, Donor of unspecified organ or tissue
Z76.1 Encounter for health supervision and care of foundling
Z76.2 Encounter for health supervision and care of other healthy infant and child
Z99.12 Encounter for respirator [ventilator] dependence during power failure

GUIDELINES

SECTION II – PRINCIPAL DIAGNOSIS
Section II.

Section II. Selection of Principal Diagnosis

The circumstances of inpatient admission always govern the selection of principal diagnosis. The principal diagnosis is defined in the Uniform Hospital Discharge Data Set (UHDDS) as "that condition established after study to be chiefly responsible for occasioning the admission of the patient to the hospital for care."

The UHDDS definitions are used by hospitals to report inpatient data elements in a standardized manner. These data elements and their definitions can be found in the July 31, 1985, Federal Register (Vol. 50, No, 147), pp. 31038-40.

Since that time the application of the UHDDS definitions has been expanded to include all non-outpatient settings (acute care, short term, long term care and psychiatric hospitals; home health agencies; rehab facilities; nursing homes, etc). The UHDDS definitions also apply to hospice services (all levels of care).

In determining principal diagnosis the coding conventions in the ICD-10-CM, the Tabular List and Alphabetic Index take precedence over these official coding guidelines. *(See Section I.A., Conventions for the ICD-10-CM)*

The importance of consistent, complete documentation in the medical record cannot be overemphasized. Without such documentation the application of all coding guidelines is a difficult, if not impossible, task.

A. Codes for symptoms, signs, and ill-defined conditions
Codes for symptoms, signs, and ill-defined conditions from Chapter 18 are not to be used as principal diagnosis when a related definitive diagnosis has been established.

B. Two or more interrelated conditions, each potentially meeting the definition for principal diagnosis.
When there are two or more interrelated conditions (such as diseases in the same ICD-10-CM chapter or manifestations characteristically associated with a certain disease) potentially meeting the definition of principal diagnosis, either condition may be sequenced first, unless the circumstances of the admission, the therapy provided, the Tabular List, or the Alphabetic Index indicate otherwise.

C. Two or more diagnoses that equally meet the definition for principal diagnosis
In the unusual instance when two or more diagnoses equally meet the criteria for principal diagnosis as determined by the circumstances of admission, diagnostic workup and/or therapy provided, and the Alphabetic Index, Tabular List, or another coding guidelines does not provide sequencing direction, any one of the diagnoses may be sequenced first.

D. Two or more comparative or contrasting conditions.
In those rare instances when two or more contrasting or comparative diagnoses are documented as "either/or" (or similar terminology), they are coded as if the diagnoses were confirmed and the diagnoses are sequenced according to the circumstances of the admission. If no further determination can be made as to which diagnosis should be principal, either diagnosis may be sequenced first.

E. A symptom(s) followed by contrasting/comparative diagnoses
Guideline has been deleted effective October 1, 2014

F. Original treatment plan not carried out
Sequence as the principal diagnosis the condition, which after study occasioned the admission to the hospital, even though treatment may not have been carried out due to unforeseen circumstances.

G. Complications of surgery and other medical care
When the admission is for treatment of a complication resulting from surgery or other medical care, the complication code is sequenced as the principal diagnosis. If the complication is classified to the T80-T88 series and the code lacks the necessary specificity in describing the complication, an additional code for the specific complication should be assigned.

H. Uncertain Diagnosis
If the diagnosis documented at the time of discharge is qualified as "probable", "suspected", "likely", "questionable", "possible", or "still to be ruled out", or other similar terms indicating uncertainty, code the condition as if it existed or was established. The bases for these guidelines are the diagnostic workup, arrangements for further workup or observation, and initial therapeutic approach that correspond most closely with the established diagnosis.

Note: This guideline is applicable only to inpatient admissions to short-term, acute, long-term care and psychiatric hospitals.

SECTION II – PRINCIPAL DIAGNOSIS
Section II. I.

I. Admission from Observation Unit

1. Admission Following Medical Observation
When a patient is admitted to an observation unit for a medical condition, which either worsens or does not improve, and is subsequently admitted as an inpatient of the same hospital for this same medical condition, the principal diagnosis would be the medical condition which led to the hospital admission.

2. Admission Following Post-Operative Observation
When a patient is admitted to an observation unit to monitor a condition (or complication) that develops following outpatient surgery, and then is subsequently admitted as an inpatient of the same hospital, hospitals should apply the Uniform Hospital Discharge Data Set (UHDDS) definition of principal diagnosis as "that condition established after study to be chiefly responsible for occasioning the admission of the patient to the hospital for care."

J. Admission from Outpatient Surgery
When a patient receives surgery in the hospital's outpatient surgery department and is subsequently admitted for continuing inpatient care at the same hospital, the following guidelines should be followed in selecting the principal diagnosis for the inpatient admission:
   • If the reason for the inpatient admission is a complication, assign the complication as the principal diagnosis.
   • If no complication, or other condition, is documented as the reason for the inpatient admission, assign the reason for the outpatient surgery as the principal diagnosis.
   • If the reason for the inpatient admission is another condition unrelated to the surgery, assign the unrelated condition as the principal diagnosis.

K. Admission/Encounters for Rehabilitation
When the purpose for the admission/encounter is rehabilitation, sequence first the code for the condition for which the service is being performed. For example, for an admission/encounter for rehabilitation right-sided dominant hemiplegia following a cerebrovascular infarction, report code I69.351, Hemiplegia and hemiparesis following cerebral infarction affecting right dominant side, as the first-listed or principal diagnosis.

If the condition for which the rehabilitation service is no longer present, report the appropriate aftercare code as the first-listed or principal diagnosis. For example, if a patient with severe degenerative osteoarthritis of the hip, underwent hip replacement and the current encounter/admission is for rehabilitation, report code Z47.1, Aftercare following joint replacement surgery, as the principal diagnosis.

See Section I.C.21.c.7, Factors influencing health status and contact with health services, Aftercare.

SECTION III – ADDITIONAL DIAGNOSES
Section III.

Section III. Reporting Additional Diagnoses

GENERAL RULES FOR OTHER (ADDITIONAL) DIAGNOSES

For reporting purposes the definition for "other diagnoses" is interpreted as additional conditions that affect patient care in terms of requiring:

    clinical evaluation; or
    therapeutic treatment; or
    diagnostic procedures; or
    extended length of hospital stay; or
    increased nursing care and/or monitoring.

The UHDDS item #11-b defines Other Diagnoses as "all conditions that coexist at the time of admission, that develop subsequently, or that affect the treatment received and/or the length of stay. Diagnoses that relate to an earlier episode which have no bearing on the current hospital stay are to be excluded." UHDDS definitions apply to inpatients in acute care, short-term, long term care and psychiatric hospital setting. The UHDDS definitions are used by acute care short-term hospitals to report inpatient data elements in a standardized manner. These data elements and their definitions can be found in the July 31, 1985, Federal Register (Vol. 50, No, 147), pp. 31038-40.

Since that time the application of the UHDDS definitions has been expanded to include all non-outpatient settings (acute care, short term, long term care and psychiatric hospitals; home health agencies; rehab facilities; nursing homes, etc). The UHDDS definitions also apply to hospice services (all levels of care).

The following guidelines are to be applied in designating "other diagnoses" when neither the Alphabetic Index nor the Tabular List in ICD-10-CM provide direction. The listing of the diagnoses in the patient record is the responsibility of the attending provider.

A. Previous conditions

If the provider has included a diagnosis in the final diagnostic statement, such as the discharge summary or the face sheet, it should ordinarily be coded. Some providers include in the diagnostic statement resolved conditions or diagnoses and status-post procedures from previous admission that have no bearing on the current stay. Such conditions are not to be reported and are coded only if required by hospital policy.

However, history codes (categories Z80-Z87) may be used as secondary codes if the historical condition or family history has an impact on current care or influences treatment.

B. Abnormal findings

Abnormal findings (laboratory, x-ray, pathologic, and other diagnostic results) are not coded and reported unless the provider indicates their clinical significance. If the findings are outside the normal range and the attending provider has ordered other tests to evaluate the condition or prescribed treatment, it is appropriate to ask the provider whether the abnormal finding should be added.

Please note: This differs from the coding practices in the outpatient setting for coding encounters for diagnostic tests that have been interpreted by a provider.

C. Uncertain Diagnosis

If the diagnosis documented at the time of discharge is qualified as "probable", "suspected", "likely", "questionable", "possible", or "still to be ruled out" or other similar terms indicating uncertainty, code the condition as if it existed or was established. The bases for these guidelines are the diagnostic workup, arrangements for further workup or observation, and initial therapeutic approach that correspond most closely with the established diagnosis.

Note: This guideline is applicable only to inpatient admissions to short-term, acute, long-term care and psychiatric hospitals.

SECTION IV – OUTPATIENT GUIDELINES
Section IV.

Section IV. Diagnostic Coding and Reporting Guidelines for Outpatient Services

These coding guidelines for outpatient diagnoses have been approved for use by hospitals/ providers in coding and reporting hospital-based outpatient services and provider-based office visits. Guidelines in Section I, Conventions, general coding guidelines and chapter-specific guidelines, should also be applied for outpatient services and office visits.

Information about the use of certain abbreviations, punctuation, symbols, and other conventions used in the ICD-10-CM Tabular List (code numbers and titles), can be found in Section IA of these guidelines, under "Conventions Used in the Tabular List." Section I.B. contains general guidelines that apply to the entire classification. Section I.C. contains chapter-specific guidelines that correspond to the chapters as they are arranged in the classification. Information about the correct sequence to use in finding a code is also described in Section I.

The terms encounter and visit are often used interchangeably in describing outpatient service contacts and, therefore, appear together in these guidelines without distinguishing one from the other.

Though the conventions and general guidelines apply to all settings, coding guidelines for outpatient and provider reporting of diagnoses will vary in a number of instances from those for inpatient diagnoses, recognizing that:

The Uniform Hospital Discharge Data Set (UHDDS) definition of principal diagnosis ~~applies only to inpatients in acute, short-term, long-term care and psychiatric hospitals~~ does not apply to hospital-based outpatient services and provider-based office visits.

Coding guidelines for inconclusive diagnoses (probable, suspected, rule out, etc.) were developed for inpatient reporting and do not apply to outpatients.

A. Selection of first-listed condition

In the outpatient setting, the term first-listed diagnosis is used in lieu of principal diagnosis.

In determining the first-listed diagnosis the coding conventions of ICD-10-CM, as well as the general and disease specific guidelines take precedence over the outpatient guidelines.

Diagnoses often are not established at the time of the initial encounter/visit. It may take two or more visits before the diagnosis is confirmed.

The most critical rule involves beginning the search for the correct code assignment through the Alphabetic Index. Never begin searching initially in the Tabular List as this will lead to coding errors.

1. Outpatient Surgery

When a patient presents for outpatient surgery (same day surgery), code the reason for the surgery as the first-listed diagnosis (reason for the encounter), even if the surgery is not performed due to a contraindication.

2. Observation Stay

When a patient is admitted for observation for a medical condition, assign a code for the medical condition as the first-listed diagnosis.

When a patient presents for outpatient surgery and develops complications requiring admission to observation, code the reason for the surgery as the first reported diagnosis (reason for the encounter), followed by codes for the complications as secondary diagnoses.

B. Codes from A00.0 through T88.9, Z00-Z99

The appropriate code(s) from A00.0 through T88.9, Z00-Z99 must be used to identify diagnoses, symptoms, conditions, problems, complaints, or other reason(s) for the encounter/visit.

C. Accurate reporting of ICD-10-CM diagnosis codes

For accurate reporting of ICD-10-CM diagnosis codes, the documentation should describe the patient's condition, using terminology which includes specific diagnoses as well as symptoms, problems, or reasons for the encounter. There are ICD-10-CM codes to describe all of these.

D. Codes that describe symptoms and signs

Codes that describe symptoms and signs, as opposed to diagnoses, are acceptable for reporting purposes when a diagnosis has not been established (confirmed) by the provider. Chapter 18 of ICD-10-CM, Symptoms, Signs, and Abnormal Clinical and Laboratory Findings Not Elsewhere Classified (codes R00-R99) contain many, but not all codes for symptoms.

E. Encounters for circumstances other than a disease or injury

ICD-10-CM provides codes to deal with encounters for circumstances other than a disease or injury. The Factors Influencing Health Status and Contact with Health Services codes (Z00-Z99) are provided to deal with occasions when circumstances other than a disease or injury are recorded as diagnosis or problems.

See Section I.C.21. Factors influencing health status and contact with health services.

SECTION IV – OUTPATIENT GUIDELINES
Section IV. F. 1.

F. Level of Detail in Coding

1. **ICD-10-CM codes with 3, 4, 5, 6 or 7 characters**
   ICD-10-CM is composed of codes with 3, 4, 5, 6 or 7 characters. Codes with three characters are included in ICD-10-CM as the heading of a category of codes that may be further subdivided by the use of fourth, fifth, sixth or seventh characters to provide greater specificity.

2. **Use of full number of characters required for a code**
   A three-character code is to be used only if it is not further subdivided. A code is invalid if it has not been coded to the full number of characters required for that code, including the 7th character, if applicable.

G. ICD-10-CM code for the diagnosis, condition, problem, or other reason for encounter/visit
List first the ICD-10-CM code for the diagnosis, condition, problem, or other reason for encounter/visit shown in the medical record to be chiefly responsible for the services provided. List additional codes that describe any coexisting conditions. In some cases the first-listed diagnosis may be a symptom when a diagnosis has not been established (confirmed) by the physician.

H. Uncertain diagnosis
Do not code diagnoses documented as "probable", "suspected," "questionable," "rule out," or "working diagnosis" or other similar terms indicating uncertainty. Rather, code the condition(s) to the highest degree of certainty for that encounter/visit, such as symptoms, signs, abnormal test results, or other reason for the visit.

Please note: This differs from the coding practices used by short-term, acute care, long-term care and psychiatric hospitals.

I. Chronic diseases
Chronic diseases treated on an ongoing basis may be coded and reported as many times as the patient receives treatment and care for the condition(s).

J. Code all documented conditions that coexist
Code all documented conditions that coexist at the time of the encounter/visit, and require or affect patient care treatment or management. Do not code conditions that were previously treated and no longer exist. However, history codes (categories Z80-Z87) may be used as secondary codes if the historical condition or family history has an impact on current care or influences treatment.

K. Patients receiving diagnostic services only
For patients receiving diagnostic services only during an encounter/visit, sequence first the diagnosis, condition, problem, or other reason for encounter/visit shown in the medical record to be chiefly responsible for the outpatient services provided during the encounter/visit. Codes for other diagnoses (e.g., chronic conditions) may be sequenced as additional diagnoses.

For encounters for routine laboratory/radiology testing in the absence of any signs, symptoms, or associated diagnosis, assign Z01.89, Encounter for other specified special examinations. If routine testing is performed during the same encounter as a test to evaluate a sign, symptom, or diagnosis, it is appropriate to assign both the Z code and the code describing the reason for the non-routine test.

For outpatient encounters for diagnostic tests that have been interpreted by a physician, and the final report is available at the time of coding, code any confirmed or definitive diagnosis(es) documented in the interpretation. Do not code related signs and symptoms as additional diagnoses.

Please note: This differs from the coding practice in the hospital inpatient setting regarding abnormal findings on test results.

L. Patients receiving therapeutic services only
For patients receiving therapeutic services only during an encounter/visit, sequence first the diagnosis, condition, problem, or other reason for encounter/visit shown in the medical record to be chiefly responsible for the outpatient services provided during the encounter/visit. Codes for other diagnoses (e.g., chronic conditions) may be sequenced as additional diagnoses.

The only exception to this rule is that when the primary reason for the admission/encounter is chemotherapy or radiation therapy, the appropriate Z code for the service is listed first, and the diagnosis or problem for which the service is being performed listed second.

M. Patients receiving preoperative evaluations only
For patients receiving preoperative evaluations only, sequence first a code from subcategory Z01.81, Encounter for pre-procedural examinations, to describe the pre-op consultations. Assign a code for the condition to describe the reason for the surgery as an additional diagnosis. Code also any findings related to the pre-op evaluation.

N. Ambulatory surgery
For ambulatory surgery, code the diagnosis for which the surgery was performed. If the postoperative diagnosis is known to be different from the preoperative diagnosis at the time the diagnosis is confirmed, select the postoperative diagnosis for coding, since it is the most definitive.

SECTION IV – OUTPATIENT GUIDELINES
Section IV. O.

O. Routine outpatient prenatal visits
See Section I.C.15. Routine outpatient prenatal visits.

P. Encounters for general medical examinations with abnormal findings
The subcategories for encounters for general medical examinations, Z00.0-, provide codes for with and without abnormal findings. Should a general medical examination result in an abnormal finding, the code for general medical examination with abnormal finding should be assigned as the first-listed diagnosis. An examination with abnormal findings refers to a condition/diagnosis that is newly identified or a change in severity of a chronic condition (such as uncontrolled hypertension, or an acute exacerbation of chronic obstructive pulmonary disease) during a routine physical examination. A secondary code for the abnormal finding should also be coded.

Q. Encounters for routine health screenings
See Section I.C.21. Factors influencing health status and contact with health services, Screening.

[2017.CM]   OFFICIAL CODING GUIDELINES – 2017 ICD-10-CM

APPENDIX I – POA GUIDELINES
Appendix I.

APPENDIX I – POA GUIDELINES
Appendix I.

GUIDELINES

Appendix I
Present on Admission Reporting Guidelines

Introduction

These guidelines are to be used as a supplement to the ICD-10-CM Official Guidelines for Coding and Reporting to facilitate the assignment of the Present on Admission (POA) indicator for each diagnosis and external cause of injury code reported on claim forms (UB-04 and 837 Institutional).

These guidelines are not intended to replace any guidelines in the main body of the ICD-10-CM Official Guidelines for Coding and Reporting. The POA guidelines are not intended to provide guidance on when a condition should be coded, but rather, how to apply the POA indicator to the final set of diagnosis codes that have been assigned in accordance with Sections I, II, and III of the official coding guidelines. Subsequent to the assignment of the ICD-10-CM codes, the POA indicator should then be assigned to those conditions that have been coded.

As stated in the Introduction to the ICD-10-CM Official Guidelines for Coding and Reporting, a joint effort between the healthcare provider and the coder is essential to achieve complete and accurate documentation, code assignment, and reporting of diagnoses and procedures. The importance of consistent, complete documentation in the medical record cannot be overemphasized. Medical record documentation from any provider involved in the care and treatment of the patient may be used to support the determination of whether a condition was present on admission or not. In the context of the official coding guidelines, the term "provider" means a physician or any qualified healthcare practitioner who is legally accountable for establishing the patient's diagnosis.

These guidelines are not a substitute for the provider's clinical judgment as to the determination of whether a condition was/was not present on admission. The provider should be queried regarding issues related to the linking of signs/symptoms, timing of test results, and the timing of findings.

Please see the CDC website for the detailed list of ICD-10-CM codes that do not require the use of a POA indicator (ftp://ftp.cdc.gov/pub/Health_Statistics/NCHS/Publications/ICD10CM/2017/). The conditions on this exempt list represent categories and/or codes for circumstances regarding the healthcare encounter or factors influencing health status that do not represent a current disease or injury or are always present on admission.

General Reporting Requirements

All claims involving inpatient admissions to general acute care hospitals or other facilities that are subject to a law or regulation mandating collection of present on admission information.

Present on admission is defined as present at the time the order for inpatient admission occurs — conditions that develop during an outpatient encounter, including emergency department, observation, or outpatient surgery, are considered as present on admission.

POA indicator is assigned to principal and secondary diagnoses (as defined in Section II of the Official Guidelines for Coding and Reporting) and the external cause of injury codes.

Issues related to inconsistent, missing, conflicting or unclear documentation must still be resolved by the provider.

If a condition would not be coded and reported based on UHDDS definitions and current official coding guidelines, then the POA indicator would not be reported.

Reporting Options

Y - Yes
N - No
U - Unknown
W — Clinically undetermined
Unreported/Not used (or "1" for Medicare usage) — (Exempt from POA reporting)

Reporting Definitions

Y = present at the time of inpatient admission
N = not present at the time of inpatient admission
U = documentation is insufficient to determine if condition is present on admission
W = provider is unable to clinically determine whether condition was present on admission or not

Timeframe for POA Identification and Documentation

There is no required timeframe as to when a provider (per the definition of "provider" used in these guidelines) must identify or document a condition to be present on admission. In some clinical situations, it may not be possible for a provider to make a definitive diagnosis (or a condition may not be recognized or reported by the patient) for a period of time after admission. In some cases it may be several days before the provider arrives at a definitive diagnosis. This does not mean that the condition was not present on admission. Determination of whether the condition was present on admission or not will be based on the applicable POA guideline as identified in this document, or on the provider's best clinical judgment.

If at the time of code assignment the documentation is unclear as to whether a condition was present on admission or not, it is appropriate to query the provider for clarification.

Assigning the POA Indicator

Condition is on the "Exempt from Reporting" list
Leave the "present on admission" field blank if the condition is on the list of ICD-10-CM codes for which this field is not applicable. This is the only circumstance in which the field may be left blank.

POA Explicitly Documented
Assign Y for any condition the provider explicitly documents as being present on admission.

Assign N for any condition the provider explicitly documents as not present at the time of admission.

Conditions diagnosed prior to inpatient admission
Assign "Y" for conditions that were diagnosed prior to admission (example: hypertension, diabetes mellitus, asthma)

Conditions diagnosed during the admission but clearly present before admission
Assign "Y" for conditions diagnosed during the admission that were clearly present but not diagnosed until after admission occurred.

Diagnoses subsequently confirmed after admission are considered present on admission if at the time of admission they are documented as suspected, possible, rule out, differential diagnosis, or constitute an underlying cause of a symptom that is present at the time of admission.

Condition develops during outpatient encounter prior to inpatient admission
Assign Y for any condition that develops during an outpatient encounter prior to a written order for inpatient admission.

Documentation does not indicate whether condition was present on admission
Assign "U" when the medical record documentation is unclear as to whether the condition was present on admission. "U" should not be routinely assigned and used only in very limited circumstances. Coders are encouraged to query the providers when the documentation is unclear.

Documentation states that it cannot be determined whether the condition was or was not present on admission
Assign "W" when the medical record documentation indicates that it cannot be clinically determined whether or not the condition was present on admission.

Chronic condition with acute exacerbation during the admission
If a single code identifies both the chronic condition and the acute exacerbation, see POA guidelines pertaining to ~~combination~~ codes that contain multiple clinical concepts.

If a single code only identifies the chronic condition and not the acute exacerbation (e.g., acute exacerbation of chronic leukemia), assign "Y."

Conditions documented as possible, probable, suspected, or rule out at the time of discharge
If the final diagnosis contains a possible, probable, suspected, or rule out diagnosis, and this diagnosis was based on signs, symptoms or clinical findings suspected at the time of inpatient admission, assign "Y."

If the final diagnosis contains a possible, probable, suspected, or rule out diagnosis, and this diagnosis was based on signs, symptoms or clinical findings that were not present on admission, assign "N".

Conditions documented as impending or threatened at the time of discharge
If the final diagnosis contains an impending or threatened diagnosis, and this diagnosis is based on symptoms or clinical findings that were present on admission, assign "Y".

If the final diagnosis contains an impending or threatened diagnosis, and this diagnosis is based on symptoms or clinical findings that were not present on admission, assign "N".

Acute and Chronic Conditions
Assign "Y" for acute conditions that are present at time of admission and N for acute conditions that are not present at time of admission.

Assign "Y" for chronic conditions, even though the condition may not be diagnosed until after admission.

If a single code identifies both an acute and chronic condition, see the POA guidelines for ~~combination~~ codes that contain multiple clinical concepts.

GUIDELINES

~~Combination~~ Codes That Contain Multiple Clinical Concepts

Assign "N" if ~~any part of the combination~~ at least one of the clinical concepts included in the code was not present on admission (e.g., COPD with acute exacerbation and the exacerbation was not present on admission; gastric ulcer that does not start bleeding until after admission; asthma patient develops status asthmaticus after admission).

Assign "Y" if all parts of the ~~combination~~ clinical concepts included in the code were present on admission (e.g., ~~patient with acute prostatitis admitted with hematuria~~ duodenal ulcer that perforates prior to admission).

If the final diagnosis includes comparative or contrasting diagnoses, and both were present, or suspected, at the time of admission, assign "Y".

For infection codes that include the causal organism, assign "Y" if the infection (or signs of the infection) ~~was~~ were present on admission, even though the culture results may not be known until after admission (e.g., patient is admitted with pneumonia and the provider documents Pseudomonas as the causal organism a few days later).

Same Diagnosis Code for Two or More Conditions

When the same ICD-10-CM diagnosis code applies to two or more conditions during the same encounter (e.g. two separate conditions classified to the same ICD-10-CM diagnosis code):

Assign "Y" if all conditions represented by the single ICD-10-CM code were present on admission (e.g. bilateral unspecified age-related cataracts).

Assign "N" if any of the conditions represented by the single ICD-10-CM code was not present on admission (e.g. traumatic secondary and recurrent hemorrhage and seroma is assigned to a single code T79.2, but only one of the conditions was present on admission).

Obstetrical conditions

Whether or not the patient delivers during the current hospitalization does not affect assignment of the POA indicator. The determining factor for POA assignment is whether the pregnancy complication or obstetrical condition described by the code was present at the time of admission or not.

If the pregnancy complication or obstetrical condition was present on admission (e.g., patient admitted in preterm labor), assign "Y".

If the pregnancy complication or obstetrical condition was not present on admission (e.g., 2nd degree laceration during delivery, postpartum hemorrhage that occurred during current hospitalization, fetal distress develops after admission), assign "N".
If the obstetrical code includes more than one diagnosis and any of the diagnoses identified by the code were not present on admission assign "N" (e.g., Category O11, Pre-existing hypertension with pre-eclampsia).

Perinatal conditions

Newborns are not considered to be admitted until after birth. Therefore, any condition present at birth or that developed in utero is considered present at admission and should be assigned "Y". This includes conditions that occur during delivery (e.g., injury during delivery, meconium aspiration, exposure to streptococcus B in the vaginal canal).

Congenital conditions and anomalies

Assign "Y" for congenital conditions and anomalies except for categories Q00-Q99, Congenital anomalies, which are on the exempt list. Congenital conditions are always considered present on admission.

External cause of injury codes

Assign "Y" for any external cause code representing an external cause of morbidity that occurred prior to inpatient admission (e.g., patient fell out of bed at home, patient fell out of bed in emergency room prior to admission).

Assign "N" for any external cause code representing an external cause of morbidity that occurred during inpatient hospitalization (e.g., patient fell out of hospital bed during hospital stay, patient experienced an adverse reaction to a medication administered after inpatient admission).

A

Aarskog's syndrome Q87.1
Abandonment — *see* Maltreatment
Abasia (-astasia) (hysterical) F44.4
Abderhalden-Kaufmann-Lignac
   syndrome (cystinosis) E72.04
Abdomen, abdominal — *see also* condition
  acute R10.0
  angina K55.1
  muscle deficiency syndrome Q79.4
Abdominalgia — *see* Pain, abdominal
Abduction contracture, hip or other joint
   — *see* Contraction, joint
Aberrant (congenital) — *see also* Malposition,
   congenital
  adrenal gland Q89.1
  artery (peripheral) Q27.8
    basilar NEC Q28.1
    cerebral Q28.3
    coronary Q24.5
    digestive system Q27.8
    eye Q15.8
    lower limb Q27.8
    precerebral Q28.1
    pulmonary Q25.79
    renal Q27.2
    retina Q14.1
    specified site NEC Q27.8
    subclavian Q27.8
    upper limb Q27.8
    vertebral Q28.1
  breast Q83.8
  endocrine gland NEC Q89.2
  hepatic duct Q44.5
  pancreas Q45.3
  parathyroid gland Q89.2
  pituitary gland Q89.2
  sebaceous glands, mucous membrane, mouth,
    congenital Q38.6
  spleen Q89.09
  subclavian artery Q27.8
  thymus (gland) Q89.2
  thyroid gland Q89.2
  vein (peripheral) NEC Q27.8
    cerebral Q28.3
    digestive system Q27.8
    lower limb Q27.8
    precerebral Q28.1
    specified site NEC Q27.8
    upper limb Q27.8
Aberration
  distantial — *see* Disturbance, visual
  mental F99
Abetalipoproteinemia E78.6
Abiotrophy R68.89
Ablatio, ablation
  retinae — *see* Detachment, retina
Ablepharia, ablepharon Q10.3
Abnormal, abnormality, abnormalities —
   see also Anomaly
  acid-base balance (mixed) E87.4
  albumin R77.0
  alphafetoprotein R77.2
  alveolar ridge K08.9
  anatomical relationship Q89.9
  apertures, congenital, diaphragm Q79.1
  auditory perception H93.29-
    diplacusis — *see* Diplacusis
    hyperacusis — *see* Hyperacusis
    recruitment — *see* Recruitment, auditory
    threshold shift — *see* Shift, auditory threshold
  autosomes Q99.9
    fragile site Q95.5
  basal metabolic rate R94.8
  biosynthesis, testicular androgen E29.1

Abnormal, abnormality, abnormalities
  (*see also* Anomaly) — *continued*
  bleeding time R79.1
  blood level (of)
    cobalt R79.0
    copper R79.0
    iron R79.0
    lithium R78.89
    magnesium R79.0
    mineral NEC R79.0
    zinc R79.0
  blood pressure
    elevated R03.0
    low reading (nonspecific) R03.1
  blood sugar R73.09
  blood-gas level R79.81
  bowel sounds R19.15
    absent R19.11
    hyperactive R19.12
  brain scan R94.02
  breathing R06.9
  caloric test R94.138
  cerebrospinal fluid R83.9
    cytology R83.6
    drug level R83.2
    enzyme level R83.0
    hormones R83.1
    immunology R83.4
    microbiology R83.5
    nonmedicinal level R83.3
    specified type NEC R83.8
  chemistry, blood R79.9
    C-reactive protein R79.82
    drugs — *see* Findings, abnormal, in blood
    gas level R79.81
    minerals R79.0
    pancytopenia D61.818
    PTT R79.1
    specified NEC R79.89
    toxins — *see* Findings, abnormal, in blood
  chest sounds (friction) (rales) R09.89
  chromosome, chromosomal Q99.9
    with more than three X chromosomes, female
      Q97.1
    analysis result R89.8
      bronchial washings R84.8
      cerebrospinal fluid R83.8
      cervix uteri NEC R87.89
      nasal secretions R84.8
      nipple discharge R89.8
      peritoneal fluid R85.89
      pleural fluid R84.8
      prostatic secretions R86.8
      saliva R85.89
      seminal fluid R86.8
      sputum R84.8
      synovial fluid R89.8
      throat scrapings R84.8
      vagina R87.89
      vulva R87.89
      wound secretions R89.8
    dicentric replacement Q93.2
    ring replacement Q93.2
    sex Q99.8
      female phenotype Q97.9
        specified NEC Q97.8
      male phenotype Q98.9
        specified NEC Q98.8
      structural male Q98.6
    specified NEC Q99.8
  clinical findings NEC R68.89
  coagulation D68.9
    newborn, transient P61.6
    profile R79.1
    time R79.1
  communication — *see* Fistula
  conjunctiva, vascular H11.41-
  coronary artery Q24.5

Abnormal, abnormality, abnormalities
  (*see also* Anomaly) — *continued*
  cortisol-binding globulin E27.8
  course, eustachian tube Q17.8
  creatinine clearance R94.4
  cytology
    anus R85.619
      atypical squamous cells cannot exclude
        high grade squamous intraepithelial
        lesion (ASC-H) R85.611
      atypical squamous cells of undetermined
        significance (ASC-US) R85.610
      cytologic evidence of malignancy R85.614
      high grade squamous intraepithelial lesion
        (HGSIL) R85.613
      human papillomavirus (HPV) DNA test
        high risk positive R85.81
        low risk postive R85.82
      inadequate smear R85.615
      low grade squamous intraepithelial lesion
        (LGSIL) R85.612
      satisfactory anal smear but lacking
        transformation zone R85.616
      specified NEC R85.618
      unsatisfactory smear R85.615
    female genital organs — *see* Abnormal,
      Papanicolaou (smear)
  dark adaptation curve H53.61
  dentofacial NEC — *see* Anomaly, dentofacial
  development, developmental Q89.9
    central nervous system Q07.9
  diagnostic imaging
    abdomen, abdominal region NEC R93.5
    biliary tract R93.2
    bladder R93.41
    breast R92.8
    central nervous system NEC R90.89
    cerebrovascular NEC R90.89
    coronary circulation R93.1
    digestive tract NEC R93.3
    gastrointestinal (tract) R93.3
    genitourinary organs R93.8
    head R93.0
    heart R93.1
    intrathoracic organ NEC R93.8
    kidney R93.42-
    limbs R93.6
    liver R93.2
    lung (field) R91.8
    musculoskeletal system NEC R93.7
    renal pelvis R93.41
    retroperitoneum R93.5
    site specified NEC R93.8
    skin and subcutaneous tissue R93.8
    skull R93.0
    ureter R93.41
    urinary organs specified NEC R93.49
  direction, teeth, fully erupted M26.30
  ear ossicles, acquired NEC H74.39-
    ankylosis — *see* Ankylosis, ear ossicles
    discontinuity — *see* Discontinuity, ossicles,
      ear
    partial loss — *see* Loss, ossicles, ear (partial)
  Ebstein Q22.5
  echocardiogram R93.1
  echoencephalogram R90.81
  echogram — *see* Abnormal, diagnostic
    imaging
  electro-oculogram [EOG] R94.110
  electrocardiogram [ECG] [EKG] R94.31
  electroencephalogram [EEG] R94.01
  electrolyte — *see* Imbalance, electrolyte
  electromyogram [EMG] R94.131
  electrophysiological intracardiac studies
    R94.39
  electroretinogram [ERG] R94.111
  erythrocytes
    congenital, with perinatal jaundice D58.9
  feces (color) (contents) (mucus) R19.5

DISEASE INDEX

Abnormal, abnormality, abnormalities
(*see also* Anomaly) — *continued*
finding — *see* Findings, abnormal, without diagnosis
fluid
  amniotic — *see* Abnormal, specimen, specified
  cerebrospinal — *see* Abnormal, cerebrospinal fluid
  peritoneal — *see* Abnormal, specimen, digestive organs
  pleural — *see* Abnormal, specimen, respiratory organs
  synovial — *see* Abnormal, specimen, specified
  thorax (bronchial washings) (pleural fluid) — *see* Abnormal, specimen, respiratory organs
  vaginal — *see* Abnormal, specimen, female genital organs
form
  teeth K00.2
  uterus — *see* Anomaly, uterus
function studies
  auditory R94.120
  bladder R94.8
  brain R94.09
  cardiovascular R94.30
  ear R94.128
  endocrine NEC R94.7
  eye NEC R94.118
  kidney R94.4
  liver R94.5
  nervous system
    central NEC R94.09
    peripheral NEC R94.138
  pancreas R94.8
  placenta R94.8
  pulmonary R94.2
  special senses NEC R94.128
  spleen R94.8
  thyroid R94.6
  vestibular R94.121
gait — *see* Gait
  hysterical F44.4
gastrin secretion E16.4
globulin R77.1
  cortisol-binding E27.8
  thyroid-binding E07.89
glomerular, minor (*see also* N00-N07 with fourth character .0) N05.0
glucagon secretion E16.3
glucose tolerance (test) (non-fasting) R73.09
gravitational (G) forces or states (effect of) T75.81
hair (color) (shaft) L67.9
  specified NEC L67.8
hard tissue formation in pulp (dental) K04.3
head movement R25.0
heart
  rate R00.9
    specified NEC R00.8
  shadow R93.1
  sounds NEC R01.2
hemoglobin (disease) (*see also* Disease, hemoglobin) D58.2
  trait — *see* Trait, hemoglobin, abnormal
histology NEC R89.7
immunological findings R89.4
  in serum R76.9
    specified NEC R76.8
increase in appetite R63.2
involuntary movement — *see* Abnormal, movement, involuntary
jaw closure M26.51
karyotype R89.8
kidney function test R94.4

Abnormal, abnormality, abnormalities
(*see also* Anomaly) — *continued*
knee jerk R29.2
leukocyte (cell) (differential) NEC D72.9
liver
loss of
  height R29.890
  weight R63.4
mammogram NEC R92.8
  calcification (calculus) R92.1
  microcalcification R92.0
Mantoux test R76.11
movement (disorder) — *see also* Disorder, movement
  head R25.0
  involuntary R25.9
    fasciculation R25.3
    of head R25.0
    spasm R25.2
    specified type NEC R25.8
    tremor R25.1
myoglobin (Aberdeen) (Annapolis) R89.7
neonatal screening P09
oculomotor study R94.113
palmar creases Q82.8
Papanicolaou (smear)
  anus R85.619
    atypical squamous cells cannot exclude high grade squamous intraepithelial lesion (ASC-H) R85.611
    atypical squamous cells of undetermined significance (ASC-US) R85.610
    cytologic evidence of malignancy R85.614
    high grade squamous intraepithelial lesion (HGSIL) R85.613
    human papillomavirus (HPV) DNA test
      high risk positive R85.81
      low risk postive R85.82
    inadequate smear R85.615
    low grade squamous intraepithelial lesion (LGSIL) R85.612
    satisfactory anal smear but lacking transformation zone R85.616
    specified NEC R85.618
    unsatisfactory smear R85.615
  bronchial washings R84.6
  cerebrospinal fluid R83.6
  cervix R87.619
    atypical squamous cells cannot exclude high grade squamous intraepithelial lesion (ASC-H) R87.611
    atypical squamous cells of undetermined significance (ASC-US) R87.610
    cytologic evidence of malignancy R87.614
    high grade squamous intraepithelial lesion (HGSIL) R87.613
    inadequate smear R87.615
    low grade squamous intraepithelial lesion (LGSIL) R87.612
    non-atypical endometrial cells R87.618
    satisfactory cervical smear but lacking transformation zone R87.616
    specified NEC R87.618
    thin preparaton R87.619
    unsatisfactory smear R87.615
  nasal secretions R84.6
  nipple discharge R89.6
  peritoneal fluid R85.69
  pleural fluid R84.6
  prostatic secretions R86.6
  saliva R85.69
  seminal fluid R86.6
  sites NEC R89.6
  sputum R84.6
  synovial fluid R89.6
  throat scrapings R84.6

Abnormal, abnormality, abnormalities
(*see also* Anomaly) — *continued*
Papanicolaou (smear) — *continued*
  vagina R87.629
    atypical squamous cells cannot exclude high grade squamous intraepithelial lesion (ASC-H) R87.621
    atypical squamous cells of undetermined significance (ASC-US) R87.620
    cytologic evidence of malignancy R87.624
    high grade squamous intraepithelial lesion (HGSIL) R87.623
    inadequate smear R87.625
    low grade squamous intraepithelial lesion (LGSIL) R87.622
    specified NEC R87.628
    thin preparation R87.629
    unsatisfactory smear R87.625
  vulva R87.69
  wound secretions R89.6
partial thromboplastin time (PTT) R79.1
pelvis (bony) — *see* Deformity, pelvis
percussion, chest (tympany) R09.89
periods (grossly) — *see* Menstruation
phonocardiogram R94.39
plantar reflex R29.2
plasma
  protein R77.9
    specified NEC R77.8
  viscosity R70.1
pleural (folds) Q34.0
posture R29.3
product of conception O02.9
  specified type NEC O02.89
prothrombin time (PT) R79.1
pulmonary
  artery, congenital Q25.79
  function, newborn P28.89
  test results R94.2
pulsations in neck R00.2
pupillary H21.56-
  function (reaction) (reflex) — *see* Anomaly, pupil, function
radiological examination — *see* Abnormal, diagnostic imaging
red blood cell(s) (morphology) (volume) R71.8
reflex — *see* Reflex
renal function test R94.4
response to nerve stimulation R94.130
retinal correspondence H53.31
retinal function study R94.111
rhythm, heart — *see also* Arrhythmia
saliva — *see* Abnormal, specimen, digestive organs
scan
  kidney R94.4
  liver R93.2
  thyroid R94.6
secretion
  gastrin E16.4
  glucagon E16.3
semen, seminal fluid — *see* Abnormal, specimen, male genital organs
serum level (of)
  acid phosphatase R74.8
  alkaline phosphatase R74.8
  amylase R74.8
  enzymes R74.9
    specified NEC R74.8
  lipase R74.8
  triacylglycerol lipase R74.8
shape
  gravid uterus — *see* Anomaly, uterus
sinus venosus Q21.1
size, tooth, teeth K00.2
spacing, tooth, teeth, fully erupted M26.30

Abnormal, abnormality, abnormalities
(see also Anomaly) — continued
specimen
digestive organs (peritoneal fluid) (saliva)
R85.9
cytology R85.69
drug level R85.2
enzyme level R85.0
histology R85.7
hormones R85.1
immunology R85.4
microbiology R85.5
nonmedicinal level R85.3
specified type NEC R85.89
female genital organs (secretions) (smears)
R87.9
cytology R87.69
cervix R87.619
human papillomavirus (HPV) DNA test
high risk positive R87.810
low risk positive R87.820
inadequate (unsatisfactory) smear
R87.615
non-atypical endometrial cells
R87.618
specified NEC R87.618
vagina R87.629
human papillomavirus (HPV) DNA test
high risk positive R87.811
low risk positive R87.821
inadequate (unsatisfactory) smear
R87.625
vulva R87.69
drug level R87.2
enzyme level R87.0
histological R87.7
hormones R87.1
immunology R87.4
microbiology R87.5
nonmedicinal level R87.3
specified type NEC R87.89
male genital organs (prostatic secretions)
(semen) R86.9
cytology R86.6
drug level R86.2
enzyme level R86.0
histological R86.7
hormones R86.1
immunology R86.4
microbiology R86.5
nonmedicinal level R86.3
specified type NEC R86.8
nipple discharge — see Abnormal,
specimen, specified
respiratory organs (bronchial washings)
(nasal secretions) (pleural fluid) (sputum)
R84.9
cytology R84.6
drug level R84.2
enzyme level R84.0
histology R84.7
hormones R84.1
immunology R84.4
microbiology R84.5
nonmedicinal level R84.3
specified type NEC R84.8
specified organ, system and tissue NOS
R89.9
cytology R89.6
drug level R89.2
enzyme level R89.0
histology R89.7
hormones R89.1
immunology R89.4
microbiology R89.5
nonmedicinal level R89.3
specified type NEC R89.8

Abnormal, abnormality, abnormalities
(see also Anomaly) — continued
specimen — continued
synovial fluid — see Abnormal, specimen,
specified
thorax (bronchial washings) (pleural fluids)
— see Abnormal, specimen, respiratory
organs
vagina (secretion) (smear) R87.629
vulva (secretion) (smear) R87.69
wound secretion — see Abnormal, specimen,
specified
spermatozoa — see Abnormal, specimen,
male genital organs
sputum (amount) (color) (odor) R09.3
stool (color) (contents) (mucus) R19.5
bloody K92.1
guaiac positive R19.5
synchondrosis Q78.8
thermography (see also Abnormal, diagnostic
imaging) R93.8
thyroid-binding globulin E07.89
tooth, teeth (form) (size) K00.2
toxicology (findings) R78.9
transport protein E88.09
tumor marker NEC R97.8
ultrasound results — see Abnormal, diagnostic
imaging
umbilical cord complicating delivery O69.9
urination NEC R39.198
urine (constituents) R82.90
bile R82.2
cytological examination R82.8
drugs R82.5
fat R82.0
glucose R81
heavy metals R82.6
hemoglobin R82.3
histological examination R82.8
ketones R82.4
microbiological examination (culture)
R82.79
myoglobin R82.1
positive culture R82.79
protein — see Proteinuria
specified substance NEC R82.99
chromoabnormality NEC R82.91
substances nonmedical R82.6
uterine hemorrhage — see Hemorrhage, uterus
vectorcardiogram R94.39
visually evoked potential (VEP) R94.112
white blood cells D72.9
specified NEC D72.89
X-ray examination — see Abnormal,
diagnostic imaging
Abnormity (any organ or part) — see Anomaly
Abocclusion M26.29
hemolytic disease (newborn) P55.1
incompatibility reaction ABO — see
Complication(s), transfusion,
incompatibility reaction, ABO
Abolition, language R48.8
Aborter, habitual or recurrent — see Loss
(of), pregnancy, recurrent
Abortion (complete) (spontaneous) O03.9
with
retained products of conception — see
Abortion, incomplete
attempted (elective) (failed) O07.4
complicated by O07.30
afibrinogenemia O07.1
cardiac arrest O07.36
chemical damage of pelvic organ(s)
O07.34
circulatory collapse O07.31
cystitis O07.38
defibrination syndrome O07.1
electrolyte imbalance O07.33

Abortion (complete) (spontaneous) O03.9 —
continued
attempted (elective) (failed) O07.4 —
continued
complicated by O07.30 — continued
embolism (air) (amniotic fluid) (blood clot)
(fat) (pulmonary) (septic) (soap)
O07.2
endometritis O07.0
genital tract and pelvic infection O07.0
hemolysis O07.1
hemorrhage (delayed) (excessive) O07.1
infection
genital tract or pelvic O07.0
urinary tract O07.38
intravascular coagulation O07.1
laceration of pelvic organ(s) O07.34
metabolic disorder O07.33
oliguria O07.32
oophoritis O07.0
parametritis O07.0
pelvic peritonitis O07.0
perforation of pelvic organ(s) O07.34
renal failure or shutdown O07.32
salpingitis or salpingo-oophoritis O07.0
sepsis O07.37
shock O07.31
specified condition NEC O07.39
tubular necrosis (renal) O07.32
uremia O07.32
urinary tract infection O07.38
venous complication NEC O07.35
embolism (air) (amniotic fluid) (blood
clot) (fat) (pulmonary) (septic) (soap)
O07.2
complicated (by) (following) O03.80
afibrinogenemia O03.6
cardiac arrest O03.86
chemical damage of pelvic organ(s) O03.84
circulatory collapse O03.81
cystitis O03.88
defibrination syndrome O03.6
electrolyte imbalance O03.83
embolism (air) (amniotic fluid) (blood clot)
(fat) (pulmonary) (septic) (soap) O03.7
endometritis O03.5
genital tract and pelvic infection O03.5
hemolysis O03.6
hemorrhage (delayed) (excessive) O03.6
infection
genital tract or pelvic O03.5
urinary tract O03.88
intravascular coagulation O03.6
laceration of pelvic organ(s) O03.84
metabolic disorder O03.83
oliguria O03.82
oophoritis O03.5
parametritis O03.5
pelvic peritonitis O03.5
perforation of pelvic organ(s) O03.84
renal failure or shutdown O03.82
salpingitis or salpingo-oophoritis O03.5
sepsis O03.87
shock O03.81
specified condition NEC O03.89
tubular necrosis (renal) O03.82
uremia O03.82
urinary tract infection O03.88
venous complication NEC O03.85
embolism (air) (amniotic fluid) (blood
clot) (fat) (pulmonary) (septic) (soap)
O03.7
failed — see Abortion, attempted
habitual or recurrent N96
with current abortion — see categories O03-
O06
care in current pregnancy O26.2-
without current pregnancy N96

DISEASE INDEX

Abortion (complete) (spontaneous) O03.9 — *continued*
  incomplete (spontaneous) O03.4
    complicated (by) (following) O03.30
      afibrinogenemia O03.1
      cardiac arrest O03.36
      chemical damage of pelvic organ(s) O03.34
      circulatory collapse O03.31
      cystitis O03.38
      defibrination syndrome O03.1
      electrolyte imbalance O03.33
      embolism (air) (amniotic fluid) (blood clot) (fat) (pulmonary) (septic) (soap) O03.2
      endometritis O03.0
      genital tract and pelvic infection O03.0
      hemolysis O03.1
      hemorrhage (delayed) (excessive) O03.1
      infection
        genital tract or pelvic O03.0
        urinary tract O03.38
      intravascular coagulation O03.1
      laceration of pelvic organ(s) O03.34
      metabolic disorder O03.33
      oliguria O03.32
      oophoritis O03.0
      parametritis O03.0
      pelvic peritonitis O03.0
      perforation of pelvic organ(s) O03.34
      renal failure or shutdown O03.32
      salpingitis or salpingo-oophoritis O03.0
      sepsis O03.37
      shock O03.31
      specified condition NEC O03.39
      tubular necrosis (renal) O03.32
      uremia O03.32
      urinary infection O03.38
      venous complication NEC O03.35
        embolism (air) (amniotic fluid) (blood clot) (fat) (pulmonary) (septic) (soap) O03.2
  induced (encounter for) Z33.2
    complicated by O04.80
      afibrinogenemia O04.6
      cardiac arrest O04.86
      chemical damage of pelvic organ(s) O04.84
      circulatory collapse O04.81
      cystitis O04.88
      defibrination syndrome O04.6
      electrolyte imbalance O04.83
      embolism (air) (amniotic fluid) (blood clot) (fat) (pulmonary) (septic) (soap) O04.7
      endometritis O04.5
      genital tract and pelvic infection O04.5
      hemolysis O04.6
      hemorrhage (delayed) (excessive) O04.6
      infection
        genital tract or pelvic O04.5
        urinary tract O04.88
      intravascular coagulation O04.6
      laceration of pelvic organ(s) O04.84
      metabolic disorder O04.83
      oliguria O04.82
      oophoritis O04.5
      parametritis O04.5
      pelvic peritonitis O04.5
      perforation of pelvic organ(s) O04.84
      renal failure or shutdown O04.82
      salpingitis or salpingo-oophoritis O04.5
      sepsis O04.87
      shock O04.81
      specified condition NEC O04.89
      tubular necrosis (renal) O04.82
      uremia O04.82
      urinary tract infection O04.88

Abortion (complete) (spontaneous) O03.9 — *continued*
  induced (encounter for) Z33.2 — *continued*
    complicated by O04.80 — *continued*
      venous complication NEC O04.85
        embolism (air) (amniotic fluid) (blood clot) (fat) (pulmonary) (septic) (soap) O04.7
  missed O02.1
  spontaneous — *see* Abortion (complete) (spontaneous)
    threatened O20.0
  threatened (spontaneous) O20.0
  tubal O00.10
    with intrauterine pregnancy O00.11
Abortus fever A23.1
Aboulomania F60.7
Abrami's disease D59.8
Abramov-Fiedler myocarditis (acute isolated myocarditis) I40.1
Abrasion T14.8
  abdomen, abdominal (wall) S30.811
  alveolar process S00.512
  ankle S90.51-
  antecubital space — *see* Abrasion, elbow
  anus S30.817
  arm (upper) S40.81-
  auditory canal — *see* Abrasion, ear
  auricle — *see* Abrasion, ear
  axilla — *see* Abrasion, arm
  back, lower S30.810
  breast S20.11-
  brow S00.81
  buttock S30.810
  calf — *see* Abrasion, leg
  canthus — *see* Abrasion, eyelid
  cheek S00.81
    internal S00.512
  chest wall — *see* Abrasion, thorax
  chin S00.81
  clitoris S30.814
  cornea S05.0-
  costal region — *see* Abrasion, thorax
  dental K03.1
  digit(s)
    foot — *see* Abrasion, toe
    hand — *see* Abrasion, finger
  ear S00.41-
  elbow S50.31-
  epididymis S30.813
  epigastric region S30.811
  epiglottis S10.11
  esophagus (thoracic) S27.818
    cervical S10.11
  eyebrow — *see* Abrasion, eyelid
  eyelid S00.21-
  face S00.81
  finger(s) S60.41-
    index S60.41-
    little S60.41-
    middle S60.41-
    ring S60.41-
  flank S30.811
  foot (except toe(s) alone) S90.81-
    toe — *see* Abrasion, toe
  forearm S50.81-
    elbow only — *see* Abrasion, elbow
  forehead S00.81
  genital organs, external
    female S30.816
    male S30.815
  groin S30.811
  gum S00.512
  hand S60.51-
  head S00.91
    ear — *see* Abrasion, ear
    eyelid — *see* Abrasion, eyelid
    lip S00.511
    nose S00.31

Abrasion — *continued*
  head S00.91 — *continued*
    oral cavity S00.512
    scalp S00.01
    specified site NEC S00.81
  heel — *see* Abrasion, foot
  hip S70.21-
  inguinal region S30.811
  interscapular region S20.419
  jaw S00.81
  knee S80.21-
  labium (majus) (minus) S30.814
  larynx S10.11
  leg (lower) S80.81-
    knee — *see* Abrasion, knee
    upper — *see* Abrasion, thigh
  lip S00.511
  lower back S30.810
  lumbar region S30.810
  malar region S00.81
  mammary — *see* Abrasion, breast
  mastoid region S00.81
  mouth S00.512
  nail
    finger — *see* Abrasion, finger
    toe — *see* Abrasion, toe
  nape S10.81
  nasal S00.31
  neck S10.91
    specified site NEC S10.81
    throat S10.11
  nose S00.31
  occipital region S00.01
  oral cavity S00.512
  orbital region — *see* Abrasion, eyelid
  palate S00.512
  palm — *see* Abrasion, hand
  parietal region S00.01
  pelvis S30.810
  penis S30.812
  perineum
    female S30.814
    male S30.810
  periocular area — *see* Abrasion, eyelid
  phalanges
    finger — *see* Abrasion, finger
    toe — *see* Abrasion, toe
  pharynx S10.11
  pinna — *see* Abrasion, ear
  popliteal space — *see* Abrasion, knee
  prepuce S30.812
  pubic region S30.810
  pudendum
    female S30.816
    male S30.815
  sacral region S30.810
  scalp S00.01
  scapular region — *see* Abrasion, shoulder
  scrotum S30.813
  shin — *see* Abrasion, leg
  shoulder S40.21-
  skin NEC T14.8
  sternal region S20.319
  submaxillary region S00.81
  submental region S00.81
  subungual
    finger(s) — *see* Abrasion, finger
    toe(s) — *see* Abrasion, toe
  supraclavicular fossa S10.81
  supraorbital S00.81
  temple S00.81
  temporal region S00.81
  testis S30.813
  thigh S70.31-
  thorax, thoracic (wall) S20.91
    back S20.41-
    front S20.31-
  throat S10.11
  thumb S60.31-

Abrasion — *continued*
toe(s) (lesser) S90.416
  great S90.41-
tongue S00.512
tooth, teeth (dentifrice) (habitual) (hard tissues) (occupational) (ritual) (traditional) K03.1
trachea S10.11
tunica vaginalis S30.813
tympanum, tympanic membrane — *see* Abrasion, ear
uvula S00.512
vagina S30.814
vocal cords S10.11
vulva S30.814
wrist S60.81-

Abrism — *see* Poisoning, food, noxious, plant

Abruptio placentae O45.9-
with
  afibrinogenemia O45.01-
  coagulation defect O45.00-
    specified NEC O45.09-
  disseminated intravascular coagulation O45.02-
  hypofibrinogenemia O45.01-
  specified NEC O45.8-

Abruption, placenta — *see* Abruptio placentae

Abscess (connective tissue) (embolic) (fistulous) (infective) (metastatic) (multiple) (pernicious) (pyogenic) (septic) L02.91
with
  diverticular disease (intestine) K57.80
    with bleeding K57.81
    large intestine K57.20
      with
        bleeding K57.21
        small intestine K57.40
          with bleeding K57.41
    small intestine K57.00
      with
        bleeding K57.01
        large intestine K57.40
          with bleeding K57.41
  lymphangitis — *code by* site under Abscess
abdomen, abdominal
  cavity K65.1
  wall L02.211
abdominopelvic K65.1
accessory sinus — *see* Sinusitis
adrenal (capsule) (gland) E27.8
alveolar K04.7
  with sinus K04.6
amebic A06.4
  brain (and liver or lung abscess) A06.6
  genitourinary tract A06.82
  liver (without mention of brain or lung abscess) A06.4
  lung (and liver) (without mention of brain abscess) A06.5
  specified site NEC A06.89
  spleen A06.89
anerobic A48.0
ankle — *see* Abscess, lower limb
anorectal K61.2
antecubital space — *see* Abscess, upper limb
antrum (chronic) (Highmore) — *see* Sinusitis, maxillary
anus K61.0
apical (tooth) K04.7
  with sinus (alveolar) K04.6
appendix K35.3
areola (acute) (chronic) (nonpuerperal) N61.1
  puerperal, postpartum or gestational — *see* Infection, nipple
arm (any part) — *see* Abscess, upper limb
artery (wall) I77.89
atheromatous I77.2
auricle, ear — *see* Abscess, ear, external

Abscess (connective tissue) (embolic) (fistulous) (infective) (metastatic) (multiple) (pernicious) (pyogenic) (septic) L02.91 — *continued*
axilla (region) L02.41-
  lymph gland or node L04.2
back (any part, except buttock) L02.212
Bartholin's gland N75.1
  with
    abortion — *see* Abortion, by type complicated by, sepsis
    ectopic or molar pregnancy O08.0
  following ectopic or molar pregnancy O08.0
Bezold's — *see* Mastoiditis, acute
bilharziasis B65.1
bladder (wall) — *see* Cystitis, specified type NEC
bone (subperiosteal) — *see also* Osteomyelitis, specified type NEC
  accessory sinus (chronic) — *see* Sinusitis
  chronic or old — *see* Osteomyelitis, chronic
  jaw (lower) (upper) M27.2
  mastoid — *see* Mastoiditis, acute, subperiosteal
  petrous — *see* Petrositis
  spinal (tuberculous) A18.01
    nontuberculous — *see* Osteomyelitis, vertebra
bowel K63.0
brain (any part) (cystic) (otogenic) G06.0
  amebic (with abscess of any other site) A06.6
  gonococcal A54.82
  pheomycotic (chromomycotic) B43.1
  tuberculous A17.81
breast (acute) (chronic) (nonpuerperal) N61.1
  newborn P39.0
  puerperal, postpartum, gestational — *see* Mastitis, obstetric, purulent
broad ligament N73.2
  acute N73.0
  chronic N73.1
Brodie's (localized) (chronic) M86.8x-
bronchi J98.09
buccal cavity K12.2
bulbourethral gland N34.0
bursa M71.00
  ankle M71.07-
  elbow M71.02-
  foot M71.07-
  hand M71.04-
  hip M71.05-
  knee M71.06-
  multiple sites M71.09
  pharyngeal J39.1
  shoulder M71.01-
  specified site NEC M71.08
  wrist M71.03-
buttock L02.31
canthus — *see* Blepharoconjunctivitis
cartilage — *see* Disorder, cartilage, specified type NEC
cecum K35.3
cerebellum, cerebellar G06.0
  sequelae G09
cerebral (embolic) G06.0
  sequelae G09
cervical (meaning neck) L02.11
  lymph gland or node L04.0
cervix (stump) (uteri) — *see* Cervicitis
cheek (external) L02.01
  inner K12.2
chest J86.9
  with fistula J86.0
  wall L02.213
chin L02.01
choroid — *see* Inflammation, chorioretinal
circumtonsillar J36

Abscess (connective tissue) (embolic) (fistulous) (infective) (metastatic) (multiple) (pernicious) (pyogenic) (septic) L02.91 — *continued*
cold (lung) (tuberculous) — *see also* Tuberculosis, abscess, lung
  articular — *see* Tuberculosis, joint
colon (wall) K63.0
colostomy K94.02
conjunctiva — *see* Conjunctivitis, acute
cornea H16.31-
corpus
  cavernosum N48.21
  luteum — *see* Oophoritis
Cowper's gland N34.0
cranium K94.02
cul-de-sac (Douglas') (posterior) — *see* Peritonitis, pelvic, female
cutaneous — *see* Abscess, by site
dental K04.7
  with sinus (alveolar) K04.6
dentoalveolar K04.7
  with sinus K04.6
diaphragm, diaphragmatic K65.1
Douglas' cul-de-sac or pouch — *see* Peritonitis, pelvic, female
Dubois A50.59
ear (middle) — *see also* Otitis, media, suppurative
  acute — *see* Otitis, media, suppurative, acute
  external H60.0-
entamebic — *see* Abscess, amebic
enterostomy K94.12
epididymis N45.4
epidural G06.2
  brain G06.0
  spinal cord G06.1
epiglottis J38.7
epiploon, epiploic K65.1
erysipelatous — *see* Erysipelas
esophagus K20.8
ethmoid (bone) (chronic) (sinus) J32.2
external auditory canal — *see* Abscess, ear, external
extradural G06.2
  brain G06.0
    sequelae G09
  spinal cord G06.1
extraperitoneal K68.19
eye — *see* Endophthalmitis, purulent
eyelid H00.03-
face (any part, except ear, eye and nose) L02.01
fallopian tube — *see* Salpingitis
fascia M72.8
fauces J39.1
fecal K63.0
femoral (region) — *see* Abscess, lower limb
filaria, filarial — *see* Infestation, filarial
finger (any) — *see also* Abscess, hand
  nail — *see* Cellulitis, finger
foot L02.61-
forehead L02.01
frontal sinus (chronic) J32.1
gallbladder K81.0
genital organ or tract
  female (external) N76.4
  male N49.9
    multiple sites N49.8
    specified NEC N49.8
gestational mammary O91.11-
gestational subareolar O91.11-
gingival — *see* Peridontitis, aggressive, localized
gland, glandular (lymph) (acute) — *see* Lymphadenitis, acute
gluteal (region) L02.31
gonorrheal — *see* Gonococcus
groin L02.214

DISEASE INDEX

Abscess (connective tissue) (embolic) (fistulous) (infective) (metastatic) (multiple) (pernicious) (pyogenic) (septic) L02.91 — *continued*
gum — *see* Peridontitis, aggressive, localized
hand L02.51-
head NEC L02.811
  face (any part, except ear, eye and nose) L02.01
heart — *see* Carditis
heel — *see* Abscess, foot
helminthic — *see* Infestation, helminth
hepatic (cholangitic) (hematogenic) (lymphogenic) (pylephlebitic) K75.0
  amebic A06.4
hip (region) — *see* Abscess, lower limb
ileocecal K35.3
ileostomy (bud) K94.12
iliac (region) L02.214
  fossa K35.3
infraclavicular (fossa) — *see* Abscess, upper limb
inguinal (region) L02.214
  lymph gland or node L04.1
intestine, intestinal NEC K63.0
  rectal K61.1
intra-abdominal (*see also* Abscess, peritoneum) K65.1
  postprocedural T81.43
    retroperitoneal K68.11
intracranial G06.0
intramammary — *see* Abscess, breast
intra-muscular, postprocedural T81.42
intraorbital — *see* Abscess, orbit
intraperitoneal K65.1
intrasphincteric (anus) K61.4
intraspinal G06.1
intratonsillar J36
ischiorectal (fossa) K61.3
jaw (bone) (lower) (upper) M27.2
joint — *see* Arthritis, pyogenic or pyemic
  spine (tuberculous) A18.01
    nontuberculous — *see* Spondylopathy, infective
kidney N15.1
  with calculus N20.0
    with hydronephrosis N13.6
  puerperal (postpartum) O86.21
knee — *see also* Abscess, lower limb
  joint M00.9
labium (majus) (minus) N76.4
lacrimal
  caruncle — *see* Inflammation, lacrimal, passages, acute
  gland — *see* Dacryoadenitis
  passages (duct) (sac) — *see* Inflammation, lacrimal, passages, acute
lacunar N34.0
larynx J38.7
lateral (alveolar) K04.7
  with sinus K04.6
leg (any part) — *see* Abscess, lower limb
lens H27.8
lingual K14.0
  tonsil J36
lip K13.0
Littre's gland N34.0
liver (cholangitic) (hematogenic) (lymphogenic) (pylephlebitic) (pyogenic) K75.0
  amebic (due to Entamoeba histolytica) (dysenteric) (tropical) A06.4
    with
      brain abscess (and liver or lung abscess) A06.6
      lung abscess A06.5
loin (region) L02.211
lower limb L02.41-
lumbar (tuberculous) A18.01
  nontuberculous L02.212

Abscess (connective tissue) (embolic) (fistulous) (infective) (metastatic) (multiple) (pernicious) (pyogenic) (septic) L02.91 — *continued*
lung (miliary) (putrid) J85.2
  with pneumonia J85.1
    due to specified organism (*see* Pneumonia, in (due to))
  amebic (with liver abscess) A06.5
    with
      brain abscess A06.6
      pneumonia A06.5
lymph, lymphatic, gland or node (acute) — *see also* Lymphadenitis, acute
mesentery I88.0
malar M27.2
mammary gland — *see* Abscess, breast
marginal, anus K61.0
mastoid — *see* Mastoiditis, acute
maxilla, maxillary M27.2
  molar (tooth) K04.7
    with sinus K04.6
  premolar K04.7
  sinus (chronic) J32.0
mediastinum J85.3
meibomian gland — *see* Hordeolum
meninges G06.2
mesentery, mesenteric K65.1
mesosalpinx — *see* Salpingitis
mons pubis L02.215
mouth (floor) K12.2
muscle — *see* Myositis, infective
myocardium I40.0
nabothian (follicle) — *see* Cervicitis
nasal J32.9
nasopharyngeal J39.1
navel L02.216
  newborn P38.9
    with mild hemorrhage P38.1
    without hemorrhage P38.9
neck (region) L02.11
  lymph gland or node L04.0
nephritic — *see* Abscess, kidney
nipple N61.1
  associated with
    lactation — *see* Pregnancy, complicated by
    pregnancy — *see* Pregnancy, complicated by
nose (external) (fossa) (septum) J34.0
  sinus (chronic) — *see* Sinusitis
omentum K65.1
operative wound T81.40
orbit, orbital — *see* Cellulitis, orbit
otogenic G06.0
ovary, ovarian (corpus luteum) — *see* Oophoritis
oviduct — *see* Oophoritis
palate (soft) K12.2
  hard M27.2
palmar (space) — *see* Abscess, hand
pancreas (duct) — *see* Pancreatitis, acute
parafrenal N48.21
parametric, parametrium N73.2
  acute N73.0
  chronic N73.1
paranephric N15.1
parapancreatic — *see* Pancreatitis, acute
parapharyngeal J39.0
pararectal K61.1
parasinus — *see* Sinusitis
parauterine (*see also* Disease, pelvis, inflammatory) N73.2
paravaginal — *see* Vaginitis
parietal region (scalp) L02.811
parodontal — *see* Peridontitis, aggressive, localized
parotid (duct) (gland) K11.3
  region K12.2
pectoral (region) L02.213

Abscess (connective tissue) (embolic) (fistulous) (infective) (metastatic) (multiple) (pernicious) (pyogenic) (septic) L02.91 — *continued*
pelvis, pelvic
  female — *see* Disease, pelvis, inflammatory
  male, peritoneal K65.1
penis N48.21
  gonococcal (accessory gland) (periurethral) A54.1
perianal K61.0
periapical K04.7
  with sinus (alveolar) K04.6
periappendicular K35.3
pericardial I30.1
pericecal K35.3
pericemental — *see* Peridontitis, aggressive, localized
pericholecystic — *see* Cholecystitis, acute
pericoronal — *see* Peridontitis, aggressive, localized
peridental — *see* Peridontitis, aggressive, localized
perimetric (*see also* Disease, pelvis, inflammatory) N73.2
perinephric, perinephritic — *see* Abscess, kidney
perineum, perineal (superficial) L02.215
  urethra N34.0
periodontal (parietal) — *see* Peridontitis, aggressive, localized
  apical K04.7
periosteum, periosteal — *see also* Osteomyelitis, specified type NEC
  with osteomyelitis — *see also* Osteomyelitis, specified type NEC
  acute — *see* Osteomyelitis, acute
  chronic — *see* Osteomyelitis, chronic
peripharyngeal J39.0
peripleuritic J86.9
  with fistula J86.0
periprostatic N41.2
perirectal K61.1
perirenal (tissue) — *see* Abscess, kidney
perisinuous (nose) — *see* Sinusitis
peritoneum, peritoneal (perforated) (ruptured) K65.1
  with appendicitis K35.3
  pelvic
    female — *see* Peritonitis, pelvic, female
    male K65.1
  postoperative T81.43
  puerperal, postpartum, childbirth O85
  tuberculous A18.31
peritonsillar J36
perityphlic K35.3
periureteral N28.89
periurethral N34.0
  gonococcal (accessory gland) (periurethral) A54.1
periuterine (*see also* Disease, pelvis, inflammatory) N73.2
perivesical — *see* Cystitis, specified type NEC
petrous bone — *see* Petrositis
phagedenic NOS L02.91
  chancroid A57
pharynx, pharyngeal (lateral) J39.1
pilonidal L05.01
pituitary (gland) E23.6
pleura J86.9
  with fistula J86.0
popliteal — *see* Abscess, lower limb
postcecal K35.3
postlaryngeal J38.7
postnasal J34.0
postoperative (any site) T81.40
  retroperitoneal K68.11
postpharyngeal J39.0
posttonsillar J36
post-typhoid A01.09

Abscess (connective tissue) (embolic) (fistulous) (infective) (metastatic) (multiple) (pernicious) (pyogenic) (septic) L02.91 — *continued*
pouch of Douglas — *see* Peritonitis, pelvic, female
premammary — *see* Abscess, breast
prepatellar — *see* Abscess, lower limb
prostate N41.2
  gonococcal (acute) (chronic) A54.22
psoas muscle K68.12
puerperal — *code by* site under Puerperal, abscess
pulmonary — *see* Abscess, lung
pulp, pulpal (dental) K04.01
  irreversible K04.02
  reversible K04.01
rectovaginal septum K63.0
rectovesical — *see* Cystitis, specified type NEC
rectum K61.1
renal — *see* Abscess, kidney
retina — *see* Inflammation, chorioretinal
retrobulbar — *see* Abscess, orbit
retrocecal K65.1
retrolaryngeal J38.7
retromammary — *see* Abscess, breast
retroperitoneal NEC K68.19
  postprocedural K68.11
retropharyngeal J39.0
retrouterine — *see* Peritonitis, pelvic, female
retrovesical — *see* Cystitis, specified type NEC
root, tooth K04.7
  with sinus (alveolar) K04.6
round ligament (*see also* Disease, pelvis, inflammatory) N73.2
rupture (spontaneous) NOS L02.91
sacrum (tuberculous) A18.01
  nontuberculous M46.28
salivary (duct) (gland) K11.3
scalp (any part) L02.811
scapular — *see* Osteomyelitis, specified type NEC
sclera — *see* Scleritis
scrofulous (tuberculous) A18.2
scrotum N49.2
seminal vesicle N49.0
septal, dental K04.7
  with sinus (alveolar) K04.6
serous — *see* Periostitis
shoulder (region) — *see* Abscess, upper limb
sigmoid K63.0
sinus (accessory) (chronic) (nasal) — *see also* Sinusitis
  intracranial venous (any) G06.0
Skene's duct or gland N34.0
skin — *see* Abscess, by site
specified site NEC L02.818
spermatic cord N49.1
sphenoidal (sinus) (chronic) J32.3
spinal cord (any part) (staphylococcal) G06.1
  tuberculous A17.81
spine (column) (tuberculous) A18.01
  epidural G06.1
  nontuberculous — *see* Osteomyelitis, vertebra
spleen D73.3
  amebic A06.89
stitch T81.48
subarachnoid G06.2
  brain G06.0
  spinal cord G06.1
subareolar — *see* Abscess, breast
subcecal K35.3
subcutaneous — *see also* Abscess, by site
  pheomycotic (chromomycotic) B43.2
  postprocedural T81.41
subdiaphragmatic K65.1

Abscess (connective tissue) (embolic) (fistulous) (infective) (metastatic) (multiple) (pernicious) (pyogenic) (septic) L02.91 — *continued*
subdural G06.2
  brain G06.0
    sequelae G09
  spinal cord G06.1
subgaleal L02.811
subhepatic K65.1
sublingual K12.2
  gland K11.3
submammary — *see* Abscess, breast
submandibular (region) (space) (triangle) K12.2
  gland K11.3
submaxillary (region) L02.01
  gland K11.3
submental L02.01
  gland K11.3
subperiosteal — *see* Osteomyelitis, specified type NEC
subphrenic K65.1
  postoperative T81.43
suburethral N34.0
sudoriparous L75.8
supraclavicular (fossa) — *see* Abscess, upper limb
suprapelvic, acute N73.0
suprarenal (capsule) (gland) E27.8
sweat gland L74.8
tear duct — *see* Inflammation, lacrimal, passages, acute
temple L02.01
temporal region L02.01
temporosphenoidal G06.0
tendon (sheath) M65.00
  ankle M65.07-
  foot M65.07-
  forearm M65.03-
  hand M65.04-
  lower leg M65.06-
  pelvic region M65.05-
  shoulder region M65.01-
  specified site NEC M65.08
  thigh M65.05-
  upper arm M65.02-
testis N45.4
thigh — *see* Abscess, lower limb
thorax J86.9
  with fistula J86.0
throat J39.1
thumb — *see also* Abscess, hand
  nail — *see* Cellulitis, finger
thymus (gland) E32.1
thyroid (gland) E06.0
toe (any) — *see also* Abscess, foot
  nail — *see* Cellulitis, toe
tongue (staphylococcal) K14.0
tonsil(s) (lingual) J36
tonsillopharyngeal J36
tooth, teeth (root) K04.7
  with sinus (alveolar) K04.6
  supporting structures NEC — *see* Peridontitis, aggressive, localized
trachea J39.8
trunk L02.219
  abdominal wall L02.211
  back L02.212
  chest wall L02.213
  groin L02.214
  perineum L02.215
  umbilicus L02.216
tubal — *see* Salpingitis
tuberculous — *see* Tuberculosis, abscess
tubo-ovarian — *see* Salpingo-oophoritis
tunica vaginalis N49.1
umbilicus L02.216

Abscess (connective tissue) (embolic) (fistulous) (infective) (metastatic) (multiple) (pernicious) (pyogenic) (septic) L02.91 — *continued*
upper
  limb L02.41-
  respiratory J39.8
urethral (gland) N34.0
urinary N34.0
uterus, uterine (wall) — *see also* Endometritis
  ligament (*see also* Disease, pelvis, inflammatory) N73.2
  neck — *see* Cervicitis
uvula K12.2
vagina (wall) — *see* Vaginitis
vaginorectal — *see* Vaginitis
vas deferens N49.1
vermiform appendix K35.3
vertebra (column) (tuberculous) A18.01
  nontuberculous — *see* Osteomyelitis, vertebra
vesical — *see* Cystitis, specified type NEC
vesico-uterine pouch — *see* Peritonitis, pelvic, female
vitreous (humor) — *see* Endophthalmitis, purulent
vocal cord J38.3
von Bezold's — *see* Mastoiditis, acute
vulva N76.4
vulvovaginal gland N75.1
web space — *see* Abscess, hand
wound T81.40
wrist — *see* Abscess, upper limb
Absence (of) (organ or part) (complete or partial)
adrenal (gland) (congenital) Q89.1
  acquired E89.6
albumin in blood E88.09
alimentary tract (congenital) Q45.8
  upper Q40.8
alveolar process (acquired) — *see* Anomaly, alveolar
ankle (acquired) Z89.44-
anus (congenital) Q42.3
  with fistula Q42.2
aorta (congenital) Q25.41
appendix, congenital Q42.8
arm (acquired) Z89.20-
  above elbow Z89.22-
    congenital (with hand present) — *see* Agenesis, arm, with hand present and hand — *see* Agenesis, forearm, and hand
  below elbow Z89.21-
    congenital (with hand present) — *see* Agenesis, arm, with hand present and hand — *see* Agenesis, forearm, and hand
  congenital — *see* Defect, reduction, upper limb
  shoulder (following explantation of shoulder joint prosthesis) (joint) (with or without presence of antibiotic-impregnated cement spacer) Z89.23-
    congenital (with hand present) — *see* Agenesis, arm, with hand present
artery (congenital) (peripheral) Q27.8
  brain Q28.3
  coronary Q24.5
  pulmonary Q25.79
  specified NEC Q27.8
  umbilical Q27.0
atrial septum (congenital) Q21.1
auditory canal (congenital) (external) Q16.1
auricle (ear), congenital Q16.0
bile, biliary duct, congenital Q44.5
bladder (acquired) Z90.6
  congenital Q64.5
bowel sounds R19.11

DISEASE INDEX

DISEASE INDEX

Absence (of) (organ or part) (complete or partial) — *continued*
brain Q00.0
  part of Q04.3
breast(s) (and nipple(s)) (acquired) Z90.1-
  congenital Q83.8
broad ligament Q50.6
bronchus (congenital) Q32.4
canaliculus lacrimalis, congenital Q10.4
cerebellum (vermis) Q04.3
cervix (acquired) (with uterus) Z90.710
  with remaining uterus Z90.712
  congenital Q51.5
chin, congenital Q18.8
cilia (congenital) Q10.3
  acquired — *see* Madarosis
clitoris (congenital) Q52.6
coccyx, congenital Q76.49
cold sense R20.8
congenital
  lumen — *see* Atresia
  organ or site NEC — *see* Agenesis
  septum — *see* Imperfect, closure
corpus callosum Q04.0
cricoid cartilage, congenital Q31.8
diaphragm (with hernia), congenital Q79.1
digestive organ(s) or tract, congenital Q45.8
  acquired NEC Z90.49
  upper Q40.8
ductus arteriosus Q28.8
duodenum (acquired) Z90.49
  congenital Q41.0
ear, congenital Q16.9
  acquired H93.8-
  auricle Q16.0
  external Q16.0
  inner Q16.5
  lobe, lobule Q17.8
  middle, except ossicles Q16.4
    ossicles Q16.3
  ossicles Q16.3
ejaculatory duct (congenital) Q55.4
endocrine gland (congenital) NEC Q89.2
  acquired E89.89
epididymis (congenital) Q55.4
  acquired Z90.79
epiglottis, congenital Q31.8
esophagus (congenital) Q39.8
  acquired (partial) Z90.49
eustachian tube (congenital) Q16.2
extremity (acquired) Z89.9
  congenital Q73.0
  knee (following explantation of knee joint prosthesis) (joint) (with or without presence of antibiotic-impregnated cement spacer) Z89.52-
  lower (above knee) Z89.619
    below knee Z89.51-
  upper — *see* Absence, arm
eye (acquired) Z90.01
  congenital Q11.1
  muscle (congenital) Q10.3
eyeball (acquired) Z90.01
eyelid (fold) (congenital) Q10.3
  acquired Z90.01
face, specified part NEC Q18.8
fallopian tube(s) (acquired) Z90.79
  congenital Q50.6
family member (causing problem in home) NEC (*see also* Disruption, family) Z63.32
femur, congenital — *see* Defect, reduction, lower limb, longitudinal, femur
fibrinogen (congenital) D68.2
  acquired D65
finger(s) (acquired) Z89.02-
  congenital — *see* Agenesis, hand
foot (acquired) Z89.43-
  congenital — *see* Agenesis, foot

Absence (of) (organ or part) (complete or partial) — *continued*
forearm (acquired) — *see* Absence, arm, below elbow
gallbladder (acquired) Z90.49
  congenital Q44.0
gamma globulin in blood D80.1
  hereditary D80.0
genital organs
  acquired (female) (male) Z90.79
  female, congenital Q52.8
    external Q52.71
    internal NEC Q52.8
  male, congenital Q55.8
genitourinary organs, congenital NEC
  female Q52.8
  male Q55.8
globe (acquired) Z90.01
  congenital Q11.1
glottis, congenital Q31.8
hand and wrist (acquired) Z89.11-
  congenital — *see* Agenesis, hand
head, part (acquired) NEC Z90.09
heat sense R20.8
hip (following explantation of hip joint prosthesis) (joint) (with or without presence of antibiotic-impregnated cement spacer) Z89.62-
hymen (congenital) Q52.4
ileum (acquired) Z90.49
  congenital Q41.2
immunoglobulin, isolated NEC D80.3
  IgA D80.2
  IgG D80.3
  IgM D80.4
incus (acquired) — *see* Loss, ossicles, ear
  congenital Q16.3
inner ear, congenital Q16.5
intestine (acquired) (small) Z90.49
  congenital Q41.9
    specified NEC Q41.8
  large Z90.49
    congenital Q42.9
      specified NEC Q42.8
iris, congenital Q13.1
jejunum (acquired) Z90.49
  congenital Q41.1
joint
  acquired
    hip (following explantation of hip joint prosthesis) (with or without presence of antibiotic-impregnated cement spacer) Z89.62-
    knee (following explantation of knee joint prosthesis) (with or without presence of antibiotic-impregnated cement spacer) Z89.52-
    shoulder (following explantation of shoulder joint prosthesis) (with or without presence of antibiotic-impregnated cement spacer) Z89.23-
  congenital NEC Q74.8
kidney(s) (acquired) Z90.5
  congenital Q60.2
    bilateral Q60.1
    unilateral Q60.0
knee (following explantation of knee joint prosthesis) (joint) (with or without presence of antibiotic-impregnated cement spacer) Z89.52-
labyrinth, membranous Q16.5
larynx (congenital) Q31.8
  acquired Z90.02
leg (acquired) (above knee) Z89.61-
  below knee (acquired) Z89.51-
  congenital — *see* Defect, reduction, lower limb
lens (acquired) — *see also* Aphakia
  congenital Q12.3
  post cataract extraction Z98.4-

Absence (of) (organ or part) (complete or partial) — *continued*
limb (acquired) — *see* Absence, extremity
lip Q38.6
liver (congenital) Q44.7
lung (fissure) (lobe) (bilateral) (unilateral) (congenital) Q33.3
  acquired (any part) Z90.2
menstruation — *see* Amenorrhea
muscle (congenital) (pectoral) Q79.8
  ocular Q10.3
neck, part Q18.8
neutrophil — *see* Agranulocytosis
nipple(s) (with breast(s)) (acquired) Z90.1-
  congenital Q83.2
nose (congenital) Q30.1
  acquired Z90.09
organ
  of Corti, congenital Q16.5
  or site, congenital NEC Q89.8
    acquired NEC Z90.89
osseous meatus (ear) Q16.4
ovary (acquired)
  bilateral Z90.722
  congenital
    bilateral Q50.02
    unilateral Q50.01
  unilateral Z90.721
oviduct (acquired)
  bilateral Z90.722
  congenital Q50.6
  unilateral Z90.721
pancreas (congenital) Q45.0
  acquired Z90.410
    complete Z90.410
    partial Z90.411
    total Z90.410
parathyroid gland (acquired) E89.2
  congenital Q89.2
patella, congenital Q74.1
penis (congenital) Q55.5
  acquired Z90.79
pericardium (congenital) Q24.8
pituitary gland (congenital) Q89.2
  acquired E89.3
prostate (acquired) Z90.79
  congenital Q55.4
pulmonary valve Q22.0
punctum lacrimale (congenital) Q10.4
radius, congenital — *see* Defect, reduction, upper limb, longitudinal, radius
rectum (congenital) Q42.1
  with fistula Q42.0
  acquired Z90.49
respiratory organ NOS Q34.9
rib (acquired) Z90.89
  congenital Q76.6
sacrum, congenital Q76.49
salivary gland(s), congenital Q38.4
scrotum, congenital Q55.29
seminal vesicles (congenital) Q55.4
  acquired Z90.79
septum
  atrial (congenital) Q21.1
  between aorta and pulmonary artery Q21.4
  ventricular (congenital) Q20.4
sex chromosome
  female phenotype Q97.8
  male phenotype Q98.8
skull bone (congenital) Q75.8
  with
    anencephaly Q00.0
    encephalocele — *see* Encephalocele
    hydrocephalus Q03.9
      with spina bifida — *see* Spina bifida, by site, with hydrocephalus
    microcephaly Q02
spermatic cord, congenital Q55.4
spine, congenital Q76.49

8

Absence (of) (organ or part) (complete or partial) — *continued*
spleen (congenital) Q89.01
　acquired Z90.81
sternum, congenital Q76.7
stomach (acquired) (partial) Z90.3
　congenital Q40.2
superior vena cava, congenital Q26.8
teeth, tooth (congenital) K00.0
　acquired (complete) K08.109
　　class I K08.101
　　class II K08.102
　　class III K08.103
　　class IV K08.104
　　due to
　　　caries K08.139
　　　　class I K08.131
　　　　class II K08.132
　　　　class III K08.133
　　　　class IV K08.134
　　　periodontal disease K08.129
　　　　class I K08.121
　　　　class II K08.122
　　　　class III K08.123
　　　　class IV K08.124
　　specified NEC K08.199
　　　class I K08.191
　　　class II K08.192
　　　class III K08.193
　　　class IV K08.194
　　trauma K08.119
　　　class I K08.111
　　　class II K08.112
　　　class III K08.113
　　　class IV K08.114
　partial K08.409
　　class I K08.401
　　class II K08.402
　　class III K08.403
　　class IV K08.404
　　due to
　　　caries K08.439
　　　　class I K08.431
　　　　class II K08.432
　　　　class III K08.433
　　　　class IV K08.434
　　　periodontal disease K08.429
　　　　class I K08.421
　　　　class II K08.422
　　　　class III K08.423
　　　　class IV K08.424
　　specified NEC K08.499
　　　class I K08.491
　　　class II K08.492
　　　class III K08.493
　　　class IV K08.494
　　trauma K08.419
　　　class I K08.411
　　　class II K08.412
　　　class III K08.413
　　　class IV K08.414
tendon (congenital) Q79.8
testis (congenital) Q55.0
　acquired Z90.79
thumb (acquired) Z89.01-
　congenital — *see* Agenesis, hand
thymus gland Q89.2
thyroid (gland) (acquired) E89.0
　cartilage, congenital Q31.8
　congenital E03.1
toe(s) (acquired) Z89.42-
　with foot — *see* Absence, foot and ankle
　congenital — *see* Agenesis, foot
　great Z89.41-
tongue, congenital Q38.3
trachea (cartilage), congenital Q32.1
transverse aortic arch, congenital Q25.49
tricuspid valve Q22.4
umbilical artery, congenital Q27.0

Absence (of) (organ or part) (complete or partial) — *continued*
upper arm and forearm with hand present, congenital — *see* Agenesis, arm, with hand present
ureter (congenital) Q62.4
　acquired Z90.6
urethra, congenital Q64.5
uterus (acquired) Z90.710
　with cervix Z90.710
　with remaining cervical stump Z90.711
　congenital Q51.0
uvula, congenital Q38.5
vagina, congenital Q52.0
vas deferens (congenital) Q55.4
　acquired Z90.79
vein (peripheral) congenital NEC Q27.8
　cerebral Q28.3
　digestive system Q27.8
　great Q26.8
　lower limb Q27.8
　portal Q26.5
　precerebral Q28.1
　specified site NEC Q27.8
　upper limb Q27.8
vena cava (inferior) (superior), congenital Q26.8
ventricular septum Q20.4
vertebra, congenital Q76.49
vulva, congenital Q52.71
wrist (acquired) Z89.12-

Absorbent system disease I87.8
Absorption
carbohydrate, disturbance K90.49
chemical — *see* Table of Drugs and Chemcials
　through placenta (newborn) P04.9
　　environmental substance P04.6
　　nutritional substance P04.5
　　obstetric anesthetic or analgesic drug P04.0
drug NEC — *see* Table of Drugs and Chemicals
　addictive
　　through placenta (newborn) P04.49
　　　cocaine P04.41
　medicinal
　　through placenta (newborn) P04.1
　through placenta (newborn) P04.1
　　obstetric anesthetic or analgesic drug P04.0
fat, disturbance K90.49
　pancreatic K90.3
noxious substance — *see* Table of Drugs and Chemicals
protein, disturbance K90.49
starch, disturbance K90.49
toxic substance — *see* Table of Drugs and Chemicals
uremic — *see* Uremia

Abstinence symptoms, syndrome
alcohol F10.239
　with delirium F10.231
cocaine F14.23
neonatal P96.1
nicotine — *see* Dependence, drug, nicotine, with, withdrawal
opioid F11.93
　with dependence F11.23
psychoactive NEC F19.939
　with
　　delirium F19.931
　　dependence F19.239
　　　with
　　　　delirium F19.231
　　　　perceptual disturbance F19.232
　　　　uncomplicated F19.230
　　perceptual disturbance F19.932
　uncomplicated F19.930

Abstinence symptoms, syndrome — *continued*
sedative F13.939
　with
　　delirium F13.931
　　dependence F13.239
　　　with
　　　　delirium F13.231
　　　　perceptual disturbance F13.232
　　　　uncomplicated F13.230
　　perceptual disturbance F13.932
　uncomplicated F13.930
stimulant NEC F15.93
　with dependence F15.23
Abulia R68.89
Abulomania F60.7
Abuse
adult — *see* Maltreatment, adult
　as reason for
　　couple seeking advice (including offender) Z63.0
alcohol (non-dependent) F10.10
　with
　　anxiety disorder F10.180
　　intoxication F10.129
　　　with delirium F10.121
　　　uncomplicated F10.120
　　mood disorder F10.14
　　other specified disorder F10.188
　　psychosis F10.159
　　　delusions F10.150
　　　hallucinations F10.151
　　sexual dysfunction F10.181
　　sleep disorder F10.182
　　unspecified disorder F10.19
　counseling and surveillance Z71.41
amphetamine (or related substance) — *see* Abuse, drug, stimulant NEC
analgesics (non-prescribed) (over the counter) F55.8
antacids F55.0
antidepressants — *see* Abuse, drug, psychoactive NEC
anxiolytic — *see* Abuse, drug, sedative
barbiturates — *see* Abuse, drug, sedative
caffeine — *see* Abuse, drug, stimulant NEC
cannabis, cannabinoids — *see* Abuse, drug, cannabis
child — *see* Maltreatment, child
cocaine — *see* Abuse, drug, cocaine
drug NEC (non-dependent) F19.10
　with sleep disorder F19.182
　amphetamine type — *see* Abuse, drug, stimulant NEC
　analgesics (non-prescribed) (over the counter) F55.8
　antacids F55.0
　antidepressants — *see* Abuse, drug, psychoactive NEC
　anxiolytics — *see* Abuse, drug, sedative
　barbiturates — *see* Abuse, drug, sedative
　caffeine — *see* Abuse, drug, stimulant NEC
　cannabis F12.10
　　with
　　　anxiety disorder F12.180
　　　intoxication F12.129
　　　　with
　　　　　delirium F12.121
　　　　　perceptual disturbance F12.122
　　　　uncomplicated F12.120
　　　other specified disorder F12.188
　　　psychosis F12.159
　　　　delusions F12.150
　　　　hallucinations F12.151
　　　unspecified disorder F12.19

DISEASE INDEX

Abuse — *continued*
  drug NEC (non-dependent) F19.10 — *continued*
    cocaine F14.10
      with
        anxiety disorder F14.180
        intoxication F14.129
          with
            delirium F14.121
            perceptual disturbance F14.122
          uncomplicated F14.120
        mood disorder F14.14
        other specified disorder F14.188
        psychosis F14.159
          delusions F14.150
          hallucinations F14.151
        sexual dysfunction F14.181
        sleep disorder F14.182
        unspecified disorder F14.19
    counseling and surveillance Z71.51
    hallucinogen F16.10
      with
        anxiety disorder F16.180
        flashbacks F16.183
        intoxication F16.129
          with
            delirium F16.121
            perceptual disturbance F16.122
          uncomplicated F16.120
        mood disorder F16.14
        other specified disorder F16.188
        perception disorder, persisting F16.183
        psychosis F16.159
          delusions F16.150
          hallucinations F16.151
        unspecified disorder F16.19
    hashish — *see* Abuse, drug, cannabis
    herbal or folk remedies F55.1
    hormones F55.3
    hypnotics — *see* Abuse, drug, sedative
    inhalant F18.10
      with
        anxiety disorder F18.180
        dementia, persisting F18.17
        intoxication F18.129
          with delirium F18.121
          uncomplicated F18.120
        mood disorder F18.14
        other specified disorder F18.188
        psychosis F18.159
          delusions F18.150
          hallucinations F18.151
        unspecified disorder F18.19
    laxatives F55.2
    LSD — *see* Abuse, drug, hallucinogen
    marihuana — *see* Abuse, drug, cannabis
    morphine type (opioids) — *see* Abuse, drug, opioid
    opioid F11.10
      with
        intoxication F11.129
          with
            delirium F11.121
            perceptual disturbance F11.122
          uncomplicated F11.120
        mood disorder F11.14
        other specified disorder F11.188
        psychosis F11.159
          delusions F11.150
          hallucinations F11.151
        sexual dysfunction F11.181
        sleep disorder F11.182
        unspecified disorder F11.19
    PCP (phencyclidine) (or related substance) — *see* Abuse, drug, hallucinogen

Abuse — *continued*
  drug NEC (non-dependent) F19.10 — *continued*
    psychoactive NEC F19.10
      with
        amnestic disorder F19.16
        anxiety disorder F19.180
        dementia F19.17
        intoxication F19.129
          with
            delirium F19.121
            perceptual disturbance F19.122
          uncomplicated F19.120
        mood disorder F19.14
        other specified disorder F19.188
        psychosis F19.159
          delusions F19.150
          hallucinations F19.151
        sexual dysfunction F19.181
        sleep disorder F19.182
        unspecified disorder F19.19
    sedative, hypnotic or anxiolytic F13.10
      with
        anxiety disorder F13.180
        intoxication F13.129
          with delirium F13.121
          uncomplicated F13.120
        mood disorder F13.14
        other specified disorder F13.188
        psychosis F13.159
          delusions F13.150
          hallucinations F13.151
        sexual dysfunction F13.181
        sleep disorder F13.182
        unspecified disorder F13.19
    solvent — *see* Abuse, drug, inhalant
    steroids F55.3
    stimulant NEC F15.10
      with
        anxiety disorder F15.180
        intoxication F15.129
          with
            delirium F15.121
            perceptual disturbance F15.122
          uncomplicated F15.120
        mood disorder F15.14
        other specified disorder F15.188
        psychosis F15.159
          delusions F15.150
          hallucinations F15.151
        sexual dysfunction F15.181
        sleep disorder F15.182
        unspecified disorder F15.19
    tranquilizers — *see* Abuse, drug, sedative
    vitamins F55.4
  hallucinogens — *see* Abuse, drug, hallucinogen
  hashish — *see* Abuse, drug, cannabis
  herbal or folk remedies F55.1
  hormones F55.3
  hypnotic — *see* Abuse, drug, sedative
  inhalant — *see* Abuse, drug, inhalant
  laxatives F55.2
  LSD — *see* Abuse, drug, hallucinogen
  marihuana — *see* Abuse, drug, cannabis
  morphine type (opioids) — *see* Abuse, drug, opioid
  non-psychoactive substance NEC F55.8
    antacids F55.0
    folk remedies F55.1
    herbal remedies F55.1
    hormones F55.3
    laxatives F55.2
    steroids F55.3
    vitamins F55.4
  opioids — *see* Abuse, drug, opioid
  PCP (phencyclidine) (or related substance) — *see* Abuse, drug, hallucinogen
  physical (adult) (child) — *see* Maltreatment

Abuse — *continued*
  psychoactive substance — *see* Abuse, drug, psychoactive NEC
  psychological (adult) (child) — *see* Maltreatment
  sedative — *see* Abuse, drug, sedative
  sexual — *see* Maltreatment
  solvent — *see* Abuse, drug, inhalant
  steroids F55.3
  vitamins F55.4
Acalculia R48.8
  developmental F81.2
Acanthamebiasis (with) B60.10
  conjunctiva B60.12
  keratoconjunctivitis B60.13
  meningoencephalitis B60.11
  other specified B60.19
Acanthocephaliasis B83.8
Acanthocheilonemiasis B74.4
Acanthocytosis E78.6
Acantholysis L11.9
Acanthosis (acquired) (nigricans) L83
  benign Q82.8
  congenital Q82.8
  seborrheic L82.1
    inflamed L82.0
  tongue K14.3
Acapnia E87.3
Acarbia E87.2
Acardia, acardius Q89.8
Acardiacus amorphus Q89.8
Acardiotrophia I51.4
Acariasis B88.0
  scabies B86
Acarodermatitis (urticarioides) B88.0
Acarophobia F40.218
Acatalasemia, acatalasia E80.3
Acathisia (drug induced) G25.71
Accelerated atrioventricular conduction I45.6
Accentuation of personality traits (type A) Z73.1
Accessory (congenital)
  adrenal gland Q89.1
  anus Q43.4
  appendix Q43.4
  atrioventricular conduction I45.6
  auditory ossicles Q16.3
  auricle (ear) Q17.0
  biliary duct or passage Q44.5
  bladder Q64.79
  blood vessels NEC Q27.9
    coronary Q24.5
  bone NEC Q79.8
  breast tissue, axilla Q83.1
  carpal bones Q74.0
  cecum Q43.4
  chromosome(s) NEC (nonsex) Q92.9
    with complex rearrangements NEC Q92.5
      seen only at prometaphase Q92.8
    13 — *see* Trisomy, 13
    18 — *see* Trisomy, 18
    21 — *see* Trisomy, 21
    partial Q92.9
    sex
      female phenotype Q97.8
  coronary artery Q24.5
  cusp(s), heart valve NEC Q24.8
    pulmonary Q22.3
  cystic duct Q44.5
  digit(s) Q69.9
  ear (auricle) (lobe) Q17.0
  endocrine gland NEC Q89.2
  eye muscle Q10.3
  eyelid Q10.3
  face bone(s) Q75.8
  fallopian tube (fimbria) (ostium) Q50.6
  finger(s) Q69.0
  foreskin N47.8

Accessory (congenital) — continued
  frontonasal process Q75.8
  gallbladder Q44.1
  genital organ(s)
    female Q52.8
      external Q52.79
      internal NEC Q52.8
    male Q55.8
  genitourinary organs NEC Q89.8
    female Q52.8
    male Q55.8
  hallux Q69.2
  heart Q24.8
    valve NEC Q24.8
      pulmonary Q22.3
  hepatic ducts Q44.5
  hymen Q52.4
  intestine (large) (small) Q43.4
  kidney Q63.0
  lacrimal canal Q10.6
  leaflet, heart valve NEC Q24.8
  ligament, broad Q50.6
  liver Q44.7
    duct Q44.5
  lobule (ear) Q17.0
  lung (lobe) Q33.1
  muscle Q79.8
  navicular of carpus Q74.0
  nervous system, part NEC Q07.8
  nipple Q83.3
  nose Q30.8
  organ or site not listed — see Anomaly, by site
  ovary Q50.31
  oviduct Q50.6
  pancreas Q45.3
  parathyroid gland Q89.2
  parotid gland (and duct) Q38.4
  pituitary gland Q89.2
  preauricular appendage Q17.0
  prepuce N47.8
  renal arteries (multiple) Q27.2
  rib Q76.6
    cervical Q76.5
  roots (teeth) K00.2
  salivary gland Q38.4
  sesamoid bones Q74.8
    foot Q74.2
    hand Q74.0
  skin tags Q82.8
  spleen Q89.09
  sternum Q76.7
  submaxillary gland Q38.4
  tarsal bones Q74.2
  teeth, tooth K00.1
  tendon Q79.8
  thumb Q69.1
  thymus gland Q89.2
  thyroid gland Q89.2
  toes Q69.2
  tongue Q38.3
  tooth, teeth K00.1
  tragus Q17.0
  ureter Q62.5
  urethra Q64.79
  urinary organ or tract NEC Q64.8
  uterus Q51.2
  vagina Q52.10
  valve, heart NEC Q24.8
    pulmonary Q22.3
  vertebra Q76.49
  vocal cords Q31.8
  vulva Q52.79
Accident
  birth — see Birth, injury
  cardiac — see Infarct, myocardium
  cerebral I63.9

Accident — continued
  cerebrovascular (embolic) (ischemic)
      (thrombotic) I63.9
    aborted I63.9
    hemorrhagic — see Hemorrhage,
        intracranial, intracerebral
    old (without sequelae) Z86.73
      with sequelae (of) — see Sequelae,
          infarction, cerebral
  coronary — see Infarct, myocardium
  craniovascular I63.9
  vascular, brain I63.9
Accidental — see condition
Accommodation (disorder) — see also
    condition
  hysterical paralysis of F44.89
  insufficiency of H52.4
  paresis — see Paresis, of accommodation
  spasm — see Spasm, of accommodation
Accouchement — see Delivery
Accreta placenta O43.21-
Accretio cordis (nonrheumatic) I31.0
Accretions, tooth, teeth K03.6
Acculturation difficulty Z60.3
Accumulation secretion, prostate N42.89
**Acephalia, acephalism, acephalus,
    acephaly** Q00.0
Acephalobrachia monster Q89.8
Acephalochirus monster Q89.8
Acephalogaster Q89.8
Acephalostomus monster Q89.8
Acephalothorax Q89.8
Acerophobia F40.298
Acetonemia R79.89
  in Type 1 diabetes E10.10
    with coma E10.11
Acetonuria R82.4
Achalasia (cardia) (esophagus) K22.0
  congenital Q39.5
  pylorus Q40.0
  sphincteral NEC K59.8
Ache(s) — see Pain
Acheilia Q38.6
Achillobursitis — see Tendinitis, Achilles
Achillodynia — see Tendinitis, Achilles
Achlorhydria, achlorhydric (neurogenic)
    K31.83
  anemia D50.8
  diarrhea K31.83
  psychogenic F45.8
  secondary to vagotomy K91.1
Achluophobia F40.228
Acholia K82.8
Acholuric jaundice (familial) (splenomegalic)
    — see also Spherocytosis
  acquired D59.8
Achondrogenesis Q77.0
Achondroplasia (osteosclerosis congenita)
    Q77.4
Achroma, cutis L80
Achromat(ism), achromatopsia (acquired)
    (congenital) H53.51
Achromia, congenital — see Albinism
Achromia parasitica B36.0
Achylia gastrica K31.89
  psychogenic F45.8
Acid
  burn — see Corrosion
  deficiency
    amide nicotinic E52
    ascorbic E54
    folic E53.8
    nicotinic E52
    pantothenic E53.8
  intoxication E87.2
  peptic disease K30
  phosphatase deficiency E83.39
  stomach K30
    psychogenic F45.8

Acidemia E87.2
  argininosuccinic E72.22
  isovaleric E71.110
  metabolic (newborn) P19.9
    first noted before onset of labor P19.0
    first noted during labor P19.1
    noted at birth P19.2
  methylmalonic E71.120
  pipecolic E72.3
  propionic E71.121
Acidity, gastric (high) K30
  psychogenic F45.8
Acidocytopenia — see Agranulocytosis
Acidocytosis D72.1
Acidopenia — see Agranulocytosis
Acidosis (lactic) (respiratory) E87.2
  in Type 1 diabetes E10.10
    with coma E10.11
  kidney, tubular N25.89
  lactic E87.2
  metabolic NEC E87.2
    with respiratory acidosis E87.4
    late, of newborn P74.0
  mixed metabolic and respiratory, newborn
      P84
  newborn P84
  renal (hyperchloremic) (tubular) N25.89
  respiratory E87.2
    complicated by
      metabolic
        acidosis E87.4
        alkalosis E87.4
Aciduria
  argininosuccinic E72.22
  glutaric (type I) E72.3
    type II E71.313
    type III E71.5-
  orotic (congenital) (hereditary) (pyrimidine
      deficiency) E79.8
    anemia D53.0
Acladiosis (skin) B36.0
Aclasis, diaphyseal Q78.6
Acleistocardia Q21.1
Aclusion — see Anomaly, dentofacial,
    malocclusion
Acne L70.9
  artificialis L70.8
  atrophica L70.2
  cachecticorum (Hebra) L70.8
  conglobata L70.1
  cystic L70.0
  decalvans L66.2
  excoriée (des jeunes filles) L70.5
  frontalis L70.2
  indurata L70.0
  infantile L70.4
  keloid L73.0
  lupoid L70.2
  necrotic, necrotica (miliaris) L70.2
  neonatal L70.4
  nodular L70.0
  occupational L70.8
  picker's L70.5
  pustular L70.0
  rodens L70.2
  rosacea L71.9
  specified NEC L70.8
  tropica L70.3
  varioliformis L70.2
  vulgaris L70.0
Acnitis (primary) A18.4
Acosta's disease T70.29
Acoustic — see condition
Acousticophobia F40.298
Acquired — see also condition
  immunodeficiency syndrome (AIDS) B20
Acrania Q00.0
Acroangiodermatitis I78.9
Acroasphyxia, chronic I73.89

DISEASE INDEX

Acrobystitis N47.7
Acrocephalopolysyndactyly Q87.0
Acrocephalosyndactyly Q87.0
Acrocephaly Q75.0
Acrochondrohyperplasia — see Syndrome, Marfan's
Acrocyanosis I73.8
  newborn P28.2
    meaning transient blue hands and feet — omit code
Acrodermatitis L30.8
  atrophicans (chronica) L90.4
  continua (Hallopeau) L40.2
  enteropathica (hereditary) E83.2
  Hallopeau's L40.2
  infantile papular L44.4
  perstans L40.2
  pustulosa continua L40.2
  recalcitrant pustular L40.2
Acrodynia — see Poisoning, mercury
Acromegaly, acromegalia E22.0
Acromelalgia I73.81
Acromicria, acromikria Q79.8
Acronyx L60.0
Acropachy, thyroid — see Thyrotoxicosis
Acroparesthesia (simple) (vasomotor) I73.89
Acropathy, thyroid — see Thyrotoxicosis
Acrophobia F40.241
Acroposthitis N47.7
Acroscleriasis, acroscleroderma, acrosclerosis — see Sclerosis, systemic
Acrosphacelus I96
Acrospiroma, eccrine — see Neoplasm, skin, benign
Acrostealgia — see Osteochondropathy
Acrotrophodynia — see Immersion
ACTH ectopic syndrome E24.3
Actinic — see condition
Actinobacillosis, actinobacillus A28.8
  mallei A24.0
  muris A25.1
Actinomyces israelii (infection) — see Actinomycosis
Actinomycetoma (foot) B47.1
Actinomycosis, actinomycotic A42.9
  with pneumonia A42.0
  abdominal A42.1
  cervicofacial A42.2
  cutaneous A42.89
  gastrointestinal A42.1
  pulmonary A42.0
  sepsis A42.7
  specified site NEC A42.89
Actinoneuritis G62.82
Action, heart
  disorder I49.9
  irregular I49.9
    psychogenic F45.8
Activated protein C resistance D68.51
Activation
  mast cell (disorder) (syndrome) D89.40
    idiopathic D89.42
    monoclonal D89.41
    secondary D89.43
    specified type NEC D89.49
Active — see condition
Acute — see also condition
  abdomen R10.0
  gallbladder — see Cholecystitis, acute
Acyanotic heart disease (congenital) Q24.9
Acystia Q64.5
Adair-Dighton syndrome (brittle bones and blue sclera, deafness) Q78.0
Adamantinoblastoma — see Ameloblastoma
Adamantinoma — see also Cyst, calcifying odontogenic
  long bones C40.90
    lower limb C40.2-
    upper limb C40.0-

Adamantinoma — see also Cyst, calcifying odontogenic — continued
  malignant C41.1
    jaw (bone) (lower) C41.1
    upper C41.0
  tibial C40.2-
Adamantoblastoma — see Ameloblastoma
Adams-Stokes(-Morgagni) disease or syndrome I45.9
Adaption reaction — see Disorder, adjustment
Addiction (see also Dependence) F19.20
  alcohol, alcoholic (ethyl) (methyl) (wood) (without remission) F10.20
    with remission F10.21
  drug — see Dependence, drug
  ethyl alcohol (without remission) F10.20
    with remission F10.21
  heroin — see Dependence, drug, opioid
  methyl alcohol (without remission) F10.20
    with remission F10.21
  methylated spirit (without remission) F10.20
    with remission F10.21
  morphine(-like substances) — see Dependence, drug, opioid
  nicotine — see Dependence, drug, nicotine
  opium and opioids — see Dependence, drug, opioid
  tobacco — see Dependence, drug, nicotine
Addison-Biermer anemia (pernicious) D51.0
Addisonian crisis E27.2
Addison's
  anemia (pernicious) D51.0
  disease (bronze) or syndrome E27.1
    tuberculous A18.7
  keloid L94.0
Addison-Schilder complex E71.528
Additional — see also Accessory
  chromosome(s) Q99.8
    21 — see Trisomy, 21
    sex — see Abnormal, chromosome, sex
Adduction contracture, hip or other joint — see Contraction, joint
Adenitis — see also Lymphadenitis
  acute, unspecified site L04.9
  axillary I88.9
    acute L04.2
    chronic or subacute I88.1
  Bartholin's gland N75.8
  bulbourethral gland — see Urethritis
  cervical I88.9
    acute L04.0
    chronic or subacute I88.1
  chancroid (Hemophilus ducreyi) A57
  chronic, unspecified site I88.1
  Cowper's gland — see Urethritis
  due to Pasteurella multocida (p. septica) A28.0
  epidemic, acute B27.09
  gangrenous L04.9
  gonorrheal NEC A54.89
  groin I88.9
    acute L04.1
    chronic or subacute I88.1
  infectious (acute) (epidemic) B27.09
  inguinal I88.9
    acute L04.1
    chronic or subacute I88.1
  lymph gland or node, except mesenteric I88.9
    acute — see Lymphadenitis, acute
    chronic or subacute I88.1
  mesenteric (acute) (chronic) (nonspecific) (subacute) I88.0
  parotid gland (suppurative) — see Sialoadenitis
  salivary gland (any) (suppurative) — see Sialoadenitis
  scrofulous (tuberculous) A18.2
  Skene's duct or gland — see Urethritis
  strumous, tuberculous A18.2

Adenitis (see also Lymphadenitis) — continued
  subacute, unspecified site I88.1
  sublingual gland (suppurative) — see Sialoadenitis
  submandibular gland (suppurative) — see Sialoadenitis
  submaxillary gland (suppurative) — see Sialoadenitis
  tuberculous — see Tuberculosis, lymph gland
  urethral gland — see Urethritis
  Wharton's duct (suppurative) — see Sialoadenitis
Adenoacanthoma — see Neoplasm, malignant, by site
Adenoameloblastoma — see Cyst, calcifying odontogenic
Adenocarcinoid (tumor) — see Neoplasm, malignant, by site
Adenocarcinoma — see also Neoplasm, malignant, by site
  acidophil
    specified site — see Neoplasm, malignant, by site
    unspecified site C75.1
  adrenal cortical C74.0-
  alveolar — see Neoplasm, lung, malignant
  apocrine
    breast — see Neoplasm, breast, malignant
    in situ
      breast D05.8-
      specified site NEC — see Neoplasm, skin, in situ
      unspecified site D04.9
    specified site NEC — see Neoplasm, skin, malignant
    unspecified site C44.99
  basal cell
    specified site — see Neoplasm, skin, malignant
    unspecified site C08.9
  basophil
    specified site — see Neoplasm, malignant, by site
    unspecified site C75.1
  bile duct type C22.1
    liver C22.1
    specified site NEC — see Neoplasm, malignant, by site
    unspecified site C22.1
  bronchiolar — see Neoplasm, lung, malignant
  bronchioloalveolar — see Neoplasm, lung, malignant
  ceruminous C44.29-
  cervix, in situ (see also Carcinoma, cervix uteri, in situ) D06.9
  chromophobe
    specified site — see Neoplasm, malignant, by site
    unspecified site C75.1
  diffuse type
    specified site — see Neoplasm, malignant, by site
    unspecified site C16.9
  duct
    infiltrating
      with Paget's disease — see Neoplasm, breast, malignant
      specified site — see Neoplasm, malignant, by site
      unspecified site (female) C50.91-
        male C50.92-
    specified site — see Neoplasm, malignant, by site
    unspecified site
      female C56.9
      male C61

Adenocarcinoma (*see also* Neoplasm, malignant, by site) — *continued*
  eosinophil
    specified site — *see* Neoplasm, malignant, by site
    unspecified site C75.1
  follicular
    with papillary C73
    moderately differentiated C73
    specified site — *see* Neoplasm, malignant, by site
    trabecular C73
    unspecified site C73
    well differentiated C73
  Hurthle cell C73
  in
    adenomatous
      polyposis coli C18.9
  infiltrating duct
    with Paget's disease — *see* Neoplasm, breast, malignant
    specified site — *see* Neoplasm, by site, malignant
    unspecified site (female) C50.91-
      male C50.92-
  inflammatory
    specified site — *see* Neoplasm, by site, malignant
    unspecified site (female) C50.91-
      male C50.92-
  intestinal type
    specified site — *see* Neoplasm, by site, malignant
    unspecified site C16.9
  intracystic papillary
  intraductal
    breast D05.1-
    noninfiltrating
      breast D05.1-
      papillary
        with invasion
          specified site — *see* Neoplasm, by site, malignant
          unspecified site (female) C50.91-
            male C50.92-
        breast D05.1-
        specified site NEC — *see* Neoplasm, in situ, by site
        unspecified site D05.1-
      specified site NEC — *see* Neoplasm, in situ, by site
      unspecified site D05.1-
    papillary
      with invasion
        specified site — *see* Neoplasm, malignant, by site
        unspecified site (female) C50.91-
          male C50.92-
      breast D05.1-
      specified site — *see* Neoplasm, in situ, by site
      unspecified site D05.1-
    specified site NEC — *see* Neoplasm, in situ, by site
    unspecified site D05.1-
  islet cell
    with exocrine, mixed
      specified site — *see* Neoplasm, malignant, by site
      unspecified site C25.9
    pancreas C25.4
    specified site NEC — *see* Neoplasm, malignant, by site
    unspecified site C25.4

Adenocarcinoma (*see also* Neoplasm, malignant, by site) — *continued*
  lobular
    in situ
      breast D05.0-
      specified site NEC — *see* Neoplasm, in situ, by site
      unspecified site D05.0-
    specified site — *see* Neoplasm, malignant, by site
    unspecified site (female) C50.91-
      male C50.92-
  mucoid — *see also* Neoplasm, malignant, by site
    cell
      specified site — *see* Neoplasm, malignant, by site
      unspecified site C75.1
  nonencapsulated sclerosing C73
  papillary
    with follicular C73
    follicular variant C73
    intraductal (noninfiltrating)
      with invasion
        specified site — *see* Neoplasm, malignant, by site
        unspecified site (female) C50.91-
          male C50.92-
      breast D05.1-
      specified site NEC — *see* Neoplasm, in situ, by site
      unspecified site D05.1-
    serous
      specified site — *see* Neoplasm, malignant, by site
      unspecified site C56.9
  papillocystic
    specified site — *see* Neoplasm, malignant, by site
    unspecified site C56.9
  pseudomucinous
    specified site — *see* Neoplasm, malignant, by site
    unspecified site C56.9
  renal cell C64-
  sebaceous — *see* Neoplasm, skin, malignant
  serous — *see also* Neoplasm, malignant, by site
    papillary
      specified site — *see* Neoplasm, malignant, by site
      unspecified site C56.9
  sweat gland — *see* Neoplasm, skin, malignant
  water-clear cell C75.0
Adenocarcinoma-in-situ — *see also* Neoplasm, in situ, by site
  breast D05.9-
Adenofibroma
  clear cell — *see* Neoplasm, benign, by site
  endometrioid D27.9
    borderline malignancy D39.10
    malignant C56-
  mucinous
    specified site — *see* Neoplasm, benign, by site
    unspecified site D27.9
  papillary
    specified site — *see* Neoplasm, benign, by site
    unspecified site D27.9
  prostate — *see* Enlargement, enlarged, prostate
  serous
    specified site — *see* Neoplasm, benign, by site
    unspecified site D27.9
  specified site — *see* Neoplasm, benign, by site
  unspecified site D27.9

Adenofibrosis
  breast — *see* Fibroadenosis, breast
  endometrioid N80.0
Adenoiditis (chronic) J35.02
  with tonsillitis J35.03
  acute J03.90
    recurrent J03.91
    specified organism NEC J03.80
      recurrent J03.81
    staphylococcal J03.80
      recurrent J03.81
    streptococcal J03.00
      recurrent J03.01
Adenoids — *see* condition
Adenolipoma — *see* Neoplasm, benign, by site
Adenolipomatosis, Launois-Bensaude E88.89
Adenolymphoma
  specified site — *see* Neoplasm, benign, by site
  unspecified site D11.9
Adenoma — *see also* Neoplasm, benign, by site
  acidophil
    specified site — *see* Neoplasm, benign, by site
    unspecified site D35.2
  acidophil-basophil, mixed
    specified site — *see* Neoplasm, benign, by site
    unspecified site D35.2
  adrenal (cortical) D35.00
    clear cell D35.00
    compact cell D35.00
    glomerulosa cell D35.00
    heavily pigmented variant D35.00
    mixed cell D35.00
  alpha-cell
    pancreas D13.7
    specified site NEC — *see* Neoplasm, benign, by site
    unspecified site D13.7
  alveolar D14.30
  apocrine
    breast D24-
    specified site NEC — *see* Neoplasm, skin, benign, by site
    unspecified site D23.9
  basal cell D11.9
  basophil
    specified site — *see* Neoplasm, benign, by site
    unspecified site D35.2
  basophil-acidophil, mixed
    specified site — *see* Neoplasm, benign, by site
    unspecified site D35.2
  beta-cell
    pancreas D13.7
    specified site NEC — *see* Neoplasm, benign, by site
    unspecified site D13.7
  bile duct D13.4
    common D13.5
    extrahepatic D13.5
    intrahepatic D13.4
    specified site NEC — *see* Neoplasm, benign, by site
    unspecified site D13.4
  black D35.00
  bronchial D38.1
    cylindroid type — *see* Neoplasm, lung, malignant
  ceruminous D23.2-
  chief cell D35.1
  chromophobe
    specified site — *see* Neoplasm, benign, by site
    unspecified site D35.2

Adenoma (see also Neoplasm, benign, by site) — continued
  colloid
    specified site — see Neoplasm, benign, by site
    unspecified site D34
  duct
  eccrine, papillary — see Neoplasm, skin, benign
  endocrine, multiple
    single specified site — see Neoplasm, uncertain behavior, by site
    two or more specified sites D44-
    unspecified site D44.9
  endometrioid — see also Neoplasm, benign
    borderline malignancy — see Neoplasm, uncertain behavior, by site
  eosinophil
    specified site — see Neoplasm, benign, by site
    unspecified site D35.2
  fetal
    specified site — see Neoplasm, benign, by site
    unspecified site D34
  follicular
    specified site — see Neoplasm, benign, by site
    unspecified site D34
  hepatocellular D13.4
  Hurthle cell D34
  islet cell
    pancreas D13.7
    specified site NEC — see Neoplasm, benign, by site
    unspecified site D13.7
  liver cell D13.4
  macrofollicular
    specified site — see Neoplasm, benign, by site
    unspecified site D34
  malignant, malignum — see Neoplasm, malignant, by site
  microcystic
    pancreas D13.6
    specified site NEC — see Neoplasm, benign, by site
    unspecified site D13.6
  microfollicular
    specified site — see Neoplasm, benign, by site
    unspecified site D34
  mucoid cell
    specified site — see Neoplasm, benign, by site
    unspecified site D35.2
  multiple endocrine
    single specified site — see Neoplasm, uncertain behavior, by site
    two or more specified sites D44-
    unspecified site D44.9
  nipple D24-
  papillary — see also Neoplasm, benign, by site
    eccrine — see Neoplasm, skin, benign, by site
  Pick's tubular
    specified site — see Neoplasm, benign, by site
    unspecified site
      female D27.9
      male D29.20
  pleomorphic
    carcinoma in — see Neoplasm, salivary gland, malignant
    specified site — see Neoplasm, malignant, by site
    unspecified site C08.9

Adenoma (see also Neoplasm, benign, by site) — continued
  polypoid — see also Neoplasm, benign
    adenocarcinoma in — see Neoplasm, malignant, by site
    adenocarcinoma in situ — see Neoplasm, in situ, by site
  prostate — see Neoplasm, benign, prostate
  rete cell D29.20
  sebaceous — see Neoplasm, skin, benign
  Sertoli cell
    specified site — see Neoplasm, benign, by site
    unspecified site
      female D27.9
      male D29.20
  skin appendage — see Neoplasm, skin, benign
  sudoriferous gland — see Neoplasm, skin, benign
  sweat gland — see Neoplasm, skin, benign
  testicular
    specified site — see Neoplasm, benign, by site
    unspecified site
      female D27.9
      male D29.20
  tubular — see also Neoplasm, benign, by site
    adenocarcinoma in — see Neoplasm, malignant, by site
    adenocarcinoma in situ — see Neoplasm, in situ, by site
    Pick's
      specified site — see Neoplasm, benign, by site
      unspecified site
        female D27.9
        male D29.20
  tubulovillous — see also Neoplasm, benign, by site
    adenocarcinoma in — see Neoplasm, malignant, by site
    adenocarcinoma in situ — see Neoplasm, in situ, by site
  villous — see Neoplasm, uncertain behavior, by site
    adenocarcinoma in — see Neoplasm, malignant, by site
    adenocarcinoma in situ — see Neoplasm, in situ, by site
  water-clear cell D35.1
Adenomatosis
  endocrine (multiple) E31.20
    single specified site — see Neoplasm, uncertain behavior, by site
  erosive of nipple D24-
  pluriendocrine — see Adenomatosis, endocrine
  pulmonary D38.1
    malignant — see Neoplasm, lung, malignant
  specified site — see Neoplasm, benign, by site
  unspecified site D12.6
Adenomatous
  goiter (nontoxic) E04.9
    with hyperthyroidism — see Hyperthyroidism, with, goiter, nodular
    toxic — see Hyperthyroidism, with, goiter, nodular
Adenomyoma — see also Neoplasm, benign, by site
  prostate — see Enlarged, prostate
Adenomyometritis N80.0
Adenomyosis N80.0
Adenopathy (lymph gland) R59.9
  generalized R59.1
  inguinal R59.0
  localized R59.0
  mediastinal R59.0
  mesentery R59.0
  syphilitic (secondary) A51.49

Adenopathy (lymph gland) R59.9 — continued
  tracheobronchial R59.0
    tuberculous A15.4
      primary (progressive) A15.7
  tuberculous — see also Tuberculosis, lymph gland
    tracheobronchial A15.4
      primary (progressive) A15.7
Adenosalpingitis — see Salpingitis
Adenosarcoma — see Neoplasm, malignant, by site
Adenosclerosis I88.8
Adenosis (sclerosing) breast — see Fibroadenosis, breast
Adenovirus, as cause of disease classified elsewhere B97.0
Adentia (complete) (partial) — see Absence, teeth
Adherent — see also Adhesions
  labia (minora) N90.89
  pericardium (nonrheumatic) I31.0
    rheumatic I09.2
  placenta (with hemorrhage) O72.0
    without hemorrhage O73.0
  prepuce, newborn N47.0
  scar (skin) L90.5
  tendon in scar L90.5
Adhesions, adhesive (postinfective) K66.0
  with intestinal obstruction K56.5
  abdominal (wall) — see Adhesions, peritoneum
  appendix K38.8
  bile duct (common) (hepatic) K83.8
  bladder (sphincter) N32.89
  bowel — see Adhesions, peritoneum
  cardiac I31.0
    rheumatic I09.2
  cecum — see Adhesions, peritoneum
  cervicovaginal N88.1
    congenital Q52.8
    postpartal O90.89
      old N88.1
  cervix N88.1
  ciliary body NEC — see Adhesions, iris
  clitoris N90.89
  colon — see Adhesions, peritoneum
  common duct K83.8
  congenital — see also Anomaly, by site
    fingers — see Syndactylism, complex, fingers
    omental, anomalous Q43.3
    peritoneal Q43.3
    tongue (to gum or roof of mouth) Q38.3
  conjunctiva (acquired) H11.21-
    congenital Q15.8
  cystic duct K82.8
  diaphragm — see Adhesions, peritoneum
  due to foreign body — see Foreign body
  duodenum — see Adhesions, peritoneum
  ear
    middle H74.1-
  epididymis N50.89
  epidural — see Adhesions, meninges
  epiglottis J38.7
  eyelid H02.59
  female pelvis N73.6
  gallbladder K82.8
  globe H44.89
  heart I31.0
    rheumatic I09.2
  ileocecal (coil) — see Adhesions, peritoneum
  ileum — see Adhesions, peritoneum
  intestine — see also Adhesions, peritoneum
    with obstruction K56.5
  intra-abdominal — see Adhesions, peritoneum

DISEASE INDEX

Adhesions, adhesive (postinfective) K66.0 — *continued*
  iris H21.50-
    anterior H21.51-
    goniosynechiae H21.52-
    posterior H21.54-
    to corneal graft T85.898
  joint — *see* Ankylosis
    knee M23.8x
    temporomandibular M26.61-
  labium (majus) (minus), congenital Q52.5
  liver — *see* Adhesions, peritoneum
  lung J98.4
  mediastinum J98.59
  meninges (cerebral) (spinal) G96.12
    congenital Q07.8
    tuberculous (cerebral) (spinal) A17.0
  mesenteric — *see* Adhesions, peritoneum
  nasal (septum) (to turbinates) J34.89
  ocular muscle — *see* Strabismus, mechanical
  omentum — *see* Adhesions, peritoneum
  ovary N73.6
    congenital (to cecum, kidney or omentum) Q50.39
  paraovarian N73.6
  pelvic (peritoneal)
    female N73.6
      postprocedural N99.4
    male — *see* Adhesions, peritoneum
    postpartal (old) N73.6
    tuberculous A18.17
  penis to scrotum (congenital) Q55.8
  periappendiceal — *see also* Adhesions, peritoneum
  pericardium (nonrheumatic) I31.0
    focal I31.8
    rheumatic I09.2
    tuberculous A18.84
  pericholecystic K82.8
  perigastric — *see* Adhesions, peritoneum
  periovarian N73.6
  periprostatic N42.89
  perirectal — *see* Adhesions, peritoneum
  perirenal N28.89
  peritoneum, peritoneal (postinfective) (postprocedural) K66.0
    with obstruction (intestinal) K56.5
    congenital Q43.3
    pelvic, female N73.6
      postprocedural N99.4
    postpartal, pelvic N73.6
    to uterus N73.6
  peritubal N73.6
  periureteral N28.89
  periuterine N73.6
  perivesical N32.89
  perivesicular (seminal vesicle) N50.89
  pleura, pleuritic J94.8
    tuberculous NEC A15.6
  pleuropericardial J94.8
  postoperative (gastrointestinal tract) K66.0
    with obstruction K91.3
    due to foreign body accidentally left in wound — *see* Foreign body, accidentally left during a procedure
    pelvic peritoneal N99.4
    urethra — *see* Stricture, urethra, postprocedural
    vagina N99.2
  postpartal, old (vulva or perineum) N90.89
  preputial, prepuce N47.5
  pulmonary J98.4
  pylorus — *see* Adhesions, peritoneum
  sciatic nerve — *see* Lesion, nerve, sciatic
  seminal vesicle N50.89
  shoulder (joint) — *see* Capsulitis, adhesive
  sigmoid flexure — *see* Adhesions, peritoneum

Adhesions, adhesive (postinfective) K66.0 — *continued*
  spermatic cord (acquired) N50.89
    congenital Q55.4
  spinal canal G96.12
  stomach — *see* Adhesions, peritoneum
  subscapular — *see* Capsulitis, adhesive
  temporomandibular M26.61-
  tendinitis — *see also* Tenosynovitis, specified type NEC
    shoulder — *see* Capsulitis, adhesive
  testis N44.8
  tongue, congenital (to gum or roof of mouth) Q38.3
    acquired K14.8
  trachea J39.8
  tubo-ovarian N73.6
  tunica vaginalis N44.8
  uterus N73.6
    internal N85.6
    to abdominal wall N73.6
  vagina (chronic) N89.5
    postoperative N99.2
  vitreomacular H43.82-
  vitreous H43.89
  vulva N90.89
Adiaspiromycosis B48.8
Adie(-Holmes) pupil or syndrome — *see* Anomaly, pupil, function, tonic pupil
Adiponecrosis neonatorum P83.8
Adiposis — *see also* Obesity
  cerebralis E23.6
  dolorosa E88.2
Adiposity — *see also* Obesity
  heart — *see* Degeneration, myocardial
  localized E65
Adiposogenital dystrophy E23.6
Adjustment
  disorder — *see* Disorder, adjustment
  implanted device — *see* Encounter (for), adjustment (of)
  prosthesis, external — *see* Fitting
  reaction — *see* Disorder, adjustment
Administration of tPA (rtPA) in a different facility within the last 24 hours prior to admission to current facility Z92.82
Admission (for) — *see also* Encounter (for)
  adjustment (of)
    artificial
      arm Z44.00-
        complete Z44.01-
        partial Z44.02-
      eye Z44.2
      leg Z44.10-
        complete Z44.11-
        partial Z44.12-
    brain neuropacemaker Z46.2
      implanted Z45.42
    breast
      implant Z45.81
      prosthesis (external) Z44.3
    colostomy belt Z46.89
    contact lenses Z46.0
    cystostomy device Z46.6
    dental prosthesis Z46.3
    device NEC
      abdominal Z46.89
      implanted Z45.89
        cardiac Z45.09
          defibrillator (with synchronous cardiace pacemaker) Z45.02
          pacemaker (cardiac resynchronization therapy (CRT-P)) Z45.018
            pulse generator Z45.010
          resynchronization therapy defibrillator (CRT-D) Z45.02

Admission (for) (*see also* Encounter (for)) — *continued*
  adjustment (of) — *continued*
    device NEC — *continued*
      implanted Z45.89 — *continued*
        hearing device Z45.328
          bone conduction Z45.320
          cochlear Z45.321
        infusion pump Z45.1
        nervous system Z45.49
          CSF drainage Z45.41
          hearing device — *see* Admission, adjustment, device, implanted, hearing device
          neuropacemaker Z45.42
          visual substitution Z45.31
        specified NEC Z45.89
        vascular access Z45.2
        visual substitution Z45.31
      nervous system Z46.2
        implanted — *see* Admission, adjustment, device, implanted, nervous system
    orthodontic Z46.4
    prosthetic Z44.9
      arm — *see* Admission, adjustment, artificial, arm
      breast Z44.3
      dental Z46.3
      eye Z44.2
      leg — *see* Admission, adjustment, artificial, leg
      specified type NEC Z44.8
    substitution
      auditory Z46.2
        implanted — *see* Admission, adjustment, device, implanted, hearing device
      nervous system Z46.2
        implanted — *see* Admission, adjustment, device, implanted, nervous system
      visual Z46.2
        implanted Z45.31
    urinary Z46.6
  hearing aid Z46.1
    implanted — *see* Admission, adjustment, device, implanted, hearing device
  ileostomy device Z46.89
  intestinal appliance or device NEC Z46.89
  neuropacemaker (brain) (peripheral nerve) (spinal cord) Z46.2
    implanted Z45.42
  orthodontic device Z46.4
  orthopedic (brace) (cast) (device) (shoes) Z46.89
  pacemaker (cardiac resynchronization therapy (CRT-P))
    cardiac Z45.018
      pulse generator Z45.010
    nervous system Z46.2
      implanted Z45.42
  portacath (port-a-cath) Z45.2
  prosthesis Z44.9
    arm — *see* Admission, adjustment, artificial, arm
    breast Z44.3
    dental Z46.3
    eye Z44.2
    leg — *see* Admission, adjustment, artificial, leg
    specified NEC Z44.8
  spectacles Z46.0
  aftercare (*see also* Aftercare) Z51.89
  postpartum
    immediately after delivery Z39.0
    routine follow-up Z39.2
  radiation therapy (antineoplastic) Z51.0

Admission (for) (*see also* Encounter (for)) — *continued*
attention to artificial opening (of) Z43.9
  artificial vagina Z43.7
  colostomy Z43.3
  cystostomy Z43.5
  enterostomy Z43.4
  gastrostomy Z43.1
  ileostomy Z43.2
  jejunostomy Z43.4
  nephrostomy Z43.6
  specified site NEC Z43.8
    intestinal tract Z43.4
    urinary tract Z43.6
  tracheostomy Z43.0
  ureterostomy Z43.6
  urethrostomy Z43.6
breast augmentation or reduction Z41.1
breast reconstruction following mastectomy Z42.1
change of
  dressing (nonsurgical) Z48.00
  neuropacemaker device (brain) (peripheral nerve) (spinal cord) Z46.2
    implanted Z45.42
  surgical dressing Z48.01
circumcision, ritual or routine (in absence of diagnosis) Z41.2
clinical research investigation (control) (normal comparison) (participant) Z00.6
contraceptive management Z30.9
cosmetic surgery NEC Z41.1
counseling — *see also* Counseling
  dietary Z71.3
  gestational carrier Z31.7
  HIV Z71.7
  human immunodeficiency virus Z71.7
  nonattending third party Z71.0
  procreative management NEC Z31.69
delivery, full-term, uncomplicated O80
  cesarean, without indication O82
desensitization to allergens Z51.6
dietary surveillance and counseling Z71.3
ear piercing Z41.3
examination at health care facility (adult) (*see also* Examination) Z00.00
  with abnormal findings Z00.01
  clinical research investigation (control) (normal comparison) (participant) Z00.6
  dental Z01.20
    with abnormal findings Z01.21
  donor (potential) Z00.5
  ear Z01.10
    with abnormal findings NEC Z01.118
  eye Z01.00
    with abnormal findings Z01.01
  general, specified reason NEC Z00.8
  hearing Z01.10
    with abnormal findings NEC Z01.118
  postpartum checkup Z39.2
  psychiatric (general) Z00.8
    requested by authority Z04.6
  vision Z01.00
    with abnormal findings Z01.01
fitting (of)
  artificial
    arm — *see* Admission, adjustment, artificial, arm
    eye Z44.2
    leg — *see* Admission, adjustment, artificial, leg
  brain neuropacemaker Z46.2
    implanted Z45.42
  breast prosthesis (external) Z44.3
  colostomy belt Z46.89
  contact lenses Z46.0
  cystostomy device Z46.6
  dental prosthesis Z46.3
  dentures Z46.3

Admission (for) (*see also* Encounter (for)) — *continued*
fitting (of) — *continued*
  device NEC
    abdominal Z46.89
    nervous system Z46.2
      implanted — *see* Admission, adjustment, device, implanted, nervous system
    orthodontic Z46.4
    prosthetic Z44.9
      breast Z44.3
      dental Z46.3
      eye Z44.2
    substitution
      auditory Z46.2
        implanted — *see* Admission, adjustment, device, implanted, hearing device
      nervous system Z46.2
        implanted — *see* Admission, adjustment, device, implanted, nervous system
      visual Z46.2
        implanted Z45.31
  hearing aid Z46.1
  ileostomy device Z46.89
  intestinal appliance or device NEC Z46.89
  neuropacemaker (brain) (peripheral nerve) (spinal cord) Z46.2
    implanted Z45.42
  orthodontic device Z46.4
  orthopedic device (brace) (cast) (shoes) Z46.89
  prosthesis Z44.9
    arm — *see* Admission, adjustment, artificial, arm
    breast Z44.3
    dental Z46.3
    eye Z44.2
    leg — *see* Admission, adjustment, artificial, leg
    specified type NEC Z44.8
  spectacles Z46.0
follow-up examination Z09
intrauterine device management Z30.431
  initial prescription Z30.014
mental health evaluation Z00.8
  requested by authority Z04.6
observation — *see* Observation
Papanicolaou smear, cervix Z12.4
  for suspected malignant neoplasm Z12.4
plastic and reconstructive surgery following medical procedure or healed injury NEC Z42.8
plastic surgery, cosmetic NEC Z41.1
postpartum observation
  immediately after delivery Z39.0
  routine follow-up Z39.2
poststerilization (for restoration) Z31.0
  aftercare Z31.42
procreative management Z31.9
prophylactic (measure) — *see also* Encounter, prophylactic measures
  organ removal Z40.00
    breast Z40.01
    ovary Z40.02
    specified organ NEC Z40.09
    testes Z40.09
  vaccination Z23
psychiatric examination (general) Z00.8
  requested by authority Z04.6
radiation therapy (antineoplastic) Z51.0
reconstructive surgery following medical procedure or healed injury NEC Z42.8
removal of
  cystostomy catheter Z43.5
  drains Z48.03
  dressing (nonsurgical) Z48.00
  intrauterine contraceptive device Z30.432

Admission (for) (*see also* Encounter (for)) — *continued*
removal of — *continued*
  implantable subdermal contraceptive Z30.46
  neuropacemaker (brain) (peripheral nerve) (spinal cord) Z46.2
    implanted Z45.42
  staples Z48.02
  surgical dressing Z48.01
  sutures Z48.02
  ureteral stent Z46.6
respirator [ventilator] use during power failure Z99.12
restoration of organ continuity (poststerilization) Z31.0
  aftercare Z31.42
sensitivity test — *see also* Test, skin
  allergy NEC Z01.82
  Mantoux Z11.1
tuboplasty following previous sterilization Z31.0
  aftercare Z31.42
vasoplasty following previous sterilization Z31.0
  aftercare Z31.42
vision examination Z01.00
  with abnormal findings Z01.01
waiting period for admission to other facility Z75.1
Adnexitis (suppurative) — *see* Salpingo-oophoritis
Adolescent X-linked adrenoleukodystrophy E71.521
Adrenal (gland) — *see* condition
Adrenalism, tuberculous A18.7
Adrenalitis, adrenitis E27.8
  autoimmune E27.1
  meningococcal, hemorrhagic A39.1
Adrenarche, premature E27.0
Adrenocortical syndrome — *see* Cushing's, syndrome
Adrenogenital syndrome E25.9
  acquired E25.8
  congenital E25.0
  salt loss E25.0
Adrenogenitalism, congenital E25.0
Adrenoleukodystrophy E71.529
  neonatal E71.511
  X-linked E71.529
    Addison only phenotype E71.528
    Addison-Schilder E71.528
    adolescent E71.521
    adrenomyeloneuropathy E71.522
    childhood cerebral E71.520
    other specified E71.528
Adrenomyeloneuropathy E71.522
Adventitious bursa — *see* Bursopathy, specified type NEC
Adverse effect — *see* Table of Drugs and Chemicals, categories T36-T50, with 6th character 5
Advice — *see* Counseling
Adynamia (episodica) (hereditary) (periodic) G72.3
Aeration lung imperfect, newborn — *see* Atelectasis
Aero-otitis media T70.0
Aerobullosis T70.3
Aerocele — *see* Embolism, air
Aerodermectasia
  subcutaneous (traumatic) T79.7
Aerodontalgia T70.29
Aeroembolism T70.3
Aerogenes capsulatus infection A48.0
Aerophagy, aerophagia (psychogenic) F45.8
Aerophobia F40.228
Aerosinusitis T70.1
Aerotitis T70.0

Affection — *see* Disease
Afibrinogenemia (*see also* Defect, coagulation) D68.8
acquired D65
congenital D68.2
following ectopic or molar pregnancy O08.1
in abortion — *see* Abortion, by type, complicated by, afibrinogenemia
puerperal O72.3
African
sleeping sickness B56.9
tick fever A68.1
trypanosomiasis B56.9
gambian B56.0
rhodesian B56.1
Aftercare (*see also* Care) Z51.89
following surgery (for) (on)
amputation Z47.81
attention to
drains Z48.03
dressings (nonsurgical) Z48.00
surgical Z48.01
sutures Z48.02
circulatory system Z48.812
delayed (planned) wound closure Z48.1
digestive system Z48.815
explantation of joint prosthesis (staged procedure)
hip Z47.32
knee Z47.33
shoulder Z47.31
genitourinary system Z48.816
joint replacement Z47.1
neoplasm Z48.3
nervous system Z48.811
oral cavity Z48.814
organ transplant
bone marrow Z48.290
heart Z48.21
heart-lung Z48.280
kidney Z48.22
liver Z48.23
lung Z48.24
multiple organs NEC Z48.288
specified NEC Z48.298
orthopedic NEC Z47.89
planned wound closure Z48.1
removal of internal fixation device Z47.2
respiratory system Z48.813
scoliosis Z47.82
sense organs Z48.810
skin and subcutaneous tissue Z48.817
specified body system
circulatory Z48.812
digestive Z48.815
genitourinary Z48.816
nervous Z48.811
oral cavity Z48.814
respiratory Z48.813
sense organs Z48.810
skin and subcutaneous tissue Z48.817
teeth Z48.814
specified NEC Z48.89
spinal Z48.89
teeth Z48.814
fracture — *code to* fracture with seventh character D
involving
removal of
drains Z48.03
dressings (nonsurgical) Z48.00
staples Z48.02
surgical dressings Z48.01
sutures Z48.02
neuropacemaker (brain) (peripheral nerve) (spinal cord) Z46.2
implanted Z45.42
orthopedic NEC Z47.89

Aftercare (*see also* Care) Z51.89 — *continued*
postprocedural — *see* Aftercare, following surgery
After-cataract — *see* Cataract, secondary
Agalactia (primary) O92.3
elective, secondary or therapeutic O92.5
Agammaglobulinemia (acquired (secondary)) (nonfamilial) D80.1
with
immunoglobulin-bearing B-lymphocytes D80.1
lymphopenia D81.9
autosomal recessive (Swiss type) D80.0
Bruton's X-linked D80.0
common variable (CVAgamma) D80.1
congenital sex-linked D80.0
hereditary D80.0
lymphopenic D81.9
Swiss type (autosomal recessive) D80.0
X-linked (with growth hormone deficiency) (Bruton) D80.0
Aganglionosis (bowel) (colon) Q43.1
Age (old) — *see* Senility
Agenesis
adrenal (gland) Q89.1
alimentary tract (complete) (partial) NEC Q45.8
upper Q40.8
anus, anal (canal) Q42.3
with fistula Q42.2
aorta Q25.41
appendix Q42.8
arm (complete) Q71.0-
with hand present Q71.1-
artery (peripheral) Q27.9
brain Q28.3
coronary Q24.5
pulmonary Q25.79
specified NEC Q27.8
umbilical Q27.0
auditory (canal) (external) Q16.1
auricle (ear) Q16.0
bile duct or passage Q44.5
bladder Q64.5
bone Q79.9
brain Q00.0
part of Q04.3
breast (with nipple present) Q83.8
with absent nipple Q83.0
bronchus Q32.4
canaliculus lacrimalis Q10.4
carpus — *see* Agenesis, hand
cartilage Q79.9
cecum Q42.8
cerebellum Q04.3
cervix Q51.5
chin Q18.8
cilia Q10.3
circulatory system, part NOS Q28.9
clavicle Q74.0
clitoris Q52.6
coccyx Q76.49
colon Q42.9
specified NEC Q42.8
corpus callosum Q04.0
cricoid cartilage Q31.8
diaphragm (with hernia) Q79.1
digestive organ(s) or tract (complete) (partial) NEC Q45.8
upper Q40.8
ductus arteriosus Q28.8
duodenum Q41.0
ear Q16.9
auricle Q16.0
lobe Q17.8
ejaculatory duct Q55.4
endocrine (gland) NEC Q89.2
epiglottis Q31.8

Agenesis — *continued*
esophagus Q39.8
eustachian tube Q16.2
eye Q11.1
adnexa Q15.8
eyelid (fold) Q10.3
face
bones NEC Q75.8
specified part NEC Q18.8
fallopian tube Q50.6
femur — *see* Defect, reduction, lower limb, longitudinal, femur
fibula — *see* Defect, reduction, lower limb, longitudinal, fibula
finger (complete) (partial) — *see* Agenesis, hand
foot (and toes) (complete) (partial) Q72.3-
forearm (with hand present) — *see* Agenesis, arm, with hand present
and hand Q71.2-
gallbladder Q44.0
gastric Q40.2
genitalia, genital (organ(s))
female Q52.8
external Q52.71
internal NEC Q52.8
male Q55.8
glottis Q31.8
hair Q84.0
hand (and fingers) (complete) (partial) Q71.3-
heart Q24.8
valve NEC Q24.8
pulmonary Q22.0
hepatic Q44.7
humerus — *see* Defect, reduction, upper limb
hymen Q52.4
ileum Q41.2
incus Q16.3
intestine (small) Q41.9
large Q42.9
specified NEC Q42.8
iris (dilator fibers) Q13.1
jaw M26.09
jejunum Q41.1
kidney(s) (partial) Q60.2
bilateral Q60.1
unilateral Q60.0
labium (majus) (minus) Q52.71
labyrinth, membranous Q16.5
lacrimal apparatus Q10.4
larynx Q31.8
leg (complete) Q72.0-
with foot present Q72.1-
lower leg (with foot present) — *see* Agenesis, leg, with foot present
and foot Q72.2-
lens Q12.3
limb (complete) Q73.0
lower — *see* Agenesis, leg
upper — *see* Agenesis, arm
lip Q38.0
liver Q44.7
lung (fissure) (lobe) (bilateral) (unilateral) Q33.3
mandible, maxilla M26.09
metacarpus — *see* Agenesis, hand
metatarsus — *see* Agenesis, foot
muscle Q79.8
eyelid Q10.3
ocular Q15.8
musculoskeletal system NEC Q79.8
nail(s) Q84.3
neck, part Q18.8
nerve Q07.8
nervous system, part NEC Q07.8
nipple Q83.2
nose Q30.1
nuclear Q07.8

Agenesis — *continued*
organ
of Corti Q16.5
or site not listed — *see* Anomaly, by site
osseous meatus (ear) Q16.1
ovary
bilateral Q50.02
unilateral Q50.01
oviduct Q50.6
pancreas Q45.0
parathyroid (gland) Q89.2
parotid gland(s) Q38.4
patella Q74.1
pelvic girdle (complete) (partial) Q74.2
penis Q55.5
pericardium Q24.8
pituitary (gland) Q89.2
prostate Q55.4
punctum lacrimale Q10.4
radioulnar — *see* Defect, reduction, upper limb
radius — *see* Defect, reduction, upper limb,
longitudinal, radius
rectum Q42.1
with fistula Q42.0
renal Q60.2
bilateral Q60.1
unilateral Q60.0
respiratory organ NEC Q34.8
rib Q76.6
roof of orbit Q75.8
round ligament Q52.8
sacrum Q76.49
salivary gland Q38.4
scapula Q74.0
scrotum Q55.29
seminal vesicles Q55.4
septum
atrial Q21.1
between aorta and pulmonary artery Q21.4
ventricular Q20.4
shoulder girdle (complete) (partial) Q74.0
skull (bone) Q75.8
with
anencephaly Q00.0
encephalocele — *see* Encephalocele
hydrocephalus Q03.9
with spina bifida — *see* Spina bifida, by
site, with hydrocephalus
microcephaly Q02
spermatic cord Q55.4
spinal cord Q06.0
spine Q76.49
spleen Q89.01
sternum Q76.7
stomach Q40.2
submaxillary gland(s) (congenital) Q38.4
tarsus — *see* Agenesis, foot
tendon Q79.8
testicle Q55.0
thymus (gland) Q89.2
thyroid (gland) E03.1
cartilage Q31.8
tibia — *see* Defect, reduction, lower limb,
longitudinal, tibia
tibiofibular — *see* Defect, reduction, lower
limb, specified type NEC
toe (and foot) (complete) (partial) — *see*
Agenesis, foot
tongue Q38.3
trachea (cartilage) Q32.1
ulna — *see* Defect, reduction, upper limb,
longitudinal, ulna
upper limb — *see* Agenesis, arm
ureter Q62.4
urethra Q64.5
urinary tract NEC Q64.8
uterus Q51.0
uvula Q38.5
vagina Q52.0

Agenesis — *continued*
vas deferens Q55.4
vein(s) (peripheral) Q27.9
brain Q28.3
great NEC Q26.8
portal Q26.5
vena cava (inferior) (superior) Q26.8
vermis of cerebellum Q04.3
vertebra Q76.49
vulva Q52.71
Ageusia R43.2
Agitated — *see* condition
Agitation R45.1
Aglossia (congenital) Q38.3
Aglossia-adactylia syndrome Q87.0
Aglycogenosis E74.00
Agnosia (body image) (other senses) (tactile)
R48.1
developmental F88
verbal R48.1
auditory R48.1
developmental F80.2
developmental F80.2
visual (object) R48.3
Agoraphobia F40.00
with panic disorder F40.01
without panic disorder F40.02
Agrammatism R48.8
Agranulocytopenia — *see* Agranulocytosis
Agranulocytosis (chronic) (cyclical) (genetic)
(infantile) (periodic) (pernicious) (*see also*
Neutropenia) D70.9
congenital D70.0
cytoreductive cancer chemotherapy sequela
D70.1
drug-induced D70.2
due to cytoreductive cancer chemotherapy
D70.1
due to infection D70.3
secondary D70.4
drug-induced D70.2
due to cytoreductive cancer chemotherapy
D70.1
Agraphia (absolute) R48.8
with alexia R48.0
developmental F81.81
Ague (dumb) — *see* Malaria
Agyria Q04.3
Ahumada-del Castillo syndrome E23.0
Aichomophobia F40.298
AIDS (related complex) B20
Ailment, heart — *see* Disease, heart
Ailurophobia F40.218
AIN — *see* Neoplasia, intraepithelial, anal
Ainhum (disease) L94.6
AIPHI (acute idiopathic pulmonary hemorrhage
in infants (over 28 days old)) R04.81
Air
anterior mediastinum J98.2
compressed, disease T70.3
conditioner lung or pneumonitis J67.7
embolism (artery) (cerebral) (any site) T79.0
with ectopic or molar pregnancy O08.2
due to implanted device NEC — *see*
Complications, by site and type,
specified NEC
following
abortion — *see* Abortion by type,
complicated by, embolism
ectopic or molar pregnancy O08.2
infusion, therapeutic injection or
transfusion T80.0
in pregnancy, childbirth or puerperium —
see Embolism, obstetric
traumatic T79.0
hunger, psychogenic F45.8
rarefied, effects of — *see* Effect, adverse, high
altitude
sickness T75.3

Airplane sickness T75.3
Akathisia (drug-induced) (treatment-induced)
G25.71
neuroleptic induced (acute) G25.71
Akinesia R29.898
Akinetic mutism R41.89
Akureyri's disease G93.3
Alactasia, congenital E73.0
Alagille's syndrome Q44.7
Alastrim B03
Albers-Schönberg syndrome Q78.2
Albert's syndrome — *see* Tendinitis, Achilles
Albinism, albino E70.30
with hematologic abnormality E70.339
Chédiak-Higashi syndrome E70.330
Hermansky-Pudlak syndrome E70.331
other specified E70.338
I E70.320
II E70.321
ocular E70.319
autosomal recessive E70.311
other specified E70.318
X-linked E70.310
oculocutaneous E70.329
other specified E70.328
tyrosinase (ty) negative E70.320
tyrosinase (ty) positive E70.321
other specified E70.39
Albinismus E70.30
Albright(-McCune)(-Sternberg)
syndrome Q78.1
Albuminous — *see* condition
Albuminuria, albuminuric (acute) (chronic)
(subacute) (*see also* Proteinuria) R80.9
complicating pregnancy — *see* Proteinuria,
gestational
with
gestational hypertension — *see* Pre-
eclampsia
pre-existing hypertension — *see*
Hypertension, complicating
pregnancy, pre-existing, with, pre-
eclampsia
gestational — *see* Proteinuria, gestational
with
gestational hypertension — *see* Pre-
eclampsia
pre-existing hypertension — *see*
Hypertension, complicating
pregnancy, pre-existing, with, pre-
eclampsia
orthostatic R80.2
postural R80.2
pre-eclamptic — *see* Pre-eclampsia
scarlatinal A38.8
Albuminurophobia F40.298
Alcaptonuria E70.29
Alcohol, alcoholic, alcohol-induced
addiction (without remission) F10.20
with remission F10.21
amnestic disorder, persisting F10.96
with dependence F10.26
anxiety disorder F10.980
bipolar and related disorder F10.94
brain syndrome, chronic F10.97
with dependence F10.27
cardiopathy I42.6
counseling and surveillance Z71.41
family member Z71.42
delirium (acute) (tremens) (withdrawal)
F10.231
with intoxication F10.921
in
abuse F10.121
dependence F10.221
dementia F10.97
with dependence F10.27
depressive disorder F10.94

Alcohol, alcoholic, alcohol-induced —
continued
  deterioration F10.97
    with dependence F10.27
  hallucinosis (acute) F10.951
    in
      abuse F10.151
      dependence F10.251
  insanity F10.959
  intoxication (acute) (without dependence)
    F10.129
    with
      delirium F10.121
      dependence F10.229
        with delirium F10.221
        uncomplicated F10.220
      uncomplicated F10.120
  jealousy F10.988
  Korsakoff's, Korsakov's, Korsakow's F10.26
  liver K70.9
    acute — *see* Disease, liver, alcoholic,
      hepatitis
  major neurocognitive disorder, amnestic-
    confabulatory type F10.96
  major neurocognitive disorder, nonamnestic-
    confabulatory type F10.97
  mania (acute) (chronic) F10.959
  mild neurocognitive disorder F10.988
  paranoia, paranoid (type) psychosis F10.950
  pellagra E52
  poisoning, accidental (acute) NEC — *see* Table
    of Drugs and Chemicals, alcohol,
    poisoning
  psychosis — *see* Psychosis, alcoholic
  psychotic disorder F10.959
  sexual dysfunction F10.981
  sleep disorder F10.982
  withdrawal (without convulsions) F10.239
    with delirium F10.231
Alcoholism (chronic) (without remission)
  F10.20
  with
    psychosis — *see* Psychosis, alcoholic
    remission F10.21
  Korsakov's F10.96
    with dependence F10.26
Alder (-Reilly) anomaly or syndrome
  (leukocyte granulation) D72.0
Aldosteronism E26.9
  familial (type I) E26.02
  glucocorticoid-remediable E26.02
  primary (due to (bilateral) adrenal
    hyperplasia) E26.09
  primary NEC E26.09
  secondary E26.1
  specified NEC E26.89
Aldosteronoma D44.10
Aldrich(-Wiskott) syndrome (eczema-
  thrombocytopenia) D82.0
Alektorophobia F40.218
Aleppo boil B55.1
Aleukemic — *see* condition
Aleukia
  congenital D70.0
  hemorrhagica D61.9
    congenital D61.09
  splenica D73.1
Alexia R48.0
  developmental F81.0
  secondary to organic lesion R48.0
Algoneurodystrophy M89.00
  ankle M89.07-
  foot M89.07-
  forearm M89.03-
  hand M89.04-
  lower leg M89.06-
  multiple sites M89.0-
  shoulder M89.01-
  specified site NEC M89.08

Algoneurodystrophy M89.00 — *continued*
  thigh M89.05-
  upper arm M89.02-
Algophobia F40.298
Alienation, mental — *see* Psychosis
Alkalemia E87.3
Alkalosis E87.3
  metabolic E87.3
    with respiratory acidosis E87.4
  respiratory E87.3
Alkaptonuria E70.29
Allen-Masters syndrome N83.8
Allergy, allergic (reaction) (to) T78.40
  air-borne substance NEC (rhinitis) J30.89
  alveolitis (extrinsic) J67.9
    due to
      Aspergillus clavatus J67.4
      Cryptostroma corticale J67.6
      organisms (fungal, thermophilic
        actinomycete) growing in ventilation
        (air conditioning) systems J67.7
    specified type NEC J67.8
  anaphylactic reaction or shock T78.2
  angioneurotic edema T78.3
  animal (dander) (epidermal) (hair) (rhinitis)
    J30.81
  bee sting (anaphylactic shock) — *see* Toxicity,
    venom, arthropod, bee
  biological — *see* Allergy, drug
  colitis (*see also* Colitis, allergic) K52.2
  dander (animal) (rhinitis) J30.81
  dandruff (rhinitis) J30.81
  dental restorative material (existing) K08.55
  dermatitis — *see* Dermatitis, contact, allergic
  diathesis — *see* History, allergy
  drug, medicament & biological (any) (external)
    (internal) T78.40
    correct substance properly administered —
      see Table of Drugs and Chemicals, by
      drug, adverse effect
    wrong substance given or taken NEC (by
      accident) — *see* Table of Drugs and
      Chemicals, by drug, poisoning
  due to pollen J30.1
  dust (house) (stock) (rhinitis) J30.89
    with asthma — *see* Asthma, allergic extrinsic
  eczema — *see* Dermatitis, contact, allergic
  epidermal (animal) (rhinitis) J30.81
  feathers (rhinitis) J30.89
  food (any) (ingested) NEC T78.1
    anaphylactic shock — *see* Shock,
      anaphylactic, due to food
    dermatitis — *see* Dermatitis, due to, food
    dietary counseling and surveillance Z71.3
    in contact with skin L23.6
    rhinitis J30.5
    status (without reaction) Z91.018
      eggs Z91.012
      milk products Z91.011
      peanuts Z91.010
      seafood Z91.013
      specified NEC Z91.018
  gastrointestinal — *see also* specific type of
    allergic reaction
    meaning colitis (*see also* Colitis, allergic)
      K52.29
    meaning gastroenteritis (*see also*
      Gastroenteritis, allergic) K52.29
    meaning other adverse food reaction not
      elsewhere classified T78.1
  grain J30.1
  grass (hay fever) (pollen) J30.1
    asthma — *see* Asthma, allergic extrinsic
  hair (animal) (rhinitis) J30.81
  history (of) — *see* History, allergy
  horse serum — *see* Allergy, serum
  inhalant (rhinitis) J30.89
    pollen J30.1
  kapok (rhinitis) J30.89

Allergy, allergic (reaction) (to) T78.40 —
continued
  medicine — *see* Allergy, drug
  milk protein (*see also* Allergy, food) Z91.011
    anaphylactic reaction T78.07
    dermatitis L27.2
    enterocolitis syndrome K52.21
    enteropathy K52.22
    gastroenteritis K52.29
    gastroesophageal reflux (*see also* Reaction,
      adverse, food) K21.9
      with esophagitis K21.0
    proctocolitis K52.82
  nasal, seasonal due to pollen J30.1
  pneumonia J82
  pollen (any) (hay fever) J30.1
    asthma — *see* Asthma, allergic extrinsic
  primrose J30.1
  primula J30.1
  proctocolitis K52.82
  purpura D69.0
  ragweed (hay fever) (pollen) J30.1
    asthma — *see* Asthma, allergic extrinsic
  rose (pollen) J30.1
  seasonal NEC J30.2
  Senecio jacobae (pollen) J30.1
  serum (*see also* Reaction, serum) T80.69
    anaphylactic shock T80.59
  shock (anaphylactic) T78.2
    due to
      adverse effect of correct medicinal
        substance properly administered
        T88.6
      administration of blood and blood
        products T80.51
      immunization T80.52
      serum NEC T80.59
      vaccination T80.52
  specific NEC T78.49
  tree (any) (hay fever) (pollen) J30.1
    asthma — *see* Asthma, allergic extrinsic
  upper respiratory J30.9
  urticaria L50.0
  vaccine — *see* Allergy, serum
  wheat — *see* Allergy, food
Allescheriasis B48.2
Alligator skin disease Q80.9
Allocheiria, allochiria R20.8
Almeida's disease — *see*
  Paracoccidioidomycosis
Alopecia (hereditaria) (seborrheica) L65.9
  androgenic L64.9
    drug-induced L64.0
    specified NEC L64.8
  areata L63.9
    ophiasis L63.2
    specified NEC L63.8
    totalis L63.0
    universalis L63.1
  cicatricial L66.9
    specified NEC L66.8
  circumscripta L63.9
  congenital, congenitalis Q84.0
  due to cytotoxic drugs NEC L65.8
  mucinosa L65.2
  postinfective NEC L65.8
  postpartum L65.0
  premature L64.8
  specific (syphilitic) A51.32
  specified NEC L65.8
  syphilitic (secondary) A51.32
  totalis (capitis) L63.0
  universalis (entire body) L63.1
  X-ray L58.1
Alpers' disease G31.81
Alpine sickness T70.29
Alport syndrome Q87.81
ALTE (apparent life threatening event) in
  newborn and infant R68.13

Alteration (of), Altered
awareness
transient R40.4
unintended under general anesthesia, during procedure T88.53
mental status R41.82
pattern of family relationships affecting child Z62.898
sensation
following
cerebrovascular disease I69.998
cerebral infarction I69.398
intracerebral hemorrhage I69.198
nontraumatic intracranial hemorrhage NEC I69.298
specified disease NEC I69.898
subarachnoid hemorrhage I69.098
Alternating — see condition
Altitude, high (effects) — see Effect, adverse, high altitude
Aluminosis (of lung) J63.0
Alveolitis
allergic (extrinsic) — see Pneumonitis, hypersensitivity
due to
Aspergillus clavatus J67.4
Cryptostroma corticale J67.6
fibrosing (cryptogenic) (idiopathic) J84.112
jaw M27.3
sicca dolorosa M27.3
Alveolus, alveolar — see condition
Alymphocytosis D72.810
thymic (with immunodeficiency) D82.1
Alymphoplasia, thymic D82.1
Alzheimer's disease or sclerosis — see Disease, Alzheimer's
Amastia (with nipple present) Q83.8
with absent nipple Q83.0
Amathophobia F40.228
Amaurosis (acquired) (congenital) — see also Blindness
fugax G45.3
hysterical F44.6
Leber's congenital H35.50
uremic — see Uremia
Amaurotic idiocy (infantile) (juvenile) (late) E75.4
Amaxophobia F40.248
Ambiguous genitalia Q56.4
Amblyopia (congenital) (ex anopsia) (partial) (suppression) H53.00-
anisometropic — see Amblyopia, refractive
deprivation H53.01-
hysterical F44.6
nocturnal — see also Blindness, night
vitamin A deficiency E50.5
refractive H53.02-
strabismic H53.03-
suspect H53.04-
tobacco H53.8
toxic NEC H53.8
uremic — see Uremia
Ameba, amebic (histolytica) — see also Amebiasis
abscess (liver) A06.4
Amebiasis A06.9
with abscess — see Abscess, amebic
acute A06.0
chronic (intestine) A06.1
with abscess — see Abscess, amebic
cutaneous A06.7
cutis A06.7
cystitis A06.81
genitourinary tract NEC A06.82
hepatic — see Abscess, liver, amebic
intestine A06.0
nondysenteric colitis A06.2
skin A06.7
specified site NEC A06.89

Ameboma (of intestine) A06.3
Amelia Q73.0
lower limb — see Agenesis, leg
upper limb — see Agenesis, arm
Ameloblastoma — see also Cyst, calcifying odontogenic
long bones C40.9-
lower limb C40.2-
upper limb C40.0-
malignant C41.1
jaw (bone) (lower) C41.1
upper C41.0
tibial C40.2-
Amelogenesis imperfecta K00.5
nonhereditaria (segmentalis) K00.4
Amenorrhea N91.2
hyperhormonal E28.8
primary N91.0
secondary N91.1
Amentia — see Disability, intellectual
Meynert's (nonalcoholic) F04
American
leishmaniasis B55.2
mountain tick fever A93.2
Ametropia — see Disorder, refraction
AMH (asymptomatic microscopic hematuria) R31.21
Amianthosis J61
Amimia R48.8
Amino-acid disorder E72.9
anemia D53.0
Aminoacidopathy E72.9
Aminoaciduria E72.9
Amnesia R41.3
anterograde R41.1
auditory R48.8
dissociative F44.0
with dissociative fugue F44.1
hysterical F44.0
postictal in epilepsy — see Epilepsy
psychogenic F44.0
retrograde R41.2
transient global G45.4
Amnes(t)ic syndrome (post-traumatic) F04
induced by
alcohol F10.96
with dependence F10.26
psychoactive NEC F19.96
with
abuse F19.16
dependence F19.26
sedative F13.96
with dependence F13.26
Amnion, amniotic — see condition
Amnionitis — see Pregnancy, complicated by
Amok F68.8
Amoral traits F60.89
Amphetamine (or other stimulant) -induced
anxiety disorder F15.980
bipolar and related disorder F15.94
delirium F15.921
depressive disorder F15.94
obsessive-compulsive and related disorder F15.988
psychotic disorder F15.959
sexual dysfunction F15.981
sleep disorder F15.982
stimulant withdrawal F15.23
Ampulla
lower esophagus K22.8
phrenic K22.8
Amputation — see also Absence, by site, acquired
neuroma (postoperative) (traumatic) — see Complications, amputation stump, neuroma

Amputation (see also Absence, by site, acquired) — continued
stump (surgical)
abnormal, painful, or with complication (late) — see Complications, amputation stump
healed or old NOS Z89.9
traumatic (complete) (partial)
arm (upper) (complete) S48.91-
at
elbow S58.01-
partial S58.02-
shoulder joint (complete) S48.01-
partial S48.02-
between
elbow and wrist (complete) S58.11-
partial S58.12-
shoulder and elbow (complete) S48.11-
partial S48.12-
partial S48.92-
breast (complete) S28.21-
partial S28.22-
clitoris (complete) S38.211
partial S38.212
ear (complete) S08.11-
partial S08.12-
finger (complete) (metacarpophalangeal) S68.11-
index S68.11-
little S68.11-
middle S68.11-
partial S68.12-
index S68.12-
little S68.12-
middle S68.12-
ring S68.12-
ring S68.11-
thumb — see Amputation, traumatic, thumb
transphalangeal (complete) S68.61-
index S68.61-
little S68.61-
middle S68.61-
partial S68.62-
index S68.62-
little S68.62-
middle S68.62-
ring S68.62-
ring S68.61-
foot (complete) S98.91-
at ankle level S98.01-
partial S98.02-
midfoot S98.31-
partial S98.32-
partial S98.92-
forearm (complete) S58.91-
at elbow level (complete) S58.01-
partial S58.02-
between elbow and wrist (complete) S58.11-
partial S58.12-
partial S58.92-
genital organ(s) (external)
female (complete) S38.211
partial S38.212
male
penis (complete) S38.221
partial S38.222
scrotum (complete) S38.231
partial S38.232
testes (complete) S38.231
partial S38.232
hand (complete) (wrist level) S68.41-
finger(s) alone — see Amputation, traumatic, finger
partial S68.42-
thumb alone — see Amputation, traumatic, thumb
transmetacarpal (complete) S68.71-
partial S68.72-

DISEASE INDEX

Amputation (see also Absence, by site, acquired) — continued
traumatic (complete) (partial) — continued
  head
    ear — see Amputation, traumatic, ear
    nose (partial) S08.812
      complete S08.811
      part S08.89
        scalp S08.0
  hip (and thigh) (complete) S78.91-
    at hip joint (complete) S78.01-
      partial S78.02-
    between hip and knee (complete) S78.11-
      partial S78.12-
    partial S78.92-
  labium (majus) (minus) (complete) S38.21-
    partial S38.21-
  leg (lower) S88.91-
    at knee level S88.01-
      partial S88.02-
    between knee and ankle S88.11-
      partial S88.12-
    partial S88.92-
  nose (partial) S08.812
    complete S08.811
  penis (complete) S38.221
    partial S38.222
  scrotum (complete) S38.231
    partial S38.232
  shoulder — see Amputation, traumatic, arm
    at shoulder joint — see Amputation, traumatic, arm, at shoulder joint
  testes (complete) S38.231
    partial S38.232
  thigh — see Amputation, traumatic, hip
  thorax, part of S28.1
    breast — see Amputation, traumatic, breast
  thumb (complete) (metacarpophalangeal) S68.01-
    partial S68.02-
    transphalangeal (complete) S68.51-
      partial S68.52-
  toe (lesser) S98.13-
    great S98.11-
      partial S98.12-
    more than one S98.21-
      partial S98.22-
    partial S98.14-
  vulva (complete) S38.211
    partial S38.212

Amputee (bilateral) (old) Z89.9
Amsterdam dwarfism Q87.1
Amusia R48.8
  developmental F80.89
Amyelencephalus, amyelencephaly Q00.0
Amyelia Q06.0
Amygdalitis — see Tonsillitis
Amygdalolith J35.8
Amyloid heart (disease) E85.4 [I43]
Amyloidosis (generalized) (primary) E85.9
  with lung involvement E85.4 [J99]
  familial E85.2
  genetic E85.2
  heart E85.4 [I43]
  hemodialysis-associated E85.3
  liver E85.4 [K77]
  localized E85.4
  neuropathic heredofamilial E85.1
  non-neuropathic heredofamilial E85.0
  organ limited E85.4
  Portuguese E85.1
  pulmonary E85.4 [J99]
  secondary systemic E85.3
  skin (lichen) (macular) E85.4 [L99]
  specified NEC E85.8
  subglottic E85.4 [J99]

Amylopectinosis (brancher enzyme deficiency) E74.03
Amylophagia — see Pica
Amyoplasia congenita Q79.8
Amyotonia M62.89
  congenita G70.2
Amyotrophia, amyotrophy, amyotrophic G71.8
  congenita Q79.8
  diabetic — see Diabetes, amyotrophy
  lateral sclerosis G12.21
  neuralgic G54.5
  spinal progressive G12.21
Anacidity, gastric K31.83
  psychogenic F45.8
Anaerosis of newborn P28.89
Analbuminemia E88.09
Analgesia — see Anesthesia
Analphalipoproteinemia E78.6
Anaphylactic
  purpura D69.0
  shock or reaction — see Shock, anaphylactic
Anaphylactoid shock or reaction — see Shock, anaphylactic
Anaphylactoid syndrome of pregnancy O88.01-
Anaphylaxis — see Shock, anaphylactic
Anaplasia cervix (see also Dysplasia, cervix) N87.9
Anaplasmosis, human A77.49
Anarthria R47.1
Anasarca R60.1
  cardiac — see Failure, heart, congestive
  lung J18.2
  newborn P83.2
  nutritional E43
  pulmonary J18.2
  renal N04.9
Anastomosis
  aneurysmal — see Aneurysm
  arteriovenous ruptured brain I60.8
  intestinal K63.89
    complicated NEC K91.89
      involving urinary tract N99.89
  retinal and choroidal vessels (congenital) Q14.8
Anatomical narrow angle H40.03-
Ancylostoma, ancylostomiasis (braziliense) (caninum) (ceylanicum) (duodenale) B76.0
  Necator americanus B76.1
Andersen's disease (glycogen storage) E74.09
Anderson-Fabry disease E75.21
Andes disease T70.29
Andrews' disease (bacterid) L08.89
Androblastoma
  benign
    specified site — see Neoplasm, benign, by site
    unspecified site
      female D27.9
      male D29.20
  malignant
    specified site — see Neoplasm, malignant, by site
    unspecified site
      female C56.9
      male C62.90
  specified site — see Neoplasm, uncertain behavior, by site
  tubular
    with lipid storage
      specified site — see Neoplasm, benign, by site
      unspecified site
        female D27.9
        male D29.20

Androblastoma — continued
  tubular — continued
    specified site — see Neoplasm, benign, by site
    unspecified site
      female D27.9
      male D29.20
  unspecified site
    female D39.10
    male D40.10
Androgen insensitivity syndrome (see also Syndrome, androgen insensitivity) E34.50
Androgen resistance syndrome (see also Syndrome, androgen insensitivity) E34.50
Android pelvis Q74.2
  with disproportion (fetopelvic) O33.3
    causing obstructed labor O65.3
Androphobia F40.290
Anectasis, pulmonary (newborn) — see Atelectasis
Anemia (essential) (general) (hemoglobin deficiency) (infantile) (primary) (profound) D64.9
  with (due to) (in)
    disorder of
      anaerobic glycolysis D55.2
      pentose phosphate pathway D55.1
    koilonychia D50.9
  achlorhydric D50.8
  achrestic D53.1
  Addison(-Biermer) (pernicious) D51.0
  agranulocytic — see Agranulocytosis
  amino-acid-deficiency D53.0
  aplastic D61.9
    congenital D61.09
    drug-induced D61.1
    due to
      drugs D61.1
      external agents NEC D61.2
      infection D61.2
      radiation D61.2
    idiopathic D61.3
    red cell (pure) D60.9
      chronic D60.0
      congenital D61.01
      specified type NEC D60.8
      transient D60.1
    specified type NEC D61.89
    toxic D61.2
  aregenerative
    congenital D61.09
  asiderotic D50.9
  atypical (primary) D64.9
  Baghdad spring D55.0
  Balantidium coli A07.0
  Biermer's (pernicious) D51.0
  blood loss (chronic) D50.0
    acute D62
  bothriocephalus B70.0 [D63.8]
  brickmaker's B76.9 [D63.8]
  cerebral I67.89
  childhood D58.9
  chlorotic D50.8
  chronic
    blood loss D50.0
    hemolytic D58.9
      idiopathic D59.9
    simple D53.9
  chronica congenita aregenerativa D61.09
  combined system disease NEC D51.0 [G32.0]
    due to dietary vitamin B12 deficiency D51.3 [G32.0]
  complicating pregnancy, childbirth or puerperium — see Pregnancy, complicated by (management affected by), anemia
  congenital P61.4
    aplastic D61.09
    due to isoimmunization NOS P55.9
    dyserythropoietic, dyshematopoietic D64.4

Anemia (essential) (general) (hemoglobin deficiency) (infantile) (primary) (profound) D64.9 — *continued*
- congenital P61.4 — *continued*
  - following fetal blood loss P61.3
  - Heinz body D58.2
  - hereditary hemolytic NOS D58.9
  - pernicious D51.0
  - spherocytic D58.0
- Cooley's (erythroblastic) D56.1
- cytogenic D51.0
- deficiency D53.9
  - 2, 3 diphosphoglycurate mutase D55.2
  - 2, 3 PG D55.2
  - 6 phosphogluconate dehydrogenase D55.1
  - 6-PGD D55.1
  - amino-acid D53.0
  - combined B12 and folate D53.1
  - enzyme D55.9
    - drug-induced (hemolytic) D59.2
    - glucose-6-phosphate dehydrogenase (G6PD) D55.0
    - glycolytic D55.2
    - nucleotide metabolism D55.3
    - related to hexose monophosphate (HMP) shunt pathway NEC D55.1
    - specified type NEC D55.8
  - erythrocytic glutathione D55.1
  - folate D52.9
    - dietary D52.0
    - drug-induced D52.1
  - folic acid D52.9
    - dietary D52.0
    - drug-induced D52.1
  - G SH D55.1
  - G6PD D55.0
  - GGS-R D55.1
  - glucose-6-phosphate dehydrogenase D55.0
  - glutathione reductase D55.1
  - glyceraldehyde phosphate dehydrogenase D55.2
  - hexokinase D55.2
  - iron D50.9
    - secondary to blood loss (chronic) D50.0
  - nutritional D53.9
    - with
      - poor iron absorption D50.8
      - specified deficiency NEC D53.8
  - phosphofructo-aldolase D55.2
  - phosphoglycerate kinase D55.2
  - PK D55.2
  - protein D53.0
  - pyruvate kinase D55.2
  - transcobalamin II D51.2
  - triose-phosphate isomerase D55.2
  - vitamin B12 NOS D51.9
    - dietary D51.3
    - due to
      - intrinsic factor deficiency D51.0
      - selective vitamin B12 malabsorption with proteinuria D51.1
    - pernicious D51.0
    - specified type NEC D51.8
- Diamond-Blackfan (congenital hypoplastic) D61.01
- dibothriocephalus B70.0 [D63.8]
- dimorphic D53.1
- diphasic D53.1
- Diphyllobothrium (Dibothriocephalus) B70.0 [D63.8]
- due to (in) (with)
  - antineoplastic chemotherapy D64.81
  - blood loss (chronic) D50.0
    - acute D62
  - chemotherapy, antineoplastic D64.81
  - chronic disease classified elsewhere NEC D63.8
  - chronic kidney disease D63.1

Anemia (essential) (general) (hemoglobin deficiency) (infantile) (primary) (profound) D64.9 — *continued*
- due to (in) (with) — *continued*
  - deficiency
    - amino-acid D53.0
    - copper D53.8
    - folate (folic acid) D52.9
      - dietary D52.0
      - drug-induced D52.1
    - molybdenum D53.8
    - protein D53.0
    - zinc D53.8
  - dietary vitamin B12 deficiency D51.3
  - disorder of
    - glutathione metabolism D55.1
    - nucleotide metabolism D55.3
  - drug — *see* Anemia, by type — *see also* Table of Drugs and Chemicals
  - end stage renal disease D63.1
  - enzyme disorder D55.9
  - fetal blood loss P61.3
  - fish tapeworm (D.latum) infestation B70.0 [D63.8]
  - hemorrhage (chronic) D50.0
    - acute D62
  - impaired absorption D50.9
  - loss of blood (chronic) D50.0
    - acute D62
  - myxedema E03.9 [D63.8]
  - Necator americanus B76.1 [D63.8]
  - prematurity P61.2
  - selective vitamin B12 malabsorption with proteinuria D51.1
  - transcobalamin II deficiency D51.2
- Dyke-Young type (secondary) (symptomatic) D59.1
- dyserythropoietic (congenital) D64.4
- dyshematopoietic (congenital) D64.4
- Egyptian B76.9 [D63.8]
- elliptocytosis — *see* Elliptocytosis
- enzyme-deficiency, drug-induced D59.2
- epidemic (*see also* Ancylostomiasis) B76.9 [D63.8]
- erythroblastic
  - familial D56.1
  - newborn (*see also* Disease, hemolytic) P55.9
  - of childhood D56.1
- erythrocytic glutathione deficiency D55.1
- erythropoietin-resistant anemia (EPO resistant anemia) D63.1
- Faber's (achlorhydric anemia) D50.9
- factitious (self-induced blood letting) D50.0
- familial erythroblastic D56.1
- Fanconi's (congenital pancytopenia) D61.09
- favism D55.0
- fish tapeworm (D. latum) infestation B70.0 [D63.8]
- folate (folic acid) deficiency D52.9
- glucose-6-phosphate dehydrogenase (G6PD) deficiency D55.0
- glutathione-reductase deficiency D55.1
- goat's milk D52.0
- granulocytic — *see* Agranulocytosis
- Heinz body, congenital D58.2
- hemolytic D58.9
  - acquired D59.9
    - with hemoglobinuria NEC D59.6
    - autoimmune NEC D59.1
    - infectious D59.4
    - specified type NEC D59.8
    - toxic D59.4
  - acute D59.9
    - due to enzyme deficiency specified type NEC D55.8
    - Lederer's D59.1
  - autoimmune D59.1
    - drug-induced D59.0

Anemia (essential) (general) (hemoglobin deficiency) (infantile) (primary) (profound) D64.9 — *continued*
- hemolytic D58.9 — *continued*
  - chronic D58.9
    - idiopathic D59.9
  - cold type (secondary) (symptomatic) D59.1
  - congenital (spherocytic) — *see* Spherocytosis
  - due to
    - cardiac conditions D59.4
    - drugs (nonautoimmune) D59.2
      - autoimmune D59.0
    - enzyme disorder D55.9
      - drug-induced D59.2
    - presence of shunt or other internal prosthetic device D59.4
  - familial D58.9
  - hereditary D58.9
    - due to enzyme disorder D55.9
      - specified type NEC D55.8
    - specified type NEC D58.8
  - idiopathic (chronic) D59.9
  - mechanical D59.4
  - microangiopathic D59.4
  - nonautoimmune D59.4
    - drug-induced D59.2
  - nonspherocytic
    - congenital or hereditary NEC D55.8
      - glucose-6-phosphate dehydrogenase deficiency D55.0
      - pyruvate kinase deficiency D55.2
    - type
      - I D55.1
      - II D55.2
    - type
      - I D55.1
      - II D55.2
  - secondary D59.4
    - autoimmune D59.1
  - specified (hereditary) type NEC D58.8
  - Stransky-Regala type (*see also* Hemoglobinopathy) D58.8
  - symptomatic D59.4
    - autoimmune D59.1
  - toxic D59.4
  - warm type (secondary) (symptomatic) D59.1
- hemorrhagic (chronic) D50.0
  - acute D62
- Herrick's D57.1
- hexokinase deficiency D55.2
- hookworm B76.9 [D63.8]
- hypochromic (idiopathic) (microcytic) (normoblastic) D50.9
  - due to blood loss (chronic) D50.0
    - acute D62
  - familial sex-linked D64.0
  - pyridoxine-responsive D64.3
  - sideroblastic, sex-linked D64.0
- hypoplasia, red blood cells D61.9
  - congenital or familial D61.01
- hypoplastic (idiopathic) D61.9
  - congenital or familial (of childhood) D61.01
- hypoproliferative (refractive) D61.9
- idiopathic D64.9
  - aplastic D61.3
  - hemolytic, chronic D59.9
- in (due to) (with)
  - chronic kidney disease D63.1
  - end stage renal disease D63.1
  - failure, kidney (renal) D63.1
  - neoplastic disease (*see also* Neoplasm) D63.0
- intertropical (*see also* Ancylostomiasis) D63.8
- iron deficiency D50.9
  - secondary to blood loss (chronic) D50.0
    - acute D62
  - specified type NEC D50.8
- Joseph-Diamond-Blackfan (congenital hypoplastic) D61.01

Anemia (essential) (general) (hemoglobin deficiency) (infantile) (primary) (profound) D64.9 — *continued*
  Lederer's (hemolytic) D59.1
  leukoerythroblastic D61.82
  macrocytic D53.9
    nutritional D52.0
    tropical D52.8
  malarial (*see also* Malaria) B54 *[D63.8]*
  malignant (progressive) D51.0
  malnutrition D53.9
  marsh (*see also* Malaria) B54 *[D63.8]*
  Mediterranean (with other hemoglobinopathy) D56.9
  megaloblastic D53.1
    combined B12 and folate deficiency D53.1
    hereditary D51.1
    nutritional D52.0
    orotic aciduria D53.0
    refractory D53.1
    specified type NEC D53.1
  megalocytic D53.1
  microcytic (hypochromic) D50.9
    due to blood loss (chronic) D50.0
      acute D62
    familial D56.8
  microdrepanocytosis D57.40
  microelliptopoikilocytic (Rietti-Greppi-Micheli) D56.9
  miner's B76.9 *[D63.8]*
  myelodysplastic D46.9
  myelofibrosis D75.81
  myelogenous D64.89
  myelopathic D64.89
  myelophthisic D61.82
  myeloproliferative D47.Z9
  newborn P61.4
    due to
      ABO (antibodies, isoimmunization, maternal/fetal incompatibility) P55.1
      Rh (antibodies, isoimmunization, maternal/fetal incompatibility) P55.0
    following fetal blood loss P61.3
    posthemorrhagic (fetal) P61.3
  nonspherocytic hemolytic — *see* Anemia, hemolytic, nonspherocytic
  normocytic (infectional) D64.9
    due to blood loss (chronic) D50.0
      acute D62
    myelophthisic D61.82
  nutritional (deficiency) D53.9
    with
      poor iron absorption D50.8
      specified deficiency NEC D53.8
    megaloblastic D52.0
  of prematurity P61.2
  orotaciduric (congenital) (hereditary) D53.0
  osteosclerotic D64.89
  ovalocytosis (hereditary) — *see* Elliptocytosis
  paludal (*see also* Malaria) B54 *[D63.8]*
  pernicious (congenital) (malignant) (progressive) D51.0
  pleochromic D64.89
    of sprue D52.8
  posthemorrhagic (chronic) D50.0
    acute D62
    newborn P61.3
  postoperative (postprocedural)
    due to (acute) blood loss D62
      chronic blood loss D50.0
    specified NEC D64.9
  postpartum O90.81
  pressure D64.89
  progressive D64.9
    malignant D51.0
    pernicious D51.0
  protein-deficiency D53.0
  pseudoleukemica infantum D64.89

Anemia (essential) (general) (hemoglobin deficiency) (infantile) (primary) (profound) D64.9 — *continued*
  pure red cell D60.9
    congenital D61.01
  pyridoxine-responsive D64.3
  pyruvate kinase deficiency D55.2
  refractory D46.4
    with
      excess of blasts D46.20
        1 (RAEB 1) D46.21
        2 (RAEB 2) D46.22
        in transformation (RAEB T) — *see* Leukemia, acute myeloblastic
      hemochromatosis D46.1
      sideroblasts (ring) (RARS) D46.1
    megaloblastic D53.1
    sideroblastic D46.1
    sideropenic D50.9
    without ring sideroblasts, so stated D46.0
    without sideroblasts without excess of blasts D46.0
  Rietti-Greppi-Micheli D56.9
  scorbutic D53.2
  secondary to
    blood loss (chronic) D50.0
      acute D62
    hemorrhage (chronic) D50.0
      acute D62
  semiplastic D61.89
  sickle-cell — *see* Disease, sickle-cell
  sideroblastic D64.3
    hereditary D64.0
    hypochromic, sex-linked D64.0
    pyridoxine-responsive NEC D64.3
    refractory D46.1
    secondary (due to)
      disease D64.1
      drugs and toxins D64.2
    specified type NEC D64.3
  sideropenic (refractory) D50.9
    due to blood loss (chronic) D50.0
      acute D62
  simple chronic D53.9
  specified type NEC D64.89
  spherocytic (hereditary) — *see* Spherocytosis
  splenic D64.89
  splenomegalic D64.89
  stomatocytosis D58.8
  syphilitic (acquired) (late) A52.79 *[D63.8]*
  target cell D64.89
  thalassemia D56.9
  thrombocytopenic — *see* Thrombocytopenia
  toxic D61.2
  tropical B76.9 *[D63.8]*
    macrocytic D52.8
  tuberculous A18.89 *[D63.8]*
  vegan D51.3
  vitamin
    B12 deficiency (dietary) pernicious D51.0
    B6-responsive D64.3
  von Jaksch's D64.89
  Witts' (achlorhydric anemia) D50.8
Anemophobia F40.228
Anencephalus, anencephaly Q00.0
Anergasia — *see* Psychosis, organic
Anesthesia, anesthetic R20.0
  complication or reaction NEC (*see also* Complications, anesthesia) T88.59
  due to
    correct substance properly administered — *see* Table of Drugs and Chemicals, by drug, adverse effect
    overdose or wrong substance given — *see* Table of Drugs and Chemicals, by drug, poisoning
    unintended awareness under general anesthesia during procedure T88.53
    personal history of Z92.84

Anesthesia, anesthetic R20.0 — *continued*
  cornea H18.81-
  dissociative F44.6
  functional (hysterical) F44.6
  hyperesthetic, thalamic G89.0
  hysterical F44.6
  local skin lesion R20.0
  sexual (psychogenic) F52.1
  shock (due to) T88.2
  skin R20.0
  testicular N50.9
Anetoderma (maculosum) (of) L90.8
  Jadassohn-Pellizzari L90.2
  Schweniger-Buzzi L90.1
Aneurin deficiency E51.9
Aneurysm (anastomotic) (artery) (cirsoid) (diffuse) (false) (fusiform) (multiple) (saccular) I72.9
  abdominal (aorta) I71.4
    ruptured I71.3
    syphilitic A52.01
  aorta, aortic (nonsyphilitic) I71.9
    abdominal I71.4
      ruptured I71.3
    arch I71.2
      ruptured I71.1
    arteriosclerotic I71.9
      ruptured I71.8
    ascending I71.2
      ruptured I71.1
    congenital Q25.43
    descending I71.9
      abdominal I71.4
        ruptured I71.3
      ruptured I71.8
      thoracic I71.2
        ruptured I71.1
    root Q25.43
    ruptured I71.8
    sinus, congenital Q25.43
    syphilitic A52.01
    thoracic I71.2
      ruptured I71.1
    thoracoabdominal I71.6
      ruptured I71.5
    thorax, thoracic (arch) I71.2
      ruptured I71.1
    transverse I71.2
      ruptured I71.1
    valve (heart) (*see also* Endocarditis, aortic) I35.8
  arteriosclerotic I72.9
    cerebral I67.1
      ruptured — *see* Hemorrhage, intracranial, subarachnoid
  arteriovenous (congenital) — *see also* Malformation, arteriovenous
    acquired I77.0
      brain I67.1
      coronary I25.41
      pulmonary I28.0
    brain Q28.2
      ruptured I60.8
    peripheral — *see* Malformation, arteriovenous, peripheral
    precerebral vessels Q28.0
    specified site NEC — *see also* Malformation, arteriovenous
      acquired I77.0
  basal — *see* Aneurysm, brain
  basilar (trunk) I72.5
  berry (congenital) (nonruptured) I67.1
    ruptured I60.7

Aneurysm (anastomotic) (artery) (cirsoid) (diffuse) (false) (fusiform) (multiple) (saccular) I72.9 — *continued*
- brain I67.1
  - arteriosclerotic I67.1
    - ruptured — *see* Hemorrhage, intracranial, subarachnoid
  - arteriovenous (congenital) (nonruptured) Q28.2
    - acquired I67.1
      - ruptured I60.8
    - ruptured I60.8
  - berry (congenital) (nonruptured) I67.1
    - ruptured (*see also* Hemorrhage, intracranial, subarachnoid) I60.7
  - congenital Q28.3
    - ruptured I60.7
  - meninges I67.1
    - ruptured I60.8
  - miliary (congenital) (nonruptured) I67.1
    - ruptured (*see also* Hemorrhage, intracranial, subarachnoid) I60.7
  - mycotic I33.0
    - ruptured — *see* Hemorrhage, intracranial, subarachnoid
  - syphilitic (hemorrhage) A52.05
- cardiac (false) (*see also* Aneurysm, heart) I25.3
- carotid artery (common) (external) I72.0
  - internal (intracranial) I67.1
    - extracranial portion I72.0
  - ruptured into brain I60.0-
  - syphilitic A52.09
    - intracranial A52.05
- cavernous sinus I67.1
  - arteriovenous (congenital) (nonruptured) Q28.3
    - ruptured I60.8
- celiac I72.8
- central nervous system, syphilitic A52.05
- cerebral — *see* Aneurysm, brain
- chest — *see* Aneurysm, thorax
- circle of Willis I67.1
  - congenital Q28.3
    - ruptured I60.6
  - ruptured I60.6
- common iliac artery I72.3
- congenital (peripheral) Q27.8
  - aorta (root) (sinus) Q25.43
  - brain Q28.3
    - ruptured I60.7
  - coronary Q24.5
  - digestive system Q27.8
  - lower limb Q27.8
  - pulmonary Q25.79
  - retina Q14.1
  - specified site NEC Q27.8
  - upper limb Q27.8
- conjunctiva — *see* Abnormality, conjunctiva, vascular
- conus arteriosus — *see* Aneurysm, heart
- coronary (arteriosclerotic) (artery) I25.41
  - arteriovenous, congenital Q24.5
  - congenital Q24.5
  - ruptured — *see* Infarct, myocardium
  - syphilitic A52.06
  - vein I25.89
- cylindroid (aorta) I71.9
  - ruptured I71.8
  - syphilitic A52.01
- ductus arteriosus Q25.0
- endocardial, infective (any valve) I33.0
- femoral (artery) (ruptured) I72.4
- gastroduodenal I72.8
- gastroepiploic I72.8
- heart (wall) (chronic or with a stated duration of over 4 weeks) I25.3
  - valve — *see* Endocarditis
- hepatic I72.8
- iliac (common) (artery) (ruptured) I72.3

Aneurysm (anastomotic) (artery) (cirsoid) (diffuse) (false) (fusiform) (multiple) (saccular) I72.9 — *continued*
- infective I72.9
  - endocardial (any valve) I33.0
  - innominate (nonsyphilitic) I72.8
    - syphilitic A52.09
- interauricular septum — *see* Aneurysm, heart
- interventricular septum — *see* Aneurysm, heart
- intrathoracic (nonsyphilitic) I71.2
  - ruptured I71.1
  - syphilitic A52.01
- lower limb I72.4
- lung (pulmonary artery) I28.1
- mediastinal (nonsyphilitic) I72.8
  - syphilitic A52.09
- miliary (congenital) I67.1
  - ruptured — *see* Hemorrhage, intracerebral, subarachnoid, intracranial
- mitral (heart) (valve) I34.8
- mural — *see* Aneurysm, heart
- mycotic I72.9
  - endocardial (any valve) I33.0
  - ruptured, brain — *see* Hemorrhage, intracerebral, subarachnoid
- myocardium — *see* Aneurysm, heart
- neck I72.0
- pancreaticoduodenal I72.8
- patent ductus arteriosus Q25.0
- peripheral NEC I72.8
  - congenital Q27.8
    - digestive system Q27.8
    - lower limb Q27.8
    - specified site NEC Q27.8
    - upper limb Q27.8
- popliteal (artery) (ruptured) I72.4
- precerebral
  - congenital (nonruptured) Q28.1
  - specified site, NEC I72.5
- pulmonary I28.1
  - arteriovenous Q25.72
    - acquired I28.0
  - syphilitic A52.09
  - valve (heart) — *see* Endocarditis, pulmonary
- racemose (peripheral) I72.9
  - congenital — *see* Aneurysm, congenital
- radial I72.1
- Rasmussen NEC A15.0
- renal (artery) I72.2
- retina — *see also* Disorder, retina, microaneurysms
  - congenital Q14.1
  - diabetic — *see* Diabetes, microaneurysms, retinal
- sinus of Valsalva Q25.49
- specified NEC I72.8
- spinal (cord) I72.8
  - syphilitic (hemorrhage) A52.09
- splenic I72.8
- subclavian (artery) (ruptured) I72.8
  - syphilitic A52.09
- superior mesenteric I72.8
- syphilitic (aorta) A52.01
  - central nervous system A52.05
  - congenital (late) A50.54 [I79.0]
  - spine, spinal A52.09
- thoracoabdominal (aorta) I71.6
  - ruptured I71.5
  - syphilitic A52.01
- thorax, thoracic (aorta) (arch) (nonsyphilitic) I71.2
  - ruptured I71.1
  - syphilitic A52.01
- traumatic (complication) (early), specified site — *see* Injury, blood vessel
- tricuspid (heart) (valve) I07.8
- ulnar I72.1
- upper limb (ruptured) I72.1
- valve, valvular — *see* Endocarditis

Aneurysm (anastomotic) (artery) (cirsoid) (diffuse) (false) (fusiform) (multiple) (saccular) I72.9 — *continued*
- venous (*see also* Varix) I86.8
  - congenital Q27.8
    - digestive system Q27.8
    - lower limb Q27.8
    - specified site NEC Q27.8
    - upper limb Q27.8
- ventricle — *see* Aneurysm, heart
- vertebral artery I72.6
- visceral NEC I72.8

Angelman syndrome Q93.5

Anger R45.4

Angiectasis, angiectopia I99.8

Angiitis I77.6
- allergic granulomatous M30.1
- hypersensitivity M31.0
- necrotizing M31.9
  - specified NEC M31.8
- nervous system, granulomatous I67.7

Angina (attack) (cardiac) (chest) (heart) (pectoris) (syndrome) (vasomotor) I20.9
- with
  - atherosclerotic heart disease — *see* Arteriosclerosis, coronary (artery)
  - documented spasm I20.1
- abdominal K55.1
- accelerated — *see* Angina, unstable
- agranulocytic — *see* Agranulocytosis
- angiospastic — *see* Angina, with, documented spasm
- aphthous B08.5
- crescendo — *see* Angina, unstable
- croupous J05.0
- cruris I73.9
- de novo effort — *see* Angina, unstable
- diphtheritic, membranous A36.0
- equivalent I20.8
- exudative, chronic J37.0
- following acute myocardial infarction I23.7
- gangrenous diphtheritic A36.0
- intestinal K55.1
- Ludovici K12.2
- Ludwig's K12.2
- malignant diphtheritic A36.0
- membranous J05.0
  - diphtheritic A36.0
  - Vincent's A69.1
- mesenteric K55.1
- monocytic — *see* Mononucleosis, infectious
- of effort — *see* Angina, specified NEC
- phlegmonous J36
  - diphtheritic A36.0
- post-infarctional I23.7
- pre-infarctional — *see* Angina, unstable
- Prinzmetal — *see* Angina, with, documented spasm
- progressive — *see* Angina, unstable
- pseudomembranous A69.1
- pultaceous, diphtheritic A36.0
- spasm-induced — *see* Angina, with, documented spasm
- specified NEC I20.8
- stable I20.8
- stenocardia — *see* Angina, specified NEC
- stridulous, diphtheritic A36.2
- tonsil J36
- trachealis J05.0
- unstable I20.0
- variant — *see* Angina, with, documented spasm
- Vincent's A69.1
- worsening effort — *see* Angina, unstable

Angioblastoma — *see* Neoplasm, connective tissue, uncertain behavior

Angiocholecystitis — *see* Cholecystitis, acute

Angiocholitis (*see also* Cholecystitis, acute) K83.0

Angiodysgenesis spinalis G95.19
Angiodysplasia (cecum) (colon) K55.20
　with bleeding K55.21
　duodenum (and stomach) K31.819
　　with bleeding K31.811
　stomach (and duodenum) K31.819
　　with bleeding K31.811
Angioedema (allergic) (any site) (with urticaria) T78.3
　hereditary D84.1
Angioendothelioma — *see* Neoplasm, uncertain behavior, by site
　benign D18.00
　　intra-abdominal D18.03
　　intracranial D18.02
　　skin D18.01
　　specified site NEC D18.09
　bone — *see* Neoplasm, bone, malignant
　Ewing's — *see* Neoplasm, bone, malignant
Angioendotheliomatosis C85.8-
Angiofibroma — *see also* Neoplasm, benign, by site
　juvenile
　　specified site — *see* Neoplasm, benign, by site
　　unspecified site D10.6
Angiohemophilia (A) (B) D68.0
Angioid streaks (choroid) (macula) (retina) H35.33
Angiokeratoma — *see* Neoplasm, skin, benign
　corporis diffusum E75.21
Angioleiomyoma — *see* Neoplasm, connective tissue, benign
Angiolipoma — *see also* Lipoma
　infiltrating — *see* Lipoma
Angioma — *see also* Hemangioma, by site
　capillary I78.1
　hemorrhagicum hereditaria I78.0
　intra-abdominal D18.03
　intracranial D18.02
　malignant — *see* Neoplasm, connective tissue, malignant
　plexiform D18.00
　　intra-abdominal D18.03
　　intracranial D18.02
　　skin D18.01
　　specified site NEC D18.09
　senile I78.1
　serpiginosum L81.7
　skin D18.01
　specified site NEC D18.09
　spider I78.1
　stellate I78.1
　venous Q28.3
Angiomatosis Q82.8
　bacillary A79.89
　encephalotrigeminal Q85.8
　hemorrhagic familial I78.0
　hereditary familial I78.0
　liver K76.4
Angiomyolipoma — *see* Lipoma
Angiomyoliposarcoma — *see* Neoplasm, connective tissue, malignant
Angiomyoma — *see* Neoplasm, connective tissue, benign
Angiomyosarcoma — *see* Neoplasm, connective tissue, malignant
Angiomyxoma — *see* Neoplasm, connective tissue, uncertain behavior
Angioneurosis F45.8
Angioneurotic edema (allergic) (any site) (with urticaria) T78.3
　hereditary D84.1
Angiopathia, angiopathy I99.9
　cerebral I67.9
　　amyloid E85.4 [I68.0]
　diabetic (peripheral) — *see* Diabetes, angiopathy

Angiopathia, angiopathy I99.9 — *continued*
　peripheral I73.9
　　diabetic — *see* Diabetes, angiopathy
　　specified type NEC I73.89
　retinae syphilitica A52.05
　retinalis (juvenilis)
　　diabetic — *see* Diabetes, retinopathy
　　proliferative — *see* Retinopathy, proliferative
Angiosarcoma — *see also* Neoplasm, connective tissue, malignant
　liver C22.3
Angiosclerosis — *see* Arteriosclerosis
Angiospasm (peripheral) (traumatic) (vessel) I73.9
　brachial plexus G54.0
　cerebral G45.9
　cervical plexus G54.2
　nerve
　　arm — *see* Mononeuropathy, upper limb
　　　axillary G54.0
　　　median — *see* Lesion, nerve, median
　　　ulnar — *see* Lesion, nerve, ulnar
　　axillary G54.0
　　leg — *see* Mononeuropathy, lower limb
　　median — *see* Lesion, nerve, median
　　plantar — *see* Lesion, nerve, plantar
　　ulnar — *see* Lesion, nerve, ulnar
Angiospastic disease or edema I73.9
Angiostrongyliasis
　due to
　　Parastrongylus
　　　cantonensis B83.2
　　　costaricensis B81.3
　intestinal B81.3
Anguillulosis — *see* Strongyloidiasis
Angulation
　cecum — *see* Obstruction, intestine
　coccyx (acquired) (*see also* subcategory) M43.8
　　congenital NEC Q76.49
　femur (acquired) — *see also* Deformity, limb, specified type NEC, thigh
　　congenital Q74.2
　intestine (large) (small) — *see* Obstruction, intestine
　sacrum (acquired) (*see also* subcategory) M43.8
　　congenital NEC Q76.49
　sigmoid (flexure) — *see* Obstruction, intestine
　spine — *see* Dorsopathy, deforming, specified NEC
　tibia (acquired) — *see also* Deformity, limb, specified type NEC, lower leg
　　congenital Q74.2
　ureter N13.5
　　with infection N13.6
　wrist (acquired) — *see also* Deformity, limb, specified type NEC, forearm
　　congenital Q74.0
Angulus infectiosus (lips) K13.0
Anhedonia R45.84
　sexual F52.0
Anhidrosis L74.4
Anhydration E86.0
Anhydremia E86.0
Anidrosis L74.4
Aniridia (congenital) Q13.1
Anisakiasis (infection) (infestation) B81.0
Anisakis larvae infestation B81.0
Aniseikonia H52.32
Anisocoria (pupil) H57.02
　congenital Q13.2
Anisocytosis R71.8
Anisometropia (congenital) H52.31
Ankle — *see* condition
Ankyloblepharon (eyelid) (acquired) — *see also* Blepharophimosis
　filiforme (adnatum) (congenital) Q10.3
　total Q10.3

Ankyloglossia Q38.1
Ankylosis (fibrous) (osseous) (joint) M24.60
　ankle M24.67-
　arthrodesis status Z98.1
　cricoarytenoid (cartilage) (joint) (larynx) J38.7
　dental K03.5
　ear ossicles H74.31-
　elbow M24.62-
　foot M24.67-
　hand M24.64-
　hip M24.65-
　incostapedial joint (infectional) — *see* Ankylosis, ear ossicles
　jaw (temporomandibular) M26.61-
　knee M24.66-
　lumbosacral (joint) M43.27
　postoperative (status) Z98.1
　produced by surgical fusion, status Z98.1
　sacro-iliac (joint) M43.28
　shoulder M24.61-
　spine (joint) — *see also* Fusion, spine
　　spondylitic — *see* Spondylitis, ankylosing
　surgical Z98.1
　temporomandibular M26.61-
　tooth, teeth (hard tissues) K03.5
　wrist M24.63-
Ankylostoma — *see* Ancylostoma
Ankylostomiasis — *see* Ancylostomiasis
Ankylurethria — *see* Stricture, urethra
Annular — *see also* condition
　detachment, cervix N88.8
　organ or site, congenital NEC — *see* Distortion
　pancreas (congenital) Q45.1
Anodontia (complete) (partial) (vera) K00.0
　acquired K08.10
Anomaly, anomalous (congenital) (unspecified type) Q89.9
　abdominal wall NEC Q79.59
　acoustic nerve Q07.8
　adrenal (gland) Q89.1
　Alder (-Reilly) (leukocyte granulation) D72.0
　alimentary tract Q45.9
　　upper Q40.9
　alveolar M26.70
　　hyperplasia M26.79
　　　mandibular M26.72
　　　maxillary M26.71
　　hypoplasia M26.79
　　　mandibular M26.74
　　　maxillary M26.73
　　ridge (process) M26.79
　　specified NEC M26.79
　ankle (joint) Q74.2
　anus Q43.9
　aorta (arch) NEC Q25.40
　　coarctation (preductal) (postductal) Q25.1
　aortic cusp or valve Q23.9
　appendix Q43.8
　apple peel syndrome Q41.1
　aqueduct of Sylvius Q03.0
　　with spina bifida — *see* Spina bifida, with hydrocephalus
　arm Q74.0
　arteriovenous NEC
　　coronary Q24.5
　　gastrointestinal Q27.33
　　　acquired — *see* Angiodysplasia
　artery (peripheral) Q27.9
　　basilar NEC Q28.1
　　cerebral Q28.3
　　coronary Q24.5
　　digestive system Q27.8
　　eye Q15.8
　　great Q25.9
　　　specified NEC Q25.8
　　lower limb Q27.8
　　peripheral Q27.9
　　　specified NEC Q27.8
　　pulmonary NEC Q25.79

Anomaly, anomalous (congenital)
  (unspecified type) Q89.9 — *continued*
    artery (peripheral) Q27.9 — *continued*
      renal Q27.2
      retina Q14.1
      specified site NEC Q27.8
      subclavian Q27.8
        origin Q25.48
      umbilical Q27.0
      upper limb Q27.8
      vertebral NEC Q28.1
    aryteno-epiglottic folds Q31.8
    atrial
      bands or folds Q20.8
      septa Q21.1
    atrioventricular
      excitation I45.6
      septum Q21.0
    auditory canal Q17.8
    auricle
      ear Q17.8
        causing impairment of hearing Q16.9
      heart Q20.8
    Axenfeld's Q15.0
    back Q89.9
    band
      atrial Q20.8
      heart Q24.8
      ventricular Q24.8
    Bartholin's duct Q38.4
    biliary duct or passage Q44.5
    bladder Q64.70
      absence Q64.5
      diverticulum Q64.6
      exstrophy Q64.10
        cloacal Q64.12
        extroversion Q64.19
        specified type NEC Q64.19
        supravesical fissure Q64.11
      neck obstruction Q64.31
      specified type NEC Q64.79
    bone Q79.9
      arm Q74.0
      face Q75.9
      leg Q74.2
      pelvic girdle Q74.2
      shoulder girdle Q74.0
      skull Q75.9
        with
          anencephaly Q00.0
          encephalocele — *see* Encephalocele
          hydrocephalus Q03.9
            with spina bifida — *see* Spina bifida,
              by site, with hydrocephalus
          microcephaly Q02
    brain (multiple) Q04.9
      vessel Q28.3
    breast Q83.9
    broad ligament Q50.6
    bronchus Q32.4
    bulbus cordis Q21.9
    bursa Q79.9
    canal of Nuck Q52.4
    canthus Q10.3
    capillary Q27.9
    cardiac Q24.9
      chambers Q20.9
        specified NEC Q20.8
      septal closure Q21.9
        specified NEC Q21.8
      valve NEC Q24.8
        pulmonary Q22.3
    cardiovascular system Q28.8
    carpus Q74.0
    caruncle, lacrimal Q10.6
    cascade stomach Q40.2
    cauda equina Q06.3
    cecum Q43.9

Anomaly, anomalous (congenital)
  (unspecified type) Q89.9 — *continued*
    cerebral Q04.9
      vessels Q28.3
    cervix Q51.9
    Chédiak-Higashi(-Steinbrinck) (congenital
      gigantism of peroxidase granules)
      E70.330
    cheek Q18.9
    chest wall Q67.8
      bones Q76.9
    chin Q18.9
    chordae tendineae Q24.8
    choroid Q14.3
      plexus Q07.8
    chromosomes, chromosomal Q99.9
      D(1) — *see* condition, chromosome 13
      E(3) — *see* condition, chromosome 18
      G — *see* condition, chromosome 21
      sex
        female phenotype Q97.8
        gonadal dysgenesis (pure) Q99.1
        Klinefelter's Q98.4
        male phenotype Q98.9
        Turner's Q96.9
      specified NEC Q99.8
    cilia Q10.3
    circulatory system Q28.9
    clavicle Q74.0
    clitoris Q52.6
    coccyx Q76.49
    colon Q43.9
    common duct Q44.5
    communication
      coronary artery Q24.5
      left ventricle with right atrium Q21.0
    concha (ear) Q17.3
    connection
      portal vein Q26.5
      pulmonary venous Q26.4
        partial Q26.3
        total Q26.2
      renal artery with kidney Q27.2
    cornea (shape) Q13.4
    coronary artery or vein Q24.5
    cranium — *see* Anomaly, skull
    cricoid cartilage Q31.8
    cystic duct Q44.5
    dental
      alveolar — *see* Anomaly, alveolar
      arch relationship M26.20
        specified NEC M26.29
    dentofacial M26.9
      alveolar — *see* Anomaly, alveolar
      dental arch relationship M26.20
        specified NEC M26.29
      functional M26.50
        specified NEC M26.59
      jaw size M26.00
        macrogenia M26.05
        mandibular
          hyperplasia M26.03
          hypoplasia M26.04
        maxillary
          hyperplasia M26.01
          hypoplasia M26.02
        microgenia M26.06
        specified type NEC M26.09
      jaw-cranial base relationship M26.10
        asymmetry M26.12
          maxillary M26.11
        specified type NEC M26.19
      malocclusion M26.4
        dental arch relationship NEC M26.29
        jaw size — *see* Anomaly, dentofacial, jaw
          size
        jaw-cranial base relationship — *see*
          Anomaly, dentofacial, jaw-cranial
          base relationship

Anomaly, anomalous (congenital)
  (unspecified type) Q89.9 — *continued*
    dentofacial M26.9 — *continued*
      specified type NEC M26.89
      temporomandibular joint M26.60-
        adhesions M26.61-
        ankylosis M26.61-
        arthralgia M26.62-
        articular disc M26.63-
        specified type NEC M26.69
      tooth position, fully erupted M26.30
        specified NEC M26.39
    dermatoglyphic Q82.8
    diaphragm (apertures) NEC Q79.1
    digestive organ(s) or tract Q45.9
      lower Q43.9
      upper Q40.9
    distance, interarch (excessive) (inadequate)
      M26.25
    distribution, coronary artery Q24.5
    ductus
      arteriosus Q25.0
      botalli Q25.0
    duodenum Q43.9
    dura (brain) Q04.9
      spinal cord Q06.9
    ear (external) Q17.9
      causing impairment of hearing Q16.9
      inner Q16.5
      middle (causing impairment of hearing)
        Q16.4
      ossicles Q16.3
    Ebstein's (heart) (tricuspid valve) Q22.5
    ectodermal Q82.9
    Eisenmenger's (ventricular septal defect)
      Q21.8
    ejaculatory duct Q55.4
    elbow Q74.0
    endocrine gland NEC Q89.2
    epididymis Q55.4
    epiglottis Q31.8
    esophagus Q39.9
    eustachian tube Q17.8
    eye Q15.9
      anterior segment Q13.9
        specified NEC Q13.89
      posterior segment Q14.9
        specified NEC Q14.8
      ptosis (eyelid) Q10.0
      specified NEC Q15.8
    eyebrow Q18.8
    eyelid Q10.3
      ptosis Q10.0
    face Q18.9
      bone(s) Q75.9
    fallopian tube Q50.6
    fascia Q79.9
    femur NEC Q74.2
    fibula NEC Q74.2
    finger Q74.0
    fixation, intestine Q43.3
    flexion (joint) NOS Q74.9
      hip or thigh Q65.89
    foot NEC Q74.2
      varus (congenital) Q66.3
    foramen
      Botalli Q21.1
      ovale Q21.1
    forearm Q74.0
    forehead Q75.8
    form, teeth K00.2
    fovea centralis Q14.1
    frontal bone — *see* Anomaly, skull
    gallbladder (position) (shape) (size) Q44.1
    Gartner's duct Q52.4
    gastrointestinal tract Q45.9

Anomaly, anomalous (congenital)
(unspecified type) Q89.9 — *continued*
genitalia, genital organ(s) or system
    female Q52.9
        external Q52.70
        internal NOS Q52.9
    male Q55.9
        hydrocele P83.5
        specified NEC Q55.8
genitourinary NEC
    female Q52.9
    male Q55.9
Gerbode Q21.0
glottis Q31.8
granulation or granulocyte, genetic
    (constitutional) (leukocyte) D72.0
gum Q38.6
gyri Q07.9
hair Q84.2
hand Q74.0
hard tissue formation in pulp K04.3
head — *see* Anomaly, skull
heart Q24.9
    auricle Q20.8
    bands or folds Q24.8
    fibroelastosis cordis I42.4
    obstructive NEC Q22.6
    patent ductus arteriosus (Botalli) Q25.0
    septum Q21.9
        auricular Q21.1
        interatrial Q21.1
        interventricular Q21.0
            with pulmonary stenosis or atresia,
                dextraposition of aorta and
                hypertrophy of right ventricle Q21.3
        specified NEC Q21.8
        ventricular Q21.0
            with pulmonary stenosis or atresia,
                dextraposition of aorta and
                hypertrophy of right ventricle Q21.3
    tetralogy of Fallot Q21.3
    valve NEC Q24.8
        aortic
            bicuspid valve Q23.1
            insufficiency Q23.1
            stenosis Q23.0
                subaortic Q24.4
        mitral
            insufficiency Q23.3
            stenosis Q23.2
        pulmonary Q22.3
            atresia Q22.0
            insufficiency Q22.2
            stenosis Q22.1
                infundibular Q24.3
                subvalvular Q24.3
        tricuspid
            atresia Q22.4
            stenosis Q22.4
    ventricle Q20.8
heel NEC Q74.2
Hegglin's D72.0
hemianencephaly Q00.0
hemicephaly Q00.0
hemicrania Q00.0
hepatic duct Q44.5
hip NEC Q74.2
hourglass stomach Q40.2
humerus Q74.0
hydatid of Morgagni
    female Q50.5
    male (epididymal) Q55.4
        testicular Q55.29
hymen Q52.4
hypersegmentation of neutrophils, hereditary
    D72.0
hypophyseal Q89.2
ileocecal (coil) (valve) Q43.9
ileum Q43.9

Anomaly, anomalous (congenital)
(unspecified type) Q89.9 — *continued*
ilium NEC Q74.2
integument Q84.9
    specified NEC Q84.8
interarch distance (excessive) (inadequate)
    M26.25
intervertebral cartilage or disc Q76.49
intestine (large) (small) Q43.9
    with anomalous adhesions, fixation or
        malrotation Q43.3
iris Q13.2
ischium NEC Q74.2
jaw — *see* Anomaly, dentofacial
    alveolar — *see* Anomaly, alveolar
jaw-cranial base relationship — *see* Anomaly,
    dentofacial, jaw-cranial base relationship
jejunum Q43.8
joint Q74.9
    specified NEC Q74.8
Jordan's D72.0
kidney(s) (calyx) (pelvis) Q63.9
    artery Q27.2
    specified NEC Q63.8
Klippel-Feil (brevicollis) Q76.1
knee Q74.1
labium (majus) (minus) Q52.70
labyrinth, membranous Q16.5
lacrimal apparatus or duct Q10.6
larynx, laryngeal (muscle) Q31.9
    web(bed) Q31.0
lens Q12.9
leukocytes, genetic D72.0
    granulation (constitutional) D72.0
lid (fold) Q10.3
ligament Q79.9
    broad Q50.6
    round Q52.8
limb Q74.9
    lower NEC Q74.2
        reduction deformity — *see* Defect,
            reduction, lower limb
    upper Q74.0
lip Q38.0
liver Q44.7
    duct Q44.5
lower limb NEC Q74.2
lumbosacral (joint) (region) Q76.49
    kyphosis — *see* Kyphosis, congenital
    lordosis — *see* Lordosis, congenital
lung (fissure) (lobe) Q33.9
mandible — *see* Anomaly, dentofacial
maxilla — *see* Anomaly, dentofacial
May (-Hegglin) D72.0
meatus urinarius NEC Q64.79
meningeal bands or folds Q07.9
    constriction of Q07.8
    spinal Q06.9
meninges Q07.9
    cerebral Q04.8
    spinal Q06.9
meningocele Q05.9
mesentery Q45.9
metacarpus Q74.0
metatarsus NEC Q74.2
middle ear Q16.4
    ossicles Q16.3
mitral (leaflets) (valve) Q23.9
    insufficiency Q23.3
    specified NEC Q23.8
    stenosis Q23.2
mouth Q38.6
Müllerian — *see also* Anomaly, by site
    uterus NEC Q51.818
multiple NEC Q89.7
muscle Q79.9
    eyelid Q10.3
musculoskeletal system, except limbs Q79.9
myocardium Q24.8

Anomaly, anomalous (congenital)
(unspecified type) Q89.9 — *continued*
nail Q84.6
narrowness, eyelid Q10.3
nasal sinus (wall) Q30.8
neck (any part) Q18.9
nerve Q07.9
    acoustic Q07.8
    optic Q07.8
nervous system (central) Q07.9
nipple Q83.9
nose, nasal (bones) (cartilage) (septum) (sinus)
    Q30.9
    specified NEC Q30.8
ocular muscle Q15.8
omphalomesenteric duct Q43.0
opening, pulmonary veins Q26.4
optic
    disc Q14.2
    nerve Q07.8
opticociliary vessels Q13.2
orbit (eye) Q10.7
organ Q89.9
    of Corti Q16.5
origin
    artery
        innominate Q25.8
        pulmonary Q25.79
        renal Q27.2
        subclavian Q25.48
osseous meatus (ear) Q16.1
ovary Q50.39
oviduct Q50.6
palate (hard) (soft) NEC Q38.5
pancreas or pancreatic duct Q45.3
papillary muscles Q24.8
parathyroid gland Q89.2
paraurethral ducts Q64.79
parotid (gland) Q38.4
patella Q74.1
Pelger-Huët (hereditary hyposegmentation)
    D72.0
pelvic girdle NEC Q74.2
pelvis (bony) NEC Q74.2
    rachitic E64.3
penis (glans) Q55.69
pericardium Q24.8
peripheral vascular system Q27.9
Peter's Q13.4
pharynx Q38.8
pigmentation L81.9
    congenital Q82.8
pituitary (gland) Q89.2
pleural (folds) Q34.0
portal vein Q26.5
    connection Q26.5
position, tooth, teeth, fully erupted M26.30
    specified NEC M26.39
precerebral vessel Q28.1
prepuce Q55.69
prostate Q55.4
pulmonary Q33.9
    artery NEC Q25.79
    valve Q22.3
        atresia Q22.0
        insufficiency Q22.2
        specified type NEC Q22.3
        stenosis Q22.1
            infundibular Q24.3
            subvalvular Q24.3
    venous connection Q26.4
        partial Q26.3
        total Q26.2
pupil Q13.2
    function H57.00
        anisocoria H57.02
        Argyll Robertson pupil H57.01
        miosis H57.03
        mydriasis H57.04

Anomaly, anomalous (congenital) (unspecified type) Q89.9 — *continued*
  pupil Q13.2 — *continued*
    function H57.00 — *continued*
      specified type NEC H57.09
      tonic pupil H57.05-
  pylorus Q40.3
  radius Q74.0
  rectum Q43.9
  reduction (extremity) (limb)
    femur (longitudinal) — *see* Defect, reduction, lower limb, longitudinal, femur
    fibula (longitudinal) — *see* Defect, reduction, lower limb, longitudinal, fibula
    lower limb — *see* Defect, reduction, lower limb
    radius (longitudinal) — *see* Defect, reduction, upper limb, longitudinal, radius
    tibia (longitudinal) — *see* Defect, reduction, lower limb, longitudinal, tibia
    ulna (longitudinal) — *see* Defect, reduction, upper limb, longitudinal, ulna
    upper limb — *see* Defect, reduction, upper limb
  refraction — *see* Disorder, refraction
  renal Q63.9
    artery Q27.2
    pelvis Q63.9
      specified NEC Q63.8
  respiratory system Q34.9
    specified NEC Q34.8
  retina Q14.1
  rib Q76.6
    cervical Q76.5
  Rieger's Q13.81
  rotation — *see* Malrotation
    hip or thigh Q65.89
  round ligament Q52.8
  sacroiliac (joint) NEC Q74.2
  sacrum NEC Q76.49
    kyphosis — *see* Kyphosis, congenital
    lordosis — *see* Lordosis, congenital
  saddle nose, syphilitic A50.57
  salivary duct or gland Q38.4
  scapula Q74.0
  scrotum — *see* Malformation, testis and scrotum
  sebaceous gland Q82.9
  seminal vesicles Q55.4
  sense organs NEC Q07.8
  sex chromosomes NEC — *see also* Anomaly, chromosomes
    female phenotype Q97.8
    male phenotype Q98.9
  shoulder (girdle) (joint) Q74.0
  sigmoid (flexure) Q43.9
  simian crease Q82.8
  sinus of Valsalva Q25.49
  skeleton generalized Q78.9
  skin (appendage) Q82.9
  skull Q75.9
    with
      anencephaly Q00.0
      encephalocele — *see* Encephalocele
      hydrocephalus Q03.9
        with spina bifida — *see* Spina bifida, by site, with hydrocephalus
      microcephaly Q02
  specified organ or site NEC Q89.8
  spermatic cord Q55.4
  spine, spinal NEC Q76.49
    column NEC Q76.49
      kyphosis — *see* Kyphosis, congenital
      lordosis — *see* Lordosis, congenital
    cord Q06.9
    nerve root Q07.8
  spleen Q89.09
    agenesis Q89.01
  stenonian duct Q38.4
  sternum NEC Q76.7

Anomaly, anomalous (congenital) (unspecified type) Q89.9 — *continued*
  stomach Q40.3
  submaxillary gland Q38.4
  tarsus NEC Q74.2
  tendon Q79.9
  testis — *see* Malformation, testis and scrotum
  thigh NEC Q74.2
  thorax (wall) Q67.8
    bony Q76.9
  throat Q38.8
  thumb Q74.0
  thymus gland Q89.2
  thyroid (gland) Q89.2
    cartilage Q31.8
  tibia NEC Q74.2
    saber A50.56
  toe Q74.2
  tongue Q38.3
  tooth, teeth K00.9
    eruption K00.6
    position, fully erupted M26.30
    spacing, fully erupted M26.30
  trachea (cartilage) Q32.1
  tragus Q17.9
  tricuspid (leaflet) (valve) Q22.9
    atresia or stenosis Q22.4
    Ebstein's Q22.5
  Uhl's (hypoplasia of myocardium, right ventricle) Q24.8
  ulna Q74.0
  umbilical artery Q27.0
  union
    cricoid cartilage and thyroid cartilage Q31.8
    thyroid cartilage and hyoid bone Q31.8
    trachea with larynx Q31.8
  upper limb Q74.0
  urachus Q64.4
  ureter Q62.8
    obstructive NEC Q62.39
      cecoureterocele Q62.32
      orthotopic ureterocele Q62.31
  urethra Q64.70
    absence Q64.5
    double Q64.74
    fistula to rectum Q64.73
    obstructive Q64.39
      stricture Q64.32
    prolapse Q64.71
    specified type NEC Q64.79
  urinary tract Q64.9
  uterus Q51.9
    with only one functioning horn Q51.4
  uvula Q38.5
  vagina Q52.4
  valleculae Q31.8
  valve (heart) NEC Q24.8
    coronary sinus Q24.5
    inferior vena cava Q24.8
    pulmonary Q22.3
    sinus coronario Q24.5
    venae cavae inferioris Q24.8
  vas deferens Q55.4
  vascular Q27.9
    brain Q28.3
    ring Q25.45
  vein(s) (peripheral) Q27.9
    brain Q28.3
    cerebral Q28.3
    coronary Q24.5
    developmental Q28.3
    great Q26.9
      specified NEC Q26.8
  vena cava (inferior) (superior) Q26.9
  venous — *see* Anomaly, vein(s)
  venous return Q26.8
  ventricular
    bands or folds Q24.8
    septa Q21.0

Anomaly, anomalous (congenital) (unspecified type) Q89.9 — *continued*
  vertebra Q76.49
    kyphosis — *see* Kyphosis, congenital
    lordosis — *see* Lordosis, congenital
  vesicourethral orifice Q64.79
  vessel(s) Q27.9
    optic papilla Q14.2
    precerebral Q28.1
  vitelline duct Q43.0
  vitreous body or humor Q14.0
  vulva Q52.70
  wrist (joint) Q74.0
Anomia R48.8
Anonychia (congenital) Q84.3
  acquired L60.8
Anophthalmos, anophthalmus (congenital) (globe) Q11.1
  acquired Z90.01
Anopia, anopsia H53.46-
  quadrant H53.46-
Anorchia, anorchism, anorchidism Q55.0
Anorexia R63.0
  hysterical F44.89
  nervosa F50.00
    atypical F50.9
    binge-eating type F50.2
      with purging F50.02
    restricting type F50.01
Anorgasmy, psychogenic (female) F52.31
  male F52.32
Anosmia R43.0
  hysterical F44.6
  postinfectional J39.8
Anosognosia R41.89
Anosteoplasia Q78.9
Anovulatory cycle N97.0
Anoxemia R09.02
  newborn P84
Anoxia (pathological) R09.02
  altitude T70.29
  cerebral G93.1
    complicating
      anesthesia (general) (local) or other sedation T88.59
        in labor and delivery O74.3
        in pregnancy O29.21-
        postpartum, puerperal O89.2
      delivery (cesarean) (instrumental) O75.4
    during a procedure G97.81
    newborn P84
    resulting from a procedure G97.82
  due to
    drowning T75.1
    high altitude T70.29
  heart — *see* Insufficiency, coronary
  intrauterine P84
  myocardial — *see* Insufficiency, coronary
  newborn P84
  spinal cord G95.11
  systemic (by suffocation) (low content in atmosphere) — *see* Asphyxia, traumatic
Anteflexion — *see* Anteversion
Antenatal
  care (normal pregnancy) Z34.90
  screening (encounter for) of mother Z36
Antepartum — *see* condition
Anterior — *see* condition
Antero-occlusion M26.220
Anteversion
  cervix — *see* Anteversion, uterus
  femur (neck), congenital Q65.89
  uterus, uterine (cervix) (postinfectional) (postpartal) (old) N85.4
    congenital Q51.818
    in pregnancy or childbirth — *see* Pregnancy, complicated by
Anthophobia F40.228
Anthracosilicosis J60

Anthracosis (lung) (occupational) J60
 lingua K14.3
Anthrax A22.9
 with pneumonia A22.1
 cerebral A22.8
 colitis A22.2
 cutaneous A22.0
 gastrointestinal A22.2
 inhalation A22.1
 intestinal A22.2
 meningitis A22.8
 pulmonary A22.1
 respiratory A22.1
 sepsis A22.7
 specified manifestation NEC A22.8
Anthropoid pelvis Q74.2
 with disproportion (fetopelvic) O33.0
Anthropophobia F40.10
 generalized F40.11
Antibodies, maternal (blood group) — *see*
 Isoimmunization, affecting management of
 pregnancy
 anti-D — *see* Isoimmunization, affecting
 management of pregnancy, Rh
 newborn P55.0
Antibody
 anticardiolipin R76.0
 with
 hemorrhagic disorder D68.312
 hypercoagulable state D68.61
 antiphosphatidylglycerol R76.0
 with
 hemorrhagic disorder D68.312
 hypercoagulable state D68.61
 antiphosphatidylinositol R76.0
 with
 hemorrhagic disorder D68.312
 hypercoagulable state D68.61
 antiphosphatidylserine R76.0
 with
 hemorrhagic disorder D68.312
 hypercoagulable state D68.61
 antiphospholipid R76.0
 with
 hemorrhagic disorder D68.312
 hypercoagulable state D68.61
Anticardiolipin syndrome D68.61
Anticoagulant, circulating (intrinsic) (*see also*
 Disorder, hemorrhagic) D68.318
 drug-induced (extrinsic) (*see also* Disorder,
 hemorrhagic) D68.32
 iatrogenic D68.32
Antidiuretic hormone syndrome E22.2
Antimonial cholera — *see* Poisoning,
 antimony
Antiphospholipid
 antibody
 with hemorrhagic disorder D68.312
 syndrome D68.61
Antisocial personality F60.2
Antithrombinemia — *see* Circulating
 anticoagulants
Antithromboplastinemia D68.318
Antithromboplastinogenemia D68.318
Antitoxin complication or reaction — *see*
 Complications, vaccination
Antlophobia F40.228
Antritis J32.0
 maxilla J32.0
 acute J01.00
 recurrent J01.01
 stomach K29.60
 with bleeding K29.61
Antrum, antral — *see* condition

Anuria R34
 calculous (impacted) (recurrent) (*see also*
 Calculus, urinary) N20.9
 following
 abortion — *see* Abortion, by type,
 complicated by, renal failure
 ectopic or molar pregnancy O08.4
 newborn P96.0
 postprocedural N99.0
 postrenal N13.8
 traumatic (following crushing) T79.5
Anus, anal — *see* condition
Anusitis K62.89
Anxiety F41.9
 depression F41.8
 episodic paroxysmal F41.0
 generalized F41.1
 hysteria F41.8
 neurosis F41.1
 panic type F41.0
 reaction F41.1
 separation, abnormal (of childhood) F93.0
 specified NEC F41.8
 state F41.1
Aorta, aortic — *see* condition
Aortectasia — *see* Ectasia, aorta
 with aneurysm — *see* Aneurysm, aorta
Aortitis (nonsyphilitic) (calcific) I77.6
 arteriosclerotic I70.0
 Doehle-Heller A52.02
 luetic A52.02
 rheumatic — *see* Endocarditis, acute,
 rheumatic
 specific (syphilitic) A52.02
 syphilitic A52.02
 congenital A50.54 *[I79.1]*
Apathetic thyroid storm — *see*
 Thyrotoxicosis
Apathy R45.3
Apeirophobia F40.228
Apepsia K30
 psychogenic F45.8
Aperistalsis, esophagus K22.0
Apertognathia M26.29
Apert's syndrome Q87.0
Aphagia R13.0
 psychogenic F50.9
Aphakia (acquired) (postoperative) H27.0-
 congenital Q12.3
Aphasia (amnestic) (global) (nominal)
 (semantic) (syntactic) R47.01
 acquired, with epilepsy (Landau-Kleffner
 syndrome) — *see* Epilepsy, specified NEC
 auditory (developmental) F80.2
 developmental (receptive type) F80.2
 expressive type F80.1
 Wernicke's F80.2
 following
 cerebrovascular disease I69.920
 cerebral infarction I69.320
 intracerebral hemorrhage I69.120
 nontraumatic intracranial hemorrhage
 NEC I69.220
 specified disease NEC I69.820
 subarachnoid hemorrhage I69.020
 primary progressive G31.01 *[F02.80]*
 with behavioral disturbance G31.01
 [F02.81]
 progressive isolated G31.01 *[F02.80]*
 with behavioral disturbance G31.01
 [F02.81]
 sensory F80.2
 syphilis, tertiary A52.19
 Wernicke's (developmental) F80.2
Aphonia (organic) R49.1
 hysterical F44.4
 psychogenic F44.4

Aphthae, aphthous — *see also* condition
 Bednar's K12.0
 cachectic K14.0
 epizootic B08.8
 fever B08.8
 oral (recurrent) K12.0
 stomatitis (major) (minor) K12.0
 thrush B37.0
 ulcer (oral) (recurrent) K12.0
 genital organ(s) NEC
 female N76.6
 male N50.89
 larynx J38.7
Apical — *see* condition
Apiphobia F40.218
Aplasia — *see also* Agenesis
 abdominal muscle syndrome Q79.4
 alveolar process (acquired) — *see* Anomaly,
 alveolar
 congenital Q38.6
 aorta (congenital) Q25.41
 axialis extracorticalis (congenita) E75.29
 bone marrow (myeloid) D61.9
 congenital D61.01
 brain Q00.0
 part of Q04.3
 bronchus Q32.4
 cementum K00.4
 cerebellum Q04.3
 cervix (congenital) Q51.5
 congenital pure red cell D61.01
 corpus callosum Q04.0
 cutis congenita Q84.8
 erythrocyte congenital D61.01
 extracortical axial E75.29
 eye Q11.1
 fovea centralis (congenital) Q14.1
 gallbladder, congenital Q44.0
 iris Q13.1
 labyrinth, membranous Q16.5
 limb (congenital) Q73.8
 lower — *see* Defect, reduction, lower limb
 upper — *see* Agenesis, arm
 lung, congenital (bilateral) (unilateral) Q33.3
 pancreas Q45.0
 parathyroid-thymic D82.1
 Pelizaeus-Merzbacher E75.29
 penis Q55.5
 prostate Q55.4
 red cell (with thymoma) D60.9
 acquired D60.9
 due to drugs D60.9
 adult D60.9
 chronic D60.0
 congenital D61.01
 constitutional D61.01
 due to drugs D60.9
 hereditary D61.01
 of infants D61.01
 primary D61.01
 pure D61.01
 due to drugs D60.9
 specified type NEC D60.8
 transient D60.1
 round ligament Q52.8
 skin Q84.8
 spermatic cord Q55.4
 spleen Q89.01
 testicle Q55.0
 thymic, with immunodeficiency D82.1
 thyroid (congenital) (with myxedema) E03.1
 uterus Q51.0
 ventral horn cell Q06.1

Apnea, apneic (of) (spells) R06.81
 newborn NEC P28.4
  obstructive P28.4
  sleep (central) (obstructive) (primary) P28.3
  prematurity P28.4
 sleep G47.30
  central (primary) G47.31
   in conditions classified elsewhere G47.37
  obstructive (adult) (pediatric) G47.33
  primary central G47.31
  specified NEC G47.39
Apneumatosis, newborn P28.0
Apocrine metaplasia (breast) — see
 Dysplasia, mammary, specified type NEC
Apophysitis (bone) — see also
 Osteochondropathy
 calcaneus M92.8
 juvenile M92.9
Apoplectiform convulsions (cerebral
 ischemia) I67.82
Apoplexia, apoplexy, apoplectic
 adrenal A39.1
 heart (auricle) (ventricle) — see Infarct,
  myocardium
 heat T67.0
 hemorrhagic (stroke) — see Hemorrhage,
  intracranial
 meninges, hemorrhagic — see Hemorrhage,
  intracranial, subarachnoid
 uremic N18.9 *[I68.8]*
Appearance
 bizarre R46.1
 specified NEC R46.89
 very low level of personal hygiene R46.0
Appendage
 epididymal (organ of Morgagni) Q55.4
 intestine (epiploic) Q43.8
 preauricular Q17.0
 testicular (organ of Morgagni) Q55.29
Appendicitis (pneumococcal) (retrocecal) K37
 with
  perforation or rupture K35.2
  peritoneal abscess K35.3
  peritonitis K35.2
   generalized (with perforation or rupture)
    K35.2
   localized (with perforation or rupture)
    K35.3
 acute (catarrhal) (fulminating) (gangrenous)
  (obstructive) (retrocecal) (suppurative)
  K35.80
  with
   peritoneal abscess K35.3
   peritonitis K35.3
    generalized (with perforation or rupture)
     K35.2
    localized (with perforation or rupture)
     K35.3
   specified NEC K35.89
 amebic A06.89
 chronic (recurrent) K36
 exacerbation — see Appendicitis, acute
 gangrenous — see Appendicitis, acute
 healed (obliterative) K36
 interval K36
 neurogenic K36
 obstructive K36
 recurrent K36
 relapsing K36
 subacute (adhesive) K36
 subsiding K36
 suppurative — see Appendicitis, acute
 tuberculous A18.32
Appendicopathia oxyurica B80
Appendix, appendicular — see also
 condition
 epididymis Q55.4

Appendix, appendicular — see also
 condition — continued
 Morgagni
  female Q50.5
  male (epididymal) Q55.4
   testicular Q55.29
 testis Q55.29
Appetite
 depraved — see Pica
 excessive R63.2
 lack or loss (see also Anorexia) R63.0
  nonorganic origin F50.89
  psychogenic F50.89
 perverted (hysterical) — see Pica
Apple peel syndrome Q41.1
Apprehension state F41.1
Apprehensiveness, abnormal F41.9
Approximal wear K03.0
Apraxia (classic) (ideational) (ideokinetic)
 (ideomotor) (motor) (verbal) R48.2
 following
  cerebrovascular disease I69.990
   cerebral infarction I69.390
   intracerebral hemorrhage I69.190
   nontraumatic intracranial hemorrhage
    NEC I69.290
   specified disease NEC I69.890
   subarachnoid hemorrhage I69.090
 oculomotor, congenital H51.8
Aptyalism K11.7
Apudoma — see Neoplasm, uncertain
 behavior, by site
Aqueous misdirection H40.83-
Arabicum elephantiasis — see Infestation,
 filarial
Arachnitis — see Meningitis
Arachnodactyly — see Syndrome, Marfan's
Arachnoiditis (acute) (adhesive) (basal) (brain)
 (cerebrospinal) — see Meningitis
Arachnophobia F40.210
Arboencephalitis, Australian A83.4
Arborization block (heart) I45.5
ARC (AIDS-related complex) B20
Arches — see condition
Arcuate uterus Q51.810
Arcuatus uterus Q51.810
Arcus (cornea) senilis — see Degeneration,
 cornea, senile
Arc-welder's lung J63.4
Areflexia R29.2
Areola — see condition
Argentaffinoma — see also Neoplasm,
 uncertain behavior, by site
 malignant — see Neoplasm, malignant, by site
 syndrome E34.0
Argininemia E72.21
Arginosuccinic aciduria E72.22
**Argyll Robertson phenomenon, pupil or
 syndrome** (syphilitic) A52.19
 atypical H57.09
 nonsyphilitic H57.09
Argyria, argyriasis
 conjunctival H11.13-
 from drug or medicament — see Table of
  Drugs and Chemicals, by substance
Argyrosis, conjunctival H11.13-
Arhinencephaly Q04.1
Ariboflavinosis E53.0
Arm — see condition
**Arnold-Chiari disease, obstruction or
 syndrome** (type II) Q07.00
 with
  hydrocephalus Q07.02
   with spina bifida Q07.03
  spina bifida Q07.01
   with hydrocephalus Q07.03
 type III — see Encephalocele
 type IV Q04.8

**Aromatic amino-acid metabolism
 disorder** E70.9
 specified NEC E70.8
Arousals, confusional G47.51
Arrest, arrested
 cardiac I46.9
  complicating
   abortion — see Abortion, by type,
    complicated by, cardiac arrest
   anesthesia (general) (local) or other
    sedation — see Table of Drugs and
    Chemicals, by drug,
    in labor and delivery O74.2
    in pregnancy O29.11-
    postpartum, puerperal O89.1
   delivery (cesarean) (instrumental) O75.4
  due to
   cardiac condition I46.2
   specified condition NEC I46.8
  intraoperative I97.71-
  newborn P29.81
  postprocedural I97.12-
   obstetric procedure O75.4
 cardiorespiratory — see Arrest, cardiac
 circulatory — see Arrest, cardiac
 deep transverse O64.0
 development or growth
  bone — see Disorder, bone, development or
   growth
  child R62.50
  tracheal rings Q32.1
 epiphyseal
  complete
   femur M89.15-
   humerus M89.12-
   tibia M89.16-
   ulna M89.13-
   forearm M89.13-
    specified NEC M89.13-
    ulna — see Arrest, epiphyseal, by type,
     ulna
   lower leg M89.16-
    specified NEC M89.168
    tibia — see Arrest, epiphyseal, by type,
     tibia
  partial
   femur M89.15-
   humerus M89.12-
   tibia M89.16-
   ulna M89.13-
  specified NEC M89.18
 granulopoiesis — see Agranulocytosis
 growth plate — see Arrest, epiphyseal
 heart — see Arrest, cardiac
 legal, anxiety concerning Z65.3
 physeal — see Arrest, epiphyseal
 respiratory R09.2
  newborn P28.81
 sinus I45.5
 spermatogenesis (complete) — see
  Azoospermia
  incomplete — see Oligospermia
 transverse (deep) O64.0
Arrhenoblastoma
 benign
  specified site — see Neoplasm, benign, by
   site
  unspecified site
   female D27.9
   male D29.20
 malignant
  specified site — see Neoplasm, malignant,
   by site
  unspecified site
   female C56.9
   male C62.90
 specified site — see Neoplasm, uncertain
  behavior, by site

Arrhenoblastoma — *continued*
  unspecified site
    female D39.10
    male D40.10
Arrhythmia (auricle) (cardiac) (juvenile)
    (nodal) (reflex) (sinus) (supraventricular)
    (transitory) (ventricle) I49.9
  block I45.9
  extrasystolic I49.49
  newborn
    bradycardia P29.12
    occurring before birth P03.819
      before onset of labor P03.810
      during labor P03.811
    tachycardia P29.11
  psychogenic F45.8
  specified NEC I49.8
  vagal R55
  ventricular re-entry I47.0
Arrillaga-Ayerza syndrome (pulmonary
    sclerosis with pulmonary hypertension)
    I27.0
Arsenical pigmentation L81.8
  from drug or medicament — *see* Table of
    Drugs and Chemicals
Arsenism — *see* Poisoning, arsenic
Arterial — *see* condition
Arteriofibrosis — *see* Arteriosclerosis
Arteriolar sclerosis — *see* Arteriosclerosis
Arteriolith — *see* Arteriosclerosis
Arteriolitis I77.6
  necrotizing, kidney I77.5
  renal — *see* Hypertension, kidney
Arteriolosclerosis — *see* Arteriosclerosis
Arterionephrosclerosis — *see* Hypertension,
    kidney
Arteriopathy I77.9
Arteriosclerosis, arteriosclerotic (diffuse)
    (obliterans) (of) (senile) (with calcification)
    I70.90
  aorta I70.0
  arteries of extremities — *see* Arteriosclerosis,
    extremities
  brain I67.2
  bypass graft
    coronary — *see* Arteriosclerosis, coronary,
      bypass graft
    extremities — *see* Arteriosclerosis,
      extremities, bypass graft
  cardiac — *see* Disease, heart, ischemic,
    atherosclerotic
  cardiopathy — *see* Disease, heart, ischemic,
    atherosclerotic
  cardiorenal — *see* Hypertension, cardiorenal
  cardiovascular — *see* Disease, heart, ischemic,
    atherosclerotic
  carotid (*see also* Occlusion, artery, carotid)
    I65.2-
  central nervous system I67.2
  cerebral I67.2
  cerebrovascular I67.2
  coronary (artery) I25.10
    bypass graft I25.810
      with
        angina pectoris I25.709
          with documented spasm I25.701
          specified type NEC I25.708
          unstable I25.700
        ischemic chest pain I25.709
      autologous artery I25.810
        with
          angina pectoris I25.729
            with documented spasm I25.721
            specified type I25.728
            unstable I25.720
          ischemic chest pain I25.729

Arteriosclerosis, arteriosclerotic (diffuse)
    (obliterans) (of) (senile) (with calcification)
    I70.90 — *continued*
  coronary (artery) I25.10 — *continued*
    bypass graft I25.810 — *continued*
      autologous vein I25.810
        with
          angina pectoris I25.719
            with documented spasm I25.711
            specified type I25.718
            unstable I25.710
          ischemic chest pain I25.719
        nonautologous biological I25.810
          with
            angina pectoris I25.739
              with documented spasm I25.731
              specified type I25.738
              unstable I25.730
            ischemic chest pain I25.739
        specified type NEC I25.810
          with
            angina pectoris I25.799
              with documented spasm I25.791
              specified type I25.798
              unstable I25.790
            ischemic chest pain I25.799
    due to
      calcified coronary lesion (severely) I25.84
      lipid rich plaque I25.83
    native vessel
      with
        angina pectoris I25.119
          with documented spasm I25.111
          specified type NEC I25.118
          unstable I25.110
        ischemic chest pain I25.119
    transplanted heart I25.811
      bypass graft I25.812
        with
          angina pectoris I25.769
            with documented spasm I25.761
            specified type I25.768
            unstable I25.760
          ischemic chest pain I25.769
      native coronary artery I25.811
        with
          angina pectoris I25.759
            with documented spasm I25.751
            specified type I25.758
            unstable I25.750
          ischemic chest pain I25.759
  extremities (native arteries) I70.209
    bypass graft I70.309
      autologous vein graft I70.409
        leg I70.409
          with
            gangrene (and intermittent
              claudication, rest pain and
              ulcer) I70.469
            intermittent claudication I70.419
            rest pain (and intermittent
              claudication) I70.429
          bilateral I70.403
            with
              gangrene (and intermittent
                claudication, rest pain and
                ulcer) I70.463
              intermittent claudication I70.413
              rest pain (and intermittent
                claudication) I70.423
              specified type NEC I70.493

Arteriosclerosis, arteriosclerotic (diffuse)
    (obliterans) (of) (senile) (with calcification)
    I70.90 — *continued*
  extremities (native arteries) I70.209 —
    continued
    bypass graft I70.309 — *continued*
      autologous vein graft I70.409 —
        continued
        leg I70.409 — *continued*
          left I70.402
            with
              gangrene (and intermittent
                claudication, rest pain and
                ulcer) I70.462
              intermittent claudication I70.412
              rest pain (and intermittent
                claudication) I70.422
              ulceration (and intermittent
                claudication and rest pain)
                I70.449
                ankle I70.443
                calf I70.442
                foot site NEC I70.445
                heel I70.444
                lower leg NEC I70.448
                midfoot I70.444
                thigh I70.441
              specified type NEC I70.492
          right I70.401
            with
              gangrene (and intermittent
                claudication, rest pain and
                ulcer) I70.461
              intermittent claudication I70.411
              rest pain (and intermittent
                claudication) I70.421
              ulceration (and intermittent
                claudication and rest pain)
                I70.439
                ankle I70.433
                calf I70.432
                foot site NEC I70.435
                heel I70.434
                lower leg NEC I70.438
                midfoot I70.434
                thigh I70.431
              specified type NEC I70.491
          specified type NEC I70.499
        specified NEC I70.408
          with
            gangrene (and intermittent
              claudication, rest pain and
              ulcer) I70.468
            intermittent claudication I70.418
            rest pain (and intermittent
              claudication) I70.428
            ulceration (and intermittent
              claudication and rest pain)
              I70.45
            specified type NEC I70.498
      leg I70.309
        with
          gangrene (and intermittent
            claudication, rest pain and ulcer)
            I70.369
          intermittent claudication I70.319
          rest pain (and intermittent
            claudication) I70.329
        bilateral I70.303
          with
            gangrene (and intermittent
              claudication, rest pain and
              ulcer) I70.363
            intermittent claudication I70.313
            rest pain (and intermittent
              claudication) I70.323
          specified type NEC I70.393

DISEASE INDEX

Arteriosclerosis, arteriosclerotic (diffuse) (obliterans) (of) (senile) (with calcification) I70.90 — *continued*
  extremities (native arteries) I70.209 — *continued*
    bypass graft I70.309 — *continued*
      leg I70.309 — *continued*
        left I70.302
          with
            gangrene (and intermittent claudication, rest pain and ulcer) I70.362
            intermittent claudication I70.312
            rest pain (and intermittent claudication) I70.322
            ulceration (and intermittent claudication and rest pain) I70.349
              ankle I70.343
              calf I70.342
              foot site NEC I70.345
              heel I70.344
              lower leg NEC I70.348
              midfoot I70.344
              thigh I70.341
            specified type NEC I70.392
        right I70.301
          with
            gangrene (and intermittent claudication, rest pain and ulcer) I70.361
            intermittent claudication I70.311
            rest pain (and intermittent claudication) I70.321
            ulceration (and intermittent claudication and rest pain) I70.339
              ankle I70.333
              calf I70.332
              foot site NEC I70.335
              heel I70.334
              lower leg NEC I70.338
              midfoot I70.334
              thigh I70.331
            specified type NEC I70.391
        specified type NEC I70.399
      nonautologous biological graft I70.509
        leg I70.509
          with
            gangrene (and intermittent claudication, rest pain and ulcer) I70.569
            intermittent claudication I70.519
            rest pain (and intermittent claudication) I70.529
          bilateral I70.503
            with
              gangrene (and intermittent claudication, rest pain and ulcer) I70.563
              intermittent claudication I70.513
              rest pain (and intermittent claudication) I70.523
              specified type NEC I70.593
          left I70.502
            with
              gangrene (and intermittent claudication, rest pain and ulcer) I70.562
              intermittent claudication I70.512
              rest pain (and intermittent claudication) I70.522

Arteriosclerosis, arteriosclerotic (diffuse) (obliterans) (of) (senile) (with calcification) I70.90 — *continued*
  extremities (native arteries) I70.209 — *continued*
    bypass graft I70.309 — *continued*
      nonautologous biological graft I70.509 — *continued*
        leg I70.509 — *continued*
          left I70.502 — *continued*
            with — *continued*
              ulceration (and intermittent claudication and rest pain) I70.549
                ankle I70.543
                calf I70.542
                foot site NEC I70.545
                heel I70.544
                lower leg NEC I70.548
                midfoot I70.544
                thigh I70.541
            specified type NEC I70.592
          right I70.501
           with
            gangrene (and intermittent claudication, rest pain and ulcer) I70.561
            intermittent claudication I70.511
            rest pain (and intermittent claudication) I70.521
            ulceration (and intermittent claudication and rest pain) I70.539
              ankle I70.533
              calf I70.532
              foot site NEC I70.535
              heel I70.534
              lower leg NEC I70.538
              midfoot I70.534
              thigh I70.531
            specified type NEC I70.591
         specified type NEC I70.599
        specified NEC I70.508
          with
            gangrene (and intermittent claudication, rest pain and ulcer) I70.568
            intermittent claudication I70.518
            rest pain (and intermittent claudication) I70.528
            ulceration (and intermittent claudication and rest pain) I70.55
          specified type NEC I70.598
      nonbiological graft I70.609
        leg I70.609
          with
            gangrene (and intermittent claudication, rest pain and ulcer) I70.669
            intermittent claudication I70.619
            rest pain (and intermittent claudication) I70.629
          bilateral I70.603
            with
              gangrene (and intermittent claudication, rest pain and ulcer) I70.663
              intermittent claudication I70.613
              rest pain (and intermittent claudication) I70.623
              specified type NEC I70.693

Arteriosclerosis, arteriosclerotic (diffuse) (obliterans) (of) (senile) (with calcification) I70.90 — *continued*
  extremities (native arteries) I70.209 — *continued*
    bypass graft I70.309 — *continued*
      nonbiological graft I70.609 — *continued*
        leg I70.609 — *continued*
          left I70.602
            with
              gangrene (and intermittent claudication, rest pain and ulcer) I70.662
              intermittent claudication I70.612
              rest pain (and intermittent claudication) I70.622
              ulceration (and intermittent claudication and rest pain) I70.649
                ankle I70.643
                calf I70.642
                foot site NEC I70.645
                heel I70.644
                lower leg NEC I70.648
                midfoot I70.644
                thigh I70.641
            specified type NEC I70.692
          right I70.601
           with
            gangrene (and intermittent claudication, rest pain and ulcer) I70.661
            intermittent claudication I70.611
            rest pain (and intermittent claudication) I70.621
            ulceration (and intermittent claudication and rest pain) I70.639
              ankle I70.633
              calf I70.632
              foot site NEC I70.635
              heel I70.634
              lower leg NEC I70.638
              midfoot I70.634
              thigh I70.631
            specified type NEC I70.691
         specified type NEC I70.699
        specified NEC I70.608
          with
            gangrene (and intermittent claudication, rest pain and ulcer) I70.668
            intermittent claudication I70.618
            rest pain (and intermittent claudication) I70.628
            ulceration (and intermittent claudication and rest pain) I70.65
          specified type NEC I70.698
      specified graft NEC I70.709
        leg I70.709
          with
            gangrene (and intermittent claudication, rest pain and ulcer) I70.769
            intermittent claudication I70.719
            rest pain (and intermittent claudication) I70.729
          bilateral I70.703
            with
              gangrene (and intermittent claudication, rest pain and ulcer) I70.763
              intermittent claudication I70.713
              rest pain (and intermittent claudication) I70.723
              specified type NEC I70.793

Arteriosclerosis, arteriosclerotic (diffuse) (obliterans) (of) (senile) (with calcification) I70.90 — *continued*
extremities (native arteries) I70.209 — *continued*
  bypass graft I70.309 — *continued*
    specified graft NEC I70.709 — *continued*
      leg I70.709 — *continued*
        left I70.702
          with
            gangrene (and intermittent claudication, rest pain and ulcer) I70.762
            intermittent claudication I70.712
            rest pain (and intermittent claudication) I70.722
            ulceration (and intermittent claudication and rest pain) I70.749
              ankle I70.743
              calf I70.742
              foot site NEC I70.745
              heel I70.744
              lower leg NEC I70.748
              midfoot I70.744
              thigh I70.741
            specified type NEC I70.792
        right I70.701
          with
            gangrene (and intermittent claudication, rest pain and ulcer) I70.761
            intermittent claudication I70.711
            rest pain (and intermittent claudication) I70.721
            ulceration (and intermittent claudication and rest pain) I70.739
              ankle I70.733
              calf I70.732
              foot site NEC I70.735
              heel I70.734
              lower leg NEC I70.738
              midfoot I70.734
              thigh I70.731
            specified type NEC I70.791
        specified type NEC I70.799
      specified NEC I70.708
        with
          gangrene (and intermittent claudication, rest pain and ulcer) I70.768
          intermittent claudication I70.718
          rest pain (and intermittent claudication) I70.728
          ulceration (and intermittent claudication and rest pain) I70.75
          specified type NEC I70.798
    specified NEC I70.308
      with
        gangrene (and intermittent claudication, rest pain and ulcer) I70.368
        intermittent claudication I70.318
        rest pain (and intermittent claudication) I70.328
        ulceration (and intermittent claudication and rest pain) I70.35
        specified type NEC I70.398
  leg I70.209
    with
      gangrene (and intermittent claudication, rest pain and ulcer) I70.269
      intermittent claudication I70.219
      rest pain (and intermittent claudication) I70.229

Arteriosclerosis, arteriosclerotic (diffuse) (obliterans) (of) (senile) (with calcification) I70.90 — *continued*
extremities (native arteries) I70.209 — *continued*
  leg I70.209 — *continued*
    bilateral I70.203
      with
        gangrene (and intermittent claudication, rest pain and ulcer) I70.263
        intermittent claudication I70.213
        rest pain (and intermittent claudication) I70.223
        specified type NEC I70.293
    left I70.202
      with
        gangrene (and intermittent claudication, rest pain and ulcer) I70.262
        intermittent claudication I70.212
        rest pain (and intermittent claudication) I70.222
        ulceration (and intermittent claudication and rest pain) I70.249
          ankle I70.243
          calf I70.242
          foot site NEC I70.245
          heel I70.244
          lower leg NEC I70.248
          midfoot I70.244
          thigh I70.241
        specified type NEC I70.292
    right I70.201
      with
        gangrene (and intermittent claudication, rest pain and ulcer) I70.261
        intermittent claudication I70.211
        rest pain (and intermittent claudication) I70.221
        ulceration (and intermittent claudication and rest pain) I70.239
          ankle I70.233
          calf I70.232
          foot site NEC I70.235
          heel I70.234
          lower leg NEC I70.238
          midfoot I70.234
          thigh I70.231
        specified type NEC I70.291
      specified type NEC I70.299
  specified site NEC I70.208
    with
      gangrene (and intermittent claudication, rest pain and ulcer) I70.268
      intermittent claudication I70.218
      rest pain (and intermittent claudication) I70.228
      ulceration (and intermittent claudication and rest pain) I70.25
      specified type NEC I70.298
generalized I70.91
heart (disease) — *see* Arteriosclerosis, coronary (artery),
kidney — *see* Hypertension, kidney
medial — *see* Arteriosclerosis, extremities
mesenteric (artery) K55.1
myocarditis I51.4
Mönckeberg's — *see* Arteriosclerosis, extremities
peripheral (of extremities) — *see* Arteriosclerosis, extremities
pulmonary (idiopathic) I27.0

Arteriosclerosis, arteriosclerotic (diffuse) (obliterans) (of) (senile) (with calcification) I70.90 — *continued*
renal (arterioles) — *see also* Hypertension, kidney
  artery I70.1
retina (vascular) I70.8 *[H35.0-]*
specified artery NEC I70.8
spinal (cord) G95.19
vertebral (artery) I67.2
Arteriospasm I73.9
Arteriovenous — *see* condition
Arteritis I77.6
allergic M31.0
aorta (nonsyphilitic) I77.6
  syphilitic A52.02
aortic arch M31.4
brachiocephalic M31.4
brain I67.7
  syphilitic A52.04
cerebral I67.7
  in
    diseases classified elsewhere I68.2
    systemic lupus erythematosus M32.19
  listerial A32.89
  syphilitic A52.04
  tuberculous A18.89
coronary (artery) I25.89
  rheumatic I01.8
    chronic I09.89
  syphilitic A52.06
cranial (left) (right), giant cell M31.6
deformans — *see* Arteriosclerosis
giant cell NEC M31.6
  with polymyalgia rheumatica M31.5
necrosing or necrotizing M31.9
  specified NEC M31.8
nodosa M30.0
obliterans — *see* Arteriosclerosis
pulmonary I28.8
rheumatic — *see* Fever, rheumatic
senile — *see* Arteriosclerosis
suppurative I77.2
syphilitic (general) A52.09
  brain A52.04
  coronary A52.06
  spinal A52.09
temporal, giant cell M31.6
young female aortic arch syndrome M31.4
Artery, arterial — *see also* condition
abscess I77.89
single umbilical Q27.0
Arthralgia (allergic) — *see also* Pain, joint
in caisson disease T70.3
temporomandibular M26.62-
Arthritis, arthritic (acute) (chronic) (nonpyogenic) (subacute) M19.90
allergic — *see* Arthritis, specified form NEC
ankylosing (crippling) (spine) — *see also* Spondylitis, ankylosing
  sites other than spine — *see* Arthritis, specified form NEC
atrophic — *see* Osteoarthritis
  spine — *see* Spondylitis, ankylosing
back — *see* Spondylopathy, inflammatory
blennorrhagic (gonococcal) A54.42
Charcot's — *see* Arthropathy, neuropathic
  diabetic — *see* Diabetes, arthropathy, neuropathic
  syringomyelic G95.0
chylous (filarial) (*see also* category M01) B74.9
climacteric (any site) NEC — *see* Arthritis, specified form NEC
crystal(-induced) — *see* Arthritis, in, crystals
deformans — *see* Osteoarthritis
degenerative — *see* Osteoarthritis

Arthritis, arthritic (acute) (chronic) (nonpyogenic) (subacute) M19.90 — *continued*
due to or associated with
  acromegaly E22.0
  brucellosis — *see* Brucellosis
  caisson disease T70.3
  diabetes — *see* Diabetes, arthropathy
  dracontiasis (*see also* category M01) B72
  enteritis NEC
    regional — *see* Enteritis, regional
  erysipelas (*see also* category M01) A46
  erythema
    epidemic A25.1
    nodosum L52
  filariasis NOS B74.9
  glanders A24.0
  helminthiasis (*see also* category M01) B83.9
  hemophilia D66 [M36.2]
  Henoch-(Schönlein) purpura D69.0 [M36.4]
  human parvovirus (*see also* category M01) B97.6
  infectious disease NEC — *see* category M01
  leprosy (*see also* category M01) (*see also* Leprosy) A30.9
  Lyme disease A69.23
  mycobacteria (*see also* category M01) A31.8
  parasitic disease NEC (*see also* category M01) B89
  paratyphoid fever (*see also* category M01) (*see also* Fever, paratyphoid) A01.4
  rat bite fever (*see also* category M01) A25.1
  regional enteritis — *see* Enteritis, regional
  respiratory disorder NOS J98.9
  serum sickness (*see also* Reaction, serum) T80.69
  syringomyelia G95.0
  typhoid fever A01.04
epidemic erythema A25.1
febrile — *see* Fever, rheumatic
gonococcal A54.42
gouty (acute) — *see* Gout
in (due to)
  acromegaly (*see also* subcategory M14.8-) E22.0
  amyloidosis (*see also* subcategory M14.8-) E85.4
  bacterial disease (*see also* category M01) A49.9
  Behçet's syndrome M35.2
  caisson disease (*see also* subcategory M14.8-) T70.3
  coliform bacilli (Escherichia coli) — *see* Arthritis, in, pyogenic organism NEC
  crystals M11.9
    dicalcium phosphate — *see* Arthritis, in, crystals, specified type NEC
    hydroxyapatite M11.0-
    pyrophosphate — *see* Arthritis, in, crystals, specified type NEC
    specified type NEC M11.80
      ankle M11.87-
      elbow M11.82-
      foot joint M11.87-
      hand joint M11.84-
      hip M11.85-
      knee M11.86-
      multiple sites M11.8-
      shoulder M11.81-
      vertebrae M11.88
      wrist M11.83-
  dermatoarthritis, lipoid E78.81
  dracontiasis (dracunculiasis) (*see also* category M01) B72
  endocrine disorder NEC (*see also* subcategory M14.8-) E34.9

Arthritis, arthritic (acute) (chronic) (nonpyogenic) (subacute) M19.90 — *continued*
in (due to) — *continued*
  enteritis, infectious NEC (*see also* category M01) A09
    specified organism NEC (*see also* category M01) A08.8
  erythema
    multiforme (*see also* subcategory M14.8-) L51.9
    nodosum (*see also* subcategory M14.8-) L52
  gout — *see* Gout
  helminthiasis NEC (*see also* category M01) B83.9
  hemochromatosis (*see also* subcategory M14.8-) E83.118
  hemoglobinopathy NEC D58.2 [M36.3]
  hemophilia NEC D66 [M36.2]
  Hemophilus influenzae M00.8- [B96.3]
  Henoch(-Schönlein) purpura D69.0 [M36.4]
  hyperparathyroidism NEC (*see also* subcategory M14.8-) E21.3
  hypersensitivity reaction NEC T78.49 [M36.4]
  hypogammaglobulinemia (*see also* subcategory M14.8-) D80.1
  hypothyroidism NEC (*see also* subcategory M14.8-) E03.9
  infection — *see* Arthritis, pyogenic or pyemic
    spine — *see* Spondylopathy, infective
  infectious disease NEC — *see* category M01
  leprosy (*see also* category M01) A30.9
  leukemia NEC C95.9- [M36.1]
  lipoid dermatoarthritis E78.81
  Lyme disease A69.23
  Mediterranean fever, familial (*see also* subcategory M14.8-) M04.1
  Meningococcus A39.83
  metabolic disorder NEC (*see also* subcategory M14.8-) E88.9
  multiple myelomatosis C90.0- [M36.1]
  mumps B26.85
  mycosis NEC (*see also* category M01) B49
  myelomatosis (multiple) C90.0- [M36.1]
  neurological disorder NEC G98.0
  ochronosis (*see also* subcategory M14.8-) E70.29
  O'nyong-nyong (*see also* category M01) A92.1
  parasitic disease NEC (*see also* category M01) B89
  paratyphoid fever (*see also* category M01) A01.4
  Pseudomonas — *see* Arthritis, pyogenic, bacterial NEC
  psoriasis L40.50
  pyogenic organism NEC — *see* Arthritis, pyogenic, bacterial NEC
  Reiter's disease — *see* Reiter's disease
  respiratory disorder NEC (*see also* subcategory M14.8-) J98.9
  reticulosis, malignant (*see also* subcategory M14.8-) C86.0
  rubella B06.82
  Salmonella (arizonae) (cholerae-suis) (enteritidis) (typhimurium) A02.23
  sarcoidosis D86.86
  specified bacteria NEC — *see* Arthritis, pyogenic, bacterial NEC
  sporotrichosis B42.82
  syringomyelia G95.0
  thalassemia NEC D56.9 [M36.3]
  tuberculosis — *see* Tuberculosis, arthritis
  typhoid fever A01.04
  urethritis, Reiter's — *see* Reiter's disease

Arthritis, arthritic (acute) (chronic) (nonpyogenic) (subacute) M19.90 — *continued*
in (due to) — *continued*
  viral disease NEC (*see also* category M01) B34.9
infectious or infective — *see also* Arthritis, pyogenic or pyemic
  spine — *see* Spondylopathy, infective
juvenile M08.90
  with systemic onset — *see* Still's disease
  ankle M08.97-
  elbow M08.92-
  foot joint M08.97-
  hand joint M08.94-
  hip M08.95-
  knee M08.96-
  multiple site M08.99
  pauciarticular M08.40
    ankle M08.47-
    elbow M08.42-
    foot joint M08.47-
    hand joint M08.44-
    hip M08.45-
    knee M08.46-
    shoulder M08.41-
    vertebrae M08.48
    wrist M08.43-
  psoriatic L40.54
  rheumatoid — *see* Arthritis, rheumatoid, juvenile
  shoulder M08.91-
  specified type NEC M08.80
    ankle M08.87-
    elbow M08.82-
    foot joint M08.87-
    hand joint M08.84-
    hip M08.85-
    knee M08.86-
    multiple site M08.89
    shoulder M08.81-
    specified joint NEC M08.88
    vertebrae M08.88
    wrist M08.83-
  wrist M08.93-
meaning osteoarthritis — *see* Osteoarthritis
meningococcal A39.83
menopausal (any site) NEC — *see* Arthritis, specified form NEC
mutilans (psoriatic) L40.52
mycotic NEC (*see also* category M01) B49
neuropathic (Charcot) — *see* Arthropathy, neuropathic
  diabetic — *see* Diabetes, arthropathy, neuropathic
  nonsyphilitic NEC G98.0
  syringomyelic G95.0
ochronotic (*see also* subcategory M14.8-) E70.29
palindromic (any site) — *see* Rheumatism, palindromic
pneumococcal M00.10
  ankle M00.17-
  elbow M00.12-
  foot joint — *see* Arthritis, pneumococcal, ankle
  hand joint M00.14-
  hip M00.15-
  knee M00.16-
  multiple site M00.19
  shoulder M00.11-
  vertebra M00.18
  wrist M00.13-
postdysenteric — *see* Arthropathy, postdysenteric
postmeningococcal A39.84
postrheumatic, chronic — *see* Arthropathy, postrheumatic, chronic

Arthritis, arthritic (acute) (chronic) (nonpyogenic) (subacute) M19.90 — *continued*
primary progressive — *see also* Arthritis, specified form NEC
  spine — *see* Spondylitis, ankylosing
psoriatic L40.50
purulent (any site except spine) — *see* Arthritis, pyogenic or pyemic
  spine — *see* Spondylopathy, infective
pyogenic or pyemic (any site except spine) M00.9
  bacterial NEC M00.80
    ankle M00.87-
    elbow M00.82-
    foot joint — *see* Arthritis, pyogenic, bacterial NEC, ankle
    hand joint M00.84-
    hip M00.85-
    knee M00.86-
    multiple site M00.89
    shoulder M00.81-
    vertebra M00.88
    wrist M00.83-
  pneumococcal — *see* Arthritis, pneumococcal
  spine — *see* Spondylopathy, infective
  staphylococcal — *see* Arthritis, staphylococcal
  streptococcal — *see* Arthritis, streptococcal NEC
  pneumococcal — *see* Arthritis, pneumococcal
reactive — *see* Reiter's disease
rheumatic — *see also* Arthritis, rheumatoid
  acute or subacute — *see* Fever, rheumatic
rheumatoid M06.9
  with
    carditis — *see* Rheumatoid, carditis
    endocarditis — *see* Rheumatoid, carditis
    heart involvement NEC — *see* Rheumatoid, carditis
    lung involvement — *see* Rheumatoid, lung
    myocarditis — *see* Rheumatoid, carditis
    myopathy — *see* Rheumatoid, myopathy
    pericarditis — *see* Rheumatoid, carditis
    polyneuropathy — *see* Rheumatoid, polyneuropathy
    rheumatoid factor — *see* Arthritis, rheumatoid, seropositive
    splenoadenomegaly and leukopenia — *see* Felty's syndrome
    vasculitis — *see* Rheumatoid, vasculitis
    visceral involvement NEC — *see* Rheumatoid, arthritis, with involvement of organs NEC
  juvenile (with or without rheumatoid factor) M08.00
    ankle M08.07-
    elbow M08.02-
    foot joint M08.07-
    hand joint M08.04-
    hip M08.05-
    knee M08.06-
    multiple site M08.09
    shoulder M08.01-
    vertebra M08.08
    wrist M08.03-
  seronegative M06.00
    ankle M06.07-
    elbow M06.02-
    foot joint M06.07-
    hand joint M06.04-
    hip M06.05-
    knee M06.06-
    multiple site M06.09
    shoulder M06.01-
    vertebra M06.08

Arthritis, arthritic (acute) (chronic) (nonpyogenic) (subacute) M19.90 — *continued*
rheumatoid M06.9 — *continued*
  seronegative M06.00 — *continued*
    wrist M06.03-
  seropositive M05.9
    specified NEC M05.80
      ankle M05.87-
      elbow M05.82-
      foot joint M05.87-
      hand joint M05.84-
      hip M05.85-
      knee M05.86-
      multiple sites M05.89
      shoulder M05.81-
      vertebra — *see* Spondylitis, ankylosing
      wrist M05.83-
    without organ involvement M05.70
      ankle M05.77-
      elbow M05.72-
      foot joint M05.77-
      hand joint M05.74-
      hip M05.75-
      knee M05.76-
      multiple sites M05.79
      shoulder M05.71-
      vertebra — *see* Spondylitis, ankylosing
      wrist M05.73-
  specified type NEC M06.80
    ankle M06.87-
    elbow M06.82-
    foot joint M06.87-
    hand joint M06.84-
    hip M06.85-
    knee M06.86-
    multiple site M06.89
    shoulder M06.81-
    vertebra M06.88
    wrist M06.83-
  spine — *see* Spondylitis, ankylosing
rubella B06.82
scorbutic (*see also* subcategory M14.8-) E54
senile or senescent — *see* Osteoarthritis
septic (any site except spine) — *see* Arthritis, pyogenic or pyemic
  spine — *see* Spondylopathy, infective
serum (nontherapeutic) (therapeutic) — *see* Arthropathy, postimmunization
specified form NEC M13.80
  ankle M13.87-
  elbow M13.82-
  foot joint M13.87-
  hand joint M13.84-
  hip M13.85-
  knee M13.86-
  multiple site M13.89
  shoulder M13.81-
  specified joint NEC M13.88
  wrist M13.83-
  spine — *see also* Spondylopathy, inflammatory
    infectious or infective NEC — *see* Spondylopathy, infective
    Marie-Strümpell — *see* Spondylitis, ankylosing
    pyogenic — *see* Spondylopathy, infective
    rheumatoid — *see* Spondylitis, ankylosing
    traumatic (old) — *see* Spondylopathy, traumatic
    tuberculous A18.01
staphylococcal M00.00
  ankle M00.07-
  elbow M00.02-
  foot joint — *see* Arthritis, staphylococcal, ankle
  hand joint M00.04-
  hip M00.05-
  knee M00.06-

Arthritis, arthritic (acute) (chronic) (nonpyogenic) (subacute) M19.90 — *continued*
staphylococcal M00.00 — *continued*
  multiple site M00.09
  shoulder M00.01-
  vertebra M00.08
  wrist M00.03-
streptococcal NEC M00.20
  ankle M00.27-
  elbow M00.22-
  foot joint — *see* Arthritis, streptococcal, ankle
  hand joint M00.24-
  hip M00.25-
  knee M00.26-
  multiple site M00.29
  shoulder M00.21-
  vertebra M00.28
  wrist M00.23-
suppurative — *see* Arthritis, pyogenic or pyemic
syphilitic (late) A52.16
  congenital A50.55 [M12.80]
syphilitica deformans (Charcot) A52.16
temporomandibular M26.69
toxic of menopause (any site) — *see* Arthritis, specified form NEC
transient — *see* Arthropathy, specified form NEC
traumatic (chronic) — *see* Arthropathy, traumatic
tuberculous A18.02
  spine A18.01
uratic — *see* Gout
urethritica (Reiter's) — *see* Reiter's disease
vertebral — *see* Spondylopathy, inflammatory
villous (any site) — *see* Arthropathy, specified form NEC

Arthrocele — *see* Effusion, joint
Arthrodesis status Z98.1
Arthrodynia — *see also* Pain, joint
Arthrodysplasia Q74.9
Arthrofibrosis, joint — *see* Ankylosis
Arthrogryposis (congenital) Q68.8
  multiplex congenita Q74.3
Arthrokatadysis M24.7
Arthropathy (*see also* Arthritis) M12.9
Charcot's — *see* Arthropathy, neuropathic
  diabetic — *see* Diabetes, arthropathy, neuropathic
  syringomyelic G95.0
cricoarytenoid J38.7
crystal(-induced) — *see* Arthritis, in, crystals
diabetic NEC — *see* Diabetes, arthropathy
distal interphalangeal, psoriatic L40.51
enteropathic M07.60
  ankle M07.67-
  elbow M07.62-
  foot joint M07.67-
  hand joint M07.64-
  hip M07.65-
  knee M07.66-
  multiple site M07.69
  shoulder M07.61-
  vertebra M07.68
  wrist M07.63-
following intestinal bypass M02.00
  ankle M02.07-
  elbow M02.02-
  foot joint M02.07-
  hand joint M02.04-
  hip M02.05-
  knee M02.06-
  multiple site M02.09
  shoulder M02.01-
  vertebra M02.08
  wrist M02.03-

Arthropathy (*see also* Arthritis) M12.9 — *continued*
gouty — *see also* Gout
  in (due to)
    Lesch-Nyhan syndrome E79.1 *[M14.8-]*
    sickle-cell disorders D57- *[M14.8-]*
hemophilic NEC D66 *[M36.2]*
  in (due to)
    hyperparathyroidism NEC E21.3 *[M14.8-]*
    metabolic disease NOS E88.9 *[M14.8-]*
in (due to)
  acromegaly E22.0 *[M14.8-]*
  amyloidosis E85.4 *[M14.8-]*
  blood disorder NOS D75.9 *[M36.3]*
  diabetes — *see* Diabetes, arthropathy
  endocrine disease NOS E34.9 *[M14.8-]*
  erythema
    multiforme L51.9 *[M14.8-]*
    nodosum L52 *[M14.8-]*
  hemochromatosis E83.118 *[M14.8-]*
  hemoglobinopathy NEC D58.2 *[M36.3]*
  hemophilia NEC D66 *[M36.2]*
  Henoch-Schönlein purpura D69.0 *[M36.4]*
  hyperthyroidism E05.90 *[M14.8-]*
  hypothyroidism E03.9 *[M14.8-]*
  infective endocarditis I33.0 *[M12.80]*
  leukemia NEC C95.9- *[M36.1]*
  malignant histiocytosis C96.A *[M36.1]*
    (follows C96.6)
  metabolic disease NOS E88.9 *[M14.8-]*
  multiple myeloma C90.0- *[M36.1]*
  neoplastic disease NOS (*see also* Neoplasm) D49.9 *[M36.1]*
  nutritional deficiency (*see also* subcategory M14.8-) E63.9
  psoriasis NOS L40.50
  sarcoidosis D86.86
  syphilis (late) A52.77
    congenital A50.55 *[M12.80]*
  thyrotoxicosis (*see also* subcategory M14.8-) E05.90
  ulcerative colitis K51.90 *[M07.60]*
  viral hepatitis (postinfectious) NEC B19.9 *[M12.80]*
  Whipple's disease (*see also* subcategory M14.8-) K90.81
Jaccoud — *see* Arthropathy, postrheumatic, chronic
juvenile — *see* Arthritis, juvenile
  psoriatic L40.54
mutilans (psoriatic) L40.52
neuropathic (Charcot) M14.60
  ankle M14.67-
  diabetic — *see* Diabetes, arthropathy, neuropathic
  elbow M14.62-
  foot joint M14.67-
  hand joint M14.64-
  hip M14.65-
  knee M14.66-
  multiple site M14.69
  nonsyphilitic NEC G98.0
  shoulder M14.61-
  syringomyelic G95.0
  vertebra M14.68
  wrist M14.63-
osteopulmonary — *see* Osteoarthropathy, hypertrophic, specified NEC
postdysenteric M02.10
  ankle M02.17-
  elbow M02.12-
  foot joint M02.17-
  hand joint M02.14-
  hip M02.15-
  knee M02.16-
  multiple site M02.19
  shoulder M02.11-
  vertebra M02.18

Arthropathy (*see also* Arthritis) M12.9 — *continued*
postdysenteric M02.10 — *continued*
  wrist M02.13-
postimmunization M02.20
  ankle M02.27-
  elbow M02.22-
  foot joint M02.27-
  hand joint M02.24-
  hip M02.25-
  knee M02.26-
  multiple site M02.29
  shoulder M02.21-
  vertebra M02.28
  wrist M02.23-
postinfectious NEC B99 *[M12.80]*
  in (due to)
    enteritis due to Yersinia enterocolitica A04.6 *[M12.80]*
    syphilis A52.77
    viral hepatitis NEC B19.9 *[M12.80]*
postrheumatic, chronic (Jaccoud) M12.00
  ankle M12.07-
  elbow M12.02-
  foot joint M12.07-
  hand joint M12.04-
  hip M12.05-
  knee M12.06-
  multiple site M12.09
  shoulder M12.01-
  specified joint NEC M12.08
  vertebrae M12.08
  wrist M12.03-
psoriatic NEC L40.59
  interphalangeal, distal L40.51
reactive M02.9
  in (due to)
    infective endocarditis I33.0 *[M02.9]*
  specified type NEC M02.80
    ankle M02.87-
    elbow M02.82-
    foot joint M02.87-
    hand joint M02.84-
    hip M02.85-
    knee M02.86-
    multiple site M02.89
    shoulder M02.81-
    vertebra M02.88
    wrist M02.83-
specified form NEC M12.80
  ankle M12.87-
  elbow M12.82-
  foot joint M12.87-
  hand joint M12.84-
  hip M12.85-
  knee M12.86-
  multiple site M12.89
  shoulder M12.81-
  specified joint NEC M12.88
  vertebrae M12.88
  wrist M12.83-
syringomyelic G95.0
tabes dorsalis A52.16
tabetic A52.16
transient — *see* Arthropathy, specified form NEC
traumatic M12.50
  ankle M12.57-
  elbow M12.52-
  foot joint M12.57-
  hand joint M12.54-
  hip M12.55-
  knee M12.56-
  multiple site M12.59
  shoulder M12.51-
  specified joint NEC M12.58
  vertebrae M12.58
  wrist M12.53-

Arthropyosis — *see* Arthritis, pyogenic or pyemic
Arthrosis (deformans) (degenerative) (localized) (*see also* Osteoarthritis) M19.90
spine — *see* Spondylosis
Arthus' phenomenon or reaction T78.41
due to
  drug — *see* Table of Drugs and Chemicals, by drug
Articular — *see* condition
Articulation, reverse (teeth) M26.24
Artificial
insemination complication — *see* Complications, artificial, fertilization
opening status (functioning) (without complication) Z93.9
  anus (colostomy) Z93.3
  colostomy Z93.3
  cystostomy Z93.50
    appendico-vesicostomy Z93.52
    cutaneous Z93.51
    specified NEC Z93.59
  enterostomy Z93.4
  gastrostomy Z93.1
  ileostomy Z93.2
  intestinal tract NEC Z93.4
  jejunostomy Z93.4
  nephrostomy Z93.6
  specified site NEC Z93.8
  tracheostomy Z93.0
  ureterostomy Z93.6
  urethrostomy Z93.6
  urinary tract NEC Z93.6
  vagina Z93.8
  vagina status Z93.8
Arytenoid — *see* condition
Asbestosis (occupational) J61
Ascariasis B77.9
with
  complications NEC B77.89
  intestinal complications B77.0
  pneumonia, pneumonitis B77.81
Ascaridosis, ascaridiasis — *see* Ascariasis
Ascaris (infection) (infestation) (lumbricoides) — *see* Ascariasis
Ascending — *see* condition
ASC-H (atypical squamous cells cannot exclude high grade squamous intraepithelial lesion on cytologic smear)
anus R85.611
cervix R87.611
vagina R87.621
Aschoff's bodies — *see* Myocarditis, rheumatic
Ascites (abdominal) R18.8
cardiac I50.9
chylous (nonfilarial) I89.8
  filarial — *see* Infestation, filarial
due to
  cirrhosis, alcoholic K70.31
  hepatitis
    alcoholic K70.11
    chronic active K71.51
  S. japonicum B65.2
heart I50.9
malignant R18.0
pseudochylous R18.8
syphilitic A52.74
tuberculous A18.31
ASC-US (atypical squamous cells of undetermined significance on cytologic smear)
anus R85.610
cervix R87.610
vagina R87.620
Aseptic — *see* condition
Asherman's syndrome N85.6
Asialia K11.7
Asiatic cholera — *see* Cholera

DISEASE INDEX

Asimultagnosia (simultanagnosia) R48.3
Askin's tumor — see Neoplasm, connective tissue, malignant
Asocial personality F60.2
Asomatognosia R41.4
Aspartylglucosaminuria E77.1
Asperger's disease or syndrome F84.5
Aspergilloma — see Aspergillosis
Aspergillosis (with pneumonia) B44.9
  bronchopulmonary, allergic B44.81
  disseminated B44.7
  generalized B44.7
  pulmonary NEC B44.1
    allergic B44.81
    invasive B44.0
  specified NEC B44.89
  tonsillar B44.2
Aspergillus (flavus) (fumigatus) (infection) (terreus) — see Aspergillosis
Aspermatogenesis — see Azoospermia
Aspermia (testis) — see Azoospermia
Asphyxia, asphyxiation (by) R09.01
  antenatal P84
  birth P84
  bunny bag — see Asphyxia, due to, mechanical threat to breathing, trapped in bed clothes
  crushing S28.0
  drowning T75.1
  gas, fumes, or vapor — see Table of Drugs and Chemicals
  inhalation — see Inhalation
  intrauterine P84
  local I73.00
    with gangrene I73.01
  mucus — see also Foreign body, respiratory tract, causing asphyxia
  newborn P84
  pathological R09.01
  postnatal P84
    mechanical — see Asphyxia, due to, mechanical threat to breathing
  prenatal P84
  reticularis R23.1
  strangulation — see Asphyxia, due to, mechanical threat to breathing
  submersion T75.1
  traumatic T71.9
    due to
      crushed chest S28.0
      foreign body (in) — see Foreign body, respiratory tract, causing asphyxia
      low oxygen content of ambient air T71.20
        due to
          being trapped in
            low oxygen environment T71.29
            in car trunk T71.221
              circumstances undetermined T71.224
              done with intent to harm by another person T71.223
              self T71.222
            in refrigerator T71.231
              circumstances undetermined T71.234
              done with intent to harm by another person T71.233
              self T71.232
        cave-in T71.21
      mechanical threat to breathing (accidental) T71.191
        circumstances undetermined T71.194
        done with intent to harm by another person T71.193
          self T71.192

Asphyxia, asphyxiation (by) R09.01 — continued
  traumatic T71.9 — continued
    due to — continued
      mechanical threat to breathing (accidental) T71.191 — continued
        hanging T71.161
          circumstances undetermined T71.164
          done with intent to harm by another person T71.163
          self T71.162
        plastic bag T71.121
          circumstances undetermined T71.124
          done with intent to harm by another person T71.123
          self T71.122
        smothering
          in furniture T71.151
            circumstances undetermined T71.154
            done with intent to harm by another person T71.153
            self T71.152
          under
            another person's body T71.141
              circumstances undetermined T71.144
              done with intent to harm T71.143
            pillow T71.111
              circumstances undetermined T71.114
              done with intent to harm by another person T71.113
              self T71.112
        trapped in bed clothes T71.131
          circumstances undetermined T71.134
          done with intent to harm by another person T71.133
          self T71.132
  vomiting, vomitus — see Foreign body, respiratory tract, causing asphyxia
Aspiration
  amniotic (clear) fluid (newborn) P24.10
    with
      pneumonia (pneumonitis) P24.11
      respiratory symptoms P24.11
  blood
    newborn (without respiratory symptoms) P24.20
      with
        pneumonia (pneumonitis) P24.21
        respiratory symptoms P24.21
      specified age NEC — see Foreign body, respiratory tract
  bronchitis J69.0
  food or foreign body (with asphyxiation) — see Asphyxia, food
  liquor (amnii) (newborn) P24.10
    with
      pneumonia (pneumonitis) P24.11
      respiratory symptoms P24.11
  meconium (newborn) (without respiratory symptoms) P24.00
    with
      pneumonitis (pneumonitis) P24.01
      respiratory symptoms P24.01
  milk (newborn) (without respiratory symptoms) P24.30
    with
      pneumonia (pneumonitis) P24.31
      respiratory symptoms P24.31
    specified age NEC — see Foreign body, respiratory tract
  mucus — see also Foreign body, by site, causing asphyxia
    newborn P24.10
      with
        pneumonia (pneumonitis) P24.11
        respiratory symptoms P24.11

Aspiration — continued
  neonatal P24.9
    specific NEC (without respiratory symptoms) P24.80
      with
        pneumonia (pneumonitis) P24.81
        respiratory symptoms P24.81
  newborn P24.9
    specific NEC (without respiratory symptoms) P24.80
      with
        pneumonia (pneumonitis) P24.81
        respiratory symptoms P24.81
  pneumonia J69.0
  pneumonitis J69.0
  syndrome of newborn — see Aspiration, by substance, with pneumonia
  vernix caseosa (newborn) P24.80
    with
      pneumonia (pneumonitis) P24.81
      respiratory symptoms P24.81
  vomitus — see also Foreign body, respiratory tract
    newborn (without respiratory symptoms) P24.30
      with
        pneumonia (pneumonitis) P24.31
        respiratory symptoms P24.31
Asplenia (congenital) Q89.01
  postsurgical Z90.81
Assam fever B55.0
Assault, sexual — see Maltreatment
Assmann's focus NEC A15.0
Astasia(-abasia) (hysterical) F44.4
Asteatosis cutis L85.3
Astereognosia, astereognosis R48.1
Asterixis R27.8
  in liver disease K71.3
Asteroid hyalitis — see Deposit, crystalline
Asthenia, asthenic R53.1
  cardiac (see also Failure, heart) I50.9
    psychogenic F45.8
  cardiovascular (see also Failure, heart) I50.9
    psychogenic F45.8
  heart (see also Failure, heart) I50.9
    psychogenic F45.8
  hysterical F44.4
  myocardial (see also Failure, heart) I50.9
    psychogenic F45.8
  nervous F48.8
  neurocirculatory F45.8
  neurotic F48.8
  psychogenic F48.8
  psychoneurotic F48.8
  psychophysiologic F48.8
  reaction (psychophysiologic) F48.8
  senile R54
Asthenopia — see also Discomfort, visual
  hysterical F44.6
  psychogenic F44.6
Asthenospermia — see Abnormal, specimen, male genital organs
Asthma, asthmatic (bronchial) (catarrh) (spasmodic) J45.909
  with
    chronic obstructive bronchitis J44.9
      with
        acute lower respiratory infection J44.0
        exacerbation (acute) J44.1
    chronic obstructive pulmonary disease J44.9
      with
        acute lower respiratory infection J44.0
        exacerbation (acute) J44.1
  exacerbation (acute) J45.901
  hay fever — see Asthma, allergic extrinsic
  rhinitis, allergic — see Asthma, allergic extrinsic
  status asthmaticus J45.902

Asthma, asthmatic (bronchial) (catarrh) (spasmodic) J45.909 — *continued*
allergic extrinsic J45.909
  with
    exacerbation (acute) J45.901
    status asthmaticus J45.902
atopic — *see* Asthma, allergic extrinsic
cardiac — *see* Failure, ventricular, left
cardiobronchial I50.1
childhood J45.909
  with
    exacerbation (acute) J45.901
    status asthmaticus J45.902
chronic obstructive J44.9
  with
    acute lower respiratory infection J44.0
    exacerbation (acute) J44.1
collier's J60
cough variant J45.991
detergent J69.8
due to
  detergent J69.8
  inhalation of fumes J68.3
eosinophilic J82
extrinsic, allergic — *see* Asthma, allergic extrinsic
grinder's J62.8
hay — *see* Asthma, allergic extrinsic
heart I50.1
idiosyncratic — *see* Asthma, nonallergic
intermittent (mild) J45.20
  with
    exacerbation (acute) J45.21
    status asthmaticus J45.22
intrinsic, nonallergic — *see* Asthma, nonallergic
Kopp's E32.8
late-onset J45.909
  with
    exacerbation (acute) J45.901
    status asthmaticus J45.902
mild intermittent J45.20
  with
    exacerbation (acute) J45.21
    status asthmaticus J45.22
mild persistent J45.30
  with
    exacerbation (acute) J45.31
    status asthmaticus J45.32
Millar's (laryngismus stridulus) J38.5
miner's J60
mixed J45.909
  with
    exacerbation (acute) J45.901
    status asthmaticus J45.902
moderate persistent J45.40
  with
    exacerbation (acute) J45.41
    status asthmaticus J45.42
nervous — *see* Asthma, nonallergic
nonallergic (intrinsic) J45.909
  with
    exacerbation (acute) J45.901
    status asthmaticus J45.902
persistent
  mild J45.30
    with
      exacerbation (acute) J45.31
      status asthmaticus J45.32
  moderate J45.40
    with
      exacerbation (acute) J45.41
      status asthmaticus J45.42
  severe J45.50
    with
      exacerbation (acute) J45.51
      status asthmaticus J45.52
platinum J45.998
pneumoconiotic NEC J64

Asthma, asthmatic (bronchial) (catarrh) (spasmodic) J45.909 — *continued*
potter's J62.8
predominantly allergic J45.909
psychogenic F54
pulmonary eosinophilic J82
red cedar J67.8
Rostan's I50.1
sandblaster's J62.8
sequoiosis J67.8
severe persistent J45.50
  with
    exacerbation (acute) J45.51
    status asthmaticus J45.52
specified NEC J45.998
stonemason's J62.8
thymic E32.8
tuberculous — *see* Tuberculosis, pulmonary
Wichmann's (laryngismus stridulus) J38.5
wood J67.8
Astigmatism (compound) (congenital) H52.20-
irregular H52.21-
regular H52.22-
Astraphobia F40.220
Astroblastoma
specified site — *see* Neoplasm, malignant, by site
unspecified site C71.9
Astrocytoma (cystic)
anaplastic
  specified site — *see* Neoplasm, malignant, by site
  unspecified site C71.9
fibrillary
  specified site — *see* Neoplasm, malignant, by site
  unspecified site C71.9
fibrous
  specified site — *see* Neoplasm, malignant, by site
  unspecified site C71.9
gemistocytic
  specified site — *see* Neoplasm, malignant, by site
  unspecified site C71.9
juvenile
  specified site — *see* Neoplasm, malignant, by site
  unspecified site C71.9
pilocytic
  specified site — *see* Neoplasm, malignant, by site
  unspecified site C71.9
piloid
  specified site — *see* Neoplasm, malignant, by site
  unspecified site C71.9
protoplasmic
  specified site — *see* Neoplasm, malignant, by site
  unspecified site C71.9
specified site NEC — *see* Neoplasm, malignant, by site
subependymal D43.2
  giant cell
    specified site — *see* Neoplasm, uncertain behavior, by site
    unspecified site D43.2
  specified site — *see* Neoplasm, uncertain behavior, by site
  unspecified site D43.2
unspecified site C71.9
Astroglioma
specified site — *see* Neoplasm, malignant, by site
unspecified site C71.9
Asymbolia R48.8

Asymmetry — *see also* Distortion
between native and reconstructed breast N65.1
face Q67.0
jaw (lower) — *see* Anomaly, dentofacial, jaw-cranial base relationship, asymmetry
Asynergia, asynergy R27.8
ventricular I51.89
Asystole (heart) — *see* Arrest, cardiac
At risk
for falling Z91.81
Ataxia, ataxy, ataxic R27.0
acute R27.8
brain (hereditary) G11.9
cerebellar (hereditary) G11.9
  with defective DNA repair G11.3
  alcoholic G31.2
  early-onset G11.1
  in
    alcoholism G31.2
    myxedema E03.9 *[G13.2]*
    neoplastic disease (*see also* Neoplasm) D49.9 *[G32.81]*
    specified disease NEC G32.81
  late-onset (Marie's) G11.2
cerebral (hereditary) G11.9
congenital nonprogressive G11.0
family, familial — *see* Ataxia, hereditary
following
  cerebrovascular disease I69.993
    cerebral infarction I69.393
    intracerebral hemorrhage I69.193
    nontraumatic intracranial hemorrhage NEC I69.293
    specified disease NEC I69.893
    subarachnoid hemorrhage I69.093
Friedreich's (heredofamilial) (cerebellar) (spinal) G11.1
gait R26.0
  hysterical F44.4
general R27.8
gluten M35.9 *[G32.81]*
  with celiac disease K90.0 *[G32.81]*
hereditary G11.9
  with neuropathy G60.2
  cerebellar — *see* Ataxia, cerebellar
  spastic G11.4
  specified NEC G11.8
  spinal (Friedreich's) G11.1
heredofamilial — *see* Ataxia, hereditary
Hunt's G11.1
hysterical F44.4
locomotor (progressive) (syphilitic) (partial) (spastic) A52.11
  diabetic — *see* Diabetes, ataxia
Marie's (cerebellar) (heredofamilial) (late-onset) G11.2
nonorganic origin F44.4
nonprogressive, congenital G11.0
psychogenic F44.4
Roussy-Lévy G60.0
Sanger-Brown's (hereditary) G11.2
spastic hereditary G11.4
spinal
  hereditary (Friedreich's) G11.1
  progressive (syphilitic) A52.11
spinocerebellar, X-linked recessive G11.1
telangiectasia (Louis-Bar) G11.3
Ataxia-telangiectasia (Louis-Bar) G11.3
Atelectasis (massive) (partial) (pressure) (pulmonary) J98.11
newborn P28.10
  due to resorption P28.11
  partial P28.19
  primary P28.0
  secondary P28.19
primary (newborn) P28.0
tuberculous — *see* Tuberculosis, pulmonary
Atelocardia Q24.9

Atelomyelia Q06.1
Atheroembolism
  of
    extremities
      lower I75.02-
      upper I75.01-
    kidney I75.81
    specified NEC I75.89
Atheroma, atheromatous (see also Arteriosclerosis) I70.90
  aorta, aortic I70.0
    valve (see also Endocarditis, aortic) I35.8
  aorto-iliac I70.0
  artery — see Arteriosclerosis
  basilar (artery) I67.2
  carotid (artery) (common) (internal) I67.2
  cerebral (arteries) I67.2
  coronary (artery) I25.10
    with angina pectoris — see Arteriosclerosis, coronary (artery),
  degeneration — see Arteriosclerosis
  heart, cardiac — see Disease, heart, ischemic, atherosclerotic
  mitral (valve) I34.8
  myocardium, myocardial — see Disease, heart, ischemic, atherosclerotic
  pulmonary valve (heart) (see also Endocarditis, pulmonary) I37.8
  tricuspid (heart) (valve) I36.8
  valve, valvular — see Endocarditis
  vertebral (artery) I67.2
Atheromatosis — see Arteriosclerosis
Atherosclerosis — see also Arteriosclerosis
  coronary
    artery I25.10
      with angina pectoris — see Arteriosclerosis, coronary (artery)
      due to
        calcified coronary lesion (severely) I25.84
        lipid rich plaque I25.83
    transplanted heart I25.811
      bypass graft I25.812
        with angina pectoris — see Arteriosclerosis, coronary (artery)
      native coronary artery I25.811
        with angina pectoris — see Arteriosclerosis, coronary (artery)
Athetosis (acquired) R25.8
  bilateral (congenital) G80.3
  congenital (bilateral) (double) G80.3
  double (congenital) G80.3
  unilateral R25.8
Athlete's
  foot B35.3
  heart I51.7
Athrepsia E41
Athyrea (acquired) — see also Hypothyroidism
  congenital E03.1
Atonia, atony, atonic
  bladder (sphincter) (neurogenic) N31.2
  capillary I78.8
  cecum K59.8
    psychogenic F45.8
  colon — see Atony, intestine
  congenital P94.2
  esophagus K22.8
  intestine K59.8
    psychogenic F45.8
  stomach K31.89
    neurotic or psychogenic F45.8
  uterus (during labor) O62.2
    with hemorrhage (postpartum) O72.1
    postpartum (with hemorrhage) O72.1
      without hemorrhage O75.89
Atopy — see History, allergy
Atransferrinemia, congenital E88.09

Atresia, atretic
  alimentary organ or tract NEC Q45.8
    upper Q40.8
  ani, anus, anal (canal) Q42.3
    with fistula Q42.2
  aorta (ring) Q25.29
  aortic (orifice) (valve) Q23.0
    arch Q25.21
    congenital with hypoplasia of ascending aorta and defective development of left ventricle (with mitral stenosis) Q23.4
    in hypoplastic left heart syndrome Q23.4
  aqueduct of Sylvius Q03.0
    with spina bifida — see Spina bifida, with hydrocephalus
  artery NEC Q27.8
    cerebral Q28.3
    coronary Q24.5
    digestive system Q27.8
    eye Q15.8
    lower limb Q27.8
    pulmonary Q25.5
    specified site NEC Q27.8
    umbilical Q27.0
    upper limb Q27.8
  auditory canal (external) Q16.1
  bile duct (common) (congenital) (hepatic) Q44.2
    acquired — see Obstruction, bile duct
  bladder (neck) Q64.39
    obstruction Q64.31
  bronchus Q32.4
  cecum Q42.8
  cervix (acquired) N88.2
    congenital Q51.828
    in pregnancy or childbirth — see Anomaly, cervix, in pregnancy or childbirth
      causing obstructed labor O65.5
  choana Q30.0
  colon Q42.9
    specified NEC Q42.8
  common duct Q44.2
  cricoid cartilage Q31.8
  cystic duct Q44.2
    acquired K82.8
      with obstruction K82.0
  digestive organs NEC Q45.8
  duodenum Q41.0
  ear canal Q16.1
  ejaculatory duct Q55.4
  epiglottis Q31.8
  esophagus Q39.0
    with tracheoesophageal fistula Q39.1
  eustachian tube Q17.8
  fallopian tube (congenital) Q50.6
    acquired N97.1
  follicular cyst N83.0-
  foramen of
    Luschka Q03.1
      with spina bifida — see Spina bifida, with hydrocephalus
    Magendie Q03.1
      with spina bifida — see Spina bifida, with hydrocephalus
  gallbladder Q44.1
  genital organ
    external
      female Q52.79
      male Q55.8
    internal
      female Q52.8
      male Q55.8
  glottis Q31.8
  gullet Q39.0
    with tracheoesophageal fistula Q39.1
  heart valve NEC Q24.8
    pulmonary Q22.0
    tricuspid Q22.4

Atresia, atretic — continued
  hymen Q52.3
    acquired (postinfective) N89.6
  ileum Q41.2
  intestine (small) Q41.9
    large Q42.9
      specified NEC Q42.8
  iris, filtration angle Q15.0
  jejunum Q41.1
  lacrimal apparatus Q10.4
  larynx Q31.8
  meatus urinarius Q64.33
  mitral valve Q23.2
    in hypoplastic left heart syndrome Q23.4
  nares (anterior) (posterior) Q30.0
  nasopharynx Q34.8
  nose, nostril Q30.0
    acquired J34.89
  organ or site NEC Q89.8
  osseous meatus (ear) Q16.1
  oviduct (congenital) Q50.6
    acquired N97.1
  parotid duct Q38.4
    acquired K11.8
  pulmonary (artery) Q25.5
    valve Q22.0
  pulmonic Q22.0
  pupil Q13.2
  rectum Q42.1
    with fistula Q42.0
  salivary duct Q38.4
    acquired K11.8
  sublingual duct Q38.4
    acquired K11.8
  submandibular duct Q38.4
    acquired K11.8
  submaxillary duct Q38.4
    acquired K11.8
  thyroid cartilage Q31.8
  trachea Q32.1
  tricuspid valve Q22.4
  ureter Q62.10
    pelvic junction Q62.11
    vesical orifice Q62.12
  ureteropelvic junction Q62.11
  ureterovesical orifice Q62.12
  urethra (valvular) Q64.39
    stricture Q64.32
  urinary tract NEC Q64.8
  uterus Q51.818
    acquired N85.8
  vagina (congenital) Q52.4
    acquired (postinfectional) (senile) N89.5
  vas deferens Q55.3
  vascular NEC Q27.8
    cerebral Q28.3
    digestive system Q27.8
    lower limb Q27.8
    specified site NEC Q27.8
    upper limb Q27.8
  vein NEC Q27.8
    digestive system Q27.8
    great Q26.8
    lower limb Q27.8
    portal Q26.5
    pulmonary Q26.3
    specified site NEC Q27.8
    upper limb Q27.8
  vena cava (inferior) (superior) Q26.8
  vesicourethral orifice Q64.31
  vulva Q52.79
    acquired N90.5
Atrichia, atrichosis — see Alopecia
At risk
  for falling Z91.81
Atrophia — see also Atrophy
  cutis senilis L90.8
    due to radiation L57.8
  gyrata of choroid and retina H31.23

Atrophia — *see also* Atrophy — *continued*
  senilis R54
    dermatological L90.8
      due to radiation (nonionizing) (solar)
        L57.8
  unguium L60.3
    congenita Q84.6
Atrophie blanche (en plaque) (de Milian)
  L95.0
Atrophoderma, atrophodermia (of) L90.9
  diffusum (idiopathic) L90.4
  maculatum L90.8
    et striatum L90.8
      due to syphilis A52.79
      syphilitic A51.39
  neuriticum L90.8
  Pasini and Pierini L90.3
  pigmentosum Q82.1
  reticulatum symmetricum faciei L66.4
  senile L90.8
    due to radiation (nonionizing) (solar) L57.8
  vermiculata (cheeks) L66.4
Atrophy, atrophic (of)
  adrenal (capsule) (gland) E27.49
    primary (autoimmune) E27.1
  alveolar process or ridge (edentulous) K08.20
  anal sphincter (disuse) N81.84
  appendix K38.8
  arteriosclerotic — *see* Arteriosclerosis
  bile duct (common) (hepatic) K83.8
  bladder N32.89
    neurogenic N31.8
  blanche (en plaque) (of Milian) L95.0
  bone (senile) NEC — *see also* Disorder, bone, specified type NEC
    due to
      tabes dorsalis (neurogenic) A52.11
  brain (cortex) (progressive) G31.9
    frontotemporal circumscribed G31.01
      [F02.80]
      with behavioral disturbance G31.01
        [F02.81]
    senile NEC G31.1
  breast N64.2
    obstetric — *see* Disorder, breast, specified type NEC
  buccal cavity K13.79
  cardiac — *see* Degeneration, myocardial
  cartilage (infectional) (joint) — *see* Disorder, cartilage, specified NEC
  cerebellar — *see* Atrophy, brain
  cerebral — *see* Atrophy, brain
  cervix (mucosa) (senile) (uteri) N88.8
    menopausal N95.8
  Charcot-Marie-Tooth G60.0
  choroid (central) (macular) (myopic) (retina) H31.10-
    diffuse secondary H31.12-
    gyrate H31.23
    senile H31.11-
  ciliary body — *see* Atrophy, iris
  conjunctiva (senile) H11.89
  corpus cavernosum N48.89
  cortical — *see* Atrophy, brain
  cystic duct K82.8
  Déjérine-Thomas G23.8
  disuse NEC — *see* Atrophy, muscle
  Duchenne-Aran G12.21
  ear H93.8-
  edentulous alveolar ridge K08.20
  endometrium (senile) N85.8
    cervix N88.8
  enteric K63.89
  epididymis N50.89
  eyeball — *see* Disorder, globe, degenerated condition, atrophy
  eyelid (senile) — *see* Disorder, eyelid, degenerative
  facial (skin) L90.9

Atrophy, atrophic (of) — *continued*
  fallopian tube (senile) N83.32-
    with ovary N83.33-
  fascioscapulohumeral (Landouzy-Déjérine) G71.0
  fatty, thymus (gland) E32.8
  gallbladder K82.8
  gastric K29.40
    with bleeding K29.41
  gastrointestinal K63.89
  glandular I89.8
  globe H44.52-
  gum (*see also* Recession, gingival) K06.0
  hair L67.8
  heart (brown) — *see* Degeneration, myocardial
  hemifacial Q67.4
    Romberg G51.8
  infantile E41
    paralysis, acute — *see* Poliomyelitis, paralytic
  intestine K63.89
  iris (essential) (progressive) H21.26-
    specified NEC H21.29
  kidney (senile) (terminal) (*see also* Sclerosis, renal) N26.1
    congenital or infantile Q60.5
      bilateral Q60.4
      unilateral Q60.3
    hydronephrotic — *see* Hydronephrosis
  lacrimal gland (primary) H04.14-
    secondary H04.15-
  Landouzy-Déjérine G71.0
  laryngitis, infective J37.0
  larynx J38.7
  Leber's optic (hereditary) H47.22
  lip K13.0
  liver (yellow) K72.90
    with coma K72.91
    acute, subacute K72.00
      with coma K72.01
    chronic K72.10
      with coma K72.11
  lung (senile) J98.4
  macular (dermatological) L90.8
    syphilitic, skin A51.39
      striated A52.79
  mandible (edentulous) K08.20
    minimal K08.21
    moderate K08.22
    severe K08.23
  maxilla K08.20
    minimal K08.24
    moderate K08.25
    severe K08.26
  muscle, muscular (diffuse) (general) (idiopathic) (primary) M62.50
    ankle M62.57-
    Duchenne-Aran G12.21
    foot M62.57-
    forearm M62.53-
    hand M62.54-
    infantile spinal G12.0
    lower leg M62.56-
    multiple sites M62.59
    myelopathic — *see* Atrophy, muscle, spinal
    myotonic G71.11
    neuritic G58.9
    neuropathic (peroneal) (progressive) G60.0
    pelvic (disuse) N81.84
    peroneal G60.0
    progressive (bulbar) G12.21
      adult G12.1
      infantile (spinal) G12.0
      spinal G12.9
        adult G12.1
        infantile G12.0
    pseudohypertrophic G71.0
    shoulder region M62.51-
    specified site NEC M62.58

Atrophy, atrophic (of) — *continued*
  muscle, muscular (diffuse) (general) (idiopathic) (primary) M62.50 — *continued*
    spinal G12.9
      adult form G12.1
      Aran-Duchenne G12.21
      childhood form, type II G12.1
      distal G12.1
      hereditary NEC G12.1
      infantile, type I (Werdnig-Hoffmann) G12.0
      juvenile form, type III (Kugelberg-Welander) G12.1
      progressive G12.21
      scapuloperoneal form G12.1
      specified NEC G12.8
    syphilitic A52.78
    thigh M62.55-
    upper arm M62.52-
  myocardium — *see* Degeneration, myocardial
  myometrium (senile) N85.8
    cervix N88.8
  myopathic NEC — *see* Atrophy, muscle
  myotonia G71.11
  nail L60.3
  nasopharynx J31.1
  nerve — *see also* Disorder, nerve
    abducens — *see* Strabismus, paralytic, sixth nerve
    accessory G52.8
    acoustic or auditory — *see* subcategory H93.3
    cranial G52.9
      eighth (auditory) — *see* subcategory H93.3
      eleventh (accessory) G52.8
      fifth (trigeminal) G50.8
      first (olfactory) G52.0
      fourth (trochlear) — *see* Strabismus, paralytic, fourth nerve
      second (optic) H47.20
      sixth (abducens) — *see* Strabismus, paralytic, sixth nerve
      tenth (pneumogastric) (vagus) G52.2
      third (oculomotor) — *see* Strabismus, paralytic, third nerve
      twelfth (hypoglossal) G52.3
    hypoglossal G52.3
    oculomotor — *see* Strabismus, paralytic, third nerve
    olfactory G52.0
    optic (papillomacular bundle)
      syphilitic (late) A52.15
        congenital A50.44
    pneumogastric G52.2
    trigeminal G50.8
    trochlear — *see* Strabismus, paralytic, fourth nerve
    vagus (pneumogastric) G52.2
  neurogenic, bone, tabetic A52.11
  nutritional E41
  old age R54
  olivopontocerebellar G23.8
  optic (nerve) H47.20
    glaucomatous H47.23-
    hereditary H47.22
    primary H47.21-
    specified type NEC H47.29-
    syphilitic (late) A52.15
      congenital A50.44
  orbit H05.31-
  ovary (senile) N83.31-
    with fallopian tube N83.33-
  oviduct (senile) — *see* Atrophy, fallopian tube
  palsy, diffuse (progressive) G12.22
  pancreas (duct) (senile) K86.89
  parotid gland K11.0
  pelvic muscle N81.84

Atrophy, atrophic (of) — *continued*
  penis N48.89
  pharynx J39.2
  pluriglandular E31.8
    autoimmune E31.0
  polyarthritis M15.9
  prostate N42.89
  pseudohypertrophic (muscle) G71.0
  renal (*see also* Sclerosis, renal) N26.1
  retina, retinal (postinfectional) H35.89
  rhinitis J31.0
  salivary gland K11.0
  scar L90.5
  sclerosis, lobar (of brain) G31.09 *[F02.80]*
    with behavioral disturbance G31.09
      [F02.81]
  scrotum N50.89
  seminal vesicle N50.89
  senile R54
    due to radiation (nonionizing) (solar) L57.8
  skin (patches) (spots) L90.9
    degenerative (senile) L90.8
    due to radiation (nonionizing) (solar) L57.8
    senile L90.8
  spermatic cord N50.89
  spinal (acute) (cord) G95.89
    muscular — *see* Atrophy, muscle, spinal
    paralysis G12.20
      acute — *see* Poliomyelitis, paralytic
      meaning progressive muscular atrophy
        G12.21
  spine (column) — *see* Spondylopathy, specified
    NEC
  spleen (senile) D73.0
  stomach K29.40
    with bleeding K29.41
  striate (skin) L90.6
    syphilitic A52.79
  subcutaneous L90.9
  sublingual gland K11.0
  submandibular gland K11.0
  submaxillary gland K11.0
  Sudeck's — *see* Algoneurodystrophy
  suprarenal (capsule) (gland) E27.49
    primary E27.1
  systemic affecting central nervous system
    in
      myxedema E03.9 *[G13.2]*
      neoplastic disease (*see also* Neoplasm)
        D49.9 *[G13.1]*
      specified disease NEC G13.8
  tarso-orbital fascia, congenital Q10.3
  testis N50.0
  thenar, partial — *see* Syndrome, carpal tunnel
  thymus (fatty) E32.8
  thyroid (gland) (acquired) E03.4
    with cretinism E03.1
    congenital (with myxedema) E03.1
  tongue (senile) K14.8
    papillae K14.4
  trachea J39.8
  tunica vaginalis N50.89
  turbinate J34.89
  tympanic membrane (nonflaccid) H73.82-
    flaccid H73.81-
  upper respiratory tract J39.8
  uterus, uterine (senile) N85.8
    cervix N88.8
    due to radiation (intended effect) N85.8
      adverse effect or misadventure N99.89
  vagina (senile) N95.2
  vas deferens N50.89
  vascular I99.8
  vertebra (senile) — *see* Spondylopathy,
    specified NEC
  vulva (senile) N90.5
  Werdnig-Hoffmann G12.0
  yellow — *see* Failure, hepatic

Attack, attacks
  with alteration of consciousness (with
    automatisms) — *see* Epilepsy, localization-
    related, symptomatic, with complex partial
    seizures
  Adams-Stokes I45.9
  akinetic — *see* Epilepsy, generalized, specified
    NEC
  angina — *see* Angina
  atonic — *see* Epilepsy, generalized, specified
    NEC
  benign shuddering G25.83
  cataleptic — *see* Catalepsy
  coronary — *see* Infarct, myocardium
  cyanotic, newborn P28.2
  drop NEC R55
  epileptic — *see* Epilepsy
  heart — *see* infarct, myocardium
  hysterical F44.9
  jacksonian — *see* Epilepsy, localization-
    related, symptomatic, with simple partial
    seizures
  myocardium, myocardial — *see* Infarct,
    myocardium
  myoclonic — *see* Epilepsy, generalized,
    specified NEC
  panic F41.0
  psychomotor — *see* Epilepsy, localization-
    related, symptomatic, with complex partial
    seizures
  salaam — *see* Epilepsy, spasms
  schizophreniform, brief F23
  shuddering, benign G25.83
  Stokes-Adams I45.9
  syncope R55
  transient ischemic (TIA) G45.9
    specified NEC G45.8
  unconsciousness R55
    hysterical F44.89
  vasomotor R55
  vasovagal (paroxysmal) (idiopathic) R55
  without alteration of consciousness — *see*
    Epilepsy, localization-related,
    symptomatic, with simple partial seizures

Attention (to)
  artificial
    opening (of) Z43.9
      digestive tract NEC Z43.4
        colon Z43.3
        ilium Z43.2
        stomach Z43.1
      specified NEC Z43.8
      trachea Z43.0
      urinary tract NEC Z43.6
        cystostomy Z43.5
        nephrostomy Z43.6
        ureterostomy Z43.6
        urethrostomy Z43.6
      vagina Z43.7
  colostomy Z43.3
  cystostomy Z43.5
  deficit disorder or syndrome F98.8
    with hyperactivity — *see* Disorder, attention-
      deficit hyperactivity
  gastrostomy Z43.1
  ileostomy Z43.2
  jejunostomy Z43.4
  nephrostomy Z43.6
  surgical dressings Z48.01
  sutures Z48.02
  tracheostomy Z43.0
  ureterostomy Z43.6
  urethrostomy Z43.6

Attrition
  gum (*see also* Recession, gingival) K06.0
  tooth, teeth (excessive) (hard tissues) K03.0

Atypical, atypism — *see also* condition
  cells (on cytolgocial smear) (endocervical)
    (endometrial) (glandular)
    cervix R87.619
    vagina R87.629
  cervical N87.9
  endometrium N85.9
    hyperplasia N85.00
  parenting situation Z62.9
Auditory — *see* condition
Aujeszky's disease B33.0
Aurantiasis, cutis E67.1
Auricle, auricular — *see also* condition
  cervical Q18.2
Auriculotemporal syndrome G50.8
Austin Flint murmur (aortic insufficiency)
  I35.1
Australian
  Q fever A78
  X disease A83.4
Autism, autistic (childhood) (infantile) F84.0
  atypical F84.9
  spectrum disorder F84.0
Autodigestion R68.89
Autoerythrocyte sensitization (syndrome)
  D69.2
Autographism L50.3
Autoimmune
  disease (systemic) M35.9
  inhibitors to clotting factors D68.311
  lymphoproliferative syndrome [ALPS] D89.82
  thyroiditis E06.3
Autointoxication R68.89
Automatism G93.89
  with temporal sclerosis G93.81
  epileptic — *see* Epilepsy, localization-related,
    symptomatic, with complex partial seizures
  paroxysmal, idiopathic — *see* Epilepsy,
    localization-related, symptomatic, with
    complex partial seizures
Autonomic, autonomous
  bladder (neurogenic) N31.2
  hysteria seizure F44.5
Autosensitivity, erythrocyte D69.2
Autosensitization, cutaneous L30.2
Autosome — *see* condition by chromosome
  involved
Autotopagnosia R48.1
Autotoxemia R68.89
Autumn — *see* condition
Avellis' syndrome G46.8
Aversion
  oral R63.3
    newborn P92-
    nonorganic origin F98.2
  sexual F52.1
Aviator's
  disease or sickness — *see* Effect, adverse, high
    altitude
  ear T70.0
Avitaminosis (multiple) (*see also* Deficiency,
  vitamin) E56.9
  B E53.9
    with
      beriberi E51.11
      pellagra E52
  B12 E53.8
  B2 E53.0
  B6 E53.1
  D E55.9
    with rickets E55.0
  G E53.0
  K E56.1
  nicotinic acid E52
AVNRT (atrioventricular nodal re-entrant
  tachycardia) I47.1
AVRT (atrioventricular nodal re-entrant
  tachycardia) I47.1

DISEASE INDEX

Avulsion (traumatic)
blood vessel — *see* Injury, blood vessel
bone — *see* Fracture, by site
cartilage — *see also* Dislocation, by site
  symphyseal (inner), complicating delivery
    O71.6
external site other than limb — *see* Wound,
  open, by site
eye S05.7-
head (intracranial)
  external site NEC S08.89
  scalp S08.0
internal organ or site — *see* Injury, by site
joint — *see also* Dislocation, by site
  capsule — *see* Sprain, by site
kidney S37.06-
ligament — *see* Sprain, by site
limb — *see also* Amputation, traumatic, by site
  skin and subcutaneous tissue — *see* Wound,
    open, by site
muscle — *see* Injury, muscle
nerve (root) — *see* Injury, nerve
scalp S08.0
skin and subcutaneous tissue — *see* Wound,
  open, by site
spleen S36.032
symphyseal cartilage (inner), complicating
  delivery O71.6
tendon — *see* Injury, muscle
tooth S03.2
Awareness of heart beat R00.2
Axenfeld's
anomaly or syndrome Q15.0
degeneration (calcareous) Q13.4
Axilla, axillary — *see also* condition
breast Q83.1
Axonotmesis — *see* Injury, nerve
Ayerza's disease or syndrome (pulmonary
  artery sclerosis with pulmonary
  hypertension) I27.0
Azoospermia (organic) N46.01
due to
  drug therapy N46.021
  efferent duct obstruction N46.023
  infection N46.022
  radiation N46.024
  specified cause NEC N46.029
  systemic disease N46.025
Azotemia R79.89
meaning uremia N19
Aztec ear Q17.3
Azygos
continuation inferior vena cava Q26.8
lobe (lung) Q33.1

B

Baastrup's disease — *see* Kissing spine
Babesiosis B60.0
Babington's disease (familial hemorrhagic
  telangiectasia) I78.0
Babinski's syndrome A52.79
Baby
crying constantly R68.11
floppy (syndrome) P94.2
Bacillary — *see* condition
Bacilluria R82.71
Bacillus — *see also* Infection, bacillus
abortus infection A23.1
anthracis infection A22.9
coli infection (*see also* Escherichia coli) B96.20
Flexner's A03.1
mallei infection A24.0
Shiga's A03.0
suipestifer infection — *see* Infection, salmonella
Back — *see* condition
Backache (postural) M54.9
sacroiliac M53.3
specified NEC M54.89
Backflow — *see* Reflux
Backward reading (dyslexia) F81.0
Bacteremia R78.81
with sepsis — *see* Sepsis
Bactericholia — *see* Cholecystitis, acute
Bacterid, bacteride (pustular) L40.3
Bacterium, bacteria, bacterial
agent NEC, as cause of disease classified
  elsewhere B96.89
in blood — *see* Bacteremia
in urine — *see* Bacteriuria
Bacteriuria, bacteruria R82.71
asymptomatic R82.71
Bacteroides
fragilis, as cause of disease classified
  elsewhere B96.6
Bad
heart — *see* Disease, heart
trip
  due to drug abuse — *see* Abuse, drug,
    hallucinogen
  due to drug dependence — *see* Dependence,
    drug, hallucinogen
Baelz's disease (cheilitis glandularis
  apostematosa) K13.0
Baerensprung's disease (eczema
  marginatum) B35.6
Bagasse disease or pneumonitis J67.1
Bagassosis J67.1
Baker's cyst — *see* Cyst, Baker's
Bakwin-Krida syndrome (metaphyseal
  dysplasia) Q78.5
Balancing side interference M26.56
Balanitis (circinata) (erosiva) (gangrenosa)
  (phagedenic) (vulgaris) N48.1
amebic A06.82
candidal B37.42
due to Haemophilus ducreyi A57
gonococcal (acute) (chronic) A54.09
xerotica obliterans N48.0
Balanoposthitis N47.6
gonococcal (acute) (chronic) A54.09
ulcerative (specific) A63.8
Balanorrhagia — *see* Balanitis
Balantidiasis, balantidiosis A07.0
Bald tongue K14.4
Baldness — *see also* Alopecia
male-pattern — *see* Alopecia, androgenic
Balkan grippe A78
Balloon disease — *see* Effect, adverse, high
  altitude
Balo's disease (concentric sclerosis) G37.5

Bamberger-Marie disease — *see*
  Osteoarthropathy, hypertrophic, specified
  type NEC
Bancroft's filariasis B74.0
Band(s)
adhesive — *see* Adhesions, peritoneum
anomalous or congenital — *see also* Anomaly,
  by site
  heart (atrial) (ventricular) Q24.8
  intestine Q43.3
  omentum Q43.3
cervix N88.1
constricting, congenital Q79.8
gallbladder (congenital) Q44.1
intestinal (adhesive) — *see* Adhesions,
  peritoneum
obstructive
  intestine K56.5
  peritoneum K56.5
periappendiceal, congenital Q43.3
peritoneal (adhesive) — *see* Adhesions,
  peritoneum
uterus N73.6
  internal N85.6
vagina N89.5
Bandemia D72.825
Bandl's ring (contraction), complicating
  delivery O62.4
Bang's disease (brucella abortus) A23.1
Bangkok hemorrhagic fever A91
Bankruptcy, anxiety concerning Z59.8
Bannister's disease T78.3
hereditary D84.1
Banti's disease or syndrome (with cirrhosis)
  (with portal hypertension) K76.6
Bar, median, prostate — *see* Enlargement,
  enlarged, prostate
Barcoo disease or rot — *see* Ulcer, skin
Barlow's disease E54
Barodontalgia T70.29
Baron Münchausen syndrome — *see*
  Disorder, factitious
Barosinusitis T70.1
Barotitis T70.0
Barotrauma T70.29
odontalgia T70.29
otitic T70.0
sinus T70.1
**Barraquer(-Simons) disease or
  syndrome** (progressive lipodystrophy)
  E88.1
Barrel chest M95.4
Barrett's
disease — *see* Barrett's, esophagus
esophagus K22.70
  with dysplasia K22.719
    high grade K22.711
    low grade K22.710
  without dysplasia K22.70
syndrome — *see* Barrett's, esophagus
ulcer K22.10
  with bleeding K22.11
  without bleeding K22.10
Barré-Guillain disease or syndrome
  G61.0
Barré-Liéou syndrome (posterior cervical
  sympathetic) M53.0
**Bársony (-Polgár) (-Teschendorf)
  syndrome** (corkscrew esophagus) K22.4
Barth syndrome E78.71
Bartholinitis (suppurating) N75.8
gonococcal (acute) (chronic) (with abscess)
  A54.1
Barton's fracture S52.56-
Bartonellosis A44.9
cutaneous A44.1
mucocutaneous A44.1
specified NEC A44.8
systemic A44.0

Bartter's syndrome E26.81
Basal — *see* condition
Basan's (hidrotic) ectodermal dysplasia Q82.4
Baseball finger — *see* Dislocation, finger
Basedow's disease (exophthalmic goiter) — *see* Hyperthyroidism, with, goiter
Basic — *see* condition
Basilar — *see* condition
Bason's (hidrotic) ectodermal dysplasia Q82.4
Basopenia — *see* Agranulocytosis
Basophilia D72.824
Basophilism (cortico-adrenal) (Cushing's) (pituitary) E24.0
Bassen-Kornzweig disease or syndrome E78.6
Bat ear Q17.5
Bateman's
  disease B08.1
  purpura (senile) D69.2
Bathing cramp T75.1
Bathophobia F40.248
Batten(-Mayou) disease E75.4
  retina E75.4 *[H36]*
Batten-Steinert syndrome G71.11
Battered — *see* Maltreatment
Battey Mycobacterium infection A31.0
Battle exhaustion F43.0
Battledore placenta O43.19-
Baumgarten-Cruveilhier cirrhosis, disease or syndrome K74.69
Bauxite fibrosis (of lung) J63.1
Bayle's disease (general paresis) A52.17
Bazin's disease (primary) (tuberculous) A18.4
Beach ear — *see* Swimmer's, ear
Beaded hair (congenital) Q84.1
Béal conjunctivitis or syndrome B30.2
Beard's disease (neurasthenia) F48.8
Beat(s)
  atrial, premature I49.1
  ectopic I49.49
  elbow — *see* Bursitis, elbow
  escaped, heart I49.49
  hand — *see* Bursitis, hand
  knee — *see* Bursitis, knee
  premature I49.40
    atrial I49.1
    auricular I49.1
    supraventricular I49.1
Beau's
  disease or syndrome — *see* Degeneration, myocardial
  lines (transverse furrows on fingernails) L60.4
Bechterev's syndrome — *see* Spondylitis, ankylosing
Becker's
  cardiomyopathy I42.8
  disease
    idiopathic mural endomyocardial disease I42.3
    myotonia congenita, recessive form G71.12
  dystrophy G71.0
  pigmented hairy nevus D22.5
Beck's syndrome (anterior spinal artery occlusion) I65.8
Beckwith-Wiedemann syndrome Q87.3
Bed confinement status Z74.01
Bed sore — *see* Ulcer, pressure, by site
Bedbug bite(s) — *see* Bite(s), by site, superficial, insect
Bedclothes, asphyxiation or suffocation by — *see* Asphyxia, traumatic, due to, mechanical, trapped
Bednar's
  aphthae K12.0
  tumor — *see* Neoplasm, malignant, by site
Bedridden Z74.01
Bedsore — *see* Ulcer, pressure, by site

Bedwetting — *see* Enuresis
Bee sting (with allergic or anaphylactic shock) — *see* Toxicity, venom, arthropod, bee
Beer drinker's heart (disease) I42.6
Begbie's disease (exophthalmic goiter) — *see* Hyperthyroidism, with, goiter
Behavior
  antisocial
    adult Z72.811
    child or adolescent Z72.810
  disorder, disturbance — *see* Disorder, conduct
  disruptive — *see* Disorder, conduct
  drug seeking Z76.5
  inexplicable R46.2
  marked evasiveness R46.5
  obsessive-compulsive R46.81
  overactivity R46.3
  poor responsiveness R46.4
  self-damaging (life-style) Z72.89
  sleep-incompatible Z72.821
  slowness R46.4
  specified NEC R46.89
  strange (and inexplicable) R46.2
  suspiciousness R46.5
  type A pattern Z73.1
  undue concern or preoccupation with stressful events R46.6
  verbosity and circumstantial detail obscuring reason for contact R46.7
Behçet's disease or syndrome M35.2
Behr's disease — *see* Degeneration, macula
Beigel's disease or morbus (white piedra) B36.2
Bejel A65
Bekhterev's syndrome — *see* Spondylitis, ankylosing
Belching — *see* Eructation
Bell's
  mania F30.8
  palsy, paralysis G51.0
    infant or newborn P11.3
  spasm G51.3
Bence Jones albuminuria or proteinuria NEC R80.3
Bends T70.3
Benedikt's paralysis or syndrome G46.3
Benign — *see also* condition
  prostatic hyperplasia — *see* Hyperplasia, prostate
Bennett's fracture (displaced) S62.21-
Benson's disease — *see* Deposit, crystalline
Bent
  back (hysterical) F44.4
  nose M95.0
    congenital Q67.4
Bereavement (uncomplicated) Z63.4
Berger's disease — *see* Nephropathy, IgA
Bergeron's disease (hysterical chorea) F44.4
Beriberi (dry) E51.11
  heart (disease) E51.12
  polyneuropathy E51.11
  wet E51.12
    involving circulatory system E51.11
Berlin's disease or edema (traumatic) S05.8x-
Berlock (berloque) dermatitis L56.2
Bernard-Horner syndrome G90.2
Bernard-Soulier disease or thrombopathia D69.1
Bernhardt(-Roth) disease — *see* Mononeuropathy, lower limb, meralgia paresthetica
Bernheim's syndrome — *see* Failure, heart, congestive
Bertielliasis B71.8
Berylliosis (lung) J63.2
Besnier-Boeck(-Schaumann) disease — *see* Sarcoidosis

Besnier's
  lupus pernio D86.3
  prurigo L20.0
Best's disease H35.50
Bestiality F65.89
Betalipoproteinemia, broad or floating E78.2
Beta-mercaptolactate-cysteine disulfiduria E72.09
Betting and gambling Z72.6
  pathological (compulsive) F63.0
Bezoar T18.9
  intestine T18.3
  stomach T18.2
Bezold's abscess — *see* Mastoiditis, acute
Bianchi's syndrome R48.8
Bicornate or bicornis uterus Q51.3
  in pregnancy or childbirth O34.0-
    causing obstructed labor O65.5
Bicuspid aortic valve Q23.1
Biedl-Bardet syndrome Q87.89
Bielschowsky(-Jansky) disease E75.4
Biermer's (pernicious) anemia or disease D51.0
Biett's disease L93.0
Bifid (congenital)
  apex, heart Q24.8
  clitoris Q52.6
  kidney Q63.8
  nose Q30.2
  patella Q74.1
  scrotum Q55.29
  toe NEC Q74.2
  tongue Q38.3
  ureter Q62.8
  uterus Q51.3
  uvula Q35.7
Biforis uterus (suprasimplex) Q51.3
Bifurcation (congenital)
  gallbladder Q44.1
  kidney pelvis Q63.8
  renal pelvis Q63.8
  rib Q76.6
  tongue, congenital Q38.3
  trachea Q32.1
  ureter Q62.8
  urethra Q64.74
  vertebra Q76.49
Big spleen syndrome D73.1
Bigeminal pulse R00.8
Bilateral — *see* condition
Bile
  duct — *see* condition
  pigments in urine R82.2
Bilharziasis — *see also* Schistosomiasis
  chyluria B65.0
  cutaneous B65.3
  galacturia B65.0
  hematochyluria B65.0
  intestinal B65.1
  lipemia B65.9
  lipuria B65.0
  oriental B65.2
  piarhemia B65.9
  pulmonary NOS B65.9 *[J99]*
    pneumonia B65.9 *[J17]*
  tropical hematuria B65.0
  vesical B65.0
Biliary — *see* condition
Bilirubin metabolism disorder E80.7
  specified NEC E80.6
Bilirubinemia, familial nonhemolytic E80.4
Bilirubinuria R82.2
Biliuria R82.2
Bilocular stomach K31.2
Binswanger's disease I67.3

Biparta, bipartite
carpal scaphoid Q74.0
patella Q74.1
vagina Q52.10
Bird
face Q75.8
fancier's disease or lung J67.2
Birth
complications in mother — *see* Delivery, complicated
compression during NOS P15.9
defect — *see* Anomaly
immature (less than 37 completed weeks) — *see* Preterm, newborn
extremely (less than 28 completed weeks) — *see* Immaturity, extreme
inattention, at or after — *see* Maltreatment, child, neglect
injury NOS P15.9
basal ganglia P11.1
brachial plexus NEC P14.3
brain (compression) (pressure) P11.2
central nervous system NOS P11.9
cerebellum P11.1
cerebral hemorrhage P10.1
external genitalia P15.5
eye P15.3
face P15.4
fracture
bone P13.9
specified NEC P13.8
clavicle P13.4
femur P13.2
humerus P13.3
long bone, except femur P13.3
radius and ulna P13.3
skull P13.0
spine P11.5
tibia and fibula P13.3
intracranial P11.2
laceration or hemorrhage P10.9
specified NEC P10.8
intraventricular hemorrhage P10.2
laceration
brain P10.1
by scalpel P15.8
peripheral nerve P14.9
liver P15.0
meninges
brain P11.1
spinal cord P11.5
nerve
brachial plexus P14.3
cranial NEC (except facial) P11.4
facial P11.3
peripheral P14.9
phrenic (paralysis) P14.2
paralysis
facial nerve P11.3
spinal P11.5
penis P15.5
rupture
spinal cord P11.5
scalp P12.9
scalpel wound P15.8
scrotum P15.5
skull NEC P13.1
fracture P13.0
specified type NEC P15.8
spinal cord P11.5
spine P11.5
spleen P15.1
sternomastoid (hematoma) P15.2
subarachnoid hemorrhage P10.3
subcutaneous fat necrosis P15.6
subdural hemorrhage P10.0
tentorial tear P10.4
testes P15.5
vulva P15.5

Birth — *continued*
lack of care, at or after — *see* Maltreatment, child, neglect
neglect, at or after — *see* Maltreatment, child, neglect
palsy or paralysis, newborn, NOS (birth injury) P14.9
premature (infant) — *see* Preterm, newborn
shock, newborn P96.89
trauma — *see* Birth, injury
weight
4000 grams to 4499 grams P08.1
4500 grams or more P08.0
low (2499 grams or less) — *see* Low, birthweight
extremely (999 grams or less) — *see* Low, birthweight, extreme
Birthmark Q82.5
Birt-Hogg-Dube syndrome Q87.89
Bisalbuminemia E88.09
Biskra's button B55.1
Bite(s) (animal) (human)
abdomen, abdominal
wall S31.159
with penetration into peritoneal cavity S31.659
epigastric region S31.152
with penetration into peritoneal cavity S31.652
left
lower quadrant S31.154
with penetration into peritoneal cavity S31.654
upper quadrant S31.151
with penetration into peritoneal cavity S31.651
periumbilic region S31.155
with penetration into peritoneal cavity S31.655
right
lower quadrant S31.153
with penetration into peritoneal cavity S31.653
upper quadrant S31.150
with penetration into peritoneal cavity S31.650
superficial NEC S30.871
insect S30.861
alveolar (process) — *see* Bite, oral cavity
amphibian (venomous) — *see* Venom, bite, amphibian
animal — *see also* Bite, by site
venomous — *see* Venom
ankle S91.05-
superficial NEC S90.57-
insect S90.56-
antecubital space — *see* Bite, elbow
anus S31.835
superficial NEC S30.877
insect S30.867
arm (upper) S41.15-
lower — *see* Bite, forearm
superficial NEC S40.87-
insect S40.86-
arthropod NEC — *see* Venom, bite, arthropod
auditory canal (external) (meatus) — *see* Bite, ear
auricle, ear — *see* Bite, ear
axilla — *see* Bite, arm
back — *see also* Bite, thorax, back
lower S31.050
with penetration into retroperitoneal space S31.051
superficial NEC S30.870
insect S30.860
bedbug — *see* Bite(s), by site, superficial, insect

Bite(s) (animal) (human) — *continued*
breast S21.05-
superficial NEC S20.17-
insect S20.16-
brow — *see* Bite, head, specified site NEC
buttock S31.805
left S31.825
right S31.815
superficial NEC S30.870
insect S30.860
calf — *see* Bite, leg
canaliculus lacrimalis — *see* Bite, eyelid
canthus, eye — *see* Bite, eyelid
centipede — *see* Toxicity, venom, arthropod, centipede
cheek (external) S01.45-
internal — *see* Bite, oral cavity
superficial NEC S00.87
insect S00.86
chest wall — *see* Bite, thorax
chigger B88.0
chin — *see* Bite, head, specified site NEC
clitoris — *see* Bite, vulva
costal region — *see* Bite, thorax
digit(s)
hand — *see* Bite, finger
toe — *see* Bite, toe
ear (canal) (external) S01.35-
superficial NEC S00.47-
insect S00.46-
elbow S51.05-
superficial NEC S50.37-
insect S50.36-
epididymis — *see* Bite, testis
epigastric region — *see* Bite, abdomen
epiglottis — *see* Bite, neck, specified site NEC
esophagus, cervical S11.25
superficial NEC S10.17
insect S10.16
eyebrow — *see* Bite, eyelid
eyelid S01.15-
superficial NEC S00.27-
insect S00.26-
face NEC — *see* Bite, head, specified site NEC
finger(s) S61.259
with
damage to nail S61.359
index S61.258
with
damage to nail S61.358
left S61.251
with
damage to nail S61.351
right S61.250
with
damage to nail S61.350
superficial NEC S60.478
insect S60.46-
little S61.25-
with
damage to nail S61.35-
superficial NEC S60.47-
insect S60.46-
middle S61.25-
with
damage to nail S61.35-
superficial NEC S60.47-
insect S60.46-
ring S61.25-
with
damage to nail S61.35-
superficial NEC S60.47-
insect S60.46-
superficial NEC S60.479
insect S60.469
thumb — *see* Bite, thumb
flank — *see* Bite, abdomen, wall
flea — *see* Bite, by site, superficial, insect

Bite(s) (animal) (human) — *continued*
- foot (except toe(s) alone) S91.35-
  - superficial NEC S90.87-
    - insect S90.86-
  - toe — *see* Bite, toe
- forearm S51.85-
  - elbow only — *see* Bite, elbow
  - superficial NEC S50.87-
    - insect S50.86-
- forehead — *see* Bite, head, specified site NEC
- genital organs, external
  - female S31.552
    - superficial NEC S30.876
      - insect S30.866
    - vagina and vulva — *see* Bite, vulva
  - male S31.551
    - penis — *see* Bite, penis
    - scrotum — *see* Bite, scrotum
    - superficial NEC S30.875
      - insect S30.865
    - testes — *see* Bite, testis
- groin — *see* Bite, abdomen, wall
- gum — *see* Bite, oral cavity
- hand S61.45-
  - finger — *see* Bite, finger
  - superficial NEC S60.57-
    - insect S60.56-
  - thumb — *see* Bite, thumb
- head S01.95
  - cheek — *see* Bite, cheek
  - ear — *see* Bite, ear
  - eyelid — *see* Bite, eyelid
  - lip — *see* Bite, lip
  - nose — *see* Bite, nose
  - oral cavity — *see* Bite, oral cavity
  - scalp — *see* Bite, scalp
  - specified site NEC S01.85
    - superficial NEC S00.87
      - insect S00.86
  - superficial NEC S00.97
    - insect S00.96
  - temporomandibular area — *see* Bite, cheek
- heel — *see* Bite, foot
- hip S71.05-
  - superficial NEC S70.27-
    - insect S70.26-
- hymen S31.45
- hypochondrium — *see* Bite, abdomen, wall
- hypogastric region — *see* Bite, abdomen, wall
- inguinal region — *see* Bite, abdomen, wall
- insect — *see* Bite, by site, superficial, insect
- instep — *see* Bite, foot
- interscapular region — *see* Bite, thorax, back
- jaw — *see* Bite, head, specified site NEC
- knee S81.05-
  - superficial NEC S80.27-
    - insect S80.26-
- labium (majus) (minus) — *see* Bite, vulva
- lacrimal duct — *see* Bite, eyelid
- larynx S11.015
  - superficial NEC S10.17
    - insect S10.16
- leg (lower) S81.85-
  - ankle — *see* Bite, ankle
  - foot — *see* Bite, foot
  - knee — *see* Bite, knee
  - superficial NEC S80.87-
    - insect S80.86-
  - toe — *see* Bite, toe
  - upper — *see* Bite, thigh
- lip S01.551
  - superficial NEC S00.571
    - insect S00.561
- lizard (venomous) — *see* Venom, bite, reptile
- loin — *see* Bite, abdomen, wall
- lower back — *see* Bite, back, lower
- lumbar region — *see* Bite, back, lower
- malar region — *see* Bite, head, specified site NEC

Bite(s) (animal) (human) — *continued*
- mammary — *see* Bite, breast
- marine animals (venomous) — *see* Toxicity, venom, marine animal
- mastoid region — *see* Bite, head, specified site NEC
- mouth — *see* Bite, oral cavity
- nail
  - finger — *see* Bite, finger
  - toe — *see* Bite, toe
- nape — *see* Bite, neck, specified site NEC
- nasal (septum) (sinus) — *see* Bite, nose
- nasopharynx — *see* Bite, head, specified site NEC
- neck S11.95
  - involving
    - cervical esophagus — *see* Bite, esophagus, cervical
    - larynx — *see* Bite, larynx
    - pharynx — *see* Bite, pharynx
    - thyroid gland S11.15
    - trachea — *see* Bite, trachea
  - specified site NEC S11.85
    - superficial NEC S10.87
      - insect S10.86
  - superficial NEC S10.97
    - insect S10.96
  - throat S11.85
    - superficial NEC S10.17
      - insect S10.16
- nose (septum) (sinus) S01.25
  - superficial NEC S00.37
    - insect S00.36
- occipital region — *see* Bite, scalp
- oral cavity S01.552
  - superficial NEC S00.572
    - insect S00.562
- orbital region — *see* Bite, eyelid
- palate — *see* Bite, oral cavity
- palm — *see* Bite, hand
- parietal region — *see* Bite, scalp
- pelvis S31.050
  - with penetration into retroperitoneal space S31.051
  - superficial NEC S30.870
    - insect S30.860
- penis S31.25
  - superficial NEC S30.872
    - insect S30.862
- perineum
  - female — *see* Bite, vulva
  - male — *see* Bite, pelvis
- periocular area (with or without lacrimal passages) — *see* Bite, eyelid
- phalanges
  - finger — *see* Bite, finger
  - toe — *see* Bite, toe
- pharynx S11.25
  - superficial NEC S10.17
    - insect S10.16
- pinna — *see* Bite, ear
- poisonous — *see* Venom
- popliteal space — *see* Bite, knee
- prepuce — *see* Bite, penis
- pubic region — *see* Bite, abdomen, wall
- rectovaginal septum — *see* Bite, vulva
- red bug B88.0
- reptile NEC — *see also* Venom, bite, reptile
  - nonvenomous — *see* Bite, by site
  - snake — *see* Venom, bite, snake
- sacral region — *see* Bite, back, lower
- sacroiliac region — *see* Bite, back, lower
- salivary gland — *see* Bite, oral cavity
- scalp S01.05
  - superficial NEC S00.07
    - insect S00.06
- scapular region — *see* Bite, shoulder

Bite(s) (animal) (human) — *continued*
- scrotum S31.35
  - superficial NEC S30.873
    - insect S30.863
- sea-snake (venomous) — *see* Toxicity, venom, snake, sea snake
- shin — *see* Bite, leg
- shoulder S41.05-
  - superficial NEC S40.27-
    - insect S40.26-
- snake — *see also* Venom, bite, snake
  - nonvenomous — *see* Bite, by site
- spermatic cord — *see* Bite, testis
- spider (venomous) — *see* Toxicity, venom, spider
  - nonvenomous — *see* Bite, by site, superficial, insect
- sternal region — *see* Bite, thorax, front
- submaxillary region — *see* Bite, head, specified site NEC
- submental region — *see* Bite, head, specified site NEC
- subungual
  - finger(s) — *see* Bite, finger
  - toe — *see* Bite, toe
- superficial — *see* Bite, by site, superficial
- supraclavicular fossa S11.85
- supraorbital — *see* Bite, head, specified site NEC
- temple, temporal region — *see* Bite, head, specified site NEC
- temporomandibular area — *see* Bite, cheek
- testis S31.35
  - superficial NEC S30.873
    - insect S30.863
- thigh S71.15-
  - superficial NEC S70.37-
    - insect S70.36-
- thorax, thoracic (wall) S21.95
  - back S21.25-
    - with penetration into thoracic cavity S21.45-
  - breast — *see* Bite, breast
  - front S21.15-
    - with penetration into thoracic cavity S21.35-
  - superficial NEC S20.97
    - back S20.47-
    - front S20.37-
    - insect S20.96
      - back S20.46-
      - front S20.36-
- throat — *see* Bite, neck, throat
- thumb S61.05-
  - with
    - damage to nail S61.15-
  - superficial NEC S60.37-
    - insect S60.36-
- thyroid S11.15
  - superficial NEC S10.87
    - insect S10.86
- toe(s) S91.15-
  - with
    - damage to nail S91.25-
  - great S91.15-
    - with
      - damage to nail S91.25-
  - lesser S91.15-
    - with
      - damage to nail S91.25-
  - superficial NEC S90.47-
    - great S90.47-
    - insect S90.46-
      - great S90.46-
- tongue S01.552
- trachea S11.025
  - superficial NEC S10.17
    - insect S10.16
- tunica vaginalis — *see* Bite, testis

DISEASE INDEX

Bite(s) (animal) (human) — *continued*
tympanum, tympanic membrane — *see* Bite, ear
umbilical region S31.155
uvula — *see* Bite, oral cavity
vagina — *see* Bite, vulva
venomous — *see* Venom
vocal cords S11.035
  superficial NEC S10.17
    insect S10.16
vulva S31.45
  superficial NEC S30.874
    insect S30.864
wrist S61.55-
  superficial NEC S60.87-
    insect S60.86-
Biting, cheek or lip K13.1
Biventricular failure (heart) I50.9
Björck (-Thorson) syndrome (malignant carcinoid) E34.0
Black
death A20.9
eye S00.1-
hairy tongue K14.3
heel (foot) S90.3-
lung (disease) J60
palm (hand) S60.22-
Blackfan-Diamond anemia or syndrome (congenital hypoplastic anemia) D61.01
Blackhead L70.0
Blackout R55
Bladder — *see* condition
Blast (air) (hydraulic) (immersion) (underwater)
blindness S05.8x-
injury
  abdomen or thorax — *see* Injury, by site
  ear (acoustic nerve trauma) — *see* Injury, nerve, acoustic, specified type NEC
  syndrome NEC T70.8
Blastoma — *see* Neoplasm, malignant, by site
pulmonary — *see* Neoplasm, lung, malignant
Blastomycosis, blastomycotic B40.9
Brazilian — *see* Paracoccidioidomycosis
cutaneous B40.3
disseminated B40.7
European — *see* Cryptococcosis
generalized B40.7
keloidal B48.0
North American B40.9
primary pulmonary B40.0
pulmonary B40.2
  acute B40.0
  chronic B40.1
skin B40.3
South American — *see* Paracoccidioidomycosis
specified NEC B40.89
Blebitis, postprocedural H59.40
stage 1 H59.41
stage 2 H59.42
stage 3 H59.43
Bleb(s) R23.8
emphysematous (lung) (solitary) J43.9
endophthalmitis H59.43
filtering (vitreous), after glaucoma surgery Z98.83
inflamed (infected), postprocedural H59.40
  stage 1 H59.41
  stage 2 H59.42
  stage 3 H59.43
lung (ruptured) J43.9
  congenital — *see* Atelectasis
  newborn P25.8
subpleural (emphysematous) J43.9
Bleeder (familial) (hereditary) — *see* Hemophilia

Bleeding — *see also* Hemorrhage
anal K62.5
anovulatory N97.0
atonic, following delivery O72.1
capillary I78.8
  puerperal O72.2
contact (postcoital) N93.0
due to uterine subinvolution N85.3
ear — *see* Otorrhagia
excessive, associated with menopausal onset N92.4
familial — *see* Defect, coagulation
following intercourse N93.0
gastrointestinal K92.2
hemorrhoids — *see* Hemorrhoids
intermenstrual (regular) N92.3
  irregular N92.1
intraoperative — *see* Complication, intraoperative, hemorrhage
irregular N92.6
menopausal N92.4
newborn, intraventricular — *see* Newborn, affected by, hemorrhage, intraventricular
nipple N64.59
nose R04.0
ovulation N92.3
postclimacteric N95.0
postcoital N93.0
postmenopausal N95.0
postoperative — *see* Complication, postprocedural, hemorrhage
preclimacteric N92.4
pre-pubertal vaginal N93.1
puberty (excessive, with onset of menstrual periods) N92.2
rectum, rectal K62.5
  newborn P54.2
tendencies — *see* Defect, coagulation
throat R04.1
tooth socket (post-extraction) K91.840
umbilical stump P51.9
uterus, uterine NEC N93.9
  climacteric N92.4
  dysfunctional or functional N93.8
  menopausal N92.4
  preclimacteric or premenopausal N92.4
  unrelated to menstrual cycle N93.9
vagina, vaginal (abnormal) N93.9
  dysfunctional or functional N93.8
  newborn P54.6
  pre-pubertal N93.1
vicarious N94.89
Blennorrhagia, blennorrhagic — *see* Gonorrhea
Blennorrhea (acute) (chronic) — *see also* Gonorrhea
inclusion (neonatal) (newborn) P39.1
lower genitourinary tract (gonococcal) A54.00
neonatorum (gonococcal ophthalmia) A54.31
Blepharelosis — *see* Entropion
Blepharitis (angularis) (ciliaris) (eyelid) (marginal) (nonulcerative) H01.009
herpes zoster B02.39
left H01.006
  lower H01.005
  upper H01.004
right H01.003
  lower H01.002
  upper H01.001
squamous H01.029
  left H01.026
    lower H01.025
    upper H01.024
  right H01.023
    lower H01.022
    upper H01.021

Blepharitis (angularis) (ciliaris) (eyelid) (marginal) (nonulcerative) H01.009 — *continued*
ulcerative H01.019
  left H01.016
    lower H01.015
    upper H01.014
  right H01.013
    lower H01.012
    upper H01.011
Blepharochalasis H02.30
congenital Q10.0
left H02.36
  lower H02.35
  upper H02.34
right H02.33
  lower H02.32
  upper H02.31
Blepharoclonus H02.59
Blepharoconjunctivitis H10.50-
angular H10.52-
contact H10.53-
ligneous H10.51-
Blepharophimosis (eyelid) H02.529
congenital Q10.3
left H02.526
  lower H02.525
  upper H02.524
right H02.523
  lower H02.522
  upper H02.521
Blepharoptosis H02.40-
congenital Q10.0
mechanical H02.41-
myogenic H02.42-
neurogenic H02.43-
paralytic H02.43-
Blepharopyorrhea, gonococcal A54.39
Blepharospasm G24.5
drug induced G24.01
Blighted ovum O02.0
Blind — *see also* Blindness
bronchus (congenital) Q32.4
loop syndrome K90.2
  congenital Q43.8
sac, fallopian tube (congenital) Q50.6
spot, enlarged — *see* Defect, visual field, localized, scotoma, blind spot area
tract or tube, congenital NEC — *see* Atresia, by site
Blindness (acquired) (congenital) (both eyes) H54.0
blast S05.8x-
color — *see* Deficiency, color vision
concussion S05.8x-
cortical H47.619
  left brain H47.612
  right brain H47.611
day H53.11
due to injury (current episode) S05.9-
  sequelae — *code to* injury with seventh character S
eclipse (total) — *see* Retinopathy, solar
emotional (hysterical) F44.6
face H53.16
hysterical F44.6
legal (both eyes) (USA definition) H54.8
mind R48.8
night H53.60
  abnormal dark adaptation curve H53.61
  acquired H53.62
  congenital H53.63
  specified type NEC H53.69
  vitamin A deficiency E50.5

Blindness (acquired) (congenital) (both eyes) H54.0 — *continued*
- one eye (other eye normal) H54.40
  - left (normal vision on right) H54.42
    - low vision on right H54.12
  - low vision, other eye H54.10
  - right (normal vision on left) H54.41
    - low vision on left H54.11
- psychic R48.8
- river B73.01
- snow — *see* Photokeratitis
- sun, solar — *see* Retinopathy, solar
- transient — *see* Disturbance, vision, subjective, loss, transient
- traumatic (current episode) S05.9-
- word (developmental) F81.0
  - acquired R48.0
  - secondary to organic lesion R48.0

Blister (nonthermal)
- abdominal wall S30.821
- alveolar process S00.522
- ankle S90.52-
- antecubital space — *see* Blister, elbow
- anus S30.827
- arm (upper) S40.82-
- auditory canal — *see* Blister, ear
- auricle — *see* Blister, ear
- axilla — *see* Blister, arm
- back, lower S30.820
- beetle dermatitis L24.89
- breast S20.12-
- brow S00.82
- calf — *see* Blister, leg
- canthus — *see* Blister, eyelid
- cheek S00.82
  - internal S00.522
- chest wall — *see* Blister, thorax
- chin S00.82
- costal region — *see* Blister, thorax
- digit(s)
  - foot — *see* Blister, toe
  - hand — *see* Blister, finger
- due to burn — *see* Burn, by site, second degree
- ear S00.42-
- elbow S50.32-
- epiglottis S10.12
- esophagus, cervical S10.12
- eyebrow — *see* Blister, eyelid
- eyelid S00.22-
- face S00.82
- fever B00.1
- finger(s) S60.429
  - index S60.42-
  - little S60.42-
  - middle S60.42-
  - ring S60.42-
- foot (except toe(s) alone) S90.82-
  - toe — *see* Blister, toe
- forearm S50.82-
  - elbow only — *see* Blister, elbow
- forehead S00.82
- fracture — *omit code*
- genital organ
  - female S30.826
  - male S30.825
- gum S00.522
- hand S60.52-
- head S00.92
  - ear — *see* Blister, ear
  - eyelid — *see* Blister, eyelid
  - lip S00.521
  - nose S00.32
  - oral cavity S00.522
  - scalp S00.02
  - specified site NEC S00.82
- heel — *see* Blister, foot
- hip S70.22-
- interscapular region S20.429

Blister (nonthermal) — *continued*
- jaw S00.82
- knee S80.22-
- larynx S10.12
- leg (lower) S80.82-
  - knee — *see* Blister, knee
  - upper — *see* Blister, thigh
- lip S00.521
- malar region S00.82
- mammary — *see* Blister, breast
- mastoid region S00.82
- mouth S00.522
- multiple, skin, nontraumatic R23.8
- nail
  - finger — *see* Blister, finger
  - toe — *see* Blister, toe
- nasal S00.32
- neck S10.92
  - specified site NEC S10.82
  - throat S10.12
- nose S00.32
- occipital region S00.02
- oral cavity S00.522
- orbital region — *see* Blister, eyelid
- palate S00.522
- palm — *see* Blister, hand
- parietal region S00.02
- pelvis S30.820
- penis S30.822
- periocular area — *see* Blister, eyelid
- phalanges
  - finger — *see* Blister, finger
  - toe — *see* Blister, toe
- pharynx S10.12
- pinna — *see* Blister, ear
- popliteal space — *see* Blister, knee
- scalp S00.02
- scapular region — *see* Blister, shoulder
- scrotum S30.823
- shin — *see* Blister, leg
- shoulder S40.22-
- sternal region S20.329
- submaxillary region S00.82
- submental region S00.82
- subungual
  - finger(s) — *see* Blister, finger
  - toe(s) — *see* Blister, toe
- supraclavicular fossa S10.82
- supraorbital S00.82
- temple S00.82
- temporal region S00.82
- testis S30.823
- thermal — *see* Burn, second degree, by site
- thigh S70.32-
- thorax, thoracic (wall) S20.92
  - back S20.42-
  - front S20.32-
- throat S10.12
- thumb S60.32-
- toe(s) S90.42-
  - great S90.42-
- tongue S00.522
- trachea S10.12
- tympanum, tympanic membrane — *see* Blister, ear
- upper arm — *see* Blister, arm (upper)
- uvula S00.522
- vagina S30.824
- vocal cords S10.12
- vulva S30.824
- wrist S60.82-

Bloating R14.0
Bloch-Sulzberger disease or syndrome Q82.3
Block, blocked
- alveolocapillary J84.10
- arborization (heart) I45.5
- arrhythmic I45.9

Block, blocked — *continued*
- atrioventricular (incomplete) (partial) I44.30
  - with atrioventricular dissociation I44.2
  - complete I44.2
    - congenital Q24.6
  - congenital Q24.6
  - first degree I44.0
  - second degree (types I and II) I44.1
  - specified NEC I44.39
  - third degree I44.2
  - types I and II I44.1
- auriculoventricular — *see* Block, atrioventricular
- bifascicular (cardiac) I45.2
- bundle-branch (complete) (false) (incomplete) I45.4
  - bilateral I45.2
  - left I44.7
    - with right bundle branch block I45.2
    - hemiblock I44.60
      - anterior I44.4
      - posterior I44.5
    - incomplete I44.7
      - with right bundle branch block I45.2
  - right I45.10
    - with
      - left bundle branch block I45.2
      - left fascicular block I45.2
    - specified NEC I45.19
  - Wilson's type I45.19
- cardiac I45.9
- conduction I45.9
  - complete I44.2
- fascicular (left) I44.60
  - anterior I44.4
  - posterior I44.5
  - right I45.0
  - specified NEC I44.69
- foramen Magendie (acquired) G91.1
  - congenital Q03.1
    - with spina bifida — *see* Spina bifida, by site, with hydrocephalus
- heart I45.9
  - bundle branch I45.4
    - bilateral I45.2
  - complete (atrioventricular) I44.2
  - congenital Q24.6
  - first degree (atrioventricular) I44.0
  - second degree (atrioventricular) I44.1
  - specified type NEC I45.5
  - third degree (atrioventricular) I44.2
- hepatic vein I82.0
- intraventricular (nonspecific) I45.4
  - bundle branch
    - bilateral I45.2
- kidney N28.9
  - postcystoscopic or postprocedural N99.0
- Mobitz (types I and II) I44.1
- myocardial — *see* Block, heart
- nodal I45.5
- organ or site, congenital NEC — *see* Atresia, by site
- portal (vein) I81
- second degree (types I and II) I44.1
- sinoatrial I45.5
- sinoauricular I45.5
- third degree I44.2
- trifascicular I45.3
- tubal N97.1
- vein NOS I82.90
- Wenckebach (types I and II) I44.1

Blockage — *see* Obstruction
Blocq's disease F44.4
Blood
- constituents, abnormal R78.9
- disease D75.9
- donor — *see* Donor, blood

DISEASE INDEX

Blood — *continued*
dyscrasia D75.9
  with
    abortion — *see* Abortion, by type, complicated by, hemorrhage
    ectopic pregnancy O08.1
    molar pregnancy O08.1
    following ectopic or molar pregnancy O08.1
    newborn P61.9
    puerperal, postpartum O72.3
flukes NEC — *see* Schistosomiasis
in
  feces K92.1
    occult R19.5
  urine — *see* Hematuria
mole O02.0
occult in feces R19.5
pressure
  decreased, due to shock following injury T79.4
  examination only Z01.30
  fluctuating I99.8
  high — *see* Hypertension
    borderline R03.0
    incidental reading, without diagnosis of hypertension R03.0
  low — *see also* Hypotension
    incidental reading, without diagnosis of hypotension R03.1
spitting — *see* Hemoptysis
staining cornea — *see* Pigmentation, cornea, stromal
transfusion
  reaction or complication — *see* Complications, transfusion
type
  A (Rh positive) Z67.10
    Rh negative Z67.11
  AB (Rh positive) Z67.30
    Rh negative Z67.31
  B (Rh positive) Z67.20
    Rh negative Z67.21
  O (Rh positive) Z67.40
    Rh negative Z67.41
  Rh (positive) Z67.90
    negative Z67.91
vessel rupture — *see* Hemorrhage
vomiting — *see* Hematemesis
Blood-forming organs, disease D75.9
Bloodgood's disease — *see* Mastopathy, cystic
Bloom(-Machacek)(-Torre) syndrome Q82.8
Blount's disease or osteochondrosis — *see* Osteochondrosis, juvenile, tibia
Blue
baby Q24.9
diaper syndrome E72.09
dome cyst (breast) — *see* Cyst, breast
dot cataract Q12.0
nevus D22.9
sclera Q13.5
  with fragility of bone and deafness Q78.0
toe syndrome I75.02-
Blueness — *see* Cyanosis
Blues, postpartal O90.6
baby O90.6
Blurring, visual H53.8
Blushing (abnormal) (excessive) R23.2
BMI — *see* Body, mass index
Boarder, hospital NEC Z76.4
accompanying sick person Z76.3
healthy infant or child Z76.2
foundling Z76.1
Bockhart's impetigo L01.02
Bodechtel-Guttman disease (subacute sclerosing panencephalitis) A81.1
Boder-Sedgwick syndrome (ataxia-telangiectasia) G11.3

Body, bodies
Aschoff's — *see* Myocarditis, rheumatic
asteroid, vitreous — *see* Deposit, crystalline
cytoid (retina) — *see* Occlusion, artery, retina
drusen (degenerative) (macula) (retinal) — *see also* Degeneration, macula, drusen
  optic disc — *see* Drusen, optic disc
foreign — *see* Foreign body
loose
  joint, except knee — *see* Loose, body, joint
    knee M23.4-
  sheath, tendon — *see* Disorder, tendon, specified type NEC
mass index (BMI)
  adult
    19 or less Z68.1
    20.0-20.9 Z68.20
    21.0-21.9 Z68.21
    22.0-22.9 Z68.22
    23.0-23.9 Z68.23
    24.0-24.9 Z68.24
    25.0-25.9 Z68.25
    26.0-26.9 Z68.26
    27.0-27.9 Z68.27
    28.0-28.9 Z68.28
    29.0-29.9 Z68.29
    30.0-30.9 Z68.30
    31.0-31.9 Z68.31
    32.0-32.9 Z68.32
    33.0-33.9 Z68.33
    34.0-34.9 Z68.34
    35.0-35.9 Z68.35
    36.0-36.9 Z68.36
    37.0-37.9 Z68.37
    38.0-38.9 Z68.38
    39.0-39.9 Z68.39
    40.0-44.9 Z68.41
    45.0-49.9 Z68.42
    50.0-59.9 Z68.43
    60.0-69.9 Z68.44
    70 and over Z68.45
  pediatric
    5th percentile to less than 85th percentile for age Z68.52
    85th percentile to less than 95th percentile for age Z68.53
    greater than or equal to ninety-fifth percentile for age Z68.54
    less than fifth percentile for age Z68.51
Mooser's A75.2
rice — *see also* Loose, body, joint
  knee M23.4-
rocking F98.4
Boeck's
disease or sarcoid — *see* Sarcoidosis
lupoid (miliary) D86.3
Boerhaave's syndrome (spontaneous esophageal rupture) K22.3
Boggy
cervix N88.8
uterus N85.8
Boil — *see also* Furuncle, by site
Aleppo B55.1
Baghdad B55.1
Delhi B55.1
lacrimal
  gland — *see* Dacryoadenitis
  passages (duct) (sac) — *see* Inflammation, lacrimal, passages, acute
Natal B55.1
orbit, orbital — *see* Abscess, orbit
tropical B55.1
Bold hives — *see* Urticaria
Bombé, iris — *see* Membrane, pupillary
Bone — *see* condition
Bonnevie-Ullrich syndrome (*see also* Turner's syndrome) Q87.1
Bonnier's syndrome — *see* subcategory H81.8

Bonvale dam fever T73.3
Bony block of joint — *see* Ankylosis
BOOP (bronchiolitis obliterans organized pneumonia) J84.89
Borderline
diabetes mellitus R73.03
hypertension R03.0
osteopenia M85.8-
pelvis, with obstruction during labor O65.1
personality F60.3
Borna disease A83.9
Bornholm disease B33.0
Boston exanthem A88.0
Botalli, ductus (patent) (persistent) Q25.0
Bothriocephalus latus infestation B70.0
Botulism (foodborne intoxication) A05.1
infant A48.51
non-foodborne A48.52
wound A48.52
Bouba — *see* Yaws
Bouchard's nodes (with arthropathy) M15.2
Bouffée délirante F23
Bouillaud's disease or syndrome (rheumatic heart disease) I01.9
Bourneville's disease Q85.1
Boutonniere deformity (finger) — *see* Deformity, finger, boutonniere
Bouveret(-Hoffmann) syndrome (paroxysmal tachycardia) I47.9
Bovine heart — *see* Hypertrophy, cardiac
Bowel — *see* condition
Bowen's
dermatosis (precancerous) — *see* Neoplasm, skin, in situ
disease — *see* Neoplasm, skin, in situ
epithelioma — *see* Neoplasm, skin, in situ
type
  epidermoid carcinoma-in-situ — *see* Neoplasm, skin, in situ
  intraepidermal squamous cell carcinoma — *see* Neoplasm, skin, in situ
Bowing
femur — *see also* Deformity, limb, specified type NEC, thigh
  congenital Q68.3
fibula — *see also* Deformity, limb, specified type NEC, lower leg
  congenital Q68.4
forearm — *see* Deformity, limb, specified type NEC, forearm
leg(s), long bones, congenital Q68.5
radius — *see* Deformity, limb, specified type NEC, forearm
tibia — *see also* Deformity, limb, specified type NEC, lower leg
  congenital Q68.4
Bowleg(s) (acquired) M21.16-
congenital Q68.5
rachitic E64.3
Boyd's dysentery A03.2
Brachial — *see* condition
Brachycardia R00.1
Brachycephaly Q75.0
Bradley's disease A08.19
Bradyarrhythmia, cardiac I49.8
Bradycardia (sinoatrial) (sinus) (vagal) R00.1
neonatal P29.12
reflex G90.09
tachycardia syndrome I49.5
Bradykinesia R25.8
Bradypnea R06.89
Bradytachycardia I49.5
Brailsford's disease or osteochondrosis — *see* Osteochondrosis, juvenile, radius
Brain — *see also* condition
death G93.82
syndrome — *see* Syndrome, brain
Branched-chain amino-acid disorder E71.2

Branchial — see condition
cartilage, congenital Q18.2
Branchiogenic remnant (in neck) Q18.0
Brandt's syndrome (acrodermatitis enteropathica) E83.2
Brash (water) R12
Bravais-jacksonian epilepsy — see Epilepsy, localization-related, symptomatic, with simple partial seizures
Braxton Hicks contractions — see False, labor
Brazilian leishmaniasis B55.2
BRBPR K62.5
Break, retina (without detachment) H33.30-
with retinal detachment — see Detachment, retina
horseshoe tear H33.31-
multiple H33.33-
round hole H33.32-
Breakdown
device, graft or implant (see also Complications, by site and type, mechanical) T85.618
arterial graft NEC — see Complication, cardiovascular device, mechanical, vascular
breast (implant) T85.41
catheter NEC T85.618
cystostomy T83.010
dialysis (renal) T82.41
intraperitoneal T85.611
Hopkins T83.018
ileostomy T83.018
infusion NEC T82.514
cranial T85.610
epidural T85.610
intrathecal T85.610
spinal T85.610
subarachnoid T85.610
subdural T85.610
nephrostomy T83.012
urethral indwelling T83.011
urinary NEC T83.018
urostomy T83.018
electronic (electrode) (pulse generator) (stimulator)
bone T84.310
cardiac T82.119
electrode T82.110
pulse generator T82.111
specified type NEC T82.118
nervous system — see Complication, prosthetic device, mechanical, electronic nervous system stimulator
urinary — see Complication, genitourinary, device, urinary, mechanical
fixation, internal (orthopedic) NEC — see Complication, fixation device, mechanical
gastrointestinal — see Complications, prosthetic device, mechanical, gastrointestinal device
genital NEC T83.418
intrauterine contraceptive device T83.31
penile prosthesis (cylinder) (implanted) (pump) (resevoir) T83.410
testicular prosthesis T83.411
heart NEC — see Complication, cardiovascular device, mechanical
intrathecal infusion pump T85.615
joint prosthesis — see Complications, joint prosthesis, internal, mechanical, by site
nervous system, specified device NEC T85.615
ocular NEC — see Complications, prosthetic device, mechanical, ocular device
orthopedic NEC — see Complication, orthopedic, device, mechanical

Breakdown — continued
device, graft or implant (see also Complications, by site and type, mechanical) T85.618 — continued
specified NEC T85.618
subcutaneous device pocket
nervous system prosthetic device, implant, or graft T85.890
other internal prosthetic device, implant, or graft T85.898
sutures, permanent T85.612
used in bone repair — see Complications, fixation device, internal (orthopedic), mechanical
urinary NEC T83.118
graft T83.21
sphincter, implanted T83.111
stent (ileal conduit) (nephroureteral) T83.113
ureteral indwelling T83.112
vascular NEC — see Complication, cardiovascular device, mechanical
ventricular intracranial shunt T85.01
nervous F48.8
perineum O90.1
respirator J95.850
specified NEC J95.859
ventilator J95.850
specified NEC J95.859
Breast — see also condition
buds E30.1
in newborn P96.89
dense R92.2
nodule N63
Breath
foul R19.6
holder, child R06.89
holding spell R06.89
shortness R06.02
Breathing
labored — see Hyperventilation
mouth R06.5
causing malocclusion M26.5
periodic R06.3
high altitude G47.32
Breathlessness R06.81
Breda's disease — see Yaws
Breech presentation (mother) O32.1
causing obstructed labor O64.1
footling O32.8
causing obstructed labor O64.8
incomplete O32.8
causing obstructed labor O64.8
Breisky's disease N90.4
Brennemann's syndrome I88.0
Brenner
tumor (benign) D27.9
borderline malignancy D39.1-
malignant C56
proliferating D39.1-
Bretonneau's disease or angina A36.0
Breus' mole O02.0
Brevicollis Q76.49
Brickmakers' anemia B76.9 [D63.8]
Bridge, myocardial Q24.5
Bright red blood per rectum (BRBPR) K62.5
Bright's disease — see also Nephritis
arteriosclerotic — see Hypertension, kidney
Brill-Symmers' disease C82.90
Brill(-Zinsser) disease (recrudescent typhus) A75.1
flea-borne A75.2
louse-borne A75.1
Brion-Kayser disease — see Fever, parathyroid
Briquet's disorder or syndrome F45.0
Brissaud's
infantilism or dwarfism E23.0
motor-verbal tic F95.2

Brittle
bones disease Q78.0
nails L60.3
congenital Q84.6
Broad — see also condition
beta disease E78.2
ligament laceration syndrome N83.8
Broad- or floating-betalipoproteinemia E78.2
Brock's syndrome (atelectasis due to enlarged lymph nodes) J98.19
Brocq-Duhring disease (dermatitis herpetiformis) L13.0
Brodie's abscess or disease M86.8x-
Broken
arches — see also Deformity, limb, flat foot
arm (meaning upper limb) — see Fracture, arm
back — see Fracture, vertebra
bone — see Fracture
implant or internal device — see Complications, by site and type, mechanical
leg (meaning lower limb) — see Fracture, leg
nose S02.2
tooth, teeth — see Fracture, tooth
Bromhidrosis, bromidrosis L75.0
Bromidism, bromism G92
chronic (dependence) F13.20
due to
correct substance properly administered — see Table of Drugs and Chemicals, by drug, adverse effect
overdose or wrong substance given or taken — see Table of Drugs and Chemicals, by drug, poisoning
Bromidrosiphobia F40.298
Bronchi, bronchial — see condition
Bronchiectasis (cylindrical) (diffuse) (fusiform) (localized) (saccular) J47.9
with
acute
bronchitis J47.0
lower respiratory infection J47.0
exacerbation (acute) J47.1
congenital Q33.4
tuberculous NEC — see Tuberculosis, pulmonary
Bronchiolectasis — see Bronchiectasis
Bronchiolitis (acute) (infective) (subacute) J21.9
with
bronchospasm or obstruction J21.9
influenza, flu or grippe — see Influenza, with, respiratory manifestations NEC
chemical (chronic) J68.4
acute J68.0
chronic (fibrosing) (obliterative) J44.9
due to
external agent — see Bronchitis, acute, due to
human metapneumovirus J21.1
respiratory syncytial virus J21.0
specified organism NEC J21.8
fibrosa obliterans J44.9
influenzal — see Influenza, with, respiratory manifestations NEC
obliterans J42
with organizing pneumonia (BOOP) J84.89
obliterative (chronic) (subacute) J44.9
due to chemicals, gases, fumes or vapors (inhalation) J68.4
due to fumes or vapors J68.4
respiratory, interstitial lung disease J84.115
Bronchitis (diffuse) (fibrinous) (hypostatic) (infective) (membranous) J40
with
influenza, flu or grippe — see Influenza, with, respiratory manifestations NEC
obstruction (airway) (lung) J44.9

DISEASE INDEX

Bronchitis (diffuse) (fibrinous) (hypostatic) (infective) (membranous) J40 — *continued*
  with — *continued*
    tracheitis (15 years of age and above) J40
      acute or subacute J20.9
      chronic J42
      under 15 years of age J20.9
  acute or subacute (with bronchospasm or obstruction) J20.9
    with
      bronchiectasis J47.0
      chronic obstructive pulmonary disease J44.0
    chemical (due to gases, fumes or vapors) J68.0
    due to
      fumes or vapors J68.0
      Haemophilus influenzae J20.1
      Mycoplasma pneumoniae J20.0
      radiation J70.0
      specified organism NEC J20.8
      Streptococcus J20.2
      virus
        coxsackie J20.3
        echovirus J20.7
        parainfluenzae J20.4
        respiratory syncytial J20.5
        rhinovirus J20.6
    viral NEC J20.8
  allergic (acute) J45.909
    with
      exacerbation (acute) J45.901
      status asthmaticus J45.902
  arachidic T17.528
  aspiration (due to fumes or vapors) J68.0
  asthmatic J45.9
    chronic J44.9
      with
        acute lower respiratory infection J44.0
        exacerbation (acute) J44.1
  capillary — *see* Pneumonia, broncho
  caseous (tuberculous) A15.5
  Castellani's A69.8
  catarrhal (15 years of age and above) J40
    acute — *see* Bronchitis, acute
    chronic J41.0
    under 15 years of age J20.9
  chemical (acute) (subacute) J68.0
    chronic J68.4
    due to fumes or vapors J68.0
      chronic J68.4
  chronic J42
    with
      airways obstruction J44.9
      tracheitis (chronic) J42
    asthmatic (obstructive) J44.9
    catarrhal J41.0
    chemical (due to fumes or vapors) J68.4
    due to
      chemicals, gases, fumes or vapors (inhalation) J68.4
      radiation J70.1
      tobacco smoking J41.0
    emphysematous J44.9
    mucopurulent J41.1
    non-obstructive J41.0
    obliterans J44.9
    obstructive J44.9
    purulent J41.1
    simple J41.0
  croupous — *see* Bronchitis, acute
  due to gases, fumes or vapors (chemical) J68.0
  emphysematous (obstructive) J44.9
  exudative — *see* Bronchitis, acute
  fetid J41.1
  grippal — *see* Influenza, with, respiratory manifestations NEC

Bronchitis (diffuse) (fibrinous) (hypostatic) (infective) (membranous) J40 — *continued*
  in those under 15 years age — *see* Bronchitis, acute
    chronic — *see* Bronchitis, chronic
  influenzal — *see* Influenza, with, respiratory manifestations NEC
  mixed simple and mucopurulent J41.8
  moulder's J62.8
  mucopurulent (chronic) (recurrent) J41.1
    acute or subacute J20.9
    simple (mixed) J41.8
  obliterans (chronic) J44.9
  obstructive (chronic) (diffuse) J44.9
  pituitous J41.1
  pneumococcal, acute or subacute J20.2
  pseudomembranous, acute or subacute — *see* Bronchitis, acute
  purulent (chronic) (recurrent) J41.1
    acute or subacute — *see* Bronchitis, acute
  putrid J41.1
  senile (chronic) J42
  simple and mucopurulent (mixed) J41.8
  smokers' J41.0
  spirochetal NEC A69.8
  subacute — *see* Bronchitis, acute
  suppurative (chronic) J41.1
    acute or subacute — *see* Bronchitis, acute
  tuberculous A15.5
  under 15 years of age — *see* Bronchitis, acute
    chronic — *see* Bronchitis, chronic
  viral NEC, acute or subacute (*see also* Bronchitis, acute) J20.8
Bronchoalveolitis J18.0
Bronchoaspergillosis B44.1
Bronchocele meaning goiter E04.0
Broncholithiasis J98.09
  tuberculous NEC A15.5
Bronchomalacia J98.09
  congenital Q32.2
Bronchomycosis NOS B49 *[J99]*
  candidal B37.1
Bronchopleuropneumonia — *see* Pneumonia, broncho
Bronchopneumonia — *see* Pneumonia, broncho
Bronchopneumonitis — *see* Pneumonia, broncho
Bronchopulmonary — *see* condition
Bronchopulmonitis — *see* Pneumonia, broncho
Bronchorrhagia (*see* Hemoptysis)
Bronchorrhea J98.09
  acute J20.9
  chronic (infective) (purulent) J42
Bronchospasm (acute) J98.01
  with
    bronchiolitis, acute J21.9
    bronchitis, acute (conditions in J20) — *see* Bronchitis, acute
  due to external agent — *see* condition, respiratory, acute, due to
  exercise induced J45.990
Bronchospirochetosis A69.8
  Castellani A69.8
Bronchostenosis J98.09
Bronchus — *see* condition
Brontophobia F40.220
Bronze baby syndrome P83.8
Brooke's tumor — *see* Neoplasm, skin, benign
Brown enamel of teeth (hereditary) K00.5
Brown-Séquard disease, paralysis or syndrome G83.81
Brown's sheath syndrome H50.61-
Bruce sepsis A23.0
Brucellosis (infection) A23.9
  abortus A23.1
  canis A23.3

Brucellosis (infection) A23.9 — *continued*
  dermatitis A23.9
  melitensis A23.0
  mixed A23.8
  sepsis A23.9
    melitensis A23.0
    specified NEC A23.8
  suis A23.2
Bruck-de Lange disease Q87.1
Bruck's disease — *see* Deformity, limb
Brugsch's syndrome Q82.8
Bruise (skin surface intact) — *see also* Contusion
  with
    open wound — *see* Wound, open
  internal organ — *see* Injury, by site
  newborn P54.5
  scalp, due to birth injury, newborn P12.3
  umbilical cord O69.5
Bruit (arterial) R09.89
  cardiac R01.1
Brush burn — *see* Abrasion, by site
Bruton's X-linked agammaglobulinemia D80.0
Bruxism
  psychogenic F45.8
  sleep related G47.63
Bubbly lung syndrome P27.0
Bubo I88.8
  blennorrhagic (gonococcal) A54.89
  chancroidal A57
  climatic A55
  due to Haemophilus ducreyi A57
  gonococcal A54.89
  indolent (nonspecific) I88.8
  inguinal (nonspecific) I88.8
    chancroidal A57
    climatic A55
    due to H. ducreyi A57
    infective I88.8
  scrofulous (tuberculous) A18.2
  soft chancre A57
  suppurating — *see* Lymphadenitis, acute
  syphilitic (primary) A51.0
    congenital A50.07
  tropical A55
  virulent (chancroidal) A57
Bubonic plague A20.0
Bubonocele — *see* Hernia, inguinal
Buccal — *see* condition
Buchanan's disease or osteochondrosis M91.0
Buchem's syndrome (hyperostosis corticalis) M85.2
Bucket-handle fracture or tear (semilunar cartilage) — *see* Tear, meniscus
Budd-Chiari syndrome (hepatic vein thrombosis) I82.0
Budgerigar fancier's disease or lung J67.2
Buds
  breast E30.1
  in newborn P96.89
Buerger's disease (thromboangiitis obliterans) I73.1
Bulbar — *see* condition
Bulbus cordis (left ventricle) (persistent) Q21.8
Bulimia (nervosa) F50.2
  atypical F50.9
  normal weight F50.9
Bulky
  stools R19.5
  uterus N85.2
Bulla(e) R23.8
  lung (emphysematous) (solitary) J43.9
  newborn P25.8
Bullet wound — *see also* Wound, open
  fracture — *code as* Fracture, by site
  internal organ — *see* Injury, by site

Bundle
branch block (complete) (false) (incomplete) — *see* Block, bundle-branch
of His — *see* condition
Bunion M21.61-
tailor's M21.62-
Bunionette M21.62-
Buphthalmia, buphthalmos (congenital) Q15.0
Burdwan fever B55.0
Bürger-Grütz disease or syndrome E78.3
Buried
penis (congenital) Q55.64
acquired N48.83
roots K08.3
Burke's syndrome K86.89
Burkitt
cell leukemia C91.0-
lymphoma (malignant) C83.7-
small noncleaved, diffuse C83.7-
spleen C83.77
undifferentiated C83.7-
tumor C83.7-
type
acute lymphoblastic leukemia C91.0-
undifferentiated C83.7-
Burn (electricity) (flame) (hot gas, liquid or hot object) (radiation) (steam) (thermal) T30.0
abdomen, abdominal (muscle) (wall) T21.02
first degree T21.12
second degree T21.22
third degree T21.32
above elbow T22.039
first degree T22.139
left T22.032
first degree T22.132
second degree T22.232
third degree T22.332
right T22.031
first degree T22.131
second degree T22.231
third degree T22.331
second degree T22.239
third degree T22.339
acid (caustic) (external) (internal) — *see* Corrosion, by site
alimentary tract NEC T28.2
esophagus T28.1
mouth T28.0
pharynx T28.0
alkaline (caustic) (external) (internal) — *see* Corrosion, by site
ankle T25.019
first degree T25.119
left T25.012
first degree T25.112
second degree T25.212
third degree T25.312
multiple with foot — *see* Burn, lower, limb, multiple, ankle and foot
right T25.011
first degree T25.111
second degree T25.211
third degree T25.311
second degree T25.219
third degree T25.319
anus — *see* Burn, buttock
arm (lower) (upper) — *see* Burn, upper, limb
axilla T22.049
first degree T22.149
left T22.042
first degree T22.142
second degree T22.242
third degree T22.342
right T22.041
first degree T22.141
second degree T22.241
third degree T22.341
second degree T22.249
third degree T22.349

Burn (electricity) (flame) (hot gas, liquid or hot object) (radiation) (steam) (thermal) T30.0 — *continued*
back (lower) T21.04
first degree T21.14
second degree T21.24
third degree T21.34
upper T21.03
first degree T21.13
second degree T21.23
third degree T21.33
blisters — *code as* Burn, second degree, by site
breast(s) — *see* Burn, chest wall
buttock(s) T21.05
first degree T21.15
second degree T21.25
third degree T21.35
calf T24.039
first degree T24.139
left T24.032
first degree T24.132
second degree T24.232
third degree T24.332
right T24.031
first degree T24.131
second degree T24.231
third degree T24.331
second degree T24.239
third degree T24.339
canthus (eye) — *see* Burn, eyelid
caustic acid or alkaline — *see* Corrosion, by site
cervix T28.3
cheek T20.06
first degree T20.16
second degree T20.26
third degree T20.36
chemical (acids) (alkalines) (caustics) (external) (internal) — *see* Corrosion, by site
chest wall T21.01
first degree T21.11
second degree T21.21
third degree T21.31
chin T20.03
first degree T20.13
second degree T20.23
third degree T20.33
colon T28.2
conjunctiva (and cornea) — *see* Burn, cornea
cornea (and conjunctiva) T26.1-
chemical — *see* Corrosion, cornea
corrosion (external) (internal) — *see* Corrosion, by site
deep necrosis of underlying tissue — *code as* Burn, third degree, by site
dorsum of hand T23.069
first degree T23.169
left T23.062
first degree T23.162
second degree T23.262
third degree T23.362
right T23.061
first degree T23.161
second degree T23.261
third degree T23.361
second degree T23.269
third degree T23.369
due to ingested chemical agent — *see* Corrosion, by site
ear (auricle) (external) (canal) T20.01
first degree T20.11
second degree T20.21
third degree T20.31

Burn (electricity) (flame) (hot gas, liquid or hot object) (radiation) (steam) (thermal) T30.0 — *continued*
elbow T22.029
first degree T22.129
left T22.022
first degree T22.122
second degree T22.222
third degree T22.322
right T22.021
first degree T22.121
second degree T22.221
third degree T22.321
second degree T22.229
third degree T22.329
epidermal loss — *code as* Burn, second degree, by site
erythema, erythematous — *code as* Burn, first degree, by site
esophagus T28.1
extent (percentage of body surface)
10-19 percent T31.10
with 0-9 percent third degree burns T31.10
with 10-19 percent third degree burns T31.11
20-29 percent T31.20
with 0-9 percent third degree burns T31.20
with 10-19 percent third degree burns T31.21
with 20-29 percent third degree burns T31.22
30-39 percent T31.30
with 0-9 percent third degree burns T31.30
with 10-19 percent third degree burns T31.31
with 20-29 percent third degree burns T31.32
with 30-39 percent third degree burns T31.33
40-49 percent T31.40
with 0-9 percent third degree burns T31.40
with 10-19 percent third degree burns T31.41
with 20-29 percent third degree burns T31.42
with 30-39 percent third degree burns T31.43
with 40-49 percent third degree burns T31.44
50-59 percent T31.50
with 0-9 percent third degree burns T31.50
with 10-19 percent third degree burns T31.51
with 20-29 percent third degree burns T31.52
with 30-39 percent third degree burns T31.53
with 40-49 percent third degree burns T31.54
with 50-59 percent third degree burns T31.55
60-69 percent T31.60
with 0-9 percent third degree burns T31.60
with 10-19 percent third degree burns T31.61
with 20-29 percent third degree burns T31.62
with 30-39 percent third degree burns T31.63
with 40-49 percent third degree burns T31.64

DISEASE INDEX

Burn (electricity) (flame) (hot gas, liquid or hot object) (radiation) (steam) (thermal) T30.0
— continued
extent (percentage of body surface) —
  continued
  60-69 percent T31.60 — continued
    with 50-59 percent third degree burns T31.65
    with 60-69 percent third degree burns T31.66
  70-79 percent T31.70
    with 0-9 percent third degree burns T31.70
    with 10-19 percent third degree burns T31.71
    with 20-29 percent third degree burns T31.72
    with 30-39 percent third degree burns T31.73
    with 40-49 percent third degree burns T31.74
    with 50-59 percent third degree burns T31.75
    with 60-69 percent third degree burns T31.76
    with 70-79 percent third degree burns T31.77
  80-89 percent T31.80
    with 0-9 percent third degree burns T31.80
    with 10-19 percent third degree burns T31.81
    with 20-29 percent third degree burns T31.82
    with 30-39 percent third degree burns T31.83
    with 40-49 percent third degree burns T31.84
    with 50-59 percent third degree burns T31.85
    with 60-69 percent third degree burns T31.86
    with 70-79 percent third degree burns T31.87
    with 80-89 percent third degree burns T31.88
  90 percent or more T31.90
    with 0-9 percent third degree burns T31.90
    with 10-19 percent third degree burns T31.91
    with 20-29 percent third degree burns T31.92
    with 30-39 percent third degree burns T31.93
    with 40-49 percent third degree burns T31.94
    with 50-59 percent third degree burns T31.95
    with 60-69 percent third degree burns T31.96
    with 70-79 percent third degree burns T31.97
    with 80-89 percent third degree burns T31.98
    with 90 percent or more third degree burns T31.99
  less than 10 percent T31.0
extremity — see Burn, limb
eye(s) and adnexa T26.4-
  with resulting rupture and destruction of eyeball T26.2-
  conjunctival sac — see Burn, cornea
  cornea — see Burn, cornea
  lid — see Burn, eyelid
  periocular area — see Burn, eyelid
  specified site NEC T26.3-
  eyeball — see Burn, eye

Burn (electricity) (flame) (hot gas, liquid or hot object) (radiation) (steam) (thermal) T30.0
— continued
eyelid(s) T26.0-
  chemical — see Corrosion, eyelid
face — see Burn, head
finger T23.029
  first degree T23.129
  left T23.022
    first degree T23.122
    second degree T23.222
    third degree T23.322
  multiple sites (without thumb) T23.039
    with thumb T23.049
      first degree T23.149
      left T23.042
        first degree T23.142
        second degree T23.242
        third degree T23.342
      right T23.041
        first degree T23.141
        second degree T23.241
        third degree T23.341
      second degree T23.249
      third degree T23.349
    first degree T23.139
    left T23.032
      first degree T23.132
      second degree T23.232
      third degree T23.332
    right T23.031
      first degree T23.131
      second degree T23.231
      third degree T23.331
    second degree T23.239
    third degree T23.339
  right T23.021
    first degree T23.121
    second degree T23.221
    third degree T23.321
  second degree T23.229
  third degree T23.329
flank — see Burn, abdominal wall
foot T25.029
  first degree T25.129
  left T25.022
    first degree T25.122
    second degree T25.222
    third degree T25.322
  multiple with ankle — see Burn, lower, limb, multiple, ankle and foot
  right T25.021
    first degree T25.121
    second degree T25.221
    third degree T25.321
  second degree T25.229
  third degree T25.329
forearm T22.019
  first degree T22.119
  left T22.012
    first degree T22.112
    second degree T22.212
    third degree T22.312
  right T22.011
    first degree T22.111
    second degree T22.211
    third degree T22.311
  second degree T22.219
  third degree T22.319
forehead T20.06
  first degree T20.16
  second degree T20.26
  third degree T20.36
fourth degree — code as Burn, third degree, by site
friction — see Burn, by site
from swallowing caustic or corrosive substance NEC — see Corrosion, by site

Burn (electricity) (flame) (hot gas, liquid or hot object) (radiation) (steam) (thermal) T30.0
— continued
full thickness skin loss — code as Burn, third degree, by site
gastrointestinal tract NEC T28.2
  from swallowing caustic or corrosive substance T28.7
genital organs
  external
    female T21.07
      first degree T21.17
      second degree T21.27
      third degree T21.37
    male T21.06
      first degree T21.16
      second degree T21.26
      third degree T21.36
  internal T28.3
    from caustic or corrosive substance T28.8
groin — see Burn, abdominal wall
hand(s) T23.009
  back — see Burn, dorsum of hand
  finger — see Burn, finger
  first degree T23.109
  left T23.002
    first degree T23.102
    second degree T23.202
    third degree T23.302
  multiple sites with wrist T23.099
    first degree T23.199
    left T23.092
      first degree T23.192
      second degree T23.292
      third degree T23.392
    right T23.091
      first degree T23.191
      second degree T23.291
      third degree T23.391
    second degree T23.299
    third degree T23.399
  palm — see Burn, palm
  right T23.001
    first degree T23.101
    second degree T23.201
    third degree T23.301
  second degree T23.209
  third degree T23.309
  thumb — see Burn, thumb
head (and face) (and neck) T20.00
  cheek — see Burn, cheek
  chin — see Burn, chin
  ear — see Burn, ear
  eye(s) only — see Burn, eye
  first degree T20.10
  forehead — see Burn, forehead
  lip — see Burn, lip
  multiple sites T20.09
    first degree T20.19
    second degree T20.29
    third degree T20.39
  neck — see Burn, neck
  nose — see Burn, nose
  scalp — see Burn, scalp
  second degree T20.20
  third degree T20.30
hip(s) — see Burn, thigh
inhalation — see Burn, respiratory tract
  caustic or corrosive substance (fumes) — see Corrosion, respiratory tract
internal organ(s) T28.40
  alimentary tract T28.2
    esophagus T28.1
  eardrum T28.41
  esophagus T28.1
  from caustic or corrosive substance (swallowing) NEC — see Corrosion, by site

Burn (electricity) (flame) (hot gas, liquid or hot object) (radiation) (steam) (thermal) T30.0 — *continued*
  internal organ(s) T28.40 — *continued*
    genitourinary T28.3
    mouth T28.0
    pharynx T28.0
    respiratory tract — *see* Burn, respiratory tract
    specified organ NEC T28.49
  interscapular region — *see* Burn, back, upper
  intestine (large) (small) T28.2
  knee T24.029
    first degree T24.129
    left T24.022
      first degree T24.122
      second degree T24.222
      third degree T24.322
    right T24.021
      first degree T24.121
      second degree T24.221
      third degree T24.321
    second degree T24.229
    third degree T24.329
  labium (majus) (minus) — *see* Burn, genital organs, external, female
  lacrimal apparatus, duct, gland or sac — *see* Burn, eye, specified site NEC
  larynx T27.0
    with lung T27.1
  leg(s) (lower) (upper) — *see* Burn, lower, limb
  lightning — *see* Burn, by site
  limb(s)
    lower (except ankle or foot alone) — *see* Burn, lower, limb
    upper — *see* Burn, upper limb
  lip(s) T20.02
    first degree T20.12
    second degree T20.22
    third degree T20.32
  lower
    back — *see* Burn, back
    limb T24.009
      ankle — *see* Burn, ankle
      calf — *see* Burn, calf
      first degree T24.109
      foot — *see* Burn, foot
      hip — *see* Burn, thigh
      knee — *see* Burn, knee
      left T24.002
        first degree T24.102
        second degree T24.202
        third degree T24.302
      multiple sites, except ankle and foot T24.099
        ankle and foot T25.099
          first degree T25.199
          left T25.092
            first degree T25.192
            second degree T25.292
            third degree T25.392
          right T25.091
            first degree T25.191
            second degree T25.291
            third degree T25.391
          second degree T25.299
          third degree T25.399
        first degree T24.199
        left T24.092
          first degree T24.192
          second degree T24.292
          third degree T24.392
        right T24.091
          first degree T24.191
          second degree T24.291
          third degree T24.391
        second degree T24.299
        third degree T24.399

Burn (electricity) (flame) (hot gas, liquid or hot object) (radiation) (steam) (thermal) T30.0 — *continued*
  lower — *continued*
    limb T24.009 — *continued*
      right T24.001
        first degree T24.101
        second degree T24.201
        third degree T24.301
      second degree T24.209
      thigh — *see* Burn, thigh
      third degree T24.309
      toe — *see* Burn, toe
  lung (with larynx and trachea) T27.1
  mouth T28.0
  neck T20.07
    first degree T20.17
    second degree T20.27
    third degree T20.37
  nose (septum) T20.04
    first degree T20.14
    second degree T20.24
    third degree T20.34
  ocular adnexa — *see* Burn, eye
  orbit region — *see* Burn, eyelid
  palm T23.059
    first degree T23.159
    left T23.052
      first degree T23.152
      second degree T23.252
      third degree T23.352
    right T23.051
      first degree T23.151
      second degree T23.251
      third degree T23.351
    second degree T23.259
    third degree T23.359
  partial thickness — *code as* Burn, unspecified degree, by site
  pelvis — *see* Burn, trunk
  penis — *see* Burn, genital organs, external, male
  perineum
    female — *see* Burn, genital organs, external, female
    male — *see* Burn, genital organs, external, male
  periocular area — *see* Burn, eyelid
  pharynx T28.0
  rectum T28.2
  respiratory tract T27.3
    larynx — *see* Burn, larynx
    specified part NEC T27.2
    trachea — *see* Burn, trachea
  sac, lacrimal — *see* Burn, eye, specified site NEC
  scalp T20.05
    first degree T20.15
    second degree T20.25
    third degree T20.35
  scapular region T22.069
    first degree T22.169
    left T22.062
      first degree T22.162
      second degree T22.262
      third degree T22.362
    right T22.061
      first degree T22.161
      second degree T22.261
      third degree T22.361
    second degree T22.269
    third degree T22.369
  sclera — *see* Burn, eye, specified site NEC
  scrotum — *see* Burn, genital organs, external, male

Burn (electricity) (flame) (hot gas, liquid or hot object) (radiation) (steam) (thermal) T30.0 — *continued*
  shoulder T22.059
    first degree T22.159
    left T22.052
      first degree T22.152
      second degree T22.252
      third degree T22.352
    right T22.051
      first degree T22.151
      second degree T22.251
      third degree T22.351
    second degree T22.259
    third degree T22.359
  stomach T28.2
  temple — *see* Burn, head
  testis — *see* Burn, genital organs, external, male
  thigh T24.019
    first degree T24.119
    left T24.012
      first degree T24.112
      second degree T24.212
      third degree T24.312
    right T24.011
      first degree T24.111
      second degree T24.211
      third degree T24.311
    second degree T24.219
    third degree T24.319
  thorax (external) — *see* Burn, trunk
  throat (meaning pharynx) T28.0
  thumb(s) T23.019
    first degree T23.119
    left T23.012
      first degree T23.112
      second degree T23.212
      third degree T23.312
    multiple sites with fingers T23.049
      first degree T23.149
      left T23.042
        first degree T23.142
        second degree T23.242
        third degree T23.342
      right T23.041
        first degree T23.141
        second degree T23.241
        third degree T23.341
      second degree T23.249
      third degree T23.349
    right T23.011
      first degree T23.111
      second degree T23.211
      third degree T23.311
    second degree T23.219
    third degree T23.319
  toe T25.039
    first degree T25.139
    left T25.032
      first degree T25.132
      second degree T25.232
      third degree T25.332
    right T25.031
      first degree T25.131
      second degree T25.231
      third degree T25.331
    second degree T25.239
    third degree T25.339
  tongue T28.0
  tonsil(s) T28.0
  trachea T27.0
    with lung T27.1
  trunk T21.00
    abdominal wall — *see* Burn, abdominal wall
    anus — *see* Burn, buttock
    axilla — *see* Burn, upper limb
    back — *see* Burn, back

DISEASE INDEX

Burn (electricity) (flame) (hot gas, liquid or hot object) (radiation) (steam) (thermal) T30.0 — continued
　trunk T21.00 — continued
　　breast — see Burn, chest wall
　　buttock — see Burn, buttock
　　chest wall — see Burn, chest wall
　　first degree T21.10
　　flank — see Burn, abdominal wall
　　genital
　　　female — see Burn, genital organs, external, female
　　　male — see Burn, genital organs, external, male
　　groin — see Burn, abdominal wall
　　interscapular region — see Burn, back, upper
　　labia — see Burn, genital organs, external, female
　　lower back — see Burn, back
　　penis — see Burn, genital organs, external, male
　　perineum
　　　female — see Burn, genital organs, external, female
　　　male — see Burn, genital organs, external, male
　　scapula region — see Burn, scapular region
　　scrotum — see Burn, genital organs, external, male
　　second degree T21.20
　　specified site NEC T21.09
　　　first degree T21.19
　　　second degree T21.29
　　　third degree T21.39
　　testes — see Burn, genital organs, external, male
　　third degree T21.30
　　upper back — see Burn, back, upper
　　vulva — see Burn, genital organs, external, female
　unspecified site with extent of body surface involved specified
　　10-19 per cent (0-9 percent third degree) T31.10
　　　with 10-19 percent third degree T31.11
　　20-29 per cent (0-9 percent third degree) T31.20
　　　with
　　　　10-19 percent third degree T31.21
　　　　20-29 percent third degree T31.22
　　30-39 per cent (0-9 percent third degree) T31.30
　　　with
　　　　10-19 percent third degree T31.31
　　　　20-29 percent third degree T31.32
　　　　30-39 percent third degree T31.33
　　40-49 per cent (0-9 percent third degree) T31.40
　　　with
　　　　10-19 percent third degree T31.41
　　　　20-29 percent third degree T31.42
　　　　30-39 percent third degree T31.43
　　　　40-49 percent third degree T31.44
　　50-59 per cent (0-9 percent third degree) T31.50
　　　with
　　　　10-19 percent third degree T31.51
　　　　20-29 percent third degree T31.52
　　　　30-39 percent third degree T31.53
　　　　40-49 percent third degree T31.54
　　　　50-59 percent third degree T31.55

Burn (electricity) (flame) (hot gas, liquid or hot object) (radiation) (steam) (thermal) T30.0 — continued
　unspecified site with extent of body surface involved specified — continued
　　60-69 per cent (0-9 percent third degree) T31.60
　　　with
　　　　10-19 percent third degree T31.61
　　　　20-29 percent third degree T31.62
　　　　30-39 percent third degree T31.63
　　　　40-49 percent third degree T31.64
　　　　50-59 percent third degree T31.65
　　　　60-69 percent third degree T31.66
　　70-79 per cent (0-9 percent third degree) T31.70
　　　with
　　　　10-19 percent third degree T31.71
　　　　20-29 percent third degree T31.72
　　　　30-39 percent third degree T31.73
　　　　40-49 percent third degree T31.74
　　　　50-59 percent third degree T31.75
　　　　60-69 percent third degree T31.76
　　　　70-79 percent third degree T31.77
　　80-89 per cent (0-9 percent third degree) T31.80
　　　with
　　　　10-19 percent third degree T31.81
　　　　20-29 percent third degree T31.82
　　　　30-39 percent third degree T31.83
　　　　40-49 percent third degree T31.84
　　　　50-59 percent third degree T31.85
　　　　60-69 percent third degree T31.86
　　　　70-79 percent third degree T31.87
　　　　80-89 percent third degree T31.88
　　90 per cent or more (0-9 percent third degree) T31.90
　　　with
　　　　10-19 percent third degree T31.91
　　　　20-29 percent third degree T31.92
　　　　30-39 percent third degree T31.93
　　　　40-49 percent third degree T31.94
　　　　50-59 percent third degree T31.95
　　　　60-69 percent third degree T31.96
　　　　70-79 percent third degree T31.97
　　　　80-89 percent third degree T31.98
　　　　90-99 percent third degree T31.99
　　less than 10 per cent T31.0
　upper limb T22.00
　　above elbow — see Burn, above elbow
　　axilla — see Burn, axilla
　　elbow — see Burn, elbow
　　first degree T22.10
　　forearm — see Burn, forearm
　　hand — see Burn, hand
　　interscapular region — see Burn, back, upper
　　multiple sites T22.099
　　　first degree T22.199
　　　left T22.092
　　　　first degree T22.192
　　　　second degree T22.292
　　　　third degree T22.392
　　　right T22.091
　　　　first degree T22.191
　　　　second degree T22.291
　　　　third degree T22.391
　　　second degree T22.299
　　　third degree T22.399
　　scapular region — see Burn, scapular region
　　second degree T22.20
　　shoulder — see Burn, shoulder
　　third degree T22.30
　　wrist — see Burn, wrist
　uterus T28.3
　vagina T28.3
　vulva — see Burn, genital organs, external, female

Burn (electricity) (flame) (hot gas, liquid or hot object) (radiation) (steam) (thermal) T30.0 — continued
　wrist T23.079
　　first degree T23.179
　　left T23.072
　　　first degree T23.172
　　　second degree T23.272
　　　third degree T23.372
　　multiple sites with hand T23.099
　　　first degree T23.199
　　　left T23.092
　　　　first degree T23.192
　　　　second degree T23.292
　　　　third degree T23.392
　　　right T23.091
　　　　first degree T23.191
　　　　second degree T23.291
　　　　third degree T23.391
　　　second degree T23.299
　　　third degree T23.399
　　right T23.071
　　　first degree T23.171
　　　second degree T23.271
　　　third degree T23.371
　　second degree T23.279
　　third degree T23.379
Burnett's syndrome E83.52
Burn-out (state) Z73.0
Burning
　feet syndrome E53.9
　sensation R20.8
　tongue K14.6
Burns' disease or osteochondrosis — see Osteochondrosis, juvenile, ulna
Bursa — see condition
Bursitis M71.9
　Achilles — see Tendinitis, Achilles
　adhesive — see Bursitis, specified NEC
　ankle — see Enthesopathy, lower limb, ankle, specified type NEC
　calcaneal — see Enthesopathy, foot, specified type NEC
　collateral ligament, tibial — see Bursitis, tibial collateral
　due to use, overuse, pressure — see also Disorder, soft tissue, due to use, specified type NEC
　　specified NEC — see Disorder, soft tissue, due to use, specified NEC
　Duplay's M75.0
　elbow NEC M70.3-
　　olecranon M70.2-
　finger — see Disorder, soft tissue, due to use, specified type NEC, hand
　foot — see Enthesopathy, foot, specified type NEC
　gonococcal A54.49
　gouty — see Gout
　hand M70.1-
　hip NEC M70.7-
　　trochanteric M70.6-
　infective NEC M71.10
　　abscess — see Abscess, bursa
　　ankle M71.17-
　　elbow M71.12-
　　foot M71.17-
　　hand M71.14-
　　hip M71.15-
　　knee M71.16-
　　multiple sites M71.19
　　shoulder M71.11-
　　specified site NEC M71.18
　　wrist M71.13-
　ischial — see Bursitis, hip
　knee NEC M70.5-
　　prepatellar M70.4-
　occupational NEC — see also Disorder, soft tissue, due to, use

DISEASE INDEX

Bursitis M71.9 — *continued*
  olecranon — *see* Bursitis, elbow, olecranon
  pharyngeal J39.1
  popliteal — *see* Bursitis, knee
  prepatellar M70.4-
  radiohumeral M77.8
  rheumatoid M06.20
    ankle M06.27-
    elbow M06.22-
    foot joint M06.27-
    hand joint M06.24-
    hip M06.25-
    knee M06.26-
    multiple site M06.29
    shoulder M06.21-
    vertebra M06.28
    wrist M06.23-
  scapulohumeral — *see* Bursitis, shoulder
  semimembranous muscle (knee) — *see* Bursitis, knee
  shoulder M75.5-
    adhesive — *see* Capsulitis, adhesive
  specified NEC M71.50
    ankle M71.57-
    due to use, overuse or pressure — *see* Disorder, soft tissue, due to, use
    elbow M71.52-
    foot M71.57-
    hand M71.54-
    hip M71.55-
    knee M71.56-
    shoulder — *see* Bursitis, shoulder
    specified site NEC M71.58
    tibial collateral M76.4-
    wrist M71.53-
  subacromial — *see* Bursitis, shoulder
  subcoracoid — *see* Bursitis, shoulder
  subdeltoid — *see* Bursitis, shoulder
  syphilitic A52.78
  Thornwaldt, Tornwaldt J39.2
  tibial collateral M76.4-
  toe — *see* Enthesopathy, foot, specified type NEC
  trochanteric (area) — *see* Bursitis, hip, trochanteric
  wrist — *see* Bursitis, hand
Bursopathy M71.9
  specified type NEC M71.80
    ankle M71.87-
    elbow M71.82-
    foot M71.87-
    hand M71.84-
    hip M71.85-
    knee M71.86-
    multiple sites M71.89
    shoulder M71.81-
    specified site NEC M71.88
    wrist M71.83-
Burst stitches or sutures (complication of surgery) T81.31
  external operation wound T81.31
  internal operation wound T81.32
Buruli ulcer A31.1
Bury's disease L95.1
Buschke's
  disease B45.3
  scleredema — *see* Sclerosis, systemic
Busse-Buschke disease B45.3
Buttock — *see* condition
Button
  Biskra B55.1
  Delhi B55.1
  oriental B55.1
Buttonhole deformity (finger) — *see* Deformity, finger, boutonniere
Bwamba fever A92.8
Byssinosis J66.0
Bywaters' syndrome T79.5

C

Cachexia R64
  cancerous R64
  cardiac — *see* Disease, heart
  dehydration E86.0
  due to malnutrition R64
  exophthalmic — *see* Hyperthyroidism
  heart — *see* Disease, heart
  hypophyseal E23.0
  hypopituitary E23.0
  lead — *see* Poisoning, lead
  malignant R64
  marsh — *see* Malaria
  nervous F48.8
  old age R54
  paludal — *see* Malaria
  pituitary E23.0
  renal N28.9
  saturnine — *see* Poisoning, lead
  senile R54
  Simmonds' E23.0
  splenica D73.0
  strumipriva E03.4
  tuberculous NEC — *see* Tuberculosis
Café, au lait spots L81.3
Caffeine-induced
  anxiety disorder F15.980
  sleep disorder F15.982
Caffey's syndrome Q78.8
Caisson disease T70.3
Cake kidney Q63.1
Caked breast (puerperal, postpartum) O92.79
Calabar swelling B74.3
Calcaneal spur — *see* Spur, bone, calcaneal
Calcaneo-apophysitis M92.8
Calcareous — *see* condition
Calcicosis J62.8
Calciferol (vitamin D) deficiency E55.9
  with rickets E55.0
Calcification
  adrenal (capsule) (gland) E27.49
    tuberculous E35 [B90.8]
  aorta I70.0
  artery (annular) — *see* Arteriosclerosis
  auricle (ear) — *see* Disorder, pinna, specified type NEC
  basal ganglia G23.8
  bladder N32.89
    due to Schistosoma hematobium B65.0
  brain (cortex) — *see* Calcification, cerebral
  bronchus J98.09
  bursa M71.40
    ankle M71.47-
    elbow M71.42-
    foot M71.47-
    hand M71.44-
    hip M71.45-
    knee M71.46-
    multiple sites M71.49
    shoulder M75.3-
    specified site NEC M71.48
    wrist M71.43-
  cardiac — *see* Degeneration, myocardial
  cerebral (cortex) G93.89
    artery I67.2
  cervix (uteri) N88.8
  choroid plexus G93.89
  conjunctiva — *see* Concretion, conjunctiva
  corpora cavernosa (penis) N48.89
  cortex (brain) — *see* Calcification, cerebral
  dental pulp (nodular) K04.2
  dentinal papilla K00.4
  fallopian tube N83.8
  falx cerebri G96.19
  gallbladder K82.8
  general E83.59

Calcification — *continued*
  heart — *see also* Degeneration, myocardial
    valve — *see* Endocarditis
  idiopathic infantile arterial (IIAC) Q28.8
  intervertebral cartilage or disc (postinfective) — *see* Disorder, disc, specified NEC
  intracranial — *see* Calcification, cerebral
  joint — *see* Disorder, joint, specified type NEC
  kidney N28.89
    tuberculous N29 [B90.1]
  larynx (senile) J38.7
  lens — *see* Cataract, specified NEC
  lung (active) (postinfectional) J98.4
    tuberculous B90.9
  lymph gland or node (postinfectional) I89.8
    tuberculous (*see also* Tuberculosis, lymph gland) B90.8
  mammographic R92.1
  massive (paraplegic) — *see* Myositis, ossificans, in, quadriplegia
  medial — *see* Arteriosclerosis, extremities
  meninges (cerebral) (spinal) G96.19
  metastatic E83.59
  muscle M61.9
    due to burns — *see* Myositis, ossificans, in, burns
    paralytic — *see* Myositis, ossificans, in, quadriplegia
    specified type NEC M61.40
      ankle M61.47-
      foot M61.47-
      forearm M61.43-
      hand M61.44-
      lower leg M61.46-
      multiple sites M61.49
      pelvic region M61.45-
      shoulder region M61.41-
      specified site NEC M61.48
      thigh M61.45-
      upper arm M61.42-
  myocardium, myocardial — *see* Degeneration, myocardial
  Mönckeberg's — *see* Arteriosclerosis, extremities
  ovary N83.8
  pancreas K86.89
  penis N48.89
  periarticular — *see* Disorder, joint, specified type NEC
  pericardium (*see also* Pericarditis) I31.1
  pineal gland E34.8
  pleura J94.8
    postinfectional J94.8
    tuberculous NEC B90.9
  pulpal (dental) (nodular) K04.2
  sclera H15.89
  spleen D73.89
  subcutaneous L94.2
  suprarenal (capsule) (gland) E27.49
  tendon (sheath) — *see also* Tenosynovitis, specified type NEC
    with bursitis, synovitis or tenosynovitis — *see* Tendinitis, calcific
  trachea J39.8
  ureter N28.89
  uterus N85.8
  vitreous — *see* Deposit, crystalline
Calcified — *see* Calcification
Calcinosis (interstitial) (tumoral) (universalis) E83.59
  with Raynaud's phenomenon, esophageal dysfunction, sclerodactyly, telangiectasia (CREST syndrome) M34.1
  circumscripta (skin) L94.2
  cutis L94.2
Calciphylaxis (*see also* Calcification, by site) E83.59

Calcium
deposits — *see* Calcification, by site
metabolism disorder E83.50
salts or soaps in vitreous — *see* Deposit, crystalline
Calciuria R82.99
Calculi — *see* Calculus
Calculosis, intrahepatic — *see* Calculus, bile duct
Calculus, calculi, calculous
ampulla of Vater — *see* Calculus, bile duct
anuria (impacted) (recurrent) (*see also* Calculus, urinary) N20.9
appendix K38.1
bile duct (common) (hepatic) K80.50
  with
    calculus of gallbladder — *see* Calculus, gallbladder and bile duct
    cholangitis K80.30
      with
        cholecystitis — *see* Calculus, bile duct, with cholecystitis
        obstruction K80.31
      acute K80.32
        with
          chronic cholangitis K80.36
            with obstruction K80.37
          obstruction K80.33
      chronic K80.34
        with
          acute cholangitis K80.36
            with obstruction K80.37
          obstruction K80.35
    cholecystitis (with cholangitis) K80.40
      with obstruction K80.41
      acute K80.42
        with
          chronic cholecystitis K80.46
            with obstruction K80.47
          obstruction K80.43
      chronic K80.44
        with
          acute cholecystitis K80.46
            with obstruction K80.47
          obstruction K80.45
    obstruction K80.51
biliary — *see also* Calculus, gallbladder
  specified NEC K80.80
    with obstruction K80.81
bilirubin, multiple — *see* Calculus, gallbladder
bladder (encysted) (impacted) (urinary) (diverticulum) N21.0
bronchus J98.09
calyx (kidney) (renal) — *see* Calculus, kidney
cholesterol (pure) (solitary) — *see* Calculus, gallbladder
common duct (bile) — *see* Calculus, bile duct
conjunctiva — *see* Concretion, conjunctiva
cystic N21.0
  duct — *see* Calculus, gallbladder
dental (subgingival) (supragingival) K03.6
diverticulum
  bladder N21.0
  kidney N20.0
epididymis N50.89

Calculus, calculi, calculous — *continued*
gallbladder K80.20
  with
    bile duct calculus — *see* Calculus, gallbladder and bile duct
    cholecystitis K80.10
      with obstruction K80.11
      acute K80.00
        with
          chronic cholecystitis K80.12
            with obstruction K80.13
          obstruction K80.01
      chronic K80.10
        with
          acute cholecystitis K80.12
            with obstruction K80.13
          obstruction K80.11
    specified NEC K80.18
      with obstruction K80.19
    obstruction K80.21
gallbladder and bile duct K80.70
  with
    cholecystitis K80.60
      with obstruction K80.61
      acute K80.62
        with
          chronic cholecystitis K80.66
            with obstruction K80.67
          obstruction K80.63
      chronic K80.64
        with
          acute cholecystitis K80.66
            with obstruction K80.67
          obstruction K80.65
    obstruction K80.71
hepatic (duct) — *see* Calculus, bile duct
hepatobiliary K80.80
  with obstruction K80.81
ileal conduit N21.8
intestinal (impaction) (obstruction) K56.49
kidney (impacted) (multiple) (pelvis) (recurrent) (staghorn) N20.0
  with calculus, ureter N20.2
  congenital Q63.8
lacrimal passages — *see* Dacryolith
liver (impacted) — *see* Calculus, bile duct
lung J98.4
mammographic R92.1
nephritic (impacted) (recurrent) — *see* Calculus, kidney
nose J34.89
pancreas (duct) K86.89
parotid duct or gland K11.5
pelvis, encysted — *see* Calculus, kidney
prostate N42.0
pulmonary J98.4
pyelitis (impacted) (recurrent) N20.0
  with hydronephrosis N13.2
pyelonephritis (impacted) (recurrent) — *see* category N20
  with hydronephrosis N13.2
renal (impacted) (recurrent) — *see* Calculus, kidney
salivary (duct) (gland) K11.5
seminal vesicle N50.89
staghorn — *see* Calculus, kidney
Stensen's duct K11.5
stomach K31.89
sublingual duct or gland K11.5
  congenital Q38.4
submandibular duct, gland or region K11.5
submaxillary duct, gland or region K11.5
suburethral N21.8
tonsil J35.8
tooth, teeth (subgingival) (supragingival) K03.6
tunica vaginalis N50.89

Calculus, calculi, calculous — *continued*
ureter (impacted) (recurrent) N20.1
  with calculus, kidney N20.2
    with hydronephrosis N13.2
      with infection N13.6
urethra (impacted) N21.1
urinary (duct) (impacted) (passage) (tract) N20.9
  with hydronephrosis N13.2
    with infection N13.6
  in (due to)
    lower N21.9
      specified NEC N21.8
vagina N89.8
vesical (impacted) N21.0
Wharton's duct K11.5
xanthine E79.8 *[N22]*
Calicectasis N28.89
Caliectasis N28.89
California
  disease B38.9
  encephalitis A83.5
Caligo cornea — *see* Opacity, cornea, central
Callositas, callosity (infected) L84
Callus (infected) L84
  bone — *see* Osteophyte
  excessive, following fracture — *code as* Sequelae of fracture
CALME (childhood asymmetric labium majus enlargement) N90.61
Calorie deficiency or malnutrition (*see also* Malnutrition) E46
Calvities — *see* Alopecia, androgenic
Calvé-Perthes disease — *see* Legg-Calvé-Perthes disease
Calvé's disease — *see* Osteochondrosis, juvenile, spine
Cameroon fever — *see* Malaria
Camptocormia (hysterical) F44.4
Camurati-Engelmann syndrome Q78.3
Canal — *see also* condition
  atrioventricular common Q21.2
Canaliculitis (lacrimal) (acute) (subacute) H04.33-
  Actinomyces A42.89
  chronic H04.42-
Canavan's disease E75.29
Canceled procedure (surgical) Z53.9
  because of
    contraindication Z53.09
      smoking Z53.01
    left against medical advice (AMA) Z53.21
    patient's decision Z53.20
      for reasons of belief or group pressure Z53.1
    specified reason NEC Z53.29
    specified reason NEC Z53.8
Cancer — *see also* Neoplasm, by site, malignant
  bile duct type liver C22.1
  blood — *see* Leukemia
  breast (*see also* Neoplasm, breast, malignant) C50.91-
  hepatocellular C22.0
  lung (*see also* Neoplasm, lung, malignant) C34.90-
  ovarian (*see also* Neoplasm ovary, malignant) C56.9-
  unspecified site (primary) C80.1
Cancer (o)phobia F45.29
Cancerous — *see* Neoplasm, malignant, by site
Cancrum oris A69.0
Candidiasis, candidal B37.9
  balanitis B37.42
  bronchitis B37.1
  cheilitis B37.83
  congenital P37.5
  cystitis B37.41
  disseminated B37.7
  endocarditis B37.6

Candidiasis, candidal B37.9 — *continued*
  enteritis B37.82
  esophagitis B37.81
  intertrigo B37.2
  lung B37.1
  meningitis B37.5
  mouth B37.0
  nails B37.2
  neonatal P37.5
  onychia B37.2
  oral B37.0
  osteomyelitis B37.89
  otitis externa B37.84
  paronychia B37.2
  perionyxis B37.2
  pneumonia B37.1
  proctitis B37.82
  pulmonary B37.1
  pyelonephritis B37.49
  sepsis B37.7
  skin B37.2
  specified site NEC B37.89
  stomatitis B37.0
  systemic B37.7
  urethritis B37.41
  urogenital site NEC B37.49
  vagina B37.3
  vulva B37.3
  vulvovaginitis B37.3
Candidid L30.2
Candidosis — *see* Candidiasis
Candiru infection or infestation B88.8
Canities (premature) L67.1
  congenital Q84.2
Canker (mouth) (sore) K12.0
  rash A38.9
Cannabinosis J66.2
Cannabis-induced
  anxiety disorder F12.980
  psychotic disorder F12.959
  sleep disorder F12.988
Canton fever A75.9
Cantrell's syndrome Q87.89
Capillariasis (intestinal) B81.1
  hepatic B83.8
Capillary — *see* condition
Caplan's syndrome — *see* Rheumatoid, lung
Capsule — *see* condition
Capsulitis (joint) — *see also* Enthesopathy
  adhesive (shoulder) M75.0-
  hepatic K65.8
  labyrinthine — *see* Otosclerosis, specified NEC
  thyroid E06.9
Caput
  crepitus Q75.8
  medusae I86.8
  succedaneum P12.81
Car sickness T75.3
Carapata (disease) A68.0
Carate — *see* Pinta
Carbon lung J60
Carbuncle L02.93
  abdominal wall L02.231
  anus K61.0
  auditory canal, external — *see* Abscess, ear, external
  auricle ear — *see* Abscess, ear, external
  axilla L02.43-
  back (any part) L02.232
  breast N61.1
  buttock L02.33
  cheek (external) L02.03
  chest wall L02.233
  chin L02.03
  corpus cavernosum N48.21
  ear (any part) (external) (middle) — *see* Abscess, ear, external
  external auditory canal — *see* Abscess, ear, external

Carbuncle L02.93 — *continued*
  eyelid — *see* Abscess, eyelid
  face NEC L02.03
  femoral (region) — *see* Carbuncle, lower limb
  finger — *see* Carbuncle, hand
  flank L02.231
  foot L02.63-
  forehead L02.03
  genital — *see* Abscess, genital
  gluteal (region) L02.33
  groin L02.234
  hand L02.53-
  head NEC L02.831
  heel — *see* Carbuncle, foot
  hip — *see* Carbuncle, lower limb
  kidney — *see* Abscess, kidney
  knee — *see* Carbuncle, lower limb
  labium (majus) (minus) N76.4
  lacrimal
    gland — *see* Dacryoadenitis
    passages (duct) (sac) — *see* Inflammation, lacrimal, passages, acute
  leg — *see* Carbuncle, lower limb
  lower limb L02.43-
  malignant A22.0
  navel L02.236
  neck L02.13
  nose (external) (septum) J34.0
  orbit, orbital — *see* Abscess, orbit
  palmar (space) — *see* Carbuncle, hand
  partes posteriores L02.33
  pectoral region L02.233
  penis N48.21
  perineum L02.235
  pinna — *see* Abscess, ear, external
  popliteal — *see* Carbuncle, lower limb
  scalp L02.831
  seminal vesicle N49.0
  shoulder — *see* Carbuncle, upper limb
  specified site NEC L02.838
  temple (region) L02.03
  thumb — *see* Carbuncle, hand
  toe — *see* Carbuncle, foot
  trunk L02.239
    abdominal wall L02.231
    back L02.232
    chest wall L02.233
    groin L02.234
    perineum L02.235
    umbilicus L02.236
  umbilicus L02.236
  upper limb L02.43-
  urethra N34.0
  vulva N76.4
Carbunculus — *see* Carbuncle
Carcinoid (tumor) — *see* Tumor, carcinoid
Carcinoidosis E34.0
Carcinoma (malignant) — *see also* Neoplasm, by site, malignant
  acidophil
    specified site — *see* Neoplasm, malignant, by site
    unspecified site C75.1
  acidophil-basophil, mixed
    specified site — *see* Neoplasm, malignant, by site
    unspecified site C75.1
  adnexal (skin) — *see* Neoplasm, skin, malignant
  adrenal cortical C74.0-
  alveolar — *see* Neoplasm, lung, malignant
    cell — *see* Neoplasm, lung, malignant
  ameloblastic C41.1
    upper jaw (bone) C41.0
  apocrine
    breast — *see* Neoplasm, breast, malignant
    specified site NEC — *see* Neoplasm, skin, malignant
    unspecified site C44.99

Carcinoma (malignant) (*see also* Neoplasm, by site, malignant) — *continued*
  basal cell (pigmented) (*see also* Neoplasm, skin, malignant) C44.91
    fibro-epithelial — *see* Neoplasm, skin, malignant
    morphea — *see* Neoplasm, skin, malignant
    multicentric — *see* Neoplasm, skin, malignant
  basal-squamous cell, mixed — *see* Neoplasm, skin, malignant
  basaloid
  basophil
    specified site — *see* Neoplasm, malignant, by site
    unspecified site C75.1
  basophil-acidophil, mixed
    specified site — *see* Neoplasm, malignant, by site
    unspecified site C75.1
  basosquamous — *see* Neoplasm, skin, malignant
  bile duct
    with hepatocellular, mixed C22.0
    liver C22.1
    specified site NEC — *see* Neoplasm, malignant, by site
    unspecified site C22.1
  branchial or branchiogenic C10.4
  bronchial or bronchogenic — *see* Neoplasm, lung, malignant
  bronchiolar — *see* Neoplasm, lung, malignant
  bronchioloalveolar — *see* Neoplasm, lung, malignant
  C cell
    specified site — *see* Neoplasm, malignant, by site
    unspecified site C73
  ceruminous C44.29-
  cervix uteri
    in situ D06.9
      endocervix D06.0
      exocervix D06.1
      specified site NEC D06.7
  chorionic
    specified site — *see* Neoplasm, malignant, by site
    unspecified site
      female C58
      male C62.90
  chromophobe
    specified site — *see* Neoplasm, malignant, by site
    unspecified site C75.1
  cloacogenic
    specified site — *see* Neoplasm, malignant, by site
    unspecified site C21.2
  diffuse type
    specified site — *see* Neoplasm, malignant, by site
    unspecified site C16.9
  duct (cell)
    with Paget's disease — *see* Neoplasm, breast, malignant
    infiltrating
      with lobular carcinoma (in situ)
        specified site — *see* Neoplasm, malignant, by site
        unspecified site (female) C50.91-
          male C50.92-
      specified site — *see* Neoplasm, malignant, by site
      unspecified site (female) C50.91-
        male C50.92-

Carcinoma (malignant) (*see also* Neoplasm, by site, malignant) — *continued*
ductal
  with lobular
    specified site — *see* Neoplasm, malignant, by site
    unspecified site (female) C50.91-
      male C50.92-
ductular, infiltrating
  specified site — *see* Neoplasm, malignant, by site
  unspecified site (female) C50.91-
    male C50.92-
embryonal
  liver C22.7
endometrioid
  specified site — *see* Neoplasm, malignant, by site
  unspecified site
    female C56.9
    male C61
eosinophil
  specified site — *see* Neoplasm, malignant, by site
  unspecified site C75.1
epidermoid — *see also* Neoplasm, skin, malignant
  in situ, Bowen's type — *see* Neoplasm, skin, in situ
fibroepithelial, basal cell — *see* Neoplasm, skin, malignant
follicular
  with papillary (mixed) C73
  moderately differentiated C73
  pure follicle C73
  specified site — *see* Neoplasm, malignant, by site
  trabecular C73
  unspecified site C73
  well differentiated C73
generalized, with unspecified primary site C80.0
glycogen-rich — *see* Neoplasm, breast, malignant
granulosa cell C56-
hepatic cell C22.0
hepatocellular C22.0
  with bile duct, mixed C22.0
  fibrolamellar C22.0
hepatocholangiolitic C22.0
Hurthle cell C73
in
  adenomatous
    polyposis coli C18.9
  pleomorphic adenoma — *see* Neoplasm, salivary glands, malignant
  situ — *see* Carcinoma-in-situ
infiltrating
  duct
    with lobular
      specified site — *see* Neoplasm, malignant, by site
      unspecified site (female) C50.91-
        male C50.92-
    with Paget's disease — *see* Neoplasm, breast, malignant
    specified site — *see* Neoplasm, malignant
    unspecified site (female) C50.91-
      male C50.92-
  ductular
    specified site — *see* Neoplasm, malignant
    unspecified site (female) C50.91-
      male C50.92-
  lobular
    specified site — *see* Neoplasm, malignant
    unspecified site (female) C50.91-
      male C50.92-

Carcinoma (malignant) (*see also* Neoplasm, by site, malignant) — *continued*
inflammatory
  specified site — *see* Neoplasm, malignant
  unspecified site (female) C50.91-
    male C50.92-
intestinal type
  specified site — *see* Neoplasm, malignant, by site
  unspecified site C16.9
intracystic
  noninfiltrating — *see* Neoplasm, in situ, by site
intraductal (noninfiltrating)
  with Paget's disease — *see* Neoplasm, breast, malignant
  breast D05.1-
  papillary
    with invasion
      specified site — *see* Neoplasm, malignant, by site
      unspecified site (female) C50.91-
        male C50.92-
    breast D05.1-
    specified site NEC — *see* Neoplasm, in situ, by site
    unspecified site (female) D05.1-
  specified site NEC — *see* Neoplasm, in situ, by site
  unspecified site (female) D05.1-
intraepidermal — *see* Neoplasm, in situ
  squamous cell, Bowen's type — *see* Neoplasm, skin, in situ
intraepithelial — *see* Neoplasm, in situ, by site
  squamous cell — *see* Neoplasm, in situ, by site
intraosseous C41.1
  upper jaw (bone) C41.0
islet cell
  with exocrine, mixed
    specified site — *see* Neoplasm, malignant, by site
    unspecified site C25.9
  pancreas C25.4
  specified site NEC — *see* Neoplasm, malignant, by site
  unspecified site C25.4
juvenile, breast — *see* Neoplasm, breast, malignant
large cell
  small cell
    specified site — *see* Neoplasm, malignant, by site
    unspecified site C34.90
Leydig cell (testis)
  specified site — *see* Neoplasm, malignant, by site
  unspecified site
    female C56.9
    male C62.90
lipid-rich (female) C50.91-
  male C50.92-
liver cell C22.0
liver NEC C22.7
lobular (infiltrating)
  with intraductal
    specified site — *see* Neoplasm, malignant, by site
    unspecified site (female) C50.91-
      male C50.92-
  noninfiltrating
    breast D05.0-
    specified site NEC — *see* Neoplasm, in situ, by site
    unspecified site D05.0-
  specified site — *see* Neoplasm, malignant, by site
  unspecified site (female) C50.91-
    male C50.92-

Carcinoma (malignant) (*see also* Neoplasm, by site, malignant) — *continued*
medullary
  with
    amyloid stroma
      specified site — *see* Neoplasm, malignant, by site
      unspecified site C73
    lymphoid stroma
      specified site — *see* Neoplasm, malignant, by site
      unspecified site (female) C50.91-
        male C50.92-
Merkel cell C4A.9 *(follows C43)*
  anal margin C4A.51 *(follows C43)*
  anal skin C4A.51 *(follows C43)*
  canthus C4A.1- *(follows C43)*
  ear and external auricular canal C4A.2- *(follows C43)*
  external auricular canal C4A.2- *(follows C43)*
  eyelid, including canthus C4A.1- *(follows C43)*
  face C4A.30 *(follows C43)*
    specified NEC C4A.39 *(follows C43)*
  hip C4A.7- *(follows C43)*
  lip C4A.0 *(follows C43)*
  lower limb, including hip C4A.7- *(follows C43)*
  neck C4A.4 *(follows C43)*
  nodal presentation C7B.1 *(follows C75)*
  nose C4A.31 *(follows C43)*
  overlapping sites C4A.8 *(follows C43)*
  perianal skin C4A.51 *(follows C43)*
  scalp C4A.4 *(follows C43)*
  secondary C7B.1 *(follows C75)*
  shoulder C4A.6- *(follows C43)*
  skin of breast C4A.52 *(follows C43)*
  trunk NEC C4A.59 *(follows C43)*
  upper limb, including shoulder C4A.6- *(follows C43)*
  visceral metastatic C7B.1 *(follows C75)*
metastatic — *see* Neoplasm, secondary, by site
metatypical — *see* Neoplasm, skin, malignant
morphea, basal cell — *see* Neoplasm, skin, malignant
mucoid
  cell
    specified site — *see* Neoplasm, malignant, by site
    unspecified site C75.1
neuroendocrine — *see also* Tumor, neuroendocrine
  high grade, any site C7A.1 *(follows C75)*
  poorly differentiated, any site C7A.1 *(follows C75)*
nonencapsulated sclerosing C73
noninfiltrating
  intracystic — *see* Neoplasm, in situ, by site
  intraductal
    breast D05.1-
    papillary
      breast D05.1-
      specified site NEC — *see* Neoplasm, in situ, by site
      unspecified site D05.1-
    specified site — *see* Neoplasm, in situ, by site
    unspecified site D05.1-
  lobular
    breast D05.0-
    specified site NEC — *see* Neoplasm, in situ, by site
    unspecified site (female) D05.0-
oat cell
  specified site — *see* Neoplasm, malignant, by site
  unspecified site C34.90
odontogenic C41.1
  upper jaw (bone) C41.0

Carcinoma (malignant) (*see also* Neoplasm, by site, malignant) — *continued*
papillary
  with follicular (mixed) C73
  follicular variant C73
  intraductal (noninfiltrating)
    with invasion
      specified site — *see* Neoplasm, malignant, by site
      unspecified site (female) C50.91-
        male C50.92-
    breast D05.1-
    specified site NEC — *see* Neoplasm, in situ, by site
    unspecified site D05.1-
  serous
    specified site — *see* Neoplasm, malignant, by site
    surface
      specified site — *see* Neoplasm, malignant, by site
      unspecified site C56.9
    unspecified site C56.9
papillocystic
  specified site — *see* Neoplasm, malignant, by site
  unspecified site C56.9
parafollicular cell
  specified site — *see* Neoplasm, malignant, by site
  unspecified site C73
pilomatrix — *see* Neoplasm, skin, malignant
pseudomucinous
  specified site — *see* Neoplasm, malignant, by site
  unspecified site C56.9
renal cell C64-
Schmincke — *see* Neoplasm, nasopharynx, malignant
Schneiderian
  specified site — *see* Neoplasm, malignant, by site
  unspecified site C30.0
sebaceous — *see* Neoplasm, skin, malignant
secondary — *see also* Neoplasm, secondary, by site
  Merkel cell C7B.1 **(follows C75)**
secretory, breast — *see* Neoplasm, breast, malignant
serous
  papillary
    specified site — *see* Neoplasm, malignant, by site
    unspecified site C56.9
  surface, papillary
    specified site — *see* Neoplasm, malignant, by site
    unspecified site C56.9
Sertoli cell
  specified site — *see* Neoplasm, malignant, by site
  unspecified site C62.90
    female C56.9
    male C62.90
skin appendage — *see* Neoplasm, skin, malignant
small cell
  fusiform cell
    specified site — *see* Neoplasm, malignant, by site
    unspecified site C34.90
  intermediate cell
    specified site — *see* Neoplasm, malignant, by site
    unspecified site C34.90
  large cell
    specified site — *see* Neoplasm, malignant, by site
    unspecified site C34.90

Carcinoma (malignant) (*see also* Neoplasm, by site, malignant) — *continued*
solid
  with amyloid stroma
    specified site — *see* Neoplasm, malignant, by site
    unspecified site C73
  microinvasive
    specified site — *see* Neoplasm, malignant, by site
    unspecified site C53.9
sweat gland — *see* Neoplasm, skin, malignant
theca cell C56-
thymic C37
unspecified site (primary) C80.1
water-clear cell C75.0
Carcinoma-in-situ — *see also* Neoplasm, in situ, by site
breast NOS D05.9-
  specified type NEC D05.8-
epidermoid — *see also* Neoplasm, in situ, by site
  with questionable stromal invasion
    cervix D06.9
    specified site NEC — *see* Neoplasm, in situ, by site
    unspecified site D06.9
  Bowen's type — *see* Neoplasm, skin, in situ
intraductal
  breast D05.1-
  specified site NEC — *see* Neoplasm, in situ, by site
  unspecified site D05.1-
lobular
  with
    infiltrating duct
      breast (female) C50.91-
        male C50.92-
      specified site NEC — *see* Neoplasm, malignant
      unspecified site (female) C50.91-
        male C50.92-
    intraductal
      breast D05.8-
      specified site NEC — *see* Neoplasm, in situ, by site
      unspecified site (female) D05.8-
  breast D05.0-
  specified site NEC — *see* Neoplasm, in situ, by site
  unspecified site D05.0-
squamous cell — *see also* Neoplasm, in situ, by site
  with questionable stromal invasion
    cervix D06.9
    specified site NEC — *see* Neoplasm, in situ, by site
    unspecified site D06.9
Carcinomaphobia F45.29
Carcinomatosis C80.0
peritonei C78.6
unspecified site (primary) (secondary) C80.0
Carcinosarcoma — *see* Neoplasm, malignant, by site
embryonal — *see* Neoplasm, malignant, by site
Cardia, cardial — *see* condition

Cardiac — *see also* condition
death, sudden — *see* Arrest, cardiac
pacemaker
  in situ Z95.0
  management or adjustment Z45.018
tamponade I31.4
Cardialgia — *see* Pain, precordial
Cardiectasis — *see* Hypertrophy, cardiac
Cardiochalasia K21.9
Cardiomalacia I51.5

Cardiomegalia glycogenica diffusa
  E74.02 [*I43*]
Cardiomegaly — *see also* Hypertrophy, cardiac
congenital Q24.8
glycogen E74.02 [*I43*]
idiopathic I51.7
Cardiomyolipossis I51.5
Cardiomyopathy (familial) (idiopathic) I42.9
alcoholic I42.6
amyloid E85.4 [*I43*]
arteriosclerotic — *see* Disease, heart, ischemic, atherosclerotic
beriberi E51.12
cobalt-beer I42.6
congenital I42.4
congestive I42.0
constrictive NOS I42.5
dilated I42.0
due to
  alcohol I42.6
  beriberi E51.12
  cardiac glycogenosis E74.02 [*I43*]
  drugs I42.7
  external agents NEC I42.7
  Friedreich's ataxia G11.1
  myotonia atrophica G71.11 [*I43*]
  progressive muscular dystrophy G71.0
glycogen storage E74.02 [*I43*]
hypertensive — *see* Hypertension, heart
hypertrophic (nonobstructive) I42.2
  obstructive I42.1
    congenital Q24.8
in
  Chagas' disease (chronic) B57.2
    acute B57.0
  sarcoidosis D86.85
ischemic I25.5
metabolic E88.9 [*I43*]
  thyrotoxic E05.90 [*I43*]
    with thyroid storm E05.91 [*I43*]
newborn I42.8
  congenital I42.4
nutritional E63.9 [*I43*]
  beriberi E51.12
obscure of Africa I42.8
peripartum O90.3
postpartum O90.3
restrictive NEC I42.5
rheumatic I09.0
secondary I42.9
stress induced I51.81
takotsubo I51.81
thyrotoxic E05.90 [*I43*]
  with thyroid storm E05.91 [*I43*]
toxic NEC I42.7
tuberculous A18.84
viral B33.24
Cardionephritis — *see* Hypertension, cardiorenal
Cardionephropathy — *see* Hypertension, cardiorenal
Cardionephrosis — *see* Hypertension, cardiorenal
Cardiopathia nigra I27.0
Cardiopathy (*see also* Disease, heart) I51.9
idiopathic I42.9
mucopolysaccharidosis E76.3 [*I52*]
Cardiopericarditis — *see* Pericarditis
Cardiophobia F45.29
Cardiorenal — *see* condition
Cardiorrhexis — *see* Infarct, myocardium
Cardiosclerosis — *see* Disease, heart, ischemic, atherosclerotic
Cardiosis — *see* Disease, heart
Cardiospasm (esophagus) (reflex) (stomach) K22.0
congenital Q39.5
  with megaesophagus Q39.5

DISEASE INDEX

Cardiostenosis — *see* Disease, heart
Cardiosymphysis I31.0
Cardiovascular — *see* condition
Carditis (acute) (bacterial) (chronic) (subacute)
    I51.89
  meningococcal A39.50
  rheumatic — *see* Disease, heart, rheumatic
  rheumatoid — *see* Rheumatoid, carditis
  viral B33.20
Care (of) (for) (following)
  child (routine) Z76.2
  family member (handicapped) (sick)
    creating problem for family Z63.6
    provided away from home for holiday relief
      Z75.5
    unavailable, due to
      absence (person rendering care) (sufferer)
        Z74.2
      inability (any reason) of person rendering
        care Z74.2
  foundling Z76.1
  holiday relief Z75.5
  improper — *see* Maltreatment
  lack of (at or after birth) (infant) — *see*
    Maltreatment, child, neglect
  lactating mother Z39.1
  palliative Z51.5
  postpartum
    immediately after delivery Z39.0
    routine follow-up Z39.2
  respite Z75.5
  unavailable, due to
    absence of person rendering care Z74.2
    inability (any reason) of person rendering
      care Z74.2
  well-baby Z76.2
Caries
  bone NEC A18.03
  dental (dentino enamel junction) (early
    childhood) (of dentine) (pre-eruptive)
    (recurrent) (to the pulp) K02.9
    arrested (coronal) (root) K02.3
    chewing surface
      limited to enamel K02.51
      penetrating into dentin K02.52
      penetrating into pulp K02.53
    coronal surface
      chewing surface
        limited to enamel K02.51
        penetrating into dentin K02.52
        penetrating into pulp K02.53
      pit and fissure surface
        limited to enamel K02.51
        penetrating into dentin K02.52
        penetrating into pulp K02.53
      smooth surface
        limited to enamel K02.61
        penetrating into dentin K02.62
        penetrating into pulp K02.63
    pit and fissure surface
      limited to enamel K02.51
      penetrating into dentin K02.52
      penetrating into pulp K02.53
    primary, cervical origin K02.52
    root K02.7
    smooth surface
      limited to enamel K02.61
      penetrating into dentin K02.62
      penetrating into pulp K02.63
  external meatus — *see* Disorder, ear, external,
    specified type NEC
  hip (tuberculous) A18.02
  initial (tooth)
    chewing surface K02.51
    pit and fissure surface K02.51
    smooth surface K02.61
  knee (tuberculous) A18.02
  labyrinth — *see* subcategory H83.8
  limb NEC (tuberculous) A18.03

Caries — *continued*
  mastoid process (chronic) — *see* Mastoiditis,
    chronic
    tuberculous A18.03
  middle ear — *see* subcategory H74.8
  nose (tuberculous) A18.03
  orbit (tuberculous) A18.03
  ossicles, ear — *see* Abnormal, ear ossicles
  petrous bone — *see* Petrositis
  root (dental) (tooth) K02.7
  sacrum (tuberculous) A18.01
  spine, spinal (column) (tuberculous) A18.01
  syphilitic A52.77
    congenital (early) A50.02 *[M90.80]*
  tooth, teeth — *see* Caries, dental
  tuberculous A18.03
  vertebra (column) (tuberculous) A18.01
Carious teeth — *see* Caries, dental
Carneous mole O02.0
Carnitine insufficiency E71.40
Carotid body or sinus syndrome G90.01
Carotidynia G90.01
Carotinemia (dietary) E67.1
Carotinosis (cutis) (skin) E67.1
Carpal tunnel syndrome — *see* Syndrome,
  carpal tunnel
Carpenter's syndrome Q87.0
Carpopedal spasm — *see* Tetany
Carr-Barr-Plunkett syndrome Q97.1
Carrier (suspected) of
  amebiasis Z22.1
  bacterial disease NEC Z22.39
    diphtheria Z22.2
    intestinal infectious NEC Z22.1
      typhoid Z22.0
    meningococcal Z22.31
    sexually transmitted Z22.4
    specified NEC Z22.39
    staphylococcal (Methicillin susceptible)
      Z22.321
      Methicillin resistant Z22.322
    streptococcal Z22.338
      group B Z22.330
        complicating pregnancy or delivery
          O99.82-
    typhoid Z22.0
  cholera Z22.1
  diphtheria Z22.2
  gastrointestinal pathogens NEC Z22.1
  genetic Z14.8
    cystic fibrosis Z14.1
    hemophilia A (asymptomatic) Z14.01
      symptomatic Z14.02
  gestational, pregnant Z33.1
  gonorrhea Z22.4
  HAA (hepatitis Australian-antigen) B18.8
  HB(c)(s)-AG B18.1
  hepatitis (viral) B18.9
    Australia-antigen (HAA) B18.8
    B surface antigen (HBsAg) B18.1
      with acute delta-(super)infection B17.0
    C B18.2
    specified NEC B18.8
  human T-cell lymphotropic virus type-1 (HTLV-
    1) infection Z22.6
  infectious organism Z22.9
    specified NEC Z22.8
  meningococci Z22.31
  Salmonella typhosa Z22.0
  serum hepatitis — *see* Carrier, hepatitis
  staphylococci (Methicillin susceptible) Z22.321
    Methicillin resistant Z22.322
  streptococci Z22.338
    group B Z22.330
      complicating pregnancy or delivery
        O99.82-
  syphilis Z22.4
  typhoid Z22.0
  venereal disease NEC Z22.4

Carrion's disease A44.0
Carter's relapsing fever (Asiatic) A68.1
Cartilage — *see* condition
Caruncle (inflamed)
  conjunctiva (acute) — *see* Conjunctivitis, acute
  labium (majus) (minus) N90.89
  lacrimal — *see* Inflammation, lacrimal,
    passages
  myrtiform N89.8
  urethral (benign) N36.2
Cascade stomach K31.2
Caseation lymphatic gland (tuberculous)
  A18.2
Cassidy (-Scholte) syndrome (malignant
  carcinoid) E34.0
Castellani's disease A69.8
Castration, traumatic, male S38.231
Casts in urine R82.99
Cat
  cry syndrome Q93.4
  ear Q17.3
  eye syndrome Q92.8
Catabolism, senile R54
Catalepsy (hysterical) F44.2
  schizophrenic F20.2
Cataplexy (idiopathic) — *see* Narcolepsy
Cataract (cortical) (immature) (incipient) H26.9
  with
    neovascularization — *see* Cataract,
      complicated
  age-related — *see* Cataract, senile
  anterior
    and posterior axial embryonal Q12.0
    pyramidal Q12.0
  associated with
    galactosemia E74.21 *[H28]*
    myotonic disorders G71.19 *[H28]*
  blue Q12.0
  central Q12.0
  cerulean Q12.0
  complicated H26.20
    with
      neovascularization H26.21-
      ocular disorder H26.22-
      glaucomatous flecks H26.23-
  congenital Q12.0
  coraliform Q12.0
  coronary Q12.0
  crystalline Q12.0
  diabetic — *see* Diabetes, cataract
  drug-induced H26.3-
  due to
    ocular disorder — *see* Cataract, complicated
    radiation H26.8
  electric H26.8
  extraction status Z98.4-
  glass-blower's H26.8
  heat ray H26.8
  heterochromic — *see* Cataract, complicated
  hypermature — *see* Cataract, senile,
    morgagnian type
  in (due to)
    chronic iridocyclitis — *see* Cataract,
      complicated
    diabetes — *see* Diabetes, cataract
    endocrine disease E34.9 *[H28]*
    eye disease — *see* Cataract, complicated
    hypoparathyroidism E20.9 *[H28]*
    malnutrition-dehydration E46 *[H28]*
    metabolic disease E88.9 *[H28]*
    myotonic disorders G71.19 *[H28]*
    nutritional disease E63.9 *[H28]*
  infantile — *see* Cataract, presenile
  irradiational — *see* Cataract, specified NEC
  juvenile — *see* Cataract, presenile
  malnutrition-dehydration E46 *[H28]*
  morgagnian — *see* Cataract, senile,
    morgagnian type
  myotonic G71.19 *[H28]*

Cataract (cortical) (immature) (incipient) H26.9
— *continued*
myxedema E03.9 *[H28]*
nuclear
  embryonal Q12.0
  sclerosis — *see* Cataract, senile, nuclear
presenile H26.00-
  combined forms H26.06-
  cortical H26.01-
    lamellar — *see* Cataract, presenile, cortical
  nuclear H26.03-
  specified NEC H26.09
  subcapsular polar (anterior) H26.04-
    posterior H26.05-
  zonular — *see* Cataract, presenile, cortical
secondary H26.40
  Soemmering's ring H26.41-
  specified NEC H26.49-
to eye disease — *see* Cataract, complicated
senile H25.9
  brunescens — *see* Cataract, senile, nuclear
  combined forms H25.81-
  coronary — *see* Cataract, senile, incipient
  cortical H25.01-
  hypermature — *see* Cataract, senile, morgagnian type
  incipient (mature) (total) H25.09-
    cortical — *see* Cataract, senile, cortical
    subcapsular — *see* Cataract, senile, subcapsular
  morgagnian type (hypermature) H25.2-
  nuclear (sclerosis) H25.1-
  polar subcapsular (anterior) (posterior) — *see* Cataract, senile, incipient
  punctate — *see* Cataract, senile, incipient
  specified NEC H25.89
  subcapsular polar (anterior) H25.03-
    posterior H25.04-
snowflake — *see* Diabetes, cataract
specified NEC H26.8
toxic — *see* Cataract, drug-induced
traumatic H26.10-
  localized H26.11-
  partially resolved H26.12-
  total H26.13-
zonular (perinuclear) Q12.0
Cataracta — *see also* Cataract
brunescens — *see* Cataract, senile, nuclear
centralis pulverulenta Q12.0
cerulea Q12.0
complicata — *see* Cataract, complicated
congenita Q12.0
coralliformis Q12.0
coronaria Q12.0
diabetic — *see* Diabetes, cataract
membranacea
  accreta — *see* Cataract, secondary
  congenita Q12.0
nigra — *see* Cataract, senile, nuclear
sunflower — *see* Cataract, complicated
Catarrh, catarrhal (acute) (febrile) (infectious)
  (inflammation) (*see also* condition) J00
bronchial — *see* Bronchitis
chest — *see* Bronchitis
chronic J31.0
due to congenital syphilis A50.03
enteric — *see* Enteritis
eustachian H68.009
fauces — *see* Pharyngitis
gastrointestinal — *see* Enteritis
gingivitis K05.00
  nonplaque induced K05.01
  plaque induced K05.00
hay — *see* Fever, hay
intestinal — *see* Enteritis
larynx, chronic J37.0
liver B15.9
  with hepatic coma B15.0
lung — *see* Bronchitis

Catarrh, catarrhal (acute) (febrile) (infectious)
  (inflammation) (*see also* condition) J00 —
  continued
middle ear, chronic — *see* Otitis, media, nonsuppurative, chronic, serous
mouth K12.1
nasal (chronic) — *see* Rhinitis
nasobronchial J31.1
nasopharyngeal (chronic) J31.1
  acute J00
pulmonary — *see* Bronchitis
spring (eye) (vernal) — *see* Conjunctivitis, acute, atopic
summer (hay) — *see* Fever, hay
throat J31.2
tubotympanal — *see also* Otitis, media, nonsuppurative
  chronic — *see* Otitis, media, nonsuppurative, chronic, serous
Catatonia (schizophrenic) F20.2
Catatonic
disorder due to known physiologic condition F06.1
schizophrenia F20.2
stupor R40.1
Cat-scratch — *see also* Abrasion
disease or fever A28.1
Cauda equina — *see* condition
Cauliflower ear M95.1-
Causalgia (upper limb) G56.4-
lower limb G57.7-
Cause
external, general effects T75.89
Caustic burn — *see* Corrosion, by site
Cavare's disease (familial periodic paralysis) G72.3
Cave-in, injury
crushing (severe) — *see* Crush
suffocation — *see* Asphyxia, traumatic, due to low oxygen, due to cave-in
Cavernitis (penis) N48.29
Cavernositis N48.29
Cavernous — *see* condition
Cavitation of lung — *see also* Tuberculosis, pulmonary
nontuberculous J98.4
Cavities, dental — *see* Caries, dental
Cavity
lung — *see* Cavitation of lung
optic papilla Q14.2
pulmonary — *see* Cavitation of lung
Cavovarus foot, congenital Q66.1
Cavus foot (congenital) Q66.7
acquired — *see* Deformity, limb, foot, specified NEC
Cazenave's disease L10.2
Cecitis K52.9
with perforation, peritonitis, or rupture K65.8
Cecum — *see* condition
Celiac
artery compression syndrome I77.4
disease (with steatorrhea) K90.0
infantilism K90.0
Cell(s), cellular — *see also* condition
in urine R82.99
Cellulitis (diffuse) (phlegmonous) (septic)
  (suppurative) L03.90
abdominal wall L03.311
anaerobic A48.0
ankle — *see* Cellulitis, lower limb
anus K61.0
arm — *see* Cellulitis, upper limb
auricle (ear) — *see* Cellulitis, ear
axilla L03.11-
back (any part) L03.312
breast (acute) (nonpuerperal) (subacute) N61.0
  nipple N61.0

Cellulitis (diffuse) (phlegmonous) (septic)
  (suppurative) L03.90 — *continued*
broad ligament
  acute N73.0
buttock L03.317
cervical (meaning neck) L03.221
cervix (uteri) — *see* Cervicitis
cheek (external) L03.211
  internal K12.2
chest wall L03.313
chronic L03.90
clostridial A48.0
corpus cavernosum N48.22
digit
  finger — *see* Cellulitis, finger
  toe — *see* Cellulitis, toe
Douglas' cul-de-sac or pouch
  acute N73.0
drainage site (following operation) T81.48
ear (external) H60.1-
eosinophilic (granulomatous) L98.3
erysipelatous — *see* Erysipelas
external auditory canal — *see* Cellulitis, ear
eyelid — *see* Abscess, eyelid
face NEC L03.211
finger (intrathecal) (periosteal) (subcutaneous)
  (subcuticular) L03.01-
foot — *see* Cellulitis, lower limb
gangrenous — *see* Gangrene
genital organ NEC
  female (external) N76.4
  male N49.9
    multiple sites N49.8
    specified NEC N49.8
gluteal (region) L03.317
gonococcal A54.89
groin L03.314
hand — *see* Cellulitis, upper limb
head NEC L03.811
  face (any part, except ear, eye and nose) L03.211
heel — *see* Cellulitis, lower limb
hip — *see* Cellulitis, lower limb
jaw (region) L03.211
knee — *see* Cellulitis, lower limb
labium (majus) (minus) — *see* Vulvitis
lacrimal passages — *see* Inflammation, lacrimal, passages
larynx J38.7
leg — *see* Cellulitis, lower limb
lip K13.0
lower limb L03.11-
  toe — *see* Cellulitis, toe
mouth (floor) K12.2
multiple sites, so stated L03.90
nasopharynx J39.1
navel L03.316
  newborn P38.9
    with mild hemorrhage P38.1
    without hemorrhage P38.9
neck (region) L03.221
nipple (acute) (nonpuerperal) (subacute) N61.0
nose (septum) (external) J34.0
orbit, orbital H05.01-
palate (soft) K12.2
pectoral (region) L03.313
pelvis, pelvic (chronic)
  female (*see also* Disease, pelvis, inflammatory) N73.2
    acute N73.0
  following ectopic or molar pregnancy O08.0
  male K65.0
penis N48.22
perineal, perineum L03.315
periorbital L03.213
perirectal K61.1
peritonsillar J36
periurethral N34.0

DISEASE INDEX

Cellulitis (diffuse) (phlegmonous) (septic) (suppurative) L03.90 — *continued*
periuterine (*see also* Disease, pelvis, inflammatory) N73.2
  acute N73.0
pharynx J39.1
preseptal L03.213
rectum K61.1
retroperitoneal K68.9
round ligament N73.2
  acute N73.0
scalp (any part) L03.811
scrotum N49.2
seminal vesicle N49.0
shoulder — *see* Cellulitis, upper limb
specified site NEC L03.818
submandibular (region) (space) (triangle) K12.2
  gland K11.3
submaxillary (region) K12.2
  gland K11.3
thigh — *see* Cellulitis, lower limb
thumb (intrathecal) (periosteal) (subcutaneous) (subcuticular) — *see* Cellulitis, finger
toe (intrathecal) (periosteal) (subcutaneous) (subcuticular) L03.03-
tonsil J36
trunk L03.319
  abdominal wall L03.311
  back (any part) L03.312
  buttock L03.317
  chest wall L03.313
  groin L03.314
  perineal, perineum L03.315
  umbilicus L03.316
tuberculous (primary) A18.4
umbilicus L03.316
upper limb L03.11-
  axilla — *see* Cellulitis, axilla
  finger — *see* Cellulitis, finger
  thumb — *see* Cellulitis, finger
vaccinal T88.0
vocal cord J38.3
vulva — *see* Vulvitis
wrist — *see* Cellulitis, upper limb
Cementoblastoma, benign — *see* Cyst, calcifying odontogenic
Cementoma — *see* Cyst, calcifying odontogenic
Cementoperiostitis — *see* Periodontitis
Cementosis K03.4
Central auditory processing disorder H93.25
Central pain syndrome G89.0
Cephalematocele, cephal(o)hematocele
newborn P52.8
  birth injury P10.8
traumatic — *see* Hematoma, brain
Cephalematoma, cephalhematoma (calcified)
newborn (birth injury) P12.0
traumatic — *see* Hematoma, brain
Cephalgia, cephalalgia — *see also* Headache
histamine G44.009
  intractable G44.001
  not intractable G44.009
trigeminal autonomic (TAC) NEC G44.099
  intractable G44.001
  not intractable G44.099
Cephalic — *see* condition
Cephalitis — *see* Encephalitis
Cephalocele — *see* Encephalocele
Cephalomenia N94.89
Cephalopelvic — *see* condition
Cerclage (with cervical incompetence) in pregnancy — *see* Incompetence, cervix, in pregnancy

Cerebellitis — *see* Encephalitis
Cerebellum, cerebellar — *see* condition
Cerebral — *see* condition
Cerebritis — *see* Encephalitis
Cerebro-hepato-renal syndrome Q87.89
Cerebromalacia — *see* Softening, brain
  sequelae of cerebrovascular disease I69.398
Cerebroside lipidosis E75.22
Cerebrospasticity (congenital) G80.1
Cerebrospinal — *see* condition
Cerebrum — *see* condition
Ceroid-lipofuscinosis, neuronal E75.4
Cerumen (accumulation) (impacted) H61.2-
Cervical — *see also* condition
auricle Q18.2
dysplasia in pregnancy — *see* Abnormal, cervix, in pregnancy or childbirth
erosion in pregnancy — *see* Abnormal, cervix, in pregnancy or childbirth
fibrosis in pregnancy — *see* Abnormal, cervix, in pregnancy or childbirth
fusion syndrome Q76.1
rib Q76.5
shortening (complicating pregnancy) O26.87-
Cervicalgia M54.2
Cervicitis (acute) (chronic) (nonvenereal) (senile (atrophic)) (subacute) (with ulceration) N72
with
  abortion — *see* Abortion, by type
    complicated by genital tract and pelvic infection
  ectopic pregnancy O08.0
  molar pregnancy O08.0
chlamydial A56.09
gonococcal A54.03
herpesviral A60.03
puerperal (postpartum) O86.11
syphilitic A52.76
trichomonal A59.09
tuberculous A18.16
Cervicocolpitis (emphysematosa) (*see also* Cervicitis) N72
Cervix — *see* condition
Cesarean delivery, previous, affecting management of pregnancy O34.219
classical (vertical) scar O34.212
low transverse scar O34.211
Céstan(-Chenais) paralysis or syndrome G46.3
Céstan-Raymond syndrome I65.8
Cestode infestation B71.9
specified type NEC B71.8
Cestodiasis B71.9
Chabert's disease A22.9
Chacaleh E53.8
Chafing L30.4
Chagas' (-Mazza) disease (chronic) B57.2
with
  cardiovascular involvement NEC B57.2
  digestive system involvement B57.30
    megacolon B57.32
    megaesophagus B57.31
    other B57.39
  megacolon B57.32
  megaesophagus B57.31
  myocarditis B57.2
  nervous system involvement B57.40
    meningitis B57.41
    meningoencephalitis B57.42
    other specified B57.49
  specified organ involvement NEC B57.5
acute (with) B57.1
  cardiovascular NEC B57.0
  myocarditis B57.0
Chagres fever B50.9
Chairridden Z74.09
Chalasia (cardiac sphincter) K21.9

Chalazion H00.19
left H00.16
  lower H00.15
  upper H00.14
right H00.13
  lower H00.12
  upper H00.11
Chalcosis — *see also* Disorder, globe, degenerative, chalcosis
cornea — *see* Deposit, cornea
crystalline lens — *see* Cataract, complicated
retina H35.89
Chalicosis (pulmonum) J62.8
Chancre (any genital site) (hard) (hunterian) (mixed) (primary) (seronegative) (seropositive) (syphilitic) A51.0
congenital A50.07
conjunctiva NEC A51.2
Ducrey's A57
extragenital A51.2
eyelid A51.2
lip A51.2
nipple A51.2
Nisbet's A57
of
  carate A67.0
  pinta A67.0
  yaws A66.0
palate, soft A51.2
phagedenic A57
simple A57
soft A57
  bubo A57
  palate A51.2
urethra A51.0
yaws A66.0
Chancroid (anus) (genital) (penis) (perineum) (rectum) (urethra) (vulva) A57
Chandler's disease (osteochondritis dissecans, hip) — *see* Osteochondritis, dissecans, hip
Change(s) (in) (of) — *see also* Removal
arteriosclerotic — *see* Arteriosclerosis
bone — *see also* Disorder, bone
  diabetic — *see* Diabetes, bone change
bowel habit R19.4
cardiorenal (vascular) — *see* Hypertension, cardiorenal
cardiovascular — *see* Disease, cardiovascular
circulatory I99.9
cognitive (mild) (organic) R41.89
color, tooth, teeth
  during formation K00.8
  posteruptive K03.7
contraceptive device Z30.433
corneal membrane H18.30
  Bowman's membrane fold or rupture H18.31-
  Descemet's membrane
    fold H18.32-
    rupture H18.33-
coronary — *see* Disease, heart, ischemic
degenerative, spine or vertebra — *see* Spondylosis
dental pulp, regressive K04.2
dressing (nonsurgical) Z48.00
  surgical Z48.01
heart — *see* Disease, heart
hip joint — *see* Derangement, joint, hip
hyperplastic larynx J38.7
hypertrophic
  nasal sinus J34.89
  turbinate, nasal J34.3
  upper respiratory tract J39.8
indwelling catheter Z46.6
inflammatory — *see also* Inflammation
  sacroiliac M46.1
job, anxiety concerning Z56.1
joint — *see* Derangement, joint

Change(s) (in) (of) (*see also* Removal) — *continued*
life — *see* Menopause
mental status R41.82
minimal (glomerular) (*see also* N00-N07 with fourth character .0) N05.0
myocardium, myocardial — *see* Degeneration, myocardial
of life — *see* Menopause
pacemaker Z45.018
    pulse generator Z45.010
personality (enduring) F68.8
    due to (secondary to)
      general medical condition F07.0
    secondary (nonspecific) F60.89
regressive, dental pulp K04.2
renal — *see* Disease, renal
retina H35.9
    myopic H44.2-
sacroiliac joint M53.3
senile (*see also* condition) R54
sensory R20.8
skin R23.9
    acute, due to ultraviolet radiation L56.9
      specified NEC L56.8
    chronic, due to nonionizing radiation L57.9
      specified NEC L57.8
    cyanosis R23.0
    flushing R23.2
    pallor R23.1
    petechiae R23.3
    specified change NEC R23.8
    swelling — *see* Mass, localized
    texture R23.4
trophic
    arm — *see* Mononeuropathy, upper limb
    leg — *see* Mononeuropathy, lower limb
vascular I99.9
vasomotor I73.9
voice R49.9
    psychogenic F44.4
    specified NEC R49.8
Changing sleep-work schedule, affecting sleep G47.26
Changuinola fever A93.1
Chapping skin T69.8
Charcot-Marie-Tooth disease, paralysis or syndrome G60.0
Charcot's
arthropathy — *see* Arthropathy, neuropathic
cirrhosis K74.3
disease (tabetic arthropathy) A52.16
joint (disease) (tabetic) A52.16
    diabetic — *see* Diabetes, with, arthropathy
    syringomyelic G95.0
syndrome (intermittent claudication) I73.9
CHARGE association Q89.8
Charley-horse (quadriceps) M62.831
traumatic (quadriceps) S76.11-
Charlouis' disease — *see* Yaws
Cheadle's disease E54
Checking (of)
cardiac pacemaker (battery) (electrode(s)) Z45.018
    pulse generator Z45.010
implantable subdermal contraceptive Z30.46
intrauterine contraceptive device Z30.431
Check-up — *see* Examination
Chédiak-Higashi(-Steinbrinck) syndrome (congenital gigantism of peroxidase granules) E70.330
Cheek — *see* condition
Cheese itch B88.0
Cheese-washer's lung J67.8
Cheese-worker's lung J67.8

Cheilitis (acute) (angular) (catarrhal) (chronic) (exfoliative) (gangrenous) (glandular) (infectional) (suppurative) (ulcerative) (vesicular) K13.0
actinic (due to sun) L56.8
    other than from sun L59.8
candidal B37.83
Cheilodynia K13.0
Cheiloschisis — *see* Cleft, lip
Cheilosis (angular) K13.0
with pellagra E52
due to
    vitamin B2 (riboflavin) deficiency E53.0
Cheiromegaly M79.89
Cheiropompholyx L30.1
Cheloid — *see* Keloid
Chemical burn — *see* Corrosion, by site
Chemodectoma — *see* Paraganglioma, nonchromaffin
Chemosis, conjunctiva — *see* Edema, conjunctiva
Chemotherapy (session) (for)
cancer Z51.11
neoplasm Z51.11
Cherubism M27.8
Chest — *see* condition
Cheyne-Stokes breathing (respiration) R06.3
Chiari's
disease or syndrome (hepatic vein thrombosis) I82.0
malformation
    type I G93.5
    type II — *see* Spina bifida
    net Q24.8
Chicago disease B40.9
Chickenpox — *see* Varicella
Chiclero ulcer or sore B55.1
Chigger (infestation) B88.0
Chignon (disease) B36.8
newborn (from vacuum extraction) (birth injury) P12.1
Chilaiditi's syndrome (subphrenic displacement, colon) Q43.3
Chilblain(s) (lupus) T69.1
Child
custody dispute Z65.3
Childbirth — *see* Delivery
Childhood
cerebral X-linked adrenoleukodystrophy E71.520
period of rapid growth Z00.2
Chill(s) R68.83
with fever R50.9
congestive in malarial regions B54
without fever R68.83
Chilomastigiasis A07.8
Chimera 46,XX/46,XY Q99.0
Chin — *see* condition
Chinese dysentery A03.9
Chionophobia F40.228
Chitral fever A93.1
Chlamydia, chlamydial A74.9
cervicitis A56.09
conjunctivitis A74.0
cystitis A56.01
endometritis A56.11
epididymitis A56.19
female
    pelvic inflammatory disease A56.11
    pelviperitonitis A56.11
orchitis A56.19
peritonitis A74.81
pharyngitis A56.4
proctitis A56.3
psittaci (infection) A70
salpingitis A56.11
sexually-transmitted infection NEC A56.8

Chlamydia, chlamydial A74.9 — *continued*
specified NEC A74.89
urethritis A56.01
vulvovaginitis A56.02
Chlamydiosis — *see* Chlamydia
Chloasma (skin) (idiopathic) (symptomatic) L81.1
eyelid H02.719
    hyperthyroid E05.90 *[H02.719]*
      with thyroid storm E05.91 *[H02.719]*
    left H02.716
      lower H02.715
      upper H02.714
    right H02.713
      lower H02.712
      upper H02.711
Chloroma C92.3-
Chlorosis D50.9
Egyptian B76.9 *[D63.8]*
miner's B76.9 *[D63.8]*
Chlorotic anemia D50.8
Chocolate cyst (ovary) N80.1
Choked
disc or disk — *see* Papilledema
on food, phlegm, or vomitus NOS — *see* Foreign body, by site
while vomiting NOS — *see* Foreign body, by site
Chokes (resulting from bends) T70.3
Choking sensation R09.89
Cholangiectasis K83.8
Cholangiocarcinoma
with hepatocellular carcinoma, combined C22.0
liver C22.1
specified site NEC — *see* Neoplasm, malignant, by site
unspecified site C22.1
Cholangiohepatitis K83.8
due to fluke infestation B66.1
Cholangiohepatoma C22.0
Cholangiolitis (acute) (chronic) (extrahepatic) (gangrenous) (intrahepatic) K83.0
paratyphoidal — *see* Fever, paratyphoid
typhoidal A01.09
Cholangioma D13.4
malignant — *see* Cholangiocarcinoma
Cholangitis (ascending) (primary) (recurrent) (sclerosing) (secondary) (stenosing) (suppurative) K83.0
with calculus, bile duct — *see* Calculus, bile duct, with cholangitis
chronic nonsuppurative destructive K74.3
Cholecystectasia K82.8
Cholecystitis K81.9
with
    calculus, stones in
      bile duct (common) (hepatic) — *see* Calculus, bile duct, with cholecystitis
      cystic duct — *see* Calculus, gallbladder, with cholecystitis
      gallbladder — *see* Calculus, gallbladder, with cholecystitis
      choledocholithiasis — *see* Calculus, bile duct, with cholecystitis
      cholelithiasis — *see* Calculus, gallbladder, with cholecystitis
acute (emphysematous) (gangrenous) (suppurative) K81.0
    with
      calculus, stones in
        cystic duct — *see* Calculus, gallbladder, with cholecystitis, acute
        gallbladder — *see* Calculus, gallbladder, with cholecystitis, acute
        choledocholithiasis — *see* Calculus, bile duct, with cholecystitis, acute

Cholecystitis K81.9 — *continued*
  acute (emphysematous) (gangrenous) (suppurative) K81.0 — *continued*
    with — *continued*
      cholelithiasis — *see* Calculus, gallbladder, with cholecystitis, acute
      chronic cholecystitis K81.2
        with gallbladder calculus K80.12
          with obstruction K80.13
  chronic K81.1
    with acute cholecystitis K81.2
      with gallbladder calculus K80.12
        with obstruction K80.13
  emphysematous (acute) — *see* Cholecystitis, acute
  gangrenous — *see* Cholecystitis, acute
  paratyphoidal, current A01.4
  suppurative — *see* Cholecystitis, acute
  typhoidal A01.09
Cholecystolithiasis — *see* Calculus, gallbladder
Choledochitis (suppurative) K83.0
Choledocholith — *see* Calculus, bile duct
Choledocholithiasis (common duct) (hepatic duct) — *see* Calculus, bile duct
  cystic — *see* Calculus, gallbladder
  typhoidal A01.09
Cholelithiasis (cystic duct) (gallbladder) (impacted) (multiple) — *see* Calculus, gallbladder
  bile duct (common) (hepatic) — *see* Calculus, bile duct
  hepatic duct — *see* Calculus, bile duct
  specified NEC K80.80
    with obstruction K80.81
Cholemia — *see also* Jaundice
  familial (simple) (congenital) E80.4
  Gilbert's E80.4
Choleperitoneum, choleperitonitis K65.3
Cholera (Asiatic) (epidemic) (malignant) A00.9
  antimonial — *see* Poisoning, antimony
  classical A00.0
  due to Vibrio cholerae 01 A00.9
    biovar cholerae A00.0
    biovar el tor A00.1
    el tor A00.1
  el tor A00.1
Cholerine — *see* Cholera
Cholestasis NEC K83.1
  with hepatocyte injury K71.0
  due to total parenteral nutrition (TPN) K76.89
  pure K71.0
Cholesteatoma (ear) (middle) (with reaction) H71.9-
  attic H71.0-
  external ear (canal) H60.4-
  mastoid H71.2-
  postmastoidectomy cavity (recurrent) — *see* Complications, postmastoidectomy, recurrent cholesteatoma
  recurrent (postmastoidectomy) — *see* Complications, postmastoidectomy, recurrent cholesteatoma
  tympanum H71.1-
Cholesteatosis, diffuse H71.3-
Cholesteremia E78.00
Cholesterin in vitreous — *see* Deposit, crystalline
Cholesterol
  deposit
    retina H35.89
    vitreous — *see* Deposit, crystalline
  elevated (high) E78.00
    with elevated (high) triglycerides E78.2
    screening for Z13.220
  imbibition of gallbladder K82.4

Cholesterolemia (essential) (pure) E78.00
  familial E78.01
  hereditary E78.01
Cholesterolosis, cholesterosis (gallbladder) K82.4
  cerebrotendinous E75.5
Cholocolic fistula K82.3
Choluria R82.2
Chondritis M94.8x9
  aurical H61.03-
  costal (Tietze's) M94.0
  external ear H61.03-
  patella, posttraumatic — *see* Chondromalacia, patella
  pinna H61.03-
  purulent M94.8x-
  tuberculous NEC A18.02
    intervertebral A18.01
Chondroblastoma — *see also* Neoplasm, bone, benign
  malignant — *see* Neoplasm, bone, malignant
Chondrocalcinosis M11.20
  ankle M11.27-
  elbow M11.22-
  familial M11.10
    ankle M11.17-
    elbow M11.12-
    foot joint M11.17-
    hand joint M11.14-
    hip M11.15-
    knee M11.16-
    multiple site M11.19
    shoulder M11.11-
    vertebrae M11.18
    wrist M11.13-
  foot joint M11.27-
  hand joint M11.24-
  hip M11.25-
  knee M11.26-
  multiple site M11.29
  shoulder M11.21-
  specified type NEC M11.20
    ankle M11.27-
    elbow M11.22-
    foot joint M11.27-
    hand joint M11.24-
    hip M11.25-
    knee M11.26-
    multiple site M11.29
    shoulder M11.21-
    vertebrae M11.28
    wrist M11.23-
  vertebrae M11.28
  wrist M11.23-
Chondrodermatitis nodularis helicis or anthelicis — *see* Perichondritis, ear
Chondrodysplasia Q78.9
  with hemangioma Q78.4
  calcificans congenita Q77.3
  fetalis Q77.4
  metaphyseal (Jansen's) (McKusick's) (Schmid's) Q78.8
  punctata Q77.3
Chondrodystrophy, chondrodystrophia (familial) (fetalis) (hypoplastic) Q78.9
  calcificans congenita Q77.3
  myotonic (congenital) G71.13
  punctata Q77.3
Chondroectodermal dysplasia Q77.6
Chondrogenesis imperfecta Q77.4
Chondrolysis M94.35-
Chondroma — *see also* Neoplasm, cartilage, benign
  juxtacortical — *see* Neoplasm, bone, benign
  periosteal — *see* Neoplasm, bone, benign
Chondromalacia (systemic) M94.20
  acromioclavicular joint M94.21-
  ankle M94.27-

Chondromalacia (systemic) M94.20 — *continued*
  elbow M94.22-
  foot joint M94.27-
  glenohumeral joint M94.21-
  hand joint M94.24-
  hip M94.25-
  knee M94.26-
    patella M22.4-
  multiple sites M94.29
  patella M22.4-
  rib M94.28
  sacroiliac joint M94.259
  shoulder M94.21-
  sternoclavicular joint M94.21-
  vertebral joint M94.28
  wrist M94.23-
Chondromatosis — *see also* Neoplasm, cartilage, uncertain behavior
  internal Q78.4
Chondromyxosarcoma — *see* Neoplasm, cartilage, malignant
Chondro-osteodysplasia (Morquio-Brailsford type) E76.219
Chondro-osteodystrophy E76.29
Chondro-osteoma — *see* Neoplasm, bone, benign
Chondropathia tuberosa M94.0
Chondrosarcoma — *see* Neoplasm, cartilage, malignant
  juxtacortical — *see* Neoplasm, bone, malignant
  mesenchymal — *see* Neoplasm, connective tissue, malignant
  myxoid — *see* Neoplasm, cartilage, malignant
Chordee (nonvenereal) N48.89
  congenital Q54.4
  gonococcal A54.09
Chorditis (fibrinous) (nodosa) (tuberosa) J38.2
Chordoma — *see* Neoplasm, vertebral (column), malignant
Chorea (chronic) (gravis) (posthemiplegic) (senile) (spasmodic) G25.5
  with
    heart involvement I02.0
      active or acute (conditions in I01-) I02.0
        rheumatic I02.9
          with valvular disorder I02.0
      rheumatic heart disease (chronic) (inactive) (quiescent) — *code to* rheumatic heart condition involved
  drug-induced G25.4
  habit F95.8
  hereditary G10
  Huntington's G10
  hysterical F44.4
  minor I02.9
    with heart involvement I02.0
  progressive G25.5
    hereditary G10
  rheumatic (chronic) I02.9
    with heart involvement I02.0
  Sydenham's I02.9
    with heart involvement — *see* Chorea, with rheumatic heart disease
  nonrheumatic G25.5
Choreoathetosis (paroxysmal) G25.5
Chorioadenoma (destruens) D39.2
Chorioamnionitis O41.12-
Chorioangioma D26.7
Choriocarcinoma — *see* Neoplasm, malignant, by site
  combined with
    embryonal carcinoma — *see* Neoplasm, malignant, by site
    other germ cell elements — *see* Neoplasm, malignant, by site
    teratoma — *see* Neoplasm, malignant, by site

Choriocarcinoma — see Neoplasm, malignant, by site — *continued*
  specified site — see Neoplasm, malignant, by site
  unspecified site
    female C58
    male C62.90
Chorioencephalitis (acute) (lymphocytic) (serous) A87.2
Chorioepithelioma — see Choriocarcinoma
Choriomeningitis (acute) (lymphocytic) (serous) A87.2
Chorionepithelioma — see Choriocarcinoma
Chorioretinitis — see also Inflammation, chorioretinal
  disseminated — see also Inflammation, chorioretinal, disseminated
    in neurosyphilis A52.19
  Egyptian B76.9 [D63.8]
  focal — see also Inflammation, chorioretinal, focal
  histoplasmic B39.9 [H32]
  in (due to)
    histoplasmosis B39.9 [H32]
    syphilis (secondary) A51.43
      late A52.71
    toxoplasmosis (acquired) B58.01
      congenital (active) P37.1 [H32]
    tuberculosis A18.53
  juxtapapillary, juxtapapillaris — see Inflammation, chorioretinal, focal, juxtapapillary
  leprous A30.9 [H32]
  miner's B76.9 [D63.8]
  progressive myopia (degeneration) H44.2-
  syphilitic (secondary) A51.43
    congenital (early) A50.01 [H32]
      late A50.32
    late A52.71
  tuberculous A18.53
Chorioretinopathy, central serous H35.71-
Choroid — see condition
Choroideremia H31.21
Choroiditis — see Chorioretinitis
Choroidopathy — see Disorder, choroid
Choroidoretinitis — see Chorioretinitis
Choroidoretinopathy, central serous — see Chorioretinopathy, central serous
Christian-Weber disease M35.6
Christmas disease D67
Chromaffinoma — see also Neoplasm, benign, by site
  malignant — see Neoplasm, malignant, by site
Chromatopsia — see Deficiency, color vision
Chromhidrosis, chromidrosis L75.1
Chromoblastomycosis — see Chromomycosis
Chromoconversion R82.91
Chromomycosis B43.9
  brain abscess B43.1
  cerebral B43.1
  cutaneous B43.0
  skin B43.0
  specified NEC B43.8
  subcutaneous abscess or cyst B43.2
Chromophytosis B36.0
Chromosome — see condition by chromosome involved
  D(1) — see condition, chromosome 13
  E(3) — see condition, chromosome 18
  G — see condition, chromosome 21
Chromotrichomycosis B36.8
Chronic — see condition
  fracture — see Fracture, pathological
Churg-Strauss syndrome M30.1
Chyle cyst, mesentery I89.8
Chylocele (nonfilarial) I89.8
  filarial (see also Infestation, filarial) B74.9 [N51]
  tunica vaginalis N50.89

Chylocele (nonfilarial) I89.8 — *continued*
  filarial (see also Infestation, filarial) B74.9 [N51]
Chylomicronemia (fasting) (with hyperprebetalipoproteinemia) E78.3
Chylopericardium I31.3
  acute I30.9
Chylothorax (nonfilarial) I89.8
  filarial (see also Infestation, filarial) B74.9 [J91.8]
Chylous — see condition
Chyluria (nonfilarial) R82.0
  due to
    bilharziasis B65.0
    Brugia (malayi) B74.1
      timori B74.2
    schistosomiasis (bilharziasis) B65.0
    Wuchereria (bancrofti) B74.0
  filarial — see Infestation, filarial
Cicatricial (deformity) — see Cicatrix
Cicatrix (adherent) (contracted) (painful) (vicious) (see also Scar) L90.5
  adenoid (and tonsil) J35.8
  alveolar process M26.79
  anus K62.89
  auricle — see Disorder, pinna, specified type NEC
  bile duct (common) (hepatic) K83.8
  bladder N32.89
  bone — see Disorder, bone, specified type NEC
  brain G93.89
  cervix (postoperative) (postpartal) N88.1
  common duct K83.8
  cornea H17.9
    tuberculous A18.59
  duodenum (bulb), obstructive K31.5
  esophagus K22.2
  eyelid — see Disorder, eyelid function
  hypopharynx J39.2
  lacrimal passages — see Obstruction, lacrimal
  larynx J38.7
  lung J98.4
  middle ear — see subcategory H74.8
  mouth K13.79
  muscle M62.89
    with contracture — see Contraction, muscle NEC
  nasopharynx J39.2
  palate (soft) K13.79
  penis N48.89
  pharynx J39.2
  prostate N42.89
  rectum K62.89
  retina — see Scar, chorioretinal
  semilunar cartilage — see Derangement, meniscus
  seminal vesicle N50.89
  skin L90.5
    infected L08.89
    postinfective L90.5
    tuberculous B90.8
    specified site NEC L90.5
  throat J39.2
  tongue K14.8
  tonsil (and adenoid) J35.8
  trachea J39.8
  tuberculous NEC B90.9
  urethra N36.8
  uterus N85.8
  vagina N89.8
    postoperative N99.2
  vocal cord J38.3
  wrist, constricting (annular) L90.5
CIDP (chronic inflammatory demyelinating polyneuropathy) G61.81
CIN — see Neoplasia, intraepithelial, cervix
CINCA (chronic infantile neurological, cutaneous and articular syndrome) M04.2

Cinchonism — see Deafness, ototoxic
  correct substance properly administered — see Table of Drugs and Chemicals, by drug, adverse effect
  overdose or wrong substance given or taken — see Table of Drugs and Chemicals, by drug, poisoning
Circle of Willis — see condition
Circular — see condition
Circulating anticoagulants (see also Disorder, hemorrhagic) D68.318
  due to drugs (see also Disorder, hemorrhagic) D68.32
  following childbirth O72.3
Circulation
  collateral, any site I99.8
  defective (lower extremity) I99.8
    congenital Q28.9
  embryonic Q28.9
  failure (peripheral) R57.9
    newborn P29.89
  fetal, persistent P29.3
  heart, incomplete Q28.9
Circulatory system — see condition
Circulus senilis (cornea) — see Degeneration, cornea, senile
Circumcision (in absence of medical indication) (ritual) (routine) Z41.2
Circumscribed — see condition
Circumvallate placenta O43.11-
Cirrhosis, cirrhotic (hepatic) (liver) K74.60
  alcoholic K70.30
    with ascites K70.31
  atrophic — see Cirrhosis, liver
  Baumgarten-Cruveilhier K74.69
  biliary (cholangiolitic) (cholangitic) (hypertrophic) (obstructive) (pericholangiolitic) K74.5
    due to
      Clonorchiasis B66.1
      flukes B66.3
    primary K74.3
    secondary K74.4
  cardiac (of liver) K76.1
  Charcot's K74.3
  cholangiolitic, cholangitic, cholostatic (primary) K74.3
  congestive K76.1
  Cruveilhier-Baumgarten K74.69
  cryptogenic (liver) K74.69
  due to
    hepatolenticular degeneration E83.01
    Wilson's disease E83.01
    xanthomatosis E78.2
  fatty K76.0
    alcoholic K70.0
  Hanot's (hypertrophic) K74.3
  hepatic — see Cirrhosis, liver
  hypertrophic K74.3
  Indian childhood K74.69
  kidney — see Sclerosis, renal
  Laennec's K70.30
    with ascites K70.31
    alcoholic K70.30
      with ascites K70.31
    nonalcoholic K74.69
  liver K74.60
    alcoholic K70.30
      with ascites K70.31
      fatty K70.0
    congenital P78.81
    syphilitic A52.74
  lung (chronic) J84.10
  macronodular K74.69
    alcoholic K70.30
      with ascites K70.31
  micronodular K74.69
    alcoholic K70.30
      with ascites K70.31

DISEASE INDEX

Cirrhosis, cirrhotic (hepatic) (liver) K74.60 — *continued*
  mixed type K74.69
  monolobular K74.3
  nephritis — *see* Sclerosis, renal
  nutritional K74.69
    alcoholic K70.30
      with ascites K70.31
  obstructive — *see* Cirrhosis, biliary
  ovarian N83.8
  pancreas (duct) K86.89
  pigmentary E83.110
  portal K74.69
    alcoholic K70.30
      with ascites K70.31
  postnecrotic K74.69
    alcoholic K70.30
      with ascites K70.31
  pulmonary J84.10
  renal — *see* Sclerosis, renal
  spleen D73.2
  stasis K76.1
  Todd's K74.3
  unilobar K74.3
  xanthomatous (biliary) K74.5
    due to xanthomatosis (familial) (metabolic) (primary) E78.2
Cistern, subarachnoid R93.0
Citrullinemia E72.23
Citrullinuria E72.23
Civatte's disease or poikiloderma L57.3
Clam digger's itch B65.3
Clammy skin R23.1
Clap — *see* Gonorrhea
Clarke-Hadfield syndrome (pancreatic infantilism) K86.89
Clark's paralysis G80.9
Clastothrix L67.8
Claude Bernard-Horner syndrome G90.2
  traumatic — *see* Injury, nerve, cervical sympathetic
Claude's disease or syndrome G46.3
Claudicatio venosa intermittens I87.8
Claudication (intermittent) I73.9
  cerebral (artery) G45.9
  spinal cord (arteriosclerotic) G95.19
    syphilitic A52.09
  venous (axillary) I87.8
Claustrophobia F40.240
Clavus (infected) L84
Clawfoot (congenital) Q66.89
  acquired — *see* Deformity, limb, clawfoot
Clawhand (acquired) — *see also* Deformity, limb, clawhand
  congenital Q68.1
Clawtoe (congenital) Q66.89
  acquired — *see* Deformity, toe, specified NEC
Clay eating — *see* Pica
Cleansing of artificial opening — *see* Attention to, artificial, opening
Cleft (congenital) — *see also* Imperfect, closure
  alveolar process M26.79
  branchial (cyst) (persistent) Q18.2
  cricoid cartilage, posterior Q31.8
  foot Q72.7
  hand Q71.6
  lip (unilateral) Q36.9
    with cleft palate Q37.9
      hard Q37.1
        with soft Q37.5
      soft Q37.3
        with hard Q37.5
    bilateral Q36.0
      with cleft palate Q37.8
        hard Q37.0
          with soft Q37.4
        soft Q37.2
          with hard Q37.4
    median Q36.1

Cleft (congenital) — *see also* Imperfect, closure — *continued*
  nose Q30.2
  palate Q35.9
    with cleft lip (unilateral) Q37.9
      bilateral Q37.8
    hard Q35.1
      with
        cleft lip (unilateral) Q37.1
          bilateral Q37.0
        soft Q35.5
          with cleft lip (unilateral) Q37.5
            bilateral Q37.4
    medial Q35.5
    soft Q35.3
      with
        cleft lip (unilateral) Q37.3
          bilateral Q37.2
        hard Q35.5
          with cleft lip (unilateral) Q37.5
            bilateral Q37.4
  penis Q55.69
  scrotum Q55.29
  thyroid cartilage Q31.8
  uvula Q35.7
Cleidocranial dysostosis Q74.0
Cleptomania F63.2
Clicking hip (newborn) R29.4
Climacteric (female) — *see also* Menopause
  arthritis (any site) NEC — *see* Arthritis, specified form NEC
  depression (single episode) F32.89
    recurrent episode F33.8
  male (symptoms) (syndrome) NEC N50.89
  melancholia (single episode) F32.89
    recurrent episode F33.8
  paranoid state F22
  polyarthritis NEC — *see* Arthritis, specified form NEC
  symptoms (female) N95.1
Clinical research investigation (clinical trial) (control subject) (normal comparison) (participant) Z00.6
Clitoris — *see* condition
Cloaca (persistent) Q43.7
Clonorchiasis, clonorchis infection (liver) B66.1
Clonus R25.8
Closed bite M26.29
Clostridium (C.) perfringens, as cause of disease classified elsewhere B96.7
Closure
  congenital, nose Q30.0
  cranial sutures, premature Q75.0
  defective or imperfect NEC — *see* Imperfect, closure
  fistula, delayed — *see* Fistula
  foramen ovale, imperfect Q21.1
  hymen N89.6
  interauricular septum, defective Q21.1
  interventricular septum, defective Q21.0
  lacrimal duct — *see also* Stenosis, lacrimal, duct
    congenital Q10.5
  nose (congenital) Q30.0
    acquired M95.0
  of artificial opening — *see* Attention to, artificial, opening
  primary angle, without glaucoma damage H40.06-
  vagina N89.5
  valve — *see* Endocarditis
  vulva N90.5
Clot (blood) — *see also* Embolism
  artery (obstruction) (occlusion) — *see* Embolism
  bladder N32.89
  brain (intradural or extradural) — *see* Occlusion, artery, cerebral
  circulation I74.9

Clot (blood) — *see also* Embolism — *continued*
  heart — *see also* Infarct, myocardium
    not resulting in infarction I51.3
  vein — *see* Thrombosis
Clouded state R40.1
  epileptic — *see* Epilepsy, specified NEC
  paroxysmal — *see* Epilepsy, specified NEC
Cloudy antrum, antra J32.0
Clouston's (hidrotic) ectodermal dysplasia Q82.4
Clubbed nail pachydermoperiostosis M89.40 *[L62]*
Clubbing of finger(s) (nails) R68.3
Clubfinger R68.3
  congenital Q68.1
Clubfoot (congenital) Q66.89
  acquired — *see* Deformity, limb, clubfoot
  equinovarus Q66.0
  paralytic — *see* Deformity, limb, clubfoot
Clubhand (congenital) (radial) Q71.4-
  acquired — *see* Deformity, limb, clubhand
Clubnail R68.3
  congenital Q84.6
Clump, kidney Q63.1
Clumsiness, clumsy child syndrome F82
Cluttering F80.81
Clutton's joints A50.51 *[M12.80]*
Coagulation, intravascular (diffuse) (disseminated) — *see also* Defibrination syndrome
  complicating abortion — *see* Abortion, by type, complicated by, intravascular coagulation
  following ectopic or molar pregnancy O08.1
Coagulopathy — *see also* Defect, coagulation
  consumption D65
  intravascular D65
  newborn P60
Coalition
  calcaneo-scaphoid Q66.89
  tarsal Q66.89
Coalminer's
  elbow — *see* Bursitis, elbow, olecranon
  lung or pneumoconiosis J60
Coalworker's lung or pneumoconiosis J60
Coarctation
  aorta (preductal) (postductal) Q25.1
  pulmonary artery Q25.71
Coated tongue K14.3
Coats' disease (exudative retinopathy) — *see* Retinopathy, exudative
Cocaine-induced
  anxiety disorder F14.980
  bipolar and related disorder F14.94
  depressive disorder F14.94
  obsessive-compulsive and related disorder F14.988
  psychotic disorder F14.959
  sexual dysfunction F14.981
  sleep disorder F14.982
Cocainism — *see* Disorder, cocaine use
Coccidioidomycosis B38.9
  cutaneous B38.3
  disseminated B38.7
  generalized B38.7
  meninges B38.4
  prostate B38.81
  pulmonary B38.2
    acute B38.0
    chronic B38.1
  skin B38.3
  specified NEC B38.89
Coccidioidosis — *see* Coccidioidomycosis
Coccidiosis (intestinal) A07.3
Coccydynia, coccygodynia M53.3
Coccyx — *see* condition
Cochin-China diarrhea K90.1
Cockayne's syndrome Q87.1

Cock's peculiar tumor L72.3
Cocked up toe — *see* Deformity, toe, specified NEC
Codman's tumor — *see* Neoplasm, bone, benign
Coenurosis B71.8
Coffee-worker's lung J67.8
Cogan's syndrome H16.32-
oculomotor apraxia H51.8
Coitus, painful (female) N94.10
male N53.12
psychogenic F52.6
Cold J00
with influenza, flu, or grippe — *see* Influenza, with, respiratory manifestations NEC
agglutinin disease or hemoglobinuria (chronic) D59.1
bronchial — *see* Bronchitis
chest — *see* Bronchitis
common (head) J00
effects of T69.9
specified effect NEC T69.8
excessive, effects of T69.9
specified effect NEC T69.8
exhaustion from T69.8
exposure to T69.9
specified effect NEC T69.8
head J00
injury syndrome (newborn) P80.0
on lung — *see* Bronchitis
rose J30.1
sensitivity, auto-immune D59.1
virus J00
Coldsore B00.1
Colibacillosis A49.8
as the cause of other disease (*see also* Escherichia coli) B96.20
generalized A41.50
Colic (bilious) (infantile) (intestinal) (recurrent) (spasmodic) R10.83
abdomen R10.83
psychogenic F45.8
appendix, appendicular K38.8
bile duct — *see* Calculus, bile duct
biliary — *see* Calculus, bile duct
common duct — *see* Calculus, bile duct
cystic duct — *see* Calculus, gallbladder
Devonshire NEC — *see* Poisoning, lead
gallbladder — *see* Calculus, gallbladder
gallstone — *see* Calculus, gallbladder
gallbladder or cystic duct — *see* Calculus, gallbladder
hepatic (duct) — *see* Calculus, bile duct
hysterical F45.8
kidney N23
lead NEC — *see* Poisoning, lead
mucous K58.9
with diarrhea K58.0
psychogenic F54
nephritic N23
painter's NEC — *see* Poisoning, lead
pancreas K86.89
psychogenic F45.8
renal N23
saturnine NEC — *see* Poisoning, lead
ureter N23
urethral N36.8
due to calculus N21.1
uterus NEC N94.89
menstrual — *see* Dysmenorrhea
worm NOS B83.9
Colicystitis — *see* Cystitis

Colitis (acute) (catarrhal) (chronic) (noninfective) (hemorrhagic) (*see also* Enteritis) K52.9
allergic K52.29
with
food protein-induced enterocolitis syndrome K52.21
proctocolitis K52.82
amebic (acute) (*see also* Amebiasis) A06.0
nondysenteric A06.2
anthrax A22.2
bacillary — *see* Infection, Shigella
balantidial A07.0
Clostridium difficile A04.7
coccidial A07.3
collagenous K52.831
cystica superficialis K52.89
dietary counseling and surveillance (for) Z71.3
dietetic (*see also* Colitis, allergic) K52.29
drug-induced K52.1
due to radiation K52.0
eosinophilic K52.82
food hypersensitivity (*see also* Colitis, allergic) K52.29
giardial A07.1
granulomatous — *see* Enteritis, regional, large intestine
indeterminate, so stated K52.3
infectious — *see* Enteritis, infectious
ischemic K55.9
acute (subacute) (*see also* Ischemia, intestine, acute) K55.039
chronic K55.1
due to mesenteric artery insufficiency K55.1
fulminant (acute) (*see also* Ischemia, intestine, acute) K55.039
left sided K51.50
with
abscess K51.514
complication K51.519
specified NEC K51.518
fistula K51.513
obstruction K51.512
rectal bleeding K51.511
lymphocytic K52.832
membranous
psychogenic F54
microscopic K52.839
specified NEC K52.838
mucous — *see* Syndrome, irritable, bowel
psychogenic F54
noninfective K52.9
specified NEC K52.89
polyposa — *see* Polyp, colon, inflammatory
protozoal A07.9
pseudomembranous A04.7
pseudomucinous — *see* Syndrome, irritable, bowel
regional — *see* Enteritis, regional, large intestine
segmental — *see* Enteritis, regional, large intestine
septic — *see* Enteritis, infectious
spastic K58.9
with diarrhea K58.0
psychogenic F54
staphylococcal A04.8
foodborne A05.0
subacute ischemic (*see also* Ischemia, intestine, acute) K55.039
thromboulcerative (*see also* Ischemia, intestine, acute) K55.039
toxic NEC K52.1
due to Clostridium difficile A04.7
transmural — *see* Enteritis, regional, large intestine
trichomonal A07.8
tuberculous (ulcerative) A18.32

Colitis (acute) (catarrhal) (chronic) (noninfective) (hemorrhagic) (*see also* Enteritis) K52.9 — *continued*
ulcerative (chronic) K51.90
with
complication K51.919
abscess K51.914
fistula K51.913
obstruction K51.912
rectal bleeding K51.911
specified complication NEC K51.918
enterocolitis — *see* Enterocolitis, ulcerative
ileocolitis — *see* Ileocolitis, ulcerative
mucosal proctocolitis — *see* Proctocolitis, mucosal
proctitis — *see* Proctitis, ulcerative
pseudopolyposis — *see* Polyp, colon, inflammatory
psychogenic F54
rectosigmoiditis — *see* Rectosigmoiditis, ulcerative
specified type NEC K51.80
with
complication K51.819
abscess K51.814
fistula K51.813
obstruction K51.812
rectal bleeding K51.811
specified complication NEC K51.818
Collagenosis, collagen disease (nonvascular) (vascular) M35.9
cardiovascular I42.8
reactive perforating L87.1
specified NEC M35.8
Collapse R55
adrenal E27.2
cardiorespiratory R57.0
cardiovascular R57.0
newborn P29.89
circulatory (peripheral) R57.9
during or after labor and delivery O75.1
following ectopic or molar pregnancy O08.3
newborn P29.89
during or
after labor and delivery O75.1
resulting from a procedure, not elsewhere classified T81.10
external ear canal — *see* Stenosis, external ear canal
general R55
heart — *see* Disease, heart
heat T67.1
hysterical F44.89
labyrinth, membranous (congenital) Q16.5
lung (massive) (*see also* Atelectasis) J98.19
pressure due to anesthesia (general) (local) or other sedation T88.2
during labor and delivery O74.1
in pregnancy O29.02-
postpartum, puerperal O89.09
myocardial — *see* Disease, heart
nervous F48.8
neurocirculatory F45.8
nose M95.0
postoperative T81.10
pulmonary (*see also* Atelectasis) J98.19
newborn — *see* Atelectasis
trachea J39.8
tracheobronchial J98.09
valvular — *see* Endocarditis
vascular (peripheral) R57.9
during or after labor and delivery O75.1
following ectopic or molar pregnancy O08.3
newborn P29.89

DISEASE INDEX

Collapse R55 — *continued*
  vertebra M48.50-
    cervical region M48.52-
    cervicothoracic region M48.53-
    in (due to)
      metastasis — *see* Collapse, vertebra, in, specified disease NEC
      osteoporosis (*see also* Osteoporosis) M80.88
        cervical region M80.88
        cervicothoracic region M80.88
        lumbar region M80.88
        lumbosacral region M80.88
        multiple sites M80.88
        occipito-atlanto-axial region M80.88
        sacrococcygeal region M80.88
        thoracic region M80.88
        thoracolumbar region M80.88
      specified disease NEC M48.50-
        cervical region M48.52-
        cervicothoracic region M48.53-
        lumbar region M48.56-
        lumbosacral region M48.57-
        occipito-atlanto-axial region M48.51-
        sacrococcygeal region M48.58-
        thoracic region M48.54-
        thoracolumbar region M48.55-
    lumbar region M48.56-
    lumbosacral region M48.57-
    occipito-atlanto-axial region M48.51-
    sacrococcygeal region M48.58-
    thoracic region M48.54-
    thoracolumbar region M48.55-
Collateral — *see also* condition
  circulation (venous) I87.8
  dilation, veins I87.8
Colles' fracture S52.53-
Collet(-Sicard) syndrome G52.7
Collier's asthma or lung J60
Collodion baby Q80.2
Colloid nodule (of thyroid) (cystic) E04.1
Coloboma (iris) Q13.0
  eyelid Q10.3
  fundus Q14.8
  lens Q12.2
  optic disc (congenital) Q14.2
    acquired H47.31-
Coloenteritis — *see* Enteritis
Colon — *see* condition
Colonization
  MRSA (Methicillin resistant Staphylococcus aureus) Z22.322
  MSSA (Methicillin susceptible Staphylococcus aureus) Z22.321
  status — *see* Carrier (suspected) of
Coloptosis K63.4
Color blindness — *see* Deficiency, color vision
Colostomy
  attention to Z43.3
  fitting or adjustment Z46.89
  malfunctioning K94.03
  status Z93.3
Colpitis (acute) — *see* Vaginitis
Colpocele N81.5
Colpocystitis — *see* Vaginitis
Colpospasm N94.2
Column, spinal, vertebral — *see* condition
Coma R40.20
  with
    motor response (none) R40.231
      abnormal R40.233
      extension R40.232
      flexion withdrawal R40.234
      localizes pain R40.235
      obeys commands R40.236

Coma R40.20 — *continued*
  with — *continued*
    opening of eyes (never) R40.211
      in response to
        pain R40.212
        sound R40.213
      spontaneous R40.214
    verbal response (none) R40.221
      confused conversation R40.224
      inappropriate words R40.223
      incomprehensible words R40.222
      oriented R40.225
  eclamptic — *see* Eclampsia
  epileptic — *see* Epilepsy
  Glasgow, scale score — *see* Glasgow coma scale
  hepatic — *see* Failure, hepatic, by type, with coma
  hyperglycemic (diabetic) — *see* Diabetes, by type, with hyperosmolarity, with coma
  hyperosmolar (diabetic) — *see* Diabetes, by type, with hyperosmolarity, with coma
  hypoglycemic (diabetic) — *see* Diabetes, by type, with hypoglycemia, with coma
    nondiabetic E15
  in diabetes — *see* Diabetes, coma
  insulin-induced — *see* Coma, hypoglycemic
  myxedematous E03.5
  newborn P91.5
  persistent vegetative state R40.3
  specified NEC, without documented Glasgow coma scale score, or with partial Glasgow coma scale score reported R40.244
Comatose — *see* Coma
Combat fatigue F43.0
Combined — *see* condition
Comedo, comedones (giant) L70.0
Comedocarcinoma — *see also* Neoplasm, breast, malignant
  noninfiltrating
    breast D05.8-
    specified site — *see* Neoplasm, in situ, by site
    unspecified site D05.8-
Comedomastitis — *see* Ectasia, mammary duct
Comminuted fracture — *code as* Fracture, closed
Common
  arterial trunk Q20.0
  atrioventricular canal Q21.2
  atrium Q21.1
  cold (head) J00
  truncus (arteriosus) Q20.0
  variable immunodeficiency — *see* Immunodeficiency, common variable
  ventricle Q20.4
Commotio, commotion (current)
  brain — *see* Injury, intracranial, concussion
  cerebri — *see* Injury, intracranial, concussion
  retinae S05.8x-
  spinal cord — *see* Injury, spinal cord, by region
  spinalis — *see* Injury, spinal cord, by region
Communication
  between
    base of aorta and pulmonary artery Q21.4
    left ventricle and right atrium Q20.5
    pericardial sac and pleural sac Q34.8
    pulmonary artery and pulmonary vein, congenital Q25.72
  congenital between uterus and digestive or urinary tract Q51.7
Compartment syndrome (deep) (posterior) (traumatic) T79.A0 *(follows T79.7)*
  abdomen T79.A3 *(follows T79.7)*
  lower extremity (hip, buttock, thigh, leg, foot, toes) T79.A2 *(follows T79.7)*

Compartment syndrome (deep) (posterior) — *continued*
  nontraumatic
    abdomen M79.A3 *(follows M79.7)*
    lower extremity (hip, buttock, thigh, leg, foot, toes) M79.A2- *(follows M79.7)*
    specified site NEC M79.A9 *(follows M79.7)*
    upper extremity (shoulder, arm, forearm, wrist, hand, fingers) M79.A1- *(follows M79.7)*
  specified site NEC T79.A9 *(follows T79.7)*
  upper extremity (shoulder, arm, forearm, wrist, hand, fingers) T79.A1 *(follows T79.7)*
Compensation
  failure — *see* Disease, heart
  neurosis, psychoneurosis — *see* Disorder, factitious
Complaint — *see also* Disease
  bowel, functional K59.9
    psychogenic F45.8
  intestine, functional K59.9
    psychogenic F45.8
  kidney — *see* Disease, renal
  miners' J60
Complete — *see* condition
Complex
  Addison-Schilder E71.528
  cardiorenal — *see* Hypertension, cardiorenal
  Costen's M26.69
  disseminated mycobacterium avium-intracellulare (DMAC) A31.2
  Eisenmenger's (ventricular septal defect) I27.89
  hypersexual F52.8
  jumped process, spine — *see* Dislocation, vertebra
  primary, tuberculous A15.7
  Schilder-Addison E71.528
  subluxation (vertebral) M99.19
    abdomen M99.19
    acromioclavicular M99.17
    cervical region M99.11
    cervicothoracic M99.11
    costochondral M99.18
    costovertebral M99.18
    head region M99.10
    hip M99.15
    lower extremity M99.16
    lumbar region M99.13
    lumbosacral M99.13
    occipitocervical M99.10
    pelvic region M99.15
    pubic M99.15
    rib cage M99.18
    sacral region M99.14
    sacrococcygeal M99.14
    sacroiliac M99.14
    specified NEC M99.19
    sternochondral M99.18
    sternoclavicular M99.17
    thoracic region M99.12
    thoracolumbar M99.12
    upper extremity M99.17
  Taussig-Bing (transposition, aorta and overriding pulmonary artery) Q20.1
Complication(s) (from) (of)
  accidental puncture or laceration during a procedure (of) — *see* Complications, intraoperative (intraprocedural), puncture or laceration
  amputation stump (surgical) (late) NEC T87.9
    dehiscence T87.81
    infection or inflammation T87.40
      lower limb T87.4-
      upper limb T87.4-
    necrosis T87.50
      lower limb T87.5-
      upper limb T87.5-

Complication(s) (from) (of) — *continued*
  amputation stump (surgical) (late) NEC T87.9
    — *continued*
    neuroma T87.30
      lower limb T87.3-
      upper limb T87.3-
    specified type NEC T87.89
  anastomosis (and bypass) — *see also*
    Complications, prosthetic device or
    implant
    intestinal (internal) NEC K91.89
      involving urinary tract N99.89
    urinary tract (involving intestinal tract)
      N99.89
    vascular — *see* Complications,
      cardiovascular device or implant
  anesthesia, anesthetic (*see also* Anesthesia,
    complication) T88.59
    brain, postpartum, puerperal O89.2
    cardiac
      in
        labor and delivery O74.2
        pregnancy O29.19-
        postpartum, puerperal O89.1
    central nervous system
      in
        labor and delivery O74.3
        pregnancy O29.29-
        postpartum, puerperal O89.2
    difficult or failed intubation T88.4
      in pregnancy O29.6-
    failed sedation (conscious) (moderate)
      during procedure T88.52
    general, unintended awareness during
      procedure T88.53
    hyperthermia, malignant T88.3
    hypothermia T88.51
    intubation failure T88.4
    malignant hyperthermia T88.3
    pulmonary
      in
        labor and delivery O74.1
        pregnancy NEC O29.09-
        postpartum, puerperal O89.09
    shock T88.2
    spinal and epidural
      in
        labor and delivery NEC O74.6
          headache O74.5
        pregnancy NEC O29.5x-
        postpartum, puerperal NEC O89.5
          headache O89.4
    unintended awareness under general
      anesthesia during procedure T88.53
  anti-reflux device — *see* Complications,
    esophageal anti-reflux device
  aortic (bifurcation) graft — *see* Complications,
    graft, vascular
  aortocoronary (bypass) graft — *see*
    Complications, coronary artery (bypass)
    graft
  aortofemoral (bypass) graft — *see*
    Complications, extremity artery (bypass)
    graft
  arteriovenous
    fistula, surgically created T82.9
      embolism T82.818
      fibrosis T82.828
      hemorrhage T82.838
      infection or inflammation T82.7
      mechanical
        breakdown T82.510
        displacement T82.520
        leakage T82.530
        malposition T82.520
        obstruction T82.590
        perforation T82.590
        protrusion T82.590

Complication(s) (from) (of) — *continued*
  arteriovenous — *continued*
    fistula, surgically created T82.9 —
      continued
      pain T82.848
      specified type NEC T82.898
      stenosis T82.858
      thrombosis T82.868
    shunt, surgically created T82.9
      embolism T82.818
      fibrosis T82.828
      hemorrhage T82.838
      infection or inflammation T82.7
      mechanical
        breakdown T82.511
        displacement T82.521
        leakage T82.531
        malposition T82.521
        obstruction T82.591
        perforation T82.591
        protrusion T82.591
      pain T82.848
      specified type NEC T82.898
      stenosis T82.858
      thrombosis T82.868
  arthroplasty — *see* Complications, joint
    prosthesis
  artificial
    fertilization or insemination N98.9
      attempted introduction (of)
        embryo in embryo transfer N98.3
        ovum following in vitro fertilization
          N98.2
      hyperstimulation of ovaries N98.1
      infection N98.0
      specified NEC N98.8
    heart T82.9
      embolism T82.817
      fibrosis T82.827
      hemorrhage T82.837
      infection or inflammation T82.7
      mechanical
        breakdown T82.512
        displacement T82.522
        leakage T82.532
        malposition T82.522
        obstruction T82.592
        perforation T82.592
        protrusion T82.592
      pain T82.847
      specified type NEC T82.897
      stenosis T82.857
      thrombosis T82.867
    opening
      cecostomy — *see* Complications, colostomy
      colostomy — *see* Complications, colostomy
      cystostomy — *see* Complications,
        cystostomy
      enterostomy — *see* Complications,
        enterostomy
      gastrostomy — *see* Complications,
        gastrostomy
      ileostomy — *see* Complications,
        enterostomy
      jejunostomy — *see* Complications,
        enterostomy
      nephrostomy — *see* Complications, stoma,
        urinary tract
      tracheostomy — *see* Complications,
        tracheostomy
      ureterostomy — *see* Complications, stoma,
        urinary tract
      urethrostomy — *see* Complications, stoma,
        urinary tract

Complication(s) (from) (of) — *continued*
  balloon implant or device
    gastrointestinal T85.9
      embolism T85.818
      fibrosis T85.828
      hemorrhage T85.838
      infection and inflammation T85.79
      pain T85.848
      specified type NEC T85.898
      stenosis T85.858
      thrombosis T85.868
    vascular (counterpulsation) T82.9
      embolism T82.818
      fibrosis T82.828
      hemorrhage T82.838
      infection or inflammation T82.7
      mechanical
        breakdown T82.513
        displacement T82.523
        leakage T82.533
        malposition T82.523
        obstruction T82.593
        perforation T82.593
        protrusion T82.593
      pain T82.848
      specified type NEC T82.898
      stenosis T82.858
      thrombosis T82.868
  bariatric procedure
    gastric band procedure K95.09
      infection K95.01
    specified procedure NEC K95.89
      infection K95.81
  bile duct implant (prosthetic) T85.9
    embolism T85.818
    fibrosis T85.828
    hemorrhage T85.838
    infection and inflammation T85.79
    mechanical
      breakdown T85.510
      displacement T85.520
      malfunction T85.510
      malposition T85.520
      obstruction T85.590
      perforation T85.590
      protrusion T85.590
      specified NEC T85.590
    pain T85.848
    specified type NEC T85.898
    stenosis T85.858
    thrombosis T85.868
  bladder device (auxiliary) — *see*
    Complications, genitourinary, device or
    implant, urinary system
  bleeding (postoperative) — *see* Complication,
    postoperative, hemorrhage
    intraoperative — *see* Complication,
      intraoperative, hemorrhage
  blood vessel graft — *see* Complications, graft,
    vascular
  bone
    device NEC T84.9
      embolism T84.81
      fibrosis T84.82
      hemorrhage T84.83
      infection or inflammation T84.7
      mechanical
        breakdown T84.318
        displacement T84.328
        malposition T84.328
        obstruction T84.398
        perforation T84.398
        protrusion T84.398
      pain T84.84
      specified type NEC T84.89
      stenosis T84.85
      thrombosis T84.86
    graft — *see* Complications, graft, bone

DISEASE INDEX

Complication(s) (from) (of) — *continued*
bone — *continued*
  growth stimulator (electrode) — *see*
    Complications, electronic stimulator
    device, bone
  marrow transplant — *see* Complications,
    transplant, bone, marrow
brain neurostimulator (electrode) — *see*
  Complications, electronic stimulator
  device, brain
breast implant (prosthetic) T85.9
  capsular contracture T85.44
  embolism T85.818
  fibrosis T85.828
  hemorrhage T85.838
  infection and inflammation T85.79
  mechanical
    breakdown T85.41
    displacement T85.42
    leakage T85.43
    malposition T85.42
    obstruction T85.49
    perforation T85.49
    protrusion T85.49
    specified NEC T85.49
  pain T85.848
  specified type NEC T85.898
  stenosis T85.858
  thrombosis T85.868
bypass — *see also* Complications, prosthetic
  device or implant
  aortocoronary — *see* Complications,
    coronary artery (bypass) graft
  arterial — *see also* Complications, graft,
    vascular
    extremity — *see* Complications, extremity
      artery (bypass) graft
cardiac — *see also* Disease, heart
  device, implant or graft T82.9
    embolism T82.817
    fibrosis T82.827
    hemorrhage T82.837
    infection or inflammation T82.7
      valve prosthesis T82.6
    mechanical
      breakdown T82.519
        specified device NEC T82.518
      displacement T82.529
        specified device NEC T82.528
      leakage T82.539
        specified device NEC T82.538
      malposition T82.529
        specified device NEC T82.528
      obstruction T82.599
        specified device NEC T82.598
      perforation T82.599
        specified device NEC T82.598
      protrusion T82.599
        specified device NEC T82.598
    pain T82.847
    specified type NEC T82.897
    stenosis T82.857
    thrombosis T82.867
cardiovascular device, graft or implant T82.9
  aortic graft — *see* Complications, graft,
    vascular
  arteriovenous
    fistula, artificial — *see* Complication,
      arteriovenous, fistula, surgically
      created
    shunt — *see* Complication, arteriovenous,
      shunt, surgically created
  artificial heart — *see* Complication, artificial,
    heart
  balloon (counterpulsation) device — *see*
    Complication, balloon implant, vascular
  carotid artery graft — *see* Complications,
    graft, vascular

Complication(s) (from) (of) — *continued*
cardiovascular device, graft or implant T82.9
  — *continued*
  coronary bypass graft — *see* Complication,
    coronary artery (bypass) graft
  dialysis catheter (vascular) — *see*
    Complication, catheter, dialysis
  electronic T82.9
    electrode T82.9
      embolism T82.817
      fibrosis T82.827
      hemorrhage T82.837
      infection T82.7
      mechanical
        breakdown T82.110
        displacement T82.120
        leakage T82.190
        obstruction T82.190
        perforation T82.190
        protrusion T82.190
        specified type NEC T82.190
      pain T82.847
      specified NEC T82.897
      stenosis T82.857
      thrombosis T82.867
    embolism T82.817
    fibrosis T82.827
    hemorrhage T82.837
    infection T82.7
    mechanical
      breakdown T82.119
      displacement T82.129
      leakage T82.199
      obstruction T82.199
      perforation T82.199
      protrusion T82.199
      specified type NEC T82.199
    pain T82.847
    pulse generator T82.9
      embolism T82.817
      fibrosis T82.827
      hemorrhage T82.837
      infection T82.7
      mechanical
        breakdown T82.111
        displacement T82.121
        leakage T82.191
        obstruction T82.191
        perforation T82.191
        protrusion T82.191
        specified type NEC T82.191
      pain T82.847
      specified NEC T82.897
      stenosis T82.857
      thrombosis T82.867
    specified condition NEC T82.897
    specified device NEC T82.9
      embolism T82.817
      fibrosis T82.827
      hemorrhage T82.837
      infection T82.7
      mechanical
        breakdown T82.118
        displacement T82.128
        leakage T82.198
        obstruction T82.198
        perforation T82.198
        protrusion T82.198
        specified type NEC T82.198
      pain T82.847
      specified NEC T82.897
      stenosis T82.857
      thrombosis T82.867
    stenosis T82.857
    thrombosis T82.867
  extremity artery graft — *see* Complication,
    extremity artery (bypass) graft
  femoral artery graft — *see* Complication,
    extremity artery (bypass) graft

Complication(s) (from) (of) — *continued*
cardiovascular device, graft or implant T82.9
  — *continued*
  heart
    transplant — *see* Complication, transplant,
      heart
    valve — *see* Complication, prosthetic
      device, heart valve
      graft — *see* Complication, heart, valve,
        graft
  heart-lung transplant — *see* Complication,
    transplant, heart, with lung
  infection or inflammation T82.7
  umbrella device — *see* Complication,
    umbrella device, vascular
  vascular graft (or anastomosis) — *see*
    Complication, graft, vascular
carotid artery (bypass) graft — *see*
  Complications, graft, vascular
catheter (device) NEC — *see also*
  Complications, prosthetic device or
  implant
  cranial infusion
    infection and inflammation T85.735
    mechanical
      breakdown T85.610
      displacement T85.620
      leakage T85.630
      malfunction T85.690
      malposition T85.620
      obstruction T85.690
      perforation T85.690
      protrusion T85.690
      specified NEC T85.690
  cystostomy T83.9
    embolism T83.81
    fibrosis T83.82
    hemorrhage T83.83
    infection and inflammation T83.510
    mechanical
      breakdown T83.010
      displacement T83.020
      leakage T83.030
      malposition T83.020
      obstruction T83.090
      perforation T83.090
      protrusion T83.090
      specified NEC T83.090
    pain T83.84
    specified type NEC T83.89
    stenosis T83.85
    thrombosis T83.86
  dialysis (vascular) T82.9
    embolism T82.818
    fibrosis T82.828
    hemorrhage T82.838
    infection and inflammation T82.7
    intraperitoneal — *see* Complications,
      catheter, intraperitoneal
    mechanical
      breakdown T82.41
      displacement T82.42
      leakage T82.43
      malposition T82.42
      obstruction T82.49
      perforation T82.49
      protrusion T82.49
    pain T82.848
    specified type NEC T82.898
    stenosis T82.858
    thrombosis T82.868
  epidural infusion T85.9
    embolism T85.810
    fibrosis T85.820
    hemorrhage T85.830
    infection and inflammation T85.735

Complication(s) (from) (of) — *continued*
catheter (device) NEC (*see also* Complications, prosthetic device or implant) — *continued*
epidural infusion T85.9 — *continued*
  mechanical
    breakdown T85.610
    displacement T85.620
    leakage T85.630
    malfunction T85.610
    malposition T85.620
    obstruction T85.690
    perforation T85.690
    protrusion T85.690
    specified NEC T85.690
  pain T85.840
  specified type NEC T85.890
  stenosis T85.850
  thrombosis T85.860
intraperitoneal dialysis T85.9
  embolism T85.818
  fibrosis T85.828
  hemorrhage T85.838
  infection and inflammation T85.71
  mechanical
    breakdown T85.611
    displacement T85.621
    leakage T85.631
    malfunction T85.611
    malposition T85.621
    obstruction T85.691
    perforation T85.691
    protrusion T85.691
    specified NEC T85.691
  pain T85.848
  specified type NEC T85.898
  stenosis T85.858
  thrombosis T85.868
intrathecal infusion
  infection and inflammation T85.735
  mechanical
    breakdown T85.610
    displacement T85.620
    leakage T85.630
    malfunction T85.690
    malposition T85.620
    obstruction T85.690
    perforation T85.690
    protrusion T85.690
    specified NEC T85.690
intravenous infusion T82.9
  embolism T82.818
  fibrosis T82.828
  hemorrhage T82.838
  infection or inflammation T82.7
  mechanical
    breakdown T82.514
    displacement T82.524
    leakage T82.534
    malposition T82.524
    obstruction T82.594
    perforation T82.594
    protrusion T82.594
  pain T82.848
  specified type NEC T82.898
  stenosis T82.858
  thrombosis T82.868
spinal infusion
  infection and inflammation T85.735
  mechanical
    breakdown T85.610
    displacement T85.620
    leakage T85.630
    malfunction T85.690
    malposition T85.620
    obstruction T85.690
    perforation T85.690
    protrusion T85.690
    specified NEC T85.690

Complication(s) (from) (of) — *continued*
catheter (device) NEC (*see also* Complications, prosthetic device or implant) — *continued*
subarachnoid infusion
  infection and inflammation T85.735
  mechanical
    breakdown T85.610
    displacement T85.620
    leakage T85.630
    malfunction T85.690
    malposition T85.620
    obstruction T85.690
    perforation T85.690
    protrusion T85.690
    specified NEC T85.690
subdural infusion T85.9
  embolism T85.810
  fibrosis T85.820
  hemorrhage T85.830
  infection and inflammation T85.735
  mechanical
    breakdown T85.610
    displacement T85.620
    leakage T85.630
    malfunction T85.610
    malposition T85.620
    obstruction T85.690
    perforation T85.690
    protrusion T85.690
    specified NEC T85.690
  pain T85.840
  specified type NEC T85.890
  stenosis T85.850
  thrombosis T85.860
urethral T83.9
  displacement T83.028
  embolism T83.81
  fibrosis T83.82
  hemorrhage T83.83
  indwelling
    breakdown T83.011
    displacement T83.021
    infection and inflammation T83.511
    leakage T83.031
    specified complication NEC T83.091
  infection and inflammation T83.511
  leakage T83.038
  malposition T83.028
  mechanical
    breakdown T83.011
  obstruction (mechanical) T83.091
  pain T83.84
  perforation T83.091
  protrusion T83.091
  specified type NEC T83.091
  stenosis T83.85
  thrombosis T83.86
urinary NEC
  breakdown T83.018
  displacement T83.028
  infection and inflammation T83.518
  leakage T83.038
  specified complication NEC T83.098
cecostomy (stoma) — *see* Complications, colostomy
cesarean delivery wound NEC O90.89
  disruption O90.0
  hematoma O90.2
  infection (following delivery) O86.0
chemotherapy (antineoplastic) NEC T88.7
chin implant (prosthetic) — *see* Complication, prosthetic device or implant, specified NEC
circulatory system I99.8
  intraoperative I97.88
  postprocedural I97.89
    following cardiac surgery I97.19-
      postcardiotomy syndrome I97.0
    hypertension I97.3
    lymphedema after mastectomy I97.2

Complication(s) (from) (of) — *continued*
circulatory system I99.8 — *continued*
  postprocedural I97.89 — *continued*
    postcardiotomy syndrome I97.0
    specified NEC I97.89
colostomy (stoma) K94.00
  hemorrhage K94.01
  infection K94.02
  malfunction K94.03
  mechanical K94.03
  specified complication NEC K94.09
contraceptive device, intrauterine — *see* Complications, intrauterine, contraceptive device
cord (umbilical) — *see* Complications, umbilical cord
corneal graft — *see* Complications, graft, cornea
coronary artery (bypass) graft T82.9
  atherosclerosis — *see* Arteriosclerosis, coronary (artery)
  embolism T82.818
  fibrosis T82.828
  hemorrhage T82.838
  infection and inflammation T82.7
  mechanical
    breakdown T82.211
    displacement T82.212
    leakage T82.213
    malposition T82.212
    obstruction T82.218
    perforation T82.218
    protrusion T82.218
    specified NEC T82.218
  pain T82.848
  specified type NEC T82.898
  stenosis T82.858
  thrombosis T82.868
counterpulsation device (balloon), intra-aortic — *see* Complications, balloon implant, vascular
cystostomy (stoma) N99.518
  catheter — *see* Complications, catheter, cystostomy
  hemorrhage N99.510
  infection N99.511
  malfunction N99.512
  specified type NEC N99.518
delivery (*see also* Complications, obstetric) O75.9
  procedure (instrumental) (manual) (surgical) O75.4
  specified NEC O75.89
dialysis (peritoneal) (renal) — *see also* Complications, infusion
  catheter (vascular) — *see* Complication, catheter, dialysis
    peritoneal, intraperitoneal — *see* Complications, catheter, intraperitoneal
dorsal column (spinal) neurostimulator — *see* Complications, electronic stimulator device, spinal cord
drug NEC T88.7
ear procedure — *see also* Disorder, ear
  intraoperative H95.88
    hematoma — *see* Complications, intraoperative, hemorrhage (hematoma) (of), ear
    hemorrhage — *see* Complications, intraoperative, hemorrhage (hematoma) (of), ear
    laceration — *see* Complications, intraoperative, puncture or laceration, ear
    specified NEC H95.88

DISEASE INDEX

Complication(s) (from) (of) — *continued*
  ear procedure — *see also* Disorder, ear —
    continued
    postoperative H95.89
      external ear canal stenosis H95.81-
      hematoma — *see* Complications,
        postprocedural, hematoma (of), ear
      hemorrhage — *see* Complications,
        postprocedural, hemorrhage (of), ear
      postmastoidectomy — *see* Complications,
        postmastoidectomy
      seroma — *see* Complications,
        postprocedural, seroma (of), mastoid
        process
      specified NEC H95.89
  ectopic pregnancy O08.9
    damage to pelvic organs O08.6
    embolism O08.2
    genital infection O08.0
    hemorrhage (delayed) (excessive) O08.1
    metabolic disorder O08.5
    renal failure O08.4
    shock O08.3
    specified type NEC O08.0
    venous complication NEC O08.7
  electronic stimulator device
    bladder (urinary) — *see* Complications,
      electronic stimulator device, urinary
    bone T84.9
      breakdown T84.310
      displacement T84.320
      embolism T84.81
      fibrosis T84.82
      hemorrhage T84.83
      infection or inflammation T84.7
      malfunction T84.310
      malposition T84.320
      mechanical NEC T84.390
      obstruction T84.390
      pain T84.84
      perforation T84.390
      protrusion T84.390
      specified type NEC T84.89
      stenosis T84.85
      thrombosis T84.86
    brain T85.9
      embolism T85.810
      fibrosis T85.820
      hemorrhage T85.830
      infection and inflammation T85.731
      mechanical
        breakdown T85.110
        displacement T85.120
        leakage T85.190
        malposition T85.120
        obstruction T85.190
        perforation T85.190
        protrusion T85.190
        specified NEC T85.190
      pain T85.840
      specified type NEC T85.890
      stenosis T85.850
      thrombosis T85.860
    cardiac (defibrillator) (pacemaker) — *see*
      Complications, cardiovascular device or
      implant, electronic
    generator (brain) (gastric) (peripheral)
      (sacral) (spinal)
      breakdown T85.113
      displacement T85.123
      leakage T85.193
      malposition T85.123
      obstruction T85.193
      perforation T85.193
      protrusion T85.193
      specified type NEC T85.193

Complication(s) (from) (of) — *continued*
  electronic stimulator device — *continued*
    muscle T84.9
      breakdown T84.418
      displacement T84.428
      embolism T84.81
      fibrosis T84.82
      hemorrhage T84.83
      infection or inflammation T84.7
      mechanical NEC T84.498
      pain T84.84
      specified type NEC T84.89
      stenosis T84.85
      thrombosis T84.86
    nervous system T85.9
      brain — *see* Complications, electronic
        stimulator device, brain
      cranial nerve — *see* Complications,
        electronic stimulator device, peripheral
        nerve
      embolism T85.810
      fibrosis T85.820
      gastric nerve — *see* Complications,
        electronic stimulator device, peripheral
        nerve
      hemorrhage T85.830
      infection and inflammation T85.738
      mechanical
        breakdown T85.118
        displacement T85.128
        leakage T85.199
        malposition T85.128
        obstruction T85.199
        perforation T85.199
        protrusion T85.199
        specified NEC T85.199
      pain T85.840
      peripheral nerve — *see* Complications,
        electronic stimulator device, peripheral
        nerve
      sacral nerve — *see* Complications,
        electronic stimulator device, peripheral
        nerve
      specified type NEC T85.890
      spinal cord — *see* Complications,
        electronic stimulator device, spinal
        cord
      stenosis T85.850
      thrombosis T85.860
      vagal nerve — *see* Complications,
        electronic stimulator device, peripheral
        nerve
    peripheral nerve T85.9
      embolism T85.810
      fibrosis T85.820
      hemorrhage T85.830
      infection and inflammation T85.732
      mechanical
        breakdown T85.111
        displacement T85.121
        leakage T85.191
        malposition T85.121
        obstruction T85.191
        perforation T85.191
        protrusion T85.191
        specified NEC T85.191
      pain T85.840
      specified type NEC T85.890
      stenosis T85.850
      thrombosis T85.860
    spinal cord T85.9
      embolism T85.810
      fibrosis T85.820
      hemorrhage T85.830
      infection and inflammation T85.733

Complication(s) (from) (of) — *continued*
  electronic stimulator device — *continued*
    spinal cord T85.9 — *continued*
      mechanical
        breakdown T85.112
        displacement T85.122
        leakage T85.192
        malposition T85.122
        obstruction T85.192
        perforation T85.192
        protrusion T85.192
        specified NEC T85.192
      pain T85.840
      specified type NEC T85.890
      stenosis T85.850
      thrombosis T85.860
    urinary T83.9
      embolism T83.81
      fibrosis T83.82
      hemorrhage T83.83
      infection and inflammation T83.598
      mechanical
        breakdown T83.110
        displacement T83.120
        malposition T83.120
        perforation T83.190
        protrusion T83.190
        specified NEC T83.190
      pain T83.84
      specified type NEC T83.89
      stenosis T83.85
      thrombosis T83.86
  electroshock therapy T88.9
    specified NEC T88.8
  endocrine E34.9
    postprocedural
      adrenal hypofunction E89.6
      hypoinsulinemia E89.1
      hypoparathyroidism E89.2
      hypopituitarism E89.3
      hypothyroidism E89.0
      ovarian failure E89.40
        asymptomatic E89.40
        symptomatic E89.41
      specified NEC E89.89
      testicular hypofunction E89.5
  endodontic treatment NEC M27.59
  enterostomy (stoma) K94.10
    hemorrhage K94.11
    infection K94.12
    malfunction K94.13
    mechanical K94.13
    specified complication NEC K94.19
  episiotomy, disruption O90.1
  esophageal anti-reflux device T85.9
    embolism T85.818
    fibrosis T85.828
    hemorrhage T85.838
    infection and inflammation T85.79
    mechanical
      breakdown T85.511
      displacement T85.521
      malfunction T85.511
      malposition T85.521
      obstruction T85.591
      perforation T85.591
      protrusion T85.591
      specified NEC T85.591
    pain T85.848
    specified type NEC T85.898
    stenosis T85.858
    thrombosis T85.868
  esophagostomy K94.30
    hemorrhage K94.31
    infection K94.32
    malfunction K94.33
    mechanical K94.33
    specified complication NEC K94.39
  extracorporeal circulation T80.90

Complication(s) (from) (of) — *continued*
  extremity artery (bypass) graft T82.9
    arteriosclerosis — *see* Arteriosclerosis,
      extremities, bypass graft
    embolism T82.818
    fibrosis T82.828
    hemorrhage T82.838
    infection and inflammation T82.7
    mechanical
      breakdown T82.318
        femoral artery T82.312
      displacement T82.328
        femoral artery T82.322
      leakage T82.338
        femoral artery T82.332
      malposition T82.328
        femoral artery T82.322
      obstruction T82.398
        femoral artery T82.392
      perforation T82.398
        femoral artery T82.392
      protrusion T82.398
        femoral artery T82.392
    pain T82.848
    specified type NEC T82.898
    stenosis T82.858
    thrombosis T82.868
  eye H57.9
    corneal graft — *see* Complications, graft,
      cornea
    implant (prosthetic) T85.9
      embolism T85.818
      fibrosis T85.828
      hemorrhage T85.838
      infection and inflammation T85.79
      mechanical
        breakdown T85.318
        displacement T85.328
        leakage T85.398
        malposition T85.328
        obstruction T85.398
        perforation T85.398
        protrusion T85.398
        specified NEC T85.398
      pain T85.848
      specified type NEC T85.898
      stenosis T85.858
      thrombosis T85.868
    intraocular lens — *see* Complications,
      intraocular lens
    orbital prosthesis — *see* Complications,
      orbital prosthesis
  female genital N94.9
    device, implant or graft NEC — *see*
      Complications, genitourinary, device or
      implant, genital tract
  femoral artery (bypass) graft — *see*
    Complication, extremity artery (bypass)
    graft
  fixation device, internal (orthopedic) T84.9
    infection and inflammation T84.60
      arm T84.61-
        humerus T84.61-
        radius T84.61-
        ulna T84.61-
      leg T84.629
        femur T84.62-
        fibula T84.62-
        tibia T84.62-
      specified site NEC T84.69
      spine T84.63

Complication(s) (from) (of) — *continued*
  fixation device, internal (orthopedic) T84.9 —
    continued
    mechanical
      breakdown
        limb T84.119
          carpal T84.210
          femur T84.11-
          fibula T84.11-
          humerus T84.11-
          metacarpal T84.210
          metatarsal T84.213
          phalanx
            foot T84.213
            hand T84.210
          radius T84.11-
          tarsal T84.213
          tibia T84.11-
          ulna T84.11-
        specified bone NEC T84.218
        spine T84.216
      displacement
        limb T84.129
          carpal T84.220
          femur T84.12-
          fibula T84.12-
          humerus T84.12-
          metacarpal T84.220
          metatarsal T84.223
          phalanx
            foot T84.223
            hand T84.220
          radius T84.12-
          tarsal T84.223
          tibia T84.12-
          ulna T84.12-
        specified bone NEC T84.228
        spine T84.226
      malposition — *see* Complications, fixation
        device, internal, mechanical,
        displacement
      obstruction — *see* Complications, fixation
        device, internal, mechanical, specified
        type NEC
      perforation — *see* Complications, fixation
        device, internal, mechanical, specified
        type NEC
      protrusion — *see* Complications, fixation
        device, internal, mechanical, specified
        type NEC
      specified type NEC
        limb T84.199
          carpal T84.290
          femur T84.19-
          fibula T84.19-
          humerus T84.19-
          metacarpal T84.290
          metatarsal T84.293
          phalanx
            foot T84.293
            hand T84.290
          radius T84.19-
          tarsal T84.293
          tibia T84.19-
          ulna T84.19-
        specified bone NEC T84.298
        vertebra T84.296
    specified type NEC T84.89
      embolism T84.81
      fibrosis T84.82
      hemorrhage T84.83
      pain T84.84
      specified complication NEC T84.89
      stenosis T84.85
      thrombosis T84.86

Complication(s) (from) (of) — *continued*
  following
    acute myocardial infarction NEC I23.8
      aneurysm (false) (of cardiac wall) (of heart
        wall) (ruptured) I23.3
      angina I23.7
      atrial
        septal defect I23.1
        thrombosis I23.6
      cardiac wall rupture I23.3
      chordae tendinae rupture I23.4
      defect
        septal
          atrial (heart) I23.1
          ventricular (heart) I23.2
      hemopericardium I23.0
      papillary muscle rupture I23.5
      rupture
        cardiac wall I23.3
          with hemopericardium I23.0
        chordae tendineae I23.4
        papillary muscle I23.5
      specified NEC I23.8
      thrombosis
        atrium I23.6
        auricular appendage I23.6
        ventricle (heart) I23.6
      ventricular
        septal defect I23.2
        thrombosis I23.6
    ectopic or molar pregnancy O08.9
      cardiac arrest O08.81
      sepsis O08.82
      specified type NEC O08.89
      urinary tract infection O08.83
    termination of pregnancy — *see* Abortion
  gastrointestinal K92.9
    bile duct prosthesis — *see* Complications,
      bile duct implant
    esophageal anti-reflux device — *see*
      Complications, esophageal anti-reflux
      device
    postoperative
      colostomy — *see* Complications, colostomy
      dumping syndrome K91.1
      enterostomy — *see* Complications,
        enterostomy
      gastrostomy — *see* Complications,
        gastrostomy
      malabsorption NEC K91.2
      obstruction K91.3
      postcholecystectomy syndrome K91.5
      specified NEC K91.89
      vomiting after GI surgery K91.0
    prosthetic device or implant
      bile duct prosthesis — *see* Complications,
        bile duct implant
      esophageal anti-reflux device — *see*
        Complications, esophageal anti-reflux
        device
      specified type NEC
        embolism T85.818
        fibrosis T85.828
        hemorrhage T85.838
        mechanical
          breakdown T85.518
          displacement T85.528
          malfunction T85.518
          malposition T85.528
          obstruction T85.598
          perforation T85.598
          protrusion T85.598
          specified NEC T85.598
        pain T85.848
        specified complication NEC T85.898
        stenosis T85.858
        thrombosis T85.868

Complication(s) (from) (of) — *continued*
gastrostomy (stoma) K94.20
  hemorrhage K94.21
  infection K94.22
  malfunction K94.23
  mechanical K94.23
  specified complication NEC K94.29
genitourinary
  device or implant T83.9
    genital tract T83.9
      infection or inflammation T83.69
      intrauterine contraceptive device — *see* Complications, intrauterine, contraceptive device
      mechanical — *see* Complications, by device, mechanical
      mesh — *see* Complications, mesh
      penile prosthesis — *see* Complications, prosthetic device, penile
      specified type NEC T83.89
        embolism T83.81
        fibrosis T83.82
        hemorrhage T83.83
        pain T83.84
        specified complication NEC T83.89
        stenosis T83.85
        thrombosis T83.86
      vaginal mesh — *see* Complications, mesh
    urinary system T83.9
      cystostomy catheter — *see* Complication, catheter, cystostomy
      electronic stimulator — *see* Complications, electronic stimulator device, urinary
      indwelling urethral catheter — *see* Complications, catheter, urethral, indwelling
      infection or inflammation T83.598
        indwelling urethral catheter T83.511
      kidney transplant — *see* Complication, transplant, kidney
      organ graft — *see* Complication, graft, urinary organ
      specified type NEC T83.89
        embolism T83.81
        fibrosis T83.82
        hemorrhage T83.83
        mechanical T83.198
          breakdown T83.118
          displacement T83.128
          malfunction T83.118
          malposition T83.128
          obstruction T83.198
          perforation T83.198
          protrusion T83.198
          specified NEC T83.198
      sphincter implant — *see* Complications, implant, urinary sphincter
      sphincter, implanted T83.191
      stent (ileal conduit) (nephroureteral) T83.193
        pain T83.84
        specified complication NEC T83.89
        stenosis T83.85
        thrombosis T83.86
        ureteral indwelling T83.192
postprocedural
  pelvic peritoneal adhesions N99.4
  renal failure N99.0
  specified NEC N99.89
  stoma — *see* Complications, stoma, urinary tract
  urethral stricture — *see* Stricture, urethra, postprocedural
vaginal
  adhesions N99.2
  vault prolapse N99.3

Complication(s) (from) (of) — *continued*
graft (bypass) (patch) — *see also* Complications, prosthetic device or implant
  aorta — *see* Complications, graft, vascular
  arterial — *see* Complication, graft, vascular
  bone T86.839
    failure T86.831
    infection T86.832
    mechanical T84.318
      breakdown T84.318
      displacement T84.328
      protrusion T84.398
      specified type NEC T84.398
    rejection T86.830
    specified type NEC T86.838
  carotid artery — *see* Complications, graft, vascular
  cornea T86.849
    failure T86.841
    infection T86.842
    mechanical T85.398
      breakdown T85.318
      displacement T85.328
      protrusion T85.398
      specified type NEC T85.398
    rejection T86.840
    retroprosthetic membrane T85.398
    specified type NEC T86.848
  femoral artery (bypass) — *see* Complication, extremity artery (bypass) graft
  genital organ or tract — *see* Complications, genitourinary, device or implant, genital tract
  muscle T84.9
    breakdown T84.410
    displacement T84.420
    embolism T84.81
    fibrosis T84.82
    hemorrhage T84.83
    infection and inflammation T84.7
    mechanical NEC T84.490
    pain T84.84
    specified type NEC T84.89
    stenosis T84.85
    thrombosis T84.86
  nerve — *see* Complication, prosthetic device or implant, specified NEC
  skin — *see* Complications, prosthetic device or implant, skin graft
  tendon T84.9
    breakdown T84.410
    displacement T84.420
    embolism T84.81
    fibrosis T84.82
    hemorrhage T84.83
    infection and inflammation T84.7
    mechanical NEC T84.490
    pain T84.84
    specified type NEC T84.89
    stenosis T84.85
    thrombosis T84.86
  urinary organ T83.9
    embolism T83.81
    fibrosis T83.82
    hemorrhage T83.83
    infection and inflammation T83.598
      indwelling urinary catheter T83.511
    mechanical
      breakdown T83.21
      displacement T83.22
      erosion T83.24
      exposure T83.25
      leakage T83.23
      malposition T83.22
      obstruction T83.29
      perforation T83.29
      protrusion T83.29
      specified NEC T83.29

Complication(s) (from) (of) — *continued*
graft (bypass) (patch) (*see also* Complications, prosthetic device or implant) — *continued*
  urinary organ T83.9 — *continued*
    pain T83.84
    specified type NEC T83.89
    stenosis T83.85
    thrombosis T83.86
  vascular T82.9
    embolism T82.818
    femoral artery — *see* Complication, extremity artery (bypass) graft
    fibrosis T82.828
    hemorrhage T82.838
    mechanical
      breakdown T82.319
        aorta (bifurcation) T82.310
        carotid artery T82.311
        specified vessel NEC T82.318
      displacement T82.329
        aorta (bifurcation) T82.320
        carotid artery T82.321
        specified vessel NEC T82.328
      leakage T82.339
        aorta (bifurcation) T82.330
        carotid artery T82.331
        specified vessel NEC T82.338
      malposition T82.329
        aorta (bifurcation) T82.320
        carotid artery T82.321
        specified vessel NEC T82.328
      obstruction T82.399
        aorta (bifurcation) T82.390
        carotid artery T82.391
        specified vessel NEC T82.398
      perforation T82.399
        aorta (bifurcation) T82.390
        carotid artery T82.391
        specified vessel NEC T82.398
      protrusion T82.399
        aorta (bifurcation) T82.390
        carotid artery T82.391
        specified vessel NEC T82.398
    pain T82.848
    specified complication NEC T82.898
    stenosis T82.858
    thrombosis T82.868
heart I51.9
  assist device
    infection and inflammation T82.7
  following acute myocardial infarction — *see* Complications, following, acute myocardial infarction
  postoperative — *see* Complications, circulatory system
  transplant — *see* Complication, transplant, heart
    and lung(s) — *see* Complications, transplant, heart, with lung
  valve
    graft (biological) T82.9
      embolism T82.817
      fibrosis T82.827
      hemorrhage T82.837
      infection and inflammation T82.7
      mechanical T82.228
        breakdown T82.221
        displacement T82.222
        leakage T82.223
        malposition T82.222
        obstruction T82.228
        perforation T82.228
        protrusion T82.228
      pain T82.847
      specified type NEC T82.897
      stenosis T82.857
      thrombosis T82.867

Complication(s) (from) (of) — *continued*
  valve — *continued*
    heart I51.9 — *continued*
      prosthesis T82.9
        embolism T82.817
        fibrosis T82.827
        hemorrhage T82.837
        infection or inflammation T82.6
        mechanical T82.09
          breakdown T82.01
          displacement T82.02
          leakage T82.03
          malposition T82.02
          obstruction T82.09
          perforation T82.09
          protrusion T82.09
        pain T82.847
        specified type NEC T82.897
          mechanical T82.09
        stenosis T82.857
        thrombosis T82.867
  hematoma
    intraoperative — *see* Complication,
      intraoperative, hemorrhage
    postprocedural — *see* Complication,
      postprocedural, hematoma
  hemodialysis — *see* Complications, dialysis
  hemorrhage
    intraoperative — *see* Complication,
      intraoperative, hemorrhage
    postprocedural — *see* Complication,
      postprocedural, hemorrhage
  ileostomy (stoma) — *see* Complications,
    enterostomy
  immunization (procedure) — *see*
    Complications, vaccination
  implant — *see also* Complications, by site and
    type
    urinary sphincter T83.9
      embolism T83.81
      fibrosis T83.82
      hemorrhage T83.83
      infection and inflammation T83.591
      mechanical
        breakdown T83.111
        displacement T83.121
        leakage T83.191
        malposition T83.121
        obstruction T83.191
        perforation T83.191
        protrusion T83.191
        specified NEC T83.191
      pain T83.84
      specified type NEC T83.89
      stenosis T83.85
      thrombosis T83.86
  infusion (procedure) T80.90
    air embolism T80.0
    blood — *see* Complications, transfusion
    catheter — *see* Complications, catheter
    infection T80.29
    pump — *see* Complications, cardiovascular,
      device or implant
    sepsis T80.29
    serum reaction (*see also* Reaction, serum)
      T80.69
      anaphylactic shock (*see also* Shock,
        anaphylactic) T80.59
    specified type NEC T80.89
  inhalation therapy NEC T81.81
  injection (procedure) T80.90
    drug reaction — *see* Reaction, drug
    infection T80.29
    sepsis T80.29
    serum (prophylactic) (therapeutic) — *see*
      Complications, vaccination
    specified type NEC T80.89
    vaccine (any) — *see* Complications,
      vaccination

Complication(s) (from) (of) — *continued*
  inoculation (any) — *see* Complications,
    vaccination
  insulin pump
    infection and inflammation T85.72
    mechanical
      breakdown T85.614
      displacement T85.624
      leakage T85.633
      malposition T85.624
      obstruction T85.694
      perforation T85.694
      protrusion T85.694
      specified NEC T85.694
  intestinal pouch NEC K91.858
  intraocular lens (prosthetic) T85.9
    embolism T85.818
    fibrosis T85.828
    hemorrhage T85.838
    infection and inflammation T85.79
    mechanical
      breakdown T85.21
      displacement T85.22
      malposition T85.22
      obstruction T85.29
      perforation T85.29
      protrusion T85.29
      specified NEC T85.29
    pain T85.848
    specified type NEC T85.898
    stenosis T85.858
    thrombosis T85.868
  intraoperative (intraprocedural)
    cardiac arrest
      during cardiac surgery I97.710
      during other surgery I97.711
    cardiac functional disturbance NEC
      during cardiac surgery I97.790
      during other surgery I97.791
    hemorrhage (hematoma) (of)
      circulatory system organ or structure
        during cardiac bypass I97.411
        during cardiac catheterization I97.410
        during other circulatory system
          procedure I97.418
        during other procedure I97.42
      digestive system organ
        during procedure on digestive system
          K91.61
        during procedure on other organ
          K91.62
      ear
        during procedure on ear and mastoid
          process H95.21
        during procedure on other organ
          H95.22
      endocrine system organ or structure
        during procedure on endocrine system
          organ or structure E36.01
        during procedure on other organ
          E36.02
      eye and adnexa
        during ophthalmic procedure H59.11-
        during other procedure H59.12-
      genitourinary organ or structure
        during procedure on genitourinary
          organ or structure N99.61
        during procedure on other organ
          N99.62
      mastoid process
        during procedure on ear and mastoid
          process H95.21
        during procedure on other organ
          H95.22

Complication(s) (from) (of) — *continued*
  intraoperative (intraprocedural) — *continued*
    hemorrhage (hematoma) (of) — *continued*
      musculoskeletal structure
        during musculoskeletal surgery
          M96.810
        during non-orthopedic surgery
          M96.811
        during orthopedic surgery M96.810
      nervous system
        during a nervous system procedure
          G97.31
        during other procedure G97.32
      respiratory system
        during other procedure J95.62
        during procedure on respiratory system
          organ or structure J95.61
      skin and subcutaneous tissue
        during a dermatologic procedure
          L76.01
        during a procedure on other organ
          L76.02
      spleen
        during a procedure on other organ
          D78.02
        during a procedure on the spleen
          D78.01
    puncture or laceration (accidental)
      (unintentional) (of)
      brain
        during a nervous system procedure
          G97.48
        during other procedure G97.49
      circulatory system organ or structure
        during circulatory system procedure
          I97.51
        during other procedure I97.52
      digestive system
        during procedure on digestive system
          K91.71
        during procedure on other organ
          K91.72
      ear
        during procedure on ear and mastoid
          process H95.31
        during procedure on other organ
          H95.32
      endocrine system organ or structure
        during procedure on endocrine system
          organ or structure E36.11
        during procedure on other organ
          E36.12
      eye and adnexa
        during ophthalmic procedure H59.21-
        during other procedure H59.22-
      genitourinary organ or structure
        during procedure on genitourinary
          organ or structure N99.71
        during procedure on other organ
          N99.72
      mastoid process
        during procedure on ear and mastoid
          process H95.31
        during procedure on other organ
          H95.32
      musculoskeletal structure
        during musculoskeletal surgery
          M96.820
        during non-orthopedic surgery
          M96.821
        during orthopedic surgery M96.820
      nervous system
        during a nervous system procedure
          G97.48
        during other procedure G97.49

Complication(s) (from) (of) — *continued*
  intraoperative (intraprocedural) — *continued*
    puncture or laceration (accidental)
      (unintentional) (of) — *continued*
      respiratory system
        during other procedure J95.72
        during procedure on respiratory system
          organ or structure J95.71
      skin and subcutaneous tissue
        during a dermatologic procedure
          L76.11
        during a procedure on other organ
          L76.12
      spleen
        during a procedure on other organ
          D78.12
        during a procedure on the spleen
          D78.11
    specified NEC
      circulatory system I97.88
      digestive system K91.81
      ear H95.88
      endocrine system E36.8
      eye and adnexa H59.88
      genitourinary system N99.81
      mastoid process H95.88
      musculoskeletal structure M96.89
      nervous system G97.81
      respiratory system J95.88
      skin and subcutaneous tissue L76.81
      spleen D78.81
  intraperitoneal catheter (dialysis) (infusion) —
    see Complications, catheter, intraperitoneal
  intrathecal infusion pump
    infection and inflammation T85.738
    mechanical
      breakdown T85.615
      displacement T85.625
      leakage T85.635
      malfunction T85.695
      malposition T85.625
      obstruction T85.695
      perforation T85.695
      protrusion T85.695
      specified NEC T85.695
  intrauterine
    contraceptive device
      embolism T83.81
      fibrosis T83.82
      hemorrhage T83.83
      infection and inflammation T83.69
      mechanical
        breakdown T83.31
        displacement T83.32
        malposition T83.32
        obstruction T83.39
        perforation T83.39
        protrusion T83.39
        specified NEC T83.39
      pain T83.84
      specified type NEC T83.89
      stenosis T83.85
      thrombosis T83.86
    procedure (fetal), to newborn P96.5
  jejunostomy (stoma) — *see* Complications,
    enterostomy
  joint prosthesis, internal T84.9
    breakage (fracture) T84.01-
    dislocation T84.02-
    fracture T84.01-
    infection or inflammation T84.50
      hip T84.5-
      knee T84.5-
      specified joint NEC T84.59
    instability T84.02-
    malposition — *see* Complications, joint
      prosthesis, mechanical, displacement

Complication(s) (from) (of) — *continued*
  joint prosthesis, internal T84.9 — *continued*
    mechanical
      breakage, broken T84.01-
      dislocation T84.02-
      fracture T84.01-
      instability T84.02-
      leakage — *see* Complications, joint
        prosthesis, mechanical, specified NEC
      loosening T84.039
        hip T84.03-
        knee T84.03-
        specified joint NEC T84.038
      obstruction — *see* Complications, joint
        prosthesis, mechanical, specified NEC
      perforation — *see* Complications, joint
        prosthesis, mechanical, specified NEC
      osteolysis T84.059
        hip T84.05-
        knee T84.05-
        other specified joint T84.058
      protrusion — *see* Complications, joint
        prosthesis, mechanical, specified NEC
      specified complication NEC T84.099
        hip T84.09-
        knee T84.09-
        other specified joint T84.098
      subluxation T84.02-
      wear of articular bearing surface T84.069
        hip T84.06-
        knee T84.06-
        other specified joint T84.068
    specified joint NEC T84.89
      embolism T84.81
      fibrosis T84.82
      hemorrhage T84.83
      pain T84.84
      specified complication NEC T84.89
      stenosis T84.85
      thrombosis T84.86
    subluxation T84.02-
  kidney transplant — *see* Complications,
    transplant, kidney
  labor O75.9
    specified NEC O75.89
  liver transplant (immune or nonimmune) — *see*
    Complications, transplant, liver
  lumbar puncture G97.1
    cerebrospinal fluid leak G97.0
    headache or reaction G97.1
  lung transplant — *see* Complications,
    transplant, lung
    and heart — *see* Complications, transplant,
      lung, with heart
  male genital N50.9
    device, implant or graft — *see*
      Complications, genitourinary, device or
      implant, genital tract
    postprocedural or postoperative — *see*
      Complications, genitourinary,
      postprocedural
      specified NEC N99.89
  mastoid (process) procedure
    intraoperative H95.88
      hematoma — *see* Complications,
        intraoperative, hematoma (of),
        mastoid process
      hemorrhage — *see* Complications,
        intraoperative, hemorrhage (of),
        mastoid process
      laceration — *see* Complications,
        intraoperative, puncture or laceration,
        mastoid process
      seroma - see Complications,
        postprocedural, seroma (of), mastoid
        process
      specified NEC H95.88

Complication(s) (from) (of) — *continued*
  mastoid (process) procedure — *continued*
    postmastoidectomy — *see* Complications,
      postmastoidectomy
    postoperative H95.89
      external ear canal stenosis H95.81-
      hematoma — *see* Complications,
        postprocedural, hematoma (of),
        mastoid process
      hemorrhage — *see* Complications,
        postprocedural, hemorrhage (of),
        mastoid process
      postmastoidectomy — *see* Complications,
        postmastoidectomy
      seroma — *see* Complications,
        postprocedural, seroma (of), mastoid
        process
      specified NEC H95.89
  mastoidectomy cavity — *see* Complications,
    postmastoidectomy
  mechanical — *see* Complications, by site and
    type, mechanical
  medical procedures (*see also* Complication(s),
    intraoperative) T88.9
  metabolic E88.9
    postoperative E89.89
    specified NEC E89.89
  molar pregnancy NOS O08.9
    damage to pelvic organs O08.6
    embolism O08.2
    genital infection O08.0
    hemorrhage (delayed) (excessive) O08.1
    metabolic disorder O08.5
    renal failure O08.4
    shock O08.3
    specified type NEC O08.0
    venous complication NEC O08.7
  musculoskeletal system — *see also*
    Complication, intraoperative
    (intraprocedural), by site
    device, implant or graft NEC — *see*
      Complications, orthopedic, device or
      implant
    internal fixation (nail) (plate) (rod) — *see*
      Complications, fixation device, internal
    joint prosthesis — *see* Complications, joint
      prosthesis
    post radiation M96.89
      kyphosis M96.2
      scoliosis M96.5
      specified complication NEC M96.89
    postoperative (postprocedural) M96.89
      with osteoporosis — *see* Osteoporosis
      fracture following insertion of device — *see*
        Fracture, following insertion of
        orthopedic implant, joint prosthesis or
        bone plate
      joint instability after prosthesis removal
        M96.89
      lordosis M96.4
      postlaminectomy syndrome NEC M96.1
      kyphosis M96.3
      pseudarthrosis M96.0
      specified complication NEC M96.89
  nephrostomy (stoma) — *see* Complications,
    stoma, urinary tract, external NEC

DISEASE INDEX

Complication(s) (from) (of) — *continued*
nervous system G98.8
  central G96.9
  device, implant or graft — *see also*
    Complication, prosthetic device or
    implant, specified NEC
    electronic stimulator (electrode(s)) — *see*
      Complications, electronic stimulator
      device
    specified NEC
      infection and inflammation T85.738
      mechanical T85.695
        breakdown T85.615
        displacement T85.625
        leakage T85.635
        malfunction T85.695
        malposition T85.625
        obstruction T85.695
        perforation T85.695
        protrusion T85.695
        specified NEC T85.695
      ventricular shunt — *see* Complications,
        ventricular shunt
  electronic stimulator (electrode(s)) — *see*
    Complications, electronic stimulator
    device
  postprocedural G97.82
    intracranial hypotension G97.2
    specified NEC G97.82
    spinal fluid leak G97.0
newborn, due to intrauterine (fetal) procedure
  P96.5
nonabsorbable (permanent) sutures — *see*
  Complication, sutures, permanent
obstetric O75.9
  procedure (instrumental) (manual) (surgical)
    specified NEC O75.4
  specified NEC O75.89
  surgical wound NEC O90.89
    hematoma O90.2
    infection O86.0
ocular lens implant — *see* Complications,
  intraocular lens
ophthalmologic
  postprocedural bleb — *see* Blebitis
orbital prosthesis T85.9
  embolism T85.818
  fibrosis T85.828
  hemorrhage T85.838
  infection and inflammation T85.79
  mechanical
    breakdown T85.31-
    displacement T85.32-
    malposition T85.32-
    obstruction T85.39-
    perforation T85.39-
    protrusion T85.39-
    specified NEC T85.39-
  pain T85.848
  specified type NEC T85.898
  stenosis T85.858
  thrombosis T85.868
organ or tissue transplant (partial) (total) — *see*
  Complications, transplant
orthopedic — *see also* Disorder, soft tissue
  device or implant T84.9
    bone
      device or implant — *see* Complication,
        bone, device NEC
      graft — *see* Complication, graft, bone
      breakdown T84.418
      displacement T84.428
      electronic bone stimulator — *see*
        Complications, electronic stimulator
        device, bone
      embolism T84.81
      fibrosis T84.82
      fixation device — *see* Complication,
        fixation device, internal

Complication(s) (from) (of) — *continued*
orthopedic — *see also* Disorder, soft tissue —
  continued
  device or implant T84.9 — *continued*
    hemorrhage T84.83
    infection or inflammation T84.7
    joint prosthesis — *see* Complication, joint
      prosthesis, internal
    malfunction T84.418
    malposition T84.428
    mechanical NEC T84.498
    muscle graft — *see* Complications, graft,
      muscle
    obstruction T84.498
    pain T84.84
    perforation T84.498
    protrusion T84.498
    specified complication NEC T84.89
    stenosis T84.85
    tendon graft — *see* Complications, graft,
      tendon
    thrombosis T84.86
  fracture (following insertion of device) — *see*
    Fracture, following insertion of
    orthopedic implant, joint prosthesis or
    bone plate
  postprocedural M96.89
    fracture — *see* Fracture, following insertion
      of orthopedic implant, joint prosthesis
      or bone plate
    postlaminectomy syndrome NEC M96.1
      kyphosis M96.3
      lordosis M96.4
    postradiation
      kyphosis M96.2
      scoliosis M96.5
    pseudarthrosis post-fusion M96.0
    specified type NEC M96.89
pacemaker (cardiac) — *see* Complications,
  cardiovascular device or implant,
  electronic
pancreas transplant — *see* Complications,
  transplant, pancreas
penile prosthesis (implant) — *see*
  Complications, prosthetic device, penile
perfusion NEC T80.90
perineal repair (obstetrical) NEC O90.89
  disruption O90.1
  hematoma O90.2
  infection (following delivery) O86.0
phototherapy T88.9
  specified NEC T88.8
postmastoidectomy NEC H95.19-
  cyst, mucosal H95.13-
  granulation H95.12-
  inflammation, chronic H95.11-
  recurrent cholesteatoma H95.0-
postoperative — *see* Complications,
  postprocedural
  circulatory — *see* Complications, circulatory
    system
  ear — *see* Complications, ear
  endocrine — *see* Complications, endocrine
  eye — *see* Complications, eye
  lumbar puncture G97.1
    cerebrospinal fluid leak G97.0
  nervous system (central) (peripheral) — *see*
    Complications, nervous system
  respiratory system — *see* Complications,
    respiratory system
postprocedural — *see also* Complications,
  surgical procedure
  cardiac arrest
    following cardiac surgery I97.120
    following other surgery I97.121
  cardiac functional disturbance NEC
    following cardiac surgery I97.190
    following other surgery I97.191

Complication(s) (from) (of) — *continued*
postprocedural — *see also* Complications,
  surgical procedure — *continued*
  cardiac insufficiency
    following cardiac surgery I97.110
    following other surgery I97.111
  chorioretinal scars following retinal surgery
    H59.81-
  following cataract surgery
    cataract (lens) fragments H59.02-
    cystoid macular edema H59.03-
    specified NEC H59.09-
    vitreous (touch) syndrome H59.01-
  heart failure
    following cardiac surgery I97.130
    following other surgery I97.131
  hematoma (of)
    circulatory system organ or structure
      following cardiac bypass I97.631
      following cardiac catheterization
        I97.630
      following other circulatory system
        procedure I97.638
      following other procedure I97.621
    digestive system
      following procedure on digestive system
        K91.870
      following procedure on other organ
        K91.871
    ear
      following other procedure H95.52
      following procedure on ear and mastoid
        process H95.51
    endocrine system
      following endocrine system procedure
        E89.820
      following other procedure E89.821
    eye and adnexa
      following ophthalmic procedure
        H59.33-
      following other procedure H59.34-
    genitourinary organ or structure
      following procedure on genitourinary
        organ or structure N99.840
      following procedure on other organ
        N99.841
    mastoid process
      following other procedure H95.52
      following procedure on ear and mastoid
        process H95.51
    musculoskeletal structure
      following musculoskeletal surgery
        M96.840
      following non-orthopedic surgery
        M96.841
      following orthopedic surgery M96.840
    nervous system
      following nervous system procedure
        G97.61
      following other procedure G97.62
    respiratory system
      following other procedure J95.861
      following procedure on respiratory
        system organ or structure J95.860
    skin and subcutaneous tissue
      following dermatologic procedure
        L76.31
      following procedure on other organ
        L76.32
    spleen
      following procedure on other organ
        D78.32
      following procedure on the spleen
        D78.31

Complication(s) (from) (of) — *continued*
  postprocedural — *see also* Complications,
    surgical procedure — *continued*
    hemorrhage (of)
      circulatory system organ or structure
        following cardiac bypass I97.611
        following cardiac catheterization
          I97.610
        following other circulatory system
          procedure I97.618
        following other procedure I97.620
      digestive system
        following procedure on digestive system
          K91.840
        following procedure on other organ
          K91.841
      ear
        following other procedure H95.42
        following procedure on ear and mastoid
          process H95.41
      endocrine system
        following endocrine system procedure
          E89.810
        following other procedure E89.811
      eye and adnexa
        following ophthalmic procedure
          H59.31-
        following other procedure H59.32-
      genitourinary organ or structure
        following procedure on genitourinary
          organ or structure N99.820
        following procedure on other organ
          N99.821
      mastoid process
        following other procedure H95.42
        following procedure on ear and mastoid
          process H95.41
      musculoskeletal structure
        following musculoskeletal surgery
          M96.830
        following non-orthopedic surgery
          M96.831
        following orthopedic surgery M96.830
      nervous system
        following nervous system procedure
          G97.51
        following other procedure G97.52
      respiratory system
        following other procedure J95.831
        following procedure on respiratory
          system organ or structure J95.830
      skin and subcutaneous tissue
        following dermatologic procedure
          L76.21
        following a procedure on other organ
          L76.22
      spleen
        following procedure on other organ
          D78.22
        following procedure on the spleen
          D78.21
    seroma (of)
      circulatory system organ or structure
        following cardiac bypass I97.641
        following cardiac catheterization
          I97.640
        following other circulatory system
          procedure I97.648
        following other procedure I97.622
      digestive system
        following procedure on digestive system
          K91.872
        following procedure on other organ
          K91.873
      ear
        following other procedure H95.54
        following procedure on ear and mastoid
          process H95.53

Complication(s) (from) (of) — *continued*
  postprocedural (*see also* Complications, surgical
    procedure) — *continued*
    seroma (of) — *continued*
      endocrine system
        following endocrine system procedure
          E89.822
        following other procedure E89.823
      eye and adnexa
        following ophthalmic procedure
          H59.35-
        following other procedure H59.36-
      genitourinary organ or structure
        following procedure on genitourinary
          organ or structure N99.842
        following procedure on other organ
          N99.843
      mastoid process
        following other procedure H95.54
        following procedure on ear and mastoid
          process H95.53
      musculoskeletal structure
        following musculoskeletal surgery
          M96.842
        following non-orthopedic surgery
          M96.843
        following orthopedic surgery M96.842
      nervous system
        following nervous system procedure
          G97.63
        following other procedure G97.64
      respiratory system
        following other procedure J95.863
        following procedure on respiratory
          system organ or structure J95.862
      skin and subcutaneous tissue
        following dermatologic procedure
          L76.33
        following procedure on other organ
          L76.34
      spleen
        following procedure on other organ
          D78.34
        following procedure on the spleen
          D78.33
    specified NEC
      circulatory system I97.89
      digestive K91.89
      ear H95.89
      endocrine E89.89
      eye and adnexa H59.89
      genitourinary N99.89
      mastoid process H95.89
      metabolic E89.89
      musculoskeletal structure M96.89
      nervous system G97.82
      respiratory system J95.89
      skin and subcutaneous tissue L76.82
      spleen D78.89
  pregnancy NEC — *see* Pregnancy, complicated
    by
  prosthetic device or implant T85.9
    bile duct — *see* Complications, bile duct
      implant
    breast — *see* Complications, breast implant
    bulking agent
      ureteral
        erosion T83.714
        exposure T83.724
      urethral
        erosion T83.713
        exposure T83.723
    cardiac and vascular NEC — *see*
      Complications, cardiovascular device or
      implant
    corneal transplant — *see* Complications,
      graft, cornea

Complication(s) (from) (of) — *continued*
  prosthetic device or implant T85.9 —
    continued
    electronic nervous system stimulator — *see*
      Complications, electronic stimulator
      device
    epidural infusion catheter — *see*
      Complications, catheter, epidural
    esophageal anti-reflux device — *see*
      Complications, esophageal anti-reflux
      device
    genital organ or tract — *see* Complications,
      genitourinary, device or implant, genital
      tract
    specified NEC T83.79
    heart valve — *see* Complications, heart,
      valve, prosthesis
    infection or inflammation T85.79
      intestine transplant T86.892
      liver transplant T86.43
      lung transplant T86.812
      pancreas transplant T86.892
      skin graft T86.822
    intraocular lens — *see* Complications,
      intraocular lens
    intraperitoneal (dialysis) catheter — *see*
      Complications, catheter, intraperitoneal
    joint — *see* Complications, joint prosthesis,
      internal
    mechanical NEC T85.698
      dialysis catheter (vascular) — *see also*
        Complication, catheter, dialysis,
        mechanical
      peritoneal — *see* Complication, catheter,
        intraperitoneal, mechanical
      gastrointestinal device T85.598
      ocular device T85.398
      subdural (infusion) catheter T85.690
      suture, permanent T85.692
        that for bone repair — *see*
          Complications, fixation device,
          internal (orthopedic), mechanical
      ventricular shunt
        breakdown T85.01
        displacement T85.02
        leakage T85.03
        malposition T85.02
        obstruction T85.09
        perforation T85.09
        protrusion T85.09
        specified NEC T85.09
    mesh
      erosion (to surrounding organ or tissue)
        T83.717
        urethral (into pelvic floor muscles)
          T83.712
        vaginal (into pelvic floor muscles)
          T83.711
      exposure (into surrounding organ or
        tissue) T83.727
        urethral (through urethral wall) T83.722
        vaginal (into vagina) (through vaginal
          wall) T83.721
    orbital — *see* Complications, orbital
      prosthesis
    penile T83.9
      embolism T83.81
      fibrosis T83.82
      hemorrhage T83.83
      infection and inflammation T83.61
      mechanical
        breakdown T83.410
        displacement T83.420
        leakage T83.490
        malposition T83.420
        obstruction T83.490
        perforation T83.490
        protrusion T83.490
        specified NEC T83.490

Complication(s) (from) (of) — *continued*
prosthetic device or implant T85.9 — *continued*
  penile T83.9 — *continued*
    pain T83.84
    specified type NEC T83.89
    stenosis T83.85
    thrombosis T83.86
  prosthetic materials NEC
    erosion (to surrounding organ or tissue) T83.718
    exposure (into surrounding organ or tissue) T83.728
  skin graft T86.829
    artificial skin or decellularized allodermis
      embolism T85.818
      fibrosis T85.828
      hemorrhage T85.838
      infection and inflammation T85.79
      mechanical
        breakdown T85.613
        displacement T85.623
        malfunction T85.613
        malposition T85.623
        obstruction T85.693
        perforation T85.693
        protrusion T85.693
        specified NEC T85.693
      pain T85.848
      specified type NEC T85.898
      stenosis T85.858
      thrombosis T85.868
    failure T86.821
    infection T86.822
    rejection T86.820
    specified NEC T86.828
  sling
    urethral (female) (male)
      erosion T83.712
      exposure T83.722
  specified NEC T85.9
    embolism T85.818
    fibrosis T85.828
    hemorrhage T85.838
    infection and inflammation T85.79
    mechanical
      breakdown T85.618
      displacement T85.628
      leakage T85.638
      malfunction T85.618
      malposition T85.628
      obstruction T85.698
      perforation T85.698
      protrusion T85.698
      specified NEC T85.698
    pain T85.848
    specified type NEC T85.898
    stenosis T85.858
    thrombosis T85.868
  subdural infusion catheter — *see* Complications, catheter, subdural
  sutures — *see* Complications, sutures
  urinary organ or tract NEC — *see* Complications, genitourinary, device or implant, urinary system
  vascular — *see* Complications, cardiovascular device or implant
  ventricular shunt — *see* Complications, ventricular shunt (device)
puerperium — *see* Puerperal
puncture, spinal G97.1
  cerebrospinal fluid leak G97.0
  headache or reaction G97.1
pyelogram N99.89
radiation
  kyphosis M96.2
  scoliosis M96.5

Complication(s) (from) (of) — *continued*
reattached
  extremity (infection) (rejection)
    lower T87.1x-
    upper T87.0x-
  specified body part NEC T87.2
reconstructed breast
  asymmetry between native and reconstructed breast N65.1
  deformity N65.0
  disproportion between native and reconstructed breast N65.1
  excess tissue N65.0
  misshappen N65.0
reimplant NEC — *see also* Complications, prosthetic device or implant
  limb (infection) (rejection) — *see* Complications, reattached, extremity
  organ (partial) (total) — *see* Complications, transplant
  prosthetic device NEC — *see* Complications, prosthetic device
renal N28.9
  allograft — *see* Complications, transplant, kidney
  dialysis — *see* Complications, dialysis
respirator
  mechancial J95.850
    specified NEC J95.859
respiratory system J98.9
  device, implant or graft — *see* Complication, prosthetic device or implant, specified NEC
  lung transplant — *see* Complications, prosthetic device or implant, lung transplant
  postoperative J95.89
    air leak J95.812
    Mendelson's syndrome (chemical pneumonitis) J95.4
    pneumothorax J95.811
    pulmonary insufficiency (acute) (after nonthoracic surgery) J95.2
      chronic J95.3
      following thoracic surgery J95.1
    respiratory failure (acute) J95.821
      acute and chronic J95.822
    specified NEC J95.89
    subglottic stenosis J95.5
    tracheostomy complication — *see* Complications, tracheostomy
  therapy T81.89
sedation during labor and delivery O74.9
  cardiac O74.2
  central nervous system O74.3
  pulmonary NEC O74.1
shunt — *see also* Complications, prosthetic device or implant
  arteriovenous — *see* Complications, arteriovenous, shunt
  ventricular (communicating) — *see* Complications, ventricular shunt
skin
  graft T86.829
    failure T86.821
    infection T86.822
    rejection T86.820
    specified type NEC T86.828
spinal
  anesthesia — *see* Complications, anesthesia, spinal
  catheter (epidural) (subdural) — *see* Complications, catheter
  puncture or tap G97.1
    cerebrospinal fluid leak G97.0
    headache or reaction G97.1

Complication(s) (from) (of) — *continued*
stent
  bile duct — *see* Complications, bile duct prosthesis
  ureteral indwelling
    breakdown T83.112
    displacement T83.122
    leakage T83.192
    malposition T83.122
    obstruction T83.192
    perforation T83.192
    protrusion T83.192
    specified NEC T83.192
  urinary NEC (ileal conduit) (nephroureteral) T83.193
    embolism T83.81
    fibrosis T83.82
    hemorrhage T83.83
    infection and inflammation T83.593
    mechanical
      breakdown T83.113
      displacement T83.123
      leakage T83.193
      malposition T83.123
      obstruction T83.193
      perforation T83.193
      protrusion T83.193
      specified NEC T83.193
    pain T83.84
    specified type NEC T83.89
    stenosis T83.85
    thrombosis T83.86
  vascular
    end stent stenosis — *see* Restenosis, stent
    in stent stenosis — *see* Restenosis, stent
stoma
  digestive tract
    colostomy — *see* Complications, colostomy
    enterostomy — *see* Complications, enterostomy
    esophagostomy — *see* Complications, esophagostomy
    gastrostomy — *see* Complications, gastrostomy
  urinary tract N99.528
    continent N99.538
      hemorrhage N99.530
      herniation N99.533
      infection N99.531
      malfunction N99.532
      specified type NEC N99.538
      stenosis N99.534
    cystostomy — *see* Complications, cystostomy
    external NOS N99.528
    hemorrhage N99.520
    herniation N99.523
    incontinent N99.528
      hemorrhage N99.520
      herniation N99.523
      infection N99.521
      malfunction N99.522
      specified type NEC N99.528
      stenosis N99.524
    infection N99.521
    malfunction N99.522
    specified type NEC N99.528
    stenosis N99.524
stomach banding — *see* Complication(s), bariatric procedure
stomach stapling — *see* Complication(s), bariatric procedure
surgical material, nonabsorbable — *see* Complication, suture, permanent
surgical procedure (on) T81.9
  amputation stump (late) — *see* Complications, amputation stump
  cardiac — *see* Complications, circulatory system

D I S E A S E   I N D E X

Complication(s) (from) (of) — *continued*
  surgical procedure (on) T81.9 — *continued*
    cholesteatoma, recurrent — *see* Complications, postmastoidectomy, recurrent cholesteatoma
    circulatory (early) — *see* Complications, circulatory system
    digestive system — *see* Complications, gastrointestinal
    dumping syndrome (postgastrectomy) K91.1
    ear — *see* Complications, ear
    elephantiasis or lymphedema I97.89
      postmastectomy I97.2
    emphysema (surgical) T81.82
    endocrine — *see* Complications, endocrine
    eye — *see* Complications, eye
    fistula (persistent postoperative) T81.83
    foreign body inadvertently left in wound (sponge) (suture) (swab) — *see* Foreign body, accidentally left during a procedure
    gastrointestinal — *see* Complications, gastrointestinal
    genitourinary NEC N99.89
    hematoma
      intraoperative — *see* Complication, intraoperative, hemorrhage
      postprocedural — *see* Complication, postprocedural, hematoma
    hemorrhage
      intraoperative — *see* Complication, intraoperative, hemorrhage
      postprocedural — *see* Complication, postprocedural, hemorrhage
    hepatic failure K91.82
    hyperglycemia (postpancreatectomy) E89.1
    hypoinsulinemia (postpancreatectomy) E89.1
    hypoparathyroidism (postparathyroidectomy) E89.2
    hypopituitarism (posthypophysectomy) E89.3
    hypothyroidism (post-thyroidectomy) E89.0
    intestinal obstruction K91.3
    intracranial hypotension following ventricular shunting (ventriculostomy) G97.2
    lymphedema I97.89
      postmastectomy I97.2
    malabsorption (postsurgical) NEC K91.2
      osteoporosis — *see* Osteoporosis, postsurgical malabsorption
    mastoidectomy cavity NEC — *see* Complications, postmastoidectomy
    metabolic E89.89
      specified NEC E89.89
    musculoskeletal — *see* Complications, musculoskeletal system
    nervous system (central) (peripheral) — *see* Complications, nervous system
    ovarian failure E89.40
      asymptomatic E89.40
      symptomatic E89.41
    peripheral vascular — *see* Complications, surgical procedure, vascular
    postcardiotomy syndrome I97.0
    postcholecystectomy syndrome K91.5
    postcommissurotomy syndrome I97.0
    postgastrectomy dumping syndrome K91.1
    postlaminectomy syndrome NEC M96.1
      kyphosis M96.3
    postmastectomy lymphedema syndrome I97.2
    postmastoidectomy cholesteatoma — *see* Complications, postmastoidectomy, recurrent cholesteatoma
    postvagotomy syndrome K91.1
    postvalvulotomy syndrome I97.0

Complication(s) (from) (of) — *continued*
  surgical procedure (on) T81.9 — *continued*
    pulmonary insufficiency (acute) J95.2
      chronic J95.3
      following thoracic surgery J95.1
    reattached body part — *see* Complications, reattached
    respiratory — *see* Complications, respiratory system
    shock (hypovolemic) T81.19
    spleen (postoperative) D78.89
      intraoperative D78.81
    stitch abscess T81.48
    subglottic stenosis (postsurgical) J95.5
    testicular hypofunction E89.5
    transplant — *see* Complications, organ or tissue transplant
    urinary NEC N99.89
    vaginal vault prolapse (posthysterectomy) N99.3
    vascular (peripheral)
      artery T81.719
        mesenteric T81.710
        renal T81.711
        specified NEC T81.718
      vein T81.72
    wound infection T81.40
  suture, permanent (wire) NEC T85.9
    with repair of bone — *see* Complications, fixation device, internal
    embolism T85.818
    fibrosis T85.828
    hemorrhage T85.838
    infection and inflammation T85.79
    mechanical
      breakdown T85.612
      displacement T85.622
      malfunction T85.612
      malposition T85.622
      obstruction T85.692
      perforation T85.692
      protrusion T85.692
      specified NEC T85.692
    pain T85.848
    specified type NEC T85.898
    stenosis T85.858
    thrombosis T85.868
  tracheostomy J95.00
    granuloma J95.09
    hemorrhage J95.01
    infection J95.02
    malfunction J95.03
    mechanical J95.03
    obstruction J95.03
    specified type NEC J95.09
    tracheo-esophageal fistula J95.04
  transfusion (blood) (lymphocytes) (plasma) T80.92
    air embolism T80.0
    circulatory overload E87.71
    febrile nonhemolytic transfusion reaction R50.84
    hemochromatosis E83.111
    hemolysis T80.89
    hemolytic reaction (antigen unspecified) T80.919
    incompatibility reaction (antigen unspecified) T80.919
      ABO T80.30
        delayed serologic (DSTR) T80.39
        hemolytic transfusion reaction (HTR) (unspecified time after transfusion) T80.319
        acute (AHTR) (less than 24 hours after transfusion) T80.310
        delayed (DHTR) (24 hours or more after transfusion) T80.311
        specified NEC T80.39

Complication(s) (from) (of) — *continued*
  transfusion (blood) (lymphocytes) (plasma) T80.92 — *continued*
    incompatibility reaction (antigen unspecified) T80.919 — *continued*
      acute (antigen unspecified) T80.910
      delayed (antigen unspecified) T80.911
      delayed serologic (DSTR) T80.89
      Non-ABO (minor antigens (Duffy) (Kell) (Kidd) (Lewis) (M) (N) (P) (S)) T80.A0
        delayed serologic (DSTR) T80.A9
        hemolytic transfusion reaction (HTR) (unspecified time after transfusion) T80.A19
        acute (AHTR) (less than 24 hours after transfusion) T80.A10
        delayed (DHTR) (24 hours or more after transfusion) T80.A11
        specified NEC T80.A9
      Rh (antigens (C) (c) (D) (E) (e)) (factor) T80.40
        delayed serologic (DSTR) T80.49
        hemolytic transfusion reaction (HTR) (unspecified time after transfusion) T80.419
        acute (AHTR) (less than 24 hours after transfusion) T80.410
        delayed (DHTR) (24 hours or more after transfusion) T80.411
        specified NEC T80.49
    infection T80.29
      acute T80.22
    reaction NEC T80.89
    sepsis T80.29
    shock T80.89
  transplant T86.90
    bone T86.839
      failure T86.831
      infection T86.832
      rejection T86.830
      specified type NEC T86.838
    bone marrow T86.00
      failure T86.02
      infection T86.03
      rejection T86.01
      specified type NEC T86.09
    cornea T86.849
      failure T86.841
      infection T86.842
      rejection T86.840
      specified type NEC T86.848
    failure T86.92
    heart T86.20
      with lung T86.30
      cardiac allograft vasculopathy T86.290
        failure T86.32
        infection T86.33
        rejection T86.31
        specified type NEC T86.39
      failure T86.22
      infection T86.23
      rejection T86.21
      specified type NEC T86.298
    infection T86.93
    intestine T86.859
      failure T86.851
      infection T86.852
      rejection T86.850
      specified type NEC T86.858
    kidney T86.10
      failure T86.12
      infection T86.13
      rejection T86.11
      specified type NEC T86.19
    liver T86.40
      failure T86.42
      infection T86.43
      rejection T86.41
      specified type NEC T86.49

Complication(s) (from) (of) — *continued*
transplant T86.90 — *continued*
  lung T86.819
    with heart T86.30
      failure T86.32
      infection T86.33
      rejection T86.31
      specified type NEC T86.39
    failure T86.811
    infection T86.812
    rejection T86.810
    specified type NEC T86.818
  malignant neoplasm C80.2
  pancreas T86.899
    failure T86.891
    infection T86.892
    rejection T86.890
    specified type NEC T86.898
  peripheral blood stem cells T86.5
  post-transplant lymphoproliferative disorder (PTLD) D47.Z1
  rejection T86.91
  skin T86.829
    failure T86.821
    infection T86.822
    rejection T86.820
    specified type NEC T86.828
  specified
    tissue T86.899
      failure T86.891
      infection T86.892
      rejection T86.890
      specified type NEC T86.898
    type NEC T86.99
  stem cell (from peripheral blood) (from umbilical cord) T86.5
  umbilical cord stem cells T86.5
trauma (early) T79.9
  specified NEC T79.8
ultrasound therapy NEC T88.9
umbilical cord NEC
  complicating delivery O69.9
    specified NEC O69.89
umbrella device, vascular T82.9
  embolism T82.818
  fibrosis T82.828
  hemorrhage T82.838
  infection or inflammation T82.7
  mechanical
    breakdown T82.515
    displacement T82.525
    leakage T82.535
    malposition T82.525
    obstruction T82.595
    perforation T82.595
    protrusion T82.595
  pain T82.848
  specified type NEC T82.898
  stenosis T82.858
  thrombosis T82.868
urethral catheter — *see* Complications, catheter, urethral, indwelling
vaccination T88.1
  anaphylaxis NEC T80.52
  arthropathy — *see* Arthropathy, postimmunization
  cellulitis T88.0
  encephalitis or encephalomyelitis G04.02
  infection (general) (local) NEC T88.0
  meningitis G03.8
  myelitis G04.02
  protein sickness T80.62
  rash T88.1
  reaction (allergic) T88.1
    serum T80.62
  sepsis T88.0

Complication(s) (from) (of) — *continued*
vaccination T88.1 — *continued*
  serum intoxication, sickness, rash, or other serum reaction NEC T80.62
    anaphylactic shock T80.52
  shock (allergic) (anaphylactic) T80.52
  vaccinia (generalized) (localized) T88.1
vas deferens device or implant — *see* Complications, genitourinary, device or implant, genital tract
vascular I99.9
  device or implant T82.9
    embolism T82.818
    fibrosis T82.828
    hemorrhage T82.838
    infection or inflammation T82.7
    mechanical
      breakdown T82.519
        specified device NEC T82.518
      displacement T82.529
        specified device NEC T82.528
      leakage T82.539
        specified device NEC T82.538
      malposition T82.529
        specified device NEC T82.528
      obstruction T82.599
        specified device NEC T82.598
      perforation T82.599
        specified device NEC T82.598
      protrusion T82.599
        specified device NEC T82.598
    pain T82.848
    specified type NEC T82.898
    stenosis T82.858
    thrombosis T82.868
  dialysis catheter — *see* Complication, catheter, dialysis
  following infusion, therapeutic injection or transfusion T80.1
  graft T82.9
    embolism T82.818
    fibrosis T82.828
    hemorrhage T82.838
    mechanical
      breakdown T82.319
        aorta (bifurcation) T82.310
        carotid artery T82.311
        specified vessel NEC T82.318
      displacement T82.329
        aorta (bifurcation) T82.320
        carotid artery T82.321
        specified vessel NEC T82.328
      leakage T82.339
        aorta (bifurcation) T82.330
        carotid artery T82.331
        specified vessel NEC T82.338
      malposition T82.329
        aorta (bifurcation) T82.320
        carotid artery T82.321
        specified vessel NEC T82.328
      obstruction T82.399
        aorta (bifurcation) T82.390
        carotid artery T82.391
        specified vessel NEC T82.398
      perforation T82.399
        aorta (bifurcation) T82.390
        carotid artery T82.391
        specified vessel NEC T82.398
      protrusion T82.399
        aorta (bifurcation) T82.390
        carotid artery T82.391
        specified vessel NEC T82.398
    pain T82.848
    specified complication NEC T82.898
    stenosis T82.858
    thrombosis T82.868
  postoperative — *see* Complications, postoperative, circulatory

Complication(s) (from) (of) — *continued*
vena cava device (filter) (sieve) (umbrella) — *see* Complications, umbrella device, vascular
ventilation therapy NEC T81.81
ventilator
  mechanical J95.850
    specified NEC J95.859
ventricular (communicating) shunt (device) T85.9
  embolism T85.810
  fibrosis T85.820
  hemorrhage T85.830
  infection and inflammation T85.730
  mechanical
    breakdown T85.01
    displacement T85.02
    leakage T85.03
    malposition T85.02
    obstruction T85.09
    perforation T85.09
    protrusion T85.09
    specified NEC T85.09
  pain T85.840
  specified type NEC T85.890
  stenosis T85.850
  thrombosis T85.860
wire suture, permanent (implanted) — *see* Complications, suture, permanent

Compressed air disease T70.3
Compression
  with injury — *code by* nature of injury
  artery I77.1
    celiac, syndrome I77.4
  brachial plexus G54.0
  brain (stem) G93.5
    due to
      contusion (diffuse) — *see* Injury, intracranial, diffuse
        focal — *see* Injury, intracranial, focal
      injury NEC — *see* Injury, intracranial, diffuse
      traumatic — *see* Injury, intracranial, diffuse
  bronchus J98.09
  cauda equina G83.4
  celiac (artery) (axis) I77.4
  cerebral — *see* Compression, brain
  cervical plexus G54.2
  cord
    spinal — *see* Compression, spinal
    umbilical — *see* Compression, umbilical cord
  cranial nerve G52.9
    eighth — *see* subcategory H93.3
    eleventh G52.8
    fifth G50.8
    first G52.0
    fourth — *see* Strabismus, paralytic, fourth nerve
    ninth G52.1
    second — *see* Disorder, nerve, optic
    seventh G52.8
    sixth — *see* Strabismus, paralytic, sixth nerve
    tenth G52.2
    third — *see* Strabismus, paralytic, third nerve
    twelfth G52.3
  diver's squeeze T70.3
  during birth (newborn) P15.9
  esophagus K22.2
  eustachian tube — *see* Obstruction, eustachian tube, cartilaginous
  facies Q67.1
  fracture
    nontraumatic NOS — *see* Collapse, vertebra
    pathological — *see* Fracture, pathological
    traumatic — *see* Fracture, traumatic
  heart — *see* Disease, heart
  intestine — *see* Obstruction, intestine

Compression — *continued*
- laryngeal nerve, recurrent G52.2
  - with paralysis of vocal cords and larynx J38.00
    - bilateral J38.02
    - unilateral J38.01
- lumbosacral plexus G54.1
- lung J98.4
- lymphatic vessel I89.0
- medulla — *see* Compression, brain
- nerve (*see also* Disorder, nerve) G58.9
  - arm NEC — *see* Mononeuropathy, upper limb
  - axillary G54.0
  - cranial — *see* Compression, cranial nerve
  - leg NEC — *see* Mononeuropathy, lower limb
  - median (in carpal tunnel) — *see* Syndrome, carpal tunnel
  - optic — *see* Disorder, nerve, optic
  - plantar — *see* Lesion, nerve, plantar
  - posterior tibial (in tarsal tunnel) — *see* Syndrome, tarsal tunnel
  - root or plexus NOS (in) G54.9
    - intervertebral disc disorder NEC — *see* Disorder, disc, with, radiculopathy
      - with myelopathy — *see* Disorder, disc, with, myelopathy
    - neoplastic disease (*see also* Neoplasm) D49.9 *[G55]*
    - spondylosis — *see* Spondylosis, with radiculopathy
  - sciatic (acute) — *see* Lesion, nerve, sciatic
  - sympathetic G90.8
  - traumatic — *see* Injury, nerve
  - ulnar — *see* Lesion, nerve, ulnar
  - upper extremity NEC — *see* Mononeuropathy, upper limb
- spinal (cord) G95.20
  - by displacement of intervertebral disc NEC — *see also* Disorder, disc, with, myelopathy
  - nerve root NOS G54.9
    - due to displacement of intervertebral disc NEC — *see* Disorder, disc, with, radiculopathy
      - with myelopathy — *see* Disorder, disc, with, myelopathy
  - specified NEC G95.29
  - spondylogenic (cervical) (lumbar, lumbosacral) (thoracic) — *see* Spondylosis, with myelopathy NEC
  - anterior — *see* Syndrome, anterior, spinal artery, compression
  - traumatic — *see* Injury, spinal cord, by region
- subcostal nerve (syndrome) — *see* Mononeuropathy, upper limb, specified NEC
- sympathetic nerve NEC G90.8
- syndrome T79.5
- trachea J39.8
- ulnar nerve (by scar tissue) — *see* Lesion, nerve, ulnar
- umbilical cord
  - complicating delivery O69.2
    - cord around neck O69.1
    - prolapse O69.0
    - specified NEC O69.2
- ureter N13.5
- vein I87.1
- vena cava (inferior) (superior) I87.1

Compulsion, compulsive
- gambling F63.0
- neurosis F42.8
- personality F60.5
- states F42.8
- swearing F42.8
  - in Gilles de la Tourette's syndrome F95.2
- tics and spasms F95.9

Concato's disease (pericardial polyserositis) A19.9
- nontubercular I31.1
- pleural — *see* Pleurisy, with effusion

Concavity chest wall M95.4
Concealed penis Q55.69
Concern (normal) about sick person in family Z63.6
Concrescence (teeth) K00.2
Concretio cordis I31.1
- rheumatic I09.2
Concretion — *see also* Calculus
- appendicular K38.1
- canaliculus — *see* Dacryolith
- clitoris N90.89
- conjunctiva H11.12-
- eyelid — *see* Disorder, eyelid, specified type NEC
- lacrimal passages — *see* Dacryolith
- prepuce (male) N47.8
- salivary gland (any) K11.5
- seminal vesicle N50.89
- tonsil J35.8
Concussion (brain) (cerebral) (current) S06.0x9
- with
  - loss of consciousness of 30 minutes or less S06.0x1
  - loss of consciousness of unspecified duration S06.0x9
- blast (air) (hydraulic) (immersion) (underwater)
  - abdomen or thorax — *see* Injury, blast, by site
  - ear with acoustic nerve injury — *see* Injury, nerve, acoustic, specified type NEC
- cauda equina S34.3
- conus medullaris S34.02
- ocular S05.8x-
- spinal (cord)
  - cervical S14.0
  - lumbar S34.01
  - sacral S34.02
  - thoracic S24.0
- syndrome F07.81
- without loss of consciousness S06.0x0
Condition — *see* Disease
Conditions arising in the perinatal period — *see* Newborn, affected by
Conduct disorder — *see* Disorder, conduct
Condyloma A63.0
- acuminatum A63.0
- gonorrheal A54.09
- latum A51.31
- syphilitic A51.31
  - congenital A50.07
- venereal, syphilitic A51.31
Conflagration — *see also* Burn
- asphyxia (by inhalation of gases, fumes or vapors) (*see also* Table of Drugs and Chemicals) T59.9-
Conflict (with) — *see also* Discord
- family Z73.9
- marital Z63.0
  - involving divorce or estrangement Z63.5
- parent-child Z62.820
  - parent-adopted child Z62.821
  - parent-biological child Z62.820
  - parent-foster child Z62.822
- social role NEC Z73.5
Confluent — *see* condition
Confusion, confused R41.0
- epileptic F05
- mental state (psychogenic) F44.89
- psychogenic F44.89
- reactive (from emotional stress, psychological trauma) F44.89
Confusional arousals G47.51
Congelation T69.9

Congenital — *see also* condition
- aortic septum Q25.49
- intrinsic factor deficiency D51.0
- malformation — *see* Anomaly
Congestion, congestive
- bladder N32.89
- bowel K63.89
- brain G93.89
- breast N64.59
- bronchial J98.09
- catarrhal J31.0
- chest R09.89
- chill, malarial — *see* Malaria
- circulatory NEC I99.8
- duodenum K31.89
- eye — *see* Hyperemia, conjunctiva
- facial, due to birth injury P15.4
- general R68.89
- glottis J37.0
- heart — *see* Failure, heart, congestive
- hepatic K76.1
- hypostatic (lung) — *see* Edema, lung
- intestine K63.89
- kidney N28.89
- labyrinth — *see* subcategory H83.8
- larynx J37.0
- liver K76.1
- lung R09.89
  - active or acute — *see* Pneumonia
- malaria, malarial — *see* Malaria
- nasal R09.81
- nose R09.81
- orbit, orbital — *see also* Exophthalmos
  - inflammatory (chronic) — *see* Inflammation, orbit
- ovary N83.8
- pancreas K86.89
- pelvic, female N94.89
- pleural J94.8
- prostate (active) N42.1
- pulmonary — *see* Congestion, lung
- renal N28.89
- retina H35.81
- seminal vesicle N50.1
- spinal cord G95.19
- spleen (chronic) D73.2
- stomach K31.89
- trachea — *see* Tracheitis
- urethra N36.8
- uterus N85.8
  - with subinvolution N85.3
- venous (passive) I87.8
- viscera R68.89
Congestive — *see* Congestion
Conical
- cervix (hypertrophic elongation) N88.4
- cornea — *see* Keratoconus
- teeth K00.2
Conjoined twins Q89.4
Conjugal maladjustment Z63.0
- involving divorce or estrangement Z63.5
Conjunctiva — *see* condition
Conjunctivitis (staphylococcal) (streptococcal) NOS H10.9
- Acanthamoeba B60.12
- acute H10.3-
  - atopic H10.1-
  - chemical (*see also* Corrosion, cornea) H10.21-
  - mucopurulent H10.02-
    - follicular H10.01-
  - pseudomembranous H10.22-
  - serous except viral H10.23-
  - viral — *see* Conjunctivitis, viral
  - toxic H10.21-
- adenoviral (acute) (follicular) B30.1
- allergic (acute) — *see* Conjunctivitis, acute, atopic
  - chronic H10.45
    - vernal H10.44

Conjunctivitis (staphylococcal) (streptococcal)
    NOS H10.9 — *continued*
  anaphylactic — *see* Conjunctivitis, acute,
      atopic
  Apollo B30.3
  atopic (acute) — *see* Conjunctivitis, acute,
      atopic
  blennorrhagic (gonococcal) (neonatorum)
      A54.31
  Béal's B30.2
  chemical (acute) (*see also* Corrosion, cornea)
      H10.21-
  chlamydial A74.0
    due to trachoma A71.1
    neonatal P39.1
  chronic (nodosa) (petrificans) (phlyctenular)
      H10.40-
    allergic H10.45
      vernal H10.44
    follicular H10.43-
    giant papillary H10.41-
    simple H10.42-
    vernal H10.44
  coxsackievirus 24 B30.3
  diphtheritic A36.86
  due to
    dust — *see* Conjunctivitis, acute, atopic
    filariasis B74.9
    mucocutaneous leishmaniasis B55.2
  enterovirus type 70 (hemorrhagic) B30.3
  epidemic (viral) B30.9
    hemorrhagic B30.3
  gonococcal (neonatorum) A54.31
  granular (trachomatous) A71.1
    sequelae (late effect) B94.0
  hemorrhagic (acute) (epidemic) B30.3
  herpes zoster B02.31
  in (due to)
    Acanthamoeba B60.12
    adenovirus (acute) (follicular) B30.1
    Chlamydia A74.0
    coxsackievirus 24 B30.3
    diphtheria A36.86
    enterovirus type 70 (hemorrhagic) B30.3
    filariasis B74.9
    gonococci A54.31
    herpes (simplex) virus B00.53
      zoster B02.31
    infectious disease NEC B99
    meningococci A39.89
    mucocutaneous leishmaniasis B55.2
    rosacea L71.9
    syphilis (late) A52.71
    zoster B02.31
  inclusion A74.0
  infantile P39.1
    gonococcal A54.31
  Koch-Weeks' — *see* Conjunctivitis, acute,
      mucopurulent
  light — *see* Conjunctivitis, acute, atopic
  ligneous — *see* Blepharoconjunctivitis, ligneous
  meningococcal A39.89
  mucopurulent — *see* Conjunctivitis, acute,
      mucopurulent
  neonatal P39.1
    gonococcal A54.31
  Newcastle B30.8
  of Béal B30.2
  parasitic
    filariasis B74.9
    mucocutaneous leishmaniasis B55.2
  Parinaud's H10.89
  petrificans H10.89
  rosacea L71.9
  specified NEC H10.89
  swimming-pool B30.1
  trachomatous A71.1
    acute A71.0
    sequelae (late effect) B94.0

Conjunctivitis (staphylococcal) (streptococcal)
    NOS H10.9 — *continued*
  traumatic NEC H10.89
  tuberculous A18.59
  tularemic A21.1
  tularensis A21.1
  viral B30.9
    due to
      adenovirus B30.1
      enterovirus B30.3
    specified NEC B30.8
Conjunctivochalasis H11.82-
Connective tissue — *see* condition
Conn's syndrome E26.01
Conradi(-Hunermann) disease Q77.3
Consanguinity Z84.3
  counseling Z71.89
Conscious simulation (of illness) Z76.5
Consecutive — *see* condition
Consolidation lung (base) — *see* Pneumonia,
    lobar
Constipation (atonic) (neurogenic) (simple)
    (spastic) K59.00
  chronic K59.09
    idiopathic K59.04
  drug-induced K59.03
  functional K59.04
  outlet dysfunction K59.02
  psychogenic F45.8
  slow transit K59.01
  specified NEC K59.09
Constitutional — *see also* condition
  substandard F60.7
Constitutionally substandard F60.7
Constriction — *see also* Stricture
  auditory canal — *see* Stenosis, external ear
      canal
  bronchial J98.09
  duodenum K31.5
  esophagus K22.2
  external
    abdomen, abdominal (wall) S30.841
    alveolar process S00.542
    ankle S90.54-
    antecubital space — *see* Constriction,
        external, forearm
    arm (upper) S40.84-
    auricle — *see* Constriction, external, ear
    axilla — *see* Constriction, external, arm
    back, lower S30.840
    breast S20.14-
    brow S00.84
    buttock S30.840
    calf — *see* Constriction, external, leg
    canthus — *see* Constriction, external, eyelid
    cheek S00.84
      internal S00.542
    chest wall — *see* Constriction, external,
        thorax
    chin S00.84
    clitoris S30.844
    costal region — *see* Constriction, external,
        thorax
    digit(s)
      foot — *see* Constriction, external, toe
      hand — *see* Constriction, external, finger
    ear S00.44-
    elbow S50.34-
    epididymis S30.843
    epigastric region S30.841
    esophagus, cervical S10.14
    eyebrow — *see* Constriction, external, eyelid
    eyelid S00.24-
    face S00.84
    finger(s) S60.44-
      index S60.44-
      little S60.44-
      middle S60.44-
      ring S60.44-

Constriction (*see also* Stricture) — *continued*
  external — *continued*
    flank S30.841
    foot (except toe(s) alone) S90.84-
      toe — *see* Constriction, external, toe
    forearm S50.84-
      elbow only — *see* Constriction, external,
          elbow
    forehead S00.84
    genital organs, external
      female S30.846
      male S30.845
    groin S30.841
    gum S00.542
    hand S60.54-
    head S00.84
      ear — *see* Constriction, external, ear
      eyelid — *see* Constriction, external, eyelid
      lip S00.541
      nose S00.34
      oral cavity S00.542
      scalp S00.04
      specified site NEC S00.84
    heel — *see* Constriction, external, foot
    hip S70.24-
    inguinal region S30.841
    interscapular region S20.449
    jaw S00.84
    knee S80.24-
    labium (majus) (minus) S30.844
    larynx S10.14
    leg (lower) S80.84-
      knee — *see* Constriction, external, knee
      upper — *see* Constriction, external, thigh
    lip S00.541
    lower back S30.840
    lumbar region S30.840
    malar region S00.84
    mammary — *see* Constriction, external,
        breast
    mastoid region S00.84
    mouth S00.542
    nail
      finger — *see* Constriction, external, finger
      toe — *see* Constriction, external, toe
    nasal S00.34
    neck S10.94
      specified site NEC S10.84
      throat S10.14
    nose S00.34
    occipital region S00.04
    oral cavity S00.542
    orbital region — *see* Constriction, external,
        eyelid
    palate S00.542
    palm — *see* Constriction, external, hand
    parietal region S00.04
    pelvis S30.840
    penis S30.842
    perineum
      female S30.844
      male S30.840
    periocular area — *see* Constriction, external,
        eyelid
    phalanges
      finger — *see* Constriction, external, finger
      toe — *see* Constriction, external, toe
    pharynx S10.14
    pinna — *see* Constriction, external, ear
    popliteal space — *see* Constriction, external,
        knee
    prepuce S30.842
    pubic region S30.840
    pudendum
      female S30.846
      male S30.845
    sacral region S30.840
    scalp S00.04

Constriction (see also Stricture) — continued
 external — continued
  scapular region — see Constriction, external, shoulder
  scrotum S30.843
  shin — see Constriction, external, leg
  shoulder S40.24-
  sternal region S20.349
  submaxillary region S00.84
  submental region S00.84
  subungual
   finger(s) — see Constriction, external, finger
   toe(s) — see Constriction, external, toe
  supraclavicular fossa S10.84
  supraorbital S00.84
  temple S00.84
  temporal region S00.84
  testis S30.843
  thigh S70.34-
  thorax, thoracic (wall) S20.94
   back S20.44-
   front S20.34-
  throat S10.14
  thumb S60.34-
  toe(s) (lesser) S90.44-
   great S90.44-
  tongue S00.542
  trachea S10.14
  tunica vaginalis S30.843
  uvula S00.542
  vagina S30.844
  vulva S30.844
  wrist S60.84-
 gallbladder — see Obstruction, gallbladder
 intestine — see Obstruction, intestine
 larynx J38.6
  congenital Q31.8
   specified NEC Q31.8
   subglottic Q31.1
 organ or site, congenital NEC — see Atresia, by site
 prepuce (acquired) (congenital) N47.1
 pylorus (adult hypertrophic) K31.1
  congenital or infantile Q40.0
  newborn Q40.0
 ring dystocia (uterus) O62.4
 spastic — see also Spasm
  ureter N13.5
 ureter N13.5
  with infection N13.6
 urethra — see Stricture, urethra
 visual field (peripheral) (functional) — see Defect, visual field
Constrictive — see condition
Consultation
 medical — see Counseling, medical
 religious Z71.81
 specified reason NEC Z71.89
 spiritual Z71.81
 without complaint or sickness Z71.9
  feared complaint unfounded Z71.1
  specified reason NEC Z71.89
Consumption — see Tuberculosis
Contact (with) — see also Exposure (to)
 acariasis Z20.7
 AIDS virus Z20.6
 air pollution Z77.110
 algae and algae toxins Z77.121
 algae bloom Z77.121
 anthrax Z20.810
 aromatic (hazardous) compounds NEC Z77.028
 aromatic amines Z77.020
 aromatic dyes NOS Z77.028
 arsenic Z77.010
 asbestos Z77.090
 bacterial disease NEC Z20.818
 benzene Z77.021

Contact (with) (see also Exposure (to)) — continued
 blue-green algae bloom Z77.121
 body fluids (potentially hazardous) Z77.21
 brown tide Z77.121
 chemicals (chiefly nonmedicinal) (hazardous) NEC Z77.098
 cholera Z20.09
 chromium compounds Z77.018
 communicable disease Z20.9
  bacterial NEC Z20.818
  specified NEC Z20.89
  viral NEC Z20.828
 cyanobacteria bloom Z77.121
 dyes Z77.098
 Escherichia coli (E. coli) Z20.01
 fiberglass — see Table of Drugs and Chemicals, fiberglass
 German measles Z20.4
 gonorrhea Z20.2
 hazardous metals NEC Z77.018
 hazardous substances NEC Z77.29
 hazards in the physical environment NEC Z77.128
 hazards to health NEC Z77.9
 HIV Z20.6
 HTLV-III/LAV Z20.6
 human immunodeficiency virus (HIV) Z20.6
 infection Z20.9
  specified NEC Z20.89
 infestation (parasitic) NEC Z20.7
 intestinal infectious disease NEC Z20.09
  Escherichia coli (E. coli) Z20.01
 lead Z77.011
 meningococcus Z20.811
 mold (toxic) Z77.120
 nickel dust Z77.018
 noise Z77.122
 parasitic disease Z20.7
 pediculosis Z20.7
 pfiesteria piscicida Z77.121
 poliomyelitis Z20.89
 pollution
  air Z77.110
  environmental NEC Z77.118
  soil Z77.112
  water Z77.111
 polycyclic aromatic hydrocarbons Z77.028
 rabies Z20.3
 radiation, naturally occurring NEC Z77.123
 radon Z77.123
 red tide (Florida) Z77.121
 rubella Z20.4
 sexually-transmitted disease Z20.2
 smallpox (laboratory) Z20.89
 syphilis Z20.2
 tuberculosis Z20.1
 uranium Z77.012
 varicella Z20.820
 venereal disease Z20.2
 viral disease NEC Z20.828
 viral hepatitis Z20.5
 water pollution Z77.111
Contamination, food — see Intoxication, foodborne
Contraception, contraceptive
 advice Z30.09
 counseling Z30.09
 device (intrauterine) (in situ) Z97.5
  causing menorrhagia T83.83
  checking Z30.431
  complications — see Complications, intrauterine, contraceptive device
  in place Z97.5
  initial prescription Z30.014
  reinsertion Z30.433
  removal Z30.432
  replacement Z30.433
 emergency (postcoital) Z30.012

Contraception, contraceptive — continued
 initial prescription Z30.019
  barrier Z30.018
  diaphragm Z30.018
  injectable Z30.013
  intrauterine device Z30.014
  pills Z30.011
  postcoital (emergency) Z30.012
  specified type NEC Z30.018
  subdermal implantable Z30.017
  transdermal patch hormonal Z30.016
  vaginal ring hormonal Z30.015
 maintenance Z30.40
  barrier Z30.49
  diaphragm Z30.49
  examination Z30.8
  injectable Z30.42
  intrauterine device Z30.431
  pills Z30.41
  specified type NEC Z30.49
  subdermal implantable Z30.46
  transdermal patch hormonal Z30.45
  vaginal ring hormonal Z30.44
 management Z30.9
  specified NEC Z30.8
 postcoital (emergency) Z30.012
 prescription Z30.019
 repeat Z30.40
 sterilization Z30.2
 surveillance (drug) — see Contraception, maintenance
Contraction(s), contracture, contracted
 Achilles tendon — see also Short, tendon, Achilles
  congenital Q66.89
 amputation stump (surgical) (flexion) (late) (next proximal joint) T87.89
 anus K59.8
 bile duct (common) (hepatic) K83.8
 bladder N32.89
  neck or sphincter N32.0
 bowel, cecum, colon or intestine, any part — see Obstruction, intestine
 Braxton Hicks — see False, labor
 breast implant, capsular T85.44
 bronchial J98.09
 burn (old) — see Cicatrix
 cervix — see Stricture, cervix
 cicatricial — see Cicatrix
 conjunctiva, trachomatous, active A71.1
  sequelae (late effect) B94.0
 Dupuytren's M72.0
 eyelid — see Disorder, eyelid function
 fascia (lata) (postural) M72.8
  Dupuytren's M72.0
  palmar M72.0
  plantar M72.2
 finger NEC — see also Deformity, finger
  congenital Q68.1
  joint — see Contraction, joint, hand
 flaccid — see Contraction, paralytic
 gallbladder K82.0
 heart valve — see Endocarditis
 hip — see Contraction, joint, hip
 hourglass
  bladder N32.89
   congenital Q64.79
  gallbladder K82.0
   congenital Q44.1
  stomach K31.89
   congenital Q40.2
   psychogenic F45.8
  uterus (complicating delivery) O62.4
 hysterical F44.4
 internal os — see Stricture, cervix

Contraction(s), contracture, contracted — *continued*

joint (abduction) (acquired) (adduction) (flexion) (rotation) M24.50
    ankle M24.57-
    congenital NEC Q68.8
        hip Q65.89
    elbow M24.52-
    foot joint M24.57-
    hand joint M24.54-
    hip M24.55-
        congenital Q65.89
    hysterical F44.4
    knee M24.56-
    shoulder M24.51-
    wrist M24.53-
kidney (granular) (secondary) N26.9
    congenital Q63.8
    hydronephritic — *see* Hydronephrosis Page N26.2
    pyelonephritic — *see* Pyelitis, chronic
    tuberculous A18.11
ligament — *see also* Disorder, ligament
    congenital Q79.8
muscle (postinfective) (postural) NEC M62.40
    with contracture of joint — *see* Contraction, joint
    ankle M62.47-
    congenital Q79.8
        sternocleidomastoid Q68.0
    extraocular — *see* Strabismus
    eye (extrinsic) — *see* Strabismus
    foot M62.47-
    forearm M62.43-
    hand M62.44-
    hysterical F44.4
    ischemic (Volkmann's) T79.6
    lower leg M62.46-
    multiple sites M62.49
    pelvic region M62.45-
    posttraumatic — *see* Strabismus, paralytic
    psychogenic F45.8
        conversion reaction F44.4
    shoulder region M62.41-
    specified site NEC M62.48
    thigh M62.45-
    upper arm M62.42-
neck — *see* Torticollis
ocular muscle — *see* Strabismus
organ or site, congenital NEC — *see* Atresia, by site
outlet (pelvis) — *see* Contraction, pelvis
palmar fascia M72.0
paralytic
    joint — *see* Contraction, joint
    muscle — *see also* Contraction, muscle NEC
    ocular — *see* Strabismus, paralytic
pelvis (acquired) (general) M95.5
    with disproportion (fetopelvic) O33.1
        causing obstructed labor O65.1
        inlet O33.2
        mid-cavity O33.3
        outlet O33.3
plantar fascia M72.2
premature
    atrium I49.1
    auriculoventricular I49.49
    heart I49.49
    junctional I49.2
    supraventricular I49.1
    ventricular I49.3
prostate N42.89
pylorus NEC — *see also* Pylorospasm
    psychogenic F45.8
rectum, rectal (sphincter) K59.8
ring (Bandl's) (complicating delivery) O62.4
scar — *see* Cicatrix
spine — *see* Dorsopathy, deforming

Contraction(s), contracture, contracted — *continued*

sternocleidomastoid (muscle), congenital Q68.0
stomach K31.89
    hourglass K31.89
        congenital Q40.2
        psychogenic F45.8
    psychogenic F45.8
tendon (sheath) M62.40
    with contracture of joint — *see* Contraction, joint
    Achilles — *see* Short, tendon, Achilles
    ankle M62.47-
        Achilles — *see* Short, tendon, Achilles
    foot M62.47-
    forearm M62.43-
    hand M62.44-
    lower leg M62.46-
    multiple sites M62.49
    neck M62.48
    pelvic region M62.45-
    shoulder region M62.41-
    specified site NEC M62.48
    thigh M62.45-
    thorax M62.48
    trunk M62.48
    upper arm M62.42-
toe — *see* Deformity, toe, specified NEC
ureterovesical orifice (postinfectional) N13.5
    with infection N13.6
urethra — *see also* Stricture, urethra
    orifice N32.0
uterus N85.8
    abnormal NEC O62.9
    clonic (complicating delivery) O62.4
    dyscoordinate (complicating delivery) O62.4
    hourglass (complicating delivery) O62.4
    hypertonic O62.4
    hypotonic NEC O62.2
    inadequate
        primary O62.0
        secondary O62.1
    incoordinate (complicating delivery) O62.4
    poor O62.2
    tetanic (complicating delivery) O62.4
vagina (outlet) N89.5
vesical N32.89
    neck or urethral orifice N32.0
visual field — *see* Defect, visual field, generalized
Volkmann's (ischemic) T79.6

Contusion (skin surface intact) T14.8
abdomen, abdominal (muscle) (wall) S30.1
adnexa, eye NEC S05.8x-
adrenal gland S37.812
alveolar process S00.532
ankle S90.0-
antecubital space — *see* Contusion, forearm
anus S30.3
arm (upper) S40.02-
    lower (with elbow) — *see* Contusion, forearm
auditory canal — *see* Contusion, ear
auricle — *see* Contusion, ear
axilla — *see* Contusion, arm, upper
back — *see also* Contusion, thorax, back
    lower S30.0
bile duct S36.13
bladder S37.22
bone NEC T14.8
brain (diffuse) — *see* Injury, intracranial, diffuse
    focal — *see* Injury, intracranial, focal
brainstem S06.38-
breast S20.0-
broad ligament S37.892
brow S00.83
buttock S30.0
canthus, eye S00.1-
cauda equina S34.3

Contusion (skin surface intact) T14.8 — *continued*

cerebellar, traumatic S06.37-
cerebral S06.33-
    left side S06.32-
    right side S06.31-
cheek S00.83
    internal S00.532
chest (wall) — *see* Contusion, thorax
chin S00.83
clitoris S30.23
colon — *see* Injury, intestine, large, contusion
common bile duct S36.13
conjunctiva S05.1-
    with foreign body (in conjunctival sac) — *see* Foreign body, conjunctival sac
conus medullaris (spine) S34.139
cornea — *see* Contusion, eyeball
    with foreign body — *see* Foreign body, cornea
corpus cavernosum S30.21
cortex (brain) (cerebral) — *see* Injury, intracranial, diffuse
    focal — *see* Injury, intracranial, focal
costal region — *see* Contusion, thorax
cystic duct S36.13
diaphragm S27.802
duodenum S36.420
ear S00.43-
elbow S50.0-
    with forearm — *see* Contusion, forearm
epididymis S30.22
epigastric region S30.1
epiglottis S10.0
esophagus (thoracic) S27.812
    cervical S10.0
eyeball S05.1-
eyebrow S00.1-
eyelid (and periocular area) S00.1-
face NEC S00.83
fallopian tube S37.529
    bilateral S37.522
    unilateral S37.521
femoral triangle S30.1
finger(s) S60.00
    with damage to nail (matrix) S60.10
    index S60.02-
        with damage to nail S60.12-
    little S60.05-
        with damage to nail S60.15-
    middle S60.03-
        with damage to nail S60.13-
    ring S60.04-
        with damage to nail S60.14-
    thumb — *see* Contusion, thumb
flank S30.1
foot (except toe(s) alone) S90.3-
    toe — *see* Contusion, toe
forearm S50.1-
    elbow only — *see* Contusion, elbow
forehead S00.83
gallbladder S36.122
genital organs, external
    female S30.202
    male S30.201
globe (eye) — *see* Contusion, eyeball
groin S30.1
gum S00.532
hand S60.22-
    finger(s) — *see* Contusion, finger
    wrist — *see* Contusion, wrist
head S00.93
    ear — *see* Contusion, ear
    eyelid — *see* Contusion, eyelid
    lip S00.531
    nose S00.33
    oral cavity S00.532
    scalp S00.03
    specified part NEC S00.83

Contusion (skin surface intact) T14.8 — continued
- heart (see also Injury, heart) S26.91
- heel — see Contusion, foot
- hepatic duct S36.13
- hip S70.0-
- ileum S36.428
- iliac region S30.1
- inguinal region S30.1
- interscapular region S20.229
- intra-abdominal organ S36.92
  - colon — see Injury, intestine, large, contusion
  - liver S36.112
  - pancreas — see Contusion, pancreas
  - rectum S36.62
  - small intestine — see Injury, intestine, small, contusion
  - specified organ NEC S36.892
  - spleen — see Contusion, spleen
  - stomach S36.32
- iris (eye) — see Contusion, eyeball
- jaw S00.83
- jejunum S36.428
- kidney S37.01-
  - major (greater than 2 cm) S37.02-
  - minor (less than 2 cm) S37.01-
- knee S80.0-
- labium (majus) (minus) S30.23
- lacrimal apparatus, gland or sac S05.8x-
- larynx S10.0
- leg (lower) S80.1-
  - knee — see Contusion, knee
- lens — see Contusion, eyeball
- lip S00.531
- liver S36.112
- lower back S30.0
- lumbar region S30.0
- lung S27.329
  - bilateral S27.322
  - unilateral S27.321
- malar region S00.83
- mastoid region S00.83
- membrane, brain — see Injury, intracranial, diffuse
  - focal — see Injury, intracranial, focal
- mesentery S36.892
- mesosalpinx S37.892
- mouth S00.532
- muscle — see Contusion, by site
- nail
  - finger — see Contusion, finger, with damage to nail
  - toe — see Contusion, toe, with damage to nail
- nasal S00.33
- neck S10.93
  - specified site NEC S10.83
  - throat S10.0
- nerve — see Injury, nerve
- newborn P54.5
- nose S00.33
- occipital
  - lobe (brain) — see Injury, intracranial, diffuse
    - focal — see Injury, intracranial, focal
  - region (scalp) S00.03
- orbit (region) (tissues) S05.1-
- ovary S37.429
  - bilateral S37.422
  - unilateral S37.421
- palate S00.532
- pancreas S36.229
  - body S36.221
  - head S36.220
  - tail S36.222

Contusion (skin surface intact) T14.8 — continued
- parietal
  - lobe (brain) — see Injury, intracranial, diffuse
    - focal — see Injury, intracranial, focal
  - region (scalp) S00.03
- pelvic organ S37.92
  - adrenal gland S37.812
  - bladder S37.22
  - fallopian tube — see Contusion, fallopian tube
  - kidney — see Contusion, kidney
  - ovary — see Contusion, ovary
  - prostate S37.822
  - specified organ NEC S37.892
  - ureter S37.12
  - urethra S37.32
  - uterus S37.62
- pelvis S30.0
- penis S30.21
- perineum
  - female S30.23
  - male S30.0
- periocular area S00.1-
- peritoneum S36.81
- periurethral tissue — see Contusion, urethra
- pharynx S10.0
- pinna — see Contusion, ear
- popliteal space — see Contusion, knee
- prepuce S30.21
- prostate S37.822
- pubic region S30.1
- pudendum
  - female S30.202
  - male S30.201
- quadriceps femoris — see Contusion, thigh
- rectum S36.62
- retroperitoneum S36.892
- round ligament S37.892
- sacral region S30.0
- scalp S00.03
  - due to birth injury P12.3
- scapular region — see Contusion, shoulder
- sclera — see Contusion, eyeball
- scrotum S30.22
- seminal vesicle S37.892
- shoulder S40.01-
- skin NEC T14.8
- small intestine — see Injury, intestine, small, contusion
- spermatic cord S30.22
- spinal cord — see Injury, spinal cord, by region
  - cauda equina S34.3
  - conus medullaris S34.139
- spleen S36.029
  - major S36.021
  - minor S36.020
- sternal region S20.219
- stomach S36.32
- subconjunctival S05.1-
- subcutaneous NEC T14.8
- submaxillary region S00.83
- submental region S00.83
- subperiosteal NEC T14.8
- subungual
  - finger — see Contusion, finger, with damage to nail
  - toe — see Contusion, toe, with damage to nail
- supraclavicular fossa S10.83
- supraorbital S00.83
- suprarenal gland S37.812
- temple (region) S00.83
- temporal
  - lobe (brain) — see Injury, intracranial, diffuse
    - focal — see Injury, intracranial, focal
  - region S00.83

Contusion (skin surface intact) T14.8 — continued
- testis S30.22
- thigh S70.1-
- thorax (wall) S20.20
  - back S20.22-
  - front S20.21-
- throat S10.0
- thumb S60.01-
  - with damage to nail S60.11-
- toe(s) (lesser) S90.12-
  - with damage to nail S90.22-
  - great S90.11-
    - with damage to nail S90.21-
    - specified type NEC S90.221
- tongue S00.532
- trachea (cervical) S10.0
  - thoracic S27.52
- tunica vaginalis S30.22
- tympanum, tympanic membrane — see Contusion, ear
- ureter S37.12
- urethra S37.32
- urinary organ NEC S37.892
- uterus S37.62
- uvula S00.532
- vagina S30.23
- vas deferens S37.892
- vesical S37.22
- vocal cord(s) S10.0
- vulva S30.23
- wrist S60.21-

Conus (congenital) (any type) Q14.8
- cornea — see Keratoconus
- medullaris syndrome G95.81

Conversion hysteria, neurosis or reaction F44.9

Converter, tuberculosis (test reaction) R76.11

Conviction (legal), anxiety concerning Z65.0
- with imprisonment Z65.1

Convulsions (idiopathic) (see also Seizure(s)) R56.9
- apoplectiform (cerebral ischemia) I67.82
- dissociative F44.5
- epileptic — see Epilepsy
- epileptiform, epileptoid — see Seizure, epileptiform
- ether (anesthetic) — see Table of Drugs and Chemicals, by drug
- febrile R56.00
  - with status epilepticus G40.901
  - complex R56.01
    - with status epilepticus G40.901
  - simple R56.00
- hysterical F44.5
- infantile P90
  - epilepsy — see Epilepsy
- jacksonian — see Epilepsy, localization-related, symptomatic, with simple partial seizures
- myoclonic G25.3
- newborn P90
- obstetrical (nephritic) (uremic) — see Eclampsia
- paretic A52.17
- post traumatic R56.1
- psychomotor — see Epilepsy, localization-related, symptomatic, with complex partial seizures
- recurrent R56.9
- reflex R25.8
- scarlatinal A38.8
- tetanus, tetanic — see Tetanus
- thymic E32.8

Convulsive — see also Convulsions

Cooley's anemia D56.1

Coolie itch B76.9

Cooper's
disease — *see* Mastopathy, cystic
hernia — *see* Hernia, abdomen, specified site NEC
Copra itch B88.0
Coprophagy F50.89
Coprophobia F40.298
Coproporphyria, hereditary E80.29
Cor
biloculare Q20.8
bovis, bovinum — *see* Hypertrophy, cardiac
pulmonale (chronic) I27.81
acute I26.09
triatriatum, triatrium Q24.2
triloculare Q20.8
biatrium Q20.4
biventriculare Q21.1
Corbus' disease (gangrenous balanitis) N48.1
Cord — *see also* condition
around neck (tightly) (with compression) complicating delivery O69.1
bladder G95.89
tabetic A52.19
Cordis ectopia Q24.8
Corditis (spermatic) N49.1
Corectopia Q13.2
Cori's disease (glycogen storage) E74.03
Corkhandler's disease or lung J67.3
Corkscrew esophagus K22.4
Corkworker's disease or lung J67.3
Corn (infected) L84
Cornea — *see also* condition
donor Z52.5
plana Q13.4
Cornelia de Lange syndrome Q87.1
Cornu cutaneum L85.8
Cornual gestation or pregnancy O00.80
with intrauterine pregnancy O00.81
Coronary (artery) — *see* condition
Coronavirus, as cause of disease classified elsewhere B97.29
SARS-associated B97.21
Corpora — *see also* condition
amylacea, prostate N42.89
cavernosa — *see* condition
Corpulence — *see* Obesity
Corpus — *see* condition
Corrected transposition Q20.5
Corrosion (injury) (acid) (caustic) (chemical) (lime) (external) (internal) T30.4
abdomen, abdominal (muscle) (wall) T21.42
first degree T21.52
second degree T21.62
third degree T21.72
above elbow T22.439
first degree T22.539
left T22.432
first degree T22.532
second degree T22.632
third degree T22.732
right T22.431
first degree T22.531
second degree T22.631
third degree T22.731
second degree T22.639
third degree T22.739
alimentary tract NEC T28.7
ankle T25.419
first degree T25.519
left T25.412
first degree T25.512
second degree T25.612
third degree T25.712
multiple with foot — *see* Corrosion, lower, limb, multiple, ankle and foot

Corrosion (injury) (acid) (caustic) (chemical) (lime) (external) (internal) T30.4 — *continued*
ankle T25.419 — *continued*
right T25.411
first degree T25.511
second degree T25.611
third degree T25.711
second degree T25.619
third degree T25.719
anus — *see* Corrosion, buttock
arm(s) (meaning upper limb(s)) — *see* Corrosion, upper limb
axilla T22.449
first degree T22.549
left T22.442
first degree T22.542
second degree T22.642
third degree T22.742
right T22.441
first degree T22.541
second degree T22.641
third degree T22.741
second degree T22.649
third degree T22.749
back (lower) T21.44
first degree T21.54
second degree T21.64
third degree T21.74
upper T21.43
first degree T21.53
second degree T21.63
third degree T21.73
blisters — *code as* Corrosion, second degree, by site
breast(s) — *see* Corrosion, chest wall
buttock(s) T21.45
first degree T21.55
second degree T21.65
third degree T21.75
calf T24.439
first degree T24.539
left T24.432
first degree T24.532
second degree T24.632
third degree T24.732
right T24.431
first degree T24.531
second degree T24.631
third degree T24.731
second degree T24.639
third degree T24.739
canthus (eye) — *see* Corrosion, eyelid
cervix T28.8
cheek T20.46
first degree T20.56
second degree T20.66
third degree T20.76
chest wall T21.41
first degree T21.51
second degree T21.61
third degree T21.71
chin T20.43
first degree T20.53
second degree T20.63
third degree T20.73
colon T28.7
conjunctiva (and cornea) — *see* Corrosion, cornea
cornea (and conjunctiva) T26.6-
deep necrosis of underlying tissue — *code as* Corrosion, third degree, by site
dorsum of hand T23.469
first degree T23.569
left T23.462
first degree T23.562
second degree T23.662
third degree T23.762

Corrosion (injury) (acid) (caustic) (chemical) (lime) (external) (internal) T30.4 — *continued*
dorsum of hand T23.469 — *continued*
right T23.461
first degree T23.561
second degree T23.661
third degree T23.761
second degree T23.669
third degree T23.769
ear (auricle) (external) (canal) T20.41
drum T28.91
first degree T20.51
second degree T20.61
third degree T20.71
elbow T22.429
first degree T22.529
left T22.422
first degree T22.522
second degree T22.622
third degree T22.722
right T22.421
first degree T22.521
second degree T22.621
third degree T22.721
second degree T22.629
third degree T22.729
entire body — *see* Corrosion, multiple body regions
epidermal loss — *code as* Corrosion, second degree, by site
epiglottis T27.4
erythema, erythematous — *code as* Corrosion, first degree, by site
esophagus T28.6
extent (percentage of body surface)
10-19 per cent (0-9 percent third degree) T32.10
with 10-19 percent third degree T32.11
20-29 per cent (0-9 percent third degree) T32.20
with
10-19 percent third degree T32.21
20-29 percent third degree T32.22
30-39 per cent (0-9 percent third degree) T32.30
with
10-19 percent third degree T32.31
20-29 percent third degree T32.32
30-39 percent third degree T32.33
40-49 per cent (0-9 percent third degree) T32.40
with
10-19 percent third degree T32.41
20-29 percent third degree T32.42
30-39 percent third degree T32.43
40-49 percent third degree T32.44
50-59 per cent (0-9 percent third degree) T32.50
with
10-19 percent third degree T32.51
20-29 percent third degree T32.52
30-39 percent third degree T32.53
40-49 percent third degree T32.54
50-59 percent third degree T32.55
60-69 per cent (0-9 percent third degree) T32.60
with
10-19 percent third degree T32.61
20-29 percent third degree T32.62
30-39 percent third degree T32.63
40-49 percent third degree T32.64
50-59 percent third degree T32.65
60-69 percent third degree T32.66

Corrosion (injury) (acid) (caustic) (chemical) (lime) (external) (internal) T30.4 — *continued*
  extent (percentage of body surface) — *continued*
    70-79 per cent (0-9 percent third degree) T32.70
      with
        10-19 percent third degree T32.71
        20-29 percent third degree T32.72
        30-39 percent third degree T32.73
        40-49 percent third degree T32.74
        50-59 percent third degree T32.75
        60-69 percent third degree T32.76
        70-79 percent third degree T32.77
    80-89 per cent (0-9 percent third degree) T32.80
      with
        10-19 percent third degree T32.81
        20-29 percent third degree T32.82
        30-39 percent third degree T32.83
        40-49 percent third degree T32.84
        50-59 percent third degree T32.85
        60-69 percent third degree T32.86
        70-79 percent third degree T32.87
        80-89 percent third degree T32.88
    90 per cent or more (0-9 percent third degree) T32.90
      with
        10-19 percent third degree T32.91
        20-29 percent third degree T32.92
        30-39 percent third degree T32.93
        40-49 percent third degree T32.94
        50-59 percent third degree T32.95
        60-69 percent third degree T32.96
        70-79 percent third degree T32.97
        80-89 percent third degree T32.98
        90-99 percent third degree T32.99
    less than 10 per cent T32.0
  extremity — *see* Corrosion, limb
  eye(s) and adnexa T26.9-
    with resulting rupture and destruction of eyeball T26.7-
    conjunctival sac — *see* Corrosion, cornea
    cornea — *see* Corrosion, cornea
    lid — *see* Corrosion, eyelid
    periocular area — *see* Corrosion eyelid
    specified site NEC T26.8-
  eyeball — *see* Corrosion, eye
  eyelid(s) T26.5-
  face — *see* Corrosion, head
  finger T23.429
    first degree T23.529
    left T23.422
      first degree T23.522
      second degree T23.622
      third degree T23.722
    multiple sites (without thumb) T23.439
      with thumb T23.449
        first degree T23.549
        left T23.442
          first degree T23.542
          second degree T23.642
          third degree T23.742
        right T23.441
          first degree T23.541
          second degree T23.641
          third degree T23.741
        second degree T23.649
        third degree T23.749
      first degree T23.539
      left T23.432
        first degree T23.532
        second degree T23.632
        third degree T23.732

Corrosion (injury) (acid) (caustic) (chemical) (lime) (external) (internal) T30.4 — *continued*
  finger T23.429 — *continued*
    multiple sites (without thumb) T23.439 — *continued*
      right T23.431
        first degree T23.531
        second degree T23.631
        third degree T23.731
      second degree T23.639
    right T23.421
      first degree T23.521
      second degree T23.621
      third degree T23.721
    second degree T23.629
    third degree T23.729
  flank — *see* Corrosion, abdomen
  foot T25.429
    first degree T25.529
    left T25.422
      first degree T25.522
      second degree T25.622
      third degree T25.722
    multiple with ankle — *see* Corrosion, lower, limb, multiple, ankle and foot
    right T25.421
      first degree T25.521
      second degree T25.621
      third degree T25.721
    second degree T25.629
    third degree T25.729
  forearm T22.419
    first degree T22.519
    left T22.412
      first degree T22.512
      second degree T22.612
      third degree T22.712
    right T22.411
      first degree T22.511
      second degree T22.611
      third degree T22.711
    second degree T22.619
    third degree T22.719
  forehead T20.46
    first degree T20.56
    second degree T20.66
    third degree T20.76
  fourth degree — *code as* Corrosion, third degree, by site
  full thickness skin loss — *code as* Corrosion, third degree, by site
  gastrointestinal tract NEC T28.7
  genital organs
    external
      female T21.47
        first degree T21.57
        second degree T21.67
        third degree T21.77
      male T21.46
        first degree T21.56
        second degree T21.66
        third degree T21.76
    internal T28.8
  groin — *see* Corrosion, abdominal wall
  hand(s) T23.409
    back — *see* Corrosion, dorsum of hand
    finger — *see* Corrosion, finger
    first degree T23.509
    left T23.402
      first degree T23.502
      second degree T23.602
      third degree T23.702

Corrosion (injury) (acid) (caustic) (chemical) (lime) (external) (internal) T30.4 — *continued*
  hand(s) T23.409 — *continued*
    multiple sites with wrist T23.499
      first degree T23.599
      left T23.492
        first degree T23.592
        second degree T23.692
        third degree T23.792
      right T23.491
        first degree T23.591
        second degree T23.691
        third degree T23.791
      second degree T23.699
      third degree T23.799
    palm — *see* Corrosion, palm
    right T23.401
      first degree T23.501
      second degree T23.601
      third degree T23.701
    second degree T23.609
    third degree T23.709
    thumb — *see* Corrosion, thumb
  head (and face) (and neck) T20.40
    cheek — *see* Corrosion, cheek
    chin — *see* Corrosion, chin
    ear — *see* Corrosion, ear
    eye(s) only — *see* Corrosion, eye
    first degree T20.50
    forehead — *see* Corrosion, forehead
    lip — *see* Corrosion, lip
    multiple sites T20.49
      first degree T20.59
      second degree T20.69
      third degree T20.79
    neck — *see* Corrosion, neck
    nose — *see* Corrosion, nose
    scalp — *see* Corrosion, scalp
    second degree T20.60
    third degree T20.70
  hip(s) — *see* Corrosion, lower, limb
  inhalation — *see* Corrosion, respiratory tract
  internal organ(s) (*see also* Corrosion, by site) T28.90
    alimentary tract T28.7
      esophagus T28.6
    esophagus T28.6
    genitourinary T28.8
    mouth T28.5
    pharynx T28.5
    specified organ NEC T28.99
  interscapular region — *see* Corrosion, back, upper
  intestine (large) (small) T28.7
  knee T24.429
    first degree T24.529
    left T24.422
      first degree T24.522
      second degree T24.622
      third degree T24.722
    right T24.421
      first degree T24.521
      second degree T24.621
      third degree T24.721
    second degree T24.629
    third degree T24.729
  labium (majus) (minus) — *see* Corrosion, genital organs, external, female
  lacrimal apparatus, duct, gland or sac — *see* Corrosion, eye, specified site NEC
  larynx T27.4
    with lung T27.5
  leg(s) (meaning lower limb(s)) — *see* Corrosion, lower limb
  limb(s)
    lower — *see* Corrosion, lower, limb
    upper — *see* Corrosion, upper limb

Corrosion (injury) (acid) (caustic) (chemical) (lime) (external) (internal) T30.4 — *continued*
lip(s) T20.42
  first degree T20.52
  second degree T20.62
  third degree T20.72
lower
  back — *see* Corrosion, back
  limb T24.409
    ankle — *see* Corrosion, ankle
    calf — *see* Corrosion, calf
    first degree T24.509
    foot — *see* Corrosion, foot
    hip — *see* Corrosion, thigh
    knee — *see* Corrosion, knee
    left T24.402
      first degree T24.502
      second degree T24.602
      third degree T24.702
    multiple sites, except ankle and foot T24.499
      ankle and foot T25.499
        first degree T25.599
        left T25.492
          first degree T25.592
          second degree T25.692
          third degree T25.792
        right T25.491
          first degree T25.591
          second degree T25.691
          third degree T25.791
        second degree T25.699
        third degree T25.799
    first degree T24.599
    left T24.492
      first degree T24.592
      second degree T24.692
      third degree T24.792
    right T24.491
      first degree T24.591
      second degree T24.691
      third degree T24.791
    second degree T24.699
    third degree T24.799
    right T24.401
      first degree T24.501
      second degree T24.601
      third degree T24.701
    second degree T24.609
    thigh — *see* Corrosion, thigh
    third degree T24.709
lung (with larynx and trachea) T27.5
mouth T28.5
neck T20.47
  first degree T20.57
  second degree T20.67
  third degree T20.77
nose (septum) T20.44
  first degree T20.54
  second degree T20.64
  third degree T20.74
ocular adnexa — *see* Corrosion, eye
orbit region — *see* Corrosion, eyelid
palm T23.459
  first degree T23.559
  left T23.452
    first degree T23.552
    second degree T23.652
    third degree T23.752
  right T23.451
    first degree T23.551
    second degree T23.651
    third degree T23.751
  second degree T23.659
  third degree T23.759
partial thickness — *code as* Corrosion, unspecified degree, by site

Corrosion (injury) (acid) (caustic) (chemical) (lime) (external) (internal) T30.4 — *continued*
pelvis — *see* Corrosion, trunk
penis — *see* Corrosion, genital organs, external, male
perineum
  female — *see* Corrosion, genital organs, external, female
  male — *see* Corrosion, genital organs, external, male
periocular area — *see* Corrosion, eyelid
pharynx T28.5
rectum T28.7
respiratory tract T27.7
  larynx — *see* Corrosion, larynx
  specified part NEC T27.6
  trachea — *see* Corrosion, larynx
sac, lacrimal — *see* Corrosion, eye, specified site NEC
scalp T20.45
  first degree T20.55
  second degree T20.65
  third degree T20.75
scapular region T22.469
  first degree T22.569
  left T22.462
    first degree T22.562
    second degree T22.662
    third degree T22.762
  right T22.461
    first degree T22.561
    second degree T22.661
    third degree T22.761
  second degree T22.669
  third degree T22.769
sclera — *see* Corrosion, eye, specified site NEC
scrotum — *see* Corrosion, genital organs, external, male
shoulder T22.459
  first degree T22.559
  left T22.452
    first degree T22.552
    second degree T22.652
    third degree T22.752
  right T22.451
    first degree T22.551
    second degree T22.651
    third degree T22.751
  second degree T22.659
  third degree T22.759
stomach T28.7
temple — *see* Corrosion, head
testis — *see* Corrosion, genital organs, external, male
thigh T24.419
  first degree T24.519
  left T24.412
    first degree T24.512
    second degree T24.612
    third degree T24.712
  right T24.411
    first degree T24.511
    second degree T24.611
    third degree T24.711
  second degree T24.619
  third degree T24.719
thorax (external) — *see* Corrosion, trunk
throat (meaning pharynx) T28.5
thumb(s) T23.419
  first degree T23.519
  left T23.412
    first degree T23.512
    second degree T23.612
    third degree T23.712

Corrosion (injury) (acid) (caustic) (chemical) (lime) (external) (internal) T30.4 — *continued*
thumb(s) T23.419 — *continued*
  multiple sites with fingers T23.449
    first degree T23.549
    left T23.442
      first degree T23.542
      second degree T23.642
      third degree T23.742
    right T23.441
      first degree T23.541
      second degree T23.641
      third degree T23.741
    second degree T23.649
    third degree T23.749
  right T23.411
    first degree T23.511
    second degree T23.611
    third degree T23.711
  second degree T23.619
  third degree T23.719
toe T25.439
  first degree T25.539
  left T25.432
    first degree T25.532
    second degree T25.632
    third degree T25.732
  right T25.431
    first degree T25.531
    second degree T25.631
    third degree T25.731
  second degree T25.639
  third degree T25.739
tongue T28.5
tonsil(s) T28.5
total body — *see* Corrosion, multiple body regions
trachea T27.4
  with lung T27.5
trunk T21.40
  abdominal wall — *see* Corrosion, abdominal wall
  anus — *see* Corrosion, buttock
  axilla — *see* Corrosion, upper limb
  back — *see* Corrosion, back
  breast — *see* Corrosion, chest wall
  buttock — *see* Corrosion, buttock
  chest wall — *see* Corrosion, chest wall
  first degree T21.50
  flank — *see* Corrosion, abdominal wall
  genital
    female — *see* Corrosion, genital organs, external, female
    male — *see* Corrosion, genital organs, external, male
  groin — *see* Corrosion, abdominal wall
  interscapular region — *see* Corrosion, back, upper
  labia — *see* Corrosion, genital organs, external, female
  lower back — *see* Corrosion, back
  penis — *see* Corrosion, genital organs, external, male
  perineum
    female — *see* Corrosion, genital organs, external, female
    male — *see* Corrosion, genital organs, external, male
  scapular region — *see* Corrosion, upper limb
  scrotum — *see* Corrosion, genital organs, external, male
  second degree T21.60
  shoulder — *see* Corrosion, upper limb
  specified site NEC T21.49
    first degree T21.59
    second degree T21.69
    third degree T21.79

DISEASE INDEX

Corrosion (injury) (acid) (caustic) (chemical) (lime) (external) (internal) T30.4 — *continued*
  trunk T21.40 — *continued*
    testes — *see* Corrosion, genital organs, external, male
    third degree T21.70
    upper back — *see* Corrosion, back, upper
    vagina T28.8
    vulva — *see* Corrosion, genital organs, external, female
  unspecified site with extent of body surface involved specified
    10-19 per cent (0-9 percent third degree) T32.10
      with 10-19 percent third degree T32.11
    20-29 per cent (0-9 percent third degree) T32.20
      with
        10-19 percent third degree T32.21
        20-29 percent third degree T32.22
    30-39 per cent (0-9 percent third degree) T32.30
      with
        10-19 percent third degree T32.31
        20-29 percent third degree T32.32
        30-39 percent third degree T32.33
    40-49 per cent (0-9 percent third degree) T32.40
      with
        10-19 percent third degree T32.41
        20-29 percent third degree T32.42
        30-39 percent third degree T32.43
        40-49 percent third degree T32.44
    50-59 per cent (0-9 percent third degree) T32.50
      with
        10-19 percent third degree T32.51
        20-29 percent third degree T32.52
        30-39 percent third degree T32.53
        40-49 percent third degree T32.54
        50-59 percent third degree T32.55
    60-69 per cent (0-9 percent third degree) T32.60
      with
        10-19 percent third degree T32.61
        20-29 percent third degree T32.62
        30-39 percent third degree T32.63
        40-49 percent third degree T32.64
        50-59 percent third degree T32.65
        60-69 percent third degree T32.66
    70-79 per cent (0-9 percent third degree) T32.70
      with
        10-19 percent third degree T32.71
        20-29 percent third degree T32.72
        30-39 percent third degree T32.73
        40-49 percent third degree T32.74
        50-59 percent third degree T32.75
        60-69 percent third degree T32.76
        70-79 percent third degree T32.77
    80-89 per cent (0-9 percent third degree) T32.80
      with
        10-19 percent third degree T32.81
        20-29 percent third degree T32.82
        30-39 percent third degree T32.83
        40-49 percent third degree T32.84
        50-59 percent third degree T32.85
        60-69 percent third degree T32.86
        70-79 percent third degree T32.87
        80-89 percent third degree T32.88

Corrosion (injury) (acid) (caustic) (chemical) (lime) (external) (internal) T30.4 — *continued*
  unspecified site with extent of body surface involved specified — *continued*
    90 per cent or more (0-9 percent third degree) T32.90
      with
        10-19 percent third degree T32.91
        20-29 percent third degree T32.92
        30-39 percent third degree T32.93
        40-49 percent third degree T32.94
        50-59 percent third degree T32.95
        60-69 percent third degree T32.96
        70-79 percent third degree T32.97
        80-89 percent third degree T32.98
        90-99 percent third degree T32.99
    less than 10 per cent T32.0
  upper limb (axilla) (scapular region) T22.40
    above elbow — *see* Corrosion, above elbow
    axilla — *see* Corrosion, axilla
    elbow — *see* Corrosion, elbow
    first degree T22.50
    forearm — *see* Corrosion, forearm
    hand — *see* Corrosion, hand
    interscapular region — *see* Corrosion, back, upper
    multiple sites T22.499
      first degree T22.599
      left T22.492
        first degree T22.592
        second degree T22.692
        third degree T22.792
      right T22.491
        first degree T22.591
        second degree T22.691
        third degree T22.791
      second degree T22.699
      third degree T22.799
    scapular region — *see* Corrosion, scapular region
    second degree T22.60
    shoulder — *see* Corrosion, shoulder
    third degree T22.70
    wrist — *see* Corrosion, hand
  uterus T28.8
  vagina T28.8
  vulva — *see* Corrosion, genital organs, external, female
  wrist T23.479
    first degree T23.579
    left T23.472
      first degree T23.572
      second degree T23.672
      third degree T23.772
    multiple sites with hand T23.499
      first degree T23.599
      left T23.492
        first degree T23.592
        second degree T23.692
        third degree T23.792
      right T23.491
        first degree T23.591
        second degree T23.691
        third degree T23.791
      second degree T23.699
      third degree T23.799
    right T23.471
      first degree T23.571
      second degree T23.671
      third degree T23.771
    second degree T23.679
    third degree T23.779

Corrosive burn — *see* Corrosion
Corsican fever — *see* Malaria
Cortical — *see* condition
Cortico-adrenal — *see* condition

Coryza (acute) J00
  with grippe or influenza — *see* Influenza, with, respiratory manifestations NEC
  syphilitic
    congenital (chronic) A50.05
Costen's syndrome or complex M26.69
Costiveness — *see* Constipation
Costochondritis M94.0
Cot death R99
Cotard's syndrome F22
Cotia virus B08.8
Cotton wool spots (retinal) H35.81
Cotungo's disease — *see* Sciatica
Cough (affected) (chronic) (epidemic) (nervous) R05
  with hemorrhage — *see* Hemoptysis
  bronchial R05
    with grippe or influenza — *see* Influenza, with, respiratory manifestations NEC
  functional F45.8
  hysterical F45.8
  laryngeal, spasmodic R05
  psychogenic F45.8
  smokers' J41.0
  tea taster's B49
Counseling (for) Z71.9
  abuse NEC
    perpetrator Z69.82
    victim Z69.81
  alcohol abuser Z71.41
    family Z71.42
  child abuse
    nonparental
      perpetrator Z69.021
      victim Z69.020
    parental
      perpetrator Z69.011
      victim Z69.010
  consanguinity Z71.89
  contraceptive Z30.09
  dietary Z71.3
  drug abuser Z71.51
    family member Z71.52
  family Z71.89
  fertility preservation (prior to cancer therapy) (prior to removal of gonads) Z31.62
  for non-attending third party Z71.0
    related to sexual behavior or orientation Z70.2
  genetic NEC Z31.5
  gestational carrier Z31.7
  health (advice) (education) (instruction) — *see* Counseling, medical
  human immunodeficiency virus (HIV) Z71.7
  impotence Z70.1
  insulin pump use Z46.81
  medical (for) Z71.9
    boarding school resident Z59.3
    consanguinity Z71.89
    feared complaint and no disease found Z71.1
    human immunodeficiency virus (HIV) Z71.7
    institutional resident Z59.3
    on behalf of another Z71.0
      related to sexual behavior or orientation Z70.2
    person living alone Z60.2
    specified reason NEC Z71.89
  natural family planning
    procreative Z31.61
    to avoid pregnancy Z30.02
  perpetrator (of)
    abuse NEC Z69.82
    child abuse
      non-parental Z69.021
      parental Z69.011
    rape NEC Z69.82
    spousal abuse Z69.12

Counseling (for) Z71.9 — *continued*
  procreative NEC Z31.69
    fertility preservation (prior to cancer therapy)
      (prior to removal of gonads) Z31.62
    using natural family planning Z31.61
  promiscuity Z70.1
  rape victim Z69.81
  religious Z71.81
  sex, sexual (related to) Z70.9
    attitude(s) Z70.0
    behavior or orientation Z70.1
    combined concerns Z70.3
    non-responsiveness Z70.1
    on behalf of third party Z70.2
    specified reason NEC Z70.8
  specified reason NEC Z71.89
  spiritual Z71.81
  spousal abuse (perpetrator) Z69.12
    victim Z69.11
  substance abuse Z71.89
    alcohol Z71.41
    drug Z71.51
    tobacco Z71.6
  tobacco use Z71.6
  use (of)
    insulin pump Z46.81
  victim (of)
    abuse Z69.81
    child abuse
      by parent Z69.010
      non-parental Z69.020
    rape NEC Z69.81
Coupled rhythm R00.8
Couvelaire syndrome or uterus
  (complicating delivery) O45.8x-
Cowper's gland — *see* condition
Cowperitis — *see* Urethritis
Cowpox B08.010
  due to vaccination T88.1
Coxa
  magna M91.4-
  plana M91.2-
  valga (acquired) — *see also* Deformity, limb,
    specified type NEC, thigh
    congenital Q65.81
    sequelae (late effect) of rickets E64.3
  vara (acquired) — *see also* Deformity, limb,
    specified type NEC, thigh
    congenital Q65.82
    sequelae (late effect) of rickets E64.3
Coxalgia, coxalgic (nontuberculous) — *see also*
  Pain, joint, hip
  tuberculous A18.02
Coxitis — *see* Monoarthritis, hip
Coxsackie (virus) (infection) B34.1
  as cause of disease classified elsewhere
    B97.11
  carditis B33.20
  central nervous system NEC A88.8
  endocarditis B33.21
  enteritis A08.39
  meningitis (aseptic) A87.0
  myocarditis B33.22
  pericarditis B33.23
  pharyngitis B08.5
  pleurodynia B33.0
  specific disease NEC B33.8
Crabs, meaning pubic lice B85.3
Crack baby P04.41
Cracked nipple N64.0
  associated with
    lactation O92.13
    pregnancy O92.11-
    puerperium O92.12
Cracked tooth K03.81
Cradle cap L21.0
Craft neurosis F48.8

Cramp(s) R25.2
  abdominal — *see* Pain, abdominal
  bathing T75.1
  colic R10.83
    psychogenic F45.8
  due to immersion T75.1
  fireman T67.2
  heat T67.2
  immersion T75.1
  intestinal — *see* Pain, abdominal
    psychogenic F45.8
  leg, sleep related G47.62
  limb (lower) (upper) NEC R25.2
    sleep related G47.62
  linotypist's F48.8
    organic G25.89
  muscle (limb) (general) R25.2
    due to immersion T75.1
    psychogenic F45.8
  occupational (hand) F48.8
    organic G25.89
  salt-depletion E87.1
  sleep related, leg G47.62
  stoker's T67.2
  swimmer's T75.1
  telegrapher's F48.8
    organic G25.89
  typist's F48.8
    organic G25.89
  uterus N94.89
    menstrual — *see* Dysmenorrhea
  writer's F48.8
    organic G25.89
Cranial — *see* condition
Craniocleidodysostosis Q74.0
Craniofenestria (skull) Q75.8
Craniolacunia (skull) Q75.8
Craniopagus Q89.4
Craniopathy, metabolic M85.2
Craniopharyngeal — *see* condition
Craniopharyngioma D44.4
Craniorachischisis (totalis) Q00.1
Cranioschisis Q75.8
Craniostenosis Q75.0
Craniosynostosis Q75.0
Craniotabes (cause unknown) M83.8
  neonatal P96.3
  rachitic E64.3
  syphilitic A50.56
Cranium — *see* condition
Craw-craw — *see* Onchocerciasis
Creaking joint — *see* Derangement, joint,
  specified type NEC
Creeping
  eruption B76.9
  palsy or paralysis G12.22
Crenated tongue K14.8
Creotoxism A05.9
Crepitus
  caput Q75.8
  joint — *see* Derangement, joint, specified type
    NEC
Crescent or conus choroid, congenital
  Q14.3
CREST syndrome M34.1
Cretin, cretinism (congenital) (endemic)
  (nongoitrous) (sporadic) E00.9
  pelvis
    with disproportion (fetopelvic) O33.0
      causing obstructed labor O65.0
  type
    hypothyroid E00.1
    mixed E00.2
    myxedematous E00.1
    neurological E00.0

Creutzfeldt-Jakob disease or syndrome
  (with dementia) A81.00
  familial A81.09
  iatrogenic A81.09
  specified NEC A81.09
  sporadic A81.09
  variant (vCJD) A81.01
Cri-du-chat syndrome Q93.4
Crib death R99
Cribriform hymen Q52.3
Crigler-Najjar disease or syndrome
  E80.5
Crime, victim of Z65.4
Crimean hemorrhagic fever A98.0
Criminalism F60.2
Crisis
  abdomen R10.0
  acute reaction F43.0
  addisonian E27.2
  adrenal (cortical) E27.2
  celiac K90.0
  Dietl's N13.8
  emotional — *see also* Disorder, adjustment
    acute reaction to stress F43.0
    specific to childhood and adolescence F93.8
  glaucomatocyclitic — *see* Glaucoma,
    secondary, inflammation
  heart — *see* Failure, heart
  nitritoid I95.2
    correct substance properly administered —
      see Table of Drugs and Chemicals, by
      drug, adverse effect
    overdose or wrong substance given or taken
      — *see* Table of Drugs and Chemicals, by
      drug, poisoning
  oculogyric H51.8
    psychogenic F45.8
  Pel's (tabetic) A52.11
  psychosexual identity F64.2
  renal N28.0
  sickle-cell D57.00
    with
      acute chest syndrome D57.01
      splenic sequestration D57.02
  state (acute reaction) F43.0
  tabetic A52.11
  thyroid — *see* Thyrotoxicosis with thyroid storm
  thyrotoxic — *see* Thyrotoxicosis with thyroid
    storm
Crocq's disease (acrocyanosis) I73.89
Crohn's disease — *see* Enteritis, regional
Crooked septum, nasal J34.2
Cross syndrome E70.328
Crossbite (anterior) (posterior) M26.24
Cross-eye — *see* Strabismus, convergent
  concomitant
Croup, croupous (catarrhal) (infectious)
  (inflammatory) (nondiphtheritic) J05.0
  bronchial J20.9
  diphtheritic A36.2
  false J38.5
  spasmodic J38.5
    diphtheritic A36.2
  stridulous J38.5
    diphtheritic A36.2
Crouzon's disease Q75.1
Crowding, tooth, teeth, fully erupted
  M26.31
CRST syndrome M34.1
Cruchet's disease A85.8
Cruelty in children — *see also* Disorder,
  conduct
Crural ulcer — *see* Ulcer, lower limb
Crush, crushed, crushing T14.8
  abdomen S38.1
  ankle S97.0-
  arm (upper) (and shoulder) S47-
  axilla — *see* Crush, arm

DISEASE INDEX

Crush, crushed, crushing — *continued*
back, lower S38.1
buttock S38.1
cheek S07.0
chest S28.0
cranium S07.1
ear S07.0
elbow S57.0-
extremity
  lower
    ankle — *see* Crush, ankle
    below knee — *see* Crush, leg
    foot — *see* Crush, foot
    hip — *see* Crush, hip
    knee — *see* Crush, knee
    thigh — *see* Crush, thigh
    toe — *see* Crush, toe
  upper
    below elbow S67.9-
    elbow — *see* Crush, elbow
    finger — *see* Crush, finger
    forearm — *see* Crush, forearm
    hand — *see* Crush, hand
    thumb — *see* Crush, thumb
    upper arm — *see* Crush, arm
    wrist — *see* Crush, wrist
face S07.0
finger(s) S67.1-
  with hand (and wrist) — *see* Crush, hand, specified site NEC
  index S67.19-
  little S67.19-
  middle S67.19-
  ring S67.19-
  thumb — *see* Crush, thumb
foot S97.8-
  toe — *see* Crush, toe
forearm S57.8-
genitalia, external
  female S38.002
    vagina S38.03
    vulva S38.03
  male S38.001
    penis S38.01
    scrotum S38.02
    testis S38.02
hand (except fingers alone) S67.2-
  with wrist S67.4-
head S07.9
  specified NEC S07.8
heel — *see* Crush, foot
hip S77.0-
  with thigh S77.2-
internal organ (abdomen, chest, or pelvis) NEC T14.8
knee S87.0-
labium (majus) (minus) S38.03
larynx S17.0
leg (lower) S87.8-
  knee — *see* Crush, knee
lip S07.0
lower
  back S38.1
  leg — *see* Crush, leg
neck S17.9
nerve — *see* Injury, nerve
nose S07.0
pelvis S38.1
penis S38.01
scalp S07.8
scapular region — *see* Crush, arm
scrotum S38.02
severe, unspecified site T14.8
shoulder (and upper arm) — *see* Crush, arm
skull S07.1
syndrome (complication of trauma) T79.5
testis S38.02

Crush, crushed, crushing — *continued*
thigh S77.1-
  with hip S77.2-
throat S17.8
thumb S67.0-
  with hand (and wrist) — *see* Crush, hand, specified site NEC
toe(s) S97.10-
  great S97.11-
  lesser S97.12-
trachea S17.0
vagina S38.03
vulva S38.03
wrist S67.3-
  with hand S67.4-
Crusta lactea L21.0
Crusts R23.4
Crutch paralysis — *see* Injury, brachial plexus
Cruveilhier's atrophy or disease G12.8
Cruveilhier-Baumgarten cirrhosis, disease or syndrome K74.69
Crying (constant) (continuous) (excessive)
child, adolescent, or adult R45.83
infant (baby) (newborn) R68.11
Cryofibrinogenemia D89.2
Cryoglobulinemia (essential) (idiopathic) (mixed) (primary) (purpura) (secondary) (vasculitis) D89.1
with lung involvement D89.1 *[J99]*
Cryptitis (anal) (rectal) K62.89
Cryptococcosis, cryptococcus (infection) (neoformans) B45.9
bone B45.3
cerebral B45.1
cutaneous B45.2
disseminated B45.7
generalized B45.7
meningitis B45.1
meningocerebralis B45.1
osseous B45.3
pulmonary B45.0
skin B45.2
specified NEC B45.8
Cryptopapillitis (anus) K62.89
Cryptophthalmos Q11.2
syndrome Q87.0
Cryptorchid, cryptorchism, cryptorchidism Q53.9
bilateral Q53.20
  abdominal Q53.21
  perineal Q53.22
unilateral Q53.10
  abdominal Q53.11
  perineal Q53.12
Cryptosporidiosis A07.2
hepatobiliary B88.8
respiratory B88.8
Cryptostromosis J67.6
Crystalluria R82.99
Cubitus
congenital Q68.8
valgus (acquired) M21.0-
  congenital Q68.8
  sequelae (late effect) of rickets E64.3
varus (acquired) M21.1-
  congenital Q68.8
  sequelae (late effect) of rickets E64.3
Cultural deprivation or shock Z60.3
Curling esophagus K22.4
Curling's ulcer — *see* Ulcer, peptic, acute
Curschmann (-Batten) (-Steinert) disease or syndrome G71.11
Curse, Ondine's — *see* Apnea, sleep
Curvature
organ or site, congenital NEC — *see* Distortion
  penis (lateral) Q55.61
Pott's (spinal) A18.01
radius, idiopathic, progressive (congenital) Q74.0

Curvature — *continued*
spine (acquired) (angular) (idiopathic) (incorrect) (postural) — *see* Dorsopathy, deforming
  congenital Q67.5
  due to or associated with
    Charcot-Marie-Tooth disease (*see also* subcategory M49.8) G60.0
    osteitis
      deformans M88.88
      fibrosa cystica (*see also* subcategory M49.8) E21.0
    tuberculosis (Pott's curvature) A18.01
  sequelae (late effect) of rickets E64.3
  tuberculous A18.01
Cushing's
syndrome or disease E24.9
  drug-induced E24.2
  iatrogenic E24.2
  pituitary-dependent E24.0
  specified NEC E24.8
ulcer — *see* Ulcer, peptic, acute
Cushingoid due to steroid therapy E24.2
correct substance properly administered — *see* Table of Drugs and Chemicals, by drug, adverse effect
overdose or wrong substance given or taken — *see* Table of Drugs and Chemicals, by drug, poisoning
Cusp, Carabelli — *omit code*
Cut (external) — *see also* Laceration
muscle — *see* Injury, muscle
Cutaneous — *see also* condition
hemorrhage R23.3
larva migrans B76.9
Cutis — *see also* condition
hyperelastica Q82.8
  acquired L57.4
laxa (hyperelastica) — *see* Dermatolysis
marmorata R23.8
osteosis L94.2
pendula — *see* Dermatolysis
rhomboidalis nuchae L57.2
verticis gyrata Q82.8
  acquired L91.8
Cyanosis R23.0
due to
  patent foramen botalli Q21.1
  persistent foramen ovale Q21.1
enterogenous D74.8
paroxysmal digital — *see* Raynaud's disease
  with gangrene I73.01
retina, retinal H35.89
Cyanotic heart disease I24.9
congenital Q24.9
Cycle
anovulatory N97.0
menstrual, irregular N92.6
Cyclencephaly Q04.9
Cyclical vomiting (*see also* Vomiting, cyclical) G43.A0 *(follows G43.7)*
psychogenic F50.89
Cyclitis (*see also* Iridocyclitis) H20.9
chronic — *see* Iridocyclitis, chronic
Fuchs' heterochromic H20.81-
granulomatous — *see* Iridocyclitis, chronic
lens-induced — *see* Iridocyclitis, lens-induced
posterior H30.2-
Cycloid personality F34.0
Cyclophoria H50.54
Cyclopia, cyclops Q87.0
Cyclopism Q87.0
Cyclosporiasis A07.4
Cyclothymia F34.0
Cyclothymic personality F34.0
Cyclotropia H50.41-

Cylindroma — see also Neoplasm, malignant, by site
eccrine dermal — see Neoplasm, skin, benign
skin — see Neoplasm, skin, benign
Cylindruria R82.99
Cynanche
diphtheritic A36.2
tonsillaris J36
Cynophobia F40.218
Cynorexia R63.2
Cyphosis — see Kyphosis
Cyprus fever — see Brucellosis
Cyst (colloid) (mucous) (simple) (retention)
adenoid (infected) J35.8
adrenal gland E27.8
congenital Q89.1
air, lung J98.4
allantoic Q64.4
alveolar process (jaw bone) M27.40
amnion, amniotic O41.8x-
aneurysmal M27.49
anterior
chamber (eye) — see Cyst, iris
nasopalatine K09.1
antrum J34.1
anus K62.89
apical (tooth) (periodontal) K04.8
appendix K38.8
arachnoid, brain (acquired) G93.0
congenital Q04.6
arytenoid J38.7
Baker's M71.2-
ruptured M66.0
tuberculous A18.02
Bartholin's gland N75.0
bile duct (common) (hepatic) K83.5
bladder (multiple) (trigone) N32.89
blue dome (breast) — see Cyst, breast
bone (local) NEC M85.60
aneurysmal M85.50
ankle M85.57-
foot M85.57-
forearm M85.53-
hand M85.54-
jaw M27.49
lower leg M85.56-
multiple site M85.59
neck M85.58
rib M85.58
shoulder M85.51-
skull M85.58
specified site NEC M85.58
thigh M85.55-
toe M85.57-
upper arm M85.52-
vertebra M85.58
solitary M85.40
ankle M85.47-
fibula M85.46-
foot M85.47-
hand M85.44-
humerus M85.42-
jaw M27.49
neck M85.48
pelvis M85.45-
radius M85.43-
rib M85.48
shoulder M85.41-
skull M85.48
specified site NEC M85.48
tibia M85.46-
toe M85.47-
ulna M85.43-
vertebra M85.48

Cyst (colloid) (mucous) (simple) (retention) — continued
bone (local) NEC M85.60 — continued
specified type NEC M85.60
ankle M85.67-
foot M85.67-
forearm M85.63-
hand M85.64-
jaw M27.40
developmental (nonodontogenic) K09.1
odontogenic K09.0
latent M27.0
lower leg M85.66-
multiple site M85.69
neck M85.68
rib M85.68
shoulder M85.61-
skull M85.68
specified site NEC M85.68
thigh M85.65-
toe M85.67-
upper arm M85.62-
vertebra M85.68
brain (acquired) G93.0
congenital Q04.6
hydatid B67.99 [G94]
third ventricle (colloid), congenital Q04.6
branchial (cleft) Q18.0
branchiogenic Q18.0
breast (benign) (blue dome) (pedunculated) (solitary) N60.0-
involution — see Dysplasia, mammary, specified type NEC
sebaceous — see Dysplasia, mammary, specified type NEC
broad ligament (benign) N83.8
bronchogenic (mediastinal) (sequestration) J98.4
congenital Q33.0
buccal K09.8
bulbourethral gland N36.8
bursa, bursal NEC M71.30
with rupture — see Rupture, synovium
ankle M71.37-
elbow M71.32-
foot M71.37-
hand M71.34-
hip M71.35-
multiple sites M71.39
pharyngeal J39.2
popliteal space — see Cyst, Baker's
shoulder M71.31-
specified site NEC M71.38
wrist M71.33-
calcifying odontogenic D16.5
upper jaw (bone) (maxilla) D16.4
canal of Nuck (female) N94.89
congenital Q52.4
canthus — see Cyst, conjunctiva
carcinomatous — see Neoplasm, malignant, by site
cauda equina G95.89
cavum septi pellucidi — see Cyst, brain
celomic (pericardium) Q24.8
cerebellopontine (angle) — see Cyst, brain
cerebellum — see Cyst, brain
cerebral — see Cyst, brain
cervical lateral Q18.0
cervix NEC N88.8
embryonic Q51.6
nabothian N88.8
chiasmal optic NEC — see Disorder, optic, chiasm
chocolate (ovary) N80.1
choledochus, congenital Q44.4
chorion O41.8x-
choroid plexus G93.0
ciliary body — see Cyst, iris
clitoris N90.7

Cyst (colloid) (mucous) (simple) (retention) — continued
colon K63.89
common (bile) duct K83.5
congenital NEC Q89.8
adrenal gland Q89.1
epiglottis Q31.8
esophagus Q39.8
fallopian tube Q50.4
kidney Q61.00
more than one (multiple) Q61.02
specified as polycystic Q61.3
adult type Q61.2
infantile type NEC Q61.19
collecting duct dilation Q61.11
solitary Q61.01
larynx Q31.8
liver Q44.6
lung Q33.0
mediastinum Q34.1
ovary Q50.1
oviduct Q50.4
periurethral (tissue) Q64.79
prepuce Q55.69
salivary gland (any) Q38.4
sublingual Q38.6
submaxillary gland Q38.6
thymus (gland) Q89.2
tongue Q38.3
ureterovesical orifice Q62.8
vulva Q52.79
conjunctiva H11.44-
cornea H18.89-
corpora quadrigemina G93.0
corpus
albicans N83.29-
luteum (hemorrhagic) (ruptured) N83.1-
Cowper's gland (benign) (infected) N36.8
cranial meninges G93.0
craniobuccal pouch E23.6
craniopharyngeal pouch E23.6
cystic duct K82.8
Cysticercus — see Cysticercosis
Dandy-Walker Q03.1
with spina bifida — see Spina bifida
dental (root) K04.8
developmental K09.0
eruption K09.0
primordial K09.0
dentigerous (mandible) (maxilla) K09.0
dermoid — see Neoplasm, benign, by site
with malignant transformation C56-
implantation
external area or site (skin) NEC L72.0
iris — see Cyst, iris, implantation
vagina N89.8
vulva N90.7
mouth K09.8
oral soft tissue K09.8
sacrococcygeal — see Cyst, pilonidal
developmental K09.1
odontogenic K09.0
oral region (nonodontogenic) K09.1
ovary, ovarian Q50.1
dura (cerebral) G93.0
spinal G96.19
ear (external) Q18.1
echinococcal — see Echinococcus
embryonic
cervix uteri Q51.6
fallopian tube Q50.4
vagina Q51.6
endometrium, endometrial (uterus) N85.8
ectopic — see Endometriosis
enterogenous Q43.8
epidermal, epidermoid (inclusion) (see also Cyst, skin) L72.0
mouth K09.8
oral soft tissue K09.8

D I S E A S E   I N D E X

Cyst (colloid) (mucous) (simple) (retention) — *continued*
- epididymis N50.3
- epiglottis J38.7
- epiphysis cerebri E34.8
- epithelial (inclusion) L72.0
- epoophoron Q50.5
- eruption K09.0
- esophagus K22.8
- ethmoid sinus J34.1
- external female genital organs NEC N90.7
- eye NEC H57.8
  - congenital Q15.8
- eyelid (sebaceous) H02.829
  - infected — *see* Hordeolum
  - left H02.826
    - lower H02.825
    - upper H02.824
  - right H02.823
    - lower H02.822
    - upper H02.821
- fallopian tube N83.8
  - congenital Q50.4
- fimbrial (twisted) Q50.4
- fissural (oral region) K09.1
- follicle (graafian) (hemorrhagic) N83.0-
  - nabothian N88.8
- follicular (atretic) (hemorrhagic) (ovarian) N83.0-
  - dentigerous K09.0
  - odontogenic K09.0
  - skin L72.9
    - specified NEC L72.8
- frontal sinus J34.1
- gallbladder K82.8
- ganglion — *see* Ganglion
- Gartner's duct Q52.4
- gingiva K09.0
- gland of Moll — *see* Cyst, eyelid
- globulomaxillary K09.1
- graafian follicle (hemorrhagic) N83.0-
- granulosal lutein (hemorrhagic) N83.1-
- hemangiomatous D18.00
  - intra-abdominal D18.03
  - intracranial D18.02
  - skin D18.01
  - specified site NEC D18.09
- hemorrhagic M27.49
- hydatid (*see also* Echinococcus) B67.90
  - brain B67.99 *[G94]*
  - liver (*see also* Cyst, liver, hydatid) B67.8
  - lung NEC B67.99 *[J99]*
  - Morgagni
    - female Q50.5
    - male (epididymal) Q55.4
      - testicular Q55.29
  - specified site NEC B67.99
- hymen N89.8
  - embryonic Q52.4
- hypopharynx J39.2
- hypophysis, hypophyseal (duct) (recurrent) E23.6
  - cerebri E23.6
- implantation (dermoid)
  - external area or site (skin) NEC L72.0
  - iris — *see* Cyst, iris, implantation
  - vagina N89.8
  - vulva N90.7
- incisive canal K09.1
- inclusion (epidermal) (epithelial) (epidermoid) (squamous) L72.0
  - not of skin — *code under* Cyst, by site
- intestine (large) (small) K63.89
- intracranial — *see* Cyst, brain
- intraligamentous — *see also* Disorder, ligament
  - knee — *see* Derangement, knee
- intrasellar E23.6

Cyst (colloid) (mucous) (simple) (retention) — *continued*
- iris H21.309
  - exudative H21.31-
  - idiopathic H21.30-
  - implantation H21.32-
  - parasitic H21.33-
  - pars plana (primary) H21.34-
    - exudative H21.35-
- jaw (bone) M27.40
  - aneurysmal M27.49
  - developmental (odontogenic) K09.0
  - fissural K09.1
  - hemorrhagic M27.49
  - traumatic M27.49
- joint NEC — *see* Disorder, joint, specified type NEC
- kidney (acquired) N28.1
  - calyceal — *see* Hydronephrosis
  - congenital Q61.00
  - more than one (multiple) Q61.02
    - specified as polycystic Q61.3
      - adult type (autosomal dominant) Q61.2
      - infantile type (autosomal recessive) NEC Q61.19
        - collecting duct dilation Q61.11
  - pyelogenic — *see* Hydronephrosis
  - simple N28.1
  - solitary (single) Q61.01
    - acquired N28.1
- labium (majus) (minus) N90.7
  - sebaceous N90.7
- lacrimal — *see also* Disorder, lacrimal system, specified NEC
  - gland H04.13-
  - passages or sac — *see* Disorder, lacrimal system, specified NEC
- larynx J38.7
- lateral periodontal K09.0
- lens H27.8
  - congenital Q12.8
- lip (gland) K13.0
- liver (idiopathic) (simple) K76.89
  - congenital Q44.6
  - hydatid B67.8
    - granulosus B67.0
    - multilocularis B67.5
- lung J98.4
  - congenital Q33.0
  - giant bullous J43.9
- lutein N83.1-
- lymphangiomatous D18.1
- lymphoepithelial, oral soft tissue K09.8
- macula — *see* Degeneration, macula, hole
- malignant — *see* Neoplasm, malignant, by site
- mammary gland — *see* Cyst, breast
- mandible M27.40
  - dentigerous K09.0
  - radicular K04.8
- maxilla M27.40
  - dentigerous K09.0
  - radicular K04.8
- medial, face and neck Q18.8
- median
  - anterior maxillary K09.1
  - palatal K09.1
- mediastinum, congenital Q34.1
- meibomian (gland) — *see* Chalazion
  - infected — *see* Hordeolum
- membrane, brain G93.0
- meninges (cerebral) G93.0
  - spinal G96.19
- meniscus, knee — *see* Derangement, knee, meniscus, cystic
- mesentery, mesenteric K66.8
  - chyle I89.8
- mesonephric duct
  - female Q50.5
  - male Q55.4

Cyst (colloid) (mucous) (simple) (retention) — *continued*
- milk N64.89
- Morgagni (hydatid)
  - female Q50.5
  - male (epididymal) Q55.4
    - testicular Q55.29
- mouth K09.8
- Müllerian duct Q50.4
  - appendix testis Q55.29
  - cervix Q51.6
  - fallopian tube Q50.4
  - female Q50.4
  - male Q55.29
  - prostatic utricle Q55.4
  - vagina (embryonal) Q52.4
- multilocular (ovary) D39.10
  - benign — *see* Neoplasm, benign, by site
- myometrium N85.8
- nabothian (follicle) (ruptured) N88.8
- nasoalveolar K09.1
- nasolabial K09.1
- nasopalatine (anterior) (duct) K09.1
- nasopharynx J39.2
- neoplastic — *see* Neoplasm, uncertain behavior, by site
  - benign — *see* Neoplasm, benign, by site
- nervous system NEC G96.8
- neuroenteric (congenital) Q06.8
- nipple — *see* Cyst, breast
- nose (turbinates) J34.1
  - sinus J34.1
- odontogenic, developmental K09.0
- omentum (lesser) K66.8
  - congenital Q45.8
- ora serrata — *see* Cyst, retina, ora serrata
- oral
  - region K09.9
    - developmental (nonodontogenic) K09.1
      - specified NEC K09.8
  - soft tissue K09.9
    - specified NEC K09.8
- orbit H05.81-
- ovary, ovarian (twisted) N83.20-
  - adherent N83.20-
  - chocolate N80.1
  - corpus
    - albicans N83.29-
    - luteum (hemorrhagic) N83.1-
  - dermoid D27.9
  - developmental Q50.1
  - due to failure of involution NEC N83.20-
  - endometrial N80.1
  - follicular (graafian) (hemorrhagic) N83.0-
  - hemorrhagic N83.20-
  - in pregnancy or childbirth O34.8-
    - with obstructed labor O65.5
  - multilocular D39.10
  - pseudomucinous D27.9
  - retention N83.29-
  - serous N83.20-
  - specified NEC N83.29-
  - theca lutein (hemorrhagic) N83.1-
  - tuberculous A18.18
- oviduct N83.8
- palate (median) (fissural) K09.1
- palatine papilla (jaw) K09.1
- pancreas, pancreatic (hemorrhagic) (true) K86.2
  - congenital Q45.2
  - false K86.3
- paralabral
  - hip M24.85-
  - shoulder S43.43-
- paramesonephric duct Q50.4
  - female Q50.4
  - male Q55.29
- paranephric N28.1
- paraphysis, cerebri, congenital Q04.6

Cyst (colloid) (mucous) (simple) (retention) — *continued*
  parasitic B89
  parathyroid (gland) E21.4
  paratubal N83.8
  paraurethral duct N36.8
  paroophoron Q50.5
  parotid gland K11.6
  parovarian Q50.5
  pelvis (female) N94.89
    in pregnancy or childbirth O34.8-
      causing obstructed labor O65.5
  penis (sebaceous) N48.89
  periapical K04.8
  pericardial, congenital Q24.8
    acquired (secondary) I31.8
  pericoronal K09.0
  periodontal K04.8
    lateral K09.0
  peripelvic (lymphatic) N28.1
  peritoneum K66.8
    chylous I89.8
  periventricular, acquired, newborn P91.1
  pharynx (wall) J39.2
  pilar L72.11
  pilonidal (infected) (rectum) L05.91
    with abscess L05.01
    malignant C44.59-
  pituitary (duct) (gland) E23.6
  placenta O43.19-
  pleura J94.8
  popliteal — *see* Cyst, Baker's
  porencephalic Q04.6
    acquired G93.0
  postanal (infected) — *see* Cyst, pilonidal
  postmastoidectomy cavity (mucosal) — *see* Complications, postmastoidectomy, cyst
  preauricular Q18.1
  prepuce N47.4
    congenital Q55.69
  primordial (jaw) K09.0
  prostate N42.83
  pseudomucinous (ovary) D27.9
  pupillary, miotic H21.27-
  radicular (residual) K04.8
  radiculodental K04.8
  ranular K11.8
  Rathke's pouch E23.6
  rectum (epithelium) (mucous) K62.89
  renal — *see* Cyst, kidney
  residual (radicular) K04.8
  retention (ovary) N83.29-
    salivary gland K11.6
  retina H33.19-
    ora serrata H33.11-
    parasitic H33.12-
  retroperitoneal K68.9
  sacrococcygeal (dermoid) — *see* Cyst, pilonidal
  salivary gland or duct (mucous extravasation or retention) K11.6
  Sampson's N80.1
  sclera H15.89
  scrotum L72.9
    sebaceous L72.3
  sebaceous (duct) (gland) L72.3
    breast — *see* Dysplasia, mammary, specified type NEC
    eyelid — *see* Cyst, eyelid
    genital organ NEC
      female N94.89
      male N50.89
    scrotum L72.3
  semilunar cartilage (knee) (multiple) — *see* Derangement, knee, meniscus, cystic
  seminal vesicle N50.89
  serous (ovary) N83.20-
  sinus (accessory) (nasal) J34.1
  Skene's gland N36.8

Cyst (colloid) (mucous) (simple) (retention) — *continued*
  skin L72.9
    breast — *see* Dysplasia, mammary, specified type NEC
    epidermal, epidermoid L72.0
    epithelial L72.0
    eyelid — *see* Cyst, eyelid
    genital organ NEC
      female N90.7
      male N50.89
    inclusion L72.0
    scrotum L72.9
    sebaceous L72.3
    sweat gland or duct L74.8
  solitary
    bone — *see* Cyst, bone, solitary
    jaw M27.40
    kidney N28.1
  spermatic cord N50.89
  sphenoid sinus J34.1
  spinal meninges G96.19
  spleen NEC D73.4
    congenital Q89.09
    hydatid (*see also* Echinococcus) B67.99 [D77]
  Stafne's M27.0
  subarachnoid intrasellar R93.0
  subcutaneous, pheomycotic (chromomycotic) B43.2
  subdural (cerebral) G93.0
    spinal cord G96.19
  sublingual gland K11.6
  submandibular gland K11.6
  submaxillary gland K11.6
  suburethral N36.8
  suprarenal gland E27.8
  suprasellar — *see* Cyst, brain
  sweat gland or duct L74.8
  synovial — *see also* Cyst, bursa
    ruptured — *see* Rupture, synovium
  tarsal — *see* Chalazion
  tendon (sheath) — *see* Disorder, tendon, specified type NEC
  testis N44.2
    tunica albuginea N44.1
  theca lutein (ovary) N83.1-
  Thornwaldt's J39.2
  thymus (gland) E32.8
  thyroglossal duct (infected) (persistent) Q89.2
  thyroid (gland) E04.1
  thyrolingual duct (infected) (persistent) Q89.2
  tongue K14.8
  tonsil J35.8
  tooth — *see* Cyst, dental
  Tornwaldt's J39.2
  trichilemmal (proliferating) L72.12
  trichodermal L72.12
  tubal (fallopian) N83.8
    inflammatory — *see* Salpingitis, chronic
  tubo-ovarian N83.8
    inflammatory N70.13
  tunica
    albuginea testis N44.1
    vaginalis N50.89
  turbinate (nose) J34.1
  Tyson's gland N48.89
  urachus, congenital Q64.4
  ureter N28.89
  ureterovesical orifice N28.89
  urethra, urethral (gland) N36.8
  uterine ligament N83.8
  uterus (body) (corpus) (recurrent) N85.8
    embryonic Q51.818
      cervix Q51.6
  vagina, vaginal (implantation) (inclusion) (squamous cell) (wall) N89.8
    embryonic Q52.4
  vallecula, vallecular (epiglottis) J38.7

Cyst (colloid) (mucous) (simple) (retention) — *continued*
  vesical (orifice) N32.89
  vitreous body H43.89
  vulva (implantation) (inclusion) N90.7
    congenital Q52.79
    sebaceous gland N90.7
  vulvovaginal gland N90.7
  wolffian
    female Q50.5
    male Q55.4

Cystadenocarcinoma — *see* Neoplasm, malignant, by site
  bile duct C22.1
  endometrioid — *see* Neoplasm, malignant, by site
    specified site — *see* Neoplasm, malignant, by site
    unspecified site
      female C56.9
      male C61
  mucinous
    papillary
      specified site — *see* Neoplasm, malignant, by site
      unspecified site C56.9
    specified site — *see* Neoplasm, malignant, by site
    unspecified site C56.9
  papillary
    mucinous
      specified site — *see* Neoplasm, malignant, by site
      unspecified site C56.9
    pseudomucinous
      specified site — *see* Neoplasm, malignant, by site
      unspecified site C56.9
    serous
      specified site — *see* Neoplasm, malignant, by site
      unspecified site C56.9
    specified site — *see* Neoplasm, malignant, by site
    unspecified site C56.9
  pseudomucinous
    papillary
      specified site — *see* Neoplasm, malignant, by site
      unspecified site C56.9
    specified site — *see* Neoplasm, malignant, by site
    unspecified site C56.9
  serous
    papillary
      specified site — *see* Neoplasm, malignant, by site
      unspecified site C56.9
    specified site — *see* Neoplasm, malignant, by site
    unspecified site C56.9

Cystadenofibroma
  clear cell — *see* Neoplasm, benign, by site
  endometrioid D27.9
    borderline malignancy D39.1-
    malignant C56-
  mucinous
    specified site — *see* Neoplasm, benign, by site
    unspecified site D27.9
  serous
    specified site — *see* Neoplasm, benign, by site
    unspecified site D27.9
  specified site — *see* Neoplasm, benign, by site
  unspecified site D27.9

Cystadenoma — *see also* Neoplasm, benign, by site
bile duct D13.4
endometrioid — *see* Neoplasm, benign, by site
    borderline malignancy — *see* Neoplasm, uncertain behavior, by site
malignant — *see* Neoplasm, malignant, by site
mucinous
    borderline malignancy
        ovary C56-
        specified site NEC — *see* Neoplasm, uncertain behavior, by site
        unspecified site C56.9
    papillary
        borderline malignancy
            ovary C56-
            specified site NEC — *see* Neoplasm, uncertain behavior, by site
            unspecified site C56.9
        specified site — *see* Neoplasm, benign, by site
        unspecified site D27.9
    specified site — *see* Neoplasm, benign, by site
    unspecified site D27.9
papillary
    borderline malignancy
        ovary C56-
        specified site NEC — *see* Neoplasm, uncertain behavior, by site
        unspecified site C56.9
    lymphomatosum
        specified site — *see* Neoplasm, benign, by site
        unspecified site D11.9
    mucinous
        borderline malignancy
            ovary C56-
            specified site NEC — *see* Neoplasm, uncertain behavior, by site
            unspecified site C56.9
        specified site — *see* Neoplasm, benign, by site
        unspecified site D27.9
    pseudomucinous
        borderline malignancy
            ovary C56-
            specified site NEC — *see* Neoplasm, uncertain behavior, by site
            unspecified site C56.9
        specified site — *see* Neoplasm, benign, by site
        unspecified site D27.9
    serous
        borderline malignancy
            ovary C56-
            specified site NEC — *see* Neoplasm, uncertain behavior, by site
            unspecified site C56.9
        specified site — *see* Neoplasm, benign, by site
        unspecified site D27.9
    specified site — *see* Neoplasm, benign, by site
    unspecified site D27.9

Cystadenoma — *see also* Neoplasm, benign, by site — *continued*
pseudomucinous
    borderline malignancy
        ovary C56-
        specified site NEC — *see* Neoplasm, uncertain behavior, by site
        unspecified site C56.9
    papillary
        borderline malignancy
            ovary C56-
            specified site NEC — *see* Neoplasm, uncertain behavior, by site
            unspecified site C56.9
        specified site — *see* Neoplasm, benign, by site
        unspecified site D27.9
    specified site — *see* Neoplasm, benign, by site
    unspecified site D27.9
serous
    borderline malignancy
        ovary C56-
        specified site NEC — *see* Neoplasm, uncertain behavior, by site
        unspecified site C56.9
    papillary
        borderline malignancy
            ovary C56-
            specified site NEC — *see* Neoplasm, uncertain behavior, by site
            unspecified site C56.9
        specified site — *see* Neoplasm, benign, by site
        unspecified site D27.9
    specified site — *see* Neoplasm, benign, by site
    unspecified site D27.9

Cystathionine synthase deficiency E72.11
Cystathioninemia E72.19
Cystathioninuria E72.19
Cystic — *see also* condition
breast (chronic) — *see* Mastopathy, cystic
corpora lutea (hemorrhagic) N83.1-
duct — *see* condition
eyeball (congenital) Q11.0
fibrosis — *see* Fibrosis, cystic
kidney (congenital) Q61.9
    adult type Q61.2
    infantile type NEC Q61.19
        collecting duct dilatation Q61.11
    medullary Q61.5
liver, congenital Q44.6
lung disease J98.4
    congenital Q33.0
mastitis, chronic — *see* Mastopathy, cystic
medullary, kidney Q61.5
meniscus — *see* Derangement, knee, meniscus, cystic
ovary N83.20-
Cysticercosis, cysticerciasis B69.9
with
    epileptiform fits B69.0
    myositis B69.81
brain B69.0
central nervous system B69.0
cerebral B69.0
ocular B69.1
specified NEC B69.89
Cysticercus cellulose infestation — *see* Cysticercosis
Cystinosis (malignant) E72.04
Cystinuria E72.01

Cystitis (exudative) (hemorrhagic) (septic) (suppurative) N30.90
with
    fibrosis — *see* Cystitis, chronic, interstitial
    hematuria N30.91
    leukoplakia — *see* Cystitis, chronic, interstitial
    malakoplakia — *see* Cystitis, chronic, interstitial
    metaplasia — *see* Cystitis, chronic, interstitial
    prostatitis N41.3
acute N30.00
    with hematuria N30.01
    of trigone N30.30
        with hematuria N30.31
allergic — *see* Cystitis, specified type NEC
amebic A06.81
bilharzial B65.9 *[N33]*
blennorrhagic (gonococcal) A54.01
bullous — *see* Cystitis, specified type NEC
calculous N21.0
chlamydial A56.01
chronic N30.20
    with hematuria N30.21
    interstitial N30.10
        with hematuria N30.11
    of trigone N30.30
        with hematuria N30.31
    specified NEC N30.20
        with hematuria N30.21
cystic(a) — *see* Cystitis, specified type NEC
diphtheritic A36.85
echinococcal
    granulosus B67.39
    multilocularis B67.69
emphysematous — *see* Cystitis, specified type NEC
encysted — *see* Cystitis, specified type NEC
eosinophilic — *see* Cystitis, specified type NEC
follicular — *see* Cystitis, of trigone
gangrenous — *see* Cystitis, specified type NEC
glandularis — *see* Cystitis, specified type NEC
gonococcal A54.01
incrusted — *see* Cystitis, specified type NEC
interstitial (chronic) — *see* Cystitis, chronic, interstitial
irradiation N30.40
    with hematuria N30.41
irritation — *see* Cystitis, specified type NEC
malignant — *see* Cystitis, specified type NEC
of trigone N30.30
    with hematuria N30.31
panmural — *see* Cystitis, chronic, interstitial
polyposa — *see* Cystitis, specified type NEC
prostatic N41.3
puerperal (postpartum) O86.22
radiation — *see* Cystitis, irradiation
specified type NEC N30.80
    with hematuria N30.81
subacute — *see* Cystitis, chronic
submucous — *see* Cystitis, chronic, interstitial
syphilitic (late) A52.76
trichomonal A59.03
tuberculous A18.12
ulcerative — *see* Cystitis, chronic, interstitial
Cystocele(-urethrocele)
female N81.10
    with prolapse of uterus — *see* Prolapse, uterus
    lateral N81.12
    midline N81.11
    paravaginal N81.12
in pregnancy or childbirth O34.8-
    causing obstructed labor O65.5
male N32.89
Cystolithiasis N21.0

Cystoma — *see also* Neoplasm, benign, by site
endometrial, ovary N80.1
mucinous
  specified site — *see* Neoplasm, benign, by
    site
  unspecified site D27.9
serous
  specified site — *see* Neoplasm, benign, by
    site
  unspecified site D27.9
simple (ovary) N83.29-
Cystoplegia N31.2
Cystoptosis N32.89
Cystopyelitis — *see* Pyelonephritis
Cystorrhagia N32.89
Cystosarcoma phyllodes D48.6-
benign D24-
malignant — *see* Neoplasm, breast, malignant
Cystostomy
attention to Z43.5
complication — *see* Complications, cystostomy
status Z93.50
  appendico-vesicostomy Z93.52
  cutaneous Z93.51
  specified NEC Z93.59
Cystourethritis — *see* Urethritis
Cystourethrocele — *see also* Cystocele
female N81.10
  with uterine prolapse — *see* Prolapse, uterus
  lateral N81.12
  midline N81.11
  paravaginal N81.12
male N32.89
Cytomegalic inclusion disease
congenital P35.1
Cytomegalovirus infection B25.9
Cytomycosis (reticuloendothelial) B39.4
Cytopenia D75.9
refractory
  with multilineage dysplasia D46.A *(follows*
    D46.2)
    and ring sideroblasts (RCMD RS) D46.B
      (follows D46.2)
Czerny's disease (periodic hydrarthrosis of
the knee) — *see* Effusion, joint, knee

D

Da Costa's syndrome F45.8
Daae (-Finsen) disease (epidemic
pleurodynia) B33.0
Dabney's grip B33.0
Dacryoadenitis, dacryadenitis H04.00-
acute H04.01-
chronic H04.02-
Dacryocystitis H04.30-
acute H04.32-
chronic H04.41-
neonatal P39.1
phlegmonous H04.31-
syphilitic A52.71
  congenital (early) A50.01
trachomatous, active A71.1
  sequelae (late effect) B94.0
Dacryocystoblenorrhea — *see* Inflammation,
lacrimal, passages, chronic
Dacryocystocele — *see* Disorder, lacrimal
system, changes
Dacryolith, dacryolithiasis H04.51-
Dacryoma — *see* Disorder, lacrimal system,
changes
Dacryopericystitis — *see* Dacryocystitis
Dacryops H04.11-
Dacryostenosis — *see also* Stenosis, lacrimal
congenital Q10.5
Dactylitis
bone — *see* Osteomyelitis
sickle-cell D57.00
  Hb C D57.219
  Hb SS D57.00
  specified NEC D57.819
skin L08.9
syphilitic A52.77
tuberculous A18.03
Dactylolysis spontanea (ainhum) L94.6
Dactylosymphysis Q70.9
fingers — *see* Syndactylism, complex, fingers
toes — *see* Syndactylism, complex, toes
Damage
arteriosclerotic — *see* Arteriosclerosis
brain (nontraumatic) G93.9
  anoxic, hypoxic G93.1
    resulting from a procedure G97.82
  child NEC G80.9
  due to birth injury P11.2
cardiorenal (vascular) — *see* Hypertension,
  cardiorenal
cerebral NEC — *see* Damage, brain
coccyx, complicating delivery O71.6
coronary — *see* Disease, heart, ischemic
eye, birth injury P15.3
liver (nontraumatic) K76.9
  alcoholic K70.9
  due to drugs — *see* Disease, liver, toxic
  toxic — *see* Disease, liver, toxic
medication T88.7
pelvic
  joint or ligament, during delivery O71.6
  organ NEC
    during delivery O71.5
    following ectopic or molar pregnancy
      O08.6
renal — *see* Disease, renal
subendocardium, subendocardial — *see*
  Degeneration, myocardial
vascular I99.9
Dana-Putnam syndrome (subacute
combined sclerosis with pernicious anemia)
— *see* Degeneration, combined
Danbolt (-Cross) syndrome (acrodermatitis
enteropathica) E83.2
Dandruff L21.0
Dandy-Walker syndrome Q03.1
with spina bifida — *see* Spina bifida

Danlos' syndrome Q79.6
Darier-Roussy sarcoid D86.3
Darier(-White) disease (congenital) Q82.8
meaning erythema annulare centrifugum L53.1
Darling's disease or histoplasmosis B39.4
Darwin's tubercle Q17.8
Dawson's (inclusion body) encephalitis
A81.1
De Beurmann(-Gougerot) disease B42.1
De la Tourette's syndrome F95.2
De Lange's syndrome Q87.1
De Morgan's spots (senile angiomas) I78.1
De Quervain's
disease (tendon sheath) M65.4
syndrome E34.51
thyroiditis (subacute granulomatous thyroiditis)
  E06.1
De Toni-Fanconi(-Debré) syndrome
E72.09
with cystinosis E72.04
Dead
fetus, retained (mother) O36.4
  early pregnancy O02.1
labyrinth — *see* subcategory H83.2
ovum, retained O02.0
Deaf nonspeaking NEC H91.3
Deafmutism (acquired) (congenital) NEC
H91.3
hysterical F44.6
syphilitic, congenital (*see also* subcategory
  H94.8) A50.09
Deafness (acquired) (complete) (hereditary)
(partial) H91.9-
with blue sclera and fragility of bone Q78.0
auditory fatigue — *see* Deafness, specified
  type NEC
aviation T70.0
  nerve injury — *see* Injury, nerve, acoustic,
    specified type NEC
boilermaker's — *see* subcategory H83.3
central — *see* Deafness, sensorineural
conductive H90.2
  and sensorineural
    mixed H90.8
      bilateral H90.6
  bilateral H90.0
  unilateral H90.1-
    with restricted hearing on the contralateral
      side H90.A- *(follows H90.8)*
congenital H90.5
  with blue sclera and fragility of bone Q78.0
due to toxic agents — *see* Deafness, ototoxic
emotional (hysterical) F44.6
functional (hysterical) F44.6
high frequency H91.9-
hysterical F44.6
low frequency H91.9-
mental R48.8
mixed conductive and sensorineural H90.8
  bilateral H90.6
  unilateral H90.7-
nerve — *see* Deafness, sensorineural
neural — *see* Deafness, sensorineural
noise-induced (*see also* subcategory) H83.3
  nerve injury — *see* Injury, nerve, acoustic,
    specified type NEC
nonspeaking H91.3
ototoxic — *see* subcategory H91.0
perceptive — *see* Deafness, sensorineural
psychogenic (hysterical) F44.6
sensorineural H90.5
  and conductive
    mixed H90.8
      bilateral H90.6
  bilateral H90.3
  unilateral H90.4-
    with restricted hearing on the contralateral
      side H90.A- *(follows H90.8)*
sensory — *see* Deafness, sensorineural

Deafness (acquired) (complete) (hereditary) (partial) H91.9- — *continued*
　specified type NEC — *see* subcategory H91.8
　sudden (idiopathic) H91.2-
　syphilitic A52.15
　transient ischemic H93.01-
　traumatic — *see* Injury, nerve, acoustic, specified type NEC
　word (developmental) H93.25
Death (cause unknown) (of) (unexplained) (unspecified cause) R99
　brain G93.82
　cardiac (sudden) (with successful resuscitation) — *code to* underlying disease
　　family history of Z82.41
　　personal history of Z86.74
　family member (assumed) Z63.4
Debility (chronic) (general) (nervous) R53.81
　congenital or neonatal NOS P96.9
　nervous R53.81
　old age R54
　senile R54
Débove's disease (splenomegaly) R16.1
Decalcification
　bone — *see* Osteoporosis
　teeth K03.89
Decapsulation, kidney N28.89
Decay
　dental — *see* Caries, dental
　senile R54
　tooth, teeth — *see* Caries, dental
Deciduitis (acute)
　following ectopic or molar pregnancy O08.0
Decline (general) — *see* Debility
　cognitive, age-associated R41.81
Decompensation
　cardiac (acute) (chronic) — *see* Disease, heart
　cardiovascular — *see* Disease, cardiovascular
　heart — *see* Disease, heart
　hepatic — *see* Failure, hepatic
　myocardial (acute) (chronic) — *see* Disease, heart
　respiratory J98.8
Decompression sickness T70.3
Decrease(d)
　absolute neutrophile count — *see* Neutropenia
　blood
　　platelets — *see* Thrombocytopenia
　　pressure R03.1
　　　due to shock following
　　　　injury T79.4
　　　　operation T81.19
　estrogen E28.39
　　postablative E89.40
　　　asymptomatic E89.40
　　　symptomatic E89.41
　fragility of erythrocytes D58.8
　function
　　lipase (pancreatic) K90.3
　　ovary in hypopituitarism E23.0
　　parenchyma of pancreas K86.89
　　pituitary (gland) (anterior) (lobe) E23.0
　　　posterior (lobe) E23.0
　functional activity R68.89
　glucose R73.09
　hematocrit R71.0
　hemoglobin R71.0
　leukocytes D72.819
　　specified NEC D72.818
　libido R68.82
　lymphocytes D72.810
　platelets D69.6
　respiration, due to shock following injury T79.4
　sexual desire R68.82
　tear secretion NEC — *see* Syndrome, dry eye

Decrease(d) — *continued*
　tolerance
　　fat K90.49
　　glucose R73.09
　　pancreatic K90.3
　　salt and water E87.8
　vision NEC H54.7
　white blood cell count D72.819
　　specified NEC D72.818
Decubitus (ulcer) — *see* Ulcer, pressure, by site
　cervix N86
Deepening acetabulum — *see* Derangement, joint, specified type NEC, hip
Defect, defective Q89.9
　3-beta-hydroxysteroid dehydrogenase E25.0
　11-hydroxylase E25.0
　21-hydroxylase E25.0
　abdominal wall, congenital Q79.59
　antibody immunodeficiency D80.9
　aorticopulmonary septum Q21.4
　atrial septal (ostium secundum type) Q21.1
　　following acute myocardial infarction (current complication) I23.1
　　ostium primum type Q21.2
　atrioventricular
　　canal Q21.2
　　septum Q21.2
　auricular septal Q21.1
　bilirubin excretion NEC E80.6
　biosynthesis, androgen (testicular) E29.1
　bulbar septum Q21.0
　catalase E80.3
　cell membrane receptor complex (CR3) D71
　circulation I99.9
　　congenital Q28.9
　　newborn Q28.9
　coagulation (factor) (*see also* Deficiency, factor) D68.9
　　with
　　　ectopic pregnancy O08.1
　　　molar pregnancy O08.1
　　acquired D68.4
　　antepartum with hemorrhage — *see* Hemorrhage, antepartum, with coagulation defect
　　due to
　　　liver disease D68.4
　　　vitamin K deficiency D68.4
　　hereditary NEC D68.2
　　intrapartum O67.0
　　newborn, transient P61.6
　　postpartum O72.3
　　specified type NEC D68.8
　complement system D84.1
　conduction (heart) I45.9
　　bone — *see* Deafness, conductive
　congenital, organ or site not listed — *see* Anomaly, by site
　coronary sinus Q21.1
　cushion, endocardial Q21.2
　degradation, glycoprotein E77.1
　dental bridge, crown, fillings — *see* Defect, dental restoration
　dental restoration K08.50
　　specified NEC K08.59
　dentin (hereditary) K00.5
　Descemet's membrane, congenital Q13.89
　developmental — *see also* Anomaly
　　cauda equina Q06.3
　diaphragm
　　with elevation, eventration or hernia — *see* Hernia, diaphragm
　　congenital Q79.1
　　　with hernia Q79.0
　　　gross (with hernia) Q79.0
　ectodermal, congenital Q82.9
　Eisenmenger's Q21.8

Defect, defective Q89.9 — *continued*
　enzyme
　　catalase E80.3
　　peroxidase E80.3
　esophagus, congenital Q39.9
　extensor retinaculum M62.89
　fibrin polymerization D68.2
　filling
　　bladder R93.41
　　kidney R93.42-
　　renal pelvis R93.41
　　stomach R93.3
　　ureter R93.41
　　urinary organs, specified NEC R93.49
　Gerbode Q21.0
　glycoprotein degradation E77.1
　Hageman (factor) D68.2
　hearing — *see* Deafness
　high grade F70
　interatrial septal Q21.1
　interauricular septal Q21.1
　interventricular septal Q21.0
　　with dextroposition of aorta, pulmonary stenosis and hypertrophy of right ventricle Q21.3
　　in tetralogy of Fallot Q21.3
　learning (specific) — *see* Disorder, learning
　lymphocyte function antigen-1 (LFA-1) D84.0
　lysosomal enzyme, post-translational modification E77.0
　major osseous M89.70
　　ankle M89.77-
　　carpus M89.74-
　　clavicle M89.71-
　　femur M89.75-
　　fibula M89.76-
　　fingers M89.74-
　　foot M89.77-
　　forearm M89.73-
　　hand M89.74-
　　humerus M89.72-
　　lower leg M89.76-
　　metacarpus M89.74-
　　metatarsus M89.77-
　　multiple sites M89.79
　　pelvic region M89.75-
　　pelvis M89.75-
　　radius M89.73-
　　scapula M89.71-
　　shoulder region M89.71-
　　specified NEC M89.78
　　tarsus M89.77-
　　thigh M89.75-
　　tibia M89.76-
　　toes M89.77-
　　ulna M89.73-
　mental — *see* Disability, intellectual
　modification, lysosomal enzymes, post-translational E77.0
　obstructive, congenital
　　renal pelvis Q62.39
　　ureter Q62.39
　　　atresia — *see* Atresia, ureter
　　　cecoureterocele Q62.32
　　　megaureter Q62.2
　　　orthotopic ureterocele Q62.31
　osseous, major M89.70
　　ankle M89.77-
　　carpus M89.74-
　　clavicle M89.71-
　　femur M89.75-
　　fibula M89.76-
　　fingers M89.74-
　　foot M89.77-
　　forearm M89.73-
　　hand M89.74-
　　humerus M89.72-
　　lower leg M89.76-
　　metacarpus M89.74-

Defect, defective Q89.9 — *continued*
osseous, major M89.70 — *continued*
metatarsus M89.77-
multiple sites M89.9
pelvic region M89.75-
pelvis M89.75-
radius M89.73-
scapula M89.71-
shoulder region M89.71-
specified NEC M89.78
tarsus M89.77-
thigh M89.75-
tibia M89.76-
toes M89.77-
ulna M89.73-
osteochondral NEC (*see also* Deformity) M95.8
ostium
primum Q21.2
secundum Q21.1
peroxidase E80.3
placental blood supply — *see* Insufficiency, placental
platelets, qualitative D69.1
constitutional D68.0
postural NEC, spine — *see* Dorsopathy, deforming
reduction
limb Q73.8
lower Q72.9-
absence — *see* Agenesis, leg
foot — *see* Agenesis, foot
longitudinal
femur Q72.4-
fibula Q72.6-
tibia Q72.5-
specified type NEC Q72.89-
split foot Q72.7-
specified type NEC Q73.8
upper Q71.9-
absence — *see* Agenesis, arm
forearm — *see* Agenesis, forearm
hand — *see* Agenesis, hand
lobster-claw hand Q71.6-
longitudinal
radius Q71.4-
ulna Q71.5-
specified type NEC Q71.89-
renal pelvis Q63.8
obstructive Q62.39
respiratory system, congenital Q34.9
restoration, dental K08.50
specified NEC K08.59
retinal nerve bundle fibers H35.89
septal (heart) NOS Q21.9
acquired (atrial) (auricular) (ventricular) (old) I51.0
atrial Q21.1
concurrent with acute myocardial infarction — *see* Infarct, myocardium
following acute myocardial infarction (current complication) I23.1
ventricular (*see also* Defect, ventricular septal) Q21.0
sinus venosus Q21.1
speech R47.9
developmental F80.9
specified NEC R47.89
Taussig-Bing (aortic transposition and overriding pulmonary artery) Q20.1
teeth, wedge K03.1
vascular (local) I99.9
congenital Q27.9
ventricular septal Q21.0
concurrent with acute myocardial infarction — *see* Infarct, myocardium
following acute myocardial infarction (current complication) I23.2
in tetralogy of Fallot Q21.3
vision NEC H54.7

Defect, defective Q89.9 — *continued*
visual field H53.40
bilateral
heteronymous H53.47
homonymous H53.46-
generalized contraction H53.48-
localized
arcuate H53.43-
scotoma (central area) H53.41-
blind spot area H53.42-
sector H53.43-
specified type NEC H53.45-
voice R49.9
specified NEC R49.8
wedge, tooth, teeth (abrasion) K03.1
Deferentitis N49.1
gonorrheal (acute) (chronic) A54.23
Defibrination (syndrome) D65
antepartum — *see* Hemorrhage, antepartum, with coagulation defect, disseminated intravascular coagulation
following ectopic or molar pregnancy O08.1
intrapartum O67.0
newborn P60
postpartum O72.3
Deficiency, deficient
3-beta hydroxysteroid dehydrogenase E25.0
5-alpha reductase (with male pseudohermaphroditism) E29.1
11-hydroxylase E25.0
21-hydroxylase E25.0
abdominal muscle syndrome Q79.4
AC globulin (congenital) (hereditary) D68.2
acquired D68.4
accelerator globulin (Ac G) (blood) D68.2
acid phosphatase E83.39
activating factor (blood) D68.2
adenosine deaminase (ADA) D81.3
aldolase (hereditary) E74.19
alpha-1-antitrypsin E88.01
amino-acids E72.9
anemia — *see* Anemia
aneurin E51.9
anti-hemophilic
factor (A) D66
B D67
C D68.1
globulin (AHG) NEC D66
antibody with
hyperimmunoglobulinemia D80.6
near-normal immunoglobins D80.6
antidiuretic hormone E23.2
antithrombin (antithrombin III) D68.59
ascorbic acid E54
attention (disorder) (syndrome) F98.8
with hyperactivity — *see* Disorder, attention-deficit hyperactivity
autoprothrombin
C D68.2
I D68.2
II D67
beta-glucuronidase E76.29
biotin E53.8
biotin-dependent carboxylase D81.819
biotinidase D81.810
brancher enzyme (amylopectinosis) E74.03
C1 esterase inhibitor (C1-INH) D84.1
calciferol E55.9
with
adult osteomalacia M83.8
rickets — *see* Rickets
calcium (dietary) E58
calorie, severe E43
with marasmus E41
and kwashiorkor E42
cardiac — *see* Insufficiency, myocardial

Deficiency, deficient — *continued*
carnitine E71.40
due to
hemodialysis E71.43
inborn errors of metabolism E71.42
Valproic acid therapy E71.43
iatrogenic E71.43
muscle palmityltransferase E71.314
primary E71.41
secondary E71.448
carotene E50.9
central nervous system G96.8
ceruloplasmin (Wilson) E83.01
choline E53.8
Christmas factor D67
chromium E61.4
clotting (blood) (*see also* Deficiency, coagulation factor) D68.9
clotting factor NEC (hereditary) (*see also* Deficiency, factor) D68.2
coagulation NOS D68.9
with
ectopic pregnancy O08.1
molar pregnancy O08.1
acquired (any) D68.4
antepartum hemorrhage — *see* Hemorrhage, antepartum, with coagulation defect
clotting factor NEC (*see also* Deficiency, factor) D68.2
due to
hyperprothrombinemia D68.4
liver disease D68.4
vitamin K deficiency D68.4
newborn, transient P61.6
postpartum O72.3
specified NEC D68.8
cognitive F09
color vision H53.50
achromatopsia H53.51
acquired H53.52
deuteranomaly H53.53
protanomaly H53.54
specified type NEC H53.59
tritanomaly H53.55
combined glucocorticoid and mineralocorticoid E27.49
contact factor D68.2
copper (nutritional) E61.0
corticoadrenal E27.40
primary E27.1
craniofacial axis Q75.0
cyanocobalamin E53.8
debrancher enzyme (limit dextrinosis) E74.03
dehydrogenase
long chain/very long chain acyl CoA E71.310
medium chain acyl CoA E71.311
short chain acyl CoA E71.312
diet E63.9
dihydropyrimidine dehydrogenase (DPD) E88.89
disaccharidase E73.9
edema — *see* Malnutrition, severe
endocrine E34.9
energy-supply — *see* Malnutrition
enzymes, circulating NEC E88.09
ergosterol E55.9
with
adult osteomalacia M83.8
rickets — *see* Rickets
essential fatty acid (EFA) E63.0
factor — *see also* Deficiency, coagulation
I (congenital) (hereditary) D68.2
II (congenital) (hereditary) D68.2
V (congenital) (hereditary) D68.2
VII (congenital) (hereditary) D68.2
VIII (congenital) (functional) (hereditary) (with functional defect) D66
with vascular defect D68.0

Deficiency, deficient — *continued*
factor — *see also* Deficiency, coagulation — *continued*
  IX (congenital) (functional) (hereditary) (with functional defect) D67
  X (congenital) (hereditary) D68.2
  XI (congenital) (hereditary) D68.1
  XII (congenital) (hereditary) D68.2
  XIII (congenital) (hereditary) D68.2
  Hageman D68.2
  multiple (congenital) D68.8
    acquired D68.4
femoral, proximal focal (congenital) — *see* Defect, reduction, lower limb, longitudinal, femur
fibrin-stabilizing factor (congenital) (hereditary) D68.2
  acquired D68.4
fibrinase D68.2
fibrinogen (congenital) (hereditary) D68.2
  acquired D65
folate E53.8
folic acid E53.8
foreskin N47.3
fructokinase E74.11
fructose 1,6-diphosphatase E74.19
fructose-1-phosphate aldolase E74.19
galactokinase E74.29
galactose-1-phosphate uridyl transferase E74.29
gammaglobulin in blood D80.1
  hereditary D80.0
glass factor D68.2
glucocorticoid E27.49
  mineralocorticoid E27.49
glucose-6-phosphatase E74.01
glucose-6-phosphate dehydrogenase anemia D55.0
glucuronyl transferase E80.5
glycogen synthetase E74.09
gonadotropin (isolated) E23.0
growth hormone (idiopathic) (isolated) E23.0
Hageman factor D68.2
hemoglobin D64.9
hepatophosphorylase E74.09
homogentisate 1,2-dioxygenase E70.29
hormone
  anterior pituitary (partial) NEC E23.0
    growth E23.0
  growth (isolated) E23.0
  pituitary E23.0
  testicular E29.1
hypoxanthine-(guanine)-phosphoribosyltransferase (HG-PRT) (total H-PRT) E79.1
immunity D84.9
  cell-mediated D84.8
    with thrombocytopenia and eczema D82.0
  combined D81.9
  humoral D80.9
  IgA (secretory) D80.2
  IgG D80.3
  IgM D80.4
immuno — *see* Immunodeficiency
immunoglobulin, selective
  A (IgA) D80.2
  G (IgG) (subclasses) D80.3
  M (IgM) D80.4
inositol (B complex) E53.8
intrinsic
  factor (congenital) D51.0
  sphincter N36.42
    with urethral hypermobility N36.43
iodine E61.8
  congenital syndrome — *see* Syndrome, iodine-deficiency, congenital
iron E61.1
  anemia D50.9
kalium E87.6
kappa-light chain D80.8

Deficiency, deficient — *continued*
labile factor (congenital) (hereditary) D68.2
  acquired D68.4
lacrimal fluid (acquired) — *see also* Syndrome, dry eye
  congenital Q10.6
lactase
  congenital E73.0
  secondary E73.1
Laki-Lorand factor D68.2
lecithin cholesterol acyltransferase E78.6
lipocaic K86.89
lipoprotein (familial) (high density) E78.6
liver phosphorylase E74.09
lysosomal alpha-1, 4 glucosidase E74.02
magnesium E61.2
major histocompatibility complex
  class I D81.6
  class II D81.7
manganese E61.3
menadione (vitamin K) E56.1
  newborn P53
mental (familial) (hereditary) — *see* Disability, intellectual
methylenetetrahydrofolate reductase (MTHFR) E72.12
mevalonate kinase M04.1
mineral NEC E61.8
mineralocorticoid E27.49
  with glucocorticoid E27.49
molybdenum (nutritional) E61.5
moral F60.2
multiple nutrient elements E61.7
muscle
  carnitine (palmityltransferase) E71.314
  phosphofructokinase E74.09
myoadenylate deaminase E79.2
myocardial — *see* Insufficiency, myocardial
myophosphorylase E74.04
NADH diaphorase or reductase (congenital) D74.0
NADH-methemoglobin reductase (congenital) D74.0
natrium E87.1
niacin (amide) (-tryptophan) E52
nicotinamide E52
nicotinic acid E52
number of teeth — *see* Anodontia
nutrient element E61.9
  multiple E61.7
  specified NEC E61.8
nutrition, nutritional E63.9
  sequelae — *see* Sequelae, nutritional deficiency
  specified NEC E63.8
of interleukin 1 receptor antagonist [DIRA] M04.8
ornithine transcarbamylase E72.4
ovarian E28.39
oxygen — *see* Anoxia
pantothenic acid E53.8
parathyroid (gland) E20.9
perineum (female) N81.89
phenylalanine hydroxylase E70.1
phosphoenolpyruvate carboxykinase E74.4
phosphofructokinase E74.19
phosphomannomutase E74.8
phosphomannose isomerase E74.8
phosphomannosyl mutase E74.8
phosphorylase kinase, liver E74.09
pituitary hormone (isolated) E23.0
plasma thromboplastin
  antecedent (PTA) D68.1
  component (PTC) D67
platelet NEC D69.1
  constitutional D68.0
polyglandular E31.8
  autoimmune E31.0
potassium (K) E87.6

Deficiency, deficient — *continued*
prepuce N47.3
proaccelerin (congenital) (hereditary) D68.2
  acquired D68.4
proconvertin factor (congenital) (hereditary) D68.2
  acquired D68.4
protein (*see also* Malnutrition) E46
  anemia D53.0
  C D68.59
  S D68.59
prothrombin (congenital) (hereditary) D68.2
  acquired D68.4
Prower factor D68.2
pseudocholinesterase E88.09
PTA (plasma thromboplastin antecedent) D68.1
PTC (plasma thromboplastin component) D67
purine nucleoside phosphorylase (PNP) D81.5
pyracin (alpha) (beta) E53.1
pyridoxal E53.1
pyridoxamine E53.1
pyridoxine (derivatives) E53.1
pyruvate
  carboxylase E74.4
  dehydrogenase E74.4
riboflavin (vitamin B2) E53.0
salt E87.1
secretion
  ovary E28.39
  salivary gland (any) K11.7
  urine R34
selenium (dietary) E59
serum antitrypsin, familial E88.01
short stature homeobox gene (SHOX)
  with
    dyschondrosteosis Q78.8
    short stature (idiopathic) E34.3
    Turner's syndrome Q96.9
sodium (Na) E87.1
SPCA (factor VII) D68.2
sphincter, intrinsic N36.42
  with urethral hypermobility N36.43
stable factor (congenital) (hereditary) D68.2
  acquired D68.4
Stuart-Prower (factor X) D68.2
sucrase E74.39
sulfatase E75.29
sulfite oxidase E72.19
thiamin, thiaminic (chloride) E51.9
  beriberi (dry) E51.11
    wet E51.12
thrombokinase D68.2
  newborn P53
thyroid (gland) — *see* Hypothyroidism
tocopherol E56.0
tooth bud K00.0
transcobalamine II (anemia) D51.2
vanadium E61.6
vascular I99.9
vasopressin E23.2
vertical ridge K06.8
viosterol — *see* Deficiency, calciferol
vitamin (multiple) NOS E56.9
  A E50.9
    with
      Bitot's spot (corneal) E50.1
      follicular keratosis E50.8
      keratomalacia E50.4
      manifestations NEC E50.8
      night blindness E50.5
      scar of cornea, xerophthalmic E50.6
      xeroderma E50.8
      xerophthalmia E50.7
      xerosis
        conjunctival E50.0
          and Bitot's spot E50.1
        cornea E50.2
          and ulceration E50.3
      sequelae E64.1

Deficiency, deficient — *continued*
  vitamin (multiple) NOS E56.9 — *continued*
    B (complex) NOS E53.9
      with
        beriberi (dry) E51.11
          wet E51.12
        pellagra E52
      B1 NOS E51.9
        beriberi (dry) E51.11
          with circulatory system manifestations E51.11
          wet E51.12
      B12 E53.8
      B2 (riboflavin) E53.0
      B6 E53.1
      C E54
        sequelae E64.2
      D E55.9
        with
          adult osteomalacia M83.8
          rickets — *see* Rickets
        25-hydroxylase E83.32
      E E56.0
      folic acid E53.8
      G E53.0
      group B E53.9
        specified NEC E53.8
      H (biotin) E53.8
      K E56.1
        of newborn P53
      nicotinic E52
      P E56.8
      PP (pellagra-preventing) E52
      specified NEC E56.8
      thiamin E51.9
        beriberi — *see* Beriberi
  zinc, dietary E60
Deficit — *see also* Deficiency
  attention and concentration R41.840
    disorder — *see* Attention, deficit
  following
    cerebral infarction I69.310
    cerebrovascular disease I69.910
      specified disease NEC I69.810
    nontraumatic
      intracerebral hemorrhage I69.110
      specified intracranial hemorrhage NEC I69.210
      subarachnoid hemorrhage I69.010
  cognitive
    communication R41.841
    emotional
      following
        cerebral infarction I69.315
        cerebrovascular disease I69.915
          specified disease NEC I69.815
        nontraumatic
          intracerebral hemorrhage I69.115
          specified intracranial hemorrhage NEC I69.215
          subarachnoid hemorrhage I69.015
    following
      cerebral infarction I69.319
      cerebrovascular disease I69.919
        specified disease NEC I69.819
      nontraumatic
        intracerebral hemorrhage I69.119
        specified intracranial hemorrhage NEC I69.219
        subarachnoid hemorrhage I69.019
    social
      following
        cerebral infarction I69.315
        cerebrovascular disease I69.915
          specified disease NEC I69.815
        nontraumatic
          intracerebral hemorrhage I69.115
          specified intracranial hemorrhage NEC I69.215
          subarachnoid hemorrhage I69.015

Deficit — *see also* Deficiency — *continued*
  cognitive NEC R41.89
    following
      cerebral infarction I69.318
      cerebrovascular disease I69.918
        specified disease NEC I69.818
      nontraumatic
        intracerebral hemorrhage I69.118
        specified intracranial hemorrhage NEC I69.218
        subarachnoid hemorrhage I69.018
  concentration R41.840
  executive function R41.844
    following
      cerebral infarction I69.314
      cerebrovascular disease I69.914
        specified disease NEC I69.814
      nontraumatic
        intracerebral hemorrhage I69.114
        specified intracranial hemorrhage NEC I69.214
        subarachnoid hemorrhage I69.014
  frontal lobe R41.844
    following
      cerebral infarction I69.314
      cerebrovascular disease I69.914
        specified disease NEC I69.814
      nontraumatic
        intracerebral hemorrhage I69.114
        specified intracranial hemorrhage NEC I69.214
        subarachnoid hemorrhage I69.014
  memory
    following
      cerebral infarction I69.311
      cerebrovascular disease I69.911
        specified disease NEC I69.811
      nontraumatic
        intracerebral hemorrhage I69.111
        specified intracranial hemorrhage NEC I69.211
        subarachnoid hemorrhage I69.011
  neurologic NEC R29.818
    ischemic
      reversible (RIND) I63.9
        prolonged (PRIND) I63.9
  oxygen R09.02
  prolonged reversible ischemic neurologic (PRIND) I63.9
  psychomotor R41.843
    following
      cerebral infarction I69.313
      cerebrovascular disease I69.913
        specified disease NEC I69.813
      nontraumatic
        intracerebral hemorrhage I69.113
        specified intracranial hemorrhage NEC I69.213
        subarachnoid hemorrhage I69.013
  visuospatial R41.842
    following
      cerebral infarction I69.312
      cerebrovascular disease I69.912
        specified disease NEC I69.812
      nontraumatic
        intracerebral hemorrhage I69.112
        specified intracranial hemorrhage NEC I69.212
        subarachnoid hemorrhage I69.012
Deflection
  radius — *see* Deformity, limb, specified type NEC, forearm
  septum (acquired) (nasal) (nose) J34.2
  spine — *see* Curvature, spine
  turbinate (nose) J34.2
Defluvium
  capillorum — *see* Alopecia
  ciliorum — *see* Madarosis
  unguium L60.8

Deformity Q89.9
  abdomen, congenital Q89.9
  abdominal wall
    acquired M95.8
    congenital Q79.59
  acquired (unspecified site) M95.9
  adrenal gland Q89.1
  alimentary tract, congenital Q45.9
    upper Q40.9
  ankle (joint) (acquired) — *see also* Deformity, limb, lower leg
    abduction — *see* Contraction, joint, ankle
    congenital Q68.8
    contraction — *see* Contraction, joint, ankle
    specified type NEC — *see* Deformity, limb, foot, specified NEC
  anus (acquired) K62.89
    congenital Q43.9
  aorta (arch) (congenital) Q25.40
    acquired I77.89
  aortic
    arch, acquired I77.89
    cusp or valve (congenital) Q23.8
      acquired (*see also* Endocarditis, aortic) I35.8
  arm (acquired) (upper) — *see also* Deformity, limb, upper arm
    congenital Q68.8
    forearm — *see* Deformity, limb, forearm
  artery (congenital) (peripheral) NOS Q27.9
    acquired I77.89
    coronary (acquired) I25.9
      congenital Q24.5
    umbilical Q27.0
  atrial septal Q21.1
  auditory canal (external) (congenital) — *see also* Malformation, ear, external
    acquired — *see* Disorder, ear, external, specified type NEC
  auricle
    ear (congenital) — *see also* Malformation, ear, external
    acquired — *see* Disorder, pinna, deformity
  back — *see* Dorsopathy, deforming
  bile duct (common) (congenital) (hepatic) Q44.5
    acquired K83.8
  biliary duct or passage (congenital) Q44.5
    acquired K83.8
  bladder (neck) (trigone) (sphincter) (acquired) N32.89
    congenital Q64.79
  bone (acquired) NOS M95.9
    congenital Q79.9
    turbinate M95.0
  brain (congenital) Q04.9
    acquired G93.89
    reduction Q04.3
  breast (acquired) N64.89
    congenital Q83.9
    reconstructed N65.0
  bronchus (congenital) Q32.4
    acquired NEC J98.09
  bursa, congenital Q79.9
  canaliculi (lacrimalis) (acquired) — *see also* Disorder, lacrimal system, changes
    congenital Q10.6
  canthus, acquired — *see* Disorder, eyelid, specified type NEC
  capillary (acquired) I78.8
  cardiovascular system, congenital Q28.9
  caruncle, lacrimal (acquired) — *see also* Disorder, lacrimal system, changes
    congenital Q10.6
  cascade, stomach K31.2
  cecum (congenital) Q43.9
    acquired K63.89
  cerebral, acquired G93.89
    congenital Q04.9

Deformity Q89.9 — *continued*
  cervix (uterus) (acquired) NEC N88.8
    congenital Q51.9
  cheek (acquired) M95.2
    congenital Q18.9
  chest (acquired) (wall) M95.4
    congenital Q67.8
    sequelae (late effect) of rickets E64.3
  chin (acquired) M95.2
    congenital Q18.9
  choroid (congenital) Q14.3
    acquired H31.8
    plexus Q07.8
      acquired G96.19
  cicatricial — *see* Cicatrix
  cilia, acquired — *see* Disorder, eyelid,
    specified type NEC
  clavicle (acquired) M95.8
    congenital Q68.8
  clitoris (congenital) Q52.6
    acquired N90.89
  clubfoot — *see* Clubfoot
  coccyx (acquired) — *see* subcategory M43.8
  colon (congenital) Q43.9
    acquired K63.89
  concha (ear), congenital — *see also*
    Malformation, ear, external
    acquired — *see* Disorder, pinna, deformity
  cornea (acquired) H18.70
    congenital Q13.4
    descemetocele — *see* Descemetocele
    ectasia — *see* Ectasia, cornea
    specified NEC H18.79-
    staphyloma — *see* Staphyloma, cornea
  coronary artery (acquired) I25.9
    congenital Q24.5
  cranium (acquired) — *see* Deformity, skull
  cricoid cartilage (congenital) Q31.8
    acquired J38.7
  cystic duct (congenital) Q44.5
    acquired K82.8
  Dandy-Walker Q03.1
    with spina bifida — *see* Spina bifida
  diaphragm (congenital) Q79.1
    acquired J98.6
  digestive organ NOS Q45.9
  ductus arteriosus Q25.0
  duodenal bulb K31.89
  duodenum (congenital) Q43.9
    acquired K31.89
  dura — *see* Deformity, meninges
  ear (acquired) — *see also* Disorder, pinna,
    deformity
    congenital (external) Q17.9
      internal Q16.5
      middle Q16.4
        ossicles Q16.3
      ossicles Q16.3
  ectodermal (congenital) NEC Q84.9
  ejaculatory duct (congenital) Q55.4
    acquired N50.89
  elbow (joint) (acquired) — *see also* Deformity,
    limb, upper arm
    congenital Q68.8
    contraction — *see* Contraction, joint, elbow
  endocrine gland NEC Q89.2
  epididymis (congenital) Q55.4
    acquired N50.89
  epiglottis (congenital) Q31.8
    acquired J38.7
  esophagus (congenital) Q39.9
    acquired K22.8
  eustachian tube (congenital) NEC Q17.8
  eye, congenital Q15.9
  eyebrow (congenital) Q18.8
  eyelid (acquired) — *see also* Disorder, eyelid,
    specified type NEC
    congenital Q10.3

Deformity Q89.9 — *continued*
  face (acquired) M95.2
    congenital Q18.9
  fallopian tube, acquired N83.8
  femur (acquired) — *see* Deformity, limb,
    specified type NEC, thigh
  fetal
    with fetopelvic disproportion O33.7
    causing obstructed labor O66.3
  finger (acquired) M20.00-
    boutonniere M20.02-
    congenital Q68.1
    flexion contracture — *see* Contraction, joint,
      hand
    mallet finger M20.01-
    specified NEC M20.09-
    swan-neck M20.03-
  flexion (joint) (acquired) (*see also* Deformity,
    limb, flexion) M21.20
    congenital NOS Q74.9
    hip Q65.89
  foot (acquired) — *see also* Deformity, limb,
    lower leg
    cavovarus (congenital) Q66.1
    congenital NOS Q66.9
      specified type NEC Q66.89
    specified type NEC — *see* Deformity, limb,
      foot, specified NEC
    valgus (congenital) Q66.6
      acquired — *see* Deformity, valgus, ankle
    varus (congenital) NEC Q66.3
      acquired — *see* Deformity, varus, ankle
  forearm (acquired) — *see also* Deformity, limb,
    forearm
    congenital Q68.8
  forehead (acquired) M95.2
    congenital Q75.8
  frontal bone (acquired) M95.2
    congenital Q75.8
  gallbladder (congenital) Q44.1
    acquired K82.8
  gastrointestinal tract (congenital) NOS Q45.9
    acquired K63.89
  genitalia, genital organ(s) or system NEC
    female (congenital) Q52.9
      acquired N94.89
      external Q52.70
    male (congenital) Q55.9
      acquired N50.89
  globe (eye) (congenital) Q15.8
    acquired H44.89
  gum, acquired NEC K06.8
  hand (acquired) — *see* Deformity, limb, hand
    congenital Q68.1
  head (acquired) M95.2
    congenital Q75.8
  heart (congenital) Q24.9
    septum Q21.9
      auricular Q21.1
      ventricular Q21.0
    valve (congenital) NEC Q24.8
      acquired — *see* Endocarditis
  heel (acquired) — *see* Deformity, foot
  hepatic duct (congenital) Q44.5
    acquired K83.8
  hip (joint) (acquired) — *see also* Deformity,
    limb, thigh
    congenital Q65.9
    due to (previous) juvenile osteochondrosis —
      see Coxa, plana
    flexion — *see* Contraction, joint, hip
  hourglass — *see* Contraction, hourglass
  humerus (acquired) M21.82-
    congenital Q74.0
  hypophyseal (congenital) Q89.2
  ileocecal (coil) (valve) (acquired) K63.89
    congenital Q43.9
  ileum (congenital) Q43.9
    acquired K63.89

Deformity Q89.9 — *continued*
  ilium (acquired) M95.5
    congenital Q74.2
  integument (congenital) Q84.9
  intervertebral cartilage or disc (acquired) —
    see Disorder, disc, specified NEC
  intestine (large) (small) (congenital) NOS
    Q43.9
    acquired K63.89
  intrinsic minus or plus (hand) — *see* Deformity,
    limb, specified type NEC, forearm
  iris (acquired) H21.89
    congenital Q13.2
  ischium (acquired) M95.5
    congenital Q74.2
  jaw (acquired) (congenital) M26.9
  joint (acquired) NEC M21.90
    congenital Q68.8
    elbow M21.92-
    hand M21.94-
    hip M21.95-
    knee M21.96-
    shoulder M21.92-
    wrist M21.93-
  kidney(s) (calyx) (pelvis) (congenital) Q63.9
    acquired N28.89
    artery (congenital) Q27.2
      acquired I77.89
  Klippel-Feil (brevicollis) Q76.1
  knee (acquired) NEC — *see also* Deformity,
    limb, lower leg
    congenital Q68.2
  labium (majus) (minus) (congenital) Q52.79
    acquired N90.89
  lacrimal passages or duct (congenital) NEC
    Q10.6
    acquired — *see* Disorder, lacrimal system,
      changes
  larynx (muscle) (congenital) Q31.8
    acquired J38.7
    web (glottic) Q31.0
  leg (upper) (acquired) NEC — *see also*
    Deformity, limb, thigh
    congenital Q68.8
    lower leg — *see* Deformity, limb, lower leg
  lens (acquired) H27.8
    congenital Q12.9
  lid (fold) (acquired) — *see also* Disorder, eyelid,
    specified type NEC
    congenital Q10.3
  ligament (acquired) — *see* Disorder, ligament
    congenital Q79.9
  limb (acquired) M21.90
    clawfoot M21.53-
    clawhand M21.51-
    clubfoot M21.54-
    clubhand M21.52-
    congenital, except reduction deformity
      Q74.9
    flat foot M21.4-
    flexion M21.20
      ankle M21.27-
      elbow M21.22-
      finger M21.24-
      hip M21.25-
      knee M21.26-
      shoulder M21.21-
      toe M21.27-
      wrist M21.23-
    foot
      claw — *see* Deformity, limb, clawfoot
      club — *see* Deformity, limb, clubfoot
      drop M21.37-
      flat — *see* Deformity, limb, flat foot
      specified NEC M21.6x-
    forearm M21.93-
    hand M21.94-
    lower leg M21.96-

Deformity Q89.9 — *continued*
limb (acquired) M21.90 — *continued*
  specified type NEC M21.80
    forearm M21.83-
    lower leg M21.86-
    thigh M21.85-
    upper arm M21.82-
  thigh M21.95-
  unequal length M21.70
    short site is
      femur M21.75-
      fibula M21.76-
      humerus M21.72-
      radius M21.73-
      tibia M21.76-
      ulna M21.73-
  upper arm M21.92-
  valgus — *see* Deformity, valgus
  varus — *see* Deformity, varus
  wrist drop M21.33-
lip (acquired) NEC K13.0
  congenital Q38.0
liver (congenital) Q44.7
  acquired K76.89
lumbosacral (congenital) (joint) (region)
    Q76.49
  acquired — *see* subcategory M43.8
  kyphosis — *see* Kyphosis, congenital
  lordosis — *see* Lordosis, congenital
lung (congenital) Q33.9
  acquired J98.4
lymphatic system, congenital Q89.9
Madelung's (radius) Q74.0
mandible (acquired) (congenital) M26.9
maxilla (acquired) (congenital) M26.9
meninges or membrane (congenital) Q07.9
  cerebral Q04.8
    acquired G96.19
  spinal cord (congenital) G96.19
    acquired G96.19
metacarpus (acquired) — *see* Deformity, limb,
    forearm
  congenital Q74.0
metatarsus (acquired) — *see* Deformity, foot
  congenital Q66.9
middle ear (congenital) Q16.4
  ossicles Q16.3
mitral (leaflets) (valve) I05.8
  parachute Q23.2
  stenosis, congenital Q23.2
mouth (acquired) K13.79
  congenital Q38.6
multiple, congenital NEC Q89.7
muscle (acquired) M62.89
  congenital Q79.9
    sternocleidomastoid Q68.0
musculoskeletal system (acquired) M95.9
  congenital Q79.9
  specified NEC M95.8
nail (acquired) L60.8
  congenital Q84.6
nasal — *see* Deformity, nose
neck (acquired) M95.3
  congenital Q18.9
    sternocleidomastoid Q68.0
nervous system (congenital) Q07.9
nipple (congenital) Q83.9
  acquired N64.89
nose (acquired) (cartilage) M95.0
  bone (turbinate) M95.0
  congenital Q30.9
    bent or squashed Q67.4
  saddle M95.0
    syphilitic A50.57
  septum (acquired) J34.2
    congenital Q30.8
  sinus (wall) (congenital) Q30.8
    acquired M95.0

Deformity Q89.9 — *continued*
nose (acquired) (cartilage) M95.0 —
    continued
  syphilitic (congenital) A50.57
    late A52.73
ocular muscle (congenital) Q10.3
  acquired — *see* Strabismus, mechanical
opticociliary vessels (congenital) Q13.2
orbit (eye) (acquired) H05.30
  atrophy — *see* Atrophy, orbit
  congenital Q10.7
  due to
    bone disease NEC H05.32-
    trauma or surgery H05.33-
  enlargement — *see* Enlargement, orbit
  exostosis — *see* Exostosis, orbit
organ of Corti (congenital) Q16.5
ovary (congenital) Q50.39
  acquired N83.8
oviduct, acquired N83.8
palate (congenital) Q38.5
  acquired M27.8
  cleft (congenital) — *see* Cleft, palate
pancreas (congenital) Q45.3
  acquired K86.89
parathyroid (gland) Q89.2
parotid (gland) (congenital) Q38.4
  acquired K11.8
patella (acquired) — *see* Disorder, patella,
    specified NEC
pelvis, pelvic (acquired) (bony) M95.5
  with disproportion (fetopelvic) O33.0
    causing obstructed labor O65.0
  congenital Q74.2
  rachitic sequelae (late effect) E64.3
penis (glans) (congenital) Q55.69
  acquired N48.89
pericardium (congenital) Q24.8
  acquired — *see* Pericarditis
pharynx (congenital) Q38.8
  acquired J39.2
pinna, acquired — *see also* Disorder, pinna,
    deformity
  congenital Q17.9
pituitary (congenital) Q89.2
posture — *see* Dorsopathy, deforming
prepuce (congenital) Q55.69
  acquired N47.8
prostate (congenital) Q55.4
  acquired N42.89
pupil (congenital) Q13.2
  acquired — *see* Abnormality, pupillary
pylorus (congenital) Q40.3
  acquired K31.89
rachitic (acquired), old or healed E64.3
radius (acquired) — *see also* Deformity, limb,
    forearm
  congenital Q68.8
rectum (congenital) Q43.9
  acquired K62.89
reduction (extremity) (limb), congenital (*see also*
    condition and site) Q73.8
  brain Q04.3
  lower — *see* Defect, reduction, lower limb
  upper — *see* Defect, reduction, upper limb
renal — *see* Deformity, kidney
respiratory system (congenital) Q34.9
rib (acquired) M95.4
  congenital Q76.6
    cervical Q76.5
rotation (joint) (acquired) — *see* Deformity,
    limb, specified site NEC
  congenital Q74.9
    hip — *see* Deformity, limb, specified type
      NEC, thigh
    congenital Q65.89
sacroiliac joint (congenital) Q74.2
  acquired — *see* subcategory M43.8

Deformity Q89.9 — *continued*
sacrum (acquired) — *see* subcategory M43.8
saddle
  back — *see* Lordosis
  nose M95.0
    syphilitic A50.57
salivary gland or duct (congenital) Q38.4
  acquired K11.8
scapula (acquired) M95.8
  congenital Q68.8
scrotum (congenital) — *see also* Malformation,
    testis and scrotum
  acquired N50.89
seminal vesicles (congenital) Q55.4
  acquired N50.89
septum, nasal (acquired) J34.2
shoulder (joint) (acquired) — *see* Deformity,
    limb, upper arm
  congenital Q74.0
  contraction — *see* Contraction, joint,
    shoulder
sigmoid (flexure) (congenital) Q43.9
  acquired K63.89
skin (congenital) Q82.9
skull (acquired) M95.2
  congenital Q75.8
    with
      anencephaly Q00.0
      encephalocele — *see* Encephalocele
      hydrocephalus Q03.9
        with spina bifida — *see* Spina bifida,
          by site, with hydrocephalus
      microcephaly Q02
soft parts, organs or tissues (of pelvis)
  in pregnancy or childbirth NEC O34.8-
    causing obstructed labor O65.5
spermatic cord (congenital) Q55.4
  acquired N50.89
  torsion — *see* Torsion, spermatic cord
spinal — *see* Dorsopathy, deforming
  column (acquired) — *see* Dorsopathy,
    deforming
  congenital Q67.5
  cord (congenital) Q06.9
    acquired G95.89
  nerve root (congenital) Q07.9
spine (acquired) — *see also* Dorsopathy,
    deforming
  congenital Q67.5
  rachitic E64.3
  specified NEC — *see* Dorsopathy,
    deforming, specified NEC
spleen
  acquired D73.89
  congenital Q89.09
Sprengel's (congenital) Q74.0
sternocleidomastoid (muscle), congenital
    Q68.0
sternum (acquired) M95.4
  congenital NEC Q76.7
stomach (congenital) Q40.3
  acquired K31.89
submandibular gland (congenital) Q38.4
submaxillary gland (congenital) Q38.4
  acquired K11.8
talipes — *see* Talipes
testis (congenital) — *see also* Malformation,
    testis and scrotum
  acquired N44.8
  torsion — *see* Torsion, testis
thigh (acquired) — *see also* Deformity, limb,
    thigh
  congenital NEC Q68.8
thorax (acquired) (wall) M95.4
  congenital Q67.8
  sequelae of rickets E64.3
thumb (acquired) — *see also* Deformity, finger
  congenital NEC Q68.1

DISEASE INDEX

Deformity Q89.9 — *continued*
thymus (tissue) (congenital) Q89.2
thyroid (gland) (congenital) Q89.2
  cartilage Q31.8
    acquired J38.7
tibia (acquired) — *see also* Deformity, limb, specified type NEC, lower leg
  congenital NEC Q68.8
  saber (syphilitic) A50.56
toe (acquired) M20.6-
  congenital Q66.9
  hallux rigidus M20.2-
  hallux valgus M20.1-
  hallux varus M20.3-
  hammer toe M20.4-
  specified NEC M20.5x-
tongue (congenital) Q38.3
  acquired K14.8
tooth, teeth K00.2
trachea (rings) (congenital) Q32.1
  acquired J39.8
transverse aortic arch (congenital) Q25.49
tricuspid (leaflets) (valve) I07.8
  atresia or stenosis Q22.4
  Ebstein's Q22.5
trunk (acquired) M95.8
  congenital Q89.9
ulna (acquired) — *see also* Deformity, limb, forearm
  congenital NEC Q68.8
urachus, congenital Q64.4
ureter (opening) (congenital) Q62.8
  acquired N28.89
urethra (congenital) Q64.79
  acquired N36.8
urinary tract (congenital) Q64.9
  urachus Q64.4
uterus (congenital) Q51.9
  acquired N85.8
uvula (congenital) Q38.5
vagina (acquired) N89.8
  congenital Q52.4
valgus NEC M21.00
  ankle M21.07-
  elbow M21.02-
  hip M21.05-
  knee M21.06-
valve, valvular (congenital) (heart) Q24.8
  acquired — *see* Endocarditis
varus NEC M21.10
  ankle M21.17-
  elbow M21.12-
  hip M21.15-
  knee M21.16-
  tibia — *see* Osteochondrosis, juvenile, tibia
vas deferens (congenital) Q55.4
  acquired N50.89
vein (congenital) Q27.9
  great Q26.9
vertebra — *see* Dorsopathy, deforming
vertical talus (congenital) Q66.80
  left foot Q66.82
  right foot Q66.81
vesicourethral orifice (acquired) N32.89
  congenital NEC Q64.79
vessels of optic papilla (congenital) Q14.2
visual field (contraction) — *see* Defect, visual field
vitreous body, acquired H43.89
vulva (congenital) Q52.79
  acquired N90.89
wrist (joint) (acquired) — *see also* Deformity, limb, forearm
  congenital Q68.8
  contraction — *see* Contraction, joint, wrist

Degeneration, degenerative
adrenal (capsule) (fatty) (gland) (hyaline) (infectional) E27.8
amyloid (*see also* Amyloidosis) E85.9
anterior cornua, spinal cord G12.29
anterior labral S43.49-
aorta, aortic I70.0
  fatty I77.89
aortic valve (heart) — *see* Endocarditis, aortic
arteriovascular — *see* Arteriosclerosis
artery, arterial (atheromatous) (calcareous) — *see also* Arteriosclerosis
  cerebral, amyloid E85.4 [I68.0]
  medial — *see* Arteriosclerosis, extremities
articular cartilage NEC — *see* Derangement, joint, articular cartilage, by site
atheromatous — *see* Arteriosclerosis
basal nuclei or ganglia G23.9
  specified NEC G23.8
bone NEC — *see* Disorder, bone, specified type NEC
brachial plexus G54.0
brain (cortical) (progressive) G31.9
  alcoholic G31.2
  arteriosclerotic I67.2
  childhood G31.9
    specified NEC G31.89
  cystic G31.89
    congenital Q04.6
  in
    alcoholism G31.2
    beriberi E51.2
    cerebrovascular disease I67.9
    congenital hydrocephalus Q03.9
      with spina bifida — *see also* Spina bifida
    Fabry-Anderson disease E75.21
    Gaucher's disease E75.22
    Hunter's syndrome E76.1
    lipidosis
      cerebral E75.4
      generalized E75.6
    mucopolysaccharidosis — *see* Mucopolysaccharidosis
    myxedema E03.9 [G32.89]
    neoplastic disease (*see also* Neoplasm) D49.6 [G32.89]
    Niemann-Pick disease E75.249 [G32.89]
    sphingolipidosis E75.3 [G32.89]
    vitamin B12 deficiency E53.8 [G32.89]
  senile NEC G31.1
breast N64.89
Bruch's membrane — *see* Degeneration, choroid
capillaries (fatty) I78.8
  amyloid E85.8 [I79.8]
cardiac — *see also* Degeneration, myocardial
  valve, valvular — *see* Endocarditis
cardiorenal — *see* Hypertension, cardiorenal
cardiovascular — *see also* Disease, cardiovascular
  renal — *see* Hypertension, cardiorenal
cerebellar NOS G31.9
  alcoholic G31.2
  primary (hereditary) (sporadic) G11.9
cerebral — *see* Degeneration, brain
cerebrovascular I67.9
  due to hypertension I67.4
cervical plexus G54.2
cervix N88.8
  due to radiation (intended effect) N88.8
    adverse effect or misadventure N99.89
chamber angle H21.21-
changes, spine or vertebra — *see* Spondylosis
chorioretinal — *see also* Degeneration, choroid
  hereditary H31.20
choroid (colloid) (drusen) H31.10-
  atrophy — *see* Atrophy, choroidal
  hereditary — *see* Dystrophy, choroidal, hereditary

Degeneration, degenerative — *continued*
ciliary body H21.22-
cochlear — *see* subcategory H83.8
combined (spinal cord) (subacute) E53.8 [G32.0]
  with anemia (pernicious) D51.0 [G32.0]
    due to dietary vitamin B12 deficiency D51.3 [G32.0]
  in (due to)
    vitamin B12 deficiency E53.8 [G32.0]
      anemia D51.9 [G32.0]
conjunctiva H11.10
  concretions — *see* Concretion, conjunctiva
  deposits — *see* Deposit, conjunctiva
  pigmentations — *see* Pigmentation, conjunctiva
  pinguecula — *see* Pinguecula
  xerosis — *see* Xerosis, conjunctiva
cornea H18.40
  calcerous H18.43
    band keratopathy H18.42-
  familial, hereditary — *see* Dystrophy, cornea
  hyaline (of old scars) H18.49
  keratomalacia — *see* Keratomalacia
  nodular H18.45-
  peripheral H18.46-
  senile H18.41-
  specified type NEC H18.49
cortical (cerebellar) (parenchymatous) G31.89
  alcoholic G31.2
  diffuse, due to arteriopathy I67.2
corticobasal G31.85
cutis L98.8
  amyloid E85.4 [L99]
dental pulp K04.2
disc disease — *see* Degeneration, intervertebral disc NEC
dorsolateral (spinal cord) — *see* Degeneration, combined
extrapyramidal G25.9
eye, macular — *see also* Degeneration, macula
  congenital or hereditary — *see* Dystrophy, retina
facet joints — *see* Spondylosis
fatty
  liver NEC K76.0
    alcoholic K70.0
grey matter (brain) (Alpers') G31.81
heart — *see also* Degeneration, myocardial
  amyloid E85.4 [I43]
  atheromatous — *see* Disease, heart, ischemic, atherosclerotic
  ischemic — *see* Disease, heart, ischemic
hepatolenticular (Wilson's) E83.01
hepatorenal K76.7
hyaline (diffuse) (generalized)
  localized — *see* Degeneration, by site
infrapatellar fat pad M79.4
intervertebral disc NOS
  with
    myelopathy — *see* Disorder, disc, with, myelopathy
    radiculitis or radiculopathy — *see* Disorder, disc, with, radiculopathy
  cervical, cervicothoracic — *see* Disorder, disc, cervical, degeneration
    with
      myelopathy — *see* Disorder, disc, cervical, with myelopathy
      neuritis, radiculitis or radiculopathy — *see* Disorder, disc, cervical, with neuritis
  lumbar region M51.36
    with
      myelopathy M51.06
      neuritis, radiculitis, radiculopathy or sciatica M51.16

Degeneration, degenerative — *continued*
intervertebral disc NOS — *continued*
  lumbosacral region M51.37
    with
      neuritis, radiculitis, radiculopathy or
        sciatica M51.17
  sacrococcygeal region M53.3
  thoracic region M51.34
    with
      myelopathy M51.04
      neuritis, radiculitis, radiculopathy
        M51.14
  thoracolumbar region M51.35
    with
      myelopathy M51.05
      neuritis, radiculitis, radiculopathy
        M51.15
intestine, amyloid E85.4
iris (pigmentary) H21.23-
ischemic — *see* Ischemia
joint disease — *see* Osteoarthritis
kidney N28.89
  amyloid E85.4 *[N29]*
  cystic, congenital Q61.9
  fatty N28.89
  polycystic Q61.3
    adult type (autosomal dominant) Q61.2
    infantile type (autosomal recessive) NEC
      Q61.19
      collecting duct dilatation Q61.11
  Kuhnt-Junius (*see also* Degeneration, macula)
    H35.32-
  lens — *see* Cataract
lenticular (familial) (progressive) (Wilson's)
  (with cirrhosis of liver) E83.01
liver (diffuse) NEC K76.89
  amyloid E85.4 *[K77]*
  cystic K76.89
    congenital Q44.6
  fatty NEC K76.0
    alcoholic K70.0
  hypertrophic K76.89
  parenchymatous, acute or subacute K72.00
    with coma K72.01
  pigmentary K76.89
  toxic (acute) K71.9
lung J98.4
lymph gland I89.8
  hyaline I89.8
macula, macular (acquired) (age-related)
  (senile) H35.30
  angioid streaks H35.33
  atrophic age-related H35.31-
  congenital or hereditary — *see* Dystrophy,
    retina
  cystoid H35.35-
  drusen H35.36-
  dry age-related H35.31-
  exudative H35.32-
  hole H35.34-
  nonexudative H35.31-
  puckering H35.37-
  toxic H35.38-
  wet age-related H35.32-
membranous labyrinth, congenital (causing
  impairment of hearing) Q16.5
meniscus — *see* Derangement, meniscus
mitral — *see* Insufficiency, mitral
Mönckeberg's — *see* Arteriosclerosis,
  extremities
motor centers, senile G31.1
multi-system G90.3
mural — *see* Degeneration, myocardial
muscle (fatty) (fibrous) (hyaline) (progressive)
  M62.89
  heart — *see* Degeneration, myocardial
myelin, central nervous system G37.9

Degeneration, degenerative — *continued*
myocardial, myocardium (fatty) (hyaline)
  (senile) I51.5
  with rheumatic fever (conditions in I00) I09.0
    active, acute or subacute I01.2
      with chorea I02.0
    inactive or quiescent (with chorea) I09.0
  hypertensive — *see* Hypertension, heart
  rheumatic — *see* Degeneration, myocardial,
    with rheumatic fever
  syphilitic A52.06
nasal sinus (mucosa) J32.9
  frontal J32.1
  maxillary J32.0
nerve — *see* Disorder, nerve
nervous system G31.9
  alcoholic G31.2
  amyloid E85.4 *[G99.8]*
  autonomic G90.9
  fatty G31.89
  specified NEC G31.89
nipple N64.89
olivopontocerebellar (hereditary) (familial)
  G23.8
osseous labyrinth — *see* subcategory H83.8
ovary N83.8
  cystic N83.20-
  microcystic N83.20-
pallidal pigmentary (progressive) G23.0
pancreas K86.89
  tuberculous A18.83
penis N48.89
pigmentary (diffuse) (general)
  localized — *see* Degeneration, by site
  pallidal (progressive) G23.0
pineal gland E34.8
pituitary (gland) E23.6
popliteal fat pad M79.4
posterolateral (spinal cord) — *see*
  Degeneration, combined
pulmonary valve (heart) I37.8
pulp (tooth) K04.2
pupillary margin H21.24-
renal — *see* Degeneration, kidney
retina H35.9
  hereditary (cerebroretinal) (congenital)
    (juvenile) (macula) (peripheral)
    (pigmentary) — *see* Dystrophy, retina
  Kuhnt-Junius (*see also* Degeneration, macula)
    H35.32-
  macula (cystic) (exudative) (hole)
    (nonexudative) (pseudohole) (senile)
    (toxic) — *see* Degeneration, macula
  peripheral H35.40
    lattice H35.41-
    microcystoid H35.42-
    paving stone H35.43-
    secondary
      pigmentary H35.45-
      vitreoretinal H35.46-
    senile reticular H35.44-
  pigmentary (primary) — *see also* Dystrophy,
    retina
    secondary — *see* Degeneration, retina,
      peripheral, secondary
  posterior pole — *see* Degeneration, macula
saccule, congenital (causing impairment of
  hearing) Q16.5
senile R54
  brain G31.1
  cardiac, heart or myocardium — *see*
    Degeneration, myocardial
  motor centers G31.1
  vascular — *see* Arteriosclerosis
sinus (cystic) — *see also* Sinusitis
  polypoid J33.1
skin L98.8
  amyloid E85.4 *[L99]*
  colloid L98.8

Degeneration, degenerative — *continued*
spinal (cord) G31.89
  amyloid E85.4 *[G32.89]*
  combined (subacute) — *see* Degeneration,
    combined
  dorsolateral — *see* Degeneration, combined
  familial NEC G31.89
  fatty G31.89
  funicular — *see* Degeneration, combined
  posterolateral — *see* Degeneration,
    combined
  subacute combined — *see* Degeneration,
    combined
  tuberculous A17.81
spleen D73.0
  amyloid E85.4 *[D77]*
stomach K31.89
striatonigral G23.2
suprarenal (capsule) (gland) E27.8
synovial membrane (pulpy) — *see* Disorder,
  synovium, specified type NEC
tapetoretinal — *see* Dystrophy, retina
thymus (gland) E32.8
  fatty E32.8
thyroid (gland) E07.89
tricuspid (heart) (valve) I07.9
tuberculous NEC — *see* Tuberculosis
turbinate J34.89
uterus (cystic) N85.8
vascular (senile) — *see* Arteriosclerosis
  hypertensive — *see* Hypertension
vitreoretinal, secondary — *see* Degeneration,
  retina, peripheral, secondary, vitreoretinal
vitreous (body) H43.81-
Wallerian — *see* Disorder, nerve
Wilson's hepatolenticular E83.01
Deglutition
  paralysis R13.0
    hysterical F44.4
  pneumonia J69.0
Degos' disease I77.89
Dehiscence (of)
  amputation stump T87.81
  cesarean wound O90.0
  closure of
    cornea T81.31
    craniotomy T81.32
    fascia (muscular) (superficial) T81.32
    internal organ or tissue T81.32
    laceration (external) (internal) T81.33
    ligament T81.32
    mucosa T81.31
    muscle or muscle flap T81.32
    ribs or rib cage T81.32
    skin and subcutaneous tissue (full-thickness)
      (superficial) T81.31
    skull T81.32
    sternum (sternotomy) T81.32
    tendon T81.32
    traumatic laceration (external) (internal)
      T81.33
  episiotomy O90.1
  operation wound NEC T81.31
    external operation wound (superficial)
      T81.31
    internal operation wound (deep) T81.32
  perineal wound (postpartum) O90.1
  traumatic injury wound repair T81.33
  wound T81.30
    traumatic repair T81.33
Dehydration E86.0
  newborn P74.1
Déjérine-Roussy syndrome G89.0
Déjérine-Sottas disease or neuropathy
  (hypertrophic) G60.0
Déjérine-Thomas atrophy G23.8
Delay, delayed
  any plane in pelvis
    complicating delivery O66.9

D I S E A S E   I N D E X

Delay, delayed — *continued*
birth or delivery NOS O63.9
closure, ductus arteriosus (Botalli) P29.3
coagulation — *see* Defect, coagulation
conduction (cardiac) (ventricular) I45.9
delivery, second twin, triplet, etc O63.2
development R62.50
  global F88
  intellectual (specific) F81.9
  language F80.9
    due to hearing loss F80.4
  learning F81.9
  pervasive F84.9
  physiological R62.50
    specified stage NEC R62.0
  reading F81.0
  sexual E30.0
  speech F80.9
    due to hearing loss F80.4
  spelling F81.81
ejaculation F52.32
gastric emptying K30
menarche E30.0
menstruation (cause unknown) N91.0
milestone R62.0
passage of meconium (newborn) P76.0
primary respiration P28.9
puberty (constitutional) E30.0
separation of umbilical cord P96.82
sexual maturation, female E30.0
sleep phase syndrome G47.21
union, fracture — *see* Fracture, by site
vaccination Z28.9
Deletion(s)
autosome Q93.9
  identified by fluorescence in situ
    hybridization (FISH) Q93.89
  identified by in situ hybridization (ISH)
    Q93.89
chromosome
  with complex rearrangements NEC Q93.7
  part of NEC Q93.5
  seen only at prometaphase Q93.89
  short arm
    22q11.2 Q93.81
    4 Q93.3
    5p Q93.4
  specified NEC Q93.89
long arm chromosome 18 or 21 Q93.89
  with complex rearrangements NEC Q93.7
microdeletions NEC Q93.88
Delhi boil or button B55.1
Delinquency (juvenile) (neurotic) F91.8
group Z72.810
Delinquent immunization status Z28.3
Delirium, delirious (acute or subacute) (not
  alcohol- or drug-induced) (with dementia)
  R41.0
alcoholic (acute) (tremens) (withdrawal)
  F10.921
  with intoxication F10.921
    in
      abuse F10.121
      dependence F10.221
due to (secondary to)
  alcohol
    intoxication F10.921
      in
        abuse F10.121
        dependence F10.221
    withdrawal F10.231
  amphetamine intoxication F15.921
    in
      abuse F15.121
      dependence F15.221

Delirium, delirious (acute or subacute) (not
  alcohol- or drug-induced) (with dementia)
  R41.0 — *continued*
due to (secondary to) — *continued*
  anxiolytic
    intoxication F13.921
      in
        abuse F13.121
        dependence F13.221
    withdrawal F13.231
  cannabis intoxication (acute) F12.921
    in
      abuse F12.121
      dependence F12.221
  cocaine intoxication (acute) F14.921
    in
      abuse F14.121
      dependence F14.221
  general medical condition F05
  hallucinogen intoxication F16.921
    in
      abuse F16.121
      dependence F16.221
  hypnotic
    intoxication F13.921
      in
        abuse F13.121
        dependence F13.221
    withdrawal F13.231
  inhalant intoxication (acute) F18.921
    in
      abuse F18.121
      dependence F18.221
  multiple etiologies F05
  opioid intoxication (acute) F11.921
    in
      abuse F11.121
      dependence F11.221
  other (or unknown) substance F19.921
  phencyclidine intoxication (acute) F16.921
    in
      abuse F16.121
      dependence F16.221
  psychoactive substance NEC intoxication
    (acute) F19.921
    in
      abuse F19.121
      dependence F19.221
  sedative
    intoxication F13.921
      in
        abuse F13.121
        dependence F13.221
    withdrawal F13.231
  unknown etiology F05
exhaustion F43.0
hysterical F44.89
postprocedural (postoperative) F05
puerperal F05
thyroid — *see* Thyrotoxicosis with thyroid storm
traumatic — *see* Injury, intracranial
tremens (alcohol-induced) F10.231
  sedative-induced F13.231
Delivery (childbirth) (labor)
arrested active phase O62.1
cesarean (for)
  abnormal
    pelvis (bony) (deformity) (major) NEC with
      disproportion (fetopelvic) O33.0
      with obstructed labor O65.0
    presentation or position O32.9
  abruptio placentae (*see also* Abruptio
    placentae) O45.9-
  acromion presentation O32.2
  atony, uterus O62.2
  breech presentation O32.1
    incomplete O32.8
  brow presentation O32.3
  cephalopelvic disproportion O33.9

Delivery (childbirth) (labor) — *continued*
cesarean (for) — *continued*
  cerclage O34.3-
  chin presentation O32.3
  cicatrix of cervix O34.4-
  contracted pelvis (general)
    inlet O33.2
    outlet O33.3
  cord presentation or prolapse O69.0
  cystocele O34.8-
  deformity (acquired) (congenital)
    pelvic organs or tissues NEC O34.8-
    pelvis (bony) NEC O33.0
  disproportion NOS O33.9
  eclampsia — *see* Eclampsia
  face presentation O32.3
  failed
    forceps O66.5
    induction of labor O61.9
      instrumental O61.1
      mechanical O61.1
      medical O61.0
      specified NEC O61.8
      surgical O61.1
    trial of labor NOS O66.40
      following previous cesarean delivery
        O66.41
    vacuum extraction O66.5
    ventouse O66.5
  fetal-maternal hemorrhage O43.01-
  hemorrhage (intrapartum) O67.9
    with coagulation defect O67.0
    specified cause NEC O67.8
  high head at term O32.4
  hydrocephalic fetus O33.6
  incarceration of uterus O34.51-
  incoordinate uterine action O62.4
  increased size, fetus O33.5
  inertia, uterus O62.2
    primary O62.0
    secondary O62.1
  lateroversion, uterus O34.59-
  mal lie O32.9
  malposition
    fetus O32.9
    pelvic organs or tissues NEC O34.8-
    uterus NEC O34.59-
  malpresentation NOS O32.9
  oblique presentation O32.2
  occurring after 37 completed weeks of
    gestation but before 39 completed
    weeks of gestation due to (spontaneous)
    onset of labor O75.82
  oversize fetus O33.5
  pelvic tumor NEC O34.8-
  placenta previa O44.0-
    complete O44.0-
      with hemorrhage O44.1-
  placental insufficiency O36.51-
  planned, occurring after 37 completed
    weeks of gestation but before 39
    completed weeks of gestation due to
    (spontaneous) onset of labor O75.82
  polyp, cervix O34.4-
    causing obstructed labor O65.5
  poor dilatation, cervix O62.0
  pre-eclampsia O14.94
    mild O14.04
    moderate O14.04
    severe O14.14
      with hemolysis, elevated liver enzymes
        and low platelet count (HELLP)
        O14.24
  previous
    cesarean delivery O34.219
      classical (vertical) scar O34.212
      low transverse scar O34.211

Delivery (childbirth) (labor) — *continued*
  cesarean (for) — *continued*
    previous — *continued*
      surgery (to)
        cervix O34.4-
        gynecological NEC O34.8-
        rectum O34.7-
        uterus O34.29
        vagina O34.6-
      prolapse
        arm or hand O32.2
        uterus O34.52-
      prolonged labor NOS O63.9
      rectocele O34.8-
      retroversion
        uterus O34.53-
      rigid
        cervix O34.4-
        pelvic floor O34.8-
        perineum O34.7-
        vagina O34.6-
        vulva O34.7-
      sacculation, pregnant uterus O34.59-
      scar(s)
        cervix O34.4-
        cesarean delivery O34.219
          classical (vertical) O34.212
          low transverse O34.211
        transmural uterine O34.29
        uterus O34.29
      Shirodkar suture in situ O34.3-
      shoulder presentation O32.2
      stenosis or stricture, cervix O34.4-
      streptococcus group B (GBS) carrier state
          O99.824
      transmural uterine scar O34.29
      transverse presentation or lie O32.2
      tumor, pelvic organs or tissues NEC O34.8-
        cervix O34.4-
      umbilical cord presentation or prolapse
          O69.0
      without indication O82
  completely normal case O80
  complicated O75.9
    by
      abnormal, abnormality (of)
        forces of labor O62.9
          specified type NEC O62.8
        glucose O99.814
        uterine contractions NOS O62.9
      abruptio placentae (*see also* Abruptio
          placentae) O45.9-
      abuse
        physical O9A.32 *(follows O99)*
        psychological O9A.52 *(follows O99)*
        sexual O9A.42 *(follows O99)*
      adherent placenta O72.0
        without hemorrhage O73.0
      alcohol use O99.314
      anemia (pre-existing) O99.02
      anesthetic death O74.8
      annular detachment of cervix O71.3
      atony, uterus O62.2
      attempted vacuum extraction and forceps
          O66.5
      Bandl's ring O62.4
      bariatric surgery status O99.844
      biliary tract disorder O26.62
      bleeding — *see* Delivery, complicated by,
          hemorrhage
      blood disorder NEC O99.12
      cervical dystocia (hypotonic) O62.2
        primary O62.0
        secondary O62.1
      circulatory system disorder O99.42
      compression of cord (umbilical) NEC
          O69.2
      condition NEC O99.89
      contraction, contracted ring O62.4

Delivery (childbirth) (labor) — *continued*
  complicated O75.9 — *continued*
    by — *continued*
      cord (umbilical)
        around neck
          with compression O69.1
          without compression O69.81
        bruising O69.5
        complication O69.9
          specified NEC O69.89
        compression NEC O69.2
        entanglement O69.2
          without compression O69.82
        hematoma O69.5
        presentation O69.0
        prolapse O69.0
        short O69.3
        thrombosis (vessels) O69.5
        vascular lesion O69.5
      Couvelaire uterus O45.8x-
      damage to (injury to) NEC
        perineum O71.82
        periurethral tissue O71.82
        vulva O71.82
      delay following rupture of membranes
          (spontaneous) — *see* Pregnancy,
          complicated by, premature rupture of
          membranes
      depressed fetal heart tones O76
      diabetes O24.92
        gestational O24.429
          diet controlled O24.420
          insulin controlled O24.424
          oral drug controlled (antidiabetic)
              (hypoglycemic) O24.425
        pre-existing O24.32
          specified NEC O24.82
          type 1 O24.02
          type 2 O24.12
      diastasis recti (abdominis) O71.89
      dilatation
        bladder O66.8
        cervix incomplete, poor or slow O62.0
      disease NEC O99.89
      disruptio uteri — *see* Delivery, complicated
          by, rupture, uterus
      drug use O99.324
      dysfunction, uterus NOS O62.9
        hypertonic O62.4
        hypotonic O62.2
          primary O62.0
          secondary O62.1
        incoordinate O62.4
      eclampsia O15.1
      embolism (pulmonary) — *see* Embolism,
          obstetric
      endocrine, nutritional or metabolic disease
          NEC O99.284
      failed
        attempted vaginal birth after previous
            cesarean delivery O66.41
        induction of labor O61.9
          instrumental O61.1
          mechanical O61.1
          medical O61.0
          specified NEC O61.8
          surgical O61.1
        trial of labor O66.40
      female genital mutilation O65.5
      fetal
        abnormal acid-base balance O68
        acidemia O68
        acidosis O68
        alkalosis O68
        death, early O02.1
        deformity O66.3
        heart rate or rhythm (abnormal) (non-
            reassuring) O76
        hypoxia O77.8

Delivery (childbirth) (labor) — *continued*
  complicated O75.9 — *continued*
    by — *continued*
      fetal — *continued*
        stress O77.9
          due to drug administration O77.1
          electrocardiographic evidence of
              O77.8
          specified NEC O77.8
          ultrasound evidence of O77.8
      fever during labor O75.2
      gastric banding status O99.844
      gastric bypass status O99.844
      gastrointestinal disease NEC O99.62
      gestational
        diabetes O24.429
          diet controlled O24.420
          insulin (and diet) controlled O24.424
          oral drug controlled (antidiabetic)
              (hypoglycemic) O24.425
        edema O12.04
          with proteinuria O12.24
        proteinuria O12.14
      gonorrhea O98.22
      hematoma O71.7
        ischial spine O71.7
        pelvic O71.7
        vagina O71.7
        vulva or perineum O71.7
      hemorrhage (uterine) O67.9
        associated with
          afibrinogenemia O67.0
          coagulation defect O67.0
          hyperfibrinolysis O67.0
          hypofibrinogenemia O67.0
        due to
          low implantation of placenta O44.5-
          low-lying placenta O44.5-
          placenta previa O44.1-
            marginal O44.3-
            partial O44.3-
          premature separation of placenta
              (normally implanted) (*see also*
              Abruptio placentae) O45.9-
          retained placenta O72.0
          uterine leiomyoma O67.8
        placenta NEC O67.8
        postpartum NEC (atonic) (immediate)
            O72.1
          with retained or trapped placenta
              O72.0
          delayed O72.2
          secondary O72.2
          third stage O72.0
      hourglass contraction, uterus O62.4
      hypertension, hypertensive (pre-existing)
          — *see* Hypertension, complicated by,
          childbirth (labor)
      hypotension O26.5-
      incomplete dilatation (cervix) O62.0
      incoordinate uterus contractions O62.4
      inertia, uterus O62.2
        during latent phase of labor O62.0
        primary O62.0
        secondary O62.1
      infection (maternal) O98.92
        carrier state NEC O99.834
        gonorrhea O98.22
        human immunodeficiency virus (HIV)
            O98.72
        sexually transmitted NEC O98.32
        specified NEC O98.82
        syphilis O98.12
        tuberculosis O98.02
        viral hepatitis O98.42
        viral NEC O98.52

Delivery (childbirth) (labor) — *continued*
complicated O75.9 — *continued*
by — *continued*
  injury (to mother) (*see also* Delivery,
    complicated, by, damage to) O71.9
    nonobstetric O9A.22 *(follows O99)*
      caused by abuse — *see* Delivery,
        complicated by, abuse
  intrauterine fetal death, early O02.1
  inversion, uterus O71.2
  laceration (perineal) O70.9
    anus (sphincter) O70.4
      with third degree laceration (*see also*
        Delivery, complicated, by,
        laceration, perineum, third
        degree) O70.20
        with mucosa O70.3
      without third degree laceration O70.4
    bladder (urinary) O71.5
    bowel O71.5
    cervix (uteri) O71.3
    fourchette O70.0
    hymen O70.0
    labia O70.0
    pelvic
      floor O70.1
      organ NEC O71.5
    perineum, perineal O70.9
      first degree O70.0
      fourth degree O70.3
      muscles O70.1
      second degree O70.1
      skin O70.0
      slight O70.0
      third degree O70.20
        with
          both external anal sphincter (EAS)
            and internal anal sphincter
            (IAS) torn (IIIc) O70.23
          less than 50% of external anal
            sphincter (EAS) thickness torn
            (IIIa) O70.21
          more than 50% external anal
            sphincter (EAS) thickness torn
            (IIIb) O70.22
        IIIa O70.21
        IIIb O70.22
        IIIc O70.23
    peritoneum (pelvic) O71.5
    rectovaginal (septum) (without perineal
      laceration) O71.4
      with perineum (*see also* Delivery,
        complicated, by, laceration,
        perineum, third degree) O70.20
        with anal or rectal mucosa O70.3
    specified NEC O71.89
    sphincter ani — *see* Delivery,
      complicated, by, laceration, anus
      (sphincter)
    urethra O71.5
    uterus O71.81
      before labor O71.81
    vagina, vaginal (deep) (high) (without
      perineal laceration) O71.4
      with perineum O70.0
      muscles, with perineum O70.1
    vulva O70.0
  liver disorder O26.62
  malignancy O9A.12 *(follows O99)*
  malnutrition O25.2
  malposition, malpresentation
    without obstruction (*see also* Delivery,
      complicated by, obstruction) O32.9
      breech O32.1
      compound O32.6
      face (brow) (chin) O32.3
      footling O32.8
      high head O32.4
      oblique O32.2

Delivery (childbirth) (labor) — *continued*
complicated O75.9 — *continued*
by — *continued*
  malposition, malpresentation
    — *continued*
    without obstruction (*see also* Delivery,
      complicated by, obstruction) O32.9
      — *continued*
      specified NEC O32.8
      transverse O32.2
      unstable lie O32.0
    placenta O44.0-
      with hemorrhage O44.1-
    uterus or cervix O65.5
  meconium in amniotic fluid O77.0
  mental disorder NEC O99.344
  metrorrhexis — *see* Delivery, complicated
    by, rupture, uterus
  nervous system disorder O99.354
  obesity (pre-existing) O99.214
  obesity surgery status O99.844
  obstetric trauma O71.9
    specified NEC O71.89
  obstructed labor
    due to
      breech (complete) (frank) presentation
        O64.1
        incomplete O64.8
      brow presenation O64.3
      buttock presentation O64.1
      chin presentation O64.2
      compound presentation O64.5
      contracted pelvis O65.1
      deep transverse arrest O64.0
      deformed pelvis O65.0
      dystocia (fetal) O66.9
        due to
          conjoined twins O66.3
          fetal
            abnormality NEC O66.3
            ascites O66.3
            hydrops O66.3
            meningomyelocele O66.3
            sacral teratoma O66.3
            tumor O66.3
          hydrocephalic fetus O66.3
        shoulder O66.0
      face presentation O64.2
      fetopelvic disproportion O65.4
      footling presentation O64.8
      impacted shoulders O66.0
      incomplete rotation of fetal head
        O64.0
      large fetus O66.2
      locked twins O66.1
      malposition O64.9
        specified NEC O64.8
      malpresentation O64.9
        specified NEC O64.8
      multiple fetuses NEC O66.6
      pelvic
        abnormality (maternal) O65.9
          organ O65.5
          specified NEC O65.8
        contraction
          inlet O65.2
          mid-cavity O65.3
          outlet O65.3
      persistent (position)
        occipitoiliac O64.0
        occipitoposterior O64.0
        occipitosacral O64.0
        occipitotransverse O64.0
      prolapsed arm O64.4
      shoulder presentation O64.4
    specified NEC O66.8
  pathological retraction ring, uterus O62.4
  penetration, pregnant uterus by instrument
    O71.1

Delivery (childbirth) (labor) — *continued*
complicated O75.9 — *continued*
by — *continued*
  perforation — *see* Delivery, complicated
    by, laceration
  placenta, placental
    ablatio (*see also* Abruptio placentae)
      O45.9-
    abnormality O43.9-
      specified NEC O43.89-
    abruptio (*see also* Abruptio placentae)
      O45.9-
    accreta O43.21-
    adherent (with hemorrhage) O72.0
      without hemorrhage O73.0
    detachment (premature) (*see also*
      Abruptio placentae) O45.9-
    disorder O43.9-
      specified NEC O43.89-
    hemorrhage NEC O67.8
    increta O43.22-
    low (implantation) (lying) O44.4-
      with hemorrhage O44.5-
    malformation O43.10-
    malposition O44.0-
      without hemorrhage O44.1-
    percreta O43.23-
    previa (central) (complete) (lateral) (total)
      O44.0-
      with hemorrhage O44.1-
      marginal O44.2-
        with hemorrhage O44.3-
      partial O44.2-
        with hemorrhage O44.3-
    retained (with hemorrhage) O72.0
      without hemorrhage O73.0
    separation (premature) O45.9-
      specified NEC O45.8x-
    vicious insertion O44.1-
  precipitate labor O62.3
  premature rupture, membranes (*see also*
    Pregnancy, complicated by, premature
    rupture of membranes) O42.90
  prolapse
    arm or hand O32.2
    cord (umbilical) O69.0
    foot or leg O32.8
    uterus O34.52-
  prolonged labor O63.9
    first stage O63.0
    second stage O63.1
  protozoal disease (maternal) O98.62
  respiratory disease NEC O99.52
  retained membranes or portions of
    placenta O72.2
    without hemorrhage O73.1
  retarded birth O63.9
  retention of secundines (with hemorrhage)
    O72.0
    without hemorrhage O73.0
    partial O72.2
      without hemorrhage O73.1
  rupture
    bladder (urinary) O71.5
    cervix O71.3
    pelvic organ NEC O71.5
    urethra O71.5
    uterus (during or after labor) O71.1
      before labor O71.0-
  separation, pubic bone (symphysis pubis)
    O71.6
  shock O75.1
  shoulder presentation O64.4
  skin disorder NEC O99.72
  spasm, cervix O62.4
  stenosis or stricture, cervix O65.5
  streptococcus group B (GBS) carrier state
    O99.824
  subluxation of symphysis (pubis) O26.72

Delivery (childbirth) (labor) — *continued*
complicated O75.9 — *continued*
  by — *continued*
    syphilis (maternal) O98.12
    tear — *see* Delivery, complicated by, laceration
    tetanic uterus O62.4
    trauma (obstetrical) (*see also* Delivery, complicated, by, damage to) O71.9
      non-obstetric O9A.22 **(follows O99)**
      periurethral O71.82
      specified NEC O71.89
    tuberculosis (maternal) O98.02
    tumor, pelvic organs or tissues NEC O65.5
    umbilical cord around neck
      with compression O69.1
      without compression O69.81
    uterine inertia O62.2
      during latent phase of labor O62.0
      primary O62.0
      secondary O62.1
    vasa previa O69.4
    velamentous insertion of cord O43.12-
  specified complication NEC O75.89
delayed NOS O63.9
  following rupture of membranes
    artificial O75.5
  second twin, triplet, etc. O63.2
forceps, low following failed vacuum extraction O66.5
missed (at or near term) O36.4
normal O80
obstructed — *see* Delivery, complicated by, obstruction
precipitate O62.3
preterm (*see also* Pregnancy, complicated by, preterm labor) O60.10
spontaneous O80
term pregnancy NOS O80
uncomplicated O80
vaginal, following previous cesarean delivery O34.219
  classical (vertical) scar O34.212
  low transverse scar O34.211
Delusions (paranoid) — *see* Disorder, delusional
Dementia (degenerative (primary)) (old age) (persisting) F03.90
  with
    aggressive behavior F03.91
    behavioral disturbance F03.91
    combative behavior F03.91
    Lewy bodies G31.83 *[F02.80]*
      with behavioral disturbance G31.83 *[F02.81]*
    Parkinsonism G31.83 *[F02.80]*
      with behavioral disturbance G31.83 *[F02.81]*
    Parkinson's disease G20 *[F02.80]*
      with behavioral disturbance G20 *[F02.81]*
    violent behavior F03.91
  alcoholic F10.97
    with dependence F10.27
  Alzheimer's type — *see* Disease, Alzheimer's
  arteriosclerotic — *see* Dementia, vascular
  atypical, Alzheimer's type — *see* Disease, Alzheimer's, specified NEC
  congenital — *see* Disability, intellectual
  frontal (lobe) G31.09 *[F02.80]*
    with behavioral disturbance G31.09 *[F02.81]*
  frontotemporal G31.09 *[F02.80]*
    with behavioral disturbance G31.09 *[F02.81]*
    specified NEC G31.09 *[F02.80]*
      with behavioral disturbance G31.09 *[F02.81]*
  in (due to)
    with behavioral disturbance G31.83 *[F02.81]*

Dementia (degenerative (primary)) (old age) (persisting) F03 — *continued*
  in (due to) — *continued*
    alcohol F10.97
      with dependence F10.27
    Alzheimer's disease — *see* Disease, Alzheimer's
    arteriosclerotic brain disease — *see* Dementia, vascular
    cerebral lipidoses E75- *[F02.80]*
      with behavioral disturbance E75-*[F02.81]*
    Creutzfeldt-Jakob disease (*see also* Creutzfeldt-Jakob disease or syndrome (with dementia)) A81.00
    epilepsy G40-*[F02.80]*
      with behavioral disturbance G40-*[F02.81]*
    hepatolenticular degeneration E83.01 *[F02.80]*
      with behavioral disturbance E83.01 *[F02.81]*
    human immunodeficiency virus (HIV) disease B20 *[F02.80]*
      with behavioral disturbance B20 *[F02.81]*
    Huntington's disease or chorea G10
    hypercalcemia E83.52 *[F02.80]*
      with behavioral disturbance E83.52 *[F02.81]*
    hypothyroidism, acquired E03.9 *[F02.80]*
      with behavioral disturbance E03.9 *[F02.81]*
      due to iodine deficiency E01.8 *[F02.80]*
        with behavioral disturbance E01.8 *[F02.81]*
    inhalants F18.97
      with dependence F18.27
    multiple
      etiologies F03
      sclerosis G35 *[F02.80]*
        with behavioral disturbance G35 *[F02.81]*
    neurosyphilis A52.17 *[F02.80]*
      with behavioral disturbance A52.17 *[F02.81]*
      juvenile A50.49 *[F02.80]*
        with behavioral disturbance A50.49 *[F02.81]*
    niacin deficiency E52 *[F02.80]*
      with behavioral disturbance E52 *[F02.81]*
    paralysis agitans G20 *[F02.80]*
      with behavioral disturbance G20 *[F02.81]*
    Parkinson's disease G20 *[F02.80]*
    pellagra E52 *[F02.80]*
      with behavioral disturbance E52 *[F02.81]*
    Pick's G31.01 *[F02.80]*
      with behavioral disturbance G31.01 *[F02.81]*
    polyarteritis nodosa M30.0 *[F02.80]*
      with behavioral disturbance M30.0 *[F02.81]*
    psychoactive drug F19.97
      with dependence F19.27
      inhalants F18.97
        with dependence F18.27
      sedatives, hypnotics or anxiolytics F13.97
        with dependence F13.27
    sedatives, hypnotics or anxiolytics F13.97
      with dependence F13.27
    systemic lupus erythematosus M32-*[F02.80]*
      with behavioral disturbance M32-*[F02.81]*
    trypanosomiasis
      African B56.9 *[F02.80]*
        with behavioral disturbance B56.9 *[F02.81]*
    unknown etiology F03
    vitamin B12 deficiency E53.8 *[F02.80]*
      with behavioral disturbance E53.8 *[F02.81]*
    volatile solvents F18.97
      with dependence F18.27
  infantile, infantilis F84.3

Dementia (degenerative (primary)) (old age) (persisting) F03 — *continued*
  Lewy body G31.83 *[F02.80]*
    with behavioral disturbance G31.83 *[F02.81]*
  multi-infarct — *see* Dementia, vascular
  paralytica, paralytic (syphilitic) A52.17 *[F02.80]*
    with behavioral disturbance A52.17 *[F02.81]*
    juvenilis A50.45
  paretic A52.17
  praecox — *see* Schizophrenia
  presenile F03
    Alzheimer's type — *see* Disease, Alzheimer's, early onset
  primary degenerative F03
  progressive, syphilitic A52.17
  senile F03
    with acute confusional state F05
    Alzheimer's type — *see* Disease, Alzheimer's, late onset
    depressed or paranoid type F03
  vascular (acute onset) (mixed) (multi-infarct) (subcortical) F01.50
    with behavioral disturbance F01.51
Demineralization, bone — *see* Osteoporosis
Demodex folliculorum (infestation) B88.0
Demophobia F40.248
Demoralization R45.3
Demyelination, demyelinization
  central nervous system G37.9
    specified NEC G37.8
  corpus callosum (central) G37.1
  disseminated, acute G36.9
    specified NEC G36.8
  global G35
  in optic neuritis G36.0
Dengue (classical) (fever) A90
  hemorrhagic A91
  sandfly A93.1
Dennie-Marfan syphilitic syndrome A50.45
Dens evaginatus, in dente or invaginatus K00.2
Dense breasts R92.2
Density
  increased, bone (disseminated) (generalized) (spotted) — *see* Disorder, bone, density and structure, specified type NEC
  lung (nodular) J98.4
Dental — *see also* condition
  examination Z01.20
    with abnormal findings Z01.21
  restoration
    aesthetically inadequate or displeasing K08.56
    defective K08.50
      specified NEC K08.59
    failure of marginal integrity K08.51
    failure of periodontal anatomical integrity K08.54
Dentia praecox K00.6
Denticles (pulp) K04.2
Dentigerous cyst K09.0
Dentin
  irregular (in pulp) K04.3
  opalescent K00.5
  secondary (in pulp) K04.3
  sensitive K03.89
Dentinogenesis imperfecta K00.5
Dentinoma — *see* Cyst, calcifying odontogenic
Dentition (syndrome) K00.7
  delayed K00.6
  difficult K00.7
  precocious K00.6
  premature K00.6
  retarded K00.6

DISEASE INDEX

Dependence (on) (syndrome) F19.20
with remission F19.21
alcohol (ethyl) (methyl) (without remission)
  F10.20
  with
    amnestic disorder, persisting F10.26
    anxiety disorder F10.280
    dementia, persisting F10.27
    intoxication F10.229
      with delirium F10.221
      uncomplicated F10.220
    mood disorder F10.24
    psychotic disorder F10.259
      with
        delusions F10.250
        hallucinations F10.251
    remission F10.21
    sexual dysfunction F10.281
    sleep disorder F10.282
    specified disorder NEC F10.288
    withdrawal F10.239
      with
        delirium F10.231
        perceptual disturbance F10.232
      uncomplicated F10.230
  counseling and surveillance Z71.41
amobarbital — see Dependence, drug,
  sedative
amphetamine(s) (type) — see Dependence,
  drug, stimulant NEC
amytal (sodium) — see Dependence, drug,
  sedative
analgesic NEC F55.8
anesthetic (agent) (gas) (general) (local) NEC
  — see Dependence, drug, psychoactive
  NEC
anxiolytic NEC — see Dependence, drug,
  sedative
barbital(s) — see Dependence, drug, sedative
barbiturate(s) (compounds) (drugs classifiable
  to T42) — see Dependence, drug, sedative
benzedrine — see Dependence, drug, stimulant
  NEC
bhang — see Dependence, drug, cannabis
bromide(s) NEC — see Dependence, drug,
  sedative
caffeine — see Dependence, drug, stimulant
  NEC
cannabis (sativa) (indica) (resin) (derivatives)
  (type) — see Dependence, drug, cannabis
chloral (betaine) (hydrate) — see Dependence,
  drug, sedative
chlordiazepoxide — see Dependence, drug,
  sedative
coca (leaf) (derivatives) — see Dependence,
  drug, cocaine
cocaine — see Dependence, drug, cocaine
codeine — see Dependence, drug, opioid
combinations of drugs F19.20
dagga — see Dependence, drug, cannabis
demerol — see Dependence, drug, opioid
dexamphetamine — see Dependence, drug,
  stimulant NEC
dexedrine — see Dependence, drug, stimulant
  NEC
dextro-nor-pseudo-ephedrine — see
  Dependence, drug, stimulant NEC
dextromethorphan — see Dependence, drug,
  opioid
dextromoramide — see Dependence, drug,
  opioid
dextrorphan — see Dependence, drug, opioid
diazepam — see Dependence, drug, sedative
dilaudid — see Dependence, drug, opioid
D-lysergic acid diethylamide — see
  Dependence, drug, hallucinogen

Dependence (on) (syndrome) F19.20 —
  continued
drug NEC F19.20
  with sleep disorder F19.282
  cannabis F12.20
    with
      anxiety disorder F12.280
      intoxication F12.229
        with
          delirium F12.221
          perceptual disturbance F12.222
        uncomplicated F12.220
      other specified disorder F12.288
      psychosis F12.259
        delusions F12.250
        hallucinations F12.251
      unspecified disorder F12.29
    in remission F12.21
  cocaine F14.20
    with
      anxiety disorder F14.280
      intoxication F14.229
        with
          delirium F14.221
          perceptual disturbance F14.222
        uncomplicated F14.220
      mood disorder F14.24
      other specified disorder F14.288
      psychosis F14.259
        delusions F14.250
        hallucinations F14.251
      sexual dysfunction F14.281
      sleep disorder F14.282
      unspecified disorder F14.29
      withdrawal F14.23
    in remission F14.21
    withdrawal symptoms in newborn P96.1
  counseling and surveillance Z71.51
  hallucinogen F16.20
    with
      anxiety disorder F16.280
      flashbacks F16.283
      intoxication F16.229
        with delirium F16.221
        uncomplicated F16.220
      mood disorder F16.24
      other specified disorder F16.288
      perception disorder, persisting F16.283
      psychosis F16.259
        delusions F16.250
        hallucinations F16.251
      unspecified disorder F16.29
    in remission F16.21
  in remission F19.21
  inhalant F18.20
    with
      anxiety disorder F18.280
      dementia, persisting F18.27
      intoxication F18.229
        with delirium F18.221
        uncomplicated F18.220
      mood disorder F18.24
      other specified disorder F18.288
      psychosis F18.259
        delusions F18.250
        hallucinations F18.251
      unspecified disorder F18.29
    in remission F18.21
  nicotine F17.200
    with disorder F17.209
      remission F17.201
      specified disorder NEC F17.208
      withdrawal F17.203
    chewing tobacco F17.220
      with disorder F17.229
        remission F17.221
        specified disorder NEC F17.228
        withdrawal F17.223

Dependence (on) (syndrome) F19.20 —
  continued
drug NEC F19.20 — continued
  nicotine F17.200 — continued
    cigarettes F17.210
      with disorder F17.219
        remission F17.211
        specified disorder NEC F17.218
        withdrawal F17.213
      specified product NEC F17.290
        with disorder F17.299
          remission F17.291
          specified disorder NEC F17.298
          withdrawal F17.293
  opioid F11.20
    with
      intoxication F11.229
        with
          delirium F11.221
          perceptual disturbance F11.222
        uncomplicated F11.220
      mood disorder F11.24
      other specified disorder F11.288
      psychosis F11.259
        delusions F11.250
        hallucinations F11.251
      sexual dysfunction F11.281
      sleep disorder F11.282
      unspecified disorder F11.29
      withdrawal F11.23
    in remission F11.21
  psychoactive NEC F19.20
    with
      amnestic disorder F19.26
      anxiety disorder F19.280
      dementia F19.27
      intoxication F19.229
        with
          delirium F19.221
          perceptual disturbance F19.222
        uncomplicated F19.220
      mood disorder F19.24
      other specified disorder F19.288
      psychosis F19.259
        delusions F19.250
        hallucinations F19.251
      sexual dysfunction F19.281
      sleep disorder F19.282
      unspecified disorder F19.29
      withdrawal F19.239
        with
          delirium F19.231
          perceptual disturbance F19.232
        uncomplicated F19.230
  sedative, hypnotic or anxiolytic F13.20
    with
      amnestic disorder F13.26
      anxiety disorder F13.280
      dementia, persisting F13.27
      intoxication F13.229
        with delirium F13.221
        uncomplicated F13.220
      mood disorder F13.24
      other specified disorder F13.288
      psychosis F13.259
        delusions F13.250
        hallucinations F13.251
      sexual dysfunction F13.281
      sleep disorder F13.282
      unspecified disorder F13.29
      withdrawal F13.239
        with
          delirium F13.231
          perceptual disturbance F13.232
        uncomplicated F13.230
    in remission F13.21

Dependence (on) (syndrome) F19.20 — *continued*
  drug NEC F19.20 — *continued*
    stimulant NEC F15.20
      with
        anxiety disorder F15.280
        intoxication F15.229
          with
            delirium F15.221
            perceptual disturbance F15.222
          uncomplicated F15.220
        mood disorder F15.24
        other specified disorder F15.288
        psychosis F15.259
          delusions F15.250
          hallucinations F15.251
        sexual dysfunction F15.281
        sleep disorder F15.282
        unspecified disorder F15.29
        withdrawal F15.23
      in remission F15.21
  ethyl
    alcohol (without remission) F10.20
      with remission F10.21
    bromide — *see* Dependence, drug, sedative
    carbamate F19.20
    chloride F19.20
    morphine — *see* Dependence, drug, opioid
  ganja — *see* Dependence, drug, cannabis
  glue (airplane) (sniffing) — *see* Dependence, drug, inhalant
  glutethimide — *see* Dependence, drug, sedative
  hallucinogenics — *see* Dependence, drug, hallucinogen
  hashish — *see* Dependence, drug, cannabis
  hemp — *see* Dependence, drug, cannabis
  heroin (salt) (any) — *see* Dependence, drug, opioid
  hypnotic NEC — *see* Dependence, drug, sedative
  Indian hemp — *see* Dependence, drug, cannabis
  inhalants — *see* Dependence, drug, inhalant
  khat — *see* Dependence, drug, stimulant NEC
  laudanum — *see* Dependence, drug, opioid
  LSD(-25) (derivatives) — *see* Dependence, drug, hallucinogen
  luminal — *see* Dependence, drug, sedative
  lysergic acid — *see* Dependence, drug, hallucinogen
  maconha — *see* Dependence, drug, cannabis
  marihuana — *see* Dependence, drug, cannabis
  meprobamate — *see* Dependence, drug, sedative
  mescaline — *see* Dependence, drug, hallucinogen
  methadone — *see* Dependence, drug, opioid
  methamphetamine(s) — *see* Dependence, drug, stimulant NEC
  methaqualone — *see* Dependence, drug, sedative
  methyl
    alcohol (without remission) F10.20
      with remission F10.21
    bromide — *see* Dependence, drug, sedative
    morphine — *see* Dependence, drug, opioid
    phenidate — *see* Dependence, drug, stimulant NEC
    sulfonal — *see* Dependence, drug, sedative
  morphine (sulfate) (sulfite) (type) — *see* Dependence, drug, opioid
  narcotic (drug) NEC — *see* Dependence, drug, opioid
  nembutal — *see* Dependence, drug, sedative
  neraval — *see* Dependence, drug, sedative
  neravan — *see* Dependence, drug, sedative
  neurobarb — *see* Dependence, drug, sedative
  nicotine — *see* Dependence, drug, nicotine

Dependence (on) (syndrome) F19.20 — *continued*
  nitrous oxide F19.20
  nonbarbiturate sedatives and tranquilizers with similar effect — *see* Dependence, drug, sedative
  on
    artificial heart (fully implantable) (mechanical) Z95.812
    aspirator Z99.0
    care provider (because of) Z74.9
      impaired mobility Z74.09
      need for
        assistance with personal care Z74.1
        continuous supervision Z74.3
      no other household member able to render care Z74.2
      specified reason NEC Z74.8
    machine Z99.89
      enabling NEC Z99.89
      specified type NEC Z99.89
    renal dialysis (hemodialysis) (peritoneal) Z99.2
    respirator Z99.11
    ventilator Z99.11
    wheelchair Z99.3
  opiate — *see* Dependence, drug, opioid
  opioids — *see* Dependence, drug, opioid
  opium (alkaloids) (derivatives) (tincture) — *see* Dependence, drug, opioid
  oxygen (long-term) (supplemental) Z99.81
  paraldehyde — *see* Dependence, drug, sedative
  paregoric — *see* Dependence, drug, opioid
  PCP (phencyclidine) (or related substance) — *see* Dependence, drug, hallucinogen
  pentobarbital — *see* Dependence, drug, sedative
  pentobarbitone (sodium) — *see* Dependence, drug, sedative
  pentothal — *see* Dependence, drug, sedative
  peyote — *see* Dependence, drug, hallucinogen
  phencyclidine (PCP) (or related substance) — *see* Dependence, drug, hallucinogen
  phenmetrazine — *see* Dependence, drug, stimulant NEC
  phenobarbital — *see* Dependence, drug, sedative
  polysubstance F19.20
  psilocibin, psilocin, psilocyn, psilocyline — *see* Dependence, drug, hallucinogen
  psychostimulant NEC — *see* Dependence, drug, stimulant NEC
  secobarbital — *see* Dependence, drug, sedative
  seconal — *see* Dependence, drug, sedative
  sedative NEC — *see* Dependence, drug, sedative
  specified drug NEC — *see* Dependence, drug
  stimulant NEC — *see* Dependence, drug, stimulant NEC
  substance NEC — *see* Dependence, drug
  supplemental oxygen Z99.81
  tobacco — *see* Dependence, drug, nicotine
    counseling and surveillance Z71.6
  tranquilizer NEC — *see* Dependence, drug, sedative
  vitamin B6 E53.1
  volatile solvents — *see* Dependence, drug, inhalant

Dependency
  care-provider Z74.9
  passive F60.7
  reactions (persistent) F60.7

Depersonalization (in neurotic state) (neurotic) (syndrome) F48.1

Depletion
  extracellular fluid E86.9
  plasma E86.1

Depletion — *continued*
  potassium E87.6
    nephropathy N25.89
  salt or sodium E87.1
    causing heat exhaustion or prostration T67.4
    nephropathy N28.9
  volume NOS E86.9

Deployment (current) (military) status Z56.82
  in theater or in support of military war, peacekeeping and humanitarian operations Z56.82
  personal history of Z91.82
    military war, peacekeeping and humanitarian deployment (current or past conflict) Z91.82
  returned from Z91.82

Depolarization, premature I49.40
  atrial I49.1
  junctional I49.2
  specified NEC I49.49
  ventricular I49.3

Deposit
  bone in Boeck's sarcoid D86.89
  calcareous, calcium — *see* Calcification
  cholesterol
    retina H35.89
    vitreous (body) (humor) — *see* Deposit, crystalline
  conjunctiva H11.11-
  cornea H18.00-
    argentous H18.02-
    due to metabolic disorder H18.03-
    Kayser-Fleischer ring H18.04-
    pigmentation — *see* Pigmentation, cornea
  crystalline, vitreous (body) (humor) H43.2-
  hemosiderin in old scars of cornea — *see* Pigmentation, cornea, stromal
  metallic in lens — *see* Cataract, specified NEC
  skin R23.8
  tooth, teeth (betel) (black) (green) (materia alba) (orange) (tobacco) K03.6
  urate, kidney — *see* Calculus, kidney

Depraved appetite — *see* Pica

Depressed
  HDL cholesterol E78.6

Depression (acute) (mental) F32.9
  agitated (single episode) F32.2
  anaclitic — *see* Disorder, adjustment
  anxiety F41.8
    persistent F34.1
  arches — *see also* Deformity, limb, flat foot
  atypical (single episode) F32.89
    recurrent episode F33.8
  basal metabolic rate R94.8
  bone marrow D75.89
  central nervous system R09.2
  cerebral R29.818
    newborn P91.4
  cerebrovascular I67.9
  chest wall M95.4
  climacteric (single episode) F32.89
    recurrent episode F33.8
  endogenous (without psychotic symptoms) F33.2
    with psychotic symptoms F33.3
  functional activity R68.89
  hysterical F44.89
  involutional (single episode) F32.89
    recurrent episode F33.8
  major F32.9
    with psychotic symptoms F32.3
    recurrent — *see* Disorder, depressive, recurrent
  manic-depressive — *see* Disorder, depressive, recurrent
  masked (single episode) F32.8
  medullary G93.89

D I S E A S E   I N D E X

Depression (acute) (mental) F32.9 — continued
- menopausal (single episode) F32.89
  - recurrent episode F33.8
- metatarsus — see Depression, arches
- monopolar F33.9
- nervous F34.1
- neurotic F34.1
- nose M95.0
- postnatal F53
- postpartum F53
- post-psychotic of schizophrenia F32.89
- post-schizophrenic F32.89
- psychogenic (reactive) (single episode) F32.9
- psychoneurotic F34.1
- psychotic (single episode) F32.3
  - recurrent F33.3
- reactive (psychogenic) (single episode) F32.9
  - psychotic (single episode) F32.3
- recurrent — see Disorder, depressive, recurrent
- respiratory center G93.89
- seasonal — see Disorder, depressive, recurrent
- senile F03
- severe, single episode F32.2
- situational F43.21
- skull Q67.4
- specified NEC (single episode) F32.89
- sternum M95.4
- visual field — see Defect, visual field
- vital (recurrent) (without psychotic symptoms) F33.2
  - with psychotic symptoms F33.3
  - single episode F32.2

Deprivation
- cultural Z60.3
- effects NOS T73.9
  - specified NEC T73.8
- emotional NEC Z65.8
  - affecting infant or child — see Maltreatment, child, psychological
- food T73.0
- protein — see Malnutrition
- sleep Z72.820
- social Z60.4
  - affecting infant or child — see Maltreatment, child, psychological
- specified NEC T73.8
- vitamins — see Deficiency, vitamin
- water T73.1

Derangement
- ankle (internal) — see Derangement, joint, ankle
- cartilage (articular) NEC — see Derangement, joint, articular cartilage, by site
  - recurrent — see Dislocation, recurrent
- cruciate ligament, anterior, current injury — see Sprain, knee, cruciate, anterior
- elbow (internal) — see Derangement, joint, elbow
- hip (joint) (internal) (old) — see Derangement, joint, hip
- joint (internal) M24.9
  - ankylosis — see Ankylosis
  - articular cartilage M24.10
    - ankle M24.17-
    - elbow M24.12-
    - foot M24.17-
    - hand M24.14-
    - hip M24.15-
    - knee NEC M23.9-
    - loose body — see Loose, body
    - shoulder M24.11-
    - wrist M24.13-
  - contracture — see Contraction, joint
  - current injury — see also Dislocation
    - knee, meniscus or cartilage — see Tear, meniscus

Derangement — continued
- joint (internal) M24.9 — continued
  - dislocation
    - pathological — see Dislocation, pathological
    - recurrent — see Dislocation, recurrent
  - knee — see Derangement, knee
  - ligament — see Disorder, ligament
  - loose body — see Loose, body
  - recurrent — see Dislocation, recurrent
  - specified type NEC M24.80
    - ankle M24.87-
    - elbow M24.82-
    - foot joint M24.87-
    - hand joint M24.84-
    - hip M24.85-
    - shoulder M24.81-
    - wrist M24.83-
  - temporomandibular M26.69
- knee (recurrent) M23.9-
  - ligament disruption, spontaneous M23.60-
    - anterior cruciate M23.61-
    - capsular M23.67-
    - instability, chronic M23.5-
    - lateral collateral M23.64-
    - medial collateral M23.63-
    - posterior cruciate M23.62-
  - loose body M23.4-
  - meniscus M23.30-
    - cystic M23.00-
      - lateral M23.002
        - anterior horn M23.04-
        - posterior horn M23.05-
        - specified NEC M23.06-
      - medial M23.005
        - anterior horn M23.01-
        - posterior horn M23.02-
        - specified NEC M23.03-
    - degenerate — see Derangement, knee, meniscus, specified NEC
    - detached — see Derangement, knee, meniscus, specified NEC
    - due to old tear or injury M23.20-
      - lateral M23.20-
        - anterior horn M23.24-
        - posterior horn M23.25-
        - specified NEC M23.26-
      - medial M23.20-
        - anterior horn M23.21-
        - posterior horn M23.22-
        - specified NEC M23.23-
    - retained — see Derangement, knee, meniscus, specified NEC
    - specified NEC M23.30-
      - lateral M23.30-
        - anterior horn M23.34-
        - posterior horn M23.35-
        - specified NEC M23.36-
      - medial M23.30-
        - anterior horn M23.31-
        - posterior horn M23.32-
        - specified NEC M23.33-
    - old M23.8x-
    - specified NEC — see subcategory M23.8
  - low back NEC — see Dorsopathy, specified NEC
- meniscus — see Derangement, knee, meniscus
- mental — see Psychosis
- patella, specified NEC — see Disorder, patella, derangement NEC
- semilunar cartilage (knee) — see Derangement, knee, meniscus, specified NEC
- shoulder (internal) — see Derangement, joint, shoulder
Dercum's disease E88.2
Derealization (neurotic) F48.1
Dermal — see condition
Dermaphytid — see Dermatophytosis

Dermatitis (eczematous) L30.9
- ab igne L59.0
- acarine B88.0
- actinic (due to sun) L57.8
  - other than from sun L59.8
- allergic — see Dermatitis, contact, allergic
- ambustionis, due to burn or scald — see Burn
- amebic A06.7
- ammonia L22
- arsenical (ingested) L27.8
- artefacta L98.1
  - psychogenic F54
- atopic L20.9
  - psychogenic F54
  - specified NEC L20.89
- autoimmune progesterone L30.8
- berlock, berloque L56.2
- blastomycotic B40.3
- blister beetle L24.89
- bullous, bullosa L13.9
  - mucosynechial, atrophic L12.1
  - seasonal L30.8
  - specified NEC L13.8
- calorica L59.0
  - due to burn or scald — see Burn
- caterpillar L24.89
- cercarial B65.3
- combustionis L59.0
  - due to burn or scald — see Burn
- congelationis T69.1
- contact (occupational) L25.9
  - allergic L23.9
    - due to
      - adhesives L23.1
      - cement L23.5
      - chemical products NEC L23.5
      - chromium L23.0
      - cosmetics L23.2
      - dander (cat) (dog) L23.81
      - drugs in contact with skin L23.3
      - dyes L23.4
      - food in contact with skin L23.6
      - hair (cat) (dog) L23.81
      - insecticide L23.5
      - metals L23.0
      - nickel L23.0
      - plants, non-food L23.7
      - plastic L23.5
      - rubber L23.5
      - specified agent NEC L23.89
  - due to
    - cement L25.3
    - chemical products NEC L25.3
    - cosmetics L25.0
    - dander (cat) (dog) L23.81
    - drugs in contact with skin L25.1
    - dyes L25.2
    - food in contact with skin L25.4
    - hair (cat) (dog) L23.81
    - plants, non-food L25.5
    - specified agent NEC L25.8
  - irritant L24.9
    - due to
      - cement L24.5
      - chemical products NEC L24.5
      - cosmetics L24.3
      - detergents L24.0
      - drugs in contact with skin L24.4
      - food in contact with skin L24.6
      - oils and greases L24.1
      - plants, non-food L24.7
      - solvents L24.2
      - specified agent NEC L24.89
- contusiformis L52
- diabetic — see E08-E13 with .620
- diaper L22
- diphtheritica A36.3
- dry skin L85.3

Dermatitis (eczematous) L30.9 — *continued*
due to
  acetone (contact) (irritant) L24.2
  acids (contact) (irritant) L24.5
  adhesive(s) (allergic) (contact) (plaster) L23.1
    irritant L24.5
  alcohol (irritant) (skin contact) (substances in
    category T51) L24.2
    taken internally L27.8
  alkalis (contact) (irritant) L24.5
  arsenic (ingested) L27.8
  carbon disulfide (contact) (irritant) L24.2
  caustics (contact) (irritant) L24.5
  cement (contact) L25.3
  cereal (ingested) L27.2
  chemical(s) NEC L25.3
    taken internally L27.8
  chlorocompounds L24.2
  chromium (contact) (irritant) L24.81
  coffee (ingested) L27.2
  cold weather L30.8
  cosmetics (contact) L25.0
    allergic L23.2
    irritant L24.3
  cyclohexanes L24.2
  dander (cat) (dog) L23.81
  Demodex species B88.0
  Dermanyssus gallinae B88.0
  detergents (contact) (irritant) L24.0
  dichromate L24.81
  drugs and medicaments (generalized)
    (internal use) L27.0
    external — *see* Dermatitis, due to, drugs,
      in contact with skin
    in contact with skin L25.1
      allergic L23.3
      irritant L24.4
    localized skin eruption L27.1
    specified substance — *see* Table of Drugs
      and Chemicals
  dyes (contact) L25.2
    allergic L23.4
    irritant L24.89
  epidermophytosis — *see* Dermatophytosis
  esters L24.2
  external irritant NEC L24.9
  fish (ingested) L27.2
  flour (ingested) L27.2
  food (ingested) L27.2
    in contact with skin L25.4
  fruit (ingested) L27.2
  furs (allergic) (contact) L23.81
  glues — *see* Dermatitis, due to, adhesives
  glycols L24.2
  greases NEC (contact) (irritant) L24.1
  hair (cat) (dog) L23.81
  hot
    objects and materials — *see* Burn
    weather or places L59.0
  hydrocarbons L24.2
  infrared rays L59.8
  ingestion, ingested substance L27.9
    chemical NEC L27.8
    drugs and medicaments — *see* Dermatitis,
      due to, drugs
    food L27.2
    specified NEC L27.8
  insecticide in contact with skin L24.5
  internal agent L27.9
    drugs and medicaments (generalized) —
      see Dermatitis, due to, drugs
    food L27.2
  irradiation — *see* Dermatitis, due to,
    radioactive substance
  ketones L24.2
  lacquer tree (allergic) (contact) L23.7
  light (sun) NEC L57.8
    acute L56.8
    other L59.8

Dermatitis (eczematous) L30.9 — *continued*
due to — *continued*
  Liponyssoides sanguineus B88.0
  low temperature L30.8
  meat (ingested) L27.2
  metals, metal salts (contact) (irritant) L24.81
  milk (ingested) L27.2
  nickel (contact) (irritant) L24.81
  nylon (contact) (irritant) L24.5
  oils NEC (contact) (irritant) L24.1
  paint solvent (contact) (irritant) L24.2
  petroleum products (contact) (irritant)
    (substances in T52.0) L24.2
  plants NEC (contact) L25.5
    allergic L23.7
    irritant L24.7
  plasters (adhesive) (any) (allergic) (contact)
    L23.1
    irritant L24.5
  plastic (contact) L25.3
  preservatives (contact) — *see* Dermatitis, due
    to, chemical, in contact with skin
  primrose (allergic) (contact) L23.7
  primula (allergic) (contact) L23.7
  radiation L59.8
    nonionizing (chronic exposure) L57.8
    sun NEC L57.8
      acute L56.8
  radioactive substance L58.9
    acute L58.0
    chronic L58.1
  radium L58.9
    acute L58.0
    chronic L58.1
  ragweed (allergic) (contact) L23.7
  Rhus (allergic) (contact) (diversiloba)
    (radicans) (toxicodendron) (venenata)
    (verniciflua) L23.7
  rubber (contact) L24.5
  Senecio jacobaea (allergic) (contact) L23.7
  solvents (contact) (irritant) (substances in
    category T52) L24.2
  specified agent NEC (contact) L25.8
    allergic L23.89
    irritant L24.89
  sunshine NEC L57.8
    acute L56.8
  tetrachlorethylene (contact) (irritant) L24.2
  toluene (contact) (irritant) L24.2
  turpentine (contact) L24.2
  ultraviolet rays (sun NEC) (chronic exposure)
    L57.8
    acute L56.8
  vaccine or vaccination L27.0
    specified substance — *see* Table of Drugs
      and Chemicals
  varicose veins — *see* Varix, leg, with,
    inflammation
  X-rays L58.9
    acute L58.0
    chronic L58.1
dyshydrotic L30.1
dysmenorrheica N94.6
escharotica — *see* Burn
exfoliative, exfoliativa (generalized) L26
  neonatorum L00
eyelid — *see also* Dermatosis, eyelid
  allergic H01.119
    left H01.116
      lower H01.115
      upper H01.114
    right H01.113
      lower H01.112
      upper H01.111
  contact — *see* Dermatitis, eyelid, allergic
  due to
    Demodex species B88.0
    herpes (zoster) B02.39
    simplex B00.59

Dermatitis (eczematous) L30.9 — *continued*
eyelid — *see also* Dermatosis, eyelid
  — *continued*
  eczematous H01.139
    left H01.136
      lower H01.135
      upper H01.134
    right H01.133
      lower H01.132
      upper H01.131
facta, factitia, factitial L98.1
  psychogenic F54
flexural NEC L20.82
friction L30.4
fungus B36.9
  specified type NEC B36.8
gangrenosa, gangrenous infantum L08.0
harvest mite B88.0
heat L59.0
herpesviral, vesicular (ear) (lip) B00.1
herpetiformis (bullous) (erythematous)
  (pustular) (vesicular) L13.0
  juvenile L12.2
  senile L12.0
hiemalis L30.8
hypostatic, hypostatica — *see* Varix, leg, with,
  inflammation
infectious eczematoid L30.3
infective L30.3
irritant — *see* Dermatitis, contact, irritant
Jacquet's (diaper dermatitis) L22
Leptus B88.0
lichenified NEC L28.0
medicamentosa (generalized) (internal use) —
  see Dermatitis, due to drugs
mite B88.0
multiformis L13.0
  juvenile L12.2
napkin L22
neurotica L13.0
nummular L30.0
papillaris capillitii L73.0
pellagrous E52
perioral L71.0
photocontact L56.2
polymorpha dolorosa L13.0
pruriginosa L13.0
pruritic NEC L30.8
psychogenic F54
purulent L08.0
pustular
  contagious B08.02
  subcorneal L13.1
pyococcal L08.0
pyogenica L08.0
repens L40.2
Ritter's (exfoliativa) L00
Schamberg's L81.7
schistosome B65.3
seasonal bullous L30.8
seborrheic L21.9
  infantile L21.1
  specified NEC L21.8
sensitization NOS L23.9
septic L08.0
solare L57.8
specified NEC L30.8
stasis I87.2
  with
    varicose ulcer — *see* Varix, leg, with ulcer,
      with inflammation
    varicose veins — *see* Varix, leg, with,
      inflammation
  due to postthrombotic syndrome — *see*
    Syndrome, postthrombotic
suppurative L08.0
traumatic NEC L30.4
trophoneurotica L13.0

DISEASE INDEX

Dermatitis (eczematous) L30.9 — *continued*
ultraviolet (sun) (chronic exposure) L57.8
　acute L56.8
varicose — *see* Varix, leg, with, inflammation
vegetans L10.1
verrucosa B43.0
vesicular, herpesviral B00.1
Dermatoarthritis, lipoid E78.81
Dermatochalasis, eyelid H02.839
left H02.836
　lower H02.835
　upper H02.834
right H02.833
　lower H02.832
　upper H02.831
Dermatofibroma (lenticulare) — *see*
　Neoplasm, skin, benign
protuberans — *see* Neoplasm, skin, uncertain
　behavior
Dermatofibrosarcoma (pigmented)
　(protuberans) — *see* Neoplasm, skin,
　malignant
Dermatographia L50.3
Dermatolysis (exfoliativa) (congenital) Q82.8
acquired L57.4
eyelids — *see* Blepharochalasis
palpebrarum — *see* Blepharochalasis
senile L57.4
Dermatomegaly NEC Q82.8
Dermatomucosomyositis M33.10
with
　myopathy M33.12
　respiratory involvement M33.11
　specified organ involvement NEC M33.19
Dermatomycosis B36.9
furfuracea B36.0
specified type NEC B36.8
Dermatomyositis (acute) (chronic) — *see also*
　Dermatopolymyositis
in (due to) neoplastic disease (*see also*
　Neoplasm) D49.9 [M36.0]
Dermatoneuritis of children — *see*
　Poisoning, mercury
Dermatophilosis A48.8
Dermatophytid L30.2
Dermatophytide — *see* Dermatophytosis
Dermatophytosis (epidermophyton) (infection)
　(Microsporum) (tinea) (Trichophyton) B35.9
beard B35.0
body B35.4
capitis B35.0
corporis B35.4
deep-seated B35.8
disseminated B35.8
foot B35.3
granulomatous B35.8
groin B35.6
hand B35.2
nail B35.1
perianal (area) B35.6
scalp B35.0
specified NEC B35.8
Dermatopolymyositis M33.90
with
　myopathy M33.92
　respiratory involvement M33.91
　specified organ involvement NEC M33.99
in neoplastic disease (*see also* Neoplasm)
　D49.9 [M36.0]
juvenile M33.00
　with
　　myopathy M33.02
　　respiratory involvement M33.01
　　specified organ involvement NEC M33.09
　specified NEC M33.10
　　myopathy M33.12
　　respiratory involvement M33.11
　　specified organ involvement NEC M33.19

Dermatopolyneuritis — *see* Poisoning,
　mercury
Dermatorrhexis Q79.6
acquired L57.4
Dermatosclerosis — *see also* Scleroderma
localized L94.0
Dermatosis L98.9
Andrews' L08.89
Bowen's — *see* Neoplasm, skin, in situ
bullous L13.9
　specified NEC L13.8
exfoliativa L26
eyelid (noninfectious)
　dermatitis — *see* Dermatitis, eyelid
　discoid lupus erythematosus — *see* Lupus,
　　erythematosus, eyelid
　xeroderma — *see* Xeroderma, acquired,
　　eyelid
factitial L98.1
febrile neutrophilic L98.2
gonococcal A54.89
herpetiformis L13.0
　juvenile L12.2
linear IgA L13.8
menstrual NEC L98.8
neutrophilic, febrile L98.2
occupational — *see* Dermatitis, contact
papulosa nigra L82.1
pigmentary L81.9
　progressive L81.7
　Schamberg's L81.7
psychogenic F54
purpuric, pigmented L81.7
pustular, subcorneal L13.1
transient acantholytic L11.1
Dermographia, dermographism L50.3
Dermoid (cyst) — *see also* Neoplasm, benign,
　by site
with malignant transformation C56-
due to radiation (nonionizing) L57.8
Dermopathy
infiltrative with thyrotoxicosis — *see*
　Thyrotoxicosis
nephrogenic fibrosing L90.8
Dermophytosis — *see* Dermatophytosis
Descemet's membrane — *see* condition
Descemetocele H18.73-
Descending — *see* condition
Descensus uteri — *see* Prolapse, uterus
Desert
rheumatism B38.0
sore — *see* Ulcer, skin
Desertion (newborn) — *see* Maltreatment
Desmoid (extra-abdominal) (tumor) — *see*
　Neoplasm, connective tissue, uncertain
　behavior
abdominal D48.1
Despondency F32.9
Desquamation, skin R23.4
Destruction, destructive — *see also* Damage
articular facet — *see also* Derangement, joint,
　specified type NEC
　knee M23.8x-
　vertebra — *see* Spondylosis
bone — *see also* Disorder, bone, specified type
　NEC
　syphilitic A52.77
joint — *see also* Derangement, joint, specified
　type NEC
　sacroiliac M53.3
rectal sphincter K62.89
septum (nasal) J34.89
tuberculous NEC — *see* Tuberculosis
tympanum, tympanic membrane
　(nontraumatic) — *see* Disorder, tympanic
　membrane, specified NEC
vertebral disc — *see* Degeneration,
　intervertebral disc

Destructiveness — *see also* Disorder, conduct
adjustment reaction — *see* Disorder, adjustment
Desultory labor O62.2
Detachment
cartilage — *see* Sprain
cervix, annular N88.8
　complicating delivery O71.3
choroid (old) (postinfectional) (simple)
　(spontaneous) H31.40-
　hemorrhagic H31.41-
　serous H31.42-
ligament — *see* Sprain
meniscus (knee) — *see also* Derangement,
　knee, meniscus, specified NEC
　current injury — *see* Tear, meniscus
　due to old tear or injury — *see*
　　Derangement, knee, meniscus, due to
　　old tear
retina (without retinal break) (serous) H33.2-
　with retinal:
　　break H33.00-
　　　giant H33.03-
　　　multiple H33.02-
　　　single H33.01-
　　dialysis H33.04-
　pigment epithelium — *see* Degeneration,
　　retina, separation of layers, pigment
　　epithelium detachment
　rhegmatogenous — *see* Detachment, retina,
　　with retinal, break
　specified NEC H33.8
　total H33.05-
　traction H33.4-
vitreous (body) H43.81
Detergent asthma J69.8
Deterioration
epileptic F06.8
general physical R53.81
heart, cardiac — *see* Degeneration,
　myocardial
mental — *see* Psychosis
myocardial, myocardium — *see* Degeneration,
　myocardial
senile (simple) R54
Deuteranomaly (anomalous trichromat)
　H53.53
Deuteranopia (complete) (incomplete) H53.53
Development
abnormal, bone Q79.9
arrested R62.50
　bone — *see* Arrest, development or growth,
　　bone
　child R62.50
　due to malnutrition E45
defective, congenital — *see also* Anomaly, by
　site
　cauda equina Q06.3
　left ventricle Q24.8
　　in hypoplastic left heart syndrome Q23.4
　valve Q24.8
　pulmonary Q22.3
delayed (*see also* Delay, development) R62.50
　arithmetical skills F81.2
　language (skills) (expressive) F80.1
　learning skill F81.9
　mixed skills F88
　motor coordination F82
　reading F81.0
　specified learning skill NEC F81.89
　speech F80.9
　spelling F81.81
　written expression F81.81
imperfect, congenital — *see also* Anomaly, by
　site
　heart Q24.9
　lungs Q33.6

Development — *continued*
  incomplete
    bronchial tree Q32.4
    organ or site not listed — *see* Hypoplasia, by
      site
    respiratory system Q34.9
  sexual, precocious NEC E30.1
  tardy, mental (*see also* Disability, intellectual)
    F79
Developmental — *see* condition
  testing, infant or child — *see* Examination,
    child
Devergie's disease (pityriasis rubra pilaris)
  L44.0
Deviation (in)
  conjugate palsy (eye) (spastic) H51.0
  esophagus (acquired) K22.8
  eye, skew H51.8
  midline (jaw) (teeth) (dental arch) M26.29
    specified site NEC — *see* Malposition
  nasal septum J34.2
    congenital Q67.4
  opening and closing of the mandible M26.53
  organ or site, congenital NEC — *see*
    Malposition, congenital
  septum (nasal) (acquired) J34.2
    congenital Q67.4
  sexual F65.9
    bestiality F65.89
    erotomania F52.8
    exhibitionism F65.2
    fetishism, fetishistic F65.0
      transvestism F65.1
    frotteurism F65.81
    masochism F65.51
    multiple F65.89
    necrophilia F65.89
    nymphomania F52.8
    pederosis F65.4
    pedophilia F65.4
    sadism, sadomasochism F65.52
    satyriasis F52.8
    specified type NEC F65.89
    transvestism F64.1
    voyeurism F65.3
  teeth, midline M26.29
  trachea J39.8
  ureter, congenital Q62.61
Devic's disease G36.0
Device
  cerebral ventricle (communicating) in situ
    Z98.2
  contraceptive — *see* Contraceptive, device
  drainage, cerebrospinal fluid, in situ Z98.2
Devil's
  grip B33.0
  pinches (purpura simplex) D69.2
Devitalized tooth K04.99
Devonshire colic — *see* Poisoning, lead
Dextraposition, aorta Q20.3
  in tetralogy of Fallot Q21.3
Dextrinosis, limit (debrancher enzyme
  deficiency) E74.03
Dextrocardia (true) Q24.0
  with
    complete transposition of viscera Q89.3
    situs inversus Q89.3
Dextrotransposition, aorta Q20.3
d-glycericacidemia E72.59
Dhat syndrome F48.8
Dhobi itch B35.6
Diabetes, diabetic (mellitus) (sugar) E11.9
  with
    amyotrophy E11.44
    arthropathy NEC E11.618
    autonomic (poly)neuropathy E11.43
    cataract E11.36
    Charcôt's joints E11.610
    chronic kidney disease E11.22

Diabetes, diabetic (mellitus) (sugar) E11.9 —
  continued
  with — *continued*
    circulatory complication NEC E11.59
    complication E11.8
      specified NEC E11.69
    dermatitis E11.620
    foot ulcer E11.621
    gangrene E11.52
    gastroparalysis E11.43
    gastroparesis E11.43
    glomerulonephrosis, intracapillary E11.21
    glomerulosclerosis, intercapillary E11.21
    hyperglycemia E11.65
    hyperosmolarity E11.00
      with coma E11.01
    hypoglycemia E11.649
      with coma E11.641
    kidney complications NEC E11.29
    Kimmelstiel-Wilson disease E11.21
    loss of protective sensation (LOPS) — *see*
      Diabetes, by type, with neuropathy
    mononeuropathy E11.41
    myasthenia E11.44
    necrobiosis lipoidica E11.620
    nephropathy E11.21
    neuralgia E11.42
    neurologic complication NEC E11.49
    neuropathic arthropathy E11.610
    neuropathy E11.40
    ophthalmic complication NEC E11.39
    oral complication NEC E11.638
    osteomyelitis E11.69
    periodontal disease E11.630
    peripheral angiopathy E11.51
      with gangrene E11.52
    polyneuropathy E11.42
    renal complication NEC E11.29
    renal tubular degeneration E11.29
    retinopathy E11.319
      with macular edema E11.311
        resolved following treatment E11.37
      nonproliferative E11.329
        with macular edema E11.321
        mild E11.329
          with macular edema E11.321
        moderate E11.339
          with macular edema E11.331
        severe E11.349
          with macular edema E11.341
      proliferative E11.359
        with
          combined traction retinal detachment
            and rhegmatogenous retinal
            detachment E11.354
          macular edema E11.351
          stable proliferative diabetic
            retinopathy E11.355
          traction retinal detachment involving
            the macula E11.352
          traction retinal detachment not
            involving the macula E11.353
    skin complication NEC E11.628
    skin ulcer NEC E11.622
  brittle — *see* Diabetes, type 1
  bronzed E83.110
  complicating pregnancy — *see* Pregnancy,
    complicated by, diabetes
  dietary counseling and surveillance Z71.3
  due to
    autoimmune process — *see* Diabetes, type 1
    immune mediated pancreatic islet beta-cell
      destruction — *see* Diabetes, type 1
  due to drug or chemical E09.9
    with
      amyotrophy E09.44
      arthropathy NEC E09.618
      autonomic (poly)neuropathy E09.43
      cataract E09.36

Diabetes, diabetic (mellitus) (sugar) E11.9 —
  continued
  due to drug or chemical E09.9 — *continued*
    with — *continued*
      Charcôt's joints E09.610
      chronic kidney disease E09.22
      circulatory complication NEC E09.59
      complication E09.8
        specified NEC E09.69
      dermatitis E09.620
      foot ulcer E09.621
      gangrene E09.52
      gastroparalysis E09.43
      gastroparesis E09.43
      glomerulonephrosis, intracapillary E09.21
      glomerulosclerosis, intercapillary E09.21
      hyperglycemia E09.65
      hyperosmolarity E09.00
        with coma E09.01
      hypoglycemia E09.649
        with coma E09.641
      ketoacidosis E09.10
        with coma E09.11
      kidney complications NEC E09.29
      Kimmelstiel-Wilson disease E09.21
      mononeuropathy E09.41
      myasthenia E09.44
      necrobiosis lipoidica E09.620
      nephropathy E09.21
      neuralgia E09.42
      neurologic complication NEC E09.49
      neuropathic arthropathy E09.610
      neuropathy E09.40
      ophthalmic complication NEC E09.39
      oral complication NEC E09.638
      periodontal disease E09.630
      peripheral angiopathy E09.51
        with gangrene E09.52
      polyneuropathy E09.42
      renal complication NEC E09.29
      renal tubular degeneration E09.29
      retinopathy E09.319
        with macular edema E09.311
          resolved following treatment E09.37
        nonproliferative E09.329
          with macular edema E09.321
          mild E09.329
            with macular edema E09.321
          moderate E09.339
            with macular edema E09.331
          severe E09.349
            with macular edema E09.341
        proliferative E09.359
          with
            combined traction retinal
              detachment and
              rhegmatogenous retinal
              detachment E09.354
            macular edema E09.351
            stable proliferative diabetic
              retinopathy E09.355
            traction retinal detachment involving
              the macula E09.352
            traction retinal detachment not
              involving the macula E09.353
      skin complication NEC E09.628
      skin ulcer NEC E09.622
  due to underlying condition E08.9
    with
      amyotrophy E08.44
      arthropathy NEC E08.618
      autonomic (poly)neuropathy E08.43
      cataract E08.36
      Charcôt's joints E08.610
      chronic kidney disease E08.22
      circulatory complication NEC E08.59
      complication E08.8
        specified NEC E08.69
      dermatitis E08.620

DISEASE INDEX

Diabetes, diabetic (mellitus) (sugar) E11.9 — *continued*
- due to underlying condition E08.9 — *continued*
  - with — *continued*
    - foot ulcer E08.621
    - gangrene E08.52
    - gastroparalysis E08.43
    - gastroparesis E08.43
    - glomerulonephrosis, intracapillary E08.21
    - glomerulosclerosis, intercapillary E08.21
    - hyperglycemia E08.65
    - hyperosmolarity E08.00
      - with coma E08.01
    - hypoglycemia E08.649
      - with coma E08.641
    - ketoacidosis E08.10
      - with coma E08.11
    - kidney complications NEC E08.29
    - Kimmelstiel-Wilson disease E08.21
    - mononeuropathy E08.41
    - myasthenia E08.44
    - necrobiosis lipoidica E08.620
    - nephropathy E08.21
    - neuralgia E08.42
    - neurologic complication NEC E08.49
    - neuropathic arthropathy E08.610
    - neuropathy E08.40
    - ophthalmic complication NEC E08.39
    - oral complication NEC E08.638
    - periodontal disease E08.630
    - peripheral angiopathy E08.51
      - with gangrene E08.52
    - polyneuropathy E08.42
    - renal complication NEC E08.29
    - renal tubular degeneration E08.29
    - retinopathy E08.319
      - with macular edema E08.311
        - resolved following treatment E08.37
      - nonproliferative E08.329
        - with macular edema E08.321
        - mild E08.329
          - with macular edema E08.321
        - moderate E08.339
          - with macular edema E08.331
        - severe E08.349
          - with macular edema E08.341
      - proliferative E08.359
        - with
          - combined traction retinal detachment and rhegmatogenous retinal detachment E08.354
          - macular edema E08.351
          - stable proliferative diabetic retinopathy E08.355
          - traction retinal detachment involving the macula E08.352
          - traction retinal detachment not involving the macula E08.353
    - skin complication NEC E08.628
    - skin ulcer NEC E08.622
- gestational (in pregnancy) O24.419
  - affecting newborn P70.0
  - diet controlled O24.410
  - in childbirth O24.429
    - diet controlled O24.420
    - insulin (and diet) controlled O24.424
    - oral drug controlled (antidiabetic) (hypoglycemic) O24.425
  - insulin (and diet) controlled O24.414
  - oral drug controlled (antidiabetic) (hypoglycemic) O24.415
  - puerperal O24.439
    - diet controlled O24.430
    - insulin (and diet) controlled O24.434
    - oral drug controlled (antidiabetic) (hypoglycemic) O24.435
- hepatogenous E13.9

Diabetes, diabetic (mellitus) (sugar) E11.9 — *continued*
- inadequately controlled — *code to* Diabetes, by type, with hyperglycemia
- idiopathic — *see* Diabetes, type 1
- insipidus E23.2
  - nephrogenic N25.1
  - pituitary E23.2
  - vasopressin resistant N25.1
- insulin dependent — *code to* type of diabetes
- juvenile-onset — *see* Diabetes, type 1
- ketosis-prone — *see* Diabetes, type 1
- latent R73.03
- neonatal (transient) P70.2
- non-insulin dependent — *code to* type of diabetes
- out of control — *code to* Diabetes, by type, with hyperglycemia
- phosphate E83.39
- poorly controlled — *code to* Diabetes, by type, with hyperglycemia
- postpancreatectomy — *see* Diabetes, specified type NEC
- postprocedural — *see* Diabetes, specified type NEC
- secondary diabetes mellitus NEC — *see* Diabetes, specified type NEC
- specified type NEC E13.9
  - with
    - amyotrophy E13.44
    - arthropathy NEC E13.618
    - autonomic (poly)neuropathy E13.43
    - cataract E13.36
    - Charcôt's joints E13.610
    - chronic kidney disease E13.22
    - circulatory complication NEC E13.59
    - complication E13.8
      - specified NEC E13.69
    - dermatitis E13.620
    - foot ulcer E13.621
    - gangrene E13.52
    - gastroparalysis E13.43
    - gastroparesis E13.43
    - glomerulonephrosis, intracapillary E13.21
    - glomerulosclerosis, intercapillary E13.21
    - hyperglycemia E13.65
    - hyperosmolarity E13.00
      - with coma E13.01
    - hypoglycemia E13.649
      - with coma E13.641
    - ketoacidosis E13.10
      - with coma E13.11
    - kidney complications NEC E13.29
    - Kimmelstiel-Wilson disease E13.21
    - mononeuropathy E13.41
    - myasthenia E13.44
    - necrobiosis lipoidica E13.620
    - nephropathy E13.21
    - neuralgia E13.42
    - neurologic complication NEC E13.49
    - neuropathic arthropathy E13.610
    - neuropathy E13.40
    - ophthalmic complication NEC E13.39
    - oral complication NEC E13.638
    - periodontal disease E13.630
    - peripheral angiopathy E13.51
      - with gangrene E13.52
    - polyneuropathy E13.42
    - renal complication NEC E13.29
    - renal tubular degeneration E13.29

Diabetes, diabetic (mellitus) (sugar) E11.9 — *continued*
- specified type NEC E13.9 — *continued*
  - with — *continued*
    - retinopathy E13.319
      - with macular edema E13.311
        - resolved following treatment E13.37
      - nonproliferative E13.329
        - with macular edema E13.321
        - mild E13.329
          - with macular edema E13.321
        - moderate E13.339
          - with macular edema E13.331
        - severe E13.349
          - with macular edema E13.341
      - proliferative E13.359
        - with
          - combined traction retinal detachment and rhegmatogenous retinal detachment E13.354
          - macular edema E13.351
          - stable proliferative diabetic retinopathy E13.355
          - traction retinal detachment involving the macula E13.352
          - traction retinal detachment not involving the macula E13.353
    - skin complication NEC E13.628
    - skin ulcer NEC E13.622
- steroid-induced — *see* Diabetes, due to, drug or chemical
- type 1 E10.9
  - with
    - amyotrophy E10.44
    - arthropathy NEC E10.618
    - autonomic (poly)neuropathy E10.43
    - cataract E10.36
    - Charcôt's joints E10.610
    - chronic kidney disease E10.22
    - circulatory complication NEC E10.59
    - complication E10.8
      - specified NEC E10.69
    - dermatitis E10.620
    - foot ulcer E10.621
    - gangrene E10.52
    - gastroparalysis E10.43
    - gastroparesis E10.43
    - glomerulonephrosis, intracapillary E10.21
    - glomerulosclerosis, intercapillary E10.21
    - hyperglycemia E10.65
    - hypoglycemia E10.649
      - with coma E10.641
    - ketoacidosis E10.10
      - with coma E10.11
    - kidney complications NEC E10.29
    - Kimmelstiel-Wilson disease E10.21
    - mononeuropathy E10.41
    - myasthenia E10.44
    - necrobiosis lipoidica E10.620
    - nephropathy E10.21
    - neuralgia E10.42
    - neurologic complication NEC E10.49
    - neuropathic arthropathy E10.610
    - neuropathy E10.40
    - ophthalmic complication NEC E10.39
    - oral complication NEC E10.638
    - periodontal disease E10.630
    - peripheral angiopathy E10.51
      - with gangrene E10.52
    - polyneuropathy E10.42
    - renal complication NEC E10.29
    - renal tubular degeneration E10.29

Diabetes, diabetic (mellitus) (sugar) E11.9 — continued
  type 1 E10.9 — continued
    with — continued
      retinopathy E10.319
        with macular edema E10.311
          resolved following treatment E10.37
        nonproliferative E10.329
          with macular edema E10.321
          mild E10.329
            with macular edema E10.321
          moderate E10.339
            with macular edema E10.331
          severe E10.349
            with macular edema E10.341
        proliferative E10.359
          with
            combined traction retinal detachment and rhegmatogenous retinal detachment E10.354
            macular edema E10.351
            stable proliferative diabetic retinopathy E10.355
            traction retinal detachment involving the macula E10.352
            traction retinal detachment not involving the macula E10.353
      skin complication NEC E10.628
      skin ulcer NEC E10.622
  type 2 E11.9
    with
      amyotrophy E11.44
      arthropathy NEC E11.618
      autonomic (poly)neuropathy E11.43
      cataract E11.36
      Charcot's joints E11.610
      chronic kidney disease E11.22
      circulatory complication NEC E11.59
      complication E11.8
        specified NEC E11.69
      dermatitis E11.620
      foot ulcer E11.621
      gangrene E11.52
      gastroparalysis E11.43
      gastroparesis E11.43
      glomerulonephrosis, intracapillary E11.21
      glomerulosclerosis, intercapillary E11.21
      hyperglycemia E11.65
      hyperosmolarity E11.00
        with coma E11.01
      hypoglycemia E11.649
        with coma E11.641
      kidney complications NEC E11.29
      Kimmelstiel-Wilson disease E11.21
      mononeuropathy E11.41
      myasthenia E11.44
      necrobiosis lipoidica E11.620
      nephropathy E11.21
      neuralgia E11.42
      neurologic complication NEC E11.49
      neuropathic arthropathy E11.610
      neuropathy E11.40
      ophthalmic complication NEC E11.39
      oral complication NEC E11.638
      periodontal disease E11.630
      peripheral angiopathy E11.51
        with gangrene E11.52
      polyneuropathy E11.42
      renal complication NEC E11.29
      renal tubular degeneration E11.29

Diabetes, diabetic (mellitus) (sugar) E11.9 — continued
  type 2 E11.9 — continued
    with — continued
      retinopathy E11.319
        with macular edema E11.311
          resolved following treatment E11.37
        nonproliferative E11.329
          with macular edema E11.321
          mild E11.329
            with macular edema E11.321
          moderate E11.339
            with macular edema E11.331
          severe E11.349
            with macular edema E11.341
        proliferative E11.359
          with
            combined traction retinal detachment and rhegmatogenous retinal detachment E11.354
            macular edema E11.351
            stable proliferative diabetic retinopathy E11.355
            traction retinal detachment involving the macula E11.352
            traction retinal detachment not involving the macula E11.353
      skin complication NEC E11.628
      skin ulcer NEC E11.622
    uncontrolled
      meaning
        hyperglycemia — see Diabetes, by type, with, hyperglycemia
        hypoglycemia — see Diabetes, by type, with, hypoglycemia
Diacyclothrombopathia D69.1
Diagnosis deferred R69
Dialysis (intermittent) (treatment)
  noncompliance (with) Z91.15
  renal (hemodialysis) (peritoneal), status Z99.2
  retina, retinal — see Detachment, retina, with retinal, dialysis
Diamond-Blackfan anemia (congenital hypoplastic) D61.01
Diamond-Gardener syndrome (autoerythrocyte sensitization) D69.2
Diaper rash L22
Diaphoresis (excessive) R61
Diaphragm — see condition
Diaphragmalgia R07.1
Diaphragmatitis, diaphragmitis J98.6
Diaphysial aclasis Q78.6
Diaphysitis — see Osteomyelitis, specified type NEC
Diarrhea, diarrheal (disease) (infantile) (inflammatory) R19.7
  achlorhydric K31.83
  allergic K52.29
    due to
      colitis — see Colitis, allergic
      enteritis — see Enteritis, allergic
  amebic (see also Amebiasis) A06.0
    with abscess — see Abscess, amebic
    acute A06.0
    chronic A06.1
    nondysenteric A06.2
  bacillary — see Dysentery, bacillary
  balantidial A07.0
  cachectic NEC K52.89
  Chilomastix A07.8
  choleriformis A00.1
  chronic (noninfectious) K52.9
  coccidial A07.3
  Cochin-China K90.1
    strongyloidiasis B78.0
  Dientamoeba A07.8
  dietetic (see also Diarrhea, allergic) K52.29
  drug-induced K52.1

Diarrhea, diarrheal (disease) (infantile) (inflammatory) R19.7 — continued
  due to
    bacteria A04.9
      specified NEC A04.8
    Campylobacter A04.5
    Capillaria philippinensis B81.1
    Clostridium difficile A04.7
    Clostridium perfringens (C) (F) A04.8
    Cryptosporidium A07.2
    drugs K52.1
    Escherichia coli A04.4
      enteroaggregative A04.4
      enterohemorrhagic A04.3
      enteroinvasive A04.2
      enteropathogenic A04.0
      enterotoxigenic A04.1
      specified NEC A04.4
    food hypersensitivity (see also Diarrhea, allergic) K52.29
    Necator americanus B76.1
    S. japonicum B65.2
    specified organism NEC A08.8
      bacterial A04.8
      viral A08.39
    Staphylococcus A04.8
    Trichuris trichiuria B79
    virus — see Enteritis, viral
    Yersinia enterocolitica A04.6
  dysenteric A09
  endemic A09
  epidemic A09
  flagellate A07.9
  Flexner's (ulcerative) A03.1
  functional K59.1
    following gastrointestinal surgery K91.89
    psychogenic F45.8
  Giardia lamblia A07.1
  giardial A07.1
  hill K90.1
  infectious A09
  malarial — see Malaria
  mite B88.0
  mycotic NEC B49
  neonatal (noninfectious) P78.3
  nervous F45.8
  neurogenic K59.1
  noninfectious K52.9
  postgastrectomy K91.1
  postvagotomy K91.1
  protozoal A07.9
    specified NEC A07.8
  psychogenic F45.8
  specified
    bacterium NEC A04.8
    virus NEC A08.39
  strongyloidiasis B78.0
  toxic K52.1
  trichomonal A07.8
  tropical K90.1
  tuberculous A18.32
  viral — see Enteritis, viral
Diastasis
  cranial bones M84.88
    congenital NEC Q75.8
  joint (traumatic) — see Dislocation
  muscle M62.00
    ankle M62.07-
    congenital Q79.8
    foot M62.07-
    forearm M62.03-
    hand M62.04-
    lower leg M62.06-
    pelvic region M62.05-
    shoulder region M62.01-
    specified site NEC M62.08
    thigh M62.05-
    upper arm M62.02-

Diastasis — *continued*
recti (abdomen)
complicating delivery O71.89
congenital Q79.59
Diastema, tooth, teeth, fully erupted M26.32
Diastematomyelia Q06.2
Diataxia, cerebral G80.4
Diathesis
allergic — *see* History, allergy
bleeding (familial) D69.9
cystine (familial) E72.00
gouty — *see* Gout
hemorrhagic (familial) D69.9
newborn NEC P53
spasmophilic R29.0
Diaz's disease or osteochondrosis
(juvenile) (talus) — *see* Osteochondrosis, juvenile, tarsus
Dibothriocephalus, dibothriocephaliasis
(latus) (infection) (infestation) B70.0
larval B70.1
Dicephalus, dicephaly Q89.4
Dichotomy, teeth K00.2
Dichromat, dichromatopsia (congenital) — *see* Deficiency, color vision
Dichuchwa A65
Dicroceliasis B66.2
Didelphia, didelphys — *see* Double uterus
Didymytis N45.1
with orchitis N45.3
Dietary
inadequacy or deficiency E63.9
surveillance and counseling Z71.3
Dietl's crisis N13.8
Dieulafoy lesion (hemorrhagic)
duodenum K31.82
esophagus K22.8
intestine (colon) K63.81
stomach K31.82
Difficult, difficulty (in)
acculturation Z60.3
feeding R63.3
newborn P92.9
breast P92.5
specified NEC P92.8
nonorganic (infant or child) F98.29
intubation, in anesthesia T88.4
mechanical, gastroduodenal stoma K91.89
causing obstruction K91.3
micturition
need to immediately re-void R39.191
position dependent R39.192
specified NEC R39.198
reading (developmental) F81.0
secondary to emotional disorders F93.9
spelling (specific) F81.81
with reading disorder F81.89
due to inadequate teaching Z55.8
swallowing — *see* Dysphagia
walking R26.2
work
conditions NEC Z56.5
schedule Z56.3
Diffuse — *see* condition
Di George's syndrome (thymic hypoplasia) D82.1
Di Guglielmo's disease C94.0-
Digestive — *see* condition
Dihydropyrimidine dehydrogenase disease (DPD) E88.89
Diktyoma — *see* Neoplasm, malignant, by site
Dilaceration, tooth K00.4
Dilatation
anus K59.8
venule — *see* Hemorrhoids
aorta (focal) (general) — *see* Ectasia, aorta
with aneurysm — *see* Aneurysm, aorta
congenital Q25.44

Dilatation — *continued*
artery — *see* Aneurysm
bladder (sphincter) N32.89
congenital Q64.79
blood vessel I99.8
bronchial J47.9
with
exacerbation (acute) J47.1
lower respiratory infection J47.0
calyx (due to obstruction) — *see* Hydronephrosis
capillaries I78.8
cardiac (acute) (chronic) — *see also* Hypertrophy, cardiac
congenital Q24.8
valve NEC Q24.8
pulmonary Q22.3
valve — *see* Endocarditis
cavum septi pellucidi Q06.8
cervix (uteri) — *see also* Incompetency, cervix
incomplete, poor, slow complicating delivery O62.0
colon K59.39
congenital Q43.1
psychogenic F45.8
toxic K59.31
common duct (acquired) K83.8
congenital Q44.5
cystic duct (acquired) K82.8
congenital Q44.5
duct, mammary — *see* Ectasia, mammary duct
duodenum K59.8
esophagus K22.8
congenital Q39.5
due to achalasia K22.0
eustachian tube, congenital Q17.8
gallbladder K82.8
gastric — *see* Dilatation, stomach
heart (acute) (chronic) — *see also* Hypertrophy, cardiac
congenital Q24.8
valve — *see* Endocarditis
ileum K59.8
psychogenic F45.8
jejunum K59.8
psychogenic F45.8
kidney (calyx) (collecting structures) (cystic) (parenchyma) (pelvis) (idiopathic) N28.89
lacrimal passages or duct — *see* Disorder, lacrimal system, changes
lymphatic vessel I89.0
mammary duct — *see* Ectasia, mammary duct
Meckel's diverticulum (congenital) Q43.0
malignant — *see* Table of Neoplasms, small intestine, malignant
myocardium (acute) (chronic) — *see* Hypertrophy, cardiac
organ or site, congenital NEC — *see* Distortion
pancreatic duct K86.89
pericardium — *see* Pericarditis
pharynx J39.2
prostate N42.89
pulmonary
artery (idiopathic) I28.8
valve, congenital Q22.3
pupil H57.04
rectum K59.39
saccule, congenital Q16.5
salivary gland (duct) K11.8
sphincter ani K62.89
stomach K31.89
acute K31.0
psychogenic F45.8
submaxillary duct K11.8
trachea, congenital Q32.1
ureter (idiopathic) N28.82
congenital Q62.2
due to obstruction N13.4
urethra (acquired) N36.8

Dilatation — *continued*
vasomotor I73.9
vein I86.8
ventricular, ventricle (acute) (chronic) — *see also* Hypertrophy, cardiac
cerebral, congenital Q04.8
venule NEC I86.8
vesical orifice N32.89
Dilated, dilation — *see* Dilatation
Diminished, diminution
hearing (acuity) — *see* Deafness
sense or sensation (cold) (heat) (tactile) (vibratory) R20.8
vision NEC H54.7
vital capacity R94.2
Diminuta taenia B71.0
Dimitri-Sturge-Weber disease Q85.8
Dimple
congenital sacral Q82.6
parasacral Q82.6
pilonidal or postanal — *see* Cyst, pilonidal
Dioctophyme renalis (infection) (infestation) B83.8
Dipetalonemiasis B74.4
Diphallus Q55.69
Diphtheria, diphtheritic (gangrenous) (hemorrhagic) A36.9
carrier (suspected) Z22.2
cutaneous A36.3
faucial A36.0
infection of wound A36.3
laryngeal A36.2
myocarditis A36.81
nasal, anterior A36.89
nasopharyngeal A36.1
neurological complication A36.89
pharyngeal A36.0
specified site NEC A36.89
tonsillar A36.0
Diphyllobothriasis (intestine) B70.0
larval B70.1
Diplacusis H93.22-
Diplegia (upper limbs) G83.0
congenital (cerebral) G80.8
facial G51.0
lower limbs G82.20
spastic G80.1
Diplococcus, diplococcal — *see* condition
Dipsomania F10.20
with
psychosis — *see* Psychosis, alcoholic
remission F10.21
Dipylidiasis B71.1
Diplopia H53.2
DIRA (deficiency of interleukin 1 receptor antagonist) M04.8
Direction, teeth, abnormal, fully erupted M26.30
Dirofilariasis B74.8
Dirt-eating child F98.3
Disability, disabilities
heart — *see* Disease, heart
intellectual F79
with
autistic features F84.9
mild (I.Q. 50-69) F70
moderate (I.Q. 35-49) F71
profound (I.Q. under 20) F73
severe (I.Q. 20-34) F72
specified level NEC F78
knowledge acquisition F81.9
learning F81.9
limiting activities Z73.6
spelling, specific F81.81
Disappearance of family member Z63.4
Disarticulation — *see* Amputation
meaning traumatic amputation — *see* Amputation, traumatic

DISEASE INDEX

Discharge (from)
  abnormal finding in — *see* Abnormal, specimen
  breast (female) (male) N64.52
  diencephalic autonomic idiopathic — *see* Epilepsy, specified NEC
  ear — *see also* Otorrhea
    blood — *see* Otorrhagia
  excessive urine R35.8
  nipple N64.52
  penile R36.9
  postnasal R09.82
  prison, anxiety concerning Z65.2
  urethral R36.9
    hematospermia R36.1
    without blood R36.0
  vaginal N89.8
Discitis, diskitis M46.40
  cervical region M46.42
  cervicothoracic region M46.43
  lumbar region M46.46
  lumbosacral region M46.47
  multiple sites M46.49
  occipito-atlanto-axial region M46.41
  pyogenic — *see* Infection, intervertebral disc, pyogenic
  sacrococcygeal region M46.48
  thoracic region M46.44
  thoracolumbar region M46.45
Discoid
  meniscus (congenital) Q68.6
  semilunar cartilage (congenital) — *see* Derangement, knee, meniscus, specified NEC
Discoloration
  nails L60.8
  teeth (posteruptive) K03.7
    during formation K00.8
Discomfort
  chest R07.89
  visual H53.14-
Discontinuity, ossicles, ear H74.2-
Discord (with)
  boss Z56.4
  classmates Z55.4
  counselor Z64.4
  employer Z56.4
  family Z63.8
  fellow employees Z56.4
  in-laws Z63.1
  landlord Z59.2
  lodgers Z59.2
  neighbors Z59.2
  probation officer Z64.4
  social worker Z64.4
  teachers Z55.4
  workmates Z56.4
Discordant connection
  atrioventricular (congenital) Q20.5
  ventriculoarterial Q20.3
Discrepancy
  centric occlusion maximum intercuspation M26.55
  leg length (acquired) — *see* Deformity, limb, unequal length
    congenital — *see* Defect, reduction, lower limb
  uterine size date O26.84-
Discrimination
  ethnic Z60.5
  political Z60.5
  racial Z60.5
  religious Z60.5
  sex Z60.5

Disease, diseased — *see also* Syndrome
  absorbent system I87.8
  acid-peptic K30
  Acosta's T70.29
  Adams-Stokes (-Morgagni) (syncope with heart block) I45.9
  Addison's anemia (pernicious) D51.0
  adenoids (and tonsils) J35.9
  adrenal (capsule) (cortex) (gland) (medullary) E27.9
    hyperfunction E27.0
    specified NEC E27.8
  ainhum L94.6
  airway
    obstructive, chronic J44.9
      due to
        cotton dust J66.0
        specific organic dusts NEC J66.8
    reactive — *see* Asthma
  akamushi (scrub typhus) A75.3
  Albers-Schönberg (marble bones) Q78.2
  Albert's — *see* Tendinitis, Achilles
  alimentary canal K63.9
  alligator-skin Q80.9
    acquired L85.0
  alpha heavy chain C88.3
  alpine T70.29
  altitude T70.20
  alveolar ridge
    edentulous K06.9
    specified NEC K06.8
  alveoli, teeth K08.9
  Alzheimer's G30.9 *[F02.80]*
    with behavioral disturbance G30.9 *[F02.81]*
    early onset G30.0 *[F02.80]*
      with behavioral disturbance G30.0 *[F02.81]*
    late onset G30.1 *[F02.80]*
      with behavioral disturbance G30.1 *[F02.81]*
    specified NEC G30.8 *[F02.80]*
      with behavioral disturbance G30.8 *[F02.81]*
  amyloid — *see* Amyloidosis
  Andersen's (glycogenosis IV) E74.09
  Andes T70.29
  Andrews' (bacterid) L08.89
  angiospastic I73.9
    cerebral G45.9
    vein I87.8
  anterior
    chamber H21.9
    horn cell G12.29
  antiglomerular basement membrane (anti-GBM) antibody M31.0
    tubulo-interstitial nephritis N12
  antral — *see* Sinusitis, maxillary
  anus K62.9
    specified NEC K62.89
  aorta (nonsyphilitic) I77.9
    syphilitic NEC A52.02
  aortic (heart) (valve) I35.9
    rheumatic I06.9
  Apollo B30.3
  aponeuroses — *see* Enthesopathy
  appendix K38.9
    specified NEC K38.8
  aqueous (chamber) H21.9
  Arnold-Chiari — *see* Arnold-Chiari disease
  arterial I77.9
    occlusive — *see* Occlusion, by site
      due to stricture or stenosis I77.1
  arteriocardiorenal — *see* Hypertension, cardiorenal
  arteriolar (generalized) (obliterative) I77.9
  arteriorenal — *see* Hypertension, kidney

Disease, diseased (*see also* Syndrome) — *continued*
  arteriosclerotic — *see also* Arteriosclerosis
    cardiovascular — *see* Disease, heart, ischemic, atherosclerotic
    coronary (artery) — *see* Disease, heart, ischemic, atherosclerotic
    heart — *see* Disease, heart, ischemic, atherosclerotic
  artery I77.9
    cerebral I67.9
    coronary I25.10
      with angina pectoris — *see* Arteriosclerosis, coronary (artery)
  arthropod-borne NOS (viral) A94
    specified type NEC A93.8
  atticoantral, chronic H66.20
    left H66.22
      with right H66.23
    right H66.21
      with left H66.23
  auditory canal — *see* Disorder, ear, external
  auricle, ear NEC — *see* Disorder, pinna
  Australian X A83.4
  autoimmune (systemic) NOS M35.9
    hemolytic (cold type) (warm type) D59.1
      drug-induced D59.0
    thyroid E06.3
  aviator's — *see* Effect, adverse, high altitude
  Ayerza's (pulmonary artery sclerosis with pulmonary hypertension) I27.0
  Babington's (familial hemorrhagic telangiectasia) I78.0
  bacterial A49.9
    specified NEC A48.8
    zoonotic A28.9
      specified type NEC A28.8
  Baelz's (cheilitis glandularis apostematosa) K13.0
  bagasse J67.1
  balloon — *see* Effect, adverse, high altitude
  Bang's (brucella abortus) A23.1
  Bannister's T78.3
  barometer makers' — *see* Poisoning, mercury
  Barraquer (-Simons') (progressive lipodystrophy) E88.1
  Barrett's — *see* Barrett's, esophagus
  Bartholin's gland N75.9
  basal ganglia G25.9
    degenerative G23.9
      specified NEC G23.8
    specified NEC G25.89
  Basedow's (exophthalmic goiter) — *see* Hyperthyroidism, with, goiter (diffuse)
  Bateman's B08.1
  Batten-Steinert G71.11
  Battey A31.0
  Beard's (neurasthenia) F48.8
  Becker
    idiopathic mural endomyocardial I42.3
    myotonia congenita G71.12
  Begbie's (exophthalmic goiter) — *see* Hyperthyroidism, with, goiter (diffuse)
  behavioral, organic F07.9
  Beigel's (white piedra) B36.2
  Benson's — *see* Deposit, crystalline
  Bernard-Soulier (thrombopathy) D69.1
  Bernhardt (-Roth) — *see* Mononeuropathy, lower limb, meralgia paresthetica
  Biermer's (pernicious anemia) D51.0
  bile duct (common) (hepatic) K83.9
    with calculus, stones — *see* Calculus, bile duct
    specified NEC K83.8
  biliary (tract) K83.9
    specified NEC K83.8
  Billroth's — *see* Spina bifida
  bird fancier's J67.2

Disease, diseased (*see also* Syndrome) — *continued*

black lung J60
bladder N32.9
  in (due to)
    schistosomiasis (bilharziasis) B65.0 *[N33]*
  specified NEC N32.89
bleeder's D66
blood D75.9
  forming organs D75.9
  vessel I99.9
Bloodgood's — *see* Mastopathy, cystic
Bodechtel-Guttmann (subacute sclerosing panencephalitis) A81.1
bone — *see also* Disorder, bone
  aluminum M83.4
  fibrocystic NEC
    jaw M27.49
bone-marrow D75.9
Borna A83.9
Bornholm (epidemic pleurodynia) B33.0
Bouchard's (myopathic dilatation of the stomach) K31.0
Bouillaud's (rheumatic heart disease) I01.9
Bourneville (-Brissaud) (tuberous sclerosis) Q85.1
Bouveret (-Hoffmann) (paroxysmal tachycardia) I47.9
bowel K63.9
  functional K59.9
    psychogenic F45.8
brain G93.9
  arterial, artery I67.9
  arteriosclerotic I67.2
  congenital Q04.9
  degenerative — *see* Degeneration, brain
  inflammatory — *see* Encephalitis
  organic G93.9
    arteriosclerotic I67.2
  parasitic NEC B71.9 *[G94]*
  senile NEC G31.1
  specified NEC G93.89
breast (*see also* Disorder, breast) N64.9
  cystic (chronic) — *see* Mastopathy, cystic
  fibrocystic — *see* Mastopathy, cystic
  Paget's
    female, unspecified side C50.91-
    male, unspecified side C50.92-
  specified NEC N64.89
Breda's — *see* Yaws
Bretonneau's (diphtheritic malignant angina) A36.0
Bright's — *see* Nephritis
  arteriosclerotic — *see* Hypertension, kidney
Brill's (recrudescent typhus) A75.1
Brill-Zinsser (recrudescent typhus) A75.1
Brion-Kayser — *see* Fever, paratyphoid
broad
  beta E78.2
  ligament (noninflammatory) N83.9
    inflammatory — *see* Disease, pelvis, inflammatory
    specified NEC N83.8
Brocq's
  meaning
    dermatitis herpetiformis L13.0
    prurigo L28.2
Brocq-Duhring (dermatitis herpetiformis) L13.0
bronchopulmonary J98.4
bronchus NEC J98.09
bronze Addison's E27.1
  tuberculous A18.7
budgerigar fancier's J67.2
Buerger's (thromboangiitis obliterans) I73.1
bullous L13.9
  chronic of childhood L12.2
  specified NEC L13.8
Bürger-Grütz (essential familial hyperlipemia) E78.3

Disease, diseased (*see also* Syndrome) — *continued*

bursa — *see* Bursopathy
caisson T70.3
California — *see* Coccidioidomycosis
capillaries I78.9
  specified NEC I78.8
Carapata A68.0
cardiac — *see* Disease, heart
cardiopulmonary, chronic I27.9
cardiorenal (hepatic) (hypertensive) (vascular) — *see* Hypertension, cardiorenal
cardiovascular (atherosclerotic) I25.10
  with angina pectoris — *see* Arteriosclerosis, coronary (artery),
  congenital Q28.9
  hypertensive — *see* Hypertension, heart
  newborn P29.9
    specified NEC P29.89
  renal (hypertensive) — *see* Hypertension, cardiorenal
  syphilitic (asymptomatic) A52.00
cartilage — *see* Disorder, cartilage
Castellani's A69.8
Castleman (unicentric) (multicentric) D47.Z2
  HHV-8-associated (*see also* Herpesvirus, human, 8) D47.Z2
cat-scratch A28.1
Cavare's (familial periodic paralysis) G72.3
cecum K63.9
celiac (adult) (infantile) (with steatorrhea) K90.0
cellular tissue L98.9
central core G71.2
cerebellar, cerebellum — *see* Disease, brain
cerebral — *see also* Disease, brain
  degenerative — *see* Degeneration, brain
cerebrospinal G96.9
cerebrovascular I67.9
  acute I67.89
    embolic I63.4-
    thrombotic I63.3-
  arteriosclerotic I67.2
  specified NEC I67.89
cervix (uteri) (noninflammatory) N88.9
  inflammatory — *see* Cervicitis
  specified NEC N88.8
Chabert's A22.9
Chandler's (osteochondritis dissecans, hip) — *see* Osteochondritis, dissecans, hip
Charlouis — *see* Yaws
Chédiak-Steinbrinck (-Higashi) (congenital gigantism of peroxidase granules) E70.330
chest J98.9
Chiari's (hepatic vein thrombosis) I82.0
Chicago B40.9
Chignon B36.8
chigo, chigoe B88.1
childhood granulomatous D71
Chinese liver fluke B66.1
chlamydial A74.9
  specified NEC A74.89
cholecystic K82.9
choroid H31.9
  specified NEC H31.8
Christmas D67
chronic bullous of childhood L12.2
chylomicron retention E78.3
ciliary body H21.9
  specified NEC H21.89
circulatory (system) NEC I99.8
  newborn P29.9
  syphilitic A52.00
    congenital A50.54
coagulation factor deficiency (congenital) — *see* Defect, coagulation
coccidioidal — *see* Coccidioidomycosis

Disease, diseased (*see also* Syndrome) — *continued*

cold
  agglutinin or hemoglobinuria D59.1
    paroxysmal D59.6
  hemagglutinin (chronic) D59.1
collagen NOS (nonvascular) (vascular) M35.9
  specified NEC M35.8
colon K63.9
  functional K59.9
    congenital Q43.2
  ischemic (*see also* Ischemia, intestine, acute) K55.039
colonic inflammatory bowel, unclassified (IBDU) K52.3
combined system — *see* Degeneration, combined
compressed air T70.3
Concato's (pericardial polyserositis) A19.9
  nontubercular I31.1
  pleural — *see* Pleurisy, with effusion
conjunctiva H11.9
  chlamydial A74.0
  specified NEC H11.89
  viral B30.9
    specified NEC B30.8
connective tissue, systemic (diffuse) M35.9
  in (due to)
    hypogammaglobulinemia D80.1 *[M36.8]*
    ochronosis E70.29 *[M36.8]*
  specified NEC M35.8
Conor and Bruch's (boutonneuse fever) A77.1
Cooper's — *see* Mastopathy, cystic
Cori's (glycogenosis III) E74.03
corkhandler's or corkworker's J67.3
cornea H18.9
  specified NEC H18.89-
coronary (artery) — *see* Disease, heart, ischemic, atherosclerotic
  congenital Q24.5
  ostial, syphilitic (aortic) (mitral) (pulmonary) A52.03
corpus cavernosum N48.9
  specified NEC N48.89
Cotugno's — *see* Sciatica
coxsackie (virus) NEC B34.1
cranial nerve NOS G52.9
Creutzfeldt-Jakob — *see* Creutzfeldt-Jakob disease or syndrome
Crocq's (acrocyanosis) I73.89
Crohn's — *see* Enteritis, regional
Curschmann G71.11
cystic
  breast (chronic) — *see* Mastopathy, cystic
  kidney, congenital Q61.9
  liver, congenital Q44.6
  lung J98.4
    congenital Q33.0
cytomegalic inclusion (generalized) B25.9
  with pneumonia B25.0
  congenital P35.1
cytomegaloviral B25.9
  specified NEC B25.8
Czerny's (periodic hydrarthrosis of the knee) — *see* Effusion, joint, knee
Daae (-Finsen) (epidemic pleurodynia) B33.0
Darling's — *see* Histoplasmosis capsulati
de Quervain's (tendon sheath) M65.4
  thyroid (subacute granulomatous thyroiditis) E06.1
Débove's (splenomegaly) R16.1
deer fly — *see* Tularemia
Degos' I77.89
demyelinating, demyelinizating (nervous system) G37.9
  multiple sclerosis G35
  specified NEC G37.8
dense deposit (*see also* N00-N07 with fourth character .6) N05.6

DISEASE INDEX

Disease, diseased (*see also* Syndrome) — *continued*

deposition, hydroxyapatite — *see* Disease, hydroxyapatite deposition
Devergie's (pityriasis rubra pilaris) L44.0
Devic's G36.0
diaphorase deficiency D74.0
diaphragm J98.6
diarrheal, infectious NEC A09
digestive system K92.9
  specified NEC K92.89
disc, degenerative — *see* Degeneration, intervertebral disc
discogenic — *see also* Displacement, intervertebral disc NEC
  with myelopathy — *see* Disorder, disc, with, myelopathy
diverticular — *see* Diverticula
Dubois (thymus) A50.59 *[E35]*
Duchenne's
  muscular dystrophy G71.0
  pseudohypertrophy, muscles G71.0
Duchenne-Griesinger G71.0
ductless glands E34.9
Duhring's (dermatitis herpetiformis) L13.0
duodenum K31.9
  specified NEC K31.89
Dupré's (meningism) R29.1
Dupuytren's (muscle contracture) M72.0
Durand-Nicholas-Favre (climatic bubo) A55
Duroziez's (congenital mitral stenosis) Q23.2
ear — *see* Disorder, ear
Eberth's — *see* Fever, typhoid
Ebola (virus) A98.4
Ebstein's heart Q22.5
Echinococcus — *see* Echinococcus
echovirus NEC B34.1
Eddowes' (brittle bones and blue sclera) Q78.0
edentulous (alveolar) ridge K06.9
  specified NEC K06.8
Edsall's T67.2
Eichstedt's (pityriasis versicolor) B36.0
Ellis-van Creveld (chondroectodermal dysplasia) Q77.6
end stage renal (ESRD) N18.6
  due to hypertension I12.0
endocrine glands or system NEC E34.9
endomyocardial (eosinophilic) I42.3
English (rickets) E55.0
enteroviral, enterovirus NEC B34.1
  central nervous system NEC A88.8
epidemic B99.9
  specified NEC B99.8
epididymis N50.9
Erb (-Landouzy) G71.0
Erdheim-Chester (ECD) E88.89
esophagus K22.9
  functional K22.4
  psychogenic F45.8
  specified NEC K22.8
Eulenburg's (congenital paramyotonia) G71.19
eustachian tube — *see* Disorder, eustachian tube
external
  auditory canal — *see* Disorder, ear, external
  ear — *see* Disorder, ear, external
extrapyramidal G25.9
  specified NEC G25.89
eye H57.9
  anterior chamber H21.9
  inflammatory NEC H57.8
  muscle (external) — *see* Strabismus
  specified NEC H57.8
  syphilitic — *see* Oculopathy, syphilitic
eyeball H44.9
  specified NEC H44.89

Disease, diseased (*see also* Syndrome) — *continued*

eyelid — *see* Disorder, eyelid
  specified NEC — *see* Disorder, eyelid, specified type NEC
eyeworm of Africa B74.3
facial nerve (seventh) G51.9
  newborn (birth injury) P11.3
Fahr (of brain) G23.8
Fahr Volhard (of kidney) I12-
fallopian tube (noninflammatory) N83.9
  inflammatory — *see* Salpingo-oophoritis
  specified NEC N83.8
familial periodic paralysis G72.3
Fanconi's (congenital pancytopenia) D61.09
fascia NEC — *see also* Disorder, muscle
  inflammatory — *see* Myositis
  specified NEC M62.89
Fauchard's (periodontitis) — *see* Periodontitis
Favre-Durand-Nicolas (climatic bubo) A55
Fede's K14.0
Feer's — *see* Poisoning, mercury
female pelvic inflammatory (*see also* Disease, pelvis, inflammatory) N73.9
  syphilitic (secondary) A51.42
  tuberculous A18.17
Fernels' (aortic aneurysm) I71.9
fibrocaseous of lung — *see* Tuberculosis, pulmonary
fibrocystic — *see* Fibrocystic disease
Fiedler's (leptospiral jaundice) A27.0
fifth B08.3
file-cutter's — *see* Poisoning, lead
fish-skin Q80.9
  acquired L85.0
Flajani (-Basedow) (exophthalmic goiter) — *see* Hyperthyroidism, with, goiter (diffuse)
flax-dresser's J66.1
fluke — *see* Infestation, fluke
foot-and-mouth B08.8
foot process N04.9
Forbes' (glycogenosis III) E74.03
Fordyce's (ectopic sebaceous glands) (mouth) Q38.6
Fordyce-Fox (apocrine miliaria) L75.2
Forestier's (rhizomelic pseudopolyarthritis) M35.3
  meaning ankylosing hyperostosis — *see* Hyperostosis, ankylosing
Fothergill's
  neuralgia — *see* Neuralgia, trigeminal
  scarlatina anginosa A38.9
Fournier (gangrene) N49.3
  female N76.89
fourth B08.8
Fox (-Fordyce) (apocrine miliaria) L75.2
Francis' — *see* Tularemia
Franklin C88.2
Frei's (climatic bubo) A55
Friedreich's
  combined systemic or ataxia G11.1
  myoclonia G25.3
frontal sinus — *see* Sinusitis, frontal
fungus NEC B49
Gaisböck's (polycythemia hypertonica) D75.1
gallbladder K82.9
  calculus — *see* Calculus, gallbladder
  cholecystitis — *see* Cholecystitis
  cholesterolosis K82.4
  fistula — *see* Fistula, gallbladder
  hydrops K82.1
  obstruction — *see* Obstruction, gallbladder
  perforation K82.2
  specified NEC K82.8
gamma heavy chain C88.2
Gamna's (siderotic splenomegaly) D73.2
Gamstorp's (adynamia episodica hereditaria) G72.3
Gandy-Nanta (siderotic splenomegaly) D73.2

Disease, diseased (*see also* Syndrome) — *continued*

ganister J62.8
gastric — *see* Disease, stomach
gastroesophageal reflux (GERD) K21.9
  with esophagitis K21.0
gastrointestinal (tract) K92.9
  amyloid E85.4
  functional K59.9
    psychogenic F45.8
  specified NEC K92.89
Gee (-Herter) (-Heubner) (-Thaysen) (nontropical sprue) K90.0
genital organs
  female N94.9
  male N50.9
Gerhardt's (erythromelalgia) I73.81
Gibert's (pityriasis rosea) L42
Gierke's (glycogenosis I) E74.01
Gilles de la Tourette's (motor-verbal tic) F95.2
gingiva K06.9
  plaque induced K05.00
  specified NEC K06.8
gland (lymph) I89.9
Glanzmann's (hereditary hemorrhagic thrombasthenia) D69.1
glass-blower's (cataract) — *see* Cataract, specified NEC
  salivary gland hypertrophy K11.1
Glisson's — *see* Rickets
globe H44.9
  specified NEC H44.89
glomerular — *see also* Glomerulonephritis
  with edema — *see* Nephrosis
  acute — *see* Nephritis, acute
  chronic — *see* Nephritis, chronic
  minimal change N05.0
  rapidly progressive N01.9
glycogen storage E74.00
  Andersen's E74.09
  Cori's E74.03
  Forbes' E74.03
  generalized E74.00
  glucose-6-phosphatase deficiency E74.01
  heart E74.02 *[I43]*
  hepatorenal E74.09
  Hers' E74.09
  liver and kidney E74.09
  McArdle's E74.04
  muscle phosphofructokinase E74.09
  myocardium E74.02 *[I43]*
  Pompe's E74.02
  Tauri's E74.09
  type 0 E74.09
  type I E74.01
  type II E74.02
  type III E74.03
  type IV E74.09
  type V E74.04
  type VI-XI E74.09
  Von Gierke's E74.01
Goldstein's (familial hemorrhagic telangiectasia) I78.0
gonococcal NOS A54.9
graft-versus-host (GVH) D89.813
  acute D89.810
  acute on chronic D89.812
  chronic D89.811
grainhandler's J67.8
granulomatous (childhood) (chronic) D71
Graves' (exophthalmic goiter) — *see* Hyperthyroidism, with, goiter (diffuse)
Griesinger's — *see* Ancylostomiasis
Grisel's M43.6
Gruby's (tinea tonsurans) B35.0
Guillain-Barré G61.0
Guinon's (motor-verbal tic) F95.2
gum K06.9
gynecological N94.9

DISEASE INDEX

Disease, diseased (*see also* Syndrome) — *continued*
H (Hartnup's) E72.02
Haff — *see* Poisoning, mercury
Hageman (congenital factor XII deficiency) D68.2
hair (color) (shaft) L67.9
  follicles L73.9
    specified NEC L73.8
Hamman's (spontaneous mediastinal emphysema) J98.2
hand, foot and mouth B08.4
Hansen's — *see* Leprosy
Hantavirus, with pulmonary manifestations B33.4
  with renal manifestations A98.5
Harada's H30.81-
Hart's (pellagra-cerebellar ataxia-renal aminoaciduria) E72.02
Hartnup (pellagra-cerebellar ataxia-renal aminoaciduria) E72.02
Hashimoto's (struma lymphomatosa) E06.3
Hb — *see* Disease, hemoglobin
heart (organic) I51.9
  with
    pulmonary edema (acute) (*see also* Failure, ventricular, left) I50.1
    rheumatic fever (conditions in I00)
      active I01.9
        with chorea I02.0
        specified NEC I01.8
      inactive or quiescent (with chorea) I09.9
        specified NEC I09.89
  amyloid E85.4 [I43]
  aortic (valve) I35.9
  arteriosclerotic or sclerotic (senile) — *see* Disease, heart, ischemic, atherosclerotic
  artery, arterial — *see* Disease, heart, ischemic, atherosclerotic
  beer drinkers' I42.6
  beriberi (wet) E51.12
  black I27.0
  congenital Q24.9
    cyanotic Q24.9
    specified NEC Q24.8
  coronary — *see* Disease, heart, ischemic
  cryptogenic I51.9
  fibroid — *see* Myocarditis
  functional I51.89
    psychogenic F45.8
  glycogen storage E74.02 [I43]
  gonococcal A54.83
  hypertensive — *see* Hypertension, heart
  hyperthyroid (*see also* Hyperthyroidism) E05.90 [I43]
    with thyroid storm E05.91 [I43]
  ischemic (chronic or with a stated duration of over 4 weeks) I25.9
    atherosclerotic (of) I25.10
      with angina pectoris — *see* Arteriosclerosis, coronary (artery)
      coronary artery bypass graft — *see* Arteriosclerosis, coronary (artery),
      cardiomyopathy I25.5
    diagnosed on ECG or other special investigation, but currently presenting no symptoms I25.6
    silent I25.6
    specified form NEC I25.89
  kyphoscoliotic I27.1
  meningococcal A39.50
    endocarditis A39.51
    myocarditis A39.52
    pericarditis A39.53
  mitral I05.9
    specified NEC I05.8
  muscular — *see* Degeneration, myocardial
  psychogenic (functional) F45.8

Disease, diseased (*see also* Syndrome) — *continued*
heart (organic) I51.9 — *continued*
  pulmonary (chronic) I27.9
    in schistosomiasis B65.9 [I52]
    specified NEC I27.89
  rheumatic (chronic) (inactive) (old) (quiescent) (with chorea) I09.9
    active or acute I01.9
      with chorea (acute) (rheumatic) (Sydenham's) I02.0
    specified NEC I09.89
  senile — *see* Myocarditis
  syphilitic A52.06
    aortic A52.03
      aneurysm A52.01
    congenital A50.54 [I52]
  thyrotoxic (*see also* Thyrotoxicosis) E05.90 [I43]
    with thyroid storm E05.91 [I43]
  valve, valvular (obstructive) (regurgitant) — *see also* Endocarditis
    congenital NEC Q24.8
    pulmonary Q22.3
  vascular — *see* Disease, cardiovascular
heavy chain NEC C88.2
  alpha C88.3
  gamma C88.2
  mu C88.2
Hebra's
  pityriasis
    maculata et circinata L42
    rubra pilaris L44.0
  prurigo L28.2
hematopoietic organs D75.9
hemoglobin or Hb
  abnormal (mixed) NEC D58.2
    with thalassemia D56.9
  AS genotype D57.3
  Bart's D56.0
  C (Hb-C) D58.2
    with other abnormal hemoglobin NEC D58.2
    elliptocytosis D58.1
    Hb-S D57.2-
    sickle-cell D57.2-
    thalassemia D56.8
  Constant Spring D58.2
  D (Hb-D) D58.2
  E (Hb-E) D58.2
  E-beta thalassemia D56.5
  elliptocytosis D58.1
  H (Hb-H) (thalassemia) D56.0
    with other abnormal hemoglobin NEC D56.9
    Constant Spring D56.0
  I thalassemia D56.9
  M D74.0
  S or SS D57.1
  SC D57.2-
  SD D57.8-
  SE D57.8-
  spherocytosis D58.0
  unstable, hemolytic D58.2
hemolytic (newborn) P55.9
  autoimmune (cold type) (warm type) D59.1
  drug-induced D59.0
  due to or with
    incompatibility
      ABO (blood group) P55.1
      blood (group) (Duffy) (K(ell)) (Kidd) (Lewis) (M) (S) NEC P55.8
      Rh (blood group) (factor) P55.0
      Rh negative mother P55.0
    specified type NEC P55.8
  unstable hemoglobin D58.2
hemorrhagic D69.9
  newborn P53
Henoch (-Schönlein) (purpura nervosa) D69.0

Disease, diseased (*see also* Syndrome) — *continued*
hepatic — *see* Disease, liver
hepatobiliary K83.9
  toxic K71.9
hepatolenticular E83.01
heredodegenerative NEC
  spinal cord G95.89
herpesviral, disseminated B00.7
Hers' (glycogenosis VI) E74.09
Herter (-Gee) (-Heubner) (nontropical sprue) K90.0
Heubner-Herter (nontropical sprue) K90.0
high fetal gene or hemoglobin thalassemia D56.9
Hildenbrand's — *see* Typhus
hip (joint) M25.9
  congenital Q65.89
  suppurative M00.9
  tuberculous A18.02
His (-Werner) (trench fever) A79.0
Hodgson's I71.2
  ruptured I71.1
Holla — *see* Spherocytosis
hookworm B76.9
  specified NEC B76.8
host-versus-graft D89.813
  acute D89.810
  acute on chronic D89.812
  chronic D89.811
human immunodeficiency virus (HIV) B20
Huntington's G10
Hutchinson's (cheiropompholyx) — *see* Hutchinson's disease
hyaline (diffuse) (generalized)
  membrane (lung) (newborn) P22.0
  adult J80
hydatid — *see* Echinococcus
hydroxyapatite deposition M11.00
  ankle M11.07-
  elbow M11.02-
  foot joint M11.07-
  hand joint M11.04-
  hip M11.05-
  knee M11.06-
  multiple site M11.09
  shoulder M11.01-
  vertebra M11.08
  wrist M11.03-
hyperkinetic — *see* Hyperkinesia
hypertensive — *see* Hypertension
hypophysis E23.7
I-cell E77.0
Iceland G93.3
immune D89.9
immunoproliferative (malignant) C88.9
  small intestinal C88.3
  specified NEC C88.8
inclusion B25.9
  salivary gland B25.9
infectious, infective B99.9
  congenital P37.9
    specified NEC P37.8
    viral P35.9
      specified type NEC P35.8
  specified NEC B99.8
inflammatory
  penis N48.29
    abscess N48.21
    cellulitis N48.22
  prepuce N47.7
    balanoposthitis N47.6
  tubo-ovarian — *see* Salpingo-oophoritis

DISEASE INDEX

Disease, diseased (see also Syndrome) — continued

intervertebral disc — see also Disorder, disc
  with myelopathy — see Disorder, disc, with, myelopathy
  cervical, cervicothoracic — see Disorder, disc, cervical
  with
    myelopathy — see Disorder, disc, cervical, with myelopathy
    neuritis, radiculitis or radiculopathy — see Disorder, disc, cervical, with neuritis
    specified NEC — see Disorder, disc, cervical, specified type NEC
  lumbar (with)
    myelopathy M51.06
    neuritis, radiculitis, radiculopathy or sciatica M51.16
    specified NEC M51.86
  lumbosacral (with)
    neuritis, radiculitis, radiculopathy or sciatica M51.17
    specified NEC M51.87
  specified NEC — see Disorder, disc, specified NEC
  thoracic (with)
    myelopathy M51.04
    neuritis, radiculitis or radiculopathy M51.14
    specified NEC M51.84
  thoracolumbar (with)
    myelopathy M51.05
    neuritis, radiculitis or radiculopathy M51.15
    specified NEC M51.85
intestine K63.9
  functional K59.9
    psychogenic F45.8
    specified NEC K59.8
  organic K63.9
  protozoal A07.9
  specified NEC K63.89
iris H21.9
  specified NEC H21.89
iron metabolism or storage E83.10
island (scrub typhus) A75.3
itai-itai — see Poisoning, cadmium
Jakob-Creutzfeldt — see Creutzfeldt-Jakob disease or syndrome
jaw M27.9
  fibrocystic M27.49
  specified NEC M27.8
jigger B88.1
joint — see also Disorder, joint
  Charcot's — see Arthropathy, neuropathic (Charcot)
  degenerative — see Osteoarthritis
    multiple M15.9
    spine — see Spondylosis
  hypertrophic — see Osteoarthritis
  sacroiliac M53.3
  specified NEC — see Disorder, joint, specified type NEC
  spine NEC — see Dorsopathy
  suppurative — see Arthritis, pyogenic or pyemic
Jourdain's (acute gingivitis) K05.00
  nonplaque induced K05.01
  plaque induced K05.00
Kaschin-Beck (endemic polyarthritis) M12.10
  ankle M12.17-
  elbow M12.12-
  foot joint M12.17-
  hand joint M12.14-
  hip M12.15-
  knee M12.16-
  multiple site M12.19
  shoulder M12.11-
  vertebra M12.18
  wrist M12.13-

Disease, diseased (see also Syndrome) — continued

Katayama B65.2
Kedani (scrub typhus) A75.3
Keshan E59
kidney (functional) (pelvis) N28.9
  chronic N18.9
    hypertensive — see Hypertension, kidney
    stage 1 N18.1
    stage 2 (mild) N18.2
    stage 3 (moderate) N18.3
    stage 4 (severe) N18.4
    stage 5 N18.5
  complicating pregnancy — see Pregnancy, complicated by, renal disease
  cystic (congenital) Q61.9
  diabetic — see E08-E13 with .22
  fibrocystic (congenital) Q61.8
  hypertensive — see Hypertension, kidney
  in (due to)
    schistosomiasis (bilharziasis) B65.9 [N29]
  multicystic Q61.4
  polycystic Q61.3
    adult type Q61.2
    childhood type NEC Q61.19
      collecting duct dilatation Q61.11
Kimmelstiel (-Wilson) (intercapillary polycystic (congenital) glomerulosclerosis) — see E08-E13 with .21
Kimura D21.9
  specified site — see Neoplasm, connective tissue, benign
Kinnier Wilson's (hepatolenticular degeneration) E83.01
kissing — see Mononucleosis, infectious
Klebs' (see also Glomerulonephritis) N05-
Klippel-Feil (brevicollis) Q76.1
Köhler-Pellegrini-Stieda (calcification, knee joint) — see Bursitis, tibial collateral
Kok Q89.8
König's (osteochondritis dissecans) — see Osteochondritis, dissecans
Korsakoff's (nonalcoholic) F04
  alcoholic F10.96
    with dependence F10.26
Kostmann's (infantile genetic agranulocytosis) D70.0
kuru A81.81
Kyasanur Forest A98.2
labyrinth, ear — see Disorder, ear, inner
lacrimal system — see Disorder, lacrimal system
Lafora's — see Epilepsy, generalized, idiopathic
Lancereaux-Mathieu (leptospiral jaundice) A27.0
Landry's G61.0
Larrey-Weil (leptospiral jaundice) A27.0
larynx J38.7
legionnaires' A48.1
  nonpneumonic A48.2
Lenegre's I44.2
lens H27.9
  specified NEC H27.8
Lev's (acquired complete heart block) I44.2
Lewy body (dementia) G31.83 [F02.80]
  with behavioral disturbance G31.83 [F02.81]
Lichtheim's (subacute combined sclerosis with pernicious anemia) D51.0
Lightwood's (renal tubular acidosis) N25.89
Lignac's (cystinosis) E72.04
lip K13.0
lipid-storage E75.6
  specified NEC E75.5
Lipschütz's N76.6

Disease, diseased (see also Syndrome) — continued

liver (chronic) (organic) K76.9
  alcoholic (chronic) K70.9
    acute — see Disease, liver, alcoholic, hepatitis
    cirrhosis K70.30
      with ascites K70.31
    failure K70.40
      with coma K70.41
    fatty liver K70.0
    fibrosis K70.2
    hepatitis K70.10
      with ascites K70.11
    sclerosis K70.2
  cystic, congenital Q44.6
  drug-induced (idiosyncratic) (toxic) (predictable) (unpredictable) — see Disease, liver, toxic
  end stage K72.90
    due to hepatitis — see Hepatitis
  fatty, nonalcoholic (NAFLD) K76.0
    alcoholic K70.0
  fibrocystic (congenital) Q44.6
  fluke
    Chinese B66.1
    oriental B66.1
    sheep B66.3
  glycogen storage E74.09 [K77]
  in (due to)
    schistosomiasis (bilharziasis) B65.9 [K77]
  inflammatory K75.9
    alcoholic K70.1
    specified NEC K75.89
  polycystic (congenital) Q44.6
  toxic K71.9
    with
      cholestasis K71.0
      cirrhosis (liver) K71.7
      fibrosis (liver) K71.7
      focal nodular hyperplasia K71.8
      hepatic granuloma K71.8
      hepatic necrosis K71.10
        with coma K71.11
      hepatitis NEC K71.6
        acute K71.2
        chronic
          active K71.50
            with ascites K71.51
          lobular K71.4
          persistent K71.3
      lupoid K71.50
        with ascites K71.51
      peliosis hepatis K71.8
      veno-occlusive disease (VOD) of liver K71.8
  veno-occlusive K76.5
Lobo's (keloid blastomycosis) B48.0
Lobstein's (brittle bones and blue sclera) Q78.0
Ludwig's (submaxillary cellulitis) K12.2
lumbosacral region M53.87
lung J98.4
  black J60
  congenital Q33.9
  cystic J98.4
    congenital Q33.0
  fibroid (chronic) — see Fibrosis, lung
  fluke B66.4
    oriental B66.4
  in
    amyloidosis E85.4 [J99]
    sarcoidosis D86.0
    Sjögren's syndrome M35.02
    systemic
      lupus erythematosus M32.13
      sclerosis M34.81

DISEASE INDEX

Disease, diseased (*see also* Syndrome) — *continued*
  lung J98.4 — *continued*
    interstitial J84.9
      of childhood, specified NEC J84.848
      respiratory bronchiolitis J84.115
      specified NEC J84.89
    obstructive (chronic) J44.9
      with
        acute
          bronchitis J44.0
          exacerbation NEC J44.1
          lower respiratory infection J44.0
        alveolitis, allergic J67.9
        asthma J44.9
        bronchiectasis J47.9
          with
            exacerbation (acute) J47.1
            lower respiratory infection J47.0
        bronchitis J44.9
          with
            exacerbation (acute) J44.1
            lower respiratory infection J44.0
        emphysema J44.9
        hypersensitivity pneumonitis J67.9
      decompensated J44.1
        with
          exacerbation (acute) J44.1
    polycystic J98.4
      congenital Q33.0
    rheumatoid (diffuse) (interstitial) — *see* Rheumatoid, lung
  Lutembacher's (atrial septal defect with mitral stenosis) Q21.1
  Lyme A69.20
  lymphatic (gland) (system) (channel) (vessel) I89.9
  lymphoproliferative D47.9
    specified NEC D47.Z9
    T-gamma D47.Z9
    X-linked D82.3
  Magitot's M27.2
  malarial — *see* Malaria
  malignant — *see also* Neoplasm, malignant, by site
  Manson's B65.1
  maple bark J67.6
  maple-syrup-urine E71.0
  Marburg (virus) A98.3
  Marion's (bladder neck obstruction) N32.0
  Marsh's (exophthalmic goiter) — *see* Hyperthyroidism, with, goiter (diffuse)
  mastoid (process) — *see* Disorder, ear, middle
  Mathieu's (leptospiral jaundice) A27.0
  Maxcy's A75.2
  McArdle (-Schmid-Pearson) (glycogenosis V) E74.04
  mediastinum J98.59
  medullary center (idiopathic) (respiratory) G93.89
  Meige's (chronic hereditary edema) Q82.0
  meningococcal — *see* Infection, meningococcal
  mental F99
    organic F09
  mesenchymal M35.9
  mesenteric embolic (*see also* Ischemia, intestine, acute) K55.039
  metabolic, metabolism E88.9
    bilirubin E80.7
  metal-polisher's J62.8
  metastatic (*see also* Neoplasm, secondary, by site) C79.9
  microvascular — *code to* condition
  microvillus
    atrophy Q43.8
    inclusion (MVD) Q43.8
  middle ear — *see* Disorder, ear, middle
  Mikulicz' (dryness of mouth, absent or decreased lacrimation) K11.8

Disease, diseased (*see also* Syndrome) — *continued*
  Milroy's (chronic hereditary edema) Q82.0
  Minamata — *see* Poisoning, mercury
  minicore G71.2
  Minor's G95.19
  Minot's (hemorrhagic disease, newborn) P53
  Minot-von Willebrand-Jürgens (angiohemophilia) D68.0
  Mitchell's (erythromelalgia) I73.81
  mitral (valve) I05.9
    nonrheumatic I34.9
  mixed connective tissue M35.1
  moldy hay J67.0
  Monge's T70.29
  Morgagni's (syndrome) (hyperostosis frontalis interna) M85.2
  Morgagni-Adams-Stokes (syncope with heart block) I45.9
  Morton's (with metatarsalgia) — *see* Lesion, nerve, plantar
  Morvan's G60.8
  motor neuron (bulbar) (familial) (mixed type) (spinal) G12.20
    amyotrophic lateral sclerosis G12.21
    progressive bulbar palsy G12.22
    specified NEC G12.29
  moyamoya I67.5
  mu heavy chain disease C88.2
  multicore G71.2
  muscle — *see also* Disorder, muscle
    inflammatory — *see* Myositis
    ocular (external) — *see* Strabismus
  musculoskeletal system, soft tissue — *see also* Disorder, soft tissue
    specified NEC — *see* Disorder, soft tissue, specified type NEC
  mushroom workers' J67.5
  mycotic B49
  myelodysplastic, not classified C94.6
  myeloproliferative, not classified C94.6
    chronic D47.1
  myocardium, myocardial (*see also* Degeneration, myocardial) I51.5
    primary (idiopathic) I42.9
  myoneural G70.9
  Naegeli's D69.1
  nails L60.9
    specified NEC L60.8
  Nairobi (sheep virus) A93.8
  nasal J34.9
  nemaline body G71.2
  nerve — *see* Disorder, nerve
  nervous system G98.8
    autonomic G90.9
    central G96.9
      specified NEC G96.8
    congenital Q07.9
    parasympathetic G90.9
    specified NEC G98.8
    sympathetic G90.9
    vegetative G90.9
  neuromuscular system G70.9
  Newcastle B30.8
  Nicolas (-Durand)-Favre (climatic bubo) A55
  nipple N64.9
    Paget's C50.01-
      female C50.01-
      male C50.02-
  Nishimoto (-Takeuchi) I67.5
  nonarthropod-borne NOS (viral) B34.9
    enterovirus NEC B34.1
  nonautoimmune hemolytic D59.4
    drug-induced D59.2
  Nonne-Milroy-Meige (chronic hereditary edema) Q82.0
  nose J34.9
  nucleus pulposus — *see* Disorder, disc
  nutritional E63.9

Disease, diseased (*see also* Syndrome) — *continued*
  oast-house-urine E72.19
  ocular
    herpesviral B00.50
    zoster B02.30
  obliterative vascular I77.1
  Ohara's — *see* Tularemia
  Opitz's (congestive splenomegaly) D73.2
  Oppenheim-Urbach (necrobiosis lipoidica diabeticorum) — *see* E08-E13 with .620
  optic nerve NEC — *see* Disorder, nerve, optic
  orbit — *see* Disorder, orbit
  Oriental liver fluke B66.1
  Oriental lung fluke B66.4
  Ormond's N13.5
  Oropouche virus A93.0
  Osler-Rendu (familial hemorrhagic telangiectasia) I78.0
  osteofibrocystic E21.0
  Otto's M24.7
  outer ear — *see* Disorder, ear, external
  ovary (noninflammatory) N83.9
    cystic N83.20-
    inflammatory — *see* Salpingo-oophoritis
    polycystic E28.2
    specified NEC N83.8
  Owren's (congenital) — *see* Defect, coagulation
  pancreas K86.9
    cystic K86.2
    fibrocystic E84.9
    specified NEC K86.89
  panvalvular I08.9
    specified NEC I08.8
  parametrium (noninflammatory) N83.9
  parasitic B89
    cerebral NEC B71.9 *[G94]*
    intestinal NOS B82.9
    mouth B37.0
    skin NOS B88.9
    specified type — *see* Infestation
    tongue B37.0
  parathyroid (gland) E21.5
    specified NEC E21.4
  Parkinson's G20
  parodontal K05.6
  Parrot's (syphilitic osteochondritis) A50.02
  Parry's (exophthalmic goiter) — *see* Hyperthyroidism, with, goiter (diffuse)
  Parson's (exophthalmic goiter) — *see* Hyperthyroidism, with, goiter (diffuse)
  Paxton's (white piedra) B36.2
  pearl-worker's — *see* Osteomyelitis, specified type NEC
  Pellegrini-Stieda (calcification, knee joint) — *see* Bursitis, tibial collateral
  pelvis, pelvic
    female NOS N94.9
      specified NEC N94.89
    gonococcal (acute) (chronic) A54.24
    inflammatory (female) N73.9
      acute N73.0
      chlamydial A56.11
      chronic N73.1
      specified NEC N73.8
      syphilitic (secondary) A51.42
        late A52.76
      tuberculous A18.17
    organ, female N94.9
    peritoneum, female NEC N94.89
  penis N48.9
    inflammatory N48.29
      abscess N48.21
      cellulitis N48.22
    specified NEC N48.89
  periapical tissues NOS K04.90
  periodontal K05.6
    specified NEC K05.5

Disease, diseased (*see also* Syndrome) — *continued*

periosteum — *see* Disorder, bone, specified type NEC
peripheral
  arterial I73.9
  autonomic nervous system G90.9
  nerves — *see* Polyneuropathy
  vascular NOS I73.9
peritoneum K66.9
  pelvic, female NEC N94.89
  specified NEC K66.8
persistent mucosal (middle ear) H66.20
  left H66.22
    with right H66.23
  right H66.21
    with left H66.23
Petit's — *see* Hernia, abdomen, specified site NEC
pharynx J39.2
  specified NEC J39.2
Phocas' — *see* Mastopathy, cystic
photochromogenic (acid-fast bacilli) (pulmonary) A31.0
  nonpulmonary A31.9
Pick's G31.01 *[F02.80]*
  with behavioral disturbance G31.01 *[F02.81]*
  brain G31.01 [F02.80]
    with behavioral disturbance G31.01 [F02.81]
  of pericardium (pericardial pseudocirrhosis of liver) I31.1
pigeon fancier's J67.2
pineal gland E34.8
pink — *see* Poisoning, mercury
Pinkus' (lichen nitidus) L44.1
pinworm B80
Piry virus A93.8
pituitary (gland) E23.7
pituitary-snuff-taker's J67.8
pleura (cavity) J94.9
  specified NEC J94.8
pneumatic drill (hammer) T75.21
Pollitzer's (hidradenitis suppurativa) L73.2
polycystic
  kidney or renal Q61.3
    adult type Q61.2
    childhood type NEC Q61.19
      collecting duct dilatation Q61.11
  liver or hepatic Q44.6
  lung or pulmonary J98.4
    congenital Q33.0
  ovary, ovaries E28.2
  spleen Q89.09
polyethylene T84.05-
Pompe's (glycogenosis II) E74.02
Posadas-Wernicke B38.9
Potain's (pulmonary edema) — *see* Edema, lung
prepuce N47.8
  inflammatory N47.7
  balanoposthitis N47.6
Pringle's (tuberous sclerosis) Q85.1
prion, central nervous system A81.9
  specified NEC A81.89
prostate N42.9
  specified NEC N42.89
protozoal B64
  acanthamebiasis — *see* Acanthamebiasis
  African trypanosomiasis — *see* African trypanosomiasis
  babesiosis B60.0
  Chagas disease — *see* Chagas disease
  intestine, intestinal A07.9
  leishmaniasis — *see* Leishmaniasis
  malaria — *see* Malaria
  naegleriasis B60.2
  pneumocystosis B59

Disease, diseased (*see also* Syndrome) — *continued*

protozoal B64 — *continued*
  specified organism NEC B60.8
  toxoplasmosis — *see* Toxoplasmosis
pseudo-Hurler's E77.0
psychiatric F99
psychotic — *see* Psychosis
Puente's (simple glandular cheilitis) K13.0
puerperal (*see also* Puerperal) O90.89
pulmonary — *see also* Disease, lung
  artery I28.9
  chronic obstructive J44.9
    with
      acute bronchitis J44.0
      exacerbation (acute) J44.1
      lower respiratory infection (acute) J44.0
    decompensated J44.1
      with
        exacerbation (acute) J44.1
  heart I27.9
    specified NEC I27.89
  hypertensive (vascular) I27.0
  valve I37.9
    rheumatic I09.89
pulp (dental) NOS K04.90
pulseless M31.4
Putnam's (subacute combined sclerosis with pernicious anemia) D51.0
Pyle (-Cohn) (metaphyseal dysplasia) Q78.5
ragpicker's or ragsorter's A22.1
Raynaud's — *see* Raynaud's disease
reactive airway — *see* Asthma
Reclus' (cystic) — *see* Mastopathy, cystic
rectum K62.9
  specified NEC K62.89
Refsum's (heredopathia atactica polyneuritiformis) G60.1
renal (functional) (pelvis) (*see also* Disease, kidney) N28.9
  with
    edema — *see* Nephrosis
    glomerular lesion — *see* Glomerulonephritis
      with edema — *see* Nephrosis
    interstitial nephritis N12
  acute N28.9
  chronic (*see also* Disease, kidney, chronic) N18.9
  cystic, congenital Q61.9
  diabetic — *see* E08-E13 with .22
  end-stage (failure) N18.6
    due to hypertension I12.0
  fibrocystic (congenital) Q61.8
  hypertensive — *see* Hypertension, kidney
  lupus M32.14
  phosphate-losing (tubular) N25.0
  polycystic (congenital) Q61.3
    adult type Q61.2
    childhood type NEC Q61.19
      collecting duct dilatation Q61.11
  rapidly progressive N01.9
  subacute N01.9
Rendu-Osler-Weber (familial hemorrhagic telangiectasia) I78.0
renovascular (arteriosclerotic) — *see* Hypertension, kidney
respiratory (tract) J98.9
  acute or subacute NOS J06.9
    due to
      chemicals, gases, fumes or vapors (inhalation) J68.3
      external agent J70.9
        specified NEC J70.8
      radiation J70.0
      smoke inhalation J70.5
  noninfectious J39.8

Disease, diseased (*see also* Syndrome) — *continued*

respiratory (tract) J98.9 — *continued*
  chronic NOS J98.9
    due to
      chemicals, gases, fumes or vapors J68.4
      external agent J70.9
        specified NEC J70.8
      radiation J70.1
  newborn P27.9
    specified NEC P27.8
  due to
    chemicals, gases, fumes or vapors J68.9
      acute or subacute NEC J68.3
      chronic J68.4
    external agent J70.9
      specified NEC J70.8
  newborn P28.9
    specified type NEC P28.89
  upper J39.9
    acute or subacute J06.9
    noninfectious NEC J39.8
    specified NEC J39.8
    streptococcal J06.9
retina, retinal H35.9
  Batten's or Batten-Mayou E75.4 *[H36]*
  specified NEC H35.89
rheumatoid — *see* Arthritis, rheumatoid
rickettsial NOS A79.9
  specified type NEC A79.89
Riga (-Fede) (cachectic aphthae) K14.0
Riggs' (compound periodontitis) — *see* Periodontitis
Ritter's L00
Rivalta's (cervicofacial actinomycosis) A42.2
Robles' (onchocerciasis) B73.01
Roger's (congenital interventricular septal defect) Q21.0
Rosenthal's (factor XI deficiency) D68.1
Ross River B33.1
Rossbach's (hyperchlorhydria) K30
Rotes Quérol — *see* Hyperostosis, ankylosing
Roth (-Bernhardt) — *see* Mononeuropathy, lower limb, meralgia paresthetica
Runeberg's (progressive pernicious anemia) D51.0
sacroiliac NEC M53.3
salivary gland or duct K11.9
  inclusion B25.9
  specified NEC K11.8
  virus B25.9
sandworm B76.9
Schimmelbusch's — *see* Mastopathy, cystic
Schmorl's — *see* Schmorl's disease or nodes
Schönlein (-Henoch) (purpura rheumatica) D69.0
Schottmüller's — *see* Fever, paratyphoid
Schultz's (agranulocytosis) — *see* Agranulocytosis
Schwalbe-Ziehen-Oppenheim G24.1
Schwartz-Jampel G71.13
sclera H15.9
  specified NEC H15.89
scrofulous (tuberculous) A18.2
scrotum N50.9
sebaceous glands L73.9
semilunar cartilage, cystic — *see also* Derangement, knee, meniscus, cystic
seminal vesicle N50.9
serum NEC (*see also* Reaction, serum) T80.69
sexually transmitted A64
  anogenital
    herpesviral infection — *see* Herpes, anogenital
    warts A63.0
  chancroid A57
  chlamydial infection — *see* Chlamydia
  gonorrhea — *see* Gonorrhea
  granuloma inguinale A58

Disease, diseased (*see also* Syndrome) — *continued*

sexually transmitted A64 — *continued*
  specified organism NEC A63.8
  syphilis — *see* Syphilis
  trichomoniasis — *see* Trichomoniasis
Sézary C84.1-
shimamushi (scrub typhus) A75.3
shipyard B30.0
sickle-cell D57.1
  with crisis (vasoocclusive pain) D57.00
    with
      acute chest syndrome D57.01
      splenic sequestration D57.02
  elliptocytosis D57.8-
  Hb-C D57.20
    with crisis (vasoocclusive pain) D57.219
      with
        acute chest syndrome D57.211
        splenic sequestration D57.212
    without crisis D57.20
  Hb-SD D57.80
    with crisis D57.819
      with
        acute chest syndrome D57.811
        splenic sequestration D57.812
  Hb-SE D57.80
    with crisis D57.819
      with
        acute chest syndrome D57.811
        splenic sequestration D57.812
  specified NEC D57.80
    with crisis D57.819
      with
        acute chest syndrome D57.811
        splenic sequestration D57.812
  spherocytosis D57.80
    with crisis D57.819
      with
        acute chest syndrome D57.811
        splenic sequestration D57.812
  thalassemia D57.40
    with crisis (vasoocclusive pain) D57.419
      with
        acute chest syndrome D57.411
        splenic sequestration D57.412
    without crisis D57.40
silo-filler's J68.8
  bronchitis J68.0
  pneumonitis J68.0
  pulmonary edema J68.1
simian B B00.4
Simons' (progressive lipodystrophy) E88.1
sin nombre virus B33.4
sinus — *see* Sinusitis
Sirkari's B55.0
sixth B08.20
  due to human herpesvirus 6 B08.21
  due to human herpesvirus 7 B08.22
skin L98.9
  due to metabolic disorder NEC E88.9 *[L99]*
  specified NEC L98.8
slim (HIV) B20
small vessel I73.9
Sneddon-Wilkinson (subcorneal pustular dermatosis) L13.1
South African creeping B88.0
spinal (cord) G95.9
  congenital Q06.9
  specified NEC G95.89
spine — *see also* Spondylopathy
  joint — *see* Dorsopathy
  tuberculous A18.01
spinocerebellar (hereditary) G11.9
  specified NEC G11.8

Disease, diseased (*see also* Syndrome) — *continued*

spleen D73.9
  amyloid E85.4 *[D77]*
  organic D73.9
  polycystic Q89.09
  postinfectional D73.89
sponge-diver's — *see* Toxicity, venom, marine animal, sea anemone
Startle Q89.8
Steinert's G71.11
Sticker's (erythema infectiosum) B08.3
Stieda's (calcification, knee joint) — *see* Bursitis, tibial collateral
Stokes' (exophthalmic goiter) — *see* Hyperthyroidism, with, goiter (diffuse)
Stokes-Adams (syncope with heart block) I45.9
stomach K31.9
  functional, psychogenic F45.8
  specified NEC K31.89
stonemason's J62.8
storage
  glycogen — *see* Disease, glycogen storage
  mucopolysaccharide — *see* Mucopolysaccharidosis
striatopallidal system NEC G25.89
Stuart's (congenital factor X deficiency) D68.2
Stuart-Prower (congenital factor X deficiency) D68.2
subcutaneous tissue — *see* Disease, skin
supporting structures of teeth K08.9
  specified NEC K08.89
suprarenal (capsule) (gland) E27.9
  hyperfunction E27.0
  specified NEC E27.8
sweat glands L74.9
  specified NEC L74.8
Sweeley-Klionsky E75.21
Swift (-Feer) — *see* Poisoning, mercury
swimming-pool granuloma A31.1
Sylvest's (epidemic pleurodynia) B33.0
sympathetic nervous system G90.9
synovium — *see* Disorder, synovium
syphilitic — *see* Syphilis
systemic tissue mast cell C96.2
tanapox (virus) B08.71
Tangier E78.6
Tarral-Besnier (pityriasis rubra pilaris) L44.0
Tauri's E74.09
tear duct — *see* Disorder, lacrimal system
tendon, tendinous — *see also* Disorder, tendon
  nodular — *see* Trigger finger
terminal vessel I73.9
testis N50.9
thalassemia Hb-S — *see* Disease, sickle-cell, thalassemia
Thaysen-Gee (nontropical sprue) K90.0
Thomsen G71.12
throat J39.2
  septic J02.0
thromboembolic — *see* Embolism
thymus (gland) E32.9
  specified NEC E32.8
thyroid (gland) E07.9
  heart (*see also* Hyperthyroidism) E05.90 *[I43]*
    with thyroid storm E05.91 *[I43]*
  specified NEC E07.89
Tietze's M94.0
tongue K14.9
  specified NEC K14.8
tonsils, tonsillar (and adenoids) J35.9
tooth, teeth K08.9
  hard tissues K03.9
    specified NEC K03.89
  pulp NEC K04.99
  specified NEC K08.89
Tourette's F95.2
trachea NEC J39.8

Disease, diseased (*see also* Syndrome) — *continued*

tricuspid I07.9
  nonrheumatic I36.9
triglyceride-storage E75.5
trophoblastic — *see* Mole, hydatidiform
tsutsugamushi A75.3
tube (fallopian) (noninflammatory) N83.9
  inflammatory — *see* Salpingitis
  specified NEC N83.8
tuberculous NEC — *see* Tuberculosis
tubo-ovarian (noninflammatory) N83.9
  inflammatory — *see* Salpingo-oophoritis
  specified NEC N83.8
tubotympanic, chronic — *see* Otitis, media, suppurative, chronic, tubotympanic
tubulo-interstitial N15.9
  specified NEC N15.8
tympanum — *see* Disorder, tympanic membrane
Uhl's Q24.8
Underwood's (sclerema neonatorum) P83.0
Unverricht (-Lundborg) — *see* Epilepsy, generalized, idiopathic
Urbach-Oppenheim (necrobiosis lipoidica diabeticorum) — *see* E08-E13 with .620
ureter N28.9
  in (due to)
    schistosomiasis (bilharziasis) B65.0 *[N29]*
urethra N36.9
  specified NEC N36.8
urinary (tract) N39.9
  bladder N32.9
    specified NEC N32.89
  specified NEC N39.8
uterus (noninflammatory) N85.9
  infective — *see* Endometritis
  inflammatory — *see* Endometritis
  specified NEC N85.8
uveal tract (anterior) H21.9
  posterior H31.9
vagabond's B85.1
vagina, vaginal (noninflammatory) N89.9
  inflammatory NEC N76.89
  specified NEC N89.8
valve, valvular I38
  multiple I08.9
    specified NEC I08.8
van Creveld-von Gierke (glycogenosis I) E74.01
vas deferens N50.9
vascular I99.9
  arteriosclerotic — *see* Arteriosclerosis
  ciliary body NEC — *see* Disorder, iris, vascular
  hypertensive — *see* Hypertension
  iris NEC — *see* Disorder, iris, vascular
  obliterative I77.1
    peripheral I73.9
  occlusive I99.8
  peripheral (occlusive) I73.9
    in diabetes mellitus — *see* E08-E13 with .51
  vasomotor I73.9
  vasospastic I73.9
vein I87.9
venereal (*see also* Disease, sexually transmitted) A64
  chlamydial NEC A56.8
    anus A56.3
    genitourinary NOS A56.2
    pharynx A56.4
    rectum A56.3
  fifth A55
  sixth A55
  specified nature or type NEC A63.8
vertebra, vertebral — *see also* Spondylopathy
  disc — *see* Disorder, disc
vibration — *see* Vibration, adverse effects

Dislocation (articular) — *continued*
  knee S83.106 — *continued*
    proximal tibia
      anteriorly S83.11-
      laterally S83.14-
      medially S83.13-
      posteriorly S83.12-
    recurrent — *see also* Derangement, knee,
        specified NEC
    specified type NEC S83.19-
  lacrimal gland H04.16-
  lens (complete) H27.10
    anterior H27.12-
    congenital Q12.1
    ocular implant — *see* Complications,
        intraocular lens
    partial H27.11-
    posterior H27.13-
    traumatic S05.8x-
  ligament — *code by* site under Dislocation
  lumbar (vertebra) — *see* Dislocation, vertebra,
      lumbar
  lumbosacral (vertebra) — *see also* Dislocation,
      vertebra, lumbar
    congenital Q76.49
  mandible S03.0-
  meniscus (knee) — *see* Tear, meniscus
    other sites — *code by* site under Dislocation
  metacarpal (bone)
    distal end — *see* Dislocation, finger
    proximal end S63.06-
  metacarpophalangeal (joint)
    finger S63.26-
      index S63.26-
      little S63.26-
      middle S63.26-
      ring S63.26-
      thumb S63.11-
  metatarsal (bone) — *see* Dislocation, foot
  metatarsophalangeal (joint(s)) — *see*
      Dislocation, toe
  midcarpal (joint) S63.03-
  midtarsal (joint) — *see* Dislocation, foot
  neck S13.20
    specified site NEC S13.29
    vertebra — *see* Dislocation, vertebra,
        cervical
  nose (septal cartilage) S03.1
  occipitoatloid S13.111
  old — *see* Derangement, joint, specified type
      NEC
  ossicles, ear — *see* Discontinuity, ossicles, ear
  partial — *see* Subluxation, by site
  patella S83.006
    congenital Q74.1
    lateral S83.01-
    recurrent (nontraumatic) M22.0-
      incomplete M22.1-
    specified type NEC S83.09-
  pathological NEC M24.30
    ankle M24.37-
    elbow M24.32-
    foot joint M24.37-
    hand joint M24.34-
    hip M24.35-
    knee M24.36-
    lumbosacral joint — *see* subcategory M53.2
    pelvic region — *see* Dislocation,
        pathological, hip
    sacroiliac — *see* subcategory M53.2
    shoulder M24.31-
    wrist M24.33-
  pelvis NEC S33.30
    specified NEC S33.39
  phalanx
    finger or hand — *see* Dislocation, finger
    foot or toe — *see* Dislocation, toe
  prosthesis, internal — *see* Complications,
      prosthetic device, by site, mechanical

Dislocation (articular) — *continued*
  radial head S53.006
    anterior S53.01-
    posterior S53.02-
    specified type NEC S53.09-
  radiocarpal (joint) S63.02-
  radiohumeral (joint) — *see* Dislocation, radial
      head
  radioulnar (joint)
    distal S63.01-
    proximal — *see* Dislocation, elbow
  radius
    distal end — *see* Dislocation, wrist
    proximal end — *see* Dislocation, radial head
  recurrent M24.40
    ankle M24.47-
    elbow M24.42-
    finger M24.44-
    foot joint M24.47-
    hand joint M24.44-
    hip M24.45-
    knee M24.46-
      patella — *see* Dislocation, patella,
          recurrent
    patella — *see* Dislocation, patella, recurrent
    sacroiliac — *see* subcategory M53.2
    shoulder M24.41-
    toe M24.47-
    vertebra (*see also* subcategory) M43.5
      atlantoaxial M43.4
        with myelopathy M43.3
    wrist M24.43-
  rib (cartilage) S23.29
  sacrococcygeal S33.2
  sacroiliac (joint) (ligament) S33.2
    congenital Q74.2
    recurrent — *see* subcategory M53.2
  sacrum S33.2
  scaphoid (bone) (hand) (wrist) — *see*
      Dislocation, wrist
    foot — *see* Dislocation, foot
  scapula — *see* Dislocation, shoulder, girdle,
      scapula
  semilunar cartilage, knee — *see* Tear, meniscus
  septal cartilage (nose) S03.1
  septum (nasal) (old) J34.2
  sesamoid bone — *code by* site under
      Dislocation
  shoulder (blade) (ligament) (joint) (traumatic)
      S43.006
    acromioclavicular — *see* Dislocation,
        acromioclavicular
    chronic — *see* Dislocation, recurrent,
        shoulder
    congenital Q68.8
    girdle S43.30-
      scapula S43.31-
      specified site NEC S43.39-
    humerus S43.00-
      anterior S43.01-
      inferior S43.03-
      posterior S43.02-
    pathological — *see* Dislocation, pathological
        NEC, shoulder
    recurrent — *see* Dislocation, recurrent,
        shoulder
    specified type NEC S43.08-
  spine
    cervical — *see* Dislocation, vertebra, cervical
    congenital Q76.49
    due to birth trauma P11.5
    lumbar — *see* Dislocation, vertebra, lumbar
    thoracic — *see* Dislocation, vertebra,
        thoracic
  spontaneous — *see* Dislocation, pathological
  sternoclavicular (joint) S43.206
    anterior S43.21-
    posterior S43.22-
  sternum S23.29

Dislocation (articular) — *continued*
  subglenoid — *see* Dislocation, shoulder
  symphysis pubis S33.4
  talus — *see* Dislocation, ankle
  tarsal (bone(s)) (joint(s)) — *see* Dislocation, foot
  tarsometatarsal (joint(s)) — *see* Dislocation, foot
  temporomandibular (joint) S03.0-
  thigh, proximal end — *see* Dislocation, hip
  thorax S23.20
    specified site NEC S23.29
    vertebra — *see* Dislocation, vertebra
  thumb S63.10-
    interphalangeal joint — *see* Dislocation,
        interphalangeal (joint), thumb
    metacarpophalangeal joint — *see*
        Dislocation, metacarpophalangeal
        (joint), thumb
  thyroid cartilage S13.29
  tibia
    distal end — *see* Dislocation, ankle
    proximal end — *see* Dislocation, knee
  tibiofibular (joint)
    distal — *see* Dislocation, ankle
    superior — *see* Dislocation, knee
  toe(s) S93.106
    great S93.10-
      interphalangeal joint S93.11-
      metatarsophalangeal joint S93.12-
    interphalangeal joint S93.119
    lesser S93.106
      interphalangeal joint S93.11-
      metatarsophalangeal joint S93.12-
    metatarsophalangeal joint S93.12-
  tooth S03.2
  trachea S23.29
  ulna
    distal end S63.07-
    proximal end — *see* Dislocation, elbow
  ulnohumeral (joint) — *see* Dislocation, elbow
  vertebra (articular process) (body) (traumatic)
    cervical S13.101
      atlantoaxial joint S13.121
      atlantooccipital joint S13.111
      atloidooccipital joint S13.111
      joint between
        C0 and C1 S13.111
        C1 and C2 S13.121
        C2 and C3 S13.131
        C3 and C4 S13.141
        C4 and C5 S13.151
        C5and C6 S13.161
        C6and C7 S13.171
        C7and T1 S13.181
      occipitoatloid joint S13.111
    congenital Q76.49
    lumbar S33.101
      joint between
        L1and L2 S33.111
        L2and L3 S33.121
        L3 and L4 S33.131
        L4and L5 S33.141
    nontraumatic — *see* Displacement,
        intervertebral disc
    partial — *see* Subluxation, by site
    recurrent NEC — *see* subcategory M43.5
    thoracic S23.101
      joint between
        T1 and T2 S23.111
        T10 and T11 S23.161
        T11 and T12 S23.163
        T12 and L1 S23.171
        T2 and T3 S23.121
        T3 and T4 S23.123
        T4 and T5 S23.131
        T5 and T6 S23.133
        T6 and T7 S23.141
        T7 and T8 S23.143
        T8 and T9 S23.151
        T9 and T10 S23.153

Dislocation (articular) — *continued*
  wrist (carpal bone) S63.006
    carpometacarpal joint — *see* Dislocation,
      carpometacarpal (joint)
    distal radioulnar joint — *see* Dislocation,
      radioulnar (joint), distal
    metacarpal bone, proximal — *see*
      Dislocation, metacarpal (bone),
      proximal end
    midcarpal — *see* Dislocation, midcarpal
      (joint)
    radiocarpal joint — *see* Dislocation,
      radiocarpal (joint)
    recurrent — *see* Dislocation, recurrent, wrist
    specified site NEC S63.09-
    ulna — *see* Dislocation, ulna, distal end
  xiphoid cartilage S23.29
Disorder (of) — *see also* Disease
  acantholytic L11.9
    specified NEC L11.8
  acute
    psychotic — *see* Psychosis, acute
    stress F43.0
  adjustment (grief) F43.20
    with
      anxiety F43.22
        with depressed mood F43.23
      conduct disturbance F43.24
        with emotional disturbance F43.25
      depressed mood F43.21
        with anxiety F43.23
      other specified symptom F43.29
  adrenal (capsule) (gland) (medullary) E27.9
    specified NEC E27.8
  adrenogenital E25.9
    drug-induced E25.8
    iatrogenic E25.8
    idiopathic E25.8
  adult personality (and behavior) F69
    specified NEC F68.8
  affective (mood) — *see* Disorder, mood
  aggressive, unsocialized F91.1
  alcohol-related F10.99
    with
      amnestic disorder, persisting F10.96
      anxiety disorder F10.980
      dementia, persisting F10.97
      intoxication F10.929
        with delirium F10.921
        uncomplicated F10.920
      mood disorder F10.94
      other specified F10.988
      psychotic disorder F10.959
        with
          delusions F10.950
          hallucinations F10.951
      sexual dysfunction F10.981
      sleep disorder F10.982
  alcohol use
    mild F10.10
      with
        alcohol-induced
          anxiety disorder F10.180
          bipolar and related disorder F10.14
          depressive disorder F10.14
          psychotic disorder F10.159
          sexual dysfunction F10.181
          sleep disorder F10.182
        alcohol intoxication F10.129
          delirium F10.121

Disorder (of) (*see also* Disease) — *continued*
  alcohol use — *continued*
    moderate or severe F10.20
      with
        alcohol-induced
          anxiety disorder F10.280
          bipolar and related disorder F10.24
          depressive disorder F10.24
          major neurocognitive disorder,
            amnestic-confabulatory type
            F10.26
          major neurocognitive disorder,
            nonamnestic-confabulatory type
            F10.27
          mild neurocognitive disorder F10.288
          psychotic disorder F10.259
          sexual dysfunction F10.281
          sleep disorder F10.282
        alcohol intoxication F10.229
          delirium F10.221
  allergic — *see* Allergy
  alveolar NEC J84.09
  amino-acid
    cystathioninuria E72.19
    cystinosis E72.04
    cystinuria E72.01
    glycinuria E72.09
    homocystinuria E72.11
    metabolism — *see* Disturbance, metabolism,
      amino-acid
    specified NEC E72.8
    neonatal, transitory P74.8
    renal transport NEC E72.09
    transport NEC E72.09
  amnesic, amnestic
    alcohol-induced F10.96
      with dependence F10.26
    due to (secondary to) general medical
      condition F04
    psychoactive NEC-induced F19.96
      with
        abuse F19.16
        dependence F19.26
    sedative, hypnotic or anxiolytic-induced
      F13.96
      with dependence F13.26
  amphetamine-type substance use
    mild F15.10
    moderate F15.20
    severe F15.20
  amphetamine (or other stimulant) use
    mild
      with
        amphetamine- (or other stimulant)
          induced
            anxiety disorder F15.180
            bipolar and related disorder F15.14
            depressive disorder F15.14
            obsessive-compulsive and related
              disorder F15.188
            psychotic disorder F15.159
            sexual dysfunction F15.181
          amphetamine, cocaine, or other
            stimulant intoxication
            with perceptual disturbances F15.122
            without perceptual disturbances
              F15.129
          intoxication delirium F15.121
    moderate or severe
      with
        amphetamine- (or other stimulant)
          induced
            anxiety disorder F15.280
            obsessive-compulsive and related
              disorder F15.288
            sexual dysfunction F15.281
            bipolar and related disorder F15.24
            depressive disorder F15.24
            psychotic disorder F15.259

Disorder (of) (*see also* Disease) — *continued*
  amphetamine (or other stimulant) use
    — *continued*
    moderate or severe — *continued*
      with — *continued*
        amphetamine, cocaine, or other
          stimulant intoxication
          with perceptual disturbances F15.222
          without perceptual disturbances
            F15.229
        intoxication delirium F15.221
  anaerobic glycolysis with anemia D55.2
  anxiety F41.9
    due to (secondary to)
      alcohol F10.980
      amphetamine F15.980
        in
          abuse F15.180
          dependence F15.280
      anxiolytic F13.980
        in
          abuse F13.180
          dependence F13.280
      caffeine F15.980
        in
          abuse F15.180
          dependence F15.280
      cannabis F12.980
        in
          abuse F12.180
          dependence F12.280
      cocaine F14.980
        in
          abuse F14.180
          dependence F14.180
      general medical condition F06.4
      hallucinogen F16.980
        in
          abuse F16.180
          dependence F16.280
      hypnotic F13.980
        in
          abuse F13.180
          dependence F13.280
      inhalant F18.980
        in
          abuse F18.180
          dependence F18.280
      phencyclidine F16.980
        in
          abuse F16.180
          dependence F16.280
      psychoactive substance NEC F19.980
        in
          abuse F19.180
          dependence F19.280
      sedative F13.980
        in
          abuse F13.180
          dependence F13.280
      volatile solvents F18.980
        in
          abuse F18.180
          dependence F18.280
    generalized F41.1
    illness F45.21
    mixed
      with depression (mild) F41.8
      specified NEC F41.3
    organic F06.4
    phobic F40.9
      of childhood F40.8
    specified NEC F41.8
  aortic valve — *see* Endocarditis, aortic
  aromatic amino-acid metabolism E70.9
    specified NEC E70.8
  arteriole NEC I77.89
  artery NEC I77.89
  articulation — *see* Disorder, joint

Disorder (of) (*see also* Disease) — *continued*
- attachment (childhood)
  - disinhibited F94.2
  - reactive F94.1
- attention-deficit hyperactivity (adolescent) (adult) (child) F90.9
  - combined type F90.2
  - hyperactive type F90.1
  - inattentive type F90.0
  - specified type NEC F90.8
- attention-deficit without hyperactivity (adolescent) (adult) (child) F98.8
- auditory processing (central) H93.25
- autism spectrum F84.0
- autistic F84.0
- autonomic nervous system G90.9
  - specified NEC G90.8
- avoidant
  - child or adolescent F40.10
  - restrictive food intake F50.89
- balance
  - acid-base E87.8
    - mixed E87.4
  - electrolyte E87.8
  - fluid NEC E87.8
- behavioral (disruptive) — *see* Disorder, conduct
- beta-amino-acid metabolism E72.8
- bile acid and cholesterol metabolism E78.70
  - Barth syndrome E78.71
  - other specified E78.79
  - Smith-Lemli-Opitz syndrome E78.72
- bilirubin excretion E80.6
- binge eating F50.81
- binocular
  - movement H51.9
    - convergence
      - excess H51.12
      - insufficiency H51.11
    - internuclear ophthalmoplegia — *see* Ophthalmoplegia, internuclear
    - palsy of conjugate gaze H51.0
    - specified type NEC H51.8
  - vision NEC — *see* Disorder, vision, binocular
- bipolar (I) F31.9
  - current episode
    - depressed F31.9
      - with psychotic features F31.5
      - without psychotic features F31.30
        - mild F31.31
        - moderate F31.32
        - severe (without psychotic features) F31.4
          - with psychotic features F31.5
    - hypomanic F31.0
    - manic F31.9
      - with psychotic features F31.2
      - without psychotic features F31.10
        - mild F31.11
        - moderate F31.12
        - severe (without psychotic features) F31.13
          - with psychotic features F31.2
    - mixed F31.60
      - mild F31.61
      - moderate F31.62
      - severe (without psychotic features) F31.63
        - with psychotic features F31.64
    - severe depression (without psychotic features) F31.4
      - with psychotic features F31.5
  - in remission (currently) F31.70
    - in full remission
      - most recent episode
        - depressed F31.76
        - hypomanic F31.72
        - manic F31.74
        - mixed F31.78

Disorder (of) (*see also* Disease) — *continued*
- bipolar (I) F31.9 — *continued*
  - in remission (currently) F31.70 — *continued*
    - in partial remission
      - most recent episode
        - depressed F31.75
        - hypomanic F31.71
        - manic F31.73
        - mixed F31.77
- bipolar (II) F31.81
- organic F06.30
- single manic episode F30.9
  - mild F30.11
  - moderate F30.12
  - severe (without psychotic symptoms) F30.13
    - with psychotic symptoms F30.2
- specified NEC F31.89
- bladder N32.9
  - functional NEC N31.9
  - in schistosomiasis B65.0 [N33]
  - specified NEC N32.89
- bleeding D68.9
- blood D75.9
  - in congenital early syphilis A50.09 [D77]
- body dysmorphic F45.22
- bone M89.9
  - continuity M84.9
    - specified type NEC M84.80
      - ankle M84.87-
      - fibula M84.86-
      - foot M84.87-
      - hand M84.84-
      - humerus M84.82-
      - neck M84.88
      - pelvis M84.859
      - radius M84.83-
      - rib M84.88
      - shoulder M84.81-
      - skull M84.88
      - thigh M84.85-
      - tibia M84.86-
      - ulna M84.83-
      - vertebra M84.88
  - density and structure M85.9
    - cyst — *see also* Cyst, bone, specified type NEC
      - aneurysmal — *see* Cyst, bone, aneurysmal
      - solitary — *see* Cyst, bone, solitary
    - diffuse idiopathic skeletal hyperostosis — *see* Hyperostosis, ankylosing
    - fibrous dysplasia (monostotic) — *see* Dysplasia, fibrous, bone
    - fluorosis — *see* Fluorosis, skeletal
    - hyperostosis of skull M85.2
    - osteitis condensans — *see* Osteitis, condensans
    - specified type NEC M85.8-
      - ankle M85.87-
      - foot M85.87-
      - forearm M85.83-
      - hand M85.84-
      - lower leg M85.86-
      - multiple sites M85.89
      - neck M85.88
      - rib M85.88
      - shoulder M85.81-
      - skull M85.88
      - thigh M85.85-
      - upper arm M85.82-
      - vertebra M85.88
  - development and growth NEC M89.20
    - carpus M89.24-
    - clavicle M89.21-
    - femur M89.25-
    - fibula M89.26-
    - finger M89.24-
    - humerus M89.22-

Disorder (of) (*see also* Disease) — *continued*
- bone M89.9 — *continued*
  - development and growth NEC M89.20 — *continued*
    - ilium M89.259
    - ischium M89.259
    - metacarpus M89.24-
    - metatarsus M89.27-
    - multiple sites M89.29
    - neck M89.28
    - radius M89.23-
    - rib M89.28
    - scapula M89.21-
    - skull M89.28
    - tarsus M89.27-
    - tibia M89.26-
    - toe M89.27-
    - ulna M89.23-
    - vertebra M89.28
    - specified type NEC M89.8x-
  - brachial plexus G54.0
  - branched-chain amino-acid metabolism E71.2
    - specified NEC E71.19
  - breast N64.9
    - agalactia — *see* Agalactia
    - associated with
      - lactation O92.70
        - specified NEC O92.79
      - pregnancy O92.20
        - specified NEC O92.29
      - puerperium O92.20
        - specified NEC O92.29
    - cracked nipple — *see* Cracked nipple
    - galactorrhea — *see* Galactorrhea
    - hypogalactia O92.4
    - lactation disorder NEC O92.79
    - mastitis — *see* Mastitis
    - nipple infection — *see* Infection, nipple
    - retracted nipple — *see* Retraction, nipple
    - specified type NEC N64.89
  - Briquet's F45.0
  - bullous, in diseases classified elsewhere L14
  - caffeine use
    - mild
      - with
        - caffeine-induced
          - anxiety disorder F15.180
          - sleep disorder F15.182
    - moderate or severe
      - with
        - caffeine-induced
          - anxiety disorder F15.280
          - sleep disorder F15.282
  - cannabis use
    - mild F12.10
      - with
        - cannabis-induced
          - anxiety disorder F12.180
          - psychotic disorder F12.159
          - sleep disorder F12.188
        - cannabis intoxication delirium F12.121
          - with perceptual disturbances F12.122
          - without perceptual disturbances F12.129
    - moderate or severe F12.20
      - with
        - cannabis-induced
          - anxiety disorder F12.280
          - psychotic disorder F12.259
          - sleep disorder F12.288
        - cannabis intoxication
          - with perceptual disturbances F12.222
          - without perceptual disturbances F12.229
        - delirium F12.221
  - carbohydrate
    - absorption, intestinal NEC E74.39
    - metabolism (congenital) E74.9
      - specified NEC E74.8

Disorder (of) (see also Disease) — continued
cardiac, functional I51.89
carnitine metabolism E71.40
cartilage M94.9
    articular NEC — see Derangement, joint,
        articular cartilage
    chondrocalcinosis — see Chondrocalcinosis
    specified type NEC M94.8x-
        articular — see Derangement, joint,
            articular cartilage
        multiple sites M94.8x0
catatonia (due to known physiological
    condition) (with another mental disorder)
    F06.1
catatonic
    due to (secondary to) known physiological
        condition F06.1
    organic F06.1
central auditory processing H93.25
cervical
    region NEC M53.82
    root (nerve) NEC G54.2
character NOS F60.9
childhood disintegrative NEC F84.3
cholesterol and bile acid metabolism E78.70
    Barth syndrome E78.71
    other specified E78.79
    Smith-Lemli-Opitz syndrome E78.72
choroid H31.9
    atrophy — see Atrophy, choroid
    degeneration — see Degeneration, choroid
    detachment — see Detachment, choroid
    dystrophy — see Dystrophy, choroid
    hemorrhage — see Hemorrhage, choroid
    rupture — see Rupture, choroid
    scar — see Scar, chorioretinal
    solar retinopathy — see Retinopathy, solar
    specified type NEC H31.8
ciliary body — see Disorder, iris
    degeneration — see Degeneration, ciliary
        body
coagulation (factor) (see also Defect,
    coagulation) D68.9
    newborn, transient P61.6
cocaine use
    mild F14.10
        with
            amphetamine, cocaine, or other
                stimulant intoxication
                with perceptual disturbances F14.122
                without perceptual disturbances
                    F14.129
            cocaine-induced
                anxiety disorder F14.180
                bipolar and related disorder F14.14
                depressive disorder F14.14
                obsessive-compulsive and related
                    disorder F14.188
                psychotic disorder F14.159
                sexual dysfunction F14.181
                sleep disorder F14.182
            cocaine intoxication delirium F14.121
    moderate or severe F14.20
        with
            amphetamine, cocaine, or other
                stimulant intoxication
                with perceptual disturbances F14.222
                without perceptual disturbances
                    F14.229
            cocaine-induced
                anxiety disorder F14.280
                bipolar and related disorder F14.24
                depressive disorder F14.24
                obsessive-compulsive and related
                    disorder F14.288
                psychotic disorder F14.259
                sexual dysfunction F14.281
                sleep disorder F14.282
            cocaine intoxication delirium F14.221

Disorder (of) (see also Disease) — continued
coccyx NEC M53.3
cognitive F09
    due to (secondary to) general medical
        condition F09
    persisting R41.89
    due to
        alcohol F10.97
            with dependence F10.27
        anxiolytics F13.97
            with dependence F13.27
        hypnotics F13.97
            with dependence F13.27
        sedatives F13.97
            with dependence F13.27
        specified substance NEC F19.97
            with
                abuse F19.17
                dependence F19.27
communication F80.9
    social pragmatic F80.82
conduct (childhood) F91.9
    adjustment reaction — see Disorder,
        adjustment
    adolescent onset type F91.2
    childhood onset type F91.1
    compulsive F63.9
    confined to family context F91.0
    depressive F91.8
    group type F91.2
    hyperkinetic — see Disorder, attention-deficit
        hyperactivity
    oppositional defiance F91.3
    socialized F91.2
    solitary aggressive type F91.1
    specified NEC F91.8
    unsocialized (aggressive) F91.1
conduction, heart I45.9
congenital glycosylation (CDG) E74.8
conjunctiva H11.9
    infection — see Conjunctivitis
connective tissue, localized L94.9
    specified NEC L94.8
conversion (functional neurological symptom
    disorder)
    with
        abnormal movement F44.4
        anesthesia or sensory loss F44.6
        attacks or seizures F44.5
        mixed symptoms F44.7
        special sensory symptoms F44.6
        speech symptoms F44.4
        swallowing symptoms F44.4
        weakness or paralysis F44.4
convulsive (secondary) — see Convulsions
cornea H18.9
    deformity — see Deformity, cornea
    degeneration — see Degeneration, cornea
    deposits — see Deposit, cornea
    due to contact lens H18.82-
        specified as edema — see Edema, cornea
    edema — see Edema, cornea
    keratitis — see Keratitis
    keratoconjunctivitis — see
        Keratoconjunctivitis
    membrane change — see Change, corneal
        membrane
    neovascularization — see
        Neovascularization, cornea
    scar — see Opacity, cornea
    specified type NEC H18.89-
    ulcer — see Ulcer, cornea
corpus cavernosum N48.9
cranial nerve — see Disorder, nerve, cranial
cyclothymic F34.0
defiant oppositional F91.3
delusional (persistent) (systematized) F22
    induced F24
depersonalization F48.1

Disorder (of) (see also Disease) — continued
depressive F32.9
    major F32.9
        with psychotic symptoms F32.3
        in remission (full) F32.5
            partial F32.4
        recurrent F33.9
        single episode F32.9
            mild F32.0
            moderate F32.1
            severe (without psychotic symptoms)
                F32.2
                with psychotic symptoms F32.3
    organic F06.31
    persistent F34.1
    recurrent F33.9
        current episode
            mild F33.0
            moderate F33.1
            severe (without psychotic symptoms)
                F33.2
                with psychotic symptoms F33.3
        in remission F33.40
            full F33.42
            partial F33.41
        specified NEC F33.8
    single episode — see Episode, depressive
    specified NEC F32.89
developmental F89
    arithmetical skills F81.2
    coordination (motor) F82
    expressive writing F81.81
    language F80.9
        expressive F80.1
        mixed receptive and expressive F80.2
        receptive type F80.2
        specified NEC F80.89
    learning F81.9
        arithmetical F81.2
        reading F81.0
    mixed F88
    motor coordination or function F82
    pervasive F84.9
        specified NEC F84.8
    phonological F80.0
    reading F81.0
    scholastic skills — see also Disorder, learning
        mixed F81.89
    specified NEC F88
    speech F80.9
        articulation F80.0
        specified NEC F80.89
    written expression F81.81
diaphragm J98.6
digestive (system) K92.9
    newborn P78.9
        specified NEC P78.89
    postprocedural — see Complication,
        gastrointestinal
    psychogenic F45.8
disc (intervertebral) M51.9
    with
        myelopathy
            cervical region M50.00
            cervicothoracic region M50.03
            high cervical region M50.01
            lumbar region M51.06
            mid-cervical region M50.020
            sacrococcygeal region M53.3
            thoracic region M51.04
            thoracolumbar region M51.05
        radiculopathy
            cervical region M50.10
            cervicothoracic region M50.13
            high cervical region M50.11
            lumbar region M51.16
            lumbosacral region M51.17
            mid-cervical region M50.120
            sacrococcygeal region M53.3

DISEASE INDEX

Disorder (of) (*see also* Disease) — *continued*
disc (intervertebral) M51.9 — *continued*
  with — *continued*
    radiculopathy — *continued*
      thoracic region M51.14
      thoracolumbar region M51.15
    cervical M50.90
      with
        myelopathy M50.00
          C2-C3 M50.01
          C3-C4 M50.01
          C4-C5 M50.021
          C5-C6 M50.022
          C6-C7 M50.023
          C7-T1 M50.03
          cervicothoracic region M50.03
          high cervical region M50.01
          mid-cervical region M50.020
        neuritis, radiculitis or radiculopathy
          M50.10
          C2-C3 M50.11
          C3-C4 M50.11
          C4-C5 M50.121
          C5-C6 M50.122
          C6-C7 M50.123
          C7-T1 M50.13
          cervicothoracic region M50.13
          high cervical region M50.11
          mid-cervical region M50.120
      C2-C3 M50.91
      C3-C4 M50.91
      C4-C5 M50.921
      C5-C6 M50.922
      C6-C7 M50.923
      C7-T1 M50.93
      cervicothoracic region M50.93
      degeneration M50.30
        C2-C3 M50.31
        C3-C4 M50.31
        C4-C5 M50.321
        C5-C6 M50.322
        C6-C7 M50.323
        C7-T1 M50.33
        cervicothoracic region M50.33
        high cervical region M50.31
        mid-cervical region M50.320
      displacement M50.20
        C2-C3 M50.21
        C3-C4 M50.21
        C4-C5 M50.221
        C5-C6 M50.222
        C6-C7 M50.223
        C7-T1 M50.23
        cervicothoracic region M50.23
        high cervical region M50.21
        mid-cervical region M50.220
      high cervical region M50.91
      mid-cervical region M50.920
      specified type NEC M50.80
        C2-C3 M50.81
        C3-C4 M50.81
        C4-C5 M50.821
        C5-C6 M50.822
        C6-C7 M50.823
        C7-T1 M50.83
        cervicothoracic region M50.83
        high cervical region M50.81
        mid-cervical region M50.820
    specified NEC
      lumbar region M51.86
      lumbosacral region M51.87
      sacrococcygeal region M53.3
      thoracic region M51.84
      thoracolumbar region M51.85
disinhibited attachment (childhood) F94.2
disintegrative, childhood NEC F84.3
disruptive F91.9
  mood dysregulation F34.81
  specified NEC F91.8

disruptive behavior F91.9
dissocial personality F60.2
dissociative F44.9
  affecting
    motor function F44.4
      and sensation F44.7
    sensation F44.6
      and motor function F44.7
  brief reactive F43.0
  due to (secondary to) general medical
    condition F06.8
  mixed F44.7
  organic F06.8
  other specified NEC F44.89
double heterozygous sickling — *see* Disease,
  sickle-cell
dream anxiety F51.5
drug induced hemorrhagic D68.32
drug related F19.99
  abuse — *see* Abuse, drug
  dependence — *see* Dependence, drug
dysmorphic body F45.22
dysthymic F34.1
ear H93.9-
  bleeding — *see* Otorrhagia
  deafness — *see* Deafness
  degenerative H93.09-
  discharge — *see* Otorrhea
  external H61.9-
    auditory canal stenosis — *see* Stenosis,
      external ear canal
    exostosis — *see* Exostosis, external ear
      canal
    impacted cerumen — *see* Impaction,
      cerumen
    otitis — *see* Otitis, externa
    perichondritis — *see* Perichondritis, ear
    pinna — *see* Disorder, pinna
    specified type NEC H61.89-
      in diseases classified elsewhere H62.8x-
  inner H83.9-
    vestibular dysfunction — *see* Disorder,
      vestibular function
  middle H74.9-
    adhesive H74.1-
    ossicle — *see* Abnormal, ear ossicles
    polyp — *see* Polyp, ear (middle)
    specified NEC, in diseases classified
      elsewhere H75.8-
  postprocedural — *see* Complications, ear,
    procedure
  specified NEC, in diseases classified
    elsewhere H94.8-
eating (adult) (psychogenic) F50.9
  anorexia — *see* Anorexia
  binge F50.81
  bulimia F50.2
  child F98.29
    pica F98.3
    rumination disorder F98.21
  pica F50.89
    childhood F98.3
electrolyte (balance) NEC E87.8
  with
    abortion — *see* Abortion by type
      complicated by specified condition
      NEC
    ectopic pregnancy O08.5
    molar pregnancy O08.5
  acidosis (metabolic) (respiratory) E87.2
  alkalosis (metabolic) (respiratory) E87.3
elimination, transepidermal L87.9
  specified NEC L87.8
emotional (persistent) F34.9
  of childhood F93.9
    specified NEC F93.8

endocrine E34.9
  postprocedural E89.89
    specified NEC E89.89
erectile (male) (organic) (*see also* Dysfunction,
  sexual, male, erectile) N52.9
  nonorganic F52.21
erythematous — *see* Erythema
esophagus K22.9
  functional K22.4
  psychogenic F45.8
eustachian tube H69.9-
  infection — *see* Salpingitis, eustachian
  obstruction — *see* Obstruction, eustachian
    tube
  patulous — *see* Patulous, eustachian tube
  specified NEC H69.8-
extrapyramidal G25.9
  in diseases classified elsewhere — *see*
    category G26
  specified type NEC G25.89
eye H57.9
  postprocedural — *see* Complication,
    postprocedural, eye
eyelid H02.9
  cyst — *see* Cyst, eyelid
  degenerative H02.70
    chloasma — *see* Chloasma, eyelid
    madarosis — *see* Madarosis
    specified type NEC H02.79
    vitiligo — *see* Vitiligo, eyelid
    xanthelasma — *see* Xanthelasma
  dermatochalasis — *see* Dermatochalasis
  edema — *see* Edema, eyelid
  elephantiasis — *see* Elephantiasis, eyelid
  foreign body, retained — *see* Foreign body,
    retained, eyelid
  function H02.59
    abnormal innervation syndrome — *see*
      Syndrome, abnormal innervation
    blepharochalasis — *see* Blepharochalasis
    blepharoclonus — *see* Blepharoclonus
    blepharophimosis — *see* Blepharophimosis
    blepharoptosis — *see* Blepharoptosis
    lagophthalmos — *see* Lagophthalmos
    lid retraction — *see* Retraction, lid
  hypertrichosis — *see* Hypertrichosis, eyelid
  specified type NEC H02.89
  vascular H02.879
    left H02.876
      lower H02.875
      upper H02.874
    right H02.873
      lower H02.872
      upper H02.871
factitious F68.10
  with predominantly
    physical symptoms F68.12
      with psychological symptoms F68.13
    psychological symptoms F68.11
      with physical symptoms F68.13
factor, coagulation — *see* Defect, coagulation
fatty acid
  metabolism E71.30
    specified NEC E71.39
  oxidation
    LCAD E71.310
    MCAD E71.311
    SCAD E71.312
    specified deficiency NEC E71.318
feeding (infant or child) (*see also* Disorder,
  eating) R63.3
feigned (with obvious motivation) Z76.5
  without obvious motivation — *see* Disorder,
    factitious
female
  hypoactive sexual desire F52.0
  orgasmic F52.31
  sexual arousal F52.22

Disorder (of) (*see also* Disease) — *continued*
  fibroblastic M72.9
    specified NEC M72.8
  fluency
    adult onset F98.5
    childhood onset F80.81
    following
      cerebral infarction I69.323
      cerebrovascular disease I69.923
        specified disease NEC I69.823
      intracerebral hemorrhage I69.123
      nontraumatic intracranial hemorrhage
        NEC I69.223
      subarachnoid hemorrhage I69.023
    in conditions classified elsewhere R47.82
  fluid balance E87.8
  follicular (skin) L73.9
    specified NEC L73.8
  fructose metabolism E74.10
    essential fructosuria E74.11
    fructokinase deficiency E74.11
    fructose-1, 6-diphosphatase deficiency
      E74.19
    hereditary fructose intolerance E74.12
    other specified E74.19
  functional polymorphonuclear neutrophils D71
  gallbladder, biliary tract and pancreas in
    diseases classified elsewhere K87
  gamma-glutamyl cycle E72.8
  gastric (functional) K31.9
    motility K30
    psychogenic F45.8
    secretion K30
  gastrointestinal (functional) NOS K92.9
    newborn P78.9
    psychogenic F45.8
  gender-identity or -role F64.9
    childhood F64.2
    effect on relationship F66
    of adolescence or adulthood F64.0
      nontranssexual F64.8
    specified NEC F64.8
    uncertainty F66
  genito-pelvic pain penetration F52.6
  genitourinary system
    female N94.9
    male N50.9
    psychogenic F45.8
  globe H44.9
    degenerated condition H44.50
      absolute glaucoma H44.51-
      atrophy H44.52-
      leucocoria H44.53-
    degenerative H44.30
      chalcosis H44.31-
      myopia H44.2-
      siderosis H44.32-
      specified type NEC H44.39-
    endophthalmitis — *see* Endophthalmitis
    foreign body, retained — *see* Foreign body,
      intraocular, old, retained
    hemophthalmos — *see* Hemophthalmos
    hypotony H44.40
      due to
        ocular fistula H44.42-
        specified disorder NEC H44.43-
      flat anterior chamber H44.41-
      primary H44.44-
    luxation — *see* Luxation, globe
    specified type NEC H44.89
  glomerular (in) N05.9
    amyloidosis E85.4 [N08]
    cryoglobulinemia D89.1 [N08]
    disseminated intravascular coagulation D65
      [N08]
    Fabry's disease E75.21 [N08]
    familial lecithin cholesterol acyltransferase
      deficiency E78.6 [N08]
    Goodpasture's syndrome M31.0

Disorder (of) (*see also* Disease) — *continued*
  glomerular (in) N05.9 — *continued*
    hemolytic-uremic syndrome D59.3
    Henoch (-Schönlein) purpura D69.0 [N08]
    malariae malaria B52.0
    microscopic polyangiitis M31.7 [N08]
    multiple myeloma C90.0- [N08]
    mumps B26.83
    schistosomiasis B65.9 [N08]
    sepsis NEC A41.- [N08]
      streptococcal A40.- [N08]
    sickle-cell disorders D57- [N08]
    strongyloidiasis B78.9 [N08]
    subacute bacterial endocarditis I33.0 [N08]
    syphilis A52.75
    systemic lupus erythematosus M32.14
    thrombotic thrombocytopenic purpura
      M31.1 [N08]
    Waldenström macroglobulinemia C88.0 [N08]
    Wegener's granulomatosis M31.31
  gluconeogenesis E74.4
  glucosaminoglycan metabolism — *see*
    Disorder, metabolism, glucosaminoglycan
  glycine metabolism E72.50
    d-glycericacidemia E72.59
    hyperhydroxyprolinemia E72.59
    hyperoxaluria E72.53
    hyperprolinemia E72.59
    non-ketotic hyperglycinemia E72.51
    oxalosis E72.53
    oxaluria E72.53
    sarcosinemia E72.59
    trimethylaminuria E72.52
  glycoprotein metabolism E77.9
    specified NEC E77.8
  habit (and impulse) F63.9
    involving sexual behavior NEC F65.9
    specified NEC F63.89
  hallucinogen use
    mild F16.10
      with
        hallucinogen-induced
          anxiety disorder F16.180
          bipolar and related disorder F16.14
          depressive disorder F16.14
          psychotic disorder F16.159
        hallucinogen intoxication delirium
          F16.121
        other hallucinogen intoxication F16.129
    moderate or severe F16.20
      with
        hallucinogen-induced
          anxiety disorder F16.280
          bipolar and related disorder F16.24
          depressive disorder F16.24
          psychotic disorder F16.259
        hallucinogen intoxication delirium
          F16.221
        other hallucinogen intoxication F16.229
  heart action I49.9
  hematological D75.9
    newborn (transient) P61.9
      specified NEC P61.8
  hematopoietic organs D75.9
  hemorrhagic NEC D69.9
    drug-induced D68.32
    due to
      extrinsic circulating anticoagulants D68.32
        increase in
          anti-IIa D68.32
          anti-Xa D68.32
      intrinsic
        circulating anticoagulants D68.318
          increase in
            antithrombin D68.318
            anti-VIIIa D68.318
            anti-IXa D68.318
            anti-XIa D68.318
    following childbirth O72.3

Disorder (of) (*see also* Disease) — *continued*
  hemostasis — *see* Defect, coagulation
  histidine metabolism E70.40
    histidinemia E70.41
    other specified E70.49
  hoarding F42.3
  hyperkinetic — *see* Disorder, attention-deficit
    hyperactivity
  hyperleucine-isoleucinemia E71.19
  hypervalinemia E71.19
  hypoactive sexual desire F52.0
  hypochondriacal F45.20
    body dysmorphic F45.22
    neurosis F45.21
    other specified F45.29
  identity
    dissociative F44.81
    illness anxiety F45.21
    of childhood F93.8
  immune mechanism (immunity) D89.9
    specified type NEC D89.89
  impaired renal tubular function N25.9
    specified NEC N25.89
  impulse (control) F63.9
  inflammatory
    pelvic, in diseases classified elsewhere — *see*
      category N74
    penis N48.29
      abscess N48.21
      cellulitis N48.22
  inhalant use
    mild F18.10
      with
        inhalant-induced
          anxiety disorder F18.180
          depressive disorder F18.14
          major neurocognitive disorder F18.17
          mild neurocognitive disorder F18.188
          psychotic disorder F18.159
        inhalant intoxication F18.129
        inhalant intoxication delirium F18.121
    moderate or severe F18.20
      with
        inhalant-induced
          anxiety disorder F18.280
          depressive disorder F18.24
          major neurocognitive disorder F18.27
          mild neurocognitive disorder F18.288
          psychotic disorder F18.259
        inhalant intoxication F18.229
        inhalant intoxication delirium F18.221
  integument, newborn P83.9
    specified NEC P83.8
  intermittent explosive F63.81
  internal secretion pancreas — *see* Increased,
    secretion, pancreas, endocrine
  intestine, intestinal
    carbohydrate absorption NEC E74.39
      postoperative K91.2
    functional NEC K59.9
      postoperative K91.89
    psychogenic F45.8
    vascular K55.9
      chronic K55.1
      specified NEC K55.8
  intraoperative (intraprocedural) — *see*
    Complications, intraoperative
  involuntary emotional expression (IEED) F48.2
  iris H21.9
    adhesions — *see* Adhesions, iris
    atrophy — *see* Atrophy, iris
    chamber angle recession — *see* Recession,
      chamber angle
    cyst — *see* Cyst, iris
    degeneration — *see* Degeneration, iris
    in diseases classified elsewhere H22
    iridodialysis — *see* Iridodialysis
    iridoschisis — *see* Iridoschisis
    miotic pupillary cyst — *see* Cyst, pupillary

DISEASE INDEX

Disorder (of) (*see also* Disease) — *continued*
  iris H21.9 — *continued*
    pupillary
      abnormality — *see* Abnormality, pupillary
      membrane — *see* Membrane, pupillary
    specified type NEC H21.89
    vascular NEC H21.1x-
  iron metabolism E83.10
    specified NEC E83.19
  isovaleric acidemia E71.110
  jaw, developmental M27.0
    temporomandibular (*see also* Anomaly, dentofacial, temporomandibular joint) M26.60-
  joint M25.9
    derangement — *see* Derangement, joint
    effusion — *see* Effusion, joint
    fistula — *see* Fistula, joint
    hemarthrosis — *see* Hemarthrosis
    instability — *see* Instability, joint
    osteophyte — *see* Osteophyte
    pain — *see* Pain, joint
    psychogenic F45.8
    specified type NEC M25.80
      ankle M25.87-
      elbow M25.82-
      foot joint M25.87-
      hand joint M25.84-
      hip M25.85-
      knee M25.86-
      shoulder M25.81-
      wrist M25.83-
    stiffness — *see* Stiffness, joint
  ketone metabolism E71.32
  kidney N28.9
    functional (tubular) N25.9
    in
      schistosomiasis B65.9 [N29]
    tubular function N25.9
      specified NEC N25.89
  lacrimal system H04.9
    changes H04.69
      fistula — *see* Fistula, lacrimal
    gland H04.19
      atrophy — *see* Atrophy, lacrimal gland
      cyst — *see* Cyst, lacrimal, gland
      dacryops — *see* Dacryops
      dislocation — *see* Dislocation, lacrimal gland
      dry eye syndrome — *see* Syndrome, dry eye
      infection — *see* Dacryoadenitis
      granuloma — *see* Granuloma, lacrimal
      inflammation — *see* Inflammation, lacrimal
      obstruction — *see* Obstruction, lacrimal
    specified NEC H04.89
  lactation NEC O92.79
  language (developmental) F80.9
    expressive F80.1
    mixed receptive and expressive F80.2
    receptive F80.2
  late luteal phase dysphoric N94.89
  learning (specific) F81.9
    acalculia R48.8
    alexia R48.0
    mathematics F81.2
    reading F81.0
    specified NEC F81.89
    spelling F81.81
    written expression F81.81
  lens H27.9
    aphakia — *see* Aphakia
    cataract — *see* Cataract
    dislocation — *see* Dislocation, lens
    specified type NEC H27.8

Disorder (of) (*see also* Disease) — *continued*
  ligament M24.20
    ankle M24.27-
    attachment, spine — *see* Enthesopathy, spinal
    elbow M24.22-
    foot joint M24.27-
    hand joint M24.24-
    hip M24.25-
    knee — *see* Derangement, knee, specified NEC
    shoulder M24.21-
    vertebra M24.28
    wrist M24.23-
  ligamentous attachments — *see also* Enthesopathy
    spine — *see* Enthesopathy, spinal
  lipid
    metabolism, congenital E78.9
    storage E75.6
      specified NEC E75.5
  lipoprotein
    deficiency (familial) E78.6
    metabolism E78.9
      specified NEC E78.89
  liver K76.9
    malarial B54 [K77]
  low back — *see also* Dorsopathy, specified NEC
  lumbosacral
    plexus G54.1
    root (nerve) NEC G54.4
  lung, interstitial, drug-induced J70.4
    acute J70.2
    chronic J70.3
  lymphoproliferative, post-transplant (PTLD) D47.Z1 **(follows D47.4)**
  lysine and hydroxylysine metabolism E72.3
  major neurocognitive — *see* Dementia, in (due to)
  male
    erectile (organic) (*see also* Dysfunction, sexual, male, erectile) N52.9
      nonorganic F52.21
    hypoactive sexual desire F52.0
    orgasmic F52.32
  manic F30.9
    organic F06.33
  mast cell activation — *see* Activation, mast cell
  mastoid — *see also* Disorder, ear, middle
    postprocedural — *see* Complications, ear, procedure
  meniscus — *see* Derangement, knee, meniscus
  menopausal N95.9
    specified NEC N95.8
  menstrual N92.6
    psychogenic F45.8
    specified NEC N92.5
  mental (or behavioral) (nonpsychotic) F99
    due to (secondary to)
      amphetamine
        due to drug abuse — *see* Abuse, drug, stimulant
        due to drug dependence — *see* Dependence, drug, stimulant
      brain disease, damage and dysfunction F09
      caffeine use
        due to drug abuse — *see* Abuse, drug, stimulant
        due to drug dependence — *see* Dependence, drug, stimulant
      cannabis use
        due to drug abuse — *see* Abuse, drug, cannabis
        due to drug dependence — *see* Dependence, drug, cannabis
      general medical condition F09

Disorder (of) (*see also* Disease) — *continued*
  mental (or behavioral) (nonpsychotic) F99 — *continued*
    due to (secondary to) — *continued*
      sedative or hypnotic use
        due to drug abuse — *see* Abuse, drug, sedative
        due to drug dependence — *see* Dependence, drug, sedative
      tobacco (nicotine) use — *see* Dependence, drug, nicotine
    following organic brain damage F07.9
      frontal lobe syndrome F07.0
      personality change F07.0
      postconcussional syndrome F07.81
      specified NEC F07.89
    infancy, childhood or adolescence F98.9
    neurotic — *see* Neurosis
    organic or symptomatic F09
    presenile, psychotic F03
    problem NEC
    psychoneurotic — *see* Neurosis
    psychotic — *see* Psychosis
    puerperal F53
    senile, psychotic NEC F03
  metabolic, amino acid, transitory, newborn P74.8
  metabolism NOS E88.9
    amino-acid E72.9
      aromatic E70.9
        albinism — *see* Albinism
        histidine E70.40
          histidinemia E70.41
          other specified E70.49
        hyperphenylalaninemia E70.1
          classical phenylketonuria E70.0
        other specified E70.8
        tryptophan E70.5
        tyrosine E70.20
          hypertyrosinemia E70.21
          other specified E70.29
      branched chain E71.2
        3-methylglutaconic aciduria E71.111
        hyperleucine-isoleucinemia E71.19
        hypervalinemia E71.19
        isovaleric acidemia E71.110
        maple syrup urine disease E71.0
        methylmalonic acidemia E71.120
        organic aciduria NEC E71.118
        other specified E71.19
        proprionate NEC E71.128
        proprionic acidemia E71.121
      glycine E72.50
        d-glycericacidemia E72.59
        hyperhydroxyprolinemia E72.59
        hyperoxaluria E72.53
        hyperprolinemia E72.59
        non-ketotic hyperglycinemia E72.51
        other specified E72.59
        sarcosinemia E72.59
        trimethylaminuria E72.52
      hydroxylysine E72.3
      lysine E72.3
      ornithine E72.4
      other specified E72.8
        beta-amino acid E72.8
        gamma-glutamyl cycle E72.8
        straight-chain E72.8
      sulfur-bearing E72.10
        homocystinuria E72.11
        methylenetetrahydrofolate reductase deficiency E72.12
        other specified E72.19
    bile acid and cholesterol metabolism E78.70
    bilirubin E80.7
      specified NEC E80.6

Disorder (of) (see also Disease) — continued
  metabolism NOS E88.9 — continued
    calcium E83.50
      hypercalcemia E83.52
      hypocalcemia E83.51
      other specified E83.59
    carbohydrate E74.9
      specified NEC E74.8
    cholesterol and bile acid metabolism E78.70
    congenital E88.9
    copper E83.00
      specified type NEC E83.09
      Wilson's disease E83.01
    cystinuria E72.01
    fructose E74.10
    galactose E74.20
    glucosaminoglycan E76.9
      mucopolysaccharidosis — see Mucopolysaccharidosis
      specified NEC E76.8
    glutamine E72.8
    glycine E72.50
    glycogen storage (hepatorenal) E74.09
    glycoprotein E77.9
      specified NEC E77.8
    glycosaminoglycan E76.9
      specified NEC E76.8
    in labor and delivery O75.89
    iron E83.10
    isoleucine E71.19
    leucine E71.19
    lipoid E78.9
    lipoprotein E78.9
      specified NEC E78.89
    magnesium E83.40
      hypermagnesemia E83.41
      hypomagnesemia E83.42
      other specified E83.49
    mineral E83.9
      specified NEC E83.89
    mitochondrial E88.40
      MELAS syndrome E88.41
      MERRF syndrome (myoclonic epilepsy associated with ragged-red fibers) E88.42
      other specified E88.49
    ornithine E72.4
    phosphatases E83.30
    phosphorus E83.30
      acid phosphatase deficiency E83.39
      hypophosphatasia E83.39
      hypophosphatemia E83.39
        familial E83.31
        other specified E83.39
        pseudovitamin D deficiency E83.32
    plasma protein NEC E88.09
    porphyrin — see Porphyria
    postprocedural E89.89
      specified NEC E89.89
    purine E79.9
      specified NEC E79.8
    pyrimidine E79.9
      specified NEC E79.8
    pyruvate E74.4
    serine E72.8
    sodium E87.8
    specified NEC E88.89
    threonine E72.8
    valine E71.19
    zinc E83.2
  methylmalonic acidemia E71.120
  micturition NEC (see also Difficulty, micturition) R39.198
    feeling of incomplete emptying R39.14
    hesitancy R39.11
    poor stream R39.12
    psychogenic F45.8
    split stream R39.13
    straining R39.16

Disorder (of) (see also Disease) — continued
  micturition NEC R39.19 — continued
    urgency R39.15
  mild neurocognitive G31.84
  mitochondrial metabolism E88.40
  mitral (valve) — see Endocarditis, mitral
  mixed
    anxiety and depressive F41.8
    of scholastic skills (developmental) F81.89
    receptive expressive language F80.2
  mood F39
    bipolar — see Disorder, bipolar
    depressive — see Disorder, depressive
    due to (secondary to)
      alcohol F10.94
      amphetamine F15.94
        in
          abuse F15.14
          dependence F15.24
      anxiolytic F13.94
        in
          abuse F13.14
          dependence F13.24
      cocaine F14.94
        in
          abuse F14.14
          dependence F14.24
      general medical condition F06.30
      hallucinogen F16.94
        in
          abuse F16.14
          dependence F16.24
      hypnotic F13.94
        in
          abuse F13.14
          dependence F13.24
      inhalant F18.94
        in
          abuse F18.14
          dependence F18.24
      opioid F11.94
        in
          abuse F11.14
          dependence F11.24
      phencyclidine (PCP) F16.94
        in
          abuse F16.14
          dependence F16.24
      physiological condition F06.30
        with
          depressive features F06.31
          major depressive-like episode F06.32
          manic features F06.33
          mixed features F06.34
      psychoactive substance NEC F19.94
        in
          abuse F19.14
          dependence F19.24
      sedative F13.94
        in
          abuse F13.14
          dependence F13.24
      volatile solvents F18.94
        in
          abuse F18.14
          dependence F18.24
    manic episode F30.9
      with psychotic symptoms F30.2
      in remission (full) F30.4
        partial F30.3
      specified type NEC F30.8
      without psychotic symptoms F30.10
        mild F30.11
        moderate F30.12
        severe F30.13
    organic F06.30
      right hemisphere F07.89

Disorder (of) (see also Disease) — continued
  mood F39 — continued
    persistent F34.9
      cyclothymia F34.0
      dysthymia F34.1
      specified type NEC F34.89
    recurrent F39
    right hemisphere organic F07.89
  movement G25.9
    drug-induced G25.70
      akathisia G25.71
      specified NEC G25.79
    hysterical F44.4
    in diseases classified elsewhere — see category G26
    periodic limb G47.61
      sleep related G47.61
    sleep related NEC G47.69
    specified NEC G25.89
    stereotyped F98.4
    treatment-induced G25.9
  multiple personality F44.81
  muscle M62.9
    attachment, spine — see Enthesopathy, spinal
    in trichinellosis — see Trichinellosis, with muscle disorder
    psychogenic F45.8
    specified type NEC M62.89
    tone, newborn P94.9
      specified NEC P94.8
  muscular
    attachments — see also Enthesopathy
      spine — see Enthesopathy, spinal
    urethra N36.44
  musculoskeletal system, soft tissue — see Disorder, soft tissue
    postprocedural M96.89
    psychogenic F45.8
  myoneural G70.9
    due to lead G70.1
    specified NEC G70.89
    toxic G70.1
  myotonic NEC G71.19
  nail, in diseases classified elsewhere L62
  neck region NEC — see Dorsopathy, specified NEC
  neonatal onset multisystemic inflammatory (NOMID) M04.2
  nerve G58.9
    abducent NEC — see Strabismus, paralytic, sixth nerve
    accessory G52.8
    acoustic — see subcategory H93.3
    auditory — see subcategory H93.3
    auriculotemporal G50.8
    axillary G54.0
    cerebral — see Disorder, nerve, cranial
    cranial G52.9
      eighth — see subcategory H93.3
      eleventh G52.8
      fifth G50.9
      first G52.0
      fourth NEC — see Strabismus, paralytic, fourth nerve
      multiple G52.7
      ninth G52.1
      second NEC — see Disorder, nerve, optic
      seventh NEC G51.8
      sixth NEC — see Strabismus, paralytic, sixth nerve
      specified NEC G52.8
      tenth G52.2
      third NEC — see Strabismus, paralytic, third nerve
      twelfth G52.3
    entrapment — see Neuropathy, entrapment
    facial G51.9
      specified NEC G51.8
    femoral — see Lesion, nerve, femoral

Disorder (of) (*see also* Disease) — *continued*
nerve G58.9 — *continued*
  glossopharyngeal NEC G52.1
  hypoglossal G52.3
  intercostal G58.0
  lateral
    cutaneous of thigh — *see*
      Mononeuropathy, lower limb,
      meralgia paresthetica
    popliteal — *see* Lesion, nerve, popliteal
  lower limb — *see* Mononeuropathy, lower
    limb
  medial popliteal — *see* Lesion, nerve,
    popliteal, medial
  median NEC — *see* Lesion, nerve, median
  multiple G58.7
  oculomotor NEC — *see* Strabismus,
    paralytic, third nerve
  olfactory G52.0
  optic NEC H47.09-
    hemorrhage into sheath — *see*
      Hemorrhage, optic nerve
    ischemic H47.01-
  peroneal — *see* Lesion, nerve, popliteal
  phrenic G58.8
  plantar — *see* Lesion, nerve, plantar
  pneumogastric G52.2
  posterior tibial — *see* Syndrome, tarsal
    tunnel
  radial — *see* Lesion, nerve, radial
  recurrent laryngeal G52.2
  root G54.9
    cervical G54.2
    lumbosacral G54.1
    specified NEC G54.8
    thoracic G54.3
  sciatic NEC — *see* Lesion, nerve, sciatic
  specified NEC G58.8
    lower limb — *see* Mononeuropathy, lower
      limb, specified NEC
    upper limb — *see* Mononeuropathy, upper
      limb, specified NEC
  sympathetic G90.9
  tibial — *see* Lesion, nerve, popliteal, medial
  trigeminal G50.9
    specified NEC G50.8
  trochlear NEC — *see* Strabismus, paralytic,
    fourth nerve
  ulnar — *see* Lesion, nerve, ulnar
  upper limb — *see* Mononeuropathy, upper
    limb
  vagus G52.2
nervous system G98.8
  autonomic (peripheral) G90.9
    specified NEC G90.8
  central G96.9
    specified NEC G96.8
  parasympathetic G90.9
  specified NEC G98.8
  sympathetic G90.9
  vegetative G90.9
neurocognitive
  major
    with
      aggressive behavior F01.51
      combative behavior F01.51
      violent behavior F01.51
    due to vascular disease, with behavioral
      disturbance F01.51
    in (due to) (other diseases classified
      elsewhere) (*see also* Dementia, in (due
      to)) F02.80
      with
        aggressive behavior F02.81
        combative behavior F02.81
        violent behavior F02.81
      without behavioral disturbance F01.50
  mild G31.84

Disorder (of) (*see also* Disease) — *continued*
neurodevelopmental F89
  specified NEC F88
neurohypophysis NEC E23.3
neurological NEC R29.818
neuromuscular G70.9
  hereditary NEC G71.9
  specified NEC G70.89
  toxic G70.1
neurotic F48.9
  specified NEC F48.8
neutrophil, polymorphonuclear D71
nicotine use — *see* Dependence, drug, nicotine
nightmare F51.5
nose J34.9
  specified NEC J34.89
obsessive-compulsive F42.9
odontogenesis NOS K00.9
opioid use
  with
    opioid-induced psychotic disorder F11.959
      with
        delusions F11.950
        hallucinations F11.951
  due to drug abuse — *see* Abuse, drug, opioid
  due to drug dependence — *see* Dependence,
    drug, opioid
  mild F11.10
    with
      opioid-induced
        anxiety disorder F11.188
        depressive disorder F11.14
        sexual dysfunction F11.181
      opioid intoxication
        with perceptual disturbances F11.122
        delirium F11.121
        without perceptual disturbances
          F11.129
  moderate or severe F11.20
    with
      opioid-induced
        anxiety disorder F11.288
        anxiety disorder F11.988
        depressive disorder F11.24
        depressive disorder F11.94
        sexual dysfunction F11.281
        sexual dysfunction F11.981
      opioid intoxication
        with perceptual disturbances F11.222
        delirium F11.221
        without perceptual disturbances
          F11.229
oppositional defiant F91.3
optic
  chiasm H47.49
    due to
      inflammatory disorder H47.41
      neoplasm H47.42
      vascular disorder H47.43
  disc H47.39-
    coloboma — *see* Coloboma, optic disc
    drusen — *see* Drusen, optic disc
    pseudopapilledema — *see*
      Pseudopapilledema
  radiations — *see* Disorder, visual, pathway
  tracts — *see* Disorder, visual, pathway
orbit H05.9
  cyst — *see* Cyst, orbit
  deformity — *see* Deformity, orbit
  edema — *see* Edema, orbit
  enophthalmos — *see* Enophthalmos
  exophthalmos — *see* Exophthalmos
  hemorrhage — *see* Hemorrhage, orbit
  inflammation — *see* Inflammation, orbit
  myopathy — *see* Myopathy, extraocular
    muscles
  retained foreign body — *see* Foreign body,
    orbit, old
  specified type NEC H05.89

Disorder (of) (*see also* Disease) — *continued*
organic
  anxiety F06.4
  catatonic F06.1
  delusional F06.2
  dissociative F06.8
  emotionally labile (asthenic) F06.8
  mood (affective) F06.30
  schizophrenia-like F06.2
orgasmic (female) F52.31
  male F52.32
ornithine metabolism E72.4
overanxious F41.1
  of childhood F93.8
pain
  with related psychological factors F45.42
  exclusively related to psychological factors
    F45.41
  genito-pelvic penetration disorder F52.6
pancreatic internal secretion E16.9
  specified NEC E16.8
panic F41.0
  with agoraphobia F40.01
papulosquamous L44.9
  in diseases classified elsewhere L45
  specified NEC L44.8
paranoid F22
  induced F24
  shared F24
parathyroid (gland) E21.5
  specified NEC E21.4
parietoalveolar NEC J84.09
paroxysmal, mixed R56.9
patella M22.9-
  chondromalacia — *see* Chondromalacia,
    patella
  derangement NEC M22.3x-
  recurrent
    dislocation — *see* Dislocation, patella,
      recurrent
    subluxation — *see* Dislocation, patella,
      recurrent, incomplete
  specified NEC M22.8x-
patellofemoral M22.2x-
pentose phosphate pathway with anemia
  D55.1
perception, due to hallucinogens F16.983
  in
    abuse F16.183
    dependence F16.283
peripheral nervous system NEC G64
peroxisomal E71.50
  biogenesis
    neonatal adrenoleukodystrophy E71.511
    specified disorder NEC E71.518
    Zellweger syndrome E71.510
  rhizomelic chondrodysplasia punctata
    E71.540
  specified form NEC E71.548
    group 1 E71.518
    group 2 E71.53
    group 3 E71.542
  X-linked adrenoleukodystrophy E71.529
    adolescent E71.521
    adrenomyeloneuropathy E71.522
    childhood E71.520
    specified form NEC E71.528
  Zellweger-like syndrome E71.541
persistent
  (somatoform) pain F45.41
  affective (mood) F34.9
personality (*see also* Personality) F60.9
  affective F34.0
  aggressive F60.3
  amoral F60.2
  anankastic F60.5
  antisocial F60.2
  anxious F60.6
  asocial F60.2

Disorder (of) (*see also* Disease) — *continued*
personality (*see also* Personality) F60.9 — *continued*
    asthenic F60.7
    avoidant F60.6
    borderline F60.3
    change (secondary) due to general medical condition F07.0
    compulsive F60.5
    cyclothymic F34.0
    dependent (passive) F60.7
    depressive F34.1
    dissocial F60.2
    emotional instability F60.3
    expansive paranoid F60.0
    explosive F60.3
    following organic brain damage F07.9
    histrionic F60.4
    hyperthymic F34.0
    hypothymic F34.1
    hysterical F60.4
    immature F60.89
    inadequate F60.7
    labile F60.3
    mixed (nonspecific) F60.89
    moral deficiency F60.2
    narcissistic F60.81
    negativistic F60.89
    obsessional F60.5
    obsessive(-compulsive) F60.5
    organic F07.9
    overconscientious F60.5
    paranoid F60.0
    passive(-dependent) F60.7
    passive-aggressive F60.89
    pathological NEC F60.9
    pseudosocial F60.2
    psychopathic F60.2
    schizoid F60.1
    schizotypal F21
    self-defeating F60.7
    specified NEC F60.89
    type A F60.5
    unstable (emotional) F60.3
pervasive, developmental F84.9
phencyclidine use
    mild F16.10
        with
            phencyclidine-induced
                anxiety disorder F16.180
                bipolar and related disorder F16.14
                depressive disorder F16.14
                psychotic disorder F16.159
            phencyclidine intoxication F16.129
            phencyclidine intoxication delirium F16.121
    moderate or severe F16.20
        with
            phencyclidine-induced
                anxiety disorder F16.280
                bipolar and related disorder F16.24
                depressive disorder F16.24
                psychotic disorder F16.259
            phencyclidine intoxication F16.229
            phencyclidine intoxication delirium F16.221
phobic anxiety, childhood F40.8
phosphate-losing tubular N25.0
pigmentation L81.9
    choroid, congenital Q14.3
    diminished melanin formation L81.6
    iron L81.8
    specified NEC L81.8
pinna (noninfective) H61.10-
    deformity, acquired H61.11-
    hematoma H61.12-
    perichondritis — *see* Perichondritis, ear
    specified type NEC H61.19-

Disorder (of) (*see also* Disease) — *continued*
pituitary gland E23.7
    iatrogenic (postprocedural) E89.3
    specified NEC E23.6
platelets D69.1
plexus G54.9
    specified NEC G54.8
polymorphonuclear neutrophils D71
porphyrin metabolism — *see* Porphyria
post-transplant lymphoproliferative D47.Z1
    (follows D47.4)
post-traumatic stress (PTSD) F43.10
    acute F43.11
    chronic F43.12
postconcussional F07.81
posthallucinogen perception F16.983
    in
        abuse F16.183
        dependence F16.283
postmenopausal N95.9
    specified NEC N95.8
postprocedural (postoperative) — *see* Complications, postprocedural
premenstrual dysphoric (PMDD) N94.81
prepuce N47.8
propionic acidemia E71.121
prostate N42.9
    specified NEC N42.89
psychogenic NOS (*see also* condition) F45.9
    anxiety F41.8
    appetite F50.9
    asthenic F48.8
    cardiovascular (system) F45.8
    compulsive F42.8
    cutaneous F54
    depressive F32.9
    digestive (system) F45.8
    dysmenorrheic F45.8
    dyspneic F45.8
    endocrine (system) F54
    eye NEC F45.8
    feeding — *see* Disorder, eating
    functional NEC F45.8
    gastric F45.8
    gastrointestinal (system) F45.8
    genitourinary (system) F45.8
    heart (function) (rhythm) F45.8
    hyperventilatory F45.8
    hypochondriacal — *see* Disorder, hypochondriacal
    intestinal F45.8
    joint F45.8
    learning F81.9
    limb F45.8
    lymphatic (system) F45.8
    menstrual F45.8
    micturition F45.8
    monoplegic NEC F44.4
    motor F44.4
    muscle F45.8
    musculoskeletal F45.8
    neurocirculatory F45.8
    obsessive F42.8
    occupational F48.8
    organ or part of body NEC F45.8
    paralytic NEC F44.4
    phobic F40.9
    physical NEC F45.8
    rectal F45.8
    respiratory (system) F45.8
    rheumatic F45.8
    sexual (function) F52.9
    skin (allergic) (eczematous) F54
    sleep F51.9
    specified part of body NEC F45.8
    stomach F45.8

Disorder (of) (*see also* Disease) — *continued*
psychological F99
    associated with
        disease classified elsewhere F54
    sexual
        development F66
        relationship F66
    uncertainty about gender identity F64.9
psychomotor NEC F44.4
    hysterical F44.4
psychoneurotic — *see also* Neurosis
    mixed NEC F48.8
psychophysiologic — *see* Disorder, somatoform
psychosexual F65.9
    development F66
    identity of childhood F64.2
psychosomatic NOS — *see* Disorder, somatoform
    multiple F45.0
    undifferentiated F45.1
psychotic — *see* Psychosis
    transient (acute) F23
puberty E30.9
    specified NEC E30.8
pulmonary (valve) — *see* Endocarditis, pulmonary
purine metabolism E79.9
pyrimidine metabolism E79.9
pyruvate metabolism E74.4
reactive attachment (childhood) F94.1
reading R48.0
    developmental (specific) F81.0
receptive language F80.2
receptor, hormonal, peripheral (*see also* Syndrome, androgen insensitivity) E34.50
recurrent brief depressive F33.8
reflex R29.2
refraction H52.7
    aniseikonia H52.32
    anisometropia H52.31
    astigmatism — *see* Astigmatism
    hypermetropia — *see* Hypermetropia
    myopia — *see* Myopia
    presbyopia H52.4
    specified NEC H52.6
relationship F68.8
    due to sexual orientation F66
REM sleep behavior G47.52
renal function, impaired (tubular) N25.9
resonance R49.9
    specified NEC R49.8
respiratory function, impaired — *see also* Failure, respiration
    postprocedural — *see* Complication, postoperative, respiratory system
    psychogenic F45.8
retina H35.9
    angioid streaks H35.33
    changes in vascular appearance H35.01-
    degeneration — *see* Degeneration, retina
    dystrophy (hereditary) — *see* Dystrophy, retina
    edema H35.81
    hemorrhage — *see* Hemorrhage, retina
    ischemia H35.82
    macular degeneration — *see* Degeneration, macula
    microaneurysms H35.04-
    microvascular abnormality NEC H35.09
    neovascularization — *see* Neovascularization, retina
    retinopathy — *see* Retinopathy
    separation of layers H35.70
        central serous chorioretinopathy H35.71-
        pigment epithelium detachment (serous) H35.72-
        hemorrhagic H35.73-
    specified type NEC H35.89
    telangiectasis — *see* Telangiectasis, retina

Disorder (of) (*see also* Disease) — *continued*
retina H35.9 — *continued*
vasculitis — *see* Vasculitis, retina
retroperitoneal K68.9
right hemisphere organic affective F07.89
rumination (infant or child) F98.21
sacrum, sacrococcygeal NEC M53.3
schizoaffective F25.9
bipolar type F25.0
depressive type F25.1
manic type F25.0
mixed type F25.0
specified NEC F25.8
schizoid of childhood F84.5
schizophreniform F20.81
brief F23
schizotypal (personality) F21
secretion, thyrocalcitonin E07.0
sedative, hypnotic, or anxiolytic use
mild F13.10
with
sedative, hypnotic, or anxiolytic-induced
anxiety disorder F13.180
bipolar and related disorder F13.14
depressive disorder F13.14
psychotic disorder F13.159
sexual dysfunction F13.181
sedative, hypnotic, or anxiolytic
intoxication F13.129
sedative, hypnotic, or anxiolytic
intoxication delirium F13.121
moderate or severe F13.20
with
sedative, hypnotic, or anxiolytic-induced
anxiety disorder F13.280
bipolar and related disorder F13.24
depressive disorder F13.24
major neurocognitive disorder F13.27
mild neurocognitive disorder F13.288
psychotic disorder F13.259
sexual dysfunction F13.281
sedative, hypnotic, or anxiolytic
intoxication F13.229
sedative, hypnotic, or anxiolytic
intoxication delirium F13.221
seizure (*see also* Epilepsy) G40.909
intractable G40.919
with status epilepticus G40.911
semantic pragmatic F80.89
with autism F84.0
sense of smell R43.1
psychogenic F45.8
separation anxiety, of childhood F93.0
sexual
arousal, female F52.22
aversion F52.1
function, psychogenic F52.9
maturation F66
nonorganic F52.9
preference (*see also* Deviation, sexual) F65.9
fetishistic transvestism F65.1
relationship F66
shyness, of childhood and adolescence F40.10
sibling rivalry F93.8
sickle-cell (sickling) (homozygous) — *see*
Disease, sickle-cell
heterozygous D57.3
specified type NEC D57.8-
trait D57.3
sinus (nasal) J34.9
specified NEC J34.89
skin L98.9
atrophic L90.9
specified NEC L90.8
granulomatous L92.9
specified NEC L92.8
hypertrophic L91.9
specified NEC L91.8
infiltrative NEC L98.6

Disorder (of) (*see also* Disease) — *continued*
skin L98.9 — *continued*
newborn P83.9
specified NEC P83.8
picking F42.4
psychogenic (allergic) (eczematous) F54
sleep G47.9
breathing-related — *see* Apnea, sleep
circadian rhythm G47.20
advance sleep phase type G47.22
delayed sleep phase type G47.21
due to
alcohol
abuse F10.182
dependence F10.282
use F10.982
amphetamines
abuse F15.182
dependence F15.282
use F15.982
caffeine
abuse F15.182
dependence F15.282
use F15.982
cocaine
abuse F14.182
dependence F14.282
use F14.982
drug NEC
abuse F19.182
dependence F19.282
use F19.982
opioid
abuse F11.182
dependence F11.282
use F11.982
psychoactive substance NEC
abuse F19.182
dependence F19.282
use F19.982
sedative, hypnotic, or anxiolytic
abuse F13.182
dependence F13.282
use F13.982
stimulant NEC
abuse F15.182
dependence F15.282
use F15.982
free running type G47.24
in conditions classified elsewhere G47.27
irregular sleep wake type G47.23
jet lag type G47.25
shift work type G47.26
specified NEC G47.29
due to
alcohol
abuse F10.182
dependence F10.282
use F10.982
amphetamine
abuse F15.182
dependence F15.282
use F15.982
anxiolytic
abuse F13.182
dependence F13.282
use F13.982
caffeine
abuse F15.182
dependence F15.282
use F15.982
cocaine
abuse F14.182
dependence F14.282
use F14.982
drug NEC
abuse F19.182
dependence F19.282
use F19.982

Disorder (of) (*see also* Disease) — *continued*
sleep G47.9 — *continued*
due to — *continued*
hypnotic
abuse F13.182
dependence F13.282
use F13.982
opioid
abuse F11.182
dependence F11.282
use F11.982
psychoactive substance NEC
abuse F19.182
dependence F19.282
use F19.982
sedative
abuse F13.182
dependence F13.282
use F13.982
stimulant NEC
abuse F15.182
dependence F15.282
use F15.982
emotional F51.9
excessive somnolence — *see* Hypersomnia
hypersomnia type — *see* Hypersomnia
initiating or maintaining — *see* Insomnia
nightmares F51.5
nonorganic F51.9
specified NEC F51.8
parasomnia type G47.50
specified NEC G47.8
terrors F51.4
walking F51.3
sleep-wake pattern or schedule — *see*
Disorder, sleep, circadian rhythm
social
anxiety of childhood F40.10
functioning in childhood F94.9
specified NEC F94.8
pragmatic F80.82
soft tissue M79.9
ankle M79.9
due to use, overuse and pressure M70.90
ankle M70.97-
bursitis — *see* Bursitis
foot M70.97-
forearm M70.93-
hand M70.94-
lower leg M70.96-
multiple sites M70.99
pelvic region M70.95-
shoulder region M70.91-
specified site NEC M70.98
specified type NEC M70.80
ankle M70.87-
foot M70.87-
forearm M70.83-
hand M70.84-
lower leg M70.86-
multiple sites M70.89
pelvic region M70.85-
shoulder region M70.81-
specified site NEC M70.88
thigh M70.85-
upper arm M70.82-
thigh M70.95-
upper arm M70.92-
foot M79.9
forearm M79.9
hand M79.9
lower leg M79.9
multiple sites M79.9
occupational — *see* Disorder, soft tissue, due
to use, overuse and pressure
pelvic region M79.9
shoulder region M79.9
specified type NEC M79.89
thigh M79.9

Disorder (of) (*see also* Disease) — *continued*
  soft tissue M79.9 — *continued*
    upper arm M79.9
  somatic symptom F45.1
  somatization F45.0
  somatoform F45.9
    pain (persistent) F45.41
    somatization (multiple) (long-lasting) F45.0
    specified NEC F45.8
    undifferentiated F45.1
  somnolence, excessive — *see* Hypersomnia
  specific
    arithmetical F81.2
    developmental, of motor F82
    reading F81.0
    speech and language F80.9
    spelling F81.81
    written expression F81.81
  speech R47.9
    articulation (functional) (specific) F80.0
    developmental F80.9
    specified NEC R47.89
  speech-sound F80.0
  spelling (specific) F81.81
  spine — *see also* Dorsopathy
    ligamentous or muscular attachments,
        peripheral — *see* Enthesopathy, spinal
    specified NEC — *see* Dorsopathy, specified
        NEC
  stereotyped, habit or movement F98.4
  stimulant use (other) (unspecified)
    mild F15.10
    moderate or severe F15.20
  stomach (functional) — *see* Disorder, gastric
  stress F43.9
    acute F43.0
    post-traumatic F43.10
      acute F43.11
      chronic F43.12
  substance use (other) (unknown)
    mild F19.10
      with substance-induced
        anxiety disorder F19.180
        bipolar and related disorder F19.14
        depressive disorder F19.14
        major neurocognitive disorder F19.17
        mild neurocognitive disorder F19.188
        obsessive-compulsive and related
            disorder F19.188
        sexual dysfunction F19.181
      substance intoxication F19.129
      substance intoxication delirium F19.121
    moderate or severe F19.20
      with substance-induced
        anxiety disorder F19.280
        bipolar and related disorder F19.24
        depressive disorder F19.24
        major neurocognitive disorder F19.27
        mild neurocognitive disorder F19.288
        obsessive-compulsive and related
            disorder F19.288
        sexual dysfunction F19.281
      substance intoxication F19.229
      substance intoxication delirium F19.221
  sulfur-bearing amino-acid metabolism E72.10
  sweat gland (eccrine) L74.9
    apocrine L75.9
      specified NEC L75.8
    specified NEC L74.8
  synovium M67.90
    acromioclavicular M67.91-
    ankle M67.97-
    elbow M67.92-
    foot M67.97-
    forearm M67.93-
    hand M67.94-
    hip M67.95-
    knee M67.96-
    multiple sites M67.99

Disorder (of) (*see also* Disease) — *continued*
  synovium M67.90 — *continued*
    rupture — *see* Rupture, synovium
    shoulder M67.91-
    specified type NEC M67.80
      acromioclavicular M67.81-
      ankle M67.87-
      elbow M67.82-
      foot M67.87-
      hand M67.84-
      hip M67.85-
      knee M67.86-
      multiple sites M67.89
      wrist M67.83-
    synovitis — *see* Synovitis
    upper arm M67.92-
    wrist M67.93-
  temperature regulation, newborn P81.9
    specified NEC P81.8
  temporomandibular joint M26.60-
  tendon M67.90
    acromioclavicular M67.91-
    ankle M67.97-
    contracture — *see* Contracture, tendon
    elbow M67.92-
    foot M67.97-
    forearm M67.93-
    hand M67.94-
    hip M67.95-
    knee M67.96-
    multiple sites M67.99
    rupture — *see* Rupture, tendon
    shoulder M67.91-
    specified type NEC M67.80
      acromioclavicular M67.81-
      ankle M67.87-
      elbow M67.82-
      foot M67.87-
      hand M67.84-
      hip M67.85-
      knee M67.86-
      multiple sites M67.89
      trunk M67.88
      wrist M67.83-
    synovitis — *see* Synovitis
    tendinitis — *see* Tendinitis
    tenosynovitis — *see* Tenosynovitis
    trunk M67.98
    upper arm M67.92-
    wrist M67.93-
  thoracic root (nerve) NEC G54.3
  thyrocalcitonin hypersecretion E07.0
  thyroid (gland) E07.9
    function NEC, neonatal, transitory P72.2
    iodine-deficiency related E01.8
    specified NEC E07.89
  tic — *see* Tic
  tobacco use
    mild Z72.0
    moderate F17.200
    severe F17.200
  tooth K08.9
    development K00.9
      specified NEC K00.8
    eruption K00.6
  Tourette's F95.2
  trance and possession F44.89
  trauma and stressor-related F43.9
    other specified F43.8
  tricuspid (valve) — *see* Endocarditis, tricuspid
  tryptophan metabolism E70.5
  tubular, phosphate-losing N25.0
  tubulo-interstitial (in)
    brucellosis A23.9 *[N16]*
    cystinosis E72.04
    diphtheria A36.84
    glycogen storage disease E74.00 *[N16]*
    leukemia NEC C95.9- *[N16]*
    lymphoma NEC C85.9- *[N16]*

Disorder (of) (*see also* Disease) — *continued*
  tubulo-interstitial (in) — *continued*
    mixed cryoglobulinemia D89.1 *[N16]*
    multiple myeloma C90.0- *[N16]*
    Salmonella infection A02.25
    sarcoidosis D86.84
    sepsis A41.9 *[N16]*
      streptococcal A40.9 *[N16]*
    systemic lupus erythematosus M32.15
    toxoplasmosis B58.83
    transplant rejection T86.91 *[N16]*
    Wilson's disease E83.01 *[N16]*
  tubulo-renal function, impaired N25.9
    specified NEC N25.89
  tympanic membrane H73.9-
    atrophy — *see* Atrophy, tympanic membrane
    infection — *see* Myringitis
    perforation — *see* Perforation, tympanum
    specified NEC H73.89-
  unsocialized aggressive F91.1
  urea cycle metabolism E72.20
    argininemia E72.21
    arginosuccinic aciduria E72.22
    citrullinemia E72.23
    ornithine transcarbamylase deficiency E72.4
    other specified E72.29
  ureter (in) N28.9
    schistosomiasis B65.0 *[N29]*
    tuberculosis A18.11
  urethra N36.9
    specified NEC N36.8
  urinary system N39.9
    specified NEC N39.8
  valve, heart
    aortic — *see* Endocarditis, aortic
    mitral — *see* Endocarditis, mitral
    pulmonary — *see* Endocarditis, pulmonary
    rheumatic
      aortic — *see* Endocarditis, aortic,
          rheumatic
      mitral — *see* Endocarditis, mitral
      pulmonary — *see* Endocarditis,
          pulmonary, rheumatic
      tricuspid — *see* Endocarditis, tricuspid
    tricuspid — *see* Endocarditis, tricuspid
  vestibular function H81.9-
    specified NEC — *see* subcategory H81.8-
    in diseases classified elsewhere H82-
  vertigo — *see* Vertigo
  vision, binocular H53.30
    abnormal retinal correspondence H53.31
    diplopia H53.2
    fusion with defective stereopsis H53.32
    simultaneous perception H53.33
    suppression H53.34
  visual
    cortex
      blindness H47.619
        left brain H47.612
        right brain H47.611
      due to
        inflammatory disorder H47.629
          left brain H47.622
          right brain H47.621
        neoplasm H47.639
          left brain H47.632
          right brain H47.631
        vascular disorder H47.649
          left brain H47.642
          right brain H47.641
    pathway H47.9
      due to
        inflammatory disorder H47.51-
        neoplasm H47.52-
        vascular disorder H47.53-
      optic chiasm — *see* Disorder, optic, chiasm

DISEASE INDEX

Disorder (of) (*see also* Disease) — *continued*
  vitreous body H43.9
    crystalline deposits — *see* Deposit, crystalline
    degeneration — *see* Degeneration, vitreous
    hemorrhage — *see* Hemorrhage, vitreous
    opacities — *see* Opacity, vitreous
    prolapse — *see* Prolapse, vitreous
    specified type NEC H43.89
  voice R49.9
    specified type NEC R49.8
  volatile solvent use
    due to drug abuse — *see* Abuse, drug, inhalant
    due to drug dependence — *see* Dependence, drug, inhalant
  white blood cells D72.9
    specified NEC D72.89
  withdrawing, child or adolescent F40.10
Disorientation R41.0
Displacement, displaced
  acquired traumatic of bone, cartilage, joint, tendon NEC — *see* Dislocation
  adrenal gland (congenital) Q89.1
  appendix, retrocecal (congenital) Q43.8
  auricle (congenital) Q17.4
  bladder (acquired) N32.89
    congenital Q64.19
  brachial plexus (congenital) Q07.8
  brain stem, caudal (congenital) Q04.8
  canaliculus (lacrimalis), congenital Q10.6
  cardia through esophageal hiatus (congenital) Q40.1
  cerebellum, caudal (congenital) Q04.8
  cervix — *see* Malposition, uterus
  colon (congenital) Q43.3
  device, implant or graft (*see also* Complications, by site and type, mechanical) T85.628
    arterial graft NEC — *see* Complication, cardiovascular device, mechanical, vascular
    breast (implant) T85.42
    catheter NEC T85.628
      dialysis (renal) T82.42
        intraperitoneal T85.621
      infusion NEC T82.524
        spinal (epidural) (subdural) T85.620
      urinary
        cystostomy T83.020
        Hopkins T83.028
        ileostomy T83.028
        indwelling T83.021
        nephrostomy T83.022
        specified NEC T83.028
        urostomy T83.028
    electronic (electrode) (pulse generator) (stimulator) — *see* Complication, electronic stimulator
    fixation, internal (orthopedic) NEC — *see* Complication, fixation device, mechanical
    gastrointestinal — *see* Complications, prosthetic device, mechanical, gastrointestinal device
    genital NEC T83.428
      intrauterine contraceptive device (string) T83.32
      penile prosthesis (cylinder) (implanted) (pump) (resevoir) T83.420
      testicular prosthesis T83.421
    heart NEC — *see* Complication, cardiovascular device, mechanical
    joint prosthesis — *see* Complications, joint prosthesis, mechanical
    ocular — *see* Complications, prosthetic device, mechanical, ocular device
    orthopedic NEC — *see* Complication, orthopedic, device or graft, mechanical
    specified NEC T85.628

Displacement, displaced — *continued*
  device, implant or graft (*see also* Complications, by site and type, mechanical) T85.628 — *continued*
    urinary NEC T83.128
      graft T83.22
      sphincter, implanted T83.121
      stent (ileal conduit) (nephroureteral) T83.123
      ureteral indwelling T83.122
    vascular NEC — *see* Complication, cardiovascular device, mechanical
    ventricular intracranial shunt T85.02
  electronic stimulator
    bone T84.320
    cardiac — *see* Complications, cardiac device, electronic
    nervous system — *see* Complication, prosthetic device, mechanical, electronic nervous system stimulator
    urinary — *see* Complications, electronic stimulator, urinary
  esophageal mucosa into cardia of stomach, congenital Q39.8
  esophagus (acquired) K22.8
    congenital Q39.8
  eyeball (acquired) (lateral) (old) — *see* Displacement, globe
    congenital Q15.8
    current — *see* Avulsion, eye
  fallopian tube (acquired) N83.4-
    congenital Q50.6
    opening (congenital) Q50.6
  gallbladder (congenital) Q44.1
  gastric mucosa (congenital) Q40.2
  globe (acquired) (old) (lateral) H05.21-
    current — *see* Avulsion, eye
  heart (congenital) Q24.8
    acquired I51.89
  hymen (upward) (congenital) Q52.4
  intervertebral disc NEC
    with myelopathy — *see* Disorder, disc, with, myelopathy
    cervical, cervicothoracic (with) M50.20
      myelopathy — *see* Disorder, disc, cervical, with myelopathy
      neuritis, radiculitis or radiculopathy — *see* Disorder, disc, cervical, with neuritis
    due to trauma — *see* Dislocation, vertebra
    lumbar region M51.26
      with
        myelopathy M51.06
        neuritis, radiculitis, radiculopathy or sciatica M51.16
    lumbosacral region M51.27
      with
        neuritis, radiculitis, radiculopathy or sciatica M51.17
    sacrococcygeal region M53.3
    thoracic region M51.24
      with
        myelopathy M51.04
        neuritis, radiculitis, radiculopathy M51.14
    thoracolumbar region M51.25
      with
        myelopathy M51.05
        neuritis, radiculitis, radiculopathy M51.15
  intrauterine device (string) T83.32
  kidney (acquired) N28.83
    congenital Q63.2
  lachrymal, lacrimal apparatus or duct (congenital) Q10.6
  lens, congenital Q12.1
  macula (congenital) Q14.1
  Meckel's diverticulum Q43.0
    malignant — *see* Table of Neoplasms, small intestine, malignant

Displacement, displaced — *continued*
  nail (congenital) Q84.6
    acquired L60.8
  opening of Wharton's duct in mouth Q38.4
  organ or site, congenital NEC — *see* Malposition, congenital
  ovary (acquired) N83.4-
    congenital Q50.39
    free in peritoneal cavity (congenital) Q50.39
    into hernial sac N83.4-
  oviduct (acquired) N83.4-
    congenital Q50.6
  parathyroid (gland) E21.4
  parotid gland (congenital) Q38.4
  punctum lacrimale (congenital) Q10.6
  sacro-iliac (joint) (congenital) Q74.2
    current injury S33.2
    old — *see* subcategory M53.2
  salivary gland (any) (congenital) Q38.4
  spleen (congenital) Q89.09
  stomach, congenital Q40.2
  sublingual duct Q38.4
  tongue (downward) (congenital) Q38.3
  tooth, teeth, fully erupted M26.30
    horizontal M26.33
    vertical M26.34
  trachea (congenital) Q32.1
  ureter or ureteric opening or orifice (congenital) Q62.62
  uterine opening of oviducts or fallopian tubes Q50.6
  uterus, uterine — *see* Malposition, uterus
  ventricular septum Q21.0
    with rudimentary ventricle Q20.4
Disproportion
  between native and reconstructed breast N65.1
  fiber-type G71.2
Disruptio uteri — *see* Rupture, uterus
Disruption (of)
  ciliary body NEC H21.89
  closure of
    cornea T81.31
    craniotomy T81.32
    fascia (muscular) (superficial) T81.32
    internal organ or tissue T81.32
    laceration (external) (internal) T81.33
    ligament T81.32
    mucosa T81.31
    muscle or muscle flap T81.32
    ribs or rib cage T81.32
    skin and subcutaneous tissue (full-thickness) (superficial) T81.31
    skull T81.32
    sternum (sternotomy) T81.32
    tendon T81.32
    traumatic laceration (external) (internal) T81.33
  family Z63.8
    due to
      absence of family member due to military deployment Z63.31
      absence of family member NEC Z63.32
      alcoholism and drug addiction in family Z63.72
      bereavement Z63.4
      death (assumed) or disappearance of family member Z63.4
      divorce or separation Z63.5
      drug addiction in family Z63.72
      return of family member from military deployment (current or past conflict) Z63.71
      stressful life events NEC Z63.79
  iris NEC H21.89

Disruption (of) — *continued*
 ligament(s) — *see also* Sprain
  knee
   current injury — *see* Dislocation, knee
   old (chronic) — *see* Derangement, knee, ligament, instability, chronic
   spontaneous NEC — *see* Derangement, knee, disruption ligament
  ossicular chain — *see* Discontinuity, ossicles, ear
 pelvic ring (stable) S32.810
  unstable S32.811
 traumatic injury wound repair T81.33
 wound T81.30
  episiotomy O90.1
  operation T81.31
   cesarean O90.0
   external operation wound (superficial) T81.31
   internal operation wound (deep) T81.32
  perineal (obstetric) O90.1
  traumatic injury repair T81.33
Dissatisfaction with
 employment Z56.9
 school environment Z55.4
Dissecting — *see* condition
Dissection
 aorta I71.00
  abdominal I71.02
  thoracic I71.01
  thoracoabdominal I71.03
 artery I77.70
  basilar (trunk) I77.75
  carotid I77.71
  cerebral (nonruptured) I67.0
   ruptured — *see* Hemorrhage, intracranial, subarachnoid
  coronary I25.42
  extremity
   lower I77.77
   upper I77.76
  iliac I77.72
  precerebral
   congenital (nonruptured) Q28.1
   specified site NEC I77.75
  renal I77.73
  specified NEC I77.79
  vertebral I77.74
 traumatic — *see* Wound, open, by site
 vascular I99.8
 wound — *see* Wound, open
Disseminated — *see* condition
Dissociation
 auriculoventricular or atrioventricular (AV) (any degree) (isorhythmic) I45.89
  with heart block I44.2
 interference I45.89
Dissociative reaction, state F44.9
Dissolution, vertebra — *see* Osteoporosis
Distension, distention
 abdomen R14.0
 bladder N32.89
 cecum K63.89
 colon K63.89
 gallbladder K82.8
 intestine K63.89
 kidney N28.89
 liver K76.89
 seminal vesicle N50.89
 stomach K31.89
  acute K31.0
  psychogenic F45.8
 ureter — *see* Dilatation, ureter
 uterus N85.8
Disto-occlusion (Division I) (Division II) M26.212
Distoma hepaticum infestation B66.3

Distomiasis B66.9
 bile passages B66.3
 hemic B65.9
 hepatic B66.3
  due to Clonorchis sinensis B66.1
 intestinal B66.5
 liver B66.3
  due to Clonorchis sinensis B66.1
 lung B66.4
 pulmonary B66.4
Distomolar (fourth molar) K00.1
Distortion(s) (congenital)
 adrenal (gland) Q89.1
 arm NEC Q68.8
 bile duct or passage Q44.5
 bladder Q64.79
 brain Q04.9
 cervix (uteri) Q51.9
 chest (wall) Q67.8
  bones Q76.8
 clavicle Q74.0
 clitoris Q52.6
 coccyx Q76.49
 common duct Q44.5
 coronary Q24.5
 cystic duct Q44.5
 ear (auricle) (external) Q17.3
  inner Q16.5
  middle Q16.4
   ossicles Q16.3
 endocrine NEC Q89.2
 eustachian tube Q17.8
 eye (adnexa) Q15.8
 face bone(s) NEC Q75.8
 fallopian tube Q50.6
 femur NEC Q68.8
 fibula NEC Q68.8
 finger(s) Q68.1
 foot Q66.9
 genitalia, genital organ(s)
  female Q52.8
   external Q52.79
   internal NEC Q52.8
 gyri Q04.8
 hand bone(s) Q68.1
 heart (auricle) (ventricle) Q24.8
  valve (cusp) Q24.8
 hepatic duct Q44.5
 humerus NEC Q68.8
 hymen Q52.4
 intrafamilial communications Z63.8
 jaw NEC M26.89
 labium (majus) (minus) Q52.79
 leg NEC Q68.8
 lens Q12.8
 liver Q44.7
 lumbar spine Q76.49
  with disproportion O33.8
   causing obstructed labor O65.0
 lumbosacral (joint) (region) Q76.49
  kyphosis — *see* Kyphosis, congenital
  lordosis — *see* Lordosis, congenital
 nerve Q07.8
 nose Q30.8
 organ
  of Corti Q16.5
  or site not listed — *see* Anomaly, by site
 ossicles, ear Q16.3
 oviduct Q50.6
 pancreas Q45.3
 parathyroid (gland) Q89.2
 pituitary (gland) Q89.2
 radius NEC Q68.8
 sacroiliac joint Q74.2
 sacrum Q76.49
 scapula Q74.0
 shoulder girdle Q74.0

Distortion(s) (congenital) — *continued*
 skull bone(s) NEC Q75.8
  with
   anencephalus Q00.0
   encephalocele — *see* Encephalocele
   hydrocephalus Q03.9
    with spina bifida — *see* Spina bifida, with hydrocephalus
   microcephaly Q02
 spinal cord Q06.8
 spine Q76.49
  kyphosis — *see* Kyphosis, congenital
  lordosis — *see* Lordosis, congenital
 spleen Q89.09
 sternum NEC Q76.7
 thorax (wall) Q67.8
  bony Q76.8
 thymus (gland) Q89.2
 thyroid (gland) Q89.2
 tibia NEC Q68.8
 toe(s) Q66.9
 tongue Q38.3
 trachea (cartilage) Q32.1
 ulna NEC Q68.8
 ureter Q62.8
 urethra Q64.79
  causing obstruction Q64.39
 uterus Q51.9
 vagina Q52.4
 vertebra Q76.49
  kyphosis — *see* Kyphosis, congenital
  lordosis — *see* Lordosis, congenital
 visual — *see also* Disturbance, vision
  shape and size H53.15
 vulva Q52.79
 wrist (bones) (joint) Q68.8
Distress
 abdomen — *see* Pain, abdominal
 acute respiratory R06.00
  syndrome (adult) (child) J80
 epigastric R10.13
 fetal P84
  complicating pregnancy — *see* Stress, fetal
 gastrointestinal (functional) K30
  psychogenic F45.8
 intestinal (functional) NOS K59.9
  psychogenic F45.8
 maternal, during labor and delivery O75.0
 respiratory (adult) (child) R06.00
  newborn P22.9
   specified NEC P22.8
  orthopnea R06.01
  psychogenic F45.8
  shortness of breath R06.02
  specified type NEC R06.09
Distribution vessel, atypical Q27.9
 coronary artery Q24.5
 precerebral Q28.1
Districhiasis L68.8
Disturbance(s) — *see also* Disease
 absorption K90.9
  calcium E58
  carbohydrate K90.49
  fat K90.49
   pancreatic K90.3
  protein K90.49
  starch K90.49
  vitamin — *see* Deficiency, vitamin
 acid-base equilibrium E87.8
  mixed E87.4
 activity and attention (with hyperkinesis) — *see* Disorder, attention-deficit hyperactivity
 amino acid transport E72.00
 assimilation, food K90.9
 auditory nerve, except deafness — *see* subcategory H93.3
 behavior — *see* Disorder, conduct
 blood clotting (mechanism) (*see also* Defect, coagulation) D68.9

Disturbance(s) (see also Disease) — continued
cerebral
 nerve — see Disorder, nerve, cranial
 status, newborn P91.9
  specified NEC P91.8
circulatory I99.9
conduct (see also Disorder, conduct) F91.9
 adjustment reaction — see Disorder,
  adjustment
 compulsive F63.9
 disruptive F91.9
 hyperkinetic — see Disorder, attention-deficit
  hyperactivity
 socialized F91.2
 specified NEC F91.8
 unsocialized F91.1
coordination R27.8
cranial nerve — see Disorder, nerve, cranial
deep sensibility — see Disturbance, sensation
digestive K30
 psychogenic F45.8
electrolyte — see also Imbalance, electrolyte
 newborn, transitory P74.4
  hyperammonemia P74.6
  potassium balance P74.3
  sodium balance P74.2
  specified type NEC P74.4
emotions specific to childhood and
  adolescence F93.9
 with
  anxiety and fearfulness NEC F93.8
  elective mutism F94.0
  oppositional disorder F91.3
  sensitivity (withdrawal) F40.10
  shyness F40.10
  social withdrawal F40.10
 involving relationship problems F93.8
 mixed F93.8
 specified NEC F93.8
endocrine (gland) E34.9
 neonatal, transitory P72.9
  specified NEC P72.8
equilibrium R42
fructose metabolism E74.10
gait — see Gait
 hysterical F44.4
 psychogenic F44.4
gastrointestinal (functional) K30
 psychogenic F45.8
habit, child F98.9
hearing, except deafness and tinnitus — see
  Abnormal, auditory perception
heart, functional (conditions in I44-I50)
 due to presence of (cardiac) prosthesis
  I97.19-
 postoperative I97.89
  cardiac surgery I97.19-
hormones E34.9
innervation uterus (parasympathetic)
  (sympathetic) N85.8
keratinization NEC
 gingiva K05.10
  nonplaque induced K05.11
  plaque induced K05.10
 lip K13.0
 oral (mucosa) (soft tissue) K13.29
 tongue K13.29
learning (specific) — see Disorder, learning
memory — see Amnesia
 mild, following organic brain damage F06.8
mental F99
 associated with diseases classified elsewhere
  F54
metabolism E88.9
 with
  abortion — see Abortion, by type with
   other specified complication
  ectopic pregnancy O08.5
  molar pregnancy O08.5

Disturbance(s) (see also Disease) — continued
metabolism E88.9 — continued
 amino-acid E72.9
  aromatic E70.9
  branched-chain E71.2
  straight-chain E72.8
  sulfur-bearing E72.10
 ammonia E72.20
 arginine E72.21
 arginosuccinic acid E72.22
 carbohydrate E74.9
 cholesterol E78.9
 citrulline E72.23
 cystathionine E72.19
 general E88.9
 glutamine E72.19
 histidine E70.40
 homocystine E72.19
 hydroxylysine E72.3
 in labor or delivery O75.89
 iron E83.10
 lipoid E78.9
 lysine E72.3
 methionine E72.19
 neonatal, transitory P74.9
  calcium and magnesium P71.9
   specified type NEC P71.8
  carbohydrate metabolism P70.9
   specified type NEC P70.8
  specified NEC P74.8
 ornithine E72.4
 phosphate E83.39
 sodium NEC E87.8
 threonine E72.8
 tryptophan E70.5
 tyrosine E70.20
 urea cycle E72.20
motor R29.2
nervous, functional R45.0
neuromuscular mechanism (eye), due to
  syphilis A52.15
nutritional E63.9
 nail L60.3
ocular motion H51.9
 psychogenic F45.8
oculogyric H51.8
 psychogenic F45.8
oculomotor H51.9
 psychogenic F45.8
olfactory nerve R43.1
optic nerve NEC — see Disorder, nerve, optic
oral epithelium, including tongue NEC K13.29
perceptual due to
 alcohol withdrawal F10.232
 amphetamine intoxication F15.922
  in
   abuse F15.122
   dependence F15.222
 anxiolytic withdrawal F13.232
 cannabis intoxication (acute) F12.922
  in
   abuse F12.122
   dependence F12.222
 cocaine intoxication (acute) F14.922
  in
   abuse F14.122
   dependence F14.222
 hypnotic withdrawal F13.232
 opioid intoxication (acute) F11.922
  in
   abuse F11.122
   dependence F11.222
 phencyclidine intoxication (acute) F16.122
 sedative withdrawal F13.232
personality (pattern) (trait) (see also Disorder,
  personality) F60.9
 following organic brain damage F07.9
polyglandular E31.9
 specified NEC E31.8

Disturbance(s) (see also Disease) — continued
potassium balance, newborn P74.3
psychogenic F45.9
psychomotor F44.4
psychophysical visual H53.16
pupillary — see Anomaly, pupil, function
reflex R29.2
rhythm, heart I49.9
salivary secretion K11.7
sensation (cold) (heat) (localization) (tactile
  discrimination) (texture) (vibratory) NEC
  R20.9
 hysterical F44.6
 skin R20.9
  anesthesia R20.0
  hyperesthesia R20.3
  hypoesthesia R20.1
  paresthesia R20.2
  specified type NEC R20.8
 smell R43.9
  and taste (mixed) R43.8
  anosmia R43.0
  parosmia R43.1
  specified NEC R43.8
 taste R43.9
  and smell (mixed) R43.8
  parageusia R43.2
  specified NEC R43.8
sensory — see Disturbance, sensation
situational (transient) — see also Disorder,
  adjustment
 acute F43.0
sleep G47.9
 nonorganic origin F51.9
smell — see Disturbance, sensation, smell
sociopathic F60.2
sodium balance, newborn P74.2
speech R47.9
 developmental F80.9
 specified NEC R47.89
stomach (functional) K31.9
sympathetic (nerve) G90.9
taste — see Disturbance, sensation, taste
temperature
 regulation, newborn P81.9
  specified NEC P81.8
 sense R20.8
  hysterical F44.6
tooth
 eruption K00.6
 formation K00.4
 structure, hereditary NEC K00.5
touch — see Disturbance, sensation
vascular I99.9
 arteriosclerotic — see Arteriosclerosis
vasomotor I73.9
vasospastic I73.9
vision, visual H53.9
 following
  cerebral infarction I69.398
  cerebrovascular disease I69.998
  intracerebral hemorrhage I69.198
  nontraumatic intracranial hemorrhage
   NEC I69.298
  specified disease NEC I69.898
  specified NEC I69.898
  subarachnoid hemorrhage I69.098
 psychophysical H53.16
 specified NEC H53.8
 subjective H53.10
  day blindness H53.11
  discomfort H53.14-
  distortions of shape and size H53.15
  loss
   sudden H53.13-
   transient H53.12-
  specified type NEC H53.19

Disturbance(s) (see also Disease) — continued
  voice R49.9
    psychogenic F44.4
    specified NEC R49.8
Diuresis R35.8
Diver's palsy, paralysis or squeeze T70.3
Diverticulitis (acute) K57.92
  bladder — see Cystitis
  ileum — see Diverticulitis, intestine, small
  intestine K57.92
    with
      abscess, perforation or peritonitis K57.80
        with bleeding K57.81
      bleeding K57.93
    congenital Q43.8
    large K57.32
      with
        abscess, perforation or peritonitis
          K57.20
          with bleeding K57.21
        bleeding K57.33
      small intestine K57.52
        with
          abscess, perforation or peritonitis
            K57.40
            with bleeding K57.41
          bleeding K57.53
    small K57.12
      with
        abscess, perforation or peritonitis
          K57.00
          with bleeding K57.01
        bleeding K57.13
      large intestine K57.52
        with
          abscess, perforation or peritonitis
            K57.40
            with bleeding K57.41
          bleeding K57.53
Diverticulosis K57.90
  with bleeding K57.91
  large intestine K57.30
    with
      bleeding K57.31
      small intestine K57.50
        with bleeding K57.51
  small intestine K57.10
    with
      bleeding K57.11
      large intestine K57.50
        with bleeding K57.51
Diverticulum, diverticula (multiple) K57.90
  appendix (noninflammatory) K38.2
  bladder (sphincter) N32.3
    congenital Q64.6
  bronchus (congenital) Q32.4
    acquired J98.09
  calyx, calyceal (kidney) N28.89
  cardia (stomach) K31.4
  cecum — see Diverticulosis, intestine, large
    congenital Q43.8
  colon — see Diverticulosis, intestine, large
    congenital Q43.8
  duodenum — see Diverticulosis, intestine, small
    congenital Q43.8
  epiphrenic (esophagus) K22.5
  esophagus (congenital) Q39.6
    acquired (epiphrenic) (pulsion) (traction)
      K22.5
  eustachian tube — see Disorder, eustachian
    tube, specified NEC
  fallopian tube N83.8
  gastric K31.4
  heart (congenital) Q24.8
  ileum — see Diverticulosis, intestine, small
  jejunum — see Diverticulosis, intestine, small
  kidney (pelvis) (calyces) N28.89
    with calculus — see Calculus, kidney

Diverticulum, diverticula (multiple) K57.90
  — continued
  Meckel's (displaced) (hypertrophic) Q43.0
    malignant — see Table of Neoplasms, small
      intestine, malignant
  midthoracic K22.5
  organ or site, congenital NEC — see Distortion
  pericardium (congenital) (cyst) Q24.8
    acquired I31.8
  pharyngoesophageal (congenital) Q39.6
    acquired K22.5
  pharynx (congenital) Q38.7
  rectosigmoid — see Diverticulosis, intestine,
    large
    congenital Q43.8
  rectum — see Diverticulosis, intestine, large
  Rokitansky's K22.5
  seminal vesicle N50.89
  sigmoid — see Diverticulosis, intestine, large
    congenital Q43.8
  stomach (acquired) K31.4
    congenital Q40.2
  trachea (acquired) J39.8
  ureter (acquired) N28.89
    congenital Q62.8
  ureterovesical orifice N28.89
  urethra (acquired) N36.1
    congenital Q64.79
  ventricle, left (congenital) Q24.8
  vesical N32.3
    congenital Q64.6
  Zenker's (esophagus) K22.5
Division
  cervix uteri (acquired) N88.8
  glans penis Q55.69
  labia minora (congenital) Q52.79
  ligament (partial or complete) (current) — see
    also Sprain
    with open wound — see Wound, open
  muscle (partial or complete) (current) — see
    also Injury, muscle
    with open wound — see Wound, open
  nerve (traumatic) — see Injury, nerve
  spinal cord — see Injury, spinal cord, by
    region
  vein I87.8
Divorce, causing family disruption Z63.5
Dix-Hallpike neurolabyrinthitis — see
  Neuronitis, vestibular
Dizziness R42
  hysterical F44.89
  psychogenic F45.8
DMAC (disseminated mycobacterium
  aviumintracellulare complex) A31.2
DNR (do not resuscitate) Z66
Doan-Wiseman syndrome (primary splenic
  neutropenia) — see Agranulocytosis
Doehle-Heller aortitis A52.02
Dog bite — see Bite
Dohle body panmyelopathic syndrome
  D72.0
Dolichocephaly Q67.2
Dolichocolon Q43.8
Dolichostenomelia — see Syndrome,
  Marfan's
Donohue's syndrome E34.8
Donor (organ or tissue) Z52.9
  blood (whole) Z52.000
    autologous Z52.010
    specified component (lymphocytes) (platelets)
      NEC Z52.008
      autologous Z52.018
      specified donor NEC Z52.098
    specified donor NEC Z52.090
  stem cells Z52.001
    autologous Z52.011
    specified donor NEC Z52.091

Donor (organ or tissue) Z52.9 — continued
  bone Z52.20
    autologous Z52.21
    marrow Z52.3
    specified type NEC Z52.29
  cornea Z52.5
  egg (Oocyte) Z52.819
    age 35 and over Z52.812
      anonymous recipient Z52.812
      designated recipient Z52.813
    under age 35 Z52.810
      anonymous recipient Z52.810
      designated recipient Z52.811
  kidney Z52.4
  liver Z52.6
  lung Z52.89
  lymphocyte — see Donor, blood, specified
    components NEC
  Oocyte — see Donor, egg
  platelets Z52.008
  potential, examination of Z00.5
  semen Z52.89
  skin Z52.10
    autologous Z52.11
    specified type NEC Z52.19
  specified organ or tissue NEC Z52.89
  sperm Z52.89
Donovanosis A58
Dorsalgia M54.9
  psychogenic F45.41
  specified NEC M54.89
Dorsopathy M53.9
  deforming M43.9
    specified NEC — see subcategory M43.8
  specified NEC M53.80
    cervical region M53.82
    cervicothoracic region M53.83
    lumbar region M53.86
    lumbosacral region M53.87
    occipito-atlanto-axial region M53.81
    sacrococcygeal region M53.88
    thoracic region M53.84
    thoracolumbar region M53.85
Double
  albumin E88.09
  aortic arch Q25.45
  auditory canal Q17.8
  auricle (heart) Q20.8
  bladder Q64.79
  cervix Q51.820
    with doubling of uterus (and vagina)
      Q51.10
      with obstruction Q51.11
  inlet ventricle Q20.4
  kidney with double pelvis (renal) Q63.0
  meatus urinarius Q64.75
  monster Q89.4
  outlet
    left ventricle Q20.2
    right ventricle Q20.1
  pelvis (renal) with double ureter Q62.5
  tongue Q38.3
  ureter (one or both sides) Q62.5
    with double pelvis (renal) Q62.5
  urethra Q64.74
  urinary meatus Q64.75
  uterus Q51.2
    with
      doubling of cervix (and vagina) Q51.10
        with obstruction Q51.11
      in pregnancy or childbirth O34.59-
        causing obstructed labor O65.5
  vagina Q52.10
    with doubling of uterus (and cervix) Q51.10
      with obstruction Q51.11
  vision H53.2
  vulva Q52.79
Douglas' pouch, cul-de-sac — see condition

DISEASE INDEX

Down syndrome Q90.9
  meiotic nondisjunction Q90.0
  mitotic nondisjunction Q90.1
  mosaicism Q90.1
  translocation Q90.2
DPD (dihydropyrimidine dehydrogenase deficiency) E88.89
Dracontiasis B72
Dracunculiasis, dracunculosis B72
Dream state, hysterical F44.89
Drepanocytic anemia — see Disease, sickle-cell
Dresbach's syndrome (elliptocytosis) D58.1
Dreschlera (hawaiiensis) (infection) B43.8
Dressler's syndrome I24.1
Drift, ulnar — see Deformity, limb, specified type NEC, forearm
Drinking (alcohol)
  excessive, to excess NEC (without dependence) F10.10
    habitual (continual) (without remission) F10.20
      with remission F10.21
Drip, postnasal (chronic) R09.82
  due to
    allergic rhinitis — see Rhinitis, allergic
    common cold J00
    gastroesophageal reflux — see Reflux, gastroesophageal
    nasopharyngitis — see Nasopharyngitis
    other know condition — code to condition
    sinusitis — see Sinusitis
Droop
  facial R29.810
    cerebrovascular disease I69.992
      cerebral infarction I69.392
      intracerebral hemorrhage I69.192
      nontraumatic intracranial hemorrhage NEC I69.292
      specified disease NEC I69.892
      subarachnoid hemorrhage I69.092
Drop (in)
  attack NEC R55
  finger — see Deformity, finger
  foot — see Deformity, limb, foot, drop
  hematocrit (precipitous) R71.0
  hemoglobin R71.0
  toe — see Deformity, toe, specified NEC
  wrist — see Deformity, limb, wrist drop
Dropped heart beats I45.9
Dropsy, dropsical — see also Hydrops
  abdomen R18.8
  brain — see Hydrocephalus
  cardiac, heart — see Failure, heart, congestive
  gangrenous — see Gangrene
  heart — see Failure, heart, congestive
  kidney — see Nephrosis
  lung — see Edema, lung
  newborn due to isoimmunization P56.0
  pericardium — see Pericarditis
Drowned, drowning (near) T75.1
Drowsiness R40.0
Drug
  abuse counseling and surveillance Z71.51
  addiction — see Dependence
  dependence — see Dependence
  habit — see Dependence
  harmful use — see Abuse, drug
  induced fever R50.2
  overdose — see Table of Drugs and Chemicals, by drug, poisoning
  poisoning — see Table of Drugs and Chemicals, by drug, poisoning
  resistant organism infection (see also Resistant, organism, to, drug) Z16.30

Drug — continued
  therapy
    long term (current) (prophylactic) — see Therapy, drug long-term (current) (prophylactic)
    short term — omit code
  wrong substance given or taken in error — see Table of Drugs and Chemicals, by drug, poisoning
Drunkenness (without dependence) F10.129
  acute in alcoholism F10.229
  chronic (without remission) F10.20
    with remission F10.21
  pathological (without dependence) F10.129
    with dependence F10.229
  sleep F51.9
Drusen
  macula (degenerative) (retina) — see Degeneration, macula, drusen
  optic disc H47.32-
Dry, dryness — see also condition
  larynx J38.7
  mouth R68.2
    due to dehydration E86.0
  nose J34.89
  socket (teeth) M27.3
  throat J39.2
DSAP L56.5
Duane's syndrome H50.81-
Dubin-Johnson disease or syndrome E80.6
Dubois' disease (thymus gland) A50.59 [E35]
Dubowitz' syndrome Q87.1
Duchenne-Aran muscular atrophy G12.21
Duchenne-Griesinger disease G71.0
Duchenne's
  disease or syndrome
    motor neuron disease G12.22
    muscular dystrophy G71.0
  locomotor ataxia (syphilitic) A52.11
  paralysis
    birth injury P14.0
    due to or associated with
      motor neuron disease G12.22
      muscular dystrophy G71.0
Ducrey's chancre A57
Duct, ductus — see condition
Duhring's disease (dermatitis herpetiformis) L13.0
Dullness, cardiac (decreased) (increased) R01.2
Dumb ague — see Malaria
Dumbness — see Aphasia
Dumdum fever B55.0
Dumping syndrome (postgastrectomy) K91.1
Duodenitis (nonspecific) (peptic) K29.80
  with bleeding K29.81
Duodenocholangitis — see Cholangitis
Duodenum, duodenal — see condition
Duplay's bursitis or periarthritis — see Tendinitis, calcific, shoulder
Duplication, duplex — see also Accessory
  alimentary tract Q45.8
  anus Q43.4
  appendix (and cecum) Q43.4
  biliary duct (any) Q44.5
  bladder Q64.79
  cecum (and appendix) Q43.4
  cervix Q51.820
  chromosome NEC
    with complex rearrangements NEC Q92.5
    seen only at prometaphase Q92.8
  cystic duct Q44.5
  digestive organs Q45.8
  esophagus Q39.8
  frontonasal process Q75.8
  intestine (large) (small) Q43.4
  kidney Q63.0

Duplication, duplex — see also Accessory — continued
  liver Q44.7
  pancreas Q45.3
  penis Q55.69
  respiratory organs NEC Q34.8
  salivary duct Q38.4
  spinal cord (incomplete) Q06.2
  stomach Q40.2
Dupré's disease (meningism) R29.1
Dupuytren's contraction or disease M72.0
Durand-Nicolas-Favre disease A55
Durotomy (inadvertent) (incidental) G97.41
Duroziez's disease (congenital mitral stenosis) Q23.2
Dutton's relapsing fever (West African) A68.1
Dwarfism E34.3
  achondroplastic Q77.4
  congenital E34.3
  constitutional E34.3
  hypochondroplastic Q77.4
  hypophyseal E23.0
  infantile E34.3
  Laron-type E34.3
  Lorain(-Levi) type E23.0
  metatropic Q77.8
  nephrotic-glycosuric (with hypophosphatemic rickets) E72.09
  nutritional E45
  pancreatic K86.89
  pituitary E23.0
  renal N25.0
  thanatophoric Q77.1
Dyke-Young anemia (secondary) (symptomatic) D59.1
Dysacusis — see Abnormal, auditory perception
Dysadrenocortism E27.9
  hyperfunction E27.0
Dysarthria R47.1
  following
    cerebral infarction I69.322
    cerebrovascular disease I69.922
      specified disease NEC I69.822
    intracerebral hemorrhage I69.122
    nontraumatic intracranial hemorrhage NEC I69.222
    subarachnoid hemorrhage I69.022
Dysautonomia (familial) G90.1
Dysbarism T70.3
Dysbasia R26.2
  angiosclerotica intermittens I73.9
  hysterical F44.4
  lordotica (progressiva) G24.1
  nonorganic origin F44.4
  psychogenic F44.4
Dysbetalipoproteinemia (familial) E78.2
Dyscalculia R48.8
  developmental F81.2
Dyschezia K59.00
Dyschondroplasia (with hemangiomata) Q78.4
Dyschromia (skin) L81.9
Dyscollagenosis M35.9
Dyscranio-pygo-phalangy Q87.0
Dyscrasia
  blood (with) D75.9
    antepartum hemorrhage — see Hemorrhage, antepartum, with coagulation defect
    intrapartum hemorrhage O67.0
    newborn P61.9
      specified type NEC P61.8
    puerperal, postpartum O72.3
  polyglandular, pluriglandular E31.9
Dysendocrinism E34.9

Dysentery, dysenteric (catarrhal) (diarrhea)
(epidemic) (hemorrhagic) (infectious)
(sporadic) (tropical) A09
abscess, liver A06.4
amebic (see also Amebiasis) A06.0
with abscess — see Abscess, amebic
acute A06.0
chronic A06.1
arthritis (see also category M01) A09
bacillary (see also category M01) A03.9
bacillary A03.9
arthritis (see also category M01) A03.9
Boyd A03.2
Flexner A03.1
Schmitz(-Stutzer) A03.0
Shiga(-Kruse) A03.0
Shigella A03.9
boydii A03.2
dysenteriae A03.0
flexneri A03.1
group A A03.0
group B A03.1
group C A03.2
group D A03.3
sonnei A03.3
specified type NEC A03.8
Sonne A03.3
specified type NEC A03.8
balantidial A07.0
Balantidium coli A07.0
Boyd's A03.2
candidal B37.82
Chilomastix A07.8
Chinese A03.9
coccidial A07.3
Dientamoeba (fragilis) A07.8
Embadomonas A07.8
Entamoeba, entamebic — see Dysentery,
amebic
Flexner's A03.1
Flexner-Boyd A03.2
Giardia lamblia A07.1
Hiss-Russell A03.1
Lamblia A07.1
leishmanial B55.0
malarial — see Malaria
metazoal B82.0
monilial B37.82
protozoal A07.9
Salmonella A02.0
schistosomal B65.1
Schmitz(-Stutzer) A03.0
Shiga(-Kruse) A03.0
Shigella NOS — see Dysentery, bacillary
Sonne A03.3
strongyloidiasis B78.0
trichomonal A07.8
viral (see also Enteritis, viral) A08.4
Dysequilibrium R42
Dysesthesia R20.8
hysterical F44.6
Dysfibrinogenemia (congenital) D68.2
Dysfunction
adrenal E27.9
hyperfunction E27.0
autonomic
due to alcohol G31.2
somatoform F45.8
bladder N31.9
neurogenic NOS — see Dysfunction,
bladder, neuromuscular
neuromuscular NOS N31.9
atonic (motor) (sensory) N31.2
autonomous N31.2
flaccid N31.2
nonreflex N31.2
reflex N31.1
specified NEC N31.8
uninhibited N31.0

Dysfunction — continued
bleeding, uterus N93.8
cerebral G93.89
colon K59.9
psychogenic F45.8
colostomy K94.03
cystic duct K82.8
cystostomy (stoma) — see Complications,
cystostomy
ejaculatory N53.19
anejaculatory orgasm N53.13
painful N53.12
premature F52.4
retarded N53.11
endocrine NOS E34.9
endometrium N85.8
enterostomy K94.13
erectile — see Dysfunction, sexual, male,
erectile
gallbladder K82.8
gastrostomy (stoma) K94.23
gland, glandular NOS E34.9
heart I51.89
hemoglobin D75.89
hepatic K76.89
hypophysis E23.7
hypothalamic NEC E23.3
ileostomy (stoma) K94.13
jejunostomy (stoma) K94.13
kidney — see Disease, renal
labyrinthine — see subcategory H83.2
left ventricular, following sudden emotional
stress I51.81
liver K76.89
male — see Dysfunction, sexual, male
orgasmic (female) F52.31
male F52.32
ovary E28.9
specified NEC E28.8
papillary muscle I51.89
parathyroid E21.4
physiological NEC R68.89
psychogenic F59
pineal gland E34.8
pituitary (gland) E23.3
platelets D69.1
polyglandular E31.9
specified NEC E31.8
psychophysiologic F59
psychosexual F52.9
with
dyspareunia F52.6
premature ejaculation F52.4
vaginismus F52.5
pylorus K31.9
rectum K59.9
psychogenic F45.8
reflex (sympathetic) — see Syndrome, pain,
complex regional I
segmental — see Dysfunction, somatic
senile R54
sexual (due to) R37
alcohol F10.981
amphetamine F15.981
in
abuse F15.181
dependence F15.281
anxiolytic F13.981
in
abuse F13.181
dependence F13.281
cocaine F14.981
in
abuse F14.181
dependence F14.281
excessive sexual drive F52.8
failure of genital response (male) F52.21
female F52.22

Dysfunction — continued
sexual (due to) R37 — continued
female N94.9
aversion F52.1
dyspareunia N94.10
psychogenic F52.6
frigidity F52.22
nymphomania F52.8
orgasmic F52.31
psychogenic F52.9
aversion F52.1
dyspareunia F52.6
frigidity F52.22
nymphomania F52.8
orgasmic F52.31
vaginismus F52.5
vaginismus N94.2
psychogenic F52.5
hypnotic F13.981
in
abuse F13.181
dependence F13.281
inhibited orgasm (female) F52.31
male F52.32
lack
of sexual enjoyment F52.1
or loss of sexual desire F52.0
male N53.9
anejaculatory orgasm N53.13
ejaculatory N53.19
painful N53.12
premature F52.4
retarded N53.11
erectile N52.9
drug induced N52.2
due to
disease classified elsewhere N52.1
drug N52.2
postoperative (postprocedural) N52.39
following
cryotherapy N52.37
interstitial seed therapy N52.36
prostate ablative therapy N52.37
prostatectomy N52.34
radical N52.31
radiation therapy N52.35
radical cystectomy N52.32
ultrasound ablative therapy N52.37
urethral surgery N52.33
psychogenic F52.21
specified cause NEC N52.8
vasculogenic
arterial insufficiency N52.01
with corporo-venous occlusive
N52.03
corporo-venous occlusive N52.02
with arterial insufficiency N52.03
impotence — see Dysfunction, sexual,
male, erectile
psychogenic F52.9
aversion F52.1
erectile F52.21
orgasmic F52.32
premature ejaculation F52.4
satyriasis F52.8
specified type NEC F52.8
specified type NEC N53.8
nonorganic F52.9
specified NEC F52.8
opioid F11.981
in
abuse F11.181
dependence F11.281
orgasmic dysfunction (female) F52.31
male F52.32
premature ejaculation F52.4

DISEASE INDEX

Dysfunction — *continued*
  sexual (due to) R37 — *continued*
    psychoactive substances NEC F19.981
      in
        abuse F19.181
        dependence F19.281
    psychogenic F52.9
    sedative F13.981
      in
        abuse F13.181
        dependence F13.281
    sexual aversion F52.1
    vaginismus (nonorganic) (psychogenic)
      F52.5
  sinoatrial node I49.5
  somatic M99.09
    abdomen M99.09
    acromioclavicular M99.07
    cervical region M99.01
    cervicothoracic M99.01
    costochondral M99.08
    costovertebral M99.08
    head region M99.00
    hip M99.05
    lower extremity M99.06
    lumbar region M99.03
    lumbosacral M99.03
    occipitocervical M99.00
    pelvic region M99.05
    pubic M99.05
    rib cage M99.08
    sacral region M99.04
    sacrococcygeal M99.04
    sacroiliac M99.04
    specified NEC M99.09
    sternochondral M99.08
    sternoclavicular M99.07
    thoracic region M99.02
    thoracolumbar M99.02
    upper extremity M99.07
  somatoform autonomic F45.8
  stomach K31.89
    psychogenic F45.8
  suprarenal E27.9
    hyperfunction E27.0
  symbolic R48.9
    specified type NEC R48.8
  temporomandibular (joint) M26.69
    joint-pain syndrome M26.62-
  testicular (endocrine) E29.9
    specified NEC E29.8
  thymus E32.9
  thyroid E07.9
  ureterostomy (stoma) — *see* Complications,
    stoma, urinary tract
  urethrostomy (stoma) — *see* Complications,
    stoma, urinary tract
  uterus, complicating delivery O62.9
    hypertonic O62.4
    hypotonic O62.2
      primary O62.0
      secondary O62.1
  ventricular I51.9
    with congestive heart failure I50.9
    left, reversible, following sudden emotional
      stress I51.81
Dysgenesis
  gonadal (due to chromosomal anomaly)
    Q96.9
    pure Q99.1
  renal Q60.5
    bilateral Q60.4
    unilateral Q60.3
  reticular D72.0
  tidal platelet D69.3

Dysgerminoma
  specified site — *see* Neoplasm, malignant, by
    site
  unspecified site
    female C56.9
    male C62.90
Dysgeusia R43.2
Dysgraphia R27.8
Dyshidrosis, dysidrosis L30.1
Dyskaryotic cervical smear R87.619
Dyskeratosis L85.8
  cervix — *see* Dysplasia, cervix
  congenital Q82.8
  uterus NEC N85.8
Dyskinesia G24.9
  biliary (cystic duct or gallbladder) K82.8
  drug induced
    orofacial G24.01
  esophagus K22.4
  hysterical F44.4
  intestinal K59.8
  nonorganic origin F44.4
  orofacial (idiopathic) G24.4
    drug induced G24.01
  psychogenic F44.4
  subacute, drug induced G24.01
  tardive G24.01
    neuroleptic induced G24.01
  trachea J39.8
  tracheobronchial J98.09
Dyslalia (developmental) F80.0
Dyslexia R48.0
  developmental F81.0
Dyslipidemia E78.5
  depressed HDL cholesterol E78.6
  elevated fasting triglycerides E78.1
Dysmaturity — *see also* Light for dates
  pulmonary (newborn) (Wilson-Mikity) P27.0
Dysmenorrhea (essential) (exfoliative) N94.6
  congestive (syndrome) N94.6
  primary N94.4
  psychogenic F45.8
  secondary N94.5
Dysmetabolic syndrome X E88.81
Dysmetria R27.8
Dysmorphism (due to)
  alcohol Q86.0
  exogenous cause NEC Q86.8
  hydantoin Q86.1
  warfarin Q86.2
Dysmorphophobia (nondelusional) F45.22
  delusional F22
Dysnomia R47.01
Dysorexia R63.0
  psychogenic F50.89
Dysostosis
  cleidocranial, cleidocranialis Q74.0
  craniofacial Q75.1
  Fairbank's (idiopathic familial generalized
    osteophytosis) Q78.9
  mandibulofacial (incomplete) Q75.4
  multiplex E76.01
  oculomandibular Q75.5
Dyspareunia (female) N94.10
  deep N94.12
  male N53.12
  nonorganic F52.6
  psychogenic F52.6
  secondary N94.19
  specified NEC N94.19
  superficial (introital) N94.11
Dyspepsia R10.13
  atonic K30
  functional (allergic) (congenital)
    (gastrointestinal) (occupational) (reflex) K30
  intestinal K59.8
  nervous F45.8
  neurotic F45.8
  psychogenic F45.8

Dysphagia R13.10
  cervical R13.19
  following
    cerebral infarction I69.391
    cerebrovascular disease I69.991
    intracerebral hemorrhage I69.191
    nontraumatic intracranial hemorrhage NEC
      I69.291
    specified disease NEC I69.891
    specified NEC I69.891
    subarachnoid hemorrhage I69.091
  functional (hysterical) F45.8
  hysterical F45.8
  nervous (hysterical) F45.8
  neurogenic R13.19
  oral phase R13.11
  oropharyngeal phase R13.12
  pharyneal phase R13.13
  pharyngoesophageal phase R13.14
  psychogenic F45.8
  sideropenic D50.1
  spastica K22.4
  specified NEC R13.19
Dysphagocytosis, congenital D71
Dysphasia R47.02
  developmental
    expressive type F80.1
    receptive type F80.2
  following
    cerebrovascular disease I69.921
      cerebral infarction I69.321
      intracerebral hemorrhage I69.121
      nontraumatic intracranial hemorrhage
        NEC I69.221
      specified disease NEC I69.821
      subarachnoid hemorrhage I69.021
Dysphonia R49.0
  functional F44.4
  hysterical F44.4
  psychogenic F44.4
  spastica J38.3
Dysphoria
  gender
    in
      adolescence and adulthood F64.0
      children F64.2
  postpartal O90.6
Dyspituitarism E23.3
Dysplasia — *see also* Anomaly
  acetabular, congenital Q65.89
  alveolar capillary, with vein misalignment
    J84.843
  anus (histologically confirmed) (mild)
    (moderate) K62.82
    severe D01.3
  arrhythmogenic right ventricular I42.8
  arterial, fibromuscular I77.3
  asphyxiating thoracic (congenital) Q77.2
  brain Q07.9
  bronchopulmonary, perinatal P27.1
  cervix (uteri) N87.9
    mild N87.0
    moderate N87.1
    severe D06.9
  chondroectodermal Q77.6
  colon D12.6
  craniometaphyseal Q78.8
  dentinal K00.5
  diaphyseal, progressive Q78.3
  dystrophic Q77.5
  ectodermal (anhidrotic) (congenital)
    (hereditary) Q82.4
    hydrotic Q82.8
  epithelial, uterine cervix — *see* Dysplasia,
    cervix
  eye (congenital) Q11.2

E

Eales' disease H35.06-
Ear — see also condition
  piercing Z41.3
  tropical NEC B36.9 [H62.40]
    in
      aspergillosis B44.89
      candidiasis B37.84
      moniliasis B37.84
  wax (impacted) H61.20
    left H61.22
      with right H61.23
    right H61.21
      with left H61.23
Earache — see subcategory H92.0
Early satiety R68.81
Eaton-Lambert syndrome — see Syndrome, Lambert-Eaton
Eberth's disease (typhoid fever) A01.00
Ebola virus disease A98.4
Ebstein's anomaly or syndrome (heart) Q22.5
Eccentro-osteochondrodysplasia E76.29
Ecchondroma — see Neoplasm, bone, benign
Ecchondrosis D48.0
Ecchymosis R58
  conjunctiva — see Hemorrhage, conjunctiva
  eye (traumatic) — see Contusion, eyeball
  eyelid (traumatic) — see Contusion, eyelid
  newborn P54.5
  spontaneous R23.3
  traumatic — see Contusion
Echinococciasis — see Echinococcus
Echinococcosis — see Echinococcus
Echinococcus (infection) B67.90
  granulosus B67.4
    bone B67.2
    liver B67.0
    lung B67.1
    multiple sites B67.32
    specified site NEC B67.39
    thyroid B67.31
  liver NOS B67.8
    granulosus B67.0
    multilocularis B67.5
  lung NEC B67.99
    granulosus B67.1
    multilocularis B67.69
  multilocularis B67.7
    liver B67.5
    multiple sites B67.61
    specified site NEC B67.69
  specified site NEC B67.99
    granulosus B67.39
    multilocularis B67.69
  thyroid NEC B67.99
    granulosus B67.31
    multilocularis B67.69 [E35]
Echinorhynchiasis B83.8
Echinostomiasis B66.8
Echolalia R48.8
Echovirus, as cause of disease classified elsewhere B97.12
Eclampsia, eclamptic (coma) (convulsions) (delirium) (with hypertension) NEC O15.9
  complicating
    labor and delivery O15.1
    postpartum O15.2
    pregnancy O15.0-
  puerperium O15.2
Economic circumstances affecting care Z59.9
Economo's disease A85.8

Ectasia, ectasis
  annuloaortic I35.8
  aorta I77.819
    with aneurysm — see Aneurysm, aorta
    abdominal I77.811
    thoracic I77.810
    thoracoabdominal I77.812
  breast — see Ectasia, mammary duct
  capillary I78.8
  cornea H18.71-
  gastric antral vascular (GAVE) K31.819
    with hemorrhage K31.811
    without hemorrhage K31.819
  mammary duct N60.4-
  salivary gland (duct) K11.8
  sclera — see Sclerectasia
Ecthyma L08.0
  contagiosum B08.02
  gangrenosum L08.0
  infectiosum B08.02
Ectocardia Q24.8
Ectodermal dysplasia (anhidrotic) Q82.4
Ectodermosis erosiva pluriorificialis L51.1
Ectopic, ectopia (congenital)
  abdominal viscera Q45.8
    due to defect in anterior abdominal wall Q79.59
  ACTH syndrome E24.3
  adrenal gland Q89.1
  anus Q43.5
  atrial beats I49.1
  beats I49.49
    atrial I49.1
    ventricular I49.3
  bladder Q64.10
  bone and cartilage in lung Q33.5
  brain Q04.8
  breast tissue Q83.8
  cardiac Q24.8
  cerebral Q04.8
  cordis Q24.8
  endometrium — see Endometriosis
  gastric mucosa Q40.2
  gestation — see Pregnancy, by site
  heart Q24.8
  hormone secretion NEC E34.2
  kidney (crossed) (pelvis) Q63.2
  lens, lentis Q12.1
  mole — see Pregnancy, by site
  organ or site NEC — see Malposition, congenital
  pancreas Q45.3
  pregnancy — see Pregnancy, ectopic
  pupil — see Abnormality, pupillary
  renal Q63.2
  sebaceous glands of mouth Q38.6
  spleen Q89.09
  testis Q53.00
    bilateral Q53.02
    unilateral Q53.01
  thyroid Q89.2
  tissue in lung Q33.5
  ureter Q62.63
  ventricular beats I49.3
  vesicae Q64.10
Ectromelia Q73.8
  lower limb — see Defect, reduction, limb, lower, specified type NEC
  upper limb — see Defect, reduction, limb, upper, specified type NEC

Ectropion H02.109
  cervix N86
    with cervicitis N72
  congenital Q10.1
  eyelid (paralytic) H02.109
    cicatricial H02.119
      left H02.116
        lower H02.115
        upper H02.114
      right H02.113
        lower H02.112
        upper H02.111
    congenital Q10.1
    left H02.106
      lower H02.105
      upper H02.104
    mechanical H02.129
      left H02.126
        lower H02.125
        upper H02.124
      right H02.123
        lower H02.122
        upper H02.121
    right H02.103
      lower H02.102
      upper H02.101
    senile H02.139
      left H02.136
        lower H02.135
        upper H02.134
      right H02.133
        lower H02.132
        upper H02.131
    spastic H02.149
      left H02.146
        lower H02.145
        upper H02.144
      right H02.143
        lower H02.142
        upper H02.141
  iris H21.89
  lip (acquired) K13.0
    congenital Q38.0
  urethra N36.8
  uvea H21.89
Eczema (acute) (chronic) (erythematous) (fissum) (rubrum) (squamous) (see also Dermatitis) L30.9
  contact — see Dermatitis, contact
  dyshydrotic L30.1
  external ear — see Otitis, externa, acute, eczematoid
  flexural L20.82
  herpeticum B00.0
  hypertrophicum L28.0
  hypostatic — see Varix, leg, with, inflammation
  impetiginous L01.1
  infantile (due to any substance) L20.83
    intertriginous L21.1
    seborrheic L21.1
  intertriginous NEC L30.4
    infantile L21.1
  intrinsic (allergic) L20.84
  lichenified NEC L28.0
  marginatum (hebrae) B35.6
  pustular L30.3
  stasis I87.2
    with varicose veins — see Varix, leg, with, inflammation
  vaccination, vaccinatum T88.1
  varicose — see Varix, leg, with, inflammation
Eczematid L30.2
Eddowes(-Spurway) syndrome Q78.0
Edema, edematous (infectious) (pitting) (toxic) R60.9
  with nephritis — see Nephrosis
  allergic T78.3
  amputation stump (surgical) (sequelae (late effect)) T87.89

Edema, edematous (infectious) (pitting) (toxic) R60.9 — *continued*
angioneurotic (allergic) (any site) (with urticaria) T78.3
  hereditary D84.1
angiospastic I73.9
Berlin's (traumatic) S05.8x-
brain (cytotoxic) (vasogenic) G93.6
  due to birth injury P11.0
  newborn (anoxia or hypoxia) P52.4
    birth injury P11.0
  traumatic — *see* Injury, intracranial, cerebral edema
cardiac — *see* Failure, heart, congestive
cardiovascular — *see* Failure, heart, congestive
cerebral — *see* Edema, brain
cerebrospinal — *see* Edema, brain
cervix (uteri) (acute) N88.8
  puerperal, postpartum O90.89
chronic hereditary Q82.0
circumscribed, acute T78.3
  hereditary D84.1
conjunctiva H11.42-
cornea H18.2-
  idiopathic H18.22-
  secondary H18.23-
    due to contact lens H18.21-
due to
  lymphatic obstruction I89.0
  salt retention E87.0
epiglottis — *see* Edema, glottis
essential, acute T78.3
  hereditary D84.1
extremities, lower — *see* Edema, legs
eyelid NEC H02.849
  left H02.846
    lower H02.845
    upper H02.844
  right H02.843
    lower H02.842
    upper H02.841
familial, hereditary Q82.0
famine — *see* Malnutrition, severe
generalized R60.1
glottis, glottic, glottidis (obstructive) (passive) J38.4
  allergic T78.3
    hereditary D84.1
heart — *see* Failure, heart, congestive
heat T67.7
hereditary Q82.0
inanition — *see* Malnutrition, severe
intracranial G93.6
iris H21.89
joint — *see* Effusion, joint
larynx — *see* Edema, glottis
legs R60.0
  due to venous obstruction I87.1
  hereditary Q82.0
localized R60.0
  due to venous obstruction I87.1
lower limbs — *see* Edema, legs
lung J81.1
  with heart condition or failure — *see* Failure, ventricular, left
  acute J81.0
  chemical (acute) J68.1
    chronic J68.1
  chronic J81.1
    due to
      chemicals, gases, fumes or vapors (inhalation) J68.1
      external agent J70.9
        specified NEC J70.8
      radiation J70.1

Edema, edematous (infectious) (pitting) (toxic) R60.9 — *continued*
lung J81.1 — *continued*
  due to
    chemicals, fumes or vapors (inhalation) J68.1
    external agent J70.9
      specified NEC J70.8
    high altitude T70.29
    near drowning T75.1
    radiation J70.0
  meaning failure, left ventricle I50.1
lymphatic I89.0
  due to mastectomy I97.2
macula H35.81
  cystoid, following cataract surgery — *see* Complications, postprocedural, following cataract surgery
  diabetic — *see* Diabetes, by type, with, retinopathy, with macular edema
malignant — *see* Gangrene, gas
Milroy's Q82.0
nasopharynx J39.2
newborn P83.30
  hydrops fetalis — *see* Hydrops, fetalis
  specified NEC P83.39
nutritional — *see also* Malnutrition, severe
  with dyspigmentation, skin and hair E40
optic disc or nerve — *see* Papilledema
orbit H05.22-
pancreas K86.89
papilla, optic — *see* Papilledema
penis N48.89
periodic T78.3
  hereditary D84.1
pharynx J39.2
pulmonary — *see* Edema, lung
Quincke's T78.3
  hereditary D84.1
renal — *see* Nephrosis
retina H35.81
  diabetic — *see* Diabetes, by type, with, retinopathy, with macular edema
salt E87.0
scrotum N50.89
seminal vesicle N50.89
spermatic cord N50.89
spinal (cord) (vascular) (nontraumatic) G95.19
starvation — *see* Malnutrition, severe
stasis — *see* Hypertension, venous, (chronic)
subglottic — *see* Edema, glottis
supraglottic — *see* Edema, glottis
testis N44.8
tunica vaginalis N50.89
vas deferens N50.89
vulva (acute) N90.89
Edentulism — *see* Absence, teeth, acquired
Edsall's disease T67.2
Educational handicap Z55.9
  specified NEC Z55.8
Edward's syndrome — *see* Trisomy, 18
Effect(s) (of) (from) — *see* Effect, adverse NEC
Effect, adverse
abnormal gravitational (G) forces or states T75.81
abuse — *see* Maltreatment
air pressure T70.9
  specified NEC T70.8
altitude (high) — *see* Effect, adverse, high altitude
anesthesia (*see also* Anesthesia) T88.59
  in labor and delivery O74.9
  local, toxic
    in labor and delivery O74.4
    in pregnancy NEC O29.3-
    postpartum, puerperal O89.3
  postpartum, puerperal O89.9

Effect, adverse — *continued*
anesthesia (*see also* Anesthesia) T88.59 — *continued*
  specified NEC T88.59
    in labor and delivery O74.8
    postpartum, puerperal O89.8
  spinal and epidural T88.59
    headache T88.59
      in labor and delivery O74.5
      postpartum, puerperal O89.4
    specified NEC
      in labor and delivery O74.6
      postpartum, puerperal O89.5
antitoxin — *see* Complications, vaccination
atmospheric pressure T70.9
  due to explosion T70.8
  high T70.3
  low — *see* Effect, adverse, high altitude
  specified effect NEC T70.8
biological, correct substance properly administered — *see* Effect, adverse, drug
blood (derivatives) (serum) (transfusion) — *see* Complications, transfusion
chemical substance — *see* Table of Drugs and Chemicals
cold (temperature) (weather) T69.9
  chilblains T69.1
  frostbite — *see* Frostbite
  specified effect NEC T69.8
drugs and medicaments T88.7
  specified drug — *see* Table of Drugs and Chemicals, by drug, adverse effect
  specified effect — *code to condition*
electric current, electricity (shock) T75.4
  burn — *see* Burn
exertion (excessive) T73.3
exposure — *see* Exposure
external cause NEC T75.89
foodstuffs T78.1
  allergic reaction — *see* Allergy, food
    causing anaphylaxis — *see* Shock, anaphylactic, due to, food
  noxious — *see* Poisoning, food, noxious
gases, fumes, or vapors T59.9-
  specified agent — *see* Table of Drugs and Chemicals
glue (airplane) sniffing
  due to drug abuse — *see* Abuse, drug, inhalant
  due to drug dependence — *see* Dependence, drug, inhalant
heat — *see* Heat
high altitude NEC T70.29
  anoxia T70.29
  on
    ears T70.0
    sinuses T70.1
  polycythemia D75.1
high pressure fluids T70.4
hot weather — *see* Heat
hunger T73.0
immersion, foot — *see* Immersion
immunization — *see* Complications, vaccination
immunological agents — *see* Complications, vaccination
infrared (radiation) (rays) NOS T66
  dermatitis or eczema L59.8
infusion — *see* Complications, infusion
lack of care of infants — *see* Maltreatment, child
lightning — *see* Lightning
medical care T88.9
  specified NEC T88.8
medicinal substance, correct, properly administered — *see* Effect, adverse, drug
motion T75.3
noise, on inner ear — *see* subcategory H83.3
overheated places — *see* Heat

Effect, adverse — *continued*
psychosocial, of work environment Z56.5
radiation (diagnostic) (infrared) (natural source) (therapeutic) (ultraviolet) (X-ray) NOS T66
dermatitis or eczema — *see* Dermatitis, due to, radiation
fibrosis of lung J70.1
pneumonitis J70.0
pulmonary manifestations
acute J70.0
chronic J70.1
skin L59.9
radioactive substance NOS
reduced temperature T69.9
immersion foot or hand — *see* Immersion
specified effect NEC T69.8
serum NEC (*see also* Reaction, serum) T80.69
specified NEC T78.8
external cause NEC T75.89
strangulation — *see* Asphyxia, traumatic
submersion T75.1
thirst T73.1
toxic — *see* Toxicity
transfusion — *see* Complications, transfusion
ultraviolet (radiation) (rays) NOS T66
burn — *see* Burn
dermatitis or eczema — *see* Dermatitis, due to, ultraviolet rays
acute L56.8
vaccine (any) — *see* Complications, vaccination
vibration — *see* Vibration, adverse effects
water pressure NEC T70.9
specified NEC T70.8
weightlessness T75.82
whole blood — *see* Complications, transfusion
work environment Z56.5
Effects, late — *see* Sequelae
Effluvium
anagen L65.1
telogen L65.0
Effort syndrome (psychogenic) F45.8
Effusion
amniotic fluid — *see* Pregnancy, complicated by, prematue rupture of membranes
brain (serous) G93.6
bronchial — *see* Bronchitis
cerebral G93.6
cerebrospinal — *see also* Meningitis
vessel G93.6
chest — *see* Effusion, pleura
chylous, chyliform (pleura) J94.0
intracranial G93.6
joint M25.40
ankle M25.47-
elbow M25.42-
foot joint M25.47-
hand joint M25.44-
hip M25.45-
knee M25.46-
shoulder M25.41-
specified joint NEC M25.48
wrist M25.43-
malignant pleural J91.0
meninges — *see* Meningitis
pericardium, pericardial (noninflammatory) I31.3
acute — *see* Pericarditis, acute
peritoneal (chronic) R18.8
pleura, pleurisy, pleuritic, pleuropericardial J90
chylous, chyliform J94.0
due to systemic lupus erythematosis M32.13
influenzal — *see* Influenza, with, respiratory manifestations NEC
malignant J91.0
newborn P28.89

Effusion — *continued*
pleura, pleurisy, pleuritic, pleuropericardial J90 — *continued*
tuberculous NEC A15.6
primary (progressive) A15.7
spinal — *see* Meningitis
thorax, thoracic — *see* Effusion, pleura
Egg shell nails L60.3
congenital Q84.6
Egyptian splenomegaly B65.1
Ehlers-Danlos syndrome Q79.6
Ehrlichiosis A77.40
due to
E. chafeensis A77.41
E. sennetsu A79.81
specified organism NEC A77.49
Eichstedt's disease B36.0
Eisenmenger's
complex or syndrome I27.89
defect Q21.8
Ejaculation
delayed F52.32
painful N53.12
premature F52.4
retarded N53.11
retrograde N53.14
semen, painful N53.12
psychogenic F52.6
Ekbom's syndrome (restless legs) G25.81
Ekman's syndrome (brittle bones and blue sclera) Q78.0
Elastic skin Q82.8
acquired L57.4
Elastofibroma — *see* Neoplasm, connective tissue, benign
Elastoma (juvenile) Q82.8
Miescher's L87.2
Elastomyofibrosis I42.4
Elastosis
actinic, solar L57.8
atrophicans (senile) L57.4
perforans serpiginosa L87.2
senilis L57.4
Elbow — *see* condition
Electric current, electricity, effects (concussion) (fatal) (nonfatal) (shock) T75.4
burn — *see* Burn
Electric feet syndrome E53.8
Electrocution T75.4
from electroshock gun (taser) T75.4
Electrolyte imbalance E87.8
with
abortion — *see* Abortion, by type, complicated by, electrolyte imbalance
ectopic pregnancy O08.5
molar pregnancy O08.5
Elephantiasis (nonfilarial) I89.0
arabicum — *see* Infestation, filarial
bancroftian B74.0
congenital (any site) (hereditary) Q82.0
due to
Brugia (malayi) B74.1
timori B74.2
mastectomy I97.2
Wuchereria (bancrofti) B74.0
eyelid H02.859
left H02.856
lower H02.855
upper H02.854
right H02.853
lower H02.852
upper H02.851
filarial, filariensis — *see* Infestation, filarial
glandular I89.0
graecorum A30.9
lymphangiectatic I89.0
lymphatic vessel I89.0
due to mastectomy I97.2
scrotum (nonfilarial) I89.0

Elephantiasis (nonfilarial) I89.0 — *continued*
streptococcal I89.0
surgical I97.89
postmastectomy I97.2
telangiectodes I89.0
vulva (nonfilarial) N90.89
Elevated, elevation
antibody titer R76.0
basal metabolic rate R94.8
blood pressure — *see also* Hypertension
reading (incidental) (isolated) (nonspecific), no diagnosis of hypertension R03.0
blood sugar R73.9
body temperature (of unknown origin) R50.9
cancer antigen 125 [CA 125] R97.1
carcinoembryonic antigen [CEA] R97.0
cholesterol E78.00
with high triglycerides E78.2
conjugate, eye H51.0
C-reactive protein (CRP) R79.82
diaphragm, congenital Q79.1
erythrocyte sedimentation rate R70.0
fasting glucose R73.01
fasting triglycerides E78.1
finding on laboratory examination — *see* Findings, abnormal, inconclusive, without diagnosis, by type of exam
GFR (glomerular filtration rate) — *see* Findings, abnormal, inconclusive, without diagnosis, by type of exam
glucose tolerance (oral) R73.02
immunoglobulin level R76.8
indoleacetic acid R82.5
lactic acid dehydrogenase (LDH) level R74.0
leukocytes D72.829
lipoprotein a level E78.8
liver function
study R94.5
test R79.89
alkaline phosphatase R74.8
aminotransferase R74.0
bilirubin R17
hepatic enzyme R74.8
lactate dehydrogenase R74.0
lymphocytes D72.820
prostate specific antigen [PSA] R97.20
Rh titer — *see* Complication(s), transfusion, incompatibility reaction, Rh (factor)
scapula, congenital Q74.0
sedimentation rate R70.0
SGOT R74.0
SGPT R74.0
transaminase level R74.0
triglycerides E78.1
with high cholesterol E78.2
tumor associated antigens [TAA] NEC R97.8
tumor specific antigens [TSA] NEC R97.8
urine level of
17-ketosteroids R82.5
catecholamine R82.5
indoleacetic acid R82.5
steroids R82.5
vanillylmandelic acid (VMA) R82.5
venous pressure I87.8
white blood cell count D72.829
specified NEC D72.828
Elliptocytosis (congenital) (hereditary) D58.1
Hb C (disease) D58.1
hemoglobin disease D58.1
sickle-cell (disease) D57.8-
trait D57.3
Ellison-Zollinger syndrome E16.4
Ellis-van Creveld syndrome (chondroectodermal dysplasia) Q77.6

Elongated, elongation (congenital) — *see also* Distortion
 bone Q79.9
 cervix (uteri) Q51.828
  acquired N88.4
  hypertrophic N88.4
 colon Q43.8
 common bile duct Q44.5
 cystic duct Q44.5
 frenulum, penis Q55.69
 labia minora (acquired) N90.69
 ligamentum patellae Q74.1
 petiolus (epiglottidis) Q31.8
 tooth, teeth K00.2
 uvula Q38.6
Eltor cholera A00.1
Emaciation (due to malnutrition) E41
Embadomoniasis A07.8
Embedded tooth, teeth K01.0
 root only K08.3
Embolic — *see* condition
Embolism (multiple) (paradoxical) I74.9
 air (any site) (traumatic) T79.0
  following
   abortion — *see* Abortion by type
    complicated by embolism
   ectopic pregnancy O08.2
   infusion, therapeutic injection or
    transfusion T80.0
   molar pregnancy O08.2
   procedure NEC
    artery T81.719
     mesenteric T81.710
     renal T81.711
     specified NEC T81.718
    vein T81.72
  in pregnancy, childbirth or puerperium —
   see Embolism, obstetric
 amniotic fluid (pulmonary) — *see also*
  Embolism, obstetric
  following
   abortion — *see* Abortion by type
    complicated by embolism
   ectopic pregnancy O08.2
   molar pregnancy O08.2
 aorta, aortic I74.10
  abdominal I74.09
   saddle I74.01
  bifurcation I74.09
  saddle I74.01
  thoracic I74.11
 artery I74.9
  auditory, internal I65.8
  basilar — *see* Occlusion, artery, basilar
  carotid (common) (internal) — *see* Occlusion,
   artery, carotid
  cerebellar (anterior inferior) (posterior
   inferior) (superior) I66.3
  cerebral — *see* Occlusion, artery, cerebral
  choroidal (anterior) I66.8
  communicating posterior I66.8
  coronary — *see also* Infarct, myocardium
   not resulting in infarction I24.0
  extremity I74.4
   lower I74.3
   upper I74.2
  hypophyseal I66.8
  iliac I74.5
  limb I74.4
   lower I74.3
   upper I74.2
  mesenteric (with gangrene) (*see also*
   Ischemia, intestine, acute) K55.059
  ophthalmic — *see* Occlusion, artery, retina
  peripheral I74.4
  pontine I66.8
  precerebral — *see* Occlusion, artery,
   precerebral
  pulmonary — *see* Embolism, pulmonary

Embolism (multiple) (paradoxical) I74.9 —
 continued
 artery I74.9 — *continued*
  renal N28.0
  retinal — *see* Occlusion, artery, retina
  septic I76
  specified NEC I74.8
  vertebral — *see* Occlusion, artery, vertebral
 basilar (artery) I65.1
 blood clot
  following
   abortion — *see* Abortion by type
    complicated by embolism
   ectopic or molar pregnancy O08.2
   in pregnancy, childbirth or puerperium —
    see Embolism, obstetric
 brain — *see also* Occlusion, artery, cerebral
  following
   abortion — *see* Abortion by type
    complicated by embolism
   ectopic or molar pregnancy O08.2
   puerperal, postpartum, childbirth — *see*
    Embolism, obstetric
 capillary I78.8
 cardiac — *see also* Infarct, myocardium
  not resulting in infarction I51.3
 carotid (artery) (common) (internal) — *see*
  Occlusion, artery, carotid
 cavernous sinus (venous) — *see* Embolism,
  intracranial venous sinus
 cerebral — *see* Occlusion, artery, cerebral
 cholesterol — *see* Atheroembolism
 coronary (artery or vein) (systemic) — *see*
  Occlusion, coronary
 due to device, implant or graft — *see also*
  Complications, by site and type, specified
  NEC
  arterial graft NEC T82.818
  breast (implant) T85.818
  catheter NEC T85.818
   dialysis (renal) T82.818
    intraperitoneal T85.818
   infusion NEC T82.818
    spinal (epidural) (subdural) T85.810
   urinary (indwelling) T83.81
  electronic (electrode) (pulse generator)
   (stimulator)
   bone T84.81
   cardiac T82.817
   nervous system (brain) (peripheral nerve)
    (spinal) T85.810
   urinary T83.81
  fixation, internal (orthopedic) NEC T84.81
  gastrointestinal (bile duct) (esophagus)
   T85.818
  genital NEC T83.81
  heart (graft) (valve) T82.817
  joint prosthesis T84.81
  ocular (corneal graft) (orbital implant)
   T85.818
  orthopedic (bone graft) NEC T86.838
  specified NEC T85.818
  urinary (graft) NEC T83.81
  vascular NEC T82.818
  ventricular intracranial shunt T85.810
 extremities
  lower — *see* Embolism, vein, lower extremity
   arterial I74.3
  upper I74.2
 eye H34.9
 fat (cerebral) (pulmonary) (systemic) T79.1
  complicating delivery — *see* Embolism,
   obstetric
  following
   abortion — *see* Abortion by type
    complicated by embolism
   ectopic or molar pregnancy O08.2

Embolism (multiple) (paradoxical) I74.9 —
 continued
 following
  abortion — *see* Abortion by type
   complicated by embolism
  ectopic or molar pregnancy O08.2
  infusion, therapeutic injection or transfusion
   air T80.0
 heart (fatty) — *see also* Infarct, myocardium
  not resulting in infarction I51.3
 hepatic (vein) I82.0
 in pregnancy, childbirth or puerperium — *see*
  Embolism, obstetric
 intestine (artery) (vein) (with gangrene) (with
  gangrene) (*see also* Ischemia, intestine,
  acute) K55.039
 intracranial — *see also* Occlusion, artery,
  cerebral
  venous sinus (any) G08
  nonpyogenic I67.6
 intraspinal venous sinuses or veins G08
  nonpyogenic G95.19
 kidney (artery) N28.0
 lateral sinus (venous) — *see* Embolism,
  intracranial, venous sinus
 leg — *see* Embolism, vein, lower extremity
  arterial I74.3
 longitudinal sinus (venous) — *see* Embolism,
  intracranial, venous sinus
 lung (massive) — *see* Embolism, pulmonary
 meninges I66.8
 mesenteric (artery) (vein) (with gangrene) (*see
  also* Ischemia, intestine, acute) K55.059
 obstetric (in) (pulmonary)
  childbirth O88.22
   air O88.02
   amniotic fluid O88.12
   blood clot O88.22
   fat O88.82
   pyemic O88.32
   septic O88.32
   specified type NEC O88.82
  pregnancy O88.21-
   air O88.01-
   amniotic fluid O88.11-
   blood clot O88.21-
   fat O88.81-
   pyemic O88.31-
   septic O88.31-
   specified type NEC O88.81-
  puerperal O88.23
   air O88.03
   amniotic fluid O88.13
   blood clot O88.23
   fat O88.83
   pyemic O88.33
   septic O88.33
   specified type NEC O88.83
 ophthalmic — *see* Occlusion, artery, retina
 penis N48.81
 peripheral artery NOS I74.4
 pituitary E23.6
 popliteal (artery) I74.3
 portal (vein) I81
 postoperative, postrprocedural
  artery T81.719
   mesenteric T81.710
   renal T81.711
   specified NEC T81.718
  vein T81.72
 precerebral artery — *see* Occlusion, artery,
  precerebral
 puerperal — *see* Embolism, obstetric

Embolism (multiple) (paradoxical) I74.9 — *continued*
  pulmonary (acute) (artery) (vein) I26.99
    with acute cor pulmonale I26.09
    chronic I27.82
    following
      abortion — *see* Abortion by type complicated by embolism
      ectopic or molar pregnancy O08.2
    healed or old Z86.711
    in pregnancy, childbirth or puerperium — *see* Embolism, obstetric
    personal history of Z86.711
    saddle I26.92
      with acute cor pulmonale I26.02
    septic I26.90
      with acute cor pulmonale I26.01
  pyemic (multiple) I76
    following
      abortion — *see* Abortion by type complicated by embolism
      ectopic or molar pregnancy O08.2
    Hemophilus influenzae A41.3
    pneumococcal A40.3
      with pneumonia J13
    puerperal, postpartum, childbirth (any organism) — *see* Embolism, obstetric
    specified organism NEC A41.89
    staphylococcal A41.2
    streptococcal A40.9
  renal (artery) N28.0
    vein I82.3
  retina, retinal — *see* Occlusion, artery, retina
  saddle
    abdominal aorta I74.01
    pulmonary artery I26.92
      with acute cor pulmonale I26.02
  septic (arterial) I76
    complicating abortion — *see* Abortion, by type, complicated by, embolism
  sinus — *see* Embolism, intracranial, venous sinus
  soap complicating abortion — *see* Abortion, by type, complicated by, embolism
  spinal cord G95.19
    pyogenic origin G06.1
  spleen, splenic (artery) I74.8
  upper extremity I74.2
  vein (acute) I82.90
    antecubital I82.61-
      chronic I82.71-
    axillary I82.A1-
      chronic I82.A2-
    basilic I82.61-
      chronic I82.71-
    brachial I82.62-
      chronic I82.72-
    brachiocephalic (innominate) I82.290
      chronic I82.291
    cephalic I82.61-
      chronic I82.71-
    chronic I82.91
    deep (DVT) I82.40-
      calf I82.4Z-
        chronic I82.5Z-
      lower leg I82.4Z-
        chronic I82.5Z-
      thigh I82.4Y-
        chronic I82.5Y-
      upper leg I82.4Y
        chronic I82.5Y-
    femoral I82.41-
      chronic I82.51-
    iliac (iliofemoral) I82.42-
      chronic I82.52-
    innominate I82.290
      chronic I82.291
    internal jugular I82.C1-
      chronic I82.C2-

Embolism (multiple) (paradoxical) I74.9 — *continued*
  vein (acute) I82.90 — *continued*
    lower extremity
      deep I82.40-
        chronic I82.50-
        specified NEC I82.49-
          chronic NEC I82.59-
      distal
        deep I82.4Z-
      proximal
        deep I82.4Y-
          chronic I82.5Y-
      superficial I82.81-
    popliteal I82.43-
      chronic I82.53-
    radial I82.62-
      chronic I82.72-
    renal I82.3
    saphenous (greater) (lesser) I82.81-
    specified NEC I82.890
      chronic NEC I82.891
    subclavian I82.B1-
      chronic I82.B2-
    thoracic NEC I82.290
      chronic I82.291
    tibial I82.44-
      chronic I82.54-
    ulnar I82.62-
      chronic I82.72-
    upper extremity I82.60-
      chronic I82.70-
      deep I82.62-
        chronic I82.72-
      superficial I82.61-
        chronic I82.71-
    vena cava
      inferior (acute) I82.220
        chronic I82.221
      superior (acute) I82.210
        chronic I82.211
    venous sinus G08
    vessels of brain — *see* Occlusion, artery, cerebral
Embolus — *see* Embolism
Embryoma — *see also* Neoplasm, uncertain behavior, by site
  benign — *see* Neoplasm, benign, by site
  kidney C64-
  liver C22.0
  malignant — *see also* Neoplasm, malignant, by site
    kidney C64-
    liver C22.0
    testis C62.9-
      descended (scrotal) C62.1-
      undescended C62.0-
  testis C62.9-
    descended (scrotal) C62.1-
    undescended C62.0-
Embryonic
  circulation Q28.9
  heart Q28.9
  vas deferens Q55.4
Embryopathia NOS Q89.9
Embryotoxon Q13.4
Emesis — *see* Vomiting
Emotional lability R45.86
Emotionality, pathological F60.3
Emotogenic disease — *see* Disorder, psychogenic
Emphysema (atrophic) (bullous) (chronic) (interlobular) (lung) (obstructive) (pulmonary) (senile) (vesicular) J43.9
  cellular tissue (traumatic) T79.7
    surgical T81.82
  centrilobular J43.2
  compensatory J98.3
  congenital (interstitial) P25.0

Emphysema (atrophic) (bullous) (chronic) (interlobular) (lung) (obstructive) (pulmonary) (senile) (vesicular) J43.9 — *continued*
  conjunctiva H11.89
  connective tissue (traumatic) T79.7
    surgical T81.82
  due to chemicals, gases, fumes or vapors J68.4
  eyelid(s) — *see* Disorder, eyelid, specified type NEC
    surgical T81.82
    traumatic T79.7
  interstitial J98.2
    congenital P25.0
    perinatal period P25.0
  laminated tissue T79.7
    surgical T81.82
  mediastinal J98.2
    newborn P25.2
  orbit, orbital — *see* Disorder, orbit, specified type NEC
  panacinar J43.1
  panlobular J43.1
  specified NEC J43.8
  subcutaneous (traumatic) T79.7
    nontraumatic J98.2
    postprocedural T81.82
    surgical T81.82
  surgical T81.82
  thymus (gland) (congenital) E32.8
  traumatic (subcutaneous) T79.7
  unilateral J43.0
Empty nest syndrome Z60.0
Empyema (acute) (chest) (double) (pleura) (supradiaphragmatic) (thorax) J86.9
  with fistula J86.0
  accessory sinus (chronic) — *see* Sinusitis
  antrum (chronic) — *see* Sinusitis, maxillary
  brain (any part) — *see* Abscess, brain
  ethmoidal (chronic) (sinus) — *see* Sinusitis, ethmoidal
  extradural — *see* Abscess, extradural
  frontal (chronic) (sinus) — *see* Sinusitis, frontal
  gallbladder K81.0
  mastoid (process) (acute) — *see* Mastoiditis, acute
  maxilla, maxillary M27.2
    sinus (chronic) — *see* Sinusitis, maxillary
  nasal sinus (chronic) — *see* Sinusitis
  sinus (accessory) (chronic) (nasal) — *see* Sinusitis
  sphenoidal (sinus) (chronic) — *see* Sinusitis, sphenoidal
  subarachnoid — *see* Abscess, extradural
  subdural — *see* Abscess, subdural
  tuberculous A15.6
  ureter — *see* Ureteritis
  ventricular — *see* Abscess, brain
En coup de sabre lesion L94.1
Enamel pearls K00.2
Enameloma K00.2
Enanthema, viral B09
Encephalitis (chronic) (hemorrhagic) (idiopathic) (nonepidemic) (spurious) (subacute) G04.90
  acute (*see also* Encephalitis, viral) A86
    disseminated G04.00
      infectious G04.01
      noninfectious G04.81
      postimmunization (postvaccination) G04.02
      postinfectious G04.01
    inclusion body A85.8
    necrotizing hemorrhagic G04.30
      postimmunization G04.32
      postinfectious G04.31
      specified NEC G04.39
  arboviral, arbovirus NEC A85.2
  arthropod-borne NEC (viral) A85.2

Encephalitis (chronic) (hemorrhagic)
(idiopathic) (nonepidemic) (spurious)
(subacute) G04.90 — *continued*
- Australian A83.4
- California (virus) A83.5
- Central European (tick-borne) A84.1
- Czechoslovakian A84.1
- Dawson's (inclusion body) A81.1
- diffuse sclerosing A81.1
- disseminated, acute G04.00
- due to
  - cat scratch disease A28.1
  - human immunodeficiency virus (HIV) disease B20 [G05.3]
  - malaria — *see* Malaria
  - rickettsiosis — *see* Rickettsiosis
  - smallpox inoculation G04.02
  - typhus — *see* Typhus
- Eastern equine A83.2
- endemic (viral) A86
- epidemic NEC (viral) A86
- equine (acute) (infectious) (viral) A83.9
  - Eastern A83.2
  - Venezuelan A92.2
  - Western A83.1
- Far Eastern (tick-borne) A84.0
- following vaccination or other immunization procedure G04.02
- herpes zoster B02.0
- herpesviral B00.4
  - due to herpesvirus 6 B10.01
  - due to herpesvirus 7 B10.09
  - specified NEC B10.09
- Ilheus (virus) A83.8
- in (due to)
  - actinomycosis A42.82
  - adenovirus A85.1
  - African trypanosomiasis B56.9 [G05.3]
  - Chagas' disease (chronic) B57.42
  - cytomegalovirus B25.8
  - enterovirus A85.0
  - herpes (simplex) virus B00.4
    - due to herpesvirus 6 B10.01
    - due to herpesvirus 7 B10.09
    - specified NEC B10.09
  - infectious disease NEC B99 [G05.3]
  - influenza — *see* Influenza, with, encephalopathy
  - listeriosis A32.12
  - measles B05.0
  - mumps B26.2
  - naegleriasis B60.2
  - parasitic disease NEC B89 [G05.3]
  - poliovirus A80.9 [G05.3]
  - rubella B06.01
  - syphilis
    - congenital A50.42
    - late A52.14
  - systemic lupus erythematosus M32.19
  - toxoplasmosis (acquired) B58.2
    - congenital P37.1
  - tuberculosis A17.82
  - zoster B02.0
- inclusion body A81.1
- infectious (acute) (virus) NEC A86
- Japanese (B type) A83.0
- La Crosse A83.5
- lead — *see* Poisoning, lead
- lethargica (acute) (infectious) A85.8
- louping ill A84.8
- lupus erythematosus, systemic M32.19
- lymphatica A87.2
- Mengo A85.8
- meningococcal A39.81
- Murray Valley A83.4
- otitic NEC H66.40 [G05.3]
- parasitic NOS B71.9
- periaxial G37.0
- periaxialis (concentrica) (diffuse) G37.5

Encephalitis (chronic) (hemorrhagic)
(idiopathic) (nonepidemic) (spurious)
(subacute) G04.90 — *continued*
- postchickenpox B01.11
- postexanthematous NEC B09
- postimmunization G04.02
- postinfectious NEC G04.01
- postmeasles B05.0
- postvaccinal G04.02
- postvaricella B01.11
- postviral NEC A86
- Powassan A84.8
- Rasmussen G04.81
- Rio Bravo A85.8
- Russian
  - autumnal A83.0
  - spring-summer (taiga) A84.0
- saturnine — *see* Poisoning, lead
- specified NEC G04.81
- St. Louis A83.3
- subacute sclerosing A81.1
- summer A83.0
- suppurative G04.81
- tick-borne A84.9
- Torula, torular (cryptococcal) B45.1
- toxic NEC G92
- trichinosis B75 [G05.3]
- type
  - B A83.0
  - C A83.3
- van Bogaert's A81.1
- Venezuelan equine A92.2
- Vienna A85.8
- viral, virus A86
  - arthropod-borne NEC A85.2
    - mosquito-borne A83.9
      - Australian X disease A83.4
      - California virus A83.5
      - Eastern equine A83.2
      - Japanese (B type) A83.0
      - Murray Valley A83.4
      - specified NEC A83.8
      - St. Louis A83.3
      - type B A83.0
      - type C A83.3
      - Western equine A83.1
    - tick-borne A84.9
      - biundulant A84.1
      - central European A84.1
      - Czechoslovakian A84.1
      - diphasic meningoencephalitis A84.1
      - Far Eastern A84.0
      - Russian spring-summer (taiga) A84.0
      - specified NEC A84.8
    - specified type NEC A85.8
  - Western equine A83.1

Encephalocele Q01.9
- frontal Q01.0
- nasofrontal Q01.1
- occipital Q01.2
- specified NEC Q01.8

Encephalocystocele — *see* Encephalocele
Encephaloduroarteriomyosynangiosis (EDAMS) I67.5
Encephalomalacia (brain) (cerebellar) (cerebral) — *see* Softening, brain
Encephalomeningitis — *see* Meningoencephalitis
Encephalomeningocele — *see* Encephalocele
Encephalomeningomyelitis — *see* Meningoencephalitis
Encephalomyelitis (*see also* Encephalitis) G04.90
- acute disseminated G04.00
  - infectious G04.01
  - noninfectious G04.81
  - postimmunization G04.02
  - postinfectious G04.01

Encephalomyelitis (*see also* Encephalitis) G04.90 — *continued*
- acute necrotizing hemorrhagic G04.30
  - postimmunization G04.32
  - postinfectious G04.31
  - specified NEC G04.39
- benign myalgic G93.3
- equine A83.9
  - Eastern A83.2
  - Venezuelan A92.2
  - Western A83.1
- in diseases classified elsewhere G05.3
- myalgic, benign G93.3
- postchickenpox B01.11
- postinfectious NEC G04.01
- postmeasles B05.0
- postvaccinal G04.02
- postvaricella B01.11
- rubella B06.01
- specified NEC G04.81
- Venezuelan equine A92.2

Encephalomyelocele — *see* Encephalocele
Encephalomyelomeningitis — *see* Meningoencephalitis
Encephalomyelopathy G96.9
Encephalomyeloradiculitis (acute) G61.0
Encephalomyeloradiculoneuritis (acute) (Guillain-Barré) G61.0
Encephalomyeloradiculopathy G96.9
Encephalopathia hyperbilirubinemica, newborn P57.9
- due to isoimmunization (conditions in P55) P57.0
Encephalopathy (acute) G93.40
- acute necrotizing hemorrhagic G04.30
  - postimmunization G04.32
  - postinfectious G04.31
  - specified NEC G04.39
- alcoholic G31.2
- anoxic — *see* Damage, brain, anoxic
- arteriosclerotic I67.2
- centrolobar progressive (Schilder) G37.0
- congenital Q07.9
- degenerative, in specified disease NEC G32.89
- demyelinating callosal G37.1
- due to
  - drugs (*see also* Table of drugs and chemicals) G92
- hepatic — *see* Failure, hepatic
- hyperbilirubinemic, newborn P57.9
  - due to isoimmunization (conditions in P55) P57.0
- hypertensive I67.4
- hypoglycemic E16.2
- hypoxic — *see* Damage, brain, anoxic
- hypoxic ischemic P91.60
  - mild P91.61
  - moderate P91.62
  - severe P91.63
- in (due to) (with)
  - birth injury P11.1
  - hyperinsulinism E16.1 [G94]
  - influenza — *see* Influenza, with, encephalopathy
  - lack of vitamin (*see also* Deficiency, vitamin) E56.9 [G32.89]
  - neoplastic disease (*see also* Neoplasm) D49.9 [G13.1]
  - serum (*see also* Reaction, serum) T80.69
  - syphilis A52.17
  - trauma (postconcussional) F07.81
    - current injury — *see* Injury, intracranial
  - vaccination G04.02
- lead — *see* Poisoning, lead
- metabolic G93.41
  - drug-induced G92
  - toxic G92

Encephalopathy (acute) G93.40 —
continued
   myoclonic, early, symptomatic — see Epilepsy,
      generalized, specified NEC
   necrotizing, subacute (Leigh) G31.82
   pellagrous E52 *[G32.89]*
   portosystemic — see Failure, hepatic
   postcontusional F07.81
      current injury — see Injury, intracranial,
         diffuse
   posthypoglycemic (coma) E16.1 *[G94]*
   postradiation G93.89
   saturnine — see Poisoning, lead
   septic G93.41
   specified NEC G93.49
   spongiform, subacute (viral) A81.09
   toxic G92
      metabolic G92
   traumatic (postconcussional) F07.81
      current injury — see Injury, intracranial
   vitamin B deficiency NEC E53.9 *[G32.89]*
      vitamin B1 E51.2
      Wernicke's E51.2
Encephalorrhagia — see Hemorrhage,
   intracranial, intracerebral
Encephalosis, posttraumatic F07.81
Enchondroma — see also Neoplasm, bone,
   benign
Enchondromatosis (cartilaginous) (multiple)
   Q78.4
Encopresis R15.9
   functional F98.1
   nonorganic origin F98.1
   psychogenic F98.1
Encounter (with health service) (for) Z76.89
   adjustment and management (of)
      breast implant Z45.81
      implanted device NEC Z45.89
      myringotomy device (stent) (tube) Z45.82
   administrative purpose only Z02.9
      examination for
         adoption Z02.82
         armed forces Z02.3
         disability determination Z02.71
         driving license Z02.4
         employment Z02.1
         insurance Z02.6
         medical certificate NEC Z02.79
         paternity testing Z02.81
         residential institution admission Z02.2
         school admission Z02.0
         sports Z02.5
         specified reason NEC Z02.89
   aftercare — see Aftercare
   antenatal screening Z36
   assisted reproductive fertility procedure cycle
      Z31.83
   blood typing Z01.83
      Rh typing Z01.83
   breast augmentation or reduction Z41.1
   breast implant exchange (different material)
      (different size) Z45.81
   breast reconstruction following mastectomy
      Z42.1
   check-up — see Examination
   chemotherapy for neoplasm Z51.11
   colonoscopy, screening Z12.11
   counseling — see Counseling
   delivery, full-term, uncomplicated O80
      cesarean, without indication O82
   desensitization to allergens Z51.6
   ear piercing Z41.3
   examination — see Examination
   expectant parent(s) (adoptive) pre-birth
      pediatrician visit Z76.81
   fertility preservation procedure (prior to cancer
      therapy) (prior to removal of gonads)
      Z31.84
   fitting (of) — see Fitting (and adjustment) (of)

Encounter (with health service) (for) Z76.89 —
continued
   genetic
      counseling Z31.5
      testing — see Test, genetic
   hearing conservation and treatment Z01.12
   immunotherapy for neoplasm Z51.12
   in vitro fertilization cycle Z31.83
   instruction (in)
      child care (postpartal) (prenatal) Z32.3
      childbirth Z32.2
      natural family planning
         procreative Z31.61
         to avoid pregnancy Z30.02
   insulin pump titration Z46.81
   joint prosthesis insertion following prior
      explantation of joint prosthesis (staged
      procedure)
      hip Z47.32
      knee Z47.33
      shoulder Z47.31
   laboratory (as part of a general medical
      examination) Z00.00
      with abnormal findings Z00.01
   mental health services (for)
      abuse NEC
         perpetrator Z69.82
         victim Z69.81
      child abuse
         nonparental
            perpetrator Z69.021
            victim Z69.020
         parental
            perpetrator Z69.011
            victim Z69.010
      spousal or partner abuse
         perpetrator Z69.12
         victim Z69.11
   observation (for) (ruled out)
      exposure to (suspected)
         anthrax Z03.810
         biological agent NEC Z03.818
   pediatrician visit, by expectant parent(s)
      (adoptive) Z76.81
   plastic and reconstructive surgery following
      medical procedure or healed injury NEC
      Z42.8
   pregnancy
      supervision of — see Pregnancy, supervision
         of
      test Z32.00
         result negative Z32.02
         result positive Z32.01
   procreative management and counseling for
      gestational carrier Z31.7
   prophylactic measures Z29.9
      antivenin Z29.12
      fluoride administration Z29.3
      immunotherapy for respiratory syncytial
         virus (RSV) Z29.11
      rabies immune globin Z29.14
      Rho (D) immune globulin Z29.13
      specified NEC Z29.8
   radiation therapy (antineoplastic) Z51.0
   radiological (as part of a general medical
      examination) Z00.00
      with abnormal findings Z00.01
   reconstructive surgery following medical
      procedure or healed injury NEC Z42.8
   removal (of) — see also Removal
      artificial
         arm Z44.00-
            complete Z44.01-
            partial Z44.02-
         eye Z44.2-
         leg Z44.10-
            complete Z44.11-
            partial Z44.12-

Encounter (with health service) (for) Z76.89 —
continued
   removal (of) — see also Removal — continued
      breast implant Z45.81
         tissue expander (without synchronous
            insertion of permanent implant)
            Z45.81
      device Z46.9
         specified NEC Z46.89
      external
         fixation device — code to fracture with
            seventh character D
         prosthesis, prosthetic device Z44.9
            breast Z44.3-
            specified NEC Z44.8
      implanted device NEC Z45.89
      insulin pump Z46.81
      internal fixation device Z47.2
      myringotomy device (stent) (tube) Z45.82
      nervous system device NEC Z46.2
         brain neuropacemaker Z46.2
         visual substitution device Z46.2
            implanted Z45.31
      non-vascular catheter Z46.82
      orthodontic device Z46.4
      stent
         ureteral Z46.6
      urinary device Z46.6
   repeat cervical smear to confirm findings of
      recent normal smear following initial
      abnormal smear Z01.42
   respirator [ventilator] use during power failure
      Z99.12
   Rh typing Z01.83
   screening — see Screening
   specified NEC Z76.89
   sterilization Z30.2
   suspected condition, ruled out
      amniotic cavity and membrane Z03.71
      cervical shortening Z03.75
      fetal anomaly Z03.73
      fetal growth Z03.74
      maternal and fetal conditions NEC Z03.79
      oligohydramnios Z03.71
      placental problem Z03.72
      polyhydramnios Z03.71
   suspected exposure (to), ruled out
      anthrax Z03.810
      biological agents NEC Z03.818
   termination of pregnancy, elective Z33.2
   testing — see Test
   therapeutic drug level monitoring Z51.81
   titration, insulin pump Z46.81
   to determine fetal viability of pregnancy
      O36.80
   training
      insulin pump Z46.81
   X-ray of chest (as part of a general medical
      examination) Z00.00
      with abnormal findings Z00.01
Encystment — see Cyst
Endarteritis (bacterial, subacute) (infective)
   I77.6
   brain I67.7
   cerebral or cerebrospinal I67.7
   deformans — see Arteriosclerosis
   embolic — see Embolism
   obliterans — see also Arteriosclerosis
      pulmonary I28.8
   pulmonary I28.8
   retina — see Vasculitis, retina
   senile — see Arteriosclerosis
   syphilitic A52.09
      brain or cerebral A52.04
      congenital A50.54 *[I79.8]*
   tuberculous A18.89
Endemic — see condition

Endocarditis (chronic) (marantic) (nonbacterial) (thrombotic) (valvular) I38
  with rheumatic fever (conditions in I00)
    active — *see* Endocarditis, acute, rheumatic
    inactive or quiescent (with chorea) I09.1
  acute or subacute I33.9
    infective I33.0
    rheumatic (aortic) (mitral) (pulmonary) (tricuspid) I01.1
      with chorea (acute) (rheumatic) (Sydenham's) I02.0
  aortic (heart) (nonrheumatic) (valve) I35.8
    with
      mitral disease I08.0
        with tricuspid (valve) disease I08.3
          active or acute I01.1
            with chorea (acute) (rheumatic) (Sydenham's) I02.0
        rheumatic fever (conditions in I00)
          active — *see* Endocarditis, acute, rheumatic
          inactive or quiescent (with chorea) I06.9
      tricuspid (valve) disease I08.2
        with mitral (valve) disease I08.3
    acute or subacute I33.9
    arteriosclerotic I35.8
    rheumatic I06.9
      with mitral disease I08.0
        with tricuspid (valve) disease I08.3
          active or acute I01.1
            with chorea (acute) (rheumatic) (Sydenham's) I02.0
        active or acute I01.1
          with chorea (acute) (rheumatic) (Sydenham's) I02.0
      specified NEC I06.8
    specified cause NEC I35.8
    syphilitic A52.03
  arteriosclerotic I38
  atypical verrucous (Libman-Sacks) M32.11
  bacterial (acute) (any valve) (subacute) I33.0
  candidal B37.6
  congenital Q24.8
  constrictive I33.0
  Coxiella burnetii A78 [I39]
  Coxsackie B33.21
  due to
    prosthetic cardiac valve T82.6
    Q fever A78 [I39]
    Serratia marcescens I33.0
    typhoid (fever) A01.02
  gonococcal A54.83
  infectious or infective (acute) (any valve) (subacute) I33.0
  lenta (acute) (any valve) (subacute) I33.0
  Libman-Sacks M32.11
  listerial A32.82
  Löffler's I42.3
  malignant (acute) (any valve) (subacute) I33.0
  meningococcal A39.51
  mitral (chronic) (double) (fibroid) (heart) (inactive) (valve) (with chorea) I05.9
    with
      aortic (valve) disease I08.0
        with tricuspid (valve) disease I08.3
          active or acute I01.1
            with chorea (acute) (rheumatic) (Sydenham's) I02.0
        rheumatic fever (conditions in I00)
          active — *see* Endocarditis, acute, rheumatic
          inactive or quiescent (with chorea) I05.9
      tricuspid (valve) disease I08.1
        with aortic (valve) disease I08.3
    active or acute I01.1
      with chorea (acute) (rheumatic) (Sydenham's) I02.0
    bacterial I33.0

Endocarditis (chronic) (marantic) (nonbacterial) (thrombotic) (valvular) I38 — *continued*
  mitral (chronic) (double) (fibroid) (heart) (inactive) (valve) (with chorea) I05.9 — *continued*
    arteriosclerotic I34.8
    nonrheumatic I34.8
      acute or subacute I33.9
    specified NEC I05.8
  monilial B37.6
  multiple valves I08.9
    specified disorders I08.8
  mycotic (acute) (any valve) (subacute) I33.0
  pneumococcal (acute) (any valve) (subacute) I33.0
  pulmonary (chronic) (heart) (valve) I37.8
    with rheumatic fever (conditions in I00)
      active — *see* Endocarditis, acute, rheumatic
      inactive or quiescent (with chorea) I09.89
        with aortic, mitral or tricuspid disease I08.8
    acute or subacute I33.9
      rheumatic I01.1
        with chorea (acute) (rheumatic) (Sydenham's) I02.0
    arteriosclerotic I37.8
    congenital Q22.2
    rheumatic (chronic) (inactive) (with chorea) I09.89
      active or acute I01.1
        with chorea (acute) (rheumatic) (Sydenham's) I02.0
    syphilitic A52.03
  purulent (acute) (any valve) (subacute) I33.0
  Q fever A78 [I39]
  rheumatic (chronic) (inactive) (with chorea) I09.1
    active or acute (aortic) (mitral) (pulmonary) (tricuspid) I01.1
      with chorea (acute) (rheumatic) (Sydenham's) I02.0
  rheumatoid — *see* Rheumatoid, carditis
  septic (acute) (any valve) (subacute) I33.0
  streptococcal (acute) (any valve) (subacute) I33.0
  subacute — *see* Endocarditis, acute
  suppurative (acute) (any valve) (subacute) I33.0
  syphilitic A52.03
  toxic I33.9
  tricuspid (chronic) (heart) (inactive) (rheumatic) (valve) (with chorea) I07.9
    with
      aortic (valve) disease I08.2
        mitral (valve) disease I08.3
      mitral (valve) disease I08.1
        aortic (valve) disease I08.3
      rheumatic fever (conditions in I00)
        active — *see* Endocarditis, acute, rheumatic
        inactive or quiescent (with chorea) I07.8
    active or acute I01.1
      with chorea (acute) (rheumatic) (Sydenham's) I02.0
    arteriosclerotic I36.8
    nonrheumatic I36.8
      acute or subacute I33.9
    specified cause, except rheumatic I36.8
  tuberculous — *see* Tuberculosis, endocarditis
  typhoid A01.02
  ulcerative (acute) (any valve) (subacute) I33.0
  vegetative (acute) (any valve) (subacute) I33.0
  verrucous (atypical) (nonbacterial) (nonrheumatic) M32.11
Endocardium, endocardial — *see also* condition
  cushion defect Q21.2

Endocervicitis — *see also* Cervicitis
  due to intrauterine (contraceptive) device T83.69
  hyperplastic N72
Endocrine — *see* condition
Endocrinopathy, pluriglandular E31.9
Endodontic
  overfill M27.52
  underfill M27.53
Endodontitis K04.01
  irreversible K04.02
  reversible K04.01
Endomastoiditis — *see* Mastoiditis
Endometrioma N80.9
Endometriosis N80.9
  appendix N80.5
  bladder N80.8
  bowel N80.5
  broad ligament N80.3
  cervix N80.0
  colon N80.5
  cul-de-sac (Douglas') N80.3
  exocervix N80.0
  fallopian tube N80.2
  female genital organ NEC N80.8
  gallbladder N80.8
  in scar of skin N80.6
  internal N80.0
  intestine N80.5
  lung N80.8
  myometrium N80.0
  ovary N80.1
  parametrium N80.3
  pelvic peritoneum N80.3
  peritoneal (pelvic) N80.3
  rectovaginal septum N80.4
  rectum N80.5
  round ligament N80.3
  skin (scar) N80.6
  specified site NEC N80.8
  stromal D39.0
  umbilicus N80.8
  uterus (internal) N80.0
  vagina N80.4
  vulva N80.8
Endometritis (decidual) (nonspecific) (purulent) (senile) (atrophic) (suppurative) N71.9
  with ectopic pregnancy O08.0
  acute N71.0
  blenorrhagic (gonococcal) (acute) (chronic) A54.24
  cervix, cervical (with erosion or ectropion) — *see also* Cervicitis
    hyperplastic N72
  chlamydial A56.11
  chronic N71.1
  following
    abortion — *see* Abortion by type complicated by genital infection
    ectopic or molar pregnancy O08.0
  gonococcal, gonorrheal (acute) (chronic) A54.24
  hyperplastic (*see also* Hyperplasia, endometrial) N85.00-
    cervix N72
  puerperal, postpartum, childbirth O86.12
  subacute N71.0
  tuberculous A18.17
Endometrium — *see* condition
Endomyocardiopathy, South African I42.3
Endomyocarditis — *see* Endocarditis
Endomyofibrosis I42.3
Endomyometritis — *see* Endometritis
Endopericarditis — *see* Endocarditis
Endoperineuritis — *see* Disorder, nerve
Endophlebitis — *see* Phlebitis
Endophthalmia — *see* Endophthalmitis, purulent

DISEASE INDEX

Endophthalmitis (acute) (infective) (metastatic) (subacute) H44.009
  bleb associated H59.4 — *see also* Bleb, inflammed (infected), postprocedural
  gonorrheal A54.39
  in (due to)
    cysticercosis B69.1
    onchocerciasis B73.01
    toxocariasis B83.0
  panuveitis — *see* Panuveitis
  parasitic H44.12-
  purulent H44.00-
    panophthalmitis — *see* Panophthalmitis
    vitreous abscess H44.02-
  specified NEC H44.19
  sympathetic — *see* Uveitis, sympathetic
Endosalpingioma D28.2
Endosalpingiosis N94.89
Endosteitis — *see* Osteomyelitis
Endothelioma, bone — *see* Neoplasm, bone, malignant
Endotheliosis (hemorrhagic infectional) D69.8
Endotoxemia — *code to* condition
Endotrachelitis — *see* Cervicitis
Engelmann(-Camurati) syndrome Q78.3
English disease — *see* Rickets
Engman's disease L30.3
Engorgement
  breast N64.59
    newborn P83.4
    puerperal, postpartum O92.79
  lung (passive) — *see* Edema, lung
  pulmonary (passive) — *see* Edema, lung
  stomach K31.89
  venous, retina — *see* Occlusion, retina, vein, engorgement
Enlargement, enlarged — *see also* Hypertrophy
  adenoids J35.2
    with tonsils J35.3
  alveolar ridge K08.89
    congenital — *see* Anomaly, alveolar
  apertures of diaphragm (congenital) Q79.1
  gingival K06.1
  heart, cardiac — *see* Hypertrophy, cardiac
  labium majus, childhood asymmetric (CALME) N90.61
  lacrimal gland, chronic H04.03-
  liver — *see* Hypertrophy, liver
  lymph gland or node R59.9
    generalized R59.1
    localized R59.0
  orbit H05.34-
  organ or site, congenital NEC — *see* Anomaly, by site
  parathyroid (gland) E21.0
  pituitary fossa R93.0
  prostate N40.0
    with lower urinary tract symptoms (LUTS) N40.1
    without lower urinary tract symtpoms (LUTS) N40.0
  sella turcica R93.0
  spleen — *see* Splenomegaly
  thymus (gland) (congenital) E32.0
  thyroid (gland) — *see* Goiter
  tongue K14.8
  tonsils J35.1
    with adenoids J35.3
  uterus N85.2
Enophthalmos H05.40-
  due to
    orbital tissue atrophy H05.41-
    trauma or surgery H05.42-
Enostosis M27.8
Entamebic, entamebiasis — *see* Amebiasis

Entanglement
  umbilical cord(s) O69.2
    with compression O69.2
      without compression O69.82
    around neck (with compression) O69.1
      without compression O69.81
    of twins in monoamniotic sac O69.2
Enteralgia — *see* Pain, abdominal
Enteric — *see* condition
Enteritis (acute) (diarrheal) (hemorrhagic) (noninfective) K52.9
  adenovirus A08.2
  aertrycke infection A02.0
  allergic K52.29
    with
      eosinophilic gastritis or gastroenteritis K52.81
      food protein-induced enterocolitis syndrome K52.21
      food protein-induced enteropathy K52.22
  amebic (acute) A06.0
    with abscess — *see* Abscess, amebic
    chronic A06.1
      with abscess — *see* Abscess, amebic
      nondysenteric A06.2
    nondysenteric A06.2
  astrovirus A08.32
  bacillary NOS A03.9
  bacterial A04.9
    specified NEC A04.8
  calicivirus A08.31
  candidal B37.82
  Chilomastix A07.8
  choleriformis A00.1
  chronic (noninfectious) K52.9
    ulcerative — *see* Colitis, ulcerative
  cicatrizing (chronic) — *see* Enteritis, regional, small intestine
  Clostridium
    botulinum (food poisoning) A05.1
    difficile A04.7
  coccidial A07.3
  coxsackie virus A08.39
  dietetic (*see also* Enteritis, allergic) K52.29
  drug-induced K52.1
  due to
    astrovirus A08.32
    calicivirus A08.31
    coxsackie virus A08.39
    drugs K52.1
    echovirus A08.39
    enterovirus NEC A08.39
    food hypersensitivity (*see also* Enteritis, allergic) K52.29
    infectious organism (bacterial) (viral) — *see* Enteritis, infectious
    torovirus A08.39
    Yersinia enterocolitica A04.6
  echovirus A08.39
  eltor A00.1
  enterovirus NEC A08.39
  eosinophilic K52.81
  epidemic (infectious) A09
  fulminant (*see also* Ischemia, intestine, acute) K55.019
  gangrenous — *see* Enteritis, infectious
  giardial A07.1
  infectious NOS A09
    due to
      adenovirus A08.2
      Aerobacter aerogenes A04.8
      Arizona (bacillus) A02.0
      bacteria NOS A04.9
        specified NEC A04.8
      Campylobacter A04.5
      Clostridium difficile A04.7
      Clostridium perfringens A04.8
      Enterobacter aerogenes A04.8
      enterovirus A08.39

Enteritis (acute) (diarrheal) (hemorrhagic) (noninfective) K52.9 — *continued*
  infectious NOS A09 — *continued*
    due to — *continued*
      Escherichia coli A04.4
        enteroaggregative A04.4
        enterohemorrhagic A04.3
        enteroinvasive A04.2
        enteropathogenic A04.0
        enterotoxigenic A04.1
        specified NEC A04.4
      specified
        bacteria NEC A04.8
        virus NEC A08.39
      Staphylococcus A04.8
      virus NEC A08.4
        specified type NEC A08.39
      Yersinia enterocolitica A04.6
      specified organism NEC A08.8
  influenzal — *see* Influenza, with, digestive manifestations
  ischemic K55.9
    acute (*see also* Ischemia, intestine, acute) K55.019
    chronic K55.1
  microsporidial A07.8
  mucomembranous, myxomembranous — *see* Syndrome, irritable bowel
  mucous — *see* Syndrome, irritable bowel
  necroticans A05.2
  necrotizing of newborn — *see* Enterocolitis, necrotizing, in newborn
  neurogenic — *see* Syndrome, irritable bowel
  newborn necrotizing — *see* Enterocolitis, necrotizing, in newborn
  noninfectious K52.9
  norovirus A08.11
  parasitic NEC B82.9
  paratyphoid (fever) — *see* Fever, paratyphoid
  protozoal A07.9
    specified NEC A07.8
  radiation K52.0
  regional (of) K50.90
    with
      complication K50.919
        abscess K50.914
        fistula K50.913
        intestinal obstruction K50.912
        rectal bleeding K50.911
        specified complication NEC K50.918
    colon — *see* Enteritis, regional, large intestine
    duodenum — *see* Enteritis, regional, small intestine
    ileum — *see* Enteritis, regional, small intestine
    jejunum — *see* Enteritis, regional, small intestine
    large bowel — *see* Enteritis, regional, large intestine
    large intestine (colon) (rectum) K50.10
      with
        complication K50.119
          abscess K50.114
          fistula K50.113
          intestinal obstruction K50.112
          rectal bleeding K50.111
          small intestine (duodenum) (ileum) (jejunum) involvement K50.80
          with
            complication K50.819
              abscess K50.814
              fistula K50.813
              intestinal obstruction K50.812
              rectal bleeding K50.811
              specified complication NEC K50.818
          specified complication NEC K50.118

Enteritis (acute) (diarrheal) (hemorrhagic) (noninfective) K52.9 — *continued*
  regional (of) K50.90 — *continued*
    rectum — *see* Enteritis, regional, large intestine
    small intestine (duodenum) (ileum) (jejunum) K50.00
      with
        complication K50.019
          abscess K50.014
          fistula K50.013
          intestinal obstruction K50.012
          large intestine (colon) (rectum) involvement K50.80
            with
              complication K50.819
                abscess K50.814
                fistula K50.813
                intestinal obstruction K50.812
                rectal bleeding K50.811
                specified complication NEC K50.818
          rectal bleeding K50.011
          specified complication NEC K50.018
  rotaviral A08.0
  Salmonella, salmonellosis (arizonae) (cholerae-suis) (enteritidis) (typhimurium) A02.0
  segmental — *see* Enteritis, regional
  septic A09
  Shigella — *see* Infection, Shigella
  small round structured NEC A08.19
  spasmodic, spastic — *see* Syndrome, irritable bowel
  staphylococcal A04.8
    due to food A05.0
  torovirus A08.39
  toxic NEC K52.1
    due to Clostridium difficile A04.7
  trichomonal A07.8
  tuberculous A18.32
  typhosa A01.00
  ulcerative (chronic) — *see* Colitis, ulcerative
  viral A08.4
    adenovirus A08.2
    enterovirus A08.39
    Rotavirus A08.0
    small round structured NEC A08.19
    specified NEC A08.39
    virus specified NEC A08.39
Enterobiasis B80
Enterobius vermicularis (infection) (infestation) B80
Enterocele — *see also* Hernia, abdomen
  pelvic, pelvis (acquired) (congenital) N81.5
  vagina, vaginal (acquired) (congenital) NEC N81.5
Enterocolitis (*see also* Enteritis) K52.9
  due to Clostridium difficile A04.7
  fulminant ischemic (*see also* Ischemia, intestine, acute) K55.059
  granulomatous — *see* Enteritis, regional
  hemorrhagic (acute) (*see also* Ischemia, intestine, acute) K55.059
    chronic K55.1
  infectious NEC A09
  ischemic K55.9
  necrotizing
    with
      perforation K55.33
      pneumatosis K55.32
        and perforation K55.33
    due to Clostridium difficile A04.7
    in newborn P77.9
      stage 1 (without pneumatosis, without perforation) P77.1
      stage 2 (with pneumatosis, without perforation) P77.2

Enterocolitis (*see also* Enteritis) K52.9 — *continued*
  necrotizing — *continued*
    in newborn P77.9 — *continued*
      stage 3 (with pneumatosis, with perforation) P77.3
    in non-newborn K55.30
      stage 1 (without pneumatosis, without perforation) K55.31
      stage 2 (with pneumatosis, without perforation) K55.32
      stage 3 (with pneumatosis, with perforation) K55.33
      without pneumatosis or perforation K55.31
  noninfectious K52.9
    newborn — *see* Enterocolitis, necrotizing, in newborn
  pseudomembranous (newborn) A04.7
  radiation K52.0
    newborn — *see* Enterocolitis, necrotizing, in newborn
  ulcerative (chronic) — *see* Pancolitis, ulcerative (chronic)
Enterogastritis — *see* Enteritis
Enteropathy K63.9
  food protein-induced enterocolitis K52.22
  gluten-sensitive K90.0
    non-celiac K90.41
  hemorrhagic, terminal (*see also* Ischemia, intestine, acute) K55.059
  protein-losing K90.49
Enteroperitonitis — *see* Peritonitis
Enteroptosis K63.4
Enterorrhagia K92.2
Enterospasm — *see also* Syndrome, irritable, bowel
  psychogenic F45.8
Enterostenosis — *see also* Obstruction, intestine K56.69
Enterostomy
  complication — *see* Complication, enterostomy
  status Z93.4
Enterovirus, as cause of disease classified elsewhere B97.10
  coxsackievirus B97.11
  echovirus B97.12
  other specified B97.19
Enthesopathy (peripheral) M77.9
  Achilles tendinitis — *see* Tendinitis, Achilles
  ankle and tarsus M77.9
    specified type NEC — *see* Enthesopathy, foot, specified type NEC
  anterior tibial syndrome M76.81-
  calcaneal spur — *see* Spur, bone, calcaneal
  elbow region M77.8
    lateral epicondylitis — *see* Epicondylitis, lateral
    medial epicondylitis — *see* Epicondylitis, medial
  foot NEC M77.9
    metatarsalgia — *see* Metatarsalgia
    specified type NEC M77.5-
  forearm M77.9
  gluteal tendinitis — *see* Tendinitis, gluteal
  hand M77.9
  hip — *see* Enthesopathy, lower limb, specified type NEC
  iliac crest spur — *see* Spur, bone, iliac crest
  iliotibial band syndrome — *see* Syndrome, iliotibial band
  knee — *see* Enthesopathy, lower limb, lower leg, specified type NEC
  lateral epicondylitis — *see* Epicondylitis, lateral
  lower limb (excluding foot) M76.9
    Achilles tendinitis — *see* Tendinitis, Achilles
    anterior tibial syndrome M76.81-
    gluteal tendinitis — *see* Tendinitis, gluteal
    iliac crest spur — *see* Spur, bone, iliac crest

Enthesopathy (peripheral) M77.9 — *continued*
  lower limb (excluding foot) M76.9 — *continued*
    iliotibial band syndrome — *see* Syndrome, iliotibial band
    patellar tendinitis — *see* Tendinitis, patellar
    pelvic region — *see* Enthesopathy, lower limb, specified type NEC
    peroneal tendinitis — *see* Tendinitis, peroneal
    posterior tibial syndrome M76.82-
    psoas tendinitis — *see* Tendinitis, psoas
    specified type NEC M76.89-
    tibial collateral bursitis — *see* Bursitis, tibial collateral
  medial epicondylitis — *see* Epicondylitis, medial
  metatarsalgia — *see* Metatarsalgia
  multiple sites M77.9
  patellar tendinitis — *see* Tendinitis, patellar
  pelvis M77.9
  periarthritis of wrist — *see* Periarthritis, wrist
  peroneal tendinitis — *see* Tendinitis, peroneal
  posterior tibial syndrome M76.82-
  psoas tendinitis — *see* Tendinitis, psoas
  shoulder M77.9
  shoulder region — *see* Lesion, shoulder
  specified site NEC M77.9
  specified type NEC M77.8
  spinal M46.00
    cervical region M46.02
    cervicothoracic region M46.03
    lumbar region M46.06
    lumbosacral region M46.07
    multiple sites M46.09
    occipito-atlanto-axial region M46.01
    sacrococcygeal region M46.08
    thoracic region M46.04
    thoracolumbar region M46.05
  tibial collateral bursitis — *see* Bursitis, tibial collateral
  upper arm M77.9
  wrist and carpus NEC M77.8
    calcaneal spur — *see* Spur, bone, calcaneal
    periarthritis of wrist — *see* Periarthritis, wrist
Entomophobia F40.218
Entomophthoromycosis B46.8
Entrance, air into vein — *see* Embolism, air
Entrapment, nerve — *see* Neuropathy, entrapment
Entropion (eyelid) (paralytic) H02.009
  cicatricial H02.019
    left H02.016
      lower H02.015
      upper H02.014
    right H02.013
      lower H02.012
      upper H02.011
  congenital Q10.2
  left H02.006
    lower H02.005
    upper H02.004
  mechanical H02.029
    left H02.026
      lower H02.025
      upper H02.024
    right H02.023
      lower H02.022
      upper H02.021
  right H02.003
    lower H02.002
    upper H02.001
  senile H02.039
    left H02.036
      lower H02.035
      upper H02.034
    right H02.033
      lower H02.032
      upper H02.031

Entropion (eyelid) (paralytic) H02.009 — *continued*
  spastic H02.049
    left H02.046
      lower H02.045
      upper H02.044
    right H02.043
      lower H02.042
      upper H02.041
Enucleated eye (traumatic, current) S05.7-
Enuresis R32
  functional F98.0
  habit disturbance F98.0
  nocturnal N39.44
    psychogenic F98.0
  nonorganic origin F98.0
  psychogenic F98.0
Eosinopenia — *see* Agranulocytosis
Eosinophilia (allergic) (hereditary) (idiopathic) (secondary) D72.1
  with
    angiolymphoid hyperplasia (ALHE) D18.01
  infiltrative J82
  Löffler's J82
  peritoneal — *see* Peritonitis, eosinophilic
  pulmonary NEC J82
  tropical (pulmonary) J82
Eosinophilia-myalgia syndrome M35.8
Ependymitis (acute) (cerebral) (chronic) (granular) — *see* Encephalomyelitis
Ependymoblastoma
  specified site — *see* Neoplasm, malignant, by site
  unspecified site C71.9
Ependymoma (epithelial) (malignant)
  anaplastic
    specified site — *see* Neoplasm, malignant, by site
    unspecified site C71.9
  benign
    specified site — *see* Neoplasm, benign, by site
    unspecified site D33.2
  myxopapillary D43.2
    specified site — *see* Neoplasm, uncertain behavior, by site
    unspecified site D43.2
  papillary D43.2
    specified site — *see* Neoplasm, uncertain behavior, by site
    unspecified site D43.2
  specified site — *see* Neoplasm, malignant, by site
  unspecified site C71.9
Ependymopathy G93.89
Ephelis, ephelides L81.2
Epiblepharon (congenital) Q10.3
Epicanthus, epicanthic fold (eyelid) (congenital) Q10.3
Epicondylitis (elbow)
  lateral M77.1-
  medial M77.0-
Epicystitis — *see* Cystitis
Epidemic — *see* condition
Epidermidalization, cervix — *see* Dysplasia, cervix
Epidermis, epidermal — *see* condition
Epidermodysplasia verruciformis B07.8
Epidermolysis
  bullosa (congenital) Q81.9
    acquired L12.30
      drug-induced L12.31
      specified cause NEC L12.35
    dystrophica Q81.2
    letalis Q81.1
    simplex Q81.0
    specified NEC Q81.8
  necroticans combustiformis L51.2

Epidermolysis — *continued*
  due to drug — *see* Table of Drugs and Chemicals, by drug
Epidermophytid — *see* Dermatophytosis
Epidermophytosis (infected) — *see* Dermatophytosis
Epididymis — *see* condition
Epididymitis (acute) (nonvenereal) (recurrent) (residual) N45.1
  with orchitis N45.3
  blennorrhagic (gonococcal) A54.23
  caseous (tuberculous) A18.15
  chlamydial A56.19
  filarial (*see also* Infestation, filarial) B74.9 [N51]
  gonococcal A54.23
  syphilitic A52.76
  tuberculous A18.15
Epididymo-orchitis (*see also* Epididymitis) N45.3
Epidural — *see* condition
Epigastrium, epigastric — *see* condition
Epigastrocele — *see* Hernia, ventral
Epiglottis — *see* condition
Epiglottitis, epiglottiditis (acute) J05.10
  with obstruction J05.11
  chronic J37.0
Epignathus Q89.4
Epilepsia partialis continua (*see also* Kozhevnikof's epilepsy) G40.1-
Epilepsy, epileptic, epilepsia (attack) (cerebral) (convulsion) (fit) (seizure) G40.909
  Note: The following terms are to be considered equivalent to intractable: pharmacoresistant (pharmacologically resistant), treatment resistant, refractory (medically) and poorly controlled
  with
    complex partial seizures — *see* Epilepsy, localization-related, symptomatic, with complex partial seizures
    grand mal seizures on awakening — *see* Epilepsy, generalized, specified NEC
    myoclonic absences — *see* Epilepsy, generalized, specified NEC
    myoclonic-astatic seizures — *see* Epilepsy, generalized, specified NEC
    simple partial seizures — *see* Epilepsy, localization-related, symptomatic, with simple partial seizures
  akinetic — *see* Epilepsy, generalized, specified NEC
  benign childhood with centrotemporal EEG spikes — *see* Epilepsy, localization-related, idiopathic
  benign myoclonic in infancy G40.80-
  Bravais-jacksonian — *see* Epilepsy, localization-related, symptomatic, with simple partial seizures
  childhood
    with occipital EEG paroxysms — *see* Epilepsy, localization-related, idiopathic
    absence G40.A09 (*follows G40.3*)
      intractable G40.A19 (*follows G40.3*)
        with status epilepticus G40.A11 (*follows G40.3*)
        without status epilepticus G40.A19 (*follows G40.3*)
      not intractable G40.A09 (*follows G40.3*)
        with status epilepticus G40.A01 (*follows G40.3*)
        without status epilepticus G40.A09 (*follows G40.3*)
  climacteric — *see* Epilepsy, specified NEC
  cysticercosis B69.0
  deterioration (mental) F06.8
  due to syphilis A52.19

Epilepsy, epileptic, epilepsia (attack) (cerebral) (convulsion) (fit) (seizure) G40.909 — *continued*
  focal — *see* Epilepsy, localization-related, symptomatic, with simple partial seizures
  generalized
    idiopathic G40.309
      intractable G40.319
        with status epilepticus G40.311
        without status epilepticus G40.319
      not intractable G40.309
        with status epilepticus G40.301
        without status epilepticus G40.309
    specified NEC G40.409
      intractable G40.419
        with status epilepticus G40.411
        without status epilepticus G40.419
      not intractable G40.409
        with status epilepticus G40.401
        without status epilepticus G40.409
  impulsive petit mal — *see* Epilepsy, juvenile myoclonic
  intractable G40.919
    with status epilepticus G40.911
    without status epilepticus G40.919
  juvenile absence G40.A09 (*follows G40.3*)
    intractable G40.A19 (*follows G40.3*)
      with status epilepticus G40.A11 (*follows G40.3*)
      without status epilepticus G40.A19 (*follows G40.3*)
    not intractable G40.A09 (*follows G40.3*)
      with status epilepticus G40.A01 (*follows G40.3*)
      without status epilepticus G40.A09 (*follows G40.3*)
  juvenile myoclonic G40.B09 (*follows G40.3*)
    intractable G40.B19 (*follows G40.3*)
      with status epilepticus G40.B11 (*follows G40.3*)
      without status epilepticus G40.B19 (*follows G40.3*)
    not intractable G40.B09 (*follows G40.3*)
      with status epilepticus G40.B01 (*follows G40.3*)
      without status epilepticus G40.B09 (*follows G40.3*)
  localization-related (focal) (partial)
    idiopathic G40.009
      with seizures of localized onset G40.009
        intractable G40.019
          with status epilepticus G40.011
          without status epilepticus G40.019
        not intractable G40.009
          with status epilepticus G40.001
          without status epilepticus G40.009
    symptomatic
      with complex partial seizures G40.209
        intractable G40.219
          with status epilepticus G40.211
          without status epilepticus G40.219
        not intractable G40.209
          with status epilepticus G40.201
          without status epilepticus G40.209
      with simple partial seizures G40.109
        intractable G40.119
          with status epilepticus G40.111
          without status epilepticus G40.119
        not intractable G40.109
          with status epilepticus G40.101
          without status epilepticus G40.109
  myoclonus, myoclonic — *see* Epilepsy, generalized, specified NEC
  progressive — *see* Epilepsy, generalized, idiopathic
  not intractable G40.909
    with status epilepticus G40.901
    without status epilepticus G40.909

Epilepsy, epileptic, epilepsia (attack) (cerebral) (convulsion) (fit) (seizure) G40.909 — *continued*
  on awakening — *see* Epilepsy, generalized, specified NEC
  parasitic NOS B71.9 *[G94]*
  partialis continua (*see also* Kozhevnikof's epilepsy) G40.1-
  peripheral — *see* Epilepsy, specified NEC
  procursiva — *see* Epilepsy, localization-related, symptomatic, with simple partial seizures
  progressive (familial) myoclonic — *see* Epilepsy, generalized, idiopathic
  reflex — *see* Epilepsy, specified NEC
  related to
    alcohol G40.509
      not intractable G40.509
        with status epilepticus G40.501
        without status epilepticus G40.509
    drugs G40.509
      not intractable G40.509
        with status epilepticus G40.501
        without status epilepticus G40.509
    external causes G40.509
      not intractable G40.509
        with status epilepticus G40.501
        without status epilepticus G40.509
    hormonal changes G40.509
      not intractable G40.509
        with status epilepticus G40.501
        without status epilepticus G40.509
    sleep deprivation G40.509
      not intractable G40.509
        with status epilepticus G40.501
        without status epilepticus G40.509
    stress G40.509
      not intractable G40.509
        with status epilepticus G40.501
        without status epilepticus G40.509
  somatomotor — *see* Epilepsy, localization-related, symptomatic, with simple partial seizures
  somatosensory — *see* Epilepsy, localization-related, symptomatic, with simple partial seizures
  spasms G40.822
    intractable G40.824
      with status epilepticus G40.823
      without status epilepticus G40.824
    not intractable G40.822
      with status epilepticus G40.821
      without status epilepticus G40.822
  specified NEC G40.802
    intractable G40.804
      with status epilepticus G40.803
      without status epilepticus G40.804
    not intractable G40.802
      with status epilepticus G40.801
      without status epilepticus G40.802
  syndromes
    generalized
      idiopathic G40.309
        intractable G40.319
          with status epilepticus G40.311
          without status epilepticus G40.319
        not intractable G40.309
          with status epilepticus G40.301
          without status epilepticus G40.309
      specified NEC G40.409
        intractable G40.419
          with status epilepticus G40.411
          without status epilepticus G40.419
        not intractable G40.409
          with status epilepticus G40.401
          without status epilepticus G40.409

Epilepsy, epileptic, epilepsia (attack) (cerebral) (convulsion) (fit) (seizure) G40.909 — *continued*
  syndromes — *continued*
    localization-related (focal) (partial)
      idiopathic G40.009
        with seizures of localized onset G40.009
          intractable G40.019
            with status epilepticus G40.011
            without status epilepticus G40.019
          not intractable G40.009
            with status epilepticus G40.001
            without status epilepticus G40.009
      symptomatic
        with complex partial seizures G40.209
          intractable G40.219
            with status epilepticus G40.211
            without status epilepticus G40.219
          not intractable G40.209
            with status epilepticus G40.201
            without status epilepticus G40.209
        with simple partial seizures G40.109
          intractable G40.119
            with status epilepticus G40.111
            without status epilepticus G40.119
          not intractable G40.109
            with status epilepticus G40.101
            without status epilepticus G40.109
      specified NEC G40.802
        intractable G40.804
          with status epilepticus G40.803
          without status epilepticus G40.804
        not intractable G40.802
          with status epilepticus G40.801
          without status epilepticus G40.802
    tonic(-clonic) — *see* Epilepsy, generalized, specified NEC
    twilight F05
    uncinate (gyrus) — *see* Epilepsy, localization-related, symptomatic, with complex partial seizures
    Unverricht (-Lundborg) (familial myoclonic) — *see* Epilepsy, generalized, idiopathic
    visceral — *see* Epilepsy, specified NEC
    visual — *see* Epilepsy, specified NEC
Epiloia Q85.1
Epimenorrhea N92.0
Epipharyngitis — *see* Nasopharyngitis
Epiphora H04.20-
  due to
    excess lacrimation H04.21-
    insufficient drainage H04.22-
Epiphyseal arrest — *see* Arrest, epiphyseal
Epiphyseolysis, epiphysiolysis — *see* Osteochondropathy
Epiphysitis — *see also* Osteochondropathy
  juvenile M92.9
  syphilitic (congenital) A50.02
Epiplocele — *see* Hernia, abdomen
Epiploitis — *see* Peritonitis
Epiplosarcomphalocele — *see* Hernia, umbilicus
Episcleritis (suppurative) H15.10-
  in (due to)
    syphilis A52.71
    tuberculosis A18.51
  nodular H15.12-
  periodica fugax H15.11-
    angioneurotic — *see* Edema, angioneurotic
  syphilitic (late) A52.71
  tuberculous A18.51
Episode
  affective, mixed F39
  depersonalization (in neurotic state) F48.1

Episode — *continued*
  depressive F32.9
    major F32.9
      mild F32.0
      moderate F32.1
      severe (without psychotic symptoms) F32.2
        with psychotic symptoms F32.3
    recurrent F33.9
      brief F33.8
    specified NEC F32.89
  hypomanic F30.8
  manic F30.9
    with
      psychotic symptoms F30.2
      remission (full) F30.4
        partial F30.3
    other specified F30.8
    recurrent F31.89
    without psychotic symptoms F30.10
      mild F30.11
      moderate F30.12
      severe (without psychotic symptoms) F30.13
        with psychotic symptoms F30.2
  psychotic F23
    organic F06.8
  schizophrenic (acute) NEC, brief F23
Epispadias (female) (male) Q64.0
Episplenitis D73.89
Epistaxis (multiple) R04.0
  hereditary I78.0
  vicarious menstruation N94.89
Epithelioma (malignant) — *see also* Neoplasm, malignant, by site
  adenoides cysticum — *see* Neoplasm, skin, benign
  basal cell — *see* Neoplasm, skin, malignant
  benign — *see* Neoplasm, benign, by site
  Bowen's — *see* Neoplasm, skin, in situ
  calcifying, of Malherbe — *see* Neoplasm, skin, benign
  external site — *see* Neoplasm, skin, malignant
  intraepidermal, Jadassohn — *see* Neoplasm, skin, benign
  squamous cell — *see* Neoplasm, malignant, by site
Epitheliomatosis pigmented Q82.1
Epitheliopathy, multifocal placoid pigment H30.14-
Epithelium, epithelial — *see* condition
Epituberculosis (with atelectasis) (allergic) A15.7
Eponychia Q84.6
Epstein's
  nephrosis or syndrome — *see* Nephrosis
  pearl K09.8
Epulis (gingiva) (fibrous) (giant cell) K06.8
Equinia A24.0
Equinovarus (congenital) (talipes) Q66.0
  acquired — *see* Deformity, limb, clubfoot
Equivalent
  convulsive (abdominal) — *see* Epilepsy, specified NEC
  epileptic (psychic) — *see* Epilepsy, localization-related, symptomatic, with complex partial seizures
Erb(-Duchenne) paralysis (birth injury) (newborn) P14.0
Erb-Goldflam disease or syndrome G70.00
  with exacerbation (acute) G70.01
  in crisis G70.01
Erb's
  disease G71.0
  palsy, paralysis (brachial) (birth) (newborn) P14.0
    spinal (spastic) syphilitic A52.17
  pseudohypertrophic muscular dystrophy G71.0

DISEASE INDEX

DISEASE INDEX

Erdheim's syndrome (acromegalic macrospondylitis) E22.0
Erection, painful (persistent) — *see* Priapism
Ergosterol deficiency (vitamin D) E55.9
  with
    adult osteomalacia M83.8
    rickets — *see* Rickets
Ergotism — *see also* Poisoning, food, noxious, plant
  from ergot used as drug (migraine therapy) — *see* Table of Drugs and Chemicals
Erosio interdigitalis blastomycetica B37.2
Erosion
  artery I77.2
    without rupture I77.89
  bone — *see* Disorder, bone, density and structure, specified NEC
  bronchus J98.09
  cartilage (joint) — *see* Disorder, cartilage, specified type NEC
  cervix (uteri) (acquired) (chronic) (congenital) N86
    with cervicitis N72
  cornea (nontraumatic) — *see* Ulcer, cornea
    recurrent H18.83-
    traumatic — *see* Abrasion, cornea
  dental (idiopathic) (occupational) (due to diet, drugs or vomiting) K03.2
  duodenum, postpyloric — *see* Ulcer, duodenum
  esophagus K22.10
    with bleeding K22.11
  gastric — *see* Ulcer, stomach
  gastrojejunal — *see* Ulcer, gastrojejunal
  implanted mesh — *see* Complications, mesh
  intestine K63.3
  lymphatic vessel I89.8
  pylorus, pyloric (ulcer) — *see* Ulcer, stomach
  spine, aneurysmal A52.09
  stomach — *see* Ulcer, stomach
  subcutaneous device pocket
    nervous system prosthetic device, implant, or graft T85.890
    other internal prosthetic device, implant, or graft T85.898
  teeth (idiopathic) (occupational) (due to diet, drugs or vomiting) K03.2
  urethra N36.8
  uterus N85.8
Erotomania F52.8
Error
  metabolism, inborn — *see* Disorder, metabolism
  refractive — *see* Disorder, refraction
Eructation R14.2
  nervous or psychogenic F45.8
Eruption
  creeping B76.9
  drug (generalized) (taken internally) L27.0
    fixed L27.1
    in contact with skin — *see* Dermatitis, due to drugs
    localized L27.1
  Hutchinson, summer L56.4
  Kaposi's varicelliform B00.0
  napkin L22
  polymorphous light (sun) L56.4
  recalcitrant pustular L13.8
  ringed R23.8
  skin (nonspecific) R21
    creeping (meaning hookworm) B76.9
    due to inoculation/vaccination (generalized) (*see also* Dermatitis, due to, vaccine) L27.0
      localized L27.1
    erysipeloid A26.0
    feigned L98.1
    Kaposi's varicelliform B00.0
    lichenoid L28.0
    meaning dermatitis — *see* Dermatitis
    toxic NEC L53.0

Eruption — *continued*
  tooth, teeth, abnormal (incomplete) (late) (premature) (sequence) K00.6
  vesicular R23.8
Erysipelas (gangrenous) (infantile) (newborn) (phlegmonous) (suppurative) A46
  external ear A46 *[H62.40]*
  puerperal, postpartum O86.89
Erysipeloid A26.9
  cutaneous (Rosenbach's) A26.0
  disseminated A26.8
  sepsis A26.7
  specified NEC A26.8
Erythema, erythematous (infectional) (inflammation) L53.9
  ab igne L59.0
  annulare (centrifugum) (rheumaticum) L53.1
  arthriticum epidemicum A25.1
  brucellum — *see* Brucellosis
  chronic figurate NEC L53.3
  chronicum migrans (Borrelia burgdorferi) A69.20
  diaper L22
  due to
    chemical NEC L53.0
      in contact with skin L24.5
    drug (internal use) — *see* Dermatitis, due to, drugs
  elevatum diutinum L95.1
  endemic E52
  epidemic, arthritic A25.1
  figuratum perstans L53.3
  gluteal L22
  heat — *code by* site under Burn, first degree
  ichthyosiforme congenitum bullous Q80.3
  in diseases classified elsewhere L54
  induratum (nontuberculous) L52
    tuberculous A18.4
  infectiosum B08.3
  intertrigo L30.4
  iris L51.9
  marginatum L53.2
    in (due to) acute rheumatic fever I00
  medicamentosum — *see* Dermatitis, due to, drugs
  migrans A26.0
    chronicum A69.20
    tongue K14.1
  multiforme (major) (minor) L51.9
    bullous, bullosum L51.1
    conjunctiva L51.1
    nonbullous L51.0
    pemphigoides L12.0
    specified NEC L51.8
  napkin L22
  neonatorum P83.8
    toxic P83.1
  nodosum L52
    tuberculous A18.4
  palmar L53.8
  pernio T69.1
  rash, newborn P83.8
  scarlatiniform (recurrent) (exfoliative) L53.8
  solare L55.0
  specified NEC L53.8
  toxic, toxicum NEC L53.0
    newborn P83.1
  tuberculous (primary) A18.4
Erythematous, erythematosus — *see* condition
Erythermalgia (primary) I73.81
Erythralgia I73.81
Erythrasma L08.1
Erythredema (polyneuropathy) — *see* Poisoning, mercury
Erythremia (acute) C94.0-
  chronic D45
  secondary D75.1

Erythroblastopenia (*see also* Aplasia, red cell) D60.9
  congenital D61.01
Erythroblastophthisis D61.09
Erythroblastosis (fetalis) (newborn) P55.9
  due to
    ABO (antibodies) (incompatibility) (isoimmunization) P55.1
    Rh (antibodies) (incompatibility) (isoimmunization) P55.0
Erythrocyanosis (crurum) I73.89
Erythrocythemia — *see* Erythremia
Erythrocytosis (megalosplenic) (secondary) D75.1
  familial D75.0
  oval, hereditary — *see* Elliptocytosis
  secondary D75.1
  stress D75.1
Erythroderma (secondary) (*see also* Erythema) L53.9
  bullous ichthyosiform, congenital Q80.3
  desquamativum L21.1
  ichthyosiform, congenital (bullous) Q80.3
  neonatorum P83.8
  psoriaticum L40.8
Erythrodysesthesia, palmar plantar (PPE) L27.1
Erythrogenesis imperfecta D61.09
Erythroleukemia C94.0-
Erythromelalgia I73.81
Erythrophagocytosis D75.89
Erythrophobia F40.298
Erythroplakia, oral epithelium, and tongue K13.29
Erythroplasia (Queyrat) D07.4
  specified site — *see* Neoplasm, skin, in situ
  unspecified site D07.4
Escherichia coli (E. coli), as cause of disease classified elsewhere B96.20
  non-O157 Shiga toxin-producing (with known O group) B96.22
  non-Shiga toxin-producing B96.29
  O157 with confirmation of Shiga toxin when H antigen is unknown, or is not H7 B96.21
  O157:H- (nonmotile) with confirmation of Shiga toxin B96.21
  O157:H7 with or without confirmation of Shiga toxin-production B96.21
  Shiga toxin-producing (with unspecified O group) (STEC) B96.23
  O157 B96.21
  O157:H7 with or without confirmation of Shiga toxin-production B96.21
  specified NEC B96.22
  specified NEC B96.29
Esophagismus K22.4
Esophagitis (acute) (alkaline) (chemical) (chronic) (infectional) (necrotic) (peptic) (postoperative) K20.9
  candidal B37.81
  due to gastrointestinal reflux disease K21.0
  eosinophilic K20.0
  reflux K21.0
  specified NEC K20.8
  tuberculous A18.83
  ulcerative K22.10
    with bleeding K22.11
Esophagocele K22.5
Esophagomalacia K22.8
Esophagospasm K22.4
Esophagostenosis K22.2
Esophagostomiasis B81.8
Esophagotracheal — *see* condition
Esophagus — *see* condition
Esophoria H50.51
  convergence, excess H51.12
  divergence, insufficiency H51.8
Esotropia — *see* Strabismus, convergent concomitant

Espundia B55.2
Essential — see condition
Esthesioneuroblastoma C30.0
Esthesioneurocytoma C30.0
Esthesioneuroepithelioma C30.0
Esthiomene A55
Estivo-autumnal malaria (fever) B50.9
Estrangement (marital) Z63.5
  parent-child NEC Z62.890
Estriasis — see Myiasis
Ethanolism — see Alcoholism
Etherism — see Dependence, drug, inhalant
Ethmoid, ethmoidal — see condition
Ethmoiditis (chronic) (nonpurulent) (purulent)
  — see also Sinusitis, ethmoidal
  influenzal — see Influenza, with, respiratory
    manifestations NEC
  Woakes' J33.1
Ethylism — see Alcoholism
Eulenburg's disease (congenital
  paramyotonia) G71.19
Eumycetoma B47.0
Eunuchoidism E29.1
  hypogonadotropic E23.0
European blastomycosis — see
  Cryptococcosis
Eustachian — see condition
Evaluation (for) (of)
  development state
    adolescent Z00.3
    period of
      delayed growth in childhood Z00.70
        with abnormal findings Z00.71
      rapid growth in childhood Z00.2
    puberty Z00.3
  growth and developmental state (period of
    rapid growth) Z00.2
    delayed growth Z00.70
      with abnormal findings Z00.71
  mental health (status) Z00.8
    requested by authority Z04.6
  period of
    delayed growth in childhood Z00.70
      with abnormal findings Z00.71
    rapid growth in childhood Z00.2
  suspected condition — see Observation
Evans syndrome D69.41
**Event, apparent life threatening in
  newborn and infant** (ALTE) R68.13
Eventration — see also Hernia, ventral
  colon into chest — see Hernia, diaphragm
  diaphragm (congenital) Q79.1
Eversion
  bladder N32.89
  cervix (uteri) N86
    with cervicitis N72
  foot NEC — see also Deformity, valgus, ankle
    congenital Q66.6
  punctum lacrimale (postinfectional) (senile)
    H04.52-
  ureter (meatus) N28.89
  urethra (meatus) N36.8
  uterus N81.4
Evidence
  cytologic
    of malignancy on anal smear R85.614
    of malignancy on cervical smear R87.614
    of malignancy on vaginal smear R87.624
Evisceration
  birth injury P15.8
  traumatic NEC
    eye — see Enucleated eye
Evulsion — see Avulsion
Ewing's sarcoma or tumor — see
  Neoplasm, bone, malignant

Examination (for) (following) (general) (of)
  (routine) Z00.00
  with abnormal findings Z00.01
  abuse, physical (alleged), ruled out
    adult Z04.71
    child Z04.72
  adolescent (development state) Z00.3
  alleged rape or sexual assault (victim), ruled
    out
    adult Z04.41
    child Z04.42
  allergy Z01.82
  annual (adult) (periodic) (physical) Z00.00
    with abnormal findings Z00.01
    gynecological Z01.419
      with abnormal findings Z01.411
  antibody response Z01.84
  blood — see Examination, laboratory
  blood pressure Z01.30
    with abnormal findings Z01.31
  cancer staging — see Neoplasm, malignant,
    by site
  cervical Papanicolaou smear Z12.4
    as part of routine gynecological examination
      Z01.419
      with abnormal findings Z01.411
  child (over 28 days old) Z00.129
    with abnormal findings Z00.121
    under 28 days old — see Newborn,
      examination
  clinical research control or normal comparison
    (control) (participant) Z00.6
  contraceptive (drug) maintenance (routine)
    Z30.8
    device (intrauterine) Z30.431
  dental Z01.20
    with abnormal findings Z01.21
  developmental — see Examination, child
  donor (potential) Z00.5
  ear Z01.10
    with abnormal findings NEC Z01.118
  eye Z01.00
    with abnormal findings Z01.01
  follow-up (routine) (following) Z09
    chemotherapy NEC Z09
      malignant neoplasm Z08
    fracture Z09
    malignant neoplasm Z08
    postpartum Z39.2
    psychotherapy Z09
    radiotherapy NEC Z09
      malignant neoplasm Z08
    surgery NEC Z09
      malignant neoplasm Z08
  following
    accident NEC Z04.3
      transport Z04.1
      work Z04.2
    assault, alleged, ruled out
      adult Z04.71
      child Z04.72
    motor vehicle accident Z04.1
    treatment (for) Z09
      combined NEC Z09
        fracture Z09
        malignant neoplasm Z08
      malignant neoplasm Z08
      mental disorder Z09
      specified condition NEC Z09
  gynecological Z01.419
    with abnormal findings Z01.411
    for contraceptive maintenance Z30.8
  health — see Examination, medical
  hearing Z01.10
    with abnormal findings NEC Z01.118
    following failed hearing screening Z01.110
  immunity status testing Z01.84

Examination (for) (following) (general) (of)
  (routine) Z00.00 — continued
  laboratory (as part of a general medical
    examination) Z00.00
    with abnormal findings Z00.01
    preprocedural Z01.812
  lactating mother Z39.1
  medical (adult) (for) (of) Z00.00
    with abnormal findings Z00.01
    administrative purpose only Z02.9
      specified NEC Z02.89
    admission to
      armed forces Z02.3
      old age home Z02.2
      prison Z02.89
      residential institution Z02.2
      school Z02.0
        following illness or medical treatment
          Z02.0
      summer camp Z02.89
    adoption Z02.82
    blood alcohol or drug level Z02.83
    camp (summer) Z02.89
    clinical research, normal subject (control)
      (participant) Z00.6
    control subject in clinical research (normal
      comparison) (participant) Z00.6
    donor (potential) Z00.5
    driving license Z02.4
    general (adult) Z00.00
      with abnormal findings Z00.01
    immigration Z02.89
    insurance purposes Z02.6
    marriage Z02.89
    medicolegal reasons NEC Z04.8
    naturalization Z02.89
    participation in sport Z02.5
    paternity testing Z02.81
    population survey Z00.8
    pre-employment Z02.1
    pre-operative — see Examination, pre-
      procedural
    pre-procedural
      cardiovascular Z01.810
      respiratory Z01.811
      specified NEC Z01.818
    preschool children
      for admission to school Z02.0
    prisoners
      for entrance into prison Z02.89
    recruitment for armed forces Z02.3
    specified NEC Z00.8
    sport competition Z02.5
  medicolegal reason NEC Z04.8
  newborn — see Newborn, examination
  pelvic (annual) (periodic) Z01.419
    with abnormal findings Z01.411
  period of rapid growth in childhood Z00.2
  periodic (adult) (annual) (routine) Z00.00
    with abnormal findings Z00.01
  physical (adult) — see also Examination,
    medical Z00.00
    sports Z02.5
  postpartum
    immediately after delivery Z39.0
    routine follow-up Z39.2
  pre-chemotherapy (antineoplastic) Z01.818
  prenatal (normal pregnancy) (see also
    Pregnancy, normal) Z34.9-
  pre-procedural (pre-operative)
    cardiovascular Z01.810
    laboratory Z01.812
    respiratory Z01.811
    specified NEC Z01.818
  prior to chemotherapy (antineoplastic)
    Z01.818
  psychiatric NEC Z00.8
    follow-up not needing further care Z09
    requested by authority Z04.6

Examination (for) (following) (general) (of) (routine) Z00.00 — *continued*
  radiological (as part of a general medical examination) Z00.00
    with abnormal findings Z00.01
  repeat cervical smear to confirm findings of recent normal smear following initial abnormal smear Z01.42
  skin (hypersensitivity) Z01.82
  special (*see also* Examination, by type) Z01.89
    specified type NEC Z01.89
  specified type or reason NEC Z04.8
  teeth Z01.20
    with abnormal findings Z01.21
  urine — *see* Examination, laboratory
  vision Z01.00
    with abnormal findings Z01.01
Exanthem, exanthema — *see also* Rash
  with enteroviral vesicular stomatitis B08.4
  Boston A88.0
  epidemic with meningitis A88.0 [G02]
  subitum B08.20
    due to human herpesvirus 6 B08.21
    due to human herpesvirus 7 B08.22
  viral, virus B09
    specified type NEC B08.8
Excess, excessive, excessively
  alcohol level in blood R78.0
  androgen (ovarian) E28.1
  attrition, tooth, teeth K03.0
  carotene, carotin (dietary) E67.1
  cold, effects of T69.9
    specified effect NEC T69.8
  convergence H51.12
  crying
    in child, adolescent, or adult R45.83
    in infant R68.11
  development, breast N62
  divergence H51.8
  drinking (alcohol) NEC (without dependence) F10.10
    habitual (continual) (without remission) F10.20
  eating R63.2
  estrogen E28.0
  fat — *see also* Obesity
    in heart — *see* Degeneration, myocardial
    localized E65
  foreskin N47.8
  gas R14.0
  glucagon E16.3
  heat — *see* Heat
  intermaxillary vertical dimension of fully erupted teeth M26.37
  interocclusal distance of fully erupted teeth M26.37
  kalium E87.5
  large
    colon K59.39
      congenital Q43.8
    infant P08.0
    organ or site, congenital NEC — *see* Anomaly, by site
  long
    organ or site, congenital NEC — *see* Anomaly, by site
  menstruation (with regular cycle) N92.0
    with irregular cycle N92.1
  napping Z72.821
  natrium E87.0
  number of teeth K00.1
  nutrient (dietary) NEC R63.2
  potassium (K) E87.5
  salivation K11.7
  secretion — *see also* Hypersecretion
    milk O92.6
    sputum R09.3
    sweat R61
  sexual drive F52.8

Excess, excessive, excessively — *continued*
  short
    organ or site, congenital NEC — *see* Anomaly, by site
    umbilical cord in labor or delivery O69.3
  skin L98.7
    and subcutaneous tissue L98.7
    eyelid (acquired) — *see* Blepharochalasis
      congenital Q10.3
  sodium (Na) E87.0
  spacing of fully erupted teeth M26.32
  sputum R09.3
  sweating R61
  thirst R63.1
    due to deprivation of water T73.1
  tuberosity of jaw M26.07
  vitamin
    A (dietary) E67.0
      administered as drug (prolonged intake) — *see* Table of Drugs and Chemicals, vitamins, adverse effect
      overdose or wrong substance given or taken — *see* Table of Drugs and Chemicals, vitamins, poisoning
    D (dietary) E67.3
      administered as drug (prolonged intake) — *see* Table of Drugs and Chemicals, vitamins, adverse effect
      overdose or wrong substance given or taken — *see* Table of Drugs and Chemicals, vitamins, poisoning
  weight
    gain R63.5
    loss R63.4
Excitability, abnormal, under minor stress (personality disorder) F60.3
Excitation
  anomalous atrioventricular I45.6
  psychogenic F30.8
  reactive (from emotional stress, psychological trauma) F30.8
Excitement
  hypomanic F30.8
  manic F30.9
  mental, reactive (from emotional stress, psychological trauma) F30.8
  state, reactive (from emotional stress, psychological trauma) F30.8
Excoriation (traumatic) — *see also* Abrasion
  neurotic L98.1
  skin picking disorder F42.4
Exfoliation
  due to erythematous conditions according to extent of body surface involved L49.0
    10-19 percent of body surface L49.1
    20-29 percent of body surface L49.2
    30-39 percent of body surface L49.3
    40-49 percent of body surface L49.4
    50-59 percent of body surface L49.5
    60-69 percent of body surface L49.6
    70-79 percent of body surface L49.7
    80-89 percent of body surface L49.8
    90-99 percent of body surface L49.9
    less than 10 percent of body surface L49.0
  teeth, due to systemic causes K08.0
Exfoliative — *see* condition
Exhaustion, exhaustive (physical NEC) R53.83
  battle F43.0
  cardiac — *see* Failure, heart
  delirium F43.0
  due to
    cold T69.8
    excessive exertion T73.3
    exposure T73.2
    neurasthenia F48.8
  heart — *see* Failure, heart

Exhaustion, exhaustive (physical NEC) R53.83 — *continued*
  heat (*see also* Heat, exhaustion) T67.5
    due to
      salt depletion T67.4
      water depletion T67.3
  maternal, complicating delivery O75.81
  mental F48.8
  myocardium, myocardial — *see* Failure, heart
  nervous F48.8
  old age R54
  psychogenic F48.8
  psychosis F43.0
  senile R54
  vital NEC Z73.0
Exhibitionism F65.2
Exocervicitis — *see* Cervicitis
Exomphalos Q79.2
  meaning hernia — *see* Hernia, umbilicus
Exophoria H50.52
  convergence, insufficiency H51.11
  divergence, excess H51.8
Exophthalmos H05.2-
  congenital Q15.8
  constant NEC H05.24-
  displacement, globe — *see* Displacement, globe
  due to thyrotoxicosis (hyperthyroidism) — *see* Hyperthyroidism, with, goiter (diffuse)
  dysthyroid — *see* Hyperthyroidism, with, goiter (diffuse)
  goiter — *see* Hyperthyroidism, with, goiter (diffuse)
  intermittent NEC H05.25-
  malignant — *see* Hyperthyroidism, with, goiter (diffuse)
  orbital
    edema — *see* Edema, orbit
    hemorrhage — *see* Hemorrhage, orbit
  pulsating NEC H05.26-
  thyrotoxic, thyrotropic — *see* Hyperthyroidism, with, goiter (diffuse)
Exostosis — *see also* Disorder, bone
  cartilaginous — *see* Neoplasm, bone, benign
  congenital (multiple) Q78.6
  external ear canal H61.81-
  gonococcal A54.49
  jaw (bone) M27.8
  multiple, congenital Q78.6
  orbit H05.35-
  osteocartilaginous — *see* Neoplasm, bone, benign
  syphilitic A52.77
Exotropia — *see* Strabismus, divergent
  concomitant
Explanation of
  investigation finding Z71.2
  medication Z71.89
Exposure (to) (*see also* Contact, with) T75.89
  acariasis Z20.7
  AIDS virus Z20.6
  air pollution Z77.110
  algae and algae toxins Z77.121
  algae bloom Z77.121
  anthrax Z20.810
  aromatic (hazardous) compounds NEC Z77.028
  aromatic amines Z77.020
  aromatic dyes NOS Z77.028
  arsenic Z77.010
  asbestos Z77.090
  bacterial disease NEC Z20.818
  benzene Z77.021
  blue-green algae bloom Z77.121
  body fluids (potentially hazardous) Z77.21
  brown tide Z77.121
  chemicals (chiefly nonmedicinal) (hazardous) NEC Z77.098
  cholera Z20.09

Exposure (to) (*see also* Contact, with) T75.89 — continued
chromium compounds Z77.018
cold, effects of T69.9
  specified effect NEC T69.8
communicable disease Z20.9
  bacterial NEC Z20.818
  specified NEC Z20.89
  viral NEC Z20.828
cyanobacteria bloom Z77.121
disaster Z65.5
discrimination Z60.5
dyes Z77.098
effects of T73.9
environmental tobacco smoke (acute) (chronic) Z77.22
Escherichia coli (E. coli) Z20.01
exhaustion due to T73.2
fiberglass — *see* Table of Drugs and Chemicals, fiberglass
German measles Z20.4
gonorrhea Z20.2
hazardous metals NEC Z77.018
hazardous substances NEC Z77.29
hazards in the physical environment NEC Z77.128
hazards to health NEC Z77.9
human immunodeficiency virus (HIV) Z20.6
human T-lymphotropic virus type-1 (HTLV-1) Z20.89
implanted
  mesh — *see* Complications, mesh
  prosthetic materials NEC — *see* Complications, prosthetic materials NEC
infestation (parasitic) NEC Z20.7
intestinal infectious disease NEC Z20.09
  Escherichia coli (E. coli) Z20.01
lead Z77.011
meningococcus Z20.811
mold (toxic) Z77.120
nickel dust Z77.018
noise Z77.122
occupational
  air contaminants NEC Z57.39
  dust Z57.2
  environmental tobacco smoke Z57.31
  extreme temperature Z57.6
  noise Z57.0
  radiation Z57.1
  risk factors Z57.9
   specified NEC Z57.8
  toxic agents (gases) (liquids) (solids) (vapors) in agriculture Z57.4
  toxic agents (gases) (liquids) (solids) (vapors) in industry NEC Z57.5
  vibration Z57.7
parasitic disease NEC Z20.7
pediculosis Z20.7
persecution Z60.5
pfiesteria piscicida Z77.121
poliomyelitis Z20.89
pollution
  air Z77.110
  environmental NEC Z77.118
  soil Z77.112
  water Z77.111
polycyclic aromatic hydrocarbons Z77.028
prenatal (drugs) (toxic chemicals) — *see* Newborn, affected by, noxious substances transmitted via placenta or breast milk
rabies Z20.3
radiation, naturally occurring NEC Z77.123
radon Z77.123
red tide (Florida) Z77.121
rubella Z20.4
second hand tobacco smoke (acute) (chronic) Z77.22
  in the perinatal period P96.81
sexually-transmitted disease Z20.2

Exposure (to) (*see also* Contact, with) T75.89 — continued
smallpox (laboratory) Z20.89
syphilis Z20.2
terrorism Z65.4
torture Z65.4
tuberculosis Z20.1
uranium Z77.012
varicella Z20.820
venereal disease Z20.2
viral disease NEC Z20.828
war Z65.5
water pollution Z77.111
Exsanguination — *see* Hemorrhage
Exstrophy
abdominal contents Q45.8
bladder Q64.10
  cloacal Q64.12
  specified type NEC Q64.19
  supravesical fissure Q64.11
Extensive — *see* condition
Extra — *see also* Accessory
marker chromosomes (normal individual) Q92.61
  in abnormal individual Q92.62
rib Q76.6
  cervical Q76.5
Extrasystoles (supraventricular) I49.49
atrial I49.1
auricular I49.1
junctional I49.2
ventricular I49.3
Extrauterine gestation or pregnancy — *see* Pregnancy, by site
Extravasation
blood R58
chyle into mesentery I89.8
pelvicalyceal N13.8
pyelosinus N13.8
urine (from ureter) R39.0
vesicant agent
  antineoplastic chemotherapy T80.810
  other agent NEC T80.818
Extremity — *see* condition, limb
Extrophy — *see* Exstrophy
Extroversion
bladder Q64.19
uterus N81.4
  complicating delivery O71.2
  postpartal (old) N81.4
Extruded tooth (teeth) M26.34
Extrusion
breast implant (prosthetic) T85.42
eye implant (globe) (ball) T85.328
intervertebral disc — *see* Displacement, intervertebral disc
ocular lens implant (prosthetic) — *see* Complications, intraocular lens
vitreous — *see* Prolapse, vitreous
Exudate
pleural — *see* Effusion, pleura
retina H35.89
Exudative — *see* condition
Eye, eyeball, eyelid — *see* condition
Eyestrain — *see* Disturbance, vision, subjective
Eyeworm disease of Africa B74.3

F

Faber's syndrome (achlorhydric anemia) D50.9
Fabry(-Anderson) disease E75.21
Faciocephalalgia, autonomic (*see also* Neuropathy, peripheral, autonomic) G90.09
Factor(s)
psychic, associated with diseases classified elsewhere F54
psychological
  affecting physical conditions F54
  or behavioral
   affecting general medical condition F54
   associated with disorders or diseases classified elsewhere F54
Fahr disease (of brain) G23.8
Fahr Volhard disease (of kidney) I12-
Failure, failed
abortion — *see* Abortion, attempted
aortic (valve) I35.8
  rheumatic I06.8
attempted abortion — *see* Abortion, attempted
biventricular I50.9
bone marrow — *see* Anemia, aplastic
cardiac — *see* Failure, heart
cardiorenal (chronic) I50.9
  hypertensive I13.2
cardiorespiratory (*see also* Failure, heart) R09.2
cardiovascular (chronic) — *see* Failure, heart
cerebrovascular I67.9
cervical dilatation in labor O62.0
circulation, circulatory (peripheral) R57.9
  newborn P29.89
compensation — *see* Disease, heart
compliance with medical treatment or regimen — *see* Noncompliance
congestive — *see* Failure, heart, congestive
dental implant (endosseous) M27.69
  due to
   failure of dental prosthesis M27.63
   lack of attached gingiva M27.62
   occlusal trauma (poor prosthetic design) M27.62
   parafunctional habits M27.62
   periodontal infection (peri-implantitis) M27.62
   poor oral hygiene M27.62
  osseointegration M27.61
   due to
    complications of systemic disease M27.61
    poor bone quality M27.61
   iatrogenic M27.61
  post-osseointegration
   biological M27.62
    due to complications of systemic disease M27.62
   iatrogenic M27.62
   mechanical M27.63
  pre-integration M27.61
  pre-osseointegration M27.61
  specified NEC M27.69
descent of head (at term) of pregnancy (mother) O32.4
endosseous dental implant — *see* Failure, dental implant
engagement of head (term of pregnancy) (mother) O32.4
erection (penile) (*see also* Dysfunction, sexual, male, erectile) N52.9
  nonorganic F52.21
examination(s), anxiety concerning Z55.2
expansion terminal respiratory units (newborn) (primary) P28.0
forceps NOS (with subsequent cesarean delivery) O66.5

D I S E A S E   I N D E X

Failure, failed — *continued*
gain weight (child over 28 days old) R62.51
  adult R62.7
  newborn P92.6
genital response (male) F52.21
  female F52.22
heart (acute) (senile) (sudden) I50.9
  with
    acute pulmonary edema — *see* Failure,
      ventricular, left
    decompensation — *see* Failure, heart,
      congestive
    dilatation — *see* Disease, heart
  arteriosclerotic I70.90
  biventricular I50.9
  combined left-right sided I50.9
  compensated I50.9
  complicating
    anesthesia (general) (local) or other
      sedation
      in labor and delivery O74.2
      in pregnancy O29.12-
      postpartum, puerperal O89.1
    delivery (cesarean) (instrumental) O75.4
  congestive (compensated) (decompensated)
    I50.9
    with rheumatic fever (conditions in I00)
      active I01.8
      inactive or quiescent (with chorea)
        I09.81
    newborn P29.0
    rheumatic (chronic) (inactive) (with chorea)
      I09.81
      active or acute I01.8
        with chorea I02.0
  decompensated I50.9
  degenerative — *see* Degeneration,
    myocardial
  diastolic (congestive) I50.30
    acute (congestive) I50.31
      and (on) chronic (congestive) I50.33
    chronic (congestive) I50.32
      and (on) acute (congestive) I50.33
    combined with systolic (congestive) I50.40
      acute (congestive) I50.41
        and (on) chronic (congestive) I50.43
      chronic (congestive) I50.42
        and (on) acute (congestive) I50.43
  due to presence of cardiac prosthesis
    I97.13-
  following cardiac surgery I97.13-
  high output NOS I50.9
  hypertensive — *see* Hypertension, heart
  left (ventricular) — *see* Failure, ventricular,
    left
  low output (syndrome) NOS I50.9
  newborn P29.0
  organic — *see* Disease, heart
  peripartum O90.3
  postprocedural I97.13-
  rheumatic (chronic) (inactive) I09.9
  right (ventricular) (secondary to left heart
    failure) — *see* Failure, heart, congestive
  systolic (congestive) I50.20
    acute (congestive) I50.21
      and (on) chronic (congestive) I50.23
    chronic (congestive) I50.22
      and (on) acute (congestive) I50.23
    combined with diastolic (congestive)
      I50.40
      acute (congestive) I50.41
        and (on) chronic (congestive) I50.43
      chronic (congestive) I50.42
        and (on) acute (congestive) I50.43
  thyrotoxic (*see also* Thyrotoxicosis) E05.90
    [I43]
    with thyroid storm E05.91 *[I43]*
  valvular — *see* Endocarditis

Failure, failed — *continued*
hepatic K72.90
  with coma K72.91
  acute or subacute K72.00
    with coma K72.01
    due to drugs K71.10
      with coma K71.11
  alcoholic (acute) (chronic) (subacute) K70.40
    with coma K70.41
  chronic K72.10
    with coma K72.11
    due to drugs (acute) (subacute) (chronic)
      K71.10
      with coma K71.11
  due to drugs (acute) (subacute) (chronic)
    K71.10
    with coma K71.11
  postprocedural K91.82
hepatorenal K76.7
induction (of labor) O61.9
  abortion — *see* Abortion, attempted
  by
    oxytocic drugs O61.0
    prostaglandins O61.0
  instrumental O61.1
  mechanical O61.1
  medical O61.0
  specified NEC O61.8
  surgical O61.1
intubation during anesthesia T88.4
  in pregnancy O29.6-
  labor and delivery O74.7
  postpartum, puerperal O89.6
involution, thymus (gland) E32.0
kidney (*see also* Disease, kidney, chronic) N19
  acute (*see also* Failure, renal, acute) N17.9
  diabetic — *see* E08-E13 with .22
lactation (complete) O92.3
  partial O92.4
Leydig's cell, adult E29.1
liver — *see* Failure, hepatic
menstruation at puberty N91.0
mitral I05.8
myocardial, myocardium (*see also* Failure,
  heart) I50.9
  chronic (*see also* Failure, heart, congestive)
    I50.9
  congestive (*see also* Failure, heart, congestive)
    I50.9
orgasm (female) (psychogenic) F52.31
  male F52.32
ovarian (primary) E28.39
  iatrogenic E89.40
    asymptomatic E89.40
    symptomatic E89.41
  postprocedural (postablative)
    (postirradiation) (postsurgical) E89.40
    asymptomatic E89.40
    symptomatic E89.41
ovulation causing infertility N97.0
polyglandular, autoimmune E31.0
prosthetic joint implant — *see* Complications,
  joint prosthesis, mechanical, breakdown,
  by site
renal N19
  with
    tubular necrosis (acute) N17.0
  acute N17.9
    with
      cortical necrosis N17.1
      medullary necrosis N17.2
      tubular necrosis N17.0
    specified NEC N17.8
  chronic N18.9
    hypertensive — *see* Hypertension, kidney
  congenital P96.0
  end stage (chronic) N18.6
    due to hypertension I12.0

Failure, failed — *continued*
renal N19 — *continued*
  following
    abortion — *see* Abortion by type
      complicated by specified condition
      NEC
    crushing T79.5
    ectopic or molar pregnancy O08.4
    labor and delivery (acute) O90.4
  hypertensive — *see* Hypertension, kidney
  postprocedural N99.0
respiration, respiratory J96.90
  with
    hypercapnia J96.92
    hypoxia J96.91
  acute J96.00
    with
      hypercapnia J96.02
      hypoxia J96.01
  acute and (on) chronic J96.20
    with
      hypercapnia J96.22
      hypoxia J96.21
  center G93.89
  chronic J96.10
    with
      hypercapnia J96.12
      hypoxia J96.11
  newborn P28.5
  postprocedural (acute) J95.821
    acute and chronic J95.822
rotation
  cecum Q43.3
  colon Q43.3
  intestine Q43.3
  kidney Q63.2
sedation (conscious) (moderate) during
  procedure T88.52
  history of Z92.83
segmentation — *see also* Fusion
  fingers — *see* Syndactylism, complex, fingers
  vertebra Q76.49
    with scoliosis Q76.3
seminiferous tubule, adult E29.1
senile (general) R54
sexual arousal (male) F52.21
  female F52.22
testicular endocrine function E29.1
to thrive (child over 28 days old) R62.51
  adult R62.7
  newborn P92.6
transplant T86.92
  bone T86.831
    marrow T86.02
  cornea T86.841
  heart T86.22
    with lung(s) T86.32
  intestine T86.851
  kidney T86.12
  liver T86.42
  lung(s) T86.811
    with heart T86.32
  pancreas T86.891
  skin (allograft) (autograft) T86.821
  specified organ or tissue NEC T86.891
  stem cell (peripheral blood) (umbilical cord)
    T86.5
trial of labor (with subsequent cesarean
  delivery) O66.40
  following previous cesarean delivery
    O66.41
tubal ligation N99.89
urinary — *see* Disease, kidney, chronic
vacuum extraction NOS (with subsequent
  cesarean delivery) O66.5
vasectomy N99.89
ventouse NOS (with subsequent cesarean
  delivery) O66.5

Failure, failed — *continued*
  ventricular (*see also* Failure, heart) I50.9
    left I50.1
      with rheumatic fever (conditions in I00)
        active I01.8
          with chorea I02.0
        inactive or quiescent (with chorea)
          I09.81
        rheumatic (chronic) (inactive) (with chorea)
          I09.81
          active or acute I01.8
            with chorea I02.0
    right (*see also* Failure, heart, congestive)
      I50.9
  vital centers, newborn P91.8
Fainting (fit) R55
Fallen arches — *see* Deformity, limb, flat foot
Falling, falls (repeated) R29.6
  any organ or part — *see* Prolapse
Fallopian
  insufflation Z31.41
  tube — *see* condition
Fallot's
  pentalogy Q21.8
  tetrad or tetralogy Q21.3
  triad or trilogy Q22.3
False — *see also* condition
  croup J38.5
  joint — *see* Nonunion, fracture
  labor (pains) O47.9
    at or after 37 completed weeks of gestation
      O47.1
    before 37 completed weeks of gestation
      O47.0-
  passage, urethra (prostatic) N36.5
  pregnancy F45.8
Family, familial — *see also* condition
  disruption Z63.8
    involving divorce or separation Z63.5
  Li-Fraumeni (syndrome) Z15.01
  planning advice Z30.09
  problem Z63.9
    specified NEC Z63.8
  retinoblastoma C69.2-
Famine (effects of) T73.0
  edema — *see* Malnutrition, severe
Fanconi (-de Toni) (-Debré) syndrome
  E72.09
  with cystinosis E72.04
Fanconi's anemia (congenital pancytopenia)
  D61.09
Farber's disease or syndrome E75.29
Farcy A24.0
Farmer's
  lung J67.0
  skin L57.8
Farsightedness — *see* Hypermetropia
Fascia — *see* condition
Fasciculation R25.3
Fasciitis M72.9
  diffuse (eosinophilic) M35.4
  infective M72.8
    necrotizing M72.6
  necrotizing M72.6
  nodular M72.4
  perirenal (with ureteral obstruction) N13.5
    with infection N13.6
  plantar M72.2
  specified NEC M72.8
  traumatic (old) M72.8
    current — *code by* site under Sprain
Fascioliasis B66.3
Fasciolopsis, fasciolopsiasis (intestinal)
  B66.5
Fascioscapulohumeral myopathy G71.0
Fast pulse R00.0

Fat
  embolism — *see* Embolism, fat
  excessive — *see also* Obesity
    in heart — *see* Degeneration, myocardial
  in stool R19.5
  localized (pad) E65
    heart — *see* Degeneration, myocardial
    knee M79.4
    retropatellar M79.4
  necrosis
    breast N64.1
    mesentery K65.4
    omentum K65.4
  pad E65
    knee M79.4
Fatigue R53.83
  auditory deafness — *see* Deafness
  chronic R53.82
  combat F43.0
  general R53.83
    psychogenic F48.8
  heat (transient) T67.6
  muscle M62.89
  myocardium — *see* Failure, heart
  neoplasm-related R53.0
  nervous, neurosis F48.8
  operational F48.8
  psychogenic (general) F48.8
  senile R54
  voice R49.8
Fatness — *see* Obesity
Fatty — *see also* condition
  apron E65
  degeneration — *see* Degeneration, fatty
  heart (enlarged) — *see* Degeneration,
    myocardial
  liver NEC K76.0
    alcoholic K70.0
    nonalcoholic K76.0
  necrosis — *see* Degeneration, fatty
Fauces — *see* condition
Fauchard's disease (periodontitis) — *see*
  Periodontitis
Faucitis J02.9
Favism (anemia) D55.0
Favus — *see* Dermatophytosis
Fazio-Londe disease or syndrome G12.1
Fear complex or reaction F40.9
Fear of — *see* Phobia
Feared complaint unfounded Z71.1
Febris, febrile — *see also* Fever
  flava (*see also* Fever, yellow) A95.9
  melitensis A23.0
  pestis — *see* Plague
  recurrens — *see* Fever, relapsing
  rubra A38.9
Fecal
  incontinence R15.9
  smearing R15.1
  soiling R15.1
  urgency R15.2
Fecalith (impaction) K56.41
  appendix K38.1
  congenital P76.8
Fede's disease K14.0
**Feeble rapid pulse due to shock
  following injury** T79.4
Feeble-minded F70
Feeding
  difficulties R63.3
  problem R63.3
    newborn P92.9
      specified NEC P92.8
    nonorganic (adult) — *see* Disorder, eating
Feeling (of)
  foreign body in throat R09.89
Feer's disease — *see* Poisoning, mercury
Feet — *see* condition
Feigned illness Z76.5

Feil-Klippel syndrome (brevicollis) Q76.1
**Feinmesser's (hidrotic) ectodermal
  dysplasia** Q82.4
Felinophobia F40.218
Felon — *see also* Cellulitis, digit
  with lymphangitis — *see* Lymphangitis, acute,
    digit
Felty's syndrome M05.00
  ankle M05.07-
  elbow M05.02-
  foot joint M05.07-
  hand joint M05.04-
  hip M05.05-
  knee M05.06-
  multiple site M05.09
  shoulder M05.01-
  vertebra — *see* Spondylitis, ankylosing
  wrist M05.03-
Female genital mutilation status (FGM)
  N90.810
  specified NEC N90.818
  type I (clitorectomy status) N90.811
  type II (clitorectomy with excision of labia
    minora status) N90.812
  type III (infibulation status) N90.813
  type IV N90.818
Female genital cutting status — *see* Female
  genital mutilation status (FGM)
Femur, femoral — *see* condition
Fenestration, fenestrated — *see also*
  Imperfect, closure
  aortico-pulmonary Q21.4
  cusps, heart valve NEC Q24.8
    pulmonary Q22.3
  pulmonic cusps Q22.3
Fernell's disease (aortic aneurysm) I71.9
Fertile eunuch syndrome E23.0
Fetid
  breath R19.6
  sweat L75.0
Fetishism F65.0
  transvestic F65.1
Fetus, fetal — *see also* condition
  alcohol syndrome (dysmorphic) Q86.0
  compressus O31.0-
  hydantoin syndrome Q86.1
  lung tissue P28.0
  papyraceous O31.0-
Fever (inanition) (of unknown origin) (persistent)
  (with chills) (with rigor) R50.9
  abortus A23.1
  Aden (dengue) A90
  African tick-borne A68.1
  American
    mountain (tick) A93.2
      spotted A77.0
  aphthous B08.8
  arbovirus, arboviral A94
    hemorrhagic A94
    specified NEC A93.8
  Argentinian hemorrhagic A96.0
  Assam B55.0
  Australian Q A78
  Bangkok hemorrhagic A91
  Barmah forest A92.8
  Bartonella A44.0
  bilious, hemoglobinuric B50.8
  blackwater B50.8
  blister B00.1
  Bolivian hemorrhagic A96.1
  Bonvale dam T73.3
  boutonneuse A77.1
  brain — *see* Encephalitis
  Brazilian purpuric A48.4
  breakbone A90
  Bullis A77.0
  Bunyamwera A92.8

DISEASE INDEX

Fever (inanition) (of unknown origin) (persistent) (with chills) (with rigor) R50.9 — *continued*
- Burdwan B55.0
- Bwamba A92.8
- Cameroon — *see* Malaria
- Canton A75.9
- catarrhal (acute) J00
  - chronic J31.0
- cat-scratch A28.1
- Central Asian hemorrhagic A98.0
- cerebral — *see* Encephalitis
- cerebrospinal meningococcal A39.0
- Chagres B50.9
- Chandipura A92.8
- Changuinola A93.1
- Charcot's (biliary) (hepatic) (intermittent) — *see* Calculus, bile duct
- Chikungunya (viral) (hemorrhagic) A92.0
- Chitral A93.1
- Colombo — *see* Fever, paratyphoid
- Colorado tick (virus) A93.2
- congestive (remittent) — *see* Malaria
- Congo virus A98.0
- continued malarial B50.9
- Corsican — *see* Malaria
- Crimean-Congo hemorrhagic A98.0
- Cyprus — *see* Brucellosis
- dandy A90
- deer fly — *see* Tularemia
- dengue (virus) A90
  - hemorrhagic A91
  - sandfly A93.1
- desert B38.0
- drug induced R50.2
- due to
  - conditions classified elsewhere R50.81
  - heat T67.0
- enteric A01.00
- enteroviral exanthematous (Boston exanthem) A88.0
- ephemeral (of unknown origin) R50.9
- epidemic hemorrhagic A98.5
- erysipelatous — *see* Erysipelas
- estivo-autumnal (malarial) B50.9
- famine A75.0
- five day A79.0
- following delivery O86.4
- Fort Bragg A27.89
- gastroenteric A01.00
- gastromalarial — *see* Malaria
- Gibraltar — *see* Brucellosis
- glandular — *see* Mononucleosis, infectious
- Guama (viral) A92.8
- Haverhill A25.1
- hay (allergic) J30.1
  - with asthma (bronchial) J45.909
    - with
      - exacerbation (acute) J45.901
      - status asthmaticus J45.902
    - due to
      - allergen other than pollen J30.89
      - pollen, any plant or tree J30.1
- heat (effects) T67.0
- hematuric, bilious B50.8
- hemoglobinuric (malarial) (bilious) B50.8
- hemorrhagic (arthropod-borne) NOS A94
  - with renal syndrome A98.5
  - arenaviral A96.9
    - specified NEC A96.8
  - Argentinian A96.0
  - Bangkok A91
  - Bolivian A96.1
  - Central Asian A98.0
  - Chikungunya A92.0
  - Crimean-Congo A98.0
  - dengue (virus) A91
  - epidemic A98.5
  - Junin (virus) A96.0

Fever (inanition) (of unknown origin) (persistent) (with chills) (with rigor) R50.9 — *continued*
- hemorrhagic (arthropod-borne) NOS A94 — *continued*
  - Korean A98.5
  - Kyasanur forest A98.2
  - Machupo (virus) A96.1
  - mite-borne A93.8
  - mosquito-borne A92.8
  - Omsk A98.1
  - Philippine A91
  - Russian A98.5
  - Singapore A91
  - Southeast Asia A91
  - Thailand A91
  - tick-borne NEC A93.8
  - viral A99
    - specified NEC A98.8
- hepatic — *see* Cholecystitis
- herpetic — *see* Herpes
- icterohemorrhagic A27.0
- Indiana A93.8
- infective B99.9
  - specified NEC B99.8
- intermittent (bilious) — *see also* Malaria
  - of unknown origin R50.9
  - pernicious B50.9
- iodide R50.2
- Japanese river A75.3
- jungle — *see also* Malaria
  - yellow A95.0
- Junin (virus) hemorrhagic A96.0
- Katayama B65.2
- kedani A75.3
- Kenya (tick) A77.1
- Kew Garden A79.1
- Korean hemorrhagic A98.5
- Lassa A96.2
- Lone Star A77.0
- Machupo (virus) hemorrhagic A96.1
- malaria, malarial — *see* Malaria
- Malta A23.9
- Marseilles A77.1
- marsh — *see* Malaria
- Mayaro (viral) A92.8
- Mediterranean (*see also* Brucellosis) A23.9
  - familial M04.1
  - tick A77.1
- meningeal — *see* Meningitis
- Meuse A79.0
- Mexican A75.2
- mianeh A68.1
- miasmatic — *see* Malaria
- mosquito-borne (viral) A92.9
  - hemorrhagic A92.8
- mountain — *see also* Brucellosis
  - meaning Rocky Mountain spotted fever A77.0
  - tick (American) (Colorado) (viral) A93.2
- Mucambo (viral) A92.8
- mud A27.9
- Neapolitan — *see* Brucellosis
- neutropenic D70.9
- newborn P81.9
  - environmental P81.0
- Nine-Mile A78
- non-exanthematous tick A93.2
- North Asian tick-borne A77.2
- O'nyong-nyong (viral) A92.1
- Omsk hemorrhagic A98.1
- Oropouche (viral) A93.0
- Oroya A44.0
- paludal — *see* Malaria
- Panama (malarial) B50.9
- Pappataci A93.1
- paratyphoid A01.4
  - A A01.1
  - B A01.2
  - C A01.3

Fever (inanition) (of unknown origin) (persistent) (with chills) (with rigor) R50.9 — *continued*
- parrot A70
- periodic (Mediterranean) M04.1
- persistent (of unknown origin) R50.9
- petechial A39.0
- pharyngoconjunctival B30.2
- Philippine hemorrhagic A91
- phlebotomus A93.1
- Piry (virus) A93.8
- Pixuna (viral) A92.8
- Plasmodium ovale B53.0
- polioviral (nonparalytic) A80.4
- Pontiac A48.2
- postimmunization R50.83
- postoperative R50.82
  - due to infection T81.40
- posttransfusion R50.84
- postvaccination R50.83
- presenting with conditions classified elsewhere R50.81
- pretibial A27.89
- puerperal O86.4
- Q A78
- quadrilateral A78
- quartan (malaria) B52.9
- Queensland (coastal) (tick) A77.3
- quintan A79.0
- rabbit — *see* Tularemia
- rat-bite A25.9
  - due to
    - Spirillum A25.0
    - Streptobacillus moniliformis A25.1
- recurrent — *see* Fever, relapsing
- relapsing (Borrelia) A68.9
  - Carter's (Asiatic) A68.1
  - Dutton's (West African) A68.1
  - Koch's A68.9
  - louse-borne A68.0
  - Novy's
    - louse-borne A68.0
    - tick-borne A68.1
  - Obermeyer's (European) A68.0
  - tick-borne A68.1
- remittent (bilious) (congestive) (gastric) — *see* Malaria
- rheumatic (active) (acute) (chronic) (subacute) I00
  - with central nervous system involvement I02.9
  - active with heart involvement — *see* category I01
  - inactive or quiescent with
    - cardiac hypertrophy I09.89
    - carditis I09.9
    - endocarditis I09.1
      - aortic (valve) I06.9
        - with mitral (valve) disease I08.0
      - mitral (valve) I05.9
        - with aortic (valve) disease I08.0
      - pulmonary (valve) I09.89
      - tricuspid (valve) I07.8
    - heart disease NEC I09.89
    - heart failure (congestive) (conditions in I50.9) I09.81
    - left ventricular failure (conditions in I50.1) I09.81
    - myocarditis, myocardial degeneration (conditions in I51.4) I09.0
    - pancarditis I09.9
    - pericarditis I09.2
- Rift Valley (viral) A92.4
- Rocky Mountain spotted A77.0
- rose J30.1
- Ross River B33.1
- Russian hemorrhagic A98.5
- San Joaquin (Valley) B38.0
- sandfly A93.1
- Sao Paulo A77.0

Fever (inanition) (of unknown origin) (persistent) (with chills) (with rigor) R50.9 — *continued*
  scarlet A38.9
  seven day (leptospirosis) (autumnal) (Japanese) A27.89
  dengue A90
  shin-bone A79.0
  Singapore hemorrhagic A91
  solar A90
  Songo A98.5
  sore B00.1
  South African tick-bite A68.1
  Southeast Asia hemorrhagic A91
  spinal — *see* Meningitis
  spirillary A25.0
  splenic — *see* Anthrax
  spotted A77.9
    American A77.0
    Brazilian A77.0
    cerebrospinal meningitis A39.0
    Colombian A77.0
    due to Rickettsia
      australis A77.3
      conorii A77.1
      rickettsii A77.0
      sibirica A77.2
      specified type NEC A77.8
    Ehrlichiosis A77.40
      due to
        E. chafeensis A77.41
        specified organism NEC A77.49
    Rocky Mountain A77.0
  steroid R50.2
  streptobacillary A25.1
  subtertian B50.9
  Sumatran mite A75.3
  sun A90
  swamp A27.9
  swine A02.8
  sylvatic, yellow A95.0
  Tahyna B33.8
  tertian — *see* Malaria, tertian
  Thailand hemorrhagic A91
  thermic T67.0
  three-day A93.1
  tick
    American mountain A93.2
    Colorado A93.2
    Kemerovo A93.8
    Mediterranean A77.1
    mountain A93.2
    nonexanthematous A93.2
    Quaranfil A93.8
  tick-bite NEC A93.8
  tick-borne (hemorrhagic) NEC A93.8
  trench A79.0
  tsutsugamushi A75.3
  typhogastric A01.00
  typhoid (abortive) (hemorrhagic) (intermittent) (malignant) A01.00
    complicated by
      arthritis A01.04
      heart involvement A01.02
      meningitis A01.01
      osteomyelitis A01.05
      pneumonia A01.03
      specified NEC A01.09
  typhomalarial — *see* Malaria
  typhus — *see* Typhus (fever)
  undulant — *see* Brucellosis
  unknown origin R50.9
  uveoparotid D86.89
  valley B38.0
  Venezuelan equine A92.2
  vesicular stomatitis A93.8
  viral hemorrhagic — *see* Fever, hemorrhagic, by type of virus
  Volhynian A79.0
  Wesselsbron (viral) A92.8

Fever (inanition) (of unknown origin) (persistent) (with chills) (with rigor) R50.9 — *continued*
  West
    African B50.8
    Nile (viral) A92.30
      with
        complications NEC A92.39
        cranial nerve disorders A92.32
        encephalitis A92.31
        encephalomyelitis A92.31
        neurologic manifestation NEC A92.32
        optic neuritis A92.32
        polyradiculitis A92.32
  Whitmore's — *see* Melioidosis
  Wolhynian A79.0
  worm B83.9
  yellow A95.9
    jungle A95.0
    sylvatic A95.0
    urban A95.1
  Zika virus A92.5
Fibrillation
  atrial or auricular (established) I48.91
    chronic I48.2
    paroxysmal I48.0
    permanent I48.2
    persistent I48.1
  cardiac I49.8
  heart I49.8
  muscular M62.89
  ventricular I49.01
Fibrin
  ball or bodies, pleural (sac) J94.1
  chamber, anterior (eye) (gelatinous exudate) — *see* Iridocyclitis, acute
Fibrinogenolysis — *see* Fibrinolysis
Fibrinogenopenia D68.8
  acquired D65
  congenital D68.2
Fibrinolysis (hemorrhagic) (acquired) D65
  antepartum hemorrhage — *see* Hemorrhage, antepartum, with coagulation defect
  following
    abortion — *see* Abortion by type
      complicated by hemorrhage
    ectopic or molar pregnancy O08.1
  intrapartum O67.0
  newborn, transient P60
  postpartum O72.3
Fibrinopenia (hereditary) D68.2
  acquired D68.4
Fibrinopurulent — *see* condition
Fibrinous — *see* condition
Fibroadenoma
  cellular intracanicular D24-
  giant D24-
  intracanalicular
    cellular D24-
    giant D24-
    specified site — *see* Neoplasm, benign, by site
    unspecified site D24-
  juvenile D24-
  pericanalicular
    specified site — *see* Neoplasm, benign, by site
    unspecified site D24-
  phyllodes D24-
  prostate D29.1
  specified site NEC — *see* Neoplasm, benign, by site
  unspecified site D24-
Fibroadenosis, breast (chronic) (cystic) (diffuse) (periodic) (segmental) N60.2-
Fibroangioma — *see also* Neoplasm, benign, by site
  juvenile
    specified site — *see* Neoplasm, benign, by site
    unspecified site D10.6

Fibrochondrosarcoma — *see* Neoplasm, cartilage, malignant
Fibrocystic
  disease — *see also* Fibrosis, cystic
    breast — *see* Mastopathy, cystic
    jaw M27.49
    kidney (congenital) Q61.8
    liver Q44.6
    pancreas E84.9
  kidney (congenital) Q61.8
Fibrodysplasia ossificans progressiva — *see* Myositis, ossificans, progressiva
Fibroelastosis (cordis) (endocardial) (endomyocardial) I42.4
Fibroid (tumor) — *see also* Neoplasm, connective tissue, benign
  disease, lung (chronic) — *see* Fibrosis, lung
  heart (disease) — *see* Myocarditis
  in pregnancy or childbirth O34.1-
    causing obstructed labor O65.5
  induration, lung (chronic) — *see* Fibrosis, lung
  lung — *see* Fibrosis, lung
  pneumonia (chronic) — *see* Fibrosis, lung
  uterus D25.9
Fibrolipoma — *see* Lipoma
Fibroliposarcoma — *see* Neoplasm, connective tissue, malignant
Fibroma — *see also* Neoplasm, connective tissue, benign
  ameloblastic — *see* Cyst, calcifying odontogenic
  bone (nonossifying) — *see* Disorder, bone, specified type NEC
    ossifying — *see* Neoplasm, bone, benign
  cementifying — *see* Neoplasm, bone, benign
  chondromyxoid — *see* Neoplasm, bone, benign
  desmoplastic — *see* Neoplasm, connective tissue, uncertain behavior
  durum — *see* Neoplasm, connective tissue, benign
  fascial — *see* Neoplasm, connective tissue, benign
  invasive — *see* Neoplasm, connective tissue, uncertain behavior
  molle — *see* Lipoma
  myxoid — *see* Neoplasm, connective tissue, benign
  nasopharynx, nasopharyngeal (juvenile) D10.6
  nonosteogenic (nonossifying) — *see* Dysplasia, fibrous
  odontogenic (central) — *see* Cyst, calcifying odontogenic
  ossifying — *see* Neoplasm, bone, benign
  periosteal — *see* Neoplasm, bone, benign
  soft — *see* Lipoma
Fibromatosis M72.9
  abdominal — *see* Neoplasm, connective tissue, uncertain behavior
  aggressive — *see* Neoplasm, connective tissue, uncertain behavior
  congenital generalized — *see* Neoplasm, connective tissue, uncertain behavior
  Dupuytren's M72.0
  gingival K06.1
  palmar (fascial) M72.0
  plantar (fascial) M72.2
  pseudosarcomatous (proliferative) (subcutaneous) M72.4
  retroperitoneal D48.3
  specified NEC M72.8
Fibromyalgia M79.7
Fibromyoma — *see also* Neoplasm, connective tissue, benign
  uterus (corpus) — *see also* Leiomyoma, uterus
    in pregnancy or childbirth — *see* Fibroid, in pregnancy or childbirth
      causing obstructed labor O65.5

DISEASE INDEX

Fibromyositis M79.7
Fibromyxolipoma D17.9
Fibromyxoma — *see* Neoplasm, connective tissue, benign
Fibromyxosarcoma — *see* Neoplasm, connective tissue, malignant
Fibro-odontoma, ameloblastic — *see* Cyst, calcifying odontogenic
Fibro-osteoma — *see* Neoplasm, bone, benign
Fibroplasia, retrolental H35.17-
Fibropurulent — *see* condition
Fibrosarcoma — *see also* Neoplasm, connective tissue, malignant
  ameloblastic C41.1
    upper jaw (bone) C41.0
  congenital — *see* Neoplasm, connective tissue, malignant
  fascial — *see* Neoplasm, connective tissue, malignant
  infantile — *see* Neoplasm, connective tissue, malignant
  odontogenic C41.1
    upper jaw (bone) C41.0
  periosteal — *see* Neoplasm, bone, malignant
Fibrosclerosis
  breast N60.3-
  multifocal M35.5
  penis (corpora cavernosa) N48.6
Fibrosis, fibrotic
  adrenal (gland) E27.8
  amnion O41.8x-
  anal papillae K62.89
  arteriocapillary — *see* Arteriosclerosis
  bladder N32.89
    interstitial — *see* Cystitis, chronic, interstitial
    localized submucosal — *see* Cystitis, chronic, interstitial
    panmural — *see* Cystitis, chronic, interstitial
  breast — *see* Fibrosclerosis, breast
  capillary (*see also* Arteriosclerosis) I70.90
    lung (chronic) — *see* Fibrosis, lung
  cardiac — *see* Myocarditis
  cervix N88.8
  chorion O41.8x-
  corpus cavernosum (sclerosing) N48.6
  cystic (of pancreas) E84.9
    with
      distal intestinal obstruction syndrome E84.19
      fecal impaction E84.19
      intestinal manifestations NEC E84.19
      pulmonary manifestations E84.0
      specified manifestations NEC E84.8
  due to device, implant or graft (*see also* Complications, by site and type, specified NEC) T85.828
    arterial graft NEC T82.828
    breast (implant) T85.828
    catheter NEC T85.828
      dialysis (renal) T82.828
        intraperitoneal T85.828
      infusion NEC T82.828
        spinal (epidural) (subdural) T85.820
      urinary (indwelling) T83.82
    electronic (electrode) (pulse generator) (stimulator)
      bone T84.82
      cardiac T82.827
      nervous system (brain) (peripheral nerve) (spinal) T85.820
      urinary T83.82
    fixation, internal (orthopedic) NEC T84.82
    gastrointestinal (bile duct) (esophagus) T85.828
    genital NEC T83.82
    heart NEC T82.827
    joint prosthesis T84.82

Fibrosis, fibrotic — *continued*
  due to device, implant or graft (*see also* Complications, by site and type, specified NEC) T85.82 — *continued*
    ocular (corneal graft) (orbital implant) NEC T85.828
    orthopedic NEC T84.82
    specified NEC T85.828
    urinary NEC T83.82
    vascular NEC T82.828
    ventricular intracranial shunt T85.820
  ejaculatory duct N50.89
  endocardium — *see* Endocarditis
  endomyocardial (tropical) I42.3
  epididymis N50.89
  eye muscle — *see* Strabismus, mechanical
  heart — *see* Myocarditis
  hepatic — *see* Fibrosis, liver
  hepatolienal (portal hypertension) K76.6
  hepatosplenic (portal hypertension) K76.6
  infrapatellar fat pad M79.4
  intrascrotal N50.89
  kidney N26.9
  liver K74.0
    with sclerosis K74.2
    alcoholic K70.2
  lung (atrophic) (chronic) (confluent) (massive) (perialveolar) (peribronchial) J84.10
    with
      anthracosilicosis J60
      anthracosis J60
      asbestosis J61
      bagassosis J67.1
      bauxite J63.1
      berylliosis J63.2
      byssinosis J66.0
      calcicosis J62.8
      chalicosis J62.8
      dust reticulation J64
      farmer's lung J67.0
      ganister disease J62.8
      graphite J63.3
      pneumoconiosis NOS J64
      siderosis J63.4
      silicosis J62.8
    capillary J84.10
    congenital P27.8
    diffuse (idiopathic) J84.10
      chemicals, gases, fumes or vapors (inhalation) J68.4
    interstitial J84.10
      acute J84.114
      talc J62.0
    following radiation J70.1
    idiopathic J84.112
    postinflammatory J84.10
    silicotic J62.8
    tuberculous — *see* Tuberculosis, pulmonary
  lymphatic gland I89.8
  median bar — *see* Hyperplasia, prostate
  mediastinum (idiopathic) J98.59
  meninges G96.19
  myocardium, myocardial — *see* Myocarditis
  ovary N83.8
  oviduct N83.8
  pancreas K86.89
  penis NEC N48.6
  pericardium I31.0
  perineum, in pregnancy or childbirth O34.7-
    causing obstructed labor O65.5
  pleura J94.1
  popliteal fat pad M79.4
  prostate (chronic) — *see* Hyperplasia, prostate
  pulmonary (*see also* Fibrosis, lung) J84.10
    congenital P27.8
    idiopathic J84.112
  rectal sphincter K62.89

Fibrosis, fibrotic — *continued*
  retroperitoneal, idiopathic (with ureteral obstruction) N13.5
    with infection N13.6
  sclerosing mesenteric (idiopathic) K65.4
  scrotum N50.89
  seminal vesicle N50.89
  senile R54
  skin L90.5
  spermatic cord N50.89
  spleen D73.89
    in schistosomiasis (bilharziasis) B65.9 *[D77]*
  subepidermal nodular — *see* Neoplasm, skin, benign
  submucous (oral) (tongue) K13.5
  testis N44.8
    chronic, due to syphilis A52.76
  thymus (gland) E32.8
  tongue, submucous K13.5
  tunica vaginalis N50.89
  uterus (non-neoplastic) N85.8
  vagina N89.8
  valve, heart — *see* Endocarditis
  vas deferens N50.89
  vein I87.8
Fibrositis (periarticular) M79.7
  nodular, chronic (Jaccoud's) (rheumatoid) — *see* Arthropathy, postrheumatic, chronic
Fibrothorax J94.1
Fibrotic — *see* Fibrosis
Fibrous — *see* condition
Fibroxanthoma — *see also* Neoplasm, connective tissue, benign
  atypical — *see* Neoplasm, connective tissue, uncertain behavior
  malignant — *see* Neoplasm, connective tissue, malignant
Fibroxanthosarcoma — *see* Neoplasm, connective tissue, malignant
Fiedler's
  disease (icterohemorrhagic leptospirosis) A27.0
  myocarditis (acute) I40.1
Fifth disease B08.3
  venereal A55
Filaria, filarial, filariasis — *see* Infestation, filarial
Filatov's disease — *see* Mononucleosis, infectious
File-cutter's disease — *see* Poisoning, lead
Filling defect
  biliary tract R93.2
  bladder R93.41
  duodenum R93.3
  gallbladder R93.2
  gastrointestinal tract R93.3
  intestine R93.3
  kidney R93.42-
  stomach R93.3
  ureter R93.41
  urinary organs, specified NEC R93.49
Fimbrial cyst Q50.4
Financial problem affecting care NOS Z59.9
  bankruptcy Z59.8
  foreclosure on loan Z59.8
Findings, abnormal, inconclusive, without diagnosis — *see also* Abnormal
  17-ketosteroids, elevated R82.5
  acetonuria R82.4
  alcohol in blood R78.0
  anisocytosis R71.8
  antenatal screening of mother O28.9
    biochemical O28.1
    chromosomal O28.5
    cytological O28.2
    genetic O28.5
    hematological O28.0
    radiological O28.4

Findings, abnormal, inconclusive, without diagnosis (see also Abnormal) — continued
  antenatal screening of mother O28.9 — continued
    specified NEC O28.8
    ultrasonic O28.3
  antibody titer, elevated R76.0
  anticardiolipin antibody R76.0
  antiphosphatidylglycerol antibody R76.0
  antiphosphatidylinositol anitbody R76.0
  antiphosphatidylserine antibody R76.0
  antiphospholipid antibody R76.0
  bacteriuria R82.71
  bicarbonate E87.8
  bile in urine R82.2
  blood sugar R73.09
    high R73.9
    low (transient) E16.2
  body fluid or substance, specified NEC R88.8
  casts, urine R82.99
  catecholamines R82.5
  cells, urine R82.99
  chloride E87.8
  cholesterol E78.9
    high E78.00
      with high triglycerides E78.2
  chyluria R82.0
  cloudy
    dialysis effluent R88.0
    urine R82.90
  creatinine clearance R94.4
  crystals, urine R82.99
  culture
    blood R78.81
    positive — see Positive, culture
  echocardiogram R93.1
  electrolyte level, urinary R82.99
  function study NEC R94.8
    bladder R94.8
    endocrine NEC R94.7
      thyroid R94.6
    kidney R94.4
    liver R94.5
    pancreas R94.8
    placenta R94.8
    pulmonary R94.2
    spleen R94.8
  gallbladder, nonvisualization R93.2
  glucose (tolerance test) (non-fasting) R73.09
  glycosuria R81
  heart
    shadow R93.1
    sounds R01.2
  hematinuria R82.3
  hematocrit drop (precipitous) R71.0
  hemoglobinuria R82.3
  human papillomavirus (HPV) DNA test positive
    cervix
      high risk R87.810
      low risk R87.820
    vagina
      high risk R87.811
      low risk R87.821
  in blood (of substance not normally found in blood) R78.9
    addictive drug NEC R78.4
    alcohol (excessive level) R78.0
    cocaine R78.2
    hallucinogen R78.3
    heavy metals (abnormal level) R78.79
    lead R78.71
    lithium (abnormal level) R78.89
    opiate drug R78.1
    psychotropic drug R78.5
    specified substance NEC R78.89
    steroid agent R78.6
  indoleacetic acid, elevated R82.5
  ketonuria R82.4

Findings, abnormal, inconclusive, without diagnosis (see also Abnormal) — continued
  lactic acid dehydrogenase (LDH) R74.0
  liver function test R79.89
  mammogram NEC R92.8
    calcification (calculus) R92.1
    inconclusive result (due to dense breasts) R92.2
    microcalcification R92.0
  mediastinal shift R93.8
  melanin, urine R82.99
  myoglobinuria R82.1
  neonatal screening P09
  nonvisualization of gallbladder R93.2
  odor of urine NOS R82.90
  Papanicolaou cervix R87.619
    non-atypical endometrial cells R87.618
  pneumoencephalogram R93.0
  poikilocytosis R71.8
  potassium (deficiency) E87.6
    excess E87.5
  PPD R76.11
  radiologic (X-ray) R93.8
    abdomen R93.5
    biliary tract R93.2
    breast R92.8
    gastrointestinal tract R93.3
    genitourinary organs R93.8
    head R93.0
    inconclusive due to excess body fat of patient R93.9
    intrathoracic organs NEC R93.1
    placenta R93.8
    retroperitoneum R93.5
    skin R93.8
    skull R93.0
    subcutaneous tissue R93.8
  red blood cell (count) (morphology) (sickling) (volume) R71.8
  scan NEC R94.8
    bladder R94.8
    bone R94.8
    kidney R94.4
    liver R93.2
    lung R94.2
    pancreas R94.8
    placental R94.8
    spleen R94.8
    thyroid R94.6
  sedimentation rate, elevated R70.0
  SGOT R74.0
  SGPT R74.0
  sodium (deficiency) E87.1
    excess E87.0
  specified body fluid NEC R88.8
  stress test R94.39
  thyroid (function) (metabolic rate) (scan) (uptake) R94.6
  transaminase (level) R74.0
  triglycerides E78.9
    high E78.1
      with high cholesterol E78.2
  tuberculin skin test (without active tuberculosis) R76.11
  urine R82.90
    acetone R82.4
    bacteria R82.71
    bile R82.2
    casts or cells R82.99
    chyle R82.0
    culture positive R82.79
    glucose R81
    hemoglobin R82.3
    ketone R82.4
    sugar R81
  vanillylmandelic acid (VMA), elevated R82.5
  vectorcardiogram (VCG) R94.39
  ventriculogram R93.0

Findings, abnormal, inconclusive, without diagnosis (see also Abnormal) — continued
  white blood cell (count) (differential) (morphology) D72.9
  xerography R92.8
Finger — see condition
Fire, Saint Anthony's — see Erysipelas
Fire-setting
  pathological (compulsive) F63.1
Fish hook stomach K31.89
Fishmeal-worker's lung J67.8
Fissure, fissured
  anus, anal K60.2
    acute K60.0
    chronic K60.1
    congenital Q43.8
  ear, lobule, congenital Q17.8
  epiglottis (congenital) Q31.8
  larynx J38.7
    congenital Q31.8
  lip K13.0
    congenital — see Cleft, lip
  nipple N64.0
    associated with
      lactation O92.13
      pregnancy O92.11-
    puerperium O92.12
  nose Q30.2
  palate (congenital) — see Cleft, palate
  skin R23.4
  spine (congenital) — see also Spina bifida
    with hydrocephalus — see Spina bifida, by site, with hydrocephalus
  tongue (acquired) K14.5
    congenital Q38.3
Fistula (cutaneous) L98.8
  abdomen (wall) K63.2
    bladder N32.2
    intestine NEC K63.2
    ureter N28.89
    uterus N82.5
  abdominorectal K63.2
  abdominosigmoidal K63.2
  abdominothoracic J86.0
  abdominouterine N82.5
    congenital Q51.7
  abdominovesical N32.2
  accessory sinuses — see Sinusitis
  actinomycotic — see Actinomycosis
  alveolar antrum — see Sinusitis, maxillary
  alveolar process K04.6
  anorectal K60.5
  antrobuccal — see Sinusitis, maxillary
  antrum — see Sinusitis, maxillary
  anus, anal (recurrent) (infectional) K60.3
    congenital Q43.6
      with absence, atresia and stenosis Q42.2
    tuberculous A18.32
  aorta-duodenal I77.2
  appendix, appendicular K38.3
  arteriovenous (acquired) (nonruptured) I77.0
    brain I67.1
      congenital Q28.2
        ruptured I60.8
      ruptured I60.8
    cerebral — see Fistula, arteriovenous, brain
    congenital (peripheral) — see also Malformation, arteriovenous
      brain Q28.2
        ruptured I60.8
      coronary Q24.5
      pulmonary Q25.72
    coronary I25.41
      congenital Q24.5
    pulmonary I28.0
      congenital Q25.72

DISEASE INDEX

Fistula (cutaneous) L98.8 — *continued*
arteriovenous (acquired) (nonruptured) I77.0
— *continued*
surgically created (for dialysis) Z99.2
complication — *see* Complication,
arteriovenous, fistula, surgically
created
traumatic — *see* Injury, blood vessel
artery I77.2
aural (mastoid) — *see* Mastoiditis, chronic
auricle — *see also* Disorder, pinna, specified
type NEC
congenital Q18.1
Bartholin's gland N82.8
bile duct (common) (hepatic) K83.3
with calculus, stones — *see* Calculus, bile
duct
biliary (tract) — *see* Fistula, bile duct
bladder (sphincter) NEC (*see also* Fistula,
vesico-) N32.2
into seminal vesicle N32.2
bone — *see also* Disorder, bone, specified type
NEC
with osteomyelitis, chronic — *see*
Osteomyelitis, chronic, with draining
sinus
brain G93.89
arteriovenous (acquired) I67.1
congenital Q28.2
branchial (cleft) Q18.0
branchiogenous Q18.0
breast N61.0
puerperal, postpartum or gestational, due to
mastitis (purulent) — *see* Mastitis,
obstetric, purulent
bronchial J86.0
bronchocutaneous, bronchomediastinal,
bronchopleural, bronchopleuromediastinal
(infective) J86.0
tuberculous NEC A15.5
bronchoesophageal J86.0
congenital Q39.2
with atresia of esophagus Q39.1
bronchovisceral J86.0
buccal cavity (infective) K12.2
cecosigmoidal K63.2
cecum K63.2
cerebrospinal (fluid) G96.0
cervical, lateral Q18.1
cervicoaural Q18.1
cervicosigmoidal N82.4
cervicovesical N82.1
cervix N82.8
chest (wall) J86.0
cholecystenteric — *see* Fistula, gallbladder
cholecystocolic — *see* Fistula, gallbladder
cholecystocolonic — *see* Fistula, gallbladder
cholecystoduodenal — *see* Fistula, gallbladder
cholecystogastric — *see* Fistula, gallbladder
cholecystointestinal — *see* Fistula, gallbladder
choledochoduodenal — *see* Fistula, bile duct
cholocolic K82.3
coccyx — *see* Sinus, pilonidal
colon K63.2
colostomy K94.09
common duct — *see* Fistula, bile duct
congenital, site not listed — *see* Anomaly, by
site
coronary, arteriovenous I25.41
congenital Q24.5
costal region J86.0
cul-de-sac, Douglas' N82.8
cystic duct — *see also* Fistula, gallbladder
congenital Q44.5
dental K04.6
diaphragm J86.0
duodenum K31.6
ear (external) (canal) — *see* Disorder, ear,
external, specified type NEC

Fistula (cutaneous) L98.8 — *continued*
enterocolic K63.2
enterocutaneous K63.2
enterouterine N82.4
congenital Q51.7
enterovaginal N82.4
congenital Q52.2
large intestine N82.3
small intestine N82.2
enterovesical N32.1
epididymis N50.89
tuberculous A18.15
esophagobronchial J86.0
congenital Q39.2
with atresia of esophagus Q39.1
esophagocutaneous K22.8
esophagopleural-cutaneous J86.0
esophagotracheal J86.0
congenital Q39.2
with atresia of esophagus Q39.1
esophagus K22.8
congenital Q39.2
with atresia of esophagus Q39.1
ethmoid — *see* Sinusitis, ethmoidal
eyeball (cornea) (sclera) — *see* Disorder,
globe, hypotony
eyelid H01.8
fallopian tube, external N82.5
fecal K63.2
congenital Q43.6
from periapical abscess K04.6
frontal sinus — *see* Sinusitis, frontal
gallbladder K82.3
with calculus, cholelithiasis, stones — *see*
Calculus, gallbladder
gastric K31.6
gastrocolic K31.6
congenital Q40.2
tuberculous A18.32
gastroenterocolic K31.6
gastroesophageal K31.6
gastrojejunal K31.6
gastrojejunocolic K31.6
genital tract (female) N82.9
specified NEC N82.8
to intestine NEC N82.4
to skin N82.5
hepatic artery-portal vein, congenital Q26.6
hepatopleural J86.0
hepatopulmonary J86.0
ileorectal or ileosigmoidal K63.2
ileovaginal N82.2
ileovesical N32.1
ileum K63.2
in ano K60.3
tuberculous A18.32
inner ear (labyrinth) — *see* subcategory H83.1
intestine NEC K63.2
intestinocolonic (abdominal) K63.2
intestinoureteral N28.89
intestinouterine N82.4
intestinovaginal N82.4
large intestine N82.3
small intestine N82.2
intestinovesical N32.1
ischiorectal (fossa) K61.3
jejunum K63.2
joint M25.10
ankle M25.17-
elbow M25.12-
foot joint M25.17-
hand joint M25.14-
hip M25.15-
knee M25.16-
shoulder M25.11-
specified joint NEC M25.18
tuberculous — *see* Tuberculosis, joint
vertebrae M25.18
wrist M25.13-

Fistula (cutaneous) L98.8 — *continued*
kidney N28.89
labium (majus) (minus) N82.8
labyrinth — *see* subcategory H83.1
lacrimal (gland) (sac) H04.61-
lacrimonasal duct — *see* Fistula, lacrimal
laryngotracheal, congenital Q34.8
larynx J38.7
lip K13.0
congenital Q38.0
lumbar, tuberculous A18.01
lung J86.0
lymphatic I89.8
mammary (gland) N61.0
mastoid (process) (region) — *see* Mastoiditis,
chronic
maxillary J32.0
medial, face and neck Q18.8
mediastinal J86.0
mediastinobronchial J86.0
mediastinocutaneous J86.0
middle ear — *see* subcategory H74.8
mouth K12.2
nasal J34.89
sinus — *see* Sinusitis
nasopharynx J39.2
nipple N64.0
nose J34.89
oral (cutaneous) K12.2
maxillary J32.0
nasal (with cleft palate) — *see* Cleft, palate
orbit, orbital — *see* Disorder, orbit, specified
type NEC
oroantral J32.0
oviduct, external N82.5
palate (hard) M27.8
pancreatic K86.89
pancreaticoduodenal K86.89
parotid (gland) K11.4
region K12.2
penis N48.89
perianal K60.3
pericardium (pleura) (sac) — *see* Pericarditis
pericecal K63.2
perineorectal K60.4
perineosigmoidal K63.2
perineum, perineal (with urethral involvement)
NEC N36.0
tuberculous A18.13
ureter N28.89
perirectal K60.4
tuberculous A18.32
peritoneum K65.9
pharyngoesophageal J39.2
pharynx J39.2
branchial cleft (congenital) Q18.0
pilonidal (infected) (rectum) — *see* Sinus,
pilonidal
pleura, pleural, pleurocutaneous,
pleuroperitoneal J86.0
tuberculous NEC A15.6
pleuropericardial I31.8
portal vein-hepatic artery, congenital Q26.6
postauricular H70.81-
postoperative, persistent T81.83
specified site — *see* Fistula, by site
preauricular (congenital) Q18.1
prostate N42.89
pulmonary J86.0
arteriovenous I28.0
congenital Q25.72
tuberculous — *see* Tuberculosis, pulmonary
pulmonoperitoneal J86.0
rectolabial N82.4
rectosigmoid (intercommunicating) K63.2
rectoureteral N28.89
rectourethral N36.0
congenital Q64.73

Fistula (cutaneous) L98.8 — *continued*
  rectouterine N82.4
    congenital Q51.7
  rectovaginal N82.3
    congenital Q52.2
    tuberculous A18.18
  rectovesical N32.1
    congenital Q64.79
  rectovesicovaginal N82.3
  rectovulval N82.4
    congenital Q52.79
  rectum (to skin) K60.4
    congenital Q43.6
      with absence, atresia and stenosis Q42.0
    tuberculous A18.32
  renal N28.89
  retroauricular — *see* Fistula, postauricular
  salivary duct or gland (any) K11.4
    congenital Q38.4
  scrotum (urinary) N50.89
    tuberculous A18.15
  semicircular canals — *see* subcategory H83.1
  sigmoid K63.2
    to bladder N32.1
  sinus — *see* Sinusitis
  skin L98.8
    to genital tract (female) N82.5
  splenocolic D73.89
  stercoral K63.2
  stomach K31.6
  sublingual gland K11.4
  submandibular gland K11.4
  submaxillary (gland) K11.4
    region K12.2
  thoracic J86.0
    duct I89.8
  thoracoabdominal J86.0
  thoracogastric J86.0
  thoracointestinal J86.0
  thorax J86.0
  thyroglossal duct Q89.2
  thyroid E07.89
  trachea, congenital (external) (internal) Q32.1
  tracheoesophageal J86.0
    congenital Q39.2
      with atresia of esophagus Q39.1
    following tracheostomy J95.04
  traumatic arteriovenous — *see* Injury, blood vessel, by site
  tuberculous — *code by* site under Tuberculosis
  typhoid A01.09
  umbilicourinary Q64.8
  urachus, congenital Q64.4
  ureter (persistent) N28.89
  ureteroabdominal N28.89
  ureterorectal N28.89
  ureterosigmoido-abdominal N28.89
  ureterovaginal N82.1
  ureterovesical N32.2
  urethra N36.0
    congenital Q64.79
    tuberculous A18.13
  urethroperineal N36.0
  urethroperineovesical N32.2
  urethrorectal N36.0
    congenital Q64.73
  urethroscrotal N50.89
  urethrovaginal N82.1
  urethrovesical N32.2
  urinary (tract) (persistent) (recurrent) N36.0
  uteroabdominal N82.5
    congenital Q51.7
  uteroenteric, uterointestinal N82.4
    congenital Q51.7
  uterorectal N82.4
    congenital Q51.7
  uteroureteric N82.1
  uterourethral Q51.7
  uterovaginal N82.8

Fistula (cutaneous) L98.8 — *continued*
  uterovesical N82.1
    congenital Q51.7
  uterus N82.8
  vagina (postpartal) (wall) N82.8
  vaginocutaneous (postpartal) N82.5
  vaginointestinal NEC N82.4
    large intestine N82.3
    small intestine N82.2
  vaginoperineal N82.5
  vasocutaneous, congenital Q55.7
  vesical NEC N32.2
  vesicoabdominal N32.2
  vesicocervicovaginal N82.1
  vesicocolic N32.1
  vesicocutaneous N32.2
  vesicoenteric N32.1
  vesicointestinal N32.1
  vesicometrorectal N82.4
  vesicoperineal N32.2
  vesicorectal N32.1
    congenital Q64.79
  vesicosigmoidal N32.1
  vesicosigmoidovaginal N82.3
  vesicoureteral N32.2
  vesicoureterovaginal N82.1
  vesicourethral N32.2
  vesicourethrorectal N32.1
  vesicouterine N82.1
    congenital Q51.7
  vesicovaginal N82.0
  vulvorectal N82.4
    congenital Q52.79

Fit R56.9
  epileptic — *see* Epilepsy
  fainting R55
  hysterical F44.5
  newborn P90

Fitting (and adjustment) (of)
  artificial
    arm — *see* Admission, adjustment, artificial, arm
    breast Z44.3
    eye Z44.2
    leg — *see* Admission, adjustment, artificial, leg
  automatic implantable cardiac defibrillator (with synchronous cardiac pacemaker) Z45.02
  brain neuropacemaker Z46.2
    implanted Z45.42
  cardiac defibrillator — *see* Fitting (and adjustment) (of), automatic implantable cardiac defibrillator
  catheter, non-vascular Z46.82
  colostomy belt Z46.89
  contact lenses Z46.0
  CRT-D (resynchronization therapy defibrillator) Z45.02
  CRT-P (cardiac resynchronization therapy pacemaker) Z45.018
    pulse generator Z45.010
  cystostomy device Z46.6
  defibrillator, cardiac — *see* Fitting (and adjustment) (of), automatic implantable cardiac defibrillator
  dentures Z46.3
  device NOS Z46.9
    abdominal Z46.89
    gastrointestinal NEC Z46.59
    implanted NEC Z45.89
    nervous system Z46.2
      implanted — *see* Admission, adjustment, device, implanted, nervous system
    orthodontic Z46.4
    orthoptic Z46.0
    orthotic Z46.89

Fitting (and adjustment) (of) — *continued*
  device NOS Z46.9 — *continued*
    prosthetic (external) Z44.9
      breast Z44.3
      dental Z46.3
      eye Z44.2
      specified NEC Z44.8
    specified NEC Z46.89
    substitution
      auditory Z46.2
        implanted — *see* Admission, adjustment, device, implanted, hearing device
      nervous system Z46.2
        implanted — *see* Admission, adjustment, device, implanted, nervous system
      visual Z46.2
        implanted Z45.31
      urinary Z46.6
  gastric lap band Z46.51
  gastrointestinal appliance NEC Z46.59
  glasses (reading) Z46.0
  hearing aid Z46.1
  ileostomy device Z46.89
  insulin pump Z46.81
  intestinal appliance NEC Z46.89
  myringotomy device (stent) (tube) Z45.82
  neuropacemaker Z46.2
    implanted Z45.42
  non-vascular catheter Z46.82
  orthodontic device Z46.4
  orthopedic device (brace) (cast) (corset) (shoes) Z46.89
  pacemaker (cardiac) (cardiac resynchronization therapy (CRT-P)) Z45.018
    nervous system (brain) (peripheral nerve) (spinal cord) Z46.2
      implanted Z45.42
    pulse generator Z45.010
  portacath (port-a-cath) Z45.2
  prosthesis (external) Z44.9
    arm — *see* Admission, adjustment, artificial, arm
    breast Z44.3
    dental Z46.3
    eye Z44.2
    leg — *see* Admission, adjustment, artificial, leg
    specified NEC Z44.8
  spectacles Z46.0
  wheelchair Z46.89

Fitz's syndrome (acute hemorrhagic pancreatitis) (*see also* Pancreatitis, acute) K85.80

Fitzhugh-Curtis syndrome
  due to
    Chlamydia trachomatis A74.81
    Neisseria gonorrhorea (gonococcal peritonitis) A54.85

Fixation
  joint — *see* Ankylosis
  larynx J38.7
  stapes — *see* Ankylosis, ear ossicles
    deafness — *see* Deafness, conductive
  uterus (acquired) — *see* Malposition, uterus
  vocal cord J38.3

Flabby ridge K06.8

Flaccid — *see also* condition
  palate, congenital Q38.5

Flail
  chest S22.5
    newborn (birth injury) P13.8
  joint (paralytic) M25.20
    ankle M25.27-
    elbow M25.22-
    foot joint M25.27-
    hand joint M25.24-
    hip M25.25-

Flail — *continued*
  joint (paralytic) M25.20 — *continued*
    knee M25.26-
    shoulder M25.21-
    specified joint NEC M25.28
    wrist M25.23-
Flajani's disease — *see* Hyperthyroidism, with, goiter (diffuse)
Flap, liver K71.3
Flashbacks (residual to hallucinogen use) F16.283
Flat
  chamber (eye) — *see* Disorder, globe, hypotony, flat anterior chamber
  chest, congenital Q67.8
  foot (acquired) (fixed type) (painful) (postural) — *see also* Deformity, limb, flat foot
    congenital (rigid) (spastic (everted)) Q66.5-
    rachitic sequelae (late effect) E64.3
  organ or site, congenital NEC — *see* Anomaly, by site
  pelvis M95.5
    with disproportion (fetopelvic) O33.0
      causing obstructed labor O65.0
    congenital Q74.2
Flatau-Schilder disease G37.0
Flatback syndrome M40.30
  lumbar region M40.36
  lumbosacral region M40.37
  thoracolumbar region M40.35
Flattening
  head, femur M89.8x5
  hip — *see* Coxa, plana
  lip (congenital) Q18.8
  nose (congenital) Q67.4
    acquired M95.0
Flatulence R14.3
  psychogenic F45.8
Flatus R14.3
  vaginalis N89.8
Flax-dresser's disease J66.1
Flea bite — *see* Injury, bite, by site, superficial, insect
Flecks, glaucomatous (subcapsular) — *see* Cataract, complicated
Fleischer(-Kayser) ring (cornea) H18.04-
Fleshy mole O02.0
Flexibilitas cerea — *see* Catalepsy
Flexion
  amputation stump (surgical) T87.89
  cervix — *see* Malposition, uterus
  contracture, joint — *see* Contraction, joint
  deformity, joint (*see also* Deformity, limb, flexion) M21.20
  hip, congenital Q65.89
  uterus — *see also* Malposition, uterus
    lateral — *see* Lateroversion, uterus
Flexner's dysentery A03.1
Flexner-Boyd dysentery A03.2
Flexure — *see* Flexion
Flint murmur (aortic insufficiency) I35.1
Floater, vitreous — *see* Opacity, vitreous
Floating
  cartilage (joint) — *see also* Loose, body, joint
    knee — *see* Derangement, knee, loose body
  gallbladder, congenital Q44.1
  kidney N28.89
    congenital Q63.8
  spleen D73.89
Flooding N92.0
Floor — *see* condition
Floppy
  baby syndrome (nonspecific) P94.2
  iris syndrome (intraoperative) (IFIS) H21.81
  nonrheumatic mitral valve syndrome I34.1

Flu — *see also* Influenza
  avian (*see also* Influenza, due to, identified novel influenza A virus) J09.x2
  bird (*see also* Influenza, due to, identified novel influenza A virus) J09.x2
  intestinal NEC A08.4
  swine (viruses that normally cause infections in pigs) (*see also* Influenza, due to, identified novel influenza A virus) J09.x2
Fluctuating blood pressure I99.8
Fluid
  abdomen R18.8
  chest J94.8
  heart — *see* Failure, heart, congestive
  joint — *see* Effusion, joint
  loss (acute) E86.9
  lung — *see* Edema, lung
  overload E87.70
    specified NEC E87.79
  peritoneal cavity R18.8
  pleural cavity J94.8
  retention R60.9
Flukes NEC — *see also* Infestation, fluke
  blood NEC — *see* Schistosomiasis
  liver B66.3
Fluor (vaginalis) N89.8
  trichomonal or due to Trichomonas (vaginalis) A59.00
Fluorosis
  dental K00.3
  skeletal M85.10
    ankle M85.17-
    foot M85.17-
    forearm M85.13-
    hand M85.14-
    lower leg M85.16-
    multiple site M85.19
    neck M85.18
    rib M85.18
    shoulder M85.11-
    skull M85.18
    specified site NEC M85.18
    thigh M85.15-
    toe M85.17-
    upper arm M85.12-
    vertebra M85.18
Flush syndrome E34.0
Flushing R23.2
  menopausal N95.1
Flutter
  atrial or auricular I48.92
    atypical I48.4
    type I I48.3
    type II I48.4
    typical I48.3
  heart I49.8
    atrial or auricular I48.92
      atypical I48.4
      type I I48.3
      type II I48.4
      typical I48.3
    ventricular I49.02
  ventricular I49.02
FNHTR (febrile nonhemolytic transfusion reaction) R50.84
Fochier's abscess — *code by* site under Abscess
Focus, Assmann's — *see* Tuberculosis, pulmonary
Fogo selvagem L10.3
Foix-Alajouanine syndrome G95.19
Fold, folds (anomalous) — *see also* Anomaly, by site
  Descemet's membrane — *see* Change, corneal membrane, Descemet's, fold
  epicanthic Q10.3
  heart Q24.8

Folie à deux F24
Follicle
  cervix (nabothian) (ruptured) N88.8
  graafian, ruptured, with hemorrhage N83.0-
  nabothian N88.8
Follicular — *see* condition
Folliculitis (superficial) L73.9
  abscedens et suffodiens L66.3
  cyst N83.0-
  decalvans L66.2
  deep — *see* Furuncle, by site
  gonococcal (acute) (chronic) A54.01
  keloid, keloidalis L73.0
  pustular L01.02
  ulerythematosa reticulata L66.4
Folliculome lipidique
  specified site — *see* Neoplasm, benign, by site
  unspecified site
    female D27.9
    male D29.20
Følling's disease E70.0
Follow-up — *see* Examination, follow-up
Fong's syndrome (hereditary osteo-onychodysplasia) Q87.2
Food
  allergy L27.2
  asphyxia (from aspiration or inhalation) — *see* Foreign body, by site
  choked on — *see* Foreign body, by site
  deprivation T73.0
    specified kind of food NEC E63.8
  intoxication — *see* Poisoning, food
  lack of T73.0
  poisoning — *see* Poisoning, food
  rejection NEC — *see* Disorder, eating
  strangulation or suffocation — *see* Foreign body, by site
  toxemia — *see* Poisoning, food
Foot — *see* condition
Foramen ovale (nonclosure) (patent) (persistent) Q21.1
Forbes' glycogen storage disease E74.03
Fordyce's disease (mouth) Q38.6
Fordyce-Fox disease L75.2
Forearm — *see* condition
Foreign body
  with
    laceration — *see* Laceration, by site, with foreign body
    puncture wound — *see* Puncture, by site, with foreign body
  accidentally left following a procedure T81.509
    aspiration T81.506
      resulting in
        adhesions T81.516
        obstruction T81.526
        perforation T81.536
        specified complication NEC T81.596
    cardiac catheterization T81.505
      resulting in
        acute reaction T81.60
          aseptic peritonitis T81.61
          specified NEC T81.69
        adhesions T81.515
        obstruction T81.525
        perforation T81.535
        specified complication NEC T81.595
    causing
      acute reaction T81.60
        aseptic peritonitis T81.61
        specified complication NEC T81.69
      adhesions T81.519
      aseptic peritonitis T81.61
      obstruction T81.529
      perforation T81.539
      specified complication NEC T81.599

DISEASE INDEX

Foreign body — *continued*
  accidentally left following a procedure
      T81.509 — *continued*
    endoscopy T81.504
      resulting in
        adhesions T81.514
        obstruction T81.524
        perforation T81.534
        specified complication NEC T81.594
    immunization T81.503
      resulting in
        adhesions T81.513
        obstruction T81.523
        perforation T81.533
        specified complication NEC T81.593
    infusion T81.501
      resulting in
        adhesions T81.511
        obstruction T81.521
        perforation T81.531
        specified complication NEC T81.591
    injection T81.503
      resulting in
        adhesions T81.513
        obstruction T81.523
        perforation T81.533
        specified complication NEC T81.593
    kidney dialysis T81.502
      resulting in
        adhesions T81.512
        obstruction T81.522
        perforation T81.532
        specified complication NEC T81.592
    packing removal T81.507
      resulting in
        acute reaction T81.60
          aseptic peritonitis T81.61
          specified NEC T81.69
        adhesions T81.517
        obstruction T81.527
        perforation T81.537
        specified complication NEC T81.597
    puncture T81.506
      resulting in
        adhesions T81.516
        obstruction T81.526
        perforation T81.536
        specified complication NEC T81.596
    specified procedure NEC T81.508
      resulting in
        acute reaction T81.60
          aseptic peritonitis T81.61
          specified NEC T81.69
        adhesions T81.518
        obstruction T81.528
        perforation T81.538
        specified complication NEC T81.598
    surgical operation T81.500
      resulting in
        acute reaction T81.60
          aseptic peritonitis T81.61
          specified NEC T81.69
        adhesions T81.510
        obstruction T81.520
        perforation T81.530
        specified complication NEC T81.590
    transfusion T81.501
      resulting in
        adhesions T81.511
        obstruction T81.521
        perforation T81.531
        specified complication NEC T81.591
  alimentary tract T18.9
    anus T18.5
    colon T18.4
    esophagus — *see* Foreign body, esophagus
    mouth T18.0
    multiple sites T18.8
    rectosigmoid (junction) T18.5

Foreign body — *continued*
  alimentary tract T18.9 — *continued*
    rectum T18.5
    small intestine T18.3
    specified site NEC T18.8
    stomach T18.2
  anterior chamber (eye) S05.5-
  auditory canal — *see* Foreign body, entering
      through orifice, ear
  bronchus T17.508
    causing
      asphyxiation T17.500
        food (bone) (seed) T17.520
        gastric contents (vomitus) T17.510
        specified type NEC T17.590
      injury NEC T17.508
        food (bone) (seed) T17.528
        gastric contents (vomitus) T17.518
        specified type NEC T17.598
  canthus — *see* Foreign body, conjunctival sac
  ciliary body (eye) S05.5-
  conjunctival sac T15.1-
  cornea T15.0-
  entering through orifice
    accessory sinus T17.0
    alimentary canal T18.9
      multiple parts T18.8
      specified part NEC T18.8
    alveolar process T18.0
    antrum (Highmore's) T17.0
    anus T18.5
    appendix T18.4
    auditory canal — *see* Foreign body, entering
        through orifice, ear
    auricle — *see* Foreign body, entering
        through orifice, ear
    bladder T19.1
    bronchioles — *see* Foreign body, respiratory
        tract, specified site NEC
    bronchus (main) — *see* Foreign body,
        bronchus
    buccal cavity T18.0
    canthus (inner) — *see* Foreign body,
        conjunctival sac
    cecum T18.4
    cervix (canal) (uteri) T19.3
    colon T18.4
    conjunctival sac — *see* Foreign body,
        conjunctival sac
    cornea — *see* Foreign body, cornea
    digestive organ or tract NOS T18.9
      multiple parts T18.8
      specified part NEC T18.8
    duodenum T18.3
    ear (external) T16-
    esophagus — *see* Foreign body, esophagus
    eye (external) NOS T15.9-
      conjunctival sac — *see* Foreign body,
          conjunctival sac
      cornea — *see* Foreign body, cornea
      specified part NEC T15.8-
    eyeball — *see also* Foreign body, entering
        through orifice, eye, specified part NEC
      with penetrating wound — *see* Puncture,
          eyeball
    eyelid — *see also* Foreign body, conjunctival
        sac
      with
        laceration — *see* Laceration, eyelid, with
            foreign body
        puncture — *see* Puncture, eyelid, with
            foreign body
        superficial injury — *see* Foreign body,
            superficial, eyelid
    gastrointestinal tract T18.9
      multiple parts T18.8
      specified part NEC T18.8

Foreign body — *continued*
  entering through orifice — *continued*
    genitourinary tract T19.9
      multiple parts T19.8
      specified part NEC T19.8
    globe — *see* Foreign body, entering through
        orifice, eyeball
    gum T18.0
    Highmore's antrum T17.0
    hypopharynx — *see* Foreign body, pharynx
    ileum T18.3
    intestine (small) T18.3
      large T18.4
    lacrimal apparatus (punctum) — *see* Foreign
        body, entering through orifice, eye,
        specified part NEC
    large intestine T18.4
    larynx — *see* Foreign body, larynx
    lung — *see* Foreign body, respiratory tract,
        specified site NEC
    maxillary sinus T17.0
    mouth T18.0
    nasal sinus T17.0
    nasopharynx — *see* Foreign body, pharynx
    nose (passage) T17.1
    nostril T17.1
    oral cavity T18.0
    palate T18.0
    penis T19.4
    pharynx — *see* Foreign body, pharynx
    piriform sinus — *see* Foreign body, pharynx
    rectosigmoid (junction) T18.5
    rectum T18.5
    respiratory tract — *see* Foreign body,
        respiratory tract
    sinus (accessory) (frontal) (maxillary) (nasal)
        T17.0
      piriform — *see* Foreign body, pharynx
    small intestine T18.3
    stomach T18.2
    suffocation by — *see* Foreign body, by site
    tear ducts or glands — *see* Foreign body,
        entering through orifice, eye, specified
        part NEC
    throat — *see* Foreign body, pharynx
    tongue T18.0
    tonsil, tonsillar (fossa) — *see* Foreign body,
        pharynx
    trachea — *see* Foreign body, trachea
    ureter T19.8
    urethra T19.0
    uterus (any part) T19.3
    vagina T19.2
    vulva T19.2
  esophagus T18.108
    causing
      injury NEC T18.108
        food (bone) (seed) T18.128
        gastric contents (vomitus) T18.118
        specified type NEC T18.198
      tracheal compression T18.100
        food (bone) (seed) T18.120
        gastric contents (vomitus) T18.110
        specified type NEC T18.190
  felling of, in throat R09.89
  fragment — *see* Retained, foreign body
      fragments (type of)
  genitourinary tract T19.9
    bladder T19.1
    multiple parts T19.8
    penis T19.4
    specified site NEC T19.8
    urethra T19.0
    uterus T19.3
    IUD Z97.5
    vagina T19.2
      contraceptive device Z97.5
    vulva T19.2

DISEASE INDEX

Foreign body — *continued*
  granuloma (old) (soft tissue) — *see also*
    Granuloma, foreign body
    skin L92.3
  in
    laceration — *see* Laceration, by site, with
      foreign body
    puncture wound — *see* Puncture, by site,
      with foreign body
    soft tissue (residual) M79.5
  inadvertently left in operation wound — *see*
    Foreign body, accidentally left during a
    procedure
  ingestion, ingested NOS T18.9
  inhalation or inspiration — *see* Foreign body,
    by site
  internal organ, not entering through a natural
    orifice — *code as* specific injury with
    foreign body
  intraocular S05.5-
    old, retained (nonmagnetic) H44.70-
      anterior chamber H44.71-
      ciliary body H44.72-
      iris H44.72-
      lens H44.73-
      magnetic H44.60-
        anterior chamber H44.61-
        ciliary body H44.62-
        iris H44.62-
        lens H44.63-
        posterior wall H44.64-
        specified site NEC H44.69-
        vitreous body H44.65-
      posterior wall H44.74-
      specified site NEC H44.79-
      vitreous body H44.75-
  iris — *see* Foreign body, intraocular
  lacrimal punctum — *see* Foreign body,
    entering through orifice, eye, specified
    part NEC
  larynx T17.308
    causing
      asphyxiation T17.300
        food (bone) (seed) T17.320
        gastric contents (vomitus) T17.310
        specified type NEC T17.390
      injury NEC T17.308
        food (bone) (seed) T17.328
        gastric contents (vomitus) T17.318
        specified type NEC T17.398
  lens — *see* Foreign body, intraocular
  ocular muscle S05.4-
    old, retained — *see* Foreign body, orbit, old
  old or residual
    soft tissue (residual) M79.5
  operation wound, left accidentally — *see*
    Foreign body, accidentally left during a
    procedure
  orbit S05.4-
    old, retained H05.5-
  pharynx T17.208
    causing
      asphyxiation T17.200
        food (bone) (seed) T17.220
        gastric contents (vomitus) T17.210
        specified type NEC T17.290
      injury NEC T17.208
        food (bone) (seed) T17.228
        gastric contents (vomitus) T17.218
        specified type NEC T17.298
  respiratory tract T17.908
    bronchioles — *see* Foreign body, respiratory
      tract, specified site NEC
    bronchus — *see* Foreign body, bronchus
    causing
      asphyxiation T17.900
        food (bone) (seed) T17.920
        gastric contents (vomitus) T17.910
        specified type NEC T17.990

Foreign body — *continued*
  respiratory tract T17.908 — *continued*
    causing — *continued*
      injury NEC T17.908
        food (bone) (seed) T17.928
        gastric contents (vomitus) T17.918
        specified type NEC T17.998
    larynx — *see* Foreign body, larynx
    lung — *see* Foreign body, respiratory tract,
      specified site NEC
    multiple parts — *see* Foreign body,
      respiratory tract, specified site NEC
    nasal sinus T17.0
    nasopharynx — *see* Foreign body, pharynx
    nose T17.1
    nostril T17.1
    pharynx — *see* Foreign body, pharynx
    specified site NEC T17.808
      causing
        asphyxiation T17.800
          food (bone) (seed) T17.820
          gastric contents (vomitus) T17.810
          specified type NEC T17.890
        injury NEC T17.808
          food (bone) (seed) T17.828
          gastric contents (vomitus) T17.818
          specified type NEC T17.898
    throat — *see* Foreign body, pharynx
    trachea — *see* Foreign body, trachea
  retained (old) (nonmagnetic) (in)
    anterior chamber (eye) — *see* Foreign body,
      intraocular, old, retained, anterior
      chamber
      magnetic — *see* Foreign body, intraocular,
        old, retained, magnetic, anterior
        chamber
    ciliary body — *see* Foreign body,
      intraocular, old, retained, ciliary body
      magnetic — *see* Foreign body, intraocular,
        old, retained, magnetic, ciliary body
    eyelid H02.819
      left H02.816
        lower H02.815
        upper H02.814
      right H02.813
        lower H02.812
        upper H02.811
    fragments — *see* Retained, foreign body
      fragments (type of)
    globe — *see* Foreign body, intraocular, old,
      retained
      magnetic — *see* Foreign body, intraocular,
        old, retained, magnetic
    intraocular — *see* Foreign body, intraocular,
      old, retained
      magnetic — *see* Foreign body, intraocular,
        old, retained, magnetic
    iris — *see* Foreign body, intraocular, old,
      retained, iris
      magnetic — *see* Foreign body, intraocular,
        old, retained, magnetic, iris
    lens — *see* Foreign body, intraocular, old,
      retained, lens
      magnetic — *see* Foreign body, intraocular,
        old, retained, magnetic, lens
    muscle — *see* Foreign body, retained, soft
      tissue
    orbit — *see* Foreign body, orbit, old
    posterior wall of globe — *see* Foreign body,
      intraocular, old, retained, posterior wall
      magnetic — *see* Foreign body, intraocular,
        old, retained, magnetic, posterior wall
    retrobulbar — *see* Foreign body, orbit, old,
      retrobulbar
    soft tissue M79.5
    vitreous — *see* Foreign body, intraocular,
      old, retained, vitreous body
      magnetic — *see* Foreign body, intraocular,
        old, retained, magnetic, vitreous body

Foreign body — *continued*
  retina S05.5-
  superficial, without open wound
    abdomen, abdominal (wall) S30.851
    alveolar process S00.552
    ankle S90.55-
    antecubital space — *see* Foreign body,
      superficial, forearm
    anus S30.857
    arm (upper) S40.85-
    auditory canal — *see* Foreign body,
      superficial, ear
    auricle — *see* Foreign body, superficial, ear
    axilla — *see* Foreign body, superficial, arm
    back, lower S30.850
    breast S20.15-
    brow S00.85
    buttock S30.850
    calf — *see* Foreign body, superficial, leg
    canthus — *see* Foreign body, superficial,
      eyelid
    cheek S00.85
      internal S00.552
    chest wall — *see* Foreign body, superficial,
      thorax
    chin S00.85
    clitoris S30.854
    costal region — *see* Foreign body,
      superficial, thorax
    digit(s)
      foot — *see* Foreign body, superficial, toe
      hand — *see* Foreign body, superficial,
        finger
    ear S00.45-
    elbow S50.35-
    epididymis S30.853
    epigastric region S30.851
    epiglottis S10.15
    esophagus, cervical S10.15
    eyebrow — *see* Foreign body, superficial,
      eyelid
    eyelid S00.25-
    face S00.85
    finger(s) S60.459
      index S60.45-
      little S60.45-
      middle S60.45-
      ring S60.45-
    flank S30.851
    foot (except toe(s) alone) S90.85-
      toe — *see* Foreign body, superficial, toe
    forearm S50.85-
      elbow only — *see* Foreign body,
        superficial, elbow
    forehead S00.85
    genital organs, external
      female S30.856
      male S30.855
    groin S30.851
    gum S00.552
    hand S60.55-
    head S00.95
      ear — *see* Foreign body, superficial, ear
      eyelid — *see* Foreign body, superficial,
        eyelid
      lip S00.551
      nose S00.35
      oral cavity S00.552
      scalp S00.05
      specified site NEC S00.85
    heel — *see* Foreign body, superficial, foot
    hip S70.25-
    inguinal region S30.851
    interscapular region S20.459
    jaw S00.85
    knee S80.25-
    labium (majus) (minus) S30.854
    larynx S10.15

Foreign body — *continued*
  superficial, without open wound — *continued*
    leg (lower) S80.85-
      knee — *see* Foreign body, superficial, knee
      upper — *see* Foreign body, superficial, thigh
    lip S00.551
    lower back S30.850
    lumbar region S30.850
    malar region S00.85
    mammary — *see* Foreign body, superficial, breast
    mastoid region S00.85
    mouth S00.552
    nail
      finger — *see* Foreign body, superficial, finger
      toe — *see* Foreign body, superficial, toe
    nape S10.85
    nasal S00.35
    neck S10.95
      specified site NEC S10.85
      throat S10.15
    nose S00.35
    occipital region S00.05
    oral cavity S00.552
    orbital region — *see* Foreign body, superficial, eyelid
    palate S00.552
    palm — *see* Foreign body, superficial, hand
    parietal region S00.05
    pelvis S30.850
    penis S30.852
    perineum
      female S30.854
      male S30.850
    periocular area — *see* Foreign body, superficial, eyelid
    phalanges
      finger — *see* Foreign body, superficial, finger
      toe — *see* Foreign body, superficial, toe
    pharynx S10.15
    pinna — *see* Foreign body, superficial, ear
    popliteal space — *see* Foreign body, superficial, knee
    prepuce S30.852
    pubic region S30.850
    pudendum
      female S30.856
      male S30.855
    sacral region S30.850
    scalp S00.05
    scapular region — *see* Foreign body, superficial, shoulder
    scrotum S30.853
    shin — *see* Foreign body, superficial, leg
    shoulder S40.25-
    sternal region S20.359
    submaxillary region S00.85
    submental region S00.85
    subungual
      finger(s) — *see* Foreign body, superficial, finger
      toe(s) — *see* Foreign body, superficial, toe
    supraclavicular fossa S10.85
    supraorbital S00.85
    temple S00.85
    temporal region S00.85
    testis S30.853
    thigh S70.35-
    thorax, thoracic (wall) S20.95
      back S20.45-
      front S20.35-
    throat S10.15
    thumb S60.35-
    toe(s) (lesser) S90.456
      great S90.45-
    tongue S00.552

Foreign body — *continued*
  superficial, without open wound — *continued*
    trachea S10.15
    tunica vaginalis S30.853
    tympanum, tympanic membrane — *see* Foreign body, superficial, ear
    uvula S00.552
    vagina S30.854
    vocal cords S10.15
    vulva S30.854
    wrist S60.85-
  swallowed T18.9
  trachea T17.408
    causing
      asphyxiation T17.400
        food (bone) (seed) T17.420
        gastric contents (vomitus) T17.410
        specified type NEC T17.490
      injury NEC T17.408
        food (bone) (seed) T17.428
        gastric contents (vomitus) T17.418
        specified type NEC T17.498
  type of fragment — *see* Retained, foreign body fragments (type of)
  vitreous (humor) S05.5-
Forestier's disease (rhizomelic pseudopolyarthritis) M35.3
  meaning ankylosing hyperostosis — *see* Hyperostosis, ankylosing
Formation
  hyalin in cornea — *see* Degeneration, cornea
  sequestrum in bone (due to infection) — *see* Osteomyelitis, chronic
  valve
    colon, congenital Q43.8
    ureter (congenital) Q62.39
Formication R20.2
Fort Bragg fever A27.89
Fossa — *see also* condition
  pyriform — *see* condition
Foster-Kennedy syndrome H47.14-
Fothergill's
  disease (trigeminal neuralgia) — *see also* Neuralgia, trigeminal
  scarlatina anginosa A38.9
Foul breath R19.6
Foundling Z76.1
Fournier disease or gangrene N49.3
  female N76.89
Fourth
  cranial nerve — *see* condition
  molar K00.1
Foville's (peduncular) disease or syndrome G46.3
Fox(-Fordyce) disease (apocrine miliaria) L75.2
Fracture, burst — *see* Fracture, traumatic, by site
Fracture, chronic — *see* Fracture, pathological
Fracture, insufficiency — *see* Fracture, pathologic, by site
Fracture, nontraumatic, NEC
  atypical
    femur M84.750-
      complete
        oblique M84.759
          left side M84.758
          right side M84.757
        transverse M84.756
          left side M84.755
          right side M84.754
      incomplete M84.753
        left side M84.752
        right side M84.751
Fracture, pathological (pathologic) — (*see also* **Fracture, traumatic**) M84.40
  ankle M84.47-
  carpus M84.44-
  clavicle M84.41-

Fracture, pathological (pathologic) — (*see also* **Fracture, traumatic**) M84.40 — *continued*
  compression (not due to trauma) (*see also* Collapse, vertebra) M48.50-
  dental implant M27.63
  dental restorative material K08.539
    with loss of material K08.531
    without loss of material K08.530
  due to
    neoplastic disease NEC (*see also* Neoplasm) M84.50
      ankle M84.57-
      carpus M84.54-
      clavicle M84.51-
      femur M84.55-
      fibula M84.56-
      finger M84.54-
      hip M84.559
      humerus M84.52-
      ilium M84.550
      ischium M84.550
      metacarpus M84.54-
      metatarsus M84.57-
      neck M84.58
      pelvis M84.550
      radius M84.53-
      rib M84.58
      scapula M84.51-
      skull M84.58
      specified site NEC M84.58
      tarsus M84.57-
      tibia M84.56-
      toe M84.57-
      ulna M84.53-
      vertebra M84.58
    osteoporosis M80.00
      disuse — *see* Osteoporosis, specified type NEC, with pathological fracture
      drug-induced — *see* Osteoporosis, drug induced, with pathological fracture
      idiopathic — *see* Osteoporosis, specified type NEC, with pathological fracture
      postmenopausal — *see* Osteoporosis, postmenopausal, with pathological fracture
      postoophorectomy — *see* Osteoporosis, postoophorectomy, with pathological fracture
      postsurgical malabsorption — *see* Osteoporosis, specified type NEC, with pathological fracture
      specified cause NEC — *see* Osteoporosis, specified type NEC, with pathological fracture
  specified disease NEC M84.60
    ankle M84.67-
    carpus M84.64-
    clavicle M84.61-
    femur M84.65-
    fibula M84.66-
    finger M84.64-
    hip M84.65-
    humerus M84.62-
    ilium M84.650
    ischium M84.650
    metacarpus M84.64-
    metatarsus M84.67-
    neck M84.68
    radius M84.63-
    rib M84.68
    scapula M84.61-
    skull M84.68
    tarsus M84.67-
    tibia M84.66-
    toe M84.67-
    ulna M84.63-
    vertebra M84.68

Fracture, pathological (pathologic) — (see also **Fracture, traumatic**) M84.40 — continued
femur M84.45-
fibula M84.46-
finger M84.44-
hip M84.459
humerus M84.42-
ilium M84.454
ischium M84.454
joint prosthesis — see Complications, joint prosthesis, mechanical, breakdown, by site
periprosthetic — see Fracture, pathological, periprosthetic
metacarpus M84.44-
metatarsus M84.47-
neck M84.48
pelvis M84.454
periprosthetic M97.9
  ankle M97.2-
  elbow M97.4-
  finger M97.8
  hip M97.0-
  knee M97.1-
  other specified joint M97.8
  shoulder M97.3-
  spinal joint M97.8
  toe joint M97.8
  wrist joint M97.8
radius M84.43-
restorative material (dental) K08.539
  with loss of material K08.531
  without loss of material K08.530
rib M84.48
scapula M84.41-
skull M84.48
tarsus M84.47-
tibia M84.46-
toe M84.47-
ulna M84.43-
vertebra M84.48
Fracture, traumatic (abduction) (adduction) (separation) (see also **Fracture, pathological**) T14.8
acetabulum S32.40-
  column
    anterior (displaced) (iliopubic) S32.43-
      nondisplaced S32.436
    posterior (displaced) (ilioischial) S32.443
      nondisplaced S32.44-
  dome (displaced) S32.48-
    nondisplaced S32.48
  specified NEC S32.49-
  transverse (displaced) S32.45-
    with associated posterior wall fracture (displaced) S32.46-
      nondisplaced S32.46-
    nondisplaced S32.45-
  wall
    anterior (displaced) S32.41-
      nondisplaced S32.41-
    medial (displaced) S32.47-
      nondisplaced S32.47-
    posterior (displaced) S32.42-
      with associated transverse fracture (displaced) S32.46-
        nondisplaced S32.46-
      nondisplaced S32.42-
acromion — see Fracture, scapula, acromial process
ankle S82.899
  bimalleolar (displaced) S82.84-
    nondisplaced S82.84-
  lateral malleolus only (displaced) S82.6-
    nondisplaced S82.6-

Fracture, traumatic (abduction) (adduction) (separation) (see also **Fracture, pathological**) T14.8 — continued
ankle S82.899 — continued
  medial malleolus (displaced) S82.5-
    associated with Maisonneuve's fracture — see Fracture, Maisonneuve's
    nondisplaced S82.5-
  talus — see Fracture, tarsal, talus
  trimalleolar (displaced) S82.85-
    nondisplaced S82.85-
arm (upper) — see also Fracture, humerus, shaft
  humerus — see Fracture, humerus
  radius — see Fracture, radius
  ulna — see Fracture, ulna
astragalus — see Fracture, tarsal, talus
atlas — see Fracture, neck, cervical vertebra, first
axis — see Fracture, neck, cervical vertebra, second
back — see Fracture, vertebra
Barton's — see Barton's fracture
base of skull — see Fracture, skull, base
basicervical (basal) (femoral) S72.0
Bennett's — see Bennett's fracture
bimalleolar — see Fracture, ankle, bimalleolar
blow-out S02.3-
bone NEC T14.8
  birth injury P13.9
  following insertion of orthopedic implant, joint prosthesis or bone plate — see Fracture, following insertion of orthopedicimplant, joint prosthesis or bone plate
  in (due to) neoplastic disease NEC — see Fracture, pathological, due to, neoplastic disease
  pathological (cause unknown) — see Fracture, pathological
breast bone — see Fracture, sternum
bucket handle (semilunar cartilage) — see Tear, meniscus
burst — see Fracture, traumatic, by site
calcaneus — see Fracture, tarsal, calcaneus
carpal bone(s) S62.10-
  capitate (displaced) S62.13-
    nondisplaced S62.13-
  cuneiform — see Fracture, carpal bone, triquetrum
  hamate (body) (displaced) S62.143
    hook process (displaced) S62.15-
      nondisplaced S62.15-
    nondisplaced S62.14-
  larger multangular — see Fracture, carpal bones, trapezium
  lunate (displaced) S62.12-
    nondisplaced S62.12-
  navicular S62.00-
    distal pole (displaced) S62.01-
      nondisplaced S62.01-
    middle third (displaced) S62.02-
      nondisplaced S62.02-
    proximal third (displaced) S62.03-
      nondisplaced S62.03-
    volar tuberosity — see Fracture, carpal bones, navicular, distal pole
  os magnum — see Fracture, carpal bones, capitate
  pisiform (displaced) S62.16-
    nondisplaced S62.16-
  semilunar — see Fracture, carpal bones, lunate
  smaller multangular — see Fracture, carpal bones, trapezoid
  trapezium (displaced) S62.17-
    nondisplaced S62.17-
  trapezoid (displaced) S62.18-
    nondisplaced S62.18-

Fracture, traumatic (abduction) (adduction) (separation) (see also **Fracture, pathological**) T14.8 — continued
carpal bone(s) S62.10- — continued
  triquetrum (displaced) S62.11-
    nondisplaced S62.11-
  unciform — see Fracture, carpal bones, hamate
cervical — see Fracture, vertebra, cervical
clavicle S42.00-
  acromial end (displaced) S42.03-
    nondisplaced S42.03-
  birth injury P13.4
  lateral end — see Fracture, clavicle, acromial end
  shaft (displaced) S42.02-
    nondisplaced S42.02-
  sternal end (anterior) (displaced) S42.01-
    nondisplaced S42.01-
    posterior S42.01-
coccyx S32.2
collapsed — see Collapse, vertebra
collar bone — see Fracture, clavicle
Colles' — see Colles' fracture
coronoid process — see Fracture, ulna, upper end, coronoid process
corpus cavernosum penis S39.840
costochondral cartilage S23.41
costochondral, costosternal junction — see Fracture, rib
cranium — see Fracture, skull
cricoid cartilage S12.8
cuboid (ankle) — see Fracture, tarsal, cuboid
cuneiform
  foot — see Fracture, tarsal, cuneiform
  wrist — see Fracture, carpal, triquetrum
delayed union — see Delay, union, fracture
dental restorative material K08.539
  with loss of material K08.531
  without loss of material K08.530
due to
  birth injury — see Birth, injury, fracture
  osteoporosis — see Osteoporosis, with fracture
Dupuytren's — see Fracture, ankle, lateral malleolus
elbow S42.40-
ethmoid (bone) (sinus) — see Fracture, skull, base
face bone S02.92
fatigue — see also Fracture, stress
  vertebra M48.40
    cervical region M48.42
    cervicothoracic region M48.43
    lumbar region M48.46
    lumbosacral region M48.47
    occipito-atlanto-axial region M48.41
    sacrococcygeal region M48.48
    thoracic region M48.44
    thoracolumbar region M48.45
femur, femoral S72.9-
  basicervical (basal) S72.0
  birth injury P13.2
  capital epiphyseal S79.01-
  condyles, epicondyles — see Fracture, femur, lower end
  distal end — see Fracture, femur, lower end
  epiphysis
    head — see Fracture, femur, upper end, epiphysis
    lower — see Fracture, femur, lower end, epiphysis
    upper — see Fracture, femur, upper end, epiphysis
  following insertion of implant, prosthesis or plate M96.66-

Fracture, traumatic (abduction) (adduction) (separation) (*see also* **Fracture, pathological**) T14.8 — *continued*
femur, femoral S72.9- — *continued*
  head — *see* Fracture, femur, upper end, head
  intertrochanteric — *see* Fracture, femur, trochanteric
  intratrochanteric — *see* Fracture, femur, trochanteric
  lower end S72.40-
    condyle (displaced) S72.41-
      lateral (displaced) S72.42-
        nondisplaced S72.42-
      medial (displaced) S72.43-
        nondisplaced S72.43-
      nondisplaced S72.41-
    epiphysis (displaced) S72.44-
      nondisplaced S72.44-
    physeal S79.10-
      Salter-Harris
        Type I S79.11-
        Type II S79.12-
        Type III S79.13-
        Type IV S79.14-
      specified NEC S79.19-
    specified NEC S72.49-
    supracondylar (displaced) S72.45-
      with intracondylar extension (displaced) S72.46-
        nondisplaced S72.46-
      nondisplaced S72.45-
    torus S72.47-
  neck — *see* Fracture, femur, upper end, neck
  pertrochanteric — *see* Fracture, femur, trochanteric
  shaft (lower third) (middle third) (upper third) S72.30-
    comminuted (displaced) S72.35-
      nondisplaced S72.35-
    oblique (displaced) S72.33-
      nondisplaced S72.33-
    segmental (displaced) S72.36-
      nondisplaced S72.36-
    specified NEC S72.39-
    spiral (displaced) S72.34-
      nondisplaced S72.34-
    transverse (displaced) S72.32-
      nondisplaced S72.32-
  specified site NEC — *see* subcategory S72.8
  subcapital (displaced) S72.01-
  subtrochanteric (region) (section) (displaced) S72.2-
    nondisplaced S72.2-
  transcervical — *see* Fracture, femur, upper end, neck
  transtrochanteric — *see* Fracture, femur, trochanteric
  trochanteric S72.10-
    apophyseal (displaced) S72.13-
      nondisplaced S72.13-
    greater trochanter (displaced) S72.11-
      nondisplaced S72.11-
    intertrochanteric (displaced) S72.14-
      nondisplaced S72.14-
    lesser trochanter (displaced) S72.12-
      nondisplaced S72.12-
  upper end S72.00-
    apophyseal (displaced) S72.13-
      nondisplaced S72.13-
    cervicotrochanteric — *see* Fracture, femur, upper end, neck, base
    epiphysis (displaced) S72.02-
      nondisplaced S72.02-
    head S72.05-
    articular (displaced) S72.06-
      nondisplaced S72.06-
    specified NEC S72.09-

Fracture, traumatic (abduction) (adduction) (separation) (*see also* **Fracture, pathological**) T14.8 — *continued*
femur, femoral S72.9- — *continued*
  upper end S72.00- — *continued*
    intertrochanteric (displaced) S72.14-
      nondisplaced S72.14-
    intracapsular S72.01-
    midcervical (displaced) S72.03-
      nondisplaced S72.03-
    neck S72.00-
      base (displaced) S72.04-
        nondisplaced S72.04-
      specified NEC S72.09-
    pertrochanteric — *see* Fracture, femur, upper end, trochanteric
    physeal S79.00-
      Salter-Harris type I S79.01-
      specified NEC S79.09-
    subcapital (displaced) S72.01-
    subtrochanteric (displaced) S72.2-
      nondisplaced S72.2-
    transcervical — *see* Fracture, femur, upper end, midcervical
    trochanteric S72.10-
      greater (displaced) S72.11-
        nondisplaced S72.11-
      lesser (displaced) S72.12-
        nondisplaced S72.12-
fibula (shaft) (styloid) S82.40-
  comminuted (displaced) S82.45-
    nondisplaced S82.45-
  following insertion of implant, prosthesis or plate M96.67-
  involving ankle or malleolus — *see* Fracture, fibula, lateral malleolus
  lateral malleolus (displaced) S82.6-
    nondisplaced S82.6-
  lower end
    physeal S89.30-
      Salter-Harris
        Type I S89.31-
        Type II S89.32-
      specified NEC S89.39-
    specified NEC S82.83-
    torus S82.82-
  oblique (displaced) S82.43-
    nondisplaced S82.43-
  segmental (displaced) S82.46-
    nondisplaced S82.46-
  specified NEC S82.49-
  spiral (displaced) S82.44-
    nondisplaced S82.44-
  transverse (displaced) S82.42-
    nondisplaced S82.42-
  upper end
    physeal S89.20-
      Salter-Harris
        Type I S89.21-
        Type II S89.22-
      specified NEC S89.29-
    specified NEC S82.83-
    torus S82.81-
finger (except thumb) S62.60-
  distal phalanx (displaced) S62.63-
    nondisplaced S62.66-
  index S62.60-
    distal phalanx (displaced) S62.63-
      nondisplaced S62.66-
    medial phalanx (displaced) S62.62-
      nondisplaced S62.65-
    proximal phalanx (displaced) S62.61-
      nondisplaced S62.64-
  little S62.60-
    distal phalanx (displaced) S62.63-
      nondisplaced S62.66-
    medial phalanx (displaced) S62.62-
      nondisplaced S62.65-

Fracture, traumatic (abduction) (adduction) (separation) (*see also* **Fracture, pathological**) T14.8 — *continued*
finger (except thumb) S62.60- — *continued*
  little S62.60- — *continued*
    proximal phalanx (displaced) S62.61-
      nondisplaced S62.64-
    medial phalanx (displaced) S62.62-
      nondisplaced S62.65-
  middle S62.60-
    distal phalanx (displaced) S62.63-
      nondisplaced S62.66-
    medial phalanx (displaced) S62.62-
      nondisplaced S62.65-
    proximal phalanx (displaced) S62.61-
      nondisplaced S62.64-
  proximal phalanx (displaced) S62.61-
    nondisplaced S62.64-
  ring S62.60-
    distal phalanx (displaced) S62.63-
      nondisplaced S62.66-
    medial phalanx (displaced) S62.62-
      nondisplaced S62.65-
    proximal phalanx (displaced) S62.61-
      nondisplaced S62.64-
  thumb — *see* Fracture, thumb
following insertion (intraoperative) (postoperative) of orthopedic implant, joint prosthesis or bone plate M96.69
  femur M96.66-
  fibula M96.67-
  humerus M96.62-
  pelvis M96.65
  radius M96.63-
  specified bone NEC M96.69
  tibia M96.67-
  ulna M96.63-
foot S92.90-
  astragalus — *see* Fracture, tarsal, talus
  calcaneus — *see* Fracture, tarsal, calcaneus
  cuboid — *see* Fracture, tarsal, cuboid
  cuneiform — *see* Fracture, tarsal, cuneiform
  metatarsal — *see* Fracture, metatarsal
  navicular — *see* Fracture, tarsal, navicular
  sesamoid S92.81-
  specified NEC S92.81-
  talus — *see* Fracture, tarsal, talus
  tarsal — *see* Fracture, tarsal
  toe — *see* Fracture, toe
forearm S52.9-
  radius — *see* Fracture, radius
  ulna — *see* Fracture, ulna
fossa (anterior) (middle) (posterior) S02.19
frontal (bone) (skull) S02.0
  sinus S02.19
glenoid (cavity) (scapula) — *see* Fracture, scapula, glenoid cavity
greenstick — *see* Fracture, by site
hallux — *see* Fracture, toe, great
hand S62.9-
  carpal — *see* Fracture, carpal bone
  finger (except thumb) — *see* Fracture, finger
  metacarpal — *see* Fracture, metacarpal
  navicular (scaphoid) (hand) — *see* Fracture, carpal bone, navicular
  thumb — *see* Fracture, thumb
healed or old
  with complications — *code by* Nature of the complication
heel bone — *see* Fracture, tarsal, calcaneus
Hill-Sachs S42.29-
hip — *see* Fracture, femur, neck
humerus S42.30-
  anatomical neck — *see* Fracture, humerus, upper end
  articular process — *see* Fracture, humerus, lower end
  capitellum — *see* Fracture, humerus, lower end, condyle, lateral

Fracture, traumatic (abduction) (adduction) (separation) (*see also* **Fracture, pathological**) T14.8 — *continued*
humerus S42.30- — *continued*
　distal end — *see* Fracture, humerus, lower end
　epiphysis
　　lower — *see* Fracture, humerus, lower end, physeal
　　upper — *see* Fracture, humerus, upper end, physeal
　external condyle — *see* Fracture, humerus, lower end, condyle, lateral
　following insertion of implant, prosthesis or plate M96.62-
　great tuberosity — *see* Fracture, humerus, upper end, greater tuberosity
　intercondylar — *see* Fracture, humerus, lower end
　internal epicondyle — *see* Fracture, humerus, lower end, epicondyle, medial
　lesser tuberosity — *see* Fracture, humerus, upper end, lesser tuberosity
　lower end S42.40-
　　condyle
　　　lateral (displaced) S42.45-
　　　　nondisplaced S42.45-
　　　medial (displaced) S42.46-
　　　　nondisplaced S42.46-
　　epicondyle
　　　lateral (displaced) S42.43-
　　　　nondisplaced S42.43-
　　　medial (displaced) S42.44-
　　　　incarcerated S42.44-
　　　　nondisplaced S42.44-
　　physeal S49.10-
　　　Salter-Harris
　　　　Type I S49.11-
　　　　Type II S49.12-
　　　　Type III S49.13-
　　　　Type IV S49.14-
　　　specified NEC S49.19-
　　specified NEC (displaced) S42.49-
　　　nondisplaced S42.49-
　　supracondylar (simple) (displaced) S42.41-
　　　with intercondylar fracture — *see* Fracture, humerus, lower end
　　　comminuted (displaced) S42.42-
　　　　nondisplaced S42.42-
　　　nondisplaced S42.41-
　　torus S42.48-
　　transcondylar (displaced) S42.47-
　　　nondisplaced S42.47-
　proximal end — *see* Fracture, humerus, upper end
　shaft S42.30-
　　comminuted (displaced) S42.35-
　　　nondisplaced S42.35-
　　greenstick S42.31-
　　oblique (displaced) S42.33-
　　　nondisplaced S42.33-
　　segmental (displaced) S42.36-
　　　nondisplaced S42.36-
　　specified NEC S42.39-
　　spiral (displaced) S42.34-
　　　nondisplaced S42.34-
　　transverse (displaced) S42.32-
　　　nondisplaced S42.32-
　supracondylar — *see* Fracture, humerus, lower end
　surgical neck — *see* Fracture, humerus, upper end, surgical neck
　trochlea — *see* Fracture, humerus, lower end, condyle, medial
　tuberosity — *see* Fracture, humerus, upper end

Fracture, traumatic (abduction) (adduction) (separation) (*see also* **Fracture, pathological**) T14.8 — *continued*
humerus S42.30- — *continued*
　upper end S42.20-
　　anatomical neck — *see* Fracture, humerus, upper end, specified NEC
　　articular head — *see* Fracture, humerus, upper end, specified NEC
　　epiphysis — *see* Fracture, humerus, upper end, physeal
　　greater tuberosity (displaced) S42.25-
　　　nondisplaced S42.25-
　　lesser tuberosity (displaced) S42.26-
　　　nondisplaced S42.26-
　　physeal S49.00-
　　　Salter-Harris
　　　　Type I S49.01-
　　　　Type II S49.02-
　　　　Type III S49.03-
　　　　Type IV S49.04-
　　　specified NEC S49.09-
　　specified NEC (displaced) S42.29-
　　　nondisplaced S42.29-
　　surgical neck (displaced) S42.21-
　　　four-part S42.24-
　　　nondisplaced S42.21-
　　　three-part S42.23-
　　　two-part (displaced) S42.22-
　　　　nondisplaced S42.22-
　　torus S42.27-
　　transepiphyseal — *see* Fracture, humerus, upper end, physeal
hyoid bone S12.8
ilium S32.30-
　with disruption of pelvic ring — *see* Disruption, pelvic ring
　avulsion (displaced) S32.31-
　　nondisplaced S32.31-
　specified NEC S32.39-
impaction, impacted — *code as* Fracture, by site
innominate bone — *see* Fracture, ilium
instep — *see* Fracture, foot
ischium S32.60-
　with disruption of pelvic ring — *see* Disruption, pelvic ring
　avulsion (displaced) S32.61-
　　nondisplaced S32.61-
　specified NEC S32.69-
jaw (bone) (lower) — *see* Fracture, mandible
　upper — *see* Fracture, maxilla
joint prosthesis — *see* Complications, joint prosthesis, mechanical, breakdown, by site
　periprosthetic — *see* Fracture, traumatic, periprosthetic
knee cap — *see* Fracture, patella
larynx S12.8
late effects — *see* Sequelae, fracture
leg (lower) S82.9-
　ankle — *see* Fracture, ankle
　femur — *see* Fracture, femur
　fibula — *see* Fracture, fibula
　malleolus — *see* Fracture, ankle
　patella — *see* Fracture, patella
　specified site NEC S82.89-
　tibia — *see* Fracture, tibia
lumbar spine — *see* Fracture, vertebra, lumbar
lumbosacral spine S32.9
Maisonneuve's (displaced) S82.86-
　nondisplaced S82.86-
malar bone (*see also* Fracture, maxilla) S02.400
　left side S02.40B *(follows S02.402)*
　right side S02.40A *(follows S02.402)*
malleolus — *see* Fracture, ankle
malunion — *see* Fracture, by site

Fracture, traumatic (abduction) (adduction) (separation) (*see also* **Fracture, pathological**) T14.8 — *continued*
mandible (lower jaw (bone)) S02.609
　alveolus S02.67-
　angle (of jaw) S02.65-
　body, unspecified S02.600
　　left side S02.602
　　right side S02.601
　condylar process S02.61-
　coronoid process S02.63-
　ramus, unspecified S02.64-
　specified site NEC S02.69-
　subcondylar process S02.62-
　symphysis S02.66
manubrium (sterni) S22.21
　dissociation from sternum S22.23
march — *see* Fracture, traumatic, stress, by site
maxilla, maxillary (bone) (sinus) (superior) (upper jaw) S02.401
　alveolus S02.42
　inferior — *see* Fracture, mandible
　LeFort I S02.411
　LeFort II S02.412
　LeFort III S02.413
　left side S02.40D *(follows S02.402)*
　right side S02.40C *(follows S02.402)*
metacarpal S62.309
　base (displaced) S62.319
　　nondisplaced S62.349
　fifth S62.30-
　　base (displaced) S62.31-
　　　nondisplaced S62.34-
　　neck (displaced) S62.33-
　　　nondisplaced S62.36-
　　shaft (displaced) S62.32-
　　　nondisplaced S62.35-
　　specified NEC S62.398
　first S62.20-
　　base NEC (displaced) S62.23-
　　　nondisplaced S62.23-
　　Bennett's — *see* Bennett's fracture
　　neck (displaced) S62.25-
　　　nondisplaced S62.25-
　　shaft (displaced) S62.24-
　　　nondisplaced S62.24-
　　specified NEC S62.29-
　fourth S62.30-
　　base (displaced) S62.31-
　　　nondisplaced S62.34-
　　neck (displaced) S62.33-
　　　nondisplaced S62.36-
　　shaft (displaced) S62.32-
　　　nondisplaced S62.35-
　　specified NEC S62.39-
　neck (displaced) S62.33-
　　nondisplaced S62.36-
　Rolando's — *see* Rolando's fracture
　second S62.30-
　　base (displaced) S62.31-
　　　nondisplaced S62.34-
　　neck (displaced) S62.33-
　　　nondisplaced S62.36-
　　shaft (displaced) S62.32-
　　　nondisplaced S62.35-
　　specified NEC S62.39-
　shaft (displaced) S62.32-
　　nondisplaced S62.35-
　specified NEC S62.399
　third S62.30-
　　base (displaced) S62.31-
　　　nondisplaced S62.34-
　　neck (displaced) S62.33-
　　　nondisplaced S62.36-
　　shaft (displaced) S62.32-
　　　nondisplaced S62.35-
　　specified NEC S62.39-

Fracture, traumatic (abduction) (adduction) (separation) (*see also* **Fracture, pathological**) T14.8 — *continued*
metastatic — *see* Fracture, pathological, due to, neoplastic disease — *see also* Neoplasm
metatarsal bone S92.30-
  fifth (displaced) S92.35-
    nondisplaced S92.35-
  first (displaced) S92.31-
    nondisplaced S92.31-
  fourth (displaced) S92.34-
    nondisplaced S92.34-
  physeal S99.10-
    Salter-Harris
      Type I S99.11-
      Type II S99.12-
      Type III S99.13-
      Type IV S99.14-
    specified NEC S99.19-
  second (displaced) S92.32-
    nondisplaced S92.32-
  third (displaced) S92.33-
    nondisplaced S92.33-
Monteggia's — *see* Monteggia's fracture
multiple
  hand (and wrist) NEC — *see* Fracture, by site
  ribs — *see* Fracture, rib, multiple
nasal (bone(s)) S02.2
navicular (scaphoid) (foot) — *see also* Fracture, tarsal, navicular
  hand — *see* Fracture, carpal, navicular
neck S12.9
  cervical vertebra S12.9
    fifth (displaced) S12.400
      nondisplaced S12.401
      specified type NEC (displaced) S12.490
        nondisplaced S12.491
    first (displaced) S12.000
      burst (stable) S12.01
        unstable S12.02
      lateral mass (displaced) S12.040
        nondisplaced S12.041
      nondisplaced S12.001
      posterior arch (displaced) S12.030
        nondisplaced S12.031
      specified type NEC (displaced) S12.090
        nondisplaced S12.091
    fourth (displaced) S12.300
      nondisplaced S12.301
      specified type NEC (displaced) S12.390
        nondisplaced S12.391
    second (displaced) S12.100
      dens (anterior) (displaced) (type II) S12.110
        nondisplaced S12.112
        posterior S12.111
      specified type NEC (displaced) S12.120
        nondisplaced S12.121
      nondisplaced S12.101
      specified type NEC (displaced) S12.190
        nondisplaced S12.191
    seventh (displaced) S12.600
      nondisplaced S12.601
      specified type NEC (displaced) S12.690
        nondisplaced S12.691
    sixth (displaced) S12.500
      nondisplaced S12.501
      specified type NEC (displaced) S12.590
        nondisplaced S12.591
    third (displaced) S12.200
      nondisplaced S12.201
      specified type NEC (displaced) S12.290
        nondisplaced S12.291
  hyoid bone S12.8
  larynx S12.8
  specified site NEC S12.8
  thyroid cartilage S12.8
  trachea S12.8

Fracture, traumatic (abduction) (adduction) (separation) (*see also* **Fracture, pathological**) T14.8 — *continued*
neoplastic NEC — *see* Fracture, pathological, due to, neoplastic disease
neural arch — *see* Fracture, vertebra
newborn — *see* Birth, injury, fracture
nontraumatic — *see* Fracture, pathological
nonunion — *see* Nonunion, fracture
nose, nasal (bone) (septum) S02.2
occiput — *see* Fracture, skull, base, occiput
odontoid process — *see* Fracture, neck, cervical vertebra, second
olecranon (process) (ulna) — *see* Fracture, ulna, upper end, olecranon process
orbit, orbital (bone) (region) S02.8-
  floor (blow-out) S02.3-
  roof S02.19
os
  calcis — *see* Fracture, tarsal, calcaneus
  magnum — *see* Fracture, carpal, capitate
  pubis — *see* Fracture, pubis
palate S02.8-
parietal bone (skull) S02.0
patella S82.00-
  comminuted (displaced) S82.04-
    nondisplaced S82.04-
  longitudinal (displaced) S82.02-
    nondisplaced S82.02-
  osteochondral (displaced) S82.01-
    nondisplaced S82.01-
  specified NEC S82.09-
  transverse (displaced) S82.03-
    nondisplaced S82.03-
pedicle (of vertebral arch) — *see* Fracture, vertebra
pelvis, pelvic (bone) S32.9
  acetabulum — *see* Fracture, acetabulum
  circle — *see* Disruption, pelvic ring
  following insertion of implant, prosthesis or plate M96.65
  ilium — *see* Fracture, ilium
  ischium — *see* Fracture, ischium
  multiple
    with disruption of pelvic ring (circle) — *see* Disruption, pelvic ring
    without disruption of pelvic ring (circle) S32.82
  pubis — *see* Fracture, pubis
  sacrum — *see* Fracture, sacrum
  specified site NEC S32.89
periprosthetic, around internal prosthetic joint M97.9
  ankle M97.2-
  elbow M97.4-
  finger M97.8
  hip M97.0-
  knee M97.1-
  shoulder M97.3-
  specified joint NEC M97.8
  spine M97.8
  toe M97.8
  wrist M97.8
phalanx
  foot — *see* Fracture, toe
  hand — *see* Fracture, finger
pisiform — *see* Fracture, carpal, pisiform
pond — *see* Fracture, skull
prosthetic device, internal — *see* Complications, prosthetic device, by site, mechanical
pubis S32.50-
  with disruption of pelvic ring — *see* Disruption, pelvic ring
  specified site NEC S32.59-
  superior rim S32.51-
radius S52.9-
  distal end — *see* Fracture, radius, lower end

Fracture, traumatic (abduction) (adduction) (separation) (*see also* **Fracture, pathological**) T14.8 — *continued*
radius S52.9- — *continued*
  following insertion of implant, prosthesis or plate M96.63-
  head — *see* Fracture, radius, upper end, head
  lower end S52.50-
    Barton's — *see* Barton's fracture
    Colles' — *see* Colles' fracture
    extraarticular NEC S52.55-
    intraarticular NEC S52.57-
    physeal S59.20-
      Salter-Harris
        Type I S59.21-
        Type II S59.22-
        Type III S59.23-
        Type IV S59.24-
      specified NEC S59.29-
    Smith's — *see* Smith's fracture
    specified NEC S52.59-
    styloid process (displaced) S52.51-
      nondisplaced S52.51-
    torus S52.52-
  neck — *see* Fracture, radius, upper end
  proximal end — *see* Fracture, radius, upper end
  shaft S52.30-
    bent bone S52.38-
    comminuted (displaced) S52.35-
      nondisplaced S52.35-
    Galeazzi's — *see* Galeazzi's fracture
    greenstick S52.31-
    oblique (displaced) S52.33-
      nondisplaced S52.33-
    segmental (displaced) S52.36-
      nondisplaced S52.36-
    specified NEC S52.39-
    spiral (displaced) S52.34-
      nondisplaced S52.34-
    transverse (displaced) S52.32-
      nondisplaced S52.32-
  upper end S52.10-
    head (displaced) S52.12-
      nondisplaced S52.12-
    neck (displaced) S52.13-
      nondisplaced S52.13-
    physeal S59.10-
      Salter-Harris
        Type I S59.11-
        Type II S59.12-
        Type III S59.13-
        Type IV S59.14-
      specified NEC S59.19-
    specified NEC S52.18-
    torus S52.11-
ramus
  inferior or superior, pubis — *see* Fracture, pubis
  mandible — *see* Fracture, mandible
restorative material (dental) K08.539
  with loss of material K08.531
  without loss of material K08.530
rib S22.3-
  with flail chest — *see* Flail, chest
  multiple S22.4-
    with flail chest — *see* Flail, chest
root, tooth — *see* Fracture, tooth
sacrum S32.10
  specified NEC S32.19
  Type
    1 S32.14
    2 S32.15
    3 S32.16
    4 S32.17

Fracture, traumatic (abduction) (adduction) (separation) (*see also* **Fracture, pathological**) T14.8 — *continued*
sacrum S32.10 — *continued*
　Zone
　　I S32.119
　　　displaced (minimally) S32.111
　　　　severely S32.112
　　　nondisplaced S32.110
　　II S32.129
　　　displaced (minimally) S32.121
　　　　severely S32.122
　　　nondisplaced S32.120
　　III S32.139
　　　displaced (minimally) S32.131
　　　　severely S32.132
　　　nondisplaced S32.130
scaphoid (hand) — *see also* Fracture, carpal, navicular
　foot — *see* Fracture, tarsal, navicular
scapula S42.10-
　acromial process (displaced) S42.12-
　　nondisplaced S42.12-
　body (displaced) S42.11-
　　nondisplaced S42.11-
　coracoid process (displaced) S42.13-
　　nondisplaced S42.13-
　glenoid cavity (displaced) S42.14-
　　nondisplaced S42.14-
　neck (displaced) S42.15-
　　nondisplaced S42.15-
　specified NEC S42.19-
semilunar bone, wrist — *see* Fracture, carpal, lunate
sequelae — *see* Sequelae, fracture
sesamoid bone
　hand — *see* Fracture, carpal
　foot S92.81-
　other — *see* Fracture, traumatic, by site
shepherd's — *see* Fracture, tarsal, talus
shoulder (girdle) S42.9-
　blade — *see* Fracture, scapula
sinus (ethmoid) (frontal) S02.19
skull S02.91
　base S02.10-
　　occiput S02.119
　　　condyle S02.113
　　　type I S02.110
　　　　left side S02.11B *(follows S02.119)*
　　　　right side S02.11A *(follows S02.119)*
　　　type II S02.111
　　　　left side S02.11D *(follows S02.119)*
　　　　right side S02.11C *(follows S02.119)*
　　　type III S02.112
　　　　left side S02.11F *(follows S02.119)*
　　　　right side S02.11E *(follows S02.119)*
　　　specified NEC S02.118
　　　　left side S02.11H *(follows S02.119)*
　　　　right side S02.11G *(follows S02.119)*
　　specified NEC S02.19
　birth injury P13.0
　frontal bone S02.0
　parietal bone S02.0
　specified site NEC S02.8-
　temporal bone S02.19
　vault S02.0
Smith's — *see* Smith's fracture
sphenoid (bone) (sinus) S02.19
spine — *see* Fracture, vertebra
spinous process — *see* Fracture, vertebra
spontaneous (cause unknown) — *see* Fracture, pathological
stave (of thumb) — *see* Fracture, metacarpal, first
sternum S22.20
　with flail chest — *see* Flail, chest
　body S22.22
　manubrium S22.21
　xiphoid (process) S22.24

Fracture, traumatic (abduction) (adduction) (separation) (*see also* **Fracture, pathological**) T14.8 — *continued*
stress M84.30
　ankle M84.37-
　carpus M84.34-
　clavicle M84.31-
　femoral neck M84.359
　femur M84.35-
　fibula M84.36-
　finger M84.34-
　hip M84.359
　humerus M84.32-
　ilium M84.350
　ischium M84.350
　metacarpus M84.34-
　metatarsus M84.37-
　neck — *see* Fracture, fatigue, vertebra
　pelvis M84.350
　radius M84.33-
　rib M84.38
　scapula M84.31-
　skull M84.38
　tarsus M84.37-
　tibia M84.36-
　toe M84.37-
　ulna M84.33-
　vertebra — *see* Fracture, fatigue, vertebra
supracondylar, elbow — *see* Fracture, humerus, lower end, supracondylar
symphysis pubis — *see* Fracture, pubis
talus (ankle bone) — *see* Fracture, tarsal, talus
tarsal bone(s) S92.20-
　astragalus — *see* Fracture, tarsal, talus
　calcaneus S92.00-
　　anterior process (displaced) S92.02-
　　　nondisplaced S92.02-
　　body (displaced) S92.01-
　　　nondisplaced S92.01-
　　extraarticular NEC (displaced) S92.05-
　　　nondisplaced S92.05-
　　intraarticular (displaced) S92.06-
　　　nondisplaced S92.06-
　　physeal S99.00-
　　　Salter-Harris
　　　　Type I S99.01-
　　　　Type II S99.02-
　　　　Type III S99.03-
　　　　Type IV S99.04-
　　　　specified NEC S99.09-
　　tuberosity (displaced) S92.04-
　　　avulsion (displaced) S92.03-
　　　　nondisplaced S92.03-
　　　nondisplaced S92.04-
　cuboid (displaced) S92.21-
　　nondisplaced S92.21-
　cuneiform
　　intermediate (displaced) S92.23-
　　　nondisplaced S92.23-
　　lateral (displaced) S92.22-
　　　nondisplaced S92.22-
　　medial (displaced) S92.24-
　　　nondisplaced S92.24-
　navicular (displaced) S92.25-
　　nondisplaced S92.25-
　scaphoid — *see* Fracture, tarsal, navicular
　talus S92.10-
　　avulsion (displaced) S92.15-
　　　nondisplaced S92.15-
　　body (displaced) S92.12-
　　　nondisplaced S92.12-
　　dome (displaced) S92.14-
　　　nondisplaced S92.14-
　　head (displaced) S92.12-
　　　nondisplaced S92.12-
　　lateral process (displaced) S92.14-
　　　nondisplaced S92.14-
　　neck (displaced) S92.11-
　　　nondisplaced S92.11-

Fracture, traumatic (abduction) (adduction) (separation) (*see also* **Fracture, pathological**) T14.8 — *continued*
tarsal bone(s) S92.20- — *continued*
　talus S92.10- — *continued*
　　posterior process (displaced) S92.13-
　　　nondisplaced S92.13-
　　specified NEC S92.19-
temporal bone (styloid) S02.19
thorax (bony) S22.9
　with flail chest — *see* Flail, chest
　rib S22.3-
　　multiple S22.4-
　　　with flail chest — *see* Flail, chest
　sternum S22.20
　　body S22.22
　　manubrium S22.21
　　xiphoid process S22.24
　vertebra (displaced) S22.009
　　burst (stable) S22.001
　　　unstable S22.002
　　eighth S22.069
　　　burst (stable) S22.061
　　　　unstable S22.062
　　　specified type NEC S22.068
　　　wedge compression S22.060
　　eleventh S22.089
　　　burst (stable) S22.081
　　　　unstable S22.082
　　　specified type NEC S22.088
　　　wedge compression S22.080
　　fifth S22.059
　　　burst (stable) S22.051
　　　　unstable S22.052
　　　specified type NEC S22.058
　　　wedge compression S22.050
　　first S22.019
　　　burst (stable) S22.011
　　　　unstable S22.012
　　　specified type NEC S22.018
　　　wedge compression S22.010
　　fourth S22.049
　　　burst (stable) S22.041
　　　　unstable S22.042
　　　specified type NEC S22.048
　　　wedge compression S22.040
　　ninth S22.079
　　　burst (stable) S22.071
　　　　unstable S22.072
　　　specified type NEC S22.078
　　　wedge compression S22.070
　　nondisplaced S22.001
　　second S22.029
　　　burst (stable) S22.021
　　　　unstable S22.022
　　　specified type NEC S22.028
　　　wedge compression S22.020
　　seventh S22.069
　　　burst (stable) S22.061
　　　　unstable S22.062
　　　specified type NEC S22.068
　　　wedge compression S22.060
　　sixth S22.059
　　　burst (stable) S22.051
　　　　unstable S22.052
　　　specified type NEC S22.058
　　　wedge compression S22.050
　　specified type NEC S22.008
　　tenth S22.079
　　　burst (stable) S22.071
　　　　unstable S22.072
　　　specified type NEC S22.078
　　　wedge compression S22.070
　　third S22.039
　　　burst (stable) S22.031
　　　　unstable S22.032
　　　specified type NEC S22.038
　　　wedge compression S22.030

Fracture, traumatic (abduction) (adduction) (separation) (*see also* **Fracture, pathological**) T14.8 — *continued*
thorax (bony) S22.9 — *continued*
  vertebra (displaced) S22.009 — *continued*
    twelfth S22.089
      burst (stable) S22.081
      unstable S22.082
      specified type NEC S22.088
      wedge compression S22.080
    wedge compression S22.000
thumb S62.50-
  distal phalanx (displaced) S62.52-
    nondisplaced S62.52-
  proximal phalanx (displaced) S62.51-
    nondisplaced S62.51-
thyroid cartilage S12.8
tibia (shaft) S82.20-
  comminuted (displaced) S82.25-
    nondisplaced S82.25-
  condyles — *see* Fracture, tibia, upper end
  distal end — *see* Fracture, tibia, lower end
  epiphysis
    lower — *see* Fracture, tibia, lower end
    upper — *see* Fracture, tibia, upper end
  following insertion of implant, prosthesis or plate M96.67-
  head (involving knee joint) — *see* Fracture, tibia, upper end
  intercondyloid eminence — *see* Fracture, tibia, upper end
  involving ankle or malleolus — *see* Fracture, ankle, medial malleolus
  lower end S82.30-
    physeal S89.10-
      Salter-Harris
        Type I S89.11-
        Type II S89.12-
        Type III S89.13-
        Type IV S89.14-
        specified NEC S89.19-
    pilon (displaced) S82.87-
      nondisplaced S82.87-
    specified NEC S82.39-
    torus S82.31-
  malleolus — *see* Fracture, ankle, medial malleolus
  oblique (displaced) S82.23-
    nondisplaced S82.23-
  pilon — *see* Fracture, tibia, lower end, pilon
  proximal end — *see* Fracture, tibia, upper end
  segmental (displaced) S82.26-
    nondisplaced S82.26-
  specified NEC S82.29-
  spine — *see* Fracture, upper end, spine
  spiral (displaced) S82.24-
    nondisplaced S82.24-
  transverse (displaced) S82.22-
    nondisplaced S82.22-
  tuberosity — *see* Fracture, tibia, upper end, tuberosity
  upper end S82.10-
    bicondylar (displaced) S82.14-
      nondisplaced S82.14-
    lateral condyle (displaced) S82.12-
      nondisplaced S82.12-
    medial condyle (displaced) S82.13-
      nondisplaced S82.13-
    physeal S89.00-
      Salter-Harris
        Type I S89.01-
        Type II S89.02-
        Type III S89.03-
        Type IV S89.04-
        specified NEC S89.09-
    plateau — *see* Fracture, tibia, upper end, bicondylar

Fracture, traumatic (abduction) (adduction) (separation) (*see also* **Fracture, pathological**) T14.8 — *continued*
tibia (shaft) S82.20- — *continued*
  upper end S82.10- — *continued*
    specified NEC S82.19-
    spine (displaced) S82.11-
      nondisplaced S82.11-
    torus S82.16-
    tuberosity (displaced) S82.15-
      nondisplaced S82.15-
toe S92.91-
  great (displaced) S92.40-
    distal phalanx (displaced) S92.42-
      nondisplaced S92.42-
    nondisplaced S92.40-
    proximal phalanx (displaced) S92.41-
      nondisplaced S92.41-
    specified NEC S92.49-
  lesser (displaced) S92.50-
    distal phalanx (displaced) S92.53-
      nondisplaced S92.53-
    medial phalanx (displaced) S92.52-
      nondisplaced S92.52-
    nondisplaced S92.50-
    proximal phalanx (displaced) S92.51-
      nondisplaced S92.51-
    specified NEC S92.59-
  physeal
    phalanx S99.20-
      Salter-Harris
        Type I S99.21-
        Type II S99.22-
        Type III S99.23-
        Type IV S99.24-
        specified NEC S99.29-
tooth (root) S02.5
trachea (cartilage) S12.8
transverse process — *see* Fracture, vertebra
trapezium or trapezoid bone — *see* Fracture, carpal
trimalleolar — *see* Fracture, ankle, trimalleolar
triquetrum (cuneiform of carpus) — *see* Fracture, carpal, triquetrum
trochanter — *see* Fracture, femur, trochanteric
tuberosity (external) — *see* Fracture, traumatic, by site
ulna (shaft) S52.20-
  bent bone S52.28-
  coronoid process — *see* Fracture, ulna, upper end, coronoid process
  distal end — *see* Fracture, ulna, lower end
  following insertion of implant, prosthesis or plate M96.63-
  head S52.00-
  lower end S52.60-
    physeal S59.00-
      Salter-Harris
        Type I S59.01-
        Type II S59.02-
        Type III S59.03-
        Type IV S59.04-
        specified NEC S59.09-
    specified NEC S52.69-
    styloid process (displaced) S52.61-
      nondisplaced S52.61-
    torus S52.62-
  proximal end — *see* Fracture, ulna, upper end
  shaft S52.20-
    comminuted (displaced) S52.25-
      nondisplaced S52.25-
    greenstick S52.21-
    Monteggia's — *see* Monteggia's fracture
    oblique (displaced) S52.23-
      nondisplaced S52.23-
    segmental (displaced) S52.26-
      nondisplaced S52.26-

Fracture, traumatic (abduction) (adduction) (separation) (*see also* **Fracture, pathological**) T14.8 — *continued*
ulna (shaft) S52.20- — *continued*
  shaft S52.20- — *continued*
    specified NEC S52.29-
    spiral (displaced) S52.24-
      nondisplaced S52.24-
    transverse (displaced) S52.22-
      nondisplaced S52.22-
  upper end S52.00-
    coronoid process (displaced) S52.04-
      nondisplaced S52.04-
    olecranon process (displaced) S52.02-
      with intraarticular extension S52.03-
      nondisplaced S52.02-
        with intraarticular extension S52.03-
    specified NEC S52.09-
    torus S52.01-
unciform — *see* Fracture, carpal, hamate
vault of skull S02.0
vertebra, vertebral (arch) (body) (column) (neural arch) (pedicle) (spinous process) (transverse process)
  atlas — *see* Fracture, neck, cervical vertebra, first
  axis — *see* Fracture, neck, cervical vertebra, second
  cervical (teardrop) S12.9
    axis — *see* Fracture, neck, cervical vertebra, second
    first (atlas) — *see* Fracture, neck, cervical vertebra, first
    second (axis) — *see* Fracture, neck, cervical vertebra, second
  chronic M84.48
  coccyx S32.2
  dorsal — *see* Fracture, thorax, vertebra
  lumbar S32.009
    burst (stable) S32.001
      unstable S32.002
    fifth S32.059
      burst (stable) S32.051
        unstable S32.052
      specified type NEC S32.058
      wedge compression S32.050
    first S32.019
      burst (stable) S32.011
        unstable S32.012
      specified type NEC S32.018
      wedge compression S32.010
    fourth S32.049
      burst (stable) S32.041
        unstable S32.042
      specified type NEC S32.048
      wedge compression S32.040
    second S32.029
      burst (stable) S32.021
        unstable S32.022
      specified type NEC S32.028
      wedge compression S32.020
    specified type NEC S32.008
    third S32.039
      burst (stable) S32.031
        unstable S32.032
      specified type NEC S32.038
      wedge compression S32.030
    wedge compression S32.000
  metastatic — *see* Collapse, vertebra, in, specified disease NEC — *see also* Neoplasm
  newborn (birth injury) P11.5
  sacrum S32.10
    specified NEC S32.19
    Type
      1 S32.14
      2 S32.15
      3 S32.16
      4 S32.17

Fracture, traumatic (abduction) (adduction) (separation) (see also **Fracture, pathological**) T14.8 — continued
  vertebra, vertebral (arch) (body) (column) (neural arch) (pedicle) (spinous process) (transverse process) — continued
    sacrum S32.10 — continued
      Zone
        I S32.119
          displaced (minimally) S32.111
            severely S32.112
          nondisplaced S32.110
        II S32.129
          displaced (minimally) S32.121
            severely S32.122
          nondisplaced S32.120
        III S32.139
          displaced (minimally) S32.131
            severely S32.132
          nondisplaced S32.130
    thoracic — see Fracture, thorax, vertebra
  vertex S02.0
  vomer (bone) S02.2
  wrist S62.10-
    carpal — see Fracture, carpal bone
    navicular (scaphoid) (hand) — see Fracture, carpal, navicular
  xiphisternum, xiphoid (process) S22.24
  zygoma S02.402
    left side S02.40F (follows S02.402)
    right side S02.40E (follows S02.402)
Fragile, fragility
  autosomal site Q95.5
  bone, congenital (with blue sclera) Q78.0
  capillary (hereditary) D69.8
  hair L67.8
  nails L60.3
  non-sex chromosome site Q95.5
  X chromosome Q99.2
Fragilitas
  crinium L67.8
  ossium (with blue sclerae) (hereditary) Q78.0
  unguium L60.3
    congenital Q84.6
Fragments, cataract (lens), following cataract surgery H59.02-
  retained foreign body — see Retained, foreign body fragments (type of)
Frailty (frail) R54
  mental R41.81
Frambesia, frambesial (tropica) — see also Yaws
  initial lesion or ulcer A66.0
  primary A66.0
Frambeside
  gummatous A66.4
  of early yaws A66.2
Frambesioma A66.1
Franceschetti-Klein(-Wildervanck) disease or syndrome Q75.4
Francis' disease — see Tularemia
Frank's essential thrombocytopenia D69.3
Franklin disease C88.2
Fraser's syndrome Q87.0
Freckle(s) L81.2
  malignant melanoma in — see Melanoma
  melanotic (Hutchinson's) — see Melanoma, in situ
  retinal D49.81
Frederickson's hyperlipoproteinemia, type
  I and V E78.3
  IIA E78.00
  IIB and III E78.2
  IV E78.1
Freeman Sheldon syndrome Q87.0
Freezing (see also Effect, adverse, cold) T69.9
Frei's disease A55

Freiberg's disease (infraction of metatarsal head or osteochondrosis) — see Osteochondrosis, juvenile, metatarsus
Fremitus, friction, cardiac R01.2
Frenum, frenulum
  external os Q51.828
  tongue (shortening) (congenital) Q38.1
Frequency micturition (nocturnal) R35.0
  psychogenic F45.8
Frey's syndrome
  auriculotemporal G50.8
  hyperhidrosis L74.52
Friction
  burn — see Burn, by site
  fremitus, cardiac R01.2
  precordial R01.2
  sounds, chest R09.89
Friderichsen-Waterhouse syndrome or disease A39.1
Friedländer's B (bacillus) NEC (see also condition) A49.8
Friedreich's
  ataxia G11.1
  combined systemic disease G11.1
  facial hemihypertrophy Q67.4
  sclerosis (cerebellum) (spinal cord) G11.1
Frigidity F52.22
Fröhlich's syndrome E23.6
Frontal — see also condition
  lobe syndrome F07.0
Frostbite (superficial) T33.90
  with
    partial thickness skin loss — see Frostbite (superficial), by site
    tissue necrosis T34.90
  abdominal wall T33.3
    with tissue necrosis T34.3
  ankle T33.81-
    with tissue necrosis T34.81-
  arm T33.4-
    with tissue necrosis T34.4-
    finger(s) — see Frostbite, finger
    hand — see Frostbite, hand
    wrist — see Frostbite, wrist
  ear T33.01-
    with tissue necrosis T34.01-
  face T33.09
    with tissue necrosis T34.09
  finger T33.53-
    with tissue necrosis T34.53-
  foot T33.82-
    with tissue necrosis T34.82-
  hand T33.52-
    with tissue necrosis T34.52-
  head T33.09
    with tissue necrosis T34.09
    ear — see Frostbite, ear
    nose — see Frostbite, nose
  hip (and thigh) T33.6-
    with tissue necrosis T34.6-
  knee T33.7-
    with tissue necrosis T34.7-
  leg T33.9-
    with tissue necrosis T34.9-
    ankle — see Frostbite, ankle
    foot — see Frostbite, foot
    knee — see Frostbite, knee
    lower T33.7-
      with tissue necrosis T34.7-
    thigh — see Frostbite, hip
    toe — see Frostbite, toe
  limb
    lower T33.99
      with tissue necrosis T34.99
    upper — see Frostbite, arm
  neck T33.1
    with tissue necrosis T34.1
  nose T33.02
    with tissue necrosis T34.02

Frostbite (superficial) T33.90 — continued
  pelvis T33.3
    with tissue necrosis T34.3
  specified site NEC T33.99
    with tissue necrosis T34.99
  thigh — see Frostbite, hip
  thorax T33.2
    with tissue necrosis T34.2
  toes T33.83-
    with tissue necrosis T34.83-
  trunk T33.99
    with tissue necrosis T34.99
  wrist T33.51-
    with tissue necrosis T34.51-
Frotteurism F65.81
Frozen (see also Effect, adverse, cold) T69.9
  pelvis (female) N94.89
    male K66.8
  shoulder — see Capsulitis, adhesive
Fructokinase deficiency E74.11
Fructose 1,6 diphosphatase deficiency E74.19
Fructosemia (benign) (essential) E74.12
Fructosuria (benign) (essential) E74.11
Fuchs'
  black spot (myopic) H44.2-
  dystrophy (corneal endothelium) H18.51
  heterochromic cyclitis — see Cyclitis, Fuchs' heterochromic
Fucosidosis E77.1
Fugue R68.89
  dissociative F44.1
  hysterical (dissociative) F44.1
  postictal in epilepsy — see Epilepsy
  reaction to exceptional stress (transient) F43.0
Fulminant, fulminating — see condition
Functional — see also condition
  bleeding (uterus) N93.8
Functioning, intellectual, borderline R41.83
Fundus — see condition
Fungemia NOS B49
Fungus, fungous
  cerebral G93.89
  disease NOS B49
  infection — see Infection, fungus
Funiculitis (acute) (chronic) (endemic) N49.1
  gonococcal (acute) (chronic) A54.23
  tuberculous A18.15
Funnel
  breast (acquired) M95.4
    congenital Q67.6
    sequelae (late effect) of rickets E64.3
  chest (acquired) M95.4
    congenital Q67.6
    sequelae (late effect) of rickets E64.3
  pelvis (acquired) M95.5
    with disproportion (fetopelvic) O33.3
      causing obstructed labor O65.3
    congenital Q74.2
FUO (fever of unknown origin) R50.9
Furfur L21.0
  microsporon B36.0
Furrier's lung J67.8
Furrowed K14.5
  nail(s) (transverse) L60.4
    congenital Q84.6
  tongue K14.5
    congenital Q38.3
Furuncle L02.92
  abdominal wall L02.221
  ankle — see Furuncle, lower limb
  antecubital space — see Furuncle, upper limb
  anus K61.0
  arm — see Furuncle, upper limb
  auditory canal, external — see Abscess, ear, external
  auricle (ear) — see Abscess, ear, external
  axilla (region) L02.42-

Furuncle L02.92 — *continued*
  back (any part) L02.222
  breast N61.1
  buttock L02.32
  cheek (external) L02.02
  chest wall L02.223
  chin L02.02
  corpus cavernosum N48.21
  ear, external — *see* Abscess, ear, external
  external auditory canal — *see* Abscess, ear, external
  eyelid — *see* Abscess, eyelid
  face L02.02
  femoral (region) — *see* Furuncle, lower limb
  finger — *see* Furuncle, hand
  flank L02.221
  foot L02.62-
  forehead L02.02
  gluteal (region) L02.32
  groin L02.224
  hand L02.52-
  head L02.821
    face L02.02
  hip — *see* Furuncle, lower limb
  kidney — *see* Abscess, kidney
  knee — *see* Furuncle, lower limb
  labium (majus) (minus) N76.4
  lacrimal
    gland — *see* Dacryoadenitis
    passages (duct) (sac) — *see* Inflammation, lacrimal, passages, acute
  leg (any part) — *see* Furuncle, lower limb
  lower limb L02.42-
  malignant A22.0
  mouth K12.2
  navel L02.226
  neck L02.12
  nose J34.0
  orbit, orbital — *see* Abscess, orbit
  palmar (space) — *see* Furuncle, hand
  partes posteriores L02.32
  pectoral region L02.223
  penis N48.21
  perineum L02.225
  pinna — *see* Abscess, ear, external
  popliteal — *see* Furuncle, lower limb
  prepatellar — *see* Furuncle, lower limb
  scalp L02.821
  seminal vesicle N49.0
  shoulder — *see* Furuncle, upper limb
  specified site NEC L02.828
  submandibular K12.2
  temple (region) L02.02
  thumb — *see* Furuncle, hand
  toe — *see* Furuncle, foot
  trunk L02.229
    abdominal wall L02.221
    back L02.222
    chest wall L02.223
    groin L02.224
    perineum L02.225
    umbilicus L02.226
  umbilicus L02.226
  upper limb L02.42-
  vulva N76.4
Furunculosis — *see* Furuncle
Fused — *see* Fusion, fused
Fusion, fused (congenital)
  astragaloscaphoid Q74.2
  atria Q21.1
  auditory canal Q16.1
  auricles, heart Q21.1
  binocular with defective stereopsis H53.32
  bone Q79.8
  cervical spine M43.22
  choanal Q30.0
  commissure, mitral valve Q23.2

Fusion, fused (congenital) — *continued*
  cusps, heart valve NEC Q24.8
    mitral Q23.2
    pulmonary Q22.1
    tricuspid Q22.4
  ear ossicles Q16.3
  fingers Q70.0-
  hymen Q52.3
  joint (acquired) — *see also* Ankylosis
    congenital Q74.8
  kidneys (incomplete) Q63.1
  labium (majus) (minus) Q52.5
  larynx and trachea Q34.8
  limb, congenital Q74.8
    lower Q74.2
    upper Q74.0
  lobes, lung Q33.8
  lumbosacral (acquired) M43.27
    arthrodesis status Z98.1
    congenital Q76.49
    postprocedural status Z98.1
  nares, nose, nasal, nostril(s) Q30.0
  organ or site not listed — *see* Anomaly, by site
  ossicles Q79.9
    auditory Q16.3
  pulmonic cusps Q22.1
  ribs Q76.6
  sacroiliac (joint) (acquired) M43.28
    arthrodesis status Z98.1
    congenital Q74.2
    postprocedural status Z98.1
  spine (acquired) NEC M43.20
    arthrodesis status Z98.1
    cervical region M43.22
    cervicothoracic region M43.23
    congenital Q76.49
    lumbar M43.26
    lumbosacral region M43.27
    occipito-atlanto-axial region M43.21
    postoperative status Z98.1
    sacrococcygeal region M43.28
    thoracic region M43.24
    thoracolumbar region M43.25
  sublingual duct with submaxillary duct at opening in mouth Q38.4
  testes Q55.1
  toes Q70.2-
  tooth, teeth K00.2
  trachea and esophagus Q39.8
  twins Q89.4
  vagina Q52.4
  ventricles, heart Q21.0
  vertebra (arch) — *see* Fusion, spine
  vulva Q52.5
Fusospirillosis (mouth) (tongue) (tonsil) A69.1
Fussy baby R68.12

Gain in weight (abnormal) (excessive) — *see also* Weight, gain
Gaisböck's disease (polycythemia hypertonica) D75.1
Gait abnormality R26.9
  ataxic R26.0
  falling R29.6
  hysterical (ataxic) (staggering) F44.4
  paralytic R26.1
  spastic R26.1
  specified type NEC R26.89
  staggering R26.0
  unsteadiness R26.81
  walking difficulty NEC R26.2
Galactocele (breast) N64.89
  puerperal, postpartum O92.79
Galactokinase deficiency E74.29
Galactophoritis N61.0
  gestational, puerperal, postpartum O91.2-
Galactorrhea O92.6
  not associated with childbirth N64.3
Galactosemia (classic) (congenital) E74.21
Galactosuria E74.29
Galacturia R82.0
  schistosomiasis (bilharziasis) B65.0
Galeazzi's fracture S52.37-
Galen's vein — *see* condition
Galeophobia F40.218
Gall duct — *see* condition
Gallbladder — *see also* condition
  acute K81.0
Gallop rhythm R00.8
Gallstone (colic) (cystic duct) (gallbladder) (impacted) (multiple) — *see also* Calculus, gallbladder
  with
    cholecystitis — *see* Calculus, gallbladder, with cholecystitis
    bile duct (common) (hepatic) — *see* Calculus, bile duct
  causing intestinal obstruction K56.3
  specified NEC K80.80
    with obstruction K80.81
Gambling Z72.6
  pathological (compulsive) F63.0
Gammopathy (of undetermined significance [MGUS]) D47.2
  associated with lymphoplasmacytic dyscrasia D47.2
  monoclonal D47.2
  polyclonal D89.0
Gamna's disease (siderotic splenomegaly) D73.1
Gamophobia F40.298
Gampsodactylia (congenital) Q66.7
Gamstorp's disease (adynamia episodica hereditaria) G72.3
Gandy-Nanta disease (siderotic splenomegaly) D73.1
Gang
  membership offenses Z72.810
Gangliocytoma D36.10
Ganglioglioma — *see* Neoplasm, uncertain behavior, by site
Ganglion (compound) (diffuse) (joint) (tendon (sheath)) M67.40
  ankle M67.47-
  foot M67.47-
  forearm M67.43-
  hand M67.44-
  lower leg M67.46-
  multiple sites M67.49
  of yaws (early) (late) A66.6
  pelvic region M67.45-
  periosteal — *see* Periostitis

Ganglion (compound) (diffuse) (joint) (tendon (sheath)) M67.40 — *continued*
 shoulder region M67.41-
 specified site NEC M67.48
 thigh region M67.45-
 tuberculous A18.09
 upper arm M67.42-
 wrist M67.43-
Ganglioneuroblastoma — *see* Neoplasm, nerve, malignant
Ganglioneuroma D36.10
 malignant — *see* Neoplasm, nerve, malignant
Ganglioneuromatosis D36.10
Ganglionitis
 fifth nerve — *see* Neuralgia, trigeminal
 gasserian (postherpetic) (postzoster) B02.21
 geniculate G51.1
  newborn (birth injury) P11.3
  postherpetic, postzoster B02.21
 herpes zoster B02.21
 postherpetic geniculate B02.21
Gangliosidosis E75.10
 GM1 E75.19
 GM2 E75.00
  other specified E75.09
  Sandhoff disease E75.01
  Tay-Sachs disease E75.02
 GM3 E75.19
 mucolipidosis IV E75.11
Gangosa A66.5
Gangrene, gangrenous (connective tissue) (dropsical) (dry) (moist) (skin) (ulcer) (*see also* Necrosis) I96
 with diabetes (mellitus) — *see* Diabetes, gangrene
 abdomen (wall) I96
 alveolar M27.3
 appendix K35.80
  with
   perforation or rupture K35.2
   peritoneal abscess K35.3
   peritonitis NEC K35.3
    generalized (with perforation or rupture) K35.2
    localized (with perforation or rupture) K35.3
 arteriosclerotic (general) (senile) — *see* Arteriosclerosis, extremities, with, gangrene
 auricle I96
 Bacillus welchii A48.0
 bladder (infectious) — *see* Cystitis, specified type NEC
 bowel, cecum, or colon — *see* Gangrene, intestine
 Clostridium perfringens or welchii A48.0
 cornea H18.89-
 corpora cavernosa N48.29
  noninfective N48.89
 cutaneous, spreading I96
 decubital — *see* Ulcer, pressure, by site
 diabetic (any site) — *see* Diabetes, gangrene
 emphysematous — *see* Gangrene, gas
 epidemic — *see* Poisoning, food, noxious, plant
 epididymis (infectional) N45.1
 erysipelas — *see* Erysipelas
 extremity (lower) (upper) I96
 Fournier N49.3
  female N76.89
 fusospirochetal A69.0
 gallbladder — *see* Cholecystitis, acute
 gas (bacillus) A48.0
  following
   abortion — *see* Abortion by type
   complicated by infection
   ectopic or molar pregnancy O08.0
 glossitis K14.0

Gangrene, gangrenous (connective tissue) (dropsical) (dry) (moist) (skin) (ulcer) (*see also* Necrosis) I96 — *continued*
 hernia — *see* Hernia, by site, with gangrene
 intestine, intestinal (hemorrhagic) (massive) (*see also* Infarct, intestine) K55.069
  with
   mesenteric embolism (*see also* Infarct, intestine) K55.069
   obstruction — *see* Obstruction, intestine
 laryngitis J04.0
 limb (lower) (upper) I96
 lung J85.0
  spirochetal A69.8
 lymphangitis I89.1
 Meleney's (synergistic) — *see* Ulcer, skin
 mesentery (*see also* Infarct, intestine) K55.069
  with
   embolism (*see also* Infarct, intestine) K55.069
   intestinal obstruction — *see* Obstruction, intestine
 mouth A69.0
 ovary — *see* Oophoritis
 pancreas — *see* Pancreatitis, acute
 penis N48.29
  noninfective N48.89
 perineum I96
 pharynx — *see also* Pharyngitis
  Vincent's A69.1
 presenile I73.1
 progressive synergistic — *see* Ulcer, skin
 pulmonary J85.0
 pulpal (dental) K04.1
 quinsy J36
 Raynaud's (symmetric gangrene) I73.01
 retropharyngeal J39.2
 scrotum N49.3
  noninfective N50.89
 senile (atherosclerotic) — *see* Arteriosclerosis, extremities, with, gangrene
 spermatic cord N49.1
  noninfective N50.89
 spine I96
 spirochetal NEC A69.8
 spreading cutaneous I96
 stomatitis A69.0
 symmetrical I73.01
 testis (infectional) N45.2
  noninfective N44.8
 throat — *see also* Pharyngitis
  diphtheritic A36.0
  Vincent's A69.1
 thyroid (gland) E07.89
 tooth (pulp) K04.1
 tuberculous NEC — *see* Tuberculosis
 tunica vaginalis N49.1
  noninfective N50.89
 umbilicus I96
 uterus — *see* Endometritis
 uvulitis K12.2
 vas deferens N49.1
  noninfective N50.89
 vulva N76.89
Ganister disease J62.8
Ganser's syndrome (hysterical) F44.89
Gardner-Diamond syndrome (autoerythrocyte sensitization) D69.2
Gargoylism E76.01
Garré's disease, osteitis (sclerosing), osteomyelitis — *see* Osteomyelitis, specified type NEC
Garrod's pad, knuckle M72.1
Gartner's duct
 cyst Q52.4
 persistent Q50.6

Gas R14.3
 asphyxiation, inhalation, poisoning, suffocation NEC — *see* Table of Drugs and Chemicals
 excessive R14.0
 gangrene A48.0
  following
   abortion — *see* Abortion by type complicated by infection
   ectopic or molar pregnancy O08.0
 on stomach R14.0
 pains R14.1
Gastralgia — *see also* Pain, abdominal
Gastrectasis K31.0
 psychogenic F45.8
Gastric — *see* condition
Gastrinoma
 malignant
  pancreas C25.4
  specified site NEC — *see* Neoplasm, malignant, by site
  unspecified site C25.4
 specified site — *see* Neoplasm, uncertain behavior
 unspecified site D37.9
Gastritis (simple) K29.70
 with bleeding K29.71
 acute (erosive) K29.00
  with bleeding K29.01
 alcoholic K29.20
  with bleeding K29.21
 allergic K29.60
  with bleeding K29.61
 atrophic (chronic) K29.40
  with bleeding K29.41
 chronic (antral) (fundal) K29.50
  with bleeding K29.51
  atrophic K29.40
   with bleeding K29.41
  superficial K29.30
   with bleeding K29.31
 dietary counseling and surveillance Z71.3
 due to diet deficiency E63.9
 eosinophilic K52.81
 giant hypertrophic K29.60
  with bleeding K29.61
 granulomatous K29.60
  with bleeding K29.61
 hypertrophic (mucosa) K29.60
  with bleeding K29.61
 nervous F54
 spastic K29.60
  with bleeding K29.61
 specified NEC K29.60
  with bleeding K29.61
 superficial chronic K29.30
  with bleeding K29.31
 tuberculous A18.83
 viral NEC A08.4
Gastrocarcinoma — *see* Neoplasm, malignant, stomach
Gastrocolic — *see* condition
Gastrodisciasis, gastrodiscoidiasis B66.8
Gastroduodenitis K29.90
 with bleeding K29.91
 virus, viral A08.4
  specified type NEC A08.39
Gastrodynia — *see* Pain, abdominal
Gastroenteritis (acute) (chronic) (noninfectious) (*see also* Enteritis) K52.9
 allergic K52.29
  with
   eosinophilic gastritis or gastroenteritis K52.81
   food protein-induced enterocolitis syndrome K52.21
   food protein-induced enteropathy K52.22
 dietetic (*see also* Gastroenteritis, allergic) K52.29

Gastroenteritis (acute) (chronic) (noninfectious) (*see also* Enteritis) K52.9 — *continued*
drug-induced K52.1
due to
  Cryptosporidium A07.2
  drugs K52.1
  food poisoning — *see* Intoxication, foodborne
  radiation K52.0
eosinophilic K52.81
epidemic (infectious) A09
food hypersensitivity (*see also* Gastroenteritis, allergic) K52.29
infectious — *see* Enteritis, infectious
influenzal — *see* Influenza, with gastroenteritis
noninfectious K52.9
  specified NEC K52.89
rotaviral A08.0
Salmonella A02.0
toxic K52.1
viral NEC A08.4
  acute infectious A08.39
    type Norwalk A08.11
  infantile (acute) A08.39
  Norwalk agent A08.11
  rotaviral A08.0
  severe of infants A08.39
  specified type NEC A08.39
Gastroenteropathy (*see also* Gastroenteritis) K52.9
acute, due to Norovirus A08.11
acute, due to Norwalk agent A08.11
infectious A09
Gastroenteroptosis K63.4
Gastroesophageal laceration-hemorrhage syndrome K22.6
Gastrointestinal — *see* condition
Gastrojejunal — *see* condition
Gastrojejunitis (*see also* Enteritis) K52.9
Gastrojejunocolic — *see* condition
Gastroliths K31.89
Gastromalacia K31.89
Gastroparalysis K31.84
diabetic — *see* Diabetes, gastroparalysis
Gastroparesis K31.84
diabetic — *see* Diabetes, by type, with gastroparesis
Gastropathy K31.9
congestive portal K31.89
erythematous K29.70
exudative K90.89
portal hypertensive K31.89
Gastroptosis K31.89
Gastrorrhagia K92.2
psychogenic F45.8
Gastroschisis (congenital) Q79.3
Gastrospasm (neurogenic) (reflex) K31.89
neurotic F45.8
psychogenic F45.8
Gastrostaxis — *see* Gastritis, with bleeding
Gastrostenosis K31.89
Gastrostomy
attention to Z43.1
status Z93.1
Gastrosuccorrhea (continuous) (intermittent) K31.89
neurotic F45.8
psychogenic F45.8
Gatophobia F40.218
Gaucher's disease or splenomegaly (adult) (infantile) E75.22
Gee(-Herter)(-Thaysen) disease (nontropical sprue) K90.0
Gélineau's syndrome G47.419
with cataplexy G47.411
Gemination, tooth, teeth K00.2

Gemistocytoma
specified site — *see* Neoplasm, malignant, by site
unspecified site C71.9
General, generalized — *see* condition
Genetic
carrier (status)
  cystic fibrosis Z14.1
  hemophilia A (asymptomatic) Z14.01
    symptomatic Z14.02
  specified NEC Z14.8
susceptibility to disease NEC Z15.89
  malignant neoplasm Z15.09
    breast Z15.01
      endometrium Z15.04
      ovary Z15.02
      prostate Z15.03
      specified NEC Z15.09
  multiple endocrine neoplasia Z15.81
Genital — *see* condition
Genito-anorectal syndrome A55
Genitourinary system — *see* condition
Genu
congenital Q74.1
extrorsum (acquired) — *see also* Deformity, varus, knee
  congenital Q74.1
  sequelae (late effect) of rickets E64.3
introrsum (acquired) — *see also* Deformity, valgus, knee
  congenital Q74.1
  sequelae (late effect) of rickets E64.3
rachitic (old) E64.3
recurvatum (acquired) — *see also* Deformity, limb, specified type NEC, lower leg
  congenital Q68.2
  sequelae (late effect) of rickets E64.3
valgum (acquired) (knock-knee) M21.06-
  congenital Q74.1
  sequelae (late effect) of rickets E64.3
varum (acquired) (bowleg) M21.16-
  congenital Q74.1
  sequelae (late effect) of rickets E64.3
Geographic tongue K14.1
Geophagia — *see* Pica
Geotrichosis B48.3
stomatitis B48.3
Gephyrophobia F40.242
Gerbode defect Q21.0
GERD (gastroesophageal reflux disease) K21.9
Gerhardt's
disease (erythromelalgia) I73.81
syndrome (vocal cord paralysis) J38.00
  bilateral J38.02
  unilateral J38.01
German measles — *see also* Rubella
exposure to Z20.4
Germinoblastoma (diffuse) C85.9-
follicular C82.9-
Germinoma — *see* Neoplasm, malignant, by site
Gerontoxon — *see* Degeneration, cornea, senile
Gerstmann's syndrome R48.8
developmental F81.2
Gerstmann-Sträussler-Scheinker syndrome (GSS) A81.82
Gestation (period) — *see also* Pregnancy
ectopic — *see* Pregnancy, by site
multiple O30.9-
  greater than quadruplets — *see* Pregnancy, multiple (gestation), specified NEC
  specified NEC — *see* Pregnancy, multiple (gestation), specified NEC
Gestational
mammary abscess O91.11-
purulent mastitis O91.11-
subareolar abscess O91.11-

Ghon tubercle, primary infection A15.7
Ghost
teeth K00.4
vessels (cornea) H16.41-
Ghoul hand A66.3
Gianotti-Crosti disease L44.4
Giant
cell
  epulis K06.8
  peripheral granuloma K06.8
esophagus, congenital Q39.5
kidney, congenital Q63.3
urticaria T78.3
  hereditary D84.1
Giardiasis A07.1
Gibert's disease or pityriasis L42
Giddiness R42
hysterical F44.89
psychogenic F45.8
Gierke's disease (glycogenosis I) E74.01
Gigantism (cerebral) (hypophyseal) (pituitary) E22.0
constitutional E34.4
Gilbert's disease or syndrome E80.4
Gilchrist's disease B40.9
Gilford-Hutchinson disease E34.8
Gilles de la Tourette's disease or syndrome (motor-verbal tic) F95.2
Gingivitis K05.10
acute (catarrhal) K05.00
  necrotizing A69.1
  nonplaque induced K05.01
  plaque induced K05.00
chronic (desquamative) (hyperplastic) (simple marginal) (pregnancy associated) (ulcerative) K05.10
  nonplaque induced K05.11
  plaque induced K05.10
expulsiva — *see* Periodontitis
necrotizing ulcerative (acute) A69.1
pellagrous E52
  acute necrotizing A69.1
Vincent's A69.1
Gingivoglossitis K14.0
Gingivopericementitis — *see* Periodontitis
Gingivosis — *see* Gingivitis, chronic
Gingivostomatitis K05.10
herpesviral B00.2
necrotizing ulcerative (acute) A69.1
Gland, glandular — *see* condition
Glanders A24.0
Glanzmann (-Naegeli) disease or thrombasthenia D69.1
Glasgow coma scale
total score
  3-8 R40.243
  9-12 R40.242
  13-15 R40.241
Glass-blower's disease (cataract) — *see* Cataract, specified NEC
Glaucoma H40.9
with
  increased episcleral venous pressure H40.81-
  pseudoexfoliation of lens — *see* Glaucoma, open angle, primary, capsular
absolute H44.51-
angle-closure (primary) H40.20-
  acute (attack) (crisis) H40.21-
  chronic H40.22-
  intermittent H40.23-
  residual stage H40.24-
borderline H40.00-
capsular (with pseudoexfoliation of lens) — *see* Glaucoma, open angle, primary, capsular
childhood Q15.0
closed angle — *see* Glaucoma, angle-closure
congenital Q15.0

DISEASE INDEX

Glaucoma H40.9 — *continued*
corticosteroid-induced — *see* Glaucoma, secondary, drugs
hypersecretion H40.82-
in (due to)
amyloidosis E85.4 *[H42]*
aniridia Q13.1 *[H42]*
concussion of globe — *see* Glaucoma, secondary, trauma
dislocation of lens — *see* Glaucoma, secondary
disorder of lens NEC — *see* Glaucoma, secondary
drugs — *see* Glaucoma, secondary, drugs
endocrine disease NOS E34.9 *[H42]*
eye
inflammation — *see* Glaucoma, secondary, inflammation
trauma — *see* Glaucoma, secondary, trauma
hypermature cataract — *see* Glaucoma, secondary
iridocyclitis — *see* Glaucoma, secondary, inflammation
lens disorder — *see* Glaucoma, secondary,
Lowe's syndrome E72.03 *[H42]*
metabolic disease NOS E88.9 *[H42]*
ocular disorders NEC — *see* Glaucoma, secondary
onchocerciasis B73.02
pupillary block — *see* Glaucoma, secondary
retinal vein occlusion — *see* Glaucoma, secondary
Rieger's anomaly Q13.81 *[H42]*
rubeosis of iris — *see* Glaucoma, secondary
tumor of globe — *see* Glaucoma, secondary
infantile Q15.0
low tension — *see* Glaucoma, open angle, primary, low-tension
malignant H40.83-
narrow angle — *see* Glaucoma, angle-closure
newborn Q15.0
noncongestive (chronic) — *see* Glaucoma, open angle
nonobstructive — *see* Glaucoma, open angle
obstructive — *see also* Glaucoma, angle-closure
due to lens changes — *see* Glaucoma, secondary
open angle H40.10-
primary H40.11-
capsular (with pseudoexfoliation of lens) H40.14-
low-tension H40.12-
pigmentary H40.13-
residual stage H40.15-
phacolytic — *see* Glaucoma, secondary
pigmentary — *see* Glaucoma, open angle, primary, pigmentary
postinfectious — *see* Glaucoma, secondary, inflammation
secondary (to) H40.5-
drugs H40.6-
inflammation H40.4-
trauma H40.3-
simple (chronic) H40.11-
simplex H40.11-
specified type NEC H40.89
suspect H40.00-
syphilitic A52.71
traumatic — *see also* Glaucoma, secondary, trauma
newborn (birth injury) P15.3
tuberculous A18.59
Glaucomatous flecks (subcapsular) — *see* Cataract, complicated
Glazed tongue K14.4
Gleet (gonococcal) A54.01
Glénard's disease K63.4

Glioblastoma (multiforme)
with sarcomatous component
specified site — *see* Neoplasm, malignant, by site
unspecified site C71.9
giant cell
specified site — *see* Neoplasm, malignant, by site
unspecified site C71.9
specified site — *see* Neoplasm, malignant, by site
unspecified site C71.9
Glioma (malignant)
astrocytic
specified site — *see* Neoplasm, malignant, by site
unspecified site C71.9
mixed
specified site — *see* Neoplasm, malignant, by site
unspecified site C71.9
nose Q30.8
specified site NEC — *see* Neoplasm, malignant, by site
subependymal D43.2
specified site — *see* Neoplasm, uncertain behavior, by site
unspecified site D43.2
unspecified site C71.9
Gliomatosis cerebri C71.0
Glioneuroma — *see* Neoplasm, uncertain behavior, by site
Gliosarcoma
specified site — *see* Neoplasm, malignant, by site
unspecified site C71.9
Gliosis (cerebral) G93.89
spinal G95.89
Glisson's disease — *see* Rickets
Globinuria R82.3
Globus (hystericus) F45.8
Glomangioma D18.00
intra-abdominal D18.03
intracranial D18.02
skin D18.01
specified site NEC D18.09
Glomangiomyoma D18.00
intra-abdominal D18.03
intracranial D18.02
skin D18.01
specified site NEC D18.09
Glomangiosarcoma — *see* Neoplasm, connective tissue, malignant
Glomerular
disease in syphilis A52.75
nephritis — *see* Glomerulonephritis
Glomerulitis — *see* Glomerulonephritis
Glomerulonephritis (*see also* Nephritis) N05.9
with
edema — *see* Nephrosis
minimal change N05.0
minor glomerular abnormality N05.0
acute N00.9
chronic N03.9
crescentic (diffuse) NEC (*see also* N00-N07 with fourth character .7) N05.7
dense deposit (*see also* N00-N07 with fourth character .6) N05.6
diffuse
crescentic (*see also* N00-N07 with fourth character .7) N05.7
endocapillary proliferative (*see also* N00-N07 with fourth character .4) N05.4
membranous (*see also* N00-N07 with fourth character .2) N05.2
mesangial proliferative (*see also* N00-N07 with fourth character .3) N05.3

Glomerulonephritis (*see also* Nephritis) N05.9 — *continued*
diffuse — *continued*
mesangiocapillary (*see also* N00-N07 with fourth character .5) N05.5
sclerosing N05.8
endocapillary proliferative (diffuse) NEC (*see also* N00-N07 with fourth character .4) N05.4
extracapillary NEC (*see also* N00-N07 with fourth character .7) N05.7
focal (and segmental) (*see also* N00-N07 with fourth character .1) N05.1
hypocomplementemic — *see* Glomerulonephritis, membranoproliferative
IgA — *see* Nephropathy, IgA
immune complex (circulating) NEC N05.8
in (due to)
amyloidosis E85.4 *[N08]*
bilharziasis B65.9 *[N08]*
cryoglobulinemia D89.1 *[N08]*
defibrination syndrome D65 *[N08]*
diabetes mellitus — *see* Diabetes, glomerulosclerosis
disseminated intravascular coagulation D65 *[N08]*
Fabry(-Anderson) disease E75.21 *[N08]*
Goodpasture's syndrome M31.0
hemolytic-uremic syndrome D59.3
Henoch(-Schönlein) purpura D69.0 *[N08]*
lecithin cholesterol acyltransferase deficiency E78.6 *[N08]*
microscopic polyangiitis M31.7 *[N08]*
multiple myeloma C90.0- *[N08]*
Plasmodium malariae B52.0
schistosomiasis B65.9 *[N08]*
sepsis A41.9 *[N08]*
streptococcal A40- *[N08]*
sickle-cell disorders D57- *[N08]*
strongyloidiasis B78.9 *[N08]*
subacute bacterial endocarditis I33.0 *[N08]*
syphilis (late) congenital A50.59 *[N08]*
systemic lupus erythematosus M32.14
thrombotic thrombocytopenic purpura M31.1 *[N08]*
typhoid fever A01.09
Waldenström macroglobulinemia C88.0 *[N08]*
Wegener's granulomatosis M31.31
latent or quiescent N03.9
lobular, lobulonodular — *see* Glomerulonephritis, membranoproliferative
membranoproliferative (diffuse) (type 1 or 3) (*see also* N00-N07 with fourth character .5) N05.5
dense deposit (type 2) NEC (*see also* N00-N07 with fourth character .6) N05.6
membranous (diffuse) NEC (*see also* N00-N07 with fourth character .2) N05.2
mesangial
IgA/IgG — *see* Nephropathy, IgA
proliferative (diffuse) NEC (*see also* N00-N07 with fourth character .3) N05.3
mesangiocapillary (diffuse) NEC (*see also* N00-N07 with fourth character .5) N05.5
necrotic, necrotizing NEC (*see also* N00-N07 with fourth character .8) N05.8
nodular — *see* Glomerulonephritis, membranoproliferative
poststreptococcal NEC N05.9
acute N00.9
chronic N03.9
rapidly progressive N01.9
proliferative NEC (*see also* N00-N07 with fourth character .8) N05.8
diffuse (lupus) M32.14

Glomerulonephritis (*see also* Nephritis)
N05.9 — *continued*
  rapidly progressive N01.9
  sclerosing, diffuse N05.8
  specified pathology NEC (*see also* N00-N07
    with fourth character .8) N05.8
  subacute N01.9
Glomerulopathy — *see* Glomerulonephritis
Glomerulosclerosis — *see also* Sclerosis, renal
  intercapillary (nodular) (with diabetes) — *see*
    Diabetes, glomerulosclerosis
  intracapillary — *see* Diabetes,
    glomerulosclerosis
Glossagra K14.6
Glossalgia K14.6
Glossitis (chronic superficial) (gangrenous)
  (Moeller's) K14.0
  areata exfoliativa K14.1
  atrophic K14.4
  benign migratory K14.1
  cortical superficial, sclerotic K14.0
  Hunter's D51.0
  interstitial, sclerous K14.0
  median rhomboid K14.2
  pellagrous E52
  superficial, chronic K14.0
Glossocele K14.8
Glossodynia K14.6
  exfoliativa K14.4
Glossoncus K14.8
Glossopathy K14.9
Glossophytia K14.3
Glossoplegia K14.8
Glossoptosis K14.8
Glossopyrosis K14.6
Glossotrichia K14.3
Glossy skin L90.8
Glottis — *see* condition
Glottitis (*see also* Laryngitis) J04.0
Glucagonoma
  pancreas
    benign D13.7
    malignant C25.4
    uncertain behavior D37.8
  specified site NEC
    benign — *see* Neoplasm, benign, by site
    malignant — *see* Neoplasm, malignant, by
      site
    uncertain behavior — *see* Neoplasm,
      uncertain behavior, by site
  unspecified site
    benign D13.7
    malignant C25.4
    uncertain behavior D37.8
Glucoglycinuria E72.51
Glucose-galactose malabsorption E74.39
Glue
  ear — *see* Otitis, media, nonsuppurative,
    chronic, mucoid
  sniffing (airplane) — *see* Abuse, drug, inhalant
    dependence — *see* Dependence, drug,
      inhalant
Glutaric aciduria E72.3
Glycinemia E72.51
Glycinuria (renal) (with ketosis) E72.09
Glycogen
  infiltration — *see* Disease, glycogen storage
  storage disease — *see* Disease, glycogen
    storage
Glycogenosis (diffuse) (generalized) — *see also*
  Disease, glycogen storage
  cardiac E74.02 [*I43*]
  diabetic, secondary — *see* Diabetes,
    glycogenosis, secondary
  pulmonary interstitial J84.842
Glycopenia E16.2
Glycosuria R81
  renal E74.8

Gnathostoma spinigerum (infection)
(infestation), gnathostomiasis
  (wandering swelling) B83.1
Goiter (plunging) (substernal) E04.9
  with
    hyperthyroidism (recurrent) — *see*
      Hyperthyroidism, with, goiter
    thyrotoxicosis — *see* Hyperthyroidism, with,
      goiter
  adenomatous — *see* Goiter, nodular
  cancerous C73
  congenital (nontoxic) E03.0
    diffuse E03.0
    parenchymatous E03.0
    transitory, with normal functioning P72.0
  cystic E04.2
    due to iodine-deficiency E01.1
  due to
    enzyme defect in synthesis of thyroid
      hormone E07.1
    iodine-deficiency (endemic) E01.2
  dyshormonogenetic (familial) E07.1
  endemic (iodine-deficiency) E01.2
    diffuse E01.0
    multinodular E01.1
  exophthalmic — *see* Hyperthyroidism, with,
    goiter
  iodine-deficiency (endemic) E01.2
    diffuse E01.0
    multinodular E01.1
    nodular E01.1
  lingual Q89.2
  lymphadenoid E06.3
  malignant C73
  multinodular (cystic) (nontoxic) E04.2
    toxic or with hyperthyroidism E05.20
      with thyroid storm E05.21
  neonatal NEC P72.0
  nodular (nontoxic) (due to) E04.9
    with
      hyperthyroidism E05.20
        with thyroid storm E05.21
      thyrotoxicosis E05.20
        with thyroid storm E05.21
    endemic E01.1
    iodine-deficiency E01.1
    sporadic E04.9
    toxic E05.20
      with thyroid storm E05.21
  nontoxic E04.9
    diffuse (colloid) E04.0
    multinodular E04.2
    simple E04.0
    specified NEC E04.8
    uninodular E04.1
  simple E04.0
  toxic — *see* Hyperthyroidism, with, goiter
  uninodular (nontoxic) E04.1
    toxic or with hyperthyroidism E05.10
      with thyroid storm E05.11
Goiter-deafness syndrome E07.1
Goldberg syndrome Q89.8
Goldberg-Maxwell syndrome E34.51
Goldblatt's hypertension or kidney I70.1
Goldenhar(-Gorlin) syndrome Q87.0
Goldflam-Erb disease or syndrome
  G70.00
  with exacerbation (acute) G70.01
  in crisis G70.01
Goldscheider's disease Q81.8
Goldstein's disease (familial hemorrhagic
  telangiectasia) I78.0
Golfer's elbow — *see* Epicondylitis, medial
Gonadoblastoma
  specified site — *see* Neoplasm, uncertain
    behavior, by site
  unspecified site
    female D39.10
    male D40.10

Gonecystitis — *see* Vesiculitis
Gongylonemiasis B83.8
Goniosynechiae — *see* Adhesions, iris,
  goniosynechiae
Gonococcemia A54.86
Gonococcus, gonococcal (disease) (infection)
  (*see also* condition) A54.9
  anus A54.6
  bursa, bursitis A54.49
  conjunctiva, conjunctivitis (neonatorum)
    A54.31
  endocardium A54.83
  eye A54.30
    conjunctivitis A54.31
    iridocyclitis A54.32
    keratitis A54.33
    newborn A54.31
    other specified A54.39
  fallopian tubes (acute) (chronic) A54.24
  genitourinary (organ) (system) (tract) (acute)
    lower A54.00
      with abscess (accessory gland)
        (periurethral) A54.1
    upper (*see also* condition) A54.29
  heart A54.83
  iridocyclitis A54.32
  joint A54.42
  lymphatic (gland) (node) A54.89
  meninges, meningitis A54.81
  musculoskeletal A54.40
    arthritis A54.42
    osteomyelitis A54.43
    other specified A54.49
    spondylopathy A54.41
  pelviperitonitis A54.24
  pelvis (acute) (chronic) A54.24
  pharynx A54.5
  proctitis A54.6
  pyosalpinx (acute) (chronic) A54.24
  rectum A54.6
  skin A54.89
  specified site NEC A54.89
  tendon sheath A54.49
  throat A54.5
  urethra (acute) (chronic) A54.01
    with abscess (accessory gland) (periurethral)
      A54.1
  vulva (acute) (chronic) A54.02
Gonocytoma
  specified site — *see* Neoplasm, uncertain
    behavior, by site
  unspecified site
    female D39.10
    male D40.10
Gonorrhea (acute) (chronic) A54.9
  Bartholin's gland (acute) (chronic) (purulent)
    A54.02
    with abscess (accessory gland) (periurethral)
      A54.1
  bladder A54.01
  cervix A54.03
  conjunctiva, conjunctivitis (neonatorum)
    A54.31
  contact Z20.2
  Cowper's gland (with abscess) A54.1
  exposure to Z20.2
  fallopian tube (acute) (chronic) A54.24
  kidney (acute) (chronic) A54.21
  lower genitourinary tract A54.00
    with abscess (accessory gland) (periurethral)
      A54.1
  ovary (acute) (chronic) A54.24
  pelvis (acute) (chronic) A54.24
    female pelvic inflammatory disease A54.24
  penis A54.09
  prostate (acute) (chronic) A54.22
  seminal vesicle (acute) (chronic) A54.23
  specified site not listed (*see also* Gonococcus)
    A54.89

Gonorrhea (acute) (chronic) A54.9 — continued
  spermatic cord (acute) (chronic) A54.23
  urethra A54.01
    with abscess (accessory gland) (periurethral) A54.1
  vagina A54.02
  vas deferens (acute) (chronic) A54.23
  vulva A54.02
Goodall's disease A08.19
Goodpasture's syndrome M31.0
Gopalan's syndrome (burning feet) E53.0
Gorlin-Chaudry-Moss syndrome Q87.0
Gottron's papules L94.4
Gougerot-Blum syndrome (pigmented purpuric lichenoid dermatitis) L81.7
Gougerot-Carteaud disease or syndrome (confluent reticulate papillomatosis) L83
Gougerot's syndrome (trisymptomatic) L81.7
Gouley's syndrome (constrictive pericarditis) I31.1
Goundou A66.6
Gout, chronic (see also Gout, gouty) M1A.9 (follows M08)
  drug-induced M1A.20 (follows M08)
    ankle M1A.27- (follows M08)
    elbow M1A.22- (follows M08)
    foot joint M1A.27- (follows M08)
    hand joint M1A.24- (follows M08)
    hip M1A.25- (follows M08)
    knee M1A.26- (follows M08)
    multiple site M1A.29- (follows M08)
    shoulder M1A.21- (follows M08)
    vertebrae M1A.28 (follows M08)
    wrist M1A.23- (follows M08)
  idiopathic M1A.00 (follows M08)
    ankle M1A.07- (follows M08)
    elbow M1A.02- (follows M08)
    foot joint M1A.07- (follows M08)
    hand joint M1A.04- (follows M08)
    hip M1A.05- (follows M08)
    knee M1A.06- (follows M08)
    multiple site M1A.09 (follows M08)
    shoulder M1A.01- (follows M08)
    vertebrae M1A.08 (follows M08)
    wrist M1A.03- (follows M08)
  in (due to) renal impairment M1A.30 (follows M08)
    ankle M1A.37- (follows M08)
    elbow M1A.32- (follows M08)
    foot joint M1A.37- (follows M08)
    hand joint M1A.34- (follows M08)
    hip M1A.35- (follows M08)
    knee M1A.36- (follows M08)
    multiple site M1A.39 (follows M08)
    shoulder M1A.31- (follows M08)
    vertebrae M1A.38 (follows M08)
    wrist M1A.33- (follows M08)
  lead-induced M1A.10 (follows M08)
    ankle M1A.17- (follows M08)
    elbow M1A.12- (follows M08)
    foot joint M1A.17- (follows M08)
    hand joint M1A.14- (follows M08)
    hip M1A.15- (follows M08)
    knee M1A.16- (follows M08)
    multiple site M1A.19 (follows M08)
    shoulder M1A.11- (follows M08)
    vertebrae M1A.18 (follows M08)
    wrist M1A.13- (follows M08)
  primary — see Gout, chronic, idiopathic
  saturnine — see Gout, chronic, lead-induced
  secondary NEC M1A.40 (follows M08)
    ankle M1A.47- (follows M08)
    elbow M1A.42- (follows M08)
    foot joint M1A.47- (follows M08)
    hand joint M1A.44- (follows M08)
    hip M1A.45- (follows M08)
    knee M1A.46- (follows M08)
    multiple site M1A.49 (follows M08)

Gout, chronic (see also Gout, gouty) M1A.9 (follows M08) — continued
  secondary NEC M1A.40 (follows M08) — continued
    shoulder M1A.41- (follows M08)
    vertebrae M1A.48 (follows M08)
    wrist M1A.43- (follows M08)
  syphilitic (see also subcategory M14.8-) A52.77
  tophi M1A.9 (follows M08)
Gout, gouty (acute) (attack) (flare) (see also Gout, chronic) M10.9
  drug-induced M10.20
    ankle M10.27-
    elbow M10.22-
    foot joint M10.27-
    hand joint M10.24-
    hip M10.25-
    knee M10.26-
    multiple site M10.29
    shoulder M10.21-
    vertebrae M10.28
    wrist M10.23-
  idiopathic M10.00
    ankle M10.07-
    elbow M10.02-
    foot joint M10.07-
    hand joint M10.04-
    hip M10.05-
    knee M10.06-
    multiple site M10.09
    shoulder M10.01-
    vertebrae M10.08
    wrist M10.03-
  in (due to) renal impairment M10.30
    ankle M10.37-
    elbow M10.32-
    foot joint M10.37-
    hand joint M10.34-
    hip M10.35-
    knee M10.36-
    multiple site M10.39
    shoulder M10.31-
    vertebrae M10.38
    wrist M10.33-
  lead-induced M10.10
    ankle M10.17-
    elbow M10.12-
    foot joint M10.17-
    hand joint M10.14-
    hip M10.15-
    knee M10.16-
    multiple site M10.19
    shoulder M10.11-
    vertebrae M10.18
    wrist M10.13-
  primary — see Gout, idiopathic
  saturnine — see Gout, lead-induced
  secondary NEC M10.40
    ankle M10.47-
    elbow M10.42-
    foot joint M10.47-
    hand joint M10.44-
    hip M10.45-
    knee M10.46-
    multiple site M10.49
    shoulder M10.41-
    vertebrae M10.48
    wrist M10.43-
  syphilitic (see also subcategory M14.8-) A52.77
  tophi — see Gout, chronic
Gower's
  muscular dystrophy G71.0
  syndrome (vasovagal attack) R55
Gradenigo's syndrome — see Otitis, media, suppurative, acute
Graefe's disease — see Strabismus, paralytic, ophthalmoplegia, progressive

Graft-versus-host disease D89.813
  acute D89.810
  acute on chronic D89.812
  chronic D89.811
Grain mite (itch) B88.0
Grainhandler's disease or lung J67.8
Grand mal — see Epilepsy, generalized, specified NEC
Grand multipara status only (not pregnant) Z64.1
  pregnant — see Pregnancy, complicated by, grand multiparity
Granite worker's lung J62.8
Granular — see also condition
  inflammation, pharynx J31.2
  kidney (contracting) — see Sclerosis, renal
  liver K74.69
Granulation tissue (abnormal) (excessive) L92.9
  postmastoidectomy cavity — see Complications, postmastoidectomy, granulation
Granulocytopenia (primary) (malignant) — see Agranulocytosis
Granuloma L92.9
  abdomen K66.8
    from residual foreign body L92.3
    pyogenicum L98.0
  actinic L57.5
  annulare (perforating) L92.0
  apical K04.5
  aural — see Otitis, externa, specified NEC
  beryllium (skin) L92.3
  bone
    eosinophilic C96.6
    from residual foreign body — see Osteomyelitis, specified type NEC
    lung C96.6
  brain (any site) G06.0
    schistosomiasis B65.9 [G07]
  canaliculus lacrimalis — see Granuloma, lacrimal
  candidal (cutaneous) B37.2
  cerebral (any site) G06.0
  coccidioidal (primary) (progressive) B38.7
    lung B38.1
    meninges B38.4
  colon K63.89
  conjunctiva H11.22-
  dental K04.5
  ear, middle — see Cholesteatoma
  eosinophilic C96.6
    bone C96.6
    lung C96.6
    oral mucosa K13.4
    skin L92.2
  eyelid H01.8
  facial(e) L92.2
  foreign body (in soft tissue) NEC M60.20
    ankle M60.27-
    foot M60.27-
    forearm M60.23-
    hand M60.24-
    in operation wound — see Foreign body, accidentally left during a procedure
    lower leg M60.26-
    pelvic region M60.25-
    shoulder region M60.21-
    skin L92.3
    specified site NEC M60.28
    subcutaneous tissue L92.3
    thigh M60.25-
    upper arm M60.22-
  gangraenescens M31.2
  genito-inguinale A58
  giant cell (central) (reparative) (jaw) M27.1
  gingiva (peripheral) K06.8
  gland (lymph) I88.8

Granuloma L92.9 — *continued*
  hepatic NEC K75.3
    in (due to)
      berylliosis J63.2 *[K77]*
      sarcoidosis D86.89
  Hodgkin C81.9
  ileum K63.89
  infectious B99.9
    specified NEC B99.8
  inguinale (Donovan) (venereal) A58
  intestine NEC K63.89
  intracranial (any site) G06.0
  intraspinal (any part) G06.1
  iridocyclitis — *see* Iridocyclitis, chronic
  jaw (bone) (central) M27.1
    reparative giant cell M27.1
  kidney (*see also* Infection, kidney) N15.8
  lacrimal H04.81-
  larynx J38.7
  lethal midline (faciale(e)) M31.2
  liver NEC — *see* Granuloma, hepatic
  lung (infectious) — *see also* Fibrosis, lung
    coccidioidal B38.1
    eosinophilic C96.6
  Majocchi's B35.8
  malignant (facial(e)) M31.2
  mandible (central) M27.1
  midline (lethal) M31.2
  monilial (cutaneous) B37.2
  nasal sinus — *see* Sinusitis
  operation wound T81.89
    foreign body — *see* Foreign body,
      accidentally left during a procedure
    stitch T81.89
    talc — *see* Foreign body, accidentally left
      during a procedure
  oral mucosa K13.4
  orbit, orbital H05.11-
  paracoccidioidal B41.8
  penis, venereal A58
  periapical K04.5
  peritoneum K66.8
    due to ova of helminths NOS (*see also*
      Helminthiasis) B83.9 *[K67]*
  postmastoidectomy cavity — *see*
    Complications, postmastoidectomy,
    recurrent cholesteatoma
  prostate N42.89
  pudendi (ulcerating) A58
  pulp, internal (tooth) K03.3
  pyogenic, pyogenicum (of) (skin) L98.0
    gingiva K06.8
    maxillary alveolar ridge K04.5
    oral mucosa K13.4
  rectum K62.89
  reticulohistiocytic D76.3
  rubrum nasi L74.8
  Schistosoma — *see* Schistosomiasis
  septic (skin) L98.0
  silica (skin) L92.3
  sinus (accessory) (infective) (nasal) — *see*
    Sinusitis
  skin L92.9
    from residual foreign body L92.3
    pyogenicum L98.0
  spine
    syphilitic (epidural) A52.19
    tuberculous A18.01
  stitch (postoperative) T81.89
  suppurative (skin) L98.0
  swimming pool A31.1
  talc — *see also* Granuloma, foreign body
    in operation wound — *see* Foreign body,
      accidentally left during a procedure
  telangiectaticum (skin) L98.0
  tracheostomy J95.09
  trichophyticum B35.8
  tropicum A66.4
  umbilicus L92.9

Granuloma L92.9 — *continued*
  urethra N36.8
  uveitis — *see* Iridocyclitis, chronic
  vagina A58
  venereum A58
  vocal cord J38.3
Granulomatosis L92.9
  lymphoid C83.8-
  miliary (listerial) A32.89
  necrotizing, respiratory M31.30
  progressive septic D71
  specified NEC L92.8
  Wegener's M31.30
    with renal involvement M31.31
Granulomatous tissue (abnormal)
  (excessive) L92.9
Granulosis rubra nasi L74.8
Graphite fibrosis (of lung) J63.3
Graphospasm F48.8
  organic G25.89
Grating scapula M89.8x1
Gravel (urinary) — *see* Calculus, urinary
Graves' disease — *see* Hyperthyroidism, with,
  goiter
Gravis — *see* condition
Grawitz tumor C64-
Gray syndrome (newborn) P93.0
Grayness, hair (premature) L67.1
  congenital Q84.2
Green sickness D50.8
Greenfield's disease
  meaning
    concentric sclerosis (encephalitis periaxialis
      concentrica) G37.5
    metachromatic leukodystrophy E75.25
Greenstick fracture — *code as* Fracture, by
  site
Grey syndrome (newborn) P93.0
Grief F43.21
  prolonged F43.29
  reaction (*see also* Disorder, adjustment) F43.20
Griesinger's disease B76.9
Grinder's lung or pneumoconiosis J62.8
Grinding, teeth
  psychogenic F45.8
  sleep related G47.63
Grip
  Dabney's B33.0
  devil's B33.0
Grippe, grippal — *see also* Influenza
  Balkan A78
  summer, of Italy A93.1
Grisel's disease M43.6
Groin — *see* condition
Grooved tongue K14.5
Ground itch B76.9
Grover's disease or syndrome L11.1
Growing pains, children R29.898
Growth (fungoid) (neoplastic) (new) — *see also*
  Neoplasm
  adenoid (vegetative) J35.8
  benign — *see* Neoplasm, benign, by site
  malignant — *see* Neoplasm, malignant, by site
  rapid, childhood Z00.2
  secondary — *see* Neoplasm, secondary, by
    site
Gruby's disease B35.0
Gubler-Millard paralysis or syndrome
  G46.3
Guerin-Stern syndrome Q74.3
Guidance, insufficient anterior (occlusal)
  M26.54
Guillain-Barré disease or syndrome
  G61.0
  sequelae G65.0
Guinea worms (infection) (infestation) B72
Guinon's disease (motor-verbal tic) F95.2
Gull's disease E03.4
Gum — *see* condition

Gumboil K04.7
  with sinus K04.6
Gumma (syphilitic) A52.79
  artery A52.09
    cerebral A52.04
  bone A52.77
    of yaws (late) A66.6
  brain A52.19
  cauda equina A52.19
  central nervous system A52.3
  ciliary body A52.71
  congenital A50.59
  eyelid A52.71
  heart A52.06
  intracranial A52.19
  iris A52.71
  kidney A52.75
  larynx A52.73
  leptomeninges A52.19
  liver A52.74
  meninges A52.19
  myocardium A52.06
  nasopharynx A52.73
  neurosyphilitic A52.3
  nose A52.73
  orbit A52.71
  palate (soft) A52.79
  penis A52.76
  pericardium A52.06
  pharynx A52.73
  pituitary A52.79
  scrofulous (tuberculous) A18.4
  skin A52.79
  specified site NEC A52.79
  spinal cord A52.19
  tongue A52.79
  tonsil A52.73
  trachea A52.73
  tuberculous A18.4
  ulcerative due to yaws A66.4
  ureter A52.75
  yaws A66.4
    bone A66.6
Gunn's syndrome Q07.8
Gunshot wound — *see also* Wound, open
  fracture — *code as* Fracture, by site
  internal organs — *see* Injury, by site
Gynandrism Q56.0
Gynandroblastoma
  specified site — *see* Neoplasm, uncertain
    behavior, by site
  unspecified site
    female D39.10
    male D40.10
Gynecological examination (periodic)
  (routine) Z01.419
  with abnormal findings Z01.411
Gynecomastia N62
Gynephobia F40.291
Gyrate scalp Q82.8

DISEASE INDEX

H

H (Hartnup's) disease E72.02
Haas' disease or osteochondrosis
(juvenile) (head of humerus) — *see*
Osteochondrosis, juvenile, humerus
Habit, habituation
bad sleep Z72.821
chorea F95.8
disturbance, child F98.9
drug — *see* Dependence, drug
irregular sleep Z72.821
laxative F55.2
spasm — *see* Tic
tic — *see* Tic
**Haemophilus (H.) influenzae, as cause of
disease classified elsewhere** B96.3
Haff disease — *see* Poisoning, mercury
**Hageman's factor defect, deficiency or
disease** D68.2
Haglund's disease or osteochondrosis
(juvenile) (os tibiale externum) — *see*
Osteochondrosis, juvenile, tarsus
Hailey-Hailey disease Q82.8
Hair — *see also* condition
plucking F63.3
in stereotyped movement disorder F98.4
tourniquet syndrome — *see also* Constriction,
external, by site
finger S60.44-
penis S30.842
thumb S60.34-
toe S90.44-
Hairball in stomach T18.2
Hair-pulling, pathological (compulsive) F63.3
Hairy black tongue K14.3
Half vertebra Q76.49
Halitosis R19.6
Hallerman-Streiff syndrome Q87.0
Hallervorden-Spatz disease G23.0
Hallopeau's acrodermatitis or disease
L40.2
Hallucination R44.3
auditory R44.0
gustatory R44.2
olfactory R44.2
specified NEC R44.2
tactile R44.2
visual R44.1
Hallucinosis (chronic) F28
alcoholic (acute) F10.951
in
abuse F10.151
dependence F10.251
drug-induced F19.951
cannabis F12.951
cocaine F14.951
hallucinogen F16.951
in
abuse F19.151
cannabis F12.151
cocaine F14.151
hallucinogen F16.151
inhalant F18.151
opioid F11.151
sedative, anxiolytic or hypnotic F13.151
stimulant NEC F15.151
dependence F19.251
cannabis F12.251
cocaine F14.251
hallucinogen F16.251
inhalant F18.251
opioid F11.251
sedative, anxiolytic or hypnotic F13.251
stimulant NEC F15.251
inhalant F18.951
opioid F11.951

Hallucinosis (chronic) F28 — *continued*
drug-induced F19.951 — *continued*
sedative, anxiolytic or hypnotic F13.951
stimulant NEC F15.951
organic F06.0
Hallux
deformity (acquired) NEC M20.5x-
limitus M20.5x-
malleus (acquired) NEC M20.3-
rigidus (acquired) M20.2-
congenital Q74.2
sequelae (late effect) of rickets E64.3
valgus (acquired) M20.1-
congenital Q66.6
varus (acquired) M20.3-
congenital Q66.3
Halo, visual H53.19
Hamartoma, hamartoblastoma Q85.9
epithelial (gingival), odontogenic, central or
peripheral — *see* Cyst, calcifying
odontogenic
Hamartosis Q85.9
Hamman-Rich syndrome J84.114
Hammer toe (acquired) NEC — *see also*
Deformity, toe, hammer toe
congenital Q66.89
sequelae (late effect) of rickets E64.3
Hand — *see* condition
Hand-foot syndrome L27.1
Handicap, handicapped
educational Z55.9
specified NEC Z55.8
**Hand-Schüller-Christian disease or
syndrome** C96.5
Hanging (asphyxia) (strangulation)
(suffocation) — *see* Asphyxia, traumatic, due
to mechanical threat
Hangnail — *see also* Cellulitis, digit
with lymphangitis — *see* Lymphangitis, acute,
digit
Hangover (alcohol) F10.129
Hanhart's syndrome Q87.0
Hanot's cirrhosis or disease K74.3
Hanot-Chauffard(-Troisier) syndrome
E83.19
Hansen's disease — *see* Leprosy
Hantaan virus disease (Korean hemorrhagic
fever) A98.5
Hantavirus disease (with renal
manifestations) (Dobrava) (Puumala) (Seoul)
A98.5
with pulmonary manifestations (Andes)
(Bayou) (Bermejo) (Black Creek Canal)
(Choclo) (Juquitiba) (Laguna negra)
(Lechiguanas) (New York) (Oran) (Sin
nombre) B33.4
Happy puppet syndrome Q93.5
Harada's disease or syndrome H30.81-
Hardening
artery — *see* Arteriosclerosis
brain G93.89
Harelip (complete) (incomplete) — *see* Cleft, lip
Harlequin (newborn) Q80.4
Harley's disease D59.6
Harmful use (of)
alcohol F10.10
anxiolytics — *see* Abuse, drug, sedative
cannabinoids — *see* Abuse, drug, cannabis
cocaine — *see* Abuse, drug, cocaine
drug — *see* Abuse, drug
hallucinogens — *see* Abuse, drug,
hallucinogen
hypnotics — *see* Abuse, drug, sedative
opioids — *see* Abuse, drug, opioid
PCP (phencyclidine) — *see* Abuse, drug,
hallucinogen
sedatives — *see* Abuse, drug, sedative
stimulants NEC — *see* Abuse, drug, stimulant
Harris' lines — *see* Arrest, epiphyseal

Hartnup's disease E72.02
Harvester's lung J67.0
Harvesting ovum for in vitro fertilization
Z31.83
Hashimoto's disease or thyroiditis E06.3
Hashitoxicosis (transient) E06.3
Hassal-Henle bodies or warts (cornea)
H18.49
Haut mal — *see* Epilepsy, generalized,
specified NEC
Haverhill fever A25.1
Hay fever (*see also* Fever, hay) J30.1
Hayem-Widal syndrome D59.8
Haygarth's nodes M15.8
Haymaker's lung J67.0
Hb (abnormal)
Bart's disease D56.0
disease — *see* Disease, hemoglobin
trait — *see* Trait
Head — *see* condition
Headache R51
allergic NEC G44.89
associated with sexual activity G44.82
chronic daily R51
cluster G44.009
chronic G44.029
intractable G44.021
not intractable G44.029
episodic G44.019
intractable G44.011
not intractable G44.019
intractable G44.001
not intractable G44.009
cough (primary) G44.83
daily chronic R51
drug-induced NEC G44.40
intractable G44.41
not intractable G44.40
exertional (primary) G44.84
histamine G44.009
intractable G44.001
not intractable G44.009
hypnic G44.81
lumbar puncture G97.1
medication overuse G44.40
intractable G44.41
not intractable G44.40
menstrual — *see* Migraine, menstrual
migraine (type) (*see also* Migraine) G43.909
nasal septum R51
neuralgiform, short lasting unilateral, with
conjunctival injection and tearing (SUNCT)
G44.059
intractable G44.051
not intractable G44.059
new daily persistent (NDPH) G44.52
orgasmic G44.82
periodic syndromes in adults and children
G43.C0 *(follows G43.7)*
with refractory migraine G43.C1 *(follows
G43.7)*
intractable G43.C19 *(follows G43.7)*
not intractable G43.C09 *(follows G43.7)*
without refractory migraine G43.C0 *(follows
G43.7)*
post-traumatic G44.309
acute G44.319
intractable G44.311
not intractable G44.319
chronic G44.329
intractable G44.321
not intractable G44.329
intractable G44.301
not intractable G44.309
postspinal puncture G97.1
pre-menstrual — *see* Migraine, menstrual
preorgasmic G44.82

Headache R51 — *continued*
  primary
    cough G44.83
    exertional G44.84
    stabbing G44.85
    thunderclap G44.53
  rebound G44.40
    intractable G44.41
    not intractable G44.40
  short lasting unilateral neuralgiform, with
    conjunctival injection and tearing (SUNCT)
    G44.059
    intractable G44.051
    not intractable G44.059
  specified syndrome NEC G44.89
  spinal and epidural anesthesia-induced
    T88.59
    in labor and delivery O74.5
    in pregnancy O29.4-
    postpartum, puerperal O89.4
  spinal fluid loss (from puncture) G97.1
  stabbing (primary) G44.85
  tension(-type) G44.209
    chronic G44.229
      intractable G44.221
      not intractable G44.229
    episodic G44.219
      intractable G44.211
      not intractable G44.219
    intractable G44.201
    not intractable G44.209
  thunderclap (primary) G44.53
  vascular NEC G44.1
Healthy
  infant
    accompanying sick mother Z76.3
    receiving care Z76.2
  person accompanying sick person Z76.3
Hearing examination Z01.10
  with abnormal findings NEC Z01.118
  following failed hearing screening Z01.110
  for hearing conservation and treatment
    Z01.12
Heart — *see* condition
Heart beat
  abnormality R00.9
    specified NEC R00.8
  awareness R00.2
  rapid R00.0
  slow R00.1
Heartburn R12
  psychogenic F45.8
Heat (effects) T67.9
  apoplexy T67.0
  burn (*see also* Burn) L55.9
  collapse T67.1
  cramps T67.2
  dermatitis or eczema L59.0
  edema T67.7
  erythema — *code by* site under Burn, first
    degree
  excessive T67.9
    specified effect NEC T67.8
  exhaustion T67.5
    anhydrotic T67.3
    due to
      salt (and water) depletion T67.4
      water depletion T67.3
        with salt depletion T67.4
  fatigue (transient) T67.6
  fever T67.0
  hyperpyrexia T67.0
  prickly L74.0
  prostration — *see* Heat, exhaustion
  pyrexia T67.0
  rash L74.0
  specified effect NEC T67.8
  stroke T67.0

Heat (effects) T67.9 — *continued*
  sunburn — *see* Sunburn
  syncope T67.1
Heavy-for-dates NEC (infant) (4000g to
  4499g) P08.1
  exceptionally (4500g or more) P08.0
Hebephrenia, hebephrenic (schizophrenia)
  F20.1
Heberden's disease or nodes (with
  arthropathy) M15.1
Hebra's
  pityriasis L26
  prurigo L28.2
Heel — *see* condition
Heerfordt's disease D86.89
Hegglin's anomaly or syndrome D72.0
Heilmeyer-Schoner disease D45
Heine-Medin disease A80.9
Heinz body anemia, congenital D58.2
Heliophobia F40.228
Heller's disease or syndrome F84.3
HELLP syndrome (hemolysis, elevated liver
  enzymes and low platelet count) O14.2-
  complicating
    childbirth O14.24
    puerperium O14.25
Helminthiasis — *see also* Infestation, helminth
  Ancylostoma B76.0
  intestinal B82.0
    mixed types (types classifiable to more than
      one of the titles B65.0-B81.3 and
      B81.8) B81.4
    specified type NEC B81.8
  mixed types (intestinal) (types classifiable to
    more than one of the titles B65.0-B81.3
    and B81.8) B81.4
  Necator (americanus) B76.1
  specified type NEC B83.8
Heloma L84
Hemangioblastoma — *see* Neoplasm,
  connective tissue, uncertain behavior
  malignant — *see* Neoplasm, connective tissue,
    malignant
Hemangioendothelioma — *see also*
  Neoplasm, uncertain behavior, by site
  benign D18.00
    intra-abdominal D18.03
    intracranial D18.02
    skin D18.01
    specified site NEC D18.09
  bone (diffuse) — *see* Neoplasm, bone,
    malignant
  epithelioid — *see also* Neoplasm, uncertain
    behavior, by site
    malignant — *see* Neoplasm, malignant, by
      site
  malignant — *see* Neoplasm, connective tissue,
    malignant
Hemangiofibroma — *see* Neoplasm, benign,
  by site
Hemangiolipoma — *see* Lipoma
Hemangioma D18.00
  arteriovenous D18.00
    intra-abdominal D18.03
    intracranial D18.02
    skin D18.01
    specified site NEC D18.09
  capillary D18.00
    intra-abdominal D18.03
    intracranial D18.02
    skin D18.01
    specified site NEC D18.09
  cavernous D18.00
    intra-abdominal D18.03
    intracranial D18.02
    skin D18.01
    specified site NEC D18.09

Hemangioma D18.00 — *continued*
  epithelioid D18.00
    intra-abdominal D18.03
    intracranial D18.02
    skin D18.01
    specified site NEC D18.09
  histiocytoid D18.00
    intra-abdominal D18.03
    intracranial D18.02
    skin D18.01
    specified site NEC D18.09
  infantile D18.00
    intra-abdominal D18.03
    intracranial D18.02
    skin D18.01
    specified site NEC D18.09
  intra-abdominal D18.03
  intracranial D18.02
  intramuscular D18.00
    intra-abdominal D18.03
    intracranial D18.02
    skin D18.01
    specified site NEC D18.09
  intrathoracic structures D18.09
  juvenile D18.00
  malignant — *see* Neoplasm, connective tissue,
    malignant
  plexiform D18.00
    intra-abdominal D18.03
    intracranial D18.02
    skin D18.01
    specified site NEC D18.09
  racemose D18.00
    intra-abdominal D18.03
    intracranial D18.02
    skin D18.01
    specified site NEC D18.09
  sclerosing — *see* Neoplasm, skin, benign
  simplex D18.00
    intra-abdominal D18.03
    intracranial D18.02
    skin D18.01
    specified site NEC D18.09
  skin D18.01
  specified site NEC D18.09
  venous D18.00
    intra-abdominal D18.03
    intracranial D18.02
    skin D18.01
    specified site NEC D18.09
  verrucous keratotic D18.00
    intra-abdominal D18.03
    intracranial D18.02
    skin D18.01
    specified site NEC D18.09
Hemangiomatosis (systemic) I78.8
  involving single site — *see* Hemangioma
Hemangiopericytoma — *see also* Neoplasm,
  connective tissue, uncertain behavior
  benign — *see* Neoplasm, connective tissue,
    benign
  malignant — *see* Neoplasm, connective tissue,
    malignant
Hemangiosarcoma — *see* Neoplasm,
  connective tissue, malignant
Hemarthrosis (nontraumatic) M25.00
  ankle M25.07-
  elbow M25.02-
  foot joint M25.07-
  hand joint M25.04-
  hip M25.05-
  in hemophilic arthropathy — *see* Arthropathy,
    hemophilic
  knee M25.06-
  shoulder M25.01-
  specified joint NEC M25.08
  traumatic — *see* Sprain, by site
  vertebrae M25.08
  wrist M25.03-

DISEASE INDEX

Hematemesis K92.0
  with ulcer — *code by* site under Ulcer, with
    hemorrhage K27.4
  newborn, neonatal P54.0
    due to swallowed maternal blood P78.2
Hematidrosis L74.8
Hematinuria — *see also* Hemoglobinuria
  malarial B50.8
Hematobilia K83.8
Hematocele
  female NEC N94.89
    with ectopic pregnancy O00.90
      with intrauterine pregnancy O00.91
    ovary N83.8
  male N50.1
Hematochezia (*see also* Melena) K92.1
Hematochyluria — *see also* Infestation, filarial
  schistosomiasis (bilharziasis) B65.0
Hematocolpos (with hematometra or
  hematosalpinx) N89.7
Hematocornea — *see* Pigmentation, cornea,
  stromal
Hematogenous — *see* condition
Hematoma (traumatic) (skin surface intact) —
  see also Contusion
  with
    injury of internal organs — *see* Injury, by site
    open wound — *see* Wound, open
  amputation stump (surgical) (late) T87.89
  aorta, dissecting I71.00
    abdominal I71.02
    thoracic I71.01
    thoracoabdominal I71.03
  aortic intramural — *see* Dissection, aorta
  arterial (complicating trauma) — *see* Injury,
    blood vessel, by site
  auricle — *see* Contusion, ear
    nontraumatic — *see* Disorder, pinna,
      hematoma
  birth injury NEC P15.8
  brain (traumatic)
    with
      cerebral laceration or contusion (diffuse)
        — *see* Injury, intracranial, diffuse
      focal — *see* Injury, intracranial, focal
    cerebellar, traumatic S06.37-
    intracerebral, traumatic — *see* Injury,
      intracranial, intracerebral hemorrhage
    newborn NEC P52.4
      birth injury P10.1
    nontraumatic — *see* Hemorrhage,
      intracranial
    subarachnoid, arachnoid, traumatic — *see*
      Injury, intracranial, subarachnoid
      hemorrhage
    subdural, traumatic — *see* Injury,
      intracranial, subdural hemorrhage
  breast (nontraumatic) N64.89
  broad ligament (nontraumatic) N83.7
    traumatic S37.892
  cerebellar, traumatic S06.37-
  cerebral — *see* Hematoma, brain
  cerebrum S06.36-
    left S06.35-
    right S06.34-
  cesarean delivery wound O90.2
  complicating delivery (perineal) (pelvic)
    (vagina) (vulva) O71.7
  corpus cavernosum (nontraumatic) N48.89
  epididymis (nontraumatic) N50.1
  epidural (traumatic) — *see* Injury, intracranial,
    epidural hemorrhage
  spinal — *see* Injury, spinal cord, by region
  episiotomy O90.2
  face, birth injury P15.4

Hematoma (traumatic) (skin surface intact) (*see
  also* Contusion) — *continued*
  genital organ NEC (nontraumatic)
    female (nonobstetric) N94.89
      traumatic S30.202
    male N50.1
      traumatic S30.201
  internal organs — *see* Injury, by site
  intracerebral, traumatic — *see* Injury,
    intracranial, intracerebral hemorrhage
  intraoperative — *see* Complications,
    intraoperative, hemorrhage
  labia (nontraumatic) (nonobstetric) N90.89
  liver (subcapsular) (nontraumatic) K76.89
    birth injury P15.0
  mediastinum — *see* Injury, intrathoracic
  mesosalpinx (nontraumatic) N83.7
    traumatic S37.898
  muscle — *code by* site under Contusion
  nontraumatic
    muscle M79.81
    soft tissue M79.81
  obstetrical surgical wound O90.2
  orbit, orbital (nontraumatic) — *see also*
    Hemorrhage, orbit
    traumatic — *see* Contusion, orbit
  pelvis (female) (nontraumatic) (nonobstetric)
    N94.89
    obstetric O71.7
    traumatic — *see* Injury, by site
  penis (nontraumatic) N48.89
    birth injury P15.5
  perianal (nontraumatic) K64.5
  perineal S30.23
    complicating delivery O71.7
  perirenal — *see* Injury, kidney
  pinna — *see* Contusion, ear
    nontraumatic — *see* Disorder, pinna,
      hematoma
  placenta O43.89-
  postoperative (postprocedural) — *see*
    Complication, postprocedural, hematoma
  retroperitoneal (nontraumatic) K66.1
    traumatic S36.892
  scrotum, superficial S30.22
    birth injury P15.5
  seminal vesicle (nontraumatic) N50.1
    traumatic S37.892
  spermatic cord (traumatic) S37.892
    nontraumatic N50.1
  spinal (cord) (meninges) — *see also* Injury,
    spinal cord, by region
    newborn (birth injury) P11.5
  spleen D73.5
    intraoperative — *see* Complications,
      intraoperative, hemorrhage, spleen
    postprocedural (postoperative) — *see*
      Complications, postprocedural,
      hemorrhage, spleen
  sternocleidomastoid, birth injury P15.2
  sternomastoid, birth injury P15.2
  subarachnoid (traumatic) — *see* Injury,
    intracranial, subarachnoid hemorrhage
    newborn (nontraumatic) P52.5
      due to birth injury P10.3
    nontraumatic — *see* Hemorrhage,
      intracranial, subarachnoid
  subdural (traumatic) — *see* Injury, intracranial,
    subdural hemorrhage
    newborn (localized) P52.8
      birth injury P10.0
    nontraumatic — *see* Hemorrhage,
      intracranial, subdural
  superficial, newborn P54.5
  testis (nontraumatic) N50.1
    birth injury P15.5
  tunica vaginalis (nontraumatic) N50.1

Hematoma (traumatic) (skin surface intact) (*see
  also* Contusion) — *continued*
  umbilical cord, complicating delivery O69.5
  uterine ligament (broad) (nontraumatic) N83.7
    traumatic S37.892
  vagina (ruptured) (nontraumatic) N89.8
    complicating delivery O71.7
  vas deferens (nontraumatic) N50.1
    traumatic S37.892
  vitreous — *see* Hemorrhage, vitreous
  vulva (nontraumatic) (nonobstetric) N90.89
    complicating delivery O71.7
    newborn (birth injury) P15.5
Hematometra N85.7
  with hematocolpos N89.7
Hematomyelia (central) G95.19
  newborn (birth injury) P11.5
  traumatic T14.8
Hematomyelitis G04.90
Hematoperitoneum — *see* Hemoperitoneum
Hematophobia F40.230
Hematopneumothorax — *see* Hemothorax
Hematopoiesis, cyclic D70.4
Hematoporphyria — *see* Porphyria
Hematorachis, hematorrhachis G95.19
  newborn (birth injury) P11.5
Hematosalpinx N83.6
  with
    hematocolpos N89.7
    hematometra N85.7
      with hematocolpos N89.7
  infectional — *see* Salpingitis
Hematospermia R36.1
Hematothorax — *see* Hemothorax
Hematuria R31.9
  benign (familial) (of childhood) — *see also*
    Hematuria, idiopathic
    essential microscopic R31.1
  due to sulphonamide, sulfonamide — *see* Table
    of Drugs and Chemicals, by drug
  endemic (*see also* Schistosomiasis) B65.0
  gross R31.0
  idiopathic N02.9
    with glomerular lesion
      crescentic (diffuse) glomerulonephritis
        N02.7
      dense deposit disease N02.6
      endocapillary proliferative
        glomerulonephritis N02.4
      focal and segmental hyalinosis or sclerosis
        N02.1
      membranoproliferative (diffuse) N02.5
      membranous (diffuse) N02.2
      mesangial proliferative (diffuse) N02.3
      mesangiocapillary (diffuse) N02.5
      minor abnormality N02.0
      proliferative NEC N02.8
      specified pathology NEC N02.8
  intermittent — *see* Hematuria, idiopathic
  malarial B50.8
  microscopic NEC (with symptoms) R31.29
    asymptomatic R31.21
    benign essential R31.1
  paroxysmal — *see also* Hematuria, idiopathic
    nocturnal D59.5
  persistent — *see* Hematuria, idiopathic
  recurrent — *see* Hematuria, idiopathic
  tropical (*see also* Schistosomiasis) B65.0
  tuberculous A18.13
Hemeralopia (day blindness) H53.11
  vitamin A deficiency E50.5
Hemi-akinesia R41.4
Hemianalgesia R20.0
Hemianencephaly Q00.0
Hemianesthesia R20.0
Hemianopia, hemianopsia (heteronymous)
  H53.47
  homonymous H53.46-
  syphilitic A52.71

Hemiathetosis R25.8
Hemiatrophy R68.89
  cerebellar G31.9
  face, facial, progressive (Romberg) G51.8
  tongue K14.8
Hemiballism(us) G25.5
Hemicardia Q24.8
Hemicephalus, hemicephaly Q00.0
Hemichorea G25.5
Hemicolitis, left — see Colitis, left sided
Hemicrania
  congenital malformation Q00.0
  continua G44.51
  meaning migraine (see also Migraine)
    G43.909
  paroxysmal G44.039
    chronic G44.049
      intractable G44.041
      not intractable G44.049
    episodic G44.039
      intractable G44.031
      not intractable G44.039
    intractable G44.031
    not intractable G44.039
Hemidystrophy — see Hemiatrophy
Hemiectromelia Q73.8
Hemihypalgesia R20.8
Hemihypesthesia R20.1
Hemi-inattention R41.4
Hemimelia Q73.8
  lower limb — see Defect, reduction, lower limb,
    specified type NEC
  upper limb — see Defect, reduction, upper
    limb, specified type NEC
Hemiparalysis — see Hemiplegia
Hemiparesis — see Hemiplegia
Hemiparesthesia R20.2
Hemiparkinsonism G20
Hemiplegia G81.9-
  alternans facialis G83.89
  ascending NEC G81.90
    spinal G95.89
  congenital (cerebral) G80.8
    spastic G80.2
  embolic (current episode) I63.4-
  flaccid G81.0-
  following
    cerebrovascular disease I69.959
      cerebral infarction I69.35-
      intracerebral hemorrhage I69.15-
      nontraumatic intracranial hemorrhage
        NEC I69.25-
      specified disease NEC I69.85-
      stroke NOS I69.35-
      subarachnoid hemorrhage I69.05-
  hysterical F44.4
  newborn NEC P91.8
    birth injury P11.9
  spastic G81.1-
    congenital G80.2
  thrombotic (current episode) I63.3-
Hemisection, spinal cord — see Injury,
  spinal cord, by region
Hemispasm (facial) R25.2
Hemisporosis B48.8
Hemitremor R25.1
Hemivertebra Q76.49
  failure of segmentation with scoliosis Q76.3
  fusion with scoliosis Q76.3
Hemochromatosis E83.119
  with refractory anemia D46.1
  due to repeated red blood cell transfusion
    E83.111
  hereditary (primary) E83.110
  primary E83.110
  specified NEC E83.118

Hemoglobin — see also condition
  abnormal (disease) — see Disease,
    hemoglobin
  AS genotype D57.3
  Constant Spring D58.2
  E-beta thalassemia D56.5
  fetal, hereditary persistence (HPFH) D56.4
  H Constant Spring D56.0
  low NOS D64.9
  S (Hb S), heterozygous D57.3
Hemoglobinemia D59.9
  due to blood transfusion T80.89
  paroxysmal D59.6
    nocturnal D59.5
Hemoglobinopathy (mixed) D58.2
  with thalassemia D56.8
  sickle-cell D57.1
    with thalassemia D57.40
      with crisis (vasoocclusive pain) D57.419
        with
          acute chest syndrome D57.411
          splenic sequestration D57.412
      without crisis D57.40
Hemoglobinuria R82.3
  with anemia, hemolytic, acquired (chronic)
    NEC D59.6
  cold (agglutinin) (paroxysmal) (with Raynaud's
    syndrome) D59.6
  due to exertion or hemolysis NEC D59.6
  intermittent D59.6
  malarial B50.8
  march D59.6
  nocturnal (paroxysmal) D59.5
  paroxysmal (cold) D59.6
    nocturnal D59.5
Hemolymphangioma D18.1
Hemolysis
  intravascular
    with
      abortion — see Abortion, by type,
        complicated by, hemorrhage
      ectopic or molar pregnancy O08.1
      hemorrhage
        antepartum — see Hemorrhage,
          antepartum, with coagulation defect
        intrapartum (see also Hemorrhage,
          complicating, delivery) O67.0
      postpartum O72.3
  neonatal (excessive) P58.9
    specified NEC P58.8
Hemolytic — see condition
Hemopericardium I31.2
  following acute myocardial infarction (current
    complication) I23.0
  newborn P54.8
  traumatic — see Injury, heart, with
    hemopericardium
Hemoperitoneum K66.1
  infectional K65.9
  traumatic S36.899
    with open wound — see Wound, open, with
      penetration into peritoneal cavity
Hemophilia (classical) (familial) (hereditary)
  D66
  A D66
  acquired D68.311
  autoimmune D68.311
  B D67
  C D68.1
  calcipriva (see also Defect, coagulation) D68.4
  nonfamilial (see also Defect, coagulation)
    D68.4
  secondary D68.311
  vascular D68.0
Hemophthalmos H44.81-
Hemopneumothorax — see also Hemothorax
  traumatic S27.2

Hemoptysis R04.2
  newborn P26.9
  tuberculous — see Tuberculosis, pulmonary
Hemorrhage, hemorrhagic (concealed) R58
  abdomen R58
  accidental antepartum — see Hemorrhage,
    antepartum
  acute idiopathic pulmonary, in infants R04.81
  adenoid J35.8
  adrenal (capsule) (gland) E27.49
    medulla E27.8
    newborn P54.4
  after delivery — see Hemorrhage, postpartum
  alveolar
    lung, newborn P26.8
    process K08.89
  alveolus K08.89
  amputation stump (surgical) T87.89
  anemia (chronic) D50.0
    acute D62
  antepartum (with) O46.90
    with coagulation defect O46.00-
      afibrinogenemia O46.01-
      disseminated intravascular coagulation
        O46.02-
      hypofibrinogenemia O46.01-
      specified defect NEC O46.09-
    before 20 weeks gestation O20.9
      specified type NEC O20.8
      threatened abortion O20.0
    due to
      abruptio placenta (see also Abruptio
        placentae) O45.9-
      leiomyoma, uterus — see Hemorrhage,
        antepartum, specified cause NEC
      placenta previa O44.1-
    specified cause NEC — see subcategory
      O46.8x-
  anus (sphincter) K62.5
  apoplexy (stroke) — see Hemorrhage,
    intracranial, intracerebral
  arachnoid — see Hemorrhage, intracranial,
    subarachnoid
  artery R58
    brain — see Hemorrhage, intracranial,
      intracerebral
  basilar (ganglion) I61.0
  bladder N32.89
  bowel K92.2
    newborn P54.3
  brain (miliary) (nontraumatic) — see
    Hemorrhage, intracranial, intracerebral
    due to
      birth injury P10.1
      syphilis A52.05
    epidural or extradural (traumatic) — see
      Injury, intracranial, epidural
      hemorrhage
    newborn P52.4
      birth injury P10.1
    subarachnoid — see Hemorrhage,
      intracranial, subarachnoid
    subdural — see Hemorrhage, intracranial,
      subdural
  brainstem (nontraumatic) I61.3
    traumatic S06.38-
  breast N64.59
  bronchial tube — see Hemorrhage, lung
  bronchopulmonary — see Hemorrhage, lung
  bronchus — see Hemorrhage, lung
  bulbar I61.5
  capillary I78.8
    primary D69.8
  cecum K92.2
  cerebellar, cerebellum (nontraumatic) I61.4
    newborn P52.6
    traumatic S06.37-

Hemorrhage, hemorrhagic (concealed) R58
— continued
cerebral, cerebrum — see also Hemorrhage,
  intracranial, intracerebral
  lobe I61.1
  newborn (anoxic) P52.4
    birth injury P10.1
cerebromeningeal I61.8
cerebrospinal — see Hemorrhage, intracranial,
  intracerebral
cervix (uteri) (stump) NEC N88.8
chamber, anterior (eye) — see Hyphema
childbirth — see Hemorrhage, complicating,
  delivery
choroid H31.30-
  expulsive H31.31-
ciliary body — see Hyphema
cochlea — see subcategory H83.8
colon K92.2
complicating
  abortion — see Abortion, by type,
    complicated by, hemorrhage
  delivery O67.9
    associated with coagulation defect
      (afibrinogenemia) (DIC)
      (hyperfibrinolysis) O67.0
    specified cause NEC O67.8
  surgical procedure — see Hemorrhage,
    intraoperative
conjunctiva H11.3-
  newborn P54.8
cord, newborn (stump) P51.9
corpus luteum (ruptured) cyst N83.1-
cortical (brain) I61.1
cranial — see Hemorrhage, intracranial
cutaneous R23.3
  due to autosensitivity, erythrocyte D69.2
  newborn P54.5
delayed
  following ectopic or molar pregnancy O08.1
  postpartum O72.2
diathesis (familial) D69.9
disease D69.9
  newborn P53
  specified type NEC D69.8
due to or associated with
  afibrinogenemia or other coagulation defect
    (conditions in categories D65-D69)
    antepartum — see Hemorrhage,
      antepartum, with coagulation defect
    intrapartum O67.0
  dental implant M27.61
  device, implant or graft (see also
    Complications, by site and type,
    specified NEC) T85.838
    arterial graft NEC T82.838
    breast T85.838
    catheter NEC T85.838
      dialysis (renal) T82.838
        intraperitoneal T85.838
      infusion NEC T82.838
        spinal (epidural) (subdural) T85.830
      urinary (indwelling) T83.83
    electronic (electrode) (pulse generator)
      (stimulator)
      bone T84.83
      cardiac T82.837
      nervous system (brain) (peripheral
        nerve) (spinal) T85.830
      urinary T83.83
    fixation, internal (orthopedic) NEC T84.83
    gastrointestinal (bile duct) (esophagus)
      T85.838
    genital NEC T83.83
    heart NEC T82.837
    joint prosthesis T84.83
    ocular (corneal graft) (orbital implant)
      NEC T85.838

Hemorrhage, hemorrhagic (concealed) R58
— continued
due to or associated with — continued
  device, implant or graft (see also
    Complications, by site and type,
    specified NEC) T85.83 — continued
    orthopedic NEC T84.83
      bone graft T86.838
    specified NEC T85.838
    urinary NEC T83.83
    vascular NEC T82.838
    ventricular intracranial shunt T85.830
duodenum, duodenal K92.2
  ulcer — see Ulcer, duodenum, with
    hemorrhage
dura mater — see Hemorrhage, intracranial,
  subdural
endotracheal — see Hemorrhage, lung
epicranial subaponeurotic (massive), birth
  injury P12.2
epidural (traumatic) — see also Injury,
  intracranial, epidural hemorrhage
  nontraumatic I62.1
esophagus K22.8
  varix I85.01
    secondary I85.11
excessive, following ectopic gestation
  (subsequent episode) O08.1
extradural (traumatic) — see Injury,
  intracranial, epidural hemorrhage
  birth injury P10.8
  newborn (anoxic) (nontraumatic) P52.8
  nontraumatic I62.1
eye NEC H57.8
  fundus — see Hemorrhage, retina
  lid — see Disorder, eyelid, specified type
    NEC
fallopian tube N83.6
fibrinogenolysis — see Fibrinolysis
fibrinolytic (acquired) — see Fibrinolysis
from
  ear (nontraumatic) — see Otorrhagia
  tracheostomy stoma J95.01
fundus, eye — see Hemorrhage, retina
funis — see Hemorrhage, umbilicus, cord
gastric — see Hemorrhage, stomach
gastroenteric K92.2
  newborn P54.3
gastrointestinal (tract) K92.2
  newborn P54.3
genital organ, male N50.1
genitourinary (tract) NOS R31.9
gingiva K06.8
globe (eye) — see Hemophthalmos
graafian follicle cyst (ruptured) N83.0-
gum K06.8
heart I51.89
hypopharyngeal (throat) R04.1
intermenstrual (regular) N92.3
  irregular N92.1
internal (organs) NEC R58
  capsule I61.0
  ear — see subcategory H83.8
  newborn P54.8
intestine K92.2
  newborn P54.3
intra-abdominal R58
intra-alveolar (lung), newborn P26.8
intracerebral (nontraumatic) — see
  Hemorrhage, intracranial, intracerebral
intracranial (nontraumatic) I62.9
  birth injury P10.9
  epidural, nontraumatic I62.1
  extradural, nontraumatic I62.1

Hemorrhage, hemorrhagic (concealed) R58
— continued
intracranial (nontraumatic) I62.9 —
  continued
  intracerebral (nontraumatic) (in) I61.9
    brain stem I61.3
    cerebellum I61.4
    hemisphere I61.2
      cortical (superficial) I61.1
      subcortical (deep) I61.0
    intraoperative
      during a nervous system procedure
        G97.31
      during other procedure G97.32
    intraventricular I61.5
    multiple localized I61.6
    newborn P52.4
      birth injury P10.1
    postprocedural
      following a nervous system procedure
        G97.51
      following other procedure G97.52
    specified NEC I61.8
    superficial I61.1
    traumatic (diffuse) — see Injury,
      intracranial, diffuse
    focal — see Injury, intracranial, focal
  newborn P52.9
    specified NEC P52.8
  subarachnoid (nontraumatic) (from) I60.9
    intracranial (cerebral) artery I60.7
      anterior communicating I60.2
      basilar I60.4
      carotid siphon and bifurcation I60.0-
      communicating I60.7
        anterior I60.2
        posterior I60.3-
      middle cerebral I60.1-
      posterior communicating I60.3-
      specified artery NEC I60.6
      vertebral I60.5-
    newborn P52.5
      birth injury P10.3
    specified NEC I60.8
    traumatic S06.6x-
  subdural (nontraumatic) I62.00
    acute I62.01
    birth injury P10.0
    chronic I62.03
    newborn (anoxic) (hypoxic) P52.8
      birth injury P10.0
    spinal G95.19
    subacute I62.02
    traumatic — see Injury, intracranial,
      subdural hemorrhage
  subgaleal P12.1
  traumatic — see Injury, intracranial, focal
    brain injury
intramedullary NEC G95.19
intraocular — see Hemophthalmos
intraoperative, intraprocedural — see
  Complication, hemorrhage (hematoma),
  intraoperative (intraprocedural), by site
intrapartum — see Hemorrhage, complicating,
  delivery
intrapelvic
  female N94.89
  male K66.1
intraperitoneal K66.1
intrapontine I61.3
intraprocedural — see Complication,
  hemorrhage (hematoma), intraoperative
  (intraprocedural), by site
intrauterine N85.7
  complicating delivery (see also Hemorrhage,
    complicating, delivery) O67.9
  postpartum — see Hemorrhage, postpartum

Hemorrhage, hemorrhagic (concealed) R58
— *continued*
intraventricular I61.5
  newborn (nontraumatic) (*see also* Newborn,
    affected by, hemorrhage) P52.3
    due to birth injury P10.2
    grade
      1 P52.0
      2 P52.1
      3 P52.21
      4 P52.22
intravesical N32.89
iris (postinfectional) (postinflammatory) (toxic)
  — *see* Hyphema
joint (nontraumatic) — *see* Hemarthrosis
kidney N28.89
knee (joint) (nontraumatic) — *see*
  Hemarthrosis, knee
labyrinth — *see* subcategory H83.8
lenticular striate artery I61.0
ligature, vessel — *see* Hemorrhage,
  postoperative
liver K76.89
lung R04.89
  newborn P26.9
    massive P26.1
    specified NEC P26.8
  tuberculous — *see* Tuberculosis, pulmonary
massive umbilical, newborn P51.0
mediastinum — *see* Hemorrhage, lung
medulla I61.3
membrane (brain) I60.8
  spinal cord — *see* Hemorrhage, spinal cord
meninges, meningeal (brain) (middle) I60.8
  spinal cord — *see* Hemorrhage, spinal cord
mesentery K66.1
metritis — *see* Endometritis
mouth K13.79
mucous membrane NEC R58
  newborn P54.8
muscle M62.89
nail (subungual) L60.8
nasal turbinate R04.0
  newborn P54.8
navel, newborn P51.9
newborn P54.9
  specified NEC P54.8
nipple N64.59
nose R04.0
  newborn P54.8
omentum K66.1
optic nerve (sheath) H47.02-
orbit, orbital H05.23-
ovary NEC N83.8
oviduct N83.6
pancreas K86.89
parathyroid (gland) (spontaneous) E21.4
parturition — *see* Hemorrhage, complicating,
  delivery
penis N48.89
pericardium, pericarditis I31.2
peritoneum, peritoneal K66.1
peritonsillar tissue J35.8
  due to infection J36
petechial R23.3
  due to autosensitivity, erythrocyte D69.2
pituitary (gland) E23.6
pleura — *see* Hemorrhage, lung
polioencephalitis, superior E51.2
polymyositis — *see* Polymyositis
pons, pontine I61.3
posterior fossa (nontraumatic) I61.8
  newborn P52.6
postmenopausal N95.0
postnasal R04.0
postoperative — *see* Complications,
  postprocedural, hemorrhage, by site

Hemorrhage, hemorrhagic (concealed) R58
— *continued*
postpartum NEC (following delivery of
  placenta) O72.1
  delayed or secondary O72.2
  retained placenta O72.0
  third stage O72.0
pregnancy — *see* Hemorrhage, antepartum
preretinal — *see* Hemorrhage, retina
prostate N42.1
puerperal — *see* Hemorrhage, postpartum
  delayed or secondary O72.2
pulmonary R04.89
  newborn P26.9
    massive P26.1
    specified NEC P26.8
  tuberculous — *see* Tuberculosis, pulmonary
purpura (primary) D69.3
rectum (sphincter) K62.5
  newborn P54.2
recurring, following initial hemorrhage at time
  of injury T79.2
renal N28.89
respiratory passage or tract R04.9
  specified NEC R04.89
retina, retinal (vessels) H35.6-
  diabetic — *see* Diabetes, retinal,
    hemorrhage
retroperitoneal R58
scalp R58
scrotum N50.1
secondary (nontraumatic) R58
  following initial hemorrhage at time of injury
    T79.2
seminal vesicle N50.1
skin R23.3
  newborn P54.5
slipped umbilical ligature P51.8
spermatic cord N50.1
spinal (cord) G95.19
  newborn (birth injury) P11.5
spleen D73.5
  intraoperative — *see* Complications,
    intraoperative, hemorrhage, spleen
  postprocedural — *see* Complications,
    postprocedural, hemorrhage, spleen
stomach K92.2
  newborn P54.3
  ulcer — *see* Ulcer, stomach, with hemorrhage
subarachnoid (nontraumatic) — *see*
  Hemorrhage, intracranial, subarachnoid
subconjunctival — *see also* Hemorrhage,
  conjunctiva
  birth injury P15.3
subcortical (brain) I61.0
subcutaneous R23.3
subdiaphragmatic R58
subdural (acute) (nontraumatic) — *see*
  Hemorrhage, intracranial, subdural
subependymal
  newborn P52.0
    with intraventricular extension P52.1
      and intracerebral extension P52.22
subgaleal P12.2
subhyaloid — *see* Hemorrhage, retina
subperiosteal — *see* Disorder, bone, specified
  type NEC
subretinal — *see* Hemorrhage, retina
subtentorial — *see* Hemorrhage, intracranial,
  subdural
subungual L60.8
suprarenal (capsule) (gland) E27.49
  newborn P54.4
tentorium (traumatic) NEC — *see* Hemorrhage,
  brain
  newborn (birth injury) P10.4
testis N50.1
third stage (postpartum) O72.0
thorax — *see* Hemorrhage, lung

Hemorrhage, hemorrhagic (concealed) R58
— *continued*
throat R04.1
thymus (gland) E32.8
thyroid (cyst) (gland) E07.89
tongue K14.8
tonsil J35.8
trachea — *see* Hemorrhage, lung
tracheobronchial R04.89
  newborn P26.0
traumatic — *code to* specific injury
  cerebellar — *see* Hemorrhage, brain
  intracranial — *see* Hemorrhage, brain
  recurring or secondary (following initial
    hemorrhage at time of injury) T79.2
tuberculous NEC (*see also* Tuberculosis,
  pulmonary) A15.0
tunica vaginalis N50.1
ulcer — *code by* site under Ulcer, with
  hemorrhage K27.4
umbilicus, umbilical
  cord
    after birth, newborn P51.9
    complicating delivery O69.5
  newborn P51.9
    massive P51.0
    slipped ligature P51.8
  stump P51.9
urethra (idiopathic) N36.8
uterus, uterine (abnormal) N93.9
  climacteric N92.4
  complicating delivery — *see* Hemorrhage,
    complicating, delivery
  dysfunctional or functional N93.8
  intermenstrual (regular) N92.3
    irregular N92.1
  postmenopausal N95.0
  postpartum — *see* Hemorrhage, postpartum
  preclimacteric or premenopausal N92.4
  prepubertal N93.8
  pubertal N92.2
vagina (abnormal) N93.9
  newborn P54.6
vas deferens N50.1
vasa previa O69.4
ventricular I61.5
vesical N32.89
viscera NEC R58
  newborn P54.8
vitreous (humor) (intraocular) H43.1-
vulva N90.89
Hemorrhoids (bleeding) (without mention of
  degree) K64.9
1st degree (grade/stage I) (without prolapse
  outside of anal canal) K64.0
2nd degree (grade/stage II) (that with
  prolapse with straining but retract
  spontaneously) K64.1
3rd degree (grade/stage III) (that with
  prolapse with straining and require
  manual replacement back inside anal
  canal) K64.2
4th degree (grade/stage IV) (with prolapsed
  tissue that cannot be manually replaced)
  K64.3
complicating
  pregnancy O22.4
  puerperium O87.2
external K64.4
  with
    thrombosis K64.5
internal (without mention of degree) K64.8
prolapsed K64.8
skin tags
  anus K64.4
  residual K64.4
specified NEC K64.8

DISEASE INDEX

Hemorrhoids (bleeding) (without mention of degree) K64.9 — *continued*
  strangulated (*see also* Hemorrhoids, by degree) K64.8
  thrombosed (*see also* Hemorrhoids, by degree) K64.5
  ulcerated (*see also* Hemorrhoids, by degree) K64.8
Hemosalpinx N83.6
  with
    hematocolpos N89.7
    hematometra N85.7
      with hematocolpos N89.7
Hemosiderosis (dietary) E83.19
  pulmonary, idiopathic E83.1- *[J84.03]*
  transfusion T80.89
Hemothorax (bacterial) (nontuberculous) J94.2
  newborn P54.8
  traumatic S27.1
    with pneumothorax S27.2
  tuberculous NEC A15.6
Henoch(-Schönlein) disease or syndrome (purpura) D69.0
Henpue, henpuye A66.6
Hepar lobatum (syphilitic) A52.74
Hepatalgia K76.89
Hepatitis K75.9
  acute B17.9
    with coma K72.01
    with hepatic failure — *see* Failure, hepatic
    alcoholic — *see* Hepatitis, alcoholic
    infectious B17.9
    non-viral K72.0
    viral B17.9
  alcoholic (acute) (chronic) K70.10
    with ascites K70.11
  amebic — *see* Abscess, liver, amebic
  anicteric, (viral) — *see* Hepatitis, viral
  antigen-associated (HAA) — *see* Hepatitis, B
  Australia-antigen (positive) — *see* Hepatitis, B
  autoimmune K75.4
  B B19.10
    with hepatic coma B19.11
    acute B16.9
      with
        delta-agent (coinfection) (without hepatic coma) B16.1
          with hepatic coma B16.0
        hepatic coma (without delta-agent coinfection) B16.2
    chronic B18.1
      with delta-agent B18.0
  bacterial NEC K75.89
  C (viral) B19.20
    with hepatic coma B19.21
    acute B17.10
      with hepatic coma B17.11
    chronic B18.2
  catarrhal (acute) B15.9
    with hepatic coma B15.0
  cholangiolitic K75.89
  cholestatic K75.89
  chronic K73.9
    active NEC K73.2
    lobular NEC K73.1
    persistent NEC K73.0
    specified NEC K73.8
  cytomegaloviral B25.1
  due to ethanol (acute) (chronic) — *see* Hepatitis, alcoholic
  epidemic B15.9
    with hepatic coma B15.0
  fulminant NEC (viral) — *see* Hepatitis, viral
  granulomatous NEC K75.3
  herpesviral B00.81
  history of
    B Z86.19
    C Z86.19

Hepatitis K75.9 — *continued*
  homologous serum — *see* Hepatitis, viral, type B
  in (due to)
    mumps B26.81
    toxoplasmosis (acquired) B58.1
      congenital (active) P37.1 *[K77]*
  infectious, infective B15.9
    acute (subacute) B17.9
    chronic B18.9
  inoculation — *see* Hepatitis, viral, type B
  interstitial (chronic) K74.69
  lupoid NEC K75.4
  malignant NEC (with hepatic failure) K72.90
    with coma K72.91
  neonatal giant cell P59.29
  neonatal (idiopathic) (toxic) P59.29
  newborn P59.29
  post-transfusion — *see* Hepatitis, viral, type B
  postimmunization — *see* Hepatitis, viral, type B
  reactive, nonspecific K75.2
  serum — *see* Hepatitis, viral, type B
  specified type NEC
    with hepatic failure — *see* Failure, hepatic
  syphilitic (late) A52.74
    congenital (early) A50.08 *[K77]*
      late A50.59 *[K77]*
    secondary A51.45
  toxic (*see also* Disease, liver, toxic) K71.6
  tuberculous A18.83
  viral, virus B19.9
    with hepatic coma B19.0
    acute B17.9
    chronic B18.9
      specified NEC B18.8
      type
        B B18.1
          with delta-agent B18.0
        C B18.2
    congenital P35.3
    coxsackie B33.8 *[K77]*
    cytomegalic inclusion B25.1
    in remission, any type — *code to* Hepatitis, chronic, by type
    non-A, non-B B17.8
    specified type NEC (with or without coma) B17.8
    type
      A B15.9
        with hepatic coma B15.0
      B B19.10
        with hepatic coma B19.11
        acute B16.9
          with
            delta-agent (coinfection) (without hepatic coma) B16.1
              with hepatic coma B16.0
            hepatic coma (without delta-agent coinfection) B16.2
        chronic B18.1
          with delta-agent B18.0
      C B19.20
        with hepatic coma B19.21
        acute B17.10
          with hepatic coma B17.11
        chronic B18.2
      E B17.2
      non-A, non-B B17.8
Hepatization lung (acute) — *see* Pneumonia, lobar
Hepatoblastoma C22.2
Hepatocarcinoma C22.0
Hepatocholangiocarcinoma C22.0
Hepatocholangioma, benign D13.4
Hepatocholangitis K75.89
Hepatolenticular degeneration E83.01
Hepatoma (malignant) C22.0
  benign D13.4
  embryonal C22.0

Hepatomegaly — *see also* Hypertrophy, liver
  with splenomegaly R16.2
  congenital Q44.7
  in mononucleosis
    gammaherpesviral B27.09
    infectious specified NEC B27.89
Hepatoptosis K76.89
Hepatorenal syndrome following labor and delivery O90.4
Hepatosis K76.89
Hepatosplenomegaly R16.2
  hyperlipemic (Bürger-Grütz type) E78.3 *[K77]*
Hereditary — *see* condition
Heredodegeneration, macular — *see* Dystrophy, retina
Heredopathia atactica polyneuritiformis G60.1
Heredosyphilis — *see* Syphilis, congenital
Herlitz' syndrome Q81.1
Hermansky-Pudlak syndrome E70.331
Hermaphrodite, hermaphroditism (true) Q56.0
  46,XX with streak gonads Q99.1
  46,XX/46,XY Q99.0
  46,XY with streak gonads Q99.1
  chimera 46,XX/46,XY Q99.0
Hernia, hernial (acquired) (recurrent) K46.9
  with
    gangrene — *see* Hernia, by site, with, gangrene
    incarceration — *see* Hernia, by site, with, obstruction
    irreducible — *see* Hernia, by site, with, obstruction
    obstruction — *see* Hernia, by site, with, obstruction
    strangulation — *see* Hernia, by site, with, obstruction
  abdomen, abdominal K46.9
    with
      gangrene (and obstruction) K46.1
      obstruction K46.0
    femoral — *see* Hernia, femoral
    incisional — *see* Hernia, incisional
    inguinal — *see* Hernia, inguinal
    specified site NEC K45.8
      with
        gangrene (and obstruction) K45.1
        obstruction K45.0
    umbilical — *see* Hernia, umbilical
    wall — *see* Hernia, ventral
  appendix — *see* Hernia, abdomen
  bladder (mucosa) (sphincter)
    congenital (female) (male) Q79.51
    female — *see* Cystocele
    male N32.89
  brain, congenital — *see* Encephalocele
  cartilage, vertebra — *see* Displacement, intervertebral disc
  cerebral, congenital — *see also* Encephalocele
    endaural Q01.8
  ciliary body (traumatic) S05.2-
  colon — *see* Hernia, abdomen
  Cooper's — *see* Hernia, abdomen, specified site NEC
  crural — *see* Hernia, femoral
  diaphragm, diaphragmatic K44.9
    with
      gangrene (and obstruction) K44.1
      obstruction K44.0
    congenital Q79.0
  direct (inguinal) — *see* Hernia, inguinal
  diverticulum, intestine — *see* Hernia, abdomen
  double (inguinal) — *see* Hernia, inguinal, bilateral
  due to adhesions (with obstruction) K56.5
  epigastric (*see also* Hernia, ventral) K43.9
  esophageal hiatus — *see* Hernia, hiatal
  external (inguinal) — *see* Hernia, inguinal

Hernia, hernial (acquired) (recurrent) K46.9
— *continued*
fallopian tube N83.4-
fascia M62.89
femoral K41.90
　with
　　gangrene (and obstruction) K41.40
　　　not specified as recurrent K41.40
　　　recurrent K41.41
　　obstruction K41.30
　　　not specified as recurrent K41.30
　　　recurrent K41.31
　bilateral K41.20
　　with
　　　gangrene (and obstruction) K41.10
　　　　not specified as recurrent K41.10
　　　　recurrent K41.11
　　　obstruction K41.00
　　　　not specified as recurrent K41.00
　　　　recurrent K41.01
　　not specified as recurrent K41.20
　　recurrent K41.21
　not specified as recurrent K41.90
　recurrent K41.91
　unilateral K41.90
　　with
　　　gangrene (and obstruction) K41.40
　　　　not specified as recurrent K41.40
　　　　recurrent K41.41
　　　obstruction K41.30
　　　　not specified as recurrent K41.30
　　　　recurrent K41.31
　　not specified as recurrent K41.90
　　recurrent K41.91
foramen magnum G93.5
　congenital Q01.8
funicular (umbilical) — *see also* Hernia,
　umbilicus
　spermatic (cord) — *see* Hernia, inguinal
gastrointestinal tract — *see* Hernia, abdomen
Hesselbach's — *see* Hernia, femoral, specified
　site NEC
hiatal (esophageal) (sliding) K44.9
　with
　　gangrene (and obstruction) K44.1
　　obstruction K44.0
　congenital Q40.1
hypogastric — *see* Hernia, ventral
incarcerated — *see also* Hernia, by site, with
　obstruction
　with gangrene — *see* Hernia, by site, with
　　gangrene
incisional K43.2
　with
　　gangrene (and obstruction) K43.1
　　obstruction K43.0
indirect (inguinal) — *see* Hernia, inguinal
inguinal (direct) (external) (funicular) (indirect)
　(internal) (oblique) (scrotal) (sliding)
　K40.90
　with
　　gangrene (and obstruction) K40.40
　　　not specified as recurrent K40.40
　　　recurrent K40.41
　　obstruction K40.30
　　　not specified as recurrent K40.30
　　　recurrent K40.31
　bilateral K40.20
　　with
　　　gangrene (and obstruction) K40.10
　　　　not specified as recurrent K40.10
　　　　recurrent K40.11
　　　obstruction K40.00
　　　　not specified as recurrent K40.00
　　　　recurrent K40.01
　　not specified as recurrent K40.20
　　recurrent K40.21
　not specified as recurrent K40.90
　recurrent K40.91

Hernia, hernial (acquired) (recurrent) K46.9
— *continued*
inguinal (direct) (external) (funicular) (indirect)
　(internal) (oblique) (scrotal) (sliding)
　K40.90 — *continued*
　unilateral K40.90
　　with
　　　gangrene (and obstruction) K40.40
　　　　not specified as recurrent K40.40
　　　　recurrent K40.41
　　　obstruction K40.30
　　　　not specified as recurrent K40.30
　　　　recurrent K40.31
　　not specified as recurrent K40.90
　　recurrent K40.91
internal — *see also* Hernia, abdomen
　inguinal — *see* Hernia, inguinal
interstitial — *see* Hernia, abdomen
intervertebral cartilage or disc — *see*
　Displacement, intervertebral disc
intestine, intestinal — *see* Hernia, by site
intra-abdominal — *see* Hernia, abdomen
iris (traumatic) S05.2-
irreducible — *see also* Hernia, by site, with
　obstruction
　with gangrene — *see* Hernia, by site, with
　　gangrene
ischiatic — *see* Hernia, abdomen, specified site
　NEC
ischiorectal — *see* Hernia, abdomen, specified
　site NEC
lens (traumatic) S05.2-
linea (alba) (semilunaris) — *see* Hernia, ventral
Littre's — *see* Hernia, abdomen
lumbar — *see* Hernia, abdomen, specified site
　NEC
lung (subcutaneous) J98.4
mediastinum J98.59
mesenteric (internal) — *see* Hernia, abdomen
midline — *see* Hernia, ventral
muscle (sheath) M62.89
nucleus pulposus — *see* Displacement,
　intervertebral disc
oblique (inguinal) — *see* Hernia, inguinal
obstructive — *see also* Hernia, by site, with
　obstruction
　with gangrene — *see* Hernia, by site, with
　　gangrene
obturator — *see* Hernia, abdomen, specified
　site NEC
omental — *see* Hernia, abdomen
ovary N83.4-
oviduct N83.4-
paraesophageal — *see also* Hernia, diaphragm
　congenital Q40.1
parastomal K43.5
　with
　　gangrene (and obstruction) K43.4
　　obstruction K43.3
paraumbilical — *see* Hernia, umbilicus
perineal — *see* Hernia, abdomen, specified
　site NEC
Petit's — *see* Hernia, abdomen, specified site
　NEC
postoperative — *see* Hernia, incisional
pregnant uterus — *see* Abnormal, uterus in
　pregnancy or childbirth
prevesical N32.89
properitoneal — *see* Hernia, abdomen,
　specified site NEC
pudendal — *see* Hernia, abdomen, specified
　site NEC
rectovaginal N81.6
retroperitoneal — *see* Hernia, abdomen,
　specified site NEC
Richter's — *see* Hernia, abdomen, with
　obstruction
Rieux's, Riex's — *see* Hernia, abdomen,
　specified site NEC

Hernia, hernial (acquired) (recurrent) K46.9
— *continued*
sac condition (adhesion) (dropsy)
　(inflammation) (laceration) (suppuration)
　— *code by* site under Hernia
sciatic — *see* Hernia, abdomen, specified site
　NEC
scrotum, scrotal — *see* Hernia, inguinal
sliding (inguinal) — *see also* Hernia, inguinal
　hiatus — *see* Hernia, hiatal
spigelian — *see* Hernia, ventral
spinal — *see* Spina bifida
strangulated — *see also* Hernia, by site, with
　obstruction
　with gangrene — *see* Hernia, by site, with
　　gangrene
subxiphoid — *see* Hernia, ventral
supra-umbilicus — *see* Hernia, ventral
tendon — *see* Disorder, tendon, specified type
　NEC
Treitz's (fossa) — *see* Hernia, abdomen,
　specified site NEC
tunica vaginalis Q55.29
umbilicus, umbilical K42.9
　with
　　gangrene (and obstruction) K42.1
　　obstruction K42.0
ureter N28.89
urethra, congenital Q64.79
urinary meatus, congenital Q64.79
uterus N81.4
　pregnant — *see* Abnormal, uterus in
　　pregnancy or childbirth
vaginal (anterior) (wall) — *see* Cystocele
Velpeau's — *see* Hernia, femoral
ventral K43.9
　with
　　gangrene (and obstruction) K43.7
　　obstruction K43.6
　incisional K43.2
　　with
　　　gangrene (and obstruction) K43.1
　　　obstruction K43.0
　　recurrent — *see* Hernia, incisional
　specified NEC K43.9
　　with
　　　gangrene (and obstruction) K43.7
　　　obstruction K43.6
vesical
　congenital (female) (male) Q79.51
　female — *see* Cystocele
　male N32.89
vitreous (into wound) S05.2-
　into anterior chamber — *see* Prolapse,
　　vitreous
Herniation — *see also* Hernia
brain (stem) G93.5
cerebral G93.5
mediastinum J98.59
nucleus pulposus — *see* Displacement,
　intervertebral disc
Herpangina B08.5
Herpes, herpesvirus, herpetic B00.9
anogenital A60.9
　perianal skin A60.1
　rectum A60.1
　urogenital tract A60.00
　　cervix A60.03
　　male genital organ NEC A60.02
　　penis A60.01
　　specified site NEC A60.09
　　vagina A60.04
　　vulva A60.04
blepharitis (zoster) B02.39
　simplex B00.59
circinatus B35.4
　bullosus L12.0
conjunctivitis (simplex) B00.53
　zoster B02.31

Herpes, herpesvirus, herpetic B00.9 — continued
  cornea B02.33
  encephalitis B00.4
    due to herpesvirus 6 B10.01
    due to herpesvirus 7 B10.09
    specified NEC B10.09
  eye (zoster) B02.30
    simplex B00.50
  eyelid (zoster) B02.39
    simplex B00.59
  facialis B00.1
  febrilis B00.1
  geniculate ganglionitis B02.21
  genital, genitalis A60.00
    female A60.09
    male A60.02
  gestational, gestationis O26.4-
  gingivostomatitis B00.2
  human B00.9
    1 — see Herpes, simplex
    2 — see Herpes, simplex
    3 — see Varicella
    4 — see Mononucleosis, Epstein-Barr (virus)
    5 — see Disease, cytomegalic inclusion
       (generalized)
    6
      encephalitis B10.01
      specified NEC B10.81
    7
      encephalitis B10.09
      specified NEC B10.82
    8 B10.89
  infection NEC B10.89
    Kaposi's sarcoma associated B10.89
  iridocyclitis (simplex) B00.51
    zoster B02.32
  iris (vesicular erythema multiforme) L51.9
  iritis (simplex) B00.51
  Kaposi's sarcoma associated B10.89
  keratitis (simplex) (dendritic) (disciform)
    (interstitial) B00.52
    zoster (interstitial) B02.33
  keratoconjunctivitis (simplex) B00.52
    zoster B02.33
  labialis B00.1
  lip B00.1
  meningitis (simplex) B00.3
    zoster B02.1
  ophthalmicus (zoster) NEC B02.30
    simplex B00.50
  penis A60.01
  perianal skin A60.1
  pharyngitis, pharyngotonsillitis B00.2
  rectum A60.1
  scrotum A60.02
  sepsis B00.7
  simplex B00.9
    complicated NEC B00.89
    congenital P35.2
    conjunctivitis B00.53
    external ear B00.1
    eyelid B00.59
    hepatitis B00.81
    keratitis (interstitial) B00.52
    myelitis B00.82
    specified complication NEC B00.89
    visceral B00.89
  stomatitis B00.2
  tonsurans B35.0
  visceral B00.89
  vulva A60.04
  whitlow B00.89
  zoster (see also condition) B02.9
    auricularis B02.21
    complicated NEC B02.8
    conjunctivitis B02.31
    disseminated B02.7
    encephalitis B02.0

Herpes, herpesvirus, herpetic B00.9 — continued
  zoster (see also condition) B02.9 — continued
    eye(lid) B02.39
    geniculate ganglionitis B02.21
    keratitis (interstitial) B02.33
    meningitis B02.1
    myelitis B02.24
    neuritis, neuralgia B02.29
    ophthalmicus NEC B02.30
    oticus B02.21
    polyneuropathy B02.23
    specified complication NEC B02.8
    trigeminal neuralgia B02.22
Herpesvirus (human) — see Herpes
Herpetophobia F40.218
Herrick's anemia — see Disease, sickle-cell
Hers' disease E74.09
Herter-Gee syndrome K90.0
Herxheimer's reaction R68.89
Hesitancy
  of micturition R39.11
  urinary R39.11
Hesselbach's hernia — see Hernia, femoral,
    specified site NEC
Heterochromia (congenital) Q13.2
  cataract — see Cataract, complicated
  cyclitis (Fuchs) — see Cyclitis, Fuchs'
    heterochromic
  hair L67.1
  iritis — see Cyclitis, Fuchs' heterochromic
  retained metallic foreign body (nonmagnetic)
    — see Foreign body, intraocular, old,
    retained
  magnetic — see Foreign body, intraocular,
    old, retained, magnetic
  uveitis — see Cyclitis, Fuchs' heterochromic
Heterophoria — see Strabismus, heterophoria
Heterophyes, heterophyiasis (small
    intestine) B66.8
Heterotopia, heterotopic — see also
    Malposition, congenital
  cerebralis Q04.8
Heterotropia — see Strabismus
Heubner-Herter disease K90.0
Hexadactylism Q69.9
HGSIL (cytology finding) (high grade squamous
    intraepithelial lesion on cytologic smear)
    (Pap smear finding)
  anus R85.613
  cervix R87.613
    biopsy (histology) finding — see Neoplasia,
      intraepithelial, cervix, grade II or grade
      III
  vagina R87.623
    biopsy (histology) finding — see Neoplasia,
      intraepithelial, vagina, grade II or grade
      III
Hibernoma — see Lipoma
Hiccup, hiccough R06.6
  epidemic B33.0
  psychogenic F45.8
Hidden penis (congenital) Q55.64
  acquired N48.83
Hidradenitis (axillaris) (suppurative) L73.2
Hidradenoma (nodular) — see also Neoplasm,
    skin, benign
  clear cell — see Neoplasm, skin, benign
  papillary — see Neoplasm, skin, benign
Hidrocystoma — see Neoplasm, skin, benign
High
  altitude effects T70.20
    anoxia T70.29
    on
      ears T70.0
      sinuses T70.1
    polycythemia D75.1

High — continued
  arch
    foot Q66.7
    palate, congenital Q38.5
  arterial tension — see Hypertension
  basal metabolic rate R94.8
  blood pressure — see also Hypertension
    borderline R03.0
    reading (incidental) (isolated) (nonspecific),
      without diagnosis of hypertension R03.0
  cholesterol E78.00
    with high triglycerides E78.2
  diaphragm (congenital) Q79.1
  expressed emotional level within family Z63.8
  head at term O32.4
  palate, congenital Q38.5
  risk
    infant NEC Z76.2
    sexual behavior (heterosexual) Z72.51
      bisexual Z72.53
      homosexual Z72.52
  temperature (of unknown origin) R50.9
  thoracic rib Q76.6
  triglycerides E78.1
    with high cholesterol E78.2
Hildenbrand's disease A75.0
Hilum — see condition
Hip — see condition
Hippel's disease Q85.8
Hippophobia F40.218
Hippus H57.09
Hirschsprung's disease or megacolon
    Q43.1
Hirsutism, hirsuties L68.0
Hirudiniasis
  external B88.3
  internal B83.4
Hiss-Russell dysentery A03.1
His-Werner disease A79.0
Histidinemia, histidinuria E70.41
Histiocytoma — see also Neoplasm, skin,
    benign
  fibrous — see also Neoplasm, skin, benign
    atypical — see Neoplasm, connective tissue,
      uncertain behavior
    malignant — see Neoplasm, connective
      tissue, malignant
Histiocytosis D76.3
  acute differentiated progressive C96.0
  Langerhans' cell NEC C96.6
    multifocal X
      multisystemic (disseminated) C96.0
      unisystemic C96.5
    pulmonary, adult (adult PLCH) J84.82
    unifocal (X) C96.6
  lipid, lipoid D76.3
    essential E75.29
  malignant C96.A
  mononuclear phagocytes NEC D76.1
    Langerhans' cells C96.6
  non-Langerhans cell D76.3
  polyostotic sclerosing D76.3
  sinus, with massive lymphadenopathy D76.3
  syndrome NEC D76.3
  X NEC C96.6
    acute (progressive) C96.0
    chronic C96.6
    multifocal C96.5
    multisystemic C96.0
    unifocal C96.6
Histoplasmosis B39.9
  with pneumonia NEC B39.2
  African B39.5
  American — see Histoplasmosis, capsulati
  capsulati B39.4
    disseminated B39.3
    generalized B39.3

Histoplasmosis B39.9 — *continued*
  capsulati B39.4 — *continued*
    pulmonary B39.2
      acute B39.0
      chronic B39.1
    Darling's B39.4
    duboisii B39.5
    lung NEC B39.2
History
  family (of) — *see also* History, personal (of)
    alcohol abuse Z81.1
    allergy NEC Z84.89
    anemia Z83.2
    arthritis Z82.61
    asthma Z82.5
    blindness Z82.1
    cardiac death (sudden) Z82.41
    carrier of genetic disease Z84.81
    chromosomal anomaly Z82.79
    chronic
      disabling disease NEC Z82.8
      lower respiratory disease Z82.5
    colonic polyps Z83.71
    congenital malformations and deformations Z82.79
      polycystic kidney Z82.71
    consanguinity Z84.3
    deafness Z82.2
    diabetes mellitus Z83.3
    disability NEC Z82.8
    disease or disorder (of)
      allergic NEC Z84.89
      behavioral NEC Z81.8
      blood and blood-forming organs Z83.2
      cardiovascular NEC Z82.49
      chronic disabling NEC Z82.8
      digestive Z83.79
      ear NEC Z83.52
      endocrine NEC Z83.49
      eye NEC Z83.518
        glaucoma Z83.511
      familial hypercholesterolemia Z83.42
      genitourinary NEC Z84.2
      glaucoma Z83.511
      hematological Z83.2
      immune mechanism Z83.2
      infectious NEC Z83.1
      ischemic heart Z82.49
      kidney Z84.1
      mental NEC Z81.8
      metabolic Z83.49
      musculoskeletal NEC Z82.69
      neurological NEC Z82.0
      nutritional Z83.49
      parasitic NEC Z83.1
      psychiatric NEC Z81.8
      respiratory NEC Z83.6
      skin and subcutaneous tissue NEC Z84.0
      specified NEC Z84.89
    drug abuse NEC Z81.3
    epilepsy Z82.0
    familial hypercholesterolemia Z83.42
    genetic disease carrier Z84.81
    glaucoma Z83.511
    hearing loss Z82.2
    human immunodeficiency virus (HIV) infection Z83.0
    Huntington's chorea Z82.0
    intellectual disability Z81.0
    leukemia Z80.6
    malignant neoplasm (of) NOS Z80.9
      bladder Z80.52
      breast Z80.3
      bronchus Z80.1
      digestive organ Z80.0
      gastrointestinal tract Z80.0

History — *continued*
  family (of) (*see also* History, personal (of)) — *continued*
    malignant neoplasm (of) NOS Z80.9 — *continued*
      genital organ Z80.49
        ovary Z80.41
        prostate Z80.42
        specified organ NEC Z80.49
        testis Z80.43
      hematopoietic NEC Z80.7
      intrathoracic organ NEC Z80.2
      kidney Z80.51
      lung Z80.1
      lymphatic NEC Z80.7
      ovary Z80.41
      prostate Z80.42
      respiratory organ NEC Z80.2
      specified site NEC Z80.8
      testis Z80.43
      trachea Z80.1
      urinary organ or tract Z80.59
        bladder Z80.52
        kidney Z80.51
    mental
      disorder NEC Z81.8
    multiple endocrine neoplasia (MEN) syndrome Z83.41
    osteoporosis Z82.62
    polycystic kidney Z82.71
    polyps (colon) Z83.71
    psychiatric disorder Z81.8
    psychoactive substance abuse NEC Z81.3
    respiratory condition NEC Z83.6
      asthma and other lower respiratory conditions Z82.5
    self-harmful behavior Z81.8
    SIDS (sudden infant death syndrome) Z84.82
    skin condition Z84.0
    specified condition NEC Z84.89
    stroke (cerebrovascular) Z82.3
    substance abuse NEC Z81.4
      alcohol Z81.1
      drug NEC Z81.3
      psychoactive NEC Z81.3
      tobacco Z81.2
    sudden
      cardiac death Z82.41
      infant death syndrome (SIDS) Z84.82
    tobacco abuse Z81.2
    violence, violent behavior Z81.8
    visual loss Z82.1
  personal (of) — *see also* History, family (of)
    abuse
      adult Z91.419
        physical and sexual Z91.410
        psychological Z91.411
      childhood Z62.819
        physical Z62.810
        psychological Z62.811
        sexual Z62.810
    alcohol dependence F10.21
    allergy (to) Z88.9
      analgesic agent NEC Z88.6
      anesthetic Z88.4
      anti-infective agent NEC Z88.3
      antibiotic agent NEC Z88.1
      contrast media Z91.041
      drugs, medicaments and biological substances Z88.9
        specified NEC Z88.8
      food Z91.018
        additives Z91.02
        eggs Z91.012
        milk products Z91.011
        peanuts Z91.010
        seafood Z91.013
        specified food NEC Z91.018

History — *continued*
  personal (of) (*see also* History, family (of)) — *continued*
    allergy (to) Z88.9 — *continued*
      insect Z91.038
        bee Z91.030
      latex Z91.040
      medicinal agents Z88.9
        specified NEC Z88.8
      narcotic agent NEC Z88.5
      nonmedicinal agents Z91.048
      penicillin Z88.0
      serum Z88.7
      specified NEC Z91.09
      sulfonamides Z88.2
      vaccine Z88.7
    anaphylactic shock Z87.892
    anaphylaxis Z87.892
    behavioral disorders Z86.59
    benign carcinoid tumor Z86.012
    benign neoplasm Z86.018
      brain Z86.011
      carcinoid Z86.012
      colonic polyps Z86.010
    brain injury (traumatic) Z87.820
    breast implant removal Z98.86
    calculi, renal Z87.442
    cancer — *see* History, personal (of), malignant neoplasm (of)
    cardiac arrest (death), successfully resuscitated Z86.74
    cerebral infarction without residual deficit Z86.73
    cervical dysplasia Z87.410
    chemotherapy for neoplastic condition Z92.21
    childhood abuse — *see* History, personal (of), abuse
    cleft lip (corrected) Z87.730
    cleft palate (corrected) Z87.730
    collapsed vertebra (healed) Z87.311
      due to osteoporosis Z87.310
    combat and operational stress reaction Z86.51
    congenital malformation (corrected) Z87.798
      circulatory system (corrected) Z87.74
      digestive system (corrected) NEC Z87.738
      ear (corrected) Z87.720
      eye (corrected) Z87.721
      face and neck (corrected) Z87.790
      genitourinary system (corrected) NEC Z87.718
      heart (corrected) Z87.74
      integument (corrected) Z87.76
      limb(s) (corrected) Z87.76
      musculoskeletal system (corrected) Z87.76
      neck (corrected) Z87.790
      nervous system (corrected) NEC Z87.728
      respiratory system (corrected) Z87.75
      sense organs (corrected) NEC Z87.728
      specified NEC Z87.798
    contraception Z92.0
    deployment (military) Z91.82
    diabetic foot ulcer Z86.31
    disease or disorder (of) Z87.898
      anaphylaxis Z87.892
      blood and blood-forming organs Z86.2
      circulatory system Z86.79
        specified condition NEC Z86.79
      connective tissue NEC Z87.39
      digestive system Z87.19
        colonic polyp Z86.010
        peptic ulcer disease Z87.11
        specified condition NEC Z87.19
      ear Z86.69
      endocrine Z86.39
        diabetic foot ulcer Z86.31
        gestational diabetes Z86.32
        specified type NEC Z86.39

DISEASE INDEX

History — *continued*
  personal (of) (*see also* History, family (of)) — *continued*
    disease or disorder (of) Z87.898 — *continued*
      eye Z86.69
      genital (track) system NEC
        female Z87.42
        male Z87.438
      hematological Z86.2
      Hodgkin Z85.71
      immune mechanism Z86.2
      infectious Z86.19
        malaria Z86.13
        methicillin resistant Staphylococcus aureus (MRSA) Z86.14
        poliomyelitis Z86.12
        specified NEC Z86.19
        tuberculosis Z86.11
      mental NEC Z86.59
      metabolic Z86.39
        diabetic foot ulcer Z86.31
        gestational diabetes Z86.32
        specified type NEC Z86.39
      musculoskeletal NEC Z87.39
      nervous system Z86.69
      nutritional Z86.39
      parasitic Z86.19
      respiratory system NEC Z87.09
      sense organs Z86.69
      skin Z87.2
      specified site or type NEC Z87.898
      subcutaneous tissue Z87.2
      trophoblastic Z87.59
      urinary system NEC Z87.448
    drug dependence — *see* Dependence, drug, by type, in remission
    drug therapy
      antineoplastic chemotherapy Z92.21
      estrogen Z92.23
      immunosupression Z92.25
      inhaled steroids Z92.240
      monoclonal drug Z92.22
      specified NEC Z92.29
      steroid Z92.241
      systemic steroids Z92.241
    dysplasia
      cervical (mild) (moderate) Z87.410
        severe (grade III) Z86.001
      prostatic Z87.430
      vaginal (mild) (moderate) Z87.411
        severe (grade III) Z86.008
      vulvar (mild) (moderate) Z87.412
        severe (grade III) Z86.008
    embolism (venous) Z86.718
      pulmonary Z86.711
    encephalitis Z86.61
    estrogen therapy Z92.23
    extracorporeal membrane oxygenation (ECMO) Z92.81
    failed conscious sedation Z92.83
    failed moderate sedation Z92.83
    fall, falling Z91.81
    fracture (healed)
      fatigue Z87.312
      fragility Z87.310
      osteoporosis Z87.310
      pathological NEC Z87.311
      stress Z87.312
      traumatic Z87.81
    gestational diabetes Z86.32
    hepatitis
      B Z86.19
      C Z86.19
    Hodgkin disease Z85.71
    hyperthermia, malignant Z88.4
    hypospadias (corrected) Z87.710
    hysterectomy Z90.710
    immunosupression therapy Z92.25

History — *continued*
  personal (of) (*see also* History, family (of)) — *continued*
    in situ neoplasm
      breast Z86.000
      cervix uteri Z86.001
      specified NEC Z86.008
    in utero procedure during pregnancy Z98.870
    in utero procedure while a fetus Z98.871
    infection NEC Z86.19
      central nervous system Z86.61
      methicillin resistant Staphylococcus aureus (MRSA) Z86.14
      urinary (recurrent) (tract) Z87.440
    injury NEC Z87.828
    irradiation Z92.3
    kidney stones Z87.442
    leukemia Z85.6
    lymphoma (non-Hodgkin) Z85.72
    malignant melanoma (skin) Z85.820
    malignant neoplasm (of) Z85.9
      accessory sinuses Z85.22
      anus NEC Z85.048
        carcinoid Z85.040
      bladder Z85.51
      bone Z85.830
      brain Z85.841
      breast Z85.3
      bronchus NEC Z85.118
        carcinoid Z85.110
      carcinoid — *see* History, personal (of), malignant neoplasm, by site, carcinoid
      cervix Z85.41
      colon NEC Z85.038
        carcinoid Z85.030
      digestive organ Z85.00
        specified NEC Z85.09
      endocrine gland NEC Z85.858
      epididymis Z85.48
      esophagus Z85.01
      eye Z85.840
      gastrointestinal tract — *see* History, malignant neoplasm, digestive organ
      genital organ
        female Z85.40
          specified NEC Z85.44
        male Z85.45
          specified NEC Z85.49
      hematopoietic NEC Z85.79
      intrathoracic organ Z85.20
      kidney NEC Z85.528
        carcinoid Z85.520
      large intestine NEC Z85.038
        carcinoid Z85.030
      larynx Z85.21
      liver Z85.05
      lung NEC Z85.118
        carcinoid Z85.110
      mediastinum Z85.29
      Merkel cell Z85.821
      middle ear Z85.22
      nasal cavities Z85.22
      nervous system NEC Z85.848
      oral cavity Z85.819
        specified site NEC Z85.818
      ovary Z85.43
      pancreas Z85.07
      pelvis Z85.53
      pharynx Z85.819
        specified site NEC Z85.818
      pleura Z85.29
      prostate Z85.46
      rectosigmoid junction NEC Z85.048
        carcinoid Z85.040
      rectum NEC Z85.048
        carcinoid Z85.040
      respiratory organ Z85.20

History — *continued*
  personal (of) (*see also* History, family (of)) — *continued*
    malignant neoplasm (of) Z85.9 — *continued*
      sinuses, accessory Z85.22
      skin NEC Z85.828
        melanoma Z85.820
        Merkel cell Z85.821
      small intestine NEC Z85.068
        carcinoid Z85.060
      soft tissue Z85.831
      specified site NEC Z85.89
      stomach NEC Z85.028
        carcinoid Z85.020
      testis Z85.47
      thymus NEC Z85.238
        carcinoid Z85.230
      thyroid Z85.850
      tongue Z85.810
      trachea Z85.12
      ureter Z85.54
      urinary organ or tract Z85.50
        specified NEC Z85.59
      uterus Z85.42
    maltreatment Z91.89
    medical treatment NEC Z92.89
    melanoma (malignant) (skin) Z85.820
    meningitis Z86.61
    mental disorder Z86.59
    Merkel cell carcinoma (skin) Z85.821
    Methicillin resistant Staphylococcus aureus (MRSA) Z86.14
    military deployment Z91.82
    military war, peacekeeping and humanitarian deployment (current or past conflict) Z91.82
    myocardial infarction (old) I25.2
    neglect (in)
      adult Z91.412
      childhood Z62.812
    neoplasm
      benign Z86.018
        brain Z86.011
        colon polyp Z86.010
      in situ
        breast Z86.000
        cervix uteri Z86.001
        specified NEC Z86.008
      malignant — *see* History of, malignant neoplasm
      uncertain behavior Z86.03
    nephrotic syndrome Z87.441
    nicotine dependence Z87.891
    noncompliance with medical treatment or regimen — *see* Noncompliance
    nutritional deficiency Z86.39
    obstetric complications Z87.59
      childbirth Z87.59
      pre-term labor Z87.51
      pregnancy Z87.59
      puerperium Z87.59
    osteoporosis fractures Z87.31
    parasuicide (attempt) Z91.5
    physical trauma NEC Z87.828
    self-harm or suicide attempt Z91.5
    pneumonia (recurrent) Z87.01
    poisoning NEC Z91.89
      self-harm or suicide attempt Z91.5
    poor personal hygiene Z91.89
    preterm labor Z87.51
    procedure during pregnancy Z98.870
    procedure while a fetus Z98.871
    prolonged reversible ischemic neurologic deficit (PRIND) Z86.73
    prostatic dysplasia Z87.430

History — *continued*
  personal (of) (*see also* History, family (of)) — *continued*
    psychological
      abuse
        adult Z91.411
        child Z62.811
      trauma, specified NEC Z91.49
    radiation therapy Z92.3
    removal
      implant
        breast Z98.86
    renal calculi Z87.442
    respiratory condition NEC Z87.09
    retained foreign body fully removed Z87.821
    risk factors NEC Z91.89
    self-harm Z91.5
    self-poisoning attempt Z91.5
    sex reassignment Z87.890
    sleep-wake cycle problem Z72.821
    specified NEC Z87.898
    steroid therapy (systemic) Z92.241
      inhaled Z92.240
    stroke without residual deficits Z86.73
    substance abuse NEC F10-F19 with fifth character 1
    sudden cardiac arrest Z86.74
    sudden cardiac death successfully resuscitated Z86.74
    suicide attempt Z91.5
    surgery NEC Z98.890
      with uterine scar Z98.891
      sex reassignment Z87.890
      transplant — *see* Transplant
    thrombophlebitis Z86.72
    thrombosis (venous) Z86.718
      pulmonary Z86.711
    tobacco dependence Z87.891
    transient ischemic attack (TIA) without residual deficits Z86.73
    trauma (physical) NEC Z87.828
      psychological NEC Z91.49
      self-harm Z91.5
    traumatic brain injury Z87.820
    unhealthy sleep-wake cycle Z72.821
    unintended awareness under general anesthesia Z92.84
    urinary (recurrent) (tract) infection(s) Z87.440
    urinary calculi Z87.442
    uterine scar from previous surgery Z98.891
    vaginal dysplasia Z87.411
    venous thrombosis or embolism Z86.718
      pulmonary Z86.711
    vulvar dysplasia Z87.412
HIV (*see also* Human, immunodeficiency virus) B20
  laboratory evidence (nonconclusive) R75
  nonconclusive test (in infants) R75
  positive, seropositive Z21
Hives (bold) — *see* Urticaria
Hoarseness R49.0
Hobo Z59.0
Hodgkin disease — *see* Lymphoma, Hodgkin
Hodgson's disease I71.2
  ruptured I71.1
Hoffa-Kastert disease E88.89
Hoffa's disease E88.89
Hoffmann's syndrome E03.9 *[G73.7]*
Hoffmann-Bouveret syndrome I47.9
Hole (round)
  macula H35.34-
  retina (without detachment) — *see* Break, retina, round hole
    with detachment — *see* Detachment, retina, with retinal, break
Holiday relief care Z75.5

Hollenhorst's plaque — *see* Occlusion, artery, retina
Hollow foot (congenital) Q66.7
  acquired — *see* Deformity, limb, foot, specified NEC
Holoprosencephaly Q04.2
Holt-Oram syndrome Q87.2
Homelessness Z59.0
Homesickness — *see* Disorder, adjustment
Homocystinemia, homocystinuria E72.11
Homogentisate 1,2-dioxygenase deficiency E70.29
Homologous serum hepatitis (prophylactic) (therapeutic) — *see* Hepatitis, viral, type B
Honeycomb lung J98.4
  congenital Q33.0
Hooded
  clitoris Q52.6
  penis Q55.69
Hookworm (anemia) (disease) (infection) (infestation) B76.9
  specified NEC B76.8
Hordeolum (eyelid) (externum) (recurrent) H00.019
  internum H00.029
    left H00.026
      lower H00.025
      upper H00.024
    right H00.023
      lower H00.022
      upper H00.021
  left H00.016
    lower H00.015
    upper H00.014
  right H00.013
    lower H00.012
    upper H00.011
Horn
  cutaneous L85.8
  nail L60.2
    congenital Q84.6
Horner(-Claude Bernard) syndrome G90.2
  traumatic — *see* Injury, nerve, cervical sympathetic
Horseshoe kidney (congenital) Q63.1
Horton's headache or neuralgia G44.099
  intractable G44.091
  not intractable G44.099
Hospital hopper syndrome — *see* Disorder, factitious
Hospitalism in children — *see* Disorder, adjustment
Hostility R45.5
  towards child Z62.3
Hot flashes
  menopausal N95.1
Hourglass (contracture) — *see also* Contraction, hourglass
  stomach K31.89
    congenital Q40.2
    stricture K31.2
Household, housing circumstance affecting care Z59.9
  specified NEC Z59.8
Housemaid's knee — *see* Bursitis, prepatellar
Hudson(-Stähli) line (cornea) — *see* Pigmentation, cornea, anterior
Human
  bite (open wound) — *see also* Bite
    intact skin surface — *see* Bite, superficial
  herpesvirus — *see* Herpes
  immunodeficiency virus (HIV) disease (infection) B20
    asymptomatic status Z21
    contact Z20.6
    counseling Z71.7

Human — *continued*
  immunodeficiency virus (HIV) disease (infection) B20 — *continued*
    dementia B20 *[F02.80]*
      with behavioral disturbance B20 *[F02.81]*
    exposure to Z20.6
    laboratory evidence R75
    type-2 (HIV 2) as cause of disease classified elsewhere B97.35
  papillomavirus (HPV)
    DNA test positive
      high risk
        cervix R87.810
        vagina R87.811
      low risk
        cervix R87.820
        vagina R87.821
    screening for Z11.51
  T-cell lymphotropic virus
    type-1 (HTLV-I) infection B33.3
      as cause of disease classified elsewhere B97.33
      carrier Z22.6
    type-2 (HTLV-II) as cause of disease classified elsewhere B97.34
Humidifier lung or pneumonitis J67.7
Humiliation (experience) in childhood Z62.898
Humpback (acquired) — *see* Kyphosis
Hunchback (acquired) — *see* Kyphosis
Hunger T73.0
  air, psychogenic F45.8
Hungry bone syndrome E83.81
Hunner's ulcer — *see* Cystitis, chronic, interstitial
Hunter's
  glossitis D51.0
  syndrome E76.1
Huntington's disease or chorea G10
  with dementia G10 *[F02.80]*
    with behavioral disturbance G10 *[F02.81]*
Hunt's
  disease or syndrome (herpetic geniculate ganglionitis) B02.21
  dyssynergia cerebellaris myoclonica G11.1
  neuralgia B02.21
Hurler(-Scheie) disease or syndrome E76.02
Hurst's disease G36.1
Hurthle cell
  adenocarcinoma C73
  adenoma D34
  carcinoma C73
  tumor D34
Hutchinson's
  disease, meaning
    angioma serpiginosum L81.7
    pompholyx (cheiropompholyx) L30.1
    prurigo estivalis L56.4
    summer eruption or summer prurigo L56.4
  melanotic freckle — *see* Melanoma, in situ
    malignant melanoma in — *see* Melanoma
  teeth or incisors (congenital syphilis) A50.52
  triad (congenital syphilis) A50.53
Hutchinson-Boeck disease or syndrome — *see* Sarcoidosis
Hutchinson-Gilford disease or syndrome E34.8
Hyalin plaque, sclera, senile H15.89
Hyaline membrane (disease) (lung) (pulmonary) (newborn) P22.0
Hyalinosis
  cutis (et mucosae) E78.89
  focal and segmental (glomerular) (*see also* N00-N07 with fourth character .1) N05.1
Hyalitis, hyalosis, asteroid — *see also* Deposit, crystalline
  syphilitic (late) A52.71

Hydatid
cyst or tumor — *see* Echinococcus
mole — *see* Hydatidiform mole
Morgagni
female Q50.5
male (epididymal) Q55.4
testicular Q55.29
Hydatidiform mole (benign) (complicating pregnancy) (delivered) (undelivered) O01.9
classical O01.0
complete O01.0
incomplete O01.1
invasive D39.2
malignant D39.2
partial O01.1
Hydatidosis — *see* Echinococcus
Hydradenitis (axillaris) (suppurative) L73.2
Hydradenoma — *see* Hidradenoma
Hydramnios O40-
Hydrancephaly, hydranencephaly Q04.3
with spina bifida — *see* Spina bifida, with hydrocephalus
Hydrargyrism NEC — *see* Poisoning, mercury
Hydrarthrosis — *see also* Effusion, joint
gonococcal A54.42
intermittent M12.40
ankle M12.47-
elbow M12.42-
foot joint M12.47-
hand joint M12.44-
hip M12.45-
knee M12.46-
multiple site M12.49
shoulder M12.41-
specified joint NEC M12.48
wrist M12.43-
of yaws (early) (late) (*see also* subcategory M14.8-) A66.6
syphilitic (late) A52.77
congenital A50.55 [M12.80]
Hydremia D64.89
Hydrencephalocele (congenital) — *see* Encephalocele
Hydrencephalomeningocele (congenital) — *see* Encephalocele
Hydroa R23.8
aestivale L56.4
vacciniforme L56.4
Hydroadenitis (axillaris) (suppurative) L73.2
Hydrocalycosis — *see* Hydronephrosis
Hydrocele (spermatic cord) (testis) (tunica vaginalis) N43.3
canal of Nuck N94.89
communicating N43.2
congenital P83.5
congenital P83.5
encysted N43.0
female NEC N94.89
infected N43.1
newborn P83.5
round ligament N94.89
specified NEC N43.2
spinalis — *see* Spina bifida
vulva N90.89
Hydrocephalus (acquired) (external) (internal) (malignant) (recurrent) G91.9
aqueduct Sylvius stricture Q03.0
causing disproportion O33.6
with obstructed labor O66.3
communicating G91.0
congenital (external) (internal) Q03.9
with spina bifida Q05.4
cervical Q05.0
dorsal Q05.1
lumbar Q05.2
lumbosacral Q05.2
sacral Q05.3
thoracic Q05.1
thoracolumbar Q05.1

Hydrocephalus (acquired) (external) (internal) (malignant) (recurrent) G91.9 — *continued*
congenital (external) (internal) Q03.9 — *continued*
specified NEC Q03.8
due to toxoplasmosis (congenital) P37.1
foramen Magendie block (acquired) G91.1
congenital (*see also* Hydrocephalus, congenital) Q03.1
in (due to)
infectious disease NEC B89 [G91.4]
neoplastic disease NEC (*see also* Neoplasm) G91.4
parasitic disease B89 [G91.4]
newborn Q03.9
with spina bifida — *see* Spina bifida, with hydrocephalus
noncommunicating G91.1
normal pressure G91.2
secondary G91.0
obstructive G91.1
otitic G93.2
post-traumatic NEC G91.3
secondary G91.4
post-traumatic G91.3
specified NEC G91.8
syphilitic, congenital A50.49
Hydrocolpos (congenital) N89.8
Hydrocystoma — *see* Neoplasm, skin, benign
Hydroencephalocele (congenital) — *see* Encephalocele
Hydroencephalomeningocele (congenital) — *see* Encephalocele
Hydrohematopneumothorax — *see* Hemothorax
Hydromeningitis — *see* Meningitis
Hydromeningocele (spinal) — *see also* Spina bifida
cranial — *see* Encephalocele
Hydrometra N85.8
Hydrometrocolpos N89.8
Hydromicrocephaly Q02
Hydromphalos (since birth) Q45.8
Hydromyelia Q06.4
Hydromyelocele — *see* Spina bifida
Hydronephrosis (atrophic) (early) (functionless) (intermittent) (primary) (secondary) NEC N13.30
with
infection N13.6
obstruction (by) (of)
renal calculus N13.2
with infection N13.6
ureteral NEC N13.1
with infection N13.6
calculus N13.2
with infection N13.6
ureteropelvic junction (congenital) Q62.0
acquired N13.0
with infection N13.6
ureteral stricture NEC N13.1
with infection N13.6
congenital Q62.0
due to acquired occlusion of ureteropelvic junction N13.0
specified type NEC N13.39
tuberculous A18.11
Hydropericarditis — *see* Pericarditis
Hydropericardium — *see* Pericarditis
Hydroperitoneum R18.8
Hydrophobia — *see* Rabies
Hydrophthalmos Q15.0
Hydropneumohemothorax — *see* Hemothorax
Hydropneumopericarditis — *see* Pericarditis
Hydropneumopericardium — *see* Pericarditis

Hydropneumothorax J94.8
traumatic — *see* Injury, intrathoracic, lung
tuberculous NEC A15.6
Hydrops R60.9
abdominis R18.8
articulorum intermittens — *see* Hydrarthrosis, intermittent
cardiac — *see* Failure, heart, congestive
causing obstructed labor (mother) O66.3
endolymphatic H81.0-
fetal — *see* Pregnancy, complicated by, hydrops, fetalis
fetalis P83.2
due to
ABO isoimmunization P56.0
alpha thalassemia D56.0
hemolytic disease P56.90
specified NEC P56.99
isoimmunization (ABO) (Rh) P56.0
other specified nonhemolytic disease NEC P83.2
Rh incompatibility P56.0
during pregnancy — *see* Pregnancy, complicated by, hydrops, fetalis
gallbladder K82.1
joint — *see* Effusion, joint
labyrinth H81.0-
newborn (idiopathic) P83.2
due to
ABO isoimmunization P56.0
alpha thalassemia D56.0
hemolytic disease P56.90
specified NEC P56.99
isoimmunization (ABO) (Rh) P56.0
Rh incompatibility P56.0
nutritional — *see* Malnutrition, severe
pericardium — *see* Pericarditis
pleura — *see* Hydrothorax
spermatic cord — *see* Hydrocele
Hydropyonephrosis N13.6
Hydrorachis Q06.4
Hydrorrhea (nasal) J34.89
pregnancy — *see* Rupture, membranes, premature
Hydrosadenitis (axillaris) (suppurative) L73.2
Hydrosalpinx (fallopian tube) (follicularis) N70.11
Hydrothorax (double) (pleura) J94.8
chylous (nonfilarial) I89.8
filarial (*see also* Infestation, filarial) B74.9 [J91.8]
traumatic — *see* Injury, intrathoracic
tuberculous NEC (non primary) A15.6
Hydroureter (*see also* Hydronephrosis) N13.4
with infection N13.6
congenital Q62.39
Hydroureteronephrosis — *see* Hydronephrosis
Hydrourethra N36.8
Hydroxykynureninuria E70.8
Hydroxylysinemia E72.3
Hydroxyprolinemia E72.59
Hygiene, sleep
abuse Z72.821
inadequate Z72.821
poor Z72.821
Hygroma (congenital) (cystic) D18.1
praepatellare, prepatellar — *see* Bursitis, prepatellar
Hymen — *see* condition
Hymenolepis, hymenolepiasis (diminuta) (infection) (infestation) (nana) B71.0
Hypalgesia R20.8
Hyperacidity (gastric) K31.89
psychogenic F45.8

DISEASE INDEX

Hyperactive, hyperactivity F90.9
　basal cell, uterine cervix — *see* Dysplasia,
　　cervix
　bowel sounds R19.12
　cervix epithelial (basal) — *see* Dysplasia,
　　cervix
　child F90.9
　　attention deficit — *see* Disorder, attention-
　　　deficit hyperactivity
　detrusor muscle N32.81
　gastrointestinal K31.89
　　psychogenic F45.8
　nasal mucous membrane J34.3
　stomach K31.89
　thyroid (gland) — *see* Hyperthyroidism
Hyperacusis H93.23-
Hyperadrenalism E27.5
Hyperadrenocorticism E24.9
　congenital E25.0
　iatrogenic E24.2
　　correct substance properly administered —
　　　see Table of Drugs and Chemicals, by
　　　drug, adverse effect
　　overdose or wrong substance given or taken
　　　— *see* Table of Drugs and Chemicals, by
　　　drug, poisoning
　not associated with Cushing's syndrome E27.0
　pituitary-dependent E24.0
Hyperaldosteronism E26.9
　familial (type I) E26.02
　glucocorticoid-remediable E26.02
　primary (due to (bilateral) adrenal
　　hyperplasia) E26.09
　primary NEC E26.09
　secondary E26.1
　specified NEC E26.89
Hyperalgesia R20.8
Hyperalimentation R63.2
　carotene, carotin E67.1
　specified NEC E67.8
　vitamin
　　A E67.0
　　D E67.3
Hyperaminoaciduria
　arginine E72.21
　cystine E72.01
　lysine E72.3
　ornithine E72.4
Hyperammonemia (congenital) E72.20
Hyperazotemia — *see* Uremia
Hyperbetalipoproteinemia (familial)
　E78.00
　with prebetalipoproteinemia E78.2
Hyperbilirubinemia
　constitutional E80.6
　familial conjugated E80.6
　neonatal (transient) — *see* Jaundice, newborn
Hypercalcemia, hypocalciuric, familial
　E83.52
Hypercalciuria, idiopathic E83.52
Hypercapnia R06.89
　newborn P84
Hypercarotenemia, hypercarotinemia
　(dietary) E67.1
Hypercementosis K03.4
Hyperchloremia E87.8
Hyperchlorhydria K31.89
　neurotic F45.8
　psychogenic F45.8
Hypercholesterinemia — *see*
　Hypercholesterolemia
Hypercholesterolemia (essential) (primary)
　(pure) E78.00
　with hyperglyceridemia, endogenous E78.2
　dietary counseling and surveillance Z71.3
　familial E78.01
　hereditary E78.01
Hyperchylia gastrica, psychogenic F45.8

Hyperchylomicronemia (familial) (primary)
　E78.3
　with hyperbetalipoproteinemia E78.3
Hypercoagulable (state) D68.59
　activated protein C resistance D68.51
　antithrombin (III) deficiency D68.59
　factor V Leiden mutation D68.51
　primary NEC D68.59
　protein C deficiency D68.59
　protein S deficiency D68.59
　prothrombin gene mutation D68.52
　secondary D68.69
　specified NEC D68.69
Hypercoagulation (state) D68.59
Hypercorticalism, pituitary-dependent
　E24.0
Hypercorticosolism — *see* Cushing's,
　syndrome
Hypercorticosteronism E24.2
　correct substance properly administered — *see*
　　Table of Drugs and Chemicals, by drug,
　　adverse effect
　overdose or wrong substance given or taken
　　— *see* Table of Drugs and Chemicals, by
　　drug, poisoning
Hypercortisonism E24.2
　correct substance properly administered — *see*
　　Table of Drugs and Chemicals, by drug,
　　adverse effect
　overdose or wrong substance given or taken
　　— *see* Table of Drugs and Chemicals, by
　　drug, poisoning
Hyperekplexia Q89.8
Hyperelectrolytemia E87.8
Hyperemesis R11.10
　with nausea R11.2
　gravidarum (mild) O21.0
　　with
　　　carbohydrate depletion O21.1
　　　dehydration O21.1
　　　electrolyte imbalance O21.1
　　　metabolic disturbance O21.1
　　　severe (with metabolic disturbance) O21.1
　projectile R11.12
　psychogenic F45.8
Hyperemia (acute) (passive) R68.89
　anal mucosa K62.89
　bladder N32.89
　cerebral I67.89
　conjunctiva H11.43-
　ear internal, acute — *see* subcategory H83.0
　enteric K59.8
　eye — *see* Hyperemia, conjunctiva
　eyelid (active) (passive) — *see* Disorder, eyelid,
　　specified type NEC
　intestine K59.8
　iris — *see* Disorder, iris, vascular
　kidney N28.89
　labyrinth — *see* subcategory H83.0
　liver (active) K76.89
　lung (passive) — *see* Edema, lung
　pulmonary (passive) — *see* Edema, lung
　renal N28.89
　retina H35.89
　stomach K31.89
Hyperesthesia (body surface) R20.3
　larynx (reflex) J38.7
　　hysterical F44.89
　pharynx (reflex) J39.2
　　hysterical F44.89
Hyperestrogenism (drug-induced)
　(iatrogenic) E28.0
Hyperexplexia Q89.8
Hyperfibrinolysis — *see* Fibrinolysis
Hyperfructosemia E74.19

Hyperfunction
　adrenal cortex, not associated with Cushing's
　　syndrome E27.0
　medulla E27.5
　　adrenomedullary E27.5
　virilism E25.9
　　congenital E25.0
　ovarian E28.8
　pancreas K86.89
　parathyroid (gland) E21.3
　pituitary (gland) (anterior) E22.9
　　specified NEC E22.8
　polyglandular E31.1
　testicular E29.0
Hypergammaglobulinemia D89.2
　polyclonal D89.0
　Waldenström D89.0
Hypergastrinemia E16.4
Hyperglobulinemia R77.1
Hyperglycemia, hyperglycemic (transient)
　R73.9
　coma — *see* Diabetes, by type, with coma
　postpancreatectomy E89.1
Hyperglyceridemia (endogenous) (essential)
　(familial) (hereditary) (pure) E78.1
　mixed E78.3
Hyperglycinemia (non-ketotic) E72.51
Hypergonadism
　ovarian E28.8
　testicular (primary) (infantile) E29.0
Hyperheparinemia D68.32
Hyperhidrosis, hyperidrosis R61
　focal
　　primary L74.519
　　　axilla L74.510
　　　face L74.511
　　　palms L74.512
　　　soles L74.513
　　secondary L74.52
　generalized R61
　localized
　　primary L74.519
　　　axilla L74.510
　　　face L74.511
　　　palms L74.512
　　　soles L74.513
　　secondary L74.52
　psychogenic F45.8
　secondary R61
　　focal L74.52
Hyperhistidinemia E70.41
Hyperhomocysteinemia E72.11
Hyperhydroxyprolinemia E72.59
Hyperinsulinism (functional) E16.1
　with
　　coma (hypoglycemic) E15
　　encephalopathy E16.1 *[G94]*
　ectopic E16.1
　therapeutic misadventure (from administration
　　of insulin) — *see* subcategory T38.3
Hyperkalemia E87.5
Hyperkeratosis (*see also* Keratosis) L85.9
　cervix N88.0
　due to yaws (early) (late) (palmar or plantar)
　　A66.3
　follicularis Q82.8
　　penetrans (in cutem) L87.0
　palmoplantaris climacterica L85.1
　pinta A67.1
　senile (with pruritus) L57.0
　universalis congenita Q80.8
　vocal cord J38.3
　vulva N90.4
Hyperkinesia, hyperkinetic (disease)
　(reaction) (syndrome) (childhood)
　(adolescence) — *see also* Disorder, attention-
　deficit hyperactivity
　heart I51.89

Hyperleucine-isoleucinemia E71.19
Hyperlipemia, hyperlipidemia E78.5
  combined E78.2
    familial E78.4
  group
    A E78.00
    B E78.1
    C E78.2
    D E78.3
  mixed E78.2
  specified NEC E78.4
Hyperlipidosis E75.6
  hereditary NEC E75.5
Hyperlipoproteinemia E78.5
  Fredrickson's type
    I E78.3
    IIa E78.00
    IIb E78.2
    III E78.2
    IV E78.1
    V E78.3
  low-density-lipoprotein-type (LDL) E78.00
  very-low-density-lipoprotein-type (VLDL) E78.1
Hyperlucent lung, unilateral J43.0
Hyperlysinemia E72.3
Hypermagnesemia E83.41
  neonatal P71.8
Hypermenorrhea N92.0
Hypermethioninemia E72.19
Hypermetropia (congenital) H52.0-
Hypermobility, hypermotility
  cecum — see Syndrome, irritable bowel
  coccyx — see subcategory M53.2
  colon — see Syndrome, irritable bowel
    psychogenic F45.8
  ileum K58.9
  intestine (see also Syndrome, irritable bowel) K58.9
    psychogenic F45.8
  meniscus (knee) — see Derangement, knee, meniscus
  scapula — see Instability, joint, shoulder
  stomach K31.89
    psychogenic F45.8
  syndrome M35.7
  urethra N36.41
    with intrinsic sphincter deficiency N36.43
Hypernasality R49.21
Hypernatremia E87.0
Hypernephroma C64-
Hyperopia — see Hypermetropia
Hyperorexia nervosa F50.2
Hyperornithinemia E72.4
Hyperosmia R43.1
Hyperosmolality E87.0
Hyperostosis (monomelic) — see also Disorder, bone, density and structure, specified NEC
  ankylosing (spine) M48.10
    cervical region M48.12
    cervicothoracic region M48.13
    lumbar region M48.16
    lumbosacral region M48.17
    multiple sites M48.19
    occipito-atlanto-axial region M48.11
    sacrococcygeal region M48.18
    thoracic region M48.14
    thoracolumbar region M48.15
  cortical (skull) M85.2
    infantile M89.8x-
  frontal, internal of skull M85.2
  interna frontalis M85.2
  skeletal, diffuse idiopathic — see Hyperostosis, ankylosing
  skull M85.2
    congenital Q75.8
  vertebral, ankylosing — see Hyperostosis, ankylosing
Hyperovarism E28.8
Hyperoxaluria (primary) E72.53

Hyperparathyroidism E21.3
  primary E21.0
  secondary (renal) N25.81
    non-renal E21.1
  specified NEC E21.2
  tertiary E21.2
Hyperpathia R20.8
Hyperperistalsis R19.2
  psychogenic F45.8
Hyperpermeability, capillary I78.8
Hyperphagia R63.2
Hyperphenylalaninemia NEC E70.1
Hyperphoria (alternating) H50.53
Hyperphosphatemia E83.39
Hyperpiesis, hyperpiesia — see Hypertension
Hyperpigmentation — see also Pigmentation
  melanin NEC L81.4
  postinflammatory L81.0
Hyperpinealism E34.8
Hyperpituitarism E22.9
Hyperplasia, hyperplastic
  adenoids J35.2
  adrenal (capsule) (cortex) (gland) E27.8
    with
      sexual precocity (male) E25.9
        congenital E25.0
      virilism, adrenal E25.9
        congenital E25.0
      virilization (female) E25.9
        congenital E25.0
    congenital E25.0
    salt-losing E25.0
  adrenomedullary E27.5
  angiolymphoid, eosinophilia (ALHE) D18.01
  appendix (lymphoid) K38.0
  artery, fibromuscular I77.3
  bone — see also Hypertrophy, bone
    marrow D75.89
  breast — see also Hypertrophy, breast
    ductal (atypical) N60.9-
  C-cell, thyroid E07.0
  cementation (tooth) (teeth) K03.4
  cervical gland R59.0
  cervix (uteri) (basal cell) (endometrium) (polypoid) — see also Dysplasia, cervix
    congenital Q51.828
  clitoris, congenital Q52.6
  denture K06.2
  endocervicitis N72
  endometrium, endometrial (adenomatous) (benign) (cystic) (glandular) (glandular-cystic) (polypoid) N85.00
    with atypia N85.02
    cervix — see Dysplasia, cervix
    complex (without atypia) N85.01
    simple (without atypia) N85.01
  epithelial L85.9
    focal, oral, including tongue K13.29
    nipple N62
    skin L85.9
    tongue K13.29
    vaginal wall N89.3
  erythroid D75.89
  fibromuscular of artery (carotid) (renal) I77.3
  genital
    female NEC N94.89
    male N50.89
  gingiva K06.1
  glandularis cystica uteri (interstitialis) (see also Hyperplasia, endometrial) N85.00-
  gum K06.1
  hymen, congenital Q52.4
  irritative, edentulous (alveolar) K06.2

Hyperplasia, hyperplastic — continued
  jaw M26.09
    alveolar M26.79
    lower M26.03
      alveolar M26.72
    upper M26.01
      alveolar M26.71
  kidney (congenital) Q63.3
  labia N90.69
    epithelial N90.3
  liver (congenital) Q44.7
    nodular, focal K76.89
  lymph gland or node R59.9
  mandible, mandibular M26.03
    alveolar M26.72
    unilateral condylar M27.8
  maxilla, maxillary M26.01
    alveolar M26.71
  myometrium, myometrial N85.2
  neuroendocrine cell, of infancy J84.841
  nose
    lymphoid J34.89
    polypoid J33.9
  oral mucosa (irritative) K13.6
  organ or site, congenital NEC — see Anomaly, by site
  ovary N83.8
  palate, papillary (irritative) K13.6
  pancreatic islet cells E16.9
    alpha E16.8
      with excess
        gastrin E16.4
        glucagon E16.3
    beta E16.1
  parathyroid (gland) E21.0
  pharynx (lymphoid) J39.2
  prostate (adenofibromatous) (nodular) N40.0
    with lower urinary tract symptoms (LUTS) N40.1
    without lower urinary tract symtpoms (LUTS) N40.0
  renal artery I77.89
  reticulo-endothelial (cell) D75.89
  salivary gland (any) K11.1
  Schimmelbusch's — see Mastopathy, cystic
  suprarenal capsule (gland) E27.8
  thymus (gland) (persistent) E32.0
  thyroid (gland) — see Goiter
  tonsils (faucial) (infective) (lingual) (lymphoid) J35.1
    with adenoids J35.3
  unilateral condylar M27.8
  uterus, uterine N85.2
    endometrium (glandular) (see also Hyperplasia, endometrial) N85.00-
  vulva N90.69
    epithelial N90.3
Hyperpnea — see Hyperventilation
Hyperpotassemia E87.5
Hyperprebetalipoproteinemia (familial) E78.1
Hyperprolactinemia E22.1
Hyperprolinemia (type I) (type II) E72.59
Hyperproteinemia E88.09
Hyperprothrombinemia, causing coagulation factor deficiency D68.4
Hyperpyrexia R50.9
  heat (effects) T67.0
  malignant, due to anesthetic T88.3
  rheumatic — see Fever, rheumatic
  unknown origin R50.9
Hyper-reflexia R29.2
Hypersalivation K11.7
Hypersecretion
  ACTH (not associated with Cushing's syndrome) E27.0
    pituitary E24.0
  adrenaline E27.5

Hypersecretion — *continued*
  adrenomedullary E27.5
  androgen (testicular) E29.0
    ovarian (drug-induced) (iatrogenic) E28.1
  calcitonin E07.0
  catecholamine E27.5
  corticoadrenal E24.9
  cortisol E24.9
  epinephrine E27.5
  estrogen E28.0
  gastric K31.89
    psychogenic F45.8
  gastrin E16.4
  glucagon E16.3
  hormone(s)
    ACTH (not associated with Cushing's
        syndrome) E27.0
      pituitary E24.0
    antidiuretic E22.2
    growth E22.0
    intestinal NEC E34.1
    ovarian androgen E28.1
    pituitary E22.9
    testicular E29.0
    thyroid stimulating E05.80
      with thyroid storm E05.81
  insulin — *see* Hyperinsulinism
  lacrimal glands — *see* Epiphora
  medulloadrenal E27.5
  milk O92.6
  ovarian androgens E28.1
  salivary gland (any) K11.7
  thyrocalcitonin E07.0
  upper respiratory J39.8
Hypersegmentation, leukocytic,
    hereditary D72.0
Hypersensitive, hypersensitiveness,
    hypersensitivity — *see also* Allergy
  carotid sinus G90.01
  colon — *see* Irritable, colon
  drug T88.7
  gastrointestinal K52.29
    immediate K52.29
    psychogenic F45.8
  labyrinth — *see* subcategory H83.2
  pain R20.8
  pneumonitis — *see* Pneumonitis, allergic
  reaction T78.40
    upper respiratory tract NEC J39.3
Hypersomnia (organic) G47.10
  due to
    alcohol
      abuse F10.182
      dependence F10.282
      use F10.982
    amphetamines
      abuse F15.182
      dependence F15.282
      use F15.982
    caffeine
      abuse F15.182
      dependence F15.282
      use F15.982
    cocaine
      abuse F14.182
      dependence F14.282
      use F14.982
    drug NEC
      abuse F19.182
      dependence F19.282
      use F19.982
    medical condition G47.14
    mental disorder F51.13
    opioid
      abuse F11.182
      dependence F11.282
      use F11.982

Hypersomnia (organic) G47.10 — *continued*
  due to — *continued*
    psychoactive substance NEC
      abuse F19.182
      dependence F19.282
      use F19.982
    sedative, hypnotic, or anxiolytic
      abuse F13.182
      dependence F13.282
      use F13.982
    stimulant NEC
      abuse F15.182
      dependence F15.282
      use F15.982
  idiopathic G47.11
    with long sleep time G47.11
    without long sleep time G47.12
  menstrual related G47.13
  nonorganic origin F51.11
    specified NEC F51.19
  not due to a substance or known physiological
      condition F51.11
    specified NEC F51.19
  primary F51.11
  recurrent G47.13
  specified NEC G47.19
Hypersplenia, hypersplenism D73.1
Hyperstimulation, ovaries (associated with
    induced ovulation) N98.1
Hypersusceptibility — *see* Allergy
Hypertelorism (ocular) (orbital) Q75.2
Hypertension, hypertensive (accelerated)
    (benign) (essential) (idiopathic) (malignant)
    (systemic) I10
  with
    heart involvement (conditions in I51.4 –
        I51.9 due to hypertension) — *see*
        Hypertension, heart
    kidney involvement — *see* Hypertension,
        kidney
  benign, intracranial G93.2
  borderline R03.0
  cardiorenal (disease) I13.10
    with heart failure I13.0
      with stage 1 through stage 4 chronic
          kidney disease I13.0
      with stage 5 or end stage renal disease
          I13.2
    without heart failure I13.10
      with stage 1 through stage 4 chronic
          kidney disease I13.10
      with stage 5 or end stage renal disease
          I13.11
  cardiovascular
    disease (arteriosclerotic) (sclerotic) — *see*
        Hypertension, heart
    renal (disease) — *see* Hypertension,
        cardiorenal
  chronic venous — *see* Hypertension, venous
      (chronic)
  complicating
    childbirth (labor) O16.4
    pre-existing O10.92
      with
        heart disease O10.12
          with renal disease O10.32
        pre-eclampsia O11.4
        renal disease O10.22
          with heart disease O10.32
      essential O10.02
      secondary O10.42

Hypertension, hypertensive (accelerated)
    (benign) (essential) (idiopathic) (malignant)
    (systemic) I10 — *continued*
  complicating — *continued*
    pregnancy O16-
      with edema (*see also* Pre-eclampsia)
          O14.9-
      gestational (pregnancy induced) (without
          proteinuria) O13-
        with proteinuria O14.9-
          mild pre-eclampsia O14.0-
          moderate pre-eclampsia O14.0-
          severe pre-eclampsia O14.1-
            with hemolysis, elevated liver
                enzymes and low platelet count
                (HELLP) O14.2-
      pre-existing O10.91-
        with
          heart disease O10.11-
            with renal disease O10.31-
          pre-eclampsia — *see* category O11
          renal disease O10.21-
            with heart disease O10.31-
          essential O10.01-
          secondary O10.41-
      transient O13.-
    puerperium, pre-existing O16.5
      pre-existing
        with
          heart disease O10.13
            with renal disease O10.33
          pre-eclampsia O11.5
          renal disease O10.23
            with heart disease O10.33
          essential O10.03
      pregnancy-induced O13.9
      secondary O10.43
  crisis I16.9
  due to
    endocrine disorders I15.2
    pheochromocytoma I15.2
    renal disorders NEC I15.1
      arterial I15.0
    renovascular disorders I15.0
    specified disease NEC I15.8
  emergency I16.2
  encephalopathy I67.4
  gestational (without significant proteinuria)
      (pregnancy-induced) (transient) O13-
    with significant proteinuria — *see* Pre-
        eclampsia
    complicating
      delivery O13.4
      puerperium O13.5
  Goldblatt's I70.1
  heart (disease) (conditions in I51.4-I51.9 due
      to hypertension) I11.9
    with
      heart failure (congestive) I11.0
      kidney disease (chronic) — *see*
          Hypertension, cardiorenal
  intracranial (benign) G93.2
  kidney I12.9
    with
      heart disease — *see* Hypertension,
          cardiorenal
      stage 1 through stage 4 chronic kidney
          disease I12.9
      stage 5 chronic kidney disease (CKD) or
          end stage renal disease (ESRD) I12.0
  lesser circulation I27.0
  maternal O16.-
  newborn P29.2
    pulmonary (persistent) P29.3
  ocular H40.05-
  pancreatic duct — *code to* underlying
      condition
    with chronic pancreatitis K86.1

D I S E A S E   I N D E X

Hypertension, hypertensive (accelerated) (benign) (essential) (idiopathic) (malignant) (systemic) I10 — *continued*
  portal (due to chronic liver disease) (idiopathic) K76.6
    gastropathy K31.89
    in (due to) schistosomiasis (bilharziasis) B65.9 *[K77]*
  postoperative I97.3
  psychogenic F45.8
  pulmonary (artery) (secondary) NEC I27.2
    with
      cor pulmonale (chronic) I27.2
        acute I26.09
      right heart ventricular strain/failure I27.2
        acute I26.09
    of newborn (persistent) P29.3
    primary (idiopathic) I27.0
  renal — *see* Hypertension, kidney
  renovascular I15.0
  secondary NEC I15.9
    due to
      endocrine disorders I15.2
      pheochromocytoma I15.2
      renal disorders NEC I15.1
        arterial I15.0
      renovascular disorders I15.0
    specified NEC I15.8
  transient, of pregnancy O13.-
  urgency I16.0
  venous (chronic)
    due to
      deep vein thrombosis — *see* Syndrome, postthrombotic
    idiopathic I87.309
      with
        inflammation I87.32-
          with ulcer I87.33-
        specified complication NEC I87.39-
        ulcer I87.31-
          with inflammation I87.33-
      asymptomatic I87.30-

Hypertensive urgency — *see* Hypertension
Hyperthecosis ovary E28.8
Hyperthermia (of unknown origin) — *see also* Hyperpyrexia
  malignant, due to anesthesia T88.3
  newborn P81.9
    environmental P81.0
Hyperthyroid (recurrent) — *see* Hyperthyroidism
Hyperthyroidism (latent) (pre-adult) (recurrent) E05.90
  with
    goiter (diffuse) E05.00
      with thyroid storm E05.01
      nodular (multinodular) E05.20
        with thyroid storm E05.21
        uninodular E05.10
          with thyroid storm E05.11
    storm E05.91
  due to ectopic thyroid tissue E05.30
    with thyroid storm E05.31
  neonatal, transitory P72.1
  specified NEC E05.80
    with thyroid storm E05.81
Hypertony, hypertonia, hypertonicity
  bladder N31.8
  congenital P94.1
  stomach K31.89
    psychogenic F45.8
  uterus, uterine (contractions) (complicating delivery) O62.4

Hypertrichosis L68.9
  congenital Q84.2
  eyelid H02.869
    left H02.866
      lower H02.865
      upper H02.864
    right H02.863
      lower H02.862
      upper H02.861
  lanuginosa Q84.2
    acquired L68.1
  localized L68.2
  specified NEC L68.8
Hypertriglyceridemia, essential E78.1
Hypertrophy, hypertrophic
  adenofibromatous, prostate — *see* Enlargement, enlarged, prostate
  adenoids (infective) J35.2
    with tonsils J35.3
  adrenal cortex E27.8
  alveolar process or ridge — *see* Anomaly, alveolar
  anal papillae K62.89
  artery I77.89
    congenital NEC Q27.8
      digestive system Q27.8
      lower limb Q27.8
      specified site NEC Q27.8
      upper limb Q27.8
  auricular — *see* Hypertrophy, cardiac
  Bartholin's gland N75.8
  bile duct (common) (hepatic) K83.8
  bladder (sphincter) (trigone) N32.89
  bone M89.30
    carpus M89.34-
    clavicle M89.31-
    femur M89.35-
    fibula M89.36-
    finger M89.34-
    humerus M89.32-
    ilium M89.359
    ischium M89.359
    metacarpus M89.34-
    metatarsus M89.37-
    multiple sites M89.39
    neck M89.38
    radius M89.33-
    rib M89.38
    scapula M89.31-
    skull M89.38
    tarsus M89.37-
    tibia M89.36-
    toe M89.37-
    ulna M89.33-
    vertebra M89.38
  brain G93.89
  breast N62
    cystic — *see* Mastopathy, cystic
    newborn P83.4
    pubertal, massive N62
    puerperal, postpartum — *see* Disorder, breast, specified type NEC
    senile (parenchymatous) N62
  cardiac (chronic) (idiopathic) I51.7
    with rheumatic fever (conditions in I00)
      active I01.8
      inactive or quiescent (with chorea) I09.89
    congenital NEC Q24.8
    fatty — *see* Degeneration, myocardial
    hypertensive — *see* Hypertension, heart
    rheumatic (with chorea) I09.89
      active or acute I01.8
        with chorea I02.0
    valve — *see* Endocarditis
  cartilage — *see* Disorder, cartilage, specified type NEC
  cecum — *see* Megacolon

Hypertrophy, hypertrophic — *continued*
  cervix (uteri) N88.8
    congenital Q51.828
    elongation N88.4
  clitoris (cirrhotic) N90.89
    congenital Q52.6
  colon — *see also* Megacolon
    congenital Q43.2
  conjunctiva, lymphoid H11.89
  corpora cavernosa N48.89
  cystic duct K82.8
  duodenum K31.89
  endometrium (glandular) (*see also* Hyperplasia, endometrial) N85.00-
    cervix N88.8
  epididymis N50.89
  esophageal hiatus (congenital) Q79.1
    with hernia — *see* Hernia, hiatal
  eyelid — *see* Disorder, eyelid, specified type NEC
  fat pad E65
    knee (infrapatellar) (popliteal) (prepatellar) (retropatellar) M79.4
  foot (congenital) Q74.2
  frenulum, frenum (tongue) K14.8
    lip K13.0
  gallbladder K82.8
  gastric mucosa K29.60
    with bleeding K29.61
  gland, glandular R59.9
    generalized R59.1
    localized R59.0
  gum (mucous membrane) K06.1
  heart (idiopathic) — *see also* Hypertrophy, cardiac
    valve (*see also* Endocarditis) I38
  hemifacial Q67.4
  hepatic — *see* Hypertrophy, liver
  hiatus (esophageal) Q79.1
  hilus gland R59.0
  hymen, congenital Q52.4
  ileum K63.89
  intestine NEC K63.89
  jejunum K63.89
  kidney (compensatory) N28.81
    congenital Q63.3
  labium (majus) (minus) N90.60
  ligament — *see* Disorder, ligament
  lingual tonsil (infective) J35.1
    with adenoids J35.3
  lip K13.0
    congenital Q18.6
  liver R16.0
    acute K76.89
    cirrhotic — *see* Cirrhosis, liver
    congenital Q44.7
    fatty — *see* Fatty, liver
  lymph, lymphatic gland R59.9
    generalized R59.1
    localized R59.0
    tuberculous — *see* Tuberculosis, lymph gland
  mammary gland — *see* Hypertrophy, breast
  Meckel's diverticulum (congenital) Q43.0
    malignant — *see* Table of Neoplasms, small intestine, malignant
  median bar — *see* Hyperplasia, prostate
  meibomian gland — *see* Chalazion
  meniscus, knee, congenital Q74.1
  metatarsal head — *see* Hypertrophy, bone, metatarsus
  metatarsus — *see* Hypertrophy, bone, metatarsus
  mucous membrane
    alveolar ridge K06.2
    gum K06.1
    nose (turbinate) J34.3
  muscle M62.89
  muscular coat, artery I77.89

Hypertrophy, hypertrophic — *continued*
myocardium — *see also* Hypertrophy, cardiac
  idiopathic I42.2
myometrium N85.2
nail L60.2
  congenital Q84.5
nasal J34.89
  alae J34.89
  bone J34.89
  cartilage J34.89
  mucous membrane (septum) J34.3
  sinus J34.89
  turbinate J34.3
nasopharynx, lymphoid (infectional) (tissue)
  (wall) J35.2
nipple N62
organ or site, congenital NEC — *see* Anomaly,
  by site
ovary N83.8
palate (hard) M27.8
  soft K13.79
pancreas, congenital Q45.3
parathyroid (gland) E21.0
parotid gland K11.1
penis N48.89
pharyngeal tonsil J35.2
pharynx J39.2
  lymphoid (infectional) (tissue) (wall) J35.2
pituitary (anterior) (fossa) (gland) E23.6
prepuce (congenital) N47.8
  female N90.89
prostate — *see* Enlargement, enlarged,
  prostate
  congenital Q55.4
pseudomuscular G71.0
pylorus (adult) (muscle) (sphincter) K31.1
  congenital or infantile Q40.0
rectal, rectum (sphincter) K62.89
rhinitis (turbinate) J31.0
salivary gland (any) K11.1
  congenital Q38.4
scaphoid (tarsal) — *see* Hypertrophy, bone,
  tarsus
scar L91.0
scrotum N50.89
seminal vesicle N50.89
sigmoid — *see* Megacolon
skin L91.9
  specified NEC L91.8
spermatic cord N50.89
spleen — *see* Splenomegaly
spondylitis — *see* Spondylosis
stomach K31.89
sublingual gland K11.1
submandibular gland K11.1
suprarenal cortex (gland) E27.8
synovial NEC M67.20
  acromioclavicular M67.21-
  ankle M67.27-
  elbow M67.22-
  foot M67.27-
  hand M67.24-
  hip M67.25-
  knee M67.26-
  multiple sites M67.29
  specified site NEC M67.28
  wrist M67.23-
tendon — *see* Disorder, tendon, specified type
  NEC
testis N44.8
  congenital Q55.29
thymic, thymus (gland) (congenital) E32.0
thyroid (gland) — *see* Goiter
toe (congenital) Q74.2
  acquired — *see also* Deformity, toe, specified
    NEC
tongue K14.8
  congenital Q38.2
  papillae (foliate) K14.3

Hypertrophy, hypertrophic — *continued*
tonsils (faucial) (infective) (lingual) (lymphoid)
  J35.1
  with adenoids J35.3
tunica vaginalis N50.89
ureter N28.89
urethra N36.8
uterus N85.2
  neck (with elongation) N88.4
  puerperal O90.89
uvula K13.79
vagina N89.8
vas deferens N50.89
vein I87.8
ventricle, ventricular (heart) — *see also*
  Hypertrophy, cardiac
  congenital Q24.8
  in tetralogy of Fallot Q21.3
verumontanum N36.8
vocal cord J38.3
vulva N90.60
  stasis (nonfilarial) N90.69
Hypertropia H50.2-
Hypertyrosinemia E70.21
Hyperuricemia (asymptomatic) E79.0
Hypervalinemia E71.19
Hyperventilation (tetany) R06.4
  hysterical F45.8
  psychogenic F45.8
  syndrome F45.8
Hypervitaminosis (dietary) NEC E67.8
  A E67.0
    administered as drug (prolonged intake) —
      see Table of Drugs and Chemicals,
      vitamins, adverse effect
    overdose or wrong substance given or taken
      — *see* Table of Drugs and Chemicals,
      vitamins, poisoning
  B6 E67.2
  D E67.3
    administered as drug (prolonged intake) —
      see Table of Drugs and Chemicals,
      vitamins, adverse effect
    overdose or wrong substance given or taken
      — *see* Table of Drugs and Chemicals,
      vitamins, poisoning
  K E67.8
    administered as drug (prolonged intake) —
      see Table of Drugs and Chemicals,
      vitamins, adverse effect
    overdose or wrong substance given or taken
      — *see* Table of Drugs and Chemicals,
      vitamins, poisoning
Hypervolemia E87.70
  specified NEC E87.79
Hypesthesia R20.1
  cornea — *see* Anesthesia, cornea
Hyphema H21.0-
  traumatic S05.1-
Hypo-osmolality E87.1
Hypo-ovarianism, hypo-ovarism E28.39
Hypoacidity, gastric K31.89
  psychogenic F45.8
Hypoadrenalism, hypoadrenia E27.40
  primary E27.1
  tuberculous A18.7
Hypoadrenocorticism E27.40
  pituitary E23.0
  primary E27.1
Hypoalbuminemia E88.09
Hypoaldosteronism E27.40
Hypoalphalipoproteinemia E78.6
Hypobarism T70.29
Hypobaropathy T70.29
Hypobetalipoproteinemia (familial) E78.6

Hypocalcemia E83.51
  dietary E58
  neonatal P71.1
    due to cow's milk P71.0
    phosphate-loading (newborn) P71.1
Hypochloremia E87.8
Hypochlorhydria K31.89
  neurotic F45.8
  psychogenic F45.8
Hypochondria, hypochondriac,
  hypochondriasis (reaction) F45.21
  sleep F51.03
Hypochondrogenesis Q77.0
Hypochondroplasia Q77.4
Hypochromasia, blood cells D50.8
Hypodontia — *see* Anodontia
Hypoeosinophilia D72.89
Hypoesthesia R20.1
Hypofibrinogenemia D68.8
  acquired D65
  congenital (hereditary) D68.2
Hypofunction
  adrenocortical E27.40
    drug-induced E27.3
    postprocedural E89.6
    primary E27.1
  adrenomedullary, postprocedural E89.6
  cerebral R29.818
  corticoadrenal NEC E27.40
  intestinal K59.8
  labyrinth — *see* subcategory H83.2
  ovary E28.39
  pituitary (gland) (anterior) E23.0
  testicular E29.1
    postprocedural (postsurgical)
      (postirradiation) (iatrogenic) E89.5
Hypogalactia O92.4
Hypogammaglobulinemia (*see also*
  Agammaglobulinemia) D80.1
  hereditary D80.0
  nonfamilial D80.1
  transient, of infancy D80.7
Hypogenitalism (congenital) — *see*
  Hypogonadism
Hypoglossia Q38.3
Hypoglycemia (spontaneous) E16.2
  coma E15
    diabetic — *see* Diabetes, coma
  diabetic — *see* Diabetes, hypoglycemia
  dietary counseling and surveillance Z71.3
  drug-induced E16.0
    with coma (nondiabetic) E15
  due to insulin E16.0
    with coma (nondiabetic) E15
      therapeutic misadventure — *see* subcategory
        T38.3
  functional, nonhyperinsulinemic E16.1
  iatrogenic E16.0
    with coma (nondiabetic) E15
  in infant of diabetic mother P70.1
    gestational diabetes P70.0
  infantile E16.1
  leucine-induced E71.19
  neonatal (transitory) P70.4
    iatrogenic P70.3
  reactive (not drug-induced) E16.1
  transitory neonatal P70.4
Hypogonadism
  female E28.39
  hypogonadotropic E23.0
  male E29.1
  ovarian (primary) E28.39
  pituitary E23.0
  testicular E29.1
Hypohidrosis, hypoidrosis L74.4
Hypoinsulinemia, postprocedural E89.1
Hypokalemia E87.6
Hypoleukocytosis — *see* Agranulocytosis
Hypolipoproteinemia (alpha) (beta) E78.6

D I S E A S E   I N D E X

Hypomagnesemia E83.42
  neonatal P71.2
Hypomania, hypomanic reaction F30.8
Hypomenorrhea — *see* Oligomenorrhea
Hypometabolism R63.8
Hypomotility
  gastrointestinal (tract) K31.89
    psychogenic F45.8
  intestine K59.8
    psychogenic F45.8
  stomach K31.89
    psychogenic F45.8
Hyponasality R49.22
Hyponatremia E87.1
Hypoparathyroidism E20.9
  familial E20.8
  idiopathic E20.0
  neonatal, transitory P71.4
  postprocedural E89.2
  specified NEC E20.8
Hypoperfusion (in)
  newborn P96.89
Hypopharyngitis — *see* Laryngopharyngitis
Hypophoria H50.53
Hypophosphatemia, hypophosphatasia
  (acquired) (congenital) (renal) E83.39
  familial E83.31
Hypophyseal, hypophysis — *see also*
  condition
  dwarfism E23.0
  gigantism E22.0
Hypopiesis — *see* Hypotension
Hypopinealism E34.8
Hypopituitarism (juvenile) E23.0
  drug-induced E23.1
  due to
    hypophysectomy E89.3
    radiotherapy E89.3
  iatrogenic NEC E23.1
  postirradiation E89.3
  postpartum O99.285
  postprocedural E89.3
Hypoplasia, hypoplastic
  adrenal (gland), congenital Q89.1
  alimentary tract, congenital Q45.8
    upper Q40.8
  anus, anal (canal) Q42.3
    with fistula Q42.2
  aorta, aortic Q25.42
    ascending, in hypoplastic left heart
      syndrome Q23.4
    valve Q23.1
      in hypoplastic left heart syndrome Q23.4
  areola, congenital Q83.8
  arm (congenital) — *see* Defect, reduction,
    upper limb
  artery (peripheral) Q27.8
    brain (congenital) Q28.3
    coronary Q24.5
    digestive system Q27.8
    lower limb Q27.8
    pulmonary Q25.79
      functional, unilateral J43.0
    retinal (congenital) Q14.1
    specified site NEC Q27.8
    umbilical Q27.0
    upper limb Q27.8
  auditory canal Q17.8
    causing impairment of hearing Q16.9
  biliary duct or passage Q44.5
  bone NOS Q79.9
    face Q75.8
    marrow D61.9
      megakaryocytic D69.49
    skull — *see* Hypoplasia, skull
  brain Q02
    gyri Q04.3
    part of Q04.3
  breast (areola) N64.82

Hypoplasia, hypoplastic — *continued*
  bronchus Q32.4
  cardiac Q24.8
  carpus — *see* Defect, reduction, upper limb,
    specified type NEC
  cartilage hair Q78.8
  cecum Q42.8
  cementum K00.4
  cephalic Q02
  cerebellum Q04.3
  cervix (uteri), congenital Q51.821
  clavicle (congenital) Q74.0
  coccyx Q76.49
  colon Q42.9
    specified NEC Q42.8
  corpus callosum Q04.0
  cricoid cartilage Q31.2
  digestive organ(s) or tract NEC Q45.8
    upper (congenital) Q40.8
  ear (auricle) (lobe) Q17.2
    middle Q16.4
  enamel of teeth (neonatal) (postnatal)
    (prenatal) K00.4
  endocrine (gland) NEC Q89.2
  endometrium N85.8
  epididymis (congenital) Q55.4
  epiglottis Q31.2
  erythroid, congenital D61.01
  esophagus (congenital) Q39.8
  eustachian tube Q17.8
  eye Q11.2
  eyelid (congenital) Q10.3
  face Q18.8
    bone(s) Q75.8
  femur (congenital) — *see* Defect, reduction,
    lower limb, specified type NEC
  fibula (congenital) — *see* Defect, reduction,
    lower limb, specified type NEC
  finger (congenital) — *see* Defect, reduction,
    upper limb, specified type NEC
  focal dermal Q82.8
  foot — *see* Defect, reduction, lower limb,
    specified type NEC
  gallbladder Q44.0
  genitalia, genital organ(s)
    female, congenital Q52.8
      external Q52.79
      internal NEC Q52.8
    in adiposogenital dystrophy E23.6
  glottis Q31.2
  hair Q84.2
  hand (congenital) — *see* Defect, reduction,
    upper limb, specified type NEC
  heart Q24.8
  humerus (congenital) — *see* Defect, reduction,
    upper limb, specified type NEC
  intestine (small) Q41.9
    large Q42.9
      specified NEC Q42.8
  jaw M26.09
    alveolar M26.79
    lower M26.04
      alveolar M26.74
    upper M26.02
      alveolar M26.73
  kidney(s) Q60.5
    bilateral Q60.4
    unilateral Q60.3
  labium (majus) (minus), congenital Q52.79
  larynx Q31.2
  left heart syndrome Q23.4
  leg (congenital) — *see* Defect, reduction, lower
    limb
  limb Q73.8
    lower (congenital) — *see* Defect, reduction,
      lower limb
    upper (congenital) — *see* Defect, reduction,
      upper limb
  liver Q44.7

Hypoplasia, hypoplastic — *continued*
  lung (lobe) (not associated with short gestation)
    Q33.6
    associated with immaturity, low birth weight,
      prematurity, or short gestation P28.0
  mammary (areola), congenital Q83.8
  mandible, mandibular M26.04
    alveolar M26.74
    unilateral condylar M27.8
  maxillary M26.02
    alveolar M26.73
  medullary D61.9
  megakaryocytic D69.49
  metacarpus — *see* Defect, reduction, upper
    limb, specified type NEC
  metatarsus — *see* Defect, reduction, lower
    limb, specified type NEC
  muscle Q79.8
  nail(s) Q84.6
  nose, nasal Q30.1
  optic nerve H47.03-
  osseous meatus (ear) Q17.8
  ovary, congenital Q50.39
  pancreas Q45.0
  parathyroid (gland) Q89.2
  parotid gland Q38.4
  patella Q74.1
  pelvis, pelvic girdle Q74.2
  penis (congenital) Q55.62
  peripheral vascular system Q27.8
    digestive system Q27.8
    lower limb Q27.8
    specified site NEC Q27.8
    upper limb Q27.8
  pituitary (gland) (congenital) Q89.2
  pulmonary (not associated with short
    gestation) Q33.6
    artery, functional J43.0
    associated with short gestation P28.0
  radioulnar — *see* Defect, reduction, upper
    limb, specified type NEC
  radius — *see* Defect, reduction, upper limb
  rectum Q42.1
    with fistula Q42.0
  respiratory system NEC Q34.8
  rib Q76.6
  right heart syndrome Q22.6
  sacrum Q76.49
  scapula Q74.0
  scrotum Q55.1
  shoulder girdle Q74.0
  skin Q82.8
  skull (bone) Q75.8
    with
      anencephaly Q00.0
      encephalocele — *see* Encephalocele
      hydrocephalus Q03.9
        with spina bifida — *see* Spina bifida, by
          site, with hydrocephalus
      microcephaly Q02
  spinal (cord) (ventral horn cell) Q06.1
  spine Q76.49
  sternum Q76.7
  tarsus — *see* Defect, reduction, lower limb,
    specified type NEC
  testis Q55.1
  thymic, with immunodeficiency D82.1
  thymus (gland) Q89.2
    with immunodeficiency D82.1
  thyroid (gland) E03.1
    cartilage Q31.2
  tibiofibular (congenital) — *see* Defect,
    reduction, lower limb, specified type NEC
  toe — *see* Defect, reduction, lower limb,
    specified type NEC
  tongue Q38.3
  Turner's K00.4
  ulna (congenital) — *see* Defect, reduction,
    upper limb

Hypoplasia, hypoplastic — *continued*
umbilical artery Q27.0
unilateral condylar M27.8
ureter Q62.8
uterus, congenital Q51.811
vagina Q52.4
vascular NEC peripheral Q27.8
brain Q28.3
digestive system Q27.8
lower limb Q27.8
specified site NEC Q27.8
upper limb Q27.8
vein(s) (peripheral) Q27.8
brain Q28.3
digestive system Q27.8
great Q26.8
lower limb Q27.8
specified site NEC Q27.8
upper limb Q27.8
vena cava (inferior) (superior) Q26.8
vertebra Q76.49
vulva, congenital Q52.79
zonule (ciliary) Q12.8
Hypopotassemia E87.6
Hypoproconvertinemia, congenital
(hereditary) D68.2
Hypoproteinemia E77.8
Hypoprothrombinemia (congenital)
(hereditary) (idiopathic) D68.2
acquired D68.4
newborn, transient P61.6
Hypoptyalism K11.7
Hypopyon (eye) (anterior chamber) — *see*
Iridocyclitis, acute, hypopyon
Hypopyrexia R68.0
Hyporeflexia R29.2
Hyposecretion
ACTH E23.0
antidiuretic hormone E23.2
ovary E28.39
salivary gland (any) K11.7
vasopressin E23.2
Hyposegmentation, leukocytic,
hereditary D72.0
Hyposiderinemia D50.9
Hypospadias Q54.9
balanic Q54.0
coronal Q54.0
glandular Q54.0
penile Q54.1
penoscrotal Q54.2
perineal Q54.3
specified NEC Q54.8
Hypospermatogenesis — *see* Oligospermia
Hyposplenism D73.0
Hypostasis pulmonary, passive — *see*
Edema, lung
Hypostatic — *see* condition
Hyposthenuria N28.89
Hypotension (arterial) (constitutional) I95.9
chronic I95.89
drug-induced I95.2
due to (of) hemodialysis I95.3
iatrogenic I95.89
idiopathic (permanent) I95.0
intra-dialytic I95.3
intracranial, following ventricular shunting
(ventriculostomy) G97.2
maternal, syndrome (following labor and
delivery) O26.5-
neurogenic, orthostatic G90.3
orthostatic (chronic) I95.1
due to drugs I95.2
neurogenic G90.3
postoperative I95.81
postural I95.1
specified NEC I95.89

Hypothermia (accidental) T68
due to anesthesia, anesthetic T88.51
low environmental temperature T68
neonatal P80.9
environmental (mild) NEC P80.8
mild P80.8
severe (chronic) (cold injury syndrome)
P80.0
specified NEC P80.8
not associated with low environmental
temperature R68.0
Hypothyroidism (acquired) E03.9
congenital (without goiter) E03.1
with goiter (diffuse) E03.0
due to
exogenous substance NEC E03.2
iodine-deficiency, acquired E01.8
subclinical E02
irradiation therapy E89.0
medicament NEC E03.2
P-aminosalicylic acid (PAS) E03.2
phenylbutazone E03.2
resorcinol E03.2
sulfonamide E03.2
surgery E89.0
thiourea group drugs E03.2
iatrogenic NEC E03.2
iodine-deficiency (acquired) E01.8
congenital — *see* Syndrome, iodine-
deficiency, congenital
subclinical E02
neonatal, transitory P72.2
postinfectious E03.3
postirradiation E89.0
postprocedural E89.0
postsurgical E89.0
specified NEC E03.8
subclinical, iodine-deficiency related E02
Hypotonia, hypotonicity, hypotony
bladder N31.2
congenital (benign) P94.2
eye — *see* Disorder, globe, hypotony
Hypotrichosis — *see* Alopecia
Hypotropia H50.2-
Hypoventilation R06.89
congenital central alveolar G47.35
sleep related
idiopathic nonobstructive alveolar G47.34
in conditions classified elsewhere G47.36
Hypovitaminosis — *see* Deficiency, vitamin
Hypovolemia E86.1
surgical shock T81.19
traumatic (shock) T79.4
Hypoxemia R09.02
newborn P84
sleep related, in conditions classified elsewhere
G47.36
Hypoxia (*see also* Anoxia) R09.02
cerebral, during a procedure NEC G97.81
postprocedural NEC G97.82
intrauterine P84
myocardial — *see* Insufficiency, coronary
newborn P84
sleep-related G47.34
Hypsarhythmia — *see* Epilepsy, generalized,
specified NEC
Hysteralgia, pregnant uterus O26.89-
Hysteria, hysterical (conversion) (dissociative
state) F44.9
anxiety F41.8
convulsions F44.5
psychosis, acute F44.9
Hysteroepilepsy F44.5

I

IBDU (colonic inflammatory bowel disease
unclassified) K52.3
Ichthyoparasitism due to Vandellia
cirrhosa B88.8
Ichthyosis (congenital) Q80.9
acquired L85.0
fetalis Q80.4
hystrix Q80.8
lamellar Q80.2
lingual K13.29
palmaris and plantaris Q82.8
simplex Q80.0
vera Q80.8
vulgaris Q80.0
X-linked Q80.1
Ichthyotoxism — *see* Poisoning, fish
bacterial — *see* Intoxication, foodborne
Icteroanemia, hemolytic (acquired) D59.9
congenital — *see* Spherocytosis
Icterus — *see also* Jaundice
conjunctiva R17
gravis, newborn P55.0
hematogenous (acquired) D59.9
hemolytic (acquired) D59.9
congenital — *see* Spherocytosis
hemorrhagic (acute) (leptospiral) (spirochetal)
A27.0
newborn P53
infectious B15.9
with hepatic coma B15.0
leptospiral A27.0
spirochetal A27.0
neonatorum — *see* Jaundice, newborn
newborn P59.9
spirochetal A27.0
Ictus solaris, solis T67.0
Id reaction (due to bacteria) L30.2
Ideation
homicidal R45.850
suicidal R45.851
Identity disorder (child) F64.9
gender role F64.2
psychosexual F64.2
Idioglossia F80.0
Idiopathic — *see* condition
Idiot, idiocy (congenital) F73
amaurotic (Bielschowsky(-Jansky)) (family)
(infantile (late)) (juvenile (late)) (Vogt-
Spielmeyer) E75.4
microcephalic Q02
IgE asthma J45.909
IIAC (idiopathic infantile arterial calcification)
Q28.8
Ileitis (chronic) (noninfectious) (*see also* Enteritis)
K52.9
backwash — *see* Pancolitis, ulcerative (chronic)
infectious A09
regional (ulcerative) — *see* Enteritis, regional,
small intestine
segmental — *see* Enteritis, regional
terminal (ulcerative) — *see* Enteritis, regional,
small intestine
Ileocolitis (*see also* Enteritis) K52.9
infectious A09
regional — *see* Enteritis, regional
Ileostomy
attention to Z43.2
malfunctioning K94.13
status Z93.2
with complication — *see* Complications,
enterostomy
Ileotyphus — *see* Typhoid
Ileum — *see* condition

Ileus (bowel) (colon) (inhibitory) (intestine) K56.7
  adynamic K56.0
  due to gallstone (in intestine) K56.3
  duodenal (chronic) K31.5
  gallstone K56.3
  mechanical NEC K56.69
  meconium P76.0
    in cystic fibrosis E84.11
    meaning meconium plug (without cystic
      fibrosis) P76.0
  myxedema K59.8
  neurogenic K56.0
    Hirschsprung's disease or megacolon Q43.1
  newborn
    due to meconium P76.0
      in cystic fibrosis E84.11
      meaning meconium plug (without cystic
        fibrosis) P76.0
    transitory P76.1
  obstructive K56.69
  paralytic K56.0
Iliac — see condition
Iliotibial band syndrome M76.3-
Illiteracy Z55.0
Illness (see also Disease) R69
  manic-depressive — see Disorder, bipolar
Imbalance R26.89
  autonomic G90.8
  constituents of food intake E63.1
  electrolyte E87.8
    with
      abortion — see Abortion, by type,
        complicated by, electrolyte imbalance
      molar pregnancy O08.5
    due to hyperemesis gravidarum O21.1
    following ectopic or molar pregnancy O08.5
    neonatal, transitory NEC P74.4
      potassium P74.3
      sodium P74.2
  endocrine E34.9
  eye muscle NOS H50.9
  hormone E34.9
  hysterical F44.4
  labyrinth — see subcategory H83.2
  posture R29.3
  protein-energy — see Malnutrition
  sympathetic G90.8
Imbecile, imbecility (I.Q. 35-49) F71
Imbedding, intrauterine device T83.39
Imbibition, cholesterol (gallbladder) K82.4
Imbrication, teeth, fully erupted M26.30
Imerslund(-Gräsbeck) syndrome D51.1
Immature — see also Immaturity
  birth (less than 37 completed weeks) — see
    Preterm, newborn
    extremely (less than 28 completed weeks) —
      see Immaturity, extreme
  personality F60.89
Immaturity (less than 37 completed weeks) —
  see also Preterm, newborn
  extreme of newborn (less than 28 completed
    weeks of gestation) (less than 196
    completed days of gestation) (unspecified
    weeks of gestation) P07.20
    gestational age
      23 completed weeks (23 weeks, 0 days
        through 23 weeks, 6 days) P07.22
      24 completed weeks (24 weeks, 0 days
        through 24 weeks, 6 days) P07.23
      25 completed weeks (25 weeks, 0 days
        through 25 weeks, 6 days) P07.24
      26 completed weeks (26 weeks, 0 days
        through 26 weeks, 6 days) P07.25
      27 completed weeks (27 weeks, 0 days
        through 27 weeks, 6 days) P07.26
      less than 23 completed weeks P07.21
  fetus or infant light-for-dates — see Light-for-
    dates

Immaturity (less than 37 completed weeks) —
  see also Preterm, newborn — continued
  lung, newborn P28.0
  organ or site NEC — see Hypoplasia
  pulmonary, newborn P28.0
  reaction F60.89
  sexual (female) (male), after puberty E30.0
Immersion T75.1
  foot T69.02-
  hand T69.01-
Immobile, immobility
  complete, due to severe physical disability or
    frailty R53.2
  intestine K59.8
  syndrome (paraplegic) M62.3
**Immune reconstitution (inflammatory)
syndrome** [IRIS] D89.3
Immunization — see also Vaccination
  ABO — see Incompatibility, ABO
    in newborn P55.1
  complication — see Complications, vaccination
  encounter for Z23
  not done (not carried out) Z28.9
    because (of)
      acute illness of patient Z28.01
      allergy to vaccine (or component) Z28.04
      caregiver refusal Z28.82
      chronic illness of patient Z28.02
      contraindication NEC Z28.09
      group pressure Z28.1
      guardian refusal Z28.82
      immune compromised state of patient
        Z28.03
      parent refusal Z28.82
      patient's belief Z28.1
      patient had disease being vaccinated
        against Z28.81
      patient refusal Z28.21
      religious beliefs of patient Z28.1
      specified reason NEC Z28.89
        of patient Z28.29
      unspecified patient reason Z28.20
  Rh factor
    affecting management of pregnancy NEC
      O36.09-
      anti-D antibody O36.01-
    from transfusion — see Complication(s),
      transfusion, incompatibility reaction, Rh
      (factor)
Immunocytoma C83.0-
Immunodeficiency D84.9
  with
    adenosine-deaminase deficiency D81.3
    antibody defects D80.9
      specified type NEC D80.8
    hyperimmunoglobulinemia D80.6
    increased immunoglobulin M (IgM) D80.5
    major defect D82.9
      specified type NEC D82.8
    partial albinism D82.8
    short-limbed stature D82.2
    thrombocytopenia and eczema D82.0
  antibody with
    hyperimmunoglobulinemia D80.6
    near-normal immunoglobulins D80.6
  autosomal recessive, Swiss type D80.0
  combined D81.9
    biotin-dependent carboxylase D81.819
      biotinidase D81.810
      holocarboxylase synthetase D81.818
      specified type NEC D81.818
    severe (SCID) D81.9
      with
        low or normal B-cell numbers D81.2
        low T-and B-cell numbers D81.1
        reticular dysgenesis D81.0
  specified type NEC D81.89

Immunodeficiency D84.9 — continued
  common variable D83.9
    with
      abnormalities of B-cell numbers and
        function D83.0
      autoantibodies to B-or T-cells D83.2
      immunoregulatory T-cell disorders D83.1
      specified type NEC D83.8
  following hereditary defective response to
    Epstein-Barr virus (EBV) D82.3
  selective, immunoglobulin
    A (IgA) D80.2
    G (IgG) (subclasses) D80.3
    M (IgM) D80.4
  severe combined (SCID) D81.9
  specified type NEC D84.8
  X-linked, with increased IgM D80.5
Immunotherapy (encounter for)
  antineoplastic Z51.12
Impaction, impacted
  bowel, colon, rectum (see also Impaction, fecal)
    K56.49
    by gallstone K56.3
  calculus — see Calculus
  cerumen (ear) (external) H61.2-
  cuspid — see Impaction, tooth
  dental (same or adjacent tooth) K01.1
  fecal, feces K56.41
  fracture — see Fracture, by site
  gallbladder — see Calculus, gallbladder
  gallstone(s) — see Calculus, gallbladder
    bile duct (common) (hepatic) — see Calculus,
      bile duct
    cystic duct — see Calculus, gallbladder
    in intestine, with obstruction (any part)
      K56.3
  intestine (calculous) NEC (see also Impaction,
    fecal) K56.49
    gallstone, with ileus K56.3
  intrauterine device (IUD) T83.39
  molar — see Impaction, tooth
  shoulder, causing obstructed labor O66.0
  tooth, teeth K01.1
  turbinate J34.89
Impaired, impairment (function)
  auditory discrimination — see Abnormal,
    auditory perception
  cognitive, mild, so stated G31.84
  dual sensory Z73.82
  fasting glucose R73.01
  glucose tolerance (oral) R73.02
  hearing — see Deafness
  heart — see Disease, heart
  kidney N28.9
    disorder resulting from N25.9
      specified NEC N25.89
  liver K72.90
    with coma K72.91
  mastication K08.89
  mild cognitive, so stated G31.84
  mobility
    ear ossicles — see Ankylosis, ear ossicles
    requiring care provider Z74.09
  myocardium, myocardial — see Insufficiency,
    myocardial
  rectal sphincter R19.8
  renal (acute) (chronic) N28.9
    disorder resulting from N25.9
      specified NEC N25.89
  vision NEC H54.7
    both eyes H54.3
Impediment, speech R47.9
  psychogenic (childhood) F98.8
  slurring R47.81
  specified NEC R47.89
Impending
  coronary syndrome I20.0
  delirium tremens F10.239
  myocardial infarction I20.0

Imperception auditory (acquired) — *see also* Deafness
  congenital H93.25
Imperfect
  aeration, lung (newborn) NEC — *see* Atelectasis
  closure (congenital)
    alimentary tract NEC Q45.8
      lower Q43.8
      upper Q40.8
    atrioventricular ostium Q21.2
    atrium (secundum) Q21.1
    branchial cleft or sinus Q18.0
    choroid Q14.3
    cricoid cartilage Q31.8
    cusps, heart valve NEC Q24.8
      pulmonary Q22.3
    ductus
      arteriosus Q25.0
      Botalli Q25.0
    ear drum (causing impairment of hearing) Q16.4
    esophagus with communication to bronchus or trachea Q39.1
    eyelid Q10.3
    foramen
      botalli Q21.1
      ovale Q21.1
    genitalia, genital organ(s) or system
      female Q52.8
        external Q52.79
        internal NEC Q52.8
      male Q55.8
    glottis Q31.8
    interatrial ostium or septum Q21.1
    interauricular ostium or septum Q21.1
    interventricular ostium or septum Q21.0
    larynx Q31.8
    lip — *see* Cleft, lip
    nasal septum Q30.3
    nose Q30.2
    omphalomesenteric duct Q43.0
    optic nerve entry Q14.2
    organ or site not listed — *see* Anomaly, by site
    ostium
      interatrial Q21.1
      interauricular Q21.1
      interventricular Q21.0
    palate — *see* Cleft, palate
    preauricular sinus Q18.1
    retina Q14.1
    roof of orbit Q75.8
    sclera Q13.5
    septum
      aorticopulmonary Q21.4
      atrial (secundum) Q21.1
      between aorta and pulmonary artery Q21.4
      heart Q21.9
      interatrial (secundum) Q21.1
      interauricular (secundum) Q21.1
      interventricular Q21.0
        in tetralogy of Fallot Q21.3
      nasal Q30.3
      ventricular Q21.0
        with pulmonary stenosis or atresia, dextraposition of aorta, and hypertrophy of right ventricle Q21.3
        in tetralogy of Fallot Q21.3
    skull Q75.0
      with
        anencephaly Q00.0
        encephalocele — *see* Encephalocele
        hydrocephalus Q03.9
          with spina bifida — *see* Spina bifida, by site, with hydrocephalus
        microcephaly Q02

Imperfect — *continued*
  closure (congenital) — *continued*
    spine (with meningocele) — *see* Spina bifida
    trachea Q32.1
    tympanic membrane (causing impairment of hearing) Q16.4
    uterus Q51.818
    vitelline duct Q43.0
  erection — *see* Dysfunction, sexual, male, erectile
  fusion — *see* Imperfect, closure
  inflation, lung (newborn) — *see* Atelectasis
  posture R29.3
  rotation, intestine Q43.3
  septum, ventricular Q21.0
Imperfectly descended testis — *see* Cryptorchid
Imperforate (congenital) — *see also* Atresia
  anus Q42.3
    with fistula Q42.2
  cervix (uteri) Q51.828
  esophagus Q39.0
    with tracheoesophageal fistula Q39.1
  hymen Q52.3
  jejunum Q41.1
  pharynx Q38.8
  rectum Q42.1
    with fistula Q42.0
  urethra Q64.39
  vagina Q52.4
Impervious (congenital) — *see also* Atresia
  anus Q42.3
    with fistula Q42.2
  bile duct Q44.2
  esophagus Q39.0
    with tracheoesophageal fistula Q39.1
  intestine (small) Q41.9
    large Q42.9
      specified NEC Q42.8
  rectum Q42.1
    with fistula Q42.0
  ureter — *see* Atresia, ureter
  urethra Q64.39
Impetiginization of dermatoses L01.1
Impetigo (any organism) (any site) (circinate) (contagiosa) (simplex) (vulgaris) L01.00
  Bockhart's L01.02
  bullous, bullosa L01.03
  external ear L01.00 *[H62.40]*
  follicularis L01.02
  furfuracea L30.5
  herpetiformis L40.1
    nonobstetrical L40.1
  neonatorum L01.03
  nonbullous L01.01
  specified type NEC L01.09
  ulcerative L01.09
Impingement (on teeth)
  soft tissue
    anterior M26.81
    posterior M26.82
Implant, endometrial N80.9
Implantation
  anomalous — *see* Anomaly, by site
    ureter Q62.63
  cyst
    external area or site (skin) NEC L72.0
    iris — *see* Cyst, iris, implantation
    vagina N89.8
    vulva N90.7
  dermoid (cyst) — *see* Implantation, cyst
Impotence (sexual) N52.9
  counseling Z70.1
  organic origin (*see also* Dysfunction, sexual, male, erectile) N52.9
  psychogenic F52.21
Impression, basilar Q75.8
Imprisonment, anxiety concerning Z65.1

Improper care (child) (newborn) — *see* Maltreatment
Improperly tied umbilical cord (causing hemorrhage) P51.8
Impulsiveness (impulsive) R45.87
Inability to swallow — *see* Aphagia
Inaccessible, inaccessibility
  health care NEC Z75.3
    due to
      waiting period Z75.2
        for admission to facility elsewhere Z75.1
    other helping agencies Z75.4
Inactive — *see* condition
Inadequate, inadequacy
  aesthetics of dental restoration K08.56
  biologic, constitutional, functional, or social F60.7
  development
    child R62.50
    genitalia
      after puberty NEC E30.0
      congenital
        female Q52.8
          external Q52.79
          internal Q52.8
        male Q55.8
    lungs Q33.6
      associated with short gestation P28.0
    organ or site not listed — *see* Anomaly, by site
  diet (causing nutritional deficiency) E63.9
  eating habits Z72.4
  environment, household Z59.1
  family support Z63.8
  food (supply) NEC Z59.4
    hunger effects T73.0
  functional F60.7
  household care, due to
    family member
      handicapped or ill Z74.2
      on vacation Z75.5
      temporarily away from home Z74.2
    technical defects in home Z59.1
    temporary absence from home of person rendering care Z74.2
  housing (heating) (space) Z59.1
  income (financial) Z59.6
  intrafamilial communication Z63.8
  material resources Z59.9
  mental — *see* Disability, intellectual
  parental supervision or control of child Z62.0
  personality F60.7
  pulmonary
    function R06.89
      newborn P28.5
    ventilation, newborn P28.5
  sample of cytologic smear
    anus R85.615
    cervix R87.615
    vagina R87.625
  social F60.7
    insurance Z59.7
    skills NEC Z73.4
  supervision of child by parent Z62.0
  teaching affecting education Z55.8
  welfare support Z59.7
Inanition R64
  with edema — *see* Malnutrition, severe
  due to
    deprivation of food T73.0
    malnutrition — *see* Malnutrition
  fever R50.9
Inappropriate
  change in quantitative human chorionic gonadotropin (hCG) in early pregnancy O02.81
  diet or eating habits Z72.4

Inappropriate — continued
  level of quantitative human chorionic
        gonadotropin (hCG) for gestational age in
        early pregnancy O02.81
  secretion
      antidiuretic hormone (ADH) (excessive) E22.2
          deficiency E23.2
      pituitary (posterior) E22.2
Inattention at or after birth — see Neglect
Incarceration, incarcerated
  enterocele K46.0
      gangrenous K46.1
  epiplocele K46.0
      gangrenous K46.1
  exomphalos K42.0
      gangrenous K42.1
  hernia — see also Hernia, by site, with
        obstruction
      with gangrene — see Hernia, by site, with
            gangrene
  iris, in wound — see Injury, eye, laceration,
        with prolapse
  lens, in wound — see Injury, eye, laceration,
        with prolapse
  omphalocele K42.0
  prison, anxiety concerning Z65.1
  rupture — see Hernia, by site
  sarcoepiplocele K46.0
      gangrenous K46.1
  sarcoepiplomphalocele K42.0
      with gangrene K42.1
  uterus N85.8
      gravid O34.51-
          causing obstructed labor O65.5
Incised wound
  external — see Laceration
  internal organs — see Injury, by site
Incision, incisional
  hernia K43.2
      with
          gangrene (and obstruction) K43.1
          obstruction K43.0
  surgical, complication — see Complications,
        surgical procedure
  traumatic
      external — see Laceration
      internal organs — see Injury, by site
Inclusion
  azurophilic leukocytic D72.0
  blennorrhea (neonatal) (newborn) P39.1
  gallbladder in liver (congenital) Q44.1
Incompatibility
  ABO
      affecting management of pregnancy O36.11-
          anti-A sensitization O36.11-
          anti-B sensitization O36.19-
          specified NEC O36.19-
      infusion or transfusion reaction — see
            Complication(s), transfusion,
            incompatibility reaction, ABO
      newborn P55.1
  blood (group) (Duffy) (K(ell)) (Kidd) (Lewis) (M)
        (S) NEC
      affecting management of pregnancy
            O36.11-
          anti-A sensitization O36.11-
          anti-B sensitization O36.19-
      infusion or transfusion reaction T80.89
      newborn P55.8
  divorce or estrangement Z63.5
  Rh (blood group) (factor) Z31.82
      affecting management of pregnancy NEC
            O36.09-
          anti-D antibody O36.01-
      infusion or transfusion reaction — see
            Complication(s), transfusion,
            incompatibility reaction, Rh (factor)
      newborn P55.0
  rhesus — see Incompatibility, Rh

**Incompetency, incompetent,
  incompetence**
  annular
      aortic (valve) — see Insufficiency, aortic
      mitral (valve) I34.0
      pulmonary valve (heart) I37.1
  aortic (valve) — see Insufficiency, aortic
  cardiac valve — see Endocarditis
  cervix, cervical (os) N88.3
      in pregnancy O34.3-
  chronotropic I45.89
      with
          autonomic dysfunction G90.8
          ischemic heart disease I25.89
          left ventricular dysfunction I51.89
          sinus node dysfunction I49.8
  esophagogastric (junction) (sphincter) K22.0
  mitral (valve) — see Insufficiency, mitral
  pelvic fundus N81.89
  pubocervical tissue N81.82
  pulmonary valve (heart) I37.1
      congenital Q22.3
  rectovaginal tissue N81.83
  tricuspid (annular) (valve) — see Insufficiency,
        tricuspid
  valvular — see Endocarditis
      congenital Q24.8
  vein, venous (saphenous) (varicose) — see
        Varix, leg
Incomplete — see also condition
  bladder, emptying R33.9
  defecation R15.0
  expansion lungs (newborn) NEC — see
        Atelectasis
  rotation, intestine Q43.3
Inconclusive
  diagnostic imaging due to excess body fat of
        patient R93.9
  findings on diagnostic imaging of breast NEC
        R92.8
  mammogram (due to dense breasts) R92.2
Incontinence R32
  anal sphincter R15.9
  coital N39.491
  feces R15.9
      nonorganic origin F98.1
  insensible (urinary) N39.42
  overflow N39.490
  postural (urinary) N39.492
  psychogenic F45.8
  rectal R15.9
  reflex N39.498
  stress (female) (male) N39.3
      and urge N39.46
  urethral sphincter R32
  urge N39.41
      and stress (female) (male) N39.46
  urine (urinary) R32
      continuous N39.45
      due to cognitive impairment, or severe
            physical disability or immobility R39.81
      functional R39.81
      insensible N39.42
      mixed (stress and urge) N39.46
      nocturnal N39.44
      nonorganic origin F98.0
      overflow N39.490
      post dribbling N39.43
      postural N39.492
      reflex N39.498
      specified NEC N39.498
      stress (female) (male) N39.3
          and urge N39.46
      total N39.498
      unaware N39.42
      urge N39.41
          and stress (female) (male) N39.46
Incontinentia pigmenti Q82.3

Incoordinate, incoordination
  esophageal-pharyngeal (newborn) — see
        Dysphagia
  muscular R27.8
  uterus (action) (contractions) (complicating
        delivery) O62.4
Increase, increased
  abnormal, in development R63.8
  androgens (ovarian) E28.1
  anticoagulants (antithrombin) (anti-VIIIa) (anti-
        IXa) (anti-Xa) (anti-XIa) — see Circulating
        anticoagulants
  cold sense R20.8
  estrogen E28.0
  function
      adrenal
          cortex — see Cushing's, syndrome
          medulla E27.5
      pituitary (gland) (anterior) (lobe) E22.9
          posterior E22.2
  heat sense R20.8
  intracranial pressure (benign) G93.2
  permeability, capillaries I78.8
  pressure, intracranial G93.2
  secretion
      gastrin E16.4
      glucagon E16.3
      pancreas, endocrine E16.9
          growth hormone-releasing hormone E16.8
          pancreatic polypeptide E16.8
          somatostatin E16.8
          vasoactive-intestinal polypeptide E16.8
  sphericity, lens Q12.4
  splenic activity D73.1
  venous pressure I87.8
      portal K76.6
Increta placenta O43.22-
Incrustation, cornea, foreign body (lead)
        (zinc) — see Foreign body, cornea
Incyclophoria H50.54
Incyclotropia — see Cyclotropia
Indeterminate sex Q56.4
India rubber skin Q82.8
Indigestion (acid) (bilious) (functional) K30
  catarrhal K31.89
  due to decomposed food NOS A05.9
  nervous F45.8
  psychogenic F45.8
Indirect — see condition
Induratio penis plastica N48.6
Induration, indurated
  brain G93.89
  breast (fibrous) N64.51
      puerperal, postpartum O92.29
  broad ligament N83.8
  chancre
      anus A51.1
      congenital A50.07
      extragenital NEC A51.2
  corpora cavernosa (penis) (plastic) N48.6
  liver (chronic) K76.89
  lung (black) (chronic) (fibroid) (see also Fibrosis,
        lung) J84.10
      essential brown J84.03
  penile (plastic) N48.6
  phlebitic — see Phlebitis
  skin R23.4
Inebriety (without dependence) — see Alcohol,
        intoxication
Inefficiency, kidney N28.9
Inelasticity, skin R23.4
Inequality, leg (length) (acquired) — see also
        Deformity, limb, unequal length
  congenital — see Defect, reduction, lower limb
  lower leg — see Deformity, limb, unequal
        length

Inertia
bladder (neurogenic) N31.2
stomach K31.89
psychogenic F45.8
uterus, uterine during labor O62.2
during latent phase of labor O62.0
primary O62.0
secondary O62.1
vesical (neurogenic) N31.2
Infancy, infantile, infantilism — *see also*
condition
celiac K90.0
genitalia, genitals (after puberty) E30.0
Herter's (nontropical sprue) K90.0
intestinal K90.0
Lorain E23.0
pancreatic K86.89
pelvis M95.5
with disproportion (fetopelvic) O33.1
causing obstructed labor O65.1
pituitary E23.0
renal N25.0
uterus — *see* Infantile, genitalia
Infant(s) — *see also* Infancy
excessive crying R68.11
irritable child R68.12
lack of care — *see* Neglect
liveborn (singleton) Z38.2
born in hospital Z38.00
by cesarean Z38.01
born outside hospital Z38.1
multiple NEC Z38.8
born in hospital Z38.68
by cesarean Z38.69
born outside hospital Z38.7
quadruplet Z38.8
born in hospital Z38.63
by cesarean Z38.64
born outside hospital Z38.7
quintuplet Z38.8
born in hospital Z38.65
by cesarean Z38.66
born outside hospital Z38.7
triplet Z38.8
born in hospital Z38.61
by cesarean Z38.62
born outside hospital Z38.7
twin Z38.5
born in hospital Z38.30
by cesarean Z38.31
born outside hospital Z38.4
of diabetic mother (syndrome of) P70.1
gestational diabetes P70.0
Infantile — *see also* condition
genitalia, genitals E30.0
os, uterine E30.0
penis E30.0
testis E29.1
uterus E30.0
Infantilism — *see* Infancy
Infarct, infarction
adrenal (capsule) (gland) E27.49
appendices epiploicae (*see also* Infarct,
intestine) K55.069
bowel (*see also* Infarct, intestine) K55.069
brain (stem) — *see* Infarct, cerebral
breast N64.89
brewer's (kidney) N28.0
cardiac — *see* Infarct, myocardium
cerebellar — *see* Infarct, cerebral
cerebral (*see also* Occlusion, artery cerebral or
precerebral, with infarction) I63.9
aborted I63.9
cortical I63.9

Infarct, infarction — *continued*
cerebral (*see also* Occlusion, artery cerebral or
precerebral, with infarction) I63.9 —
continued
due to
cerebral venous thrombosis, nonpyogenic
I63.6
embolism
cerebral arteries I63.4-
precerebral arteries I63.1-
occlusion NEC
cerebral arteries I63.5-
precerebral arteries I63.2-
stenosis NEC
cerebral arteries I63.5-
precerebral arteries I63.2-
thrombosis
cerebral artery I63.3-
precerebral artery I63.0-
intraoperative
during cardiac surgery I97.810
during other surgery I97.811
postprocedural
following cardiac surgery I97.820
following other surgery I97.821
specified NEC I63.8
colon (acute) (agnogenic) (embolic)
(hemorrhagic) (nonocclusive)
(nonthrombotic) (occlusive) (segmental)
(thrombotic) (with gangrene) (*see also*
Infarct, intestine) K55.049
coronary artery — *see* Infarct, myocardium
embolic — *see* Embolism
fallopian tube N83.8
gallbladder K82.8
heart — *see* Infarct, myocardium
hepatic K76.3
hypophysis (anterior lobe) E23.6
impending (myocardium) I20.0
intestine (acute) (agnogenic) (embolic)
(hemorrhagic) (nonocclusive)
(nonthrombotic) (occlusive) (thrombotic)
(with gangrene) K55.069
diffuse K55.062
focal K55.061
large K55.049
diffuse K55.042
focal K55.041
small K55.029
diffuse K55.022
focal K55.021
kidney N28.0
liver K76.3
lung (embolic) (thrombotic) — *see* Embolism,
pulmonary
lymph node I89.8
mesentery, mesenteric (embolic) (thrombotic)
(with gangrene) (*see also* Infarct, intestine)
K55.069
muscle (ischemic) M62.20
ankle M62.27-
foot M62.27-
forearm M62.23-
hand M62.24-
lower leg M62.26-
pelvic region M62.25-
shoulder region M62.21-
specified site NEC M62.28
thigh M62.25-
upper arm M62.22-
myocardium, myocardial (acute) (with stated
duration of 4 weeks or less) I21.3
diagnosed on ECG, but presenting no
symptoms I25.2
healed or old I25.2
intraoperative
during cardiac surgery I97.790
during other surgery I97.791
non-Q wave I21.4

Infarct, infarction — *continued*
myocardium, myocardial (acute) (with stated
duration of 4 weeks or less) I21.3 —
continued
non-ST elevation (NSTEMI) I21.4
subsequent I22.2
nontransmural I21.4
past (diagnosed on ECG or other
investigation, but currently presenting no
symptoms) I25.2
postprocedural
following cardiac surgery I97.190
following other surgery I97.191
Q wave (*see also* Infarct, myocardium, by
site) I21.3
ST elevation (STEMI) I21.3
anterior (anteroapical) (anterolateral)
(anteroseptal) (Q wave) (wall) I21.09
subsequent I22.0
inferior (diaphragmatic) (inferolateral)
(inferoposterior) (wall) NEC I21.19
subsequent I22.1
inferoposterior transmural (Q wave)
I21.11
involving
coronary artery of anterior wall NEC
I21.09
coronary artery of inferior wall NEC
I21.19
diagonal coronary artery I21.02
left anterior descending coronary artery
I21.02
left circumflex coronary artery I21.21
left main coronary artery I21.01
oblique marginal coronary artery
I21.21
right coronary artery I21.11
lateral (apical-lateral) (basal-lateral) (high)
I21.29
subsequent I22.8
posterior (posterobasal) (posterolateral)
(posteroseptal) (true) I21.29
subsequent I22.8
septal I21.29
subsequent I22.8
specified NEC I21.29
subsequent I22.8
subsequent I22.9
subsequent (recurrent) (reinfarction) I22.9
anterior (anteroapical) (anterolateral)
(anteroseptal) (wall) I22.0
diaphragmatic (wall) I22.1
inferior (diaphragmatic) (inferolateral)
(inferoposterior) (wall) I22.1
lateral (apical-lateral) (basal-lateral) (high)
I22.8
non-ST elevation (NSTEMI) I22.2
posterior (posterobasal) (posterolateral)
(posteroseptal) (true) I22.8
septal I22.8
specified NEC I22.8
ST elevation I22.9
anterior (anteroapical) (anterolateral)
(anteroseptal) (wall) I22.0
inferior (diaphragmatic) (inferolateral)
(inferoposterior) (wall) I22.1
specified NEC I22.8
subendocardial I22.2
transmural I22.9
anterior (anteroapical) (anterolateral)
(anteroseptal) (wall) I22.0
diaphragmatic (wall) I22.1
inferior (diaphragmatic) (inferolateral)
(inferoposterior) (wall) I22.1
lateral (apical-lateral) (basal-lateral)
(high) I22.8
posterior (posterobasal) (posterolateral)
(posteroseptal) (true) I22.8
specified NEC I22.8

DISEASE INDEX

Infarct, infarction — *continued*
myocardium, myocardial (acute) (with stated duration of 4 weeks or less) I21.3 — *continued*
  syphilitic A52.06
  transmural I21.3
    anterior (anteroapical) (anterolateral) (anteroseptal) (Q wave) (wall) NEC I21.09
    inferior (diaphragmatic) (inferolateral) (inferoposterior) (Q wave) (wall) NEC I21.19
    inferoposterior (Q wave) I21.11
    lateral (apical-lateral) (basal-lateral) (high) NEC I21.29
    posterior (posterobasal) (posterolateral) (posteroseptal) (true) NEC I21.29
    septal NEC I21.29
    specified NEC I21.29
  nontransmural I21.4
  omentum (*see also* Infarct, intestine) K55.069
  ovary N83.8
  pancreas K86.89
  papillary muscle — *see* Infarct, myocardium
  parathyroid gland E21.4
  pituitary (gland) E23.6
  placenta O43.81-
  prostate N42.89
  pulmonary (artery) (vein) (hemorrhagic) — *see* Embolism, pulmonary
  renal (embolic) (thrombotic) N28.0
  retina, retinal (artery) — *see* Occlusion, artery, retina
  spinal (cord) (acute) (embolic) (nonembolic) G95.11
  spleen D73.5
    embolic or thrombotic I74.8
  subendocardial (acute) (nontransmural) I21.4
  suprarenal (capsule) (gland) E27.49
  testis N50.1
  thrombotic — *see also* Thrombosis
    artery, arterial — *see* Embolism
  thyroid (gland) E07.89
  ventricle (heart) — *see* Infarct, myocardium
Infecting — *see* condition
Infection, infected, infective (opportunistic) B99.9
  with
    drug resistant organism — *see* Resistance (to), drug — *see also* specific organism
    lymphangitis — *see* Lymphangitis
    organ dysfunction (acute) R65.20
      with septic shock R65.21
  abscess (skin) — *code by* site under Abscess
  Absidia — *see* Mucormycosis
  Acanthamoeba — *see* Acanthamebiasis
  Acanthocheilonema (perstans) (streptocerca) B74.4
  accessory sinus (chronic) — *see* Sinusitis
  achorion — *see* Dermatophytosis
  Acremonium falciforme B47.0
  acromioclavicular M00.9
  Actinobacillus (actinomycetem-comitans) A28.8
    mallei A24.0
    muris A25.1
  Actinomadura B47.1
  Actinomyces (israelii) (*see also* Actinomycosis) A42.9
  Actinomycetales — *see* Actinomycosis
  actinomycotic NOS — *see* Actinomycosis
  adenoid (and tonsil) J03.90
    chronic J35.02
  adenovirus NEC
    as cause of disease classified elsewhere B97.0
    unspecified nature or site B34.0
  aerogenes capsulatus A48.0
  aertrycke — *see* Infection, salmonella

Infection, infected, infective (opportunistic) B99.9 — *continued*
  alimentary canal NOS — *see* Enteritis, infectious
  Allescheria boydii B48.2
  Alternaria B48.8
  alveolus, alveolar (process) K04.7
  Ameba, amebic (histolytica) — *see* Amebiasis
  amniotic fluid, sac or cavity O41.10-
    chorioamnionitis O41.12-
    placentitis O41.14-
  amputation stump (surgical) — *see* Complication, amputation stump, infection
  Ancylostoma (duodenalis) B76.0
  Anisakiasis, Anisakis larvae B81.0
  anthrax — *see* Anthrax
  antrum (chronic) — *see* Sinusitis, maxillary
  anus, anal (papillae) (sphincter) K62.89
  arbovirus (arbor virus) A94
    specified type NEC A93.8
  artificial insemination N98.0
  Ascaris lumbricoides — *see* Ascariasis
  Ascomycetes B47.0
  Aspergillus (flavus) (fumigatus) (terreus) — *see* Aspergillosis
  atypical
    acid-fast (bacilli) — *see* Mycobacterium, atypical
    mycobacteria — *see* Mycobacterium, atypical
    virus A81.9
      specified type NEC A81.89
  auditory meatus (external) — *see* Otitis, externa, infective
  auricle (ear) — *see* Otitis, externa, infective
  axillary gland (lymph) L04.2
  Bacillus A49.9
    abortus A23.1
    anthracis — *see* Anthrax
    Ducrey's (any location) A57
    Flexner's A03.1
    Friedländer's NEC A49.8
    gas (gangrene) A48.0
    mallei A24.0
    melitensis A23.0
    paratyphoid, paratyphosus A01.4
      A A01.1
      B A01.2
      C A01.3
    Shiga(-Kruse) A03.0
    suipestifer — *see* Infection, salmonella
    swimming pool A31.1
    typhosa A01.00
    welchii — *see* Gangrene, gas
  bacterial NOS A49.9
    as cause of disease classified elsewhere B96.89
      Bacteroides fragilis [B. fragilis] B96.6
      Clostridium perfringens [C. perfringens] B96.7
      Enterobacter sakazakii B96.89
      Enterococcus B95.2
      Escherichia coli [E. coli] (*see also* Escherichia coli) B96.20
      Helicobacter pylori [H.pylori] B96.81
      Hemophilus influenzae [H. influenzae] B96.3
      Klebsiella pneumoniae [K. pneumoniae] B96.1
      Mycoplasma pneumoniae [M. pneumoniae] B96.0
      Proteus (mirabilis) (morganii) B96.4
      Pseudomonas (aeruginosa) (mallei) (pseudomallei) B96.5
      Staphylococcus B95.8
        aureus (methicillin susceptible) (MSSA) B95.61
        methicillin resistant (MRSA) B95.62
        specified NEC B95.7

Infection, infected, infective (opportunistic) B99.9 — *continued*
  bacterial NOS A49.9 — *continued*
    as cause of disease classified elsewhere B96.89 — *continued*
      Streptococcus B95.5
        group A B95.0
        group B B95.1
        pneumoniae B95.3
        specified NEC B95.4
      Vibrio vulnificus B96.82
    specified NEC A48.8
  Bacterium
    paratyphosum A01.4
      A A01.1
      B A01.2
      C A01.3
    typhosum A01.00
  Bacteroides NEC A49.8
    fragilis, as cause of disease classified elsewhere B96.6
  Balantidium coli A07.0
  Bartholin's gland N75.8
  Basidiobolus B46.8
  bile duct (common) (hepatic) — *see* Cholangitis
  bladder — *see* Cystitis
  Blastomyces, blastomycotic — *see also* Blastomycosis
    brasiliensis — *see* Paracoccidioidomycosis
    dermatitidis — *see* Blastomycosis
    European — *see* Cryptococcosis
    Loboi B48.0
    North American B40.9
    South American — *see* Paracoccidioidomycosis
  bleb, postprocedure — *see* Blebitis
  bone — *see* Osteomyelitis
  Bordetella — *see* Whooping cough
  Borrelia bergdorfi A69.20
  brain (*see also* Encephalitis) G04.90
    membranes — *see* Meningitis
    septic G06.0
    meninges — *see* Meningitis, bacterial
  branchial cyst Q18.0
  breast — *see* Mastitis
  bronchus — *see* Bronchitis
  Brucella A23.9
    abortus A23.1
    canis A23.3
    melitensis A23.0
    mixed A23.8
    specified NEC A23.8
    suis A23.2
  Brugia (malayi) B74.1
    timori B74.2
  bursa — *see* Bursitis, infective
  buttocks (skin) L08.9
  Campylobacter, intestinal A04.5
    as cause of disease classified elsewhere B96.81
  Candida (albicans) (tropicalis) — *see* Candidiasis
  candiru B88.8
  Capillaria (intestinal) B81.1
    hepatica B83.8
    philippinensis B81.1
  cartilage — *see* Disorder, cartilage, specified type NEC
  cat liver fluke B66.0
  catheter-related bloodstream (CRBSI) T80.211
  cellulitis — *code by* site under Cellulitis
  central line-associated T80.219
    bloodstream (CLABSI) T80.211
    specified NEC T80.218
  Cephalosporium falciforme B47.0
  cerebrospinal — *see* Meningitis
  cervical gland (lymph) L04.0
  cervix — *see* Cervicitis
  cesarean delivery wound (puerperal) O86.0

Infection, infected, infective (opportunistic)
B99.9 — *continued*
cestodes — *see* Infestation, cestodes
chest J22
Chilomastix (intestinal) A07.8
Chlamydia, chlamydial A74.9
  anus A56.3
  genitourinary tract A56.2
    lower A56.00
    specified NEC A56.19
  lymphogranuloma A55
  pharynx A56.4
  psittaci A70
  rectum A56.3
  sexually transmitted NEC A56.8
cholera — *see* Cholera
Cladosporium
  bantianum (brain abscess) B43.1
  carrionii B43.0
  castellanii B36.1
  trichoides (brain abscess) B43.1
  werneckii B36.1
Clonorchis (sinensis) (liver) B66.1
Clostridium NEC
  bifermentans A48.0
  botulinum (food poisoning) A05.1
    infant A48.51
    wound A48.52
  difficile
    as cause of disease classified elsewhere
      B96.89
    foodborne (disease) A04.7
    gas gangrene A48.0
    necrotizing enterocolitis A04.7
    sepsis A41.4
  gas-forming NEC A48.0
  histolyticum A48.0
  novyi, causing gas gangrene A48.0
  oedematiens A48.0
  perfringens
    as cause of disease classified elsewhere
      B96.7
    due to food A05.2
    foodborne (disease) A05.2
    gas gangrene A48.0
    sepsis A41.4
  septicum, causing gas gangrene A48.0
  sordellii, causing gas gangrene A48.0
  welchii
    as cause of disease classified elsewhere
      B96.7
    foodborne (disease) A05.2
    gas gangrene A48.0
    necrotizing enteritis A05.2
    sepsis A41.4
Coccidioides (immitis) — *see*
  Coccidioidomycosis
colon — *see* Enteritis, infectious
colostomy K94.02
common duct — *see* Cholangitis
congenital P39.9
  Candida (albicans) P37.5
  cytomegalovirus P35.1
  hepatitis, viral P35.3
  herpes simplex P35.2
  infectious or parasitic disease P37.9
    specified NEC P37.8
  listeriosis (disseminated) P37.2
  malaria NEC P37.4
    falciparum P37.3
  Plasmodium falciparum P37.3
  poliomyelitis P35.8
  rubella P35.0
  skin P39.4
  toxoplasmosis (acute) (subacute) (chronic)
    P37.1
  tuberculosis P37.0
  urinary (tract) P39.3
  vaccinia P35.8

Infection, infected, infective (opportunistic)
B99.9 — *continued*
congenital P39.9 — *continued*
  virus P35.9
    specified type NEC P35.8
Conidiobolus B46.8
coronavirus NEC B34.2
  as cause of disease classified elsewhere
    B97.29
  severe acute respiratory syndrome (SARS
    associated) B97.21
corpus luteum — *see* Salpingo-oophoritis
Corynebacterium diphtheriae — *see* Diphtheria
cotia virus B08.8
Coxiella burnetii A78
coxsackie — *see* Coxsackie
Cryptococcus neoformans — *see*
  Cryptococcosis
Cryptosporidium A07.2
Cunninghamella — *see* Mucormycosis
cyst — *see* Cyst
cystic duct (see also Cholecystitis) K81.9
Cysticercus cellulosae — *see* Cysticercosis
cytomegalovirus, cytomegaloviral B25.9
  congenital P35.1
  maternal, maternal care for (suspected)
    damage to fetus O35.3
  mononucleosis B27.10
    with
      complication NEC B27.19
      meningitis B27.12
      polyneuropathy B27.11
delta-agent (acute), in hepatitis B carrier B17.0
dental (pulpal origin) K04.7
Deuteromycetes B47.0
Dicrocoelium dendriticum B66.2
Dipetalonema (perstans) (streptocerca) B74.4
diphtherial — *see* Diphtheria
Diphyllobothrium (adult) (latum) (pacificum)
  B70.0
  larval B70.1
Diplogonoporus (grandis) B71.8
Dipylidium caninum B67.4
Dirofilaria B74.8
Dracunculus medinensis B72
Drechslera (hawaiiensis) B43.8
Ducrey Haemophilus (any location) A57
due to or resulting from
  artificial insemination N98.0
  central venous catheter T80.219
    bloodstream T80.211
    exit or insertion site T80.212
    localized T80.212
    port or reservoir T80.212
    specified NEC T80.218
    tunnel T80.212
  device, implant or graft (see also
    Complications, by site and type,
    infection or inflammation) T85.79
    arterial graft NEC T82.7
    breast (implant) T85.79
    catheter NEC T85.79
      dialysis (renal) T82.7
        intraperitoneal T85.71
      infusion NEC T82.7
        cranial T85.735
        intrathecal T85.735
        spinal (epidural) (subdural) T85.735
        subarachnoid T85.735
      urinary T83.518
        cystostomy T83.510
        Hopkins T83.518
        ileostomy T83.518
        nephrostomy T83.512
        specified NEC T83.518
        urethral indwelling T83.511
        urostomy T83.518

Infection, infected, infective (opportunistic)
B99.9 — *continued*
due to or resulting from — *continued*
  device, implant or graft (see also
    Complications, by site and type,
    infection or inflammation) T85.79 —
    continued
    electronic (electrode) (pulse generator)
      (stimulator)
      bone T84.7
      cardiac T82.7
      nervous system T85.738
        brain T85.731
        cranial nerve T85.732
        gastric nerve T85.732
        generator pocket T85.734
        neurostimulator generator T85.734
        peripheral nerve T85.732
        sacral nerve T85.732
        spinal cord T85.733
        vagal nerve T85.732
      urinary T83.590
    fixation, internal (orthopedic) NEC — *see*
      Complication, fixation device,
      infection
    gastrointestinal (bile duct) (esophagus)
      T85.79
      neurostimulator electrode (lead) T85.732
    genital NEC T83.69
    heart NEC T82.7
      valve (prosthesis) T82.6
      graft T82.7
    joint prosthesis — *see* Complication, joint
      prosthesis, infection
    ocular (corneal graft) (orbital implant)
      NEC T85.79
    orthopedic NEC T84.7
    penile (cylinder) (pump) (resevoir) T83.61
    specified NEC T85.79
    testicular T83.62
    urinary NEC T83.598
      ileal conduit stent T83.593
      implanted neurostimulation T83.590
      implanted sphincter T83.591
      indwelling ureteral stent T83.592
      nephroureteral stent T83.593
      specified stent NEC T83.593
    vascular NEC T82.7
    ventricular intracranial (communicating)
      shunt T85.730
  Hickman catheter T80.219
    bloodstream T80.211
    localized T80.212
    specified NEC T80.218
  immunization or vaccination T88.0
  infusion, injection or transfusion NEC
    T80.29
    acute T80.22
  injury NEC — *code by* site under Wound,
    open
  peripherally inserted central catheter (PICC)
    T80.219
    bloodstream T80.211
    localized T80.212
    specified NEC T80.218
  portacath (port-a-cath) T80.219
    bloodstream T80.211
    localized T80.212
    specified NEC T80.218
  pulmonary artery catheter — *see* Infection,
    due to or resulting from, central venous
    catheter
  surgery T81.40
  Swan Ganz catheter — *see* Infection, due to
    or resulting from, central venous catheter
  triple lumen catheter T80.219
    bloodstream T80.211
    localized T80.212
    specified NEC T80.218

Infection, infected, infective (opportunistic)
B99.9 — *continued*
due to or resulting from — *continued*
umbilical venous catheter T80.219
bloodstream T80.211
localized T80.212
specified NEC T80.218
during labor NEC O75.3
ear (middle) — *see also* Otitis media
external — *see* Otitis, externa, infective
inner — *see* subcategory H83.0
Eberthella typhosa A01.00
Echinococcus — *see* Echinococcus
echovirus
as cause of disease classified elsewhere
B97.12
unspecified nature or site B34.1
endocardium I33.0
endocervix — *see* Cervicitis
Entamoeba — *see* Amebiasis
enteric — *see* Enteritis, infectious
Enterobacter sakazakii B96.89
Enterobius vermicularis B80
enterostomy K94.12
enterovirus B34.1
as cause of disease classified elsewhere
B97.10
coxsackievirus B97.11
echovirus B97.12
specified NEC B97.19
Entomophthora B46.8
Epidermophyton — *see* Dermatophytosis
epididymis — *see* Epididymitis
episiotomy (puerperal) O86.0
Erysipelothrix (insidiosa) (rhusiopathiae) — *see*
Erysipeloid
erythema infectiosum B08.3
Escherichia (E.) coli NEC A49.8
as cause of disease classified elsewhere (*see*
also Escherichia coli) B96.20
congenital P39.8
sepsis P36.4
generalized A41.51
intestinal — *see* Enteritis, infectious, due to,
Escherichia coli
ethmoidal (chronic) (sinus) — *see* Sinusitis,
ethmoidal
eustachian tube (ear) — *see* Salpingitis,
eustachian
external auditory canal (meatus) NEC — *see*
Otitis, externa, infective
eye (purulent) — *see* Endophthalmitis, purulent
eyelid — *see* Inflammation, eyelid
fallopian tube — *see* Salpingo-oophoritis
Fasciola (gigantica) (hepatica) (indica) B66.3
Fasciolopsis (buski) B66.5
filarial — *see* Infestation, filarial
finger (skin) L08.9
nail L03.01-
fungus B35.1
fish tapeworm B70.0
larval B70.1
flagellate, intestinal A07.9
fluke — *see* Infestation, fluke
focal
teeth (pulpal origin) K04.7
tonsils J35.01
Fonsecaea (compactum) (pedrosoi) B43.0
food — *see* Intoxication, foodborne
foot (skin) L08.9
dermatophytic fungus B35.3
Francisella tularensis — *see* Tularemia
frontal (sinus) (chronic) — *see* Sinusitis, frontal
fungus NOS B49
beard B35.0
dermatophytic — *see* Dermatophytosis
foot B35.3
groin B35.6
hand B35.2

Infection, infected, infective (opportunistic)
B99.9 — *continued*
fungus NOS B49 — *continued*
nail B35.1
pathogenic to compromised host only B48.8
perianal (area) B35.6
scalp B35.0
skin B36.9
foot B35.3
hand B35.2
toenails B35.1
Fusarium B48.8
gallbladder — *see* Cholecystitis
gas bacillus — *see* Gangrene, gas
gastrointestinal — *see* Enteritis, infectious
generalized NEC — *see* Sepsis
generator pocket, implanted electronic
neurostimulator T85.734
genital organ or tract
female — *see* Disease, pelvis, inflammatory
male N49.9
multiple sites N49.8
specified NEC N49.8
Ghon tubercle, primary A15.7
Giardia lamblia A07.1
gingiva (chronic) K05.10
acute K05.00
nonplaque induced K05.01
plaque induced K05.00
nonplaque induced K05.11
plaque induced K05.10
glanders A24.0
glenosporopsis B48.0
Gnathostoma (spinigerum) B83.1
Gongylonema B83.8
gonococcal — *see* Gonococcus
gram-negative bacilli NOS A49.9
guinea worm B72
gum (chronic) K05.10
acute K05.00
nonplaque induced K05.01
plaque induced K05.00
nonplaque induced K05.11
plaque induced K05.10
Haemophilus — *see* Infection, Hemophilus
heart — *see* Carditis
Helicobacter pylori A04.8
as cause of disease classified elsewhere
B96.81
helminths B83.9
intestinal B82.0
mixed (types classifiable to more than one
of the titles B65.0-B81.3 and B81.8)
B81.4
specified type NEC B81.8
specified type NEC B83.8
Hemophilus
aegyptius, systemic A48.4
ducrey (any location) A57
generalized A41.3
influenzae NEC A49.2
as cause of disease classified elsewhere
B96.3
herpes (simplex) — *see also* Herpes
congenital P35.2
disseminated B00.7
zoster B02.9
herpesvirus, herpesviral — *see* Herpes
Heterophyes (heterophyes) B66.8
hip (joint) NEC M00.9
due to internal joint prosthesis
left T84.52
right T84.51
skin NEC L08.9
Histoplasma — *see* Histoplasmosis
American B39.4
capsulatum B39.4
hookworm B76.9

Infection, infected, infective (opportunistic)
B99.9 — *continued*
human
papilloma virus A63.0
T-cell lymphotropic virus type-1 (HTLV-1)
B33.3
hydrocele N43.0
Hymenolepis B71.0
hypopharynx — *see* Pharyngitis
inguinal (lymph) glands L04.1
due to soft chancre A57
intervertebral disc, pyogenic M46.30
cervical region M46.32
cervicothoracic region M46.33
lumbar region M46.36
lumbosacral region M46.37
multiple sites M46.39
occipito-atlanto-axial region M46.31
sacrococcygeal region M46.38
thoracic region M46.34
thoracolumbar region M46.35
intestine, intestinal — *see* Enteritis, infectious
specified NEC A08.8
intra-amniotic affecting newborn NEC P39.2
Isospora belli or hominis A07.3
Japanese B encephalitis A83.0
jaw (bone) (lower) (upper) M27.2
joint NEC M00.9
due to internal joint prosthesis T84.50
kidney (cortex) (hematogenous) N15.9
with calculus N20.0
with hydronephrosis N13.6
following ectopic gestation O08.83
pelvis and ureter (cystic) N28.85
puerperal (postpartum) O86.21
specified NEC N15.8
Klebsiella (K.) pneumoniae NEC A49.8
as cause of disease classified elsewhere
B96.1
knee (joint) NEC M00.9
due to internal joint prosthesis
left T84.54
right T84.53
skin NEC L08.9
Koch's — *see* Tuberculosis
labia (majora) (minora) (acute) — *see* Vulvitis
lacrimal
gland — *see* Dacryoadenitis
passages (duct) (sac) — *see* Inflammation,
lacrimal, passages
lancet fluke B66.2
larynx NEC J38.7
leg (skin) NOS L08.9
Legionella pneumophila A48.1
nonpneumonic A48.2
Leishmania — *see also* Leishmaniasis
aethiopica B55.1
braziliensis B55.2
chagasi B55.0
donovani B55.0
infantum B55.0
major B55.1
mexicana B55.1
tropica B55.1
lentivirus, as cause of disease classified
elsewhere B97.31
Leptosphaeria senegalensis B47.0
Leptospira interrogans A27.9
autumnalis A27.89
canicola A27.89
hebdomadis A27.89
icterohaemorrhagiae A27.0
pomona A27.89
specified type NEC A27.89
leptospirochetal NEC — *see* Leptospirosis
Listeria monocytogenes — *see also* Listeriosis
congenital P37.2

Infection, infected, infective (opportunistic)
  B99.9 — *continued*
  Loa loa B74.3
    with conjunctival infestation B74.3
    eyelid B74.3
  Loboa loboi B48.0
  local, skin (staphylococcal) (streptococcal)
    L08.9
    abscess — *code by* site under Abscess
    cellulitis — *code by* site under Cellulitis
    specified NEC L08.89
    ulcer — *see* Ulcer, skin
  Loefflerella mallei A24.0
  lung (*see also* Pneumonia) J18.9
    atypical Mycobacterium A31.0
    spirochetal A69.8
    tuberculous — *see* Tuberculosis, pulmonary
    virus — *see* Pneumonia, viral
  lymph gland — *see also* Lymphadenitis, acute
    mesenteric I88.0
  lymphoid tissue, base of tongue or posterior
    pharynx, NEC (chronic) J35.03
  Madurella (grisea) (mycetomii) B47.0
  major
    following ectopic or molar pregnancy O08.0
    puerperal, postpartum, childbirth O85
  Malassezia furfur B36.0
  Malleomyces
    mallei A24.0
    pseudomallei (whitmori) — *see* Melioidosis
  mammary gland N61.0
  Mansonella (ozzardi) (perstans) (streptocerca)
    B74.4
  mastoid — *see* Mastoiditis
  maxilla, maxillary M27.2
    sinus (chronic) — *see* Sinusitis, maxillary
  mediastinum J98.51
  Medina (worm) B72
  meibomian cyst or gland — *see* Hordeolum
  meninges — *see* Meningitis, bacterial
  meningococcal (*see also* condition) A39.9
    adrenals A39.1
    brain A39.81
    cerebrospinal A39.0
    conjunctiva A39.89
    endocardium A39.51
    heart A39.50
      endocardium A39.51
      myocardium A39.52
      pericardium A39.53
    joint A39.83
    meninges A39.0
    meningococcemia A39.4
      acute A39.2
      chronic A39.3
    myocardium A39.52
    pericardium A39.53
    retrobulbar neuritis A39.82
    specified site NEC A39.89
  mesenteric lymph nodes or glands NEC I88.0
  Metagonimus B66.8
  metatarsophalangeal M00.9
  methicillin
    resistant Staphylococcus aureus (MRSA)
      A49.02
    susceptible Staphylococcus aureus (MSSA)
      A49.01
  Microsporum, microsporic — *see*
    Dermatophytosis
  mixed flora (bacterial) NEC A49.8
  Monilia — *see* Candidiasis
  Monosporium apiospermum B48.2
  mouth, parasitic B37.0
  Mucor — *see* Mucormycosis
  muscle NEC — *see* Myositis, infective
  mycelium NOS B49
  mycetoma B47.9
    actinomycotic NEC B47.1
    mycotic NEC B47.0

Infection, infected, infective (opportunistic)
  B99.9 — *continued*
  Mycobacterium, mycobacterial — *see*
    Mycobacterium
  Mycoplasma NEC A49.3
    pneumoniae, as cause of disease classified
      elsewhere B96.0
  mycotic NOS B49
    pathogenic to compromised host only B48.8
    skin NOS B36.9
  myocardium NEC I40.0
  nail (chronic)
    with lymphangitis — *see* Lymphangitis,
      acute, digit
    finger L03.01-
      fungus B35.1
      ingrowing L60.0
    toe L03.03-
      fungus B35.1
  nasal sinus (chronic) — *see* Sinusitis
  nasopharynx — *see* Nasopharyngitis
  navel L08.82
  Necator americanus B76.1
  Neisseria — *see* Gonococcus
  Neotestudina rosatii B47.0
  newborn P39.9
    intra-amniotic NEC P39.2
    skin P39.4
    specified type NEC P39.8
  nipple N61.0
    associated with
      lactation O91.03
      pregnancy O91.01-
      puerperium O91.02
  Nocardia — *see* Nocardiosis
  obstetrical surgical wound (puerperal) O86.0
  Oesophagostomum (apiostomum) B81.8
  Oestrus ovis — *see* Myiasis
  Oidium albicans B37.9
  Onchocerca (volvulus) — *see* Onchocerciasis
  oncovirus, as cause of disease classified
    elsewhere B97.32
  operation wound T81.40
  Opisthorchis (felineus) (viverrini) B66.0
  orbit, orbital — *see* Inflammation, orbit
  orthopoxvirus NEC B08.09
  ovary — *see* Salpingo-oophoritis
  Oxyuris vermicularis B80
  pancreas (acute) — *see* Pancreatitis, acute
    abscess — *see* Pancreatitis, acute
    specified NEC (*see also* Pancreatitis, acute)
      K85.80
  papillomavirus, as cause of disease classified
    elsewhere B97.7
  papovavirus NEC B34.4
  Paracoccidioides brasiliensis — *see*
    Paracoccidioidomycosis
  Paragonimus (westermani) B66.4
  parainfluenza virus B34.8
  parameningococcus NOS A39.9
  parapoxvirus B08.60
    specified NEC B08.69
  parasitic B89
  Parastrongylus
    cantonensis B83.2
    costaricensis B81.3
    paratyphoid A01.4
      Type A A01.1
      Type B A01.2
      Type C A01.3
  paraurethral ducts N34.2
  parotid gland — *see* Sialoadenitis
  parvovirus NEC B34.3
    as cause of disease classified elsewhere
      B97.6
  Pasteurella NEC A28.0
    multocida A28.0
    pestis — *see* Plague
    pseudotuberculosis A28.0

Infection, infected, infective (opportunistic)
  B99.9 — *continued*
  Pasteurella NEC A28.0 — *continued*
    septica (cat bite) (dog bite) A28.0
    tularensis — *see* Tularemia
  pelvic, female — *see* Disease, pelvis,
    inflammatory
  Penicillium (marneffei) B48.4
  penis (glans) (retention) NEC N48.29
  periapical K04.5
  peridental, periodontal K05.20
    generalized — *see* Peridontitis, aggressive,
      generalized
    localized — *see* Peridontitis, aggressive,
      localized
  perinatal period P39.9
    specified type NEC P39.8
  perineal repair (puerperal) O86.0
  periorbital — *see* Inflammation, orbit
  perirectal K62.89
  perirenal — *see* Infection, kidney
  peritoneal — *see* Peritonitis
  periureteral N28.89
  Petriellidium boydii B48.2
  pharynx — *see also* Pharyngitis
    coxsackievirus B08.5
    posterior, lymphoid (chronic) J35.03
  Phialophora
    gougerotii (subcutaneous abscess or cyst)
      B43.2
    jeanselmei (subcutaneous abscess or cyst)
      B43.2
    verrucosa (skin) B43.0
  Piedraia hortae B36.3
  pinta A67.9
    intermediate A67.1
    late A67.2
    mixed A67.3
    primary A67.0
  pinworm B80
  pityrosporum furfur B36.0
  pleuro-pneumonia-like organism (PPLO) NEC
    A49.3
    as cause of disease classified elsewhere
      B96.0
  pneumococcus, pneumococcal NEC A49.1
    as cause of disease classified elsewhere
      B95.3
    generalized (purulent) A40.3
      with pneumonia J13
  Pneumocystis carinii (pneumonia) B59
  Pneumocystis jiroveci (pneumonia) B59
  port or reservoir T80.212
  postoperative T81.40
  postoperative wound T81.40
  postprocedural T81.40
    deep incisional surgical site T81.42
    organ and space surgical site T81.43
    sepsis T81.49
    specified surgical site NEC T81.48
    superficial incisional surgical site T81.41
  postvaccinal T88.0
  prepuce NEC N47.7
    with penile inflammation N47.6
  prion — *see* Disease, prion, central nervous
    system
  prostate (capsule) — *see* Prostatitis
  Proteus (mirabilis) (morganii) (vulgaris) NEC
    A49.8
    as cause of disease classified elsewhere
      B96.4
  protozoal NEC B64
    intestinal A07.9
      specified NEC A07.8
    specified NEC B60.8
  Pseudoallescheria boydii B48.2

DISEASE INDEX

Infection, infected, infective (opportunistic)
B99.9 — *continued*
Pseudomonas NEC A49.8
  as cause of disease classified elsewhere B96.5
  mallei A24.0
  pneumonia J15.1
  pseudomallei — *see* Melioidosis
puerperal O86.4
  genitourinary tract NEC O86.89
  major or generalized O85
  minor O86.4
  specified NEC O86.89
pulmonary — *see* Infection, lung
purulent — *see* Abscess
Pyrenochaeta romeroi B47.0
Q fever A78
rectum (sphincter) K62.89
renal — *see also* Infection, kidney
  pelvis and ureter (cystic) N28.85
reovirus, as cause of disease classified elsewhere B97.5
respiratory (tract) NEC J98.8
  acute J22
  chronic J98.8
  influenzal (upper) (acute) — *see* Influenza, with, respiratory manifestations NEC
  lower (acute) J22
    chronic — *see* Bronchitis, chronic
  rhinovirus J00
  syncytial virus, as cause of disease classified elsewhere B97.4
  upper (acute) NOS J06.9
    chronic J39.8
    streptococcal J06.9
    viral NOS J06.9
resulting from
  presence of internal prosthesis, implant, graft — *see* Complications, by site and type, infection
retortamoniasis A07.8
retroperitoneal NEC K68.9
retrovirus B33.3
  as cause of disease classified elsewhere B97.30
    human
     immunodeficiency, type 2 (HIV 2) B97.35
     T-cell lymphotropic
      type I (HTLV-I) B97.33
      type II (HTLV-II) B97.34
    lentivirus B97.31
    oncovirus B97.32
    specified NEC B97.39
Rhinosporidium (seeberi) B48.1
rhinovirus
  as cause of disease classified elsewhere B97.89
  unspecified nature or site B34.8
Rhizopus — *see* Mucormycosis
rickettsial NOS A79.9
roundworm (large) NEC B82.0
  Ascariasis (*see also* Ascariasis) B77.9
rubella — *see* Rubella
Saccharomyces — *see* Candidiasis
salivary duct or gland (any) — *see* Sialoadenitis
Salmonella (aertrycke) (arizonae) (callinarum) (cholerae-suis) (enteritidis) (suipestifer) (typhimurium) A02.9
  with
    (gastro)enteritis A02.0
    sepsis A02.1
    specified manifestation NEC A02.8
  due to food (poisoning) A02.9
  hirschfeldii A01.3
  localized A02.20
    arthritis A02.23
    meningitis A02.21

Infection, infected, infective (opportunistic)
B99.9 — *continued*
Salmonella (aertrycke) (arizonae) (callinarum) (cholerae-suis) (enteritidis) (suipestifer) (typhimurium) A02.9 — *continued*
  localized A02.20 — *continued*
    osteomyelitis A02.24
    pneumonia A02.22
    pyelonephritis A02.25
    specified NEC A02.29
  paratyphi A01.4
    A A01.1
    B A01.2
    C A01.3
  schottmuelleri A01.2
  typhi, typhosa — *see* Typhoid
Sarcocystis A07.8
scabies B86
Schistosoma — *see* Infestation, Schistosoma
scrotum (acute) NEC N49.2
seminal vesicle — *see* Vesiculitis
septic
  localized, skin — *see* Abscess
sheep liver fluke B66.3
Shigella A03.9
  boydii A03.2
  dysenteriae A03.0
  flexneri A03.1
  group
    A A03.0
    B A03.1
    C A03.2
    D A03.3
  Schmitz (-Stutzer) A03.0
  schmitzii A03.0
  shigae A03.0
  sonnei A03.3
  specified NEC A03.8
shoulder (joint) NEC M00.9
  due to internal joint prosthesis T84.59
  skin NEC L08.9
sinus (accessory) (chronic) (nasal) — *see also* Sinusitis
  pilonidal — *see* Sinus, pilonidal
  skin NEC L08.89
Skene's duct or gland — *see* Urethritis
skin (local) (staphylococcal) (streptococcal) L08.9
  abscess — *code by* site under Abscess
  cellulitis — *code by* site under Cellulitis
  due to fungus B36.9
    specified type NEC B36.8
  mycotic B36.9
    specified type NEC B36.8
  newborn P39.4
  ulcer — *see* Ulcer, skin
slow virus A81.9
  specified NEC A81.89
Sparganum (mansoni) (proliferum) (baxteri) B70.1
specific — *see also* Syphilis
  to perinatal period — *see* Infection, congenital
specified NEC B99.8
spermatic cord NEC N49.1
sphenoidal (sinus) — *see* Sinusitis, sphenoidal
spinal cord NOS (*see also* Myelitis) G04.91
  abscess G06.1
  meninges — *see* Meningitis
  streptococcal G04.89
Spirillum A25.0
spirochetal NOS A69.9
  lung A69.8
  specified NEC A69.8
Spirometra larvae B70.1
spleen D73.89
Sporotrichum, Sporothrix (schenckii) — *see* Sporotrichosis

Infection, infected, infective (opportunistic)
B99.9 — *continued*
staphylococcal, unspecified site
  as cause of disease classified elsewhere B95.8
    aureus (methicillin susceptible) (MSSA) B95.61
     methicillin resistant (MRSA) B95.62
    specified NEC B95.7
  aureus (methicillin susceptible) (MSSA) A49.01
    methicillin resistant (MRSA) A49.02
  food poisoning A05.0
  generalized (purulent) A41.2
  pneumonia — *see* Pneumonia, staphylococcal
Stellantchasmus falcatus B66.8
streptobacillus moniliformis A25.1
streptococcal NEC A49.1
  as cause of disease classified elsewhere B95.5
  B genitourinary complicating
    childbirth O98.82
    pregnancy O98.81-
    puerperium O98.83
  congenital
    sepsis P36.10
     group B P36.0
    specified NEC P36.19
  generalized (purulent) A40.9
Streptomyces B47.1
Strongyloides (stercoralis) — *see* Strongyloidiasis
stump (amputation) (surgical) — *see* Complication, amputation stump, infection
subcutaneous tissue, local L08.9
suipestifer — *see* Infection, salmonella
swimming pool bacillus A31.1
Taenia — *see* Infestation, Taenia
Taeniarhynchus saginatus B68.1
tapeworm — *see* Infestation, tapeworm
tendon (sheath) — *see* Tenosynovitis, infective NEC
Ternidens diminutus B81.8
testis — *see* Orchitis
threadworm B80
throat — *see* Pharyngitis
thyroglossal duct K14.8
toe (skin) L08.9
  cellulitis L03.03-
    fungus B35.1
  nail L03.03-
    fungus B35.1
tongue NEC K14.0
  parasitic B37.0
tonsil (and adenoid) (faucial) (lingual) (pharyngeal) — *see* Tonsillitis
tooth, teeth K04.7
  periapical K04.7
  peridental, periodontal K05.20
    generalized — *see* Peridontitis, aggressive, generalized
    localized — *see* Peridontitis, aggressive, localized
  pulp K04.01
    irreversible K04.02
    reversible K04.01
  socket M27.3
TORCH — *see* Infection, congenital without active infection P00.2
Torula histolytica — *see* Cryptococcosis
Toxocara (canis) (cati) (felis) B83.0
Toxoplasma gondii — *see* Toxoplasma
trachea, chronic J42
trematode NEC — *see* Infestation, fluke
trench fever A79.0
Treponema pallidum — *see* Syphilis
Trichinella (spiralis) B75

Infection, infected, infective (opportunistic)
  B99.9 — continued
  Trichomonas A59.9
    cervix A59.09
    intestine A07.8
    prostate A59.02
    specified site NEC A59.8
    urethra A59.03
    urogenitalis A59.00
    vagina A59.01
    vulva A59.01
  Trichophyton, trichophytic — see
      Dermatophytosis
  Trichosporon (beigelii) cutaneum B36.2
  Trichostrongylus B81.2
  Trichuris (trichiura) B79
  Trombicula (irritans) B88.0
  Trypanosoma
    brucei
      gambiense B56.0
      rhodesiense B56.1
    cruzi — see Chagas' disease
    tubal — see Salpingo-oophoritis
    tuberculous NEC — see Tuberculosis
    tubo-ovarian — see Salpingo-oophoritis
    tunica vaginalis N49.1
    tunnel T80.212
    tympanic membrane NEC — see Myringitis
    typhoid (abortive) (ambulant) (bacillus) — see
      Typhoid
    typhus A75.9
      flea-borne A75.2
      mite-borne A75.3
      recrudescent A75.1
      tick-borne A77.9
        African A77.1
        North Asian A77.2
    umbilicus L08.82
    ureter N28.86
    urethra — see Urethritis
    urinary (tract) N39.0
      bladder — see Cystitis
      complicating
        pregnancy O23.4-
          specified type NEC O23.3-
        kidney — see Infection, kidney
        newborn P39.3
        puerperal (postpartum) O86.20
        tuberculous A18.13
        urethra — see Urethritis
    uterus, uterine — see Endometritis
    vaccination T88.0
    vaccinia not from vaccination B08.011
    vagina (acute) — see Vaginitis
    varicella B01.9
    varicose veins — see Varix
    vas deferens NEC N49.1
    vesical — see Cystitis
    Vibrio
      cholerae A00.0
        El Tor A00.1
      parahaemolyticus (food poisoning) A05.3
      vulnificus
        as cause of disease classified elsewhere
          B96.82
        foodborne intoxication A05.5
    Vincent's (gum) (mouth) (tonsil) A69.1
    virus, viral NOS B34.9
      adenovirus
        as cause of disease classified elsewhere
          B97.0
        unspecified nature or site B34.0
      arborvirus, arbovirus arthropod-borne A94
        as cause of disease classified elsewhere
          B97.89
        adenovirus B97.0
        coronavirus B97.29
          SARS-associated B97.21
        coxsackievirus B97.11

Infection, infected, infective (opportunistic)
  B99.9 — continued
  virus, viral NOS B34.9 — continued
    as cause of disease classified elsewhere
      B97.89 — continued
      echovirus B97.12
      enterovirus B97.10
        coxsackievirus B97.11
        echovirus B97.12
        specified NEC B97.19
      human
        immunodeficiency, type 2 (HIV 2)
          B97.35
        metapneumovirus B97.81
        T-cell lymphotropic,
          type I (HTLV-I) B97.33
          type II (HTLV-II) B97.34
      papillomavirus B97.7
      parvovirus B97.6
      reovirus B97.5
      respiratory syncytial B97.4
      retrovirus B97.30
        human
          immunodeficiency, type 2 (HIV 2)
            B97.35
          T-cell lymphotropic,
            type I (HTLV-I) B97.33
            type II (HTLV-II) B97.34
        lentivirus B97.31
        oncovirus B97.32
        specified NEC B97.39
      specified NEC B97.89
    central nervous system A89
      atypical A81.9
        specified NEC A81.89
      enterovirus NEC A88.8
        meningitis A87.0
      slow virus A81.9
        specified NEC A81.89
      specified NEC A88.8
    chest J98.8
    cotia B08.8
    coxsackie (see also Infection, coxsackie) B34.1
      as cause of disease classified elsewhere
        B97.11
    ECHO
      as cause of disease classified elsewhere
        B97.12
      unspecified nature or site B34.1
    encephalitis, tick-borne A84.9
    enterovirus, as cause of disease classified
        elsewhere B97.10
      coxsackievirus B97.11
      echovirus B97.12
      specified NEC B97.19
    exanthem NOS B09
    human metapneumovirus as cause of
        disease classified elsewhere B97.81
    human papilloma as cause of disease
        classified elsewhere B97.7
    intestine — see Enteritis, viral
    respiratory syncytial
      as cause of disease classified elsewhere
        B97.4
      bronchopneumonia J12.1
      common cold syndrome J00
      nasopharyngitis (acute) J00
    rhinovirus
      as cause of disease classified elsewhere
        B97.89
      unspecified nature or site B34.8
    slow A81.9
      specified NEC A81.89
    specified type NEC B33.8
      as cause of disease classified elsewhere
        B97.89
      unspecified nature or site B34.8
    unspecified nature or site B34.9
    West Nile — see Virus, West Nile

Infection, infected, infective (opportunistic)
  B99.9 — continued
  vulva (acute) — see Vulvitis
  West Nile — see Virus, West Nile
  whipworm B79
  worms B83.9
    specified type NEC B83.8
  Wuchereria (bancrofti) B74.0
    malayi B74.1
  yatapoxvirus B08.70
    specified NEC B08.79
  yeast (see also Candidiasis) B37.9
  yellow fever — see Fever, yellow
  Yersinia
    enterocolitica (intestinal) A04.6
    pestis — see Plague
    pseudotuberculosis A28.2
  Zeis' gland — see Hordeolum
  Zika virus A92.5
  zoonotic bacterial NOS A28.9
  Zopfia senegalensis B47.0
Infective, infectious — see condition
Infertility
  female N97.9
    age-related N97.8
    associated with
      anovulation N97.0
      cervical (mucus) disease or anomaly
        N88.3
      congenital anomaly
        cervix N88.3
        fallopian tube N97.1
        uterus N97.2
        vagina N97.8
      dysmucorrhea N88.3
      fallopian tube disease or anomaly N97.1
      pituitary-hypothalamic origin E23.0
      specified origin NEC N97.8
      Stein-Leventhal syndrome E28.2
      uterine disease or anomaly N97.2
      vaginal disease or anomaly N97.8
    due to
      cervical anomaly N88.3
      fallopian tube anomaly N97.1
      ovarian failure E28.39
      Stein-Leventhal syndrome E28.2
      uterine anomaly N97.2
      vaginal anomaly N97.8
    nonimplantation N97.2
    origin
      cervical N88.3
      tubal (block) (occlusion) (stenosis) N97.1
      uterine N97.2
      vaginal N97.8
  male N46.9
    azoospermia N46.01
      extratesticular cause N46.029
        drug therapy N46.021
        efferent duct obstruction N46.023
        infection N46.022
        radiation N46.024
        specified cause NEC N46.029
        systemic disease N46.025
    oligospermia N46.11
      extratesticular cause N46.129
        drug therapy N46.121
        efferent duct obstruction N46.123
        infection N46.122
        radiation N46.124
        specified cause NEC N46.129
        systemic disease N46.125
    specified type NEC N46.8
Infestation B88.9
  Acanthocheilonema (perstans) (streptocerca)
    B74.4
  Acariasis B88.0
    demodex folliculorum B88.0
    sarcoptes scabiei B86
    trombiculae B88.0

DISEASE INDEX

Infestation B88.9 — *continued*
  Schistosoma B65.9 — *continued*
    specified type NEC B65.8
    spindale B65.8
  screw worms — *see* Myiasis
  skin NOS B88.9
  Sparganum (mansoni) (proliferum) (baxteri)
      B70.1
    larval B70.1
  specified type NEC B88.8
  Spirometra larvae B70.1
  Stellantchasmus falcatus B66.8
  Strongyloides stercoralis — *see* Strongyloidiasis
  Taenia B68.9
    diminuta B71.0
    echinococcus — *see* Echinococcus
    mediocanellata B68.1
    nana B71.0
    saginata B68.1
    solium (intestinal form) B68.0
      larval form — *see* Cysticercosis
  Taeniarhynchus saginatus B68.1
  tapeworm B71.9
    beef B68.1
    broad B70.0
      larval B70.1
    dog B67.4
    dwarf B71.0
    fish B70.0
      larval B70.1
    pork B68.0
    rat B71.0
  Ternidens diminutus B81.8
  Tetranychus molestissimus B88.0
  threadworm B80
  tongue B37.0
  Toxocara (canis) (cati) (felis) B83.0
  trematode(s) NEC — *see* Infestation, fluke
  Trichinella (spiralis) B75
  Trichocephalus B79
  Trichomonas — *see* Trichomoniasis
  Trichostrongylus B81.2
  Trichuris (trichiura) B79
  Trombicula (irritans) B88.0
  Tunga penetrans B88.1
  Uncinaria americana B76.1
  Vandellia cirrhosa B88.8
  whipworm B79
  worms B83.9
    intestinal B82.0
  Wuchereria (bancrofti) B74.0

Infiltrate, infiltration
  amyloid (generalized) (localized) — *see*
      Amyloidosis
  calcareous NEC R89.7
    localized — *see* Degeneration, by site
  calcium salt R89.7
  cardiac
    fatty — *see* Degeneration, myocardial
    glycogenic E74.02 *[I43]*
  corneal — *see* Edema, cornea
  eyelid — *see* Inflammation, eyelid
  glycogen, glycogenic — *see* Disease, glycogen
      storage
  heart, cardiac
    fatty — *see* Degeneration, myocardial
    glycogenic E74.02 *[I43]*
  inflammatory in vitreous H43.89
  kidney N28.89
  leukemic — *see* Leukemia
  liver K76.89
    fatty — *see* Fatty, liver NEC
    glycogen (*see also* Disease, glycogen storage)
      E74.03 *[K77]*
  lung R91.8
    eosinophilic J82
  lymphatic (*see also* Leukemia, lymphatic)
      C91.9-
    gland I88.9

Infiltrate, infiltration — *continued*
  muscle, fatty M62.89
  myocardium, myocardial
    fatty — *see* Degeneration, myocardial
    glycogenic E74.02 *[I43]*
  on chest x-ray R91.8
  pulmonary R91.8
    with eosinophilia J82
  skin (lymphocytic) L98.6
  thymus (gland) (fatty) E32.8
  urine R39.0
  vesicant agent
    antineoplastic chemotherapy T80.810
    other agent NEC T80.818
  vitreous body H43.89

Infirmity R68.89
  senile R54

Inflammation, inflamed, inflammatory
  (with exudation)
  abducent (nerve) — *see* Strabismus, paralytic,
      sixth nerve
  accessory sinus (chronic) — *see* Sinusitis
  adrenal (gland) E27.8
  alveoli, teeth M27.3
    scorbutic E54
  anal canal, anus K62.89
  antrum (chronic) — *see* Sinusitis, maxillary
  appendix — *see* Appendicitis
  arachnoid — *see* Meningitis
  areola N61.0
    puerperal, postpartum or gestational — *see*
        Infection, nipple
  areolar tissue NOS L08.9
  artery — *see* Arteritis
  auditory meatus (external) — *see* Otitis,
      externa
  Bartholin's gland N75.8
  bile duct (common) (hepatic) or passage — *see*
      Cholangitis
  bladder — *see* Cystitis
  bone — *see* Osteomyelitis
  brain — *see also* Encephalitis
    membrane — *see* Meningitis
  breast N61.0
    puerperal, postpartum, gestational — *see*
        Mastitis, obstetric
  broad ligament — *see* Disease, pelvis,
      inflammatory
  bronchi — *see* Bronchitis
  catarrhal J00
  cecum — *see* Appendicitis
  cerebral — *see also* Encephalitis
    membrane — *see* Meningitis
  cerebrospinal
    meningococcal A39.0
  cervix (uteri) — *see* Cervicitis
  chest J98.8
  chorioretinal H30.9-
    cyclitis — *see* Cyclitis
    disseminated H30.10-
      generalized H30.13-
      peripheral H30.12-
      posterior pole H30.11-
    epitheliopathy — *see* Epitheliopathy
    focal H30.00-
      juxtapapillary H30.01-
      macular H30.04-
      paramacular — *see* Inflammation,
          chorioretinal, focal, macular
      peripheral H30.03-
      posterior pole H30.02-
    specified type NEC H30.89-
  choroid — *see* Inflammation, chorioretinal
  chronic, postmastoidectomy cavity — *see*
      Complications, postmastoidectomy,
      inflammation
  colon — *see* Enteritis
  connective tissue (diffuse) NEC — *see* Disorder,
      soft tissue, specified type NEC

Inflammation, inflamed, inflammatory
  (with exudation) — *continued*
  cornea — *see* Keratitis
  corpora cavernosa N48.29
  cranial nerve — *see* Disorder, nerve, cranial
  Douglas' cul-de-sac or pouch (chronic) N73.0
  due to device, implant or graft — *see also*
      Complications, by site and type, infection
      or inflammation
    arterial graft T82.7
    breast (implant) T85.79
    catheter T85.79
      dialysis (renal) T82.7
        intraperitoneal T85.71
      infusion T82.7
        cranial T85.735
        intrathecal T85.735
        spinal (epidural) (subdural) T85.735
        subarachnoid T85.735
      urinary T83.518
        cystostomy T83.510
        Hopkins T83.518
        ileostomy T83.518
        nephrostomy T83.512
        specified NEC T83.518
        urethral indwelling T83.511
        urostomy T83.518
    electronic (electrode) (pulse generator)
        (stimulator)
      bone T84.7
      cardiac T82.7
      nervous system T85.738
        brain T85.731
        cranial nerve T85.732
        gastric nerve T85.732
        neurostimulator generator T85.734
        peripheral nerve T85.732
        sacral nerve T85.732
        spinal cord T85.733
        vagal nerve T85.732
      urinary T83.590
    fixation, internal (orthopedic) NEC — *see*
        Complication, fixation device, infection
    gastrointestinal (bile duct) (esophagus)
        T85.79
      neurostimulator electrode (lead) T85.732
    genital NEC T83.69
    heart NEC T82.7
      valve (prosthesis) T82.6
      graft T82.7
    joint prosthesis — *see* Complication, joint
        prosthesis, infection
    ocular (corneal graft) (orbital implant) NEC
        T85.79
    orthopedic NEC T84.7
    penile (cylinder) (pump) (resevoir) T83.61
    specified NEC T85.79
    testicular T83.62
    urinary NEC T83.598
      ileal conduit stent T83.593
      implanted neurostimulation T83.590
      implanted sphincter T83.591
      indwelling ureteral stent T83.592
      nephroureteral stent T83.593
      specified stent NEC T83.593
    vascular NEC T82.7
    ventricular intracranial (communicating)
        shunt T85.730
  duodenum K29.80
    with bleeding K29.81
  dura mater — *see* Meningitis
  ear (middle) — *see also* Otitis, media
    external — *see* Otitis, externa
    inner — *see* subcategory H83.0
  epididymis — *see* Epididymitis
  esophagus K20.9
  ethmoidal (sinus) (chronic) — *see* Sinusitis,
      ethmoidal

Inflammation, inflamed, inflammatory
(with exudation) — *continued*
eustachian tube (catarrhal) — *see* Salpingitis, eustachian
eyelid H01.9
abscess — *see* Abscess, eyelid
blepharitis — *see* Blepharitis
chalazion — *see* Chalazion
dermatosis (noninfectious) — *see* Dermatosis, eyelid
hordeolum — *see* Hordeolum
specified NEC H01.8
fallopian tube — *see* Salpingo-oophoritis
fascia — *see* Myositis
follicular, pharynx J31.2
frontal (sinus) (chronic) — *see* Sinusitis, frontal
gallbladder — *see* Cholecystitis
gastric — *see* Gastritis
gastrointestinal — *see* Enteritis
genital organ (internal) (diffuse)
female — *see* Disease, pelvis, inflammatory
male N49.9
multiple sites N49.8
specified NEC N49.8
gland (lymph) — *see* Lymphadenitis
glottis — *see* Laryngitis
granular, pharynx J31.2
gum K05.10
nonplaque induced K05.11
plaque induced K05.10
heart — *see* Carditis
hepatic duct — *see* Cholangitis
ileoanal (internal) pouch K91.850
ileum — *see also* Enteritis
regional or terminal — *see* Enteritis, regional
intestinal pouch K91.850
intestine (any part) — *see* Enteritis
jaw (acute) (bone) (chronic) (lower) (suppurative) (upper) M27.2
joint NEC — *see* Arthritis
sacroiliac M46.1
kidney — *see* Nephritis
knee (joint) M13.169
tuberculous A18.02
labium (majus) (minus) — *see* Vulvitis
lacrimal
gland — *see* Dacryoadenitis
passages (duct) (sac) — *see also* Dacryocystitis
canaliculitis — *see* Canaliculitis, lacrimal
larynx — *see* Laryngitis
leg NOS L08.9
lip K13.0
liver (capsule) — *see also* Hepatitis
chronic K73.9
suppurative K75.0
lung (acute) — *see also* Pneumonia
chronic J98.4
lymph gland or node — *see* Lymphadenitis
lymphatic vessel — *see* Lymphangitis
maxilla, maxillary M27.2
sinus (chronic) — *see* Sinusitis, maxillary
membranes of brain or spinal cord — *see* Meningitis
meninges — *see* Meningitis
mouth K12.1
muscle — *see* Myositis
myocardium — *see* Myocarditis
nasal sinus (chronic) — *see* Sinusitis
nasopharynx — *see* Nasopharyngitis
navel L08.82
nerve NEC — *see* Neuralgia
nipple N61.0
puerperal, postpartum or gestational — *see* Infection, nipple
nose — *see* Rhinitis
oculomotor (nerve) — *see* Strabismus, paralytic, third nerve
optic nerve — *see* Neuritis, optic

Inflammation, inflamed, inflammatory
(with exudation) — *continued*
orbit (chronic) H05.10
acute H05.00
abscess — *see* Abscess, orbit
cellulitis — *see* Cellulitis, orbit
osteomyelitis — *see* Osteomyelitis, orbit
periostitis — *see* Periostitis, orbital
tenonitis — *see* Tenonitis, eye
granuloma — *see* Granuloma, orbit
myositis — *see* Myositis, orbital
ovary — *see* Salpingo-oophoritis
oviduct — *see* Salpingo-oophoritis
pancreas (acute) — *see* Pancreatitis
parametrium N73.0
parotid region L08.9
pelvis, female — *see* Disease, pelvis, inflammatory
penis (corpora cavernosa) N48.29
perianal K62.89
pericardium — *see* Pericarditis
perineum (female) (male) L08.9
perirectal K62.89
peritoneum — *see* Peritonitis
periuterine — *see* Disease, pelvis, inflammatory
perivesical — *see* Cystitis
petrous bone (acute) (chronic) — *see* Petrositis
pharynx (acute) — *see* Pharyngitis
pia mater — *see* Meningitis
pleura — *see* Pleurisy
polyp, colon (*see also* Polyp, colon, inflammatory) K51.40
prostate — *see also* Prostatitis
specified type NEC N41.8
rectosigmoid — *see* Rectosigmoiditis
rectum (*see also* Proctitis) K62.89
respiratory, upper (*see also* Infection, respiratory, upper) J06.9
acute, due to radiation J70.0
chronic, due to external agent — *see* condition, respiratory, chronic, due to
due to
chemicals, gases, fumes or vapors (inhalation) J68.2
radiation J70.1
retina — *see* Chorioretinitis
retrocecal — *see* Appendicitis
retroperitoneal — *see* Peritonitis
salivary duct or gland (any) (suppurative) — *see* Sialoadenitis
scorbutic, alveoli, teeth E54
scrotum N49.2
seminal vesicle — *see* Vesiculitis
sigmoid — *see* Enteritis
sinus — *see* Sinusitis
Skene's duct or gland — *see* Urethritis
skin L08.9
spermatic cord N49.1
sphenoidal (sinus) — *see* Sinusitis, sphenoidal
spinal
cord — *see* Encephalitis
membrane — *see* Meningitis
nerve — *see* Disorder, nerve
spine — *see* Spondylopathy, inflammatory
spleen (capsule) D73.89
stomach — *see* Gastritis
subcutaneous tissue L08.9
suprarenal (gland) E27.8
synovial — *see* Tenosynovitis
tendon (sheath) NEC — *see* Tenosynovitis
testis — *see* Orchitis
throat (acute) — *see* Pharyngitis
thymus (gland) E32.8
thyroid (gland) — *see* Thyroiditis
tongue K14.0
tonsil — *see* Tonsillitis
trachea — *see* Tracheitis

Inflammation, inflamed, inflammatory
(with exudation) — *continued*
trochlear (nerve) — *see* Strabismus, paralytic, fourth nerve
tubal — *see* Salpingo-oophoritis
tuberculous NEC — *see* Tuberculosis
tubo-ovarian — *see* Salpingo-oophoritis
tunica vaginalis N49.1
tympanic membrane — *see* Tympanitis
umbilicus, umbilical L08.82
uterine ligament — *see* Disease, pelvis, inflammatory
uterus (catarrhal) — *see* Endometritis
uveal tract (anterior) NOS — *see also* Iridocyclitis
posterior — *see* Chorioretinitis
vagina — *see* Vaginitis
vas deferens N49.1
vein — *see also* Phlebitis
intracranial or intraspinal (septic) G08
thrombotic I80.9
leg — *see* Phlebitis, leg
lower extremity — *see* Phlebitis, leg
vocal cord J38.3
vulva — *see* Vulvitis
Wharton's duct (suppurative) — *see* Sialoadenitis
Inflation, lung, imperfect (newborn) — *see* Atelectasis
Influenza (bronchial) (epidemic) (respiratory (upper)) (unidentified influenza virus) J11.1
with
digestive manifestations J11.2
encephalopathy J11.81
enteritis J11.2
gastroenteritis J11.2
gastrointestinal manifestations J11.2
laryngitis J11.1
myocarditis J11.82
otitis media J11.83
pharyngitis J11.1
pneumonia J11.00
specified type J11.08
respiratory manifestations NEC J11.1
specified manifestation NEC J11.89
A/H5N1 (*see also* Influenza, due to, identified novel influenza A virus) J09.x2
avian (*see also* Influenza, due to, identified novel influenza A virus) J09.x2
bird (*see also* Influenza, due to, identified novel influenza A virus) J09.x2
due to
avian (*see also* Influenza, due to, identified novel influenza A virus) J09.x2
identified influenza virus NEC J10.1
with
digestive manifestations J10.2
encephalopathy J10.81
enteritis J10.2
gastroenteritis J10.2
gastrointestinal manifestations J10.2
laryngitis J10.1
myocarditis J10.82
otitis media J10.83
pharyngitis J10.1
pneumonia (unspecified type) J10.00
with same identified influenza virus J10.01
specified type NEC J10.08
respiratory manifestations NEC J10.1
specified manifestation NEC J10.89
identified novel influenza A virus J09.x2
with
digestive manifestations J09.x3
encephalopathy J09.x9
enteritis J09.x3
gastroenteritis J09.x3
gastrointestinal manifestations J09.x3
laryngitis J09.x2

Influenza (bronchial) (epidemic) (respiratory (upper)) (unidentified influenza virus) J11.1
due to — *continued*
  identified novel influenza A virus J09.x2 — *continued*
    with — *continued*
      myocarditis J09.x9
      otitis media J09.x9
      pharyngitis J09.x2
      pneumonia J09.x1
      respiratory manifestations NEC J09.x2
      specified manifestation NEC J09.x9
      upper respiratory symptoms J09.x2
  novel (2009) H1N1 influenza (*see also* Influenza, due to, identified influenza virus NEC) J10.1
  novel influenza A/H1N1 (*see also* Influenza, due to, identified influenza virus NEC) J10.1
  of other animal origin, not bird or swine (*see also* Influenza, due to, identified novel influenza A virus) J09.x2
  swine (viruses that normally cause infections in pigs) (*see also* Influenza, due to, identified novel influenza A virus) J09.x2
Influenzal — *see* Influenza
Influenza-like disease — *see* Influenza
Infraction, Freiberg's (metatarsal head) — *see* Osteochondrosis, juvenile, metatarsus
Infraeruption of tooth (teeth) M26.34
Infusion complication, misadventure, or reaction — *see* Complications, infusion
Ingestion
chemical — *see* Table of Drugs and Chemicals, by substance, poisoning
drug or medicament
  correct substance properly administered — *see* Table of Drugs and Chemicals, by drug, adverse effect
  overdose or wrong substance given or taken — *see* Table of Drugs and Chemicals, by drug, poisoning
foreign body — *see* Foreign body, alimentary tract
tularemia A21.3
Ingrowing
hair (beard) L73.1
nail (finger) (toe) L60.0
Inguinal — *see also* condition
testicle Q53.9
  bilateral Q53.21
  unilateral Q53.11
Inhalant-induced
anxiety disorder F18.980
depressive disorder F18.94
major neurocognitive disorder F18.97
mild neurocognitive disorder F18.988
psychotic disorder F18.959
Inhalation
anthrax A22.1
flame T27.3
food or foreign body — *see* Foreign body, by site
gases, fumes, or vapors NEC T59.9-
  specified agent — *see* Table of Drugs and Chemicals, by substance
liquid or vomitus — *see* Asphyxia
meconium (newborn) P24.00
  with
    with respiratory symptoms P24.01
    pneumonia (pneumonitis) P24.01
mucus — *see* Asphyxia, mucus
oil or gasoline (causing suffocation) — *see* Foreign body, by site
smoke J70.5
  due to chemicals, gases, fumes and vapors J68.9
steam — *see* Toxicity, vapors

Inhalation — *continued*
stomach contents or secretions — *see* Foreign body, by site
  due to anesthesia (general) (local) or other sedation T88.59
    in labor and delivery O74.0
    in pregnancy O29.01-
    postpartum, puerperal O89.01
Inhibition, orgasm
female F52.31
male F52.32
Inhibitor, systemic lupus erythematosus (presence of) D68.62
Iniencephalus, iniencephaly Q00.2
Injection, traumatic jet (air) (industrial) (water) (paint or dye) T70.4
Injury (*see also* specified injury type) T14.90
abdomen, abdominal S39.91
  blood vessel — *see* Injury, blood vessel, abdomen
  cavity — *see* Injury, intra-abdominal
  contusion S30.1
  internal — *see* Injury, intra-abdominal
  intra-abdominal organ — *see* Injury, intra-abdominal
  nerve — *see* Injury, nerve, abdomen
  open — *see* Wound, open, abdomen
  specified NEC S39.81
  superficial — *see* Injury, superficial, abdomen
Achilles tendon S86.00-
  laceration S86.02-
  specified type NEC S86.09-
  strain S86.01-
acoustic, resulting in deafness — *see* Injury, nerve, acoustic
adrenal (gland) S37.819
  contusion S37.812
  laceration S37.813
  specified type NEC S37.818
alveolar (process) S09.93
ankle S99.91-
  contusion — *see* Contusion, ankle
  dislocation — *see* Dislocation, ankle
  fracture — *see* Fracture, ankle
  nerve — *see* Injury, nerve, ankle
  open — *see* Wound, open, ankle
  specified type NEC S99.81-
  sprain — *see* Sprain, ankle
  superficial — *see* Injury, superficial, ankle
anterior chamber, eye — *see* Injury, eye, specified NEC
anus — *see* Injury, abdomen
aorta (thoracic) S25.00
  abdominal S35.00
    laceration (minor) (superficial) S35.01
      major S35.02
    specified type NEC S35.09
  laceration (minor) (superficial) S25.01
    major S25.02
  specified type NEC S25.09
arm (upper) S49.9-
  blood vessel — *see* Injury, blood vessel, arm
  contusion — *see* Contusion, arm, upper
  fracture — *see* Fracture, humerus
  lower — *see* Injury, forearm
  muscle — *see* Injury, muscle, shoulder
  nerve — *see* Injury, nerve, arm
  open — *see* Wound, open, arm
  specified type NEC S49.8-
  superficial — *see* Injury, superficial, arm
artery (complicating trauma) — *see also* Injury, blood vessel, by site
  cerebral or meningeal — *see* Injury, intracranial
auditory canal (external) (meatus) S09.91
auricle, auris, ear S09.91
axilla — *see* Injury, shoulder
back — *see* Injury, back, lower

Injury (*see also* specified injury type) T14.90 — *continued*
bile duct S36.13
birth (*see also* Birth, injury) P15.9
bladder (sphincter) S37.20
  at delivery O71.5
  contusion S37.22
  laceration S37.23
  obstetrical trauma O71.5
  specified type NEC S37.29
blast (air) (hydraulic) (immersion) (underwater) NEC T14.8
  acoustic nerve trauma — *see* Injury, nerve, acoustic
  bladder — *see* Injury, bladder
  brain — *see* Concussion
  colon — *see* Injury, intestine, large, blast injury
  ear (primary) S09.31-
    secondary S09.39-
  generalized T70.8
  lung — *see* Injury, intrathoracic, lung, blast injury
  multiple body organs T70.8
  peritoneum S36.81
  rectum S36.61
  retroperitoneum S36.898
  small intestine S36.419
    duodenum S36.410
    specified site NEC S36.418
  specified
    intra-abdominal organ NEC S36.898
    pelvic organ NEC S37.899
blood vessel NEC T14.8
  abdomen S35.9-
    aorta — *see* Injury, aorta, abdominal
    celiac artery — *see* Injury, blood vessel, celiac artery
    iliac vessel — *see* Injury, blood vessel, iliac
    laceration S35.91
    mesenteric vessel — *see* Injury, mesenteric
    portal vein — *see* Injury, blood vessel, portal vein
    renal vessel — *see* Injury, blood vessel, renal
    specified vessel NEC S35.8x-
    splenic vessel — *see* Injury, blood vessel, splenic
    vena cava — *see* Injury, vena cava, inferior
  ankle — *see* Injury, blood vessel, foot
  aorta (abdominal) (thoracic) — *see* Injury, aorta
  arm (upper) NEC S45.90-
    forearm — *see* Injury, blood vessel, forearm
    laceration S45.91-
    specified
      site NEC S45.80-
        laceration S45.81-
        specified type NEC S45.89-
      type NEC S45.99-
    superficial vein S45.30-
      laceration S45.31-
      specified type NEC S45.39-
    axillary
      artery S45.00-
        laceration S45.01-
        specified type NEC S45.09-
      vein S45.20-
        laceration S45.21-
        specified type NEC S45.29-
    azygos vein — *see* Injury, blood vessel, thoracic, specified site NEC
    brachial
      artery S45.10-
        laceration S45.11-
        specified type NEC S45.19-

Injury (*see also* specified injury type) T14.90 — continued
  blood vessel NEC T14.8 — *continued*
    brachial — *continued*
      vein S45.20-
        laceration S45.219
        specified type NEC S45.29-
    carotid artery (common) (external) (internal, extracranial) S15.00-
      internal, intracranial S06.8-
      laceration (minor) (superficial) S15.01-
        major S15.02-
      specified type NEC S15.09-
    celiac artery S35.219
      branch S35.299
        laceration (minor) (superficial) S35.291
          major S35.292
        specified NEC S35.298
      laceration (minor) (superficial) S35.211
        major S35.212
      specified type NEC S35.218
    cerebral — *see* Injury, intracranial
    deep plantar — *see* Injury, blood vessel, plantar artery
    digital (hand) — *see* Injury, blood vessel, finger
    dorsal
      artery (foot) S95.00-
        laceration S95.01-
        specified type NEC S95.09-
      vein (foot) S95.20-
        laceration S95.21-
        specified type NEC S95.29-
    due to accidental laceration during procedure — *see* Laceration, accidental complicating surgery
    extremity — *see* Injury, blood vessel, limb
    femoral
      artery (common) (superficial) S75.00-
        laceration (minor) (superficial) S75.01-
          major S75.02-
        specified type NEC S75.09-
      vein (hip level) (thigh level) S75.10-
        laceration (minor) (superficial) S75.11-
          major S75.12-
        specified type NEC S75.19-
    finger S65.50-
      index S65.50-
        laceration S65.51-
        specified type NEC S65.59-
      laceration S65.51-
      little S65.50-
        laceration S65.51-
        specified type NEC S65.59-
      middle S65.50-
      specified type NEC S65.59-
      thumb — *see* Injury, blood vessel, thumb
    foot S95.90-
      dorsal
        artery — *see* Injury, blood vessel, dorsal, artery
        vein — *see* Injury, blood vessel, dorsal, vein
      laceration S95.91-
      plantar artery — *see* Injury, blood vessel, plantar artery
      specified
        site NEC S95.80-
          laceration S95.81-
          specified type NEC S95.89-
        specified type NEC S95.99-
    forearm S55.90-
      laceration S55.91-
      radial artery — *see* Injury, blood vessel, radial artery

Injury (*see also* specified injury type) T14.90 — continued
  blood vessel NEC T14.8 — *continued*
    forearm S55.90- — *continued*
      specified
        site NEC S55.80-
          laceration S55.81-
          specified type NEC S55.89-
        type NEC S55.99-
    ulnar artery — *see* Injury, blood vessel, ulnar artery
      vein S55.20-
        laceration S55.21-
        specified type NEC S55.29-
    gastric
      artery — *see* Injury, mesenteric, artery, branch
      vein — *see* Injury, blood vessel, abdomen
    gastroduodenal artery — *see* Injury, mesenteric, artery, branch
    greater saphenous vein (lower leg level) S85.30-
      hip (and thigh) level S75.20-
        laceration (minor) (superficial) S75.21-
          major S75.22-
        specified type NEC S75.29-
      laceration S85.31-
      specified type NEC S85.39-
    hand (level) S65.90-
      finger — *see* Injury, blood vessel, finger
      laceration S65.91-
      palmar arch — *see* Injury, blood vessel, palmar arch
      radial artery — *see* Injury, blood vessel, radial artery, hand
      specified
        site NEC S65.80-
          laceration S65.81-
          specified type NEC S65.89-
        type NEC S65.99-
      thumb — *see* Injury, blood vessel, thumb
      ulnar artery — *see* Injury, blood vessel, ulnar artery, hand
    head S09.0
      intracranial — *see* Injury, intracranial
      multiple S09.0
    hepatic
      artery — *see* Injury, mesenteric, artery
      vein — *see* Injury, vena cava, inferior
    hip S75.90-
      femoral artery — *see* Injury, blood vessel, femoral, artery
      femoral vein — *see* Injury, blood vessel, femoral, vein
      greater saphenous vein — *see* Injury, blood vessel, greater saphenous, hip level
      laceration S75.91-
      specified
        site NEC S75.80-
          laceration S75.81-
          specified type NEC S75.89-
        type NEC S75.99-
    hypogastric (artery) (vein) — *see* Injury, blood vessel, iliac
    iliac S35.5-
      artery S35.51-
      specified vessel NEC S35.5-
      uterine vessel — *see* Injury, blood vessel, uterine
      vein S35.51-
    innominate — *see* Injury, blood vessel, thoracic, innominate
    intercostal (artery) (vein) — *see* Injury, blood vessel, thoracic, intercostal

Injury (*see also* specified injury type) T14.90 — continued
  blood vessel NEC T14.8 — *continued*
    jugular vein (external) S15.20-
      internal S15.30-
        laceration (minor) (superficial) S15.31-
          major S15.32-
        specified type NEC S15.39-
      laceration (minor) (superficial) S15.21-
        major S15.22-
      specified type NEC S15.29-
    leg (level) (lower) S85.90-
      greater saphenous — *see* Injury, blood vessel, greater saphenous
      laceration S85.91-
      lesser saphenous — *see* Injury, blood vessel, lesser saphenous
      peroneal artery — *see* Injury, blood vessel, peroneal artery
      popliteal
        artery — *see* Injury, blood vessel, popliteal, artery
        vein — *see* Injury, blood vessel, popliteal, vein
      specified
        site NEC S85.80-
          laceration S85.81-
          specified type NEC S85.89-
        type NEC S85.99-
      thigh — *see* Injury, blood vessel, hip
      tibial artery — *see* Injury, blood vessel, tibial artery
    lesser saphenous vein (lower leg level) S85.40-
      laceration S85.41-
      specified type NEC S85.49-
    limb
      lower — *see* Injury, blood vessel, leg
      upper — *see* Injury, blood vessel, arm
    lower back — *see* Injury, blood vessel, abdomen
    specified NEC — *see* Injury, blood vessel, abdomen, specified, site NEC
    mammary (artery) (vein) — *see* Injury, blood vessel, thoracic, specified site NEC
    mesenteric (inferior) (superior)
      artery — *see* Injury, mesenteric, artery
      vein — *see* Injury, mesenteric, vein
    neck S15.9
      specified site NEC S15.8
    ovarian (artery) (vein) — *see* subcategory S35.8
    palmar arch (superficial) S65.20-
      deep S65.30-
        laceration S65.31-
        specified type NEC S65.39-
      laceration S65.21-
      specified type NEC S65.29-
    pelvis — *see* Injury, blood vessel, abdomen
    specified NEC — *see* Injury, blood vessel, abdomen, specified, site NEC
    peroneal artery S85.20-
      laceration S85.21-
      specified type NEC S85.29-
    plantar artery (deep) (foot) S95.10-
      laceration S95.11-
      specified type NEC S95.19-
    popliteal
      artery S85.00-
        laceration S85.01-
        specified type NEC S85.09-
      vein S85.50-
        laceration S85.51-
        specified type NEC S85.59-
    portal vein S35.319
      laceration S35.311
      specified type NEC S35.318
    precerebral — *see* Injury, blood vessel, neck

Injury (*see also* specified injury type) T14.90 — *continued*
blood vessel NEC T14.8 — *continued*
pulmonary (artery) (vein) — *see* Injury, blood vessel, thoracic, pulmonary
radial artery (forearm level) S55.10-
 hand and wrist (level) S65.10-
  laceration S65.11-
  specified type NEC S65.19-
 laceration S55.11-
 specified type NEC S55.19-
renal
 artery S35.40-
  laceration S35.41-
  specified NEC S35.49-
 vein S35.40-
  laceration S35.41-
  specified NEC S35.49-
saphenous vein (greater) (lower leg level) — *see* Injury, blood vessel, greater saphenous
 hip and thigh level — *see* Injury, blood vessel, greater saphenous, hip level
 lesser — *see* Injury, blood vessel, lesser saphenous
shoulder
 specified NEC — *see* Injury, blood vessel, arm, specified site NEC
 superficial vein — *see* Injury, blood vessel, arm, superficial vein
specified NEC T14.8
splenic
 artery — *see* Injury, blood vessel, celiac artery, branch
 vein S35.329
  laceration S35.321
  specified NEC S35.328
subclavian — *see* Injury, blood vessel, thoracic, innominate
thigh — *see* Injury, blood vessel, hip
thoracic S25.90
 aorta S25.00
  laceration (minor) (superficial) S25.01
  major S25.02
  specified type NEC S25.09
 azygos vein — *see* Injury, blood vessel, thoracic, specified, site NEC
 innominate
  artery S25.10-
   laceration (minor) (superficial) S25.11-
   major S25.12-
   specified type NEC S25.19-
  vein S25.30-
   laceration (minor) (superficial) S25.31-
   major S25.32-
   specified type NEC S25.39-
 intercostal S25.50-
  laceration S25.51-
  specified type NEC S25.59-
 laceration S25.91
 mammary vessel — *see* Injury, blood vessel, thoracic, specified, site NEC
 pulmonary S25.40-
  laceration (minor) (superficial) S25.41-
  major S25.42-
  specified type NEC S25.49-
 specified
  site NEC S25.80-
   laceration S25.81-
   specified type NEC S25.89-
  type NEC S25.99
 subclavian — *see* Injury, blood vessel, thoracic, innominate
 vena cava (superior) S25.20
  laceration (minor) (superficial) S25.21
  major S25.22
  specified type NEC S25.29

Injury (*see also* specified injury type) T14.90 — *continued*
blood vessel NEC T14.8 — *continued*
thumb S65.40-
 laceration S65.41-
 specified type NEC S65.49-
tibial artery S85.10-
 anterior S85.13-
  laceration S85.14-
  specified injury NEC S85.15-
 laceration S85.11-
 posterior S85.16-
  laceration S85.17-
  specified injury NEC S85.18-
 specified injury NEC S85.12-
ulnar artery (forearm level) S55.00-
 hand and wrist (level) S65.00-
  laceration S65.01-
  specified type NEC S65.09-
 laceration S55.01-
 specified type NEC S55.09-
upper arm (level) — *see* Injury, blood vessel, arm
 superficial vein — *see* Injury, blood vessel, arm, superficial vein
uterine S35.5-
 artery S35.53-
 vein S35.53-
vena cava — *see* Injury, vena cava
vertebral artery S15.10-
 laceration (minor) (superficial) S15.11-
  major S15.12-
 specified type NEC S15.19-
wrist (level) — *see* Injury, blood vessel, hand
brachial plexus S14.3
 newborn P14.3
brain (traumatic) S06.9-
 diffuse (axonal) S06.2x-
 focal S06.30-
brainstem S06.38-
breast NOS S29.9
broad ligament — *see* Injury, pelvic organ, specified site NEC
bronchus, bronchi — *see* Injury, intrathoracic, bronchus
brow S09.90
buttock S39.92
canthus, eye S05.90
cardiac plexus — *see* Injury, nerve, thorax, sympathetic
cauda equina S34.3
cavernous sinus — *see* Injury, intracranial
cecum — *see* Injury, colon
celiac ganglion or plexus — *see* Injury, nerve, lumbosacral, sympathetic
cerebellum — *see* Injury, intracranial
cerebral — *see* Injury, intracranial
cervix (uteri) — *see* Injury, uterus
cheek (wall) S09.93
chest — *see* Injury, thorax
childbirth (newborn) — *see also* Birth, injury
 maternal NEC O71.9
chin S09.93
choroid (eye) — *see* Injury, eye, specified site NEC
clitoris S39.94
coccyx — *see also* Injury, back, lower
 complicating delivery O71.6
colon — *see* Injury, intestine, large
common bile duct — *see* Injury, liver
conjunctiva (superficial) — *see* Injury, eye, conjunctiva
conus medullaris — *see* Injury, spinal, sacral cord
cord
 spermatic (pelvic region) S37.898
  scrotal region S39.848
 spinal — *see* Injury, spinal cord, by region

Injury (*see also* specified injury type) T14.90 — *continued*
cornea — *see* Injury, eye, specified site NEC
 abrasion — *see* Injury, eye, cornea, abrasion
cortex (cerebral) — *see also* Injury, intracranial
 visual — *see* Injury, nerve, optic
costal region NEC S29.9
costochondral NEC S29.9
cranial
 cavity — *see* Injury, intracranial
 nerve — *see* Injury, nerve, cranial
crushing — *see* Crush
cutaneous sensory nerve
cystic duct — *see* Injury, liver
deep tissue — *see* Contusion, by site
 meaning pressure ulcer — *see* Ulcer, pressure, unstageable, by site
delivery (newborn) P15.9
 maternal NEC O71.9
Descemet's membrane — *see* Injury, eyeball, penetrating
diaphragm — *see* Injury, intrathoracic, diaphragm
duodenum — *see* Injury, intestine, small, duodenum
ear (auricle) (external) (canal) S09.91
 abrasion — *see* Abrasion, ear
 bite — *see* Bite, ear
 blister — *see* Blister, ear
 bruise — *see* Contusion, ear
 contusion — *see* Contusion, ear
 external constriction — *see* Constriction, external, ear
 hematoma — *see* Hematoma, ear
 inner — *see* Injury, ear, middle
 laceration — *see* Laceration, ear
 middle S09.30-
  blast — *see* Injury, blast, ear
  specified NEC S09.39-
 puncture — *see* Puncture, ear
 superficial — *see* Injury, superficial, ear
eighth cranial nerve (acoustic or auditory) — *see* Injury, nerve, acoustic
elbow S59.90-
 contusion — *see* Contusion, elbow
 dislocation — *see* Dislocation, elbow
 fracture — *see* Fracture, ulna, upper end
 open — *see* Wound, open, elbow
 specified NEC S59.80-
 sprain — *see* Sprain, elbow
 superficial — *see* Injury, superficial, elbow
eleventh cranial nerve (accessory) — *see* Injury, nerve, accessory
epididymis S39.94
epigastric region S39.91
epiglottis NEC S19.89
esophageal plexus — *see* Injury, nerve, thorax, sympathetic
esophagus (thoracic part) — *see also* Injury, intrathoracic, esophagus
 cervical NEC S19.85
eustachian tube S09.30-
eye S05.9-
 avulsion S05.7-
 ball — *see* Injury, eyeball
 conjunctiva S05.0-
 cornea
  abrasion S05.0-
  laceration S05.3-
   with prolapse S05.2-
 lacrimal apparatus S05.8x-
 orbit penetration S05.4-
 specified site NEC S05.8x-

Injury (*see also* specified injury type) T14.90 — *continued*
  eyeball S05.8x-
    contusion S05.1-
    penetrating S05.6-
      with
        foreign body S05.5-
          prolapse or loss of intraocular tissue S05.2-
        without prolapse or loss of intraocular tissue S05.3-
    specified type NEC S05.8-
  eyebrow S09.93
  eyelid S09.93
    abrasion — *see* Abrasion, eyelid
    contusion — *see* Contusion, eyelid
    open — *see* Wound, open, eyelid
  face S09.93
  fallopian tube S37.509
    bilateral S37.502
      blast injury S37.512
      contusion S37.522
      laceration S37.532
      specified type NEC S37.592
    blast injury (primary) S37.519
      bilateral S37.512
      secondary — *see* Injury, fallopian tube, specified type NEC
      unilateral S37.511
    contusion S37.529
      bilateral S37.522
      unilateral S37.521
    laceration S37.539
      bilateral S37.532
      unilateral S37.531
    specified type NEC S37.599
      bilateral S37.592
      unilateral S37.591
    unilateral S37.501
      blast injury S37.511
      contusion S37.521
      laceration S37.531
      specified type NEC S37.591
  fascia — *see* Injury, muscle
  fifth cranial nerve (trigeminal) — *see* Injury, nerve, trigeminal
  finger (nail) S69.9-
    blood vessel — *see* Injury, blood vessel, finger
    contusion — *see* Contusion, finger
    dislocation — *see* Dislocation, finger
    fracture — *see* Fracture, finger
    muscle — *see* Injury, muscle, finger
    nerve — *see* Injury, nerve, digital, finger
    open — *see* Wound, open, finger
    specified NEC S69.8-
    sprain — *see* Sprain, finger
    superficial — *see* Injury, superficial, finger
  first cranial nerve (olfactory) — *see* Injury, nerve, olfactory
  flank — *see* Injury, abdomen
  foot S99.92-
    blood vessel — *see* Injury, blood vessel, foot
    contusion — *see* Contusion, foot
    dislocation — *see* Dislocation, foot
    fracture — *see* Fracture, foot
    muscle — *see* Injury, muscle, foot
    open — *see* Wound, open, foot
    specified type NEC S99.82-
    sprain — *see* Sprain, foot
    superficial — *see* Injury, superficial, foot
  forceps NOS P15.9
  forearm S59.91-
    blood vessel — *see* Injury, blood vessel, forearm
    contusion — *see* Contusion, forearm
    fracture — *see* Fracture, forearm
    muscle — *see* Injury, muscle, forearm
    nerve — *see* Injury, nerve, forearm

Injury (*see also* specified injury type) T14.90 — *continued*
  forearm S59.91- — *continued*
    open — *see* Wound, open, forearm
    specified NEC S59.81-
    superficial — *see* Injury, superficial, forearm
  forehead S09.90
  fourth cranial nerve (trochlear) — *see* Injury, nerve, trochlear
  gallbladder S36.129
    contusion S36.122
    laceration S36.123
    specified NEC S36.128
  ganglion
    celiac, coeliac — *see* Injury, nerve, lumbosacral, sympathetic
    gasserian — *see* Injury, nerve, trigeminal
    stellate — *see* Injury, nerve, thorax, sympathetic
    thoracic sympathetic — *see* Injury, nerve, thorax, sympathetic
  gasserian ganglion — *see* Injury, nerve, trigeminal
  gastric artery — *see* Injury, blood vessel, celiac artery, branch
  gastroduodenal artery — *see* Injury, blood vessel, celiac artery, branch
  gastrointestinal tract — *see* Injury, intra-abdominal
    with open wound into abdominal cavity — *see* Wound, open, with penetration into peritoneal cavity
    colon — *see* Injury, intestine, large
    rectum — *see* Injury, intestine, large, rectum
    with open wound into abdominal cavity S36.61
    small intestine — *see* Injury, intestine, small
    specified site NEC — *see* Injury, intra-abdominal, specified, site NEC
    stomach — *see* Injury, stomach
  genital organ(s)
    external S39.94
      specified NEC S39.848
    internal S37.90
      fallopian tube — *see* Injury, fallopian tube
      ovary — *see* Injury, ovary
      prostate — *see* Injury, prostate
      seminal vesicle — *see* Injury, pelvis, organ, specified site NEC
      uterus — *see* Injury, uterus
      vas deferens — *see* Injury, pelvis, organ, specified site NEC
    obstetrical trauma O71.9
  gland
    lacrimal laceration — *see* Injury, eye, specified site NEC
    salivary S09.93
    thyroid NEC S19.84
  globe (eye) S05.90
    specified NEC S05.8x-
  groin — *see* Injury, abdomen
  gum S09.90
  hand S69.9-
    blood vessel — *see* Injury, blood vessel, hand
    contusion — *see* Contusion, hand
    fracture — *see* Fracture, hand
    muscle — *see* Injury, muscle, hand
    nerve — *see* Injury, nerve, hand
    open — *see* Wound, open, hand
    specified NEC S69.8-
    sprain — *see* Sprain, hand
    superficial — *see* Injury, superficial, hand
  head S09.90
    with loss of consciousness S06.9-
    specified NEC S09.8

Injury (*see also* specified injury type) T14.90 — *continued*
  heart S26.90
    with hemopericardium S26.00
      contusion S26.01
      laceration (mild) S26.020
        major S26.022
        moderate S26.021
      specified type NEC S26.09
    contusion S26.91
    laceration S26.92
    specified type NEC S26.99
    without hemopericardium S26.10
      contusion S26.11
      laceration S26.12
      specified type NEC S26.19
  heel — *see* Injury, foot
  hepatic
    artery — *see* Injury, blood vessel, celiac artery, branch
    duct — *see* Injury, liver
    vein — *see* Injury, vena cava, inferior
  hip S79.91-
    blood vessel — *see* Injury, blood vessel, hip
    contusion — *see* Contusion, hip
    dislocation — *see* Dislocation, hip
    fracture — *see* Fracture, femur, neck
    muscle — *see* Injury, muscle, hip
    nerve — *see* Injury, nerve, hip
    open — *see* Wound, open, hip
    specified NEC S79.81-
    sprain — *see* Sprain, hip
    superficial — *see* Injury, superficial, hip
  hymen S39.94
  hypogastric
    blood vessel — *see* Injury, blood vessel, iliac
    plexus — *see* Injury, nerve, lumbosacral, sympathetic
  ileum — *see* Injury, intestine, small
  iliac region S39.91
  instrumental (during surgery) — *see* Laceration, accidental complicating surgery
    birth injury — *see* Birth, injury
    nonsurgical — *see* Injury, by site
    obstetrical O71.9
      bladder O71.5
      cervix O71.3
      high vaginal O71.4
      perineal NOS O70.9
      urethra O71.5
      uterus O71.5
        with rupture or perforation O71.1
  internal T14.8
    aorta — *see* Injury, aorta
    bladder (sphincter) — *see* Injury, bladder
      with
        ectopic or molar pregnancy O08.6
        following ectopic or molar pregnancy O08.6
        obstetrical trauma O71.5
    bronchus, bronchi — *see* Injury, intrathoracic, bronchus
    cecum — *see* Injury, intestine, large
    cervix (uteri) — *see also* Injury, uterus
      with ectopic or molar pregnancy O08.6
      following ectopic or molar pregnancy O08.6
      obstetrical trauma O71.3
    chest — *see* Injury, intrathoracic
    gastrointestinal tract — *see* Injury, intra-abdominal
    heart — *see* Injury, heart
    intestine NEC — *see* Injury, intestine
    intrauterine — *see* Injury, uterus
    mesentery — *see* Injury, intra-abdominal, specified, site NEC

Injury (see also specified injury type) T14.90 — continued
  internal T14.8 — continued
    pelvis, pelvic (organ) S37.90
      following ectopic or molar pregnancy (subsequent episode) O08.6
      obstetrical trauma NEC O71.5
      rupture or perforation O71.1
      specified NEC S39.83
    rectum — see Injury, intestine, large, rectum
    stomach — see Injury, stomach
    ureter — see Injury, ureter
    urethra (sphincter) following ectopic or molar pregnancy O08.6
    uterus — see Injury, uterus
  interscapular area — see Injury, thorax
  intestine
    large S36.509
      ascending (right) S36.500
        blast injury (primary) S36.510
          secondary S36.590
        contusion S36.520
        laceration S36.530
        specified type NEC S36.590
      blast injury (primary) S36.519
        ascending (right) S36.510
        descending (left) S36.512
        rectum S36.61
        sigmoid S36.513
        specified site NEC S36.518
        transverse S36.511
      contusion S36.529
        ascending (right) S36.520
        descending (left) S36.522
        rectum S36.62
        sigmoid S36.523
        specified site NEC S36.528
        transverse S36.521
      descending (left) S36.502
        blast injury (primary) S36.512
          secondary S36.592
        contusion S36.522
        laceration S36.532
        specified type NEC S36.592
      laceration S36.539
        ascending (right) S36.530
        descending (left) S36.532
        rectum S36.63
        sigmoid S36.533
        specified site NEC S36.538
        transverse S36.531
      rectum S36.60
        blast injury (primary) S36.61
          secondary S36.69
        contusion S36.62
        laceration S36.63
        specified type NEC S36.69
      sigmoid S36.503
        blast injury (primary) S36.513
          secondary S36.593
        contusion S36.523
        laceration S36.533
        specified type NEC S36.593
      specified
        site NEC S36.508
          blast injury (primary) S36.518
            secondary S36.598
          contusion S36.528
          laceration S36.538
          specified type NEC S36.598
        type NEC S36.599
          ascending (right) S36.590
          descending (left) S36.592
          rectum S36.69
          sigmoid S36.593
          specified site NEC S36.598
          transverse S36.591

Injury (see also specified injury type) T14.90 — continued
  intestine — continued
    large S36.509 — continued
      transverse S36.501
        blast injury (primary) S36.511
          secondary S36.591
        contusion S36.521
        laceration S36.531
        specified type NEC S36.591
    small S36.409
      blast injury (primary) S36.419
        duodenum S36.410
        secondary S36.499
          duodenum S36.490
          specified site NEC S36.498
        specified site NEC S36.418
      contusion S36.429
        duodenum S36.420
        specified site NEC S36.428
      duodenum S36.400
        blast injury (primary) S36.410
          secondary S36.490
        contusion S36.420
        laceration S36.430
        specified NEC S36.490
      laceration S36.439
        duodenum S36.430
        specified site NEC S36.438
      specified
        site NEC S36.408
        type NEC S36.499
          duodenum S36.490
          specified site NEC S36.498
  intra-abdominal S36.90
    adrenal gland — see Injury, adrenal gland
    bladder — see Injury, bladder
    colon — see Injury, intestine, large
    contusion S36.92
    fallopian tube — see Injury, fallopian tube
    gallbladder — see Injury, gallbladder
    intestine — see Injury, intestine
    kidney — see Injury, kidney
    laceration S36.93
    liver — see Injury, liver
    ovary — see Injury, ovary
    pancreas — see Injury, pancreas
    pelvic NOS S37.90
    peritoneum — see Injury, intra-abdominal, specified, site NEC
    prostate — see Injury, prostate
    rectum — see Injury, intestine, large, rectum
    retroperitoneum — see Injury, intra-abdominal, specified, site NEC
    seminal vesicle — see Injury, pelvis, organ, specified site NEC
    small intestine — see Injury, intestine, small
    specified
      pelvic S37.90
        specified
          site NEC S37.899
            specified type NEC S37.898
          type NEC S37.99
      site NEC S36.899
        contusion S36.892
        laceration S36.893
        specified type NEC S36.898
      type NEC S36.99
    spleen — see Injury, spleen
    stomach — see Injury, stomach
    ureter — see Injury, ureter
    urethra — see Injury, urethra
    uterus — see Injury, uterus
    vas deferens — see Injury, pelvis, organ, specified site NEC

Injury (see also specified injury type) T14.90 — continued
  intracranial (traumatic) S06.9-
    cerebellar hemorrhage, traumatic — see Injury, intracranial, focal
    cerebral edema, traumatic S06.1x-
      diffuse S06.1x-
      focal S06.1x-
    diffuse (axonal) S06.2x-
    epidural hemorrhage (traumatic) S06.4x-
    focal brain injury S06.30-
      contusion — see Contusion, cerebral
      laceration — see Laceration, cerebral
      intracerebral hemorrhage, traumatic S06.36-
        left side S06.35-
        right side S06.34-
      subarachnoid hemorrhage, traumatic S06.6x-
      subdural hemorrhage, traumatic S06.5x-
  intraocular — see Injury, eyeball, penetrating
  intrathoracic S27.9
    bronchus S27.409
      bilateral S27.402
      blast injury (primary) S27.419
        bilateral S27.412
        secondary — see Injury, intrathoracic, bronchus, specified type NEC
        unilateral S27.411
      contusion S27.429
        bilateral S27.422
        unilateral S27.421
      laceration S27.439
        bilateral S27.432
        unilateral S27.431
      specified type NEC S27.499
        bilateral S27.492
        unilateral S27.491
      unilateral S27.401
    diaphragm S27.809
      contusion S27.802
      laceration S27.803
      specified type NEC S27.808
    esophagus (thoracic) S27.819
      contusion S27.812
      laceration S27.813
      specified type NEC S27.818
    heart — see Injury, heart
    hemopneumothorax S27.2
    hemothorax S27.1
    lung S27.309
      aspiration J69.0
      bilateral S27.302
      blast injury (primary) S27.319
        bilateral S27.312
        secondary — see Injury, intrathoracic, lung, specified type NEC
        unilateral S27.311
      contusion S27.329
        bilateral S27.322
        unilateral S27.321
      laceration S27.339
        bilateral S27.332
        unilateral S27.331
      specified type NEC S27.399
        bilateral S27.392
        unilateral S27.391
      unilateral S27.301
    pleura S27.60
      laceration S27.63
      specified type NEC S27.69
    pneumothorax S27.0
    specified organ NEC S27.899
      contusion S27.892
      laceration S27.893
      specified type NEC S27.898
    thoracic duct — see Injury, intrathoracic, specified organ NEC

Injury (see also specified injury type) T14.90 — continued
intrathoracic S27.9 — continued
thymus gland — see Injury, intrathoracic, specified organ NEC
trachea, thoracic S27.50
blast (primary) S27.51
contusion S27.52
laceration S27.53
specified type NEC S27.59
iris — see Injury, eye, specified site NEC
penetrating — see Injury, eyeball, penetrating
jaw S09.93
jejunum — see Injury, intestine, small
joint NOS T14.8
old or residual — see Disorder, joint, specified type NEC
kidney S37.00-
acute (nontraumatic) N17.9
contusion — see Contusion, kidney
laceration — see Laceration, kidney
specified NEC S37.09-
knee S89.9-
contusion — see Contusion, knee
dislocation — see Dislocation, knee
meniscus (lateral) (medial) — see Sprain, knee, specified site NEC
old injury or tear — see Derangement, knee, meniscus, due to old injury
open — see Wound, open, knee
specified NEC S89.8-
sprain — see Sprain, knee
superficial — see Injury, superficial, knee
labium (majus) (minus) S39.94
labyrinth, ear S09.30-
lacrimal apparatus, duct, gland, or sac — see Injury, eye, specified site NEC
larynx NEC S19.81
leg (lower) S89.9-
blood vessel — see Injury, blood vessel, leg
contusion — see Contusion, leg
fracture — see Fracture, leg
muscle — see Injury, muscle, leg
nerve — see Injury, nerve, leg
open — see Wound, open, leg
specified NEC S89.8-
superficial — see Injury, superficial, leg
lens, eye — see Injury, eye, specified site NEC
penetrating — see Injury, eyeball, penetrating
limb NEC T14.8
lip S09.93
liver S36.119
contusion S36.112
laceration S36.113
major (stellate) S36.116
minor S36.114
moderate S36.115
specified NEC S36.118
lower back S39.92
specified NEC S39.82
lumbar, lumbosacral (region) S39.92
plexus — see Injury, lumbosacral plexus
lumbosacral plexus S34.4
lung — see also Injury, intrathoracic, lung
aspiration J69.0
transfusion-related (TRALI) J95.84
lymphatic thoracic duct — see Injury, intrathoracic, specified organ NEC
malar region S09.93
mastoid region S09.90
maxilla S09.93
mediastinum — see Injury, intrathoracic, specified organ NEC
membrane, brain — see Injury, intracranial
meningeal artery — see Injury, intracranial, subdural hemorrhage
meninges (cerebral) — see Injury, intracranial

Injury (see also specified injury type) T14.90 — continued
mesenteric
artery
branch S35.299
laceration (minor) (superficial) S35.291
major S35.292
specified NEC S35.298
inferior S35.239
laceration (minor) (superficial) S35.231
major S35.232
specified NEC S35.238
superior S35.229
laceration (minor) (superficial) S35.221
major S35.222
specified NEC S35.228
plexus (inferior) (superior) — see Injury, nerve, lumbosacral, sympathetic
vein
inferior S35.349
laceration S35.341
specified NEC S35.348
superior S35.339
laceration S35.331
specified NEC S35.338
mesentery — see Injury, intra-abdominal, specified site NEC
mesosalpinx — see Injury, pelvic organ, specified site NEC
middle ear S09.30-
midthoracic region NOS S29.9
mouth S09.93
multiple NOS T07
muscle (and fascia) (and tendon)
abdomen S39.001
laceration S39.021
specified type NEC S39.091
strain S39.011
abductor
thumb, forearm level — see Injury, muscle, thumb, abductor
adductor
thigh S76.20-
laceration S76.22-
specified type NEC S76.29-
strain S76.21-
ankle — see Injury, muscle, foot
anterior muscle group, at leg level (lower) S86.20-
laceration S86.22-
specified type NEC S86.29-
strain S86.21-
arm (upper) — see Injury, muscle, shoulder
biceps (parts NEC) S46.20-
laceration S46.22-
long head S46.10-
laceration S46.12-
specified type NEC S46.19-
strain S46.11-
specified type NEC S46.29-
strain S46.21-
extensor
finger(s) (other than thumb) — see Injury, muscle, finger by site, extensor
forearm level, specified NEC — see Injury, muscle, forearm, extensor
thumb — see Injury, muscle, thumb, extensor
toe (large) (ankle level) (foot level) — see Injury, muscle, toe, extensor
finger
extensor (forearm level) S56.40-
hand level S66.309
laceration S66.329
specified type NEC S66.399
strain S66.319
laceration S56.429
specified type NEC S56.499
strain S56.419

Injury (see also specified injury type) T14.90 — continued
muscle (and fascia) (and tendon) — continued
finger — continued
flexor (forearm level) S56.10-
hand level S66.109
laceration S66.129
specified type NEC S66.199
strain S66.119
laceration S56.129
specified type NEC S56.199
strain S56.119
index
extensor (forearm level)
hand level S66.308
laceration S66.32-
specified type NEC S66.39-
strain S66.31-
specified type NEC S56.492-
flexor (forearm level)
hand level S66.108
laceration S66.12-
specified type NEC S66.19-
strain S66.11-
specified type NEC S56.19-
strain S56.11-
intrinsic S66.50-
laceration S66.52-
specified type NEC S66.59-
strain S66.51-
intrinsic S66.509
laceration S66.529
specified type NEC S66.599
strain S66.519
little
extensor (forearm level)
hand level S66.30-
laceration S66.32-
specified type NEC S66.39-
strain S66.31-
laceration S56.42-
specified type NEC S56.49-
strain S56.41-
flexor (forearm level)
hand level S66.10-
laceration S66.12-
specified type NEC S66.19-
strain S66.11-
laceration S56.12-
specified type NEC S56.19-
strain S56.11-
intrinsic S66.50-
laceration S66.52-
specified type NEC S66.59-
strain S66.51-
middle
extensor (forearm level)
hand level S66.30-
laceration S66.32-
specified type NEC S66.39-
strain S66.31-
laceration S56.42-
specified type NEC S56.49-
strain S56.41-
flexor (forearm level)
hand level S66.10-
laceration S66.12-
specified type NEC S66.19-
strain S66.11-
laceration S56.12-
specified type NEC S56.19-
strain S56.11-
intrinsic S66.50-
laceration S66.52-
specified type NEC S66.59-
strain S66.51-

Injury (*see also* specified injury type) T14.90 — *continued*
 muscle (and fascia) (and tendon) — *continued*
  finger — *continued*
   ring
    extensor (forearm level)
     hand level S66.30-
      laceration S66.32-
      specified type NEC S66.39-
      strain S66.31-
     laceration S56.42-
     specified type NEC S56.49-
     strain S56.41-
    flexor (forearm level)
     hand level S66.10-
      laceration S66.12-
      specified type NEC S66.19-
      strain S66.11-
     laceration S56.12-
     specified type NEC S56.19-
     strain S56.11-
    intrinsic S66.50-
     laceration S66.52-
     specified type NEC S66.59-
     strain S66.51-
 flexor
  finger(s) (other than thumb) — *see* Injury, muscle, finger
  forearm level, specified NEC — *see* Injury, muscle, forearm, flexor
  thumb — *see* Injury, muscle, thumb, flexor
  toe (long) (ankle level) (foot level) — *see* Injury, muscle, toe, flexor
 foot S96.90-
  intrinsic S96.20-
   laceration S96.22-
   specified type NEC S96.29-
   strain S96.21-
  laceration S96.92-
  long extensor, toe — *see* Injury, muscle, toe, extensor
  long flexor, toe — *see* Injury, muscle, toe, flexor
  specified
   site NEC S96.80-
    laceration S96.82-
    specified type NEC S96.89-
    strain S96.81-
   type NEC S96.99-
  strain S96.91-
 forearm (level) S56.90-
  extensor S56.50-
   laceration S56.52-
   specified type NEC S56.59-
   strain S56.51-
  flexor S56.20-
   laceration S56.22-
   specified type NEC S56.29-
   strain S56.21-
  laceration S56.92-
  specified S56.99-
   site NEC S56.80-
    laceration S56.82-
    strain S56.81-
    type NEC S56.89-
  strain S56.91-
 hand (level) S66.90-
  laceration S66.92-
  specified
   site NEC S66.80-
    laceration S66.82-
    specified type NEC S66.89-
    strain S66.81-
   type NEC S66.99-
  strain S66.91-

Injury (*see also* specified injury type) T14.90 — *continued*
 muscle (and fascia) (and tendon) — *continued*
  head S09.10
   laceration S09.12
   specified type NEC S09.19
   strain S09.11
  hip NEC S76.00-
   laceration S76.02-
   specified type NEC S76.09-
   strain S76.01-
  intrinsic
   ankle and foot level — *see* Injury, muscle, foot, intrinsic
   finger (other than thumb) — *see* Injury, muscle, finger by site, intrinsic
   foot (level) — *see* Injury, muscle, foot, intrinsic
   thumb — *see* Injury, muscle, thumb, intrinsic
  leg (level) (lower) S86.90-
   Achilles tendon — *see* Injury, Achilles tendon
   anterior muscle group — *see* Injury, muscle, anterior muscle group
   laceration S86.92-
   peroneal muscle group — *see* Injury, muscle, peroneal muscle group
   posterior muscle group — *see* Injury, muscle, posterior muscle group, leg level
   specified
    site NEC S86.80-
     laceration S86.82-
     specified type NEC S86.89-
     strain S86.81-
    type NEC S86.99-
   strain S86.91-
  long
   extensor toe, at ankle and foot level — *see* Injury, muscle, toe, extensor
   flexor, toe, at ankle and foot level — *see* Injury, muscle, toe, flexor
   head, biceps — *see* Injury, muscle, biceps, long head
  lower back S39.002
   laceration S39.022
   specified type NEC S39.092
   strain S39.012
  neck (level) S16.9
   laceration S16.2
   specified type NEC S16.8
   strain S16.1
  pelvis S39.003
   laceration S39.023
   specified type NEC S39.093
   strain S39.013
  peroneal muscle group, at leg level (lower) S86.30-
   laceration S86.32-
   specified type NEC S86.39-
   strain S86.31-
  posterior muscle (group)
   leg level (lower) S86.10-
    laceration S86.12-
    specified type NEC S86.19-
    strain S86.11-
   thigh level S76.30-
    laceration S76.32-
    specified type NEC S76.39-
    strain S76.31-
  quadriceps (thigh) S76.10-
   laceration S76.12-
   specified type NEC S76.19-
   strain S76.11-
  shoulder S46.90-
   laceration S46.92-
   rotator cuff — *see* Injury, rotator cuff

Injury (*see also* specified injury type) T14.90 — *continued*
 muscle (and fascia) (and tendon) — *continued*
  shoulder S46.90- — *continued*
   specified site NEC S46.80-
    laceration S46.82-
    specified type NEC S46.89-
    strain S46.81-
   specified type NEC S46.99-
   strain S46.91-
  thigh NEC (level) S76.90-
   adductor — *see* Injury, muscle, adductor, thigh
   laceration S76.92-
   posterior muscle (group) — *see* Injury, muscle, posterior muscle, thigh level
   quadriceps — *see* Injury, muscle, quadriceps
   specified
    site NEC S76.80-
     laceration S76.82-
     specified type NEC S76.89-
     strain S76.81-
    type NEC S76.99-
   strain S76.91-
  thorax (level) S29.009
   back wall S29.002
   front wall S29.001
   laceration S29.029
    back wall S29.022
    front wall S29.021
   specified type NEC S29.099
    back wall S29.092
    front wall S29.091
   strain S29.019
    back wall S29.012
    front wall S29.011
  thumb
   abductor (forearm level) S56.30-
    laceration S56.32-
    specified type NEC S56.39-
    strain S56.31-
   extensor (forearm level) S56.30-
    hand level S66.20-
     laceration S66.22-
     specified type NEC S66.29-
     strain S66.21-
    laceration S56.32-
    specified type NEC S56.39-
    strain S56.31-
   flexor (forearm level) S56.00-
    hand level S66.00-
     laceration S66.02-
     specified type NEC S66.09-
     strain S66.01-
    laceration S56.02-
    specified type NEC S56.09-
    strain S56.01-
    wrist level — *see* Injury, muscle, thumb, flexor, hand level
   intrinsic S66.40-
    laceration S66.42-
    specified type NEC S66.49-
    strain S66.41-
  toe — *see also* Injury, muscle, foot
   extensor, long S96.10-
    laceration S96.12-
    specified type NEC S96.19-
    strain S96.11-
   flexor, long S96.00-
    laceration S96.02-
    specified type NEC S96.09-
    strain S96.01-
  triceps S46.30-
   laceration S46.32-
   specified type NEC S46.39-
   strain S46.31-
  wrist (and hand) level — *see* Injury, muscle, hand

Injury (see also specified injury type) T14.90 — continued

musculocutaneous nerve — see Injury, nerve, musculocutaneous
myocardium — see Injury, heart
nape — see Injury, neck
nasal (septum) (sinus) S09.92
nasopharynx S09.92
neck S19.9
  specified NEC S19.80
    specified site NEC S19.89
nerve NEC T14.8
  abdomen S34.9
    peripheral S34.6
    specified site NEC S34.8
  abducens S04.4-
    contusion S04.4-
    laceration S04.4-
    specified type NEC S04.4-
  abducent — see Injury, nerve, abducens
  accessory S04.7-
    contusion S04.7-
    laceration S04.7-
    specified type NEC S04.7-
  acoustic S04.6-
    contusion S04.6-
    laceration S04.6-
    specified type NEC S04.6-
  ankle S94.9-
    cutaneous sensory S94.3-
    specified site NEC — see subcategory S94.8
  anterior crural, femoral — see Injury, nerve, femoral
  arm (upper) S44.9-
    axillary — see Injury, nerve, axillary
    cutaneous — see Injury, nerve, cutaneous, arm
    median — see Injury, nerve, median, upper arm
    musculocutaneous — see Injury, nerve, musculocutaneous
    radial — see Injury, nerve, radial, upper arm
    specified site NEC — see subcategory S44.8
    ulnar — see Injury, nerve, ulnar, arm
  auditory — see Injury, nerve, acoustic
  axillary S44.3-
  brachial plexus — see Injury, brachial plexus
  cervical sympathetic S14.5
  cranial S04.9
    contusion S04.9
    eighth (acoustic or auditory) — see Injury, nerve, acoustic
    eleventh (accessory) — see Injury, nerve, accessory
    fifth (trigeminal) — see Injury, nerve, trigeminal
    first (olfactory) — see Injury, nerve, olfactory
    fourth (trochlear) — see Injury, nerve, trochlear
    laceration S04.9
    ninth (glossopharyngeal) — see Injury, nerve, glossopharyngeal
    second (optic) — see Injury, nerve, optic
    seventh (facial) — see Injury, nerve, facial
    sixth (abducent) — see Injury, nerve, abducens
    specified
      nerve NEC S04.89-
        contusion S04.89-
        laceration S04.89-
        specified type NEC S04.89-
      type NEC S04.9
    tenth (pneumogastric or vagus) — see Injury, nerve, vagus

Injury (see also specified injury type) T14.90 — continued

nerve NEC T14.8 — continued
  cranial S04.9 — continued
    third (oculomotor) — see Injury, nerve, oculomotor
    twelfth (hypoglossal) — see Injury, nerve, hypoglossal
  cutaneous sensory
    ankle (level) S94.3-
    arm (upper) (level) S44.5-
    foot (level) — see Injury, nerve, cutaneous sensory, ankle
    forearm (level) S54.3-
    hip (level) S74.2-
    leg (lower level) S84.2-
    shoulder (level) — see Injury, nerve, cutaneous sensory, arm
    thigh (level) — see Injury, nerve, cutaneous sensory, hip
  deep peroneal — see Injury, nerve, peroneal, foot
  digital
    finger S64.4-
      index S64.49-
      little S64.49-
      middle S64.49-
      ring S64.49-
    thumb S64.3-
    toe — see Injury, nerve, ankle, specified site NEC
  eighth cranial (acoustic or auditory) — see Injury, nerve, acoustic
  eleventh cranial (accessory) — see Injury, nerve, accessory
  facial S04.5-
    contusion S04.5-
    laceration S04.5-
    newborn P11.3
    specified type NEC S04.5-
  femoral (hip level) (thigh level) S74.1-
  fifth cranial (trigeminal) — see Injury, nerve, trigeminal
  finger (digital) — see Injury, nerve, digital, finger
  first cranial (olfactory) — see Injury, nerve, olfactory
  foot S94.9-
    cutaneous sensory S94.3-
    deep peroneal S94.2-
    lateral plantar S94.0-
    medial plantar S94.1-
    specified site NEC — see subcategory S94.8
  forearm (level) S54.9-
    cutaneous sensory — see Injury, nerve, cutaneous sensory, forearm
    median — see Injury, nerve, median
    radial — see Injury, nerve, radial
    specified site NEC — see subcategory S54.8
    ulnar — see Injury, nerve, ulnar
  fourth cranial (trochlear) — see Injury, nerve, trochlear
  glossopharyngeal S04.89-
    specified type NEC S04.89-
  hand S64.9-
    median — see Injury, nerve, median, hand
    radial — see Injury, nerve, radial, hand
    specified NEC — see subcategory S64.8
    ulnar — see Injury, nerve, ulnar, hand
  hip (level) S74.9-
    cutaneous sensory — see Injury, nerve, cutaneous sensory, hip
    femoral — see Injury, nerve, femoral
    sciatic — see Injury, nerve, sciatic
    specified site NEC — see subcategory S74.8

Injury (see also specified injury type) T14.90 — continued

nerve NEC T14.8 — continued
  hypoglossal S04.89-
    specified type NEC S04.89-
  lateral plantar S94.0-
  leg (lower) S84.9-
    cutaneous sensory — see Injury, nerve, cutaneous sensory, leg
    peroneal — see Injury, nerve, peroneal
    specified site NEC — see subcategory S84.8
    tibial — see Injury, nerve, tibial
    upper — see Injury, nerve, thigh
  lower
    back — see Injury, nerve, abdomen, specified site NEC
    peripheral — see Injury, nerve, abdomen, peripheral
    limb — see Injury, nerve, leg
  lumbar plexus — see Injury, nerve, lumbosacral, sympathetic
  lumbar spinal — see Injury, nerve, spinal, lumbar
  lumbosacral
    plexus — see Injury, nerve, lumbosacral, sympathetic
    sympathetic S34.5
  medial plantar S94.1-
  median (forearm level) S54.1-
    hand (level) S64.1-
    upper arm (level) S44.1-
    wrist (level) — see Injury, nerve, median, hand
  musculocutaneous S44.4-
  musculospiral (upper arm level) — see Injury, nerve, radial, upper arm
  neck S14.9
    peripheral S14.4
    specified site NEC S14.8
    sympathetic S14.5
  ninth cranial (glossopharyngeal) — see Injury, nerve, glossopharyngeal
  oculomotor S04.1-
    contusion S04.1-
    laceration S04.1-
    specified type NEC S04.1-
  olfactory S04.81-
    specified type NEC S04.81-
  optic S04.01-
    contusion S04.01-
    laceration S04.01-
    specified type NEC S04.01-
  pelvic girdle — see Injury, nerve, hip
  pelvis — see Injury, nerve, abdomen, specified site NEC
  peripheral — see Injury, nerve, abdomen, peripheral
  peripheral NEC T14.8
    abdomen — see Injury, nerve, abdomen, peripheral
    lower back — see Injury, nerve, abdomen, peripheral
    neck — see Injury, nerve, neck, peripheral
    pelvis — see Injury, nerve, abdomen, peripheral
    specified NEC T14.8
  peroneal (lower leg level) S84.1-
    foot S94.2-
  plexus
    brachial — see Injury, brachial plexus
    celiac, coeliac — see Injury, nerve, lumbosacral, sympathetic
    mesenteric, inferior — see Injury, nerve, lumbosacral, sympathetic
    sacral — see Injury, lumbosacral plexus

Injury (see also specified injury type) T14.90 — continued
- nerve NEC T14.8 — continued
  - plexus — continued
    - spinal
      - brachial — see Injury, brachial plexus
      - lumbosacral — see Injury, lumbosacral plexus
  - pneumogastric — see Injury, nerve, vagus
  - radial (forearm level) S54.2-
    - hand (level) S64.2-
    - upper arm (level) S44.2-
    - wrist (level) — see Injury, nerve, radial, hand
  - root — see Injury, nerve, spinal, root
  - sacral plexus — see Injury, lumbosacral plexus
  - sacral spinal — see Injury, nerve, spinal, sacral
  - sciatic (hip level) (thigh level) S74.0-
  - second cranial (optic) — see Injury, nerve, optic
  - seventh cranial (facial) — see Injury, nerve, facial
  - shoulder — see Injury, nerve, arm
  - sixth cranial (abducent) — see Injury, nerve, abducens
  - spinal
    - plexus — see Injury, nerve, plexus, spinal
    - root
      - cervical S14.2
      - dorsal S24.2
      - lumbar S34.21
      - sacral S34.22
      - thoracic — see Injury, nerve, spinal, root, dorsal
  - splanchnic — see Injury, nerve, lumbosacral, sympathetic
  - sympathetic NEC — see Injury, nerve, lumbosacral, sympathetic
    - cervical — see Injury, nerve, cervical sympathetic
  - tenth cranial (pneumogastric or vagus) — see Injury, nerve, vagus
  - thigh (level) — see Injury, nerve, hip
    - cutaneous sensory — see Injury, nerve, cutaneous sensory, hip
    - femoral — see Injury, nerve, femoral
    - sciatic — see Injury, nerve, sciatic
    - specified NEC — see Injury, nerve, hip
  - third cranial (oculomotor) — see Injury, nerve, oculomotor
  - thorax S24.9
    - peripheral S24.3
    - specified site NEC S24.8
    - sympathetic S24.4
  - thumb, digital — see Injury, nerve, digital, thumb
  - tibial (lower leg level) (posterior) S84.0-
  - toe — see Injury, nerve, ankle
  - trigeminal S04.3-
    - contusion S04.3-
    - laceration S04.3-
    - specified type NEC S04.3-
  - trochlear S04.2-
    - contusion S04.2-
    - laceration S04.2-
    - specified type NEC S04.2-
  - twelfth cranial (hypoglossal) — see Injury, nerve, hypoglossal
  - ulnar (forearm level) S54.0-
    - arm (upper) (level) S44.0-
    - hand (level) S64.0-
    - wrist (level) — see Injury, nerve, ulnar, hand
  - vagus S04.89-
    - specified type NEC S04.89-
  - wrist (level) — see Injury, nerve, hand

Injury (see also specified injury type) T14.90 — continued
- ninth cranial nerve (glossopharyngeal) — see Injury, nerve, glossopharyngeal
- nose (septum) S09.92
- obstetrical O71.9
  - specified NEC O71.89
- occipital (region) (scalp) S09.90
  - lobe — see Injury, intracranial
- optic chiasm S04.02
- optic radiation S04.03-
- optic tract and pathways S04.03-
- orbit, orbital (region) — see Injury, eye
  - penetrating (with foreign body) — see Injury, eye, orbit, penetrating
  - specified NEC — see Injury, eye, specified site NEC
- ovary, ovarian S37.409
  - bilateral S37.402
    - contusion S37.422
    - laceration S37.432
    - specified type NEC S37.492
  - blood vessel — see Injury, blood vessel, ovarian
  - contusion S37.429
    - bilateral S37.422
    - unilateral S37.421
  - laceration S37.439
    - bilateral S37.432
    - unilateral S37.431
  - specified type NEC S37.499
    - bilateral S37.492
    - unilateral S37.491
  - unilateral S37.401
    - contusion S37.421
    - laceration S37.431
    - specified type NEC S37.491
- palate (hard) (soft) S09.93
- pancreas S36.209
  - body S36.201
    - contusion S36.221
    - laceration S36.231
      - major S36.261
      - minor S36.241
      - moderate S36.251
    - specified type NEC S36.291
  - contusion S36.229
  - head S36.200
    - contusion S36.220
    - laceration S36.230
      - major S36.260
      - minor S36.240
      - moderate S36.250
    - specified type NEC S36.290
  - laceration S36.239
    - major S36.269
    - minor S36.249
    - moderate S36.259
  - specified type NEC S36.299
  - tail S36.202
    - contusion S36.222
    - laceration S36.232
      - major S36.262
      - minor S36.242
      - moderate S36.252
    - specified type NEC S36.292
- parietal (region) (scalp) S09.90
  - lobe — see Injury, intracranial
- patellar ligament (tendon) S76.10-
  - laceration S76.12-
  - specified NEC S76.19-
  - strain S76.11-
- pelvis, pelvic (floor) S39.93
  - complicating delivery O70.1
  - joint or ligament, complicating delivery O71.6
  - organ S37.90
    - with ectopic or molar pregnancy O08.6
    - complication of abortion — see Abortion

Injury (see also specified injury type) T14.90 — continued
- pelvis, pelvic (floor) S39.93 — continued
  - organ S37.90 — continued
    - contusion S37.92
    - following ectopic or molar pregnancy O08.6
    - laceration S37.93
    - obstetrical trauma NEC O71.5
    - specified
      - site NEC S37.899
        - contusion S37.892
        - laceration S37.893
        - specified type NEC S37.898
      - type NEC S37.99
    - specified NEC S39.83
- penis S39.94
- perineum S39.94
- peritoneum S36.81
  - laceration S36.893
- periurethral tissue — see Injury, urethra
  - complicating delivery O71.82
- phalanges
  - foot — see Injury, foot
  - hand — see Injury, hand
- pharynx NEC S19.85
- pleura — see Injury, intrathoracic, pleura
- plexus
  - brachial — see Injury, brachial plexus
  - cardiac — see Injury, nerve, thorax, sympathetic
  - celiac, coeliac — see Injury, nerve, lumbosacral, sympathetic
  - esophageal — see Injury, nerve, thorax, sympathetic
  - hypogastric — see Injury, nerve, lumbosacral, sympathetic
  - lumbar, lumbosacral — see Injury, lumbosacral plexus
  - mesenteric — see Injury, nerve, lumbosacral, sympathetic
  - pulmonary — see Injury, nerve, thorax, sympathetic
- postcardiac surgery (syndrome) I97.0
- prepuce S39.94
- prostate S37.829
  - contusion S37.822
  - laceration S37.823
  - specified type NEC S37.828
- pubic region S39.94
- pudendum S39.94
- pulmonary plexus — see Injury, nerve, thorax, sympathetic
- rectovaginal septum NEC S39.83
- rectum — see Injury, intestine, large, rectum
- retina — see Injury, eye, specified site NEC
  - penetrating — see Injury, eyeball, penetrating
- retroperitoneal — see Injury, intra-abdominal, specified site NEC
- rotator cuff (muscle(s)) (tendon(s)) S46.00-
  - laceration S46.02-
  - specified type NEC S46.09-
  - strain S46.01-
- round ligament — see Injury, pelvic organ, specified site NEC
- sacral plexus — see Injury, lumbosacral plexus
- salivary duct or gland S09.93
- scalp S09.90
  - newborn (birth injury) P12.9
    - due to monitoring (electrode) (sampling incision) P12.4
    - specified NEC P12.89
    - caput succedaneum P12.81
- scapular region — see Injury, shoulder
- sclera — see Injury, eye, specified site NEC
  - penetrating — see Injury, eyeball, penetrating
- scrotum S39.94

Injury (*see also* specified injury type) T14.90 — *continued*
  second cranial nerve (optic) — *see* Injury, nerve, optic
  seminal vesicle — *see* Injury, pelvic organ, specified site NEC
  seventh cranial nerve (facial) — *see* Injury, nerve, facial
  shoulder S49.9-
    blood vessel — *see* Injury, blood vessel, arm
    contusion — *see* Contusion, shoulder
    dislocation — *see* Dislocation, shoulder
    fracture — *see* Fracture, shoulder
    muscle — *see* Injury, muscle, shoulder
    nerve — *see* Injury, nerve, shoulder
    open — *see* Wound, open, shoulder
    specified type NEC S49.8-
    sprain — *see* Sprain, shoulder girdle
    superficial — *see* Injury, superficial, shoulder
  sinus
    cavernous — *see* Injury, intracranial
    nasal S09.92
  sixth cranial nerve (abducent) — *see* Injury, nerve, abducens
  skeleton, birth injury P13.9
    specified part NEC P13.8
  skin NEC T14.8
    surface intact — *see* Injury, superficial
  skull NEC S09.90
  specified NEC T14.8
  spermatic cord (pelvic region) S37.898
    scrotal region S39.848
  spinal (cord)
    cervical (neck) S14.109
      anterior cord syndrome S14.139
        C1 level S14.131
        C2 level S14.132
        C3 level S14.133
        C4 level S14.134
        C5 level S14.135
        C6 level S14.136
        C7 level S14.137
        C8 level S14.138
      Brown-Séquard syndrome S14.149
        C1 level S14.141
        C2 level S14.142
        C3 level S14.143
        C4 level S14.144
        C5 level S14.145
        C6 level S14.146
        C7 level S14.147
        C8 level S14.148
      C1 level S14.101
      C2 level S14.102
      C3 level S14.103
      C4 level S14.104
      C5 level S14.105
      C6 level S14.106
      C7 level S14.107
      C8 level S14.108
      central cord syndrome S14.129
        C1 level S14.121
        C2 level S14.122
        C3 level S14.123
        C4 level S14.124
        C5 level S14.125
        C6 level S14.126
        C7 level S14.127
        C8 level S14.128
      complete lesion S14.119
        C1 level S14.111
        C2 level S14.112
        C3 level S14.113
        C4 level S14.114
        C5 level S14.115
        C6 level S14.116
        C7 level S14.117
        C8 level S14.118
      concussion S14.0

Injury (*see also* specified injury type) T14.90 — *continued*
  spinal (cord) — *continued*
    cervical (neck) S14.109 — *continued*
      edema S14.0
      incomplete lesion specified NEC S14.159
        C1 level S14.151
        C2 level S14.152
        C3 level S14.153
        C4 level S14.154
        C5 level S14.155
        C6 level S14.156
        C7 level S14.157
        C8 level S14.158
      posterior cord syndrome S14.159
        C1 level S14.151
        C2 level S14.152
        C3 level S14.153
        C4 level S14.154
        C5 level S14.155
        C6 level S14.156
        C7 level S14.157
        C8 level S14.158
    dorsal — *see* Injury, spinal, thoracic
    lumbar S34.109
      complete lesion S34.119
        L1 level S34.111
        L2 level S34.112
        L3 level S34.113
        L4 level S34.114
        L5 level S34.115
      concussion S34.01
      edema S34.01
      incomplete lesion S34.129
        L1 level S34.121
        L2 level S34.122
        L3 level S34.123
        L4 level S34.124
        L5 level S34.125
      L1 level S34.101
      L2 level S34.102
      L3 level S34.103
      L4 level S34.104
      L5 level S34.105
    nerve root NEC
      cervical — *see* Injury, nerve, spinal, root, cervical
      dorsal — *see* Injury, nerve, spinal, root, dorsal
      lumbar S34.21
      sacral S34.22
      thoracic — *see* Injury, nerve, spinal, root, dorsal
    plexus
      brachial — *see* Injury, brachial plexus
      lumbosacral — *see* Injury, lumbosacral plexus
    sacral S34.139
      complete lesion S34.131
      incomplete lesion S34.132
    thoracic S24.109
      anterior cord syndrome S24.139
        T1 level S24.131
        T11-T12 level S24.134
        T2-T6 level S24.132
        T7-T10 level S24.133
      Brown-Séquard syndrome S24.149
        T1 level S24.141
        T11-T12 level S24.144
        T2-T6 level S24.142
        T7-T10 level S24.143
      complete lesion S24.119
        T1 level S24.111
        T11-T12 level S24.114
        T2-T6 level S24.112
        T7-T10 level S24.113
      concussion S24.0
      edema S24.0

Injury (*see also* specified injury type) T14.90 — *continued*
  spinal (cord) — *continued*
    thoracic S24.109 — *continued*
      incomplete lesion specified NEC S24.159
        T1 level S24.151
        T11-T12 level S24.154
        T2-T6 level S24.152
        T7-T10 level S24.153
      posterior cord syndrome S24.159
        T1 level S24.151
        T11-T12 level S24.154
        T2-T6 level S24.152
        T7-T10 level S24.153
      T1 level S24.101
      T11-T12 level S24.104
      T2-T6 level S24.102
      T7-T10 level S24.103
  splanchnic nerve — *see* Injury, nerve, lumbosacral, sympathetic
  spleen S36.00
    contusion S36.029
      major S36.021
      minor S36.020
    laceration S36.039
      major (massive) (stellate) S36.032
      moderate S36.031
      superficial (capsular) (minor) S36.030
    specified type NEC S36.09
  splenic artery — *see* Injury, blood vessel, celiac artery, branch
  stellate ganglion — *see* Injury, nerve, thorax, sympathetic
  sternal region S29.9
  stomach S36.30
    contusion S36.32
    laceration S36.33
    specified type NEC S36.39
  subconjunctival — *see* Injury, eye, conjunctiva
  subcutaneous NEC T14.8
  submaxillary region S09.93
  submental region S09.93
  subungual
    fingers — *see* Injury, hand
    toes — *see* Injury, foot
  superficial NEC T14.8
    abdomen, abdominal (wall) S30.92
      abrasion S30.811
      bite S30.871
        insect S30.861
      contusion S30.1
      external constriction S30.841
      foreign body S30.851
    abrasion — *see* Abrasion, by site
    adnexa, eye NEC — *see* Injury, eye, specified site NEC
    alveolar process — *see* Injury, superficial, oral cavity
    ankle S90.91-
      abrasion — *see* Abrasion, ankle
      bite — *see* Bite, ankle
      blister — *see* Blister, ankle
      contusion — *see* Contusion, ankle
      external constriction — *see* Constriction, external, ankle
      foreign body — *see* Foreign body, superficial, ankle
    anus S30.98
    arm (upper) S40.92-
      abrasion — *see* Abrasion, arm
      bite — *see* Bite, superficial, arm
      blister — *see* Blister, arm (upper)
      contusion — *see* Contusion, arm
      external constriction — *see* Constriction, external, arm
      foreign body — *see* Foreign body, superficial, arm

Injury (*see also* specified injury type) T14.90 — *continued*
  superficial NEC T14.8 — *continued*
    auditory canal (external) (meatus) — *see* Injury, superficial, ear
    auricle — *see* Injury, superficial, ear
    axilla — *see* Injury, superficial, arm
    back — *see also* Injury, superficial, thorax, back
      lower S30.91
        abrasion S30.810
        contusion S30.0
        external constriction S30.840
        superficial
          bite NEC S30.870
            insect S30.860
          foreign body S30.850
    bite NEC — *see* Bite, superficial NEC, by site
    blister — *see* Blister, by site
    breast S20.10-
      abrasion — *see* Abrasion, breast
      bite — *see* Bite, superficial, breast
      contusion — *see* Contusion, breast
      external constriction — *see* Constriction, external, breast
      foreign body — *see* Foreign body, superficial, breast
    brow — *see* Injury, superficial, head, specified NEC
    buttock S30.91
    calf — *see* Injury, superficial, leg
    canthus, eye — *see* Injury, superficial, periocular area
    cheek (external) — *see* Injury, superficial, head, specified NEC
      internal — *see* Injury, superficial, oral cavity
    chest wall — *see* Injury, superficial, thorax
    chin — *see* Injury, superficial, head NEC
    clitoris S30.95
    conjunctiva — *see* Injury, eye, conjunctiva
      with foreign body (in conjunctival sac) — *see* Foreign body, conjunctival sac
    contusion — *see* Contusion, by site
    costal region — *see* Injury, superficial, thorax
    digit(s)
      hand — *see* Injury, superficial, finger
    ear (auricle) (canal) (external) S00.40-
      abrasion — *see* Abrasion, ear
      bite — *see* Bite, superficial, ear
      contusion — *see* Contusion, ear
      external constriction — *see* Constriction, external, ear
      foreign body — *see* Foreign body, superficial, ear
    elbow S50.90-
      abrasion — *see* Abrasion, elbow
      bite — *see* Bite, superficial, elbow
      blister — *see* Blister, elbow
      contusion — *see* Contusion, elbow
      external constriction — *see* Constriction, external, elbow
      foreign body — *see* Foreign body, superficial, elbow
    epididymis S30.94
    epigastric region S30.92
    epiglottis — *see* Injury, superficial, throat
    esophagus
      cervical — *see* Injury, superficial, throat
    external constriction — *see* Constriction, external, by site
    extremity NEC T14.8
    eyeball NEC — *see* Injury, eye, specified site NEC
    eyebrow — *see* Injury, superficial, periocular area

Injury (*see also* specified injury type) T14.90 — *continued*
  superficial NEC T14.8 — *continued*
    eyelid S00.20-
      abrasion — *see* Abrasion, eyelid
      bite — *see* Bite, superficial, eyelid
      contusion — *see* Contusion, eyelid
      external constriction — *see* Constriction, external, eyelid
      foreign body — *see* Foreign body, superficial, eyelid
    face NEC — *see* Injury, superficial, head, specified NEC
    finger(s) S60.949
      abrasion — *see* Abrasion, finger
      bite — *see* Bite, superficial, finger
      blister — *see* Blister, finger
      contusion — *see* Contusion, finger
      external constriction — *see* Constriction, external, finger
      foreign body — *see* Foreign body, superficial, finger
      index S60.94-
      insect bite — *see* Bite, by site, superficial, insect
      little S60.94-
      middle S60.94-
      ring S60.94-
    flank S30.92
    foot S90.92-
      abrasion — *see* Abrasion, foot
      bite — *see* Bite, foot
      blister — *see* Blister, foot
      contusion — *see* Contusion, foot
      external constriction — *see* Constriction, external, foot
      foreign body — *see* Foreign body, superficial, foot
    forearm S50.91-
      abrasion — *see* Abrasion, forearm
      bite — *see* Bite, forearm, superficial
      blister — *see* Blister, forearm
      contusion — *see* Contusion, forearm
      elbow only — *see* Injury, superficial, elbow
      external constriction — *see* Constriction, external, forearm
      foreign body — *see* Foreign body, superficial, forearm
    forehead — *see* Injury, superficial, head NEC
    foreign body — *see* Foreign body, superficial
    genital organs, external
      female S30.97
      male S30.96
    globe (eye) — *see* Injury, eye, specified site NEC
    groin S30.92
    gum — *see* Injury, superficial, oral cavity
    hand S60.92-
      abrasion — *see* Abrasion, hand
      bite — *see* Bite, superficial, hand
      contusion — *see* Contusion, hand
      external constriction — *see* Constriction, external, hand
      foreign body — *see* Foreign body, superficial, hand
    head S00.90
      ear — *see* Injury, superficial, ear
      eyelid — *see* Injury, superficial, eyelid
      nose S00.30
      oral cavity S00.502
      scalp S00.00
      specified site NEC S00.80
    heel — *see* Injury, superficial, foot

Injury (*see also* specified injury type) T14.90 — *continued*
  superficial NEC T14.8 — *continued*
    hip S70.91-
      abrasion — *see* Abrasion, hip
      bite — *see* Bite, superficial, hip
      blister — *see* Blister, hip
      contusion — *see* Contusion, hip
      external constriction — *see* Constriction, external, hip
      foreign body — *see* Foreign body, superficial, hip
    iliac region — *see* Injury, superficial, abdomen
    inguinal region — *see* Injury, superficial, abdomen
    insect bite — *see* Bite, by site, superficial, insect
    interscapular region — *see* Injury, superficial, thorax, back
    jaw — *see* Injury, superficial, head, specified NEC
    knee S80.91-
      abrasion — *see* Abrasion, knee
      bite — *see* Bite, superficial, knee
      blister — *see* Blister, knee
      contusion — *see* Contusion, knee
      external constriction — *see* Constriction, external, knee
      foreign body — *see* Foreign body, superficial, knee
    labium (majus) (minus) S30.95
    lacrimal (apparatus) (gland) (sac) — *see* Injury, eye, specified site NEC
    larynx — *see* Injury, superficial, throat
    leg (lower) S80.92-
      abrasion — *see* Abrasion, leg
      bite — *see* Bite, superficial, leg
      contusion — *see* Contusion, leg
      external constriction — *see* Constriction, external, leg
      foreign body — *see* Foreign body, superficial, leg
      knee — *see* Injury, superficial, knee
    limb NEC T14.8
    lip S00.501
    lower back S30.91
    lumbar region S30.91
    malar region — *see* Injury, superficial, head, specified NEC
    mammary — *see* Injury, superficial, breast
    mastoid region — *see* Injury, superficial, head, specified NEC
    mouth — *see* Injury, superficial, oral cavity
    muscle NEC T14.8
    nail NEC T14.8
      finger — *see* Injury, superficial, finger
      toe — *see* Injury, superficial, toe
    nasal (septum) — *see* Injury, superficial, nose
    neck S10.90
      specified site NEC S10.80
    nose (septum) S00.30
    occipital region — *see* Injury, superficial, scalp
    oral cavity S00.502
    orbital region — *see* Injury, superficial, periocular area
    palate — *see* Injury, superficial, oral cavity
    palm — *see* Injury, superficial, hand
    parietal region — *see* Injury, superficial, scalp
    pelvis S30.91
      girdle — *see* Injury, superficial, hip
    penis S30.93
    perineum
      female S30.95
      male S30.91

Injury (*see also* specified injury type) T14.90 — *continued*
  superficial NEC T14.8 — *continued*
    periocular area S00.20-
      abrasion — *see* Abrasion, eyelid
      bite — *see* Bite, superficial, eyelid
      contusion — *see* Contusion, eyelid
      external constriction — *see* Constriction, external, eyelid
      foreign body — *see* Foreign body, superficial, eyelid
    phalanges
      finger — *see* Injury, superficial, finger
      toe — *see* Injury, superficial, toe
    pharynx — *see* Injury, superficial, throat
    pinna — *see* Injury, superficial, ear
    popliteal space — *see* Injury, superficial, knee
    prepuce S30.93
    pubic region S30.91
    pudendum
      female S30.97
      male S30.96
    sacral region S30.91
    scalp S00.00
    scapular region — *see* Injury, superficial, shoulder
    sclera — *see* Injury, eye, specified site NEC
    scrotum S30.94
    shin — *see* Injury, superficial, leg
    shoulder S40.91-
      abrasion — *see* Abrasion, shoulder
      bite — *see* Bite, superficial, shoulder
      blister — *see* Blister, shoulder
      contusion — *see* Contusion, shoulder
      external constriction — *see* Constriction, external, shoulder
      foreign body — *see* Foreign body, superficial, shoulder
    skin NEC T14.8
    sternal region — *see* Injury, superficial, thorax, front
    subconjunctival — *see* Injury, eye, specified site NEC
    subcutaneous NEC T14.8
    submaxillary region — *see* Injury, superficial, head, specified NEC
    submental region — *see* Injury, superficial, head, specified NEC
    subungual
      finger(s) — *see* Injury, superficial, finger
      toe(s) — *see* Injury, superficial, toe
    supraclavicular fossa — *see* Injury, superficial, neck
    supraorbital — *see* Injury, superficial, head, specified NEC
    temple — *see* Injury, superficial, head, specified NEC
    temporal region — *see* Injury, superficial, head, specified NEC
    testis S30.94
    thigh S70.92-
      abrasion — *see* Abrasion, thigh
      bite — *see* Bite, superficial, thigh
      blister — *see* Blister, thigh
      contusion — *see* Contusion, thigh
      external constriction — *see* Constriction, external, thigh
      foreign body — *see* Foreign body, superficial, thigh
    thorax, thoracic (wall) S20.90
      abrasion — *see* Abrasion, thorax
      back S20.40-
      bite — *see* Bite, thorax, superficial
      blister — *see* Blister, thorax
      contusion — *see* Contusion, thorax
      external constriction — *see* Constriction, external, thorax

Injury (*see also* specified injury type) T14.90 — *continued*
  superficial NEC T14.8 — *continued*
    thorax, thoracic (wall) S20.90 — *continued*
      foreign body — *see* Foreign body, superficial, thorax
      front S20.30-
    throat S10.10
      abrasion S10.11
      bite S10.17
        insect S10.16
      blister S10.12
      contusion S10.0
      external constriction S10.14
      foreign body S10.15
    thumb S60.93-
      abrasion — *see* Abrasion, thumb
      bite — *see* Bite, superficial, thumb
      blister — *see* Blister, thumb
      contusion — *see* Contusion, thumb
      external constriction — *see* Constriction, external, thumb
      foreign body — *see* Foreign body, superficial, thumb
      insect bite — *see* Bite, by site, superficial, insect
      specified type NEC S60.39-
    toe(s) S90.93-
      abrasion — *see* Abrasion, toe
      bite — *see* Bite, toe
      blister — *see* Blister, toe
      contusion — *see* Contusion, toe
      external constriction — *see* Constriction, external, toe
      foreign body — *see* Foreign body, superficial, toe
      great S90.93-
    tongue — *see* Injury, superficial, oral cavity
    tooth, teeth — *see* Injury, superficial, oral cavity
    trachea S10.10
    tunica vaginalis S30.94
    tympanum, tympanic membrane — *see* Injury, superficial, ear
    uvula — *see* Injury, superficial, oral cavity
    vagina S30.95
    vocal cords — *see* Injury, superficial, throat
    vulva S30.95
    wrist S60.91-
  supraclavicular region — *see* Injury, neck
  supraorbital S09.93
  suprarenal gland (multiple) — *see* Injury, adrenal
  surgical complication (external or internal site) — *see* Laceration, accidental complicating surgery
  temple S09.90
  temporal region S09.90
  tendon — *see also* Injury, muscle, by site
    abdomen — *see* Injury, muscle, abdomen
    Achilles — *see* Injury, Achilles tendon
    lower back — *see* Injury, muscle, lower back
    pelvic organs — *see* Injury, muscle, pelvis
  tenth cranial nerve (pneumogastric or vagus) — *see* Injury, nerve, vagus
  testis S39.94
  thigh S79.92-
    blood vessel — *see* Injury, blood vessel, hip
    contusion — *see* Contusion, thigh
    fracture — *see* Fracture, femur
    muscle — *see* Injury, muscle, thigh
    nerve — *see* Injury, nerve, thigh
    open — *see* Wound, open, thigh
    specified NEC S79.82-
    superficial — *see* Injury, superficial, thigh
  third cranial nerve (oculomotor) — *see* Injury, nerve, oculomotor

Injury (*see also* specified injury type) T14.90 — *continued*
  thorax, thoracic S29.9
    blood vessel — *see* Injury, blood vessel, thorax
    cavity — *see* Injury, intrathoracic
    dislocation — *see* Dislocation, thorax
    external (wall) S29.9
      contusion — *see* Contusion, thorax
      nerve — *see* Injury, nerve, thorax
      open — *see* Wound, open, thorax
      specified NEC S29.8
      sprain — *see* Sprain, thorax
      superficial — *see* Injury, superficial, thorax
    fracture — *see* Fracture, thorax
    internal — *see* Injury, intrathoracic
    intrathoracic organ — *see* Injury, intrathoracic
    sympathetic ganglion — *see* Injury, nerve, thorax, sympathetic
  throat (*see also* Injury, neck) S19.9
  thumb S69.9-
    blood vessel — *see* Injury, blood vessel, thumb
    contusion — *see* Contusion, thumb
    dislocation — *see* Dislocation, thumb
    fracture — *see* Fracture, thumb
    muscle — *see* Injury, muscle, thumb
    nerve — *see* Injury, nerve, digital, thumb
    open — *see* Wound, open, thumb
    specified NEC S69.8-
    sprain — *see* Sprain, thumb
    superficial — *see* Injury, superficial, thumb
  thymus (gland) — *see* Injury, intrathoracic, specified organ NEC
  thyroid (gland) NEC S19.84
  toe S99.92-
    contusion — *see* Contusion, toe
    dislocation — *see* Dislocation, toe
    fracture — *see* Fracture, toe
    muscle — *see* Injury, muscle, toe
    open — *see* Wound, open, toe
    specified type NEC S99.82-
    sprain — *see* Sprain, toe
    superficial — *see* Injury, superficial, toe
  tongue S09.93
  tonsil S09.93
  tooth S09.93
  trachea (cervical) NEC S19.82
    thoracic — *see* Injury, intrathoracic, trachea, thoracic
  transfusion-related acute lung (TRALI) J95.84
  tunica vaginalis S39.94
  twelfth cranial nerve (hypoglossal) — *see* Injury, nerve, hypoglossal
  ureter S37.10
    contusion S37.12
    laceration S37.13
    specified type NEC S37.19
  urethra (sphincter) S37.30
    at delivery O71.5
    contusion S37.32
    laceration S37.33
    specified type NEC S37.39
  urinary organ S37.90
    contusion S37.92
    laceration S37.93
    specified
      site NEC S37.899
        contusion S37.892
        laceration S37.893
        specified type NEC S37.898
      type NEC S37.99
  uterus, uterine S37.60
    with ectopic or molar pregnancy O08.6
    blood vessel — *see* Injury, blood vessel, iliac
    contusion S37.62

Injury (see also specified injury type) T14.90 — continued
  uterus, uterine S37.60 — continued
    laceration S37.63
      cervix at delivery O71.3
    rupture associated with obstetrics — see
      Rupture, uterus
    specified type NEC S37.69
  uvula S09.93
  vagina S39.93
    abrasion S30.814
    bite S31.45
      insect S30.864
      superficial NEC S30.874
    contusion S30.23
    crush S38.03
    during delivery — see Laceration, vagina,
      during delivery
    external constriction S30.844
    insect bite S30.864
    laceration S31.41
      with foreign body S31.42
    open wound S31.40
    puncture S31.43
      with foreign body S31.44
    superficial S30.95
      foreign body S30.854
  vas deferens — see Injury, pelvic organ,
    specified site NEC
  vascular NEC T14.8
  vein — see Injury, blood vessel
  vena cava (superior) S25.20
    inferior S35.10
      laceration (minor) (superficial) S35.11
        major S35.12
      specified type NEC S35.19
    laceration (minor) (superficial) S25.21
      major S25.22
    specified type NEC S25.29
  vesical (sphincter) — see Injury, bladder
  visual cortex S04.04-
  vitreous (humor) S05.90
    specified NEC S05.8x-
  vocal cord NEC S19.83
  vulva S39.94
    abrasion S30.814
    bite S31.45
      insect S30.864
      superficial NEC S30.874
    contusion S30.23
    crush S38.03
    during delivery — see Laceration, perineum,
      female, during delivery
    external constriction S30.844
    insect bite S30.864
    laceration S31.41
      with foreign body S31.42
    open wound S31.40
    puncture S31.43
      with foreign body S31.44
    superficial S30.95
      foreign body S30.854
  whiplash (cervical spine) S13.4
  wrist S69.9-
    blood vessel — see Injury, blood vessel,
      hand
    contusion — see Contusion, wrist
    dislocation — see Dislocation, wrist
    fracture — see Fracture, wrist
    muscle — see Injury, muscle, hand
    nerve — see Injury, nerve, hand
    open — see Wound, open, wrist
    specified NEC S69.8-
    sprain — see Sprain, wrist
    superficial — see Injury, superficial, wrist
Inoculation — see also Vaccination
  complication or reaction — see Complications,
    vaccination

Insanity, insane — see also Psychosis
  adolescent — see Schizophrenia
  confusional F28
    acute or subacute F05
  delusional F22
  senile F03
Insect
  bite — see Bite, by site, superficial, insect
  venomous, poisoning NEC (by) — see Venom,
    arthropod
Insensitivity
  adrenocorticotropin hormone (ACTH) E27.49
  androgen E34.50
    complete E34.51
    partial E34.52
Insertion
  cord (umbilical) lateral or velamentous
    O43.12-
  intrauterine contraceptive device (encounter
    for) — see Intrauterine contraceptive
    device
Insolation (sunstroke) T67.0
Insomnia (organic) G47.00
  adjustment F51.02
  adjustment disorder F51.02
  behavioral, of childhood Z73.819
    combined type Z73.812
    limit setting type Z73.811
    sleep-onset association type Z73.810
  childhood Z73.819
  chronic F51.04
    somatized tension F51.04
  conditioned F51.04
  due to
    alcohol
      abuse F10.182
      dependence F10.282
      use F10.982
    amphetamines
      abuse F15.182
      dependence F15.282
      use F15.982
    anxiety disorder F51.05
    caffeine
      abuse F15.182
      dependence F15.282
      use F15.982
    cocaine
      abuse F14.182
      dependence F14.282
      use F14.982
    depression F51.05
    drug NEC
      abuse F19.182
      dependence F19.282
      use F19.982
    medical condition G47.01
    mental disorder NEC F51.05
    opioid
      abuse F11.182
      dependence F11.282
      use F11.982
    psychoactive substance NEC
      abuse F19.182
      dependence F19.282
      use F19.982
    sedative, hypnotic, or anxiolytic
      abuse F13.182
      dependence F13.282
      use F13.982
    stimulant NEC
      abuse F15.182
      dependence F15.282
      use F15.982
  fatal familial (FFI) A81.83
  idiopathic F51.01
  learned F51.3
  nonorganic origin F51.01

Insomnia (organic) G47.00 — continued
  not due to a substance or known physiological
    condition F51.01
  specified NEC F51.09
  paradoxical F51.03
  primary F51.01
  psychiatric F51.05
  psychophysiologic F51.04
  related to psychopathology F51.05
  short-term F51.02
  specified NEC G47.09
  stress-related F51.02
  transient F51.02
  without objective findings F51.02
Inspiration
  food or foreign body — see Foreign body, by
    site
  mucus — see Asphyxia, mucus
Inspissated bile syndrome (newborn) P59.1
Instability
  emotional (excessive) F60.3
  joint (post-traumatic) M25.30
    ankle M25.37-
    due to old ligament injury — see Disorder,
      ligament
    elbow M25.32-
    flail — see Flail, joint
    foot M25.37-
    hand M25.34-
    hip M25.35-
    knee M25.36-
    lumbosacral — see subcategory M53.2
    prosthesis — see Complications, joint
      prosthesis, mechanical, displacement, by
      site
    sacroiliac — see subcategory M53.2
    secondary to
      old ligament injury — see Disorder,
        ligament
      removal of joint prosthesis M96.89
    shoulder (region) M25.31-
    spine — see subcategory M53.2
    wrist M25.33-
  knee (chronic) M23.5-
  lumbosacral — see subcategory M53.2
  nervous F48.8
  personality (emotional) F60.3
  spine — see Instability, joint, spine
  vasomotor R55
Institutional syndrome (childhood) F94.2
Institutionalization, affecting child
  Z62.22
  disinhibited attachment F94.2
Insufficiency, insufficient
  accommodation, old age H52.4
  adrenal (gland) E27.40
    primary E27.1
  adrenocortical E27.40
    drug-induced E27.3
    iatrogenic E27.3
    primary E27.1
  anatomic crown height K08.89
  anterior (occlusal) guidance M26.54
  anus K62.89
  aortic (valve) I35.1
    with
      mitral (valve) disease I08.0
        with tricuspid (valve) disease I08.3
      stenosis I35.2
      tricuspid (valve) disease I08.2
        with mitral (valve) disease I08.3
    congenital Q23.1

Insufficiency, insufficient — *continued*
 aortic (valve) I35.1 — *continued*
  rheumatic I06.1
   with
    mitral (valve) disease I08.0
     with tricuspid (valve) disease I08.3
    stenosis I06.2
     with mitral (valve) disease I08.0
      with tricuspid (valve) disease I08.3
    tricuspid (valve) disease I08.2
     with mitral (valve) disease I08.3
  specified cause NEC I35.1
  syphilitic A52.03
 arterial I77.1
  basilar G45.0
  carotid (hemispheric) G45.1
  cerebral I67.81
  coronary (acute or subacute) I24.8
  mesenteric K55.1
  peripheral I73.9
  precerebral (multiple) (bilateral) G45.2
  vertebral G45.0
 arteriovenous I99.8
 biliary K83.8
 cardiac — *see also* Insufficiency, myocardial
  due to presence of (cardiac) prosthesis I97.11-
  postprocedural I97.11-
 cardiorenal, hypertensive I13.2
 cardiovascular — *see* Disease, cardiovascular
 cerebrovascular (acute) I67.81
  with transient focal neurological signs and symptoms G45.8
 circulatory NEC I99.8
  newborn P29.89
 clinical crown length K08.89
 convergence H51.11
 coronary (acute or subacute) I24.8
  chronic or with a stated duration of over 4 weeks I25.89
 corticoadrenal E27.40
  primary E27.1
 dietary E63.9
 divergence H51.8
 food T73.0
 gastroesophageal K22.8
 gonadal
  ovary E28.39
  testis E29.1
 heart — *see also* Insufficiency, myocardial
  newborn P29.0
  valve — *see* Endocarditis
 hepatic — *see* Failure, hepatic
 idiopathic autonomic G90.09
 interocclusal distance of fully erupted teeth (ridge) M26.36
 kidney N28.9
  acute N28.9
  chronic N18.9
 lacrimal (secretion) H04.12-
  passages — *see* Stenosis, lacrimal
 liver — *see* Failure, hepatic
 lung — *see* Insufficiency, pulmonary
 mental (congenital) — *see* Disability, intellectual
 mesenteric K55.1
 mitral (valve) I34.0
  with
   aortic valve disease I08.0
    with tricuspid (valve) disease I08.3
   obstruction or stenosis I05.2
    with aortic valve disease I08.0
   tricuspid (valve) disease I08.1
    with aortic (valve) disease I08.3
  congenital Q23.3

Insufficiency, insufficient — *continued*
 mitral (valve) I34.0 — *continued*
  rheumatic I05.1
   with
    aortic valve disease I08.0
     with tricuspid (valve) disease I08.3
    obstruction or stenosis I05.2
     with aortic valve disease I08.0
      with tricuspid (valve) disease I08.3
    tricuspid (valve) disease I08.1
     with aortic (valve) disease I08.3
   active or acute I01.1
    with chorea, rheumatic (Sydenham's) I02.0
  specified cause, except rheumatic I34.0
 muscle — *see also* Disease, muscle
  heart — *see* Insufficiency, myocardial
  ocular NEC H50.9
 myocardial, myocardium (with arteriosclerosis) I50.9
  with
   rheumatic fever (conditions in I00) I09.0
    active, acute or subacute I01.2
     with chorea I02.0
    inactive or quiescent (with chorea) I09.0
  congenital Q24.8
  hypertensive — *see* Hypertension, heart
  newborn P29.0
  rheumatic I09.0
   active, acute, or subacute I01.2
  syphilitic A52.06
 nourishment T73.0
 pancreatic K86.89
  exocrine K86.81
 parathyroid (gland) E20.9
 peripheral vascular (arterial) I73.9
 pituitary E23.0
 placental (mother) O36.51-
 platelets D69.6
 prenatal care affecting management of pregnancy O09.3-
 progressive pluriglandular E31.0
 pulmonary J98.4
  acute, following surgery (nonthoracic) J95.2
   thoracic J95.1
  chronic, following surgery J95.3
  following
   shock J98.4
   trauma J98.4
  newborn P28.5
  valve I37.1
   with stenosis I37.2
   congenital Q22.2
   rheumatic I09.89
    with aortic, mitral or tricuspid (valve) disease I08.8
 pyloric K31.89
 renal (acute) N28.9
  chronic N18.9
 respiratory R06.89
  newborn P28.5
 rotation — *see* Malrotation
 sleep syndrome F51.12
 social insurance Z59.7
 suprarenal E27.40
  primary E27.1
 tarso-orbital fascia, congenital Q10.3
 testis E29.1
 thyroid (gland) (acquired) E03.9
  congenital E03.1

Insufficiency, insufficient — *continued*
 tricuspid (valve) (rheumatic) I07.1
  with
   aortic (valve) disease I08.2
    with mitral (valve) disease I08.3
   mitral (valve) disease I08.1
    with aortic (valve) disease I08.3
   obstruction or stenosis I07.2
    with aortic (valve) disease I08.2
     with mitral (valve) disease I08.3
  congenital Q22.8
  nonrheumatic I36.1
   with stenosis I36.2
 urethral sphincter R32
 valve, valvular (heart) — *see* Endocarditis
  congenital Q24.8
 vascular I99.8
  intestine K55.9
   acute (*see also* Ischemia, intestine, acute) K55.059
  mesenteric K55.1
  peripheral I73.9
  renal — *see* Hypertension, kidney
 velopharyngeal
  acquired K13.79
  congenital Q38.8
 venous (chronic) (peripheral) I87.2
 ventricular — *see* Insufficiency, myocardial
 welfare support Z59.7
Insufflation, fallopian Z31.41
Insular — *see* condition
Insulinoma
 pancreas
  benign D13.7
  malignant C25.4
  uncertain behavior D37.8
 specified site
  benign — *see* Neoplasm, by site, benign
  malignant — *see* Neoplasm, by site, malignant
  uncertain behavior — *see* Neoplasm, by site, uncertain behavior
 unspecified site
  benign D13.7
  malignant C25.4
  uncertain behavior D37.8
Insuloma — *see* Insulinoma
Interference
 balancing side M26.56
 non-working side M26.56
Intermenstrual — *see* condition
Intermittent — *see* condition
Internal — *see* condition
Interrogation
 cardiac defibrillator (automatic) (implantable) Z45.02
 cardiac pacemaker Z45.018
 cardiac (event) (loop) recorder Z45.09
 infusion pump (implanted) (intrathecal) Z45.1
 neurostimulator Z46.2
Interruption
 aortic arch Q25.21
 bundle of His I44.30
 phase-shift, sleep cycle — *see* Disorder, sleep, circadian rhythm
 sleep phase-shift, or 24 hour sleep-wake cycle — *see* Disorder, sleep, circadian rhythm
Interstitial — *see* condition
Intertrigo L30.4
 labialis K13.0
Intervertebral disc — *see* condition
Intestine, intestinal — *see* condition
Intolerance
 carbohydrate K90.49
 disaccharide, hereditary E73.0
 fat NEC K90.49
  pancreatic K90.3
 food K90.49
  dietary counseling and surveillance Z71.3

Intolerance — *continued*
  fructose E74.10
    hereditary E74.12
  glucose(-galactose) E74.39
  gluten K90.41
  lactose E73.9
    specified NEC E73.8
  lysine E72.3
  milk NEC K90.49
    lactose E73.9
  protein K90.49
  starch NEC K90.49
  sucrose(-isomaltose) E74.31
Intoxicated NEC (without dependence) — *see* Alcohol, intoxication
Intoxication
  acid E87.2
  alcoholic (acute) (without dependence) — *see* Alcohol, intoxication
  alimentary canal K52.1
  amphetamine (without dependence) — *see* Abuse, drug, stimulant, with intoxication
    with dependence — *see* Dependence, drug, stimulant, with intoxication
  anxiolytic (acute) (without dependence) — *see* Abuse, drug, sedative, with intoxication
    with dependence — *see* Dependence, drug, sedative, with intoxication
  caffeine F15.929
    with dependence — *see* Dependence, drug, stimulant, with intoxication
  cannabinoids (acute) (without dependence) — *see* Use, cannabis, with intoxication
    with
      abuse — *see* Abuse, drug, cannabis, with intoxication
      dependence — *see* Dependence, drug, cannabis, with intoxication
  chemical — *see* Table of Drugs and Chemicals
    via placenta or breast milk — *see* Absorption, chemical, through placenta
  cocaine (acute) (without dependence) — *see* Abuse, drug, cocaine, with intoxication
    with dependence — *see* Dependence, drug, cocaine, with intoxication
  drug
    acute (without dependence) — *see* Abuse, drug, by type with intoxication
      with dependence — *see* Dependence, drug, by type with intoxication
    addictive
      via placenta or breast milk — *see* Absorption, drug, addictive, through placenta
    newborn P93.8
      gray baby syndrome P93.0
    overdose or wrong substance given or taken — *see* Table of Drugs and Chemicals, by drug, poisoning
  enteric K52.1
  foodborne A05.9
    bacterial A05.9
    classical (Clostridium botulinum) A05.1
    due to
      Bacillus cereus A05.4
      bacterium A05.9
        specified NEC A05.8
      Clostridium
        botulinum A05.1
        perfringens A05.2
        welchii A05.2
      Salmonella A02.9
        with
          (gastro)enteritis A02.0
          localized infection(s) A02.20
            arthritis A02.23
            meningitis A02.21
            osteomyelitis A02.24
            pneumonia A02.22

Intoxication — *continued*
  foodborne A05.9 — *continued*
    due to — *continued*
      Salmonella A02.9 — *continued*
        with — *continued*
          localized infection(s) A02.20 — *continued*
            pyelonephritis A02.25
            specified NEC A02.29
          sepsis A02.1
          specified manifestation NEC A02.8
      Staphylococcus A05.0
      Vibrio
        parahaemolyticus A05.3
        vulnificus A05.5
      enterotoxin, staphylococcal A05.0
    noxious — *see* Poisoning, food, noxious
  gastrointestinal K52.1
  hallucinogenic (without dependence) — *see* Abuse, drug, hallucinogen, with intoxication
    with dependence — *see* Dependence, drug, hallucinogen, with intoxication
  hypnotic (acute) (without dependence) — *see* Abuse, drug, sedative, with intoxication
    with dependence — *see* Dependence, drug, sedative, with intoxication
  inhalant (acute) (without dependence) — *see* Abuse, drug, inhalant, with intoxication
    with dependence — *see* Dependence, drug, inhalant, with intoxication
  meaning
    inebriation — *see* category F10
    poisoning — *see* Table of Drugs and Chemicals
  methyl alcohol (acute) (without dependence) — *see* Alcohol, intoxication
  opioid (acute) (without dependence) — *see* Abuse, drug, opioid, with intoxication
    with dependence — *see* Dependence, drug, opioid, with intoxication
  pathologic NEC (without dependence) — *see* Alcohol, intoxication
  phencyclidine (without dependence) — *see* Abuse, drug, hallucinogen NEC, with intoxication
    with dependence — *see* Dependence, drug, hallucinogen, with intoxication
  potassium (K) E87.5
  psychoactive substance NEC (without dependence) — *see* Abuse, drug, hallucinogen, with intoxication
    with dependence — *see* Dependence, drug, hallucinogen, with intoxication
  sedative (acute) (without dependence) — *see* Abuse, drug, sedative, with intoxication
    with dependence — *see* Dependence, drug, sedative, with intoxication
  serum (*see also* Reaction, serum) T80.69
  uremic — *see* Uremia
  volatile solvents (acute) (without dependence) — *see* Abuse, drug, inhalant, with intoxication
    with dependence — *see* Dependence, drug, inhalant, with intoxication
  water E87.79
Intracranial — *see* condition
Intrahepatic gallbladder Q44.1
Intraligamentous — *see* condition
Intrathoracic — *see also* condition
  kidney Q63.2
Intrauterine contraceptive device
  checking Z30.431
  in situ Z97.5
  insertion Z30.430
    immediately following removal Z30.433
  management Z30.431
  reinsertion Z30.433

Intrauterine contraceptive device — *continued*
  removal Z30.432
  replacement Z30.433
  retention in pregnancy O26.3-
Intraventricular — *see* condition
Intrinsic deformity — *see* Deformity
Intubation, difficult or failed T88.4
Intumescence, lens (eye) (cataract) — *see* Cataract
Intussusception (bowel) (colon) (enteric) (ileocecal) (ileocolic) (intestine) (rectum) K56.1
  appendix K38.8
  congenital Q43.8
  ureter (with obstruction) N13.5
Invagination (bowel, colon, intestine or rectum) K56.1
Inversion
  albumin-globulin (A-G) ratio E88.09
  bladder N32.89
  cecum — *see* Intussusception
  cervix N88.8
  chromosome in normal individual Q95.1
  circadian rhythm — *see* Disorder, sleep, circadian rhythm
  nipple N64.59
    congenital Q83.8
    gestational — *see* Retraction, nipple
    puerperal, postpartum — *see* Retraction, nipple
  nyctohemeral rhythm — *see* Disorder, sleep, circadian rhythm
  optic papilla Q14.2
  organ or site, congenital NEC — *see* Anomaly, by site
  sleep rhythm — *see* Disorder, sleep, circadian rhythm
  testis (congenital) Q55.29
  uterus (chronic) (postinfectional) (postpartal, old) N85.5
    postpartum O71.2
  vagina (posthysterectomy) N99.3
  ventricular Q20.5
Investigation (*see also* Examination) Z04.9
  clinical research subject (control) (normal comparison) (participant) Z00.6
Involuntary movement, abnormal R25.9
Involution, involutional — *see also* condition
  breast, cystic — *see* Dysplasia, mammary, specified type NEC
  depression (single episode) F32.89
    recurrent episode F33.9
  melancholia (single episode) F32.89
    recurrent episode F33.8
  ovary, senile — *see* Atrophy, ovary
  thymus failure E32.8
I.Q.
  20-34 F72
  35-49 F71
  50-69 F70
  under 20 F73
IRDS (type I) P22.0
  type II P22.1
Irideremia Q13.1
Iridis rubeosis — *see* Disorder, iris, vascular
Iridochoroiditis (panuveitis) — *see* Panuveitis
Iridocyclitis H20.9
  acute H20.0-
    hypopyon H20.05-
    primary H20.01-
    recurrent H20.02-
    secondary (noninfectious) H20.04-
      infectious H20.03-
  chronic H20.1-
  due to allergy — *see* Iridocyclitis, acute, secondary
  endogenous — *see* Iridocyclitis, acute, primary

Iridocyclitis H20.9- — *continued*
  Fuchs' — *see* Cyclitis, Fuchs' heterochromic
  gonococcal A54.32
  granulomatous — *see* Iridocyclitis, chronic
  herpes, herpetic (simplex) B00.51
    zoster B02.32
  hypopyon — *see* Iridocyclitis, acute, hypopyon
  in (due to)
    ankylosing spondylitis M45.9
    gonococcal infection A54.32
    herpes (simplex) virus B00.51
      zoster B02.32
    infectious disease NOS B99
    parasitic disease NOS B89 *[H22]*
    sarcoidosis D86.83
    syphilis A51.43
    tuberculosis A18.54
    zoster B02.32
  lens-induced H20.2-
  nongranulomatous — *see* Iridocyclitis, acute
  recurrent — *see* Iridocyclitis, acute, recurrent
  rheumatic — *see* Iridocyclitis, chronic
  subacute — *see* Iridocyclitis, acute
  sympathetic — *see* Uveitis, sympathetic
  syphilitic (secondary) A51.43
  tuberculous (chronic) A18.54
  Vogt-Koyanagi H20.82-
Iridocyclochoroiditis (panuveitis) — *see*
    Panuveitis
Iridodialysis H21.53-
Iridodonesis H21.89
Iridoplegia (complete) (partial) (reflex) H57.09
Iridoschisis H21.25-
Iris — *see also* condition
  bombé — *see* Membrane, pupillary
Iritis — *see also* Iridocyclitis
  chronic — *see* Iridocyclitis, chronic
  diabetic — *see* E08-E13 with .39
  due to
    herpes simplex B00.51
    leprosy A30.9 *[H22]*
  gonococcal A54.32
  gouty (*see also* Gout, by type) M10.9 *[H22]*
  granulomatous — *see* Iridocyclitis, chronic
  lens induced — *see* Iridocyclitis, lens-induced
  papulosa (syphilitic) A52.71
  rheumatic — *see* Iridocyclitis, chronic
  syphilitic (secondary) A51.43
    congenital (early) A50.01
    late A52.71
  tuberculous A18.54
Iron — *see* condition
Iron-miner's lung J63.4
Irradiated enamel (tooth, teeth) K03.89
Irradiation effects, adverse T66
Irreducible, irreducibility — *see* condition
Irregular, irregularity
  action, heart I49.9
  alveolar process K08.89
  bleeding N92.6
  breathing R06.89
  contour of cornea (acquired) — *see* Deformity,
    cornea
    congenital Q13.4
  contour, reconstructed breast N65.0
  dentin (in pulp) K04.3
  eye movements H55.89
    nystagmus — *see* Nystagmus
    saccadic H55.81
  labor O62.2
  menstruation (cause unknown) N92.6
  periods N92.6
  prostate N42.9
  pupil — *see* Abnormality, pupillary
  reconstructed breast N65.0
  respiratory R06.89
  septum (nasal) J34.2

Irregular, irregularity — *continued*
  shape, organ or site, congenital NEC — *see*
    Distortion
  sleep-wake pattern (rhythm) G47.23
Irritable, irritability R45.4
  bladder N32.89
  bowel (syndrome) K58.9
    with
      constipation K58.1
      diarrhea K58.0
    mixed K58.2
    psychogenic F45.8
    specified NEC K58.8
  bronchial — *see* Bronchitis
  cerebral, in newborn P91.3
  colon (*see also* Irritable, bowel) K58.9
    with diarrhea K58.0
    psychogenic F45.8
  duodenum K59.8
  heart (psychogenic) F45.8
  hip — *see* Derangement, joint, specified type
    NEC, hip
  ileum K59.8
  infant R68.12
  jejunum K59.8
  rectum K59.8
  stomach K31.89
    psychogenic F45.8
  sympathetic G90.8
  urethra N36.8
Irritation
  anus K62.89
  axillary nerve G54.0
  bladder N32.89
  brachial plexus G54.0
  bronchial — *see* Bronchitis
  cervical plexus G54.2
  cervix — *see* Cervicitis
  choroid, sympathetic — *see* Endophthalmitis
  cranial nerve — *see* Disorder, nerve, cranial
  gastric K31.89
    psychogenic F45.8
  globe, sympathetic — *see* Uveitis, sympathetic
  labyrinth — *see* subcategory H83.2
  lumbosacral plexus G54.1
  meninges (traumatic) — *see* Injury, intracranial
    nontraumatic — *see* Meningismus
  nerve — *see* Disorder, nerve
  nervous R45.0
  penis N48.89
  perineum NEC L29.3
  peripheral autonomic nervous system G90.8
  peritoneum — *see* Peritonitis
  pharynx J39.2
  plantar nerve — *see* Lesion, nerve, plantar
  spinal (cord) (traumatic) — *see also* Injury,
    spinal cord, by region
    nerve G58.9
      root NEC — *see* Radiculopathy
    nontraumatic — *see* Myelopathy
  stomach K31.89
    psychogenic F45.8
  sympathetic nerve NEC G90.8
  ulnar nerve — *see* Lesion, nerve, ulnar
  vagina N89.8
Ischemia, ischemic I99.8
  bowel (transient)
    acute (*see also* Ischemia, intestine, acute)
      K55.059
    chronic K55.1
    due to mesenteric artery insufficiency K55.1
  brain — *see* Ischemia, cerebral
  cardiac (*see* Disease, heart, ischemic)
  cardiomyopathy I25.5

Ischemia, ischemic I99.8 — *continued*
  cerebral (chronic) (generalized) I67.82
    arteriosclerotic I67.2
    intermittent G45.9
    newborn P91.0
    recurrent focal G45.8
    transient G45.9
  colon chronic (due to mesenteric artery
    insufficiency) K55.1
  coronary — *see* Disease, heart, ischemic
  demand (coronary) (*see also* Angina) I24.8
  heart (chronic or with a stated duration of over
    4 weeks) I25.9
    acute or with a stated duration of 4 weeks or
      less I24.9
    subacute I24.9
  infarction, muscle — *see* Infarct, muscle
  intestine (large) (small) (transient) K55.9
    acute K55.059
      diffuse K55.052
      focal K55.051
      large K55.039
        diffuse K55.032
        focal K55.031
      small K55.019
        diffuse K55.012
        focal K55.011
    chronic K55.1
    due to mesenteric artery insufficiency K55.1
  kidney N28.0
  mesenteric, acute (*see also* Ischemia, intestine,
    acute) K55.059
  muscle, traumatic T79.6
  myocardium, myocardial (chronic or with a
    stated duration of over 4 weeks) I25.9
    acute, without myocardial infarction I51.3
    silent (asymptomatic) I25.6
    transient of newborn P29.4
  renal N28.0
  retina, retinal — *see* Occlusion, artery, retina
  small bowel
    acute K55.019
      diffuse K55.012
      focal K55.011
    chronic K55.1
    due to mesenteric artery insufficiency K55.1
  spinal cord G95.11
  subendocardial — *see* Insufficiency, coronary
  supply (coronary) (*see also* Angina) I25.9
    due to vasospasm I20.1
Ischial spine — *see* condition
Ischialgia — *see* Sciatica
Ischiopagus Q89.4
Ischium, ischial — *see* condition
Ischuria R34
Iselin's disease or osteochondrosis — *see*
    Osteochondrosis, juvenile, metatarsus
Islands of
  parotid tissue in
    lymph nodes Q38.6
    neck structures Q38.6
  submaxillary glands in
    fascia Q38.6
    lymph nodes Q38.6
    neck muscles Q38.6
Islet cell tumor, pancreas D13.7

Isoimmunization NEC — *see also* Incompatibility
affecting management of pregnancy (ABO) (with hydrops fetalis) O36.11-
  anti-A sensitization O36.11-
  anti-B sensitization O36.19-
  anti-c sensitization O36.09-
  anti-C sensitization O36.09-
  anti-e sensitization O36.09-
  anti-E sensitization O36.09-
  Rh NEC O36.09-
    anti-D antibody O36.01-
  specified NEC O36.19-
newborn P55.9
  with
    hydrops fetalis P56.0
    kernicterus P57.0
  ABO (blood groups) P55.1
  Rhesus (Rh) factor P55.0
  specified type NEC P55.8
Isolation, isolated
dwelling Z59.8
family Z63.79
social Z60.4
Isoleucinosis E71.19
Isomerism atrial appendages (with asplenia or polysplenia) Q20.6
Isosporiasis, isosporosis A07.3
Isovaleric acidemia E71.110
Issue of
medical certificate Z02.79
  for disability determination Z02.71
repeat prescription (appliance) (glasses) (medicinal substance, medicament, medicine) Z76.0
  contraception — *see* Contraception
Itch, itching — *see also* Pruritus
baker's L23.6
barber's B35.0
bricklayer's L24.5
cheese B88.0
clam digger's B65.3
coolie B76.9
copra B88.0
dew B76.9
dhobi B35.6
filarial — *see* Infestation, filarial
grain B88.0
grocer's B88.0
ground B76.9
harvest B88.0
jock B35.6
Malabar B35.5
  beard B35.0
  foot B35.3
  scalp B35.0
meaning scabies B86
Norwegian B86
perianal L29.0
poultrymen's B88.0
sarcoptic B86
scabies B86
scrub B88.0
straw B88.0
swimmer's B65.3
water B76.9
winter L29.8
Ivemark's syndrome (asplenia with congenital heart disease) Q89.01
Ivory bones Q78.2
Ixodiasis NEC B88.8

J

Jaccoud's syndrome — *see* Arthropathy, postrheumatic, chronic
Jackson's
membrane Q43.3
paralysis or syndrome G83.89
veil Q43.3
Jacquet's dermatitis (diaper dermatitis) L22
Jadassohn's
blue nevus — *see* Nevus
intraepidermal epithelioma — *see* Neoplasm, skin, benign
Jadassohn-Pellizari's disease or anetoderma L90.2
Jaffe-Lichtenstein (-Uehlinger) syndrome — *see* Dysplasia, fibrous, bone NEC
Jakob-Creutzfeldt disease or syndrome — *see* Creutzfeldt-Jakob disease or syndrome
Jaksch-Luzet disease D64.89
Jamaican
neuropathy G92
paraplegic tropical ataxic-spastic syndrome G92
Janet's disease F48.8
Janiceps Q89.4
Jansky-Bielschowsky amaurotic idiocy E75.4
Japanese
B-type encephalitis A83.0
river fever A75.3
Jaundice (yellow) R17
acholuric (familial) (splenomegalic) — *see also* Spherocytosis
  acquired D59.8
breast-milk (inhibitor) P59.3
catarrhal (acute) B15.9
  with hepatic coma B15.0
cholestatic (benign) R17
due to or associated with
  delayed conjugation P59.8
    associated with (due to) preterm delivery P59.0
  preterm delivery P59.0
epidemic (catarrhal) B15.9
  with hepatic coma B15.0
  leptospiral A27.0
  spirochetal A27.0
familial nonhemolytic (congenital) (Gilbert) E80.4
  Crigler-Najjar E80.5
febrile (acute) B15.9
  with hepatic coma B15.0
  leptospiral A27.0
  spirochetal A27.0
hematogenous D59.9
hemolytic (acquired) D59.9
  congenital — *see* Spherocytosis
hemorrhagic (acute) (leptospiral) (spirochetal) A27.0
infectious (acute) (subacute) B15.9
  with hepatic coma B15.0
  leptospiral A27.0
  spirochetal A27.0
leptospiral (hemorrhagic) A27.0
malignant (without coma) K72.90
  with coma K72.91
neonatal — *see* Jaundice, newborn

Jaundice (yellow) R17 — *continued*
newborn P59.9
due to or associated with
  ABO
    antibodies P55.1
    incompatibility, maternal/fetal P55.1
    isoimmunization P55.1
  absence or deficiency of enzyme system for bilirubin conjugation (congenital) P59.8
  bleeding P58.1
  breast milk inhibitors to conjugation P59.3
    associated with preterm delivery P59.0
  bruising P58.0
  Crigler-Najjar syndrome E80.5
  delayed conjugation P59.8
    associated with preterm delivery P59.0
  drugs or toxins
    given to newborn P58.42
    transmitted from mother P58.41
  excessive hemolysis P58.9
    due to
      bleeding P58.1
      bruising P58.0
      drugs or toxins
        given to newborn P58.42
        transmitted from mother P58.41
      infection P58.2
      polycythemia P58.3
      swallowed maternal blood P58.5
    specified type NEC P58.8
  galactosemia E74.21
  Gilbert syndrome E80.4
  hemolytic disease P55.9
    ABO isoimmunization P55.1
    Rh isoimmunization P55.0
    specified NEC P55.8
  hepatocellular damage P59.20
    specified NEC P59.29
  hereditary hemolytic anemia P58.8
  hypothyroidism, congenital E03.1
  incompatibility, maternal/fetal NOS P55.9
  infection P58.2
  inspissated bile syndrome P59.1
  isoimmunization NOS P55.9
  mucoviscidosis E84.9
  polycythemia P58.3
  preterm delivery P59.0
  Rh
    antibodies P55.0
    incompatibility, maternal/fetal P55.0
    isoimmunization P55.0
  specified cause NEC P59.8
  swallowed maternal blood P58.5
spherocytosis (congenital) D58.0
nonhemolytic congenital familial (Gilbert) E80.4
nuclear, newborn (*see also* Kernicterus of newborn) P57.9
obstructive (*see also* Obstruction, bile duct) K83.1
post-immunization — *see* Hepatitis, viral, type, B
post-transfusion — *see* Hepatitis, viral, type, B
regurgitation (*see also* Obstruction, bile duct) K83.1
serum (homologous) (prophylactic) (therapeutic) — *see* Hepatitis, viral, type, B
spirochetal (hemorrhagic) A27.0
symptomatic R17
newborn P59.9
Jaw — *see* condition
Jaw-winking phenomenon or syndrome Q07.8

DISEASE INDEX

Jealousy
  alcoholic F10.988
  childhood F93.8
  sibling F93.8
Jejunitis — *see* Enteritis
Jejunostomy status Z93.4
Jejunum, jejunal — *see* condition
Jensen's disease — *see* Inflammation, chorioretinal, focal, juxtapapillary
Jerks, myoclonic G25.3
Jervell-Lange-Nielsen syndrome I45.81
Jeune's disease Q77.2
Jigger disease B88.1
Job's syndrome (chronic granulomatous disease) D71
Joint — *see also* condition
  mice — *see* Loose, body, joint
    knee M23.4-
Jordan's anomaly or syndrome D72.0
Joseph-Diamond-Blackfan anemia (congenital hypoplastic) D61.01
Jungle yellow fever A95.0
Jüngling's disease — *see* Sarcoidosis
Juvenile — *see* condition

K

Kahler's disease C90.0-
Kakke E51.11
Kala-azar B55.0
Kallmann's syndrome E23.0
Kanner's syndrome (autism) — *see* Psychosis, childhood
Kaposi's
  dermatosis (xeroderma pigmentosum) Q82.1
  lichen ruber L44.0
    acuminatus L44.0
  sarcoma
    colon C46.4
    connective tissue C46.1
    gastrointestinal organ C46.4
    lung C46.5-
    lymph node (multiple) C46.3
    palate (hard) (soft) C46.2
    rectum C46.4
    skin (multiple sites) C46.0
    specified site NEC C46.7
    stomach C46.4
    unspecified site C46.9
  varicelliform eruption B00.0
    vaccinia T88.1
Kartagener's syndrome or triad (sinusitis, bronchiectasis, situs inversus) Q89.3
Karyotype
  with abnormality except iso (Xq) Q96.2
  45,X Q96.0
  46,X
    iso (Xq) Q96.1
  46,XX Q98.3
    with streak gonads Q50.32
    hermaphrodite (true) Q99.1
    male Q98.3
  46,XY
    with streak gonads Q56.1
    female Q97.3
    hermaphrodite (true) Q99.1
  47,XXX Q97.0
  47,XXY Q98.0
  47,XYY Q98.5
Kaschin-Beck disease — *see* Disease, Kaschin-Beck
Katayama's disease or fever B65.2
Kawasaki's syndrome M30.3
Kayser-Fleischer ring (cornea) (pseudosclerosis) H18.04-
Kaznelson's syndrome (congenital hypoplastic anemia) D61.01
Kearns-Sayre syndrome H49.81-
Kedani fever A75.3
Kelis L91.0
Kelly (-Patterson) syndrome (sideropenic dysphagia) D50.1
Keloid, cheloid L91.0
  acne L73.0
  Addison's L94.0
  cornea — *see* Opacity, cornea
  Hawkin's L91.0
  scar L91.0
Keloma L91.0
Kenya fever A77.1
Keratectasia — *see also* Ectasia, cornea
  congenital Q13.4
Keratinization of alveolar ridge mucosa
  excessive K13.23
  minimal K13.22
Keratinized residual ridge mucosa
  excessive K13.23
  minimal K13.22

Keratitis (nodular) (nonulcerative) (simple) (zonular) H16.9
  with ulceration (central) (marginal) (perforated) (ring) — *see* Ulcer, cornea
  actinic — *see* Photokeratitis
  arborescens (herpes simplex) B00.52
  areolar H16.11-
  bullosa H16.8
  deep H16.309
    specified type NEC H16.399
  dendritic(a) (herpes simplex) B00.52
  disciform(is) (herpes simplex) B00.52
    varicella B01.81
  filamentary H16.12-
  gonococcal (congenital or prenatal) A54.33
  herpes, herpetic (simplex) B00.52
    zoster B02.33
  in (due to)
    acanthamebiasis B60.13
    adenovirus B30.0
    exanthema (*see also* Exanthem) B09
    herpes (simplex) virus B00.52
    measles B05.81
    syphilis A50.31
    tuberculosis A18.52
    zoster B02.33
  interstitial (nonsyphilitic) H16.30-
    diffuse H16.32-
    herpes, herpetic (simplex) B00.52
      zoster B02.33
    sclerosing H16.33-
    specified type NEC H16.39-
    syphilitic (congenital) (late) A50.31
    tuberculous A18.52
  macular H16.11-
  nummular H16.11-
  oyster shuckers' H16.8
  parenchymatous — *see* Keratitis, interstitial
  petrificans H16.8
  postmeasles B05.81
  punctata
    leprosa A30.9 *[H16.14-]*
    syphilitic (profunda) A50.31
  punctate H16.14-
  purulent H16.8
  rosacea L71.8
  sclerosing H16.33-
  specified type NEC H16.8
  stellate H16.11-
  striate H16.11-
  superficial H16.10-
    with conjunctivitis — *see* Keratoconjunctivitis
    due to light — *see* Photokeratitis
  suppurative H16.8
  syphilitic (congenital) (prenatal) A50.31
  trachomatous A71.1
    sequelae B94.0
  tuberculous A18.52
  vesicular H16.8
  xerotic (*see also* Keratomalacia) H16.8
    vitamin A deficiency E50.4
Kerato-uveitis — *see* Iridocyclitis
Keratoacanthoma L85.8
Keratocele — *see* Descemetocele
Keratoconjunctivitis H16.20-
  Acanthamoeba B60.13
  adenoviral B30.0
  epidemic B30.0
  exposure H16.21-
  herpes, herpetic (simplex) B00.52
    zoster B02.33
  in exanthema (*see also* Exanthem) B09
  infectious B30.0
  lagophthalmic — *see* Keratoconjunctivitis, specified type NEC
  neurotrophic H16.23-
  phlyctenular H16.25-
  postmeasles B05.81
  shipyard B30.0

Keratoconjunctivitis H16.20- — *continued*
  sicca (Sjogren's) M35.0-
    not Sjogren's H16.22-
  specified type NEC H16.29-
  tuberculous (phlyctenular) A18.52
  vernal H16.26-
Keratoconus H18.60-
  congenital Q13.4
  stable H18.61-
  unstable H18.62-
Keratocyst (dental) (odontogenic) — *see* Cyst,
  calcifying odontogenic
Keratoderma, keratodermia (congenital)
  (palmaris et plantaris) (symmetrical) Q82.8
  acquired L85.1
    in diseases classified elsewhere L86
  climactericum L85.1
  gonococcal A54.89
  gonorrheal A54.89
  punctata L85.2
  Reiter's — *see* Reiter's disease
Keratodermatocele — *see* Descemetocele
Keratoglobus H18.79
  congenital Q15.8
    with glaucoma Q15.0
Keratohemia — *see* Pigmentation, cornea,
  stromal
Keratoiritis — *see also* Iridocyclitis
  syphilitic A50.39
  tuberculous A18.54
Keratoma L57.0
  palmaris and plantaris hereditarium Q82.8
  senile L57.0
Keratomalacia H18.44-
  vitamin A deficiency E50.4
Keratomegaly Q13.4
Keratomycosis B49
  nigrans, nigricans (palmaris) B36.1
Keratopathy H18.9
  band H18.42-
  bullous H18.1-
  bullous (aphakic), following cataract surgery
    H59.01-
Keratoscleritis, tuberculous A18.52
Keratosis L57.0
  actinic L57.0
  arsenical L85.8
  congenital, specified NEC Q80.8
  female genital NEC N94.89
  follicularis Q82.8
    acquired L11.0
    congenita Q82.8
    et parafollicularis in cutem penetrans L87.0
    spinulosa (decalvans) Q82.8
    vitamin A deficiency E50.8
  gonococcal A54.89
  male genital (external) N50.89
  nigricans L83
  obturans, external ear (canal) — *see*
    Cholesteatoma, external ear
  palmaris et plantaris (inherited) (symmetrical)
    Q82.8
    acquired L85.1
  penile N48.89
  pharynx J39.2
  pilaris, acquired L85.8
  punctata (palmaris et plantaris) L85.2
  scrotal N50.89
  seborrheic L82.1
    inflamed L82.0
  senile L57.0
  solar L57.0
  tonsillaris J35.8
  vagina N89.4
  vegetans Q82.8
  vitamin A deficiency E50.8
  vocal cord J38.3
Kerion (celsi) B35.0

Kernicterus of newborn (not due to
  isoimmunization) P57.9
  due to isoimmunization (conditions in P55.0-
    P55.9) P57.0
  specified type NEC P57.8
Kerunoparalysis T75.09
Keshan disease E59
Ketoacidosis E87.2
  diabetic — *see* Diabetes, by type, with
    ketoacidosis
Ketonuria R82.4
Ketosis NEC E88.89
  diabetic — *see* Diabetes, by type, with
    ketoacidosis
Kew Garden fever A79.1
Kidney — *see* condition
Kienböck's disease — *see also*
  Osteochondrosis, juvenile, hand, carpal
  lunate
  adult M93.1
Kimmelstiel (-Wilson) disease — *see*
  Diabetes, Kimmelstiel (-Wilson) disease
Kimura disease D21.9
  specified site — *see* Neoplasm, connective
    tissue, benign
Kink, kinking
  artery I77.1
  hair (acquired) L67.8
  ileum or intestine — *see* Obstruction, intestine
  Lane's — *see* Obstruction, intestine
  organ or site, congenital NEC — *see* Anomaly,
    by site
  ureter (pelvic junction) N13.5
    with
      hydronephrosis N13.1
        with infection N13.6
      pyelonephritis (chronic) N11.1
    congenital Q62.39
  vein(s) I87.8
    caval I87.1
    peripheral I87.1
Kinnier Wilson's disease (hepatolenticular
  degeneration) E83.01
Kissing spine M48.20
  cervical region M48.22
  cervicothoracic region M48.23
  lumbar region M48.26
  lumbosacral region M48.27
  occipito-atlanto-axial region M48.21
  thoracic region M48.24
  thoracolumbar region M48.25
Klatskin's tumor C24.0
Klauder's disease A26.8
Klebs' disease (*see also* Glomerulonephritis)
  N05-
Klebsiella (K.) pneumoniae, as cause of
  disease classified elsewhere B96.1
Klein(e)-Levin syndrome G47.13
Kleptomania F63.2
Klinefelter's syndrome Q98.4
  karyotype 47,XXY Q98.0
  male with more than two X chromosomes Q98.1
Klippel-Feil deficiency, disease, or
  syndrome (brevicollis) Q76.1
Klippel's disease I67.2
Klippel-Trenaunay (-Weber) syndrome
  Q87.2
Klumpke(-Déjerine) palsy, paralysis
  (birth) (newborn) P14.1
Knee — *see* condition
Knock knee (acquired) M21.06-
  congenital Q74.1
Knot(s)
  intestinal, syndrome (volvulus) K56.2
  surfer S89.8-
  umbilical cord (true) O69.2
Knotting (of)
  hair L67.8
  intestine K56.2

Knuckle pad (Garrod's) M72.1
Koch's
  infection — *see* Tuberculosis
  relapsing fever A68.9
Koch-Weeks' conjunctivitis — *see*
  Conjunctivitis, acute, mucopurulent
Köebner's syndrome Q81.8
Köenig's disease (osteochondritis dissecans)
  — *see* Osteochondritis, dissecans
Köhler's disease
  patellar — *see* Osteochondrosis, juvenile,
    patella
  tarsal navicular — *see* Osteochondrosis,
    juvenile, tarsus
Köhler-Pellegrini-Steida disease or
  syndrome (calcification, knee joint) — *see*
  Bursitis, tibial collateral
Koilonychia L60.3
  congenital Q84.6
Kojevnikov's, epilepsy — *see* Kozhevnikof's
  epilepsy
Kozhevnikof's epilepsy G40.109
  intractable G40.119
    with status epilepticus G40.111
    without status epilepticus G40.119
  not intractable G40.109
    with status epilepticus G40.101
    without status epilepticus G40.109
Koplik's spots B05.9
Kopp's asthma E32.8
Korsakoff's (Wernicke) disease,
  psychosis or syndrome (alcoholic)
  F10.96
  with dependence F10.26
  drug-induced
    due to drug abuse — *see* Abuse, drug, by
      type, with amnestic disorder
    due to drug dependence — *see*
      Dependence, drug, by type, with
      amnestic disorder
  nonalcoholic F04
Korsakov's disease, psychosis or
  syndrome — *see* Korsakoff's disease
Korsakow's disease, psychosis or
  syndrome — *see* Korsakoff's disease
Kostmann's disease or syndrome (infantile
  genetic agranulocytosis) — *see*
  Agranulocytosis
Krabbe's
  disease E75.23
  syndrome, congenital muscle hypoplasia
    Q79.8
Kraepelin-Morel disease — *see*
  Schizophrenia
Kraft-Weber-Dimitri disease Q85.8
Kraurosis
  ani K62.89
  penis N48.0
  vagina N89.8
  vulva N90.4
Kreotoxism A05.9
Krukenberg's
  spindle — *see* Pigmentation, cornea, posterior
  tumor C79.6-
Kufs' disease E75.4
Kugelberg-Welander disease G12.1
Kuhnt-Junius degeneration (*see also*
  Degeneration, macula) H35.32-
Kümmell's disease or spondylitis — *see*
  Spondylopathy, traumatic
Kupffer cell sarcoma C22.3
Kuru A81.81
Kussmaul's
  disease M30.0
  respiration E87.2
    in diabetic acidosis — *see* Diabetes, by type,
      with ketoacidosis
Kwashiorkor E40
  marasmic, marasmus type E42

DISEASE INDEX

Kyasanur Forest disease A98.2
Kyphoscoliosis, kyphoscoliotic (acquired)
(see also Scoliosis) M41.9
  congenital Q67.5
  heart (disease) I27.1
  sequelae of rickets E64.3
  tuberculous A18.01
Kyphosis, kyphotic (acquired) M40.209
  cervical region M40.202
  cervicothoracic region M40.203
  congenital Q76.419
    cervical region Q76.412
    cervicothoracic region Q76.413
    occipito-atlanto-axial region Q76.411
    thoracic region Q76.414
    thoracolumbar region Q76.415
  Morquio-Brailsford type (spinal) (see also
    subcategory M49.8) E76.219
  postlaminectomy M96.3
  postradiation therapy M96.2
  postural (adolescent) M40.00
    cervicothoracic region M40.03
    thoracic region M40.04
    thoracolumbar region M40.05
  secondary NEC M40.10
    cervical region M40.12
    cervicothoracic region M40.13
    thoracic region M40.14
    thoracolumbar region M40.15
  sequelae of rickets E64.3
  specified type NEC M40.299
    cervical region M40.292
    cervicothoracic region M40.293
    thoracic region M40.294
    thoracolumbar region M40.295
  syphilitic, congenital A50.56
  thoracic region M40.204
  thoracolumbar region M40.205
  tuberculous A18.01
Kyrle disease L87.0

L

Labia, labium — see condition
Labile
  blood pressure R09.89
  vasomotor system I73.9
Labioglossal paralysis G12.29
Labium leporinum — see Cleft, lip
Labor — see Delivery
Labored breathing — see Hyperventilation
Labyrinthitis (circumscribed) (destructive)
  (diffuse) (inner ear) (latent) (purulent)
  (suppurative) (see also subcategory) H83.0
  syphilitic A52.79
Laceration
  with abortion — see Abortion, by type,
    complicated by laceration of pelvic organs
  abdomen, abdominal
    wall S31.119
      with
        foreign body S31.129
        penetration into peritoneal cavity
          S31.619
          with foreign body S31.629
      epigastric region S31.112
        with
          foreign body S31.122
          penetration into peritoneal cavity
            S31.612
            with foreign body S31.622
      left
        lower quadrant S31.114
          with
            foreign body S31.124
            penetration into peritoneal cavity
              S31.614
              with foreign body S31.624
        upper quadrant S31.111
          with
            foreign body S31.121
            penetration into peritoneal cavity
              S31.611
              with foreign body S31.621
      periumbilic region S31.115
        with
          foreign body S31.125
          penetration into peritoneal cavity
            S31.615
            with foreign body S31.625
      right
        lower quadrant S31.113
          with
            foreign body S31.123
            penetration into peritoneal cavity
              S31.613
              with foreign body S31.623
        upper quadrant S31.110
          with
            foreign body S31.120
            penetration into peritoneal cavity
              S31.610
              with foreign body S31.620
  accidental, complicating surgery — see
    Complications, surgical, accidental
    puncture or laceration
  Achilles tendon S86.02-
  adrenal gland S37.813
  alveolar (process) — see Laceration, oral cavity
  ankle S91.01-
    with
      foreign body S91.02-
  antecubital space — see Laceration, elbow
  anus (sphincter) S31.831
    with
      ectopic or molar pregnancy O08.6
      foreign body S31.832

Laceration — continued
  anus (sphincter) S31.831 — continued
    complicating delivery — see Delivery,
      complicated, by, laceration, anus
      (sphincter)
    following ectopic or molar pregnancy O08.6
    nontraumatic, nonpuerperal — see Fissure,
      anus
  arm (upper) S41.11-
    with foreign body S41.12-
    lower — see Laceration, forearm
  auditory canal (external) (meatus) —
    Laceration, ear
  auricle, ear — see Laceration, ear
  axilla — see Laceration, arm
  back — see also Laceration, thorax, back
    lower S31.010
      with
        foreign body S31.020
          with penetration into retroperitoneal
            space S31.021
        penetration into retroperitoneal space
          S31.011
  bile duct S36.13
  bladder S37.23
    with ectopic or molar pregnancy O08.6
    following ectopic or molar pregnancy O08.6
    obstetrical trauma O71.5
  blood vessel — see Injury, blood vessel
  bowel — see also Laceration, intestine
    with ectopic or molar pregnancy O08.6
    complicating abortion — see Abortion, by
      type, complicated by, specified
      condition NEC
    following ectopic or molar pregnancy O08.6
    obstetrical trauma O71.5
  brain (any part) (cortex) (diffuse) (membrane)
    — see also Injury, intracranial, diffuse
    during birth P10.8
      with hemorrhage P10.1
    focal — see Injury, intracranial, focal brain
      injury
  brainstem S06.38-
  breast S21.01-
    with foreign body S21.02-
  broad ligament S37.893
    with ectopic or molar pregnancy O08.6
    following ectopic or molar pregnancy O08.6
    laceration syndrome N83.8
    obstetrical trauma O71.6
    syndrome (laceration) N83.8
  buttock S31.801
    with foreign body S31.802
    left S31.821
      with foreign body S31.822
    right S31.811
      with foreign body S31.812
  calf — see Laceration, leg
  canaliculus lacrimalis — see Laceration, eyelid
  canthus, eye — see Laceration, eyelid
  capsule, joint — see Sprain
  causing eversion of cervix uteri (old) N86
  central (perineal), complicating delivery O70.9
  cerebellum, traumatic S06.37-
  cerebral S06.33-
    during birth P10.8
      with hemorrhage P10.1
    left side S06.32-
    right side S06.31-
  cervix (uteri)
    with ectopic or molar pregnancy O08.6
    following ectopic or molar pregnancy O08.6
    nonpuerperal, nontraumatic N88.1
    obstetrical trauma (current) O71.3
    old (postpartal) N88.1
    traumatic S37.63
  cheek (external) S01.41-
    with foreign body S01.42-
    internal — see Laceration, oral cavity

DISEASE INDEX

DISEASE INDEX

Laceration — *continued*
 intracranial NEC — *see also* Injury,
 intracranial, diffuse
 birth injury P10.9
 jaw — *see* Laceration, head, specified site NEC
 jejunum S36.438
 joint capsule — *see* Sprain, by site
 kidney S37.03-
 major (greater than 3 cm) (massive) (stellate)
 S37.06-
 minor (less than 1 cm) S37.04-
 moderate (1 to 3 cm) S37.05-
 multiple S37.06-
 knee S81.01-
 with foreign body S81.02-
 labium (majus) (minus) — *see* Laceration, vulva
 lacrimal duct — *see* Laceration, eyelid
 large intestine — *see* Laceration, intestine,
 large
 larynx S11.011
 with foreign body S11.012
 leg (lower) S81.819
 with foreign body S81.829
 foot — *see* Laceration, foot
 knee — *see* Laceration, knee
 left S81.812
 with foreign body S81.822
 right S81.811
 with foreign body S81.821
 upper — *see* Laceration, thigh
 ligament — *see* Sprain
 lip S01.511
 with foreign body S01.521
 liver S36.113
 major (stellate) S36.116
 minor S36.114
 moderate S36.115
 loin — *see* Laceration, abdomen, wall
 lower back — *see* Laceration, back, lower
 lumbar region — *see* Laceration, back, lower
 lung S27.339
 bilateral S27.332
 unilateral S27.331
 malar region — *see* Laceration, head, specified
 site NEC
 mammary — *see* Laceration, breast
 mastoid region — *see* Laceration, head,
 specified site NEC
 meninges — *see* Injury, intracranial, diffuse
 meniscus — *see* Tear, meniscus
 mesentery S36.893
 mesosalpinx S37.893
 mouth — *see* Laceration, oral cavity
 muscle — *see* Injury, muscle, by site, laceration
 nail
 finger — *see* Laceration, finger, with damage
 to nail
 toe — *see* Laceration, toe, with damage to
 nail
 nasal (septum) (sinus) — *see* Laceration, nose
 nasopharynx — *see* Laceration, head,
 specified site NEC
 neck S11.91
 with foreign body S11.92
 involving
 cervical esophagus S11.21
 with foreign body S11.22
 larynx — *see* Laceration, larynx
 pharynx — *see* Laceration, pharynx
 thyroid gland — *see* Laceration, thyroid
 gland
 trachea — *see* Laceration, trachea
 specified site NEC S11.81
 with foreign body S11.82
 nerve — *see* Injury, nerve
 nose (septum) (sinus) S01.21
 with foreign body S01.22
 ocular NOS S05.3-
 adnexa NOS S01.11-

Laceration — *continued*
 oral cavity S01.512
 with foreign body S01.522
 orbit (eye) — *see* Wound, open, ocular, orbit
 ovary S37.439
 bilateral S37.432
 unilateral S37.431
 palate — *see* Laceration, oral cavity
 palm — *see* Laceration, hand
 pancreas S36.239
 body S36.231
 major S36.261
 minor S36.241
 moderate S36.251
 head S36.230
 major S36.260
 minor S36.240
 moderate S36.250
 major S36.269
 minor S36.249
 moderate S36.259
 tail S36.232
 major S36.262
 minor S36.242
 moderate S36.252
 pelvic S31.010
 with
 foreign body S31.020
 penetration into retroperitoneal cavity
 S31.021
 penetration into retroperitoneal cavity
 S31.011
 floor — *see also* Laceration, back, lower
 with ectopic or molar pregnancy O08.6
 complicating delivery O70.1
 following ectopic or molar pregnancy
 O08.6
 old (postpartal) N81.89
 organ S37.93
 with ectopic or molar pregnancy O08.6
 adrenal gland S37.813
 bladder S37.23
 fallopian tube — *see* Laceration, fallopian
 tube
 following ectopic or molar pregnancy
 O08.6
 kidney — *see* Laceration, kidney
 obstetrical trauma O71.5
 ovary — *see* Laceration, ovary
 prostate S37.823
 specified site NEC S37.893
 ureter S37.13
 urethra S37.33
 uterus S37.63
 penis S31.21
 with foreign body S31.22
 perineum
 female S31.41
 with
 ectopic or molar pregnancy O08.6
 foreign body S31.42
 during delivery O70.9
 first degree O70.0
 fourth degree O70.3
 second degree O70.1
 third degree (*see also* Delivery,
 complicated, by, laceration,
 perineum, third degree) O70.20
 old (postpartal) N81.89
 postpartal N81.89
 secondary (postpartal) O90.1
 male S31.119
 with foreign body S31.129
 periocular area (with or without lacrimal
 passages) — *see* Laceration, eyelid
 peritoneum S36.893
 periumbilic region — *see* Laceration,
 abdomen, wall, periumbilic
 periurethral tissue — *see* Laceration, urethra

Laceration — *continued*
 phalanges
 finger — *see* Laceration, finger
 toe — *see* Laceration, toe
 pharynx S11.21
 with foreign body S11.22
 pinna — *see* Laceration, ear
 popliteal space — *see* Laceration, knee
 prepuce — *see* Laceration, penis
 prostate S37.823
 pubic region S31.119
 with foreign body S31.129
 pudendum — *see* Laceration, genital organs,
 external
 rectovaginal septum — *see* Laceration, vagina
 rectum S36.63
 retroperitoneum S36.893
 round ligament S37.893
 sacral region — *see* Laceration, back, lower
 sacroiliac region — *see* Laceration, back,
 lower
 salivary gland — *see* Laceration, oral cavity
 scalp S01.01
 with foreign body S01.02
 scapular region — *see* Laceration, shoulder
 scrotum S31.31
 with foreign body S31.32
 seminal vesicle S37.893
 shin — *see* Laceration, leg
 shoulder S41.019
 with foreign body S41.029
 left S41.012
 with foreign body S41.022
 right S41.011
 with foreign body S41.021
 small intestine — *see* Laceration, intestine,
 small
 spermatic cord — *see* Laceration, testis
 spinal cord (meninges) — *see also* Injury, spinal
 cord, by region
 due to injury at birth P11.5
 newborn (birth injury) P11.5
 spleen S36.039
 major (massive) (stellate) S36.032
 moderate S36.031
 superficial (minor) S36.030
 sternal region — *see* Laceration, thorax, front
 stomach S36.33
 submaxillary region — *see* Laceration, head,
 specified site NEC
 submental region — *see* Laceration, head,
 specified site NEC
 subungual
 finger(s) — *see* Laceration, finger, with
 damage to nail
 toe(s) — *see* Laceration, toe, with damage to
 nail
 suprarenal gland — *see* Laceration, adrenal
 gland
 temple, temporal region — *see* Laceration,
 head, specified site NEC
 temporomandibular area — *see* Laceration,
 cheek
 tendon — *see* Injury, muscle, by site, laceration
 Achilles S86.02-
 tentorium cerebelli — *see* Injury, intracranial,
 diffuse
 testis S31.31
 with foreign body S31.32
 thigh S71.11-
 with foreign body S71.12-
 thorax, thoracic (wall) S21.91
 with foreign body S21.92
 back S21.22-
 with penetration into thoracic cavity
 S21.42-
 front S21.12-
 with penetration into thoracic cavity
 S21.32-

Laceration — *continued*
thorax, thoracic (wall) S21.91 — *continued*
  back S21.21-
    with
      foreign body S21.22-
        with penetration into thoracic cavity S21.42-
        penetration into thoracic cavity S21.41-
    breast — *see* Laceration, breast
  front S21.11-
    with
      foreign body S21.12-
        with penetration into thoracic cavity S21.32-
        penetration into thoracic cavity S21.31-
  thumb S61.019
    with
      damage to nail S61.119
        with
          foreign body S61.129
      foreign body S61.029
    left S61.012
      with
        damage to nail S61.112
          with
            foreign body S61.122
        foreign body S61.022
    right S61.011
      with
        damage to nail S61.111
          with
            foreign body S61.121
        foreign body S61.021
  thyroid gland S11.11
    with foreign body S11.12
  toe(s) S91.119
    with
      damage to nail S91.219
        with
          foreign body S91.229
      foreign body S91.129
    great S91.113
      with
        damage to nail S91.213
          with
            foreign body S91.223
        foreign body S91.123
      left S91.112
        with
          damage to nail S91.212
            with
              foreign body S91.222
          foreign body S91.122
      right S91.111
        with
          damage to nail S91.211
            with
              foreign body S91.221
          foreign body S91.121
    lesser S91.116
      with
        damage to nail S91.216
          with
            foreign body S91.226
        foreign body S91.126
      left S91.115
        with
          damage to nail S91.215
            with
              foreign body S91.225
          foreign body S91.125
      right S91.114
        with
          damage to nail S91.214
            with
              foreign body S91.224
          foreign body S91.124

Laceration — *continued*
tongue — *see* Laceration, oral cavity
trachea S11.021
  with foreign body S11.022
tunica vaginalis — *see* Laceration, testis
tympanum, tympanic membrane — *see* Laceration, ear, drum
umbilical region S31.115
  with foreign body S31.125
ureter S37.13
urethra S37.33
  with or following ectopic or molar pregnancy O08.6
  obstetrical trauma O71.5
urinary organ NEC S37.893
uterus S37.63
  with ectopic or molar pregnancy O08.6
  following ectopic or molar pregnancy O08.6
  nonpuerperal, nontraumatic N85.8
  obstetrical trauma NEC O71.81
  old (postpartal) N85.8
uvula — *see* Laceration, oral cavity
vagina S31.41
  with
    ectopic or molar pregnancy O08.6
    foreign body S31.42
  during delivery O71.4
    with perineal laceration — *see* Laceration, perineum, female, during delivery
  following ectopic or molar pregnancy O08.6
  nonpuerperal, nontraumatic N89.8
  old (postpartal) N89.8
vas deferens S37.893
vesical — *see* Laceration, bladder
vocal cords S11.031
  with foreign body S11.032
vulva S31.41
  with
    ectopic or molar pregnancy O08.6
    foreign body S31.42
  complicating delivery O70.0
  following ectopic or molar pregnancy O08.6
  nonpuerperal, nontraumatic N90.89
  old (postpartal) N90.89
wrist S61.519
  with
    foreign body S61.529
  left S61.512
    with
      foreign body S61.522
  right S61.511
    with
      foreign body S61.521

Lack of
achievement in school Z55.3
adequate
  food Z59.4
  intermaxillary vertical dimension of fully erupted teeth M26.36
  sleep Z72.820
appetite (*see also* Anorexia) R63.0
awareness R41.9
care
  in home Z74.2
  of infant (at or after birth) T76.02
    confirmed T74.02
cognitive functions R41.9
coordination R27.9
  ataxia R27.0
  specified type NEC R27.8
development (physiological) R62.50
  failure to thrive (child over 28 days old) R62.51
    adult R62.7
    newborn P92.6
  short stature R62.52
  specified type NEC R62.59
energy R53.83
financial resources Z59.6

Lack of — *continued*
food T73.0
growth R62.52
heating Z59.1
housing (permanent) (temporary) Z59.0
  adequate Z59.1
learning experiences in childhood Z62.898
leisure time (affecting life-style) Z73.2
material resources Z59.9
memory — *see also* Amnesia
  mild, following organic brain damage F06.8
ovulation N97.0
parental supervision or control of child Z62.0
person able to render necessary care Z74.2
physical exercise Z72.3
play experience in childhood Z62.898
posterior occlusal support M26.57
relaxation (affecting life-style) Z73.2
sexual
  desire F52.0
  enjoyment F52.1
shelter Z59.0
sleep (adequate) Z72.820
supervision of child by parent Z62.0
support, posterior occlusal M26.57
water T73.1
Lacrimal — *see* condition
Lacrimation, abnormal — *see* Epiphora
Lacrimonasal duct — *see* condition
Lactation, lactating (breast) (puerperal, postpartum)
associated
  cracked nipple O92.13
  retracted nipple O92.03
defective O92.4
disorder NEC O92.79
excessive O92.6
failed (complete) O92.3
  partial O92.4
mastitis NEC — *see* Mastitis, obstetric
mother (care and/or examination) Z39.1
nonpuerperal N64.3
Lacticemia, excessive E87.2
Lacunar skull Q75.8
Laennec's cirrhosis K70.30
with ascites K70.31
nonalcoholic K74.69
Lafora's disease — *see* Epilepsy, generalized, idiopathic
Lag, lid (nervous) — *see* Retraction, lid
Lagophthalmos (eyelid) (nervous) H02.209
cicatricial H02.219
  left H02.216
    lower H02.215
    upper H02.214
  right H02.213
    lower H02.212
    upper H02.211
keratoconjunctivitis — *see* Keratoconjunctivitis
left H02.206
  lower H02.205
  upper H02.204
mechanical H02.229
  left H02.226
    lower H02.225
    upper H02.224
  right H02.223
    lower H02.222
    upper H02.221
paralytic H02.239
  left H02.236
    lower H02.235
    upper H02.234
  right H02.233
    lower H02.232
    upper H02.231
right H02.203
  lower H02.202
  upper H02.201

Leiomyoma — *see also* Neoplasm, connective tissue, benign
  bizarre — *see* Neoplasm, connective tissue, benign
  cellular — *see* Neoplasm, connective tissue, benign
  epithelioid — *see* Neoplasm, connective tissue, benign
  uterus (cervix) (corpus) D25.9
    intramural D25.1
    submucous D25.0
    subserosal D25.2
  vascular — *see* Neoplasm, connective tissue, benign
Leiomyoma, leiomyomatosis (intravascular) — *see* Neoplasm, connective tissue, uncertain behavior
Leiomyosarcoma — *see also* Neoplasm, connective tissue, malignant
  epithelioid — *see* Neoplasm, connective tissue, malignant
  myxoid — *see* Neoplasm, connective tissue, malignant
Leishmaniasis B55.9
  American (mucocutaneous) B55.2
    cutaneous B55.1
  Asian Desert B55.1
  Brazilian B55.2
  cutaneous (any type) B55.1
  dermal — *see also* Leishmaniasis, cutaneous
    post-kala-azar B55.0
  eyelid B55.1
  infantile B55.0
  Mediterranean B55.0
  mucocutaneous (American) (New World) B55.2
  naso-oral B55.2
  nasopharyngeal B55.2
  old world B55.1
  tegumentaria diffusa B55.1
  visceral B55.0
Leishmanoid, dermal — *see also* Leishmaniasis, cutaneous
  post-kala-azar B55.0
Lenegre's disease I44.2
Lengthening, leg — *see* Deformity, limb, unequal length
Lennert's lymphoma — *see* Lymphoma, Lennert's
Lennox-Gastaut syndrome G40.812
  intractable G40.814
    with status epilepticus G40.813
    without status epilepticus G40.814
  not intractable G40.812
    with status epilepticus G40.811
    without status epilepticus G40.812
Lens — *see* condition
Lenticonus (anterior) (posterior) (congenital) Q12.8
Lenticular degeneration, progressive E83.01
Lentiglobus (posterior) (congenital) Q12.8
Lentigo (congenital) L81.4
  maligna — *see also* Melanoma, in situ
    melanoma — *see* Melanoma
Lentivirus, as cause of disease classified elsewhere B97.31
Leontiasis
  ossium M85.2
  syphilitic (late) A52.78
    congenital A50.59
Lepothrix A48.8
Lepra — *see* Leprosy
Leprechaunism E34.8
Leprosy A30-
  with muscle disorder A30.9 *[M63.80]*
    ankle A30.9 *[M63.8-]*
    foot A30.9 *[M63.8-]*
    forearm A30.9 *[M63.8-]*

Leprosy A30- — *continued*
  with muscle disorder A30.9 *[M63.80]* — *continued*
    hand A30.9 *[M63.8-]*
    lower leg A30.9 *[M63.8-]*
    multiple sites A30.9 *[M63.8-]*
    pelvic region A30.9 *[M63.8-]*
    shoulder region A30.9 *[M63.8-]*
    specified site NEC A30.9 *[M63.8-]*
    thigh A30.9 *[M63.8-]*
    upper arm A30.9 *[M63.8-]*
  anesthetic A30.9
  BB A30.3
  BL A30.4
  borderline (infiltrated) (neuritic) A30.3
    lepromatous A30.4
    tuberculoid A30.2
  BT A30.2
  dimorphous (infiltrated) (neuritic) A30.3
  I A30.0
  indeterminate (macular) (neuritic) A30.0
  lepromatous (diffuse) (infiltrated) (macular) (neuritic) (nodular) A30.5
  LL A30.5
  macular (early) (neuritic) (simple) A30.9
  maculoanesthetic A30.9
  mixed A30.3
  neural A30.9
  nodular A30.5
  primary neuritic A30.3
  specified type NEC A30.8
  TT A30.1
  tuberculoid (major) (minor) A30.1
Leptocytosis, hereditary D56.9
Leptomeningitis (chronic) (circumscribed) (hemorrhagic) (nonsuppurative) — *see* Meningitis
Leptomeningopathy G96.19
Leptospiral — *see* condition
Leptospirochetal — *see* condition
Leptospirosis A27.9
  canicola A27.89
  due to Leptospira interrogans serovar icterohaemorrhagiae A27.0
  icterohemorrhagica A27.0
  pomona A27.89
  Weil's disease A27.0
Leptus dermatitis B88.0
Leri's pleonosteosis Q78.8
Leri-Weill syndrome Q77.8
Leriche's syndrome (aortic bifurcation occlusion) I74.09
Lermoyez' syndrome — *see* Vertigo, peripheral NEC
Lesch-Nyhan syndrome E79.1
Leser-Trélat disease L82.1
  inflamed L82.0
Lesion(s) (nontraumatic)
  abducens nerve — *see* Strabismus, paralytic, sixth nerve
  alveolar process K08.9
  angiocentric immunoproliferative D47.Z9
  anorectal K62.9
  aortic (valve) I35.9
  auditory nerve — *see* subcategory H93.3
  basal ganglion G25.9
  bile duct — *see* Disease, bile duct
  biomechanical M99.9
    specified type NEC M99.89
      abdomen M99.89
      acromioclavicular M99.87
      cervical region M99.81
      cervicothoracic M99.81
      costochondral M99.88
      costovertebral M99.88
      head region M99.80
      hip M99.85
      lower extremity M99.86
      lumbar region M99.83

Lesion(s) (nontraumatic) — *continued*
  biomechanical M99.9 — *continued*
    specified type NEC M99.89 — *continued*
      lumbosacral M99.83
      occipitocervical M99.80
      pelvic region M99.85
      pubic M99.85
      rib cage M99.88
      sacral region M99.84
      sacrococcygeal M99.84
      sacroiliac M99.84
      specified NEC M99.89
      sternochondral M99.88
      sternoclavicular M99.87
      thoracic region M99.82
      thoracolumbar M99.82
      upper extremity M99.87
  bladder N32.9
  bone — *see* Disorder, bone
  brachial plexus G54.0
  brain G93.9
    congenital Q04.9
    vascular I67.9
      degenerative I67.9
      hypertensive I67.4
  buccal cavity K13.79
  calcified — *see* Calcification
  canthus — *see* Disorder, eyelid
  carate — *see* Pinta, lesions
  cardia K31.9
  cardiac (*see also* Disease, heart) I51.9
    congenital Q24.9
    valvular — *see* Endocarditis
  cauda equina G83.4
  cecum K63.9
  cerebral — *see* Lesion, brain
  cerebrovascular I67.9
    degenerative I67.9
    hypertensive I67.4
  cervical (nerve) root NEC G54.2
  chiasmal — *see* Disorder, optic, chiasm
  chorda tympani G51.8
  coin, lung R91.1
  colon K63.9
  combined periodontic-endodontic K05.5
  congenital — *see* Anomaly, by site
  conjunctiva H11.9
  conus medullaris — *see* Injury, conus medullaris
  coronary artery — *see* Ischemia, heart
  cranial nerve G52.9
    eighth — *see* Disorder, ear
    eleventh G52.9
    fifth G50.9
    first G52.0
    fourth — *see* Strabismus, paralytic, fourth nerve
    seventh G51.9
    sixth — *see* Strabismus, paralytic, sixth nerve
    tenth G52.2
    twelfth G52.3
  cystic — *see* Cyst
  degenerative — *see* Degeneration
  duodenum K31.9
  edentulous (alveolar) ridge, associated with trauma, due to traumatic occlusion K06.2
  en coup de sabre L94.1
  eyelid — *see* Disorder, eyelid
  gasserian ganglion G50.8
  gastric K31.9
  gastroduodenal K31.9
  gastrointestinal K63.9
  gingiva, associated with trauma K06.2
  glomerular
    focal and segmental (*see also* N00-N07 with fourth character .1) N05.1
    minimal change (*see also* N00-N07 with fourth character .0) N05.0
  heart (organic) — *see* Disease, heart

Lesion(s) (nontraumatic) — *continued*
  hyperchromic, due to pinta (carate) A67.1
  hyperkeratotic — *see* Hyperkeratosis
  hypothalamic E23.7
  ileocecal K63.9
  ileum K63.9
  iliohypogastric nerve G57.8-
  inflammatory — *see* Inflammation
  intestine K63.9
  intracerebral — *see* Lesion, brain
  intrachiasmal (optic) — *see* Disorder, optic, chiasm
  intracranial, space-occupying R90.0
  joint — *see* Disorder, joint
    sacroiliac (old) M53.3
  keratotic — *see* Keratosis
  kidney — *see* Disease, renal
  laryngeal nerve (recurrent) G52.2
  lip K13.0
  liver K76.9
  lumbosacral
    plexus G54.1
    root (nerve) NEC G54.4
  lung (coin) R91.1
  maxillary sinus J32.0
  mitral I05.9
  Morel-Lavallée — *see* Hematoma, by site
  motor cortex NEC G93.89
  mouth K13.79
  nerve G58.9
    femoral G57.2-
    median G56.1-
      carpal tunnel syndrome — *see* Syndrome, carpal tunnel
    plantar G57.6-
    popliteal (lateral) G57.3-
      medial G57.4-
    radial G56.3-
    sciatic G57.0-
    spinal — *see* Injury, nerve, spinal
    ulnar G56.2-
  nervous system, congenital Q07.9
  nonallopathic — *see* Lesion, biomechanical
  nose (internal) J34.89
  obstructive — *see* Obstruction
  obturator nerve G57.8-
  oral mucosa K13.70
  organ or site NEC — *see* Disease, by site
  osteolytic — *see* Osteolysis
  peptic K27.9
  periodontal, due to traumatic occlusion K05.5
  pharynx J39.2
  pigment, pigmented (skin) L81.9
  pinta — *see* Pinta, lesions
  polypoid — *see* Polyp
  prechiasmal (optic) — *see* Disorder, optic, chiasm
  primary (*see also* Syphilis, primary) A51.0
    carate A67.0
    pinta A67.0
    yaws A66.0
  pulmonary J98.4
    valve I37.9
  pylorus K31.9
  rectosigmoid K63.9
  retina, retinal H35.9
  sacroiliac (joint) (old) M53.3
  salivary gland K11.9
    benign lymphoepithelial K11.8
  saphenous nerve G57.8-
  sciatic nerve G57.0-
  secondary — *see* Syphilis, secondary
  shoulder (region) M75.9-
    specified NEC M75.8-
  sigmoid K63.9
  sinus (accessory) (nasal) J34.89
  skin L98.9
    suppurative L08.0
  SLAP S43.43-

Lesion(s) (nontraumatic) — *continued*
  spinal cord G95.9
    congenital Q06.9
  spleen D73.89
  stomach K31.9
  superior glenoid labrum S43.43-
  syphilitic — *see* Syphilis
  tertiary — *see* Syphilis, tertiary
  thoracic root (nerve) NEC G54.3
  tonsillar fossa J35.9
  tooth, teeth K08.9
    white spot
      chewing surface K02.51
      pit and fissure surface K02.51
      smooth surface K02.61
  traumatic — *see* specific type of injury by site
  tricuspid (valve) I07.9
    nonrheumatic I36.9
  trigeminal nerve G50.9
  ulcerated or ulcerative — *see* Ulcer, skin
  uterus N85.9
  vagus nerve G52.2
  valvular — *see* Endocarditis
  vascular I99.9
    affecting central nervous system I67.9
    following trauma NEC T14.8
    umbilical cord, complicating delivery O69.5
  warty — *see* Verruca
  white spot (tooth)
    chewing surface K02.51
    pit and fissure surface K02.51
    smooth surface K02.61
Lethargic — *see* condition
Lethargy R53.83
Letterer-Siwe's disease C96.0
Leukemia, leukemic C95.9-
  acute basophilic C94.8-
  acute bilineal C95.0-
  acute erythroid C94.0-
  acute lymphoblastic C91.0-
  acute megakaryoblastic C94.2-
  acute megakaryocytic C94.2-
  acute mixed lineage C95.0-
  acute monoblastic (monoblastic/monocytic) C93.0-
  acute monocytic (monoblastic/monocytic) C93.0-
  acute myeloblastic (minimal differentiation) (with maturation) C92.0-
  acute myeloid
    with
      11q23-abnormality C92.6-
      dysplasia of remaining hematopoesis and/or myelodysplastic disease in its history C92.A- *(follows C92.6)*
      multilineage dysplasia C92.A- *(follows C92.6)*
      variation of MLL-gene C92.6-
    M6(a)(b) C94.0-
    M7 C94.2-
  acute myelomonocytic C92.5-
  acute promyelocytic C92.4-
  adult T-cell (HTLV-1-associated) (acute variant) (chronic variant) (lymphomatoid variant) (smouldering variant) C91.5-
  aggressive NK-cell C94.8-
  AML (1/ETO) (M0) (M1) (M2) (without a FAB classification) C92.0-
  AML M3 C92.4-
  AML M4 (Eo with inv(16) or t(16;16)) C92.5-
  AML M5 C93.0-
  AML M5a C93.0-
  AML M5b C93.0-
  AML Me with t(15;17) and variants C92.4-
  atypical chronic myeloid, BCR/ABL-negative C92.2-
  biphenotypic acute C95.0-
  blast cell C95.0-
  Burkitt-type, mature B-cell C91.A- *(follows C91.6)*

Leukemia, leukemic C95.9- — *continued*
  chronic lymphocytic, of B-cell type C91.1-
  chronic monocytic C93.1-
  chronic myelogenous (Philadelphia chromosome (Ph1) positive) (t(9;22)) (q34;q11) (with crisis of blast cells) C92.1-
  chronic myeloid, BCR/ABL-positive C92.1-
    atypical, BCR/ABL-negative C92.2-
  chronic myelomonocytic C93.1-
  chronic neutrophilic D47.1
  CMML (-1) (-2) (with eosinophilia) C93.1-
  granulocytic (*see also* Category C92) C92.9-
  hairy cell C91.4-
  juvenile myelomonocytic C93.3-
  lymphoid C91.9-
    specified NEC C91.Z- *(follows C91.6)*
  mast cell C94.3-
  mature B-cell, Burkitt-type C91.A- *(follows C91.6)*
  monocytic (subacute) C93.9-
    specified NEC C93.Z- *(follows C93.3)*
  myelogenous (*see also* Category C92) C92.9-
  myeloid C92.9-
    specified NEC C92.Z- *(follows C92.6)*
  plasma cell C90.1-
  plasmacytic C90.1-
  prolymphocytic
    of B-cell type C91.3-
    of T-cell type C91.6-
  specified NEC C94.8-
  stem cell, of unclear lineage C95.0-
  subacute lymphocytic C91.9-
  T-cell large granular lymphocytic C91.Z- *(follows C91.6)*
  unspecified cell type C95.9-
    acute C95.0-
    chronic C95.1-
Leukemoid reaction (*see also* Reaction, leukemoid) D72.823-
Leukoaraiosis (hypertensive) I67.81
Leukoariosis — *see* Leukoaraiosis
Leukocoria — *see* Disorder, globe, degenerated condition, leucocoria
Leukocytopenia D72.819
Leukocytosis D72.829
  eosinophilic D72.1
Leukoderma, leukodermia NEC L81.5
  syphilitic A51.39
    late A52.79
Leukodystrophy E75.29
Leukoedema, oral epithelium K13.29
Leukoencephalitis G04.81
  acute (subacute) hemorrhagic G36.1
    postimmunization or postvaccinal G04.02
  postinfectious G04.01
  subacute sclerosing A81.1
  van Bogaert's (sclerosing) A81.1
Leukoencephalopathy (*see also* Encephalopathy) G93.49
  Binswanger's I67.3
  heroin vapor G92
  metachromatic E75.25
  multifocal (progressive) A81.2
  postimmunization and postvaccinal G04.02
  progressive multifocal A81.2
  reversible, posterior G93.6
  van Bogaert's (sclerosing) A81.1
  vascular, progressive I67.3
Leukoerythroblastosis D75.9
Leukokeratosis — *see also* Leukoplakia
  mouth K13.21
  nicotina palati K13.24
  oral mucosa K13.21
  tongue K13.21
  vocal cord J38.3
Leukokraurosis vulva(e) N90.4
Leukoma (cornea) — *see also* Opacity, cornea
  adherent H17.0-
  interfering with central vision — *see* Opacity, cornea, central

Leukomalacia, cerebral, newborn P91.2
  periventricular P91.2
Leukomelanopathy, hereditary D72.0
Leukonychia (punctata) (striata) L60.8
  congenital Q84.4
Leukopathia unguium L60.8
  congenital Q84.4
Leukopenia D72.819
  basophilic D72.818
  chemotherapy (cancer) induced D70.1
  congenital D70.0
  cyclic D70.0
  drug induced NEC D70.2
    due to cytoreductive cancer chemotherapy D70.1
  eosinophilic D72.818
  familial D70.0
  infantile genetic D70.0
  malignant D70.9
  periodic D70.0
  transitory neonatal P61.5
Leukopenic — see condition
Leukoplakia
  anus K62.89
  bladder (postinfectional) N32.89
  buccal K13.21
  cervix (uteri) N88.0
  esophagus K22.8
  gingiva K13.21
  hairy (oral mucosa) (tongue) K13.3
  kidney (pelvis) N28.89
  larynx J38.7
  lip K13.21
  mouth K13.21
  oral epithelium, including tongue (mucosa) K13.21
  palate K13.21
  pelvis (kidney) N28.89
  penis (infectional) N48.0
  rectum K62.89
  syphilitic (late) A52.79
  tongue K13.21
  ureter (postinfectional) N28.89
  urethra (postinfectional) N36.8
  uterus N85.8
  vagina N89.4
  vocal cord J38.3
  vulva N90.4
Leukorrhea N89.8
  due to Trichomonas (vaginalis) A59.00
  trichomonal A59.00
Leukosarcoma C85.9-
Levocardia (isolated) Q24.1
  with situs inversus Q89.3
Levotransposition Q20.5
Lev's disease or syndrome (acquired complete heart block) I44.2
Levulosuria — see Fructosuria
Levurid L30.2
Lewy body(ies) (dementia) (disease) G31.83
Leyden-Moebius dystrophy G71.0
Leydig cell
  carcinoma
    specified site — see Neoplasm, malignant, by site
    unspecified site
      female C56.9
      male C62.9-
  tumor
    benign
      specified site — see Neoplasm, benign, by site
      unspecified site
        female D27-
        male D29.2-

Leydig cell — continued
  tumor — continued
    malignant
      specified site — see Neoplasm, malignant, by site
      unspecified site
        female C56-
        male C62.9-
    specified site — see Neoplasm, uncertain behavior, by site
    unspecified site
      female D39.1-
      male D40.1-
Leydig-Sertoli cell tumor
  specified site — see Neoplasm, benign, by site
  unspecified site
    female D27-
    male D29.2-
LGSIL (low grade squamous intraepithelial lesion on cytologic smear of)
  anus R85.612
  cervix R87.612
  vagina R87.622
Liar, pathologic F60.2
Libido
  decreased R68.82
Libman-Sacks disease M32.11
Lice (infestation) B85.2
  body (Pediculus corporis) B85.1
  crab B85.3
  head (Pediculus capitis) B85.0
  mixed (classifiable to more than one of the titles B85.0-B85.3) B85.4
  pubic (Phthirus pubis) B85.3
Lichen L28.0
  albus L90.0
    penis N48.0
    vulva N90.4
  amyloidosis E85.4 [L99]
  atrophicus L90.0
    penis N48.0
    vulva N90.4
  congenital Q82.8
  myxedematosus L98.5
  nitidus L44.1
  pilaris Q82.8
    acquired L85.8
  planopilaris L66.1
  planus (chronicus) L43.9
    annularis L43.8
    bullous L43.1
    follicular L66.1
    hypertrophic L43.0
    moniliformis L44.3
    of Wilson L43.9
    specified NEC L43.8
    subacute (active) L43.3
    tropicus L43.3
  ruber
    acuminatus L44.0
    moniliformis L44.3
    planus L43.9
  sclerosus (et atrophicus) L90.0
    penis N48.0
    vulva N90.4
  scrofulosus (primary) (tuberculous) A18.4
  simplex (chronicus) (circumscriptus) L28.0
  striatus L44.2
  urticatus L28.2
Lichenification L28.0
Lichenoides tuberculosis (primary) A18.4
Lichtheim's disease or syndrome — see Degeneration, combined
Lien migrans D73.89
Ligament — see condition
Light
  for gestational age — see Light for dates
  headedness R42

Light-for-dates (infant) P05.00
  with weight of
    499 grams or less P05.01
    500-749 grams P05.02
    750-999 grams P05.03
    1000-1249 grams P05.04
    1250-1499 grams P05.05
    1500-1749 grams P05.06
    1750-1999 grams P05.07
    2000-2499 grams P05.08
    2500 grams and over P05.09
  affecting management of pregnancy O36.59-
  and small-for-dates — see Small for dates
  specified NEC P05.09
Lightning (effects) (stroke) (struck by) T75.00
  burn — see Burn
  foot E53.8
  shock T75.01
  specified effect NEC T75.09
Lightwood-Albright syndrome N25.89
Lightwood's disease or syndrome (renal tubular acidosis) N25.89
Lignac(-de Toni) (-Fanconi) (-Debré) disease or syndrome E72.09
  with cystinosis E72.04
Ligneous thyroiditis E06.5
Likoff's syndrome I20.8
Limb — see condition
Limbic epilepsy personality syndrome F07.0
Limitation, limited
  activities due to disability Z73.6
  cardiac reserve — see Disease, heart
  eye muscle duction, traumatic — see Strabismus, mechanical
  mandibular range of motion M26.52
Lindau(-von Hippel) disease Q85.8
Line(s)
  Beau's L60.4
  Harris' — see Arrest, epiphyseal
  Hudson's (cornea) — see Pigmentation, cornea, anterior
  Stähli's (cornea) — see Pigmentation, cornea, anterior
Linea corneae senilis — see Change, cornea, senile
Lingua
  geographica K14.1
  nigra (villosa) K14.3
  plicata K14.5
  tylosis K13.29
Lingual — see condition
Linguatulosis B88.8
Linitis (gastric) plastica C16.9
Lip — see condition
Lipedema — see Edema
Lipemia — see also Hyperlipidemia
  retina, retinalis E78.3
Lipidosis E75.6
  cerebral (infantile) (juvenile) (late) E75.4
  cerebroretinal E75.4
  cerebroside E75.22
  cholesterol (cerebral) E75.5
  glycolipid E75.21
  hepatosplenomegalic E78.3
  sphingomyelin — see Niemann-Pick disease or syndrome
  sulfatide E75.29
Lipoadenoma — see Neoplasm, benign, by site
Lipoblastoma — see Lipoma
Lipoblastomatosis — see Lipoma
Lipochondrodystrophy E76.01
Lipochrome histiocytosis (familial) D71
Lipodermatosclerosis — see Varix, leg, with, inflammation
  ulcerated — see Varix, leg, with, ulcer, with inflammation by site
Lipodystrophia progressiva E88.1

DISEASE INDEX

Lipodystrophy (progressive) E88.1
  insulin E88.1
  intestinal K90.81
  mesenteric K65.4
Lipofibroma — see Lipoma
Lipofuscinosis, neuronal (with ceroidosis) E75.4
Lipogranuloma, sclerosing L92.8
Lipogranulomatosis E78.89
Lipoid — see also condition
  histiocytosis D76.3
    essential E75.29
  nephrosis N04.9
  proteinosis of Urbach E78.89
Lipoidemia — see Hyperlipidemia
Lipoidosis — see Lipidosis
Lipoma D17.9
  fetal D17.9
    fat cell D17.9
  infiltrating D17.9
  intramuscular D17.9
  pleomorphic D17.9
  site classification
    arms (skin) (subcutaneous) D17.2-
    connective tissue D17.30
      intra-abdominal D17.5
      intrathoracic D17.4
      peritoneum D17.79
      retroperitoneum D17.79
      specified site NEC D17.39
      spermatic cord D17.6
    face (skin) (subcutaneous) D17.0
    genitourinary organ NEC D17.72
    head (skin) (subcutaneous) D17.0
    intra-abdominal D17.5
    intrathoracic D17.4
    kidney D17.71
    legs (skin) (subcutaneous) D17.2-
    neck (skin) (subcutaneous) D17.0
    peritoneum D17.79
    retroperitoneum D17.79
    skin D17.30
      specified site NEC D17.39
    specified site NEC D17.79
    spermatic cord D17.6
    subcutaneous D17.30
      specified site NEC D17.39
    trunk (skin) (subcutaneous) D17.1
    unspecified D17.9
  spindle cell D17.9
Lipomatosis E88.2
  dolorosa (Dercum) E88.2
  fetal — see Lipoma
  Launois-Bensaude E88.89
Lipomyoma — see Lipoma
Lipomyxoma — see Lipoma
Lipomyxosarcoma — see Neoplasm, connective tissue, malignant
Lipoprotein metabolism disorder E78.9
Lipoproteinemia E78.5
  broad-beta E78.2
  floating-beta E78.2
  hyper-pre-beta E78.1
Liposarcoma — see also Neoplasm, connective tissue, malignant
  dedifferentiated — see Neoplasm, connective tissue, malignant
  differentiated type — see Neoplasm, connective tissue, malignant
  embryonal — see Neoplasm, connective tissue, malignant
  mixed type — see Neoplasm, connective tissue, malignant
  myxoid — see Neoplasm, connective tissue, malignant
  pleomorphic — see Neoplasm, connective tissue, malignant
  round cell — see Neoplasm, connective tissue, malignant

Liposarcoma — see also Neoplasm, connective tissue, malignant — continued
  well differentiated type — see Neoplasm, connective tissue, malignant
Liposynovitis prepatellaris E88.89
Lipping, cervix N86
Lipschütz disease or ulcer N76.6
Lipuria R82.0
  schistosomiasis (bilharziasis) B65.0
Lisping F80.0
Lissauer's paralysis A52.17
Lissencephalia, lissencephaly Q04.3
Listeriosis, listerellosis A32.9
  congenital (disseminated) P37.2
  cutaneous A32.0
  neonatal, newborn (disseminated) P37.2
  oculoglandular A32.81
  specified NEC A32.89
Lithemia E79.0
Lithiasis — see Calculus
Lithosis J62.8
Lithuria R82.99
Litigation, anxiety concerning Z65.3
Little leaguer's elbow — see Epicondylitis, medial
Little's disease G80.9
Littre's
  gland — see condition
  hernia — see Hernia, abdomen
Littritis — see Urethritis
Livedo (annularis) (racemosa) (reticularis) R23.1
Liver — see condition
Living alone (problems with) Z60.2
  with handicapped person Z74.2
Lloyd's syndrome — see Adenomatosis, endocrine
Loa loa, loaiasis, loasis B74.3
Lobar — see condition
Lobomycosis B48.0
Lobo's disease B48.0
Lobotomy syndrome F07.0
Lobstein(-Ekman) disease or syndrome Q78.0
Lobster-claw hand Q71.6-
Lobulation (congenital) — see also Anomaly, by site
  kidney, Q63.1
  liver, abnormal Q44.7
  spleen Q89.09
Lobule, lobular — see condition
Local, localized — see condition
Locked twins causing obstructed labor O66.1
Locked-in state G83.5
Locking
  joint — see Derangement, joint, specified type NEC
  knee — see Derangement, knee
Lockjaw — see Tetanus
Löffler's
  endocarditis I42.3
  eosinophilia J82
  pneumonia J82
  syndrome (eosinophilic pneumonitis) J82
Loiasis (with conjunctival infestation) (eyelid) B74.3
Lone Star fever A77.0
Long
  labor O63.9
    first stage O63.0
    second stage O63.1
  QT syndrome I45.81

Long-term (current) (prophylactic) drug therapy (use of)
  agents affecting estrogen receptors and estrogen levels NEC Z79.818
  anastrozole (Arimidex) Z79.811
  anti-inflammatory, non-steroidal (NSAID) Z79.1
  antibiotics Z79.2
    short-term use — omit code
  anticoagulants Z79.01
  antiplatelet Z79.02
  antithrombotics Z79.02
  aromatase inhibitors Z79.811
  aspirin Z79.82
  birth control pill or patch Z79.3
  bisphosphonates Z79.83
  contraceptive, oral Z79.3
  drug, specified NEC Z79.899
  estrogen receptor downregulators Z79.818
  Evista Z79.810
  exemestane (Aromasin) Z79.811
  Fareston Z79.810
  fulvestrant (Faslodex) Z79.818
  gonadotropin-releasing hormone (GnRH) agonist Z79.818
  goserelin acetate (Zoladex) Z79.818
  hormone replacement (postmenopausal) Z79.890
  insulin Z79.4
  letrozole (Femara) Z79.811
  leuprolide acetate (leuprorelin) (Lupron) Z79.818
  megestrol acetate (Megace) Z79.818
  methadone for pain management Z79.891
  Nolvadex Z79.810
  non-steroidal anti-inflammatories (NSAID) Z79.1
  opiate analgesic Z79.891
  oral
    antidiabetic Z79.84
    contraceptive Z79.3
    hypoglycemic Z79.84
  raloxifene (Evista) Z79.810
  selective estrogen receptor modulators (SERMs) Z79.810
  steroids
    inhaled Z79.51
    systemic Z79.52
  tamoxifen (Nolvadex) Z79.810
  toremifene (Fareston) Z79.810
Longitudinal stripes or grooves, nails L60.8
  congenital Q84.6
Loop
  intestine — see Volvulus
  vascular on papilla (optic) Q14.2
Loose — see also condition
  body
    joint M24.00
      ankle M24.07-
      elbow M24.02-
      hand M24.04-
      hip M24.05-
      knee M23.4-
      shoulder (region) M24.01-
      specified site NEC M24.08
      toe M24.07-
      vertebra M24.08
      wrist M24.03-
    knee M23.4-
    sheath, tendon — see Disorder, tendon, specified type NEC
  cartilage — see Loose, body, joint
  skin and subcutaneous tissue (following bariatric surgery weight loss) (following dietary weight loss) L98.7
  tooth, teeth K08.89

Loosening
  aseptic
    joint prosthesis — *see* Complications, joint
      prosthesis, mechanical, loosening, by
      site
    epiphysis — *see* Osteochondropathy
  mechanical
    joint prosthesis — *see* Complications, joint
      prosthesis, mechanical, loosening, by
      site
Looser-Milkman(-Debray) syndrome
  M83.8
Lop ear (deformity) Q17.3
Lorain(-Levi) short stature syndrome
  E23.0
Lordosis M40.50
  acquired — *see* Lordosis, specified type NEC
  congenital Q76.429
    lumbar region Q76.426
    lumbosacral region Q76.427
    sacral region Q76.428
    sacrococcygeal region Q76.428
    thoracolumbar region Q76.425
  lumbar region M40.56
  lumbosacral region M40.57
  postsurgical M96.4
  postural — *see* Lordosis, specified type NEC
  rachitic (late effect) (sequelae) E64.3
  sequelae of rickets E64.3
  specified type NEC M40.40
    lumbar region M40.46
    lumbosacral region M40.47
    thoracolumbar region M40.45
  thoracolumbar region M40.55
  tuberculous A18.01
Loss (of)
  appetite (*see also* Anorexia) R63.0
    hysterical F50.89
    nonorganic origin F50.89
    psychogenic F50.89
  blood — *see* Hemorrhage
  bone — *see* Loss, substance of, bone
  consciousness, transient R55
    traumatic — *see* Injury, intracranial
  control, sphincter, rectum R15.9
    nonorganic origin F98.1
  elasticity, skin R23.4
  family (member) in childhood Z62.898
  fluid (acute) E86.9
  function of labyrinth — *see* subcategory H83.2
  hair, nonscarring — *see* Alopecia
  hearing — *see also* Deafness
    central NOS H90.5
    conductive H90.2
      bilateral H90.0
      unilateral
        with
          restricted hearing on the contralateral
            side H90.A1- *(follows H90.8)*
          unrestricted hearing on the
            contralateral side H90.1-
    mixed conductive and sensorineural hearing
      loss H90.8
      bilateral H90.6
        unilateral
          with
            restricted hearing on the
              contralateral side H90.A3-
                (follows H90.8)
            unrestricted hearing on the
              contralateral side H90.7-
    neural NOS H90.5
    perceptive NOS H90.5

Loss (of) — *continued*
  hearing — *see also* Deafness — *continued*
    sensorineural NOS H90.5
      bilateral H90.3
      unilateral
        with
          restricted hearing on the contralateral
            side H90.A2- *(follows H90.8)*
          unrestricted hearing on the
            contralateral side H90.4-
    sensory NOS H90.5
  height R29.890
  limb or member, traumatic, current — *see*
    Amputation, traumatic
  love relationship in childhood Z62.898
  memory — *see also* Amnesia
    mild, following organic brain damage F06.8
  mind — *see* Psychosis
  occlusal vertical dimension of fully erupted
    teeth M26.37
  organ or part — *see* Absence, by site,
    acquired
  ossicles, ear (partial) H74.32-
  parent in childhood Z63.4
  pregnancy, recurrent N96
    care in current pregnancy O26.2-
    without current pregnancy N96
  recurrent pregnancy — *see* Loss, pregnancy,
    recurrent
  self-esteem, in childhood Z62.898
  sense of
    smell — *see* Disturbance, sensation, smell
    taste — *see* Disturbance, sensation, taste
    touch R20.8
  sensory R44.9
    dissociative F44.6
  sexual desire F52.0
  sight (acquired) (complete) (congenital) — *see*
    Blindness
  substance of
    bone — *see* Disorder, bone, density and
      structure, specified NEC
      horizontal alveolar K06.3
    cartilage — *see* Disorder, cartilage, specified
      type NEC
    auricle (ear) — *see* Disorder, pinna,
      specified type NEC
    vitreous (humor) H15.89
  tooth, teeth — *see* Absence, teeth, acquired
  vision, visual H54.7
    both eyes H54.3
    one eye H54.60
      left (normal vision on right) H54.62
      right (normal vision on left) H54.61
    specified as blindness — *see* Blindness
    subjective
      sudden H53.13-
      transient H53.12-
  vitreous — *see* Prolapse, vitreous
  voice — *see* Aphonia
  weight (abnormal) (cause unknown) R63.4
Louis-Bar syndrome (ataxia-telangiectasia)
  G11.3
Louping ill (encephalitis) A84.8
Louse, lousiness — *see* Lice
Low
  achiever, school Z55.3
  back syndrome M54.5
  basal metabolic rate R94.8
  birthweight (2499 grams or less) P07.10
    with weight of
      1000-1249 grams P07.14
      1250-1499 grams P07.15
      1500-1749 grams P07.16
      1750-1999 grams P07.17
      2000-2499 grams P07.18

Low — *continued*
  birthweight (2499 grams or less) P07.10 —
      continued
    extreme (999 grams or less) P07.00
      with weight of
        499 grams or less P07.01
        500-749 grams P07.02
        750-999 grams P07.03
    for gestational age — *see* Light for dates
  blood pressure — *see also* Hypotension
    reading (incidental) (isolated) (nonspecific)
      R03.1
  cardiac reserve — *see* Disease, heart
  function — *see also* Hypofunction
    kidney N28.9
  hematocrit D64.9
  hemoglobin D64.9
  income Z59.6
  level of literacy Z55.0
  lying
    kidney N28.89
    organ or site, congenital — *see* Malposition,
      congenital
  output syndrome (cardiac) — *see* Failure, heart
  platelets (blood) — *see* Thrombocytopenia
  reserve, kidney N28.89
  salt syndrome E87.1
  self esteem R45.81
  set ears Q17.4
  vision H54.2
    one eye (other eye normal) H54.50
      left (normal vision on right) H54.52
      other eye blind — *see* Blindness
      right (normal vision on left) H54.51
Low-density-lipoprotein-type (LDL)
  hyperlipoproteinemia E78.00
Lowe's syndrome E72.03
Lown-Ganong-Levine syndrome I45.6
LSD reaction (acute) (without dependence)
  F16.90
  with dependence F16.20
L-shaped kidney Q63.8
Ludwig's angina or disease K12.2
Lues (venerea), luetic — *see* Syphilis
Luetscher's syndrome (dehydration) E86.0
Lumbago, lumbalgia M54.5
  with sciatica M54.4-
    due to intervertebral disc disorder M51.17
  due to displacement, intervertebral disc
    M51.27
  with sciatica M51.17
Lumbar — *see* condition
Lumbarization, vertebra, congenital
  Q76.49
Lumbermen's itch B88.0
Lump — *see* Mass
Lunacy — *see* Psychosis
Lung — *see* condition
Lupoid (miliary) of Boeck D86.3
Lupus
  anticoagulant D68.62
    with
      hemorrhagic disorder D68.312
      hypercoagulable state D68.62
    finding without diagnosis R76.0
  discoid (local) L93.0
  erythematosus (discoid) (local) L93.0
    disseminated — *see* Lupus, erythematosus,
      systemic
  eyelid H01.129
    left H01.126
      lower H01.125
      upper H01.124
    right H01.123
      lower H01.122
      upper H01.121
  profundus L93.2
  specified NEC L93.2
  subacute cutaneous L93.1

Lupus — *continued*
erythematosus (discoid) (local) L93.0 —
        continued
    systemic M32.9
        with organ or system involvement M32.10
            endocarditis M32.11
            lung M32.13
            pericarditis M32.12
            renal (glomerular) M32.14
                tubulo-interstitial M32.15
            specified organ or system NEC M32.19
        drug-induced M32.0
        inhibitor (presence of) D68.62
            with
                hemorrhagic disorder D68.312
                hypercoagulable state D68.62
            finding without diagnosis R76.0
        specified NEC M32.8
exedens A18.4
hydralazine M32.0
    correct substance properly administered —
        see Table of Drugs and Chemicals, by
        drug, adverse effect
    overdose or wrong substance given or taken
        — *see* Table of Drugs and Chemicals, by
        drug, poisoning
nephritis (chronic) M32.14
nontuberculous, not disseminated L93.0
panniculitis L93.2
pernio (Besnier) D86.3
systemic — *see* Lupus, erythematosus, systemic
tuberculous A18.4
    eyelid A18.4
    vulgaris A18.4
        eyelid A18.4
Luteinoma D27-
Lutembacher's disease or syndrome
    (atrial septal defect with mitral stenosis)
    Q21.1
Luteoma D27-
Lutz(-Splendore-de Almeida) disease —
    see Paracoccidioidomycosis
Luxation — *see also* Dislocation
    eyeball (nontraumatic) — *see* Luxation, globe
        birth injury P15.3
    globe, nontraumatic H44.82-
    lacrimal gland — *see* Dislocation, lacrimal
        gland
    lens (old) (partial) (spontaneous)
        congenital Q12.1
        syphilitic A50.39
Lycanthropy F22
Lyell's syndrome L51.2
    due to drug L51.2
        correct substance properly administered —
            see Table of Drugs and Chemicals, by
            drug, adverse effect
        overdose or wrong substance given or taken
            — *see* Table of Drugs and Chemicals, by
            drug, poisoning
Lyme disease A69.20
Lymph
    gland or node — *see* condition
    scrotum — *see* Infestation, filarial
Lymphadenitis I88.9
    with ectopic or molar pregnancy O08.0
    acute L04.9
        axilla L04.2
        face L04.0
        head L04.0
        hip L04.3
        limb
            lower L04.3
            upper L04.2
        neck L04.0
        shoulder L04.2
        specified site NEC L04.8
        trunk L04.1
    anthracosis (occupational) J60

Lymphadenitis I88.9 — *continued*
    any site, except mesenteric I88.9
        chronic I88.1
        subacute I88.1
    breast
        gestational — *see* Mastitis, obstetric
        puerperal, postpartum (nonpurulent)
            O91.22
    chancroidal (congenital) A57
    chronic I88.1
        mesenteric I88.0
    due to
        Brugia (malayi) B74.1
            timori B74.2
        chlamydial lymphogranuloma A55
        diphtheria (toxin) A36.89
        lymphogranuloma venereum A55
        Wuchereria bancrofti B74.0
    following ectopic or molar pregnancy O08.0
    gonorrheal A54.89
    infective — *see* Lymphadenitis, acute
    mesenteric (acute) (chronic) (nonspecific)
        (subacute) I88.0
        due to Salmonella typhi A01.09
        tuberculous A18.39
    mycobacterial A31.8
    purulent — *see* Lymphadenitis, acute
    pyogenic — *see* Lymphadenitis, acute
    regional, nonbacterial I88.8
    septic — *see* Lymphadenitis, acute
    subacute, unspecified site I88.1
    suppurative — *see* Lymphadenitis, acute
    syphilitic (early) (secondary) A51.49
        late A52.79
    tuberculous — *see* Tuberculosis, lymph gland
    venereal (chlamydial) A55
Lymphadenoid goiter E06.3
Lymphadenopathy (generalized) R59.1
    angioimmunoblastic, with dysproteinemia
        (AILD) C86.5
    due to toxoplasmosis (acquired) B58.89
        congenital (acute) (subacute) (chronic) P37.1
    localized R59.0
    syphilitic (early) (secondary) A51.49
Lymphadenosis R59.1
Lymphangiectasis I89.0
    conjunctiva H11.89
    postinfectional I89.0
    scrotum I89.0
**Lymphangiectatic elephantiasis,
    nonfilarial** I89.0
Lymphangioendothelioma D18.1
    malignant — *see* Neoplasm, connective tissue,
        malignant
Lymphangioleiomyomatosis J84.81
Lymphangioma D18.1
    capillary D18.1
    cavernous D18.1
    cystic D18.1
    malignant — *see* Neoplasm, connective tissue,
        malignant
Lymphangiomyoma D18.1
Lymphangiomyomatosis J84.81
Lymphangiosarcoma — *see* Neoplasm,
    connective tissue, malignant
Lymphangitis I89.1
    with
        abscess — *code by* site under Abscess
        cellulitis — *code by* site under Cellulitis
        ectopic or molar pregnancy O08.0
    acute L03.91
        abdominal wall L03.321
        ankle — *see* Lymphangitis, acute, lower limb
        arm — *see* Lymphangitis, acute, upper limb
        auricle (ear) — *see* Lymphangitis, acute, ear
        axilla L03.12-
        back (any part) L03.322
        buttock L03.327
        cervical (meaning neck) L03.222

Lymphangitis I89.1 — *continued*
    acute L03.91 — *continued*
        cheek (external) L03.212
        chest wall L03.323
        digit
            finger — *see* Lymphangitis, acute, finger
            toe — *see* Lymphangitis, acute, toe
        ear (external) H60.1-
        external auditory canal — *see* Lymphangitis,
            acute, ear
        eyelid — *see* Abscess, eyelid
        face NEC L03.212
        finger (intrathecal) (periosteal)
            (subcutaneous) (subcuticular) L03.02-
        foot — *see* Lymphangitis, acute, lower limb
        gluteal (region) L03.327
        groin L03.324
        hand — *see* Lymphangitis, acute, upper limb
        head NEC L03.891
            face (any part, except ear, eye and nose)
                L03.212
        heel — *see* Lymphangitis, acute, lower limb
        hip — *see* Lymphangitis, acute, lower limb
        jaw (region) L03.212
        knee — *see* Lymphangitis, acute, lower limb
        leg — *see* Lymphangitis, acute, lower limb
        lower limb L03.12-
            toe — *see* Lymphangitis, acute, toe
        navel L03.326
        neck (region) L03.222
        orbit, orbital — *see* Cellulitis, orbit
        pectoral (region) L03.323
        perineal, perineum L03.325
        scalp (any part) L03.891
        shoulder — *see* Lymphangitis, acute, upper
            limb
        specified site NEC L03.898
        thigh — *see* Lymphangitis, acute, lower limb
        thumb (intrathecal) (periosteal)
            (subcutaneous) (subcuticular) — *see*
            Lymphangitis, acute, finger
        toe (intrathecal) (periosteal) (subcutaneous)
            (subcuticular) L03.04-
        trunk L03.329
            abdominal wall L03.321
            back (any part) L03.322
            buttock L03.327
            chest wall L03.323
            groin L03.324
            perineal, perineum L03.325
            umbilicus L03.326
        umbilicus L03.326
        upper limb L03.12-
            axilla — *see* Lymphangitis, acute, axilla
            finger — *see* Lymphangitis, acute, finger
            thumb — *see* Lymphangitis, acute, finger
            wrist — *see* Lymphangitis, acute, upper limb
    breast
        gestational — *see* Mastitis, obstetric
    chancroidal A57
    chronic (any site) I89.1
    due to
        Brugia (malayi) B74.1
            timori B74.2
        Wuchereria bancrofti B74.0
    following ectopic or molar pregnancy O08.89
    penis
        acute N48.29
        gonococcal (acute) (chronic) A54.09
    puerperal, postpartum, childbirth O86.89
    strumous, tuberculous A18.2
    subacute (any site) I89.1
    tuberculous — *see* Tuberculosis, lymph gland
Lymphatic (vessel) — *see* condition
Lymphatism E32.8
Lymphectasia I89.0

Maintenance (encounter for)
antineoplastic chemotherapy Z51.11
antineoplastic radiation therapy Z51.0
methadone F11.20
Majocchi's
disease L81.7
granuloma B35.8
Major — *see* condition
Mal de los pintos — *see* Pinta
Mal de mer T75.3
Malabar itch (any site) B35.5
Malabsorption K90.9
calcium K90.89
carbohydrate K90.49
disaccharide E73.9
fat K90.49
galactose E74.20
glucose(-galactose) E74.39
intestinal K90.9
specified NEC K90.89
isomaltose E74.31
lactose E73.9
methionine E72.19
monosaccharide E74.39
postgastrectomy K91.2
postsurgical K91.2
protein K90.49
starch K90.49
sucrose E74.39
syndrome K90.9
postsurgical K91.2
Malacia, bone (adult) M83.9
juvenile — *see* Rickets
Malacoplakia
bladder N32.89
pelvis (kidney) N28.89
ureter N28.89
urethra N36.8
Malacosteon, juvenile — *see* Rickets
Maladaptation — *see* Maladjustment
Maladie de Roger Q21.0
Maladjustment
conjugal Z63.0
involving divorce or estrangement Z63.5
educational Z55.4
family Z63.9
marital Z63.0
involving divorce or estrangement Z63.5
occupational NEC Z56.89
simple, adult — *see* Disorder, adjustment
situational — *see* Disorder, adjustment
social Z60.9
due to
acculturation difficulty Z60.3
discrimination and persecution (perceived) Z60.5
exclusion and isolation Z60.4
life-cycle (phase of life) transition Z60.0
rejection Z60.4
specified reason NEC Z60.8
Malaise R53.81
Malakoplakia — *see* Malacoplakia
Malaria, malarial (fever) B54
with
blackwater fever B50.8
hemoglobinuric (bilious) B50.8
hemoglobinuria B50.8
accidentally induced (therapeutically) — *code by type under Malaria*
algid B50.9
cerebral B50.0 *[G94]*
clinically diagnosed (without parasitological confirmation) B54
congenital NEC P37.4
falciparum P37.3
congestion, congestive B54
continued (fever) B50.9
estivo-autumnal B50.9

Malaria, malarial (fever) B54 — *continued*
falciparum B50.9
with complications NEC B50.8
cerebral B50.0 *[G94]*
severe B50.8
hemorrhagic B54
malariae B52.9
with
complications NEC B52.8
glomerular disorder B52.0
malignant (tertian) — *see* Malaria, falciparum
mixed infections — *code to first listed type in B50-B53*
ovale B53.0
parasitologically confirmed NEC B53.8
pernicious, acute — *see* Malaria, falciparum
Plasmodium (P.)
falciparum NEC — *see* Malaria, falciparum
malariae NEC B52.9
with Plasmodium
falciparum (and or vivax) — *see* Malaria, falciparum
vivax — *see also* Malaria, vivax
and falciparum — *see* Malaria, falciparum
ovale B53.0
with Plasmodium malariae — *see also* Malaria, malariae
and vivax — *see also* Malaria, vivax
and falciparum — *see* Malaria, falciparum
simian B53.1
with Plasmodium malariae — *see also* Malaria, malariae
and vivax — *see also* Malaria, vivax
and falciparum — *see* Malaria, falciparum
vivax NEC B51.9
with Plasmodium falciparum — *see* Malaria, falciparum
quartan — *see* Malaria, malariae
quotidian — *see* Malaria, falciparum
recurrent B54
remittent B54
specified type NEC (parasitologically confirmed) B53.8
spleen B54
subtertian (fever) — *see* Malaria, falciparum
tertian (benign) — *see also* Malaria, vivax
malignant B50.9
tropical B50.9
typhoid B54
vivax B51.9
with
complications NEC B51.8
ruptured spleen B51.0
Malassez's disease (cystic) N50.89
Malassimilation K90.9
Maldescent, testis Q53.9
bilateral Q53.20
abdominal Q53.21
perineal Q53.22
unilateral Q53.10
abdominal Q53.11
perineal Q53.12
Maldevelopment — *see also* Anomaly
brain Q07.9
colon Q43.9
hip Q74.2
congenital dislocation Q65.2
bilateral Q65.1
unilateral Q65.0-
mastoid process Q75.8
middle ear Q16.4
except ossicles Q16.4
ossicles Q16.3
ossicles Q16.3
spine Q76.49
toe Q74.2

Male type pelvis Q74.2
with disproportion (fetopelvic) O33.3
causing obstructed labor O65.3
Malformation (congenital) — *see also* Anomaly
adrenal gland Q89.1
affecting multiple systems with skeletal changes NEC Q87.5
alimentary tract Q45.9
specified type NEC Q45.8
upper Q40.9
specified type NEC Q40.8
aorta Q25.40
absence Q25.41
aneurysm, congenital Q25.43
aplasia Q25.41
atresia Q25.29
aortic arch Q25.21
coarctation (preductal) (postductal) Q25.1
dilatation, congenital Q25.44
hypoplasia Q25.42
patent ductus arteriosus Q25.0
specified type NEC Q25.49
stenosis Q25.1
supravalvular Q25.3
aortic valve Q23.9
specified NEC Q23.8
arteriovenous, aneurysmatic (congenital) Q27.30
brain Q28.2
cerebral Q28.2
peripheral Q27.30
digestive system Q27.33
lower limb Q27.32
other specified site Q27.39
renal vessel Q27.34
upper limb Q27.31
precerebral vessels (nonruptured) Q28.0
auricle
ear (congenital) Q17.3
acquired H61.119
left H61.112
with right H61.113
right H61.111
with left H61.113
bile duct Q44.5
bladder Q64.79
aplasia Q64.5
diverticulum Q64.6
exstrophy — *see* Exstrophy, bladder
neck obstruction Q64.31
bone Q79.9
face Q75.9
specified type NEC Q75.8
skull Q75.9
specified type NEC Q75.8
brain (multiple) Q04.9
arteriovenous Q28.2
specified type NEC Q04.8
branchial cleft Q18.2
breast Q83.9
specified type NEC Q83.8
broad ligament Q50.6
bronchus Q32.4
bursa Q79.9
cardiac
chambers Q20.9
specified type NEC Q20.8
septum Q21.9
specified type NEC Q21.8
cerebral Q04.9
vessels Q28.3
cervix uteri Q51.9
specified type NEC Q51.828
Chiari
Type I G93.5
Type II Q07.01
choroid (congenital) Q14.3
plexus Q07.8
circulatory system Q28.9

DISEASE INDEX

Malformation (congenital) (*see also* Anomaly) — continued
cochlea Q16.5
cornea Q13.4
coronary vessels Q24.5
corpus callosum (congenital) Q04.0
diaphragm Q79.1
digestive system NEC, specified type NEC Q45.8
dura Q07.9
  brain Q04.9
  spinal Q06.9
ear Q17.9
  causing impairment of hearing Q16.9
  external Q17.9
    accessory auricle Q17.0
    causing impairment of hearing Q16.9
    absence of
      auditory canal Q16.1
      auricle Q16.0
    macrotia Q17.1
    microtia Q17.2
    misplacement Q17.4
    misshapen NEC Q17.3
    prominence Q17.5
    specified type NEC Q17.8
  inner Q16.5
  middle Q16.4
    absence of eustachian tube Q16.2
    ossicles (fusion) Q16.3
  ossicles Q16.3
  specified type NEC Q17.8
epididymis Q55.4
esophagus Q39.9
  specified type NEC Q39.8
eye Q15.9
  lid Q10.3
  specified NEC Q15.8
fallopian tube Q50.6
genital organ — *see* Anomaly, genitalia
great
  artery Q25.9
    aorta — *see* Malformation, aorta
    pulmonary artery — *see* Malformation, pulmonary, artery
    specified type NEC Q25.8
  vein Q26.9
    anomalous
      portal venous connection Q26.5
      pulmonary venous connection Q26.4
        partial Q26.3
        total Q26.2
    persistent left superior vena cava Q26.1
    portal vein-hepatic artery fistula Q26.6
    specified type NEC Q26.8
    vena cava stenosis, congenital Q26.0
gum Q38.6
hair Q84.2
heart Q24.9
  specified type NEC Q24.8
integument Q84.9
  specified type NEC Q84.8
internal ear Q16.5
intestine Q43.9
  specified type NEC Q43.8
iris Q13.2
joint Q74.9
  ankle Q74.2
  lumbosacral Q76.49
  sacroiliac Q74.2
  specified type NEC Q74.8
kidney Q63.9
  accessory Q63.0
  giant Q63.3
  horseshoe Q63.1
  hydronephrosis Q62.0
  malposition Q63.2
  specified type NEC Q63.8
lacrimal apparatus Q10.6

Malformation (congenital) (*see also* Anomaly) — continued
lingual Q38.3
lip Q38.0
liver Q44.7
lung Q33.9
meninges or membrane (congenital) Q07.9
  cerebral Q04.8
  spinal (cord) Q06.9
middle ear Q16.4
  ossicles Q16.3
mitral valve Q23.9
  specified NEC Q23.8
Mondini's (congenital) (malformation, cochlea) Q16.5
mouth (congenital) Q38.6
multiple types NEC Q89.7
musculoskeletal system Q79.9
myocardium Q24.8
nail Q84.6
nervous system (central) Q07.9
nose Q30.9
  specified type NEC Q30.8
optic disc Q14.2
orbit Q10.7
ovary Q50.39
palate Q38.5
parathyroid gland Q89.2
pelvic organs or tissues NEC
  in pregnancy or childbirth O34.8-
    causing obstructed labor O65.5
penis Q55.69
  aplasia Q55.5
  curvature (lateral) Q55.61
  hypoplasia Q55.62
pericardium Q24.8
peripheral vascular system Q27.9
  specified type NEC Q27.8
pharynx Q38.8
precerebral vessels Q28.1
prostate Q55.4
pulmonary
  arteriovenous Q25.72
  artery Q25.9
    atresia Q25.5
    specified type NEC Q25.79
    stenosis Q25.6
  valve Q22.3
renal artery Q27.2
respiratory system Q34.9
retina Q14.1
scrotum — *see* Malformation, testis and scrotum
seminal vesicles Q55.4
sense organs NEC Q07.9
skin Q82.9
specified NEC Q89.8
spinal
  cord Q06.9
  nerve root Q07.8
spine Q76.49
  kyphosis — *see* Kyphosis, congenital
  lordosis — *see* Lordosis, congenital
spleen Q89.09
stomach Q40.3
  specified type NEC Q40.2
teeth, tooth K00.9
tendon Q79.9
testis and scrotum Q55.20
  aplasia Q55.0
  hypoplasia Q55.1
  polyorchism Q55.21
  retractile testis Q55.22
  scrotal transposition Q55.23
  specified NEC Q55.29
thorax, bony Q76.9
throat Q38.8
thyroid gland Q89.2

Malformation (congenital) (*see also* Anomaly) — continued
tongue (congenital) Q38.3
  hypertrophy Q38.2
  tie Q38.1
trachea Q32.1
tricuspid valve Q22.9
  specified type NEC Q22.8
umbilical cord NEC (complicating delivery) O69.89
umbilicus Q89.9
ureter Q62.8
  agenesis Q62.4
  duplication Q62.5
  malposition — *see* Malposition, congenital, ureter
  obstructive defect — *see* Defect, obstructive, ureter
  vesico-uretero-renal reflux Q62.7
urethra Q64.79
  aplasia Q64.5
  duplication Q64.74
  posterior valves Q64.2
  prolapse Q64.71
  stricture Q64.32
urinary system Q64.9
uterus Q51.9
  specified type NEC Q51.818
vagina Q52.4
vas deferens Q55.4
  atresia Q55.3
vascular system, peripheral Q27.9
venous — *see* Anomaly, vein(s)
vulva Q52.70
Malfunction — *see also* Dysfunction
cardiac electronic device T82.119
  electrode T82.110
  pulse generator T82.111
  specified type NEC T82.118
catheter device NEC T85.618
  cystostomy T83.010
  dialysis (renal) (vascular) T82.41
    intraperitoneal T85.611
  infusion NEC T82.514
    cranial T85.610
    epidural T85.610
    intrathecal T85.610
    spinal T85.610
    subarachnoid T85.610
    subdural T85.610
  urinary (*see also* Breakdown, device, catheter) T83.018
colostomy K94.03
  valve K94.03
cystostomy (stoma) N99.512
  catheter T83.010
enteric stoma K94.13
enterostomy K94.13
esophagostomy K94.33
gastroenteric K31.89
gastrostomy K94.23
ileostomy K94.13
  valve K94.13
intrathecal infusion pump T85.615
jejunostomy K94.13
nervous system device, implant or graft, specified NEC T85.615
pacemaker — *see* Malfunction, cardiac electronic device
prosthetic device, internal — *see* Complications, prosthetic device, by site, mechanical
tracheostomy J95.03
urinary device NEC — *see* Complication, genitourinary, device, urinary, mechanical
valve
  colostomy K94.03
  heart T82.09
    ileostomy K94.13

Malfunction — *see also* Dysfunction — *continued*
  vascular graft or shunt NEC — *see* Complication, cardiovascular device, mechanical, vascular
  ventricular (communicating shunt) T85.01
Malherbe's tumor — *see* Neoplasm, skin, benign
Malibu disease L98.8
Malignancy — *see also* Neoplasm, malignant, by site
  unspecified site (primary) C80.1
Malignant — *see* condition
Malingerer, malingering Z76.5
Mallet finger (acquired) — *see* Deformity, finger, mallet finger
  congenital Q74.0
  sequelae of rickets E64.3
Malleus A24.0
Mallory's bodies R89.7
Mallory-Weiss syndrome K22.6
Malnutrition E46
  degree
    first E44.1
    mild (protein) E44.1
    moderate (protein) E44.0
    second E44.0
    severe (protein-energy) E43
      intermediate form E42
        with
          kwashiorkor (and marasmus) E42
          marasmus E41
    third E43
  following gastrointestinal surgery K91.2
  intrauterine
    light-for-dates — *see* Light for dates
    small-for-dates — *see* Small for dates
  lack of care, or neglect (child) (infant) T76.02
    confirmed T74.02
  malignant E40
  protein E46
    calorie E46
      mild E44.1
      moderate E44.0
      severe E43
        intermediate form E42
          with
            kwashiorkor (and marasmus) E42
            marasmus E41
    energy E46
      mild E44.1
      moderate E44.0
      severe E43
        intermediate form E42
          with
            kwashiorkor (and marasmus) E42
            marasmus E41
    severe (protein-energy) E43
      with
        kwashiorkor (and marasmus) E42
        marasmus E41
Malocclusion (teeth) M26.4
  Angle's M26.219
    class I M26.211
    class II M26.212
    class III M26.213
  due to
    abnormal swallowing M26.59
    mouth breathing M26.59
    tongue, lip or finger habits M26.59
    temporomandibular (joint) M26.69
Malposition
  cervix — *see* Malposition, uterus
  congenital
    adrenal (gland) Q89.1
    alimentary tract Q45.8
      lower Q43.8
      upper Q40.8
    aorta Q25.49

Malposition — *continued*
  congenital — *continued*
    appendix Q43.8
    arterial trunk Q20.0
    artery (peripheral) Q27.8
      coronary Q24.5
      digestive system Q27.8
      lower limb Q27.8
      pulmonary Q25.79
      specified site NEC Q27.8
      upper limb Q27.8
    auditory canal Q17.8
      causing impairment of hearing Q16.9
    auricle (ear) Q17.4
      causing impairment of hearing Q16.9
      cervical Q18.2
    biliary duct or passage Q44.5
    bladder (mucosa) — *see* Exstrophy, bladder
    brachial plexus Q07.8
    brain tissue Q04.8
    breast Q83.8
    bronchus Q32.4
    cecum Q43.8
    clavicle Q74.0
    colon Q43.8
    digestive organ or tract NEC Q45.8
      lower Q43.8
      upper Q40.8
    ear (auricle) (external) Q17.4
      ossicles Q16.3
    endocrine (gland) NEC Q89.2
    epiglottis Q31.8
    eustachian tube Q17.8
    eye Q15.8
    facial features Q18.8
    fallopian tube Q50.6
    finger(s) Q68.1
      supernumerary Q69.0
    foot Q66.9
    gallbladder Q44.1
    gastrointestinal tract Q45.8
    genitalia, genital organ(s) or tract
      female Q52.8
        external Q52.79
        internal NEC Q52.8
      male Q55.8
    glottis Q31.8
    hand Q68.1
    heart Q24.8
      dextrocardia Q24.0
        with complete transposition of viscera Q89.3
    hepatic duct Q44.5
    hip (joint) Q65.89
    intestine (large) (small) Q43.8
      with anomalous adhesions, fixation or malrotation Q43.3
    joint NEC Q68.8
    kidney Q63.2
    larynx Q31.8
    limb Q68.8
      lower Q68.8
      upper Q68.8
    liver Q44.7
    lung (lobe) Q33.8
    nail(s) Q84.6
    nerve Q07.8
    nervous system NEC Q07.8
    nose, nasal (septum) Q30.8
    organ or site not listed — *see* Anomaly, by site
    ovary Q50.39
    pancreas Q45.3
    parathyroid (gland) Q89.2
    patella Q74.1
    peripheral vascular system Q27.8
    pituitary (gland) Q89.2
    respiratory organ or system NEC Q34.8

Malposition — *continued*
  congenital — *continued*
    rib (cage) Q76.6
      supernumerary in cervical region Q76.5
    scapula Q74.0
    shoulder Q74.0
    spinal cord Q06.8
    spleen Q89.09
    sternum NEC Q76.7
    stomach Q40.2
    symphysis pubis Q74.2
    thymus (gland) Q89.2
    thyroid (gland) (tissue) Q89.2
      cartilage Q31.8
    toe(s) Q66.9
      supernumerary Q69.2
    tongue Q38.3
    trachea Q32.1
    ureter Q62.60
      deviation Q62.61
      displacement Q62.62
      ectopia Q62.63
      specified type NEC Q62.69
    uterus Q51.818
    vein(s) (peripheral) Q27.8
      great Q26.8
    vena cava (inferior) (superior) Q26.8
  device, implant or graft (*see also* Complications, by site and type, mechanical) T85.628
    arterial graft NEC — *see* Complication, cardiovascular device, mechanical, vascular
    breast (implant) T85.42
    catheter NEC T85.628
      cystostomy T83.020
      dialysis (renal) T82.42
        intraperitoneal T85.621
      infusion NEC T82.524
        spinal (epidural) (subdural) T85.620
      urinary (*see also* Displacement, device, catheter, urinary) T83.028
    electronic (electrode) (pulse generator) (stimulator)
      bone T84.320
      cardiac T82.129
      electrode T82.120
      pulse generator T82.121
      specified type NEC T82.128
      nervous system — *see* Complication, prosthetic device, mechanical, electronic nervous system stimulator
      urinary — *see* Complication, genitourinary, device, urinary, mechanical
    fixation, internal (orthopedic) NEC — *see* Complication, fixation device, mechanical
    gastrointestinal — *see* Complications, prosthetic device, mechanical, gastrointestinal device
    genital NEC T83.428
      intrauterine contraceptive device (string) T83.32
      penile prosthesis (cylinder) (implanted) (pump) (resevoir) T83.420
      testicular prosthesis T83.421
    heart NEC — *see* Complication, cardiovascular device, mechanical
    joint prosthesis — *see* Complication, joint prosthesis, mechanical
    ocular NEC — *see* Complications, prosthetic device, mechanical, ocular device
    orthopedic NEC — *see* Complication, orthopedic, device, mechanical
    specified NEC T85.628
    urinary NEC — *see also* Complication, genitourinary, device, urinary, mechanical
      graft T83.22

Malposition — *continued*
device, implant or graft (*see also* Complications, by site and type, mechanical) T85.628 — *continued*
  vascular NEC — *see* Complication, cardiovascular device, mechanical
  ventricular intracranial shunt T85.02
fetus — *see* Pregnancy, complicated by (management affected by), presentation, fetal
gallbladder K82.8
gastrointestinal tract, congenital Q45.8
heart, congenital NEC Q24.8
joint prosthesis — *see* Complications, joint prosthesis, mechanical, displacement, by site
stomach K31.89
  congenital Q40.2
tooth, teeth, fully erupted M26.30
uterus (acute) (acquired) (adherent) (asymptomatic) (postinfectional) (postpartal, old) N85.4
  anteflexion or anteversion N85.4
    congenital Q51.818
  flexion N85.4
    lateral — *see* Lateroversion, uterus
  inversion N85.5
  lateral (flexion) (version) — *see* Lateroversion, uterus
    in pregnancy or childbirth — *see* subcategory O34.5
  retroflexion or retroversion — *see* Retroversion, uterus
Malposture R29.3
Malrotation
cecum Q43.3
colon Q43.3
intestine Q43.3
kidney Q63.2
Malta fever — *see* Brucellosis
Maltreatment
adult
  abandonment
    confirmed T74.01
    suspected T76.01
  confirmed T74.91
  history of Z91.419
  neglect
    confirmed T74.01
    suspected T76.01
  physical abuse
    confirmed T74.11
    suspected T76.11
  psychological abuse
    confirmed T74.31
    history of Z91.411
    suspected T76.31
  sexual abuse
    confirmed T74.21
    suspected T76.21
    suspected T76.91
child
  abandonment
    confirmed T74.02
    suspected T76.02
  confirmed T74.92
  history of — *see* History, personal (of), abuse
  neglect
    confirmed T74.02
    history of — *see* History, personal (of), abuse
    suspected T76.02
  physical abuse
    confirmed T74.12
    history of — *see* History, personal (of), abuse
    suspected T76.12

Maltreatment — *continued*
child — *continued*
  psychological abuse
    confirmed T74.32
    history of — *see* History, personal (of), abuse
    suspected T76.32
  sexual abuse
    confirmed T74.22
    history of — *see* History, personal (of), abuse
    suspected T76.22
  suspected T76.92
  personal history of Z91.89
Maltworker's lung J67.4
Malunion, fracture — *see* Fracture, by site
Mammillitis N61.0
puerperal, postpartum O91.02
Mammitis — *see* Mastitis
Mammogram (examination) Z12.39
routine Z12.31
Mammoplasia N62
Management (of)
bone conduction hearing device (implanted) Z45.320
cardiac pacemaker NEC Z45.018
cerebrospinal fluid drainage device Z45.41
cochlear device (implanted) Z45.321
contraceptive Z30.9
  specified NEC Z30.8
implanted device Z45.9
  specified NEC Z45.89
infusion pump Z45.1
procreative Z31.9
  male factor infertility in female Z31.81
  specified NEC Z31.89
prosthesis (external) (*see also* Fitting) Z44.9
  implanted Z45.9
    specified NEC Z45.89
renal dialysis catheter Z49.01
vascular access device Z45.2
Mangled — *see* specified injury by site
Mania (monopolar) — *see also* Disorder, mood, manic episode
with psychotic symptoms F30.2
Bell's F30.8
chronic (recurrent) F31.89
hysterical F44.89
puerperal F30.8
recurrent F31.89
without psychotic symptoms F30.10
  mild F30.11
  moderate F30.12
  severe F30.13
Manic-depressive insanity, psychosis, or syndrome — *see* Disorder, bipolar
Mannosidosis E77.1
Manson's
disease B65.1
schistosomiasis B65.1
Mansonelliasis, mansonellosis B74.4
Manual — *see* condition
Maple-bark-stripper's lung (disease) J67.6
Maple-syrup-urine disease E71.0
Marable's syndrome (celiac artery compression) O77.4
Marasmus E41
due to malnutrition E41
intestinal E41
nutritional E41
senile R54
tuberculous NEC — *see* Tuberculosis
Marble
bones Q78.2
skin R23.8
Marburg virus disease A98.3

March
fracture — *see* Fracture, traumatic, stress, by site
hemoglobinuria D59.6
Marchesani(-Weill) syndrome Q87.0
Marchiafava(-Bignami) syndrome or disease G37.1
Marchiafava-Micheli syndrome D59.5
Marcus Gunn's syndrome Q07.8
Marfan's syndrome — *see* Syndrome, Marfan's
Marie-Bamberger disease — *see* Osteoarthropathy, hypertrophic, specified NEC
Marie-Charcot-Tooth neuropathic muscular atrophy G60.0
Marie's
cerebellar ataxia (late-onset) G11.2
disease or syndrome (acromegaly) E22.0
Marie-Strümpell arthritis, disease or spondylitis — *see* Spondylitis, ankylosing
Marion's disease (bladder neck obstruction) N32.0
Marital conflict Z63.0
Mark
port wine Q82.5
raspberry Q82.5
strawberry Q82.5
stretch L90.6
tattoo L81.8
Marker heterochromatin — *see* Extra, marker chromosomes
Maroteaux-Lamy syndrome (mild) (severe) E76.29
Marrow (bone)
arrest D61.9
poor function D75.89
Marseilles fever A77.1
Marsh fever — *see* Malaria
Marsh's disease (exophthalmic goiter) E05.00
with storm E05.01
Marshall's (hidrotic) ectodermal dysplasia Q82.4
Masculinization (female) with adrenal hyperplasia E25.9
congenital E25.0
Masculinovoblastoma D27-
Masochism (sexual) F65.51
Mason's lung J62.8
Mass
abdominal R19.00
  epigastric R19.06
  generalized R19.07
  left lower quadrant R19.04
  left upper quadrant R19.02
  periumbilic R19.05
  right lower quadrant R19.03
  right upper quadrant R19.01
  specified site NEC R19.09
breast N63
chest R22.2
cystic — *see* Cyst
ear H93.8-
head R22.0
intra-abdominal (diffuse) (generalized) — *see* Mass, abdominal
kidney N28.89
liver R16.0
localized (skin) R22.9
  chest R22.2
  head R22.0
  limb
    lower R22.4-
    upper R22.3-
  neck R22.1
  trunk R22.2
lung R91.8
malignant — *see* Neoplasm, malignant, by site
neck R22.1

DISEASE INDEX

Mass — *continued*
pelvic (diffuse) (generalized) — *see* Mass, abdominal
specified organ NEC — *see* Disease, by site
splenic R16.1
substernal thyroid — *see* Goiter
superficial (localized) R22.9
umbilical (diffuse) (generalized) R19.09
Massive — *see* condition
Mast cell
disease, systemic tissue D47.0
leukemia C94.3-
sarcoma C96.2
tumor D47.0
malignant C96.2
Mastalgia N64.4
Masters-Allen syndrome N83.8
Mastitis (acute) (diffuse) (nonpuerperal) (subacute) N61.0
with abscess N61.1
chronic (cystic) — *see* Mastopathy, cystic
cystic (Schimmelbusch's type) — *see* Mastopathy, cystic
fibrocystic — *see* Mastopathy, cystic
infective N61.0
newborn P39.0
interstitial, gestational or puerperal — *see* Mastitis, obstetric
neonatal (noninfective) P83.4
infective P39.0
obstetric (interstitial) (nonpurulent)
associated with
lactation O91.23
pregnancy O91.21-
puerperium O91.22
purulent
associated with
lactation O91.13
pregnancy O91.11-
puerperium O91.12
periductal — *see* Ectasia, mammary duct
phlegmonous — *see* Mastopathy, cystic
plasma cell — *see* Ectasia, mammary duct
without abscess N61.0
Mastocytoma D47.0
malignant C96.2
Mastocytosis Q82.2
aggressive systemic C96.2
indolent systemic D47.0
malignant C96.2
systemic, associated with clonal hematopoetic non-mast-cell disease (SM-AHNMD) D47.0
Mastodynia N64.4
Mastoid — *see* condition
Mastoidalgia — *see* subcategory H92.0
Mastoiditis (coalescent) (hemorrhagic) (suppurative) H70.9-
acute, subacute H70.00-
complicated NEC H70.09-
subperiosteal H70.01-
chronic (necrotic) (recurrent) H70.1-
in (due to)
infectious disease NEC B99 [H75.-]
parasitic disease NEC B89 [H75.-]
tuberculosis A18.03
petrositis — *see* Petrositis
postauricular fistula — *see* Fistula, postauricular
specified NEC H70.89-
tuberculous A18.03
Mastopathy, mastopathia N64.9
chronica cystica — *see* Mastopathy, cystic
cystic (chronic) (diffuse) N60.1-
with epithelial proliferation N60.3-
diffuse cystic — *see* Mastopathy, cystic
estrogenic, oestrogenica N64.89
ovarian origin N64.89
Mastoplasia, mastoplastia N62

Masturbation (excessive) F98.8
Maternal care (for) — *see* Pregnancy (complicated by) (management affected by)
Mathieu's disease (leptospiral jaundice) A27.0
Mauclaire's disease or osteochondrosis — *see* Osteochondrosis, juvenile, hand, metacarpal
Maxcy's disease A75.2
Maxilla, maxillary — *see* condition
May(-Hegglin) anomaly or syndrome D72.0
McArdle(-Schmid)(-Pearson) disease (glycogen storage) E74.04
McCune-Albright syndrome Q78.1
McQuarrie's syndrome (idiopathic familial hypoglycemia) E16.2
Meadow's syndrome Q86.1
Measles (black) (hemorrhagic) (suppressed) B05.9
with
complications NEC B05.89
encephalitis B05.0
intestinal complications B05.4
keratitis (keratoconjunctivitis) B05.81
meningitis B05.1
otitis media B05.3
pneumonia B05.2
French — *see* Rubella
German — *see* Rubella
Liberty — *see* Rubella
Meat-wrappers' asthma J68.9
Meatitis, urethral — *see* Urethritis
Meatus, meatal — *see* condition
Meckel's diverticulitis, diverticulum (displaced) (hypertrophic) Q43.0
malignant — *see* Table of Neoplasms, small intestine, malignant
Meckel-Gruber syndrome Q61.9
Meconium
ileus, newborn P76.0
in cystic fibrosis E84.11
meaning meconium plug (without cystic fibrosis) P76.0
obstruction, newborn P76.0
due to fecaliths P76.0
in mucoviscidosis E84.11
peritonitis P78.0
plug syndrome (newborn) NEC P76.0
Median — *see also* condition
arcuate ligament syndrome I77.4
bar (prostate) (vesical orifice) — *see* Hyperplasia, prostate
rhomboid glossitis K14.2
Mediastinal shift R93.8
Mediastinitis (acute) (chronic) J98.51
syphilitic A52.73
tuberculous A15.8
Mediastinopericarditis — *see also* Pericarditis
acute I30.9
adhesive I31.0
chronic I31.8
rheumatic I09.2
Mediastinum, mediastinal — *see* condition
Medicine poisoning — *see* Table of Drugs and Chemicals, by drug, poisoning
Mediterranean
fever — *see* Brucellosis
familial M04.1
tick A77.1
kala-azar B55.0
leishmaniasis B55.0
tick fever A77.1
Medulla — *see* condition
Medullary cystic kidney Q61.5
Medullated fibers
optic (nerve) Q14.8
retina Q14.1

Medulloblastoma
desmoplastic C71.6
specified site — *see* Neoplasm, malignant, by site
unspecified site C71.6
Medulloepithelioma — *see also* Neoplasm, malignant, by site
teratoid — *see* Neoplasm, malignant, by site
Medullomyoblastoma
specified site — *see* Neoplasm, malignant, by site
unspecified site C71.6
Meekeren-Ehlers-Danlos syndrome Q79.6
Megacolon (acquired) (functional) (not Hirschsprung's disease) (in) K59.39
Chagas' disease B57.32
congenital, congenitum (aganglionic) Q43.1
Hirschsprung's (disease) Q43.1
toxic NEC K59.31
due to Clostridium difficile A04.7
Megaesophagus (functional) K22.0
congenital Q39.5
in (due to) Chagas' disease B57.31
Megalencephaly Q04.5
Megalerythema (epidemic) B08.3
Megaloappendix Q43.8
Megalocephalus, megalocephaly NEC Q75.3
Megalocornea Q15.8
with glaucoma Q15.0
Megalocytic anemia D53.91
Megalodactylia (fingers) (thumbs) (congenital) Q74.0
toes Q74.2
Megaloduodenum Q43.8
Megaloesophagus (functional) K22.0
congenital Q39.5
Megalogastria (acquired) K31.89
congenital Q40.2
Megalophthalmos Q11.3
Megalopsia H53.15
Megalosplenia — *see* Splenomegaly
Megaloureter N28.82
congenital Q62.2
Megarectum K62.89
Megasigmoid K59.39
congenital Q43.2
Megaureter N28.82
congenital Q62.2
Megavitamin-B6 syndrome E67.2
Megrim — *see* Migraine
Meibomian
cyst, infected — *see* Hordeolum
gland — *see* condition
sty, stye — *see* Hordeolum
Meibomitis — *see* Hordeolum
Meige's syndrome Q82.0
Meige-Milroy disease (chronic hereditary edema) Q82.0
Melalgia, nutritional E53.8
Melancholia F32.9
climacteric (single episode) F32.89
recurrent episode F33.8
hypochondriac F45.29
intermittent (single episode) F32.89
recurrent episode F33.8
involutional (single episode) F32.89
recurrent episode F33.8
menopausal (single episode) F32.89
recurrent episode F33.8
puerperal F32.89
reactive (emotional stress or trauma) F32.3
recurrent F33.9
senile F03
stuporous (single episode) F32.89
recurrent episode F33.8
Melanemia R79.89

Melanoameloblastoma — *see* Neoplasm, bone, benign
Melanoblastoma — *see* Melanoma
Melanocarcinoma — *see* Melanoma
Melanocytoma, eyeball D31.9-
Melanocytosis, neurocutaneous Q82.8
Melanoderma, melanodermia L81.4
Melanodontia, infantile K03.89
Melanodontoclasia K03.89
Melanoepithelioma — *see* Melanoma
Melanoma (malignant) C43.9
  acral lentiginous, malignant — *see* Melanoma, skin, by site
  amelanotic — *see* Melanoma, skin, by site
  balloon cell — *see* Melanoma, skin, by site
  benign — *see* Nevus
  desmoplastic, malignant — *see* Melanoma, skin, by site
  epithelioid cell — *see* Melanoma, skin, by site
    with spindle cell, mixed — *see* Melanoma, skin, by site
  in
    giant pigmented nevus — *see* Melanoma, skin, by site
    Hutchinson's melanotic freckle — *see* Melanoma, skin, by site
    junctional nevus — *see* Melanoma, skin, by site
    precancerous melanosis — *see* Melanoma, skin, by site
  in situ D03.9
    abdominal wall D03.59
    ala nasi D03.39
    ankle D03.7-
    anus, anal (margin) (skin) D03.51
    arm D03.6-
    auditory canal D03.2-
    auricle (ear) D03.2-
    auricular canal (external) D03.2-
    axilla, axillary fold D03.59
    back D03.59
    breast D03.52
    brow D03.39
    buttock D03.59
    canthus (eye) D03.1-
    cheek (external) D03.39
    chest wall D03.59
    chin D03.39
    choroid D03.8
    conjunctiva D03.8
    ear (external) D03.2-
    external meatus (ear) D03.2-
    eye D03.8
    eyebrow D03.39
    eyelid (lower) (upper) D03.1-
    face D03.30
      specified NEC D03.39
    female genital organ (external) NEC D03.8
    finger D03.6-
    flank D03.59
    foot D03.7-
    forearm D03.6-
    forehead D03.39
    foreskin D03.8
    gluteal region D03.59
    groin D03.59
    hand D03.6-
    heel D03.7-
    helix D03.2-
    hip D03.7-
    interscapular region D03.59
    iris D03.8
    jaw D03.39
    knee D03.7-
    labium (majus) (minus) D03.8
    lacrimal gland D03.8
    leg D03.7-
    lip (lower) (upper) D03.0
    lower limb NEC D03.7-

Melanoma (malignant) C43.9 — *continued*
  in situ D03.9 — *continued*
    male genital organ (external) NEC D03.8
    nail D03.9
      finger D03.6-
      toe D03.7-
    neck D03.4
    nose (external) D03.39
    orbit D03.8
    penis D03.8
    perianal skin D03.51
    perineum D03.51
    pinna D03.2-
    popliteal fossa or space D03.7-
    prepuce D03.8
    pudendum D03.8
    retina D03.8
    retrobulbar D03.8
    scalp D03.4
    scrotum D03.8
    shoulder D03.6-
    specified site NEC D03.8
    submammary fold D03.52
    temple D03.39
    thigh D03.7-
    toe D03.7-
    trunk NEC D03.59
    umbilicus D03.59
    upper limb NEC D03.6-
    vulva D03.8
  juvenile — *see* Nevus
  malignant, of soft parts except skin — *see* Neoplasm, connective tissue, malignant
  metastatic
    breast C79.81
    genital organ C79.82
    specified site NEC C79.89
  neurotropic, malignant — *see* Melanoma, skin, by site
  nodular — *see* Melanoma, skin, by site
  regressing, malignant — *see* Melanoma, skin, by site
  skin C43.9
    abdominal wall C43.59
    ala nasi C43.31
    ankle C43.7-
    anus, anal (skin) C43.51
    arm C43.6-
    auditory canal (external) C43.2-
    auricle (ear) C43.2-
    auricular canal (external) C43.2-
    axilla, axillary fold C43.59
    back C43.59
    breast (female) (male) C43.52
    brow C43.39
    buttock C43.59
    canthus (eye) C43.1-
    cheek (external) C43.39
    chest wall C43.59
    chin C43.39
    ear (external) C43.2-
    elbow C43.6-
    external meatus (ear) C43.2-
    eyebrow C43.39
    eyelid (lower) (upper) C43.1-
    face C43.30
      specified NEC C43.39
    female genital organ (external) NEC C51.9
    finger C43.6-
    flank C43.59
    foot C43.7-
    forearm C43.6-
    forehead C43.39
    foreskin C60.0
    glabella C43.39
    gluteal region C43.59
    groin C43.59
    hand C43.6-
    heel C43.7-

Melanoma (malignant) C43.9 — *continued*
  skin C43.9 — *continued*
    helix C43.2-
    hip C43.7-
    interscapular region C43.59
    jaw (external) C43.39
    knee C43.7-
    labium C51.9
      majus C51.0
      minus C51.1
    leg C43.7-
    lip (lower) (upper) C43.0
    lower limb NEC C43.7-
    male genital organ (external) NEC C63.9
    nail
      finger C43.6-
      toe C43.7-
    nasolabial groove C43.39
    nates C43.59
    neck C43.4
    nose (external) C43.31
    overlapping site C43.8
    palpebra C43.1-
    penis C60.9
    perianal skin C43.51
    perineum C43.51
    pinna C43.2-
    popliteal fossa or space C43.7-
    prepuce C60.0
    pudendum C51.9
    scalp C43.4
    scrotum C63.2
    shoulder C43.6-
    skin NEC C43.9
    submammary fold C43.52
    temple C43.39
    thigh C43.7-
    toe C43.7-
    trunk NEC C43.59
    umbilicus C43.59
    upper limb NEC C43.6-
    vulva C51.9
      overlapping sites C51.8
  spindle cell
    with epithelioid, mixed — *see* Melanoma, skin, by site
    type A C69.4-
    type B C69.4-
  superficial spreading — *see* Melanoma, skin, by site
Melanosarcoma — *see also* Melanoma
  epithelioid cell — *see* Melanoma
Melanosis L81.4
  addisonian E27.1
    tuberculous A18.7
  adrenal E27.1
  colon K63.89
  conjunctiva — *see* Pigmentation, conjunctiva
    congenital Q13.89
  cornea (presenile) (senile) — *see also* Pigmentation, cornea
    congenital Q13.4
  eye NEC H57.8
    congenital Q15.8
  lenticularis progressiva Q82.1
  liver K76.89
  precancerous — *see also* Melanoma, in situ
    malignant melanoma in — *see* Melanoma
  Riehl's L81.4
  sclera H15.89
    congenital Q13.89
  suprarenal E27.1
  tar L81.4
  toxic L81.4
Melanuria R82.99
MELAS syndrome E88.41
Melasma L81.1
  adrenal (gland) E27.1
  suprarenal (gland) E27.1

Melena K92.1
with ulcer — *code by* site under Ulcer, with hemorrhage K27.4
due to swallowed maternal blood P78.2
newborn, neonatal P54.1
due to swallowed maternal blood P78.2
Meleney's
gangrene (cutaneous) — *see* Ulcer, skin
ulcer (chronic undermining) — *see* Ulcer, skin
Melioidosis A24.9
acute A24.1
chronic A24.2
fulminating A24.1
pneumonia A24.1
pulmonary (chronic) A24.2
acute A24.1
subacute A24.2
sepsis A24.1
specified NEC A24.3
subacute A24.2
Melitensis, febris A23.0
Melkersson(-Rosenthal) syndrome G51.2
Mellitus, diabetes — *see* Diabetes
Melorheostosis (bone) — *see* Disorder, bone, density and structure, specified NEC
Meloschisis Q18.4
Melotia Q17.4
Membrana
capsularis lentis posterior Q13.89
epipapillaris Q14.2
Membranacea placenta O43.19-
Membranaceous uterus N85.8
Membrane(s), membranous — *see also* condition
cyclitic — *see* Membrane, pupillary
folds, congenital — *see* Web
Jackson's Q43.3
over face of newborn P28.9
premature rupture — *see* Rupture, membranes, premature
pupillary H21.4-
persistent Q13.89
retained (with hemorrhage) (complicating delivery) O72.2
without hemorrhage O73.1
secondary cataract — *see* Cataract, secondary
unruptured (causing asphyxia) — *see* Asphyxia, newborn
vitreous — *see* Opacity, vitreous, membranes and strands
Membranitis — *see* Chorioamnionitis
Memory disturbance, lack or loss — *see also* Amnesia
mild, following organic brain damage F06.8
Menadione deficiency E56.1
Menarche
delayed E30.0
precocious E30.1
Mendacity, pathologic F60.2
Mendelson's syndrome (due to anesthesia) J95.4
in labor and delivery O74.0
in pregnancy O29.01-
obstetric O74.0
postpartum, puerperal O89.01
Ménétrier's disease or syndrome K29.60
with bleeding K29.61
Ménière's disease, syndrome or vertigo H81.0-
Meninges, meningeal — *see* condition
Meningioma — *see also* Neoplasm, meninges, benign
angioblastic — *see* Neoplasm, meninges, benign
angiomatous — *see* Neoplasm, meninges, benign
endotheliomatous — *see* Neoplasm, meninges, benign

Meningioma — *see also* Neoplasm, meninges, benign — *continued*
fibroblastic — *see* Neoplasm, meninges, benign
fibrous — *see* Neoplasm, meninges, benign
hemangioblastic — *see* Neoplasm, meninges, benign
hemangiopericytic — *see* Neoplasm, meninges, benign
malignant — *see* Neoplasm, meninges, malignant
meningiothelial — *see* Neoplasm, meninges, benign
meningotheliomatous — *see* Neoplasm, meninges, benign
mixed — *see* Neoplasm, meninges, benign
multiple — *see* Neoplasm, meninges, uncertain behavior
papillary — *see* Neoplasm, meninges, uncertain behavior
psammomatous — *see* Neoplasm, meninges, benign
syncytial — *see* Neoplasm, meninges, benign
transitional — *see* Neoplasm, meninges, benign
Meningiomatosis (diffuse) — *see* Neoplasm, meninges, uncertain behavior
Meningism — *see* Meningismus
Meningismus (infectional) (pneumococcal) R29.1
due to serum or vaccine R29.1
influenzal — *see* Influenza, with, manifestations NEC
Meningitis (basal) (basic) (brain) (cerebral) (cervical) (congestive) (diffuse) (hemorrhagic) (infantile) (membranous)(metastatic) (nonspecific) (pontine) (progressive) (simple) (spinal) (subacute) (sympathetic) (toxic) G03.9
abacterial G03.0
actinomycotic A42.81
adenoviral A87.1
arbovirus A87.8
aseptic (acute) G03.0
bacterial G00.9
Escherichia coli (E. coli) G00.8
Friedländer (bacillus) G00.8
gram-negative G00.9
H. influenzae G00.0
Klebsiella G00.8
pneumococcal G00.1
specified organism NEC G00.8
staphylococcal G00.3
streptococcal (acute) G00.2
benign recurrent (Mollaret) G03.2
candidal B37.5
caseous (tuberculous) A17.0
cerebrospinal A39.0
chronic NEC G03.1
clear cerebrospinal fluid NEC G03.0
coxsackievirus A87.0
cryptococcal B45.1
diplococcal (gram positive) A39.0
echovirus A87.0
enteroviral A87.0
eosinophilic B83.2
epidemic NEC A39.0
Escherichia coli (E. coli) G00.8
fibrinopurulent G00.9
specified organism NEC G00.8
Friedländer (bacillus) G00.8
gonococcal A54.81
gram-negative cocci G00.9
gram-positive cocci G00.9
H. influenzae G00.0
Haemophilus (influenzae) G00.0

Meningitis (basal) (basic) (brain) (cerebral) (cervical) (congestive) (diffuse) (hemorrhagic) (infantile) (membranous)(metastatic) (nonspecific) (pontine) (progressive) (simple) (spinal) (subacute) (sympathetic) (toxic) G03.9 — *continued*
in (due to)
adenovirus A87.1
African trypanosomiasis B56.9 *[G02]*
anthrax A22.8
bacterial disease NEC A48.8 *[G01]*
Chagas' disease (chronic) B57.41
chickenpox B01.0
coccidioidomycosis B38.4
Diplococcus pneumoniae G00.1
enterovirus A87.0
herpes (simplex) virus B00.3
zoster B02.1
infectious mononucleosis B27.92
leptospirosis A27.81
Listeria monocytogenes A32.11
Lyme disease A69.21
measles B05.1
mumps (virus) B26.1
neurosyphilis (late) A52.13
parasitic disease NEC B89 *[G02]*
poliovirus A80.9 *[G02]*
preventive immunization, inoculation or vaccination G03.8
rubella B06.02
Salmonella infection A02.21
specified cause NEC G03.8
Streptococcal pneumoniae G00.1
typhoid fever A01.01
varicella B01.0
viral disease NEC A87.8
whooping cough A37.90
zoster B02.1
infectious G00.9
influenzal (H. influenzae) G00.0
Klebsiella G00.8
leptospiral (aseptic) A27.81
lymphocytic (acute) (benign) (serous) A87.2
meningococcal A39.0
Mima polymorpha G00.8
Mollaret (benign recurrent) G03.2
monilial B37.5
mycotic NEC B49 *[G02]*
Neisseria A39.0
nonbacterial G03.0
nonpyogenic NEC G03.0
ossificans G96.19
pneumococcal streptococcus pneumoniae G00.1
poliovirus A80.9 *[G02]*
postmeasles B05.1
purulent G00.9
specified organism NEC G00.8
pyogenic G00.9
specified organism NEC G00.8
Salmonella (arizonae) (Cholerae-Suis) (enteritidis) (typhimurium) A02.21
septic G00.9
specified organism NEC G00.8
serosa circumscripta NEC G03.0
serous NEC G93.2
specified organism NEC G00.8
sporotrichosis B42.81
staphylococcal G00.3
sterile G03.0
Streptococcal (acute) G00.2
pneumoniae G00.1
suppurative G00.9
specified organism NEC G00.8
syphilitic (late) (tertiary) A52.13
acute A51.41
congenital A50.41
secondary A51.41
Torula histolytica (cryptococcal) B45.1

Meningitis (basal) (basic) (brain) (cerebral) (cervical) (congestive) (diffuse) (hemorrhagic) (infantile) (membranous)(metastatic) (nonspecific) (pontine) (progressive) (simple) (spinal) (subacute) (sympathetic) (toxic) G03.9 — *continued*
  traumatic (complication of injury) T79.8
  tuberculous A17.0
  typhoid A01.01
  viral NEC A87.9
  Yersinia pestis A20.3
Meningocele (spinal) — *see also* Spina bifida
  with hydrocephalus — *see* Spina bifida, by site, with hydrocephalus
  acquired (traumatic) G96.19
  cerebral — *see* Encephalocele
Meningocerebritis — *see* Meningoencephalitis
Meningococcemia A39.4
  acute A39.2
  chronic A39.3
Meningococcus, meningococcal (*see also* condition) A39.9
  adrenalitis, hemorrhagic A39.1
  carrier (suspected) of Z22.31
  meningitis (cerebrospinal) A39.0
Meningoencephalitis (*see also* Encephalitis) G04.90
  acute NEC (*see also* Encephalitis, viral) A86
  bacterial NEC G04.2
  California A83.5
  diphasic A84.1
  eosinophilic B83.2
  epidemic A39.81
  herpesviral, herpetic B00.4
    due to herpesvirus 6 B10.01
    due to herpesvirus 7 B10.09
    specified NEC B10.09
  in (due to)
    blastomycosis NEC B40.81
    diseases classified elsewhere G05.3
    free-living amebae B60.2
    H. influenzae G00.0
    Hemophilus influenzae (H .influenzae) G00.0
    herpes B00.4
      due to herpesvirus 6 B10.01
      due to herpesvirus 7 B10.09
      specified NEC B10.09
    Lyme disease A69.22
    mercury — *see* subcategory T56.1
    mumps B26.2
    Naegleria (amebae) (organisms) (fowleri) B60.2
    Parastrongylus cantonensis B83.2
    toxoplasmosis (acquired) B58.2
      congenital P37.1
  infectious (acute) (viral) A86
  influenzal (H. influenzae) G00.0
  Listeria monocytogenes A32.12
  lymphocytic (serous) A87.2
  mumps B26.2
  parasitic NEC B89 *[G05.3]*
  pneumococcal G04.2
  primary amebic B60.2
  specific (syphilitic) A52.14
  specified organism NEC G04.81
  staphylococcal G04.2
  streptococcal G04.2
  syphilitic A52.14
  toxic NEC G92
    due to mercury — *see* subcategory T56.1
  tuberculous A17.82
  virus NEC A86
Meningoencephalocele — *see also* Encephalocele
  syphilitic A52.19
    congenital A50.49

Meningoencephalomyelitis — *see also* Meningoencephalitis
  acute NEC (viral) A86
    disseminated G04.00
      postimmunization or postvaccination G04.02
      postinfectious G04.01
  due to
    actinomycosis A42.82
    Torula B45.1
    Toxoplasma or toxoplasmosis (acquired) B58.2
      congenital P37.1
  postimmunization or postvaccination G04.02
Meningoencephalomyelopathy G96.9
Meningoencephalopathy G96.9
Meningomyelitis — *see also* Meningoencephalitis
  bacterial NEC G04.2
  blastomycotic NEC B40.81
  cryptococcal B45.1
  in diseases classified elsewhere G05.4
  meningococcal A39.81
  syphilitic A52.14
  tuberculous A17.82
Meningomyelocele — *see also* Spina bifida
  syphilitic A52.19
Meningomyeloneuritis — *see* Meningoencephalitis
Meningoradiculitis — *see* Meningitis
Meningovascular — *see* condition
Menkes' disease or syndrome E83.09
  meaning maple-syrup-urine disease E71.0
Menometrorrhagia N92.1
Menopause, menopausal (asymptomatic) (state) Z78.0
  arthritis (any site) NEC — *see* Arthritis, specified form NEC
  bleeding N92.4
  depression (single episode) F32.89
    agitated (single episode) F32.2
      recurrent episode F33.9
    psychotic (single episode) F32.89
      recurrent episode F33.9
    recurrent episode F33.8
    melancholia (single episode) F32.89
      recurrent episode F33.8
  paranoid state F22
  premature E28.319
    asymptomatic E28.319
      postirradiation E89.40
      postsurgical E89.40
    symptomatic E28.310
      postirradiation E89.41
      postsurgical E89.41
  psychosis NEC F28
  symptomatic N95.1
  toxic polyarthritis NEC — *see* Arthritis, specified form NEC
Menorrhagia (primary) N92.0
  climacteric N92.4
    menopausal N92.4
  menopausal N92.4
  postclimacteric N95.0
  postmenopausal N95.0
  preclimacteric or premenopausal N92.4
  pubertal (menses retained) N92.2
Menostaxis N92.0
Menses, retention N94.89
Menstrual — *see* Menstruation
Menstruation
  absent — *see* Amenorrhea
  anovulatory N97.0
  cycle, irregular N92.6
  delayed N91.0
  disorder N93.9
    psychogenic F45.8
  during pregnancy O20.8

Menstruation — *continued*
  excessive (with regular cycle) N92.0
    with irregular cycle N92.1
    at puberty N92.2
  frequent N92.0
  infrequent — *see* Oligomenorrhea
  irregular N92.6
    specified NEC N92.5
  latent N92.5
  membranous N92.5
  painful (*see also* Dysmenorrhea) N94.6
    primary N94.4
    psychogenic F45.8
    secondary N94.5
  passage of clots N92.0
  precocious E30.1
  protracted N92.5
  rare — *see* Oligomenorrhea
  retained N94.89
  retrograde N92.5
  scanty — *see* Oligomenorrhea
  suppression N94.89
  vicarious (nasal) N94.89
Mental — *see also* condition
  deficiency — *see* Disability, intellectual
  deterioration — *see* Psychosis
  disorder — *see* Disorder, mental
  exhaustion F48.8
  insufficiency (congenital) — *see* Disability, intellectual
  observation without need for further medical care Z03.89
  retardation — *see* Disability, intellectual
  subnormality — *see* Disability, intellectual
  upset — *see* Disorder, mental
Meralgia paresthetica G57.1-
Mercurial — *see* condition
Mercurialism — *see* subcategory T56.1
MERFF syndrome (myoclonic epilepsy associated with ragged-red fiber) E88.42
Merkel cell tumor — *see* Carcinoma, Merkel cell
Merocele — *see* Hernia, femoral
Meromelia
  lower limb — *see* Defect, reduction, lower limb
    intercalary
    femur — *see* Defect, reduction, lower limb, specified type NEC
      tibiofibular (complete) (incomplete) — *see* Defect, reduction, lower limb
  upper limb — *see* Defect, reduction, upper limb
    intercalary, humeral, radioulnar — *see* Agenesis, arm, with hand present
Merzbacher-Pelizaeus disease E75.29
Mesaortitis — *see* Aortitis
Mesarteritis — *see* Arteritis
Mesencephalitis — *see* Encephalitis
Mesenchymoma — *see also* Neoplasm, connective tissue, uncertain behavior
  benign — *see* Neoplasm, connective tissue, benign
  malignant — *see* Neoplasm, connective tissue, malignant
Mesenteritis
  retractile K65.4
  sclerosing K65.4
Mesentery, mesenteric — *see* condition
Mesio-occlusion M26.213
Mesiodens, mesiodentes K00.1
Mesocolon — *see* condition
Mesonephroma (malignant) — *see* Neoplasm, malignant, by site
  benign — *see* Neoplasm, benign, by site
Mesophlebitis — *see* Phlebitis
Mesostromal dysgenesia Q13.89

Mesothelioma (malignant) C45.9
  benign
    mesentery D19.1
    mesocolon D19.1
    omentum D19.1
    peritoneum D19.1
    pleura D19.0
    specified site NEC D19.7
    unspecified site D19.9
  biphasic C45.9
    benign
      mesentery D19.1
      mesocolon D19.1
      omentum D19.1
      peritoneum D19.1
      pleura D19.0
      specified site NEC D19.7
      unspecified site D19.9
  cystic D48.4
  epithelioid C45.9
    benign
      mesentery D19.1
      mesocolon D19.1
      omentum D19.1
      peritoneum D19.1
      pleura D19.0
      specified site NEC D19.7
      unspecified site D19.9
  fibrous C45.9
    benign
      mesentery D19.1
      mesocolon D19.1
      omentum D19.1
      peritoneum D19.1
      pleura D19.0
      specified site NEC D19.7
      unspecified site D19.9
  site classification
    liver C45.7
    lung C45.7
    mediastinum C45.7
    mesentery C45.1
    mesocolon C45.1
    omentum C45.1
    pericardium C45.2
    peritoneum C45.1
    pleura C45.0
      parietal C45.0
    retroperitoneum C45.7
    specified site NEC C45.7
    unspecified C45.9
Metabolic syndrome E88.81
Metagonimiasis B66.8
Metagonimus infestation (intestine) B66.8
Metal
  pigmentation L81.8
  polisher's disease J62.8
Metamorphopsia H53.15
Metaplasia
  apocrine (breast) — see Dysplasia, mammary, specified type NEC
  cervix (squamous) — see Dysplasia, cervix
  endometrium (squamous) (uterus) N85.8
  esophagus K22.7-
  kidney (pelvis) (squamous) N28.89
  myelogenous D73.1
  myeloid (agnogenic) (megakaryocytic) D73.1
  spleen D73.1
  squamous cell, bladder N32.89
Metastasis, metastatic
  abscess — see Abscess
  calcification E83.59
  cancer
    from specified site — see Neoplasm, malignant, by site
    to specified site — see Neoplasm, secondary, by site
  deposits (in) — see Neoplasm, secondary, by site

Metastasis, metastatic — continued
  disease (see also Neoplasm, secondary, by site) C79.9
  spread (to) — see Neoplasm, secondary, by site
Metastrongyliasis B83.8
Metatarsalgia M77.4-
  anterior G57.6-
  Morton's G57.6-
Metatarsus, metatarsal — see also condition
  adductus, congenital Q66.22
  valgus (abductus), congenital Q66.6
  varus (congenital) Q66.22
    primus Q66.21
Methadone use — see Use, opioid
Methemoglobinemia D74.9
  acquired (with sulfhemoglobinemia) D74.8
  congenital D74.0
  enzymatic (congenital) D74.0
  Hb M disease D74.0
  hereditary D74.0
  toxic D74.8
Methemoglobinuria — see Hemoglobinuria
Methioninemia E72.19
Methylmalonic acidemia E71.120
Metritis (catarrhal) (hemorrhagic) (septic) (suppurative) — see also Endometritis
  cervical — see Cervicitis
Metropathia hemorrhagica N93.8
Metroperitonitis — see Peritonitis, pelvic, female
Metrorrhagia N92.1
  climacteric N92.4
  menopausal N92.4
  postpartum NEC (atonic) (following delivery of placenta) O72.1
    delayed or secondary O72.2
  preclimacteric or premenopausal N92.4
  psychogenic F45.8
Metrorrhexis — see Rupture, uterus
Metrosalpingitis N70.91
Metrostaxis N93.8
Metrovaginitis — see Endometritis
Meyer-Schwickerath and Weyers syndrome Q87.0
Meynert's amentia (nonalcoholic) F04
  alcoholic F10.96
    with dependence F10.26
Mibelli's disease (porokeratosis) Q82.8
Mice, joint — see Loose, body, joint
  knee M23.4-
Micrencephalon, micrencephaly Q02
Microalbuminuria R80.9
Microaneurysm, retinal — see also Disorder, retina, microaneurysms
  diabetic — see E08-E13 with .31
Microangiopathy (peripheral) I73.9
  thrombotic M31.1
Microcalcifications, breast R92.0
Microcephalus, microcephalic, microcephaly Q02
  due to toxoplasmosis (congenital) P37.1
Microcheilia Q18.7
Microcolon (congenital) Q43.8
Microcornea (congenital) Q13.4
Microcytic — see condition
Microdeletions NEC Q93.88
Microdontia K00.2
Microdrepanocytosis D57.40
  with crisis (vasoocclusive pain) D57.419
  with
    acute chest syndrome D57.411
    splenic sequestration D57.412
Microembolism
  atherothrombotic — see Atheroembolism
  retinal — see Occlusion, artery, retina
Microencephalon Q02
Microfilaria streptocerca infestation — see Onchocerciasis

Microgastria (congenital) Q40.2
Microgenia M26.06
Microgenitalia, congenital
  female Q52.8
  male Q55.8
Microglioma — see Lymphoma, non-Hodgkin, specified NEC
Microglossia (congenital) Q38.3
Micrognathia, micrognathism (congenital) (mandibular) (maxillary) M26.09
Microgyria (congenital) Q04.3
Microinfarct of heart — see Insufficiency, coronary
Microlentia (congenital) Q12.8
Microlithiasis, alveolar, pulmonary J84.02
Micromastia N64.82
Micromyelia (congenital) Q06.8
Micropenis Q55.62
Microphakia (congenital) Q12.8
Microphthalmos, microphthalmia (congenital) Q11.2
  due to toxoplasmosis P37.1
Micropsia H53.15
Microscopic polyangiitis (polyarteritis) M31.7
Microsporidiosis B60.8
  intestinal A07.8
Microsporon furfur infestation B36.0
Microsporosis — see also Dermatophytosis
  nigra B36.1
Microstomia (congenital) Q18.5
Microtia (congenital) (external ear) Q17.2
Microtropia H50.40
Microvillus inclusion disease (MVD) (MVID) Q43.8
Micturition
  disorder NEC (see also Difficulty, micturition) R39.198
    psychogenic F45.8
  frequency R35.0
    psychogenic F45.8
  hesitancy R39.11
  incomplete emptying R39.14
  nocturnal R35.1
  painful R30.9
    dysuria R30.0
    psychogenic F45.8
    tenesmus R30.1
  poor stream R39.12
  position dependent R39.192
  split stream R39.13
  straining R39.16
  urgency R39.15
Mid plane — see condition
Middle
  ear — see condition
  lobe (right) syndrome J98.19
Miescher's elastoma L87.2
Mietens' syndrome Q87.2
Migraine (idiopathic) G43.909
  with aura (acute-onset) (prolonged) (typical) (without headache) G43.109
    with refractory migraine G43.119
      with status migrainosus G43.111
      without status migrainosus G43.919
    intractable G43.119
      with status migrainosus G43.111
      without status migrainosus G43.119
    not intractable G43.109
      with status migrainosus G43.101
      without status migrainosus G43.109

Migraine (idiopathic) G43.909 — *continued*
with aura (acute-onset) (prolonged) (typical) (without headache) G43.109 — *continued*
  persistent G43.509
    with cerebral infarction G43.609
      with refractory migraine G43.619
        with status migrainosus G43.611
        without status migrainosus G43.619
      intractable G43.619
        with status migrainosus G43.611
        without status migrainosus G43.619
      not intractable G43.609
        with status migrainosus G43.601
        without status migrainosus G43.609
      without refractory migraine G43.609
        with status migrainosus G43.601
        without status migrainosus G43.609
    without cerebral infarction G43.509
      with refractory migraine G43.519
        with status migrainosus G43.511
        without status migrainosus G43.519
      intractable G43.519
        with status migrainosus G43.511
        without status migrainosus G43.519
      not intractable G43.509
        with status migrainosus G43.501
        without status migrainosus G43.509
      without refractory migraine G43.509
        with status migrainosus G43.501
        without status migrainosus G43.509
  without mention of refractory migraine G43.109
    with status migrainosus G43.101
    without status migrainosus G43.109
  with refractory migraine G43.919
    with status migrainosus G43.911
    without status migrainosus G43.919
  abdominal G43.D0 *(follows G43.7)*
    with refractory migraine G43.D1 *(follows G43.7)*
    intractable G43.D1 *(follows G43.7)*
    not intractable G43.D0 *(follows G43.7)*
    without refractory migraine G43.D0 *(follows G43.7)*
  basilar — *see* Migraine, with aura
  classical — *see* Migraine, with aura
  common — *see* Migraine, without aura
  complicated G43.109
  equivalents — *see* Migraine, with aura
  familiar — *see* Migraine, hemiplegic
  hemiplegic G43.409
    with refractory migraine G43.419
      with status migrainosus G43.411
      without status migrainosus G43.419
    intractable G43.419
      with status migrainosus G43.411
      without status migrainosus G43.419
    not intractable G43.409
      with status migrainosus G43.401
      without status migrainosus G43.409
    without refractory migraine G43.409
      with status migrainosus G43.401
      without status migrainosus G43.409
  intractable G43.919
    with status migrainosus G43.911
    without status migrainosus G43.919
  menstrual G43.829
    with refractory migraine G43.839
      with status migrainosus G43.831
      without status migrainosus G43.839
    intractable G43.839
      with status migrainosus G43.831
      without status migrainosus G43.839
    not intractable G43.829
      with status migrainosus G43.821
      without status migrainosus G43.829

Migraine (idiopathic) G43.909 — *continued*
menstrual G43.829 — *continued*
    without refractory migraine G43.829
      with status migrainosus G43.821
      without status migrainosus G43.829
  menstrually related — *see* Migraine, menstrual
  not intractable G43.909
    with status migrainosus G43.901
    without status migrainosus G43.919
  ophthalmoplegic G43.B0 *(follows G43.7)*
    with refractory migraine G43.B1 *(follows G43.7)*
    intractable G43.B1 *(follows G43.7)*
    not intractable G43.B0 *(follows G43.7)*
    without refractory migraine G43.B0 *(follows G43.7)*
  persistent aura (with, without) cerebral infarction — *see* Migraine, with aura, persistent
  preceded or accompanied by transient focal neurological phenomena — *see* Migraine, with aura
  pre-menstrual — *see* Migraine, menstrual
  pure menstrual — *see* Migraine, menstrual
  retinal — *see* Migraine, with aura
  specified NEC G43.809
    intractable G43.819
      with status migrainosus G43.811
      without status migrainosus G43.819
    not intractable G43.809
      with status migrainosus G43.801
      without status migrainosus G43.809
  sporadic — *see* Migraine, hemiplegic
  transformed — *see* Migraine, without aura, chronic
  triggered seizures — *see* Migraine, with aura
  without aura G43.009
    with refractory migraine G43.019
      with status migrainosus G43.011
      without status migrainosus G43.019
    chronic G43.709
      with refractory migraine G43.719
        with status migrainosus G43.711
        without status migrainosus G43.719
      intractable
        with status migrainosus G43.711
        without status migrainosus G43.719
      not intractable
        with status migrainosus G43.701
        without status migrainosus G43.709
      without refractory migraine G43.709
        with status migrainosus G43.701
        without status migrainosus G43.709
    intractable
      with status migrainosus G43.011
      without status migrainosus G43.019
    not intractable
      with status migrainosus G43.001
      without status migrainosus G43.009
    without mention of refractory migraine G43.009
      with status migrainosus G43.001
      without status migrainosus G43.009
    without refractory migraine G43.909
      with status migrainosus G43.901
      without status migrainosus G43.909
Migrant, social Z59.0
Migration, anxiety concerning Z60.3
Migratory, migrating — *see also* condition
  person Z59.0
  testis Q55.29
Mikity-Wilson disease or syndrome P27.0
Mikulicz' disease or syndrome K11.8

Miliaria L74.3
  alba L74.1
  apocrine L75.2
  crystallina L74.1
  profunda L74.2
  rubra L74.0
  tropicalis L74.2
Miliary — *see* condition
Milium L72.0
  colloid L57.8
Milk
  crust L21.0
  excessive secretion O92.6
  poisoning — *see* Poisoning, food, noxious
  retention O92.79
  sickness — *see* Poisoning, food, noxious
  spots I31.0
Milk-alkali disease or syndrome E83.52
Milk-leg (deep vessels) (nonpuerperal) — *see* Embolism, vein, lower extremity
  complicating pregnancy O22.3-
  puerperal, postpartum, childbirth O87.1
Milkman's disease or syndrome M83.8
Milky urine — *see* Chyluria
Millar's asthma J38.5
Millard-Gubler(-Foville) paralysis or syndrome G46.3
Miller Fisher syndrome G61.0
Mills' disease — *see* Hemiplegia
Millstone maker's pneumoconiosis J62.8
Milroy's disease (chronic hereditary edema) Q82.0
Minamata disease T56.1-
Miners' asthma or lung J60
Minkowski-Chauffard syndrome — *see* Spherocytosis
Minor — *see* condition
Minor's disease (hematomyelia) G95.19
Minot's disease (hemorrhagic disease), newborn P53
Minot-von Willebrand-Jurgens disease or syndrome (angiohemophilia) D68.0
Minus (and plus) hand (intrinsic) — *see* Deformity, limb, specified type NEC, forearm
Miosis (pupil) H57.03
Mirizzi's syndrome (hepatic duct stenosis) K83.1
Mirror writing F81.0
Misadventure (of) (prophylactic) (therapeutic) (*see also* Complications) T88.9
  administration of insulin (by accident) — *see* subcategory T38.3
  infusion — *see* Complications, infusion
  local applications (of fomentations, plasters, etc.) T88.9
    burn or scald — *see* Burn
    specified NEC T88.8
  medical care (early) (late) T88.9
    adverse effect of drugs or chemicals — *see* Table of Drugs and Chemicals
    specified NEC T88.8
  surgical procedure (early) (late) — *see* Complications, surgical procedure
  transfusion — *see* Complications, transfusion
  vaccination or other immunological procedure — *see* Complications, vaccination
Miscarriage O03.9
Misdirection, aqueous H40.83-
Misperception, sleep state F51.02
Misplaced, misplacement
  ear Q17.4
  kidney (acquired) N28.89
    congenital Q63.2
  organ or site, congenital NEC — *see* Malposition, congenital
Missed
  abortion O02.1
  delivery O36.4

DISEASE INDEX

Missing — *see also* Absence
  string of intrauterine contraceptive device
    T83.32
Misuse of drugs F19.99
Mitchell's disease (erythromelalgia) I73.81
Mite(s) (infestation) B88.9
  diarrhea B88.0
  grain (itch) B88.0
  hair follicle (itch) B88.0
  in sputum B88.0
Mitral — *see* condition
Mittelschmerz N94.0
Mixed — *see* condition
MNGIE (mitochondrial neurogastrointestinal
    encephalopathy) syndrome E88.49
MNN (multifocal motor neuropathy) G61.82
Mobile, mobility
  cecum Q43.3
  excessive — *see* Hypermobility
  gallbladder, congenital Q44.1
  kidney N28.89
  organ or site, congenital NEC — *see*
    Malposition, congenital
Mobitz heart block (atrioventricular) I44.1
Moebius, Möbius
  disease (ophthalmoplegic migraine) — *see*
    Migraine, ophthalmoplegic
  syndrome Q87.0
    congenital oculofacial paralysis (with other
      anomalies) Q87.0
    ophthalmoplegic migraine — *see* Migraine,
      ophthalmoplegic
Moeller's glossitis K14.0
Mohr's syndrome (Types I and II) Q87.0
Mola destruens D39.2
Molar pregnancy O02.0
Molarization of premolars K00.2
Molding, head (during birth) — *omit code*
Mole (pigmented) — *see also* Nevus
  blood O02.0
  Breus' O02.0
  cancerous — *see* Melanoma
  carneous O02.0
  destructive D39.2
  fleshy O02.0
  hydatid, hydatidiform (benign) (complicating
    pregnancy) (delivered) (undelivered)
    O01.9
    classical O01.0
    complete O01.0
    incomplete O01.1
    invasive D39.2
    malignant D39.2
    partial O01.1
  intrauterine O02.0
  invasive (hydatidiform) D39.2
  malignant
    meaning
      malignant hydatidiform mole D39.2
      melanoma — *see* Melanoma
  nonhydatidiform O02.0
  nonpigmented — *see* Nevus
  pregnancy NEC O02.0
  skin — *see* Nevus
  tubal O00.10
    with intrauterine pregnancy O00.11
  vesicular — *see* Mole, hydatidiform
Molimen, molimina (menstrual) N94.3
Molluscum contagiosum (epitheliale) B08.1
Mönckeberg's arteriosclerosis, disease,
  or sclerosis — *see* Arteriosclerosis,
    extremities
Mondini's malformation (cochlea) Q16.5
Mondor's disease I80.8
Monge's disease T70.29
Monilethrix (congenital) Q84.1
Moniliasis (*see also* Candidiasis) B37.9
  neonatal P37.5

Monitoring (encounter for)
  therapeutic drug level Z51.81
Monkey malaria B53.1
Monkeypox B04
Monoarthritis M13.10
  ankle M13.17-
  elbow M13.12-
  foot joint M13.17-
  hand joint M13.14-
  hip M13.15-
  knee M13.16-
  shoulder M13.11-
  wrist M13.13-
Monoblastic — *see* condition
Monochromat(ism), monochromatopsia
  (acquired) (congenital) H53.51
Monocytic — *see* condition
Monocytopenia D72.818
Monocytosis (symptomatic) D72.821
Monomania — *see* Psychosis
Mononeuritis G58.9
  cranial nerve — *see* Disorder, nerve, cranial
  femoral nerve G57.2-
  lateral
    cutaneous nerve of thigh G57.1-
    popliteal nerve G57.3-
  lower limb G57.9-
    specified nerve NEC G57.8-
  medial popliteal nerve G57.4-
  median nerve G56.1-
  multiplex G58.7
  plantar nerve G57.6-
  posterior tibial nerve G57.5-
  radial nerve G56.3-
  sciatic nerve G57.0-
  specified NEC G58.8
  tibial nerve G57.4-
  ulnar nerve G56.2-
  upper limb G56.9-
    specified nerve NEC G56.8-
  vestibular — *see* subcategory H93.3
Mononeuropathy G58.9
  carpal tunnel syndrome — *see* Syndrome,
    carpal tunnel
  diabetic NEC — *see* E08-E13 with .41
  femoral nerve — *see* Lesion, nerve, femoral
  ilioinguinal nerve G57.8-
  in diseases classified elsewhere — *see*
    category G59
  intercostal G58.0
  lower limb G57.9-
    causalgia — *see* Causalgia, lower limb
    femoral nerve — *see* Lesion, nerve, femoral
    meralgia paresthetica G57.1-
    plantar nerve — *see* Lesion, nerve, plantar
    popliteal nerve — *see* Lesion, nerve,
      popliteal
    sciatic nerve — *see* Lesion, nerve, sciatic
    specified NEC G57.8-
    tarsal tunnel syndrome — *see* Syndrome,
      tarsal tunnel
  median nerve — *see* Lesion, nerve, median
  multiplex G58.7
  obturator nerve G57.8-
  popliteal nerve — *see* Lesion, nerve, popliteal
  radial nerve — *see* Lesion, nerve, radial
  saphenous nerve G57.8-
  specified NEC G58.8
  tarsal tunnel syndrome — *see* Syndrome, tarsal
    tunnel
  tuberculous A17.83
  ulnar nerve — *see* Lesion, nerve, ulnar
  upper limb G56.9-
    carpal tunnel syndrome — *see* Syndrome,
      carpal tunnel
    causalgia — *see* Causalgia
    median nerve — *see* Lesion, nerve, median
    radial nerve — *see* Lesion, nerve, radial
    specified site NEC G56.8-

Mononeuropathy G58.9 — *continued*
  upper limb G56.9- — *continued*
    ulnar nerve — *see* Lesion, nerve, ulnar
Mononucleosis, infectious B27.90
  with
    complication NEC B27.99
    meningitis B27.92
    polyneuropathy B27.91
  cytomegaloviral B27.10
    with
      complication NEC B27.19
      meningitis B27.12
      polyneuropathy B27.11
  Epstein-Barr (virus) B27.00
    with
      complication NEC B27.09
      meningitis B27.02
      polyneuropathy B27.01
  gammaherpesviral B27.00
    with
      complication NEC B27.09
      meningitis B27.02
      polyneuropathy B27.01
  specified NEC B27.80
    with
      complication NEC B27.89
      meningitis B27.82
      polyneuropathy B27.81
Monoplegia G83.3-
  congenital (cerebral) G80.8
    spastic G80.1
  embolic (current episode) I63.4-
  following
    cerebrovascular disease
      cerebral infarction
        lower limb I69.34-
        upper limb I69.33-
      intracerebral hemorrhage
        lower limb I69.14-
        upper limb I69.13-
      lower limb I69.94-
      nontraumatic intracranial hemorrhage NEC
        lower limb I69.24-
        upper limb I69.23-
      specified disease NEC
        lower limb I69.84-
        upper limb I69.83-
      stroke NOS
        lower limb I69.34-
        upper limb I69.33-
      subarachnoid hemorrhage
        lower limb I69.04-
        upper limb I69.03-
      upper limb I69.93-
  hysterical (transient) F44.4
  lower limb G83.1-
  psychogenic (conversion reaction) F44.4
  thrombotic (current episode) I63.3-
  transient R29.818
  upper limb G83.2-
Monorchism, monorchidism Q55.0
Monosomy (*see also* Deletion, chromosome)
  Q93.9
  specified NEC Q93.89
  whole chromosome
    meiotic nondisjunction Q93.0
    mitotic nondisjunction Q93.1
    mosaicism Q93.1
  X Q96.9
Monster, monstrosity (single) Q89.7
  acephalic Q00.0
  twin Q89.4
Monteggia's fracture(-dislocation)
  S52.27-
Moore's syndrome — *see* Epilepsy, specified
  NEC
Mooren's ulcer (cornea) — *see* Ulcer, cornea,
  Mooren's
Mooser's bodies A75.2

DISEASE INDEX

Mooser-Neill reaction A75.2
Morbidity not stated or unknown R69
Morbilli — *see* Measles
Morbus — *see also* Disease
  angelicus, anglorum E55.0
  Beigel B36.2
  caducus — *see* Epilepsy
  celiacus K90.0
  comitialis — *see* Epilepsy
  cordis (*see also* Disease, heart) I51.9
    valvulorum — *see* Endocarditis
  coxae senilis M16.9
    tuberculous A18.02
  hemorrhagicus neonatorum P53
  maculosus neonatorum P54.5
Morel-Kraepelin disease — *see* Schizophrenia
Morel-Moore syndrome M85.2
Morel(-Stewart)(-Morgagni) syndrome M85.2
Morgagni's
  cyst, organ, hydatid, or appendage
    female Q50.5
    male (epididymal) Q55.4
      testicular Q55.29
  syndrome M85.2
Morgagni-Stewart-Morel syndrome M85.2
Morgagni-Stokes-Adams syndrome I45.9
Morgagni-Turner(-Albright) syndrome Q96.9
Moria F07.0
Moron (I.Q. 50-69) F70
Morphea L94.0
Morphinism (without remission) F11.20
  with remission F11.21
Morphinomania (without remission) F11.20
  with remission F11.21
Morquio(-Ullrich)(-Brailsford) disease or syndrome — *see* Mucopolysaccharidosis
Mortification (dry) (moist) — *see* Gangrene
Morton's metatarsalgia (neuralgia) (neuroma) (syndrome) G57.6-
Morvan's disease or syndrome G60.8
Mosaicism, mosaic (autosomal) (chromosomal)
  45,X/46,XX Q96.3
  45,X/other cell lines NEC with abnormal sex chromosome Q96.4
  sex chromosome
    female Q97.8
    lines with various numbers of X chromosomes Q97.2
    male Q98.7
    XY Q96.3
Moschowitz' disease M31.1
Mother yaw A66.0
Motion sickness (from travel, any vehicle) (from roundabouts or swings) T75.3
Mottled, mottling, teeth (enamel) (endemic) (nonendemic) K00.3
Mounier-Kuhn syndrome Q32.4
  with bronchiectasis J47.9
    exacerbation (acute) J47.1
    lower respiratory infection J47.0
  acquired J98.09
    with bronchiectasis J47.9
      with
        exacerbation (acute) J47.1
        lower respiratory infection J47.0
Mountain
  sickness T70.29
    with polycythemia , acquired (acute) D75.1
  tick fever A93.2
Mouse, joint — *see* Loose, body, joint
  knee M23.4-
Mouth — *see* condition

Movable
  coccyx — *see* subcategory M53.2
  kidney N28.89
    congenital Q63.8
  spleen D73.89
Movements, dystonic R25.8
Moyamoya disease I67.5
MRSA (methicillin resistant Staphylococcus aureus)
  infection A49.02
    as the cause of diseases classified elsewhere B95.62
  sepsis A41.02
MSSA (methicillin susceptible Staphylococcus aureus)
  infection A49.01
    as the cause of diseases classified elsewhere B95.61
  sepsis A41.01
Mucha-Habermann disease L41.0
Mucinosis (cutaneous) (focal) (papular) (reticular erythematous) (skin) L98.5
  oral K13.79
Mucocele
  appendix K38.8
  buccal cavity K13.79
  gallbladder K82.1
  lacrimal sac, chronic H04.43-
  nasal sinus J34.1
  nose J34.1
  salivary gland (any) K11.6
  sinus (accessory) (nasal) J34.1
  turbinate (bone) (middle) (nasal) J34.1
  uterus N85.8
Mucolipidosis
  I E77.1
  II, III E77.0
  IV E75.11
Mucopolysaccharidosis E76.3
  beta-gluduronidase deficiency E76.29
  cardiopathy E76.3 [I52]
  Hunter's syndrome E76.1
  Hurler's syndrome E76.01
  Hurler-Scheie syndrome E76.02
  Maroteaux-Lamy syndrome E76.29
  Morquio syndrome E76.219
    A E76.210
    B E76.211
    classic E76.210
  Sanfilippo syndrome E76.22
  Scheie's syndrome E76.03
  specified NEC E76.29
  type
    I
      Hurler's syndrome E76.01
      Hurler-Scheie syndrome E76.02
      Scheie's syndrome E76.03
    II E76.1
    III E76.22
    IV E76.219
    IVA E76.210
    IVB E76.211
    VI E76.29
    VII E76.29
Mucormycosis B46.5
  cutaneous B46.3
  disseminated B46.4
  gastrointestinal B46.2
  generalized B46.4
  pulmonary B46.0
  rhinocerebral B46.1
  skin B46.3
  subcutaneous B46.3

Mucositis (ulcerative) K12.30
  due to drugs NEC K12.32
  gastrointestinal K92.81
  mouth (oral) (oropharyngeal) K12.30
    due to antineoplastic therapy K12.31
    due to drugs NEC K12.32
    due to radiation K12.33
    specified NEC K12.39
    viral K12.39
  nasal J34.81
  oral cavity — *see* Mucositis, mouth
  oral soft tissues — *see* Mucositis, mouth
  vagina and vulva N76.81
Mucositis necroticans agranulocytica — *see* Agranulocytosis
Mucous — *see also* condition
  patches (syphilitic) A51.39
    congenital A50.07
Mucoviscidosis E84.9
  with meconium obstruction E84.11
Mucus
  asphyxia or suffocation — *see* Asphyxia, mucus
  in stool R19.5
  plug — *see* Asphyxia, mucus
Muguet B37.0
Mulberry molars (congenital syphilis) A50.52
Müllerian mixed tumor
  specified site — *see* Neoplasm, malignant, by site
  unspecified site C54.9
Multicystic kidney (development) Q61.4
Multiparity (grand) Z64.1
  affecting management of pregnancy, labor and delivery (supervision only) O09.4-
  requiring contraceptive management — *see* Contraception
Multipartita placenta O43.19-
Multiple, multiplex — *see also* condition
  digits (congenital) Q69.9
  endocrine neoplasia — *see* Neoplasia, endocrine, multiple (MEN)
  personality F44.81
Mumps B26.9
  arthritis B26.85
  complication NEC B26.89
  encephalitis B26.2
  hepatitis B26.81
  meningitis (aseptic) B26.1
  meningoencephalitis B26.2
  myocarditis B26.82
  oophoritis B26.89
  orchitis B26.0
  pancreatitis B26.3
  polyneuropathy B26.84
Mumu (*see also* Infestation, filarial) B74.9 [N51]
Münchhausen's syndrome — *see* Disorder, factitious
Münchmeyer's syndrome — *see* Myositis, ossificans, progressiva
Mural — *see* condition
Murmur (cardiac) (heart) (organic) R01.1
  abdominal R19.15
  aortic (valve) — *see* Endocarditis, aortic
  benign R01.0
  diastolic — *see* Endocarditis
  Flint I35.1
  functional R01.0
  Graham Steell I37.1
  innocent R01.0
  mitral (valve) — *see* Insufficiency, mitral
  nonorganic R01.0
  presystolic, mitral — *see* Insufficiency, mitral
  pulmonic (valve) I37.8
  systolic R01.1
  tricuspid (valve) I07.9
  valvular — *see* Endocarditis
Murri's disease (intermittent hemoglobinuria) D59.6

D I S E A S E   I N D E X

Muscle, muscular — *see also* condition
  carnitine (palmityltransferase) deficiency
    E71.314
Musculoneuralgia — *see* Neuralgia
Mushroom-workers' (pickers') disease or
  lung J67.5
Mushrooming hip — *see* Derangement, joint,
  specified NEC, hip
Mutation(s)
  factor V Leiden D68.51
  prothrombin gene D68.52
  surfactant, of lung J84.83
Mutism — *see also* Aphasia
  deaf (acquired) (congenital) NEC H91.3
  elective (adjustment reaction) (childhood)
    F94.0
  hysterical F44.4
  selective (childhood) F94.0
MVD (microvillus inclusion disease) Q43.8
MVID (microvillus inclusion disease) Q43.8
Myalgia M79.1
  epidemic (cervical) B33.0
  traumatic NEC T14.8
Myasthenia G70.9
  congenital G70.2
  cordis — *see* Failure, heart
  developmental G70.2
  gravis G70.00
    with exacerbation (acute) G70.01
    in crisis G70.01
    neonatal, transient P94.0
    pseudoparalytica G70.00
      with exacerbation (acute) G70.01
      in crisis G70.01
  stomach, psychogenic F45.8
  syndrome
    in
      diabetes mellitus — *see* E08-E13 with .44
      neoplastic disease (*see also* Neoplasm)
        D49.9 *[G73.3]*
      pernicious anemia D51.0 *[G73.3]*
      thyrotoxicosis E05.90 *[G73.3]*
        with thyroid storm E05.91 *[G73.3]*
Myasthenic M62.81
Mycelium infection B49
Mycetismus — *see* Poisoning, food, noxious,
  mushroom
Mycetoma B47.9
  actinomycotic B47.1
  bone (mycotic) B47.9 *[M90.80]*
  eumycotic B47.0
  foot B47.9
    actinomycotic B47.1
    mycotic B47.0
  madurae NEC B47.9
    mycotic B47.0
  maduromycotic B47.0
  mycotic B47.0
  nocardial B47.1
Mycobacteriosis — *see* Mycobacterium
Mycobacterium, mycobacterial (infection)
  A31.9
  anonymous A31.9
  atypical A31.9
    cutaneous A31.1
    pulmonary A31.0
      tuberculous — *see* Tuberculosis, pulmonary
    specified site NEC A31.8
  avium (intracellulare complex) A31.0
  balnei A31.1
  Battey A31.0
  chelonei A31.8
  cutaneous A31.1
  extrapulmonary systemic A31.8
  fortuitum A31.8
  intracellulare (Battey bacillus) A31.0
  kakaferifu A31.8
  kansasii (yellow bacillus) A31.0
  kasongo A31.8

Mycobacterium, mycobacterial (infection)
  A31.9 — *continued*
  leprae (*see also* Leprosy) A30.9
  luciflavum A31.1
  marinum (M. balnei) A31.1
  nonspecific — *see* Mycobacterium, atypical
  pulmonary (atypical) A31.0
    tuberculous — *see* Tuberculosis, pulmonary
  scrofulaceum A31.8
  simiae A31.8
  systemic, extrapulmonary A31.8
  szulgai A31.8
  terrae A31.8
  triviale A31.8
  tuberculosis (human, bovine) —
    seeTuberculosis
  ulcerans A31.1
  xenopi A31.8
**Mycoplasma (M.) pneumoniae, as cause
  of disease classified elsewhere** B96.0
Mycosis, mycotic B49
  cutaneous NEC B36.9
  ear B36.9
    in
      aspergillosis B44.89
      candidiasis B37.84
      moniliasis B37.84
  fungoides (extranodal) (solid organ) C84.0-
  mouth B37.0
  nails B35.1
  opportunistic B48.8
  skin NEC B36.9
  specified NEC B48.8
  stomatitis B37.0
  vagina, vaginitis (candidal) B37.3
Mydriasis (pupil) H57.04
Myelatelia Q06.1
Myelinolysis, pontine, central G37.2
Myelitis (acute) (ascending) (childhood)
  (chronic) (descending) (diffuse)
  (disseminated) (idiopathic) (pressure)
  (progressive) (spinal cord) (subacute) (*see
  also* Encephalitis) G04.91
  herpes simplex B00.82
  herpes zoster B02.24
  in diseases classified elsewhere G05.4
  necrotizing, subacute G37.4
  optic neuritis in G36.0
  postchickenpox B01.12
  postherpetic B02.24
  postimmunization G04.02
  postinfectious NEC G04.89
  postvaccinal G04.02
  specified NEC G04.89
  syphilitic (transverse) A52.14
  toxic G92
  transverse (in demyelinating diseases of central
    nervous system) G37.3
  tuberculous A17.82
  varicella B01.12
**Myelo-osteo-musculodysplasia
  hereditaria** Q79.8
Myeloblastic — *see* condition
Myeloblastoma
  granular cell — *see also* Neoplasm, connective
    tissue
    malignant — *see* Neoplasm, connective
      tissue, malignant
  tongue D10.1
Myelocele — *see* Spina bifida
Myelocystocele — *see* Spina bifida
Myelocytic — *see* condition
Myelodysplasia D46.9
  specified NEC D46.Z
  spinal cord (congenital) Q06.1

Myelodysplastic syndrome D46.9
  with
    5q deletion D46.C
    isolated del(5q) chromosomal abnormality
      D46.C
  specified NEC D46.Z
Myeloencephalitis — *see* Encephalitis
Myelofibrosis D75.81
  with myeloid metaplasia D47.4
  acute C94.4-
  idiopathic (chronic) D47.4
  primary D47.1
  secondary D75.81
    in myeloproliferative disease D47.4
Myelogenous — *see* condition
Myeloid — *see* condition
Myelokathexis D70.9
Myeloleukodystrophy E75.29
Myelolipoma — *see* Lipoma
Myeloma (multiple) C90.0-
  monostatic C90.3
    plasma cell C90.0-
  plasma cell C90.0-
  solitary (*see also* Plasmacytoma, solitary)
    C90.3-
Myelomalacia G95.89
Myelomatosis C90.0-
Myelomeningitis — *see* Meningoencephalitis
Myelomeningocele (spinal cord) — *see* Spina
  bifida
Myelopathic
  anemia D64.89
  muscle atrophy — *see* Atrophy, muscle, spinal
  pain syndrome G89.0
Myelopathy (spinal cord) G95.9
  drug-induced G95.89
  in (due to)
    degeneration or displacement, intervertebral
      disc NEC — *see* Disorder, disc, with,
      myelopathy
    infection — *see* Encephalitis
    intervertebral disc disorder — *see also*
      Disorder, disc, with, myelopathy
    mercury — *see* subcategory T56.1
    neoplastic disease (*see also* Neoplasm)
      D49.9 *[G99.2]*
    pernicious anemia D51.0 *[G99.2]*
    spondylosis — *see* Spondylosis, with
      myelopathy NEC
  necrotic (subacute) (vascular) G95.19
  radiation-induced G95.89
  spondylogenic NEC — *see* Spondylosis, with
    myelopathy NEC
  toxic G95.89
  transverse, acute G37.3
  vascular G95.19
  vitamin B12 E53.8 *[G32.0]*
Myelophthisis D61.82
Myeloradiculitis G04.91
Myeloradiculodysplasia (spinal) Q06.1
Myelosarcoma C92.3-
Myelosclerosis D75.89
  with myeloid metaplasia D47.4
  disseminated, of nervous system G35
  megakaryocytic D47.4
    with myeloid metaplasia D47.4
Myelosis
  acute C92.0-
  aleukemic C92.9-
  chronic D47.1
  erythremic (acute) C94.0-
  megakaryocytic C94.2-
  nonleukemic D72.828
  subacute C92.9-

Myiasis (cavernous) B87.9
  aural B87.4
  creeping B87.0
  cutaneous B87.0
  dermal B87.0
  ear (external) (middle) B87.4
  eye B87.2
  genitourinary B87.81
  intestinal B87.82
  laryngeal B87.3
  nasopharyngeal B87.3
  ocular B87.2
  orbit B87.2
  skin B87.0
  specified site NEC B87.89
  traumatic B87.1
  wound B87.1
Myoadenoma, prostate — *see* Hyperplasia,
    prostate
Myoblastoma
  granular cell — *see also* Neoplasm, connective
      tissue, benign
    malignant — *see* Neoplasm, connective
        tissue, malignant
  tongue D10.1
Myocardial — *see* condition
Myocardiopathy (congestive) (constrictive)
    (familial) (hypertrophic nonobstructive)
    (idiopathic) (infiltrative) (obstructive)
    (primary) (restrictive) (sporadic) (*see also*
    Cardiomyopathy) I42.9
  alcoholic I42.6
  cobalt-beer I42.6
  glycogen storage E74.02 *[I43]*
  hypertrophic obstructive I42.1
  in (due to)
    beriberi E51.12
    cardiac glycogenosis E74.02 *[I43]*
    Friedreich's ataxia G11.1 *[I43]*
    myotonia atrophica G71.11 *[I43]*
    progressive muscular dystrophy G71.0 *[I43]*
  obscure (African) I42.8
  secondary I42.9
  thyrotoxic E05.90 *[I43]*
    with storm E05.91 *[I43]*
  toxic NEC I42.7
Myocarditis (with arteriosclerosis) (chronic)
    (fibroid) (interstitial) (old) (progressive)
    (senile) I51.4
  with
    rheumatic fever (conditions in I00) I09.0
      active — *see* Myocarditis, acute, rheumatic
      inactive or quiescent (with chorea) I09.0
  active I40.9
    rheumatic I01.2
      with chorea (acute) (rheumatic)
          (Sydenham's) I02.0
  acute or subacute (interstitial) I40.9
    due to
      streptococcus (beta-hemolytic) I01.2
    idiopathic I40.1
    rheumatic I01.2
      with chorea (acute) (rheumatic)
          (Sydenham's) I02.0
    specified NEC I40.8
  aseptic of newborn B33.22
  bacterial (acute) I40.0
  Coxsackie (virus) B33.22
  diphtheritic A36.81
  eosinophilic I40.1
  epidemic of newborn (Coxsackie) B33.22
  Fiedler's (acute) (isolated) I40.1
  giant cell (acute) (subacute) I40.1
  gonococcal A54.83
  granulomatous (idiopathic) (isolated)
      (nonspecific) I40.1
  hypertensive — *see* Hypertension, heart
  idiopathic (granulomatous) I40.1

Myocarditis (with arteriosclerosis) (chronic)
    (fibroid) (interstitial) (old) (progressive)
    (senile) I51.4 — *continued*
  in (due to)
    diphtheria A36.81
    epidemic louse-borne typhus A75.0 *[I41]*
    Lyme disease A69.29
    sarcoidosis D86.85
    scarlet fever A38.1
    toxoplasmosis (acquired) B58.81
    typhoid A01.02
    typhus NEC A75.9 *[I41]*
  infective I40.0
  influenzal — *see* Influenza, with, myocarditis
  isolated (acute) I40.1
  meningococcal A39.52
  mumps B26.82
  nonrheumatic, active I40.9
  parenchymatous I40.9
  pneumococcal I40.0
  rheumatic (chronic) (inactive) (with chorea)
      I09.0
    active or acute I01.2
      with chorea (acute) (rheumatic)
          (Sydenham's) I02.0
  rheumatoid — *see* Rheumatoid, carditis
  septic I40.0
  staphylococcal I40.0
  suppurative I40.0
  syphilitic (chronic) A52.06
  toxic I40.8
    rheumatic — *see* Myocarditis, acute,
        rheumatic
  tuberculous A18.84
  typhoid A01.02
  valvular — *see* Endocarditis
  virus, viral I40.0
    of newborn (Coxsackie) B33.22
Myocardium, myocardial — *see* condition
Myocardosis — *see* Cardiomyopathy
Myoclonus, myoclonic, myoclonia (familial)
    (essential) (multifocal) (simplex) G25.3
  drug-induced G25.3
  epilepsy (*see also* Epilepsy, generalized,
      specified NEC) G40.4-
    familial (progressive) G25.3
  epileptica G40.409
    with status epilepticus G40.401
  facial G51.3
  familial progressive G25.3
  Friedreich's G25.3
  jerks G25.3
  massive G25.3
  palatal G25.3
  pharyngeal G25.3
Myocytolysis I51.5
Myodiastasis — *see* Diastasis, muscle
Myoendocarditis — *see* Endocarditis
Myoepithelioma — *see* Neoplasm, benign, by
    site
Myofasciitis (acute) — *see* Myositis
Myofibroma — *see also* Neoplasm, connective
    tissue, benign
  uterus (cervix) (corpus) — *see* Leiomyoma
Myofibromatosis D48.1
  infantile Q89.8
Myofibrosis M62.89
  heart — *see* Myocarditis
  scapulohumeral — *see* Lesion, shoulder,
      specified NEC
Myofibrositis M79.7
  scapulohumeral — *see* Lesion, shoulder,
      specified NEC
Myoglobulinuria, myoglobinuria (primary)
    R82.1
Myokymia, facial G51.4
Myolipoma — *see* Lipoma

Myoma — *see also* Neoplasm, connective tissue,
    benign
  malignant — *see* Neoplasm, connective tissue,
    malignant
  prostate D29.1
  uterus (cervix) (corpus) — *see* Leiomyoma
Myomalacia M62.89
Myometritis — *see* Endometritis
Myometrium — *see* condition
Myonecrosis, clostridial A48.0
Myopathy G72.9
  acute
    necrotizing G72.81
    quadriplegic G72.81
  alcoholic G72.1
  benign congenital G71.2
  central core G71.2
  centronuclear G71.2
  congenital (benign) G71.2
  critical illness G72.81
  distal G71.0
  drug-induced G72.0
  endocrine NEC E34.9 *[G73.7]*
  extraocular muscles H05.82-
  facioscapulohumeral G71.0
  hereditary G71.9
    specified NEC G71.8
  immune NEC G72.49
  in (due to)
    Addison's disease E27.1 *[G73.7]*
    alcohol G72.1
    amyloidosis E85.0 *[G73.7]*
    cretinism E00.9 *[G73.7]*
    Cushing's syndrome E24.9 *[G73.7]*
    drugs G72.0
    endocrine disease NEC E34.9 *[G73.7]*
    giant cell arteritis M31.6 *[G73.7]*
    glycogen storage disease E74.00 *[G73.7]*
    hyperadrenocorticism E24.9 *[G73.7]*
    hyperparathyroidism NEC E21.3 *[G73.7]*
    hypoparathyroidism E20.9 *[G73.7]*
    hypopituitarism E23.0 *[G73.7]*
    hypothyroidism E03.9 *[G73.7]*
    infectious disease NEC B99 *[G73.7]*
    lipid storage disease E75.6 *[G73.7]*
    metabolic disease NEC E88.9 *[G73.7]*
    myxedema E03.9 *[G73.7]*
    parasitic disease NEC B89 *[G73.7]*
    polyarteritis nodosa M30.0 *[G73.7]*
    rheumatoid arthritis — *see* Rheumatoid,
        myopathy
    sarcoidosis D86.87
    scleroderma M34.82
    sicca syndrome M35.03
    Sjögren's syndrome M35.03
    systemic lupus erythematosus M32.19
    thyrotoxicosis (hyperthyroidism) E05.90
        [G73.7]
      with thyroid storm E05.91 *[G73.7]*
    toxic agent NEC G72.2
  inflammatory NEC G72.49
  intensive care (ICU) G72.81
  limb-girdle G71.0
  mitochondrial NEC G71.3
  myotubular G71.2
  mytonic, proximal (PROMM) G71.11
  nemaline G71.2
  ocular G71.0
  oculopharyngeal G71.0
  of critical illness G72.81
  primary G71.9
    specified NEC G71.8
  progressive NEC G72.89
  proximal myotonic (PROMM) G71.11
  rod G71.2
  scapulohumeral G71.0
  specified NEC G72.89
  toxic G72.2

Myopericarditis — *see also* Pericarditis
  chronic rheumatic I09.2
Myopia (axial) (congenital) H52.1-
  degenerative (malignant) H44.2-
  malignant H44.2-
  pernicious H44.2-
  progressive high (degenerative) H44.2-
Myosarcoma — *see* Neoplasm, connective
    tissue, malignant
Myosis (pupil) H57.03
  stromal (endolymphatic) D39.0
Myositis M60.9
  clostridial A48.0
  due to posture — *see* Myositis, specified type
    NEC
  epidemic B33.0
  fibrosa or fibrous (chronic), Volkmann's T79.6
  foreign body granuloma — *see* Granuloma,
      foreign body
  in (due to)
    bilharziasis B65.9 *[M63.8-]*
    cysticercosis B69.81
    leprosy A30.9 *[M63.8-]*
    mycosis B49 *[M63.8-]*
    sarcoidosis D86.87
    schistosomiasis B65.9 *[M63.8-]*
    syphilis
      late A52.78
      secondary A51.49
    toxoplasmosis (acquired) B58.82
    trichinellosis B75 *[M63.8-]*
    tuberculosis A18.09
  inclusion body [IBM] G72.41
  infective M60.009
    arm M60.002
      left M60.001
      right M60.000
    leg M60.005
      left M60.004
      right M60.003
    lower limb M60.005
      ankle M60.07-
      foot M60.07-
      lower leg M60.06-
      thigh M60.05-
      toe M60.07-
    multiple sites M60.09
    specified site NEC M60.08
    upper limb M60.002
      finger M60.04-
      forearm M60.03-
      hand M60.04-
      shoulder region M60.01-
      upper arm M60.02-
  interstitial M60.10
    ankle M60.17-
    foot M60.17-
    forearm M60.13-
    hand M60.14-
    lower leg M60.16-
    multiple sites M60.19
    shoulder region M60.11-
    specified site NEC M60.18
    thigh M60.15-
    upper arm M60.12-
  mycotic B49 *[M63.8-]*
  orbital, chronic H05.12-

Myositis M60.9 — *continued*
  ossificans or ossifying (circumscripta) — *see
    also* Ossification, muscle, specified NEC
    in (due to)
      burns M61.30
        ankle M61.37-
        foot M61.37-
        forearm M61.33-
        hand M61.34-
        lower leg M61.36-
        multiple sites M61.39
        pelvic region M61.35-
        shoulder region M61.31-
        specified site NEC M61.38
        thigh M61.35-
        upper arm M61.32-
      quadriplegia or paraplegia M61.20
        ankle M61.27-
        foot M61.27-
        forearm M61.23-
        hand M61.24-
        lower leg M61.26-
        multiple sites M61.29
        pelvic region M61.25-
        shoulder region M61.21-
        specified site NEC M61.28
        thigh M61.25-
        upper arm M61.22-
    progressiva M61.10
      ankle M61.17-
      finger M61.14-
      foot M61.17-
      forearm M61.13-
      hand M61.14-
      lower leg M61.16-
      multiple sites M61.19
      pelvic region M61.15-
      shoulder region M61.11-
      specified site NEC M61.18
      thigh M61.15-
      toe M61.17-
      upper arm M61.12-
    traumatica M61.00
      ankle M61.07-
      foot M61.07-
      forearm M61.03-
      hand M61.04-
      lower leg M61.06-
      multiple sites M61.09
      pelvic region M61.05-
      shoulder region M61.01-
      specified site NEC M61.08
      thigh M61.05-
      upper arm M61.02-
  purulent — *see* Myositis, infective
  specified type NEC M60.80
    ankle M60.87-
    foot M60.87-
    forearm M60.83-
    hand M60.84-
    lower leg M60.86-
    multiple sites M60.89
    pelvic region M60.85-
    shoulder region M60.81-
    specified site NEC M60.88
    thigh M60.85-
    upper arm M60.82-
  suppurative — *see* Myositis, infective
  traumatic (old) — *see* Myositis, specified type
    NEC

Myospasia impulsiva F95.2
Myotonia (acquisita) (intermittens) M62.89
  atrophica G71.11
  chondrodystrophic G71.13
  congenita (acetazolamide responsive)
    (dominant) (recessive) G71.12
  drug-induced G71.14
  dystrophica G71.11
  fluctuans G71.19
  levior G71.12
  permanens G71.19
  symptomatic G71.19
Myotonic pupil — *see* Anomaly, pupil,
    function, tonic pupil
Myriapodiasis B88.2
Myringitis H73.2-
  with otitis media — *see* Otitis, media
  acute H73.00-
    bullous H73.01-
    specified NEC H73.09-
  bullous — *see* Myringitis, acute, bullous
  chronic H73.1-
Mysophobia F40.228
Mytilotoxism — *see* Poisoning, fish
Myxadenitis labialis K13.0
Myxedema (adult) (idiocy) (infantile) (juvenile)
    (*see also* Hypothyroidism) E03.9
  circumscribed E05.90
    with storm E05.91
  coma E03.5
  congenital E00.1
  cutis L98.5
  localized (pretibial) E05.90
    with storm E05.91
  papular L98.5
Myxochondrosarcoma — *see* Neoplasm,
    cartilage, malignant
Myxofibroma — *see* Neoplasm, connective
    tissue, benign
  odontogenic — *see* Cyst, calcifying
    odontogenic
Myxofibrosarcoma — *see* Neoplasm,
    connective tissue, malignant
Myxolipoma D17.9
Myxoliposarcoma — *see* Neoplasm,
    connective tissue, malignant
Myxoma — *see also* Neoplasm, connective
    tissue, benign
  nerve sheath — *see* Neoplasm, nerve, benign
  odontogenic — *see* Cyst, calcifying
    odontogenic
Myxosarcoma — *see* Neoplasm, connective
    tissue, malignant

N

Naegeli's
  disease Q82.8
  leukemia, monocytic C93.1-
Naegleriasis (with meningoencephalitis)
    B60.2
Naffziger's syndrome G54.0
Naga sore — *see* Ulcer, skin
Nägele's pelvis M95.5
  with disproportion (fetopelvic) O33.0
    causing obstructed labor O65.0
Nail — *see also* condition
  biting F98.8
  patella syndrome Q87.2
Nanism, nanosomia — *see* Dwarfism
Nanophyetiasis B66.8
Nanukayami A27.89
Napkin rash L22
Narcolepsy G47.419
  with cataplexy G47.411
  in conditions classified elsewhere G47.429
    with cataplexy G47.421
Narcosis R06.89
Narcotism — *see* Dependence
NARP (neuropathy, ataxia and retinitis
    pigmentosa) syndrome E88.49
Narrow
  anterior chamber angle H40.03-
  gingival width (of periodontal soft tissue)
      K05.5
  pelvis — *see* Contraction, pelvis
Narrowing — *see also* Stenosis
  artery I77.1
    auditory, internal I65.8
    basilar — *see* Occlusion, artery, basilar
    carotid — *see* Occlusion, artery, carotid
    cerebellar — *see* Occlusion, artery,
        cerebellar
    cerebral — *see* Occlusion artery, cerebral
    choroidal — *see* Occlusion, artery, cerebral,
        specified NEC
    communicating posterior — *see* Occlusion,
        artery, cerebral, specified NEC
    coronary — *see also* Disease, heart,
        ischemic, atherosclerotic
      congenital Q24.5
      syphilitic A50.54 [I52]
      due to syphilis NEC A52.06
    hypophyseal — *see* Occlusion, artery,
        cerebral, specified NEC
    pontine — *see* Occlusion, artery, cerebral,
        specified NEC
    precerebral — *see* Occlusion, artery,
        precerebral
    vertebral — *see* Occlusion, artery, vertebral
  auditory canal (external) — *see* Stenosis,
      external ear canal
  eustachian tube — *see* Obstruction, eustachian
      tube
  eyelid — *see* Disorder, eyelid function
  larynx J38.6
  mesenteric artery (*see also* Ischemia, intestine,
      acute) K55.059
  palate M26.89
  palpebral fissure — *see* Disorder, eyelid
      function
  ureter N13.5
    with infection N13.6
  urethra — *see* Stricture, urethra
Narrowness, abnormal, eyelid Q10.3
Nasal — *see* condition
Nasolachrymal, nasolacrimal — *see*
    condition
Nasopharyngeal — *see also* condition
  pituitary gland Q89.2
  torticollis M43.6

Nasopharyngitis (acute) (infective)
    (streptococcal) (subacute) J00
  chronic (suppurative) (ulcerative) J31.1
Nasopharynx, nasopharyngeal — *see*
    condition
Natal tooth, teeth K00.6
Nausea (without vomiting) R11.0
  with vomiting R11.2
  gravidarum — *see* Hyperemesis, gravidarum
  marina T75.3
  navalis T75.3
Navel — *see* condition
Neapolitan fever — *see* Brucellosis
Near drowning T75.1
Near-syncope R55
Nearsightedness — *see* Myopia
Nebula, cornea — *see* Opacity, cornea
Necator americanus infestation B76.1
Necatoriasis B76.1
Neck — *see* condition
Necrobiosis R68.89
  lipoidica NEC L92.1
  with diabetes — *see* E08-E13 with .620
Necrolysis, toxic epidermal L51.2
  due to drug
    correct substance properly administered —
        see Table of Drugs and Chemicals, by
        drug, adverse effect
    overdose or wrong substance given or taken
        — *see* Table of Drugs and Chemicals, by
        drug, poisoning
Necrophilia F65.89
Necrosis, necrotic (ischemic) — *see also*
    Gangrene
  adrenal (capsule) (gland) E27.49
  amputation stump (surgical) (late) T87.50
    arm T87.5-
    leg T87.5-
  antrum J32.0
  aorta (hyaline) — *see also* Aneurysm, aorta
    cystic medial — *see* Dissection, aorta
  artery I77.5
  bladder (aseptic) (sphincter) N32.89
  bone (*see also* Osteonecrosis) M87.9
    aseptic or avascular — *see* Osteonecrosis
      idiopathic M87.00
    ethmoid J32.2
    jaw M27.2
    tuberculous — *see* Tuberculosis, bone
  brain I67.89
  breast (aseptic) (fat) (segmental) N64.1
  bronchus J98.09
  central nervous system NEC I67.89
  cerebellar I67.89
  cerebral I67.89
  colon (*see also* Infarct, intestine) K55.049
  cornea H18.89-
  cortical (acute) (renal) N17.1
  cystic medial (aorta) — *see* Dissection, aorta
  dental pulp K04.1
  esophagus K22.8
  ethmoid (bone) J32.2
  eyelid — *see* Disorder, eyelid, degenerative
  fat, fatty (generalized) — *see also* Disorder, soft
      tissue, specified type NEC
    abdominal wall K65.4
    breast (aseptic) (segmental) N64.1
    localized — *see* Degeneration, by site, fatty
    mesentery K65.4
    omentum K65.4
    pancreas K86.89
    peritoneum K65.4
    skin (subcutaneous), newborn P83.0
    subcutaneous, due to birth injury P15.6
  gallbladder — *see* Cholecystitis, acute
  heart — *see* Infarct, myocardium
  hip, aseptic or avascular — *see* Osteonecrosis,
      by type, femur

Necrosis, necrotic (ischemic) — *see also*
    Gangrene — *continued*
  intestine (acute) (hemorrhagic) (massive) (*see*
      also Infarct, intestine) K55.069
  jaw M27.2
  kidney (bilateral) N28.0
    acute N17.9
    cortical (acute) (bilateral) N17.1
      with ectopic or molar pregnancy O08.4
    medullary (bilateral) (in acute renal failure)
        (papillary) N17.2
    papillary (bilateral) (in acute renal failure)
        N17.2
    tubular N17.0
      with ectopic or molar pregnancy O08.4
      complicating
        abortion — *see* Abortion, by type,
            complicated by, tubular necrosis
        ectopic or molar pregnancy O08.4
        pregnancy — *see* Pregnancy,
            complicated by, diseases of,
            specified type or system NEC
      following ectopic or molar pregnancy
          O08.4
      traumatic T79.5
  larynx J38.7
  liver (with hepatic failure) (cell) — *see* Failure,
      hepatic
    hemorrhagic, central K76.2
  lung J85.0
  lymphatic gland — *see* Lymphadenitis, acute
  mammary gland (fat) (segmental) N64.1
  mastoid (chronic) — *see* Mastoiditis, chronic
  medullary (acute) (renal) N17.2
  mesentery (*see also* Infarct, intestine) K55.069
    fat K65.4
  mitral valve — *see* Insufficiency, mitral
  myocardium, myocardial — *see* Infarct,
      myocardium
  nose J34.0
  omentum (with mesenteric infarction) (*see also*
      Infarct, intestine) K55.069
    fat K65.4
  orbit, orbital — *see* Osteomyelitis, orbit
  ossicles, ear — *see* Abnormal, ear ossicles
  ovary N70.92
  pancreas (aseptic) (duct) (fat) K86.89
    acute (infective) — *see* Pancreatitis, acute
    infective — *see* Pancreatitis, acute
  papillary (acute) (renal) N17.2
  perineum N90.89
  peritoneum (with mesenteric infarction) (*see also*
      Infarct, intestine) K55.069
    fat K65.4
  pharynx J02.9
    in granulocytopenia — *see* Neutropenia
      Vincent's A69.1
  phosphorus — *see* subcategory T54.2
  pituitary (gland) E23.0
    postpartum O99.285
    Sheehan O99.285
  pressure — *see* Ulcer, pressure, by site
  pulmonary J85.0
  pulp (dental) K04.1
  radiation — *see* Necrosis, by site
  radium — *see* Necrosis, by site
  renal — *see* Necrosis, kidney
  sclera H15.89
  scrotum N50.89
  skin or subcutaneous tissue NEC I96
  spine, spinal (column) — *see also*
      Osteonecrosis, by type, vertebra
    cord G95.19
  spleen D73.5
  stomach K31.89
  stomatitis (ulcerative) A69.0
  subcutaneous fat, newborn P83.8
  subendocardial (acute) I21.4
    chronic I25.89

Necrosis, necrotic (ischemic) — *see also*
  Gangrene — *continued*
  suprarenal (capsule) (gland) E27.49
  testis N50.89
  thymus (gland) E32.8
  tonsil J35.8
  trachea J39.8
  tuberculous NEC — *see* Tuberculosis
  tubular (acute) (anoxic) (renal) (toxic) N17.0
    postprocedural N99.0
  vagina N89.8
  vertebra — *see also* Osteonecrosis, by type,
    vertebra
    tuberculous A18.01
  vulva N90.89
  X-ray — *see* Necrosis, by site
Necrospermia — *see* Infertility, male
Need (for)
  care provider because (of)
    assistance with personal care Z74.1
    continuous supervision required Z74.3
    impaired mobility Z74.09
    no other household member able to render
      care Z74.2
    specified reason NEC Z74.8
  immunization — *see* Vaccination
  vaccination — *see* Vaccination
Neglect
  adult
    confirmed T74.01
    history of Z91.412
    suspected T76.01
  child (childhood)
    confirmed T74.02
    history of Z62.812
    suspected T76.02
  emotional, in childhood Z62.898
  hemispatial R41.4
  left-sided R41.4
  sensory R41.4
  visuospatial R41.4
Neisserian infection NEC — *see* Gonococcus
Nelaton's syndrome G60.8
Nelson's syndrome E24.1
Nematodiasis (intestinal) B82.0
  Ancylostoma B76.0
Neonatal — *see also* Newborn
  acne L70.4
  bradycardia P29.12
  screening, abnormal findings on P09
  tachycardia P29.11
  tooth, teeth K00.6
Neonatorum — *see* condition
Neoplasia
  endocrine, multiple (MEN) E31.20
    type I E31.21
    type IIA E31.22
    type IIB E31.23
  intraepithelial (histologically confirmed)
    anal (AIN) (histologically confirmed) K62.82
      grade I K62.82
      grade II K62.82
      severe D01.3
    cervical glandular (histologically confirmed)
      D06.9
    cervix (uteri) (CIN) (histologically confirmed)
      N87.9
      glandular D06.9
      grade I N87.0
      grade II N87.1
      grade III (severe dysplasia) (*see also*
        Carcinoma, cervix uteri, in situ) D06.9
    prostate (histologically confirmed) (PIN)
      N42.31
      grade I N42.31
      grade II N42.31
      grade III (severe dysplasia) D07.5

Neoplasia — *continued*
  intraepithelial (histologically confirmed) —
    continued
    vagina (histologically confirmed) (VAIN)
      N89.3
      grade I N89.0
      grade II N89.1
      grade III (severe dysplasia) D07.2
    vulva (histologically confirmed) (VIN) N90.3
      grade I N90.0
      grade II N90.1
      grade III (severe dysplasia) D07.1
Neoplasm, neoplastic — *see also* Table of
  Neoplasms
  lipomatous, benign — *see* Lipoma

NEOPLASM TABLE

ICD-10-CM Table of Neoplasms

The list below gives the code numbers for neoplasms by anatomical site. For each site there are six possible code numbers according to whether the neoplasm in question is malignant, benign, in situ, of uncertain behavior, or of unspecified nature. The description of the neoplasm will often indicate which of the six columns is appropriate; e.g., malignant melanoma of skin, benign fibroadenoma of breast, carcinoma in situ of cervix uteri.

Where such descriptors are not present, the remainder of the Index should be consulted where guidance is given to the appropriate column for each morphological (histological) variety listed; e.g., Mesonephroma — see Neoplasm, malignant; Embryoma — see also Neoplasm, uncertain behavior; Disease, Bowen's — see Neoplasm, skin, in situ. However, the guidance in the Index can be overridden if one of the descriptors mentioned above is present; e.g., malignant adenoma of colon is coded to C18.9 and not to D12.6 as the adjective "malignant" overrides the Index entry "Adenoma — see also Neoplasm, benign."

Codes listed with a dash -, following the code have a required additional character for laterality. The tabular list must be reviewed for the complete code.

Neoplasm Table	Malignant Primary	Malignant Secondary	Ca In situ	Benign	Uncertain Behavior	Unspecified Behavior
Neoplasm, neoplastic	C80.1	C79.9	D09.9	D36.9	D48.9	D49.9
abdomen, abdominal	C76.2	C79.8-	D09.8	D36.7	D48.7	D49.89
cavity	C76.2	C79.8-	D09.8	D36.7	D48.7	D49.89
organ	C76.2	C79.8-	D09.8	D36.7	D48.7	D49.89
viscera	C76.2	C79.8-	D09.8	D36.7	D48.7	D49.89
wall — see also Neoplasm,						
abdomen, wall, skin	C44.509	C79.2-	D04.5	D23.5	D48.5	D49.2
connective tissue	C49.4	C79.8-	—	D21.4	D48.1	D49.2
skin	C44.509	—	—	—	—	—
basal cell carcinoma	C44.519	—	—	—	—	—
specified type NEC	C44.599	—	—	—	—	—
squamous cell						
carcinoma	C44.529	—	—	—	—	—
abdominopelvic	C76.8	C79.8-	—	D36.7	D48.7	D49.89
accessory sinus — see						
Neoplasm, sinus						
acoustic nerve	C72.4-	C79.49	—	D33.3	D43.3	D49.7
adenoid (pharynx) (tissue)	C11.1	C79.89	D00.08	D10.6	D37.05	D49.0
adipose tissue — see also						
Neoplasm, connective						
tissue	C49.4	C79.89	—	D21.9	D48.1	D49.2
adnexa (uterine)	C57.4	C79.89	D07.39	D28.7	D39.8	D49.59
adrenal	C74.9-	C79.7-	D09.3	D35.0-	D44.1-	D49.7
capsule	C74.9-	C79.7-	D09.3	D35.0-	D44.1-	D49.7
cortex	C74.0-	C79.7-	D09.3	D35.0-	D44.1-	D49.7
gland	C74.9-	C79.7-	D09.3	D35.0-	D44.1-	D49.7
medulla	C74.1-	C79.7-	D09.3	D35.0-	D44.1-	D49.7
ala nasi (external) — see also						
Neoplasm, skin, nose	C44.301	C79.2	D04.39	D23.39	D48.5	D49.2
alimentary canal or tract NEC	C26.9	C78.80	D01.9	D13.9	D37.9	D49.0
alveolar	C03.9	C79.89	D00.03	D10.39	D37.09	D49.0
mucosa	C03.9	C79.89	D00.03	D10.39	D37.09	D49.0
lower	C03.1	C79.89	D00.03	D10.39	D37.09	D49.0
upper	C03.0	C79.89	D00.03	D10.39	D37.09	D49.0

Neoplasm Table	Malignant Primary	Malignant Secondary	Ca In situ	Benign	Uncertain Behavior	Unspecified Behavior
Neoplasm, neoplastic - continued						
alveolar - continued	C03.9	C79.89	D00.03	D10.39	D37.09	D49.0
ridge or process	C41.1	C79.51	—	D16.5-	D48.0	D49.2
carcinoma	C03.9	C79.8-	—	—	—	—
lower	C03.1	C79.8-	—	—	—	—
upper	C03.0	C79.8-	—	—	—	—
lower	C41.1	C79.51	—	D16.5-	D48.0	D49.2
mucosa	C03.9	C79.89	D00.03	D10.39	D37.09	D49.0
lower	C03.1	C79.89	D00.03	D10.39	D37.09	D49.0
upper	C03.0	C79.89	D00.03	D10.39	D37.09	D49.0
upper	C41.0	C79.51	—	D16.4-	D48.0	D49.2
sulcus	C06.1	C79.89	D00.02	D10.39	D37.09	D49.0
alveolus	C03.9	C79.89	D00.03	D10.39	D37.09	D49.0
lower	C03.1	C79.89	D00.03	D10.39	D37.09	D49.0
upper	C03.0	C79.89	D00.03	D10.39	D37.09	D49.0
ampulla of Vater	C24.1	C78.89	D01.5	D13.5	D37.6	D49.0
ankle NEC	C76.5-	C79.89	D04.7-	D36.7	D48.7	D49.89
anorectum, anorectal						
(junction)	C21.8	C78.5	D01.3	D12.9	D37.8	D49.0
antecubital fossa or space	C76.4-	C79.89	D04.6-	D36.7	D48.7	D49.89
antrum (Highmore)						
(maxillary)	C31.0	C78.39	D02.3	D14.0	D38.5	D49.1
pyloric	C16.3	C78.89	D00.2	D13.1	D37.1	D49.0
tympanicum	C30.1	C78.39	D02.3	D14.0	D38.5	D49.1
anus, anal	C21.0	C78.5	D01.3	D12.9	D37.8	D49.0
canal	C21.1	C78.5	D01.3	D12.9	D37.8	D49.0
cloacogenic zone	C21.2	C78.5	D01.3	D12.9	D37.8	D49.0
margin — see also						
Neoplasm, anus, skin	C44.500	C79.2	D04.5	D23.5	D48.5	D49.2
overlapping lesion with						
rectosigmoid junction						
or rectum	C21.8	—	—	—	—	—
skin	C44.500	C79.2	D04.5	D23.5	D48.5	D49.2
basal cell carcinoma	C44.510	—	—	—	—	—
specified type NEC	C44.590	—	—	—	—	—
squamous cell						
carcinoma	C44.520	—	—	—	—	—
sphincter	C21.1	C78.5	D01.3	D12.9	D37.8	D49.0
aorta (thoracic)	C49.3	C79.89	—	D21.3	D48.1	D49.2
abdominal	C49.4	C79.89	—	D21.4	D48.1	D49.2
aortic body	C75.5	C79.89	—	D35.6	D44.7	D49.7
aponeurosis	C49.9	C79.89	—	D21.9	D48.1	D49.2
palmar	C49.1-	C79.89	—	D21.1-	D48.1	D49.2
plantar	C49.2-	C79.89	—	D21.2-	D48.1	D49.2
appendix	C18.1	C78.5	D01.0	D12.1	D37.3	D49.0
arachnoid	C70.9	C79.49	—	D32.9	D42.9	D49.7
cerebral	C70.0	C79.32	—	D32.0	D42.0	D49.7
spinal	C70.1	C79.49	—	D32.1	D42.1	D49.7
areola	C50.0-	C79.81	D05.-	D24.-	D48.6-	D49.3
arm NEC	C76.4-	C79.89	D04.6-	D36.7	D48.7	D49.89
artery — see Neoplasm,						
connective tissue						
aryepiglottic fold	C13.1	C79.89	D00.08	D10.7	D37.05	D49.0
hypopharyngeal aspect	C13.1	C79.89	D00.08	D10.7	D37.05	D49.0
laryngeal aspect	C32.1	C78.39	D02.0	D14.1	D38.0	D49.1
marginal zone	C13.1	C79.89	D00.08	D10.7	D37.05	D49.0
arytenoid (cartilage)	C32.3	C78.39	D02.0	D14.1	D38.0	D49.1
fold — see Neoplasm,						
aryepiglottic						
associated with transplanted						
organ	C80.2	—	—	—	—	—
atlas	C41.2	C79.51	—	D16.6	D48.0	D49.2
atrium, cardiac	C38.0	C79.89	—	D15.1	D48.7	D49.89

NEOPLASM TABLE

Neoplasm Table	Malignant Primary	Malignant Secondary	Ca In situ	Benign	Uncertain Behavior	Unspecified Behavior
Neoplasm, neoplastic - *continued*						
auditory						
canal (external) (skin)	C44.20-	C79.2	D04.2-	D23.2-	D48.5	D49.2
internal	C30.1	C78.39	D02.3	D14.0	D38.5	D49.1
nerve	C72.4-	C79.49	—	D33.3	D43.3	D49.7
tube	C30.1	C78.39	D02.3	D14.0	D38.5	D49.1
opening	C11.2	C79.89	D00.08	D10.6	D37.05	D49.0
auricle, ear — *see also*						
Neoplasm, skin, ear	C44.20-	C79.2	D04.2-	D23.2-	D48.5	D49.2
auricular canal (external) —						
see also Neoplasm, skin,						
ear	C44.20-	C79.2	D04.2-	D23.2-	D48.5	D49.2
internal	C30.1	C78.39	D02.3	D14.0	D38.5	D49.2
autonomic nerve or nervous						
system NEC (*see*						
Neoplasm, nerve,						
peripheral)						
axilla, axillary	C76.1	C79.89	D09.8	D36.7	D48.7	D49.89
fold — *see also*						
Neoplasm, skin, trunk	C44.509	C79.2	D04.5	D23.5	D48.5	D49.2
back NEC	C76.8	C79.89	D04.5	D36.7	D48.7	D49.89
Bartholin's gland	C51.0	C79.82	D07.1	D28.0	D39.8	D49.59
basal ganglia	C71.0	C79.31	—	D33.0	D43.0	D49.6
basis pedunculi	C71.7	C79.31	—	D33.1	D43.1	D49.6
bile or biliary (tract)	C24.9	C78.89	D01.5	D13.5	D37.6	D49.0
canaliculi (biliferi)						
(intrahepatic)	C22.1	C78.7	D01.5	D13.4	D37.6	D49.0
canals, interlobular	C22.1	C78.89	D01.5	D13.4	D37.6	D49.0
duct or passage (common)						
(cystic) (extrahepatic)	C24.0	C78.89	D01.5	D13.5	D37.6	D49.0
interlobular	C22.1	C78.89	D01.5	D13.4	D37.6	D49.0
intrahepatic	C22.1	C78.7	D01.5	D13.4	D37.6	D49.0
and extrahepatic	C24.8	C78.89	D01.5	D13.5	D37.6	D49.0
bladder (urinary)	C67.9	C79.11	D09.0	D30.3	D41.4	D49.4
dome	C67.1	C79.11	D09.0	D30.3	D41.4	D49.4
neck	C67.5	C79.11	D09.0	D30.3	D41.4	D49.4
orifice	C67.9	C79.11	D09.0	D30.3	D41.4	D49.4
ureteric	C67.6	C79.11	D09.0	D30.3	D41.4	D49.4
urethral	C67.5	C79.11	D09.0	D30.3	D41.4	D49.4
overlapping lesion	C67.8	—	—	—	—	—
sphincter	C67.8	C79.11	D09.0	D30.3	D41.4	D49.4
trigone	C67.0	C79.11	D09.0	D30.3	D41.4	D49.4
urachus	C67.7	C79.11	D09.0	D30.3	D41.4	D49.4
wall	C67.9	C79.11	D09.0	D30.3	D41.4	D49.4
anterior	C67.3	C79.11	D09.0	D30.3	D41.4	D49.4
lateral	C67.2	C79.11	D09.0	D30.3	D41.4	D49.4
posterior	C67.4	C79.11	D09.0	D30.3	D41.4	D49.4
blood vessel — *see* Neoplasm,						
connective tissue						
bone (periosteum)	C41.9	C79.51	—	D16.9-	D48.0	D49.2
acetabulum	C41.4	C79.51	—	D16.8-	D48.0	D49.2
ankle	C40.3-	C79.51	—	D16.3-	—	—
arm NEC	C40.0-	C79.51	—	D16.0-	—	—
astragalus	C40.3-	C79.51	—	D16.3-	—	—
atlas	C41.2	C79.51	—	D16.6-	D48.0	D49.2
axis	C41.2	C79.51	—	D16.6-	D48.0	D49.2
back NEC	C41.2	C79.51	—	D16.6-	D48.0	D49.2
calcaneus	C40.3-	C79.51	—	D16.3-	—	—
calvarium	C41.0	C79.51	—	D16.4-	D48.0	D49.2
carpus (any)	C40.1-	C79.51	—	D16.1-	—	—
cartilage NEC	C41.9	C79.51	—	D16.9-	D48.0	D49.2
clavicle	C41.3	C79.51	—	D16.7-	D48.0	D49.2
clivus	C41.0	C79.51	—	D16.4-	D48.0	D49.2
coccygeal vertebra	C41.4	C79.51	—	D16.8-	D48.0	D49.2

Neoplasm Table	Malignant Primary	Malignant Secondary	Ca In situ	Benign	Uncertain Behavior	Unspecified Behavior
Neoplasm, neoplastic - *continued*						
bone (periosteum) - *continued*	C41.9	C79.51	—	D16.9-	D48.0	D49.2
coccyx	C41.4	C79.51	—	D16.8-	D48.0	D49.2
costal cartilage	C41.3	C79.51	—	D16.7-	D48.0	D49.2
costovertebral joint	C41.3	C79.51	—	D16.7-	D48.0	D49.2
cranial	C41.0	C79.51	—	D16.4-	D48.0	D49.2
cuboid	C40.3-	C79.51	—	D16.3-	—	—
cuneiform	C41.9	C79.51	—	D16.9-	D48.0	D49.2
elbow	C40.0-	C79.51	—	D16.0-	—	—
ethmoid (labyrinth)	C41.0	C79.51	—	D16.4-	D48.0	D49.2
face	C41.0	C79.51	—	D16.4-	D48.0	D49.2
femur (any part)	C40.2-	C79.51	—	D16.2-	—	—
fibula (any part)	C40.2-	C79.51	—	D16.2-	—	—
finger (any)	C40.1-	C79.51	—	D16.1-	—	—
foot	C40.3-	C79.51	—	D16.3-	—	—
forearm	C40.0-	C79.51	—	D16.0-	—	—
frontal	C41.0	C79.51	—	D16.4-	D48.0	D49.2
hand	C40.1-	C79.51	—	D16.1-	—	—
heel	C40.3-	C79.51	—	D16.3-	—	—
hip	C41.4	C79.51	—	D16.8-	D48.0	D49.2
humerus (any part)	C40.0-	C79.51	—	D16.0-	—	—
hyoid	C41.0	C79.51	—	D16.4-	D48.0	D49.2
ilium	C41.4	C79.51	—	D16.8-	D48.0	D49.2
innominate	C41.4	C79.51	—	D16.8-	D48.0	D49.2
intervertebral cartilage or						
disc	C41.2	C79.51	—	D16.6-	D48.0	D49.2
ischium	C41.4	C79.51	—	D16.8-	D48.0	D49.2
jaw (lower)	C41.1	C79.51	—	D16.5-	D48.0	D49.2
knee	C40.2-	C79.51	—	D16.2-	—	—
leg NEC	C40.2-	C79.51	—	D16.2-	—	—
limb NEC	C40.9-	C79.51	—	D16.9-	—	—
lower (long bones)	C40.2-	C79.51	—	D16.2-	—	—
short bones	C40.3-	C79.51	—	D16.3-	—	—
upper (long bones)	C40.0-	C79.51	—	D16.0-	—	—
short bones	C40.1-	C79.51	—	D16.1-	—	—
malar	C41.0	C79.51	—	D16.4-	D48.0	D49.2
mandible	C41.1	C79.51	—	D16.5-	D48.0	D49.2
marrow NEC (any bone)	C96.9	C79.52	—	—	D47.9	D49.89
mastoid	C41.0	C79.51	—	D16.4-	D48.0	D49.2
maxilla, maxillary						
(superior)	C41.0	C79.51	—	D16.4-	D48.0	D49.2
inferior	C41.1	C79.51	—	D16.5-	D48.0	D49.2
metacarpus (any)	C40.1-	C79.51	—	D16.1-	—	—
metatarsus (any)	C40.3-	C79.51	—	D16.3-	—	—
overlapping sites	C40.8-	—	—	—	—	—
navicular						
ankle	C40.3-	C79.51	—	—	—	—
hand	C40.1-	C79.51	—	—	—	—
nose, nasal	C41.0	C79.51	—	D16.4-	D48.0	D49.2
occipital	C41.0	C79.51	—	D16.4-	D48.0	D49.2
orbit	C41.0	C79.51	—	D16.4-	D48.0	D49.2
parietal	C41.0	C79.51	—	D16.4-	D48.0	D49.2
patella	C40.2-	C79.51	—	D16.2-	—	—
pelvic	C41.4	C79.51	—	D16.8	D48.0	D49.2
phalanges						
foot	C40.3-	C79.51	—	—	—	—
hand	C40.1-	C79.51	—	—	—	—
pubic	C41.4	C79.51	—	D16.8	D48.0	D49.2
radius (any part)	C40.0-	C79.51	—	D16.0-	—	—
rib	C41.3	C79.51	—	D16.7	D48.0	D49.2
sacral vertebra	C41.4	C79.51	—	D16.8	D48.0	D49.2
sacrum	C41.4	C79.51	—	D16.8	D48.0	D49.2

NEOPLASM TABLE

Neoplasm Table	Malignant Primary	Malignant Secondary	Ca In situ	Benign	Uncertain Behavior	Unspecified Behavior
Neoplasm, neoplastic - continued						
bone (periosteum) - continued	C41.9	C79.51	—	D16.9-	D48.0	D49.2
scaphoid	—	—				
of ankle	C40.3-	C79.51	—	—	—	—
of hand	C40.1-	C79.51	—	—	—	—
scapula (any part)	C40.0-	C79.51	—	D16.0-	—	—
sella turcica	C41.0	C79.51	—	D16.4-	D48.0	D49.2
shoulder	C40.0-	C79.51	—	D16.0-	—	—
skull	C41.0	C79.51	—	D16.4-	D48.0	D49.2
sphenoid	C41.0	C79.51	—	D16.4-	D48.0	D49.2
spine, spinal (column)	C41.2	C79.51	—	D16.6	D48.0	D49.2
coccyx	C41.4	C79.51	—	D16.8	D48.0	D49.2
sacrum	C41.4	C79.51	—	D16.8	D48.0	D49.2
sternum	C41.3	C79.51	—	D16.7	D48.0	D49.2
tarsus (any)	C40.3-	C79.51	—	—	—	—
temporal	C41.0	C79.51	—	D16.4-	D48.0	D49.2
thumb	C40.1-	C79.51	—	—	—	—
tibia (any part)	C40.2-	C79.51	—	—	—	—
toe (any)	C40.3-	C79.51	—	—	—	—
trapezium	C40.1-	C79.51	—	—	—	—
trapezoid	C40.1-	C79.51	—	—	—	—
turbinate	C41.0	C79.51	—	D16.4-	D48.0	D49.2
ulna (any part)	C40.0-	C79.51	—	D16.0-	—	—
unciform	C40.1-	C79.51	—	—	—	—
vertebra (column)	C41.2	C79.51	—	D16.6	D48.0	D49.2
coccyx	C41.4	C79.51	—	D16.8	D48.0	D49.2
sacrum	C41.4	C79.51	—	D16.8	D48.0	D49.2
vomer	C41.0	C79.51	—	D16.4-	D48.0	D49.2
wrist	C40.1-	C79.51	—	—	—	—
xiphoid process	C41.3	C79.51	—	D16.7	D48.0	D49.2
zygomatic	C41.0	C79.51	—	D16.4-	D48.0	D49.2
book-leaf (mouth) [ventral surface of tongue and floor of mouth]	C06.89	C79.89	D00.00	D10.39	D37.09	D49.0
bowel — see Neoplasm, intestine						
brachial plexus	C47.1-	C79.89	—	D36.12	D48.2	D49.2
brain NEC	C71.9	C79.31	—	D33.2	D43.2	D49.6
basal ganglia	C71.0	C79.31	—	D33.0	D43.0	D49.6
cerebellopontine angle	C71.6	C79.31	—	D33.1	D43.1	D49.6
cerebellum NOS	C71.6	C79.31	—	D33.1	D43.1	D49.6
cerebrum	C71.0	C79.31	—	D33.0	D43.0	D49.6
choroid plexus	C71.7	C79.31	—	D33.1	D43.1	D49.6
corpus callosum	C71.8	C79.31	—	D33.2	D43.2	D49.6
corpus striatum	C71.0	C79.31	—	D33.0	D43.0	D49.6
cortex (cerebral)	C71.0	C79.31	—	D33.0	D43.0	D49.6
frontal lobe	C71.1	C79.31	—	D33.0	D43.0	D49.6
globus pallidus	C71.0	C79.31	—	D33.0	D43.0	D49.6
hippocampus	C71.2	C79.31	—	D33.0	D43.0	D49.6
hypothalamus	C71.0	C79.31	—	D33.0	D43.0	D49.6
internal capsule	C71.0	C79.31	—	D33.0	D43.0	D49.6
medulla oblongata	C71.7	C79.31	—	D33.1	D43.1	D49.6
meninges	C70.0	C79.32	—	D32.0	D42.0	D49.7
midbrain	C71.7	C79.31	—	D33.1	D43.1	D49.6
occipital lobe	C71.4	C79.31	—	D33.0	D43.0	D49.6
overlapping lesion	C71.8	C79.31	—	—	—	—
parietal lobe	C71.3	C79.31	—	D33.0	D43.0	D49.6
peduncle	C71.7	C79.31	—	D33.1	D43.1	D49.6
pons	C71.7	C79.31	—	D33.1	D43.1	D49.6
stem	C71.7	C79.31	—	D33.1	D43.1	D49.6
tapetum	C71.8	C79.31	—	D33.2	D43.2	D49.6
temporal lobe	C71.0	C79.31	—	D33.0	D43.0	D49.6
thalamus	C71.0	C79.31	—	D33.0	D43.0	D49.6
uncus	C71.2	C79.31	—	D33.0	D43.0	D49.6
Neoplasm, neoplastic - continued						
brain NEC - continued	C71.9	C79.31	—	D33.2	D43.2	D49.6
ventricle (floor)	C71.5	C79.31	—	D33.0	D43.0	D49.6
fourth	C71.7	C79.31	—	D33.1	D43.1	D49.6
branchial (cleft) (cyst) (vestiges)	C10.4	C79.89	D00.08	D10.5	D37.05	D49.0
breast (connective tissue) (glandular tissue) (soft parts)	C50.9-	C79.81	D05.-	D24.-	D48.6-	D49.3
areola	C50.0-	C79.81	D05.-	D24.-	D48.6-	D49.3
axillary tail	C50.6-	C79.81	D05.-	D24.-	D48.6-	D49.3
central portion	C50.1-	C79.81	D05.-	D24.-	D48.6-	D49.3
inner	C50.8-	C79.81	D05.-	D24.-	D48.6-	D49.3
lower	C50.8-	C79.81	D05.-	D24.-	D48.6-	D49.3
lower-inner quadrant	C50.3-	C79.81	D05.-	D24.-	D48.6-	D49.3
lower-outer quadrant	C50.5-	C79.81	D05.-	D24.-	D48.6-	D49.3
mastectomy site (skin) — see also Neoplasm, breast, skin	C44.501	C79.2	—	—	—	—
specified as breast tissue	C50.8-	C79.81	—	—	—	—
midline	C50.8-	C79.81	D05.-	D24.-	D48.6-	D49.3
nipple	C50.0-	C79.81	D05.-	D24.-	D48.6-	D49.3
outer	C50.8-	C79.81	D05.-	D24.-	D48.6-	D49.3
overlapping lesion	C50.8-	—	—	—	—	—
skin	C44.501	C79.2	D04.5	D23.5	D48.5	D49.2
basal cell carcinoma	C44.511	—	—	—	—	—
specified type NEC	C44.591	—	—	—	—	—
squamous cell carcinoma	C44.521	—	—	—	—	—
tail (axillary)	C50.6-	C79.81	D05.-	D24.-	D48.6-	D49.3
upper	C50.8-	C79.81	D05.-	D24.-	D48.6-	D49.3
upper-inner quadrant	C50.2-	C79.81	D05.-	D24.-	D48.6-	D49.3
upper-outer quadrant	C50.4-	C79.81	D05.-	D24.-	D48.6-	D49.3
broad ligament	C57.1	C79.82	D07.39	D28.2	D39.8	D49.59
bronchiogenic, bronchogenic (lung)	C34.9-	C78.0-	D02.2-	D14.3-	D38.1	D49.1
bronchiole	C34.9-	C78.0-	D02.2-	D14.3-	D38.1	D49.1
bronchus	C34.9-	C78.0-	D02.2-	D14.3-	D38.1	D49.1
carina	C34.0-	C78.0-	D02.2-	D14.3-	D38.1	D49.1
lower lobe of lung	C34.3-	C78.0-	D02.2-	D14.3-	D38.1	D49.1
main	C34.0-	C78.0-	D02.2-	D14.3-	D38.1	D49.1
middle lobe of lung	C34.2	C78.0-	D02.21	D14.31	D38.1	D49.1
overlapping lesion	C34.8-					
upper lobe of lung	C34.1-	C78.0-	D02.2-	D14.3-	D38.1	D49.1
brow	C44.309	C79.2	D04.39	D23.39	D48.5	D49.2
basal cell carcinoma	C44.319	—				
specified type NEC	C44.399	—				
squamous cell carcinoma	C44.329					
buccal (cavity)	C06.9	C79.89	D00.00	D10.39	D37.09	D49.0
commissure	C06.0	C79.89	D00.02	D10.39	D37.09	D49.0
groove (lower) (upper)	C06.1	C79.89	D00.02	D10.39	D37.09	D49.0
mucosa	C06.0	C79.89	D00.02	D10.39	D37.09	D49.0
sulcus (lower) (upper)	C06.1	C79.89	D00.02	D10.39	D37.09	D49.0
bulbourethral gland	C68.0	C79.19	D09.19	D30.4	D41.3	D49.59
bursa — see Neoplasm, connective tissue						
buttock NEC	C76.3	C79.89	D04.5	D36.7	D48.7	D49.89
calf	C76.5-	C79.89	D04.7-	D36.7	D48.7	D49.89
calvarium	C41.0	C79.51	—	D16.4-	D48.0	D49.2
calyx, renal	C65.-	C79.0	D09.19	D30.1-	D41.1-	D49.51

NEOPLASM TABLE

Neoplasm Table	Malignant Primary	Malignant Secondary	Ca In situ	Benign	Uncertain Behavior	Unspecified Behavior
Neoplasm, neoplastic - *continued*						
canal						
anal	C21.1	C78.5	D01.3	D12.9	D37.8	D49.0
auditory (external) — *see also* Neoplasm, skin, ear	C44.20-	C79.2	D04.2-	D23.2-	D48.5	D49.2
auricular (external) — *see also* Neoplasm, skin, ear	C44.20-	C79.2	D04.2-	D23.2-	D48.5	D49.2
canaliculi, biliary (biliferi) (intrahepatic)	C22.1	C78.7	D01.5	D13.4	D37.6	D49.0
canthus (eye) (inner) (outer)	C44.10-	C79.2	D04.1-	D23.1-	D48.5	D49.2
basal cell carcinoma	C44.11-	—	—	—	—	—
specified type NEC	C44.19-	—	—	—	—	—
squamous cell carcinoma	C44.12-	—	—	—	—	—
capillary — *see* Neoplasm, connective tissue						
caput coli	C18.0	C78.5	D01.0	D12.0	D37.4	D49.0
carcinoid — *see* Tumor, carcinoid						
cardia (gastric)	C16.0	C78.89	D00.2	D13.1	D37.1	D49.0
cardiac orifice (stomach)	C16.0	C78.89	D00.2	D13.1	D37.1	D49.0
cardio-esophageal junction	C16.0	C78.89	D00.2	D13.1	D37.1	D49.0
cardio-esophagus	C16.0	C78.89	D00.2	D13.1	D37.1	D49.0
carina (bronchus)	C34.0-	C78.0-	D02.2-	D14.3-	D38.1	D49.1
carotid (artery)	C49.0	C79.89	—	D21.0	D48.1	D49.2
body	C75.4	C79.89	—	D35.5	D44.6	D49.7
carpus (any bone)	C40.1-	C79.51	—	D16.1-	—	—
cartilage (articular) (joint) NEC — *see also* Neoplasm, bone	C41.9	C79.51	—	D16.9-	D48.0	D49.2
arytenoid	C32.3	C78.39	D02.0	D14.1	D38.0	D49.1
auricular	C49.0	C79.89	—	D21.0	D48.1	D49.2
bronchi	C34.0-	C78.39	—	D14.3-	D38.1	D49.1
costal	C41.3	C79.51	—	D16.7	D48.0	D49.2
cricoid	C32.3	C78.39	D02.0	D14.1	D38.0	D49.1
cuneiform	C32.3	C78.39	D02.0	D14.1	D38.0	D49.1
ear (external)	C49.0	C79.89	—	D21.0	D48.1	D49.2
ensiform	C41.3	C79.51	—	D16.7	D48.0	D49.2
epiglottis	C32.1	C78.39	D02.0	D14.1	D38.0	D49.1
anterior surface	C10.1	C79.89	D00.08	D10.5	D37.05	D49.0
eyelid	C49.0	C79.89	—	D21.0	D48.1	D49.2
intervertebral	C41.2	C79.51	—	D16.6	D48.0	D49.2
larynx, laryngeal	C32.3	C78.39	D02.0	D14.1	D38.0	D49.1
nose, nasal	C30.0	C78.39	D02.3	D14.0	D38.5	D49.1
pinna	C49.0	C79.89	—	D21.0	D48.1	D49.2
rib	C41.3	C79.51	—	D16.7	D48.0	D49.2
semilunar (knee)	C40.2-	C79.51	—	D16.2-	D48.0	D49.2
thyroid	C32.3	C78.39	D02.0	D14.1	D38.0	D49.1
trachea	C33	C78.39	D02.1	D14.2	D38.1	D49.1
cauda equina	C72.1	C79.49	—	D33.4	D43.4	D49.7
cavity						
buccal	C06.9	C79.89	D00.00	D10.30	D37.09	D49.0
nasal	C30.0	C78.39	D02.3	D14.0	D38.5	D49.1
oral	C06.9	C79.89	D00.00	D10.30	D37.09	D49.0
peritoneal	C48.2	C78.6	—	D20.1	D48.4	D49.0
tympanic	C30.1	C78.39	D02.3	D14.0	D38.5	D49.1
cecum	C18.0	C78.5	D01.0	D12.0	D37.4	D49.0
central nervous system	C72.9	C79.40	—	—	—	—
Neoplasm, neoplastic - *continued*						
cerebellopontine (angle)	C71.6	C79.31	—	D33.1	D43.1	D49.6
cerebellum, cerebellar	C71.6	C79.31	—	D33.1	D43.1	D49.6
cerebrum, cerebral (cortex) (hemisphere) (white matter)	C71.0	C79.31	—	D33.0	D43.0	D49.6
meninges	C70.0	C79.32	—	D32.0	D42.0	D49.7
peduncle	C71.7	C79.31	—	D33.1	D43.1	D49.6
ventricle	C71.5	C79.31	—	D33.0	D43.0	D49.6
fourth	C71.7	C79.31	—	D33.1	D43.1	D49.6
cervical region	C76.0	C79.89	D09.8	D36.7	D48.7	D49.89
cervix (cervical) (uteri) (uterus)	C53.9	C79.82	D06.9	D26.0	D39.0	D49.59
canal	C53.0	C79.82	D06.0	D26.0	D39.0	D49.59
endocervix (canal) (gland)	C53.0	C79.82	D06.0	D26.0	D39.0	D49.59
exocervix	C53.1	C79.82	D06.1	D26.0	D39.0	D49.59
external os	C53.1	C79.82	D06.1	D26.0	D39.0	D49.59
internal os	C53.0	C79.82	D06.0	D26.0	D39.0	D49.59
nabothian gland	C53.0	C79.82	D06.0	D26.0	D39.0	D49.59
overlapping lesion	C53.8	—	—	—	—	—
squamocolumnar junction	C53.8	C79.82	D06.7	D26.0	D39.0	D49.59
stump	C53.8	C79.82	D06.7	D26.0	D39.0	D49.59
cheek	C76.0	C79.89	D09.8	D36.7	D48.7	D49.89
external	C44.309	C79.2	D04.39	D23.39	D48.5	D49.2
basal cell carcinoma	C44.319	—	—	—	—	—
specified type NEC	C44.399	—	—	—	—	—
squamous cell carcinoma	C44.329	—	—	—	—	—
inner aspect	C06.0	C79.89	D00.02	D10.39	D37.09	D49.0
internal	C06.0	C79.89	D00.02	D10.39	D37.09	D49.0
mucosa	C06.0	C79.89	D00.02	D10.39	D37.09	D49.0
chest (wall) NEC	C76.1	C79.89	D09.8	D36.7	D48.7	D49.89
chiasma opticum	C72.3-	C79.49	—	D33.3	D43.3	D49.7
chin	C44.309	C79.2	D04.39	D23.39	D48.5	D49.2
basal cell carcinoma	C44.319	—	—	—	—	—
specified type NEC	C44.399	—	—	—	—	—
squamous cell carcinoma	C44.329	—	—	—	—	—
choana	C11.3	C79.89	D00.08	D10.6	D37.05	D49.0
cholangiole	C22.1	C78.89	D01.5	D13.4	D37.6	D49.0
choledochal duct	C24.0	C78.89	D01.5	D13.5	D37.6	D49.0
choroid	C69.3-	C79.49	D09.2-	D31.3	D48.7	D49.81
plexus	C71.5	C79.31	—	D33.0	D43.0	D49.6
ciliary body	C69.4-	C79.49	D09.2-	D31.4-	D48.7	D49.89
clavicle	C41.3	C79.51	—	D16.7	D48.0	D49.2
clitoris	C51.2	C79.82	D07.1	D28.0	D39.8	D49.59
clivus	C41.0	C79.51	—	D16.4-	D48.0	D49.2
cloacogenic zone	C21.2	C78.5	D01.3	D12.9	D37.8	D49.0
coccygeal						
body or glomus	C49.5	C79.89	—	D21.5	D48.1	D49.2
vertebra	C41.4	C79.51	—	D16.8	D48.0	D49.2
coccyx	C41.4	C79.51	—	D16.8	D48.0	D49.2
colon — *see also* Neoplasm, intestine, large	C18.9	C78.5	—	—	—	—
with rectum	C19	C78.5	D01.1	D12.7	D37.5	D49.0
column, spinal — *see* Neoplasm, spine						
columnella — *see also* Neoplasm, skin, face	C44.390	C79.2	D04.39	D23.39	D48.5	D49.2
commissure						
labial, lip	C00.6	C79.89	D00.01	D10.39	D37.01	D49.0
laryngeal	C32.0	C78.39	D02.0	D14.1	D38.0	D49.1

Neoplasm Table	Malignant Primary	Malignant Secondary	Ca In situ	Benign	Uncertain Behavior	Unspecified Behavior
Neoplasm, neoplastic - *continued*						
common (bile) duct	C24.0	C78.89	D01.5	D13.5	D37.6	D49.0
concha — *see also*						
Neoplasm, skin, ear	C44.20-	C79.2	D04.2-	D23.2-	D48.5	D49.2
nose	C30.0	C78.39	D02.3	D14.0	D38.5	D49.1
conjunctiva	C69.0-	C79.49	D09.2-	D31.0-	D48.7	D49.89
connective tissue NEC	C49.9	C79.89	—	D21.9	D48.1	D49.2

Connective tissue Notes:

Note: For neoplasms of connective tissue (blood vessel, bursa, fascia, ligament, muscle, peripheral nerves, sympathetic and parasympathetic nerves and ganglia, synovia, tendon, etc.) or of morphological types that indicate connective tissue, code according to the list under "Neoplasm, connective tissue". For sites that do not appear in this list, code to neoplasm of that site; e.g., fibrosarcoma, pancreas (C25.9)

Note: Morphological types that indicate connective tissue appear in their proper place in the alphabetic index with the instruction "see Neoplasm, connective tissue ...."

Neoplasm Table	Malignant Primary	Malignant Secondary	Ca In situ	Benign	Uncertain Behavior	Unspecified Behavior
abdomen	C49.4	C79.89	—	D21.4	D48.1	D49.2
abdominal wall	C49.4	C79.89	—	D21.4	D48.1	D49.2
ankle	C49.2-	C79.89	—	D21.2-	D48.1	D49.2
antecubital fossa or space	C49.1-	C79.89	—	D21.1-	D48.1	D49.2
arm	C49.1-	C79.89	—	D21.1-	D48.1	D49.2
auricle (ear)	C49.0	C79.89	—	D21.0	D48.1	D49.2
axilla	C49.3	C79.89	—	D21.3	D48.1	D49.2
back	C49.6	C79.89	—	D21.6	D48.1	D49.2
breast — *see* Neoplasm, breast						
buttock	C49.5	C79.89	—	D21.5	D48.1	D49.2
calf	C49.2-	C79.89	—	D21.2-	D48.1	D49.2
cervical region	C49.0	C79.89	—	D21.0	D48.1	D49.2
cheek	C49.0	C79.89	—	D21.0	D48.1	D49.2
chest (wall)	C49.3	C79.89	—	D21.3	D48.1	D49.2
chin	C49.0	C79.89	—	D21.0	D48.1	D49.2
diaphragm	C49.3	C79.89	—	D21.3	D48.1	D49.2
ear (external)	C49.0	C79.89	—	D21.0	D48.1	D49.2
elbow	C49.1-	C79.89	—	D21.1-	D48.1	D49.2
extrarectal	C49.5	C79.89	—	D21.5	D48.1	D49.2
extremity	C49.9	C79.89	—	D21.9	D48.1	D49.2
lower	C49.2-	C79.89	—	D21.2-	D48.1	D49.2
upper	C49.1-	C79.89	—	D21.1-	D48.1	D49.2
eyelid	C49.0	C79.89	—	D21.0	D48.1	D49.2
face	C49.0	C79.89	—	D21.0	D48.1	D49.2
finger	C49.1-	C79.89	—	D21.1-	D48.1	D49.2
flank	C49.6	C79.89	—	D21.6	D48.1	D49.2
foot	C49.2-	C79.89	—	D21.2-	D48.1	D49.2
forearm	C49.1-	C79.89	—	D21.1-	D48.1	D49.2
forehead	C49.0	C79.89	—	D21.0	D48.1	D49.2
gastric	C49.4	C79.89	—	D21.4	D48.1	D49.2
gastrointestinal	C49.4	C79.89	—	D21.4	D48.1	D49.2
gluteal region	C49.5	C79.89	—	D21.5	D48.1	D49.2
great vessels NEC	C49.3	C79.89	—	D21.3	D48.1	D49.2
groin	C49.5	C79.89	—	D21.5	D48.1	D49.2
hand	C49.1-	C79.89	—	D21.1-	D48.1	D49.2
head	C49.0	C79.89	—	D21.0	D48.1	D49.2
heel	C49.2-	C79.89	—	D21.2-	D48.1	D49.2
hip	C49.2-	C79.89	—	D21.2-	D48.1	D49.2
hypochondrium	C49.4	C79.89	—	D21.4	D48.1	D49.2
iliopsoas muscle	C49.5	C79.89	—	D21.5	D48.1	D49.2

Neoplasm Table	Malignant Primary	Malignant Secondary	Ca In situ	Benign	Uncertain Behavior	Unspecified Behavior
Neoplasm, neoplastic - *continued*						
connective tissue NEC - *continued*						
infraclavicular region	C49.3	C79.89	—	D21.3	D48.1	D49.2
inguinal (canal) (region)	C49.5	C79.89	—	D21.5	D48.1	D49.2
intestinal	C49.4	C79.89	—	D21.4	D48.1	D49.2
intrathoracic	C49.3	C79.89	—	D21.3	D48.1	D49.2
ischiorectal fossa	C49.5	C79.89	—	D21.5	D48.1	D49.2
jaw	C03.9	C79.89	D00.03	D10.39	D48.1	D49.0
knee	C49.2-	C79.89	—	D21.2-	D48.1	D49.2
leg	C49.2-	C79.89	—	D21.2-	D48.1	D49.2
limb NEC	C49.9	C79.89	—	D21.9	D48.1	D49.2
lower	C49.2-	C79.89	—	D21.2-	D48.1	D49.2
upper	C49.1-	C79.89	—	D21.1-	D48.1	D49.2
nates	C49.5	C79.89	—	D21.5	D48.1	D49.2
neck	C49.0	C79.89	—	D21.0	D48.1	D49.2
orbit	C69.6-	C79.49	D09.2-	D31.6-	D48.1	D49.89
overlapping lesion	C49.8	—	—	—	—	—
pararectal	C49.5	C79.89	—	D21.5	D48.1	D49.2
para-urethral	C49.5	C79.89	—	D21.5	D48.1	D49.2
paravaginal	C49.5	C79.89	—	D21.5	D48.1	D49.2
pelvis (floor)	C49.5	C79.89	—	D21.5	D48.1	D49.2
pelvo-abdominal	C49.8	C79.89	—	D21.6	D48.1	D49.2
perineum	C49.5	C79.89	—	D21.5	D48.1	D49.2
perirectal (tissue)	C49.5	C79.89	—	D21.5	D48.1	D49.2
periurethral (tissue)	C49.5	C79.89	—	D21.5	D48.1	D49.2
popliteal fossa or space	C49.2-	C79.89	—	D21.2-	D48.1	D49.2
presacral	C49.5	C79.89	—	D21.5	D48.1	D49.2
psoas muscle	C49.4	C79.89	—	D21.4	D48.1	D49.2
pterygoid fossa	C49.0	C79.89	—	D21.0	D48.1	D49.2
rectovaginal septum or wall	C49.5	C79.89	—	D21.5	D48.1	D49.2
rectovesical	C49.5	C79.89	—	D21.5	D48.1	D49.2
retroperitoneum	C48.0	C78.6	—	D20.0	D48.3	D49.0
sacrococcygeal region	C49.5	C79.89	—	D21.5	D48.1	D49.2
scalp	C49.0	C79.89	—	D21.0	D48.1	D49.2
scapular region	C49.3	C79.89	—	D21.3	D48.1	D49.2
shoulder	C49.1-	C79.89	—	D21.1-	D48.1	D49.2
skin (dermis) NEC — *see also* Neoplasm, skin, by site	C44.90	C79.2	D04.9	D23.9	D48.5	D49.2
stomach	C49.4	C79.89	—	D21.4	D48.1	D49.2
submental	C49.0	C79.89	—	D21.0	D48.1	D49.2
supraclavicular region	C49.0	C79.89	—	D21.0	D48.1	D49.2
temple	C49.0	C79.89	—	D21.0	D48.1	D49.2
temporal region	C49.0	C79.89	—	D21.0	D48.1	D49.2
thigh	C49.2-	C79.89	—	D21.2-	D48.1	D49.2
thoracic (duct) (wall)	C49.3	C79.89	—	D21.3	D48.1	D49.2
thorax	C49.3	C79.89	—	D21.3	D48.1	D49.2
thumb	C49.1-	C79.89	—	D21.1-	D48.1	D49.2
toe	C49.2-	C79.89	—	D21.2-	D48.1	D49.2
trunk	C49.6	C79.89	—	D21.6	D48.1	D49.2
umbilicus	C49.4	C79.89	—	D21.4	D48.1	D49.2
vesicorectal	C49.5	C79.89	—	D21.5	D48.1	D49.2
wrist	C49.1-	C79.89	—	D21.1-	D48.1	D49.2
conus medullaris	C72.0	C79.49	—	D33.4	D43.4	D49.7
cord (true) (vocal)	C32.0	C78.39	D02.0	D14.1	D38.0	D49.1
false	C32.1	C78.39	D02.0	D14.1	D38.0	D49.1
spermatic	C63.1-	C79.82	D07.69	D29.8	D40.8	D49.59
spinal (cervical) (lumbar) (thoracic)	C72.0	C79.49	—	D33.4	D43.4	D49.7
cornea (limbus)	C69.1-	C79.49	D09.2-	D31.1-	D48.7	D49.89

Neoplasm Table	Malignant Primary	Malignant Secondary	Ca In situ	Benign	Uncertain Behavior	Unspecified Behavior
Neoplasm, neoplastic - *continued*						
corpus						
albicans	C56.-	C79.6-	D07.39	D27.-	D39.1-	D49.59
callosum, brain	C71.0	C79.31	—	D33.2	D43.2	D49.6
cavernosum	C60.2	C79.82	D07.4	D29.0	D40.8	D49.59
gastric	C16.2	C78.89	D00.2	D13.1	D37.1	D49.0
overlapping sites	C54.8	—	—	—	—	—
penis	C60.2	C79.82	D07.4	D29.0	D40.8	D49.59
striatum, cerebrum	C71.0	C79.31	—	D33.0	D43.0	D49.6
uteri	C54.9	C79.82	D07.0	D26.1	D39.0	D49.59
isthmus	C54.0	C79.82	D07.0	D26.1	D39.0	D49.59
cortex						
adrenal	C74.0-	C79.7-	D09.3	D35.0-	D44.1-	D49.7
cerebral	C71.0	C79.31	—	D33.0	D43.0	D49.6
costal cartilage	C41.3	C79.51	—	D16.7	D48.0	D49.2
costovertebral joint	C41.3	C79.51	—	D16.7	D48.0	D49.2
Cowper's gland	C68.0	C79.19	D09.19	D30.4	D41.3	D49.59
cranial (fossa, any)	C71.9	C79.31	—	D33.2	D43.2	D49.6
meninges	C70.0	C79.32	—	D32.0	D42.0	D49.7
nerve	C72.50	C79.49	—	D33.3	D43.3	D49.7
specified NEC	C72.59	C79.49	—	D33.3	D43.3	D49.7
craniobuccal pouch	C75.2	C79.89	D09.3	D35.2	D44.3	D49.7
craniopharyngeal (duct) (pouch)	C75.2	C79.89	D09.3	D35.3	D44.4	D49.7
cricoid	C13.0	C79.89	D00.08	D10.7	D37.05	D49.0
cartilage	C32.3	C78.39	D02.0	D14.1	D38.0	D49.1
cricopharynx	C13.0	C79.89	D00.08	D10.7	D37.05	D49.0
crypt of Morgagni	C21.8	C78.5	D01.3	D12.9	D37.8	D49.0
crystalline lens	C69.4-	C79.49	D09.2-	D31.4-	D48.7	D49.89
cul-de-sac (Douglas')	C48.1	C78.6	—	D20.1	D48.4	D49.0
cuneiform cartilage	C32.3	C78.39	D02.0	D14.1	D38.0	D49.1
cutaneous — *see* Neoplasm, skin						
cutis — *see* Neoplasm, skin						
cystic (bile) duct (common)	C24.0	C78.89	D01.5	D13.5	D37.6	D49.0
dermis — *see* Neoplasm, skin						
diaphragm	C49.3	C79.89	—	D21.3	D48.1-	D49.2
digestive organs, system, tube, or tract NEC	C26.9	C78.89	D01.9	D13.9	D37.9	D49.0
disc, intervertebral	C41.2	C79.51	—	D16.6	D48.0	D49.2
disease, generalized	C80.0	—	—	—	—	—
disseminated	C80.0	—	—	—	—	—
Douglas' cul-de-sac or pouch	C48.1	C78.6	—	D20.1	D48.4	D49.0
duodenojejunal junction	C17.8	C78.4	D01.49	D13.39	D37.2	D49.0
duodenum	C17.0	C78.4	D01.49	D13.2	D37.2	D49.0
dura (cranial) (mater)	C70.9	C79.49	—	D32.9	D42.9	D49.7
cerebral	C70.0	C79.32	—	D32.0	D42.0	D49.7
spinal	C70.1	C79.49	—	D32.1	D42.1	D49.7
ear (external) — *see also* Neoplasm, skin, ear	C44.20-	C79.2	D04.2-	D23.2-	D48.5	D49.2
auricle or auris — *see also* Neoplasm, skin, ear	C44.20-	C79.2	D04.2-	D23.2-	D48.5	D49.2
canal, external — *see also* Neoplasm, skin, ear	C44.20-	C79.2	D04.2-	D23.2-	D48.5	D49.2
cartilage	C49.0	C79.89	—	D21.0	D48.1	D49.2
external meatus — *see also* Neoplasm, skin, ear	C44.20-	C79.2	D04.2-	D23.2-	D48.5	D49.2
inner	C30.1	C78.39	D02.3	D14.0	D38.5	D49.1
lobule — *see also* Neoplasm, skin, ear	C44.20-	C79.2	D04.2-	D23.2-	D48.5	D49.2
middle	C30.1	C78.39	D02.3	D14.0	D38.5	D49.1
overlapping lesion with accessory sinuses	C31.8	—	—	—	—	—
ear (external) — *see also* Neoplasm, skin, ear - *continued*	C44.20-	C79.2	D04.2-	D23.2-	D48.5	D49.2
skin	C44.20-	C79.2	D04.2-	D23.2-	D48.5	D49.2
basal cell carcinoma	C44.21-	—	—	—	—	—
specified type NEC	C44.29-	—	—	—	—	—
squamous cell carcinoma	C44.22-	—	—	—	—	—
earlobe	C44.20-	C79.2	D04.2-	D23.2-	D48.5	D49.2
basal cell carcinoma	C44.21-	—	—	—	—	—
specified type NEC	C44.29-	—	—	—	—	—
squamous cell carcinoma	C44.22-	—	—	—	—	—
ejaculatory duct	C63.7	C79.82	D07.69	D29.8	D40.8	D49.59
elbow NEC	C76.4-	C79.89	D04.6-	D36.7	D48.7	D49.89
endocardium	C38.0	C79.89	—	D15.1	D48.7	D49.89
endocervix (canal) (gland)	C53.0	C79.82	D06.0	D26.0	D39.0	D49.59
endocrine gland NEC	C75.9	C79.89	D09.3	D35.9	D44.9	D49.7
pluriglandular	C75.8	C79.89	D09.3	D35.7	D44.9	D49.7
endometrium (gland) (stroma)	C54.1	C79.82	D07.0	D26.1	D39.0	D49.59
ensiform cartilage	C41.3	C79.51	—	D16.7	D48.0	D49.2
enteric — *see* Neoplasm, intestine						
ependyma (brain)	C71.5	C79.31	—	D33.0	D43.0	D49.6
fourth ventricle	C71.7	C79.31	—	D33.1	D43.1	D49.6
epicardium	C38.0	C79.89	—	D15.1	D48.7	D49.89
epididymis	C63.0-	C79.82	D07.69	D29.3-	D40.8	D49.59
epidural	C72.9	C79.49	—	D33.9	D43.9	D49.7
epiglottis	C32.1	C78.39	D02.0	D14.1	D38.0	D49.1
anterior aspect or surface	C10.1	C79.89	D00.08	D10.5	D37.05	D49.0
cartilage	C32.3	C78.39	D02.0	D14.1	D38.0	D49.1
free border (margin)	C10.1	C79.89	D00.08	D10.5	D37.05	D49.0
junctional region	C10.8	C79.89	D00.08	D10.5	D37.05	D49.0
posterior (laryngeal) surface	C32.1	C78.39	D02.0	D14.1	D38.0	D49.1
suprahyoid portion	C32.1	C78.39	D02.0	D14.1	D38.0	D49.1
esophagogastric junction	C16.0	C78.89	D00.2	D13.1	D37.1	D49.0
esophagus	C15.9	C78.89	D00.1	D13.0	D37.8	D49.0
abdominal	C15.5	C78.89	D00.1	D13.0	D37.8	D49.0
cervical	C15.3	C78.89	D00.1	D13.0	D37.8	D49.0
distal (third)	C15.5	C78.89	D00.1	D13.0	D37.8	D49.0
lower (third)	C15.5	C78.89	D00.1	D13.0	D37.8	D49.0
middle (third)	C15.4	C78.89	D00.1	D13.0	D37.8	D49.0
overlapping lesion	C15.8	—	—	—	—	—
proximal (third)	C15.3	C78.89	D00.1	D13.0	D37.8	D49.0
thoracic	C15.4	C78.89	D00.1	D13.0	D37.8	D49.0
upper (third)	C15.3	C78.89	D00.1	D13.0	D37.8	D49.0
ethmoid (sinus)	C31.1	C78.39	D02.3	D14.0	D38.5	D49.1
bone or labyrinth	C41.0	C79.51	—	D16.4-	D48.0	D49.2
eustachian tube	C30.1	C78.39	D02.3	D14.0	D38.5	D49.1
exocervix	C53.1	C79.82	D06.1	D26.0	D39.0	D49.59
external						
meatus (ear) — *see also* Neoplasm, skin, ear	C44.20-	C79.2	D04.2-	D23.2-	D48.5	D49.2
os, cervix uteri	C53.1	C79.82	D06.1	D26.0	D39.0	D49.59
extradural	C72.9	C79.49	—	D33.9	D43.9	D49.7
extrahepatic (bile) duct	C24.0	C78.89	D01.5	D13.5	D37.6	D49.0
overlapping lesion with gallbladder	C24.8	—	—	—	—	—
extraocular muscle	C69.6-	C79.49	D09.2-	D31.6-	D48.7	D49.89
extrarectal	C76.3	C79.89	D09.8	D36.7	D48.7	D49.89

Neoplasm Table	Malignant Primary	Malignant Secondary	Ca In situ	Benign	Uncertain Behavior	Unspecified Behavior
Neoplasm, neoplastic - *continued*						
extremity	C76.8	C79.89	D04.8	D36.7	D48.7	D49.89
lower	C76.5-	C79.89	D04.7-	D36.7	D48.7	D49.89
upper	C76.4-	C79.89	D04.6-	D36.7	D48.7	D49.89
eye NEC	C69.9-	C79.49	D09.2	D31.9-	D48.7	D49.89
overlapping sites	C69.8	—	—	—	—	—
eyeball	C69.9-	C79.49	D09.2-	D31.9-	D48.7	D49.89
eyebrow	C44.309	C79.2	D04.39	D23.39	D48.5	D49.2
basal cell carcinoma	C44.319	—	—	—	—	—
specified type NEC	C44.399	—	—	—	—	—
squamous cell carcinoma	C44.329	—	—	—	—	—
eyelid (lower) (skin) (upper)	C44.10-	—	—	—	—	—
basal cell carcinoma	C44.11-	—	—	—	—	—
cartilage	C49.0	C79.89	—	D21.0	D48.1	D49.2
specified type NEC	C44.19-	—	—	—	—	—
squamous cell carcinoma	C44.12-	—	—	—	—	—
face NEC	C76.0	C79.89	D04.39	D36.7	D48.7	D49.89
fallopian tube (accessory)	C57.0-	C79.82	D07.39	D28.2	D39.8	D49.59
falx (cerebella) (cerebri)	C70.0	C79.32		D32.0	D42.0	D49.7
fascia — *see also* Neoplasm, connective tissue						
palmar	C49.1-	C79.89	—	D21.1-	D48.1	D49.2
plantar	C49.2-	C79.89	—	D21.2-	D48.1	D49.2
fatty tissue — *see* Neoplasm, connective tissue						
fauces, faucial NEC	C10.9	C79.89	D00.08	D10.5	D37.05	D49.0
pillars	C09.1	C79.89	D00.08	D10.5	D37.05	D49.0
tonsil	C09.9	C79.89	D00.08	D10.4	D37.05	D49.0
femur (any part)	C40.2-	—	—	D16.2-	—	—
fetal membrane	C58	C79.82	D07.0	D26.7	D39.2	D49.59
fibrous tissue — *see* Neoplasm, connective tissue						
fibula (any part)	C40.2-	C79.51	—	D16.2-	—	—
filum terminale	C72.0	C79.49	—	D33.4	D43.4	D49.7
finger NEC	C76.4-	C79.89	D04.6-	D36.7	D48.7	D49.89
flank NEC	C76.8	C79.89	D04.5	D36.7	D48.7	D49.89
follicle, nabothian	C53.0	C79.82	D06.0	D26.0	D39.0	D49.59
foot NEC	C76.5-	C79.89	D04.7-	D36.7	D48.7	D49.89
forearm NEC	C76.4-	C79.89	D04.6-	D36.7	D48.7	D49.89
forehead (skin)	C44.309	C79.2	D04.39	D23.39	D48.5	D49.2
basal cell carcinoma	C44.319	—	—	—	—	—
specified type NEC	C44.399	—	—	—	—	—
squamous cell carcinoma	C44.329	—	—	—	—	—
foreskin	C60.0	C79.82	D07.4	D29.0	D40.8	D49.59
fornix						
pharyngeal	C11.3	C79.89	D00.08	D10.6	D37.05	D49.0
vagina	C52	C79.82	D07.2	D28.1	D39.8	D49.59
fossa (of)						
anterior (cranial)	C71.9	C79.31	—	D33.2	D43.2	D49.6
cranial	C71.9	C79.31	—	D33.2	D43.2	D49.6
ischiorectal	C76.3	C79.89	D09.8	D36.7	D48.7	D49.89
middle (cranial)	C71.9	C79.31	—	D33.2	D43.2	D49.6
piriform	C12	C79.89	D00.08	D10.7	D37.05	D49.0
pituitary	C75.1	C79.89	D09.3	D35.2	D44.3	D49.7
posterior (cranial)	C71.9	C79.31	—	D33.2	D43.2	D49.6
pterygoid	C49.0	C79.89	—	D21.0	D48.1	D49.2
pyriform	C12	C79.89	D00.08	D10.7	D37.05	D49.0
Rosenmüller	C11.2	C79.89	D00.08	D10.6	D37.05	D49.0
tonsillar	C09.0	C79.89	D00.08	D10.5	D37.05	D49.0
fourchette	C51.9	C79.82	D07.1	D28.0	D39.8	D49.59

Neoplasm Table	Malignant Primary	Malignant Secondary	Ca In situ	Benign	Uncertain Behavior	Unspecified Behavior
Neoplasm, neoplastic - *continued*						
frenulum						
labii — *see* Neoplasm, lip, internal						
linguae	C02.2	C79.89	D00.07	D10.1	D37.02	D49.0
frontal						
bone	C41.0	C79.51	—	D16.4-	D48.0	D49.2
lobe, brain	C71.1	C79.31	—	D33.0	D43.0	D49.6
pole	C71.1	C79.31	—	D33.0	D43.0	D49.6
sinus	C31.2	C78.39	D02.3	D14.0	D38.5	D49.1
fundus						
stomach	C16.1	C78.89	D00.2	D13.1	D37.1	D49.0
uterus	C54.3	C79.82	D07.0	D26.1	D39.0	D49.59
gall duct (extrahepatic)	C24.0	C78.89	D01.5	D13.5	D37.6	D49.0
intrahepatic	C22.1	C78.7	D01.5	D13.4	D37.6	D49.0
gallbladder	C23	C78.89	D01.5	D13.5	D37.6	D49.0
overlapping lesion with extrahepatic bile ducts	C24.8	—	—	—	—	—
ganglia — *see also* Neoplasm, nerve, peripheral	C47.9	C79.89	—	D36.10	D48.2	D49.2
basal	C71.0	C79.31	—	D33.0	D43.0	D49.6
cranial nerve	C72.50	C79.49	—	D33.3	D43.3	D49.7
Gartner's duct	C52	C79.82	D07.2	D28.1	D39.8	D49.59
gastric — *see* Neoplasm, stomach						
gastrocolic	C26.9	C78.89	D01.9	D13.9	D37.9	D49.0
gastroesophageal junction	C16.0	C78.89	D00.2	D13.1	D37.1	D49.0
gastrointestinal (tract) NEC	C26.9	C78.89	D01.9	D13.9	D37.9	D49.0
generalized	C80.0	—	—	—	—	—
genital organ or tract						
female NEC	C57.9	C79.82	D07.30	D28.9	D39.9	D49.59
overlapping lesion	C57.8	—	—	—	—	—
specified site NEC	C57.7	C79.82	D07.39	D28.7	D39.8	D49.59
male NEC	C63.9	C79.82	D07.60	D29.9	D40.9	D49.59
overlapping lesion	C63.8	—	—	—	—	—
specified site NEC	C63.7	C79.82	D07.69	D29.8	D40.8	D49.59
genitourinary tract						
female	C57.9	C79.82	D07.30	D28.9	D39.9	D49.59
male	C63.9	C79.82	D07.60	D29.9	D40.9	D49.59
gingiva (alveolar) (marginal)	C03.9	C79.89	D00.03	D10.39	D37.09	D49.0
lower	C03.1	C79.89	D00.03	D10.39	D37.09	D49.0
mandibular	C03.1	C79.89	D00.03	D10.39	D37.09	D49.0
maxillary	C03.0	C79.89	D00.03	D10.39	D37.09	D49.0
upper	C03.0	C79.89	D00.03	D10.39	D37.09	D49.0
gland, glandular (lymphatic) (system) — *see also* Neoplasm, lymph gland						
endocrine NEC	C75.9	C79.89	D09.3	D35.9	D44.9	D49.7
salivary — *see* Neoplasm, salivary gland						
glans penis	C60.1	C79.82	D07.4	D29.0	D40.8	D49.59
globus pallidus	C71.0	C79.31	—	D33.0	D43.0	D49.6
glomus						
coccygeal	C49.5	C79.89	—	D21.5	D48.1	D49.2
jugularis	C75.5	C79.89	—	D35.6	D44.7	D49.7
glosso-epiglottic fold (s)	C10.1	C79.89	D00.08	D10.5	D37.05	D49.0
glossopalatine fold	C09.1	C79.89	D00.08	D10.5	D37.05	D49.0
glossopharyngeal sulcus	C09.0	C79.89	D00.08	D10.5	D37.05	D49.0
glottis	C32.0	C78.39	D02.0	D14.1	D38.0	D49.1
gluteal region	C76.3	C79.89	D04.5	D36.7	D48.7	D49.89
great vessels NEC	C49.3	C79.89	—	D21.3	D48.1	D49.2
groin NEC	C76.3	C79.89	D04.5	D36.7	D48.7	D49.89

NEOPLASM TABLE

Neoplasm Table	Malignant Primary	Malignant Secondary	Ca In situ	Benign	Uncertain Behavior	Unspecified Behavior
Neoplasm, neoplastic - *continued*						
gum	C03.9	C79.89	D00.03	D10.39	D37.09	D49.0
lower	C03.1	C79.89	D00.03	D10.39	D37.09	D49.0
upper	C03.0	C79.89	D00.03	D10.39	D37.09	D49.0
hand NEC	C76.4-	C79.89	D04.6-	D36.7	D48.7	D49.89
head NEC	C76.0	C79.89	D04.4	D36.7	D48.7	D49.89
heart	C38.0	C79.89	—	D15.1	D48.7	D49.89
heel NEC	C76.5-	C79.89	D04.7-	D36.7	D48.7	D49.89
helix — *see also* Neoplasm, skin, ear	C44.20-	C79.2	D04.2-	D23.2-	D48.5	D49.2
hematopoietic, hemopoietic tissue NEC	C96.9	—	—	—	—	—
specified NEC	C96.Z	—	—	—	—	—
hemisphere, cerebral	C71.0	C79.31	—	D33.0	D43.0	D49.6
hemorrhoidal zone	C21.1	C78.5	D01.3	D12.9	D37.8	D49.0
hepatic — *see also* Index to disease, by histology	C22.9	C78.7	D01.5	D13.4	D37.6	D49.0
duct (bile)	C24.0	C78.89	D01.5	D13.5	D37.6	D49.0
flexure (colon)	C18.3	C78.5	D01.0	D12.3	D37.4	D49.0
primary	C22.8	C78.7	D01.5	D13.4	D37.6	D49.0
hepatobiliary	C24.9	C78.89	D01.5	D13.5	D37.6	D49.0
hepatoblastoma	C22.2	C78.7	D01.5	D13.4	D37.6	D49.0
hepatoma	C22.0	C78.7	D01.5	D13.4	D37.6	D49.0
hilus of lung	C34.0-	C78.0-	D02.2-	D14.3-	D38.1	D49.1
hip NEC	C76.5-	C79.89	D04.7-	D36.7	D48.7	D49.89
hippocampus, brain	C71.2	C79.31	—	D33.0	D43.0	D49.6
humerus (any part)	C40.0-	C79.51	—	D16.0-		
hymen	C52	C79.82	D07.2	D28.1	D39.8	D49.59
hypopharynx, hypopharyngeal NEC	C13.9	C79.89	D00.08	D10.7	D37.05	D49.0
overlapping lesion	C13.8	—		—		—
postcricoid region	C13.0	C79.89	D00.08	D10.7	D37.05	D49.0
posterior wall	C13.2	C79.89	D00.08	D10.7	D37.05	D49.0
pyriform fossa (sinus)	C12	C79.89	D00.08	D10.7	D37.05	D49.0
hypophysis	C75.1	C79.89	D09.3	D35.2	D44.3	D49.7
hypothalamus	C71.0	C79.31	—	D33.0	D43.0	D49.6
ileocecum, ileocecal (coil) (junction) (valve)	C18.0	C78.5	D01.0	D12.0	D37.4	D49.0
ileum	C17.2	C78.4	D01.49	D13.39	D37.2	D49.0
ilium	C41.4	C79.51	—	D16.8	D48.0	D49.2
immunoproliferative NEC	C88.9	—	—	—	—	—
infraclavicular (region)	C76.1	C79.89	D04.5	D36.7	D48.7	D49.89
inguinal (region)	C76.3	C79.89	D04.5	D36.7	D48.7	D49.89
insula	C71.0	C79.31	—	D33.0	D43.0	D49.6
insular tissue (pancreas)	C25.4	C78.89	D01.7	D13.7	D37.8	D49.0
brain	C71.0	C79.31	—	D33.0	D43.0	D49.6
interarytenoid fold	C13.1	C79.89	D00.08	D10.7	D37.05	D49.0
hypopharyngeal aspect	C13.1	C79.89	D00.08	D10.7	D37.05	D49.0
laryngeal aspect	C32.1	C78.39	D02.0	D14.1	D38.0	D49.1
marginal zone	C13.1	C79.89	D00.08	D10.7	D37.05	D49.0
interdental papillae	C03.9	C79.89	D00.03	D10.39	D37.09	D49.0
lower	C03.1	C79.89	D00.03	D10.39	D37.09	D49.0
upper	C03.0	C79.89	D00.03	D10.39	D37.09	D49.0
internal						
capsule	C71.0	C79.31	—	D33.0	D43.0	D49.6
os (cervix)	C53.0	C79.82	D06.0	D26.0	D39.0	D49.59
intervertebral cartilage or disc	C41.2	C79.51	—	D16.6	D48.0	D49.2
intestine, intestinal	C26.0	C78.80	D01.40	D13.9	D37.8	D49.0
large	C18.9	C78.5	D01.	D12.6	D37.4	D49.0
appendix	C18.1	C78.5	D01.0	D12.1	D37.3	D49.0
caput coli	C18.0	C78.5	D01.0	D12.0	D37.4	D49.0
cecum	C18.0	C78.5	D01.0	D12.0	D37.4	D49.0
colon	C18.9	C78.5	D01.0	D12.6	D37.4	D49.0
and rectum	C19	C78.5	D01.1	D12.7	D37.5	D49.0
ascending	C18.2	C78.5	D01.0	D12.2	D37.4	D49.0
caput	C18.0	C78.5	D01.0	D12.0	D37.4	D49.0
descending	C18.6	C78.5	D01.0	D12.4	D37.4	D49.0
distal	C18.6	C78.5	D01.0	D12.4	D37.4	D49.0
left	C18.6	C78.5	D01.0	D12.4	D37.4	D49.0
overlapping lesion	C18.8	—		—		—
pelvic	C18.7	C78.5	D01.0	D12.5	D37.4	D49.0
right	C18.2	C78.5	D01.0	D12.2	D37.4	D49.0
sigmoid (flexure)	C18.7	C78.5	D01.0	D12.5	D37.4	D49.0
transverse	C18.4	C78.5	D01.0	D12.3	D37.4	D49.0
hepatic flexure	C18.3	C78.5	D01.0	D12.3	D37.4	D49.0
ileocecum, ileocecal (coil) (valve)	C18.0	C78.5	D01.0	D12.0	D37.4	D49.0
overlapping lesion	C18.8	—		—		—
sigmoid flexure (lower) (upper)	C18.7	C78.5	D01.0	D12.5	D37.4	D49.0
splenic flexure	C18.5	C78.5	D01.0	D12.3	D37.4	D49.0
small	C17.9	C78.4	D01.40	D13.30	D37.2	D49.0
duodenum	C17.0	C78.4	D01.49	D13.2	D37.2	D49.0
ileum	C17.2	C78.4	D01.49	D13.39	D37.2	D49.0
jejunum	C17.1	C78.4	D01.49	D13.39	D37.2	D49.0
overlapping lesion	C17.8	—		—		—
tract NEC	C26.0	C78.89	D01.40	D13.9	D37.8	D49.0
intra-abdominal	C76.2	C79.89	D09.8	D36.7	D48.7	D49.89
intracranial NEC	C71.9	C79.31	—	D33.2	D43.2	D49.6
intrahepatic (bile) duct	C22.1	C78.7	D01.5	D13.4	D37.6	D49.0
intraocular	C69.9-	C79.49	D09.2-	D31.9-	D48.7	D49.89
intraorbital	C69.6-	C79.49	D09.2-	D31.6-	D48.7	D49.89
intrasellar	C75.1	C79.89	D09.3	D35.2	D44.3	D49.7
intrathoracic (cavity) (organs)	C76.1	C79.89	D09.8	D15.9	D48.7	D49.89
specified NEC	C76.1	C79.89	D09.8	D15.7		
iris	C69.4-	C79.49	D09.2-	D31.4-	D48.7	D49.89
ischiorectal (fossa)	C76.3	C79.89	D09.8	D36.7	D48.7	D49.89
ischium	C41.4	C79.51	—	D16.8	D48.0	D49.2
island of Reil	C71.0	C79.31	—	D33.0	D43.0	D49.6
islands or islets of Langerhans	C25.4	C78.89	D01.7	D13.7	D37.8	D49.0
isthmus uteri	C54.0	C79.82	D07.0	D26.1	D39.0	D49.59
jaw	C76.0	C79.89	D09.8	D36.7	D48.7	D49.89
bone	C41.1	C79.51	—	D16.5-	D48.0	D49.2
lower	C41.1	C79.51	—	D16.5-	—	—
upper	C41.0	C79.51	—	D16.4-	—	—
carcinoma (any type) (lower) (upper)	C76.0	C79.89				
skin — *see also* Neoplasm, skin, face	C44.309	C79.2	D04.39	D23.39	D48.5	D49.2
soft tissues	C03.9	C79.89	D00.03	D10.39	D37.09	D49.0
lower	C03.1	C79.89	D00.03	D10.39	D37.09	D49.0
upper	C03.0	C79.89	D00.03	D10.39	D37.09	D49.0
jejunum	C17.1	C78.4	D01.49	D13.39	D37.2	D49.0

Neoplasm, neoplastic - continued

Neoplasm Table	Malignant Primary	Malignant Secondary	Ca In situ	Benign	Uncertain Behavior	Unspecified Behavior
joint NEC — see also Neoplasm, bone	C41.9	C79.51	—	D16.9-	D48.0	D49.2
acromioclavicular	C40.0-	C79.51	—	D16.0-	—	—
bursa or synovial membrane — see Neoplasm, connective tissue						
costovertebral	C41.3	C79.51	—	D16.7	D48.0	D49.2
sternocostal	C41.3	C79.51	—	D16.7	D48.0	D49.2
temporomandibular	C41.1	C79.51	—	D16.5-	D48.0	D49.2
junction						
anorectal	C21.8	C78.5	D01.3	D12.9	D37.8	D49.0
cardioesophageal	C16.0	C78.89	D00.2	D13.1	D37.1	D49.0
esophagogastric	C16.0	C78.89	D00.2	D13.1	D37.1	D49.0
gastroesophageal	C16.0	C78.89	D00.2	D13.1	D37.1	D49.0
hard and soft palate	C05.9	C79.89	D00.00	D10.39	D37.09	D49.0
ileocecal	C18.0	C78.5	D01.0	D12.0	D37.4	D49.0
pelvirectal	C19	C78.5	D01.1	D12.7	D37.5	D49.0
pelviureteric	C65.-	C79.0-	D09.19	D30.1-	D41.1-	D49.59
rectosigmoid	C19	C78.5	D01.1	D12.7	D37.5	D49.0
squamocolumnar, of cervix	C53.8	C79.82	D06.7	D26.0	D39.0	D49.59
Kaposi's sarcoma — see Kaposi's, sarcoma						
kidney (parenchymal)	C64.-	C79.0-	D09.19	D30.0-	D41.0-	D49.51-
calyx	C65.-	C79.0-	D09.19	D30.1-	D41.1-	D49.51-
hilus	C65.-	C79.0-	D09.19	D30.1-	D41.1-	D49.51-
pelvis	C65.-	C79.0-	D09.19	D30.1-	D41.1-	D49.51-
knee NEC	C76.5-	C79.89	D04.7-	D36.7	D48.7	D49.89
labia (skin)	C51.9	C79.82	D07.1	D28.0	D39.8	D49.59
majora	C51.0	C79.82	D07.1	D28.0	D39.8	D49.59
minora	C51.1	C79.82	D07.1	D28.0	D39.8	D49.59
labial — see also Neoplasm, lip	C00.9	C79.89	D00.01	D10.0	D37.01	D49.0
sulcus (lower) (upper)	C06.1	C79.89	D00.02	D10.39	D37.09	D49.0
labium (skin)	C51.9	C79.82	D07.1	D28.0	D39.8	D49.59
majus	C51.0	C79.82	D07.1	D28.0	D39.8	D49.59
minus	C51.1	C79.82	D07.1	D28.0	D39.8	D49.59
lacrimal						
canaliculi	C69.5-	C79.49	D09.2-	D31.5-	D48.7	D49.89
duct (nasal)	C69.5-	C79.49	D09.2-	D31.5-	D48.7	D49.89
gland	C69.5-	C79.49	D09.2-	D31.5-	D48.7	D49.89
punctum	C69.5-	C79.49	D09.2-	D31.5-	D48.7	D49.89
sac	C69.5-	C79.49	D09.2-	D31.5-	D48.7	D49.89
Langerhans, islands or islets	C25.4	C78.89	D01.7	D13.7	D37.8	D49.0
laryngopharynx	C13.9	C79.89	D00.08	D10.7	D37.05	D49.0
larynx, laryngeal NEC	C32.9	C78.39	D02.0	D14.1	D38.0	D49.1
aryepiglottic fold	C32.1	C78.39	D02.0	D14.1	D38.0	D49.1
cartilage (arytenoid) (cricoid) (cuneiform) (thyroid)	C32.3	C78.39	D02.0	D14.1	D38.0	D49.1
commissure (anterior) (posterior)	C32.0	C78.39	D02.0	D14.1	D38.0	D49.1
extrinsic NEC	C32.1	C78.39	D02.0	D14.1	D38.0	D49.1
meaning hypopharynx	C13.9	C79.89	D00.08	D10.7	D37.05	D49.0
interarytenoid fold	C32.1	C78.39	D02.0	D14.1	D38.0	D49.1
intrinsic	C32.0	C78.39	D02.0	D14.1	D38.0	D49.1
overlapping lesion	C32.8	—	—	—	—	—
ventricular band	C32.1	C78.39	D02.0	D14.1	D38.0	D49.1
leg NEC	C76.5-	C79.89	D04.7-	D36.7	D48.7	D49.89
lens, crystalline	C69.4-	C79.49	D09.2-	D31.4-	D48.7	D49.89
lid (lower) (upper)	C44.10-	C79.2	D04.1-	D23.1-	D48.5	D49.2
basal cell carcinoma	C44.11-	—	—	—	—	—
specified type NEC	C44.19-	—	—	—	—	—
squamous cell carcinoma	C44.12-	—	—	—	—	—

Neoplasm, neoplastic - continued

Neoplasm Table	Malignant Primary	Malignant Secondary	Ca In situ	Benign	Uncertain Behavior	Unspecified Behavior
ligament — see also Neoplasm, connective tissue						
broad	C57.1	C79.82	D07.39	D28.2	D39.8	D49.59
Mackenrodt's	C57.7	C79.82	D07.39	D28.7	D39.8	D49.59
non-uterine — see Neoplasm, connective tissue						
round	C57.2	C79.82	—	D28.2	D39.8	D49.59
sacro-uterine	C57.3	C79.82	—	D28.2	D39.8	D49.59
uterine	C57.3	C79.82	—	D28.2	D39.8	D49.59
utero-ovarian	C57.7	C79.82	D07.39	D28.2	D39.8	D49.59
uterosacral	C57.3	C79.82	—	D28.2	D39.8	D49.59
limb	C76.8	C79.89	D04.8	D36.7	D48.7	D49.89
lower	C76.5-	C79.89	D04.7-	D36.7	D48.7	D49.89
upper	C76.4-	C79.89	D04.6-	D36.7	D48.7	D49.89
limbus of cornea	C69.1-	C79.49	D09.2-	D31.1-	D48.7	D49.89
lingual NEC — see also Neoplasm, tongue	C02.9	C79.89	D00.07	D10.1	D37.02	D49.0
lingula, lung	C34.1-	C78.0-	D02.2-	D14.3-	D38.1	D49.1
lip	C00.9	C79.89	D00.01	D10.0	D37.01	D49.0
buccal aspect — see Neoplasm, lip, internal						
commissure	C00.6	C79.89	D00.01	D10.0	D37.01	D49.0
external	C00.2	C79.89	D00.01	D10.0	D37.01	D49.0
lower	C00.1	C79.89	D00.01	D10.0	D37.01	D49.0
upper	C00.0	C79.89	D00.01	D10.0	D37.01	D49.0
frenulum — see Neoplasm, lip, internal						
inner aspect — see Neoplasm, lip, internal						
internal	C00.5	C79.89	D00.01	D10.0	D37.01	D49.0
lower	C00.4	C79.89	D00.01	D10.0	D37.01	D49.0
upper	C00.3	C79.89	D00.01	D10.0	D37.01	D49.0
lipstick area	C00.2	C79.89	D00.01	D10.0	D37.01	D49.0
lower	C00.1	C79.89	D00.01	D10.0	D37.01	D49.0
upper	C00.0	C79.89	D00.01	D10.0	D37.01	D49.0
lower	C00.1	C79.89	D00.01	D10.0	D37.01	D49.0
internal	C00.4	C79.89	D00.01	D10.0	D37.01	D49.0
mucosa — see Neoplasm, lip, internal						
oral aspect — see Neoplasm, lip, internal						
overlapping lesion	C00.8	—	—	—	—	—
with oral cavity or pharynx	C14.8					
skin (commissure) (lower) (upper)	C44.00	C79.2	D04.0	D23.0	D48.5	D49.2
basal cell carcinoma	C44.01	—	—	—	—	—
specified type NEC	C44.09	—	—	—	—	—
squamous cell carcinoma	C44.02	—	—	—	—	—
upper	C00.0	C79.89	D00.01	D10.0	D37.01	D49.0
internal	C00.3	C79.89	D00.01	D10.0	D37.01	D49.0
vermilion border	C00.2	C79.89	D00.01	D10.0	D37.01	D49.0
lower	C00.1	C79.89	D00.01	D10.0	D37.01	D49.0
upper	C00.0	C79.89	D00.01	D10.0	D37.01	D49.0
lipomatous — see Lipoma, by site						
liver — see also Index to disease, by histology	C22.9	C78.7	D01.5	D13.4	D37.6	D49.0
primary	C22.8	C78.7	D01.5	D13.4	D37.6	D49.0

NEOPLASM TABLE

Neoplasm Table	Malignant Primary	Malignant Secondary	Ca In situ	Benign	Uncertain Behavior	Unspecified Behavior
Neoplasm, neoplastic - *continued*						
lumbosacral plexus	C47.5	C79.89	—	D36.16	D48.2	D49.2
lung	C34.9-	C78.0-	D02.2-	D14.3-	D38.1	D49.1
azygos lobe	C34.1-	C78.0-	D02.2-	D14.3-	D38.1	D49.1
carina	C34.0-	C78.0-	D02.2-	D14.3-	D38.1	D49.1
hilus	C34.0-	C78.0-	D02.2-	D14.3-	D38.1	D49.1
lingula	C34.1-	C78.0-	D02.2-	D14.3-	D38.1	D49.1
lobe NEC	C34.9-	C78.0-	D02.2-	D14.3-	D38.1	D49.1
lower lobe	C34.3-	C78.0-	D02.2-	D14.3-	D38.1	D49.1
main bronchus	C34.0-	C78.0-	D02.2-	D14.3-	D38.1	D49.1
mesothelioma — *see* Mesothelioma						
middle lobe	C34.2	C78.0-	D02.21	D14.31	D38.1	D49.1
overlapping lesion	C34.8-	—	—	—	—	—
upper lobe	C34.1-	C78.0-	D02.2-	D14.3-	D38.1	D49.1
lymph, lymphatic channel						
NEC	C49.9	C79.89	—	D21.9	D48.1	D49.2
gland (secondary)	—	C77.9	—	D36.0	D48.7	D49.89
abdominal	—	C77.2	—	D36.0	D48.7	D49.89
aortic	—	C77.2	—	D36.0	D48.7	D49.89
arm	—	C77.3	—	D36.0	D48.7	D49.89
auricular (anterior) (posterior)	—	C77.0	—	D36.0	D48.7	D49.89
axilla, axillary	—	C77.3	—	D36.0	D48.7	D49.89
brachial	—	C77.3	—	D36.0	D48.7	D49.89
bronchial	—	C77.1	—	D36.0	D48.7	D49.89
bronchopulmonary	—	C77.1	—	D36.0	D48.7	D49.89
celiac	—	C77.2	—	D36.0	D48.7	D49.89
cervical	—	C77.0	—	D36.0	D48.7	D49.89
cervicofacial	—	C77.0	—	D36.0	D48.7	D49.89
Cloquet	—	C77.4	—	D36.0	D48.7	D49.89
colic	—	C77.2	—	D36.0	D48.7	D49.89
common duct	—	C77.2	—	D36.0	D48.7	D49.89
cubital	—	C77.3	—	D36.0	D48.7	D49.89
diaphragmatic	—	C77.1	—	D36.0	D48.7	D49.89
epigastric, inferior	—	C77.1	—	D36.0	D48.7	D49.89
epitrochlear	—	C77.3	—	D36.0	D48.7	D49.89
esophageal	—	C77.1	—	D36.0	D48.7	D49.89
face	—	C77.0	—	D36.0	D48.7	D49.89
femoral	—	C77.4	—	D36.0	D48.7	D49.89
gastric	—	C77.2	—	D36.0	D48.7	D49.89
groin	—	C77.4	—	D36.0	D48.7	D49.89
head	—	C77.0	—	D36.0	D48.7	D49.89
hepatic	—	C77.2	—	D36.0	D48.7	D49.89
hilar (pulmonary)	—	C77.1	—	D36.0	D48.7	D49.89
splenic	—	C77.2	—	D36.0	D48.7	D49.89
hypogastric	—	C77.5	—	D36.0	D48.7	D49.89
ileocolic	—	C77.2	—	D36.0	D48.7	D49.89
iliac	—	C77.5	—	D36.0	D48.7	D49.89
infraclavicular	—	C77.3	—	D36.0	D48.7	D49.89
inguina, inguinal	—	C77.4	—	D36.0	D48.7	D49.89
innominate	—	C77.1	—	D36.0	D48.7	D49.89
intercostal	—	C77.1	—	D36.0	D48.7	D49.89
intestinal	—	C77.2	—	D36.0	D48.7	D49.89
intrabdominal	—	C77.2	—	D36.0	D48.7	D49.89
intrapelvic	—	C77.5	—	D36.0	D48.7	D49.89
intrathoracic	—	C77.1	—	D36.0	D48.7	D49.89
jugular	—	C77.0	—	D36.0	D48.7	D49.89
leg	—	C77.4	—	D36.0	D48.7	D49.89
limb						
lower	—	C77.4	—	D36.0	D48.7	D49.89
upper	—	C77.3	—	D36.0	D48.7	D49.89
lower limb	—	C77.4	—	D36.0	D48.7	D49.89
Neoplasm, neoplastic - *continued*						
lymph, lymphatic channel						
NEC - *continued*	C49.9	C79.89	—	D21.9	D48.1	D49.2
gland (secondary) - *continued*	—	C77.9	—	D36.0	D48.7	D49.89
lumbar	—	C77.2	—	D36.0	D48.7	D49.89
mandibular	—	C77.0	—	D36.0	D48.7	D49.89
mediastinal	—	C77.1	—	D36.0	D48.7	D49.89
mesenteric (inferior) (superior)	—	C77.2	—	D36.0	D48.7	D49.89
midcolic	—	C77.2	—	D36.0	D48.7	D49.89
multiple sites in categories C77.0-C77.5	—	C77.8	—	D36.0	D48.7	D49.89
neck	—	C77.0	—	D36.0	D48.7	D49.89
obturator	—	C77.5	—	D36.0	D48.7	D49.89
occipital	—	C77.0	—	D36.0	D48.7	D49.89
pancreatic	—	C77.2	—	D36.0	D48.7	D49.89
para-aortic	—	C77.2	—	D36.0	D48.7	D49.89
paracervical	—	C77.5	—	D36.0	D48.7	D49.89
parametrial	—	C77.5	—	D36.0	D48.7	D49.89
parasternal	—	C77.1	—	D36.0	D48.7	D49.89
parotid	—	C77.0	—	D36.0	D48.7	D49.89
pectoral	—	C77.3	—	D36.0	D48.7	D49.89
pelvic	—	C77.5	—	D36.0	D48.7	D49.89
peri-aortic	—	C77.2	—	D36.0	D48.7	D49.89
peripancreatic	—	C77.2	—	D36.0	D48.7	D49.89
popliteal	—	C77.4	—	D36.0	D48.7	D49.89
porta hepatis	—	C77.2	—	D36.0	D48.7	D49.89
portal	—	C77.2	—	D36.0	D48.7	D49.89
preauricular	—	C77.0	—	D36.0	D48.7	D49.89
prelaryngeal	—	C77.0	—	D36.0	D48.7	D49.89
presymphysial	—	C77.5	—	D36.0	D48.7	D49.89
pretracheal	—	C77.0	—	D36.0	D48.7	D49.89
primary (any site) NEC	C96.9	—	—	—	—	—
pulmonary (hiler)	—	C77.1	—	D36.0	D48.7	D49.89
pyloric	—	C77.2	—	D36.0	D48.7	D49.89
retroperitoneal	—	C77.2	—	D36.0	D48.7	D49.89
retropharyngeal	—	C77.0	—	D36.0	D48.7	D49.89
Rosenmüller's	—	C77.4	—	D36.0	D48.7	D49.89
sacral	—	C77.5	—	D36.0	D48.7	D49.89
scalene	—	C77.0	—	D36.0	D48.7	D49.89
site NEC	—	C77.9	—	D36.0	D48.7	D49.89
splenic (hilar)	—	C77.2	—	D36.0	D48.7	D49.89
subclavicular	—	C77.3	—	D36.0	D48.7	D49.89
subinguinal	—	C77.4	—	D36.0	D48.7	D49.89
sublingual	—	C77.0	—	D36.0	D48.7	D49.89
submandibular	—	C77.0	—	D36.0	D48.7	D49.89
submaxillary	—	C77.0	—	D36.0	D48.7	D49.89
submental	—	C77.0	—	D36.0	D48.7	D49.89
subscapular	—	C77.3	—	D36.0	D48.7	D49.89
supraclavicular	—	C77.0	—	D36.0	D48.7	D49.89
thoracic	—	C77.1	—	D36.0	D48.7	D49.89
tibial	—	C77.4	—	D36.0	D48.7	D49.89
tracheal	—	C77.1	—	D36.0	D48.7	D49.89
tracheobronchial	—	C77.1	—	D36.0	D48.7	D49.89
upper limb	—	C77.3	—	D36.0	D48.7	D49.89
Virchow's	—	C77.0	—	D36.0	D48.7	D49.89
node — *see also* Neoplasm, lymph gland						
primary NEC	C96.9	—	—	—	—	—
vessel — *see also* Neoplasm, connective tissue	C49.9	C79.89	—	D21.9	D48.1	D49.2

Neoplasm Table	Malignant Primary	Malignant Secondary	Ca In situ	Benign	Uncertain Behavior	Unspecified Behavior	Neoplasm Table	Malignant Primary	Malignant Secondary	Ca In situ	Benign	Uncertain Behavior	Unspecified Behavior
Neoplasm, neoplastic - *continued*							**Neoplasm, neoplastic** - *continued*						
Mackenrodt's ligament	C57.7	C79.82	D07.39	D28.7	D39.8	D49.59	mesothelial tissue — *see* Mesothelioma						
malar	C41.0	C79.51	—	D16.4-	D48.0	D49.2	mesothelioma — *see* Mesothelioma						
region — *see* Neoplasm, cheek							mesovarium	C57.1	C79.82	D07.39	D28.2	D39.8	D49.59
mammary gland — *see* Neoplasm, breast							metacarpus (any bone)	C40.1-	C79.51	—	D16.1-	—	—
mandible	C41.1	C79.51	—	D16.5-	D48.0	D49.2	metastatic NEC — *see also* Neoplasm, by site,						
alveolar							secondary	—	C79.9				
mucosa (carcinoma)	C03.1	C79.89	D00.03	D10.39	D37.09	D49.0	metatarsus (any bone)	C40.3-	C79.51	—	D16.3-	—	—
ridge or process	C41.1	C79.51	—	D16.5-	D48.0	D49.2	midbrain	C71.7	C79.31	—	D33.1	D43.1	D49.6
marrow (bone) NEC	C96.9	C79.52	—	—	D47.9	D49.89	milk duct — *see* Neoplasm, breast						
mastectomy site (skin) — *see also* Neoplasm, breast,							mons						
skin	C44.501	C79.2	—	—	—	—	pubis	C51.9	C79.82	D07.1	D28.0	D39.8	D49.59
specified as breast tissue	C50.8	C79.81	—	—	—	—	veneris	C51.9	C79.82	D07.1	D28.0	D39.8	D49.59
mastoid (air cells) (antrum) (cavity)	C30.1	C78.39	D02.3	D14.0	D38.5	D49.1	motor tract	C72.9	C79.49	—	D33.9	D43.9	D49.7
bone or process	C41.0	C79.51	—	D16.4-	D48.0	D49.2	brain	C71.9	C79.31	—	D33.2	D43.2	D49.6
maxilla, maxillary (superior)	C41.0	C79.51	—	D16.4-	D48.0	D49.2	cauda equina	C72.1	C79.49	—	D33.4	D43.4	D49.7
alveolar							spinal	C72.0	C79.49	—	D33.4	D43.4	D49.7
mucosa	C03.0	C79.89	D00.03	D10.39	D37.09	D49.0	mouth	C06.9	C79.89	D00.00	D10.30	D37.09	D49.0
ridge or process (carcinoma)	C41.0	C79.51	—	D16.4-	D48.0	D49.2	book-leaf	C06.89	C79.89	—	—	—	—
antrum	C31.0	C78.39	D02.3	D14.0	D38.5	D49.1	floor	C04.9	C79.89	D00.06	D10.2	D37.09	D49.0
carcinoma	C03.0	C79.51	—	—	—	—	anterior portion	C04.0	C79.89	D00.06	D10.2	D37.09	D49.0
inferior — *see* Neoplasm, mandible							lateral portion	C04.1	C79.89	D00.06	D10.2	D37.09	D49.0
sinus	C31.0	C78.39	D02.3	D14.0	D38.5	D49.1	overlapping lesion	C04.8	—	—	—	—	—
meatus external (ear) — *see also* Neoplasm, skin, ear	C44.20-	C79.2	D04.2-	D23.2-	D48.5	D49.2	overlapping NEC	C06.80	—	—	—	—	—
Meckel diverticulum, malignant	C17.3	C78.4	D01.49	D13.39	D37.2	D49.0	roof	C05.9	C79.89	D00.00	D10.39	D37.09	D49.0
mediastinum, mediastinal	C38.3	C78.1	—	D15.2	D38.3	D49.89	specified part NEC	C06.89	C79.89	D00.00	D10.39	D37.09	D49.0
anterior	C38.1	C78.1	—	D15.2	D38.3	D49.89	vestibule	C06.1	C79.89	D00.00	D10.39	D37.09	D49.0
posterior	C38.2	C78.1	—	D15.2	D38.3	D49.89	mucosa						
medulla							alveolar (ridge or process)	C03.9	C79.89	D00.03	D10.39	D37.09	D49.0
adrenal	C74.1-	C79.7-	D09.3	D35.0-	D44.1-	D49.7	lower	C03.1	C79.89	D00.03	D10.39	D37.09	D49.0
oblongata	C71.7	C79.31	—	D33.1	D43.1	D49.6	upper	C03.0	C79.89	D00.03	D10.39	D37.09	D49.0
meibomian gland	C44.10-	C79.2	D04.1-	D23.1-	D48.5	D49.2	buccal	C06.0	C79.89	D00.02	D10.39	D37.09	D49.0
basal cell carcinoma	C44.11-	—	—	—	—	—	cheek	C06.0	C79.89	D00.02	D10.39	D37.09	D49.0
specified type NEC	C44.19-	—	—	—	—	—	lip — *see* Neoplasm, lip, internal						
squamous cell carcinoma	C44.12-	—	—	—	—	—	nasal	C30.0	C78.39	D02.3	D14.0	D38.5	D49.1
melanoma — *see* Melanoma							oral	C06.0	C79.89	D00.02	D10.39	D37.09	D49.0
meninges	C70.9	C79.49	—	D32.9	D42.9	D49.7	Müllerian duct						
brain	C70.0	C79.32	—	D32.0	D42.0	D49.7	female	C57.7	C79.82	D07.39	D28.7	D39.8	D49.59
cerebral	C70.0	C79.32	—	D32.0	D42.0	D49.7	male	C63.7	C79.82	D07.69	D29.8	D40.8	D49.59
crainial	C70.0	C79.32	—	D32.0	D42.0	D49.7	muscle — *see also* Neoplasm, connective tissue						
intracranial	C70.0	C79.32	—	D32.0	D42.0	D49.7	extraocular	C69.6-	C79.49	D09.2-	D31.6-	D48.7	D49.89
spinal (cord)	C70.1	C79.49	—	D32.1	D42.1	D49.7	myocardium	C38.0	C79.89	—	D15.1	D48.7	D49.89
meniscus, knee joint (lateral) (medial)	C40.2-	C79.51	—	D16.2-	D48.0	D49.2	myometrium	C54.2	C79.82	D07.0	D26.1	D39.0	D49.59
Merkel cell — *see* Carcinoma, Merkel cell							myopericardium	C38.0	C79.89	—	D15.1	D48.7	D49.89
mesentery, mesenteric	C48.1	C78.6	—	D20.1	D48.4	D49.0	nabothian gland (follicle)	C53.0	C79.82	D06.0	D26.0	D39.0	D49.59
mesoappendix	C48.1	C78.6	—	D20.1	D48.4	D49.0	nail — *see also* Neoplasm, skin, limb	C44.90	C79.2	D04.9	D23.9	D48.5	D49.2
mesocolon	C48.1	C78.6	—	D20.1	D48.4	D49.0	finger — *see also* Neoplasm, skin, limb, upper	C44.60-	C79.2	D04.6-	D23.6-	D48.5	D49.2
mesopharynx — *see* Neoplasm, oropharynx							toe — *see also* Neoplasm, skin, limb, lower	C44.70-	C79.2	D04.7-	D23.7-	D48.5	D49.2
mesosalpinx	C57.1	C79.82	D07.39	D28.2	D39.8	D49.59	nares, naris (anterior) (posterior)	C30.0	C78.39	D02.3	D14.0	D38.5	D49.1

NEOPLASM TABLE

Neoplasm Table	Malignant Primary	Malignant Secondary	Ca In situ	Benign	Uncertain Behavior	Unspecified Behavior
Neoplasm, neoplastic - *continued*						
nasal — *see* Neoplasm, nose						
nasolabial groove — *see also* Neoplasm, skin, face	C44.309	C79.2	D04.39	D23.39	D48.5	D49.2
nasolacrimal duct	C69.5-	C79.49	D09.2-	D31.5-	D48.7	D49.89
nasopharynx, nasopharyngeal	C11.9	C79.89	D00.08	D10.6	D37.05	D49.0
floor	C11.3	C79.89	D00.08	D10.6	D37.05	D49.0
overlapping lesion	C11.8	—	—	—	—	—
roof	C11.0	C79.89	D00.08	D10.6	D37.05	D49.0
wall	C11.9	C79.89	D00.08	D10.6	D37.05	D49.0
anterior	C11.3	C79.89	D00.08	D10.6	D37.05	D49.0
lateral	C11.2	C79.89	D00.08	D10.6	D37.05	D49.0
posterior	C11.1	C79.89	D00.08	D10.6	D37.05	D49.0
superior	C11.0	C79.89	D00.08	D10.6	D37.05	D49.0
nates — *see also* Neoplasm, skin, trunk	C44.509	C79.2	D04.5	D23.5	D48.5	D49.2
neck NEC	C76.0	C79.89	D09.8	D36.7	D48.7	D49.89
skin	C44.40	—	—	—	—	—
basal cell carcinoma	C44.41	—	—	—	—	—
specified type NEC	C44.49	—	—	—	—	—
squamous cell carcinoma	C44.42	—	—	—	—	—
nerve (ganglion)	C47.9	C79.89	—	D36.10	D48.2	D49.2
abducens	C72.59	C79.49	—	D33.3	D43.3	D49.7
accessory (spinal)	C72.59	C79.49	—	D33.3	D43.3	D49.7
acoustic	C72.4-	C79.49	—	D33.3	D43.3	D49.7
auditory	C72.4-	C79.49	—	D33.3	D43.3	D49.7
autonomic NEC — *see also* Neoplasm, nerve, peripheral	C47.9	C79.89	—	D36.10	D48.2	D49.2
brachial	C47.1-	C79.89	—	D36.12	D48.2	D49.2
cranial	C72.50	C79.49	—	D33.3	D43.3	D49.7
specified NEC	C72.59	C79.49	—	D33.3	D43.3	D49.7
facial	C72.59	C79.49	—	D33.3	D43.3	D49.7
femoral	C47.2-	C79.89	—	D36.13	D48.2	D49.2
ganglion NEC — *see also* Neoplasm, nerve, peripheral	C47.9	C79.89	—	D36.10	D48.2	D49.2
glossopharyngeal	C72.59	C79.49	—	D33.3	D43.3	D49.7
hypoglossal	C72.59	C79.49	—	D33.3	D43.3	D49.7
intercostal	C47.3	C79.89	—	D36.14	D48.2	D49.2
lumbar	C47.6	C79.89	—	D36.17	D48.2	D49.2
median	C47.1-	C79.89	—	D36.12	D48.2	D49.2
obturator	C47.2-	C79.89	—	D36.13	D48.2	D49.2
oculomotor	C72.59	C79.49	—	D33.3	D43.3	D49.7
olfactory	C47.2-	C79.49	—	D33.3	D43.3	D49.7
optic	C72.3-	C79.49	—	D33.3	D43.3	D49.7
parasympathetic NEC	C47.9	C79.89	—	D36.10	D48.2	D49.2
peripheral NEC	C47.9	C79.89	—	D36.10	D48.2	D49.2
abdomen	C47.4	C79.89	—	D36.15	D48.2	D49.2
abdominal wall	C47.4	C79.89	—	D36.15	D48.2	D49.2
ankle	C47.2-	C79.89	—	D36.13	D48.2	D49.2
antecubital fossa or space	C47.1-	C79.89	—	D36.12	D48.2	D49.2
arm	C47.1-	C79.89	—	D36.12	D48.2	D49.2
auricle (ear)	C47.0	C79.89	—	D36.11	D48.2	D49.2
axilla	C47.3	C79.89	—	D36.12	D48.2	D49.2
back	C47.6	C79.89	—	D36.17	D48.2	D49.2
buttock	C47.5	C79.89	—	D36.16	D48.2	D49.2
calf	C47.2-	C79.89	—	D36.13	D48.2	D49.2
cervical region	C47.0	C79.89	—	D36.11	D48.2	D49.2
cheek	C47.0	C79.89	—	D36.11	D48.2	D49.2
chest (wall)	C47.3	C79.89	—	D36.14	D48.2	D49.2
chin	C47.0	C79.89	—	D36.11	D48.2	D49.2
ear (external)	C47.0	C79.89	—	D36.11	D48.2	D49.2
elbow	C47.1-	C79.89	—	D36.12	D48.2	D49.2
Neoplasm, neoplastic - *continued*						
nerve (ganglion) - *continued*	C47.9	C79.89	—	D36.10	D48.2	D49.2
peripheral NEC - *continued*	C47.9	C79.89	—	D36.10	D48.2	D49.2
extrarectal	C47.5	C79.89	—	D36.16	D48.2	D49.2
extremity	C47.9	C79.89	—	D36.10	D48.2	D49.2
lower	C47.2-	C79.89	—	D36.13	D48.2	D49.2
upper	C47.1-	C79.89	—	D36.12	D48.2	D49.2
eyelid	C47.0	C79.89	—	D36.11	D48.2	D49.2
face	C47.0	C79.89	—	D36.11	D48.2	D49.2
finger	C47.1-	C79.89	—	D36.12	D48.2	D49.2
flank	C47.6	C79.89	—	D36.17	D48.2	D49.2
foot	C47.2-	C79.89	—	D36.13	D48.2	D49.2
forearm	C47.1-	C79.89	—	D36.12	D48.2	D49.2
forehead	C47.0	C79.89	—	D36.11	D48.2	D49.2
gluteal region	C47.5	C79.89	—	D36.16	D48.2	D49.2
groin	C47.5	C79.89	—	D36.16	D48.2	D49.2
hand	C47.1-	C79.89	—	D36.12	D48.2	D49.2
head	C47.0	C79.89	—	D36.11	D48.2	D49.2
heel	C47.2-	C79.89	—	D36.13	D48.2	D49.2
hip	C47.2-	C79.89	—	D36.13	D48.2	D49.2
infraclavicular region	C47.3	C79.89	—	D36.14	D48.2	D49.2
inguinal (canal) (region)	C47.5	C79.89	—	D36.16	D48.2	D49.2
intrathoracic	C47.3	C79.89	—	D36.14	D48.2	D49.2
ischiorectal fossa	C47.5	C79.89	—	D36.16	D48.2	D49.2
knee	C47.2-	C79.89	—	D36.13	D48.2	D49.2
leg	C47.2-	C79.89	—	D36.13	D48.2	D49.2
limb NEC	C47.9	C79.89	—	D36.10	D48.2	D49.2
lower	C47.2	C79.89	—	D36.13	D48.2	D49.2
upper	C47.1	C79.89	—	D36.12	D48.2	D49.2
nates	C47.5	C79.89	—	D36.16	D48.2	D49.2
neck	C47.0	C79.89	—	D36.11	D48.2	D49.2
orbit	C69.6-	C79.49	—	D31.6-	D48.7	D49.2
pararectal	C47.5	C79.89	—	D36.16	D48.2	D49.2
paraurethral	C47.5	C79.89	—	D36.16	D48.2	D49.2
paravaginal	C47.5	C79.89	—	D36.16	D48.2	D49.2
pelvis (floor)	C47.5	C79.89	—	D36.16	D48.2	D49.2
pelvoabdominal	C47.8	C79.89	—	D36.17	D48.2	D49.2
perineum	C47.5	C79.89	—	D36.16	D48.2	D49.2
perirectal (tissue)	C47.5	C79.89	—	D36.16	D48.2	D49.2
periurethral (tissue)	C47.5	C79.89	—	D36.16	D48.2	D49.2
popliteal fossa or space	C47.2-	C79.89	—	D36.13	D48.2	D49.2
presacral	C47.5	C79.89	—	D36.16	D48.2	D49.2
pterygoid fossa	C47.0	C79.89	—	D36.11	D48.2	D49.2
rectovaginal septum or wall	C47.5	C79.89	—	D36.16	D48.2	D49.2
rectovesical	C47.5	C79.89	—	D36.16	D48.2	D49.2
sacrococcygeal region	C47.5	C79.89	—	D36.16	D48.2	D49.2
scalp	C47.0	C79.89	—	D36.11	D48.2	D49.2
scapular region	C47.3	C79.89	—	D36.14	D48.2	D49.2
shoulder	C47.1-	C79.89	—	D36.12	D48.2	D49.2
submental	C47.0	C79.89	—	D36.11	D48.2	D49.2
supraclavicular region	C47.0	C79.89	—	D36.11	D48.2	D49.2
temple	C47.0	C79.89	—	D36.11	D48.2	D49.2
temporal region	C47.0	C79.89	—	D36.11	D48.2	D49.2
thigh	C47.2-	C79.89	—	D36.13	D48.2	D49.2
thoracic (duct) (wall)	C47.3	C79.89	—	D36.14	D48.2	D49.2
thorax	C47.3	C79.89	—	D36.14	D48.2	D49.2
thumb	C47.1-	C79.89	—	D36.12	D48.2	D49.2
toe	C47.2-	C79.89	—	D36.13	D48.2	D49.2
trunk	C47.6	C79.89	—	D36.17	D48.2	D49.2
umbilicus	C47.4	C79.89	—	D36.15	D48.2	D49.2
vesicorectal	C47.5	C79.89	—	D36.16	D48.2	D49.2
wrist	C47.1-	C79.89	—	D36.12	D48.2	D49.2

NEOPLASM TABLE

Neoplasm Table	Malignant Primary	Malignant Secondary	Ca In situ	Benign	Uncertain Behavior	Unspecified Behavior
Neoplasm, neoplastic - continued						
nerve (ganglion) - continued ..	C47.9	C79.89	—	D36.10	D48.2	D49.2
radial	C47.1-	C79.89	—	D36.12	D48.2	D49.2
sacral	C47.5	C79.89	—	D36.16	D48.2	D49.2
sciatic	C47.2-	C79.89	—	D36.13	D48.2	D49.2
spinal NEC	C47.9	C79.89	—	D36.10	D48.2	D49.2
accessory	C72.59	C79.49	—	D33.3	D43.3	D49.7
sympathetic NEC — see also Neoplasm, nerve, peripheral	C47.9	C79.89	—	D36.10	D48.2	D49.2
trigeminal	C72.59	C79.49	—	D33.3	D43.3	D49.7
trochlear	C72.59	C79.49	—	D33.3	D43.3	D49.7
ulnar	C47.1-	C79.89	—	D36.12	D48.2	D49.2
vagus	C72.59	C79.49	—	D33.3	D43.3	D49.7
nervous system (central)	C72.9	C79.40	—	D33.9	D43.9	D49.7
autonomic — see Neoplasm, nerve, peripheral						
parasympathetic — see Neoplasm, nerve, peripheral						
specified site NEC	—	C79.49	—	D33.7	D43.8	—
sympathetic — see Neoplasm, nerve, peripheral						
nevus — see Nevus						
nipple	C50.0-	C79.81	D05.-	D24.-	—	—
nose, nasal	C76.0	C79.89	D09.8	D36.7	D48.7	D49.89
ala (external) (nasi) — see also Neoplasm, nose, skin	C44.301	C79.2	D04.39	D23.39	D48.5	D49.2
bone	C41.0	C79.51	—	D16.4-	D48.0	D49.2
cartilage	C30.0	C78.39	D02.3	D14.0	D38.5	D49.1
cavity	C30.0	C78.39	D02.3	D14.0	D38.5	D49.1
choana	C11.3	C79.89	D00.08	D10.6	D37.05	D49.0
external (skin) — see also Neoplasm, nose, skin	C44.301	C79.2	D04.39	D23.39	D48.5	D49.2
fossa	C30.0	C78.39	D02.3	D14.0	D38.5	D49.1
internal	C30.0	C78.39	D02.3	D14.0	D38.5	D49.1
mucosa	C30.0	C78.39	D02.3	D14.0	D38.5	D49.1
septum	C30.0	C78.39	D02.3	D14.0	D38.5	D49.1
posterior margin	C11.3	C79.89	D00.08	D10.6	D37.05	D49.0
sinus — see Neoplasm, sinus						
skin	C44.301	C79.2	D04.39	D23.39	D48.5	D49.2
basal cell carcinoma	C44.311	—	—	—	—	—
specified type NEC	C44.391	—	—	—	—	—
squamous cell carcinoma	C44.321	—	—	—	—	—
turbinate (mucosa)	C30.0	C78.39	D02.3	D14.0	D38.5	D49.1
bone	C41.0	C79.51	—	D16.4-	D48.0	D49.2
vestibule	C30.0	C78.39	D02.3	D14.0	D38.5	D49.1
nostril	C30.0	C78.39	D02.3	D14.0	D38.5	D49.1
nucleus pulposus	C41.2	C79.51	—	D16.6	D48.0	D49.2
occipital						
bone	C41.0	C79.51	—	D16.4-	D48.0	D49.2
lobe or pole, brain	C71.4	C79.31	—	D33.0	D43.0	D49.6
odontogenic — see Neoplasm, jaw bone						
olfactory nerve or bulb	C72.2-	C79.49	—	D33.3	D43.3	D49.7
olive (brain)	C71.7	C79.31	—	D33.1	D43.1	D49.6
omentum	C48.1	C78.6	—	D20.1	D48.4	D49.0

Neoplasm Table	Malignant Primary	Malignant Secondary	Ca In situ	Benign	Uncertain Behavior	Unspecified Behavior
Neoplasm, neoplastic - continued						
operculum (brain)	C71.0	C79.31	—	D33.0	D43.0	D49.6
optic nerve, chiasm, or tract	C72.3-	C79.49	—	D33.3	D43.3	D49.7
oral (cavity)	C06.9	C79.89	D00.00	D10.30	D37.09	D49.0
ill-defined	C14.8	C79.89	D00.00	D10.30	D37.09	D49.0
mucosa	C06.0	C79.89	D00.02	D10.39	D37.09	D49.0
orbit	C69.6-	C79.49	D09.2-	D31.6-	D48.7	D49.89
autonomic nerve	C69.6-	C79.49	—	D31.6-	D48.7	D49.2
bone	C41.0	C79.51	—	D16.4-	D48.0	D49.2
eye	C69.6-	C79.49	D09.2-	D31.6-	D48.7	D49.89
peripheral nerves	C69.6-	C79.49	—	D31.6-	D48.7	D49.2
soft parts	C69.6-	C79.49	D09.2-	D31.6-	D48.7	D49.89
organ of Zuckerkandl	C75.5	C79.89	—	D35.6	D44.7	D49.7
oropharynx	C10.9	C79.89	D00.08	D10.5	D37.05	D49.0
branchial cleft (vestige)	C10.4	C79.89	D00.08	D10.5	D37.05	D49.0
junctional region	C10.8	C79.89	D00.08	D10.5	D37.05	D49.0
lateral wall	C10.2	C79.89	D00.08	D10.5	D37.05	D49.0
overlapping lesion	C10.8	—	—	—	—	—
pillars or fauces	C09.1	C79.89	D00.08	D10.5	D37.05	D49.0
posterior wall	C10.3	C79.89	D00.08	D10.5	D37.05	D49.0
vallecula	C10.0	C79.89	D00.08	D10.5	D37.05	D49.0
os						
external	C53.1	C79.82	D06.1	D26.0	D39.0	D49.59
internal	C53.0	C79.82	D06.0	D26.0	D39.0	D49.59
ovary	C56.-	C79.6-	D07.39	D27.-	D39.1-	D49.59
oviduct	C57.0-	C79.82	D07.39	D28.2	D39.8	D49.59
palate	C05.9	C79.89	D00.00	D10.39	D37.09	D49.0
hard	C05.0	C79.89	D00.05	D10.39	D37.09	D49.0
junction of hard and soft palate	C05.9	C79.89	D00.00	D10.39	D37.09	D49.0
overlapping lesions	C05.8	—	—	—	—	—
soft	C05.1	C79.89	D00.04	D10.39	D37.09	D49.0
nasopharyngeal surface	C11.3	C79.89	D00.08	D10.6	D37.05	D49.0
posterior surface	C11.3	C79.89	D00.08	D10.6	D37.05	D49.0
superior surface	C11.3	C79.89	D00.08	D10.6	D37.05	D49.0
palatoglossal arch	C09.1	C79.89	D00.00	D10.5	D37.09	D49.0
palatopharyngeal arch	C09.1	C79.89	D00.00	D10.5	D37.09	D49.0
pallium	C71.0	C79.31	—	D33.0	D43.0	D49.6
palpebra	C44.10-	C79.2	D04.1-	D23.1-	D48.5	D49.2
basal cell carcinoma	C44.11-	—	—	—	—	—
specified type NEC	C44.19-	—	—	—	—	—
squamous cell carcinoma	C44.12-	—	—	—	—	—
pancreas	C25.9	C78.89	D01.7	D13.6	D37.8	D49.0
body	C25.1	C78.89	D01.7	D13.6	D37.8	D49.0
duct (of Santorini) (of Wirsung)	C25.3	C78.89	D01.7	D13.6	D37.8	D49.0
ectopic tissue	C25.7	C78.89	—	D13.6	D37.8	D49.0
head	C25.0	C78.89	D01.7	D13.6	D37.8	D49.0
islet cells	C25.4	C78.89	D01.7	D13.7	D37.8	D49.0
neck	C25.7	C78.89	D01.7	D13.6	D37.8	D49.0
overlapping lesion	C25.8	—	—	—	—	—
tail	C25.2	C78.89	D01.7	D13.6	D37.8	D49.0
para-aortic body	C75.5	C79.89	—	D35.6	D44.7	D49.7
paraganglion NEC	C75.5	C79.89	—	D35.6	D44.7	D49.7
parametrium	C57.3	C79.82	—	D28.2	D39.8	D49.59
paranephric	C48.0	C78.6	—	D20.0	D48.3	D49.0
pararectal	C76.3	C79.89	—	D36.7	D48.7	D49.89
parasagittal (region)	C76.0	C79.89	D09.8	D36.7	D48.7	D49.89
parasellar	C72.9	C79.49	—	D33.9	D43.8	D49.7
parathyroid (gland)	C75.0	C79.89	D09.3	D35.1	D44.2	D49.7
paraurethral	C76.3	C79.89	—	D36.7	D48.7	D49.89
gland	C68.1	C79.19	D09.19	D30.8	D41.8	D49.59

Neoplasm Table	Malignant Primary	Malignant Secondary	Ca In situ	Benign	Uncertain Behavior	Unspecified Behavior
Neoplasm, neoplastic - *continued*						
paravaginal	C76.3	C79.89	—	D36.7	D48.7	D49.89
parenchyma, kidney	C64.-	C79.0-	D09.19	D30.0-	D41.0-	D49.51-
parietal						
bone	C41.0	C79.51	—	D16.4-	D48.0	D49.2
lobe, brain	C71.3	C79.31	—	D33.0	D43.0	D49.6
paroophoron	C57.1	C79.82	D07.39	D28.2	D39.8	D49.59
parotid (duct) (gland)	C07	C79.89	D00.00	D11.0	D37.030	D49.0
parovarium	C57.1	C79.82	D07.39	D28.2	D39.8	D49.59
patella	C40.20	C79.51	—	—	—	—
peduncle, cerebral	C71.7	C79.31	—	D33.1	D43.1	D49.6
pelvirectal junction	C19	C78.5	D01.1	D12.7	D37.5	D49.0
pelvis, pelvic	C76.3	C79.89	D09.8	D36.7	D48.7	D49.89
bone	C41.4	C79.51	—	D16.8	D48.0	D49.2
floor	C76.3	C79.89	D09.8	D36.7	D48.7	D49.89
renal	C65.-	C79.0-	D09.19	D30.1-	D41.1-	D49.51-
viscera	C76.3	C79.89	D09.8	D36.7	D48.7	D49.89
wall	C76.3	C79.89	D09.8	D36.7	D48.7	D49.89
pelvo-abdominal	C76.8	C79.89	D09.8	D36.7	D48.7	D49.89
penis	C60.9	C79.82	D07.4	D29.0	D40.8	D49.59
body	C60.2	C79.82	D07.4	D29.0	D40.8	D49.59
corpus (cavernosum)	C60.2	C79.82	D07.4	D29.0	D40.8	D49.59
glans	C60.1	C79.82	D07.4	D29.0	D40.8	D49.59
overlapping sites	C60.8					
skin NEC	C60.9	C79.82	D07.4	D29.0	D40.8	D49.59
periadrenal (tissue)	C48.0	C78.6	—	D20.0	D48.3	D49.0
perianal (skin) — *see also*						
Neoplasm, anus, skin	C44.500	C79.2	D04.5	D23.5	D48.5	D49.2
pericardium	C38.0	C79.89	—	D15.1	D48.7	D49.89
perinephric	C48.0	C78.6	—	D20.0	D48.3	D49.0
perineum	C76.3	C79.89	D09.8	D36.7	D48.7	D49.89
periodontal tissue NEC	C03.9	C79.89	D00.03	D10.39	D37.09	D49.0
periosteum — *see Neoplasm, bone*						
peripancreatic	C48.0	C78.6	—	D20.0	D48.3	D49.0
peripheral nerve NEC	C47.9	C79.89	—	D36.10	D48.2	D49.2
perirectal (tissue)	C76.3	C79.89	—	D36.7	D48.7	D49.89
perirenal (tissue)	C48.0	C78.6	—	D20.0	D48.3	D49.0
peritoneum, peritoneal (cavity)	C48.2	C78.6	—	D20.1	D48.4	D49.0
benign mesothelial tissue — *see Mesothelioma, benign*						
overlapping lesion	C48.8	—	—	—	—	—
with digestive organs	C26.9					
parietal	C48.1	C78.6	—	D20.1	D48.4	D49.0
pelvic	C48.1	C78.6	—	D20.1	D48.4	D49.0
specified part NEC	C48.1	C78.6	—	D20.1	D48.4	D49.0
peritonsillar (tissue)	C76.0	C79.89	D09.8	D36.7	D48.7	D49.89
periurethral tissue	C76.3	C79.89	—	D36.7	D48.7	D49.89
phalanges						
foot	C40.3-	C79.51	—	D16.3-	—	—
hand	C40.1-	C79.51	—	D16.1-	—	—
pharynx, pharyngeal	C14.0	C79.89	D00.08	D10.9	D37.05	D49.0
bursa	C11.1	C79.89	D00.08	D10.6	D37.05	D49.0
fornix	C11.3	C79.89	D00.08	D10.6	D37.05	D49.0
recess	C11.2	C79.89	D00.08	D10.6	D37.05	D49.0
region	C14.0	C79.89	D00.08	D10.9	D37.05	D49.0
tonsil	C11.1	C79.89	D00.08	D10.6	D37.05	D49.0
wall (lateral) (posterior)	C14.0	C79.89	D00.08	D10.9	D37.05	D49.0

Neoplasm Table	Malignant Primary	Malignant Secondary	Ca In situ	Benign	Uncertain Behavior	Unspecified Behavior
Neoplasm, neoplastic - *continued*						
pia mater	C70.9	C79.40	—	D32.9	D42.9	D49.7
cerebral	C70.0	C79.32	—	D32.0	D42.0	D49.7
cranial	C70.0	C79.32	—	D32.0	D42.0	D49.7
spinal	C70.1	C79.49	—	D32.1	D42.1	D49.7
pillars of fauces	C09.1	C79.89	D00.08	D10.5	D37.05	D49.0
pineal (body) (gland)	C75.3	C79.89	D09.3	D35.4	D44.5	D49.7
pinna (ear) NEC — *see also*						
Neoplasm, skin, ear	C44.20-	C79.2	D04.2-	D23.2-	D48.5	D49.2
piriform fossa or sinus	C12	C79.89	D00.08	D10.7	D37.05	D49.0
pituitary (body) (fossa) (gland) (lobe)	C75.1	C79.89	D09.3	D35.2	D44.3	D49.7
placenta	C58	C79.82	D07.0	D26.7	D39.2	D49.59
pleura, pleural (cavity)	C38.4	C78.2	—	D19.0	D38.2	D49.1
overlapping lesion with heart or mediastinum	C38.8	—	—	—	—	—
parietal	C38.4	C78.2	—	D19.0	D38.2	D49.1
visceral	C38.4	C78.2	—	D19.0	D38.2	D49.1
plexus						
brachial	C47.1-	C79.89	—	D36.12	D48.2	D49.2
cervical	C47.0	C79.89	—	D36.11	D48.2	D49.2
choroid	C71.5	C79.31	—	D33.0	D43.0	D49.6
lumbosacral	C47.5	C79.89	—	D36.16	D48.2	D49.2
sacral	C47.5	C79.89	—	D36.16	D48.2	D49.2
pluriendocrine	C75.8	C79.89	D09.3	D35.7	D44.9	D49.7
pole						
frontal	C71.1	C79.31	—	D33.0	D43.0	D49.6
occipital	C71.4	C79.31	—	D33.0	D43.0	D49.6
pons (varolii)	C71.7	C79.31	—	D33.1	D43.1	D49.6
popliteal fossa or space	C76.5-	C79.89	D04.7-	D36.7	D48.7	D49.89
postcricoid (region)	C13.0	C79.89	D00.08	D10.7	D37.05	D49.0
posterior fossa (cranial)	C71.9	C79.31	—	D33.2	D43.2	D49.6
postnasal space	C11.9	C79.89	D00.08	D10.6	D37.05	D49.0
prepuce	C60.0	C79.82	D07.4	D29.0	D40.8	D49.59
prepylorus	C16.4	C78.89	D00.2	D13.1	D37.1	D49.0
presacral (region)	C76.3	C79.89	—	D36.7	D48.7	D49.89
prostate (gland)	C61	C79.82	D07.5	D29.1	D40.0	D49.59
utricle	C68.0	C79.19	D09.19	D30.4	D41.3	D49.59
pterygoid fossa	C49.0	C79.89	—	D21.0	D48.1	D49.2
pubic bone	C41.4	C79.51	—	D16.8	D48.0	D49.2
pudenda, pudendum (female)	C51.9	C79.82	D07.1	D28.0	D39.8	D49.59
pulmonary — *see also*						
Neoplasm, lung	C34.9-	C78.0-	D02.2-	D14.3-	D38.1	D49.1
putamen	C71.0	C79.31	—	D33.0	D43.0	D49.6
pyloric						
antrum	C16.3	C78.89	D00.2	D13.1	D37.1	D49.0
canal	C16.4	C78.89	D00.2	D13.1	D37.1	D49.0
pylorus	C16.4	C78.89	D00.2	D13.1	D37.1	D49.0
pyramid (brain)	C71.7	C79.31	—	D33.1	D43.1	D49.6
pyriform fossa or sinus	C12	C79.89	D00.08	D10.7	D37.05	D49.0
radius (any part)	C40.0-	C79.51	—	D16.0-	—	—
Rathke's pouch	C75.1	C79.89	D09.3	D35.2	D44.3	D49.7
rectosigmoid (junction)	C19	C78.5	D01.1	D12.7	D37.5	D49.0
overlapping lesion with anus or rectum	C21.8	—	—	—	—	—
rectouterine pouch	C48.1	C78.6	—	D20.1	D48.4	D49.0
rectovaginal septum or wall	C76.3	C79.89	D09.8	D36.7	D48.7	D49.89
rectovesical septum	C76.3	C79.89	D09.8	D36.7	D48.7	D49.89

NEOPLASM TABLE

Neoplasm Table	Malignant Primary	Malignant Secondary	Ca In situ	Benign	Uncertain Behavior	Unspecified Behavior
Neoplasm, neoplastic - *continued*						
rectum (ampulla)	C20	C78.5	D01.2	D12.8	D37.5	D49.0
and colon	C19	C78.5	D01.1	D12.7	D37.5	D49.0
overlapping lesion with anus or rectosigmoid junction	C21.8	—	—	—	—	—
renal	C64.-	C79.0-	D09.19	D30.0-	D41.0-	D49.51-
calyx	C65.-	C79.0-	D09.19	D30.1-	D41.1-	D49.51-
hilus	C65.-	C79.0-	D09.19	D30.1-	D41.1-	D49.51-
parenchyma	C64.-	C79.0-	D09.19	D30.0-	D41.0-	D49.51-
pelvis	C65.-	C79.0-	D09.19	D30.1-	D41.1-	D49.51-
respiratory						
organs or system NEC	C39.9	C78.30	D02.4	D14.4	D38.6	D49.1
tract NEC	C39.9	C78.30	D02.4	D14.4	D38.5	D49.1
upper	C39.0	C78.30	D02.4	D14.4	D38.5	D49.1
retina	C69.2-	C79.49	D09.2-	D31.2-	D48.7	D49.81
retrobulbar	C69.6-	C79.49	—	D31.6-	D48.7	D49.89
retrocecal	C48.0	C78.6	—	D20.0	D48.3	D49.0
retromolar (area) (triangle) (trigone)	C06.2	C79.89	D00.00	D10.39	D37.09	D49.0
retro-orbital	C76.0	C79.89	D09.8	D36.7	D48.7	D49.89
retroperitoneal (space) (tissue)	C48.0	C78.6	—	D20.0	D48.3	D49.0
retroperitoneum	C48.0	C78.6	—	D20.0	D48.3	D49.0
retropharyngeal	C14.0	C79.89	D00.08	D10.9	D37.05	D49.0
retrovesical (septum)	C76.3	C79.89	D09.8	D36.7	D48.7	D49.89
rhinencephalon	C71.0	C79.31	—	D33.0	D43.0	D49.6
rib	C41.3	C79.51	—	D16.7	D48.0	D49.2
Rosenmüller's fossa	C11.2	C79.89	D00.08	D10.6	D37.05	D49.0
round ligament	C57.2	C79.82	—	D28.2	D39.8	D49.59
sacrococcyx, sacrococcygeal	C41.4	C79.51	—	D16.8	D48.0	D49.2
region	C76.3	C79.89	D09.8	D36.7	D48.7	D49.89
sacrouterine ligament	C57.3	C79.82	—	D28.2	D39.8	D49.59
sacrum, sacral (vertebra)	C41.4	C79.51	—	D16.8	D48.0	D49.2
salivary gland or duct (major)	C08.9	C79.89	D00.00	D11.9	D37.039	D49.0
minor NEC	C06.9	C79.89	D00.00	D10.39	D37.04	D49.0
overlapping lesion	C08.9	—	—	—	—	—
parotid	C07	C79.89	D00.00	D11.0	D37.030	D49.0
pluriglandular	C08.9	C79.89	D00.00	D11.9	D37.039	D49.0
sublingual	C08.1	C79.89	D00.00	D11.7	D37.031	D49.0
submandibular	C08.0	C79.89	D00.00	D11.7	D37.032	D49.0
submaxillary	C08.0	C79.89	D00.00	D11.7	D37.032	D49.0
salpinx (uterine)	C57.0-	C79.82	D07.39	D28.2	D39.8	D49.59
Santorini's duct	C25.3	C78.89	D01.7	D13.6	D37.8	D49.0
scalp	C44.40	C79.2	D04.4	D23.4	D48.5	D49.2
basal cell carcinoma	C44.41	—	—	—	—	—
specified type NEC	C44.49	—	—	—	—	—
squamous cell carcinoma	C44.42	—	—	—	—	—
scapula (any part)	C40.0-	C79.51	—	D16.0-	—	—
scapular region	C76.1	C79.89	D09.8	D36.7	D48.7	D49.89
scar NEC — *see also* Neoplasm, skin, by site	C44.90	C79.2	D04.9	D23.9	D48.5	D49.2
sciatic nerve	C47.2-	C79.89	—	D36.13	D48.2	D49.2
sclera	C69.4-	C79.49	D09.2-	D31.4-	D48.7	D49.89
scrotum (skin)	C63.2	C79.82	D07.61	D29.4	D40.8	D49.59
sebaceous gland — *see* Neoplasm, skin						
sella turcica	C75.1	C79.89	D09.3	D35.2	D44.3	D49.7
bone	C41.0	C79.51	—	D16.4-	D48.0	D49.2
semilunar cartilage (knee)	C40.2-	C79.51	—	D16.2-	D48.0	D49.2
seminal vesicle	C63.7	C79.82	D07.69	D29.8	D40.8	D49.59

Neoplasm Table	Malignant Primary	Malignant Secondary	Ca In situ	Benign	Uncertain Behavior	Unspecified Behavior
Neoplasm, neoplastic - *continued*						
septum						
nasal	C30.0	C78.39	D02.3	D14.0	D38.5	D49.1
posterior margin	C11.3	C79.89	D00.08	D10.6	D37.05	D49.0
rectovaginal	C76.3	C79.89	D09.8	D36.7	D48.7	D49.89
rectovesical	C76.3	C79.89	D09.8	D36.7	D48.7	D49.89
urethrovaginal	C57.9	C79.82	D07.30	D28.9	D39.9	D49.59
vesicovaginal	C57.9	C79.82	D07.30	D28.9	D39.9	D49.59
shoulder NEC	C76.4-	C79.89	D04.6-	D36.7	D48.7	D49.89
sigmoid flexure (lower) (upper)	C18.7	C78.5	D01.0	D12.5	D37.4	D49.0
sinus (accessory)	C31.9	C78.39	D02.3	D14.0	D38.5	D49.1
bone (any)	C41.0	C79.51	—	D16.4-	D48.0	D49.2
ethmoidal	C31.1	C78.39	D02.3	D14.0	D38.5	D49.1
frontal	C31.2	C78.39	D02.3	D14.0	D38.5	D49.1
maxillary	C31.0	C78.39	D02.3	D14.0	D38.5	D49.1
nasal, paranasal NEC	C31.9	C78.39	D02.3	D14.0	D38.5	D49.1
overlapping lesion	C31.8	—	—	—	—	—
pyriform	C12	C79.89	D00.08	D10.7	D37.05	D49.0
sphenoid	C31.3	C78.39	D02.3	D14.0	D38.5	D49.1
skeleton, skeletal NEC	C41.9	C79.51	—	D16.9-	D48.0	D49.2
Skene's gland	C68.1	C79.19	D09.19	D30.8	D41.8	D49.59
skin NOS	C44.90	C79.2	D04.9	D23.9	D48.5	D49.2
abdominal wall	C44.509	C79.2	D04.5	D23.5	D48.5	D49.2
basal cell carcinoma	C44.519	—	—	—	—	—
specified type NEC	C44.599	—	—	—	—	—
squamous cell carcinoma	C44.529	—	—	—	—	—
ala nasi — *see also* Neoplasm, nose, skin	C44.301	C79.2	D04.39	D23.39	D48.5	D49.2
ankle — *see also* Neoplasm, skin, limb, lower	C44.70-	C79.2	D04.7-	D23.7-	D48.5	D49.2
antecubital space — *see also* Neoplasm, skin, limb, upper	C44.60-	C79.2	D04.6-	D23.6-	D48.5	D49.2
anus	C44.500	C79.2	D04.5	D23.5	D48.5	D49.2
basal cell carcinoma	C44.510	—	—	—	—	—
specified type NEC	C44.590	—	—	—	—	—
squamous cell carcinoma	C44.520	—	—	—	—	—
arm — *see also* Neoplasm, skin, limb, upper	C44.60-	C79.2	D04.6-	D23.6-	D48.5	D49.2
auditory canal (external) — *see also* Neoplasm, skin, ear	C44.20-	C79.2	D04.2-	D23.2-	D48.5	D49.2
auricle (ear) — *see also* Neoplasm, skin, ear	C44.20-	C79.2	D04.2-	D23.2-	D48.5	D49.2
auricular canal (external) — *see also* Neoplasm, skin, ear	C44.20-	C79.2	D04.2-	D23.2-	D48.5	D49.2
axilla, axillary fold — *see also* Neoplasm, skin, trunk	C44.509	C79.2	D04.5	D23.5	D48.5	D49.2
back — *see also* Neoplasm, skin, trunk	C44.509	C79.2	D04.5	D23.5	D48.5	D49.2
basal cell carcinoma	C44.91	—	—	—	—	—
breast	C44.501	C79.2	D04.5	D23.5	D48.5	D49.2
basal cell carcinoma	C44.511	—	—	—	—	—
specified type NEC	C44.591	—	—	—	—	—
squamous cell carcinoma	C44.521	—	—	—	—	—
brow — *see also* Neoplasm, skin, face	C44.309	C79.2	D04.39	D23.39	D48.5	D49.2
buttock — *see also* Neoplasm, skin, trunk	C44.509	C79.2	D04.5	D23.5	D48.5	D49.2

NEOPLASM TABLE

Neoplasm Table	Malignant Primary	Malignant Secondary	Ca In situ	Benign	Uncertain Behavior	Unspecified Behavior
Neoplasm, neoplastic - *continued*						
skin NOS - *continued*	C44.90	C79.2	D04.9	D23.9	D48.5	D49.2
calf — *see also* Neoplasm, skin, limb, lower	C44.70-	C79.2	D04.7-	D23.7-	D48.5	D49.2
canthus (eye) (inner) (outer)	C44.10-	C79.2	D04.1-	D23.1-	D48.5	D49.2
basal cell carcinoma	C44.11-	—	—	—	—	—
specified type NEC	C44.19-	—	—	—	—	—
squamous cell carcinoma	C44.12-	—	—	—	—	—
cervical region — *see also* Neoplasm, skin, neck	C44.40	C79.2	D04.4	D23.4	D48.5	D49.2
cheek (external) — *see also* Neoplasm, skin, face	C44.309	C79.2	D04.39	D23.39	D48.5	D49.2
chest (wall) — *see also* Neoplasm, skin, trunk	C44.509	C79.2	D04.5	D23.5	D48.5	D49.2
chin — *see also* Neoplasm, skin, face	C44.309	C79.2	D04.39	D23.39	D48.5	D49.2
clavicular area — *see also* Neoplasm, skin, trunk	C44.509	C79.2	D04.5	D23.5	D48.5	D49.2
clitoris	C51.2	C79.82	D07.1	D28.0	D39.8	D49.59
columnella — *see also* Neoplasm, skin, face	C44.309	C79.2	D04.39	D23.39	D48.5	D49.2
concha — *see also* Neoplasm, skin, ear	C44.20-	C79.2	D04.2-	D23.2-	D48.5	D49.2
ear (external)	C44.20-	C79.2	D04.2-	D23.2-	D48.5	D49.2
basal cell carcinoma	C44.21-	—	—	—	—	—
specified type NEC	C44.29-	—	—	—	—	—
squamous cell carcinoma	C44.22-	—	—	—	—	—
elbow — *see also* Neoplasm, skin, limb, upper	C44.60-	C79.2	D04.6-	D23.6-	D48.5	D49.2
eyebrow — *see also* Neoplasm, skin, face	C44.309	C79.2	D04.39	D23.39	D48.5	D49.2
eyelid	C44.10-	C79.2	D04.1-	D23.1-	D48.5	D49.2
basal cell carcinoma	C44.11-	—	—	—	—	—
specified type NEC	C44.19-	—	—	—	—	—
squamous cell carcinoma	C44.12-	—	—	—	—	—
face NOS	C44.300	C79.2	D04.30	D23.30	D48.5	D49.2
basal cell carcinoma	C44.310	—	—	—	—	—
specified type NEC	C44.390	—	—	—	—	—
squamous cell carcinoma	C44.320	—	—	—	—	—
female genital organs (external)	C51.9	C79.82	D07.1	D28.0	D39.8	D49.59
clitoris	C51.2	C79.82	D07.1	D28.0	D39.8	D49.59
labium NEC	C51.9	C79.82	D07.1	D28.0	D39.8	D49.59
majus	C51.0	C79.82	D07.1	D28.0	D39.8	D49.59
minus	C51.1	C79.82	D07.1	D28.0	D39.8	D49.59
pudendum	C51.9	C79.82	D07.1	D28.0	D39.8	D49.59
vulva	C51.9	C79.82	D07.1	D28.0	D39.8	D49.59
finger — *see also* Neoplasm, skin, limb, upper	C44.60-	C79.2	D04.6-	D23.6-	D48.5	D49.2
flank — *see also* Neoplasm, skin, trunk	C44.509	C79.2	D04.5	D23.5	D48.5	D49.2
foot — *see also* Neoplasm, skin, limb, lower	C44.70-	C79.2	D04.7-	D23.7-	D48.5	D49.2
forearm — *see also* Neoplasm, skin, limb, upper	C44.60-	C79.2	D04.6-	D23.6-	D48.5	D49.2
forehead — *see also* Neoplasm, skin, face	C44.309	C79.2	D04.39	D23.39	D48.5	D49.2
glabella — *see also* Neoplasm, skin, face	C44.309	C79.2	D04.39	D23.39	D48.5	D49.2
gluteal region — *see also* Neoplasm, skin, trunk	C44.509	C79.2	D04.5	D23.5	D48.5	D49.2
Neoplasm, neoplastic - *continued*						
skin NOS - *continued*	C44.90	C79.2	D04.9	D23.9	D48.5	D49.2
groin — *see also* Neoplasm, skin, trunk	C44.509	C79.2	D04.5	D23.5	D48.5	D49.2
hand — *see also* Neoplasm, skin, limb, upper	C44.60-	C79.2	D04.6-	D23.6-	D48.5	D49.2
head NEC — *see also* Neoplasm, skin, scalp	C44.40	C79.2	D04.4	D23.4	D48.5	D49.2
heel — *see also* Neoplasm, skin, limb, lower	C44.70-	C79.2	D04.7-	D23.7-	D48.5	D49.2
helix — *see also* Neoplasm, skin, ear	C44.20-	C79.2	D04.2-	D23.2-	D48.5	D49.2
hip — *see also* Neoplasm, skin, limb, lower	C44.70-	C79.2	D04.7-	D23.7-	D48.5	D49.2
infraclavicular region — *see also* Neoplasm, skin, trunk	C44.509	C79.2	D04.5	D23.5	D48.5	D49.2
inguinal region — *see also* Neoplasm, skin, trunk	C44.509	C79.2	D04.5	D23.5	D48.5	D49.2
jaw — *see also* Neoplasm, skin, face	C44.309	C79.2	D04.39	D23.39	D48.5	D49.2
Kaposi's sarcoma — *see* Kaposi's, sarcoma, skin						
knee — *see also* Neoplasm, skin, limb, lower	C44.70-	C79.2	D04.7-	D23.7-	D48.5	D49.2
labia						
majora	C51.0	C79.82	D07.1	D28.0	D39.8	D49.59
minora	C51.1	C79.82	D07.1	D28.0	D39.8	D49.59
leg — *see also* Neoplasm, skin, limb, lower	C44.70-	C79.2	D04.7-	D23.7-	D48.5	D49.2
lid (lower) (upper)	C44.10-	C79.2	D04.1-	D23.1-	D48.5	D49.2
basal cell carcinoma	C44.11-	—	—	—	—	—
specified type NEC	C44.19-	—	—	—	—	—
squamous cell carcinoma	C44.12-	—	—	—	—	—
limb NEC	C44.90	C79.2	D04.9	D23.9	D48.5	D49.2
basal cell carcinoma	C44.91	—	—	—	—	—
lower	C44.70-	C79.2	D04.7-	D23.7-	D48.5	D49.2
basal cell carcinoma	C44.71-	—	—	—	—	—
specified type NEC	C44.79-	—	—	—	—	—
squamous cell carcinoma	C44.72-	—	—	—	—	—
upper	C44.60-	C79.2	D04.6-	D23.6-	D48.5	D49.2
basal cell carcinoma	C44.61-	—	—	—	—	—
specified type NEC	C44.69-	—	—	—	—	—
squamous cell carcinoma	C44.62-	—	—	—	—	—
lip (lower) (upper)	C44.00	C79.2	D04.0	D23.0	D48.5	D49.2
basal cell carcinoma	C44.01	—	—	—	—	—
specified type NEC	C44.09	—	—	—	—	—
squamous cell carcinoma	C44.02	—	—	—	—	—
male genital organs	C63.9	C79.82	D07.60	D29.9	D40.8	D49.59
penis	C60.9	C79.82	D07.4	D29.0	D40.8	D49.59
prepuce	C60.0	C79.82	D07.4	D29.0	D40.8	D49.59
scrotum	C63.2	C79.82	D07.61	D29.4	D40.8	D49.59
mastectomy site (skin) — *see also* Neoplasm, skin, breast	C44.501	C79.2	—	—	—	—
specified as breast tissue	C50.8-	C79.81	—	—	—	—
meatus, acoustic (external) — *see also* Neoplasm, skin, ear	C44.20-	C79.2	D04.2-	D23.2-	D48.5	D49.2

Neoplasm, neoplastic - continued

Neoplasm Table	Malignant Primary	Malignant Secondary	Ca In situ	Benign	Uncertain Behavior	Unspecified Behavior
skin NOS - continued	C44.90	C79.2	D04.9	D23.9	D48.5	D49.2
melanotic — see Melanoma						
Merkel cell — see Carcinoma, Merkel cell						
nates — see also Neoplasm, skin, trunk	C44.509	C79.2	D04.5	D23.5	D48.5	D49.2
neck	C44.40	C79.2	D04.4	D23.4	D48.5	D49.2
basal cell carcinoma	C44.41	—	—	—	—	—
specified type NEC	C44.49	—	—	—	—	—
squamous cell carcinoma	C44.42	—	—	—	—	—
nevus — see Nevus, skin						
nose (external) — see also Neoplasm, nose, skin	C44.301	C79.2	D04.39	D23.39	D48.5	D49.2
overlapping lesion	C44.80					
basal cell carcinoma	C44.81					
specified type NEC	C44.89					
squamous cell carcinoma	C44.82					
palm — see also Neoplasm, skin, limb, upper	C44.60-	C79.2	D04.6-	D23.6-	D48.5	D49.2
palpebra	C44.10-	C79.2	D04.1-	D23.1-	D48.5	D49.2
basal cell carcinoma	C44.11-					
specified type NEC	C44.19-					
squamous cell carcinoma	C44.12-					
penis NEC	C60.9	C79.82	D07.4	D29.0	D40.8	D49.59
perianal — see also Neoplasm, skin, anus	C44.500	C79.2	D04.5	D23.5	D48.5	D49.2
perineum — see also Neoplasm, skin, anus	C44.500	C79.2	D04.5	D23.5	D48.5	D49.2
pinna — see also Neoplasm, skin, ear	C44.20-	C79.2	D04.2-	D23.2-	D48.5	D49.2
plantar — see also Neoplasm, skin, limb, lower	C44.70-	C79.2	D04.7-	D23.7-	D48.5	D49.2
popliteal fossa or space — see also Neoplasm, skin, limb, lower	C44.70-	C79.2	D04.7-	D23.7-	D48.5	D49.2
prepuce	C60.0	C79.82	D07.4	D29.0	D40.8	D49.59
pubes — see also Neoplasm, skin, trunk	C44.509	C79.2	D04.5	D23.5	D48.5	D49.2
sacrococcygeal region — see also Neoplasm, skin, trunk	C44.509	C79.2	D04.5	D23.5	D48.5	D49.2
scalp	C44.40	C79.2	D04.4	D23.4	D48.5	D49.2
basal cell carcinoma	C44.41	—	—	—	—	—
specified type NEC	C44.49	—	—	—	—	—
squamous cell carcinoma	C44.42	—	—	—	—	—
scapular region — see also Neoplasm, skin, trunk	C44.509	C79.2	D04.5	D23.5	D48.5	D49.2
scrotum	C63.2	C79.82	D07.61	D29.4	D40.8	D49.59
shoulder — see also Neoplasm, skin, limb, upper	C44.60-	C79.2	D04.6-	D23.6-	D48.5	D49.2
sole (foot) — see also Neoplasm, skin, limb, lower	C44.70-	C79.2	D04.7-	D23.7-	D48.5	D49.2
specified sites NEC	C44.80	C79.2	D04.8	D23.9	D48.5	D49.2
basal cell carcinoma	C44.81	—	—	—	—	—
specified type NEC	C44.89	—	—	—	—	—
squamous cell carcinoma	C44.82	—	—	—	—	—
specified type NEC	C44.99	—	—	—	—	—

Neoplasm Table	Malignant Primary	Malignant Secondary	Ca In situ	Benign	Uncertain Behavior	Unspecified Behavior
skin NOS - continued	C44.90	C79.2	D04.9	D23.9	D48.5	D49.2
squamous cell carcinoma	C44.92	—				
submammary fold — see also Neoplasm, skin, trunk	C44.509	C79.2	D04.5	D23.5	D48.5	D49.2
supraclavicular region — see also Neoplasm, skin, neck	C44.40	C79.2	D04.4	D23.4	D48.5	D49.2
temple — see also Neoplasm, skin, face	C44.309	C79.2	D04.39	D23.39	D48.5	D49.2
thigh — see also Neoplasm, skin, limb, lower	C44.70-	C79.2	D04.7-	D23.7-	D48.5	D49.2
thoracic wall — see also Neoplasm, skin, trunk	C44.509	C79.2	D04.5	D23.5	D48.5	D49.2
thumb — see also Neoplasm, skin, limb, upper	C44.60-	C79.2	D04.6-	D23.6-	D48.5	D49.2
toe — see also Neoplasm, skin, limb, lower	C44.70-	C79.2	D04.7-	D23.7-	D48.5	D49.2
tragus — see also Neoplasm, skin, ear	C44.20-	C79.2	D04.2-	D23.2-	D48.5	D49.2
trunk	C44.509	C79.2	D04.5	D23.5	D48.5	D49.2
basal cell carcinoma	C44.519					
specified type NEC	C44.599					
squamous cell carcinoma	C44.529					
umbilicus — see also Neoplasm, skin, trunk	C44.509	C79.2	D04.5	D23.5	D48.5	D49.2
vulva	C51.9	C79.82	D07.1	D28.0	D39.8	D49.59
overlapping lesion	C51.8	—				
wrist — see also Neoplasm, skin, limb, upper	C44.60-	C79.2	D04.6-	D23.6-	D48.5	D49.2
skull	C41.0	C79.51	—	D16.4-	D48.0	D49.2
soft parts or tissues — see Neoplasm, connective tissue						
specified site NEC	C76.8	C79.89	D09.8	D36.7	D48.7	D49.89
spermatic cord	C63.1-	C79.82	D07.69	D29.8	D40.8	D49.59
sphenoid	C31.3	C78.39	D02.3	D14.0	D38.5	D49.1
bone	C41.0	C79.51	—	D16.4-	D48.0	D49.2
sinus	C31.3	C78.39	D02.3	D14.0	D38.5	D49.1
sphincter						
anal	C21.1	C78.5	D01.3	D12.9	D37.8	D49.0
of Oddi	C24.0	C78.89	D01.5	D13.5	D37.6	D49.0
spine, spinal (column)	C41.2	C79.51	—	D16.6	D48.0	D49.2
bulb	C71.7	C79.31	—	D33.1	D43.1	D49.6
coccyx	C41.4	C79.51	—	D16.8	D48.0	D49.2
cord (cervical) (lumbar) (sacral) (thoracic)	C72.0	C79.49	—	D33.4	D43.4	D49.7
dura mater	C70.1	C79.49	—	D32.1	D42.1	D49.7
lumbosacral	C41.2	C79.51	—	D16.6	D48.0	D49.2
marrow NEC	C96.9	C79.52	—		D47.9	D49.89
membrane	C70.1	C79.49	—	D32.1	D42.1	D49.7
meninges	C70.1	C79.49	—	D32.1	D42.1	D49.7
nerve (root)	C47.9	C79.89	—	D36.10	D48.2	D49.2
pia mater	C70.1	C79.49	—	D32.1	D42.1	D49.7
root	C47.9	C79.89	—	D36.10	D48.2	D49.2
sacrum	C41.4	C79.51	—	D16.8	D48.0	D49.2
spleen, splenic NEC	C26.1	C78.89	D01.7	D13.9	D37.8	D49.0
flexure (colon)	C18.5	C78.5	D01.0	D12.3	D37.4	D49.0
stem, brain	C71.7	C79.31	—	D33.1	D43.1	D49.6
Stensen's duct	C07	C79.89	D00.00	D11.0	D37.030	D49.0
sternum	C41.3	C79.51	—	D16.7	D48.0	D49.2

NEOPLASM TABLE

Neoplasm, neoplastic - *continued*

Neoplasm Table	Malignant Primary	Malignant Secondary	Ca In situ	Benign	Uncertain Behavior	Unspecified Behavior
stomach	C16.9	C78.89	D00.2	D13.1	D37.1	D49.0
antrum (pyloric)	C16.3	C78.89	D00.2	D13.1	D37.1	D49.0
body	C16.2	C78.89	D00.2	D13.1	D37.1	D49.0
cardia	C16.0	C78.89	D00.2	D13.1	D37.1	D49.0
cardiac orifice	C16.0	C78.89	D00.2	D13.1	D37.1	D49.0
corpus	C16.2	C78.89	D00.2	D13.1	D37.1	D49.0
fundus	C16.1	C78.89	D00.2	D13.1	D37.1	D49.0
greater curvature NEC	C16.6	C78.89	D00.2	D13.1	D37.1	D49.0
lesser curvature NEC	C16.5	C78.89	D00.2	D13.1	D37.1	D49.0
overlapping lesion	C16.8	—	—	—	—	—
prepylorus	C16.4	C78.89	D00.2	D13.1	D37.1	D49.0
pylorus	C16.4	C78.89	D00.2	D13.1	D37.1	D49.0
wall NEC	C16.9	C78.89	D00.2	D13.1	D37.1	D49.0
anterior NEC	C16.8	C78.89	D00.2	D13.1	D37.1	D49.0
posterior NEC	C16.8	C78.89	D00.2	D13.1	D37.1	D49.0
stroma, endometrial	C54.1	C79.82	D07.0	D26.1	D39.0	D49.59
stump, cervical	C53.8	C79.82	D06.7	D26.0	D39.0	D49.59
subcutaneous (nodule) (tissue) NEC — *see* Neoplasm, connective tissue						
subdural	C70.9	C79.32	—	D32.9	D42.9	D49.7
subglottis, subglottic	C32.2	C78.39	D02.0	D14.1	D38.0	D49.1
sublingual	C04.9	C79.89	D00.06	D10.2	D37.09	D49.0
gland or duct	C08.1	C79.89	D00.00	D11.7	D37.031	D49.0
submandibular gland	C08.0	C79.89	D00.00	D11.7	D37.032	D49.0
submaxillary gland or duct	C08.0	C79.89	D00.00	D11.7	D37.032	D49.0
submental	C76.0	C79.89	D09.8	D36.7	D48.7	D49.89
subpleural	C34.9-	C78.0-	D02.2-	D14.3-	D38.1	D49.1
substernal	C38.1	C78.1		D15.2	D38.3	D49.89
sudoriferous, sudoriparous gland, site unspecified	C44.90	C79.2	D04.9	D23.9	D48.5	D49.2
specified site — *see* Neoplasm, skin						
supraclavicular region	C76.0	C79.89	D09.8	D36.7	D48.7	D49.89
supraglottis	C32.1	C78.39	D02.0	D14.1	D38.0	D49.1
suprarenal	C74.9-	C79.7-	D09.3	D35.0-	D44.1-	D49.7
capsule	C74.9-	C79.7-	D09.3	D35.0-	D44.1-	D49.7
cortex	C74.0-	C79.7-	D09.3	D35.0-	D44.1-	D49.7
gland	C74.9-	C79.7-	D09.3	D35.0-	D44.1-	D49.7
medulla	C74.1-	C79.7-	D09.3	D35.0-	D44.1-	D49.7
suprasellar (region)	C71.9	C79.31	—	D33.2	D43.2	D49.6
supratentorial (brain) NEC	C71.0	C79.31	—	D33.0	D43.0	D49.6
sweat gland (apocrine) (eccrine), site unspecified	C44.90	C79.2	D04.9	D23.9	D48.5	D49.2
specified site — *see* Neoplasm, skin						
sympathetic nerve or nervous system NEC	C47.9	C79.89	—	D36.10	D48.2	D49.2
symphysis pubis	C41.4	C79.51	—	D16.8	D48.0	D49.2
synovial membrane — *see* Neoplasm, connective tissue						
tapetum, brain	C71.8	C79.31	—	D33.2	D43.2	D49.6
tarsus (any bone)	C40.3-	C79.51	—	D16.3-	—	—
temple (skin) — *see also* Neoplasm, skin, face	C44.309	C79.2	D04.39	D23.39	D48.5	D49.2

Neoplasm, neoplastic - *continued*

Neoplasm Table	Malignant Primary	Malignant Secondary	Ca In situ	Benign	Uncertain Behavior	Unspecified Behavior
temporal						
bone	C41.0	C79.51	—	D16.4-	D48.0	D49.2
lobe or pole	C71.2	C79.31	—	D33.0	D43.0	D49.6
region	C76.0	C79.89	D09.8	D36.7	D48.7	D49.89
skin — *see also* Neoplasm, skin, face	C44.309	C79.2	D04.39	D23.39	D48.5	D49.2
tendon (sheath) — *see* Neoplasm, connective tissue						
tentorium (cerebelli)	C70.0	C79.32	—	D32.0	D42.0	D49.7
testis, testes	C62.9-	C79.82	D07.69	D29.2-	D40.1-	D49.59
descended	C62.1-	C79.82	D07.69	D29.2-	D40.1-	D49.59
ectopic	C62.0-	C79.82	D07.69	D29.2-	D40.1-	D49.59
retained	C62.0-	C79.82	D07.69	D29.2-	D40.1-	D49.59
scrotal	C62.1-	C79.82	D07.69	D29.2-	D40.1-	D49.59
undescended	C62.0-	C79.82	D07.69	D29.2-	D40.1-	D49.59
unspecified whether descended or undescended	C62.9-	C79.82	D07.69	D29.2-	D40.1-	D49.59
thalamus	C71.0	C79.31	—	D33.0	D43.0	D49.6
thigh NEC	C76.5-	C79.89	D04.7-	D36.7	D48.7	D49.89
thorax, thoracic (cavity) (organs NEC)	C76.1	C79.89	D09.8	D36.7	D48.7	D49.89
duct	C49.3	C79.89	—	D21.3	D48.1	D49.2
wall NEC	C76.1	C79.89	D09.8	D36.7	D48.7	D49.89
throat	C14.0	C79.89	D00.08	D10.9	D37.05	D49.0
thumb NEC	C76.4-	C79.89	D04.6-	D36.7	D48.7	D49.89
thymus (gland)	C37	C79.89	D09.3	D15.0	D38.4	D49.89
thyroglossal duct	C73	C79.89	D09.3	D34	D44.0	D49.7
thyroid (gland)	C73	C79.89	D09.3	D34	D44.0	D49.7
cartilage	C32.3	C78.39	D02.0	D14.1	D38.0	D49.1
tibia (any part)	C40.2-	C79.51	—	D16.2-	—	—
toe NEC	C76.5-	C79.89	D04.7-	D36.7	D48.7	D49.89
tongue	C02.9	C79.89	D00.07	D10.1	D37.02	D49.0
anterior (two-thirds) NEC	C02.3	C79.89	D00.07	D10.1	D37.02	D49.0
dorsal surface	C02.0	C79.89	D00.07	D10.1	D37.02	D49.0
ventral surface	C02.2	C79.89	D00.07	D10.1	D37.02	D49.0
base (dorsal surface)	C01	C79.89	D00.07	D10.1	D37.02	D49.0
border (lateral)	C02.1	C79.89	D00.07	D10.1	D37.02	D49.0
dorsal surface NEC	C02.0	C79.89	D00.07	D10.1	D37.02	D49.0
fixed part NEC	C01	C79.89	D00.07	D10.1	D37.02	D49.0
foreamen cecum	C02.0	C79.89	D00.07	D10.1	D37.02	D49.0
frenulum linguae	C02.2	C79.89	D00.07	D10.1	D37.02	D49.0
junctional zone	C02.8	C79.89	D00.07	D10.1	D37.02	D49.0
margin (lateral)	C02.1	C79.89	D00.07	D10.1	D37.02	D49.0
midline NEC	C02.0	C79.89	D00.07	D10.1	D37.02	D49.0
mobile part NEC	C02.3	C79.89	D00.07	D10.1	D37.02	D49.0
overlapping lesion	C02.8	—	—	—	—	—
posterior (third)	C01	C79.89	D00.07	D10.1	D37.02	D49.0
root	C01	C79.89	D00.07	D10.1	D37.02	D49.0
surface (dorsal)	C02.0	C79.89	D00.07	D10.1	D37.02	D49.0
base	C01	C79.89	D00.07	D10.1	D37.02	D49.0
ventral	C02.2	C79.89	D00.07	D10.1	D37.02	D49.0
tip	C02.1	C79.89	D00.07	D10.1	D37.02	D49.0
tonsil	C02.4	C79.89	D00.07	D10.1	D37.02	D49.0
tonsil	C09.9	C79.89	D00.08	D10.4	D37.05	D49.0
fauces, faucial	C09.9	C79.89	D00.08	D10.4	D37.05	D49.0
lingual	C02.4	C79.89	D00.07	D10.1	D37.02	D49.0
overlapping sites	C09.8	—	—	—	—	—
palatine	C09.9	C79.89	D00.08	D10.4	D37.05	D49.0
pharyngeal	C11.1	C79.89	D00.08	D10.6	D37.05	D49.0
pillar (anterior) (posterior)	C09.1	C79.89	D00.08	D10.5	D37.05	D49.0

Neoplasm Table	Malignant Primary	Malignant Secondary	Ca In situ	Benign	Uncertain Behavior	Unspecified Behavior
Neoplasm, neoplastic - *continued*						
tonsillar fossa	C09.0	C79.89	D00.08	D10.5	D37.05	D49.0
tooth socket NEC	C03.9	C79.89	D00.03	D10.39	D37.09	D49.0
trachea (cartilage) (mucosa)	C33	C78.39	D02.1	D14.2	D38.1	D49.1
overlapping lesion with bronchus or lung	C34.8-	—	—	—	—	—
tracheobronchial	C34.8-	C78.39	D02.1	D14.2	D38.1	D49.1
overlapping lesion with lung	C34.8-	—	—	—	—	—
tragus — *see also* Neoplasm, skin, ear	C44.20-	C79.2	D04.2-	D23.2-	D48.5	D49.2
trunk NEC	C76.8	C79.89	D04.5	D36.7	D48.7	D49.89
tubo-ovarian	C57.8	C79.82	D07.39	D28.7	D39.8	D49.59
tunica vaginalis	C63.7	C79.82	D07.69	D29.8	D40.8	D49.59
turbinate (bone)	C41.0	C79.51		D16.4-	D48.0	D49.2
nasal	C30.0	C78.39	D02.3	D14.0	D38.5	D49.1
tympanic cavity	C30.1	C78.39	D02.3	D14.0	D38.5	D49.1
ulna (any part)	C40.0-	C79.51		D16.0-		
umbilicus, umbilical — *see also* Neoplasm, skin, trunk	C44.509	C79.2	D04.5	D23.5	D48.5	D49.2
uncus, brain	C71.2	C79.31	—	D33.0	D43.0	D49.6
unknown site or unspecified	C80.1	C79.9	D09.9	D36.9	D48.9	D49.9
urachus	C67.7	C79.11	D09.0	D30.3	D41.4	D49.4
ureter, ureteral	C66.-	C79.19	D09.19	D30.2-	D41.2-	D49.59
orifice (bladder)	C67.6	C79.11	D09.0	D30.3	D41.4	D49.4
ureter-bladder (junction)	C67.6	C79.11	D09.0	D30.3	D41.4	D49.4
urethra, urethral (gland)	C68.0	C79.19	D09.19	D30.4	D41.3	D49.59
orifice, internal	C67.5	C79.11	D09.0	D30.3	D41.4	D49.4
urethrovaginal (septum)	C57.9	C79.82	D07.30	D28.9	D39.8	D49.59
urinary organ or system	C68.9	C79.10	D09.10	D30.9	D41.9	D49.59
bladder — *see* Neoplasm, bladder						
overlapping lesion	C68.8	—	—	—	—	—
specified sites NEC	C68.8	C79.19	D09.19	D30.8	D41.8	D49.59
utero-ovarian	C57.8	C79.82	D07.39	D28.7	D39.8	D49.59
ligament	C57.1	C79.82	D07.39	D28.2	D39.8	D49.59
uterosacral ligament	C57.3	C79.82	—	D28.2	D39.8	D49.59
uterus, uteri, uterine	C55	C79.82	D07.0	D26.9	D39.0	D49.59
adnexa NEC	C57.4	C79.82	D07.39	D28.7	D39.8	D49.59
body	C54.9	C79.82	D07.0	D26.1	D39.0	D49.59
cervix	C53.9	C79.82	D06.9	D26.0	D39.0	D49.59
cornu	C54.9	C79.82	D07.0	D26.1	D39.0	D49.59
corpus	C54.9	C79.82	D07.0	D26.1	D39.0	D49.59
endocervix (canal) (gland)	C53.0	C79.82	D06.0	D26.0	D39.0	D49.59
endometrium	C54.1	C79.82	D07.0	D26.1	D39.0	D49.59
exocervix	C53.1	C79.82	D06.1	D26.0	D39.0	D49.59
external os	C53.1	C79.82	D06.1	D26.0	D39.0	D49.59
fundus	C54.3	C79.82	D07.0	D26.1	D39.0	D49.59
internal os	C53.0	C79.82	D06.0	D26.0	D39.0	D49.59
isthmus	C54.0	C79.82	D07.0	D26.1	D39.0	D49.59
ligament	C57.3	C79.82	—	D28.2	D39.8	D49.59
broad	C57.1	C79.82	D07.39	D28.2	D39.8	D49.59
round	C57.2	C79.82	—	D28.2	D39.8	D49.59
lower segment	C54.0	C79.82	D07.0	D26.1	D39.0	D49.59
myometrium	C54.2	C79.82	D07.0	D26.1	D39.0	D49.59
overlapping sites	C54.8	—	—	—	—	—
squamocolumnar junction	C53.8	C79.82	D06.7	D26.0	D39.0	D49.59
tube	C57.0-	C79.82	D07.39	D28.2	D39.8	D49.59
utricle, prostatic	C68.0	C79.19	D09.19	D30.4	D41.3	D49.59
uveal tract	C69.4-	C79.49	D09.2-	D31.4-	D48.7	D49.89
uvula	C05.2	C79.89	D00.04	D10.39	D37.09	D49.09

Neoplasm Table	Malignant Primary	Malignant Secondary	Ca In situ	Benign	Uncertain Behavior	Unspecified Behavior
Neoplasm, neoplastic - *continued*						
vagina, vaginal (fornix) (vault) (wall)	C52	C79.82	D07.2	D28.1	D39.8	D49.59
vaginovesical	C57.9	C79.82	D07.30	D28.9	D39.9	D49.59
septum	C57.9	C79.82	D07.30	D28.9	D39.9	D49.59
vallecula (epiglottis)	C10.0	C79.89	D00.08	D10.5	D37.05	D49.0
vas deferens	C63.1-	C79.82	D07.69	D29.8	D40.8	D49.59
vascular — *see* Neoplasm, connective tissue						
Vater's ampulla	C24.1	C78.89	D01.5	D13.5	D37.6	D49.0
vein, venous — *see* Neoplasm, connective tissue						
vena cava (abdominal) (inferior)	C49.4	C79.89	—	D21.4	D48.1	D49.2
superior	C49.3	C79.89	—	D21.3	D48.1	D49.2
ventricle (cerebral) (floor) (lateral) (third)	C71.5	C79.31	—	D33.0	D43.0	D49.6
cardiac (left) (right)	C38.0	C79.89	—	D15.1	D48.7	D49.89
fourth	C71.7	C79.31	—	D33.1	D43.1	D49.6
ventricular band of larynx	C32.1	C78.39	D02.0	D14.1	D38.0	D49.1
ventriculus — *see* Neoplasm, stomach						
vermillion border — *see* Neoplasm, lip						
vermis, cerebellum	C71.6	C79.31	—	D33.1	D43.1	D49.6
vertebra (column)	C41.2	C79.51	—	D16.6	D48.0	D49.2
coccyx	C41.4	C79.51	—	D16.8-	D48.0	D49.2
marrow NEC	C96.9	C79.52	—	—	D47.9	D49.89
sacrum	C41.4	C79.51	—	D16.8-	D48.0	D49.2
vesical — *see* Neoplasm, bladder						
vesicle, seminal	C63.7	C79.82	D07.69	D29.8	D40.8	D49.59
vesicocervical tissue	C57.9	C79.82	D07.30	D28.9	D39.9	D49.59
vesicorectal	C76.3	C79.82	D09.8	D36.7	D48.7	D49.89
vesicovaginal	C57.9	C79.82	D07.30	D28.9	D39.9	D49.59
septum	C57.9	C79.82	D07.30	D28.9	D39.8	D49.59
vessel (blood) — *see* Neoplasm, connective tissue						
vestibular gland, greater	C51.0	C79.82	D07.1	D28.0	D39.8	D49.59
vestibule						
mouth	C06.1	C79.89	D00.00	D10.39	D37.09	D49.0
nose	C30.0	C78.39	D02.3	D14.0	D38.5	D49.1
Virchow's gland	C77.0	C77.0	—	D36.0	D48.7	D49.89
viscera NEC	C76.8	C79.89	D09.8	D36.7	D48.7	D49.89
vocal cords (true)	C32.0	C78.39	D02.0	D14.1	D38.0	D49.1
false	C32.1	C78.39	D02.0	D14.1	D38.0	D49.1
vomer	C41.0	C79.51	—	D16.4-	D48.0	D49.2
vulva	C51.9	C79.82	D07.1	D28.0	D39.8	D49.59
vulvovaginal gland	C51.0	C79.82	D07.1	D28.0	D39.8	D49.59
Waldeyer's ring	C14.2	C79.89	D00.08	D10.9	D37.05	D49.0
Wharton's duct	C08.0	C79.89	D00.00	D11.7	D37.032	D49.0
white matter (central) (cerebral)	C71.0	C79.31	—	D33.0	D43.0	D49.6
windpipe	C33	C78.39	D02.1	D14.2	D38.1	D49.1
Wirsung's duct	C25.3	C78.89	D01.7	D13.6	D37.8	D49.0
wolffian (body) (duct)						
female	C57.7	C79.82	D07.39	D28.7	D39.8	D49.59
male	C63.7	C79.82	D07.69	D29.8	D40.8	D49.59
womb — *see* Neoplasm, uterus						
wrist NEC	C76.4-	C79.89	D04.6-	D36.7	D48.7	D49.89
xiphoid process	C41.3	C79.51	—	D16.7	D48.0	D49.2
Zuckerkandl organ	C75.5	C79.89	—	D35.6	D44.7	D49.7

NEOPLASM TABLE

NOTES

Neovascularization
ciliary body — *see* Disorder, iris, vascular
cornea H16.40-
  deep H16.44-
  ghost vessels — *see* Ghost, vessels
  localized H16.43-
  pannus — *see* Pannus
iris — *see* Disorder, iris, vascular
retina H35.05-
Nephralgia N23
Nephritis, nephritic (albuminuric) (azotemic)
(congenital) (disseminated) (epithelial)
(familial) (focal) (granulomatous)
(hemorrhagic) (infantile) (nonsuppurative,
excretory) (uremic) N05.9
with
  dense deposit disease N05.6
  diffuse
    crescentic glomerulonephritis N05.7
    endocapillary proliferative
      glomerulonephritis N05.4
    membranous glomerulonephritis N05.2
    mesangial proliferative glomerulonephritis
      N05.3
    mesangiocapillary glomerulonephritis
      N05.5
  edema — *see* Nephrosis
  focal and segmental glomerular lesions
    N05.1
  foot process disease N04.9
  glomerular lesion
    diffuse sclerosing N05.8
    hypocomplementemic — *see* Nephritis,
      membranoproliferative
    IgA — *see* Nephropathy, IgA
    lobular, lobulonodular — *see* Nephritis,
      membranoproliferative
    nodular — *see* Nephritis,
      membranoproliferative
  lesion of
    glomerulonephritis, proliferative N05.8
    renal necrosis N05.9
  minor glomerular abnormality N05.0
  specified morphological changes NEC
    N05.8
acute N00.9
  with
    dense deposit disease N00.6
    diffuse
      crescentic glomerulonephritis N00.7
      endocapillary proliferative
        glomerulonephritis N00.4
      membranous glomerulonephritis N00.2
      mesangial proliferative
        glomerulonephritis N00.3
      mesangiocapillary glomerulonephritis
        N00.5
    focal and segmental glomerular lesions
      N00.1
    minor glomerular abnormality N00.0
    specified morphological changes NEC
      N00.8
amyloid E85.4 *[N08]*
antiglomerular basement membrane (anti-
  GBM) antibody NEC
  in Goodpasture's syndrome M31.0
antitubular basement membrane (tubulo-
  interstitial) NEC N12
  toxic — *see* Nephropathy, toxic
arteriolar — *see* Hypertension, kidney
arteriosclerotic — *see* Hypertension, kidney
ascending — *see* Nephritis, tubulo-interstitial
atrophic N03.9
Balkan (endemic) N15.0
calculous, calculus — *see* Calculus, kidney
cardiac — *see* Hypertension, kidney
cardiovascular — *see* Hypertension, kidney

Nephritis, nephritic (albuminuric) (azotemic)
(congenital) (disseminated) (epithelial)
(familial) (focal) (granulomatous)
(hemorrhagic) (infantile) (nonsuppurative,
excretory) (uremic) N05.9 — *continued*
chronic N03.9
  with
    dense deposit disease N03.6
    diffuse
      crescentic glomerulonephritis N03.7
      endocapillary proliferative
        glomerulonephritis N03.4
      membranous glomerulonephritis N03.2
      mesangial proliferative
        glomerulonephritis N03.3
      mesangiocapillary glomerulonephritis
        N03.5
    focal and segmental glomerular lesions
      N03.1
    minor glomerular abnormality N03.0
    specified morphological changes NEC
      N03.8
  arteriosclerotic — *see* Hypertension, kidney
cirrhotic N26.9
complicating pregnancy O26.83-
croupous N00.9
degenerative — *see* Nephrosis
diffuse sclerosing N05.8
due to
  diabetes mellitus — *see* E08-E13 with .21
  subacute bacterial endocarditis I33.0
  systemic lupus erythematosus (chronic)
    M32.14
  typhoid fever A01.09
gonococcal (acute) (chronic) A54.21
hypocomplementemic — *see* Nephritis,
  membranoproliferative
IgA — *see* Nephropathy, IgA
immune complex (circulating) NEC N05.8
infective — *see* Nephritis, tubulo-interstitial
interstitial — *see* Nephritis, tubulo-interstitial
lead N14.3
membranoproliferative (diffuse) (type 1 or 3)
  (*see also* N00-N07 with fourth character
  .5) N05.5
  type 2 (*see also* N00-N07 with fourth
    character .6) N05.6
minimal change N05.0
necrotic, necrotizing NEC (*see also* N00-N07
  with fourth character .8) N05.8
nephrotic — *see* Nephrosis
nodular — *see* Nephritis,
  membranoproliferative
polycystic Q61.3
  adult type Q61.2
  autosomal
    dominant Q61.2
    recessive NEC Q61.19
  childhood type NEC Q61.19
  infantile type NEC Q61.19
poststreptococcal N05.9
  acute N00.9
  chronic N03.9
  rapidly progressive N01.9
proliferative NEC (*see also* N00-N07 with
  fourth character .8) N05.8
purulent — *see* Nephritis, tubulo-interstitial
rapidly progressive N01.9
  with
    dense deposit disease N01.6
    diffuse
      crescentic glomerulonephritis N01.7
      endocapillary proliferative
        glomerulonephritis N01.4
      membranous glomerulonephritis N01.2
      mesangial proliferative
        glomerulonephritis N01.3
      mesangiocapillary glomerulonephritis
        N01.5

Nephritis, nephritic (albuminuric) (azotemic)
(congenital) (disseminated) (epithelial)
(familial) (focal) (granulomatous)
(hemorrhagic) (infantile) (nonsuppurative,
excretory) (uremic) N05.9 — *continued*
rapidly progressive N01.9 — *continued*
  with — *continued*
    focal and segmental glomerular lesions
      N01.1
    minor glomerular abnormality N01.0
    specified morphological changes NEC
      N01.8
salt losing or wasting NEC N28.89
saturnine N14.3
sclerosing, diffuse N05.8
septic — *see* Nephritis, tubulo-interstitial
specified pathology NEC (*see also* N00-N07
  with fourth character .8) N05.8
subacute N01.9
suppurative — *see* Nephritis, tubulo-interstitial
syphilitic (late) A52.75
  congenital A50.59 *[N08]*
  early (secondary) A51.44
toxic — *see* Nephropathy, toxic
tubal, tubular — *see* Nephritis, tubulo-
  interstitial
tuberculous A18.11
tubulo-interstitial (in) N12
  acute (infectious) N10
  chronic (infectious) N11.9
    nonobstructive N11.8
      reflux-associated N11.0
    obstructive N11.1
    specified NEC N11.8
  due to
    brucellosis A23.9 *[N16]*
    cryoglobulinemia D89.1 *[N16]*
    glycogen storage disease E74.00 *[N16]*
    Sjögren's syndrome M35.04
vascular — *see* Hypertension, kidney
war N00.9
Nephroblastoma (epithelial) (mesenchymal)
  C64-
Nephrocalcinosis E83.59 *[N29]*
Nephrocystitis, pustular — *see* Nephritis,
  tubulo-interstitial
Nephrolithiasis (congenital) (pelvis)
  (recurrent) — *see also* Calculus, kidney
Nephroma C64-
  mesoblastic D41.0-
Nephronephritis — *see* Nephrosis
Nephronophthisis Q61.5
Nephropathia epidemica A98.5
Nephropathy (*see also* Nephritis) N28.9
with
  edema — *see* Nephrosis
  glomerular lesion — *see* Glomerulonephritis
amyloid, hereditary E85.0
analgesic N14.0
  with medullary necrosis, acute N17.2
Balkan (endemic) N15.0
chemical — *see* Nephropathy, toxic
diabetic — *see* E08-E13 with .21
drug-induced N14.2
  specified NEC N14.1
focal and segmental hyalinosis or sclerosis
  N02.1
heavy metal-induced N14.3
hereditary NEC N07.9
  with
    dense deposit disease N07.6
    diffuse
      crescentic glomerulonephritis N07.7
      endocapillary proliferative
        glomerulonephritis N07.4
      membranous glomerulonephritis N07.2
      mesangial proliferative
        glomerulonephritis N07.3

Nephropathy (see also Nephritis) N28.9 — continued
  hereditary NEC N07.9 — continued
    with — continued
      diffuse — continued
        mesangiocapillary glomerulonephritis N07.5
        focal and segmental glomerular lesions N07.1
        minor glomerular abnormality N07.0
        specified morphological changes NEC N07.8
  hypercalcemic N25.89
  hypertensive — see Hypertension, kidney
  hypokalemic (vacuolar) N25.89
  IgA N02.8
    with glomerular lesion N02.9
      focal and segmental hyalinosis or sclerosis N02.1
      membranoproliferative (diffuse) N02.5
      membranous (diffuse) N02.2
      mesangial proliferative (diffuse) N02.3
      mesangiocapillary (diffuse) N02.5
      proliferative NEC N02.8
      specified pathology NEC N02.8
  lead N14.3
  membranoproliferative (diffuse) N02.5
  membranous (diffuse) N02.2
  mesangial (IgA/IgG) — see Nephropathy, IgA
    proliferative (diffuse) N02.3
  mesangiocapillary (diffuse) N02.5
  obstructive N13.8
  phenacetin N17.2
  phosphate-losing N25.0
  potassium depletion N25.89
  pregnancy-related O26.83-
  proliferative NEC (see also N00-N07 with fourth character .8) N05.8
  protein-losing N25.89
  saturnine N14.3
  sickle-cell D57- [N08]
  toxic NEC N14.4
    due to
      drugs N14.2
      analgesic N14.0
        specified NEC N14.1
      heavy metals N14.3
  vasomotor N17.0
  water-losing N25.89
Nephroptosis N28.83
Nephropyosis — see Abscess, kidney
Nephrorrhagia N28.89
Nephrosclerosis (arteriolar) (arteriosclerotic) (chronic) (hyaline) — see also Hypertension, kidney
  hyperplastic — see Hypertension, kidney
  senile N26.9
Nephrosis, nephrotic (Epstein's) (syndrome) (congenital) N04.9
  with
    foot process disease N04.9
    glomerular lesion N04.1
    hypocomplementemic N04.5
  acute N04.9
  anoxic — see Nephrosis, tubular
  chemical — see Nephrosis, tubular
  cholemic K76.7
  diabetic — see E08-E13 with .21
  Finnish type (congenital) Q89.8
  hemoglobin N10
  hemoglobinuric — see Nephrosis, tubular
  in
    amyloidosis E85.4 [N08]
    diabetes mellitus — see E08-E13 with .21
    epidemic hemorrhagic fever A98.5
    malaria (malariae) B52.0
  ischemic — see Nephrosis, tubular
  lipoid N04.9
  lower nephron — see Nephrosis, tubular

Nephrosis, nephrotic (Epstein's) (syndrome) (congenital) N04.9 — continued
  malarial (malariae) B52.0
  minimal change N04.0
  myoglobin N10
  necrotizing — see Nephrosis, tubular
  osmotic (sucrose) N25.89
  radiation N04.9
  syphilitic (late) A52.75
  toxic — see Nephrosis, tubular
  tubular (acute) N17.0
    postprocedural N99.0
    radiation N04.9
Nephrosonephritis, hemorrhagic (endemic) A98.5
Nephrostomy
  attention to Z43.6
  status Z93.6
Nerve — see also condition
  injury — see Injury, nerve, by body site
Nerves R45.0
Nervous (see also condition) R45.0
  heart F45.8
  stomach F45.8
  tension R45.0
Nervousness R45.0
Nesidioblastoma
  pancreas D13.7
  specified site NEC — see Neoplasm, benign, by site
  unspecified site D13.7
Nettleship's syndrome Q82.2
Neumann's disease or syndrome L10.1
Neuralgia, neuralgic (acute) M79.2
  accessory (nerve) G52.8
  acoustic (nerve) — see subcategory H93.3
  auditory (nerve) — see subcategory H93.3
  ciliary G44.009
    intractable G44.001
    not intractable G44.009
  cranial
    nerve — see also Disorder, nerve, cranial
      fifth or trigeminal — see Neuralgia, trigeminal
      postherpetic, postzoster B02.29
  ear — see subcategory H92.0
  facialis vera G51.1
  Fothergill's — see Neuralgia, trigeminal
  glossopharyngeal (nerve) G52.1
  Horton's G44.099
    intractable G44.091
    not intractable G44.099
  Hunt's B02.21
  hypoglossal (nerve) G52.3
  infraorbital — see Neuralgia, trigeminal
  malarial — see Malaria
  migrainous G44.009
    intractable G44.001
    not intractable G44.009
  Morton's G57.6-
  nerve, cranial — see Disorder, nerve, cranial
  nose G52.0
  occipital M54.81
  olfactory G52.0
  penis N48.9
  perineum R10.2
  postherpetic NEC B02.29
    trigeminal B02.22
  pubic region R10.2
  scrotum R10.2
  Sluder's G44.89
  specified nerve NEC G58.8
  spermatic cord R10.2
  sphenopalatine (ganglion) G90.09
  trifacial — see Neuralgia, trigeminal
  trigeminal G50.0
    postherpetic, postzoster B02.22
  vagus (nerve) G52.2

Neuralgia, neuralgic (acute) M79.2 — continued
  writer's F48.8
  organic G25.89
Neurapraxia — see Injury, nerve
Neurasthenia F48.8
  cardiac F45.8
  gastric F45.8
  heart F45.8
Neurilemmoma — see also Neoplasm, nerve, benign
  acoustic (nerve) D33.3
  malignant — see also Neoplasm, nerve, malignant
    acoustic (nerve) C72.4-
Neurilemmosarcoma — see Neoplasm, nerve, malignant
Neurinoma — see Neoplasm, nerve, benign
Neurinomatosis — see Neoplasm, nerve, uncertain behavior
Neuritis (rheumatoid) M79.2
  abducens (nerve) — see Strabismus, paralytic, sixth nerve
  accessory (nerve) G52.8
  acoustic (nerve) (see also subcategory) H93.3
    in (due to)
      infectious disease NEC B99 [H94.-]
      parasitic disease NEC B89 [H94.-]
    syphilitic A52.15
  alcoholic G62.1
    with psychosis — see Psychosis, alcoholic
  amyloid, any site E85.4 [G63]
  auditory (nerve) — see subcategory H93.3
  brachial — see Radiculopathy
    due to displacement, intervertebral disc — see Disorder, disc, cervical, with neuritis
  cranial nerve
    due to Lyme disease A69.22
    eighth or acoustic or auditory — see subcategory H93.3
    eleventh or accessory G52.8
    fifth or trigeminal G51.0
    first or olfactory G52.0
    fourth or trochlear — see Strabismus, paralytic, fourth nerve
    second or optic — see Neuritis, optic
    seventh or facial G51.8
      newborn (birth injury) P11.3
    sixth or abducent — see Strabismus, paralytic, sixth nerve
    tenth or vagus G52.2
    third or oculomotor — see Strabismus, paralytic, third nerve
    twelfth or hypoglossal G52.3
  Déjérine-Sottas G60.0
  diabetic (mononeuropathy) — see E08-E13 with .41
    polyneuropathy — see E08-E13 with .42
  due to
    beriberi E51.11
    displacement, prolapse or rupture, intervertebral disc — see Disorder, disc, with, radiculopathy
    herniation, nucleus pulposus M51.9 [G55]
  endemic E51.11
  facial G51.8
    newborn (birth injury) P11.3
  general — see Polyneuropathy
  geniculate ganglion G51.1
    due to herpes (zoster) B02.21
  gouty (see also Gout, by type) M10.9 [G63]
  hypoglossal (nerve) G52.3
  ilioinguinal (nerve) G57.9-
  infectious (multiple) NEC G61.0
  interstitial hypertrophic progressive G60.0
  lumbar M54.16
  lumbosacral M54.17

Neuritis (rheumatoid) M79.2 — *continued*
  multiple — *see also* Polyneuropathy
    endemic E51.11
    infective, acute G61.0
  multiplex endemica E51.11
  nerve root — *see* Radiculopathy
  oculomotor (nerve) — *see* Strabismus,
    paralytic, third nerve
  olfactory nerve G52.0
  optic (nerve) (hereditary) (sympathetic) H46.9
    with demyelination G36.0
    in myelitis G36.0
    nutritional H46.2
    papillitis — *see* Papillitis, optic
    retrobulbar H46.1-
    specified type NEC H46.8
    toxic H46.3
  peripheral (nerve) G62.9
    multiple — *see* Polyneuropathy
    single — *see* Mononeuritis
  pneumogastric (nerve) G52.2
  postherpetic, postzoster B02.29
  progressive hypertrophic interstitial G60.0
  retrobulbar — *see also* Neuritis, optic,
    retrobulbar
    in (due to)
      late syphilis A52.15
      meningococcal infection A39.82
    meningococcal A39.82
    syphilitic A52.15
  sciatic (nerve) — *see also* Sciatica
    due to displacement of intervertebral disc —
      see Disorder, disc, with, radiculopathy
  serum (*see also* Reaction, serum) T80.69
  shoulder-girdle G54.5
  specified nerve NEC G58.8
  spinal (nerve) root — *see* Radiculopathy
  syphilitic A52.15
  thenar (median) G56.1-
  thoracic M54.14
  toxic NEC G62.2
  trochlear (nerve) — *see* Strabismus, paralytic,
    fourth nerve
  vagus (nerve) G52.2
Neuroastrocytoma — *see* Neoplasm,
  uncertain behavior, by site
Neuroavitaminosis E56.9 *[G99.8]*
Neuroblastoma
  olfactory C30.0
  specified site — *see* Neoplasm, malignant, by
    site
  unspecified site C74.90
Neurochorioretinitis — *see* Chorioretinitis
Neurocirculatory asthenia F45.8
Neurocysticercosis B69.0
Neurocytoma — *see* Neoplasm, benign, by
  site
Neurodermatitis (circumscribed)
  (circumscripta) (local) L28.0
  atopic L20.81
  diffuse (Brocq) L20.81
  disseminated L20.81
Neuroencephalomyelopathy, optic G36.0
Neuroepithelioma — *see also* Neoplasm,
  malignant, by site
  olfactory C30.0
Neurofibroma — *see also* Neoplasm, nerve,
  benign
  melanotic — *see* Neoplasm, nerve, benign
  multiple — *see* Neurofibromatosis
  plexiform — *see* Neoplasm, nerve, benign
Neurofibromatosis (multiple) (nonmalignant)
  Q85.00
  acoustic Q85.02
  malignant — *see* Neoplasm, nerve, malignant
  specified NEC Q85.09
  type 1 (von Recklinghausen) Q85.01
  type 2 Q85.02

Neurofibrosarcoma — *see* Neoplasm, nerve,
  malignant
Neurogenic — *see also* condition
  bladder (*see also* Dysfunction, bladder,
    neuromuscular) N31.9
    cauda equina syndrome G83.4
  bowel NEC K59.2
  heart F45.8
Neuroglioma — *see* Neoplasm, uncertain
  behavior, by site
Neurolabyrinthitis (of Dix and Hallpike) —
  see Neuronitis, vestibular
Neurolathyrism — *see* Poisoning, food,
  noxious, plant
Neuroleprosy A30.9
Neuroma — *see also* Neoplasm, nerve, benign
  acoustic (nerve) D33.3
  amputation (stump) (traumatic) (surgical
    complication) (late) T87.3-
    arm T87.3-
    leg T87.3-
  digital (toe) G57.6-
  interdigital G58.8
    lower limb (toe) G57.8-
    upper limb G56.8-
  intermetatarsal G57.8-
  Morton's G57.6-
  nonneoplastic
    arm G56.9-
    leg G57.9-
    lower extremity G57.9-
    upper extremity G56.9-
  optic (nerve) D33.3
  plantar G57.6-
  plexiform — *see* Neoplasm, nerve, benign
  surgical (nonneoplastic)
    arm G56.9-
    leg G57.9-
    lower extremity G57.9-
    upper extremity G56.9-
Neuromyalgia — *see* Neuralgia
Neuromyasthenia (epidemic) (postinfectious)
  G93.3
Neuromyelitis G36.9
  ascending G61.0
  optica G36.0
Neuromyopathy G70.9
  paraneoplastic D49.9 *[G13.0]*
Neuromyotonia (Isaacs) G71.19
Neuronevus — *see* Nevus
Neuronitis G58.9
  ascending (acute) G57.2-
  vestibular H81.2-
Neuroparalytic — *see* condition
Neuropathy, neuropathic G62.9
  acute motor G62.81
  alcoholic G62.1
    with psychosis — *see* Psychosis, alcoholic
  arm G56.9-
  autonomic, peripheral — *see* Neuropathy,
    peripheral, autonomic
  axillary G56.9-
  bladder N31.9
    atonic (motor) (sensory) N31.2
    autonomous N31.2
    flaccid N31.2
    nonreflex N31.2
    reflex N31.1
    uninhibited N31.0
  brachial plexus G54.0
  cervical plexus G54.2
  chronic
    progressive segmentally demyelinating
      G62.89
    relapsing demyelinating G62.89
  Déjérine-Sottas G60.0
  diabetic — *see* E08-E13 with .40
    mononeuropathy — *see* E08-E13 with .41
    polyneuropathy — *see* E08-E13 with .42

Neuropathy, neuropathic G62.9 —
  continued
  entrapment G58.9
    iliohypogastric nerve G57.8-
    ilioinguinal nerve G57.8-
    lateral cutaneous nerve of thigh G57.1-
    median nerve G56.0-
    obturator nerve G57.8-
    peroneal nerve G57.3-
    posterior tibial nerve G57.5-
    saphenous nerve G57.8-
    ulnar nerve G56.2-
  facial nerve G51.9
  hereditary G60.9
    motor and sensory (types I-IV) G60.0
    sensory G60.8
    specified NEC G60.8
  hypertrophic G60.0
    Charcot-Marie-Tooth G60.0
    Déjérine-Sottas G60.0
    interstitial progressive G60.0
    of infancy G60.0
    Refsum G60.1
  idiopathic G60.9
    progressive G60.3
    specified NEC G60.8
  in association with hereditary ataxia G60.2
  intercostal G58.0
  ischemic — *see* Disorder, nerve
  Jamaica (ginger) G62.2
  leg NEC G57.9-
  lower extremity G57.9-
  lumbar plexus G54.1
  median nerve G56.1-
  motor and sensory — *see also* Polyneuropathy
    hereditary (types I-IV) G60.0
  multifocal motor (MMN) G61.82
  multiple (acute) (chronic) — *see* Polyneuropathy
  optic (nerve) — *see also* Neuritis, optic
    ischemic H47.01-
  paraneoplastic (sensorial) (Denny Brown)
    D49.9 *[G13.0]*
  peripheral (nerve) (*see also* Polyneuropathy)
    G62.9
    autonomic G90.9
      idiopathic G90.09
      in (due to)
        amyloidosis E85.4 *[G99.0]*
        diabetes mellitus — *see* E08-E13 with
          .43
        endocrine disease NEC E34.9 *[G99.0]*
        gout M10.00 *[G99.0]*
        hyperthyroidism E05.90 *[G99.0]*
          with thyroid storm E05.91 *[G99.0]*
        metabolic disease NEC E88.9 *[G99.0]*
    idiopathic G60.9
      progressive G60.3
    in (due to)
      antitetanus serum G62.0
      arsenic G62.2
      drugs NEC G62.0
      lead G62.2
      organophosphate compounds G62.2
      toxic agent NEC G62.2
  plantar nerves G57.6-
  progressive
    hypertrophic interstitial G60.0
    inflammatory G62.81
  radicular NEC — *see* Radiculopathy
  sacral plexus G54.1
  sciatic G57.0-
  serum G61.1
  toxic NEC G62.2
  trigeminal sensory G50.8
  ulnar nerve G56.2-
  uremic N18.9 *[G63]*
  vitamin B12 E53.8 *[G63]*
    with anemia (pernicious) D51.0 *[G63]*
      due to dietary deficiency D51.3 *[G63]*

Neurophthisis — *see also* Disorder, nerve
  peripheral, diabetic — *see* E08-E13 with .42
Neuroretinitis — *see* Chorioretinitis
Neuroretinopathy, hereditary optic
  H47.22
Neurosarcoma — *see* Neoplasm, nerve,
  malignant
Neurosclerosis — *see* Disorder, nerve
Neurosis, neurotic F48.9
  anankastic F42.8
  anxiety (state) F41.1
    panic type F41.0
  asthenic F48.8
  bladder F45.8
  cardiac (reflex) F45.8
  cardiovascular F45.8
  character F60.9
  colon F45.8
  compensation F68.1
  compulsive, compulsion F42.8
  conversion F44.9
  craft F48.8
  cutaneous F45.8
  depersonalization F48.1
  depressive (reaction) (type) F34.1
  environmental F48.8
  excoriation L98.1
  fatigue F48.8
  functional — *see* Disorder, somatoform
  gastric F45.8
  gastrointestinal F45.8
  heart F45.8
  hypochondriacal F45.21
  hysterical F44.9
  incoordination F45.8
    larynx F45.8
    vocal cord F45.8
  intestine F45.8
  larynx (sensory) F45.8
    hysterical F44.4
  mixed NEC F48.8
  musculoskeletal F45.8
  obsessional F42.8
  obsessive-compulsive F42.8
  occupational F48.8
  ocular NEC F45.8
  organ — *see* Disorder, somatoform
  pharynx F45.8
  phobic F40.9
  posttraumatic (situational) F43.10
    acute F43.11
    chronic F43.12
  psychasthenic (type) F48.8
  railroad F48.8
  rectum F45.8
  respiratory F45.8
  rumination F45.8
  sexual F65.9
  situational F48.8
  social F40.10
    generalized F40.11
  specified type NEC F48.8
  state F48.9
    with depersonalization episode F48.1
  stomach F45.8
  traumatic F43.10
    acute F43.11
    chronic F43.12
  vasomotor F45.8
  visceral F45.8
  war F48.8
Neurospongioblastosis diffusa Q85.1
Neurosyphilis (arrested) (early) (gumma) (late)
  (latent) (recurrent) (relapse) A52.3
  with ataxia (cerebellar) (locomotor) (spastic)
    (spinal) A52.19
  aneurysm (cerebral) A52.05
  arachnoid (adhesive) A52.13
  arteritis (any artery) (cerebral) A52.04

Neurosyphilis (arrested) (early) (gumma) (late)
  (latent) (recurrent) (relapse) A52.3 —
  continued
  asymptomatic A52.2
  congenital A50.40
  dura (mater) A52.13
  general paresis A52.17
  hemorrhagic A52.05
  juvenile (asymptomatic) (meningeal) A50.40
  leptomeninges (aseptic) A52.13
  meningeal, meninges (adhesive) A52.13
  meningitis A52.13
  meningovascular (diffuse) A52.13
  optic atrophy A52.15
  parenchymatous (degenerative) A52.19
  paresis, paretic A52.17
    juvenile A50.45
  remission in (sustained) A52.3
  serological (without symptoms) A52.2
  specified nature or site NEC A52.19
  tabes, tabetic (dorsalis) A52.11
    juvenile A50.45
  taboparesis A52.17
    juvenile A50.45
  thrombosis (cerebral) A52.05
  vascular (cerebral) NEC A52.05
Neurothekeoma — *see* Neoplasm, nerve,
  benign
Neurotic — *see* Neurosis
Neurotoxemia — *see* Toxemia
Neutroclusion M26.211
Neutropenia, neutropenic (chronic)
  (genetic) (idiopathic) (immune) (infantile)
  (malignant) (pernicious) (splenic) D70.9
  congenital (primary) D70.0
  cyclic D70.4
  cytoreductive cancer chemotherapy sequela
    D70.1
  drug-induced D70.2
    due to cytoreductive cancer chemotherapy
      D70.1
  due to infection D70.3
  fever D70.9
  neonatal, transitory (isoimmune) (maternal
    transfer) P61.5
  periodic D70.4
  secondary (cyclic) (periodic) (splenic) D70.4
    drug-induced D70.2
      due to cytoreductive cancer chemotherapy
        D70.1
  toxic D70.8
Neutrophilia, hereditary giant D72.0
Nevocarcinoma — *see* Melanoma
Nevus D22.9
  achromic — *see* Neoplasm, skin, benign
  amelanotic — *see* Neoplasm, skin, benign
  angiomatousD18.00
    intra-abdominal D18.03
    intracranial D18.02
    skin D18.01
    specified site NEC D18.09
  araneus I78.1
  balloon cell — *see* Neoplasm, skin, benign
  bathing trunk D48.5
  blue — *see* Neoplasm, skin, benign
    cellular — *see* Neoplasm, skin, benign
    giant — *see* Neoplasm, skin, benign
    Jadassohn's — *see* Neoplasm, skin, benign
    malignant — *see* Melanoma
  capillary D18.00
    intra-abdominal D18.03
    intracranial D18.02
    skin D18.01
    specified site NEC D18.09
  cavernous D18.00
    intra-abdominal D18.03
    intracranial D18.02
    skin D18.01
    specified site NEC D18.09

Nevus D22.9 — *continued*
  cellular — *see* Neoplasm, skin, benign
    blue — *see* Neoplasm, skin, benign
  choroid D31.3-
  comedonicus Q82.5
  conjunctiva D31.0-
  dermal — *see* Neoplasm, skin, benign
    with epidermal nevus — *see* Neoplasm, skin,
      benign
  dysplastic — *see* Neoplasm, skin, benign
  eye D31.9-
  flammeus Q82.5
  hemangiomatous D18.00
    intra-abdominal D18.03
    intracranial D18.02
    skin D18.01
    specified site NEC D18.09
  iris D31.4-
  lacrimal gland D31.5-
  lymphatic D18.1
  magnocellular
    specified site — *see* Neoplasm, benign, by
      site
    unspecified site D31.40
  malignant — *see* Melanoma
  meaning hemangioma D18.00
    intra-abdominal D18.03
    intracranial D18.02
    skin D18.01
    specified site NEC D18.09
  mouth (mucosa) D10.30
    specified site NEC D10.39
    white sponge Q38.6
  multiplex Q85.1
  non-neoplastic I78.1
  oral mucosa D10.30
    specified site NEC D10.39
    white sponge Q38.6
  orbit D31.6-
  pigmented
    giant (*see also* Neoplasm, skin, uncertain
      behavior) D48.5
      malignant melanoma in — *see* Melanoma
  portwine Q82.5
  retina D31.2-
  retrobulbar D31.6-
  sanguineous Q82.5
  senile I78.1
  skin D22.9
    abdominal wall D22.5
    ala nasi D22.39
    ankle D22.7-
    anus, anal D22.5
    arm D22.6-
    auditory canal (external) D22.2-
    auricle (ear) D22.2-
    auricular canal (external) D22.2-
    axilla, axillary fold D22.5
    back D22.5
    breast D22.5
    brow D22.39
    buttock D22.5
    canthus (eye) D22.1-
    cheek (external) D22.39
    chest wall D22.5
    chin D22.39
    ear (external) D22.2-
    external meatus (ear) D22.2-
    eyebrow D22.39
    eyelid (lower) (upper) D22.1-
    face D22.30
      specified NEC D22.39
    female genital organ (external) NEC D28.0
    finger D22.6-
    flank D22.5
    foot D22.7-
    forearm D22.6-
    forehead D22.39
    foreskin D29.0

Nevus D22.9 — *continued*
skin D22.9 — *continued*
genital organ (external) NEC
female D28.0
male D29.9
gluteal region D22.5
groin D22.5
hand D22.6-
heel D22.7-
helix D22.2-
hip D22.7-
interscapular region D22.5
jaw D22.39
knee D22.7-
labium (majus) (minus) D28.0
leg D22.7-
lip (lower) (upper) D22.0
lower limb D22.7-
male genital organ (external) D29.9
nail D22.9
finger D22.6-
toe D22.7-
nasolabial groove D22.39
nates D22.5
neck D22.4
nose (external) D22.39
palpebra D22.1-
penis D29.0
perianal skin D22.5
perineum D22.5
pinna D22.2-
popliteal fossa or space D22.7-
prepuce D29.0
pudendum D28.0
scalp D22.4
scrotum D29.4
shoulder D22.6-
submammary fold D22.5
temple D22.39
thigh D22.7-
toe D22.7-
trunk NEC D22.5
umbilicus D22.5
upper limb D22.6-
vulva D28.0
specified site NEC — *see* Neoplasm, by site, benign
spider I78.1
stellar I78.1
strawberry Q82.5
Sutton's — *see* Neoplasm, skin, benign
unius lateris Q82.5
Unna's Q82.5
vascular Q82.5
verrucous Q82.5
Newborn (infant) (liveborn) (singleton) Z38.2
abstinence syndrome P96.1
acne L70.4
affected by
abnormalities of membranes P02.9
specified NEC P02.8
abruptio placenta P02.1
amino-acid metabolic disorder, transitory P74.8
amniocentesis (while in utero) P00.6
amnionitis P02.7
apparent life threatening event (ALTE) R68.13
bleeding (into)
cerebral cortex P52.22
germinal matrix P52.0
ventricles P52.1
breech delivery P03.0
cardiac arrest P29.81
cardiomyopathy I42.8
congenital I42.4
cerebral ischemia P91.0
cesarean delivery P03.4
chemotherapy agents P04.1

Newborn (infant) (liveborn) (singleton) Z38.2
— *continued*
affected by — *continued*
chorioamnionitis P02.7
cocaine (crack) P04.41
complications of labor and delivery P03.9
specified NEC P03.89
compression of umbilical cord NEC P02.5
contracted pelvis P03.1
delivery P03.9
cesarean P03.4
forceps P03.2
vacuum extractor P03.3
entanglement (knot) in umbilical cord P02.5
environmental chemicals P04.6
fetal (intrauterine)
growth retardation P05.9
malnutrition not light or small for gestational age P05.2
forceps delivery P03.2
heart rate abnormalities
bradycardia P29.12
intrauterine P03.819
before onset of labor P03.810
during labor P03.811
tachycardia P29.11
hemorrhage (antepartum) P02.1
cerebellar (nontraumatic) P52.6
intracerebral (nontraumatic) P52.4
intracranial (nontraumatic) P52.9
specified NEC P52.8
intraventricular (nontraumatic) P52.3
grade 1 P52.0
grade 2 P52.1
grade 3 P52.21
grade 4 P52.22
posterior fossa (nontraumatic) P52.6
subarachnoid (nontraumatic) P52.5
subependymal P52.0
with intracerebral extension P52.22
with intraventricular extension P52.1
with enlargment of ventricles P52.21
without intraventricular extension P52.0
hypoxic ischemic encephalopathy [HIE] P91.60
mild P91.61
moderate P91.62
severe P91.63
induction of labor P03.89
intestinal perforation P78.0
intrauterine (fetal) blood loss P50.9
due to (from)
cut end of co-twin cord P50.5
hemorrhage into
co-twin P50.3
maternal circulation P50.4
placenta P50.2
ruptured cord blood P50.1
vasa previa P50.0
specified NEC P50.8
intrauterine (fetal) hemorrhage P50.9
intrauterine (in utero) procedure P96.5
malpresentation (malposition) NEC P03.1
maternal (complication of) (use of)
alcohol P04.3
analgesia (maternal) P04.0
anesthesia (maternal) P04.0
blood loss P02.1
circulatory disease P00.3
condition P00.9
specified NEC P00.89
delivery P03.9
Cesarean P03.4
forceps P03.2
vacuum extractor P03.3
diabetes mellitus (pre-existing) P70.1
disorder P00.9
specified NEC P00.89
drugs (addictive) (illegal) NEC P04.49

Newborn (infant) (liveborn) (singleton) Z38.2
— *continued*
affected by — *continued*
maternal (complication of) (use of) — *continued*
ectopic pregnancy P01.4
gestational diabetes P70.0
hemorrhage P02.1
hypertensive disorder P00.0
incompetent cervix P01.0
infectious disease P00.2
injury P00.5
labor and delivery P03.9
malpresentation before labor P01.7
maternal death P01.6
medical procedure P00.7
medication P04.1
multiple pregnancy P01.5
nutritional disorder P00.4
oligohydramnios P01.2
parasitic disease P00.2
periodontal disease P00.81
placenta previa P02.0
polyhydramnios P01.3
precipitate delivery P03.5
pregnancy P01.9
specified P01.8
premature rupture of membranes P01.1
renal disease P00.1
respiratory disease P00.3
surgical procedure P00.6
urinary tract disease P00.1
uterine contraction (abnormal) P03.6
meconium peritonitis P78.0
medication (legal) (maternal use) (prescribed) P04.1
membrane abnormalities P02.9
specified NEC P02.8
membranitis P02.7
methamphetamine(s) P04.49
mixed metabolic and respiratory acidosis P84
neonatal abstinence syndrome P96.1
noxious substances transmitted via placenta or breast milk P04.9
specified NEC P04.8
nutritional supplements P04.5
placenta previa P02.0
placental
abnormality (functional) (morphological) P02.20
specified NEC P02.29
dysfunction P02.29
infarction P02.29
insufficiency P02.29
separation NEC P02.1
transfusion syndromes P02.3
placentitis P02.7
precipitate delivery P03.5
prolapsed cord P02.4
respiratory arrest P28.81
slow intrauterine growth P05.9
tobacco P04.2
twin to twin transplacental transfusion P02.3
umbilical cord (tightly) around neck P02.5
umbilical cord condition P02.60
short cord P02.69
specified NEC P02.69
uterine contractions (abnormal) P03.6
vasa previa P02.69
from intrauterine blood loss P50.0
apnea P28.4
obstructive P28.4
primary P28.3
sleep (central) (obstructive) (primary) P28.3
born in hospital Z38.00
by cesarean Z38.01
born outside hospital Z38.1
breast buds P96.89

Newborn (infant) (liveborn) (singleton) Z38.2
— *continued*
breast engorgement P83.4
check-up — *see* Newborn, examination
convulsion P90
dehydration P74.1
examination
  8 to 28 days old Z00.111
  under 8 days old Z00.110
fever P81.9
  environmentally-induced P81.0
hyperbilirubinemia P59.9
  of prematurity P59.0
hypernatremia P74.2
hyponatremia P74.2
infection P39.9
  candidal P37.5
  specified NEC P39.8
  urinary tract P39.3
jaundice P59.9
  due to
    breast milk inhibitor P59.3
    hepatocellular damage P59.20
      specified NEC P59.29
    preterm delivery P59.0
  of prematurity P59.0
  specified NEC P59.8
late metabolic acidosis P74.0
mastitis P39.0
  infective P39.0
  noninfective P83.4
multiple born NEC Z38.8
  born in hospital Z38.68
    by cesarean Z38.69
  born outside hospital Z38.7
omphalitis P38.9
  with mild hemorrhage P38.1
  without hemorrhage P38.9
post-term P08.21
prolonged gestation (over 42 completed weeks) P08.22
quadruplet Z38.8
  born in hospital Z38.63
    by cesarean Z38.64
  born outside hospital Z38.7
quintuplet Z38.8
  born in hospital Z38.65
    by cesarean Z38.66
  born outside hospital Z38.7
seizure P90
sepsis (congenital) P36.9
  due to
    anaerobes NEC P36.5
    Escherichia coli P36.4
    Staphylococcus P36.30
      aureus P36.2
      specified NEC P36.39
    Streptococcus P36.10
      group B P36.0
      specified NEC P36.19
    specified NEC P36.8
triplet Z38.8
  born in hospital Z38.61
    by cesarean Z38.62
  born outside hospital Z38.7
twin Z38.5
  born in hospital Z38.30
    by cesarean Z38.31
  born outside hospital Z38.4
vomiting P92.09
  bilious P92.01
weight check Z00.111
Newcastle conjunctivitis or disease B30.8
Nezelof's syndrome (pure alymphocytosis) D81.4
Niacin(amide) deficiency E52
Nicolas(-Durand)-Favre disease A55
Nicotine — *see* Tobacco
Nicotinic acid deficiency E52

Niemann-Pick disease or syndrome E75.249
specified NEC E75.248
type
  A E75.240
  B E75.241
  C E75.242
  D E75.243
Night
blindness — *see* Blindness, night
sweats R61
terrors (child) F51.4
Nightmares (REM sleep type) F51.5
NIHSS (National Institutes of Health Stroke Scale) score R29.7-
Nipple — *see* condition
Nisbet's chancre A57
Nishimoto (-Takeuchi) disease I67.5
Nitritoid crisis or reaction — *see* Crisis, nitritoid
Nitrosohemoglobinemia D74.8
Njovera A65
Nocardiosis, nocardiasis A43.9
cutaneous A43.1
lung A43.0
pneumonia A43.0
pulmonary A43.0
specified site NEC A43.8
Nocturia R35.1
psychogenic F45.8
Nocturnal — *see* condition
Nodal rhythm I49.8
Node(s) — *see also* Nodule
Bouchard's (with arthropathy) M15.2
Haygarth's M15.8
Heberden's (with arthropathy) M15.1
larynx J38.7
lymph — *see* condition
milker's B08.03
Osler's I33.0
Schmorl's — *see* Schmorl's disease
singer's J38.2
teacher's J38.2
tuberculous — *see* Tuberculosis, lymph gland
vocal cord J38.2
Nodule(s), nodular
actinomycotic — *see* Actinomycosis
breast NEC N63
colloid (cystic), thyroid E04.1
cutaneous — *see* Swelling, localized
endometrial (stromal) D26.1
Haygarth's M15.8
inflammatory — *see* Inflammation
juxta-articular
  syphilitic A52.77
  yaws A66.7
larynx J38.7
lung, solitary (subsegmental branch of the bronchial tree) R91.1
  multiple R91.8
milker's B08.03
prostate N40.2
  with lower urinary tract symptoms (LUTS) N40.3
  without lower urinary tract symptoms (LUTS) N40.2
pulmonary, solitary (subsegmental branch of the bronchial tree) R91.1
retrocardiac R09.89
rheumatoid M06.30
  ankle M06.37-
  elbow M06.32-
  foot joint M06.37-
  hand joint M06.34-
  hip M06.35-
  knee M06.36-
  multiple site M06.39
  shoulder M06.31-
  vertebra M06.38

Nodule(s), nodular — *continued*
rheumatoid M06.30 — *continued*
  wrist M06.33-
scrotum (inflammatory) N49.2
singer's J38.2
solitary, lung (subsegmental branch of the bronchial tree) R91.1
  multiple R91.8
subcutaneous — *see* Swelling, localized
teacher's J38.2
thyroid (cold) (gland) (nontoxic) E04.1
  with thyrotoxicosis E05.20
    with thyroid storm E05.21
  toxic or with hyperthyroidism E05.20
    with thyroid storm E05.21
vocal cord J38.2
Noma (gangrenous) (hospital) (infective) A69.0
auricle I96
mouth A69.0
pudendi N76.89
vulvae N76.89
Nomad, nomadism Z59.0
NOMID (neonatal onset multisystemic inflammatory disorder) M04.2
Nonautoimmune hemolytic anemia D59.4
drug-induced D59.2
Nonclosure — *see also* Imperfect, closure
ductus arteriosus (Botallo's) Q25.0
foramen
  botalli Q21.1
  ovale Q21.1
Noncompliance Z91.19
with
  dialysis Z91.15
  dietary regimen Z91.11
  medical treatment Z91.19
  medication regimen NEC Z91.14
    underdosing (*see also* Table of Drugs and Chemicals, categories T36-T50, with final character 6) Z91.14
      intentional NEC Z91.128
        due to financial hardship of patient Z91.120
      unintentional NEC Z91.138
        due to patient's age related debility Z91.130
  renal dialysis Z91.15
Nondescent (congenital) — *see also* Malposition, congenital
cecum Q43.3
colon Q43.3
testicle Q53.9
  bilateral Q53.20
    abdominal Q53.21
    perineal Q53.22
  unilateral Q53.10
    abdominal Q53.11
    perineal Q53.12
Nondevelopment
brain Q02
  part of Q04.3
organ or site, congenital NEC — *see* Hypoplasia
Nonengagement
head NEC O32.4
  in labor, causing obstructed labor O64.8
Nonexanthematous tick fever A93.2
Nonexpansion, lung (newborn) P28.0
Nonfunctioning
cystic duct (*see also* Disease, gallbladder) K82.8
gallbladder (*see also* Disease, gallbladder) K82.8
kidney N28.9
labyrinth — *see* subcategory H83.2
Non-Hodgkin lymphoma NEC — *see* Lymphoma, non-Hodgkin
Nonimplantation, ovum N97.2

Noninsufflation, fallopian tube N97.1
Non-ketotic hyperglycinemia E72.51
Nonne-Milroy syndrome Q82.0
Nonovulation N97.0
Nonpatent fallopian tube N97.1
Nonpneumatization, lung NEC P28.0
Nonrotation — see Malrotation
Nonsecretion, urine — see Anuria
Nonunion
    fracture — see Fracture, by site
    joint, following fusion or arthrodesis M96.0
    organ or site, congenital NEC — see Imperfect,
        closure
    symphysis pubis, congenital Q74.2
Nonvisualization, gallbladder R93.2
Nonvital, nonvitalized tooth K04.99
Non-working side interference M26.56
Noonan's syndrome Q87.1
Normocytic anemia (infectional) due to blood loss (chronic) D50.0
    acute D62
Norrie's disease (congenital) Q15.8
North American blastomycosis B40.9
Norwegian itch B86
Nose, nasal — see condition
Nosebleed R04.0
Nosomania F45.21
Nosophobia F45.22
Nose-picking F98.8
Nostalgia F43.20
Notch of iris Q13.2
Notching nose, congenital (tip) Q30.2
Nothnagel's
    syndrome — see Strabismus, paralytic, third
        nerve
    vasomotor acroparesthesia I73.89
Novy's relapsing fever A68.9
    louse-borne A68.0
    tick-borne A68.1
Noxious
    foodstuffs, poisoning by — see Poisoning,
        food, noxious, plant
    substances transmitted through placenta or
        breast milk P04.9
Nucleus pulposus — see condition
Numbness R20.0
Nuns' knee — see Bursitis, prepatellar
Nursemaid's elbow S53.03-
Nutcracker esophagus K22.4
Nutmeg liver K76.1
Nutrient element deficiency E61.9
    specified NEC E61.8
Nutrition deficient or insufficient (see also Malnutrition) E46
    due to
        insufficient food T73.0
        lack of
            care (child) T76.02
                adult T76.01
            food T73.0
Nutritional stunting E45
Nyctalopia (night blindness) — see Blindness, night
Nycturia R35.1
    psychogenic F45.8
Nymphomania F52.8
Nystagmus H55.00
    benign paroxysmal — see Vertigo, benign
        paroxysmal
    central positional H81.4-
    congenital H55.01
    dissociated H55.04
    latent H55.02
    miners' H55.09
    positional
        benign paroxysmal H81.4-
        central H81.4-
    specified form NEC H55.09
    visual deprivation H55.03

O

Obermeyer's relapsing fever (European) A68.0
Obesity E66.9
    with alveolar hypoventilation E66.2
    adrenal E27.8
    complicating
        childbirth O99.214
        pregnancy O99.21-
        puerperium O99.215
    constitutional E66.8
    dietary counseling and surveillance Z71.3
    drug-induced E66.1
    due to
        drug E66.1
        excess calories E66.09
            morbid E66.01
            severe E66.01
    endocrine E66.8
    endogenous E66.8
    exogenous E66.09
    familial E66.8
    glandular E66.8
    hypothyroid — see Hypothyroidism
    hypoventilation syndrome (OHS) E66.2
    morbid E66.01
        with
            alveolar hypoventilation E66.2
            obesity hypoventilation syndrome (OHS) E66.2
        due to excess calories E66.01
    nutritional E66.09
    pituitary E23.6
    severe E66.01
    specified type NEC E66.8
Oblique — see condition
Obliteration
    appendix (lumen) K38.8
    artery I77.1
    bile duct (noncalculous) K83.1
    common duct (noncalculous) K83.1
    cystic duct — see Obstruction, gallbladder
    disease, arteriolar I77.1
    endometrium N85.8
    eye, anterior chamber — see Disorder, globe, hypotony
    fallopian tube N97.1
    lymphatic vessel I89.0
        due to mastectomy I97.2
    organ or site, congenital NEC — see Atresia, by site
    ureter N13.5
        with infection N13.6
    urethra — see Stricture, urethra
    vein I87.8
    vestibule (oral) K08.89
Observation (following) (for) (without need for further medical care) Z04.9
    accident NEC Z04.3
        at work Z04.2
        transport Z04.1
    adverse effect of drug Z03.6
    alleged rape or sexual assault (victim), ruled out
        adult Z04.41
        child Z04.42
    criminal assault Z04.8
    development state
        adolescent Z00.3
        period of rapid growth in childhood Z00.2
        puberty Z00.3
    disease, specified NEC Z03.89
    following work accident Z04.2
    growth and development state — see Observation, development state
    injuries (accidental) NEC — see also Observation, accident

Observation (following) (for) (without need for further medical care) Z04.9 — continued
    newborn (for)
        suspected condition, related to exposure from the mother or birth process — see Newborn, affected by, maternal
        ruled out Z05.9
            cardiac Z05.0
            connective tissue Z05.73
            gastrointestinal Z05.5
            genetic Z05.41
            genitourinary Z05.6
            immunologic Z05.43
            infectious Z05.1
            metabolic Z05.42
            musculoskeletal Z05.72
            neurological Z05.2
            respiratory Z05.3
            skin and subcutaneous tissue Z05.71
            specified condition NEC Z05.8
    postpartum
        immediately after delivery Z39.0
        routine follow-up Z39.2
    pregnancy (normal) (without complication) Z34.9-
        high risk O09.9-
    suicide attempt, alleged NEC Z03.89
        self-poisoning Z03.6
    suspected, ruled out — see also Suspected condition, ruled out
        abuse, physical
            adult Z04.71
            child Z04.72
        accident at work Z04.2
        adult battering victim Z04.71
        child battering victim Z04.72
        condition NEC Z03.89
            newborn (see also Observation, newborn (for), suspected condition, ruled out) Z05.9
        drug poisoning or adverse effect Z03.6
        exposure (to)
            anthrax Z03.810
            biological agent NEC Z03.818
        inflicted injury NEC Z04.8
        suicide attempt, alleged Z03.89
            self-poisoning Z03.6
        toxic effects from ingested substance (drug) (poison) Z03.6
    toxic effects from ingested substance (drug) (poison) Z03.6
Obsession, obsessional state F42.8
    mixed thoughts and acts F42.2
Obsessive-compulsive neurosis or reaction F42.8
Obstetric embolism, septic — see Embolism, obstetric, septic
Obstetrical trauma (complicating delivery) O71.9
    with or following ectopic or molar pregnancy O08.6
    specified type NEC O71.89
Obstipation — see Constipation
Obstruction, obstructed, obstructive
    airway J98.8
        with
            allergic alveolitis J67.9
            asthma J45.909
                with
                    exacerbation (acute) J45.901
                    status asthmaticus J45.902
            bronchiectasis J47.9
                with
                    exacerbation (acute) J47.1
                    lower respiratory infection J47.0
            bronchitis (chronic) J44.9
            emphysema J43.9

DISEASE INDEX

Obstruction, obstructed, obstructive —
continued
airway J98.8 — *continued*
  chronic J44.9
    with
      allergic alveolitis — *see* Pneumonitis,
        hypersensitivity
      bronchiectasis J47.9
        with
          exacerbation (acute) J47.1
          lower respiratory infection J47.0
  due to
    foreign body — *see* Foreign body, by site,
      causing asphyxia
    inhalation of fumes or vapors J68.9
    laryngospasm J38.5
ampulla of Vater K83.1
aortic (heart) (valve) — *see* Stenosis, aortic
aortoiliac I74.09
aqueduct of Sylvius G91.1
  congenital Q03.0
    with spina bifida — *see* Spina bifida, by
      site, with hydrocephalus
Arnold-Chiari — *see* Arnold-Chiari disease
artery (*see also* Embolism, artery) I74.9
  basilar (complete) (partial) — *see* Occlusion,
    artery, basilar
  carotid (complete) (partial) — *see* Occlusion,
    artery, carotid
  cerebellar — *see* Occlusion, artery,
    cerebellar
  cerebral (anterior) (middle) (posterior) — *see*
    Occlusion, artery, cerebral
  precerebral — *see* Occlusion, artery,
    precerebral
  renal N28.0
  retinal NEC — *see* Occlusion, artery, retina
  stent — *see* Restenosis, stent
  vertebral (complete) (partial) — *see*
    Occlusion, artery, vertebral
band (intestinal) K56.69
bile duct or passage (common) (hepatic)
  (noncalculous) K83.1
  with calculus K80.51
  congenital (causing jaundice) Q44.3
biliary (duct) (tract) K83.1
  gallbladder K82.0
bladder-neck (acquired) N32.0
  congenital Q64.31
  due to hyperplasia (hypertrophy) of prostate
    — *see* Hyperplasia, prostate
bowel — *see* Obstruction, intestine
bronchus J98.09
canal, ear — *see* Stenosis, external ear canal
cardia K22.2
caval veins (inferior) (superior) I87.1
cecum — *see* Obstruction, intestine
circulatory I99.8
colon — *see* Obstruction, intestine
common duct (noncalculous) K83.1
coronary (artery) — *see* Occlusion, coronary
cystic duct — *see also* Obstruction, gallbladder
  with calculus K80.21
device, implant or graft (*see also* Complications,
  by site and type, mechanical) T85.698
  arterial graft NEC — *see* Complication,
    cardiovascular device, mechanical,
    vascular
  catheter NEC T85.628
    cystostomy T83.090
    dialysis (renal) T82.49
      intraperitoneal T85.691
    Hopkins T83.098
    ileostomy T83.098
    infusion NEC T82.594
      spinal (epidural) (subdural) T85.690
    nephrostomy T83.092
    urethral indwelling T83.091
    urinary T83.098

Obstruction, obstructed, obstructive —
continued
device, implant or graft (*see also* Complications,
  by site and type, mechanical) T85.698 —
  continued
  catheter NEC T85.628 — *continued*
    urostomy T83.098
  due to infection T85.79
  gastrointestinal — *see* Complications,
    prosthetic device, mechanical,
    gastrointestinal device
  genital NEC T83.498
    intrauterine contraceptive device T83.39
    penile prosthesis (cylinder) (implanted)
      (pump) (resevoir) T83.490
    testicular prosthesis T83.491
  heart NEC — *see* Complication,
    cardiovascular device, mechanical
  joint prosthesis — *see* Complications, joint
    prosthesis, mechanical, specified NEC,
    by site
  orthopedic NEC — *see* Complication,
    orthopedic, device, mechanical
  specified NEC T85.628
  urinary NEC — *see also* Complication,
    genitourinary, device, urinary,
    mechanical
    graft T83.29
  vascular NEC — *see* Complication,
    cardiovascular device, mechanical
  ventricular intracranial shunt T85.09
  due to foreign body accidentally left in
    operative wound T81.529
duodenum K31.5
ejaculatory duct N50.89
esophagus K22.2
eustachian tube (complete) (partial) H68.10-
  cartilagenous (extrinsic) H68.13-
    intrinsic H68.12-
  osseous H68.11-
fallopian tube (bilateral) N97.1
fecal K56.41
  with hernia — *see* Hernia, by site, with
    obstruction
foramen of Monro (congenital) Q03.8
  with spina bifida — *see* Spina bifida, by site,
    with hydrocephalus
foreign body — *see* Foreign body
gallbladder K82.0
  with calculus, stones K80.21
  congenital Q44.1
gastric outlet K31.1
gastrointestinal — *see* Obstruction, intestine
hepatic K76.89
  duct (noncalculous) K83.1
hepatobiliary K83.1
ileum — *see* Obstruction, intestine
iliofemoral (artery) I74.5
intestine K56.60
  with
    adhesions (intestinal) (peritoneal) K56.5
  adynamic K56.0
  by gallstone K56.3
  congenital (small) Q41.9
    large Q42.9
      specified part NEC Q42.8
  neurogenic K56.0
    Hirschsprung's disease or megacolon Q43.1
  newborn P76.9
    due to
      fecaliths P76.8
      inspissated milk P76.2
      meconium (plug) P76.0
        in mucoviscidosis E84.11
    specified NEC P76.8
  postoperative K91.3
  reflex K56.0
  specified NEC K56.69
  volvulus K56.2

Obstruction, obstructed, obstructive —
continued
intracardiac ball valve prosthesis T82.09
jejunum — *see* Obstruction, intestine
joint prosthesis — *see* Complications, joint
  prosthesis, mechanical, specified NEC, by
  site
kidney (calices) N28.89
labor — *see* Delivery
lacrimal (passages) (duct)
  by
    dacryolith — *see* Dacryolith
    stenosis — *see* Stenosis, lacrimal
  congenital Q10.5
  neonatal H04.53-
lacrimonasal duct — *see* Obstruction, lacrimal
lacteal, with steatorrhea K90.2
laryngitis — *see* Laryngitis
larynx NEC J38.6
  congenital Q31.8
lung J98.4
  disease, chronic J44.9
lymphatic I89.0
meconium (plug)
  newborn P76.0
    due to fecaliths P76.0
    in mucoviscidosis E84.11
mitral — *see* Stenosis, mitral
nasal J34.89
nasolacrimal duct — *see also* Obstruction,
  lacrimal
  congenital Q10.5
nasopharynx J39.2
nose J34.89
organ or site, congenital NEC — *see* Atresia,
  by site
pancreatic duct K86.89
parotid duct or gland K11.8
pelviureteral junction N13.5
  with hydronephrosis N13.0
  congenital Q62.39
pharynx J39.2
portal (circulation) (vein) I81
prostate — *see also* Hyperplasia, prostate
  valve (urinary) N32.0
pulmonary valve (heart) I37.0
pyelonephritis (chronic) N11.1
pylorus
  adult K31.1
  congenital or infantile Q40.0
rectosigmoid — *see* Obstruction, intestine
rectum K62.4
renal N28.89
  outflow N13.8
  pelvis, congenital Q62.39
respiratory J98.8
  chronic J44.9
retinal (vessels) H34.9
salivary duct (any) K11.8
  with calculus K11.5
sigmoid — *see* Obstruction, intestine
sinus (accessory) (nasal) J34.89
Stensen's duct K11.8
stomach NEC K31.89
  acute K31.0
  congenital Q40.2
  due to pylorospasm K31.3
submandibular duct K11.8
submaxillary gland K11.8
  with calculus K11.5
thoracic duct I89.0
thrombotic — *see* Thrombosis
trachea J39.8
tracheostomy airway J95.03
tricuspid (valve) — *see* Stenosis, tricuspid
upper respiratory, congenital Q34.8

Obstruction, obstructed, obstructive —
continued
ureter (functional) (pelvic junction) NEC N13.5
    with
        hydronephrosis N13.1
            with infection N13.6
        pyelonephritis (chronic) N11.1
    congenital Q62.39
    due to calculus — see Calculus, ureter
urethra NEC N36.8
    congenital Q64.39
urinary (moderate) N13.9
    due to hyperplasia (hypertrophy) of prostate
        — see Hyperplasia, prostate
    organ or tract (lower) N13.9
    prostatic valve N32.0
    specified NEC N13.8
uropathy N13.9
uterus N85.8
vagina N89.5
valvular — see Endocarditis
vein, venous I87.1
    caval (inferior) (superior) I87.1
    thrombotic — see Thrombosis
vena cava (inferior) (superior) I87.1
vesical NEC N32.0
vesicourethral orifice N32.0
    congenital Q64.31
vessel NEC I99.8
    stent — see Restenosis, stent
Obturator — see condition
Occlusal wear, teeth K03.0
Occlusio pupillae — see Membrane, pupillary
Occlusion, occluded
anus K62.4
    congenital Q42.3
        with fistula Q42.2
aortoiliac (chronic) I74.09
aqueduct of Sylvius G91.1
    congenital Q03.0
        with spina bifida — see Spina bifida, by
            site, with hydrocephalus
artery (see also Embolism, artery) I74.9
    auditory, internal I65.8
    basilar I65.1
        with
            infarction I63.22
                due to
                    embolism I63.12
                    thrombosis I63.02
    brain or cerebral I66.9
        with infarction (due to) I63.5-
            embolism I63.4-
            thrombosis I63.3-
    carotid I65.2-
        with
            infarction I63.23-
                due to
                    embolism I63.13-
                    thrombosis I63.03-
    cerebellar (anterior inferior) (posterior
        inferior) (superior) I66.3
        with infarction I63.54-
            due to
                embolism I63.44-
                thrombosis I63.34-
    cerebral I66.9
        with infarction I63.50
            due to
                embolism I63.40
                    specified NEC I63.49
                thrombosis I63.30
                    specified NEC I63.39
        anterior I66.1-
            with infarction I63.52-
                due to
                    embolism I63.42-
                    thrombosis I63.32-

Occlusion, occluded — continued
artery (see also Embolism, artery) I74.9 —
    continued
    cerebral I66.9 — continued
        middle I66.0-
            with infarction I63.51-
                due to
                    embolism I63.41-
                    thrombosis I63.31-
        posterior I66.2-
            with infarction I63.53-
                due to
                    embolism I63.43-
                    thrombosis I63.33-
        specified NEC I66.8
            with infarction I63.59
                due to
                    embolism I63.4-
                    thrombosis I63.3-
    choroidal (anterior) — see Occlusion, artery,
        precerebral, specified NEC
    communicating posterior — see Occlusion,
        artery, cerebral, specified NEC
    complete
        coronary I25.82
        extremities I70.92
    coronary (acute) (thrombotic) (without
        myocardial infarction) I24.0
        with myocardial infarction — see
            Infarction, myocardium
        chronic total I25.82
        complete I25.82
        healed or old I25.2
        total (chronic) I25.82
    hypophyseal — see Occlusion, artery,
        precerebral, specified NEC
    iliac I74.5
    lower extremities due to stenosis or stricture
        I77.1
    mesenteric (embolic) (thrombotic) (see also
        Infarct, intestine) K55.069
    perforating — see Occlusion, artery,
        cerebral, specified NEC
    peripheral I77.9
        thrombotic or embolic I74.4
    pontine — see Occlusion, artery, cerebral,
        specified NEC
    precerebral I65.9
        with infarction I63.20
            due to
                embolism I63.10
                    specified NEC I63.19
                thrombosis I63.00
                    specified NEC I63.09
                specified NEC I63.29
        basilar — see Occlusion, artery, basilar
        carotid — see Occlusion, artery, carotid
        puerperal O88.23
        specified NEC I65.8
            with infarction I63.29
                due to
                    embolism I63.19
                    thrombosis I63.00
        vertebral — see Occlusion, artery,
            vertebral
    renal N28.0
    retinal
        branch H34.23-
        central H34.1-
        partial H34.21-
        transient H34.0-
    spinal — see Occlusion, artery, precerebral,
        vertebral
    total (chronic)
        coronary I25.82
        extremities I70.92

Occlusion, occluded — continued
artery (see also Embolism, artery) I74.9 —
    continued
    vertebral I65.0-
        with
            infarction I63.21-
                due to
                    embolism I63.11-
                    thrombosis I63.01-
basilar artery — see Occlusion, artery, basilar
bile duct (common) (hepatic) (noncalculous)
    K83.1
bowel — see Obstruction, intestine
carotid (artery) (common) (internal) — see
    Occlusion, artery, carotid
centric (of teeth) M26.59
    maximum intercuspation discrepancy
        M26.55
cerebellar (artery) — see Occlusion, artery,
    cerebellar
cerebral (artery) — see Occlusion, artery,
    cerebral
cerebrovascular — see also Occlusion, artery,
    cerebral
    with infarction I63.5-
cervical canal — see Stricture, cervix
cervix (uteri) — see Stricture, cervix
choanal Q30.0
choroidal (artery) — see Occlusion, artery,
    precerebral, specified NEC
colon — see Obstruction, intestine
communicating posterior artery — see
    Occlusion, artery, precerebral, specified
    NEC
coronary (artery) (vein) (thrombotic) — see also
    Infarct, myocardium
    chronic total I25.82
    healed or old I25.2
    not resulting in infarction I24.0
    total (chronic) I25.82
cystic duct — see Obstruction, gallbladder
embolic — see Embolism
fallopian tube N97.1
    congenital Q50.6
gallbladder — see also Obstruction,
    gallbladder
    congenital (causing jaundice) Q44.1
gingiva, traumatic K06.2
hymen N89.6
    congenital Q52.3
hypophyseal (artery) — see Occlusion, artery,
    precerebral, specified NEC
iliac artery I74.5
intestine — see Obstruction, intestine
lacrimal passages — see Obstruction, lacrimal
lung J98.4
lymph or lymphatic channel I89.0
mammary duct N64.89
mesenteric artery (embolic) (thrombotic) (see
    also Infarct, intestine) K55.069
nose J34.89
    congenital Q30.0
organ or site, congenital NEC — see Atresia,
    by site
oviduct N97.1
    congenital Q50.6
peripheral arteries
    due to stricture or stenosis I77.1
    upper extremity I74.2
pontine (artery) — see Occlusion, artery,
    precerebral, specified NEC
posterior lingual, of mandibular teeth M26.29
precerebral artery — see Occlusion, artery,
    precerebral
punctum lacrimale — see Obstruction, lacrimal
pupil — see Membrane, pupillary
pylorus, adult (see also Stricture, pylorus) K31.1
renal artery N28.0

Occlusion, occluded — *continued*
retina, retinal
artery — *see* Occlusion, artery, retinal
vein (central) H34.81-
engorgement H34.82-
tributary H34.83-
vessels H34.9
spinal artery — *see* Occlusion, artery,
precerebral, vertebral
teeth (mandibular) (posterior lingual) M26.29
thoracic duct I89.0
thrombotic — *see* Thrombosis, artery
traumatic
edentulous (alveolar) ridge K06.2
gingiva K06.2
periodontal K05.5
tubal N97.1
ureter (complete) (partial) N13.5
congenital Q62.10
ureteropelvic junction N13.5
congenital Q62.11
ureterovesical orifice N13.5
congenital Q62.12
urethra — *see* Stricture, urethra
uterus N85.8
vagina N89.5
vascular NEC I99.8
vein — *see* Thrombosis
retinal — *see* Occlusion, retinal, vein
vena cava (inferior) (superior) — *see*
Embolism, vena cava
ventricle (brain) NEC G91.1
vertebral (artery) — *see* Occlusion, artery,
vertebral
vessel (blood) I99.8
vulva N90.5
Occult
blood in feces (stools) R19.5
Occupational
problems NEC Z56.89
Ochlophobia — *see* Agoraphobia
Ochronosis (endogenous) E70.29
Ocular muscle — *see* condition
Oculogyric crisis or disturbance H51.8
psychogenic F45.8
Oculomotor syndrome H51.9
Oculopathy
syphilitic NEC A52.71
congenital
early A50.01
late A50.30
early (secondary) A51.43
late A52.71
Oddi's sphincter spasm K83.4
Odontalgia K08.89
Odontoameloblastoma — *see* Cyst,
calcifying odontogenic
Odontoclasia K03.89
Odontodysplasia, regional K00.4
Odontogenesis imperfecta K00.5
Odontoma (ameloblastic) (complex)
(compound) (fibroameloblastic) — *see* Cyst,
calcifying odontogenic
Odontomyelitis (closed) (open) K04.01
irreversible K04.02
reversible K04.01
Odontorrhagia K08.89
Odontosarcoma, ameloblastic C41.1
upper jaw (bone) C41.0
Oestriasis — *see* Myiasis
Oguchi's disease H53.63
Ohara's disease — *see* Tularemia
OHS (obesity hypoventilation syndrome) E66.2
Oidiomycosis — *see* Candidiasis
Oidium albicans infection — *see*
Candidiasis
Old age (without mention of debility) R54
dementia F03

Old (previous) myocardial infarction
I25.2
Olfactory — *see* condition
Oligemia — *see* Anemia
Oligoastrocytoma
specified site — *see* Neoplasm, malignant, by
site
unspecified site C71.9
Oligocythemia D64.9
Oligodendroblastoma
specified site — *see* Neoplasm, malignant
unspecified site C71.9
Oligodendroglioma
anaplastic type
specified site — *see* Neoplasm, malignant,
by site
unspecified site C71.9
specified site — *see* Neoplasm, malignant, by
site
unspecified site C71.9
Oligodontia — *see* Anodontia
Oligoencephalon Q02
Oligohidrosis L74.4
Oligohydramnios O41.0-
Oligohydrosis L74.4
Oligomenorrhea N91.5
primary N91.3
secondary N91.4
Oligophrenia — *see also* Disability, intellectual
phenylpyruvic E70.0
Oligospermia N46.11
due to
drug therapy N46.121
efferent duct obstruction N46.123
infection N46.122
radiation N46.124
specified cause NEC N46.129
systemic disease N46.125
Oligotrichia — *see* Alopecia
Oliguria R34
postprocedural N99.0
with, complicating or following ectopic or
molar pregnancy O08.4
Ollier's disease Q78.4
Omenotocele — *see* Hernia, abdomen,
specified site NEC
Omentitis — *see* Peritonitis
Omentum, omental — *see* condition
Omphalitis (congenital) (newborn) P38.9
with mild hemorrhage P38.1
not of newborn L08.82
tetanus A33
without hemorrhage P38.9
Omphalocele Q79.2
Omphalomesenteric duct, persistent
Q43.0
Omphalorrhagia, newborn P51.9
Omsk hemorrhagic fever A98.1
Onanism (excessive) F98.8
Onchocerciasis, onchocercosis B73.1
with
eye disease B73.00
endophthalmitis B73.01
eyelid B73.09
glaucoma B73.02
specified NEC B73.09
eye NEC B73.00
eyelid B73.09
Oncocytoma — *see* Neoplasm, benign, by site
Oncovirus, as cause of disease classified
elsewhere B97.32
Ondine's curse — *see* Apnea, sleep
Oneirophrenia F23
Onychauxis L60.2
congenital Q84.5

Onychia — *see also* Cellulitis, digit
with lymphangitis — *see* Lymphangitis, acute,
digit
candidal B37.2
dermatophytic B35.1
Onychitis — *see also* Cellulitis, digit
with lymphangitis — *see* Lymphangitis, acute,
digit
Onychocryptosis L60.0
Onychodystrophy L60.3
congenital Q84.6
Onychogryphosis, onychogryposis L60.2
Onycholysis L60.1
Onychomadesis L60.8
Onychomalacia L60.3
Onychomycosis (finger) (toe) B35.1
Onycho-osteodysplasia Q87.2
Onychophagia F98.8
Onychophosis L60.8
Onychoptosis L60.8
Onychorrhexis L60.3
congenital Q84.6
Onychoschizia L60.3
Onyxis (finger) (toe) L60.0
Onyxitis — *see also* Cellulitis, digit
with lymphangitis — *see* Lymphangitis, acute,
digit
Oophoritis (cystic) (infectional) (interstitial)
N70.92
with salpingitis N70.93
acute N70.02
with salpingitis N70.03
chronic N70.12
with salpingitis N70.13
complicating abortion — *see* Abortion, by
type, complicated by, oophoritis
Oophorocele N83.4-
Opacity, opacities
cornea H17-
central H17.1-
congenital Q13.3
degenerative — *see* Degeneration, cornea
hereditary — *see* Dystrophy, cornea
inflammatory — *see* Keratitis
minor H17.81-
peripheral H17.82-
sequelae of trachoma (healed) B94.0
specified NEC H17.89
enamel (teeth) (fluoride) (nonfluoride) K00.3
lens — *see* Cataract
snowball — *see* Deposit, crystalline
vitreous (humor) NEC H43.39-
congenital Q14.0
membranes and strands H43.31-
Opalescent dentin (hereditary) K00.5
Open, opening
abnormal, organ or site, congenital — *see*
Imperfect, closure
angle
borderline
findings
high risk H40.02-
low risk H40.01-
intraocular pressure H40.00-
cupping of discs H40.01-
glaucoma (primary) — *see* Glaucoma, open
angle
bite
anterior M26.220
posterior M26.221
false — *see* Imperfect, closure
margin on tooth restoration K08.51
restoration margins of tooth K08.51
wound — *see* Wound, open
Operational fatigue F48.8
Operative — *see* condition
Operculitis — *see* Periodontitis
Operculum — *see* Break, retina
Ophiasis L63.2

Ophthalmia (*see also* Conjunctivitis) H10.9
  actinic rays — *see* Photokeratitis
  allergic (acute) — *see* Conjunctivitis, acute,
    atopic
  blennorrhagic (gonococcal) (neonatorum)
    A54.31
  diphtheritic A36.86
  Egyptian A71.1
  electrica — *see* Photokeratitis
  gonococcal (neonatorum) A54.31
  metastatic — *see* Endophthalmitis, purulent
  migraine — *see* Migraine, ophthalmoplegic
  neonatorum, newborn P39.1
    gonococcal A54.31
  nodosa H16.24-
  purulent — *see* Conjunctivitis, acute,
    mucopurulent
  spring — *see* Conjunctivitis, acute, atopic
  sympathetic — *see* Uveitis, sympathetic
Ophthalmitis — *see* Ophthalmia
Ophthalmocele (congenital) Q15.8
Ophthalmoneuromyelitis G36.0
Ophthalmoplegia — *see also* Strabismus,
    paralytic
  anterior internuclear — *see* Ophthalmoplegia,
    internuclear
  ataxia-areflexia G61.0
  diabetic — *see* E08-E13 with .39
  exophthalmic E05.00
    with thyroid storm E05.01
  external H49.88-
    progressive H49.4-
      with pigmentary retinopathy — *see*
        Kearns-Sayre syndrome
    total H49.3-
  internal (complete) (total) H52.51-
  internuclear H51.2-
  migraine — *see* Migraine, ophthalmoplegic
  Parinaud's H49.88-
  progressive external — *see* Ophthalmoplegia,
    external, progressive
  supranuclear, progressive G23.1
  total (external) — *see* Ophthalmoplegia,
    external, total
Opioid(s)
  abuse — *see* Abuse, drug, opioids
  dependence — *see* Dependence, drug, opioids
  induced, without use disorder
    anxiety disorder F11.988
    delirium F11.921
    depressive disorder F11.94
    sexual dysfunction F11.981
    sleep disorder F11.982
Opisthognathism M26.09
Opisthorchiasis (felineus) (viverrini) B66.0
Opitz' disease D73.2
Opiumism — *see* Dependence, drug, opioid
Oppenheim's disease G70.2
Oppenheim-Urbach disease (necrobiosis
    lipoidica diabeticorum) — *see* E08-E13 with
    .620
Optic nerve — *see* condition
Orbit — *see* condition
Orchioblastoma C62.9-
Orchitis (gangrenous) (nonspecific) (septic)
    (suppurative) N45.2
  blennorrhagic (gonococcal) (acute) (chronic)
    A54.23
  chlamydial A56.19
  filarial (*see also* Infestation, filarial) B74.9
    [N51]
  gonococcal (acute) (chronic) A54.23
  mumps B26.0
  syphilitic A52.76
  tuberculous A18.15
Orf (virus disease) B08.02

Organic — *see also* condition
  brain syndrome F09
  heart — *see* Disease, heart
  mental disorder F09
  psychosis F09
Orgasm
  anejaculatory N53.13
Oriental
  bilharziasis B65.2
  schistosomiasis B65.2
Orifice — *see* condition
**Origin of both great vessels from right
    ventricle** Q20.1
Ormond's disease (with ureteral obstruction)
    N13.5
  with infection N13.6
Ornithine metabolism disorder E72.4
Ornithinemia (Type I) (Type II) E72.4
Ornithosis A70
Orotaciduria, oroticaciduria (congenital)
    (hereditary) (pyrimidine deficiency) E79.8
  anemia D53.0
Orthodontics
  adjustment Z46.4
  fitting Z46.4
Orthopnea R06.01
Orthopoxvirus B08.09
  specified NEC B08.09
Os, uterus — *see* condition
**Osgood-Schlatter disease or
    osteochondrosis** — *see* Osteochondrosis,
    juvenile, tibia
Osler's nodes I33.0
Osler(-Weber)-Rendu disease I78.0
Osmidrosis L75.0
Osseous — *see* condition
Ossification
  artery — *see* Arteriosclerosis
  auricle (ear) — *see* Disorder, pinna, specified
    type NEC
  bronchial J98.09
  cardiac — *see* Degeneration, myocardial
  cartilage (senile) — *see* Disorder, cartilage,
    specified type NEC
  coronary (artery) — *see* Disease, heart,
    ischemic, atherosclerotic
  diaphragm J98.6
  ear, middle — *see* Otosclerosis
  falx cerebri G96.19
  fontanel, premature Q75.0
  heart — *see also* Degeneration, myocardial
    valve — *see* Endocarditis
  larynx J38.7
  ligament — *see* Disorder, tendon, specified
    type NEC
    posterior longitudinal — *see* Spondylopathy,
      specified NEC
  meninges (cerebral) (spinal) G96.19
  multiple, eccentric centers — *see* Disorder,
    bone, development or growth
  muscle — *see also* Calcification, muscle
    due to burns — *see* Myositis, ossificans, in,
      burns
    paralytic — *see* Myositis, ossificans, in,
      quadriplegia
    progressive — *see* Myositis, ossificans,
      progressiva
  specified NEC M61.50
    ankle M61.57-
    foot M61.57-
    forearm M61.53-
    hand M61.54-
    lower leg M61.56-
    multiple sites M61.59
    pelvic region M61.55-
    shoulder region M61.51-
    specified site NEC M61.58
    thigh M61.55-
    upper arm M61.52-

Ossification — *continued*
  muscle — *see also* Calcification, muscle —
      continued
    traumatic — *see* Myositis, ossificans,
      traumatica
  myocardium, myocardial — *see* Degeneration,
    myocardial
  penis N48.89
  periarticular — *see* Disorder, joint, specified
    type NEC
  pinna — *see* Disorder, pinna, specified type
    NEC
  rider's bone — *see* Ossification, muscle,
    specified NEC
  sclera H15.89
  subperiosteal, post-traumatic M89.8x-
  tendon — *see* Disorder, tendon, specified type
    NEC
  trachea J39.8
  tympanic membrane — *see* Disorder, tympanic
    membrane, specified NEC
  vitreous (humor) — *see* Deposit, crystalline
Osteitis — *see also* Osteomyelitis
  alveolar M27.3
  condensans M85.30
    ankle M85.37- ·
    foot M85.37-
    forearm M85.33-
    hand M85.34-
    lower leg M85.36-
    multiple site M85.39
    neck M85.38
    rib M85.38
    shoulder M85.31-
    skull M85.38
    specified site NEC M85.38
    thigh M85.35-
    toe M85.37-
    upper arm M85.32-
    vertebra M85.38
  deformans M88.9
    in (due to)
      malignant neoplasm of bone C41.9
        [M90.60]
      neoplastic disease (*see also* Neoplasm)
        D49.9 [M90.60]
      carpus D49.9 [M90.6-]
      clavicle D49.9 [M90.6-]
      femur D49.9 [M90.6-]
      fibula D49.9 [M90.6-]
      finger D49.9 [M90.6-]
      humerus D49.9 [M90.6-]
      ilium D49.9 [M90.6-]
      ischium D49.9 [M90.6-]
      metacarpus D49.9 [M90.6-]
      metatarsus D49.9 [M90.6-]
      multiple sites D49.9 [M90.69]
      neck D49.9 [M90.68]
      radius D49.9 [M90.6-]
      rib D49.9 [M90.68]
      scapula D49.9 [M90.6-]
      skull D49.9 [M90.68]
      tarsus D49.9 [M90.6-]
      tibia D49.9 [M90.6-]
      toe D49.9 [M90.6-]
      ulna D49.9 [M90.6-]
      vertebra D49.9 [M90.68]
    skull M88.0
    specified NEC — *see* Paget's disease, bone,
      by site
    vertebra M88.1
  due to yaws A66.6
  fibrosa NEC — *see* Cyst, bone, by site
    circumscripta — *see* Dysplasia, fibrous, bone
      NEC
    cystica (generalisata) E21.0
    disseminata Q78.1
    osteoplastica E21.0
  fragilitans Q78.0

Osteitis (see also Osteomyelitis) — continued
Garr's (sclerosing) — see Osteomyelitis, specified type NEC
jaw (acute) (chronic) (lower) (suppurative) (upper) M27.2
parathyroid E21.0
petrous bone (acute) (chronic) — see Petrositis
sclerotic, nonsuppurative — see Osteomyelitis, specified type NEC
tuberculosa A18.09
  cystica D86.89
  multiplex cystoides D86.89
Osteoarthritis M19.90
ankle M19.07-
elbow M19.02-
foot joint M19.07-
generalized M15.9
  erosive M15.4
  primary M15.0
  specified NEC M15.8
hand joint M19.04-
  first carpometacarpal joint M18.9
hip M16.1-
  bilateral M16.0
  due to hip dysplasia (unilateral) M16.3-
    bilateral M16.2
interphalangeal
  distal (Heberden) M15.1
  proximal (Bouchard) M15.2
knee M17.9
  bilateral M17.0
post-traumatic NEC M19.92
  ankle M19.17-
  elbow M19.12-
  foot joint M19.17-
  hand joint M19.14-
    first carpometacarpal joint M18.3-
      bilateral M18.2
  hip M16.5-
    bilateral M16.4
  knee M17.3-
    bilateral M17.2
  shoulder M19.11-
  wrist M19.13-
primary M19.91
  ankle M19.07-
  elbow M19.02-
  foot joint M19.07-
  hand joint M19.04-
    first carpometacarpal joint M18.1-
      bilateral M18.0
  hip M16.1-
    bilateral M16.0
  knee M17.1-
    bilateral M17.0
  shoulder M19.01-
  spine — see Spondylosis
  wrist M19.03-
secondary M19.93
  ankle M19.27-
  elbow M19.22-
  foot joint M19.27-
  hand joint M19.24-
    first carpometacarpal joint M18.5-
      bilateral M18.4
  hip M16.7
    bilateral M16.6
  knee M17.5
    bilateral M17.4
  multiple M15.3
  shoulder M19.21-
  spine — see Spondylosis
  wrist M19.23-
shoulder M19.01-
spine — see Spondylosis
wrist M19.03-
Osteoarthropathy (hypertrophic) M19.90
ankle — see Osteoarthritis, primary, ankle
elbow — see Osteoarthritis, primary, elbow

Osteoarthropathy (hypertrophic) M19.90 — continued
foot joint — see Osteoarthritis, primary, foot
hand joint — see Osteoarthritis, primary, hand joint
knee joint — see Osteoarthritis, primary, knee
multiple site — see Osteoarthritis, primary, multiple joint
pulmonary — see also Osteoarthropathy, specified type NEC
  hypertrophic — see Osteoarthropathy, hypertrophic, specified type NEC
  secondary — see Osteoarthropathy, specified type NEC
secondary hypertrophic — see Osteoarthropathy, specified type NEC
shoulder — see Osteoarthritis, primary, shoulder
specified joint NEC — see Osteoarthritis, primary, specified joint NEC
specified type NEC M89.40
  carpus M89.44-
  clavicle M89.41-
  femur M89.45-
  fibula M89.46-
  finger M89.44-
  humerus M89.42-
  ilium M89.459
  ischium M89.459
  metacarpus M89.44-
  metatarsus M89.47-
  multiple sites M89.49
  neck M89.48
  radius M89.43-
  rib M89.48
  scapula M89.41-
  skull M89.48
  tarsus M89.47-
  tibia M89.46-
  toe M89.47-
  ulna M89.43-
  vertebra M89.48
spine — see Spondylosis
wrist — see Osteoarthritis, primary, wrist
Osteoarthrosis (degenerative) (hypertrophic) (joint) — see also Osteoarthritis
deformans alkaptonurica E70.29 [M36.8]
erosive M15.4
generalized M15.9
  primary M15.0
polyarticular M15.9
spine — see Spondylosis
Osteoblastoma — see Neoplasm, bone, benign
aggressive — see Neoplasm, bone, uncertain behavior
Osteochondritis — see also Osteochondropathy, by site
Brailsford's — see Osteochondrosis, juvenile, radius
dissecans M93.20
  ankle M93.27-
  elbow M93.22-
  foot M93.27-
  hand M93.24-
  hip M93.25-
  knee M93.26-
  multiple sites M93.29
  shoulder joint M93.21-
  specified site NEC M93.28
  wrist M93.23-
juvenile M92.9
  patellar — see Osteochondrosis, juvenile, patella
syphilitic (congenital) (early) A50.02 [M90.80]
  ankle A50.02 [M90.8-]
  elbow A50.02 [M90.8-]
  foot A50.02 [M90.8-]
  forearm A50.02 [M90.8-]

Osteochondritis — see also Osteochondropathy, by site — continued
syphilitic (congenital) (early) A50.02 [M90.80] — continued
  hand A50.02 [M90.8-]
  hip A50.02 [M90.8-]
  knee A50.02 [M90.8-]
  multiple sites A50.02 [M90.89]
  shoulder joint A50.02 [M90.8-]
  specified site NEC A50.02 [M90.88]
Osteochondroarthrosis deformans endemica — see Disease, Kaschin-Beck
Osteochondrodysplasia Q78.9
with defects of growth of tubular bones and spine Q77.9
specified NEC Q77.8
specified NEC Q78.8
Osteochondrodystrophy E78.9
Osteochondrolysis — see Osteochondritis, dissecans
Osteochondroma — see Neoplasm, bone, benign
Osteochondromatosis D48.0
syndrome Q78.4
Osteochondromyxosarcoma — see Neoplasm, bone, malignant
Osteochondropathy M93.90
ankle M93.97-
elbow M93.92-
foot M93.97-
hand M93.94-
hip M93.95-
Kienböck's disease of adults M93.1
knee M93.96-
multiple joints M93.99
osteochondritis dissecans — see Osteochondritis, dissecans
osteochondrosis — see Osteochondrosis
shoulder region M93.91-
slipped upper femoral epiphysis — see Slipped, epiphysis, upper femoral
specified joint NEC M93.98
specified type NEC M93.80
  ankle M93.87-
  elbow M93.82-
  foot M93.87-
  hand M93.84-
  hip M93.85-
  knee M93.86-
  multiple joints M93.89
  shoulder region M93.81-
  specified joint NEC M93.88
  wrist M93.83-
syphilitic, congenital
  early A50.02 [M90.80]
  late A50.56 [M90.80]
wrist M93.93-
Osteochondrosarcoma — see Neoplasm, bone, malignant
Osteochondrosis — see also Osteochondropathy, by site
acetabulum (juvenile) M91.0
adult — see Osteochondropathy, specified type NEC, by site
astragalus (juvenile) — see Osteochondrosis, juvenile, tarsus
Blount's — see Osteochondrosis, juvenile, tibia
Buchanan's M91.0
Burns' — see Osteochondrosis, juvenile, ulna
calcaneus (juvenile) — see Osteochondrosis, juvenile, tarsus
capitular epiphysis (femur) (juvenile) — see Legg-Calvé-Perthes disease
carpal (juvenile) (lunate) (scaphoid) — see Osteochondrosis, juvenile, hand, carpal lunate
adult M93.1
coxae juvenilis — see Legg-Calvé-Perthes disease

Osteochondrosis (*see also* Osteochondropathy, by site) — *continued*
  deformans juvenilis, coxae — *see* Legg-Calvé-Perthes disease
  Diaz's — *see* Osteochondrosis, juvenile, tarsus
  dissecans (knee) (shoulder) — *see* Osteochondritis, dissecans
  femoral capital epiphysis (juvenile) — *see* Legg-Calvé-Perthes disease
  femur (head), juvenile — *see* Legg-Calvé-Perthes disease
  fibula (juvenile) — *see* Osteochondrosis, juvenile, fibula
  foot NEC (juvenile) M92.8
  Freiberg's — *see* Osteochondrosis, juvenile, metatarsus
  Haas' (juvenile) — *see* Osteochondrosis, juvenile, humerus
  Haglund's — *see* Osteochondrosis, juvenile, tarsus
  hip (juvenile) — *see* Legg-Calvé-Perthes disease
  humerus (capitulum) (head) (juvenile) — *see* Osteochondrosis, juvenile, humerus
  ilium, iliac crest (juvenile) M91.0
  ischiopubic synchondrosis M91.0
  Iselin's — *see* Osteochondrosis, juvenile, metatarsus
  juvenile, juvenilis M92.9
    after congenital dislocation of hip reduction — *see* Osteochondrosis, juvenile, hip, specified NEC
    arm — *see* Osteochondrosis, juvenile, upper limb NEC
    capitular epiphysis (femur) — *see* Legg-Calvé-Perthes disease
    clavicle, sternal epiphysis — *see* Osteochondrosis, juvenile, upper limb NEC
    coxae — *see* Legg-Calvé-Perthes disease
    deformans M92.9
    fibula M92.5-
    foot NEC M92.8
    hand M92.20-
      carpal lunate M92.21-
      metacarpal head M92.22-
      specified site NEC M92.29-
    head of femur — *see* Legg-Calvé-Perthes disease
    hip and pelvis M91.9-
      coxa plana — *see* Coxa, plana
      femoral head — *see* Legg-Calvé-Perthes disease
      pelvis M91.0
      pseudocoxalgia — *see* Pseudocoxalgia
      specified NEC M91.8-
    humerus M92.0-
    limb
      lower NEC M92.8
      upper NEC — *see* Osteochondrosis, juvenile, upper limb NEC
    medial cuneiform bone — *see* Osteochondrosis, juvenile, tarsus
    metatarsus M92.7-
    patella M92.4-
    radius M92.1-
    specified site NEC M92.8
    spine M42.00
      cervical region M42.02
      cervicothoracic region M42.03
      lumbar region M42.06
      lumbosacral region M42.07
      multiple sites M42.09
      occipito-atlanto-axial region M42.01
      sacrococcygeal region M42.08
      thoracic region M42.04
      thoracolumbar region M42.05
    tarsus M92.6-
    tibia M92.5-
    ulna M92.1-

Osteochondrosis (*see also* Osteochondropathy, by site) — *continued*
  juvenile, juvenilis M92.9 — *continued*
    upper limb NEC M92.3-
      vertebra (body) (epiphyseal plates) (Calvé's) (Scheuermann's) — *see* Osteochondrosis, juvenile, spine
    Kienböck's — *see* Osteochondrosis, juvenile, hand, carpal lunate
      adult M93.1
    Köhler's
      patellar — *see* Osteochondrosis, juvenile, patella
      tarsal navicular — *see* Osteochondrosis, juvenile, tarsus
    Legg-Perthes(-Calvé)(-Waldenström) — *see* Legg-Calvé-Perthes disease
    limb
      lower NEC (juvenile) M92.8
      upper NEC (juvenile) — *see* Osteochondrosis, juvenile, upper limb NEC
    lunate bone (carpal) (juvenile) — *see also* Osteochondrosis, juvenile, hand, carpal lunate
      adult M93.1
    Mauclaire's — *see* Osteochondrosis, juvenile, hand, metacarpal
    metacarpal (head) (juvenile) — *see* Osteochondrosis, juvenile, hand, metacarpal
    metatarsus (fifth) (head) (juvenile) (second) — *see* Osteochondrosis, juvenile, metatarsus
    navicular (juvenile) — *see* Osteochondrosis, juvenile, tarsus
    os
      calcis (juvenile) — *see* Osteochondrosis, juvenile, tarsus
      tibiale externum (juvenile) — *see* Osteochondrosis, juvenile, tarsus
    Osgood-Schlatter — *see* Osteochondrosis, juvenile, tibia
    Panner's — *see* Osteochondrosis, juvenile, humerus
    patellar center (juvenile) (primary) (secondary) — *see* Osteochondrosis, juvenile, patella
    pelvis (juvenile) M91.0
    Pierson's M91.0
    radius (head) (juvenile) — *see* Osteochondrosis, juvenile, radius
    Scheuermann's — *see* Osteochondrosis, juvenile, spine
    Sever's — *see* Osteochondrosis, juvenile, tarsus
    Sinding-Larsen — *see* Osteochondrosis, juvenile, patella
    spine M42.9
      adult M42.10
        cervical region M42.12
        cervicothoracic region M42.13
        lumbar region M42.16
        lumbosacral region M42.17
        multiple sites M42.19
        occipito-atlanto-axial region M42.11
        sacrococcygeal region M42.18
        thoracic region M42.14
        thoracolumbar region M42.15
      juvenile — *see* Osteochondrosis, juvenile, spine
    symphysis pubis (juvenile) M91.0
    syphilitic (congenital) A50.02
    talus (juvenile) — *see* Osteochondrosis, juvenile, tarsus
    tarsus (navicular) (juvenile) — *see* Osteochondrosis, juvenile, tarsus
    tibia (proximal) (tubercle) (juvenile) — *see* Osteochondrosis, juvenile, tibia
    tuberculous — *see* Tuberculosis, bone
    ulna (lower) (juvenile) — *see* Osteochondrosis, juvenile, ulna

Osteochondrosis (*see also* Osteochondropathy, by site) — *continued*
  van Neck's M91.0
  vertebral — *see* Osteochondrosis, spine
Osteoclastoma D48.0
  malignant — *see* Neoplasm, bone, malignant
Osteodynia — *see* Disorder, bone, specified type NEC
Osteodystrophy Q78.9
  azotemic N25.0
  congenital Q78.9
  parathyroid, secondary E21.1
  renal N25.0
Osteofibroma — *see* Neoplasm, bone, benign
Osteofibrosarcoma — *see* Neoplasm, bone, malignant
Osteogenesis imperfecta Q78.0
Osteogenic — *see* condition
Osteolysis M89.50
  carpus M89.54-
  clavicle M89.51-
  femur M89.55-
  fibula M89.56-
  finger M89.54-
  humerus M89.52-
  ilium M89.559
  ischium M89.559
  joint prosthesis (periprosthetic) — *see* Complications, joint prosthesis, mechanical, periprosthetic, osteolysis, by site
  metacarpus M89.54-
  metatarsus M89.57-
  multiple sites M89.59
  neck M89.58
  periprosthetic — *see* Complications, joint prosthesis, mechanical, periprosthetic, osteolysis, by site
  radius M89.53-
  rib M89.58
  scapula M89.51-
  skull M89.58
  tarsus M89.57-
  tibia M89.56-
  toe M89.57-
  ulna M89.53-
  vertebra M89.58
Osteoma — *see also* Neoplasm, bone, benign
  osteoid — *see also* Neoplasm, bone, benign
    giant — *see* Neoplasm, bone, benign
Osteomalacia M83.9
  adult M83.9
    drug-induced NEC M83.5
    due to
      malabsorption (postsurgical) M83.2
      malnutrition M83.3
    specified NEC M83.8
  aluminium-induced M83.4
  infantile — *see* Rickets
  juvenile — *see* Rickets
  oncogenic E83.89
  pelvis M83.8
  puerperal M83.0
  senile M83.1
  vitamin-D-resistant in adults E83.31 *[M90.-]*
    carpus E83.31 *[M90.8-]*
    clavicle E83.31 *[M90.8-]*
    femur E83.31 *[M90.8-]*
    fibula E83.31 *[M90.8-]*
    finger E83.31 *[M90.8-]*
    humerus E83.31 *[M90.8-]*
    ilium E83.31 *[M90.859]*
    ischium E83.31 *[M90.859]*
    metacarpus E83.31 *[M90.8-]*
    metatarsus E83.31 *[M90.8-]*
    multiple sites E83.31 *[M90.89]*
    neck E83.31 *[M90.88]*
    radius E83.31 *[M90.8-]*
    rib E83.31 *[M90.88]*

D I S E A S E   I N D E X

Osteomalacia M83.9 — *continued*
 vitamin-D-resistant in adults E83.31 *[M90.-]*
  — *continued*
   scapula E83.31 *[M90.819]*
   skull E83.31 *[M90.88]*
   tarsus E83.31 *[M90.879]*
   tibia E83.31 *[M90.869]*
   toe E83.31 *[M90.879]*
   ulna E83.31 *[M90.839]*
   vertebra E83.31 *[M90.88]*
Osteomyelitis (general) (infective) (localized)
 (neonatal) (purulent) (septic) (staphylococcal)
 (streptococcal) (suppurative) (with periostitis)
 M86.9
 acute M86.10
  carpus M86.14-
  clavicle M86.11-
  femur M86.15-
  fibula M86.16-
  finger M86.14-
  hematogenous M86.00
   carpus M86.04-
   clavicle M86.01-
   femur M86.05-
   fibula M86.06-
   finger M86.04-
   humerus M86.02-
   ilium M86.059
   ischium M86.059
   mandible M27.2
   metacarpus M86.04-
   metatarsus M86.07-
   multiple sites M86.09
   neck M86.08
   orbit H05.02-
   petrous bone — *see* Petrositis
   radius M86.03-
   rib M86.08
   scapula M86.01-
   skull M86.08
   tarsus M86.07-
   tibia M86.06-
   toe M86.07-
   ulna M86.03-
   vertebra — *see* Osteomyelitis, vertebra
  humerus M86.12-
  ilium M86.159
  ischium M86.159
  mandible M27.2
  metacarpus M86.14-
  metatarsus M86.17-
  multiple sites M86.19
  neck M86.18
  orbit H05.02-
  petrous bone — *see* Petrositis
  radius M86.13-
  rib M86.18
  scapula M86.11-
  skull M86.18
  tarsus M86.17-
  tibia M86.16-
  toe M86.17-
  ulna M86.13-
  vertebra — *see* Osteomyelitis, vertebra
 chronic (or old) M86.60
  with draining sinus M86.40
   carpus M86.44-
   clavicle M86.41-
   femur M86.45-
   fibula M86.46-
   finger M86.44-
   humerus M86.42-
   ilium M86.459
   ischium M86.459
   mandible M27.2
   metacarpus M86.44-
   metatarsus M86.47-
   multiple sites M86.49
   neck M86.48

Osteomyelitis (general) (infective) (localized)
 (neonatal) (purulent) (septic) (staphylococcal)
 (streptococcal) (suppurative) (with periostitis)
 M86.9 — *continued*
 chronic (or old) M86.60 — *continued*
  with draining sinus M86.40 — *continued*
   orbit H05.02-
   petrous bone — *see* Petrositis
   radius M86.43-
   rib M86.48
   scapula M86.41-
   skull M86.48
   tarsus M86.47-
   tibia M86.46-
   toe M86.47-
   ulna M86.43-
   vertebra — *see* Osteomyelitis, vertebra
  carpus M86.64-
  clavicle M86.61-
  femur M86.65-
  fibula M86.66-
  finger M86.64-
  hematogenous NEC M86.50
   carpus M86.54-
   clavicle M86.51-
   femur M86.55-
   fibula M86.56-
   finger M86.54-
   humerus M86.52-
   ilium M86.559
   ischium M86.559
   mandible M27.2
   metacarpus M86.54-
   metatarsus M86.57-
   multifocal M86.30
    carpus M86.34-
    clavicle M86.31-
    femur M86.35-
    fibula M86.36-
    finger M86.34-
    humerus M86.32-
    ilium M86.359
    ischium M86.359
    metacarpus M86.34-
    metatarsus M86.37-
    multiple sites M86.39
    neck M86.38
    radius M86.33-
    rib M86.38
    scapula M86.31-
    skull M86.38
    tarsus M86.37-
    tibia M86.36-
    toe M86.37-
    ulna M86.33-
    vertebra — *see* Osteomyelitis, vertebra
   multiple sites M86.59
   neck M86.58
   orbit H05.02-
   petrous bone — *see* Petrositis
   radius M86.53-
   rib M86.58
   scapula M86.51-
   skull M86.58
   tarsus M86.57-
   tibia M86.56-
   toe M86.57-
   ulna M86.53-
   vertebra — *see* Osteomyelitis, vertebra
  humerus M86.62-
  ilium M86.659
  ischium M86.659
  mandible M27.2
  metacarpus M86.64-
  metatarsus M86.67-
  multifocal — *see* Osteomyelitis, chronic,
   hematogenous, multifocal
  multiple sites M86.69
  neck M86.68

Osteomyelitis (general) (infective) (localized)
 (neonatal) (purulent) (septic) (staphylococcal)
 (streptococcal) (suppurative) (with periostitis)
 M86.9 — *continued*
 chronic (or old) M86.60 — *continued*
  orbit H05.02-
  petrous bone — *see* Petrositis
  radius M86.63-
  rib M86.68
  scapula M86.61-
  skull M86.68
  tarsus M86.67-
  tibia M86.66-
  toe M86.67-
  ulna M86.63-
  vertebra — *see* Osteomyelitis, vertebra
 echinococcal B67.2
 Garr's — *see* Osteomyelitis, specified type
  NEC
 in diabetes mellitus — *see* E08-E13 with .69
 jaw (acute) (chronic) (lower) (neonatal)
  (suppurating) (upper) M27.2
 nonsuppurating — *see* Osteomyelitis, specified
  type NEC
 orbit H05.02-
 petrous bone — *see* Petrositis
 Salmonella (arizonae) (cholerae-suis)
  (enteritidis) (typhimurium) A02.24
 sclerosing, nonsuppurative — *see*
  Osteomyelitis, specified type NEC
 specified type NEC (*see also* subcategory)
  M86.8x-
  mandible M27.2
  orbit H05.02-
  petrous bone — *see* Petrositis
  vertebra — *see* Osteomyelitis, vertebra
 subacute M86.20
  carpus M86.24-
  clavicle M86.21-
  femur M86.25-
  fibula M86.26-
  finger M86.24-
  humerus M86.22-
  mandible M27.2
  metacarpus M86.24-
  metatarsus M86.27-
  multiple sites M86.29
  neck M86.28
  orbit H05.02-
  petrous bone — *see* Petrositis
  radius M86.23-
  rib M86.28
  scapula M86.21-
  skull M86.28
  tarsus M86.27-
  tibia M86.26-
  toe M86.27-
  ulna M86.23-
  vertebra — *see* Osteomyelitis, vertebra
 syphilitic A52.77
  congenital (early) A50.02 *[M90.80]*
 tuberculous — *see* Tuberculosis, bone
 typhoid A01.05
 vertebra M46.20
  cervical region M46.22
  cervicothoracic region M46.23
  lumbar region M46.26
  lumbosacral region M46.27
  occipito-atlanto-axial region M46.21
  sacrococcygeal region M46.28
  thoracic region M46.24
  thoracolumbar region M46.25
Osteomyelofibrosis D47.4
Osteomyelosclerosis D75.89
Osteonecrosis M87.9
 due to
  drugs — *see* Osteonecrosis, secondary, due
   to, drugs

Osteonecrosis M87.9 — *continued*
  due to — *continued*
    trauma — *see* Osteonecrosis, secondary,
      due to, trauma
  idiopathic aseptic M87.00
    ankle M87.07-
    carpus M87.03-
    clavicle M87.01-
    femur M87.05-
    fibula M87.06-
    finger M87.04-
    humerus M87.02-
    ilium M87.050
    ischium M87.050
    metacarpus M87.04-
    metatarsus M87.07-
    multiple sites M87.09
    neck M87.08
    pelvis M87.050
    radius M87.03-
    rib M87.08
    scapula M87.01-
    skull M87.08
    tarsus M87.07-
    tibia M87.06-
    toe M87.07-
    ulna M87.03-
    vertebra M87.08
  secondary NEC M87.30
    carpus M87.33-
    clavicle M87.31-
    due to
      drugs M87.10
        carpus M87.13-
        clavicle M87.11-
        femur M87.15-
        fibula M87.16-
        finger M87.14-
        humerus M87.12-
        ilium M87.159
      drugs M87.10
        ischium M87.159
        jaw M87.180
        metacarpus M87.14-
        metatarsus M87.17-
        multiple sites M87.19
        neck M87.18
        radius M87.13-
        rib M87.18
        scapula M87.11-
        skull M87.18
        tarsus M87.17-
        tibia M87.16-
        toe M87.17-
        ulna M87.13-
        vertebra M87.18
      hemoglobinopathy NEC D58.2 [M90.50]
        carpus D58.2 [M90.5-]
        clavicle D58.2 [M90.5-]
        femur D58.2 [M90.5-]
        fibula D58.2 [M90.5-]
        finger D58.2 [M90.5-]
        humerus D58.2 [M90.5-]
        ilium D58.2 [M90.5-]
        ischium D58.2 [M90.5-]
        metacarpus D58.2 [M90.5-]
        metatarsus D58.2 [M90.5-]
        multiple sites D58.2 [M90.58]
        neck D58.2 [M90.58]
        radius D58.2 [M90.5-]
        rib D58.2 [M90.58]
        scapula D58.2 [M90.5-]
        skull D58.2 [M90.58]
        tarsus D58.2 [M90.5-]
        tibia D58.2 [M90.5-]
        toe D58.2 [M90.5-]
        ulna D58.2 [M90.5-]
        vertebra D58.2 [M90.58]

Osteonecrosis M87.9 — *continued*
  secondary NEC M87.30 — *continued*
    due to — *continued*
      trauma (previous) M87.20
        carpus M87.23-
        clavicle M87.21-
        femur M87.25-
        fibula M87.26-
        finger M87.24-
        humerus M87.22-
        ilium M87.25-
        ischium M87.25-
        metacarpus M87.24-
        metatarsus M87.27-
        multiple sites M87.29
        neck M87.28
        radius M87.23-
        rib M87.28
        scapula M87.21-
        skull M87.28
        tarsus M87.27-
        tibia M87.26-
        toe M87.27-
        ulna M87.23-
        vertebra M87.28
    femur M87.35-
    fibula M87.36-
    finger M87.34-
    humerus M87.32-
    ilium M87.350
    in
      caisson disease T70.3 [M90.50]
        carpus T70.3 [M90.5-]
        clavicle T70.3 [M90.5-]
        femur T70.3 [M90.5-]
        fibula T70.3 [M90.5-]
        finger T70.3 [M90.5-]
        humerus T70.3 [M90.5-]
        ilium T70.3 [M90.5-]
        ischium T70.3 [M90.5-]
        metacarpus T70.3 [M90.5-]
        metatarsus T70.3 [M90.5-]
        multiple sites T70.3 [M90.59]
        neck T70.3 [M90.58]
        radius T70.3 [M90.5-]
        rib T70.3 [M90.58]
        scapula T70.3 [M90.5-]
        skull T70.3 [M90.58]
        tarsus T70.3 [M90.5-]
        tibia T70.3 [M90.5-]
        toe T70.3 [M90.5-]
        ulna T70.3 [M90.5-]
        vertebra T70.3 [M90.58]
    ischium M87.350
    metacarpus M87.34-
    metatarsus M87.37-
    multiple site M87.39
    neck M87.38
    radius M87.33-
    rib M87.38
    scapula M87.319
    skull M87.38
    tarsus M87.379
    tibia M87.366
    toe M87.379
    ulna M87.33-
    vertebra M87.38
  specified type NEC M87.80
    carpus M87.83-
    clavicle M87.81-
    femur M87.85-
    fibula M87.86-
    finger M87.84-
    humerus M87.82-
    ilium M87.85-
    ischium M87.85-
    metacarpus M87.84-
    metatarsus M87.87-
    multiple sites M87.89

Osteonecrosis M87.9 — *continued*
  specified type NEC M87.80 — *continued*
    neck M87.88
    radius M87.83-
    rib M87.88
    scapula M87.81-
    skull M87.88
    tarsus M87.87-
    tibia M87.86-
    toe M87.87-
    ulna M87.83-
    vertebra M87.88
Osteo-onycho-arthro-dysplasia Q87.2
Osteo-onychodysplasia, hereditary Q87.2
Osteopathia condensans disseminata
  Q78.8
Osteopathy — *see also* Osteomyelitis,
  Osteonecrosis, Osteoporosis
  after poliomyelitis M89.60
    carpus M89.64-
    clavicle M89.61-
    femur M89.65-
    fibula M89.66-
    finger M89.64-
    humerus M89.62-
    ilium M89.659
    ischium M89.659
    metacarpus M89.64-
    metatarsus M89.67-
    multiple sites M89.69
    neck M89.68
    radius M89.63-
    rib M89.68
    scapula M89.61-
    skull M89.68
    tarsus M89.67-
    tibia M89.66-
    toe M89.67-
    ulna M89.63-
    vertebra M89.68
  in (due to)
    renal osteodystrophy N25.0
    specified diseases classified elsewhere — *see*
      subcategory M90.8
Osteopenia M85.8-
  borderline M85.8-
Osteoperiostitis — *see* Osteomyelitis,
  specified type NEC
Osteopetrosis (familial) Q78.2
Osteophyte M25.70
  ankle M25.77-
  elbow M25.72-
  foot joint M25.77-
  hand joint M25.74-
  hip M25.75-
  knee M25.76-
  shoulder M25.71-
  spine M25.78
  vertebrae M25.78
  wrist M25.73-
Osteopoikilosis Q78.8
Osteoporosis (female) (male) M81.0
  with current pathological fracture M80.00
  age-related M81.0
    with current pathologic fracture M80.00
      carpus M80.04-
      clavicle M80.01-
      fibula M80.06-
      finger M80.04-
      humerus M80.02-
      ilium M80.05-
      ischium M80.05-
      metacarpus M80.04-
      metatarsus M80.07-
      pelvis M80.05-
      radius M80.03-
      scapula M80.01-
      tarsus M80.07-
      tibia M80.06-

Osteoporosis (female) (male) M81.0 — continued
  age-related M81.0 — continued
    with current pathologic fracture M80.00 — continued
      toe M80.07-
      ulna M80.03-
      vertebra M80.08
  disuse M81.8
    with current pathological fracture M80.80
      carpus M80.84-
      clavicle M80.81-
      fibula M80.86-
      finger M80.84-
      humerus M80.82-
      ilium M80.85-
      ischium M80.85-
      metacarpus M80.84-
      metatarsus M80.87-
      pelvis M80.85-
      radius M80.83-
      scapula M80.81-
      tarsus M80.87-
      tibia M80.86-
      toe M80.87-
      ulna M80.83-
      vertebra M80.88
  drug-induced — see Osteoporosis, specified type NEC
  idiopathic — see Osteoporosis, specified type NEC
  involutional — see Osteoporosis, age-related
  Lequesne M81.6
  localized M81.6
  post-traumatic — see Osteoporosis, specified type NEC
  postmenopausal M81.0
    with pathological fracture M80.00
      carpus M80.04-
      clavicle M80.01-
      fibula M80.06-
      finger M80.04-
      humerus M80.02-
      ilium M80.05-
      ischium M80.05-
      metacarpus M80.04-
      metatarsus M80.07-
      pelvis M80.05-
      radius M80.03-
      scapula M80.01-
      tarsus M80.07-
      tibia M80.06-
      toe M80.07-
      ulna M80.03-
      vertebra M80.08
  postoophorectomy — see Osteoporosis, specified type NEC
  postsurgical malabsorption — see Osteoporosis, specified type NEC
  senile — see Osteoporosis, age-related
  specified type NEC M81.8
    with pathological fracture M80.80
      carpus M80.84-
      clavicle M80.81-
      fibula M80.86-
      finger M80.84-
      humerus M80.82-
      ilium M80.85-
      ischium M80.85-
      metacarpus M80.84-
      metatarsus M80.87-
      pelvis M80.85-
      radius M80.83-
      scapula M80.81-
      tarsus M80.87-
      tibia M80.86-
      toe M80.87-
      ulna M80.83-
      vertebra M80.88

Osteopsathyrosis (idiopathica) Q78.0
Osteoradionecrosis, jaw (acute) (chronic) (lower) (suppurative) (upper) M27.2
Osteosarcoma (any form) — see Neoplasm, bone, malignant
Osteosclerosis Q78.2
  acquired M85.8-
  congenita Q77.4
  fragilitas (generalisata) Q78.2
  myelofibrosis D75.81
Osteosclerotic anemia D64.89
Osteosis
  cutis L94.2
  renal fibrocystic N25.0
Österreicher-Turner syndrome Q87.2
Ostium
  atrioventriculare commune Q21.2
  primum (arteriosum) (defect) (persistent) Q21.2
  secundum (arteriosum) (defect) (patent) (persistent) Q21.1
Ostrum-Furst syndrome Q75.8
Otalgia — see subcategory H92.0
Otitis (acute) H66.90
  with effusion — see also Otitis, media, nonsuppurative
    purulent — see Otitis, media, suppurative
  adhesive — see subcategory H74.1
  chronic — see also Otitis, media, chronic
    with effusion — see also Otitis, media, nonsuppurative, chronic
  externa H60.9-
    abscess — see Abscess, ear, external
    acute (noninfective) H60.50-
      actinic H60.51-
      chemical H60.52-
      contact H60.53-
      eczematoid H60.54-
      infective — see Otitis, externa, infective
      reactive H60.55-
      specified NEC H60.59-
    cellulitis — see Cellulitis, ear
    chronic H60.6-
    diffuse — see Otitis, externa, infective, diffuse
    hemorrhagic — see Otitis, externa, infective, hemorrhagic
    in (due to)
      aspergillosis B44.89
      candidiasis B37.84
      erysipelas A46 [H62.40]
      herpes (simplex) virus infection B00.1
        zoster B02.8
      impetigo L01.00 [H62.40]
      infectious disease NEC B99 [H62.-]
      mycosis NEC B36.9 [H62.40]
      parasitic disease NEC B89 [H62.40]
      viral disease NEC B34.9 [H62.40]
      zoster B02.8
    infective NEC H60.39-
      abscess — see Abscess, ear, external
      cellulitis — see Cellulitis, ear
      diffuse H60.31-
      hemorrhagic H60.32-
      swimmer's ear — see Swimmer's, ear
    malignant H60.2-
    mycotic NEC B36.9 [H62.40]
      in
        aspergillosis B44.89
        candidiasis B37.84
        moniliasis B37.84
    necrotizing — see Otitis, externa, malignant
    Pseudomonas aeruginosa — see Otitis, externa, malignant
    reactive — see Otitis, externa, acute, reactive
    specified NEC — see subcategory H60.8

Otitis (acute) H66.90 — continued
  externa H60.9- — continued
    tropical NEC B36.9 [H62.40]
      in
        aspergillosis B44.89
        candidiasis B37.84
        moniliasis B37.84
  insidiosa — see Otosclerosis
  interna — see subcategory H83.0
  media (hemorrhagic) (staphylococcal) (streptococcal) H66.9-
    with effusion (nonpurulent) — see Otitis, media, nonsuppurative
    acute, subacute H66.90
      allergic — see Otitis, media, nonsuppurative, acute, allergic
      exudative — see Otitis, media, suppurative, acute
      mucoid — see Otitis, media, nonsuppurative, acute
      necrotizing — see also Otitis, media, suppurative, acute
        in
          measles B05.3
          scarlet fever A38.0
      nonsuppurative NEC — see Otitis, media, nonsuppurative, acute
      purulent — see Otitis, media, suppurative, acute
      sanguinous — see Otitis, media, nonsuppurative, acute
      secretory — see Otitis, media, nonsuppurative, acute, serous
      seromucinous — see Otitis, media, nonsuppurative, acute
      serous — see Otitis, media, nonsuppurative, acute, serous
      suppurative — see Otitis, media, suppurative, acute
    allergic — see Otitis, media, nonsuppurative
    catarrhal — see Otitis, media, nonsuppurative
    chronic H66.90
      with effusion (nonpurulent) — see Otitis, media, nonsuppurative, chronic
      allergic — see Otitis, media, nonsuppurative, chronic, allergic
      benign suppurative — see Otitis, media, suppurative, chronic, tubotympanic
      catarrhal — see Otitis, media, nonsuppurative, chronic, serous
      exudative — see Otitis, media, nonsuppurative, chronic
      mucinous — see Otitis, media, nonsuppurative, chronic, mucoid
      mucoid — see Otitis, media, nonsuppurative, chronic, mucoid
      nonsuppurative NEC — see Otitis, media, nonsuppurative, chronic
      purulent — see Otitis, media, suppurative, chronic
      secretory — see Otitis, media, nonsuppurative, chronic, mucoid
      seromucinous — see Otitis, media, nonsuppurative, chronic
      serous — see Otitis, media, nonsuppurative, chronic, serous
      suppurative — see Otitis, media, suppurative, chronic
      transudative — see Otitis, media, nonsuppurative, chronic, mucoid
    exudative — see Otitis, media, suppurative
    in (due to) (with)
      influenza — see Influenza, with, otitis media
      measles B05.3
      scarlet fever A38.0
      tuberculosis A18.6
      viral disease NEC B34- [H67-]

Otitis (acute) H66.90 — *continued*
media (hemorrhagic) (staphylococcal)
(streptococcal) H66.9- — *continued*
mucoid — *see* Otitis, media, nonsuppurative
nonsuppurative H65.9-
acute or subacute NEC H65.19-
allergic H65.11-
recurrent H65.11-
recurrent H65.19-
secretory — *see* Otitis, media,
nonsuppurative, serous
serous H65.0-
recurrent H65.0-
chronic H65.49-
allergic H65.41-
mucoid H65.3-
serous H65.2-
postmeasles B05.3
purulent — *see* Otitis, media, suppurative
secretory — *see* Otitis, media,
nonsuppurative
seromucinous — *see* Otitis, media,
nonsuppurative
serous — *see* Otitis, media, nonsuppurative
suppurative H66.4-
acute H66.00-
with rupture of ear drum H66.01-
recurrent H66.00-
with rupture of ear drum H66.01-
chronic (*see also* subcategory) H66.3
atticoantral H66.2-
benign — *see* Otitis, media, suppurative,
chronic, tubotympanic
tubotympanic H66.1-
transudative — *see* Otitis, media,
nonsuppurative
tuberculous A18.6
Otocephaly Q18.2
Otolith syndrome — *see* subcategory H81.8
Otomycosis (diffuse) NEC B36.9 *[H62.40]*
in
aspergillosis B44.89
candidiasis B37.84
moniliasis B37.84
Otoporosis — *see* Otosclerosis
Otorrhagia (nontraumatic) H92.2-
traumatic — *code by* Type of injury
Otorrhea H92.1-
cerebrospinal G96.0
Otosclerosis (general) H80.9-
cochlear (endosteal) H80.2-
involving
otic capsule — *see* Otosclerosis, cochlear
oval window
nonobliterative H80.0-
obliterative H80.1-
round window — *see* Otosclerosis, cochlear
nonobliterative — *see* Otosclerosis, involving,
oval window, nonobliterative
obliterative — *see* Otosclerosis, involving, oval
window, obliterative
specified NEC H80.8-
Otospongiosis — *see* Otosclerosis
Otto's disease or pelvis M24.7
Outcome of delivery Z37.9
multiple births Z37.9
all liveborn Z37.50
quadruplets Z37.52
quintuplets Z37.53
sextuplets Z37.54
specified number NEC Z37.59
triplets Z37.51
all stillborn Z37.7
some liveborn Z37.60
quadruplets Z37.62
quintuplets Z37.63
sextuplets Z37.64
specified number NEC Z37.69
triplets Z37.61

Outcome of delivery Z37.9 — *continued*
single NEC Z37.9
liveborn Z37.0
stillborn Z37.1
twins NEC Z37.9
both liveborn Z37.2
both stillborn Z37.4
one liveborn, one stillborn Z37.3
Outlet — *see* condition
Ovalocytosis (congenital) (hereditary) — *see*
Elliptocytosis
Ovarian — *see* condition
Ovariocele N83.4-
Ovaritis (cystic) — *see* Oophoritis
Ovary, ovarian — *see also* condition
resistant syndrome E28.39
vein syndrome N13.8
Overactive — *see also* Hyperfunction
adrenal cortex NEC E27.0
bladder N32.81
hypothalamus E23.3
thyroid — *see* Hyperthyroidism
Overactivity R46.3
child — *see* Disorder, attention-deficit
hyperactivity
Overbite (deep) (excessive) (horizontal)
(vertical) M26.29
Overbreathing — *see* Hyperventilation
Overconscientious personality F60.5
Overdevelopment — *see* Hypertrophy
Overdistension — *see* Distension
Overdose, overdosage (drug) — *see* Table of
Drugs and Chemicals, by drug, poisoning
Overeating R63.2
nonorganic origin F50.89
psychogenic F50.89
Overexertion (effects) (exhaustion) T73.3
Overexposure (effects) T73.9
exhaustion T73.2
Overfeeding — *see* Overeating
newborn P92.4
Overfill, endodontic M27.52
Overgrowth, bone — *see* Hypertrophy, bone
**Overhanging of dental restorative
material** (unrepairable) K08.52
Overheated (places) (effects) — *see* Heat
Overjet (excessive horizontal) M26.23
Overlaid, overlying (suffocation) — *see*
Asphyxia, traumatic, due to mechanical
threat
Overlap, excessive horizontal (teeth)
M26.23
Overlapping toe (acquired) — *see also*
Deformity, toe, specified NEC
congenital (fifth toe) Q66.89
Overload
circulatory, due to transfusion (blood) (blood
components) (TACO) E87.71
fluid E87.70
due to transfusion (blood) (blood
components) E87.71
specified NEC E87.79
iron, due to repeated red blood cell
transfusions E83.111
potassium (K) E87.5
sodium (Na) E87.0
Overnutrition — *see* Hyperalimentation
Overproduction — *see also* Hypersecretion
ACTH E27.0
catecholamine E27.5
growth hormone E22.0
Overprotection, child by parent Z62.1
Overriding
aorta Q25.49
finger (acquired) — *see* Deformity, finger
congenital Q68.1
toe (acquired) — *see also* Deformity, toe,
specified NEC
congenital Q66.89

Overstrained R53.83
heart — *see* Hypertrophy, cardiac
Overuse, muscle NEC M70.8-
Overweight E66.3
Overworked R53.83
Oviduct — *see* condition
Ovotestis Q56.0
Ovulation (cycle)
failure or lack of N97.0
pain N94.0
Ovum — *see* condition
Owren's disease or syndrome
(parahemophilia) D68.2
Ox heart — *see* Hypertrophy, cardiac
Oxalosis E72.53
Oxaluria E72.53
Oxycephaly, oxycephalic Q75.0
syphilitic, congenital A50.02
Oxyuriasis B80
Oxyuris vermicularis (infestation) B80
Ozena J31.0

P

Pachyderma, pachydermia L85.9
 larynx (verrucosa) J38.7
Pachydermatocele (congenital) Q82.8
Pachydermoperiostosis — see also
 Osteoarthropathy, hypertrophic, specified
 type NEC
 clubbed nail M89.40 [L62]
Pachygyria Q04.3
Pachymeningitis (adhesive) (basal) (brain)
 (cervical) (chronic) (circumscribed) (external)
 (fibrous) (hemorrhagic) (hypertrophic)
 (internal) (purulent) (spinal) (suppurative) —
 see Meningitis
Pachyonychia (congenital) Q84.5
Pacinian tumor — see Neoplasm, skin, benign
Pad, knuckle or Garrod's M72.1
Paget's disease
 with infiltrating duct carcinoma — see
 Neoplasm, breast, malignant
 bone M88.9
 carpus M88.84-
 clavicle M88.81-
 femur M88.85-
 fibula M88.86-
 finger M88.84-
 humerus M88.82-
 ilium M88.85-
 in neoplastic disease — see Osteitis,
 deformans, in neoplastic disease
 ischium M88.85-
 metacarpus M88.84-
 metatarsus M88.87-
 multiple sites M88.89
 neck M88.88
 radius M88.83-
 rib M88.88
 scapula M88.81-
 skull M88.0
 tarsus M88.87-
 tibia M88.86-
 toe M88.87-
 ulna M88.83-
 vertebra M88.88
 breast (female) C50.01-
 male C50.02-
 extramammary — see also Neoplasm, skin,
 malignant
 anus C21.0
 margin C44.590
 skin C44.590
 intraductal carcinoma — see Neoplasm,
 breast, malignant
 malignant — see Neoplasm, skin, malignant
 breast (female) C50.01-
 male C50.02-
 unspecified site (female) C50.01-
 male C50.02-
 mammary — see Paget's disease, breast
 nipple — see Paget's disease, breast
 osteitis deformans — see Paget's disease, bone
Paget-Schroetter syndrome I82.890
Pain(s) (see also Painful) R52
 abdominal R10.9
 colic R10.83
 generalized R10.84
 with acute abdomen R10.0
 lower R10.30
 left quadrant R10.32
 pelvic or perineal R10.2
 periumbilical R10.33
 right quadrant R10.31
 rebound — see Tenderness, abdominal,
 rebound
 severe with abdominal rigidity R10.0
 tenderness — see Tenderness, abdominal

Pain(s) (see also Painful) R52 — continued
 abdominal R10.9 — continued
 upper R10.10
 epigastric R10.13
 left quadrant R10.12
 right quadrant R10.11
 acute R52
 due to trauma G89.11
 neoplasm related G89.3
 post-thoracotomy G89.12
 postprocedural NEC G89.18
 specified by site — code to Pain, by site
 adnexa (uteri) R10.2
 anginoid — see Pain, precordial
 anus K62.89
 arm — see Pain, limb, upper
 axillary (axilla) M79.62-
 back (postural) M54.9
 bladder R39.89
 associated with micturition — see Micturition,
 painful
 chronic R39.82
 bone — see Disorder, bone, specified type
 NEC
 breast N64.4
 broad ligament R10.2
 cancer associated (acute) (chronic) G89.3
 cecum — see Pain, abdominal
 cervicobrachial M53.1
 chest (central) R07.9
 anterior wall R07.89
 atypical R07.89
 ischemic I20.9
 musculoskeletal R07.89
 non-cardiac R07.89
 on breathing R07.1
 pleurodynia R07.81
 precordial R07.2
 wall (anterior) R07.89
 chronic G89.29
 associated with significant psychosocial
 dysfunction G89.4
 due to trauma G89.21
 neoplasm related G89.3
 post-thoracotomy G89.22
 postoperative NEC G89.28
 postprocedural NEC G89.28
 specified NEC G89.29
 coccyx M53.3
 colon — see Pain, abdominal
 coronary — see Angina
 costochondral R07.1
 diaphragm R07.1
 due to cancer G89.3
 due to device, implant or graft (see also
 Complications, by site and type, specified
 NEC) T85.848
 arterial graft NEC T82.848
 breast (implant) T85.848
 catheter NEC T85.848
 dialysis (renal) T82.848
 intraperitoneal T85.848
 infusion NEC T82.848
 spinal (epidural) (subdural) T85.840
 urinary (indwelling) T83.84
 electronic (electrode) (pulse generator)
 (stimulator)
 bone T84.84
 cardiac T82.847
 nervous system (brain) (peripheral nerve)
 (spinal) T85.840
 urinary T83.84
 fixation, internal (orthopedic) NEC T84.84
 gastrointestinal (bile duct) (esophagus)
 T85.848
 genital NEC T83.84
 heart NEC T82.847
 infusion NEC T85.848
 joint prosthesis T84.84

Pain(s) (see also Painful) R52 — continued
 due to device, implant or graft (see also
 Complications, by site and type, specified
 NEC) T85.848 — continued
 ocular (corneal graft) (orbital implant) NEC
 T85.848
 orthopedic NEC T84.84
 specified NEC T85.848
 urinary NEC T83.84
 vascular NEC T82.848
 ventricular intracranial shunt T85.840
 due to malignancy (primary) (secondary)
 G89.3
 ear — see subcategory H92.0
 epigastric, epigastrium R10.13
 eye — see Pain, ocular
 face, facial R51
 atypical G50.1
 female genital organs NEC N94.89
 finger — see Pain, limb, upper
 flank — see Pain, abdominal
 foot — see Pain, limb, lower
 gallbladder K82.9
 gas (intestinal) R14.1
 gastric — see Pain, abdominal
 generalized NOS R52
 genital organ
 female N94.89
 male N50.89
 groin — see Pain, abdominal, lower
 hand — see Pain, limb, upper
 head — see Headache
 heart — see Pain, precordial
 infra-orbital — see Neuralgia, trigeminal
 intercostal R07.82
 intermenstrual N94.0
 jaw R68.84
 joint M25.50
 ankle M25.57-
 elbow M25.52-
 finger M25.54-
 foot M25.57-
 hand M25.54-
 hip M25.55-
 knee M25.56-
 shoulder M25.51-
 toe M25.57-
 wrist M25.53-
 kidney N23
 laryngeal R07.0
 leg — see Pain, limb, lower
 limb M79.609
 lower M79.60-
 foot M79.67-
 lower leg M79.66-
 thigh M79.65-
 toe M79.67-
 upper M79.60-
 axilla M79.62-
 finger M79.64-
 forearm M79.63-
 hand M79.64-
 upper arm M79.62-
 loin M54.5
 low back M54.5
 lumbar region M54.5
 mandibular R68.84
 mastoid — see subcategory H92.0
 maxilla R68.84
 menstrual (see also Dysmenorrhea) N94.6
 metacarpophalangeal (joint) — see Pain, joint,
 hand
 metatarsophalangeal (joint) — see Pain, joint,
 foot
 mouth K13.79
 muscle — see Myalgia
 musculoskeletal (see also Pain, by site) M79.1
 myofascial M79.1

Pain(s) (*see also* Painful) R52 — *continued*
  nasal J34.89
  nasopharynx J39.2
  neck NEC M54.2
  nerve NEC — *see* Neuralgia
  neuromuscular — *see* Neuralgia
  nose J34.89
  ocular H57.1-
  ophthalmic — *see* Pain, ocular
  orbital region — *see* Pain, ocular
  ovary N94.89
  over heart — *see* Pain, precordial
  ovulation N94.0
  pelvic (female) R10.2
  penis N48.89
  pericardial — *see* Pain, precordial
  perineal, perineum R10.2
  pharynx J39.2
  pleura, pleural, pleuritic R07.81
  post-thoracotomy G89.12
  postoperative NOS G89.18
  postprocedural NOS G89.18
  precordial (region) R07.2
  premenstrual N94.3
  psychogenic (persistent) (any site) F45.41
  radicular (spinal) — *see* Radiculopathy
  rectum K62.89
  respiration R07.1
  retrosternal R07.2
  rheumatoid, muscular — *see* Myalgia
  rib R07.81
  root (spinal) — *see* Radiculopathy
  round ligament (stretch) R10.2
  sacroiliac M53.3
  sciatic — *see* Sciatica
  scrotum N50.82
  seminal vesicle N50.89
  shoulder M25.51-
  spermatic cord N50.89
  spinal root — *see* Radiculopathy
  spine M54.9
    cervical M54.2
    low back M54.5
      with sciatica M54.4-
    thoracic M54.6
  stomach — *see* Pain, abdominal
  substernal R07.2
  temporomandibular (joint) M26.62-
  testis N50.81-
  thoracic spine M54.6
    with radicular and visceral pain M54.14
  throat R07.0
  tibia — *see* Pain, limb, lower
  toe — *see* Pain, limb, lower
  tongue K14.6
  tooth K08.89
  trigeminal — *see* Neuralgia, trigeminal
  tumor associated G89.3
  ureter N23
  urinary (organ) (system) N23
  uterus NEC N94.89
  vagina R10.2
  vertebrogenic (syndrome) M54.89
  vesical R39.89
    associated with micturition — *see* Micturition, painful
  vulva R10.2
Painful — *see also* Pain
  coitus
    female N94.10
    male N53.12
    psychogenic F52.6
  ejaculation (semen) N53.12
    psychogenic F52.6
  erection — *see* Priapism
  feet syndrome E53.8
  joint replacement (hip) (knee) T84.84
  menstruation — *see* Dysmenorrhea
    psychogenic F45.8

Painful — *see also* Pain - *continued*
  micturition — *see* Micturition, painful
  respiration R07.1
  scar NEC L90.5
  wire sutures T81.89
Painter's colic — *see* subcategory T56.0
Palate — *see* condition
Palatoplegia K13.79
Palatoschisis — *see* Cleft, palate
Palilalia R48.8
Palliative care Z51.5
Pallor R23.1
  optic disc, temporal — *see* Atrophy, optic
Palmar — *see also* condition
  fascia — *see* condition
Palpable
  cecum K63.89
  kidney N28.89
  ovary N83.8
  prostate N42.9
  spleen — *see* Splenomegaly
Palpitations (heart) R00.2
  psychogenic F45.8
Palsy (*see also* Paralysis) G83.9
  atrophic diffuse (progressive) G12.22
  Bell's — *see also* Palsy, facial
    newborn P11.3
  brachial plexus NEC G54.0
    newborn (birth injury) P14.3
  brain — *see* Palsy, cerebral
  bulbar (progressive) (chronic) G12.22
    of childhood (Fazio-Londe) G12.1
    pseudo NEC G12.29
    supranuclear (progressive) G23.1
  cerebral (congenital) G80.9
    ataxic G80.4
    athetoid G80.3
    choreathetoid G80.3
    diplegic G80.8
      spastic G80.1
    dyskinetic G80.3
      athetoid G80.3
      choreathetoid G80.3
      distonic G80.3
    dystonic G80.3
    hemiplegic G80.8
      spastic G80.2
    mixed G80.8
    monoplegic G80.8
      spastic G80.1
    paraplegic G80.8
      spastic G80.1
    quadriplegic G80.8
      spastic G80.0
    spastic G80.1
      diplegic G80.1
      hemiplegic G80.2
      monoplegic G80.1
      quadriplegic G80.0
      specified NEC G80.1
      tetrapelgic G80.0
    specified NEC G80.8
    syphilitic A52.12
      congenital A50.49
    tetraplegic G80.8
      spastic G80.0
  cranial nerve — *see also* Disorder, nerve, cranial
    multiple G52.7
      in
        infectious disease B99 *[G53]*
        neoplastic disease (*see also* Neoplasm) D49.9 *[G53]*
        parasitic disease B89 *[G53]*
        sarcoidosis D86.82
  creeping G12.22
  diver's T70.3
  Erb's P14.0

Palsy (*see also* Paralysis) G83.9 — *continued*
  facial G51.0
    newborn (birth injury) P11.3
  glossopharyngeal G52.1
  Klumpke(-Déjérine) P14.1
  lead — *see* subcategory T56.0
  median nerve (tardy) G56.1-
  nerve G58.9
    specified NEC G58.8
  peroneal nerve (acute) (tardy) G57.3-
  progressive supranuclear G23.1
  pseudobulbar NEC G12.29
  radial nerve (acute) G56.3-
  seventh nerve — *see also* Palsy, facial
    newborn P11.3
  shaking — *see* Parkinsonism
  spastic (cerebral) (spinal) G80.1
  ulnar nerve (tardy) G56.2-
  wasting G12.29
Paludism — *see* Malaria
Panangiitis M30.0
Panaris, panaritium — *see also* Cellulitis, digit
  with lymphangitis — *see* Lymphangitis, acute, digit
Panarteritis nodosa M30.0
  brain or cerebral I67.7
Pancake heart R93.1
  with cor pulmonale (chronic) I27.81
Pancarditis (acute) (chronic) I51.89
  rheumatic I09.89
    active or acute I01.8
Pancoast's syndrome or tumor C34.1-
Pancolitis, ulcerative (chronic) K51.00
  with
    abscess K51.014
    complication K51.019
    fistula K51.013
    obstruction K51.012
    rectal bleeding K51.011
    specified complication NEC K51.018
Pancreas, pancreatic — *see* condition
Pancreatitis (annular) (apoplectic) (calcareous) (edematous) (hemorrhagic) (malignant) (recurrent) (subacute) (suppurative) K85.90
  with necrosis (uninfected) K85.91
    infected K85.92
  acute (without necrosis or infection) K85.90
    with necrosis (uninfected) K85.91
      infected K85.92
    alcohol-induced (without necrosis or infection) K85.20
      with necrosis (uninfected) K85.21
        infected K85.22
    biliary (without necrosis or infection) K85.10
      with necrosis (uninfected) K85.11
        infected K85.12
    drug-induced (without necrosis or infection) K85.30
      with necrosis (uninfected) K85.31
        infected K85.32
    gallstone (without necrosis or infection) K85.10
      with necrosis (uninfected) K85.11
        infected K85.12
    idiopathic (without necrosis or infection) K85.00
      with necrosis (uninfected) K85.01
        infected K85.02
    specified NEC (without necrosis or infection) K85.80
      with necrosis (uninfected) K85.81
        infected K85.82
  chronic (infectious) K86.1
    alcohol-induced K86.0
    recurrent K86.1
    relapsing K86.1
  cystic (chronic) K86.1
  cytomegaloviral B25.2

D I S E A S E   I N D E X

Pancreatitis (annular) (apoplectic) (calcareous) (edematous) (hemorrhagic) (malignant) (recurrent) (subacute) (suppurative) K85.9 — *continued*
  fibrous (chronic) K86.1
  gallstone (without necrosis or infection) K85.10
    with necrosis (uninfected) K85.11
      infected K85.12
  gangrenous — *see* Pancreatitis, acute
  interstitial (chronic) K86.1
    acute (*see also* Pancreatitis, acute) K85.80
  mumps B26.3
  recurrent (chronic) K86.1
  relapsing, chronic K86.1
  syphilitic A52.74
Pancreatoblastoma — *see* Neoplasm, pancreas, malignant
Pancreolithiasis K86.89
Pancytolysis D75.89
Pancytopenia (acquired) D61.818
  with
    malformations D61.09
    myelodysplastic syndrome — *see* Syndrome, myelodysplastic
  antineoplastic chemotherapy induced D61.810
  congenital D61.09
  drug-induced NEC D61.811
Panencephalitis, subacute, sclerosing A81.1
Panhematopenia D61.9
  congenital D61.09
  constitutional D61.09
  splenic, primary D73.1
Panhemocytopenia D61.9
  congenital D61.09
  constitutional D61.09
Panhypogonadism E29.1
Panhypopituitarism E23.0
  prepubertal E23.0
Panic (attack) (state) F41.0
  reaction to exceptional stress (transient) F43.0
Panmyelopathy, familial, constitutional D61.09
Panmyelophthisis D61.82
  congenital D61.09
Panmyelosis (acute) (with myelofibrosis) C94.4-
Panner's disease — *see* Osteochondrosis, juvenile, humerus
Panneuritis endemica E51.11
Panniculitis (nodular) (nonsuppurative) M79.3
  back M54.00
    cervical region M54.02
    cervicothoracic region M54.03
    lumbar region M54.06
    lumbosacral region M54.07
    multiple sites M54.09
    occipito-atlanto-axial region M54.01
    sacrococcygeal region M54.08
    thoracic region M54.04
    thoracolumbar region M54.05
  lupus L93.2
  mesenteric K65.4
  neck M54.02
    cervicothoracic region M54.03
    occipito-atlanto-axial region M54.01
  relapsing M35.6
Panniculus adiposus (abdominal) E65
Pannus (allergic) (cornea) (degenerativus) (keratic) H16.42-
  abdominal (symptomatic) E65
  trachomatosus, trachomatous (active) A71.1
Panophthalmitis H44.01-
Pansinusitis (chronic) (hyperplastic) (nonpurulent) (purulent) J32.4
  acute J01.40
    recurrent J01.41
  tuberculous A15.8
Panuveitis (sympathetic) H44.11-

Panvalvular disease I08.9
  specified NEC I08.8
PAPA (pyogenic arthritis, pyoderma gangrenosum, and acne syndrome) M04.8
Papanicolaou smear, cervix Z12.4
  as part of routine gynecological examination Z01.419
    with abnormal findings Z01.411
  for suspected neoplasm Z12.4
  nonspecific abnormal finding R87.619
  routine Z01.419
    with abnormal findings Z01.411
Papilledema (choked disc) H47.10
  associated with
    decreased ocular pressure H47.12
    increased intracranial pressure H47.11
    retinal disorder H47.13
  Foster-Kennedy syndrome H47.14-
Papillitis H46.00
  anus K62.89
  chronic lingual K14.4
  necrotizing, kidney N17.2
  optic H46.0-
  rectum K62.89
  renal, necrotizing N17.2
  tongue K14.0
Papilloma — *see also* Neoplasm, benign, by site
  acuminatum (female) (male) (anogenital) A63.0
  basal cell L82.1
    inflamed L82.0
  benign pinta (primary) A67.0
  bladder (urinary) (transitional cell) D41.4
  choroid plexus (lateral ventricle) (third ventricle) D33.0
    anaplastic C71.5
    fourth ventricle D33.1
    malignant C71.5
  renal pelvis (transitional cell) D41.1-
    benign D30.1-
  Schneiderian
    specified site — *see* Neoplasm, benign, by site
    unspecified site D14.0
  serous surface
    borderline malignancy
      specified site — *see* Neoplasm, uncertain behavior, by site
      unspecified site D39.10
    specified site — *see* Neoplasm, benign, by site
    unspecified site D27.9
  transitional (cell)
    bladder (urinary) D41.4
    inverted type — *see* Neoplasm, uncertain behavior, by site
    renal pelvis D41.1-
    ureter D41.2-
  ureter (transitional cell) D41.2-
    benign D30.2-
  urothelial — *see* Neoplasm, uncertain behavior, by site
  villous — *see* Neoplasm, uncertain behavior, by site
    adenocarcinoma in — *see* Neoplasm, malignant, by site
    in situ — *see* Neoplasm, in situ
  yaws, plantar or palmar A66.1
Papillomata, multiple, of yaws A66.1
Papillomatosis — *see also* Neoplasm, benign, by site
  confluent and reticulated L83
  cystic, breast — *see* Mastopathy, cystic
  ductal, breast — *see* Mastopathy, cystic
  intraductal (diffuse) — *see* Neoplasm, benign, by site
  subareolar duct D24-

Papillomavirus, as cause of disease classified elsewhere B97.7
Papillon-Léage and Psaume syndrome Q87.0
Papule(s) R23.8
  carate (primary) A67.0
  fibrous, of nose D22.39
  Gottron's L94.4
  pinta (primary) A67.0
Papulosis
  lymphomatoid C86.6
  malignant I77.89
Papyraceous fetus O31.0-
Para-albuminemia E88.09
Paracephalus Q89.7
Parachute mitral valve Q23.2
Paracoccidioidomycosis B41.9
  disseminated B41.7
  generalized B41.7
  mucocutaneous-lymphangitic B41.8
  pulmonary B41.0
  specified NEC B41.8
  visceral B41.8
Paradentosis K05.4
Paraffinoma T88.8
Paraganglioma D44.7
  adrenal D35.0-
    malignant C74.1-
  aortic body D44.7
    malignant C75.5
  carotid body D44.6
    malignant C75.4
  chromaffin — *see also* Neoplasm, benign, by site
    malignant — *see* Neoplasm, malignant, by site
  extra-adrenal D44.7
    malignant C75.5
      specified site — *see* Neoplasm, malignant, by site
      unspecified site C75.5
    specified site — *see* Neoplasm, uncertain behavior, by site
    unspecified site D44.7
  gangliocytic D13.2
    specified site — *see* Neoplasm, benign, by site
    unspecified site D13.2
  glomus jugulare D44.7
    malignant C75.5
  jugular D44.7
  malignant C75.5
    specified site — *see* Neoplasm, malignant, by site
    unspecified site C75.5
  nonchromaffin D44.7
    malignant C75.5
      specified site — *see* Neoplasm, malignant, by site
      unspecified site C75.5
    specified site — *see* Neoplasm, uncertain behavior, by site
    unspecified site D44.7
  parasympathetic D44.7
    specified site — *see* Neoplasm, uncertain behavior, by site
    unspecified site D44.7
  specified site — *see* Neoplasm, uncertain behavior, by site
  sympathetic D44.7
    specified site — *see* Neoplasm, uncertain behavior, by site
    unspecified site D44.7
  unspecified site D44.7
Parageusia R43.2
  psychogenic F45.8
Paragonimiasis B66.4

Paragranuloma, Hodgkin — *see*
  Lymphoma, Hodgkin, classical, specified
  type NEC
Parahemophilia (*see also* Defect, coagulation)
  D68.2
Parakeratosis R23.4
  variegata L41.0
Paralysis, paralytic (complete) (incomplete)
  G83.9
  with
    syphilis A52.17
  abducens, abducent (nerve) — *see* Strabismus,
    paralytic, sixth nerve
  abductor, lower extremity G57.9-
  accessory nerve G52.8
  accommodation — *see also* Paresis, of
    accommodation
    hysterical F44.89
  acoustic nerve (except Deafness) — *see*
    subcategory H93.3
  agitans (*see also* Parkinsonism) G20
    arteriosclerotic G21.4
  alternating (oculomotor) G83.89
  amyotrophic G12.21
  ankle G57.9-
  anus (sphincter) K62.89
  arm — *see* Monoplegia, upper limb
  ascending (spinal), acute G61.0
  association G12.29
  asthenic bulbar G70.00
    with exacerbation (acute) G70.01
    in crisis G70.01
  ataxic (hereditary) G11.9
    general (syphilitic) A52.17
  atrophic G58.9
    infantile, acute — *see* Poliomyelitis, paralytic
    progressive G12.22
    spinal (acute) — *see* Poliomyelitis, paralytic
  axillary G54.0
  Babinski-Nageotte's G83.89
  Bell's G51.0
    newborn P11.3
  Benedikt's G46.3
  birth injury P14.9
    spinal cord P11.5
  bladder (neurogenic) (sphincter) N31.2
  bowel, colon or intestine K56.0
  brachial plexus G54.0
    birth injury P14.3
    newborn (birth injury) P14.3
  brain G83.9
    diplegia G83.0
    triplegia G83.89
  bronchial J98.09
  Brown-Séquard G83.81
  bulbar (chronic) (progressive) G12.22
    infantile — *see* Poliomyelitis, paralytic
    poliomyelitic — *see* Poliomyelitis, paralytic
    pseudo G12.29
  bulbospinal G70.00
    with exacerbation (acute) G70.01
    in crisis G70.01
  cardiac (*see also* Failure, heart) I50.9
  cerebrocerebellar, diplegic G80.1
  cervical
    plexus G54.2
    sympathetic G90.09
  Céstan-Chenais G46.3
  Charcot-Marie-Tooth type G60.0
  Clark's G80.9
  colon K56.0
  compressed air T70.3
  compression
    arm G56.9-
    leg G57.9-
      lower extremity G57.9-
      upper extremity G56.9-
  congenital (cerebral) — *see* Palsy, cerebral

Paralysis, paralytic (complete) (incomplete)
  G83.9 — *continued*
  conjugate movement (gaze) (of eye) H51.0
    cortical (nuclear) (supranuclear) H51.0
  cordis — *see* Failure, heart
  cranial or cerebral nerve G52.9
  creeping G12.22
  crossed leg G83.89
  crutch — *see* Injury, brachial plexus
  deglutition R13.0
    hysterical F44.4
  dementia A52.17
  descending (spinal) NEC G12.29
  diaphragm (flaccid) J98.6
    due to accidental dissection of phrenic nerve
      during procedure — *see* Puncture,
      accidental complicating surgery
  digestive organs NEC K59.8
  diplegic — *see* Diplegia
  diver's T70.3
  divergence (nuclear) H51.8
  Duchenne's
    birth injury P14.0
    due to or associated with
      motor neuron disease G12.22
      muscular dystrophy G71.0
    due to intracranial or spinal birth injury — *see*
      Palsy, cerebral
  embolic (current episode) I63.4-
  Erb's syphilitic spastic spinal A52.17
  Erb(-Duchenne) (birth) (newborn) P14.0
  esophagus K22.8
  eye muscle (extrinsic) H49.9
    intrinsic — *see also* Paresis, of
      accommodation
  facial (nerve) G51.0
    birth injury P11.3
    congenital P11.3
    following operation NEC — *see* Puncture,
      accidental complicating surgery
    newborn (birth injury) P11.3
  familial (recurrent) (periodic) G72.3
    spastic G11.4
  fauces J39.2
  finger G56.9-
  gait R26.1
  gastric nerve (nondiabetic) G52.2
  gaze, conjugate H51.0
  general (progressive) (syphilitic) A52.17
    juvenile A50.45
  glottis J38.00
    bilateral J38.02
    unilateral J38.01
  gluteal G54.1
  Gubler(-Millard) G46.3
  hand — *see* Monoplegia, upper limb
  heart — *see* Arrest, cardiac
  hemiplegic — *see* Hemiplegia
  hyperkalemic periodic (familial) G72.3
  hypoglossal (nerve) G52.3
  hypokalemic periodic G72.3
  hysterical F44.4
  ileus K56.0
  infantile (*see also* Poliomyelitis, paralytic)
    A80.30
    bulbar — *see* Poliomyelitis, paralytic
    cerebral — *see* Palsy, cerebral
    spastic — *see* Palsy, cerebral, spastic
    infective — *see* Poliomyelitis, paralytic
  inferior nuclear G83.9
  internuclear — *see* Ophthalmoplegia,
    internuclear
  intestine K56.0
  iris H57.09
    due to diphtheria (toxin) A36.89
  ischemic, Volkmann's (complicating trauma)
    T79.6
  Jackson's G83.89
  jake — *see* Poisoning, food, noxious, plant

Paralysis, paralytic (complete) (incomplete)
  G83.9 — *continued*
  Jamaica ginger (jake) G62.2
  juvenile general A50.45
  Klumpke(-Déjérine) (birth) (newborn) P14.1
  labioglossal (laryngeal) (pharyngeal) G12.29
  Landry's G61.0
  laryngeal nerve (recurrent) (superior)
    (unilateral) J38.00
    bilateral J38.02
    unilateral J38.01
  larynx J38.00
    bilateral J38.02
    due to diphtheria (toxin) A36.2
    unilateral J38.01
  lateral G12.21
  lead — *see* subcategory T56.0
  left side — *see* Hemiplegia
  leg G83.1-
    both — *see* Paraplegia
    crossed G83.89
    hysterical F44.4
    psychogenic F44.4
    transient or transitory R29.818
      traumatic NEC — *see* Injury, nerve, leg
  levator palpebrae superioris — *see*
    Blepharoptosis, paralytic
  limb — *see* Monoplegia
  lip K13.0
  Lissauer's A52.17
  lower limb — *see* Monoplegia, lower limb
    both — *see* Paraplegia
  lung J98.4
  median nerve G56.1-
  medullary (tegmental) G83.89
  mesencephalic NEC G83.89
    tegmental G83.89
  middle alternating G83.89
  Millard-Gubler-Foville G46.3
  monoplegic — *see* Monoplegia
  motor G83.9
  muscle, muscular NEC G72.89
    due to nerve lesion G58.9
    eye (extrinsic) H49.9
      intrinsic — *see* Paresis, of accommodation
      oblique — *see* Strabismus, paralytic, fourth
        nerve
    iris sphincter H21.9
  ischemic (Volkmann's) (complicating trauma)
    T79.6
  progressive G12.21
  pseudohypertrophic G71.0
  musculocutaneous nerve G56.9-
  musculospiral G56.9-
  nerve — *see also* Disorder, nerve
    abducent — *see* Strabismus, paralytic, sixth
      nerve
    accessory G52.8
    auditory (except Deafness) — *see*
      subcategory H93.3
    birth injury P14.9
    cranial or cerebral G52.9
    facial G51.0
      birth injury P11.3
      congenital P11.3
      newborn (birth injury) P11.3
    fourth or trochlear — *see* Strabismus,
      paralytic, fourth nerve
    newborn (birth injury) P14.9
    oculomotor — *see* Strabismus, paralytic,
      third nerve
    phrenic (birth injury) P14.2
    radial G56.3-
    seventh or facial G51.0
      newborn (birth injury) P11.3
    sixth or abducent — *see* Strabismus,
      paralytic, sixth nerve
  syphilitic A52.15

Paralysis, paralytic (complete) (incomplete) G83.9 — *continued*
  nerve — *see also* Disorder, nerve — *continued*
    third or oculomotor — *see* Strabismus, paralytic, third nerve
    trigeminal G50.9
    trochlear — *see* Strabismus, paralytic, fourth nerve
    ulnar G56.2-
  normokalemic periodic G72.3
  ocular H49.9
    alternating G83.89
  oculofacial, congenital (Moebius) Q87.0
  oculomotor (external bilateral) (nerve) — *see* Strabismus, paralytic, third nerve
  palate (soft) K13.79
  paratrigeminal G50.9
  periodic (familial) (hyperkalemic) (hypokalemic) (myotonic) (normokalemic) (potassium sensitive) (secondary) G72.3
  peripheral autonomic nervous system — *see* Neuropathy, peripheral, autonomic
  peroneal (nerve) G57.3-
  pharynx J39.2
  phrenic nerve G56.8-
  plantar nerve(s) G57.6-
  pneumogastric nerve G52.2
  poliomyelitis (current) — *see* Poliomyelitis, paralytic
  popliteal nerve G57.3-
  postepileptic transitory G83.84
  progressive (atrophic) (bulbar) (spinal) G12.22
    general A52.17
    infantile acute — *see* Poliomyelitis, paralytic
    supranuclear G23.1
  pseudobulbar G12.29
  pseudohypertrophic (muscle) G71.0
  psychogenic F44.4
  quadriceps G57.9-
  quadriplegic — *see* Tetraplegia
  radial nerve G56.3-
  rectus muscle (eye) H49.9
  recurrent isolated sleep G47.53
  respiratory (muscle) (system) (tract) R06.81
    center NEC G93.89
    congenital P28.89
    newborn P28.89
  right side — *see* Hemiplegia
  saturnine — *see* subcategory T56.0
  sciatic nerve G57.0-
  senile G83.9
  shaking — *see* Parkinsonism
  shoulder G56.9-
  sleep, recurrent isolated G47.53
  spastic G83.9
    cerebral — *see* Palsy, cerebral, spastic
    congenital (cerebral) — *see* Palsy, cerebral, spastic
    familial G11.4
    hereditary G11.4
    quadriplegic G80.0
    syphilitic (spinal) A52.17
  sphincter, bladder — *see* Paralysis, bladder
  spinal (cord) G83.9
    accessory nerve G52.8
    acute — *see* Poliomyelitis, paralytic
    ascending acute G61.0
    atrophic (acute) — *see also* Poliomyelitis, paralytic
      spastic, syphilitic A52.17
    congenital NEC — *see* Palsy, cerebral
    hereditary G95.89
    infantile — *see* Poliomyelitis, paralytic
    progressive G12.21
    sequelae NEC G83.89
  sternomastoid G52.8

Paralysis, paralytic (complete) (incomplete) G83.9 — *continued*
  stomach K31.84
    diabetic — *see* Diabetes, by type, with gastroparesis
    nerve G52.2
      diabetic — *see* Diabetes, by type, with gastroparesis
  stroke — *see* Infarct, brain
  subcapsularis G56.8-
  supranuclear (progressive) G23.1
  sympathetic G90.8
    cervical G90.09
    nervous system — *see* Neuropathy, peripheral, autonomic
  syndrome G83.9
    specified NEC G83.89
  syphilitic spastic spinal (Erb's) A52.17
  thigh G57.9-
  throat J39.2
    diphtheritic A36.0
    muscle J39.2
  thrombotic (current episode) I63.3-
  thumb G56.9-
  tick — *see* Toxicity, venom, arthropod, specified NEC
  Todd's (postepileptic transitory paralysis) G83.84
  toe G57.6-
  tongue K14.8
  transient R29.5
    arm or leg NEC R29.818
    traumatic NEC — *see* Injury, nerve
  trapezius G52.8
  traumatic, transient NEC — *see* Injury, nerve
  trembling — *see* Parkinsonism
  triceps brachii G56.9-
  trigeminal nerve G50.9
  trochlear (nerve) — *see* Strabismus, paralytic, fourth nerve
  ulnar nerve G56.2-
  upper limb — *see* Monoplegia, upper limb
  uremic N18.9 *[G99.8]*
  uveoparotitic D86.89
  uvula K13.79
    postdiphtheritic A36.0
  vagus nerve G52.2
  vasomotor NEC G90.8
  velum palati K13.79
  vesical — *see* Paralysis, bladder
  vestibular nerve (except Vertigo) — *see* subcategory H93.3
  vocal cords J38.00
    bilateral J38.02
    unilateral J38.01
  Volkmann's (complicating trauma) T79.6
  wasting G12.29
  Weber's G46.3
  wrist G56.9-
Paramedial urethrovesical orifice Q64.79
Paramenia N92.6
Parametritis (*see also* Disease, pelvis, inflammatory) N73.2
  acute N73.0
  complicating abortion — *see* Abortion, by type, complicated by, parametritis
Parametrium, parametric — *see* condition
Paramnesia — *see* Amnesia
Paramolar K00.1
Paramyloidosis E85.8
Paramyoclonus multiplex G25.3
Paramyotonia (congenita) G71.19
Parangi — *see* Yaws
Paranoia (querulans) F22
  senile F03
Paranoid
  dementia (senile) F03
    praecox — *see* Schizophrenia
  personality F60.0

Paranoid — *continued*
  psychosis (climacteric) (involutional) (menopausal) F22
    psychogenic (acute) F23
    senile F03
  reaction (acute) F23
    chronic F22
  schizophrenia F20.0
  state (climacteric) (involutional) (menopausal) (simple) F22
    senile F03
  tendencies F60.0
  traits F60.0
  trends F60.0
  type, psychopathic personality F60.0
Paraparesis — *see* Paraplegia
Paraphasia R47.02
Paraphilia F65.9
Paraphimosis (congenital) N47.2
  chancroidal A57
Paraphrenia, paraphrenic (late) F22
  schizophrenia F20.0
Paraplegia (lower) G82.20
  ataxic — *see* Degeneration, combined, spinal cord
  complete G82.21
  congenital (cerebral) G80.8
    spastic G80.1
  familial spastic G11.4
  functional (hysterical) F44.4
  hereditary, spastic G11.4
  hysterical F44.4
  incomplete G82.22
  Pott's A18.01
  psychogenic F44.4
  spastic
    Erb's spinal, syphilitic A52.17
    hereditary G11.4
    tropical G04.1
  syphilitic (spastic) A52.17
  tropical spastic G04.1
Parapoxvirus B08.60
  specified NEC B08.69
Paraproteinemia D89.2
  benign (familial) D89.2
  monoclonal D47.2
  secondary to malignant disease D47.2
Parapsoriasis L41.9
  en plaques L41.4
  guttata L41.1
  large plaque L41.4
  retiform, retiformis L41.5
  small plaque L41.3
  specified NEC L41.8
  varioliformis (acuta) L41.0
Parasitic — *see also* condition
  disease NEC B89
  stomatitis B37.0
  sycosis (beard) (scalp) B35.0
  twin Q89.4
Parasitism B89
  intestinal B82.9
  skin B88.9
  specified — *see* Infestation
Parasitophobia F40.218
Parasomnia G47.50
  due to
    alcohol
      abuse F10.182
      dependence F10.282
      use F10.982
    amphetamines
      abuse F15.182
      dependence F15.282
      use F15.982
    caffeine
      abuse F15.182
      dependence F15.282
      use F15.982

DISEASE INDEX

Parasomnia G47.50 — *continued*
  due to — *continued*
    cocaine
      abuse F14.182
      dependence F14.282
      use F14.982
    drug NEC
      abuse F19.182
      dependence F19.282
      use F19.982
    opioid
      abuse F11.182
      dependence F11.282
      use F11.982
    psychoactive substance NEC
      abuse F19.182
      dependence F19.282
      use F19.982
    sedative, hypnotic, or anxiolytic
      abuse F13.182
      dependence F13.282
      use F13.982
    stimulant NEC
      abuse F15.182
      dependence F15.282
      use F15.982
  in conditions classified elsewhere G47.54
  nonorganic origin F51.8
  organic G47.50
  specified NEC G47.59
Paraspadias Q54.9
Paraspasmus facialis G51.8
Parasuicide (attempt)
  history of (personal) Z91.5
  in family Z81.8
Parathyroid gland — *see* condition
Parathyroid tetany E20.9
Paratrachoma A74.0
Paratyphilitis — *see* Appendicitis
Paratyphoid (fever) — *see* Fever, paratyphoid
Paratyphus — *see* Fever, paratyphoid
Paraurethral duct Q64.79
  nonorganic origin F51.5
Paraurethritis — *see also* Urethritis
  gonococcal (acute) (chronic) (with abscess)
    A54.1
Paravaccinia NEC B08.04
Paravaginitis — *see* Vaginitis
Parencephalitis — *see also* Encephalitis
  sequelae G09
Parent-child conflict — *see* Conflict, parent-
  child
  estrangement NEC Z62.890
Paresis — *see also* Paralysis
  accommodation — *see* Paresis, of
    accommodation
  Bernhardt's G57.1-
  bladder (sphincter) — *see also* Paralysis,
    bladder
    tabetic A52.17
  bowel, colon or intestine K56.0
  extrinsic muscle, eye H49.9
  general (progressive) (syphilitic) A52.17
    juvenile A50.45
  heart — *see* Failure, heart
  insane (syphilitic) A52.17
  juvenile (general) A50.45
  of accommodation H52.52-
  peripheral progressive (idiopathic) G60.3
  pseudohypertrophic G71.0
  senile G83.9
  syphilitic (general) A52.17
    congenital A50.45
  vesical NEC N31.2
Paresthesia — *see also* Disturbance, sensation
  Bernhardt G57.1-
Paretic — *see* condition

Parinaud's
  conjunctivitis H10.89
  oculoglandular syndrome H10.89
  ophthalmoplegia H49.88-
**Parkinson's disease, syndrome or
    tremor** — *see* Parkinsonism
Parkinsonism (idiopathic) (primary) G20
  with neurogenic orthostatic hypotension
    (symptomatic) G90.3
  arteriosclerotic G21.4
  dementia G31.83 *[F02.80]*
    with behavioral disturbance G31.83
      [F02.81]
  due to
    drugs NEC G21.19
      neuroleptic G21.11
  neuroleptic induced G21.11
  postencephalitic G21.3
  secondary G21.9
    due to
      arteriosclerosis G21.4
      drugs NEC G21.19
        neuroleptic G21.11
      encephalitis G21.3
      external agents NEC G21.2
      syphilis A52.19
    specified NEC G21.8
  syphilitic A52.19
  treatment-induced NEC G21.19
  vascular G21.4
Parodontitis — *see* Periodontitis
Parodontosis K05.4
Paronychia — *see also* Cellulitis, digit
  with lymphangitis — *see* Lymphangitis, acute,
    digit
  candidal (chronic) B37.2
  tuberculous (primary) A18.4
Parorexia (psychogenic) F50.89
Parosmia R43.1
  psychogenic F45.8
Parotid gland — *see* condition
Parotitis, parotiditis (allergic) (nonspecific
    toxic) (purulent) (septic) (suppurative) — *see
    also* Sialoadenitis
  epidemic — *see* Mumps
  infectious — *see* Mumps
  postoperative K91.89
  surgical K91.89
Parrot fever A70
Parrot's disease (early congenital syphilitic
    pseudoparalysis) A50.02
Parry-Romberg syndrome G51.8
Parry's disease or syndrome E05.00
  with thyroid storm E05.01
Pars planitis — *see* Cyclitis
Parson's disease (exophthalmic goiter)
    E05.00
  with thyroid storm E05.01
Parsonage(-Aldren)-Turner syndrome
    G54.5
Particolored infant Q82.8
Parturition — *see* Delivery
Parulis K04.7
  with sinus K04.6
**Parvovirus, as cause of disease classified
    elsewhere** B97.6
Pasini and Pierini's atrophoderma L90.3
Passage
  false, urethra N36.5
  meconium (newborn) during delivery P03.82
  of sounds or bougies — *see* Attention to,
    artificial, opening
Passive — *see* condition
  smoking Z77.22
Pasteurella septica A28.0
Pasteurellosis — *see* Infection, Pasteurella
PAT (paroxysmal atrial tachycardia) I47.1
Patau's syndrome — *see* Trisomy, 13

Patches
  mucous (syphilitic) A51.39
    congenital A50.07
  smokers' (mouth) K13.24
Patellar — *see* condition
Patent — *see also* Imperfect, closure
  canal of Nuck Q52.4
  cervix N88.3
  ductus arteriosus or Botallo's Q25.0
  foramen
    botalli Q21.1
    ovale Q21.1
  interauricular septum Q21.1
  interventricular septum Q21.0
  omphalomesenteric duct Q43.0
  os (uteri) — *see* Patent, cervix
  ostium secundum Q21.1
  urachus Q64.4
  vitelline duct Q43.0
**Paterson(-Brown)(-Kelly) syndrome or
    web** D50.1
Pathologic, pathological — *see also*
    condition
  asphyxia R09.01
  fire-setting F63.1
  gambling F63.0
  ovum O02.0
  resorption, tooth K03.3
  stealing F63.2
Pathology (of) — *see* Disease
  periarticular, associated with previous
    endodontic treatment NEC M27.59
Pattern, sleep-wake, irregular G47.23
Patulous — *see also* Imperfect, closure
    (congenital)
  alimentary tract Q45.8
    lower Q43.8
    upper Q40.8
  eustachian tube H69.0-
Pause, sinoatrial I49.5
Paxton's disease B36.2
Pearl(s)
  enamel K00.2
  Epstein's K09.8
Pearl-worker's disease — *see* Osteomyelitis,
    specified type NEC
Pectenosis K62.4
Pectoral — *see* condition
Pectus
  carinatum (congenital) Q67.7
    acquired M95.4
    rachitic sequelae (late effect) E64.3
  excavatum (congenital) Q67.6
    acquired M95.4
    rachitic sequelae (late effect) E64.3
  recurvatum (congenital) Q67.6
Pedatrophia E41
Pederosis F65.4
Pediculosis (infestation) B85.2
  capitis (head-louse) (any site) B85.0
  corporis (body-louse) (any site) B85.1
  eyelid B85.0
  mixed (classifiable to more than one of the
    titles B85.0-B85.3) B85.4
  pubis (pubic louse) (any site) B85.3
  vestimenti B85.1
  vulvae B85.3
Pediculus (infestation) — *see* Pediculosis
Pedophilia F65.4
Peg-shaped teeth K00.2
Pelade — *see* Alopecia, areata
Pelger-Huët anomaly or syndrome D72.0
Peliosis (rheumatica) D69.0
  hepatis K76.4
    with toxic liver disease K71.8
Pelizaeus-Merzbacher disease E75.29
Pellagra (alcoholic) (with polyneuropathy) E52
**Pellagra-cerebellar-ataxia-renal
    aminoaciduria syndrome** E72.02

Pellegrini (-Stieda) disease or syndrome — see Bursitis, tibial collateral
Pellizzi's syndrome E34.8
Pel's crisis A52.11
Pelvic — see also condition
  examination (periodic) (routine) Z01.419
    with abnormal findings Z01.411
  kidney, congenital Q63.2
Pelviolithiasis — see Calculus, kidney
Pelviperitonitis — see also Peritonitis, pelvic
  gonococcal A54.24
  puerperal O85
Pelvis — see condition or type
Pemphigoid L12.9
  benign, mucous membrane L12.1
  bullous L12.0
  cicatricial L12.1
  juvenile L12.2
  ocular L12.1
  specified NEC L12.8
Pemphigus L10.9
  benign familial (chronic) Q82.8
  Brazilian L10.3
  circinatus L13.0
  conjunctiva L12.1
  drug-induced L10.5
  erythematosus L10.4
  foliaceous L10.2
  gangrenous — see Gangrene
  neonatorum L01.03
  ocular L12.1
  paraneoplastic L10.81
  specified NEC L10.89
  syphilitic (congenital) A50.06
  vegetans L10.1
  vulgaris L10.0
  wildfire L10.3
Pendred's syndrome E07.1
Pendulous
  abdomen, in pregnancy — see Pregnancy, complicated by, abnormal, pelvic organs or tissues NEC
  breast N64.89
Penetrating wound — see also Puncture
  with internal injury — see Injury, by site
  eyeball — see Puncture, eyeball
  orbit (with or without foreign body) — see Puncture, orbit
  uterus by instrument with or following ectopic or molar pregnancy O08.6
Penicillosis B48.4
Penis — see condition
Penitis N48.29
Pentalogy of Fallot Q21.8
Pentasomy X syndrome Q97.1
Pentosuria (essential) E74.8
Percreta placenta O43.23-
Peregrinating patient — see Disorder, factitious
Perforation, perforated (nontraumatic) (of)
  accidental during procedure (blood vessel) (nerve) (organ) — see Complication, accidental puncture or laceration
  antrum — see Sinusitis, maxillary
  appendix K35.2
    with localized peritonitis K35.3
  atrial septum, multiple Q21.1
  attic, ear — see Perforation, tympanum, attic
  bile duct (common) (hepatic) K83.2
    cystic K82.2
  bladder (urinary)
    with or following ectopic or molar pregnancy O08.6
    obstetrical trauma O71.5
    traumatic S37.29
      at delivery O71.5

Perforation, perforated (nontraumatic) (of) — continued
  bowel K63.1
    with or following ectopic or molar pregnancy O08.6
    newborn P78.0
    obstetrical trauma O71.5
    traumatic — see Laceration, intestine
  broad ligament N83.8
    with or following ectopic or molar pregnancy O08.6
    obstetrical trauma O71.6
  by
    device, implant or graft (see also Complications, by site and type, mechanical) T85.628
      arterial graft NEC — see Complication, cardiovascular device, mechanical, vascular
      breast (implant) T85.49
      catheter NEC T85.698
        cystostomy T83.090
        dialysis (renal) T82.49
          intraperitoneal T85.691
        infusion NEC T82.594
          spinal (epidural) (subdural) T85.690
        urinary (see also Complications, catheter, urinary) T83.098
      electronic (electrode) (pulse generator) (stimulator)
        bone T84.390
        cardiac T82.199
          electrode T82.190
          pulse generator T82.191
          specified type NEC T82.198
        nervous system — see Complication, prosthetic device, mechanical, electronic nervous system stimulator
        urinary — see Complication, genitourinary, device, urinary, mechanical
      fixation, internal (orthopedic) NEC — see Complication, fixation device, mechanical
      gastrointestinal — see Complications, prosthetic device, mechanical, gastrointestinal device
      genital NEC T83.498
        intrauterine contraceptive device T83.39
        penile prosthesis T83.490
      heart NEC — see Complication, cardiovascular device, mechanical
      joint prosthesis — see Complications, joint prosthesis, mechanical, specified NEC, by site
      ocular NEC — see Complications, prosthetic device, mechanical, ocular device
      orthopedic NEC — see Complication, orthopedic, device, mechanical
      specified NEC T85.628
      urinary NEC — see also Complication, genitourinary, device, urinary, mechanical
        graft T83.29
      vascular NEC — see Complication, cardiovascular device, mechanical
      ventricular intracranial shunt T85.09
    foreign body left accidentally in operative wound T81.539
    instrument (any) during a procedure, accidental — see Puncture, accidental complicating surgery
  cecum K35.2
    with localized peritonitis K35.3
  cervix (uteri) N88.8
    with or following ectopic or molar pregnancy O08.6
    obstetrical trauma O71.3

Perforation, perforated (nontraumatic) (of) — continued
  colon K63.1
    newborn P78.0
    obstetrical trauma O71.5
    traumatic — see Laceration, intestine, large
  common duct (bile) K83.2
  cornea (due to ulceration) — see Ulcer, cornea, perforated
  cystic duct K82.2
  diverticulum (intestine) K57.80
    with bleeding K57.81
    large intestine K57.20
      with
        bleeding K57.21
        small intestine K57.40
          with bleeding K57.41
      small intestine K57.00
      with
        bleeding K57.01
        large intestine K57.40
          with bleeding K57.41
  ear drum — see Perforation, tympanum
  esophagus K22.3
  ethmoidal sinus — see Sinusitis, ethmoidal
  frontal sinus — see Sinusitis, frontal
  gallbladder K82.2
  heart valve — see Endocarditis
  ileum K63.1
    newborn P78.0
    obstetrical trauma O71.5
    traumatic — see Laceration, intestine, small
  instrumental, surgical (accidental) (blood vessel) (nerve) (organ) — see Puncture, accidental complicating surgery
  intestine NEC K63.1
    with ectopic or molar pregnancy O08.6
    newborn P78.0
    obstetrical trauma O71.5
    traumatic — see Laceration, intestine
    ulcerative NEC K63.1
      newborn P78.0
  jejunum, jejunal K63.1
    obstetrical trauma O71.5
    traumatic — see Laceration, intestine, small
    ulcer — see Ulcer, gastrojejunal, with perforation
  joint prosthesis — see Complications, joint prosthesis, mechanical, specified NEC, by site
  mastoid (antrum) (cell) — see Disorder, mastoid, specified NEC
  maxillary sinus — see Sinusitis, maxillary
  membrana tympani — see Perforation, tympanum
  nasal
    septum J34.89
      congenital Q30.3
      syphilitic A52.73
    sinus J34.89
      congenital Q30.8
      due to sinusitis — see Sinusitis
  palate (see also Cleft, palate) Q35.9
    syphilitic A52.79
  palatine vault (see also Cleft, palate, hard) Q35.1
    syphilitic A52.79
      congenital A50.59
  pars flaccida (ear drum) — see Perforation, tympanum, attic
  pelvic
    floor S31.030
      with
        ectopic or molar pregnancy O08.6
        penetration into retroperitoneal space S31.031
        retained foreign body S31.040
          with penetration into retroperitoneal space S31.041

Perforation, perforated (nontraumatic) (of)
— continued
pelvic — continued
    floor S31.030 — continued
        following ectopic or molar pregnancy
            O08.6
        obstetrical trauma O70.1
    organ S37.99
        adrenal gland S37.818
        bladder — see Perforation, bladder
        fallopian tube S37.599
            bilateral S37.592
            unilateral S37.591
        kidney S37.09-
            obstetrical trauma O71.5
        ovary S37.499
            bilateral S37.492
            unilateral S37.491
        prostate S37.828
        specified organ NEC S37.898
        ureter — see Perforation, ureter
        urethra — see Perforation, urethra
        uterus — see Perforation, uterus
    perineum — see Laceration, perineum
    pharynx J39.2
    rectum K63.1
        newborn P78.0
        obstetrical trauma O71.5
        traumatic S36.63
    root canal space due to endodontic treatment
        M27.51
    sigmoid K63.1
        newborn P78.0
        obstetrical trauma O71.5
        traumatic S36.533
    sinus (accessory) (chronic) (nasal) J34.89
    sphenoidal sinus — see Sinusitis, sphenoidal
    surgical (accidental) (by instrument) (blood
        vessel) (nerve) (organ) — see Puncture,
        accidental complicating surgery
    traumatic
        external — see Puncture
        eye — see Puncture, eyeball
        internal organ — see Injury, by site
    tympanum, tympanic (membrane) (persistent
        post-traumatic) (postinflammatory) H72.9-
        attic H72.1-
            multiple — see Perforation, tympanum,
                multiple
            total — see Perforation, tympanum, total
        central H72.0-
            multiple — see Perforation, tympanum,
                multiple
            total — see Perforation, tympanum, total
        marginal NEC — see subcategory H72.2
        multiple H72.81-
            pars flaccida — see Perforation, tympanum,
                attic
        total H72.82-
        traumatic, current episode S09.2-
    typhoid, gastrointestinal — see Typhoid
    ulcer — see Ulcer, by site, with perforation
    ureter N28.89
        traumatic S37.19
    urethra N36.8
        with ectopic or molar pregnancy O08.6
        following ectopic or molar pregnancy O08.6
        obstetrical trauma O71.5
        traumatic S37.39
            at delivery O71.5
    uterus
        with ectopic or molar pregnancy O08.6
        by intrauterine contraceptive device T83.39
        following ectopic or molar pregnancy O08.6
        obstetrical trauma O71.1
        traumatic S37.69
            obstetric O71.1
    uvula K13.79
        syphilitic A52.79

Perforation, perforated (nontraumatic) (of)
— continued
vagina
    obstetrical trauma O71.4
    other trauma — see Puncture, vagina
Periadenitis mucosa necrotica recurrens
    K12.0
Periappendicitis (acute) — see Appendicitis
Periarteritis nodosa (disseminated)
    (infectious) (necrotizing) M30.0
Periarthritis (joint) — see also Enthesopathy
    Duplay's M75.0-
    gonococcal A54.42
    humeroscapularis — see Capsulitis, adhesive
    scapulohumeral — see Capsulitis, adhesive
    shoulder — see Capsulitis, adhesive
    wrist M77.2-
Periarthrosis (angioneural) — see
    Enthesopathy
Pericapsulitis, adhesive (shoulder) — see
    Capsulitis, adhesive
Pericarditis (with decompensation) (with
    effusion) I31.9
    with rheumatic fever (conditions in I00)
        active — see Pericarditis, rheumatic
        inactive or quiescent I09.2
    acute (hemorrhagic) (nonrheumatic) (Sicca)
        I30.9
        with chorea (acute) (rheumatic) (Sydenham's)
            I02.0
        benign I30.8
        nonspecific I30.0
        rheumatic I01.0
            with chorea (acute) (Sydenham's) I02.0
    adhesive or adherent (chronic) (external)
        (internal) I31.0
        acute — see Pericarditis, acute
        rheumatic I09.2
    bacterial (acute) (subacute) (with serous or
        seropurulent effusion) I30.1
    calcareous I31.1
    cholesterol (chronic) I31.8
        acute I30.9
    chronic (nonrheumatic) I31.9
        rheumatic I09.2
    constrictive (chronic) I31.1
    coxsackie B33.23
    fibrinocaseous (tuberculous) A18.84
    fibrinopurulent I30.1
    fibrinous I30.8
    fibrous I31.0
    gonococcal A54.83
    idiopathic I30.0
    in systemic lupus erythematosus M32.12
    infective I30.1
    meningococcal A39.53
    neoplastic (chronic) I31.8
        acute I30.9
    obliterans, obliterating I31.0
    plastic I31.0
    pneumococcal I30.1
    postinfarction I24.1
    purulent I30.1
    rheumatic (active) (acute) (with effusion) (with
        pneumonia) I01.0
        with chorea (acute) (rheumatic) (Sydenham's)
            I02.0
        chronic or inactive (with chorea) I09.2
    rheumatoid — see Rheumatoid, carditis
    septic I30.1
    serofibrinous I30.8
    staphylococcal I30.1
    streptococcal I30.1
    suppurative I30.1
    syphilitic A52.06
    tuberculous A18.84
    uremic N18.9 *[I32]*
    viral I30.1
Pericardium, pericardial — see condition

Pericellulitis — see Cellulitis
Pericementitis (chronic) (suppurative) — see
    also Periodontitis
    acute K05.20
        generalized — see Peridontitis, aggressive,
            generalized
        localized — see Peridontitis, aggressive,
            localized
Perichondritis
    auricle — see Perichondritis, ear
    bronchus J98.09
    ear (external) H61.00-
        acute H61.01-
        chronic H61.02-
    external auditory canal — see Perichondritis,
        ear
    larynx J38.7
        syphilitic A52.73
        typhoid A01.09
    nose J34.89
    pinna — see Perichondritis, ear
    trachea J39.8
Periclasia K05.4
Pericoronitis — see Periodontitis
Pericystitis N30.90
    with hematuria N30.91
Peridiverticulitis (intestine) K57.92
    cecum — see Diverticulitis, intestine, large
    colon — see Diverticulitis, intestine, large
    duodenum — see Diverticulitis, intestine, small
    intestine — see Diverticulitis, intestine
    jejunum — see Diverticulitis, intestine, small
    rectosigmoid — see Diverticulitis, intestine,
        large
    rectum — see Diverticulitis, intestine, large
    sigmoid — see Diverticulitis, intestine, large
Periendocarditis — see Endocarditis
Periepididymitis N45.1
Perifolliculitis L01.02
    abscedens, caput, scalp L66.3
    capitis, abscedens (et suffodiens) L66.3
    superficial pustular L01.02
Perihepatitis K65.8
Perilabyrinthitis (acute) — see subcategory
    H83.0
Perimeningitis — see Meningitis
Perimetritis — see Endometritis
Perimetrosalpingitis — see Salpingo-
    oophoritis
Perineocele N81.81
Perinephric, perinephritic — see condition
Perinephritis — see also Infection, kidney
    purulent — see Abscess, kidney
Perineum, perineal — see condition
Perineuritis NEC — see Neuralgia
Periodic — see condition
Periodontitis (chronic) (complex) (compound)
    (local) (simplex) K05.30
    acute K05.20
        generalized K05.229
            moderate K05.222
            severe K05.223
            slight K05.221
        localized K05.219
            moderate K05.212
            severe K05.213
            slight K05.211
    apical K04.5
        acute (pulpal origin) K04.4
    generalized K05.329
        moderate K05.322
        severe K05.323
        slight K05.321
    localized K05.319
        moderate K05.312
        severe K05.313
        slight K05.311
Periodontoclasia K05.4
Periodontosis (juvenile) K05.4

Periods — see also Menstruation
  heavy N92.0
  irregular N92.6
  shortened intervals (irregular) N92.1
Perionychia — see also Cellulitis, digit
  with lymphangitis — see Lymphangitis, acute,
    digit
Perioophoritis — see Salpingo-oophoritis
Periorchitis N45.2
Periosteum, periosteal — see condition
Periostitis (albuminosa) (circumscribed)
  (diffuse) (infective) (monomelic) — see also
  Osteomyelitis
  alveolar M27.3
  alveolodental M27.3
  dental M27.3
  gonorrheal A54.43
  jaw (lower) (upper) M27.2
  orbit H05.03-
  syphilitic A52.77
    congenital (early) A50.02 [M90.80]
    secondary A51.46
  tuberculous — see Tuberculosis, bone
  yaws (hypertrophic) (early) (late) A66.6
    [M90.80]
Periostosis (hyperplastic) — see also Disorder,
  bone, specified type NEC
  with osteomyelitis — see Osteomyelitis,
    specified type NEC
Peripartum
  cardiomyopathy O90.3
Periphlebitis — see Phlebitis
Periproctitis K62.89
Periprostatitis — see Prostatitis
Perirectal — see condition
Perirenal — see condition
Perisalpingitis — see Salpingo-oophoritis
Perisplenitis (infectional) D73.89
Peristalsis, visible or reversed R19.2
Peritendinitis — see Enthesopathy
Peritoneum, peritoneal — see condition
Peritonitis (adhesive) (bacterial) (fibrinous)
  (hemorrhagic) (idiopathic) (localized)
  (perforative) (primary) (with adhesions) (with
  effusion) K65.9
  with or following
    abscess K65.1
    appendicitis K35.3
      with perforation or rupture K35.2
      generalized K35.2
      localized K35.3
    diverticular disease (intestine) K57.80
      with bleeding K57.81
      ectopic or molar pregnancy O08.0
      large intestine K57.20
        with
          bleeding K57.21
          small intestine K57.40
            with bleeding K57.41
      small intestine K57.00
        with
          bleeding K57.01
          large intestine K57.40
            with bleeding K57.41
  acute (generalized) K65.0
  aseptic T81.61
  bile, biliary K65.3
  chemical T81.61
  chlamydial A74.81
  chronic proliferative K65.8
  complicating abortion — see Abortion, by
    type, complicated by, pelvic peritonitis
  congenital P78.1
  diaphragmatic K65.0
  diffuse K65.0
  diphtheritic A36.89
  disseminated K65.0

Peritonitis (adhesive) (bacterial) (fibrinous)
  (hemorrhagic) (idiopathic) (localized)
  (perforative) (primary) (with adhesions) (with
  effusion) K65.9 — continued
  due to
    bile K65.3
    foreign
      body or object accidentally left during a
        procedure (instrument) (sponge)
        (swab) T81.599
      substance accidentally left during a
        procedure (chemical) (powder) (talc)
        T81.61
    talc T81.61
    urine K65.8
  eosinophilic K65.8
    acute K65.0
  fibrocaseous (tuberculous) A18.31
  fibropurulent K65.0
  following ectopic or molar pregnancy O08.0
  general(ized) K65.0
  gonococcal A54.85
  meconium (newborn) P78.0
  neonatal P78.1
    meconium P78.0
  pancreatic K65.0
  paroxysmal, familial E85.0
    benign E85.0
  pelvic
    female N73.5
      acute N73.3
      chronic N73.4
        with adhesions N73.6
    male K65.0
  periodic, familial E85.0
  proliferative, chronic K65.8
  puerperal, postpartum, childbirth O85
  purulent K65.0
  septic K65.0
  specified NEC K65.8
  spontaneous bacterial K65.2
  subdiaphragmatic K65.0
  subphrenic K65.0
  suppurative K65.0
  syphilitic A52.74
    congenital (early) A50.08 [K67]
  talc T81.61
  tuberculous A18.31
  urine K65.8
Peritonsillar — see condition
Peritonsillitis J36
Perityphlitis K37
Periureteritis N28.89
Periurethral — see condition
Periurethritis (gangrenous) — see Urethritis
Periuterine — see condition
Perivaginitis — see Vaginitis
Perivasculitis, retinal H35.06-
Perivasitis (chronic) N49.1
Perivesiculitis (seminal) — see Vesiculitis
Perlèche NEC K13.0
  due to
    candidiasis B37.83
    moniliasis B37.83
    riboflavin deficiency E53.0
    vitamin B2 (riboflavin) deficiency E53.0
Pernicious — see condition
Pernio, perniosis T69.1
Perpetrator (of abuse) — see Index to External
  Causes of Injury, Perpetrator
Persecution
  delusion F22
  social Z60.5
Perseveration (tonic) R48.8
Persistence, persistent (congenital)
  anal membrane Q42.3
    with fistula Q42.2
  arteria stapedia Q16.3
  atrioventricular canal Q21.2

Persistence, persistent (congenital) —
  continued
  branchial cleft Q18.0
  bulbus cordis in left ventricle Q21.8
  canal of Cloquet Q14.0
  capsule (opaque) Q12.8
  cilioretinal artery or vein Q14.8
  cloaca Q43.7
  communication — see Fistula, congenital
  convolutions
    aortic arch Q25.46
    fallopian tube Q50.6
    oviduct Q50.6
    uterine tube Q50.6
  double aortic arch Q25.45
  ductus arteriosus (Botalli) Q25.0
  fetal
    circulation P29.3
    form of cervix (uteri) Q51.828
    hemoglobin, hereditary (HPFH) D56.4
  foramen
    Botalli Q21.1
    ovale Q21.1
  Gartner's duct Q52.4
  hemoglobin, fetal (hereditary) (HPFH) D56.4
  hyaloid
    artery (generally incomplete) Q14.0
    system Q14.8
  hymen, in pregnancy or childbirth — see
    Pregnancy, complicated by, abnormal,
    vulva
  lanugo Q84.2
  left
    posterior cardinal vein Q26.8
    root with right arch of aorta Q25.49
    superior vena cava Q26.1
  Meckel's diverticulum Q43.0
    malignant — see Table of Neoplasms, small
      intestine, malignant
  mucosal disease (middle ear) — see Otitis,
    media, suppurative, chronic, tubotympanic
  nail(s), anomalous Q84.6
  omphalomesenteric duct Q43.0
  organ or site not listed — see Anomaly, by site
  ostium
    atrioventriculare commune Q21.2
    primum Q21.2
    secundum Q21.1
  ovarian rests in fallopian tube Q50.6
  pancreatic tissue in intestinal tract Q43.8
  primary (deciduous)
    teeth K00.6
    vitreous hyperplasia Q14.0
  pupillary membrane Q13.89
  rhesus (Rh) titer — see Complication(s),
    transfusion, incompatibility reaction, Rh
    (factor)
  right aortic arch Q25.47
  sinus
    urogenitalis
      female Q52.8
      male Q55.8
    venosus with imperfect incorporation in right
      auricle Q26.8
  thymus (gland) (hyperplasia) E32.0
  thyroglossal duct Q89.2
  thyrolingual duct Q89.2
  truncus arteriosus or communis Q20.0
  tunica vasculosa lentis Q12.2
  umbilical sinus Q64.4
  urachus Q64.4
  vitelline duct Q43.0
Person (with)
  admitted for clinical research, as a control
    subject (normal comparison) (participant)
    Z00.6
  awaiting admission to adequate facility
    elsewhere Z75.1

Person (with) — *continued*
  concern (normal) about sick person in family
      Z63.6
  consulting on behalf of another Z71.0
  feigning illness Z76.5
  living (in)
    alone Z60.2
    boarding school Z59.3
    residential institution Z59.3
    without
      adequate housing (heating) (space) Z59.1
      housing (permanent) (temporary) Z59.0
      person able to render necessary care
          Z74.2
      shelter Z59.0
  on waiting list Z75.1
  sick or handicapped in family Z63.6
Personality (disorder) F60.9
  accentuation of traits (type A pattern) Z73.1
  affective F34.0
  aggressive F60.3
  amoral F60.2
  anacastic, anankastic F60.5
  antisocial F60.2
  anxious F60.6
  asocial F60.2
  asthenic F60.7
  avoidant F60.6
  borderline F60.3
  change due to organic condition (enduring)
      F07.0
  compulsive F60.5
  cycloid F34.0
  cyclothymic F34.0
  dependent F60.7
  depressive F34.1
  dissocial F60.2
  dual F44.81
  eccentric F60.89
  emotionally unstable F60.3
  expansive paranoid F60.0
  explosive F60.3
  fanatic F60.0
  haltose type F60.89
  histrionic F60.4
  hyperthymic F34.0
  hypothymic F34.1
  hysterical F60.4
  immature F60.89
  inadequate F60.7
  labile (emotional) F60.3
  mixed (nonspecific) F60.89
  morally defective F60.2
  multiple F44.81
  narcissistic F60.81
  obsessional F60.5
  obsessive(-compulsive) F60.5
  organic F07.0
  overconscientious F60.5
  paranoid F60.0
  passive-aggressive F60.89
  passive(-dependent) F60.7
  pathologic F60.9
  pattern defect or disturbance F60.9
  pseudopsychopathic (organic) F07.0
  pseudoretarded (organic) F07.0
  psychoinfantile F60.4
  psychoneurotic NEC F60.89
  psychopathic F60.2
  querulant F60.0
  sadistic F60.89
  schizoid F60.1
  self-defeating F60.7
  sensitive paranoid F60.0
  sociopathic (amoral) (antisocial) (asocial)
      (dissocial) F60.2
  specified NEC F60.89
  type A Z73.1
  unstable (emotional) F60.3

Perthes' disease — *see* Legg-Calvé-Perthes
    disease
Pertussis (*see also* Whooping cough) A37.90
Perversion, perverted
  appetite F50.89
    psychogenic F50.89
  function
    pituitary gland E23.2
      posterior lobe E22.2
  sense of smell and taste R43.8
    psychogenic F45.8
  sexual — *see* Deviation, sexual
Pervious, congenital — *see also* Imperfect,
    closure
  ductus arteriosus Q25.0
Pes (congenital) — *see also* Talipes
  acquired — *see also* Deformity, limb, foot,
      specified NEC
    planus — *see* Deformity, limb, flat foot
  adductus Q66.89
  cavus Q66.7
  deformity NEC, acquired — *see* Deformity,
      limb, foot, specified NEC
  planus (acquired) (any degree) — *see also*
      Deformity, limb, flat foot
    rachitic sequelae (late effect) E64.3
  valgus Q66.6
Pest, pestis — *see* Plague
Petechia, petechiae R23.3
  newborn P54.5
Petechial typhus A75.9
Peter's anomaly Q13.4
Petit mal seizure — *see* Epilepsy,
    generalized, specified NEC
Petit's hernia — *see* Hernia, abdomen,
    specified site NEC
Petrellidosis B48.2
Petrositis H70.20-
  acute H70.21-
  chronic H70.22-
Peutz-Jeghers disease or syndrome
    Q85.8
Peyronie's disease N48.6
PFAPA (periodic fever, aphthous stomatitis,
    pharyngitis, and adenopathy syndrome)
    M04.8
Pfeiffer's disease — *see* Mononucleosis,
    infectious
Phagedena (dry) (moist) (sloughing) — *see also*
    Gangrene
  geometric L88
  penis N48.29
  tropical — *see* Ulcer, skin
  vulva N76.6
Phagedenic — *see* condition
Phakoma H35.89
Phakomatosis (*see also* specific eponymous
    syndromes) Q85.9
  Bourneville's Q85.1
  specified NEC Q85.8
Phantom limb syndrome (without pain)
    G54.7
  with pain G54.6
Pharyngeal pouch syndrome D82.1
Pharyngitis (acute) (catarrhal) (gangrenous)
    (infective) (malignant) (membranous)
    (phlegmonous) (pseudomembranous)
    (simple) (subacute) (suppurative) (ulcerative)
    (viral) J02.9
  with influenza, flu, or grippe — *see* Influenza,
      with, pharyngitis
  aphthous B08.5
  atrophic J31.2
  chlamydial A56.4
  chronic (atrophic) (granular) (hypertrophic)
      J31.2
  coxsackievirus B08.5
  diphtheritic A36.0
  enteroviral vesicular B08.5

Pharyngitis (acute) (catarrhal) (gangrenous)
    (infective) (malignant) (membranous)
    (phlegmonous) (pseudomembranous)
    (simple) (subacute) (suppurative) (ulcerative)
    (viral) J02.9 — *continued*
  follicular (chronic) J31.2
  fusospirochetal A69.1
  gonococcal A54.5
  granular (chronic) J31.2
  herpesviral B00.2
  hypertrophic J31.2
  infectional, chronic J31.2
  influenzal — *see* Influenza, with, respiratory
      manifestations NEC
  lymphonodular, acute (enteroviral) B08.8
  pneumococcal J02.8
  purulent J02.9
  putrid J02.9
  septic J02.0
  sicca J31.2
  specified organism NEC J02.8
  staphylococcal J02.8
  streptococcal J02.0
  syphilitic, congenital (early) A50.03
  tuberculous A15.8
  vesicular, enteroviral B08.5
  viral NEC J02.8
Pharyngoconjunctivitis, viral B30.2
Pharyngolaryngitis (acute) J06.0
  chronic J37.0
Pharyngoplegia J39.2
Pharyngotonsillitis, herpesviral B00.2
Pharyngotracheitis, chronic J42
Pharynx, pharyngeal — *see* condition
Phencyclidine-induced
  anxiety disorder F16.980
  bipolar and related disorder F16.94
  depressive disorder F16.94
  psychotic disorder F16.959
Phenomenon
  Arthus' — *see* Arthus' phenomenon
  jaw-winking Q07.8
  lupus erythematosus (LE) cell M32.9
  Raynaud's (secondary) I73.00
    with gangrene I73.01
  vasomotor R55
  vasospastic I73.9
  vasovagal R55
  Wenckebach's I44.1
Phenylketonuria E70.1
  classical E70.0
  maternal E70.1
Pheochromoblastoma
  specified site — *see* Neoplasm, malignant, by
      site
  unspecified site C74.10
Pheochromocytoma
  malignant
    specified site — *see* Neoplasm, malignant,
        by site
    unspecified site C74.10
  specified site — *see* Neoplasm, benign, by site
  unspecified site D35.00
Pheohyphomycosis — *see* Chromomycosis
Pheomycosis — *see* Chromomycosis
Phimosis (congenital) (due to infection) N47.1
  chancroidal A57
Phlebectasia — *see also* Varix
  congenital Q27.4
Phlebitis (infective) (pyemic) (septic)
    (suppurative) I80.9
  antepartum — *see* Thrombophlebitis,
      antepartum
  blue — *see* Phlebitis, leg, deep
  breast, superficial I80.8
  cavernous (venous) sinus — *see* Phlebitis,
      intracranial (venous) sinus
  cerebral (venous) sinus — *see* Phlebitis,
      intracranial (venous) sinus

Phlebitis (infective) (pyemic) (septic) (suppurative) I80.9 — *continued*
 chest wall, superficial I80.8
 cranial (venous) sinus — *see* Phlebitis, intracranial (venous) sinus
 deep (vessels) — *see* Phlebitis, leg, deep
 due to implanted device — *see* Complications, by site and type, specified NEC
 during or resulting from a procedure T81.72
 femoral vein (superficial) I80.1-
 femoropopliteal vein I80.0-
 gestational — *see* Phlebopathy, gestational
 hepatic veins I80.8
 iliofemoral — *see* Phlebitis, femoral vein
 intracranial (venous) sinus (any) G08
  nonpyogenic I67.6
 intraspinal venous sinuses and veins G08
  nonpyogenic G95.19
 lateral (venous) sinus — *see* Phlebitis, intracranial (venous) sinus
 leg I80.3
  antepartum — *see* Thrombophlebitis, antepartum
  deep (vessels) NEC I80.20-
   iliac I80.21-
   popliteal vein I80.22-
   specified vessel NEC I80.29-
   tibial vein I80.23-
  femoral vein (superficial) I80.1-
  superficial (vessels) I80.0-
 longitudinal sinus — *see* Phlebitis, intracranial (venous) sinus
 lower limb — *see* Phlebitis, leg
 migrans, migrating (superficial) I82.1
 pelvic
  with ectopic or molar pregnancy O08.0
  following ectopic or molar pregnancy O08.0
  puerperal, postpartum O87.1
 popliteal vein — *see* Phlebitis, leg, deep, popliteal
 portal (vein) K75.1
 postoperative T81.72
 pregnancy — *see* Thrombophlebitis, antepartum
 puerperal, postpartum, childbirth O87.0
  deep O87.1
  pelvic O87.1
  superficial O87.0
 retina — *see* Vasculitis, retina
 saphenous (accessory) (great) (long) (small) — *see* Phlebitis, leg, superficial
 sinus (meninges) — *see* Phlebitis, intracranial (venous) sinus
 specified site NEC I80.8
 syphilitic A52.09
 tibial vein — *see* Phlebitis, leg, deep, tibial
 ulcerative I80.9
  leg — *see* Phlebitis, leg
 umbilicus I80.8
 uterus (septic) — *see* Endometritis
 varicose (leg) (lower limb) — *see* Varix, leg, with, inflammation
Phlebofibrosis I87.8
Phleboliths I87.8
Phlebopathy
 gestational O22.9-
 puerperal O87.9
Phlebosclerosis I87.8
Phlebothrombosis — *see also* Thrombosis
 antepartum — *see* Thrombophlebitis, antepartum
 pregnancy — *see* Thrombophlebitis, antepartum
 puerperal — *see* Thrombophlebitis, puerperal
Phlebotomus fever A93.1
Phlegmasia
 alba dolens O87.1
  nonpuerperal — *see* Phlebitis, femoral vein
 cerulea dolens — *see* Phlebitis, leg, deep

Phlegmon — *see* Abscess
Phlegmonous — *see* condition
Phlyctenulosis (allergic) (keratoconjunctivitis) (nontuberculous) — *see also* Keratoconjunctivitis
 cornea — *see* Keratoconjunctivitis
 tuberculous A18.52
Phobia, phobic F40.9
 animal F40.218
  spiders F40.210
 examination F40.298
 reaction F40.9
 simple F40.298
 social F40.10
  generalized F40.11
 specific (isolated) F40.298
  animal F40.218
   spiders F40.210
  blood F40.230
  injection F40.231
  injury F40.233
  men F40.290
  natural environment F40.228
   thunderstorms F40.220
  situational F40.248
   bridges F40.242
   closed in spaces F40.240
   flying F40.243
   heights F40.241
  specified focus NEC F40.298
  transfusion F40.231
  women F40.291
 specified NEC F40.8
  medical care NEC F40.232
 state F40.9
Phocas' disease — *see* Mastopathy, cystic
Phocomelia Q73.1
 lower limb — *see* Agenesis, leg, with foot present
 upper limb — *see* Agenesis, arm, with hand present
Phoria H50.50
Phosphate-losing tubular disorder N25.0
Phosphatemia E83.39
Phosphaturia E83.39
Photodermatitis (sun) L56.8
 chronic L57.8
 due to drug L56.8
 light other than sun L59.8
Photokeratitis H16.13-
Photophobia H53.14
Photophthalmia — *see* Photokeratitis
Photopsia H53.19
Photoretinitis — *see* Retinopathy, solar
Photosensitivity, photosensitization (sun) skin L56.8
 light other than sun L59.8
Phrenitis — *see* Encephalitis
Phrynoderma (vitamin A deficiency) E50.8
Phthiriasis (pubis) B85.3
 with any infestation classifiable to B85.0-B85.2 B85.4
Phthirus infestation — *see* Phthiriasis
Phthisis — *see also* Tuberculosis
 bulbi (infectional) — *see* Disorder, globe, degenerated condition, atrophy
 eyeball (due to infection) — *see* Disorder, globe, degenerated condition, atrophy
Phycomycosis — *see* Zygomycosis
Physalopteriasis B81.8
Physical restraint status Z78.1
Phytobezoar T18.9
 intestine T18.3
 stomach T18.2
Pian — *see* Yaws
Pianoma A66.1
Pica F50.89
 in adults F50.89
 infant or child F98.3

Picking, nose F98.8
Pick-Niemann disease — *see* Niemann-Pick disease or syndrome
Pick's
 cerebral atrophy G31.01 *[F02.80]*
  with behavioral disturbance G31.01 *[F02.81]*
 disease or syndrome (brain) G31.01 *[F02.80]*
  with behavioral disturbance G31.01 *[F02.81]*
  brain G31.01 *[F02.80]*
   with behavioral disturbance G31.01 *[F02.81]*
  pericardium (pericardial pseudocirrhosis of liver) I31.1
 syndrome
  brain G31.01 *[F02.80]*
   with behavioral disturbance G31.01 *[F02.81]*
  of heart (pericardial pseudocirrhosis of liver) I31.1
Pickwickian syndrome E66.2
Piebaldism E70.39
Piedra (beard) (scalp) B36.8
 black B36.3
 white B36.2
Pierre Robin deformity or syndrome Q87.0
Pierson's disease or osteochondrosis M91.0
Pig-bel A05.2
Pigeon
 breast or chest (acquired) M95.4
  congenital Q67.7
  rachitic sequelae (late effect) E64.3
 breeder's disease or lung J67.2
 fancier's disease or lung J67.2
 toe — *see* Deformity, toe, specified NEC
Pigmentation (abnormal) (anomaly) L81.9
 conjunctiva H11.13-
 cornea (anterior) H18.01-
  posterior H18.05-
  stromal H18.06-
 diminished melanin formation NEC L81.6
 iron L81.8
 lids, congenital Q82.8
 limbus corneae — *see* Pigmentation, cornea
 metals L81.8
 optic papilla, congenital Q14.2
 retina, congenital (grouped) (nevoid) Q14.1
 scrotum, congenital Q82.8
 tattoo L81.8
Piles (*see also* Hemorrhoids) K64.9
Pili
 annulati or torti (congenital) Q84.1
 incarnati L73.1
Pill roller hand (intrinsic) — *see* Parkinsonism
Pilomatrixoma — *see* Neoplasm, skin, benign
 malignant — *see* Neoplasm, skin, malignant
Pilonidal — *see* condition
Pimple R23.8
PIN — *see* Neoplasia, intraepithelial, prostate
Pinched nerve — *see* Neuropathy, entrapment
Pindborg tumor — *see* Cyst, calcifying odontogenic
Pineal body or gland — *see* condition
Pinealoblastoma C75.3
Pinealoma D44.5
 malignant C75.3
Pineoblastoma C75.3
Pineocytoma D44.5
Pinguecula H11.15-
Pingueculitis H10.81-
Pinhole meatus (*see also* Stricture, urethra) N35.9
Pink
 disease — *see* subcategory T56.1
 eye — *see* Conjunctivitis, acute, mucopurulent
Pinkus' disease (lichen nitidus) L44.1

Pinpoint
 meatus — *see* Stricture, urethra
 os (uteri) — *see* Stricture, cervix
Pins and needles R20.2
Pinta A67.9
 cardiovascular lesions A67.2
 chancre (primary) A67.0
 erythematous plaques A67.1
 hyperchromic lesions A67.1
 hyperkeratosis A67.1
 lesions A67.9
  cardiovascular A67.2
  hyperchromic A67.1
  intermediate A67.1
  late A67.2
  mixed A67.3
  primary A67.0
  skin (achromic) (cicatricial) (dyschromic)
   A67.2
   hyperchromic A67.1
   mixed (achromic and hyperchromic)
    A67.3
 papule (primary) A67.0
 skin lesions (achromic) (cicatricial)
  (dyschromic) A67.2
  hyperchromic A67.1
  mixed (achromic and hyperchromic) A67.3
 vitiligo A67.2
Pintids A67.1
Pinworm (disease) (infection) (infestation) B80
Piroplasmosis B60.0
Pistol wound — *see* Gunshot wound
Pitchers' elbow — *see* Derangement, joint,
 specified type NEC, elbow
Pithecoid pelvis Q74.2
 with disproportion (fetopelvic) O33.0
  causing obstructed labor O65.0
Pithiatism F48.8
Pitted — *see* Pitting
Pitting (*see also* Edema) R60.9
 lip R60.0
 nail L60.8
 teeth K00.4
Pituitary gland — *see* condition
Pituitary-snuff-taker's disease J67.8
Pityriasis (capitis) L21.0
 alba L30.5
 circinata (et maculata) L42
 furfuracea L21.0
 Hebra's L26
 lichenoides L41.0
  chronica L41.1
  et varioliformis (acuta) L41.0
 maculata (et circinata) L30.5
 nigra B36.1
 pilaris, Hebra's L44.0
 rosea L42
 rotunda L44.8
 rubra (Hebra) pilaris L44.0
 simplex L30.5
 specified type NEC L30.5
 streptogenes L30.5
 versicolor (scrotal) B36.0
Placenta, placental — *see* Pregnancy,
 complicated by (care of) (management
 affected by), specified condition
Placentitis O41.14-
Plagiocephaly Q67.3
Plague A20.9
 abortive A20.8
 ambulatory A20.8
 asymptomatic A20.8
 bubonic A20.0
 cellulocutaneous A20.1
 cutaneobubonic A20.1
 lymphatic gland A20.0
 meningitis A20.3
 pharyngeal A20.8
 pneumonic (primary) (secondary) A20.2

Plague A20.9 — *continued*
 pulmonary, pulmonic A20.2
 septicemic A20.7
 tonsillar A20.8
  septicemic A20.7
Planning, family
 contraception Z30.9
 procreation Z31.69
Plaque(s)
 artery, arterial — *see* Arteriosclerosis
 calcareous — *see* Calcification
 coronary, lipid rich I25.83
 epicardial I31.8
 erythematous, of pinta A67.1
 Hollenhorst's — *see* Occlusion, artery, retina
 lipid rich, coronary I25.83
 pleural (without asbestos) J92.9
  with asbestos J92.0
 tongue K13.29
Plasmacytoma C90.3-
 extramedullary C90.2-
 medullary C90.0-
 solitary C90.3-
Plasmacytopenia D72.818
Plasmacytosis D72.822
Plaster ulcer — *see* Ulcer, pressure, by site
Plateau iris syndrome (post-iridectomy)
 (postprocedural) (without glaucoma) H21.82
 with glaucoma H40.22-
Platybasia Q75.8
Platyonychia (congenital) Q84.6
 acquired L60.8
Platypelloid pelvis M95.5
 with disproportion (fetopelvic) O33.0
  causing obstructed labor O65.0
 congenital Q74.2
Platyspondylisis Q76.49
Plaut(-Vincent) disease (*see also* Vincent's)
 A69.1
Plethora R23.2
 newborn P61.1
Pleura, pleural — *see* condition
Pleuralgia R07.81
Pleurisy (acute) (adhesive) (chronic) (costal)
 (diaphragmatic) (double) (dry) (fibrinous)
 (fibrous) (interlobar) (latent) (plastic)
 (primary) (residual) (sicca) (sterile)
 (subacute) (unresolved) R09.1
 with
  adherent pleura J86.0
  effusion J90
   chylous, chyliform J94.0
   tuberculous (non primary) A15.6
    primary (progressive) A15.7
  tuberculosis — *see* Pleurisy, tuberculous (non
   primary)
 encysted — *see* Pleurisy, with effusion
 exudative — *see* Pleurisy, with effusion
 fibrinopurulent, fibropurulent — *see* Pyothorax
 hemorrhagic — *see* Hemothorax
 pneumococcal J90
 purulent — *see* Pyothorax
 septic — *see* Pyothorax
 serofibrinous — *see* Pleurisy, with effusion
 seropurulent — *see* Pyothorax
 serous — *see* Pleurisy, with effusion
 staphylococcal J86.9
 streptococcal J90
 suppurative — *see* Pyothorax
 traumatic (post) (current) — *see* Injury,
  intrathoracic, pleura
 tuberculous (with effusion) (non primary) A15.6
  primary (progressive) A15.7
Pleuritis sicca — *see* Pleurisy
Pleurobronchopneumonia — *see*
 Pneumonia, broncho-
Pleurodynia R07.81
 epidemic B33.0
 viral B33.0

Pleuropericarditis — *see also* Pericarditis
 acute I30.9
Pleuropneumonia (acute) (bilateral) (double)
 (septic) (*see also* Pneumonia) J18.8
 chronic — *see* Fibrosis, lung
Pleuro-pneumonia-like-organism
 (PPLO), as cause of disease classified
 elsewhere B96.0
Pleurorrhea — *see* Pleurisy, with effusion
Plexitis, brachial G54.0
Plica
 polonica B85.0
 syndrome, knee M67.5-
 tonsil J35.8
Plicated tongue K14.5
Plug
 bronchus NEC J98.09
 meconium (newborn) NEC syndrome P76.0
 mucus — *see* Asphyxia, mucus
Plumbism — *see* subcategory T56.0
Plummer's disease E05.20
 with thyroid storm E05.21
Plummer-Vinson syndrome D50.1
Pluricarential syndrome of infancy E40
Plus (and minus) hand (intrinsic) — *see*
 Deformity, limb, specified type NEC,
 forearm
Pneumathemia — *see* Air, embolism
Pneumatic hammer (drill) syndrome
 T75.21
Pneumatocele (lung) J98.4
 intracranial G93.89
 tension J44.9
Pneumatosis
 cystoides intestinalis K63.89
 intestinalis K63.89
 peritonei K66.8
Pneumaturia R39.89
Pneumoblastoma — *see* Neoplasm, lung,
 malignant
Pneumocephalus G93.89
Pneumococcemia A40.3
Pneumococcus, pneumococcal — *see*
 condition
Pneumoconiosis (due to) (inhalation of) J64
 with tuberculosis (any type in A15) J65
 aluminum J63.0
 asbestos J61
 bagasse, bagassosis J67.1
 bauxite J63.1
 beryllium J63.2
 coal miners' (simple) J60
 coalworkers' (simple) J60
 collier's J60
 cotton dust J66.0
 diatomite (diatomaceous earth) J62.8
 dust
  inorganic NEC J63.6
  lime J62.8
  marble J62.8
  organic NEC J66.8
 fumes or vapors (from silo) J68.9
 graphite J63.3
 grinder's J62.8
 kaolin J62.8
 mica J62.8
 millstone maker's J62.8
 miner's J60
 mineral fibers NEC J61
 moldy hay J67.0
 potter's J62.8
 rheumatoid — *see* Rheumatoid, lung
 sandblaster's J62.8
 silica, silicate NEC J62.8
  with carbon J60
 stonemason's J62.8
 talc (dust) J62.0
Pneumocystis carinii pneumonia B59
Pneumocystis jiroveci (pneumonia) B59

Pneumocystosis (with pneumonia) B59
Pneumohemopericardium I31.2
Pneumohemothorax J94.2
  traumatic S27.2
Pneumohydropericardium — *see*
  Pericarditis
Pneumohydrothorax — *see* Hydrothorax
Pneumomediastinum J98.2
  congenital or perinatal P25.2
Pneumomycosis B49 [J99]
Pneumonia (acute) (double) (migratory)
  (purulent) (septic) (unresolved) J18.9
  with
    influenza — *see* Influenza, with, pneumonia
    lung abscess J85.1
      due to specified organism — *see*
        Pneumonia, in (due to)
  adenoviral J12.0
  adynamic J18.2
  alba A50.04
  allergic (eosinophilic) J82
  alveolar — *see* Pneumonia, lobar
  anaerobes J15.8
  anthrax A22.1
  apex, apical — *see* Pneumonia, lobar
  Ascaris B77.81
  aspiration J69.0
    due to
      aspiration of microorganisms
        bacterial J15.9
        viral J12.9
      food (regurgitated) J69.0
      gastric secretions J69.0
      milk (regurgitated) J69.0
      oils, essences J69.1
      solids, liquids NEC J69.8
      vomitus J69.0
    newborn P24.81
      amniotic fluid (clear) P24.11
      blood P24.21
      food (regurgitated) P24.31
      liquor (amnii) P24.11
      meconium P24.01
      milk P24.31
      mucus P24.11
      specified NEC P24.81
      stomach contents P24.31
    postprocedural J95.4
  atypical NEC J18.9
  bacillus J15.9
    specified NEC J15.8
  bacterial J15.9
    specified NEC J15.8
  Bacteroides (fragilis) (oralis) (melaninogenicus)
    J15.8
  basal, basic, basilar — *see* Pneumonia, by
    type
  bronchiolitis obliterans organized (BOOP)
    J84.89
  broncho-, bronchial (confluent) (croupous)
    (diffuse) (disseminated) (hemorrhagic)
    (involving lobes) (lobar) (terminal) J18.0
    allergic (eosinophilic) J82
    aspiration — *see* Pneumonia, aspiration
    bacterial J15.9
      specified NEC J15.8
    chronic — *see* Fibrosis, lung
    diplococcal J13
    Eaton's agent J15.7
    Escherichia coli (E. coli) J15.5
    Friedländer's bacillus J15.0
    Hemophilus influenzae J14
    hypostatic J18.2
    inhalation — *see also* Pneumonia, aspiration
      due to fumes or vapors (chemical) J68.0
      of oils or essences J69.1
    Klebsiella (pneumoniae) J15.0
    lipid, lipoid J69.1
      endogenous J84.89

Pneumonia (acute) (double) (migratory)
  (purulent) (septic) (unresolved) J18.9 —
  continued
  broncho-, bronchial (confluent) (croupous)
    (diffuse) (disseminated) (hemorrhagic)
    (involving lobes) (lobar) (terminal) J18.0
    — *continued*
    Mycoplasma (pneumoniae) J15.7
    pleuro-pneumonia-like-organisms (PPLO)
      J15.7
    pneumococcal J13
    Proteus J15.6
    Pseudomonas J15.1
    Serratia marcescens J15.6
    specified organism NEC J16.8
    staphylococcal — *see* Pneumonia,
      staphylococcal
    streptococcal NEC J15.4
      group B J15.3
      pneumoniae J13
    viral, virus — *see* Pneumonia, viral
  Butyrivibrio (fibrisolvens) J15.8
  Candida B37.1
  caseous — *see* Tuberculosis, pulmonary
  catarrhal — *see* Pneumonia, broncho
  chlamydial J16.0
    congenital P23.1
  cholesterol J84.89
  cirrhotic (chronic) — *see* Fibrosis, lung
  Clostridium (haemolyticum) (novyi) J15.8
  confluent — *see* Pneumonia, broncho
  congenital (infective) P23.9
    due to
      bacterium NEC P23.6
      Chlamydia P23.1
      Escherichia coli P23.4
      Haemophilus influenzae P23.6
      infective organism NEC P23.8
      Klebsiella pneumoniae P23.6
      Mycoplasma P23.6
      Pseudomonas P23.5
      Staphylococcus P23.2
      Streptococcus (except group B) P23.6
        group B P23.3
      viral agent P23.0
      specified NEC P23.8
  croupous — *see* Pneumonia, lobar
  cryptogenic organizing J84.116
  cytomegalic inclusion B25.0
  cytomegaloviral B25.0
  deglutition — *see* Pneumonia, aspiration
  desquamative interstitial J84.117
  diffuse — *see* Pneumonia, broncho
  diplococcal, diplococcus (broncho-) (lobar) J13
  disseminated (focal) — *see* Pneumonia,
    broncho
  Eaton's agent J15.7
  embolic, embolism — *see* Embolism,
    pulmonary
  Enterobacter J15.6
  eosinophilic J82
  Escherichia coli (E. coli) J15.5
  Eubacterium J15.8
  fibrinous — *see* Pneumonia, lobar
  fibroid, fibrous (chronic) — *see* Fibrosis, lung
  Friedländer's bacillus J15.0
  Fusobacterium (nucleatum) J15.8
  gangrenous J85.0
  giant cell (measles) B05.2
  gonococcal A54.84
  gram-negative bacteria NEC J15.6
    anaerobic J15.8
  Hemophilus influenzae (broncho) (lobar) J14
  human metapneumovirus J12.3
  hypostatic (broncho) (lobar) J18.2
  in (due to)
    actinomycosis A42.0
    adenovirus J12.0
    anthrax A22.1

Pneumonia (acute) (double) (migratory)
  (purulent) (septic) (unresolved) J18.9 —
  continued
  in (due to) — *continued*
    ascariasis B77.81
    aspergillosis B44.9
    Bacillus anthracis A22.1
    Bacterium anitratum J15.6
    candidiasis B37.1
    chickenpox B01.2
    Chlamydia J16.0
      neonatal P23.1
    coccidioidomycosis B38.2
      acute B38.0
      chronic B38.1
    cytomegalovirus disease B25.0
    Diplococcus (pneumoniae) J13
    Eaton's agent J15.7
    Enterobacter J15.6
    Escherichia coli (E. coli) J15.5
    Friedländer's bacillus J15.0
    fumes and vapors (chemical) (inhalation)
      J68.0
    gonorrhea A54.84
    Hemophilus influenzae (H. influenzae) J14
    Herellea J15.6
    histoplasmosis B39.2
      acute B39.0
      chronic B39.1
    human metapneumovirus J12.3
    Klebsiella (pneumoniae) J15.0
    measles B05.2
    Mycoplasma (pneumoniae) J15.7
    nocardiosis, nocardiasis A43.0
    ornithosis A70
    parainfluenza virus J12.2
    pleuro-pneumonia-like-organism (PPLO)
      J15.7
    pneumococcus J13
    pneumocystosis (Pneumocystis carinii)
      (Pneumocystis jiroveci) B59
    Proteus J15.6
    Pseudomonas NEC J15.1
      pseudomallei A24.1
    psittacosis A70
    Q fever A78
    respiratory syncytial virus J12.1
    rheumatic fever I00 [J17]
    rubella B06.81
    Salmonella (infection) A02.22
      typhi A01.03
    schistosomiasis B65.9 [J17]
    Serratia marcescens J15.6
    specified
      bacterium NEC J15.8
      organism NEC J16.8
      spirochetal NEC A69.8
    Staphylococcus J15.20
      aureus (methicillin susceptible) (MSSA)
        J15.211
        methicillin resistant (MRSA) J15.212
      specified NEC J15.29
    Streptococcus J15.4
      group B J15.3
      pneumoniae J13
      specified NEC J15.4
    toxoplasmosis B58.3
    tularemia A21.2
    typhoid (fever) A01.03
    varicella B01.2
    virus — *see* Pneumonia, viral
    whooping cough A37.91
      due to
        Bordetella parapertussis A37.11
        Bordetella pertussis A37.01
        specified NEC A37.81
    Yersinia pestis A20.2
  inhalation of food or vomit — *see* Pneumonia,
    aspiration

Pneumonia (acute) (double) (migratory) (purulent) (septic) (unresolved) J18.9 — *continued*
interstitial J84.9
chronic J84.111
desquamative J84.117
due to
collagen vascular disease J84.17
known underlying cause J84.17
idiopathic NOS J84.111
in diseases classified elsewhere J84.17
lymphocytic (due to collagen vacular disease) (in diseases classified elsewhere) J84.17
lymphoid J84.2
non-specific J84.89
due to
collagen vascular disease J84.17
known underlying cause J84.17
idiopathic J84.113
in diseases classified elsewhere J84.17
plasma cell B59
pseudomonas J15.1
usual J84.112
due to collagen vascular disease J84.17
idiopathic J84.112
in diseases classified elsewhere J84.17
Klebsiella (pneumoniae) J15.0
lipid, lipoid (exogenous) J69.1
endogenous J84.89
lobar (disseminated) (double) (interstitial) J18.1
bacterial J15.9
specified NEC J15.8
chronic — *see* Fibrosis, lung
Escherichia coli (E. coli) J15.5
Friedländer's bacillus J15.0
Hemophilus influenzae J14
hypostatic J18.2
Klebsiella (pneumoniae) J15.0
pneumococcal J13
Proteus J15.6
Pseudomonas J15.1
specified organism NEC J16.8
staphylococcal — *see* Pneumonia, staphylococcal
streptococcal NEC J15.4
Streptococcus pneumoniae J13
viral, virus — *see* Pneumonia, viral
lobular — *see* Pneumonia, broncho
lymphoid interstitial J84.2
Löffler's J82
massive — *see* Pneumonia, lobar
meconium P24.01
MRSA (Methicillin resistant Staphylococcus aureus) J15.212
MSSA (methicillin susceptible Staphylococcus aureus) J15.211
Mycoplasma (pneumoniae) J15.7
necrotic J85.0
neonatal P23.9
aspiration — *see* Aspiration, by substance, with pneumonia
nitrogen dioxide J68.0
organizing J84.89
due to
collagen vascular disease J84.17
known underlying cause J84.17
in diseases classified elsewhere J84.17
orthostatic J18.2
parainfluenza virus J12.2
parenchymatous — *see* Fibrosis, lung
passive J18.2
patchy — *see* Pneumonia, broncho
Peptococcus J15.8
Peptostreptococcus J15.8
plasma cell (of infants) B59
pleurolobar — *see* Pneumonia, lobar
pleuro-pneumonia-like organism (PPLO) J15.7

Pneumonia (acute) (double) (migratory) (purulent) (septic) (unresolved) J18.9 — *continued*
pneumococcal (broncho) (lobar) J13
Pneumocystis (carinii) (jiroveci) B59
postinfectional NEC B99 *[J17]*
postmeasles B05.2
Proteus J15.6
Pseudomonas J15.1
psittacosis A70
radiation J70.0
respiratory syncytial virus J12.1
resulting from a procedure J95.89
rheumatic I00 *[J17]*
Salmonella (arizonae) (cholerae-suis) (enteritidis) (typhimurium) A02.22
typhi A01.03
typhoid fever A01.03
SARS-associated coronavirus J12.81
segmented, segmental — *see* Pneumonia, broncho-
Serratia marcescens J15.6
specified NEC J18.8
bacterium NEC J15.8
organism NEC J16.8
virus NEC J12.89
spirochetal NEC A69.8
staphylococcal (broncho) (lobar) J15.20
aureus (methicillin susceptible) (MSSA) J15.211
methicillin resistant (MRSA) J15.212
specified NEC J15.29
static, stasis J18.2
streptococcal NEC (broncho) (lobar) J15.4
group
A J15.4
B J15.3
specified NEC J15.4
Streptococcus pneumoniae J13
syphilitic, congenital (early) A50.04
traumatic (complication) (early) (secondary) T79.8
tuberculous (any) — *see* Tuberculosis, pulmonary
tularemic A21.2
varicella B01.2
Veillonella J15.8
ventilator associated J95.851
viral, virus (broncho) (interstitial) (lobar) J12.9
adenoviral J12.0
congenital P23.0
human metapneumovirus J12.3
parainfluenza J12.2
respiratory syncytial J12.1
SARS-associated coronavirus J12.81
specified NEC J12.89
white (congenital) A50.04
Pneumonic — *see* condition
Pneumonitis (acute) (primary) — *see also* Pneumonia
air-conditioner J67.7
allergic (due to) J67.9
organic dust NEC J67.8
red cedar dust J67.8
sequoiosis J67.8
wood dust J67.8
aspiration J69.0
due to
anesthesia J95.4
during
labor and delivery O74.0
pregnancy O29.01-
puerperium O89.01
fumes or gases J68.0
obstetric O74.0
chemical (due to gases, fumes or vapors) (inhalation) J68.0
due to anesthesia J95.4
cholesterol J84.89

Pneumonitis (acute) (primary) — *see also* Pneumonia — *continued*
chronic — *see* Fibrosis, lung
congenital rubella P35.0
crack (cocaine) J68.0
due to
beryllium J68.0
cadmium J68.0
crack (cocaine) J68.0
detergent J69.8
fluorocarbon-polymer J68.0
food, vomit (aspiration) J69.0
fumes or vapors J68.0
gases, fumes or vapors (inhalation) J68.0
inhalation
blood J69.8
essences J69.1
food (regurgitated), milk, vomit J69.0
oils, essences J69.1
saliva J69.0
solids, liquids NEC J69.8
manganese J68.0
nitrogen dioxide J68.0
oils, essences J69.1
solids, liquids NEC J69.8
toxoplasmosis (acquired) B58.3
congenital P37.1
vanadium J68.0
ventilator J95.851
eosinophilic J82
hypersensitivity J67.9
air conditioner lung J67.7
bagassosis J67.1
bird fancier's lung J67.2
farmer's lung J67.0
maltworker's lung J67.4
maple bark-stripper's lung J67.6
mushroom worker's lung J67.5
specified organic dust NEC J67.8
suberosis J67.3
interstitial (chronic) J84.89
acute J84.114
lymphoid J84.2
non-specific J84.89
idiopathic J84.113
lymphoid, interstitial J84.2
meconium P24.01
postanesthetic J95.4
correct substance properly administered — *see* Table of Drugs and Chemcials, by drug, adverse effect
in labor and delivery O74.0
in pregnancy O29.01-
obstetric O74.0
overdose or wrong substance given or taken (by accident) — *see* Table of Drugs and Chemicals, by drug, poisoning
postpartum, puerperal O89.01
postoperative J95.4
obstetric O74.0
radiation J70.0
rubella, congenital P35.0
ventilation (air-conditioning) J67.7
ventilator associated J95.851
wood-dust J67.8
Pneumonoconiosis — *see* Pneumoconiosis
Pneumoparotid K11.8
Pneumopathy NEC J98.4
alveolar J84.09
due to organic dust NEC J66.8
parietoalveolar J84.09
Pneumopericarditis — *see also* Pericarditis
acute I30.9
Pneumopericardium — *see also* Pericarditis
congenital P25.3
newborn P25.3
traumatic (post) — *see* Injury, heart
Pneumophagia (psychogenic) F45.8

Pneumopleurisy, pneumopleuritis (see also Pneumonia) J18.8
Pneumopyopericardium I30.1
Pneumopyothorax — see Pyopneumothorax
  with fistula J86.0
Pneumorrhagia — see also Hemorrhage, lung
  tuberculous — see Tuberculosis, pulmonary
Pneumothorax NOS J93.9
  acute J93.8
  chronic J93.81
  congenital P25.1
  perinatal period P25.1
  postprocedural J95.811
  specified NEC J93.83
  spontaneous NOS J93.83
    newborn P25.1
    primary J93.11
    secondary J93.12
    tension J93.0
  tense valvular, infectional J93.0
  tension (spontaneous) J93.0
  traumatic S27.0
    with hemothorax S27.2
  tuberculous — see Tuberculosis, pulmonary
Podagra (see also Gout) M10.9
Podencephalus Q01.9
Poikilocytosis R71.8
Poikiloderma L81.6
  Civatte's L57.3
  congenital Q82.8
  vasculare atrophicans L94.5
Poikilodermatomyositis M33.10
  with
    myopathy M33.12
    respiratory involvement M33.11
    specified organ involvement NEC M33.19
Pointed ear (congenital) Q17.3
Poison ivy, oak, sumac or other plant dermatitis (allergic) (contact) L23.7
Poisoning (acute) — see also Table of Drugs and Chemicals
  algae and toxins T65.82-
  Bacillus B (aertrycke) (cholerae (suis)) (paratyphosus) (suipestifer) A02.9
    botulinus A05.1
  bacterial toxins A05.9
  berries, noxious — see Poisoning, food, noxious, berries
  botulism A05.1
  ciguatera fish T61.0-
  Clostridium botulinum A05.1
  death-cap (Amanita phalloides) (Amanita verna) — see Poisoning, food, noxious, mushrooms
  drug — see Table of Drugs and Chemicals, by drug, poisoning
  epidemic, fish (noxious) — see Poisoning, seafood
    bacterial A05.9
  fava bean D55.0
  fish (noxious) T61.9-
    bacterial — see Intoxication, foodborne, by agent
    ciguatera fish — see Poisoning, ciguatera fish
    scombroid fish — see Poisoning, scombroid fish
    specified type NEC T61.77-
  food (acute) (diseased) (infected) (noxious) NEC T62.9-
    bacterial — see Intoxication, foodborne, by agent
    due to
      Bacillus (aertrycke) (choleraesuis) (paratyphosus) (suipestifer) A02.9
        botulinus A05.1
      Clostridium (perfringens) (Welchii) A05.2

Poisoning (acute) (see also Table of Drugs and Chemicals) — continued
  food (acute) (diseased) (infected) (noxious) NEC T62.9- — continued
    due to — continued
      salmonella (aertrycke) (callinarum) (choleraesuis) (enteritidis) (paratyphi) (suipestifer) A02.9
        with
          gastroenteritis A02.0
          sepsis A02.1
      staphylococcus A05.0
      Vibrio
        parahaemolyticus A05.3
        vulnificus A05.5
    noxious or naturally toxic T62.9-
      berries — see subcategory T62.1-
      fish — see Poisoning, seafood
      mushrooms — see subcategory T62.0x-
      plants NEC — see subcategory T62.2x-
      seafood — see Poisoning, seafood
      specified NEC — see subcategory T62.8x-
  ichthyotoxism — see Poisoning, seafood
  kreotoxism, food A05.9
  latex T65.81-
  lead T56.0-
  mushroom — see Poisoning, food, noxious, mushroom
  mussels — see also Poisoning, shellfish
    bacterial — see Intoxication, foodborne, by agent
  nicotine (tobacco) T65.2-
  noxious foodstuffs — see Poisoning, food, noxious
  plants, noxious — see Poisoning, food, noxious, plants NEC
  ptomaine — see Poisoning, food
  radiation J70.0
  Salmonella (arizonae) (cholerae-suis) (enteritidis) (typhimurium) A02.9
  scombroid fish T61.1-
  seafood (noxious) T61.9-
    bacterial — see Intoxication, foodborne, by agent
    fish — see Poisoning, fish
    shellfish — see Poisoning, shellfish
    specified NEC — see subcategory T61.8x-
  shellfish (amnesic) (azaspiracid) (diarrheic) (neurotoxic) (noxious) (paralytic) T61.78-
    bacterial — see Intoxication, foodborne, by agent
    ciguatera mollusk — see Poisoning, ciguatera fish
  specified substance NEC T65.891
  Staphylococcus, food A05.0
  tobacco (nicotine) T65.2-
  water E87.79
Poker spine — see Spondylitis, ankylosing
Poland syndrome Q79.8
Polioencephalitis (acute) (bulbar) A80.9
  inferior G12.22
  influenzal — see Influenza, with, encephalopathy
  superior hemorrhagic (acute) (Wernicke's) E51.2
  Wernicke's E51.2
Polioencephalomyelitis (acute) (anterior) A80.9
  with beriberi E51.2
Polioencephalopathy, superior hemorrhagic E51.2
  with
  beriberi E51.11
  pellagra E52
Poliomeningoencephalitis — see Meningoencephalitis

Poliomyelitis (acute) (anterior) (epidemic) A80.9
  with paralysis (bulbar) — see Poliomyelitis, paralytic
  abortive A80.4
  ascending (progressive) — see Poliomyelitis, paralytic
  bulbar (paralytic) — see Poliomyelitis, paralytic
  congenital P35.8
  nonepidemic A80.9
  nonparalytic A80.4
  paralytic A80.30
    specified NEC A80.39
    vaccine-associated A80.0
    wild virus
      imported A80.1
      indigenous A80.2
  spinal, acute A80.9
Poliosis (eyebrow) (eyelashes) L67.1
  circumscripta, acquired L67.1
Pollakiuria R35.0
  psychogenic F45.8
Pollinosis J30.1
Pollitzer's disease L73.2
Polyadenitis — see also Lymphadenitis
  malignant A20.0
Polyalgia M79.89
Polyangiitis M30.0
  microscopic M31.7
  overlap syndrome M30.8
Polyarteritis
  microscopic M31.7
  nodosa M30.0
    with lung involvement M30.1
    juvenile M30.2
    related condition NEC M30.8
Polyarthralgia — see Pain, joint
Polyarthritis, polyarthropathy (see also Arthritis) M13.0
  due to or associated with other specified conditions — see Arthritis
  epidemic (Australian) (with exanthema) B33.1
  infective — see Arthritis, pyogenic or pyemic
  inflammatory M06.4
  juvenile (chronic) (seronegative) M08.3
  migratory — see Fever, rheumatic
  rheumatic, acute — see Fever, rheumatic
Polyarthrosis M15.9
  post-traumatic M15.3
  primary M15.0
  specified NEC M15.8
Polycarential syndrome of infancy E40
Polychondritis (atrophic) (chronic) — see also Disorder, cartilage, specified type NEC
  relapsing M94.1
Polycoria Q13.2
Polycystic (disease)
  degeneration, kidney Q61.3
    autosomal dominant (adult type) Q61.2
    autosomal recessive (infantile type) NEC Q61.19
  kidney Q61.3
    autosomal
      dominant Q61.2
      recessive NEC Q61.19
    autosomal dominant (adult type) Q61.2
    autosomal recessive (childhood type) NEC Q61.19
    infantile type NEC Q61.19
  liver Q44.6
  lung J98.4
    congenital Q33.0
  ovary, ovaries E28.2
  spleen Q89.09
Polycythemia (secondary) D75.1
  acquired D75.1
  benign (familial) D75.0

Polycythemia (secondary) D75.1— *continued*
  due to
    donor twin P61.1
    erythropoietin D75.1
    fall in plasma volume D75.1
    high altitude D75.1
    maternal-fetal transfusion P61.1
    stress D75.1
  emotional D75.1
  erythropoietin D75.1
  familial (benign) D75.0
  Gaisböck's (hypertonica) D75.1
  high altitude D75.1
  hypertonica D75.1
  hypoxemic D75.1
  neonatorum P61.1
  nephrogenous D75.1
  relative D75.1
  secondary D75.1
  spurious D75.1
  stress D75.1
  vera D45
Polycytosis cryptogenica D75.1
Polydactylism, polydactyly Q69.9
  toes Q69.2
Polydipsia R63.1
Polydystrophy, pseudo-Hurler E77.0
Polyembryoma — *see* Neoplasm, malignant, by site
Polyglandular
  deficiency E31.0
  dyscrasia E31.9
  dysfunction E31.9
  syndrome E31.8
Polyhydramnios O40-
Polymastia Q83.1
Polymenorrhea N92.0
Polymyalgia M35.3
  arteritica, giant cell M31.5
  rheumatica M35.3
    with giant cell arteritis M31.5
Polymyositis (acute) (chronic) (hemorrhagic) M33.20
  with
    myopathy M33.22
    respiratory involvement M33.21
    skin involvement — *see* Dermatopolymyositis
    specified organ involvement NEC M33.29
  ossificans (generalisata) (progressiva) — *see* Myositis, ossificans, progressiva
Polyneuritis, polyneuritic — *see also* Polyneuropathy
  acute (post-)infective G61.0
  alcoholic G62.1
  cranialis G52.7
  demyelinating, chronic inflammatory (CIDP) G61.81
  diabetic — *see* Diabetes, polyneuropathy
  diphtheritic A36.83
  due to lack of vitamin NEC E56.9 *[G63]*
  endemic E51.11
  erythredema — *see* subcategory T56.1
  febrile, acute G61.0
  hereditary ataxic G60.1
  idiopathic, acute G61.0
  infective (acute) G61.0
  inflammatory, chronic demyelinating (CIDP) G61.81
  nutritional E63.9 *[G63]*
  postinfective (acute) G61.0
  specified NEC G62.89
Polyneuropathy (peripheral) G62.9
  alcoholic G62.1
  amyloid (Portuguese) E85.1 *[G63]*
  arsenical G62.2
  critical illness G62.81
  demyelinating, chronic inflammatory (CIDP) G61.81
  diabetic — *see* Diabetes, polyneuropathy

Polyneuropathy (peripheral) G62.9 — *continued*
  drug-induced G62.0
  hereditary G60.9
    specified NEC G60.8
  idiopathic G60.9
    progressive G60.3
  in (due to)
    alcohol G62.1
      sequelae G65.2
    amyloidosis, familial (Portuguese) E85.1 *[G63]*
    antitetanus serum G61.1
    arsenic G62.2
      sequelae G65.2
    avitaminosis NEC E56.9 *[G63]*
    beriberi E51.11
    collagen vascular disease NEC M35.9 *[G63]*
    deficiency (of)
      B(-complex) vitamins E53.9 *[G63]*
      vitamin B6 E53.1 *[G63]*
    diabetes — *see* Diabetes, polyneuropathy
    diphtheria A36.83
    drug or medicament G62.0
      correct substance properly administered — *see* Table of Drugs and Chemicals, by drug, adverse effect
      overdose or wrong substance given or taken — *see* Table of Drugs and Chemicals, by drug, poisoning
    endocrine disease NEC E34.9 *[G63]*
    herpes zoster B02.23
    hypoglycemia E16.2 *[G63]*
    infectious
      disease NEC B99 *[G63]*
      mononucleosis B27.91
    lack of vitamin NEC E56.9 *[G63]*
    lead G62.2
      sequelae G65.2
    leprosy A30.9 *[G63]*
    Lyme disease A69.22
    metabolic disease NEC E88.9 *[G63]*
    microscopic polyangiitis M31.7 *[G63]*
    mumps B26.84
    neoplastic disease (*see also* Neoplasm) D49.9 *[G63]*
    nutritional deficiency NEC E63.9 *[G63]*
    organophosphate compounds G62.2
      sequelae G65.2
    parasitic disease NEC B89 *[G63]*
    pellagra E52 *[G63]*
    polyarteritis nodosa M30.0
    porphyria E80.20 *[G63]*
    radiation G62.82
    rheumatoid arthritis — *see* Rheumatoid, polyneuropathy
    sarcoidosis D86.89
    serum G61.1
    syphilis (late) A52.15
      congenital A50.43
    systemic
      connective tissue disorder M35.9 *[G63]*
      lupus erythematosus M32.19
    toxic agent NEC G62.2
      sequelae G65.2
    triorthocresyl phosphate G62.2
      sequelae G65.2
    tuberculosis A17.89
    uremia N18.9 *[G63]*
    vitamin B12 deficiency E53.8 *[G63]*
      with anemia (pernicious) D51.0 *[G63]*
        due to dietary deficiency D51.3 *[G63]*
    zoster B02.23
  inflammatory G61.9
    chronic demyelinating (CIDP) G61.81
    sequelae G65.1
    specified NEC G61.89

Polyneuropathy (peripheral) G62.9 — *continued*
  lead G62.2
    sequelae G65.2
  nutritional NEC E63.9 *[G63]*
  postherpetic (zoster) B02.23
  progressive G60.3
  radiation-induced G62.82
  sensory (hereditary) (idiopathic) G60.8
  specified NEC G62.89
  syphilitic (late) A52.15
    congenital A50.43
Polyopia H53.8
Polyorchism, polyorchidism Q55.21
Polyosteoarthritis (*see also* Osteoarthritis, generalized) M15.9-
  post-traumatic M15.3
  specified NEC M15.8
Polyostotic fibrous dysplasia Q78.1
Polyotia Q17.0
Polyp, polypus
  accessory sinus J33.8
  adenocarcinoma in — *see* Neoplasm, malignant, by site
  adenocarcinoma in situ in — *see* Neoplasm, in situ, by site
  adenoid tissue J33.0
  adenomatous — *see also* Neoplasm, benign, by site
    adenocarcinoma in — *see* Neoplasm, malignant, by site
    adenocarcinoma in situ in — *see* Neoplasm, in situ, by site
    carcinoma in — *see* Neoplasm, malignant, by site
    carcinoma in situ in — *see* Neoplasm, in situ, by site
    multiple — *see* Neoplasm, benign
      adenocarcinoma in — *see* Neoplasm, malignant, by site
      adenocarcinoma in situ in — *see* Neoplasm, in situ, by site
  antrum J33.8
  anus, anal (canal) K62.0
  Bartholin's gland N84.3
  bladder D41.4
  carcinoma in — *see* Neoplasm, malignant, by site
  carcinoma in situ in — *see* Neoplasm, in situ, by site
  cecum D12.0
  cervix (uteri) N84.1
    in pregnancy or childbirth — *see* Pregnancy, complicated by, abnormal, cervix
    mucous N84.1
    nonneoplastic N84.1
  choanal J33.0
  cholesterol K82.4
  clitoris N84.3
  colon K63.5
    adenomatous D12.6
    ascending D12.2
    cecum D12.0
    descending D12.4
    inflammatory K51.40
      with
        abscess K51.414
        complication K51.419
          specified NEC K51.418
        fistula K51.413
        intestinal obstruction K51.412
        rectal bleeding K51.411
    sigmoid D12.5
    transverse D12.3
  corpus uteri N84.0
  dental K04.01
    irreversible K04.02
    reversible K04.01
  duodenum K31.7

Polyp, polypus — continued
ear (middle) H74.4-
endometrium N84.0
ethmoidal (sinus) J33.8
fallopian tube N84.8
female genital tract N84.9
  specified NEC N84.8
frontal (sinus) J33.8
gallbladder K82.4
gingiva, gum K06.8
labia, labium (majus) (minus) N84.3
larynx (mucous) J38.1
  adenomatous D14.1
malignant — see Neoplasm, malignant, by site
maxillary (sinus) J33.8
middle ear — see Polyp, ear (middle)
myometrium N84.0
nares
  anterior J33.9
  posterior J33.0
nasal (mucous) J33.9
  cavity J33.0
  septum J33.0
nasopharyngeal J33.0
nose (mucous) J33.9
oviduct N84.8
pharynx J39.2
placenta O90.89
prostate — see Enlargement, enlarged, prostate
pudenda, pudendum N84.3
pulpal (dental) K04.01
  irreversible K04.02
  reversible K04.01
rectum (nonadenomatous) K62.1
  adenomatous — see Polyp, adenomatous
septum (nasal) J33.0
sinus (accessory) (ethmoidal) (frontal) (maxillary) (sphenoidal) J33.8
sphenoidal (sinus) J33.8
stomach K31.7
  adenomatous D13.1
tube, fallopian N84.8
turbinate, mucous membrane J33.8
umbilical, newborn P83.6
ureter N28.89
urethra N36.2
uterus (body) (corpus) (mucous) N84.0
  cervix N84.1
  in pregnancy or childbirth — see Pregnancy, complicated by, tumor, uterus
vagina N84.2
vocal cord (mucous) J38.1
vulva N84.3
Polyphagia R63.2
Polyploidy Q92.7
Polypoid — see condition
Polyposis — see also Polyp
coli (adenomatous) D12.6
  adenocarcinoma in C18.9
  adenocarcinoma in situ in — see Neoplasm, in situ, by site
  carcinoma in C18.9
colon (adenomatous) D12.6
familial D12.6
  adenocarcinoma in situ in — see Neoplasm, in situ, by site
intestinal (adenomatous) D12.6
malignant lymphomatous C83.1-
multiple, adenomatous (see also Neoplasm, benign) D36.9
Polyradiculitis — see Polyneuropathy
Polyradiculoneuropathy (acute) (postinfective) (segmentally demyelinating) G61.0
Polyserositis
due to pericarditis I31.1
pericardial I31.1
periodic, familial E85.0

Polyserositis — continued
tuberculous A19.9
  acute A19.1
  chronic A19.8
Polysplenia syndrome Q89.09
Polysyndactyly (see also Syndactylism, syndactyly) Q70.4
Polytrichia L68.3
Polyunguia Q84.6
Polyuria R35.8
nocturnal R35.1
psychogenic F45.8
Pompe's disease (glycogen storage) E74.02
Pompholyx L30.1
Poncet's disease (tuberculous rheumatism) A18.09
Pond fracture — see Fracture, skull
Ponos B55.0
Pons, pontine — see condition
Poor
aesthetic of existing restoration of tooth K08.56
contractions, labor O62.2
gingival margin to tooth restoration K08.51
personal hygiene R46.0
prenatal care, affecting management of pregnancy — see Pregnancy, complicated by, insufficient, prenatal care
sucking reflex (newborn) R29.2
urinary stream R39.12
vision NEC H54.7
Poradenitis, nostras inguinalis or venerea A55
Porencephaly (congenital) (developmental) (true) Q04.6
acquired G93.0
nondevelopmental G93.0
traumatic (post) F07.89
Porocephaliasis B88.8
Porokeratosis Q82.8
Poroma, eccrine — see Neoplasm, skin, benign
Porphyria (South African) E80.20
acquired E80.20
acute intermittent (hepatic) (Swedish) E80.21
cutanea tarda (hereditary) (symptomatic) E80.1
due to drugs E80.20
  correct substance properly administered — see Table of Drugs and Chemicals, by drug, adverse effect
  overdose or wrong substance given or taken — see Table of Drugs and Chemicals, by drug, poisoning
erythropoietic (congenital) (hereditary) E80.0
hepatocutaneous type E80.1
secondary E80.20
toxic NEC E80.20
variegata E80.20
Porphyrinuria — see Porphyria
Porphyruria — see Porphyria
Port wine nevus, mark, or stain Q82.5
Portal — see condition
Posadas-Wernicke disease B38.9
Positive
culture (nonspecific)
  blood R78.81
  bronchial washings R84.5
  cerebrospinal fluid R83.5
  cervix uteri R87.5
  nasal secretions R84.5
  nipple discharge R89.5
  nose R84.5
    staphylococcus (methicillin susceptible) Z22.321
     methicillin resistant Z22.322
  peritoneal fluid R85.5
  pleural fluid R84.5
  prostatic secretions R86.5
  saliva R85.5

Positive — continued
culture (nonspecific) — continued
  seminal fluid R86.5
  sputum R84.5
  synovial fluid R89.5
  throat scrapings R84.5
  urine R82.79
  vagina R87.5
  vulva R87.5
  wound secretions R89.5
PPD (skin test) R76.11
serology for syphilis A53.0
  with signs or symptoms — code as Syphilis, by site and stage
  false R76.8
skin test, tuberculin (without active tuberculosis) R76.11
test, human immunodeficiency virus (HIV) R75
VDRL A53.0
  with signs or symptoms — code by site and stage under Syphilis A53.9
Wassermann reaction A53.0
Postcardiotomy syndrome I97.0
Postcaval ureter Q62.62
Postcholecystectomy syndrome K91.5
Postclimacteric bleeding N95.0
Postcommissurotomy syndrome I97.0
Postconcussional syndrome F07.81
Postcontusional syndrome F07.81
Postcricoid region — see condition
Post-dates (40-42 weeks) (pregnancy) (mother) O48.0
more than 42 weeks gestation O48.1
Postencephalitic syndrome F07.89
Posterior — see condition
Posterolateral sclerosis (spinal cord) — see Degeneration, combined
Postexanthematous — see condition
Postfebrile — see condition
Postgastrectomy dumping syndrome K91.1
Posthemiplegic chorea — see Monoplegia
Posthemorrhagic anemia (chronic) D50.0
acute D62
newborn P61.3
Postherpetic neuralgia (zoster) B02.29
trigeminal B02.22
Posthitis N47.7
Postimmunization complication or reaction — see Complications, vaccination
Postinfectious — see condition
Postlaminectomy syndrome NEC M96.1
Postleukotomy syndrome F07.0
Postmastectomy lymphedema (syndrome) I97.2
Postmaturity, postmature (over 42 weeks)
maternal (over 42 weeks gestation) O48.1
newborn P08.22
Postmeasles complication NEC (see also condition) B05.89
Postmenopausal
endometrium (atrophic) N95.8
  suppurative (see also Endometritis) N71.9
osteoporosis — see Osteoporosis, postmenopausal
Postnasal drip R09.82
due to
  allergic rhinitis — see Rhinitis, allergic
  common cold J00
  gastroesophageal reflux — see Reflux, gastroesophageal
  nasopharyngitis — see Nasopharyngitis
  other know condition — code to condition
  sinusitis — see Sinusitis
Postnatal — see condition
Postoperative (postprocedural) — see Complication, postoperative
pneumothorax, therapeutic Z98.3
state NEC Z98.890

Postpancreatectomy hyperglycemia E89.1
Postpartum — see Puerperal
Postphlebitic syndrome — see Syndrome, postthrombotic
Postpolio (myelitic) syndrome G14
Postpoliomyelitic — see also condition
  osteopathy — see Osteopathy, after poliomyelitis
Postprocedural — see also Postoperative
  hypoinsulinemia E89.1
Postschizophrenic depression F32.89
Postsurgery status — see also Status (post)
  pneumothorax, therapeutic Z98.3
Post-term (40-42 weeks) (pregnancy) (mother) O48.0
  infant P08.21
  more than 42 weeks gestation (mother) O48.1
Post-traumatic brain syndrome, nonpsychotic F07.81
Post-typhoid abscess A01.09
Postures, hysterical F44.2
Postvaccinal reaction or complication — see Complications, vaccination
Postvalvulotomy syndrome I97.0
Potain's
  disease (pulmonary edema) — see Edema, lung
  syndrome (gastrectasis with dyspepsia) K31.0
Potter's
  asthma J62.8
  facies Q60.6
  lung J62.8
  syndrome (with renal agenesis) Q60.6
Pott's
  curvature (spinal) A18.01
  disease or paraplegia A18.01
  spinal curvature A18.01
  tumor, puffy — see Osteomyelitis, specified type NEC
Pouch
  bronchus Q32.4
  Douglas' — see condition
  esophagus, esophageal, congenital Q39.6
    acquired K22.5
  gastric K31.4
  Hartmann's K82.8
  pharynx, pharyngeal (congenital) Q38.7
Pouchitis K91.850
Poultrymen's itch B88.0
Poverty NEC Z59.6
  extreme Z59.5
Poxvirus NEC B08.8
Prader-Willi syndrome Q87.1
Preauricular appendage or tag Q17.0
Prebetalipoproteinemia (acquired) (essential) (familial) (hereditary) (primary) (secondary) E78.1
  with chylomicronemia E78.3
Precipitate labor or delivery O62.3
Preclimacteric bleeding (menorrhagia) N92.4
Precocious
  adrenarche E30.1
  menarche E30.1
  menstruation E30.1
  pubarche E30.1
  puberty E30.1
    central E22.8
  sexual development NEC E30.1
  thelarche E30.8
Precocity, sexual (constitutional) (cryptogenic) (female) (idiopathic) (male) E30.1
  with adrenal hyperplasia E25.9
    congenital E25.0
Precordial pain R07.2
Predeciduous teeth K00.2

Prediabetes, prediabetic R73.03
  complicating
    pregnancy — see Pregnancy, complicated by, diseases of, specified type or system NEC
    puerperium O99.89
Predislocation status of hip at birth Q65.6
Pre-eclampsia O14.9-
  with pre-existing hypertension — see Hypertension, complicating pregnancy, pre-existing, with, pre-eclampsia
  complicating
    childbirth O14.94
    puerperium O14.95
  mild O14.0-
    complicating
      childbirth O14.04
      puerperium O14.05
  moderate O14.0-
    complicating
      childbirth O14.04
      puerperium O14.05
  severe O14.1-
    with hemolysis, elevated liver enzymes and low platelet count (HELLP) O14.2-
    complicating
      childbirth O14.24
      puerperium O14.25
    complicating
      childbirth O14.14
      puerperium O14.15
Pre-eruptive color change, teeth, tooth K00.8
Pre-excitation atrioventricular conduction I45.6
Pre-glaucoma H40.00-
Pregnancy (childbirth) (labor) (puerperium) — see also Delivery and Puerperal
Note — The tabular must be reviewed for assignment of the appropriate character indicating the trimester of the pregnancy
Note — The tabular must be reviewed for assignment of the appropriate seventh character for multiple gestation codes in Chapter 15
  abdominal (ectopic) O00.00
    with intrauterine pregnancy O00.01
    with viable fetus O36.7-
  ampullar O00.10
    with intrauterine pregnancy O00.11
  biochemical O02.81
  broad ligament O00.80
    with intrauterine pregnancy O00.81
  cervical O00.80
    with intrauterine pregnancy O00.81
  chemical O02.81
  complicated by (care of) (management affected by)
    abnormal, abnormality
      cervix O34.4-
        causing obstructed labor O65.5
      cord (umbilical) O69.9
      findings on antenatal screening of mother O28.9
        biochemical O28.1
        chromosomal O28.5
        cytological O28.2
        genetic O28.5
        hematological O28.0
        radiological O28.4
        specified NEC O28.8
        ultrasonic O28.3
      glucose (tolerance) NEC O99.810
      pelvic organs O34.9-
        specified NEC O34.8-
          causing obstructed labor O65.5
      pelvis (bony) (major) NEC O33.0
      perineum O34.7-

Pregnancy (childbirth) (labor) (puerperium) (see also Delivery and Puerperal) — continued
  complicated by (care of) (management affected by) — continued
    abnormal, abnormality — continued
      position
        placenta O44.0-
          with hemorrhage O44.1-
        uterus O34.59-
      uterus O34.59-
        causing obstructed labor O65.5
        congenital O34.0-
      vagina O34.6-
        causing obstructed labor O65.5
      vulva O34.7-
        causing obstructed labor O65.5
    abruptio placentae — see Abruptio placentae
    abscess or cellulitis
      bladder O23.1-
      breast O91.11-
      genital organ or tract O23.9-
    abuse
      physical O9A.31- *(follows O99)*
      psychological O9A.51- *(follows O99)*
      sexual O9A.41- *(follows O99)*
    adverse effect anesthesia O29.9-
      aspiration pneumonitis O29.01-
      cardiac arrest O29.11-
      cardiac complication NEC O29.19-
      cardiac failure O29.12-
      central nervous system complication NEC O29.29-
      cerebral anoxia O29.21-
      failed or difficult intubation O29.6-
      inhalation of stomach contents or secretions NOS O29.01-
      local, toxic reaction O29.3x
      Mendelson's syndrome O29.01-
      pressure collapse of lung O29.02-
      pulmonary complications NEC O29.09-
      specified NEC O29.8x-
      spinal and epidural type NEC O29.5x
        induced headache O29.4-
    albuminuria (see also Proteinuria, gestational) O12.1-
    alcohol use O99.31-
    amnionitis O41.12-
    anaphylactoid syndrome of pregnancy O88.01-
    anemia (conditions in D50-D64) (pre-existing) O99.01-
      complicating the puerperium O99.03
    antepartum hemorrhage O46.9-
      with coagulation defect — see Hemorrhage, antepartum, with coagulation defect
      specified NEC O46.8x-
    appendicitis O99.61-
    atrophy (yellow) (acute) liver (subacute) O26.61-
    bariatric surgery status O99.84-
    bicornis or bicornuate uterus O34.0-
    biliary tract problems O26.61-
    breech presentation O32.1
    cardiovascular diseases (conditions in I00-I09, I20-I52, I70-I99) O99.41-
    cerebrovascular disorders (conditions in I60-I69) O99.41-
    cervical shortening O26.87-
    cervicitis O23.51-
    chloasma (gravidarum) O26.89-
    cholecystitis O99.61-
    cholestasis (intrahepatic) O26.61-
    chorioamnionitis O41.12-
    circulatory system disorder (conditions in I00-I09, I20-I99) O99.41-
    compound presentation O32.6
    conjoined twins O30.02-

DISEASE INDEX

Pregnancy (childbirth) (labor) (puerperium) (*see also* Delivery and Puerperal) — *continued*
complicated by (care of) (management affected by) — *continued*
connective system disorders (conditions in M00-M99) O99.89
contracted pelvis (general) O33.1
  inlet O33.2
  outlet O33.3
convulsions (eclamptic) (uremic) (*see also* Eclampsia) O15.9-
cracked nipple O92.11-
cystitis O23.1-
cystocele O34.8-
death of fetus (near term) O36.4
  early pregnancy O02.1
  of one fetus or more in multiple gestation O31.2-
deciduitis O41.14-
decreased fetal movement O36.81-
dental problems O99.61-
diabetes (mellitus) O24.91-
  gestational (pregnancy induced) — *see* Diabetes, gestational
  pre-existing O24.31-
    specified NEC O24.81-
    type 1 O24.01-
    type 2 O24.11-
digestive system disorders (conditions in K00-K93) O99.61-
diseases of — *see* Pregnancy, complicated by, specified body system disease
  biliary tract O26.61-
  blood NEC (conditions in D65-D77) O99.11-
  liver O26.61-
  specified NEC O99.89
disorders of — *see* Pregnancy, complicated by, specified body system disorder
  amniotic fluid and membranes O41.9-
    specified NEC O41.8x-
  biliary tract O26.61-
  ear and mastoid process (conditions in H60-H95) O99.89
  eye and adnexa (conditions in H00-H59) O99.89
  liver O26.61-
  skin (conditions in L00-L99) O99.71-
  specified NEC O99.89
displacement, uterus NEC O34.59-
  causing obstructed labor O65.5
disproportion (due to) O33.9
  fetal (ascites) (hydrops) (meningomyelocele) (sacral teratoma) (tumor) deformities NEC O33.7
  generally contracted pelvis O33.1
  hydrocephalic fetus O33.6
  inlet contraction of pelvis O33.2
  mixed maternal and fetal origin O33.4
  specified NEC O33.8
double uterus O34.0-
  causing obstructed labor O65.5
drug use (conditions in F11-F19) O99.32-
eclampsia, eclamptic (coma) (convulsions) (delirium) (nephritis) (uremia) (*see also* Eclampsia) O15-
ectopic pregnancy — *see* Pregnancy, ectopic
edema O12.0-
  with
    gestational hypertension, mild (*see also* Pre-eclampsia) O14.0-
    proteinuria O12.2-
effusion, amniotic fluid — *see* Pregnancy, complicated by, premature rupture of membranes
elderly
  multigravida O09.52-
  primigravida O09.51-

Pregnancy (childbirth) (labor) (puerperium) (*see also* Delivery and Puerperal) — *continued*
complicated by (care of) (management affected by) — *continued*
embolism (*see also* Embolism, obstetric, pregnancy) O88.-
endocrine diseases NEC O99.28-
endometritis O86.12
excessive weight gain O26.0-
exhaustion O26.81-
  during labor and delivery O75.81
face presentation O32.3
failed induction of labor O61.9
  instrumental O61.1
  mechanical O61.1
  medical O61.0
  specified NEC O61.8
  surgical O61.1
failed or difficult intubation for anesthesia O29.6-
false labor (pains) O47.9
  at or after 37 completed weeks of pregnancy O47.1
  before 37 completed weeks of pregnancy O47.0-
fatigue O26.81-
  during labor and delivery O75.81
fatty metamorphosis of liver O26.61-
female genital mutilation O34.8- *[N90.8-]*
fetal (maternal care for)
  abnormality or damage O35.9
    acid-base balance O68
    specified type NEC O35.8
  acidemia O68
  acidosis O68
  alkalosis O68
  anemia and thrombocytopenia O36.82-
  anencephaly O35.0
  chromosomal abnormality (conditions in Q90-Q99) O35.1
  conjoined twins O30.02-
  damage from
    amniocentesis O35.7
    biopsy procedures O35.7
    drug addiction O35.5
    hematological investigation O35.7
    intrauterine contraceptive device O35.7
    maternal
      alcohol addiction O35.4
      cytomegalovirus infection O35.3
      disease NEC O35.8
      drug addiction O35.5
      listeriosis O35.8
      rubella O35.3
      toxoplasmosis O35.8
      viral infection O35.3
    medical procedure NEC O35.7
    radiation O35.6
  death (near term) O36.4
    early pregnancy O02.1
  decreased movement O36.81-
  disproportion due to deformity (fetal) O33.7
  excessive growth (large for dates) O36.6-
  growth retardation O36.59-
    light for dates O36.59-
    small for dates O36.59-
  heart rate irregularity (bradycardia) (decelerations) (tachycardia) O76
  hereditary disease O35.2
  hydrocephalus O35.0
  intrauterine death O36.4
  poor growth O36.59-
    light for dates O36.59-
    small for dates O36.59-
  problem O36.9-
    specified NEC O36.89-
  reduction (elective) O31.3-
  selective termination O31.3-

Pregnancy (childbirth) (labor) (puerperium) (*see also* Delivery and Puerperal) — *continued*
complicated by (care of) (management affected by) — *continued*
fetal (maternal care for) — *continued*
  spina bifida O35.0
  thrombocytopenia O36.82-
fibroid (tumor) (uterus) O34.1-
fissure of nipple O92.11-
gallstones O99.61-
gastric banding status O99.84-
gastric bypass status O99.84-
genital herpes (asymptomatic) (history of) (inactive) O98.51-
genital tract infection O23.9-
glomerular diseases (conditions in N00-N07) O26.83-
  with hypertension, pre-existing — *see* Hypertension, complicating, pregnancy, pre-existing, with, renal disease
gonorrhea O98.21-
grand multiparity O09.4
habitual aborter — *see* Pregnancy, complicated by, recurrent pregnancy loss
HELLP syndrome (hemolysis, elevated liver enzymes and low platelet count) O14.2-
hemorrhage
  antepartum — *see* Hemorrhage, antepartum
  before 20 completed weeks gestation O20.9
    specified NEC O20.8
  due to premature separation, placenta (*see also* Abruptio placentae) O45.9-
  early O20.9
    specified NEC O20.8
  threatened abortion O20.0
hemorrhoids O22.4-
hepatitis (viral) O98.41-
herniation of uterus O34.59-
high
  head at term O32.4
  risk — *see* Supervision (of) (for), high-risk
history of in utero procedure during previous pregnancy O09.82-
HIV O98.71-
human immunodeficiency virus (HIV) disease O98.71-
hydatidiform mole (*see also* Mole, hydatidiform) O01.9-
hydramnios O40-
hydrocephalic fetus (disproportion) O33.6
hydrops
  amnii O40-
  fetalis O36.2-
    associated with isoimmunization (*see also* Pregnancy, complicated by, isoimmunization) O36.11-
hydrorrhea O42.90
hyperemesis (gravidarum) (mild) (*see also* Hyperemesis, gravidarum) O21.0-
hypertension — *see* Hypertension, complicating pregnancy
hypertensive
  heart and renal disease, pre-existing — *see* Hypertension, complicating, pregnancy, pre-existing, with, heart disease,with renal disease
  heart disease, pre-existing — *see* Hypertension, complicating, pregnancy, pre-existing, with, heart disease
  renal disease, pre-existing — *see* Hypertension, complicating, pregnancy, pre-existing, with, renal disease
hypotension O26.5-

Pregnancy (childbirth) (labor) (puerperium) (*see also* Delivery and Puerperal) — *continued*
complicated by (care of) (management affected by) — *continued*
immune disorders NEC (conditions in D80-D89) O99.11-
incarceration, uterus O34.51-
incompetent cervix O34.3-
inconclusive fetal viability O36.80
infection(s) O98.91-
  amniotic fluid or sac O41.10-
  bladder O23.1-
  carrier state NEC O99.830
    streptococcus B O99.820
  genital organ or tract O23.9-
    specified NEC O23.59-
  genitourinary tract O23.9-
  gonorrhea O98.21-
  hepatitis (viral) O98.41-
  HIV O98.71-
  human immunodeficiency virus (HIV) O98.71-
  kidney O23.0-
  nipple O91.01-
  parasitic disease O98.91-
    specified NEC O98.81-
  protozoal disease O98.61-
  sexually transmitted NEC O98.31-
  specified type NEC O98.81-
  syphilis O98.11-
  tuberculosis O98.01-
  urethra O23.2-
  urinary (tract) O23.4-
    specified NEC O23.3-
  viral disease O98.51-
injury or poisoning (conditions in S00-T88) O9A.21- *(follows O99)*
  due to abuse
    physical O9A.31- *(follows O99)*
    psychological O9A.51- *(follows O99)*
    sexual O9A.41- *(follows O99)*
insufficient
  prenatal care O09.3-
  weight gain O26.1-
insulin resistance O26.89-
intrauterine fetal death (near term) O36.4
  early pregnancy O02.1
  multiple gestation (one fetus or more) O31.2-
isoimmunization O36.11-
  anti-A sensitization O36.11-
  anti-B sensitization O36.19-
  Rh O36.09-
    anti-D antibody O36.01-
    specified NEC O36.19-
laceration of uterus NEC O71.81
malformation
  placenta, placental (vessel) O43.10-
    specified NEC O43.19-
  uterus (congenital) O34.0-
malnutrition (conditions in E40-E46) O25.1-
maternal hypotension syndrome O26.5-
mental disorders (conditions in F01-F09, F20-F99) O99.34-
  alcohol use O99.31-
  drug use O99.32-
  smoking O99.33-
mentum presentation O32.3
metabolic disorders O99.28-
missed
  abortion O02.1
  delivery O36.4
multiple gestations O30.9-
  conjoined twins O30.02-
  quadruplet — *see* Pregnancy, quadruplet
  specified complication NEC O31.8x-
  specified number of multiples NEC — *see* Pregnancy, multiple (gestation), specified NEC

Pregnancy (childbirth) (labor) (puerperium) (*see also* Delivery and Puerperal) — *continued*
complicated by (care of) (management affected by) — *continued*
multiple gestations O30.9- — *continued*
  triplet — *see* Pregnancy, triplet
  twin — *see* Pregnancy, twin
musculoskeletal condition (conditions is M00-M99) O99.89
necrosis, liver (conditions in K72) O26.61-
neoplasm
  benign
    cervix O34.4-
    corpus uteri O34.1-
    uterus O34.1-
  malignant O9A.11- *(follows O99)*
nephropathy NEC O26.83-
nervous system condition (conditions in G00-G99) O99.35-
nutritional diseases NEC O99.28-
obesity (pre-existing) O99.21-
obesity surgery status O99.84-
oblique lie or presentation O32.2
older mother — *see* Pregnancy, complicated by, elderly
oligohydramnios O41.0-
  with premature rupture of membranes (*see also* Pregnancy, complicated by, premature rupture of membranes) O42-
onset (spontaneous) of labor after 37 completed weeks of gestation but before 39 completed weeks gestation, with delivery by (planned) cesarean section O75.82
oophoritis O23.52-
overdose, drug (*see also* Table of Drugs and Chemicals, by drug, poisoning) O9A.21- *(follows O99)*
oversize fetus O33.5
papyraceous fetus O31.0-
pelvic inflammatory disease O99.89
periodontal disease O99.61-
peripheral neuritis O26.82-
peritoneal (pelvic) adhesions O99.89
phlebitis O22.9-
phlebopathy O22.9-
phlebothrombosis (superficial) O22.2-
  deep O22.3-
placenta accreta O43.21-
placenta increta O43.22-
placenta percreta O43.23-
placenta previa O44.0-
  complete O44.0-
    with hemorrhage O44.1-
  marginal O44.2-
    with hemorrhage O44.3-
  partial O44.2-
    with hemorrhage O44.3-
placental disorder O43.9-
  specified NEC O43.89-
placental dysfunction O43.89-
placental infarction O43.81-
placental insufficiency O36.51-
placental transfusion syndromes
  fetomaternal O43.01-
  fetus to fetus O43.02-
  maternofetal O43.01-
placentitis O41.14-
pneumonia O99.51-
poisoning (*see also* Table of Drugs and Chemicals) O9A.21- *(follows O99)*
polyhydramnios O40-
polymorphic eruption of pregnancy O26.86
poor obstetric history NEC O09.29-
postmaturity (post-term) (40 to 42 weeks) O48.0
  more than 42 completed weeks gestation (prolonged) O48.1

Pregnancy (childbirth) (labor) (puerperium) (*see also* Delivery and Puerperal) — *continued*
complicated by (care of) (management affected by) — *continued*
pre-eclampsia O14.9-
  mild O14.0-
  moderate O14.0-
  severe O14.1-
    with hemolysis, elevated liver enzymes and low platelet count (HELLP) O14.2-
premature labor — *see* Pregnancy, complicated by, preterm labor
premature rupture of membranes O42.90
  with onset of labor
    after 24 hours O42.10
      at or after 37 weeks gestation, onset of labor more than 24 hours following rupture O42.12
      pre-term (before 37 completed weeks of gestation) O42.11-
    within 24 hours O42.00
      at or after 37 weeks gestation, onset of labor within 24 hours of rupture O42.02
      pre-term (before 37 completed weeks of gestation) O42.01-
  at or after 37 weeks gestation, unspecified as to length of time between rupture and onset of labor O42.92
  full-term, unspecified as to length of time between rupture and onset of labor O42.92
  pre-term (before 37 completed weeks of gestation) O42.91-
premature separation of placenta (*see also* Abruptio placentae) O45.9-
presentation, fetal — *see* Delivery, complicated by, malposition
preterm delivery O60.10
preterm labor
  with delivery O60.10
    preterm O60.10
    term O60.20
  without delivery O60.00
    second trimester O60.02
    third trimester O60.03
  second trimester
    with preterm delivery
      second trimester O60.12
      third trimester O60.13
    with term delivery O60.22
    without delivery O60.02
  third trimester
    with term delivery O60.23
    with third trimester preterm delivery O60.14
    without delivery O60.03
previous history of — *see* Pregnancy, supervision of, high-risk
prolapse, uterus O34.52-
proteinuria (gestational) (*see also* Proteinuria, gestational) O12.1-
  with edema O12.2-
pruritic urticarial papules and plaques of pregnancy (PUPPP) O26.86
pruritus (neurogenic) O26.89-
psychosis or psychoneurosis (puerperal) F53
ptyalism O26.89-
PUPPP (pruritic urticarial papules and plaques of pregnancy) O26.86
pyelitis O23.0-
recurrent pregnancy loss O26.2-
renal disease or failure NEC O26.83-
  with secondary hypertension, pre-existing — *see* Hypertension, complicating, pregnancy, pre-existing, secondary

DISEASE INDEX

Pregnancy (childbirth) (labor) (puerperium) (*see also* Delivery and Puerperal) — *continued*
complicated by (care of) (management affected by) — *continued*
  renal disease or failure NEC O26.83- — *continued*
    hypertensive, pre-existing — *see* Hypertension, complicating, pregnancy, pre-existing, with, renal disease
  respiratory condition (conditions in J00-J99) O99.51-
  retained, retention
    dead ovum O02.0
    intrauterine contraceptive device O26.3-
  retroversion, uterus O34.53-
  Rh immunization, incompatibility or sensitization NEC O36.09-
    anti-D antibody O36.01-
  rupture
    amnion (premature) (*see also* Pregnancy, complicated by, premature rupture of membranes) O42-
    membranes (premature) (*see also* Pregnancy, complicated by, premature rupture of membranes) O42-
    uterus (during labor) O71.1
      before onset of labor O71.0-
  salivation (excessive) O26.89-
  salpingitis O23.52-
  salpingo-oophoritis O23.52-
  sepsis (conditions in A40, A41) O98.81-
  size date discrepancy (uterine) O26.84-
  skin condition (conditions in L00-L99) O99.71-
  smoking (tobacco) O99.33-
  social problem O09.7-
  specified condition NEC O26.89-
  spotting O26.85-
  streptococcus group B (GBS) carrier state O99.820
  subluxation of symphysis (pubis) O26.71-
  syphilis (conditions in A50-A53) O98.11-
  threatened
    abortion O20.0
    labor O47.9
      at or after 37 completed weeks of gestation O47.1
      before 37 completed weeks of gestation O47.0-
  thrombophlebitis (superficial) O22.2-
  thrombosis O22.9-
    cerebral venous O22.5-
    cerebrovenous sinus O22.5-
    deep O22.3-
  tobacco use disorder (smoking) O99.33-
  torsion of uterus O34.59-
  toxemia O14.9-
  transverse lie or presentation O32.2
  tuberculosis (conditions in A15-A19) O98.01-
  tumor (benign)
    cervix O34.4-
    malignant O9A.11- *(follows O99)*
    uterus O34.1-
  unstable lie O32.0
  upper respiratory infection O99.51-
  urethritis O23.2-
  uterine size date discrepancy O26.84-
  vaginitis or vulvitis O23.59-
  varicose veins (lower extremities) O22.0-
    genitals O22.1-
    legs O22.0-
    perineal O22.1-
    vaginal or vulval O22.1-
  venereal disease NEC (conditions in A63.8) O98.31-
  venous disorders O22.9-
    specified NEC O22.8x-

Pregnancy (childbirth) (labor) (puerperium) (*see also* Delivery and Puerperal) — *continued*
complicated by (care of) (management affected by) — *continued*
  very young mother — *see* Pregnancy, complicated by, young mother
  viral diseases (conditions in A80-B09, B25-B34) O98.51-
  vomiting O21.9
    due to diseases classified elsewhere O21.8
    hyperemesis gravidarum (mild) (*see also* Hyperemesis, gravidarum) O21.0-
    late (occurring after 20 weeks of gestation) O21.2
  young mother
    multigravida O09.62-
    primigravida O09.61-
complicated NOS O26.9-
concealed O09.3-
continuing following
  elective fetal reduction of one or more fetus O31.3-
  intrauterine death of one or more fetus O31.2-
  spontaneous abortion of one or more fetus O31.1-
cornual O00.80
  with intrauterine pregnancy O00.81
ectopic (ruptured) O00.90
  with intrauterine pregnancy O00.91
  abdominal O00.00
    with
      intrauterine pregnancy O00.01
      viable fetus O36.7-
  cervical O00.80
    with intrauterine pregnancy O00.81
  complicated (by) O08.9
    afibrinogenemia O08.1
    cardiac arrest O08.81
    chemical damage of pelvic organ(s) O08.6
    circulatory collapse O08.3
    defibrination syndrome O08.1
    electrolyte imbalance O08.5
    embolism (amniotic fluid) (blood clot) (pulmonary) (septic) O08.2
    endometritis O08.0
    genital tract and pelvic infection O08.0
    hemorrhage (delayed) (excessive) O08.1
    infection
      genital tract or pelvic O08.0
      kidney O08.83
      urinary tract O08.83
    intravascular coagulation O08.1
    laceration of pelvic organ(s) O08.6
    metabolic disorder O08.5
    oliguria O08.4
    oophoritis O08.0
    parametritis O08.0
    pelvic peritonitis O08.0
    perforation of pelvic organ(s) O08.6
    renal failure or shutdown O08.4
    salpingitis or salpingo-oophoritis O08.0
    sepsis O08.82
    shock O08.83
      septic O08.82
    specified condition NEC O08.89
    tubular necrosis (renal) O08.4
    uremia O08.4
    urinary infection O08.83
    venous complication NEC O08.7
      embolism O08.2
  cornual O00.80
    with intrauterine pregnancy O00.81
  intraligamentous O00.80
    with intrauterine pregnancy O00.81
  mural O00.80
    with intrauterine pregnancy O00.81

Pregnancy (childbirth) (labor) (puerperium) (*see also* Delivery and Puerperal) — *continued*
ectopic (ruptured) O00.90 — *continued*
  ovarian O00.20
    with intrauterine pregnancy O00.21
  specified site NEC O00.80
    with intrauterine pregnancy O00.81
  tubal (ruptured) O00.10
    with intrauterine pregnancy O00.11
examination (normal) Z34.9-
  first Z34.0-
  high-risk — *see* Pregnancy, supervision of, high-risk
  specified Z34.8-
extrauterine — *see* Pregnancy, ectopic
fallopian O00.10
  with intrauterine pregnancy O00.11
false F45.8
gestational carrier Z33.3
hidden O09.3-
high-risk — *see* Pregnancy, supervision of, high-risk
incidental finding Z33.1
interstitial O00.80
  with intrauterine pregnancy O00.81
intraligamentous O00.80
  with intrauterine pregnancy O00.81
intramural O00.80
  with intrauterine pregnancy O00.81
intraperitoneal O00.00
  with intrauterine pregnancy O00.01
isthmian O00.10
  with intrauterine pregnancy O00.11
mesometric (mural) O00.80
  with intrauterine pregnancy O00.81
molar NEC O02.0
  complicated (by) O08.9
    afibrinogenemia O08.1
    cardiac arrest O08.81
    chemical damage of pelvic organ(s) O08.6
    circulatory collapse O08.3
    defibrination syndrome O08.1
    electrolyte imbalance O08.5
    embolism (amniotic fluid) (blood clot) (pulmonary) (septic) O08.2
    endometritis O08.0
    genital tract and pelvic infection O08.0
    hemorrhage (delayed) (excessive) O08.1
    infection
      genital tract or pelvic O08.0
      kidney O08.83
      urinary tract O08.83
    intravascular coagulation O08.1
    laceration of pelvic organ(s) O08.6
    metabolic disorder O08.5
    oliguria O08.4
    oophoritis O08.0
    parametritis O08.0
    pelvic peritonitis O08.0
    perforation of pelvic organ(s) O08.6
    renal failure or shutdown O08.4
    salpingitis or salpingo-oophoritis O08.0
    sepsis O08.82
    shock O08.3
      septic O08.82
    specified condition NEC O08.89
    tubular necrosis (renal) O08.4
    uremia O08.4
    urinary infection O08.83
    venous complication NEC O08.7
      embolism O08.2
  hydatidiform (*see also* Mole, hydatidiform) O01.9-
multiple (gestation) O30.9-
  greater than quadruplets — *see* Pregnancy, multiple (gestation), specified NEC

Pregnancy (childbirth) (labor) (puerperium) (*see also* Delivery and Puerperal) — *continued*
multiple (gestation) O30.9- — *continued*
  specified NEC O30.80-
    with
      two or more monoamniotic fetuses O30.82-
      two or more monochorionic fetuses O30.81-
    two or more monoamniotic fetuses O30.82-
    two or more monochorionic fetuses O30.81-
    unable to determine number of placenta and number of amniotic sacs O30.89-
    unspecified number of placenta and unspecified number of amniotic sacs O30.80-
  mural O00.80
    with intrauterine pregnancy O00.81
  normal (supervision of) Z34.9-
    first Z34.0-
    high-risk — *see* Pregnancy, supervision of, high-risk
    specified Z34.8-
  ovarian O00.20
    with intrauterine pregnancy O00.21
  postmature (40 to 42 weeks) O48.0
    more than 42 weeks gestation O48.1
  post-term (40 to 42 weeks) O48.0
  prenatal care only Z34.9-
    first Z34.0-
    high-risk — *see* Pregnancy, supervision of, high-risk
    specified Z34.8-
  prolonged (more than 42 weeks gestation) O48.1
  quadruplet O30.20-
    with
      two or more monoamniotic fetuses O30.22-
      two or more monochorionic fetuses O30.21-
    two or more monoamniotic fetuses O30.22-
    two or more monochorionic fetuses O30.21-
    unable to determine number of placenta and number of amniotic sacs O30.29-
    unspecified number of placenta and unspecified number of amniotic sacs O30.20-
  quintuplet — *see* Pregnancy, multiple (gestation), specified NEC
  sextuplet — *see* Pregnancy, multiple (gestation), specified NEC
  supervision of
    concealed pregnancy O09.3-
    elderly mother
      multigravida O09.52-
      primigravida O09.51-
    hidden pregnancy O09.3-
    high-risk O09.9-
      due to (history of)
        ectopic pregnancy O09.1-
        elderly — *see* Pregnancy, supervision of, elderly mother
        grand multiparity O09.4
        in utero procedure during previous pregnancy O09.82-
        in vitro fertilization O09.81-
        infertility O09.0-
        insufficient prenatal care O09.3-
        molar pregnancy O09.A- *(follows O09.1)*
        multiple previous pregnancies O09.4-
        older mother — *see* Pregnancy, supervision of, elderly mother
        poor reproductive or obstetric history NEC O09.29-
        pre-term labor O09.21-

Pregnancy (childbirth) (labor) (puerperium) (*see also* Delivery and Puerperal) — *continued*
supervision of — *continued*
  high-risk O09.9- — *continued*
    due to (history of) — *continued*
      previous
        neonatal death O09.29-
        social problems O09.7-
      specified NEC O09.89-
      very young mother — *see* Pregnancy, supervision of, young mother
    resulting from in vitro fertilization O09.81-
  normal Z34.9-
    first Z34.0-
    specified NEC Z34.8-
  young mother
    multigravida O09.62-
    primigravida O09.61-
  triplet O30.10-
    with
      two or more monoamniotic fetuses O30.12-
      two or more monochrorionic fetuses O30.11-
    two or more monoamniotic fetuses O30.12-
    two or more monochrorionic fetuses O30.11-
    unable to determine number of placenta and number of amniotic sacs O30.19-
    unspecified number of placenta and unspecified number of amniotic sacs O30.10-
  tubal (with abortion) (with rupture) O00.10
    with intrauterine pregnancy O00.11
  twin O30.00-
    conjoined O30.02-
    dichorionic/diamniotic (two placenta, two amniotic sacs) O30.04-
    monochorionic/diamniotic (one placenta, two amniotic sacs) O30.03-
    monochorionic/monoamniotic (one placenta, one amniotic sac) O30.01-
    unable to determine number of placenta and number of amniotic sacs O30.09-
    unspecified number of placenta and unspecified number of amniotic sacs O30.00-
  unwanted Z64.0
  weeks of gestation
    8 weeks Z3A.08 *(follows Z36)*
    9 weeks Z3A.09 *(follows Z36)*
    10 weeks Z3A.10 *(follows Z36)*
    11 weeks Z3A.11 *(follows Z36)*
    12 weeks Z3A.12 *(follows Z36)*
    13 weeks Z3A.13 *(follows Z36)*
    14 weeks Z3A.14 *(follows Z36)*
    15 weeks Z3A.15 *(follows Z36)*
    16 weeks Z3A.16 *(follows Z36)*
    17 weeks Z3A.17 *(follows Z36)*
    18 weeks Z3A.18 *(follows Z36)*
    19 weeks Z3A.19 *(follows Z36)*
    20 weeks Z3A.20 *(follows Z36)*
    21 weeks Z3A.21 *(follows Z36)*
    22 weeks Z3A.22 *(follows Z36)*
    23 weeks Z3A.23 *(follows Z36)*
    24 weeks Z3A.24 *(follows Z36)*
    25 weeks Z3A.25 *(follows Z36)*
    26 weeks Z3A.26 *(follows Z36)*
    27 weeks Z3A.27 *(follows Z36)*
    28 weeks Z3A.28 *(follows Z36)*
    29 weeks Z3A.29 *(follows Z36)*
    30 weeks Z3A.30 *(follows Z36)*
    31 weeks Z3A.31 *(follows Z36)*
    32 weeks Z3A.32 *(follows Z36)*
    33 weeks Z3A.33 *(follows Z36)*
    34 weeks Z3A.34 *(follows Z36)*
    35 weeks Z3A.35 *(follows Z36)*
    36 weeks Z3A.36 *(follows Z36)*
    37 weeks Z3A.37 *(follows Z36)*

Pregnancy (childbirth) (labor) (puerperium) (*see also* Delivery and Puerperal) — *continued*
weeks of gestation — *continued*
  38 weeks Z3A.38 *(follows Z36)*
  39 weeks Z3A.39 *(follows Z36)*
  40 weeks Z3A.40 *(follows Z36)*
  41 weeks Z3A.41 *(follows Z36)*
  42 weeks Z3A.42 *(follows Z36)*
  greater than 42 weeks Z3A.49 *(follows Z36)*
  less than 8 weeks Z3A.01 *(follows Z36)*
  not specified Z3A.00 *(follows Z36)*
Preiser's disease — *see* Osteonecrosis, secondary, due to, trauma, metacarpus
Pre-kwashiorkor — *see* Malnutrition, severe
Preleukemia (syndrome) D46.9
Preluxation, hip, congenital Q65.6
Premature — *see also* condition
  adrenarche E27.0
  aging E34.8
  beats I49.40
    atrial I49.1
    auricular I49.1
    supraventricular I49.1
  birth NEC — *see* Preterm, newborn
  closure, foramen ovale Q21.8
  contraction
    atrial I49.1
    atrioventricular I49.2
    auricular I49.1
    auriculoventricular I49.49
    heart (extrasystole) I49.49
    junctional I49.2
    ventricular I49.3
  delivery (*see also* Pregnancy, complicated by, preterm labor) O60.10
  ejaculation F52.4
  infant NEC — *see* Preterm, newborn
    light-for-dates — *see* Light for dates
  labor — *see* Pregnancy, complicated by, preterm labor
  lungs P28.0
  menopause E28.319
    asymptomatic E28.319
    symptomatic E28.310
  newborn
    extreme (less than 28 completed weeks) — *see* Immaturity, extreme
    less than 37 completed weeks — *see* Preterm, newborn
  puberty E30.1
  rupture membranes or amnion — *see* Pregnancy, complicated by, premature rupture of membranes
  senility E34.8
  thelarche E30.8
  ventricular systole I49.3
Prematurity NEC (less than 37 completed weeks) — *see* Preterm, newborn
  extreme (less than 28 completed weeks) — *see* Immaturity, extreme
Premenstrual
  dysphoric disorder (PMDD) F32.81
  tension (syndrome) N94.3
Premolarization, cuspids K00.2
Prenatal
  care, normal pregnancy — *see* Pregnancy, normal
  screening of mother Z36
  teeth K00.6
Preparatory care for subsequent treatment NEC
  for dialysis Z49.01
    peritoneal Z49.02
Prepartum — *see* condition
Preponderance, left or right ventricular I51.7
Prepuce — *see* condition
PRES (posterior reversible encephalopathy syndrome) I67.83

Preterm — *continued*
  newborn (infant) P07.30 — *continued*
    gestational age — *continued*
      32 completed weeks (32 weeks, 0 days
        through 32 weeks, 6 days) P07.35
      33 completed weeks (33 weeks, 0 days
        through 33 weeks, 6 days) P07.36
      34 completed weeks (34 weeks, 0 days
        through 34 weeks, 6 days) P07.37
      35 completed weeks (35 weeks, 0 days
        through 35 weeks, 6 days) P07.38
      36 completed weeks (36 weeks, 0 days
        through 36 weeks, 6 days) P07.39
Previa
  placenta (total) (with hemorrhage) O44.0-
    with hemorrhage O44.1-
    complete O44.0-
      with hemorrhage O44.1-
    low (see also Delivery, complicated, by,
      placenta, low) O44.4-
      with hemorrhage O44.5-
    marginal O44.2-
      with hemorrhage O44.3-
    partial O44.2-
      with hemorrhage O44.3-
  vasa O69.4
Priapism N48.30
  due to
    disease classified elsewhere N48.32
    drug N48.33
    specified cause NEC N48.39
    trauma N48.31
Prickling sensation (skin) R20.2
Prickly heat L74.0
Primary — *see* condition
Primigravida
  elderly, affecting management of pregnancy,
    labor and delivery (supervision only) —
    see Pregnancy, complicated by, elderly,
    primigravida
  older, affecting management of pregnancy,
    labor and delivery (supervision only) —
    see Pregnancy, complicated by, elderly,
    primigravida
  very young, affecting management of
    pregnancy, labor and delivery
    (supervision only) — *see* Pregnancy,
    complicated by, young mother,
    primigravida
Primipara
  elderly, affecting management of pregnancy,
    labor and delivery (supervision only) —
    see Pregnancy, complicated by, elderly,
    primigravida
  older, affecting management of pregnancy,
    labor and delivery (supervision only) —
    see Pregnancy, complicated by, elderly,
    primigravida
  very young, affecting management of
    pregnancy, labor and delivery
    (supervision only) — *see* Pregnancy,
    complicated by, young mother,
    primigravida
Primus varus (bilateral) Q66.2
PRIND (prolonged reversible ischemic
  neurologic deficit) I63.9
Pringle's disease (tuberous sclerosis) Q85.1
Prinzmetal angina I20.1
Prizefighter ear — *see* Cauliflower ear
Problem (with) (related to)
  academic Z55.8
  acculturation Z60.3
  adjustment (to)
    change of job Z56.1
    life-cycle transition Z60.0
    pension Z60.0
    retirement Z60.0
  adopted child Z62.821
  alcoholism in family Z63.72

Problem (with) (related to) — *continued*
  atypical parenting situation Z62.9
  bankruptcy Z59.8
  behavioral (adult) F69
    drug seeking Z76.5
  birth of sibling affecting child Z62.898
  care (of)
    provider dependency Z74.9
      specified NEC Z74.8
    sick or handicapped person in family or
      household Z63.6
  child
    abuse (affecting the child) — *see*
      Maltreatment, child
    custody or support proceedings Z65.3
    in care of non-parental family member
      Z62.21
    in foster care Z62.21
    in welfare custody Z62.21
    living in orphanage or group home Z62.22
  child-rearing Z62.9
    specified NEC Z62.898
  communication (developmental) F80.9
  conflict or discord (with)
    boss Z56.4
    classmates Z55.4
    counselor Z64.4
    employer Z56.4
    family Z63.9
      specified NEC Z63.8
    probation officer Z64.4
    social worker Z64.4
    teachers Z55.4
    workmates Z56.4
  conviction in legal proceedings Z65.0
    with imprisonment Z65.1
  counselor Z64.4
  creditors Z59.8
  digestive K92.9
  drug addict in family Z63.72
  ear — *see* Disorder, ear
  economic Z59.9
    affecting care Z59.9
    specified NEC Z59.8
  education Z55.9
    specified NEC Z55.8
  employment Z56.9
    change of job Z56.1
    discord Z56.4
    environment Z56.5
    sexual harassment Z56.81
    specified NEC Z56.89
    stress NEC Z56.6
    stressful schedule Z56.3
    threat of job loss Z56.2
    unemployment Z56.0
  enuresis, child F98.0
  eye H57.9
  failed examinations (school) Z55.2
  falling Z91.81
  family (*see also* Disruption, family) Z63.9-
    specified NEC Z63.8
  feeding (elderly) (infant) R63.3
    newborn P92.9
      breast P92.5
      overfeeding P92.4
      slow P92.2
      specified NEC P92.8
      underfeeding P92.3
    nonorganic F50.89
  finance Z59.9
    specified NEC Z59.8
  foreclosure on loan Z59.8
  foster child Z62.822
  frightening experience(s) in childhood
    Z62.898
  genital NEC
    female N94.9
    male N50.9

Problem (with) (related to) — *continued*
  health care Z75.9
    specified NEC Z75.8
  hearing — *see* Deafness
  homelessness Z59.0
  housing Z59.9
    inadequate Z59.1
    isolated Z59.8
    specified NEC Z59.8
  identity (of childhood) F93.8
  illegitimate pregnancy (unwanted) Z64.0
  illiteracy Z55.0
  impaired mobility Z74.09
  imprisonment or incarceration Z65.1
  inadequate teaching affecting education Z55.8
  inappropriate (excessive) parental pressure
    Z62.6
  influencing health status NEC Z78.9
  in-law Z63.1
  institutionalization, affecting child Z62.22
  intrafamilial communication Z63.8
  jealousy, child F93.8
  landlord Z59.2
  language (developmental) F80.9
  learning (developmental) F81.9
  legal Z65.3
    conviction without imprisonment Z65.0
    imprisonment Z65.1
    release from prison Z65.2
  life-management Z73.9
    specified NEC Z73.89
  life-style Z72.9
    gambling Z72.6
    high-risk sexual behavior (heterosexual)
      Z72.51
      bisexual Z72.53
      homosexual Z72.52
    inappropriate eating habits Z72.4
    self-damaging behavior NEC Z72.89
    specified NEC Z72.89
    tobacco use Z72.0
  literacy Z55.9
    low level Z55.0
    specified NEC Z55.8
  living alone Z60.2
  lodgers Z59.2
  loss of love relationship in childhood Z62.898
  marital Z63.0
    involving
      divorce Z63.5
      estrangement Z63.5
      gender identity F66
  mastication K08.89
  medical
    care, within family Z63.6
    facilities Z75.9
      specified NEC Z75.8
  mental F48.9
  multiparity Z64.1
  negative life events in childhood Z62.9
    altered pattern of family relationships
      Z62.898
    frightening experience Z62.898
    loss of
      love relationship Z62.898
      self-esteem Z62.898
    physical abuse (alleged) — *see*
      Maltreatment, child
    removal from home Z62.29
    specified event NEC Z62.898
  neighbor Z59.2
  neurological NEC R29.818
  new step-parent affecting child Z62.898
  none (feared complaint unfounded) Z71.1
  occupational NEC Z56.89
  parent-child — *see* Conflict, parent-child
  personal hygiene Z91.89
  personality F69
  phase-of-life transition, adjustment Z60.0

Problem (with) (related to) — *continued*
  presence of sick or disabled person in family
     or household Z63.79
    needing care Z63.6
  primary support group (family) Z63.9
    specified NEC Z63.8
  probation officer Z64.4
  psychiatric F99
  psychosexual (development) F66
  psychosocial Z65.9
    specified NEC Z65.8
  relationship Z63.9
    childhood F93.8
  release from prison Z65.2
  removal from home affecting child Z62.29
  seeking and accepting known hazardous and
    harmful
     behavioral or psychological interventions
      Z65.8
     chemical, nutritional or physical
      interventions Z65.8
  sexual function (nonorganic) F52.9
  sight H54.7
  sleep disorder, child F51.9
  smell — *see* Disturbance, sensation, smell
  social
    environment Z60.9
     specified NEC Z60.8
    exclusion and rejection Z60.4
    worker Z64.4
  speech R47.9
    developmental F80.9
    specified NEC R47.89
  swallowing — *see* Dysphagia
  taste — *see* Disturbance, sensation, taste
  tic, child F95.0
  underachievement in school Z55.3
  unemployment Z56.0
    threatened Z56.2
  unwanted pregnancy Z64.0
  upbringing Z62.9
    specified NEC Z62.898
  urinary N39.9
  voice production R47.89
  work schedule (stressful) Z56.3
Procedure (surgical)
  converted
    arthroscopic to open Z53.33
    laparoscopic to open Z53.31
    specified procedure NEC to open Z53.39
    thoracoscopic to open Z53.32
  for purpose other than remedying health state
    Z41.9
    specified NEC Z41.8
  not done Z53.9
    because of
     administrative reasons Z53.8
     contraindication Z53.09
      smoking Z53.01
     patient's decision Z53.20
      for reasons of belief or group pressure
       Z53.1
      left against medical advice (AMA)
       Z53.21
      specified reason NEC Z53.29
     specified reason NEC Z53.8
Procidentia (uteri) N81.3
Proctalgia K62.89
  fugax K59.4
  spasmodic K59.4
Proctitis K62.89
  amebic (acute) A06.0
  chlamydial A56.3
  gonococcal A54.6
  granulomatous — *see* Enteritis, regional, large
    intestine
  herpetic A60.1
  radiation K62.7
  tuberculous A18.32

Proctitis K62.89 — *continued*
  ulcerative (chronic) K51.20
    with
     complication K51.219
      abscess K51.214
      fistula K51.213
      obstruction K51.212
      rectal bleeding K51.211
      specified NEC K51.218
Proctocele
  female (without uterine prolapse) N81.6
    with uterine prolapse N81.2
     complete N81.3
  male K62.3
Proctocolitis
  food-induced eosinophilic K52.82
  food protein-induced K52.82
  milk protein-induced K52.82
  mucosal — *see* Rectosigmoiditis, ulcerative
Proctocolitis, mucosal — *see*
  Rectosigmoiditis, ulcerative
Proctoptosis K62.3
Proctorrhagia K62.5
Proctosigmoiditis K63.89
  ulcerative (chronic) — *see* Rectosigmoiditis,
    ulcerative
Proctospasm K59.4
  psychogenic F45.8
Profichet's disease — *see* Disorder, soft
  tissue, specified type NEC
Progeria E34.8
Prognathism (mandibular) (maxillary)
  M26.19
Progonoma (melanotic) — *see* Neoplasm,
  benign, by site
Progressive — *see* condition
Prolactinoma
  specified site — *see* Neoplasm, benign, by site
  unspecified site D35.2
Prolapse, prolapsed
  anus, anal (canal) (sphincter) K62.2
  arm or hand O32.2
    causing obstructed labor O64.4
  bladder (mucosa) (sphincter) (acquired)
    congenital Q79.4
    female — *see* Cystocele
    male N32.89
  breast implant (prosthetic) T85.49
  cecostomy K94.09
  cecum K63.4
  cervix, cervical (hypertrophied) N81.2
    anterior lip, obstructing labor O65.5
    congenital Q51.828
    postpartal, old N81.2
    stump N81.85
  ciliary body (traumatic) — *see* Laceration,
    eye(ball), with prolapse or loss of
    interocular tissue
  colon (pedunculated) K63.4
  colostomy K94.09
  disc (intervertebral) — *see* Displacement,
    intervertebral disc
  eye implant (orbital) T85.398
    lens (ocular) — *see* Complications,
     intraocular lens
  fallopian tube N83.4-
  gastric (mucosa) K31.89
  genital, female N81.9
    specified NEC N81.89
  globe, nontraumatic — *see* Luxation, globe
  ileostomy bud K94.19
  intervertebral disc — *see* Displacement,
    intervertebral disc
  intestine (small) K63.4
  iris (traumatic) — *see* Laceration, eye(ball),
    with prolapse or loss of interocular tissue
    nontraumatic H21.89
  kidney N28.83
    congenital Q63.2

Prolapse, prolapsed — *continued*
  laryngeal muscles or ventricle J38.7
  liver K76.89
  meatus urinarius N36.8
  mitral (valve) I34.1
  ocular lens implant — *see* Complications,
    intraocular lens
  organ or site, congenital NEC — *see*
    Malposition, congenital
  ovary N83.4-
  pelvic floor, female N81.89
  perineum, female N81.89
  rectum (mucosa) (sphincter) K62.3
    due to trichuris trichuria B79
  spleen D73.89
  stomach K31.89
  umbilical cord
    complicating delivery O69.0
  urachus, congenital Q64.4
  ureter N28.89
    with obstruction N13.5
     with infection N13.6
  ureterovesical orifice N28.89
  urethra (acquired) (infected) (mucosa) N36.8
    congenital Q64.71
  urinary meatus N36.8
    congenital Q64.72
  uterovaginal N81.4
    complete N81.3
    incomplete N81.2
  uterus (with prolapse of vagina) N81.4
    complete N81.3
    congenital Q51.818
    first degree N81.2
    in pregnancy or childbirth — *see* Pregnancy,
     complicated by, abnormal, uterus
    incomplete N81.2
    postpartal (old) N81.4
    second degree N81.2
    third degree N81.3
  uveal (traumatic) — *see* Laceration, eye(ball),
    with prolapse or loss of interocular tissue
  vagina (anterior) (wall) — *see* Cystocele
    with prolapse of uterus N81.4
     complete N81.3
     incomplete N81.2
    posterior wall N81.6
    posthysterectomy N99.3
  vitreous (humor) H43.0-
    in wound — *see* Laceration, eye(ball), with
     prolapse or loss of interocular tissue
  womb — *see* Prolapse, uterus
Prolapsus, female N81.9
  specified NEC N81.89
Proliferation(s)
  primary cutaneous CD30-positive large T-cell
    C86.6
  prostate, atypical small acinar N42.32
Proliferative — *see* condition
Prolonged, prolongation (of)
  bleeding (time) (idiopathic) R79.1
  coagulation (time) R79.1
  gestation (over 42 completed weeks)
    mother O48.1
    newborn P08.22
  interval I44.0
  labor O63.9
    first stage O63.0
    second stage O63.1
  partial thromboplastin time (PTT) R79.1
  pregnancy (more than 42 weeks gestation)
    O48.1
  prothrombin time R79.1
  QT interval I45.81
  uterine contractions in labor O62.4

Prominence, prominent
with disproportion (fetopelvic) O33.0
causing obstructed labor O65.0
auricle (congenital) (ear) Q17.5
ischial spine or sacral promontory
nose (congenital) acquired M95.0
Promiscuity — *see* High, risk, sexual behavior
Pronation
ankle — *see* Deformity, limb, foot, specified NEC
foot — *see also* Deformity, limb, foot, specified NEC
congenital Q74.2
Prophylactic
administration of
antibiotics, long-term Z79.2
short-term use — *omit code*
drug (*see also* Long-term (current) drug therapy (use of)) Z79.899-
medication Z79.899
organ removal (for neoplasia management) Z40.00
breast Z40.01
ovary Z40.02
specified site NEC Z40.09
surgery Z40.9
for risk factors related to malignant neoplasm — *see* Prophylactic, organ removal
specified NEC Z40.8
vaccination Z23
Propionic acidemia E71.121
Proptosis (ocular) — *see also* Exophthalmos
thyroid — *see* Hyperthyroidism, with goiter
Prosecution, anxiety concerning Z65.3
Prosopagnosia R48.3
Prostadynia N42.81
Prostate, prostatic — *see* condition
Prostatism — *see* Hyperplasia, prostate
Prostatitis (congestive) (suppurative) (with cystitis) N41.9
acute N41.0
cavitary N41.8
chronic N41.1
diverticular N41.8
due to Trichomonas (vaginalis) A59.02
fibrous N41.1
gonococcal (acute) (chronic) A54.22
granulomatous N41.4
hypertrophic N41.1
subacute N41.1
trichomonal A59.02
tuberculous A18.14
Prostatocystitis N41.3
Prostatorrhea N42.89
Prostatosis N42.82
Prostration R53.83
heat — *see also* Heat, exhaustion
anhydrotic T67.3
due to
salt (and water) depletion T67.4
water depletion T67.3
nervous F48.8
senile R54
Protanomaly (anomalous trichromat) H53.54
Protanopia (complete) (incomplete) H53.54
Protection (against) (from) — *see* Prophylactic
Protein
deficiency NEC — *see* Malnutrition
malnutrition — *see* Malnutrition
sickness (*see also* Reaction, serum) T80.69
Proteinemia R77.9
Proteinosis
alveolar (pulmonary) J84.01
lipid or lipoid (of Urbach) E78.89
Proteinuria R80.9
Bence Jones R80.3
complicating pregnancy — *see* Proteinuria, gestational

Proteinuria R80.9 — *continued*
gestational
complicating
childbirth O12.14
pregnancy O12.1-
with edema O12.2-
puerperium O12.15
idiopathic R80.0
isolated R80.0
with glomerular lesion N06.9
dense deposit disease N06.6
diffuse
crescentic glomerulonephritis N06.7
endocapillary proliferative glomerulonephritis N06.4
mesangiocapillary glomerulonephritis N06.5
focal and segmental hyalinosis or sclerosis N06.1
membranous (diffuse) N06.2
mesangial proliferative (diffuse) N06.3
minimal change N06.0
specified pathology NEC N06.8
orthostatic R80.2
with glomerular lesion — *see* Proteinuria, isolated, with glomerular lesion
persistent R80.1
with glomerular lesion — *see* Proteinuria, isolated, with glomerular lesion
postural R80.2
with glomerular lesion — *see* Proteinuria, isolated, with glomerular lesion
pre-eclamptic — *see* Pre-eclampsia
puerperal O12.15
specified type NEC R80.8
Proteolysis, pathologic D65
Proteus (mirabilis) (morganii), as cause of disease classified elsewhere B96.4
Prothrombin gene mutation D68.52
Protoporphyria, erythropoietic E80.0
Protozoal — *see also* condition
disease B64
specified NEC B60.8
Protrusion, protrusio
acetabuli M24.7
acetabulum (into pelvis) M24.7
device, implant or graft (*see also* Complications, by site and type, mechanical) T85.698
arterial graft NEC — *see* Complication, cardiovascular device, mechanical, vascular
breast (implant) T85.49
catheter NEC T85.698
cystostomy T83.090
dialysis (renal) T82.49
intraperitoneal T85.691
infusion NEC T82.594
spinal (epidural) (subdural) T85.690
urinary (*see also* Complications, catheter, urinary) T83.098
electronic (electrode) (pulse generator) (stimulator)
bone T84.390
nervous system — *see* Complication, prosthetic device, mechanical, electronic nervous system stimulator
fixation, internal (orthopedic) NEC — *see* Complication, fixation device, mechanical
gastrointestinal — *see* Complications, prosthetic device, mechanical, gastrointestinal device
genital NEC T83.498
intrauterine contraceptive device T83.39
penile prosthesis (cylinder) (implanted) (pump) (resevoir) T83.490
testicular prosthesis T83.491

Protrusion, protrusio — *continued*
heart NEC — *see* Complication, cardiovascular device, mechanical
joint prosthesis — *see* Complications, joint prosthesis, mechanical, specified NEC, by site
ocular NEC — *see* Complications, prosthetic device, mechanical, ocular device
orthopedic NEC — *see* Complication, orthopedic, device, mechanical
specified NEC T85.628
urinary NEC — *see also* Complication, genitourinary, device, urinary, mechanical
graft T83.29
vascular NEC — *see* Complication, cardiovascular device, mechanical
ventricular intracranial shunt T85.09
intervertebral disc — *see* Displacement, intervertebral disc
joint prosthesis — *see* Complications, joint prosthesis, mechanical, specified NEC, by site
nucleus pulposus — *see* Displacement, intervertebral disc
Prune belly (syndrome) Q79.4
Prurigo (ferox) (gravis) (Hebrae) (Hebra's) (mitis) (simplex) L28.2
Besnier's L20.0
estivalis L56.4
nodularis L28.1
psychogenic F45.8
Pruritus, pruritic (essential) L29.9
ani, anus L29.0
psychogenic F45.8
anogenital L29.3
psychogenic F45.8
due to onchocerca volvulus B73.1
gravidarum — *see* Pregnancy, complicated by, specified pregnancy-related condition NEC
hiemalis L29.8
neurogenic (any site) F45.8
perianal L29.0
psychogenic (any site) F45.8
scroti, scrotum L29.1
psychogenic F45.8
senile, senilis L29.8
specified NEC L29.8
psychogenic F45.8
Trichomonas A59.9
vulva, vulvae L29.2
psychogenic F45.8
Pseudarthrosis, pseudoarthrosis (bone) — *see* Nonunion, fracture
clavicle, congenital Q74.0
joint, following fusion or arthrodesis M96.0
Pseudoaneurysm — *see* Aneurysm
Pseudoangina (pectoris) — *see* Angina
Pseudoangioma I81
Pseudoarteriosus Q28.8
Pseudoarthrosis — *see* Pseudarthrosis
Pseudobulbar affect (PBA) F48.2
Pseudochromhidrosis L67.8
Pseudocirrhosis, liver, pericardial I31.1
Pseudocowpox B08.03
Pseudocoxalgia M91.3-
Pseudocroup J38.5
Pseudo-Cushing's syndrome, alcohol-induced E24.4
Pseudocyesis F45.8
Pseudocyst
lung J98.4
pancreas K86.3
retina — *see* Cyst, retina
Pseudoelephantiasis neuroarthritica Q82.0
Pseudoexfoliation, capsule (lens) — *see* Cataract, specified NEC

DISEASE INDEX

Pseudofolliculitis barbae L73.1
Pseudoglioma H44.89
Pseudohemophilia (Bernuth's) (hereditary)
 (type B) D68.0
 Type A D69.8
 vascular D69.8
Pseudohermaphroditism Q56.3
 adrenal E25.8
 female Q56.2
  with adrenocortical disorder E25.8
  without adrenocortical disorder Q56.2
  adrenal (congenital) E25.0
 male Q56.1
  with
   5-alpha-reductase deficiency E29.1
   adrenocortical disorder E25.8
   androgen resistance E34.51
   cleft scrotum Q56.1
   feminizing testis E34.51
  without gonadal disorder Q56.1
  adrenal E25.8
Pseudo-Hurler's polydystrophy E77.0
Pseudohydrocephalus G93.2
Pseudohypertrophic muscular dystrophy
 (Erb's) G71.0
Pseudohypertrophy, muscle G71.0
Pseudohypoparathyroidism E20.1
Pseudoinsomnia F51.03
Pseudoleukemia, infantile D64.89
Pseudo-obstruction intestine (acute)
 (chronic) (idiopathic) (intermittent secondary)
 (primary) K59.8
Pseudomembranous — see condition
Pseudomeningocele (cerebral) (infective)
 (post-traumatic) G96.19
 postprocedural (spinal) G97.82
Pseudomenses (newborn) P54.6
Pseudomenstruation (newborn) P54.6
Pseudomonas
 aeruginosa, as cause of disease classified
  elsewhere B96.5
 mallei infection A24.0
  as cause of disease classified elsewhere
   B96.5
 pseudomallei, as cause of disease classified
  elsewhere B96.5
Pseudomyotonia G71.19
Pseudomyxoma peritonei C78.6
Pseudoneuritis, optic (nerve) (disc) (papilla),
 congenital Q14.2
Pseudopapilledema H47.33-
 congenital Q14.2
Pseudoparalysis
 arm or leg R29.818
 atonic, congenital P94.2
Pseudopelade L66.0
Pseudophakia Z96.1
Pseudopolyarthritis, rhizomelic M35.3
Pseudopolycythemia D75.1
Pseudopseudohypoparathyroidism E20.1
Pseudopterygium H11.81-
Pseudoptosis (eyelid) — see Blepharochalasis
Pseudopuberty, precocious
 female heterosexual E25.8
 male isosexual E25.8
Pseudorickets (renal) N25.0
Pseudorubella B08.20
Pseudosclerema, newborn P83.8
Pseudosclerosis (brain)
 Jakob's — see Creutzfeldt-Jakob disease or
  syndrome
 of Westphal (Strümpell) E83.01
 spastic — see Creutzfeldt-Jakob disease or
  syndrome
Pseudotetanus — see Convulsions
Pseudotetany R29.0
 hysterical F44.5
Pseudotruncus arteriosus Q25.49

Pseudotuberculosis A28.2
 enterocolitis A04.8
 pasteurella (infection) A28.0
Pseudotumor
 cerebri G93.2
 orbital H05.11-
Pseudoxanthoma elasticum Q82.8
Psilosis (sprue) (tropical) K90.1
 nontropical K90.0
Psittacosis A70
Psoitis M60.88
Psoriasis L40.9
 arthropathic L40.50
  arthritis mutilans L40.52
  distal interphalangeal L40.51
  juvenile L40.54
  other specified L40.59
  spondylitis L40.53
 buccal K13.29
 flexural L40.8
 guttate L40.4
 mouth K13.29
 nummular L40.0
 plaque L40.0
 psychogenic F54
 pustular (generalized) L40.1
  palmaris et plantaris L40.3
 specified NEC L40.8
 vulgaris L40.0
Psychasthenia F48.8
Psychiatric disorder or problem F99
Psychogenic — see also condition
 factors associated with physical conditions F54
**Psychological and behavioral factors
 affecting medical condition** F59
Psychoneurosis, psychoneurotic — see also
 Neurosis
 anxiety (state) F41.1
 depersonalization F48.1
 hypochondriacal F45.21
 hysteria F44.9
 neurasthenic F48.8
 personality NEC F60.89
Psychopathy, psychopathic
 affectionless F94.2
 autistic F84.5
 constitution, post-traumatic F07.81
 personality — see Disorder, personality
 sexual — see Deviation, sexual
 state F60.2
**Psychosexual identity disorder of
 childhood** F64.2
Psychosis, psychotic F29
 acute (transient) F23
  hysterical F44.9
 affective — see Disorder, mood
 alcoholic F10.959
  with
   abuse F10.159
   anxiety disorder F10.980
    with
     abuse F10.180
     dependence F10.280
   delirium tremens F10.231
   delusions F10.950
    with
     abuse F10.150
     dependence F10.250
   dementia F10.97
    with dependence F10.27
   dependence F10.259
   hallucinosis F10.951
    with
     abuse F10.151
     dependence F10.251
   mood disorder F10.94
    with
     abuse F10.14
     dependence F10.24

Psychosis, psychotic F29 — continued
 alcoholic F10.959 — continued
  with — continued
   paranoia F10.950
    with
     abuse F10.150
     dependence F10.250
   persisting amnesia F10.96
    with dependence F10.26
   amnestic confabulatory F10.96
    with dependence F10.26
   delirium tremens F10.231
   Korsakoff's, Korsakov's, Korsakow's F10.26
   paranoid type F10.950
    with
     abuse F10.150
     dependence F10.250
 anergastic — see Psychosis, organic
 arteriosclerotic (simple type) (uncomplicated)
  F01.50
  with behavioral disturbance F01.51
 childhood F84.0
  atypical F84.8
 climacteric — see Psychosis, involutional
 confusional F29
  acute or subacute F05
  reactive F23
 cycloid F23
 depressive — see Disorder, depressive
 disintegrative (childhood) F84.3
 drug-induced — see F11-F19 with .x59
  paranoid and hallucinatory states — see
   F11-F19 with .x50 or .x51
 due to or associated with
  addiction, drug — see F11-F19 with .x59
  dependence
   alcohol F10.259
   drug — see F11-F19 with .x59
  epilepsy F06.8
  Huntington's chorea F06.8
  ischemia, cerebrovascular (generalized)
   F06.8
  multiple sclerosis F06.8
  physical disease F06.8
  presenile dementia F03
  senile dementia F03
  vascular disease (arteriosclerotic) (cerebral)
   F01.50
   with behavioral disturbance F01.51
 epileptic F06.8
 episode F23
  due to or associated with physical condition
   F06.8
 exhaustive F43.0
 hallucinatory, chronic F28
 hypomanic F30.8
 hysterical (acute) F44.9
 induced F24
 infantile F84.0
  atypical F84.8
 infective (acute) (subacute) F05
 involutional F28
  depressive — see Disorder, depressive
  melancholic — see Disorder, depressive
  paranoid (state) F22
 Korsakoff's, Korsakov's, Korsakow's
  (nonalcoholic) F04
  alcoholic F10.96
   in dependence F10.26
  induced by other psychoactive substance —
   see categories F11-F19 with .x5x
 mania, manic (single episode) F30.2
  recurrent type F31.89
 manic-depressive — see Disorder, bipolar
 menopausal — see Psychosis, involutional
 mixed schizophrenic and affective F25.8
 multi-infarct (cerebrovascular) F01.50
  with behavioral disturbance F01.51

Psychosis, psychotic F29 — *continued*
  nonorganic F29
    specified NEC F28
  organic F09
    due to or associated with
      arteriosclerosis (cerebral) — *see* Psychosis, arteriosclerotic
      cerebrovascular disease, arteriosclerotic — *see* Psychosis, arteriosclerotic
      childbirth — *see* Psychosis, puerperal
      Creutzfeldt-Jakob disease or syndrome — *see* Creutzfeldt-Jakob disease or syndrome
      dependence, alcohol F10.259
      disease
        alcoholic liver F10.259
        brain, arteriosclerotic — *see* Psychosis, arteriosclerotic
        cerebrovascular F01.50
          with behavioral disturbance F01.51
        Creutzfeldt-Jakob — *see* Creutzfeldt-Jakob disease or syndrome
        endocrine or metabolic F06.8
          acute or subacute F05
        liver, alcoholic F10.259
      epilepsy transient (acute) F05
      infection
        brain (intracranial) F06.8
          acute or subacute F05
      intoxication
        alcoholic (acute) F10.259
        drug F19 with .x59 F11-
      ischemia, cerebrovascular (generalized) — *see* Psychosis, arteriosclerotic
      puerperium — *see* Psychosis, puerperal
      trauma, brain (birth) (from electric current) (surgical) F06.8
        acute or subacute F05
    infective F06.8
      acute or subacute F05
    post-traumatic F06.8
      acute or subacute F05
  paranoiac F22
  paranoid (climacteric) (involutional) (menopausal) F22
  psychogenic (acute) F23
  schizophrenic F20.0
  senile F03
  postpartum F53
  presbyophrenic (type) F03
  presenile F03
  psychogenic (paranoid) F23
    depressive F32.3
  puerperal F53
    specified type — *see* Psychosis, by type
  reactive (brief) (transient) (emotional stress) (psychological trauma) F23
    depressive F32.3
      recurrent F33.3
    excitative type F30.8
  schizoaffective F25.9
    depressive type F25.1
    manic type F25.0
  schizophrenia, schizophrenic — *see* Schizophrenia
  schizophrenia-like, in epilepsy F06.2
  schizophreniform F20.81
    affective type F25.9
    brief F23
    confusional type F23
    depressive type F25.1
    manic type F25.0
    mixed type F25.0
  senile NEC F03
    depressed or paranoid type F03
    simple deterioration F03
    specified type — *code to* condition
  shared F24
  situational (reactive) F23

Psychosis, psychotic F29 — *continued*
  symbiotic (childhood) F84.3
  symptomatic F09
Psychosomatic — *see* Disorder, psychosomatic
Psychosyndrome, organic F07.9
Psychotic episode due to or associated with physical condition F06.8
Pterygium (eye) H11.00-
  amyloid H11.01-
  central H11.02-
  colli Q18.3
  double H11.03-
  peripheral
    progressive H11.05-
    stationary H11.04-
  recurrent H11.06-
Ptilosis (eyelid) — *see* Madarosis
Ptomaine (poisoning) — *see* Poisoning, food
Ptosis — *see also* Blepharoptosis
  adiposa (false) — *see* Blepharoptosis
  breast N64.81
  cecum K63.4
  colon K63.4
  congenital (eyelid) Q10.0
    specified site NEC — *see* Anomaly, by site
  eyelid — *see* Blepharoptosis
    congenital Q10.0
  gastric K31.89
  intestine K63.4
  kidney N28.83
  liver K76.89
  renal N28.83
  splanchnic K63.4
  spleen D73.89
  stomach K31.89
  viscera K63.4
PTP D69.51
Ptyalism (periodic) K11.7
  hysterical F45.8
  pregnancy — *see* Pregnancy, complicated by, specified pregnancy-related condition NEC
  psychogenic F45.8
Ptyalolithiasis K11.5
Pubarche, precocious E30.1
Pubertas praecox E30.1
Puberty (development state) Z00.3
  bleeding (excessive) N92.2
  delayed E30.0
  precocious (constitutional) (cryptogenic) (idiopathic) E30.1
    central E22.8
    due to
      ovarian hyperfunction E28.1
        estrogen E28.0
      testicular hyperfunction E29.0
  premature E30.1
    due to
      adrenal cortical hyperfunction E25.8
      pineal tumor E34.8
      pituitary (anterior) hyperfunction E22.8
Puckering, macula — *see* Degeneration, macula, puckering
Pudenda, pudendum — *see* condition
Puente's disease (simple glandular cheilitis) K13.0
Puerperal, puerperium (complicated by, complications)
  abnormal glucose (tolerance test) O99.815
  abscess
    areola O91.02
      associated with lactation O91.03
    Bartholin's gland O86.19
    breast O91.12
      associated with lactation O91.13
    cervix (uteri) O86.11
    genital organ NEC O86.19
    kidney O86.21

Puerperal, puerperium (complicated by, complications) — *continued*
  abscess — *continued*
    mammary O91.12
      associated with lactation O91.13
    nipple O91.02
      associated with lactation O91.03
    peritoneum O85
    subareolar O91.12
      associated with lactation O91.13
    urinary tract — *see* Puerperal, infection, urinary
    uterus O86.12
    vagina (wall) O86.13
    vaginorectal O86.13
    vulvovaginal gland O86.13
  adnexitis O86.19
  afibrinogenemia, or other coagulation defect O72.3
  albuminuria (acute) (subacute) — *see* Proteinuria, gestational
  alcohol use O99.315
  anemia O90.81
    pre-existing (pre-pregnancy) O99.03
  anesthetic death O89.8
  apoplexy O99.43
  bariatric surgery status O99.845
  blood disorder NEC O99.13
  blood dyscrasia O72.3
  cardiomyopathy O90.3
  cerebrovascular disorder (conditions in I60-I69) O99.43
  cervicitis O86.11
  circulatory system disorder O99.43
  coagulopathy (any) O72.3
  complications O90.9
    specified NEC O90.89
  convulsions — *see* Eclampsia
  cystitis O86.22
  cystopyelitis O86.29
  delirium NEC F05
  diabetes O24.93
    gestational — *see* Puerperal, gestational diabetes
    pre-existing O24.33
      specified NEC O24.83
      type 1 O24.03
      type 2 O24.13
  digestive system disorder O99.63
  disease O90.9
    breast NEC O92.29
    cerebrovascular (acute) O99.43
    nonobstetric NEC O99.89
    tubo-ovarian O86.19
    Valsuani's O99.03
  disorder O90.9
    biliary tract O26.63
    lactation O92.70
    liver O26.63
    nonobstetric NEC O99.89
  disruption
    cesarean wound O90.0
    episiotomy wound O90.1
    perineal laceration wound O90.1
  drug use O99.325
  eclampsia (with pre-existing hypertension) O15.2
  embolism (pulmonary) (blood clot) — *see* Embolism, obstetric, puerperal
  endocrine, nutritional or metabolic disease NEC O99.285
  endophlebitis — *see* Puerperal, phlebitis
  endotrachelitis O86.11
  failure
    lactation (complete) O92.3
      partial O92.4
    renal, acute O90.4
  fever (of unknown origin) O86.4
    septic O85

Puerperal, puerperium (complicated by, complications) — *continued*
fissure, nipple O92.12
  associated with lactation O92.13
fistula
  breast (due to mastitis) O91.12
    associated with lactation O91.13
  nipple O91.02
    associated with lactation O91.03
galactophoritis O91.22
  associated with lactation O91.23
galactorrhea O92.6
gastric banding status O99.845
gastric bypass status O99.845
gastrointestinal disease NEC O99.63
gestational
  diabetes O24.439
    diet controlled O24.430
    insulin (and diet) controlled O24.434
    oral drug controlled (antidiabetic) (hypoglycemic) O24.435
  edema O12.05
    with proteinuria O12.25
  proteinuria O12.15
gonorrhea O98.23
hematoma, subdural O99.43
hemiplegia, cerebral O99.355
  due to cerbrovascular disorder O99.43
hemorrhage O72.1
  brain O99.43
  bulbar O99.43
  cerebellar O99.43
  cerebral O99.43
  cortical O99.43
  delayed or secondary O72.2
  extradural O99.43
  internal capsule O99.43
  intracranial O99.43
  intrapontine O99.43
  meningeal O99.43
  pontine O99.43
  retained placenta O72.0
  subarachnoid O99.43
  subcortical O99.43
  subdural O99.43
  third stage O72.0
  uterine, delayed O72.2
  ventricular O99.43
hemorrhoids O87.2
hepatorenal syndrome O90.4
hypertension — *see* Hypertension, complicating, puerperium
hypertrophy, breast O92.29
induration breast (fibrous) O92.29
infection O86.4
  cervix O86.11
  generalized O85
  genital tract NEC O86.19
    obstetric surgical wound O86.0
  kidney (bacillus coli) O86.21
  maternal O98.93
    carrier state NEC O99.835
    gonorrhea O98.23
    human immunodeficiency virus (HIV) O98.73
    protozoal O98.63
    sexually transmitted NEC O98.33
    specified NEC O98.83
    streptococcus group B (GBS) carrier state O99.825
    syphilis O98.13
    tuberculosis O98.03
    viral hepatitis O98.43
    viral NEC O98.53
  nipple O91.02
    associated with lactation O91.03
  peritoneum O85
  renal O86.21
  specified NEC O86.89

Puerperal, puerperium (complicated by, complications) — *continued*
infection O86.4 — *continued*
  urinary (asymptomatic) (tract) NEC O86.20
    bladder O86.22
    kidney O86.21
    specified site NEC O86.29
    urethra O86.22
  vagina O86.13
  vein — *see* Puerperal, phlebitis
ischemia, cerebral O99.43
lymphangitis O86.89
  breast O91.22
    associated with lactation O91.23
malignancy O9A.13 *(follows O99)*
malnutrition O25.3
mammillitis O91.02
  associated with lactation O91.03
mammitis O91.22
  associated with lactation O91.23
mania F30.8
mastitis O91.22
  associated with lactation O91.23
  purulent O91.12
    associated with lactation O91.13
melancholia — *see* Disorder, depressive
mental disorder NEC O99.345
metroperitonitis O85
metrorrhagia — *see* Hemorrhage, postpartum
metrosalpingitis O86.19
metrovaginitis O86.13
milk leg O87.1
monoplegia, cerebral O99.43
mood disturbance O90.6
necrosis, liver (acute) (subacute) (conditions in subcategory K72.0) O26.63
  with renal failure O90.4
nervous system disorder O99.355
neuritis O90.89
obesity (pre-existing prior to pregnancy) O99.215
obesity surgery status O99.845
occlusion, precerebral artery O99.43
paralysis
  bladder (sphincter) O90.89
  cerebral O99.43
paralytic stroke O99.43
parametritis O85
paravaginitis O86.13
pelviperitonitis O85
perimetritis O86.12
perimetrosalpingitis O86.19
perinephritis O86.21
periphlebitis — *see* Puerperal phlebitis
peritoneal infection O85
peritonitis (pelvic) O85
perivaginitis O86.13
phlebitis O87.0
  deep O87.1
  pelvic O87.1
  superficial O87.0
phlebothrombosis, deep O87.1
phlegmasia alba dolens O87.1
placental polyp O90.89
pneumonia, embolic — *see* Embolism, obstetric, puerperal
pre-eclampsia — *see* Pre-eclampsia
psychosis F53
pyelitis O86.21
pyelocystitis O86.29
pyelonephritis O86.21
pyelonephrosis O86.21
pyemia O85
pyocystitis O86.29
pyohemia O85
pyometra O86.12
pyonephritis O86.21
pyosalpingitis O86.19
pyrexia (of unknown origin) O86.4

Puerperal, puerperium (complicated by, complications) — *continued*
renal
  disease NEC O90.89
  failure O90.4
respiratory disease NEC O99.53
retention
  decidua — *see* Retention, decidua
  placenta O72.0
  secundines — *see* Retention, secundines
retracted nipple O92.02
salpingo-ovaritis O86.19
salpingoperitonitis O85
secondary perineal tear O90.1
sepsis O85
sepsis (pelvic) O85
septic thrombophlebitis O86.81
skin disorder NEC O99.73
specified condition NEC O99.89
stroke O99.43
subinvolution (uterus) O90.89
subluxation of symphysis (pubis) O26.73
suppuration — *see* Puerperal, abscess
tetanus A34
thelitis O91.02
  associated with lactation O91.03
thrombocytopenia O72.3
thrombophlebitis (superficial) O87.0
  deep O87.1
  pelvic O87.1
  septic O86.81
thrombosis (venous) — *see* Thrombosis, puerperal
thyroiditis O90.5
toxemia (eclamptic) (pre-eclamptic) (with convulsions) O15.2
trauma, non-obstetric O9A.23 *(follows O99)*
  caused by abuse (physical) (suspected) O9A.33 *(follows O99)*
    confirmed O9A.33 *(follows O99)*
    psychological (suspected) O9A.53 *(follows O99)*
      confirmed O9A.53 *(follows O99)*
    sexual (suspected) O9A.43 *(follows O99)*
      confirmed O9A.43 *(follows O99)*
uremia (due to renal failure) O90.4
urethritis O86.22
vaginitis O86.13
varicose veins (legs) O87.4
  vulva or perineum O87.8
venous O87.9
vulvitis O86.13
vulvovaginitis O86.13
white leg O87.1
Puerperium — *see* Puerperal
Pulmolithiasis J98.4
Pulmonary — *see* condition
Pulpitis (acute) (anachoretic) (chronic) (hyperplastic) (putrescent) (suppurative) (ulcerative) K04.01
irreversible K04.02
reversible K04.01
Pulpless tooth K04.99
Pulse
alternating R00.8
bigeminal R00.8
fast R00.0
feeble, rapid due to shock following injury T79.4
rapid R00.0
weak R09.89
Pulsus alternans or trigeminus R00.8
Punch drunk F07.81
Punctum lacrimale occlusion — *see* Obstruction, lacrimal

Puncture
abdomen, abdominal
  wall S31.139
    with
      foreign body S31.149
      penetration into peritoneal cavity S31.639
        with foreign body S31.649
    epigastric region S31.132
      with
        foreign body S31.142
        penetration into peritoneal cavity S31.632
          with foreign body S31.642
    left
      lower quadrant S31.134
        with
          foreign body S31.144
          penetration into peritoneal cavity S31.634
            with foreign body S31.644
      upper quadrant S31.131
        with
          foreign body S31.141
          penetration into peritoneal cavity S31.631
            with foreign body S31.641
    periumbilic region S31.135
      with
        foreign body S31.145
        penetration into peritoneal cavity S31.635
          with foreign body S31.645
    right
      lower quadrant S31.133
        with
          foreign body S31.143
          penetration into peritoneal cavity S31.633
            with foreign body S31.643
      upper quadrant S31.130
        with
          foreign body S31.140
          penetration into peritoneal cavity S31.630
            with foreign body S31.640
accidental, complicating surgery — see Complication, accidental puncture or laceration
alveolar (process) — see Puncture, oral cavity
ankle S91.039
  with
    foreign body S91.049
  left S91.032
    with
      foreign body S91.042
  right S91.031
    with
      foreign body S91.041
anus S31.833
  with foreign body S31.834
arm (upper) S41.139
  with foreign body S41.149
  left S41.132
    with foreign body S41.142
  lower — see Puncture, forearm
  right S41.131
    with foreign body S41.141
auditory canal (external) (meatus) — see Puncture, ear
auricle, ear — see Puncture, ear
axilla — see Puncture, arm

Puncture — *continued*
back — *see also* Puncture, thorax, back
  lower S31.030
    with
      foreign body S31.040
        with penetration into retroperitoneal space S31.041
      penetration into retroperitoneal space S31.031
bladder (traumatic) S37.29
  nontraumatic N32.89
breast S21.039
  with foreign body S21.049
  left S21.032
    with foreign body S21.042
  right S21.031
    with foreign body S21.041
buttock S31.803
  with foreign body S31.804
  left S31.823
    with foreign body S31.824
  right S31.813
    with foreign body S31.814
by
  device, implant or graft — see Complications, by site and type, mechanical
  foreign body left accidentally in operative wound T81.539
  instrument (any) during a procedure, accidental — see Puncture, accidental complicating surgery
calf — see Puncture, leg
canaliculus lacrimalis — see Puncture, eyelid
canthus, eye — see Puncture, eyelid
cervical esophagus S11.23
  with foreign body S11.24
cheek (external) S01.439
  with foreign body S01.449
  internal — see Puncture, oral cavity
  left S01.432
    with foreign body S01.442
  right S01.431
    with foreign body S01.441
chest wall — see Puncture, thorax
chin — see Puncture, head, specified site NEC
clitoris — see Puncture, vulva
costal region — see Puncture, thorax
digit(s)
  foot — see Puncture, toe
  hand — see Puncture, finger
ear (canal) (external) S01.339
  with foreign body S01.349
  drum S09.2-
  left S01.332
    with foreign body S01.342
  right S01.331
    with foreign body S01.341
elbow S51.039
  with
    foreign body S51.049
  left S51.032
    with
      foreign body S51.042
  right S51.031
    with
      foreign body S51.041
epididymis — see Puncture, testis
epigastric region — see Puncture, abdomen, wall, epigastric
epiglottis S11.83
  with foreign body S11.84
esophagus
  cervical S11.23
    with foreign body S11.24
  thoracic S27.818
eyeball S05.6-
  with foreign body S05.5-
eyebrow — see Puncture, eyelid

Puncture — *continued*
eyelid S01.13-
  with foreign body S01.14-
  left S01.132
    with foreign body S01.142
  right S01.131
    with foreign body S01.141
face NEC — see Puncture, head, specified site NEC
finger(s) S61.239
  with
    damage to nail S61.339
      with
        foreign body S61.349
    foreign body S61.249
  index S61.238
    with
      damage to nail S61.338
        with
          foreign body S61.348
      foreign body S61.248
    left S61.231
      with
        damage to nail S61.331
          with
            foreign body S61.341
        foreign body S61.241
    right S61.230
      with
        damage to nail S61.330
          with
            foreign body S61.340
        foreign body S61.240
  little S61.238
    with
      damage to nail S61.338
        with
          foreign body S61.348
      foreign body S61.248
    left S61.237
      with
        damage to nail S61.337
          with
            foreign body S61.347
        foreign body S61.247
    right S61.236
      with
        damage to nail S61.336
          with
            foreign body S61.346
        foreign body S61.246
  middle S61.238
    with
      damage to nail S61.338
        with
          foreign body S61.348
      foreign body S61.248
    left S61.233
      with
        damage to nail S61.333
          with
            foreign body S61.343
        foreign body S61.243
    right S61.232
      with
        damage to nail S61.332
          with
            foreign body S61.342
        foreign body S61.242
  ring S61.238
    with
      damage to nail S61.338
        with
          foreign body S61.348
      foreign body S61.248

DISEASE INDEX

Puncture — *continued*
  finger(s) S61.239 — *continued*
    ring S61.238 — *continued*
      left S61.235
        with
          damage to nail S61.335
            with
              foreign body S61.345
          foreign body S61.245
      right S61.234
        with
          damage to nail S61.334
            with
              foreign body S61.344
          foreign body S61.244
  flank S31.139
    with foreign body S31.149
  foot (except toe(s) alone) S91.339
    with foreign body S91.349
    left S91.332
      with foreign body S91.342
    right S91.331
      with foreign body S91.341
    toe — *see* Puncture, toe
  forearm S51.839
    with
      foreign body S51.849
    elbow only — *see* Puncture, elbow
    left S51.832
      with
        foreign body S51.842
    right S51.831
      with
        foreign body S51.841
  forehead — *see* Puncture, head, specified site NEC
  genital organs, external
    female S31.532
      with foreign body S31.542
      vagina — *see* Puncture, vagina
      vulva — *see* Puncture, vulva
    male S31.531
      with foreign body S31.541
      penis — *see* Puncture, penis
      scrotum — *see* Puncture, scrotum
      testis — *see* Puncture, testis
  groin — *see* Puncture, abdomen, wall
  gum — *see* Puncture, oral cavity
  hand S61.439
    with
      foreign body S61.449
    finger — *see* Puncture, finger
    left S61.432
      with
        foreign body S61.442
    right S61.431
      with
        foreign body S61.441
    thumb — *see* Puncture, thumb
  head S01.93
    with foreign body S01.94
    cheek — *see* Puncture, cheek
    ear — *see* Puncture, ear
    eyelid — *see* Puncture, eyelid
    lip — *see* Puncture, oral cavity
    nose — *see* Puncture, nose
    oral cavity — *see* Puncture, oral cavity
    scalp S01.03
      with foreign body S01.04
    specified site NEC S01.83
      with foreign body S01.84
    temporomandibular area — *see* Puncture, cheek
  heart S26.99
    with hemopericardium S26.09
    without hemopericardium S26.19
  heel — *see* Puncture, foot

Puncture — *continued*
  hip S71.039
    with foreign body S71.049
    left S71.032
      with foreign body S71.042
    right S71.031
      with foreign body S71.041
  hymen — *see* Puncture, vagina
  hypochondrium — *see* Puncture, abdomen, wall
  hypogastric region — *see* Puncture, abdomen, wall
  inguinal region — *see* Puncture, abdomen, wall
  instep — *see* Puncture, foot
  internal organs — *see* Injury, by site
  interscapular region — *see* Puncture, thorax, back
  intestine
    large
      colon S36.599
        ascending S36.590
        descending S36.592
        sigmoid S36.593
        specified site NEC S36.598
        transverse S36.591
      rectum S36.69
    small S36.499
      duodenum S36.490
      specified site NEC S36.498
  intra-abdominal organ S36.99
    gallbladder S36.128
    intestine — *see* Puncture, intestine
    liver S36.118
    pancreas — *see* Puncture, pancreas
    peritoneum S36.81
    specified site NEC S36.898
    spleen S36.09
    stomach S36.39
  jaw — *see* Puncture, head, specified site NEC
  knee S81.039
    with foreign body S81.049
    left S81.032
      with foreign body S81.042
    right S81.031
      with foreign body S81.041
  labium (majus) (minus) — *see* Puncture, vulva
  lacrimal duct — *see* Puncture, eyelid
  larynx S11.013
    with foreign body S11.014
  leg (lower) S81.839
    with foreign body S81.849
    foot — *see* Puncture, foot
    knee — *see* Puncture, knee
    left S81.832
      with foreign body S81.842
    right S81.831
      with foreign body S81.841
    upper — *see* Puncture, thigh
  lip S01.531
    with foreign body S01.541
  loin — *see* Puncture, abdomen, wall
  lower back — *see* Puncture, back, lower
  lumbar region — *see* Puncture, back, lower
  malar region — *see* Puncture, head, specified site NEC
  mammary — *see* Puncture, breast
  mastoid region — *see* Puncture, head, specified site NEC
  mouth — *see* Puncture, oral cavity
  nail
    finger — *see* Puncture, finger, with damage to nail
    toe — *see* Puncture, toe, with damage to nail
  nasal (septum) (sinus) — *see* Puncture, nose
  nasopharynx — *see* Puncture, head, specified site NEC

Puncture — *continued*
  neck S11.93
    with foreign body S11.94
    involving
      cervical esophagus — *see* Puncture, cervical esophagus
      larynx — *see* Puncture, larynx
      pharynx — *see* Puncture, pharynx
      thyroid gland — *see* Puncture, thyroid gland
      trachea — *see* Puncture, trachea
    specified site NEC S11.83
      with foreign body S11.84
  nose (septum) (sinus) S01.23
    with foreign body S01.24
  ocular — *see* Puncture, eyeball
  oral cavity S01.532
    with foreign body S01.542
  orbit S05.4-
  palate — *see* Puncture, oral cavity
  palm — *see* Puncture, hand
  pancreas S36.299
    body S36.291
    head S36.290
    tail S36.292
  pelvis — *see* Puncture, back, lower
  penis S31.23
    with foreign body S31.24
  perineum
    female S31.43
      with foreign body S31.44
    male S31.139
      with foreign body S31.149
  periocular area (with or without lacrimal passages) — *see* Puncture, eyelid
  phalanges
    finger — *see* Puncture, finger
    toe — *see* Puncture, toe
  pharynx S11.23
    with foreign body S11.24
  pinna — *see* Puncture, ear
  popliteal space — *see* Puncture, knee
  prepuce — *see* Puncture, penis
  pubic region S31.139
    with foreign body S31.149
  pudendum — *see* Puncture, genital organs, external
  rectovaginal septum — *see* Puncture, vagina
  sacral region — *see* Puncture, back, lower
  sacroiliac region — *see* Puncture, back, lower
  salivary gland — *see* Puncture, oral cavity
  scalp S01.03
    with foreign body S01.04
  scapular region — *see* Puncture, shoulder
  scrotum S31.33
    with foreign body S31.34
  shin — *see* Puncture, leg
  shoulder S41.039
    with foreign body S41.049
    left S41.032
      with foreign body S41.042
    right S41.031
      with foreign body S41.041
  spermatic cord — *see* Puncture, testis
  sternal region — *see* Puncture, thorax, front
  submaxillary region — *see* Puncture, head, specified site NEC
  submental region — *see* Puncture, head, specified site NEC
  subungual
    finger(s) — *see* Puncture, finger, with damage to nail
    toe — *see* Puncture, toe, with damage to nail
  supraclavicular fossa — *see* Puncture, neck, specified site NEC
  temple, temporal region — *see* Puncture, head, specified site NEC
  temporomandibular area — *see* Puncture, cheek

Puncture — *continued*
testis S31.33
  with foreign body S31.34
thigh S71.139
  with foreign body S71.149
  left S71.132
    with foreign body S71.142
  right S71.131
    with foreign body S71.141
thorax, thoracic (wall) S21.93
  with foreign body S21.94
  back S21.23-
    with
      foreign body S21.24-
        with penetration S21.44
      penetration S21.43
  breast — *see* Puncture, breast
  front S21.13-
    with
      foreign body S21.14-
        with penetration S21.34
      penetration S21.33
throat — *see* Puncture, neck
thumb S61.039
  with
    damage to nail S61.139
      with
        foreign body S61.149
    foreign body S61.049
  left S61.032
    with
      damage to nail S61.132
        with
          foreign body S61.142
      foreign body S61.042
  right S61.031
    with
      damage to nail S61.131
        with
          foreign body S61.141
      foreign body S61.041
thyroid gland S11.13
  with foreign body S11.14
toe(s) S91.139
  with
    damage to nail S91.239
      with
        foreign body S91.249
    foreign body S91.149
  great S91.133
    with
      damage to nail S91.233
        with
          foreign body S91.243
      foreign body S91.143
    left S91.132
      with
        damage to nail S91.232
          with
            foreign body S91.242
        foreign body S91.142
    right S91.131
      with
        damage to nail S91.231
          with
            foreign body S91.241
        foreign body S91.141
  lesser S91.136
    with
      damage to nail S91.236
        with
          foreign body S91.246
      foreign body S91.146
    left S91.135
      with
        damage to nail S91.235
          with
            foreign body S91.245
        foreign body S91.145

Puncture — *continued*
toe(s) S91.139 — *continued*
  lesser S91.136 — *continued*
    right S91.134
      with
        damage to nail S91.234
          with
            foreign body S91.244
        foreign body S91.144
tongue — *see* Puncture, oral cavity
trachea S11.023
  with foreign body S11.024
tunica vaginalis — *see* Puncture, testis
tympanum, tympanic membrane S09.2-
umbilical region S31.135
  with foreign body S31.145
uvula — *see* Puncture, oral cavity
vagina S31.43
  with foreign body S31.44
vocal cords S11.033
  with foreign body S11.034
vulva S31.43
  with foreign body S31.44
wrist S61.539
  with
    foreign body S61.549
  left S61.532
    with
      foreign body S61.542
  right S61.531
    with
      foreign body S61.541
PUO (pyrexia of unknown origin) R50.9
Pupillary membrane (persistent) Q13.89
Pupillotonia — *see* Anomaly, pupil, function, tonic pupil
Purpura D69.2
  abdominal D69.0
  allergic D69.0
  anaphylactoid D69.0
  annularis telangiectodes L81.7
  arthritic D69.0
  autoerythrocyte sensitization D69.2
  autoimmune D69.0
  bacterial D69.0
  Bateman's (senile) D69.2
  capillary fragility (hereditary) (idiopathic) D69.8
  cryoglobulinemic D89.1
  Devil's pinches D69.2
  fibrinolytic — *see* Fibrinolysis
  fulminans, fulminous D65
  gangrenous D65
  hemorrhagic, hemorrhagica D69.3
    not due to thrombocytopenia D69.0
  Henoch(-Schönlein) (allergic) D69.0
  hypergammaglobulinemic (benign) (Waldenström) D89.0
  idiopathic (thrombocytopenic) D69.3
    nonthrombocytopenic D69.0
  immune thrombocytopenic D69.3
  infectious D69.0
  malignant D69.0
  neonatorum P54.5
  nervosa D69.0
  newborn P54.5
  nonthrombocytopenic D69.2
    hemorrhagic D69.0
    idiopathic D69.0
  nonthrombopenic D69.2
  peliosis rheumatica D69.0
  posttransfusion (post-transfusion) (from (fresh) whole blood or blood products) D69.51
  primary D69.49
  red cell membrane sensitivity D69.2
  rheumatica D69.0
  Schönlein(-Henoch) (allergic) D69.0
  scorbutic E54 [D77]
  senile D69.2

Purpura D69.2 — *continued*
  simplex D69.2
  symptomatica D69.0
  telangiectasia annularis L81.7
  thrombocytopenic D69.49
    congenital D69.42
    hemorrhagic D69.3
    hereditary D69.42
    idiopathic D69.3
    immune D69.3
    neonatal, transitory P61.0
    thrombotic M31.1
  thrombohemolytic — *see* Fibrinolysis
  thrombolytic — *see* Fibrinolysis
  thrombopenic D69.49
  thrombotic, thrombocytopenic M31.1
  toxic D69.0
  vascular D69.0
  visceral symptoms D69.0
Purpuric spots R23.3
Purulent — *see* condition
Pus
  in
    stool R19.5
    urine N39.0
  tube (rupture) — *see* Salpingo-oophoritis
Pustular rash L08.0
Pustule (nonmalignant) L08.9
  malignant A22.0
Pustulosis palmaris et plantaris L40.3
Putnam(-Dana) disease or syndrome — *see* Degeneration, combined
Putrescent pulp (dental) K04.1
Pyarthritis, pyarthrosis — *see* Arthritis, pyogenic or pyemic
  tuberculous — *see* Tuberculosis, joint
Pyelectasis — *see* Hydronephrosis
Pyelitis (congenital) (uremic) — *see also* Pyelonephritis
  with
    calculus — *see* category N20
      with hydronephrosis N13.2
    contracted kidney N11.9
  acute N10
  chronic N11.9
    with calculus — *see* category N20
      with hydronephrosis N13.2
  cystica N28.84
  puerperal (postpartum) O86.21
  tuberculous A18.11
Pyelocystitis — *see* Pyelonephritis
Pyelonephritis — *see also* Nephritis, tubulo-interstitial
  with
    calculus — *see* category N20
      with hydronephrosis N13.2
    contracted kidney N11.9
  acute N10
  calculous — *see* category N20
    with hydronephrosis N13.2
  chronic N11.9
    with calculus — *see* category N20
      with hydronephrosis N13.2
    associated with ureteral obstruction or stricture N11.1
    nonobstructive N11.8
      with reflux (vesicoureteral) N11.0
    obstructive N11.1
    specified NEC N11.8
  in (due to)
    brucellosis A23.9 [N16]
    cryoglobulinemia (mixed) D89.1 [N16]
    cystinosis E72.04
    diphtheria A36.84
    glycogen storage disease E74.09 [N16]
    leukemia NEC C95.9- [N16]
    lymphoma NEC C85.90 [N16]
    multiple myeloma C90.0- [N16]
    obstruction N11.1

Pyelonephritis — *see also* Nephritis, tubulo-
  interstitial — *continued*
  in (due to) — *continued*
    Salmonella infection A02.25
    sarcoidosis D86.84
    sepsis A41.9 [N16]
    Sjögren's disease M35.04
    toxoplasmosis B58.83
    transplant rejection T86.91 [N16]
    Wilson's disease E83.01 [N16]
  nonobstructive N12
    with reflux (vesicoureteral) N11.0
      chronic N11.8
  syphilitic A52.75
Pyelonephrosis (obstructive) N11.1
  chronic N11.9
Pyelophlebitis I80.8
Pyeloureteritis cystica N28.85
Pyemia, pyemic (fever) (infection) (purulent)
    — *see also* Sepsis
  joint — *see* Arthritis, pyogenic or pyemic
  liver K75.1
  pneumococcal A40.3
  portal K75.1
  postvaccinal T88.0
  puerperal, postpartum, childbirth O85
  specified organism NEC A41.89
  tuberculous — *see* Tuberculosis, miliary
Pygopagus Q89.4
Pyknoepilepsy (idiopathic) — *see* Pyknolepsy
Pyknolepsy
  intractable G40.A19
    with status epilepticus G40.A11
    without status epilepticus G40.A19
  not intractable G40.A09
    with status epilepticus G40.A01
    without status epilepticus G40.A09
Pylephlebitis K75.1
Pyle's syndrome Q78.5
Pylethrombophlebitis K75.1
Pylethrombosis K75.1
Pyloritis K29.90
  with bleeding K29.91
Pylorospasm (reflex) NEC K31.3
  congenital or infantile Q40.0
  neurotic F45.8
  newborn Q40.0
  psychogenic F45.8
Pylorus, pyloric — *see* condition
Pyoarthrosis — *see* Arthritis, pyogenic or
    pyemic
Pyocele
  mastoid — *see* Mastoiditis, acute
  sinus (accessory) — *see* Sinusitis
  turbinate (bone) J32.9
  urethra (*see also* Urethritis) N34.0
Pyocolpos — *see* Vaginitis
Pyocystitis N30.80
  with hematuria N30.81
Pyoderma, pyodermia L08.0
  gangrenosum L88
  newborn P39.4
  phagedenic L88
  vegetans L08.81
Pyodermatitis L08.0
  vegetans L08.81
Pyogenic — *see* condition
Pyohydronephrosis N13.6
Pyometra, pyometrium, pyometritis — *see*
    Endometritis
Pyomyositis (tropical) — *see* Myositis, infective
Pyonephritis N12
Pyonephrosis N13.6
  tuberculous A18.11
Pyo-oophoritis — *see* Salpingo-oophoritis
Pyo-ovarium — *see* Salpingo-oophoritis
Pyopericarditis, pyopericardium I30.1
Pyophlebitis — *see* Phlebitis
Pyopneumopericardium I30.1

Pyopneumothorax (infective) J86.9
  with fistula J86.0
  tuberculous NEC A15.6
Pyosalpinx, pyosalpingitis — *see also*
    Salpingo-oophoritis
Pyothorax J86.9
  with fistula J86.0
  tuberculous NEC A15.6
Pyoureter N28.89
  tuberculous A18.11
Pyramidopallidonigral syndrome G20
Pyrexia (of unknown origin) R50.9
  atmospheric T67.0
  during labor NEC O75.2
  heat T67.0
  newborn P81.9
    environmentally-induced P81.0
  persistent R50.9
  puerperal O86.4
Pyroglobulinemia NEC E88.09
Pyromania F63.1
Pyrosis R12
Pyuria (bacterial) N39.0

Q

Q fever A78
  with pneumonia A78
Quadricuspid aortic valve Q23.8
Quadrilateral fever A78
Quadriparesis — *see* Quadriplegia
  meaning muscle weakness M62.81
Quadriplegia G82.50
  complete
    C1-C4 level G82.51
    C5-C7 level G82.53
  congenital (cerebral) (spinal) G80.8
    spastic G80.0
  embolic (current episode) I63.4-
  incomplete
    C1-C4 level G82.52
    C5-C7 level G82.54
  thrombotic (current episode) I63.3-
  traumatic — *code to* injury with seventh
      character S
    current episode — *see* Injury, spinal (cord),
        cervical
Quadruplet, pregnancy — *see* Pregnancy,
    quadruplet
Quarrelsomeness F60.3
Queensland fever A77.3
Quervain's disease M65.4
  thyroid E06.1
Queyrat's erythroplasia D07.4
  penis D07.4
  specified site — *see* Neoplasm, skin, in situ
  unspecified site D07.4
Quincke's disease or edema T78.3
  hereditary D84.1
Quinsy (gangrenous) J36
Quintan fever A79.0
Quintuplet, pregnancy — *see* Pregnancy,
    quintuplet

R

Rabbit fever — *see* Tularemia
Rabies A82.9
  contact Z20.3
  exposure to Z20.3
  inoculation reaction — *see* Complications, vaccination
  sylvatic A82.0
  urban A82.1
Rachischisis — *see* Spina bifida
Rachitic — *see also* condition
  deformities of spine (late effect) (sequelae) E64.3
  pelvis (late effect) (sequelae) E64.3
    with disproportion (fetopelvic) O33.0
      causing obstructed labor O65.0
Rachitis, rachitism (acute) (tarda) — *see also* Rickets
  renalis N25.0
  sequelae E64.3
Radial nerve — *see* condition
Radiation
  burn — *see* Burn
  effects NOS T66
  sickness NOS T66
  therapy, encounter for Z51.0
Radiculitis (pressure) (vertebrogenic) — *see* Radiculopathy
Radiculomyelitis — *see also* Encephalitis
  toxic, due to
    Clostridium tetani A35
    Corynebacterium diphtheriae A36.82
Radiculopathy M54.10
  cervical region M54.12
  cervicothoracic region M54.13
  due to
    disc disorder
      C3 M50.11
      C4 M50.11
      C5 M50.121
      C6 M50.122
      C7 M50.123
      C8 M50.13
    displacement of intervertebral disc — *see* Disorder, disc, with, radiculopathy
  leg M54.1-
  lumbar region M54.16
  lumbosacral region M54.17
  occipito-atlanto-axial region M54.11
  postherpetic B02.29
  sacrococcygeal region M54.18
  syphilitic A52.11
  thoracic region (with visceral pain) M54.14
  thoracolumbar region M54.15
Radiodermal burns (acute, chronic, or occupational) — *see* Burn
Radiodermatitis L58.9
  acute L58.0
  chronic L58.1
Radiotherapy session Z51.0
RAEB (refractory anemia with excess blasts) D46.2-
Rage, meaning rabies — *see* Rabies
Ragpicker's disease A22.1
Ragsorter's disease A22.1
Raillietiniasis B71.8
Railroad neurosis F48.8
Railway spine F48.8
Raised — *see also* Elevated
  antibody titer R76.0
Rake teeth, tooth M26.39
Rales R09.89
Ramifying renal pelvis Q63.8
Ramsay-Hunt disease or syndrome (*see also* Hunt's disease) B02.21
  meaning dyssynergia cerebellaris myoclonica G11.1

Ranula K11.6
  congenital Q38.4
Rape
  adult
    confirmed T74.21
    suspected T76.21
  alleged, observation or examination, ruled out
    adult Z04.41
    child Z04.42
  child
    confirmed T74.22
    suspected T76.22
Rapid
  feeble pulse, due to shock, following injury T79.4
  heart (beat) R00.0
    psychogenic F45.8
  second stage (delivery) O62.3
  time-zone change syndrome — *see* Disorder, sleep, circadian rhythm, psychogenic
Rarefaction, bone — *see* Disorder, bone, density and structure, specified NEC
Rash (toxic) R21
  canker A38.9
  diaper L22
  drug (internal use) L27.0
    contact (*see also* Dermatitis, due to, drugs, external) L25.1
  following immunization T88.1
  food — *see* Dermatitis, due to, food
  heat L74.0
  napkin (psoriasiform) L22
  nettle — *see* Urticaria
  pustular L08.0
  rose R21
    epidemic B06.9
  scarlet A38.9
  serum (*see also* Reaction, serum) T80.69
  wandering tongue K14.1
Rasmussen aneurysm — *see* Tuberculosis, pulmonary
Rasmussen encephalitis G04.81
Rat-bite fever A25.9
  due to Streptobacillus moniliformis A25.1
  spirochetal (morsus muris) A25.0
Rathke's pouch tumor D44.3
Raymond (-Céstan) syndrome I65.8
Raynaud's disease, phenomenon or syndrome (secondary) I73.00
  with gangrene (symmetric) I73.01
RDS (newborn) (type I) P22.0
  type II P22.1
Reaction — *see also* Disorder
  adaptation — *see* Disorder, adjustment
  adjustment (anxiety) (conduct disorder) (depressiveness) (distress) — *see* Disorder, adjustment
    with
      mutism, elective (child) (adolescent) F94.0
  adverse
    food (any) (ingested) NEC T78.1
      anaphylactic — *see* Shock, anaphylactic, due to food
  affective — *see* Disorder, mood
  allergic — *see* Allergy
  anaphylactic — *see* Shock, anaphylactic
  anaphylactoid — *see* Shock, anaphylactic
  anesthesia — *see* Anesthesia, complication
  antitoxin (prophylactic) (therapeutic) — *see* Complications, vaccination
  anxiety F41.1
  Arthus — *see* Arthus' phenomenon
  asthenic F48.8
  combat and operational stress F43.0
  compulsive F42.8
  conversion F44.9
  crisis, acute F43.0
  deoxyribonuclease (DNA) (DNase) hypersensitivity D69.2

Reaction (*see also* Disorder) — *continued*
  depressive (single episode) F32.9
    affective (single episode) F31.4
      recurrent episode F33.9
    neurotic F34.1
    psychoneurotic F34.1
    psychotic F32.3
    recurrent — *see* Disorder, depressive, recurrent
  dissociative F44.9
  drug NEC T88.7
    addictive — *see* Dependence, drug
      transmitted via placenta or breast milk — *see* Absorption, drug, addictive, through placenta
    allergic — *see* Allergy, drug
    lichenoid L43.2
    newborn P93.8
      gray baby syndrome P93.0
    overdose or poisoning (by accident) — *see* Table of Drugs and Chemicals, by drug, poisoning
    photoallergic L56.1
    phototoxic L56.0
    withdrawal — *see* Dependence, by drug, with, withdrawal
      infant of dependent mother P96.1
      newborn P96.1
    wrong substance given or taken (by accident) — *see* Table of Drugs and Chemicals, by drug, poisoning
  fear F40.9
    child (abnormal) F93.8
  febrile nonhemolytic transfusion (FNHTR) R50.84
  fluid loss, cerebrospinal G97.1
  foreign
    body NEC — *see* Granuloma, foreign body
      in operative wound (inadvertently left) — *see* Foreign body, accidentally left during a procedure
    substance accidentally left during a procedure (chemical) (powder) (talc) T81.60
      aseptic peritonitis T81.61
      body or object (instrument) (sponge) (swab) — *see* Foreign body, accidentally left during a procedure
      specified reaction NEC T81.69
  grief — *see* Disorder, adjustment
  Herxheimer's R68.89
  hyperkinetic — *see* Hyperkinesia
  hypochondriacal F45.20
  hypoglycemic, due to insulin E16.0
    with coma (diabetic) — *see* Diabetes, coma nondiabetic E15
    therapeutic misadventure — *see* subcategory T38.3
  hypomanic F30.8
  hysterical F44.9
  immunization — *see* Complications, vaccination
  incompatibility
    ABO blood group (infusion) (transfusion) — *see* Complication(s), transfusion, incompatibility reaction, ABO
      delayed serologic T80.39
    minor blood group (Duffy) (E) (K(ell)) (Kidd) (Lewis) (M) (N) (P) (S) T80.89
    Rh (factor) (infusion) (transfusion) — *see* Complication(s), transfusion, incompatibility reaction, Rh (factor)
  inflammatory — *see* Infection
  infusion — *see* Complications, infusion
  inoculation (immune serum) — *see* Complications, vaccination
  insulin T38.3-
  involutional psychotic — *see* Disorder, depressive

Reaction (see also Disorder) — continued
  leukemoid D72.823
    basophilic D72.823
    lymphocytic D72.823
    monocytic D72.823
    myelocytic D72.823
    neutrophilic D72.823
  LSD (acute)
    due to drug abuse — see Abuse, drug, hallucinogen
    due to drug dependence — see Dependence, drug, hallucinogen
  lumbar puncture G97.1
  manic-depressive — see Disorder, bipolar
  neurasthenic F48.8
  neurogenic — see Neurosis
  neurotic F48.9
  neurotic-depressive F34.1
  nitritoid — see Crisis, nitritoid
  nonspecific
    to
      cell mediated immunity measurement of gamma interferon anitgen response without active tuberculosis R76.12
      Quanti-FERON-TB test (QFT) without active tuberculosis R76.12
      tuberculin test (see also Reaction, tuberculin skin test) R76.11
  obsessive-compulsive F42.8
  organic, acute or subacute — see Delirium
  paranoid (acute) F23
    chronic F22
    senile F03
  passive dependency F60.7
  phobic F40.9
  post-traumatic stress, uncomplicated Z73.3
  psychogenic F99
  psychoneurotic — see also Neurosis
    compulsive F42.8
    depersonalization F48.1
    depressive F34.1
    hypochondriacal F45.20
    neurasthenic F48.8
    obsessive F42.8
  psychophysiologic — see Disorder, somatoform
  psychosomatic — see Disorder, somatoform
  psychotic — see Psychosis
  scarlet fever toxin — see Complications, vaccination
  schizophrenic F23
    acute (brief) (undifferentiated) F23
    latent F21
    undifferentiated (acute) (brief) F23
  serological for syphilis — see Serology for syphilis
  serum T80.69
    anaphylactic (immediate) (see also Shock, anaphylactic) T80.59
    specified reaction NEC
      due to
        administration of blood and blood products T80.61
        immunization T80.62
        serum specified NEC T80.69
        vaccination T80.62
  situational — see Disorder, adjustment
  somatization — see Disorder, somatoform
  spinal puncture G97.1
  stress (severe) F43.9
    acute (agitation) ("daze") (disorientation) (disturbance of consciousness) (flight reaction) (fugue) F43.0
    specified NEC F43.8
  surgical procedure — see Complications, surgical procedure
  tetanus antitoxin — see Complications, vaccination

Reaction (see also Disorder) — continued
  toxic, to local anesthesia T88.59
    in labor and delivery O74.4
    in pregnancy O29.3x-
    postpartum, puerperal O89.3
  toxin-antitoxin — see Complications, vaccination
  transfusion (blood) (bone marrow) (lymphocytes) (allergic) — see Complications, transfusion
  tuberculin skin test, abnormal R76.11
  vaccination (any) — see Complications, vaccination
  withdrawing, child or adolescent F93.8
Reactive airway disease — see Asthma
Reactive depression — see Reaction, depressive
Rearrangement
  chromosomal
    balanced (in) Q95.9
      abnormal individual (autosomal) Q95.2
      non-sex (autosomal) chromosomes Q95.2
      sex/non-sex chromosomes Q95.3
      specified NEC Q95.8
Recalcitrant patient — see Noncompliance
Recanalization, thrombus — see Thrombosis
Recession, receding
  chamber angle (eye) H21.55-
  chin M26.09
  gingival (generalized) (localized) (postinfective) (postoperative) K06.00
    Miller Class I K06.01
    Miller Class II K06.02
    Miller Class III K06.03
    Miller Class IV K06.04
Recklinghausen disease Q85.01
  bones E21.0
Reclus' disease (cystic) — see Mastopathy, cystic
Recrudescent typhus (fever) A75.1
Recruitment, auditory H93.21-
Rectalgia K62.89
Rectitis K62.89
Rectocele
  female (without uterine prolapse) N81.6
    with uterine prolapse N81.4
      incomplete N81.2
  in pregnancy — see Pregnancy, complicated by, abnormal, pelvic organs or tissues NEC
  male K62.3
Rectosigmoid junction — see condition
Rectosigmoiditis K63.89
  ulcerative (chronic) K51.30
    with
      complication K51.319
        abscess K51.314
        fistula K51.313
        obstruction K51.312
        rectal bleeding K51.311
        specified NEC K51.318
Rectourethral — see condition
Rectovaginal — see condition
Rectovesical — see condition
Rectum, rectal — see condition
Recurrent — see condition
  pregnancy loss — see Loss (of), pregnancy, recurrent
Red bugs B88.0
Red-cedar lung or pneumonitis J67.8
Red tide (see also Table of Drugs and Chemicals) T65.82-
Reduced
  mobility Z74.09
  ventilatory or vital capacity R94.2

Redundant, redundancy
  anus (congenital) Q43.8
  clitoris N90.89
  colon (congenital) Q43.8
  foreskin (congenital) N47.8
  intestine (congenital) Q43.8
  labia N90.69
  organ or site, congenital NEC — see Accessory
  panniculus (abdominal) E65
  prepuce (congenital) N47.8
  pylorus K31.89
  rectum (congenital) Q43.8
  scrotum N50.89
  sigmoid (congenital) Q43.8
  skin L98.7
    and subcutaneous tissue L98.7
    of face L57.4
      eyelids — see Blepharochalasis
  stomach K31.89
Reduplication — see Duplication
Reflex R29.2
  hyperactive gag J39.2
  pupillary, abnormal — see Anomaly, pupil, function
  vasoconstriction I73.9
  vasovagal R55
Reflux K21.9
  acid K21.9
  esophageal K21.9
    with esophagitis K21.0
    newborn P78.83
  gastroesophageal K21.9
    with esophagitis K21.0
  mitral — see Insufficiency, mitral
  ureteral — see Reflux, vesicoureteral
  vesicoureteral (with scarring) N13.70
    with
      nephropathy N13.729
        with hydroureter N13.739
          bilateral N13.732
          unilateral N13.731
        bilateral N13.722
        unilateral N13.721
      without hydroureter N13.729
        bilateral N13.722
        unilateral N13.721
    pyelonephritis (chronic) N11.0
    congenital Q62.7
    without nephropathy N13.71
Reforming, artificial openings — see Attention to, artificial, opening
Refractive error — see Disorder, refraction
Refsum's disease or syndrome G60.1
Refusal of
  food, psychogenic F50.89
  treatment (because of) Z53.20
    left against medical advice (AMA) Z53.21
    patient's decision NEC Z53.29
    reasons of belief or group pressure Z53.1
Regional — see condition
Regurgitation R11.10
  aortic (valve) — see Insufficiency, aortic
  food — see also Vomiting
    with reswallowing — see Rumination
    newborn P92.1
  gastric contents — see Vomiting
  heart — see Endocarditis
  mitral (valve) — see Insufficiency, mitral
    congenital Q23.3
  myocardial — see Endocarditis
  pulmonary (valve) (heart) I37.1
    congenital Q22.2
    syphilitic A52.03
  tricuspid — see Insufficiency, tricuspid
  valve, valvular — see Endocarditis
    congenital Q24.8
  vesicoureteral — see Reflux, vesicoureteral
Reichmann's disease or syndrome K31.89
Reifenstein syndrome E34.52

Reinsertion
  implantable subdermal contraceptive Z30.46
  intrauterine contraceptive device Z30.433
Reiter's disease, syndrome, or urethritis
  M02.30
  ankle M02.37-
  elbow M02.32-
  foot joint M02.37-
  hand joint M02.34-
  hip M02.35-
  knee M02.36-
  multiple site M02.39
  shoulder M02.31-
  vertebra M02.38
  wrist M02.33-
Rejection
  food, psychogenic F50.89
  transplant T86.91
    bone T86.830
      marrow T86.01
    cornea T86.840
    heart T86.21
      with lung(s) T86.31
    intestine T86.850
    kidney T86.11
    liver T86.41
    lung(s) T86.810
      with heart T86.31
    organ (immune or nonimmune cause)
      T86.91
    pancreas T86.890
    skin (allograft) (autograft) T86.820
    specified NEC T86.890
    stem cell (peripheral blood) (umbilical cord)
      T86.5
Relapsing fever A68.9
  Carter's (Asiatic) A68.1
  Dutton's (West African) A68.1
  Koch's A68.9
  louse-borne (epidemic) A68.0
  Novy's (American) A68.1
  Obermeyers's (European) A68.0
  Spirillum A68.9
  tick-borne (endemic) A68.1
Relationship
  occlusal
    open anterior M26.220
    open posterior M26.221
Relaxation
  anus (sphincter) K62.89
    psychogenic F45.8
  arch (foot) — see also Deformity, limb, flat foot
  back ligaments — see Instability, joint, spine
  bladder (sphincter) N31.2
  cardioesophageal K21.9
  cervix — see Incompetency, cervix
  diaphragm J98.6
  joint (capsule) (ligament) (paralytic) — see
    Flail, joint
    congenital NEC Q74.8
  lumbosacral (joint) — see subcategory M53.2
  pelvic floor N81.89
  perineum N81.89
  posture R29.3
  rectum (sphincter) K62.89
  sacroiliac (joint) — see subcategory M53.2
  scrotum N50.89
  urethra (sphincter) N36.44
  vesical N31.2
Release from prison, anxiety concerning
  Z65.2
Remains
  canal of Cloquet Q14.0
  capsule (opaque) Q14.8
Remittent fever (malarial) B54
Remnant
  canal of Cloquet Q14.0
  capsule (opaque) Q14.8

Remnant — continued
  cervix, cervical stump (acquired)
    (postoperative) N88.8
  cystic duct, postcholecystectomy K91.5
  fingernail L60.8
    congenital Q84.6
  meniscus, knee — see Derangement, knee,
    meniscus, specified NEC
  thyroglossal duct Q89.2
  tonsil J35.8
    infected (chronic) J35.01
  urachus Q64.4
Removal (from) (of)
  artificial
    arm Z44.00-
      complete Z44.01-
      partial Z44.02-
    eye Z44.2-
    leg Z44.10-
      complete Z44.11-
      partial Z44.12-
  breast implant Z45.81
  cardiac pulse generator (battery) (end-of-life)
    Z45.010
  catheter (urinary) (indwelling) Z46.6
    from artificial opening — see Attention to,
      artificial, opening
    non-vascular Z46.82
    vascular NEC Z45.2
  device Z46.9
    contraceptive Z30.432
      implantable subdermal Z30.46
    implanted NEC Z45.89
    specified NEC Z46.89
  drains Z48.03
  dressing (nonsurgical) Z48.00
    surgical Z48.01
  external
    fixation device — code to fracture with
      seventh character D
    prosthesis, prosthetic device Z44.9
      breast Z44.3-
      specified NEC Z44.8
  home in childhood (to foster home or
    institution) Z62.29
  ileostomy Z43.2
  insulin pump Z46.81
  myringotomy device (stent) (tube) Z45.82
  nervous system device NEC Z46.2
    brain neuropacemaker Z46.2
    visual substitution device Z46.2
      implanted Z45.31
  non-vascular catheter Z46.82
  organ, prophylactic (for neoplasia manage-
    ment) — see Prophylactic, organ removal
  orthodontic device Z46.4
  staples Z48.02
  stent
    ureteral Z46.6
  suture Z48.02
  urinary device Z46.6
  vascular access device or catheter Z45.2
Ren
  arcuatus Q63.1
  mobile, mobilis N28.89
    congenital Q63.8
  unguliformis Q63.1
Renal — see condition
Rendu-Osler-Weber disease or
  syndrome I78.0
Reninoma D41.0-
Renon-Delille syndrome E23.3
Reovirus, as cause of disease classified
  elsewhere B97.5
Repeated falls NEC R29.6
Replaced chromosome by dicentric ring
  Q93.2

Replacement by artificial or mechanical
  device or prosthesis of
  bladder Z96.0
  blood vessel NEC Z95.828
  bone NEC Z96.7
  cochlea Z96.21
  coronary artery Z95.5
  eustachian tube Z96.29
  eye globe Z97.0
  heart Z95.812
    valve Z95.2
      prosthetic Z95.2
      specified NEC Z95.4
      xenogenic Z95.3
  intestine Z96.89
  joint Z96.60
    hip — see Presence, hip joint implant
    knee — see Presence, knee joint implant
    specified site NEC Z96.698
  larynx Z96.3
  lens Z96.1
  limb(s) — see Presence, artificial, limb
  mandible NEC (for tooth root implant(s)) Z96.5
  organ NEC Z96.89
  peripheral vessel NEC Z95.828
  stapes Z96.29
  teeth Z97.2
  tendon Z96.7
  tissue NEC Z96.89
  tooth root(s) Z96.5
  vessel NEC Z95.828
    coronary (artery) Z95.5
Request for expert evidence Z04.8
Reserve, decreased or low
  cardiac — see Disease, heart
  kidney N28.89
Residual — see also condition
  ovary syndrome N99.83
  state, schizophrenic F20.5
  urine R39.198
Resistance, resistant (to)
  activated protein C D68.51
  complicating pregnancy O26.89
  insulin E88.81
  organism(s)
    to
      drug Z16.30
        aminoglycosides Z16.29
        amoxicillin Z16.11
        ampicillin Z16.11
        antibiotic(s) Z16.20
          multiple Z16.24
          specified NEC Z16.29
        antifungal Z16.32
        antimicrobial (single) Z16.30
          multiple Z16.35
          specified NEC Z16.39
        antimycobacterial (single) Z16.341
          multiple Z16.342
        antiparasitic Z16.31
        antiviral Z16.33
        beta lactam antibiotics Z16.10
          specified NEC Z16.19
        cephalosporins Z16.19
        extended beta lactamase (ESBL) Z16.12
        fluoroquinolones Z16.23
        macrolides Z16.29
        methicillin — see MRSA
        multiple drugs (MDRO)
          antibiotics Z16.24
          antimicrobial Z16.35
          antimycobacterial (single) Z16.341
        penicillins Z16.11
        quinine (and related compounds)
          Z16.31
        quinolones Z16.23
        sulfonamides Z16.29
        tetracyclines Z16.29

Resistance

DISEASE INDEX

Retinitis — *see also* Inflammation, chorioretinal
— *continued*
  juxtapapillaris — *see* Inflammation,
    chorioretinal, focal, juxtapapillary
  luetic — *see* Retinitis, syphilitic
  pigmentosa H35.52
  proliferans — *see* Disorder, globe,
    degenerative, specified type NEC
  proliferating — *see* Disorder, globe,
    degenerative, specified type NEC
  renal N18.9 [H32]
  syphilitic (early) (secondary) A51.43
    central, recurrent A52.71
    congenital (early) A50.01 [H32]
    late A52.71
  tuberculous A18.53
Retinoblastoma C69.2-
  differentiated C69.2-
  undifferentiated C69.2-
Retinochoroiditis — *see also* Inflammation,
  chorioretinal
  disseminated — *see* Inflammation,
    chorioretinal, disseminated
    syphilitic A52.71
  focal — *see* Inflammation, chorioretinal
  juxtapapillaris — *see* Inflammation,
    chorioretinal, focal, juxtapapillary
Retinopathy (background) H35.00
  arteriosclerotic I70.8 [H35.0-]
  atherosclerotic I70.8 [H35.0-]
  central serous — *see* Chorioretinopathy, central
    serous
  Coats H35.02-
  diabetic — *see* Diabetes, retinopathy
  exudative H35.02-
  hypertensive H35.03-
  in (due to)
    diabetes — *see* Diabetes, retinopathy
    sickle-cell disorders D57-[H36]
  of prematurity H35.10-
    stage 0 H35.11-
    stage 1 H35.12-
    stage 2 H35.13-
    stage 3 H35.14-
    stage 4 H35.15-
    stage 5 H35.16-
  pigmentary, congenital — *see* Dystrophy,
    retina
  proliferative NEC H35.2-
    diabetic — *see* Diabetes, retinopathy,
      proliferative
    sickle-cell D57-[H36]
  solar H31.02-
Retinoschisis H33.10-
  congenital Q14.1
  specified type NEC H33.19-
Retortamoniasis A07.8
Retractile testis Q55.22
Retraction
  cervix — *see* Retroversion, uterus
  drum (membrane) — *see* Disorder, tympanic
    membrane, specified NEC
  finger — *see* Deformity, finger
  lid H02.539
    left H02.536
      lower H02.535
      upper H02.534
    right H02.533
      lower H02.532
      upper H02.531
  lung J98.4
  mediastinum J98.59
  nipple N64.53
    associated with
      lactation O92.03
      pregnancy O92.01-
      puerperium O92.02
    congenital Q83.8
  palmar fascia M72.0

Retraction — *continued*
  pleura — *see* Pleurisy
  ring, uterus (Bandl's) (pathological) O62.4
  sternum (congenital) Q76.7
    acquired M95.4
  uterus — *see* Retroversion, uterus
  valve (heart) — *see* Endocarditis
Retrobulbar — *see* condition
Retrocecal — *see* condition
Retrocession — *see* Retroversion
Retrodisplacement — *see* Retroversion
Retroflection, retroflexion — *see*
  Retroversion
Retrognathia, retrognathism (mandibular)
  (maxillary) M26.19
Retrograde menstruation N92.5
Retroperineal — *see* condition
Retroperitoneal — *see* condition
Retroperitonitis K68.9
Retropharyngeal — *see* condition
Retroplacental — *see* condition
Retroposition — *see* Retroversion
Retroprosthetic membrane T85.398
Retrosternal thyroid (congenital) Q89.2
Retroversion, retroverted
  cervix — *see* Retroversion, uterus
  female NEC — *see* Retroversion, uterus
  iris H21.89
  testis (congenital) Q55.29
  uterus (acquired) (acute) (any degree)
    (asymptomatic) (cervix) (postinfectional)
    (postpartal, old) N85.4
    congenital Q51.818
    in pregnancy O34.53-
Retrovirus, as cause of disease classified
  elsewhere B97.30
  human
    immunodeficiency, type 2 (HIV 2) B97.35
    T-cell lymphotropic
      type I (HTLV-I) B97.33
      type II (HTLV-II) B97.34
  lentivirus B97.31
  oncovirus B97.32
  specified NEC B97.39
Retrusion, premaxilla (developmental)
  M26.09
Rett's disease or syndrome F84.2
Reverse peristalsis R19.2
Reye's syndrome G93.7
Rh (factor)
  hemolytic disease (newborn) P55.0
  incompatibility, immunization or sensitization
    affecting management of pregnancy NEC
    O36.09-
      anti-D antibody O36.01-
    newborn P55.0
    transfusion reaction — *see* Complication(s),
      transfusion, incompatibility reaction, Rh
      (factor)
  negative mother affecting newborn P55.0
  titer elevated — *see* Complication(s),
    transfusion, incompatibility reaction, Rh
    (factor)
  transfusion reaction — *see* Complication(s),
    transfusion, incompatibility reaction, Rh
    (factor)
Rhabdomyolysis (idiopathic) NEC M62.82
  traumatic T79.6
Rhabdomyoma — *see also* Neoplasm,
  connective tissue, benign
  adult — *see* Neoplasm, connective tissue,
    benign
  fetal — *see* Neoplasm, connective tissue,
    benign
  glycogenic — *see* Neoplasm, connective tissue,
    benign
Rhabdomyosarcoma (any type) — *see*
  Neoplasm, connective tissue, malignant
Rhabdosarcoma — *see* Rhabdomyosarcoma

Rhesus (factor) incompatibility — *see* Rh,
  incompatibility
Rheumatic (acute) (subacute) (chronic)
  adherent pericardium I09.2
  coronary arteritis I01.9
  degeneration, myocardium I09.0
  fever (acute) — *see* Fever, rheumatic
  heart — *see* Disease, heart, rheumatic
  myocardial degeneration — *see* Degeneration,
    myocardium
  myocarditis (chronic) (inactive) (with chorea)
    I09.0
    with chorea (acute) (rheumatic) (Sydenham's)
      I02.0
    active or acute I01.2
  pancarditis, acute I01.8
    with chorea (acute (rheumatic) Sydenham's)
      I02.0
  pericarditis (active) (acute) (with effusion) (with
    pneumonia) I01.0
    with chorea (acute) (rheumatic) (Sydenham's)
      I02.0
    chronic or inactive I09.2
  pneumonia I00 [J17]
  torticollis M43.6
  typhoid fever A01.09
Rheumatism (articular) (neuralgic)
  (nonarticular) M79.0
  gout — *see* Arthritis, rheumatoid
  intercostal, meaning Tietze's disease M94.0
  palindromic (any site) M12.30
    ankle M12.37-
    elbow M12.32-
    foot joint M12.37-
    hand joint M12.34-
    hip M12.35-
    knee M12.36-
    multiple site M12.39
    shoulder M12.31-
    specified joint NEC M12.38
    vertebrae M12.38
    wrist M12.33-
  sciatic M54.4-
Rheumatoid — *see also* condition
  arthritis — *see also* Arthritis, rheumatoid
    with involvement of organs NEC M05.60
      ankle M05.67-
      elbow M05.62-
      foot joint M05.67-
      hand joint M05.64-
      hip M05.65-
      knee M05.66-
      multiple site M05.69
      shoulder M05.61-
      vertebra — *see* Spondylitis, ankylosing
      wrist M05.63-
    seronegative — *see* Arthritis, rheumatoid,
      seronegative
    seropositive — *see* Arthritis, rheumatoid,
      seropositive
  carditis M05.30
    ankle M05.37-
    elbow M05.32-
    foot joint M05.37-
    hand joint M05.34-
    hip M05.35-
    knee M05.36-
    multiple site M05.39
    shoulder M05.31-
    vertebra — *see* Spondylitis, ankylosing
    wrist M05.33-
  endocarditis — *see* Rheumatoid, carditis
  lung (disease) M05.10
    ankle M05.17-
    elbow M05.12-
    foot joint M05.17-
    hand joint M05.14-
    hip M05.15-
    knee M05.16-

Rheumatoid (see also condition) — continued
lung (disease) M05.10 — continued
  multiple site M05.19
  shoulder M05.11-
  vertebra — see Spondylitis, ankylosing
  wrist M05.13-
myocarditis — see Rheumatoid, carditis
myopathy M05.40
  ankle M05.47-
  elbow M05.42-
  foot joint M05.47-
  hand joint M05.44-
  hip M05.45-
  knee M05.46-
  multiple site M05.49
  shoulder M05.41-
  vertebra — see Spondylitis, ankylosing
  wrist M05.43-
pericarditis — see Rheumatoid, carditis
polyarthritis — see Arthritis, rheumatoid
polyneuropathy M05.50
  ankle M05.57-
  elbow M05.52-
  foot joint M05.57-
  hand joint M05.54-
  hip M05.55-
  knee M05.56-
  multiple site M05.59
  shoulder M05.51-
  vertebra — see Spondylitis, ankylosing
  wrist M05.53-
vasculitis M05.20
  ankle M05.27-
  elbow M05.22-
  foot joint M05.27-
  hand joint M05.24-
  hip M05.25-
  knee M05.26-
  multiple site M05.29
  shoulder M05.21-
  vertebra — see Spondylitis, ankylosing
  wrist M05.23-
Rhinitis (atrophic) (catarrhal) (chronic)
  (croupous) (fibrinous) (granulomatous)
  (hyperplastic) (hypertrophic) (membranous)
  (obstructive) (purulent) (suppurative)
  (ulcerative) J31.0
with
  sore throat — see Nasopharyngitis
acute J00
allergic J30.9
  with asthma J45.909
    with
      exacerbation (acute) J45.901
      status asthmaticus J45.902
  due to
    food J30.5
    pollen J30.1
  nonseasonal J30.89
  perennial J30.89
  seasonal NEC J30.2
  specified NEC J30.89
infective J00
pneumococcal J00
syphilitic A52.73
  congenital A50.05 [J99]
tuberculous A15.8
vasomotor J30.0
Rhinoantritis (chronic) — see Sinusitis,
  maxillary
Rhinodacryolith — see Dacryolith
Rhinolith (nasal sinus) J34.89
Rhinomegaly J34.89
Rhinopharyngitis (acute) (subacute) — see
  also Nasopharyngitis
chronic J31.1
destructive ulcerating A66.5
mutilans A66.5
Rhinophyma L71.1

Rhinorrhea J34.89
cerebrospinal (fluid) G96.0
paroxysmal — see Rhinitis, allergic
spasmodic — see Rhinitis, allergic
Rhinosalpingitis — see Salpingitis, eustachian
Rhinoscleroma A48.8
Rhinosporidiosis B48.1
Rhinovirus infection NEC B34.8
Rhizomelic chondrodysplasia punctata
  E71.540
Rhythm
atrioventricular nodal I49.8
disorder I49.9
  coronary sinus I49.8
  ectopic I49.8
  nodal I49.8
escape I49.9
heart, abnormal I49.9
idioventricular I44.2
nodal I49.8
sleep, inversion G47.2-
  nonorganic origin — see Disorder, sleep,
    circadian rhythm, psychogenic
Rhytidosis facialis L98.8
Rib — see also condition
cervical Q76.5
Riboflavin deficiency E53.0
Rice bodies — see also Loose, body, joint
knee M23.4-
Richter syndrome — see Leukemia, chronic
  lymphocytic, B-cell type
Richter's hernia — see Hernia, abdomen,
  with obstruction
Ricinism — see Poisoning, food, noxious, plant
Rickets (active) (acute) (adolescent) (chest wall)
  (congenital) (current) (infantile) (intestinal)
  E55.0
adult — see Osteomalacia
celiac K90.0
hypophosphatemic with nephrotic-glycosuric
  dwarfism E72.09
inactive E64.3
kidney N25.0
renal N25.0
sequelae, any E64.3
vitamin-D-resistant E83.31 [M90.80]
Rickettsial disease A79.9
specified type NEC A79.89
Rickettsialpox (Rickettsia akari) A79.1
Rickettsiosis A79.9
due to
  Ehrlichia sennetsu A79.81
  Rickettsia akari (rickettsialpox) A79.1
specified type NEC A79.89
tick-borne A77.9
vesicular A79.1
Rider's bone — see Ossification, muscle,
  specified NEC
Ridge, alveolus — see also condition
flabby K06.8
Ridged ear, congenital Q17.3
Riedel's
lobe, liver Q44.7
struma, thyroiditis or disease E06.5
Rieger's anomaly or syndrome Q13.81
Riehl's melanosis L81.4
Rietti-Greppi-Micheli anemia D56.9
Rieux's hernia — see Hernia, abdomen,
  specified site NEC
Riga (-Fede) disease K14.0
Riggs' disease — see Periodontitis
Right aortic arch Q25.47
Right middle lobe syndrome J98.11
Rigid, rigidity — see also condition
abdominal R19.30
  with severe abdominal pain R10.0
  epigastric R19.36
  generalized R19.37
  left lower quadrant R19.34

Rigid, rigidity — see also condition —
  continued
abdominal R19.30 — continued
  left upper quadrant R19.32
  periumbilic R19.35
  right lower quadrant R19.33
  right upper quadrant R19.31
articular, multiple, congenital Q68.8
cervix (uteri) in pregnancy — see Pregnancy,
  complicated by, abnormal, cervix
hymen (acquired) (congenital) N89.6
nuchal R29.1
pelvic floor in pregnancy — see Pregnancy,
  complicated by, abnormal, pelvic organs
  or tissues NEC
perineum or vulva in pregnancy — see
  Pregnancy, complicated by, abnormal,
  vulva
spine — see Dorsopathy, specified NEC
vagina in pregnancy — see Pregnancy,
  complicated by, abnormal, vagina
Rigors R68.89
with fever R50.9
Riley-Day syndrome G90.1
RIND (reversible ischemic neurologic deficit)
  I63.9
Ring(s)
aorta (vascular) Q25.45
Bandl's O62.4
contraction, complicating delivery O62.4
esophageal, lower (muscular) K22.2
Fleischer's (cornea) H18.04-
hymenal, tight (acquired) (congenital) N89.6
Kayser-Fleischer (cornea) H18.04-
retraction, uterus, pathological O62.4
Schatzki's (esophagus) (lower) K22.2
  congenital Q39.3
Soemmerring's — see Cataract, secondary
vascular (congenital) Q25.8
  aorta Q25.45
Ringed hair (congenital) Q84.1
Ringworm B35.9
beard B35.0
black dot B35.0
body B35.4
Burmese B35.5
corporeal B35.4
foot B35.3
groin B35.6
hand B35.2
honeycomb B35.0
nails B35.1
perianal (area) B35.6
scalp B35.0
specified NEC B35.8
Tokelau B35.5
Rise, venous pressure I87.8
Rising, PSA following treatment for
  malignant neoplasm of prostate
  R97.21
Risk, suicidal
meaning personal history of attempted suicide
  Z91.5
meaning suicidal ideation — see Ideation,
  suicidal
Ritter's disease L00
Rivalry, sibling Z62.891
Rivalta's disease A42.2
River blindness B73.01
Robert's pelvis Q74.2
with disproportion (fetopelvic) O33.0
  causing obstructed labor O65.0
Robin(-Pierre) syndrome Q87.0
Robinow-Silvermann-Smith syndrome
  Q87.1
Robinson's (hidrotic) ectodermal
  dysplasia or syndrome Q82.4
Robles' disease B73.01
Rocky Mountain (spotted) fever A77.0

Roetheln — *see* Rubella
Roger's disease Q21.0
Rokitansky-Aschoff sinuses (gallbladder) K82.8
Rolando's fracture (displaced) S62.22-
nondisplaced S62.22-
Romano-Ward (prolonged QT interval) syndrome I45.81
Romberg's disease or syndrome G51.8
Roof, mouth — *see* condition
Rosacea L71.9
acne L71.9
keratitis L71.8
specified NEC L71.8
Rosary, rachitic E55.0
Rose
cold J30.1
fever J30.1
rash R21
epidemic B06.9
Rosenbach's erysipeloid A26.0
Rosenthal's disease or syndrome D68.1
Roseola B09
infantum B08.20
due to human herpesvirus 6 B08.21
due to human herpesvirus 7 B08.22
Ross River disease or fever B33.1
Rossbach's disease K31.89
psychogenic F45.8
Rostan's asthma (cardiac) — *see* Failure, ventricular, left
Rotation
anomalous, incomplete or insufficient, intestine Q43.3
cecum (congenital) Q43.3
colon (congenital) Q43.3
spine, incomplete or insufficient — *see* Dorsopathy, deforming, specified NEC
tooth, teeth, fully erupted M26.35
vertebra, incomplete or insufficient — *see* Dorsopathy, deforming, specified NEC
Rotes Quérol disease or syndrome — *see* Hyperostosis, ankylosing
Roth(-Bernhardt) disease or syndrome — *see* Meralgia paraesthetica
Rothmund(-Thomson) syndrome Q82.8
Rotor's disease or syndrome E80.6
Round
back (with wedging of vertebrae) — *see* Kyphosis
sequelae (late effect) of rickets E64.3
worms (large) (infestation) NEC B82.0
Ascariasis (*see also* Ascariasis) B77.9
Roussy-Lévy syndrome G60.0
Rubella (German measles) B06.9
complication NEC B06.09
neurological B06.00
congenital P35.0
contact Z20.4
exposure to Z20.4
maternal
care for (suspected) damage to fetus O35.3
manifest rubella in infant P35.0
suspected damage to fetus affecting management of pregnancy O35.3
specified complications NEC B06.89
Rubeola (meaning measles) — *see* Measles
meaning rubella — *see* Rubella
Rubeosis, iris — *see* Disorder, iris, vascular
Rubinstein-Taybi syndrome Q87.2
Rudimentary (congenital) — *see also* Agenesis
arm — *see* Defect, reduction, upper limb
bone Q79.9
cervix uteri Q51.828
eye Q11.2
lobule of ear Q17.3
patella Q74.1
respiratory organs in thoracopagus Q89.4
tracheal bronchus Q32.4

Rudimentary (congenital) — *see also* Agenesis — *continued*
uterus Q51.818
in male Q56.1
vagina Q52.0
Ruled out condition — *see* Observation, suspected
Rumination R11.10
with nausea R11.2
disorder of infancy F98.21
neurotic F42.8
newborn P92.1
obsessional F42.8
psychogenic F42.8
Runeberg's disease D51.0
Runny nose R09.89
Rupia (syphilitic) A51.39
congenital A50.06
tertiary A52.79
Rupture, ruptured
abscess (spontaneous) — *code by* site under Abscess
aneurysm — *see* Aneurysm
anus (sphincter) — *see* Laceration, anus
aorta, aortic I71.8
abdominal I71.3
arch I71.1
ascending I71.1
descending I71.8
abdominal I71.3
thoracic I71.1
syphilitic A52.01
thoracoabdominal I71.5
thorax, thoracic I71.1
transverse I71.1
traumatic — *see* Injury, aorta, laceration, major
valve or cusp (*see also* Endocarditis, aortic) I35.8
appendix (with peritonitis) K35.2
with localized peritonitis K35.3
arteriovenous fistula, brain I60.8
artery I77.2
brain — *see* Hemorrhage, intracranial, intracerebral
coronary — *see* Infarct, myocardium
heart — *see* Infarct, myocardium
pulmonary I28.8
traumatic (complication) — *see* Injury, blood vessel
bile duct (common) (hepatic) K83.2
cystic K82.2
bladder (sphincter) (nontraumatic) (spontaneous) N32.89
following ectopic or molar pregnancy O08.6
obstetrical trauma O71.5
traumatic S37.29
blood vessel — *see also* Hemorrhage
brain — *see* Hemorrhage, intracranial, intracerebral
heart — *see* Infarct, myocardium
traumatic (complication) — *see* Injury, blood vessel, laceration, major, by site
bone — *see* Fracture
bowel (nontraumatic) K63.1
brain
aneurysm (congenital) — *see also* Hemorrhage, intracranial, subarachnoid
syphilitic A52.05
hemorrhagic — *see* Hemorrhage, intracranial, intracerebral
capillaries I78.8
cardiac (auricle) (ventricle) (wall) I23.3
with hemopericardium I23.0
infectional I40.9
traumatic — *see* Injury, heart
cartilage (articular) (current) — *see also* Sprain
knee S83.3-
semilunar — *see* Tear, meniscus

Rupture, ruptured — *continued*
cecum (with peritonitis) K65.0
with peritoneal abscess K35.3
traumatic S36.598
celiac artery, traumatic — *see* Injury, blood vessel, celiac artery, laceration, major
cerebral aneurysm (congenital) (*see* Hemorrhage, intracranial, subarachnoid)
cervix (uteri)
with ectopic or molar pregnancy O08.6
following ectopic or molar pregnancy O08.6
obstetrical trauma O71.3
traumatic S37.69
chordae tendineae NEC I51.1
concurrent with acute myocardial infarction — *see* Infarct, myocardium
following acute myocardial infarction (current complication) I23.4
choroid (direct) (indirect) (traumatic) H31.32-
circle of Willis I60.6
colon (nontraumatic) K63.1
traumatic — *see* Injury, intestine, large
cornea (traumatic) — *see* Injury, eye, laceration
coronary (artery) (thrombotic) — *see* Infarct, myocardium
corpus luteum (infected) (ovary) N83.1-
cyst — *see* Cyst
cystic duct K82.2
Descemet's membrane — *see* Change, corneal membrane, Descemet's, rupture
traumatic — *see* Injury, eye, laceration
diaphragm, traumatic — *see* Injury, intrathoracic, diaphragm
disc — *see* Rupture, intervertebral disc
diverticulum (intestine) K57.80
with bleeding K57.81
bladder N32.3
large intestine K57.20
with
bleeding K57.21
small intestine K57.40
with bleeding K57.41
small intestine K57.00
with
bleeding K57.01
large intestine K57.40
with bleeding K57.41
duodenal stump K31.89
ear drum (nontraumatic) — *see also* Perforation, tympanum
traumatic S09.2-
due to blast injury — *see* Injury, blast, ear
esophagus K22.3
eye (without prolapse or loss of intraocular tissue) — *see* Injury, eye, laceration
fallopian tube NEC (nonobstetric) (nontraumatic) N83.8
due to pregnancy O00.10
with intrauterine pregnancy O00.11
fontanel P13.1
gallbladder K82.2
traumatic S36.128
gastric — *see also* Rupture, stomach
vessel K92.2
globe (eye) (traumatic) — *see* Injury, eye, laceration
graafian follicle (hematoma) N83.0-
heart — *see* Rupture, cardiac
hymen (nontraumatic) (nonintentional) N89.8
internal organ, traumatic — *see* Injury, by site
intervertebral disc — *see* Displacement, intervertebral disc
traumatic — *see* Rupture, traumatic, intervertebral disc
intestine NEC (nontraumatic) K63.1
traumatic — *see* Injury, intestine
iris — *see also* Abnormality, pupillary
traumatic — *see* Injury, eye, laceration

Rupture, ruptured — *continued*
joint capsule, traumatic — *see* Sprain
kidney (traumatic) S37.06-
  birth injury P15.8
  nontraumatic N28.89
lacrimal duct (traumatic) — *see* Injury, eye,
  specified site NEC
lens (cataract) (traumatic) — *see* Cataract,
  traumatic
ligament, traumatic — *see* Rupture, traumatic,
  ligament, by site
liver S36.116
  birth injury P15.0
lymphatic vessel I89.8
marginal sinus (placental) (with hemorrhage)
  — *see* Hemorrhage, antepartum, specified
  cause NEC
membrana tympani (nontraumatic) — *see*
  Perforation, tympanum
membranes (spontaneous)
  artificial
    delayed delivery following O75.5
  delayed delivery following — *see* Pregnancy,
    complicated by, premature rupture of
    membranes
meningeal artery I60.8
meniscus (knee) — *see also* Tear, meniscus
  old — *see* Derangement, meniscus
  site other than knee — *code as* Sprain
mesenteric artery, traumatic — *see* Injury,
  mesenteric, artery, laceration, major
mesentery (nontraumatic) K66.8
  traumatic — *see* Injury, intra-abdominal,
    specified, site NEC
mitral (valve) I34.8
muscle (traumatic) — *see also* Strain
  diastasis — *see* Diastasis, muscle
  nontraumatic M62.10
    ankle M62.17-
    foot M62.17-
    forearm M62.13-
    hand M62.14-
    lower leg M62.16-
    pelvic region M62.15-
    shoulder region M62.11-
    specified site NEC M62.18
    thigh M62.15-
    upper arm M62.12-
  traumatic — *see* Strain, by site
musculotendinous junction NEC, nontraumatic
  — *see* Rupture, tendon, spontaneous
mycotic aneurysm causing cerebral
  hemorrhage — *see* Hemorrhage,
  intracranial, subarachnoid
myocardium, myocardial — *see* Rupture,
  cardiac
  traumatic — *see* Injury, heart
nontraumatic, meaning hernia — *see* Hernia
obstructed — *see* Hernia, by site, obstructed
operation wound — *see* Disruption, wound,
  operation
ovary, ovarian N83.8
  corpus luteum cyst N83.1-
  follicle (graafian) N83.0-
oviduct (nonobstetric) (nontraumatic) N83.8
  due to pregnancy O00.10
    with intrauterine pregnancy O00.11
pancreas (nontraumatic) K86.89
  traumatic S36.299
papillary muscle NEC I51.2
  following acute myocardial infarction
    (current complication) I23.5
pelvic
  floor, complicating delivery O70.1
  organ NEC, obstetrical trauma O71.5
perineum (nonobstetric) (nontraumatic) N90.89
  complicating delivery — *see* Delivery,
    complicated, by, laceration, anus
    (sphincter)

Rupture, ruptured — *continued*
postoperative wound — *see* Disruption,
  wound, operation
prostate (traumatic) S37.828
pulmonary
  artery I28.8
  valve (heart) I37.8
  vein I28.8
  vessel I28.8
pus tube — *see* Salpingitis
pyosalpinx — *see* Salpingitis
rectum (nontraumatic) K63.1
  traumatic S36.69
retina, retinal (traumatic) (without detachment)
  — *see also* Break, retina
  with detachment — *see* Detachment, retina,
    with retinal, break
rotator cuff (nontraumatic) M75.10-
  complete M75.12-
  incomplete M75.11-
sclera — *see* Injury, eye, laceration
sigmoid (nontraumatic) K63.1
  traumatic S36.593
spinal cord — *see also* Injury, spinal cord, by
  region
  due to injury at birth P11.5
  newborn (birth injury) P11.5
spleen (traumatic) S36.09
  birth injury P15.1
  congenital (birth injury) P15.1
  due to P. vivax malaria B51.0
  nontraumatic D73.5
  spontaneous D73.5
splenic vein R58
  traumatic — *see* Injury, blood vessel, splenic
    vein
stomach (nontraumatic) (spontaneous) K31.89
  traumatic S36.39
supraspinatus (complete) (incomplete)
  (nontraumatic) — *see* Tear, rotator cuff
symphysis pubis
  obstetric O71.6
  traumatic S33.4
synovium (cyst) M66.10
  ankle M66.17-
  elbow M66.12-
  finger M66.14-
  foot M66.17-
  forearm M66.13-
  hand M66.14-
  pelvic region M66.15-
  shoulder region M66.11-
  specified site NEC M66.18
  thigh M66.15-
  toe M66.17-
  upper arm M66.12-
  wrist M66.13-
tendon (traumatic) — *see* Strain
  nontraumatic (spontaneous) M66.9
    ankle M66.87-
    extensor M66.20
      ankle M66.27-
      foot M66.27-
      forearm M66.23-
      hand M66.24-
      lower leg M66.26-
      multiple sites M66.29
      pelvic region M66.25-
      shoulder region M66.21-
      specified site NEC M66.28
      thigh M66.25-
      upper arm M66.22-
    flexor M66.30
      ankle M66.37-
      foot M66.37-
      forearm M66.33-
      hand M66.34-
      lower leg M66.36-
      multiple sites M66.39

Rupture, ruptured — *continued*
tendon (traumatic) — *see* Strain — *continued*
  nontraumatic (spontaneous) M66.9 —
    continued
    flexor M66.30 — *continued*
      pelvic region M66.35-
      shoulder region M66.31-
      specified site NEC M66.38
      thigh M66.35-
      upper arm M66.32-
    foot M66.87-
    forearm M66.83-
    hand M66.84-
    lower leg M66.86-
    multiple sites M66.89
    pelvic region M66.85-
    shoulder region M66.81-
    specified
      site NEC M66.88
      tendon M66.80
    thigh M66.85-
    upper arm M66.82-
thoracic duct I89.8
tonsil J35.8
traumatic
  aorta — *see* Injury, aorta, laceration, major
  diaphragm — *see* Injury, intrathoracic,
    diaphragm
  external site — *see* Wound, open, by site
  eye — *see* Injury, eye, laceration
  internal organ — *see* Injury, by site
  intervertebral disc
    cervical S13.0
    lumbar S33.0
    thoracic S23.0
  kidney S37.06-
  ligament — *see also* Sprain
    ankle — *see* Sprain, ankle
    carpus — *see* Rupture, traumatic, ligament,
      wrist
    collateral (hand) — *see* Rupture, traumatic,
      ligament, finger, collateral
    finger (metacarpophalangeal)
      (interphalangeal) S63.40-
    collateral S63.41-
      index S63.41-
      little S63.41-
      middle S63.41-
      ring S63.41-
    index S63.40-
    little S63.40-
    middle S63.40-
    palmar S63.42-
      index S63.42-
      little S63.42-
      middle S63.42-
      ring S63.42-
    ring S63.40-
    specified site NEC S63.499
      index S63.49-
      little S63.49-
      middle S63.49-
      ring S63.49-
    volar plate S63.43-
      index S63.43-
      little S63.43-
      middle S63.43-
      ring S63.43-
    foot — *see* Sprain, foot
    radial collateral S53.2-
    radiocarpal — *see* Rupture, traumatic,
      ligament, wrist, radiocarpal
    ulnar collateral S53.3-
    ulnocarpal — *see* Rupture, traumatic,
      ligament, wrist, ulnocarpal

Rupture, ruptured — *continued*
 traumatic — *continued*
  wrist S63.30-
   collateral S63.31-
   radiocarpal S63.32-
   specified site NEC S63.39-
   ulnocarpal (palmar) S63.33-
  liver S36.116
  membrana tympani — *see* Rupture, ear
    drum, traumatic
  muscle or tendon — *see* Strain
  myocardium — *see* Injury, heart
  pancreas S36.299
  rectum S36.69
  sigmoid S36.593
  spleen S36.09
  stomach S36.39
  symphysis pubis S33.4
  tympanum, tympanic (membrane) — *see*
    Rupture, ear drum, traumatic
  ureter S37.19
  uterus S37.69
  vagina — *see* Injury, vagina
  vena cava — *see* Injury, vena cava,
    laceration, major
 tricuspid (heart) (valve) I07.8
 tube, tubal (nonobstetric) (nontraumatic)
   N83.8
  abscess — *see* Salpingitis
  due to pregnancy O00.10
   with intrauterine pregnancy O00.11
 tympanum, tympanic (membrane)
   (nontraumatic) (*see also* Perforation,
   tympanic membrane) H72.9-
  traumatic — *see* Rupture, ear drum,
    traumatic
 umbilical cord, complicating delivery O69.89
 ureter (traumatic) S37.19
  nontraumatic N28.89
 urethra (nontraumatic) N36.8
  with ectopic or molar pregnancy O08.6
  following ectopic or molar pregnancy O08.6
  obstetrical trauma O71.5
  traumatic S37.39
 uterosacral ligament (nonobstetric)
   (nontraumatic) N83.8
 uterus (traumatic) S37.69
  before labor O71.0-
  during or after labor O71.1
  nonpuerperal, nontraumatic N85.8
  pregnant (during labor) O71.1
   before labor O71.0-
 vagina — *see* Injury, vagina
 valve, valvular (heart) — *see* Endocarditis
 varicose vein — *see* Varix
 varix — *see* Varix
 vena cava R58
  traumatic — *see* Injury, vena cava,
    laceration, major
 vesical (urinary) N32.89
 vessel (blood) R58
  pulmonary I28.8
  traumatic — *see* Injury, blood vessel
 viscus R19.8
 vulva complicating delivery O70.0
Russell-Silver syndrome Q87.1
**Russian spring-summer type
 encephalitis** A84.0
Rust's disease (tuberculous cervical
 spondylitis) A18.01
Ruvalcaba-Myhre-Smith syndrome
 E71.440
Rytand-Lipsitch syndrome I44.2

S

Saber, sabre shin or tibia (syphilitic)
 A50.56 [M90.-]
Sac lacrimal — *see* condition
Saccharomyces infection B37.9
Saccharopinuria E72.3
Saccular — *see* condition
Sacculation
 aorta (nonsyphilitic) — *see* Aneurysm, aorta
 bladder N32.3
 intralaryngeal (congenital) (ventricular) Q31.3
 larynx (congenital) (ventricular) Q31.3
 organ or site, congenital — *see* Distortion
 pregnant uterus — *see* Pregnancy, complicated
   by, abnormal, uterus
 ureter N28.89
 urethra N36.1
 vesical N32.3
**Sachs' amaurotic familial idiocy or
 disease** E75.02
Sachs-Tay disease E75.02
Sacks-Libman disease M32.11
Sacralgia M53.3
Sacralization Q76.49
Sacrodynia M53.3
Sacroiliac joint — *see* condition
Sacroiliitis NEC M46.1
Sacrum — *see* condition
Saddle
 back — *see* Lordosis
 embolus
  abdominal aorta I74.01
  pulmonary artery I26.92
   with acute cor pulmonale I26.02
 injury — *code to* condition
 nose M95.0
  due to syphilis A50.57
Sadism (sexual) F65.52
Sadness, postpartal O90.6
Sadomasochism F65.50
Saemisch's ulcer (cornea) — *see* Ulcer,
 cornea, central
Sagging
 skin and subcutaneous tissue (following bariatric
   surgery weight loss) (following dietary
   weight loss) L98.7
Sahib disease B55.0
Sailors' skin L57.8
Saint
 Anthony's fire — *see* Erysipelas
 triad — *see* Hernia, diaphragm
 Vitus' dance — *see* Chorea, Sydenham's
Salaam
 attack(s) — *see* Epilepsy, spasms
 tic R25.8
Salicylism
 abuse F55.8
 overdose or wrong substance given — *see*
   Table of Drugs and Chemicals, by drug,
   poisoning
Salivary duct or gland — *see* condition
Salivation, excessive K11.7
Salmonella — *see* Infection, Salmonella
Salmonellosis A02.0
Salpingitis (catarrhal) (fallopian tube)
 (nodular) (pseudofollicular) (purulent) (septic)
 N70.91
 with oophoritis N70.93
 acute N70.01
  with oophoritis N70.03
 chlamydial A56.11
 chronic N70.11
  with oophoritis N70.13
 complicating abortion — *see* Abortion, by
   type, complicated by, salpingitis
 ear — *see* Salpingitis, eustachian

Salpingitis (catarrhal) (fallopian tube)
 (nodular) (pseudofollicular) (purulent) (septic)
 N70.91 — *continued*
 eustachian (tube) H68.00-
  acute H68.01-
  chronic H68.02-
 follicularis N70.11
  with oophoritis N70.13
 gonococcal (acute) (chronic) A54.24
 interstitial, chronic N70.11
  with oophoritis N70.13
 isthmica nodosa N70.11
  with oophoritis N70.13
 specific (gonococcal) (acute) (chronic) A54.24
 tuberculous (acute) (chronic) A18.17
 venereal (gonococcal) (acute) (chronic)
   A54.24
Salpingocele N83.4-
Salpingo-oophoritis (catarrhal) (purulent)
 (ruptured) (septic) (suppurative) N70.93
 acute N70.03
  with ectopic or molar pregnancy O08.0
  following ectopic or molar pregnancy O08.0
  gonococcal A54.24
 chronic N70.13
 following ectopic or molar pregnancy O08.0
 gonococcal (acute) (chronic) A54.24
 puerperal O86.19
 specific (gonococcal) (acute) (chronic) A54.24
 subacute N70.03
 tuberculous (acute) (chronic) A18.17
 venereal (gonococcal) (acute) (chronic) A54.24
Salpingo-ovaritis — *see* Salpingo-oophoritis
Salpingoperitonitis — *see* Salpingo-
 oophoritis
Salzmann's nodular dystrophy — *see*
 Degeneration, cornea, nodular
Sampson's cyst or tumor N80.1
San Joaquin (Valley) fever B38.0
**Sandblaster's asthma, lung or
 pneumoconiosis** J62.8
Sander's disease (paranoia) F22
Sandfly fever A93.1
Sandhoff's disease E75.01
**Sanfilippo (Type B) (Type C) (Type D)
 syndrome** E76.22
Sanger-Brown ataxia G11.2
Sao Paulo fever or typhus A77.0
Saponification, mesenteric K65.8
Sarcocele (benign)
 syphilitic A52.76
  congenital A50.59
Sarcocystosis A07.8
Sarcoepiplocele — *see* Hernia
Sarcoepiplomphalocele Q79.2
Sarcoid — *see also* Sarcoidosis
 arthropathy D86.86
 Boeck's D86.9
 Darier-Roussy D86.3
 iridocyclitis D86.83
 meningitis D86.81
 myocarditis D86.85
 myositis D86.87
 pyelonephritis D86.84
 Spiegler-Fendt L08.89
Sarcoidosis D86.9
 with
  cranial nerve palsies D86.82
  hepatic granuloma D86.89
  polyarthritis D86.86
  tubulo-interstitial nephropathy D86.84
 combined sites NEC D86.89
 lung D86.0
  and lymph nodes D86.2
 lymph nodes D86.1
  and lung D86.2
 meninges D86.81
 skin D86.3
 specified type NEC D86.89

Sarcoma (of) — *see also* Neoplasm, connective tissue, malignant
alveolar soft part — *see* Neoplasm, connective tissue, malignant
ameloblastic C41.1
upper jaw (bone) C41.0
botryoid — *see* Neoplasm, connective tissue, malignant
botryoides — *see* Neoplasm, connective tissue, malignant
cerebellar C71.6
circumscribed (arachnoidal) C71.6
circumscribed (arachnoidal) cerebellar C71.6
clear cell — *see also* Neoplasm, connective tissue, malignant
kidney C64-
dendritic cells (accessory cells) C96.4
embryonal — *see* Neoplasm, connective tissue, malignant
endometrial (stromal) C54.1
isthmus C54.0
epithelioid (cell) — *see* Neoplasm, connective tissue, malignant
Ewing's — *see* Neoplasm, bone, malignant
follicular dendritic cell C96.4
germinoblastic (diffuse) — *see* Lymphoma, diffuse large cell
follicular — *see* Lymphoma, follicular, specified NEC
giant cell (except of bone) — *see also* Neoplasm, connective tissue, malignant
bone — *see* Neoplasm, bone, malignant
glomoid — *see* Neoplasm, connective tissue, malignant
granulocytic C92.3-
hemangioendothelial — *see* Neoplasm, connective tissue, malignant
hemorrhagic, multiple — *see* Sarcoma, Kaposi's
histiocytic C96.A **(follows C96.6)**
Hodgkin — *see* Lymphoma, Hodgkin
immunoblastic (diffuse) — *see* Lymphoma, diffuse large cell
interdigitating dendritic cell C96.4
Kaposi's
colon C46.4
connective tissue C46.1
gastrointestinal organ C46.4
lung C46.5-
lymph node(s) C46.3
palate (hard) (soft) C46.2
rectum C46.4
skin C46.0
specified site NEC C46.7
stomach C46.4
unspecified site C46.9
Kupffer cell C22.3
Langerhans cell C96.4
leptomeningeal — *see* Neoplasm, meninges, malignant
liver NEC C22.4
lymphangioendothelial — *see* Neoplasm, connective tissue, malignant
lymphoblastic — *see* Lymphoma, lymphoblastic (diffuse)
lymphocytic — *see* Lymphoma, small cell B-cell
mast cell C96.2
melanotic — *see* Melanoma
meningeal — *see* Neoplasm, meninges, malignant
meningothelial — *see* Neoplasm, meninges, malignant
mesenchymal — *see also* Neoplasm, connective tissue, malignant
mixed — *see* Neoplasm, connective tissue, malignant
mesothelial — *see* Mesothelioma

Sarcoma (of) (*see also* Neoplasm, connective tissue, malignant) — *continued*
monstrocellular
specified site — *see* Neoplasm, malignant, by site
unspecified site C71.9
myeloid C92.3-
neurogenic — *see* Neoplasm, nerve, malignant
odontogenic C41.1
upper jaw (bone) C41.0
osteoblastic — *see* Neoplasm, bone, malignant
osteogenic — *see also* Neoplasm, bone, malignant
juxtacortical — *see* Neoplasm, bone, malignant
periosteal — *see* Neoplasm, bone, malignant
periosteal — *see also* Neoplasm, bone, malignant
osteogenic — *see* Neoplasm, bone, malignant
pleomorphic cell — *see* Neoplasm, connective tissue, malignant
reticulum cell (diffuse) — *see* Lymphoma, diffuse large cell
nodular — *see* Lymphoma, follicular
pleomorphic cell type — *see* Lymphoma, diffuse large cell
rhabdoid — *see* Neoplasm, malignant, by site
round cell — *see* Neoplasm, connective tissue, malignant
small cell — *see* Neoplasm, connective tissue, malignant
soft tissue — *see* Neoplasm, connective tissue, malignant
spindle cell — *see* Neoplasm, connective tissue, malignant
stromal (endometrial) C54.1
isthmus C54.0
synovial — *see also* Neoplasm, connective tissue, malignant
biphasic — *see* Neoplasm, connective tissue, malignant
epithelioid cell — *see* Neoplasm, connective tissue, malignant
spindle cell — *see* Neoplasm, connective tissue, malignant
Sarcomatosis
meningeal — *see* Neoplasm, meninges, malignant
specified site NEC — *see* Neoplasm, connective tissue, malignant
unspecified site C80.1
Sarcopenia (age-related) M62.84
Sarcosinemia E72.59
Sarcosporidiosis (intestinal) A07.8
Satiety, early R68.81
Saturnine — *see* condition
Saturnism
overdose or wrong substance given or taken — *see* Table of Drugs and Chemicals, by drug, poisoning
Satyriasis F52.8
Sauriasis — *see* Ichthyosis
SBE (subacute bacterial endocarditis) I33.0
Scabies (any site) B86
Scabs R23.4
Scaglietti-Dagnini syndrome E22.0
Scald — *see* Burn
Scalenus anticus (anterior) syndrome G54.0
Scales R23.4
Scaling, skin R23.4
Scalp — *see* condition
Scapegoating affecting child Z62.3
Scaphocephaly Q75.0
Scapulalgia M89.8x1
Scapulohumeral myopathy G71.0

Scar, scarring (*see also* Cicatrix) L90.5
adherent L90.5
atrophic L90.5
cervix
in pregnancy or childbirth — *see* Pregnancy, complicated by, abnormal cervix
cheloid L91.0
chorioretinal H31.00-
posterior pole macula H31.01-
postsurgical H59.81-
solar retinopathy H31.02-
specified type NEC H31.09-
choroid — *see* Scar, chorioretinal
conjunctiva H11.24-
cornea H17.9
xerophthalmic — *see also* Opacity, cornea
vitamin A deficiency E50.6
duodenum, obstructive K31.5
hypertrophic L91.0
keloid L91.0
labia N90.89
lung (base) J98.4
macula — *see* Scar, chorioretinal, posterior pole
muscle M62.89
myocardium, myocardial I25.2
painful L90.5
posterior pole (eye) — *see* Scar, chorioretinal, posterior pole
retina — *see* Scar, chorioretinal
trachea J39.8
transmural uterine, in pregnancy O34.29
uterus N85.8
in pregnancy O34.29
vagina N89.8
postoperative N99.2
vulva N90.89
Scarabiasis B88.2
Scarlatina (anginosa) (maligna) (ulcerosa) A38.9
myocarditis (acute) A38.1
old — *see* Myocarditis
otitis media A38.0
Scarlet fever (albuminuria) (angina) A38.9
Schamberg's disease (progressive pigmentary dermatosis) L81.7
Schatzki's ring (acquired) (esophagus) (lower) K22.2
congenital Q39.3
Schaufenster krankheit I20.8
Schaumann's
benign lymphogranulomatosis D86.1
disease or syndrome — *see* Sarcoidosis
Scheie's syndrome E76.03
Schenck's disease B42.1
Scheuermann's disease or osteochondrosis — *see* Osteochondrosis, juvenile, spine
Schilder(-Flatau) disease G37.0
Schilling-type monocytic leukemia C93.0-
Schimmelbusch's disease, cystic mastitis, or hyperplasia — *see* Mastopathy, cystic
Schistosoma infestation — *see* Infestation, Schistosoma
Schistosomiasis B65.9
with muscle disorder B65.9 *[M63.80]*
ankle B65.9 *[M63.8-]*
foot B65.9 *[M63.8-]*
forearm B65.9 *[M63.8-]*
hand B65.9 *[M63.8-]*
lower leg B65.9 *[M63.8-]*
multiple sites B65.9 *[M63.89]*
pelvic region B65.9 *[M63.8-]*
shoulder region B65.9 *[M63.8-]*
specified site NEC B65.9 *[M63.88]*
thigh B65.9 *[M63.8-]*
upper arm B65.9 *[M63.8-]*
Asiatic B65.2
bladder B65.0

Schistosomiasis B65.9 — *continued*
  chestermani B65.8
  colon B65.1
  cutaneous B65.3
  due to
    S. haematobium B65.0
    S. japonicum B65.2
    S. mansoni B65.1
    S. mattheii B65.8
  Eastern B65.2
  genitourinary tract B65.0
  intestinal B65.1
  lung NEC B65.9 [J99]
    pneumonia B65.9 [J17]
  Manson's (intestinal) B65.1
  oriental B65.2
  pulmonary NEC B65.9 [J99]
    pneumonia B65.9
  Schistosoma
    haematobium B65.0
    japonicum B65.2
    mansoni B65.1
  specified type NEC B65.8
  urinary B65.0
  vesical B65.0
Schizencephaly Q04.6
Schizoaffective psychosis F25.9
Schizodontia K00.2
Schizoid personality F60.1
Schizophrenia, schizophrenic F20.9
  acute (brief) (undifferentiated) F23
  atypical (form) F20.3
  borderline F21
  catalepsy F20.2
  catatonic (type) (excited) (withdrawn) F20.2
  cenesthopathic, cenesthesiopathic F20.89
  childhood type F84.5
  chronic undifferentiated F20.5
  cyclic F25.0
  disorganized (type) F20.1
  flexibilitas cerea F20.2
  hebephrenic (type) F20.1
  incipient F21
  latent F21
  negative type F20.5
  paranoid (type) F20.0
  paraphrenic F20.0
  post-psychotic depression F32.89
  prepsychotic F21
  prodromal F21
  pseudoneurotic F21
  pseudopsychopathic F21
  reaction F23
  residual (state) (type) F20.5
  restzustand F20.5
  schizoaffective (type) — *see* Psychosis, schizoaffective
  simple (type) F20.89
  simplex F20.89
  specified type NEC F20.89
  stupor F20.2
  syndrome of childhood F84.5
  undifferentiated (type) F20.3
    chronic F20.5
Schizothymia (persistent) F60.1
Schlatter-Osgood disease or osteochondrosis — *see* Osteochondrosis, juvenile, tibia
Schlatter's tibia — *see* Osteochondrosis, juvenile, tibia
Schmidt's syndrome (polyglandular, autoimmune) E31.0
Schmincke's carcinoma or tumor — *see* Neoplasm, nasopharynx, malignant
Schmitz(-Stutzer) dysentery A03.0

Schmorl's disease or nodes
  lumbar region M51.46
  lumbosacral region M51.47
  sacrococcygeal region M53.3
  thoracic region M51.44
  thoracolumbar region M51.45
Schneiderian
  papilloma — *see* Neoplasm, nasopharynx, benign
    specified site — *see* Neoplasm, benign, by site
    unspecified site D14.0
  specified site — *see* Neoplasm, malignant, by site
  unspecified site C30.0
Scholte's syndrome (malignant carcinoid) E34.0
Scholz(-Bielchowsky-Henneberg) disease or syndrome E75.25
Schönlein(-Henoch) disease or purpura (primary) (rheumatic) D69.0
Schottmuller's disease A01.4
Schroeder's syndrome (endocrine hypertensive) E27.0
Schüller-Christian disease or syndrome C96.5
Schultze's type acroparesthesia, simple I73.89
Schultz's disease or syndrome — *see* Agranulocytosis
Schwalbe-Ziehen-Oppenheim disease G24.1
Schwannoma — *see also* Neoplasm, nerve, benign
  malignant — *see also* Neoplasm, nerve, malignant
    with rhabdomyoblastic differentiation — *see* Neoplasm, nerve, malignant
  melanocytic (9560/0) — *see* Neoplasm, nerve, benign
  pigmented — *see* Neoplasm, nerve, benign
Schwannomatosis Q85.03
Schwartz-Bartter syndrome E22.2
Schwartz(-Jampel) syndrome G71.13
Schweniger-Buzzi anetoderma L90.1
Sciatic — *see* condition
Sciatica (infective)
  with lumbago M54.4-
    due to intervertebral disc disorder — *see* Disorder, disc, with, radiculopathy
  due to displacement of intervertebral disc (with lumbago) — *see* Disorder, disc, with, radiculopathy
  wallet M54.3-
Scimitar syndrome Q26.8
Sclera — *see* condition
Sclerectasia H15.84-
Scleredema
  adultorum — *see* Sclerosis, systemic
  Buschke's — *see* Sclerosis, systemic
  newborn P83.8
Sclerema (adiposum) (edematosum) (neonatorum) (newborn) P83.0
  adultorum — *see* Sclerosis, systemic
Scleriasis — *see* Scleroderma
Scleritis H15.00-
  with corneal involvement H15.04-
  anterior H15.01-
  brawny H15.02-
  in (due to) zoster B02.34
  posterior H15.03-
  specified type NEC H15.09-
  syphilitic A52.71
  tuberculous (nodular) A18.51
Sclerochoroiditis H31.8
Scleroconjunctivitis — *see* Scleritis
Sclerocystic ovary syndrome E28.2
Sclerodactyly, sclerodactylia L94.3

Scleroderma, sclerodermia (acrosclerotic) (diffuse) (generalized) (progressive) (pulmonary) (*see also* Sclerosis, systemic) M34.9-
  circumscribed L94.0
  linear L94.1
  localized L94.0
  newborn P83.8
  systemic M34.9
Sclerokeratitis H16.8
  tuberculous A18.52
Scleroma nasi A48.8
Scleromalacia (perforans) H15.05-
Scleromyxedema L98.5
Sclérose en plaques G35
Sclerosis, sclerotic
  adrenal (gland) E27.8
  Alzheimer's — *see* Disease, Alzheimer's
  amyotrophic (lateral) G12.21
  aorta, aortic I70.0
    valve — *see* Endocarditis, aortic
  artery, arterial, arteriolar, arteriovascular — *see* Arteriosclerosis
  ascending multiple G35
  brain (generalized) (lobular) G37.9
    artery, arterial I67.2
    diffuse G37.0
    disseminated G35
    insular G35
    Krabbe's E75.23
    miliary G35
    multiple G35
    presenile (Alzheimer's) — *see* Disease, Alzheimer's, early onset
    senile (arteriosclerotic) I67.2
    stem, multiple G35
    tuberous Q85.1
  bulbar, multiple G35
  bundle of His I44.39
  cardiac — *see* Disease, heart, ischemic, atherosclerotic
  cardiorenal — *see* Hypertension, cardiorenal
  cardiovascular — *see also* Disease, cardiovascular
    renal — *see* Hypertension, cardiorenal
  cerebellar — *see* Sclerosis, brain
  cerebral — *see* Sclerosis, brain
  cerebrospinal (disseminated) (multiple) G35
  cerebrovascular I67.2
  choroid — *see* Degeneration, choroid
  combined (spinal cord) — *see also* Degeneration, combined
    multiple G35
  concentric (Balo) G37.5
  cornea — *see* Opacity, cornea
  coronary (artery) I25.10
    with angina pectoris — *see* Arteriosclerosis, coronary (artery),
  corpus cavernosum
    female N90.89
    male N48.6
  diffuse (brain) (spinal cord) G37.0
  disseminated G35
  dorsal G35
  dorsolateral (spinal cord) — *see* Degeneration, combined
  endometrium N85.5
  extrapyramidal G25.9
  eye, nuclear (senile) — *see* Cataract, senile, nuclear
  focal and segmental (glomerular) (*see also* N00-N07 with fourth character .1) N05.1
  Friedreich's (spinal cord) G11.1
  funicular (spermatic cord) N50.89
  general (vascular) — *see* Arteriosclerosis
  gland (lymphatic) I89.8
  hepatic K74.1
    alcoholic K70.2

Sclerosis, sclerotic — *continued*
  hereditary
    cerebellar G11.9
    spinal (Friedreich's ataxia) G11.1
  hippocampal G93.81
  insular G35
  kidney — *see* Sclerosis, renal
  larynx J38.7
  lateral (amyotrophic) (descending) (primary)
    (spinal) G12.21
  lens, senile nuclear — *see* Cataract, senile,
    nuclear
  liver K74.1
    with fibrosis K74.2
      alcoholic K70.2
    alcoholic K70.2
    cardiac K76.1
  lung — *see* Fibrosis, lung
  mastoid — *see* Mastoiditis, chronic
  mesial temporal G93.81
  mitral I05.8
  Mönckeberg's (medial) — *see* Arteriosclerosis,
    extremities
  multiple (brain stem) (cerebral) (generalized)
    (spinal cord) G35
  myocardium, myocardial — *see* Disease,
    heart, ischemic, atherosclerotic
  nuclear (senile), eye — *see* Cataract, senile,
    nuclear
  ovary N83.8
  pancreas K86.89
  penis N48.6
  peripheral arteries — *see* Arteriosclerosis,
    extremities
  plaques G35
  pluriglandular E31.8
  polyglandular E31.8
  posterolateral (spinal cord) — *see*
    Degeneration, combined
  presenile (Alzheimer's) — *see* Disease,
    Alzheimer's, early onset
  primary, lateral G12.29
  progressive, systemic M34.0
  pulmonary — *see* Fibrosis, lung
    artery I27.0
    valve (heart) — *see* Endocarditis, pulmonary
  renal N26.9
    with
      cystine storage disease E72.09
      hypertensive heart disease (conditions in
        I11) — *see* Hypertension, cardiorenal
    arteriolar (hyaline) (hyperplastic) — *see*
      Hypertension, kidney
  retina (senile) (vascular) H35.00
  senile (vascular) — *see* Arteriosclerosis
  spinal (cord) (progressive) G95.89
    ascending G61.0
    combined — *see also* Degeneration,
      combined
      multiple G35
      syphilitic A52.11
    disseminated G35
    dorsolateral — *see* Degeneration, combined
    hereditary (Friedreich's) (mixed form) G11.1
    lateral (amyotrophic) G12.21
    multiple G35
    posterior (syphilitic) A52.11
  stomach K31.89
  subendocardial, congenital I42.4
  systemic M34.9
    with
      lung involvement M34.81
      myopathy M34.82
      polyneuropathy M34.83
    drug-induced M34.2
    due to chemicals NEC M34.2
    progressive M34.0
    specified NEC M34.89

Sclerosis, sclerotic — *continued*
  temporal (mesial) G93.81
  tricuspid (heart) (valve) I07.8
  tuberous (brain) Q85.1
  tympanic membrane — *see* Disorder, tympanic
    membrane, specified NEC
  valve, valvular (heart) — *see* Endocarditis
  vascular — *see* Arteriosclerosis
  vein I87.8
Scoliosis (acquired) (postural) M41.9
  adolescent (idiopathic) — *see* Scoliosis,
    idiopathic, adolescent
  congenital Q67.5
    due to bony malformation Q76.3
    failure of segmentation (hemivertebra)
      Q76.3
    hemivertebra fusion Q76.3
    postural Q67.5
  idiopathic M41.20
    adolescent M41.129
      cervical region M41.122
      cervicothoracic region M41.123
      lumbar region M41.126
      lumbosacral region M41.127
      thoracic region M41.124
      thoracolumbar region M41.125
    cervical region M41.22
    cervicothoracic region M41.23
    infantile M41.00
      cervical region M41.02
      cervicothoracic region M41.03
      lumbar region M41.06
      lumbosacral region M41.07
      sacrococcygeal region M41.08
      thoracic region M41.04
      thoracolumbar region M41.05
    juvenile M41.119
      cervical region M41.112
      cervicothoracic region M41.113
      lumbar region M41.116
      lumbosacral region M41.117
      thoracic region M41.114
      thoracolumbar region M41.115
    lumbar region M41.26
    lumbosacral region M41.27
    thoracic region M41.24
    thoracolumbar region M41.25
  infantile — *see* Scoliosis, idiopathic, infantile
  neuromuscular M41.40
    cervical region M41.42
    cervicothoracic region M41.43
    lumbar region M41.46
    lumbosacral region M41.47
    occipito-atlanto-axial region M41.41
    thoracic region M41.44
    thoracolumbar region M41.45
  paralytic — *see* Scoliosis, neuromuscular
  postradiation therapy M96.5
  rachitic (late effect or sequelae) E64.3
    [M49.80]
    cervical region E64.3 *[M49.82]*
    cervicothoracic region E64.3 *[M49.83]*
    lumbar region E64.3 *[M49.86]*
    lumbosacral region E64.3 *[M49.87]*
    multiple sites E64.3 *[M49.89]*
    occipito-atlanto-axial region E64.3
      [M49.81]
    sacrococcygeal region E64.3 *[M49.88]*
    thoracic region E64.3 *[M49.84]*
    thoracolumbar region E64.3 *[M49.85]*
  sciatic M54.4-
  secondary (to) NEC M41.50
    cerebral palsy, Friedreich's ataxia,
      poliomyelitis, neuromuscular disorders
      — *see* Scoliosis, neuromuscular
    cervical region M41.52
    cervicothoracic region M41.53
    lumbar region M41.56
    lumbosacral region M41.57

Scoliosis (acquired) (postural) M41.9 —
continued
  secondary (to) NEC M41.50 — *continued*
    thoracic region M41.54
    thoracolumbar region M41.55
    specified form NEC M41.80
      cervical region M41.82
      cervicothoracic region M41.83
      lumbar region M41.86
      lumbosacral region M41.87
      thoracic region M41.84
      thoracolumbar region M41.85
    thoracogenic M41.30
      thoracic region M41.34
      thoracolumbar region M41.35
    tuberculous A18.01
Scoliotic pelvis
  with disproportion (fetopelvic) O33.0
    causing obstructed labor O65.0
Scorbutus, scorbutic — *see also* Scurvy
  anemia D53.2
Score, NIHSS (National Institutes of Health
  Stroke Scale) R29.7-
Scotoma (arcuate) (Bjerrum) (central) (ring) —
  see also Defect, visual field, localized,
  scotoma
  scintillating H53.19
Scratch — *see* Abrasion
Scratchy throat R09.89
Screening (for) Z13.9
  alcoholism Z13.89
  anemia Z13.0
  anomaly, congenital Z13.89
  antenatal, of mother Z36
  arterial hypertension Z13.6
  arthropod-borne viral disease NEC Z11.59
  bacteriuria, asymptomatic Z13.89
  behavioral disorder Z13.89
  brain injury, traumatic Z13.850
  bronchitis, chronic Z13.83
  brucellosis Z11.2
  cardiovascular disorder Z13.6
  cataract Z13.5
  chlamydial diseases Z11.8
  cholera Z11.0
  chromosomal abnormalities (nonprocreative)
    NEC Z13.79
  colonoscopy Z12.11
  congenital
    dislocation of hip Z13.89
    eye disorder Z13.5
    malformation or deformation Z13.89
  contamination NEC Z13.88
  cystic fibrosis Z13.228
  dengue fever Z11.59
  dental disorder Z13.84
  depression Z13.89
  developmental handicap Z13.42
    in early childhood Z13.42
    infant Z13.41
  diabetes mellitus Z13.1
  diphtheria Z11.2
  disability, intellectual Z13.42
    infant Z13.41
  disease or disorder Z13.9
    bacterial NEC Z11.2
      intestinal infectious Z11.0
      respiratory tuberculosis Z11.1
    blood or blood-forming organ Z13.0
    cardiovascular Z13.6
    Chagas' Z11.6
    chlamydial Z11.8
    dental Z13.89
    developmental Z13.42
      in child Z13.42
      infant Z13.41
    digestive tract NEC Z13.818
      lower GI Z13.811
      upper GI Z13.810

Screening (for) Z13.9 — *continued*
  disease or disorder Z13.9 — *continued*
    ear Z13.5
    endocrine Z13.29
    eye Z13.5
    genitourinary Z13.89
    heart Z13.6
    human immunodeficiency virus (HIV)
      infection Z11.4
    immunity Z13.0
    infection
      intestinal Z11.0
        specified NEC Z11.6
    infectious Z11.9
    mental Z13.89
    metabolic Z13.228
    neurological Z13.89
    nutritional Z13.21
      metabolic Z13.228
        lipoid disorders Z13.220
    protozoal Z11.6
      intestinal Z11.0
    respiratory Z13.83
    rheumatic Z13.828
    rickettsial Z11.8
    sexually-transmitted NEC Z11.3
      human immunodeficiency virus (HIV)
        Z11.4
    sickle-cell (trait) Z13.0
    skin Z13.89
    specified NEC Z13.89
    spirochetal Z11.8
    thyroid Z13.29
    vascular Z13.6
    venereal Z11.3
    viral NEC Z11.59
      human immunodeficiency virus (HIV)
        Z11.4
      intestinal Z11.0
  elevated titer Z13.89
  emphysema Z13.83
  encephalitis, viral (mosquito-or tick-borne)
    Z11.59
  exposure to contaminants (toxic) Z13.88
  fever
    dengue Z11.59
    hemorrhagic Z11.59
    yellow Z11.59
  filariasis Z11.6
  galactosemia Z13.228
  gastrointestinal condition Z13.818
  genetic (nonprocreative)
    disease carrier status (nonprocreative)
      Z13.71
    for procreative management — *see* Testing,
      genetic, for procreative management
    specified NEC (nonprocreative) Z13.79
  genitourinary condition Z13.89
  glaucoma Z13.5
  gonorrhea Z11.3
  gout Z13.89
  helminthiasis (intestinal) Z11.6
  hematopoietic malignancy Z12.89
  hemoglobinopathies NEC Z13.0
  hemorrhagic fever Z11.59
  Hodgkin disease Z12.89
  human immunodeficiency virus (HIV) Z11.4
  human papillomavirus Z11.51
  hypertension Z13.6
  immunity disorders Z13.0
  infection
    mycotic Z11.8
    parasitic Z11.8
  ingestion of radioactive substance Z13.88
  intellectual disability Z13.42
    infant Z13.41
  intestinal
    helminthiasis Z11.6
    infectious disease Z11.0

Screening (for) Z13.9 — *continued*
  leishmaniasis Z11.6
  leprosy Z11.2
  leptospirosis Z11.8
  leukemia Z12.89
  lymphoma Z12.89
  malaria Z11.6
  malnutrition Z13.29
    metabolic Z13.228
    nutritional Z13.21
  measles Z11.59
  mental disorder Z13.89
  metabolic errors, inborn Z13.228
  multiphasic Z13.89
  musculoskeletal disorder Z13.828
    osteoporosis Z13.820
  mycoses Z11.8
  myocardial infarction (acute) Z13.6
  neoplasm (malignant) (of) Z12.9
    bladder Z12.6
    blood Z12.89
    breast Z12.39
      routine mammogram Z12.31
    cervix Z12.4
    colon Z12.11
    genitourinary organs NEC Z12.79
      bladder Z12.6
      cervix Z12.4
      ovary Z12.73
      prostate Z12.5
      testis Z12.71
      vagina Z12.72
    hematopoietic system Z12.89
    intestinal tract Z12.10
      colon Z12.11
      rectum Z12.12
      small intestine Z12.13
    lung Z12.2
    lymph (glands) Z12.89
    nervous system Z12.82
    oral cavity Z12.81
    prostate Z12.5
    rectum Z12.12
    respiratory organs Z12.2
    skin Z12.83
    small intestine Z12.13
    specified site NEC Z12.89
    stomach Z12.0
  nephropathy Z13.89
  nervous system disorders NEC Z13.858
  neurological condition Z13.89
  osteoporosis Z13.820
  parasitic infestation Z11.9
    specified NEC Z11.8
  phenylketonuria Z13.228
  plague Z11.2
  poisoning (chemical) (heavy metal) Z13.88
  poliomyelitis Z11.59
  postnatal, chromosomal abnormalities Z13.89
  prenatal, of mother Z36
  protozoal disease Z11.6
    intestinal Z11.0
  pulmonary tuberculosis Z11.1
  radiation exposure Z13.88
  respiratory condition Z13.83
  respiratory tuberculosis Z11.1
  rheumatoid arthritis Z13.828
  rubella Z11.59
  schistosomiasis Z11.6
  sexually-transmitted disease NEC Z11.3
    human immunodeficiency virus (HIV) Z11.4
  sickle-cell disease or trait Z13.0
  skin condition Z13.89
  sleeping sickness Z11.6
  special Z13.9
    specified NEC Z13.89
  syphilis Z11.3
  tetanus Z11.2
  trachoma Z11.8

Screening (for) Z13.9 — *continued*
  traumatic brain injury Z13.850
  trypanosomiasis Z11.6
  tuberculosis, respiratory Z11.1
  venereal disease Z11.3
  viral encephalitis (mosquito-or tick-borne)
    Z11.59
  whooping cough Z11.2
  worms, intestinal Z11.6
  yaws Z11.8
  yellow fever Z11.59
Scrofula, scrofulosis (tuberculosis of cervical
  lymph glands) A18.2
Scrofulide (primary) (tuberculous) A18.4
Scrofuloderma, scrofulodermia (any site)
  (primary) A18.4
Scrofulosus lichen (primary) (tuberculous)
  A18.4
Scrofulous — *see* condition
Scrotal tongue K14.5
Scrotum — *see* condition
Scurvy, scorbutic E54
  anemia D53.2
  gum E54
  infantile E54
  rickets E55.0 *[M90.80]*
Sealpox B08.62
Seasickness T75.3
Seatworm (infection) (infestation) B80
Sebaceous — *see also* condition
  cyst — *see* Cyst, sebaceous
Seborrhea, seborrheic L21.9
  capillitii R23.8
  capitis L21.0
  dermatitis L21.9
    infantile L21.1
  eczema L21.9
    infantile L21.1
  sicca L21.0
Seckel's syndrome Q87.1
Seclusion, pupil — *see* Membrane, pupillary
Second hand tobacco smoke exposure
  (acute) (chronic) Z77.22
  in the perinatal period P96.81
Secondary
  dentin (in pulp) K04.3
  neoplasm, secondaries — *see* Table of
    Neoplasms, secondary
Secretion
  antidiuretic hormone, inappropriate E22.2
  catecholamine, by pheochromocytoma E27.5
  hormone
    antidiuretic, inappropriate (syndrome) E22.2
    by
      carcinoid tumor E34.0
      pheochromocytoma E27.5
    ectopic NEC E34.2
  urinary
    excessive R35.8
    suppression R34
Section
  nerve, traumatic — *see* Injury, nerve
Sedative, hypnotic, or anxiolytic-induced
  anxiety disorder F13.980
  bipolar and related disorder F13.94
  delirium F13.921
  depressive disorder F13.94
  major neurocognitive disorder F13.97
  mild neurocognitive disorder F13.988
  psychotic disorder F13.959
  sexual dysfunction F13.981
  sleep disorder F13.982
Segmentation, incomplete (congenital) —
  see also Fusion
  bone NEC Q78.8
  lumbosacral (joint) (vertebra) Q76.49
Seitelberger's syndrome (infantile
  neuraxonal dystrophy) G31.89

Seizure(s) (see also Convulsions) R56.9
 akinetic — see Epilepsy, generalized, specified NEC
 atonic — see Epilepsy, generalized, specified NEC
 autonomic (hysterical) F44.5
 convulsive — see Convulsions
 cortical (focal) (motor) — see Epilepsy, localization-related, symptomatic, with simple partial seizures
 disorder (see also Eplepsy) G40.909
 due to stroke — see Sequelae (of), disease, cerebrovascular, by type, specified NEC
 epileptic — see Epilepsy
 febrile (simple) R56.00
  with status epilepticus G40.901
  complex (atypical) (complicated) R56.01
   with status epilepticus G40.901
 grand mal G40.409
  intractable G40.419
   with status epilepticus G40.411
   without status epilepticus G40.419
  not intractable G40.409
   with status epilepticus G40.401
   without status epilepticus G40.409
 heart — see Disease, heart
 hysterical F44.5
 intractable G40.919
  with status epilepticus G40.911
 Jacksonian (focal) (motor type) (sensory type) — see Epilepsy, localization-related, symptomatic, with simple partial seizures
 newborn P90
 nonspecific epileptic
  atonic — see Epilepsy, generalized, specified NEC
  clonic — see Epilepsy, generalized, specified NEC
  myoclonic — see Epilepsy, generalized, specified NEC
  tonic — see Epilepsy, generalized, specified NEC
  tonic-clonic — see Epilepsy, generalized, specified NEC
 partial, developing into secondarily generalized seizures
  complex — see Epilepsy, localization-related, symptomatic, with complex partial seizures
  simple — see Epilepsy, localization-related, symptomatic, with simple partial seizures
 petit mal G40.409
  intractable G40.419
   with status epilepticus G40.411
   without status epilepticus G40.419
  not intractable G40.409
   with status epilepticus G40.401
   without status epilepticus G40.409
 post traumatic R56.1
 recurrent G40.909
 specified NEC G40.89
 uncinate — see Epilepsy, localization-related, symptomatic, with complex partial seizures
Selenium deficiency, dietary E59
Self-damaging behavior (life-style) Z72.89
Self-harm (attempted)
 history (personal) Z91.5
  in family Z81.8
Self-mutilation (attempted)
 history (personal) Z91.5
  in family Z81.8
Self-poisoning
 history (personal) Z91.5
  in family Z81.8
 observation following (alleged) attempt Z03.6
Semicoma R40.1
Seminal vesiculitis N49.0

Seminoma C62.9-
 specified site — see Neoplasm, malignant, by site
Senear-Usher disease or syndrome L10.4
Senectus R54
Senescence (without mention of psychosis) R54
Senile, senility (see also condition) R41.81
 with
  acute confusional state F05
  mental changes NOS F03
  psychosis NEC — see Psychosis, senile
 asthenia R54
 cervix (atrophic) N88.8
 debility R54
 endometrium (atrophic) N85.8
 fallopian tube (atrophic) — see Atrophy, fallopian tube
 heart (failure) R54
 ovary (atrophic) — see Atrophy, ovary
 premature E34.8
 vagina, vaginitis (atrophic) N95.2
 wart L82.1
Sensation
 burning (skin) R20.8
  tongue K14.6
 loss of R20.8
 prickling (skin) R20.2
 tingling (skin) R20.2
Sense loss
 smell — see Disturbance, sensation, smell
 taste — see Disturbance, sensation, taste
 touch R20.8
Sensibility disturbance (cortical) (deep) (vibratory) R20.9
Sensitive, sensitivity — see also Allergy
 carotid sinus G90.01
 child (excessive) F93.8
 cold, autoimmune D59.1
 dentin K03.89
 gluten (non-celiac) K90.41
 latex Z91.040
 methemoglobin D74.8
 tuberculin, without clinical or radiological symptoms R76.11
 visual
  glare H53.71
  impaired contrast H53.72
Sensitiver Beziehungswahn F22
Sensitization, auto-erythrocytic D69.2
Separation
 anxiety, abnormal (of childhood) F93.0
 apophysis, traumatic — code as Fracture, by site
 choroid — see Detachment, choroid
 epiphysis, epiphyseal
  nontraumatic — see also Osteochondropathy, specified type NEC
   upper femoral — see Slipped, epiphysis, upper femoral
  traumatic — code as Fracture, by site
 fracture — see Fracture
 infundibulum cardiac from right ventricle by a partition Q24.3
 joint (traumatic) (current) — code by site under Dislocation
 pubic bone, obstetrical trauma O71.6
 retina, retinal — see Detachment, retina
 symphysis pubis, obstetrical trauma O71.6
 tracheal ring, incomplete, congenital Q32.1
Sepsis (generalized) (unspecified organism) A41.9
 with
  organ dysfunction (acute) (multiple) R65.20
   with septic shock R65.21
 actinomycotic A42.7
 adrenal hemorrhage syndrome (meningococcal) A39.1
 anaerobic A41.4
 Bacillus anthracis A22.7

Sepsis (generalized) (unspecified organism) A41.9 — continued
 Brucella (see also Brucellosis) A23.9
 candidal B37.7
 cryptogenic A41.9
 due to device, implant or graft T85.79
  arterial graft NEC T82.7
  breast (implant) T85.79
  catheter NEC T85.79
   dialysis (renal) T82.7
    intraperitoneal T85.71
   infusion NEC T82.7
    spinal (cranial) (epidural) (intrathecal) (spinal) (subarachnoid) (subdural) T85.735
   urethral indwelling T83.511
   urinary T83.518
  ectopic or molar pregnancy O08.82
  electronic (electrode) (pulse generator) (stimulator)
   bone T84.7
   cardiac T82.7
   nervous system T85.738
    brain T85.731
    neurostimulator generator T85.734
    peripheral nerve T85.732
    spinal cord T85.733
   urinary T83.590
  fixation, internal (orthopedic) — see Complication, fixation device, infection
  gastrointestinal (bile duct) (esophagus) T85.79
  neurostimulator electrode (lead) T85.732
  genital T83.69
  heart NEC T82.7
   valve (prosthesis) T82.6
    graft T82.7
  joint prosthesis — see Complication, joint prosthesis, infection
  ocular (corneal graft) (orbital implant) T85.79
  orthopedic NEC T84.7
   fixation device, internal — see Complication, fixation device, infection
  specified NEC T85.79
  vascular T82.7
  ventricular intracranial (communicating) shunt T85.730
 during labor O75.3
 Enterococcus A41.81
 Erysipelothrix (rhusiopathiae) (erysipeloid) A26.7
 Escherichia coli (E. coli) A41.5
 extraintestinal yersiniosis A28.2
 following
  abortion (subsequent episode) O08.0
   current episode — see Abortion
  ectopic or molar pregnancy O08.82
  immunization T88.0
  infusion, therapeutic injection or transfusion NEC T80.29
 gangrenous A41.9
 gonococcal A54.86
 Gram-negative (organism) A41.5
  anaerobic A41.4
 Haemophilus influenzae A41.3
 herpesviral B00.7
 intra-abdominal K65.1
 intraocular — see Endophthalmitis, purulent
 Listeria monocytogenes A32.7
 localized — code to specific localized infection
  in operation wound T81.49
  skin — see Abscess
 malleus A24.0
 melioidosis A24.1
 meningeal — see Meningitis

Sepsis (generalized) (unspecified organism)
  A41.9 — *continued*
  meningococcal A39.4
    acute A39.2
    chronic A39.3
  MSSA (methicillin susceptible Staphylococcus aureus) A41.01
  newborn P36.9
    due to
      anaerobes NEC P36.5
      Escherichia coli P36.4
      Staphylococcus P36.30
        aureus P36.2
        specified NEC P36.39
      Streptococcus P36.10
        group B P36.0
        specified NEC P36.19
      specified NEC P36.8
  Pasteurella multocida A28.0
  pelvic, puerperal, postpartum, childbirth O85
  pneumococcal A40.3
  postprocedural T81.49
  puerperal, postpartum, childbirth (pelvic) O85
  Salmonella (arizonae) (cholerae-suis) (enteritidis) (typhimurium) A02.1
  severe R65.20
    with septic shock R65.21
  Shigella (*see also* Dysentery, bacillary) A03.9
  skin, localized — *see* Abscess
  specified organism NEC A41.89
  Staphylococcus, staphylococcal A41.2
    aureus (methicillin susceptible) (MSSA) A41.01
      methicillin resistant (MRSA) A41.02
    coagulase-negative A41.1
    specified NEC A41.1
  Streptococcus, streptococcal A40.9
    agalactiae A40.1
    group
      A A40.0
      B A40.1
      D A41.81
    neonatal P36.10
      group B P36.0
      specified NEC P36.19
    pneumoniae A40.3
    pyogenes A40.0
    specified NEC A40.8
  tracheostomy stoma J95.02
  tularemic A21.7
  umbilical, umbilical cord (newborn) — *see* Sepsis, newborn
  Yersinia pestis A20.7
Septate — *see* Septum
Septic — *see* condition
  arm — *see* Cellulitis, upper limb
    with lymphangitis — *see* Lymphangitis, acute, upper limb
  embolus — *see* Embolism
  finger — *see* Cellulitis, digit
    with lymphangitis — *see* Lymphangitis, acute, digit
  foot — *see* Cellulitis, lower limb
    with lymphangitis — *see* Lymphangitis, acute, lower limb
  gallbladder (acute) K81.0
  hand — *see* Cellulitis, upper limb
    with lymphangitis — *see* Lymphangitis, acute, upper limb
  joint — *see* Arthritis, pyogenic or pyemic
  leg — *see* Cellulitis, lower limb
    with lymphangitis — *see* Lymphangitis, acute, lower limb
  nail — *see also* Cellulitis, digit
    with lymphangitis — *see* Lymphangitis, acute, digit
  sore — *see also* Abscess
    throat J02.0
      streptococcal J02.0

Septic — *see* condition — *continued*
  spleen (acute) D73.89
  teeth, tooth (pulpal origin) K04.4
  throat — *see* Pharyngitis
  thrombus — *see* Thrombosis
  toe — *see* Cellulitis, digit
    with lymphangitis — *see* Lymphangitis, acute, digit
  tonsils, chronic J35.01
    with adenoiditis J35.03
  uterus — *see* Endometritis
Septicemia A41.9
  meaning sepsis — *see* Sepsis
Septum, septate (congenital) — *see also* Anomaly, by site
  anal Q42.3
    with fistula Q42.2
  aqueduct of Sylvius Q03.0
    with spina bifida — *see* Spina bifida, by site, with hydrocephalus
  uterus (complete) (partial) Q51.2
  vagina Q52.10
    in pregnancy — *see* Pregnancy, complicated by, abnormal vagina
      causing obstructed labor O65.5
    longitudinal Q52.129
      microperforate
        left side Q52.124
        right side Q52.123
      nonobstruction Q52.120
      obstructing Q52.129
        left side Q52.122
        right side Q52.121
    transverse Q52.11
Sequelae (of) — *see also* condition
  abscess, intracranial or intraspinal (conditions in G06) G09
  amputation — *code to* injury with seventh character S
  burn and corrosion — *code to* injury with seventh character S
  calcium deficiency E64.8
  cerebrovascular disease — *see* Sequelae, disease, cerebrovascular
  childbirth O94
  contusion — *code to* injury with seventh character S
  corrosion — *see* Sequelae, burn and corrosion
  crushing injury — *code to* injury with seventh character S
  disease
    cerebrovascular I69.90
      alteration of sensation I69.998
      aphasia I69.920
      apraxia I69.990
      ataxia I69.993
      cognitive deficits I69.91
      disturbance of vision I69.998
      dysarthria I69.922
      dysphagia I69.991
      dysphasia I69.921
      facial droop I69.992
      facial weakness I69.992
      fluency disorder I69.923
      hemiplegia I69.95-
      hemorrhage
        intracerebral — *see* Sequelae, hemorrhage, intracerebral
        intracranial, nontraumatic NEC — *see* Sequelae, hemorrhage, intracranial, nontraumatic
        subarachnoid — *see* Sequelae, hemorrhage, subarachnoid
      language deficit I69.928
      monoplegia
        lower limb I69.84-
        upper limb I69.93-
      paralytic syndrome I69.96-
      specified effect NEC I69.998

Sequelae (of) (*see also* condition) — *continued*
  disease — *continued*
    cerebrovascular I69.90 — *continued*
      specified type NEC I69.80
        alteration of sensation I69.898
        aphasia I69.820
        apraxia I69.890
        ataxia I69.893
        cognitive deficits I69.81
        disturbance of vision I69.898
        dysarthria I69.822
        dysphagia I69.891
        dysphasia I69.821
        facial droop I69.892
        facial weakness I69.892
        fluency disorder I69.823
        hemiplegia I69.85-
        language deficit I69.828
        monoplegia
          lower limb I69.84-
          upper limb I69.83-
        paralytic syndrome I69.86-
        specified effect NEC I69.898
        speech deficit I69.928
        speech deficit I69.828
        stroke NOS — *see* Sequelae, stroke NOS
  dislocation — *code to* injury with seventh character S
  encephalitis or encephalomyelitis (conditions in G04) G09
    in infectious disease NEC B94.8
    viral B94.1
  external cause — *code to* injury with seventh character S
  foreign body entering natural orifice — *code to* injury with seventh character S
  fracture — *code to* injury with seventh character S
  frostbite — *code to* injury with seventh character S
  Hansen's disease B92
  hemorrhage
    intracerebral I69.10
      alteration of sensation I69.198
      aphasia I69.120
      apraxia I69.190
      ataxia I69.193
      cognitive deficits I69.11
      disturbance of vision I69.198
      dysarthria I69.122
      dysphagia I69.191
      dysphasia I69.121
      facial droop I69.192
      facial weakness I69.192
      fluency disorder I69.123
      hemiplegia I69.15-
      language deficit NEC I69.128
      monoplegia
        lower limb I69.14-
        upper limb I69.13-
      paralytic syndrome I69.16-
      specified effect NEC I69.198
      speech deficit NEC I69.128
    intracranial, nontraumatic NEC I69.20
      alteration of sensation I69.298
      aphasia I69.220
      apraxia I69.290
      ataxia I69.293
      cognitive deficits I69.21
      disturbance of vision I69.298
      dysarthria I69.222
      dysphagia I69.291
      dysphasia I69.221
      facial droop I69.292
      facial weakness I69.292
      fluency disorder I69.223
      hemiplegia I69.25-
      language deficit NEC I69.228

Sequelae (of) (see also condition) — continued
hemorrhage — continued
  intracranial, nontraumatic NEC I69.20 —
    continued
    monoplegia
      lower limb I69.24-
      upper limb I69.23-
    paralytic syndrome I69.26-
    specified effect NEC I69.298
    speech deficit NEC I69.228
  subarachnoid I69.00
    alteration of sensation I69.098
    aphasia I69.020
    apraxia I69.090
    ataxia I69.093
    cognitive deficits — see subcategory
      I69.01-
    disturbance of vision I69.098
    dysarthria I69.022
    dysphagia I69.091
    dysphasia I69.021
    facial droop I69.092
    facial weakness I69.092
    fluency disorder I69.023
    hemiplegia I69.05-
    language deficit NEC I69.028
    monoplegia
      lower limb I69.04-
      upper limb I69.03-
    paralytic syndrome I69.06-
    specified effect NEC I69.098
    speech deficit NEC I69.028
hepatitis, viral B94.2
hyperalimentation E68
infarction
  cerebral I69.30
    alteration of sensation I69.398
    aphasia I69.320
    apraxia I69.390
    ataxia I69.393
    cognitive deficits I69.31
    disturbance of vision I69.398
    dysarthria I69.322
    dysphagia I69.391
    dysphasia I69.321
    facial droop I69.392
    facial weakness I69.392
    fluency disorder I69.323
    hemiplegia I69.35-
    language deficit NEC I69.328
    monoplegia
      lower limb I69.34-
      upper limb I69.33-
    paralytic syndrome I69.36-
    specified effect NEC I69.398
    speech deficit NEC I69.328
infection, pyogenic, intracranial or intraspinal
  G09
infectious disease B94.9
  specified NEC B94.8
injury — code to injury with seventh character
  S
leprosy B92
meningitis
  bacterial (conditions in G00) G09
  other or unspecified cause (conditions in
    G03) G09
muscle (and tendon) injury — code to injury
  with seventh character S
myelitis — see Sequelae, encephalitis
niacin deficiency E64.8
nutritional deficiency E64.9
  specified NEC E64.8
obstetrical condition O94
parasitic disease B94.9
phlebitis or thrombophlebitis of intracranial or
  intraspinal venous sinuses and veins
  (conditions in G08) G09

Sequelae (of) (see also condition) — continued
poisoning — code to poisoning with seventh
  character S
  nonmedicinal substance — see Sequelae,
    toxic effect, nonmedicinal substance
poliomyelitis (acute) B91
pregnancy O94
protein-energy malnutrition E64.0
puerperium O94
rickets E64.3
selenium deficiency E64.8
sprain and strain — code to injury with seventh
  character S
stroke NOS I69.30
  alteration in sensation I69.398
  aphasia I69.320
  apraxia I69.390
  ataxia I69.393
  cognitive deficits I69.31
  disturbance of vision I69.398
  dysarthria I69.322
  dysphagia I69.391
  dysphasia I69.321
  facial droop I69.392
  facial weakness I69.392
  hemiplegia I69.35-
  language deficit NEC I69.328
  monoplegia
    lower limb I69.34-
    upper limb I69.33-
  paralytic syndrome I69.36-
  specified effect NEC I69.398
  speech deficit NEC I69.328
tendon and muscle injury — code to injury
  with seventh character S
thiamine deficiency E64.8
trachoma B94.0
tuberculosis B90.9
  bones and joints B90.2
  central nervous system B90.0
  genitourinary B90.1
  pulmonary (respiratory) B90.9
  specified organs NEC B90.8
viral
  encephalitis B94.1
  hepatitis B94.2
vitamin deficiency NEC E64.8
  A E64.1
  B E64.8
  C E64.2
wound, open — code to injury with seventh
  character S
Sequestration — see also Sequestrum
disk — see Displacement, intervertebral disk
lung, congenital Q33.2
Sequestrum
bone — see Osteomyelitis, chronic
dental M27.2
jaw bone M27.2
orbit — see Osteomyelitis, orbit
sinus (accessory) (nasal) — see Sinusitis
Sequoiosis lung or pneumonitis J67.8
Serology for syphilis
doubtful
  with signs or symptoms — code by site and
    stage under Syphilis
  follow-up of latent syphilis — see Syphilis,
    latent
negative, with signs or symptoms — code by
  site and stage under Syphilis
positive A53.0
  with signs or symptoms — code by site and
    stage under Syphilis
reactivated A53.0
Seroma — see also Hematoma
postprocedural — see Complication,
  postprocedural, seroma
traumatic, secondary and recurrent T79.2
Seropurulent — see condition

Serositis, multiple K65.8
pericardial I31.1
peritoneal K65.8
Serous — see condition
Sertoli cell
adenoma
  specified site — see Neoplasm, benign, by
    site
  unspecified site
    female D27.9
    male D29.20
carcinoma
  specified site — see Neoplasm, malignant,
    by site
  unspecified site (male) C62.9-
    female C56.9
tumor
  with lipid storage
    specified site — see Neoplasm, benign, by
      site
    unspecified site
      female D27.9
      male D29.20
  specified site — see Neoplasm, benign, by
    site
  unspecified site
    female D27.9
    male D29.20
Sertoli-Leydig cell tumor — see Neoplasm,
  benign, by site
specified site — see Neoplasm, benign, by site
unspecified site
  female D27.9
  male D29.20
Serum
allergy, allergic reaction (see also Reaction,
  serum) T80.69
  shock (see also Shock, anaphylactic) T80.59
arthritis T80.6
complication or reaction NEC (see also
  Reaction, serum) T80.69
disease NEC (see also Reaction, serum) T80.69
hepatitis — see also Hepatitis, viral, type B
  carrier (suspected) of B18.1
intoxication (see also Reaction, serum) T80.69
neuritis (see also Reaction, serum) T80.69
neuropathy G61.1
poisoning NEC (see also Reaction, serum)
  T80.69
rash NEC (see also Reaction, serum) T80.69
reaction NEC (see also Reaction, serum) T80.69
sickness NEC (see also Reaction, serum) T80.69
urticaria (see also Reaction, serum) T80.69
Sesamoiditis M25.8-
Sever's disease or osteochondrosis — see
  Osteochondrosis, juvenile, tarsus
Severe sepsis R65.20
with septic shock R65.21
Sex
chromosome mosaics Q97.8
  lines with various numbers of X
    chromosomes Q97.2
education Z70.8
reassignment surgery status Z87.890
Sextuplet pregnancy — see Pregnancy,
  sextuplet
Sexual
function, disorder of (psychogenic) F52.9
immaturity (female) (male) E30.0
impotence (psychogenic) organic origin NEC
  — see Dysfunction, sexual, male
precocity (constitutional) (cryptogenic) (female)
  (idiopathic) (male) E30.1
Sexuality, pathologic — see Deviation, sexual
Sézary disease C84.1-
Shadow, lung R91.8
Shaking palsy or paralysis — see
  Parkinsonism

DISEASE INDEX

Shallowness, acetabulum — see Derangement, joint, specified type NEC, hip
Shaver's disease J63.1
Sheath (tendon) — see condition
Sheathing, retinal vessels H35.01
Shedding
 nail L60.8
 premature, primary (deciduous) teeth K00.6
Sheehan's disease or syndrome E23.0
Shelf, rectal K62.89
Shell teeth K00.5
Shellshock (current) F43.0
 lasting state — see Disorder, post-traumatic stress
Shield kidney Q63.1
Shift
 auditory threshold (temporary) H93.24-
 mediastinal R93.8
Shifting sleep-work schedule (affecting sleep) G47.26
Shiga(-Kruse) dysentery A03.0
Shiga's bacillus A03.0
Shigella (dysentery) — see Dysentery, bacillary
Shigellosis A03.9
 Group A A03.0
 Group B A03.1
 Group C A03.2
 Group D A03.3
Shin splints S86.89
Shingles — see Herpes, zoster
Shipyard disease or eye B30.0
Shirodkar suture, in pregnancy — see Pregnancy, complicated by, incompetent cervix
Shock R57.9
 with ectopic or molar pregnancy O08.3
 adrenal (cortical) (Addisonian) E27.2
 adverse food reaction (anaphylactic) — see Shock, anaphylactic, due to food
 allergic — see Shock, anaphylactic
 anaphylactic T78.2
  chemical — see Table of Drugs and Chemicals
  due to drug or medicinal substance
   correct substance properly administered T88.6
   overdose or wrong substance given or taken (by accident) — see Table of Drugs and Chemicals, by drug, poisoning
  due to food (nonpoisonous) T78.00
   additives T78.06
   dairy products T78.07
   eggs T78.08
   fish T78.03
    shellfish T78.02
   fruit T78.04
   milk T78.07
   nuts T78.05
    multiple types T78.05
    peanuts T78.01
   peanuts T78.01
   seeds T78.05
   specified type NEC T78.09
   vegetable T78.04
  following sting(s) — see Venom
  immunization T80.52
  serum T80.59
   blood and blood products T80.51
   immunization T80.52
   specified NEC T80.59
   vaccination T80.52
 anaphylactoid — see Shock, anaphylactic
 anesthetic
  correct substance properly administered T88.2

Shock R57.9 — continued
 anesthetic — continued
  overdose or wrong substance given or taken — see Table of Drugs and Chemicals, by drug, poisoning
  specified anesthetic — see Table of Drugs and Chemicals, by drug, poisoning
 cardiogenic R57.0
 chemical substance — see Table of Drugs and Chemicals
 complicating ectopic or molar pregnancy O08.3
 culture — see Disorder, adjustment
 drug
  due to correct substance properly administered T88.6
  overdose or wrong substance given or taken (by accident) — see Table of Drugs and Chemicals, by drug, poisoning
 during or after labor and delivery O75.1
 electric T75.4
  (taser) T75.4
 endotoxic R65.21
  postprocedural (resulting from a procedure, not elsewhere classified) T81.12
 following
  ectopic or molar pregnancy O08.3
  injury (immediate) (delayed) T79.4
  labor and delivery O75.1
 food (anaphylactic) — see Shock, anaphylactic, due to food
 from electroshock gun (taser) T75.4
 gram-negative R65.21
  postprocedural (resulting from a procedure, not elsewhere classified) T81.12
 hematologic R57.8
 hemorrhagic
  surgery (intraoperative) (postoperative) T81.19
  trauma T79.4
 hypovolemic R57.1
  surgical T81.19
  traumatic T79.4
 insulin E15
  therapeutic misadventure — see subcategory T38.3
 kidney N17.0
  traumatic (following crushing) T79.5
 lightning T75.01
 liver K72.00
 lung J80
 obstetric O75.1
  with ectopic or molar pregnancy O08.3
  following ectopic or molar pregnancy O08.3
 pleural (surgical) T81.19
  due to trauma T79.4
 postprocedural (postoperative) T81.10
  with ectopic or molar pregnancy O08.3
  cardiogenic T81.11
  endotoxic T81.12
  following ectopic or molar pregnancy O08.3
  gram-negative T81.12
  hypovolemic T81.19
  septic T81.12
  specified type NEC T81.19
 psychic F43.0
 septic (due to severe sepsis) R65.21
 specified NEC R57.8
 surgical T81.10
 taser gun (taser) T75.4
 therapeutic misadventure NEC T81.10
 thyroxin
  overdose or wrong substance given or taken — see Table of Drugs and Chemicals, by drug, poisoning
 toxic, syndrome A48.3
 transfusion — see Complications, transfusion
 traumatic (immediate) (delayed) T79.4
Shoemaker's chest M95.4

Short, shortening, shortness
 arm (acquired) — see also Deformity, limb, unequal length
  congenital Q71.81-
  forearm — see Deformity, limb, unequal length
 bowel syndrome K91.2
 breath R06.02
 cervical (complicating pregnancy) O26.87-
  non-gravid uterus N88.3
 common bile duct, congenital Q44.5
 cord (umbilical), complicating delivery O69.3
 cystic duct, congenital Q44.5
 esophagus (congenital) Q39.8
 femur (acquired) — see Deformity, limb, unequal length, femur
  congenital — see Defect, reduction, lower limb, longitudinal, femur
 frenum, frenulum, linguae (congenital) Q38.1
 hip (acquired) — see also Deformity, limb, unequal length
  congenital Q65.89
 leg (acquired) — see also Deformity, limb, unequal length
  congenital Q72.81-
  lower leg — see also Deformity, limb, unequal length
 limbed stature, with immunodeficiency D82.2
 lower limb (acquired) — see also Deformity, limb, unequal length
  congenital Q72.81-
 organ or site, congenital NEC — see Distortion
 palate, congenital Q38.5
 radius (acquired) — see also Deformity, limb, unequal length
  congenital — see Defect, reduction, upper limb, longitudinal, radius
 rib syndrome Q77.2
 stature (child) (hereditary) (idiopathic) NEC R62.52
  constitutional E34.3
  due to endocrine disorder E34.3
  Laron-type E34.3
 tendon — see also Contraction, tendon
  with contracture of joint — see Contraction, joint
  Achilles (acquired) M67.0-
   congenital Q66.89
  congenital Q79.8
 thigh (acquired) — see also Deformity, limb, unequal length, femur
  congenital — see Defect, reduction, lower limb, longitudinal, femur
 tibialis anterior (tendon) — see Contraction, tendon
 umbilical cord
  complicating delivery O69.3
 upper limb, congenital — see Defect, reduction, upper limb, specified type NEC
 urethra N36.8
 uvula, congenital Q38.5
 vagina (congenital) Q52.4
Shortsightedness — see Myopia
Shoshin (acute fulminating beriberi) E51.11
Shoulder — see condition
Shovel-shaped incisors K00.2
Shower, thromboembolic — see Embolism
Shunt
 arterial-venous (dialysis) Z99.2
 arteriovenous, pulmonary (acquired) I28.0
  congenital Q25.72
 cerebral ventricle (communicating) in situ Z98.2
 surgical, prosthetic, with complications — see Complications, cardiovascular, device or implant
Shutdown, renal N28.9
Shy-Drager syndrome G90.3

Sialadenitis, sialadenosis (any gland) (chronic) (periodic) (suppurative) — *see* Sialoadenitis
Sialectasia K11.8
Sialidosis E77.1
Sialitis, silitis (any gland) (chronic) (suppurative) — *see* Sialoadenitis
Sialoadenitis (any gland) (periodic) (suppurative) K11.20
  acute K11.21
    recurrent K11.22
  chronic K11.23
Sialoadenopathy K11.9
Sialoangitis — *see* Sialoadenitis
Sialodochitis (fibrinosa) — *see* Sialoadenitis
Sialodocholithiasis K11.5
Sialolithiasis K11.5
Sialometaplasia, necrotizing K11.8
Sialorrhea — *see also* Ptyalism
  periodic — *see* Sialoadenitis
Sialosis K11.7
Siamese twin Q89.4
Sibling rivalry Z62.891
Sicard's syndrome G52.7
Sicca syndrome M35.00
  with
    keratoconjunctivitis M35.01
    lung involvement M35.02
    myopathy M35.03
    renal tubulo-interstitial disorders M35.04
    specified organ involvement NEC M35.09
Sick R69
  or handicapped person in family Z63.79
    needing care at home Z63.6
  sinus (syndrome) I49.5
Sick-euthyroid syndrome E07.81
Sickle-cell
  anemia — *see* Disease, sickle-cell
  trait D57.3
Sicklemia — *see also* Disease, sickle-cell
  trait D57.3
Sickness
  air (travel) T75.3
  airplane T75.3
  alpine T70.29
  altitude T70.20
  Andes T70.29
  aviator's T70.29
  balloon T70.29
  car T75.3
  compressed air T70.3
  decompression T70.3
  green D50.8
  milk — *see* Poisoning, food, noxious
  motion T75.3
  mountain T70.29
    acute D75.1
  protein (*see also* Reaction, serum) T80.69
  radiation T66
  roundabout (motion) T75.3
  sea T75.3
  serum NEC (*see also* Reaction, serum) T80.69
  sleeping (African) B56.9
    by Trypanosoma B56.9
      brucei
        gambiense B56.0
        rhodesiense B56.1
      East African B56.1
      Gambian B56.0
      Rhodesian B56.1
      West African B56.0
  swing (motion) T75.3
  train (railway) (travel) T75.3
  travel (any vehicle) T75.3
Sideropenia — *see* Anemia, iron deficiency
Siderosilicosis J62.8
Siderosis (lung) J63.4
  eye (globe) — *see* Disorder, globe, degenerative, siderosis

Siemens' syndrome (ectodermal dysplasia) Q82.8
Sighing R06.89
  psychogenic F45.8
Sigmoid — *see also* condition
  flexure — *see* condition
  kidney Q63.1
Sigmoiditis (*see also* Enteritis) K52.9
  infectious A09
  noninfectious K52.9
Silversköld's syndrome Q78.9
Silicosiderosis J62.8
Silicosis, silicotic (simple) (complicated) J62.8
  with tuberculosis J65
Silicotuberculosis J65
Silo-fillers' disease J68.8
  bronchitis J68.0
  pneumonitis J68.0
  pulmonary edema J68.1
Silver's syndrome Q87.1
Simian malaria B53.1
Simmonds' cachexia or disease E23.0
Simons' disease or syndrome (progressive lipodystrophy) E88.1
Simple, simplex — *see* condition
Simulation, conscious (of illness) Z76.5
Simultanagnosia (asimultagnosia) R48.3
Sin Nombre virus disease (Hantavirus) (cardio)-pulmonary syndrome) B33.4
Sinding-Larsen disease or osteochondrosis — *see* Osteochondrosis, juvenile, patella
Singapore hemorrhagic fever A91
Singer's node or nodule J38.2
Single
  atrium Q21.2
  coronary artery Q24.5
  umbilical artery Q27.0
  ventricle Q20.4
Singultus R06.6
  epidemicus B33.0
Sinus — *see also* Fistula
  abdominal K63.89
  arrest I45.5
  arrhythmia I49.8
  bradycardia R00.1
  branchial cleft (internal) (external) Q18.0
  coccygeal — *see* Sinus, pilonidal
  dental K04.6
  dermal (congenital) Q06.8
    with abscess Q06.8
    coccygeal, pilonidal — *see* Sinus, coccygeal
  infected, skin NEC L08.89
  marginal, ruptured or bleeding — *see* Hemorrhage, antepartum, specified cause NEC
  medial, face and neck Q18.8
  pause I45.5
  pericranii Q01.9
  pilonidal (infected) (rectum) L05.92
    with abscess L05.02
  preauricular Q18.1
  rectovaginal N82.3
  Rokitansky-Aschoff (gallbladder) K82.8
  sacrococcygeal (dermoid) (infected) — *see* Sinus, pilonidal
  tachycardia R00.0
    paroxysmal I47.1
  tarsi syndrome M25.57-
  testis N50.89
  tract (postinfective) — *see* Fistula
  urachus Q64.4
Sinusitis (accessory) (chronic) (hyperplastic) (nasal) (nonpurulent) (purulent) J32.9
  acute J01.90
    ethmoidal J01.20
      recurrent J01.21
    frontal J01.10
      recurrent J01.11

Sinusitis (accessory) (chronic) (hyperplastic) (nasal) (nonpurulent) (purulent) J32.9 — *continued*
  acute J01.90 — *continued*
    involving more than one sinus, other than pansinusitis J01.80
      recurrent J01.81
    maxillary J01.00
      recurrent J01.01
    pansinusitis J01.40
      recurrent J01.41
    recurrent J01.91
    specified NEC J01.80
      recurrent J01.81
    sphenoidal J01.30
      recurrent J01.31
  allergic — *see* Rhinitis, allergic
  due to high altitude T70.1
  ethmoidal J32.2
    acute J01.20
      recurrent J01.21
  frontal J32.1
    acute J01.10
      recurrent J01.11
  influenzal — *see* Influenza, with, respiratory manifestations NEC
  involving more than one sinus but not pansinusitis J32.8
    acute J01.80
      recurrent J01.81
  maxillary J32.0
    acute J01.00
      recurrent J01.01
  sphenoidal J32.3
    acute J01.30
      recurrent J01.31
  tuberculous, any sinus A15.8
Sinusitis-bronchiectasis-situs inversus (syndrome) (triad) Q89.3
Sipple's syndrome E31.22
Sirenomelia (syndrome) Q87.2
Siriasis T67.0
Sirkari's disease B55.0
Siti A65
Situation, psychiatric F99
Situational
  disturbance (transient) — *see* Disorder, adjustment
    acute F43.0
  maladjustment — *see* Disorder, adjustment
  reaction — *see* Disorder, adjustment
    acute F43.0
Situs inversus or transversus (abdominalis) (thoracic) Q89.3
Sixth disease B08.20
  due to human herpesvirus 6 B08.21
  due to human herpesvirus 7 B08.22
Sjögren-Larsson syndrome Q87.1
Sjögren's syndrome or disease — *see* Sicca syndrome
Skeletal — *see* condition
Skene's gland — *see* condition
Skenitis — *see* Urethritis
Skerljevo A65
Skevas-Zerfus disease — *see* Toxicity, venom, marine animal, sea anemone
Skin — *see also* condition
  clammy R23.1
  donor — *see* Donor, skin
  hidebound M35.9
Slate-dressers' or slate-miners' lung J62.8
Sleep
  apnea — *see* Apnea, sleep
  deprivation Z72.820
  disorder or disturbance G47.9
    child F51.9
      nonorganic origin F51.9
    specified NEC G47.8

Sleep — *continued*
disturbance G47.9
nonorganic origin F51.9
drunkenness F51.9
rhythm inversion G47.2-
terrors F51.4
walking F51.3
hysterical F44.89
Sleep hygiene
abuse Z72.821
inadequate Z72.821
poor Z72.821
Sleeping sickness — *see* Sickness, sleeping
Sleeplessness — *see* Insomnia
menopausal N95.1
Sleep-wake schedule disorder G47.20
Slim disease (in HIV infection) B20
Slipped, slipping
epiphysis (traumatic) — *see also*
Osteochondropathy, specified type NEC
capital femoral (traumatic)
acute (on chronic) S79.01-
current traumatic — *code as* Fracture, by site
upper femoral (nontraumatic) M93.00-
acute M93.01-
on chronic M93.03-
chronic M93.02-
intervertebral disc — *see* Displacement,
intervertebral disc
ligature, umbilical P51.8
patella — *see* Disorder, patella, derangement
NEC
rib M89.8x8
sacroiliac joint — *see* subcategory M53.2
tendon — *see* Disorder, tendon
ulnar nerve, nontraumatic — *see* Lesion, nerve,
ulnar
vertebra NEC — *see* Spondylolisthesis
Slocumb's syndrome E27.0
Sloughing (multiple) (phagedena) (skin) — *see*
also Gangrene
abscess — *see* Abscess
appendix K38.8
fascia — *see* Disorder, soft tissue, specified
type NEC
scrotum N50.89
tendon — *see* Disorder, tendon
transplanted organ — *see* Rejection, transplant
ulcer — *see* Ulcer, skin
Slow
feeding, newborn P92.2
flow syndrome, coronary I20.8
heart(beat) R00.1
Slowing, urinary stream R39.198
Sluder's neuralgia (syndrome) G44.89
Slurred, slurring speech R47.81
Small(ness)
for gestational age — *see* Small for dates
introitus, vagina N89.6
kidney (unknown cause) N27.9
bilateral N27.1
unilateral N27.0
ovary (congenital) Q50.39
pelvis
with disproportion (fetopelvic) O33.1
causing obstructed labor O65.1
uterus N85.8
white kidney N03.9
Small-and-light-for-dates — *see* Small for
dates
Small-for-dates (infant) P05.10
with weight of
99 grams or less P05.11
500-749 grams P05.12
4750-999 grams P05.13
1000-1249 grams P05.14
1250-1499 grams P05.15
1500-1749 grams P05.16
1750-1999 grams P05.17

Small-for-dates (infant) P05.10 — *continued*
with weight of — *continued*
2000-2499 grams P05.18
2500 grams and over P05.19
specified NEC P05.19
Smallpox B03
Smearing, fecal R15.1
Smith-Lemli-Opitz syndrome E78.72
Smith's fracture S52.54-
Smoker — *see* Dependence, drug, nicotine
Smoker's
bronchitis J41.0
cough J41.0
palate K13.24
throat J31.2
tongue K13.24
Smoking
passive Z77.22
Smothering spells R06.81
Snaggle teeth, tooth M26.39
Snapping
finger — *see* Trigger finger
hip — *see* Derangement, joint, specified type
NEC, hip
involving the iliotibial band M76.3-
knee — *see* Derangement, knee
involving the iliotibial band M76.3-
Sneddon-Wilkinson disease or syndrome
(sub-corneal pustular dermatosis) L13.1
Sneezing (intractable) R06.7
Sniffing
cocaine
abuse — *see* Abuse, drug, cocaine
dependence — *see* Dependence, drug,
cocaine
gasoline
abuse — *see* Abuse, drug, inhalant
dependence — *see* Dependence, drug,
inhalant
glue (airplane)
abuse — *see* Abuse, drug, inhalant
drug dependence — *see* Dependence, drug,
inhalant
Sniffles
newborn P28.89
Snoring R06.83
Snow blindness — *see* Photokeratitis
Snuffles (non-syphilitic) R06.5
newborn P28.89
syphilitic (infant) A50.05 *[J99]*
Social
exclusion Z60.4
due to discrimination or persecution
(perceived) Z60.5
migrant Z59.0
acculturation difficulty Z60.3
rejection Z60.4
due to discrimination or persecution Z60.5
role conflict NEC Z73.5
skills inadequacy NEC Z73.4
transplantation Z60.3
Sodoku A25.0
Soemmerring's ring — *see* Cataract,
secondary
Soft — *see also* condition
nails L60.3
Softening
bone — *see* Osteomalacia
brain (necrotic) (progressive) G93.89
congenital Q04.8
embolic I63.4-
hemorrhagic — *see* Hemorrhage,
intracranial, intracerebral
occlusive I63.5-
thrombotic I63.3-
cartilage M94.2-
patella M22.4-
cerebellar — *see* Softening, brain
cerebral — *see* Softening, brain

Softening — *continued*
cerebrospinal — *see* Softening, brain
myocardial, heart — *see* Degeneration,
myocardial
spinal cord G95.89
stomach K31.89
Soldier's
heart F45.8
patches I31.0
Solitary
cyst, kidney N28.1
kidney, congenital Q60.0
Solvent abuse — *see* Abuse, drug, inhalant
dependence — *see* Dependence, drug,
inhalant
Somatization reaction, somatic reaction
— *see* Disorder, somatoform
Somnambulism F51.3
hysterical F44.89
Somnolence R40.0
nonorganic origin F51.11
Sonne dysentery A03.3
Soor B37.0
Sore
bed — *see* Ulcer, pressure, by site
chiclero B55.1
Delhi B55.1
desert — *see* Ulcer, skin
eye H57.1-
Lahore B55.1
mouth K13.79
canker K12.0
muscle M79.1
Naga — *see* Ulcer, skin
of skin — *see* Ulcer, skin
oriental B55.1
pressure — *see* Ulcer, pressure, by site
skin L98.9
soft A57
throat (acute) — *see also* Pharyngitis
with influenza, flu, or grippe — *see*
Influenza, with, respiratory
manifestations NEC
chronic J31.2
coxsackie (virus) B08.5
diphtheritic A36.0
herpesviral B00.2
influenzal — *see* Influenza, with, respiratory
manifestations NEC
septic J02.0
streptococcal (ulcerative) J02.0
viral NEC J02.8
coxsackie B08.5
tropical — *see* Ulcer, skin
veldt — *see* Ulcer, skin
Soto's syndrome (cerebral gigantism) Q87.3
South African cardiomyopathy syndrome
I42.8
Southeast Asian hemorrhagic fever A91
Spacing
abnormal, tooth, teeth, fully erupted M26.30
excessive, tooth, fully erupted M26.32
Spade-like hand (congenital) Q68.1
Spading nail L60.8
congenital Q84.6
Spanish collar N47.1
Sparganosis B70.1
Spasm(s), spastic, spasticity (*see also*
condition) R25.2
accommodation — *see* Spasm, of
accommodation
ampulla of Vater K83.4
anus, ani (sphincter) (reflex) K59.4
psychogenic F45.8
artery I73.9
cerebral G45.9
Bell's G51.3

Spasm(s), spastic, spasticity (see also condition) R25.2 — continued
  bladder (sphincter, external or internal) N32.89
    psychogenic F45.8
  bronchus, bronchiole J98.01
  cardia K22.0
  cardiac I20.1
  carpopedal — see Tetany
  cerebral (arteries) (vascular) G45.9
  cervix, complicating delivery O62.4
  ciliary body (of accommodation) — see Spasm, of accommodation
  colon (see also Irritable, bowel) K58.9
    with diarrhea K58.0
    psychogenic F45.8
  common duct K83.8
  compulsive — see Tic
  conjugate H51.8
  coronary (artery) I20.1
  diaphragm (reflex) R06.6
    epidemic B33.0
    psychogenic F45.8
  duodenum K59.8
  epidemic diaphragmatic (transient) B33.0
  esophagus (diffuse) K22.4
    psychogenic F45.8
  facial G51.3
  fallopian tube N83.8
  gastrointestinal (tract) K31.89
    psychogenic F45.8
  glottis J38.5
    hysterical F44.4
    psychogenic F45.8
      conversion reaction F44.4
    reflex through recurrent laryngeal nerve J38.5
  habit — see Tic
  heart I20.1
  hemifacial (clonic) G51.3
  hourglass — see Contraction, hourglass
  hysterical F44.4
  infantile — see Epilepsy, spasms
  inferior oblique, eye H51.8
  intestinal (see also Syndrome, irritable bowel) K58.9
    psychogenic F45.8
  larynx, laryngeal J38.5
    hysterical F44.4
    psychogenic F45.8
      conversion reaction F44.4
  levator palpebrae superioris — see Disorder, eyelid function
  muscle NEC M62.838
    back M62.830
  nerve, trigeminal G51.0
  nervous F45.8
  nodding F98.4
  occupational F48.8
  oculogyric H51.8
    psychogenic F45.8
  of accommodation H52.53-
  ophthalmic artery — see Occlusion, artery, retina
  perineal, female N94.89
  peroneo-extensor — see also Deformity, limb, flat foot
  pharynx (reflex) J39.2
    hysterical F45.8
    psychogenic F45.8
  psychogenic F45.8
  pylorus NEC K31.3
    adult hypertrophic K31.89
    congenital or infantile Q40.0
    psychogenic F45.8
  rectum (sphincter) K59.4
    psychogenic F45.8
  retinal (artery) — see Occlusion, artery, retina

Spasm(s), spastic, spasticity (see also condition) R25.2 — continued
  sigmoid (see also Syndrome, irritable bowel) K58.9
    psychogenic F45.8
  sphincter of Oddi K83.4
  stomach K31.89
    neurotic F45.8
  throat J39.2
    hysterical F45.8
    psychogenic F45.8
  tic F95.9
    chronic F95.1
    transient of childhood F95.0
  tongue K14.8
  torsion (progressive) G24.1
  trigeminal nerve — see Neuralgia, trigeminal
  ureter N13.5
  urethra (sphincter) N35.9
  uterus N85.8
    complicating labor O62.4
  vagina N94.2
    psychogenic F52.5
  vascular I73.9
  vasomotor I73.9
  vein NEC I87.8
  viscera — see Pain, abdominal
Spasmodic — see condition
Spasmophilia — see Tetany
Spasmus nutans F98.4
Spastic, spasticity — see also Spasm
  child (cerebral) (congenital) (paralysis) G80.1
Speaker's throat R49.8
Specific, specified — see condition
Speech
  defect, disorder, disturbance, impediment R47.9
    psychogenic, in childhood and adolescence F98.8
    slurring R47.81
    specified NEC R47.89
Spencer's disease A08.19
Spens' syndrome (syncope with heart block) I45.9
Sperm counts (fertility testing) Z31.41
  postvasectomy Z30.8
    reversal Z31.42
Spermatic cord — see condition
Spermatocele N43.40
  congenital Q55.4
  multiple N43.42
  single N43.41
Spermatocystitis N49.0
Spermatocytoma C62.9-
  specified site — see Neoplasm, malignant, by site
Spermatorrhea N50.89
Sphacelus — see Gangrene
Sphenoidal — see condition
Sphenoiditis (chronic) — see Sinusitis, sphenoidal
Sphenopalatine ganglion neuralgia G90.09
Sphericity, increased, lens (congenital) Q12.4
Spherocytosis (congenital) (familial) (hereditary) D58.0
  hemoglobin disease D58.0
  sickle-cell (disease) D57.8-
Spherophakia Q12.4
Sphincter — see condition
Sphincteritis, sphincter of Oddi — see Cholangitis
Sphingolipidosis E75.3
  specified NEC E75.29
Sphingomyelinosis E75.3
Spicule tooth K00.2

Spider
  bite — see Toxicity, venom, spider
  fingers — see Syndrome, Marfan's
  nevus I78.1
  toes — see Syndrome, Marfan's
  vascular I78.1
Spiegler-Fendt
  benign lymphocytoma L98.8
  sarcoid L08.89
Spielmeyer-Vogt disease E75.4
Spina bifida (aperta) Q05.9
  with hydrocephalus NEC Q05.4
  cervical Q05.5
    with hydrocephalus Q05.0
  dorsal Q05.6
    with hydrocephalus Q05.1
  lumbar Q05.7
    with hydrocephalus Q05.2
  lumbosacral Q05.7
    with hydrocephalus Q05.2
  occulta Q76.0
  sacral Q05.8
    with hydrocephalus Q05.3
  thoracic Q05.6
    with hydrocephalus Q05.1
  thoracolumbar Q05.6
    with hydrocephalus Q05.1
Spindle, Krukenberg's — see Pigmentation, cornea, posterior
Spine, spinal — see condition
Spiradenoma (eccrine) — see Neoplasm, skin, benign
Spirillosis A25.0
Spirillum
  minus A25.0
  obermeieri infection A68.0
Spirochetal — see condition
Spirochetosis A69.9
  arthritic, arthritica A69.9
  bronchopulmonary A69.8
  icterohemorrhagic A27.0
  lung A69.8
Spirometrosis B70.1
Spitting blood — see Hemoptysis
Splanchnoptosis K63.4
Spleen, splenic — see condition
Splenectasis — see Splenomegaly
Splenitis (interstitial) (malignant) (nonspecific) D73.89
  malarial (see also Malaria) B54 [D77]
  tuberculous A18.85
Splenocele D73.89
Splenomegaly, splenomegalia (Bengal) (cryptogenic) (idiopathic) (tropical) R16.1
  with hepatomegaly R16.2
  cirrhotic D73.2
  congenital Q89.09
  congestive, chronic D73.2
  Egyptian B65.1
  Gaucher's E75.22
  malarial (see also Malaria) B54 [D77]
  neutropenic D73.81
  Niemann-Pick — see Niemann-Pick disease or syndrome
  siderotic D73.2
  syphilitic A52.79
    congenital (early) A50.08 [D77]
Splenopathy D73.9
Splenoptosis D73.89
Splenosis D73.89
Splinter — see Foreign body, superficial, by site
Split, splitting
  foot Q72.7-
  hand Q71.6
  heart sounds R01.2
  lip, congenital — see Cleft, lip
  nails L60.3
  urinary stream R39.13
Spondylarthrosis — see Spondylosis

Spondylitis (chronic) — *see also*
Spondylopathy, inflammatory
ankylopoietica — *see* Spondylitis, ankylosing
ankylosing (chronic) M45.9
  with lung involvement M45.9 *[J99]*
  cervical region M45.2
  cervicothoracic region M45.3
  juvenile M08.1
  lumbar region M45.6
  lumbosacral region M45.7
  multiple sites M45.0
  occipito-atlanto-axial region M45.1
  sacrococcygeal region M45.8
  thoracic region M45.4
  thoracolumbar region M45.5
atrophic (ligamentous) — *see* Spondylitis,
  ankylosing
deformans (chronic) — *see* Spondylosis
gonococcal A54.41
gouty (*see also* Gout, by type, vertebrae)
  M10.08
in (due to)
  brucellosis A23.9 *[M49.80]*
    cervical region A23.9 *[M49.82]*
    cervicothoracic region A23.9 *[M49.83]*
    lumbar region A23.9 *[M49.86]*
    lumbosacral region A23.9 *[M49.87]*
    multiple sites A23.9 *[M49.89]*
    occipito-atlanto-axial region A23.9
      [M49.81]
    sacrococcygeal region A23.9 *[M49.88]*
    thoracic region A23.9 *[M49.84]*
    thoracolumbar region A23.9 *[M49.85]*
  enterobacteria (*see also* subcategory M49.8)
    A04.9
  tuberculosis A18.01
infectious NEC — *see* Spondylopathy, infective
juvenile ankylosing (chronic) M08.1
Kümmell's — *see* Spondylopathy, traumatic
Marie-Strümpell — *see* Spondylitis, ankylosing
muscularis — *see* Spondylopathy, specified
  NEC
psoriatic L40.53
rheumatoid — *see* Spondylitis, ankylosing
rhizomelica — *see* Spondylitis, ankylosing
sacroiliac NEC M46.1
senescent, senile — *see* Spondylosis
traumatic (chronic) or post-traumatic — *see*
  Spondylopathy, traumatic
tuberculous A18.01
typhosa A01.05
Spondylolisthesis (acquired) (degenerative)
  M43.10
with disproportion (fetopelvic) O33.0
  causing obstructed labor O65.0
cervical region M43.12
cervicothoracic region M43.13
congenital Q76.2
lumbar region M43.16
lumbosacral region M43.17
multiple sites M43.19
occipito-atlanto-axial region M43.11
sacrococcygeal region M43.18
thoracic region M43.14
thoracolumbar region M43.15
traumatic (old) M43.10
  acute
    fifth cervical (displaced) S12.430
      nondisplaced S12.431
      specified type NEC (displaced) S12.450
        nondisplaced S12.451
      type III S12.44
    fourth cervical (displaced) S12.330
      nondisplaced S12.331
      specified type NEC (displaced) S12.350
        nondisplaced S12.351
      type III S12.34

Spondylolisthesis (acquired) (degenerative)
  M43.10 — *continued*
traumatic (old) M43.10 — *continued*
  acute — *continued*
    second cervical (displaced) S12.130
      nondisplaced S12.131
      specified type NEC (displaced) S12.150
        nondisplaced S12.151
      type III S12.14
    seventh cervical (displaced) S12.630
      nondisplaced S12.631
      specified type NEC (displaced) S12.650
        nondisplaced S12.651
      type III S12.64
    sixth cervical (displaced) S12.530
      nondisplaced S12.531
      specified type NEC (displaced) S12.550
        nondisplaced S12.551
      type III S12.54
    third cervical (displaced) S12.230
      nondisplaced S12.231
      specified type NEC (displaced) S12.250
        nondisplaced S12.251
      type III S12.24
Spondylolysis (acquired) M43.00
cervical region M43.02
cervicothoracic region M43.03
congenital Q76.2
lumbar region M43.06
lumbosacral region M43.07
  with disproportion (fetopelvic) O33.0
    causing obstructed labor O65.8
multiple sites M43.09
occipito-atlanto-axial region M43.01
sacrococcygeal region M43.08
thoracic region M43.04
thoracolumbar region M43.05
Spondylopathy M48.9
infective NEC M46.50
  cervical region M46.52
  cervicothoracic region M46.53
  lumbar region M46.56
  lumbosacral region M46.57
  multiple sites M46.59
  occipito-atlanto-axial region M46.51
  sacrococcygeal region M46.58
  thoracic region M46.54
  thoracolumbar region M46.55
inflammatory M46.90
  cervical region M46.92
  cervicothoracic region M46.93
  lumbar region M46.96
  lumbosacral region M46.97
  multiple sites M46.99
  occipito-atlanto-axial region M46.91
  sacrococcygeal region M46.98
  specified type NEC M46.80
    cervical region M46.82
    cervicothoracic region M46.83
    lumbar region M46.86
    lumbosacral region M46.87
    multiple sites M46.89
    occipito-atlanto-axial region M46.81
    sacrococcygeal region M46.88
    thoracic region M46.84
    thoracolumbar region M46.85
  thoracic region M46.94
  thoracolumbar region M46.95
neuropathic, in
  syringomyelia and syringobulbia G95.0
  tabes dorsalis A52.11
specified NEC — *see* subcategory M48.8
traumatic M48.30
  cervical region M48.32
  cervicothoracic region M48.33
  lumbar region M48.36
  lumbosacral region M48.37
  occipito-atlanto-axial region M48.31
  sacrococcygeal region M48.38

Spondylopathy M48.9 — *continued*
traumatic M48.30 — *continued*
  thoracic region M48.34
  thoracolumbar region M48.35
Spondylosis M47.9
with
  disproportion (fetopelvic) O33.0
    causing obstructed labor O65.0
  myelopathy NEC M47.10
    cervical region M47.12
    cervicothoracic region M47.13
    lumbar region M47.16
    occipito-atlanto-axial region M47.11
    thoracic region M47.14
    thoracolumbar region M47.15
  radiculopathy M47.20
    cervical region M47.22
    cervicothoracic region M47.23
    lumbar region M47.26
    lumbosacral region M47.27
    occipito-atlanto-axial region M47.21
    sacrococcygeal region M47.28
    thoracic region M47.24
    thoracolumbar region M47.25
specified NEC M47.899
  cervical region M47.892
  cervicothoracic region M47.893
  lumbar region M47.896
  lumbosacral region M47.897
  occipito-atlanto-axial region M47.891
  sacrococcygeal region M47.898
  thoracic region M47.894
  thoracolumbar region M47.895
traumatic — *see* Spondylopathy, traumatic
without myelopathy or radiculopathy M47.819
  cervical region M47.812
  cervicothoracic region M47.813
  lumbar region M47.816
  lumbosacral region M47.817
  occipito-atlanto-axial region M47.811
  sacrococcygeal region M47.818
  thoracic region M47.814
  thoracolumbar region M47.815
Sponge
inadvertently left in operation wound — *see*
  Foreign body, accidentally left during a
  procedure
kidney (medullary) Q61.5
Sponge-diver's disease — *see* Toxicity,
  venom, marine animal, sea anemone
Spongioblastoma (any type) — *see*
  Neoplasm, malignant, by site
  specified site — *see* Neoplasm, malignant, by
    site
  unspecified site C71.9
Spongioneuroblastoma — *see* Neoplasm,
  malignant, by site
Spontaneous — *see also* condition
fracture (cause unknown) — *see* Fracture,
  pathological
Spoon nail L60.3
congenital Q84.6
Sporadic — *see* condition
Sporothrix schenckii infection — *see*
  Sporotrichosis
Sporotrichosis B42.9
arthritis B42.82
disseminated B42.7
generalized B42.7
lymphocutaneous (fixed) (progressive) B42.1
pulmonary B42.0
specified NEC B42.89
Spots, spotting (in) (of)
Bitot's — *see also* Pigmentation, conjunctiva
  in the young child E50.1
  vitamin A deficiency E50.1
café, au lait L81.3
Cayenne pepper I78.1

DISEASE INDEX

Spots, spotting (in) (of) — *continued*
cotton wool, retina — *see* Occlusion, artery, retina
de Morgan's (senile angiomas) I78.1
Fuchs' black (myopic) H44.2-
intermenstrual (regular) N92.0
  irregular N92.1
Koplik's B05.9
liver L81.4
pregnancy O26.85-
purpuric R23.3
ruby I78.1
Spotted fever — *see* Fever, spotted N92.3
Sprain (joint) (ligament)
acromioclavicular joint or ligament S43.5-
ankle S93.40-
  calcaneofibular ligament S93.41-
  deltoid ligament S93.42-
  internal collateral ligament — *see* Sprain, ankle, specified ligament NEC
  specified ligament NEC S93.49-
  talofibular ligament — *see* Sprain, ankle, specified ligament NEC
  tibiofibular ligament S93.43-
anterior longitudinal, cervical S13.4
atlas, atlanto-axial, atlanto-occipital S13.4
breast bone — *see* Sprain, sternum
calcaneofibular — *see* Sprain, ankle
carpal — *see* Sprain, wrist
carpometacarpal — *see* Sprain, hand, specified site NEC
cartilage
  costal S23.41
  semilunar (knee) — *see* Sprain, knee, specified site NEC
    with current tear — *see* Tear, meniscus
  thyroid region S13.5
  xiphoid — *see* Sprain, sternum
cervical, cervicodorsal, cervicothoracic S13.4
chondrosternal S23.421
coracoclavicular S43.8-
coracohumeral S43.41-
coronary, knee — *see* Sprain, knee, specified site NEC
costal cartilage S23.41
cricoarytenoid articulation or ligament S13.5
cricothyroid articulation S13.5
cruciate, knee — *see* Sprain, knee, cruciate
deltoid, ankle — *see* Sprain, ankle
dorsal (spine) S23.3
elbow S53.40-
  radial collateral ligament S53.43-
  radiohumeral S53.41-
  rupture
    radial collateral ligament — *see* Rupture, traumatic, ligament, radial collateral
    ulnar collateral ligament — *see* Rupture, traumatic, ligament, ulnar collateral
  specified type NEC S53.49-
  ulnar collateral ligament S53.44-
  ulnohumeral S53.42-
femur, head — *see* Sprain, hip
fibular collateral, knee — *see* Sprain, knee, collateral
fibulocalcaneal — *see* Sprain, ankle
finger(s) S63.61-
  index S63.61-
  interphalangeal (joint) S63.63-
    index S63.63-
    little S63.63-
    middle S63.63-
    ring S63.63-
  little S63.61-
  metacarpophalangeal (joint) S63.65-
  middle S63.61-
  ring S63.61-
  specified site NEC S63.69-
    index S63.69-
    little S63.69-

Sprain (joint) (ligament) — *continued*
finger(s) S63.61- — *continued*
  specified site NEC S63.69- — *continued*
    middle S63.69-
    ring S63.69-
foot S93.60-
  specified ligament NEC S93.69-
  tarsal ligament S93.61-
  tarsometatarsal ligament S93.62-
  toe — *see* Sprain, toe
hand S63.9-
  finger — *see* Sprain, finger
  specified site NEC — *see* subcategory S63.8
  thumb — *see* Sprain, thumb
head S03.9
hip S73.10-
  iliofemoral ligament S73.11-
  ischiocapsular (ligament) S73.12-
  specified NEC S73.19-
iliofemoral — *see* Sprain, hip
innominate
  acetabulum — *see* Sprain, hip
  sacral junction S33.6
internal
  collateral, ankle — *see* Sprain, ankle
  semilunar cartilage — *see* Sprain, knee, specified site NEC
interphalangeal
  finger — *see* Sprain, finger, interphalangeal (joint)
  toe — *see* Sprain, toe, interphalangeal joint
ischiocapsular — *see* Sprain, hip
ischiofemoral — *see* Sprain, hip
jaw (articular disc) (cartilage) (meniscus) S03.4-
  old M26.69
knee S83.9-
  collateral ligament S83.40-
    lateral (fibular) S83.42-
    medial (tibial) S83.41-
  cruciate ligament S83.50-
    anterior S83.51-
    posterior S83.52-
  lateral (fibular) collateral ligament S83.42-
  medial (tibial) collateral ligament S83.41-
  patellar ligament S76.11-
  specified site NEC S83.8x-
  superior tibiofibular joint (ligament) S83.6-
lateral collateral, knee — *see* Sprain, knee, collateral
lumbar (spine) S33.5
lumbosacral S33.9
mandible (articular disc) S03.4-
  old M26.69
medial collateral, knee — *see* Sprain, knee, collateral
meniscus
  jaw S03.4-
    old M26.69
  knee — *see* Sprain, knee, specified site NEC
    with current tear — *see* Tear, meniscus
    old — *see* Derangement, knee, meniscus, due to old tear
  mandible S03.4-
    old M26.69
metacarpal (distal) (proximal) — *see* Sprain, hand, specified site NEC
metacarpophalangeal — *see* Sprain, finger, metacarpophalangeal (joint)
metatarsophalangeal — *see* Sprain, toe, metatarsophalangeal joint
midcarpal — *see* Sprain, hand, specified site NEC
midtarsal — *see* Sprain, foot, specified site NEC
neck S13.9
  anterior longitudinal cervical ligament S13.4
  atlanto-axial joint S13.4
  atlanto-occipital joint S13.4

Sprain (joint) (ligament) — *continued*
neck S13.9 — *continued*
  cervical spine S13.4
  cricoarytenoid ligament S13.5
  cricothyroid ligament S13.5
  specified site NEC S13.8
  thyroid region (cartilage) S13.5
nose S03.8
orbicular, hip — *see* Sprain, hip
patella — *see* Sprain, knee, specified site NEC
patellar ligament S76.11-
pelvis NEC S33.8
phalanx
  finger — *see* Sprain, finger
  toe — *see* Sprain, toe
pubofemoral — *see* Sprain, hip
radiocarpal — *see* Sprain, wrist
radiohumeral — *see* Sprain, elbow
radius, collateral — *see* Rupture, traumatic, ligament, radial collateral
rib (cage) S23.41
rotator cuff (capsule) S43.42-
sacroiliac (region)
  chronic or old — *see* subcategory M53.2
  joint S33.6
scaphoid (hand) — *see* Sprain, hand, specified site NEC
scapula(r) — *see* Sprain, shoulder girdle, specified site NEC
semilunar cartilage (knee) — *see* Sprain, knee, specified site NEC
  with current tear — *see* Tear, meniscus
  old — *see* Derangement, knee, meniscus, due to old tear
shoulder joint S43.40-
  acromioclavicular joint (ligament) — *see* Sprain, acromioclavicular joint
  blade — *see* Sprain, shoulder, girdle, specified site NEC
  coracoclavicular ligament (ligament) — *see* Sprain, coracoclavicular joint
  coracohumeral ligament — *see* Sprain, coracohumeral joint
  girdle S43.9-
    specified site NEC S43.8-
  rotator cuff — *see* Sprain, rotator cuff
  specified site NEC S43.49-
  sternoclavicular joint (ligament) — *see* Sprain, sternoclavicular joint
spine
  cervical S13.4
  lumbar S33.5
  thoracic S23.3
sternoclavicular joint S43.6-
sternum S23.429
  chondrosternal joint S23.421
  specified site NEC S23.428
  sternoclavicular (joint) (ligament) S23.420
symphysis
  jaw S03.4-
    old M26.69
  mandibular S03.4-
    old M26.69
talofibular — *see* Sprain, ankle
tarsal — *see* Sprain, foot, specified site NEC
tarsometatarsal — *see* Sprain, foot, specified site NEC
temporomandibular S03.4-
  old M26.69
thorax S23.9
  ribs S23.41
  specified site NEC S23.8
  spine S23.3
  sternum — *see* Sprain, sternum
thumb S63.60-
  interphalangeal (joint) S63.62-
  metacarpophalangeal (joint) S63.64-
  specified site NEC S63.68-
thyroid cartilage or region S13.5

Sprain (joint) (ligament) — *continued*
  tibia (proximal end) — *see* Sprain, knee,
    specified site NEC
  tibial collateral, knee — *see* Sprain, knee,
    collateral
  tibiofibular
    distal — *see* Sprain, ankle
    superior — *see* Sprain, knee, specified site
      NEC
  toe(s) S93.50-
    great S93.50-
    interphalangeal joint S93.51-
      great S93.51-
      lesser S93.51-
    lesser S93.50-
    metatarsophalangeal joint S93.52-
      great S93.52-
      lesser S93.52-
  ulna, collateral — *see* Rupture, traumatic,
    ligament, ulnar collateral
  ulnohumeral — *see* Sprain, elbow
  wrist S63.50-
    carpal S63.51-
    radiocarpal S63.52-
    specified site NEC S63.59-
  xiphoid cartilage — *see* Sprain, sternum
Sprengel's deformity (congenital) Q74.0
Sprue (tropical) K90.1
  celiac K90.0
  idiopathic K90.49
  meaning thrush B37.0
  nontropical K90.0
Spur, bone — *see also* Enthesopathy
  calcaneal M77.3-
  iliac crest M76.2-
  nose (septum) J34.89
Spurway's syndrome Q78.0
Sputum
  abnormal (amount) (color) (odor) (purulent)
    R09.3
  blood-stained R04.2
  excessive (cause unknown) R09.3
Squamous — *see also* condition
  epithelium in
    cervical canal (congenital) Q51.828
    uterine mucosa (congenital) Q51.818
Squashed nose M95.0
  congenital Q67.4
Squeeze, diver's T70.3
Squint — *see also* Strabismus
  accommodative — *see* Strabismus, convergent
    concomitant
St. Hubert's disease A82.9
Stab — *see also* Laceration
  internal organs — *see* Injury, by site
Stafne's cyst or cavity M27.0
Staggering gait R26.0
  hysterical F44.4
Staghorn calculus — *see* Calculus, kidney
Stähli's line (cornea) (pigment) — *see*
  Pigmentation, cornea, anterior
Stain, staining
  meconium (newborn) P96.83
  port wine Q82.5
  tooth, teeth (hard tissues) (extrinsic) K03.6
    due to
      accretions K03.6
      deposits (betel) (black) (green) (materia
        alba) (orange) (soft) (tobacco) K03.6
      metals (copper) (silver) K03.7
      nicotine K03.6
      pulpal bleeding K03.7
      tobacco K03.6
    intrinsic K00.8
Stammering (*see also* Disorder, fluency) F80.81

Standstill
  auricular I45.5
  cardiac — *see* Arrest, cardiac
  sinoatrial I45.5
  ventricular — *see* Arrest, cardiac
Stannosis J63.5
Stanton's disease — *see* Melioidosis
Staphylitis (acute) (catarrhal) (chronic)
  (gangrenous) (membranous) (suppurative)
  (ulcerative) K12.2
Staphylococcal scalded skin syndrome
  L00
Staphylococcemia A41.2
Staphylococcus, staphylococcal — *see also*
  condition
  as cause of disease classified elsewhere B95.8
    aureus (methicillin susceptible) (MSSA)
      B95.61
      methicillin resistant (MRSA) B95.62
    specified NEC, as cause of disease classified
      elsewhere B95.7
Staphyloma (sclera)
  cornea H18.72-
  equatorial H15.81-
  localized (anterior) H15.82-
  posticum H15.83-
  ring H15.85-
Stargardt's disease — *see* Dystrophy, retina
Starvation (inanition) (due to lack of food)
  T73.0
  edema — *see* Malnutrition, severe
Stasis
  bile (noncalculous) K83.1
  bronchus J98.09
    with infection — *see* Bronchitis
  cardiac — *see* Failure, heart, congestive
  cecum K59.8
  colon K59.8
  dermatitis I87.2
    with
      varicose ulcer — *see* Varix, leg, with ulcer,
        with inflammation
      varicose veins — *see* Varix, leg, with,
        inflammation
    due to postthrombotic syndrome — *see*
      Syndrome, postthrombotic
  duodenal K31.5
  eczema — *see* Varix, leg, with, inflammation
  edema — *see* Hypertension, venous (chronic),
    idiopathic
  foot T69.0-
  ileocecal coil K59.8
  ileum K59.8
  intestinal K59.8
  jejunum K59.8
  kidney N19
  liver (cirrhotic) K76.1
  lymphatic I89.8
  pneumonia J18.2
  pulmonary — *see* Edema, lung
  rectal K59.8
  renal N19
    tubular N17.0
  ulcer — *see* Varix, leg, with, ulcer
    without varicose veins I87.2
  urine — *see* Retention, urine
  venous I87.8
State (of)
  affective and paranoid, mixed, organic
    psychotic F06.8
  agitated R45.1
    acute reaction to stress F43.0
  anxiety (neurotic) F41.1
  apprehension F41.1
  burn-out Z73.0
  climacteric, female Z78.0
    symptomatic N95.1
  compulsive F42.8
    mixed with obsessional thoughts F42.2

State (of) — *continued*
  confusional (psychogenic) F44.89
    acute — *see also* Delirium
      with
        arteriosclerotic dementia F01.50
          with behavioral disturbance F01.51
        senility or dementia F05
    alcoholic F10.231
    epileptic F05
    reactive (from emotional stress,
      psychological trauma) F44.89
    subacute — *see* Delirium
  convulsive — *see* Convulsions
  crisis F43.0
  depressive F32.9
    neurotic F34.1
  dissociative F44.9
  emotional shock (stress) R45.7
  hypercoagulation — *see* Hypercoagulable
  locked-in G83.5
  menopausal Z78.0
    symptomatic N95.1
  neurotic F48.9
    with depersonalization F48.1
  obsessional F42.8
  oneiroid (schizophrenia-like) F23
  organic
    hallucinatory (nonalcoholic) F06.0
    paranoid(-hallucinatory) F06.2
  panic F41.0
  paranoid F22
    climacteric F22
    involutional F22
    menopausal F22
    organic F06.2
    senile F03
    simple F22
  persistent vegetative R40.3
  phobic F40.9
  postleukotomy F07.0
  pregnant
    gestational carrier Z33.3
    incidental Z33.1
  psychogenic, twilight F44.89
  psychopathic (constitutional) F60.2
  psychotic, organic — *see also* Psychosis,
    organic
    mixed paranoid and affective F06.8
    senile or presenile F03
    transient NEC F06.8
      with
        depression F06.31
        hallucinations F06.0
  residual schizophrenic F20.5
  restlessness R45.1
  stress (emotional) R45.7
  tension (mental) F48.9
    specified NEC F48.8
  transient organic psychotic NEC F06.8
    depressive type F06.31
    hallucinatory type F06.0
  twilight
    epileptic F05
    psychogenic F44.89
  vegetative, persistent R40.3
  vital exhaustion Z73.0
  withdrawal — *see* Withdrawal, state
Status (post) — *see also* Presence (of)
  absence, epileptic — *see* Epilepsy, by type,
    with status epilepticus
  administration of tPA (rtPA) in a different
    facility within the last 24 hours prior to
    admission to current facility Z92.82
  adrenalectomy (unilateral) (bilateral) E89.6
  anastomosis Z98.0
  anginosus I20.9

Status (post) (*see also* Presence (of)) — continued
- angioplasty (peripheral) Z98.62
  - with implant Z95.820
  - coronary artery Z98.61
    - with implant Z95.5
- aortocoronary bypass Z95.1
- arthrodesis Z98.1
- artificial opening (of) Z93.9
  - gastrointestinal tract Z93.4
  - specified NEC Z93.8
  - urinary tract Z93.6
  - vagina Z93.8
- asthmaticus — *see* Asthma, by type, with status asthmaticus
- awaiting organ transplant Z76.82
- bariatric surgery Z98.84
- bed confinement Z74.01
- bleb, filtering (vitreous), after glaucoma surgery Z98.83
- breast implant Z98.82
  - removal Z98.86
- cataract extraction Z98.4-
- cholecystectomy Z90.49
- clitorectomy N90.811
  - with excision of labia minora N90.812
- colectomy (complete) (partial) Z90.49
- colonization — *see* Carrier (suspected) of
- colostomy Z93.3
- convulsivus idiopathicus — *see* Epilepsy, by type, with status epilepticus
- coronary artery angioplasty — *see* Status, angioplasty, coronary artery
- cystectomy (urinary bladder) Z90.6
- cystostomy Z93.50
  - appendico-vesicostomy Z93.52
  - cutaneous Z93.51
  - specified NEC Z93.59
- delinquent immunization Z28.3
- dental Z98.818
  - crown Z98.811
  - fillings Z98.811
  - restoration Z98.811
  - sealant Z98.810
  - specified NEC Z98.818
- deployment (current) (military) Z56.82
- dialysis (hemodialysis) (peritoneal) Z99.2
- do not resuscitate (DNR) Z66
- donor — *see* Donor
- embedded fragments — *see* Retained, foreign body fragments (type of)
- embedded splinter — *see* Retained, foreign body fragments (type of)
- enterostomy Z93.4
- epileptic, epilepticus (*see also* Epilepsy, by type, with status epilepticus) G40.901
- estrogen receptor
  - negative Z17.1
  - positive Z17.0
- female genital cutting — *see* Female genital mutilation status
- female genital mutilation — *see* Female genital mutilation status
- filtering (vitreous) bleb after glaucoma surgery Z98.83
- gastrectomy (complete) (partial) Z90.3
- gastric banding Z98.84
- gastric bypass for obesity Z98.84
- gastrostomy Z93.1
- human immunodeficiency virus (HIV) infection, asymptomatic Z21
- hysterectomy (complete) (total) Z90.710
  - partial (with remaining cervial stump) Z90.711
- ileostomy Z93.2
- implant
  - breast Z98.82
- infibulation N90.813
- intestinal bypass Z98.0

Status (post) (*see also* Presence (of)) — continued
- jejunostomy Z93.4
- lapsed immunization schedule Z28.3
- laryngectomy Z90.02
- lymphaticus E32.8
- malignancy
  - castrate resistant prostate Z19.2
  - hormone resistant Z19.2
  - hormone sensitive Z19.1
- marmoratus G80.3
- mastectomy (unilateral) (bilateral) Z90.1-
- military deployment status (current) Z56.82
  - in theater or in support of military war, peacekeeping and humanitarian operations Z56.82
- nephrectomy (unilateral) (bilateral) Z90.5
- nephrostomy Z93.6
- obesity surgery Z98.84
- oophorectomy
  - bilateral Z90.722
  - unilateral Z90.721
- organ replacement
  - by artificial or mechanical device or prosthesis of
    - artery Z95.828
    - bladder Z96.0
    - blood vessel Z95.828
    - breast Z97.8
    - eye globe Z97.0
    - heart Z95.812
      - valve Z95.2
    - intestine Z97.8
    - joint Z96.60
      - hip — *see* Presence, hip joint implant
      - knee — *see* Presence, knee joint implant
      - specified site NEC Z96.698
    - kidney Z97.8
    - larynx Z96.3
    - lens Z96.1
    - limbs — *see* Presence, artificial, limb
    - liver Z97.8
    - lung Z97.8
    - pancreas Z97.8
  - by organ transplant (heterologous) (homologous) — *see* Transplant
- pacemaker
  - brain Z96.89
  - cardiac Z95.0
  - specified NEC Z96.89
- pancreatectomy Z90.410
  - complete Z90.410
  - partial Z90.411
  - total Z90.410
- physical restraint Z78.1
- pneumonectomy (complete) (partial) Z90.2
- pneumothorax, therapeutic Z98.3
- postcommotio cerebri F07.81
- postoperative (postprocedural) NEC Z98.890
  - breast implant Z98.82
  - dental Z98.818
    - crown Z98.811
    - fillings Z98.811
    - restoration Z98.811
    - sealant Z98.810
    - specified NEC Z98.818
  - pneumothorax, therapeutic Z98.3
  - uterine scar Z98.891
- postpartum (routine follow-up) Z39.2
  - care immediately after delivery Z39.0
- postsurgical (postprocedural) NEC Z98.890
  - pneumothorax, therapeutic Z98.3
- pregnancy, incidental Z33.1
- prosthesis coronary angioplasty Z95.5
- pseudophakia Z96.1
- renal dialysis (hemodialysis) (peritoneal) Z99.2
- retained foreign body — *see* Retained, foreign body fragments (type of)

Status (post) (*see also* Presence (of)) — continued
- reversed jejunal transposition (for bypass) Z98.0
- salpingo-oophorectomy
  - bilateral Z90.722
  - unilateral Z90.721
- sex reassignment surgery status Z87.890
- shunt
  - arteriovenous (for dialysis) Z99.2
  - cerebrospinal fluid Z98.2
  - ventricular (communicating) (for drainage) Z98.2
- splenectomy Z90.81
- thymicolymphaticus E32.8
- thymicus E32.8
- thymolymphaticus E32.8
- thyroidectomy (hypothyroidism) E89.0
- tooth (teeth) extraction (*see also* Absence, teeth, acquired) K08.409
- tPA (rtPA) administration in a different facility within the last 24 hours prior to admission to current facility Z92.82
- tracheostomy Z93.0
- transplant — *see* Transplant
  - organ removed Z98.85
- tubal ligation Z98.51
- underimmunization Z28.3
- ureterostomy Z93.6
- urethrostomy Z93.6
- vagina, artificial Z93.8
- vasectomy Z98.52
- wheelchair confinement Z99.3

Stealing
- child problem F91.8
  - in company with others Z72.810
- pathological (compulsive) F63.2

Steam burn — *see* Burn

Steatocystoma multiplex L72.2

Steatohepatitis (nonalcoholic) (NASH) K75.81

Steatoma L72.3
- eyelid (cystic) — *see* Dermatosis, eyelid
  - infected — *see* Hordeolum

Steatorrhea (chronic) K90.9
- with lacteal obstruction K90.2
- idiopathic (adult) (infantile) K90.9
- pancreatic K90.3
- primary K90.0
- tropical K90.1

Steatosis E88.89
- heart — *see* Degeneration, myocardial
- kidney N28.89
- liver NEC K76.0

Steele-Richardson-Olszewski disease or syndrome G23.1

Stein-Leventhal syndrome E28.2

Stein's syndrome E28.2

Steinbrocker's syndrome G90.8

Steinert's disease G71.11

STEMI (*see also* Infarct, myocardium, ST elevation) I21.3

Stenocardia I20.8

Stenocephaly Q75.8

Stenosis, stenotic (cicatricial) — *see also* Stricture
- ampulla of Vater K83.1
- anus, anal (canal) (sphincter) K62.4
  - and rectum K62.4
  - congenital Q42.3
    - with fistula Q42.2
- aorta (ascending) (supraventricular) (congenital) Q25.1
  - arteriosclerotic I70.0
  - calcified I70.0
  - supravalvular Q25.3

Stenosis, stenotic (cicatricial) (*see also* Stricture) — *continued*
  aortic (valve) I35.0
    with insufficiency I35.2
    congenital Q23.0
    rheumatic I06.0
      with
        incompetency, insufficiency or regurgitation I06.2
          with mitral (valve) disease I08.0
            with tricuspid (valve) disease I08.3
          mitral (valve) disease I08.0
            with tricuspid (valve) disease I08.3
          tricuspid (valve) disease I08.2
            with mitral (valve) disease I08.3
    specified cause NEC I35.0
    syphilitic A52.03
  aqueduct of Sylvius (congenital) Q03.0
    with spina bifida — *see* Spina bifida, by site, with hydrocephalus
    acquired G91.1
  artery NEC (*see also* Arteriosclerosis) I77.1
    celiac I77.4
    cerebral — *see* Occlusion, artery, cerebral
    extremities — *see* Arteriosclerosis, extremities
    precerebral — *see* Occlusion, artery, precerebral
    pulmonary (congenital) Q25.6
      acquired I28.8
    renal I70.1
    stent
      coronary T82.855
      peripheral T82.856
  bile duct (common) (hepatic) K83.1
    congenital Q44.3
  bladder-neck (acquired) N32.0
    congenital Q64.31
  brain G93.89
  bronchus J98.09
    congenital Q32.3
    syphilitic A52.72
  cardia (stomach) K22.2
    congenital Q39.3
  cardiovascular — *see* Disease, cardiovascular
  caudal M48.08
  cervix, cervical (canal) N88.2
    congenital Q51.828
    in pregnancy or childbirth — *see* Pregnancy, complicated by, abnormal cervix
  colon — *see also* Obstruction, intestine
    congenital Q42.9
      specified NEC Q42.8
  colostomy K94.03
  common (bile) duct K83.1
    congenital Q44.3
  coronary (artery) — *see* Disease, heart, ischemic, atherosclerotic
  cystic duct — *see* Obstruction, gallbladder
  due to presence of device, implant or graft (*see also* Complications, by site and type, specified NEC) T85.858
    arterial graft NEC T82.858
    breast (implant) T85.858
    catheter T85.858
      dialysis (renal) T82.858
        intraperitoneal T85.858
      infusion NEC T82.858
        spinal (epidural) (subdural) T85.858
      urinary (indwelling) T83.85
    fixation, internal (orthopedic) NEC T84.85
    gastrointestinal (bile duct) (esophagus) T85.858
    genital NEC T83.85
    heart NEC T82.857
    joint prosthesis T84.85
    ocular (corneal graft) (orbital implant) NEC T85.858
    orthopedic NEC T84.85
    specified NEC T85.858

Stenosis, stenotic (cicatricial) (*see also* Stricture) — *continued*
  due to presence of device, implant or graft (*see also* Complications, by site and type, specified NEC) T85.858 — *continued*
    urinary NEC T83.85
    vascular NEC T82.858
    ventricular intracranial shunt T85.850
  duodenum K31.5
    congenital Q41.0
  ejaculatory duct NEC N50.89
  endocervical os — *see* Stenosis, cervix
  enterostomy K94.13
  esophagus K22.2
    congenital Q39.3
    syphilitic A52.79
      congenital A50.59 [K23]
  eustachian tube — *see* Obstruction, eustachian tube
  external ear canal (acquired) H61.30-
    congenital Q16.1
    due to
      inflammation H61.32-
      trauma H61.31-
    postprocedural H95.81-
    specified cause NEC H61.39-
  gallbladder — *see* Obstruction, gallbladder
  glottis J38.6
  heart valve (congenital) Q24.8
    aortic Q23.0
    mitral Q23.2
    pulmonary Q22.1
    tricuspid Q22.4
  hepatic duct K83.1
  hymen N89.6
  hypertrophic subaortic (idiopathic) I42.1
  ileum K56.69
    congenital Q41.2
  infundibulum cardia Q24.3
  intervertebral foramina — *see also* Lesion, biomechanical, specified NEC
    connective tissue M99.79
      abdomen M99.79
      cervical region M99.71
      cervicothoracic M99.71
      head region M99.70
      lumbar region M99.73
      lumbosacral M99.73
      occipitocervical M99.70
      sacral region M99.74
      sacrococcygeal M99.74
      sacroiliac M99.74
      specified NEC M99.79
      thoracic region M99.72
      thoracolumbar M99.72
    disc M99.79
      abdomen M99.79
      cervical region M99.71
      cervicothoracic M99.71
      head region M99.70
      lower extremity M99.76
      lumbar region M99.73
      lumbosacral M99.73
      occipitocervical M99.70
      pelvic M99.75
      rib cage M99.78
      sacral region M99.74
      sacrococcygeal M99.74
      sacroiliac M99.74
      specified NEC M99.79
      thoracic region M99.72
      thoracolumbar M99.72
      upper extremity M99.77
    osseous M99.69
      abdomen M99.69
      cervical region M99.61
      cervicothoracic M99.61
      head region M99.60
      lower extremity M99.66

Stenosis, stenotic (cicatricial) (*see also* Stricture) — *continued*
  intervertebral foramina — *see also* Lesion, biomechanical, specified NEC — *continued*
    osseous M99.69 — *continued*
      lumbar region M99.63
      lumbosacral M99.63
      occipitocervical M99.60
      pelvic M99.65
      rib cage M99.68
      sacral region M99.64
      sacrococcygeal M99.64
      sacroiliac M99.64
      specified NEC M99.69
      thoracic region M99.62
      thoracolumbar M99.62
      upper extremity M99.67
    subluxation — *see* Stenosis, intervertebral foramina, osseous
  intestine — *see also* Obstruction, intestine
    congenital (small) Q41.9
      large Q42.9
        specified NEC Q42.8
      specified NEC Q41.8
  jejunum K56.69
    congenital Q41.1
  lacrimal (passage)
    canaliculi H04.54-
    congenital Q10.5
    duct H04.55-
    punctum H04.56-
    sac H04.57-
  lacrimonasal duct — *see* Stenosis, lacrimal, duct
    congenital Q10.5
  larynx J38.6
    congenital NEC Q31.8
      subglottic Q31.1
    syphilitic A52.73
      congenital A50.59 [J99]
  mitral (chronic) (inactive) (valve) I05.0
    with
      aortic valve disease I08.0
      incompetency, insufficiency or regurgitation I05.2
    active or acute I01.1
      with rheumatic or Sydenham's chorea I02.0
    congenital Q23.2
    specified cause, except rheumatic I34.2
    syphilitic A52.03
  myocardium, myocardial — *see also* Degeneration, myocardial
    hypertrophic subaortic (idiopathic) I42.1
  nares (anterior) (posterior) J34.89
    congenital Q30.0
  nasal duct — *see also* Stenosis, lacrimal, duct
    congenital Q10.5
  nasolacrimal duct — *see also* Stenosis, lacrimal, duct
    congenital Q10.5
  neural canal — *see also* Lesion, biomechanical, specified NEC
    connective tissue M99.49
      abdomen M99.49
      cervical region M99.41
      cervicothoracic M99.41
      head region M99.40
      lower extremity M99.46
      lumbar region M99.43
      lumbosacral M99.43
      occipitocervical M99.40
      pelvic M99.45
      rib cage M99.48
      sacral region M99.44
      sacrococcygeal M99.44
      sacroiliac M99.44
      specified NEC M99.49

Stenosis, stenotic (cicatricial) (*see also* Stricture) — *continued*
  neural canal — *see also* Lesion, biomechanical, specified NEC — *continued*
    connective tissue M99.49 — *continued*
      thoracic region M99.42
      thoracolumbar M99.42
      upper extremity M99.47
    intervertebral disc M99.59
      abdomen M99.59
      cervical region M99.51
      cervicothoracic M99.51
      head region M99.50
      lower extremity M99.56
      lumbar region M99.53
      lumbosacral M99.53
      occipitocervical M99.50
      pelvic M99.55
      rib cage M99.58
      sacral region M99.54
      sacrococcygeal M99.54
      sacroiliac M99.54
      specified NEC M99.59
      thoracic region M99.52
      thoracolumbar M99.52
      upper extremity M99.57
    osseous M99.39
      abdomen M99.39
      cervical region M99.31
      cervicothoracic M99.31
      head region M99.30
      lower extremity M99.36
      lumbar region M99.33
      lumbosacral M99.33
      occipitocervical M99.30
      pelvic M99.35
      rib cage M99.38
      sacral region M99.34
      sacrococcygeal M99.34
      sacroiliac M99.34
      specified NEC M99.39
      thoracic region M99.32
      thoracolumbar M99.32
      upper extremity M99.37
    subluxation M99.29
      cervical region M99.21
      cervicothoracic M99.21
      head region M99.20
      lower extremity M99.26
      lumbar region M99.23
      lumbosacral M99.23
      occipitocervical M99.20
      pelvic M99.25
      rib cage M99.28
      sacral region M99.24
      sacrococcygeal M99.24
      sacroiliac M99.24
      specified NEC M99.29
      thoracic region M99.22
      thoracolumbar M99.22
      upper extremity M99.27
  organ or site, congenital NEC — *see* Atresia, by site
  papilla of Vater K83.1
  pulmonary (artery) (congenital) Q25.6
    with ventricular septal defect, transposition of aorta, and hypertrophy of right ventricle Q21.3
    acquired I28.8
    in tetralogy of Fallot Q21.3
    infundibular Q24.3
    subvalvular Q24.3
    supravalvular Q25.6
    valve I37.0
      with insufficiency I37.2
      congenital Q22.1
      rheumatic I09.89
        with aortic, mitral or tricuspid (valve) disease I08.8

Stenosis, stenotic (cicatricial) (*see also* Stricture) — *continued*
  pulmonary (artery) (congenital) Q25.6 — *continued*
    vein, acquired I28.8
    vessel NEC I28.8
  pulmonic (congenital) Q22.1
    infundibular Q24.3
    subvalvular Q24.3
  pylorus (hypertrophic) (acquired) K31.1
    adult K31.1
    congenital Q40.0
    infantile Q40.0
  rectum (sphincter) — *see* Stricture, rectum
  renal artery I70.1
    congenital Q27.1
  salivary duct (any) K11.8
  sphincter of Oddi K83.1
  spinal M48.00
    cervical region M48.02
    cervicothoracic region M48.03
    lumbar region M48.06
    lumbosacral region M48.07
    occipito-atlanto-axial region M48.01
    sacrococcygeal region M48.08
    thoracic region M48.04
    thoracolumbar region M48.05
  stent
    vascular
      end stent
        adjacent to stent — *see* Arteriosclerosis
        within the stent
          coronary T82.855
          peripheral T82.856
      in stent
        coronary vessel T82.855
        peripheral vessel T82.856
  stomach, hourglass K31.2
  subaortic (congenital) Q24.4
    hypertrophic (idiopathic) I42.1
  subglottic J38.6
    congenital Q31.1
    postprocedural J95.5
  trachea J39.8
    congenital Q32.1
    syphilitic A52.73
    tuberculous NEC A15.5
  tracheostomy J95.03
  tricuspid (valve) I07.0
    with
      aortic (valve) disease I08.2
      incompetency, insufficiency or regurgitation I07.2
        with aortic (valve) disease I08.2
          with mitral (valve) disease I08.3
      mitral (valve) disease I08.1
        with aortic (valve) disease I08.3
    congenital Q22.4
    nonrheumatic I36.0
      with insufficiency I36.2
  tubal N97.1
  ureter — *see* Atresia, ureter
  ureteropelvic junction, congenital Q62.11
  ureterovesical orifice, congenital Q62.12
  urethra (valve) — *see also* Stricture, urethra
    congenital Q64.32
  urinary meatus, congenital Q64.33
  vagina N89.5
    congenital Q52.4
    in pregnancy — *see* Pregnancy, complicated by, abnormal vagina
      causing obstructed labor O65.5
  valve (cardiac) (heart) (*see also* Endocarditis) I38
    congenital Q24.8
      aortic Q23.0
      mitral Q23.2
      pulmonary Q22.1
      tricuspid Q22.4

Stenosis, stenotic (cicatricial) (*see also* Stricture) — *continued*
  vena cava (inferior) (superior) I87.1
    congenital Q26.0
  vesicourethral orifice Q64.31
  vulva N90.5
Stent jail T82.897
Stercolith (impaction) K56.41
  appendix K38.1
Stercoraceous, stercoral ulcer K63.3
  anus or rectum K62.6
Stereotypies NEC F98.4
Sterility — *see* Infertility
Sterilization — *see* Encounter (for), sterilization
Sternalgia — *see* Angina
Sternopagus Q89.4
Sternum bifidum Q76.7
Steroid
  effects (adverse) (adrenocortical) (iatrogenic)
    cushingoid E24.2
      correct substance properly administered — *see* Table of Drugs and Chemicals, by drug, adverse effect
      overdose or wrong substance given or taken — *see* Table of Drugs and Chemicals, by drug, poisoning
    diabetes — *see* category E09
      correct substance properly administered — *see* Table of Drugs and Chemicals, by drug, adverse effect
      overdose or wrong substance given or taken — *see* Table of Drugs and Chemicals, by drug, poisoning
    fever R50.2
    insufficiency E27.3
      correct substance properly administered — *see* Table of Drugs and Chemicals, by drug, adverse effect
      overdose or wrong substance given or taken — *see* Table of Drugs and Chemicals, by drug, poisoning
  responder H40.04-
Stevens-Johnson disease or syndrome L51.1
  toxic epidermal necrolysis overlap L51.3
Stewart-Morel syndrome M85.2
Sticker's disease B08.3
Sticky eye — *see* Conjunctivitis, acute, mucopurulent
Stieda's disease — *see* Bursitis, tibial collateral
Stiff neck — *see* Torticollis
Stiff-man syndrome G25.82
Stiffness, joint NEC M25.60-
  ankle M25.67-
  ankylosis — *see* Ankylosis, joint
  contracture — *see* Contraction, joint
  elbow M25.62-
  foot M25.67-
  hand M25.64-
  hip M25.65-
  knee M25.66-
  shoulder M25.61-
  wrist M25.63-
Stigmata congenital syphilis A50.59
Still's disease or syndrome (juvenile) M08.20
  adult-onset M06.1
  ankle M08.27-
  elbow M08.22-
  foot joint M08.27-
  hand joint M08.24-
  hip M08.25-
  knee M08.26-
  multiple site M08.29
  shoulder M08.21-
  vertebra M08.28
  wrist M08.23-
Still-Felty syndrome — *see* Felty's syndrome

Stillbirth P95
Stimulation, ovary E28.1
Sting (venomous) (with allergic or anaphylactic shock) — *see* Table of Drugs and Chemicals, by animal or substance, poisoning
Stippled epiphyses Q78.8
Stitch
  abscess T81.48
  burst (in operation wound) — *see* Disruption, wound, operation
Stokes' disease E05.00
  with thyroid storm E05.01
Stokes-Adams disease or syndrome I45.9
Stokvis(-Talma) disease D74.8
Stoma malfunction
  colostomy K94.03
  enterostomy K94.13
  gastrostomy K94.23
  ileostomy K94.13
  tracheostomy J95.03
Stomach — *see* condition
Stomatitis (denture) (ulcerative) K12.1
  angular K13.0
    due to dietary or vitamin deficiency E53.0
  aphthous K12.0
  bovine B08.61
  candidal B37.0
  catarrhal K12.1
  diphtheritic A36.89
  due to
    dietary deficiency E53.0
    thrush B37.0
    vitamin deficiency
      B group NEC E53.9
      B2 (riboflavin) E53.0
  epidemic B08.8
  epizootic B08.8
  follicular K12.1
  gangrenous A69.0
  Geotrichum B48.3
  herpesviral, herpetic B00.2
  herpetiformis K12.0
  malignant K12.1
  membranous acute K12.1
  monilial B37.0
  mycotic B37.0
  necrotizing ulcerative A69.0
  parasitic B37.0
  septic K12.1
  spirochetal A69.1
  suppurative (acute) K12.2
  ulceromembranous A69.1
  vesicular K12.1
    with exanthem (enteroviral) B08.4
    virus disease A93.8
  Vincent's A69.1
Stomatocytosis D58.8
Stomatomycosis B37.0
Stomatorrhagia K13.79
Stone(s) — *see also* Calculus
  bladder (diverticulum) N21.0
  cystine E72.09
  heart syndrome I50.1
  kidney N20.0
  prostate N42.0
  pulpal (dental) K04.2
  renal N20.0
  salivary gland or duct (any) K11.5
  urethra (impacted) N21.1
  urinary (duct) (impacted) (passage) N20.9
    bladder (diverticulum) N21.0
    lower tract N21.9
    specified NEC N21.8
  xanthine E79.8 [N22]
Stonecutter's lung J62.8
Stonemason's asthma, disease, lung or pneumoconiosis J62.8

Stoppage
  heart — *see* Arrest, cardiac
  urine — *see* Retention, urine
Storm, thyroid — *see* Thyrotoxicosis
Strabismus (congenital) (nonparalytic) H50.9
  concomitant H50.40
    convergent — *see* Strabismus, convergent concomitant
    divergent — *see* Strabismus, divergent concomitant
  convergent concomitant H50.00
    accommodative component H50.43
    alternating H50.05
      with
        A pattern H50.06
        specified nonconcomitances NEC H50.08
        V pattern H50.07
    monocular H50.01-
      with
        A pattern H50.02-
        specified nonconcomitances NEC H50.04-
        V pattern H50.03-
      intermittent H50.31-
        alternating H50.32
  cyclotropia H50.41
  divergent concomitant H50.10
    alternating H50.15
      with
        A pattern H50.16
        specified noncomitances NEC H50.18
        V pattern H50.17
    monocular H50.11-
      with
        A pattern H50.12-
        specified noncomitances NEC H50.14-
        V pattern H50.13-
      intermittent H50.33
        alternating H50.34
  Duane's syndrome H50.81-
  due to adhesions, scars H50.69
  heterophoria H50.50
    alternating H50.55
    cyclophoria H50.54
    esophoria H50.51
    exophoria H50.52
    vertical H50.53
  heterotropia H50.40
    intermittent H50.30
  hypertropia H50.2-
  hypotropia — *see* Hypertropia
  latent H50.50
  mechanical H50.60
    Brown's sheath syndrome H50.61-
    specified type NEC H50.69
  monofixation syndrome H50.42
  paralytic H49.9
    abducens nerve H49.2-
    fourth nerve H49.1-
    Kearns-Sayre syndrome H49.81-
    ophthalmoplegia (external)
      progressive H49.4-
        with pigmentary retinopathy H49.81-
      total H49.3-
    sixth nerve H49.2-
    specified type NEC H49.88-
    third nerve H49.0-
    trochlear nerve H49.1-
  specified type NEC H50.89
  vertical H50.2-
Strain
  back S39.012
  cervical S16.1
  eye NEC — *see* Disturbance, vision, subjective
  heart — *see* Disease, heart
  low back S39.012
  mental NOS Z73.3
    work-related Z56.6

Strain — *continued*
  muscle (tendon) — *see* Injury, muscle, by site, strain
  neck S16.1
  physical NOS Z73.3
    work-related Z56.6
  postural — *see also* Disorder, soft tissue, due to use
  psychological NEC Z73.3
  tendon — *see* Injury, muscle, by site, strain
Straining, on urination R39.16
Strand, vitreous — *see* Opacity, vitreous, membranes and strands
Strangulation, strangulated — *see also* Asphyxia, traumatic
  appendix K38.8
  bladder-neck N32.0
  bowel or colon K56.2
  food or foreign body — *see* Foreign body, by site
  hemorrhoids — *see* Hemorrhoids, with complication
  hernia — *see also* Hernia, by site, with obstruction
    with gangrene — *see* Hernia, by site, with gangrene
  intestine (large) (small) K56.2
    with hernia — *see also* Hernia, by site, with obstruction
      with gangrene — *see* Hernia, by site, with gangrene
  mesentery K56.2
  mucus — *see* Asphyxia, mucus
  omentum K56.2
  organ or site, congenital NEC — *see* Atresia, by site
  ovary — *see* Torsion, ovary
  penis N48.89
    foreign body T19.4
  rupture — *see* Hernia, by site, with obstruction
  stomach due to hernia — *see also* Hernia, by site, with obstruction
    with gangrene — *see* Hernia, by site, with gangrene
  vesicourethral orifice N32.0
Strangury R30.0
Straw itch B88.0
Strawberry
  gallbladder K82.4
  mark Q82.5
  tongue (red) (white) K14.3
Streak(s)
  macula, angioid H35.33
  ovarian Q50.32
Strephosymbolia F81.0
  secondary to organic lesion R48.8
Streptobacillary fever A25.1
Streptobacillosis A25.1
Streptobacillus moniliformis A25.1
Streptococcus, streptococcal — *see also* condition
  as cause of disease classified elsewhere B95.5
  group
    A, as cause of disease classified elsewhere B95.0
    B, as cause of disease classified elsewhere B95.1
    D, as cause of disease classified elsewhere B95.2
  pneumoniae, as cause of disease classified elsewhere B95.3
  specified NEC, as cause of disease classified elsewhere B95.4
Streptomycosis B47.1
Streptotrichosis A48.8

DISEASE INDEX

Stress F43.9
  family — *see* Disruption, family
  fetal P84
    complicating pregnancy O77.9
      due to drug administration O77.1
  mental NEC Z73.3
    work-related Z56.6
  physical NEC Z73.3
    work-related Z56.6
  polycythemia D75.1
  reaction (*see also* Reaction, stress) F43.9
  work schedule Z56.3
Stretching, nerve — *see* Injury, nerve
Striae albicantes, atrophicae or
  distensae (cutis) L90.6
Stricture — *see also* Stenosis
  ampulla of Vater K83.1
  anus (sphincter) K62.4
    congenital Q42.3
      with fistula Q42.2
    infantile Q42.3
      with fistula Q42.2
  aorta (ascending) (congenital) Q25.1
    arteriosclerotic I70.0
    calcified I70.0
    supravalvular, congenital Q25.3
  aortic (valve) — *see* Stenosis, aortic
  aqueduct of Sylvius (congenital) Q03.0
    with spina bifida — *see* Spina bifida, by site,
      with hydrocephalus
    acquired G91.1
  artery I77.1
    basilar — *see* Occlusion, artery, basilar
    carotid — *see* Occlusion, artery, carotid
    celiac I77.4
    congenital (peripheral) Q27.8
      cerebral Q28.3
      coronary Q24.5
      digestive system Q27.8
      lower limb Q27.8
      retinal Q14.1
      specified site NEC Q27.8
      umbilical Q27.0
      upper limb Q27.8
    coronary — *see* Disease, heart, ischemic,
      atherosclerotic
      congenital Q24.5
    precerebral — *see* Occlusion, artery,
      precerebral
    pulmonary (congenital) Q25.6
      acquired I28.8
    renal I70.1
    vertebral — *see* Occlusion, artery, vertebral
  auditory canal (external) (congenital)
    acquired — *see* Stenosis, external ear canal
  bile duct (common) (hepatic) K83.1
    congenital Q44.3
    postoperative K91.89
  bladder N32.89
    neck N32.0
  bowel — *see* Obstruction, intestine
  brain G93.89
  bronchus J98.09
    congenital Q32.3
    syphilitic A52.72
  cardia (stomach) K22.2
    congenital Q39.3
  cardiac — *see* Disease, heart
    orifice (stomach) K22.2
  cecum — *see* Obstruction, intestine
  cervix, cervical (canal) N88.2
    congenital Q51.828
    in pregnancy — *see* Pregnancy, complicated
      by, abnormal cervix
      causing obstructed labor O65.5
  colon — *see also* Obstruction, intestine
    congenital Q42.9
      specified NEC Q42.8
  colostomy K94.03

Stricture (*see also* Stenosis) — *continued*
  common (bile) duct K83.1
  coronary (artery) — *see* Disease, heart,
    ischemic, atherosclerotic
  cystic duct — *see* Obstruction, gallbladder
  digestive organs NEC, congenital Q45.8
  duodenum K31.5
    congenital Q41.0
  ear canal (external) (congenital) Q16.1
    acquired — *see* Stricture, auditory canal,
      acquired
  ejaculatory duct N50.89
  enterostomy K94.13
  esophagus K22.2
    congenital Q39.3
    syphilitic A52.79
      congenital A50.59 *[K23]*
  eustachian tube — *see also* Obstruction,
    eustachian tube
    congenital Q17.8
  fallopian tube N97.1
    gonococcal A54.24
    tuberculous A18.17
  gallbladder — *see* Obstruction, gallbladder
  glottis J38.6
  heart — *see also* Disease, heart
    valve (*see also* Endocarditis) I38
      aortic Q23.0
      mitral Q23.4
      pulmonary Q22.1
      tricuspid Q22.4
  hepatic duct K83.1
  hourglass, of stomach K31.2
  hymen N89.6
  hypopharynx J39.2
  ileum K56.69
    congenital Q41.2
  intestine — *see also* Obstruction, intestine
    congenital (small) Q41.9
      large Q42.9
        specified NEC Q42.8
      specified NEC Q41.8
    ischemic K55.1
  jejunum K56.69
    congenital Q41.1
  lacrimal passages — *see also* Stenosis, lacrimal
    congenital Q10.5
  larynx J38.6
    congenital NEC Q31.8
      subglottic Q31.1
    syphilitic A52.73
      congenital A50.59 *[J99]*
  meatus
    ear (congenital) Q16.1
      acquired — *see* Stricture, auditory canal,
        acquired
    osseous (ear) (congenital) Q16.1
      acquired — *see* Stricture, auditory canal,
        acquired
    urinarius — *see also* Stricture, urethra
      congenital Q64.33
  mitral (valve) — *see* Stenosis, mitral
  myocardium, myocardial I51.5
    hypertrophic subaortic (idiopathic) I42.1
  nares (anterior) (posterior) J34.89
    congenital Q30.0
  nasal duct — *see also* Stenosis, lacrimal, duct
    congenital Q10.5
  nasolacrimal duct — *see also* Stenosis, lacrimal,
    duct
    congenital Q10.5
  nasopharynx J39.2
    syphilitic A52.73
  nose J34.89
    congenital Q30.0
  nostril (anterior) (posterior) J34.89
    congenital Q30.0
    syphilitic A52.73
      congenital A50.59 *[J99]*

Stricture (*see also* Stenosis) — *continued*
  organ or site, congenital NEC — *see* Atresia,
    by site
  os uteri — *see* Stricture, cervix
  osseous meatus (ear) (congenital) Q16.1
    acquired — *see* Stricture, auditory canal,
      acquired
  oviduct — *see* Stricture, fallopian tube
  pelviureteric junction (congenital) Q62.11
    acquired, with hydronephrosis N13.0
  penis, by foreign body T19.4
  pharynx J39.2
  prostate N42.89
  pulmonary, pulmonic
    artery (congenital) Q25.6
      acquired I28.8
      noncongenital I28.8
    infundibulum (congenital) Q24.3
    valve I37.0
      congenital Q22.1
    vein, acquired I28.8
    vessel NEC I28.8
  punctum lacrimale — *see also* Stenosis,
    lacrimal, punctum
    congenital Q10.5
  pylorus (hypertrophic) K31.1
    adult K31.1
    congenital Q40.0
    infantile Q40.0
  rectosigmoid K56.69
  rectum (sphincter) K62.4
    congenital Q42.1
      with fistula Q42.0
    due to
      chlamydial lymphogranuloma A55
      irradiation K91.89
      lymphogranuloma venereum A55
    gonococcal A54.6
    inflammatory (chlamydial) A55
    syphilitic A52.74
    tuberculous A18.32
  renal artery I70.1
    congenital Q27.1
  salivary duct or gland (any) K11.8
  sigmoid (flexure) — *see* Obstruction, intestine
  spermatic cord N50.89
  stoma (following) (of)
    colostomy K94.03
    enterostomy K94.13
    gastrostomy K94.23
    ileostomy K94.13
    tracheostomy J95.03
  stomach K31.89
    congenital Q40.2
    hourglass K31.2
  subaortic Q24.4
    hypertrophic (acquired) (idiopathic) I42.1
  subglottic J38.6
  syphilitic NEC A52.79
  trachea J39.8
    congenital Q32.1
    syphilitic A52.73
    tuberculous NEC A15.5
  tracheostomy J95.03
  tricuspid (valve) — *see* Stenosis, tricuspid
  tunica vaginalis N50.89
  ureter (postoperative) N13.5
    with
      hydronephrosis N13.1
        with infection N13.6
      pyelonephritis (chronic) N11.1
    congenital — *see* Atresia, ureter
    tuberculous A18.11
  ureteropelvic junction (congenital) Q62.11
    acquired, with hydronephrosis N13.0
  ureterovesical orifice N13.5
    with infection N13.6

Stricture (*see also* Stenosis) — *continued*
  urethra (organic) (spasmodic) N35.9
    associated with schistosomiasis B65.0 *[N37]*
    congenital Q64.39
      valvular (posterior) Q64.2
    due to
      infection — *see* Stricture, urethra,
        postinfective
      trauma — *see* Stricture, urethra, post-
        traumatic
    gonococcal, gonorrheal A54.01
    infective NEC — *see* Stricture, urethra,
      postinfective
    late effect (sequelae) of injury — *see*
      Stricture, urethra, post-traumatic
    post-traumatic
      female N35.028
        due to childbirth N35.021
      male N35.014
        anterior urethra N35.013
        bulbous urethra N35.011
        meatal N35.010
        membranous urethra N35.012
    postcatheterization — *see* Stricture, urethra,
      postprocedural
    postinfective NEC
      female N35.12
      male N35.119
        anterior urethra N35.114
        bulbous urethra N35.112
        meatal N35.111
        membranous urethra N35.113
    postobstetric N35.021
    postoperative — *see* Stricture, urethra,
      postprocedural
    postprocedural
      female N99.12
      male N99.114
        anterior bulbous urethra N99.113
        bulbous urethra N99.111
        fossa navicularis N99.115
        meatal N99.110
        membranous urethra N99.112
    sequela (late effect) of
      childbirth N35.021
      injury — *see* Stricture, urethra, post-
        traumatic
    specified cause NEC N35.8
    syphilitic A52.76
    traumatic — *see* Stricture, urethra, post-
      traumatic
    valvular (posterior), congenital Q64.2
  urinary meatus — *see* Stricture, urethra
  uterus, uterine (synechiae) N85.6
  os (external) (internal) — *see* Stricture, cervix
  vagina (outlet) — *see* Stenosis, vagina
  valve (cardiac) (heart) — *see also* Endocarditis
    congenital
      aortic Q23.0
      mitral Q23.2
      pulmonary Q22.1
      tricuspid Q22.4
  vas deferens N50.89
    congenital Q55.4
  vein I87.1
  vena cava (inferior) (superior) NEC I87.1
    congenital Q26.0
  vesicourethral orifice N32.0
    congenital Q64.31
  vulva (acquired) N90.5
Stridor R06.1
  congenital (larynx) P28.89
Stridulous — *see* condition
Stroke (apoplectic) (brain) (embolic) (ischemic)
  (paralytic) (thrombotic) I63.9
  epileptic — *see* Epilepsy
  heat T67.0
  in evolution I63.9

Stroke (apoplectic) (brain) (embolic) (ischemic)
  (paralytic) (thrombotic) I63.9 — *continued*
  intraoperative
    during cardiac surgery I97.810
    during other surgery I97.811
  lightning — *see* Lightning
  meaning
    cerebral hemorrhage — *code to*
      Hemorrhage, intracranial
    cerebral infarction — *code to* Infarction,
      cerebral
  postprocedural
    following cardiac surgery I97.820
    following other surgery I97.821
  unspecified (NOS) I63.9
Stromatosis, endometrial D39.0
Strongyloidiasis, strongyloidosis B78.9
  cutaneous B78.1
  disseminated B78.7
  intestinal B78.0
Strophulus pruriginosus L28.2
Struck by lightning — *see* Lightning
Struma — *see also* Goiter
  Hashimoto E06.3
  lymphomatosa E06.3
  nodosa (simplex) E04.9
    endemic E01.2
      multinodular E01.1
    multinodular E04.2
      iodine-deficiency related E01.1
    toxic or with hyperthyroidism E05.20
      with thyroid storm E05.21
    multinodular E05.20
      with thyroid storm E05.21
    uninodular E05.10
      with thyroid storm E05.11
    toxicosa E05.20
      with thyroid storm E05.21
    multinodular E05.20
      with thyroid storm E05.21
    uninodular E05.10
      with thyroid storm E05.11
    uninodular E04.1
  ovarii D27-
  Riedel's E06.5
Strumipriva cachexia E03.4
Strümpell-Marie spine — *see* Spondylitis,
  ankylosing
Strümpell-Westphal pseudosclerosis
  E83.01
Stuart deficiency disease (factor X) D68.2
Stuart-Prower factor deficiency (factor X)
  D68.2
Student's elbow — *see* Bursitis, elbow,
  olecranon
Stump — *see* Amputation
Stunting, nutritional E45
Stupor (catatonic) R40.1
  depressive (single episode) F32.89
    recurrent episode F33.8
  dissociative F44.2
  manic F30.2
  manic-depressive F31.89
  psychogenic (anergic) F44.2
  reaction to exceptional stress (transient) F43.0
Sturge (-Weber) (-Dimitri) (-Kalischer)
  disease or syndrome Q85.8
Stuttering F80.81
  adult onset F98.5
  childhood onset F80.81
  following cerebrovascular disease — *see*
    Disorder, fluency, following
    cerebrovascular disease
  in conditions classified elsewhere R47.82
Sty, stye (external) (internal) (meibomian)
  (zeisian) — *see* Hordeolum
Subacidity, gastric K31.89
  psychogenic F45.8
Subacute — *see* condition

Subarachnoid — *see* condition
Subcortical — *see* condition
Subcostal syndrome, nerve compression
  — *see* Mononeuropathy, upper limb,
  specified site NEC
Subcutaneous, subcuticular — *see* condition
Subdural — *see* condition
Subendocardium — *see* condition
Subependymoma
  specified site — *see* Neoplasm, uncertain
    behavior, by site
  unspecified site D43.2
Suberosis J67.3
Subglossitis — *see* Glossitis
Subhemophilia D66
Subinvolution
  breast (postlactational) (postpuerperal)
    N64.89
  puerperal O90.89
  uterus (chronic) (nonpuerperal) N85.3
    puerperal O90.89
Sublingual — *see* condition
Sublinguitis — *see* Sialoadenitis
Subluxatable hip Q65.6
Subluxation — *see also* Dislocation
  acromioclavicular S43.11-
  ankle S93.0-
  atlantoaxial, recurrent M43.4
    with myelopathy M43.3
  carpometacarpal (joint) NEC S63.05-
    thumb S63.04-
  complex, vertebral — *see* Complex,
    subluxation
  congenital — *see also* Malposition, congenital
    hip — *see* Dislocation, hip, congenital,
      partial
    joint (excluding hip)
      lower limb Q68.8
      shoulder Q68.8
      upper limb Q68.8
  elbow (traumatic) S53.10-
    anterior S53.11-
    lateral S53.14-
    medial S53.13-
    posterior S53.12-
    specified type NEC S53.19-
  finger S63.20-
    index S63.20-
    interphalangeal S63.22-
      distal S63.24-
        index S63.24-
        little S63.24-
        middle S63.24-
        ring S63.24-
      index S63.22-
      little S63.22-
      middle S63.22-
      proximal S63.23-
        index S63.23-
        little S63.23-
        middle S63.23-
        ring S63.23-
      ring S63.22-
    little S63.20-
    metacarpophalangeal S63.21-
      index S63.21-
      little S63.21-
      middle S63.21-
      ring S63.21-
    middle S63.20-
    ring S63.20-
  foot S93.30-
    specified site NEC S93.33-
    tarsal joint S93.31-
    tarsometatarsal joint S93.32-
    toe — *see* Subluxation, toe

Subluxation (see also Dislocation) — continued
hip S73.00-
  anterior S73.03-
    obturator S73.02-
  central S73.04-
  posterior S73.01-
interphalangeal (joint)
  finger S63.22-
    distal joint S63.24-
      index S63.24-
      little S63.24-
      middle S63.24-
      ring S63.24-
    index S63.22-
    little S63.22-
    middle S63.22-
    proximal joint S63.23-
      index S63.23-
      little S63.23-
      middle S63.23-
      ring S63.23-
    ring S63.22-
  thumb S63.12-
    distal joint S63.14-
    proximal joint S63.13-
  toe S93.13-
    great S93.13-
    lesser S93.13-
joint prosthesis — see Complications, joint prosthesis, mechanical, displacement, by site
knee S83.10-
  cap — see Subluxation, patella
  patella — see Subluxation, patella
  proximal tibia
    anteriorly S83.11-
    laterally S83.14-
    medially S83.13-
    posteriorly S83.12-
  specified type NEC S83.19-
lens — see Dislocation, lens, partial
ligament, traumatic — see Sprain, by site
metacarpal (bone)
  proximal end S63.06-
metacarpophalangeal (joint)
  finger S63.21-
    index S63.21-
    little S63.21-
    middle S63.21-
    ring S63.21-
  thumb S63.11-
metatarsophalangeal joint S93.14-
  great toe S93.14-
  lesser toe S93.14-
midcarpal (joint) S63.03-
patella S83.00-
  lateral S83.01-
  recurrent (nontraumatic) — see Dislocation, patella, recurrent, incomplete
  specified type NEC S83.09-
pathological — see Dislocation, pathological
radial head S53.00-
  anterior S53.01-
  nursemaid's elbow S53.03-
  posterior S53.02-
  specified type NEC S53.09-
radiocarpal (joint) S63.02-
radioulnar (joint)
  distal S63.01-
  proximal — see Subluxation, elbow
shoulder
  congenital Q68.8
  girdle S43.30-
    scapula S43.31-
    specified site NEC S43.39-
  traumatic S43.00-
    anterior S43.01-
    inferior S43.03-
    posterior S43.02-

Subluxation (see also Dislocation) — continued
shoulder — continued
  traumatic S43.00- — continued
    specified type NEC S43.08-
sternoclavicular (joint) S43.20-
  anterior S43.21-
  posterior S43.22-
symphysis (pubis)
thumb S63.103
  interphalangeal joint — see Subluxation, interphalangeal (joint), thumb
  metacarpophalangeal joint — see Subluxation, metacarpophalangeal (joint), thumb
toe(s) S93.10-
  great S93.10-
    interphalangeal joint S93.13-
    metatarsophalangeal joint S93.14-
  interphalangeal joint S93.13-
  lesser S93.10-
    interphalangeal joint S93.13-
    metatarsophalangeal joint S93.14-
  metatarsophalangeal joint S93.149
ulna
  distal end S63.07-
  proximal end — see Subluxation, elbow
ulnohumeral joint — see Subluxation, elbow
vertebral
  recurrent NEC — see subcategory M43.5
  traumatic
    cervical S13.100
      atlantoaxial joint S13.120
      atlantooccipital joint S13.110
      atloidooccipital joint S13.110
      joint between
        C0 and C1 S13.110
        C1 and C2 S13.120
        C2 and C3 S13.130
        C3 and C4 S13.140
        C4 and C5 S13.150
        C5and C6 S13.160
        C6and C7 S13.170
        C7and T1 S13.180
      occipitoatloid joint S13.110
    lumbar S33.100
      joint between
        L1and L2 S33.110
        L2and L3 S33.120
        L3 and L4 S33.130
        L4and L5 S33.140
    thoracic S23.100
      joint between
        T10 and T11 S23.160
        T11 and T12 S23.162
        T12 and L1 S23.170
        T1and T2 S23.110
        T2and T3 S23.120
        T3 and T4 S23.122
        T4 and T5 S23.130
        T5 and T6 S23.132
        T6 and T7 S23.140
        T7 and T8 S23.142
        T8 and T9 S23.150
        T9 and T10 S23.152
wrist (carpal bone) S63.00-
  carpometacarpal joint — see Subluxation, carpometacarpal (joint)
  distal radioulnar joint — see Subluxation, radioulnar (joint), distal
  metacarpal bone, proximal — see Subluxation, metacarpal (bone), proximal end
  midcarpal — see Subluxation, midcarpal (joint)
  radiocarpal joint — see Subluxation, radiocarpal (joint)
  recurrent — see Dislocation, recurrent, wrist
specified site NEC S63.09-
ulna — see Subluxation, ulna, distal end

Submaxillary — see condition
Submersion (fatal) (nonfatal) T75.1
Submucous — see condition
Subnormal, subnormality
  accommodation (old age) H52.4
  mental — see Disability, intellectual
  temperature (accidental) T68
Subphrenic — see condition
Subscapular nerve — see condition
Subseptus uterus Q51.2
Subsiding appendicitis K36
Substance (other psychoactive) -induced
  anxiety disorder F19.980
  bipolar and related disorder F19.94
  delirium F19.921
  depressive disorder F19.94
  major neurocognitive disorder F19.97
  mild neurocognitive disorder F19.988
  obsessive-compulsive and related disorder F19.988
  psychotic disorder F19.959
  sexual dysfunction F19.981
  sleep disorder F19.982
Substernal thyroid E04.9
  congenital Q89.2
Substitution disorder F44.9
Subtentorial — see condition
Subthyroidism (acquired) — see also Hypothyroidism
  congenital E03.1
Succenturiate placenta O43.19-
Sucking thumb, child (excessive) F98.8
Sudamen, sudamina L74.1
Sudanese kala-azar B55.0
Sudden
  hearing loss — see Deafness, sudden
  heart failure — see Failure, heart
Sudeck's atrophy, disease, or syndrome — see Algoneurodystrophy
Suffocation — see Asphyxia, traumatic
Sugar
  blood
    high (transient) R73.9
    low (transient) E16.2
  in urine R81
Suicide, suicidal (attempted) T14.91
  by poisoning — see Table of Drugs and Chemicals
  history of (personal) Z91.5
    in family Z81.8
  ideation — see Ideation, suicidal
  risk
    meaning personal history of attempted suicide Z91.5
    meaning suicidal ideation — see Ideation, suicidal
  tendencies
    meaning personal history of attempted suicide Z91.5
    meaning suicidal ideation — see Ideation, suicidal
  trauma — see nature of injury by site
Suipestifer infection — see Infection, salmonella
Sulfhemoglobinemia, sulphemoglobinemia (acquired) (with methemoglobinemia) D74.8
Sumatran mite fever A75.3
Summer — see condition
Sunburn L55.9
  due to
    tanning bed (acute) L56.8
      chronic L57.8
    ultraviolet radiation (acute) L56.8
      chronic L57.8
  first degree L55.0
  second degree L55.1
  third degree L55.2

SUNCT (short lasting unilateral neuralgiform headache with conjunctival injection and tearing) G44.059
  intractable G44.051
  not intractable G44.059
Sunken acetabulum — see Derangement, joint, specified type NEC, hip
Sunstroke T67.0
Superfecundation — see Pregnancy, multiple
Superfetation — see Pregnancy, multiple
Superinvolution (uterus) N85.8
Supernumerary (congenital)
  aortic cusps Q23.8
  auditory ossicles Q16.3
  bone Q79.8
  breast Q83.1
  carpal bones Q74.0
  cusps, heart valve NEC Q24.8
    aortic Q23.8
    mitral Q23.2
    pulmonary Q22.3
  digit(s) Q69.9
  ear (lobule) Q17.0
  fallopian tube Q50.6
  finger Q69.0
  hymen Q52.4
  kidney Q63.0
  lacrimonasal duct Q10.6
  lobule (ear) Q17.0
  mitral cusps Q23.2
  muscle Q79.8
  nipple(s) Q83.3
  organ or site not listed — see Accessory
  ossicles, auditory Q16.3
  ovary Q50.31
  oviduct Q50.6
  pulmonary, pulmonic cusps Q22.3
  rib Q76.6
    cervical or first (syndrome) Q76.5
  roots (of teeth) K00.2
  spleen Q89.09
  tarsal bones Q74.2
  teeth K00.1
  testis Q55.29
  thumb Q69.1
  toe Q69.2
  uterus Q51.2
  vagina Q52.1
  vertebra Q76.49
Supervision (of)
  contraceptive — see Prescription, contraceptives
  dietary (for) Z71.3
    allergy (food) Z71.3
    colitis Z71.3
    diabetes mellitus Z71.3
    food allergy or intolerance Z71.3
    gastritis Z71.3
    hypercholesterolemia Z71.3
    hypoglycemia Z71.3
    intolerance (food) Z71.3
    obesity Z71.3
    specified NEC Z71.3
  healthy infant or child Z76.2
    foundling Z76.1
  high-risk pregnancy — see Pregnancy, complicated by, high, risk
  lactation Z39.1
  pregnancy — see Pregnancy, supervision of
Supplemental teeth K00.1
Suppression
  binocular vision H53.34
  lactation O92.5
  menstruation N94.89
  ovarian secretion E28.39
  renal N28.9
  urine, urinary secretion R34

Suppuration, suppurative — see also condition
  accessory sinus (chronic) — see Sinusitis
  adrenal gland
  antrum (chronic) — see Sinusitis, maxillary
  bladder — see Cystitis
  brain G06.0
    sequelae G09
  breast N61.1
    puerperal, postpartum or gestational — see Mastitis, obstetric, purulent
  dental periosteum M27.3
  ear (middle) — see also Otitis, media
    external NEC — see Otitis, externa, infective
    internal — see subcategory H83.0
  ethmoidal (chronic) (sinus) — see Sinusitis, ethmoidal
  fallopian tube — see Salpingo-oophoritis
  frontal (chronic) (sinus) — see Sinusitis, frontal
  gallbladder (acute) K81.0
  gum K05.20
    generalized — see Peridontitis, aggressive, generalized
    localized — see Peridontitis, aggressive, localized
  intracranial G06.0
  joint — see Arthritis, pyogenic or pyemic
  labyrinthine — see subcategory H83.0
  lung — see Abscess, lung
  mammary gland N61.1
    puerperal, postpartum O91.12
    associated with lactation O91.13
  maxilla, maxillary M27.2
    sinus (chronic) — see Sinusitis, maxillary
  muscle — see Myositis, infective
  nasal sinus (chronic) — see Sinusitis
  pancreas, acute (see also Pancreatitis, acute) K85.80
  parotid gland — see Sialoadenitis
  pelvis, pelvic
    female — see Disease, pelvis, inflammatory
    male K65.0
  pericranial — see Osteomyelitis
  salivary duct or gland (any) — see Sialoadenitis
  sinus (accessory) (chronic) (nasal) — see Sinusitis
  sphenoidal sinus (chronic) — see Sinusitis, sphenoidal
  thymus (gland) E32.1
  thyroid (gland) E06.0
  tonsil — see Tonsillitis
  uterus — see Endometritis
Supraeruption of tooth (teeth) M26.34
Supraglottitis J04.30
  with obstruction J04.31
Suprarenal (gland) — see condition
Suprascapular nerve — see condition
Suprasellar — see condition
Surfer's knots or nodules S89.8-
Surgical
  emphysema T81.82
  procedures, complication or misadventure — see Complications, surgical procedures
  shock T81.10
Surveillance (of) (for) — see also Observation
  alcohol abuse Z71.41
  contraceptive — see Prescription, contraceptives
  dietary Z71.3
  drug abuse Z71.51
Susceptibility to disease, genetic Z15.89
  malignant neoplasm Z15.09
    breast Z15.01
    endometrium Z15.04
    ovary Z15.02
    prostate Z15.03
    specified NEC Z15.09
  multiple endocrine neoplasia Z15.81

Suspected condition, ruled out — see also Observation, suspected
  amniotic cavity and membrane Z03.71
  cervical shortening Z03.75
  fetal anomaly Z03.73
  fetal growth Z03.74
  maternal and fetal conditions NEC Z03.79
  newborn (see also Observation, newborn, suspected condition ruled out) Z05.9
  oligohydramnios Z03.71
  placental problem Z03.72
  polyhydramnios Z03.71
Suspended uterus
  in pregnancy or childbirth — see Pregnancy, complicated by, abnormal uterus
Sutton's nevus D22.9
Suture
  burst (in operation wound) T81.31
    external operation wound T81.31
    internal operation wound T81.32
  inadvertently left in operation wound — see Foreign body, accidentally left during a procedure
  removal Z48.02
Swab inadvertently left in operation wound — see Foreign body, accidentally left during a procedure
Swallowed, swallowing
  difficulty — see Dysphagia
  foreign body — see Foreign body, alimentary tract
Swan-neck deformity (finger) — see Deformity, finger, swan-neck
Swearing, compulsive F42.8
  in Gilles de la Tourette's syndrome F95.2
Sweat, sweats
  fetid L75.0
  night R61
Sweating, excessive R61
Sweeley-Klionsky disease E75.21
Sweet's disease or dermatosis L98.2
Swelling (of) R60.9
  abdomen, abdominal (not referable to any particular organ) — see Mass, abdominal
  ankle — see Effusion, joint, ankle
  arm M79.89
    forearm M79.89
  breast N63
  Calabar B74.3
  cervical gland R59.0
  chest, localized R22.2
  ear H93.8-
  extremity (lower) (upper) — see Disorder, soft tissue, specified type NEC
  finger M79.89
  foot M79.89
  glands R59.9
    generalized R59.1
    localized R59.0
  hand M79.89
  head (localized) R22.0
  inflammatory — see Inflammation
  intra-abdominal — see Mass, abdominal
  joint — see Effusion, joint
  leg M79.89
    lower M79.89
  limb — see Disorder, soft tissue, specified type NEC
  localized (skin) R22.9
    chest R22.2
    head R22.0
    limb
      lower — see Mass, localized, limb, lower
      upper — see Mass, localized, limb, upper
    neck R22.1
    trunk R22.2
  neck (localized) R22.1
  pelvic — see Mass, abdominal
  scrotum N50.89

Swelling (of) R60.9 — *continued*
  splenic — *see* Splenomegaly
  testis N50.89
  toe M79.89
  umbilical R19.09
  wandering, due to Gnathostoma (spinigerum) B83.1
  white — *see* Tuberculosis, arthritis
Swift(-Feer) disease
  overdose or wrong substance given or taken — *see* Table of Drugs and Chemicals, by drug, poisoning
Swimmer's
  cramp T75.1
  ear H60.33-
  itch B65.3
Swimming in the head R42
Swollen — *see* Swelling
Swyer syndrome Q99.1
Sycosis L73.8
  barbae (not parasitic) L73.8
  contagiosa (mycotic) B35.0
  lupoides L73.8
  mycotic B35.0
  parasitic B35.0
  vulgaris L73.8
Sydenham's chorea — *see* Chorea, Sydenham's
Sylvatic yellow fever A95.0
Sylvest's disease B33.0
Symblepharon H11.23-
  congenital Q10.3
Symond's syndrome G93.2
Sympathetic — *see* condition
Sympatheticotonia G90.8
Sympathicoblastoma
  specified site — *see* Neoplasm, malignant, by site
  unspecified site C74.90
Sympathogonioma — *see* Sympathicoblastoma
Symphalangy (fingers) (toes) Q70.9
Symptoms NEC R68.89
  breast NEC N64.59
  development NEC R63.8
  factitious, self-induced — *see* Disorder, factitious
  genital organs, female R10.2
  involving
    abdomen NEC R19.8
    appearance NEC R46.89
    awareness R41.9
      altered mental status R41.82
      amnesia — *see* Amnesia
      borderline intellectual functioning R41.83
      coma — *see* Coma
      disorientation R41.0
      neurologic neglect syndrome R41.4
      senile cognitive decline R41.81
      specified symptom NEC R41.89
    behavior NEC R46.89
    cardiovascular system NEC R09.89
    chest NEC R09.89
    circulatory system NEC R09.89
    cognitive functions R41.9
      altered mental status R41.82
      amnesia — *see* Amnesia
      borderline intellectual functioning R41.83
      coma — *see* Coma
      disorientation R41.0
      neurologic neglect syndrome R41.4
      senile cognitive decline R41.81
      specified symptom NEC R41.89
    development NEC R62.50
    digestive system NEC R19.8
    emotional state NEC R45.89
      emotional lability R45.86
    food and fluid intake R63.8

Symptoms NEC R68.89 — *continued*
  involving — *continued*
    general perceptions and sensations R44.9
      specified NEC R44.8
    musculoskeletal system R29.91
      specified NEC R29.898
    nervous system R29.90
      specified NEC R29.818
    pelvis NEC R19.8
    respiratory system NEC R09.89
    skin and integument R23.9
    urinary system R39.9
  menopausal N95.1
  metabolism NEC R63.8
  neurotic F48.8
  of infancy R68.19
  pelvis NEC, female R10.2
  skin and integument NEC R23.9
  subcutaneous tissue NEC R23.9
Sympus Q74.2
Syncephalus Q89.4
Synchondrosis
  abnormal (congenital) Q78.8
  ischiopubic M91.0
Synchysis (scintillans) (senile) (vitreous body) H43.89
Syncope (near) (pre-) R55
  anginosa I20.8
  bradycardia R00.1
  cardiac R55
  carotid sinus G90.01
  due to spinal (lumbar) puncture G97.1
  heart R55
  heat T67.1
  laryngeal R05
  psychogenic F48.8
  tussive R05
  vasoconstriction R55
  vasodepressor R55
  vasomotor R55
  vasovagal R55
Syndactylism, syndactyly Q70.9
  complex (with synostosis)
    fingers Q70.0-
    toes Q70.2-
  simple (without synostosis)
    fingers Q70.1-
    toes Q70.3-
Syndrome — *see also* Disease
  48,XXXX Q97.1
  49,XXXXX Q97.1
  5q minus NOS D46.C
  abdominal
    acute R10.0
    muscle deficiency Q79.4
  abnormal innervation H02.519
    left H02.516
      lower H02.515
      upper H02.514
    right H02.513
      lower H02.512
      upper H02.511
  abstinence, neonatal P96.1
  acid pulmonary aspiration, obstetric O74.0
  acquired immunodeficiency — *see* Human, immunodeficiency virus (HIV) disease
  acute abdominal R10.0
  acute respiratory distress (adult) (child) J80
    idiopathic J84.114
  Adair-Dighton Q78.0
  Adams-Stokes(-Morgagni) I45.9
  adiposogenital E23.6
  adrenal
    hemorrhage (meningococcal) A39.1
    meningococcic A39.1
  adrenocortical — *see* Cushing's, syndrome
  adrenogenital E25.9
    congenital, associated with enzyme deficiency E25.0

Syndrome (*see also* Disease) — *continued*
  afferent loop NEC K91.89
  Alagille's Q44.7
  alcohol withdrawal (without convulsions) — *see* Dependence, alcohol, with, withdrawal
  Alder's D72.0
  Aldrich(-Wiskott) D82.0
  alien hand R41.4
  Alport Q87.81
  alveolar hypoventilation E66.2
  alveolocapillary block J84.10
  amnesic, amnestic (confabulatory) (due to) — *see* Disorder, amnesic
  amyostatic (Wilson's disease) E83.01
  androgen insensitivity E34.50
    complete E34.51
    partial E34.52
  androgen resistance (*see also* Syndrome, androgen insensitivity) E34.50
  Angelman Q93.5
  anginal — *see* Angina
  ankyloglossia superior Q38.1
  anterior
    chest wall R07.89
    cord G83.82
    spinal artery G95.19
      compression M47.019
        cervical region M47.012
        cervicothoracic region M47.013
        lumbar region M47.016
        occipito-atlanto-axial region M47.011
        thoracic region M47.014
        thoracolumbar region M47.015
    tibial M76.81-
  antibody deficiency D80.9
    agammaglobulinemic D80.1
      hereditary D80.0
    congenital D80.0
    hypogammaglobulinemic D80.1
      hereditary D80.0
  anticardiolipin (-antibody) D68.61
  antiphospholipid (-antibody) D68.61
  aortic
    arch M31.4
    bifurcation I74.09
  aortomesenteric duodenum occlusion K31.5
  apical ballooning (transient left ventricular) I51.81
  arcuate ligament I77.4
  argentaffin, argintaffinoma E34.0
  Arnold-Chiari — *see* Arnold-Chiari disease
  Arrillaga-Ayerza I27.0
  arterial tortuosity Q87.82
  arteriovenous steal T82.898-
  Asherman's N85.6
  aspiration, of newborn — *see* Aspiration, by substance, with pneumonia
    meconium P24.01
  ataxia-telangiectasia G11.3
  auriculotemporal G50.8
  autoerythrocyte sensitization (Gardner-Diamond) D69.2
  autoimmune lymphoproliferative [ALPS] D89.82
  autoimmune polyglandular E31.0
  autoinflammatory M04.9
    specified type NEC M04.8
  autosomal — *see* Abnormal, autosomes
  Avellis' G46.8
  Ayerza(-Arrillaga) I27.0
  Babinski-Nageotte G83.89
  Bakwin-Krida Q78.5
  bare lymphocyte D81.6
  Barrett's — *see* Barrett's, esophagus
  Barré-Guillain G61.0
  Barré-Liéou M53.0
  Barsony-Polgar K22.4
  Barsony-Teschendorf K22.4
  Barth E78.71

Syndrome (see also Disease) — continued
Bartter's E26.81
basal cell nevus Q87.89
Basedow's E05.00
  with thyroid storm E05.01
basilar artery G45.0
Batten-Steinert G71.11
battered
  baby or child — see Maltreatment, child,
    physical abuse
  spouse — see Maltreatment, adult, physical
    abuse
Beals Q87.40
Beau's I51.5
Beck's I65.8
Benedikt's G46.3
Béquez César (-Steinbrinck-Chédiak-Higashi)
  E70.330
Bernhardt-Roth — see Meralgia paresthetica
Bernheim's I50.9
big spleen D73.1
bilateral polycystic ovarian E28.2
Bing-Horton's — see Horton's headache
Birt-Hogg-Dube syndrome Q87.89
Björck(-Thorsen) E34.0
black
  lung J60
  widow spider bite — see Toxicity, venom,
    spider, black widow
Blackfan-Diamond D61.01
Blau M04.8
blind loop K90.2
  congenital Q43.8
  postsurgical K91.2
blue sclera Q78.0
blue toe I75.02-
Boder-Sedgewick G11.3
Boerhaave's K22.3
Borjeson Forssman Lehmann Q89.8
Bouillaud's I01.9
Bourneville(-Pringle) Q85.1
Bouveret(-Hoffman) I47.9
brachial plexus G54.0
bradycardia-tachycardia I49.5
brain (nonpsychotic) F09
  with psychosis, psychotic reaction F09
  acute or subacute — see Delirium
  congenital — see Disability, intellectual
  organic F09
    post-traumatic (nonpsychotic) F07.81
      psychotic F09
  personality change F07.0
  post-traumatic, nonpsychotic F07.81
  postcontusional F07.81
  psycho-organic F09
  psychotic F06.8
brain stem stroke G46.3
Brandt's (acrodermatitis enteropathica) E83.2
broad ligament laceration N83.8
Brock's J98.11
bronze baby P83.8
Brown-Sequard G83.81
bubbly lung P27.0
Buchem's M85.2
Budd-Chiari I82.0
bulbar (progressive) G12.22
Bürger-Grütz E78.3
Burke's K86.89
Burnett's (milk-alkali) E83.52
burning feet E53.9
Bywaters' T79.5
Call-Fleming I67.841
carbohydrate-deficient glycoprotein (CDGS)
  E77.8
carcinogenic thrombophlebitis I82.1
carcinoid E34.0
cardiac asthma I50.1
cardiacos negros I27.0
cardiofaciocutaneous Q87.89

Syndrome (see also Disease) — continued
cardiopulmonary-obesity E66.2
cardiorenal — see Hypertension, cardiorenal
cardiorespiratory distress (idiopathic),
  newborn P22.0
cardiovascular renal — see Hypertension,
  cardiorenal
carotid
  artery (hemispheric) (internal) G45.1
  body G90.01
  sinus G90.01
carpal tunnel G56.0-
Cassidy(-Scholte) E34.0
cat cry Q93.4
cat eye Q92.8
cauda equina G83.4
causalgia — see Causalgia
celiac K90.0
  artery compression I77.4
  axis I77.4
central pain G89.0
cerebellar
  hereditary G11.9
  stroke G46.4
cerebellomedullary malformation — see Spina
  bifida
cerebral
  artery
    anterior G46.1
    middle G46.0
    posterior G46.2
  gigantism E22.0
cervical (root) M53.1
  disc — see Disorder, disc, cervical, with
    neuritis
  fusion Q76.1
  posterior, sympathicus M53.0
  rib Q76.5
  sympathetic paralysis G90.2
cervicobrachial (diffuse) M53.1
cervicocranial M53.0
cervicodorsal outlet G54.2
cervicothoracic outlet G54.0
Céstan(-Raymond) I65.8
Charcot's (angina cruris) (intermittent
  claudication) I73.9
Charcot-Weiss-Baker G90.09
CHARGE Q89.8
Chédiak-Higashi(-Steinbrinck) E70.330
chest wall R07.1
Chiari's (hepatic vein thrombosis) I82.0
Chilaiditi's Q43.3
child maltreatment — see Maltreatment, child
chondrocostal junction M94.0
chondroectodermal dysplasia Q77.6
chromosome 4 short arm deletion Q93.3
chromosome 5 short arm deletion Q93.4
chronic
  infantile neurological, cutaneous and
    articular (CINCA) M04.2
  pain G89.4
    personality F68.8
Clarke-Hadfield K86.89
Clerambault's automatism G93.89
Clouston's (hidrotic ectodermal dysplasia)
  Q82.4
clumsiness, clumsy child F82
cluster headache G44.009
  intractable G44.001
  not intractable G44.009
Coffin-Lowry Q89.8
cold injury (newborn) P80.0
combined immunity deficiency D81.9
compartment (deep) (posterior) (traumatic)
  T79.A0 (follows T79.7)
  abdomen T79.A3 (follows T79.7)
  lower extremity (hip, buttock, thigh, leg, foot,
    toes) T79.A2 (follows T79.7)

Syndrome (see also Disease) — continued
compartment (deep) (posterior) (traumatic)
  T79.A0 (follows T79.7) — continued
  nontraumatic
    abdomen M79.A3 (follows M79.7)
    lower extremity (hip, buttock, thigh, leg,
      foot, toes) M79.A2- (follows M79.7)
    specified site NEC M79.A9 (follows M79.7)
    upper extremity (shoulder, arm, forearm,
      wrist, hand, fingers) M79.A1- (follows
      M79.7)
  postprocedural — see Syndrome,
    compartment, nontraumatic
  specified site NEC T79.A9 (follows T79.7)
  upper extremity (shoulder, arm, forearm,
    wrist, hand, fingers) T79.A1 (follows
    T79.7)
complex regional pain — see Syndrome, pain,
  complex regional
compression T79.5
  anterior spinal — see Syndrome, anterior,
    spinal artery, compression
  cauda equina G83.4
  celiac artery I77.4
  vertebral artery M47.029
    cervical region M47.022
    occipito-atlanto-axial region M47.021
concussion F07.81
congenital
  affecting multiple systems NEC Q87.89
  central alveolar hypoventilation G47.35
  facial diplegia Q87.0
  muscular hypertrophy-cerebral Q87.89
  oculo-auriculovertebral Q87.0
  oculofacial diplegia (Moebius) Q87.0
  rubella (manifest) P35.0
congestion-fibrosis (pelvic), female N94.89
congestive dysmenorrhea N94.6
Conn's E26.01
connective tissue M35.9
  overlap NEC M35.1
conus medullaris G95.81
cord
  anterior G83.82
  posterior G83.83
coronary
  acute NEC I24.9
  insufficiency or intermediate I20.0
  slow flow I20.8
Costen's (complex) M26.69
costochondral junction M94.0
costoclavicular G54.0
costovertebral E22.0
Cowden Q85.8
craniovertebral M53.0
Creutzfeldt-Jakob — see Creutzfeldt-Jakob
  disease or syndrome
crib death R99
cricopharyngeal — see Dysphagia
cri-du-chat Q93.4
croup J05.0
CRPS I — see Syndrome, pain, complex
  regional I
crush T79.5
cryopyrin-associated periodic M04.2
cryptophthalmos Q87.0
cubital tunnel — see Lesion, nerve, ulnar
Curschmann (-Batten) (-Steinert) G71.11
Cushing's E24.9
  alcohol-induced E24.4
  drug-induced E24.2
  due to
    alcohol
      drugs E24.2
    ectopic ACTH E24.3
    overproduction of pituitary ACTH E24.0
  overdose or wrong substance given or taken
    — see Table of Drugs and Chemicals, by
    drug, poisoning

DISEASE INDEX

Syndrome (*see also* Disease) — *continued*
Cushing's E24.9 — *continued*
 pituitary-dependent E24.0
 specified type NEC E24.8
cystic duct stump K91.5
Dana-Putnam D51.0
Danbolt (-Cross) (acrodermatitis enteropathica) E83.2
Dandy-Walker Q03.1
 with spina bifida Q07.01
Danlos' Q79.6
De Quervain E34.51
de Toni-Fanconi (-Debré) E72.09
 with cystinosis E72.04
defibrination — *see also* Fibrinolysis
 with
 antepartum hemorrhage — *see* Hemorrhage, antepartum, with coagulation defect
 intrapartum hemorrhage — *see* Hemorrhage, complicating, delivery
 newborn P60
 postpartum O72.3
Degos' I77.89
Déjérine-Roussy G89.0
delayed sleep phase G47.21
demyelinating G37.9
dependence — *see* F10-F19 with fourth character .2
depersonalization(-derealization) F48.1
diabetes mellitus in newborn infant P70.2
diabetes mellitus-hypertension-nephrosis — *see* Diabetes, nephrosis
diabetes-nephrosis — *see* Diabetes, nephrosis
diabetic amyotrophy — *see* Diabetes, amyotrophy
dialysis associated steal T82.898-
Diamond-Blackfan D61.01
Diamond-Gardener D69.2
DIC (diffuse or disseminated intravascular coagulopathy) D65
di George's D82.1
Dighton's Q78.0
disequilibrium E87.2
Döhle body-panmyelopathic D72.0
dorsolateral medullary G46.4
double athetosis G80.3
Down (*see also* Down syndrome) Q90.9
Dresbach's (elliptocytosis) D58.1
Dressler's (postmyocardial infarction) I24.1
 postcardiotomy I97.0
drug withdrawal, infant of dependent mother P96.1
dry eye H04.12-
due to abnormality
 chromosomal Q99.9
 sex
 female phenotype Q97.9
 male phenotype Q98.9
 specified NEC Q99.8
dumping (postgastrectomy) K91.1
 nonsurgical K31.89
Dupré's (meningism) R29.1
dysmetabolic X E88.81
dyspraxia, developmental F82
Eagle-Barrett Q79.4
Eaton-Lambert — *see* Syndrome, Lambert-Eaton
Ebstein's Q22.5
ectopic ACTH E24.3
eczema-thrombocytopenia D82.0
Eddowes' Q78.0
effort (psychogenic) F45.8
Ehlers-Danlos Q79.6
Eisenmenger's I27.89
Ekman's Q78.0
electric feet E53.8
Ellis-van Creveld Q77.6
empty nest Z60.0

Syndrome (*see also* Disease) — *continued*
endocrine-hypertensive E27.0
entrapment — *see* Neuropathy, entrapment
eosinophilia-myalgia M35.8
epileptic — *see also* Epilepsy, by type
 absence G40.A09 *(follows G40.3)*
 intractable G40.A19 *(follows G40.3)*
 with status epilepticus G40.A11 *(follows G40.3)*
 without status epilepticus G40.A19 *(follows G40.3)*
 not intractable G40.A09 *(follows G40.3)*
 with status epilepticus G40.A01 *(follows G40.3)*
 without status epilepticus G40.A09 *(follows G40.3)*
Erdheim-Chester (ECD) E88.89
Erdheim's E22.0
erythrocyte fragmentation D59.4
Evans D69.41
exhaustion F48.8
extrapyramidal G25.9
 specified NEC G25.89
eye retraction — *see* Strabismus
eyelid-malar-mandible Q87.0
Faber's D50.9
facial pain, paroxysmal G50.0
Fallot's Q21.3
familial cold autoinflammatory M04.2
familial eczema-thrombocytopenia (Wiskott-Aldrich) D82.0
Fanconi (-de Toni) (-Debré) E72.09
 with cystinosis E72.04
Fanconi's (anemia) (congenital pancytopenia) D61.09
fatigue
 chronic R53.82
 psychogenic F48.8
faulty bowel habit K59.39
Feil-Klippel (brevicollis) Q76.1
Felty's — *see* Felty's syndrome
fertile eunuch E23.0
fetal
 alcohol (dysmorphic) Q86.0
 hydantoin Q86.1
Fiedler's I40.1
first arch Q87.0
fish odor E72.8
Fisher's G61.0
Fitz's (*see also* Pancreatitis, acute) K85.80
Fitzhugh-Curtis
 due to
 Chlamydia trachomatis A74.81
 Neisseria gonorrhorea (gonococcal peritonitis) A54.85
Flajani (-Basedow) E05.00
 with thyroid storm E05.01
flatback — *see* Flatback syndrome
floppy
 baby P94.2
 iris (intraoeprative) (IFIS) H21.81
 mitral valve I34.1
flush E34.0
Foix-Alajouanine G95.19
Fong's Q87.2
food protein-induced enterocolitis K52.21
foramen magnum G93.5
Foster-Kennedy H47.14-
Foville's (peduncular) G46.3
fragile X Q99.2
Franceschetti Q75.4
Frey's
 auriculotemporal G50.8
 hyperhidrosis L74.52
Friderichsen-Waterhouse A39.1
Froin's G95.89
frontal lobe F07.0
Fukuhara E88.49

Syndrome (*see also* Disease) — *continued*
functional
 bowel K59.9
 prepubertal castrate E29.1
Gaisböck's D75.1
ganglion (basal ganglia brain) G25.9
 geniculi G51.1
Gardner-Diamond D69.2
gastroesophageal
 junction K22.0
 laceration-hemorrhage K22.6
gastrojejunal loop obstruction K91.89
Gee-Herter-Heubner K90.0
Gelineau's G47.419
 with cataplexy G47.411
genito-anorectal A55
Gerstmann-Sträussler-Scheinker (GSS) A81.82
Gianotti-Crosti L44.4
giant platelet (Bernard-Soulier) D69.1
Gilles de la Tourette's F95.2
goiter-deafness E07.1
Goldberg Q89.8
Goldberg-Maxwell E34.51
Good's D83.8
Gopalan' (burning feet) E53.8
Gorlin's Q87.89
Gougerot-Blum L81.7
Gouley's I31.1
Gower's R55
gray or grey (newborn) P93.0
 platelet D69.1
Gubler-Millard G46.3
Guillain-Barré (-Strohl) G61.0
gustatory sweating G50.8
Hadfield-Clarke K86.89
hair tourniquet — *see* Constriction, external, by site
Hamman's J98.19
hand-foot L27.1
hand-shoulder G90.8
hantavirus (cardio)-pulmonary (HPS) (HCPS) B33.4
happy puppet Q93.5
Harada's H30.81-
Hayem-Faber D50.9
headache NEC G44.89
 complicated NEC G44.59
Heberden's I20.8
Hedinger's E34.0
Hegglin's D72.0
HELLP (hemolysis, elevated liver enzymes and low platelet count) O14.2-
 complicating
 childbirth O14.24
 puerperium O14.25
hemolytic-uremic D59.3
hemophagocytic, infection-associated D76.2
Henoch-Schönlein D69.0
hepatic flexure K59.8
hepatopulmonary K76.81
hepatorenal K76.7
 following delivery O90.4
 postoperative or postprocedural K91.83
 postpartum, puerperal O90.4
hepatourologic K76.7
Herter (-Gee) (nontropical sprue) K90.0
Heubner-Herter K90.0
Heyd's K76.7
Hilger's G90.09
histamine-like (fish poisoning) — *see* Poisoning, fish
histiocytic D76.3
histiocytosis NEC D76.3
HIV infection, acute B20
Hoffmann-Werdnig G12.0
Hollander-Simons E88.1
Hoppe-Goldflam G70.00
 with exacerbation (acute) G70.01
 in crisis G70.01

Syndrome (*see also* Disease) — *continued*
Horner's G90.2
hungry bone E83.81
hunterian glossitis D51.0
Hutchinson's triad A50.53
hyperabduction G54.0
hyperammonemia-hyperornithinemia-
    homocitrullinemia E72.4
hypereosinophilic (idiopathic) D72.1
hyperimmunoglobulin D M04.1
hyperimmunoglobulin E (IgE) D82.4
hyperkalemic E87.5
hyperkinetic — *see* Hyperkinesia
hypermobility M35.7
hypernatremia E87.0
hyperosmolarity E87.0
hyperperfusion G97.82
hypersplenic D73.1
hypertransfusion, newborn P61.1
hyperventilation F45.8
hyperviscosity (of serum)
    polycythemic D75.1
    sclerothymic D58.8
hypoglycemic (familial) (neonatal) E16.2
hypokalemic E87.6
hyponatremic E87.1
hypopituitarism E23.0
hypoplastic left-heart Q23.4
hypopotassemia E87.6
hyposmolality E87.1
hypotension, maternal O26.5-
hypothenar hammer I73.89
hypoventilation, obesity (OHS) E66.2
ICF (intravascular coagulation-fibrinolysis) D65
idiopathic
    cardiorespiratory distress, newborn P22.0
    nephrotic (infantile) N04.9
iliotibial band M76.3-
immobility, immobilization (paraplegic) M62.3
immune reconstitution D89.3
immune reconstitution inflammatory [IRIS]
    D89.3
immunity deficiency, combined D81.9
immunodeficiency
    acquired — *see* Human, immunodeficiency
        virus (HIV) disease
    combined D81.9
impending coronary I20.0
impingement, shoulder M75.4-
inappropriate secretion of antidiuretic
    hormone E22.2
infant
    gestational diabetes P70.0
    of diabetic mother P70.1
infantilism (pituitary) E23.0
inferior vena cava I87.1
inspissated bile (newborn) P59.1
institutional (childhood) F94.2
insufficient sleep F51.12
intermediate coronary (artery) I20.0
interspinous ligament — *see* Spondylopathy,
    specified NEC
intestinal
    carcinoid E34.0
    knot K56.2
intravascular coagulation-fibrinolysis (ICF) D65
iodine-deficiency, congenital E00.9
    type
        mixed E00.2
        myxedematous E00.1
        neurological E00.0
IRDS (idiopathic respiratory distress, newborn)
    P22.0

Syndrome (*see also* Disease) — *continued*
irritable
    bowel K58.9
        with
            constipation K58.1
            diarrhea K58.0
        mixed K58.2
        psychogenic F45.8
        specified NEC K58.8
    heart (psychogenic) F45.8
    weakness F48.8
ischemic
    bowel (transient) K55.9
        chronic K55.1
        due to mesenteric artery insufficiency
            K55.1
    steal T82.898
IVC (intravascular coagulopathy) D65
Ivemark's Q89.01
Jaccoud's — *see* Arthropathy, postrheumatic,
    chronic
Jackson's G83.89
Jakob-Creutzfeldt — *see* Creutzfeldt-Jakob
    disease or syndrome
jaw-winking Q07.8
Jervell-Lange-Nielsen I45.81
jet lag G47.25
Job's D71
Joseph-Diamond-Blackfan D61.01
jugular foramen G52.7
Kabuki Q89.8
Kanner's (autism) F84.0
Kartagener's Q89.3
Kelly's D50.1
Kimmelstiel-Wilson — *see* Diabetes, specified
    type, with Kimmelstiel-Wilson disease
Klein(e)-Levine G47.13
Klippel-Feil (brevicollis) Q76.1
Köhler-Pellegrini-Steida — *see* Bursitis, tibial
    collateral
König's K59.8
Korsakoff (-Wernicke) (nonalcoholic) F04
    alcoholic F10.26
Kostmann's D70.0
Krabbe's congenital muscle hypoplasia Q79.8
labyrinthine — *see* subcategory H83.2
lacunar NEC G46.7
Lambert-Eaton G70.80
    in
        neoplastic disease G73.1
        specified disease NEC G70.81
Landau-Kleffner — *see* Epilepsy, specified NEC
Larsen's Q74.8
lateral
    cutaneous nerve of thigh G57.1-
    medullary G46.4
Launois' E22.0
lazy
    leukocyte D70.8
    posture M62.3
Lemiere I80.8
Lennox-Gastaut G40.812
    intractable G40.814
        with status epilepticus G40.813
        without status epilepticus G40.814
    not intractable G40.812
        with status epilepticus G40.811
        without status epilepticus G40.812
lenticular, progressive E83.01
Leopold-Levi's E05.90
Lev's I44.2
Li-Fraumeni Z15.01
Lichtheim's D51.0
Lightwood's N25.89
Lignac (de Toni) (-Fanconi) (-Debré) E72.09
    with cystinosis E72.04
Likoff's I20.8
limbic epilepsy personality F07.0
liver-kidney K76.7

Syndrome (*see also* Disease) — *continued*
lobotomy F07.0
Loffler's J82
long arm 18 or 21 deletion Q93.89
long QT I45.81
Louis-Barré G11.3
low
    atmospheric pressure T70.29
    back M54.5
    output (cardiac) I50.9
lower radicular, newborn (birth injury) P14.8
Luetscher's (dehydration) E86.0
Lupus anticoagulant D68.62
Lutembacher's Q21.1
macrophage activation D76.1
    due to infection D76.2
magnesium-deficiency R29.0
Majeed M04.8
Mal de Debarquement R42
malformation, congenital, due to
    alcohol Q86.0
    exogenous cause NEC Q86.8
    hydantoin Q86.1
    warfarin Q86.2
malignant
    carcinoid E34.0
    neuroleptic G21.0
Mallory-Weiss K22.6
mandibulofacial dysostosis Q75.4
manic-depressive — *see* Disorder, bipolar
maple-syrup-urine E71.0
Marable's I77.4
Marfan's Q87.40
    with
        cardiovascular manifestations Q87.418
            aortic dilation Q87.410
        ocular manifestations Q87.42
        skeletal manifestations Q87.43
Marie's (acromegaly) E22.0
mast cell activation — *see* Activation, mast cell
maternal hypotension — *see* Syndrome,
    hypotension, maternal
May (-Hegglin) D72.0
McArdle (-Schmidt) (-Pearson) E74.04
McQuarrie's E16.2
meconium plug (newborn) P76.0
median arcuate ligament I77.4
Meekeren-Ehlers-Danlos Q79.6
megavitamin-B6 E67.2
Meige G24.4
MELAS E88.41
Mendelson's O74.0
MERFF (myoclonic epilepsy associated with
    ragged-red fibers) E88.42
mesenteric
    artery (superior) K55.1
    vascular insufficiency K55.1
metabolic E88.81
metastatic carcinoid E34.0
micrognathia-glossoptosis Q87.0
midbrain NEC G93.89
middle lobe (lung) J98.19
middle radicular G54.0
migraine (*see also* Migraine) G43.909-
Mikulicz' K11.8
milk-alkali E83.52
Millard-Gubler G46.3
Miller-Dieker Q93.88
Miller-Fisher G61.0
Minkowski-Chauffard D58.0
Mirizzi's K83.1
MNGIE (mitochondrial neurogastrointestinal
    encephalopathy) E88.49
Möbius, ophthalmoplegic migraine — *see*
    Migraine, ophthalmoplegic
monofixation H50.42
Morel-Moore M85.2
Morel-Morgagni M85.2
Morgagni (-Morel) (-Stewart) M85.2

Syndrome (see also Disease) — continued
Morgagni-Adams-Stokes I45.9
Mounier-Kuhn Q32.4
  with bronchiectasis J47.9
    with
      exacerbation (acute) J47.1
      lower respiratory infection J47.0
  acquired J98.09
    with bronchiectasis J47.9
      with
        exacerbation (acute) J47.1
        lower respiratory infection J47.0
Muckle-Wells M04.2
mucocutaneous lymph node (acute febrile)
  (MCLS) M30.3
multiple endocrine neoplasia (MEN) — see
  Neoplasia, endocrine, multiple (MEN)
multiple operations — see Disorder, factitious
myasthenic G70.9
  in
    diabetes mellitus — see Diabetes,
      amyotrophy
    endocrine disease NEC E34.9 [G73.3]
    neoplastic disease (see also Neoplasm)
      D49.9 [G73.3]
    thyrotoxicosis (hyperthyroidism) E05.90
      [G73.3]
      with thyroid storm E05.91 [G73.3]
myelodysplastic D46.9
  with
    5q deletion D46.C *(follows D46.2)*
    isolated del(5q) chromosomal abnormality
      D46.C *(follows D46.2)*
  lesions, low grade D46.20
  specified NEC D46.Z *(follows D46.4)*
myelopathic pain G89.0
myeloproliferative (chronic) D47.1
myofascial pain M79.1
Naffziger's G54.0
nail patella Q87.2
NARP (Neuropathy, Ataxia and Retinitis
  pigmentosa) E88.49
neonatal abstinence P96.1
nephritic — see also Nephritis
  with edema — see Nephrosis
  acute N00.9
  chronic N03.9
  rapidly progressive N01.9
nephrotic (congenital) (see also Nephrosis)
  N04.9
  with
    dense deposit disease N04.6
    diffuse
      crescentic glomerulonephritis N04.7
      endocapillary proliferative
        glomerulonephritis N04.4
      membranous glomerulonephritis N04.2
      mesangial proliferative
        glomerulonephritis N04.3
      mesangiocapillary glomerulonephritis
        N04.5
    focal and segmental glomerular lesions
      N04.1
    minor glomerular abnormality N04.0
    specified morphological changes NEC
      N04.8
  diabetic — see Diabetes, nephrosis
neurologic neglect R41.4
Nezelof's D81.4
Nonne-Milroy-Meige Q82.0
Nothnagel's vasomotor acroparesthesia I73.89
obesity hypoventilation (OHS) E66.2
oculomotor H51.9
ophthalmoplegia-cerebellar ataxia — see
  Strabismus, paralytic, third nerve
oral allergy T78.1
oral-facial-digital Q87.0

Syndrome (see also Disease) — continued
organic
  affective F06.30
  amnesic (not alcohol-or drug-induced) F04
  brain F09
  depressive F06.31
  hallucinosis F06.0
  personality F07.0
Ormond's N13.5
oro-facial-digital Q87.0
os trigonum Q68.8
Osler-Weber-Rendu I78.0
osteoporosis-osteomalacia M83.8
Osterreicher-Turner Q87.2
oto-palatal-digital Q87.0
otolith — see subcategory H81.8
outlet (thoracic) G54.0
ovary
  polycystic E28.2
  resistant E28.39
  sclerocystic E28.2
Owren's D68.2
Paget-Schroetter I82.890
pain — see also Pain
  complex regional I G90.50
    lower limb G90.52-
    specified site NEC G90.59
    upper limb G90.51-
  complex regional II — see Causalgia
painful
  bruising D69.2
  feet E53.8
  prostate N42.81
paralysis agitans — see Parkinsonism
paralytic G83.9
  specified NEC G83.89
Parinaud's H51.0
Parkinson's — see Parkinsonism
parkinsonian — see Parkinsonism
paroxysmal facial pain G50.0
Parry's E05.00
  with thyroid storm E05.01
Parsonage(-Aldren)-Turner G54.5
patella clunk M25.86-
Paterson(-Brown) (-Kelly) D50.1
pectoral girdle I77.89
pectoralis minor I77.89
Pelger-Huet D72.0
pellagra-cerebellar ataxia-renal aminoaciduria
  E72.02
pellagroid E52
Pellegrini-Stieda — see Bursitis, tibial collateral
pelvic congestion-fibrosis, female N94.89
penta X Q97.1
peptic ulcer — see Ulcer, peptic
perabduction I77.89
periodic fever M04.1
periodic fever, aphthous stomatitis,
  pharyngitis, and adenopathy [PFAPA]
  M04.8
periodic headache, in adults and children —
  see Headache, periodic syndromes in
  adults and children
periurethral fibrosis N13.5
phantom limb (without pain) G54.7
  with pain G54.6
pharyngeal pouch D82.1
Pick's — see Disease, Pick's
Pickwickian E66.2
PIE (pulmonary infiltration with eosinophilia)
  J82
pigmentary pallidal degeneration (progressive)
  G23.0
pineal E34.8
pituitary E22.0
placental transfusion — see Pregnancy,
  complicated by, placental transfusion
  syndromes
plantar fascia M72.2

Syndrome (see also Disease) — continued
plateau iris (post-iridectomy) (postprocedural)
  H21.82
Plummer-Vinson D50.1
pluricarential of infancy E40
plurideficiency E40
pluriglandular (compensatory) E31.8
  autoimmune E31.0
pneumatic hammer T75.21
polyangiitis overlap M30.8
polycarential of infancy E40
polyglandular E31.8
  autoimmune E31.0
polysplenia Q89.09
pontine NEC G93.89
popliteal
  artery entrapment I77.89
  web Q87.89
post chemoembolization — code to associated
  conditions
postcardiac injury
  postcardiotomy I97.0
  postmyocardial infarction I24.1
postcardiotomy I97.0
postcholecystectomy K91.5
postcommissurotomy I97.0
postconcussional F07.81
postcontusional F07.81
postencephalitic F07.89
posterior
  cervical sympathetic M53.0
  cord G83.83
  fossa compression G93.5
  reversible encephalopathy (PRES) I67.83
postgastrectomy (dumping) K91.1
postgastric surgery K91.1
postinfarction I24.1
postlaminectomy NEC M96.1
postleukotomy F07.0
postmastectomy lymphedema I97.2
postmyocardial infarction I24.1
postoperative NEC T81.9
  blind loop K90.2
postpartum panhypopituitary (Sheehan) E23.0
postpolio (myelitic) G14
postthrombotic I87.009
  with
    inflammation I87.02-
      with ulcer I87.03-
    specified complication NEC I87.09-
    ulcer I87.01-
      with inflammation I87.03-
  asymptomatic I87.00-
postvagotomy K91.1
postvalvulotomy I97.0
postviral NEC G93.3
  fatigue G93.3
Potain's K31.0
potassium intoxication E87.5
precerebral artery (multiple) (bilateral) G45.2
preinfarction I20.0
preleukemic D46.9
premature senility E34.8
premenstrual dysphoric F32.89
premenstrual tension N94.3
Prinzmetal-Massumi R07.1
prune belly Q79.4
pseudocarpal tunnel (sublimis) — see
  Syndrome, carpal tunnel
pseudoparalytica G70.00
  with exacerbation (acute) G70.01
  in crisis G70.01
pseudo-Turner's Q87.1
psycho-organic (nonpsychotic severity) F07.9
  acute or subacute F05
  depressive type F06.31
  hallucinatory type F06.0
  nonpsychotic severity F07.0
  specified NEC F07.89

Syndrome (*see also* Disease) — *continued*
pulmonary
  arteriosclerosis I27.0
  dysmaturity (Wilson-Mikity) P27.0
  hypoperfusion (idiopathic) P22.0
  renal (hemorrhagic) (Goodpasture's) M31.0
pure
  motor lacunar G46.5
  sensory lacunar G46.6
Putnam-Dana D51.0
pyogenic arthritis, pyoderma gangrenosum, and acne [PAPA] M04.8
pyramidopallidonigral G20
pyriformis — *see* Lesion, nerve, sciatic
QT interval prolongation I45.81
radicular NEC — *see* Radiculopathy
  upper limbs, newborn (birth injury) P14.3
rapid time-zone change G47.25
Rasmussen G04.81
Raymond (-Céstan) I65.8
Raynaud's I73.00
  with gangrene I73.01
RDS (respiratory distress syndrome, newborn) P22.0
reactive airways dysfunction J68.3
Refsum's G60.1
Reifenstein E34.52
renal glomerulohyalinosis-diabetic — *see* Diabetes, nephrosis
Rendu-Osler-Weber I78.0
residual ovary N99.83
resistant ovary E28.39
respiratory
  distress
    acute J80
      adult J80
      child J80
      idiopathic J84.114
      newborn (idiopathic) (type I) P22.0
      type II P22.1
restless legs G25.81
retinoblastoma (familial) C69.2
retroperitoneal fibrosis N13.5
retroviral seroconversion (acute) Z21
Reye's G93.7
Richter — *see* Leukemia, chronic lymphocytic, B-cell type
Ridley's I50.1
right
  heart, hypoplastic Q22.6
  ventricular obstruction — *see* Failure, heart, congestive
Romano-Ward (prolonged QT interval) I45.81
rotator cuff, shoulder (*see also* Tear, rotator cuff) M75.10-
Rotes Quérol — *see* Hyperostosis, ankylosing
Roth — *see* Meralgia paresthetica
rubella (congenital) P35.0
Ruvalcaba-Myhre-Smith E71.440
Rytand-Lipsitch I44.2
salt
  depletion E87.1
    due to heat NEC T67.8
      causing heat exhaustion or prostration T67.4
  low E87.1
salt-losing N28.89
Scaglietti-Dagnini E22.0
scalenus anticus (anterior) G54.0
scapulocostal — *see* Mononeuropathy, upper limb, specified site NEC
scapuloperoneal G71.0
schizophrenic, of childhood NEC F84.5
Schnitzler D47.2
Scholte's E34.0
Schroeder's E27.0
Schüller-Christian C96.5
Schwachman's — *see* Syndrome, Shwachman's
Schwartz (-Jampel) G71.13

Syndrome (*see also* Disease) — *continued*
Schwartz-Bartter E22.2
scimitar Q26.8
sclerocystic ovary E28.2
Seitelberger's G31.89
septicemic adrenal hemorrhage A39.1
seroconversion, retroviral (acute) Z21
serous meningitis G93.2
severe acute respiratory (SARS) J12.81
shaken infant T74.4
shock (traumatic) T79.4
  kidney N17.0
    following crush injury T79.5
  toxic A48.3
shock-lung J80
Shone's — *code to* specific anomalies
short
  bowel K91.2
  rib Q77.2
shoulder-hand — *see* Algoneurodystrophy
Shwachman's D70.4
sicca — *see* Sicca syndrome
sick
  cell E87.1
  sinus I49.5
sick-euthyroid E07.81
sideropenic D50.1
Siemens' ectodermal dysplasia Q82.4
Silfversköld's Q78.9
Simons' E88.1
sinus tarsi M25.57-
sinusitis-bronchiectasis-situs inversus Q89.3
Sipple's E31.22
sirenomelia Q87.2
Slocumb's E27.0
slow flow, coronary I20.8
Sluder's G44.89
Smith-Magenis Q93.88
Sneddon-Wilkinson L13.1
Soto's Q87.3
South African cardiomyopathy I42.8
spasmodic
  upward movement, eyes H51.8
  winking F95.8
Spen's I45.9
splenic
  agenesis Q89.01
  flexure K59.8
  neutropenia D73.81
Spurway's Q78.0
staphylococcal scalded skin L00
steal
  arteriovenous T82.898-
  ischemic T82.898-
  subclavian G45.8
Stein-Leventhal E28.2
Stein's E28.2
Stevens-Johnson syndrome L51.1
  toxic epidermal necrolysis overlap L51.3
Stewart-Morel M85.2
Stickler Q89.8
stiff baby Q89.8
stiff man G25.82
Still-Felty — *see* Felty's syndrome
Stokes (-Adams) I45.9
stone heart I50.1
straight back, congenital Q76.49
subclavian steal G45.8
subcoracoid-pectoralis minor G54.0
subcostal nerve compression I77.89
subphrenic interposition Q43.3
superior
  cerebellar artery I63.8
  mesenteric artery K55.1
  semi-circular canal dehiscence H83.8x-
  vena cava I87.1
supine hypotensive (maternal) — *see* Syndrome, hypotension, maternal
suprarenal cortical E27.0

Syndrome (*see also* Disease) — *continued*
supraspinatus (*see also* Tear, rotator cuff) M75.10-
Susac G93.49
swallowed blood P78.2
sweat retention L74.0
Swyer Q99.1
Symond's G93.2
sympathetic
  cervical paralysis G90.2
  pelvic, female N94.89
systemic inflammatory response (SIRS), of non-infectious origin (without organ dysfunction) R65.10
  with acute organ dysfunction R65.11
tachycardia-bradycardia I49.5
takotsubo I51.81
TAR (thrombocytopenia with absent radius) Q87.2
tarsal tunnel G57.5-
teething K00.7
tegmental G93.89
telangiectasic-pigmentation-cataract Q82.8
temporal pyramidal apex — *see* Otitis, media, suppurative, acute
temporomandibular joint-pain-dysfunction M26.62-
Terry's H44.2-
testicular feminization (*see also* Syndrome, androgen insensitivity) E34.51
thalamic pain (hyperesthetic) G89.0
thoracic outlet (compression) G54.0
Thorson-Björck E34.0
thrombocytopenia with absent radius (TAR) Q87.2
thyroid-adrenocortical insufficiency E31.0
tibial
  anterior M76.81-
  posterior M76.82-
Tietze's M94.0
time-zone (rapid) G47.25
Toni-Fanconi E72.09
  with cystinosis E72.04
Touraine's Q79.8
tourniquet — *see* Constriction, external, by site
toxic shock A48.3
transient left ventricular apical ballooning I51.81
traumatic vasospastic T75.22
Treacher Collins Q75.4
triple X, female Q97.0
trisomy Q92.9
  13 Q91.7
    meiotic nondisjunction Q91.4
    mitotic nondisjunction Q91.5
    mosaicism Q91.5
    translocation Q91.6
  18 Q91.3
    meiotic nondisjunction Q91.0
    mitotic nondisjunction Q91.1
    mosaicism Q91.1
    translocation Q91.2
  20(q) (p) Q92.8
  21 Q90.9
    meiotic nondisjunction Q90.0
    mitotic nondisjunction Q90.1
    mosaicism Q90.1
    translocation Q90.2
  22 Q92.8
tropical wet feet T69.0-
Trousseau's I82.1
tumor lysis (following antineoplastic chemotherapy) (spontaneous) NEC E88.3
tumor necrosis factor receptor associated periodic (TRAPS) M04.1
Twiddler's (due to)
  automatic implantable defibrillator T82.198
  cardiac pacemaker T82.198

Syndrome (see also Disease) — continued
Unverricht (-Lundborg) — see Epilepsy, generalized, idiopathic
upward gaze H51.8
uremia, chronic (see also Disease, kidney, chronic) N18.9
urethral N34.3
urethro-oculo-articular — see Reiter's disease
urohepatic K76.7
vago-hypoglossal G52.7
van Buchem's M85.2
van der Hoeve's Q78.0
vascular NEC in cerebrovascular disease G46.8
vasoconstriction, reversible cerebrovascular I67.841
vasomotor I73.9
vasospastic (traumatic) T75.22
vasovagal R55
VATER Q87.2
velo-cardio-facial Q93.81
vena cava (inferior) (superior) (obstruction) I87.1
vertebral
   artery G45.0
      compression — see Syndrome, anterior, spinal artery, compression
   steal G45.0
vertebro-basilar artery G45.0
vertebrogenic (pain) M54.89
vertiginous — see Disorder, vestibular function
Vinson-Plummer D50.1
virus B34.9
visceral larva migrans B83.0
visual disorientation H53.8
vitamin B6 deficiency E53.1
vitreal corneal H59.01-
vitreous (touch) H59.01-
Vogt-Koyanagi H20.82-
Volkmann's T79.6
von Schroetter's I82.890
von Willebrand (-Jürgen) D68.0
Waldenström-Kjellberg D50.1
Wallenberg's G46.3
water retention E87.79
Waterhouse (-Friderichsen) A39.1
Weber-Gubler G46.3
Weber-Leyden G46.3
Weber's G46.3
Wegener's M31.30
   with
      kidney involvement M31.31
      lung involvement M31.30
         with kidney involvement M31.31
Weingarten's (tropical eosinophilia) J82
Weiss-Baker G90.09
Werdnig-Hoffman G12.0
Wermer's E31.21
Werner's E34.8
Wernicke-Korsakoff (nonalcoholic) F04
   alcoholic F10.26
West's — see Epilepsy, spasms
Westphal-Strümpell E83.01
wet
   feet (maceration) (tropical) T69.0-
   lung, newborn P22.1
whiplash S13.4
whistling face Q87.0
Wilkie's K55.1
Wilkinson-Sneddon L13.1
Willebrand (-Jürgens) D68.0
Wilson's (hepatolenticular degeneration) E83.01
Wiskott-Aldrich D82.0
withdrawal — see Withdrawal, state
   drug
      infant of dependent mother P96.1
      therapeutic use, newborn P96.2
Woakes' (ethmoiditis) J33.1

Syndrome (see also Disease) — continued
Wright's (hyperabduction) I77.89
X I20.9
XXXX Q97.1
XXXXX Q97.1
XXXXY Q98.1
XXY Q98.0
yellow nail L60.5
Zahorsky's B08.5
Zellweger syndrome E71.510
Zellweger-like syndrome E71.541
Synechia (anterior) (iris) (posterior) (pupil) — see also Adhesions, iris
   intra-uterine (traumatic) N85.6
Synesthesia R20.8
Syngamiasis, syngamosis B83.3
Synodontia K00.2
Synorchidism, synorchism Q55.1
Synostosis (congenital) Q78.8
   astragalo-scaphoid Q74.2
   radioulnar Q74.0
Synovial sarcoma — see Neoplasm, connective tissue, malignant
Synovioma (malignant) — see also Neoplasm, connective tissue, malignant
   benign — see Neoplasm, connective tissue, benign
Synoviosarcoma — see Neoplasm, connective tissue, malignant
Synovitis (see also Tenosynovitis) M65.9
   crepitant
      hand M70.0-
      wrist M70.03-
   gonococcal A54.49
   gouty — see Gout
   in (due to)
      crystals M65.8-
      gonorrhea A54.49
      syphilis (late) A52.78
      use, overuse, pressure — see Disorder, soft tissue, due to use
   infective NEC — see Tenosynovitis, infective NEC
   specified NEC — see Tenosynovitis, specified type NEC
   syphilitic A52.78
      congenital (early) A50.02
   toxic — see Synovitis, transient
   transient M67.3-
      ankle M67.37-
      elbow M67.32-
      foot joint M67.37-
      hand joint M67.34-
      hip M67.35-
      knee M67.36-
      multiple site M67.39
      pelvic region M67.35-
      shoulder M67.31-
      specified joint NEC M67.38
      wrist M67.33-
   traumatic, current — see Sprain
   tuberculous — see Tuberculosis, synovitis
   villonodular (pigmented) M12.2-
      ankle M12.27-
      elbow M12.22-
      foot joint M12.27-
      hand joint M12.24-
      hip M12.25-
      knee M12.26-
      multiple site M12.29
      pelvic region M12.25-
      shoulder M12.21-
      specified joint NEC M12.28
      vertebrae M12.28
      wrist M12.23-
Syphilid A51.39
   congenital A50.06
   newborn A50.06
   tubercular (late) A52.79

Syphilis, syphilitic (acquired) A53.9
abdomen (late) A52.79
acoustic nerve A52.15
adenopathy (secondary) A51.49
adrenal (gland) (with cortical hypofunction) A52.79
age under 2 years NOS — see also Syphilis, congenital, early
   acquired A51.9
alopecia (secondary) A51.32
anemia (late) A52.79 [D63.8]
aneurysm (aorta) (ruptured) A52.01
   central nervous system A52.05
   congenital A50.54 [I79.0]
anus (late) A52.74
   primary A51.1
   secondary A51.39
aorta (arch) (abdominal) (thoracic) A52.02
   aneurysm A52.01
aortic (insufficiency) (regurgitation) (stenosis) A52.03
   aneurysm A52.01
arachnoid (adhesive) (cerebral) (spinal) A52.13
asymptomatic — see Syphilis, latent
ataxia (locomotor) A52.11
atrophoderma maculatum A51.39
auricular fibrillation A52.06
bladder (late) A52.76
bone A52.77
   secondary A51.46
brain A52.17
breast (late) A52.79
bronchus (late) A52.72
bubo (primary) A51.0
bulbar palsy A52.19
bursa (late) A52.78
cardiac decompensation A52.06
cardiovascular A52.00
central nervous system (late) (recurrent) (relapse) (tertiary) A52.3
   with
      ataxia A52.11
      general paralysis A52.17
         juvenile A50.45
      paresis (general) A52.17
         juvenile A50.45
      tabes (dorsalis) A52.11
         juvenile A50.45
      taboparesis A52.17
         juvenile A50.45
   aneurysm A52.05
   congenital A50.40
   juvenile A50.40
   remission in (sustained) A52.3
   serology doubtful, negative, or positive A52.3
   specified nature or site NEC A52.19
   vascular A52.05
cerebral A52.17
   meningovascular A52.13
   nerves (multiple palsies) A52.15
   sclerosis A52.17
   thrombosis A52.05
cerebrospinal (tabetic type) A52.12
cerebrovascular A52.05
cervix (late) A52.76
chancre (multiple) A51.0
   extragenital A51.2
   Rollet's A51.0
Charcôt's joint A52.16
chorioretinitis A51.43
   congenital A50.01
   late A52.71
   prenatal A50.01
choroiditis — see Syphilitic chorioretinitis
choroidoretinitis — see Syphilitic chorioretinitis
ciliary body (secondary) A51.43
   late A52.71

Syphilis, syphilitic (acquired) A53.9 — continued
colon (late) A52.74
combined spinal sclerosis A52.11
condyloma (latum) A51.31
congenital A50.9
  with
    paresis (general) A50.45
    tabes (dorsalis) A50.45
    taboparesis A50.45
  chorioretinitis, choroiditis A50.01 [H32]
  early, or less than 2 years after birth NEC A50.2
    with manifestations — see Syphilis, congenital, early, symptomatic
    latent (without manifestations) A50.1
      negative spinal fluid test A50.1
      serology positive A50.1
    symptomatic A50.09
      cutaneous A50.06
      mucocutaneous A50.07
      oculopathy A50.01
      osteochondropathy A50.02
      pharyngitis A50.03
      pneumonia A50.04
      rhinitis A50.05
      visceral A50.08
  interstitial keratitis A50.31
  juvenile neurosyphilis A50.45
  late, or 2 years or more after birth NEC A50.7
    chorioretinitis, choroiditis A50.32
    interstitial keratitis A50.31
    juvenile neurosyphilis A50.45
    latent (without manifestations) A50.6
      negative spinal fluid test A50.6
      serology positive A50.6
    symptomatic or with manifestations NEC A50.59
      arthropathy A50.55
      cardiovascular A50.54
      Clutton's joints A50.51
      Hutchinson's teeth A50.52
      Hutchinson's triad A50.53
      osteochondropathy A50.56
      saddle nose A50.57
conjugal A53.9
  tabes A52.11
conjunctiva (late) A52.71
contact Z20.2
cord bladder A52.19
cornea, late A52.71
coronary (artery) (sclerosis) A52.06
coryza, congenital A50.05
cranial nerve A52.15
  multiple palsies A52.15
cutaneous — see Syphilis, skin
dacryocystitis (late) A52.71
degeneration, spinal cord A52.12
dementia paralytica A52.17
  juvenilis A50.45
destruction of bone A52.77
dilatation, aorta A52.01
due to blood transfusion A53.9
dura mater A52.13
ear A52.79
  inner A52.79
    nerve (eighth) A52.15
    neurorecurrence A52.15
early A51.9
  cardiovascular A52.00
  central nervous system A52.3
  latent (without manifestations) (less than 2 years after infection) A51.5
    negative spinal fluid test A51.5
    serological relapse after treatment A51.5
    serology positive A51.5
  relapse (treated, untreated) A51.9
  skin A51.39

Syphilis, syphilitic (acquired) A53.9 — continued
early A51.9 — continued
  symptomatic A51.9
    extragenital chancre A51.2
    primary, except extragenital chancre A51.0
    secondary (see also Syphilis, secondary) A51.39
      relapse (treated, untreated) A51.49
    ulcer A51.39
eighth nerve (neuritis) A52.15
endemic A65
endocarditis A52.03
  aortic A52.03
  pulmonary A52.03
epididymis (late) A52.76
epiglottis (late) A52.73
epiphysitis (congenital) (early) A50.02
episcleritis (late) A52.71
esophagus A52.79
eustachian tube A52.73
exposure to Z20.2
eye A52.71
eyelid (late) (with gumma) A52.71
fallopian tube (late) A52.76
fracture A52.77
gallbladder (late) A52.74
gastric (polyposis) (late) A52.74
general A53.9
  paralysis A52.17
    juvenile A50.45
  genital (primary) A51.0
  glaucoma A52.71
  gumma NEC A52.79
    cardiovascular system A52.00
    central nervous system A52.3
    congenital A50.59
  heart (block) (decompensation) (disease) (failure) A52.06 [I52]
    valve NEC A52.03
hemianesthesia A52.19
hemianopsia A52.71
hemiparesis A52.17
hemiplegia A52.17
hepatic artery A52.09
hepatis A52.74
hepatomegaly, congenital A50.08
hereditaria tarda — see Syphilis, congenital, late
hereditary — see Syphilis, congenital
Hutchinson's teeth A50.52
hyalitis A52.71
inactive — see Syphilis, latent
infantum — see Syphilis, congenital
inherited — see Syphilis, congenital
internal ear A52.79
intestine (late) A52.74
iris, iritis (secondary) A51.43
  late A52.71
joint (late) A52.77
keratitis (congenital) (interstitial) (late) A50.31
kidney (late) A52.75
lacrimal passages (late) A52.71
larynx (late) A52.73
late A52.9
  cardiovascular A52.00
  central nervous system A52.3
  kidney A52.75
  latent or 2 years or more after infection (without manifestations) A52.8
    negative spinal fluid test A52.8
    serology positive A52.8
  paresis A52.17
  specified site NEC A52.79
  symptomatic or with manifestations A52.79
  tabes A52.11

Syphilis, syphilitic (acquired) A53.9 — continued
latent A53.0
  with signs or symptoms — code by site and stage under Syphilis
  central nervous system A52.2
  date of infection unspecified A53.0
  early, or less than 2 years after infection A51.5
  follow-up of latent syphilis A53.0
    date of infection unspecified A53.0
    late, or 2 years or more after infection A52.8
  late, or 2 years or more after infection A52.8
  positive serology (only finding) A53.0
    date of infection unspecified A53.0
    early, or less than 2 years after infection A51.5
    late, or 2 years or more after infection A52.8
lens (late) A52.71
leukoderma A51.39
  late A52.79
lienitis A52.79
lip A51.39
  chancre (primary) A51.2
  late A52.79
Lissauer's paralysis A52.17
liver A52.74
locomotor ataxia A52.11
lung A52.72
lymph gland (early) (secondary) A51.49
  late A52.79
lymphadenitis (secondary) A51.49
macular atrophy of skin A51.39
  striated A52.79
mediastinum (late) A52.73
meninges (adhesive) (brain) (spinal cord) A52.13
meningitis A52.13
  acute (secondary) A51.41
  congenital A50.41
meningoencephalitis A52.14
meningovascular A52.13
  congenital A50.41
mesarteritis A52.09
  brain A52.04
middle ear A52.77
mitral stenosis A52.03
monoplegia A52.17
mouth (secondary) A51.39
  late A52.79
mucocutaneous (secondary) A51.39
  late A52.79
mucous
  membrane (secondary) A51.39
    late A52.79
  patches A51.39
    congenital A50.07
mulberry molars A50.52
muscle A52.78
myocardium A52.06
nasal sinus (late) A52.73
neonatorum — see Syphilis, congenital
nephrotic syndrome (secondary) A51.44
nerve palsy (any cranial nerve) A52.15
  multiple A52.15
nervous system, central A52.3
neuritis A52.15
  acoustic A52.15
neurorecidive of retina A52.19
neuroretinitis A52.19
newborn — see Syphilis, congenital
nodular superficial (late) A52.79
nonvenereal A65
nose (late) A52.73
  saddle back deformity A50.57
occlusive arterial disease A52.09

DISEASE INDEX

Syphilis, syphilitic (acquired) A53.9 — *continued*
oculopathy A52.71
ophthalmic (late) A52.71
optic nerve (atrophy) (neuritis) (papilla) A52.15
orbit (late) A52.71
organic A53.9
osseous (late) A52.77
osteochondritis (congenital) (early) A50.02 *[M90.80]*
osteoporosis A52.77
ovary (late) A52.76
oviduct (late) A52.76
palate (late) A52.79
pancreas (late) A52.74
paralysis A52.17
　general A52.17
　　juvenile A50.45
paresis (general) A52.17
　juvenile A50.45
paresthesia A52.19
Parkinson's disease or syndrome A52.19
paroxysmal tachycardia A52.06
pemphigus (congenital) A50.06
penis (chancre) A51.0
　late A52.76
pericardium A52.06
perichondritis, larynx (late) A52.73
periosteum (late) A52.77
　congenital (early) A50.02 *[M90.80]*
　early (secondary) A51.46
peripheral nerve A52.79
petrous bone (late) A52.77
pharynx (late) A52.73
　secondary A51.39
pituitary (gland) A52.79
pleura (late) A52.73
pneumonia, white A50.04
pontine lesion A52.17
portal vein A52.09
primary A51.0
　anal A51.1
　and secondary — *see* Syphilis, secondary
　central nervous system A52.3
　extragenital chancre NEC A51.2
　fingers A51.2
　genital A51.0
　lip A51.2
　specified site NEC A51.2
　tonsils A51.2
prostate (late) A52.76
ptosis (eyelid) A52.71
pulmonary (late) A52.72
　artery A52.09
pyelonephritis (late) A52.75
recently acquired, symptomatic A51.9
rectum (late) A52.74
respiratory tract (late) A52.73
retina, late A52.71
retrobulbar neuritis A52.15
salpingitis A52.76
sclera (late) A52.71
sclerosis
　cerebral A52.17
　coronary A52.06
　multiple A52.11
scotoma (central) A52.71
scrotum (late) A52.76
secondary (and primary) A51.49
　adenopathy A51.49
　anus A51.39
　bone A51.46
　chorioretinitis, choroiditis A51.43
　hepatitis A51.45
　liver A51.45
　lymphadenitis A51.49
　meningitis (acute) A51.41
　mouth A51.39

Syphilis, syphilitic (acquired) A53.9 — *continued*
secondary (and primary) A51.49 — *continued*
　mucous membranes A51.39
　periosteum, periostitis A51.46
　pharynx A51.39
　relapse (treated, untreated) A51.49
　skin A51.39
　specified form NEC A51.49
　tonsil A51.39
　ulcer A51.39
　viscera NEC A51.49
　vulva A51.39
seminal vesicle (late) A52.76
seronegative with signs or symptoms — *code by site and stage under Syphilis*
seropositive
　with signs or symptoms — *code by* site and stage under Syphilis
　follow-up of latent syphilis — *see* Syphilis, latent
　only finding — *see* Syphilis, latent
seventh nerve (paralysis) A52.15
sinus, sinusitis (late) A52.73
skeletal system A52.77
skin (with ulceration) (early) (secondary) A51.39
　late or tertiary A52.79
small intestine A52.74
spastic spinal paralysis A52.17
spermatic cord (late) A52.76
spinal (cord) A52.12
spleen A52.79
splenomegaly A52.79
spondylitis A52.77
staphyloma A52.71
stigmata (congenital) A50.59
stomach A52.74
synovium A52.78
tabes dorsalis (late) A52.11
　juvenile A50.45
tabetic type A52.11
　juvenile A50.45
taboparesis A52.17
　juvenile A50.45
tachycardia A52.06
tendon (late) A52.78
tertiary A52.9
　with symptoms NEC A52.79
　cardiovascular A52.00
　central nervous system A52.3
　multiple NEC A52.79
　specified site NEC A52.79
testis A52.76
thorax A52.73
throat A52.73
thymus (gland) (late) A52.79
thyroid (late) A52.79
tongue (late) A52.79
tonsil (lingual) (late) A52.73
　primary A51.2
　secondary A51.39
trachea (late) A52.73
tunica vaginalis (late) A52.76
ulcer (any site) (early) (secondary) A51.39
　late A52.79
　perforating A52.79
　　foot A52.11
urethra (late) A52.76
urogenital (late) A52.76
uterus (late) A52.76
uveal tract (secondary) A51.43
　late A52.71
uveitis (secondary) A51.43
　late A52.71
uvula (late) (perforated) A52.79
vagina A51.0
　late A52.76

Syphilis, syphilitic (acquired) A53.9 — *continued*
valvulitis NEC A52.03
vascular A52.00
　brain (cerebral) A52.05
ventriculi A52.74
vesicae urinariae (late) A52.76
viscera (abdominal) (late) A52.74
　secondary A51.49
vitreous (opacities) (late) A52.71
　hemorrhage A52.71
vulva A51.0
　late A52.76
　secondary A51.39
Syphiloma A52.79
cardiovascular system A52.00
central nervous system A52.3
circulatory system A52.00
congenital A50.59
Syphilophobia F45.29
Syringadenoma — *see also* Neoplasm, skin, benign
papillary — *see* Neoplasm, skin, benign
Syringobulbia G95.0
Syringocystadenoma — *see* Neoplasm, skin, benign
papillary — *see* Neoplasm, skin, benign
Syringoma — *see also* Neoplasm, skin, benign
chondroid — *see* Neoplasm, skin, benign
Syringomyelia G95.0
Syringomyelitis — *see* Encephalitis
Syringomyelocele — *see* Spina bifida
Syringopontia G95.0
System, systemic — *see also* condition
disease, combined — *see* Degeneration, combined
inflammatory response syndrome (SIRS) of non-infectious origin (without organ dysfunction) R65.10
　with acute organ dysfunction R65.11
lupus erythematosus M32.9
　inhibitor present D68.62

T

Tabacism, tabacosis, tabagism — *see also*
　　Poisoning, tobacco
　　meaning dependence (without remission)
　　　F17.200
　　with
　　　disorder F17.299
　　　　remission F17.211
　　　　specified disorder NEC F17.298
　　　withdrawal F17.203
Tabardillo A75.9
　　flea-borne A75.2
　　louse-borne A75.0
Tabes, tabetic A52.10
　　with
　　　central nervous system syphilis A52.10
　　　Charcot's joint A52.16
　　　cord bladder A52.19
　　　crisis, viscera (any) A52.19
　　　paralysis, general A52.17
　　　paresis (general) A52.17
　　　perforating ulcer (foot) A52.19
　　arthropathy (Charcot) A52.16
　　bladder A52.19
　　bone A52.11
　　cerebrospinal A52.12
　　congenital A50.45
　　conjugal A52.10
　　dorsalis A52.11
　　　juvenile A50.49
　　juvenile A50.49
　　latent A52.19
　　mesenterica A18.39
　　paralysis, insane, general A52.17
　　spasmodic A52.17
　　syphilis (cerebrospinal) A52.12
Taboparalysis A52.17
Taboparesis (remission) A52.17
　　juvenile A50.45
TAC (trigeminal autonomic cephalgia) NEC
　　G44.099
　　intractable G44.091
　　not intractable G44.099
Tache noir S60.22-
Tachyalimentation K91.2
Tachyarrhythmia, tachyrhythmia — *see*
　　Tachycardia
Tachycardia R00.0
　　atrial (paroxysmal) I47.1
　　auricular I47.1
　　AV nodal re-entry (re-entrant) I47.1
　　junctional (paroxysmal) I47.1
　　newborn P29.11
　　nodal (paroxysmal) I47.1
　　non-paroxysmal AV nodal I45.89
　　paroxysmal (sustained) (nonsustained) I47.9
　　　with sinus bradycardia I49.5
　　　atrial (PAT) I47.1
　　　atrioventricular (AV) (re-entrant) I47.1
　　　　psychogenic F54
　　　junctional I47.1
　　　　ectopic I47.1
　　　nodal I47.1
　　　psychogenic (atrial) (supraventricular)
　　　　(ventricular) F54
　　　supraventricular (sustained) I47.1
　　　　psychogenic F54
　　　ventricular I47.2
　　　　psychogenic F54
　　psychogenic F45.8
　　sick sinus I49.5
　　sinoauricular NOS R00.0
　　　paroxysmal I47.1
　　sinus [sinusal] NOS R00.0
　　　paroxysmal I47.1
　　supraventricular I47.1

Tachycardia R00.0 — *continued*
　　ventricular (paroxysmal) (sustained) I47.2
　　　psychogenic F54
Tachygastria K31.89
Tachypnea R06.82
　　hysterical F45.8
　　newborn (idiopathic) (transitory) P22.1
　　psychogenic F45.8
　　transitory, of newborn P22.1
TACO (transfusion associated circulatory
　　overload) E87.71
Taenia (infection) (infestation) B68.9
　　diminuta B71.0
　　echinococcal infestation B67.90
　　mediocanellata B68.1
　　nana B71.0
　　saginata B68.1
　　solium (intestinal form) B68.0
　　　larval form — *see* Cysticercosis
Taeniasis (intestine) — *see* Taenia
Tag (hypertrophied skin) (infected) L91.8
　　adenoid J35.8
　　anus K64.4
　　hemorrhoidal K64.4
　　hymen N89.8
　　perineal N90.89
　　preauricular Q17.0
　　sentinel K64.4
　　skin L91.8
　　　accessory (congenital) Q82.8
　　　anus K64.4
　　　congenital Q82.8
　　　preauricular Q17.0
　　tonsil J35.8
　　urethra, urethral N36.8
　　vulva N90.89
Tahyna fever B33.8
Takahara's disease E80.3
Takayasu's disease or syndrome M31.4
Talcosis (pulmonary) J62.0
Talipes (congenital) Q66.89
　　acquired, planus — *see* Deformity, limb, flat
　　　foot
　　asymmetric Q66.89
　　calcaneovalgus Q66.4
　　calcaneovarus Q66.1
　　calcaneus Q66.89
　　cavus Q66.7
　　equinovalgus Q66.6
　　equinovarus Q66.0
　　equinus Q66.89
　　percavus Q66.7
　　planovalgus Q66.6
　　planus (acquired) (any degree) — *see also*
　　　Deformity, limb, flat foot
　　　congenital Q66.5-
　　　due to rickets (sequelae) E64.3
　　valgus Q66.6
　　varus Q66.3
Tall stature, constitutional E34.4
Talma's disease M62.89
Talon noir S90.3-
　　hand S60.22-
　　heel S90.3-
　　toe S90.1-
Tamponade, heart I31.4
Tanapox (virus disease) B08.71
Tangier disease E78.6
Tantrum, child problem F91.8
Tapeworm (infection) (infestation) — *see*
　　Infestation, tapeworm
Tapia's syndrome G52.7
TAR (thrombocytopenia with absent radius)
　　syndrome Q87.2
Tarral-Besnier disease L44.0
Tarsal tunnel syndrome — *see* Syndrome,
　　tarsal tunnel
Tarsalgia — *see* Pain, limb, lower

Tarsitis (eyelid) H01.8
　　syphilitic A52.71
　　tuberculous A18.4
Tartar (teeth) (dental calculus) K03.6
Tattoo (mark) L81.8
Tauri's disease E74.09
Taurodontism K00.2
Taussig-Bing syndrome Q20.1
Taybi's syndrome Q87.2
Tay-Sachs amaurotic familial idiocy or
　　disease E75.02
TBI (traumatic brain injury) S06.9
Teacher's node or nodule J38.2
Tear, torn (traumatic) — *see also* Laceration
　　with abortion — *see* Abortion
　　annular fibrosis M51.35
　　anus, anal (sphincter) S31.831
　　　complicating delivery
　　　　with third degree perineal laceration (*see*
　　　　　also Delivery, complicated, by,
　　　　　laceration, perineum, third degree)
　　　　　O70.20
　　　　　with mucosa O70.3
　　　　without third degree perineal laceration
　　　　　O70.4
　　　nontraumatic (healed) (old) K62.81
　　articular cartilage, old — *see* Derangement,
　　　joint, articular cartilage, by site
　　bladder
　　　with ectopic or molar pregnancy O08.6
　　　following ectopic or molar pregnancy O08.6
　　　obstetrical O71.5
　　　traumatic — *see* Injury, bladder
　　bowel
　　　with ectopic or molar pregnancy O08.6
　　　following ectopic or molar pregnancy O08.6
　　　obstetrical trauma O71.5
　　broad ligament
　　　with ectopic or molar pregnancy O08.6
　　　following ectopic or molar pregnancy O08.6
　　　obstetrical trauma O71.6
　　bucket handle (knee) (meniscus) — *see* Tear,
　　　meniscus
　　capsule, joint — *see* Sprain
　　cartilage — *see also* Sprain
　　　articular, old — *see* Derangement, joint,
　　　　articular cartilage, by site
　　cervix
　　　with ectopic or molar pregnancy O08.6
　　　following ectopic or molar pregnancy O08.6
　　　obstetrical trauma (current) O71.3
　　　old N88.1
　　　traumatic — *see* Injury, uterus
　　dural G97.41
　　　nontraumatic G96.11
　　internal organ — *see* Injury, by site
　　knee cartilage
　　　articular (current) S83.3-
　　　old — *see* Derangement, knee, meniscus,
　　　　due to old tear
　　ligament — *see* Sprain
　　meniscus (knee) (current injury) S83.209
　　　bucket-handle S83.20-
　　　lateral
　　　　bucket-handle S83.25-
　　　　complex S83.27-
　　　　peripheral S83.26-
　　　　specified type NEC S83.28-
　　　medial
　　　　bucket-handle S83.21-
　　　　complex S83.23-
　　　　peripheral S83.22-
　　　　specified type NEC S83.24-
　　　old — *see* Derangement, knee, meniscus,
　　　　due to old tear
　　　site other than knee — *code as* Sprain
　　　specified type NEC S83.20-
　　muscle — *see* Strain

DISEASE INDEX

DISEASE INDEX

Tear, torn (traumatic) (*see also* Laceration) — *continued*
- pelvic
  - floor, complicating delivery O70.1
  - organ NEC, obstetrical trauma O71.5
    - with ectopic or molar pregnancy O08.6
    - following ectopic or molar pregnancy O08.6
- perineal, secondary O90.1
- periurethral tissue, obstetrical trauma O71.82
  - with ectopic or molar pregnancy O08.6
  - following ectopic or molar pregnancy O08.6
- rectovaginal septum — *see* Laceration, vagina
- retina, retinal (without detachment) (horseshoe) — *see also* Break, retina, horseshoe
  - with detachment — *see* Detachment, retina, with retinal, break
- rotator cuff (nontraumatic) M75.10-
  - complete M75.12-
  - incomplete M75.11-
  - traumatic S46.01-
    - capsule S43.42-
- semilunar cartilage, knee — *see* Tear, meniscus
- supraspinatus (complete) (incomplete) (nontraumatic) (*see also* Tear, rotator cuff) M75.10-
- tendon — *see* Strain
- tentorial, at birth P10.4
- umbilical cord
  - complicating delivery O69.89
- urethra
  - with ectopic or molar pregnancy O08.6
  - following ectopic or molar pregnancy O08.6
  - obstetrical trauma O71.5
- uterus — *see* Injury, uterus
- vagina — *see* Laceration, vagina
- vessel, from catheter — *see* Puncture, accidental complicating surgery
- vulva, complicating delivery O70.0

Tear-stone — *see* Dacryolith
Teeth — *see also* condition
- grinding
  - psychogenic F45.8
  - sleep related G47.63
Teething (syndrome) K00.7
Telangiectasia, telangiectasis (verrucous) I78.1
- ataxic (cerebellar) (Louis-Bar) G11.3
- familial I78.0
- hemorrhagic, hereditary (congenital) (senile) I78.0
- hereditary, hemorrhagic (congenital) (senile) I78.0
- juxtafoveal H35.07-
- macular H35.07-
- parafoveal H35.07-
- retinal (idiopathic) (juxtafoveal) (macular) (parafoveal) H35.07-
- spider I78.1
Telephone scatologia F65.89
Telescoped bowel or intestine K56.1
- congenital Q43.8
Temperature
- body, high (of unknown origin) R50.9
- cold, trauma from T69.9
  - newborn P80.0
  - specified effect NEC T69.8
Temple — *see* condition
Temporal — *see* condition
Temporomandibular joint pain-dysfunction syndrome M26.62-
Temporosphenoidal — *see* condition
Tendency
- bleeding — *see* Defect, coagulation
- suicide
  - meaning personal history of attempted suicide Z91.5
  - meaning suicidal ideation — *see* Ideation, suicidal

Tendency — *continued*
- to fall R29.6
Tenderness, abdominal R10.819
- epigastric R10.816
- generalized R10.817
- left lower quadrant R10.814
- left upper quadrant R10.812
- periumbilic R10.815
- rebound R10.829
  - epigastric R10.826
  - generalized R10.827
  - left lower quadrant R10.824
  - left upper quadrant R10.822
  - periumbilic R10.825
  - right lower quadrant R10.823
  - right upper quadrant R10.821
- right lower quadrant R10.813
- right upper quadrant R10.811
Tendinitis, tendonitis — *see also* Enthesopathy
- Achilles M76.6-
- adhesive — *see* Tenosynovitis, specified type NEC
  - shoulder — *see* Capsulitis, adhesive
- bicipital M75.2-
- calcific M65.2-
  - ankle M65.27-
  - foot M65.27-
  - forearm M65.23-
  - hand M65.24-
  - lower leg M65.26-
  - multiple sites M65.29
  - pelvic region M65.25-
  - shoulder M75.3-
  - specified site NEC M65.28
  - thigh M65.25-
  - upper arm M65.22-
- due to use, overuse, pressure — *see also* Disorder, soft tissue, due to use
  - specified NEC — *see* Disorder, soft tissue, due to use, specified NEC
- gluteal M76.0-
- patellar M76.5-
- peroneal M76.7-
- psoas M76.1-
- tibial (posterior) M76.82-
  - anterior M76.81-
- trochanteric — *see* Bursitis, hip, trochanteric
Tendon — *see* condition
Tendosynovitis — *see* Tenosynovitis
Tenesmus (rectal) R19.8
- vesical R30.1
Tennis elbow — *see* Epicondylitis, lateral
Tenonitis — *see also* Tenosynovitis
- eye (capsule) H05.04-
Tenontosynovitis — *see* Tenosynovitis
Tenontothecitis — *see* Tenosynovitis
Tenophyte — *see* Disorder, synovium, specified type NEC
Tenosynovitis (*see also* Synovitis) M65.9
- adhesive — *see* Tenosynovitis, specified type NEC
  - shoulder — *see* Capsulitis, adhesive
- bicipital (calcifying) — *see* Tendinitis, bicipital
- gonococcal A54.49
- in (due to)
  - crystals M65.8-
  - gonorrhea A54.49
  - syphilis (late) A52.78
  - use, overuse, pressure — *see also* Disorder, soft tissue, due to use
    - specified NEC — *see* Disorder, soft tissue, due to use, specified NEC
- infective NEC M65.1-
  - ankle M65.17-
  - foot M65.17-
  - forearm M65.13-
  - hand M65.14-
  - lower leg M65.16-

Tenosynovitis (*see also* Synovitis) M65.9 — *continued*
- infective NEC M65.1- — *continued*
  - multiple sites M65.19
  - pelvic region M65.15-
  - shoulder region M65.11-
  - specified site NEC M65.18
  - thigh M65.15-
  - upper arm M65.12-
- radial styloid M65.4
- shoulder region M65.81-
  - adhesive — *see* Capsulitis, adhesive
- specified type NEC M65.88
  - ankle M65.87-
  - foot M65.87-
  - forearm M65.83-
  - hand M65.84-
  - lower leg M65.86-
  - multiple sites M65.89
  - pelvic region M65.85-
  - shoulder region M65.81-
  - specified site NEC M65.88
  - thigh M65.85-
  - upper arm M65.82-
- tuberculous — *see* Tuberculosis, tenosynovitis
Tenovaginitis — *see* Tenosynovitis
Tension
- arterial, high — *see also* Hypertension
  - without diagnosis of hypertension R03.0
- headache G44.209
  - intractable G44.201
  - not intractable G44.209
- nervous R45.0
- pneumothorax J93.0
- premenstrual N94.3
- state (mental) F48.9
Tentorium — *see* condition
Teratencephalus Q89.8
Teratism Q89.7
Teratoblastoma (malignant) — *see* Neoplasm, malignant, by site
Teratocarcinoma — *see also* Neoplasm, malignant, by site
- liver C22.7
Teratoma (solid) — *see also* Neoplasm, uncertain behavior, by site
- with embryonal carcinoma, mixed — *see* Neoplasm, malignant, by site
- with malignant transformation — *see* Neoplasm, malignant, by site
- adult (cystic) — *see* Neoplasm, benign, by site
- benign — *see* Neoplasm, benign, by site
- combined with choriocarcinoma — *see* Neoplasm, malignant, by site
- cystic (adult) — *see* Neoplasm, benign, by site
- differentiated — *see* Neoplasm, benign, by site
- embryonal — *see also* Neoplasm, malignant, by site
  - liver C22.7
- immature — *see* Neoplasm, malignant, by site
- liver C22.7
  - adult, benign, cystic, differentiated type or mature D13.4
- malignant — *see also* Neoplasm, malignant, by site
  - anaplastic — *see* Neoplasm, malignant, by site
  - intermediate — *see* Neoplasm, malignant, by site
  - specified site — *see* Neoplasm, malignant, by site
  - unspecified site C62.90
  - undifferentiated — *see* Neoplasm, malignant, by site
- mature — *see* Neoplasm, uncertain behavior, by site
  - malignant — *see* Neoplasm, by site, malignant, by site

DISEASE INDEX

Teratoma (solid) (*see also* Neoplasm, uncertain behavior, by site) — *continued*
  ovary D27-
    embryonal, immature or malignant C56-
    solid — *see* Neoplasm, uncertain behavior, by site
  testis C62.9-
    adult, benign, cystic, differentiated type or mature D29.2-
    scrotal C62.1-
    undescended C62.0-
Termination
  anomalous — *see also* Malposition, congenital
    right pulmonary vein Q26.3
  pregnancy, elective Z33.2
Ternidens diminutus infestation B81.8
Ternidensiasis B81.8
Terror(s) night (child) F51.4
Terrorism, victim of Z65.4
Terry's syndrome H44.2-
Tertiary — *see* condition
Test, tests, testing (for)
  adequacy (for dialysis)
    hemodialysis Z49.31
    peritoneal Z49.32
  blood pressure Z01.30
    abnormal reading — *see* Blood, pressure
  blood typing Z01.83
    Rh typing Z01.83
  blood-alcohol Z04.8
    positive — *see* Findings, abnormal, in blood
  blood-drug Z04.8
    positive — *see* Findings, abnormal, in blood
  cardiac pulse generator (battery) Z45.010
  fertility Z31.41
  genetic
    disease carrier status for procreative management
      female Z31.430
      male Z31.440
    male partner of patient with recurrent pregnancy loss Z31.441
    procreative management NEC
      female Z31.438
      male Z31.448
  hearing Z01.10
    with abnormal findings NEC Z01.118
  HIV (human immunodeficiency virus)
    nonconclusive (in infants) R75
    positive Z21
    seropositive Z21
  immunity status Z01.84
  intelligence NEC Z01.89
  laboratory (as part of a general medical examination) Z00.00
    with abnormal finding Z00.01
    for medicolegal reason NEC Z04.8
  male partner of patient with recurrent pregnancy loss Z31.441
  Mantoux (for tuberculosis) Z11.1
    abnormal result R76.11
  pregnancy, positive first pregnancy — *see* Pregnancy, normal, first
  procreative Z31.49
    fertility Z31.41
  skin, diagnostic
    allergy Z01.82
      special screening examination — *see* Screening, by name of disease
    Mantoux Z11.1
    tuberculin Z11.1
    specified NEC Z01.89
    tuberculin Z11.1
      abnormal result R76.11
  vision Z01.00
    with abnormal findings Z01.01
  Wassermann Z11.3
    positive — *see* Serology for syphilis, positive

Testicle, testicular, testis — *see also* condition
  feminization syndrome (*see also* Syndrome, androgen insensitivity) E34.51
  migrans Q55.29
Tetanus, tetanic (cephalic) (convulsions) A35
  with
    abortion A34
    ectopic or molar pregnancy O08.0
  following ectopic or molar pregnancy O08.0
  inoculation reaction (due to serum) — *see* Complications, vaccination
  neonatorum A33
  obstetrical A34
  puerperal, postpartum, childbirth A34
Tetany (due to) R29.0
  alkalosis E87.3
  associated with rickets E55.0
  convulsions R29.0
    hysterical F44.5
  functional (hysterical) F44.5
  hyperkinetic R29.0
    hysterical F44.5
  hyperpnea R06.4
    hysterical F44.5
    psychogenic F45.8
  hyperventilation (*see also* Hyperventilation) R06.4
    hysterical F44.5
  neonatal (without calcium or magnesium deficiency) P71.3
  parathyroid (gland) E20.9
  parathyroprival E89.2
  post- (para)thyroidectomy E89.2
  postoperative E89.2
  pseudotetany R29.0
  psychogenic (conversion reaction) F44.5
Tetralogy of Fallot Q21.3
Tetraplegia (chronic) (*see also* Quadriplegia) G82.50
Thailand hemorrhagic fever A91
Thalassanemia — *see* Thalassemia
Thalassemia (anemia) (disease) D56.9
  with other hemoglobinopathy D56.8
  alpha (major) (severe) (triple gene defect) D56.0
    minor D56.3
    silent carrier D56.3
    trait D56.3
  beta (severe) D56.1
    homozygous D56.1
    major D56.1
    minor D56.3
    trait D56.3
  delta-beta (homozygous) D56.2
    minor D56.3
    trait D56.3
  dominant D56.8
  hemoglobin
    C D56.8
    E-beta D56.5
  intermedia D56.1
  major D56.1
  minor D56.3
  mixed D56.8
  sickle-cell — *see* Disease, sickle-cell, thalassemia
  specified type NEC D56.8
  trait D56.3
  variants D56.8
Thanatophoric dwarfism or short stature Q77.1
Thaysen-Gee disease (nontropical sprue) K90.0
Thaysen's disease K90.0
Thecoma D27-
  luteinized D27-
  malignant C56-
Thelarche, premature E30.8
Thelaziasis B83.8

Thelitis N61.0
  puerperal, postpartum or gestational — *see* Infection, nipple
Therapeutic — *see* condition
Therapy
  drug, long-term (current) (prophylactic)
    agents affecting estrogen receptors and estrogen levels NEC Z79.818
    anastrozole (Arimidex) Z79.811
    anti-inflammatory Z79.1
    antibiotics Z79.2
      short-term use — *omit code*
    anticoagulants Z79.01
    antiplatelet Z79.02
    antithrombotics Z79.02
    aromatase inhibitors Z79.811
    aspirin Z79.82
    birth control pill or patch Z79.3
    bisphosphonates Z79.83
    contraceptive, oral Z79.3
    drug, specified NEC Z79.899
    estrogen receptor downregulators Z79.818
    Evista Z79.810
    exemestane (Aromasin) Z79.811
    Fareston Z79.810
    fulvestrant (Faslodex) Z79.818
    gonadotropin-releasing hormone (GnRH) agonist Z79.818
    goserelin acetate (Zoladex) Z79.818
    hormone replacement (postmenopausal) Z79.890
    insulin Z79.4
    letrozole (Femara) Z79.811
    leuprolide acetate (leuprorelin) (Lupron) Z79.818
    megestrol acetate (Megace) Z79.818
    methadone
      for pain management Z79.891
      maintenance therapy F11.20
    Nolvadex Z79.810
    opiate analgesic Z79.891
    oral contraceptive Z79.3
    raloxifene (Evista) Z79.810
    selective estrogen receptor modulators (SERMs) Z79.810
    short term — *omit code*
    steroids
      inhaled Z79.51
      systemic Z79.52
    tamoxifen (Nolvadex) Z79.810
    toremifene (Fareston) Z79.810
Thermic — *see* condition
Thermography (abnormal) (*see also* Abnormal, diagnostic imaging) R93.8
  breast R92.8
Thermoplegia T67.0
Thesaurismosis, glycogen — *see* Disease, glycogen storage
Thiamin deficiency E51.9
  specified NEC E51.8
Thiaminic deficiency with beriberi E51.11
Thibierge-Weissenbach syndrome — *see* Sclerosis, systemic
Thickening
  bone — *see* Hypertrophy, bone
  breast N64.59
  endometrium R93.8
  epidermal L85.9
    specified NEC L85.8
  hymen N89.6
  larynx J38.7
  nail L60.2
    congenital Q84.5
  periosteal — *see* Hypertrophy, bone
  pleura J92.9
    with asbestos J92.0
  skin R23.4
  subepiglottic J38.7
  tongue K14.8

Thickening — *continued*
  valve, heart — *see* Endocarditis
Thigh — *see* condition
Thinning vertebra — *see* Spondylopathy,
    specified NEC
Thirst, excessive R63.1
  due to deprivation of water T73.1
Thomsen disease G71.12
Thoracic — *see also* condition
  kidney Q63.2
  outlet syndrome G54.0
Thoracogastroschisis (congenital) Q79.8
Thoracopagus Q89.4
Thorax — *see* condition
Thorn's syndrome N28.89
Thorson-Björck syndrome E34.0
Threadworm (infection) (infestation) B80
Threatened
  abortion O20.0
    with subsequent abortion O03.9
  job loss, anxiety concerning Z56.2
  labor (without delivery) O47.9
    at or after 37 completed weeks of gestation
      O47.1
    before 37 completed weeks of gestation
      O47.0-
  loss of job, anxiety concerning Z56.2
  miscarriage O20.0
  unemployment, anxiety concerning Z56.2
Three-day fever A93.1
Threshers' lung J67.0
Thrix annulata (congenital) Q84.1
Throat — *see* condition
Thrombasthenia (Glanzmann) (hemorrhagic)
    (hereditary) D69.1
Thromboangiitis I73.1
  obliterans (general) I73.1
    cerebral I67.89
    vessels
      brain I67.89
      spinal cord I67.89
Thromboarteritis — *see* Arteritis
Thromboasthenia (Glanzmann)
    (hemorrhagic) (hereditary) D69.1
Thrombocytasthenia (Glanzmann) D69.1
Thrombocythemia (essential) (hemorrhagic)
    (idiopathic) (primary) D47.3
Thrombocytopathy (dystrophic)
    (granulopenic) D69.1
Thrombocytopenia, thrombocytopenic
    D69.6
  with absent radius (TAR) Q87.2
  congenital D69.42
  dilutional D69.59
  due to
    drugs D69.59
    extracorporeal circulation of blood D69.59
    (massive) blood transfusion D69.59
    platelet alloimmunization D69.59
  essential D69.3
  heparin induced (HIT) D75.82
  hereditary D69.42
  idiopathic D69.3
  neonatal, transitory P61.0
    due to
      exchange transfusion P61.0
      idiopathic maternal thrombocytopenia
        P61.0
      isoimmunization P61.0
  primary NEC D69.49
    idiopathic D69.3
  puerperal, postpartum O72.3
  secondary D69.59
  transient neonatal P61.0
Thrombocytosis, essential D47.3
  primary D47.3
Thromboembolism — *see* Embolism

Thrombopathy (Bernard-Soulier) D69.1
  constitutional D68.0
  Willebrand-Jurgens D68.0
Thrombopenia — *see* Thrombocytopenia
Thrombophilia D68.59
  primary NEC D68.59
  secondary NEC D68.69
  specified NEC D68.69
Thrombophlebitis I80.9
  antepartum O22.2-
    deep O22.3-
    superficial O22.2-
  cavernous (venous) sinus G08
    complicating pregnancy O22.5-
    nonpyogenic I67.6
  cerebral (sinus) (vein) G08
    nonpyogenic I67.6
    sequelae G09
  due to implanted device — *see* Complications,
    by site and type, specified NEC
  during or resulting from a procedure NEC
    T81.72
  femoral vein (superficial) I80.1-
  femoropopliteal vein I80.0-
  hepatic (vein) I80.8
  idiopathic, recurrent I82.1
  iliofemoral I80.1-
  intracranial venous sinus (any) G08
    nonpyogenic I67.6
    sequelae G09
  intraspinal venous sinuses and veins G08
    nonpyogenic G95.19
  lateral (venous) sinus G08
    nonpyogenic I67.6
  leg I80.299
    superficial I80.0-
  longitudinal (venous) sinus G08
    nonpyogenic I67.6
  lower extremity I80.299
  migrans, migrating I82.1
  pelvic
    with ectopic or molar pregnancy O08.0
    following ectopic or molar pregnancy O08.0
    puerperal O87.1
  popliteal vein — *see* Phlebitis, leg, deep,
    popliteal
  portal (vein) K75.1
  postoperative T81.72
  pregnancy — *see* Thrombophlebitis,
    antepartum
  puerperal, postpartum, childbirth O87.0
    deep O87.1
    pelvic O87.1
    septic O86.81
    superficial O87.0
  saphenous (greater) (lesser) I80.0-
  sinus (intracranial) G08
    nonpyogenic I67.6
  specified site NEC I80.8
  tibial vein I80.23-
Thrombosis, thrombotic (bland) (multiple)
    (progressive) (silent) (vessel) I82.90
  anal K64.5
  antepartum — *see* Thrombophlebitis,
    antepartum
  aorta, aortic I74.10
    abdominal I74.09
      saddle I74.01
    bifurcation I74.09
    saddle I74.09
    specified site NEC I74.19
    terminal I74.09
    thoracic I74.11
    valve — *see* Endocarditis, aortic
  apoplexy I63.3-
  artery, arteries (postinfectional) I74.9
    auditory, internal — *see* Occlusion, artery,
      precerebral, specified NEC
    basilar — *see* Occlusion, artery, basilar

Thrombosis, thrombotic (bland) (multiple)
    (progressive) (silent) (vessel) I82.90 —
    continued
  artery, arteries (postinfectional) I74.9 —
    continued
    carotid (common) (internal) — *see* Occlusion,
      artery, carotid
    cerebellar (anterior inferior) (posterior
      inferior) (superior) — *see* Occlusion,
      artery, cerebellar
    cerebral — *see* Occlusion, artery, cerebral
    choroidal (anterior) — *see* Occlusion, artery,
      cerebral, specified NEC
    communicating, posterior — *see* Occlusion,
      artery, cerebral, specified NEC
    coronary — *see also* Infarct, myocardium
      not resulting in infarction I24.0
    hepatic I74.8
    hypophyseal — *see* Occlusion, artery,
      cerebral, specified NEC
    iliac I74.5
    limb I74.4
      lower I74.3
      upper I74.2
    meningeal, anterior or posterior — *see*
      Occlusion, artery, cerebral, specified
      NEC
    mesenteric (with gangrene) (*see also* Infarct,
      intestine) K55.069
    ophthalmic — *see* Occlusion, artery, retina
    pontine — *see* Occlusion, artery, cerebral,
      specified NEC
    precerebral — *see* Occlusion, artery,
      precerebral
    pulmonary (iatrogenic) — *see* Embolism,
      pulmonary
    renal N28.0
    retinal — *see* Occlusion, artery, retina
    spinal, anterior or posterior G95.11
    traumatic NEC T14.8
    vertebral — *see* Occlusion, artery, vertebral
  atrium, auricular — *see also* Infarct,
    myocardium
    following acute myocardial infarction
      (current complication) I23.6
    not resulting in infarction I51.3
  basilar (artery) — *see* Occlusion, artery,
    basilar
  brain (artery) (stem) — *see also* Occlusion,
    artery, cerebral
    due to syphilis A52.05
    puerperal O99.43
    sinus — *see* Thrombosis, intracranial venous
      sinus
  capillary I78.8
  cardiac — *see also* Infarct, myocardium
    not resulting in infarction I51.3
    valve — *see* Endocarditis
  carotid (artery) (common) (internal) — *see*
    Occlusion, artery, carotid
  cavernous (venous) sinus — *see* Thrombosis,
    intracranial venous sinus
  cerebellar artery (anterior inferior) (posterior
    inferior) (superior) I66.3
  cerebral (artery) — *see* Occlusion, artery,
    cerebral
  cerebrovenous sinus — *see also* Thrombosis,
    intracranial venous sinus
    puerperium O87.3
  chronic I82.91
  coronary (artery) (vein) — *see also* Infarct,
    myocardium
    not resulting in infarction I24.0
  corpus cavernosum N48.89
  cortical I66.9
  deep — *see* Embolism, vein, lower extremity

Thrombosis, thrombotic (bland) (multiple) (progressive) (silent) (vessel) I82.90 — *continued*
　due to device, implant or graft (*see also* Complications, by site and type, specified NEC) T85.868
　　arterial graft NEC T82.868
　　breast (implant) T85.868
　　catheter NEC T85.868
　　　dialysis (renal) T82.868
　　　　intraperitoneal T85.868
　　　infusion NEC T82.868
　　　　spinal (epidural) (subdural) T85.860
　　　urinary (indwelling) T83.86
　　electronic (electrode) (pulse generator) (stimulator)
　　　bone T84.86
　　　cardiac T82.867
　　　nervous system (brain) (peripheral nerve) (spinal) T85.860
　　　urinary T83.86
　　fixation, internal (orthopedic) NEC T84.86
　　gastrointestinal (bile duct) (esophagus) T85.868
　　genital NEC T83.86
　　heart T82.867
　　joint prosthesis T84.86
　　ocular (corneal graft) (orbital implant) NEC T85.868
　　orthopedic NEC T84.868
　　specified NEC T85.868
　　urinary NEC T83.86
　　vascular NEC T82.868
　　ventricular intracranial shunt T85.860
　during the puerperium — *see* Thrombosis, puerperal
　endocardial — *see also* Infarct, myocardium
　　not resulting in infarction I51.3
　eye — *see* Occlusion, retina
　genital organ
　　female NEC N94.89
　　　pregnancy — *see* Thrombophlebitis, antepartum
　　male N50.1
　gestational — *see* Phlebopathy, gestational
　heart (chamber) — *see also* Infarct, myocardium
　　not resulting in infarction I51.3
　hepatic (vein) I82.0
　　artery I74.8
　history (of) Z86.718
　intestine (with gangrene) (*see also* Infarct, intestine) K55.069
　intracardiac NEC (apical) (atrial) (auricular) (ventricular) (old) I51.3
　intracranial (arterial) I66.9
　　venous sinus (any) G08
　　　nonpyogenic origin I67.6
　　　puerperium O87.3
　intramural — *see also* Infarct, myocardium
　　not resulting in infarction I51.3
　intraspinal venous sinuses and veins G08
　　nonpyogenic G95.19
　kidney (artery) N28.0
　lateral (venous) sinus — *see* Thrombosis, intracranial venous sinus
　leg — *see* Thrombosis, vein, lower extremity
　　arterial I74.3
　liver (venous) I82.0
　　artery I74.8
　　portal vein I81
　longitudinal (venous) sinus — *see* Thrombosis, intracranial venous sinus
　lower limb — *see* Thrombosis, vein, lower extremity
　lung (iatrogenic) (postoperative) — *see* Embolism, pulmonary
　meninges (brain) (arterial) I66.8

Thrombosis, thrombotic (bland) (multiple) (progressive) (silent) (vessel) I82.90 — *continued*
　mesenteric (artery) (with gangrene) (*see also* Infarct, intestine) K55.069
　　vein (inferior) (superior) I81
　mitral I34.8
　mural — *see also* Infarct, myocardium
　　due to syphilis A52.06
　　not resulting in infarction I51.3
　omentum (with gangrene) (*see also* Infarct, intestine) K55.069
　ophthalmic — *see* Occlusion, retina
　pampiniform plexus (male) N50.1
　parietal — *see also* Infarct, myocardium
　　not resulting in infarction I24.0
　penis, superficial vein N48.81
　perianal venous K64.5
　peripheral arteries I74.4
　　upper I74.2
　personal history (of) Z86.718
　portal I81
　　due to syphilis A52.09
　precerebral artery — *see* Occlusion, artery, precerebral
　puerperal, postpartum O87.0
　　brain (artery) O99.43
　　　venous (sinus) O87.3
　　cardiac O99.43
　　cerebral (artery) O99.43
　　　venous (sinus) O87.3
　　superficial O87.0
　pulmonary (artery) (iatrogenic) (postoperative) (vein) — *see* Embolism, pulmonary
　renal (artery) N28.0
　　vein I82.3
　resulting from presence of device, implant or graft — *see* Complications, by site and type, specified NEC
　retina, retinal — *see* Occlusion, retina
　scrotum N50.1
　seminal vesicle N50.1
　sigmoid (venous) sinus — *see* Thrombosis, intracranial venous sinus
　sinus, intracranial (any) — *see* Thrombosis, intracranial venous sinus
　specified site NEC I82.890
　　chronic I82.891
　spermatic cord N50.1
　spinal cord (arterial) G95.11
　　due to syphilis A52.09
　　pyogenic origin G06.1
　spleen, splenic D73.5
　　artery I74.8
　testis N50.1
　traumatic NEC T14.8
　tricuspid I07.8
　tumor — *see* Neoplasm, unspecified behavior, by site
　tunica vaginalis N50.1
　umbilical cord (vessels), complicating delivery O69.5
　vas deferens N50.1
　vein (acute) I82.90
　　antecubital I82.61-
　　　chronic I82.71-
　　axillary I82.A1- *(follows I82.7)*
　　　chronic I82.A2- *(follows I82.7)*
　　basilic I82.61-
　　　chronic I82.71-
　　brachial I82.62-
　　　chronic I82.72-
　　brachiocephalic (innominate) I82.290
　　　chronic I82.291
　　cephalic I82.61-
　　　chronic I82.71-
　　cerebral, nonpyogenic I67.6
　　chronic I82.91

Thrombosis, thrombotic (bland) (multiple) (progressive) (silent) (vessel) I82.90 — *continued*
　vein (acute) I82.90 — *continued*
　　deep (DVT) I82.40-
　　　calf I82.4Z- *(follows I82.49)*
　　　　chronic I82.5Z- *(follows I82.59)*
　　　lower leg I82.4Z- *(follows I82.49)*
　　　　chronic I82.5Z- *(follows I82.59)*
　　　thigh I82.4Y- *(follows I82.49)*
　　　　chronic I82.5Y- *(follows I82.59)*
　　　upper leg I82.4Y- *(follows I82.49)*
　　　　chronic I82.5Y- *(follows I82.59)*
　　femoral I82.41-
　　　chronic I82.51-
　　iliac (iliofemoral) I82.42-
　　　chronic I82.52-
　　innominate I82.290
　　　chronic I82.291
　　internal jugular I82.C1- *(follows I82.7)*
　　　chronic I82.C2- *(follows I82.7)*
　　lower extremity
　　　deep I82.40-
　　　　chronic I82.50-
　　　　specified NEC I82.49-
　　　　　chronic NEC I82.59-
　　　distal
　　　　deep I82.4Z- *(follows I82.49)*
　　　proximal
　　　　deep I82.4Y- *(follows I82.49)*
　　　　　chronic I82.5Y- *(follows I82.59)*
　　　superficial I82.81-
　　perianal K64.5
　　popliteal I82.43-
　　　chronic I82.53-
　　radial I82.62-
　　　chronic I82.72-
　　renal I82.3
　　saphenous (greater) (lesser) I82.81-
　　specified NEC I82.890
　　　chronic NEC I82.891
　　subclavian I82.B1- *(follows I82.7)*
　　　chronic I82.B2- *(follows I82.7)*
　　thoracic NEC I82.290
　　　chronic I82.291
　　tibial I82.44-
　　　chronic I82.54-
　　ulnar I82.62-
　　　chronic I82.72-
　　upper extremity I82.60-
　　　chronic I82.70-
　　　deep I82.62-
　　　　chronic I82.72-
　　　superficial I82.61-
　　　　chronic I82.71-
　vena cava
　　inferior I82.220
　　　chronic I82.221
　　superior I82.210
　　　chronic I82.211
　ventricle — *see also* Infarct, myocardium
　　following acute myocardial infarction (current complication) I23.6
　　not resulting in infarction I24.0
　venous, perianal K64.5
Thrombus — *see* Thrombosis
Thrush — *see also* Candidiasis
　newborn P37.5
　oral B37.0
　vaginal B37.3
Thumb — *see also* condition
　sucking (child problem) F98.8
Thymitis E32.8
Thymoma (benign) D15.0
　malignant C37
Thymus, thymic (gland) — *see* condition
Thyrocele — *see* Goiter

Thyroglossal — *see also* condition
  cyst Q89.2
  duct, persistent Q89.2
Thyroid (gland) (body) — *see also* condition
  hormone resistance E07.89
  lingual Q89.2
  nodule (cystic) (nontoxic) (single) E04.1
Thyroiditis E06.9
  acute (nonsuppurative) (pyogenic)
      (suppurative) E06.0
  autoimmune E06.3
  chronic (nonspecific) (sclerosing) E06.5
      with thyrotoxicosis, transient E06.2
    fibrous E06.5
    lymphadenoid E06.3
    lymphocytic E06.3
    lymphoid E06.3
  de Quervain's E06.1
  drug-induced E06.4
  fibrous (chronic) E06.5
  giant-cell (follicular) E06.1
  granulomatous (de Quervain) (subacute)
      E06.1
  Hashimoto's (struma lymphomatosa) E06.3
  iatrogenic E06.4
  ligneous E06.5
  lymphocytic (chronic) E06.3
  lymphoid E06.3
  lymphomatous E06.3
  nonsuppurative E06.1
  postpartum, puerperal O90.5
  pseudotuberculous E06.1
  pyogenic E06.0
  radiation E06.4
  Riedel's E06.5
  subacute (granulomatous) E06.1
  suppurative E06.0
  tuberculous A18.81
  viral E06.1
  woody E06.5
Thyrolingual duct, persistent Q89.2
Thyromegaly E01.0
Thyrotoxic
  crisis — *see* Thyrotoxicosis
  heart disease or failure (*see also* Thyrotoxicosis)
      E05.90 [*I43*]
      with thyroid storm E05.91 [*I43*]
  storm — *see* Thyrotoxicosis
Thyrotoxicosis (recurrent) E05.90
  with
    goiter (diffuse) E05.00
      with thyroid storm E05.01
      adenomatous uninodular E05.10
        with thyroid storm E05.11
      multinodular E05.20
        with thyroid storm E05.21
      nodular E05.20
        with thyroid storm E05.21
      uninodular E05.10
        with thyroid storm E05.11
    infiltrative
      dermopathy E05.00
        with thyroid storm E05.01
      ophthalmopathy E05.00
        with thyroid storm E05.01
    single thyroid nodule E05.10
      with thyroid storm E05.11
  due to
    ectopic thyroid nodule or tissue E05.30
      with thyroid storm E05.31
    ingestion of (excessive) thyroid material
        E05.40
      with thyroid storm E05.41
    overproduction of thyroid-stimulating
        hormone E05.80
      with thyroid storm E05.81
    specified cause NEC E05.80
      with thyroid storm E05.81

Thyrotoxicosis (recurrent) E05.90 —
    continued
  factitia E05.40
    with thyroid storm E05.41
  heart E05.90 [*I43*]
    with thyroid storm E05.91 [*I43*]
    failure E05.90 [*I43*]
  neonatal (transient) P72.1
  transient with chronic thyroiditis E06.2
Tibia vara — *see* Osteochondrosis, juvenile,
    tibia
Tic (disorder) F95.9
  breathing F95.8
  child problem F95.0
  compulsive F95.1
  de la Tourette F95.2
  degenerative (generalized) (localized) G25.69
    facial G25.69
  disorder
    chronic
      motor F95.1
      vocal F95.1
      combined vocal and multiple motor F95.2
    transient F95.0
  douloureux G50.0
    atypical G50.1
    postherpetic, postzoster B02.22
  drug-induced G25.61
  eyelid F95.8
  habit F95.9
    chronic F95.1
    transient of childhood F95.0
  lid, transient of childhood F95.0
  motor-verbal F95.2
  occupational F48.8
  orbicularis F95.8
    transient of childhood F95.0
  organic origin G25.69
  postchoreic G25.69
  provisional F95.0
  psychogenic, compulsive F95.1
  salaam R25.8
  spasm (motor or vocal) F95.9
    chronic F95.1
    transient of childhood F95.0
  specified NEC F95.8
Tick-borne — *see* condition
Tietze's disease or syndrome M94.0
Tight, tightness
  anus K62.89
  chest R07.89
  fascia (lata) M62.89
  foreskin (congenital) N47.1
  hymen, hymenal ring N89.6
  introitus (acquired) (congenital) N89.6
  rectal sphincter K62.89
  tendon — *see* Short, tendon
  urethral sphincter N35.9
Tilting vertebra — *see* Dorsopathy,
    deforming, specified NEC
Timidity, child F93.8
Tin-miner's lung J63.5
Tinea (intersecta) (tarsi) B35.9
  amiantacea L44.8
  asbestina B35.0
  barbae B35.0
  beard B35.0
  black dot B35.0
  blanca B36.2
  capitis B35.0
  corporis B35.4
  cruris B35.6
  flava B36.0
  foot B35.3
  furfuracea B36.0
  imbricata (Tokelau) B35.5
  kerion B35.0
  manuum B35.2
  microsporic — *see* Dermatophytosis

Tinea (intersecta) (tarsi) B35.9 — *continued*
  nigra B36.1
  nodosa — *see* Piedra
  pedis B35.3
  scalp B35.0
  specified site NEC B35.8
  sycosis B35.0
  tonsurans B35.0
  trichophytic — *see* Dermatophytosis
  unguium B35.1
  versicolor B36.0
Tingling sensation (skin) R20.2
Tinnitus NOS H93.1-
  audible H93.1-
  aurium H93.1-
  pulsatile H93.A- *(follows H93.1)*
  subjective H93.1-
Tipped tooth (teeth) M26.33
Tipping
  pelvis M95.5
    with disproportion (fetopelvic) O33.0
      causing obstructed labor O65.0
  tooth (teeth), fully erupted M26.33
Tiredness R53.83
Tissue — *see* condition
Tobacco (nicotine)
  abuse — *see* Tobacco, use
  dependence — *see* Dependence, drug, nicotine
  harmful use Z72.0
  heart — *see* Tobacco, toxic effect
  maternal use, affecting newborn P04.2
  toxic effect — *see* Table of Drugs and
      Chemicals, by substance, poisoning
    chewing tobacco — *see* Table of Drugs and
        Chemicals, by substance, poisoning
    cigarettes — *see* Table of Drugs and
        Chemicals, by substance, poisoning
  use Z72.0
    complicating
      childbirth O99.334
      pregnancy O99.33-
      puerperium O99.335
    counseling and surveillance Z71.6
    history Z87.891
  withdrawal state (*see also* Dependence, drug,
      nicotine) F17.203
Tocopherol deficiency E56.0
Todd's
  cirrhosis K74.3
  paralysis (postepileptic) (transitory) G83.84
Toe — *see* condition
Toilet, artificial opening — *see* Attention to,
    artificial, opening
Tokelau (ringworm) B35.5
Tollwut — *see* Rabies
Tommaselli's disease R31.9
  correct substance properly administered — *see*
      Table of Drugs and Chemicals, by drug,
      adverse effect
  overdose or wrong substance given or taken
      — *see* Table of Drugs and Chemicals, by
      drug, poisoning
Tongue — *see also* condition
  tie Q38.1
Tonic pupil — *see* Anomaly, pupil, function,
    tonic pupil
Toni-Fanconi syndrome (cystinosis) E72.09
  with cystinosis E72.04
Tonsil — *see* condition

Tonsillitis (acute) (catarrhal) (croupous) (follicular) (gangrenous) (infective) (lacunar) (lingual) (malignant) (membranous) (parenchymatous) (phlegmonous) (pseudomembranous) (purulent) (septic) (subacute) (suppurative) (toxic) (ulcerative) (vesicular) (viral) J03.90
  chronic J35.01
    with adenoiditis J35.03
  diphtheritic A36.0
  hypertrophic J35.01
    with adenoiditis J35.03
  recurrent J03.91
  specified organism NEC J03.80
    recurrent J03.81
  staphylococcal J03.80
    recurrent J03.81
  streptococcal J03.00
    recurrent J03.01
  tuberculous A15.8
  Vincent's A69.1
Tooth, teeth — *see* condition
Toothache K08.89
Topagnosis R20.8
Tophi — *see* Gout, chronic
TORCH infection — *see* Infection, congenital without active infection P00.2
Torn — *see* Tear
Tornwaldt's cyst or disease J39.2
Torsion
  accessory tube — *see* Torsion, fallopian tube
  adnexa (female) — *see* Torsion, fallopian tube
  aorta, acquired I77.1
  appendix epididymis N44.04
  appendix testis N44.03
  bile duct (common) (hepatic) K83.8
    congenital Q44.5
  bowel, colon or intestine K56.2
  cervix — *see* Malposition, uterus
  cystic duct K82.8
  dystonia — *see* Dystonia, torsion
  epididymis (appendix) N44.04
  fallopian tube N83.52-
    with ovary N83.53
  gallbladder K82.8
    congenital Q44.1
  hydatid of Morgagni
    female N83.52-
    male N44.03
  kidney (pedicle) (leading to infarction) N28.0
  Meckel's diverticulum (congenital) Q43.0
    malignant — *see* Table of Neoplasms, small intestine, malignant
  mesentery K56.2
  omentum K56.2
  organ or site, congenital NEC — *see* Anomaly, by site
  ovary (pedicle) N83.51-
    with fallopian tube N83.53
    congenital Q50.2
  oviduct — *see* Torsion, fallopian tube
  penis (acquired) N48.82
    congenital Q55.69
  spasm — *see* Dystonia, torsion
  spermatic cord N44.02
    extravaginal N44.01
    intravaginal N44.02
  spleen D73.5
  testis, testicle N44.00
    appendix N44.03
  tibia — *see* Deformity, limb, specified type NEC, lower leg
  uterus — *see* Malposition, uterus
Torticollis (intermittent) (spastic) M43.6
  congenital (sternomastoid) Q68.0
  due to birth injury P15.8
  hysterical F44.4
  ocular R29.891

Torticollis (intermittent) (spastic) M43.6 — *continued*
  psychogenic F45.8
    conversion reaction F44.4
  rheumatic M43.6
  rheumatoid M06.88
  spasmodic G24.3
  traumatic, current S13.4
Tortipelvis G24.1
Tortuous
  aortic arch Q25.46
  artery I77.1
  organ or site, congenital NEC — *see* Distortion
  retinal vessel, congenital Q14.1
  ureter N13.8
  urethra N36.8
  vein — *see* Varix
Torture, victim of Z65.4
Torula, torular (histolytica) (infection) — *see* Cryptococcosis
Torulosis — *see* Cryptococcosis
Torus (mandibularis) (palatinus) M27.0
  fracture — *see* Fracture, by site, torus
Touraine's syndrome Q79.8
Tourette's syndrome F95.2
Tourniquet syndrome — *see* Constriction, external, by site
Tower skull Q75.0
  with exophthalmos Q87.0
Toxemia R68.89
  bacterial — *see* Sepsis
  burn — *see* Burn
  eclamptic (with pre-existing hypertension) — *see* Eclampsia
  erysipelatous — *see* Erysipelas
  fatigue R68.89
  food — *see* Poisoning, food
  gastrointestinal K52.1
  intestinal K52.1
  kidney — *see* Uremia
  malarial — *see* Malaria
  myocardial — *see* Myocarditis, toxic
  of pregnancy — *see* Pre-eclampsia
  pre-eclamptic — *see* Pre-eclampsia
  small intestine K52.1
  staphylococcal, due to food A05.0
  stasis R68.89
  uremic — *see* Uremia
  urinary — *see* Uremia
Toxemica cerebropathia psychica (nonalcoholic) F04
  alcoholic — *see* Alcohol, amnestic disorder
Toxic (poisoning) (*see also* condition) T65.91
  effect — *see* Table of Drugs and Chemicals, by substance, poisoning
  shock syndrome A48.3
  thyroid (gland) — *see* Thyrotoxicosis
Toxicemia — *see* Toxemia
Toxicity — *see* Table of Drugs and Chemicals, by substance, poisoning
  fava bean D55.0
  food, noxious — *see* Poisoning, food
  from drug or nonmedicinal substance — *see* Table of Drugs and Chemicals, by drug
Toxicosis — *see also* Toxemia
  capillary, hemorrhagic D69.0
Toxinfection, gastrointestinal K52.1
Toxocariasis B83.0
Toxoplasma, toxoplasmosis (acquired) B58.9
  with
    hepatitis B58.1
    meningoencephalitis B58.2
    ocular involvement B58.00
    other organ involvement B58.89
    pneumonia, pneumonitis B58.3
  congenital (acute) (subacute) (chronic) P37.1
  maternal, manifest toxoplasmosis in infant (acute) (subacute) (chronic) P37.1

tPA (rtPA) administration in a different facility within the last 24 hours prior to admission to current facility Z92.82
Trabeculation, bladder N32.89
Trachea — *see* condition
Tracheitis (catarrhal) (infantile) (membranous) (plastic) (septal) (suppurative) (viral) J04.10
  with
    bronchitis (15 years of age and above) J40
      acute or subacute — *see* Bronchitis, acute
      chronic J42
      tuberculous NEC A15.5
      under 15 years of age J20.9
    laryngitis (acute) J04.2
      chronic J37.1
      tuberculous NEC A15.5
  acute J04.10
    with obstruction J04.11
  chronic J42
    with
      bronchitis (chronic) J42
      laryngitis (chronic) J37.1
  diphtheritic (membranous) A36.89
  due to external agent — *see* Inflammation, respiratory, upper, due to
  syphilitic A52.73
  tuberculous A15.5
Trachelitis (nonvenereal) — *see* Cervicitis
Tracheobronchial — *see* condition
Tracheobronchitis (15 years of age and above) — *see also* Bronchitis
  due to
    Bordetella bronchiseptica A37.80
      with pneumonia A37.81
    Francisella tularensis A21.8
Tracheobronchomegaly Q32.4
  with bronchiectasis J47.9
    with
      exacerbation (acute) J47.1
      lower respiratory infection J47.0
  acquired J98.09
    with bronchiectasis J47.9
      with
        exacerbation (acute) J47.1
        lower respiratory infection J47.0
Tracheobronchopneumonitis — *see* Pneumonia, broncho-
Tracheocele (external) (internal) J39.8
  congenital Q32.1
Tracheomalacia J39.8
  congenital Q32.0
Tracheopharyngitis (acute) J06.9
  chronic J42
  due to external agent — *see* Inflammation, respiratory, upper, due to
Tracheostenosis J39.8
Tracheostomy
  complication — *see* Complication, tracheostomy
  status Z93.0
    attention to Z43.0
    malfunctioning J95.03
Trachoma, trachomatous A71.9
  active (stage) A71.1
  contraction of conjunctiva A71.1
  dubium A71.0
  healed or sequelae B94.0
  initial (stage) A71.0
  pannus A71.1
  Türck's J37.0
Traction, vitreomacular H43.82-
Train sickness T75.3
Trait(s)
  Hb-S D57.3
  hemoglobin
    abnormal NEC D58.2
      with thalassemia D56.3
    C — *see* Disease, hemoglobin C
    S (Hb-S) D57.3

DISEASE INDEX

Trait(s) — *continued*
Lepore D56.3
personality, accentuated Z73.1
sickle-cell D57.3
  with elliptocytosis or spherocytosis D57.3
type A personality Z73.1
Tramp Z59.0
Trance R41.89
hysterical F44.89
Transaminasemia R74.0
Transection
abdomen (partial) S38.3
aorta (incomplete) — *see also* Injury, aorta
  complete — *see* Injury, aorta, laceration, major
carotid artery (incomplete) — *see also* Injury, blood vessel, carotid, laceration
  complete — *see* Injury, blood vessel, carotid, laceration, major
celiac artery (incomplete) S35.211
  branch (incomplete) S35.291
    complete S35.292
  complete S35.212
innominate
  artery (incomplete) — *see also* Injury, blood vessel, thoracic, innominate, artery, laceration
    complete — *see* Injury, blood vessel, thoracic, innominate, artery, laceration, major
  vein (incomplete) — *see also* Injury, blood vessel, thoracic, innominate, vein, laceration
    complete — *see* Injury, blood vessel, thoracic, innominate, vein, laceration, major
jugular vein (external) (incomplete) — *see also* Injury, blood vessel, jugular vein, laceration
  complete — *see* Injury, blood vessel, jugular vein, laceration, major
  internal (incomplete) — *see also* Injury, blood vessel, jugular vein, internal, laceration
    complete — *see* Injury, blood vessel, jugular vein, internal, laceration, major
mesenteric artery (incomplete) — *see also* Injury, mesenteric, artery, laceration
  complete — *see* Injury, mesenteric artery, laceration, major
pulmonary vessel (incomplete) — *see also* Injury, blood vessel, thoracic, pulmonary, laceration
  complete — *see* Injury, blood vessel, thoracic, pulmonary, laceration, major
subclavian — *see* Transection, innominate
vena cava (incomplete) — *see also* Injury, vena cava
  complete — *see* Injury, vena cava, laceration, major
vertebral artery (incomplete) — *see also* Injury, blood vessel, vertebral, laceration
  complete — *see* Injury, blood vessel, vertebral, laceration, major
Transfusion
associated (red blood cell) hemochromatosis E83.111
blood
  ABO incompatible — *see* Complication(s), transfusion, incompatibility reaction, ABO
  minor blood group (Duffy) (E) (K(ell)) (Kidd) (Lewis) (M) (N) (P) (S) T80.89
  reaction or complication — *see* Complications, transfusion
fetomaternal (mother) — *see* Pregnancy, complicated by, placenta, transfusion syndrome

Transfusion — *continued*
maternofetal (mother) — *see* Pregnancy, complicated by, placenta, transfusion syndrome
placental (syndrome) (mother) — *see* Pregnancy, complicated by, placenta, transfusion syndrome
reaction (adverse) — *see* Complications, transfusion
related acute lung injury (TRALI) J95.84
twin-to-twin — *see* Pregnancy, complicated by, placenta, transfusion syndrome, fetus to fetus
Transient (meaning homeless) (*see also* condition) Z59.0
Translocation
balanced autosomal Q95.9
  in normal individual Q95.0
chromosomes NEC Q99.8
  balanced and insertion in normal individual Q95.0
Down syndrome Q90.2
trisomy
  13 Q91.6
  18 Q91.2
  21 Q90.2
Translucency, iris — *see* Degeneration, iris
Transmission of chemical substances through the placenta — *see* Absorption, chemical, through placenta
Transparency, lung, unilateral J43.0
Transplant(ed) (status) Z94.9
awaiting organ Z76.82
bone Z94.6
  marrow Z94.81
candidate Z76.82
complication — *see* Complication, transplant
cornea Z94.7
heart Z94.1
  and lung(s) Z94.3
  valve Z95.2
    prosthetic Z95.2
    specified NEC Z95.4
    xenogenic Z95.3
intestine Z94.82
kidney Z94.0
liver Z94.4
lung(s) Z94.2
  and heart Z94.3
organ (failure) (infection) (rejection) Z94.9
  removal status Z98.85
pancreas Z94.83
skin Z94.5
social Z60.3
specified organ or tissue NEC Z94.89
stem cells Z94.84
tissue Z94.9
Transplants, ovarian, endometrial N80.1
Transposed — *see* Transposition
Transposition (congenital) — *see also* Malposition, congenital
abdominal viscera Q89.3
aorta (dextra) Q20.3
appendix Q43.8
colon Q43.8
corrected Q20.5
great vessels (complete) (partial) Q20.3
heart Q24.0
  with complete transposition of viscera Q89.3
intestine (large) (small) Q43.8
reversed jejunal (for bypass) (status) Z98.0
scrotum Q55.23
stomach Q40.2
  with general transposition of viscera Q89.3
tooth, teeth, fully erupted M26.30
vessels, great (complete) (partial) Q20.3
viscera (abdominal) (thoracic) Q89.3
Transsexualism F64.0

Transverse — *see also* condition
arrest (deep), in labor O64.0
lie (mother) O32.2
  causing obstructed labor O64.8
Transvestism, transvestitism (dual-role) F64.1
fetishistic F65.1
Trapped placenta (with hemorrhage) O72.0
without hemorrhage O73.0
TRAPS (tumor necrosis factor receptor associated periodic syndrome) M04.1
Trauma, traumatism — *see also* Injury
acoustic — *see* subcategory H83.3
birth — *see* Birth, injury
complicating ectopic or molar pregnancy O08.6
during delivery O71.9
following ectopic or molar pregnancy O08.6
obstetric O71.9
  specified NEC O71.89
occlusal
  primary K08.81
  secondary K08.82
Traumatic — *see also* condition
brain injury S06.9
Treacher Collins syndrome Q75.4
Treitz's hernia — *see* Hernia, abdomen, specified site NEC
Trematode infestation — *see* Infestation, fluke
Trematodiasis — *see* Infestation, fluke
Trembling paralysis — *see* Parkinsonism
Tremor(s) R25.1
drug induced G25.1
essential (benign) G25.0
familial G25.0
hereditary G25.0
hysterical F44.4
intention G25.2
medication induced postural G25.1
mercurial — *see* subcategory T56.1
Parkinson's — *see* Parkinsonism
psychogenic (conversion reaction) F44.4
senilis R54
specified type NEC G25.2
Trench
fever A79.0
foot — *see* Immersion, foot
mouth A69.1
Treponema pallidum infection — *see* Syphilis
Treponematosis
due to
  T. pallidum — *see* Syphilis
  T. pertenue — *see* Yaws
Triad
Hutchinson's (congenital syphilis) A50.53
Kartagener's Q89.3
Saint's — *see* Hernia, diaphragm
Trichiasis (eyelid) H02.059
with entropion — *see* Entropion
left H02.056
  lower H02.055
  upper H02.054
right H02.053
  lower H02.052
  upper H02.051
Trichinella spiralis (infection) (infestation) B75
Trichinellosis, trichiniasis, trichinelliasis, trichinosis B75
with muscle disorder B75 *[M63.80]*
  ankle B75 *[M63.8-]*
  foot B75 *[M63.8-]*
  forearm B75 *[M63.8-]*
  hand B75 *[M63.8-]*
  lower leg B75 *[M63.8-]*
  multiple sites B75 *[M63.89]*
  pelvic region B75 *[M63.8-]*

Trichinellosis, trichiniasis, trichinelliasis, trichinosis B75 — *continued*
with muscle disorder B75 [M63.80] — *continued*
shoulder region B75 [M63.8-]
specified site NEC B75 [M63.88]
thigh B75 [M63.8-]
upper arm B75 [M63.8-]
Trichobezoar T18.9
intestine T18.3
stomach T18.2
Trichocephaliasis, trichocephalosis B79
Trichocephalus infestation B79
Trichoclasis L67.8
Trichoepithelioma — *see also* Neoplasm, skin, benign
malignant — *see* Neoplasm, skin, malignant
Trichofolliculoma — *see* Neoplasm, skin, benign
Tricholemmoma — *see* Neoplasm, skin, benign
Trichomoniasis A59.9
bladder A59.03
cervix A59.09
intestinal A07.8
prostate A59.02
seminal vesicles A59.09
specified site NEC A59.8
urethra A59.03
urogenitalis A59.00
vagina A59.01
vulva A59.01
Trichomycosis
axillaris A48.8
nodosa, nodularis B36.8
Trichonodosis L67.8
Trichophytid, trichophyton infection — *see* Dermatophytosis
Trichophytobezoar T18.9
intestine T18.3
stomach T18.2
Trichophytosis — *see* Dermatophytosis
Trichoptilosis L67.8
Trichorrhexis (nodosa) (invaginata) L67.0
Trichosis axillaris A48.8
Trichosporosis nodosa B36.2
Trichostasis spinulosa (congenital) Q84.1
Trichostrongyliasis, trichostrongylosis (small intestine) B81.2
Trichostrongylus infection B81.2
Trichotillomania F63.3
Trichromat, trichromatopsia, anomalous (congenital) H53.55
Trichuriasis B79
Trichuris trichiura (infection) (infestation) (any site) B79
Tricuspid (valve) — *see* condition
Trifid — *see also* Accessory
kidney (pelvis) Q63.8
tongue Q38.3
Trigeminal neuralgia — *see* Neuralgia, trigeminal
Trigeminy R00.8
Trigger finger (acquired) M65.30
congenital Q74.0
index finger M65.32-
little finger M65.35-
middle finger M65.33-
ring finger M65.34-
thumb M65.31-
Trigonitis (bladder) (chronic) (pseudomembranous) N30.30
with hematuria N30.31
Trigonocephaly Q75.0
Trilocular heart — *see* Cor triloculare
Trimethylaminuria E72.52
Tripartite placenta O43.19-
Triphalangeal thumb Q74.0

Triple — *see also* Accessory
kidneys Q63.0
uteri Q51.818
X, female Q97.0
Triplegia G83.89
congenital G80.8
Triplet (newborn) — *see also* Newborn, triplet
complicating pregnancy — *see* Pregnancy, triplet
Triplication — *see* Accessory
Triploidy Q92.7
Trismus R25.2
neonatorum A33
newborn A33
Trisomy (syndrome) Q92.9
13 (partial) Q91.7
meiotic nondisjunction Q91.4
mitotic nondisjunction Q91.5
mosaicism Q91.5
translocation Q91.6
18 (partial) Q91.3
meiotic nondisjunction Q91.0
mitotic nondisjunction Q91.1
mosaicism Q91.1
translocation Q91.2
20 Q92.8
21 (partial) Q90.9
meiotic nondisjunction Q90.0
mitotic nondisjunction Q90.1
mosaicism Q90.1
translocation Q90.2
22 Q92.8
autosomes Q92.9
chromosome specified NEC Q92.8
partial Q92.2
due to unbalanced translocation Q92.5
specified NEC Q92.8
whole (nonsex chromosome)
meiotic nondisjunction Q92.0
mitotic nondisjunction Q92.1
mosaicism Q92.1
due to
dicentrics — *see* Extra, marker chromosomes
extra rings — *see* Extra, marker chromosomes
isochromosomes — *see* Extra, marker chromosomes
specified NEC Q92.8
whole chromosome Q92.9
meiotic nondisjunction Q92.0
mitotic nondisjunction Q92.1
mosaicism Q92.1
partial Q92.9
specified NEC Q92.8
Tritanomaly, tritanopia H53.55
Trombiculosis, trombiculiasis, trombidiosis B88.0
Trophedema (congenital) (hereditary) Q82.0
Trophoblastic disease (see also Mole, hydatidiform) O01.9
Tropholymphedema Q82.0
Trophoneurosis NEC G96.8
disseminated M34.9
Tropical — *see* condition
Trouble — *see also* Disease
heart — *see* Disease, heart
kidney — *see* Disease, renal
nervous R45.0
sinus — *see* Sinusitis
Trousseau's syndrome (thrombophlebitis migrans) I82.1
Truancy, childhood
from school Z72.810
Truncus
arteriosus (persistent) Q20.0
communis Q20.0
Trunk — *see* condition

Trypanosomiasis
African B56.9
by Trypanosoma brucei
gambiense B56.0
rhodesiense B56.1
American — *see* Chagas' disease
Brazilian — *see* Chagas' disease
by Trypanosoma
brucei gambiense B56.0
brucei rhodesiense B56.1
cruzi — *see* Chagas' disease
gambiensis, Gambian B56.0
rhodesiensis, Rhodesian B56.1
South American — *see* Chagas' disease
where
African trypanosomiasis is prevalent B56.9
Chagas' disease is prevalent B57.2
T-shaped incisors K00.2
Tsutsugamushi (disease) (fever) A75.3
Tube, tubal, tubular — *see* condition
Tubercle — *see also* Tuberculosis
brain, solitary A17.81
Darwin's Q17.8
Ghon, primary infection A15.7
Tuberculid, tuberculide (indurating, subcutaneous) (lichenoid) (miliary) (papulonecrotic) (primary) (skin) A18.4
Tuberculoma — *see also* Tuberculosis
brain A17.81
meninges (cerebral) (spinal) A17.1
spinal cord A17.81
Tuberculosis, tubercular, tuberculous (calcification) (calcified) (caseous) (chromogenic acid-fast bacilli) (degeneration) (fibrocaseous) (fistula) (interstitial) (isolated circumscribed lesions) (necrosis) (parenchymatous) (ulcerative) A15.9
with pneumoconiosis (any condition in J60-J64) J65
abdomen (lymph gland) A18.39
abscess (respiratory) A15.9
bone A18.03
hip A18.02
knee A18.02
sacrum A18.01
specified site NEC A18.03
spinal A18.01
vertebra A18.01
brain A17.81
breast A18.89
Cowper's gland A18.15
dura (mater) (cerebral) (spinal) A17.81
epidural (cerebral) (spinal) A17.81
female pelvis A18.17
frontal sinus A15.8
genital organs NEC A18.10
genitourinary A18.10
gland (lymphatic) — *see* Tuberculosis, lymph gland
hip A18.02
intestine A18.32
ischiorectal A18.32
joint NEC A18.02
hip A18.02
knee A18.02
specified NEC A18.02
vertebral A18.01
kidney A18.11
knee A18.02
latent R76.11
lumbar (spine) A18.01
lung — *see* Tuberculosis, pulmonary
meninges (cerebral) (spinal) A17.0
muscle A18.09
perianal (fistula) A18.32
perinephritic A18.11
perirectal A18.32
rectum A18.32

Tuberculosis, tubercular, tuberculous
(calcification) (calcified) (caseous)
(chromogenic acid-fast bacilli)
(degeneration) (fibrocaseous) (fistula)
(interstitial) (isolated circumscribed lesions)
(necrosis) (parenchymatous) (ulcerative)
A15.9 — *continued*
abscess (respiratory) A15.9 — *continued*
   retropharyngeal A15.8
   sacrum A18.01
   scrofulous A18.2
   scrotum A18.15
   skin (primary) A18.4
   spinal cord A17.81
   spine or vertebra (column) A18.01
   subdiaphragmatic A18.31
   testis A18.15
   urinary A18.13
   uterus A18.17
accessory sinus — *see* Tuberculosis, sinus
Addison's disease A18.7
adenitis — *see* Tuberculosis, lymph gland
adenoids A15.8
adenopathy — *see* Tuberculosis, lymph gland
adherent pericardium A18.84
adnexa (uteri) A18.17
adrenal (capsule) (gland) A18.7
alimentary canal A18.32
anemia A18.89
ankle (joint) (bone) A18.02
anus A18.32
apex, apical — *see* Tuberculosis, pulmonary
appendicitis, appendix A18.32
arachnoid A17.0
artery, arteritis A18.89
   cerebral A18.89
arthritis (chronic) (synovial) A18.02
   spine or vertebra (column) A18.01
articular — *see* Tuberculosis, joint
ascites A18.31
asthma — *see* Tuberculosis, pulmonary
axilla, axillary (gland) A18.2
bladder A18.12
bone A18.03
   hip A18.02
   knee A18.02
   limb NEC A18.03
   sacrum A18.01
   spine or vertebral column A18.01
bowel (miliary) A18.32
brain A17.81
breast A18.89
broad ligament A18.17
bronchi, bronchial, bronchus A15.5
   ectasia, ectasis (bronchiectasis) — *see*
      Tuberculosis, pulmonary
   fistula A15.5
      primary (progressive) A15.7
   gland or node A15.4
      primary (progressive) A15.7
   lymph gland or node A15.4
      primary (progressive) A15.7
bronchiectasis — *see* Tuberculosis, pulmonary
bronchitis A15.5
bronchopleural A15.6
bronchopneumonia, bronchopneumonic — *see*
   Tuberculosis, pulmonary
bronchorrhagia A15.5
bronchotracheal A15.5
bronze disease A18.7
buccal cavity A18.83
bulbourethral gland A18.15
bursa A18.09
cachexia A15.9
cardiomyopathy A18.84
caries — *see* Tuberculosis, bone
cartilage A18.02
   intervertebral A18.01
catarrhal — *see* Tuberculosis, respiratory

Tuberculosis, tubercular, tuberculous
(calcification) (calcified) (caseous)
(chromogenic acid-fast bacilli)
(degeneration) (fibrocaseous) (fistula)
(interstitial) (isolated circumscribed lesions)
(necrosis) (parenchymatous) (ulcerative)
A15.9 — *continued*
cecum A18.32
cellulitis (primary) A18.4
cerebellum A17.81
cerebral, cerebrum A17.81
cerebrospinal A17.81
   meninges A17.0
cervical (lymph gland or node) A18.2
cervicitis, cervix (uteri) A18.16
chest — *see* Tuberculosis, respiratory
chorioretinitis A18.53
choroid, choroiditis A18.53
ciliary body A18.54
colitis A18.32
collier's J65
colliquativa (primary) A18.4
colon A18.32
complex, primary A15.7
congenital P37.0
conjunctiva A18.59
contact Z20.1
cornea (ulcer) A18.52
Cowper's gland A18.15
coxae A18.02
coxalgia A18.02
cul-de-sac of Douglas A18.17
curvature, spine A18.01
cutis (colliquativa) (primary) A18.4
cyst, ovary A18.18
cystitis A18.12
dactylitis A18.03
diarrhea A18.32
diffuse — *see* Tuberculosis, miliary
digestive tract A18.32
disseminated — *see* Tuberculosis, miliary
duodenum A18.32
dura (mater) (cerebral) (spinal) A17.0
   abscess (cerebral) (spinal) A17.81
dysentery A18.32
ear (inner) (middle) A18.6
   bone A18.03
   external (primary) A18.4
   skin (primary) A18.4
elbow A18.02
emphysema — *see* Tuberculosis, pulmonary
empyema A15.6
encephalitis A17.82
endarteritis A18.89
endocarditis A18.84
   aortic A18.84
   mitral A18.84
   pulmonary A18.84
   tricuspid A18.84
endocrine glands NEC A18.82
endometrium A18.17
enteric, enterica, enteritis A18.32
enterocolitis A18.32
epididymis, epididymitis A18.15
epidural abscess (cerebral) (spinal) A17.81
epiglottis A15.5
episcleritis A18.51
erythema (induratum) (nodosum) (primary)
   A18.4
esophagus A18.83
eustachian tube A18.6
exposure (to) Z20.1
exudative — *see* Tuberculosis, pulmonary
eye A18.50
eyelid (primary) (lupus) A18.4
fallopian tube (acute) (chronic) A18.17
fascia A18.09
fauces A15.8

Tuberculosis, tubercular, tuberculous
(calcification) (calcified) (caseous)
(chromogenic acid-fast bacilli)
(degeneration) (fibrocaseous) (fistula)
(interstitial) (isolated circumscribed lesions)
(necrosis) (parenchymatous) (ulcerative)
A15.9 — *continued*
female pelvic inflammatory disease A18.17
finger A18.03
first infection A15.7
gallbladder A18.83
ganglion A18.09
gastritis A18.83
gastrocolic fistula A18.32
gastroenteritis A18.32
gastrointestinal tract A18.32
general, generalized — *see* Tuberculosis,
   miliary
genital organs A18.10
genitourinary A18.10
genu A18.02
glandula suprarenalis A18.7
glandular, general A18.2
glottis A15.5
grinder's J65
gum A18.83
hand A18.03
heart A18.84
hematogenous — *see* Tuberculosis, miliary
hemoptysis — *see* Tuberculosis, pulmonary
hemorrhage NEC — *see* Tuberculosis,
   pulmonary
hemothorax A15.6
hepatitis A18.83
hilar lymph nodes A15.4
   primary (progressive) A15.7
hip (joint) (disease) (bone) A18.02
hydropneumothorax A15.6
hydrothorax A15.6
hypoadrenalism A18.7
hypopharynx A15.8
ileocecal (hyperplastic) A18.32
ileocolitis A18.32
ileum A18.32
iliac spine (superior) A18.03
immunological findings only A15.7
indurativa (primary) A18.4
infantile A15.7
infection A15.9
   without clinical manifestations A15.7
infraclavicular gland A18.2
inguinal gland A18.2
inguinalis A18.2
intestine (any part) A18.32
iridocyclitis A18.54
iris, iritis A18.54
ischiorectal A18.32
jaw A18.03
jejunum A18.32
joint A18.02
   vertebral A18.01
keratitis (interstitial) A18.52
keratoconjunctivitis A18.52
kidney A18.11
knee (joint) A18.02
kyphosis, kyphoscoliosis A18.01
laryngitis A15.5
larynx A15.5
latent R76.11
leptomeninges, leptomeningitis (cerebral)
   (spinal) A17.0
lichenoides (primary) A18.4
linguae A18.83
lip A18.83
liver A18.83
lordosis A18.01
lung — *see* Tuberculosis, pulmonary
lupus vulgaris A18.4

Tuberculosis, tubercular, tuberculous
(calcification) (calcified) (caseous)
(chromogenic acid-fast bacilli)
(degeneration) (fibrocaseous) (fistula)
(interstitial) (isolated circumscribed lesions)
(necrosis) (parenchymatous) (ulcerative)
A15.9 — *continued*
lymph gland or node (peripheral) A18.2
abdomen A18.39
bronchial A15.4
primary (progressive) A15.7
cervical A18.2
hilar A15.4
primary (progressive) A15.7
intrathoracic A15.4
primary (progressive) A15.7
mediastinal A15.4
primary (progressive) A15.7
mesenteric A18.39
retroperitoneal A18.39
tracheobronchial A15.4
primary (progressive) A15.7
lymphadenitis — *see* Tuberculosis, lymph gland
lymphangitis — *see* Tuberculosis, lymph gland
lymphatic (gland) (vessel) — *see* Tuberculosis,
lymph gland
mammary gland A18.89
marasmus A15.9
mastoiditis A18.03
mediastinal lymph gland or node A15.4
primary (progressive) A15.7
mediastinitis A15.8
primary (progressive) A15.7
mediastinum A15.8
primary (progressive) A15.7
medulla A17.81
melanosis, Addisonian A18.7
meninges, meningitis (basilar) (cerebral)
(cerebrospinal) (spinal) A17.0
meningoencephalitis A17.82
mesentery, mesenteric (gland or node) A18.39
miliary A19.9
acute A19.2
multiple sites A19.1
single specified site A19.0
chronic A19.8
specified NEC A19.8
millstone makers' J65
miner's J65
molder's J65
mouth A18.83
multiple A19.9
acute A19.1
chronic A19.8
muscle A18.09
myelitis A17.82
myocardium, myocarditis A18.84
nasal (passage) (sinus) A15.8
nasopharynx A15.8
neck gland A18.2
nephritis A18.11
nerve (mononeuropathy) A17.83
nervous system A17.9
nose (septum) A15.8
ocular A18.50
omentum A18.31
oophoritis (acute) (chronic) A18.17
optic (nerve trunk) (papilla) A18.59
orbit A18.59
orchitis A18.15
organ, specified NEC A18.89
osseous — *see* Tuberculosis, bone
osteitis — *see* Tuberculosis, bone
osteomyelitis — *see* Tuberculosis, bone
otitis media A18.6
ovary, ovaritis (acute) (chronic) A18.17
oviduct (acute) (chronic) A18.17
pachymeningitis A17.0
palate (soft) A18.83

Tuberculosis, tubercular, tuberculous
(calcification) (calcified) (caseous)
(chromogenic acid-fast bacilli)
(degeneration) (fibrocaseous) (fistula)
(interstitial) (isolated circumscribed lesions)
(necrosis) (parenchymatous) (ulcerative)
A15.9 — *continued*
pancreas A18.83
papulonecrotic(a) (primary) A18.4
parathyroid glands A18.82
paronychia (primary) A18.4
parotid gland or region A18.83
pelvis (bony) A18.03
penis A18.15
peribronchitis A15.5
pericardium, pericarditis A18.84
perichondritis, larynx A15.5
periostitis — *see* Tuberculosis, bone
perirectal fistula A18.32
peritoneum NEC A18.31
peritonitis A18.31
pharynx, pharyngitis A15.8
phlyctenulosis (keratoconjunctivitis) A18.52
phthisis NEC — *see* Tuberculosis, pulmonary
pituitary gland A18.82
pleura, pleural, pleurisy, pleuritis (fibrinous)
(obliterative) (purulent) (simple plastic)
(with effusion) A15.6
primary (progressive) A15.7
pneumonia, pneumonic — *see* Tuberculosis,
pulmonary
pneumothorax (spontaneous) (tense valvular)
— *see* Tuberculosis, pulmonary
polyneuropathy A17.89
polyserositis A19.9
acute A19.1
chronic A19.8
potter's J65
prepuce A18.15
primary (complex) A15.7
proctitis A18.32
prostate, prostatitis A18.14
pulmonalis — *see* Tuberculosis, pulmonary
pulmonary (cavitated) (fibrotic) (infiltrative)
(nodular) A15.0
childhood type or first infection A15.7
primary (complex) A15.7
pyelitis A18.11
pyelonephritis A18.11
pyemia — *see* Tuberculosis, miliary
pyonephrosis A18.11
pyopneumothorax A15.6
pyothorax A15.6
rectum (fistula) (with abscess) A18.32
reinfection stage — *see* Tuberculosis,
pulmonary
renal A18.11
renis A18.11
respiratory A15.9
primary A15.7
specified site NEC A15.8
retina, retinitis A18.53
retroperitoneal (lymph gland or node) A18.39
rheumatism NEC A18.09
rhinitis A15.8
sacroiliac (joint) A18.01
sacrum A18.01
salivary gland A18.83
salpingitis (acute) (chronic) A18.17
sandblaster's J65
sclera A18.51
scoliosis A18.01
scrofulous A18.2
scrotum A18.15
seminal tract or vesicle A18.15
senile A15.9
septic — *see* Tuberculosis, miliary
shoulder (joint) A18.02
blade A18.03

Tuberculosis, tubercular, tuberculous
(calcification) (calcified) (caseous)
(chromogenic acid-fast bacilli)
(degeneration) (fibrocaseous) (fistula)
(interstitial) (isolated circumscribed lesions)
(necrosis) (parenchymatous) (ulcerative)
A15.9 — *continued*
sigmoid A18.32
sinus (any nasal) A15.8
bone A18.03
epididymis A18.15
skeletal NEC A18.03
skin (any site) (primary) A18.4
small intestine A18.32
soft palate A18.83
spermatic cord A18.15
spine, spinal (column) A18.01
cord A17.81
medulla A17.81
membrane A17.0
meninges A17.0
spleen, splenitis A18.85
spondylitis A18.01
sternoclavicular joint A18.02
stomach A18.83
stonemason's J65
subcutaneous tissue (cellular) (primary) A18.4
subcutis (primary) A18.4
subdeltoid bursa A18.83
submaxillary (region) A18.83
supraclavicular gland A18.2
suprarenal (capsule) (gland) A18.7
swelling, joint (*see also* category M01) (*see also*
Tuberculosis, joint) A18.02
symphysis pubis A18.02
synovitis A18.09
articular A18.02
spine or vertebra A18.01
systemic — *see* Tuberculosis, miliary
tarsitis A18.4
tendon (sheath) — *see* Tuberculosis,
tenosynovitis
tenosynovitis A18.09
spine or vertebra A18.01
testis A18.15
throat A15.8
thymus gland A18.82
thyroid gland A18.81
tongue A18.83
tonsil, tonsillitis A15.8
trachea, tracheal A15.5
lymph gland or node A15.4
primary (progressive) A15.7
tracheobronchial A15.5
lymph gland or node A15.4
primary (progressive) A15.7
tubal (acute) (chronic) A18.17
tunica vaginalis A18.15
ulcer (skin) (primary) A18.4
bowel or intestine A18.32
specified NEC — *code under* Tuberculosis,
by site
unspecified site A15.9
ureter A18.11
urethra, urethral (gland) A18.13
urinary organ or tract A18.13
uterus A18.17
uveal tract A18.54
uvula A18.83
vagina A18.18
vas deferens A18.15
verruca, verrucosa (cutis) (primary) A18.4
vertebra (column) A18.01
vesiculitis A18.15
vulva A18.18
wrist (joint) A18.02

Tuberculum
- Carabelli — *see* Note at K00.2
- occlusal — *see* Note at K00.2
- paramolare K00.2

Tuberosity, enitre maxillary M26.07
Tuberous sclerosis (brain) Q85.1
Tubo-ovarian — *see* condition
Tuboplasty, after previous sterilization Z31.0
- aftercare Z31.42

Tubotympanitis, catarrhal (chronic) — *see* Otitis, media, nonsuppurative, chronic, serous

Tularemia A21.9
- with
  - conjunctivitis A21.1
  - pneumonia A21.2
- abdominal A21.3
- bronchopneumonic A21.2
- conjunctivitis A21.1
- cryptogenic A21.3
- enteric A21.3
- gastrointestinal A21.3
- generalized A21.7
- ingestion A21.3
- intestinal A21.3
- oculoglandular A21.1
- ophthalmic A21.1
- pneumonia (any), pneumonic A21.2
- pulmonary A21.2
- sepsis A21.7
- specified NEC A21.8
- typhoidal A21.7
- ulceroglandular A21.0

Tularensis conjunctivitis A21.1
Tumefaction — *see also* Swelling
- liver — *see* Hypertrophy, liver

Tumor — *see also* Neoplasm, unspecified behavior, by site
- acinar cell — *see* Neoplasm, uncertain behavior, by site
- acinic cell — *see* Neoplasm, uncertain behavior, by site
- adenocarcinoid — *see* Neoplasm, malignant, by site
- adenomatoid — *see also* Neoplasm, benign, by site
  - odontogenic — *see* Cyst, calcifying odontogenic
- adnexal (skin) — *see* Neoplasm, skin, benign, by site
- adrenal
  - cortical (benign) D35.0-
    - malignant C74.0-
  - rest — *see* Neoplasm, benign, by site
- alpha-cell
  - malignant
    - pancreas C25.4
    - specified site NEC — *see* Neoplasm, malignant, by site
    - unspecified site C25.4
  - pancreas D13.7
  - specified site NEC — *see* Neoplasm, benign, by site
  - unspecified site D13.7
- aneurysmal — *see* Aneurysm
- aortic body D44.7
  - malignant C75.5
- Askin's — *see* Neoplasm, connective tissue, malignant
- basal cell (*see also* Neoplasm, skin, uncertain behavior) D48.5
- Bednar — *see* Neoplasm, skin, malignant
- benign (unclassified) — *see* Neoplasm, benign, by site

Tumor (*see also* Neoplasm, unspecified behavior, by site) — *continued*
- beta-cell
  - malignant
    - pancreas C25.4
    - specified site NEC — *see* Neoplasm, malignant, by site
    - unspecified site C25.4
  - pancreas D13.7
  - specified site NEC — *see* Neoplasm, benign, by site
  - unspecified site D13.7
- Brenner D27.9
  - borderline malignancy D39.1-
  - malignant C56-
  - proliferating D39.1-
- bronchial alveolar, intravascular D38.1
- Brooke's — *see* Neoplasm, skin, benign
- brown fat — *see* Lipoma
- Burkitt — *see* Lymphoma, Burkitt
- calcifying epithelial odontogenic — *see* Cyst, calcifying odontogenic
- carcinoid
  - benign D3A.00 *(follows D36)*
    - appendix D3A.020 *(follows D36)*
    - ascending colon D3A.022 *(follows D36)*
    - bronchus (lung) D3A.090 *(follows D36)*
    - cecum D3A.021 *(follows D36)*
    - colon D3A.029 *(follows D36)*
    - descending colon D3A.024 *(follows D36)*
    - duodenum D3A.010 *(follows D36)*
    - foregut NOS D3A.094 *(follows D36)*
    - hindgut NOS D3A.096 *(follows D36)*
    - ileum D3A.012 *(follows D36)*
    - jejunum D3A.011 *(follows D36)*
    - kidney D3A.093 *(follows D36)*
    - large intestine D3A.029 *(follows D36)*
    - lung (bronchus) D3A.090 *(follows D36)*
    - midgut NOS D3A.095 *(follows D36)*
    - rectum D3A.026 *(follows D36)*
    - sigmoid colon D3A.025 *(follows D36)*
    - small intestine D3A.019 *(follows D36)*
    - specified NEC D3A.098 *(follows D36)*
    - stomach D3A.092 *(follows D36)*
    - thymus D3A.091 *(follows D36)*
    - transverse colon D3A.023 *(follows D36)*
  - malignant C7A.00 *(follows C75)*
    - appendix C7A.020 *(follows C75)*
    - ascending colon C7A.022 *(follows C75)*
    - bronchus (lung) C7A.090 *(follows C75)*
    - cecum C7A.021 *(follows C75)*
    - colon C7A.029 *(follows C75)*
    - descending colon C7A.024 *(follows C75)*
    - duodenum C7A.010 *(follows C75)*
    - foregut NOS C7A.094 *(follows C75)*
    - hindgut NOS C7A.096 *(follows C75)*
    - ileum C7A.012 *(follows C75)*
    - jejunum C7A.011 *(follows C75)*
    - kidney C7A.093 *(follows C75)*
    - large intestine C7A.029 *(follows C75)*
    - lung (bronchus) C7A.090 *(follows C75)*
    - midgut NOS C7A.095 *(follows C75)*
    - rectum C7A.026 *(follows C75)*
    - sigmoid colon C7A.025 *(follows C75)*
    - small intestine C7A.019 *(follows C75)*
    - specified NEC C7A.098 *(follows C75)*
    - stomach C7A.092 *(follows C75)*
    - thymus C7A.091 *(follows C75)*
    - transverse colon C7A.023 *(follows C75)*
  - mesentary metastasis C7B.04 *(follows C75)*
  - secondary C7B.00 *(follows C75)*
    - bone C7B.03 *(follows C75)*
    - distant lymph nodes C7B.01 *(follows C75)*
    - liver C7B.02 *(follows C75)*
    - peritoneum C7B.04 *(follows C75)*
    - specified NEC C7B.09 *(follows C75)*
  - carotid body D44.6
    - malignant C75.4

Tumor (*see also* Neoplasm, unspecified behavior, by site) — *continued*
- cells — *see also* Neoplasm, unspecified behavior, by site
  - benign — *see* Neoplasm, benign, by site
  - malignant — *see* Neoplasm, malignant, by site
  - uncertain whether benign or malignant — *see* Neoplasm, uncertain behavior, by site
- cervix, in pregnancy or childbirth — *see* Pregnancy, complicated by, tumor, cervix
- chondromatous giant cell — *see* Neoplasm, bone, benign
- chromaffin — *see also* Neoplasm, benign, by site
  - malignant — *see* Neoplasm, malignant, by site
- Cock's peculiar L72.3
- Codman's — *see* Neoplasm, bone, benign
- dentigerous, mixed — *see* Cyst, calcifying odontogenic
- dermoid — *see* Neoplasm, benign, by site
  - with malignant transformation C56-
- desmoid (extra-abdominal) — *see also* Neoplasm, connective tissue, uncertain behavior
  - abdominal — *see* Neoplasm, connective tissue, uncertain behavior
- embolus — *see* Neoplasm, secondary, by site
- embryonal (mixed) — *see also* Neoplasm, uncertain behavior, by site
  - liver C22.7
- endodermal sinus
  - specified site — *see* Neoplasm, malignant, by site
  - unspecified site
    - female C56-
    - male C62.90
- epithelial
  - benign — *see* Neoplasm, benign, by site
  - malignant — *see* Neoplasm, malignant, by site
- Ewing's — *see* Neoplasm, bone, malignant, by site
- fatty — *see* Lipoma
- fibroid — *see* Leiomyoma
- G cell
  - malignant
    - pancreas C25.4
    - specified site NEC — *see* Neoplasm, malignant, by site
    - unspecified site C25.4
  - specified site — *see* Neoplasm, uncertain behavior, by site
  - unspecified site D37.8
- germ cell — *see also* Neoplasm, malignant, by site
  - mixed — *see* Neoplasm, malignant, by site
- ghost cell, odontogenic — *see* Cyst, calcifying odontogenic
- giant cell — *see also* Neoplasm, uncertain behavior, by site
  - bone D48.0
    - malignant — *see* Neoplasm, bone, malignant
  - chondromatous — *see* Neoplasm, bone, benign
  - malignant — *see* Neoplasm, malignant, by site
  - soft parts — *see* Neoplasm, connective tissue, uncertain behavior
    - malignant — *see* Neoplasm, connective tissue, malignant

Tumor (see also Neoplasm, unspecified behavior, by site) — continued
- glomus D18.00
  - intra-abdominal D18.03
  - intracranial D18.02
  - jugulare D44.7
    - malignant C75.5
  - skin D18.01
  - specified site NEC D18.09
- gonadal stromal — see Neoplasm, uncertain behavior, by site
- granular cell — see also Neoplasm, connective tissue, benign
  - malignant — see Neoplasm, connective tissue, malignant
- granulosa cell D39.1-
  - juvenile D39.1-
  - malignant C56-
- granulosa cell-theca cell D39.1-
  - malignant C56-
- Grawitz's C64-
- hemorrhoidal — see Hemorrhoids
- hilar cell D27-
- hilus cell D27-
- Hurthle cell (benign) D34
  - malignant C73
- hydatid — see Echinococcus
- hypernephroid — see also Neoplasm, uncertain behavior, by site
- interstitial cell — see also Neoplasm, uncertain behavior, by site
  - benign — see Neoplasm, benign, by site
  - malignant — see Neoplasm, malignant, by site
- intravascular bronchial alveolar D38.1
- islet cell — see Neoplasm, benign, by site
  - malignant — see Neoplasm, malignant, by site
    - pancreas C25.4
    - specified site NEC — see Neoplasm, malignant, by site
    - unspecified site C25.4
  - pancreas D13.7
  - specified site NEC — see Neoplasm, benign, by site
  - unspecified site D13.7
- juxtaglomerular D41.0-
- Klatskin's C24.0
- Krukenberg's C79.6-
- Leydig cell — see Neoplasm, uncertain behavior, by site
  - benign — see Neoplasm, benign, by site
    - specified site — see Neoplasm, benign, by site
    - unspecified site
      - female D27.9
      - male D29.20
  - malignant — see Neoplasm, malignant, by site
    - specified site — see Neoplasm, malignant, by site
    - unspecified site
      - female C56.9
      - male C62.90
  - specified site — see Neoplasm, uncertain behavior, by site
  - unspecified site
    - female D39.10
    - male D40.10
- lipid cell, ovary D27-
- lipoid cell, ovary D27-
- malignant (see also Neoplasm, malignant, by site) C80.1
  - fusiform cell (type) C80.1
  - giant cell (type) C80.1
  - localized, plasma cell — see Plasmacytoma, solitary
  - mixed NEC C80.1
  - small cell (type) C80.1

Tumor (see also Neoplasm, unspecified behavior, by site) — continued
- malignant (see also Neoplasm, malignant, by site) C80.1 — continued
  - spindle cell (type) C80.1
  - unclassified C80.1
- mast cell D47.0
  - malignant C96.2
- melanotic, neuroectodermal — see Neoplasm, benign, by site
- Merkel cell — see Carcinoma, Merkel cell
- mesenchymal
  - malignant — see Neoplasm, connective tissue, malignant
  - mixed — see Neoplasm, connective tissue, uncertain behavior
- mesodermal, mixed — see also Neoplasm, malignant, by site
  - liver C22.4
- mesonephric — see also Neoplasm, uncertain behavior, by site
  - malignant — see Neoplasm, malignant, by site
- metastatic
  - from specified site — see Neoplasm, malignant, by site
  - of specified site — see Neoplasm, malignant, by site
  - to specified site — see Neoplasm, secondary, by site
- mixed NEC — see also Neoplasm, benign, by site
  - malignant — see Neoplasm, malignant, by site
- mucinous of low malignant potential
  - specified site — see Neoplasm, malignant, by site
  - unspecified site C56.9
- mucocarcinoid
  - specified site — see Neoplasm, malignant, by site
  - unspecified site C18.1
- mucoepidermoid — see Neoplasm, uncertain behavior, by site
- Müllerian, mixed
  - specified site — see Neoplasm, malignant, by site
  - unspecified site C54.9
- myoepithelial — see Neoplasm, benign, by site
- neuroectodermal (peripheral) — see Neoplasm, malignant, by site
  - primitive
    - specified site — see Neoplasm, malignant, by site
    - unspecified site C71.9
- neuroendocrine D3A.8 (follows D36)
  - malignant poorly differentiated C7A.1 (follows C75)
  - secondary NEC C7B.8 (follows C75)
  - specified NEC C7A.8 (follows C75)
- neurogenic olfactory C30.0
- nonencapsulated sclerosing C73
- odontogenic (adenomatoid) (benign) (calcifying epithelial) (keratocystic) (squamous) — see Cyst, calcifying odontogenic
  - malignant C41.1
    - upper jaw (bone) C41.0
- ovarian stromal D39.1-
- ovary, in pregnancy — see Pregnancy, complicated by
- pacinian — see Neoplasm, skin, benign
- Pancoast's — see Pancoast's syndrome
- papillary — see also Papilloma
  - cystic D37.9
  - mucinous of low malignant potential C56-
    - specified site — see Neoplasm, malignant, by site
    - unspecified site C56.9

Tumor (see also Neoplasm, unspecified behavior, by site) — continued
- papillary — see also Papilloma — continued
  - serous of low malignant potential
    - specified site — see Neoplasm, malignant, by site
    - unspecified site C56.9
- pelvic, in pregnancy or childbirth — see Pregnancy, complicated by
- phantom F45.8
- phyllodes D48.6-
  - benign D24-
  - malignant — see Neoplasm, breast, malignant
- Pindborg — see Cyst, calcifying odontogenic
- placental site trophoblastic D39.2
- plasma cell (malignant) (localized) — see Plasmacytoma, solitary
- polyvesicular vitelline
  - specified site — see Neoplasm, malignant, by site
  - unspecified site
    - female C56.9
    - male C62.90
- Pott's puffy — see Osteomyelitis, specified NEC
- Rathke's pouch D44.3
- retinal anlage — see Neoplasm, benign, by site
- salivary gland type, mixed — see Neoplasm, salivary gland, benign
  - malignant — see Neoplasm, salivary gland, malignant
- Sampson's N80.1
- Schmincke's — see Neoplasm, nasopharynx, malignant
- sclerosing stromal D27-
- sebaceous — see Cyst, sebaceous
- secondary — see Neoplasm, secondary, by site
  - carcinoid C7B.00 (follows C75)
    - bone C7B.03 (follows C75)
    - distant lymph nodes C7B.01 (follows C75)
    - liver C7B.02 (follows C75)
    - peritoneum C7B.04 (follows C75)
    - specified NEC C7B.09 (follows C75)
  - neuroendocrine NEC C7B.8 (follows C75)
- serous of low malignant potential
  - specified site — see Neoplasm, malignant, by site
  - unspecified site C56.9
- Sertoli cell — see Neoplasm, benign, by site
  - with lipid storage
    - specified site — see Neoplasm, benign, by site
    - unspecified site
      - female D27.9
      - male D29.20
  - specified site — see Neoplasm, benign, by site
  - unspecified site
    - female D27.9
    - male D29.20
- Sertoli-Leydig cell — see Neoplasm, benign, by site
  - specified site — see Neoplasm, benign, by site
  - unspecified site
    - female D27.9
    - male D29.20
- sex cord(-stromal) — see Neoplasm, uncertain behavior, by site
  - with annular tubules D39.1-
- skin appendage — see Neoplasm, skin, benign
- smooth muscle — see Neoplasm, connective tissue, uncertain behavior

DISEASE INDEX

Tumor (*see also* Neoplasm, unspecified behavior, by site) — *continued*
  soft tissue
    benign — *see* Neoplasm, connective tissue, benign
    malignant — *see* Neoplasm, connective tissue, malignant
  sternomastoid (congenital) Q68.0
  stromal
    endometrial D39.0
    gastric D48.1
      benign D21.4
      malignant C16.9
      uncertain behavior D48.1
    gastrointestinal C49.A- *(follows C49.9)*
      benign D21.4
      esophagus C49.A1 *(follows C49.9)*
      large intestine C49.A4 *(follows C49.9)*
      malignant C49.A0 *(follows C49.9)*
        colon C49.A4 *(follows C49.9)*
        duodenum C49.A3 *(follows C49.9)*
        esophagus C49.A1 *(follows C49.9)*
        ileum C49.A3 *(follows C49.9)*
        jejunum C49.A3 *(follows C49.9)*
        Meckel diverticulum C49.A3 *(follows C49.9)*
        large intestine C49.A4 *(follows C49.9)*
        omentum C49.A9 *(follows C49.9)*
        peritoneum C49.A9 *(follows C49.9)*
        rectum C49.A5 *(follows C49.9)*
        small intestine C49.A3 *(follows C49.9)*
        specified site NEC C49.A9 *(follows C49.9)*
        stomach C49.A2 *(follows C49.9)*
      large intestine C49.A4 *(follows C49.9)*
      rectum C49.A5 *(follows C49.9)*
      small intestine C49.A3 *(follows C49.9)*
      specified site NEC C49.A9 *(follows C49.9)*
      stomach C49.A2 *(follows C49.9)*
      uncertain behavior D48.1
    intestine
      benign D21.4
      malignant
        large C49.A4 *(follows C49.9)*
        small C49.A3 *(follows C49.9)*
      uncertain behavior D48.1
    ovarian D39.1-
    stomach C49.A2 *(follows C49.9)*
      benign D21.4
      malignant C49.A2 *(follows C49.9)*
      uncertain behavior D48.1
  sweat gland — *see also* Neoplasm, skin, uncertain behavior
    benign — *see* Neoplasm, skin, benign
    malignant — *see* Neoplasm, skin, malignant
  syphilitic, brain A52.17
  testicular D40.10
  testicular stromal D40.1-
  theca cell D27-
  theca cell-granulosa cell D39.1-
  Triton, malignant — *see* Neoplasm, nerve, malignant
  trophoblastic, placental site D39.2
  turban D23.4
  uterus (body), in pregnancy or childbirth — *see* Pregnancy, complicated by, tumor, uterus
  vagina, in pregnancy or childbirth — *see* Pregnancy, complicated by
  varicose — *see* Varix
  von Recklinghausen's — *see* Neurofibromatosis
  vulva or perineum, in pregnancy or childbirth — *see* Pregnancy, complicated by
    causing obstructed labor O65.5
  Warthin's — *see* Neoplasm, salivary gland, benign
  Wilms' C64-

Tumor (*see also* Neoplasm, unspecified behavior, by site) — *continued*
  yolk sac — *see* Neoplasm, malignant, by site
    specified site — *see* Neoplasm, malignant, by site
    unspecified site
      female C56.9
      male C62.90
Tumor lysis syndrome (following antineoplastic chemotherapy) (spontaneous) NEC E88.3
Tumorlet — *see* Neoplasm, uncertain behavior, by site
Tungiasis B88.1
Tunica vasculosa lentis Q12.2
Turban tumor D23.4
Türck's trachoma J37.0
Turner's
  hypoplasia (tooth) K00.4
  syndrome Q96.9
    specified NEC Q96.8
  tooth K00.4
Turner-Kieser syndrome Q87.2
Turner-like syndrome Q87.1
Turner-Ullrich syndrome Q96.9
Tussis convulsiva — *see* Whooping cough
Twiddler's syndrome (due to)
  automatic implantable defibrillator T82.198
  cardiac pacemaker T82.198
Twilight state
  epileptic F05
  psychogenic F44.89
Twin (newborn) — *see also* Newborn, twin
  conjoined Q89.4
  pregnancy — *see* Pregnancy, twin, conjoined
Twinning, teeth K00.2
Twist, twisted
  bowel, colon or intestine K56.2
  hair (congenital) Q84.1
  mesentery K56.2
  omentum K56.2
  organ or site, congenital NEC — *see* Anomaly, by site
  ovarian pedicle — *see* Torsion, ovary
Twitching R25.3
Tylosis (acquired) L84
  buccalis K13.29
  linguae K13.29
  palmaris et plantaris (congenital) (inherited) Q82.8
    acquired L85.1
Tympanism R14.0
Tympanites (abdominal) (intestinal) R14.0
Tympanitis — *see* Myringitis
Tympanosclerosis — *see* subcategory H74.0
Tympanum — *see* condition
Tympany
  abdomen R14.0
  chest R09.89
Type A behavior pattern Z73.1
Typhlitis — *see* Appendicitis
Typhoenteritis — *see* Typhoid
Typhoid (abortive) (ambulant) (any site) (clinical) (fever) (hemorrhagic) (infection) (intermittent) (malignant) (rheumatic) (Widal negative) A01.00
  with pneumonia A01.03
  abdominal A01.09
  arthritis A01.04
  carrier (suspected) of Z22.0
  cholecystitis (current) A01.09
  endocarditis A01.02
  heart involvement A01.02
  inoculation reaction — *see* Complications, vaccination

Typhoid (abortive) (ambulant) (any site) (clinical) (fever) (hemorrhagic) (infection) (intermittent) (malignant) (rheumatic) (Widal negative) A01.00 — *continued*
  meningitis A01.01
  mesenteric lymph nodes A01.09
  myocarditis A01.02
  osteomyelitis A01.05
  perichondritis, larynx A01.09
  pneumonia A01.03
  specified NEC A01.09
  spine A01.05
  ulcer (perforating) A01.09
Typhomalaria (fever) — *see* Malaria
Typhomania A01.00
Typhoperitonitis A01.09
Typhus (fever) A75.9
  abdominal, abdominalis — *see* Typhoid
  African tick A77.1
  amarillic A95.9
  brain A75.9 *[G94]*
  cerebral A75.9 *[G94]*
  classical A75.0
  due to Rickettsia
    prowazekii A75.0
      recrudescent A75.1
    tsutsugamushi A75.3
    typhi A75.2
  endemic (flea-borne) A75.2
  epidemic (louse-borne) A75.0
  exanthematic NEC A75.0
  exanthematicus SAI A75.0
    brillii SAI A75.1
    mexicanus SAI A75.2
    typhus murinus A75.2
  flea-borne A75.2
  India tick A77.1
  Kenya (tick) A77.1
  louse-borne A75.0
  Mexican A75.2
  mite-borne A75.3
  murine A75.2
  North Asian tick-borne A77.2
  petechial A75.9
  Queensland tick A77.3
  rat A75.2
  recrudescent A75.1
  recurrens — *see* Fever, relapsing
  Sao Paulo A77.0
  scrub (China) (India) (Malaysia) (New Guinea) A75.3
  shop (of Malaysia) A75.2
  Siberian tick A77.2
  tick-borne A77.9
  tropical (mite-borne) A75.3
Tyrosinemia E70.21
  newborn, transitory P74.5
Tyrosinosis E70.21
Tyrosinuria E70.29

U

Uhl's anomaly or disease Q24.8
Ulcer, ulcerated, ulcerating, ulceration, ulcerative
  alveolar process M27.3
  amebic (intestine) A06.1
    skin A06.7
  anastomotic — *see* Ulcer, gastrojejunal
  anorectal K62.6
  antral — *see* Ulcer, stomach
  anus (sphincter) (solitary) K62.6
  aorta — *see* Aneurysm
  aphthous (oral) (recurrent) K12.0
    genital organ(s)
      female N76.6
      male N50.89
  artery I77.2
  atrophic — *see* Ulcer, skin
    decubitus — *see* Ulcer, pressure, by site
  back L98.429
    with
      bone necrosis L98.424
      exposed fat layer L98.422
      muscle necrosis L98.423
      skin breakdown only L98.421
  Barrett's (esophagus) K22.10
    with bleeding K22.11
  bile duct (common) (hepatic) K83.8
  bladder (solitary) (sphincter) NEC N32.89
    bilharzial B65.9 *[N33]*
    in schistosomiasis (bilharzial) B65.9 *[N33]*
    submucosal — *see* Cystitis, interstitial
    tuberculous A18.12
  bleeding K27.4
  bone — *see* Osteomyelitis, specified type NEC
  bowel — *see* Ulcer, intestine
  breast N61.1
  bronchus J98.09
  buccal (cavity) (traumatic) K12.1
  Buruli A31.1
  buttock L98.419
    with
      bone necrosis L98.414
      exposed fat layer L98.412
      muscle necrosis L98.413
      skin breakdown only L98.411
  cancerous — *see* Neoplasm, malignant, by site
  cardia K22.10
    with bleeding K22.11
  cardioesophageal (peptic) K22.10
    with bleeding K22.11
  cecum — *see* Ulcer, intestine
  cervix (uteri) (decubitus) (trophic) N86
    with cervicitis N72
  chancroidal A57
  chiclero B55.1
  chronic (cause unknown) — *see* Ulcer, skin
  Cochin-China B55.1
  colon — *see* Ulcer, intestine
  conjunctiva H10.89
  cornea H16.00-
    with hypopyon H16.03-
    central H16.01-
    dendritic (herpes simplex) B00.52
    marginal H16.04-
    Mooren's H16.05-
    mycotic H16.06-
    perforated H16.07-
    ring H16.02-
    tuberculous (phlyctenular) A18.52
  corpus cavernosum (chronic) N48.5
  crural — *see* Ulcer, lower limb
  Curling's — *see* Ulcer, peptic, acute
  Cushing's — *see* Ulcer, peptic, acute
  cystic duct K82.8
  cystitis (interstitial) — *see* Cystitis, interstitial

Ulcer, ulcerated, ulcerating, ulceration, ulcerative — *continued*
  decubitus — *see* Ulcer, pressure, by site
  dendritic, cornea (herpes simplex) B00.52
  diabetes, diabetic — *see* Diabetes, ulcer
  Dieulafoy's K25.0
  due to
    infection NEC — *see* Ulcer, skin
    radiation NEC L59.8
    trophic disturbance (any region) — *see* Ulcer, skin
    X-ray L58.1
  duodenum, duodenal (eroded) (peptic) K26.9
    with
      hemorrhage K26.4
        and perforation K26.6
      perforation K26.5
    acute K26.3
      with
        hemorrhage K26.0
          and perforation K26.2
        perforation K26.1
    chronic K26.7
      with
        hemorrhage K26.4
          and perforation K26.6
        perforation K26.5
  dysenteric A09
  elusive — *see* Cystitis, interstitial
  endocarditis (acute) (chronic) (subacute) I28.8
  epiglottis J38.7
  esophagus (peptic) K22.10
    with bleeding K22.11
    due to
      aspirin K22.10
        with bleeding K22.11
      gastrointestinal reflux disease K21.0
      ingestion of chemical or medicament K22.10
        with bleeding K22.11
    fungal K22.10
      with bleeding K22.11
    infective K22.10
      with bleeding K22.11
    varicose — *see* Varix, esophagus
  eyelid (region) H01.8
  fauces J39.2
  Fenwick (-Hunner) (solitary) — *see* Cystitis, interstitial
  fistulous — *see* Ulcer, skin
  foot (indolent) (trophic) — *see* Ulcer, lower limb
  frambesial, initial A66.0
  frenum (tongue) K14.0
  gallbladder or duct K82.8
  gangrenous — *see* Gangrene
  gastric — *see* Ulcer, stomach
  gastrocolic — *see* Ulcer, gastrojejunal
  gastroduodenal — *see* Ulcer, peptic
  gastroesophageal — *see* Ulcer, stomach
  gastrointestinal — *see* Ulcer, gastrojejunal
  gastrojejunal (peptic) K28.9
    with
      hemorrhage K28.4
        and perforation K28.6
      perforation K28.5
    acute K28.3
      with
        hemorrhage K28.0
          and perforation K28.2
        perforation K28.1
    chronic K28.7
      with
        hemorrhage K28.4
          and perforation K28.6
        perforation K28.5
  gastrojejunocolic — *see* Ulcer, gastrojejunal
  gingiva K06.8

Ulcer, ulcerated, ulcerating, ulceration, ulcerative — *continued*
  gingivitis K05.10
    nonplaque induced K05.11
    plaque induced K05.10
  glottis J38.7
  granuloma of pudenda A58
  gum K06.8
  gumma, due to yaws A66.4
  heel — *see* Ulcer, lower limb
  hemorrhoid (*see also* Hemorrhoids, by degree) K64.8
  Hunner's — *see* Cystitis, interstitial
  hypopharynx J39.2
  hypopyon (chronic) (subacute) — *see* Ulcer, cornea, with hypopyon
  hypostaticum — *see* Ulcer, varicose
  ileum — *see* Ulcer, intestine
  intestine, intestinal K63.3
    with perforation K63.1
    amebic A06.1
    duodenal — *see* Ulcer, duodenum
    granulocytopenic (with hemorrhage) — *see* Neutropenia
    marginal — *see* Ulcer, gastrojejunal
    perforating K63.1
      newborn P78.0
    primary, small intestine K63.3
    rectum K62.6
    stercoraceous, stercoral K63.3
    tuberculous A18.32
    typhoid (fever) — *see* Typhoid
    varicose I86.8
  jejunum, jejunal — *see* Ulcer, gastrojejunal
  keratitis — *see* Ulcer, cornea
  knee — *see* Ulcer, lower limb
  labium (majus) (minus) N76.6
  laryngitis — *see* Laryngitis
  larynx (aphthous) (contact) J38.7
    diphtheritic A36.2
  leg — *see* Ulcer, lower limb
  lip K13.0
  Lipschütz's N76.6
  lower limb (atrophic) (chronic) (neurogenic) (perforating) (pyogenic) (trophic) (tropical) L97.909
    with
      bone necrosis L97.904
      exposed fat layer L97.902
      muscle necrosis L97.903
      skin breakdown only L97.901
    ankle L97.309
      with
        bone necrosis L97.304
        exposed fat layer L97.302
        muscle necrosis L97.303
        skin breakdown only L97.301
      left L97.329
        with
          bone necrosis L97.324
          exposed fat layer L97.322
          muscle necrosis L97.323
          skin breakdown only L97.321
      right L97.319
        with
          bone necrosis L97.314
          exposed fat layer L97.312
          muscle necrosis L97.313
          skin breakdown only L97.311
    calf L97.209
      with
        bone necrosis L97.204
        exposed fat layer L97.202
        muscle necrosis L97.203
        skin breakdown only L97.201

DISEASE INDEX

Ulcer, ulcerated, ulcerating, ulceration, ulcerative — *continued*
lower limb (atrophic) (chronic) (neurogenic) (perforating) (pyogenic) (trophic) (tropical) L97.909 — *continued*
  calf L97.209 — *continued*
    left L97.229
      with
        bone necrosis L97.224
        exposed fat layer L97.222
        muscle necrosis L97.223
        skin breakdown only L97.221
    right L97.219
      with
        bone necrosis L97.214
        exposed fat layer L97.212
        muscle necrosis L97.213
        skin breakdown only L97.211
  decubitus — *see* Ulcer, pressure, by site
  foot specified NEC L97.509
    with
      bone necrosis L97.504
      exposed fat layer L97.502
      muscle necrosis L97.503
      skin breakdown only L97.501
    left L97.529
      with
        bone necrosis L97.524
        exposed fat layer L97.522
        muscle necrosis L97.523
        skin breakdown only L97.521
    right L97.519
      with
        bone necrosis L97.514
        exposed fat layer L97.512
        muscle necrosis L97.513
        skin breakdown only L97.511
  heel L97.409
    with
      bone necrosis L97.404
      exposed fat layer L97.402
      muscle necrosis L97.403
      skin breakdown only L97.401
    left L97.429
      with
        bone necrosis L97.424
        exposed fat layer L97.422
        muscle necrosis L97.423
        skin breakdown only L97.421
    right L97.419
      with
        bone necrosis L97.414
        exposed fat layer L97.412
        muscle necrosis L97.413
        skin breakdown only L97.411
    left L97.929
      with
        bone necrosis L97.924
        exposed fat layer L97.922
        muscle necrosis L97.923
        skin breakdown only L97.921
  leprous A30.1
  lower leg NOS L97.909
    with
      bone necrosis L97.904
      exposed fat layer L97.902
      muscle necrosis L97.903
      skin breakdown only L97.901
    left L97.929
      with
        bone necrosis L97.924
        exposed fat layer L97.922
        muscle necrosis L97.923
        skin breakdown only L97.921

Ulcer, ulcerated, ulcerating, ulceration, ulcerative — *continued*
lower limb (atrophic) (chronic) (neurogenic) (perforating) (pyogenic) (trophic) (tropical) L97.909 — *continued*
  lower leg NOS L97.909 — *continued*
    right L97.919
      with
        bone necrosis L97.914
        exposed fat layer L97.912
        muscle necrosis L97.913
        skin breakdown only L97.911
  specified site NEC L97.809
    with
      bone necrosis L97.804
      exposed fat layer L97.802
      muscle necrosis L97.803
      skin breakdown only L97.801
    left L97.829
      with
        bone necrosis L97.824
        exposed fat layer L97.822
        muscle necrosis L97.823
        skin breakdown only L97.821
    right L97.819
      with
        bone necrosis L97.814
        exposed fat layer L97.812
        muscle necrosis L97.813
        skin breakdown only L97.811
  midfoot L97.409
    with
      bone necrosis L97.404
      exposed fat layer L97.402
      muscle necrosis L97.403
      skin breakdown only L97.401
    left L97.429
      with
        bone necrosis L97.424
        exposed fat layer L97.422
        muscle necrosis L97.423
        skin breakdown only L97.421
    right L97.419
      with
        bone necrosis L97.414
        exposed fat layer L97.412
        muscle necrosis L97.413
        skin breakdown only L97.411
  right L97.919
    with
      bone necrosis L97.914
      exposed fat layer L97.912
      muscle necrosis L97.913
      skin breakdown only L97.911
  syphilitic A52.19
  thigh L97.109
    with
      bone necrosis L97.104
      exposed fat layer L97.102
      muscle necrosis L97.103
      skin breakdown only L97.101
    left L97.129
      with
        bone necrosis L97.124
        exposed fat layer L97.122
        muscle necrosis L97.123
        skin breakdown only L97.121
    right L97.119
      with
        bone necrosis L97.114
        exposed fat layer L97.112
        muscle necrosis L97.113
        skin breakdown only L97.111

Ulcer, ulcerated, ulcerating, ulceration, ulcerative — *continued*
lower limb (atrophic) (chronic) (neurogenic) (perforating) (pyogenic) (trophic) (tropical) L97.909 — *continued*
  toe L97.509
    with
      bone necrosis L97.504
      exposed fat layer L97.502
      muscle necrosis L97.503
      skin breakdown only L97.501
    left L97.529
      with
        bone necrosis L97.524
        exposed fat layer L97.522
        muscle necrosis L97.523
        skin breakdown only L97.521
    right L97.519
      with
        bone necrosis L97.514
        exposed fat layer L97.512
        muscle necrosis L97.513
        skin breakdown only L97.511
  varicose — *see* Varix, leg, with, ulcer
  luetic — *see* Ulcer, syphilitic
  lung J98.4
    tuberculous — *see* Tuberculosis, pulmonary
  malignant — *see* Neoplasm, malignant, by site
  marginal NEC — *see* Ulcer, gastrojejunal
  meatus (urinarius) N34.2
  Meckel's diverticulum Q43.0
    malignant — *see* Table of Neoplasms, small intestine, malignant
  Meleney's (chronic undermining) — *see* Ulcer, skin
  Mooren's (cornea) — *see* Ulcer, cornea, Mooren's
  mycobacterial (skin) A31.1
  nasopharynx J39.2
  neck, uterus N86
  neurogenic NEC — *see* Ulcer, skin
  nose, nasal (passage) (infective) (septum) J34.0
    skin — *see* Ulcer, skin
    spirochetal A69.8
    varicose (bleeding) I86.8
  oral mucosa (traumatic) K12.1
  palate (soft) K12.1
  penis (chronic) N48.5
  peptic (site unspecified) K27.9
    with
      hemorrhage K27.4
        and perforation K27.6
      perforation K27.5
    acute K27.3
      with
        hemorrhage K27.0
          and perforation K27.2
        perforation K27.1
    chronic K27.7
      with
        hemorrhage K27.4
          and perforation K27.6
        perforation K27.5
  esophagus K22.10
    with bleeding K22.11
  newborn P78.82
  perforating K27.5
    skin — *see* Ulcer, skin
  peritonsillar J35.8
  phagedenic (tropical) — *see* Ulcer, skin
  pharynx J39.2
  phlebitis — *see* Phlebitis
  plaster — *see* Ulcer, pressure, by site
  popliteal space — *see* Ulcer, lower limb
  postpyloric — *see* Ulcer, duodenum
  prepuce N47.7
  prepyloric — *see* Ulcer, stomach

Ulcer, ulcerated, ulcerating, ulceration, ulcerative — continued
- pressure (pressure area) L89.9-
  - ankle L89.5-
  - back L89.1-
  - buttock L89.3-
  - coccyx L89.15-
  - contiguous site of back, buttock, hip L89.4-
  - elbow L89.0-
  - face L89.81-
  - head L89.81-
  - heel L89.6-
  - hip L89.2-
  - sacral region (tailbone) L89.15-
  - specified site NEC L89.89-
  - stage 1 (healing) (pre-ulcer skin changes limited to persistent focal edema)
    - ankle L89.5-
    - back L89.1-
    - buttock L89.3-
    - coccyx L89.15-
    - contiguous site of back, buttock, hip L89.4-
    - elbow L89.0-
    - face L89.81-
    - head L89.81-
    - heel L89.6-
    - hip L89.2-
    - sacral region (tailbone) L89.15-
    - specified site NEC L89.89-
  - stage 2 (healing) (abrasion, blister, partial thickness skin loss involving epidermis and/or dermis)
    - ankle L89.5-
    - back L89.1-
    - buttock L89.3-
    - coccyx L89.15-
    - contiguous site of back, buttock, hip L89.4-
    - elbow L89.0-
    - face L89.81-
    - head L89.81-
    - heel L89.6-
    - hip L89.2-
    - sacral region (tailbone) L89.15-
    - specified site NEC L89.89-
  - stage 3 (healing) (full thickness skin loss involving damage or necrosis of subcutaneous tissue)
    - ankle L89.5-
    - back L89.1-
    - buttock L89.3-
    - coccyx L89.15-
    - contiguous site of back, buttock, hip L89.4-
    - elbow L89.0-
    - face L89.81-
    - head L89.81-
    - heel L89.6-
    - hip L89.2-
    - sacral region (tailbone) L89.15-
    - specified site NEC L89.89-
  - stage 4 (healing) (necrosis of soft tissues through to underlying muscle, tendon, or bone)
    - ankle L89.5-
    - back L89.1-
    - buttock L89.3-
    - coccyx L89.15-
    - contiguous site of back, buttock, hip L89.4-
    - elbow L89.0-
    - face L89.81-
    - head L89.81-
    - heel L89.6-
    - hip L89.2-
    - sacral region (tailbone) L89.15-
    - specified site NEC L89.89-

Ulcer, ulcerated, ulcerating, ulceration, ulcerative — continued
- pressure (pressure area) L89.9- — continued
  - unspecified stage
    - ankle L89.5-
    - back L89.1-
    - buttock L89.3-
    - coccyx L89.15-
    - contiguous site of back, buttock, hip L89.4-
    - elbow L89.0-
    - face L89.81-
    - head L89.81-
    - heel L89.6-
    - hip L89.2-
    - sacral region (tailbone) L89.15-
    - specified site NEC L89.89-
  - unstageable
    - ankle L89.5-
    - back L89.1-
    - buttock L89.3-
    - coccyx L89.15-
    - contiguous site of back, buttock, hip L89.4-
    - elbow L89.0-
    - face L89.81-
    - head L89.81-
    - heel L89.6-
    - hip L89.2-
    - sacral region (tailbone) L89.15-
    - specified site NEC L89.89-
- primary of intestine K63.3
  - with perforation K63.1
- prostate N41.9
- pyloric — see Ulcer, stomach
- rectosigmoid K63.3
  - with perforation K63.1
- rectum (sphincter) (solitary) K62.6
  - stercoraceous, stercoral K62.6
- retina — see Inflammation, chorioretinal
- rodent — see also Neoplasm, skin, malignant
- sclera — see Scleritis
- scrofulous (tuberculous) A18.2
- scrotum N50.89
  - tuberculous A18.15
  - varicose I86.1
- seminal vesicle N50.89
- sigmoid — see Ulcer, intestine
- skin (atrophic) (chronic) (neurogenic) (non-healing) (perforating) (pyogenic) (trophic) (tropical) L98.499
  - with gangrene — see Gangrene
  - amebic A06.7
  - back — see Ulcer, back
  - buttock — see Ulcer, buttock
  - decubitus — see Ulcer, pressure
  - lower limb — see Ulcer, lower limb
  - mycobacterial A31.1
  - specified site NEC L98.499
    - with
      - bone necrosis L98.494
      - exposed fat layer L98.492
      - muscle necrosis L98.493
      - skin breakdown only L98.491
  - tuberculous (primary) A18.4
  - varicose — see Ulcer, varicose
- sloughing — see Ulcer, skin
- solitary, anus or rectum (sphincter) K62.6
- sore throat J02.9
  - streptococcal J02.0
- spermatic cord N50.89
- spine (tuberculous) A18.01
- stasis (venous) — see Varix, leg, with, ulcer
  - without varicose veins I87.2
- stercoraceous, stercoral K63.3
  - with perforation K63.1
  - anus or rectum K62.6
- stoma, stomal — see Ulcer, gastrojejunal

Ulcer, ulcerated, ulcerating, ulceration, ulcerative — continued
- stomach (eroded) (peptic) (round) K25.9
  - with
    - hemorrhage K25.4
      - and perforation K25.6
    - perforation K25.5
  - acute K25.3
    - with
      - hemorrhage K25.0
        - and perforation K25.2
      - perforation K25.1
  - chronic K25.7
    - with
      - hemorrhage K25.4
        - and perforation K25.6
      - perforation K25.5
- stomal — see Ulcer, gastrojejunal
- stomatitis K12.1
- stress — see Ulcer, peptic
- strumous (tuberculous) A18.2
- submucosal, bladder — see Cystitis, interstitial
- syphilitic (any site) (early) (secondary) A51.39
  - late A52.79
    - perforating A52.79
      - foot A52.11
- testis N50.89
- thigh — see Ulcer, lower limb
- throat J39.2
  - diphtheritic A36.0
- toe — see Ulcer, lower limb
- tongue (traumatic) K14.0
- tonsil J35.8
  - diphtheritic A36.0
- trachea J39.8
- trophic — see Ulcer, skin
- tropical — see Ulcer, skin
- tuberculous — see Tuberculosis, ulcer
- tunica vaginalis N50.89
- turbinate J34.89
- typhoid (perforating) — see Typhoid
- unspecified site — see Ulcer, skin
- urethra (meatus) — see Urethritis
- uterus N85.8
  - cervix N86
    - with cervicitis N72
  - neck N86
    - with cervicitis N72
- vagina N76.5
  - in Behçet's disease M35.2 [N77.0]
  - pessary N89.8
- valve, heart I33.0
- varicose (lower limb, any part) — see also Varix, leg, with, ulcer
  - broad ligament I86.2
  - esophagus — see Varix, esophagus
  - inflamed or infected — see Varix, leg, with, ulcer, with inflammation
  - nasal septum I86.8
  - perineum I86.3
  - scrotum I86.1
  - specified site NEC I86.8
  - sublingual I86.0
  - vulva I86.3
- vas deferens N50.89
- vulva (acute) (infectional) N76.6
  - in (due to)
    - Behçet's disease M35.2 [N77.0]
    - herpesviral (herpes simplex) infection A60.04
    - tuberculosis A18.18
- vulvobuccal, recurring N76.6
- X-ray L58.1
- yaws A66.4

Ulcerosa scarlatina A38.8
Ulcus — *see also* Ulcer
  cutis tuberculosum A18.4
  duodeni — *see* Ulcer, duodenum
  durum (syphilitic) A51.0
    extragenital A51.2
  gastrojejunale — *see* Ulcer, gastrojejunal
  hypostaticum — *see* Ulcer, varicose
  molle (cutis) (skin) A57
  serpens corneae — *see* Ulcer, cornea, central
  ventriculi — *see* Ulcer, stomach
Ulegyria Q04.8
Ulerythema
  ophryogenes, congenital Q84.2
  sycosiforme L73.8
Ullrich(-Bonnevie)(-Turner) syndrome (*see also* Turner's syndrome) Q87.1
Ullrich-Feichtiger syndrome Q87.0
Ulnar — *see* condition
Ulorrhagia, ulorrhea K06.8
Umbilicus, umbilical — *see* condition
Unacceptable
  contours of tooth K08.54
  morphology of tooth K08.54
Unavailability (of)
  bed at medical facility Z75.1
  health service-related agencies Z75.4
  medical facilities (at) Z75.3
    due to
      investigation by social service agency Z75.2
      lack of services at home Z75.0
      remoteness from facility Z75.3
      waiting list Z75.1
    home Z75.0
    outpatient clinic Z75.3
  schooling Z55.1
  social service agencies Z75.4
Uncinaria americana infestation B76.1
Uncinariasis B76.9
Uncongenial work Z56.5
Unconscious(ness) — *see* Coma
Under observation — *see* Observation
Underachievement in school Z55.3
Underdevelopment — *see also* Undeveloped
  nose Q30.1
  sexual E30.0
Underdosing (*see also* Table of Drugs and Chemicals, categories T36-T50, with final character 6) Z91.14
  intentional NEC Z91.128
    due to financial hardship of patient Z91.120
  unintentional NEC Z91.138
    due to patient's age related debility Z91.130
Underfeeding, newborn P92.3
Underfill, endodontic M27.53
Underimmunization status Z28.3
Undernourishment — *see* Malnutrition
Undernutrition — *see* Malnutrition
Underweight R63.6
  for gestational age — *see* Light for dates
Underwood's disease P83.0
Undescended — *see also* Malposition, congenital
  cecum Q43.3
  colon Q43.3
  testicle — *see* Cryptorchid
Undeveloped, undevelopment — *see also* Hypoplasia
  brain (congenital) Q02
  cerebral (congenital) Q02
  heart Q24.8
  lung Q33.6
  testis E29.1
  uterus E30.0
Undiagnosed (disease) R69
Undulant fever — *see* Brucellosis
Unemployment, anxiety concerning Z56.0
  threatened Z56.2

Unequal length (acquired) (limb) — *see also* Deformity, limb, unequal length
  leg — *see also* Deformity, limb, unequal length
    congenital Q72.9-
Unextracted dental root K08.3
Unguis incarnatus L60.0
Unhappiness R45.2
Unicornate uterus Q51.4
Unilateral — *see also* condition
  development, breast N64.89
  organ or site, congenital NEC — *see* Agenesis, by site
Unilocular heart Q20.8
Union, abnormal — *see also* Fusion
  larynx and trachea Q34.8
Universal mesentery Q43.3
Unrepairable overhanging of dental restorative materials K08.52
Unsatisfactory
  restoration of tooth K08.50
    specified NEC K08.59
  sample of cytologic smear
    anus R85.615
    cervix R87.615
    vagina R87.625
  surroundings Z59.1
  work Z56.5
Unsoundness of mind — *see* Psychosis
Unstable
  back NEC — *see* Instability, joint, spine
  hip (congenital) Q65.6
    acquired — *see* Derangement, joint, specified type NEC, hip
  joint — *see* Instability, joint
    secondary to removal of joint prosthesis M96.89
  lie (mother) O32.0
  lumbosacral joint (congenital)
    acquired — *see* subcategory M53.2
    sacroiliac — *see* subcategory M53.2
    spine NEC — *see* Instability, joint, spine
Unsteadiness on feet R26.81
Untruthfulness, child problem F91.8
Unverricht(-Lundborg) disease or epilepsy — *see* Epilepsy, generalized, idiopathic
Unwanted pregnancy Z64.0
Upbringing, institutional Z62.22
  away from parents NEC Z62.29
  in care of non-parental family member Z62.21
  in foster care Z62.21
  in orphanage or group home Z62.22
  in welfare custody Z62.21
Upper respiratory — *see* condition
Upset
  gastric K30
  gastrointestinal K30
    psychogenic F45.8
  intestinal (large) (small) K59.9
    psychogenic F45.8
  menstruation N93.9
  mental F48.9
  stomach K30
    psychogenic F45.8
Urachus — *see also* condition
  patent or persistent Q64.4
Urbach-Oppenheim disease (necrobiosis lipoidica diabeticorum) — *see* E08-E13 with .620
Urbach's lipoid proteinosis E78.89
Urbach-Wiethe disease E78.89
Urban yellow fever A95.1
Urea
  blood, high — *see* Uremia
  cycle metabolism disorder — *see* Disorder, urea cycle metabolism

Uremia, uremic N19
  with
    ectopic or molar pregnancy O08.4
    polyneuropathy N18.9 *[G63]*
  chronic (*see also* Disease, kidney, chronic) N18.9
    due to hypertension — *see* Hypertensive, kidney
  complicating
    ectopic or molar pregnancy O08.4
  congenital P96.0
  extrarenal R39.2
  following ectopic or molar pregnancy O08.4
  newborn P96.0
  prerenal R39.2
Ureter, ureteral — *see* condition
Ureteralgia N23
Ureterectasis — *see* Hydroureter
Ureteritis N28.89
  cystica N28.86
  due to calculus N20.1
    with calculus, kidney N20.2
      with hydronephrosis N13.2
  gonococcal (acute) (chronic) A54.21
  nonspecific N28.89
Ureterocele N28.89
  congenital (orthotopic) Q62.31
  ectopic Q62.32
Ureterolith, ureterolithiasis — *see* Calculus, ureter
Ureterostomy
  attention to Z43.6
  status Z93.6
Urethra, urethral — *see* condition
Urethralgia R39.89
Urethritis (anterior) (posterior) N34.2
  calculous N21.1
  candidal B37.41
  chlamydial A56.01
  diplococcal (gonococcal) A54.01
    with abscess (accessory gland) (periurethral) A54.1
  gonococcal A54.01
    with abscess (accessory gland) (periurethral) A54.1
  nongonococcal N34.1
    Reiter's — *see* Reiter's disease
  nonspecific N34.1
  nonvenereal N34.1
  postmenopausal N34.2
  puerperal O86.22
  Reiter's — *see* Reiter's disease
  specified NEC N34.2
  trichomonal or due to Trichomonas (vaginalis) A59.03
Urethrocele N81.0
  with
    cystocele — *see* Cystocele
    prolapse of uterus — *see* Prolapse, uterus
Urethrolithiasis (with colic or infection) N21.1
Urethrorectal — *see* condition
Urethrorrhagia N36.8
Urethrorrhea R36.9
Urethrostomy
  attention to Z43.6
  status Z93.6
Urethrotrigonitis — *see* Trigonitis
Urethrovaginal — *see* condition
Urgency
  fecal R15.2
  hypertensive — *see* Hypertension
  urinary R39.15
Urhidrosis, uridrosis L74.8
Uric acid in blood (increased) E79.0
Uricacidemia (asymptomatic) E79.0
Uricemia (asymptomatic) E79.0
Uricosuria R82.99
Urinary — *see* condition

Urination
 frequent R35.0
 painful R30.9
Urine
 blood in — *see* Hematuria
 discharge, excessive R35.8
 enuresis, nonorganic origin F98.0
 extravasation R39.0
 frequency R35.0
 incontinence R32
  nonorganic origin F98.0
 intermittent stream R39.198
 pus in N39.0
 retention or stasis R33.9
  organic R33.8
   drug-induced R33.0
  psychogenic F45.8
 secretion
  deficient R34
  excessive R35.8
  frequency R35.0
 stream
  intermittent R39.198
  slowing R39.198
  splitting R39.13
  weak R39.12
Urinemia — *see* Uremia
Urinoma, urethra N36.8
Uroarthritis, infectious (Reiter's) — *see* Reiter's disease
Urodialysis R34
Urolithiasis — *see* Calculus, urinary
Uronephrosis — *see* Hydronephrosis
Uropathy N39.9
 obstructive N13.9
  specified NEC N13.8
 reflux N13.9
  specified NEC N13.8
 vesicoureteral reflux-associated — *see* Reflux, vesicoureteral
Urosepsis — *code to* condition
Urticaria L50.9
 with angioneurotic edema T78.3
  hereditary D84.1
 allergic L50.0
 cholinergic L50.5
 chronic L50.8
 cold, familial L50.2
 contact L50.6
 dermatographic L50.3
 due to
  cold or heat L50.2
  drugs L50.0
  food L50.0
  inhalants L50.0
  plants L50.6
  serum (*see also* Reaction, serum) T80.69
 factitial L50.3
 familial cold M04.2
 giant T78.3
  hereditary D84.1
 gigantea T78.3
 idiopathic L50.1
 larynx T78.3
  hereditary D84.1
 neonatorum P83.8
 nonallergic L50.1
 papulosa (Hebra) L28.2
 pigmentosa Q82.2
 recurrent periodic L50.8
 serum (*see also* Reaction, serum) T80.69
 solar L56.3
 specified type NEC L50.8
 thermal (cold) (heat) L50.2
 vibratory L50.4
 xanthelasmoidea Q82.2

Use (of)
 alcohol Z72.89
  with
   intoxication F10.929
   sleep disorder F10.982
  harmful — *see* Abuse, alcohol
 amphetamines — *see* Use, stimulant NEC
 caffeine — *see* Use, stimulant NEC
 cannabis F12.90
  with
   anxiety disorder F12.980
   intoxication F12.929
    with
     delirium F12.921
     perceptual disturbance F12.922
    uncomplicated F12.920
   other specified disorder F12.988
   psychosis F12.959
    delusions F12.950
    hallucinations F12.951
   unspecified disorder F12.99
 cocaine F14.90
  with
   anxiety disorder F14.980
   intoxication F14.929
    with
     delirium F14.921
     perceptual disturbance F14.922
    uncomplicated F14.920
   other specified disorder F14.988
   psychosis F14.959
    delusions F14.950
    hallucinations F14.951
   sexual dysfunction F14.981
   sleep disorder F14.982
   unspecified disorder F14.99
  harmful — *see* Abuse, drug, cocaine
 drug(s) NEC F19.90
  with sleep disorder F19.982
  harmful — *see* Abuse, drug, by type
 hallucinogen NEC F16.90
  with
   anxiety disorder F16.980
   intoxication F16.929
    with
     delirium F16.921
    uncomplicated F16.920
   mood disorder F16.94
   other specified disorder F16.988
   perception disorder (flashbacks) F16.983
   psychosis F16.959
    delusions F16.950
    hallucinations F16.951
   unspecified disorder F16.99
  harmful — *see* Abuse, drug, hallucinogen NEC
 inhalants F18.90
  with
   anxiety disorder F18.980
   intoxication F18.929
    with delirium F18.921
    uncomplicated F18.920
   mood disorder F18.94
   other specified disorder F18.988
   persisting dementia F18.97
   psychosis F18.959
    delusions F18.950
    hallucinations F18.951
   unspecified disorder F18.99
  harmful — *see* Abuse, drug, inhalant
 methadone — *see* Use, opioid
 nonprescribed drugs F19.90
  harmful — *see* Abuse, non-psychoactive substance

Use (of) — *continued*
 opioid F11.90
  with
   disorder F11.99
    mood F11.94
    sleep F11.982
    specified type NEC F11.988
   intoxication F11.929
    with
     delirium F11.921
     perceptual disturbance F11.922
    uncomplicated F11.920
   withdrawal F11.93
  harmful — *see* Abuse, drug, opioid
 patent medicines F19.90
  harmful — *see* Abuse, non-psychoactive substance
 psychoactive drug NEC F19.90
  with
   anxiety disorder F19.980
   intoxication F19.929
    with
     delirium F19.921
     perceptual disturbance F19.922
    uncomplicated F19.920
   mood disorder F19.94
   other specified disorder F19.988
   persisting
    amnestic disorder F19.96
    dementia F19.97
   psychosis F19.959
    delusions F19.950
    hallucinations F19.951
   sexual dysfunction F19.981
   sleep disorder F19.982
   unspecified disorder F19.99
   withdrawal F19.939
    with
     delirium F19.931
     perceptual disturbance F19.932
    uncomplicated F19.930
  harmful — *see* Abuse, drug NEC, psychoactive NEC
 sedative, hypnotic, or anxiolytic F13.90
  with
   anxiety disorder F13.980
   intoxication F13.929
    with
     delirium F13.921
    uncomplicated F13.920
   other specified disorder F13.988
   persisting
    amnestic disorder F13.96
    dementia F13.97
   psychosis F13.959
    delusions F13.950
    hallucinations F13.951
   sexual dysfunction F13.981
   sleep disorder F13.982
   unspecified disorder F13.99
  harmful — *see* Abuse, drug, sedative, hypnotic, or anxiolytic
 stimulant NEC F15.90
  with
   anxiety disorder F15.980
   intoxication F15.929
    with
     delirium F15.921
     perceptual disturbance F15.922
    uncomplicated F15.920
   mood disorder F15.94
   other specified disorder F15.988
   psychosis F15.959
    delusions F15.950
    hallucinations F15.951
   sexual dysfunction F15.981
   sleep disorder F15.982
   unspecified disorder F15.99

V

D I S E A S E I N D E X

Use (of) — *continued*
　stimulant NEC F15.90 — *continued*
　　with — *continued*
　　　withdrawal F15.93
　　　harmful — *see* Abuse, drug, stimulant NEC
　　tobacco Z72.0
　　　with dependence — *see* Dependence, drug, nicotine
　　volatile solvents (*see also* Use, inhalant) F18.90
　　　harmful — *see* Abuse, drug, inhalant
Usher-Senear disease or syndrome L10.4
Uta B55.1
Uteromegaly N85.2
Uterovaginal — *see* condition
Uterovesical — *see* condition
Uveal — *see* condition
Uveitis (anterior) — *see also* Iridocyclitis
　acute — *see* Iridocyclitis, acute
　chronic — *see* Iridocyclitis, chronic
　due to toxoplasmosis (acquired) B58.09
　　congenital P37.1
　granulomatous — *see* Iridocyclitis, chronic
　heterochromic — *see* Cyclitis, Fuchs' heterochromic
　lens-induced — *see* Iridocyclitis, lens-induced
　posterior — *see* Chorioretinitis
　sympathetic H44.13-
　syphilitic (secondary) A51.43
　　congenital (early) A50.01
　　late A52.71
　tuberculous A18.54
Uveoencephalitis — *see* Inflammation, chorioretinal
Uveokeratitis — *see* Iridocyclitis
Uveoparotitis D86.89
Uvula — *see* condition
Uvulitis (acute) (catarrhal) (chronic) (membranous) (suppurative) (ulcerative) K12.2

Vaccination (prophylactic)
　complication or reaction — *see* Complications, vaccination
　delayed Z28.9
　encounter for Z23
　not done — *see* Immunization, not done, because (of)
Vaccinia (generalized) (localized) T88.1
　congenital P35.8
　without vaccination B08.011
Vacuum, in sinus (accessory) (nasal) J34.89
Vagabond's disease B85.1
Vagabond, vagabondage Z59.0
Vagina, vaginal — *see* condition
Vaginalitis (tunica) (testis) N49.1
Vaginismus (reflex) N94.2
　functional F52.5
　nonorganic F52.5
　psychogenic F52.5
　secondary N94.2
Vaginitis (acute) (circumscribed) (diffuse) (emphysematous) (nonvenereal) (ulcerative) N76.0
　with ectopic or molar pregnancy O08.0
　amebic A06.82
　atrophic, postmenopausal N95.2
　bacterial N76.0
　blennorrhagic (gonococcal) A54.02
　candidal B37.3
　chlamydial A56.02
　chronic N76.1
　due to Trichomonas (vaginalis) A59.01
　following ectopic or molar pregnancy O08.0
　gonococcal A54.02
　　with abscess (accessory gland) (periurethral) A54.1
　granuloma A58
　in (due to)
　　candidiasis B37.3
　　herpesviral (herpes simplex) infection A60.04
　　pinworm infection B80 [N77.1]
　monilial B37.3
　mycotic (candidal) B37.3
　postmenopausal atrophic N95.2
　puerperal (postpartum) O86.13
　senile (atrophic) N95.2
　subacute or chronic N76.1
　syphilitic (early) A51.0
　　late A52.76
　trichomonal A59.01
　tuberculous A18.18
Vaginosis — *see* Vaginitis
Vagotonia G52.2
Vagrancy Z59.0
VAIN — *see* Neoplasia, intraepithelial, vagina
Vallecula — *see* condition
Valley fever B38.0
Valsuani's disease — *see* Anemia, obstetric
Valve, valvular (formation) — *see also* condition
　cerebral ventricle (communicating) in situ Z98.2
　cervix, internal os Q51.828
　congenital NEC — *see* Atresia, by site
　ureter (pelvic junction) (vesical orifice) Q62.39
　urethra (congenital) (posterior) Q64.2
Valvulitis (chronic) — *see* Endocarditis
Valvulopathy — *see* Endocarditis
Van Bogaert's leukoencephalopathy (sclerosing) (subacute) A81.1
Van Bogaert-Scherer-Epstein disease or syndrome E75.5
Van Buchem's syndrome M85.2
Van Creveld-von Gierke disease E74.01

Van der Hoeve(-de Kleyn) syndrome Q78.0
Van der Woude's syndrome Q38.0
Van Neck's disease or osteochondrosis M91.0
Vanishing lung J44.9
Vapor asphyxia or suffocation T59.9
　specified agent — *see* Table of Drugs and Chemicals
Variance, lethal ball, prosthetic heart valve T82.09
Variants, thalassemic D56.8
Variations in hair color L67.1
Varicella B01.9
　with
　　complications NEC B01.89
　　encephalitis B01.11
　　encephalomyelitis B01.11
　　meningitis B01.0
　　myelitis B01.12
　　pneumonia B01.2
　congenital P35.8
Varices — *see* Varix
Varicocele (scrotum) (thrombosed) I86.1
　ovary I86.2
　perineum I86.3
　spermatic cord (ulcerated) I86.1
Varicose
　aneurysm (ruptured) I77.0
　dermatitis — *see* Varix, leg, with, inflammation
　eczema — *see* Varix, leg, with, inflammation
　phlebitis — *see* Varix, with, inflammation
　tumor — *see* Varix
　ulcer (lower limb, any part) — *see also* Varix, leg, with, ulcer
　　anus (*see also* Hemorrhoids) K64.8
　　esophagus — *see* Varix, esophagus
　　inflamed or infected — *see* Varix, leg, with, ulcer, with inflammation
　　nasal septum I86.8
　　perineum I86.3
　　scrotum I86.1
　　specified site NEC I86.8
　vein — *see* Varix
　vessel — *see* Varix, leg
Varicosis, varicosities, varicosity — *see* Varix
Variola (major) (minor) B03
Varioloid B03
Varix (lower limb) (ruptured) I83.90
　with
　　edema I83.899
　　inflammation I83.10
　　　with ulcer (venous) I83.209
　　pain I83.819
　　specified complication NEC I83.899
　　stasis dermatitis I83.10
　　　with ulcer (venous) I83.209
　　swelling I83.899
　　ulcer I83.009
　　　with inflammation I83.209
　aneurysmal I77.0
　asymptomatic I83.9-
　bladder I86.2
　broad ligament I86.2
　complicating
　　childbirth (lower extremity) O87.4
　　　anus or rectum O87.2
　　　genital (vagina, vulva or perineum) O87.8
　　pregnancy (lower extremity) O22.0-
　　　anus or rectum O22.4-
　　　genital (vagina, vulva or perineum) O22.1-
　　puerperium (lower extremity) O87.4
　　　anus or rectum O87.2
　　　genital (vagina, vulva, perineum) O87.8
　congenital (any site) Q27.8

Varix (lower limb) (ruptured) I83.90 — *continued*
esophagus (idiopathic) (primary) (ulcerated) I85.00
bleeding I85.01
congenital Q27.8
in (due to)
alcoholic liver disease I85.10
bleeding I85.11
cirrhosis of liver I85.10
bleeding I85.11
portal hypertension I85.10
bleeding I85.11
schistosomiasis I85.10
bleeding I85.11
toxic liver disease I85.10
bleeding I85.11
secondary I85.10
bleeding I85.11
gastric I86.4
inflamed or infected I83.10
ulcerated I83.209
labia (majora) I86.3
leg (asymptomatic) I83.90
with
edema I83.899
inflammation I83.10
with ulcer — *see* Varix, leg, with, ulcer, with inflammation by site
pain I83.819
specified complication NEC I83.899
swelling I83.899
ulcer I83.009
with inflammation I83.209
ankle I83.003
with inflammation I83.203
calf I83.002
with inflammation I83.202
foot NEC I83.005
with inflammation I83.205
heel I83.004
with inflammation I83.204
lower leg NEC I83.008
with inflammation I83.208
midfoot I83.004
with inflammation I83.204
thigh I83.001
with inflammation I83.201
bilateral (asymptomatic) I83.93
with
edema I83.893
pain I83.813
specified complication NEC I83.893
swelling I83.893
ulcer I83.009
with inflammation I83.209
left (asymptomatic) I83.92
with
edema I83.892
inflammation I83.12
with ulcer — *see* Varix, leg, with, ulcer, with inflammation by site
pain I83.812
specified complication NEC I83.892
swelling I83.892
ulcer I83.029
with inflammation I83.229
ankle I83.023
with inflammation I83.223
calf I83.022
with inflammation I83.222
foot NEC I83.025
with inflammation I83.225
heel I83.024
with inflammation I83.224
lower leg NEC I83.028
with inflammation I83.228

Varix (lower limb) (ruptured) I83.90 — *continued*
leg (asymptomatic) I83.90 — *continued*
left (asymptomatic) I83.92 — *continued*
with — *continued*
ulcer I83.029 — *continued*
midfoot I83.024
with inflammation I83.224
thigh I83.021
with inflammation I83.221
right (asymptomatic) I83.91
with
edema I83.891
inflammation I83.11
with ulcer — *see* Varix, leg, with, ulcer, with inflammation by site
pain I83.811
specified complication NEC I83.891
swelling I83.891
ulcer I83.019
with inflammation I83.219
ankle I83.013
with inflammation I83.213
calf I83.012
with inflammation I83.212
foot NEC I83.015
with inflammation I83.215
heel I83.014
with inflammation I83.214
lower leg NEC I83.018
with inflammation I83.218
midfoot I83.014
with inflammation I83.214
thigh I83.011
with inflammation I83.211
nasal septum I86.8
orbit I86.8
congenital Q27.8
ovary I86.2
papillary I78.1
pelvis I86.2
perineum I86.3
pharynx I86.8
placenta O43.89-
renal papilla I86.8
retina H35.09
scrotum (ulcerated) I86.1
sigmoid colon I86.8
specified site NEC I86.8
spinal (cord) (vessels) I86.8
spleen, splenic (vein) (with phlebolith) I86.8
stomach I86.4
sublingual I86.0
ulcerated I83.009
inflamed or infected I83.209
uterine ligament I86.2
vagina I86.8
vocal cord I86.8
vulva I86.3
Vas deferens — *see* condition
Vas deferentitis N49.1
Vasa previa O69.4
hemorrhage from, affecting newborn P50.0
Vascular — *see also* condition
loop on optic papilla Q14.2
spasm I73.9
spider I78.1
Vascularization, cornea — *see* Neovascularization, cornea
Vasculitis I77.6
allergic D69.0
cryoglobulinemic D89.1
disseminated I77.6
hypocomplementemic M31.8
kidney I77.89
livedoid L95.0
nodular L95.8
retina H35.06-

Vasculitis I77.6 — *continued*
rheumatic — *see* Fever, rheumatic
rheumatoid — *see* Rheumatoid, vasculitis
skin (limited to) L95.9
specified NEC L95.8
Vasculopathy, necrotizing M31.9
cardiac allograft T86.290
specified NEC M31.8
Vasitis (nodosa) N49.1
tuberculous A18.15
Vasodilation I73.9
Vasomotor — *see* condition
Vasoplasty, after previous sterilization Z31.0
aftercare Z31.42
Vasospasm (vasoconstriction) I73.9
cerebral (artery) (cerebrovascular) I67.848
reversible I67.841
coronary I20.1
nerve
arm — *see* Mononeuropathy, upper limb
brachial plexus G54.0
cervical plexus G54.2
leg — *see* Mononeuropathy, lower limb
peripheral NOS I73.9
retina (artery) — *see* Occlusion, artery, retina
Vasospastic — *see* condition
Vasovagal attack (paroxysmal) R55
psychogenic F45.8
VATER syndrome Q87.2
Vater's ampulla — *see* condition
Vegetation, vegetative
adenoid (nasal fossa) J35.8
endocarditis (acute) (any valve) (subacute) I33.0
heart (mycotic) (valve) I33.0
Veil
Jackson's Q43.3
Vein, venous — *see* condition
Veldt sore — *see* Ulcer, skin
Velpeau's hernia — *see* Hernia, femoral
Venereal
bubo A55
disease A64
granuloma inguinale A58
lymphogranuloma (Durand-Nicolas-Favre) A55
Venofibrosis I87.8
Venom, venomous — *see* Table of Drugs and Chemicals, by animal or substance, poisoning
Venous — *see* condition
Ventilator lung, newborn P27.8
Ventral — *see* condition
Ventricle, ventricular — *see also* condition
escape I49.3
inversion Q20.5
Ventriculitis (cerebral) (*see also* Encephalitis) G04.90
Ventriculostomy status Z98.2
Vernet's syndrome G52.7
Verneuil's disease (syphilitic bursitis) A52.78
Verruca (due to HPV) (filiformis) (simplex) (viral) (vulgaris) B07.9
acuminata A63.0
necrogenica (primary) (tuberculosa) A18.4
plana B07.8
plantaris B07.0
seborrheica L82.1
inflamed L82.0
senile (seborrheic) L82.1
inflamed L82.0
tuberculosa (primary) A18.4
venereal A63.0
Verrucosities — *see* Verruca
Verruga peruana, peruviana A44.1

Version
with extraction
cervix — *see* Malposition, uterus
uterus (postinfectional) (postpartal, old) — *see*
Malposition, uterus
Vertebra, vertebral — *see* condition
Vertical talus (congenital) Q66.80
left foot Q66.82
right foot Q66.81
Vertigo R42
auditory — *see* Vertigo, aural
aural H81.31-
benign paroxysmal (positional) H81.1-
central (origin) H81.4-
cerebral H81.4-
Dix and Hallpike (epidemic) — *see* Neuronitis,
vestibular
due to infrasound T75.23
epidemic A88.1
Dix and Hallpike — *see* Neuronitis,
vestibular
Pedersen's — *see* Neuronitis, vestibular
vestibular neuronitis — *see* Neuronitis,
vestibular
hysterical F44.89
infrasound T75.23
labyrinthine — *see* subcategory H81.0
laryngeal R05
malignant positional H81.4-
menopausal N95.1
Ménière's — *see* subcategory H81.0
otogenic — *see* Vertigo, aural
paroxysmal positional, benign — *see* Vertigo,
benign paroxysmal
Pedersen's (epidemic) — *see* Neuronitis,
vestibular
peripheral NEC H81.39-
positional
benign paroxysmal — *see* Vertigo, benign
paroxysmal
malignant H81.4-
Very-low-density-lipoprotein-type (VLDL)
hyperlipoproteinemia E78.1
Vesania — *see* Psychosis
Vesical — *see* condition
Vesicle
cutaneous R23.8
seminal — *see* condition
skin R23.8
Vesicocolic — *see* condition
Vesicoperineal — *see* condition
Vesicorectal — *see* condition
Vesicourethrorectal — *see* condition
Vesicovaginal — *see* condition
Vesicular — *see* condition
Vesiculitis (seminal) N49.0
amebic A06.82
gonorrheal (acute) (chronic) A54.23
trichomonal A59.09
tuberculous A18.15
Vestibulitis (ear) (*see also* subcategory) H83.0
nose (external) J34.89
vulvar N94.810
Vestibulopathy, acute peripheral
(recurrent) — *see* Neuronitis, vestibular
Vestige, vestigial — *see also* Persistence
branchial Q18.0
structures in vitreous Q14.0
Vibration
adverse effects T75.20
pneumatic hammer syndrome T75.21
specified effect NEC T75.29
vasospastic syndrome T75.22
vertigo from infrasound T75.23
exposure (occupational) Z57.7
vertigo T75.23
Vibriosis A28.9

Victim (of)
crime Z65.4
disaster Z65.5
terrorism Z65.4
torture Z65.4
war Z65.5
Vidal's disease L28.0
Villaret's syndrome G52.7
Villous — *see* condition
VIN — *see* Neoplasia, intraepithelial, vulva
Vincent's infection (angina) (gingivitis) A69.1
stomatitis NEC A69.1
Vinson-Plummer syndrome D50.1
Violence, physical R45.6
Viosterol deficiency — *see* Deficiency,
calciferol
Vipoma — *see* Neoplasm, malignant, by site
Viremia B34.9
Virilism (adrenal) E25.9
congenital E25.0
Virilization (female) (suprarenal) E25.9
congenital E25.0
isosexual E28.2
Virulent bubo A57
Virus, viral — *see also* condition
as cause of disease classified elsewhere
B97.89
cytomegalovirus B25.9
human immunodeficiency (HIV) — *see* Human,
immunodeficiency virus (HIV) disease
infection — *see* Infection, virus
specified NEC B34.8
swine influenza (viruses that normally cause
infections in pigs) (*see also* Influenza, due
to, identified novel influenza A virus)
J09.x2
West Nile (fever) A92.30
with
complications NEC A92.39
cranial nerve disorders A92.32
encephalitis A92.31
encephalomyelitis A92.31
neurologic manifestation NEC A92.32
optic neuritis A92.32
polyradiculitis A92.32
Viscera, visceral — *see* condition
Visceroptosis K63.4
Visible peristalsis R19.2
Vision, visual
binocular, suppression H53.34
blurred, blurring H53.8
hysterical F44.6
defect, defective NEC H54.7
disorientation (syndrome) H53.8
disturbance H53.9
hysterical F44.6
double H53.2
examination Z01.00
with abnormal findings Z01.01
field, limitation (defect) — *see* Defect, visual
field
hallucinations R44.1
halos H53.19
loss — *see* Loss, vision
sudden — *see* Disturbance, vision,
subjective, loss, sudden
low (both eyes) — *see* Low, vision
perception, simultaneous without fusion
H53.33
Vitality, lack or want of R53.83
newborn P96.89
Vitamin deficiency — *see* Deficiency, vitamin
Vitelline duct, persistent Q43.0

Vitiligo L80
eyelid H02.739
left H02.736
lower H02.735
upper H02.734
right H02.733
lower H02.732
upper H02.731
pinta A67.2
vulva N90.89
Vitreal corneal syndrome H59.01-
Vitreoretinopathy, proliferative — *see also*
Retinopathy, proliferative
with retinal detachment — *see* Detachment,
retina, traction
Vitreous — *see also* condition
touch syndrome — *see* Complication,
postprocedural, following cataract surgery
Vocal cord — *see* condition
Vogt-Koyanagi syndrome H20.82-
Vogt's disease or syndrome G80.3
**Vogt-Spielmeyer amaurotic idiocy or
disease** E75.4
Voice
change R49.9
specified NEC R49.8
loss — *see* Aphonia
Volhynian fever A79.0
**Volkmann's ischemic contracture or
paralysis** (complicating trauma) T79.6
Volvulus (bowel) (colon) (intestine) K56.2
with perforation K56.2
congenital Q43.8
duodenum K31.5
fallopian tube — *see* Torsion, fallopian tube
oviduct — *see* Torsion, fallopian tube
stomach (due to absence of gastrocolic
ligament) K31.89
Vomiting R11.10
with nausea R11.2
asphyxia — *see* Foreign body, by site, causing
asphyxia, gastric contents
bilious (cause unknown) R11.14
following gastro-intestinal surgery K91.0
in newborn P92.01
blood — *see* Hematemesis
causing asphyxia, choking, or suffocation —
see Foreign body, by site
cyclical G43.A0 *(follows G43.7)*
with refractory migraine G43.A1 *(follows
G43.7)*
intractable G43.A1 *(follows G43.7)*
not intractable G43.A0 *(follows G43.7)*
psychogenic F50.89
without refractory migraine G43.A0 *(follows
G43.7)*
fecal mater R11.13
following gastrointestinal surgery K91.0
psychogenic F50.89
functional K31.89
hysterical F50.89
nervous F50.89
neurotic F50.89
newborn NEC P92.09
bilious P92.01
periodic R11.10
psychogenic F50.89
projectile R11.12
psychogenic F50.89
uremic — *see* Uremia
without nausea R11.11
Vomito negro — *see* Fever, yellow
Von Bezold's abscess — *see* Mastoiditis,
acute
Von Economo-Cruchet disease A85.8
Von Eulenburg's disease G71.19
Von Gierke's disease E74.01

Von Hippel(-Lindau) disease or syndrome Q85.8
Von Jaksch's anemia or disease D64.89
Von Recklinghausen
disease (neurofibromatosis) Q85.01
bones E21.0
Von Schroetter's syndrome I82.890
Von Willebrand(-Jurgens)(-Minot) disease or syndrome D68.0
Von Zumbusch's disease L40.1
Voyeurism F65.3
Vrolik's disease Q78.0
Vulva — *see* condition
Vulvismus N94.2
Vulvitis (acute) (allergic) (atrophic) (hypertrophic) (intertriginous) (senile) N76.2
with ectopic or molar pregnancy O08.0
adhesive, congenital Q52.79
blennorrhagic (gonococcal) A54.02
candidal B37.3
chlamydial A56.02
due to Haemophilus ducreyi A57
following ectopic or molar pregnancy O08.0
gonococcal A54.02
with abscess (accessory gland) (periurethral) A54.1
herpesviral A60.04
leukoplakia N90.4
monilial B37.3
puerperal (postpartum) O86.19
subacute or chronic N76.3
syphilitic (early) A51.0
late A52.76
trichomonal A59.01
tuberculous A18.18
Vulvodynia N94.819
specified NEC N94.818
Vulvorectal — *see* condition
Vulvovaginitis (acute) — *see* Vaginitis

W

Waiting list, person on Z75.1
for organ transplant Z76.82
undergoing social agency investigation Z75.2
Waldenström
hypergammaglobulinemia D89.0
syndrome or macroglobulinemia C88.0
Waldenström-Kjellberg syndrome D50.1
Walking
difficulty R26.2
psychogenic F44.4
sleep F51.3
hysterical F44.89
Wall, abdominal — *see* condition
Wallenberg's disease or syndrome G46.3
Wallgren's disease I87.8
Wandering
gallbladder, congenital Q44.1
in diseases classified elsewhere Z91.83
kidney, congenital Q63.8
organ or site, congenital NEC — *see* Malposition, congenital, by site
pacemaker (heart) I49.8
spleen D73.89
War neurosis F48.8
Wart (due to HPV) (filiform) (infectious) (viral) B07.9
anogenital region (venereal) A63.0
common B07.8
external genital organs (venereal) A63.0
flat B07.8
Hassal-Henle's (of cornea) H18.49
Peruvian A44.1
plantar B07.0
prosector (tuberculous) A18.4
seborrheic L82.1
inflamed L82.0
senile (seborrheic) L82.1
inflamed L82.0
tuberculous A18.4
venereal A63.0
Warthin's tumor — *see* Neoplasm, salivary gland, benign
Wassilieff's disease A27.0
Wasting
disease R64
due to malnutrition E41
extreme (due to malnutrition) E41
muscle NEC — *see* Atrophy, muscle
Water
clefts (senile cataract) — *see* Cataract, senile, incipient
deprivation of T73.1
intoxication E87.79
itch B76.9
lack of T73.1
loading E87.70
on
brain — *see* Hydrocephalus
chest J94.8
poisoning E87.79
Waterbrash R12
Water-losing nephritis N25.89
Waterhouse(-Friderichsen) syndrome or disease (meningococcal) A39.1
Watermelon stomach K31.819
with hemorrhage K31.811
without hemorrhage K31.819
Watsoniasis B66.8
Wax in ear — *see* Impaction, cerumen
Weak, weakening, weakness (generalized) R53.1
arches (acquired) — *see also* Deformity, limb, flat foot
bladder (sphincter) R32

Weak, weakening, weakness (generalized) R53.1 — *continued*
facial R29.810
following
cerebrovascular disease I69.992
cerebral infarction I69.392
intracerebral hemorrhage I69.192
nontraumatic intracranial hemorrhage NEC I69.292
specified disease NEC I69.892
stroke I69.392
subarachnoid hemorrhage I69.092
foot (double) — *see* Weak, arches
heart, cardiac — *see* Failure, heart
mind F70
muscle M62.81
myocardium — *see* Failure, heart
newborn P96.89
pelvic fundus N81.89
pubocervical tissue N81.82
rectovaginal tissue N81.83
senile R54
urinary stream R39.12
valvular — *see* Endocarditis
Wear, worn (with normal or routine use)
articular bearing surface of internal joint prosthesis — *see* Complications, joint prosthesis, mechanical, wear of articularbearing surfaces, by site
device, implant or graft — *see* Complications, by site, mechanical complication
tooth, teeth (approximal) (hard tissues) (interproximal) (occlusal) K03.0
Weather, weathered
effects of
cold T69.9
specified effect NEC T69.8
hot — *see* Heat
skin L57.8
Weaver's syndrome Q87.3
Web, webbed (congenital)
duodenal Q43.8
esophagus Q39.4
fingers Q70.1-
larynx (glottic) (subglottic) Q31.0
neck (pterygium colli) Q18.3
Paterson-Kelly D50.1
popliteal syndrome Q87.89
toes Q70.3-
Weber-Christian disease M35.6
Weber-Cockayne syndrome (epidermolysis bullosa) Q81.8
Weber-Gubler syndrome G46.3
Weber-Leyden syndrome G46.3
Weber-Osler syndrome I78.0
Weber's paralysis or syndrome G46.3
Wedge-shaped or wedging vertebra — *see* Collapse, vertebra NEC
Wegener's granulomatosis or syndrome M31.30
with
kidney involvement M31.31
lung involvement M31.30
with kidney involvement M31.31
Wegner's disease A50.02
Weight
1000-2499 grams at birth (low) — *see* Low, birthweight
999 grams or less at birth (extremely low) — *see* Low, birthweight, extreme
and length below 10th percentile for gestational age P05.1-
below but length above 10th percentile for gestational age P05.0-
gain (abnormal) (excessive) R63.5
in pregnancy — *see* Pregnancy, complicated by, excessive weight gain
low — *see* Pregnancy, complicated by, insufficient, weight gain

DISEASE INDEX

DISEASE INDEX

Weight — *continued*
  loss (abnormal) (cause unknown) R63.4
Weightlessness (effect of) T75.82
Weil (I)-Marchesani syndrome Q87.1
Weil's disease A27.0
Weingarten's syndrome J82
Weir Mitchell's disease I73.81
Weiss-Baker syndrome G90.09
Wells' disease L98.3
Wen — *see* Cyst, sebaceous
Wenckebach's block or phenomenon
  I44.1
Werdnig-Hoffmann syndrome (muscular
  atrophy) G12.0
Werlhof's disease D69.3
Wermer's disease or syndrome E31.21
Werner-His disease A79.0
Werner's disease or syndrome E34.8
Wernicke-Korsakoff's syndrome or
  psychosis (alcoholic) F10.96
  with dependence F10.26
  drug-induced
    due to drug abuse — *see* Abuse, drug, by
      type, with amnestic disorder
    due to drug dependence — *see* Dependence,
      drug, by type, with amnestic disorder
  nonalcoholic F04
Wernicke-Posadas disease B38.9
Wernicke's
  developmental aphasia F80.2
  disease or syndrome E51.2
  encephalopathy E51.2
  polioencephalitis, superior E51.2
West African fever B50.8
Westphal-Strümpell syndrome E83.01
West's syndrome — *see* Epilepsy, spasms
Wet
  feet, tropical (maceration) (syndrome) — *see*
    Immersion, foot
  lung (syndrome), newborn P22.1
Wharton's duct — *see* condition
Wheal — *see* Urticaria
Wheezing R06.2
Whiplash injury S13.4
Whipple's disease (*see also* subcategory
  M14.8-) K90.81
Whipworm (disease) (infection) (infestation)
  B79
Whistling face Q87.0
White — *see also* condition
  kidney, small N03.9
  leg, puerperal, postpartum, childbirth O87.1
  mouth B37.0
  patches of mouth K13.29
  spot lesions, teeth
    chewing surface K02.51
    pit and fissure surface K02.51
    smooth surface K02.61
Whitehead L70.0
Whitlow — *see also* Cellulitis, digit
  with lymphangitis — *see* Lymphangitis, acute,
    digit
  herpesviral B00.89
Whitmore's disease or fever — *see*
  Melioidosis
Whooping cough A37.90
  with pneumonia A37.91
  due to Bordetella
    bronchiseptica A37.81
    parapertussis A37.11
    pertussis A37.01
    specified organism NEC A37.81
  due to
    Bordetella
      bronchiseptica A37.80
        with pneumonia A37.81
      parapertussis A37.10
        with pneumonia A37.11

Whooping cough A37.90 — *continued*
  due to — *continued*
    Bordetella — *continued*
      pertussis A37.00
        with pneumonia A37.01
      specified NEC A37.80
        with pneumonia A37.81
Wichman's asthma J38.5
Wide cranial sutures, newborn P96.3
Widening aorta — *see* Ectasia, aorta
  with aneurysm — *see* Aneurysm, aorta
Wilkie's disease or syndrome K55.1
Wilkinson-Sneddon disease or syndrome
  L13.1
Willebrand (-Jürgens) thrombopathy
  D68.0
Willige-Hunt disease or syndrome G23.1
Wilms' tumor C64-
Wilson-Mikity syndrome P27.0
Wilson's
  disease or syndrome E83.01
  hepatolenticular degeneration E83.01
  lichen ruber L43.9
Window — *see also* Imperfect, closure
  aorticopulmonary Q21.4
Winter — *see* condition
Wiskott-Aldrich syndrome D82.0
Withdrawal state — *see also* Dependence,
  drug by type, with withdrawal
  alcohol
    with perceptual disturbances F10.232
    without perceptual disturbances F10.239
  caffeine F15.93
  cannabis F12.288
  newborn
    correct therapeutic substance properly
      administered P96.2
    infant of dependent mother P96.1
    therapeutic substance, neonatal P96.2
Witts' anemia D50.8
Witzelsucht F07.0
Woakes' ethmoiditis or syndrome J33.1
Wolff-Hirschorn syndrome Q93.3
Wolff-Parkinson-White syndrome I45.6
Wolhynian fever A79.0
Wolman's disease E75.5
Wood lung or pneumonitis J67.8
Woolly, wooly hair (congenital) (nevus)
  Q84.1
Woolsorter's disease A22.1
Word
  blindness (congenital) (developmental) F81.0
  deafness (congenital) (developmental) H93.25
Worm-eaten soles A66.3
Worm(s) (infection) (infestation) — *see also*
  Infestation, helminth
  guinea B72
  in intestine NEC B82.0
Worn out — *see* Exhaustion
  cardiac
    defibrillator (with synchronous cardiac
      pacemaker) Z45.02
    pacemaker
      battery Z45.010
      lead Z45.018
  device, implant or graft — *see* Complications,
    by site, mechanical
Worried well Z71.1
Worries R45.82

Wound, open
abdomen, abdominal
  wall S31.109
    with penetration into peritoneal cavity
      S31.609
    bite — *see* Bite, abdomen, wall
    epigastric region S31.102
      with penetration into peritoneal cavity
        S31.602
      bite — *see* Bite, abdomen, wall,
        epigastric region
      laceration — *see* Laceration, abdomen,
        wall, epigastric region
      puncture — *see* Puncture, abdomen,
        wall, epigastric region
    laceration — *see* Laceration, abdomen,
      wall
    left
      lower quadrant S31.104
        with penetration into peritoneal cavity
          S31.604
        bite — *see* Bite, abdomen, wall, left,
          lower quadrant
        laceration — *see* Laceration,
          abdomen, wall, left, lower
          quadrant
        puncture — *see* Puncture, abdomen,
          wall, left, lower quadrant
      upper quadrant S31.101
        with penetration into peritoneal cavity
          S31.601
        bite — *see* Bite, abdomen, wall, left,
          upper quadrant
        laceration — *see* Laceration,
          abdomen, wall, left, upper
          quadrant
        puncture — *see* Puncture, abdomen,
          wall, left, upper quadrant
    periumbilic region S31.105
      with penetration into peritoneal cavity
        S31.605
      bite — *see* Bite, abdomen, wall,
        periumbilic region
      laceration — *see* Laceration, abdomen,
        wall, periumbilic region
      puncture — *see* Puncture, abdomen,
        wall, periumbilic region
    puncture — *see* Puncture, abdomen, wall
    right
      lower quadrant S31.103
        with penetration into peritoneal cavity
          S31.603
        bite — *see* Bite, abdomen, wall, right,
          lower quadrant
        laceration — *see* Laceration,
          abdomen, wall, right, lower
          quadrant
        puncture — *see* Puncture, abdomen,
          wall, right, lower quadrant
      upper quadrant S31.100
        with penetration into peritoneal cavity
          S31.600
        bite — *see* Bite, abdomen, wall, right,
          upper quadrant
        laceration — *see* Laceration,
          abdomen, wall, right, upper
          quadrant
        puncture — *see* Puncture, abdomen,
          wall, right, upper quadrant
alveolar (process) — *see* Wound, open, oral
  cavity
ankle S91.00-
  bite — *see* Bite, ankle
  laceration — *see* Laceration, ankle
  puncture — *see* Puncture, ankle
antecubital space — *see* Wound, open, elbow
anterior chamber, eye — *see* Wound, open,
  ocular

Wound, open — *continued*

anus S31.839
  bite S31.835
  laceration — *see* Laceration, anus
  puncture — *see* Puncture, anus
arm (upper) S41.10-
  with amputation — *see* Amputation, traumatic, arm
  bite — *see* Bite, arm
  forearm — *see* Wound, open, forearm
  laceration — *see* Laceration, arm
  puncture — *see* Puncture, arm
auditory canal (external) (meatus) — *see* Wound, open, ear
auricle, ear — *see* Wound, open, ear
axilla — *see* Wound, open, arm
back — *see also* Wound, open, thorax, back
  lower S31.000
    with penetration into retroperitoneal space S31.001
    bite — *see* Bite, back, lower
    laceration — *see* Laceration, back, lower
    puncture — *see* Puncture, back, lower
bite — *see* Bite
blood vessel — *see* Injury, blood vessel
breast S21.00-
  with amputation — *see* Amputation, traumatic, breast
  bite — *see* Bite, breast
  laceration — *see* Laceration, breast
  puncture — *see* Puncture, breast
buttock S31.809
  bite — *see* Bite, buttock
  laceration — *see* Laceration, buttock
  left S31.829
  puncture — *see* Puncture, buttock
  right S31.819
calf — *see* Wound, open, leg
canaliculus lacrimalis — *see* Wound, open, eyelid
canthus, eye — *see* Wound, open, eyelid
cervical esophagus S11.20
  bite S11.25
  laceration — *see* Laceration, esophagus, traumatic, cervical
  puncture — *see* Puncture, cervical esophagus
cheek (external) S01.40-
  bite — *see* Bite, cheek
  internal — *see* Wound, open, oral cavity
  laceration — *see* Laceration, cheek
  puncture — *see* Puncture, cheek
chest wall — *see* Wound, open, thorax
chin — *see* Wound, open, head, specified site NEC
choroid — *see* Wound, open, ocular
ciliary body (eye) — *see* Wound, open, ocular
clitoris S31.40
  with amputation — *see* Amputation, traumatic, clitoris
  bite S31.45
  laceration — *see* Laceration, vulva
  puncture — *see* Puncture, vulva
conjunctiva — *see* Wound, open, ocular
cornea — *see* Wound, open, ocular
costal region — *see* Wound, open, thorax
Descemet's membrane — *see* Wound, open, ocular
digit(s)
  foot — *see* Wound, open, toe
  hand — *see* Wound, open, finger
ear (canal) (external) S01.30-
  with amputation — *see* Amputation, traumatic, ear
  bite — *see* Bite, ear
  drum S09.2-
  laceration — *see* Laceration, ear
  puncture — *see* Puncture, ear

Wound, open — *continued*

elbow S51.00-
  bite — *see* Bite, elbow
  laceration — *see* Laceration, elbow
  puncture — *see* Puncture, elbow
epididymis — *see* Wound, open, testis
epigastric region S31.102
  with penetration into peritoneal cavity S31.602
  bite — *see* Bite, abdomen, wall, epigastric region
  laceration — *see* Laceration, abdomen, wall, epigastric region
  puncture — *see* Puncture, abdomen, wall, epigastric region
epiglottis — *see* Wound, open, neck, specified site NEC
esophagus (thoracic) S27.819
  cervical — *see* Wound, open, cervical esophagus
  laceration S27.813
  specified type NEC S27.818
eye — *see* Wound, open, ocular
eyeball — *see* Wound, open, ocular
eyebrow — *see* Wound, open, eyelid
eyelid S01.10-
  bite — *see* Bite, eyelid
  laceration — *see* Laceration, eyelid
  puncture — *see* Puncture, eyelid
face NEC — *see* Wound, open, head, specified site NEC
finger(s) S61.209
  with
    amputation — *see* Amputation, traumatic, finger
    damage to nail S61.309
  bite — *see* Bite, finger
  index S61.208
    with
      damage to nail S61.308
    left S61.201
      with
        damage to nail S61.301
    right S61.200
      with
        damage to nail S61.300
  laceration — *see* Laceration, finger
  little S61.208
    with
      damage to nail S61.308
    left S61.207
      with damage to nail S61.307
    right S61.206
      with damage to nail S61.306
  middle S61.208
    with
      damage to nail S61.308
    left S61.203
      with damage to nail S61.303
    right S61.202
      with damage to nail S61.302
  puncture — *see* Puncture, finger
  ring S61.208
    with
      damage to nail S61.308
    left S61.205
      with damage to nail S61.305
    right S61.204
      with damage to nail S61.304
flank — *see* Wound, open, abdomen, wall
foot (except toe(s) alone) S91.30-
  with amputation — *see* Amputation, traumatic, foot
  bite — *see* Bite, foot
  laceration — *see* Laceration, foot
  puncture — *see* Puncture, foot
  toe — *see* Wound, open, toe

Wound, open — *continued*

forearm S51.80-
  with
    amputation — *see* Amputation, traumatic, forearm
  bite — *see* Bite, forearm
  elbow only — *see* Wound, open, elbow
  laceration — *see* Laceration, forearm
  puncture — *see* Puncture, forearm
forehead — *see* Wound, open, head, specified site NEC
genital organs, external
  with amputation — *see* Amputation, traumatic, genital organs
  bite — *see* Bite, genital organ
  female S31.502
    vagina S31.40
    vulva S31.40
  laceration — *see* Laceration, genital organ
  male S31.501
    penis S31.20
    scrotum S31.30
    testes S31.30
  puncture — *see* Puncture, genital organ
globe (eye) — *see* Wound, open, ocular
groin — *see* Wound, open, abdomen, wall
gum — *see* Wound, open, oral cavity
hand S61.40-
  with
    amputation — *see* Amputation, traumatic, hand
  bite — *see* Bite, hand
  finger(s) — *see* Wound, open, finger
  laceration — *see* Laceration, hand
  puncture — *see* Puncture, hand
  thumb — *see* Wound, open, thumb
head S01.90
  bite — *see* Bite, head
  cheek — *see* Wound, open, cheek
  ear — *see* Wound, open, ear
  eyelid — *see* Wound, open, eyelid
  laceration — *see* Laceration, head
  lip — *see* Wound, open, lip
  nose S01.20
  oral cavity — *see* Wound, open, oral cavity
  puncture — *see* Puncture, head
  scalp — *see* Wound, open, scalp
  specified site NEC S01.80
  temporomandibular area — *see* Wound, open, cheek
heel — *see* Wound, open, foot
hip S71.00-
  with amputation — *see* Amputation, traumatic, hip
  bite — *see* Bite, hip
  laceration — *see* Laceration, hip
  puncture — *see* Puncture, hip
hymen S31.40
  bite — *see* Bite, vulva
  laceration — *see* Laceration, vagina
  puncture — *see* Puncture, vagina
hypochondrium S31.109
  bite — *see* Bite, hypochondrium
  laceration — *see* Laceration, hypochondrium
  puncture — *see* Puncture, hypochondrium
hypogastric region S31.109
  bite — *see* Bite, hypogastric region
  laceration — *see* Laceration, hypogastric region
  puncture — *see* Puncture, hypogastric region
iliac (region) — *see* Wound, open, inguinal region
inguinal region S31.109
  bite — *see* Bite, abdomen, wall, lower quadrant
  laceration — *see* Laceration, inguinal region
  puncture — *see* Puncture, inguinal region
instep — *see* Wound, open, foot

Wound, open — *continued*

interscapular region — *see* Wound, open, thorax, back
intraocular — *see* Wound, open, ocular
iris — *see* Wound, open, ocular
jaw — *see* Wound, open, head, specified site NEC
knee S81.00-
  bite — *see* Bite, knee
  laceration — *see* Laceration, knee
  puncture — *see* Puncture, knee
labium (majus) (minus) — *see* Wound, open, vulva
laceration — *see* Laceration, by site
lacrimal duct — *see* Wound, open, eyelid
larynx S11.019
  bite — *see* Bite, larynx
  laceration — *see* Laceration, larynx
  puncture — *see* Puncture, larynx
left
  lower quadrant S31.104
    with penetration into peritoneal cavity S31.604
    bite — *see* Bite, abdomen, wall, left, lower quadrant
    laceration — *see* Laceration, abdomen, wall, left, lower quadrant
    puncture — *see* Puncture, abdomen, wall, left, lower quadrant
  upper quadrant S31.101
    with penetration into peritoneal cavity S31.601
    bite — *see* Bite, abdomen, wall, left, upper quadrant
    laceration — *see* Laceration, abdomen, wall, left, upper quadrant
    puncture — *see* Puncture, abdomen, wall, left, upper quadrant
leg (lower) S81.80-
  with amputation — *see* Amputation, traumatic, leg
  ankle — *see* Wound, open, ankle
  bite — *see* Bite, leg
  foot — *see* Wound, open, foot
  knee — *see* Wound, open, knee
  laceration — *see* Laceration, leg
  puncture — *see* Puncture, leg
  toe — *see* Wound, open, toe
  upper — *see* Wound, open, thigh
lip S01.501
  bite — *see* Bite, lip
  laceration — *see* Laceration, lip
  puncture — *see* Puncture, lip
loin S31.109
  bite — *see* Bite, abdomen, wall
  laceration — *see* Laceration, loin
  puncture — *see* Puncture, loin
lower back — *see* Wound, open, back, lower
lumbar region — *see* Wound, open, back, lower
malar region — *see* Wound, open, head, specified site NEC
mammary — *see* Wound, open, breast
mastoid region — *see* Wound, open, head, specified site NEC
mouth — *see* Wound, open, oral cavity
nail
  finger — *see* Wound, open, finger, with damage to nail
  toe — *see* Wound, open, toe, with damage to nail
nape (neck) — *see* Wound, open, neck
nasal (septum) (sinus) — *see* Wound, open, nose
nasopharynx — *see* Wound, open, head, specified site NEC

Wound, open — *continued*

neck S11.90
  bite — *see* Bite, neck
  involving
    cervical esophagus S11.20
    larynx — *see* Wound, open, larynx
    pharynx S11.20
    thyroid S11.10
    trachea (cervical) S11.029
      bite — *see* Bite, trachea
      laceration S11.021
        with foreign body S11.022
      puncture S11.023
        with foreign body S11.024
  laceration — *see* Laceration, neck
  puncture — *see* Puncture, neck
  specified site NEC S11.80
  specified type NEC S11.89
nose (septum) (sinus) S01.20
  with amputation — *see* Amputation, traumatic, nose
  bite — *see* Bite, nose
  laceration — *see* Laceration, nose
  puncture — *see* Puncture, nose
ocular S05.90
  avulsion (traumatic enucleation) S05.7-
  eyeball S05.6-
    with foreign body S05.5-
  eyelid — *see* Wound, open, eyelid
  laceration and rupture S05.3-
    with prolapse or loss of intraocular tissue S05.2-
  orbit (penetrating) (with or without foreign body) S05.4-
  periocular area — *see* Wound, open, eyelid
  specified NEC S05.8x-
oral cavity S01.502
  bite S01.552
  laceration — *see* Laceration, oral cavity
  puncture — *see* Puncture, oral cavity
orbit — *see* Wound, open, ocular, orbit
palate — *see* Wound, open, oral cavity
palm — *see* Wound, open, hand
pelvis, pelvic — *see also* Wound, open, back, lower
  girdle — *see* Wound, open, hip
penetrating — *see* Puncture, by site
penis S31.20
  with amputation — *see* Amputation, traumatic, penis
  bite S31.25
  laceration — *see* Laceration, penis
  puncture — *see* Puncture, penis
perineum
  bite — *see* Bite, perineum
  female S31.502
  laceration — *see* Laceration, perineum
  male S31.501
  puncture — *see* Puncture, perineum
periocular area (with or without lacrimal passages) — *see* Wound, open, eyelid
periumbilic region S31.105
  with penetration into peritoneal cavity S31.605
  bite — *see* Bite, abdomen, wall, periumbilic region
  laceration — *see* Laceration, abdomen, wall, periumbilic region
  puncture — *see* Puncture, abdomen, wall, periumbilic region
phalanges
  finger — *see* Wound, open, finger
  toe — *see* Wound, open, toe
pharynx S11.20
pinna — *see* Wound, open, ear
popliteal space — *see* Wound, open, knee
prepuce — *see* Wound, open, penis
pubic region — *see* Wound, open, back, lower

Wound, open — *continued*

pudendum — *see* Wound, open, genital organs, external
puncture wound — *see* Puncture
rectovaginal septum — *see* Wound, open, vagina
right
  lower quadrant S31.103
    with penetration into peritoneal cavity S31.603
    bite — *see* Bite, abdomen, wall, right, lower quadrant
    laceration — *see* Laceration, abdomen, wall, right, lower quadrant
    puncture — *see* Puncture, abdomen, wall, right, lower quadrant
  upper quadrant S31.100
    with penetration into peritoneal cavity S31.600
    bite — *see* Bite, abdomen, wall, right, upper quadrant
    laceration — *see* Laceration, abdomen, wall, right, upper quadrant
    puncture — *see* Puncture, abdomen, wall, right, upper quadrant
sacral region — *see* Wound, open, back, lower
sacroiliac region — *see* Wound, open, back, lower
salivary gland — *see* Wound, open, oral cavity
scalp S01.00
  bite S01.05
  laceration — *see* Laceration, scalp
  puncture — *see* Puncture, scalp
scalpel, newborn (birth injury) P15.8
scapular region — *see* Wound, open, shoulder
sclera — *see* Wound, open, ocular
scrotum S31.30
  with amputation — *see* Amputation, traumatic, scrotum
  bite S31.35
  laceration — *see* Laceration, scrotum
  puncture — *see* Puncture, scrotum
shin — *see* Wound, open, leg
shoulder S41.00-
  with amputation — *see* Amputation, traumatic, arm
  bite — *see* Bite, shoulder
  laceration — *see* Laceration, shoulder
  puncture — *see* Puncture, shoulder
skin NOS T14.8
spermatic cord — *see* Wound, open, testis
sternal region — *see* Wound, open, thorax, front wall
submaxillary region — *see* Wound, open, head, specified site NEC
submental region — *see* Wound, open, head, specified site NEC
subungual
  finger(s) — *see* Wound, open, finger
  toe(s) — *see* Wound, open, toe
supraclavicular region — *see* Wound, open, neck, specified site NEC
temple, temporal region — *see* Wound, open, head, specified site NEC
temporomandibular area — *see* Wound, open, cheek
testis S31.30
  with amputation — *see* Amputation, traumatic, testes
  bite S31.35
  laceration — *see* Laceration, testis
  puncture — *see* Puncture, testis
thigh S71.10-
  with amputation — *see* Amputation, traumatic, hip
  bite — *see* Bite, thigh
  laceration — *see* Laceration, thigh
  puncture — *see* Puncture, thigh

Wound, open — *continued*
  thorax, thoracic (wall) S21.90
    back S21.20-
      with penetration S21.40
    bite — *see* Bite, thorax
    breast — *see* Wound, open, breast
    front S21.10-
      with penetration S21.30
    laceration — *see* Laceration, thorax
    puncture — *see* Puncture, thorax
  throat — *see* Wound, open, neck
  thumb S61.009
    with
      amputation — *see* Amputation, traumatic, thumb
      damage to nail S61.109
    bite — *see* Bite, thumb
    laceration — *see* Laceration, thumb
    left S61.002
      with
        damage to nail S61.102
    puncture — *see* Puncture, thumb
    right S61.001
      with
        damage to nail S61.101
  thyroid (gland) — *see* Wound, open, neck, thyroid
  toe(s) S91.109
    with
      amputation — *see* Amputation, traumatic, toe
      damage to nail S91.209
    bite — *see* Bite, toe
    great S91.103
      with
        damage to nail S91.203
      left S91.102
        with
          damage to nail S91.202
      right S91.101
        with
          damage to nail S91.201
    laceration — *see* Laceration, toe
    lesser S91.106
      with
        damage to nail S91.206
      left S91.105
        with
          damage to nail S91.205
      right S91.104
        with
          damage to nail S91.204
    puncture — *see* Puncture, toe
  tongue — *see* Wound, open, oral cavity
  trachea (cervical region) — *see* Wound, open, neck, trachea
  tunica vaginalis — *see* Wound, open, testis
  tympanum, tympanic membrane S09.2-
    laceration — *see* Laceration, ear, drum
    puncture — *see* Puncture, tympanum
  umbilical region — *see* Wound, open, abdomen, wall, periumbilic region
  uvula — *see* Wound, open, oral cavity
  vagina S31.40
    bite S31.45
    laceration — *see* Laceration, vagina
    puncture — *see* Puncture, vagina
  vitreous (humor) — *see* Wound, open, ocular
  vocal cord S11.039
    bite — *see* Bite, vocal cord
    laceration S11.031
      with foreign body S11.032
    puncture S11.033
      with foreign body S11.034

Wound, open — *continued*
  vulva S31.40
    with amputation — *see* Amputation, traumatic, vulva
    bite S31.45
    laceration — *see* Laceration, vulva
    puncture — *see* Puncture, vulva
  wrist S61.50-
    bite — *see* Bite, wrist
    laceration — *see* Laceration, wrist
    puncture — *see* Puncture, wrist
Wound, superficial — *see* Injury — *see also* specified injury type
Wright's syndrome G54.0
Wrist — *see* condition
Wrong drug (by accident) (given in error) — *see* Table of Drugs and Chemicals, by drug, poisoning
Wry neck — *see* Torticollis
Wuchereria (bancrofti) infestation B74.0
Wuchereriasis B74.0
Wuchernde Struma Langhans C73

X

X-ray (of)
  abnormal findings — *see* Abnormal, diagnostic imaging
  breast (mammogram) (routine) Z12.31
  chest
    routine (as part of a general medical examination) Z00.00
      with abnormal findings Z00.01
  routine (as part of a general medical examination) Z00.00
    with abnormal findings Z00.01
Xanthelasma (eyelid) (palpebrarum) H02.60
  left H02.66
    lower H02.65
    upper H02.64
  right H02.63
    lower H02.62
    upper H02.61
Xanthelasmatosis (essential) E78.2
Xanthinuria, hereditary E79.8
Xanthoastrocytoma
  specified site — *see* Neoplasm, malignant, by site
  unspecified site C71.9
Xanthofibroma — *see* Neoplasm, connective tissue, benign
Xanthogranuloma D76.3
Xanthoma(s), xanthomatosis (primary) (familial) (hereditary) E75.5
  with
    hyperlipoproteinemia
      Type I E78.3
      Type III E78.2
      Type IV E78.1
      Type V E78.3
  bone (generalisata) C96.5
  cerebrotendinous E75.5
  cutaneotendinous E75.5
  disseminatum (skin) E78.2
  eruptive E78.2
  hypercholesterinemic E78.00
  hypercholesterolemic E78.00
  hyperlipidemic E78.5
  joint E75.5
  multiple (skin) E78.2
  tendon (sheath) E75.5
  tuberosum E78.2
  tuberous E78.2
  tubo-eruptive E78.2
  verrucous, oral mucosa K13.4
Xanthosis R23.8
Xenophobia F40.10
Xeroderma — *see also* Ichthyosis
  acquired L85.0
    eyelid H01.149
      left H01.146
        lower H01.145
        upper H01.144
      right H01.143
        lower H01.142
        upper H01.141
  pigmentosum Q82.1
  vitamin A deficiency E50.8
Xerophthalmia (vitamin A deficiency) E50.7
  unrelated to vitamin A deficiency — *see* Keratoconjunctivitis

DISEASE INDEX

Xerosis
conjunctiva H11.14-
with Bitot's spots — *see also* Pigmentation,
conjunctiva
vitamin A deficiency E50.1
vitamin A deficiency E50.0
cornea H18.89-
with ulceration — *see* Ulcer, cornea
vitamin A deficiency E50.3
vitamin A deficiency E50.2
cutis L85.3
skin L85.3
Xerostomia K11.7
Xiphopagus Q89.4
XO syndrome Q96.9
XXXXY syndrome Q98.1
XXY syndrome Q98.0

Y

Yaba pox (virus disease) B08.72
Yatapoxvirus B08.70
specified NEC B08.79
Yawning R06.89
psychogenic F45.8
Yaws A66.9
bone lesions A66.6
butter A66.1
chancre A66.0
cutaneous, less than five years after infection
A66.2
early (cutaneous) (macular) (maculopapular)
(micropapular) (papular) A66.2
frambeside A66.2
skin lesions NEC A66.2
eyelid A66.2
ganglion A66.6
gangosis, gangosa A66.5
gumma, gummata A66.4
bone A66.6
gummatous
frambeside A66.4
osteitis A66.6
periostitis A66.6
hydrarthrosis (*see also* subcategory M14.8-)
A66.6
hyperkeratosis (early) (late) A66.3
initial lesions A66.0
joint lesions (*see also* subcategory M14.8-)
A66.6
juxta-articular nodules A66.7
late nodular (ulcerated) A66.4
latent (without clinical manifestations) (with
positive serology) A66.8
mother A66.0
mucosal A66.7
multiple papillomata A66.1
nodular, late (ulcerated) A66.4
osteitis A66.6
papilloma, plantar or palmar A66.1
periostitis (hypertrophic) A66.6
specified NEC A66.7
ulcers A66.4
wet crab A66.1
Yeast infection (*see also* Candidiasis) B37.9
Yellow
atrophy (liver) — *see* Failure, hepatic
fever — *see* Fever, yellow
jack — *see* Fever, yellow
jaundice — *see* Jaundice
nail syndrome L60.5
Yersiniosis — *see also* Infection, Yersinia
extraintestinal A28.2
intestinal A04.6

Z

Zahorsky's syndrome (herpangina) B08.5
Zellweger's syndrome Q87.89
Zenker's diverticulum (esophagus) K22.5
Ziehen-Oppenheim disease G24.1
Zieve's syndrome K70.0
Zika NOS A92.5
Zinc
deficiency, dietary E60
metabolism disorder E83.2
Zollinger-Ellison syndrome E16.4
Zona — *see* Herpes, zoster
Zoophobia F40.218
Zoster (herpes) — *see* Herpes, zoster
Zygomycosis B46.9
specified NEC B46.8
Zymotic — *see* condition

DRUGS & CHEMICALS

Table of Drugs & Chemicals	Accidental (Unintentional)	Self-Harm (Intentional)	Assault	Undetermined	Adverse Effect	Underdosing
14-hydroxydihydro-morphinone	T40.2x1-	T40.2x2-	T40.2x3-	T40.2x4-	T40.2x5-	T40.2x6-
1-propanol	T51.3x1-	T51.3x2-	T51.3x3-	T51.3x4-	—	—
2,4,5-T (trichloro-phenoxyacetic acid)	T60.1x1-	T60.1x2-	T60.1x3-	T60.1x4-	—	—
2,4-D (dichlorophen-oxyacetic acid)	T60.3x1-	T60.3x2-	T60.3x3-	T60.3x4-	—	—
2,4-toluene diisocyanate	T65.0x1-	T65.0x2-	T65.0x3-	T65.0x4-	—	—
2-propanol	T51.2x1-	T51.2x2-	T51.2x3-	T51.2x4-	—	—
ABOB	T37.5x1-	T37.5x2-	T37.5x3-	T37.5x4-	T37.5x5-	T37.5x6-
Abrine	T62.2x1-	T62.2x2-	T62.2x3-	T62.2x4-	—	—
Abrus (seed)	T62.2x1-	T62.2x2-	T62.2x3-	T62.2x4-	—	—
Absinthe	T51.0x1-	T51.0x2-	T51.0x3-	T51.0x4-	—	—
beverage	T51.0x1-	T51.0x2-	T51.0x3-	T51.0x4-	—	—
Acaricide	T60.8x1-	T60.8x2-	T60.8x3-	T60.8x4-	—	—
Acebutolol	T44.7x1-	T44.7x2-	T44.7x3-	T44.7x4-	T44.7x5-	T44.7x6-
Acecarbromal	T42.6x1-	T42.6x2-	T42.6x3-	T42.6x4-	T42.6x5-	T42.6x6-
Aceclidine	T44.1x1-	T44.1x2-	T44.1x3-	T44.1x4-	T44.1x5-	T44.1x6-
Acedapsone	T37.0x1-	T37.0x2-	T37.0x3-	T37.0x4-	T37.0x5-	T37.0x6-
Acefylline piperazine	T48.6x1-	T48.6x2-	T48.6x3-	T48.6x4-	T48.6x5-	T48.6x6-
Acemorphan	T40.2x1-	T40.2x2-	T40.2x3-	T40.2x4-	T40.2x5-	T40.2x6-
Acenocoumarin	T45.511-	T45.512-	T45.513-	T45.514-	T45.515-	T45.516-
Acenocoumarol	T45.511-	T45.512-	T45.513-	T45.514-	T45.515-	T45.516-
Acepifylline	T48.6x1-	T48.6x2-	T48.6x3-	T48.6x4-	T48.6x5-	T48.6x6-
Acepromazine	T43.3x1-	T43.3x2-	T43.3x3-	T43.3x4-	T43.3x5-	T43.3x6-
Acesulfamethoxypyridazine	T37.0x1-	T37.0x2-	T37.0x3-	T37.0x4-	T37.0x5-	T37.0x6-
Acetal	T52.8x1-	T52.8x2-	T52.8x3-	T52.8x4-	—	—
Acetaldehyde (vapor)	T52.8x1-	T52.8x2-	T52.8x3-	T52.8x4-	—	—
liquid	T65.891-	T65.892-	T65.893-	T65.894-	—	—
P-Acetamidophenol	T39.1x1-	T39.1x2-	T39.1x3-	T39.1x4-	T39.1x5-	T39.1x6-
Acetaminophen	T39.1x1-	T39.1x2-	T39.1x3-	T39.1x4-	T39.1x5-	T39.1x6-
Acetaminosalol	T39.1x1-	T39.1x2-	T39.1x3-	T39.1x4-	T39.1x5-	T39.1x6-
Acetanilide	T39.1x1-	T39.1x2-	T39.1x3-	T39.1x4-	T39.1x5-	T39.1x6-
Acetarsol	T37.3x1-	T37.3x2-	T37.3x3-	T37.3x4-	T37.3x5-	T37.3x6-
Acetazolamide	T50.2x1-	T50.2x2-	T50.2x3-	T50.2x4-	T50.2x5-	T50.2x6-
Acetiamine	T45.2x1-	T45.2x2-	T45.2x3-	T45.2x4-	T45.2x5-	T45.2x6-
Acetic						
acid	T54.2x1-	T54.2x2-	T54.2x3-	T54.2x4-	—	—
with sodium acetate (ointment)	T49.3x1-	T49.3x2-	T49.3x3-	T49.3x4-	T49.3x5-	T49.3x6-
ester (solvent) (vapor)	T52.8x1-	T52.8x2-	T52.8x3-	T52.8x4-	—	—
irrigating solution	T50.3x1-	T50.3x2-	T50.3x3-	T50.3x4-	T50.3x5-	T50.3x6-
medicinal (lotion)	T49.2x1-	T49.2x2-	T49.2x3-	T49.2x4-	T49.2x5-	T49.2x6-
anhydride	T65.891-	T65.892-	T65.893-	T65.894-	—	—
ether (vapor)	T52.8x1-	T52.8x2-	T52.8x3-	T52.8x4-	—	—
Acetohexamide	T38.3x1-	T38.3x2-	T38.3x3-	T38.3x4-	T38.3x5-	T38.3x6-
Acetohydroxamic acid	T50.991-	T50.992-	T50.993-	T50.994-	T50.995-	T50.996-
Acetomenaphthone	T45.7x1-	T45.7x2-	T45.7x3-	T45.7x4-	T45.7x5-	T45.7x6-
Acetomorphine	T40.1x1-	T40.1x2-	T40.1x3-	T40.1x4-	—	—
Acetone (oils)	T52.4x1-	T52.4x2-	T52.4x3-	T52.4x4-	—	—
chlorinated	T52.4x1-	T52.4x2-	T52.4x3-	T52.4x4-	—	—
vapor	T52.4x1-	T52.4x2-	T52.4x3-	T52.4x4-	—	—
Acetonitrile	T52.8x1-	T52.8x2-	T52.8x3-	T52.8x4-	—	—
Acetophenazine	T43.3x1-	T43.3x2-	T43.3x3-	T43.3x4-	T43.3x5-	T43.3x6-
Acetophenetedin	T39.1x1-	T39.1x2-	T39.1x3-	T39.1x4-	T39.1x5-	T39.1x6-
Acetophenone	T52.4x1-	T52.4x2-	T52.4x3-	T52.4x4-	—	—
Acetorphine	T40.2x1-	T40.2x2-	T40.2x3-	T40.2x4-	—	—
Acetosulfone (sodium)	T37.1x1-	T37.1x2-	T37.1x3-	T37.1x4-	T37.1x5-	T37.1x6-
Acetrizoate (sodium)	T50.8x1-	T50.8x2-	T50.8x3-	T50.8x4-	T50.8x5-	T50.8x6-
Acetrizoic acid	T50.8x1-	T50.8x2-	T50.8x3-	T50.8x4-	T50.8x5-	T50.8x6-
Acetyl						
bromide	T53.6x1-	T53.6x2-	T53.6x3-	T53.6x4-	—	—
chloride	T53.6x1-	T53.6x2-	T53.6x3-	T53.6x4-	—	—

Table of Drugs & Chemicals	Accidental (Unintentional)	Self-Harm (Intentional)	Assault	Undetermined	Adverse Effect	Underdosing
Acetylcarbromal	T42.6x1-	T42.6x2-	T42.6x3-	T42.6x4-	T42.6x5-	T42.6x6-
Acetylcholine						
chloride	T44.1x1-	T44.1x2-	T44.1x3-	T44.1x4-	T44.1x5-	T44.1x6-
derivative	T44.1x1-	T44.1x2-	T44.1x3-	T44.1x4-	T44.1x5-	T44.1x6-
Acetylcysteine	T48.4x1-	T48.4x2-	T48.4x3-	T48.4x4-	T48.4x5-	T48.4x6-
Acetyldigitoxin	T46.0x1-	T46.0x2-	T46.0x3-	T46.0x4-	T46.0x5-	T46.0x6-
Acetyldigoxin	T46.0x1-	T46.0x2-	T46.0x3-	T46.0x4-	T46.0x5-	T46.0x6-
Acetyldihydrocodeine	T40.2x1-	T40.2x2-	T40.2x3-	T40.2x4-	—	—
Acetyldihydrocodeinone	T40.2x1-	T40.2x2-	T40.2x3-	T40.2x4-	—	—
Acetylene (gas)	T59.891-	T59.892-	T59.893-	T59.894-	—	—
dichloride	T53.6x1-	T53.6x2-	T53.6x3-	T53.6x4-	—	—
incomplete combustion of	T58.11x-	T58.12x-	T58.13x-	T58.14x-	—	—
industrial	T59.891-	T59.892-	T59.893-	T59.894-	—	—
tetrachloride	T53.6x1-	T53.6x2-	T53.6x3-	T53.6x4-	—	—
vapor	T53.6x1-	T53.6x2-	T53.6x3-	T53.6x4-	—	—
Acetylpheneturide	T42.6x1-	T42.6x2-	T42.6x3-	T42.6x4-	T42.6x5-	T42.6x6-
Acetylphenylhydrazine	T39.8x1-	T39.8x2-	T39.8x3-	T39.8x4-	T39.8x5-	T39.8x6-
Acetylsalicylic acid (salts)	T39.011-	T39.012-	T39.013-	T39.014-	T39.015-	T39.016-
enteric coated	T39.011-	T39.012-	T39.013-	T39.014-	T39.015-	T39.016-
Acetylsulfamethoxypyrida-zine	T37.0x1-	T37.0x2-	T37.0x3-	T37.0x4-	T37.0x5-	T37.0x6-
Achromycin	T36.4x1-	T36.4x2-	T36.4x3-	T36.4x4-	T36.4x5-	T36.4x6-
ophthalmic preparation	T49.5x1-	T49.5x2-	T49.5x3-	T49.5x4-	T49.5x5-	T49.5x6-
topical NEC	T49.0x1-	T49.0x2-	T49.0x3-	T49.0x4-	T49.0x5-	T49.0x6-
Aciclovir	T37.5x1-	T37.5x2-	T37.5x3-	T37.5x4-	T37.5x5-	T37.5x6
Acid (corrosive) NEC	T54.2x1-	T54.2x2-	T54.2x3-	T54.2x4-	—	—
Acidifying agent NEC	T50.901-	T50.902-	T50.903-	T50.904-	T50.905-	T50.906-
Acipimox	T46.6x1-	T46.6x2-	T46.6x3-	T46.6x4-	T46.6x5-	T46.6x6-
Acitretin	T50.991-	T50.992-	T50.993-	T50.994-	T50.995-	T50.996-
Aclarubicin	T45.1x1-	T45.1x2-	T45.1x3-	T45.1x4-	T45.1x5-	T45.1x6-
Aclatonium napadisilate	T48.1x1-	T48.1x2-	T48.1x3-	T48.1x4-	T48.1x5-	T48.1x6-
Aconite (wild)	T46.991-	T46.992-	T46.993-	T46.994-	T46.995-	T46.996-
Aconitine	T46.991-	T46.992-	T46.993-	T46.994-	T46.995-	T46.996-
Aconitum ferox	T46.991-	T46.992-	T46.993-	T46.994-	T46.995-	T46.996-
Acridine	T65.6x1-	T65.6x2-	T65.6x3-	T65.6x4-	—	—
vapor	T59.891-	T59.892-	T59.893-	T59.894-	—	—
Acriflavine	T37.91x-	T37.92x-	T37.93x-	T37.94x-	T37.95x-	T37.96x-
Acriflavinium chloride	T49.0x1-	T49.0x2-	T49.0x3-	T49.0x4-	T49.0x5-	T49.0x6-
Acrinol	T49.0x1-	T49.0x2-	T49.0x3-	T49.0x4-	T49.0x5-	T49.0x6-
Acrisorcin	T49.0x1-	T49.0x2-	T49.0x3-	T49.0x4-	T49.0x5-	T49.0x6-
Acrivastine	T45.0x1-	T45.0x2-	T45.0x3-	T45.0x4-	T45.0x5-	T45.0x6-
Acrolein (gas)	T59.891-	T59.892-	T59.893-	T59.894-	—	—
liquid	T54.1x1-	T54.1x2-	T54.1x3-	T54.1x4-	—	—
Acrylamide	T65.891-	T65.892-	T65.893-	T65.894-	—	—
Acrylic resin	T49.3x1-	T49.3x2-	T49.3x3-	T49.3x4-	T49.3x5-	T49.3x6-
Acrylonitrile	T65.891-	T65.892-	T65.893-	T65.894-	—	—
Actaea spicata	T62.2x1-	T62.2x2-	T62.2x3-	T62.2x4-	—	—
berry	T62.1x1-	T62.1x2-	T62.1x3-	T62.1x4-	—	—
Acterol	T37.3x1-	T37.3x2-	T37.3x3-	T37.3x4-	T37.3x5-	T37.3x6-
ACTH	T38.811-	T38.812-	T38.813-	T38.814-	T38.815-	T38.816-
Actinomycin C	T45.1x1-	T45.1x2-	T45.1x3-	T45.1x4-	T45.1x5-	T45.1x6-
Actinomycin D	T45.1x1-	T45.1x2-	T45.1x3-	T45.1x4-	T45.1x5-	T45.1x6-
Activated charcoal — see also Charcoal,						
medicinal	T47.6x1-	T47.6x2-	T47.6x3-	T47.6x4-	T47.6x5-	T47.6x6-
Acyclovir	T37.5x1-	T37.5x2-	T37.5x3-	T37.5x4-	T37.5x5-	T37.5x6-
Adenine	T45.2x1-	T45.2x2-	T45.2x3-	T45.2x4-	T45.2x5-	T45.2x6-
arabinoside	T37.5x1-	T37.5x2-	T37.5x3-	T37.5x4-	T37.5x5-	T37.5x6-
Adenosine (phosphate)	T46.2x1-	T46.2x2-	T46.2x3-	T46.2x4-	T46.2x5-	T46.2x6-
ADH	T38.891-	T38.892-	T38.893-	T38.894-	T38.895-	T38.896-
Adhesive NEC	T65.891-	T65.892-	T65.893-	T65.894-	—	—
Adicillin	T36.0x1-	T36.0x2-	T36.0x3-	T36.0x4-	T36.0x5-	T36.0x6-

Table of Drugs & Chemicals	POISONING Accidental (Unintentional)	Self-Harm (Intentional)	Assault	Undetermined	Adverse Effect	Underdosing
Adiphenine	T44.3x1-	T44.3x2-	T44.3x3-	T44.3x4-	T44.3x5-	T44.3x6-
Adipiodone	T50.8x1-	T50.8x2-	T50.8x3-	T50.8x4-	T50.8x5-	T50.8x6-
Adjunct, pharmaceutical	T50.901-	T50.902-	T50.903-	T50.904-	T50.905-	T50.906-
Adrenal (extract, cortex or medulla) (glucocorticoids) (hormones) (mineralocorticoids)	T38.0x1-	T38.0x2-	T38.0x3-	T38.0x4-	T38.0x5-	T38.0x6-
ENT agent	T49.6x1-	T49.6x2-	T49.6x3-	T49.6x4-	T49.6x5-	T49.6x6-
ophthalmic preparation	T49.5x1-	T49.5x2-	T49.5x3-	T49.5x4-	T49.5x5-	T49.5x6-
topical NEC	T49.0x1-	T49.0x2-	T49.0x3-	T49.0x4-	T49.0x5-	T49.0x6-
Adrenaline	T44.5x1-	T44.5x2-	T44.5x3-	T44.5x4-	T44.5x5-	T44.5x6-
Adrenalin − see Adrenaline						
Adrenergic NEC	T44.901-	T44.902-	T44.903-	T44.904-	T44.905-	T44.906-
blocking agent NEC	T44.8x1-	T44.8x2-	T44.8x3-	T44.8x4-	T44.8x5-	T44.8x6-
beta, heart	T44.7x1-	T44.7x2-	T44.7x3-	T44.7x4-	T44.7x5-	T44.7x6-
specified NEC	T44.991-	T44.992-	T44.993-	T44.994-	T44.995-	T44.996-
Adrenochrome						
derivative	T46.991-	T46.992-	T46.993-	T46.994-	T46.995-	T46.996-
(mono) semicarbazone	T46.991-	T46.992-	T46.993-	T46.994-	T46.995-	T46.996-
Adrenocorticotrophic						
hormone	T38.811-	T38.812-	T38.813-	T38.814-	T38.815-	T38.816-
Adrenocorticotrophin	T38.811-	T38.812-	T38.813-	T38.814-	T38.815-	T38.816-
Adriamycin	T45.1x1-	T45.1x2-	T45.1x3-	T45.1x4-	T45.1x5-	T45.1x6-
Aerosol spray NEC	T65.91x-	T65.92x-	T65.93x-	T65.94x-	—	—
Aerosporin	T36.8x1-	T36.8x2-	T36.8x3-	T36.8x4-	T36.8x5-	T36.8x6-
ENT agent	T49.6x1-	T49.6x2-	T49.6x3-	T49.6x4-	T49.6x5-	T49.6x6-
ophthalmic preparation	T49.5x1-	T49.5x2-	T49.5x3-	T49.5x4-	T49.5x5-	T49.5x6-
topical NEC	T49.0x1-	T49.0x2-	T49.0x3-	T49.0x4-	T49.0x5-	T49.0x6-
Aethusa cynapium	T62.2x1-	T62.2x2-	T62.2x3-	T62.2x4-	—	—
Afghanistan black	T40.7x1-	T40.7x2-	T40.7x3-	T40.7x4-	T40.7x5-	T40.7x6-
Aflatoxin	T64.01x-	T64.02x-	T64.03x-	T64.04x-	—	—
Afloqualone	T42.8x1-	T42.8x2-	T42.8x3-	T42.8x4-	T42.8x5-	T42.8x6-
African boxwood	T62.2x1-	T62.2x2-	T62.2x3-	T62.2x4-	—	—
Agar	T47.4x1-	T47.4x2-	T47.4x3-	T47.4x4-	T47.4x5-	T47.4x6-
Agonist						
predominantly						
alpha-adrenoreceptor	T44.4x1-	T44.4x2-	T44.4x3-	T44.4x4-	T44.4x5-	T44.4x6-
beta-adrenoreceptor	T44.5x1-	T44.5x2-	T44.5x3-	T44.5x4-	T44.5x5-	T44.5x6-
Agricultural agent NEC	T65.91x-	T65.92x-	T65.93x-	T65.94x-	—	—
Agrypnal	T42.3x1-	T42.3x2-	T42.3x3-	T42.3x4-	T42.3x5-	T42.3x6-
AHLG	T50.Z11-	T50.Z12-	T50.Z13-	T50.Z14-	T50.Z15-	T50.Z16-
Air contaminant(s), source/type NOS	T65.91x-	T65.92x-	T65.93x-	T65.94x-	—	—
Ajmaline	T46.2x1-	T46.2x2-	T46.2x3-	T46.2x4-	T46.2x5-	T46.2x6-
Akee	T62.1x1-	T62.1x2-	T62.1x3-	T62.1x4-	—	—
Akrinol	T49.0x1-	T49.0x2-	T49.0x3-	T49.0x4-	T49.0x5-	T49.0x6-
Akritoin	T37.8x1-	T37.8x2-	T37.8x3-	T37.8x4-	T37.8x5-	T37.8x6-
Alacepril	T46.4x1-	T46.4x2-	T46.4x3-	T46.4x4-	T46.4x5-	T46.4x6-
Alantolactone	T37.4x1-	T37.4x2-	T37.4x3-	T37.4x4-	T37.4x5-	T37.4x6-
Albamycin	T36.8x1-	T36.8x2-	T36.8x3-	T36.8x4-	T36.8x5-	T36.8x6-
Albendazole	T37.4x1-	T37.4x2-	T37.4x3-	T37.4x4-	T37.4x5-	T37.4x6-
Albumin						
bovine	T45.8x1-	T45.8x2-	T45.8x3-	T45.8x4-	T45.8x5-	T45.8x6-
human serum	T45.8x1-	T45.8x2-	T45.8x3-	T45.8x4-	T45.8x5-	T45.8x6-
salt-poor	T45.8x1-	T45.8x2-	T45.8x3-	T45.8x4-	T45.8x5-	T45.8x6-
normal human serum	T45.8x1-	T45.8x2-	T45.8x3-	T45.8x4-	T45.8x5-	T45.8x6-
Albuterol	T48.6x1-	T48.6x2-	T48.6x3-	T48.6x4-	T48.6x5-	T48.6x6-
Albutoin	T42.0x1-	T42.0x2-	T42.0x3-	T42.0x4-	T42.0x5-	T42.0x6-
Alclometasone	T49.0x1-	T49.0x2-	T49.0x3-	T49.0x4-	T49.0x5-	T49.0x6-
Alcohol	T51.91x-	T51.92x-	T51.93x-	T51.94x-	—	—
absolute	T51.0x1-	T51.0x2-	T51.0x3-	T51.0x4-	—	—
beverage	T51.0x1-	T51.0x2-	T51.0x3-	T51.0x4-	—	—
allyl	T51.8x1-	T51.8x2-	T51.8x3-	T51.8x4-	—	—
antifreeze	T51.1x1-	T51.1x2-	T51.1x3-	T51.1x4-	—	—

Table of Drugs & Chemicals	POISONING Accidental (Unintentional)	Self-Harm (Intentional)	Assault	Undetermined	Adverse Effect	Underdosing
Alcohol - continued	T51.91x-	T51.92x-	T51.93x-	T51.94x-	—	—
amyl	T51.3x1-	T51.3x2-	T51.3x3-	T51.3x4-	—	—
beverage	T51.0x1-	T51.0x2-	T51.0x3-	T51.0x4-	—	—
butyl	T51.3x1-	T51.3x2-	T51.3x3-	T51.3x4-	—	—
dehydrated	T51.0x1-	T51.0x2-	T51.0x3-	T51.0x4-	—	—
beverage	T51.0x1-	T51.0x2-	T51.0x3-	T51.0x4-	—	—
denatured	T51.0x1-	T51.0x2-	T51.0x3-	T51.0x4-	—	—
deterrent NEC	T50.6x1-	T50.6x2-	T50.6x3-	T50.6x4-	T50.6x5-	T50.6x6-
diagnostic (gastric function)	T50.8x1-	T50.8x2-	T50.8x3-	T50.8x4-	T50.8x5-	T50.8x6-
ethyl	T51.0x1-	T51.0x2-	T51.0x3-	T51.0x4-	—	—
beverage	T51.0x1-	T51.0x2-	T51.0x3-	T51.0x4-	—	—
grain	T51.0x1-	T51.0x2-	T51.0x3-	T51.0x4-	—	—
beverage	T51.0x1-	T51.0x2-	T51.0x3-	T51.0x4-	—	—
industrial	T51.0x1-	T51.0x2-	T51.0x3-	T51.0x4-	—	—
isopropyl	T51.2x1-	T51.2x2-	T51.2x3-	T51.2x4-	—	—
methyl	T51.1x1-	T51.1x2-	T51.1x3-	T51.1x4-	—	—
preparation for consumption	T51.0x1-	T51.0x2-	T51.0x3-	T51.0x4-	—	—
propyl	T51.3x1-	T51.3x2-	T51.3x3-	T51.3x4-	—	—
secondary	T51.2x1-	T51.2x2-	T51.2x3-	T51.2x4-	—	—
radiator	T51.1x1-	T51.1x2-	T51.1x3-	T51.1x4-	—	—
rubbing	T51.2x1-	T51.2x2-	T51.2x3-	T51.2x4-	—	—
specified type NEC	T51.8x1-	T51.8x2-	T51.8x3-	T51.8x4-	—	—
surgical	T51.0x1-	T51.0x2-	T51.0x3-	T51.0x4-	—	—
vapor (from any type of alcohol)	T59.891-	T59.892-	T59.893-	T59.894-	—	—
wood	T51.1x1-	T51.1x2-	T51.1x3-	T51.1x4-	—	—
Alcuronium (chloride)	T48.1x1-	T48.1x2-	T48.1x3-	T48.1x4-	T48.1x5-	T48.1x6-
Aldactone	T50.0x1-	T50.0x2-	T50.0x3-	T50.0x4-	T50.0x5-	T50.0x6-
Aldesulfone sodium	T37.1x1-	T37.1x2-	T37.1x3-	T37.1x4-	T37.1x5-	T37.1x6-
Aldicarb	T60.0x1-	T60.0x2-	T60.0x3-	T60.0x4-	—	—
Aldomet	T46.5x1-	T46.5x2-	T46.5x3-	T46.5x4-	T46.5x5-	T46.5x6-
Aldosterone	T50.0x1-	T50.0x2-	T50.0x3-	T50.0x4-	T50.0x5-	T50.0x6-
Aldrin (dust)	T60.1x1-	T60.1x2-	T60.1x3-	T60.1x4-	—	—
Aleve — see Naproxen						
Alexitol sodium	T47.1x1-	T47.1x2-	T47.1x3-	T47.1x4-	T47.1x5-	T47.1x6-
Alfacalcidol	T45.2x1-	T45.2x2-	T45.2x3-	T45.2x4-	T45.2x5-	T45.2x6-
Alfadolone	T41.1x1-	T41.1x2-	T41.1x3-	T41.1x4-	T41.1x5-	T41.1x6-
Alfaxalone	T41.1x1-	T41.1x2-	T41.1x3-	T41.1x4-	T41.1x5-	T41.1x6-
Alfentanil	T40.4x1-	T40.4x2-	T40.4x3-	T40.4x4-	T40.4x5-	T40.4x6-
Alfuzosin (hydrochloride)	T44.8x1-	T44.8x2-	T44.8x3-	T44.8x4-	T44.8x5-	T44.8x6-
Algae (harmful) (toxin)	T65.821-	T65.822-	T65.823-	T65.824-	—	—
Algeldrate	T47.1x1-	T47.1x2-	T47.1x3-	T47.1x4-	T47.1x5-	T47.1x6-
Algin	T47.8x1-	T47.8x2-	T47.8x3-	T47.8x4-	T47.8x5-	T47.8x6-
Alglucerase	T45.3x1-	T45.3x2-	T45.3x3-	T45.3x4-	T45.3x5-	T45.3x6-
Alidase	T45.3x1-	T45.3x2-	T45.3x3-	T45.3x4-	T45.3x5-	T45.3x6-
Alimemazine	T43.3x1-	T43.3x2-	T43.3x3-	T43.3x4-	T43.3x5-	T43.3x6-
Aliphatic thiocyanates	T65.0x1-	T65.0x2-	T65.0x3-	T65.0x4-	—	—
Alizapride	T45.0x1-	T45.0x2-	T45.0x3-	T45.0x4-	T45.0x5-	T45.0x6-
Alkali (caustic)	T54.3x1-	T54.3x2-	T54.3x3-	T54.3x4-	—	—
Alkaline antiseptic solution (aromatic)	T49.6x1-	T49.6x2-	T49.6x3-	T49.6x4-	T49.6x5-	T49.6x6-
Alkalinizing agents (medicinal)	T50.901-	T50.902-	T50.903-	T50.904-	T50.905-	T50.906-
Alkalizing agent NEC	T50.901-	T50.902-	T50.903-	T50.904-	T50.905-	T50.906-
Alka-seltzer	T39.011-	T39.012-	T39.013-	T39.014-	T39.015-	T39.016-
Alkavervir	T46.5x1-	T46.5x2-	T46.5x3-	T46.5x4-	T46.5x5-	T46.5x6-
Alkonium (bromide)	T49.0x1-	T49.0x2-	T49.0x3-	T49.0x4-	T49.0x5-	T49.0x6-
Alkylating drug NEC	T45.1x1-	T45.1x2-	T45.1x3-	T45.1x4-	T45.1x5-	T45.1x6-
antimyeloproliferative	T45.1x1-	T45.1x2-	T45.1x3-	T45.1x4-	T45.1x5-	T45.1x6-
lymphatic	T45.1x1-	T45.1x2-	T45.1x3-	T45.1x4-	T45.1x5-	T45.1x6-
Alkylisocyanate	T65.0x1-	T65.0x2-	T65.0x3-	T65.0x4-	—	—
Allantoin	T49.4x1-	T49.4x2-	T49.4x3-	T49.4x4-	T49.4x5-	T49.4x6-
Allegron	T43.011-	T43.012-	T43.013-	T43.014-	T43.015-	T43.016-

DRUGS & CHEMICALS

Table of Drugs & Chemicals	Accidental (Unintentional)	Self-Harm (Intentional)	Assault	Undetermined	Adverse Effect	Underdosing
Allethrin	T49.0x1-	T49.0x2-	T49.0x3-	T49.0x4-	T49.0x5-	T49.0x6-
Allobarbital	T42.3x1-	T42.3x2-	T42.3x3-	T42.3x4-	T42.3x5-	T42.3x6-
Allopurinol	T50.4x1-	T50.4x2-	T50.4x3-	T50.4x4-	T50.4x5-	T50.4x6-
Allyl						
alcohol	T51.8x1-	T51.8x2-	T51.8x3-	T51.8x4-	—	—
disulfide	T46.6x1-	T46.6x2-	T46.6x3-	T46.6x4-	T46.6x5-	T46.6x6-
Allylestrenol	T38.5x1-	T38.5x2-	T38.5x3-	T38.5x4-	T38.5x5-	T38.5x6-
Allylisopropylacetylurea	T42.6x1-	T42.6x2-	T42.6x3-	T42.6x4-	T42.6x5-	T42.6x6-
Allylisopropylmalonylurea	T42.3x1-	T42.3x2-	T42.3x3-	T42.3x4-	T42.3x5-	T42.3x6-
Allylthiourea	T49.3x1-	T49.3x2-	T49.3x3-	T49.3x4-	T49.3x5-	T49.3x6-
Allyltribromide	T42.6x1-	T42.6x2-	T42.6x3-	T42.6x4-	T42.6x5-	T42.6x6-
Allypropymal	T42.3x1-	T42.3x2-	T42.3x3-	T42.3x4-	T42.3x5-	T42.3x6-
Almagate	T47.1x1-	T47.1x2-	T47.1x3-	T47.1x4-	T47.1x5-	T47.1x6-
Almasilate	T47.1x1-	T47.1x2-	T47.1x3-	T47.1x4-	T47.1x5-	T47.1x6-
Almitrine	T50.7x1-	T50.7x2-	T50.7x3-	T50.7x4-	T50.7x5-	T50.7x6-
Aloes	T47.2x1-	T47.2x2-	T47.2x3-	T47.2x4-	T47.2x5-	T47.2x6-
Aloglutamol	T47.1x1-	T47.1x2-	T47.1x3-	T47.1x4-	T47.1x5-	T47.1x6-
Aloin	T47.2x1-	T47.2x2-	T47.2x3-	T47.2x4-	T47.2x5-	T47.2x6-
Aloxidone	T42.2x1-	T42.2x2-	T42.2x3-	T42.2x4-	T42.2x5-	T42.2x6-
Alpha						
acetyldigoxin	T46.0x1-	T46.0x2-	T46.0x3-	T46.0x4-	T46.0x5-	T46.0x6-
adrenergic blocking drug	T44.6x1-	T44.6x2-	T44.6x3-	T44.6x4-	T44.6x5-	T44.6x6-
amylase	T45.3x1-	T45.3x2-	T45.3x3-	T45.3x4-	T45.3x5-	T45.3x6-
tocoferol (acetate)	T45.2x1-	T45.2x2-	T45.2x3-	T45.2x4-	T45.2x5-	T45.2x6-
Alphadolone	T41.1x1-	T41.1x2-	T41.1x3-	T41.1x4-	T41.1x5-	T41.1x6-
Alphaprodine	T40.4x1-	T40.4x2-	T40.4x3-	T40.4x4-	T40.4x5-	T40.4x6-
Alphaxalone	T41.1x1-	T41.1x2-	T41.1x3-	T41.1x4-	T41.1x5-	T41.1x6-
Alprazolam	T42.4x1-	T42.4x2-	T42.4x3-	T42.4x4-	T42.4x5-	T42.4x6-
Alprenolol	T44.7x1-	T44.7x2-	T44.7x3-	T44.7x4-	T44.7x5-	T44.7x6-
Alprostadil	T46.7x1-	T46.7x2-	T46.7x3-	T46.7x4-	T46.7x5-	T46.7x6-
Alsactide	T38.811-	T38.812-	T38.813-	T38.814-	T38.815-	T38.816-
Alseroxylon	T46.5x1-	T46.5x2-	T46.5x3-	T46.5x4-	T46.5x5-	T46.5x6-
Alteplase	T45.611-	T45.612-	T45.613-	T45.614-	T45.615-	T45.616-
Altizide	T50.2x1-	T50.2x2-	T50.2x3-	T50.2x4-	T50.2x5-	T50.2x6-
Altretamine	T45.1x1-	T45.1x2-	T45.1x3-	T45.1x4-	T45.1x5-	T45.1x6-
Alum (medicinal)	T49.4x1-	T49.4x2-	T49.4x3-	T49.4x4-	T49.4x5-	T49.4x6-
nonmedicinal						
(ammonium)						
(potassium)	T56.891-	T56.892-	T56.893-	T56.894-	—	—
Aluminium, aluminum						
acetate	T49.2x1-	T49.2x2-	T49.2x3-	T49.2x4-	T49.2x5-	T49.2x6-
solution	T49.0x1-	T49.0x2-	T49.0x3-	T49.0x4-	T49.0x5-	T49.0x6-
aspirin	T39.011-	T39.012-	T39.013-	T39.014-	T39.015-	T39.016-
bis (acetylsalicylate)	T39.011-	T39.012-	T39.013-	T39.014-	T39.015-	T39.016-
carbonate (gel, basic)	T47.1x1-	T47.1x2-	T47.1x3-	T47.1x4-	T47.1x5-	T47.1x6-
chlorhydroxide-complex	T47.1x1-	T47.1x2-	T47.1x3-	T47.1x4-	T47.1x5-	T47.1x6-
chloride	T49.2x1-	T49.2x2-	T49.2x3-	T49.2x4-	T49.2x5-	T49.2x6-
clofibrate	T46.6x1-	T46.6x2-	T46.6x3-	T46.6x4-	T46.6x5-	T46.6x6-
diacetate	T49.2x1-	T49.2x2-	T49.2x3-	T49.2x4-	T49.2x5-	T49.2x6-
glycinate	T47.1x1-	T47.1x2-	T47.1x3-	T47.1x4-	T47.1x5-	T47.1x6-
hydroxide (gel)	T47.1x1-	T47.1x2-	T47.1x3-	T47.1x4-	T47.1x5-	T47.1x6-
hydroxide-magnesium						
carb. gel	T47.1x1-	T47.1x2-	T47.1x3-	T47.1x4-	T47.1x5-	T47.1x6-
magnesium silicate	T47.1x1-	T47.1x2-	T47.1x3-	T47.1x4-	T47.1x5-	T47.1x6-
nicotinate	T46.7x1-	T46.7x2-	T46.7x3-	T46.7x4-	T46.7x5-	T46.7x6-
ointment (surgical)						
(topical)	T49.3x1-	T49.3x2-	T49.3x3-	T49.3x4-	T49.3x5-	T49.3x6-
phosphate	T47.1x1-	T47.1x2-	T47.1x3-	T47.1x4-	T47.1x5-	T47.1x6-
salicylate	T39.091-	T39.092-	T39.093-	T39.094-	T39.095-	T39.096-
silicate	T47.1x1-	T47.1x2-	T47.1x3-	T47.1x4-	T47.1x5-	T47.1x6-
sodium silicate	T47.1x1-	T47.1x2-	T47.1x3-	T47.1x4-	T47.1x5-	T47.1x6-
subacetate	T49.2x1-	T49.2x2-	T49.2x3-	T49.2x4-	T49.2x5-	T49.2x6-
sulfate	T49.0x1-	T49.0x2-	T49.0x3-	T49.0x4-	T49.0x5-	T49.0x6-
tannate	T47.6x1-	T47.6x2-	T47.6x3-	T47.6x4-	T47.6x5-	T47.6x6-
topical NEC	T49.3x1-	T49.3x2-	T49.3x3-	T49.3x4-	T49.3x5-	T49.3x6-

Table of Drugs & Chemicals	Accidental (Unintentional)	Self-Harm (Intentional)	Assault	Undetermined	Adverse Effect	Underdosing
Alurate	T42.3x1-	T42.3x2-	T42.3x3-	T42.3x4-	T42.3x5-	T42.3x6-
Alverine	T44.3x1-	T44.3x2-	T44.3x3-	T44.3x4-	T44.3x5-	T44.3x6-
Alvodine	T40.2x1-	T40.2x2-	T40.2x3-	T40.2x4-	T40.2x5-	T40.2x6-
Amanita phalloides	T62.0x1-	T62.0x2-	T62.0x3-	T62.0x4-	—	—
Amanitine	T62.0x1-	T62.0x2-	T62.0x3-	T62.0x4-	—	—
Amantadine	T42.8x1-	T42.8x2-	T42.8x3-	T42.8x4-	T42.8x5-	T42.8x6-
Ambazone	T49.6x1-	T49.6x2-	T49.6x3-	T49.6x4-	T49.6x5-	T49.6x6-
Ambenonium (chloride)	T44.0x1-	T44.0x2-	T44.0x3-	T44.0x4-	T44.0x5-	T44.0x6-
Ambroxol	T48.4x1-	T48.4x2-	T48.4x3-	T48.4x4-	T48.4x5-	T48.4x6-
Ambuphylline	T48.6x1-	T48.6x2-	T48.6x3-	T48.6x4-	T48.6x5-	T48.6x6-
Ambutonium bromide	T44.3x1-	T44.3x2-	T44.3x3-	T44.3x4-	T44.3x5-	T44.3x6-
Amcinonide	T49.0x1-	T49.0x2-	T49.0x3-	T49.0x4-	T49.0x5-	T49.0x6-
Amdinocilline	T36.0x1-	T36.0x2-	T36.0x3-	T36.0x4-	T36.0x5-	T36.0x6-
Ametazole	T50.8x1-	T50.8x2-	T50.8x3-	T50.8x4-	T50.8x5-	T50.8x6-
Amethocaine	T41.3x1-	T41.3x2-	T41.3x3-	T41.3x4-	T41.3x5-	T41.3x6-
regional	T41.3x1-	T41.3x2-	T41.3x3-	T41.3x4-	T41.3x5-	T41.3x6-
spinal	T41.3x1-	T41.3x2-	T41.3x3-	T41.3x4-	T41.3x5-	T41.3x6-
Amethopterin	T45.1x1-	T45.1x2-	T45.1x3-	T45.1x4-	T45.1x5-	T45.1x6-
Amezinium metilsulfate	T44.991-	T44.992-	T44.993-	T44.994-	T44.995-	T44.996-
Amfebutamone	T43.291-	T43.292-	T43.293-	T43.294-	T43.295-	T43.296-
Amfepramone	T50.5x1-	T50.5x2-	T50.5x3-	T50.5x4-	T50.5x5-	T50.5x6-
Amfetamine	T43.621-	T43.622-	T43.623-	T43.624-	T43.625-	T43.626-
Amfetaminil	T43.621-	T43.622-	T43.623-	T43.624-	T43.625-	T43.626-
Amfomycin	T36.8x1-	T36.8x2-	T36.8x3-	T36.8x4-	T36.8x5-	T36.8x6-
Amidefrine mesilate	T48.5x1-	T48.5x2-	T48.5x3-	T48.5x4-	T48.5x5-	T48.5x6-
Amidone	T40.3x1-	T40.3x2-	T40.3x3-	T40.3x4-	T40.3x5-	T40.3x6-
Amidopyrine	T39.2x1-	T39.2x2-	T39.2x3-	T39.2x4-	T39.2x5-	T39.2x6-
Amidotrizoate	T50.8x1-	T50.8x2-	T50.8x3-	T50.8x4-	T50.8x5-	T50.8x6-
Amiflamine	T43.1x1-	T43.1x2-	T43.1x3-	T43.1x4-	T43.1x5-	T43.1x6-
Amikacin	T36.5x1-	T36.5x2-	T36.5x3-	T36.5x4-	T36.5x5-	T36.5x6-
Amikhelline	T46.3x1-	T46.3x2-	T46.3x3-	T46.3x4-	T46.3x5-	T46.3x6-
Amiloride	T50.2x1-	T50.2x2-	T50.2x3-	T50.2x4-	T50.2x5-	T50.2x6-
Aminacrine	T49.0x1-	T49.0x2-	T49.0x3-	T49.0x4-	T49.0x5-	T49.0x6-
Amineptine	T43.011-	T43.012-	T43.013-	T43.014-	T43.015-	T43.016-
Aminitrozole	T37.3x1-	T37.3x2-	T37.3x3-	T37.3x4-	T37.3x5-	T37.3x6-
Amino acids	T50.3x1-	T50.3x2-	T50.3x3-	T50.3x4-	T50.3x5-	T50.3x6-
Aminoacetic acid						
(derivatives)	T50.3x1-	T50.3x2-	T50.3x3-	T50.3x4-	T50.3x5-	T50.3x6-
Aminoacridine	T49.0x1-	T49.0x2-	T49.0x3-	T49.0x4-	T49.0x5-	T49.0x6-
Aminobenzoic acid (-p)	T49.3x1-	T49.3x2-	T49.3x3-	T49.3x4-	T49.3x5-	T49.3x6-
4-Aminobutyric acid	T43.8x1-	T43.8x2-	T43.8x3-	T43.8x4-	T43.8x5-	T43.8x6-
Aminocaproic acid	T45.621-	T45.622-	T45.623-	T45.624-	T45.625-	T45.626-
Aminoethylisothiourium	T45.8x1-	T45.8x2-	T45.8x3-	T45.8x4-	T45.8x5-	T45.8x6-
Aminofenazone	T39.2x1-	T39.2x2-	T39.2x3-	T39.2x4-	T39.2x5-	T39.2x6-
Aminoglutethimide	T45.1x1-	T45.1x2-	T45.1x3-	T45.1x4-	T45.1x5-	T45.1x6-
Aminohippuric acid	T50.8x1-	T50.8x2-	T50.8x3-	T50.8x4-	T50.8x5-	T50.8x6-
Aminomethylbenzoic acid	T45.691-	T45.692-	T45.693-	T45.694-	T45.695-	T45.696-
Aminometradine	T50.2x1-	T50.2x2-	T50.2x3-	T50.2x4-	T50.2x5-	T50.2x6-
Aminopentamide	T44.3x1-	T44.3x2-	T44.3x3-	T44.3x4-	T44.3x5-	T44.3x6-
Aminophenazone	T39.2x1-	T39.2x2-	T39.2x3-	T39.2x4-	T39.2x5-	T39.2x6-
Aminophenol	T54.0x1-	T54.0x2-	T54.0x3-	T54.0x4-	—	—
4-Aminophenol derivatives	T39.1x1-	T39.1x2-	T39.1x3-	T39.1x4-	T39.1x5-	T39.1x6-
Aminophenylpyridone	T43.591-	T43.592-	T43.593-	T43.594-	T43.595-	T43.596-
Aminophylline	T48.6x1-	T48.6x2-	T48.6x3-	T48.6x4-	T48.6x5-	T48.6x6-
Aminopterin sodium	T45.1x1-	T45.1x2-	T45.1x3-	T45.1x4-	T45.1x5-	T45.1x6-
Aminopyrine	T39.2x1-	T39.2x2-	T39.2x3-	T39.2x4-	T39.2x5-	T39.2x6-
8-Aminoquinoline drugs	T37.2x1-	T37.2x2-	T37.2x3-	T37.2x4-	T37.2x5-	T37.2x6-
Aminorex	T50.5x1-	T50.5x2-	T50.5x3-	T50.5x4-	T50.5x5-	T50.5x6-
Aminosalicylic acid	T37.1x1-	T37.1x2-	T37.1x3-	T37.1x4-	T37.1x5-	T37.1x6-
Aminosalylum	T37.1x1-	T37.1x2-	T37.1x3-	T37.1x4-	T37.1x5-	T37.1x6-
Amiodarone	T46.2x1-	T46.2x2-	T46.2x3-	T46.2x4-	T46.2x5-	T46.2x6-

DRUGS & CHEMICALS

Table of Drugs & Chemicals	Poisoning Accidental (Unintentional)	Poisoning Self-Harm (Intentional)	Poisoning Assault	Poisoning Undetermined	Adverse Effect	Underdosing
Amiphenazole	T50.7x1-	T50.7x2-	T50.7x3-	T50.7x4-	T50.7x5-	T50.7x6-
Amiquinsin	T46.5x1-	T46.5x2-	T46.5x3-	T46.5x4-	T46.5x5-	T46.5x6-
Amisometradine	T50.2x1-	T50.2x2-	T50.2x3-	T50.2x4-	T50.2x5-	T50.2x6-
Amisulpride	T43.591-	T43.592-	T43.593-	T43.594-	T43.595-	T43.596-
Amitriptyline	T43.011-	T43.012-	T43.013-	T43.014-	T43.015-	T43.016-
Amitriptylinoxide	T43.011-	T43.012-	T43.013-	T43.014-	T43.015-	T43.016-
Amlexanox	T48.6x1-	T48.6x2-	T48.6x3-	T48.6x4-	T48.6x5-	T48.6x6-
Ammonia (fumes) (gas) (vapor)	T59.891-	T59.892-	T59.893-	T59.894-	—	—
aromatic spirit	T48.991-	T48.992-	T48.993-	T48.994-	T48.995-	T48.996-
liquid (household)	T54.3x1-	T54.3x2-	T54.3x3-	T54.3x4-	—	—
Ammoniated mercury	T49.0x1-	T49.0x2-	T49.0x3-	T49.0x4-	T49.0x5-	T49.0x6-
Ammonium						
acid tartrate	T49.5x1-	T49.5x2-	T49.5x3-	T49.5x4-	T49.5x5-	T49.5x6-
bromide	T42.6x1-	T42.6x2-	T42.6x3-	T42.6x4-	T42.6x5-	T42.6x6-
carbonate	T54.3x1-	T54.3x2-	T54.3x3-	T54.3x4-	—	—
chloride	T50.991-	T50.992-	T50.993-	T50.994-	T50.995-	T50.996-
expectorant	T48.4x1-	T48.4x2-	T48.4x3-	T48.4x4-	T48.4x5-	T48.4x6-
compounds (household) NEC	T54.3x1-	T54.3x2-	T54.3x3-	T54.3x4-	—	—
fumes (any usage)	T59.891-	T59.892-	T59.893-	T59.894-	—	—
industrial	T54.3x1-	T54.3x2-	T54.3x3-	T54.3x4-	—	—
ichthyosulronate	T49.4x1-	T49.4x2-	T49.4x3-	T49.4x4-	T49.4x5-	T49.4x6-
mandelate	T37.91x-	T37.92x-	T37.93x-	T37.94x-	T37.95x-	T37.96x-
sulfamate	T60.3x1-	T60.3x2-	T60.3x3-	T60.3x4-	—	—
sulfonate resin	T47.8x1-	T47.8x2-	T47.8x3-	T47.8x4-	T47.8x5-	T47.8x6-
Amobarbital (sodium)	T42.3x1-	T42.3x2-	T42.3x3-	T42.3x4-	T42.3x5-	T42.3x6-
Amodiaquine	T37.2x1-	T37.2x2-	T37.2x3-	T37.2x4-	T37.2x5-	T37.2x6-
Amopyroquin (e)	T37.2x1-	T37.2x2-	T37.2x3-	T37.2x4-	T37.2x5-	T37.2x6-
Amoxapine	T43.011-	T43.012-	T43.013-	T43.014-	T43.015-	T43.016-
Amoxicillin	T36.0x1-	T36.0x2-	T36.0x3-	T36.0x4-	T36.0x5-	T36.0x6-
Amperozide	T43.591-	T43.592-	T43.593-	T43.594-	T43.595-	T43.596-
Amphenidone	T43.591-	T43.592-	T43.593-	T43.594-	T43.595-	T43.596-
Amphetamine NEC	T43.621-	T43.622-	T43.623-	T43.624-	T43.625-	T43.626-
Amphomycin	T36.8x1-	T36.8x2-	T36.8x3-	T36.8x4-	T36.8x5-	T36.8x6-
Amphotalide	T37.4x1-	T37.4x2-	T37.4x3-	T37.4x4-	T37.4x5-	T37.4x6-
Amphotericin B	T36.7x1-	T36.7x2-	T36.7x3-	T36.7x4-	T36.7x5-	T36.7x6-
topical	T49.0x1-	T49.0x2-	T49.0x3-	T49.0x4-	T49.0x5-	T49.0x6-
Ampicillin	T36.0x1-	T36.0x2-	T36.0x3-	T36.0x4-	T36.0x5-	T36.0x6-
Amprotropine	T44.3x1-	T44.3x2-	T44.3x3-	T44.3x4-	T44.3x5-	T44.3x6-
Amsacrine	T45.1x1-	T45.1x2-	T45.1x3-	T45.1x4-	T45.1x5-	T45.1x6-
Amygdaline	T62.2x1-	T62.2x2-	T62.2x3-	T62.2x4-	—	—
Amyl						
acetate	T52.8x1-	T52.8x2-	T52.8x3-	T52.8x4-	—	—
vapor	T59.891-	T59.892-	T59.893-	T59.894-	—	—
alcohol	T51.3x1-	T51.3x2-	T51.3x3-	T51.3x4-	—	—
chloride	T53.6x1-	T53.6x2-	T53.6x3-	T53.6x4-	—	—
formate	T52.8x1-	T52.8x2-	T52.8x3-	T52.8x4-	—	—
nitrite	T46.3x1-	T46.3x2-	T46.3x3-	T46.3x4-	T46.3x5-	T46.3x6-
propionate	T65.891-	T65.892-	T65.893-	T65.894-	—	—
Amylase	T47.5x1-	T47.5x2-	T47.5x3-	T47.5x4-	T47.5x5-	T47.5x6-
Amyleine, regional	T41.3x1-	T41.3x2-	T41.3x3-	T41.3x4-	T41.3x5-	T41.3x6-
Amylene						
dichloride	T53.6x1-	T53.6x2-	T53.6x3-	T53.6x4-	—	—
hydrate	T51.3x1-	T51.3x2-	T51.3x3-	T51.3x4-	—	—
Amylmetacresol	T49.6x1-	T49.6x2-	T49.6x3-	T49.6x4-	T49.6x5-	T49.6x6-
Amylobarbitone	T42.3x1-	T42.3x2-	T42.3x3-	T42.3x4-	T42.3x5-	T42.3x6-
Amylocaine, regional	T41.3x1-	T41.3x2-	T41.3x3-	T41.3x4-	T41.3x5-	T41.3x6-
infiltration (subcutaneous)	T41.3x1-	T41.3x2-	T41.3x3-	T41.3x4-	T41.3x5-	T41.3x6-
nerve block (peripheral) (plexus)	T41.3x1-	T41.3x2-	T41.3x3-	T41.3x4-	T41.3x5-	T41.3x6-
spinal	T41.3x1-	T41.3x2-	T41.3x3-	T41.3x4-	T41.3x5-	T41.3x6-
topical (surface)	T41.3x1-	T41.3x2-	T41.3x3-	T41.3x4-	T41.3x5-	T41.3x6-
Amylopectin	T47.6x1-	T47.6x2-	T47.6x3-	T47.6x4-	T47.6x5-	T47.6x6-
Amytal (sodium)	T42.3x1-	T42.3x2-	T42.3x3-	T42.3x4-	T42.3x5-	T42.3x6-
Anabolic steroid	T38.7x1-	T38.7x2-	T38.7x3-	T38.7x4-	T38.7x5-	T38.7x6-
Analeptic NEC	T50.7x1-	T50.7x2-	T50.7x3-	T50.7x4-	T50.7x5-	T50.7x6-
Analgesic	T39.91x-	T39.92x-	T39.93x-	T39.94x-	T39.95x-	T39.96x-
anti-inflammatory NEC	T39.91x-	T39.92x-	T39.93x-	T39.94x-	T39.95x-	T39.96x-
propionic acid derivative	T39.311-	T39.312-	T39.313-	T39.314-	T39.315-	T39.316-
antirheumatic NEC	T39.4x1-	T39.4x2-	T39.4x3-	T39.4x4-	T39.4x5-	T39.4x6-
aromatic NEC	T39.1x1-	T39.1x2-	T39.1x3-	T39.1x4-	T39.1x5-	T39.1x6-
narcotic NEC	T40.601-	T40.602-	T40.603-	T40.604-	T40.605-	T40.606-
combination	T40.601-	T40.602-	T40.603-	T40.604-	T40.605-	T40.606-
obstetric	T40.601-	T40.602-	T40.603-	T40.604-	T40.605-	T40.606-
non-narcotic NEC	T39.91x-	T39.92x-	T39.93x-	T39.94x-	T39.95x-	T39.96x-
combination	T39.91x-	T39.92x-	T39.93x-	T39.94x-	T39.95x-	T39.96x-
pyrazole	T39.2x1-	T39.2x2-	T39.2x3-	T39.2x4-	T39.2x5-	T39.2x6-
specified NEC	T39.8x1-	T39.8x2-	T39.8x3-	T39.8x4-	T39.8x5-	T39.8x6-
Analgin	T39.2x1-	T39.2x2-	T39.2x3-	T39.2x4-	T39.2x5-	T39.2x6-
Anamirta cocculus	T62.1x1-	T62.1x2-	T62.1x3-	T62.1x4-	—	—
Ancillin	T36.0x1-	T36.0x2-	T36.0x3-	T36.0x4-	T36.0x5-	T36.0x6-
Ancrod	T45.691-	T45.692-	T45.693-	T45.694-	T45.695-	T45.696-
Androgen	T38.7x1-	T38.7x2-	T38.7x3-	T38.7x4-	T38.7x5-	T38.7x6-
Androgen-estrogen mixture	T38.7x1-	T38.7x2-	T38.7x3-	T38.7x4-	T38.7x5-	T38.7x6-
Androstalone	T38.7x1-	T38.7x2-	T38.7x3-	T38.7x4-	T38.7x5-	T38.7x6-
Androstanolone	T38.7x1-	T38.7x2-	T38.7x3-	T38.7x4-	T38.7x5-	T38.7x6-
Androsterone	T38.7x1-	T38.7x2-	T38.7x3-	T38.7x4-	T38.7x5-	T38.7x6-
Anemone pulsatilla	T62.2x1-	T62.2x2-	T62.2x3-	T62.2x4-	—	—
Anesthesia						
caudal	T41.3x1-	T41.3x2-	T41.3x3-	T41.3x4-	T41.3x5-	T41.3x6-
endotracheal	T41.0x1-	T41.0x2-	T41.0x3-	T41.0x4-	T41.0x5-	T41.0x6-
epidural	T41.3x1-	T41.3x2-	T41.3x3-	T41.3x4-	T41.3x5-	T41.3x6-
inhalation	T41.0x1-	T41.0x2-	T41.0x3-	T41.0x4-	T41.0x5-	T41.0x6-
local	T41.3x1-	T41.3x2-	T41.3x3-	T41.3x4-	T41.3x5-	T41.3x6-
mucosal	T41.3x1-	T41.3x2-	T41.3x3-	T41.3x4-	T41.3x5-	T41.3x6-
muscle relaxation	T48.1x1-	T48.1x2-	T48.1x3-	T48.1x4-	T48.1x5-	T48.1x6-
nerve blocking	T41.3x1-	T41.3x2-	T41.3x3-	T41.3x4-	T41.3x5-	T41.3x6-
plexus blocking	T41.3x1-	T41.3x2-	T41.3x3-	T41.3x4-	T41.3x5-	T41.3x6-
potentiated	T41.201-	T41.202-	T41.203-	T41.204-	T41.205-	T41.206-
rectal	T41.201-	T41.202-	T41.203-	T41.204-	T41.205-	T41.206-
general	T41.201-	T41.202-	T41.203-	T41.204-	T41.205-	T41.206-
local	T41.3x1-	T41.3x2-	T41.3x3-	T41.3x4-	T41.3x5-	T41.3x6-
regional	T41.3x1-	T41.3x2-	T41.3x3-	T41.3x4-	T41.3x5-	T41.3x6-
surface	T41.3x1-	T41.3x2-	T41.3x3-	T41.3x4-	T41.3x5-	T41.3x6-
Anesthetic NEC — see also Anesthesia	T41.41x-	T41.42x-	T41.43x-	T41.44x-	T41.45x-	T41.46x-
with muscle relaxant	T41.201-	T41.202-	T41.203-	T41.204-	T41.205-	T41.206-
general	T41.201-	T41.202-	T41.203-	T41.204-	T41.205-	T41.206-
local	T41.3x1-	T41.3x2-	T41.3x3-	T41.3x4-	T41.3x5-	T41.3x6-
gaseous NEC	T41.0x1-	T41.0x2-	T41.0x3-	T41.0x4-	T41.0x5-	T41.0x6-
general NEC	T41.201-	T41.202-	T41.203-		T41.205-	T41.206-
halogenated hydrocarbon derivatives NEC	T41.0x1-	T41.0x2-	T41.0x3-	T41.0x4-	T41.0x5-	T41.0x6-
infiltration NEC	T41.3x1-	T41.3x2-	T41.3x3-	T41.3x4-	T41.3x5-	T41.3x6-
intravenous NEC	T41.1x1-	T41.1x2-	T41.1x3-	T41.1x4-	T41.1x5-	T41.1x6-
local NEC	T41.3x1-	T41.3x2-	T41.3x3-	T41.3x4-	T41.3x5-	T41.3x6-
rectal	T41.201-	T41.202-	T41.203-	T41.204-	T41.205-	T41.206-
general	T41.201-	T41.202-	T41.203-	T41.204-	T41.205-	T41.206-
local	T41.3x1-	T41.3x2-	T41.3x3-	T41.3x4-	T41.3x5-	T41.3x6-
regional NEC	T41.3x1-	T41.3x2-	T41.3x3-	T41.3x4-	T41.3x5-	T41.3x6-
spinal NEC	T41.3x1-	T41.3x2-	T41.3x3-	T41.3x4-	T41.3x5-	T41.3x6-
thiobarbiturate	T41.1x1-	T41.1x2-	T41.1x3-	T41.1x4-	T41.1x5-	T41.1x6-
topical	T41.3x1-	T41.3x2-	T41.3x3-	T41.3x4-	T41.3x5-	T41.3x6-

Table of Drugs & Chemicals	POISONING Accidental (Unintentional)	Self-Harm (Intentional)	Assault	Undetermined	Adverse Effect	Underdosing
Aneurine	T45.2x1-	T45.2x2-	T45.2x3-	T45.2x4-	T45.2x5-	T45.2x6-
Angio-Conray	T50.8x1-	T50.8x2-	T50.8x3-	T50.8x4-	T50.8x5-	T50.8x6-
Angiotensin	T44.5x1-	T44.5x2-	T44.5x3-	T44.5x4-	T44.5x5-	T44.5x6-
Angiotensinamide	T44.991-	T44.992-	T44.993-	T44.994-	T44.995-	T44.996-
Anhydrohydroxy-progesterone	T38.5x1-	T38.5x2-	T38.5x3-	T38.5x4-	T38.5x5-	T38.5x6-
Anhydron	T50.2x1-	T50.2x2-	T50.2x3-	T50.2x4-	T50.2x5-	T50.2x6-
Anileridine	T40.4x1-	T40.4x2-	T40.4x3-	T40.4x4-	T40.4x5-	T40.4x6-
Aniline (dye) (liquid)	T65.3x1-	T65.3x2-	T65.3x3-	T65.3x4-	—	—
analgesic	T39.1x1-	T39.1x2-	T39.1x3-	T39.1x4-	T39.1x5-	T39.1x6-
derivatives, therapeutic NEC	T39.1x1-	T39.1x2-	T39.1x3-	T39.1x4-	T39.1x5-	T39.1x6-
vapor	T65.3x1-	T65.3x2-	T65.3x3-	T65.3x4-	—	—
Aniscoropine	T44.3x1-	T44.3x2-	T44.3x3-	T44.3x4-	T44.3x5-	T44.3x6-
Anise oil	T47.5x1-	T47.5x2-	T47.5x3-	T47.5x4-	T47.5x5-	T47.5x6-
Anisidine	T65.3x1-	T65.3x2-	T65.3x3-	T65.3x4-	—	—
Anisindione	T45.511-	T45.512-	T45.513-	T45.514-	T45.515-	T45.516-
Anisotropine methyl-bromide	T44.3x1-	T44.3x2-	T44.3x3-	T44.3x4-	T44.3x5-	T44.3x6-
Anistreplase	T45.611-	T45.612-	T45.613-	T45.614-	T45.615-	T45.616-
Anorexiant (central)	T50.5x1-	T50.5x2-	T50.5x3-	T50.5x4-	T50.5x5-	T50.5x6-
Anorexic agents	T50.5x1-	T50.5x2-	T50.5x3-	T50.5x4-	T50.5x5-	T50.5x6-
Ansamycin	T36.6x1-	T36.6x2-	T36.6x3-	T36.6x4-	T36.6x5-	T36.6x6-
Ant (bite) (sting)	T63.421-	T63.422-	T63.423-	T63.424-		
Ant poison — see Insecticide						
Antabuse	T50.6x1-	T50.6x2-	T50.6x3-	T50.6x4-	T50.6x5-	T50.6x6-
Antacid NEC	T47.1x1-	T47.1x2-	T47.1x3-	T47.1x4-	T47.1x5-	T47.1x6-
Antagonist						
aldosterone	T50.0x1-	T50.0x2-	T50.0x3-	T50.0x4-	T50.0x5-	T50.0x6-
alpha-adrenoreceptor	T44.6x1-	T44.6x2-	T44.6x3-	T44.6x4-	T44.6x5-	T44.6x6-
anticoagulant	T45.7x1-	T45.7x2-	T45.7x3-	T45.7x4-	T45.7x5-	T45.7x6-
beta-adrenoreceptor	T44.7x1-	T44.7x2-	T44.7x3-	T44.7x4-	T44.7x5-	T44.7x6-
extrapyramidal NEC	T44.3x1-	T44.3x2-	T44.3x3-	T44.3x4-	T44.3x5-	T44.3x6-
folic acid	T45.1x1-	T45.1x2-	T45.1x3-	T45.1x4-	T45.1x5-	T45.1x6-
heavy metal	T45.8x1-	T45.8x2-	T45.8x3-	T45.8x4-	T45.8x5-	T45.8x6-
H2 receptor	T47.0x1-	T47.0x2-	T47.0x3-	T47.0x4-	T47.0x5-	T47.0x6-
narcotic analgesic	T50.7x1-	T50.7x2-	T50.7x3-	T50.7x4-	T50.7x5-	T50.7x6-
opiate	T50.7x1-	T50.7x2-	T50.7x3-	T50.7x4-	T50.7x5-	T50.7x6-
pyrimidine	T45.1x1-	T45.1x2-	T45.1x3-	T45.1x4-	T45.1x5-	T45.1x6-
serotonin	T46.5x1-	T46.5x2-	T46.5x3-	T46.5x4-	T46.5x5-	T46.5x6-
Antazolin(e)	T45.0x1-	T45.0x2-	T45.0x3-	T45.0x4-	T45.0x5-	T45.0x6-
Anterior pituitary hormone NEC	T38.811-	T38.812-	T38.813-	T38.814-	T38.815-	T38.816-
Anthelmintic NEC	T37.4x1-	T37.4x2-	T37.4x3-	T37.4x4-	T37.4x5-	T37.4x6-
Anthiolimine	T37.4x1-	T37.4x2-	T37.4x3-	T37.4x4-	T37.4x5-	T37.4x6-
Anthralin	T49.4x1-	T49.4x2-	T49.4x3-	T49.4x4-	T49.4x5-	T49.4x6-
Anthramycin	T45.1x1-	T45.1x2-	T45.1x3-	T45.1x4-	T45.1x5-	T45.1x6-
Antiadrenergic NEC	T44.8x1-	T44.8x2-	T44.8x3-	T44.8x4-	T44.8x5-	T44.8x6-
Antiallergic NEC	T45.0x1-	T45.0x2-	T45.0x3-	T45.0x4-	T45.0x5-	T45.0x6-
Antiandrogen NEC	T38.6x1-	T38.6x2-	T38.6x3-	T38.6x4-	T38.6x5-	T38.6x6-
Anti-anemic (drug) (preparation)	T45.8x1-	T45.8x2-	T45.8x3-	T45.8x4-	T45.8x5-	T45.8x6-
Antianxiety drug NEC	T43.501-	T43.502-	T43.503-	T43.504-	T43.505-	T43.506-
Antiaris toxicaria	T65.891-	T65.892-	T65.893-	T65.894-	—	—
Antiarteriosclerotic drug	T46.6x1-	T46.6x2-	T46.6x3-	T46.6x4-	T46.6x5-	T46.6x6-
Antiasthmatic drug NEC	T48.6x1-	T48.6x2-	T48.6x3-	T48.6x4-	T48.6x5-	T48.6x6-
Antibiotic NEC	T36.91x-	T36.92x-	T36.93x-	T36.94x-	T36.95x-	T36.96x-
aminoglycoside	T36.5x1-	T36.5x2-	T36.5x3-	T36.5x4-	T36.5x5-	T36.5x6-
anticancer	T45.1x1-	T45.1x2-	T45.1x3-	T45.1x4-	T45.1x5-	T45.1x6-
antifungal	T36.7x1-	T36.7x2-	T36.7x3-	T36.7x4-	T36.7x5-	T36.7x6-
antimycobacterial	T36.5x1-	T36.5x2-	T36.5x3-	T36.5x4-	T36.5x5-	T36.5x6-
antineoplastic	T45.1x1-	T45.1x2-	T45.1x3-	T45.1x4-	T45.1x5-	T45.1x6-
cephalosporin (group)	T36.1x1-	T36.1x2-	T36.1x3-	T36.1x4-	T36.1x5-	T36.1x6-
chloramphenicol (group)	T36.2x1-	T36.2x2-	T36.2x3-	T36.2x4-	T36.2x5-	T36.2x6-
ENT	T49.6x1-	T49.6x2-	T49.6x3-	T49.6x4-	T49.6x5-	T49.6x6-
Antibiotic NEC - continued	T36.91x-	T36.92x-	T36.93x-	T36.94x-	T36.95x-	T36.96x-
eye	T49.5x1-	T49.5x2-	T49.5x3-	T49.5x4-	T49.5x5-	T49.5x6-
fungicidal (local)	T49.0x1-	T49.0x2-	T49.0x3-	T49.0x4-	T49.0x5-	T49.0x6-
intestinal	T36.8x1-	T36.8x2-	T36.8x3-	T36.8x4-	T36.8x5-	T36.8x6-
b-lactam NEC	T36.1x1-	T36.1x2-	T36.1x3-	T36.1x4-	T36.1x5-	T36.1x6-
local	T49.0x1-	T49.0x2-	T49.0x3-	T49.0x4-	T49.0x5-	T49.0x6-
macrolides	T36.3x1-	T36.3x2-	T36.3x3-	T36.3x4-	T36.3x5-	T36.3x6-
polypeptide	T36.8x1-	T36.8x2-	T36.8x3-	T36.8x4-	T36.8x5-	T36.8x6-
specified NEC	T36.8x1-	T36.8x2-	T36.8x3-	T36.8x4-	T36.8x5-	T36.8x6-
tetracycline (group)	T36.4x1-	T36.4x2-	T36.4x3-	T36.4x4-	T36.4x5-	T36.4x6-
throat	T49.6x1-	T49.6x2-	T49.6x3-	T49.6x4-	T49.6x5-	T49.6x6-
Anticancer agents NEC	T45.1x1-	T45.1x2-	T45.1x3-	T45.1x4-	T45.1x5-	T45.1x6-
Anticholesterolemic drug NEC	T46.6x1-	T46.6x2-	T46.6x3-	T46.6x4-	T46.6x5-	T46.6x6-
Anticholinergic NEC	T44.3x1-	T44.3x2-	T44.3x3-	T44.3x4-	T44.3x5-	T44.3x6-
Anticholinesterase	T44.0x1-	T44.0x2-	T44.0x3-	T44.0x4-	T44.0x5-	T44.0x6-
organophosphorus	T44.0x1-	T44.0x2-	T44.0x3-	T44.0x4-	T44.0x5-	T44.0x6-
insecticide	T60.0x1-	T60.0x2-	T60.0x3-	T60.0x4-	—	—
nerve gas	T59.891-	T59.892-	T59.893-	T59.894-	—	—
reversible	T44.0x1-	T44.0x2-	T44.0x3-	T44.0x4-	T44.0x5-	T44.0x6-
ophthalmological	T49.5x1-	T49.5x2-	T49.5x3-	T49.5x4-	T49.5x5-	T49.5x6-
Anticoagulant NEC	T45.511-	T45.512-	T45.513-	T45.514-	T45.515-	T45.516-
antagonist	T45.7x1-	T45.7x2-	T45.7x3-	T45.7x4-	T45.7x5-	T45.7x6-
Anti-common-cold drug NEC	T48.5x1-	T48.5x2-	T48.5x3-	T48.5x4-	T48.5x5-	T48.5x6-
Anticonvulsant	T42.71x-	T42.72x-	T42.73x-	T42.74x-	T42.75x-	T42.76x-
barbiturate	T42.3x1-	T42.3x2-	T42.3x3-	T42.3x4-	T42.3x5-	T42.3x6-
combination (with barbiturate)	T42.3x1-	T42.3x2-	T42.3x3-	T42.3x4-	T42.3x5-	T42.3x6-
hydantoin	T42.0x1-	T42.0x2-	T42.0x3-	T42.0x4-	T42.0x5-	T42.0x6-
hypnotic NEC	T42.6x1-	T42.6x2-	T42.6x3-	T42.6x4-	T42.6x5-	T42.6x6-
oxazolidinedione	T42.2x1-	T42.2x2-	T42.2x3-	T42.2x4-	T42.2x5-	T42.2x6-
pyrimidinedione	T42.6x1-	T42.6x2-	T42.6x3-	T42.6x4-	T42.6x5-	T42.6x6-
specified NEC	T42.6x1-	T42.6x2-	T42.6x3-	T42.6x4-	T42.6x5-	T42.6x6-
succinimide	T42.2x1-	T42.2x2-	T42.2x3-	T42.2x4-	T42.2x5-	T42.2x6-
Anti-D immunoglobulin (human)	T50.Z11-	T50.Z12-	T50.Z13-	T50.Z14-	T50.Z15-	T50.Z16-
Antidepressant	T43.201-	T43.202-	T43.203-	T43.204-	T43.205-	T43.206-
monoamine oxidase inhibitor	T43.1x1-	T43.1x2-	T43.1x3-	T43.1x4-	T43.1x5-	T43.1x6-
selective serotonin norepinephrine reuptake inhibitor	T43.211-	T43.212-	T43.213-	T43.214-	T43.215-	T43.216-
selective serotonin reuptake inhibitor	T43.221-	T43.222-	T43.223-	T43.224-	T43.225-	T43.226-
specified NEC	T43.291-	T43.292-	T43.293-	T43.294-	T43.295-	T43.296-
triazolopyridine	T43.211-	T43.212-	T43.213-	T43.214-	T43.215-	T43.216-
tetracyclic	T43.021-	T43.022-	T43.023-	T43.024-	T43.025-	T43.026-
tricyclic	T43.011-	T43.012-	T43.013-	T43.014-	T43.015-	T43.016-
Antidiabetic NEC	T38.3x1-	T38.3x2-	T38.3x3-	T38.3x4-	T38.3x5-	T38.3x6-
biguanide	T38.3x1-	T38.3x2-	T38.3x3-	T38.3x4-	T38.3x5-	T38.3x6-
and sulfonyl combined	T38.3x1-	T38.3x2-	T38.3x3-	T38.3x4-	T38.3x5-	T38.3x6-
combined	T38.3x1-	T38.3x2-	T38.3x3-	T38.3x4-	T38.3x5-	T38.3x6-
sulfonylurea	T38.3x1-	T38.3x2-	T38.3x3-	T38.3x4-	T38.3x5-	T38.3x6-
Antidiarrheal drug NEC	T47.6x1-	T47.6x2-	T47.6x3-	T47.6x4-	T47.6x5-	T47.6x6-
absorbent	T47.6x1-	T47.6x2-	T47.6x3-	T47.6x4-	T47.6x5-	T47.6x6-
Antidiphtheria serum	T50.Z11-	T50.Z12-	T50.Z13-	T50.Z14-	T50.Z15-	T50.Z16-
Antidiuretic hormone	T38.891-	T38.892-	T38.893-	T38.894-	T38.895-	T38.896-
Antidote NEC	T50.6x1-	T50.6x2-	T50.6x3-	T50.6x4-	T50.6x5-	T50.6x6-
heavy metal	T45.8x1-	T45.8x2-	T45.8x3-	T45.8x4-	T45.8x5-	T45.8x6-
Antidysrhythmic NEC	T46.2x1-	T46.2x2-	T46.2x3-	T46.2x4-	T46.2x5-	T46.2x6-

DRUGS & CHEMICALS

Table of Drugs & Chemicals	POISONING Accidental (Unintentional)	Self-Harm (Intentional)	Assault	Undetermined	Adverse Effect	Underdosing
Antiemetic drug	T45.0x1-	T45.0x2-	T45.0x3-	T45.0x4-	T45.0x5-	T45.0x6-
Antiepilepsy agent	T42.71x-	T42.72x-	T42.73x-	T42.74x-	T42.75x-	T42.76x-
combination	T42.5x1-	T42.5x2-	T42.5x3-	T42.5x4-	T42.5x5-	T42.5x6-
mixed	T42.5x1-	T42.5x2-	T42.5x3-	T42.5x4-	T42.5x5-	T42.5x6-
specified, NEC	T42.6x1-	T42.6x2-	T42.6x3-	T42.6x4-	T42.6x5-	T42.6x6-
Antiestrogen NEC	T38.6x1-	T38.6x2-	T38.6x3-	T38.6x4-	T38.6x5-	T38.6x6-
Antifertility pill	T38.4x1-	T38.4x2-	T38.4x3-	T38.4x4-	T38.4x5-	T38.4x6-
Antifibrinolytic drug	T45.621-	T45.622-	T45.623-	T45.624-	T45.625-	T45.626-
Antifilarial drug	T37.4x1-	T37.4x2-	T37.4x3-	T37.4x4-	T37.4x5-	T37.4x6-
Antiflatulent	T47.5x1-	T47.5x2-	T47.5x3-	T47.5x4-	T47.5x5-	T47.5x6-
Antifreeze	T65.91x-	T65.92x-	T65.93x-	T65.94x-	—	—
alcohol	T51.1x1-	T51.1x2-	T51.1x3-	T51.1x4-	—	—
ethylene glycol	T51.8x1-	T51.8x2-	T51.8x3-	T51.8x4-	—	—
Antifungal						
antibiotic (systemic)	T36.7x1-	T36.7x2-	T36.7x3-	T36.7x4-	T36.7x5-	T36.7x6-
anti-infective NEC	T37.91x-	T37.92x-	T37.93x-	T37.94x-	T37.95x-	T37.96x-
disinfectant, local	T49.0x1-	T49.0x2-	T49.0x3-	T49.0x4-	T49.0x5-	T49.0x6-
nonmedicinal (spray)	T60.3x1-	T60.3x2-	T60.3x3-	T60.3x4-	—	—
topical	T49.0x1-	T49.0x2-	T49.0x3-	T49.0x4-	T49.0x5-	T49.0x6-
Anti-gastric-secretion drug NEC	T47.1x1-	T47.1x2-	T47.1x3-	T47.1x4-	T47.1x5-	T47.1x6-
Antigonadotrophin NEC	T38.6x1-	T38.6x2-	T38.6x3-	T38.6x4-	T38.6x5-	T38.6x6-
Antihallucinogen	T43.501-	T43.502-	T43.503-	T43.504-	T43.505-	T43.506-
Antihelmintics	T37.4x1-	T37.4x2-	T37.4x3-	T37.4x4-	T37.4x5-	T37.4x6-
Antihemophilic						
factor	T45.8x1-	T45.8x2-	T45.8x3-	T45.8x4-	T45.8x5-	T45.8x6-
fraction	T45.8x1-	T45.8x2-	T45.8x3-	T45.8x4-	T45.8x5-	T45.8x6-
globulin concentrate	T45.7x1-	T45.7x2-	T45.7x3-	T45.7x4-	T45.7x5-	T45.7x6-
human plasma	T45.8x1-	T45.8x2-	T45.8x3-	T45.8x4-	T45.8x5-	T45.8x6-
plasma, dried	T45.7x1-	T45.7x2-	T45.7x3-	T45.7x4-	T45.7x5-	T45.7x6-
Antihemorrhoidal preparation	T49.2x1-	T49.2x2-	T49.2x3-	T49.2x4-	T49.2x5-	T49.2x6-
Antiheparin drug	T45.7x1-	T45.7x2-	T45.7x3-	T45.7x4-	T45.7x5-	T45.7x6-
Antihistamine	T45.0x1-	T45.0x2-	T45.0x3-	T45.0x4-	T45.0x5-	T45.0x6-
Antihookworm drug	T37.4x1-	T37.4x2-	T37.4x3-	T37.4x4-	T37.4x5-	T37.4x6-
Anti-human lymphocytic globulin	T50.Z11-	T50.Z12-	T50.Z13-	T50.Z14-	T50.Z15-	T50.Z16-
Antihyperlipidemic drug	T46.6x1-	T46.6x2-	T46.6x3-	T46.6x4-	T46.6x5-	T46.6x6-
Antihypertensive drug NEC	T46.5x1-	T46.5x2-	T46.5x3-	T46.5x4-	T46.5x5-	T46.5x6-
Anti-infective NEC	T37.91x-	T37.92x-	T37.93x-	T37.94x-	T37.95x-	T37.96x-
antibiotics	T36.91x-	T36.92x-	T36.93x-	T36.94x-	T36.95x-	T36.96x-
specified NEC	T36.8x1-	T36.8x2-	T36.8x3-	T36.8x4-	T36.8x5-	T36.8x6-
anthelmintic	T37.4x1-	T37.4x2-	T37.4x3-	T37.4x4-	T37.4x5-	T37.4x6-
antimalarial	T37.2x1-	T37.2x2-	T37.2x3-	T37.2x4-	T37.2x5-	T37.2x6-
antimycobacterial NEC	T37.1x1-	T37.1x2-	T37.1x3-	T37.1x4-	T37.1x5-	T37.1x6-
antibiotics	T36.5x1-	T36.5x2-	T36.5x3-	T36.5x4-	T36.5x5-	T36.5x6-
antiprotozoal NEC	T37.3x1-	T37.3x2-	T37.3x3-	T37.3x4-	T37.3x5-	T37.3x6-
blood	T37.2x1-	T37.2x2-	T37.2x3-	T37.2x4-	T37.2x5-	T37.2x6-
antiviral	T37.5x1-	T37.5x2-	T37.5x3-	T37.5x4-	T37.5x5-	T37.5x6-
arsenical	T37.8x1-	T37.8x2-	T37.8x3-	T37.8x4-	T37.8x5-	T37.8x6-
bismuth, local	T49.0x1-	T49.0x2-	T49.0x3-	T49.0x4-	T49.0x5-	T49.0x6-
ENT	T49.6x1-	T49.6x2-	T49.6x3-	T49.6x4-	T49.6x5-	T49.6x6-
eye NEC	T49.5x1-	T49.5x2-	T49.5x3-	T49.5x4-	T49.5x5-	T49.5x6-
heavy metals NEC	T37.8x1-	T37.8x2-	T37.8x3-	T37.8x4-	T37.8x5-	T37.8x6-
local NEC	T49.0x1-	T49.0x2-	T49.0x3-	T49.0x4-	T49.0x5-	T49.0x6-
specified NEC	T49.0x1-	T49.0x2-	T49.0x3-	T49.0x4-	T49.0x5-	T49.0x6-
mixed	T37.91x-	T37.92x-	T37.93x-	T37.94x-	T37.95x-	T37.96x-
ophthalmic preparation	T49.5x1-	T49.5x2-	T49.5x3-	T49.5x4-	T49.5x5-	T49.5x6-
topical NEC	T49.0x1-	T49.0x2-	T49.0x3-	T49.0x4-	T49.0x5-	T49.0x6-
Anti-inflammatory drug NEC	T39.391-	T39.392-	T39.393-	T39.394-	T39.395-	T39.396-
local	T49.0x1-	T49.0x2-	T49.0x3-	T49.0x4-	T49.0x5-	T49.0x6-
nonsteroidal NEC	T39.391-	T39.392-	T39.393-	T39.394-	T39.395-	T39.396-
propionic acid derivative	T39.311-	T39.312-	T39.313-	T39.314-	T39.315-	T39.316-
specified NEC	T39.391-	T39.392-	T39.393-	T39.394-	T39.395-	T39.396-
Antikaluretic	T50.3x1-	T50.3x2-	T50.3x3-	T50.3x4-	T50.3x5-	T50.3x6-
Antiknock (tetraethyl lead)	T56.0x1-	T56.0x2-	T56.0x3-	T56.0x4-	—	—
Antilipemic drug NEC	T46.6x1-	T46.6x2-	T46.6x3-	T46.6x4-	T46.6x5-	T46.6x6-
Antimalarial	T37.2x1-	T37.2x2-	T37.2x3-	T37.2x4-	T37.2x5-	T37.2x6-
prophylactic NEC	T37.2x1-	T37.2x2-	T37.2x3-	T37.2x4-	T37.2x5-	T37.2x6-
pyrimidine derivative	T37.2x1-	T37.2x2-	T37.2x3-	T37.2x4-	T37.2x5-	T37.2x6-
Antimetabolite	T45.1x1-	T45.1x2-	T45.1x3-	T45.1x4-	T45.1x5-	T45.1x6-
Antimitotic agent	T45.1x1-	T45.1x2-	T45.1x3-	T45.1x4-	T45.1x5-	T45.1x6-
Antimony (compounds) (vapor) NEC	T56.891-	T56.892-	T56.893-	T56.894-	—	—
anti-infectives	T37.8x1-	T37.8x2-	T37.8x3-	T37.8x4-	T37.8x5-	T37.8x6-
dimercaptosuccinate	T37.3x1-	T37.3x2-	T37.3x3-	T37.3x4-	T37.3x5-	T37.3x6-
hydride	T56.891-	T56.892-	T56.893-	T56.894-	—	—
pesticide (vapor)	T60.8x1-	T60.8x2-	T60.8x3-	T60.8x4-	—	—
potassium (sodium) tartrate	T37.8x1-	T37.8x2-	T37.8x3-	T37.8x4-	T37.8x5-	T37.8x6-
tartrated	T37.8x1-	T37.8x2-	T37.8x3-	T37.8x4-	T37.8x5-	T37.8x6-
sodium dimercapto-succinate	T37.3x1-	T37.3x2-	T37.3x3-	T37.3x4-	T37.3x5-	T37.3x6-
Antimuscarinic NEC	T44.3x1-	T44.3x2-	T44.3x3-	T44.3x4-	T44.3x5-	T44.3x6-
Antimycobacterial drug NEC	T37.1x1-	T37.1x2-	T37.1x3-	T37.1x4-	T37.1x5-	T37.1x6-
antibiotics	T36.5x1-	T36.5x2-	T36.5x3-	T36.5x4-	T36.5x5-	T36.5x6-
combination	T37.1x1-	T37.1x2-	T37.1x3-	T37.1x4-	T37.1x5-	T37.1x6-
Antinausea drug	T45.0x1-	T45.0x2-	T45.0x3-	T45.0x4-	T45.0x5-	T45.0x6-
Antinematode drug	T37.4x1-	T37.4x2-	T37.4x3-	T37.4x4-	T37.4x5-	T37.4x6-
Antineoplastic NEC	T45.1x1-	T45.1x2-	T45.1x3-	T45.1x4-	T45.1x5-	T45.1x6-
antibiotics	T45.1x1-	T45.1x2-	T45.1x3-	T45.1x4-	T45.1x5-	T45.1x6-
alkaloidal	T45.1x1-	T45.1x2-	T45.1x3-	T45.1x4-	T45.1x5-	T45.1x6-
combination	T45.1x1-	T45.1x2-	T45.1x3-	T45.1x4-	T45.1x5-	T45.1x6-
estrogen	T38.5x1-	T38.5x2-	T38.5x3-	T38.5x4-	T38.5x5-	T38.5x6-
steroid	T38.7x1-	T38.7x2-	T38.7x3-	T38.7x4-	T38.7x5-	T38.7x6-
Antiparasitic drug (systemic)	T37.91x-	T37.92x-	T37.93x-	T37.94x-	T37.95x-	T37.96x-
local	T49.0x1-	T49.0x2-	T49.0x3-	T49.0x4-	T49.0x5-	T49.0x6-
specified NEC	T37.8x1-	T37.8x2-	T37.8x3-	T37.8x4-	T37.8x5-	T37.8x6-
Antiparkinsonism drug NEC	T42.8x1-	T42.8x2-	T42.8x3-	T42.8x4-	T42.8x5-	T42.8x6-
Antiperspirant NEC	T49.2x1-	T49.2x2-	T49.2x3-	T49.2x4-	T49.2x5-	T49.2x6-
Antiphlogistic NEC	T39.4x1-	T39.4x2-	T39.4x3-	T39.4x4-	T39.4x5-	T39.4x6-
Antiplatyhelmintic drug	T37.4x1-	T37.4x2-	T37.4x3-	T37.4x4-	T37.4x5-	T37.4x6-
Antiprotozoal drug NEC	T37.3x1-	T37.3x2-	T37.3x3-	T37.3x4-	T37.3x5-	T37.3x6-
blood	T37.2x1-	T37.2x2-	T37.2x3-	T37.2x4-	T37.2x5-	T37.2x6-
local	T49.0x1-	T49.0x2-	T49.0x3-	T49.0x4-	T49.0x5-	T49.0x6-
Antipruritic drug NEC	T49.1x1-	T49.1x2-	T49.1x3-	T49.1x4-	T49.1x5-	T49.1x6-
Antipsychotic drug NEC	T43.501-	T43.502-	T43.503-	T43.504-	T43.505-	T43.506-
specified NEC	T43.591-	T43.592-	T43.593-	T43.594-	T43.595-	T43.596-
Antipyretic	T39.91x-	T39.92x-	T39.93x-	T39.94x-	T39.95x-	T39.96x-
specified NEC	T39.8x1-	T39.8x2-	T39.8x3-	T39.8x4-	T39.8x5-	T39.8x6-
Antipyrine	T39.2x1-	T39.2x2-	T39.2x3-	T39.2x4-	T39.2x5-	T39.2x6-
Antirabies hyperimmune serum	T50.Z11-	T50.Z12-	T50.Z13-	T50.Z14-	T50.Z15-	T50.Z16-
Antirheumatic NEC	T39.4x1-	T39.4x2-	T39.4x3-	T39.4x4-	T39.4x5-	T39.4x6-
Antirigidity drug NEC	T42.8x1-	T42.8x2-	T42.8x3-	T42.8x4-	T42.8x5-	T42.8x6-
Antischistosomal drug	T37.4x1-	T37.4x2-	T37.4x3-	T37.4x4-	T37.4x5-	T37.4x6-
Antiscorpion sera	T50.Z11-	T50.Z12-	T50.Z13-	T50.Z14-	T50.Z15-	T50.Z16-
Antiseborrheics	T49.4x1-	T49.4x2-	T49.4x3-	T49.4x4-	T49.4x5-	T49.4x6-
Antiseptics (external) (medicinal)	T49.0x1-	T49.0x2-	T49.0x3-	T49.0x4-	T49.0x5-	T49.0x6-

DRUGS & CHEMICALS

Table of Drugs & Chemicals	POISONING Accidental (Unintentional)	Self-Harm (Intentional)	Assault	Undetermined	Adverse Effect	Underdosing
Antistine	T45.0x1-	T45.0x2-	T45.0x3-	T45.0x4-	T45.0x5-	T45.0x6-
Antitapeworm drug	T37.4x1-	T37.4x2-	T37.4x3-	T37.4x4-	T37.4x5-	T37.4x6-
Antitetanus immunoglobulin	T50.Z11	T50.Z12-	T50.Z13-	T50.Z14-	T50.Z15-	T50.Z16-
Antithyroid drug NEC	T38.2x1-	T38.2x2-	T38.2x3-	T38.2x4-	T38.2x5-	T38.2x6-
Antitoxin	T50.Z11-	T50.Z12-	T50.Z13-	T50.Z14-	T50.Z15-	T50.Z16-
diphtheria	T50.Z11-	T50.Z12-	T50.Z13-	T50.Z14-	T50.Z15-	T50.Z16-
gas gangrene	T50.Z11-	T50.Z12-	T50.Z13-	T50.Z14-	T50.Z15-	T50.Z16-
tetanus	T50.Z11-	T50.Z12-	T50.Z13-	T50.Z14-	T50.Z15-	T50.Z16-
Antitrichomonal drug	T37.3x1-	T37.3x2-	T37.3x3-	T37.3x4-	T37.3x5-	T37.3x6-
Antituberculars	T37.1x1-	T37.1x2-	T37.1x3-	T37.1x4-	T37.1x5-	T37.1x6-
antibiotics	T36.5x1-	T36.5x2-	T36.5x3-	T36.5x4-	T36.5x5-	T36.5x6-
Antitussive NEC	T48.3x1-	T48.3x2-	T48.3x3-	T48.3x4-	T48.3x5-	T48.3x6-
codeine mixture	T40.2x1-	T40.2x2-	T40.2x3-	T40.2x4-	T40.2x5-	T40.2x6-
opiate	T40.2x1-	T40.2x2-	T40.2x3-	T40.2x4-	T40.2x5-	T40.2x6-
Antivaricose drug	T46.8x1-	T46.8x2-	T46.8x3-	T46.8x4-	T46.8x5-	T46.8x6-
Antivenin, antivenom (sera)	T50.Z11-	T50.Z12-	T50.Z13-	T50.Z14-	T50.Z15-	T50.Z16-
crotaline	T50.Z11-	T50.Z12-	T50.Z13-	T50.Z14-	T50.Z15-	T50.Z16-
spider bite	T50.Z11-	T50.Z12-	T50.Z13-	T50.Z14-	T50.Z15-	T50.Z16-
Antivertigo drug	T45.0x1-	T45.0x2-	T45.0x3-	T45.0x4-	T45.0x5-	T45.0x6-
Antiviral drug NEC	T37.5x1-	T37.5x2-	T37.5x3-	T37.5x4-	T37.5x5-	T37.5x6-
eye	T49.5x1-	T49.5x2-	T49.5x3-	T49.5x4-	T49.5x5-	T49.5x6-
Antiwhipworm drug	T37.4x1-	T37.4x2-	T37.4x3-	T37.4x4-	T37.4x5-	T37.4x6-
Antrol — see also by specific chemical substance	T60.91x-	T60.92x-	T60.93x-	T60.94x-	—	—
fungicide	T60.91x-	T60.92x-	T60.93x-	T60.94x-	—	—
ANTU (alpha naphthylthiourea)	T60.4x1-	T60.4x2-	T60.4x3-	T60.4x4-	—	—
Apalcillin	T36.0x1-	T36.0x2-	T36.0x3-	T36.0x4-	T36.0x5-	T36.0x6-
APC	T48.5x1-	T48.5x2-	T48.5x3-	T48.5x4-	T48.5x5-	T48.5x6-
Aplonidine	T44.4x1-	T44.4x2-	T44.4x3-	T44.4x4-	T44.4x5-	T44.4x6-
Apomorphine	T47.7x1-	T47.7x2-	T47.7x3-	T47.7x4-	T47.7x5-	T47.7x6-
Appetite depressants, central	T50.5x1-	T50.5x2-	T50.5x3-	T50.5x4-	T50.5x5-	T50.5x6-
Apraclonidine (hydrochloride)	T44.4x1-	T44.4x2-	T44.4x3-	T44.4x4-	T44.4x5-	T44.4x6-
Apresoline	T46.5x1-	T46.5x2-	T46.5x3-	T46.5x4-	T46.5x5-	T46.5x6-
Aprindine	T46.2x1-	T46.2x2-	T46.2x3-	T46.2x4-	T46.2x5-	T46.2x6-
Aprobarbital	T42.3x1-	T42.3x2-	T42.3x3-	T42.3x4-	T42.3x5-	T42.3x6-
Apronalide	T42.6x1-	T42.6x2-	T42.6x3-	T42.6x4-	T42.6x5-	T42.6x6-
Aprotinin	T45.621-	T45.622-	T45.623-	T45.624-	T45.625-	T45.626-
Aptocaine	T41.3x1-	T41.3x2-	T41.3x3-	T41.3x4-	T41.3x5-	T41.3x6-
Aqua fortis	T54.2x1-	T54.2x2-	T54.2x3-	T54.2x4-	—	—
Ara-A	T37.5x1-	T37.5x2-	T37.5x3-	T37.5x4-	T37.5x5-	T37.5x6-
Ara-C	T45.1x1-	T45.1x2-	T45.1x3-	T45.1x4-	T45.1x5-	T45.1x6-
Arachis oil	T49.3x1-	T49.3x2-	T49.3x3-	T49.3x4-	T49.3x5-	T49.3x6-
cathartic	T47.4x1-	T47.4x2-	T47.4x3-	T47.4x4-	T47.4x5-	T47.4x6-
Aralen	T37.2x1-	T37.2x2-	T37.2x3-	T37.2x4-	T37.2x5-	T37.2x6-
Arecoline	T44.1x1-	T44.1x2-	T44.1x3-	T44.1x4-	T44.1x5-	T44.1x6-
Arginine	T50.991-	T50.992-	T50.993-	T50.994-	T50.995-	T50.996-
glutamate	T50.991-	T50.992-	T50.993-	T50.994-	T50.995-	T50.996-
Argyrol	T49.0x1-	T49.0x2-	T49.0x3-	T49.0x4-	T49.0x5-	T49.0x6-
ENT agent	T49.6x1-	T49.6x2-	T49.6x3-	T49.6x4-	T49.6x5-	T49.6x6-
ophthalmic preparation	T49.5x1-	T49.5x2-	T49.5x3-	T49.5x4-	T49.5x5-	T49.5x6-
Aristocort	T38.0x1-	T38.0x2-	T38.0x3-	T38.0x4-	T38.0x5-	T38.0x6-
ENT agent	T49.6x1-	T49.6x2-	T49.6x3-	T49.6x4-	T49.6x5-	T49.6x6-
ophthalmic preparation	T49.5x1-	T49.5x2-	T49.5x3-	T49.5x4-	T49.5x5-	T49.5x6-
topical NEC	T49.0x1-	T49.0x2-	T49.0x3-	T49.0x4-	T49.0x5-	T49.0x6-
Aromatics, corrosive	T54.1x1-	T54.1x2-	T54.1x3-	T54.1x4-	—	—
disinfectants	T54.1x1-	T54.1x2-	T54.1x3-	T54.1x4-	—	—
Arsenate of lead	T57.0x1-	T57.0x2-	T57.0x3-	T57.0x4-	—	—
herbicide	T57.0x1-	T57.0x2-	T57.0x3-	T57.0x4-	—	—
Arsenic, arsenicals (compounds) (dust) (vapor) NEC	T57.0x1-	T57.0x2-	T57.0x3-	T57.0x4-	—	—
anti-infectives	T37.8x1-	T37.8x2-	T37.8x3-	T37.8x4-	T37.8x5-	T37.8x6-
pesticide (dust) (fumes)	T57.0x1-	T57.0x2-	T57.0x3-	T57.0x4-	—	—
Arsine (gas)	T57.0x1-	T57.0x2-	T57.0x3-	T57.0x4-	—	—
Arsphenamine (silver)	T37.8x1-	T37.8x2-	T37.8x3-	T37.8x4-	T37.8x5-	T37.8x6-
Arsthinol	T37.3x1-	T37.3x2-	T37.3x3-	T37.3x4-	T37.3x5-	T37.3x6-
Artane	T44.3x1-	T44.3x2-	T44.3x3-	T44.3x4-	T44.3x5-	T44.3x6-
Arthropod (venomous) NEC	T63.481-	T63.482-	T63.483-	T63.484-		
Articaine	T41.3x1-	T41.3x2-	T41.3x3-	T41.3x4-	T41.3x5-	T41.3x6-
Asbestos	T57.8x1-	T57.8x2-	T57.8x3-	T57.8x4-		
Ascaridole	T37.4x1-	T37.4x2-	T37.4x3-	T37.4x4-	T37.4x5-	T37.4x6-
Ascorbic acid	T45.2x1-	T45.2x2-	T45.2x3-	T45.2x4-	T45.2x5-	T45.2x6-
Asiaticoside	T49.0x1-	T49.0x2-	T49.0x3-	T49.0x4-	T49.0x5-	T49.0x6-
Asparaginase	T45.1x1-	T45.1x2-	T45.1x3-	T45.1x4-	T45.1x5-	T45.1x6-
Aspidium (oleoresin)	T37.4x1-	T37.4x2-	T37.4x3-	T37.4x4-	T37.4x5-	T37.4x6-
Aspirin (aluminum) (soluble)	T39.011-	T39.012-	T39.013-	T39.014-	T39.015-	T39.016-
Aspoxicillin	T36.0x1-	T36.0x2-	T36.0x3-	T36.0x4-	T36.0x5-	T36.0x6-
Astemizole	T45.0x1-	T45.0x2-	T45.0x3-	T45.0x4-	T45.0x5-	T45.0x6-
Astringent (local) specified NEC	T49.2x1-	T49.2x2-	T49.2x3-	T49.2x4-	T49.2x5-	T49.2x6-
	T49.2x1-	T49.2x2-	T49.2x3-	T49.2x4-	T49.2x5-	T49.2x6-
Astromicin	T36.5x1-	T36.5x2-	T36.5x3-	T36.5x4-	T36.5x5-	T36.5x6-
Ataractic drug NEC	T43.501-	T43.502-	T43.503-	T43.504-	T43.505-	T43.506-
Atenolol	T44.7x1-	T44.7x2-	T44.7x3-	T44.7x4-	T44.7x5-	T44.7x6-
Atonia drug, intestinal	T47.4x1-	T47.4x2-	T47.4x3-	T47.4x4-	T47.4x5-	T47.4x6-
Atophan	T50.4x1-	T50.4x2-	T50.4x3-	T50.4x4-	T50.4x5-	T50.4x6-
Atracurium besilate	T48.1x1-	T48.1x2-	T48.1x3-	T48.1x4-	T48.1x5-	T48.1x6-
Atropine	T44.3x1-	T44.3x2-	T44.3x3-	T44.3x4-	T44.3x5-	T44.3x6-
derivative	T44.3x1-	T44.3x2-	T44.3x3-	T44.3x4-	T44.3x5-	T44.3x6-
methonitrate	T44.3x1-	T44.3x2-	T44.3x3-	T44.3x4-	T44.3x5-	T44.3x6-
Attapulgite	T47.6x1-	T47.6x2-	T47.6x3-	T47.6x4-	T47.6x5-	T47.6x6-
Auramine	T65.891-	T65.892-	T65.893-	T65.894-	—	—
dye	T65.6x1-	T65.6x2-	T65.6x3-	T65.6x4-	—	—
fungicide	T60.3x1-	T60.3x2-	T60.3x3-	T60.3x4-	—	—
Auranofin	T39.4x1-	T39.4x2-	T39.4x3-	T39.4x4-	T39.4x5-	T39.4x6-
Aurantiin	T46.991-	T46.992-	T46.993-	T46.994-	T46.995-	T46.996-
Aureomycin	T36.4x1-	T36.4x2-	T36.4x3-	T36.4x4-	T36.4x5-	T36.4x6-
ophthalmic preparation	T49.5x1-	T49.5x2-	T49.5x3-	T49.5x4-	T49.5x5-	T49.5x6-
topical NEC	T49.0x1-	T49.0x2-	T49.0x3-	T49.0x4-	T49.0x5-	T49.0x6-
Aurothioglucose	T39.4x1-	T39.4x2-	T39.4x3-	T39.4x4-	T39.4x5-	T39.4x6-
Aurothioglycanide	T39.4x1-	T39.4x2-	T39.4x3-	T39.4x4-	T39.4x5-	T39.4x6-
Aurothiomalate sodium	T39.4x1-	T39.4x2-	T39.4x3-	T39.4x4-	T39.4x5-	T39.4x6-
Aurotioprol	T39.4x1-	T39.4x2-	T39.4x3-	T39.4x4-	T39.4x5-	T39.4x6-
Automobile fuel	T52.0x1-	T52.0x2-	T52.0x3-	T52.0x4-	—	—
Autonomic nervous system agent NEC	T44.901-	T44.902-	T44.903-	T44.904-	T44.905-	T44.906-
Avlosulfon	T37.1x1-	T37.1x2-	T37.1x3-	T37.1x4-	T37.1x5-	T37.1x6-
Avomine	T42.6x1-	T42.6x2-	T42.6x3-	T42.6x4-	T42.6x5-	T42.6x6-
Axerophthol	T45.2x1-	T45.2x2-	T45.2x3-	T45.2x4-	T45.2x5-	T45.2x6-
Azacitidine	T45.1x1-	T45.1x2-	T45.1x3-	T45.1x4-	T45.1x5-	T45.1x6-
Azacyclonol	T43.591-	T43.592-	T43.593-	T43.594-	T43.595-	T43.596-
Azadirachta	T60.2x1-	T60.2x2-	T60.2x3-	T60.2x4-	—	—
Azanidazole	T37.3x1-	T37.3x2-	T37.3x3-	T37.3x4-	T37.3x5-	T37.3x6-
Azapetine	T46.7x1-	T46.7x2-	T46.7x3-	T46.7x4-	T46.7x5-	T46.7x6-
Azapropazone	T39.2x1-	T39.2x2-	T39.2x3-	T39.2x4-	T39.2x5-	T39.2x6-
Azaribine	T45.1x1-	T45.1x2-	T45.1x3-	T45.1x4-	T45.1x5-	T45.1x6-
Azaserine	T45.1x1-	T45.1x2-	T45.1x3-	T45.1x4-	T45.1x5-	T45.1x6-
Azatadine	T45.0x1-	T45.0x2-	T45.0x3-	T45.0x4-	T45.0x5-	T45.0x6-
Azatepa	T45.1x1-	T45.1x2-	T45.1x3-	T45.1x4-	T45.1x5-	T45.1x6-
Azathioprine	T45.1x1-	T45.1x2-	T45.1x3-	T45.1x4-	T45.1x5-	T45.1x6-

DRUGS & CHEMICALS

Table of Drugs & Chemicals	POISONING Accidental (Unintentional)	Self-Harm (Intentional)	Assault	Undetermined	Adverse Effect	Underdosing
Azelaic acid	T49.0x1-	T49.0x2-	T49.0x3-	T49.0x4-	T49.0x5-	T49.0x6-
Azelastine	T45.0x1-	T45.0x2-	T45.0x3-	T45.0x4-	T45.0x5-	T45.0x6-
Azidocillin	T36.0x1-	T36.0x2-	T36.0x3-	T36.0x4-	T36.0x5-	T36.0x6-
Azidothymidine	T37.5x1-	T37.5x2-	T37.5x3-	T37.5x4-	T37.5x5-	T37.5x6-
Azinphos (ethyl) (methyl)	T60.0x1-	T60.0x2-	T60.0x3-	T60.0x4-	—	—
Aziridine (chelating)	T54.1x1-	T54.1x2-	T54.1x3-	T54.1x4-	—	—
Azithromycin	T36.3x1-	T36.3x2-	T36.3x3-	T36.3x4-	T36.3x5-	T36.3x6-
Azlocillin	T36.0x1-	T36.0x2-	T36.0x3-	T36.0x4-	T36.0x5-	T36.0x6-
Azobenzene smoke	T65.3x1-	T65.3x2-	T65.3x3-	T65.3x4-	—	—
acaricide	T60.8x1-	T60.8x2-	T60.8x3-	T60.8x4-	—	—
Azosulfamide	T37.0x1-	T37.0x2-	T37.0x3-	T37.0x4-	T37.0x5-	T37.0x6-
AZT	T37.5x1-	T37.5x2-	T37.5x3-	T37.5x4-	T37.5x5-	T37.5x6-
Aztreonam	T36.1x1-	T36.1x2-	T36.1x3-	T36.1x4-	T36.1x5-	T36.1x6-
Azulfidine	T37.0x1-	T37.0x2-	T37.0x3-	T37.0x4-	T37.0x5-	T37.0x6-
Azuresin	T50.8x1-	T50.8x2-	T50.8x3-	T50.8x4-	T50.8x5-	T50.8x6-
Bacampicillin	T36.0x1-	T36.0x2-	T36.0x3-	T36.0x4-	T36.0x5-	T36.0x6-
b-acetyldigoxin	T46.0x1-	T46.0x2-	T46.0x3-	T46.0x4-	T46.0x5-	T46.0x6-
Bacillus						
lactobacillus	T47.8x1-	T47.8x2-	T47.8x3-	T47.8x4-	T47.8x5-	T47.8x6-
subtilis	T47.6x1-	T47.6x2-	T47.6x3-	T47.6x4-	T47.6x5-	T47.6x6-
Bacimycin	T49.0x1-	T49.0x2-	T49.0x3-	T49.0x4-	T49.0x5-	T49.0x6-
ophthalmic preparation	T49.5x1-	T49.5x2-	T49.5x3-	T49.5x4-	T49.5x5-	T49.5x6-
Bacitracin zinc	T49.0x1-	T49.0x2-	T49.0x3-	T49.0x4-	T49.0x5-	T49.0x6-
with neomycin	T49.0x1-	T49.0x2-	T49.0x3-	T49.0x4-	T49.0x5-	T49.0x6-
ENT agent	T49.6x1-	T49.6x2-	T49.6x3-	T49.6x4-	T49.6x5-	T49.6x6-
ophthalmic preparation	T49.5x1-	T49.5x2-	T49.5x3-	T49.5x4-	T49.5x5-	T49.5x6-
topical NEC	T49.0x1-	T49.0x2-	T49.0x3-	T49.0x4-	T49.0x5-	T49.0x6-
Baclofen	T42.8x1-	T42.8x2-	T42.8x3-	T42.8x4-	T42.8x5-	T42.8x6-
Baking soda	T50.991-	T50.992-	T50.993-	T50.994-	T50.995-	T50.996-
BAL	T45.8x1-	T45.8x2-	T45.8x3-	T45.8x4-	T45.8x5-	T45.8x6-
Bambuterol	T48.6x1-	T48.6x2-	T48.6x3-	T48.6x4-	T48.6x5-	T48.6x6-
Bamethan (sulfate)	T46.7x1-	T46.7x2-	T46.7x3-	T46.7x4-	T46.7x5-	T46.7x6-
Bamifylline	T48.6x1-	T48.6x2-	T48.6x3-	T48.6x4-	T48.6x5-	T48.6x6-
Bamipine	T45.0x1-	T45.0x2-	T45.0x3-	T45.0x4-	T45.0x5-	T45.0x6-
Baneberry — see Actaea spicata						
Banewort — see Belladonna						
Barbenyl	T42.3x1-	T42.3x2-	T42.3x3-	T42.3x4-	T42.3x5-	T42.3x6-
Barbexaclone	T42.6x1-	T42.6x2-	T42.6x3-	T42.6x4-	T42.6x5-	T42.6x6-
Barbital	T42.3x1-	T42.3x2-	T42.3x3-	T42.3x4-	T42.3x5-	T42.3x6-
sodium	T42.3x1-	T42.3x2-	T42.3x3-	T42.3x4-	T42.3x5-	T42.3x6-
Barbitone	T42.3x1-	T42.3x2-	T42.3x3-	T42.3x4-	T42.3x5-	T42.3x6-
Barbiturate NEC	T42.3x1-	T42.3x2-	T42.3x3-	T42.3x4-	T42.3x5-	T42.3x6-
with tranquilizer	T42.3x1-	T42.3x2-	T42.3x3-	T42.3x4-	T42.3x5-	T42.3x6-
anesthetic (intravenous)	T41.1x1-	T41.1x2-	T41.1x3-	T41.1x4-	T41.1x5-	T41.1x6-
Barium (carbonate) (chloride) (sulfite)	T57.8x1-	T57.8x2-	T57.8x3-	T57.8x4-	—	—
diagnostic agent	T50.8x1-	T50.8x2-	T50.8x3-	T50.8x4-	T50.8x5-	T50.8x6-
pesticide	T60.4x1-	T60.4x2-	T60.4x3-	T60.4x4-	—	—
rodenticide	T60.4x1-	T60.4x2-	T60.4x3-	T60.4x4-	—	—
sulfate (medicinal)	T50.8x1-	T50.8x2-	T50.8x3-	T50.8x4-	T50.8x5-	T50.8x6-
Barrier cream	T49.3x1-	T49.3x2-	T49.3x3-	T49.3x4-	T49.3x5-	T49.3x6-
Basic fuchsin	T49.0x1-	T49.0x2-	T49.0x3-	T49.0x4-	T49.0x5-	T49.0x6-
Battery acid or fluid	T54.2x1-	T54.2x2-	T54.2x3-	T54.2x4-	—	—
Bay rum	T51.8x1-	T51.8x2-	T51.8x3-	T51.8x4-	—	—
b-benzalbutyramide	T46.6x1-	T46.6x2-	T46.6x3-	T46.6x4-	T46.6x5-	T46.6x6-
BCG (vaccine)	T50.A91-	T50.A92-	T50.A93-	T50.A94-	T50.A95	T50.A96-
BCNU	T45.1x1-	T45.1x2-	T45.1x3-	T45.1x4-	T45.1x5-	T45.1x6-
Bearsfoot	T62.2x1-	T62.2x2-	T62.2x3-	T62.2x4-	—	—
Beclamide	T42.6x1-	T42.6x2-	T42.6x3-	T42.6x4-	T42.6x5-	T42.6x6-
Beclomethasone	T44.5x1-	T44.5x2-	T44.5x3-	T44.5x4-	T44.5x5-	T44.5x6-
Bee (sting) (venom)	T63.441-	T63.442-	T63.443-	T63.444-	—	—
Befunolol	T49.5x1-	T49.5x2-	T49.5x3-	T49.5x4-	T49.5x5-	T49.5x6-

Table of Drugs & Chemicals	POISONING Accidental (Unintentional)	Self-Harm (Intentional)	Assault	Undetermined	Adverse Effect	Underdosing
Bekanamycin	T36.5x1-	T36.5x2-	T36.5x3-	T36.5x4-	T36.5x5-	T36.5x6-
Belladonna — see also Nightshade						
alkaloids	T44.3x1-	T44.3x2-	T44.3x3-	T44.3x4-	T44.3x5-	T44.3x6-
extract	T44.3x1-	T44.3x2-	T44.3x3-	T44.3x4-	T44.3x5-	T44.3x6-
herb	T44.3x1-	T44.3x2-	T44.3x3-	T44.3x4-	T44.3x5-	T44.3x6-
Bemegride	T50.7x1-	T50.7x2-	T50.7x3-	T50.7x4-	T50.7x5-	T50.7x6-
Benactyzine	T44.3x1-	T44.3x2-	T44.3x3-	T44.3x4-	T44.3x5-	T44.3x6-
Benadryl	T45.0x1-	T45.0x2-	T45.0x3-	T45.0x4-	T45.0x5-	T45.0x6-
Benaprizine	T44.3x1-	T44.3x2-	T44.3x3-	T44.3x4-	T44.3x5-	T44.3x6-
Benazepril	T46.4x1-	T46.4x2-	T46.4x3-	T46.4x4-	T46.4x5-	T46.4x6-
Bencyclane	T46.7x1-	T46.7x2-	T46.7x3-	T46.7x4-	T46.7x5-	T46.7x6-
Bendazol	T46.3x1-	T46.3x2-	T46.3x3-	T46.3x4-	T46.3x5-	T46.3x6-
Bendrofluazide	T50.2x1-	T50.2x2-	T50.2x3-	T50.2x4-	T50.2x5-	T50.2x6-
Bendroflumethiazide	T50.2x1-	T50.2x2-	T50.2x3-	T50.2x4-	T50.2x5-	T50.2x6-
Benemid	T50.4x1-	T50.4x2-	T50.4x3-	T50.4x4-	T50.4x5-	T50.4x6-
Benethamine penicillin	T36.0x1-	T36.0x2-	T36.0x3-	T36.0x4-	T36.0x5-	T36.0x6-
Benexate	T47.1x1-	T47.1x2-	T47.1x3-	T47.1x4-	T47.1x5-	T47.1x6-
Benfluorex	T46.6x1-	T46.6x2-	T46.6x3-	T46.6x4-	T46.6x5-	T46.6x6-
Benfotiamine	T45.2x1-	T45.2x2-	T45.2x3-	T45.2x4-	T45.2x5-	T45.2x6-
Benisone	T49.0x1-	T49.0x2-	T49.0x3-	T49.0x4-	T49.0x5-	T49.0x6-
Benomyl	T60.0x1-	T60.0x2-	T60.0x3-	T60.0x4-	—	—
Benoquin	T49.8x1-	T49.8x2-	T49.8x3-	T49.8x4-	T49.8x5-	T49.8x6-
Benoxinate	T41.3x1-	T41.3x2-	T41.3x3-	T41.3x4-	T41.3x5-	T41.3x6-
Benperidol	T43.4x1-	T43.4x2-	T43.4x3-	T43.4x4-	T43.4x5-	T43.4x6-
Benproperine	T48.3x1-	T48.3x2-	T48.3x3-	T48.3x4-	T48.3x5-	T48.3x6-
Benserazide	T42.8x1-	T42.8x2-	T42.8x3-	T42.8x4-	T42.8x5-	T42.8x6-
Bentazepam	T42.4x1-	T42.4x2-	T42.4x3-	T42.4x4-	T42.4x5-	T42.4x6-
Bentiromide	T50.8x1-	T50.8x2-	T50.8x3-	T50.8x4-	T50.8x5-	T50.8x6-
Bentonite	T49.3x1-	T49.3x2-	T49.3x3-	T49.3x4-	T49.3x5-	T49.3x6-
Benzalbutyramide	T46.6x1-	T46.6x2-	T46.6x3-	T46.6x4-	T46.6x5-	T46.6x6-
Benzalkonium (chloride)	T49.0x1-	T49.0x2-	T49.0x3-	T49.0x4-	T49.0x5-	T49.0x6-
ophthalmic preparation	T49.5x1-	T49.5x2-	T49.5x3-	T49.5x4-	T49.5x5-	T49.5x6-
Benzamidosalicylate (calcium)	T37.1x1-	T37.1x2-	T37.1x3-	T37.1x4-	T37.1x5-	T37.1x6-
Benzamine	T41.3x1-	T41.3x2-	T41.3x3-	T41.3x4-	T41.3x5-	T41.3x6-
lactate	T49.1x1-	T49.1x2-	T49.1x3-	T49.1x4-	T49.1x5-	T49.1x6-
Benzamphetamine	T50.5x1-	T50.5x2-	T50.5x3-	T50.5x4-	T50.5x5-	T50.5x6-
Benzapril hydrochloride	T46.5x1-	T46.5x2-	T46.5x3-	T46.5x4-	T46.5x5-	T46.5x6-
Benzathine benzylpenicillin	T36.0x1-	T36.0x2-	T36.0x3-	T36.0x4-	T36.0x5-	T36.0x6-
Benzathine penicillin	T36.0x1-	T36.0x2-	T36.0x3-	T36.0x4-	T36.0x5-	T36.0x6-
Benzatropine	T42.8x1-	T42.8x2-	T42.8x3-	T42.8x4-	T42.8x5-	T42.8x6-
Benzbromarone	T50.4x1-	T50.4x2-	T50.4x3-	T50.4x4-	T50.4x5-	T50.4x6-
Benzcarbimine	T45.1x1-	T45.1x2-	T45.1x3-	T45.1x4-	T45.1x5-	T45.1x6-
Benzedrex	T44.991-	T44.992-	T44.993-	T44.994-	T44.995-	T44.996-
Benzedrine (amphetamine)	T43.621-	T43.622-	T43.623-	T43.624-	T43.625-	T43.626-
Benzenamine	T65.3x1-	T65.3x2-	T65.3x3-	T65.3x4-	—	—
Benzene	T52.1x1-	T52.1x2-	T52.1x3-	T52.1x4-	—	—
homologues (acetyl) (dimethyl) (methyl) (solvent)	T52.2x1-	T52.2x2-	T52.2x3-	T52.2x4-	—	—
Benzethonium (chloride)	T49.0x1-	T49.0x2-	T49.0x3-	T49.0x4-	T49.0x5-	T49.0x6-
Benzfetamine	T50.5x1-	T50.5x2-	T50.5x3-	T50.5x4-	T50.5x5-	T50.5x6-
Benzhexol	T44.3x1-	T44.3x2-	T44.3x3-	T44.3x4-	T44.3x5-	T44.3x6-
Benzhydramine (chloride)	T45.0x1-	T45.0x2-	T45.0x3-	T45.0x4-	T45.0x5-	T45.0x6-
Benzidine	T65.891-	T65.892-	T65.893-	T65.894-	—	—
Benzilonium bromide	T44.3x1-	T44.3x2-	T44.3x3-	T44.3x4-	T44.3x5-	T44.3x6-
Benzimidazole	T60.3x1-	T60.3x2-	T60.3x3-	T60.3x4-	—	—
Benzin (e) — see Ligroin						
Benziodarone	T46.3x1-	T46.3x2-	T46.3x3-	T46.3x4-	T46.3x5-	T46.3x6-
Benznidazole	T37.3x1-	T37.3x2-	T37.3x3-	T37.3x4-	T37.3x5-	T37.3x6-
Benzocaine	T41.3x1-	T41.3x2-	T41.3x3-	T41.3x4-	T41.3x5-	T41.3x6-
Benzodiapin	T42.4x1-	T42.4x2-	T42.4x3-	T42.4x4-	T42.4x5-	T42.4x6-

DRUGS & CHEMICALS

Table of Drugs & Chemicals	Accidental (Unintentional)	Self-Harm (Intentional)	Assault	Undetermined	Adverse Effect	Underdosing
Benzodiazepine NEC	T42.4x1-	T42.4x2-	T42.4x3-	T42.4x4-	T42.4x5-	T42.4x6-
Benzoic acid	T49.0x1-	T49.0x2-	T49.0x3-	T49.0x4-	T49.0x5-	T49.0x6-
with salicylic acid	T49.0x1-	T49.0x2-	T49.0x3-	T49.0x4-	T49.0x5-	T49.0x6-
Benzoin (tincture)	T48.5x1-	T48.5x2-	T48.5x3-	T48.5x4-	T48.5x5-	T48.5x6-
Benzol (benzene)	T52.1x1-	T52.1x2-	T52.1x3-	T52.1x4-	—	—
vapor	T52.0x1-	T52.0x2-	T52.0x3-	T52.0x4-	—	—
Benzomorphan	T40.2x1-	T40.2x2-	T40.2x3-	T40.2x4-	T40.2x5-	T40.2x6-
Benzonatate	T48.3x1-	T48.3x2-	T48.3x3-	T48.3x4-	T48.3x5-	T48.3x6-
Benzophenones	T49.3x1-	T49.3x2-	T49.3x3-	T49.3x4-	T49.3x5-	T49.3x6-
Benzopyrone	T46.991-	T46.992-	T46.993-	T46.994-	T46.995-	T46.996-
Benzothiadiazides	T50.2x1-	T50.2x2-	T50.2x3-	T50.2x4-	T50.2x5-	T50.2x6-
Benzoxonium chloride	T49.0x1-	T49.0x2-	T49.0x3-	T49.0x4-	T49.0x5-	T49.0x6-
Benzoyl peroxide	T49.0x1-	T49.0x2-	T49.0x3-	T49.0x4-	T49.0x5-	T49.0x6-
Benzoylpas calcium	T37.1x1-	T37.1x2-	T37.1x3-	T37.1x4-	T37.1x5-	T37.1x6-
Benzperidin	T43.591-	T43.592-	T43.593-	T43.594-	T43.595-	T43.596-
Benzperidol	T43.591-	T43.592-	T43.593-	T43.594-	T43.595-	T43.596-
Benzphetamine	T50.5x1-	T50.5x2-	T50.5x3-	T50.5x4-	T50.5x5-	T50.5x6-
Benzpyrinium bromide	T44.1x1-	T44.1x2-	T44.1x3-	T44.1x4-	T44.1x5-	T44.1x6-
Benzquinamide	T45.0x1-	T45.0x2-	T45.0x3-	T45.0x4-	T45.0x5-	T45.0x6-
Benzthiazide	T50.2x1-	T50.2x2-	T50.2x3-	T50.2x4-	T50.2x5-	T50.2x6-
Benztropine						
anticholinergic	T44.3x1-	T44.3x2-	T44.3x3-	T44.3x4-	T44.3x5-	T44.3x6-
antiparkinson	T42.8x1-	T42.8x2-	T42.8x3-	T42.8x4-	T42.8x5-	T42.8x6-
Benzydamine	T49.0x1-	T49.0x2-	T49.0x3-	T49.0x4-	T49.0x5-	T49.0x6-
Benzyl						
acetate	T52.8x1-	T52.8x2-	T52.8x3-	T52.8x4-	—	—
alcohol	T49.0x1-	T49.0x2-	T49.0x3-	T49.0x4-	T49.0x5-	T49.0x6-
benzoate	T49.0x1-	T49.0x2-	T49.0x3-	T49.0x4-	T49.0x5-	T49.0x6-
Benzoic acid	T49.0x1-	T49.0x2-	T49.0x3-	T49.0x4-	T49.0x5-	T49.0x6-
morphine	T40.2x1-	T40.2x2-	T40.2x3-	T40.2x4-	—	—
nicotinate	T46.6x1-	T46.6x2-	T46.6x3-	T46.6x4-	T46.6x5-	T46.6x6-
penicillin	T36.0x1-	T36.0x2-	T36.0x3-	T36.0x4-	T36.0x5-	T36.0x6-
Benzylhydrochlorthiazide	T50.2x1-	T50.2x2-	T50.2x3-	T50.2x4-	T50.2x5-	T50.2x6-
Benzylpenicillin	T36.0x1-	T36.0x2-	T36.0x3-	T36.0x4-	T36.0x5-	T36.0x6-
Benzylthiouracil	T38.2x1-	T38.2x2-	T38.2x3-	T38.2x4-	T38.2x5-	T38.2x6-
Bephenium hydroxy-naphthoate	T37.4x1-	T37.4x2-	T37.4x3-	T37.4x4-	T37.4x5-	T37.4x6-
Bepridil	T46.1x1-	T46.1x2-	T46.1x3-	T46.1x4-	T46.1x5-	T46.1x6-
Bergamot oil	T65.891-	T65.892-	T65.893-	T65.894-	—	—
Bergapten	T50.991-	T50.992-	T50.993-	T50.994-	T50.995-	T50.996-
Berries, poisonous	T62.1x1-	T62.1x2-	T62.1x3-	T62.1x4-	—	—
Beryllium (compounds)	T56.7x1-	T56.7x2-	T56.7x3-	T56.7x4-	—	—
Beta adrenergic blocking agent, heart	T44.7x1-	T44.7x2-	T44.7x3-	T44.7x4-	T44.7x5-	T44.7x6-
Betacarotene	T45.2x1-	T45.2x2-	T45.2x3-	T45.2x4-	T45.2x5-	T45.2x6-
Beta-Chlor	T42.6x1-	T42.6x2-	T42.6x3-	T42.6x4-	T42.6x5-	T42.6x6-
Betahistine	T46.7x1-	T46.7x2-	T46.7x3-	T46.7x4-	T46.7x5-	T46.7x6-
Betaine	T47.5x1-	T47.5x2-	T47.5x3-	T47.5x4-	T47.5x5-	T47.5x6-
Betamethasone	T49.0x1-	T49.0x2-	T49.0x3-	T49.0x4-	T49.0x5-	T49.0x6-
topical	T49.0x1-	T49.0x2-	T49.0x3-	T49.0x4-	T49.0x5-	T49.0x6-
Betamicin	T36.8x1-	T36.8x2-	T36.8x3-	T36.8x4-	T36.8x5-	T36.8x6-
Betanidine	T46.5x1-	T46.5x2-	T46.5x3-	T46.5x4-	T46.5x5-	T46.5x6-
Betaxolol	T44.7x1-	T44.7x2-	T44.7x3-	T44.7x4-	T44.7x5-	T44.7x6-
Betazole	T50.8x1-	T50.8x2-	T50.8x3-	T50.8x4-	T50.8x5-	T50.8x6-
Bethanechol	T44.1x1-	T44.1x2-	T44.1x3-	T44.1x4-	T44.1x5-	T44.1x6-
chloride	T44.1x1-	T44.1x2-	T44.1x3-	T44.1x4-	T44.1x5-	T44.1x6-
Bethanidine	T46.5x1-	T46.5x2-	T46.5x3-	T46.5x4-	T46.5x5-	T46.5x6-
Betoxycaine	T41.3x1-	T41.3x2-	T41.3x3-	T41.3x4-	T41.3x5-	T41.3x6-
Betula oil	T49.3x1-	T49.3x2-	T49.3x3-	T49.3x4-	T49.3x5-	T49.3x6-
b-eucaine	T49.1x1-	T49.1x2-	T49.1x3-	T49.1x4-	T49.1x5-	T49.1x6-
Bevantolol	T44.7x1-	T44.7x2-	T44.7x3-	T44.7x4-	T44.7x5-	T44.7x6-
Bevonium metilsulfate	T44.3x1-	T44.3x2-	T44.3x3-	T44.3x4-	T44.3x5-	T44.3x6-
Bezafibrate	T46.6x1-	T46.6x2-	T46.6x3-	T46.6x4-	T46.6x5-	T46.6x6-
Bezitramide	T40.4x1-	T40.4x2-	T40.4x3-	T40.4x4-	T40.4x5-	T40.4x6-
b-galactosidase	T47.5x1-	T47.5x2-	T47.5x3-	T47.5x4-	T47.5x5-	T47.5x6-
BHA	T50.991-	T50.992-	T50.993-	T50.994-	T50.995-	T50.996-
Bhang	T40.7x1-	T40.7x2-	T40.7x3-	T40.7x4-	T40.7x5-	T40.7x6-
BHC (medicinal)	T49.0x1-	T49.0x2-	T49.0x3-	T49.0x4-	T49.0x5-	T49.0x6-
nonmedicinal (vapor)	T53.6x1-	T53.6x2-	T53.6x3-	T53.6x4-	—	—
Bialamicol	T37.3x1-	T37.3x2-	T37.3x3-	T37.3x4-	T37.3x5-	T37.3x6-
Bibenzonium bromide	T48.3x1-	T48.3x2-	T48.3x3-	T48.3x4-	T48.3x5-	T48.3x6-
Bibrocathol	T49.5x1-	T49.5x2-	T49.5x3-	T49.5x4-	T49.5x5-	T49.5x6-
Bichloride of mercury — see Mercury, chloride						
Bichromates (calcium) (potassium) (sodium) (crystals)	T57.8x1-	T57.8x2-	T57.8x3-	T57.8x4-		
fumes	T56.2x1-	T56.2x2-	T56.2x3-	T56.2x4-	—	—
Biclotymol	T49.6x1-	T49.6x2-	T49.6x3-	T49.6x4-	T49.6x5-	T49.6x6-
Bicuculline	T50.7x1-	T50.7x2-	T50.7x3-	T50.7x4-	T50.7x5-	T50.7x6-
Bifemelane	T43.291-	T43.292-	T43.293-	T43.294-	T43.295-	T43.296-
Biguanide derivatives, oral	T38.3x1-	T38.3x2-	T38.3x3-	T38.3x4-	T38.3x5-	T38.3x6-
Bile salts	T47.5x1-	T47.5x2-	T47.5x3-	T47.5x4-	T47.5x5-	T47.5x6-
Biligrafin	T50.8x1-	T50.8x2-	T50.8x3-	T50.8x4-	T50.8x5-	T50.8x6-
Bilopaque	T50.8x1-	T50.8x2-	T50.8x3-	T50.8x4-	T50.8x5-	T50.8x6-
Binifibrate	T46.6x1-	T46.6x2-	T46.6x3-	T46.6x4-	T46.6x5-	T46.6x6-
Binitrobenzol	T65.3x1-	T65.3x2-	T65.3x3-	T65.3x4-		
Bioflavonoid(s)	T46.991-	T46.992-	T46.993-	T46.994-	T46.995-	T46.996-
Biological substance NEC	T50.901-	T50.902-	T50.903-	T50.904-	T50.905-	T50.906-
Biotin	T45.2x1-	T45.2x2-	T45.2x3-	T45.2x4-	T45.2x5-	T45.2x6-
Biperiden	T44.3x1-	T44.3x2-	T44.3x3-	T44.3x4-	T44.3x5-	T44.3x6-
Bisacodyl	T47.2x1-	T47.2x2-	T47.2x3-	T47.2x4-	T47.2x5-	T47.2x6-
Bisbentiamine	T45.2x1-	T45.2x2-	T45.2x3-	T45.2x4-	T45.2x5-	T45.2x6-
Bisbutiamine	T45.2x1-	T45.2x2-	T45.2x3-	T45.2x4-	T45.2x5-	T45.2x6-
Bisdequalinium (salts) (diacetate)	T49.6x1-	T49.6x2-	T49.6x3-	T49.6x4-	T49.6x5-	T49.6x6-
Bishydroxycoumarin	T45.511-	T45.512-	T45.513-	T45.514-	T45.515-	T45.516-
Bismarsen	T37.8x1-	T37.8x2-	T37.8x3-	T37.8x4-	T37.8x5-	T37.8x6-
Bismuth salts	T47.6x1-	T47.6x2-	T47.6x3-	T47.6x4-	T47.6x5-	T47.6x6-
aluminate	T47.1x1-	T47.1x2-	T47.1x3-	T47.1x4-	T47.1x5-	T47.1x6-
anti-infectives	T37.8x1-	T37.8x2-	T37.8x3-	T37.8x4-	T37.8x5-	T37.8x6-
formic iodide	T49.0x1-	T49.0x2-	T49.0x3-	T49.0x4-	T49.0x5-	T49.0x6-
glycolylarsenate	T49.0x1-	T49.0x2-	T49.0x3-	T49.0x4-	T49.0x5-	T49.0x6-
nonmedicinal (compounds) NEC	T65.91x-	T65.92x-	T65.93x-	T65.94x-	—	—
subcarbonate	T47.6x1-	T47.6x2-	T47.6x3-	T47.6x4-	T47.6x5-	T47.6x6-
subsalicylate	T37.8x1-	T37.8x2-	T37.8x3-	T37.8x4-	T37.8x5-	T37.8x6-
sulfarsphenamine	T37.8x1-	T37.8x2-	T37.8x3-	T37.8x4-	T37.8x5-	T37.8x6-
Bisoprolol	T44.7x1-	T44.7x2-	T44.7x3-	T44.7x4-	T44.7x5-	T44.7x6-
Bisoxatin	T47.2x1-	T47.2x2-	T47.2x3-	T47.2x4-	T47.2x5-	T47.2x6-
Bisulepin (hydrochloride)	T45.0x1-	T45.0x2-	T45.0x3-	T45.0x4-	T45.0x5-	T45.0x6-
Bithionol	T37.8x1-	T37.8x2-	T37.8x3-	T37.8x4-	T37.8x5-	T37.8x6-
anthelminthic	T37.4x1-	T37.4x2-	T37.4x3-	T37.4x4-	T37.4x5-	T37.4x6-
Bitolterol	T48.6x1-	T48.6x2-	T48.6x3-	T48.6x4-	T48.6x5-	T48.6x6-
Bitoscanate	T37.4x1-	T37.4x2-	T37.4x3-	T37.4x4-	T37.4x5-	T37.4x6-
Bitter almond oil	T62.8x1-	T62.8x2-	T62.8x3-	T62.8x4-	—	—
Bittersweet	T62.2x1-	T62.2x2-	T62.2x3-	T62.2x4-	—	—
Black						
flag	T60.91x-	T60.92x-	T60.93x-	T60.94x-	—	—
henbane	T62.2x1-	T62.2x2-	T62.2x3-	T62.2x4-	—	—
leaf (40)	T60.91x-	T60.92x-	T60.93x-	T60.94x-	—	—
widow spider (bite)	T63.311-	T63.312-	T63.313-	T63.314-	—	—
antivenin	T50.Z11-	T50.Z12-	T50.Z13-	T50.Z14-	T50.Z15-	T50.Z16-
Blast furnace gas (carbon monoxide from)	T58.8x1-	T58.8x2-	T58.8x3-	T58.8x4-	—	—

DRUGS & CHEMICALS

Table of Drugs & Chemicals	POISONING Accidental (Unintentional)	Self-Harm (Intentional)	Assault	Undetermined	Adverse Effect	Underdosing
Bleach	T54.91x-	T54.92x-	T54.93x-	T54.94x-	—	—
Bleaching agent (medicinal)	T49.4x1-	T49.4x2-	T49.4x3-	T49.4x4-	T49.4x5-	T49.4x6-
Bleomycin	T45.1x1-	T45.1x2-	T45.1x3-	T45.1x4-	T45.1x5-	T45.1x6-
Blockain	T41.3x1-	T41.3x2-	T41.3x3-	T41.3x4-	T41.3x5-	T41.3x6-
infiltration (subcutaneous)	T41.3x1-	T41.3x2-	T41.3x3-	T41.3x4-	T41.3x5-	T41.3x6-
nerve block (peripheral) (plexus)	T41.3x1-	T41.3x2-	T41.3x3-	T41.3x4-	T41.3x5-	T41.3x6-
topical (surface)	T41.3x1-	T41.3x2-	T41.3x3-	T41.3x4-	T41.3x5-	T41.3x6-
Blockers, calcium channel	T46.1x1-	T46.1x2-	T46.1x3-	T46.1x4-	T46.1x5-	T46.1x6-
Blood (derivatives) (natural) (plasma) (whole)	T45.8x1-	T45.8x2-	T45.8x3-	T45.8x4-	T45.8x5-	T45.8x6-
dried	T45.8x1-	T45.8x2-	T45.8x3-	T45.8x4-	T45.8x5-	T45.8x6-
drug affecting NEC	T45.91x-	T45.92x-	T45.93x-	T45.94x-	T45.95x-	T45.96x-
expander NEC	T45.8x1-	T45.8x2-	T45.8x3-	T45.8x4-	T45.8x5-	T45.8x6-
fraction NEC	T45.8x1-	T45.8x2-	T45.8x3-	T45.8x4-	T45.8x5-	T45.8x6-
substitute (macromolecular)	T45.8x1-	T45.8x2-	T45.8x3-	T45.8x4-	T45.8x5-	T45.8x6-
Blue velvet	T40.2x1-	T40.2x2-	T40.2x3-	T40.2x4-	—	—
Bone meal	T62.8x1-	T62.8x2-	T62.8x3-	T62.8x4-	—	—
Bonine	T45.0x1-	T45.0x2-	T45.0x3-	T45.0x4-	T45.0x5-	T45.0x6-
Bopindolol	T44.7x1-	T44.7x2-	T44.7x3-	T44.7x4-	T44.7x5-	T44.7x6-
Boracic acid	T49.0x1-	T49.0x2-	T49.0x3-	T49.0x4-	T49.0x5-	T49.0x6-
ENT agent	T49.6x1-	T49.6x2-	T49.6x3-	T49.6x4-	T49.6x5-	T49.6x6-
ophthalmic preparation	T49.5x1-	T49.5x2-	T49.5x3-	T49.5x4-	T49.5x5-	T49.5x6-
Borane complex	T57.8x1-	T57.8x2-	T57.8x3-	T57.8x4-	—	—
Borate (s)	T57.8x1-	T57.8x2-	T57.8x3-	T57.8x4-	—	—
buffer	T50.991-	T50.992-	T50.993-	T50.994-	T50.995-	T50.996-
cleanser	T54.91x-	T54.92x-	T54.93x-	T54.94x-	—	—
sodium	T57.8x1-	T57.8x2-	T57.8x3-	T57.8x4-	—	—
Borax (cleanser)	T54.91x-	T54.92x-	T54.93x-	T54.94x-	—	—
Bordeaux mixture	T60.3x1-	T60.3x2-	T60.3x3-	T60.3x4-	—	—
Boric acid	T49.0x1-	T49.0x2-	T49.0x3-	T49.0x4-	T49.0x5-	T49.0x6-
ENT agent	T49.6x1-	T49.6x2-	T49.6x3-	T49.6x4-	T49.6x5-	T49.6x6-
ophthalmic preparation	T49.5x1-	T49.5x2-	T49.5x3-	T49.5x4-	T49.5x5-	T49.5x6-
Bornaprine	T44.3x1-	T44.3x2-	T44.3x3-	T44.3x4-	T44.3x5-	T44.3x6-
Boron	T57.8x1-	T57.8x2-	T57.8x3-	T57.8x4-	—	—
hydride NEC	T57.8x1-	T57.8x2-	T57.8x3-	T57.8x4-	—	—
fumes or gas	T57.8x1-	T57.8x2-	T57.8x3-	T57.8x4-	—	—
trifluoride	T59.891-	T59.892-	T59.893-	T59.894-	—	—
Botox	T48.291-	T48.292-	T48.293-	T48.294-	T48.295-	T48.296-
Botulinus anti-toxin (type A, B)	T50.Z11-	T50.Z12-	T50.Z13-	T50.Z14-	T50.Z15-	T50.Z16-
Brake fluid vapor	T59.891-	T59.892-	T59.893-	T59.894-	—	—
Brallobarbital	T42.3x1-	T42.3x2-	T42.3x3-	T42.3x4-	T42.3x5-	T42.3x6-
Bran (wheat)	T47.4x1-	T47.4x2-	T47.4x3-	T47.4x4-	T47.4x5-	T47.4x6-
Brass (fumes)	T56.891-	T56.892-	T56.893-	T56.894-	—	—
Brasso	T52.0x1-	T52.0x2-	T52.0x3-	T52.0x4-	—	—
Bretylium tosilate	T46.2x1-	T46.2x2-	T46.2x3-	T46.2x4-	T46.2x5-	T46.2x6-
Brevital (sodium)	T41.1x1-	T41.1x2-	T41.1x3-	T41.1x4-	T41.1x5-	T41.1x6-
Brinase	T45.3x1-	T45.3x2-	T45.3x3-	T45.3x4-	T45.3x5-	T45.3x6-
British antilewisite	T45.8x1-	T45.8x2-	T45.8x3-	T45.8x4-	T45.8x5-	T45.8x6-
Brodifacoum	T60.4x1-	T60.4x2-	T60.4x3-	T60.4x4-	—	—
Bromal (hydrate)	T42.6x1-	T42.6x2-	T42.6x3-	T42.6x4-	T42.6x5-	T42.6x6-
Bromazepam	T42.4x1-	T42.4x2-	T42.4x3-	T42.4x4-	T42.4x5-	T42.4x6-
Bromazine	T45.0x1-	T45.0x2-	T45.0x3-	T45.0x4-	T45.0x5-	T45.0x6-
Brombenzylcyanide	T59.3x1-	T59.3x2-	T59.3x3-	T59.3x4-	—	—
Bromelains	T45.3x1-	T45.3x2-	T45.3x3-	T45.3x4-	T45.3x5-	T45.3x6-
Bromethalin	T60.4x1-	T60.4x2-	T60.4x3-	T60.4x4-	—	—
Bromhexine	T48.4x1-	T48.4x2-	T48.4x3-	T48.4x4-	T48.4x5-	T48.4x6-
Bromide salts	T42.6x1-	T42.6x2-	T42.6x3-	T42.6x4-	T42.6x5-	T42.6x6-
Bromindione	T45.511-	T45.512-	T45.513-	T45.514-	T45.515-	T45.516-

Table of Drugs & Chemicals	POISONING Accidental (Unintentional)	Self-Harm (Intentional)	Assault	Undetermined	Adverse Effect	Underdosing
Bromine						
compounds (medicinal)	T42.6x1-	T42.6x2-	T42.6x3-	T42.6x4-	T42.6x5-	T42.6x6-
sedative	T42.6x1-	T42.6x2-	T42.6x3-	T42.6x4-	T42.6x5-	T42.6x6-
vapor	T59.891-	T59.892-	T59.893-	T59.894-	—	—
Bromisoval	T42.6x1-	T42.6x2-	T42.6x3-	T42.6x4-	T42.6x5-	T42.6x6-
Bromisovalum	T42.6x1-	T42.6x2-	T42.6x3-	T42.6x4-	T42.6x5-	T42.6x6-
Bromobenzylcyanide	T59.3x1-	T59.3x2-	T59.3x3-	T59.3x4-	—	—
Bromochlorosalicylanilide	T49.0x1-	T49.0x2-	T49.0x3-	T49.0x4-	T49.0x5-	T49.0x6-
Bromocriptine	T42.8x1-	T42.8x2-	T42.8x3-	T42.8x4-	T42.8x5-	T42.8x6-
Bromodiphenhydramine	T45.0x1-	T45.0x2-	T45.0x3-	T45.0x4-	T45.0x5-	T45.0x6-
Bromoform	T42.6x1-	T42.6x2-	T42.6x3-	T42.6x4-	T42.6x5-	T42.6x6-
Bromophenol blue reagent	T50.991-	T50.992-	T50.993-	T50.994-	T50.995-	T50.996-
Bromopride	T47.8x1-	T47.8x2-	T47.8x3-	T47.8x4-	T47.8x5-	T47.8x6-
Bromosalicylchloranitide	T49.0x1-	T49.0x2-	T49.0x3-	T49.0x4-	T49.0x5-	T49.0x6-
Bromosalicylhydroxamic acid	T37.1x1-	T37.1x2-	T37.1x3-	T37.1x4-	T37.1x5-	T37.1x6-
Bromo-seltzer	T39.1x1-	T39.1x2-	T39.1x3-	T39.1x4-	T39.1x5-	T39.1x6-
Bromoxynil	T60.3x1-	T60.3x2-	T60.3x3-	T60.3x4-	—	—
Bromperidol	T43.4x1-	T43.4x2-	T43.4x3-	T43.4x4-	T43.4x5-	T43.4x6-
Brompheniramine	T45.0x1-	T45.0x2-	T45.0x3-	T45.0x4-	T45.0x5-	T45.0x6-
Bromsulfophthalein	T50.8x1-	T50.8x2-	T50.8x3-	T50.8x4-	T50.8x5-	T50.8x6-
Bromural	T42.6x1-	T42.6x2-	T42.6x3-	T42.6x4-	T42.6x5-	T42.6x6-
Bromvaletone	T42.6x1-	T42.6x2-	T42.6x3-	T42.6x4-	T42.6x5-	T42.6x6-
Bronchodilator NEC	T48.6x1-	T48.6x2-	T48.6x3-	T48.6x4-	T48.6x5-	T48.6x6-
Brotizolam	T42.4x1-	T42.4x2-	T42.4x3-	T42.4x4-	T42.4x5-	T42.4x6-
Brovincamine	T46.7x1-	T46.7x2-	T46.7x3-	T46.7x4-	T46.7x5-	T46.7x6-
Brown recluse spider (bite) (venom)	T63.331-	T63.332-	T63.333-	T63.334-	—	—
Brown spider (bite) (venom)	T63.391-	T63.392-	T63.393-	T63.394-	—	—
Broxaterol	T48.6x1-	T48.6x2-	T48.6x3-	T48.6x4-	T48.6x5-	T48.6x6-
Broxuridine	T45.1x1-	T45.1x2-	T45.1x3-	T45.1x4-	T45.1x5-	T45.1x6-
Broxyquinoline	T37.8x1-	T37.8x2-	T37.8x3-	T37.8x4-	T37.8x5-	T37.8x6-
Bruceine	T48.291-	T48.292-	T48.293-	T48.294-	T48.295-	T48.296-
Brucia	T62.2x1-	T62.2x2-	T62.2x3-	T62.2x4-	—	—
Brucine	T65.1x1-	T65.1x2-	T65.1x3-	T65.1x4-	—	—
Brunswick green — *see* Copper						
Bruten — *see* Ibuprofen						
Bryonia	T47.2x1-	T47.2x2-	T47.2x3-	T47.2x4-	T47.2x5-	T47.2x6-
b-sitosterol(s)	T46.6x1-	T46.6x2-	T46.6x3-	T46.6x4-	T46.6x5-	T46.6x6-
Buclizine	T45.0x1-	T45.0x2-	T45.0x3-	T45.0x4-	T45.0x5-	T45.0x6-
Buclosamide	T49.0x1-	T49.0x2-	T49.0x3-	T49.0x4-	T49.0x5-	T49.0x6-
Budesonide	T44.5x1-	T44.5x2-	T44.5x3-	T44.5x4-	T44.5x5-	T44.5x6-
Budralazine	T46.5x1-	T46.5x2-	T46.5x3-	T46.5x4-	T46.5x5-	T46.5x6-
Bufferin	T39.011-	T39.012-	T39.013-	T39.014-	T39.015-	T39.016-
Buflomedil	T46.7x1-	T46.7x2-	T46.7x3-	T46.7x4-	T46.7x5-	T46.7x6-
Buformin	T38.3x1-	T38.3x2-	T38.3x3-	T38.3x4-	T38.3x5-	T38.3x6-
Bufotenine	T40.991-	T40.992-	T40.993-	T40.994-	—	—
Bufrolin	T48.6x1-	T48.6x2-	T48.6x3-	T48.6x4-	T48.6x5-	T48.6x6-
Bufylline	T48.6x1-	T48.6x2-	T48.6x3-	T48.6x4-	T48.6x5-	T48.6x6-
Bulk filler	T50.5x1-	T50.5x2-	T50.5x3-	T50.5x4-	T50.5x5-	T50.5x6-
cathartic	T47.4x1-	T47.4x2-	T47.4x3-	T47.4x4-	T47.4x5-	T47.4x6-
Bumetanide	T50.1x1-	T50.1x2-	T50.1x3-	T50.1x4-	T50.1x5-	T50.1x6-
Bunaftine	T46.2x1-	T46.2x2-	T46.2x3-	T46.2x4-	T46.2x5-	T46.2x6-
Bunamiodyl	T50.8x1-	T50.8x2-	T50.8x3-	T50.8x4-	T50.8x5-	T50.8x6-
Bunazosin	T44.6x1-	T44.6x2-	T44.6x3-	T44.6x4-	T44.6x5-	T44.6x6-
Bunitrolol	T44.7x1-	T44.7x2-	T44.7x3-	T44.7x4-	T44.7x5-	T44.7x6-
Buphenine	T46.7x1-	T46.7x2-	T46.7x3-	T46.7x4-	T46.7x5-	T46.7x6-
Bupivacaine	T41.3x1-	T41.3x2-	T41.3x3-	T41.3x4-	T41.3x5-	
infiltration (subcutaneous)	T41.3x1-	T41.3x2-	T41.3x3-	T41.3x4-	T41.3x5-	
nerve block (peripheral) (plexus)	T41.3x1-	T41.3x2-	T41.3x3-	T41.3x4-	T41.3x5-	T41.3x6-
spinal	T41.3x1-	T41.3x2-	T41.3x3-	T41.3x4-	T41.3x5-	T41.3x6-

Table of Drugs & Chemicals	POISONING				Adverse Effect	Underdosing	Table of Drugs & Chemicals	POISONING				Adverse Effect	Underdosing
	Accidental (Unintentional)	Self-Harm (Intentional)	Assault	Undetermined				Accidental (Unintentional)	Self-Harm (Intentional)	Assault	Undetermined		
Bupranolol	T44.7x1-	T44.7x2-	T44.7x3-	T44.7x4-	T44.7x5-	T44.7x6-	Cabergoline	T42.8x1-	T42.8x2-	T42.8x3-	T42.8x4-	T42.8x5-	T42.8x6-
Buprenorphine	T40.4x1-	T40.4x2-	T40.4x3-	T40.4x4-	T40.4x5-	T40.4x6-	Cacodyl, cacodylic acid	T57.0x1-	T57.0x2-	T57.0x3-	T57.0x4-	—	—
Bupropion	T43.291-	T43.292-	T43.293-	T43.294-	T43.295-	T43.296-	Cactinomycin	T45.1x1-	T45.1x2-	T45.1x3-	T45.1x4-	T45.1x5-	T45.1x6-
Burimamide	T47.1x1-	T47.1x2-	T47.1x3-	T47.1x4-	T47.1x5-	T47.1x6-	Cade oil	T49.4x1-	T49.4x2-	T49.4x3-	T49.4x4-	T49.4x5-	T49.4x6-
Buserelin	T38.891-	T38.892-	T38.893-	T38.894-	T38.895-	T38.896-	Cadexomer iodine	T49.0x1-	T49.0x2-	T49.0x3-	T49.0x4-	T49.0x5-	T49.0x6-
Buspirone	T43.591-	T43.592-	T43.593-	T43.594-	T43.595-	T43.596-	Cadmium (chloride) (fumes) (oxide)	T56.3x1-	T56.3x2-	T56.3x3-	T56.3x4-		
Busulfan, busulphan	T45.1x1-	T45.1x2-	T45.1x3-	T45.1x4-	T45.1x5-	T45.1x6-	sulfide (medicinal) NEC	T49.4x1-	T49.4x2-	T49.4x3-	T49.4x4-	T49.4x5-	T49.4x6-
Butabarbital (sodium)	T42.3x1-	T42.3x2-	T42.3x3-	T42.3x4-	T42.3x5-	T42.3x6-	Cadralazine	T46.5x1-	T46.5x2-	T46.5x3-	T46.5x4-	T46.5x5-	T46.5x6-
Butabarbitone	T42.3x1-	T42.3x2-	T42.3x3-	T42.3x4-	T42.3x5-	T42.3x6-	Caffeine	T43.611-	T43.612-	T43.613-	T43.614-	T43.615-	T43.616-
Butabarpal	T42.3x1-	T42.3x2-	T42.3x3-	T42.3x4-	T42.3x5-	T42.3x6-	Calabar bean	T62.2x1-	T62.2x2-	T62.2x3-	T62.2x4-	—	—
Butacaine	T41.3x1-	T41.3x2-	T41.3x3-	T41.3x4-	T41.3x5-	T41.3x6-	Caladium seguinum	T62.2x1-	T62.2x2-	T62.2x3-	T62.2x4-	—	—
Butalamine	T46.7x1-	T46.7x2-	T46.7x3-	T46.7x4-	T46.7x5-	T46.7x6-	Calamine (lotion)	T49.3x1-	T49.3x2-	T49.3x3-	T49.3x4-	T49.3x5-	T49.3x6-
Butalbital	T42.3x1-	T42.3x2-	T42.3x3-	T42.3x4-	T42.3x5-	T42.3x6-	Calcifediol	T45.2x1-	T45.2x2-	T45.2x3-	T45.2x4-	T45.2x5-	T45.2x6-
Butallylonal	T42.3x1-	T42.3x2-	T42.3x3-	T42.3x4-	T42.3x5-	T42.3x6-	Calciferol	T45.2x1-	T45.2x2-	T45.2x3-	T45.2x4-	T45.2x5-	T45.2x6-
Butamben	T41.3x1-	T41.3x2-	T41.3x3-	T41.3x4-	T41.3x5-	T41.3x6-	Calcitonin	T50.991-	T50.992-	T50.993-	T50.994-	T50.995-	T50.996-
Butamirate	T48.3x1-	T48.3x2-	T48.3x3-	T48.3x4-	T48.3x5-	T48.3x6-	Calcitriol	T45.2x1-	T45.2x2-	T45.2x3-	T45.2x4-	T45.2x5-	T45.2x6-
Butane (distributed in mobile container)	T59.891-	T59.892-	T59.893-	T59.894-			Calcium	T50.3x1-	T50.3x2-	T50.3x3-	T50.3x4-	T50.3x5-	T50.3x6-
distributed through pipes	T59.891-	T59.892-	T59.893-	T59.894-			actylsalicylate	T39.011-	T39.012-	T39.013-	T39.014-	T39.015-	T39.016-
incomplete combustion	T58.11x-	T58.12x-	T58.13x-	T58.14x-			benzamidosalicylate	T37.1x1-	T37.1x2-	T37.1x3-	T37.1x4-	T37.1x5-	T37.1x6-
Butanilicaine	T41.3x1-	T41.3x2-	T41.3x3-	T41.3x4-	T41.3x5-	T41.3x6-	bromide	T42.6x1-	T42.6x2-	T42.6x3-	T42.6x4-	T42.6x5-	T42.6x6-
Butanol	T51.3x1-	T51.3x2-	T51.3x3-	T51.3x4-			bromolactobionate	T42.6x1-	T42.6x2-	T42.6x3-	T42.6x4-	T42.6x5-	T42.6x6-
Butanone, 2-butanone	T52.4x1-	T52.4x2-	T52.4x3-	T52.4x4-			carbaspirin	T39.011-	T39.012-	T39.013-	T39.014-	T39.015-	T39.016-
Butantrone	T49.4x1-	T49.4x2-	T49.4x3-	T49.4x4-	T49.4x5-	T49.4x6-	carbimide	T50.6x1-	T50.6x2-	T50.6x3-	T50.6x4-	T50.6x5-	T50.6x6-
Butaperazine	T43.3x1-	T43.3x2-	T43.3x3-	T43.3x4-	T43.3x5-	T43.3x6-	carbonate	T47.1x1-	T47.1x2-	T47.1x3-	T47.1x4-	T47.1x5-	T47.1x6-
Butazolidin	T39.2x1-	T39.2x2-	T39.2x3-	T39.2x4-	T39.2x5-	T39.2x6-	chloride	T50.991-	T50.992-	T50.993-	T50.994-	T50.995-	T50.996-
Butetamate	T48.6x1-	T48.6x2-	T48.6x3-	T48.6x4-	T48.6x5-	T48.6x6-	anhydrous	T50.991-	T50.992-	T50.993-	T50.994-	T50.995-	T50.996-
Butethal	T42.3x1-	T42.3x2-	T42.3x3-	T42.3x4-	T42.3x5-	T42.3x6-	cyanide	T57.8x1-	T57.8x2-	T57.8x3-	T57.8x4-	—	—
Butethamate	T44.3x1-	T44.3x2-	T44.3x3-	T44.3x4-	T44.3x5-	T44.3x6-	dioctyl sulfosuccinate	T47.4x1-	T47.4x2-	T47.4x3-	T47.4x4-	T47.4x5-	T47.4x6-
Buthalitone (sodium)	T41.1x1-	T41.1x2-	T41.1x3-	T41.1x4-	T41.1x5-	T41.1x6-	disodium edathamil	T45.8x1-	T45.8x2-	T45.8x3-	T45.8x4-	T45.8x5-	T45.8x6-
Butisol (sodium)	T42.3x1-	T42.3x2-	T42.3x3-	T42.3x4-	T42.3x5-	T42.3x6-	disodium edetate	T45.8x1-	T45.8x2-	T45.8x3-	T45.8x4-	T45.8x5-	T45.8x6-
Butizide	T50.2x1-	T50.2x2-	T50.2x3-	T50.2x4-	T50.2x5-	T50.2x6-	dobesilate	T46.991-	T46.992-	T46.993-	T46.994-	T46.995-	T46.996-
Butobarbital	T42.3x1-	T42.3x2-	T42.3x3-	T42.3x4-	T42.3x5-	T42.3x6-	EDTA	T45.8x1-	T45.8x2-	T45.8x3-	T45.8x4-	T45.8x5-	T45.8x6-
sodium	T42.3x1-	T42.3x2-	T42.3x3-	T42.3x4-	T42.3x5-	T42.3x6-	ferrous citrate	T45.4x1-	T45.4x2-	T45.4x3-	T45.4x4-	T45.4x5-	T45.4x6-
Butobarbitone	T42.3x1-	T42.3x2-	T42.3x3-	T42.3x4-	T42.3x5-	T42.3x6-	folinate	T45.8x1-	T45.8x2-	T45.8x3-	T45.8x4-	T45.8x5-	T45.8x6-
Butoconazole (nitrate)	T49.0x1-	T49.0x2-	T49.0x3-	T49.0x4-	T49.0x5-	T49.0x6-	glubionate	T50.3x1-	T50.3x2-	T50.3x3-	T50.3x4-	T50.3x5-	T50.3x6-
Butorphanol	T40.4x1-	T40.4x2-	T40.4x3-	T40.4x4-	T40.4x5-	T40.4x6-	gluconate	T50.3x1-	T50.3x2-	T50.3x3-	T50.3x4-	T50.3x5-	T50.3x6-
Butriptyline	T43.011-	T43.012-	T43.013-	T43.014-	T43.015-	T43.016-	gluconogalactogluc-onate	T50.3x1-	T50.3x2-	T50.3x3-	T50.3x4-	T50.3x5-	T50.3x6-
Butropium bromide	T44.3x1-	T44.3x2-	T44.3x3-	T44.3x4-	T44.3x5-	T44.3x6-	hydrate, hydroxide	T54.3x1-	T54.3x2-	T54.3x3-	T54.3x4-	—	—
Butter of antimony — see Antimony							hypochlorite	T54.3x1-	T54.3x2-	T54.3x3-	T54.3x4-	—	—
Buttercups	T62.2x1-	T62.2x2-	T62.2x3-	T62.2x4-	—	—	iodide	T48.4x1-	T48.4x2-	T48.4x3-	T48.4x4-	T48.4x5-	T48.4x6-
Butyl							ipodate	T50.8x1-	T50.8x2-	T50.8x3-	T50.8x4-	T50.8x5-	T50.8x6-
acetate (secondary)	T52.8x1-	T52.8x2-	T52.8x3-	T52.8x4-			lactate	T50.3x1-	T50.3x2-	T50.3x3-	T50.3x4-	T50.3x5-	T50.3x6-
alcohol	T51.3x1-	T51.3x2-	T51.3x3-	T51.3x4-			leucovorin	T45.8x1-	T45.8x2-	T45.8x3-	T45.8x4-	T45.8x5-	T45.8x6-
aminobenzoate	T41.3x1-	T41.3x2-	T41.3x3-	T41.3x4-	T41.3x5-	T41.3x6-	mandelate	T37.91x-	T37.92x-	T37.93x-	T37.94x-	T37.95x-	T37.96x-
butyrate	T52.8x1-	T52.8x2-	T52.8x3-	T52.8x4-			oxide	T54.3x1-	T54.3x2-	T54.3x3-	T54.3x4-	—	—
carbinol	T51.3x1-	T51.3x2-	T51.3x3-	T51.3x4-			pantothenate	T45.2x1-	T45.2x2-	T45.2x3-	T45.2x4-	T45.2x5-	T45.2x6-
carbitol	T52.3x1-	T52.3x2-	T52.3x3-	T52.3x4-			phosphate	T50.3x1-	T50.3x2-	T50.3x3-	T50.3x4-	T50.3x5-	T50.3x6-
cellosolve	T52.3x1-	T52.3x2-	T52.3x3-	T52.3x4-			salicylate	T39.091-	T39.092-	T39.093-	T39.094-	T39.095-	T39.096-
chloral (hydrate)	T42.6x1-	T42.6x2-	T42.6x3-	T42.6x4-	T42.6x5-	T42.6x6-	salts	T50.3x1-	T50.3x2-	T50.3x3-	T50.3x4-	T50.3x5-	T50.3x6-
formate	T52.8x1-	T52.8x2-	T52.8x3-	T52.8x4-			Calculus-dissolving drug	T50.991-	T50.992-	T50.993-	T50.994-	T50.995-	T50.996-
lactate	T52.8x1-	T52.8x2-	T52.8x3-	T52.8x4-			Calomel	T49.0x1-	T49.0x2-	T49.0x3-	T49.0x4-	T49.0x5-	T49.0x6-
propionate	T52.8x1-	T52.8x2-	T52.8x3-	T52.8x4-			Caloric agent	T50.3x1-	T50.3x2-	T50.3x3-	T50.3x4-	T50.3x5-	T50.3x6-
scopolamine bromide	T44.3x1-	T44.3x2-	T44.3x3-	T44.3x4-	T44.3x5-	T44.3x6-	Calusterone	T38.7x1-	T38.7x2-	T38.7x3-	T38.7x4-	T38.7x5-	T38.7x6-
thiobarbital sodium	T41.1x1-	T41.1x2-	T41.1x3-	T41.1x4-	T41.1x5-	T41.1x6-	Camazepam	T42.4x1-	T42.4x2-	T42.4x3-	T42.4x4-	T42.4x5-	T42.4x6-
Butylated hydroxy-anisole	T50.991-	T50.992-	T50.993-	T50.994-	T50.995-	T50.996-	Camomile	T49.0x1-	T49.0x2-	T49.0x3-	T49.0x4-	T49.0x5-	T49.0x6-
Butylchloral hydrate	T42.6x1-	T42.6x2-	T42.6x3-	T42.6x4-	T42.6x5-	T42.6x6-	Camoquin	T37.2x1-	T37.2x2-	T37.2x3-	T37.2x4-	T37.2x5-	T37.2x6-
Butyltoluene	T52.2x1-	T52.2x2-	T52.2x3-	T52.2x4-			Camphor						
Butyn	T41.3x1-	T41.3x2-	T41.3x3-	T41.3x4-	T41.3x5-	T41.3x6-	insecticide	T60.2x1-	T60.2x2-	T60.2x3-	T60.2x4-	—	—
Butyrophenone (-based tranquilizers)	T43.4x1-	T43.4x2-	T43.4x3-	T43.4x4-	T43.4x5-	T43.4x6-	medicinal	T49.8x1-	T49.8x2-	T49.8x3-	T49.8x4-	T49.8x5-	T49.8x6-
							Camylofin	T44.3x1-	T44.3x2-	T44.3x3-	T44.3x4-	T44.3x5-	T44.3x6-
							Cancer chemotherapy drug regimen	T45.1x1-	T45.1x2-	T45.1x3-	T45.1x4-	T45.1x5-	T45.1x6-

DRUGS & CHEMICALS

DRUGS & CHEMICALS

Table of Drugs & Chemicals	POISONING				Adverse Effect	Underdosing
	Accidental (Unintentional)	Self-Harm (Intentional)	Assault	Undetermined		
Candeptin	T49.0x1-	T49.0x2-	T49.0x3-	T49.0x4-	T49.0x5-	T49.0x6-
Candicidin	T49.0x1-	T49.0x2-	T49.0x3-	T49.0x4-	T49.0x5-	T49.0x6-
Cannabinol	T40.7x1-	T40.7x2-	T40.7x3-	T40.7x4-	T40.7x5-	T40.7x6-
Cannabis (derivatives)	T40.7x1-	T40.7x2-	T40.7x3-	T40.7x4-	T40.7x5-	T40.7x6-
Canned heat	T51.1x1-	T51.1x2-	T51.1x3-	T51.1x4-	—	—
Canrenoic acid	T50.0x1-	T50.0x2-	T50.0x3-	T50.0x4-	T50.0x5-	T50.0x6-
Canrenone	T50.0x1-	T50.0x2-	T50.0x3-	T50.0x4-	T50.0x5-	T50.0x6-
Cantharides, cantharidin, cantharis	T49.8x1-	T49.8x2-	T49.8x3-	T49.8x4-	T49.8x5-	T49.8x6-
Canthaxanthin	T50.991-	T50.992-	T50.993-	T50.994-	T50.995-	T50.996-
Capillary-active drug NEC	T46.901-	T46.902-	T46.903-	T46.904-	T46.905-	T46.906-
Capreomycin	T36.8x1-	T36.8x2-	T36.8x3-	T36.8x4-	T36.8x5-	T36.8x6-
Capsicum	T49.4x1-	T49.4x2-	T49.4x3-	T49.4x4-	T49.4x5-	T49.4x6-
Captafol	T60.3x1-	T60.3x2-	T60.3x3-	T60.3x4-	—	—
Captan	T60.3x1-	T60.3x2-	T60.3x3-	T60.3x4-	—	—
Captodiame, captodiamine	T43.591-	T43.592-	T43.593-	T43.594-	T43.595-	T43.596-
Captopril	T46.4x1-	T46.4x2-	T46.4x3-	T46.4x4-	T46.4x5-	T46.4x6-
Caramiphen	T44.3x1-	T44.3x2-	T44.3x3-	T44.3x4-	T44.3x5-	T44.3x6-
Carazolol	T44.7x1-	T44.7x2-	T44.7x3-	T44.7x4-	T44.7x5-	T44.7x6-
Carbachol	T44.1x1-	T44.1x2-	T44.1x3-	T44.1x4-	T44.1x5-	T44.1x6-
Carbacrylamine (resin)	T50.3x1-	T50.3x2-	T50.3x3-	T50.3x4-	T50.3x5-	T50.3x6-
Carbamate (insecticide)	T60.0x1-	T60.0x2-	T60.0x3-	T60.0x4-		
Carbamate (sedative)	T42.6x1-	T42.6x2-	T42.6x3-	T42.6x4-	T42.6x5-	T42.6x6-
herbicide	T60.0x1-	T60.0x2-	T60.0x3-	T60.0x4-		
insecticide	T60.0x1-	T60.0x2-	T60.0x3-	T60.0x4-		
Carbamazepine	T42.1x1-	T42.1x2-	T42.1x3-	T42.1x4-	T42.1x5-	T42.1x6-
Carbamide	T47.3x1-	T47.3x2-	T47.3x3-	T47.3x4-	T47.3x5-	T47.3x6-
peroxide	T49.0x1-	T49.0x2-	T49.0x3-	T49.0x4-	T49.0x5-	T49.0x6-
topical	T49.8x1-	T49.8x2-	T49.8x3-	T49.8x4-	T49.8x5-	T49.8x6-
Carbamylcholine chloride	T44.1x1-	T44.1x2-	T44.1x3-	T44.1x4-	T44.1x5-	T44.1x6-
Carbaril	T60.0x1-	T60.0x2-	T60.0x3-	T60.0x4-	—	
Carbarsone	T37.3x1-	T37.3x2-	T37.3x3-	T37.3x4-	T37.3x5-	T37.3x6-
Carbaryl	T60.0x1-	T60.0x2-	T60.0x3-	T60.0x4-	—	
Carbaspirin	T39.011-	T39.012-	T39.013-	T39.014-	T39.015-	T39.016-
Carbazochrome (salicylate) (sodium sulfonate)	T49.4x1-	T49.4x2-	T49.4x3-	T49.4x4-	T49.4x5-	T49.4x6-
Carbenicillin	T36.0x1-	T36.0x2-	T36.0x3-	T36.0x4-	T36.0x5-	T36.0x6-
Carbenoxolone	T47.1x1-	T47.1x2-	T47.1x3-	T47.1x4-	T47.1x5-	T47.1x6-
Carbetapentane	T48.3x1-	T48.3x2-	T48.3x3-	T48.3x4-	T48.3x5-	T48.3x6-
Carbethyl salicylate	T39.091-	T39.092-	T39.093-	T39.094-	T39.095-	T39.096-
Carbidopa (with levodopa)	T42.8x1-	T42.8x2-	T42.8x3-	T42.8x4-	T42.8x5-	T42.8x6-
Carbimazole	T38.2x1-	T38.2x2-	T38.2x3-	T38.2x4-	T38.2x5-	T38.2x6-
Carbinol	T51.1x1-	T51.1x2-	T51.1x3-	T51.1x4-	—	—
Carbinoxamine	T45.0x1-	T45.0x2-	T45.0x3-	T45.0x4-	T45.0x5-	T45.0x6-
Carbiphene	T39.8x1-	T39.8x2-	T39.8x3-	T39.8x4-	T39.8x5-	T39.8x6-
Carbitol	T52.3x1-	T52.3x2-	T52.3x3-	T52.3x4-	—	—
Carbo medicinalis	T47.6x1-	T47.6x2-	T47.6x3-	T47.6x4-	T47.6x5-	T47.6x6-
Carbocaine	T41.3x1-	T41.3x2-	T41.3x3-	T41.3x4-	T41.3x5-	T41.3x6-
infiltration (subcutaneous)	T41.3x1-	T41.3x2-	T41.3x3-	T41.3x4-	T41.3x5-	T41.3x6-
nerve block (peripheral) (plexus)	T41.3x1-	T41.3x2-	T41.3x3-	T41.3x4-	T41.3x5-	T41.3x6-
topical (surface)	T41.3x1-	T41.3x2-	T41.3x3-	T41.3x4-	T41.3x5-	T41.3x6-
Carbocisteine	T48.4x1-	T48.4x2-	T48.4x3-	T48.4x4-	T48.4x5-	T48.4x6-
Carbocromen	T46.3x1-	T46.3x2-	T46.3x3-	T46.3x4-	T46.3x5-	T46.3x6-
Carbol fuchsin	T49.0x1-	T49.0x2-	T49.0x3-	T49.0x4-	T49.0x5-	T49.0x6-
Carbolic acid — see also Phenol	T54.0x1-	T54.0x2-	T54.0x3-	T54.0x4-	—	—
Carbolonium (bromide)	T48.1x1-	T48.1x2-	T48.1x3-	T48.1x4-	T48.1x5-	T48.1x6-
Carbomycin	T36.8x1-	T36.8x2-	T36.8x3-	T36.8x4-	T36.8x5-	T36.8x6-

Table of Drugs & Chemicals	POISONING				Adverse Effect	Underdosing
	Accidental (Unintentional)	Self-Harm (Intentional)	Assault	Undetermined		
Carbon						
bisulfide (liquid)	T65.4x1-	T65.4x2-	T65.4x3-	T65.4x4-	—	—
vapor	T65.4x1-	T65.4x2-	T65.4x3-	T65.4x4-	—	—
dioxide (gas)	T59.7x1-	T59.7x2-	T59.7x3-	T59.7x4-	—	—
medicinal	T41.5x1-	T41.5x2-	T41.5x3-	T41.5x4-	T41.5x5-	T41.5x6-
nonmedicinal	T59.7x1-	T59.7x2-	T59.7x3-	T59.7x4-	—	—
snow	T49.4x1-	T49.4x2-	T49.4x3-	T49.4x4-	T49.4x5-	T49.4x6-
disulfide (liquid)	T65.4x1-	T65.4x2-	T65.4x3-	T65.4x4-	—	—
vapor	T65.4x1-	T65.4x2-	T65.4x3-	T65.4x4-	—	—
monoxide (from incomplete combustion)	T58.91x-	T58.92x-	T58.93x-	T58.94x-	—	—
blast furnace gas	T58.8x1-	T58.8x2-	T58.8x3-	T58.8x4-	—	—
butane (distributed in mobile container)	T58.11x-	T58.12x-	T58.13x-	T58.14x-	—	—
distributed through pipes	T58.11x-	T58.12x-	T58.13x-	T58.14x-	—	—
charcoal fumes	T58.2x1-	T58.2x2-	T58.2x3-	T58.2x4-	—	—
coal	T58.2x1-	T58.2x2-	T58.2x3-	T58.2x4-	—	—
gas (piped)	T58.11x-	T58.12x-	T58.13x-	T58.14x-	—	—
solid (in domestic stoves, fireplaces)	T58.2x1-	T58.2x2-	T58.2x3-	T58.2x4-	—	—
coke (in domestic stoves, fireplaces)	T58.2x1-	T58.2x2-	T58.2x3-	T58.2x4-	—	—
exhaust gas (motor) not in transit	T58.01x-	T58.02x-	T58.03x-	T58.04x-	—	—
combustion engine, any not in watercraft	T58.01x-	T58.02x-	T58.03x-	T58.04x-	—	—
farm tractor, not in transit	T58.01x-	T58.02x-	T58.03x-	T58.04x-	—	—
gas engine	T58.01x-	T58.02x-	T58.03x-	T58.04x-	—	—
motor pump	T58.01x-	T58.02x-	T58.03x-	T58.04x-	—	—
motor vehicle, not in transit	T58.01x-	T58.02x-	T58.03x-	T58.04x-	—	—
fuel (in domestic use)	T58.2x1-	T58.2x2-	T58.2x3-	T58.2x4-	—	—
gas (piped)	T58.11x-	T58.12x-	T58.13x-	T58.14x-	—	—
in mobile container	T58.11x-	T58.12x-	T58.13x-	T58.14x-	—	—
utility	T58.11x-	T58.12x-	T58.13x-	T58.14x-	—	—
in mobile container	T58.11x-	T58.12x-	T58.13x-	T58.14x-	—	—
piped (natural)	T58.11x-	T58.12x-	T58.13x-	T58.14x-	—	—
illuminating gas	T58.11x-	T58.12x-	T58.13x-	T58.14x-	—	—
industrial fuels or gases, any	T58.8x1-	T58.8x2-	T58.8x3-	T58.8x4-	—	—
kerosene (in domestic stoves, fireplaces)	T58.2x1-	T58.2x2-	T58.2x3-	T58.2x4-	—	—
kiln gas or vapor	T58.8x1-	T58.8x2-	T58.8x3-	T58.8x4-	—	—
motor exhaust gas, not in transit	T58.01x-	T58.02x-	T58.03x-	T58.04x-	—	—
piped gas (manufactured) (natural)	T58.11x-	T58.12x-	T58.13x-	T58.14x-	—	—
producer gas	T58.8x1-	T58.8x2-	T58.8x3-	T58.8x4-	—	—
propane (distributed in mobile container)	T58.11x-	T58.12x-	T58.13x-	T58.14x-	—	—
distributed through pipes	T58.11x-	T58.12x-	T58.13x-	T58.14x-	—	—
specified source NEC	T58.8x1-	T58.8x2-	T58.8x3-	T58.8x4-	—	—
stove gas	T58.11x-	T58.12x-	T58.13x-	T58.14x-	—	—
piped	T58.11x-	T58.12x-	T58.13x-	T58.14x-	—	—
utility gas	T58.11x-	T58.12x-	T58.13x-	T58.14x-	—	—
piped	T58.11x-	T58.12x-	T58.13x-	T58.14x-	—	—

DRUGS & CHEMICALS

Table of Drugs & Chemicals	POISONING Accidental (Unintentional)	Self-Harm (Intentional)	Assault	Undetermined	Adverse Effect	Underdosing
Carbon - continued monoxide (from incomplete combustion) - continued	T58.91x-	T58.92x-	T58.93x-	T58.94x-	—	—
water gas	T58.11x-	T58.12x-	T58.13x-	T58.14x-	—	—
wood (in domestic stoves, fireplaces)	T58.2x1-	T58.2x2-	T58.2x3-	T58.2x4-	—	—
tetrachloride (vapor) NEC	T53.0x1-	T53.0x2-	T53.0x3-	T53.0x4-	—	—
liquid (cleansing agent) NEC	T53.0x1-	T53.0x2-	T53.0x3-	T53.0x4-	—	—
solvent	T53.0x1-	T53.0x2-	T53.0x3-	T53.0x4-	—	—
Carbonic acid gas	T59.7x1-	T59.7x2-	T59.7x3-	T59.7x4-	—	—
anhydrase inhibitor NEC	T50.2x1-	T50.2x2-	T50.2x3-	T50.2x4-	T50.2x5-	T50.2x6-
Carbophenothion	T60.0x1-	T60.0x2-	T60.0x3-	T60.0x4-	—	—
Carboplatin	T45.1x1-	T45.1x2-	T45.1x3-	T45.1x4-	T45.1x5-	T45.1x6-
Carboprost	T48.0x1-	T48.0x2-	T48.0x3-	T48.0x4-	T48.0x5-	T48.0x6-
Carboquone	T45.1x1-	T45.1x2-	T45.1x3-	T45.1x4-	T45.1x5-	T45.1x6-
Carbowax	T49.3x1-	T49.3x2-	T49.3x3-	T49.3x4-	T49.3x5-	T49.3x6-
Carboxymethyl-cellulose	T47.4x1-	T47.4x2-	T47.4x3-	T47.4x4-	T47.4x5-	T47.4x6-
S-Carboxymethyl-cysteine	T48.4x1-	T48.4x2-	T48.4x3-	T48.4x4-	T48.4x5-	T48.4x6-
Carbrital	T42.3x1-	T42.3x2-	T42.3x3-	T42.3x4-	T42.3x5-	T42.3x6-
Carbromal	T42.6x1-	T42.6x2-	T42.6x3-	T42.6x4-	T42.6x5-	T42.6x6-
Carbutamide	T38.3x1-	T38.3x2-	T38.3x3-	T38.3x4-	T38.3x5-	T38.3x6-
Carbuterol	T48.6x1-	T48.6x2-	T48.6x3-	T48.6x4-	T48.6x5-	T48.6x6-
Cardiac depressants	T46.2x1-	T46.2x2-	T46.2x3-	T46.2x4-	T46.2x5-	T46.2x6-
rhythm regulator	T46.2x1-	T46.2x2-	T46.2x3-	T46.2x4-	T46.2x5-	T46.2x6-
specified NEC	T46.2x1-	T46.2x2-	T46.2x3-	T46.2x4-	T46.2x5-	T46.2x6-
Cardiografin	T50.8x1-	T50.8x2-	T50.8x3-	T50.8x4-	T50.8x5-	T50.8x6-
Cardio-green	T50.8x1-	T50.8x2-	T50.8x3-	T50.8x4-	T50.8x5-	T50.8x6-
Cardiotonic (glycoside) NEC	T46.0x1-	T46.0x2-	T46.0x3-	T46.0x4-	T46.0x5-	T46.0x6-
Cardiovascular drug NEC	T46.901-	T46.902-	T46.903-	T46.904-	T46.905-	T46.906-
Cardrase	T50.2x1-	T50.2x2-	T50.2x3-	T50.2x4-	T50.2x5-	T50.2x6-
Carfecillin	T36.0x1-	T36.0x2-	T36.0x3-	T36.0x4-	T36.0x5-	T36.0x6-
Carfenazine	T43.3x1-	T43.3x2-	T43.3x3-	T43.3x4-	T43.3x5-	T43.3x6-
Carfusin	T49.0x1-	T49.0x2-	T49.0x3-	T49.0x4-	T49.0x5-	T49.0x6-
Carindacillin	T36.0x1-	T36.0x2-	T36.0x3-	T36.0x4-	T36.0x5-	T36.0x6-
Carisoprodol	T42.8x1-	T42.8x2-	T42.8x3-	T42.8x4-	T42.8x5-	T42.8x6-
Carmellose	T47.4x1-	T47.4x2-	T47.4x3-	T47.4x4-	T47.4x5-	T47.4x6-
Carminative	T47.5x1-	T47.5x2-	T47.5x3-	T47.5x4-	T47.5x5-	T47.5x6-
Carmofur	T45.1x1-	T45.1x2-	T45.1x3-	T45.1x4-	T45.1x5-	T45.1x6-
Carmustine	T45.1x1-	T45.1x2-	T45.1x3-	T45.1x4-	T45.1x5-	T45.1x6-
Carotene	T45.2x1-	T45.2x2-	T45.2x3-	T45.2x4-	T45.2x5-	T45.2x6-
Carphenazine	T43.3x1-	T43.3x2-	T43.3x3-	T43.3x4-	T43.3x5-	T43.3x6-
Carpipramine	T42.4x1-	T42.4x2-	T42.4x3-	T42.4x4-	T42.4x5-	T42.4x6-
Carprofen	T39.311-	T39.312-	T39.313-	T39.314-	T39.315-	T39.316-
Carpronium chloride	T44.3x1-	T44.3x2-	T44.3x3-	T44.3x4-	T44.3x5-	T44.3x6-
Carrageenan	T47.8x1-	T47.8x2-	T47.8x3-	T47.8x4-	T47.8x5-	T47.8x6-
Carteolol	T44.7x1-	T44.7x2-	T44.7x3-	T44.7x4-	T44.7x5-	T44.7x6-
Carter's Little Pills	T47.2x1-	T47.2x2-	T47.2x3-	T47.2x4-	T47.2x5-	T47.2x6-
Cascara (sagrada)	T47.2x1-	T47.2x2-	T47.2x3-	T47.2x4-	T47.2x5-	T47.2x6-
Cassava	T62.2x1-	T62.2x2-	T62.2x3-	T62.2x4-	—	—
Castellani's paint	T49.0x1-	T49.0x2-	T49.0x3-	T49.0x4-	T49.0x5-	T49.0x6-
Castor bean	T62.2x1-	T62.2x2-	T62.2x3-	T62.2x4-	—	—
oil	T47.2x1-	T47.2x2-	T47.2x3-	T47.2x4-	T47.2x5-	T47.2x6-
Catalase	T45.3x1-	T45.3x2-	T45.3x3-	T45.3x4-	T45.3x5-	T45.3x6-
Caterpillar (sting)	T63.431-	T63.432-	T63.433-	T63.434-	—	—
Catha (edulis) (tea)	T43.691-	T43.692-	T43.693-	T43.694-	—	—
Cathartic NEC	T47.4x1-	T47.4x2-	T47.4x3-	T47.4x4-	T47.4x5-	T47.4x6-
anthracene derivative	T47.2x1-	T47.2x2-	T47.2x3-	T47.2x4-	T47.2x5-	T47.2x6-
bulk	T47.4x1-	T47.4x2-	T47.4x3-	T47.4x4-	T47.4x5-	T47.4x6-
contact	T47.2x1-	T47.2x2-	T47.2x3-	T47.2x4-	T47.2x5-	T47.2x6-
emollient NEC	T47.4x1-	T47.4x2-	T47.4x3-	T47.4x4-	T47.4x5-	T47.4x6-
irritant NEC	T47.2x1-	T47.2x2-	T47.2x3-	T47.2x4-	T47.2x5-	T47.2x6-
mucilage	T47.4x1-	T47.4x2-	T47.4x3-	T47.4x4-	T47.4x5-	T47.4x6-
saline	T47.3x1-	T47.3x2-	T47.3x3-	T47.3x4-	T47.3x5-	T47.3x6-
vegetable	T47.2x1-	T47.2x2-	T47.2x3-	T47.2x4-	T47.2x5-	T47.2x6-
Cathine	T50.5x1-	T50.5x2-	T50.5x3-	T50.5x4-	T50.5x5-	T50.5x6-
Cathomycin	T36.8x1-	T36.8x2-	T36.8x3-	T36.8x4-	T36.8x5-	T36.8x6-
Cation exchange resin	T50.3x1-	T50.3x2-	T50.3x3-	T50.3x4-	T50.3x5-	T50.3x6-
Caustic(s) NEC	T54.91x-	T54.92x-	T54.93x-	T54.94x-	—	—
alkali	T54.3x1-	T54.3x2-	T54.3x3-	T54.3x4-	—	—
hydroxide	T54.3x1-	T54.3x2-	T54.3x3-	T54.3x4-	—	—
potash	T54.3x1-	T54.3x2-	T54.3x3-	T54.3x4-	—	—
specified NEC	T54.91x-	T54.92x-	T54.93x-	T54.94x-	—	—
soda	T54.3x1-	T54.3x2-	T54.3x3-	T54.3x4-	—	—
Ceepryn	T49.0x1-	T49.0x2-	T49.0x3-	T49.0x4-	T49.0x5-	T49.0x6-
ENT agent	T49.6x1-	T49.6x2-	T49.6x3-	T49.6x4-	T49.6x5-	T49.6x6-
lozenges	T49.6x1-	T49.6x2-	T49.6x3-	T49.6x4-	T49.6x5-	T49.6x6-
Cefacetrile	T36.1x1-	T36.1x2-	T36.1x3-	T36.1x4-	T36.1x5-	T36.1x6-
Cefaclor	T36.1x1-	T36.1x2-	T36.1x3-	T36.1x4-	T36.1x5-	T36.1x6-
Cefadroxil	T36.1x1-	T36.1x2-	T36.1x3-	T36.1x4-	T36.1x5-	T36.1x6-
Cefalexin	T36.1x1-	T36.1x2-	T36.1x3-	T36.1x4-	T36.1x5-	T36.1x6-
Cefaloglycin	T36.1x1-	T36.1x2-	T36.1x3-	T36.1x4-	T36.1x5-	T36.1x6-
Cefaloridine	T36.1x1-	T36.1x2-	T36.1x3-	T36.1x4-	T36.1x5-	T36.1x6-
Cefalosporins	T36.1x1-	T36.1x2-	T36.1x3-	T36.1x4-	T36.1x5-	T36.1x6-
Cefalotin	T36.1x1-	T36.1x2-	T36.1x3-	T36.1x4-	T36.1x5-	T36.1x6-
Cefamandole	T36.1x1-	T36.1x2-	T36.1x3-	T36.1x4-	T36.1x5-	T36.1x6-
Cefamycin antibiotic	T36.1x1-	T36.1x2-	T36.1x3-	T36.1x4-	T36.1x5-	T36.1x6-
Cefapirin	T36.1x1-	T36.1x2-	T36.1x3-	T36.1x4-	T36.1x5-	T36.1x6-
Cefatrizine	T36.1x1-	T36.1x2-	T36.1x3-	T36.1x4-	T36.1x5-	T36.1x6-
Cefazedone	T36.1x1-	T36.1x2-	T36.1x3-	T36.1x4-	T36.1x5-	T36.1x6-
Cefazolin	T36.1x1-	T36.1x2-	T36.1x3-	T36.1x4-	T36.1x5-	T36.1x6-
Cefbuperazone	T36.1x1-	T36.1x2-	T36.1x3-	T36.1x4-	T36.1x5-	T36.1x6-
Cefetamet	T36.1x1-	T36.1x2-	T36.1x3-	T36.1x4-	T36.1x5-	T36.1x6-
Cefixime	T36.1x1-	T36.1x2-	T36.1x3-	T36.1x4-	T36.1x5-	T36.1x6-
Cefmenoxime	T36.1x1-	T36.1x2-	T36.1x3-	T36.1x4-	T36.1x5-	T36.1x6-
Cefmetazole	T36.1x1-	T36.1x2-	T36.1x3-	T36.1x4-	T36.1x5-	T36.1x6-
Cefminox	T36.1x1-	T36.1x2-	T36.1x3-	T36.1x4-	T36.1x5-	T36.1x6-
Cefonicid	T36.1x1-	T36.1x2-	T36.1x3-	T36.1x4-	T36.1x5-	T36.1x6-
Cefoperazone	T36.1x1-	T36.1x2-	T36.1x3-	T36.1x4-	T36.1x5-	T36.1x6-
Ceforanide	T36.1x1-	T36.1x2-	T36.1x3-	T36.1x4-	T36.1x5-	T36.1x6-
Cefotaxime	T36.1x1-	T36.1x2-	T36.1x3-	T36.1x4-	T36.1x5-	T36.1x6-
Cefotetan	T36.1x1-	T36.1x2-	T36.1x3-	T36.1x4-	T36.1x5-	T36.1x6-
Cefotiam	T36.1x1-	T36.1x2-	T36.1x3-	T36.1x4-	T36.1x5-	T36.1x6-
Cefoxitin	T36.1x1-	T36.1x2-	T36.1x3-	T36.1x4-	T36.1x5-	T36.1x6-
Cefpimizole	T36.1x1-	T36.1x2-	T36.1x3-	T36.1x4-	T36.1x5-	T36.1x6-
Cefpiramide	T36.1x1-	T36.1x2-	T36.1x3-	T36.1x4-	T36.1x5-	T36.1x6-
Cefradine	T36.1x1-	T36.1x2-	T36.1x3-	T36.1x4-	T36.1x5-	T36.1x6-
Cefroxadine	T36.1x1-	T36.1x2-	T36.1x3-	T36.1x4-	T36.1x5-	T36.1x6-
Cefsulodin	T36.1x1-	T36.1x2-	T36.1x3-	T36.1x4-	T36.1x5-	T36.1x6-
Ceftazidime	T36.1x1-	T36.1x2-	T36.1x3-	T36.1x4-	T36.1x5-	T36.1x6-
Cefteram	T36.1x1-	T36.1x2-	T36.1x3-	T36.1x4-	T36.1x5-	T36.1x6-
Ceftezole	T36.1x1-	T36.1x2-	T36.1x3-	T36.1x4-	T36.1x5-	T36.1x6-
Ceftizoxime	T36.1x1-	T36.1x2-	T36.1x3-	T36.1x4-	T36.1x5-	T36.1x6-
Ceftriaxone	T36.1x1-	T36.1x2-	T36.1x3-	T36.1x4-	T36.1x5-	T36.1x6-
Cefuroxime	T36.1x1-	T36.1x2-	T36.1x3-	T36.1x4-	T36.1x5-	T36.1x6-
Cefuzonam	T36.1x1-	T36.1x2-	T36.1x3-	T36.1x4-	T36.1x5-	T36.1x6-
Celestone	T38.0x1-	T38.0x2-	T38.0x3-	T38.0x4-	T38.0x5-	T38.0x6-
topical	T49.0x1-	T49.0x2-	T49.0x3-	T49.0x4-	T49.0x5-	T49.0x6-

DRUGS & CHEMICALS

Table of Drugs & Chemicals	POISONING Accidental (Unintentional)	Self-Harm (Intentional)	Assault	Undetermined	Adverse Effect	Underdosing
Celiprolol	T44.7x1-	T44.7x2-	T44.7x3-	T44.7x4-	T44.7x5-	T44.7x6-
Cell stimulants and proliferants	T49.8x1-	T49.8x2-	T49.8x3-	T49.8x4-	T49.8x5-	T49.8x6-
Cellosolve	T52.91x-	T52.92x-	T52.93x-	T52.94x-	—	—
Cellulose						
cathartic	T47.4x1-	T47.4x2-	T47.4x3-	T47.4x4-	T47.4x5-	T47.4x6-
hydroxyethyl	T47.4x1-	T47.4x2-	T47.4x3-	T47.4x4-	T47.4x5-	T47.4x6-
nitrates (topical)	T49.3x1-	T49.3x2-	T49.3x3-	T49.3x4-	T49.3x5-	T49.3x6-
oxidized	T49.4x1-	T49.4x2-	T49.4x3-	T49.4x4-	T49.4x5-	T49.4x6-
Centipede (bite)	T63.411-	T63.412-	T63.413-	T63.414-		
Central nervous system						
depressants	T42.71x-	T42.72x-	T42.73x-	T42.74x-	T42.75x-	T42.76x-
anesthetic (general)						
NEC	T41.201-	T41.202-	T41.203-	T41.204-	T41.205-	T41.206-
gases NEC	T41.0x1-	T41.0x2-	T41.0x3-	T41.0x4-	T41.0x5-	T41.0x6-
intravenous	T41.1x1-	T41.1x2-	T41.1x3-	T41.1x4-	T41.1x5-	T41.1x6-
barbiturates	T42.3x1-	T42.3x2-	T42.3x3-	T42.3x4-	T42.3x5-	T42.3x6-
benzodiazepines	T42.4x1-	T42.4x2-	T42.4x3-	T42.4x4-	T42.4x5-	T42.4x6-
bromides	T42.6x1-	T42.6x2-	T42.6x3-	T42.6x4-	T42.6x5-	T42.6x6-
cannabis sativa	T40.7x1-	T40.7x2-	T40.7x3-	T40.7x4-	T40.7x5-	T40.7x6-
chloral hydrate	T42.6x1-	T42.6x2-	T42.6x3-	T42.6x4-	T42.6x5-	T42.6x6-
ethanol	T51.0x1-	T51.0x2-	T51.0x3-	T51.0x4-	—	—
hallucinogenics	T40.901-	T40.902-	T40.903-	T40.904-	T40.905-	T40.906-
hypnotics	T42.71x-	T42.72x-	T42.73x-	T42.74x-	T42.75x-	T42.76x-
specified NEC	T42.6x1-	T42.6x2-	T42.6x3-	T42.6x4-	T42.6x5-	T42.6x6-
muscle relaxants	T42.8x1-	T42.8x2-	T42.8x3-	T42.8x4-	T42.8x5-	T42.8x6-
paraldehyde	T42.6x1-	T42.6x2-	T42.6x3-	T42.6x4-	T42.6x5-	T42.6x6-
sedatives; sedative-hypnotics	T42.71x-	T42.72x-	T42.73x-	T42.74x-	T42.75x-	T42.76x-
mixed NEC	T42.6x1-	T42.6x2-	T42.6x3-	T42.6x4-	T42.6x5-	T42.6x6-
specified NEC	T42.6x1-	T42.6x2-	T42.6x3-	T42.6x4-	T42.6x5-	T42.6x6-
muscle-tone depressants	T42.8x1-	T42.8x2-	T42.8x3-	T42.8x4-	T42.8x5-	T42.8x6-
stimulants	T43.601-	T43.602-	T43.603-	T43.604-	T43.605-	T43.606-
amphetamines	T43.621-	T43.622-	T43.623-	T43.624-	T43.625-	T43.626-
analeptics	T50.7x1-	T50.7x2-	T50.7x3-	T50.7x4-	T50.7x5-	T50.7x6-
antidepressants	T43.201-	T43.202-	T43.203-	T43.204-	T43.205-	T43.206-
opiate antagonists	T50.7x1-	T50.7x2-	T50.7x3-	T50.7x4-	T50.7x5-	T50.7x6-
specified NEC	T43.691-	T43.692-	T43.693-	T43.694-	T43.695-	T43.696-
Cephalexin	T36.1x1-	T36.1x2-	T36.1x3-	T36.1x4-	T36.1x5-	T36.1x6-
Cephaloglycin	T36.1x1-	T36.1x2-	T36.1x3-	T36.1x4-	T36.1x5-	T36.1x6-
Cephaloridine	T36.1x1-	T36.1x2-	T36.1x3-	T36.1x4-	T36.1x5-	T36.1x6-
Cephalosporins	T36.1x1-	T36.1x2-	T36.1x3-	T36.1x4-	T36.1x5-	T36.1x6-
N (adicillin)	T36.0x1-	T36.0x2-	T36.0x3-	T36.0x4-	T36.0x5-	T36.0x6-
Cephalothin	T36.1x1-	T36.1x2-	T36.1x3-	T36.1x4-	T36.1x5-	T36.1x6-
Cephalotin	T36.1x1-	T36.1x2-	T36.1x3-	T36.1x4-	T36.1x5-	T36.1x6-
Cephradine	T36.1x1-	T36.1x2-	T36.1x3-	T36.1x4-	T36.1x5-	T36.1x6-
Cerbera (odallam)	T62.2x1-	T62.2x2-	T62.2x3-	T62.2x4-	—	—
Cerberin	T46.0x1-	T46.0x2-	T46.0x3-	T46.0x4-	T46.0x5-	T46.0x6-
Cerebral stimulants	T43.601-	T43.602-	T43.603-	T43.604-	T43.605-	T43.606-
psychotherapeutic	T43.601-	T43.602-	T43.603-	T43.604-	T43.605-	T43.606-
specified NEC	T43.691-	T43.692-	T43.693-	T43.694-	T43.695-	T43.696-
Cerium oxalate	T45.0x1-	T45.0x2-	T45.0x3-	T45.0x4-	T45.0x5-	T45.0x6-
Cerous oxalate	T45.0x1-	T45.0x2-	T45.0x3-	T45.0x4-	T45.0x5-	T45.0x6-
Ceruletide	T50.8x1-	T50.8x2-	T50.8x3-	T50.8x4-	T50.8x5-	T50.8x6-
Cetalkonium (chloride)	T49.0x1-	T49.0x2-	T49.0x3-	T49.0x4-	T49.0x5-	T49.0x6-
Cethexonium chloride	T49.0x1-	T49.0x2-	T49.0x3-	T49.0x4-	T49.0x5-	T49.0x6-
Cetiedil	T46.7x1-	T46.7x2-	T46.7x3-	T46.7x4-	T46.7x5-	T46.7x6-
Cetirizine	T45.0x1-	T45.0x2-	T45.0x3-	T45.0x4-	T45.0x5-	T45.0x6-
Cetomacrogol	T50.991-	T50.992-	T50.993-	T50.994-	T50.995-	T50.996-
Cetotiamine	T45.2x1-	T45.2x2-	T45.2x3-	T45.2x4-	T45.2x5-	T45.2x6-
Cetoxime	T45.0x1-	T45.0x2-	T45.0x3-	T45.0x4-	T45.0x5-	T45.0x6-
Cetraxate	T47.1x1-	T47.1x2-	T47.1x3-	T47.1x4-	T47.1x5-	T47.1x6-
Cetrimide	T49.0x1-	T49.0x2-	T49.0x3-	T49.0x4-	T49.0x5-	T49.0x6-

Table of Drugs & Chemicals	POISONING Accidental (Unintentional)	Self-Harm (Intentional)	Assault	Undetermined	Adverse Effect	Underdosing
Cetrimonium (bromide)	T49.0x1-	T49.0x2-	T49.0x3-	T49.0x4-	T49.0x5-	T49.0x6-
Cetylpyridinium chloride	T49.0x1-	T49.0x2-	T49.0x3-	T49.0x4-	T49.0x5-	T49.0x6-
ENT agent	T49.6x1-	T49.6x2-	T49.6x3-	T49.6x4-	T49.6x5-	T49.6x6-
lozenges	T49.6x1-	T49.6x2-	T49.6x3-	T49.6x4-	T49.6x5-	T49.6x6-
Cevadilla — see Sabadilla						
Cevitamic acid	T45.2x1-	T45.2x2-	T45.2x3-	T45.2x4-	T45.2x5-	T45.2x6-
Ch'an su	T46.0x1-	T46.0x2-	T46.0x3-	T46.0x4-	T46.0x5-	T46.0x6-
Chalk, precipitated	T47.1x1-	T47.1x2-	T47.1x3-	T47.1x4-	T47.1x5-	T47.1x6-
Chamomile	T49.0x1-	T49.0x2-	T49.0x3-	T49.0x4-	T49.0x5-	T49.0x6-
Charcoal	T47.6x1-	T47.6x2-	T47.6x3-	T47.6x4-	T47.6x5-	T47.6x6-
activated — see also						
Charcoal, medicinal	T47.6x1-	T47.6x2-	T47.6x3-	T47.6x4-	T47.6x5-	T47.6x6-
fumes (carbon monoxide)	T58.2x1-	T58.2x2-		T58.2x4-	—	—
industrial	T58.8x1-	T58.8x2-		T58.8x4-	—	—
medicinal (activated)	T47.6x1-	T47.6x2-	T47.6x3-	T47.6x4-	T47.6x5-	T47.6x6-
antidiarrheal	T47.6x1-	T47.6x2-	T47.6x3-	T47.6x4-	T47.6x5-	T47.6x6-
poison control	T47.8x1-	T47.8x2-	T47.8x3-	T47.8x4-	T47.8x5-	T47.8x6-
specified use other than for diarrhea	T47.8x1-	T47.8x2-	T47.8x3-	T47.8x4-	T47.8x5-	T47.8x6-
topical	T49.8x1-	T49.8x2-	T49.8x3-	T49.8x4-	T49.8x5-	T49.8x6-
Chaulmosulfone	T37.1x1-	T37.1x2-	T37.1x3-	T37.1x4-	T37.1x5-	T37.1x6-
Chelating agent NEC	T50.6x1-	T50.6x2-	T50.6x3-	T50.6x4-	T50.6x5-	T50.6x6-
Chelidonium majus	T62.2x1-	T62.2x2-	T62.2x3-	T62.2x4-	—	—
Chemical substance NEC	T65.91x-	T65.92x-	T65.93x-	T65.94x-	—	—
Chenodeoxycholic acid	T47.5x1-	T47.5x2-	T47.5x3-	T47.5x4-	T47.5x5-	T47.5x6-
Chenodiol	T47.5x1-	T47.5x2-	T47.5x3-	T47.5x4-	T47.5x5-	T47.5x6-
Chenopodium	T37.4x1-	T37.4x2-	T37.4x3-	T37.4x4-	T37.4x5-	T37.4x6-
Cherry laurel	T62.2x1-	T62.2x2-	T62.2x3-	T62.2x4-	—	—
Chinidin(e)	T46.2x1-	T46.2x2-	T46.2x3-	T46.2x4-	T46.2x5-	T46.2x6-
Chiniofon	T37.8x1-	T37.8x2-	T37.8x3-	T37.8x4-	T37.8x5-	T37.8x6-
Chlophedianol	T48.3x1-	T48.3x2-	T48.3x3-	T48.3x4-	T48.3x5-	T48.3x6-
Chloral	T42.6x1-	T42.6x2-	T42.6x3-	T42.6x4-	T42.6x5-	T42.6x6-
derivative	T42.6x1-	T42.6x2-	T42.6x3-	T42.6x4-	T42.6x5-	T42.6x6-
hydrate	T42.6x1-	T42.6x2-	T42.6x3-	T42.6x4-	T42.6x5-	T42.6x6-
Chloralamide	T42.6x1-	T42.6x2-	T42.6x3-	T42.6x4-	T42.6x5-	T42.6x6-
Chloralodol	T42.6x1-	T42.6x2-	T42.6x3-	T42.6x4-	T42.6x5-	T42.6x6-
Chloralose	T60.4x1-	T60.4x2-	T60.4x3-	T60.4x4-	—	—
Chlorambucil	T45.1x1-	T45.1x2-	T45.1x3-	T45.1x4-	T45.1x5-	T45.1x6-
Chloramine	T57.8x1-	T57.8x2-	T57.8x3-	T57.8x4-	—	—
T	T49.0x1-	T49.0x2-	T49.0x3-	T49.0x4-	T49.0x5-	T49.0x6-
topical	T49.0x1-	T49.0x2-	T49.0x3-	T49.0x4-	T49.0x5-	T49.0x6-
Chloramphenicol	T36.2x1-	T36.2x2-	T36.2x3-	T36.2x4-	T36.2x5-	T36.2x6-
ENT agent	T49.6x1-	T49.6x2-	T49.6x3-	T49.6x4-	T49.6x5-	T49.6x6-
ophthalmic preparation	T49.5x1-	T49.5x2-	T49.5x3-	T49.5x4-	T49.5x5-	T49.5x6-
topical NEC	T49.0x1-	T49.0x2-	T49.0x3-	T49.0x4-	T49.0x5-	T49.0x6-
Chlorate (potassium) (sodium) NEC	T60.3x1-	T60.3x2-	T60.3x3-	T60.3x4-	—	—
herbicide	T60.3x1-	T60.3x2-	T60.3x3-	T60.3x4-	—	—
Chlorazanil	T50.2x1-	T50.2x2-	T50.2x3-	T50.2x4-	T50.2x5-	T50.2x6-
Chlorbenzene, chlorbenzol	T53.7x1-	T53.7x2-	T53.7x3-	T53.7x4-		
Chlorbenzoxamine	T44.3x1-	T44.3x2-	T44.3x3-	T44.3x4-	T44.3x5-	T44.3x6-
Chlorbutol	T42.6x1-	T42.6x2-	T42.6x3-	T42.6x4-	T42.6x5-	T42.6x6-
Chlorcyclizine	T45.0x1-	T45.0x2-	T45.0x3-	T45.0x4-	T45.0x5-	T45.0x6-
Chlordan(e) (dust)	T60.1x1-	T60.1x2-	T60.1x3-	T60.1x4-		
Chlordantoin	T49.0x1-	T49.0x2-	T49.0x3-	T49.0x4-	T49.0x5-	T49.0x6-
Chlordiazepoxide	T42.4x1-	T42.4x2-	T42.4x3-	T42.4x4-	T42.4x5-	T42.4x6-
Chlordiethyl benzamide	T49.3x1-	T49.3x2-	T49.3x3-	T49.3x4-	T49.3x5-	T49.3x6-
Chloresium	T49.8x1-	T49.8x2-	T49.8x3-	T49.8x4-	T49.8x5-	T49.8x6-
Chlorethiazol	T42.6x1-	T42.6x2-	T42.6x3-	T42.6x4-	T42.6x5-	T42.6x6-
Chlorethyl — see Ethyl chloride						
Chloretone	T42.6x1-	T42.6x2-	T42.6x3-	T42.6x4-	T42.6x5-	T42.6x6-
Chlorex	T53.6x1-	T53.6x2-	T53.6x3-	T53.6x4-	—	—
insecticide	T60.1x1-	T60.1x2-	T60.1x3-	T60.1x4-	—	—

Table of Drugs & Chemicals	POISONING Accidental (Unintentional)	Self-Harm (Intentional)	Assault	Undetermined	Adverse Effect	Underdosing
Chlorfenvinphos	T60.0x1-	T60.0x2-	T60.0x3-	T60.0x4-	—	—
Chlorhexadol	T42.6x1-	T42.6x2-	T42.6x3-	T42.6x4-	T42.6x5-	T42.6x6-
Chlorhexamide	T45.1x1-	T45.1x2-	T45.1x3-	T45.1x4-	T45.1x5-	T45.1x6-
Chlorhexidine	T49.0x1-	T49.0x2-	T49.0x3-	T49.0x4-	T49.0x5-	T49.0x6-
Chlorhydroxyquinolin	T49.0x1-	T49.0x2-	T49.0x3-	T49.0x4-	T49.0x5-	T49.0x6-
Chloride of lime (bleach)	T54.3x1-	T54.3x2-	T54.3x3-	T54.3x4-	—	—
Chlorimipramine	T43.011-	T43.012-	T43.013-	T43.014-	T43.015-	T43.016-
Chlorinated						
camphene	T53.6x1-	T53.6x2-	T53.6x3-	T53.6x4-	—	—
diphenyl	T53.7x1-	T53.7x2-	T53.7x3-	T53.7x4-	—	—
hydrocarbons NEC	T53.91x-	T53.92x-	T53.93x-	T53.94x-	—	—
solvents	T53.91x-	T53.92x-	T53.93x-	T53.94x-	—	—
lime (bleach)	T54.3x1-	T54.3x2-	T54.3x3-	T54.3x4-	—	—
and boric acid solution	T49.0x1-	T49.0x2-	T49.0x3-	T49.0x4-	T49.0x5-	T49.0x6-
naphthalene (insecticide)	T60.1x1-	T60.1x2-	T60.1x3-	T60.1x4-	—	—
industrial (non-pesticide)	T53.7x1-	T53.7x2-	T53.7x3-	T53.7x4-	—	—
pesticide NEC	T60.8x1-	T60.8x2-	T60.8x3-	T60.8x4-	—	—
soda — see also Sodium hypochlorite						
solution	T49.0x1-	T49.0x2-	T49.0x3-	T49.0x4-	T49.0x5-	T49.0x6-
Chlorine (fumes) (gas)	T59.4x1-	T59.4x2-	T59.4x3-	T59.4x4-	—	—
bleach	T54.3x1-	T54.3x2-	T54.3x3-	T54.3x4-	—	—
compound gas NEC	T59.4x1-	T59.4x2-	T59.4x3-	T59.4x4-	—	—
disinfectant	T59.4x1-	T59.4x2-	T59.4x3-	T59.4x4-	—	—
releasing agents NEC	T59.4x1-	T59.4x2-	T59.4x3-	T59.4x4-	—	—
Chlorisondamine chloride	T46.991-	T46.992-	T46.993-	T46.994-	T46.995-	T46.996-
Chlormadinone	T38.5x1-	T38.5x2-	T38.5x3-	T38.5x4-	T38.5x5-	T38.5x6-
Chlormephos	T60.0x1-	T60.0x2-	T60.0x3-	T60.0x4-	—	—
Chlormerodrin	T50.2x1-	T50.2x2-	T50.2x3-	T50.2x4-	T50.2x5-	T50.2x6-
Chlormethiazole	T42.6x1-	T42.6x2-	T42.6x3-	T42.6x4-	T42.6x5-	T42.6x6-
Chlormethine	T45.1x1-	T45.1x2-	T45.1x3-	T45.1x4-	T45.1x5-	T45.1x6-
Chlormethylenecycline	T36.4x1-	T36.4x2-	T36.4x3-	T36.4x4-	T36.4x5-	T36.4x6-
Chlormezanone	T42.6x1-	T42.6x2-	T42.6x3-	T42.6x4-	T42.6x5-	T42.6x6-
Chloroacetic acid	T60.3x1-	T60.3x2-	T60.3x3-	T60.3x4-	—	—
Chloroacetone	T59.3x1-	T59.3x2-	T59.3x3-	T59.3x4-	—	—
Chloroacetophenone	T59.3x1-	T59.3x2-	T59.3x3-	T59.3x4-	—	—
Chloroaniline	T53.7x1-	T53.7x2-	T53.7x3-	T53.7x4-	—	—
Chlorobenzene, chlorobenzol	T53.7x1-	T53.7x2-	T53.7x3-	T53.7x4-	—	—
Chlorobromomethane (fire extinguisher)	T53.6x1-	T53.6x2-	T53.6x3-	T53.6x4-	—	—
Chlorobutanol	T49.0x1-	T49.0x2-	T49.0x3-	T49.0x4-	T49.0x5-	T49.0x6-
Chlorocresol	T49.0x1-	T49.0x2-	T49.0x3-	T49.0x4-	T49.0x5-	T49.0x6-
Chlorodehydro-methyltestosterone	T38.7x1-	T38.7x2-	T38.7x3-	T38.7x4-	T38.7x5-	T38.7x6-
Chlorodinitrobenzene	T53.7x1-	T53.7x2-	T53.7x3-	T53.7x4-	—	—
dust or vapor	T53.7x1-	T53.7x2-	T53.7x3-	T53.7x4-	—	—
Chlorodiphenyl	T53.7x1-	T53.7x2-	T53.7x3-	T53.7x4-	—	—
Chloroethane — see Ethyl chloride						
Chloroethylene	T53.6x1-	T53.6x2-	T53.6x3-	T53.6x4-	—	—
Chlorofluorocarbons	T53.5x1-	T53.5x2-	T53.5x3-	T53.5x4-	—	—
Chloroform (fumes) (vapor)	T53.1x1-	T53.1x2-	T53.1x3-	T53.1x4-	—	—
anesthetic	T41.0x1-	T41.0x2-	T41.0x3-	T41.0x4-	T41.0x5-	T41.0x6-
solvent	T53.1x1-	T53.1x2-	T53.1x3-	T53.1x4-	—	—
water, concentrated	T41.0x1-	T41.0x2-	T41.0x3-	T41.0x4-	T41.0x5-	T41.0x6-
Chloroguanide	T37.2x1-	T37.2x2-	T37.2x3-	T37.2x4-	T37.2x5-	T37.2x6-
Chloromycetin	T36.2x1-	T36.2x2-	T36.2x3-	T36.2x4-	T36.2x5-	T36.2x6-
ENT agent	T49.6x1-	T49.6x2-	T49.6x3-	T49.6x4-	T49.6x5-	T49.6x6-
ophthalmic preparation	T49.5x1-	T49.5x2-	T49.5x3-	T49.5x4-	T49.5x5-	T49.5x6-
otic solution	T49.6x1-	T49.6x2-	T49.6x3-	T49.6x4-	T49.6x5-	T49.6x6-
topical NEC	T49.0x1-	T49.0x2-	T49.0x3-	T49.0x4-	T49.0x5-	T49.0x6-

Table of Drugs & Chemicals	POISONING Accidental (Unintentional)	Self-Harm (Intentional)	Assault	Undetermined	Adverse Effect	Underdosing
Chloronitrobenzene	T53.7x1-	T53.7x2-	T53.7x3-	T53.7x4-	—	—
dust or vapor	T53.7x1-	T53.7x2-	T53.7x3-	T53.7x4-	—	—
Chlorophacinone	T60.4x1-	T60.4x2-	T60.4x3-	T60.4x4-	—	—
Chlorophenol	T53.7x1-	T53.7x2-	T53.7x3-	T53.7x4-	—	—
Chlorophenothane	T60.1x1-	T60.1x2-	T60.1x3-	T60.1x4-	—	—
Chlorophyll	T50.991-	T50.992-	T50.993-	T50.994-	T50.995-	T50.996-
Chloropicrin (fumes)	T53.6x1-	T53.6x2-	T53.6x3-	T53.6x4-	—	—
fumigant	T60.8x1-	T60.8x2-	T60.8x3-	T60.8x4-	—	—
fungicide	T60.3x1-	T60.3x2-	T60.3x3-	T60.3x4-	—	—
pesticide	T60.8x1-	T60.8x2-	T60.8x3-	T60.8x4-	—	—
Chloroprocaine	T41.3x1-	T41.3x2-	T41.3x3-	T41.3x4-	T41.3x5-	T41.3x6-
infiltration (subcutaneous)	T41.3x1-	T41.3x2-	T41.3x3-	T41.3x4-	T41.3x5-	T41.3x6-
nerve block (peripheral) (plexus)	T41.3x1-	T41.3x2-	T41.3x3-	T41.3x4-	T41.3x5-	T41.3x6-
spinal	T41.3x1-	T41.3x2-	T41.3x3-	T41.3x4-	T41.3x5-	T41.3x6-
Chloroptic	T49.5x1-	T49.5x2-	T49.5x3-	T49.5x4-	T49.5x5-	T49.5x6-
Chloropurine	T45.1x1-	T45.1x2-	T45.1x3-	T45.1x4-	T45.1x5-	T45.1x6-
Chloropyramine	T45.0x1-	T45.0x2-	T45.0x3-	T45.0x4-	T45.0x5-	T45.0x6-
Chloropyrifos	T60.1x1-	T60.1x2-	T60.1x3-	T60.1x4-	—	—
Chloropyrilene	T45.0x1-	T45.0x2-	T45.0x3-	T45.0x4-	T45.0x5-	T45.0x6-
Chloroquine	T37.2x1-	T37.2x2-	T37.2x3-	T37.2x4-	T37.2x5-	T37.2x6-
Chlorothalonil	T60.3x1-	T60.3x2-	T60.3x3-	T60.3x4-	—	—
Chlorothen	T45.0x1-	T45.0x2-	T45.0x3-	T45.0x4-	T45.0x5-	T45.0x6-
Chlorothiazide	T50.2x1-	T50.2x2-	T50.2x3-	T50.2x4-	T50.2x5-	T50.2x6-
Chlorothymol	T49.4x1-	T49.4x2-	T49.4x3-	T49.4x4-	T49.4x5-	T49.4x6-
Chlorotrianisene	T38.5x1-	T38.5x2-	T38.5x3-	T38.5x4-	T38.5x5-	T38.5x6-
Chlorovinyldichloro-arsine, not in war	T57.0x1-	T57.0x2-	T57.0x3-	T57.0x4-	—	—
Chloroxine	T49.4x1-	T49.4x2-	T49.4x3-	T49.4x4-	T49.4x5-	T49.4x6-
Chloroxylenol	T49.0x1-	T49.0x2-	T49.0x3-	T49.0x4-	T49.0x5-	T49.0x6-
Chlorphenamine	T45.0x1-	T45.0x2-	T45.0x3-	T45.0x4-	T45.0x5-	T45.0x6-
Chlorphenesin	T42.8x1-	T42.8x2-	T42.8x3-	T42.8x4-	T42.8x5-	T42.8x6-
topical (antifungal)	T49.0x1-	T49.0x2-	T49.0x3-	T49.0x4-	T49.0x5-	T49.0x6-
Chlorpheniramine	T45.0x1-	T45.0x2-	T45.0x3-	T45.0x4-	T45.0x5-	T45.0x6-
Chlorphenoxamine	T45.0x1-	T45.0x2-	T45.0x3-	T45.0x4-	T45.0x5-	T45.0x6-
Chlorphentermine	T50.5x1-	T50.5x2-	T50.5x3-	T50.5x4-	T50.5x5-	T50.5x6-
Chlorprocaine — see Chloroprocaine						
Chlorproguanil	T37.2x1-	T37.2x2-	T37.2x3-	T37.2x4-	T37.2x5-	T37.2x6-
Chlorpromazine	T43.3x1-	T43.3x2-	T43.3x3-	T43.3x4-	T43.3x5-	T43.3x6-
Chlorpropamide	T38.3x1-	T38.3x2-	T38.3x3-	T38.3x4-	T38.3x5-	T38.3x6-
Chlorprothixene	T43.4x1-	T43.4x2-	T43.4x3-	T43.4x4-	T43.4x5-	T43.4x6-
Chlorquinaldol	T49.0x1-	T49.0x2-	T49.0x3-	T49.0x4-	T49.0x5-	T49.0x6-
Chlorquinol	T49.0x1-	T49.0x2-	T49.0x3-	T49.0x4-	T49.0x5-	T49.0x6-
Chlortalidone	T50.2x1-	T50.2x2-	T50.2x3-	T50.2x4-	T50.2x5-	T50.2x6-
Chlortetracycline	T36.4x1-	T36.4x2-	T36.4x3-	T36.4x4-	T36.4x5-	T36.4x6-
Chlorthalidone	T50.2x1-	T50.2x2-	T50.2x3-	T50.2x4-	T50.2x5-	T50.2x6-
Chlorthion	T60.0x1-	T60.0x2-	T60.0x3-	T60.0x4-	—	—
Chlorthiophos	T60.0x1-	T60.0x2-	T60.0x3-	T60.0x4-	—	—
Chlortrianisene	T38.5x1-	T38.5x2-	T38.5x3-	T38.5x4-	T38.5x5-	T38.5x6-
Chlor-Trimeton	T45.0x1-	T45.0x2-	T45.0x3-	T45.0x4-	T45.0x5-	T45.0x6-
Chlorzoxazone	T42.8x1-	T42.8x2-	T42.8x3-	T42.8x4-	T42.8x5-	T42.8x6-
Choke damp	T59.7x1-	T59.7x2-	T59.7x3-	T59.7x4-	—	—
Cholagogues	T47.5x1-	T47.5x2-	T47.5x3-	T47.5x4-	T47.5x5-	T47.5x6-
Cholebrine	T50.8x1-	T50.8x2-	T50.8x3-	T50.8x4-	T50.8x5-	T50.8x6-
Cholecalciferol	T45.2x1-	T45.2x2-	T45.2x3-	T45.2x4-	T45.2x5-	T45.2x6-
Cholecystokinin	T50.8x1-	T50.8x2-	T50.8x3-	T50.8x4-	T50.8x5-	T50.8x6-
Cholera vaccine	T50.A91-	T50.A92-	T50.A93-	T50.A94-	T50.A95-	T50.A96-
Choleretic	T47.5x1-	T47.5x2-	T47.5x3-	T47.5x4-	T47.5x5-	T47.5x6-
Cholesterol-lowering agents	T46.6x1-	T46.6x2-	T46.6x3-	T46.6x4-	T46.6x5-	T46.6x6-
Cholestyramine (resin)	T46.6x1-	T46.6x2-	T46.6x3-	T46.6x4-	T46.6x5-	T46.6x6-

DRUGS & CHEMICALS

Table of Drugs & Chemicals	POISONING Accidental (Unintentional)	Self-Harm (Intentional)	Assault	Undetermined	Adverse Effect	Underdosing
Cholic acid	T47.5x1-	T47.5x2-	T47.5x3-	T47.5x4-	T47.5x5-	T47.5x6-
Choline	T48.6x1-	T48.6x2-	T48.6x3-	T48.6x4-	T48.6x5-	T48.6x6-
chloride	T50.991-	T50.992-	T50.993-	T50.994-	T50.995-	T50.996-
dihydrogen citrate	T50.991-	T50.992-	T50.993-	T50.994-	T50.995-	T50.996-
salicylate	T39.091-	T39.092-	T39.093-	T39.094-	T39.095-	T39.096-
theophyllinate	T48.6x1-	T48.6x2-	T48.6x3-	T48.6x4-	T48.6x5-	T48.6x6-
Cholinergic (drug) NEC	T44.1x1-	T44.1x2-	T44.1x3-	T44.1x4-	T44.1x5-	T44.1x6-
muscle tone enhancer	T44.1x1-	T44.1x2-	T44.1x3-	T44.1x4-	T44.1x5-	T44.1x6-
organophosphorus	T44.0x1-	T44.0x2-	T44.0x3-	T44.0x4-	T44.0x5-	T44.0x6-
insecticide	T60.0x1-	T60.0x2-	T60.0x3-	T60.0x4-	—	—
nerve gas	T59.891-	T59.892-	T59.893-	T59.894-	—	—
trimethyl ammonium propanediol	T44.1x1-	T44.1x2-	T44.1x3-	T44.1x4-	T44.1x5-	T44.1x6-
Cholinesterase reactivator	T50.6x1-	T50.6x2-	T50.6x3-	T50.6x4-	T50.6x5-	T50.6x6-
Cholografin	T50.8x1-	T50.8x2-	T50.8x3-	T50.8x4-	T50.8x5-	T50.8x6-
Chorionic gonadotropin	T38.891-	T38.892-	T38.893-	T38.894-	T38.895-	T38.896-
Chromate	T56.2x1-	T56.2x2-	T56.2x3-	T56.2x4-	—	—
dust or mist	T56.2x1-	T56.2x2-	T56.2x3-	T56.2x4-	—	—
lead — see also Lead	T56.0x1-	T56.0x2-	T56.0x3-	T56.0x4-	—	—
paint	T56.0x1-	T56.0x2-	T56.0x3-	T56.0x4-	—	—
Chromic						
acid	T56.2x1-	T56.2x2-	T56.2x3-	T56.2x4-	—	—
dust or mist	T56.2x1-	T56.2x2-	T56.2x3-	T56.2x4-	—	—
phosphate 32P	T45.1x1-	T45.1x2-	T45.1x3-	T45.1x4-	T45.1x5-	T45.1x6-
Chromium	T56.2x1-	T56.2x2-	T56.2x3-	T56.2x4-	—	—
compounds — see Chromate						
sesquioxide	T50.8x1-	T50.8x2-	T50.8x3-	T50.8x4-	T50.8x5-	T50.8x6-
Chromomycin A3	T45.1x1-	T45.1x2-	T45.1x3-	T45.1x4-	T45.1x5-	T45.1x6-
Chromonar	T46.3x1-	T46.3x2-	T46.3x3-	T46.3x4-	T46.3x5-	T46.3x6-
Chromyl chloride	T56.2x1-	T56.2x2-	T56.2x3-	T56.2x4-	—	—
Chrysarobin	T49.4x1-	T49.4x2-	T49.4x3-	T49.4x4-	T49.4x5-	T49.4x6-
Chrysazin	T47.2x1-	T47.2x2-	T47.2x3-	T47.2x4-	T47.2x5-	T47.2x6-
Chymar	T45.3x1-	T45.3x2-	T45.3x3-	T45.3x4-	T45.3x5-	T45.3x6-
ophthalmic preparation	T49.5x1-	T49.5x2-	T49.5x3-	T49.5x4-	T49.5x5-	T49.5x6-
Chymopapain	T45.3x1-	T45.3x2-	T45.3x3-	T45.3x4-	T45.3x5-	T45.3x6-
Chymotrypsin	T45.3x1-	T45.3x2-	T45.3x3-	T45.3x4-	T45.3x5-	T45.3x6-
ophthalmic preparation	T49.5x1-	T49.5x2-	T49.5x3-	T49.5x4-	T49.5x5-	T49.5x6-
Cianidanol	T50.991-	T50.992-	T50.993-	T50.994-	T50.995-	T50.996-
Cianopramine	T43.011-	T43.012-	T43.013-	T43.014-	T43.015-	T43.016-
Cibenzoline	T46.2x1-	T46.2x2-	T46.2x3-	T46.2x4-	T46.2x5-	T46.2x6-
Ciclacillin	T36.0x1-	T36.0x2-	T36.0x3-	T36.0x4-	T36.0x5-	T36.0x6-
Ciclobarbital — see Hexobarbital						
Ciclonicate	T46.7x1-	T46.7x2-	T46.7x3-	T46.7x4-	T46.7x5-	T46.7x6-
Ciclopirox (olamine)	T49.0x1-	T49.0x2-	T49.0x3-	T49.0x4-	T49.0x5-	T49.0x6-
Ciclosporin	T45.1x1-	T45.1x2-	T45.1x3-	T45.1x4-	T45.1x5-	T45.1x6-
Cicuta maculata or virosa	T62.2x1-	T62.2x2-	T62.2x3-	T62.2x4-	—	—
Cicutoxin	T62.2x1-	T62.2x2-	T62.2x3-	T62.2x4-	—	—
Cigarette lighter fluid	T52.0x1-	T52.0x2-	T52.0x3-	T52.0x4-	—	—
Cigarettes (tobacco)	T65.221-	T65.222-	T65.223-	T65.224-	—	—
Ciguatoxin	T61.01x-	T61.02x-	T61.03x-	T61.04x-	—	—
Cilazapril	T46.4x1-	T46.4x2-	T46.4x3-	T46.4x4-	T46.4x5-	T46.4x6-
Cimetidine	T47.0x1-	T47.0x2-	T47.0x3-	T47.0x4-	T47.0x5-	T47.0x6-
Cimetropium bromide	T44.3x1-	T44.3x2-	T44.3x3-	T44.3x4-	T44.3x5-	T44.3x6-
Cinchocaine	T41.3x1-	T41.3x2-	T41.3x3-	T41.3x4-	T41.3x5-	T41.3x6-
topical (surface)	T41.3x1-	T41.3x2-	T41.3x3-	T41.3x4-	T41.3x5-	T41.3x6-
Cinchona	T37.2x1-	T37.2x2-	T37.2x3-	T37.2x4-	T37.2x5-	T37.2x6-
Cinchonine alkaloids	T37.2x1-	T37.2x2-	T37.2x3-	T37.2x4-	T37.2x5-	T37.2x6-
Cinchophen	T50.4x1-	T50.4x2-	T50.4x3-	T50.4x4-	T50.4x5-	T50.4x6-
Cinepazide	T46.7x1-	T46.7x2-	T46.7x3-	T46.7x4-	T46.7x5-	T46.7x6-
Cinnamedrine	T48.5x1-	T48.5x2-	T48.5x3-	T48.5x4-	T48.5x5-	T48.5x6-
Cinnarizine	T45.0x1-	T45.0x2-	T45.0x3-	T45.0x4-	T45.0x5-	T45.0x6-

Table of Drugs & Chemicals	POISONING Accidental (Unintentional)	Self-Harm (Intentional)	Assault	Undetermined	Adverse Effect	Underdosing
Cinoxacin	T37.8x1-	T37.8x2-	T37.8x3-	T37.8x4-	T37.8x5-	T37.8x6-
Ciprofibrate	T46.6x1-	T46.6x2-	T46.6x3-	T46.6x4-	T46.6x5-	T46.6x6-
Ciprofloxacin	T36.8x1-	T36.8x2-	T36.8x3-	T36.8x4-	T36.8x5-	T36.8x6-
Cisapride	T47.8x1-	T47.8x2-	T47.8x3-	T47.8x4-	T47.8x5-	T47.8x6-
Cisplatin	T45.1x1-	T45.1x2-	T45.1x3-	T45.1x4-	T45.1x5-	T45.1x6-
Citalopram	T43.221-	T43.222-	T43.223-	T43.224-	T43.225-	T43.226-
Citanest	T41.3x1-	T41.3x2-	T41.3x3-	T41.3x4-	T41.3x5-	T41.3x6-
infiltration (subcutaneous)	T41.3x1-	T41.3x2-	T41.3x3-	T41.3x4-	T41.3x5-	T41.3x6-
nerve block (peripheral) (plexus)	T41.3x1-	T41.3x2-	T41.3x3-	T41.3x4-	T41.3x5-	T41.3x6-
Citric acid	T47.5x1-	T47.5x2-	T47.5x3-	T47.5x4-	T47.5x5-	T47.5x6-
Citrovorum (factor)	T45.8x1-	T45.8x2-	T45.8x3-	T45.8x4-	T45.8x5-	T45.8x6-
Claviceps purpurea	T62.2x1-	T62.2x2-	T62.2x3-	T62.2x4-	—	—
Clavulanic acid	T36.1x1-	T36.1x2-	T36.1x3-	T36.1x4-	T36.1x5-	T36.1x6-
Cleaner, cleansing agent, type not specified	T65.891-	T65.892-	T65.893-	T65.894-	—	—
of paint or varnish	T52.91x-	T52.92x-	T52.93x-	T52.94x-	—	—
specified type NEC	T65.891-	T65.892-	T65.893-	T65.894-	—	—
Clebopride	T47.8x1-	T47.8x2-	T47.8x3-	T47.8x4-	T47.8x5-	T47.8x6-
Clefamide	T37.3x1-	T37.3x2-	T37.3x3-	T37.3x4-	T37.3x5-	T37.3x6-
Clemastine	T45.0x1-	T45.0x2-	T45.0x3-	T45.0x4-	T45.0x5-	T45.0x6-
Clematis vitalba	T62.2x1-	T62.2x2-	T62.2x3-	T62.2x4-	—	—
Clemizole	T45.0x1-	T45.0x2-	T45.0x3-	T45.0x4-	T45.0x5-	T45.0x6-
penicillin	T36.0x1-	T36.0x2-	T36.0x3-	T36.0x4-	T36.0x5-	T36.0x6-
Clenbuterol	T48.6x1-	T48.6x2-	T48.6x3-	T48.6x4-	T48.6x5-	T48.6x6-
Clidinium bromide	T44.3x1-	T44.3x2-	T44.3x3-	T44.3x4-	T44.3x5-	T44.3x6-
Clindamycin	T36.8x1-	T36.8x2-	T36.8x3-	T36.8x4-	T36.8x5-	T36.8x6-
Clinofibrate	T46.6x1-	T46.6x2-	T46.6x3-	T46.6x4-	T46.6x5-	T46.6x6-
Clioquinol	T37.8x1-	T37.8x2-	T37.8x3-	T37.8x4-	T37.8x5-	T37.8x6-
Cliradon	T40.2x1-	T40.2x2-	T40.2x3-	T40.2x4-	—	—
Clobazam	T42.4x1-	T42.4x2-	T42.4x3-	T42.4x4-	T42.4x5-	T42.4x6-
Clobenzorex	T50.5x1-	T50.5x2-	T50.5x3-	T50.5x4-	T50.5x5-	T50.5x6-
Clobetasol	T49.0x1-	T49.0x2-	T49.0x3-	T49.0x4-	T49.0x5-	T49.0x6-
Clobetasone	T49.0x1-	T49.0x2-	T49.0x3-	T49.0x4-	T49.0x5-	T49.0x6-
Clobutinol	T48.3x1-	T48.3x2-	T48.3x3-	T48.3x4-	T48.3x5-	T48.3x6-
Clocortolone	T38.0x1-	T38.0x2-	T38.0x3-	T38.0x4-	T38.0x5-	T38.0x6-
Clodantoin	T49.0x1-	T49.0x2-	T49.0x3-	T49.0x4-	T49.0x5-	T49.0x6-
Clodronic acid	T50.991-	T50.992-	T50.993-	T50.994-	T50.995-	T50.996-
Clofazimine	T37.1x1-	T37.1x2-	T37.1x3-	T37.1x4-	T37.1x5-	T37.1x6-
Clofedanol	T48.3x1-	T48.3x2-	T48.3x3-	T48.3x4-	T48.3x5-	T48.3x6-
Clofenamide	T50.2x1-	T50.2x2-	T50.2x3-	T50.2x4-	T50.2x5-	T50.2x6-
Clofenotane	T49.0x1-	T49.0x2-	T49.0x3-	T49.0x4-	T49.0x5-	T49.0x6-
Clofezone	T39.2x1-	T39.2x2-	T39.2x3-	T39.2x4-	T39.2x5-	T39.2x6-
Clofibrate	T46.6x1-	T46.6x2-	T46.6x3-	T46.6x4-	T46.6x5-	T46.6x6-
Clofibride	T46.6x1-	T46.6x2-	T46.6x3-	T46.6x4-	T46.6x5-	T46.6x6-
Cloforex	T50.5x1-	T50.5x2-	T50.5x3-	T50.5x4-	T50.5x5-	T50.5x6-
Clomethiazole	T42.6x1-	T42.6x2-	T42.6x3-	T42.6x4-	T42.6x5-	T42.6x6-
Clometocillin	T36.0x1-	T36.0x2-	T36.0x3-	T36.0x4-	T36.0x5-	T36.0x6-
Clomifene	T38.5x1-	T38.5x2-	T38.5x3-	T38.5x4-	T38.5x5-	T38.5x6-
Clomiphene	T38.5x1-	T38.5x2-	T38.5x3-	T38.5x4-	T38.5x5-	T38.5x6-
Clomipramine	T43.011-	T43.012-	T43.013-	T43.014-	T43.015-	T43.016-
Clomocycline	T36.4x1-	T36.4x2-	T36.4x3-	T36.4x4-	T36.4x5-	T36.4x6-
Clonazepam	T42.4x1-	T42.4x2-	T42.4x3-	T42.4x4-	T42.4x5-	T42.4x6-
Clonidine	T46.5x1-	T46.5x2-	T46.5x3-	T46.5x4-	T46.5x5-	T46.5x6-
Clonixin	T39.8x1-	T39.8x2-	T39.8x3-	T39.8x4-	T39.8x5-	T39.8x6-
Clopamide	T50.2x1-	T50.2x2-	T50.2x3-	T50.2x4-	T50.2x5-	T50.2x6-
Clopenthixol	T43.4x1-	T43.4x2-	T43.4x3-	T43.4x4-	T43.4x5-	T43.4x6-
Cloperastine	T48.3x1-	T48.3x2-	T48.3x3-	T48.3x4-	T48.3x5-	T48.3x6-
Clophedianol	T48.3x1-	T48.3x2-	T48.3x3-	T48.3x4-	T48.3x5-	T48.3x6-
Cloponone	T36.2x1-	T36.2x2-	T36.2x3-	T36.2x4-	T36.2x5-	T36.2x6-
Cloprednol	T38.0x1-	T38.0x2-	T38.0x3-	T38.0x4-	T38.0x5-	T38.0x6-
Cloral betaine	T42.6x1-	T42.6x2-	T42.6x3-	T42.6x4-	T42.6x5-	T42.6x6-

DRUGS & CHEMICALS

Table of Drugs & Chemicals	POISONING				Adverse Effect	Underdosing
	Accidental (Unintentional)	Self-Harm (Intentional)	Assault	Undetermined		
Cloramfenicol	T36.2x1-	T36.2x2-	T36.2x3-	T36.2x4-	T36.2x5-	T36.2x6-
Clorazepate (dipotassium)	T42.4x1-	T42.4x2-	T42.4x3-	T42.4x4-	T42.4x5-	T42.4x6-
Clorexolone	T50.2x1-	T50.2x2-	T50.2x3-	T50.2x4-	T50.2x5-	T50.2x6-
Clorfenamine	T45.0x1-	T45.0x2-	T45.0x3-	T45.0x4-	T45.0x5-	T45.0x6-
Clorgiline	T43.1x1-	T43.1x2-	T43.1x3-	T43.1x4-	T43.1x5-	T43.1x6-
Clorotepine	T44.3x1-	T44.3x2-	T44.3x3-	T44.3x4-	T44.3x5-	T44.3x6-
Clorox (bleach)	T54.91x-	T54.92x-	T54.93x-	T54.94x-	—	—
Clorprenaline	T48.6x1-	T48.6x2-	T48.6x3-	T48.6x4-	T48.6x5-	T48.6x6-
Clortermine	T50.5x1-	T50.5x2-	T50.5x3-	T50.5x4-	T50.5x5-	T50.5x6-
Clotiapine	T43.591-	T43.592-	T43.593-	T43.594-	T43.595-	T43.596-
Clotiazepam	T42.4x1-	T42.4x2-	T42.4x3-	T42.4x4-	T42.4x5-	T42.4x6-
Clotibric acid	T46.6x1-	T46.6x2-	T46.6x3-	T46.6x4-	T46.6x5-	T46.6x6-
Clotrimazole	T49.0x1-	T49.0x2-	T49.0x3-	T49.0x4-	T49.0x5-	T49.0x6-
Cloxacillin	T36.0x1-	T36.0x2-	T36.0x3-	T36.0x4-	T36.0x5-	T36.0x6-
Cloxazolam	T42.4x1-	T42.4x2-	T42.4x3-	T42.4x4-	T42.4x5-	T42.4x6-
Cloxiquine	T49.0x1-	T49.0x2-	T49.0x3-	T49.0x4-	T49.0x5-	T49.0x6-
Clozapine	T42.4x1-	T42.4x2-	T42.4x3-	T42.4x4-	T42.4x5-	T42.4x6-
Coagulant NEC	T45.7x1-	T45.7x2-	T45.7x3-	T45.7x4-	T45.7x5-	T45.7x6-
Coal (carbon monoxide from) — see also Carbon, monoxide, coal	T58.2x1-	T58.2x2-	T58.2x3-	T58.2x4-	—	—
oil — see Kerosene						
tar	T49.1x1-	T49.1x2-	T49.1x3-	T49.1x4-	T49.1x5-	T49.1x6-
fumes	T59.891-	T59.892-	T59.893-	T59.894-	—	—
medicinal (ointment)	T49.4x1-	T49.4x2-	T49.4x3-	T49.4x4-	T49.4x5-	T49.4x6-
analgesics NEC	T39.2x1-	T39.2x2-	T39.2x3-	T39.2x4-	T39.2x5-	T39.2x6-
naphtha (solvent)	T52.0x1-	T52.0x2-	T52.0x3-	T52.0x4-	—	—
Cobalamine	T45.2x1-	T45.2x2-	T45.2x3-	T45.2x4-	T45.2x5-	T45.2x6-
Cobalt (nonmedicinal) (fumes) (industrial)	T56.891-	T56.892-	T56.893-	T56.894-	—	—
medicinal (trace) (chloride)	T45.8x1-	T45.8x2-	T45.8x3-	T45.8x4-	T45.8x5-	T45.8x6-
Cobra (venom)	T63.041-	T63.042-	T63.043-	T63.044-	—	—
Coca (leaf)	T40.5x1-	T40.5x2-	T40.5x3-	T40.5x4-	T40.5x5-	T40.5x6-
Cocaine	T40.5x1-	T40.5x2-	T40.5x3-	T40.5x4-	T40.5x5-	T40.5x6-
topical anesthetic	T41.3x1-	T41.3x2-	T41.3x3-	T41.3x4-	T41.3x5-	T41.3x6-
Cocarboxylase	T45.3x1-	T45.3x2-	T45.3x3-	T45.3x4-	T45.3x5-	T45.3x6-
Coccidioidin	T50.8x1-	T50.8x2-	T50.8x3-	T50.8x4-	T50.8x5-	T50.8x6-
Cocculus indicus	T62.1x1-	T62.1x2-	T62.1x3-	T62.1x4-	—	—
Cochineal	T65.6x1-	T65.6x2-	T65.6x3-	T65.6x4-	—	—
medicinal products	T50.991-	T50.992-	T50.993-	T50.994-	T50.995-	T50.996-
Codeine	T40.2x1-	T40.2x2-	T40.2x3-	T40.2x4-	T40.2x5-	T40.2x6-
Cod-liver oil	T45.2x1-	T45.2x2-	T45.2x3-	T45.2x4-	T45.2x5-	T45.2x6-
Coenzyme A	T50.991-	T50.992-	T50.993-	T50.994-	T50.995-	T50.996-
Coffee	T62.8x1-	T62.8x2-	T62.8x3-	T62.8x4-	—	—
Cogalactoiso-merase	T50.991-	T50.992-	T50.993-	T50.994-	T50.995-	T50.996-
Cogentin	T44.3x1-	T44.3x2-	T44.3x3-	T44.3x4-	T44.3x5-	T44.3x6-
Coke fumes or gas (carbon monoxide)	T58.2x1-	T58.2x2-	T58.2x3-	T58.2x4-	—	—
industrial use	T58.8x1-	T58.8x2-	T58.8x3-	T58.8x4-	—	—
Colace	T47.4x1-	T47.4x2-	T47.4x3-	T47.4x4-	T47.4x5-	T47.4x6-
Colaspase	T45.1x1-	T45.1x2-	T45.1x3-	T45.1x4-	T45.1x5-	T45.1x6-
Colchicine	T50.4x1-	T50.4x2-	T50.4x3-	T50.4x4-	T50.4x5-	T50.4x6-
Colchicum	T62.2x1-	T62.2x2-	T62.2x3-	T62.2x4-	—	—
Cold cream	T49.3x1-	T49.3x2-	T49.3x3-	T49.3x4-	T49.3x5-	T49.3x6-
Colecalciferol	T45.2x1-	T45.2x2-	T45.2x3-	T45.2x4-	T45.2x5-	T45.2x6-
Colestipol	T46.6x1-	T46.6x2-	T46.6x3-	T46.6x4-	T46.6x5-	T46.6x6-
Colestyramine	T46.6x1-	T46.6x2-	T46.6x3-	T46.6x4-	T46.6x5-	T46.6x6-
Colimycin	T36.8x1-	T36.8x2-	T36.8x3-	T36.8x4-	T36.8x5-	T36.8x6-
Colistimethate	T36.8x1-	T36.8x2-	T36.8x3-	T36.8x4-	T36.8x5-	T36.8x6-
Colistin	T36.8x1-	T36.8x2-	T36.8x3-	T36.8x4-	T36.8x5-	T36.8x6-
sulfate (eye preparation)	T49.5x1-	T49.5x2-	T49.5x3-	T49.5x4-	T49.5x5-	T49.5x6-
Collagen	T50.991-	T50.992-	T50.993-	T50.994-	T50.995-	T50.996-
Collagenase	T49.4x1-	T49.4x2-	T49.4x3-	T49.4x4-	T49.4x5-	T49.4x6-
Collodion	T49.3x1-	T49.3x2-	T49.3x3-	T49.3x4-	T49.3x5-	T49.3x6-
Colocynth	T47.2x1-	T47.2x2-	T47.2x3-	T47.2x4-	T47.2x5-	T47.2x6-
Colophony adhesive	T49.3x1-	T49.3x2-	T49.3x3-	T49.3x4-	T49.3x5-	T49.3x6-
Colorant — see also Dye	T50.991-	T50.992-	T50.993-	T50.994-	T50.995-	T50.996-
Coloring matter — see Dye(s)						
Combustion gas (after combustion) — see Carbon, monoxide						
prior to combustion	T59.891-	T59.892-	T59.893-	T59.894-	—	—
Compazine	T43.3x1-	T43.3x2-	T43.3x3-	T43.3x4-	T43.3x5-	T43.3x6-
Compound						
1080 (sodium fluoroacetate)	T60.4x1-	T60.4x2-	T60.4x3-	T60.4x4-	—	—
269 (endrin)	T60.1x1-	T60.1x2-	T60.1x3-	T60.1x4-	—	—
497 (dieldrin)	T60.1x1-	T60.1x2-	T60.1x3-	T60.1x4-	—	—
3422 (parathion)	T60.0x1-	T60.0x2-	T60.0x3-	T60.0x4-	—	—
3911 (phorate)	T60.0x1-	T60.0x2-	T60.0x3-	T60.0x4-	—	—
3956 (toxaphene)	T60.1x1-	T60.1x2-	T60.1x3-	T60.1x4-	—	—
4049 (malathion)	T60.0x1-	T60.0x2-	T60.0x3-	T60.0x4-	—	—
4069 (malathion)	T60.0x1-	T60.0x2-	T60.0x3-	T60.0x4-	—	—
4124 (dicapthon)	T60.0x1-	T60.0x2-	T60.0x3-	T60.0x4-	—	—
E (cortisone)	T38.0x1-	T38.0x2-	T38.0x3-	T38.0x4-	T38.0x5-	T38.0x6-
F (hydrocortisone)	T38.0x1-	T38.0x2-	T38.0x3-	T38.0x4-	T38.0x5-	T38.0x6-
Congener, anabolic	T38.7x1-	T38.7x2-	T38.7x3-	T38.7x4-	T38.7x5-	T38.7x6-
Congo red	T50.8x1-	T50.8x2-	T50.8x3-	T50.8x4-	T50.8x5-	T50.8x6-
Coniine, conine	T62.2x1-	T62.2x2-	T62.2x3-	T62.2x4-	—	—
Conium (maculatum)	T62.2x1-	T62.2x2-	T62.2x3-	T62.2x4-	—	—
Conjugated estrogenic substances	T38.5x1-	T38.5x2-	T38.5x3-	T38.5x4-	T38.5x5-	T38.5x6-
Contac	T48.5x1-	T48.5x2-	T48.5x3-	T48.5x4-	T48.5x5-	T48.5x6-
Contact lens solution	T49.5x1-	T49.5x2-	T49.5x3-	T49.5x4-	T49.5x5-	T49.5x6-
Contraceptive (oral)	T38.4x1-	T38.4x2-	T38.4x3-	T38.4x4-	T38.4x5-	T38.4x6-
vaginal	T49.8x1-	T49.8x2-	T49.8x3-	T49.8x4-	T49.8x5-	T49.8x6-
Contrast medium, radiography	T50.8x1-	T50.8x2-	T50.8x3-	T50.8x4-	T50.8x5-	T50.8x6-
Convallaria glycosides	T46.0x1-	T46.0x2-	T46.0x3-	T46.0x4-	T46.0x5-	T46.0x6-
Convallaria majalis	T62.2x1-	T62.2x2-	T62.2x3-	T62.2x4-	—	—
berry	T62.1x1-	T62.1x2-	T62.1x3-	T62.1x4-	—	—
Copper (dust) (fumes) (nonmedicinal) NEC	T56.4x1-	T56.4x2-	T56.4x3-	T56.4x4-	—	—
arsenate, arsenite	T57.0x1-	T57.0x2-	T57.0x3-	T57.0x4-	—	—
insecticide	T60.2x1-	T60.2x2-	T60.2x3-	T60.2x4-	—	—
emetic	T47.7x1-	T47.7x2-	T47.7x3-	T47.7x4-	T47.7x5-	T47.7x6-
fungicide	T60.3x1-	T60.3x2-	T60.3x3-	T60.3x4-	—	—
gluconate	T49.0x1-	T49.0x2-	T49.0x3-	T49.0x4-	T49.0x5-	T49.0x6-
insecticide	T60.2x1-	T60.2x2-	T60.2x3-	T60.2x4-	—	—
medicinal (trace)	T45.8x1-	T45.8x2-	T45.8x3-	T45.8x4-	T45.8x5-	T45.8x6-
oleate	T49.0x1-	T49.0x2-	T49.0x3-	T49.0x4-	T49.0x5-	T49.0x6-
sulfate	T56.4x1-	T56.4x2-	T56.4x3-	T56.4x4-	—	—
cupric	T56.4x1-	T56.4x2-	T56.4x3-	T56.4x4-	—	—
fungicide	T60.3x1-	T60.3x2-	T60.3x3-	T60.3x4-	—	—
medicinal						
ear	T49.6x1-	T49.6x2-	T49.6x3-	T49.6x4-	T49.6x5-	T49.6x6-
emetic	T47.7x1-	T47.7x2-	T47.7x3-	T47.7x4-	T47.7x5-	T47.7x6-
eye	T49.5x1-	T49.5x2-	T49.5x3-	T49.5x4-	T49.5x5-	T49.5x6-
cuprous	T56.4x1-	T56.4x2-	T56.4x3-	T56.4x4-	—	—
fungicide	T60.3x1-	T60.3x2-	T60.3x3-	T60.3x4-	—	—
medicinal						
ear	T49.6x1-	T49.6x2-	T49.6x3-	T49.6x4-	T49.6x5-	T49.6x6-
emetic	T47.7x1-	T47.7x2-	T47.7x3-	T47.7x4-	T47.7x5-	T47.7x6-
eye	T49.5x1-	T49.5x2-	T49.5x3-	T49.5x4-	T49.5x5-	T49.5x6-

DRUGS & CHEMICALS

Table of Drugs & Chemicals	POISONING Accidental (Unintentional)	Self-Harm (Intentional)	Assault	Undetermined	Adverse Effect	Underdosing
Copperhead snake (bite) (venom)	T63.061-	T63.062-	T63.063-	T63.064-	—	—
Coral (sting)	T63.691-	T63.692-	T63.693-	T63.694-	—	—
snake (bite) (venom)	T63.021-	T63.022-	T63.023-	T63.024-	—	—
Corbadrine	T49.6x1-	T49.6x2-	T49.6x3-	T49.6x4-	T49.6x5-	T49.6x6-
Cordite	T65.891-	T65.892-	T65.893-	T65.894-	—	—
vapor	T59.891-	T59.892-	T59.893-	T59.894-	—	—
Cordran	T49.0x1-	T49.0x2-	T49.0x3-	T49.0x4-	T49.0x5-	T49.0x6-
Corn cures	T49.4x1-	T49.4x2-	T49.4x3-	T49.4x4-	T49.4x5-	T49.4x6-
Corn starch	T49.3x1-	T49.3x2-	T49.3x3-	T49.3x4-	T49.3x5-	T49.3x6-
Cornhusker's lotion	T49.3x1-	T49.3x2-	T49.3x3-	T49.3x4-	T49.3x5-	T49.3x6-
Coronary vasodilator NEC	T46.3x1-	T46.3x2-	T46.3x3-	T46.3x4-	T46.3x5-	T46.3x6-
Corrosive NEC	T54.91x-	T54.92x-	T54.93x-	T54.94x-	—	—
acid NEC	T54.2x1-	T54.2x2-	T54.2x2-	T54.2x4-	—	—
aromatics	T54.1x1-	T54.1x2-	T54.1x3-	T54.1x4-	—	—
disinfectant	T54.1x1-	T54.1x2-	T54.1x3-	T54.1x4-	—	—
fumes NEC	T54.91x-	T54.92x-	T54.93x-	T54.94x-	—	—
specified NEC	T54.91x-	T54.92x-	T54.93x-	T54.94x-	—	—
sublimate	T56.1x1-	T56.1x2-	T56.1x3-	T56.1x4-	—	—
Cortate	T38.0x1-	T38.0x2-	T38.0x3-	T38.0x4-	T38.0x5-	T38.0x6-
Cort-Dome	T38.0x1-	T38.0x2-	T38.0x3-	T38.0x4-	T38.0x5-	T38.0x6-
ENT agent	T49.6x1-	T49.6x2-	T49.6x3-	T49.6x4-	T49.6x5-	T49.6x6-
ophthalmic preparation	T49.5x1-	T49.5x2-	T49.5x3-	T49.5x4-	T49.5x5-	T49.5x6-
topical NEC	T49.0x1-	T49.0x2-	T49.0x3-	T49.0x4-	T49.0x5-	T49.0x6-
Cortef	T38.0x1-	T38.0x2-	T38.0x3-	T38.0x4-	T38.0x5-	T38.0x6-
ENT agent	T49.6x1-	T49.6x2-	T49.6x3-	T49.6x4-	T49.6x5-	T49.6x6-
ophthalmic preparation	T49.5x1-	T49.5x2-	T49.5x3-	T49.5x4-	T49.5x5-	T49.5x6-
topical NEC	T49.0x1-	T49.0x2-	T49.0x3-	T49.0x4-	T49.0x5-	T49.0x6-
Corticosteroid	T38.0x1-	T38.0x2-	T38.0x3-	T38.0x4-	T38.0x5-	T38.0x6-
ENT agent	T49.6x1-	T49.6x2-	T49.6x3-	T49.6x4-	T49.6x5-	T49.6x6-
mineral	T50.0x1-	T50.0x2-	T50.0x3-	T50.0x4-	T50.0x5-	T50.0x6-
ophthalmic	T49.5x1-	T49.5x2-	T49.5x3-	T49.5x4-	T49.5x5-	T49.5x6-
topical NEC	T49.0x1-	T49.0x2-	T49.0x3-	T49.0x4-	T49.0x5-	T49.0x6-
Corticotropin	T38.811-	T38.812-	T38.813-	T38.814-	T38.815-	T38.816-
Cortisol	T49.0x1-	T49.0x2-	T49.0x3-	T49.0x4-	T49.0x5-	T49.0x6-
ENT agent	T49.6x1-	T49.6x2-	T49.6x3-	T49.6x4-	T49.6x5-	T49.6x6-
ophthalmic preparation	T49.5x1-	T49.5x2-	T49.5x3-	T49.5x4-	T49.5x5-	T49.5x6-
topical NEC	T49.0x1-	T49.0x2-	T49.0x3-	T49.0x4-	T49.0x5-	T49.0x6-
Cortisone (acetate)	T38.0x1-	T38.0x2-	T38.0x3-	T38.0x4-	T38.0x5-	T38.0x6-
ENT agent	T49.6x1-	T49.6x2-	T49.6x3-	T49.6x4-	T49.6x5-	T49.6x6-
ophthalmic preparation	T49.5x1-	T49.5x2-	T49.5x3-	T49.5x4-	T49.5x5-	T49.5x6-
topical NEC	T49.0x1-	T49.0x2-	T49.0x3-	T49.0x4-	T49.0x5-	T49.0x6-
Cortivazol	T38.0x1-	T38.0x2-	T38.0x3-	T38.0x4-	T38.0x5-	T38.0x6-
Cortogen	T38.0x1-	T38.0x2-	T38.0x3-	T38.0x4-	T38.0x5-	T38.0x6-
ENT agent	T49.6x1-	T49.6x2-	T49.6x3-	T49.6x4-	T49.6x5-	T49.6x6-
ophthalmic preparation	T49.5x1-	T49.5x2-	T49.5x3-	T49.5x4-	T49.5x5-	T49.5x6-
Cortone	T38.0x1-	T38.0x2-	T38.0x3-	T38.0x4-	T38.0x5-	T38.0x6-
ENT agent	T49.6x1-	T49.6x2-	T49.6x3-	T49.6x4-	T49.6x5-	T49.6x6-
ophthalmic preparation	T49.5x1-	T49.5x2-	T49.5x3-	T49.5x4-	T49.5x5-	T49.5x6-
Cortril	T38.0x1-	T38.0x2-	T38.0x3-	T38.0x4-	T38.0x5-	T38.0x6-
ENT agent	T49.6x1-	T49.6x2-	T49.6x3-	T49.6x4-	T49.6x5-	T49.6x6-
ophthalmic preparation	T49.5x1-	T49.5x2-	T49.5x3-	T49.5x4-	T49.5x5-	T49.5x6-
topical NEC	T49.0x1-	T49.0x2-	T49.0x3-	T49.0x4-	T49.0x5-	T49.0x6-
Corynebacterium parvum	T45.1x1-	T45.1x2-	T45.1x3-	T45.1x4-	T45.1x5-	T45.1x6-
Cosmetic preparation	T49.8x1-	T49.8x2-	T49.8x3-	T49.8x4-	T49.8x5-	T49.8x6-
Cosmetics	T49.8x1-	T49.8x2-	T49.8x3-	T49.8x4-	T49.8x5-	T49.8x6-
Cosyntropin	T38.811-	T38.812-	T38.813-	T38.814-	T38.815-	T38.816-
Cotarnine	T45.7x1-	T45.7x2-	T45.7x3-	T45.7x4-	T45.7x5-	T45.7x6-
Co-trimoxazole	T36.8x1-	T36.8x2-	T36.8x3-	T36.8x4-	T36.8x5-	T36.8x6-
Cottonseed oil	T49.3x1-	T49.3x2-	T49.3x3-	T49.3x4-	T49.3x5-	T49.3x6-
Cough mixture (syrup)	T48.4x1-	T48.4x2-	T48.4x3-	T48.4x4-	T48.4x5-	T48.4x6-
containing opiates	T40.2x1-	T40.2x2-	T40.2x3-	T40.2x4-	T40.2x5-	T40.2x6-
expectorants	T48.4x1-	T48.4x2-	T48.4x3-	T48.4x4-	T48.4x5-	T48.4x6-
Coumadin	T45.511-	T45.512-	T45.513-	T45.514-	T45.515-	T45.516-
rodenticide	T60.4x1-	T60.4x2-	T60.4x3-	T60.4x4-	—	—
Coumaphos	T60.0x1-	T60.0x2-	T60.0x3-	T60.0x4-	—	—
Coumarin	T45.511-	T45.512-	T45.513-	T45.514-	T45.515-	T45.516-
Coumetarol	T45.511-	T45.512-	T45.513-	T45.514-	T45.515-	T45.516-
Cowbane	T62.2x1-	T62.2x2-	T62.2x3-	T62.2x4-	—	—
Cozyme	T45.2x1-	T45.2x2-	T45.2x3-	T45.2x4-	T45.2x5-	T45.2x6-
Crack	T40.5x1-	T40.5x2-	T40.5x3-	T40.5x4-	—	—
Crataegus extract	T46.0x1-	T46.0x2-	T46.0x3-	T46.0x4-	T46.0x5-	T46.0x6-
Creolin	T54.1x1-	T54.1x2-	T54.1x3-	T54.1x4-	—	—
disinfectant	T54.1x1-	T54.1x2-	T54.1x3-	T54.1x4-	—	—
Creosol (compound)	T49.0x1-	T49.0x2-	T49.0x3-	T49.0x4-	T49.0x5-	T49.0x6-
Creosote (coal tar) (beechwood)	T49.0x1-	T49.0x2-	T49.0x3-	T49.0x4-	T49.0x5-	T49.0x6-
medicinal (expectorant)	T48.4x1-	T48.4x2-	T48.4x3-	T48.4x4-	T48.4x5-	T48.4x6-
syrup	T48.4x1-	T48.4x2-	T48.4x3-	T48.4x4-	T48.4x5-	T48.4x6-
Cresol(s)	T49.0x1-	T49.0x2-	T49.0x3-	T49.0x4-	T49.0x5-	T49.0x6-
and soap solution	T49.0x1-	T49.0x2-	T49.0x3-	T49.0x4-	T49.0x5-	T49.0x6-
Cresyl acetate	T49.0x1-	T49.0x2-	T49.0x3-	T49.0x4-	T49.0x5-	T49.0x6-
Cresylic acid	T49.0x1-	T49.0x2-	T49.0x3-	T49.0x4-	T49.0x5-	T49.0x6-
Crimidine	T60.4x1-	T60.4x2-	T60.4x3-	T60.4x4-	—	—
Croconazole	T37.8x1-	T37.8x2-	T37.8x3-	T37.8x4-	T37.8x5-	T37.8x6-
Cromoglicic acid	T48.6x1-	T48.6x2-	T48.6x3-	T48.6x4-	T48.6x5-	T48.6x6-
Cromolyn	T48.6x1-	T48.6x2-	T48.6x3-	T48.6x4-	T48.6x5-	T48.6x6-
Cromonar	T46.3x1-	T46.3x2-	T46.3x3-	T46.3x4-	T46.3x5-	T46.3x6-
Cropropamide	T39.8x1-	T39.8x2-	T39.8x3-	T39.8x4-	T39.8x5-	T39.8x6-
with crotethamide	T50.7x1-	T50.7x2-	T50.7x3-	T50.7x4-	T50.7x5-	T50.7x6-
Crotamiton	T49.0x1-	T49.0x2-	T49.0x3-	T49.0x4-	T49.0x5-	T49.0x6-
Crotethamide	T39.8x1-	T39.8x2-	T39.8x3-	T39.8x4-	T39.8x5-	T39.8x6-
with cropropamide	T50.7x1-	T50.7x2-	T50.7x3-	T50.7x4-	T50.7x5-	T50.7x6-
Croton (oil)	T47.2x1-	T47.2x2-	T47.2x3-	T47.2x4-	T47.2x5-	T47.2x6-
chloral	T42.6x1-	T42.6x2-	T42.6x3-	T42.6x4-	T42.6x5-	T42.6x6-
Crude oil	T52.0x1-	T52.0x2-	T52.0x3-	T52.0x4-	—	—
Cryogenine	T39.8x1-	T39.8x2-	T39.8x3-	T39.8x4-	T39.8x5-	T39.8x6-
Cryolite (vapor)	T60.1x1-	T60.1x2-	T60.1x3-	T60.1x4-	—	—
insecticide	T60.1x1-	T60.1x2-	T60.1x3-	T60.1x4-	—	—
Cryptenamine (tannates)	T46.5x1-	T46.5x2-	T46.5x3-	T46.5x4-	T46.5x5-	T46.5x6-
Crystal violet	T49.0x1-	T49.0x2-	T49.0x3-	T49.0x4-	T49.0x5-	T49.0x6-
Cuckoopint	T62.2x1-	T62.2x2-	T62.2x3-	T62.2x4-	—	—
Cumetharol	T45.511-	T45.512-	T45.513-	T45.514-	T45.515-	T45.516-
Cupric						
acetate	T60.3x1-	T60.3x2-	T60.3x3-	T60.3x4-	—	—
acetoarsenite	T57.0x1-	T57.0x2-	T57.0x3-	T57.0x4-	—	—
arsenate	T57.0x1-	T57.0x2-	T57.0x3-	T57.0x4-	—	—
gluconate	T49.0x1-	T49.0x2-	T49.0x3-	T49.0x4-	T49.0x5-	T49.0x6-
oleate	T49.0x1-	T49.0x2-	T49.0x3-	T49.0x4-	T49.0x5-	T49.0x6-
sulfate	T56.4x1-	T56.4x2-	T56.4x3-	T56.4x4-	—	—
Cuprous sulfate — see also Copper sulfate	T56.4x1-	T56.4x2-	T56.4x3-	T56.4x4-	—	—
Curare, curarine	T48.1x1-	T48.1x2-	T48.1x3-	T48.1x4-	T48.1x5-	T48.1x6-
Cyamemazine	T43.3x1-	T43.3x2-	T43.3x3-	T43.3x4-	T43.3x5-	T43.3x6-
Cyamopsis tetragono-loba	T46.6x1-	T46.6x2-	T46.6x3-	T46.6x4-	T46.6x5-	T46.6x6-
Cyanacetyl hydrazide	T37.1x1-	T37.1x2-	T37.1x3-	T37.1x4-	T37.1x5-	T37.1x6-
Cyanic acid (gas)	T59.891-	T59.892-	T59.893-	T59.894-	—	—
Cyanide (s) (compounds) (potassium) (sodium) NEC	T65.0x1-	T65.0x2-	T65.0x3-	T65.0x4-	—	—
dust or gas (inhalation) NEC	T57.3x1-	T57.3x2-	T57.3x3-	T57.3x4-	—	—
fumigant	T65.0x1-	T65.0x2-	T65.0x3-	T65.0x4-	—	—
hydrogen	T57.3x1-	T57.3x2-	T57.3x3-	T57.3x4-	—	—
mercuric — see Mercury						
pesticide (dust) (fumes)	T65.0x1-	T65.0x2-	T65.0x3-	T65.0x4-	—	—

Table of Drugs & Chemicals	Poisoning				Adverse Effect	Underdosing
	Accidental (Unintentional)	Self-Harm (Intentional)	Assault	Undetermined		
Cyanoacrylate adhesive	T49.3x1-	T49.3x2-	T49.3x3-	T49.3x4-	T49.3x5-	T49.3x6-
Cyanocobalamin	T45.8x1-	T45.8x2-	T45.8x3-	T45.8x4-	T45.8x5-	T45.8x6-
Cyanogen (chloride) (gas) NEC	T59.891-	T59.892-	T59.893-	T59.894-	—	—
Cyclacillin	T36.0x1-	T36.0x2-	T36.0x3-	T36.0x4-	T36.0x5-	T36.0x6-
Cyclaine	T41.3x1-	T41.3x2-	T41.3x3-	T41.3x4-	T41.3x5-	T41.3x6-
Cyclamate	T50.991-	T50.992-	T50.993-	T50.994-	T50.995-	T50.996-
Cyclamen europaeum	T62.2x1-	T62.2x2-	T62.2x3-	T62.2x4-	—	—
Cyclandelate	T46.7x1-	T46.7x2-	T46.7x3-	T46.7x4-	T46.7x5-	T46.7x6-
Cyclazocine	T50.7x1-	T50.7x2-	T50.7x3-	T50.7x4-	T50.7x5-	T50.7x6-
Cyclizine	T45.0x1-	T45.0x2-	T45.0x3-	T45.0x4-	T45.0x5-	T45.0x6-
Cyclobarbital	T42.3x1-	T42.3x2-	T42.3x3-	T42.3x4-	T42.3x5-	T42.3x6-
Cyclobarbitone	T42.3x1-	T42.3x2-	T42.3x3-	T42.3x4-	T42.3x5-	T42.3x6-
Cyclobenzaprine	T48.1x1-	T48.1x2-	T48.1x3-	T48.1x4-	T48.1x5-	T48.1x6-
Cyclodrine	T44.3x1-	T44.3x2-	T44.3x3-	T44.3x4-	T44.3x5-	T44.3x6-
Cycloguanil embonate	T37.2x1-	T37.2x2-	T37.2x3-	T37.2x4-	T37.2x5-	T37.2x6-
Cyclohexane	T52.8x1-	T52.8x2-	T52.8x3-	T52.8x4-	—	—
Cyclohexanol	T51.8x1-	T51.8x2-	T51.8x3-	T51.8x4-	—	—
Cyclohexanone	T52.4x1-	T52.4x2-	T52.4x3-	T52.4x4-	—	—
Cycloheximide	T60.3x1-	T60.3x2-	T60.3x3-	T60.3x4-	—	—
Cyclohexyl acetate	T52.8x1-	T52.8x2-	T52.8x3-	T52.8x4-	—	—
Cycloleucin	T45.1x1-	T45.1x2-	T45.1x3-	T45.1x4-	T45.1x5-	T45.1x6-
Cyclomethycaine	T41.3x1-	T41.3x2-	T41.3x3-	T41.3x4-	T41.3x5-	T41.3x6-
Cyclopentamine	T44.4x1-	T44.4x2-	T44.4x3-	T44.4x4-	T44.4x5-	T44.4x6-
Cyclopenthiazide	T50.2x1-	T50.2x2-	T50.2x3-	T50.2x4-	T50.2x5-	T50.2x6-
Cyclopentolate	T44.3x1-	T44.3x2-	T44.3x3-	T44.3x4-	T44.3x5-	T44.3x6-
Cyclophosphamide	T45.1x1-	T45.1x2-	T45.1x3-	T45.1x4-	T45.1x5-	T45.1x6-
Cycloplegic drug	T49.5x1-	T49.5x2-	T49.5x3-	T49.5x4-	T49.5x5-	T49.5x6-
Cyclopropane	T41.291-	T41.292-	T41.293-	T41.294-	T41.295-	T41.296-
Cyclopyrabital	T39.8x1-	T39.8x2-	T39.8x3-	T39.8x4-	T39.8x5-	T39.8x6-
Cycloserine	T37.1x1-	T37.1x2-	T37.1x3-	T37.1x4-	T37.1x5-	T37.1x6-
Cyclosporin	T45.1x1-	T45.1x2-	T45.1x3-	T45.1x4-	T45.1x5-	T45.1x6-
Cyclothiazide	T50.2x1-	T50.2x2-	T50.2x3-	T50.2x4-	T50.2x5-	T50.2x6-
Cycrimine	T44.3x1-	T44.3x2-	T44.3x3-	T44.3x4-	T44.3x5-	T44.3x6-
Cyhalothrin	T60.1x1-	T60.1x2-	T60.1x3-	T60.1x4-	—	—
Cymarin	T46.0x1-	T46.0x2-	T46.0x3-	T46.0x4-	T46.0x5-	T46.0x6-
Cypermethrin	T60.1x1-	T60.1x2-	T60.1x3-	T60.1x4-	—	—
Cyphenothrin	T60.2x1-	T60.2x2-	T60.2x3-	T60.2x4-	—	—
Cyproheptadine	T45.0x1-	T45.0x2-	T45.0x3-	T45.0x4-	T45.0x5-	T45.0x6-
Cyproterone	T38.6x1-	T38.6x2-	T38.6x3-	T38.6x4-	T38.6x5-	T38.6x6-
Cysteamine	T50.6x1-	T50.6x2-	T50.6x3-	T50.6x4-	T50.6x5-	T50.6x6-
Cytarabine	T45.1x1-	T45.1x2-	T45.1x3-	T45.1x4-	T45.1x5-	T45.1x6-
Cytisus laburnum	T62.2x1-	T62.2x2-	T62.2x3-	T62.2x4-	—	—
scoparius	T62.2x1-	T62.2x2-	T62.2x3-	T62.2x4-	—	—
Cytochrome C	T47.5x1-	T47.5x2-	T47.5x3-	T47.5x4-	T47.5x5-	T47.5x6-
Cytomel	T38.1x1-	T38.1x2-	T38.1x3-	T38.1x4-	T38.1x5-	T38.1x6-
Cytosine arabinoside	T45.1x1-	T45.1x2-	T45.1x3-	T45.1x4-	T45.1x5-	T45.1x6-
Cytoxan	T45.1x1-	T45.1x2-	T45.1x3-	T45.1x4-	T45.1x5-	T45.1x6-
Cytozyme	T45.7x1-	T45.7x2-	T45.7x3-	T45.7x4-	T45.7x5-	T45.7x6-
2,4-D	T60.3x1-	T60.3x2-	T60.3x3-	T60.3x4-	—	—
Dacarbazine	T45.1x1-	T45.1x2-	T45.1x3-	T45.1x4-	T45.1x5-	T45.1x6-
Dactinomycin	T45.1x1-	T45.1x2-	T45.1x3-	T45.1x4-	T45.1x5-	T45.1x6-
DADPS	T37.1x1-	T37.1x2-	T37.1x3-	T37.1x4-	T37.1x5-	T37.1x6-
Dakin's solution	T49.0x1-	T49.0x2-	T49.0x3-	T49.0x4-	T49.0x5-	T49.0x6-
Dalapon (sodium)	T60.3x1-	T60.3x2-	T60.3x3-	T60.3x4-	—	—
Dalmane	T42.4x1-	T42.4x2-	T42.4x3-	T42.4x4-	T42.4x5-	T42.4x6-
Danazol	T38.6x1-	T38.6x2-	T38.6x3-	T38.6x4-	T38.6x5-	T38.6x6-
Danilone	T45.511-	T45.512-	T45.513-	T45.514-	T45.515-	T45.516-
Danthron	T47.2x1-	T47.2x2-	T47.2x3-	T47.2x4-	T47.2x5-	T47.2x6-
Dantrolene	T42.8x1-	T42.8x2-	T42.8x3-	T42.8x4-	T42.8x5-	T42.8x6-
Dantron	T47.2x1-	T47.2x2-	T47.2x3-	T47.2x4-	T47.2x5-	T47.2x6-

Table of Drugs & Chemicals	Poisoning				Adverse Effect	Underdosing
	Accidental (Unintentional)	Self-Harm (Intentional)	Assault	Undetermined		
Daphne (gnidium) (mezereum)	T62.2x1-	T62.2x2-	T62.2x3-	T62.2x4-	—	—
berry	T62.1x1-	T62.1x2-	T62.1x3-	T62.1x4-	—	—
Dapsone	T37.1x1-	T37.1x2-	T37.1x3-	T37.1x4-	T37.1x5-	T37.1x6-
Daraprim	T37.2x1-	T37.2x2-	T37.2x3-	T37.2x4-	T37.2x5-	T37.2x6-
Darnel	T62.2x1-	T62.2x2-	T62.2x3-	T62.2x4-	—	—
Darvon	T39.8x1-	T39.8x2-	T39.8x3-	T39.8x4-	T39.8x5-	T39.8x6-
Daunomycin	T45.1x1-	T45.1x2-	T45.1x3-	T45.1x4-	T45.1x5-	T45.1x6-
Daunorubicin	T45.1x1-	T45.1x2-	T45.1x3-	T45.1x4-	T45.1x5-	T45.1x6-
DBI	T38.3x1-	T38.3x2-	T38.3x3-	T38.3x4-	T38.3x5-	T38.3x6-
D-Con	T60.91x-	T60.92x-	T60.93x-	T60.94x-	—	—
insecticide	T60.2x1-	T60.2x2-	T60.2x3-	T60.2x4-	—	—
rodenticide	T60.4x1-	T60.4x2-	T60.4x3-	T60.4x4-	—	—
DDAVP	T38.891-	T38.892-	T38.893-	T38.894-	T38.895-	T38.896-
DDE (bis(chlorophenyl)-dichloroethylene)	T60.2x1-	T60.2x2-	T60.2x3-	T60.2x4-	—	—
DDS	T37.1x1-	T37.1x2-	T37.1x3-	T37.1x4-	T37.1x5-	T37.1x6-
DDT (dust)	T60.1x1-	T60.1x2-	T60.1x3-	T60.1x4-	—	—
Deadly nightshade — see also Belladonna	T62.2x1-	T62.2x2-	T62.2x3-	T62.2x4-	—	—
berry	T62.1x1-	T62.1x2-	T62.1x3-	T62.1x4-	—	—
Deamino-D-arginine vasopressin	T38.891-	T38.892-	T38.893-	T38.894-	T38.895-	T38.896-
Deanol (aceglumate)	T50.991-	T50.992-	T50.993-	T50.994-	T50.995-	T50.996-
Debrisoquine	T46.5x1-	T46.5x2-	T46.5x3-	T46.5x4-	T46.5x5-	T46.5x6-
Decaborane	T57.8x1-	T57.8x2-	T57.8x3-	T57.8x4-	—	—
fumes	T59.891-	T59.892-	T59.893-	T59.894-	—	—
Decadron	T38.0x1-	T38.0x2-	T38.0x3-	T38.0x4-	T38.0x5-	T38.0x6-
ENT agent	T49.6x1-	T49.6x2-	T49.6x3-	T49.6x4-	T49.6x5-	T49.6x6-
ophthalmic preparation	T49.5x1-	T49.5x2-	T49.5x3-	T49.5x4-	T49.5x5-	T49.5x6-
topical NEC	T49.0x1-	T49.0x2-	T49.0x3-	T49.0x4-	T49.0x5-	T49.0x6-
Decahydronaphthalene	T52.8x1-	T52.8x2-	T52.8x3-	T52.8x4-	—	—
Decalin	T52.8x1-	T52.8x2-	T52.8x3-	T52.8x4-	—	—
Decamethonium (bromide)	T48.1x1-	T48.1x2-	T48.1x3-	T48.1x4-	T48.1x5-	T48.1x6-
Decholin	T47.5x1-	T47.5x2-	T47.5x3-	T47.5x4-	T47.5x5-	T47.5x6-
Declomycin	T36.4x1-	T36.4x2-	T36.4x3-	T36.4x4-	T36.4x5-	T36.4x6-
Decongestant, nasal (mucosa)	T48.5x1-	T48.5x2-	T48.5x3-	T48.5x4-	T48.5x5-	T48.5x6-
combination	T48.5x1-	T48.5x2-	T48.5x3-	T48.5x4-	T48.5x5-	T48.5x6-
Deet	T60.8x1-	T60.8x2-	T60.8x3-	T60.8x4-	—	—
Deferoxamine	T45.8x1-	T45.8x2-	T45.8x3-	T45.8x4-	T45.8x5-	T45.8x6-
Deflazacort	T38.0x1-	T38.0x2-	T38.0x3-	T38.0x4-	T38.0x5-	T38.0x6-
Deglycyrrhizinized extract of licorice	T48.4x1-	T48.4x2-	T48.4x3-	T48.4x4-	T48.4x5-	T48.4x6-
Dehydrocholic acid	T47.5x1-	T47.5x2-	T47.5x3-	T47.5x4-	T47.5x5-	T47.5x6-
Dehydroemetine	T37.3x1-	T37.3x2-	T37.3x3-	T37.3x4-	T37.3x5-	T37.3x6-
Dekalin	T52.8x1-	T52.8x2-	T52.8x3-	T52.8x4-	—	—
Delalutin	T38.5x1-	T38.5x2-	T38.5x3-	T38.5x4-	T38.5x5-	T38.5x6-
Delorazepam	T42.4x1-	T42.4x2-	T42.4x3-	T42.4x4-	T42.4x5-	T42.4x6-
Delphinium	T62.2x1-	T62.2x2-	T62.2x3-	T62.2x4-	—	—
Deltamethrin	T60.1x1-	T60.1x2-	T60.1x3-	T60.1x4-	—	—
Deltasone	T38.0x1-	T38.0x2-	T38.0x3-	T38.0x4-	T38.0x5-	T38.0x6-
Deltra	T38.0x1-	T38.0x2-	T38.0x3-	T38.0x4-	T38.0x5-	T38.0x6-
Delvinal	T42.3x1-	T42.3x2-	T42.3x3-	T42.3x4-	T42.3x5-	T42.3x6-
Demecarium (bromide)	T49.5x1-	T49.5x2-	T49.5x3-	T49.5x4-	T49.5x5-	T49.5x6-
Demeclocycline	T36.4x1-	T36.4x2-	T36.4x3-	T36.4x4-	T36.4x5-	T36.4x6-
Demecolcine	T45.1x1-	T45.1x2-	T45.1x3-	T45.1x4-	T45.1x5-	T45.1x6-
Demegestone	T38.5x1-	T38.5x2-	T38.5x3-	T38.5x4-	T38.5x5-	T38.5x6-
Demelanizing agents	T49.8x1-	T49.8x2-	T49.8x3-	T49.8x4-	T49.8x5-	T49.8x6-
Demephion -O and -S	T60.0x1-	T60.0x2-	T60.0x3-	T60.0x4-	—	—
Demerol	T40.2x1-	T40.2x2-	T40.2x3-	T40.2x4-	T40.2x5-	T40.2x6-
Demethylchlortetracycline	T36.4x1-	T36.4x2-	T36.4x3-	T36.4x4-	T36.4x5-	T36.4x6-
Demethyltetracycline	T36.4x1-	T36.4x2-	T36.4x3-	T36.4x4-	T36.4x5-	T36.4x6-

DRUGS & CHEMICALS

Table of Drugs & Chemicals	Accidental (Unintentional)	Self-Harm (Intentional)	Assault	Undetermined	Adverse Effect	Underdosing
Demeton -O and -S	T60.0x1-	T60.0x2-	T60.0x3-	T60.0x4-	—	—
Demulcent (external)	T49.3x1-	T49.3x2-	T49.3x3-	T49.3x4-	T49.3x5-	T49.3x6-
specified NEC	T49.3x1-	T49.3x2-	T49.3x3-	T49.3x4-	T49.3x5-	T49.3x6-
Demulen	T38.4x1-	T38.4x2-	T38.4x3-	T38.4x4-	T38.4x5-	T38.4x6-
Denatured alcohol	T51.0x1-	T51.0x2-	T51.0x3-	T51.0x4-	—	—
Dendrid	T49.5x1-	T49.5x2-	T49.5x3-	T49.5x4-	T49.5x5-	T49.5x6-
Dental drug, topical application NEC	T49.7x1-	T49.7x2-	T49.7x3-	T49.7x4-	T49.7x5-	T49.7x6-
Dentifrice	T49.7x1-	T49.7x2-	T49.7x3-	T49.7x4-	T49.7x5-	T49.7x6-
Deodorant spray (feminine hygiene)	T49.8x1-	T49.8x2-	T49.8x3-	T49.8x4-	T49.8x5-	T49.8x6-
Deoxycortone	T50.0x1-	T50.0x2-	T50.0x3-	T50.0x4-	T50.0x5-	T50.0x6-
2-Deoxy-5-fluorouridine	T45.1x1-	T45.1x2-	T45.1x3-	T45.1x4-	T45.1x5-	T45.1x6-
5-Deoxy-5-fluorouridine	T45.1x1-	T45.1x2-	T45.1x3-	T45.1x4-	T45.1x5-	T45.1x6-
Deoxyribonuclease (pancreatic)	T45.3x1-	T45.3x2-	T45.3x3-	T45.3x4-	T45.3x5-	T45.3x6-
Depilatory	T49.4x1-	T49.4x2-	T49.4x3-	T49.4x4-	T49.4x5-	T49.4x6-
Deprenalin	T42.8x1-	T42.8x2-	T42.8x3-	T42.8x4-	T42.8x5-	T42.8x6-
Deprenyl	T42.8x1-	T42.8x2-	T42.8x3-	T42.8x4-	T42.8x5-	T42.8x6-
Depressant, appetite	T50.5x1-	T50.5x2-	T50.5x3-	T50.5x4-	T50.5x5-	T50.5x6-
Depressant appetite, central	T50.5x1-	T50.5x2-	T50.5x3-	T50.5x4-	T50.5x5-	T50.5x6-
cardiac	T46.2x1-	T46.2x2-	T46.2x3-	T46.2x4-	T46.2x5-	T46.2x6-
central nervous system (anesthetic) — see also Central nervous system, depressants	T42.71x-	T42.72x-	T42.73x-	T42.74x-	T42.75x-	T42.76x-
general anesthetic	T41.201-	T41.202-	T41.203-	T41.204-	T41.205-	T41.206-
muscle tone	T42.8x1-	T42.8x2-	T42.8x3-	T42.8x4-	T42.8x5-	T42.8x6-
muscle tone, central	T42.8x1-	T42.8x2-	T42.8x3-	T42.8x4-	T42.8x5-	T42.8x6-
psychotherapeutic	T43.501-	T43.502-	T43.503-	T43.504-	T43.505-	T43.506-
Deptropine	T45.0x1-	T45.0x2-	T45.0x3-	T45.0x4-	T45.0x5-	T45.0x6-
Dequalinium (chloride)	T49.0x1-	T49.0x2-	T49.0x3-	T49.0x4-	T49.0x5-	T49.0x6-
Derris root	T60.2x1-	T60.2x2-	T60.2x3-	T60.2x4-	—	—
Deserpidine	T46.5x1-	T46.5x2-	T46.5x3-	T46.5x4-	T46.5x5-	T46.5x6-
Desferrioxamine	T45.8x1-	T45.8x2-	T45.8x3-	T45.8x4-	T45.8x5-	T45.8x6-
Desipramine	T43.011-	T43.012-	T43.013-	T43.014-	T43.015-	T43.016-
Deslanoside	T46.0x1-	T46.0x2-	T46.0x3-	T46.0x4-	T46.0x5-	T46.0x6-
Desloughing agent	T49.4x1-	T49.4x2-	T49.4x3-	T49.4x4-	T49.4x5-	T49.4x6-
Desmethylimipramine	T43.011-	T43.012-	T43.013-	T43.014-	T43.015-	T43.016-
Desmopressin	T38.891-	T38.892-	T38.893-	T38.894-	T38.895-	T38.896-
Desocodeine	T40.2x1-	T40.2x2-	T40.2x3-	T40.2x4-	T40.2x5-	T40.2x6-
Desogestrel	T38.5x1-	T38.5x2-	T38.5x3-	T38.5x4-	T38.5x5-	T38.5x6-
Desomorphine	T40.2x1-	T40.2x2-	T40.2x3-	T40.2x4-	—	—
Desonide	T49.0x1-	T49.0x2-	T49.0x3-	T49.0x4-	T49.0x5-	T49.0x6-
Desoximetasone	T49.0x1-	T49.0x2-	T49.0x3-	T49.0x4-	T49.0x5-	T49.0x6-
Desoxycorticosteroid	T50.0x1-	T50.0x2-	T50.0x3-	T50.0x4-	T50.0x5-	T50.0x6-
Desoxycortone	T50.0x1-	T50.0x2-	T50.0x3-	T50.0x4-	T50.0x5-	T50.0x6-
Desoxyephedrine	T43.621-	T43.622-	T43.623-	T43.624-	T43.625-	T43.626-
Detaxtran	T46.6x1-	T46.6x2-	T46.6x3-	T46.6x4-	T46.6x5-	T46.6x6-
Detergent	T49.2x1-	T49.2x2-	T49.2x3-	T49.2x4-	T49.2x5-	T49.2x6-
external medication	T49.2x1-	T49.2x2-	T49.2x3-	T49.2x4-	T49.2x5-	T49.2x6-
local	T49.2x1-	T49.2x2-	T49.2x3-	T49.2x4-	T49.2x5-	T49.2x6-
medicinal	T49.2x1-	T49.2x2-	T49.2x3-	T49.2x4-	T49.2x5-	T49.2x6-
nonmedicinal	T55.1x1-	T55.1x2-	T55.1x3-	T55.1x4-	—	—
specified NEC	T55.1x1-	T55.1x2-	T55.1x3-	T55.1x4-	—	—
Deterrent, alcohol	T50.6x1-	T50.6x2-	T50.6x3-	T50.6x4-	T50.6x5-	T50.6x6-
Detoxifying agent	T50.6x1-	T50.6x2-	T50.6x3-	T50.6x4-	T50.6x5-	T50.6x6-
Detrothyronine	T38.1x1-	T38.1x2-	T38.1x3-	T38.1x4-	T38.1x5-	T38.1x6-
Dettol (external medication)	T49.0x1-	T49.0x2-	T49.0x3-	T49.0x4-	T49.0x5-	T49.0x6-
Dexamethasone	T38.0x1-	T38.0x2-	T38.0x3-	T38.0x4-	T38.0x5-	T38.0x6-
ENT agent	T49.6x1-	T49.6x2-	T49.6x3-	T49.6x4-	T49.6x5-	T49.6x6-
ophthalmic preparation	T49.5x1-	T49.5x2-	T49.5x3-	T49.5x4-	T49.5x5-	T49.5x6-
topical NEC	T49.0x1-	T49.0x2-	T49.0x3-	T49.0x4-	T49.0x5-	T49.0x6-
Dexamfetamine	T43.621-	T43.622-	T43.623-	T43.624-	T43.625-	T43.626-
Dexamphetamine	T43.621-	T43.622-	T43.623-	T43.624-	T43.625-	T43.626-
Dexbrompheniramine	T45.0x1-	T45.0x2-	T45.0x3-	T45.0x4-	T45.0x5-	T45.0x6-
Dexchlorpheniramine	T45.0x1-	T45.0x2-	T45.0x3-	T45.0x4-	T45.0x5-	T45.0x6-
Dexedrine	T43.621-	T43.622-	T43.623-	T43.624-	T43.625-	T43.626-
Dexetimide	T44.3x1-	T44.3x2-	T44.3x3-	T44.3x4-	T44.3x5-	T44.3x6-
Dexfenfluramine	T50.5x1-	T50.5x2-	T50.5x3-	T50.5x4-	T50.5x5-	T50.5x6-
Dexpanthenol	T45.2x1-	T45.2x2-	T45.2x3-	T45.2x4-	T45.2x5-	T45.2x6-
Dextran (40) (70) (150)	T45.8x1-	T45.8x2-	T45.8x3-	T45.8x4-	T45.8x5-	T45.8x6-
Dextriferron	T45.4x1-	T45.4x2-	T45.4x3-	T45.4x4-	T45.4x5-	T45.4x6-
Dextro calcium pantothenate	T45.2x1-	T45.2x2-	T45.2x3-	T45.2x4-	T45.2x5-	T45.2x6-
Dextro pantothenyl alcohol	T45.2x1-	T45.2x2-	T45.2x3-	T45.2x4-	T45.2x5-	T45.2x6-
Dextroamphetamine	T43.621-	T43.622-	T43.623-	T43.624-	T43.625-	T43.626-
Dextromethorphan	T48.3x1-	T48.3x2-	T48.3x3-	T48.3x4-	T48.3x5-	T48.3x6-
Dextromoramide	T40.4x1-	T40.4x2-	T40.4x3-	T40.4x4-	—	—
topical	T49.8x1-	T49.8x2-	T49.8x3-	T49.8x4-	T49.8x5-	T49.8x6-
Dextropropoxyphene	T40.4x1-	T40.4x2-	T40.4x3-	T40.4x4-	T40.4x5-	T40.4x6-
Dextrorphan	T40.2x1-	T40.2x2-	T40.2x3-	T40.2x4-	T40.2x5-	T40.2x6-
Dextrose	T50.3x1-	T50.3x2-	T50.3x3-	T50.3x4-	T50.3x5-	T50.3x6-
concentrated solution, intravenous	T46.8x1-	T46.8x2-	T46.8x3-	T46.8x4-	T46.8x5-	T46.8x6-
Dextrothyroxin	T38.1x1-	T38.1x2-	T38.1x3-	T38.1x4-	T38.1x5-	T38.1x6-
Dextrothyroxine sodium	T38.1x1-	T38.1x2-	T38.1x3-	T38.1x4-	T38.1x5-	T38.1x6-
DFP	T44.0x1-	T44.0x2-	T44.0x3-	T44.0x4-	T44.0x5-	T44.0x6-
DHE	T37.3x1-	T37.3x2-	T37.3x3-	T37.3x4-	T37.3x5-	T37.3x6-
45	T46.5x1-	T46.5x2-	T46.5x3-	T46.5x4-	T46.5x5-	T46.5x6-
Diabinese	T38.3x1-	T38.3x2-	T38.3x3-	T38.3x4-	T38.3x5-	T38.3x6-
Diacetone alcohol	T52.4x1-	T52.4x2-	T52.4x3-	T52.4x4-	—	—
Diacetyl monoxime	T50.991-	T50.992-	T50.993-	T50.994-	—	—
Diacetylmorphine	T40.1x1-	T40.1x2-	T40.1x3-	T40.1x4-	—	—
Diachylon plaster	T49.4x1-	T49.4x2-	T49.4x3-	T49.4x4-	T49.4x5-	T49.4x6-
Diaethylstilboestrolum	T38.5x1-	T38.5x2-	T38.5x3-	T38.5x4-	T38.5x5-	T38.5x6-
Diagnostic agent NEC	T50.8x1-	T50.8x2-	T50.8x3-	T50.8x4-	T50.8x5-	T50.8x6-
Dial (soap)	T49.2x1-	T49.2x2-	T49.2x3-	T49.2x4-	T49.2x5-	T49.2x6-
sedative	T42.3x1-	T42.3x2-	T42.3x3-	T42.3x4-	T42.3x5-	T42.3x6-
Dialkyl carbonate	T52.91x-	T52.92x-	T52.93x-	T52.94x-	—	—
Diallylbarbituric acid	T42.3x1-	T42.3x2-	T42.3x3-	T42.3x4-	T42.3x5-	T42.3x6-
Diallymal	T42.3x1-	T42.3x2-	T42.3x3-	T42.3x4-	T42.3x5-	T42.3x6-
Dialysis solution (intraperitoneal)	T50.3x1-	T50.3x2-	T50.3x3-	T50.3x4-	T50.3x5-	T50.3x6-
Diaminodiphenylsulfone	T37.1x1-	T37.1x2-	T37.1x3-	T37.1x4-	T37.1x5-	T37.1x6-
Diamorphine	T40.1x1-	T40.1x2-	T40.1x3-	T40.1x4-	—	—
Diamox	T50.2x1-	T50.2x2-	T50.2x3-	T50.2x4-	T50.2x5-	T50.2x6-
Diamthazole	T49.0x1-	T49.0x2-	T49.0x3-	T49.0x4-	T49.0x5-	T49.0x6-
Dianthone	T47.2x1-	T47.2x2-	T47.2x3-	T47.2x4-	T47.2x5-	T47.2x6-
Diaphenylsulfone	T37.0x1-	T37.0x2-	T37.0x3-	T37.0x4-	T37.0x5-	T37.0x6-
Diasone (sodium)	T37.1x1-	T37.1x2-	T37.1x3-	T37.1x4-	T37.1x5-	T37.1x6-
Diastase	T47.5x1-	T47.5x2-	T47.5x3-	T47.5x4-	T47.5x5-	T47.5x6-
Diatrizoate	T50.8x1-	T50.8x2-	T50.8x3-	T50.8x4-	T50.8x5-	T50.8x6-
Diazepam	T42.4x1-	T42.4x2-	T42.4x3-	T42.4x4-	T42.4x5-	T42.4x6-
Diazinon	T60.0x1-	T60.0x2-	T60.0x3-	T60.0x4-	—	—
Diazomethane (gas)	T59.891-	T59.892-	T59.893-	T59.894-	—	—
Diazoxide	T46.5x1-	T46.5x2-	T46.5x3-	T46.5x4-	T46.5x5-	T46.5x6-
Dibekacin	T36.5x1-	T36.5x2-	T36.5x3-	T36.5x4-	T36.5x5-	T36.5x6-
Dibenamine	T44.6x1-	T44.6x2-	T44.6x3-	T44.6x4-	T44.6x5-	T44.6x6-
Dibenzepin	T43.011-	T43.012-	T43.013-	T43.014-	T43.015-	T43.016-
Dibenzheptropine	T45.0x1-	T45.0x2-	T45.0x3-	T45.0x4-	T45.0x5-	T45.0x6-
Dibenzyline	T44.6x1-	T44.6x2-	T44.6x3-	T44.6x4-	T44.6x5-	T44.6x6-
Diborane (gas)	T59.891-	T59.892-	T59.893-	T59.894-	—	—
Dibromochloropropane	T60.8x1-	T60.8x2-	T60.8x3-	T60.8x4-	—	—

DRUGS & CHEMICALS

Table of Drugs & Chemicals	POISONING Accidental (Unintentional)	Self-Harm (Intentional)	Assault	Undetermined	Adverse Effect	Underdosing
Dibromodulcitol	T45.1x1-	T45.1x2-	T45.1x3-	T45.1x4-	T45.1x5-	T45.1x6-
Dibromoethane	T53.6x1-	T53.6x2-	T53.6x3-	T53.6x4-	—	—
Dibromomannitol	T45.1x1-	T45.1x2-	T45.1x3-	T45.1x4-	T45.1x5-	T45.1x6-
Dibromopropamidine isethionate	T49.0x1-	T49.0x2-	T49.0x3-	T49.0x4-	T49.0x5-	T49.0x6-
Dibrompropamidine	T49.0x1-	T49.0x2-	T49.0x3-	T49.0x4-	T49.0x5-	T49.0x6-
Dibucaine	T41.3x1-	T41.3x2-	T41.3x3-	T41.3x4-	T41.3x5-	T41.3x6-
topical (surface)	T41.3x1-	T41.3x2-	T41.3x3-	T41.3x4-	T41.3x5-	T41.3x6-
Dibunate sodium	T48.3x1-	T48.3x2-	T48.3x3-	T48.3x4-	T48.3x5-	T48.3x6-
Dibutoline sulfate	T44.3x1-	T44.3x2-	T44.3x3-	T44.3x4-	T44.3x5-	T44.3x6-
Dicamba	T60.3x1-	T60.3x2-	T60.3x3-	T60.3x4-	—	—
Dicapthon	T60.0x1-	T60.0x2-	T60.0x3-	T60.0x4-	—	—
Dichlobenil	T60.3x1-	T60.3x2-	T60.3x3-	T60.3x4-	—	—
Dichlone	T60.3x1-	T60.3x2-	T60.3x3-	T60.3x4-	—	—
Dichloralphenozone	T42.6x1-	T42.6x2-	T42.6x3-	T42.6x4-	T42.6x5-	T42.6x6-
Dichlorbenzidine	T65.3x1-	T65.3x2-	T65.3x3-	T65.3x4-	—	—
Dichlorhydrin	T52.8x1-	T52.8x2-	T52.8x3-	T52.8x4-	—	—
Dichlorhydroxyquinoline	T37.8x1-	T37.8x2-	T37.8x3-	T37.8x4-	T37.8x5-	T37.8x6-
Dichlorobenzene	T53.7x1-	T53.7x2-	T53.7x3-	T53.7x4-	—	—
Dichlorobenzyl alcohol	T49.6x1-	T49.6x2-	T49.6x3-	T49.6x4-	T49.6x5-	T49.6x6-
Dichlorodifluoromethane	T53.5x1-	T53.5x2-	T53.5x3-	T53.5x4-	—	—
Dichloroethane	T52.8x1-	T52.8x2-	T52.8x3-	T52.8x4-	—	—
Sym-Dichloroethyl ether	T53.6x1-	T53.6x2-	T53.6x3-	T53.6x4-	—	—
Dichloroethyl sulfide, not in war	T59.891-	T59.892-	T59.893-	T59.894-	—	—
Dichloroethylene	T53.6x1-	T53.6x2-	T53.6x3-	T53.6x4-	—	—
Dichloroformoxine, not in war	T59.891-	T59.892-	T59.893-	T59.894-	—	—
Dichlorohydrin, alpha-dichlorohydrin	T52.8x1-	T52.8x2-	T52.8x3-	T52.8x4-	—	—
Dichloromethane (solvent)	T53.4x1-	T53.4x2-	T53.4x3-	T53.4x4-	—	—
vapor	T53.4x1-	T53.4x2-	T53.4x3-	T53.4x4-	—	—
Dichloronaphthoquinone	T60.3x1-	T60.3x2-	T60.3x3-	T60.3x4-	—	—
Dichlorophen	T37.4x1-	T37.4x2-	T37.4x3-	T37.4x4-	T37.4x5-	T37.4x6-
2,4-Dichlorophenoxyacetic acid	T60.3x1-	T60.3x2-	T60.3x3-	T60.3x4-	—	—
Dichloropropene	T60.3x1-	T60.3x2-	T60.3x3-	T60.3x4-	—	—
Dichloropropionic acid	T60.3x1-	T60.3x2-	T60.3x3-	T60.3x4-	—	—
Dichlorphenamide	T50.2x1-	T50.2x2-	T50.2x3-	T50.2x4-	T50.2x5-	T50.2x6-
Dichlorvos	T60.0x1-	T60.0x2-	T60.0x3-	T60.0x4-	—	—
Diclofenac	T39.391-	T39.392-	T39.393-	T39.394-	T39.395-	T39.396-
Diclofenamide	T50.2x1-	T50.2x2-	T50.2x3-	T50.2x4-	T50.2x5-	T50.2x6-
Diclofensine	T43.291-	T43.292-	T43.293-	T43.294-	T43.295-	T43.296-
Diclonixine	T39.8x1-	T39.8x2-	T39.8x3-	T39.8x4-	T39.8x5-	T39.8x6-
Dicloxacillin	T36.0x1-	T36.0x2-	T36.0x3-	T36.0x4-	T36.0x5-	T36.0x6-
Dicophane	T49.0x1-	T49.0x2-	T49.0x3-	T49.0x4-	T49.0x5-	T49.0x6-
Dicoumarol, dicoumarin, dicumarol	T45.511-	T45.512-	T45.513-	T45.514-	T45.515-	T45.516-
Dicrotophos	T60.0x1-	T60.0x2-	T60.0x3-	T60.0x4-	—	—
Dicyanogen (gas)	T65.0x1-	T65.0x2-	T65.0x3-	T65.0x4-	—	—
Dicyclomine	T44.3x1-	T44.3x2-	T44.3x3-	T44.3x4-	T44.3x5-	T44.3x6-
Dicycloverine	T44.3x1-	T44.3x2-	T44.3x3-	T44.3x4-	T44.3x5-	T44.3x6-
Dideoxycytidine	T37.5x1-	T37.5x2-	T37.5x3-	T37.5x4-	T37.5x5-	T37.5x6-
Dideoxyinosine	T37.5x1-	T37.5x2-	T37.5x3-	T37.5x4-	T37.5x5-	T37.5x6-
Dieldrin (vapor)	T60.1x1-	T60.1x2-	T60.1x3-	T60.1x4-	—	—
Diemal	T42.3x1-	T42.3x2-	T42.3x3-	T42.3x4-	T42.3x5-	T42.3x6-
Dienestrol	T38.5x1-	T38.5x2-	T38.5x3-	T38.5x4-	T38.5x5-	T38.5x6-
Dienoestrol	T38.5x1-	T38.5x2-	T38.5x3-	T38.5x4-	T38.5x5-	T38.5x6-
Dietetic drug NEC	T50.901-	T50.902-	T50.903-	T50.904-	T50.905-	T50.906-
Diethazine	T42.8x1-	T42.8x2-	T42.8x3-	T42.8x4-	T42.8x5-	T42.8x6-

Table of Drugs & Chemicals	POISONING Accidental (Unintentional)	Self-Harm (Intentional)	Assault	Undetermined	Adverse Effect	Underdosing
Diethyl						
barbituric acid	T42.3x1-	T42.3x2-	T42.3x3-	T42.3x4-	T42.3x5-	T42.3x6-
carbamazine	T37.4x1-	T37.4x2-	T37.4x3-	T37.4x4-	T37.4x5-	T37.4x6-
carbinol	T51.3x1-	T51.3x2-	T51.3x3-	T51.3x4-	—	—
carbonate	T52.8x1-	T52.8x2-	T52.8x3-	T52.8x4-	—	—
ether (vapor) — *see also* Ether	T41.0x1-	T41.0x2-	T41.0x3-	T41.0x4-	T41.0x5-	T41.0x6-
oxide	T52.8x1-	T52.8x2-	T52.8x3-	T52.8x4-	—	—
propion	T50.5x1-	T50.5x2-	T50.5x3-	T50.5x4-	T50.5x5-	T50.5x6-
stilbestrol	T38.5x1-	T38.5x2-	T38.5x3-	T38.5x4-	T38.5x5-	T38.5x6-
toluamide (nonmedicinal)	T60.8x1-	T60.8x2-	T60.8x3-	T60.8x4-	—	—
medicinal	T49.3x1-	T49.3x2-	T49.3x3-	T49.3x4-	T49.3x5-	T49.3x6-
Diethylcarbamazine	T37.4x1-	T37.4x2-	T37.4x3-	T37.4x4-	T37.4x5-	T37.4x6-
Diethylene						
dioxide	T52.8x1-	T52.8x2-	T52.8x3-	T52.8x4-	—	—
glycol (monoacetate) (monobutyl ether) (monoethyl ether)	T52.3x1-	T52.3x2-	T52.3x3-	T52.3x4-	—	—
Diethylhexylphthalate	T65.891-	T65.892-	T65.893-	T65.894-	—	—
Diethylpropion	T50.5x1-	T50.5x2-	T50.5x3-	T50.5x4-	T50.5x5-	T50.5x6-
Diethylstilbestrol	T38.5x1-	T38.5x2-	T38.5x3-	T38.5x4-	T38.5x5-	T38.5x6-
Diethylstilboestrol	T38.5x1-	T38.5x2-	T38.5x3-	T38.5x4-	T38.5x5-	T38.5x6-
Diethylsulfone-diethylmethane	T42.6x1-	T42.6x2-	T42.6x3-	T42.6x4-	T42.6x5-	T42.6x6-
Diethyltoluamide	T49.0x1-	T49.0x2-	T49.0x3-	T49.0x4-	T49.0x5-	—
Diethyltryptamine (DET)	T40.991-	T40.992-	T40.993-	T40.994-	—	—
Difebarbamate	T42.3x1-	T42.3x2-	T42.3x3-	T42.3x4-	T42.3x5-	T42.3x6-
Difencloxazine	T40.2x1-	T40.2x2-	T40.2x3-	T40.2x4-	T40.2x5-	T40.2x6-
Difenidol	T45.0x1-	T45.0x2-	T45.0x3-	T45.0x4-	T45.0x5-	T45.0x6-
Difenoxin	T47.6x1-	T47.6x2-	T47.6x3-	T47.6x4-	T47.6x5-	T47.6x6-
Difetarsone	T37.3x1-	T37.3x2-	T37.3x3-	T37.3x4-	T37.3x5-	T37.3x6-
Diffusin	T45.3x1-	T45.3x2-	T45.3x3-	T45.3x4-	T45.3x5-	T45.3x6-
Diflorasone	T49.0x1-	T49.0x2-	T49.0x3-	T49.0x4-	T49.0x5-	T49.0x6-
Diflos	T44.0x1-	T44.0x2-	T44.0x3-	T44.0x4-	T44.0x5-	T44.0x6-
Diflubenzuron	T60.1x1-	T60.1x2-	T60.1x3-	T60.1x4-	—	—
Diflucortolone	T49.0x1-	T49.0x2-	T49.0x3-	T49.0x4-	T49.0x5-	T49.0x6-
Diflunisal	T39.091-	T39.092-	T39.093-	T39.094-	T39.095-	T39.096-
Difluoromethyldopa	T42.8x1-	T42.8x2-	T42.8x3-	T42.8x4-	T42.8x5-	T42.8x6-
Difluorophate	T44.0x1-	T44.0x2-	T44.0x3-	T44.0x4-	T44.0x5-	T44.0x6-
Digestant NEC	T47.5x1-	T47.5x2-	T47.5x3-	T47.5x4-	T47.5x5-	T47.5x6-
Digitalin(e)	T46.0x1-	T46.0x2-	T46.0x3-	T46.0x4-	T46.0x5-	T46.0x6-
Digitalis (leaf) (glycoside)	T46.0x1-	T46.0x2-	T46.0x3-	T46.0x4-	T46.0x5-	T46.0x6-
lanata	T46.0x1-	T46.0x2-	T46.0x3-	T46.0x4-	T46.0x5-	T46.0x6-
purpurea	T46.0x1-	T46.0x2-	T46.0x3-	T46.0x4-	T46.0x5-	T46.0x6-
Digitoxin	T46.0x1-	T46.0x2-	T46.0x3-	T46.0x4-	T46.0x5-	T46.0x6-
Digitoxose	T46.0x1-	T46.0x2-	T46.0x3-	T46.0x4-	T46.0x5-	T46.0x6-
Digoxin	T46.0x1-	T46.0x2-	T46.0x3-	T46.0x4-	T46.0x5-	T46.0x6-
Digoxine	T46.0x1-	T46.0x2-	T46.0x3-	T46.0x4-	T46.0x5-	T46.0x6-
Dihydralazine	T46.5x1-	T46.5x2-	T46.5x3-	T46.5x4-	T46.5x5-	T46.5x6-
Dihydrazine	T46.5x1-	T46.5x2-	T46.5x3-	T46.5x4-	T46.5x5-	T46.5x6-
Dihydrocodeine	T40.2x1-	T40.2x2-	T40.2x3-	T40.2x4-	T40.2x5-	T40.2x6-
Dihydrocodein-one	T40.2x1-	T40.2x2-	T40.2x3-	T40.2x4-	T40.2x5-	T40.2x6-
Dihydroergocornine	T46.7x1-	T46.7x2-	T46.7x3-	T46.7x4-	T46.7x5-	T46.7x6-
Dihydroergocristine (mesilate)	T46.7x1-	T46.7x2-	T46.7x3-	T46.7x4-	T46.7x5-	T46.7x6-
Dihydroergokryptine	T46.7x1-	T46.7x2-	T46.7x3-	T46.7x4-	T46.7x5-	T46.7x6-
Dihydroergotamine	T46.5x1-	T46.5x2-	T46.5x3-	T46.5x4-	T46.5x5-	T46.5x6-
Dihydroergotoxine	T46.7x1-	T46.7x2-	T46.7x3-	T46.7x4-	T46.7x5-	T46.7x6-
mesilate	T46.7x1-	T46.7x2-	T46.7x3-	T46.7x4-	T46.7x5-	T46.7x6-
Dihydrohydroxycodein-one	T40.2x1-	T40.2x2-	T40.2x3-	T40.2x4-	T40.2x5-	T40.2x6-
Dihydrohydroxymorphinone	T40.2x1-	T40.2x2-	T40.2x3-	T40.2x4-	T40.2x5-	T40.2x6-
Dihydroisocodeine	T40.2x1-	T40.2x2-	T40.2x3-	T40.2x4-	T40.2x5-	T40.2x6-

DRUGS & CHEMICALS

Table of Drugs & Chemicals	POISONING				Adverse Effect	Underdosing
	Accidental (Unintentional)	Self-Harm (Intentional)	Assault	Undetermined		
Dihydromorphine	T40.2x1-	T40.2x2-	T40.2x3-	T40.2x4-	—	—
Dihydromorphinone	T40.2x1-	T40.2x2-	T40.2x3-	T40.2x4-	T40.2x5-	T40.2x6-
Dihydrostreptomycin	T36.5x1-	T36.5x2-	T36.5x3-	T36.5x4-	T36.5x5-	T36.5x6-
Dihydrotachysterol	T45.2x1-	T45.2x2-	T45.2x3-	T45.2x4-	T45.2x5-	T45.2x6-
Dihydroxyaluminum aminoacetate	T47.1x1-	T47.1x2-	T47.1x3-	T47.1x4-	T47.1x5-	T47.1x6-
Dihydroxyaluminum sodium carbonate	T47.1x1-	T47.1x2-	T47.1x3-	T47.1x4-	T47.1x5-	T47.1x6-
Dihydroxyanthraquinone	T47.2x1-	T47.2x2-	T47.2x3-	T47.2x4-	T47.2x5-	T47.2x6-
Dihydroxycodeinone	T40.2x1-	T40.2x2-	T40.2x3-	T40.2x4-	T40.2x5-	T40.2x6-
Dihydroxypropyl theophylline	T50.2x1-	T50.2x2-	T50.2x3-	T50.2x4-	T50.2x5-	T50.2x6-
Diiodohydroxyquin	T37.8x1-	T37.8x2-	T37.8x3-	T37.8x4-	T37.8x5-	T37.8x6-
topical	T49.0x1-	T49.0x2-	T49.0x3-	T49.0x4-	T49.0x5-	T49.0x6-
Diiodohydroxyquinoline	T37.8x1-	T37.8x2-	T37.8x3-	T37.8x4-	T37.8x5-	T37.8x6-
Diiodotyrosine	T38.2x1-	T38.2x2-	T38.2x3-	T38.2x4-	T38.2x5-	T38.2x6-
Diisopromine	T44.3x1-	T44.3x2-	T44.3x3-	T44.3x4-	T44.3x5-	T44.3x6-
Diisopropylamine	T46.3x1-	T46.3x2-	T46.3x3-	T46.3x4-	T46.3x5-	T46.3x6-
Diisopropylfluorophosphonate	T44.0x1-	T44.0x2-	T44.0x3-	T44.0x4-	T44.0x5-	T44.0x6-
Dilantin	T42.0x1-	T42.0x2-	T42.0x3-	T42.0x4-	T42.0x5-	T42.0x6-
Dilaudid	T40.2x1-	T40.2x2-	T40.2x3-	T40.2x4-	T40.2x5-	T40.2x6-
Dilazep	T46.3x1-	T46.3x2-	T46.3x3-	T46.3x4-	T46.3x5-	T46.3x6-
Dill	T47.5x1-	T47.5x2-	T47.5x3-	T47.5x4-	T47.5x5-	T47.5x6-
Diloxanide	T37.3x1-	T37.3x2-	T37.3x3-	T37.3x4-	T37.3x5-	T37.3x6-
Diltiazem	T46.1x1-	T46.1x2-	T46.1x3-	T46.1x4-	T46.1x5-	T46.1x6-
Dimazole	T49.0x1-	T49.0x2-	T49.0x3-	T49.0x4-	T49.0x5-	T49.0x6-
Dimefline	T50.7x1-	T50.7x2-	T50.7x3-	T50.7x4-	T50.7x5-	T50.7x6-
Dimefox	T60.0x1-	T60.0x2-	T60.0x3-	T60.0x4-	—	—
Dimemorfan	T48.3x1-	T48.3x2-	T48.3x3-	T48.3x4-	T48.3x5-	T48.3x6-
Dimenhydrinate	T45.0x1-	T45.0x2-	T45.0x3-	T45.0x4-	T45.0x5-	T45.0x6-
Dimercaprol (British anti-lewisite)	T45.8x1-	T45.8x2-	T45.8x3-	T45.8x4-	T45.8x5-	T45.8x6-
Dimercaptopropanol	T45.8x1-	T45.8x2-	T45.8x3-	T45.8x4-	T45.8x5-	T45.8x6-
Dimestrol	T38.5x1-	T38.5x2-	T38.5x3-	T38.5x4-	T38.5x5-	T38.5x6-
Dimetane	T45.0x1-	T45.0x2-	T45.0x3-	T45.0x4-	T45.0x5-	T45.0x6-
Dimethicone	T47.1x1-	T47.1x2-	T47.1x3-	T47.1x4-	T47.1x5-	T47.1x6-
Dimethindene	T45.0x1-	T45.0x2-	T45.0x3-	T45.0x4-	T45.0x5-	T45.0x6-
Dimethisoquin	T49.1x1-	T49.1x2-	T49.1x3-	T49.1x4-	T49.1x5-	T49.1x6-
Dimethisterone	T38.5x1-	T38.5x2-	T38.5x3-	T38.5x4-	T38.5x5-	T38.5x6-
Dimethoate	T60.0x1-	T60.0x2-	T60.0x3-	T60.0x4-	—	—
Dimethocaine	T41.3x1-	T41.3x2-	T41.3x3-	T41.3x4-	T41.3x5-	T41.3x6-
Dimethoxanate	T48.3x1-	T48.3x2-	T48.3x3-	T48.3x4-	T48.3x5-	T48.3x6-
Dimethyl arsine, arsinic acid	T57.0x1-	T57.0x2-	T57.0x3-	T57.0x4-	—	—
carbinol	T51.2x1-	T51.2x2-	T51.2x3-	T51.2x4-	—	—
carbonate	T52.8x1-	T52.8x2-	T52.8x3-	T52.8x4-	—	—
diguanide	T38.3x1-	T38.3x2-	T38.3x3-	T38.3x4-	T38.3x5-	T38.3x6-
ketone	T52.4x1-	T52.4x2-	T52.4x3-	T52.4x4-	—	—
vapor	T52.4x1-	T52.4x2-	T52.4x3-	T52.4x4-	—	—
meperidine	T40.2x1-	T40.2x2-	T40.2x3-	T40.2x4-	T40.2x5-	T40.2x6-
parathion	T60.0x1-	T60.0x2-	T60.0x3-	T60.0x4-	—	—
phthlate	T49.3x1-	T49.3x2-	T49.3x3-	T49.3x4-	T49.3x5-	T49.3x6-
polysiloxane	T47.8x1-	T47.8x2-	T47.8x3-	T47.8x4-	T47.8x5-	T47.8x6-
sulfate (fumes)	T59.891-	T59.892-	T59.893-	T59.894-	—	—
liquid	T65.891-	T65.892-	T65.893-	T65.894-	—	—
sulfoxide (nonmedicinal)	T52.8x1-	T52.8x2-	T52.8x3-	T52.8x4-	—	—
medicinal	T49.4x1-	T49.4x2-	T49.4x3-	T49.4x4-	T49.4x5-	T49.4x6-
tryptamine	T40.991-	T40.992-	T40.993-	T40.994-	—	—
tubocurarine	T48.1x1-	T48.1x2-	T48.1x3-	T48.1x4-	T48.1x5-	T48.1x6-
Dimethylamine sulfate	T49.4x1-	T49.4x2-	T49.4x3-	T49.4x4-	T49.4x5-	T49.4x6-
Dimethylformamide	T52.8x1-	T52.8x2-	T52.8x3-	T52.8x4-	—	—
Dimethyltubocurarinium chloride	T48.1x1-	T48.1x2-	T48.1x3-	T48.1x4-	T48.1x5-	T48.1x6-

Table of Drugs & Chemicals	POISONING				Adverse Effect	Underdosing
	Accidental (Unintentional)	Self-Harm (Intentional)	Assault	Undetermined		
Dimeticone	T47.1x1-	T47.1x2-	T47.1x3-	T47.1x4-	T47.1x5-	T47.1x6-
Dimetilan	T60.0x1-	T60.0x2-	T60.0x3-	T60.0x4-	—	—
Dimetindene	T45.0x1-	T45.0x2-	T45.0x3-	T45.0x4-	T45.0x5-	T45.0x6-
Dimetotiazine	T43.3x1-	T43.3x2-	T43.3x3-	T43.3x4-	T43.3x5-	T43.3x6-
Dimorpholamine	T50.7x1-	T50.7x2-	T50.7x3-	T50.7x4-	T50.7x5-	T50.7x6-
Dimoxyline	T46.3x1-	T46.3x2-	T46.3x3-	T46.3x4-	T46.3x5-	T46.3x6-
Dinitro (-ortho-)cresol (pesticide) (spray)	T65.3x1-	T65.3x2-	T65.3x3-	T65.3x4-	—	—
Dinitrobenzene	T65.3x1-	T65.3x2-	T65.3x3-	T65.3x4-	—	—
vapor	T59.891-	T59.892-	T59.893-	T59.894-	—	—
Dinitrobenzol	T65.3x1-	T65.3x2-	T65.3x3-	T65.3x4-	—	—
vapor	T59.891-	T59.892-	T59.893-	T59.894-	—	—
Dinitrobutylphenol	T65.3x1-	T65.3x2-	T65.3x3-	T65.3x4-	—	—
Dinitrocyclohexylphenol	T65.3x1-	T65.3x2-	T65.3x3-	T65.3x4-	—	—
Dinitrophenol	T65.3x1-	T65.3x2-	T65.3x3-	T65.3x4-	—	—
Dinoprost	T48.0x1-	T48.0x2-	T48.0x3-	T48.0x4-	T48.0x5-	T48.0x6-
Dinoprostone	T48.0x1-	T48.0x2-	T48.0x3-	T48.0x4-	T48.0x5-	T48.0x6-
Dinoseb	T60.3x1-	T60.3x2-	T60.3x3-	T60.3x4-	—	—
Dioctyl sulfosuccinate (calcium) (sodium)	T47.4x1-	T47.4x2-	T47.4x3-	T47.4x4-	T47.4x5-	T47.4x6-
Diodone	T50.8x1-	T50.8x2-	T50.8x3-	T50.8x4-	T50.8x5-	T50.8x6-
Diodoquin	T37.8x1-	T37.8x2-	T37.8x3-	T37.8x4-	T37.8x5-	T37.8x6-
Dionin	T40.2x1-	T40.2x2-	T40.2x3-	T40.2x4-	T40.2x5-	T40.2x6-
Diosmin	T46.991-	T46.992-	T46.993-	T46.994-	T46.995-	T46.996-
Dioxane	T52.8x1-	T52.8x2-	T52.8x3-	T52.8x4-	—	—
Dioxathion	T60.0x1-	T60.0x2-	T60.0x3-	T60.0x4-	—	—
Dioxin	T53.7x1-	T53.7x2-	T53.7x3-	T53.7x4-	—	—
Dioxopromethazine	T43.3x1-	T43.3x2-	T43.3x3-	T43.3x4-	T43.3x5-	T43.3x6-
Dioxyline	T46.3x1-	T46.3x2-	T46.3x3-	T46.3x4-	T46.3x5-	T46.3x6-
Dipentene	T52.8x1-	T52.8x2-	T52.8x3-	T52.8x4-	—	—
Diperodon	T41.3x1-	T41.3x2-	T41.3x3-	T41.3x4-	T41.3x5-	T41.3x6-
Diphacinone	T60.4x1-	T60.4x2-	T60.4x3-	T60.4x4-	—	—
Diphemanil	T44.3x1-	T44.3x2-	T44.3x3-	T44.3x4-	T44.3x5-	T44.3x6-
metilsulfate	T44.3x1-	T44.3x2-	T44.3x3-	T44.3x4-	T44.3x5-	T44.3x6-
Diphenadione	T45.511-	T45.512-	T45.513-	T45.514-	T45.515-	T45.516-
rodenticide	T60.4x1-	T60.4x2-	T60.4x3-	T60.4x4-	—	—
Diphenhydramine	T45.0x1-	T45.0x2-	T45.0x3-	T45.0x4-	T45.0x5-	T45.0x6-
Diphenidol	T45.0x1-	T45.0x2-	T45.0x3-	T45.0x4-	T45.0x5-	T45.0x6-
Diphenoxylate	T47.6x1-	T47.6x2-	T47.6x3-	T47.6x4-	T47.6x5-	T47.6x6-
Diphenylamine	T65.3x1-	T65.3x2-	T65.3x3-	T65.3x4-	—	—
Diphenylbutazone	T39.2x1-	T39.2x2-	T39.2x3-	T39.2x4-	T39.2x5-	T39.2x6-
Diphenylchloroarsine, not in war	T57.0x1-	T57.0x2-	T57.0x3-	T57.0x4-	—	—
Diphenylhydantoin	T42.0x1-	T42.0x2-	T42.0x3-	T42.0x4-	T42.0x5-	T42.0x6-
Diphenylmethane dye	T52.1x1-	T52.1x2-	T52.1x3-	T52.1x4-	—	—
Diphenylpyraline	T45.0x1-	T45.0x2-	T45.0x3-	T45.0x4-	T45.0x5-	T45.0x6-
Diphtheria antitoxin	T50.Z11-	T50.Z12-	T50.Z13-	T50.Z14-	T50.Z15-	T50.Z16-
toxoid	T50.A91-	T50.A92-	T50.A93-	T50.A94-	T50.A95-	T50.A96-
with tetanus toxoid	T50.A21-	T50.A22-	T50.A23-	T50.A24-	T50.A25-	T50.A26-
with pertussis component	T50.A11-	T50.A12-	T50.A13-	T50.A14-	T50.A15-	T50.A16-
vaccine	T50.A91-	T50.A92-	T50.A93-	T50.A94-	T50.A95-	T50.A96-
combination including pertussis	T50.A11-	T50.A12-	T50.A13-	T50.A14-	T50.A15-	T50.A16-
without pertussis	T50.A21-	T50.A22-	T50.A23-	T50.A24-	T50.A25-	T50.A26-
Diphylline	T50.2x1-	T50.2x2-	T50.2x3-	T50.2x4-	T50.2x5-	T50.2x6-
Dipipanone	T40.4x1-	T40.4x2-	T40.4x3-	T40.4x4-	—	—
Dipivefrine	T49.5x1-	T49.5x2-	T49.5x3-	T49.5x4-	T49.5x5-	T49.5x6-
Diplovax	T50.B91-	T50.B92-	T50.B93-	T50.B94-	T50.B95-	T50.B96-
Diprophylline	T50.2x1-	T50.2x2-	T50.2x3-	T50.2x4-	T50.2x5-	T50.2x6-
Dipropyline	T48.291-	T48.292-	T48.293-	T48.294-	T48.295-	T48.296-
Dipyridamole	T46.3x1-	T46.3x2-	T46.3x3-	T46.3x4-	T46.3x5-	T46.3x6-
Dipyrone	T39.2x1-	T39.2x2-	T39.2x3-	T39.2x4-	T39.2x5-	T39.2x6-

DRUGS & CHEMICALS

Table of Drugs & Chemicals	POISONING Accidental (Unintentional)	Self-Harm (Intentional)	Assault	Undetermined	Adverse Effect	Underdosing
Diquat (dibromide)	T60.3x1-	T60.3x2-	T60.3x3-	T60.3x4-	—	—
Disinfectant	T65.891-	T65.892-	T65.893-	T65.894-	—	—
alkaline	T54.3x1-	T54.3x2-	T54.3x3-	T54.3x4-	—	—
aromatic	T54.1x1-	T54.1x2-	T54.1x3-	T54.1x4-	—	—
intestinal	T37.8x1-	T37.8x2-	T37.8x3-	T37.8x4-	T37.8x5-	T37.8x6-
Disipal	T42.8x1-	T42.8x2-	T42.8x3-	T42.8x4-	T42.8x5-	T42.8x6-
Disodium edetate	T50.6x1-	T50.6x2-	T50.6x3-	T50.6x4-	T50.6x5-	T50.6x6-
Disoprofol	T41.291-	T41.292-	T41.293-	T41.294-	T41.295-	T41.296-
Distigmine (bromide)	T44.0x1-	T44.0x2-	T44.0x3-	T44.0x4-	T44.0x5-	T44.0x6-
Disulfamide	T50.2x1-	T50.2x2-	T50.2x3-	T50.2x4-	T50.2x5-	T50.2x6-
Disulfanilamide	T37.0x1-	T37.0x2-	T37.0x3-	T37.0x4-	T37.0x5-	T37.0x6-
Disulfiram	T50.6x1-	T50.6x2-	T50.6x3-	T50.6x4-	T50.6x5-	T50.6x6-
Disulfoton	T60.0x1-	T60.0x2-	T60.0x3-	T60.0x4-	—	—
Dithiazanine iodide	T37.4x1-	T37.4x2-	T37.4x3-	T37.4x4-	T37.4x5-	T37.4x6-
Dithiocarbamate	T60.0x1-	T60.0x2-	T60.0x3-	T60.0x4-	—	—
Dithranol	T49.4x1-	T49.4x2-	T49.4x3-	T49.4x4-	T49.4x5-	T49.4x6-
Diucardin	T50.2x1-	T50.2x2-	T50.2x3-	T50.2x4-	T50.2x5-	T50.2x6-
Diupres	T50.2x1-	T50.2x2-	T50.2x3-	T50.2x4-	T50.2x5-	T50.2x6-
Diuretic NEC	T50.2x1-	T50.2x2-	T50.2x3-	T50.2x4-	T50.2x5-	T50.2x6-
benzothiadiazine	T50.2x1-	T50.2x2-	T50.2x3-	T50.2x4-	T50.2x5-	T50.2x6-
carbonic acid anhydrase inhibitors	T50.2x1-	T50.2x2-	T50.2x3-	T50.2x4-	T50.2x5-	T50.2x6-
furfuryl NEC	T50.2x1-	T50.2x2-	T50.2x3-	T50.2x4-	T50.2x5-	T50.2x6-
loop (high-ceiling)	T50.1x1-	T50.1x2-	T50.1x3-	T50.1x4-	T50.1x5-	T50.1x6-
mercurial NEC	T50.2x1-	T50.2x2-	T50.2x3-	T50.2x4-	T50.2x5-	T50.2x6-
osmotic	T50.2x1-	T50.2x2-	T50.2x3-	T50.2x4-	T50.2x5-	T50.2x6-
purine NEC	T50.2x1-	T50.2x2-	T50.2x3-	T50.2x4-	T50.2x5-	T50.2x6-
saluretic NEC	T50.2x1-	T50.2x2-	T50.2x3-	T50.2x4-	T50.2x5-	T50.2x6-
sulfonamide	T50.2x1-	T50.2x2-	T50.2x3-	T50.2x4-	T50.2x5-	T50.2x6-
thiazide NEC	T50.2x1-	T50.2x2-	T50.2x3-	T50.2x4-	T50.2x5-	T50.2x6-
xanthine	T50.2x1-	T50.2x2-	T50.2x3-	T50.2x4-	T50.2x5-	T50.2x6-
Diurgin	T50.2x1-	T50.2x2-	T50.2x3-	T50.2x4-	T50.2x5-	T50.2x6-
Diuril	T50.2x1-	T50.2x2-	T50.2x3-	T50.2x4-	T50.2x5-	T50.2x6-
Diuron	T60.3x1-	T60.3x2-	T60.3x3-	T60.3x4-	—	—
Divalproex	T42.6x1-	T42.6x2-	T42.6x3-	T42.6x4-	T42.6x5-	T42.6x6-
Divinyl ether	T41.0x1-	T41.0x2-	T41.0x3-	T41.0x4-	T41.0x5-	T41.0x6-
Dixanthogen	T49.0x1-	T49.0x2-	T49.0x3-	T49.0x4-	T49.0x5-	T49.0x6-
Dixyrazine	T43.3x1-	T43.3x2-	T43.3x3-	T43.3x4-	T43.3x5-	T43.3x6-
D-lysergic acid diethylamide	T40.8x1-	T40.8x2-	T40.8x3-	T40.8x4-	—	—
DMCT	T36.4x1-	T36.4x2-	T36.4x3-	T36.4x4-	T36.4x5-	T36.4x6-
DMSO — see Dimethyl sulfoxide						
DNBP	T60.3x1-	T60.3x2-	T60.3x3-	T60.3x4-	—	—
DNOC	T65.3x1-	T65.3x2-	T65.3x3-	T65.3x4-	—	—
Dobutamine	T44.5x1-	T44.5x2-	T44.5x3-	T44.5x4-	T44.5x5-	T44.5x6-
DOCA	T38.0x1-	T38.0x2-	T38.0x3-	T38.0x4-	T38.0x5-	T38.0x6-
Docusate sodium	T47.4x1-	T47.4x2-	T47.4x3-	T47.4x4-	T47.4x5-	T47.4x6-
Dodicin	T49.0x1-	T49.0x2-	T49.0x3-	T49.0x4-	T49.0x5-	T49.0x6-
Dofamium chloride	T49.0x1-	T49.0x2-	T49.0x3-	T49.0x4-	T49.0x5-	T49.0x6-
Dolophine	T40.3x1-	T40.3x2-	T40.3x3-	T40.3x4-	T40.3x5-	T40.3x6-
Doloxene	T39.8x1-	T39.8x2-	T39.8x3-	T39.8x4-	T39.8x5-	T39.8x6-
Domestic gas (after combustion) — see Gas, utility						
prior to combustion	T59.891-	T59.892-	T59.893-	T59.894-	—	—
Domiodol	T48.4x1-	T48.4x2-	T48.4x3-	T48.4x4-	T48.4x5-	T48.4x6-
Domiphen (bromide)	T49.0x1-	T49.0x2-	T49.0x3-	T49.0x4-	T49.0x5-	T49.0x6-
Domperidone	T45.0x1-	T45.0x2-	T45.0x3-	T45.0x4-	T45.0x5-	T45.0x6-
Dopa	T42.8x1-	T42.8x2-	T42.8x3-	T42.8x4-	T42.8x5-	T42.8x6-
Dopamine	T44.991-	T44.992-	T44.993-	T44.994-	T44.995-	T44.996-
Doriden	T42.6x1-	T42.6x2-	T42.6x3-	T42.6x4-	T42.6x5-	T42.6x6-
Dormiral	T42.3x1-	T42.3x2-	T42.3x3-	T42.3x4-	T42.3x5-	T42.3x6-
Dormison	T42.6x1-	T42.6x2-	T42.6x3-	T42.6x4-	T42.6x5-	T42.6x6-
Dornase	T48.4x1-	T48.4x2-	T48.4x3-	T48.4x4-	T48.4x5-	T48.4x6-
Dorsacaine	T41.3x1-	T41.3x2-	T41.3x3-	T41.3x4-	T41.3x5-	T41.3x6-
Dosulepin	T43.011-	T43.012-	T43.013-	T43.014-	T43.015-	T43.016-
Dothiepin	T43.011-	T43.012-	T43.013-	T43.014-	T43.015-	T43.016-
Doxantrazole	T48.6x1-	T48.6x2-	T48.6x3-	T48.6x4-	T48.6x5-	T48.6x6-
Doxapram	T50.7x1-	T50.7x2-	T50.7x3-	T50.7x4-	T50.7x5-	T50.7x6-
Doxazosin	T44.6x1-	T44.6x2-	T44.6x3-	T44.6x4-	T44.6x5-	T44.6x6-
Doxepin	T43.011-	T43.012-	T43.013-	T43.014-	T43.015-	T43.016-
Doxifluridine	T45.1x1-	T45.1x2-	T45.1x3-	T45.1x4-	T45.1x5-	T45.1x6-
Doxorubicin	T45.1x1-	T45.1x2-	T45.1x3-	T45.1x4-	T45.1x5-	T45.1x6-
Doxycycline	T36.4x1-	T36.4x2-	T36.4x3-	T36.4x4-	T36.4x5-	T36.4x6-
Doxylamine	T45.0x1-	T45.0x2-	T45.0x3-	T45.0x4-	T45.0x5-	T45.0x6-
Dramamine	T45.0x1-	T45.0x2-	T45.0x3-	T45.0x4-	T45.0x5-	T45.0x6-
Drano (drain cleaner)	T54.3x1-	T54.3x2-	T54.3x3-	T54.3x4-	—	—
Dressing, live pulp	T49.7x1-	T49.7x2-	T49.7x3-	T49.7x4-	T49.7x5-	T49.7x6-
Drocode	T40.2x1-	T40.2x2-	T40.2x3-	T40.2x4-	T40.2x5-	T40.2x6-
Dromoran	T40.2x1-	T40.2x2-	T40.2x3-	T40.2x4-	T40.2x5-	T40.2x6-
Dromostanolone	T38.7x1-	T38.7x2-	T38.7x3-	T38.7x4-	T38.7x5-	T38.7x6-
Dronabinol	T40.7x1-	T40.7x2-	T40.7x3-	T40.7x4-	T40.7x5-	T40.7x6-
Droperidol	T43.591-	T43.592-	T43.593-	T43.594-	T43.595-	T43.596-
Dropropizine	T48.3x1-	T48.3x2-	T48.3x3-	T48.3x4-	T48.3x5-	T48.3x6-
Drostanolone	T38.7x1-	T38.7x2-	T38.7x3-	T38.7x4-	T38.7x5-	T38.7x6-
Drotaverine	T44.3x1-	T44.3x2-	T44.3x3-	T44.3x4-	T44.3x5-	T44.3x6-
Drotrecogin alfa	T45.511-	T45.512-	T45.513-	T45.514-	T45.515-	T45.516-
Drug NEC	T50.901-	T50.902-	T50.903-	T50.904-	T50.905-	T50.906-
specified NEC	T50.991-	T50.992-	T50.993-	T50.994-	T50.995-	T50.996-
DTIC	T45.1x1-	T45.1x2-	T45.1x3-	T45.1x4-	T45.1x5-	T45.1x6-
Duboisine	T44.3x1-	T44.3x2-	T44.3x3-	T44.3x4-	T44.3x5-	T44.3x6-
Dulcolax	T47.2x1-	T47.2x2-	T47.2x3-	T47.2x4-	T47.2x5-	T47.2x6-
Duponol (C) (EP)	T49.2x1-	T49.2x2-	T49.2x3-	T49.2x4-	T49.2x5-	T49.2x6-
Durabolin	T38.7x1-	T38.7x2-	T38.7x3-	T38.7x4-	T38.7x5-	T38.7x6-
Dyclone	T41.3x1-	T41.3x2-	T41.3x3-	T41.3x4-	T41.3x5-	T41.3x6-
Dyclonine	T41.3x1-	T41.3x2-	T41.3x3-	T41.3x4-	T41.3x5-	T41.3x6-
Dydrogesterone	T38.5x1-	T38.5x2-	T38.5x3-	T38.5x4-	T38.5x5-	T38.5x6-
Dye NEC	T65.6x1-	T65.6x2-	T65.6x3-	T65.6x4-	—	—
antiseptic	T49.0x1-	T49.0x2-	T49.0x3-	T49.0x4-	T49.0x5-	T49.0x6-
diagnostic agents	T50.8x1-	T50.8x2-	T50.8x3-	T50.8x4-	T50.8x5-	T50.8x6-
pharmaceutical NEC	T50.901-	T50.902-	T50.903-	T50.904-	T50.905-	T50.906-
Dyflos	T44.0x1-	T44.0x2-	T44.0x3-	T44.0x4-	T44.0x5-	T44.0x6-
Dymelor	T38.3x1-	T38.3x2-	T38.3x3-	T38.3x4-	T38.3x5-	T38.3x6-
Dynamite	T65.3x1-	T65.3x2-	T65.3x3-	T65.3x4-	—	—
fumes	T59.891-	T59.892-	T59.893-	T59.894-	—	—
Dyphylline	T44.3x1-	T44.3x2-	T44.3x3-	T44.3x4-	T44.3x5-	T44.3x6-
Ear drug NEC	T49.6x1-	T49.6x2-	T49.6x3-	T49.6x4-	T49.6x5-	T49.6x6-
Ear preparations	T49.6x1-	T49.6x2-	T49.6x3-	T49.6x4-	T49.6x5-	T49.6x6-
Echothiophate, echothiopate, ecothiopate	T49.5x1-	T49.5x2-	T49.5x3-	T49.5x4-	T49.5x5-	T49.5x6-
Econazole	T49.0x1-	T49.0x2-	T49.0x3-	T49.0x4-	T49.0x5-	T49.0x6-
Ecothiopate iodide	T49.5x1-	T49.5x2-	T49.5x3-	T49.5x4-	T49.5x5-	T49.5x6-
Ecstasy	T43.621-	T43.622-	T43.623-	T43.624-	T43.625-	T43.626-
Ectylurea	T42.6x1-	T42.6x2-	T42.6x3-	T42.6x4-	T42.6x5-	T42.6x6-
Edathamil disodium	T45.8x1-	T45.8x2-	T45.8x3-	T45.8x4-	T45.8x5-	T45.8x6-
Edecrin	T50.1x1-	T50.1x2-	T50.1x3-	T50.1x4-	T50.1x5-	T50.1x6-
Edetate, disodium (calcium)	T45.8x1-	T45.8x2-	T45.8x3-	T45.8x4-	T45.8x5-	T45.8x6-
Edoxudine	T49.5x1-	T49.5x2-	T49.5x3-	T49.5x4-	T49.5x5-	T49.5x6-
Edrophonium	T44.0x1-	T44.0x2-	T44.0x3-	T44.0x4-	T44.0x5-	T44.0x6-
chloride	T44.0x1-	T44.0x2-	T44.0x3-	T44.0x4-	T44.0x5-	T44.0x6-
EDTA	T50.6x1-	T50.6x2-	T50.6x3-	T50.6x4-	T50.6x5-	T50.6x6-
Eflornithine	T37.2x1-	T37.2x2-	T37.2x3-	T37.2x4-	T37.2x5-	T37.2x6-
Efloxate	T46.3x1-	T46.3x2-	T46.3x3-	T46.3x4-	T46.3x5-	T46.3x6-

DRUGS & CHEMICALS

Table of Drugs & Chemicals	POISONING Accidental (Unintentional)	Self-Harm (Intentional)	Assault	Undetermined	Adverse Effect	Underdosing
Elase	T49.8x1-	T49.8x2-	T49.8x3-	T49.8x4-	T49.8x5-	T49.8x6-
Elastase	T47.5x1-	T47.5x2-	T47.5x3-	T47.5x4-	T47.5x5-	T47.5x6-
Elaterium	T47.2x1-	T47.2x2-	T47.2x3-	T47.2x4-	T47.2x5-	T47.2x6-
Elcatonin	T50.991-	T50.992-	T50.993-	T50.994-	T50.995-	T50.996-
Elder	T62.2x1-	T62.2x2-	T62.2x3-	T62.2x4-	—	—
berry, (unripe)	T62.1x1-	T62.1x2-	T62.1x3-	T62.1x4-	—	—
Electrolyte balance drug	T50.3x1-	T50.3x2-	T50.3x3-	T50.3x4-	T50.3x5-	T50.3x6-
Electrolytes NEC	T50.3x1-	T50.3x2-	T50.3x3-	T50.3x4-	T50.3x5-	T50.3x6-
Electrolytic agent NEC	T50.3x1-	T50.3x2-	T50.3x3-	T50.3x4-	T50.3x5-	T50.3x6-
Elemental diet	T50.901-	T50.902-	T50.903-	T50.904-	T50.905-	T50.906-
Elliptinium acetate	T45.1x1-	T45.1x2-	T45.1x3-	T45.1x4-	T45.1x5-	T45.1x6-
Embramine	T45.0x1-	T45.0x2-	T45.0x3-	T45.0x4-	T45.0x5-	T45.0x6-
Emepronium (salts)	T44.3x1-	T44.3x2-	T44.3x3-	T44.3x4-	T44.3x5-	T44.3x6-
bromide	T44.3x1-	T44.3x2-	T44.3x3-	T44.3x4-	T44.3x5-	T44.3x6-
Emetic NEC	T47.7x1-	T47.7x2-	T47.7x3-	T47.7x4-	T47.7x5-	T47.7x6-
Emetine	T37.3x1-	T37.3x2-	T37.3x3-	T37.3x4-	T37.3x5-	T37.3x6-
Emollient NEC	T49.3x1-	T49.3x2-	T49.3x3-	T49.3x4-	T49.3x5-	T49.3x6-
Emorfazone	T39.8x1-	T39.8x2-	T39.8x3-	T39.8x4-	T39.8x5-	T39.8x6-
Emylcamate	T43.591-	T43.592-	T43.593-	T43.594-	T43.595-	T43.596-
Enalapril	T46.4x1-	T46.4x2-	T46.4x3-	T46.4x4-	T46.4x5-	T46.4x6-
Enalaprilat	T46.4x1-	T46.4x2-	T46.4x3-	T46.4x4-	T46.4x5-	T46.4x6-
Encainide	T46.2x1-	T46.2x2-	T46.2x3-	T46.2x4-	T46.2x5-	T46.2x6-
Endocaine	T41.3x1-	T41.3x2-	T41.3x3-	T41.3x4-	T41.3x5-	T41.3x6-
Endosulfan	T60.2x1-	T60.2x2-	T60.2x3-	T60.2x4-	—	—
Endothall	T60.3x1-	T60.3x2-	T60.3x3-	T60.3x4-	—	—
Endralazine	T46.5x1-	T46.5x2-	T46.5x3-	T46.5x4-	T46.5x5-	T46.5x6-
Endrin	T60.1x1-	T60.1x2-	T60.1x3-	T60.1x4-	—	—
Enflurane	T41.0x1-	T41.0x2-	T41.0x3-	T41.0x4-	T41.0x5-	T41.0x6-
Enhexymal	T42.3x1-	T42.3x2-	T42.3x3-	T42.3x4-	T42.3x5-	T42.3x6-
Enocitabine	T45.1x1-	T45.1x2-	T45.1x3-	T45.1x4-	T45.1x5-	T45.1x6-
Enovid	T38.4x1-	T38.4x2-	T38.4x3-	T38.4x4-	T38.4x5-	T38.4x6-
Enoxacin	T36.8x1-	T36.8x2-	T36.8x3-	T36.8x4-	T36.8x5-	T36.8x6-
Enoxaparin (sodium)	T45.511-	T45.512-	T45.513-	T45.514-	T45.515-	T45.516-
Enpiprazole	T43.591-	T43.592-	T43.593-	T43.594-	T43.595-	T43.596-
Enprofylline	T48.6x1-	T48.6x2-	T48.6x3-	T48.6x4-	T48.6x5-	T48.6x6-
Enprostil	T47.1x1-	T47.1x2-	T47.1x3-	T47.1x4-	T47.1x5-	T47.1x6-
ENT preparations (anti-infectives)	T49.6x1-	T49.6x2-	T49.6x3-	T49.6x4-	T49.6x5-	T49.6x6-
Enterogastrone	T38.891-	T38.892-	T38.893-	T38.894-	T38.895-	T38.896-
Enviomycin	T36.8x1-	T36.8x2-	T36.8x3-	T36.8x4-	T36.8x5-	T36.8x6-
Enzodase	T45.3x1-	T45.3x2-	T45.3x3-	T45.3x4-	T45.3x5-	T45.3x6-
Enzyme NEC	T45.3x1-	T45.3x2-	T45.3x3-	T45.3x4-	T45.3x5-	T45.3x6-
depolymerizing	T49.8x1-	T49.8x2-	T49.8x3-	T49.8x4-	T49.8x5-	T49.8x6-
fibrolytic	T45.3x1-	T45.3x2-	T45.3x3-	T45.3x4-	T45.3x5-	T45.3x6-
gastric	T47.5x1-	T47.5x2-	T47.5x3-	T47.5x4-	T47.5x5-	T47.5x6-
intestinal	T47.5x1-	T47.5x2-	T47.5x3-	T47.5x4-	T47.5x5-	T47.5x6-
local action	T49.4x1-	T49.4x2-	T49.4x3-	T49.4x4-	T49.4x5-	T49.4x6-
proteolytic	T49.4x1-	T49.4x2-	T49.4x3-	T49.4x4-	T49.4x5-	T49.4x6-
thrombolytic	T45.3x1-	T45.3x2-	T45.3x3-	T45.3x4-	T45.3x5-	T45.3x6-
EPAB	T41.3x1-	T41.3x2-	T41.3x3-	T41.3x4-	T41.3x5-	T41.3x6-
Epanutin	T42.0x1-	T42.0x2-	T42.0x3-	T42.0x4-	T42.0x5-	T42.0x6-
Ephedra	T44.991-	T44.992-	T44.993-	T44.994-	T44.995-	T44.996-
Ephedrine	T44.991-	T44.992-	T44.993-	T44.994-	T44.995-	T44.996-
Epichlorhydrin, epichlorohydrin	T52.8x1-	T52.8x2-	T52.8x3-	T52.8x4-	—	—
Epicillin	T36.0x1-	T36.0x2-	T36.0x3-	T36.0x4-	T36.0x5-	T36.0x6-
Epiestriol	T38.5x1-	T38.5x2-	T38.5x3-	T38.5x4-	T38.5x5-	T38.5x6-
Epilim — *see* Sodium valproate						
Epimestrol	T38.5x1-	T38.5x2-	T38.5x3-	T38.5x4-	T38.5x5-	T38.5x6-
Epinephrine	T44.5x1-	T44.5x2-	T44.5x3-	T44.5x4-	T44.5x5-	T44.5x6-
Epirubicin	T45.1x1-	T45.1x2-	T45.1x3-	T45.1x4-	T45.1x5-	T45.1x6-
Epitiostanol	T38.7x1-	T38.7x2-	T38.7x3-	T38.7x4-	T38.7x5-	T38.7x6-
Epitizide	T50.2x1-	T50.2x2-	T50.2x3-	T50.2x4-	T50.2x5-	T50.2x6-
EPN	T60.0x1-	T60.0x2-	T60.0x3-	T60.0x4-	—	—
EPO	T45.8x1-	T45.8x2-	T45.8x3-	T45.8x4-	T45.8x5-	T45.8x6-
Epoetin alpha	T45.8x1-	T45.8x2-	T45.8x3-	T45.8x4-	T45.8x5-	T45.8x6-
Epomediol	T50.991-	T50.992-	T50.993-	T50.994-	T50.995-	T50.996-
Epoprostenol	T45.521-	T45.522-	T45.523-	T45.524-	T45.525-	T45.526-
Epoxy resin	T65.891-	T65.892-	T65.893-	T65.894-	—	—
Eprazinone	T48.4x1-	T48.4x2-	T48.4x3-	T48.4x4-	T48.4x5-	T48.4x6-
Epsilon amino-caproic acid	T45.621-	T45.622-	T45.623-	T45.624-	T45.625-	T45.626-
Epsom salt	T47.3x1-	T47.3x2-	T47.3x3-	T47.3x4-	T47.3x5-	T47.3x6-
Eptazocine	T40.4x1-	T40.4x2-	T40.4x3-	T40.4x4-	T40.4x5-	T40.4x6-
Equanil	T43.591-	T43.592-	T43.593-	T43.594-	T43.595-	T43.596-
Equisetum	T62.2x1-	T62.2x2-	T62.2x3-	T62.2x4-	—	—
diuretic	T50.2x1-	T50.2x2-	T50.2x3-	T50.2x4-	T50.2x5-	T50.2x6-
Ergobasine	T48.0x1-	T48.0x2-	T48.0x3-	T48.0x4-	T48.0x5-	T48.0x6-
Ergocalciferol	T45.2x1-	T45.2x2-	T45.2x3-	T45.2x4-	T45.2x5-	T45.2x6-
Ergoloid mesylates	T46.7x1-	T46.7x2-	T46.7x3-	T46.7x4-	T46.7x5-	T46.7x6-
Ergometrine	T48.0x1-	T48.0x2-	T48.0x3-	T48.0x4-	T48.0x5-	T48.0x6-
Ergonovine	T48.0x1-	T48.0x2-	T48.0x3-	T48.0x4-	T48.0x5-	T48.0x6-
Ergot NEC	T64.81x-	T64.82x-	T64.83x-	T64.84x-	—	—
derivative	T48.0x1-	T48.0x2-	T48.0x3-	T48.0x4-	T48.0x5-	T48.0x6-
medicinal (alkaloids)	T48.0x1-	T48.0x2-	T48.0x3-	T48.0x4-	T48.0x5-	T48.0x6-
prepared	T48.0x1-	T48.0x2-	T48.0x3-	T48.0x4-	T48.0x5-	T48.0x6-
Ergotamine	T46.5x1-	T46.5x2-	T46.5x3-	T46.5x4-	T46.5x5-	T46.5x6-
Ergotocine	T48.0x1-	T48.0x2-	T48.0x3-	T48.0x4-	T48.0x5-	T48.0x6-
Ergotrate	T48.0x1-	T48.0x2-	T48.0x3-	T48.0x4-	T48.0x5-	T48.0x6-
Eritrityl tetranitrate	T46.3x1-	T46.3x2-	T46.3x3-	T46.3x4-	T46.3x5-	T46.3x6-
Erythrityl tetranitrate	T46.3x1-	T46.3x2-	T46.3x3-	T46.3x4-	T46.3x5-	T46.3x6-
Erythrol tetranitrate	T46.3x1-	T46.3x2-	T46.3x3-	T46.3x4-	T46.3x5-	T46.3x6-
Erythromycin (salts)	T36.3x1-	T36.3x2-	T36.3x3-	T36.3x4-	T36.3x5-	T36.3x6-
ophthalmic preparation	T49.5x1-	T49.5x2-	T49.5x3-	T49.5x4-	T49.5x5-	T49.5x6-
topical NEC	T49.0x1-	T49.0x2-	T49.0x3-	T49.0x4-	T49.0x5-	T49.0x6-
Erythropoietin	T45.8x1-	T45.8x2-	T45.8x3-	T45.8x4-	T45.8x5-	T45.8x6-
human	T45.8x1-	T45.8x2-	T45.8x3-	T45.8x4-	T45.8x5-	T45.8x6-
Escin	T46.991-	T46.992-	T46.993-	T46.994-	T46.995-	T46.996-
Esculin	T45.2x1-	T45.2x2-	T45.2x3-	T45.2x4-	T45.2x5-	T45.2x6-
Esculoside	T45.2x1-	T45.2x2-	T45.2x3-	T45.2x4-	T45.2x5-	T45.2x6-
ESDT (ether-soluble tar distillate)	T49.1x1-	T49.1x2-	T49.1x3-	T49.1x4-	T49.1x5-	T49.1x6-
Eserine	T49.5x1-	T49.5x2-	T49.5x3-	T49.5x4-	T49.5x5-	T49.5x6-
Esflurbiprofen	T39.311-	T39.312-	T39.313-	T39.314-	T39.315-	T39.316-
Eskabarb	T42.3x1-	T42.3x2-	T42.3x3-	T42.3x4-	T42.3x5-	T42.3x6-
Eskalith	T43.8x1-	T43.8x2-	T43.8x3-	T43.8x4-	T43.8x5-	T43.8x6-
Esmolol	T44.7x1-	T44.7x2-	T44.7x3-	T44.7x4-	T44.7x5-	T44.7x6-
Estanozolol	T38.7x1-	T38.7x2-	T38.7x3-	T38.7x4-	T38.7x5-	T38.7x6-
Estazolam	T42.4x1-	T42.4x2-	T42.4x3-	T42.4x4-	T42.4x5-	T42.4x6-
Estradiol	T38.5x1-	T38.5x2-	T38.5x3-	T38.5x4-	T38.5x5-	T38.5x6-
with testosterone	T38.7x1-	T38.7x2-	T38.7x3-	T38.7x4-	T38.7x5-	T38.7x6-
benzoate	T38.5x1-	T38.5x2-	T38.5x3-	T38.5x4-	T38.5x5-	T38.5x6-
Estramustine	T45.1x1-	T45.1x2-	T45.1x3-	T45.1x4-	T45.1x5-	T45.1x6-
Estriol	T38.5x1-	T38.5x2-	T38.5x3-	T38.5x4-	T38.5x5-	T38.5x6-
Estrogen	T38.5x1-	T38.5x2-	T38.5x3-	T38.5x4-	T38.5x5-	T38.5x6-
with progesterone	T38.5x1-	T38.5x2-	T38.5x3-	T38.5x4-	T38.5x5-	T38.5x6-
conjugated	T38.5x1-	T38.5x2-	T38.5x3-	T38.5x4-	T38.5x5-	T38.5x6-
Estrone	T38.5x1-	T38.5x2-	T38.5x3-	T38.5x4-	T38.5x5-	T38.5x6-
Estropipate	T38.5x1-	T38.5x2-	T38.5x3-	T38.5x4-	T38.5x5-	T38.5x6-
Etacrynate sodium	T50.1x1-	T50.1x2-	T50.1x3-	T50.1x4-	T50.1x5-	T50.1x6-
Etacrynic acid	T50.1x1-	T50.1x2-	T50.1x3-	T50.1x4-	T50.1x5-	T50.1x6-
Etafedrine	T48.6x1-	T48.6x2-	T48.6x3-	T48.6x4-	T48.6x5-	T48.6x6-
Etafenone	T46.3x1-	T46.3x2-	T46.3x3-	T46.3x4-	T46.3x5-	T46.3x6-
Etambutol	T37.1x1-	T37.1x2-	T37.1x3-	T37.1x4-	T37.1x5-	T37.1x6-

Table of Drugs & Chemicals	POISONING				Adverse Effect	Underdosing
	Accidental (Unintentional)	Self-Harm (Intentional)	Assault	Undetermined		
Etamiphyllin	T48.6x1-	T48.6x2-	T48.6x3-	T48.6x4-	T48.6x5-	T48.6x6-
Etamivan	T50.7x1-	T50.7x2-	T50.7x3-	T50.7x4-	T50.7x5-	T50.7x6-
Etamsylate	T45.7x1-	T45.7x2-	T45.7x3-	T45.7x4-	T45.7x5-	T45.7x6-
Etebenecid	T50.4x1-	T50.4x2-	T50.4x3-	T50.4x4-	T50.4x5-	T50.4x6-
Ethacridine	T49.0x1-	T49.0x2-	T49.0x3-	T49.0x4-	T49.0x5-	T49.0x6-
Ethacrynic acid	T50.1x1-	T50.1x2-	T50.1x3-	T50.1x4-	T50.1x5-	T50.1x6-
Ethadione	T42.2x1-	T42.2x2-	T42.2x3-	T42.2x4-	T42.2x5-	T42.2x6-
Ethambutol	T37.1x1-	T37.1x2-	T37.1x3-	T37.1x4-	T37.1x5-	T37.1x6-
Ethamide	T50.2x1-	T50.2x2-	T50.2x3-	T50.2x4-	T50.2x5-	T50.2x6-
Ethamivan	T50.7x1-	T50.7x2-	T50.7x3-	T50.7x4-	T50.7x5-	T50.7x6-
Ethamsylate	T45.7x1-	T45.7x2-	T45.7x3-	T45.7x4-	T45.7x5-	T45.7x6-
Ethanol	T51.0x1-	T51.0x2-	T51.0x3-	T51.0x4-	—	—
beverage	T51.0x1-	T51.0x2-	T51.0x3-	T51.0x4-	—	—
Ethanolamine oleate	T46.8x1-	T46.8x2-	T46.8x3-	T46.8x4-	T46.8x5-	T46.8x6-
Ethaverine	T44.3x1-	T44.3x2-	T44.3x3-	T44.3x4-	T44.3x5-	T44.3x6-
Ethchlorvynol	T42.6x1-	T42.6x2-	T42.6x3-	T42.6x4-	T42.6x5-	T42.6x6-
Ethebenecid	T50.4x1-	T50.4x2-	T50.4x3-	T50.4x4-	T50.4x5-	T50.4x6-
Ether (vapor)	T41.0x1-	T41.0x2-	T41.0x3-	T41.0x4-	T41.0x5-	T41.0x6-
anesthetic	T41.0x1-	T41.0x2-	T41.0x3-	T41.0x4-	T41.0x5-	T41.0x6-
divinyl	T41.0x1-	T41.0x2-	T41.0x3-	T41.0x4-	T41.0x5-	T41.0x6-
ethyl (medicinal)	T41.0x1-	T41.0x2-	T41.0x3-	T41.0x4-	T41.0x5-	T41.0x6-
nonmedicinal	T52.8x1-	T52.8x2-	T52.8x3-	T52.8x4-	—	—
petroleum — see Ligroin						
solvent	T52.8x1-	T52.8x2-	T52.8x3-	T52.8x4-	—	—
Ethiazide	T50.2x1-	T50.2x2-	T50.2x3-	T50.2x4-	T50.2x5-	T50.2x6-
Ethidium chloride (vapor)	T59.891-	T59.892-	T59.893-	T59.894-	—	—
Ethinamate	T42.6x1-	T42.6x2-	T42.6x3-	T42.6x4-	T42.6x5-	T42.6x6-
Ethinylestradiol, ethinyloestradiol	T38.5x1-	T38.5x2-	T38.5x3-	T38.5x4-	T38.5x5-	T38.5x6-
with						
levonorgestrel	T38.4x1-	T38.4x2-	T38.4x3-	T38.4x4-	T38.4x5-	T38.4x6-
norethisterone	T38.4x1-	T38.4x2-	T38.4x3-	T38.4x4-	T38.4x5-	T38.4x6-
Ethiodized oil (131 I)	T50.8x1-	T50.8x2-	T50.8x3-	T50.8x4-	T50.8x5-	T50.8x6-
Ethion	T60.0x1-	T60.0x2-	T60.0x3-	T60.0x4-	—	—
Ethionamide	T37.1x1-	T37.1x2-	T37.1x3-	T37.1x4-	T37.1x5-	T37.1x6-
Ethioniamide	T37.1x1-	T37.1x2-	T37.1x3-	T37.1x4-	T37.1x5-	T37.1x6-
Ethisterone	T38.5x1-	T38.5x2-	T38.5x3-	T38.5x4-	T38.5x5-	T38.5x6-
Ethobral	T42.3x1-	T42.3x2-	T42.3x3-	T42.3x4-	T42.3x5-	T42.3x6-
Ethocaine (infiltration) (topical)	T41.3x1-	T41.3x2-	T41.3x3-	T41.3x4-	T41.3x5-	T41.3x6-
nerve block (peripheral) (plexus)	T41.3x1-	T41.3x2-	T41.3x3-	T41.3x4-	T41.3x5-	T41.3x6-
spinal	T41.3x1-	T41.3x2-	T41.3x3-	T41.3x4-	T41.3x5-	T41.3x6-
Ethoheptazine	T40.4x1-	T40.4x2-	T40.4x3-	T40.4x4-	T40.4x5-	T40.4x6-
Ethopropazine	T44.3x1-	T44.3x2-	T44.3x3-	T44.3x4-	T44.3x5-	T44.3x6-
Ethosuximide	T42.2x1-	T42.2x2-	T42.2x3-	T42.2x4-	T42.2x5-	T42.2x6-
Ethotoin	T42.0x1-	T42.0x2-	T42.0x3-	T42.0x4-	T42.0x5-	T42.0x6-
Ethoxazene	T37.91x-	T37.92x-	T37.93x-	T37.94x-	T37.95x-	T37.96x-
Ethoxazorutoside	T46.991-	T46.992-	T46.993-	T46.994-	T46.995-	T46.996-
2-Ethoxyethanol	T52.3x1-	T52.3x2-	T52.3x3-	T52.3x4-	—	—
Ethoxzolamide	T50.2x1-	T50.2x2-	T50.2x3-	T50.2x4-	T50.2x5-	T50.2x6-
Ethyl						
acetate	T52.8x1-	T52.8x2-	T52.8x3-	T52.8x4-	—	—
alcohol	T51.0x1-	T51.0x2-	T51.0x3-	T51.0x4-	—	—
beverage	T51.0x1-	T51.0x2-	T51.0x3-	T51.0x4-	—	—
aldehyde (vapor)	T59.891-	T59.892-	T59.893-	T59.894-	—	—
liquid	T52.8x1-	T52.8x2-	T52.8x3-	T52.8x4-	—	—
aminobenzoate	T41.3x1-	T41.3x2-	T41.3x3-	T41.3x4-	T41.3x5-	T41.3x6-
aminophenothiazine	T43.3x1-	T43.3x2-	T43.3x3-	T43.3x4-	T43.3x5-	T43.3x6-
benzoate	T52.8x1-	T52.8x2-	T52.8x3-	T52.8x4-	—	—
biscoumacetate	T45.511-	T45.512-	T45.513-	T45.514-	T45.515-	T45.516-
bromide (anesthetic)	T41.0x1-	T41.0x2-	T41.0x3-	T41.0x4-	T41.0x5-	T41.0x6-
carbamate	T45.1x1-	T45.1x2-	T45.1x3-	T45.1x4-	T45.1x5-	T45.1x6-
carbinol	T51.3x1-	T51.3x2-	T51.3x3-	T51.3x4-	—	—
carbonate	T52.8x1-	T52.8x2-	T52.8x3-	T52.8x4-	—	—

Table of Drugs & Chemicals	POISONING				Adverse Effect	Underdosing
	Accidental (Unintentional)	Self-Harm (Intentional)	Assault	Undetermined		
Ethyl - continued						
chaulmoograte	T37.1x1-	T37.1x2-	T37.1x3-	T37.1x4-	T37.1x5-	T37.1x6-
chloride (anesthetic)	T41.0x1-	T41.0x2-	T41.0x3-	T41.0x4-	T41.0x5-	T41.0x6-
anesthetic (local)	T41.3x1-	T41.3x2-	T41.3x3-	T41.3x4-	T41.3x5-	T41.3x6-
inhaled	T41.0x1-	T41.0x2-	T41.0x3-	T41.0x4-	T41.0x5-	T41.0x6-
local	T49.4x1-	T49.4x2-	T49.4x3-	T49.4x4-	T49.4x5-	T49.4x6-
solvent	T53.6x1-	T53.6x2-	T53.6x3-	T53.6x4-	—	—
dibunate	T48.3x1-	T48.3x2-	T48.3x3-	T48.3x4-	T48.3x5-	T48.3x6-
dichloroarsine (vapor)	T57.0x1-	T57.0x2-	T57.0x3-	T57.0x4-	—	—
estranol	T38.7x1-	T38.7x2-	T38.7x3-	T38.7x4-	T38.7x5-	T38.7x6-
ether — see also Ether						
formate NEC (solvent)	T52.0x1-	T52.0x2-	T52.0x3-	T52.0x4-	—	—
fumarate	T49.4x1-	T49.4x2-	T49.4x3-	T49.4x4-	T49.4x5-	T49.4x6-
hydroxyisobutyrate NEC (solvent)	T52.8x1-	T52.8x2-	T52.8x3-	T52.8x4-	—	—
iodoacetate	T59.3x1-	T59.3x2-	T59.3x3-	T59.3x4-	—	—
lactate NEC (solvent)	T52.8x1-	T52.8x2-	T52.8x3-	T52.8x4-	—	—
loflazepate	T42.4x1-	T42.4x2-	T42.4x3-	T42.4x4-	T42.4x5-	T42.4x6-
mercuric chloride	T56.1x1-	T56.1x2-	T56.1x3-	T56.1x4-	—	—
methylcarbinol	T51.8x1-	T51.8x2-	T51.8x3-	T51.8x4-	—	—
morphine	T40.2x1-	T40.2x2-	T40.2x3-	T40.2x4-	T40.2x5-	T40.2x6-
noradrenaline	T48.6x1-	T48.6x2-	T48.6x3-	T48.6x4-	T48.6x5-	T48.6x6-
oxybutyrate NEC (solvent)	T52.8x1-	T52.8x2-	T52.8x3-	T52.8x4-	—	—
Ethylene (gas)	T59.891-	T59.892-	T59.893-	T59.894-	—	—
anesthetic (general)	T41.0x1-	T41.0x2-	T41.0x3-	T41.0x4-	T41.0x5-	T41.0x6-
chlorohydrin	T52.8x1-	T52.8x2-	T52.8x3-	T52.8x4-	—	—
vapor	T53.6x1-	T53.6x2-	T53.6x3-	T53.6x4-	—	—
dichloride	T52.8x1-	T52.8x2-	T52.8x3-	T52.8x4-	—	—
vapor	T53.6x1-	T53.6x2-	T53.6x3-	T53.6x4-	—	—
dinitrate	T52.3x1-	T52.3x2-	T52.3x3-	T52.3x4-	—	—
glycol(s)	T52.8x1-	T52.8x2-	T52.8x3-	T52.8x4-	—	—
dinitrate	T52.3x1-	T52.3x2-	T52.3x3-	T52.3x4-	—	—
monobutyl ether	T52.3x1-	T52.3x2-	T52.3x3-	T52.3x4-	—	—
imine	T54.1x1-	T54.1x2-	T54.1x3-	T54.1x4-	—	—
oxide (fumigant) (nonmedicinal)	T59.891-	T59.892-	T59.893-	T59.894-	—	—
medicinal	T49.0x1-	T49.0x2-	T49.0x3-	T49.0x4-	T49.0x5-	T49.0x6-
Ethylenediamine theophylline	T48.6x1-	T48.6x2-	T48.6x3-	T48.6x4-	T48.6x5-	T48.6x6-
Ethylenediaminetetra-acetic acid	T50.6x1-	T50.6x2-	T50.6x3-	T50.6x4-	T50.6x5-	T50.6x6-
Ethylenedinitrilotetra-acetate	T50.6x1-	T50.6x2-	T50.6x3-	T50.6x4-	T50.6x5-	T50.6x6-
Ethylestrenol	T38.7x1-	T38.7x2-	T38.7x3-	T38.7x4-	T38.7x5-	T38.7x6-
Ethylhydroxycellulose	T47.4x1-	T47.4x2-	T47.4x3-	T47.4x4-	T47.4x5-	T47.4x6-
Ethylidene						
chloride NEC	T53.6x1-	T53.6x2-	T53.6x3-	T53.6x4-	—	—
diacetate	T60.3x1-	T60.3x2-	T60.3x3-	T60.3x4-	—	—
dicoumarin	T45.511-	T45.512-	T45.513-	T45.514-	T45.515-	T45.516-
dicoumarol	T45.511-	T45.512-	T45.513-	T45.514-	T45.515-	T45.516-
diethyl ether	T52.0x1-	T52.0x2-	T52.0x3-	T52.0x4-	—	—
Ethylmorphine	T40.2x1-	T40.2x2-	T40.2x3-	T40.2x4-	T40.2x5-	T40.2x6-
Ethylnorepinephrine	T48.6x1-	T48.6x2-	T48.6x3-	T48.6x4-	T48.6x5-	T48.6x6-
Ethylparachlorphen-oxyisobutyrate	T46.6x1-	T46.6x2-	T46.6x3-	T46.6x4-	T46.6x5-	T46.6x6-
Ethynodiol	T38.4x1-	T38.4x2-	T38.4x3-	T38.4x4-	T38.4x5-	T38.4x6-
with mestranol diacetate	T38.4x1-	T38.4x2-	T38.4x3-	T38.4x4-	T38.4x5-	T38.4x6-
Etidocaine	T41.3x1-	T41.3x2-	T41.3x3-	T41.3x4-	T41.3x5-	T41.3x6-
infiltration (subcutaneous)	T41.3x1-	T41.3x2-	T41.3x3-	T41.3x4-	T41.3x5-	T41.3x6-
nerve (peripheral) (plexus)	T41.3x1-	T41.3x2-	T41.3x3-	T41.3x4-	T41.3x5-	T41.3x6-

Table of Drugs & Chemicals	POISONING Accidental (Unintentional)	Self-Harm (Intentional)	Assault	Undetermined	Adverse Effect	Underdosing
Etidronate	T50.991-	T50.992-	T50.993-	T50.994-	T50.995-	T50.996-
Etidronic acid (disodium salt)	T50.991-	T50.992-	T50.993-	T50.994-	T50.995-	T50.996-
Etifoxine	T42.6x1-	T42.6x2-	T42.6x3-	T42.6x4-	T42.6x5-	T42.6x6-
Etilefrine	T44.4x1-	T44.4x2-	T44.4x3-	T44.4x4-	T44.4x5-	T44.4x6-
Etilfen	T42.3x1-	T42.3x2-	T42.3x3-	T42.3x4-	T42.3x5-	T42.3x6-
Etinodiol	T38.4x1-	T38.4x2-	T38.4x3-	T38.4x4-	T38.4x5-	T38.4x6-
Etiroxate	T46.6x1-	T46.6x2-	T46.6x3-	T46.6x4-	T46.6x5-	T46.6x6-
Etizolam	T42.4x1-	T42.4x2-	T42.4x3-	T42.4x4-	T42.4x5-	T42.4x6-
Etodolac	T39.391-	T39.392-	T39.393-	T39.394-	T39.395-	T39.396-
Etofamide	T37.3x1-	T37.3x2-	T37.3x3-	T37.3x4-	T37.3x5-	T37.3x6-
Etofibrate	T46.6x1-	T46.6x2-	T46.6x3-	T46.6x4-	T46.6x5-	T46.6x6-
Etofylline	T46.7x1-	T46.7x2-	T46.7x3-	T46.7x4-	T46.7x5-	T46.7x6-
clofibrate	T46.6x1-	T46.6x2-	T46.6x3-	T46.6x4-	T46.6x5-	T46.6x6-
Etoglucid	T45.1x1-	T45.1x2-	T45.1x3-	T45.1x4-	T45.1x5-	T45.1x6-
Etomidate	T41.1x1-	T41.1x2-	T41.1x3-	T41.1x4-	T41.1x5-	T41.1x6-
Etomide	T39.8x1-	T39.8x2-	T39.8x3-	T39.8x4-	T39.8x5-	T39.8x6-
Etomidoline	T44.3x1-	T44.3x2-	T44.3x3-	T44.3x4-	T44.3x5-	T44.3x6-
Etoposide	T45.1x1-	T45.1x2-	T45.1x3-	T45.1x4-	T45.1x5-	T45.1x6-
Etorphine	T40.2x1-	T40.2x2-	T40.2x3-	T40.2x4-	T40.2x5-	T40.2x6-
Etoval	T42.3x1-	T42.3x2-	T42.3x3-	T42.3x4-	T42.3x5-	T42.3x6-
Etozolin	T50.1x1-	T50.1x2-	T50.1x3-	T50.1x4-	T50.1x5-	T50.1x6-
Etretinate	T50.991-	T50.992-	T50.993-	T50.994-	T50.995-	T50.996-
Etryptamine	T43.691-	T43.692-	T43.693-	T43.694-	T43.695-	T43.696-
Etybenzatropine	T44.3x1-	T44.3x2-	T44.3x3-	T44.3x4-	T44.3x5-	T44.3x6-
Etynodiol	T38.4x1-	T38.4x2-	T38.4x3-	T38.4x4-	T38.4x5-	T38.4x6-
Eucaine	T41.3x1-	T41.3x2-	T41.3x3-	T41.3x4-	T41.3x5-	T41.3x6-
Eucalyptus oil	T49.7x1-	T49.7x2-	T49.7x3-	T49.7x4-	T49.7x5-	T49.7x6-
Eucatropine	T49.5x1-	T49.5x2-	T49.5x3-	T49.5x4-	T49.5x5-	T49.5x6-
Eucodal	T40.2x1-	T40.2x2-	T40.2x3-	T40.2x4-	T40.2x5-	T40.2x6-
Euneryl	T42.3x1-	T42.3x2-	T42.3x3-	T42.3x4-	T42.3x5-	T42.3x6-
Euphthalmine	T44.3x1-	T44.3x2-	T44.3x3-	T44.3x4-	T44.3x5-	T44.3x6-
Eurax	T49.0x1-	T49.0x2-	T49.0x3-	T49.0x4-	T49.0x5-	T49.0x6-
Euresol	T49.4x1-	T49.4x2-	T49.4x3-	T49.4x4-	T49.4x5-	T49.4x6-
Euthroid	T38.1x1-	T38.1x2-	T38.1x3-	T38.1x4-	T38.1x5-	T38.1x6-
Evans blue	T50.8x1-	T50.8x2-	T50.8x3-	T50.8x4-	T50.8x5-	T50.8x6-
Evipal	T42.3x1-	T42.3x2-	T42.3x3-	T42.3x4-	T42.3x5-	T42.3x6-
sodium	T41.1x1-	T41.1x2-	T41.1x3-	T41.1x4-	T41.1x5-	T41.1x6-
Evipan	T42.3x1-	T42.3x2-	T42.3x3-	T42.3x4-	T42.3x5-	T42.3x6-
sodium	T41.1x1-	T41.1x2-	T41.1x3-	T41.1x4-	T41.1x5-	T41.1x6-
Exalamide	T49.0x1-	T49.0x2-	T49.0x3-	T49.0x4-	T49.0x5-	T49.0x6-
Exalgin	T39.1x1-	T39.1x2-	T39.1x3-	T39.1x4-	T39.1x5-	T39.1x6-
Excipients, pharmaceutical	T50.901-	T50.902-	T50.903-	T50.904-	T50.905-	T50.906-
Exhaust gas (engine) (motor vehicle)	T58.01x-	T58.02x-	T58.03x-	T58.04x-	—	—
Ex-Lax (phenolphthalein)	T47.2x1-	T47.2x2-	T47.2x3-	T47.2x4-	T47.2x5-	T47.2x6-
Expectorant NEC	T48.4x1-	T48.4x2-	T48.4x3-	T48.4x4-	T48.4x5-	T48.4x6-
Extended insulin zinc suspension	T38.3x1-	T38.3x2-	T38.3x3-	T38.3x4-	T38.3x5-	T38.3x6-
External medications (skin) (mucous membrane)	T49.91x-	T49.92x-	T49.93x-	T49.94x-	T49.95x-	T49.96x-
dental agent	T49.7x1-	T49.7x2-	T49.7x3-	T49.7x4-	T49.7x5-	T49.7x6-
ENT agent	T49.6x1-	T49.6x2-	T49.6x3-	T49.6x4-	T49.6x5-	T49.6x6-
ophthalmic preparation	T49.5x1-	T49.5x2-	T49.5x3-	T49.5x4-	T49.5x5-	T49.5x6-
specified NEC	T49.8x1-	T49.8x2-	T49.8x3-	T49.8x4-	T49.8x5-	T49.8x6-
Extrapyramidal antagonist NEC	T44.3x1-	T44.3x2-	T44.3x3-	T44.3x4-	T44.3x5-	T44.3x6-
Eye agents (anti-infective)	T49.5x1-	T49.5x2-	T49.5x3-	T49.5x4-	T49.5x5-	T49.5x6-
Eye drug NEC	T49.5x1-	T49.5x2-	T49.5x3-	T49.5x4-	T49.5x5-	T49.5x6-
FAC (fluorouracil + doxorubicin + cyclophosphamide)	T45.1x1-	T45.1x2-	T45.1x3-	T45.1x4-	T45.1x5-	T45.1x6-
Factor						
I (fibrinogen)	T45.8x1-	T45.8x2-	T45.8x3-	T45.8x4-	T45.8x5-	T45.8x6-
III (thromboplastin)	T45.8x1-	T45.8x2-	T45.8x3-	T45.8x4-	T45.8x5-	T45.8x6-
VIII (antihemophilic Factor) (concentrate)	T45.8x1-	T45.8x2-	T45.8x3-	T45.8x4-	T45.8x5-	T45.8x6-
IX complex	T45.7x1-	T45.7x2-	T45.7x3-	T45.7x4-	T45.7x5-	T45.7x6-
human	T45.8x1-	T45.8x2-	T45.8x3-	T45.8x4-	T45.8x5-	T45.8x6-
Famotidine	T47.0x1-	T47.0x2-	T47.0x3-	T47.0x4-	T47.0x5-	T47.0x6-
Fat suspension, intravenous	T50.991-	T50.992-	T50.993-	T50.994-	T50.995-	T50.996-
Fazadinium bromide	T48.1x1-	T48.1x2-	T48.1x3-	T48.1x4-	T48.1x5-	T48.1x6-
Febarbamate	T42.3x1-	T42.3x2-	T42.3x3-	T42.3x4-	T42.3x5-	T42.3x6-
Fecal softener	T47.4x1-	T47.4x2-	T47.4x3-	T47.4x4-	T47.4x5-	T47.4x6-
Fedrilate	T48.3x1-	T48.3x2-	T48.3x3-	T48.3x4-	T48.3x5-	T48.3x6-
Felodipine	T46.1x1-	T46.1x2-	T46.1x3-	T46.1x4-	T46.1x5-	T46.1x6-
Felypressin	T38.891-	T38.892-	T38.893-	T38.894-	T38.895-	T38.896-
Femoxetine	T43.221-	T43.222-	T43.223-	T43.224-	T43.225-	T43.226-
Fenalcomine	T46.3x1-	T46.3x2-	T46.3x3-	T46.3x4-	T46.3x5-	T46.3x6-
Fenamisal	T37.1x1-	T37.1x2-	T37.1x3-	T37.1x4-	T37.1x5-	T37.1x6-
Fenazone	T39.2x1-	T39.2x2-	T39.2x3-	T39.2x4-	T39.2x5-	T39.2x6-
Fenbendazole	T37.4x1-	T37.4x2-	T37.4x3-	T37.4x4-	T37.4x5-	T37.4x6-
Fenbutrazate	T50.5x1-	T50.5x2-	T50.5x3-	T50.5x4-	T50.5x5-	T50.5x6-
Fencamfamine	T43.691-	T43.692-	T43.693-	T43.694-	T43.695-	T43.696-
Fendiline	T46.1x1-	T46.1x2-	T46.1x3-	T46.1x4-	T46.1x5-	T46.1x6-
Fenetylline	T43.691-	T43.692-	T43.693-	T43.694-	T43.695-	T43.696-
Fenflumizole	T39.391-	T39.392-	T39.393-	T39.394-	T39.395-	T39.396-
Fenfluramine	T50.5x1-	T50.5x2-	T50.5x3-	T50.5x4-	T50.5x5-	T50.5x6-
Fenobarbital	T42.3x1-	T42.3x2-	T42.3x3-	T42.3x4-	T42.3x5-	T42.3x6-
Fenofibrate	T46.6x1-	T46.6x2-	T46.6x3-	T46.6x4-	T46.6x5-	T46.6x6-
Fenoprofen	T39.311-	T39.312-	T39.313-	T39.314-	T39.315-	T39.316-
Fenoterol	T48.6x1-	T48.6x2-	T48.6x3-	T48.6x4-	T48.6x5-	T48.6x6-
Fenoverine	T44.3x1-	T44.3x2-	T44.3x3-	T44.3x4-	T44.3x5-	T44.3x6-
Fenoxazoline	T48.5x1-	T48.5x2-	T48.5x3-	T48.5x4-	T48.5x5-	T48.5x6-
Fenproporex	T50.5x1-	T50.5x2-	T50.5x3-	T50.5x4-	T50.5x5-	T50.5x6-
Fenquizone	T50.2x1-	T50.2x2-	T50.2x3-	T50.2x4-	T50.2x5-	T50.2x6-
Fentanyl	T40.4x1-	T40.4x2-	T40.4x3-	T40.4x4-	T40.4x5-	T40.4x6-
Fentazin	T43.3x1-	T43.3x2-	T43.3x3-	T43.3x4-	T43.3x5-	T43.3x6-
Fenthion	T60.0x1-	T60.0x2-	T60.0x3-	T60.0x4-	—	—
Fenticlor	T49.0x1-	T49.0x2-	T49.0x3-	T49.0x4-	T49.0x5-	T49.0x6-
Fenylbutazone	T39.2x1-	T39.2x2-	T39.2x3-	T39.2x4-	T39.2x5-	T39.2x6-
Feprazone	T39.2x1-	T39.2x2-	T39.2x3-	T39.2x4-	T39.2x5-	T39.2x6-
Fer de lance (bite) (venom)	T63.061-	T63.062-	T63.063-	T63.064-	—	—
Ferric — see also Iron						
chloride	T45.4x1-	T45.4x2-	T45.4x3-	T45.4x4-	T45.4x5-	T45.4x6-
citrate	T45.4x1-	T45.4x2-	T45.4x3-	T45.4x4-	T45.4x5-	T45.4x6-
hydroxide						
colloidal	T45.4x1-	T45.4x2-	T45.4x3-	T45.4x4-	T45.4x5-	T45.4x6-
polymaltose	T45.4x1-	T45.4x2-	T45.4x3-	T45.4x4-	T45.4x5-	T45.4x6-
pyrophosphate	T45.4x1-	T45.4x2-	T45.4x3-	T45.4x4-	T45.4x5-	T45.4x6-
Ferritin	T45.4x1-	T45.4x2-	T45.4x3-	T45.4x4-	T45.4x5-	T45.4x6-
Ferrocholinate	T45.4x1-	T45.4x2-	T45.4x3-	T45.4x4-	T45.4x5-	T45.4x6-
Ferrodextrane	T45.4x1-	T45.4x2-	T45.4x3-	T45.4x4-	T45.4x5-	T45.4x6-
Ferropolimaler	T45.4x1-	T45.4x2-	T45.4x3-	T45.4x4-	T45.4x5-	T45.4x6-
Ferrous — see also Iron						
phosphate	T45.4x1-	T45.4x2-	T45.4x3-	T45.4x4-	T45.4x5-	T45.4x6-
salt	T45.4x1-	T45.4x2-	T45.4x3-	T45.4x4-	T45.4x5-	T45.4x6-
with folic acid	T45.4x1-	T45.4x2-	T45.4x3-	T45.4x4-	T45.4x5-	T45.4x6-
Ferrous fumarate, gluconate, lactate, salt NEC, sulfate (medicinal)	T45.4x1-	T45.4x2-	T45.4x3-	T45.4x4-	T45.4x5-	T45.4x6-
Ferrovanadium (fumes)	T59.891-	T59.892-	T59.893-	T59.894-	—	—
Ferrum — see Iron						
Fertilizers NEC	T65.891-	T65.892-	T65.893-	T65.894-	—	—
with herbicide mixture	T60.3x1-	T60.3x2-	T60.3x3-	T60.3x4-	—	—

Table of Drugs & Chemicals	POISONING				Adverse Effect	Underdosing
	Accidental (Unintentional)	Self-Harm (Intentional)	Assault	Undetermined		
Fetoxilate	T47.6x1-	T47.6x2-	T47.6x3-	T47.6x4-	T47.6x5-	T47.6x6-
Fiber, dietary	T47.4x1-	T47.4x2-	T47.4x3-	T47.4x4-	T47.4x5-	T47.4x6-
Fiberglass	T65.831-	T65.832-	T65.833-	T65.834-	—	—
Fibrinogen (human)	T45.8x1-	T45.8x2-	T45.8x3-	T45.8x4-	T45.8x5-	T45.8x6-
Fibrinolysin (human)	T45.691-	T45.692-	T45.693-	T45.694-	T45.695-	T45.696-
Fibrinolysis						
affecting drug	T45.601-	T45.602-	T45.603-	T45.604-	T45.605-	T45.606-
inhibitor NEC	T45.621-	T45.622-	T45.623-	T45.624-	T45.625-	T45.626-
Fibrinolytic drug	T45.611-	T45.612-	T45.613-	T45.614-	T45.615-	T45.616-
Filix mas	T37.4x1-	T37.4x2-	T37.4x3-	T37.4x4-	T37.4x5-	T37.4x6-
Filtering cream	T49.3x1-	T49.3x2-	T49.3x3-	T49.3x4-	T49.3x5-	T49.3x6-
Fiorinal	T39.011-	T39.012-	T39.013-	T39.014-	T39.015-	T39.016-
Firedamp	T59.891-	T59.892-	T59.893-	T59.894-	—	—
Fish, noxious, nonbacterial	T61.91x-	T61.92x-	T61.93x-	T61.94x-	—	—
ciguatera	T61.01x-	T61.02x-	T61.03x-	T61.04x-	—	—
scombroid	T61.11x-	T61.12x-	T61.13x-	T61.14x-	—	—
shell	T61.781-	T61.782-	T61.783-	T61.784-	—	—
specified NEC	T61.771-	T61.772-	T61.773-	T61.774-	—	—
Flagyl	T37.3x1-	T37.3x2-	T37.3x3-	T37.3x4-	T37.3x5-	T37.3x6-
Flavine adenine dinucleotide	T45.2x1-	T45.2x2-	T45.2x3-	T45.2x4-	T45.2x5-	T45.2x6-
Flavodic acid	T46.991-	T46.992-	T46.993-	T46.994-	T46.995-	T46.996-
Flavoxate	T44.3x1-	T44.3x2-	T44.3x3-	T44.3x4-	T44.3x5-	T44.3x6-
Flaxedil	T48.1x1-	T48.1x2-	T48.1x3-	T48.1x4-	T48.1x5-	T48.1x6-
Flaxseed (medicinal)	T49.3x1-	T49.3x2-	T49.3x3-	T49.3x4-	T49.3x5-	T49.3x6-
Flecainide	T46.2x1-	T46.2x2-	T46.2x3-	T46.2x4-	T46.2x5-	T46.2x6-
Fleroxacin	T36.8x1-	T36.8x2-	T36.8x3-	T36.8x4-	T36.8x5-	T36.8x6-
Floctafenine	T39.8x1-	T39.8x2-	T39.8x3-	T39.8x4-	T39.8x5-	T39.8x6-
Flomax	T44.6x1-	T44.6x2-	T44.6x3-	T44.6x4-	T44.6x5-	T44.6x6-
Flomoxef	T36.1x1-	T36.1x2-	T36.1x3-	T36.1x4-	T36.1x5-	T36.1x6-
Flopropione	T44.3x1-	T44.3x2-	T44.3x3-	T44.3x4-	T44.3x5-	T44.3x6-
Florantyrone	T47.5x1-	T47.5x2-	T47.5x3-	T47.5x4-	T47.5x5-	T47.5x6-
Floraquin	T37.8x1-	T37.8x2-	T37.8x3-	T37.8x4-	T37.8x5-	T37.8x6-
Florinef	T38.0x1-	T38.0x2-	T38.0x3-	T38.0x4-	T38.0x5-	T38.0x6-
ENT agent	T49.6x1-	T49.6x2-	T49.6x3-	T49.6x4-	T49.6x5-	T49.6x6-
ophthalmic preparation	T49.5x1-	T49.5x2-	T49.5x3-	T49.5x4-	T49.5x5-	T49.5x6-
topical NEC	T49.0x1-	T49.0x2-	T49.0x3-	T49.0x4-	T49.0x5-	T49.0x6-
Flowers of sulfur	T49.4x1-	T49.4x2-	T49.4x3-	T49.4x4-	T49.4x5-	T49.4x6-
Floxuridine	T45.1x1-	T45.1x2-	T45.1x3-	T45.1x4-	T45.1x5-	T45.1x6-
Fluanisone	T43.4x1-	T43.4x2-	T43.4x3-	T43.4x4-	T43.4x5-	T43.4x6-
Flubendazole	T37.4x1-	T37.4x2-	T37.4x3-	T37.4x4-	T37.4x5-	T37.4x6-
Fluclorolone acetonide	T49.0x1-	T49.0x2-	T49.0x3-	T49.0x4-	T49.0x5-	T49.0x6-
Flucloxacillin	T36.0x1-	T36.0x2-	T36.0x3-	T36.0x4-	T36.0x5-	T36.0x6-
Fluconazole	T37.8x1-	T37.8x2-	T37.8x3-	T37.8x4-	T37.8x5-	T37.8x6-
Flucytosine	T37.8x1-	T37.8x2-	T37.8x3-	T37.8x4-	T37.8x5-	T37.8x6-
Fludeoxyglucose (18F)	T50.8x1-	T50.8x2-	T50.8x3-	T50.8x4-	T50.8x5-	T50.8x6-
Fludiazepam	T42.4x1-	T42.4x2-	T42.4x3-	T42.4x4-	T42.4x5-	T42.4x6-
Fludrocortisone	T50.0x1-	T50.0x2-	T50.0x3-	T50.0x4-	T50.0x5-	T50.0x6-
ENT agent	T49.6x1-	T49.6x2-	T49.6x3-	T49.6x4-	T49.6x5-	T49.6x6-
ophthalmic preparation	T49.5x1-	T49.5x2-	T49.5x3-	T49.5x4-	T49.5x5-	T49.5x6-
topical NEC	T49.0x1-	T49.0x2-	T49.0x3-	T49.0x4-	T49.0x5-	T49.0x6-
Fludroxycortide	T49.0x1-	T49.0x2-	T49.0x3-	T49.0x4-	T49.0x5-	T49.0x6-
Flufenamic acid	T39.391-	T39.392-	T39.393-	T39.394-	T39.395-	T39.396-
Fluindione	T45.511-	T45.512-	T45.513-	T45.514-	T45.515-	T45.516-
Flumequine	T37.8x1-	T37.8x2-	T37.8x3-	T37.8x4-	T37.8x5-	T37.8x6-
Flumethasone	T49.0x1-	T49.0x2-	T49.0x3-	T49.0x4-	T49.0x5-	T49.0x6-
Flumethiazide	T50.2x1-	T50.2x2-	T50.2x3-	T50.2x4-	T50.2x5-	T50.2x6-
Flumidin	T37.5x1-	T37.5x2-	T37.5x3-	T37.5x4-	T37.5x5-	T37.5x6-
Flunarizine	T46.7x1-	T46.7x2-	T46.7x3-	T46.7x4-	T46.7x5-	T46.7x6-
Flunidazole	T37.8x1-	T37.8x2-	T37.8x3-	T37.8x4-	T37.8x5-	T37.8x6-
Flunisolide	T48.6x1-	T48.6x2-	T48.6x3-	T48.6x4-	T48.6x5-	T48.6x6-
Flunitrazepam	T42.4x1-	T42.4x2-	T42.4x3-	T42.4x4-	T42.4x5-	T42.4x6-

Table of Drugs & Chemicals	POISONING				Adverse Effect	Underdosing
	Accidental (Unintentional)	Self-Harm (Intentional)	Assault	Undetermined		
Fluocinolone (acetonide)	T49.0x1-	T49.0x2-	T49.0x3-	T49.0x4-	T49.0x5-	T49.0x6-
Fluocinonide	T49.0x1-	T49.0x2-	T49.0x3-	T49.0x4-	T49.0x5-	T49.0x6-
Fluocortin (butyl)	T49.0x1-	T49.0x2-	T49.0x3-	T49.0x4-	T49.0x5-	T49.0x6-
Fluocortolone	T49.0x1-	T49.0x2-	T49.0x3-	T49.0x4-	T49.0x5-	T49.0x6-
Fluohydrocortisone	T38.0x1-	T38.0x2-	T38.0x3-	T38.0x4-	T38.0x5-	T38.0x6-
ENT agent	T49.6x1-	T49.6x2-	T49.6x3-	T49.6x4-	T49.6x5-	T49.6x6-
ophthalmic preparation	T49.5x1-	T49.5x2-	T49.5x3-	T49.5x4-	T49.5x5-	T49.5x6-
topical NEC	T49.0x1-	T49.0x2-	T49.0x3-	T49.0x4-	T49.0x5-	T49.0x6-
Fluonid	T49.0x1-	T49.0x2-	T49.0x3-	T49.0x4-	T49.0x5-	T49.0x6-
Fluopromazine	T43.3x1-	T43.3x2-	T43.3x3-	T43.3x4-	T43.3x5-	T43.3x6-
Fluoracetate	T60.8x1-	T60.8x2-	T60.8x3-	T60.8x4-	—	—
Fluorescein	T50.8x1-	T50.8x2-	T50.8x3-	T50.8x4-	T50.8x5-	T50.8x6-
Fluorhydrocortisone	T50.0x1-	T50.0x2-	T50.0x3-	T50.0x4-	T50.0x5-	T50.0x6-
Fluoride (nonmedicinal) (pesticide) (sodium) NEC	T60.8x1-	T60.8x2-	T60.8x3-	T60.8x4-	—	—
hydrogen — see Hydrofluoric acid						
medicinal NEC	T50.991-	T50.992-	T50.993-	T50.994-	T50.995-	T50.996-
dental use	T49.7x1-	T49.7x2-	T49.7x3-	T49.7x4-	T49.7x5-	T49.7x6-
not pesticide NEC	T54.91x-	T54.92x-	T54.93x-	T54.94x-	—	—
stannous	T49.7x1-	T49.7x2-	T49.7x3-	T49.7x4-	T49.7x5-	T49.7x6-
Fluorinated corticosteroids	T38.0x1-	T38.0x2-	T38.0x3-	T38.0x4-	T38.0x5-	T38.0x6-
Fluorine (gas)	T59.5x1-	T59.5x2-	T59.5x3-	T59.5x4-	—	—
salt — see Fluoride(s)						
Fluoristan	T49.7x1-	T49.7x2-	T49.7x3-	T49.7x4-	T49.7x5-	T49.7x6-
Fluormetholone	T49.0x1-	T49.0x2-	T49.0x3-	T49.0x4-	T49.0x5-	T49.0x6-
Fluoroacetate	T60.8x1-	T60.8x2-	T60.8x3-	T60.8x4-	—	—
Fluorocarbon monomer	T53.6x1-	T53.6x2-	T53.6x3-	T53.6x4-	—	—
Fluorocytosine	T37.8x1-	T37.8x2-	T37.8x3-	T37.8x4-	T37.8x5-	T37.8x6-
Fluorodeoxyuridine	T45.1x1-	T45.1x2-	T45.1x3-	T45.1x4-	T45.1x5-	T45.1x6-
Fluorometholone	T49.0x1-	T49.0x2-	T49.0x3-	T49.0x4-	T49.0x5-	T49.0x6-
ophthalmic preparation	T49.5x1-	T49.5x2-	T49.5x3-	T49.5x4-	T49.5x5-	T49.5x6-
Fluorophosphate insecticide	T60.0x1-	T60.0x2-	T60.0x3-	T60.0x4-	—	—
Fluorosol	T46.3x1-	T46.3x2-	T46.3x3-	T46.3x4-	T46.3x5-	T46.3x6-
Fluorouracil	T45.1x1-	T45.1x2-	T45.1x3-	T45.1x4-	T45.1x5-	T45.1x6-
Fluorphenylalanine	T49.5x1-	T49.5x2-	T49.5x3-	T49.5x4-	T49.5x5-	T49.5x6-
Fluothane	T41.0x1-	T41.0x2-	T41.0x3-	T41.0x4-	T41.0x5-	T41.0x6-
Fluoxetine	T43.221-	T43.222-	T43.223-	T43.224-	T43.225-	T43.226-
Fluoxymesterone	T38.7x1-	T38.7x2-	T38.7x3-	T38.7x4-	T38.7x5-	T38.7x6-
Flupenthixol	T43.4x1-	T43.4x2-	T43.4x3-	T43.4x4-	T43.4x5-	T43.4x6-
Flupentixol	T43.4x1-	T43.4x2-	T43.4x3-	T43.4x4-	T43.4x5-	T43.4x6-
Fluphenazine	T43.3x1-	T43.3x2-	T43.3x3-	T43.3x4-	T43.3x5-	T43.3x6-
Fluprednidene	T49.0x1-	T49.0x2-	T49.0x3-	T49.0x4-	T49.0x5-	T49.0x6-
Fluprednisolone	T38.0x1-	T38.0x2-	T38.0x3-	T38.0x4-	T38.0x5-	T38.0x6-
Fluradoline	T39.8x1-	T39.8x2-	T39.8x3-	T39.8x4-	T39.8x5-	T39.8x6-
Flurandrenolide	T49.0x1-	T49.0x2-	T49.0x3-	T49.0x4-	T49.0x5-	T49.0x6-
Flurandrenolone	T49.0x1-	T49.0x2-	T49.0x3-	T49.0x4-	T49.0x5-	T49.0x6-
Flurazepam	T42.4x1-	T42.4x2-	T42.4x3-	T42.4x4-	T42.4x5-	T42.4x6-
Flurbiprofen	T39.311-	T39.312-	T39.313-	T39.314-	T39.315-	T39.316-
Flurobate	T49.0x1-	T49.0x2-	T49.0x3-	T49.0x4-	T49.0x5-	T49.0x6-
Fluroxene	T41.0x1-	T41.0x2-	T41.0x3-	T41.0x4-	T41.0x5-	T41.0x6-
Fluspirilene	T43.591-	T43.592-	T43.593-	T43.594-	T43.595-	T43.596-
Flutamide	T38.6x1-	T38.6x2-	T38.6x3-	T38.6x4-	T38.6x5-	T38.6x6-
Flutazolam	T42.4x1-	T42.4x2-	T42.4x3-	T42.4x4-	T42.4x5-	T42.4x6-
Fluticasone propionate	T49.1x1-	T49.1x2-	T49.1x3-	T49.1x4-	T49.1x5-	T49.1x6-
Flutoprazepam	T42.4x1-	T42.4x2-	T42.4x3-	T42.4x4-	T42.4x5-	T42.4x6-
Flutropium bromide	T48.6x1-	T48.6x2-	T48.6x3-	T48.6x4-	T48.6x5-	T48.6x6-
Fluvoxamine	T43.221-	T43.222-	T43.223-	T43.224-	T43.225-	T43.226-
Folacin	T45.8x1-	T45.8x2-	T45.8x3-	T45.8x4-	T45.8x5-	T45.8x6-

DRUGS & CHEMICALS

Table of Drugs & Chemicals	POISONING Accidental (Unintentional)	Self-Harm (Intentional)	Assault	Undetermined	Adverse Effect	Underdosing
Folic acid	T45.8x1-	T45.8x2-	T45.8x3-	T45.8x4-	T45.8x5-	T45.8x6-
with ferrous salt	T45.2x1-	T45.2x2-	T45.2x3-	T45.2x4-	T45.2x5-	T45.2x6-
antagonist	T45.1x1-	T45.1x2-	T45.1x3-	T45.1x4-	T45.1x5-	T45.1x6-
Folinic acid	T45.8x1-	T45.8x2-	T45.8x3-	T45.8x4-	T45.8x5-	T45.8x6-
Folium stramoniae	T48.6x1-	T48.6x2-	T48.6x3-	T48.6x4-	T48.6x5-	T48.6x6-
Follicle-stimulating hormone, human	T38.811-	T38.812-	T38.813-	T38.814-	T38.815-	T38.816-
Folpet	T60.3x1-	T60.3x2-	T60.3x3-	T60.3x4-	—	—
Fominoben	T48.3x1-	T48.3x2-	T48.3x3-	T48.3x4-	T48.3x5-	T48.3x6-
Food, foodstuffs, noxious, nonbacterial, NEC	T62.91x-	T62.92x-	T62.93x-	T62.94x-	—	—
berries	T62.1x1-	T62.1x2-	T62.1x3-	T62.1x4-	—	—
fish — see also Fish	T61.91x-	T61.92x-	T61.93x-	T61.94x-	—	—
mushrooms	T62.0x1-	T62.0x2-	T62.0x3-	T62.0x4-	—	—
plants	T62.2x1-	T62.2x2-	T62.2x3-	T62.2x4-	—	—
seafood	T61.91x-	T61.92x-	T61.93x-	T61.94x-	—	—
specified NEC	T61.8x1-	T61.8x2-	T61.8x3-	T61.8x4-	—	—
seeds	T62.2x1-	T62.2x2-	T62.2x3-	T62.2x4-	—	—
shellfish	T61.781-	T61.782-	T61.783-	T61.784-	—	—
specified NEC	T62.8x1-	T62.8x2-	T62.8x3-	T62.8x4-	—	—
Fool's parsley	T62.2x1-	T62.2x2-	T62.2x3-	T62.2x4-	—	—
Formaldehyde (solution), gas or vapor	T59.2x1-	T59.2x2-	T59.2x3-	T59.2x4-	—	—
fungicide	T60.3x1-	T60.3x2-	T60.3x3-	T60.3x4-	—	—
Formalin	T59.2x1-	T59.2x2-	T59.2x3-	T59.2x4-	—	—
fungicide	T60.3x1-	T60.3x2-	T60.3x3-	T60.3x4-	—	—
vapor	T59.2x1-	T59.2x2-	T59.2x3-	T59.2x4-	—	—
Formic acid	T54.2x1-	T54.2x2-	T54.2x3-	T54.2x4-	—	—
vapor	T59.891-	T59.892-	T59.893-	T59.894-	—	—
Foscarnet sodium	T37.5x1-	T37.5x2-	T37.5x3-	T37.5x4-	T37.5x5-	T37.5x6-
Fosfestrol	T38.5x1-	T38.5x2-	T38.5x3-	T38.5x4-	T38.5x5-	T38.5x6-
Fosfomycin	T36.8x1-	T36.8x2-	T36.8x3-	T36.8x4-	T36.8x5-	T36.8x6-
Fosfonet sodium	T37.5x1-	T37.5x2-	T37.5x3-	T37.5x4-	T37.5x5-	T37.5x6-
Fosinopril	T46.4x1-	T46.4x2-	T46.4x3-	T46.4x4-	T46.4x5-	T46.4x6-
sodium	T46.4x1-	T46.4x2-	T46.4x3-	T46.4x4-	T46.4x5-	T46.4x6-
Fowler's solution	T57.0x1-	T57.0x2-	T57.0x3-	T57.0x4-	—	—
Foxglove	T62.2x1-	T62.2x2-	T62.2x3-	T62.2x4-	—	—
Framycetin	T36.5x1-	T36.5x2-	T36.5x3-	T36.5x4-	T36.5x5-	T36.5x6-
Frangula	T47.2x1-	T47.2x2-	T47.2x3-	T47.2x4-	T47.2x5-	T47.2x6-
extract	T47.2x1-	T47.2x2-	T47.2x3-	T47.2x4-	T47.2x5-	T47.2x6-
Frei antigen	T50.8x1-	T50.8x2-	T50.8x3-	T50.8x4-	T50.8x5-	T50.8x6-
Freon	T53.5x1-	T53.5x2-	T53.5x3-	T53.5x4-	—	—
Fructose	T50.3x1-	T50.3x2-	T50.3x3-	T50.3x4-	T50.3x5-	T50.3x6-
Frusemide	T50.1x1-	T50.1x2-	T50.1x3-	T50.1x4-	T50.1x5-	T50.1x6-
FSH	T38.811-	T38.812-	T38.813-	T38.814-	T38.815-	T38.816-
Ftorafur	T45.1x1-	T45.1x2-	T45.1x3-	T45.1x4-	T45.1x5-	T45.1x6-
Fuel						
automobile	T52.0x1-	T52.0x2-	T52.0x3-	T52.0x4-	—	—
exhaust gas, not in transit	T58.01x-	T58.02x-	T58.03x-	T58.04x-	—	—
vapor NEC	T52.0x1-	T52.0x2-	T52.0x3-	T52.0x4-	—	—
gas (domestic use) — see also Carbon, monoxide, fuel, utility	T59.891-	T59.892-	T59.893-	T59.894-	—	—
utility	T59.891-	T59.892-	T59.893-	T59.894-	—	—
incomplete combustion of — see Carbon, monoxide, fuel, utility						
in mobile container	T59.891-	T59.892-	T59.893-	T59.894-	—	—
piped (natural)	T59.891-	T59.892-	T59.893-	T59.894-	—	—
industrial, incomplete combustion	T58.8x1-	T58.8x2-	T58.8x3-	T58.8x4-	—	—
Fugillin	T36.8x1-	T36.8x2-	T36.8x3-	T36.8x4-	T36.8x5-	T36.8x6-
Fulminate of mercury	T56.1x1-	T56.1x2-	T56.1x3-	T56.1x4-	—	—
Fulvicin	T36.7x1-	T36.7x2-	T36.7x3-	T36.7x4-	T36.7x5-	T36.7x6-
Fumadil	T36.8x1-	T36.8x2-	T36.8x3-	T36.8x4-	T36.8x5-	T36.8x6-
Fumagillin	T36.8x1-	T36.8x2-	T36.8x3-	T36.8x4-	T36.8x5-	T36.8x6-
Fumaric acid	T49.4x1-	T49.4x2-	T49.4x3-	T49.4x4-	T49.4x5-	T49.4x6-
Fumes (from)	T59.91x-	T59.92x-	T59.93x-	T59.94x-	—	—
carbon monoxide — see Carbon, monoxide						
charcoal (domestic use) — see Charcoal, fumes						
chloroform — see Chloroform						
coke (in domestic stoves, fireplaces) — see Coke fumes						
corrosive NEC	T54.91x-	T54.92x-	T54.93x-	T54.94x-	—	—
ether — see Ether						
freons	T53.5x1-	T53.5x2-	T53.5x3-	T53.5x4-	—	—
hydrocarbons	T59.891-	T59.892-	T59.893-	T59.894-	—	—
petroleum (liquefied) distributed through pipes (pure or mixed with air)	T59.891-	T59.892-	T59.893-	T59.894-	—	—
lead — see Lead						
metal — see Metals, or the specified metal						
nitrogen dioxide	T59.0x1-	T59.0x2-	T59.0x3-	T59.0x4-	—	—
pesticides — see Pesticides						
petroleum (liquefied) distributed through pipes (pure or mixed with air)	T59.891-	T59.892-	T59.893-	T59.894-	—	—
polyester	T59.891-	T59.892-	T59.893-	T59.894-	—	—
specified source NEC — see also substance, specified	T59.891-	T59.892-	T59.893-	T59.894-	—	—
sulfur dioxide	T59.1x1-	T59.1x2-	T59.1x3-	T59.1x4-	—	—
Fumigant NEC	T60.91x-	T60.92x-	T60.93x-	T60.94x-	—	—
Fungi, noxious, used as food	T62.0x1-	T62.0x2-	T62.0x3-	T62.0x4-	—	—
Fungicide NEC (nonmedicinal)	T60.3x1-	T60.3x2-	T60.3x3-	T60.3x4-	—	—
Fungizone	T36.7x1-	T36.7x2-	T36.7x3-	T36.7x4-	T36.7x5-	T36.7x6-
topical	T49.0x1-	T49.0x2-	T49.0x3-	T49.0x4-	T49.0x5-	T49.0x6-
Furacin	T49.0x1-	T49.0x2-	T49.0x3-	T49.0x4-	T49.0x5-	T49.0x6-
Furadantin	T37.91x-	T37.92x-	T37.93x-	T37.94x-	T37.95x-	T37.96x-
Furazolidone	T37.8x1-	T37.8x2-	T37.8x3-	T37.8x4-	T37.8x5-	T37.8x6-
Furazolium chloride	T49.0x1-	T49.0x2-	T49.0x3-	T49.0x4-	T49.0x5-	T49.0x6-
Furfural	T52.8x1-	T52.8x2-	T52.8x3-	T52.8x4-	—	—
Furnace (coal burning) (domestic), gas from	T58.2x1-	T58.2x2-	T58.2x3-	T58.2x4-	—	—
industrial	T58.8x1-	T58.8x2-	T58.8x3-	T58.8x4-	—	—
Furniture polish	T65.891-	T65.892-	T65.893-	T65.894-	—	—
Furosemide	T50.1x1-	T50.1x2-	T50.1x3-	T50.1x4-	T50.1x5-	T50.1x6-
Furoxone	T37.91x-	T37.92x-	T37.93x-	T37.94x-	T37.95x-	T37.96x-
Fursultiamine	T45.2x1-	T45.2x2-	T45.2x3-	T45.2x4-	T45.2x5-	T45.2x6-
Fusafungine	T36.8x1-	T36.8x2-	T36.8x3-	T36.8x4-	T36.8x5-	—
Fusel oil (any) (amyl) (butyl) (propyl), vapor	T51.3x1-	T51.3x2-	T51.3x3-	T51.3x4-	—	—
Fusidate (ethanolamine) (sodium)	T36.8x1-	T36.8x2-	T36.8x3-	T36.8x4-	T36.8x5-	T36.8x6-
Fusidic acid	T36.8x1-	T36.8x2-	T36.8x3-	T36.8x4-	T36.8x5-	T36.8x6-
Fytic acid, nonasodium	T50.6x1-	T50.6x2-	T50.6x3-	T50.6x4-	T50.6x5-	T50.6x6-

Table of Drugs & Chemicals	POISONING				Adverse Effect	Underdosing
	Accidental (Unintentional)	Self-Harm (Intentional)	Assault	Undetermined		
GABA	T43.8x1-	T43.8x2-	T43.8x3-	T43.8x4-	T43.8x5-	T43.8x6-
Gadopentetic acid	T50.8x1-	T50.8x2-	T50.8x3-	T50.8x4-	T50.8x5-	T50.8x6-
Galactose	T50.3x1-	T50.3x2-	T50.3x3-	T50.3x4-	T50.3x5-	T50.3x6-
b-Galactosidase	T47.5x1-	T47.5x2-	T47.5x3-	T47.5x4-	T47.5x5-	T47.5x6-
Galantamine	T44.0x1-	T44.0x2-	T44.0x3-	T44.0x4-	T44.0x5-	T44.0x6-
Gallamine (triethiodide)	T48.1x1-	T48.1x2-	T48.1x3-	T48.1x4-	T48.1x5-	T48.1x6-
Gallium citrate	T50.991	T50.992	T50.993	T50.994	T50.995	T50.996
Gallopamil	T46.1x1-	T46.1x2-	T46.1x3-	T46.1x4-	T46.1x5-	T46.1x6-
Gamboge	T47.2x1-	T47.2x2-	T47.2x3-	T47.2x4-	T47.2x5-	T47.2x6-
Gamimune	T50.Z11	T50.Z12	T50.Z13	T50.Z14	T50.Z15	T50.Z16
Gamma globulin	T50.Z11	T50.Z12	T50.Z13	T50.Z14	T50.Z15	T50.Z16
Gamma-aminobutyric acid	T43.8x1-	T43.8x2-	T43.8x3-	T43.8x4-	T43.8x5-	T43.8x6-
Gamma-benzene hexachloride (medicinal)	T49.0x1-	T49.0x2-	T49.0x3-	T49.0x4-	T49.0x5-	T49.0x6-
nonmedicinal, vapor	T53.6x1-	T53.6x2-	T53.6x3-	T53.6x4-	—	—
Gamma-BHC (medicinal) — see also Gamma-benzene hexachloride	T49.0x1-	T49.0x2-	T49.0x3-	T49.0x4-	T49.0x5-	T49.0x6-
Gamulin	T50.Z11	T50.Z12	T50.Z13	T50.Z14	T50.Z15	T50.Z16
Ganciclovir (sodium)	T37.5x1-	T37.5x2-	T37.5x3-	T37.5x4-	T37.5x5-	T37.5x6-
Ganglionic blocking drug NEC	T44.2x1-	T44.2x2-	T44.2x3-	T44.2x4-	T44.2x5-	T44.2x6-
specified NEC	T44.2x1-	T44.2x2-	T44.2x3-	T44.2x4-	T44.2x5-	T44.2x6-
Ganja	T40.7x1-	T40.7x2-	T40.7x3-	T40.7x4-	T40.7x5-	T40.7x6-
Garamycin	T36.5x1-	T36.5x2-	T36.5x3-	T36.5x4-	T36.5x5-	T36.5x6-
ophthalmic preparation	T49.5x1-	T49.5x2-	T49.5x3-	T49.5x4-	T49.5x5-	T49.5x6-
topical NEC	T49.0x1-	T49.0x2-	T49.0x3-	T49.0x4-	T49.0x5-	T49.0x6-
Gardenal	T42.3x1-	T42.3x2-	T42.3x3-	T42.3x4-	T42.3x5-	T42.3x6-
Gardepanyl	T42.3x1-	T42.3x2-	T42.3x3-	T42.3x4-	T42.3x5-	T42.3x6-
Gas	T59.91x-	T59.92x-	T59.93x-	T59.94x-	—	—
acetylene	T59.891-	T59.892-	T59.893-	T59.894-	—	—
incomplete combustion of	T58.11x-	T58.12x-	T58.13x-	T58.14x-	—	—
air contaminants, source or type not specified	T59.91x-	T59.92x-	T59.93x-	T59.94x-	—	—
anesthetic	T41.0x1-	T41.0x2-	T41.0x3-	T41.0x4-	T41.0x5-	T41.0x6-
blast furnace	T58.8x1-	T58.8x2-	T58.8x3-	T58.8x4-	—	—
butane — see Butane						
carbon monoxide — see Carbon, monoxide						
chlorine	T59.4x1-	T59.4x2-	T59.4x3-	T59.4x4-	—	—
coal	T58.2x1-	T58.2x2-	T58.2x3-	T58.2x4-	—	—
cyanide	T57.3x1-	T57.3x2-	T57.3x3-	T57.3x4-	—	—
dicyanogen	T65.0x1-	T65.0x2-	T65.0x3-	T65.0x4-	—	—
domestic — see Domestic gas						
exhaust	T58.01x-	T58.02x-	T58.03x-	T58.04x-	—	—
from utility (for cooking, heating, or lighting) (after combustion) — see Carbon, monoxide, fuel, utility						
prior to combustion	T59.891-	T59.892-	T59.893-	T59.894-	—	—
from wood- or coal-burning stove or fireplace	T58.2x1-	T58.2x2-	T58.2x3-	T58.2x4-	—	—

Table of Drugs & Chemicals	POISONING				Adverse Effect	Underdosing
	Accidental (Unintentional)	Self-Harm (Intentional)	Assault	Undetermined		
Gas - continued	T59.91x-	T59.92x-	T59.93x-	T59.94x-	—	—
fuel (domestic use) (after combustion) — see also Carbon, monoxide, fuel						
industrial use	T58.8x1-	T58.8x2-	T58.8x3-	T58.8x4-	—	—
prior to combustion	T59.891-	T59.892-	T59.893-	T59.894-	—	—
utility	T59.891-	T59.892-	T59.893-	T59.894-	—	—
incomplete combustion of — see Carbon, monoxide, fuel, utility						
in mobile container	T59.891-	T59.892-	T59.893-	T59.894-	—	—
piped (natural)	T59.891-	T59.892-	T59.893-	T59.894-	—	—
garage	T58.01x-	T58.02x-	T58.03x-	T58.04x-	—	—
hydrocarbon NEC	T59.891-	T59.892-	T59.893-	T59.894-	—	—
incomplete combustion of — see Carbon, monoxide, fuel, utility						
liquefied — see Butane						
piped	T59.891-	T59.892-	T59.893-	T59.894-	—	—
hydrocyanic acid	T65.0x1-	T65.0x2-	T65.0x3-	T65.0x4-	—	—
illuminating (after combustion)	T58.11x-	T58.12x-	T58.13x-	T58.14x-	—	—
prior to combustion	T59.891-	T59.892-	T59.893-	T59.894-	—	—
incomplete combustion, any — see Carbon, monoxide						
kiln	T58.8x1-	T58.8x2-	T58.8x3-	T58.8x4-	—	—
lacrimogenic	T59.3x1-	T59.3x2-	T59.3x3-	T59.3x4-	—	—
liquefied petroleum — see Butane						
marsh	T59.891-	T59.892-	T59.893-	T59.894-	—	—
motor exhaust, not in transit	T58.01x-	T58.02x-	T58.03x-	T58.04x-	—	—
mustard, not in war	T59.891-	T59.892-	T59.893-	T59.894-	—	—
natural	T59.891-	T59.892-	T59.893-	T59.894-	—	—
nerve, not in war	T59.91x-	T59.92x-	T59.93x-	T59.94x-	—	—
oil	T52.0x1-	T52.0x2-	T52.0x3-	T52.0x4-	—	—
petroleum (liquefied) (distributed in mobile containers)	T59.891-	T59.892-	T59.893-	T59.894-	—	—
piped (pure or mixed with air)	T59.891-	T59.892-	T59.893-	T59.894-	—	—
piped (manufactured) (natural) NEC	T59.891-	T59.892-	T59.893-	T59.894-	—	—
producer	T58.8x1-	T58.8x2-	T58.8x3-	T58.8x4-	—	—
propane — see Propane						
refrigerant (chlorofluoro-carbon)	T53.5x1-	T53.5x2-	T53.5x3-	T53.5x4-	—	—
not chlorofluoro-carbon	T59.891-	T59.892-	T59.893-	T59.894-	—	—
sewer	T59.91x-	T59.92x-	T59.93x-	T59.94x-	—	—
specified source NEC	T59.91x-	T59.92x-	T59.93x-	T59.94x-	—	—
stove (after combustion)	T58.11x-	T58.12x-	T58.13x-	T58.14x-	—	—
prior to combustion	T59.891-	T59.892-	T59.893-	T59.894-	—	—
tear	T59.3x1-	T59.3x2-	T59.3x3-	T59.3x4-	—	—
therapeutic	T41.5x1-	T41.5x2-	T41.5x3-	T41.5x4-	T41.5x5-	T41.5x6-

DRUGS & CHEMICALS

DRUGS & CHEMICALS

Table of Drugs & Chemicals	POISONING Accidental (Unintentional)	Self-Harm (Intentional)	Assault	Undetermined	Adverse Effect	Underdosing
Gas - continued	T59.91x-	T59.92x-	T59.93x-	T59.94x-	—	—
utility (for cooking, heating, or lighting) (piped) NEC	T59.891-	T59.892-	T59.893-	T59.894-	—	—
incomplete combustion of — see Carbon, monoxide, fuel, utilty						
in mobile container	T59.891-	T59.892-	T59.893-	T59.894-	—	—
piped (natural)	T59.891-	T59.892-	T59.893-	T59.894-	—	—
water	T58.11x-	T58.12x-	T58.13x-	T58.14x-	—	—
incomplete combustion of — see Carbon, monoxide, fuel, utility						
Gaseous substance — see Gas						
Gasoline	T52.0x1-	T52.0x2-	T52.0x3-	T52.0x4-	—	—
vapor	T52.0x1-	T52.0x2-	T52.0x3-	T52.0x4-	—	—
Gastric enzymes	T47.5x1-	T47.5x2-	T47.5x3-	T47.5x4-	T47.5x5-	T47.5x6-
Gastrografin	T50.8x1-	T50.8x2-	T50.8x3-	T50.8x4-	T50.8x5-	T50.8x6-
Gastrointestinal drug	T47.91x-	T47.92x-	T47.93x-	T47.94x-	T47.95x-	T47.96x-
biological	T47.8x1-	T47.8x2-	T47.8x3-	T47.8x4-	T47.8x5-	T47.8x6-
specified NEC	T47.8x1-	T47.8x2-	T47.8x3-	T47.8x4-	T47.8x5-	T47.8x6-
Gaultheria procumbens	T62.2x1-	T62.2x2-	T62.2x3-	T62.2x4-	—	—
Gefarnate	T44.3x1-	T44.3x2-	T44.3x3-	T44.3x4-	T44.3x5-	T44.3x6-
Gelatin (intravenous)	T45.8x1-	T45.8x2-	T45.8x3-	T45.8x4-	T45.8x5-	T45.8x6-
absorbable (sponge)	T45.7x1-	T45.7x2-	T45.7x3-	T45.7x4-	T45.7x5-	T45.7x6-
Gelfilm	T49.8x1-	T49.8x2-	T49.8x3-	T49.8x4-	T49.8x5-	T49.8x6-
Gelfoam	T45.7x1-	T45.7x2-	T45.7x3-	T45.7x4-	T45.7x5-	T45.7x6-
Gelsemine	T50.991-	T50.992-	T50.993-	T50.994-	T50.995-	T50.996-
Gelsemium (sempervirens)	T62.2x1-	T62.2x2-	T62.2x3-	T62.2x4-	—	—
Gemeprost	T48.0x1-	T48.0x2-	T48.0x3-	T48.0x4-	T48.0x5-	T48.0x6-
Gemfibrozil	T46.6x1-	T46.6x2-	T46.6x3-	T46.6x4-	T46.6x5-	T46.6x6-
Gemonil	T42.3x1-	T42.3x2-	T42.3x3-	T42.3x4-	T42.3x5-	T42.3x6-
Gentamicin	T36.5x1-	T36.5x2-	T36.5x3-	T36.5x4-	T36.5x5-	T36.5x6-
ophthalmic preparation	T49.5x1-	T49.5x2-	T49.5x3-	T49.5x4-	T49.5x5-	T49.5x6-
topical NEC	T49.0x1-	T49.0x2-	T49.0x3-	T49.0x4-	T49.0x5-	T49.0x6-
Gentian	T47.5x1-	T47.5x2-	T47.5x3-	T47.5x4-	T47.5x5-	T47.5x6-
violet	T49.0x1-	T49.0x2-	T49.0x3-	T49.0x4-	T49.0x5-	T49.0x6-
Gepefrine	T44.4x1-	T44.4x2-	T44.4x3-	T44.4x4-	T44.4x5-	T44.4x6-
Gestonorone caproate	T38.5x1-	T38.5x2-	T38.5x3-	T38.5x4-	T38.5x5-	T38.5x6-
Gexane	T49.0x1-	T49.0x2-	T49.0x3-	T49.0x4-	T49.0x5-	T49.0x6-
Gila monster (venom)	T63.111-	T63.112-	T63.113-	T63.114-	—	—
Ginger	T47.5x1-	T47.5x2-	T47.5x3-	T47.5x4-	T47.5x5-	T47.5x6-
Jamaica — see Jamaica, ginger						
Gitalin	T46.0x1-	T46.0x2-	T46.0x3-	T46.0x4-	T46.0x5-	T46.0x6-
amorphous	T46.0x1-	T46.0x2-	T46.0x3-	T46.0x4-	T46.0x5-	T46.0x6-
Gitaloxin	T46.0x1-	T46.0x2-	T46.0x3-	T46.0x4-	T46.0x5-	T46.0x6-
Gitoxin	T46.0x1-	T46.0x2-	T46.0x3-	T46.0x4-	T46.0x5-	T46.0x6-
Glafenine	T39.8x1-	T39.8x2-	T39.8x3-	T39.8x4-	T39.8x5-	T39.8x6-
Glandular extract (medicinal) NEC	T50.Z91-	T50.Z92-	T50.Z93-	T50.Z94-	T50.Z95-	T50.Z96-
Glaucarubin	T37.3x1-	T37.3x2-	T37.3x3-	T37.3x4-	T37.3x5-	T37.3x6-
Glibenclamide	T38.3x1-	T38.3x2-	T38.3x3-	T38.3x4-	T38.3x5-	T38.3x6-
Glibornuride	T38.3x1-	T38.3x2-	T38.3x3-	T38.3x4-	T38.3x5-	T38.3x6-
Gliclazide	T38.3x1-	T38.3x2-	T38.3x3-	T38.3x4-	T38.3x5-	T38.3x6-
Glimidine	T38.3x1-	T38.3x2-	T38.3x3-	T38.3x4-	T38.3x5-	T38.3x6-
Glipizide	T38.3x1-	T38.3x2-	T38.3x3-	T38.3x4-	T38.3x5-	T38.3x6-
Gliquidone	T38.3x1-	T38.3x2-	T38.3x3-	T38.3x4-	T38.3x5-	T38.3x6-
Glisolamide	T38.3x1-	T38.3x2-	T38.3x3-	T38.3x4-	T38.3x5-	T38.3x6-
Glisoxepide	T38.3x1-	T38.3x2-	T38.3x3-	T38.3x4-	T38.3x5-	T38.3x6-

Table of Drugs & Chemicals	POISONING Accidental (Unintentional)	Self-Harm (Intentional)	Assault	Undetermined	Adverse Effect	Underdosing
Globin zinc insulin	T38.3x1-	T38.3x2-	T38.3x3-	T38.3x4-	T38.3x5-	T38.3x6-
Globulin						
antilymphocytic	T50.Z11-	T50.Z12-	T50.Z13-	T50.Z14-	T50.Z15-	T50.Z16-
antirhesus	T50.Z11-	T50.Z12-	T50.Z13-	T50.Z14-	T50.Z15-	T50.Z16-
antivenin	T50.Z11-	T50.Z12-	T50.Z13-	T50.Z14-	T50.Z15-	T50.Z16-
antiviral	T50.Z11-	T50.Z12-	T50.Z13-	T50.Z14-	T50.Z15-	T50.Z16-
Glucagon	T38.3x1-	T38.3x2-	T38.3x3-	T38.3x4-	T38.3x5-	T38.3x6-
Glucocorticoids	T38.0x1-	T38.0x2-	T38.0x3-	T38.0x4-	T38.0x5-	T38.0x6-
Glucocorticosteroid	T38.0x1-	T38.0x2-	T38.0x3-	T38.0x4-	T38.0x5-	T38.0x6-
Gluconic acid	T50.991-	T50.992-	T50.993-	T50.994-	T50.995-	T50.996-
Glucosamine sulfate	T39.4x1-	T39.4x2-	T39.4x3-	T39.4x4-	T39.4x5-	T39.4x6-
Glucose	T50.3x1-	T50.3x2-	T50.3x3-	T50.3x4-	T50.3x5-	T50.3x6-
with sodium chloride	T50.3x1-	T50.3x2-	T50.3x3-	T50.3x4-	T50.3x5-	T50.3x6-
Glucosulfone sodium	T37.1x1-	T37.1x2-	T37.1x3-	T37.1x4-	T37.1x5-	T37.1x6-
Glucurolactone	T47.8x1-	T47.8x2-	T47.8x3-	T47.8x4-	T47.8x5-	T47.8x6-
Glue NEC	T52.8x1-	T52.8x2-	T52.8x3-	T52.8x4-	—	—
Glutamic acid	T47.5x1-	T47.5x2-	T47.5x3-	T47.5x4-	T47.5x5-	T47.5x6-
Glutaral (medicinal)	T49.0x1-	T49.0x2-	T49.0x3-	T49.0x4-	T49.0x5-	T49.0x6-
nonmedicinal	T65.891-	T65.892-	T65.893-	T65.894-	—	—
Glutaraldehyde (nonmedicinal)	T65.891-	T65.892-	T65.893-	T65.894-	—	—
medicinal	T49.0x1-	T49.0x2-	T49.0x3-	T49.0x4-	T49.0x5-	T49.0x6-
Glutathione	T50.6x1-	T50.6x2-	T50.6x3-	T50.6x4-	T50.6x5-	T50.6x6-
Glutethimide	T42.6x1-	T42.6x2-	T42.6x3-	T42.6x4-	T42.6x5-	T42.6x6-
Glyburide	T38.3x1-	T38.3x2-	T38.3x3-	T38.3x4-	T38.3x5-	T38.3x6-
Glycerin	T47.4x1-	T47.4x2-	T47.4x3-	T47.4x4-	T47.4x5-	T47.4x6-
Glycerol	T47.4x1-	T47.4x2-	T47.4x3-	T47.4x4-	T47.4x5-	T47.4x6-
borax	T49.6x1-	T49.6x2-	T49.6x3-	T49.6x4-	T49.6x5-	T49.6x6-
intravenous	T50.3x1-	T50.3x2-	T50.3x3-	T50.3x4-	T50.3x5-	T50.3x6-
iodinated	T48.4x1-	T48.4x2-	T48.4x3-	T48.4x4-	T48.4x5-	T48.4x6-
Glycerophosphate	T50.991-	T50.992-	T50.993-	T50.994-	T50.995-	T50.996-
Glyceryl						
gualacolate	T48.4x1-	T48.4x2-	T48.4x3-	T48.4x4-	T48.4x5-	T48.4x6-
nitrate	T46.3x1-	T46.3x2-	T46.3x3-	T46.3x4-	T46.3x5-	T46.3x6-
triacetate (topical)	T49.0x1-	T49.0x2-	T49.0x3-	T49.0x4-	T49.0x5-	T49.0x6-
trinitrate	T46.3x1-	T46.3x2-	T46.3x3-	T46.3x4-	T46.3x5-	T46.3x6-
Glycine	T50.3x1-	T50.3x2-	T50.3x3-	T50.3x4-	T50.3x5-	T50.3x6-
Glyclopyramide	T38.3x1-	T38.3x2-	T38.3x3-	T38.3x4-	T38.3x5-	T38.3x6-
Glycobiarsol	T37.3x1-	T37.3x2-	T37.3x3-	T37.3x4-	T37.3x5-	T37.3x6-
Glycols (ether)	T52.3x1-	T52.3x2-	T52.3x3-	T52.3x4-	—	—
Glyconiazide	T37.1x1-	T37.1x2-	T37.1x3-	T37.1x4-	T37.1x5-	T37.1x6-
Glycopyrrolate	T44.3x1-	T44.3x2-	T44.3x3-	T44.3x4-	T44.3x5-	T44.3x6-
Glycopyrronium	T44.3x1-	T44.3x2-	T44.3x3-	T44.3x4-	T44.3x5-	T44.3x6-
bromide	T44.3x1-	T44.3x2-	T44.3x3-	T44.3x4-	T44.3x5-	T44.3x6-
Glycoside, cardiac (stimulant)	T46.0x1-	T46.0x2-	T46.0x3-	T46.0x4-	T46.0x5-	T46.0x6-
Glycyclamide	T38.3x1-	T38.3x2-	T38.3x3-	T38.3x4-	T38.3x5-	T38.3x6-
Glycyrrhiza extract	T48.4x1-	T48.4x2-	T48.4x3-	T48.4x4-	T48.4x5-	T48.4x6-
Glycyrrhizic acid	T48.4x1-	T48.4x2-	T48.4x3-	T48.4x4-	T48.4x5-	T48.4x6-
Glycyrrhizinate potassium	T48.4x1-	T48.4x2-	T48.4x3-	T48.4x4-	T48.4x5-	T48.4x6-
Glymidine sodium	T38.3x1-	T38.3x2-	T38.3x3-	T38.3x4-	T38.3x5-	T38.3x6-
Glyphosate	T60.3x1-	T60.3x2-	T60.3x3-	T60.3x4-	—	—
Glyphylline	T48.6x1-	T48.6x2-	T48.6x3-	T48.6x4-	T48.6x5-	T48.6x6-
Gold						
colloidal (l98Au)	T45.1x1-	T45.1x2-	T45.1x3-	T45.1x4-	T45.1x5-	T45.1x6-
salts	T39.4x1-	T39.4x2-	T39.4x3-	T39.4x4-	T39.4x5-	T39.4x6-
Golden sulfide of antimony	T56.891-	T56.892-	T56.893-	T56.894-	—	—
Goldylocks	T62.2x1-	T62.2x2-	T62.2x3-	T62.2x4-	—	—
Gonadal tissue extract	T38.901-	T38.902-	T38.903-	T38.904-	T38.905-	T38.906-
female	T38.5x1-	T38.5x2-	T38.5x3-	T38.5x4-	T38.5x5-	T38.5x6-
male	T38.7x1-	T38.7x2-	T38.7x3-	T38.7x4-	T38.7x5-	T38.7x6-
Gonadorelin	T38.891-	T38.892-	T38.893-	T38.894-	T38.895-	T38.896-

DRUGS & CHEMICALS

Table of Drugs & Chemicals	POISONING Accidental (Unintentional)	Self-Harm (Intentional)	Assault	Undetermined	Adverse Effect	Underdosing
Gonadotropin	T38.891-	T38.892-	T38.893-	T38.894-	T38.895-	T38.896-
chorionic	T38.891-	T38.892-	T38.893-	T38.894-	T38.895-	T38.896-
pituitary	T38.811-	T38.812-	T38.813-	T38.814-	T38.815-	T38.816-
Goserelin	T45.1x1-	T45.1x2-	T45.1x3-	T45.1x4-	T45.1x5-	T45.1x6-
Grain alcohol	T51.0x1-	T51.0x2-	T51.0x3-	T51.0x4-	—	—
Gramicidin	T49.0x1-	T49.0x2-	T49.0x3-	T49.0x4-	T49.0x5-	T49.0x6-
Granisetron	T45.0x1-	T45.0x2-	T45.0x3-	T45.0x4-	T45.0x5-	T45.0x6-
Gratiola officinalis	T62.2x1-	T62.2x2-	T62.2x3-	T62.2x4-	—	—
Grease	T65.891-	T65.892-	T65.893-	T65.894-	—	—
Green hellebore	T62.2x1-	T62.2x2-	T62.2x3-	T62.2x4-	—	—
Green soap	T49.2x1-	T49.2x2-	T49.2x3-	T49.2x4-	T49.2x5-	T49.2x6-
Grifulvin	T36.7x1-	T36.7x2-	T36.7x3-	T36.7x4-	T36.7x5-	T36.7x6-
Griseofulvin	T36.7x1-	T36.7x2-	T36.7x3-	T36.7x4-	T36.7x5-	T36.7x6-
Growth hormone	T38.811-	T38.812-	T38.813-	T38.814-	T38.815-	T38.816-
Guaiac reagent	T50.991-	T50.992-	T50.993-	T50.994-	T50.995-	T50.996-
Guaiacol derivatives	T48.4x1-	T48.4x2-	T48.4x3-	T48.4x4-	T48.4x5-	T48.4x6-
Guaifenesin	T48.4x1-	T48.4x2-	T48.4x3-	T48.4x4-	T48.4x5-	T48.4x6-
Guaimesal	T48.4x1-	T48.4x2-	T48.4x3-	T48.4x4-	T48.4x5-	T48.4x6-
Guaiphenesin	T48.4x1-	T48.4x2-	T48.4x3-	T48.4x4-	T48.4x5-	T48.4x6-
Guamecycline	T36.4x1-	T36.4x2-	T36.4x3-	T36.4x4-	T36.4x5-	T36.4x6-
Guanabenz	T46.5x1-	T46.5x2-	T46.5x3-	T46.5x4-	T46.5x5-	T46.5x6-
Guanacline	T46.5x1-	T46.5x2-	T46.5x3-	T46.5x4-	T46.5x5-	T46.5x6-
Guanadrel	T46.5x1-	T46.5x2-	T46.5x3-	T46.5x4-	T46.5x5-	T46.5x6-
Guanatol	T37.2x1-	T37.2x2-	T37.2x3-	T37.2x4-	T37.2x5-	T37.2x6-
Guanethidine	T46.5x1-	T46.5x2-	T46.5x3-	T46.5x4-	T46.5x5-	T46.5x6-
Guanfacine	T46.5x1-	T46.5x2-	T46.5x3-	T46.5x4-	T46.5x5-	T46.5x6-
Guano	T65.891-	T65.892-	T65.893-	T65.894-	—	—
Guanochlor	T46.5x1-	T46.5x2-	T46.5x3-	T46.5x4-	T46.5x5-	T46.5x6-
Guanoclor	T46.5x1-	T46.5x2-	T46.5x3-	T46.5x4-	T46.5x5-	T46.5x6-
Guanoctine	T46.5x1-	T46.5x2-	T46.5x3-	T46.5x4-	T46.5x5-	T46.5x6-
Guanoxabenz	T46.5x1-	T46.5x2-	T46.5x3-	T46.5x4-	T46.5x5-	T46.5x6-
Guanoxan	T46.5x1-	T46.5x2-	T46.5x3-	T46.5x4-	T46.5x5-	T46.5x6-
Guar gum (medicinal)	T46.6x1-	T46.6x2-	T46.6x3-	T46.6x4-	T46.6x5-	T46.6x6-
Hachimycin	T36.7x1-	T36.7x2-	T36.7x3-	T36.7x4-	T36.7x5-	T36.7x6-
Hair						
dye	T49.4x1-	T49.4x2-	T49.4x3-	T49.4x4-	T49.4x5-	T49.4x6-
preparation NEC	T49.4x1-	T49.4x2-	T49.4x3-	T49.4x4-	T49.4x5-	T49.4x6-
Halazepam	T42.4x1-	T42.4x2-	T42.4x3-	T42.4x4-	T42.4x5-	T42.4x6-
Halcinolone	T49.0x1-	T49.0x2-	T49.0x3-	T49.0x4-	T49.0x5-	T49.0x6-
Halcinonide	T49.0x1-	T49.0x2-	T49.0x3-	T49.0x4-	T49.0x5-	T49.0x6-
Halethazole	T49.0x1-	T49.0x2-	T49.0x3-	T49.0x4-	T49.0x5-	T49.0x6-
Hallucinogen NEC	T40.901-	T40.902-	T40.903-	T40.904-	T40.905-	T40.906-
Halofantrine	T37.2x1-	T37.2x2-	T37.2x3-	T37.2x4-	T37.2x5-	T37.2x6-
Halofenate	T46.6x1-	T46.6x2-	T46.6x3-	T46.6x4-	T46.6x5-	T46.6x6-
Halometasone	T49.0x1-	T49.0x2-	T49.0x3-	T49.0x4-	T49.0x5-	T49.0x6-
Haloperidol	T43.4x1-	T43.4x2-	T43.4x3-	T43.4x4-	T43.4x5-	T43.4x6-
Haloprogin	T49.0x1-	T49.0x2-	T49.0x3-	T49.0x4-	T49.0x5-	T49.0x6-
Halotex	T49.0x1-	T49.0x2-	T49.0x3-	T49.0x4-	T49.0x5-	T49.0x6-
Halothane	T41.0x1-	T41.0x2-	T41.0x3-	T41.0x4-	T41.0x5-	T41.0x6-
Haloxazolam	T42.4x1-	T42.4x2-	T42.4x3-	T42.4x4-	T42.4x5-	T42.4x6-
Halquinols	T49.0x1-	T49.0x2-	T49.0x3-	T49.0x4-	T49.0x5-	T49.0x6-
Hamamelis	T49.2x1-	T49.2x2-	T49.2x3-	T49.2x4-	T49.2x5-	T49.2x6-
Haptendextran	T45.8x1-	T45.8x2-	T45.8x3-	T45.8x4-	T45.8x5-	T45.8x6-
Harmonyl	T46.5x1-	T46.5x2-	T46.5x3-	T46.5x4-	T46.5x5-	T46.5x6-
Hartmann's solution	T50.3x1-	T50.3x2-	T50.3x3-	T50.3x4-	T50.3x5-	T50.3x6-
Hashish	T40.7x1-	T40.7x2-	T40.7x3-	T40.7x4-	T40.7x5-	T40.7x6-
Hawaiian Woodrose seeds	T40.991-	T40.992-	T40.993-	T40.994-	—	—
HCB	T60.3x1-	T60.3x2-	T60.3x3-	T60.3x4-	—	—
HCH	T53.6x1-	T53.6x2-	T53.6x3-	T53.6x4-	—	—
medicinal	T49.0x1-	T49.0x2-	T49.0x3-	T49.0x4-	T49.0x5-	T49.0x6-
HCN	T57.3x1-	T57.3x2-	T57.3x3-	T57.3x4-	—	—
Headache cures, drugs, powders NEC	T50.901-	T50.902-	T50.903-	T50.904-	T50.905-	T50.906-
Heavenly Blue (morning glory)	T40.991-	T40.992-	T40.993-	T40.994-	—	—
Heavy metal antidote	T45.8x1-	T45.8x2-	T45.8x3-	T45.8x4-	T45.8x5-	T45.8x6-
Hedaquinium	T49.0x1-	T49.0x2-	T49.0x3-	T49.0x4-	T49.0x5-	T49.0x6-
Hedge hyssop	T62.2x1-	T62.2x2-	T62.2x3-	T62.2x4-	—	—
Heet	T49.8x1-	T49.8x2-	T49.8x3-	T49.8x4-	T49.8x5-	T49.8x6-
Helenin	T37.4x1-	T37.4x2-	T37.4x3-	T37.4x4-	T37.4x5-	T37.4x6-
Helium (nonmedicinal) NEC	T59.891-	T59.892-	T59.893-	T59.894-	—	—
medicinal	T48.991-	T48.992-	T48.993-	T48.994-	T48.995-	T48.996-
Hellebore (black) (green) (white)	T62.2x1-	T62.2x2-	T62.2x3-	T62.2x4-	—	—
Hematin	T45.8x1-	T45.8x2-	T45.8x3-	T45.8x4-	T45.8x5-	T45.8x6-
Hematinic preparation	T45.8x1-	T45.8x2-	T45.8x3-	T45.8x4-	T45.8x5-	T45.8x6-
Hematological agent	T45.91x-	T45.92x-	T45.93x-	T45.94x-	T45.95x-	T45.96x-
specified NEC	T45.8x1-	T45.8x2-	T45.8x3-	T45.8x4-	T45.8x5-	T45.8x6-
Hemlock	T62.2x1-	T62.2x2-	T62.2x3-	T62.2x4-	—	—
Hemostatic	T45.621-	T45.622-	T45.623-	T45.624-	T45.625-	T45.626-
drug, systemic	T45.621-	T45.622-	T45.623-	T45.624-	T45.625-	T45.626-
Hemostyptic	T49.4x1-	T49.4x2-	T49.4x3-	T49.4x4-	T49.4x5-	T49.4x6-
Henbane	T62.2x1-	T62.2x2-	T62.2x3-	T62.2x4-	—	—
Heparin (sodium)	T45.511-	T45.512-	T45.513-	T45.514-	T45.515-	T45.516-
action reverser	T45.7x1-	T45.7x2-	T45.7x3-	T45.7x4-	T45.7x5-	T45.7x6-
Heparin-fraction	T45.511-	T45.512-	T45.513-	T45.514-	T45.515-	T45.516-
Heparinoid (systemic)	T45.511-	T45.512-	T45.513-	T45.514-	T45.515-	T45.516-
Hepatic secretion stimulant	T47.8x1-	T47.8x2-	T47.8x3-	T47.8x4-	T47.8x5-	T47.8x6-
Hepatitis B						
immune globulin	T50.Z11-	T50.Z12-	T50.Z13-	T50.Z14-	T50.Z15-	T50.Z16-
vaccine	T50.B91-	T50.B92-	T50.B93-	T50.B94-	T50.B95-	T50.B96-
Hepronicate	T46.7x1-	T46.7x2-	T46.7x3-	T46.7x4-	T46.7x5-	T46.7x6-
Heptabarb	T42.3x1-	T42.3x2-	T42.3x3-	T42.3x4-	T42.3x5-	T42.3x6-
Heptabarbital	T42.3x1-	T42.3x2-	T42.3x3-	T42.3x4-	T42.3x5-	T42.3x6-
Heptabarbitone	T42.3x1-	T42.3x2-	T42.3x3-	T42.3x4-	T42.3x5-	T42.3x6-
Heptachlor	T60.1x1-	T60.1x2-	T60.1x3-	T60.1x4-	—	—
Heptalgin	T40.2x1-	T40.2x2-	T40.2x3-	T40.2x4-	T40.2x5-	T40.2x6-
Heptaminol	T46.3x1-	T46.3x2-	T46.3x3-	T46.3x4-	T46.3x5-	T46.3x6-
Herbicide NEC	T60.3x1-	T60.3x2-	T60.3x3-	T60.3x4-		
Heroin	T40.1x1-	T40.1x2-	T40.1x3-	T40.1x4-	—	
Herplex	T49.5x1-	T49.5x2-	T49.5x3-	T49.5x4-	T49.5x5-	T49.5x6-
HES	T45.8x1-	T45.8x2-	T45.8x3-	T45.8x4-	T45.8x5-	T45.8x6-
Hesperidin	T46.991-	T46.992-	T46.993-	T46.994-	T46.995-	T46.996-
Hetacillin	T36.0x1-	T36.0x2-	T36.0x3-	T36.0x4-	T36.0x5-	T36.0x6-
Hetastarch	T45.8x1-	T45.8x2-	T45.8x3-	T45.8x4-	T45.8x5-	T45.8x6-
HETP	T60.0x1-	T60.0x2-	T60.0x3-	T60.0x4-	—	—
Hexachlorobenzene (vapor)	T60.3x1-	T60.3x2-	T60.3x3-	T60.3x4-	—	—
Hexachlorocyclohexane	T53.6x1-	T53.6x2-	T53.6x3-	T53.6x4-	—	—
Hexachlorophene	T49.0x1-	T49.0x2-	T49.0x3-	T49.0x4-	T49.0x5-	T49.0x6-
Hexadiline	T46.3x1-	T46.3x2-	T46.3x3-	T46.3x4-	T46.3x5-	T46.3x6-
Hexadimethrine (bromide)	T45.7x1-	T45.7x2-	T45.7x3-	T45.7x4-	T45.7x5-	T45.7x6-
Hexadylamine	T46.3x1-	T46.3x2-	T46.3x3-	T46.3x4-	T46.3x5-	T46.3x6-
Hexaethyl tetraphos-phate	T60.0x1-	T60.0x2-	T60.0x3-	T60.0x4-	—	—
Hexafluorenium bromide	T48.1x1-	T48.1x2-	T48.1x3-	T48.1x4-	T48.1x5-	T48.1x6-
Hexafluronium (bromide)	T48.1x1-	T48.1x2-	T48.1x3-	T48.1x4-	T48.1x5-	T48.1x6-
Hexa-germ	T49.2x1-	T49.2x2-	T49.2x3-	T49.2x4-	T49.2x5-	T49.2x6-
Hexahydrobenzol	T52.8x1-	T52.8x2-	T52.8x3-	T52.8x4-	—	—
Hexahydrocresol(s)	T51.8x1-	T51.8x2-	T51.8x3-	T51.8x4-	—	—
arsenide	T57.0x1-	T57.0x2-	T57.0x3-	T57.0x4-	—	—
arseniurated	T57.0x1-	T57.0x2-	T57.0x3-	T57.0x4-	—	—
cyanide	T57.3x1-	T57.3x2-	T57.3x3-	T57.3x4-	—	—
gas	T59.891-	T59.892-	T59.893-	T59.894-	—	—
fluoride (liquid)	T57.8x1-	T57.8x2-	T57.8x3-	T57.8x4-	—	—
vapor	T59.891-	T59.892-	T59.893-	T59.894-	—	—
phophorated	T60.0x1-	T60.0x2-	T60.0x3-	T60.0x4-	—	—
sulfate	T57.8x1-	T57.8x2-	T57.8x3-	T57.8x4-	—	—
sulfide (gas)	T59.6x1-	T59.6x2-	T59.6x3-	T59.6x4-	—	—
arseniurated	T57.0x1-	T57.0x2-	T57.0x3-	T57.0x4-	—	—
sulfurated	T57.8x1-	T57.8x2-	T57.8x3-	T57.8x4-	—	—
Hexahydrophenol	T51.8x1-	T51.8x2-	T51.8x3-	T51.8x4-		

DRUGS & CHEMICALS

Table of Drugs & Chemicals	POISONING Accidental (Unintentional)	Self-Harm (Intentional)	Assault	Undetermined	Adverse Effect	Underdosing
Hexalen	T51.8x1-	T51.8x2-	T51.8x3-	T51.8x4-	—	—
Hexamethonium bromide ..	T44.2x1-	T44.2x2-	T44.2x3-	T44.2x4-	T44.2x5-	T44.2x6-
Hexamethylene	T52.8x1-	T52.8x2-	T52.8x3-	T52.8x4-	—	—
Hexamethylmelamine	T45.1x1-	T45.1x2-	T45.1x3-	T45.1x4-	T45.1x5-	T45.1x6-
Hexamidine	T49.0x1-	T49.0x2-	T49.0x3-	T49.0x4-	T49.0x5-	T49.0x6-
Hexamine (mandelate)	T37.8x1-	T37.8x2-	T37.8x3-	T37.8x4-	T37.8x5-	T37.8x6-
Hexanone, 2-hexanone	T52.4x1-	T52.4x2-	T52.4x3-	T52.4x4-	—	—
Hexanuorenium	T48.1x1-	T48.1x2-	T48.1x3-	T48.1x4-	T48.1x5-	T48.1x6-
Hexapropymate	T42.6x1-	T42.6x2-	T42.6x3-	T42.6x4-	T42.6x5-	T42.6x6-
Hexasonium iodide	T44.3x1-	T44.3x2-	T44.3x3-	T44.3x4-	T44.3x5-	T44.3x6-
Hexcarbacholine bromide ..	T48.1x1-	T48.1x2-	T48.1x3-	T48.1x4-	T48.1x5-	T48.1x6-
Hexemal	T42.3x1-	T42.3x2-	T42.3x3-	T42.3x4-	T42.3x5-	T42.3x6-
Hexestrol	T38.5x1-	T38.5x2-	T38.5x3-	T38.5x4-	T38.5x5-	T38.5x6-
Hexethal (sodium)	T42.3x1-	T42.3x2-	T42.3x3-	T42.3x4-	T42.3x5-	T42.3x6-
Hexetidine	T37.8x1-	T37.8x2-	T37.8x3-	T37.8x4-	T37.8x5-	T37.8x6-
Hexobarbital	T42.3x1-	T42.3x2-	T42.3x3-	T42.3x4-	T42.3x5-	T42.3x6-
rectal	T41.291-	T41.292-	T41.293-	T41.294-	T41.295-	T41.296-
sodium	T41.1x1-	T41.1x2-	T41.1x3-	T41.1x4-	T41.1x5-	T41.1x6-
Hexobendine	T46.3x1-	T46.3x2-	T46.3x3-	T46.3x4-	T46.3x5-	T46.3x6-
Hexocyclium	T44.3x1-	T44.3x2-	T44.3x3-	T44.3x4-	T44.3x5-	T44.3x6-
metilsulfate	T44.3x1-	T44.3x2-	T44.3x3-	T44.3x4-	T44.3x5-	T44.3x6-
Hexoestrol	T38.5x1-	T38.5x2-	T38.5x3-	T38.5x4-	T38.5x5-	T38.5x6-
Hexone	T52.4x1-	T52.4x2-	T52.4x3-	T52.4x4-	—	—
Hexoprenaline	T48.6x1-	T48.6x2-	T48.6x3-	T48.6x4-	T48.6x5-	T48.6x6-
Hexylcaine	T41.3x1-	T41.3x2-	T41.3x3-	T41.3x4-	T41.3x5-	T41.3x6-
Hexylresorcinol	T52.2x1-	T52.2x2-	T52.2x3-	T52.2x4-	—	—
HGH (human growth hormone)	T38.811-	T38.812-	T38.813-	T38.814-	T38.815-	T38.816-
Hinkle's pills	T47.2x1-	T47.2x2-	T47.2x3-	T47.2x4-	T47.2x5-	T47.2x6-
Histalog	T50.8x1-	T50.8x2-	T50.8x3-	T50.8x4-	T50.8x5-	T50.8x6-
Histamine (phosphate)	T50.8x1-	T50.8x2-	T50.8x3-	T50.8x4-	T50.8x5-	T50.8x6-
Histoplasmin	T50.8x1-	T50.8x2-	T50.8x3-	T50.8x4-	T50.8x5-	T50.8x6-
Holly berries	T62.2x1-	T62.2x2-	T62.2x3-	T62.2x4-	—	—
Homatropine	T44.3x1-	T44.3x2-	T44.3x3-	T44.3x4-	T44.3x5-	T44.3x6-
methylbromide	T44.3x1-	T44.3x2-	T44.3x3-	T44.3x4-	T44.3x5-	T44.3x6-
Homochlorcyclizine	T45.0x1-	T45.0x2-	T45.0x3-	T45.0x4-	T45.0x5-	T45.0x6-
Homosalate	T49.3x1-	T49.3x2-	T49.3x3-	T49.3x4-	T49.3x5-	T49.3x6-
Homo-tet	T50.Z11-	T50.Z12-	T50.Z13-	T50.Z14-	T50.Z15-	T50.Z16-
Hormone	T38.801-	T38.802-	T38.803-	T38.804-	T38.805-	T38.806-
adrenal cortical steroids..	T38.0x1-	T38.0x2-	T38.0x3-	T38.0x4-	T38.0x5-	T38.0x6-
androgenic	T38.7x1-	T38.7x2-	T38.7x3-	T38.7x4-	T38.7x5-	T38.7x6-
anterior pituitary NEC	T38.811-	T38.812-	T38.813-	T38.814-	T38.815-	T38.816-
antidiabetic agents	T38.3x1-	T38.3x2-	T38.3x3-	T38.3x4-	T38.3x5-	T38.3x6-
antidiuretic	T38.891-	T38.892-	T38.893-	T38.894-	T38.895-	T38.896-
cancer therapy	T45.1x1-	T45.1x2-	T45.1x3-	T45.1x4-	T45.1x5-	T45.1x6-
follicle stimulating	T38.811-	T38.812-	T38.813-	T38.814-	T38.815-	T38.816-
gonadotropic	T38.891-	T38.892-	T38.893-	T38.894-	T38.895-	T38.896-
pituitary	T38.811-	T38.812-	T38.813-	T38.814-	T38.815-	T38.816-
growth	T38.811-	T38.812-	T38.813-	T38.814-	T38.815-	T38.816-
luteinizing	T38.811-	T38.812-	T38.813-	T38.814-	T38.815-	T38.816-
ovarian	T38.5x1-	T38.5x2-	T38.5x3-	T38.5x4-	T38.5x5-	T38.5x6-
oxytocic	T48.0x1-	T48.0x2-	T48.0x3-	T48.0x4-	T48.0x5-	T48.0x6-
parathyroid (derivatives)	T50.991-	T50.992-	T50.993-	T50.994-	T50.995-	T50.996-
pituitary (posterior) NEC	T38.891-	T38.892-	T38.893-	T38.894-	T38.895-	T38.896-
anterior	T38.811-	T38.812-	T38.813-	T38.814-	T38.815-	T38.816-
specified, NEC	T38.891-	T38.892-	T38.893-	T38.894-	T38.895-	T38.896-
thyroid	T38.1x1-	T38.1x2-	T38.1x3-	T38.1x4-	T38.1x5-	T38.1x6-
Hornet (sting)	T63.451-	T63.452-	T63.453-	T63.454-	—	—
Horse anti-human lymphocytic serum	T50.Z11-	T50.Z12-	T50.Z13-	T50.Z14-	T50.Z15-	T50.Z16-
Horticulture agent NEC	T65.91x-	T65.92x-	T65.93x-	T65.94x-	—	—
with pesticide	T60.91x-	T60.92x-	T60.93x-	T60.94x-	—	—
Human						
albumin	T45.8x1-	T45.8x2-	T45.8x3-	T45.8x4-	T45.8x5-	T45.8x6-
growth hormone (HGH)	T38.811-	T38.812-	T38.813-	T38.814-	T38.815-	T38.816-
immune serum	T50.Z11-	T50.Z12-	T50.Z13-	T50.Z14-	T50.Z15-	T50.Z16-
Hyaluronidase	T45.3x1-	T45.3x2-	T45.3x3-	T45.3x4-	T45.3x5-	T45.3x6-
Hyazyme	T45.3x1-	T45.3x2-	T45.3x3-	T45.3x4-	T45.3x5-	T45.3x6-
Hycodan	T40.2x1-	T40.2x2-	T40.2x3-	T40.2x4-	T40.2x5-	T40.2x6-
Hydantoin derivative NEC ..	T42.0x1-	T42.0x2-	T42.0x3-	T42.0x4-	T42.0x5-	T42.0x6-
Hydeltra	T38.0x1-	T38.0x2-	T38.0x3-	T38.0x4-	T38.0x5-	T38.0x6-
Hydergine	T44.6x1-	T44.6x2-	T44.6x3-	T44.6x4-	T44.6x5-	T44.6x6-
Hydrabamine penicillin	T36.0x1-	T36.0x2-	T36.0x3-	T36.0x4-	T36.0x5-	T36.0x6-
Hydralazine	T46.5x1-	T46.5x2-	T46.5x3-	T46.5x4-	T46.5x5-	T46.5x6-
Hydrargaphen	T49.0x1-	T49.0x2-	T49.0x3-	T49.0x4-	T49.0x5-	T49.0x6-
Hydrargyri amino-chloridum	T49.0x1-	T49.0x2-	T49.0x3-	T49.0x4-	T49.0x5-	T49.0x6-
Hydrastine	T48.291-	T48.292-	T48.293-	T48.294-	T48.295-	T48.296-
Hydrazine	T54.1x1-	T54.1x2-	T54.1x3-	T54.1x4-	—	—
monoamine oxidase inhibitors	T43.1x1-	T43.1x2-	T43.1x3-	T43.1x4-	T43.1x5-	T43.1x6-
Hydrazoic acid, azides	T54.2x1-	T54.2x2-	T54.2x3-	T54.2x4-	—	—
Hydriodic acid	T48.4x1-	T48.4x2-	T48.4x3-	T48.4x4-	T48.4x5-	T48.4x6-
Hydrocarbon gas	T59.891-	T59.892-	T59.893-	T59.894-	—	—
incomplete combustion of — see Carbon, monoxide, fuel, utility						
liquefied (mobile container)	T59.891-	T59.892-	T59.893-	T59.894-	—	—
piped (natural)	T59.891-	T59.892-	T59.893-	T59.894-	—	—
Hydrochloric acid (liquid)	T54.2x1-	T54.2x2-	T54.2x3-	T54.2x4-	—	—
medicinal (digestant)	T47.5x1-	T47.5x2-	T47.5x3-	T47.5x4-	T47.5x5-	T47.5x6-
vapor	T59.891-	T59.892-	T59.893-	T59.894-	—	—
Hydrochlorothiazide	T50.2x1-	T50.2x2-	T50.2x3-	T50.2x4-	T50.2x5-	T50.2x6-
Hydrocodone	T40.2x1-	T40.2x2-	T40.2x3-	T40.2x4-	T40.2x5-	T40.2x6-
Hydrocortisone (derivatives)	T38.0x1-	T38.0x2-	T38.0x3-	T38.0x4-	T38.0x5-	T38.0x6-
aceponate	T49.0x1-	T49.0x2-	T49.0x3-	T49.0x4-	T49.0x5-	T49.0x6-
ENT agent	T49.6x1-	T49.6x2-	T49.6x3-	T49.6x4-	T49.6x5-	T49.6x6-
ophthalmic preparation ..	T49.5x1-	T49.5x2-	T49.5x3-	T49.5x4-	T49.5x5-	T49.5x6-
topical NEC	T49.0x1-	T49.0x2-	T49.0x3-	T49.0x4-	T49.0x5-	T49.0x6-
Hydrocortone	T38.0x1-	T38.0x2-	T38.0x3-	T38.0x4-	T38.0x5-	T38.0x6-
ENT agent	T49.6x1-	T49.6x2-	T49.6x3-	T49.6x4-	T49.6x5-	T49.6x6-
ophthalmic preparation ..	T49.5x1-	T49.5x2-	T49.5x3-	T49.5x4-	T49.5x5-	T49.5x6-
topical NEC	T49.0x1-	T49.0x2-	T49.0x3-	T49.0x4-	T49.0x5-	T49.0x6-
Hydrocyanic acid (liquid)	T57.3x1-	T57.3x2-	T57.3x3-	T57.3x4-	—	—
gas	T65.0x1-	T65.0x2-	T65.0x3-	T65.0x4-	—	—
Hydroflumethiazide	T50.2x1-	T50.2x2-	T50.2x3-	T50.2x4-	T50.2x5-	T50.2x6-
Hydrofluoric acid (liquid)	T54.2x1-	T54.2x2-	T54.2x3-	T54.2x4-	—	—
vapor	T59.891-	T59.892-	T59.893-	T59.894-	—	—
Hydrogen	T59.891-	T59.892-	T59.893-	T59.894-	—	—
arsenide	T57.0x1-	T57.0x2-	T57.0x3-	T57.0x4-	—	—
arseniureted	T57.0x1-	T57.0x2-	T57.0x3-	T57.0x4-	—	—
chloride	T57.8x1-	T57.8x2-	T57.8x3-	T57.8x4-	—	—
cyanide (salts)	T57.3x1-	T57.3x2-	T57.3x3-	T57.3x4-	—	—
gas	T57.3x1-	T57.3x2-	T57.3x3-	T57.3x4-	—	—
fluoride	T59.5x1-	T59.5x2-	T59.5x3-	T59.5x4-	—	—
vapor	T59.5x1-	T59.5x2-	T59.5x3-	T59.5x4-	—	—
peroxide	T49.0x1-	T49.0x2-	T49.0x3-	T49.0x4-	T49.0x5-	T49.0x6-
phosphureted	T57.1x1-	T57.1x2-	T57.1x3-	T57.1x4-	—	—
sulfide	T59.6x1-	T59.6x2-	T59.6x3-	T59.6x4-	—	—
arseniureted	T57.0x1-	T57.0x2-	T57.0x3-	T57.0x4-	—	—
sulfureted	T59.6x1-	T59.6x2-	T59.6x3-	T59.6x4-	—	—

DRUGS & CHEMICALS

Table of Drugs & Chemicals	POISONING Accidental (Unintentional)	POISONING Self-Harm (Intentional)	POISONING Assault	POISONING Undetermined	Adverse Effect	Underdosing
Hydromethylpyridine	T46.7x1-	T46.7x2-	T46.7x3-	T46.7x4-	T46.7x5-	T46.7x6-
Hydromorphinol	T40.2x1-	T40.2x2-	T40.2x3-	T40.2x4-	—	—
Hydromorphinone	T40.2x1-	T40.2x2-	T40.2x3-	T40.2x4-	T40.2x5-	T40.2x6-
Hydromorphone	T40.2x1-	T40.2x2-	T40.2x3-	T40.2x4-	T40.2x5-	T40.2x6-
Hydromox	T50.2x1-	T50.2x2-	T50.2x3-	T50.2x4-	T50.2x5-	T50.2x6-
Hydrophilic lotion	T49.3x1-	T49.3x2-	T49.3x3-	T49.3x4-	T49.3x5-	T49.3x6-
Hydroquinidine	T46.2x1-	T46.2x2-	T46.2x3-	T46.2x4-	T46.2x5-	T46.2x6-
Hydroquinone	T52.2x1-	T52.2x2-	T52.2x3-	T52.2x4-	—	—
vapor	T59.891-	T59.892-	T59.893-	T59.894-	—	—
Hydrosulfuric acid (gas)	T59.6x1-	T59.6x2-	T59.6x3-	T59.6x4-	—	—
Hydrotalcite	T47.1x1-	T47.1x2-	T47.1x3-	T47.1x4-	T47.1x5-	T47.1x6-
Hydrous wool fat	T49.3x1-	T49.3x2-	T49.3x3-	T49.3x4-	T49.3x5-	T49.3x6-
Hydroxide, caustic	T54.3x1-	T54.3x2-	T54.3x3-	T54.3x4-	—	—
Hydroxocobalamin	T45.8x1-	T45.8x2-	T45.8x3-	T45.8x4-	T45.8x5-	T45.8x6-
Hydroxyamphetamine	T49.5x1-	T49.5x2-	T49.5x3-	T49.5x4-	T49.5x5-	T49.5x6-
Hydroxycarbamide	T45.1x1-	T45.1x2-	T45.1x3-	T45.1x4-	T45.1x5-	T45.1x6-
Hydroxychloroquine	T37.8x1-	T37.8x2-	T37.8x3-	T37.8x4-	T37.8x5-	T37.8x6-
Hydroxydihydrocodeinone	T40.2x1-	T40.2x2-	T40.2x3-	T40.2x4-	T40.2x5-	T40.2x6-
Hydroxyestrone	T38.5x1-	T38.5x2-	T38.5x3-	T38.5x4-	T38.5x5-	T38.5x6-
Hydroxyethyl starch	T45.8x1-	T45.8x2-	T45.8x3-	T45.8x4-	T45.8x5-	T45.8x6-
Hydroxymethylpenta-none..	T52.4x1-	T52.4x2-	T52.4x3-	T52.4x4-	—	—
Hydroxyphenamate	T43.591-	T43.592-	T43.593-	T43.594-	T43.595-	T43.596-
Hydroxyphenylbutazone	T39.2x1-	T39.2x2-	T39.2x3-	T39.2x4-	T39.2x5-	T39.2x6-
Hydroxyprogesterone	T38.5x1-	T38.5x2-	T38.5x3-	T38.5x4-	T38.5x5-	T38.5x6-
caproate	T38.5x1-	T38.5x2-	T38.5x3-	T38.5x4-	T38.5x5-	T38.5x6-
Hydroxyquinoline (derivatives) NEC	T37.8x1-	T37.8x2-	T37.8x3-	T37.8x4-	T37.8x5-	T37.8x6-
Hydroxystilbamidine	T37.3x1-	T37.3x2-	T37.3x3-	T37.3x4-	T37.3x5-	T37.3x6-
Hydroxytoluene (nonmedicinal)	T54.0x1-	T54.0x2-	T54.0x3-	T54.0x4-	—	—
medicinal	T49.0x1-	T49.0x2-	T49.0x3-	T49.0x4-	T49.0x5-	T49.0x6-
Hydroxyurea	T45.1x1-	T45.1x2-	T45.1x3-	T45.1x4-	T45.1x5-	T45.1x6-
Hydroxyzine	T43.591-	T43.592-	T43.593-	T43.594-	T43.595-	T43.596-
Hyoscine	T44.3x1-	T44.3x2-	T44.3x3-	T44.3x4-	T44.3x5-	T44.3x6-
Hyoscyamine	T44.3x1-	T44.3x2-	T44.3x3-	T44.3x4-	T44.3x5-	T44.3x6-
Hyoscyamus	T44.3x1-	T44.3x2-	T44.3x3-	T44.3x4-	T44.3x5-	T44.3x6-
dry extract	T44.3x1-	T44.3x2-	T44.3x3-	T44.3x4-	T44.3x5-	T44.3x6-
Hypaque	T50.8x1-	T50.8x2-	T50.8x3-	T50.8x4-	T50.8x5-	T50.8x6-
Hypertussis	T50.Z11-	T50.Z12-	T50.Z13-	T50.Z14-	T50.Z15-	T50.Z16-
Hypnotic	T42.71x-	T42.72x-	T42.73x-	T42.74x-	T42.75x-	T42.76x-
anticonvulsant	T42.71x-	T42.72x-	T42.73x-	T42.74x-	T42.75x-	T42.76x-
specified NEC	T42.6x1-	T42.6x2-	T42.6x3-	T42.6x4-	T42.6x5-	T42.6x6-
Hypochlorite	T49.0x1-	T49.0x2-	T49.0x3-	T49.0x4-	T49.0x5-	T49.0x6-
Hypophysis, posterior	T38.891-	T38.892-	T38.893-	T38.894-	T38.895-	T38.896-
Hypotensive NEC	T46.5x1-	T46.5x2-	T46.5x3-	T46.5x4-	T46.5x5-	T46.5x6-
Hypromellose	T49.5x1-	T49.5x2-	T49.5x3-	T49.5x4-	T49.5x5-	T49.5x6-
Ibacitabine	T37.5x1-	T37.5x2-	T37.5x3-	T37.5x4-	T37.5x5-	T37.5x6-
Ibopamine	T44.991-	T44.992-	T44.993-	T44.994-	T44.995-	T44.996-
Ibufenac	T39.311-	T39.312-	T39.313-	T39.314-	T39.315-	T39.316-
Ibuprofen	T39.311-	T39.312-	T39.313-	T39.314-	T39.315-	T39.316-
Ibuproxam	T39.311-	T39.312-	T39.313-	T39.314-	T39.315-	T39.316-
Ibuterol	T48.6x1-	T48.6x2-	T48.6x3-	T48.6x4-	T48.6x5-	T48.6x6-
Ichthammol	T49.0x1-	T49.0x2-	T49.0x3-	T49.0x4-	T49.0x5-	T49.0x6-
Ichthyol	T49.4x1-	T49.4x2-	T49.4x3-	T49.4x4-	T49.4x5-	T49.4x6-
Idarubicin	T45.1x1-	T45.1x2-	T45.1x3-	T45.1x4-	T45.1x5-	T45.1x6-
Idrocilamide	T42.8x1-	T42.8x2-	T42.8x3-	T42.8x4-	T42.8x5-	T42.8x6-
Ifenprodil	T46.7x1-	T46.7x2-	T46.7x3-	T46.7x4-	T46.7x5-	T46.7x6-
Ifosfamide	T45.1x1-	T45.1x2-	T45.1x3-	T45.1x4-	T45.1x5-	T45.1x6-
Iletin	T38.3x1-	T38.3x2-	T38.3x3-	T38.3x4-	T38.3x5-	T38.3x6-
Ilex	T62.2x1-	T62.2x2-	T62.2x3-	T62.2x4-	—	—
Illuminating gas (after combustion)	T58.11x-	T58.12x-	T58.13x-	T58.14x-	—	—
prior to combustion	T59.891-	T59.892-	T59.893-	T59.894-	—	—
Ilopan	T45.2x1-	T45.2x2-	T45.2x3-	T45.2x4-	T45.2x5-	T45.2x6-
Iloprost	T46.7x1-	T46.7x2-	T46.7x3-	T46.7x4-	T46.7x5-	T46.7x6-
Ilotycin	T36.3x1-	T36.3x2-	T36.3x3-	T36.3x4-	T36.3x5-	T36.3x6-
ophthalmic preparation	T49.5x1-	T49.5x2-	T49.5x3-	T49.5x4-	T49.5x5-	T49.5x6-
topical NEC	T49.0x1-	T49.0x2-	T49.0x3-	T49.0x4-	T49.0x5-	T49.0x6-
Imidazole-4-carboxamide	T45.1x1-	T45.1x2-	T45.1x3-	T45.1x4-	T45.1x5-	T45.1x6-
Iminostilbene	T42.1x1-	T42.1x2-	T42.1x3-	T42.1x4-	T42.1x5-	T42.1x6-
Imipenem	T36.0x1-	T36.0x2-	T36.0x3-	T36.0x4-	T36.0x5-	T36.0x6-
Imipramine	T43.011-	T43.012-	T43.013-	T43.014-	T43.015-	T43.016-
Immu-G	T50.Z11-	T50.Z12-	T50.Z13-	T50.Z14-	T50.Z15-	T50.Z16-
Immuglobin	T50.Z11-	T50.Z12-	T50.Z13-	T50.Z14-	T50.Z15-	T50.Z16-
Immune globulin	T50.Z11-	T50.Z12-	T50.Z13-	T50.Z14-	T50.Z15-	T50.Z16-
serum globulin	T50.Z11-	T50.Z12-	T50.Z13-	T50.Z14-	T50.Z15-	T50.Z16-
Immunoglobin human (intravenous) (normal)	T50.Z11-	T50.Z12-	T50.Z13-	T50.Z14-	T50.Z15-	T50.Z16-
unmodified	T50.Z11-	T50.Z12-	T50.Z13-	T50.Z14-	T50.Z15-	T50.Z16-
Immunosuppressive drug	T45.1x1-	T45.1x2-	T45.1x3-	T45.1x4-	T45.1x5-	T45.1x6-
Immu-tetanus	T50.Z11-	T50.Z12-	T50.Z13-	T50.Z14-	T50.Z15-	T50.Z16-
Indalpine	T43.221-	T43.222-	T43.223-	T43.224-	T43.225-	T43.226-
Indanazoline	T48.5x1-	T48.5x2-	T48.5x3-	T48.5x4-	T48.5x5-	T48.5x6-
Indandione (derivatives)	T45.511-	T45.512-	T45.513-	T45.514-	T45.515-	T45.516-
Indapamide	T46.5x1-	T46.5x2-	T46.5x3-	T46.5x4-	T46.5x5-	T46.5x6-
Indendione (derivatives)	T45.511-	T45.512-	T45.513-	T45.514-	T45.515-	T45.516-
Indenolol	T44.7x1-	T44.7x2-	T44.7x3-	T44.7x4-	T44.7x5-	T44.7x6-
Inderal	T44.7x1-	T44.7x2-	T44.7x3-	T44.7x4-	T44.7x5-	T44.7x6-
Indian hemp	T40.7x1-	T40.7x2-	T40.7x3-	T40.7x4-	T40.7x5-	T40.7x6-
tobacco	T62.2x1-	T62.2x2-	T62.2x3-	T62.2x4-	—	—
Indigo carmine	T50.8x1-	T50.8x2-	T50.8x3-	T50.8x4-	T50.8x5-	T50.8x6-
Indobufen	T45.521-	T45.522-	T45.523-	T45.524-	T45.525-	T45.526-
Indocin	T39.2x1-	T39.2x2-	T39.2x3-	T39.2x4-	T39.2x5-	T39.2x6-
Indocyanine green	T50.8x1-	T50.8x2-	T50.8x3-	T50.8x4-	T50.8x5-	T50.8x6-
Indometacin	T39.391-	T39.392-	T39.393-	T39.394-	T39.395-	T39.396-
Indomethacin	T39.391-	T39.392-	T39.393-	T39.394-	T39.395-	T39.396-
farnesil	T39.4x1-	T39.4x2-	T39.4x3-	T39.4x4-	T39.4x5-	T39.4x6-
Indoramin	T44.6x1-	T44.6x2-	T44.6x3-	T44.6x4-	T44.6x5-	T44.6x6-
Industrial alcohol	T51.0x1-	T51.0x2-	T51.0x3-	T51.0x4-	—	—
fumes	T59.891-	T59.892-	T59.893-	T59.894-	—	—
solvents (fumes) (vapors)	T52.91x-	T52.92x-	T52.93x-	T52.94x-	—	—
Influenza vaccine	T50.B91-	T50.B92-	T50.B93-	T50.B94-	T50.B95-	T50.B96-
Ingested substance NEC	T65.91x-	T65.92x-	T65.93x-	T65.94x-	—	—
INH	T37.1x1-	T37.1x2-	T37.1x3-	T37.1x4-	T37.1x5-	T37.1x6-
Inhalation, gas (noxious) — see Gas						
Inhibitor angiotensin-converting enzyme	T46.4x1-	T46.4x2-	T46.4x3-	T46.4x4-	T46.4x5-	T46.4x6-
carbonic anhydrase	T50.2x1-	T50.2x2-	T50.2x3-	T50.2x4-	T50.2x5-	T50.2x6-
fibrinolysis	T45.621-	T45.622-	T45.623-	T45.624-	T45.625-	T45.626-
monoamine oxidase NEC	T43.1x1-	T43.1x2-	T43.1x3-	T43.1x4-	T43.1x5-	T43.1x6-
hydrazine	T43.1x1-	T43.1x2-	T43.1x3-	T43.1x4-	T43.1x5-	T43.1x6-
postsynaptic	T43.8x1-	T43.8x2-	T43.8x3-	T43.8x4-	T43.8x5-	T43.8x6-
prothrombin synthesis	T45.511-	T45.512-	T45.513-	T45.514-	T45.515-	T45.516-
Ink	T65.891-	T65.892-	T65.893-	T65.894-	—	—
Inorganic substance	T57.91x-	T57.92x-	T57.93x-	T57.94x-	—	—
Inosine pranobex	T37.5x1-	T37.5x2-	T37.5x3-	T37.5x4-	T37.5x5-	T37.5x6-
Inositol	T50.991-	T50.992-	T50.993-	T50.994-	T50.995-	T50.996-
nicotinate	T46.7x1-	T46.7x2-	T46.7x3-	T46.7x4-	T46.7x5-	T46.7x6-
Inproquone	T45.1x1-	T45.1x2-	T45.1x3-	T45.1x4-	T45.1x5-	T45.1x6-

DRUGS & CHEMICALS

Table of Drugs & Chemicals	POISONING Accidental (Unintentional)	POISONING Self-Harm (Intentional)	Assault	Undetermined	Adverse Effect	Underdosing
Insect (sting), venomous	T63.481-	T63.482-	T63.483-	T63.484-	—	—
ant	T63.421-	T63.422-	T63.423-	T63.424-	—	—
bee	T63.441-	T63.442-	T63.443-	T63.444-	—	—
caterpillar	T63.431-	T63.432-	T63.433-	T63.434-	—	—
hornet	T63.451-	T63.452-	T63.453-	T63.454-	—	—
wasp	T63.461-	T63.462-	T63.463-	T63.464-	—	—
Insecticide NEC	T60.91x-	T60.92x-	T60.93x-	T60.94x-	—	—
carbamate	T60.0x1-	T60.0x2-	T60.0x3-	T60.0x4-	—	—
chlorinated	T60.1x1-	T60.1x2-	T60.1x3-	T60.1x4-	—	—
mixed	T60.91x-	T60.92x-	T60.93x-	T60.94x-	—	—
organochlorine	T60.1x1-	T60.1x2-	T60.1x3-	T60.1x4-	—	—
organophosphorus	T60.0x1-	T60.0x2-	T60.0x3-	T60.0x4-	—	—
Insular tissue extract	T38.3x1-	T38.3x2-	T38.3x3-	T38.3x4-	T38.3x5-	T38.3x6-
Insulin (amorphous) (globin) (isophane) (Lente) (NPH) (Semilente) (Ultralente) (zinc)	T38.3x1-	T38.3x2-	T38.3x3-	T38.3x4-	T38.3x5-	T38.3x6-
defalan	T38.3x1-	T38.3x2-	T38.3x3-	T38.3x4-	T38.3x5-	T38.3x6-
human	T38.3x1-	T38.3x2-	T38.3x3-	T38.3x4-	T38.3x5-	T38.3x6-
injection, soluble	T38.3x1-	T38.3x2-	T38.3x3-	T38.3x4-	T38.3x5-	T38.3x6-
biphasic	T38.3x1-	T38.3x2-	T38.3x3-	T38.3x4-	T38.3x5-	T38.3x6-
intermediate acting	T38.3x1-	T38.3x2-	T38.3x3-	T38.3x4-	T38.3x5-	T38.3x6-
protamine zinc	T38.3x1-	T38.3x2-	T38.3x3-	T38.3x4-	T38.3x5-	T38.3x6-
slow acting	T38.3x1-	T38.3x2-	T38.3x3-	T38.3x4-	T38.3x5-	T38.3x6-
zinc						
protamine injection	T38.3x1-	T38.3x2-	T38.3x3-	T38.3x4-	T38.3x5-	T38.3x6-
suspension (amorphous) (crystalline)	T38.3x1-	T38.3x2-	T38.3x3-	T38.3x4-	T38.3x5-	T38.3x6-
Interferon (alpha) (beta) (gamma)	T37.5x1-	T37.5x2-	T37.5x3-	T37.5x4-	T37.5x5-	T37.5x6-
Intestinal motility control drug	T47.6x1-	T47.6x2-	T47.6x3-	T47.6x4-	T47.6x5-	T47.6x6-
biological	T47.8x1-	T47.8x2-	T47.8x3-	T47.8x4-	T47.8x5-	T47.8x6-
Intranarcon	T41.1x1-	T41.1x2-	T41.1x3-	T41.1x4-	T41.1x5-	T41.1x6-
Intravenous						
amino acids	T50.991-	T50.992-	T50.993-	T50.994-	T50.995-	T50.996-
fat suspension	T50.991-	T50.992-	T50.993-	T50.994-	T50.995-	T50.996-
Inulin	T50.8x1-	T50.8x2-	T50.8x3-	T50.8x4-	T50.8x5-	T50.8x6-
Invert sugar	T50.3x1-	T50.3x2-	T50.3x3-	T50.3x4-	T50.3x5-	T50.3x6-
Inza — see Naproxen						
Iobenzamic acid	T50.8x1-	T50.8x2-	T50.8x3-	T50.8x4-	T50.8x5-	T50.8x6-
Iocarmic acid	T50.8x1-	T50.8x2-	T50.8x3-	T50.8x4-	T50.8x5-	T50.8x6-
Iocetamic acid	T50.8x1-	T50.8x2-	T50.8x3-	T50.8x4-	T50.8x5-	T50.8x6-
Iodamide	T50.8x1-	T50.8x2-	T50.8x3-	T50.8x4-	T50.8x5-	T50.8x6-
Iodide NEC — see also						
Iodine	T49.0x1-	T49.0x2-	T49.0x3-	T49.0x4-	T49.0x5-	T49.0x6-
mercury (ointment)	T49.0x1-	T49.0x2-	T49.0x3-	T49.0x4-	T49.0x5-	T49.0x6-
methylate	T49.0x1-	T49.0x2-	T49.0x3-	T49.0x4-	T49.0x5-	T49.0x6-
potassium (expectorant) NEC	T48.4x1-	T48.4x2-	T48.4x3-	T48.4x4-	T48.4x5-	T48.4x6-
Iodinated						
contrast medium	T50.8x1-	T50.8x2-	T50.8x3-	T50.8x4-	T50.8x5-	T50.8x6-
glycerol	T48.4x1-	T48.4x2-	T48.4x3-	T48.4x4-	T48.4x5-	T48.4x6-
human serum albumin (131I)	T50.8x1-	T50.8x2-		T50.8x4-	T50.8x5-	T50.8x6-
Iodine (antiseptic, external) (tincture) NEC	T49.0x1-	T49.0x2-	T49.0x3-	T49.0x4-	T49.0x5-	T49.0x6-
125 — see also Radiation sickness, and Exposure to radioactive isotopes	T50.8x1-	T50.8x2-	T50.8x3-	T50.8x4-	T50.8x5-	T50.8x6-
therapeutic	T50.991-	T50.992-	T50.993-	T50.994-	T50.995-	T50.996-
131 — see also Radiation sickness, and Exposure to radioactive isotopes	T50.8x1-	T50.8x2-	T50.8x3-	T50.8x4-	T50.8x5-	T50.8x6-
therapeutic	T38.2x1-	T38.2x2-	T38.2x3-	T38.2x4-	T38.2x5-	T38.2x6-
diagnostic	T50.8x1-	T50.8x2-	T50.8x3-	T50.8x4-	T50.8x5-	T50.8x6-
for thyroid conditions (antithyroid)	T38.2x1-	T38.2x2-	T38.2x3-	T38.2x4-	T38.2x5-	T38.2x6-
solution	T49.0x1-	T49.0x2-	T49.0x3-	T49.0x4-	T49.0x5-	T49.0x6-
vapor	T59.891-	T59.892-	T59.893-	T59.894-	—	—
Iodipamide	T50.8x1-	T50.8x2-	T50.8x3-	T50.8x4-	T50.8x5-	T50.8x6-
Iodized (poppy seed) oil	T50.8x1-	T50.8x2-	T50.8x3-	T50.8x4-	T50.8x5-	T50.8x6-
Iodobismitol	T37.8x1-	T37.8x2-	T37.8x3-	T37.8x4-	T37.8x5-	T37.8x6-
Iodochlorhydroxyquin	T37.8x1-	T37.8x2-	T37.8x3-	T37.8x4-	T37.8x5-	T37.8x6-
topical	T49.0x1-	T49.0x2-	T49.0x3-	T49.0x4-	T49.0x5-	T49.0x6-
Iodochlorhydroxyquinoline	T37.8x1-	T37.8x2-	T37.8x3-	T37.8x4-	T37.8x5-	T37.8x6-
Iodocholesterol (131I)	T50.8x1-	T50.8x2-	T50.8x3-	T50.8x4-	T50.8x5-	T50.8x6-
Iodoform	T49.0x1-	T49.0x2-	T49.0x3-	T49.0x4-	T49.0x5-	T49.0x6-
Iodohippuric acid	T50.8x1-	T50.8x2-	T50.8x3-	T50.8x4-	T50.8x5-	T50.8x6-
Iodopanoic acid	T50.8x1-	T50.8x2-	T50.8x3-	T50.8x4-	T50.8x5-	T50.8x6-
Iodophthalein (sodium)	T50.8x1-	T50.8x2-	T50.8x3-	T50.8x4-	T50.8x5-	T50.8x6-
Iodopyracet	T50.8x1-	T50.8x2-	T50.8x3-	T50.8x4-	T50.8x5-	T50.8x6-
Iodoquinol	T37.8x1-	T37.8x2-	T37.8x3-	T37.8x4-	T37.8x5-	T37.8x6-
Iodoxamic acid	T50.8x1-	T50.8x2-	T50.8x3-	T50.8x4-	T50.8x5-	T50.8x6-
Iofendylate	T50.8x1-	T50.8x2-	T50.8x3-	T50.8x4-	T50.8x5-	T50.8x6-
Ioglycamic acid	T50.8x1-	T50.8x2-	T50.8x3-	T50.8x4-	T50.8x5-	T50.8x6-
Iohexol	T50.8x1-	T50.8x2-	T50.8x3-	T50.8x4-	T50.8x5-	T50.8x6-
Ion exchange resin						
anion	T47.8x1-	T47.8x2-	T47.8x3-	T47.8x4-	T47.8x5-	T47.8x6-
cation	T50.3x1-	T50.3x2-	T50.3x3-	T50.3x4-	T50.3x5-	T50.3x6-
cholestyramine	T46.6x1-	T46.6x2-	T46.6x3-	T46.6x4-	T46.6x5-	T46.6x6-
intestinal	T47.8x1-	T47.8x2-	T47.8x3-	T47.8x4-	T47.8x5-	T47.8x6-
Iopamidol	T50.8x1-	T50.8x2-	T50.8x3-	T50.8x4-	T50.8x5-	T50.8x6-
Iopanoic acid	T50.8x1-	T50.8x2-	T50.8x3-	T50.8x4-	T50.8x5-	T50.8x6-
Iophenoic acid	T50.8x1-	T50.8x2-	T50.8x3-	T50.8x4-	T50.8x5-	T50.8x6-
Iopodate, sodium	T50.8x1-	T50.8x2-	T50.8x3-	T50.8x4-	T50.8x5-	T50.8x6-
Iopodic acid	T50.8x1-	T50.8x2-	T50.8x3-	T50.8x4-	T50.8x5-	T50.8x6-
Iopromide	T50.8x1-	T50.8x2-	T50.8x3-	T50.8x4-	T50.8x5-	T50.8x6-
Iopydol	T50.8x1-	T50.8x2-	T50.8x3-	T50.8x4-	T50.8x5-	T50.8x6-
Iotalamic acid	T50.8x1-	T50.8x2-	T50.8x3-	T50.8x4-	T50.8x5-	T50.8x6-
Iothalamate	T50.8x1-	T50.8x2-	T50.8x3-	T50.8x4-	T50.8x5-	T50.8x6-
Iothiouracil	T38.2x1-	T38.2x2-	T38.2x3-	T38.2x4-	T38.2x5-	T38.2x6-
Iotrol	T50.8x1-	T50.8x2-	T50.8x3-	T50.8x4-	T50.8x5-	T50.8x6-
Iotrolan	T50.8x1-	T50.8x2-	T50.8x3-	T50.8x4-	T50.8x5-	T50.8x6-
Iotroxate	T50.8x1-	T50.8x2-	T50.8x3-	T50.8x4-	T50.8x5-	T50.8x6-
Iotroxic acid	T50.8x1-	T50.8x2-	T50.8x3-	T50.8x4-	T50.8x5-	T50.8x6-
Ioversol	T50.8x1-	T50.8x2-	T50.8x3-	T50.8x4-	T50.8x5-	T50.8x6-
Ioxaglate	T50.8x1-	T50.8x2-	T50.8x3-	T50.8x4-	T50.8x5-	T50.8x6-
Ioxaglic acid	T50.8x1-	T50.8x2-	T50.8x3-	T50.8x4-	T50.8x5-	T50.8x6-
Ioxitalamic acid	T50.8x1-	T50.8x2-	T50.8x3-	T50.8x4-	T50.8x5-	T50.8x6-
Ipecac	T47.7x1-	T47.7x2-	T47.7x3-	T47.7x4-	T47.7x5-	T47.7x6-
Ipecacuanha	T48.4x1-	T48.4x2-	T48.4x3-	T48.4x4-	T48.4x5-	T48.4x6-
Ipodate, calcium	T50.8x1-	T50.8x2-	T50.8x3-	T50.8x4-	T50.8x5-	T50.8x6-
Ipral	T42.3x1-	T42.3x2-	T42.3x3-	T42.3x4-	T42.3x5-	T42.3x6-
Ipratropium (bromide)	T48.6x1-	T48.6x2-	T48.6x3-	T48.6x4-	T48.6x5-	T48.6x6-

DRUGS & CHEMICALS

Table of Drugs & Chemicals	POISONING				Adverse Effect	Underdosing
	Accidental (Unintentional)	Self-Harm (Intentional)	Assault	Undetermined		
Ipriflavone	T46.3x1-	T46.3x2-	T46.3x3-	T46.3x4-	T46.3x5-	T46.3x6-
Iprindole	T43.011-	T43.012-	T43.013-	T43.014-	T43.015-	T43.016-
Iproclozide	T43.1x1-	T43.1x2-	T43.1x3-	T43.1x4-	T43.1x5-	T43.1x6-
Iprofenin	T50.8x1-	T50.8x2-	T50.8x3-	T50.8x4-	T50.8x5-	T50.8x6-
Iproheptine	T49.2x1-	T49.2x2-	T49.2x3-	T49.2x4-	T49.2x5-	T49.2x6-
Iproniazid	T43.1x1-	T43.1x2-	T43.1x3-	T43.1x4-	T43.1x5-	T43.1x6-
Iproplatin	T45.1x1-	T45.1x2-	T45.1x3-	T45.1x4-	T45.1x5-	T45.1x6-
Iproveratril	T46.1x1-	T46.1x2-	T46.1x3-	T46.1x4-	T46.1x5-	T46.1x6-
Iron (compounds) (medicinal) NEC	T45.4x1-	T45.4x2-	T45.4x3-	T45.4x4-	T45.4x5-	T45.4x6-
ammonium	T45.4x1-	T45.4x2-	T45.4x3-	T45.4x4-	T45.4x5-	T45.4x6-
dextran injection	T45.4x1-	T45.4x2-	T45.4x3-	T45.4x4-	T45.4x5-	T45.4x6-
nonmedicinal	T56.891-	T56.892-	T56.893-	T56.894-	—	—
salts	T45.4x1-	T45.4x2-	T45.4x3-	T45.4x4-	T45.4x5-	T45.4x6-
sorbitex	T45.4x1-	T45.4x2-	T45.4x3-	T45.4x4-	T45.4x5-	T45.4x6-
sorbitol citric acid complex	T45.4x1-	T45.4x2-	T45.4x3-	T45.4x4-	T45.4x5-	T45.4x6-
Irrigating fluid (vaginal)	T49.8x1-	T49.8x2-	T49.8x3-	T49.8x4-	T49.8x5-	T49.8x6-
eye	T49.5x1-	T49.5x2-	T49.5x3-	T49.5x4-	T49.5x5-	T49.5x6-
Isepamicin	T36.5x1-	T36.5x2-	T36.5x3-	T36.5x4-	T36.5x5-	T36.5x6-
Isoaminile (citrate)	T48.3x1-	T48.3x2-	T48.3x3-	T48.3x4-	T48.3x5-	T48.3x6-
Isoamyl nitrite	T46.3x1-	T46.3x2-	T46.3x3-	T46.3x4-	T46.3x5-	T46.3x6-
Isobenzan	T60.1x1-	T60.1x2-	T60.1x3-	T60.1x4-	—	—
Isobutyl acetate	T52.8x1-	T52.8x2-	T52.8x3-	T52.8x4-	—	—
Isocarboxazid	T43.1x1-	T43.1x2-	T43.1x3-	T43.1x4-	T43.1x5-	T43.1x6-
Isoconazole	T49.0x1-	T49.0x2-	T49.0x3-	T49.0x4-	T49.0x5-	T49.0x6-
Isocyanate	T65.0x1-	T65.0x2-	T65.0x3-	T65.0x4-	—	—
Isoephedrine	T44.991-	T44.992-	T44.993-	T44.994-	T44.995-	T44.996-
Isoetarine	T48.6x1-	T48.6x2-	T48.6x3-	T48.6x4-	T48.6x5-	T48.6x6-
Isoethadione	T42.2x1-	T42.2x2-	T42.2x3-	T42.2x4-	T42.2x5-	T42.2x6-
Isoetharine	T44.5x1-	T44.5x2-	T44.5x3-	T44.5x4-	T44.5x5-	T44.5x6-
Isoflurane	T41.0x1-	T41.0x2-	T41.0x3-	T41.0x4-	T41.0x5-	T41.0x6-
Isoflurophate	T44.0x1-	T44.0x2-	T44.0x3-	T44.0x4-	T44.0x5-	T44.0x6-
Isomaltose, ferric complex	T45.4x1-	T45.4x2-	T45.4x3-	T45.4x4-	T45.4x5-	T45.4x6-
Isometheptene	T44.3x1-	T44.3x2-	T44.3x3-	T44.3x4-	T44.3x5-	T44.3x6-
Isoniazid	T37.1x1-	T37.1x2-	T37.1x3-	T37.1x4-	T37.1x5-	T37.1x6-
with rifampicin	T36.6x1-	T36.6x2-	T36.6x3-	T36.6x4-	T36.6x5-	T36.6x6-
thioacetazone	T37.1x1-	T37.1x2-	T37.1x3-	T37.1x4-	T37.1x5-	T37.1x6-
Isonicotinic acid hydrazide	T37.1x1-	T37.1x2-	T37.1x3-	T37.1x4-	T37.1x5-	T37.1x6-
Isonipecaine	T40.4x1-	T40.4x2-	T40.4x3-	T40.4x4-	T40.4x5-	T40.4x6-
Isopentaquine	T37.2x1-	T37.2x2-	T37.2x3-	T37.2x4-	T37.2x5-	T37.2x6-
Isophane insulin	T38.3x1-	T38.3x2-	T38.3x3-	T38.3x4-	T38.3x5-	T38.3x6-
Isophorone	T65.891-	T65.892-	T65.893-	T65.894-	—	—
Isophosphamide	T45.1x1-	T45.1x2-	T45.1x3-	T45.1x4-	T45.1x5-	T45.1x6-
Isopregnenone	T38.5x1-	T38.5x2-	T38.5x3-	T38.5x4-	T38.5x5-	T38.5x6-
Isoprenaline	T48.6x1-	T48.6x2-	T48.6x3-	T48.6x4-	T48.6x5-	T48.6x6-
Isopromethazine	T43.3x1-	T43.3x2-	T43.3x3-	T43.3x4-	T43.3x5-	T43.3x6-
Isopropamide	T44.3x1-	T44.3x2-	T44.3x3-	T44.3x4-	T44.3x5-	T44.3x6-
iodide	T44.3x1-	T44.3x2-	T44.3x3-	T44.3x4-	T44.3x5-	T44.3x6-
Isopropanol	T51.2x1-	T51.2x2-	T51.2x3-	T51.2x4-	—	—
Isopropyl acetate	T52.8x1-	T52.8x2-	T52.8x3-	T52.8x4-	—	—
alcohol	T51.2x1-	T51.2x2-	T51.2x3-	T51.2x4-	—	—
medicinal	T49.4x1-	T49.4x2-	T49.4x3-	T49.4x4-	T49.4x5-	T49.4x6-
ether	T52.8x1-	T52.8x2-	T52.8x3-	T52.8x4-	—	—
Isopropylaminophenazone	T39.2x1-	T39.2x2-	T39.2x3-	T39.2x4-	T39.2x5-	T39.2x6-
Isoproterenol	T48.6x1-	T48.6x2-	T48.6x3-	T48.6x4-	T48.6x5-	T48.6x6-
Isosorbide dinitrate	T46.3x1-	T46.3x2-	T46.3x3-	T46.3x4-	T46.3x5-	T46.3x6-
Isothipendyl	T45.0x1-	T45.0x2-	T45.0x3-	T45.0x4-	T45.0x5-	T45.0x6-
Isotretinoin	T50.991-	T50.992-	T50.993-	T50.994-	T50.995-	T50.996-
Isoxazolyl penicillin	T36.0x1-	T36.0x2-	T36.0x3-	T36.0x4-	T36.0x5-	T36.0x6-
Isoxicam	T39.391-	T39.392-	T39.393-	T39.394-	T39.395-	T39.396-
Isoxsuprine	T46.7x1-	T46.7x2-	T46.7x3-	T46.7x4-	T46.7x5-	T46.7x6-
Ispagula	T47.4x1-	T47.4x2-	T47.4x3-	T47.4x4-	T47.4x5-	T47.4x6-
husk	T47.4x1-	T47.4x2-	T47.4x3-	T47.4x4-	T47.4x5-	T47.4x6-
Isradipine	T46.1x1-	T46.1x2-	T46.1x3-	T46.1x4-	T46.1x5-	T46.1x6-
I-thyroxine sodium	T38.1x1-	T38.1x2-	T38.1x3-	T38.1x4-	T38.1x5-	T38.1x6-
Itraconazole	T37.8x1-	T37.8x2-	T37.8x3-	T37.8x4-	T37.8x5-	T37.8x6-
Itramin tosilate	T46.3x1-	T46.3x2-	T46.3x3-	T46.3x4-	T46.3x5-	T46.3x6-
Ivermectin	T37.4x1-	T37.4x2-	T37.4x3-	T37.4x4-	T37.4x5-	T37.4x6-
Izoniazid	T37.1x1-	T37.1x2-	T37.1x3-	T37.1x4-	T37.1x5-	T37.1x6-
with thioacetazone	T37.1x1-	T37.1x2-	T37.1x3-	T37.1x4-	T37.1x5-	T37.1x6-
Jalap	T47.2x1-	T47.2x2-	T47.2x3-	T47.2x4-	T47.2x5-	T47.2x6-
Jamaica dogwood (bark)	T39.8x1-	T39.8x2-	T39.8x3-	T39.8x4-	T39.8x5-	
ginger	T65.891-	T65.892-	T65.893-	T65.894-	—	—
root	T62.2x1-	T62.2x2-	T62.2x3-	T62.2x4-	—	—
Jatropha	T62.2x1-	T62.2x2-	T62.2x3-	T62.2x4-	—	—
curcas	T62.2x1-	T62.2x2-	T62.2x3-	T62.2x4-	—	—
Jectofer	T45.4x1-	T45.4x2-	T45.4x3-	T45.4x4-	T45.4x5-	T45.4x6-
Jellyfish (sting)	T63.621-	T63.622-	T63.623-	T63.624-	—	—
Jequirity (bean)	T62.2x1-	T62.2x2-	T62.2x3-	T62.2x4-	—	—
Jimson weed (stramonium)	T62.2x1-	T62.2x2-	T62.2x3-	T62.2x4-	—	—
seeds	T62.2x1-	T62.2x2-	T62.2x3-	T62.2x4-	—	—
Josamycin	T36.3x1-	T36.3x2-	T36.3x3-	T36.3x4-	T36.3x5-	T36.3x6-
Juniper tar	T49.1x1-	T49.1x2-	T49.1x3-	T49.1x4-	T49.1x5-	T49.1x6-
Kallidinogenase	T46.7x1-	T46.7x2-	T46.7x3-	T46.7x4-	T46.7x5-	T46.7x6-
Kallikrein	T46.7x1-	T46.7x2-	T46.7x3-	T46.7x4-	T46.7x5-	T46.7x6-
Kanamycin	T36.5x1-	T36.5x2-	T36.5x3-	T36.5x4-	T36.5x5-	T36.5x6-
Kantrex	T36.5x1-	T36.5x2-	T36.5x3-	T36.5x4-	T36.5x5-	T36.5x6-
Kaolin	T47.6x1-	T47.6x2-	T47.6x3-	T47.6x4-	T47.6x5-	T47.6x6-
light	T47.6x1-	T47.6x2-	T47.6x3-	T47.6x4-	T47.6x5-	T47.6x6-
Karaya (gum)	T47.4x1-	T47.4x2-	T47.4x3-	T47.4x4-	T47.4x5-	T47.4x6-
Kebuzone	T39.2x1-	T39.2x2-	T39.2x3-	T39.2x4-	T39.2x5-	T39.2x6-
Kelevan	T60.1x1-	T60.1x2-	T60.1x3-	T60.1x4-	—	—
Kemithal	T41.1x1-	T41.1x2-	T41.1x3-	T41.1x4-	T41.1x5-	T41.1x6-
Kenacort	T38.0x1-	T38.0x2-	T38.0x3-	T38.0x4-	T38.0x5-	T38.0x6-
Keratolytic drug NEC	T49.4x1-	T49.4x2-	T49.4x3-	T49.4x4-	T49.4x5-	T49.4x6-
anthracene	T49.4x1-	T49.4x2-	T49.4x3-	T49.4x4-	T49.4x5-	T49.4x6-
Keratoplastic NEC	T49.4x1-	T49.4x2-	T49.4x3-	T49.4x4-	T49.4x5-	T49.4x6-
Kerosene, kerosine (fuel) (solvent) NEC	T52.0x1-	T52.0x2-	T52.0x3-	T52.0x4-	—	—
insecticide	T52.0x1-	T52.0x2-	T52.0x3-	T52.0x4-	—	—
vapor	T52.0x1-	T52.0x2-	T52.0x3-	T52.0x4-	—	—
Ketamine	T41.291-	T41.292-	T41.293-	T41.294-	T41.295-	T41.296-
Ketazolam	T42.4x1-	T42.4x2-	T42.4x3-	T42.4x4-	T42.4x5-	T42.4x6-
Ketazon	T39.2x1-	T39.2x2-	T39.2x3-	T39.2x4-	T39.2x5-	T39.2x6-
Ketobemidone	T40.4x1-	T40.4x2-	T40.4x3-	T40.4x4-	—	—
Ketoconazole	T49.0x1-	T49.0x2-	T49.0x3-	T49.0x4-	T49.0x5-	T49.0x6-
Ketols	T52.4x1-	T52.4x2-	T52.4x3-	T52.4x4-	—	—
Ketone oils	T52.4x1-	T52.4x2-	T52.4x3-	T52.4x4-	—	—
Ketoprofen	T39.311-	T39.312-	T39.313-	T39.314-	T39.315-	T39.316-
Ketorolac	T39.8x1-	T39.8x2-	T39.8x3-	T39.8x4-	T39.8x5-	T39.8x6-
Ketotifen	T45.0x1-	T45.0x2-	T45.0x3-	T45.0x4-	T45.0x5-	T45.0x6-
Khat	T43.691-	T43.692-	T43.693-	T43.694-	—	—
Khellin	T46.3x1-	T46.3x2-	T46.3x3-	T46.3x4-	T46.3x5-	T46.3x6-
Khelloside	T46.3x1-	T46.3x2-	T46.3x3-	T46.3x4-	T46.3x5-	T46.3x6-
Kiln gas or vapor (carbon monoxide)	T58.8x1-	T58.8x2-	T58.8x3-	T58.8x4-	—	—
Kitasamycin	T36.3x1-	T36.3x2-	T36.3x3-	T36.3x4-	T36.3x5-	T36.3x6-
Konsyl	T47.4x1-	T47.4x2-	T47.4x3-	T47.4x4-	T47.4x5-	T47.4x6-
Kosam seed	T62.2x1-	T62.2x2-	T62.2x3-	T62.2x4-	—	—
Krait (venom)	T63.091-	T63.092-	T63.093-	T63.094-	—	—
Kwell (insecticide)	T60.1x1-	T60.1x2-	T60.1x3-	T60.1x4-	—	—
anti-infective (topical)	T49.0x1-	T49.0x2-	T49.0x3-	T49.0x4-	T49.0x5-	T49.0x6-

Table of Drugs & Chemicals	POISONING				Adverse Effect	Underdosing	Table of Drugs & Chemicals	POISONING				Adverse Effect	Underdosing
	Accidental (Unintentional)	Self-Harm (Intentional)	Assault	Undetermined				Accidental (Unintentional)	Self-Harm (Intentional)	Assault	Undetermined		
Labetalol	T44.8x1-	T44.8x2-	T44.8x3-	T44.8x4-	T44.8x5-	T44.8x6-	Lead (dust) (fumes) (vapor)						
Laburnum (seeds)	T62.2x1-	T62.2x2-	T62.2x3-	T62.2x4-	—	—	NEC - *continued*	T56.0x1-	T56.0x2-	T56.0x3-	T56.0x4-	—	—
leaves	T62.2x1-	T62.2x2-	T62.2x3-	T62.2x4-	—	—	paint	T56.0x1-	T56.0x2-	T56.0x3-	T56.0x4-	—	—
Lachesine	T49.5x1-	T49.5x2-	T49.5x3-	T49.5x4-	T49.5x5-	T49.5x6-	salts	T56.0x1-	T56.0x2-	T56.0x3-	T56.0x4-	—	—
Lacidipine	T46.5x1-	T46.5x2-	T46.5x3-	T46.5x4-	T46.5x5-	T46.5x6-	specified compound NEC	T56.0x1-	T56.0x2-	T56.0x3-	T56.0x4-	—	—
Lacquer	T65.6x1-	T65.6x2-	T65.6x3-	T65.6x4-	—	—	tetra-ethyl	T56.0x1-	T56.0x2-	T56.0x3-	T56.0x4-	—	—
Lacrimogenic gas	T59.3x1-	T59.3x2-	T59.3x3-	T59.3x4-	—	—	Lebanese red	T40.7x1-	T40.7x2-	T40.7x3-	T40.7x4-	T40.7x5-	T40.7x6-
Lactated potassic saline	T50.3x1-	T50.3x2-	T50.3x3-	T50.3x4-	T50.3x5-	T50.3x6-	Lefetamine	T39.8x1-	T39.8x2-	T39.8x3-	T39.8x4-	T39.8x5-	T39.8x6-
Lactic acid	T49.8x1-	T49.8x2-	T49.8x3-	T49.8x4-	T49.8x5-	T49.8x6-	Lenperone	T43.4x1-	T43.4x2-	T43.4x3-	T43.4x4-	T43.4x5-	T43.4x6-
Lactobacillus							Lente lietin (insulin)	T38.3x1-	T38.3x2-	T38.3x3-	T38.3x4-	T38.3x5-	T38.3x6-
acidophilus	T47.6x1-	T47.6x2-	T47.6x3-	T47.6x4-	T47.6x5-	T47.6x6-	Leptazol	T50.7x1-	T50.7x2-	T50.7x3-	T50.7x4-	T50.7x5-	T50.7x6-
compound	T47.6x1-	T47.6x2-	T47.6x3-	T47.6x4-	T47.6x5-	T47.6x6-	Leptophos	T60.0x1-	T60.0x2-	T60.0x3-	T60.0x4-	—	—
bifidus, lyophilized	T47.6x1-	T47.6x2-	T47.6x3-	T47.6x4-	T47.6x5-	T47.6x6-	Leritine	T40.2x1-	T40.2x2-	T40.2x3-	T40.2x4-	T40.2x5-	T40.2x6-
bulgaricus	T47.6x1-	T47.6x2-	T47.6x3-	T47.6x4-	T47.6x5-	T47.6x6-	Letosteine	T48.4x1-	T48.4x2-	T48.4x3-	T48.4x4-	T48.4x5-	T48.4x6-
sporogenes	T47.6x1-	T47.6x2-	T47.6x3-	T47.6x4-	T47.6x5-	T47.6x6-	Letter	T38.1x1-	T38.1x2-	T38.1x3-	T38.1x4-	T38.1x5-	T38.1x6-
Lactoflavin	T45.2x1-	T45.2x2-	T45.2x3-	T45.2x4-	T45.2x5-	T45.2x6-	Lettuce opium	T42.6x1-	T42.6x2-	T42.6x3-	T42.6x4-	T42.6x5-	T42.6x6-
Lactose (as excipient)	T50.901-	T50.902-	T50.903-	T50.904-	T50.905-	T50.906-	Leucinocaine	T41.3x1-	T41.3x2-	T41.3x3-	T41.3x4-	T41.3x5-	T41.3x6-
Lactuca (virosa) (extract)	T42.6x1-	T42.6x2-	T42.6x3-	T42.6x4-	T42.6x5-	T42.6x6-	Leucocianidol	T46.991-	T46.992-	T46.993-	T46.994-	T46.995-	T46.996-
Lactucarium	T42.6x1-	T42.6x2-	T42.6x3-	T42.6x4-	T42.6x5-	T42.6x6-	Leucovorin (factor)	T45.8x1-	T45.8x2-	T45.8x3-	T45.8x4-	T45.8x5-	T45.8x6-
Lactulose	T47.3x1-	T47.3x2-	T47.3x3-	T47.3x4-	T47.3x5-	T47.3x6-	Leukeran	T45.1x1-	T45.1x2-	T45.1x3-	T45.1x4-	T45.1x5-	T45.1x6-
Laevo— *see* Levo-							Leuprolide	T38.891-	T38.892-	T38.893-	T38.894-	T38.895-	T38.896-
Lanatosides	T46.0x1-	T46.0x2-	T46.0x3-	T46.0x4-	T46.0x5-	T46.0x6-	Levalbuterol	T48.6x1-	T48.6x2-	T48.6x3-	T48.6x4-	T48.6x5-	T48.6x6-
Lanolin	T49.3x1-	T49.3x2-	T49.3x3-	T49.3x4-	T49.3x5-	T49.3x6-	Levallorphan	T50.7x1-	T50.7x2-	T50.7x3-	T50.7x4-	T50.7x5-	T50.7x6-
Largactil	T43.3x1-	T43.3x2-	T43.3x3-	T43.3x4-	T43.3x5-	T43.3x6-	Levamisole	T37.4x1-	T37.4x2-	T37.4x3-	T37.4x4-	T37.4x5-	T37.4x6-
Larkspur	T62.2x1-	T62.2x2-	T62.2x3-	T62.2x4-	—	—	Levanil	T42.6x1-	T42.6x2-	T42.6x3-	T42.6x4-	T42.6x5-	T42.6x6-
Laroxyl	T43.011-	T43.012-	T43.013-	T43.014-	T43.015-	T43.016-	Levarterenol	T44.4x1-	T44.4x2-	T44.4x3-	T44.4x4-	T44.4x5-	T44.4x6-
Lasix	T50.1x1-	T50.1x2-	T50.1x3-	T50.1x4-	T50.1x5-	T50.1x6-	Levdropropizine	T48.3x1-	T48.3x2-	T48.3x3-	T48.3x4-	T48.3x5-	T48.3x6-
Lassar's paste	T49.4x1-	T49.4x2-	T49.4x3-	T49.4x4-	T49.4x5-	T49.4x6-	Levobunolol	T49.5x1-	T49.5x2-	T49.5x3-	T49.5x4-	T49.5x5-	T49.5x6-
Latamoxef	T36.1x1-	T36.1x2-	T36.1x3-	T36.1x4-	T36.1x5-	T36.1x6-	Levocabastine						
Latex	T65.811-	T65.812-	T65.813-	T65.814-	—	—	(hydrochloride)	T45.0x1-	T45.0x2-	T45.0x3-	T45.0x4-	T45.0x5-	T45.0x6-
Lathyrus (seed)	T62.2x1-	T62.2x2-	T62.2x3-	T62.2x4-	—	—	Levocarnitine	T50.991-	T50.992-	T50.993-	T50.994-	T50.995-	T50.996-
Laudanum	T40.0x1-	T40.0x2-	T40.0x3-	T40.0x4-	T40.0x5-	T40.0x6-	Levodopa	T42.8x1-	T42.8x2-	T42.8x3-	T42.8x4-	T42.8x5-	T42.8x6-
Laudexium	T48.1x1-	T48.1x2-	T48.1x3-	T48.1x4-	T48.1x5-	T48.1x6-	with carbidopa	T42.8x1-	T42.8x2-	T42.8x3-	T42.8x4-	T42.8x5-	T42.8x6-
Laughing gas	T41.0x1-	T41.0x2-	T41.0x3-	T41.0x4-	T41.0x5-	T41.0x6-	Levo-dromoran	T40.2x1-	T40.2x2-	T40.2x3-	T40.2x4-	T40.2x5-	T40.2x6-
Laurel, black or cherry	T62.2x1-	T62.2x2-	T62.2x3-	T62.2x4-	—	—	Levoglutamide	T50.991-	T50.992-	T50.993-	T50.994-	T50.995-	T50.996-
Laurolinium	T49.0x1-	T49.0x2-	T49.0x3-	T49.0x4-	T49.0x5-	T49.0x6-	Levoid	T38.1x1-	T38.1x2-	T38.1x3-	T38.1x4-	T38.1x5-	T38.1x6-
Lauryl sulfoacetate	T49.2x1-	T49.2x2-	T49.2x3-	T49.2x4-	T49.2x5-	T49.2x6-	Levo-iso-methadone	T40.3x1-	T40.3x2-	T40.3x3-	T40.3x4-	T40.3x5-	T40.3x6-
Laxative NEC	T47.4x1-	T47.4x2-	T47.4x3-	T47.4x4-	T47.4x5-	T47.4x6-	Levomepromazine	T43.3x1-	T43.3x2-	T43.3x3-	T43.3x4-	T43.3x5-	T43.3x6-
osmotic	T47.3x1-	T47.3x2-	T47.3x3-	T47.3x4-	T47.3x5-	T47.3x6-	Levonordefrin	T49.6x1-	T49.6x2-	T49.6x3-	T49.6x4-	T49.6x5-	T49.6x6-
saline	T47.3x1-	T47.3x2-	T47.3x3-	T47.3x4-	T47.3x5-	T47.3x6-	Levonorgestrel	T38.4x1-	T38.4x2-	T38.4x3-	T38.4x4-	T38.4x5-	T38.4x6-
stimulant	T47.2x1-	T47.2x2-	T47.2x3-	T47.2x4-	T47.2x5-	T47.2x6-	with ethinylestradiol	T38.5x1-	T38.5x2-	T38.5x3-	T38.5x4-	T38.5x5-	T38.5x6-
L-dopa	T42.8x1-	T42.8x2-	T42.8x3-	T42.8x4-	T42.8x5-	T42.8x6-	Levopromazine	T43.3x1-	T43.3x2-	T43.3x3-	T43.3x4-	T43.3x5-	T43.3x6-
Lead (dust) (fumes) (vapor)							Levoprome	T42.6x1-	T42.6x2-	T42.6x3-	T42.6x4-	T42.6x5-	T42.6x6-
NEC	T56.0x1-	T56.0x2-	T56.0x3-	T56.0x4-	—	—	Levopropoxyphene	T40.4x1-	T40.4x2-	T40.4x3-	T40.4x4-	T40.4x5-	T40.4x6-
acetate	T49.2x1-	T49.2x2-	T49.2x3-	T49.2x4-	T49.2x5-	T49.2x6-	Levopropylhexedrine	T50.5x1-	T50.5x2-	T50.5x3-	T50.5x4-	T50.5x5-	T50.5x6-
alkyl (fuel additive)	T56.0x1-	T56.0x2-	T56.0x3-	T56.0x4-	—	—	Levoproxyphylline	T48.6x1-	T48.6x2-	T48.6x3-	T48.6x4-	T48.6x5-	T48.6x6-
anti-infectives	T37.8x1-	T37.8x2-	T37.8x3-	T37.8x4-	T37.8x5-	T37.8x6-	Levorphanol	T40.4x1-	T40.4x2-	T40.4x3-	T40.4x4-	T40.4x5-	T40.4x6-
antiknock compound (tetraethyl)	T56.0x1-	T56.0x2-	T56.0x3-	T56.0x4-	—	—	Levothyroxine	T38.1x1-	T38.1x2-	T38.1x3-	T38.1x4-	T38.1x5-	T38.1x6-
arsenate, arsenite (dust) (herbicide) (insecticide) (vapor)	T57.0x1-	T57.0x2-	T57.0x3-	T57.0x4-	—	—	sodium	T38.1x1-	T38.1x2-	T38.1x3-	T38.1x4-	T38.1x5-	T38.1x6-
carbonate	T56.0x1-	T56.0x2-	T56.0x3-	T56.0x4-	—	—	Levsin	T44.3x1-	T44.3x2-	T44.3x3-	T44.3x4-	T44.3x5-	T44.3x6-
paint	T56.0x1-	T56.0x2-	T56.0x3-	T56.0x4-	—	—	Levulose	T50.3x1-	T50.3x2-	T50.3x3-	T50.3x4-	T50.3x5-	T50.3x6-
chromate	T56.0x1-	T56.0x2-	T56.0x3-	T56.0x4-	—	—	Lewisite (gas), not in war	T57.0x1-	T57.0x2-	T57.0x3-	T57.0x4-	—	—
paint	T56.0x1-	T56.0x2-	T56.0x3-	T56.0x4-	—	—	Librium	T42.4x1-	T42.4x2-	T42.4x3-	T42.4x4-	T42.4x5-	T42.4x6-
dioxide	T56.0x1-	T56.0x2-	T56.0x3-	T56.0x4-	—	—	Lidex	T49.0x1-	T49.0x2-	T49.0x3-	T49.0x4-	T49.0x5-	T49.0x6-
inorganic	T56.0x1-	T56.0x2-	T56.0x3-	T56.0x4-	—	—	Lidocaine	T41.3x1-	T41.3x2-	T41.3x3-	T41.3x4-	T41.3x5-	T41.3x6-
iodide	T56.0x1-	T56.0x2-	T56.0x3-	T56.0x4-	—	—	regional	T41.3x1-	T41.3x2-	T41.3x3-	T41.3x4-	T41.3x5-	T41.3x6-
pigment (paint)	T56.0x1-	T56.0x2-	T56.0x3-	T56.0x4-	—	—	spinal	T41.3x1-	T41.3x2-	T41.3x3-	T41.3x4-	T41.3x5-	T41.3x6-
monoxide (dust)	T56.0x1-	T56.0x2-	T56.0x3-	T56.0x4-	—	—	Lidofenin	T50.8x1-	T50.8x2-	T50.8x3-	T50.8x4-	T50.8x5-	T50.8x6-
paint	T56.0x1-	T56.0x2-	T56.0x3-	T56.0x4-	—	—	Lidoflazine	T46.1x1-	T46.1x2-	T46.1x3-	T46.1x4-	T46.1x5-	T46.1x6-
organic	T56.0x1-	T56.0x2-	T56.0x3-	T56.0x4-	—	—	Lighter fluid	T52.0x1-	T52.0x2-	T52.0x3-	T52.0x4-	—	—
oxide	T56.0x1-	T56.0x2-	T56.0x3-	T56.0x4-	—	—	Lignin hemicellulose	T47.6x1-	T47.6x2-	T47.6x3-	T47.6x4-	T47.6x5-	T47.6x6-
paint	T56.0x1-	T56.0x2-	T56.0x3-	T56.0x4-	—	—							

Table of Drugs & Chemicals	Accidental (Unintentional)	Self-Harm (Intentional)	Assault	Undetermined	Adverse Effect	Underdosing
Lignocaine	T41.3x1-	T41.3x2-	T41.3x3-	T41.3x4-	T41.3x5-	T41.3x6-
regional	T41.3x1-	T41.3x2-	T41.3x3-	T41.3x4-	T41.3x5-	T41.3x6-
spinal	T41.3x1-	T41.3x2-	T41.3x3-	T41.3x4-	T41.3x5-	T41.3x6-
Ligroin(e) (solvent)	T52.0x1-	T52.0x2-	T52.0x3-	T52.0x4-	—	—
vapor	T59.891-	T59.892-	T59.893-	T59.894-	—	—
Ligustrum vulgare	T62.2x1-	T62.2x2-	T62.2x3-	T62.2x4-	—	—
Lily of the valley	T62.2x1-	T62.2x2-	T62.2x3-	T62.2x4-	—	—
Lime (chloride)	T54.3x1-	T54.3x2-	T54.3x3-	T54.3x4-	—	—
Limonene	T52.8x1-	T52.8x2-	T52.8x3-	T52.8x4-	—	—
Lincomycin	T36.8x1-	T36.8x2-	T36.8x3-	T36.8x4-	T36.8x5-	T36.8x6-
Lindane (insecticide) (nonmedicinal) (vapor)	T53.6x1-	T53.6x2-	T53.6x3-	T53.6x4-	—	—
medicinal	T49.0x1-	T49.0x2-	T49.0x3-	T49.0x4-	T49.0x5-	T49.0x6-
Liniments NEC	T49.91x-	T49.92x-	T49.93x-	T49.94x-	T49.95x-	T49.96x-
Linoleic acid	T46.6x1-	T46.6x2-	T46.6x3-	T46.6x4-	T46.6x5-	T46.6x6-
Linolenic acid	T46.6x1-	T46.6x2-	T46.6x3-	T46.6x4-	T46.6x5-	T46.6x6-
Linseed	T47.4x1-	T47.4x2-	T47.4x3-	T47.4x4-	T47.4x5-	T47.4x6-
Liothyronine	T38.1x1-	T38.1x2-	T38.1x3-	T38.1x4-	T38.1x5-	T38.1x6-
Liotrix	T38.1x1-	T38.1x2-	T38.1x3-	T38.1x4-	T38.1x5-	T38.1x6-
Lipancreatin	T47.5x1-	T47.5x2-	T47.5x3-	T47.5x4-	T47.5x5-	T47.5x6-
Lipo-alprostadil	T46.7x1-	T46.7x2-	T46.7x3-	T46.7x4-	T46.7x5-	T46.7x6-
Lipo-Lutin	T38.5x1-	T38.5x2-	T38.5x3-	T38.5x4-	T38.5x5-	T38.5x6-
Lipotropic drug NEC	T50.901-	T50.902-	T50.903-	T50.904-	T50.905-	T50.906-
Liquefied petroleum gases	T59.891-	T59.892-	T59.893-	T59.894-	—	—
piped (pure or mixed with air)	T59.891-	T59.892-	T59.893-	T59.894-	—	—
Liquid						
paraffin	T47.4x1-	T47.4x2-	T47.4x3-	T47.4x4-	T47.4x5-	T47.4x6-
petrolatum	T47.4x1-	T47.4x2-	T47.4x3-	T47.4x4-	T47.4x5-	T47.4x6-
topical	T49.3x1-	T49.3x2-	T49.3x3-	T49.3x4-	T49.3x5-	T49.3x6-
specified NEC	T65.891-	T65.892-	T65.893-	T65.894-	—	—
substance	T65.91x-	T65.92x-	T65.93x-	T65.94x-	—	—
Liquor creosolis compositus	T65.891-	T65.892-	T65.893-	T65.894-	—	—
Liquorice	T48.4x1-	T48.4x2-	T48.4x3-	T48.4x4-	T48.4x5-	T48.4x6-
extract	T47.8x1-	T47.8x2-	T47.8x3-	T47.8x4-	T47.8x5-	T47.8x6-
Lisinopril	T46.4x1-	T46.4x2-	T46.4x3-	T46.4x4-	T46.4x5-	T46.4x6-
Lisuride	T42.8x1-	T42.8x2-	T42.8x3-	T42.8x4-	T42.8x5-	T42.8x6-
Lithane	T43.8x1-	T43.8x2-	T43.8x3-	T43.8x4-	T43.8x5-	T43.8x6-
Lithium	T56.891-	T56.892-	T56.893-	T56.894-	—	—
gluconate	T43.591-	T43.592-	T43.593-	T43.594-	T43.595-	T43.596-
salts (carbonate)	T43.591-	T43.592-	T43.593-	T43.594-	T43.595-	T43.596-
Lithonate	T43.8x1-	T43.8x2-	T43.8x3-	T43.8x4-	T43.8x5-	T43.8x6-
Liver						
extract	T45.8x1-	T45.8x2-	T45.8x3-	T45.8x4-	T45.8x5-	T45.8x6-
for parenteral use	T45.8x1-	T45.8x2-	T45.8x3-	T45.8x4-	T45.8x5-	T45.8x6-
fraction 1	T45.8x1-	T45.8x2-	T45.8x3-	T45.8x4-	T45.8x5-	T45.8x6-
hydrolysate	T45.8x1-	T45.8x2-	T45.8x3-	T45.8x4-	T45.8x5-	T45.8x6-
Lizard (bite) (venom)	T63.121-	T63.122-	T63.123-	T63.124-	—	—
LMD	T45.8x1-	T45.8x2-	T45.8x3-	T45.8x4-	T45.8x5-	T45.8x6-
Lobelia	T62.2x1-	T62.2x2-	T62.2x3-	T62.2x4-	—	—
Lobeline	T50.7x1-	T50.7x2-	T50.7x3-	T50.7x4-	T50.7x5-	T50.7x6-
Local action drug NEC	T49.8x1-	T49.8x2-	T49.8x3-	T49.8x4-	T49.8x5-	T49.8x6-
Locorten	T49.0x1-	T49.0x2-	T49.0x3-	T49.0x4-	T49.0x5-	T49.0x6-
Lofepramine	T43.011-	T43.012-	T43.013-	T43.014-	T43.015-	T43.016-
Lolium temulentum	T62.2x1-	T62.2x2-	T62.2x3-	T62.2x4-	—	—
Lomotil	T47.6x1-	T47.6x2-	T47.6x3-	T47.6x4-	T47.6x5-	T47.6x6-
Lomustine	T45.1x1-	T45.1x2-	T45.1x3-	T45.1x4-	T45.1x5-	T45.1x6-
Lonidamine	T45.1x1-	T45.1x2-	T45.1x3-	T45.1x4-	T45.1x5-	T45.1x6-
Loperamide	T47.6x1-	T47.6x2-	T47.6x3-	T47.6x4-	T47.6x5-	T47.6x6-
Loprazolam	T42.4x1-	T42.4x2-	T42.4x3-	T42.4x4-	T42.4x5-	T42.4x6-
Lorajmine	T46.2x1-	T46.2x2-	T46.2x3-	T46.2x4-	T46.2x5-	T46.2x6-
Loratidine	T45.0x1-	T45.0x2-	T45.0x3-	T45.0x4-	T45.0x5-	T45.0x6-
Lorazepam	T42.4x1-	T42.4x2-	T42.4x3-	T42.4x4-	T42.4x5-	T42.4x6-
Lorcainide	T46.2x1-	T46.2x2-	T46.2x3-	T46.2x4-	T46.2x5-	T46.2x6-
Lormetazepam	T42.4x1-	T42.4x2-	T42.4x3-	T42.4x4-	T42.4x5-	T42.4x6-
Lotions NEC	T49.91x-	T49.92x-	T49.93x-	T49.94x-	T49.95x-	T49.96x-
Lotusate	T42.3x1-	T42.3x2-	T42.3x3-	T42.3x4-	T42.3x5-	T42.3x6-
Lovastatin	T46.6x1-	T46.6x2-	T46.6x3-	T46.6x4-	T46.6x5-	T46.6x6-
Lowila	T49.2x1-	T49.2x2-	T49.2x3-	T49.2x4-	T49.2x5-	T49.2x6-
Loxapine	T43.591-	T43.592-	T43.593-	T43.594-	T43.595-	T43.596-
Lozenges (throat)	T49.6x1-	T49.6x2-	T49.6x3-	T49.6x4-	T49.6x5-	T49.6x6-
LSD	T40.8x1-	T40.8x2-	T40.8x3-	T40.8x4-	—	—
L-Tryptophan — see Amino acid						
Lubricant, eye	T49.5x1-	T49.5x2-	T49.5x3-	T49.5x4-	T49.5x5-	T49.5x6-
Lubricating oil NEC	T52.0x1-	T52.0x2-	T52.0x3-	T52.0x4-	—	—
Lucanthone	T37.4x1-	T37.4x2-	T37.4x3-	T37.4x4-	T37.4x5-	T37.4x6-
Luminal	T42.3x1-	T42.3x2-	T42.3x3-	T42.3x4-	T42.3x5-	T42.3x6-
Lung irritant (gas) NEC	T59.91x-	T59.92x-	T59.93x-	T59.94x-	—	—
Luteinizing hormone	T38.811-	T38.812-	T38.813-	T38.814-	T38.815-	T38.816-
Lutocylol	T38.5x1-	T38.5x2-	T38.5x3-	T38.5x4-	T38.5x5-	T38.5x6-
Lutromone	T38.5x1-	T38.5x2-	T38.5x3-	T38.5x4-	T38.5x5-	T38.5x6-
Lututrin	T48.291-	T48.292-	T48.293-	T48.294-	T48.295-	T48.296-
Lye (concentrated)	T54.3x1-	T54.3x2-	T54.3x3-	T54.3x4-	—	—
Lygranum (skin test)	T50.8x1-	T50.8x2-	T50.8x3-	T50.8x4-	T50.8x5-	T50.8x6-
Lymecycline	T36.4x1-	T36.4x2-	T36.4x3-	T36.4x4-	T36.4x5-	T36.4x6-
Lymphogranuloma venereum antigen	T50.8x1-	T50.8x2-	T50.8x3-	T50.8x4-	T50.8x5-	T50.8x6-
Lynestrenol	T38.4x1-	T38.4x2-	T38.4x3-	T38.4x4-	T38.4x5-	T38.4x6-
Lyovac Sodium Edecrin	T50.1x1-	T50.1x2-	T50.1x3-	T50.1x4-	T50.1x5-	T50.1x6-
Lypressin	T38.891-	T38.892-	T38.893-	T38.894-	T38.895-	T38.896-
Lysergic acid diethylamide	T40.8x1-	T40.8x2-	T40.8x3-	T40.8x4-	—	—
Lysergide	T40.8x1-	T40.8x2-	T40.8x3-	T40.8x4-	—	—
Lysine vasopressin	T38.891-	T38.892-	T38.893-	T38.894-	T38.895-	T38.896-
Lysol	T54.1x1-	T54.1x2-	T54.1x3-	T54.1x4-	—	—
Lysozyme	T49.0x1-	T49.0x2-	T49.0x3-	T49.0x4-	T49.0x5-	T49.0x6-
Lytta (vitatta)	T49.8x1-	T49.8x2-	T49.8x3-	T49.8x4-	T49.8x5-	T49.8x6-
Mace	T59.3x1-	T59.3x2-	T59.3x3-	T59.3x4-	—	—
Macrogol	T50.991-	T50.992-	T50.993-	T50.994-	T50.995-	T50.996-
Macrolide						
anabolic drug	T38.7x1-	T38.7x2-	T38.7x3-	T38.7x4-	T38.7x5-	T38.7x6-
antibiotic	T36.3x1-	T36.3x2-	T36.3x3-	T36.3x4-	T36.3x5-	T36.3x6-
Mafenide	T49.0x1-	T49.0x2-	T49.0x3-	T49.0x4-	T49.0x5-	T49.0x6-
Magaldrate	T47.1x1-	T47.1x2-	T47.1x3-	T47.1x4-	T47.1x5-	T47.1x6-
Magic mushroom	T40.991-	T40.992-	T40.993-	T40.994-	—	—
Magnamycin	T36.8x1-	T36.8x2-	T36.8x3-	T36.8x4-	T36.8x5-	T36.8x6-
Magnesia magma	T47.1x1-	T47.1x2-	T47.1x3-	T47.1x4-	T47.1x5-	T47.1x6-
Magnesium NEC	T56.891-	T56.892-	T56.893-	T56.894-	—	—
carbonate	T47.1x1-	T47.1x2-	T47.1x3-	T47.1x4-	T47.1x5-	T47.1x6-
citrate	T47.4x1-	T47.4x2-	T47.4x3-	T47.4x4-	T47.4x5-	T47.4x6-
hydroxide	T47.1x1-	T47.1x2-	T47.1x3-	T47.1x4-	T47.1x5-	T47.1x6-
oxide	T47.1x1-	T47.1x2-	T47.1x3-	T47.1x4-	T47.1x5-	T47.1x6-
peroxide	T49.0x1-	T49.0x2-	T49.0x3-	T49.0x4-	T49.0x5-	T49.0x6-
salicylate	T39.091-	T39.092-	T39.093-	T39.094-	T39.095-	T39.096-
silicofluoride	T50.3x1-	T50.3x2-	T50.3x3-	T50.3x4-	T50.3x5-	T50.3x6-
sulfate	T47.4x1-	T47.4x2-	T47.4x3-	T47.4x4-	T47.4x5-	T47.4x6-
thiosulfate	T45.0x1-	T45.0x2-	T45.0x3-	T45.0x4-	T45.0x5-	T45.0x6-
trisilicate	T47.1x1-	T47.1x2-	T47.1x3-	T47.1x4-	T47.1x5-	T47.1x6-
Malathion (medicinal)	T49.0x1-	T49.0x2-	T49.0x3-	T49.0x4-	T49.0x5-	T49.0x6-
insecticide	T60.0x1-	T60.0x2-	T60.0x3-	T60.0x4-	—	—
Male fern extract	T37.4x1-	T37.4x2-	T37.4x3-	T37.4x4-	T37.4x5-	T37.4x6-
M-AMSA	T45.1x1-	T45.1x2-	T45.1x3-	T45.1x4-	T45.1x5-	T45.1x6-
Mandelic acid	T37.8x1-	T37.8x2-	T37.8x3-	T37.8x4-	T37.8x5-	T37.8x6-
Manganese (dioxide) (salts)	T57.2x1-	T57.2x2-	T57.2x3-	T57.2x4-	—	—
medicinal	T50.991-	T50.992-	T50.993-	T50.994-	T50.995-	T50.996-

DRUGS & CHEMICALS

Table of Drugs & Chemicals	Poisoning				Adverse Effect	Underdosing
	Accidental (Unintentional)	Self-Harm (Intentional)	Assault	Undetermined		
Mannitol	T47.3x1-	T47.3x2-	T47.3x3-	T47.3x4-	T47.3x5-	T47.3x6-
hexanitrate	T46.3x1-	T46.3x2-	T46.3x3-	T46.3x4-	T46.3x5-	T46.3x6-
Mannomustine	T45.1x1-	T45.1x2-	T45.1x3-	T45.1x4-	T45.1x5-	T45.1x6-
MAO inhibitors	T43.1x1-	T43.1x2-	T43.1x3-	T43.1x4-	T43.1x5-	T43.1x6-
Mapharsen	T37.8x1-	T37.8x2-	T37.8x3-	T37.8x4-	T37.8x5-	T37.8x6-
Maphenide	T49.0x1-	T49.0x2-	T49.0x3-	T49.0x4-	T49.0x5-	T49.0x6-
Maprotiline	T43.021-	T43.022-	T43.023-	T43.024-	T43.025-	T43.026-
Marcaine	T41.3x1-	T41.3x2-	T41.3x3-	T41.3x4-	T41.3x5-	T41.3x6-
infiltration (subcutaneous)	T41.3x1-	T41.3x2-	T41.3x3-	T41.3x4-	T41.3x5-	T41.3x6-
nerve block (peripheral) (plexus)	T41.3x1-	T41.3x2-	T41.3x3-	T41.3x4-	T41.3x5-	T41.3x6-
Marezine	T45.0x1-	T45.0x2-	T45.0x3-	T45.0x4-	T45.0x5-	T45.0x6-
Marihuana	T40.7x1-	T40.7x2-	T40.7x3-	T40.7x4-	T40.7x5-	T40.7x6-
Marijuana	T40.7x1-	T40.7x2-	T40.7x3-	T40.7x4-	T40.7x5-	T40.7x6-
Marine (sting)	T63.691-	T63.692-	T63.693-	T63.694-	—	—
animals (sting)	T63.691-	T63.692-	T63.693-	T63.694-	—	—
plants (sting)	T63.711-	T63.712-	T63.713-	T63.714-	—	—
Marplan	T43.1x1-	T43.1x2-	T43.1x3-	T43.1x4-	T43.1x5-	T43.1x6-
Marsh gas	T59.891-	T59.892-	T59.893-	T59.894-	—	—
Marsilid	T43.1x1-	T43.1x2-	T43.1x3-	T43.1x4-	T43.1x5-	T43.1x6-
Matulane	T45.1x1-	T45.1x2-	T45.1x3-	T45.1x4-	T45.1x5-	T45.1x6-
Mazindol	T50.5x1-	T50.5x2-	T50.5x3-	T50.5x4-	T50.5x5-	T50.5x6-
MCPA	T60.3x1-	T60.3x2-	T60.3x3-	T60.3x4-	—	—
MDMA	T43.621-	T43.622-	T43.623-	T43.624-	T43.625-	T43.626-
Meadow saffron	T62.2x1-	T62.2x2-	T62.2x3-	T62.2x4-	—	—
Measles virus vaccine (attenuated)	T50.B91-	T50.B92-	T50.B93-	T50.B94-	T50.B95-	T50.B96-
Meat, noxious	T62.8x1-	T62.8x2-	T62.8x3-	T62.8x4-	—	—
Meballymal	T42.3x1-	T42.3x2-	T42.3x3-	T42.3x4-	T42.3x5-	T42.3x6-
Mebanazine	T43.1x1-	T43.1x2-	T43.1x3-	T43.1x4-	T43.1x5-	T43.1x6-
Mebaral	T42.3x1-	T42.3x2-	T42.3x3-	T42.3x4-	T42.3x5-	T42.3x6-
Mebendazole	T37.4x1-	T37.4x2-	T37.4x3-	T37.4x4-	T37.4x5-	T37.4x6-
Mebeverine	T44.3x1-	T44.3x2-	T44.3x3-	T44.3x4-	T44.3x5-	T44.3x6-
Mebhydrolin	T45.0x1-	T45.0x2-	T45.0x3-	T45.0x4-	T45.0x5-	T45.0x6-
Mebumal	T42.3x1-	T42.3x2-	T42.3x3-	T42.3x4-	T42.3x5-	T42.3x6-
Mebutamate	T43.591-	T43.592-	T43.593-	T43.594-	T43.595-	T43.596-
Mecamylamine	T44.2x1-	T44.2x2-	T44.2x3-	T44.2x4-	T44.2x5-	T44.2x6-
Mechlorethamine	T45.1x1-	T45.1x2-	T45.1x3-	T45.1x4-	T45.1x5-	T45.1x6-
Mecillinam	T36.0x1-	T36.0x2-	T36.0x3-	T36.0x4-	T36.0x5-	T36.0x6-
Meclizine (hydrochloride)	T45.0x1-	T45.0x2-	T45.0x3-	T45.0x4-	T45.0x5-	T45.0x6-
Meclocycline	T36.4x1-	T36.4x2-	T36.4x3-	T36.4x4-	T36.4x5-	T36.4x6-
Meclofenamate	T39.391-	T39.392-	T39.393-	T39.394-	T39.395-	T39.396-
Meclofenamic acid	T39.391-	T39.392-	T39.393-	T39.394-	T39.395-	T39.396-
Meclofenoxate	T43.691-	T43.692-	T43.693-	T43.694-	T43.695-	T43.696-
Meclozine	T45.0x1-	T45.0x2-	T45.0x3-	T45.0x4-	T45.0x5-	T45.0x6-
Mecobalamin	T45.8x1-	T45.8x2-	T45.8x3-	T45.8x4-	T45.8x5-	T45.8x6-
Mecoprop	T60.3x1-	T60.3x2-	T60.3x3-	T60.3x4-	—	—
Mecrilate	T49.3x1-	T49.3x2-	T49.3x3-	T49.3x4-	T49.3x5-	T49.3x6-
Mecysteine	T48.4x1-	T48.4x2-	T48.4x3-	T48.4x4-	T48.4x5-	T48.4x6-
Medazepam	T42.4x1-	T42.4x2-	T42.4x3-	T42.4x4-	T42.4x5-	T42.4x6-
Medicament NEC	T50.901-	T50.902-	T50.903-	T50.904-	T50.905-	T50.906-
Medinal	T42.3x1-	T42.3x2-	T42.3x3-	T42.3x4-	T42.3x5-	T42.3x6-
Medomin	T42.3x1-	T42.3x2-	T42.3x3-	T42.3x4-	T42.3x5-	T42.3x6-
Medrogestone	T38.5x1-	T38.5x2-	T38.5x3-	T38.5x4-	T38.5x5-	T38.5x6-
Medroxalol	T44.8x1-	T44.8x2-	T44.8x3-	T44.8x4-	T44.8x5-	T44.8x6-
Medroxyprogesterone acetate (depot)	T38.5x1-	T38.5x2-	T38.5x3-	T38.5x4-	T38.5x5-	T38.5x6-
Medrysone	T49.0x1-	T49.0x2-	T49.0x3-	T49.0x4-	T49.0x5-	T49.0x6-
Mefenamic acid	T39.391-	T39.392-	T39.393-	T39.394-	T39.395-	T39.396-
Mefenorex	T50.5x1-	T50.5x2-	T50.5x3-	T50.5x4-	T50.5x5-	T50.5x6-
Mefloquine	T37.2x1-	T37.2x2-	T37.2x3-	T37.2x4-	T37.2x5-	T37.2x6-

Table of Drugs & Chemicals	Poisoning				Adverse Effect	Underdosing
	Accidental (Unintentional)	Self-Harm (Intentional)	Assault	Undetermined		
Mefruside	T50.2x1-	T50.2x2-	T50.2x3-	T50.2x4-	T50.2x5-	T50.2x6-
Megahallucinogen	T40.901-	T40.902-	T40.903-	T40.904-	T40.905-	T40.906-
Megestrol	T38.5x1-	T38.5x2-	T38.5x3-	T38.5x4-	T38.5x5-	T38.5x6-
Meglumine antimoniate	T37.8x1-	T37.8x2-	T37.8x3-	T37.8x4-	T37.8x5-	T37.8x6-
diatrizoate	T50.8x1-	T50.8x2-	T50.8x3-	T50.8x4-	T50.8x5-	T50.8x6-
iodipamide	T50.8x1-	T50.8x2-	T50.8x3-	T50.8x4-	T50.8x5-	T50.8x6-
iotroxate	T50.8x1-	T50.8x2-	T50.8x3-	T50.8x4-	T50.8x5-	T50.8x6-
MEK (methyl ethyl ketone)	T52.4x1-	T52.4x2-	T52.4x3-	T52.4x4-	—	—
Meladinin	T49.3x1-	T49.3x2-	T49.3x3-	T49.3x4-	T49.3x5-	T49.3x6-
Meladrazine	T44.3x1-	T44.3x2-	T44.3x3-	T44.3x4-	T44.3x5-	T44.3x6-
Melaleuca alternifolia oil	T49.0x1-	T49.0x2-	T49.0x3-	T49.0x4-	T49.0x5-	T49.0x6-
Melanizing agents	T49.3x1-	T49.3x2-	T49.3x3-	T49.3x4-	T49.3x5-	T49.3x6-
Melanocyte-stimulating hormone	T38.891-	T38.892-	T38.893-	T38.894-	T38.895-	T38.896-
Melarsonyl potassium	T37.3x1-	T37.3x2-	T37.3x3-	T37.3x4-	T37.3x5-	T37.3x6-
Melarsoprol	T37.3x1-	T37.3x2-	T37.3x3-	T37.3x4-	T37.3x5-	T37.3x6-
Melia azedarach	T62.2x1-	T62.2x2-	T62.2x3-	T62.2x4-	—	—
Melitracen	T43.011-	T43.012-	T43.013-	T43.014-	T43.015-	T43.016-
Mellaril	T43.3x1-	T43.3x2-	T43.3x3-	T43.3x4-	T43.3x5-	T43.3x6-
Meloxine	T49.3x1-	T49.3x2-	T49.3x3-	T49.3x4-	T49.3x5-	T49.3x6-
Melperone	T43.4x1-	T43.4x2-	T43.4x3-	T43.4x4-	T43.4x5-	T43.4x6-
Melphalan	T45.1x1-	T45.1x2-	T45.1x3-	T45.1x4-	T45.1x5-	T45.1x6-
Memantine	T43.8x1-	T43.8x2-	T43.8x3-	T43.8x4-	T43.8x5-	T43.8x6-
Menadiol	T45.7x1-	T45.7x2-	T45.7x3-	T45.7x4-	T45.7x5-	T45.7x6-
sodium sulfate	T45.7x1-	T45.7x2-	T45.7x3-	T45.7x4-	T45.7x5-	T45.7x6-
Menadione	T45.7x1-	T45.7x2-	T45.7x3-	T45.7x4-	T45.7x5-	T45.7x6-
sodium bisulfite	T45.7x1-	T45.7x2-	T45.7x3-	T45.7x4-	T45.7x5-	T45.7x6-
Menaphthone	T45.7x1-	T45.7x2-	T45.7x3-	T45.7x4-	T45.7x5-	T45.7x6-
Menaquinone	T45.7x1-	T45.7x2-	T45.7x3-	T45.7x4-	T45.7x5-	T45.7x6-
Menatetrenone	T45.7x1-	T45.7x2-	T45.7x3-	T45.7x4-	T45.7x5-	T45.7x6-
Meningococcal vaccine	T50.A91-	T50.A92-	T50.A93-	T50.A94-	T50.A95-	T50.A96-
Menningovax (-AC) (-C)	T50.A91-	T50.A92-	T50.A93-	T50.A94-	T50.A95-	T50.A96-
Menotropins	T38.811-	T38.812-	T38.813-	T38.814-	T38.815-	T38.816-
Menthol	T48.5x1-	T48.5x2-	T48.5x3-	T48.5x4-	T48.5x5-	T48.5x6-
Mepacrine	T37.2x1-	T37.2x2-	T37.2x3-	T37.2x4-	T37.2x5-	T37.2x6-
Meparfynol	T42.6x1-	T42.6x2-	T42.6x3-	T42.6x4-	T42.6x5-	T42.6x6-
Mepartricin	T36.7x1-	T36.7x2-	T36.7x3-	T36.7x4-	T36.7x5-	T36.7x6-
Mepazine	T43.3x1-	T43.3x2-	T43.3x3-	T43.3x4-	T43.3x5-	T43.3x6-
Mepenzolate	T44.3x1-	T44.3x2-	T44.3x3-	T44.3x4-	T44.3x5-	T44.3x6-
bromide	T44.3x1-	T44.3x2-	T44.3x3-	T44.3x4-	T44.3x5-	T44.3x6-
Meperidine	T40.4x1-	T40.4x2-	T40.4x3-	T40.4x4-	T40.4x5-	T40.4x6-
Mephebarbital	T42.3x1-	T42.3x2-	T42.3x3-	T42.3x4-	T42.3x5-	T42.3x6-
Mephenamin(e)	T42.8x1-	T42.8x2-	T42.8x3-	T42.8x4-	T42.8x5-	T42.8x6-
Mephenesin	T42.8x1-	T42.8x2-	T42.8x3-	T42.8x4-	T42.8x5-	T42.8x6-
Mephenhydramine	T45.0x1-	T45.0x2-	T45.0x3-	T45.0x4-	T45.0x5-	T45.0x6-
Mephenoxalone	T42.8x1-	T42.8x2-	T42.8x3-	T42.8x4-	T42.8x5-	T42.8x6-
Mephentermine	T44.991-	T44.992-	T44.993-	T44.994-	T44.995-	T44.996-
Mephenytoin	T42.0x1-	T42.0x2-	T42.0x3-	T42.0x4-	T42.0x5-	T42.0x6-
with phenobarbital	T42.3x1-	T42.3x2-	T42.3x3-	T42.3x4-	T42.3x5-	T42.3x6-
Mephobarbital	T42.3x1-	T42.3x2-	T42.3x3-	T42.3x4-	T42.3x5-	T42.3x6-
Mephosfolan	T60.0x1-	T60.0x2-	T60.0x3-	T60.0x4-	—	—
Mepindolol	T44.7x1-	T44.7x2-	T44.7x3-	T44.7x4-	T44.7x5-	T44.7x6-
Mepiperphenidol	T44.3x1-	T44.3x2-	T44.3x3-	T44.3x4-	T44.3x5-	T44.3x6-
Mepitiostane	T38.7x1-	T38.7x2-	T38.7x3-	T38.7x4-	T38.7x5-	T38.7x6-
Mepivacaine	T41.3x1-	T41.3x2-	T41.3x3-	T41.3x4-	T41.3x5-	T41.3x6-
epidural	T41.3x1-	T41.3x2-	T41.3x3-	T41.3x4-	T41.3x5-	T41.3x6-
Meprednisone	T38.0x1-	T38.0x2-	T38.0x3-	T38.0x4-	T38.0x5-	T38.0x6-
Meprobam	T43.591-	T43.592-	T43.593-	T43.594-	T43.595-	T43.596-
Meprobamate	T43.591-	T43.592-	T43.593-	T43.594-	T43.595-	T43.596-
Meproscillarin	T46.0x1-	T46.0x2-	T46.0x3-	T46.0x4-	T46.0x5-	T46.0x6-

DRUGS & CHEMICALS

Table of Drugs & Chemicals	POISONING Accidental (Unintentional)	Self-Harm (Intentional)	Assault	Undetermined	Adverse Effect	Underdosing
Meprylcaine	T41.3x1-	T41.3x2-	T41.3x3-	T41.3x4-	T41.3x5-	T41.3x6-
Meptazinol	T39.8x1-	T39.8x2-	T39.8x3-	T39.8x4-	T39.8x5-	T39.8x6-
Mepyramine	T45.0x1-	T45.0x2-	T45.0x3-	T45.0x4-	T45.0x5-	T45.0x6-
Mequitazine	T43.3x1-	T43.3x2-	T43.3x3-	T43.3x4-	T43.3x5-	T43.3x6-
Meralluride	T50.2x1-	T50.2x2-	T50.2x3-	T50.2x4-	T50.2x5-	T50.2x6-
Merbaphen	T50.2x1-	T50.2x2-	T50.2x3-	T50.2x4-	T50.2x5-	T50.2x6-
Merbromin	T49.0x1-	T49.0x2-	T49.0x3-	T49.0x4-	T49.0x5-	T49.0x6-
Mercaptobenzothiazole salts	T49.0x1-	T49.0x2-	T49.0x3-	T49.0x4-	T49.0x5-	T49.0x6-
Mercaptomerin	T50.2x1-	T50.2x2-	T50.2x3-	T50.2x4-	T50.2x5-	T50.2x6-
Mercaptopurine	T45.1x1-	T45.1x2-	T45.1x3-	T45.1x4-	T45.1x5-	T45.1x6-
Mercumatilin	T50.2x1-	T50.2x2-	T50.2x3-	T50.2x4-	T50.2x5-	T50.2x6-
Mercuramide	T50.2x1-	T50.2x2-	T50.2x3-	T50.2x4-	T50.2x5-	T50.2x6-
Mercurochrome	T49.0x1-	T49.0x2-	T49.0x3-	T49.0x4-	T49.0x5-	T49.0x6-
Mercurophylline	T50.2x1-	T50.2x2-	T50.2x3-	T50.2x4-	T50.2x5-	T50.2x6-
Mercury, mercurial, mercuric, mercurous (compounds) (cyanide) (fumes) (nonmedicinal) (vapor) NEC	T56.1x1-	T56.1x2-	T56.1x3-	T56.1x4-	—	—
ammoniated	T49.0x1-	T49.0x2-	T49.0x3-	T49.0x4-	T49.0x5-	T49.0x6-
anti-infective local	T49.0x1-	T49.0x2-	T49.0x3-	T49.0x4-	T49.0x5-	T49.0x6-
systemic	T37.8x1-	T37.8x2-	T37.8x3-	T37.8x4-	T37.8x5-	T37.8x6-
topical	T49.0x1-	T49.0x2-	T49.0x3-	T49.0x4-	T49.0x5-	T49.0x6-
chloride (ammoniated)	T49.0x1-	T49.0x2-	T49.0x3-	T49.0x4-	T49.0x5-	T49.0x6-
fungicide	T56.1x1-	T56.1x2-	T56.1x3-	T56.1x4-	—	—
diuretic NEC	T50.2x1-	T50.2x2-	T50.2x3-	T50.2x4-	T50.2x5-	T50.2x6-
fungicide	T56.1x1-	T56.1x2-	T56.1x3-	T56.1x4-	—	—
organic (fungicide)	T56.1x1-	T56.1x2-	T56.1x3-	T56.1x4-	—	—
oxide, yellow	T49.0x1-	T49.0x2-	T49.0x3-	T49.0x4-	T49.0x5-	T49.0x6-
Mersalyl	T50.2x1-	T50.2x2-	T50.2x3-	T50.2x4-	T50.2x5-	T50.2x6-
Merthiolate	T49.0x1-	T49.0x2-	T49.0x3-	T49.0x4-	T49.0x5-	T49.0x6-
ophthalmic preparation	T49.5x1-	T49.5x2-	T49.5x3-	T49.5x4-	T49.5x5-	T49.5x6-
Meruvax	T50.B91-	T50.B92-	T50.B93-	T50.B94-	T50.B95-	T50.B96-
Mesalazine	T47.8x1-	T47.8x2-	T47.8x3-	T47.8x4-	T47.8x5-	T47.8x6-
Mescal buttons	T40.991-	T40.992-	T40.993-	T40.994-	—	—
Mescaline	T40.991-	T40.992-	T40.993-	T40.994-	—	—
Mesna	T48.4x1-	T48.4x2-	T48.4x3-	T48.4x4-	T48.4x5-	T48.4x6-
Mesoglycan	T46.6x1-	T46.6x2-	T46.6x3-	T46.6x4-	T46.6x5-	T46.6x6-
Mesoridazine	T43.3x1-	T43.3x2-	T43.3x3-	T43.3x4-	T43.3x5-	T43.3x6-
Mestanolone	T38.7x1-	T38.7x2-	T38.7x3-	T38.7x4-	T38.7x5-	T38.7x6-
Mesterolone	T38.7x1-	T38.7x2-	T38.7x3-	T38.7x4-	T38.7x5-	T38.7x6-
Mestranol	T38.5x1-	T38.5x2-	T38.5x3-	T38.5x4-	T38.5x5-	T38.5x6-
Mesulergine	T42.8x1-	T42.8x2-	T42.8x3-	T42.8x4-	T42.8x5-	T42.8x6-
Mesulfen	T49.0x1-	T49.0x2-	T49.0x3-	T49.0x4-	T49.0x5-	T49.0x6-
Mesuximide	T42.2x1-	T42.2x2-	T42.2x3-	T42.2x4-	T42.2x5-	T42.2x6-
Metabutethamine	T41.3x1-	T41.3x2-	T41.3x3-	T41.3x4-	T41.3x5-	T41.3x6-
Metactesylacetate	T49.0x1-	T49.0x2-	T49.0x3-	T49.0x4-	T49.0x5-	T49.0x6-
Metacycline	T36.4x1-	T36.4x2-	T36.4x3-	T36.4x4-	T36.4x5-	T36.4x6-
Metaldehyde (snail killer) NEC	T60.8x1-	T60.8x2-	T60.8x3-	T60.8x4-	—	—
Metals (heavy) (nonmedicinal)	T56.91x-	T56.92x-	T56.93x-	T56.94x-	—	—
dust, fumes, or vapor NEC	T56.91x-	T56.92x-	T56.93x-	T56.94x-	—	—
light NEC	T56.91x-	T56.92x-	T56.93x-	T56.94x-	—	—
dust, fumes, or vapor NEC	T56.91x-	T56.92x-	T56.93x-	T56.94x-	—	—
specified NEC	T56.891-	T56.892-	T56.893-	T56.894-	—	—
thallium	T56.811-	T56.812-	T56.813-	T56.814-	—	—
Metamfetamine	T43.621-	T43.622-	T43.623-	T43.624-	T43.625-	T43.626-
Metamizole sodium	T39.2x1-	T39.2x2-	T39.2x3-	T39.2x4-	T39.2x5-	T39.2x6-
Metampicillin	T36.0x1-	T36.0x2-	T36.0x3-	T36.0x4-	T36.0x5-	T36.0x6-
Metamucil	T47.4x1-	T47.4x2-	T47.4x3-	T47.4x4-	T47.4x5-	T47.4x6-
Metandienone	T38.7x1-	T38.7x2-	T38.7x3-	T38.7x4-	T38.7x5-	T38.7x6-
Metandrostenolone	T38.7x1-	T38.7x2-	T38.7x3-	T38.7x4-	T38.7x5-	T38.7x6-
Metaphen	T49.0x1-	T49.0x2-	T49.0x3-	T49.0x4-	T49.0x5-	T49.0x6-
Metaphos	T60.0x1-	T60.0x2-	T60.0x3-	T60.0x4-	—	—
Metapramine	T43.011-	T43.012-	T43.013-	T43.014-	T43.015-	T43.016-
Metaproterenol	T48.291-	T48.292-	T48.293-	T48.294-	T48.295-	T48.296-
Metaraminol	T44.4x1-	T44.4x2-	T44.4x3-	T44.4x4-	T44.4x5-	T44.4x6-
Metaxalone	T42.8x1-	T42.8x2-	T42.8x3-	T42.8x4-	T42.8x5-	T42.8x6-
Metenolone	T38.7x1-	T38.7x2-	T38.7x3-	T38.7x4-	T38.7x5-	T38.7x6-
Metergoline	T42.8x1-	T42.8x2-	T42.8x3-	T42.8x4-	T42.8x5-	T42.8x6-
Metescufylline	T46.991-	T46.992-	T46.993-	T46.994-	T46.995-	T46.996-
Metetoin	T42.0x1-	T42.0x2-	T42.0x3-	T42.0x4-	T42.0x5-	T42.0x6-
Metformin	T38.3x1-	T38.3x2-	T38.3x3-	T38.3x4-	T38.3x5-	T38.3x6-
Methacholine	T44.1x1-	T44.1x2-	T44.1x3-	T44.1x4-	T44.1x5-	T44.1x6-
Methacycline	T36.4x1-	T36.4x2-	T36.4x3-	T36.4x4-	T36.4x5-	T36.4x6-
Methadone	T40.3x1-	T40.3x2-	T40.3x3-	T40.3x4-	T40.3x5-	T40.3x6-
Methallenestril	T38.5x1-	T38.5x2-	T38.5x3-	T38.5x4-	T38.5x5-	T38.5x6-
Methallenoestril	T38.5x1-	T38.5x2-	T38.5x3-	T38.5x4-	T38.5x5-	T38.5x6-
Methamphetamine	T43.621-	T43.622-	T43.623-	T43.624-	T43.625-	T43.626-
Methampyrone	T39.2x1-	T39.2x2-	T39.2x3-	T39.2x4-	T39.2x5-	T39.2x6-
Methandienone	T38.7x1-	T38.7x2-	T38.7x3-	T38.7x4-	T38.7x5-	T38.7x6-
Methandriol	T38.7x1-	T38.7x2-	T38.7x3-	T38.7x4-	T38.7x5-	T38.7x6-
Methandrostenolone	T38.7x1-	T38.7x2-	T38.7x3-	T38.7x4-	T38.7x5-	T38.7x6-
Methane	T59.891-	T59.892-	T59.893-	T59.894-	—	—
Methanethiol	T59.891-	T59.892-	T59.893-	T59.894-	—	—
Methaniazide	T37.1x1-	T37.1x2-	T37.1x3-	T37.1x4-	T37.1x5-	T37.1x6-
Methanol (vapor)	T51.1x1-	T51.1x2-	T51.1x3-	T51.1x4-	—	—
Methantheline	T44.3x1-	T44.3x2-	T44.3x3-	T44.3x4-	T44.3x5-	T44.3x6-
Methanthelinium bromide	T44.3x1-	T44.3x2-	T44.3x3-	T44.3x4-	T44.3x5-	T44.3x6-
Methaphenilene	T45.0x1-	T45.0x2-	T45.0x3-	T45.0x4-	T45.0x5-	T45.0x6-
Methapyrilene	T45.0x1-	T45.0x2-	T45.0x3-	T45.0x4-	T45.0x5-	T45.0x6-
Methaqualone (compound)	T42.6x1-	T42.6x2-	T42.6x3-	T42.6x4-	T42.6x5-	T42.6x6-
Metharbital	T42.3x1-	T42.3x2-	T42.3x3-	T42.3x4-	T42.3x5-	T42.3x6-
Methazolamide	T50.2x1-	T50.2x2-	T50.2x3-	T50.2x4-	T50.2x5-	T50.2x6-
Methdilazine	T43.3x1-	T43.3x2-	T43.3x3-	T43.3x4-	T43.3x5-	T43.3x6-
Methedrine	T43.621-	T43.622-	T43.623-	T43.624-	T43.625-	T43.626-
Methenamine (mandelate)	T37.8x1-	T37.8x2-	T37.8x3-	T37.8x4-	T37.8x5-	T37.8x6-
Methenolone	T38.7x1-	T38.7x2-	T38.7x3-	T38.7x4-	T38.7x5-	T38.7x6-
Methergine	T48.0x1-	T48.0x2-	T48.0x3-	T48.0x4-	T48.0x5-	T48.0x6-
Methetoin	T42.0x1-	T42.0x2-	T42.0x3-	T42.0x4-	T42.0x5-	T42.0x6-
Methiacil	T38.2x1-	T38.2x2-	T38.2x3-	T38.2x4-	T38.2x5-	T38.2x6-
Methicillin	T36.0x1-	T36.0x2-	T36.0x3-	T36.0x4-	T36.0x5-	T36.0x6-
Methimazole	T38.2x1-	T38.2x2-	T38.2x3-	T38.2x4-	T38.2x5-	T38.2x6-
Methiodal sodium	T50.8x1-	T50.8x2-	T50.8x3-	T50.8x4-	T50.8x5-	T50.8x6-
Methionine	T50.991-	T50.992-	T50.993-	T50.994-	T50.995-	T50.996-
Methisazone	T37.5x1-	T37.5x2-	T37.5x3-	T37.5x4-	T37.5x5-	T37.5x6-
Methisoprinol	T37.5x1-	T37.5x2-	T37.5x3-	T37.5x4-	T37.5x5-	T37.5x6-
Methitural	T42.3x1-	T42.3x2-	T42.3x3-	T42.3x4-	T42.3x5-	T42.3x6-
Methixene	T44.3x1-	T44.3x2-	T44.3x3-	T44.3x4-	T44.3x5-	T44.3x6-
Methobarbital, methobarbitone	T42.3x1-	T42.3x2-	T42.3x3-	T42.3x4-	T42.3x5-	T42.3x6-
Methocarbamol	T42.8x1-	T42.8x2-	T42.8x3-	T42.8x4-	T42.8x5-	T42.8x6-
skeletal muscle relaxant	T48.1x1-	T48.1x2-	T48.1x3-	T48.1x4-	T48.1x5-	T48.1x6-
Methohexital	T41.1x1-	T41.1x2-	T41.1x3-	T41.1x4-	T41.1x5-	T41.1x6-
Methohexitone	T41.1x1-	T41.1x2-	T41.1x3-	T41.1x4-	T41.1x5-	T41.1x6-
Methoin	T42.0x1-	T42.0x2-	T42.0x3-	T42.0x4-	T42.0x5-	T42.0x6-
Methopholine	T39.8x1-	T39.8x2-	T39.8x3-	T39.8x4-	T39.8x5-	T39.8x6-
Methopromazine	T43.3x1-	T43.3x2-	T43.3x3-	T43.3x4-	T43.3x5-	T43.3x6-
Methorate	T48.3x1-	T48.3x2-	T48.3x3-	T48.3x4-	T48.3x5-	T48.3x6-
Methoserpidine	T46.5x1-	T46.5x2-	T46.5x3-	T46.5x4-	T46.5x5-	T46.5x6-
Methotrexate	T45.1x1-	T45.1x2-	T45.1x3-	T45.1x4-	T45.1x5-	T45.1x6-
Methotrimeprazine	T43.3x1-	T43.3x2-	T43.3x3-	T43.3x4-	T43.3x5-	T43.3x6-
Methoxa-Dome	T49.3x1-	T49.3x2-	T49.3x3-	T49.3x4-	T49.3x5-	T49.3x6-

DRUGS & CHEMICALS

Table of Drugs & Chemicals	Accidental (Unintentional)	Self-Harm (Intentional)	Assault	Undetermined	Adverse Effect	Underdosing
Methoxamine	T44.4x1-	T44.4x2-	T44.4x3-	T44.4x4-	T44.4x5-	T44.4x6-
Methoxsalen	T50.991-	T50.992-	T50.993-	T50.994-	T50.995-	T50.996-
Methoxyaniline	T65.3x1-	T65.3x2-	T65.3x3-	T65.3x4-	—	—
Methoxybenzyl penicillin	T36.0x1-	T36.0x2-	T36.0x3-	T36.0x4-	T36.0x5-	T36.0x6-
Methoxychlor	T53.7x1-	T53.7x2-	T53.7x3-	T53.7x4-	—	—
Methoxy-DDT	T53.7x1-	T53.7x2-	T53.7x3-	T53.7x4-	—	—
2-Methoxyethanol	T52.3x1-	T52.3x2-	T52.3x3-	T52.3x4-	—	—
Methoxyflurane	T41.0x1-	T41.0x2-	T41.0x3-	T41.0x4-	T41.0x5-	T41.0x6-
Methoxyphenamine	T48.6x1-	T48.6x2-	T48.6x3-	T48.6x4-	T48.6x5-	T48.6x6-
Methoxypromazine	T43.3x1-	T43.3x2-	T43.3x3-	T43.3x4-	T43.3x5-	T43.3x6-
5-Methoxypsoralen (5-MOP)	T50.991-	T50.992-	T50.993-	T50.994-	T50.995-	T50.996-
8-Methoxypsoralen (8-MOP)	T50.991-	T50.992-	T50.993-	T50.994-	T50.995-	T50.996-
Methscopolamine bromide	T44.3x1-	T44.3x2-	T44.3x3-	T44.3x4-	T44.3x5-	T44.3x6-
Methsuximide	T42.2x1-	T42.2x2-	T42.2x3-	T42.2x4-	T42.2x5-	T42.2x6-
Methyclothiazide	T50.2x1-	T50.2x2-	T50.2x3-	T50.2x4-	T50.2x5-	T50.2x6-
Methyl						
acetate	T52.4x1-	T52.4x2-	T52.4x3-	T52.4x4-	—	—
acetone	T52.4x1-	T52.4x2-	T52.4x3-	T52.4x4-	—	—
acrylate	T65.891-	T65.892-	T65.893-	T65.894-	—	—
alcohol	T51.1x1-	T51.1x2-	T51.1x3-	T51.1x4-	—	—
aminophenol	T65.3x1-	T65.3x2-	T65.3x3-	T65.3x4-	—	—
amphetamine	T43.621-	T43.622-	T43.623-	T43.624-	T43.625-	T43.626-
androstanolone	T38.7x1-	T38.7x2-	T38.7x3-	T38.7x4-	T38.7x5-	T38.7x6-
atropine	T44.3x1-	T44.3x2-	T44.3x3-	T44.3x4-	T44.3x5-	T44.3x6-
benzene	T52.2x1-	T52.2x2-	T52.2x3-	T52.2x4-	—	—
benzoate	T52.8x1-	T52.8x2-	T52.8x3-	T52.8x4-	—	—
benzol	T52.2x1-	T52.2x2-	T52.2x3-	T52.2x4-	—	—
bromide (gas)	T59.891-	T59.892-	T59.893-	T59.894-	—	—
fumigant	T60.8x1-	T60.8x2-	T60.8x3-	T60.8x4-	—	—
butanol	T51.3x1-	T51.3x2-	T51.3x3-	T51.3x4-	—	—
carbonate	T52.8x1-	T52.8x2-	T52.8x3-	T52.8x4-	—	—
carbinol	T51.1x1-	T51.1x2-	T51.1x3-	T51.1x4-	—	—
CCNU	T45.1x1-	T45.1x2-	T45.1x3-	T45.1x4-	T45.1x5-	T45.1x6-
cellosolve	T52.91x-	T52.92x-	T52.93x-	T52.94x-	—	—
cellulose	T47.4x1-	T47.4x2-	T47.4x3-	T47.4x4-	T47.4x5-	T47.4x6-
chloride (gas)	T59.891-	T59.892-	T59.893-	T59.894-	—	—
chloroformate	T59.3x1-	T59.3x2-	T59.3x3-	T59.3x4-	—	—
cyclohexane	T52.8x1-	T52.8x2-	T52.8x3-	T52.8x4-	—	—
cyclohexanol	T51.8x1-	T51.8x2-	T51.8x3-	T51.8x4-	—	—
cyclohexanone	T52.8x1-	T52.8x2-	T52.8x3-	T52.8x4-	—	—
cyclohexyl acetate	T52.8x1-	T52.8x2-	T52.8x3-	T52.8x4-	—	—
demeton	T60.0x1-	T60.0x2-	T60.0x3-	T60.0x4-	—	—
dihydromorphinone	T40.2x1-	T40.2x2-	T40.2x3-	T40.2x4-	T40.2x5-	T40.2x6-
ergometrine	T48.0x1-	T48.0x2-	T48.0x3-	T48.0x4-	T48.0x5-	T48.0x6-
ergonovine	T48.0x1-	T48.0x2-	T48.0x3-	T48.0x4-	T48.0x5-	T48.0x6-
ethyl ketone	T52.4x1-	T52.4x2-	T52.4x3-	T52.4x4-	—	—
glucamine antimonate	T37.8x1-	T37.8x2-	T37.8x3-	T37.8x4-	T37.8x5-	T37.8x6-
hydrazine	T65.891-	T65.892-	T65.893-	T65.894-	—	—
iodide	T65.891-	T65.892-	T65.893-	T65.894-	—	—
isobutyl ketone	T52.4x1-	T52.4x2-	T52.4x3-	T52.4x4-	—	—
isothiocyanate	T60.3x1-	T60.3x2-	T60.3x3-	T60.3x4-	—	—
mercaptan	T59.891-	T59.892-	T59.893-	T59.894-	—	—
morphine NEC	T40.2x1-	T40.2x2-	T40.2x3-	T40.2x4-	T40.2x5-	T40.2x6-
nicotinate	T49.4x1-	T49.4x2-	T49.4x3-	T49.4x4-	T49.4x5-	T49.4x6-
paraben	T49.0x1-	T49.0x2-	T49.0x3-	T49.0x4-	T49.0x5-	T49.0x6-
parafynol	T42.6x1-	T42.6x2-	T42.6x3-	T42.6x4-	T42.6x5-	T42.6x6-
parathion	T60.0x1-	T60.0x2-	T60.0x3-	T60.0x4-	—	—
propylcarbinol	T51.3x1-	T51.3x2-	T51.3x3-	T51.3x4-	—	—
peridol	T43.4x1-	T43.4x2-	T43.4x3-	T43.4x4-	T43.4x5-	T43.4x6-
phenidate	T43.631-	T43.632-	T43.633-	T43.634-	T43.635-	T43.636-
prednisolone	T38.0x1-	T38.0x2-	T38.0x3-	T38.0x4-	T38.0x5-	T38.0x6-
ENT agent	T49.6x1-	T49.6x2-	T49.6x3-	T49.6x4-	T49.6x5-	T49.6x6-
ophthalmic preparation	T49.5x1-	T49.5x2-	T49.5x3-	T49.5x4-	T49.5x5-	T49.5x6-
topical NEC	T49.0x1-	T49.0x2-	T49.0x3-	T49.0x4-	T49.0x5-	T49.0x6-

Table of Drugs & Chemicals	Accidental (Unintentional)	Self-Harm (Intentional)	Assault	Undetermined	Adverse Effect	Underdosing
Methyl - *continued*						
rosaniline NEC	T49.0x1-	T49.0x2-	T49.0x3-	T49.0x4-	T49.0x5-	T49.0x6-
salicylate	T49.2x1-	T49.2x2-	T49.2x3-	T49.2x4-	T49.2x5-	T49.2x6-
sulfate (fumes)	T59.891-	T59.892-	T59.893-	T59.894-	—	—
liquid	T52.8x1-	T52.8x2-	T52.8x3-	T52.8x4-	—	—
sulfonal	T42.6x1-	T42.6x2-	T42.6x3-	T42.6x4-	T42.6x5-	T42.6x6-
testosterone	T38.7x1-	T38.7x2-	T38.7x3-	T38.7x4-	T38.7x5-	T38.7x6-
thiouracil	T38.2x1-	T38.2x2-	T38.2x3-	T38.2x4-	T38.2x5-	T38.2x6-
Methylamphetamine	T43.621-	T43.622-	T43.623-	T43.624-	T43.625-	T43.626-
Methylated spirit	T51.1x1-	T51.1x2-	T51.1x3-	T51.1x4-	—	—
Methylatropine nitrate	T44.3x1-	T44.3x2-	T44.3x3-	T44.3x4-	T44.3x5-	T44.3x6-
Methylbenactyzium bromide	T44.3x1-	T44.3x2-	T44.3x3-	T44.3x4-	T44.3x5-	T44.3x6-
Methylbenzethonium chloride	T49.0x1-	T49.0x2-	T49.0x3-	T49.0x4-	T49.0x5-	T49.0x6-
Methylcellulose	T47.4x1-	T47.4x2-	T47.4x3-	T47.4x4-	T47.4x5-	T47.4x6-
laxative	T47.4x1-	T47.4x2-	T47.4x3-	T47.4x4-	T47.4x5-	T47.4x6-
Methylchlorophenoxy-acetic acid	T60.3x1-	T60.3x2-	T60.3x3-	T60.3x4-	—	—
Methyldopa	T46.5x1-	T46.5x2-	T46.5x3-	T46.5x4-	T46.5x5-	T46.5x6-
Methyldopate	T46.5x1-	T46.5x2-	T46.5x3-	T46.5x4-	T46.5x5-	T46.5x6-
Methylene						
blue	T50.6x1-	T50.6x2-	T50.6x3-	T50.6x4-	T50.6x5-	T50.6x6-
chloride or dichloride (solvent) NEC	T53.4x1-	T53.4x2-	T53.4x3-	T53.4x4-	—	—
Methylenedioxyamphetamine	T43.621-	T43.622-	T43.623-	T43.624-	T43.625-	T43.626-
Methylenedioxymethamphetamine	T43.621-	T43.622-	T43.623-	T43.624-	T43.625-	T43.626-
Methylergometrine	T48.0x1-	T48.0x2-	T48.0x3-	T48.0x4-	T48.0x5-	T48.0x6-
Methylergonovine	T48.0x1-	T48.0x2-	T48.0x3-	T48.0x4-	T48.0x5-	T48.0x6-
Methylestrenolone	T38.5x1-	T38.5x2-	T38.5x3-	T38.5x4-	T38.5x5-	T38.5x6-
Methylethyl cellulose	T50.991-	T50.992-	T50.993-	T50.994-	T50.995-	T50.996-
Methylhexabital	T42.3x1-	T42.3x2-	T42.3x3-	T42.3x4-	T42.3x5-	T42.3x6-
Methylmorphine	T40.2x1-	T40.2x2-	T40.2x3-	T40.2x4-	T40.2x5-	T40.2x6-
Methylparaben (ophthalmic)	T49.5x1-	T49.5x2-	T49.5x3-	T49.5x4-	T49.5x5-	T49.5x6-
Methylparafynol	T42.6x1-	T42.6x2-	T42.6x3-	T42.6x4-	T42.6x5-	T42.6x6-
Methylpentynol, methylpenthynol	T42.6x1-	T42.6x2-	T42.6x3-	T42.6x4-	T42.6x5-	T42.6x6-
Methylphenidate	T43.631-	T43.632-	T43.633-	T43.634-	T43.635-	T43.636-
Methylphenobarbital	T42.3x1-	T42.3x2-	T42.3x3-	T42.3x4-	T42.3x5-	T42.3x6-
Methylpolysiloxane	T47.1x1-	T47.1x2-	T47.1x3-	T47.1x4-	T47.1x5-	T47.1x6-
Methylprednisolone — *see* Methyl, prednisolone						
Methylrosaniline	T49.0x1-	T49.0x2-	T49.0x3-	T49.0x4-	T49.0x5-	T49.0x6-
Methylrosanilinium chloride	T49.0x1-	T49.0x2-	T49.0x3-	T49.0x4-	T49.0x5-	T49.0x6-
Methyltestosterone	T38.7x1-	T38.7x2-	T38.7x3-	T38.7x4-	T38.7x5-	T38.7x6-
Methylthionine chloride	T50.6x1-	T50.6x2-	T50.6x3-	T50.6x4-	T50.6x5-	T50.6x6-
Methylthioninium chloride	T50.6x1-	T50.6x2-	T50.6x3-	T50.6x4-	T50.6x5-	T50.6x6-
Methylthiouracil	T38.2x1-	T38.2x2-	T38.2x3-	T38.2x4-	T38.2x5-	T38.2x6-
Methyprylon	T42.6x1-	T42.6x2-	T42.6x3-	T42.6x4-	T42.6x5-	T42.6x6-
Methysergide	T46.5x1-	T46.5x2-	T46.5x3-	T46.5x4-	T46.5x5-	T46.5x6-
Metiamide	T47.1x1-	T47.1x2-	T47.1x3-	T47.1x4-	T47.1x5-	T47.1x6-
Meticillin	T36.0x1-	T36.0x2-	T36.0x3-	T36.0x4-	T36.0x5-	T36.0x6-
Meticrane	T50.2x1-	T50.2x2-	T50.2x3-	T50.2x4-	T50.2x5-	T50.2x6-
Metildigoxin	T46.0x1-	T46.0x2-	T46.0x3-	T46.0x4-	T46.0x5-	T46.0x6-
Metipranolol	T49.5x1-	T49.5x2-	T49.5x3-	T49.5x4-	T49.5x5-	T49.5x6-
Metirosine	T46.5x1-	T46.5x2-	T46.5x3-	T46.5x4-	T46.5x5-	T46.5x6-
Metisazone	T37.5x1-	T37.5x2-	T37.5x3-	T37.5x4-	T37.5x5-	T37.5x6-
Metixene	T44.3x1-	T44.3x2-	T44.3x3-	T44.3x4-	T44.3x5-	T44.3x6-
Metizoline	T48.5x1-	T48.5x2-	T48.5x3-	T48.5x4-	T48.5x5-	T48.5x6-
Metoclopramide	T45.0x1-	T45.0x2-	T45.0x3-	T45.0x4-	T45.0x5-	T45.0x6-
Metofenazate	T43.3x1-	T43.3x2-	T43.3x3-	T43.3x4-	T43.3x5-	T43.3x6-

DRUGS & CHEMICALS

Table of Drugs & Chemicals	POISONING Accidental (Unintentional)	POISONING Self-Harm (Intentional)	POISONING Assault	POISONING Undetermined	Adverse Effect	Underdosing
Metofoline	T39.8x1-	T39.8x2-	T39.8x3-	T39.8x4-	T39.8x5-	T39.8x6-
Metolazone	T50.2x1-	T50.2x2-	T50.2x3-	T50.2x4-	T50.2x5-	T50.2x6-
Metopon	T40.2x1-	T40.2x2-	T40.2x3-	T40.2x4-	T40.2x5-	T40.2x6-
Metoprine	T45.1x1-	T45.1x2-	T45.1x3-	T45.1x4-	T45.1x5-	T45.1x6-
Metoprolol	T44.7x1-	T44.7x2-	T44.7x3-	T44.7x4-	T44.7x5-	T44.7x6-
Metrifonate	T60.0x1-	T60.0x2-	T60.0x3-	T60.0x4-	—	—
Metrizamide	T50.8x1-	T50.8x2-	T50.8x3-	T50.8x4-	T50.8x5-	T50.8x6-
Metrizoic acid	T50.8x1-	T50.8x2-	T50.8x3-	T50.8x4-	T50.8x5-	T50.8x6-
Metronidazole	T37.8x1-	T37.8x2-	T37.8x3-	T37.8x4-	T37.8x5-	T37.8x6-
Metycaine	T41.3x1-	T41.3x2-	T41.3x3-	T41.3x4-	T41.3x5-	T41.3x6-
infiltration (subcutaneous)	T41.3x1-	T41.3x2-	T41.3x3-	T41.3x4-	T41.3x5-	T41.3x6-
nerve block (peripheral) (plexus)	T41.3x1-	T41.3x2-	T41.3x3-	T41.3x4-	T41.3x5-	T41.3x6-
topical (surface)	T41.3x1-	T41.3x2-	T41.3x3-	T41.3x4-	T41.3x5-	T41.3x6-
Metyrapone	T50.8x1-	T50.8x2-	T50.8x3-	T50.8x4-	T50.8x5-	T50.8x6-
Mevinphos	T60.0x1-	T60.0x2-	T60.0x3-	T60.0x4-	—	—
Mexazolam	T42.4x1-	T42.4x2-	T42.4x3-	T42.4x4-	T42.4x5-	T42.4x6-
Mexenone	T49.3x1-	T49.3x2-	T49.3x3-	T49.3x4-	T49.3x5-	T49.3x6-
Mexiletine	T46.2x1-	T46.2x2-	T46.2x3-	T46.2x4-	T46.2x5-	T46.2x6-
Mezereon	T62.2x1-	T62.2x2-	T62.2x3-	T62.2x4-	—	—
berries	T62.1x1-	T62.1x2-	T62.1x3-	T62.1x4-	—	—
Mezlocillin	T36.0x1-	T36.0x2-	T36.0x3-	T36.0x4-	T36.0x5-	T36.0x6-
Mianserin	T43.021-	T43.022-	T43.023-	T43.024-	T43.025-	T43.026-
Micatin	T49.0x1-	T49.0x2-	T49.0x3-	T49.0x4-	T49.0x5-	T49.0x6-
Miconazole	T49.0x1-	T49.0x2-	T49.0x3-	T49.0x4-	T49.0x5-	T49.0x6-
Micronomicin	T36.5x1-	T36.5x2-	T36.5x3-	T36.5x4-	T36.5x5-	T36.5x6-
Midazolam	T42.4x1-	T42.4x2-	T42.4x3-	T42.4x4-	T42.4x5-	T42.4x6-
Midecamycin	T36.3x1-	T36.3x2-	T36.3x3-	T36.3x4-	T36.3x5-	T36.3x6-
Mifepristone	T38.6x1-	T38.6x2-	T38.6x3-	T38.6x4-	T38.6x5-	T38.6x6-
Milk of magnesia	T47.1x1-	T47.1x2-	T47.1x3-	T47.1x4-	T47.1x5-	T47.1x6-
Millipede (tropical) (venomous)	T63.411-	T63.412-	T63.413-	T63.414-	—	—
Miltown	T43.591-	T43.592-	T43.593-	T43.594-	T43.595-	T43.596-
Milverine	T44.3x1-	T44.3x2-	T44.3x3-	T44.3x4-	T44.3x5-	T44.3x6-
Minaprine	T43.291-	T43.292-	T43.293-	T43.294-	T43.295-	T43.296-
Minaxolone	T41.291-	T41.292-	T41.293-	T41.294-	T41.295-	T41.296-
Mineral acids	T54.2x1-	T54.2x2-	T54.2x3-	T54.2x4-	—	—
oil (laxative) (medicinal)	T47.4x1-	T47.4x2-	T47.4x3-	T47.4x4-	T47.4x5-	T47.4x6-
emulsion	T47.2x1-	T47.2x2-	T47.2x3-	T47.2x4-	T47.2x5-	T47.2x6-
nonmedicinal	T52.0x1-	T52.0x2-	T52.0x3-	T52.0x4-	—	—
topical	T49.3x1-	T49.3x2-	T49.3x3-	T49.3x4-	T49.3x5-	T49.3x6-
salt NEC	T50.3x1-	T50.3x2-	T50.3x3-	T50.3x4-	T50.3x5-	T50.3x6-
spirits	T52.0x1-	T52.0x2-	T52.0x3-	T52.0x4-	—	—
Mineralocorticosteroid	T50.0x1-	T50.0x2-	T50.0x3-	T50.0x4-	T50.0x5-	T50.0x6-
Minocycline	T36.4x1-	T36.4x2-	T36.4x3-	T36.4x4-	T36.4x5-	T36.4x6-
Minoxidil	T46.7x1-	T46.7x2-	T46.7x3-	T46.7x4-	T46.7x5-	T46.7x6-
Miokamycin	T36.3x1-	T36.3x2-	T36.3x3-	T36.3x4-	T36.3x5-	T36.3x6-
Miotic drug	T49.5x1-	T49.5x2-	T49.5x3-	T49.5x4-	T49.5x5-	T49.5x6-
Mipafox	T60.0x1-	T60.0x2-	T60.0x3-	T60.0x4-	—	—
Mirex	T60.1x1-	T60.1x2-	T60.1x3-	T60.1x4-	—	—
Mirtazapine	T43.021-	T43.022-	T43.023-	T43.024-	T43.025-	T43.026-
Misonidazole	T37.3x1-	T37.3x2-	T37.3x3-	T37.3x4-	T37.3x5-	T37.3x6-
Misoprostol	T47.1x1-	T47.1x2-	T47.1x3-	T47.1x4-	T47.1x5-	T47.1x6-
Mithramycin	T45.1x1-	T45.1x2-	T45.1x3-	T45.1x4-	T45.1x5-	T45.1x6-
Mitobronitol	T45.1x1-	T45.1x2-	T45.1x3-	T45.1x4-	T45.1x5-	T45.1x6-
Mitoguazone	T45.1x1-	T45.1x2-	T45.1x3-	T45.1x4-	T45.1x5-	T45.1x6-
Mitolactol	T45.1x1-	T45.1x2-	T45.1x3-	T45.1x4-	T45.1x5-	T45.1x6-
Mitomycin	T45.1x1-	T45.1x2-	T45.1x3-	T45.1x4-	T45.1x5-	T45.1x6-
Mitopodozide	T45.1x1-	T45.1x2-	T45.1x3-	T45.1x4-	T45.1x5-	T45.1x6-
Mitotane	T45.1x1-	T45.1x2-	T45.1x3-	T45.1x4-	T45.1x5-	T45.1x6-
Mitoxantrone	T45.1x1-	T45.1x2-	T45.1x3-	T45.1x4-	T45.1x5-	T45.1x6-
Mivacurium chloride	T48.1x1-	T48.1x2-	T48.1x3-	T48.1x4-	T48.1x5-	T48.1x6-
Miyari bacteria	T47.6x1-	T47.6x2-	T47.6x3-	T47.6x4-	T47.6x5-	T47.6x6-
Moclobemide	T43.1x1-	T43.1x2-	T43.1x3-	T43.1x4-	T43.1x5-	T43.1x6-
Moderil	T46.5x1-	T46.5x2-	T46.5x3-	T46.5x4-	T46.5x5-	T46.5x6-
Mofebutazone	T39.2x1-	T39.2x2-	T39.2x3-	T39.2x4-	T39.2x5-	T39.2x6-
Mogadon — see Nitrazepam						
Molindone	T43.591-	T43.592-	T43.593-	T43.594-	T43.595-	T43.596-
Molsidomine	T46.3x1-	T46.3x2-	T46.3x3-	T46.3x4-	T46.3x5-	T46.3x6-
Mometasone	T49.0x1-	T49.0x2-	T49.0x3-	T49.0x4-	T49.0x5-	T49.0x6-
Monistat	T49.0x1-	T49.0x2-	T49.0x3-	T49.0x4-	T49.0x5-	T49.0x6-
Monkshood	T62.2x1-	T62.2x2-	T62.2x3-	T62.2x4-	—	—
Monoamine oxidase inhibitor NEC	T43.1x1-	T43.1x2-	T43.1x3-	T43.1x4-	T43.1x5-	T43.1x6-
hydrazine	T43.1x1-	T43.1x2-	T43.1x3-	T43.1x4-	T43.1x5-	T43.1x6-
Monobenzone	T49.4x1-	T49.4x2-	T49.4x3-	T49.4x4-	T49.4x5-	T49.4x6-
Monochloroacetic acid	T60.3x1-	T60.3x2-	T60.3x3-	T60.3x4-	—	—
Monochlorobenzene	T53.7x1-	T53.7x2-	T53.7x3-	T53.7x4-	—	—
Monoethanolamine	T46.8x1-	T46.8x2-	T46.8x3-	T46.8x4-	T46.8x5-	T46.8x6-
oleate	T46.8x1-	T46.8x2-	T46.8x3-	T46.8x4-	T46.8x5-	T46.8x6-
Monooctanoin	T50.991-	T50.992-	T50.993-	T50.994-	T50.995-	T50.996-
Monophenylbutazone	T39.2x1-	T39.2x2-	T39.2x3-	T39.2x4-	T39.2x5-	T39.2x6-
Monosodium glutamate	T65.891-	T65.892-	T65.893-	T65.894-	—	—
Monosulfiram	T49.0x1-	T49.0x2-	T49.0x3-	T49.0x4-	T49.0x5-	T49.0x6-
Monoxide, carbon — see Carbon, monoxide						
Monoxidine hydrochloride	T46.1x1-	T46.1x2-	T46.1x3-	T46.1x4-	T46.1x5-	T46.1x6-
Monuron	T60.3x1-	T60.3x2-	T60.3x3-	T60.3x4-	—	—
Moperone	T43.4x1-	T43.4x2-	T43.4x3-	T43.4x4-	T43.4x5-	T43.4x6-
Mopidamol	T45.1x1-	T45.1x2-	T45.1x3-	T45.1x4-	T45.1x5-	T45.1x6-
MOPP (mechlorethamine + vincristine + prednisone + procarba-zine)	T45.1x1-	T45.1x2-	T45.1x3-	T45.1x4-	T45.1x5-	T45.1x6-
Morfin	T40.2x1-	T40.2x2-	T40.2x3-	T40.2x4-	T40.2x5-	T40.2x6-
Morinamide	T37.1x1-	T37.1x2-	T37.1x3-	T37.1x4-	T37.1x5-	T37.1x6-
Morning glory seeds	T40.991-	T40.992-	T40.993-	T40.994-	—	—
Moroxydine	T37.5x1-	T37.5x2-	T37.5x3-	T37.5x4-	T37.5x5-	T37.5x6-
Morphazinamide	T37.1x1-	T37.1x2-	T37.1x3-	T37.1x4-	T37.1x5-	T37.1x6-
Morphine	T40.2x1-	T40.2x2-	T40.2x3-	T40.2x4-	T40.2x5-	T40.2x6-
antagonist	T50.7x1-	T50.7x2-	T50.7x3-	T50.7x4-	T50.7x5-	T50.7x6-
Morpholinylethylmorphine	T40.2x1-	T40.2x2-	T40.2x3-	T40.2x4-	—	—
Morsuximide	T42.2x1-	T42.2x2-	T42.2x3-	T42.2x4-	T42.2x5-	T42.2x6-
Mosapramine	T43.591-	T43.592-	T43.593-	T43.594-	T43.595-	T43.596-
Moth balls — see also Pesticides	T60.2x1-	T60.2x2-	T60.2x3-	T60.2x4-	—	—
naphthalene	T60.2x1-	T60.2x2-	T60.2x3-	T60.2x4-	—	—
paradichlorobenzene	T60.1x1-	T60.1x2-	T60.1x3-	T60.1x4-	—	—
Motor exhaust gas	T58.01x-	T58.02x-	T58.03x-	T58.04x-	—	—
Mouthwash (antiseptic) (zinc chloride)	T49.6x1-	T49.6x2-	T49.6x3-	T49.6x4-	T49.6x5-	T49.6x6-
Moxastine	T45.0x1-	T45.0x2-	T45.0x3-	T45.0x4-	T45.0x5-	T45.0x6-
Moxaverine	T44.3x1-	T44.3x2-	T44.3x3-	T44.3x4-	T44.3x5-	T44.3x6-
Moxisylyte	T46.7x1-	T46.7x2-	T46.7x3-	T46.7x4-	T46.7x5-	T46.7x6-
Mucilage, plant	T47.4x1-	T47.4x2-	T47.4x3-	T47.4x4-	T47.4x5-	T47.4x6-
Mucolytic drug	T48.4x1-	T48.4x2-	T48.4x3-	T48.4x4-	T48.4x5-	T48.4x6-
Mucomyst	T48.4x1-	T48.4x2-	T48.4x3-	T48.4x4-	T48.4x5-	T48.4x6-
Mucous membrane agents (external)	T49.91x-	T49.92x-	T49.93x-	T49.94x-	T49.95x-	T49.96x-
specified NEC	T49.8x1-	T49.8x2-	T49.8x3-	T49.8x4-	T49.8x5-	T49.8x6-

DRUGS & CHEMICALS

Table of Drugs & Chemicals	POISONING Accidental (Unintentional)	Self-Harm (Intentional)	Assault	Undetermined	Adverse Effect	Underdosing
Mumps						
immune globulin (human)	T50.Z11-	T50.Z12-	T50.Z13-	T50.Z14-	T50.Z15-	T50.Z16-
skin test antigen	T50.8x1-	T50.8x2-	T50.8x3-	T50.8x4-	T50.8x5-	T50.8x6-
vaccine	T50.B91-	T50.B92-	T50.B93-	T50.B94-	T50.B95-	T50.B96-
Mumpsvax	T50.B91-	T50.B92-	T50.B93-	T50.B94-	T50.B95-	T50.B96-
Mupirocin	T49.0x1-	T49.0x2-	T49.0x3-	T49.0x4-	T49.0x5-	T49.0x6-
Muriatic acid — see Hydrochloric acid						
Muromonab-CD3	T45.1x1-	T45.1x2-	T45.1x3-	T45.1x4-	T45.1x5-	T45.1x6-
Muscle affecting agents NEC	T48.201-	T48.202-	T48.203-	T48.204-	T48.205-	T48.206-
oxytocic	T48.0x1-	T48.0x2-	T48.0x3-	T48.0x4-	T48.0x5-	T48.0x6-
relaxants	T48.201-	T48.202-	T48.203-	T48.204-	T48.205-	T48.206-
central nervous system	T42.8x1-	T42.8x2-	T42.8x3-	T42.8x4-	T42.8x5-	T42.8x6-
skeletal	T48.1x1-	T48.1x2-	T48.1x3-	T48.1x4-	T48.1x5-	T48.1x6-
smooth	T44.3x1-	T44.3x2-	T44.3x3-	T44.3x4-	T44.3x5-	T44.3x6-
Muscle relaxant — see Relaxant, muscle						
Muscle-action drug NEC	T48.201-	T48.202-	T48.203-	T48.204-	T48.205-	T48.206-
Muscle-tone depressant, central NEC	T42.8x1-	T42.8x2-	T42.8x3-	T42.8x4-	T42.8x5-	T42.8x6-
specified NEC	T42.8x1-	T42.8x2-	T42.8x3-	T42.8x4-	T42.8x5-	T42.8x6-
Mushroom, noxious	T62.0x1-	T62.0x2-	T62.0x3-	T62.0x4-	—	—
Mussel, noxious	T61.781-	T61.782-	T61.783-	T61.784-		
Mustard (emetic)	T47.7x1-	T47.7x2-	T47.7x3-	T47.7x4-	T47.7x5-	T47.7x6-
black	T47.7x1-	T47.7x2-	T47.7x3-	T47.7x4-	T47.7x5-	T47.7x6-
gas, not in war	T59.91x-	T59.92x-	T59.93x-	T59.94x-		
nitrogen	T45.1x1-	T45.1x2-	T45.1x3-	T45.1x4-	T45.1x5-	T45.1x6-
Mustine	T45.1x1-	T45.1x2-	T45.1x3-	T45.1x4-	T45.1x5-	T45.1x6-
M-vac	T45.1x1-	T45.1x2-	T45.1x3-	T45.1x4-	T45.1x5-	T45.1x6-
Mycifradin	T36.5x1-	T36.5x2-	T36.5x3-	T36.5x4-	T36.5x5-	T36.5x6-
topical	T49.0x1-	T49.0x2-	T49.0x3-	T49.0x4-	T49.0x5-	T49.0x6-
Mycitracin	T36.8x1-	T36.8x2-	T36.8x3-	T36.8x4-	T36.8x5-	T36.8x6-
ophthalmic preparation	T49.5x1-	T49.5x2-	T49.5x3-	T49.5x4-	T49.5x5-	T49.5x6-
Mycostatin	T36.7x1-	T36.7x2-	T36.7x3-	T36.7x4-	T36.7x5-	T36.7x6-
topical	T49.0x1-	T49.0x2-	T49.0x3-	T49.0x4-	T49.0x5-	T49.0x6-
Mycotoxins	T64.81x-	T64.82x-	T64.83x-	T64.84x-	—	—
aflatoxin	T64.01x-	T64.02x-	T64.03x-	T64.04x-	—	—
specified NEC	T64.81x-	T64.82x-	T64.83x-	T64.84x-	—	—
Mydriacyl	T44.3x1-	T44.3x2-	T44.3x3-	T44.3x4-	T44.3x5-	T44.3x6-
Mydriatic drug	T49.5x1-	T49.5x2-	T49.5x3-	T49.5x4-	T49.5x5-	T49.5x6-
Myelobromal	T45.1x1-	T45.1x2-	T45.1x3-	T45.1x4-	T45.1x5-	T45.1x6-
Myleran	T45.1x1-	T45.1x2-	T45.1x3-	T45.1x4-	T45.1x5-	T45.1x6-
Myochrysin(e)	T39.2x1-	T39.2x2-	T39.2x3-	T39.2x4-	T39.2x5-	T39.2x6-
Myoneural blocking agents	T48.1x1-	T48.1x2-	T48.1x3-	T48.1x4-	T48.1x5-	T48.1x6-
Myralact	T49.0x1-	T49.0x2-	T49.0x3-	T49.0x4-	T49.0x5-	T49.0x6-
Myristica fragrans	T62.2x1-	T62.2x2-	T62.2x3-	T62.2x4-	—	—
Myristicin	T65.891-	T65.892-	T65.893-	T65.894-		
Mysoline	T42.3x1-	T42.3x2-	T42.3x3-	T42.3x4-	T42.3x5-	T42.3x6-
Nabilone	T40.7x1-	T40.7x2-	T40.7x3-	T40.7x4-	T40.7x5-	T40.7x6-
Nabumetone	T39.391-	T39.392-	T39.393-	T39.394-	T39.395-	T39.396-
Nadolol	T44.7x1-	T44.7x2-	T44.7x3-	T44.7x4-	T44.7x5-	T44.7x6-
Nafcillin	T36.0x1-	T36.0x2-	T36.0x3-	T36.0x4-	T36.0x5-	T36.0x6-
Nafoxidine	T38.6x1-	T38.6x2-	T38.6x3-	T38.6x4-	T38.6x5-	T38.6x6-
Naftazone	T46.991-	T46.992-	T46.993-	T46.994-	T46.995-	T46.996-
Naftidrofuryl (oxalate)	T46.7x1-	T46.7x2-	T46.7x3-	T46.7x4-	T46.7x5-	T46.7x6-
Naftifine	T49.0x1-	T49.0x2-	T49.0x3-	T49.0x4-	T49.0x5-	T49.0x6-
Nail polish remover	T52.91x-	T52.92x-	T52.93x-	T52.94x-	—	—
Nalbuphine	T40.4x1-	T40.4x2-	T40.4x3-	T40.4x4-	T40.4x5-	T40.4x6-
Naled	T60.0x1-	T60.0x2-	T60.0x3-	T60.0x4-	—	—
Nalidixic acid	T37.8x1-	T37.8x2-	T37.8x3-	T37.8x4-	T37.8x5-	T37.8x6-
Nalorphine	T50.7x1-	T50.7x2-	T50.7x3-	T50.7x4-	T50.7x5-	T50.7x6-
Naloxone	T50.7x1-	T50.7x2-	T50.7x3-	T50.7x4-	T50.7x5-	T50.7x6-
Naltrexone	T50.7x1-	T50.7x2-	T50.7x3-	T50.7x4-	T50.7x5-	T50.7x6-
Namenda	T43.8x1-	T43.8x2-	T43.8x3-	T43.8x4-	T43.8x5-	T43.8x6-
Nandrolone	T38.7x1-	T38.7x2-	T38.7x3-	T38.7x4-	T38.7x5-	T38.7x6-
Naphazoline	T48.5x1-	T48.5x2-	T48.5x3-	T48.5x4-	T48.5x5-	T48.5x6-
Naphtha (painters') (petroleum)	T52.0x1-	T52.0x2-	T52.0x3-	T52.0x4-	—	—
solvent	T52.0x1-	T52.0x2-	T52.0x3-	T52.0x4-	—	—
vapor	T52.0x1-	T52.0x2-	T52.0x3-	T52.0x4-	—	—
Naphthalene (non-chlorinated)	T60.2x1-	T60.2x2-	T60.2x3-	T60.2x4-	—	—
chlorinated	T60.1x1-	T60.1x2-	T60.1x3-	T60.1x4-	—	—
vapor	T60.1x1-	T60.1x2-	T60.1x3-	T60.1x4-	—	—
insecticide or moth repellent	T60.2x1-	T60.2x2-	T60.2x3-	T60.2x4-	—	—
chlorinated	T60.1x1-	T60.1x2-	T60.1x3-	T60.1x4-	—	—
vapor	T60.2x1-	T60.2x2-	T60.2x3-	T60.2x4-	—	—
chlorinated	T60.1x1-	T60.1x2-	T60.1x3-	T60.1x4-	—	—
Naphthol	T65.891-	T65.892-	T65.893-	T65.894-		
Naphthylamine	T65.891-	T65.892-	T65.893-	T65.894-		
Naphthylthiourea (ANTU)	T60.4x1-	T60.4x2-	T60.4x3-	T60.4x4-	—	
Naprosyn — see Naproxen						
Naproxen	T39.311-	T39.312-	T39.313-	T39.314-	T39.315-	T39.316-
Narcotic (drug)	T40.601-	T40.602-	T40.603-	T40.604-	T40.605-	T40.606-
analgesic NEC	T40.601-	T40.602-	T40.603-	T40.604-	T40.605-	T40.606-
antagonist	T50.7x1-	T50.7x2-	T50.7x3-	T50.7x4-	T50.7x5-	T50.7x6-
specified NEC	T40.691-	T40.692-	T40.693-	T40.694-	T40.695-	T40.696-
synthetic	T40.4x1-	T40.4x2-	T40.4x3-	T40.4x4-	T40.4x5-	T40.4x6-
Narcotine	T48.3x1-	T48.3x2-	T48.3x3-	T48.3x4-	T48.3x5-	T48.3x6-
Nardil	T43.1x1-	T43.1x2-	T43.1x3-	T43.1x4-	T43.1x5-	T43.1x6-
Nasal drug NEC	T49.6x1-	T49.6x2-	T49.6x3-	T49.6x4-	T49.6x5-	T49.6x6-
Natamycin	T49.0x1-	T49.0x2-	T49.0x3-	T49.0x4-	T49.0x5-	T49.0x6-
Natrium cyanide — see Cyanide(s)						
Natural						
blood (product)	T45.8x1-	T45.8x2-	T45.8x3-	T45.8x4-	T45.8x5-	T45.8x6-
gas (piped)	T59.891-	T59.892-	T59.893-	T59.894-		
incomplete combustion	T58.11x-	T58.12x-	T58.13x-	T58.14x-	—	—
Nealbarbital	T42.3x1-	T42.3x2-	T42.3x3-	T42.3x4-	T42.3x5-	T42.3x6-
Nectadon	T48.3x1-	T48.3x2-	T48.3x3-	T48.3x4-	T48.3x5-	T48.3x6-
Nedocromil	T48.6x1-	T48.6x2-	T48.6x3-	T48.6x4-	T48.6x5-	T48.6x6-
Nefopam	T39.8x1-	T39.8x2-	T39.8x3-	T39.8x4-	T39.8x5-	T39.8x6-
Nematocyst (sting)	T63.691-	T63.692-	T63.693-	T63.694-	—	—
Nembutal	T42.3x1-	T42.3x2-	T42.3x3-	T42.3x4-	T42.3x5-	T42.3x6-
Nemonapride	T43.591-	T43.592-	T43.593-	T43.594-	T43.595-	T43.596-
Neoarsphenamine	T37.8x1-	T37.8x2-	T37.8x3-	T37.8x4-	T37.8x5-	T37.8x6-
Neocinchophen	T50.4x1-	T50.4x2-	T50.4x3-	T50.4x4-	T50.4x5-	T50.4x6-
Neomycin (derivatives)	T36.5x1-	T36.5x2-	T36.5x3-	T36.5x4-	T36.5x5-	T36.5x6-
with bacitracin	T49.0x1-	T49.0x2-	T49.0x3-	T49.0x4-	T49.0x5-	T49.0x6-
neostigmine	T44.0x1-	T44.0x2-	T44.0x3-	T44.0x4-	T44.0x5-	T44.0x6-
ENT agent	T49.6x1-	T49.6x2-	T49.6x3-	T49.6x4-	T49.6x5-	T49.6x6-
ophthalmic preparation	T49.5x1-	T49.5x2-	T49.5x3-	T49.5x4-	T49.5x5-	T49.5x6-
topical NEC	T49.0x1-	T49.0x2-	T49.0x3-	T49.0x4-	T49.0x5-	T49.0x6-
Neonal	T42.3x1-	T42.3x2-	T42.3x3-	T42.3x4-	T42.3x5-	T42.3x6-
Neoprontosil	T37.0x1-	T37.0x2-	T37.0x3-	T37.0x4-	T37.0x5-	T37.0x6-
Neosalvarsan	T37.8x1-	T37.8x2-	T37.8x3-	T37.8x4-	T37.8x5-	T37.8x6-
Neosilversalvarsan	T37.8x1-	T37.8x2-	T37.8x3-	T37.8x4-	T37.8x5-	T37.8x6-
Neosporin	T36.8x1-	T36.8x2-	T36.8x3-	T36.8x4-	T36.8x5-	T36.8x6-
ENT agent	T49.6x1-	T49.6x2-	T49.6x3-	T49.6x4-	T49.6x5-	T49.6x6-
ophthalmic preparation	T49.5x1-	T49.5x2-	T49.5x3-	T49.5x4-	T49.5x5-	T49.5x6-
topical NEC	T49.0x1-	T49.0x2-	T49.0x3-	T49.0x4-	T49.0x5-	T49.0x6-

Table of Drugs & Chemicals	POISONING Accidental (Unintentional)	Self-Harm (Intentional)	Assault	Undetermined	Adverse Effect	Underdosing
Neostigmine bromide	T44.0x1-	T44.0x2-	T44.0x3-	T44.0x4-	T44.0x5-	T44.0x6-
Neraval	T42.3x1-	T42.3x2-	T42.3x3-	T42.3x4-	T42.3x5-	T42.3x6-
Neravan	T42.3x1-	T42.3x2-	T42.3x3-	T42.3x4-	T42.3x5-	T42.3x6-
Nerium oleander	T62.2x1-	T62.2x2-	T62.2x3-	T62.2x4-	—	—
Nerve gas, not in war	T59.91x-	T59.92x-	T59.93x-	T59.94x-	—	—
Nesacaine	T41.3x1-	T41.3x2-	T41.3x3-	T41.3x4-	T41.3x5-	T41.3x6-
infiltration (subcutaneous)	T41.3x1-	T41.3x2-	T41.3x3-	T41.3x4-	T41.3x5-	T41.3x6-
nerve block (peripheral) (plexus)	T41.3x1-	T41.3x2-	T41.3x3-	T41.3x4-	T41.3x5-	T41.3x6-
Netilmicin	T36.5x1-	T36.5x2-	T36.5x3-	T36.5x4-	T36.5x5-	T36.5x6-
Neurobarb	T42.3x1-	T42.3x2-	T42.3x3-	T42.3x4-	T42.3x5-	T42.3x6-
Neuroleptic drug NEC	T43.501-	T43.502-	T43.503-	T43.504-	T43.505-	T43.506-
Neuromuscular blocking drug	T48.1x1-	T48.1x2-	T48.1x3-	T48.1x4-	T48.1x5-	T48.1x6-
Neutral insulin injection	T38.3x1-	T38.3x2-	T38.3x3-	T38.3x4-	T38.3x5-	T38.3x6-
Neutral spirits	T51.0x1-	T51.0x2-	T51.0x3-	T51.0x4-	—	—
beverage	T51.0x1-	T51.0x2-	T51.0x3-	T51.0x4-	—	—
Niacin	T46.7x1-	T46.7x2-	T46.7x3-	T46.7x4-	T46.7x5-	T46.7x6-
Niacinamide	T45.2x1-	T45.2x2-	T45.2x3-	T45.2x4-	T45.2x5-	T45.2x6-
Nialamide	T43.1x1-	T43.1x2-	T43.1x3-	T43.1x4-	T43.1x5-	T43.1x6-
Niaprazine	T42.6x1-	T42.6x2-	T42.6x3-	T42.6x4-	T42.6x5-	T42.6x6-
Nicametate	T46.7x1-	T46.7x2-	T46.7x3-	T46.7x4-	T46.7x5-	T46.7x6-
Nicardipine	T46.1x1-	T46.1x2-	T46.1x3-	T46.1x4-	T46.1x5-	T46.1x6-
Nicergoline	T46.7x1-	T46.7x2-	T46.7x3-	T46.7x4-	T46.7x5-	T46.7x6-
Nickel (carbonyl) (tetra-carbonyl) (fumes) (vapor)	T56.891-	T56.892-	T56.893-	T56.894-	—	—
Nickelocene	T56.891-	T56.892-	T56.893-	T56.894-	—	—
Niclosamide	T37.4x1-	T37.4x2-	T37.4x3-	T37.4x4-	T37.4x5-	T37.4x6-
Nicofuranose	T46.7x1-	T46.7x2-	T46.7x3-	T46.7x4-	T46.7x5-	T46.7x6-
Nicomorphine	T40.2x1-	T40.2x2-	T40.2x3-	T40.2x4-	—	—
Nicorandil	T46.3x1-	T46.3x2-	T46.3x3-	T46.3x4-	T46.3x5-	T46.3x6-
Nicotiana (plant)	T62.2x1-	T62.2x2-	T62.2x3-	T62.2x4-	—	—
Nicotinamide	T45.2x1-	T45.2x2-	T45.2x3-	T45.2x4-	T45.2x5-	T45.2x6-
Nicotine (insecticide) (spray) (sulfate) NEC	T60.2x1-	T60.2x2-	T60.2x3-	T60.2x4-	—	—
from tobacco	T65.291-	T65.292-	T65.293-	T65.294-	—	—
cigarettes	T65.221-	T65.222-	T65.223-	T65.224-	—	—
not insecticide	T65.291-	T65.292-	T65.293-	T65.294-	—	—
Nicotinic acid	T46.7x1-	T46.7x2-	T46.7x3-	T46.7x4-	T46.7x5-	T46.7x6-
Nicotinyl alcohol	T46.7x1-	T46.7x2-	T46.7x3-	T46.7x4-	T46.7x5-	T46.7x6-
Nicoumalone	T45.511-	T45.512-	T45.513-	T45.514-	T45.515-	T45.516-
Nifedipine	T46.1x1-	T46.1x2-	T46.1x3-	T46.1x4-	T46.1x5-	T46.1x6-
Nifenazone	T39.2x1-	T39.2x2-	T39.2x3-	T39.2x4-	T39.2x5-	T39.2x6-
Nifuraldezone	T37.91x-	T37.92x-	T37.93x-	T37.94x-	T37.95x-	T37.96x-
Nifuratel	T37.8x1-	T37.8x2-	T37.8x3-	T37.8x4-	T37.8x5-	T37.8x6-
Nifurtimox	T37.3x1-	T37.3x2-	T37.3x3-	T37.3x4-	T37.3x5-	T37.3x6-
Nifurtoinol	T37.8x1-	T37.8x2-	T37.8x3-	T37.8x4-	T37.8x5-	T37.8x6-
Nightshade, deadly (solanum) — see also Belladonna	T62.2x1-	T62.2x2-	T62.2x3-	T62.2x4-	—	—
berry	T62.1x1-	T62.1x2-	T62.1x3-	T62.1x4-	—	—
Nikethamide	T50.7x1-	T50.7x2-	T50.7x3-	T50.7x4-	T50.7x5-	T50.7x6-
Nilstat	T36.7x1-	T36.7x2-	T36.7x3-	T36.7x4-	T36.7x5-	T36.7x6-
topical	T49.0x1-	T49.0x2-	T49.0x3-	T49.0x4-	T49.0x5-	T49.0x6-
Nilutamide	T38.6x1-	T38.6x2-	T38.6x3-	T38.6x4-	T38.6x5-	T38.6x6-
Nimesulide	T39.391-	T39.392-	T39.393-	T39.394-	T39.395-	T39.396-
Nimetazepam	T42.4x1-	T42.4x2-	T42.4x3-	T42.4x4-	T42.4x5-	T42.4x6-
Nimodipine	T46.1x1-	T46.1x2-	T46.1x3-	T46.1x4-	T46.1x5-	T46.1x6-
Nimorazole	T37.3x1-	T37.3x2-	T37.3x3-	T37.3x4-	T37.3x5-	T37.3x6-
Nimustine	T45.1x1-	T45.1x2-	T45.1x3-	T45.1x4-	T45.1x5-	T45.1x6-
Niridazole	T37.4x1-	T37.4x2-	T37.4x3-	T37.4x4-	T37.4x5-	T37.4x6-
Nisentil	T40.2x1-	T40.2x2-	T40.2x3-	T40.2x4-	T40.2x5-	T40.2x6-
Nisoldipine	T46.1x1-	T46.1x2-	T46.1x3-	T46.1x4-	T46.1x5-	T46.1x6-
Nitramine	T65.3x1-	T65.3x2-	T65.3x3-	T65.3x4-	—	—
Nitrate, organic	T46.3x1-	T46.3x2-	T46.3x3-	T46.3x4-	T46.3x5-	T46.3x6-
Nitrazepam	T42.4x1-	T42.4x2-	T42.4x3-	T42.4x4-	T42.4x5-	T42.4x6-
Nitrefazole	T50.6x1-	T50.6x2-	T50.6x3-	T50.6x4-	T50.6x5-	T50.6x6-
Nitrendipine	T46.1x1-	T46.1x2-	T46.1x3-	T46.1x4-	T46.1x5-	T46.1x6-
Nitric						
acid (liquid)	T54.2x1-	T54.2x2-	T54.2x3-	T54.2x4-	—	—
vapor	T59.891-	T59.892-	T59.893-	T59.894-	—	—
oxide (gas)	T59.0x1-	T59.0x2-	T59.0x3-	T59.0x4-	—	—
Nitrimidazine	T37.3x1-	T37.3x2-	T37.3x3-	T37.3x4-	T37.3x5-	T37.3x6-
Nitrite, amyl (medicinal) (vapor)	T46.3x1-	T46.3x2-	T46.3x3-	T46.3x4-	T46.3x5-	T46.3x6-
Nitroaniline	T65.3x1-	T65.3x2-	T65.3x3-	T65.3x4-	—	—
vapor	T59.891-	T59.892-	T59.893-	T59.894-	—	—
Nitrobenzene, nitrobenzol	T65.3x1-	T65.3x2-	T65.3x3-	T65.3x4-	—	—
vapor	T65.3x1-	T65.3x2-	T65.3x3-	T65.3x4-	—	—
Nitrocellulose	T65.891-	T65.892-	T65.893-	T65.894-	—	—
lacquer	T65.891-	T65.892-	T65.893-	T65.894-	—	—
Nitrodiphenyl	T65.3x1-	T65.3x2-	T65.3x3-	T65.3x4-	—	—
Nitrofural	T49.0x1-	T49.0x2-	T49.0x3-	T49.0x4-	T49.0x5-	T49.0x6-
Nitrofurantoin	T37.8x1-	T37.8x2-	T37.8x3-	T37.8x4-	T37.8x5-	T37.8x6-
Nitrofurazone	T49.0x1-	T49.0x2-	T49.0x3-	T49.0x4-	T49.0x5-	T49.0x6-
Nitrogen	T59.0x1-	T59.0x2-	T59.0x3-	T59.0x4-	—	—
mustard	T45.1x1-	T45.1x2-	T45.1x3-	T45.1x4-	T45.1x5-	T45.1x6-
Nitroglycerin, nitro-glycerol (medicinal)	T46.3x1-	T46.3x2-	T46.3x3-	T46.3x4-	T46.3x5-	T46.3x6-
nonmedicinal	T65.5x1-	T65.5x2-	T65.5x3-	T65.5x4-	—	—
fumes	T65.5x1-	T65.5x2-	T65.5x3-	T65.5x4-	—	—
Nitroglycol	T52.3x1-	T52.3x2-	T52.3x3-	T52.3x4-	—	—
Nitrohydrochloric acid	T54.2x1-	T54.2x2-	T54.2x3-	T54.2x4-	—	—
Nitromersol	T49.0x1-	T49.0x2-	T49.0x3-	T49.0x4-	T49.0x5-	T49.0x6-
Nitronaphthalene	T65.891-	T65.892-	T65.893-	T65.894-	—	—
Nitrophenol	T54.0x1-	T54.0x2-	T54.0x3-	T54.0x4-	—	—
Nitropropane	T52.8x1-	T52.8x2-	T52.8x3-	T52.8x4-	—	—
Nitroprusside	T46.5x1-	T46.5x2-	T46.5x3-	T46.5x4-	T46.5x5-	T46.5x6-
Nitrosodimethylamine	T65.3x1-	T65.3x2-	T65.3x3-	T65.3x4-	—	—
Nitrothiazol	T37.4x1-	T37.4x2-	T37.4x3-	T37.4x4-	T37.4x5-	T37.4x6-
Nitrotoluene, nitrotoluol	T65.3x1-	T65.3x2-	T65.3x3-	T65.3x4-	—	—
vapor	T65.3x1-	T65.3x2-	T65.3x3-	T65.3x4-	—	—
Nitrous						
acid (liquid)	T54.2x1-	T54.2x2-	T54.2x3-	T54.2x4-	—	—
fumes	T59.891-	T59.892-	T59.893-	T59.894-	—	—
ether spirit	T46.3x1-	T46.3x2-	T46.3x3-	T46.3x4-	T46.3x5-	T46.3x6-
oxide	T41.0x1-	T41.0x2-	T41.0x3-	T41.0x4-	T41.0x5-	T41.0x6-
Nitroxoline	T37.8x1-	T37.8x2-	T37.8x3-	T37.8x4-	T37.8x5-	T37.8x6-
Nitrozone	T49.0x1-	T49.0x2-	T49.0x3-	T49.0x4-	T49.0x5-	T49.0x6-
Nizatidine	T47.0x1-	T47.0x2-	T47.0x3-	T47.0x4-	T47.0x5-	T47.0x6-
Nizofenone	T43.8x1-	T43.8x2-	T43.8x3-	T43.8x4-	T43.8x5-	T43.8x6-
Noctec	T42.6x1-	T42.6x2-	T42.6x3-	T42.6x4-	T42.6x5-	T42.6x6-
Noludar	T42.6x1-	T42.6x2-	T42.6x3-	T42.6x4-	T42.6x5-	T42.6x6-
Nomegestrol	T38.5x1-	T38.5x2-	T38.5x3-	T38.5x4-	T38.5x5-	T38.5x6-
Nomifensine	T43.291-	T43.292-	T43.293-	T43.294-	T43.295-	T43.296-
Nonoxinol	T49.8x1-	T49.8x2-	T49.8x3-	T49.8x4-	T49.8x5-	T49.8x6-
Nonylphenoxy (polyethoxy-ethanol)	T49.8x1-	T49.8x2-	T49.8x3-	T49.8x4-	T49.8x5-	T49.8x6-
Noptil	T42.3x1-	T42.3x2-	T42.3x3-	T42.3x4-	T42.3x5-	T42.3x6-
Noradrenaline	T44.4x1-	T44.4x2-	T44.4x3-	T44.4x4-	T44.4x5-	T44.4x6-
Noramidopyrine	T39.2x1-	T39.2x2-	T39.2x3-	T39.2x4-	T39.2x5-	T39.2x6-
methanesulfonate sodium	T39.2x1-	T39.2x2-	T39.2x3-	T39.2x4-	T39.2x5-	T39.2x6-

DRUGS & CHEMICALS

DRUGS & CHEMICALS

Table of Drugs & Chemicals	POISONING				Adverse Effect	Underdosing
	Accidental (Unintentional)	Self-Harm (Intentional)	Assault	Undetermined		
Norbormide	T60.4x1-	T60.4x2-	T60.4x3-	T60.4x4-	—	—
Nordazepam	T42.4x1-	T42.4x2-	T42.4x3-	T42.4x4-	T42.4x5-	T42.4x6-
Norepinephrine	T44.4x1-	T44.4x2-	T44.4x3-	T44.4x4-	T44.4x5-	T44.4x6-
Norethandrolone	T38.7x1-	T38.7x2-	T38.7x3-	T38.7x4-	T38.7x5-	T38.7x6-
Norethindrone	T38.4x1-	T38.4x2-	T38.4x3-	T38.4x4-	T38.4x5-	T38.4x6-
Norethisterone (acetate) (enantate)	T38.4x1-	T38.4x2-	T38.4x3-	T38.4x4-	T38.4x5-	T38.4x6-
with ethinylestradiol	T38.5x1-	T38.5x2-	T38.5x3-	T38.5x4-	T38.5x5-	T38.5x6-
Noretynodrel	T38.5x1-	T38.5x2-	T38.5x3-	T38.5x4-	T38.5x5-	T38.5x6-
Norfenefrine	T44.4x1-	T44.4x2-	T44.4x3-	T44.4x4-	T44.4x5-	T44.4x6-
Norfloxacin	T36.8x1-	T36.8x2-	T36.8x3-	T36.8x4-	T36.8x5-	T36.8x6-
Norgestrel	T38.4x1-	T38.4x2-	T38.4x3-	T38.4x4-	T38.4x5-	T38.4x6-
Norgestrienone	T38.4x1-	T38.4x2-	T38.4x3-	T38.4x4-	T38.4x5-	T38.4x6-
Norlestrin	T38.4x1-	T38.4x2-	T38.4x3-	T38.4x4-	T38.4x5-	T38.4x6-
Norlutin	T38.4x1-	T38.4x2-	T38.4x3-	T38.4x4-	T38.4x5-	T38.4x6-
Normal serum albumin (human), salt-poor	T45.8x1-	T45.8x2-	T45.8x3-	T45.8x4-	T45.8x5-	T45.8x6-
Normethandrone	T38.5x1-	T38.5x2-	T38.5x3-	T38.5x4-	T38.5x5-	T38.5x6-
Normison — see Benzodiazepines						
Normorphine	T40.2x1-	T40.2x2-	T40.2x3-	T40.2x4-	—	—
Norpseudoephedrine	T50.5x1-	T50.5x2-	T50.5x3-	T50.5x4-	T50.5x5-	T50.5x6-
Nortestosterone (furanpropionate)	T38.7x1-	T38.7x2-	T38.7x3-	T38.7x4-	T38.7x5-	T38.7x6-
Nortriptyline	T43.011-	T43.012-	T43.013-	T43.014-	T43.015-	T43.016-
Noscapine	T48.3x1-	T48.3x2-	T48.3x3-	T48.3x4-	T48.3x5-	T48.3x6-
Nose preparations	T49.6x1-	T49.6x2-	T49.6x3-	T49.6x4-	T49.6x5-	T49.6x6-
Novobiocin	T36.5x1-	T36.5x2-	T36.5x3-	T36.5x4-	T36.5x5-	T36.5x6-
Novocain (infiltration) (topical)	T41.3x1-	T41.3x2-	T41.3x3-	T41.3x4-	T41.3x5-	T41.3x6-
nerve block (peripheral) (plexus)	T41.3x1-	T41.3x2-	T41.3x3-	T41.3x4-	T41.3x5-	T41.3x6-
spinal	T41.3x1-	T41.3x2-	T41.3x3-	T41.3x4-	T41.3x5-	T41.3x6-
Noxious foodstuff	T62.91x-	T62.92x-	T62.93x-	T62.94x-	—	—
specified NEC	T62.8x1-	T62.8x2-	T62.8x3-	T62.8x4-	—	—
Noxiptiline	T43.011-	T43.012-	T43.013-	T43.014-	T43.015-	T43.016-
Noxytiolin	T49.0x1-	T49.0x2-	T49.0x3-	T49.0x4-	T49.0x5-	T49.0x6-
NPH lletin (insulin)	T38.3x1-	T38.3x2-	T38.3x3-	T38.3x4-	T38.3x5-	T38.3x6-
Numorphan	T40.2x1-	T40.2x2-	T40.2x3-	T40.2x4-	T40.2x5-	T40.2x6-
Nunol	T42.3x1-	T42.3x2-	T42.3x3-	T42.3x4-	T42.3x5-	T42.3x6-
Nupercaine (spinal anesthetic)	T41.3x1-	T41.3x2-	T41.3x3-	T41.3x4-	T41.3x5-	T41.3x6-
topical (surface)	T41.3x1-	T41.3x2-	T41.3x3-	T41.3x4-	T41.3x5-	T41.3x6-
Nutmeg oil (liniment)	T49.3x1-	T49.3x2-	T49.3x3-	T49.3x4-	T49.3x5-	T49.3x6-
Nutritional supplement	T50.901-	T50.902-	T50.903-	T50.904-	T50.905-	T50.906-
Nux vomica	T65.1x1-	T65.1x2-	T65.1x3-	T65.1x4-		
Nydrazid	T37.1x1-	T37.1x2-	T37.1x3-	T37.1x4-	T37.1x5-	T37.1x6-
Nylidrin	T46.7x1-	T46.7x2-	T46.7x3-	T46.7x4-	T46.7x5-	T46.7x6-
Nystatin	T36.7x1-	T36.7x2-	T36.7x3-	T36.7x4-	T36.7x5-	T36.7x6-
topical	T49.0x1-	T49.0x2-	T49.0x3-	T49.0x4-	T49.0x5-	T49.0x6-
Nytol	T45.0x1-	T45.0x2-	T45.0x3-	T45.0x4-	T45.0x5-	T45.0x6-
Obidoxime chloride	T50.6x1-	T50.6x2-	T50.6x3-	T50.6x4-	T50.6x5-	T50.6x6-
Octafonium (chloride)	T49.3x1-	T49.3x2-	T49.3x3-	T49.3x4-	T49.3x5-	T49.3x6-
Octamethyl pyrophosphoramide	T60.0x1-	T60.0x2-	T60.0x3-	T60.0x4-	—	—
Octanoin	T50.991-	T50.992-	T50.993-	T50.994-	T50.995-	T50.996-
Octatropine methyl bromide	T44.3x1-	T44.3x2-	T44.3x3-	T44.3x4-	T44.3x5-	T44.3x6-
Octotiamine	T45.2x1-	T45.2x2-	T45.2x3-	T45.2x4-	T45.2x5-	T45.2x6-
Octoxinol (9)	T49.8x1-	T49.8x2-	T49.8x3-	T49.8x4-	T49.8x5-	T49.8x6-
Octreotide	T38.991-	T38.992-	T38.993-	T38.994-	T38.995-	T38.996-
Octyl nitrite	T46.3x1-	T46.3x2-	T46.3x3-	T46.3x4-	T46.3x5-	T46.3x6-
Oestradiol	T38.5x1-	T38.5x2-	T38.5x3-	T38.5x4-	T38.5x5-	T38.5x6-
Oestriol	T38.5x1-	T38.5x2-	T38.5x3-	T38.5x4-	T38.5x5-	T38.5x6-
Oestrogen	T38.5x1-	T38.5x2-	T38.5x3-	T38.5x4-	T38.5x5-	T38.5x6-
Oestrone	T38.5x1-	T38.5x2-	T38.5x3-	T38.5x4-	T38.5x5-	T38.5x6-
Ofloxacin	T36.8x1-	T36.8x2-	T36.8x3-	T36.8x4-	T36.8x5-	T36.8x6-
Oil (of)	T65.891-	T65.892-	T65.893-	T65.894-	—	—
bitter almond	T62.8x1-	T62.8x2-	T62.8x3-	T62.8x4-	—	—
cloves	T49.7x1-	T49.7x2-	T49.7x3-	T49.7x4-	T49.7x5-	T49.7x6-
colors	T65.6x1-	T65.6x2-	T65.6x3-	T65.6x4-	—	—
fumes	T59.891-	T59.892-	T59.893-	T59.894-	—	—
lubricating	T52.0x1-	T52.0x2-	T52.0x3-	T52.0x4-	—	—
Niobe	T52.8x1-	T52.8x2-	T52.8x3-	T52.8x4-	—	—
vitriol (liquid)	T54.2x1-	T54.2x2-	T54.2x3-	T54.2x4-	—	—
fumes	T54.2x1-	T54.2x2-	T54.2x3-	T54.2x4-	—	—
wintergreen (bitter) NEC	T49.3x1-	T49.3x2-	T49.3x3-	T49.3x4-	T49.3x5-	T49.3x6-
Oily preparation (for skin)	T49.3x1-	T49.3x2-	T49.3x3-	T49.3x4-	T49.3x5-	T49.3x6-
Ointment NEC	T49.3x1-	T49.3x2-	T49.3x3-	T49.3x4-	T49.3x5-	T49.3x6-
Olanzapine	T43.591-	T43.592-	T43.593-	T43.594-	T43.595-	T43.596-
Oleander	T62.2x1-	T62.2x2-	T62.2x3-	T62.2x4-	—	—
Oleandomycin	T36.3x1-	T36.3x2-	T36.3x3-	T36.3x4-	T36.3x5-	T36.3x6-
Oleandrin	T46.0x1-	T46.0x2-	T46.0x3-	T46.0x4-	T46.0x5-	T46.0x6-
Oleic acid	T46.6x1-	T46.6x2-	T46.6x3-	T46.6x4-	T46.6x5-	T46.6x6-
Oleovitamin A	T45.2x1-	T45.2x2-	T45.2x3-	T45.2x4-	T45.2x5-	T45.2x6-
Oleum ricini	T47.2x1-	T47.2x2-	T47.2x3-	T47.2x4-	T47.2x5-	T47.2x6-
Olive oil (medicinal) NEC	T47.4x1-	T47.4x2-	T47.4x3-	T47.4x4-	T47.4x5-	T47.4x6-
Olivomycin	T45.1x1-	T45.1x2-	T45.1x3-	T45.1x4-	T45.1x5-	T45.1x6-
Olsalazine	T47.8x1-	T47.8x2-	T47.8x3-	T47.8x4-	T47.8x5-	T47.8x6-
Omeprazole	T47.1x1-	T47.1x2-	T47.1x3-	T47.1x4-	T47.1x5-	T47.1x6-
OMPA	T60.0x1-	T60.0x2-	T60.0x3-	T60.0x4-	—	—
Oncovin	T45.1x1-	T45.1x2-	T45.1x3-	T45.1x4-	T45.1x5-	T45.1x6-
Ondansetron	T45.0x1-	T45.0x2-	T45.0x3-	T45.0x4-	T45.0x5-	T45.0x6-
Ophthaine	T41.3x1-	T41.3x2-	T41.3x3-	T41.3x4-	T41.3x5-	T41.3x6-
Ophthetic	T41.3x1-	T41.3x2-	T41.3x3-	T41.3x4-	T41.3x5-	T41.3x6-
Opiate NEC	T40.601-	T40.602-	T40.603-	T40.604-	T40.605-	T40.606-
antagonists	T50.7x1-	T50.7x2-	T50.7x3-	T50.7x4-	T50.7x5-	T50.7x6-
Opioid NEC	T40.2x1-	T40.2x2-	T40.2x3-	T40.2x4-	T40.2x5-	T40.2x6-
Opipramol	T43.011-	T43.012-	T43.013-	T43.014-	T43.015-	T43.016-
Opium alkaloids (total)	T40.0x1-	T40.0x2-	T40.0x3-	T40.0x4-	T40.0x5-	T40.0x6-
standardized powdered	T40.0x1-	T40.0x2-	T40.0x3-	T40.0x4-	T40.0x5-	T40.0x6-
tincture (camphorated)	T40.0x1-	T40.0x2-	T40.0x3-	T40.0x4-	T40.0x5-	T40.0x6-
Oracon	T38.4x1-	T38.4x2-	T38.4x3-	T38.4x4-	T38.4x5-	T38.4x6-
Oragrafin	T50.8x1-	T50.8x2-	T50.8x3-	T50.8x4-	T50.8x5-	T50.8x6-
Oral contraceptives	T38.4x1-	T38.4x2-	T38.4x3-	T38.4x4-	T38.4x5-	T38.4x6-
Oral rehydration salts	T50.3x1-	T50.3x2-	T50.3x3-	T50.3x4-	T50.3x5-	T50.3x6-
Orazamide	T50.991-	T50.992-	T50.993-	T50.994-	T50.995-	T50.996-
Orciprenaline	T48.291-	T48.292-	T48.293-	T48.294-	T48.295-	T48.296-
Organidin	T48.4x1-	T48.4x2-	T48.4x3-	T48.4x4-	T48.4x5-	T48.4x6-
Organonitrate NEC	T46.3x1-	T46.3x2-	T46.3x3-	T46.3x4-	T46.3x5-	T46.3x6-
Organophosphates	T60.0x1-	T60.0x2-	T60.0x3-	T60.0x4-	—	—
Orimune	T50.B91-	T50.B92-	T50.B93-	T50.B94-	T50.B95-	T50.B96-
Orinase	T38.3x1-	T38.3x2-	T38.3x3-	T38.3x4-	T38.3x5-	T38.3x6-
Ormeloxifene	T38.6x1-	T38.6x2-	T38.6x3-	T38.6x4-	T38.6x5-	T38.6x6-
Ornidazole	T37.3x1-	T37.3x2-	T37.3x3-	T37.3x4-	T37.3x5-	T37.3x6-
Ornithine aspartate	T50.991-	T50.992-	T50.993-	T50.994-	T50.995-	T50.996-
Ornoprostil	T47.1x1-	T47.1x2-	T47.1x3-	T47.1x4-	T47.1x5-	T47.1x6-
Orphenadrine (hydrochloride)	T42.8x1-	T42.8x2-	T42.8x3-	T42.8x4-	T42.8x5-	T42.8x6-
Ortal (sodium)	T42.3x1-	T42.3x2-	T42.3x3-	T42.3x4-	T42.3x5-	T42.3x6-
Orthoboric acid	T49.0x1-	T49.0x2-	T49.0x3-	T49.0x4-	T49.0x5-	T49.0x6-
ENT agent	T49.6x1-	T49.6x2-	T49.6x3-	T49.6x4-	T49.6x5-	T49.6x6-
ophthalmic preparation	T49.5x1-	T49.5x2-	T49.5x3-	T49.5x4-	T49.5x5-	T49.5x6-
Orthocaine	T41.3x1-	T41.3x2-	T41.3x3-	T41.3x4-	T41.3x5-	T41.3x6-
Orthodichlorobenzene	T53.7x1-	T53.7x2-	T53.7x3-	T53.7x4-		

Table of Drugs & Chemicals	POISONING				Adverse Effect	Underdosing
	Accidental (Unintentional)	Self-Harm (Intentional)	Assault	Undetermined		
Ortho-Novum	T38.4x1-	T38.4x2-	T38.4x3-	T38.4x4-	T38.4x5-	T38.4x6-
Orthotolidine (reagent)	T54.2x1-	T54.2x2-	T54.2x3-	T54.2x4-	—	—
Osmic acid (liquid)	T54.2x1-	T54.2x2-	T54.2x3-	T54.2x4-	—	—
fumes	T54.2x1-	T54.2x2-	T54.2x3-	T54.2x4-	—	—
Osmotic diuretics	T50.2x1-	T50.2x2-	T50.2x3-	T50.2x4-	T50.2x5-	T50.2x6-
Otilonium bromide	T44.3x1-	T44.3x2-	T44.3x3-	T44.3x4-	T44.3x5-	T44.3x6-
Otorhinolaryngological drug NEC	T49.6x1-	T49.6x2-	T49.6x3-	T49.6x4-	T49.6x5-	T49.6x6-
Ouabain(e)	T46.0x1-	T46.0x2-	T46.0x3-	T46.0x4-	T46.0x5-	T46.0x6-
Ovarian						
hormone	T38.5x1-	T38.5x2-	T38.5x3-	T38.5x4-	T38.5x5-	T38.5x6-
stimulant	T38.5x1-	T38.5x2-	T38.5x3-	T38.5x4-	T38.5x5-	T38.5x6-
Ovral	T38.4x1-	T38.4x2-	T38.4x3-	T38.4x4-	T38.4x5-	T38.4x6-
Ovulen	T38.4x1-	T38.4x2-	T38.4x3-	T38.4x4-	T38.4x5-	T38.4x6-
Ox bile extract	T47.5x1-	T47.5x2-	T47.5x3-	T47.5x4-	T47.5x5-	T47.5x6-
Oxacillin	T36.0x1-	T36.0x2-	T36.0x3-	T36.0x4-	T36.0x5-	T36.0x6-
Oxalic acid	T54.2x1-	T54.2x2-	T54.2x3-	T54.2x4-	—	—
ammonium salt	T50.991-	T50.992-	T50.993-	T50.994-	T50.995-	T50.996-
Oxamniquine	T37.4x1-	T37.4x2-	T37.4x3-	T37.4x4-	T37.4x5-	T37.4x6-
Oxanamide	T43.591-	T43.592-	T43.593-	T43.594-	T43.595-	T43.596-
Oxandrolone	T38.7x1-	T38.7x2-	T38.7x3-	T38.7x4-	T38.7x5-	T38.7x6-
Oxantel	T37.4x1-	T37.4x2-	T37.4x3-	T37.4x4-	T37.4x5-	T37.4x6-
Oxapium iodide	T44.3x1-	T44.3x2-	T44.3x3-	T44.3x4-	T44.3x5-	T44.3x6-
Oxaprotiline	T43.021-	T43.022-	T43.023-	T43.024-	T43.025-	T43.026-
Oxaprozin	T39.311-	T39.312-	T39.313-	T39.314-	T39.315-	T39.316-
Oxatomide	T45.0x1-	T45.0x2-	T45.0x3-	T45.0x4-	T45.0x5-	T45.0x6-
Oxazepam	T42.4x1-	T42.4x2-	T42.4x3-	T42.4x4-	T42.4x5-	T42.4x6-
Oxazimedrine	T50.5x1-	T50.5x2-	T50.5x3-	T50.5x4-	T50.5x5-	T50.5x6-
Oxazolam	T42.4x1-	T42.4x2-	T42.4x3-	T42.4x4-	T42.4x5-	T42.4x6-
Oxazolidine derivatives	T42.2x1-	T42.2x2-	T42.2x3-	T42.2x4-	T42.2x5-	T42.2x6-
Oxazolidinedione (derivative)	T42.2x1-	T42.2x2-	T42.2x3-	T42.2x4-	T42.2x5-	T42.2x6-
Oxcarbazepine	T42.1x1-	T42.1x2-	T42.1x3-	T42.1x4-	T42.1x5-	T42.1x6-
Oxedrine	T44.4x1-	T44.4x2-	T44.4x3-	T44.4x4-	T44.4x5-	T44.4x6-
Oxeladin (citrate)	T48.3x1-	T48.3x2-	T48.3x3-	T48.3x4-	T48.3x5-	T48.3x6-
Oxendolone	T38.5x1-	T38.5x2-	T38.5x3-	T38.5x4-	T38.5x5-	T38.5x6-
Oxetacaine	T41.3x1-	T41.3x2-	T41.3x3-	T41.3x4-	T41.3x5-	T41.3x6-
Oxethazine	T41.3x1-	T41.3x2-	T41.3x3-	T41.3x4-	T41.3x5-	T41.3x6-
Oxetorone	T39.8x1-	T39.8x2-	T39.8x3-	T39.8x4-	T39.8x5-	T39.8x6-
Oxiconazole	T49.0x1-	T49.0x2-	T49.0x3-	T49.0x4-	T49.0x5-	T49.0x6-
Oxidizing agent NEC	T54.91x-	T54.92x-	T54.93x-	T54.94x-	—	—
Oxipurinol	T50.4x1-	T50.4x2-	T50.4x3-	T50.4x4-	T50.4x5-	T50.4x6-
Oxitriptan	T43.291-	T43.292-	T43.293-	T43.294-	T43.295-	T43.296-
Oxitropium bromide	T48.6x1-	T48.6x2-	T48.6x3-	T48.6x4-	T48.6x5-	T48.6x6-
Oxodipine	T46.1x1-	T46.1x2-	T46.1x3-	T46.1x4-	T46.1x5-	T46.1x6-
Oxolamine	T48.3x1-	T48.3x2-	T48.3x3-	T48.3x4-	T48.3x5-	T48.3x6-
Oxolinic acid	T37.8x1-	T37.8x2-	T37.8x3-	T37.8x4-	T37.8x5-	T37.8x6-
Oxomemazine	T43.3x1-	T43.3x2-	T43.3x3-	T43.3x4-	T43.3x5-	T43.3x6-
Oxophenarsine	T37.3x1-	T37.3x2-	T37.3x3-	T37.3x4-	T37.3x5-	T37.3x6-
Oxprenolol	T44.7x1-	T44.7x2-	T44.7x3-	T44.7x4-	T44.7x5-	T44.7x6-
Oxsoralen	T49.3x1-	T49.3x2-	T49.3x3-	T49.3x4-	T49.3x5-	T49.3x6-
Oxtriphylline	T48.6x1-	T48.6x2-	T48.6x3-	T48.6x4-	T48.6x5-	T48.6x6-
Oxybate sodium	T41.291-	T41.292-	T41.293-	T41.294-	T41.295-	T41.296-
Oxybuprocaine	T41.3x1-	T41.3x2-	T41.3x3-	T41.3x4-	T41.3x5-	T41.3x6-
Oxybutynin	T44.3x1-	T44.3x2-	T44.3x3-	T44.3x4-	T44.3x5-	T44.3x6-
Oxychlorosene	T49.0x1-	T49.0x2-	T49.0x3-	T49.0x4-	T49.0x5-	T49.0x6-
Oxycodone	T40.2x1-	T40.2x2-	T40.2x3-	T40.2x4-	T40.2x5-	T40.2x6-
Oxyfedrine	T46.3x1-	T46.3x2-	T46.3x3-	T46.3x4-	T46.3x5-	T46.3x6-
Oxygen	T41.5x1-	T41.5x2-	T41.5x3-	T41.5x4-	T41.5x5-	T41.5x6-
Oxylone	T49.0x1-	T49.0x2-	T49.0x3-	T49.0x4-	T49.0x5-	T49.0x6-
ophthalmic preparation	T49.5x1-	T49.5x2-	T49.5x3-	T49.5x4-	T49.5x5-	T49.5x6-
Oxymesterone	T38.7x1-	T38.7x2-	T38.7x3-	T38.7x4-	T38.7x5-	T38.7x6-
Oxymetazoline	T48.5x1-	T48.5x2-	T48.5x3-	T48.5x4-	T48.5x5-	T48.5x6-
Oxymetholone	T38.7x1-	T38.7x2-	T38.7x3-	T38.7x4-	T38.7x5-	T38.7x6-
Oxymorphone	T40.2x1-	T40.2x2-	T40.2x3-	T40.2x4-	T40.2x5-	T40.2x6-
Oxypertine	T43.591-	T43.592-	T43.593-	T43.594-	T43.595-	T43.596-
Oxyphenbutazone	T39.2x1-	T39.2x2-	T39.2x3-	T39.2x4-	T39.2x5-	T39.2x6-
Oxyphencyclimine	T44.3x1-	T44.3x2-	T44.3x3-	T44.3x4-	T44.3x5-	T44.3x6-
Oxyphenisatine	T47.2x1-	T47.2x2-	T47.2x3-	T47.2x4-	T47.2x5-	T47.2x6-
Oxyphenonium bromide	T44.3x1-	T44.3x2-	T44.3x3-	T44.3x4-	T44.3x5-	T44.3x6-
Oxypolygelatin	T45.8x1-	T45.8x2-	T45.8x3-	T45.8x4-	T45.8x5-	T45.8x6-
Oxyquinoline (derivatives)	T37.8x1-	T37.8x2-	T37.8x3-	T37.8x4-	T37.8x5-	T37.8x6-
Oxytetracycline	T36.4x1-	T36.4x2-	T36.4x3-	T36.4x4-	T36.4x5-	T36.4x6-
Oxytocic drug NEC	T48.0x1-	T48.0x2-	T48.0x3-	T48.0x4-	T48.0x5-	T48.0x6-
Oxytocin (synthetic)	T48.0x1-	T48.0x2-	T48.0x3-	T48.0x4-	T48.0x5-	T48.0x6-
Ozone	T59.891-	T59.892-	T59.893-	T59.894-	—	—
PABA	T49.3x1-	T49.3x2-	T49.3x3-	T49.3x4-	T49.3x5-	T49.3x6-
Packed red cells	T45.8x1-	T45.8x2-	T45.8x3-	T45.8x4-	T45.8x5-	T45.8x6-
Padimate	T49.3x1-	T49.3x2-	T49.3x3-	T49.3x4-	T49.3x5-	T49.3x6-
Paint NEC	T65.6x1-	T65.6x2-	T65.6x3-	T65.6x4-	—	—
cleaner	T52.91x-	T52.92x-	T52.93x-	T52.94x-	—	—
fumes NEC	T59.891-	T59.892-	T59.893-	T59.894-	—	—
lead (fumes)	T56.0x1-	T56.0x2-	T56.0x3-	T56.0x4-	—	—
solvent NEC	T52.8x1-	T52.8x2-	T52.8x3-	T52.8x4-	—	—
stripper	T52.8x1-	T52.8x2-	T52.8x3-	T52.8x4-	—	—
Palfium	T40.2x1-	T40.2x2-	T40.2x3-	T40.2x4-	—	—
Palm kernel oil	T50.991-	T50.992-	T50.993-	T50.994-	T50.995-	T50.996-
Paludrine	T37.2x1-	T37.2x2-	T37.2x3-	T37.2x4-	T37.2x5-	T37.2x6-
PAM (pralidoxime)	T50.6x1-	T50.6x2-	T50.6x3-	T50.6x4-	T50.6x5-	T50.6x6-
Pamaquine (naphthoute)	T37.2x1-	T37.2x2-	T37.2x3-	T37.2x4-	T37.2x5-	T37.2x6-
Panadol	T39.1x1-	T39.1x2-	T39.1x3-	T39.1x4-	T39.1x5-	T39.1x6-
Pancreatic digestive secretion stimulant	T47.8x1-	T47.8x2-	T47.8x3-	T47.8x4-	T47.8x5-	T47.8x6-
dornase	T45.3x1-	T45.3x2-	T45.3x3-	T45.3x4-	T45.3x5-	T45.3x6-
Pancreatin	T47.5x1-	T47.5x2-	T47.5x3-	T47.5x4-	T47.5x5-	T47.5x6-
Pancrelipase	T47.5x1-	T47.5x2-	T47.5x3-	T47.5x4-	T47.5x5-	T47.5x6-
Pancuronium (bromide)	T48.1x1-	T48.1x2-	T48.1x3-	T48.1x4-	T48.1x5-	T48.1x6-
Pangamic acid	T45.2x1-	T45.2x2-	T45.2x3-	T45.2x4-	T45.2x5-	T45.2x6-
Panthenol	T45.2x1-	T45.2x2-	T45.2x3-	T45.2x4-	T45.2x5-	T45.2x6-
topical	T49.8x1-	T49.8x2-	T49.8x3-	T49.8x4-	T49.8x5-	T49.8x6-
Pantopon	T40.0x1-	T40.0x2-	T40.0x3-	T40.0x4-	T40.0x5-	T40.0x6-
Pantothenic acid	T45.2x1-	T45.2x2-	T45.2x3-	T45.2x4-	T45.2x5-	T45.2x6-
Panwarfin	T45.511-	T45.512-	T45.513-	T45.514-	T45.515-	T45.516-
Papain	T47.5x1-	T47.5x2-	T47.5x3-	T47.5x4-	T47.5x5-	T47.5x6-
digestant	T47.5x1-	T47.5x2-	T47.5x3-	T47.5x4-	T47.5x5-	T47.5x6-
Papaveretum	T40.0x1-	T40.0x2-	T40.0x3-	T40.0x4-	T40.0x5-	T40.0x6-
Papaverine	T44.3x1-	T44.3x2-	T44.3x3-	T44.3x4-	T44.3x5-	T44.3x6-
Para-acetamidophenol	T39.1x1-	T39.1x2-	T39.1x3-	T39.1x4-	T39.1x5-	T39.1x6-
Para-aminobenzoic acid	T49.3x1-	T49.3x2-	T49.3x3-	T49.3x4-	T49.3x5-	T49.3x6-
Para-aminophenol derivatives	T39.1x1-	T39.1x2-	T39.1x3-	T39.1x4-	T39.1x5-	T39.1x6-
Para-aminosalicylic acid	T37.1x1-	T37.1x2-	T37.1x3-	T37.1x4-	T37.1x5-	T37.1x6-
Paracetaldehyde	T42.6x1-	T42.6x2-	T42.6x3-	T42.6x4-	T42.6x5-	T42.6x6-
Paracetamol	T39.1x1-	T39.1x2-	T39.1x3-	T39.1x4-	T39.1x5-	T39.1x6-
Parachlorophenol (camphorated)	T49.0x1-	T49.0x2-	T49.0x3-	T49.0x4-	T49.0x5-	T49.0x6-
Paracodin	T40.2x1-	T40.2x2-	T40.2x3-	T40.2x4-	T40.2x5-	T40.2x6-
Paradione	T42.2x1-	T42.2x2-	T42.2x3-	T42.2x4-	T42.2x5-	T42.2x6-
Paraffin(s) (wax)	T52.0x1-	T52.0x2-	T52.0x3-	T52.0x4-	—	—
liquid (medicinal)	T47.4x1-	T47.4x2-	T47.4x3-	T47.4x4-	T47.4x5-	T47.4x6-
nonmedicinal	T52.0x1-	T52.0x2-	T52.0x3-	T52.0x4-	—	—

Table of Drugs & Chemicals	POISONING Accidental (Unintentional)	POISONING Self-Harm (Intentional)	POISONING Assault	POISONING Undetermined	Adverse Effect	Underdosing
Paraformaldehyde	T60.3x1-	T60.3x2-	T60.3x3-	T60.3x4-	—	—
Paraldehyde	T42.6x1-	T42.6x2-	T42.6x3-	T42.6x4-	T42.6x5-	T42.6x6-
Paramethadione	T42.2x1-	T42.2x2-	T42.2x3-	T42.2x4-	T42.2x5-	T42.2x6-
Paramethasone	T38.0x1-	T38.0x2-	T38.0x3-	T38.0x4-	T38.0x5-	T38.0x6-
acetate	T49.0x1-	T49.0x2-	T49.0x3-	T49.0x4-	T49.0x5-	T49.0x6-
Paraoxon	T60.0x1-	T60.0x2-	T60.0x3-	T60.0x4-	—	—
Paraquat	T60.3x1-	T60.3x2-	T60.3x3-	T60.3x4-	—	—
Parasympatholytic NEC	T44.3x1-	T44.3x2-	T44.3x3-	T44.3x4-	T44.3x5-	T44.3x6-
Parasympathomimetic drug NEC	T44.1x1-	T44.1x2-	T44.1x3-	T44.1x4-	T44.1x5-	T44.1x6-
Parathion	T60.0x1-	T60.0x2-	T60.0x3-	T60.0x4-	—	—
Parathormone	T50.991-	T50.992-	T50.993-	T50.994-	T50.995-	T50.996-
Parathyroid extract	T50.991-	T50.992-	T50.993-	T50.994-	T50.995-	T50.996-
Paratyphoid vaccine	T50.A91-	T50.A92-	T50.A93-	T50.A94-	T50.A95-	T50.A96-
Paredrine	T44.4x1-	T44.4x2-	T44.4x3-	T44.4x4-	T44.4x5-	T44.4x6-
Paregoric	T40.0x1-	T40.0x2-	T40.0x3-	T40.0x4-	T40.0x5-	T40.0x6-
Pargyline	T46.5x1-	T46.5x2-	T46.5x3-	T46.5x4-	T46.5x5-	T46.5x6-
Paris green	T57.0x1-	T57.0x2-	T57.0x3-	T57.0x4-	—	—
insecticide	T57.0x1-	T57.0x2-	T57.0x3-	T57.0x4-	—	—
Parnate	T43.1x1-	T43.1x2-	T43.1x3-	T43.1x4-	T43.1x5-	T43.1x6-
Paromomycin	T36.5x1-	T36.5x2-	T36.5x3-	T36.5x4-	T36.5x5-	T36.5x6-
Paroxypropione	T45.1x1-	T45.1x2-	T45.1x3-	T45.1x4-	T45.1x5-	T45.1x6-
Parzone	T40.2x1-	T40.2x2-	T40.2x3-	T40.2x4-	T40.2x5-	T40.2x6-
PAS	T37.1x1-	T37.1x2-	T37.1x3-	T37.1x4-	T37.1x5-	T37.1x6-
Pasiniazid	T37.1x1-	T37.1x2-	T37.1x3-	T37.1x4	T37.1x5-	T37.1x6-
PBB (polybrominated biphenyls)	T65.891-	T65.892-	T65.893-	T65.894-	—	—
PCB	T65.891-	T65.892-	T65.893-	T65.894-	—	—
PCP						
meaning pentachlorophenol	T60.1x1-	T60.1x2-	T60.1x3-	T60.1x4-	—	—
fungicide	T60.3x1-	T60.3x2-	T60.3x3-	T60.3x4-	—	—
herbicide	T60.3x1-	T60.3x2-	T60.3x3-	T60.3x4-	—	—
insecticide	T60.1x1-	T60.1x2-	T60.1x3-	T60.1x4-	—	—
meaning phencyclidine	T40.991-	T40.992-	T40.993-	T40.994-		—
Peach kernel oil (emulsion)	T47.4x1-	T47.4x2-	T47.4x3-	T47.4x4-	T47.4x5-	T47.4x6-
Peanut oil (emulsion) NEC	T47.4x1-	T47.4x2-	T47.4x3-	T47.4x4-	T47.4x5-	T47.4x6-
topical	T49.3x1-	T49.3x2-	T49.3x3-	T49.3x4-	T49.3x5-	T49.3x6-
Pearly Gates (morning glory seeds)	T40.991-	T40.992-	T40.993-	T40.994-	—	—
Pecazine	T43.3x1-	T43.3x2-	T43.3x3-	T43.3x4-	T43.3x5-	T43.3x6-
Pectin	T47.6x1-	T47.6x2-	T47.6x3-	T47.6x4-	T47.6x5-	T47.6x6-
Pefloxacin	T37.8x1-	T37.8x2-	T37.8x3-	T37.8x4-	T37.8x5-	T37.8x6-
Pegademase, bovine	T50.Z91-	T50.Z92-	T50.Z93-	T50.Z94-	T50.Z95-	T50.Z96-
Pelletierine tannate	T37.4x1-	T37.4x2-	T37.4x3-	T37.4x4-	T37.4x5-	T37.4x6-
Pemirolast (potassium)	T48.6x1-	T48.6x2-	T48.6x3-	T48.6x4-	T48.6x5-	T48.6x6-
Pemoline	T50.7x1-	T50.7x2-	T50.7x3-	T50.7x4-	T50.7x5-	T50.7x6-
Pempidine	T44.2x1-	T44.2x2-	T44.2x3-	T44.2x4-	T44.2x5-	T44.2x6-
Penamecillin	T36.0x1-	T36.0x2-	T36.0x3-	T36.0x4-	T36.0x5-	T36.0x6-
Penbutolol	T44.7x1-	T44.7x2-	T44.7x3-	T44.7x4-	T44.7x5-	T44.7x6-
Penethamate	T36.0x1-	T36.0x2-	T36.0x3-	T36.0x4-	T36.0x5-	T36.0x6-
Penfluridol	T43.591-	T43.592-	T43.593-	T43.594-	T43.595-	T43.596-
Penflutizide	T50.2x1-	T50.2x2-	T50.2x3-	T50.2x4-	T50.2x5-	T50.2x6-
Pengitoxin	T46.0x1-	T46.0x2-	T46.0x3-	T46.0x4-	T46.0x5-	T46.0x6-
Penicillamine	T50.6x1-	T50.6x2-	T50.6x3-	T50.6x4-	T50.6x5-	T50.6x6-
Penicillin (any)	T36.0x1-	T36.0x2-	T36.0x3-	T36.0x4-	T36.0x5-	T36.0x6-
Penicillinase	T45.3x1-	T45.3x2-	T45.3x3-	T45.3x4-	T45.3x5-	T45.3x6-
Penicilloyl polylysine	T50.8x1-	T50.8x2-	T50.8x3-	T50.8x4-	T50.8x5-	T50.8x6-
Penimepicycline	T36.4x1-	T36.4x2-	T36.4x3-	T36.4x4-	T36.4x5-	T36.4x6-
Pentachloroethane	T53.6x1-	T53.6x2-	T53.6x3-	T53.6x4-	—	—
Pentachloronaphthalene	T53.7x1-	T53.7x2-	T53.7x3-	T53.7x4-	—	—
Pentachlorophenol (pesticide)	T60.1x1-	T60.1x2-	T60.1x3-	T60.1x4-	—	—
fungicide	T60.3x1-	T60.3x2-	T60.3x3-	T60.3x4-	—	—
herbicide	T60.3x1-	T60.3x2-	T60.3x3-	T60.3x4-	—	—
insecticide	T60.1x1-	T60.1x2-	T60.1x3-	T60.1x4-	—	—
Pentaerythritol	T46.3x1-	T46.3x2-	T46.3x3-	T46.3x4-	T46.3x5-	T46.3x6-
chloral	T42.6x1-	T42.6x2-	T42.6x3-	T42.6x4-	T42.6x5-	T42.6x6-
tetranitrate NEC	T46.3x1-	T46.3x2-	T46.3x3-	T46.3x4-	T46.3x5-	T46.3x6-
Pentaerythrityl tetranitrate	T46.3x1-	T46.3x2-	T46.3x3-	T46.3x4-	T46.3x5-	T46.3x6-
Pentagastrin	T50.8x1-	T50.8x2-	T50.8x3-	T50.8x4-	T50.8x5-	T50.8x6-
Pentalin	T53.6x1-	T53.6x2-	T53.6x3-	T53.6x4-		
Pentamethonium bromide	T44.2x1-	T44.2x2-	T44.2x3-	T44.2x4-	T44.2x5-	T44.2x6-
Pentamidine	T37.3x1-	T37.3x2-	T37.3x3-	T37.3x4-	T37.3x5-	T37.3x6-
Pentanol	T51.3x1-	T51.3x2-	T51.3x3-	T51.3x4-		
Pentapyrrolinium (bitartrate)	T44.2x1-	T44.2x2-	T44.2x3-	T44.2x4-	T44.2x5-	T44.2x6-
Pentaquine	T37.2x1-	T37.2x2-	T37.2x3-	T37.2x4-	T37.2x5-	T37.2x6-
Pentazocine	T40.4x1-	T40.4x2-	T40.4x3-	T40.4x4-	T40.4x5-	T40.4x6-
Pentetrazole	T50.7x1-	T50.7x2-	T50.7x3-	T50.7x4-	T50.7x5-	T50.7x6-
Penthienate bromide	T44.3x1-	T44.3x2-	T44.3x3-	T44.3x4-	T44.3x5-	T44.3x6-
Pentifylline	T46.7x1-	T46.7x2-	T46.7x3-	T46.7x4-	T46.7x5-	T46.7x6-
Pentobarbital	T42.3x1-	T42.3x2-	T42.3x3-	T42.3x4-	T42.3x5-	T42.3x6-
sodium	T42.3x1-	T42.3x2-	T42.3x3-	T42.3x4-	T42.3x5-	T42.3x6-
Pentobarbitone	T42.3x1-	T42.3x2-	T42.3x3-	T42.3x4-	T42.3x5-	T42.3x6-
Pentolonium tartrate	T44.2x1-	T44.2x2-	T44.2x3-	T44.2x4-	T44.2x5-	T44.2x6-
Pentosan polysulfate (sodium)	T39.8x1-	T39.8x2-	T39.8x3-	T39.8x4-	T39.8x5-	T39.8x6-
Pentostatin	T45.1x1-	T45.1x2-	T45.1x3-	T45.1x4-	T45.1x5-	T45.1x6-
Pentothal	T41.1x1-	T41.1x2-	T41.1x3-	T41.1x4-	T41.1x5-	T41.1x6-
Pentoxifylline	T46.7x1-	T46.7x2-	T46.7x3-	T46.7x4-	T46.7x5-	T46.7x6-
Pentoxyverine	T48.3x1-	T48.3x2-	T48.3x3-	T48.3x4-	T48.3x5-	T48.3x6-
Pentrinat	T46.3x1-	T46.3x2-	T46.3x3-	T46.3x4-	T46.3x5-	T46.3x6-
Pentylenetetrazole	T50.7x1-	T50.7x2-	T50.7x3-	T50.7x4-	T50.7x5-	T50.7x6-
Pentylsalicylamide	T37.1x1-	T37.1x2-	T37.1x3-	T37.1x4-	T37.1x5-	T37.1x6-
Pentymal	T42.3x1-	T42.3x2-	T42.3x3-	T42.3x4-	T42.3x5-	T42.3x6-
Peplomycin	T45.1x1-	T45.1x2-	T45.1x3-	T45.1x4-	T45.1x5-	T45.1x6-
Peppermint (oil)	T47.5x1-	T47.5x2-	T47.5x3-	T47.5x4-	T47.5x5-	T47.5x6-
Pepsin	T47.5x1-	T47.5x2-	T47.5x3-	T47.5x4-	T47.5x5-	T47.5x6-
digestant	T47.5x1-	T47.5x2-	T47.5x3-	T47.5x4-	T47.5x5-	T47.5x6-
Pepstatin	T47.1x1-	T47.1x2-	T47.1x3-	T47.1x4-	T47.1x5-	T47.1x6-
Peptavlon	T50.8x1-	T50.8x2-	T50.8x3-	T50.8x4-	T50.8x5-	T50.8x6-
Perazine	T43.3x1-	T43.3x2-	T43.3x3-	T43.3x4-	T43.3x5-	T43.3x6-
Percaine (spinal)	T41.3x1-	T41.3x2-	T41.3x3-	T41.3x4-	T41.3x5-	T41.3x6-
topical (surface)	T41.3x1-	T41.3x2-	T41.3x3-	T41.3x4-	T41.3x5-	T41.3x6-
Perchloroethylene	T53.3x1-	T53.3x2-	T53.3x3-	T53.3x4-	—	—
vapor	T53.3x1-	T53.3x2-	T53.3x3-	T53.3x4-		
medicinal	T37.4x1-	T37.4x2-	T37.4x3-	T37.4x4-	T37.4x5-	T37.4x6-
Percodan	T40.2x1-	T40.2x2-	T40.2x3-	T40.2x4-	T40.2x5-	T40.2x6-
Percogesic — see also Acetaminophen						
Percorten	T38.0x1-	T38.0x2-	T38.0x3-	T38.0x4-	T38.0x5-	T38.0x6-
Pergolide	T42.8x1-	T42.8x2-	T42.8x3-	T42.8x4-	T42.8x5-	T42.8x6-
Pergonal	T38.811-	T38.812-	T38.813-	T38.814-	T38.815-	T38.816-
Perhexilene	T46.3x1-	T46.3x2-	T46.3x3-	T46.3x4-	T46.3x5-	T46.3x6-
Perhexiline (maleate)	T46.3x1-	T46.3x2-	T46.3x3-	T46.3x4-	T46.3x5-	T46.3x6-
Periactin	T45.0x1-	T45.0x2-	T45.0x3-	T45.0x4-	T45.0x5-	T45.0x6-
Periciazine	T43.3x1-	T43.3x2-	T43.3x3-	T43.3x4-	T43.3x5-	T43.3x6-
Periclor	T42.6x1-	T42.6x2-	T42.6x3-	T42.6x4-	T42.6x5-	T42.6x6-
Perindopril	T46.4x1-	T46.4x2-	T46.4x3-	T46.4x4-	T46.4x5-	T46.4x6-
Perisoxal	T39.8x1-	T39.8x2-	T39.8x3-	T39.8x4-	T39.8x5-	T39.8x6-

Table of Drugs & Chemicals	POISONING				Adverse Effect	Underdosing
	Accidental (Unintentional)	Self-Harm (Intentional)	Assault	Undetermined		
Peritoneal dialysis solution	T50.3x1-	T50.3x2-	T50.3x3-	T50.3x4-	T50.3x5-	T50.3x6-
Peritrate	T46.3x1-	T46.3x2-	T46.3x3-	T46.3x4-	T46.3x5-	T46.3x6-
Perlapine	T42.4x1-	T42.4x2-	T42.4x3-	T42.4x4-	T42.4x5-	T42.4x6-
Permanganate	T65.891-	T65.892-	T65.893-	T65.894-	—	—
Permethrin	T60.1x1-	T60.1x2-	T60.1x3-	T60.1x4-	—	—
Pernocton	T42.3x1-	T42.3x2-	T42.3x3-	T42.3x4-	T42.3x5-	T42.3x6-
Pernoston	T42.3x1-	T42.3x2-	T42.3x3-	T42.3x4-	T42.3x5-	T42.3x6-
Peronine	T40.2x1-	T40.2x2-	T40.2x3-	T40.2x4-	—	—
Perphenazine	T43.3x1-	T43.3x2-	T43.3x3-	T43.3x4-	T43.3x5-	T43.3x6-
Pertofrane	T43.011-	T43.012-	T43.013-	T43.014-	T43.015-	T43.016-
Pertussis						
immune serum (human)	T50.Z11-	T50.Z12-	T50.Z13-	T50.Z14-	T50.Z15-	T50.Z16-
vaccine (with diphtheria toxoid) (with tetanus toxoid)	T50.A11-	T50.A12-	T50.A13-	T50.A14-	T50.A15-	T50.A16-
Peruvian balsam	T49.0x1-	T49.0x2-	T49.0x3-	T49.0x4-	T49.0x5-	T49.0x6-
Peruvoside	T46.0x1-	T46.0x2-	T46.0x3-	T46.0x4-	T46.0x5-	T46.0x6-
Pesticide (dust) (fumes) (vapor) NEC	T60.91x-	T60.92x-	T60.93x-	T60.94x-	—	—
arsenic	T57.0x1-	T57.0x2-	T57.0x3-	T57.0x4-	—	—
chlorinated	T60.1x1-	T60.1x2-	T60.1x3-	T60.1x4-	—	—
cyanide	T65.0x1-	T65.0x2-	T65.0x3-	T65.0x4-	—	—
kerosene	T52.0x1-	T52.0x2-	T52.0x3-	T52.0x4-	—	—
mixture (of compounds)	T60.91x-	T60.92x-	T60.93x-	T60.94x-	—	—
naphthalene	T60.2x1-	T60.2x2-	T60.2x3-	T60.2x4-	—	—
organochlorine (compounds)	T60.1x1-	T60.1x2-	T60.1x3-	T60.1x4-	—	—
petroleum (distillate) (products) NEC	T60.8x1-	T60.8x2-	T60.8x3-	T60.8x4-	—	—
specified ingredient NEC	T60.8x1-	T60.8x2-	T60.8x3-	T60.8x4-	—	—
strychnine	T65.1x1-	T65.1x2-	T65.1x3-	T65.1x4-	—	—
thallium	T60.4x1-	T60.4x2-	T60.4x3-	T60.4x4-	—	—
Pethidine	T40.4x1-	T40.4x2-	T40.4x3-	T40.4x4-	T40.4x5-	T40.4x6-
Petrichloral	T42.6x1-	T42.6x2-	T42.6x3-	T42.6x4-	T42.6x5-	T42.6x6-
Petrol	T52.0x1-	T52.0x2-	T52.0x3-	T52.0x4-	—	—
vapor	T52.0x1-	T52.0x2-	T52.0x3-	T52.0x4-	—	—
Petrolatum	T49.3x1-	T49.3x2-	T49.3x3-	T49.3x4-	T49.3x5-	T49.3x6-
hydrophilic	T49.3x1-	T49.3x2-	T49.3x3-	T49.3x4-	T49.3x5-	T49.3x6-
liquid	T47.4x1-	T47.4x2-	T47.4x3-	T47.4x4-	T47.4x5-	T47.4x6-
topical	T49.3x1-	T49.3x2-	T49.3x3-	T49.3x4-	T49.3x5-	T49.3x6-
nonmedicinal	T52.0x1-	T52.0x2-	T52.0x3-	T52.0x4-	—	—
red veterinary	T49.3x1-	T49.3x2-	T49.3x3-	T49.3x4-	T49.3x5-	T49.3x6-
white	T49.3x1-	T49.3x2-	T49.3x3-	T49.3x4-	T49.3x5-	T49.3x6-
Petroleum (products) NEC	T52.0x1-	T52.0x2-	T52.0x3-	T52.0x4-	—	—
benzine (s) — see Ligroin						
ether — see Ligroin						
jelly — see Petrolatum						
naphtha — see Ligroin						
pesticide	T60.8x1-	T60.8x2-	T60.8x3-	T60.8x4-	—	—
solids	T52.0x1-	T52.0x2-	T52.0x3-	T52.0x4-	—	—
solvents	T52.0x1-	T52.0x2-	T52.0x3-	T52.0x4-	—	—
vapor	T52.0x1-	T52.0x2-	T52.0x3-	T52.0x4-	—	—
Peyote	T40.991-	T40.992-	T40.993-	T40.994-	—	—
Phanodorm, phanodorn	T42.3x1-	T42.3x2-	T42.3x3-	T42.3x4-	T42.3x5-	T42.3x6-
Phanquinone	T37.3x1-	T37.3x2-	T37.3x3-	T37.3x4-	T37.3x5-	T37.3x6-
Phanquone	T37.3x1-	T37.3x2-	T37.3x3-	T37.3x4-	T37.3x5-	T37.3x6-
Pharmaceutical						
adjunct NEC	T50.901-	T50.902-	T50.903-	T50.904-	T50.905-	T50.906-
excipient NEC	T50.901-	T50.902-	T50.903-	T50.904-	T50.905-	T50.906-
sweetener	T50.901-	T50.902-	T50.903-	T50.904-	T50.905-	T50.906-
viscous agent	T50.901-	T50.902-	T50.903-	T50.904-	T50.905-	T50.906-

Table of Drugs & Chemicals	POISONING				Adverse Effect	Underdosing
	Accidental (Unintentional)	Self-Harm (Intentional)	Assault	Undetermined		
Phemitone	T42.3x1-	T42.3x2-	T42.3x3	T42.3x4-	T42.3x5-	T42.3x6-
Phenacaine	T41.3x1-	T41.3x2-	T41.3x3-	T41.3x4-	T41.3x5-	T41.3x6-
Phenacemide	T42.6x1-	T42.6x2-	T42.6x3-	T42.6x4-	T42.6x5-	T42.6x6-
Phenacetin	T39.1x1-	T39.1x2-	T39.1x3-	T39.1x4-	T39.1x5-	T39.1x6-
Phenadoxone	T40.2x1-	T40.2x2-	T40.2x3-	T40.2x4-	—	—
Phenaglycodol	T43.591-	T43.592-	T43.593-	T43.594-	T43.595-	T43.596-
Phenantoin	T42.0x1-	T42.0x2-	T42.0x3-	T42.0x4-	T42.0x5-	T42.0x6-
Phenaphthazine reagent	T50.991-	T50.992-	T50.993-	T50.994-	T50.995-	T50.996-
Phenazocine	T40.4x1-	T40.4x2-	T40.4x3-	T40.4x4-	T40.4x5-	T40.4x6-
Phenazone	T39.2x1-	T39.2x2-	T39.2x3-	T39.2x4-	T39.2x5-	T39.2x6-
Phenazopyridine	T39.8x1-	T39.8x2-	T39.8x3-	T39.8x4-	T39.8x5-	T39.8x6-
Phenbenicillin	T36.0x1-	T36.0x2-	T36.0x3-	T36.0x4-	T36.0x5-	T36.0x6-
Phenbutrazate	T50.5x1-	T50.5x2-	T50.5x3-	T50.5x4-	T50.5x5-	T50.5x6-
Phencyclidine	T40.991-	T40.992-	T40.993-	T40.994-	T40.995-	T40.996-
Phendimetrazine	T50.5x1-	T50.5x2-	T50.5x3-	T50.5x4-	T50.5x5-	T50.5x6-
Phenelzine	T43.1x1-	T43.1x2-	T43.1x3-	T43.1x4-	T43.1x5-	T43.1x6-
Phenemal	T42.3x1-	T42.3x2-	T42.3x3-	T42.3x4-	T42.3x5-	T42.3x6-
Phenergan	T42.6x1-	T42.6x2-	T42.6x3-	T42.6x4-	T42.6x5-	T42.6x6-
Pheneticillin	T36.0x1-	T36.0x2-	T36.0x3-	T36.0x4-	T36.0x5-	T36.0x6-
Pheneturide	T42.6x1-	T42.6x2-	T42.6x3-	T42.6x4-	T42.6x5-	T42.6x6-
Phenformin	T38.3x1-	T38.3x2-	T38.3x3-	T38.3x4-	T38.3x5-	T38.3x6-
Phenglutarimide	T44.3x1-	T44.3x2-	T44.3x3-	T44.3x4-	T44.3x5-	T44.3x6-
Phenicarbazide	T39.8x1-	T39.8x2-	T39.8x3-	T39.8x4-	T39.8x5-	T39.8x6-
Phenindamine	T45.0x1-	T45.0x2-	T45.0x3-	T45.0x4-	T45.0x5-	T45.0x6-
Phenindione	T45.511-	T45.512-	T45.513-	T45.514-	T45.515-	T45.516-
Pheniprazine	T43.1x1-	T43.1x2-	T43.1x3-	T43.1x4-	T43.1x5-	T43.1x6-
Pheniramine	T45.0x1-	T45.0x2-	T45.0x3-	T45.0x4-	T45.0x5-	T45.0x6-
Phenisatin	T47.2x1-	T47.2x2-	T47.2x3-	T47.2x4-	T47.2x5-	T47.2x6-
Phenmetrazine	T50.5x1-	T50.5x2-	T50.5x3-	T50.5x4-	T50.5x5-	T50.5x6-
Phenobal	T42.3x1-	T42.3x2-	T42.3x3-	T42.3x4-	T42.3x5-	T42.3x6-
Phenobarbital	T42.3x1-	T42.3x2-	T42.3x3-	T42.3x4-	T42.3x5-	T42.3x6-
with						
mephenytoin	T42.3x1-	T42.3x2-	T42.3x3-	T42.3x4-	T42.3x5-	T42.3x6-
phenytoin	T42.3x1-	T42.3x2-	T42.3x3-	T42.3x4-	T42.3x5-	T42.3x6-
sodium	T42.3x1-	T42.3x2-	T42.3x3-	T42.3x4-	T42.3x5-	T42.3x6-
Phenobarbitone	T42.3x1-	T42.3x2-	T42.3x3-	T42.3x4-	T42.3x5-	T42.3x6-
Phenobutiodil	T50.8x1-	T50.8x2-	T50.8x3-	T50.8x4-	T50.8x5-	T50.8x6-
Phenoctide	T49.0x1-	T49.0x2-	T49.0x3-	T49.0x4-	T49.0x5-	T49.0x6-
Phenol	T49.0x1-	T49.0x2-	T49.0x3-	T49.0x4-	T49.0x5-	T49.0x6-
disinfectant	T54.0x1-	T54.0x2-	T54.0x3-	T54.0x4-	—	—
in oil injection	T46.8x1-	T46.8x2-	T46.8x3-	T46.8x4-	T46.8x5-	T46.8x6-
medicinal	T49.1x1-	T49.1x2-	T49.1x3-	T49.1x4-	T49.1x5-	T49.1x6-
nonmedicinal NEC	T54.0x1-	T54.0x2-	T54.0x3-	T54.0x4-	—	—
pesticide	T60.8x1-	T60.8x2-	T60.8x3-	T60.8x4-	—	—
red	T50.8x1-	T50.8x2-	T50.8x3-	T50.8x4-	T50.8x5-	T50.8x6-
Phenolic preparation	T49.1x1-	T49.1x2-	T49.1x3-	T49.1x4-	T49.1x5-	T49.1x6-
Phenolphthalein	T47.2x1-	T47.2x2-	T47.2x3-	T47.2x4-	T47.2x5-	T47.2x6-
Phenolsulfonphthalein	T50.8x1-	T50.8x2-	T50.8x3-	T50.8x4-	T50.8x5-	T50.8x6-
Phenomorphan	T40.2x1-	T40.2x2-	T40.2x3-	T40.2x4-	—	—
Phenonyl	T42.3x1-	T42.3x2-	T42.3x3-	T42.3x4-	T42.3x5-	T42.3x6-
Phenoperidine	T40.4x1-	T40.4x2-	T40.4x3-	T40.4x4-	—	—
Phenopyrazone	T46.991-	T46.992-	T46.993-	T46.994-	T46.995-	T46.996-
Phenoquin	T50.4x1-	T50.4x2-	T50.4x3-	T50.4x4-	T50.4x5-	T50.4x6-
Phenothiazine (psychotropic) NEC	T43.3x1-	T43.3x2-	T43.3x3-	T43.3x4-	T43.3x5-	T43.3x6-
insecticide	T60.2x1-	T60.2x2-	T60.2x3-	T60.2x4-	—	—
Phenothrin	T49.0x1-	T49.0x2-	T49.0x3-	T49.0x4-	T49.0x5-	T49.0x6-
Phenoxybenzamine	T46.7x1-	T46.7x2-	T46.7x3-	T46.7x4-	T46.7x5-	T46.7x6-
Phenoxyethanol	T49.0x1-	T49.0x2-	T49.0x3-	T49.0x4-	T49.0x5-	T49.0x6-
Phenoxymethyl penicillin	T36.0x1-	T36.0x2-	T36.0x3-	T36.0x4-	T36.0x5-	T36.0x6-
Phenprobamate	T42.8x1-	T42.8x2-	T42.8x3-	T42.8x4-	T42.8x5-	T42.8x6-

DRUGS & CHEMICALS

Table of Drugs & Chemicals	POISONING Accidental (Unintentional)	Self-Harm (Intentional)	Assault	Undetermined	Adverse Effect	Underdosing
Phenprocoumon	T45.511-	T45.512-	T45.513-	T45.514-	T45.515-	T45.516-
Phensuximide	T42.2x1-	T42.2x2-	T42.2x3-	T42.2x4-	T42.2x5-	T42.2x6-
Phentermine	T50.5x1-	T50.5x2-	T50.5x3-	T50.5x4-	T50.5x5-	T50.5x6-
Phenthicillin	T36.0x1-	T36.0x2-	T36.0x3-	T36.0x4-	T36.0x5-	T36.0x6-
Phentolamine	T46.7x1-	T46.7x2-	T46.7x3-	T46.7x4-	T46.7x5-	T46.7x6-
Phenyl						
butazone	T39.2x1-	T39.2x2-	T39.2x3-	T39.2x4-	T39.2x5-	T39.2x6-
enediamine	T65.3x1-	T65.3x2-	T65.3x3-	T65.3x4-	—	—
hydrazine	T65.3x1-	T65.3x2-	T65.3x3-	T65.3x4-	—	—
antineoplastic	T45.1x1-	T45.1x2-	T45.1x3-	T45.1x4-	T45.1x5-	T45.1x6-
mercuric compounds — *see* Mercury						
salicylate	T49.3x1-	T49.3x2-	T49.3x3-	T49.3x4-	T49.3x5-	T49.3x6-
Phenylalanine mustard	T45.1x1-	T45.1x2-	T45.1x3-	T45.1x4-	T45.1x5-	T45.1x6-
Phenylbutazone	T39.2x1-	T39.2x2-	T39.2x3-	T39.2x4-	T39.2x5-	T39.2x6-
Phenylenediamine	T65.3x1-	T65.3x2-	T65.3x3-	T65.3x4-	—	—
Phenylephrine	T44.4x1-	T44.4x2-	T44.4x3-	T44.4x4-	T44.4x5-	T44.4x6-
Phenylethylbiguanide	T38.3x1-	T38.3x2-	T38.3x3-	T38.3x4-	T38.3x5-	T38.3x6-
Phenylmercuric						
acetate	T49.0x1-	T49.0x2-	T49.0x3-	T49.0x4-	T49.0x5-	T49.0x6-
borate	T49.0x1-	T49.0x2-	T49.0x3-	T49.0x4-	T49.0x5-	T49.0x6-
nitrate	T49.0x1-	T49.0x2-	T49.0x3-	T49.0x4-	T49.0x5-	T49.0x6-
Phenylmethylbarbitone	T42.3x1-	T42.3x2-	T42.3x3-	T42.3x4-	T42.3x5-	T42.3x6-
Phenylpropanol	T47.5x1-	T47.5x2-	T47.5x3-	T47.5x4-	T47.5x5-	T47.5x6-
Phenylpropanolamine	T44.991-	T44.992-	T44.993-	T44.994-	T44.995-	T44.996-
Phenylsulfthion	T60.0x1-	T60.0x2-	T60.0x3-	T60.0x4-	—	—
Phenyltoloxamine	T45.0x1-	T45.0x2-	T45.0x3-	T45.0x4-	T45.0x5-	T45.0x6-
Phenyramidol, phenyramidon	T39.8x1-	T39.8x2-	T39.8x3-	T39.8x4-	T39.8x5-	T39.8x6-
Phenytoin	T42.0x1-	T42.0x2-	T42.0x3-	T42.0x4-	T42.0x5-	T42.0x6-
with phenobarbital	T42.3x1-	T42.3x2-	T42.3x3-	T42.3x4-	T42.3x5-	T42.3x6-
pHisoHex	T49.2x1-	T49.2x2-	T49.2x3-	T49.2x4-	T49.2x5-	T49.2x6-
Pholcodine	T48.3x1-	T48.3x2-	T48.3x3-	T48.3x4-	T48.3x5-	T48.3x6-
Pholedrine	T46.991-	T46.992-	T46.993-	T46.994-	T46.995-	T46.996-
Phorate	T60.0x1-	T60.0x2-	T60.0x3-	T60.0x4-	—	—
Phosdrin	T60.0x1-	T60.0x2-	T60.0x3-	T60.0x4-	—	—
Phosfolan	T60.0x1-	T60.0x2-	T60.0x3-	T60.0x4-	—	—
Phosgene (gas)	T59.891-	T59.892-	T59.893-	T59.894-	—	—
Phosphamidon	T60.0x1-	T60.0x2-	T60.0x3-	T60.0x4-	—	—
Phosphate	T65.891-	T65.892-	T65.893-	T65.894-	—	—
laxative	T47.4x1-	T47.4x2-	T47.4x3-	T47.4x4-	T47.4x5-	T47.4x6-
organic	T60.0x1-	T60.0x2-	T60.0x3-	T60.0x4-	—	—
solvent	T52.91x-	T52.92x-	T52.93x-	T52.94x-	—	—
tricresyl	T65.891-	T65.892-	T65.893-	T65.894-	—	—
Phosphine	T57.1x1-	T57.1x2-	T57.1x3-	T57.1x4-	—	—
fumigant	T57.1x1-	T57.1x2-	T57.1x3-	T57.1x4-	—	—
Phospholine	T49.5x1-	T49.5x2-	T49.5x3-	T49.5x4-	T49.5x5-	T49.5x6-
Phosphoric acid	T54.2x1-	T54.2x2-	T54.2x3-	T54.2x4-	—	—
Phosphorus (compound) NEC	T57.1x1-	T57.1x2-	T57.1x3-	T57.1x4-	—	—
pesticide	T60.0x1-	T60.0x2-	T60.0x3-	T60.0x4-	—	—
Phthalates	T65.891-	T65.892-	T65.893-	T65.894-	—	—
Phthalic anhydride	T65.891-	T65.892-	T65.893-	T65.894-	—	—
Phthalimidoglutarimide	T42.6x1-	T42.6x2-	T42.6x3-	T42.6x4-	T42.6x5-	T42.6x6-
Phthalylsulfathiazole	T37.0x1-	T37.0x2-	T37.0x3-	T37.0x4-	T37.0x5-	T37.0x6-
Phylloquinone	T45.7x1-	T45.7x2-	T45.7x3-	T45.7x4-	T45.7x5-	T45.7x6-
Physeptone	T40.3x1-	T40.3x2-	T40.3x3-	T40.3x4-	T40.3x5-	T40.3x6-
Physostigma venenosum	T62.2x1-	T62.2x2-	T62.2x3-	T62.2x4-	—	—
Physostigmine	T49.5x1-	T49.5x2-	T49.5x3-	T49.5x4-	T49.5x5-	T49.5x6-
Phytolacca decandra	T62.2x1-	T62.2x2-	T62.2x3-	T62.2x4-	—	—
berries	T62.1x1-	T62.1x2-	T62.1x3-	T62.1x4-	—	—
Phytomenadione	T45.7x1-	T45.7x2-	T45.7x3-	T45.7x4-	T45.7x5-	T45.7x6-
Phytonadione	T45.7x1-	T45.7x2-	T45.7x3-	T45.7x4-	T45.7x5-	T45.7x6-
Picoperine	T48.3x1-	T48.3x2-	T48.3x3-	T48.3x4-	T48.3x5-	T48.3x6-
Picosulfate (sodium)	T47.2x1-	T47.2x2-	T47.2x3-	T47.2x4-	T47.2x5-	T47.2x6-
Picric (acid)	T54.2x1-	T54.2x2-	T54.2x3-	T54.2x4-	—	—
Picrotoxin	T50.7x1-	T50.7x2-	T50.7x3-	T50.7x4-	T50.7x5-	T50.7x6-
Piketoprofen	T49.0x1-	T49.0x2-	T49.0x3-	T49.0x4-	T49.0x5-	T49.0x6-
Pilocarpine	T44.1x1-	T44.1x2-	T44.1x3-	T44.1x4-	T44.1x5-	T44.1x6-
Pilocarpus (jaborandi) extract	T44.1x1-	T44.1x2-	T44.1x3-	T44.1x4-	T44.1x5-	T44.1x6-
Pilsicainide (hydrochloride)	T46.2x1-	T46.2x2-	T46.2x3-	T46.2x4-	T46.2x5-	T46.2x6-
Pimaricin	T36.7x1-	T36.7x2-	T36.7x3-	T36.7x4-	T36.7x5-	T36.7x6-
Pimeclone	T50.7x1-	T50.7x2-	T50.7x3-	T50.7x4-	T50.7x5-	T50.7x6-
Pimelic ketone	T52.8x1-	T52.8x2-	T52.8x3-	T52.8x4-	—	—
Pimethixene	T45.0x1-	T45.0x2-	T45.0x3-	T45.0x4-	T45.0x5-	T45.0x6-
Piminodine	T40.2x1-	T40.2x2-	T40.2x3-	T40.2x4-	T40.2x5-	T40.2x6-
Pimozide	T43.591-	T43.592-	T43.593-	T43.594-	T43.595-	T43.596-
Pinacidil	T46.5x1-	T46.5x2-	T46.5x3-	T46.5x4-	T46.5x5-	T46.5x6-
Pinaverium bromide	T44.3x1-	T44.3x2-	T44.3x3-	T44.3x4-	T44.3x5-	T44.3x6-
Pinazepam	T42.4x1-	T42.4x2-	T42.4x3-	T42.4x4-	T42.4x5-	T42.4x6-
Pindolol	T44.7x1-	T44.7x2-	T44.7x3-	T44.7x4-	T44.7x5-	T44.7x6-
Pindone	T60.4x1-	T60.4x2-	T60.4x3-	T60.4x4-	—	—
Pine oil (disinfectant)	T65.891-	T65.892-	T65.893-	T65.894-	—	—
Pinkroot	T37.4x1-	T37.4x2-	T37.4x3-	T37.4x4-	T37.4x5-	T37.4x6-
Pipadone	T40.2x1-	T40.2x2-	T40.2x3-	T40.2x4-	—	—
Pipamazine	T45.0x1-	T45.0x2-	T45.0x3-	T45.0x4-	T45.0x5-	T45.0x6-
Pipamperone	T43.4x1-	T43.4x2-	T43.4x3-	T43.4x4-	T43.4x5-	T43.4x6-
Pipazetate	T48.3x1-	T48.3x2-	T48.3x3-	T48.3x4-	T48.3x5-	T48.3x6-
Pipemidic acid	T37.8x1-	T37.8x2-	T37.8x3-	T37.8x4-	T37.8x5-	T37.8x6-
Pipenzolate bromide	T44.3x1-	T44.3x2-	T44.3x3-	T44.3x4-	T44.3x5-	T44.3x6-
Piper cubeba	T62.2x1-	T62.2x2-	T62.2x3-	T62.2x4-	—	—
Piperacetazine	T43.3x1-	T43.3x2-	T43.3x3-	T43.3x4-	T43.3x5-	T43.3x6-
Piperacillin	T36.0x1-	T36.0x2-	T36.0x3-	T36.0x4-	T36.0x5-	T36.0x6-
Piperazine	T37.4x1-	T37.4x2-	T37.4x3-	T37.4x4-	T37.4x5-	T37.4x6-
estrone sulfate	T38.5x1-	T38.5x2-	T38.5x3-	T38.5x4-	T38.5x5-	T38.5x6-
Piperidione	T48.3x1-	T48.3x2-	T48.3x3-	T48.3x4-	T48.3x5-	T48.3x6-
Piperidolate	T44.3x1-	T44.3x2-	T44.3x3-	T44.3x4-	T44.3x5-	T44.3x6-
Piperocaine	T41.3x1-	T41.3x2-	T41.3x3-	T41.3x4-	T41.3x5-	T41.3x6-
infiltration (subcutaneous)	T41.3x1-	T41.3x2-	T41.3x3-	T41.3x4-	T41.3x5-	T41.3x6-
nerve block (peripheral) (plexus)	T41.3x1-	T41.3x2-	T41.3x3-	T41.3x4-	T41.3x5-	T41.3x6-
topical (surface)	T41.3x1-	T41.3x2-	T41.3x3-	T41.3x4-	T41.3x5-	T41.3x6-
Piperonyl butoxide	T60.8x1-	T60.8x2-	T60.8x3-	T60.8x4-	—	—
Pipethanate	T44.3x1-	T44.3x2-	T44.3x3-	T44.3x4-	T44.3x5-	T44.3x6-
Pipobroman	T45.1x1-	T45.1x2-	T45.1x3-	T45.1x4-	T45.1x5-	T45.1x6-
Pipotiazine	T43.3x1-	T43.3x2-	T43.3x3-	T43.3x4-	T43.3x5-	T43.3x6-
Pipoxizine	T45.0x1-	T45.0x2-	T45.0x3-	T45.0x4-	T45.0x5-	T45.0x6-
Pipradrol	T43.691-	T43.692-	T43.693-	T43.694-	T43.695-	T43.696-
Piprinhydrinate	T45.0x1-	T45.0x2-	T45.0x3-	T45.0x4-	T45.0x5-	T45.0x6-
Pirarubicin	T45.1x1-	T45.1x2-	T45.1x3-	T45.1x4-	T45.1x5-	T45.1x6-
Pirazinamide	T37.1x1-	T37.1x2-	T37.1x3-	T37.1x4-	T37.1x5-	T37.1x6-
Pirbuterol	T48.6x1-	T48.6x2-	T48.6x3-	T48.6x4-	T48.6x5-	T48.6x6-
Pirenzepine	T47.1x1-	T47.1x2-	T47.1x3-	T47.1x4-	T47.1x5-	T47.1x6-
Piretanide	T50.1x1-	T50.1x2-	T50.1x3-	T50.1x4-	T50.1x5-	T50.1x6-
Piribedil	T42.8x1-	T42.8x2-	T42.8x3-	T42.8x4-	T42.8x5-	T42.8x6-
Piridoxilate	T46.3x1-	T46.3x2-	T46.3x3-	T46.3x4-	T46.3x5-	T46.3x6-
Piritramide	T40.4x1-	T40.4x2-	T40.4x3-	T40.4x4-	—	—
Piromidic acid	T37.8x1-	T37.8x2-	T37.8x3-	T37.8x4-	T37.8x5-	T37.8x6-
Piroxicam	T39.391-	T39.392-	T39.393-	T39.394-	T39.395-	T39.396-
beta-cyclodextrin complex	T39.8x1-	T39.8x2-	T39.8x3-	T39.8x4-	T39.8x5-	T39.8x6-

DRUGS & CHEMICALS

Table of Drugs & Chemicals	Poisoning Accidental (Unintentional)	Poisoning Self-Harm (Intentional)	Poisoning Assault	Poisoning Undetermined	Adverse Effect	Underdosing
Pirozadil	T46.6x1-	T46.6x2-	T46.6x3-	T46.6x4-	T46.6x5-	T46.6x6-
Piscidia (bark) (erythrina)	T39.8x1-	T39.8x2-	T39.8x3-	T39.8x4-	T39.8x5-	T39.8x6-
Pitch	T65.891-	T65.892-	T65.893-	T65.894-	—	—
Pitkin's solution	T41.3x1-	T41.3x2-	T41.3x3-	T41.3x4-	T41.3x5-	T41.3x6-
Pitocin	T48.0x1-	T48.0x2-	T48.0x3-	T48.0x4-	T48.0x5-	T48.0x6-
Pitressin (tannate)	T38.891-	T38.892-	T38.893-	T38.894-	T38.895-	T38.896-
Pituitary extracts (posterior)	T38.891-	T38.892-	T38.893-	T38.894-	T38.895-	T38.896-
anterior	T38.811-	T38.812-	T38.813-	T38.814-	T38.815-	T38.816-
Pituitrin	T38.891-	T38.892-	T38.893-	T38.894-	T38.895-	T38.896-
Pivampicillin	T36.0x1-	T36.0x2-	T36.0x3-	T36.0x4-	T36.0x5-	T36.0x6-
Pivmecillinam	T36.0x1-	T36.0x2-	T36.0x3-	T36.0x4-	T36.0x5-	T36.0x6-
Placental hormone	T38.891-	T38.892-	T38.893-	T38.894-	T38.895-	T38.896-
Placidyl	T42.6x1-	T42.6x2-	T42.6x3-	T42.6x4-	T42.6x5-	T42.6x6-
Plague vaccine	T50.A91-	T50.A92-	T50.A93-	T50.A94-	T50.A95-	T50.A96-
Plant food or fertilizer NEC	T65.891-	T65.892-	T65.893-	T65.894-	—	—
containing herbicide	T60.3x1-	T60.3x2-	T60.3x3-	T60.3x4-	—	—
noxious, used as food	T62.2x1-	T62.2x2-	T62.2x3-	T62.2x4-	—	—
berries	T62.1x1-	T62.1x2-	T62.1x3-	T62.1x4-	—	—
seeds	T62.2x1-	T62.2x2-	T62.2x3-	T62.2x4-	—	—
specified type NEC	T62.2x1-	T62.2x2-	T62.2x3-	T62.2x4-	—	—
Plasma	T45.8x1-	T45.8x2-	T45.8x3-	T45.8x4-	T45.8x5-	T45.8x6-
expander NEC	T45.8x1-	T45.8x2-	T45.8x3-	T45.8x4-	T45.8x5-	T45.8x6-
protein fraction (human)	T45.8x1-	T45.8x2-	T45.8x3-	T45.8x4-	T45.8x5-	T45.8x6-
Plasmanate	T45.8x1-	T45.8x2-	T45.8x3-	T45.8x4-	T45.8x5-	T45.8x6-
Plasminogen (tissue) activator	T45.611-	T45.612-	T45.613-	T45.614-	T45.615-	T45.616-
Plaster dressing	T49.3x1-	T49.3x2-	T49.3x3-	T49.3x4-	T49.3x5-	T49.3x6-
Plastic dressing	T49.3x1-	T49.3x2-	T49.3x3-	T49.3x4-	T49.3x5-	T49.3x6-
Plegicil	T43.3x1-	T43.3x2-	T43.3x3-	T43.3x4-	T43.3x5-	T43.3x6-
Plicamycin	T45.1x1-	T45.1x2-	T45.1x3-	T45.1x4-	T45.1x5-	T45.1x6-
Podophyllotoxin	T49.8x1-	T49.8x2-	T49.8x3-	T49.8x4-	T49.8x5-	T49.8x6-
Podophyllum (resin)	T49.4x1-	T49.4x2-	T49.4x3-	T49.4x4-	T49.4x5-	T49.4x6-
Poison NEC	T65.91x-	T65.92x-	T65.93x-	T65.94x-	—	—
Poisonous berries	T62.1x1-	T62.1x2-	T62.1x3-	T62.1x4-	—	—
Pokeweed (any part)	T62.2x1-	T62.2x2-	T62.2x3-	T62.2x4-	—	—
Poldine metilsulfate	T44.3x1-	T44.3x2-	T44.3x3-	T44.3x4-	T44.3x5-	T44.3x6-
Polidexide (sulfate)	T46.6x1-	T46.6x2-	T46.6x3-	T46.6x4-	T46.6x5-	T46.6x6-
Polidocanol	T46.8x1-	T46.8x2-	T46.8x3-	T46.8x4-	T46.8x5-	T46.8x6-
Poliomyelitis vaccine	T50.B91-	T50.B92-	T50.B93-	T50.B94-	T50.B95-	T50.B96-
Polish (car) (floor) (furniture) (metal) (porcelain) (silver)	T65.891-	T65.892-	T65.893-	T65.894-		
abrasive	T65.891-	T65.892-	T65.893-	T65.894-	—	—
porcelain	T65.891-	T65.892-	T65.893-	T65.894-	—	—
Poloxalkol	T47.4x1-	T47.4x2-	T47.4x3-	T47.4x4-	T47.4x5-	T47.4x6-
Poloxamer	T47.4x1-	T47.4x2-	T47.4x3-	T47.4x4-	T47.4x5-	T47.4x6-
Polyaminostyrene resins	T50.3x1-	T50.3x2-	T50.3x3-	T50.3x4-	T50.3x5-	T50.3x6-
Polycarbophil	T47.4x1-	T47.4x2-	T47.4x3-	T47.4x4-	T47.4x5-	T47.4x6-
Polychlorinated biphenyl	T65.891-	T65.892-	T65.893-	T65.894-	—	—
Polycycline	T36.4x1-	T36.4x2-	T36.4x3-	T36.4x4-	T36.4x5-	T36.4x6-
Polyester fumes	T59.891-	T59.892-	T59.893-	T59.894-	—	—
Polyester resin hardener	T52.91x-	T52.92x-	T52.93x-	T52.94x-	—	—
fumes	T59.891-	T59.892-	T59.893-	T59.894-	—	—
Polyestradiol phosphate	T38.5x1-	T38.5x2-	T38.5x3-	T38.5x4-	T38.5x5-	T38.5x6-
Polyethanolamine alkyl sulfate	T49.2x1-	T49.2x2-	T49.2x3-	T49.2x4-	T49.2x5-	T49.2x6-
Polyethylene adhesive	T49.3x1-	T49.3x2-	T49.3x3-	T49.3x4-	T49.3x5-	T49.3x6-
Polyferose	T45.4x1-	T45.4x2-	T45.4x3-	T45.4x4-	T45.4x5-	T45.4x6-
Polygeline	T45.8x1-	T45.8x2-	T45.8x3-	T45.8x4-	T45.8x5-	T45.8x6-
Polymyxin	T36.8x1-	T36.8x2-	T36.8x3-	T36.8x4-	T36.8x5-	T36.8x6-
B	T36.8x1-	T36.8x2-	T36.8x3-	T36.8x4-	T36.8x5-	T36.8x6-
ENT agent	T49.6x1-	T49.6x2-	T49.6x3-	T49.6x4-	T49.6x5-	T49.6x6-
ophthalmic preparation	T49.5x1-	T49.5x2-	T49.5x3-	T49.5x4-	T49.5x5-	T49.5x6-
topical NEC	T49.0x1-	T49.0x2-	T49.0x3-	T49.0x4-	T49.0x5-	T49.0x6-
E sulfate (eye preparation)	T49.5x1-	T49.5x2-	T49.5x3-	T49.5x4-	T49.5x5-	T49.5x6-
Polynoxylin	T49.0x1-	T49.0x2-	T49.0x3-	T49.0x4-	T49.0x5-	T49.0x6-
Polyoestradiol phosphate	T38.5x1-	T38.5x2-	T38.5x3-	T38.5x4-	T38.5x5-	T38.5x6-
Polyoxymethyleneurea	T49.0x1-	T49.0x2-	T49.0x3-	T49.0x4-	T49.0x5-	T49.0x6-
Polysilane	T47.8x1-	T47.8x2-	T47.8x3-	T47.8x4-	T47.8x5-	T47.8x6-
Polytetrafluoroethylene (inhaled)	T59.891-	T59.892-	T59.893-	T59.894-	—	—
Polythiazide	T50.2x1-	T50.2x2-	T50.2x3-	T50.2x4-	T50.2x5-	T50.2x6-
Polyvidone	T45.8x1-	T45.8x2-	T45.8x3-	T45.8x4-	T45.8x5-	T45.8x6-
Polyvinylpyrrolidone	T45.8x1-	T45.8x2-	T45.8x3-	T45.8x4-	T45.8x5-	T45.8x6-
Pontocaine (hydrochloride) (infiltration) (topical)	T41.3x1-	T41.3x2-	T41.3x3-	T41.3x4-	T41.3x5-	T41.3x6-
nerve block (peripheral) (plexus)	T41.3x1-	T41.3x2-	T41.3x3-	T41.3x4-	T41.3x5-	T41.3x6-
spinal	T41.3x1-	T41.3x2-	T41.3x3-	T41.3x4-	T41.3x5-	T41.3x6-
Porfiromycin	T45.1x1-	T45.1x2-	T45.1x3-	T45.1x4-	T45.1x5-	T45.1x6-
Posterior pituitary hormone NEC	T38.891-	T38.892-	T38.893-	T38.894-	T38.895-	T38.896-
Pot	T40.7x1-	T40.7x2-	T40.7x3-	T40.7x4-	T40.7x5-	T40.7x6-
Potash (caustic)	T54.3x1-	T54.3x2-	T54.3x3-	T54.3x4-	—	—
Potassic saline injection (lactated)	T50.3x1-	T50.3x2-	T50.3x3-	T50.3x4-	T50.3x5-	T50.3x6-
Potassium (salts) NEC	T50.3x1-	T50.3x2-	T50.3x3-	T50.3x4-	T50.3x5-	T50.3x6-
aminobenzoate	T45.8x1-	T45.8x2-	T45.8x3-	T45.8x4-	T45.8x5-	T45.8x6-
aminosalicylate	T37.1x1-	T37.1x2-	T37.1x3-	T37.1x4-	T37.1x5-	T37.1x6-
antimony 'tartrate'	T37.8x1-	T37.8x2-	T37.8x3-	T37.8x4-	T37.8x5-	T37.8x6-
arsenite (solution)	T57.0x1-	T57.0x2-	T57.0x3-	T57.0x4-	—	—
bichromate	T56.2x1-	T56.2x2-	T56.2x3-	T56.2x4-	—	—
bisulfate	T47.3x1-	T47.3x2-	T47.3x3-	T47.3x4-	T47.3x5-	T47.3x6-
bromide	T42.6x1-	T42.6x2-	T42.6x3-	T42.6x4-	T42.6x5-	T42.6x6-
canrenoate	T50.0x1-	T50.0x2-	T50.0x3-	T50.0x4-	T50.0x5-	T50.0x6-
carbonate	T54.3x1-	T54.3x2-	T54.3x3-	T54.3x4-	—	—
chlorate NEC	T65.891-	T65.892-	T65.893-	T65.894-	—	—
chloride	T50.3x1-	T50.3x2-	T50.3x3-	T50.3x4-	T50.3x5-	T50.3x6-
citrate	T50.991-	T50.992-	T50.993-	T50.994-	T50.995-	T50.996-
cyanide	T65.0x1-	T65.0x2-	T65.0x3-	T65.0x4-	—	—
ferric hexacyanoferrate (medicinal)	T50.6x1-	T50.6x2-	T50.6x3-	T50.6x4-	T50.6x5-	T50.6x6-
nonmedicinal	T65.891-	T65.892-	T65.893-	T65.894-	—	—
fluoride	T57.8x1-	T57.8x2-	T57.8x3-	T57.8x4-	—	—
glucaldrate	T47.1x1-	T47.1x2-	T47.1x3-	T47.1x4-	T47.1x5-	T47.1x6-
hydroxide	T54.3x1-	T54.3x2-	T54.3x3-	T54.3x4-	—	—
iodate	T49.0x1-	T49.0x2-	T49.0x3-	T49.0x4-	T49.0x5-	T49.0x6-
iodide	T48.4x1-	T48.4x2-	T48.4x3-	T48.4x4-	T48.4x5-	T48.4x6-
nitrate	T57.8x1-	T57.8x2-	T57.8x3-	T57.8x4-	—	—
oxalate	T65.891-	T65.892-	T65.893-	T65.894-	—	—
perchlorate (nonmedicinal) NEC	T65.891-	T65.892-	T65.893-	T65.894-	—	—
antithyroid	T38.2x1-	T38.2x2-	T38.2x3-	T38.2x4-	T38.2x5-	T38.2x6-
medicinal	T38.2x1-	T38.2x2-	T38.2x3-	T38.2x4-	T38.2x5-	T38.2x6-
permanganate (nonmedicinal)	T65.891-	T65.892-	T65.893-	T65.894-	—	—
medicinal	T49.0x1-	T49.0x2-	T49.0x3-	T49.0x4-	T49.0x5-	T49.0x6-
sulfate	T47.2x1-	T47.2x2-	T47.2x3-	T47.2x4-	T47.2x5-	T47.2x6-

Table of Drugs & Chemicals	POISONING				Adverse Effect	Underdosing
	Accidental (Unintentional)	Self-Harm (Intentional)	Assault	Undetermined		
Potassium-removing resin ..	T50.3x1-	T50.3x2-	T50.3x3-	T50.3x4-	T50.3x5-	T50.3x6-
Potassium-retaining drug ..	T50.3x1-	T50.3x2-	T50.3x3-	T50.3x4-	T50.3x5-	T50.3x6-
Povidone	T45.8x1-	T45.8x2-	T45.8x3-	T45.8x4-	T45.8x5-	T45.8x6-
iodine	T49.0x1-	T49.0x2-	T49.0x3-	T49.0x4-	T49.0x5-	T49.0x6-
Practolol	T44.7x1-	T44.7x2-	T44.7x3-	T44.7x4-	T44.7x5-	T44.7x6-
Prajmalium bitartrate	T46.2x1-	T46.2x2-	T46.2x3-	T46.2x4-	T46.2x5-	T46.2x6-
Pralidoxime (iodide)	T50.6x1-	T50.6x2-	T50.6x3-	T50.6x4-	T50.6x5-	T50.6x6-
chloride	T50.6x1-	T50.6x2-	T50.6x3-	T50.6x4-	T50.6x5-	T50.6x6-
Pramiverine	T44.3x1-	T44.3x2-	T44.3x3-	T44.3x4-	T44.3x5-	T44.3x6-
Pramocaine	T49.1x1-	T49.1x2-	T49.1x3-	T49.1x4-	T49.1x5-	T49.1x6-
Pramoxine	T49.1x1-	T49.1x2-	T49.1x3-	T49.1x4-	T49.1x5-	T49.1x6-
Prasterone	T38.7x1-	T38.7x2-	T38.7x3-	T38.7x4-	T38.7x5-	T38.7x6-
Pravastatin	T46.6x1-	T46.6x2-	T46.6x3-	T46.6x4-	T46.6x5-	T46.6x6-
Prazepam	T42.4x1-	T42.4x2-	T42.4x3-	T42.4x4-	T42.4x5-	T42.4x6-
Praziquantel	T37.4x1-	T37.4x2-	T37.4x3-	T37.4x4-	T37.4x5-	T37.4x6-
Prazitone	T43.291-	T43.292-	T43.293-	T43.294-	T43.295-	T43.296-
Prazosin	T44.6x1-	T44.6x2-	T44.6x3-	T44.6x4-	T44.6x5-	T44.6x6-
Prednicarbate	T49.0x1-	T49.0x2-	T49.0x3-	T49.0x4-	T49.0x5-	T49.0x6-
Prednimustine	T45.1x1-	T45.1x2-	T45.1x3-	T45.1x4-	T45.1x5-	T45.1x6-
Prednisolone	T38.0x1-	T38.0x2-	T38.0x3-	T38.0x4-	T38.0x5-	T38.0x6-
ENT agent	T49.6x1-	T49.6x2-	T49.6x3-	T49.6x4-	T49.6x5-	T49.6x6-
ophthalmic preparation ..	T49.5x1-	T49.5x2-	T49.5x3-	T49.5x4-	T49.5x5-	T49.5x6-
steaglate	T49.0x1-	T49.0x2-	T49.0x3-	T49.0x4-	T49.0x5-	T49.0x6-
topical NEC	T49.0x1-	T49.0x2-	T49.0x3-	T49.0x4-	T49.0x5-	T49.0x6-
Prednisone	T38.0x1-	T38.0x2-	T38.0x3-	T38.0x4-	T38.0x5-	T38.0x6-
Prednylidene	T38.0x1-	T38.0x2-	T38.0x3-	T38.0x4-	T38.0x5-	T38.0x6-
Pregnandiol	T38.5x1-	T38.5x2-	T38.5x3-	T38.5x4-	T38.5x5-	T38.5x6-
Pregneninolone	T38.5x1-	T38.5x2-	T38.5x3-	T38.5x4-	T38.5x5-	T38.5x6-
Preludin	T43.691-	T43.692-	T43.693-	T43.694-	T43.695-	T43.696-
Premarin	T38.5x1-	T38.5x2-	T38.5x3-	T38.5x4-	T38.5x5-	T38.5x6-
Premedication anesthetic	T41.201-	T41.202-	T41.203-	T41.204-	T41.205-	T41.206-
Prenalterol	T44.5x1-	T44.5x2-	T44.5x3-	T44.5x4-	T44.5x5-	T44.5x6-
Prenoxdiazine	T48.3x1-	T48.3x2-	T48.3x3-	T48.3x4-	T48.3x5-	T48.3x6-
Prenylamine	T46.3x1-	T46.3x2-	T46.3x3-	T46.3x4-	T46.3x5-	T46.3x6-
Preparation, local	T49.4x1-	T49.4x2-	T49.4x3-	T49.4x4-	T49.4x5-	T49.4x6-
Preparation H	T49.8x1-	T49.8x2-	T49.8x3-	T49.8x4-	T49.8x5-	T49.8x6-
Preservative (nonmedicinal)	T65.891-	T65.892-	T65.893-	T65.894-	—	—
medicinal	T50.901-	T50.902-	T50.903-	T50.904-	T50.905-	T50.906-
wood	T60.91x-	T60.92x-	T60.93x-	T60.94x-	—	—
Prethcamide	T50.7x1-	T50.7x2-	T50.7x3-	T50.7x4-	T50.7x5-	T50.7x6-
Pride of China	T62.2x1-	T62.2x2-	T62.2x3-	T62.2x4-	—	—
Pridinol	T44.3x1-	T44.3x2-	T44.3x3-	T44.3x4-	T44.3x5-	T44.3x6-
Prifinium bromide	T44.3x1-	T44.3x2-	T44.3x3-	T44.3x4-	T44.3x5-	T44.3x6-
Prilocaine	T41.3x1-	T41.3x2-	T41.3x3-	T41.3x4-	T41.3x5-	T41.3x6-
infiltration (subcutaneous)	T41.3x1-	T41.3x2-	T41.3x3-	T41.3x4-	T41.3x5-	T41.3x6-
nerve block (peripheral) (plexus)	T41.3x1-	T41.3x2-	T41.3x3-	T41.3x4-	T41.3x5-	T41.3x6-
regional	T41.3x1-	T41.3x2-	T41.3x3-	T41.3x4-	T41.3x5-	T41.3x6-
Primaquine	T37.2x1-	T37.2x2-	T37.2x3-	T37.2x4-	T37.2x5-	T37.2x6-
Primidone	T42.6x1-	T42.6x2-	T42.6x3-	T42.6x4-	T42.6x5-	T42.6x6-
Primula (veris)	T62.2x1-	T62.2x2-	T62.2x3-	T62.2x4-	—	—
Prinadol	T40.2x1-	T40.2x2-	T40.2x3-	T40.2x4-	T40.2x5-	T40.2x6-
Priscol, Priscoline	T44.6x1-	T44.6x2-	T44.6x3-	T44.6x4-	T44.6x5-	T44.6x6-
Pristinamycin	T36.3x1-	T36.3x2-	T36.3x3-	T36.3x4-	T36.3x5-	T36.3x6-
Privet	T62.2x1-	T62.2x2-	T62.2x3-	T62.2x4-	—	—
berries	T62.1x1-	T62.1x2-	T62.1x3-	T62.1x4-	—	—
Privine	T44.4x1-	T44.4x2-	T44.4x3-	T44.4x4-	T44.4x5-	T44.4x6-
Pro-Banthine	T44.3x1-	T44.3x2-	T44.3x3-	T44.3x4-	T44.3x5-	T44.3x6-
Probarbital	T42.3x1-	T42.3x2-	T42.3x3-	T42.3x4-	T42.3x5-	T42.3x6-
Probenecid	T50.4x1-	T50.4x2-	T50.4x3-	T50.4x4-	T50.4x5-	T50.4x6-

Table of Drugs & Chemicals	POISONING				Adverse Effect	Underdosing
	Accidental (Unintentional)	Self-Harm (Intentional)	Assault	Undetermined		
Probucol	T46.6x1-	T46.6x2-	T46.6x3-	T46.6x4-	T46.6x5-	T46.6x6-
Procainamide	T46.2x1-	T46.2x2-	T46.2x3-	T46.2x4-	T46.2x5-	T46.2x6-
Procaine	T41.3x1-	T41.3x2-	T41.3x3-	T41.3x4-	T41.3x5-	T41.3x6-
benzylpenicillin	T36.0x1-	T36.0x2-	T36.0x3-	T36.0x4-	T36.0x5-	T36.0x6-
nerve block (periphreal) (plexus)	T41.3x1-	T41.3x2-	T41.3x3-	T41.3x4-	T41.3x5-	T41.3x6-
penicillin G	T36.0x1-	T36.0x2-	T36.0x3-	T36.0x4-	T36.0x5-	T36.0x6-
regional	T41.3x1-	T41.3x2-	T41.3x3-	T41.3x4-	T41.3x5-	T41.3x6-
spinal	T41.3x1-	T41.3x2-	T41.3x3-	T41.3x4-	T41.3x5-	T41.3x6-
Procalmidol	T43.591-	T43.592-	T43.593-	T43.594-	T43.595-	T43.596-
Procarbazine	T45.1x1-	T45.1x2-	T45.1x3-	T45.1x4-	T45.1x5-	T45.1x6-
Procaterol	T44.5x1-	T44.5x2-	T44.5x3-	T44.5x4-	T44.5x5-	T44.5x6-
Prochlorperazine	T43.3x1-	T43.3x2-	T43.3x3-	T43.3x4-	T43.3x5-	T43.3x6-
Procyclidine	T44.3x1-	T44.3x2-	T44.3x3-	T44.3x4-	T44.3x5-	T44.3x6-
Producer gas	T58.8x1-	T58.8x2-	T58.8x3-	T58.8x4-	—	—
Profadol	T40.4x1-	T40.4x2-	T40.4x3-	T40.4x4-	T40.4x5-	T40.4x6-
Profenamine	T44.3x1-	T44.3x2-	T44.3x3-	T44.3x4-	T44.3x5-	T44.3x6-
Profenil	T44.3x1-	T44.3x2-	T44.3x3-	T44.3x4-	T44.3x5-	T44.3x6-
Proflavine	T49.0x1-	T49.0x2-	T49.0x3-	T49.0x4-	T49.0x5-	T49.0x6-
Progabide	T42.6x1-	T42.6x2-	T42.6x3-	T42.6x4-	T42.6x5-	T42.6x6-
Progesterone	T38.5x1-	T38.5x2-	T38.5x3-	T38.5x4-	T38.5x5-	T38.5x6-
Progestin	T38.5x1-	T38.5x2-	T38.5x3-	T38.5x4-	T38.5x5-	T38.5x6-
oral contraceptive	T38.4x1-	T38.4x2-	T38.4x3-	T38.4x4-	T38.4x5-	T38.4x6-
Progestogen NEC	T38.5x1-	T38.5x2-	T38.5x3-	T38.5x4-	T38.5x5-	T38.5x6-
Progestone	T38.5x1-	T38.5x2-	T38.5x3-	T38.5x4-	T38.5x5-	T38.5x6-
Proglumide	T47.1x1-	T47.1x2-	T47.1x3-	T47.1x4-	T47.1x5-	T47.1x6-
Proguanil	T37.2x1-	T37.2x2-	T37.2x3-	T37.2x4-	T37.2x5-	T37.2x6-
Prolactin	T38.811-	T38.812-	T38.813-	T38.814-	T38.815-	T38.816-
Prolintane	T43.691-	T43.692-	T43.693-	T43.694-	T43.695-	T43.696-
Proloid	T38.1x1-	T38.1x2-	T38.1x3-	T38.1x4-	T38.1x5-	T38.1x6-
Proluton	T38.5x1-	T38.5x2-	T38.5x3-	T38.5x4-	T38.5x5-	T38.5x6-
Promacetin	T37.1x1-	T37.1x2-	T37.1x3-	T37.1x4-	T37.1x5-	T37.1x6-
Promazine	T43.3x1-	T43.3x2-	T43.3x3-	T43.3x4-	T43.3x5-	T43.3x6-
Promedol	T40.2x1-	T40.2x2-	T40.2x3-	T40.2x4-		
Promegestone	T38.5x1-	T38.5x2-	T38.5x3-	T38.5x4-	T38.5x5-	T38.5x6-
Promethazine (teoclate)	T43.3x1-	T43.3x2-	T43.3x3-	T43.3x4-	T43.3x5-	T43.3x6-
Promin	T37.1x1-	T37.1x2-	T37.1x3-	T37.1x4-	T37.1x5-	T37.1x6-
Pronase	T45.3x1-	T45.3x2-	T45.3x3-	T45.3x4-	T45.3x5-	T45.3x6-
Pronestyl (hydrochloride) ..	T46.2x1-	T46.2x2-	T46.2x3-	T46.2x4-	T46.2x5-	T46.2x6-
Pronetalol	T44.7x1-	T44.7x2-	T44.7x3-	T44.7x4-	T44.7x5-	T44.7x6-
Prontosil	T37.0x1-	T37.0x2-	T37.0x3-	T37.0x4-	T37.0x5-	T37.0x6-
Propachlor	T60.3x1-	T60.3x2-	T60.3x3-	T60.3x4-	—	—
Propafenone	T46.2x1-	T46.2x2-	T46.2x3-	T46.2x4-	T46.2x5-	T46.2x6-
Propallylonal	T42.3x1-	T42.3x2-	T42.3x3-	T42.3x4-	T42.3x5-	T42.3x6-
Propamidine	T49.0x1-	T49.0x2-	T49.0x3-	T49.0x4-	T49.0x5-	T49.0x6-
Propane (distributed in mobile container)	T59.891-	T59.892-	T59.893-	T59.894-	—	—
distributed through pipes	T59.891-	T59.892-	T59.893-	T59.894-	—	—
incomplete combustion ..	T58.11x-	T58.12x-	T58.13x-	T58.14x-	—	—
Propanidid	T41.291-	T41.292-	T41.293-	T41.294-	T41.295-	T41.296-
Propanil	T60.3x1-	T60.3x2-	T60.3x3-	T60.3x4-	—	—
1-Propanol	T51.3x1-	T51.3x2-	T51.3x3-	T51.3x4-	—	—
2-Propanol	T51.2x1-	T51.2x2-	T51.2x3-	T51.2x4-	—	—
Propantheline	T44.3x1-	T44.3x2-	T44.3x3-	T44.3x4-	T44.3x5-	T44.3x6-
bromide	T44.3x1-	T44.3x2-	T44.3x3-	T44.3x4-	T44.3x5-	T44.3x6-
Proparacaine	T41.3x1-	T41.3x2-	T41.3x3-	T41.3x4-	T41.3x5-	T41.3x6-
Propatylnitrate	T46.3x1-	T46.3x2-	T46.3x3-	T46.3x4-	T46.3x5-	T46.3x6-
Propicillin	T36.0x1-	T36.0x2-	T36.0x3-	T36.0x4-	T36.0x5-	T36.0x6-
Propiolactone	T49.0x1-	T49.0x2-	T49.0x3-	T49.0x4-	T49.0x5-	T49.0x6-
Propiomazine	T45.0x1-	T45.0x2-	T45.0x3-	T45.0x4-	T45.0x5-	T45.0x6-
Propion gel	T49.0x1-	T49.0x2-	T49.0x3-	T49.0x4-	T49.0x5-	T49.0x6-

DRUGS & CHEMICALS

Table of Drugs & Chemicals	POISONING				Adverse Effect	Underdosing
	Accidental (Unintentional)	Self-Harm (Intentional)	Assault	Undetermined		
Propionaldehyde (medicinal)	T42.6x1-	T42.6x2-	T42.6x3-	T42.6x4-	T42.6x5-	T42.6x6-
Propionate (calcium) (sodium)	T49.0x1-	T49.0x2-	T49.0x3-	T49.0x4-	T49.0x5-	T49.0x6-
Propitocaine	T41.3x1-	T41.3x2-	T41.3x3-	T41.3x4-	T41.3x5-	T41.3x6-
infiltration (subcutaneous)	T41.3x1-	T41.3x2-	T41.3x3-	T41.3x4-	T41.3x5-	T41.3x6-
nerve block (peripheral) (plexus)	T41.3x1-	T41.3x2-	T41.3x3-	T41.3x4-	T41.3x5-	T41.3x6-
Propofol	T41.291-	T41.292-	T41.293-	T41.294-	T41.295-	T41.296-
Propoxur	T60.0x1-	T60.0x2-	T60.0x3-	T60.0x4-	—	—
Propoxycaine	T41.3x1-	T41.3x2-	T41.3x3-	T41.3x4-	T41.3x5-	T41.3x6-
infiltration (subcutaneous)	T41.3x1-	T41.3x2-	T41.3x3-	T41.3x4-	T41.3x5-	T41.3x6-
nerve block (peripheral) (plexus)	T41.3x1-	T41.3x2-	T41.3x3-	T41.3x4-	T41.3x5-	T41.3x6-
topical (surface)	T41.3x1-	T41.3x2-	T41.3x3-	T41.3x4-	T41.3x5-	T41.3x6-
Propoxyphene	T40.4x1-	T40.4x2-	T40.4x3-	T40.4x4-	T40.4x5-	T40.4x6-
Propranolol	T44.7x1-	T44.7x2-	T44.7x3-	T44.7x4-	T44.7x5-	T44.7x6-
Propyl						
alcohol	T51.3x1-	T51.3x2-	T51.3x3-	T51.3x4-	—	—
carbinol	T51.3x1-	T51.3x2-	T51.3x3-	T51.3x4-	—	—
hexadrine	T44.4x1-	T44.4x2-	T44.4x3-	T44.4x4-	T44.4x5-	T44.4x6-
iodone	T50.8x1-	T50.8x2-	T50.8x3-	T50.8x4-	T50.8x5-	T50.8x6-
thiouracil	T38.2x1-	T38.2x2-	T38.2x3-	T38.2x4-	T38.2x5-	T38.2x6-
Propylaminophenothiazine	T43.3x1-	T43.3x2-	T43.3x3-	T43.3x4-	T43.3x5-	T43.3x6-
Propylene	T59.891-	T59.892-	T59.893-	T59.894-	—	—
Propylhexedrine	T48.5x1-	T48.5x2-	T48.5x3-	T48.5x4-	T48.5x5-	T48.5x6-
Propyliodone	T50.8x1-	T50.8x2-	T50.8x3-	T50.8x4-	T50.8x5-	T50.8x6-
Propylparaben (ophthalmic)	T49.5x1-	T49.5x2-	T49.5x3-	T49.5x4-	T49.5x5-	T49.5x6-
Propylthiouracil	T38.2x1-	T38.2x2-	T38.2x3-	T38.2x4-	T38.2x5-	T38.2x6-
Propyphenazone	T39.2x1-	T39.2x2-	T39.2x3-	T39.2x4-	T39.2x5-	T39.2x6-
Proquazone	T39.391-	T39.392-	T39.393-	T39.394-	T39.395-	T39.396-
Proscillaridin	T46.0x1-	T46.0x2-	T46.0x3-	T46.0x4-	T46.0x5-	T46.0x6-
Prostacyclin	T45.521-	T45.522-	T45.523-	T45.524-	T45.525-	T45.526-
Prostaglandin (I2)	T45.521-	T45.522-	T45.523-	T45.524-	T45.525-	T45.526-
E1	T46.7x1-	T46.7x2-	T46.7x3-	T46.7x4-	T46.7x5-	T46.7x6-
E2	T48.0x1-	T48.0x2-	T48.0x3-	T48.0x4-	T48.0x5-	T48.0x6-
F2 alpha	T48.0x1-	T48.0x2-	T48.0x3-	T48.0x4-	T48.0x5-	T48.0x6-
Prostigmin	T44.0x1-	T44.0x2-	T44.0x3-	T44.0x4-	T44.0x5-	T44.0x6-
Prosultiamine	T45.2x1-	T45.2x2-	T45.2x3-	T45.2x4-	T45.2x5-	T45.2x6-
Protamine sulfate	T45.7x1-	T45.7x2-	T45.7x3-	T45.7x4-	T45.7x5-	T45.7x6-
zinc insulin	T38.3x1-	T38.3x2-	T38.3x3-	T38.3x4-	T38.3x5-	T38.3x6-
Protease	T47.5x1-	T47.5x2-	T47.5x3-	T47.5x4-	T47.5x5-	T47.5x6-
Protectant, skin NEC	T49.3x1-	T49.3x2-	T49.3x3-	T49.3x4-	T49.3x5-	T49.3x6-
Protein hydrolysate	T50.991-	T50.992-	T50.993-	T50.994-	T50.995-	T50.996-
Prothiaden — see Dothiepin hydrochloride						
Prothionamide	T37.1x1-	T37.1x2-	T37.1x3-	T37.1x4-	T37.1x5-	T37.1x6-
Prothipendyl	T43.591-	T43.592-	T43.593-	T43.594-	T43.595-	T43.596-
Prothoate	T60.0x1-	T60.0x2-	T60.0x3-	T60.0x4-	—	—
Prothrombin						
activator	T45.7x1-	T45.7x2-	T45.7x3-	T45.7x4-	T45.7x5-	T45.7x6-
synthesis inhibitor	T45.511-	T45.512-	T45.513-	T45.514-	T45.515-	T45.516-
Protionamide	T37.1x1-	T37.1x2-	T37.1x3-	T37.1x4-	T37.1x5-	T37.1x6-
Protirelin	T38.891-	T38.892-	T38.893-	T38.894-	T38.895-	T38.896-
Protokylol	T48.6x1-	T48.6x2-	T48.6x3-	T48.6x4-	T48.6x5-	T48.6x6-
Protopam	T50.6x1-	T50.6x2-	T50.6x3-	T50.6x4-	T50.6x5-	T50.6x6-
Protoveratrine(s) (A) (B)	T46.5x1-	T46.5x2-	T46.5x3-	T46.5x4-	T46.5x5-	T46.5x6-
Protriptyline	T43.011-	T43.012-	T43.013-	T43.014-	T43.015-	T43.016-
Provera	T38.5x1-	T38.5x2-	T38.5x3-	T38.5x4-	T38.5x5-	T38.5x6-
Provitamin A	T45.2x1-	T45.2x2-	T45.2x3-	T45.2x4-	T45.2x5-	T45.2x6-
Proxibarbal	T42.3x1-	T42.3x2-	T42.3x3-	T42.3x4-	T42.3x5-	T42.3x6-
Proxymetacaine	T41.3x1-	T41.3x2-	T41.3x3-	T41.3x4-	T41.3x5-	T41.3x6-
Proxyphylline	T48.6x1-	T48.6x2-	T48.6x3-	T48.6x4-	T48.6x5-	T48.6x6-
Prozac — see Fluoxetine hydrochloride						
Prunus						
laurocerasus	T62.2x1-	T62.2x2-	T62.2x3-	T62.2x4-	—	—
virginiana	T62.2x1-	T62.2x2-	T62.2x3-	T62.2x4-	—	—
Prussian blue						
commercial	T65.891-	T65.892-	T65.893-	T65.894-	—	—
therapeutic	T50.6x1-	T50.6x2-	T50.6x3-	T50.6x4-	T50.6x5-	T50.6x6-
Prussic acid	T65.0x1-	T65.0x2-	T65.0x3-	T65.0x4-	—	—
vapor	T57.3x1-	T57.3x2-	T57.3x3-	T57.3x4-	—	—
Pseudoephedrine	T44.991-	T44.992-	T44.993-	T44.994-	T44.995-	T44.996-
Psilocin	T40.991-	T40.992-	T40.993-	T40.994-		
Psilocybin	T40.991-	T40.992-	T40.993-	T40.994-		
Psilocybine	T40.991-	T40.992-	T40.993-	T40.994-		
Psoralene (nonmedicinal)	T65.891-	T65.892-	T65.893-	T65.894-		
Psoralens (medicinal)	T50.991-	T50.992-	T50.993-	T50.994-	T50.995-	T50.996-
PSP (phenolsulfon-phthalein)	T50.8x1-	T50.8x2-	T50.8x3-	T50.8x4-	T50.8x5-	T50.8x6-
Psychodysleptic drug NEC	T40.901-	T40.902-	T40.903-	T40.904-	T40.905-	T40.906-
Psychostimulant	T43.601-	T43.602-	T43.603-	T43.604-	T43.605-	T43.606-
amphetamine	T43.621-	T43.622-	T43.623-	T43.624-	T43.625-	T43.626-
caffeine	T43.611-	T43.612-	T43.613-	T43.614-	T43.615-	T43.616-
methylphenidate	T43.631-	T43.632-	T43.633-	T43.634-	T43.635-	T43.636-
specified NEC	T43.691-	T43.692-	T43.693-	T43.694-	T43.695-	T43.696-
Psychotherapeutic drug NEC	T43.91x-	T43.92x-	T43.93x-	T43.94x-	T43.95x-	T43.96x-
antidepressants — see also Antidepressant	T43.201-	T43.202-	T43.203-	T43.204-	T43.205-	T43.206-
specified NEC	T43.8x1-	T43.8x2-	T43.8x3-	T43.8x4-	T43.8x5-	T43.8x6-
tranquilizers NEC	T43.501-	T43.502-	T43.503-	T43.504-	T43.505-	T43.506-
Psychotomimetic agents	T40.901-	T40.902-	T40.903-	T40.904-	T40.905-	T40.906-
Psychotropic drug NEC	T43.91x-	T43.92x-	T43.93x-	T43.94x-	T43.95x-	T43.96x-
specified NEC	T43.8x1-	T43.8x2-	T43.8x3-	T43.8x4-	T43.8x5-	T43.8x6-
Psyllium hydrophilic mucilloid	T47.4x1-	T47.4x2-	T47.4x3-	T47.4x4-	T47.4x5-	T47.4x6-
Pteroylglutamic acid	T45.8x1-	T45.8x2-	T45.8x3-	T45.8x4-	T45.8x5-	T45.8x6-
Pteroyltriglutamate	T45.1x1-	T45.1x2-	T45.1x3-	T45.1x4-	T45.1x5-	T45.1x6-
PTFE — see Polytetrafluoroethylene						
Pulp						
devitalizing paste	T49.7x1-	T49.7x2-	T49.7x3-	T49.7x4-	T49.7x5-	T49.7x6-
dressing	T49.7x1-	T49.7x2-	T49.7x3-	T49.7x4-	T49.7x5-	T49.7x6-
Pulsatilla	T62.2x1-	T62.2x2-	T62.2x3-	T62.2x4-	—	—
Pumpkin seed extract	T37.4x1-	T37.4x2-	T37.4x3-	T37.4x4-	T37.4x5-	T37.4x6-
Purex (bleach)	T54.91x-	T54.92x-	T54.93x-	T54.94x-	—	—
Purgative NEC — see also Cathartic	T47.4x1-	T47.4x2-	T47.4x3-	T47.4x4-	T47.4x5-	T47.4x6-
Purine analogue (antineoplastic)	T45.1x1-	T45.1x2-	T45.1x3-	T45.1x4-	T45.1x5-	T45.1x6-
Purine diuretics	T50.2x1-	T50.2x2-	T50.2x3-	T50.2x4-	T50.2x5-	T50.2x6-
Purinethol	T45.1x1-	T45.1x2-	T45.1x3-	T45.1x4-	T45.1x5-	T45.1x6-
PVP	T45.8x1-	T45.8x2-	T45.8x3-	T45.8x4-	T45.8x5-	T45.8x6-
Pyrabital	T39.8x1-	T39.8x2-	T39.8x3-	T39.8x4-	T39.8x5-	T39.8x6-
Pyramidon	T39.2x1-	T39.2x2-	T39.2x3-	T39.2x4-	T39.2x5-	T39.2x6-
Pyrantel	T37.4x1-	T37.4x2-	T37.4x3-	T37.4x4-	T37.4x5-	T37.4x6-
Pyrathiazine	T45.0x1-	T45.0x2-	T45.0x3-	T45.0x4-	T45.0x5-	T45.0x6-
Pyrazinamide	T37.1x1-	T37.1x2-	T37.1x3-	T37.1x4-	T37.1x5-	T37.1x6-
Pyrazinoic acid (amide)	T37.1x1-	T37.1x2-	T37.1x3-	T37.1x4-	T37.1x5-	T37.1x6-
Pyrazole (derivatives)	T39.2x1-	T39.2x2-	T39.2x3-	T39.2x4-	T39.2x5-	T39.2x6-
Pyrazolone analgesic NEC	T39.2x1-	T39.2x2-	T39.2x3-	T39.2x4-	T39.2x5-	T39.2x6-

Table of Drugs & Chemicals	POISONING Accidental (Unintentional)	Self-Harm (Intentional)	Assault	Undetermined	Adverse Effect	Underdosing
Pyrethrin, pyrethrum (nonmedicinal)	T60.2x1-	T60.2x2-	T60.2x3-	T60.2x4-	—	—
Pyrethrum extract	T49.0x1-	T49.0x2-	T49.0x3-	T49.0x4-	T49.0x5-	T49.0x6-
Pyribenzamine	T45.0x1-	T45.0x2-	T45.0x3-	T45.0x4-	T45.0x5-	T45.0x6-
Pyridine	T52.8x1-	T52.8x2-	T52.8x3-	T52.8x4-	—	—
aldoxime methiodide	T50.6x1-	T50.6x2-	T50.6x3-	T50.6x4-	T50.6x5-	T50.6x6-
aldoxime methyl chloride	T50.6x1-	T50.6x2-	T50.6x3-	T50.6x4-	T50.6x5-	T50.6x6-
vapor	T59.891-	T59.892-	T59.893-	T59.894-		
Pyridium	T39.8x1-	T39.8x2-	T39.8x3-	T39.8x4-	T39.8x5-	T39.8x6-
Pyridostigmine bromide	T44.0x1-	T44.0x2-	T44.0x3-	T44.0x4-	T44.0x5-	T44.0x6-
Pyridoxal phosphate	T45.2x1-	T45.2x2-	T45.2x3-	T45.2x4-	T45.2x5-	T45.2x6-
Pyridoxine	T45.2x1-	T45.2x2-	T45.2x3-	T45.2x4-	T45.2x5-	T45.2x6-
Pyrilamine	T45.0x1-	T45.0x2-	T45.0x3-	T45.0x4-	T45.0x5-	T45.0x6-
Pyrimethamine	T37.2x1-	T37.2x2-	T37.2x3-	T37.2x4-	T37.2x5-	T37.2x6-
with sulfadoxine	T37.2x1-	T37.2x2-	T37.2x3-	T37.2x4-	T37.2x5-	T37.2x6-
Pyrimidine antagonist	T45.1x1-	T45.1x2-	T45.1x3-	T45.1x4-	T45.1x5-	T45.1x6-
Pyriminil	T60.4x1-	T60.4x2-	T60.4x3-	T60.4x4-	—	—
Pyrithione zinc	T49.4x1-	T49.4x2-	T49.4x3-	T49.4x4-	T49.4x5-	T49.4x6-
Pyrithyldione	T42.6x1-	T42.6x2-	T42.6x3-	T42.6x4-	T42.6x5-	T42.6x6-
Pyrogallic acid	T49.0x1-	T49.0x2-	T49.0x3-	T49.0x4-	T49.0x5-	T49.0x6-
Pyrogallol	T49.0x1-	T49.0x2-	T49.0x3-	T49.0x4-	T49.0x5-	T49.0x6-
Pyroxylin	T49.3x1-	T49.3x2-	T49.3x3-	T49.3x4-	T49.3x5-	T49.3x6-
Pyrrobutamine	T45.0x1-	T45.0x2-	T45.0x3-	T45.0x4-	T45.0x5-	T45.0x6-
Pyrrolizidine alkaloids	T62.8x1-	T62.8x2-	T62.8x3-	T62.8x4-	—	—
Pyrvinium chloride	T37.4x1-	T37.4x2-	T37.4x3-	T37.4x4-	T37.4x5-	T37.4x6-
PZI	T38.3x1-	T38.3x2-	T38.3x3-	T38.3x4-	T38.3x5-	T38.3x6-
Quaalude	T42.6x1-	T42.6x2-	T42.6x3-	T42.6x4-	T42.6x5-	T42.6x6-
Quarternary ammonium						
anti-infective	T49.0x1-	T49.0x2-	T49.0x3-	T49.0x4-	T49.0x5-	T49.0x6-
ganglion blocking	T44.2x1-	T44.2x2-	T44.2x3-	T44.2x4-	T44.2x5-	T44.2x6-
parasympatholytic	T44.3x1-	T44.3x2-	T44.3x3-	T44.3x4-	T44.3x5-	T44.3x6-
Quazepam	T42.4x1-	T42.4x2-	T42.4x3-	T42.4x4-	T42.4x5-	T42.4x6-
Quicklime	T54.3x1-	T54.3x2-	T54.3x3-	T54.3x4-	—	—
Quillaja extract	T48.4x1-	T48.4x2-	T48.4x3-	T48.4x4-	T48.4x5-	T48.4x6-
Quinacrine	T37.2x1-	T37.2x2-	T37.2x3-	T37.2x4-	T37.2x5-	T37.2x6-
Quinaglute	T46.2x1-	T46.2x2-	T46.2x3-	T46.2x4-	T46.2x5-	T46.2x6-
Quinalbarbital	T42.3x1-	T42.3x2-	T42.3x3-	T42.3x4-	T42.3x5-	T42.3x6-
Quinalbarbitone sodium	T42.3x1-	T42.3x2-	T42.3x3-	T42.3x4-	T42.3x5-	T42.3x6-
Quinalphos	T60.0x1-	T60.0x2-	T60.0x3-	T60.0x4-	—	—
Quinapril	T46.4x1-	T46.4x2-	T46.4x3-	T46.4x4-	T46.4x5-	T46.4x6-
Quinestradiol	T38.5x1-	T38.5x2-	T38.5x3-	T38.5x4-	T38.5x5-	T38.5x6-
Quinestradol	T38.5x1-	T38.5x2-	T38.5x3-	T38.5x4-	T38.5x5-	T38.5x6-
Quinestrol	T38.5x1-	T38.5x2-	T38.5x3-	T38.5x4-	T38.5x5-	T38.5x6-
Quinethazone	T50.2x1-	T50.2x2-	T50.2x3-	T50.2x4-	T50.2x5-	T50.2x6-
Quingestanol	T38.4x1-	T38.4x2-	T38.4x3-	T38.4x4-	T38.4x5-	T38.4x6-
Quinidine	T46.2x1-	T46.2x2-	T46.2x3-	T46.2x4-	T46.2x5-	T46.2x6-
Quinine	T37.2x1-	T37.2x2-	T37.2x3-	T37.2x4-	T37.2x5-	T37.2x6-
Quiniobine	T37.8x1-	T37.8x2-	T37.8x3-	T37.8x4-	T37.8x5-	T37.8x6-
Quinisocaine	T49.1x1-	T49.1x2-	T49.1x3-	T49.1x4-	T49.1x5-	T49.1x6-
Quinocide	T37.2x1-	T37.2x2-	T37.2x3-	T37.2x4-	T37.2x5-	T37.2x6-
Quinoline (derivatives) NEC	T37.8x1-	T37.8x2-	T37.8x3-	T37.8x4-	T37.8x5-	T37.8x6-
Quinupramine	T43.011-	T43.012-	T43.013-	T43.014-	T43.015-	T43.016-
Quotane	T41.3x1-	T41.3x2-	T41.3x3-	T41.3x4-	T41.3x5-	T41.3x6-
Rabies						
immune globulin (human)	T50.Z11-	T50.Z12-	T50.Z13-	T50.Z14-	T50.Z15-	T50.Z16-
vaccine	T50.B91-	T50.B92-	T50.B93-	T50.B94-	T50.B95-	T50.B96-
Racemoramide	T40.2x1-	T40.2x2-	T40.2x3-	T40.2x4-	—	—
Racemorphan	T40.2x1-	T40.2x2-	T40.2x3-	T40.2x4-	T40.2x5-	T40.2x6-
Racepinefrin	T44.5x1-	T44.5x2-	T44.5x3-	T44.5x4-	T44.5x5-	T44.5x6-
Raclopride	T43.591-	T43.592-	T43.593-	T43.594-	T43.595-	T43.596-

Table of Drugs & Chemicals	POISONING Accidental (Unintentional)	Self-Harm (Intentional)	Assault	Undetermined	Adverse Effect	Underdosing
Radiator alcohol	T51.1x1-	T51.1x2-	T51.1x3-	T51.1x4-	—	—
Radioactive drug NEC	T50.8x1-	T50.8x2-	T50.8x3-	T50.8x4-	T50.8x5-	T50.8x6-
Radio-opaque (drugs) (materials)	T50.8x1-	T50.8x2-	T50.8x3-	T50.8x4-	T50.8x5-	T50.8x6-
Ramifenazone	T39.2x1-	T39.2x2-	T39.2x3-	T39.2x4-	T39.2x5-	T39.2x6-
Ramipril	T46.4x1-	T46.4x2-	T46.4x3-	T46.4x4-	T46.4x5-	T46.4x6-
Ranitidine	T47.0x1-	T47.0x2-	T47.0x3-	T47.0x4-	T47.0x5-	T47.0x6-
Ranunculus	T62.2x1-	T62.2x2-	T62.2x3-	T62.2x4-	—	—
Rat poison NEC	T60.4x1-	T60.4x2-	T60.4x3-	T60.4x4-	—	—
Rattlesnake (venom)	T63.011-	T63.012-	T63.013-	T63.014-	—	—
Raubasine	T46.7x1-	T46.7x2-	T46.7x3-	T46.7x4-	T46.7x5-	T46.7x6-
Raudixin	T46.5x1-	T46.5x2-	T46.5x3-	T46.5x4-	T46.5x5-	T46.5x6-
Rautensin	T46.5x1-	T46.5x2-	T46.5x3-	T46.5x4-	T46.5x5-	T46.5x6-
Rautina	T46.5x1-	T46.5x2-	T46.5x3-	T46.5x4-	T46.5x5-	T46.5x6-
Rautotal	T46.5x1-	T46.5x2-	T46.5x3-	T46.5x4-	T46.5x5-	T46.5x6-
Rauwiloid	T46.5x1-	T46.5x2-	T46.5x3-	T46.5x4-	T46.5x5-	T46.5x6-
Rauwoldin	T46.5x1-	T46.5x2-	T46.5x3-	T46.5x4-	T46.5x5-	T46.5x6-
Rauwolfia (alkaloids)	T46.5x1-	T46.5x2-	T46.5x3-	T46.5x4-	T46.5x5-	T46.5x6-
Razoxane	T45.1x1-	T45.1x2-	T45.1x3-	T45.1x4-	T45.1x5-	T45.1x6-
Realgar	T57.0x1-	T57.0x2-	T57.0x3-	T57.0x4-	—	—
Recombinant (R) — see specific protein						
Red blood cells, packed	T45.8x1-	T45.8x2-	T45.8x3-	T45.8x4-	T45.8x5-	T45.8x6-
Red squill (scilliroside)	T60.4x1-	T60.4x2-	T60.4x3-	T60.4x4-		
Reducing agent, industrial NEC	T65.891-	T65.892-	T65.893-	T65.894-		
Refrigerant gas (chlorofluoro-carbon)	T53.5x1-	T53.5x2-	T53.5x3-	T53.5x4-	—	—
not chlorofluoro-carbon	T59.891-	T59.892-	T59.893-	T59.894-	—	—
Regroton	T50.2x1-	T50.2x2-	T50.2x3-	T50.2x4-	T50.2x5-	T50.2x6-
Rehydration salts (oral)	T50.3x1-	T50.3x2-	T50.3x3-	T50.3x4-	T50.3x5-	T50.3x6-
Rela	T42.8x1-	T42.8x2-	T42.8x3-	T42.8x4-	T42.8x5-	T42.8x6-
Relaxant, muscle						
anesthetic	T48.1x1-	T48.1x2-	T48.1x3-	T48.1x4-	T48.1x5-	T48.1x6-
central nervous system	T42.8x1-	T42.8x2-	T42.8x3-	T42.8x4-	T42.8x5-	T42.8x6-
skeletal NEC	T48.1x1-	T48.1x2-	T48.1x3-	T48.1x4-	T48.1x5-	T48.1x6-
smooth NEC	T44.3x1-	T44.3x2-	T44.3x3-	T44.3x4-	T44.3x5-	T44.3x6-
Remoxipride	T43.591-	T43.592-	T43.593-	T43.594-	T43.595-	T43.596-
Renese	T50.2x1-	T50.2x2-	T50.2x3-	T50.2x4-	T50.2x5-	T50.2x6-
Renografin	T50.8x1-	T50.8x2-	T50.8x3-	T50.8x4-	T50.8x5-	T50.8x6-
Replacement solution	T50.3x1-	T50.3x2-	T50.3x3-	T50.3x4-	T50.3x5-	T50.3x6-
Reproterol	T48.6x1-	T48.6x2-	T48.6x3-	T48.6x4-	T48.6x5-	T48.6x6-
Rescinnamine	T46.5x1-	T46.5x2-	T46.5x3-	T46.5x4-	T46.5x5-	T46.5x6-
Reserpin(e)	T46.5x1-	T46.5x2-	T46.5x3-	T46.5x4-	T46.5x5-	T46.5x6-
Resorcin, resorcinol (nonmedicinal)	T65.891-	T65.892-	T65.893-	T65.894-		
medicinal	T49.4x1-	T49.4x2-	T49.4x3-	T49.4x4-	T49.4x5-	T49.4x6-
Respaire	T48.4x1-	T48.4x2-	T48.4x3-	T48.4x4-	T48.4x5-	T48.4x6-
Respiratory drug NEC	T48.901-	T48.902-	T48.903-	T48.904-	T48.905-	T48.906-
antiasthmatic NEC	T48.6x1-	T48.6x2-	T48.6x3-	T48.6x4-	T48.6x5-	T48.6x6-
anti-common-cold NEC	T48.5x1-	T48.5x2-	T48.5x3-	T48.5x4-	T48.5x5-	T48.5x6-
expectorant NEC	T48.4x1-	T48.4x2-	T48.4x3-	T48.4x4-	T48.4x5-	T48.4x6-
stimulant	T48.901-	T48.902-	T48.903-	T48.904-	T48.905-	T48.906-
Retinoic acid	T49.0x1-	T49.0x2-	T49.0x3-	T49.0x4-	T49.0x5-	T49.0x6-
Retinol	T45.2x1-	T45.2x2-	T45.2x3-	T45.2x4-	T45.2x5-	T45.2x6-
Rh (D) immune globulin (human)	T50.Z11-	T50.Z12-	T50.Z13-	T50.Z14-	T50.Z15-	T50.Z16-
Rhodine	T39.011-	T39.012-	T39.013-	T39.014-	T39.015-	T39.016-
RhoGAM	T50.Z11-	T50.Z12-	T50.Z13-	T50.Z14-	T50.Z15-	T50.Z16-
Rhubarb						
dry extract	T47.2x1-	T47.2x2-	T47.2x3-	T47.2x4-	T47.2x5-	T47.2x6-
tincture, compound	T47.2x1-	T47.2x2-	T47.2x3-	T47.2x4-	T47.2x5-	T47.2x6-

DRUGS & CHEMICALS

Table of Drugs & Chemicals	POISONING — Accidental (Unintentional)	POISONING — Self-Harm (Intentional)	POISONING — Assault	POISONING — Undetermined	Adverse Effect	Underdosing
Ribavirin	T37.5x1-	T37.5x2-	T37.5x3-	T37.5x4-	T37.5x5-	T37.5x6-
Riboflavin	T45.2x1-	T45.2x2-	T45.2x3-	T45.2x4-	T45.2x5-	T45.2x6-
Ribostamycin	T36.5x1-	T36.5x2-	T36.5x3-	T36.5x4-	T36.5x5-	T36.5x6-
Ricin	T62.2x1-	T62.2x2-	T62.2x3-	T62.2x4-	—	—
Ricinus communis	T62.2x1-	T62.2x2-	T62.2x3-	T62.2x4-	—	—
Rickettsial vaccine NEC	T50.A91-	T50.A92-	T50.A93-	T50.A94-	T50.A95-	T50.A96-
Rifabutin	T36.6x1-	T36.6x2-	T36.6x3-	T36.6x4-	T36.6x5-	T36.6x6-
Rifamide	T36.6x1-	T36.6x2-	T36.6x3-	T36.6x4-	T36.6x5-	T36.6x6-
Rifampicin	T36.6x1-	T36.6x2-	T36.6x3-	T36.6x4-	T36.6x5-	T36.6x6-
with isoniazid	T37.1x1-	T37.1x2-	T37.1x3-	T37.1x4-	T37.1x5-	T37.1x6-
Rifampin	T36.6x1-	T36.6x2-	T36.6x3-	T36.6x4-	T36.6x5-	T36.6x6-
Rifamycin	T36.6x1-	T36.6x2-	T36.6x3-	T36.6x4-	T36.6x5-	T36.6x6-
Rifaximin	T36.6x1-	T36.6x2-	T36.6x3-	T36.6x4-	T36.6x5-	T36.6x6-
Rimantadine	T37.5x1-	T37.5x2-	T37.5x3-	T37.5x4-	T37.5x5-	T37.5x6-
Rimazolium metilsulfate	T39.8x1-	T39.8x2-	T39.8x3-	T39.8x4-	T39.8x5-	T39.8x6-
Rimifon	T37.1x1-	T37.1x2-	T37.1x3-	T37.1x4-	T37.1x5-	T37.1x6-
Rimiterol	T48.6x1-	T48.6x2-	T48.6x3-	T48.6x4-	T48.6x5-	T48.6x6-
Ringer (lactate) solution	T50.3x1-	T50.3x2-	T50.3x3-	T50.3x4-	T50.3x5-	T50.3x6-
Ristocetin	T36.8x1-	T36.8x2-	T36.8x3-	T36.8x4-	T36.8x5-	T36.8x6-
Ritalin	T43.631-	T43.632-	T43.633-	T43.634-	T43.635-	T43.636-
Ritodrine	T44.5x1-	T44.5x2-	T44.5x3-	T44.5x4-	T44.5x5-	T44.5x6-
Roach killer — see Insecticide						
Rociverine	T44.3x1-	T44.3x2-	T44.3x3-	T44.3x4-	T44.3x5-	T44.3x6-
Rocky Mountain spotted fever vaccine	T50.A91-	T50.A92-	T50.A93-	T50.A94-	T50.A95-	T50.A96-
Rodenticide NEC	T60.4x1-	T60.4x2-	T60.4x3-	T60.4x4-		
Rohypnol	T42.4x1-	T42.4x2-	T42.4x3-	T42.4x4-	T42.4x5-	T42.4x6-
Rokitamycin	T36.3x1-	T36.3x2-	T36.3x3-	T36.3x4-	T36.3x5-	T36.3x6-
Rolaids	T47.1x1-	T47.1x2-	T47.1x3-	T47.1x4-	T47.1x5-	T47.1x6-
Rolitetracycline	T36.4x1-	T36.4x2-	T36.4x3-	T36.4x4-	T36.4x5-	T36.4x6-
Romilar	T48.3x1-	T48.3x2-	T48.3x3-	T48.3x4-	T48.3x5-	T48.3x6-
Ronifibrate	T46.6x1-	T46.6x2-	T46.6x3-	T46.6x4-	T46.6x5-	T46.6x6-
Rosaprostol	T47.1x1-	T47.1x2-	T47.1x3-	T47.1x4-	T47.1x5-	T47.1x6-
Rose bengal sodium (131I)	T50.8x1-	T50.8x2-	T50.8x3-	T50.8x4-	T50.8x5-	T50.8x6-
Rose water ointment	T49.3x1-	T49.3x2-	T49.3x3-	T49.3x4-	T49.3x5-	T49.3x6-
Rosoxacin	T37.8x1-	T37.8x2-	T37.8x3-	T37.8x4-	T37.8x5-	T37.8x6-
Rotenone	T60.2x1-	T60.2x2-	T60.2x3-	T60.2x4-		
Rotoxamine	T45.0x1-	T45.0x2-	T45.0x3-	T45.0x4-	T45.0x5-	T45.0x6-
Rough-on-rats	T60.4x1-	T60.4x2-	T60.4x3-	T60.4x4-		
Roxatidine	T47.0x1-	T47.0x2-	T47.0x3-	T47.0x4-	T47.0x5-	T47.0x6-
Roxithromycin	T36.3x1-	T36.3x2-	T36.3x3-	T36.3x4-	T36.3x5-	T36.3x6-
Rt-PA	T45.611-	T45.612-	T45.613-	T45.614-	T45.615-	T45.616-
Rubbing alcohol	T51.2x1-	T51.2x2-	T51.2x3-	T51.2x4-		
Rubefacient	T49.4x1-	T49.4x2-	T49.4x3-	T49.4x4-	T49.4x5-	T49.4x6-
Rubella vaccine	T50.B91-	T50.B92-	T50.B93-	T50.B94-	T50.B95-	T50.B96-
Rubeola vaccine	T50.B91-	T50.B92-	T50.B93-	T50.B94-	T50.B95-	T50.B96-
Rubidium chloride Rb82	T50.8x1-	T50.8x2-	T50.8x3-	T50.8x4-	T50.8x5-	T50.8x6-
Rubidomycin	T45.1x1-	T45.1x2-	T45.1x3-	T45.1x4-	T45.1x5-	T45.1x6-
Rue	T62.2x1-	T62.2x2-	T62.2x3-	T62.2x4-		
Rufocromomycin	T45.1x1-	T45.1x2-	T45.1x3-	T45.1x4-	T45.1x5-	T45.1x6-
Russel's viper venin	T45.7x1-	T45.7x2-	T45.7x3-	T45.7x4-	T45.7x5-	T45.7x6-
Ruta (graveolens)	T62.2x1-	T62.2x2-	T62.2x3-	T62.2x4-		
Rutinum	T46.991-	T46.992-	T46.993-	T46.994-	T46.995-	T46.996-
Rutoside	T46.991-	T46.992-	T46.993-	T46.994-	T46.995-	T46.996-
Sabadilla (plant)	T62.2x1-	T62.2x2-	T62.2x3-	T62.2x4-		
pesticide	T60.2x1-	T60.2x2-	T60.2x3-	T60.2x4-		
Saccharated iron oxide	T45.8x1-	T45.8x2-	T45.8x3-	T45.8x4-	T45.8x5-	T45.8x6-
Saccharin	T50.901-	T50.902-	T50.903-	T50.904-	T50.905-	T50.906-
Saccharomyces boulardii	T47.6x1-	T47.6x2-	T47.6x3-	T47.6x4-	T47.6x5-	T47.6x6-
Safflower oil	T46.6x1-	T46.6x2-	T46.6x3-	T46.6x4-	T46.6x5-	T46.6x6-
Safrazine	T43.1x1-	T43.1x2-	T43.1x3-	T43.1x4-	T43.1x5-	T43.1x6-
Salazosulfapyridine	T37.0x1-	T37.0x2-	T37.0x3-	T37.0x4-	T37.0x5-	T37.0x6-
Salbutamol	T48.6x1-	T48.6x2-	T48.6x3-	T48.6x4-	T48.6x5-	T48.6x6-
Salicylamide	T39.091-	T39.092-	T39.093-	T39.094-	T39.095-	T39.096-
Salicylate NEC	T39.091-	T39.092-	T39.093-	T39.094-	T39.095-	T39.096-
methyl	T49.3x1-	T49.3x2-	T49.3x3-	T49.3x4-	T49.3x5-	T49.3x6-
theobromine calcium	T50.2x1-	T50.2x2-	T50.2x3-	T50.2x4-	T50.2x5-	T50.2x6-
Salicylazosulfapyridine	T37.0x1-	T37.0x2-	T37.0x3-	T37.0x4-	T37.0x5-	T37.0x6-
Salicylhydroxamic acid	T49.0x1-	T49.0x2-	T49.0x3-	T49.0x4-	T49.0x5-	T49.0x6-
Salicylic acid	T49.4x1-	T49.4x2-	T49.4x3-	T49.4x4-	T49.4x5-	T49.4x6-
with benzoic acid	T49.4x1-	T49.4x2-	T49.4x3-	T49.4x4-	T49.4x5-	T49.4x6-
congeners	T39.091-	T39.092-	T39.093-	T39.094-	T39.095-	T39.096-
derivative	T39.091-	T39.092-	T39.093-	T39.094-	T39.095-	T39.096-
salts	T39.091-	T39.092-	T39.093-	T39.094-	T39.095-	T39.096-
Salinazid	T37.1x1-	T37.1x2-	T37.1x3-	T37.1x4-	T37.1x5-	T37.1x6-
Salmeterol	T48.6x1-	T48.6x2-	T48.6x3-	T48.6x4-	T48.6x5-	T48.6x6-
Salol	T49.3x1-	T49.3x2-	T49.3x3-	T49.3x4-	T49.3x5-	T49.3x6-
Salsalate	T39.091-	T39.092-	T39.093-	T39.094-	T39.095-	T39.096-
Salt substitute	T50.901-	T50.902-	T50.903-	T50.904-	T50.905-	T50.906-
Salt-replacing drug	T50.901-	T50.902-	T50.903-	T50.904-	T50.905-	T50.906-
Salt-retaining mineralocorticoid	T50.0x1-	T50.0x2-	T50.0x3-	T50.0x4-	T50.0x5-	T50.0x6-
Saluretic NEC	T50.2x1-	T50.2x2-	T50.2x3-	T50.2x4-	T50.2x5-	T50.2x6-
Saluron	T50.2x1-	T50.2x2-	T50.2x3-	T50.2x4-	T50.2x5-	T50.2x6-
Salvarsan 606 (neosilver) (silver)	T37.8x1-	T37.8x2-	T37.8x3-	T37.8x4-	T37.8x5-	T37.8x6-
Sambucus canadensis	T62.2x1-	T62.2x2-	T62.2x3-	T62.2x4-	—	—
berry	T62.1x1-	T62.1x2-	T62.1x3-	T62.1x4-	—	—
Sandril	T46.5x1-	T46.5x2-	T46.5x3-	T46.5x4-	T46.5x5-	T46.5x6-
Sanguinaria canadensis	T62.2x1-	T62.2x2-	T62.2x3-	T62.2x4-		
Saniflush (cleaner)	T54.2x1-	T54.2x2-	T54.2x3-	T54.2x4-		
Santonin	T37.4x1-	T37.4x2-	T37.4x3-	T37.4x4-	T37.4x5-	T37.4x6-
Santyl	T49.8x1-	T49.8x2-	T49.8x3-	T49.8x4-	T49.8x5-	T49.8x6-
Saralasin	T46.5x1-	T46.5x2-	T46.5x3-	T46.5x4-	T46.5x5-	T46.5x6-
Sarcolysin	T45.1x1-	T45.1x2-	T45.1x3-	T45.1x4-	T45.1x5-	T45.1x6-
Sarkomycin	T45.1x1-	T45.1x2-	T45.1x3-	T45.1x4-	T45.1x5-	T45.1x6-
Saroten	T43.011-	T43.012-	T43.013-	T43.014-	T43.015-	T43.016-
Saturnine — see Lead						
Savin (oil)	T49.4x1-	T49.4x2-	T49.4x3-	T49.4x4-	T49.4x5-	T49.4x6-
Scammony	T47.2x1-	T47.2x2-	T47.2x3-	T47.2x4-	T47.2x5-	T47.2x6-
Scarlet red	T49.8x1-	T49.8x2-	T49.8x3-	T49.8x4-	T49.8x5-	T49.8x6-
Scheele's green	T57.0x1-	T57.0x2-	T57.0x3-	T57.0x4-		
insecticide	T57.0x1-	T57.0x2-	T57.0x3-	T57.0x4-		
Schizontozide (blood) (tissue)	T37.2x1-	T37.2x2-	T37.2x3-	T37.2x4-	T37.2x5-	T37.2x6-
Schradan	T60.0x1-	T60.0x2-	T60.0x3-	T60.0x4-		
Schweinfurth green	T57.0x1-	T57.0x2-	T57.0x3-	T57.0x4-		
insecticide	T57.0x1-	T57.0x2-	T57.0x3-	T57.0x4-		
Scilla, rat poison	T60.4x1-	T60.4x2-	T60.4x3-	T60.4x4-		
Scillaren	T60.4x1-	T60.4x2-	T60.4x3-	T60.4x4-		
Sclerosing agent	T46.8x1-	T46.8x2-	T46.8x3-	T46.8x4-	T46.8x5-	T46.8x6-
Scombrotoxin	T61.11x-	T61.12x-	T61.13x-	T61.14x-		
Scopolamine	T44.3x1-	T44.3x2-	T44.3x3-	T44.3x4-	T44.3x5-	T44.3x6-
Scopolia extract	T44.3x1-	T44.3x2-	T44.3x3-	T44.3x4-	T44.3x5-	T44.3x6-
Scouring powder	T65.891-	T65.892-	T65.893-	T65.894-		
Sea anemone (sting)	T63.631-	T63.632-	T63.633-	T63.634-		
cucumber (sting)	T63.691-	T63.692-	T63.693-	T63.694-		
snake (bite) (venom)	T63.091-	T63.092-	T63.093-	T63.094-		
urchin spine (puncture)	T63.691-	T63.692-	T63.693-	T63.694-		

DRUGS & CHEMICALS

Table of Drugs & Chemicals	POISONING Accidental (Unintentional)	POISONING Self-Harm (Intentional)	POISONING Assault	POISONING Undetermined	Adverse Effect	Underdosing
Seafood	T61.91x-	T61.92x-	T61.93x-	T61.94x-	—	—
specified NEC	T61.8x1-	T61.8x2-	T61.8x3-	T61.8x4-	—	—
Secbutabarbital	T42.3x1-	T42.3x2-	T42.3x3-	T42.3x4-	T42.3x5-	T42.3x6-
Secbutabarbitone	T42.3x1-	T42.3x2-	T42.3x3-	T42.3x4-	T42.3x5-	T42.3x6-
Secnidazole	T37.3x1-	T37.3x2-	T37.3x3-	T37.3x4-	T37.3x5-	T37.3x6-
Secobarbital	T42.3x1-	T42.3x2-	T42.3x3-	T42.3x4-	T42.3x5-	T42.3x6-
Seconal	T42.3x1-	T42.3x2-	T42.3x3-	T42.3x4-	T42.3x5-	T42.3x6-
Secretin	T50.8x1-	T50.8x2-	T50.8x3-	T50.8x4-	T50.8x5-	T50.8x6-
Sedative NEC	T42.71x-	T42.72x-	T42.73x-	T42.74x-	T42.75x-	T42.76x-
mixed NEC	T42.6x1-	T42.6x2-	T42.6x3-	T42.6x4-	T42.6x5-	T42.6x6-
Sedormid	T42.6x1-	T42.6x2-	T42.6x3-	T42.6x4-	T42.6x5-	T42.6x6-
Seed disinfectant or dressing	T60.8x1-	T60.8x2-	T60.8x3-	T60.8x4-	—	—
Seeds (poisonous)	T62.2x1-	T62.2x2-	T62.2x3-	T62.2x4-	—	—
Selegiline	T42.8x1-	T42.8x2-	T42.8x3-	T42.8x4-	T42.8x5-	T42.8x6-
Selenium NEC	T56.891-	T56.892-	T56.893-	T56.894-	—	—
disulfide or sulfide	T49.4x1-	T49.4x2-	T49.4x3-	T49.4x4-	T49.4x5-	T49.4x6-
fumes	T59.891-	T59.892-	T59.893-	T59.894-	—	—
sulfide	T49.4x1-	T49.4x2-	T49.4x3-	T49.4x4-	T49.4x5-	T49.4x6-
Selenomethionine (75Se)	T50.8x1-	T50.8x2-	T50.8x3-	T50.8x4-	T50.8x5-	T50.8x6-
Selsun	T49.4x1-	T49.4x2-	T49.4x3-	T49.4x4-	T49.4x5-	T49.4x6-
Semustine	T45.1x1-	T45.1x2-	T45.1x3-	T45.1x4-	T45.1x5-	T45.1x6-
Senega syrup	T48.4x1-	T48.4x2-	T48.4x3-	T48.4x4-	T48.4x5-	T48.4x6-
Senna	T47.2x1-	T47.2x2-	T47.2x3-	T47.2x4-	T47.2x5-	T47.2x6-
Sennoside A + B	T47.2x1-	T47.2x2-	T47.2x3-	T47.2x4-	T47.2x5-	T47.2x6-
Septisol	T49.2x1-	T49.2x2-	T49.2x3-	T49.2x4-	T49.2x5-	T49.2x6-
Seractide	T38.811-	T38.812-	T38.813-	T38.814-	T38.815-	T38.816-
Serax	T42.4x1-	T42.4x2-	T42.4x3-	T42.4x4-	T42.4x5-	T42.4x6-
Serenesil	T42.6x1-	T42.6x2-	T42.6x3-	T42.6x4-	T42.6x5-	T42.6x6-
Serenium (hydrochloride)	T37.91x-	T37.92x-	T37.93x-	T37.94x-	T37.95x-	T37.96x-
Serepax — see Oxazepam						
Sermorelin	T38.891-	T38.892-	T38.893-	T38.894-	T38.895-	T38.896-
Sernyl	T41.1x1-	T41.1x2-	T41.1x3-	T41.1x4-	T41.1x5-	T41.1x6-
Serotonin	T50.991-	T50.992-	T50.993-	T50.994-	T50.995-	T50.996-
Serpasil	T46.5x1-	T46.5x2-	T46.5x3-	T46.5x4-	T46.5x5-	T46.5x6-
Serrapeptase	T45.3x1-	T45.3x2-	T45.3x3-	T45.3x4-	T45.3x5-	T45.3x6-
Serum						
antibotulinus	T50.Z11-	T50.Z12-	T50.Z13-	T50.Z14-	T50.Z15-	T50.Z16-
anticytotoxic	T50.Z11-	T50.Z12-	T50.Z13-	T50.Z14-	T50.Z15-	T50.Z16-
antidiphtheria	T50.Z11-	T50.Z12-	T50.Z13-	T50.Z14-	T50.Z15-	T50.Z16-
antimeningococcus	T50.Z11-	T50.Z12-	T50.Z13-	T50.Z14-	T50.Z15-	T50.Z16-
anti-Rh	T50.Z11-	T50.Z12-	T50.Z13-	T50.Z14-	T50.Z15-	T50.Z16-
anti-snake-bite	T50.Z11-	T50.Z12-	T50.Z13-	T50.Z14-	T50.Z15-	T50.Z16-
antitetanic	T50.Z11-	T50.Z12-	T50.Z13-	T50.Z14-	T50.Z15-	T50.Z16-
antitoxic	T50.Z11-	T50.Z12-	T50.Z13-	T50.Z14-	T50.Z15-	T50.Z16-
complement (inhibitor)	T45.8x1-	T45.8x2-	T45.8x3-	T45.8x4-	T45.8x5-	T45.8x6-
convalescent	T50.Z11-	T50.Z12-	T50.Z13-	T50.Z14-	T50.Z15-	T50.Z16-
hemolytic complement	T45.8x1-	T45.8x2-	T45.8x3-	T45.8x4-	T45.8x5-	T45.8x6-
immune (human)	T50.Z11-	T50.Z12-	T50.Z13-	T50.Z14-	T50.Z15-	T50.Z16-
protective NEC	T50.Z11-	T50.Z12-	T50.Z13-	T50.Z14-	T50.Z15-	T50.Z16-
Setastine	T45.0x1-	T45.0x2-	T45.0x3-	T45.0x4-	T45.0x5-	T45.0x6-
Setoperone	T43.591-	T43.592-	T43.593-	T43.594-	T43.595-	T43.596-
Sewer gas	T59.91x-	T59.92x-	T59.93x-	T59.94x-	—	—
Shampoo	T55.0x1-	T55.0x2-	T55.0x3-	T55.0x4-	—	—
Shellfish, noxious, nonbacterial	T61.781-	T61.782-	T61.783-	T61.784-	—	—
Sildenafil	T46.7x1-	T46.7x2-	T46.7x3-	T46.7x4-	T46.7x5-	T46.7x6-
Silibinin	T50.991-	T50.992-	T50.993-	T50.994-	T50.995-	T50.996-
Silicone NEC	T65.891-	T65.892-	T65.893-	T65.894-	—	—
medicinal	T49.3x1-	T49.3x2-	T49.3x3-	T49.3x4-	T49.3x5-	T49.3x6-
Silvadene	T49.0x1-	T49.0x2-	T49.0x3-	T49.0x4-	T49.0x5-	T49.0x6-
Silver	T49.0x1-	T49.0x2-	T49.0x3-	T49.0x4-	T49.0x5-	T49.0x6-
anti-infectives	T49.0x1-	T49.0x2-	T49.0x3-	T49.0x4-	T49.0x5-	T49.0x6-
arsphenamine	T37.8x1-	T37.8x2-	T37.8x3-	T37.8x4-	T37.8x5-	T37.8x6-
colloidal	T49.0x1-	T49.0x2-	T49.0x3-	T49.0x4-	T49.0x5-	T49.0x6-
nitrate	T49.0x1-	T49.0x2-	T49.0x3-	T49.0x4-	T49.0x5-	T49.0x6-
ophthalmic preparation	T49.5x1-	T49.5x2-	T49.5x3-	T49.5x4-	T49.5x5-	T49.5x6-
toughened (keratolytic)	T49.4x1-	T49.4x2-	T49.4x3-	T49.4x4-	T49.4x5-	T49.4x6-
nonmedicinal (dust)	T56.891-	T56.892-	T56.893-	T56.894-	—	—
protein	T49.5x1-	T49.5x2-	T49.5x3-	T49.5x4-	T49.5x5-	T49.5x6-
salvarsan	T37.8x1-	T37.8x2-	T37.8x3-	T37.8x4-	T37.8x5-	T37.8x6-
sulfadiazine	T49.4x1-	T49.4x2-	T49.4x3-	T49.4x4-	T49.4x5-	T49.4x6-
Silymarin	T50.991-	T50.992-	T50.993-	T50.994-	T50.995-	T50.996-
Simaldrate	T47.1x1-	T47.1x2-	T47.1x3-	T47.1x4-	T47.1x5-	T47.1x6-
Simazine	T60.3x1-	T60.3x2-	T60.3x3-	T60.3x4-	—	—
Simethicone	T47.1x1-	T47.1x2-	T47.1x3-	T47.1x4-	T47.1x5-	T47.1x6-
Simfibrate	T46.6x1-	T46.6x2-	T46.6x3-	T46.6x4-	T46.6x5-	T46.6x6-
Simvastatin	T46.6x1-	T46.6x2-	T46.6x3-	T46.6x4-	T46.6x5-	T46.6x6-
Sincalide	T50.8x1-	T50.8x2-	T50.8x3-	T50.8x4-	T50.8x5-	T50.8x6-
Sinequan	T43.011-	T43.012-	T43.013-	T43.014-	T43.015-	T43.016-
Singoserp	T46.5x1-	T46.5x2-	T46.5x3-	T46.5x4-	T46.5x5-	T46.5x6-
Sintrom	T45.511-	T45.512-	T45.513-	T45.514-	T45.515-	T45.516-
Sisomicin	T36.5x1-	T36.5x2-	T36.5x3-	T36.5x4-	T36.5x5-	T36.5x6-
Sitosterols	T46.6x1-	T46.6x2-	T46.6x3-	T46.6x4-	T46.6x5-	T46.6x6-
Skeletal muscle relaxants	T48.1x1-	T48.1x2-	T48.1x3-	T48.1x4-	T48.1x5-	T48.1x6-
Skin						
agents (external)	T49.91x-	T49.92x-	T49.93x-	T49.94x-	T49.95x-	T49.96x-
specified NEC	T49.8x1-	T49.8x2-	T49.8x3-	T49.8x4-	T49.8x5-	T49.8x6-
test antigen	T50.8x1-	T50.8x2-	T50.8x3-	T50.8x4-	T50.8x5-	T50.8x6-
Sleep-eze	T45.0x1-	T45.0x2-	T45.0x3-	T45.0x4-	T45.0x5-	T45.0x6-
Sleeping draught, pill	T42.71x-	T42.72x-	T42.73x-	T42.74x-	T42.75x-	T42.76x-
Smallpox vaccine	T50.B11-	T50.B12-	T50.B13-	T50.B14-	T50.B15-	T50.B16-
Smelter fumes NEC	T56.91x-	T56.92x-	T56.93x-	T56.94x-	—	—
Smog	T59.1x1-	T59.1x2-	T59.1x3-	T59.1x4-	—	—
Smoke NEC	T59.811-	T59.812-	T59.813-	T59.814-	—	—
Smooth muscle relaxant	T44.3x1-	T44.3x2-	T44.3x3-	T44.3x4-	T44.3x5-	T44.3x6-
Snail killer NEC	T60.8x1-	T60.8x2-	T60.8x3-	T60.8x4-	—	—
Snake venom or bite	T63.001-	T63.002-	T63.003-	T63.004-	—	—
hemocoagulase	T45.7x1-	T45.7x2-	T45.7x3-	T45.7x4-	T45.7x5-	T45.7x6-
Snuff	T65.211-	T65.212-	T65.213-	T65.214-	—	—
Soap (powder) (product)	T55.0x1-	T55.0x2-	T55.0x3-	T55.0x4-	—	—
enema	T47.4x1-	T47.4x2-	T47.4x3-	T47.4x4-	T47.4x5-	T47.4x6-
medicinal, soft	T49.2x1-	T49.2x2-	T49.2x3-	T49.2x4-	T49.2x5-	T49.2x6-
superfatted	T49.2x1-	T49.2x2-	T49.2x3-	T49.2x4-	T49.2x5-	T49.2x6-
Sobrerol	T48.4x1-	T48.4x2-	T48.4x3-	T48.4x4-	T48.4x5-	T48.4x6-
Soda (caustic)	T54.3x1-	T54.3x2-	T54.3x3-	T54.3x4-	—	—
bicarb	T47.1x1-	T47.1x2-	T47.1x3-	T47.1x4-	T47.1x5-	T47.1x6-
chlorinated — see Sodium, hypochlorite						
Sodium						
l-triiodothyronine	T38.1x1-	T38.1x2-	T38.1x3-	T38.1x4-	T38.1x5-	T38.1x6-
acetosulfone	T37.1x1-	T37.1x2-	T37.1x3-	T37.1x4-	T37.1x5-	T37.1x6-
acetrizoate	T50.8x1-	T50.8x2-	T50.8x3-	T50.8x4-	T50.8x5-	T50.8x6-
acid phosphate	T50.3x1-	T50.3x2-	T50.3x3-	T50.3x4-	T50.3x5-	T50.3x6-
alginate	T47.8x1-	T47.8x2-	T47.8x3-	T47.8x4-	T47.8x5-	T47.8x6-
amidotrizoate	T50.8x1-	T50.8x2-	T50.8x3-	T50.8x4-	T50.8x5-	T50.8x6-
aminopterin	T45.1x1-	T45.1x2-	T45.1x3-	T45.1x4-	T45.1x5-	T45.1x6-
amylosulfate	T47.8x1-	T47.8x2-	T47.8x3-	T47.8x4-	T47.8x5-	T47.8x6-
amytal	T42.3x1-	T42.3x2-	T42.3x3-	T42.3x4-	T42.3x5-	T42.3x6-
antimony gluconate	T37.3x1-	T37.3x2-	T37.3x3-	T37.3x4-	T37.3x5-	T37.3x6-
arsenate	T57.0x1-	T57.0x2-	T57.0x3-	T57.0x4-	—	—
aurothiomalate	T39.4x1-	T39.4x2-	T39.4x3-	T39.4x4-	T39.4x5-	T39.4x6-
aurothiosulfate	T39.4x1-	T39.4x2-	T39.4x3-	T39.4x4-	T39.4x5-	T39.4x6-
barbiturate	T42.3x1-	T42.3x2-	T42.3x3-	T42.3x4-	T42.3x5-	T42.3x6-
basic phosphate	T47.4x1-	T47.4x2-	T47.4x3-	T47.4x4-	T47.4x5-	T47.4x6-
bicarbonate	T47.1x1-	T47.1x2-	T47.1x3-	T47.1x4-	T47.1x5-	T47.1x6-

DRUGS & CHEMICALS

Table of Drugs & Chemicals	POISONING				Adverse Effect	Underdosing
	Accidental (Unintentional)	Self-Harm (Intentional)	Assault	Undetermined		
Sodium - *continued*						
bichromate	T57.8x1-	T57.8x2-	T57.8x3-	T57.8x4-	—	—
biphosphate	T50.3x1-	T50.3x2-	T50.3x3-	T50.3x4-	T50.3x5-	T50.3x6-
bisulfate	T65.891-	T65.892-	T65.893-	T65.894-	—	—
borate						
cleanser	T57.8x1-	T57.8x2-	T57.8x3-	T57.8x4-	—	—
eye	T49.5x1-	T49.5x2-	T49.5x3-	T49.5x4-	T49.5x5-	T49.5x6-
therapeutic	T49.8x1-	T49.8x2-	T49.8x3-	T49.8x4-	T49.8x5-	T49.8x6-
bromide	T42.6x1-	T42.6x2-	T42.6x3-	T42.6x4-	T42.6x5-	T42.6x6-
cacodylate (nonmedicinal)						
NEC	T50.8x1-	T50.8x2-	T50.8x3-	T50.8x4-	T50.8x5-	T50.8x6-
anti-infective	T37.8x1-	T37.8x2-	T37.8x3-	T37.8x4-	T37.8x5-	T37.8x6-
herbicide	T60.3x1-	T60.3x2-	T60.3x3-	T60.3x4-	—	—
calcium edetate	T45.8x1-	T45.8x2-	T45.8x3-	T45.8x4-	T45.8x5-	T45.8x6-
carbonate NEC	T54.3x1-	T54.3x2-	T54.3x3-	T54.3x4-	—	—
chlorate NEC	T65.891-	T65.892-	T65.893-	T65.894-	—	—
herbicide	T54.91x-	T54.92x-	T54.93x-	T54.94x-	—	—
chloride	T50.3x1-	T50.3x2-	T50.3x3-	T50.3x4-	T50.3x5-	T50.3x6-
with glucose	T50.3x1-	T50.3x2-	T50.3x3-	T50.3x4-	T50.3x5-	T50.3x6-
chromate	T65.891-	T65.892-	T65.893-	T65.894-	—	—
citrate	T50.991-	T50.992-	T50.993-	T50.994-	T50.995-	T50.996-
cromoglicate	T48.6x1-	T48.6x2-	T48.6x3-	T48.6x4-	T48.6x5-	T48.6x6-
cyanide	T65.0x1-	T65.0x2-	T65.0x3-	T65.0x4-	—	—
cyclamate	T50.3x1-	T50.3x2-	T50.3x3-	T50.3x4-	T50.3x5-	T50.3x6-
dehydrocholate	T45.8x1-	T45.8x2-	T45.8x3-	T45.8x4-	T45.8x5-	T45.8x6-
diatrizoate	T50.8x1-	T50.8x2-	T50.8x3-	T50.8x4-	T50.8x5-	T50.8x6-
dibunate	T48.4x1-	T48.4x2-	T48.4x3-	T48.4x4-	T48.4x5-	T48.4x6-
dioctyl sulfosuccinate	T47.4x1-	T47.4x2-	T47.4x3-	T47.4x4-	T47.4x5-	T47.4x6-
dipantoyl ferrate	T45.8x1-	T45.8x2-	T45.8x3-	T45.8x4-	T45.8x5-	T45.8x6-
edetate	T45.8x1-	T45.8x2-	T45.8x3-	T45.8x4-	T45.8x5-	T45.8x6-
ethacrynate	T50.1x1-	T50.1x2-	T50.1x3-	T50.1x4-	T50.1x5-	T50.1x6-
feredetate	T45.8x1-	T45.8x2-	T45.8x3-	T45.8x4-	T45.8x5-	T45.8x6-
fluoride — *see* Fluoride						
fluoroacetate (dust)						
(pesticide)	T60.4x1-	T60.4x2-	T60.4x3-	T60.4x4-	—	—
free salt	T50.3x1-	T50.3x2-	T50.3x3-	T50.3x4-	T50.3x5-	T50.3x6-
fusidate	T36.8x1-	T36.8x2-	T36.8x3-	T36.8x4-	T36.8x5-	T36.8x6-
glucaldrate	T47.1x1-	T47.1x2-	T47.1x3-	T47.1x4-	T47.1x5-	T47.1x6-
glucosulfone	T37.1x1-	T37.1x2-	T37.1x3-	T37.1x4-	T37.1x5-	T37.1x6-
glutamate	T45.8x1-	T45.8x2-	T45.8x3-	T45.8x4-	T45.8x5-	T45.8x6-
hydrogen carbonate	T50.3x1-	T50.3x2-	T50.3x3-	T50.3x4-	T50.3x5-	T50.3x6-
hydroxide	T54.3x1-	T54.3x2-	T54.3x3-	T54.3x4-	—	—
hypochlorite (bleach) NEC	T54.3x1-	T54.3x2-	T54.3x3-	T54.3x4-	—	—
disinfectant	T54.3x1-	T54.3x2-	T54.3x3-	T54.3x4-	—	—
medicinal (anti-infective) (external)	T49.0x1-	T49.0x2-	T49.0x3-	T49.0x4-	T49.0x5-	T49.0x6-
vapor	T54.3x1-	T54.3x2-	T54.3x3-	T54.3x4-	—	—
hyposulfite	T49.0x1-	T49.0x2-	T49.0x3-	T49.0x4-	T49.0x5-	T49.0x6-
indigotin disulfonate	T50.8x1-	T50.8x2-	T50.8x3-	T50.8x4-	T50.8x5-	T50.8x6-
iodide	T50.991-	T50.992-	T50.993-	T50.994-	T50.995-	T50.996-
I-131	T50.8x1-	T50.8x2-	T50.8x3-	T50.8x4-	T50.8x5-	T50.8x6-
therapeutic	T38.2x1-	T38.2x2-	T38.2x3-	T38.2x4-	T38.2x5-	T38.2x6-
iodohippurate (131I)	T50.8x1-	T50.8x2-	T50.8x3-	T50.8x4-	T50.8x5-	T50.8x6-
iopodate	T50.8x1-	T50.8x2-	T50.8x3-	T50.8x4-	T50.8x5-	T50.8x6-
iothalamate	T50.8x1-	T50.8x2-	T50.8x3-	T50.8x4-	T50.8x5-	T50.8x6-
iron edetate	T45.4x1-	T45.4x2-	T45.4x3-	T45.4x4-	T45.4x5-	T45.4x6-
lactate (compound solution)	T45.8x1-	T45.8x2-	T45.8x3-	T45.8x4-	T45.8x5-	T45.8x6-
lauryl (sulfate)	T49.2x1-	T49.2x2-	T49.2x3-	T49.2x4-	T49.2x5-	T49.2x6-
(L)-triiodothyronine	T38.1x1-	T38.1x2-	T38.1x3-	T38.1x4-	T38.1x5-	T38.1x6-
Sodium - *continued*						
magnesium citrate	T50.991-	T50.992-	T50.993-	T50.994-	T50.995-	T50.996-
mersalate	T50.2x1-	T50.2x2-	T50.2x3-	T50.2x4-	T50.2x5-	T50.2x6-
metasilicate	T65.891-	T65.892-	T65.893-	T65.894-	—	—
metrizoate	T50.8x1-	T50.8x2-	T50.8x3-	T50.8x4-	T50.8x5-	T50.8x6-
monofluoroacetate (pesticide)	T60.1x1-	T60.1x2-	T60.1x3-	T60.1x4-	—	—
morrhuate	T46.8x1-	T46.8x2-	T46.8x3-	T46.8x4-	T46.8x5-	T46.8x6-
nafcillin	T36.0x1-	T36.0x2-	T36.0x3-	T36.0x4-	T36.0x5-	T36.0x6-
nitrate (oxidizing agent)	T65.891-	T65.892-	T65.893-	T65.894-	—	—
nitrite	T50.6x1-	T50.6x2-	T50.6x3-	T50.6x4-	T50.6x5-	T50.6x6-
nitroferricyanide	T46.5x1-	T46.5x2-	T46.5x3-	T46.5x4-	T46.5x5-	T46.5x6-
nitroprusside	T46.5x1-	T46.5x2-	T46.5x3-	T46.5x4-	T46.5x5-	T46.5x6-
oxalate	T65.891-	T65.892-	T65.893-	T65.894-	—	—
oxide/peroxide	T65.891-	T65.892-	T65.893-	T65.894-	—	—
oxybate	T41.291-	T41.292-	T41.293-	T41.294-	T41.295-	T41.296-
para-aminohippurate	T50.8x1-	T50.8x2-	T50.8x3-	T50.8x4-	T50.8x5-	T50.8x6-
perborate (nonmedicinal)						
NEC	T65.891-	T65.892-	T65.893-	T65.894-	—	—
medicinal	T49.0x1-	T49.0x2-	T49.0x3-	T49.0x4-	T49.0x5-	T49.0x6-
soap	T55.0x1-	T55.0x2-	T55.0x3-	T55.0x4-	—	—
percarbonate — *see* Sodium, perborate						
pertechnetate Tc99m	T50.8x1-	T50.8x2-	T50.8x3-	T50.8x4-	T50.8x5-	T50.8x6-
phosphate						
cellulose	T45.8x1-	T45.8x2-	T45.8x3-	T45.8x4-	T45.8x5-	T45.8x6-
dibasic	T47.2x1-	T47.2x2-	T47.2x3-	T47.2x4-	T47.2x5-	T47.2x6-
monobasic	T47.2x1-	T47.2x2-	T47.2x3-	T47.2x4-	T47.2x5-	T47.2x6-
phytate	T50.6x1-	T50.6x2-	T50.6x3-	T50.6x4-	T50.6x5-	T50.6x6-
picosulfate	T47.2x1-	T47.2x2-	T47.2x3-	T47.2x4-	T47.2x5-	T47.2x6-
polyhydroxyaluminium monocarbonate	T47.1x1-	T47.1x2-	T47.1x3-	T47.1x4-	T47.1x5-	T47.1x6-
polystyrene sulfonate	T50.3x1-	T50.3x2-	T50.3x3-	T50.3x4-	T50.3x5-	T50.3x6-
propionate	T49.0x1-	T49.0x2-	T49.0x3-	T49.0x4-	T49.0x5-	T49.0x6-
propyl hydroxybenzoate	T50.991-	T50.992-	T50.993-	T50.994-	T50.995-	T50.996-
psylliate	T46.8x1-	T46.8x2-	T46.8x3-	T46.8x4-	T46.8x5-	T46.8x6-
removing resins	T50.3x1-	T50.3x2-	T50.3x3-	T50.3x4-	T50.3x5-	T50.3x6-
salicylate	T39.091-	T39.092-	T39.093-	T39.094-	T39.095-	T39.096-
salt NEC	T50.3x1-	T50.3x2-	T50.3x3-	T50.3x4-	T50.3x5-	T50.3x6-
selenate	T60.2x1-	T60.2x2-	T60.2x3-	T60.2x4-	—	—
stibogluconate	T37.3x1-	T37.3x2-	T37.3x3-	T37.3x4-	T37.3x5-	T37.3x6-
sulfate	T47.4x1-	T47.4x2-	T47.4x3-	T47.4x4-	T47.4x5-	T47.4x6-
sulfoxone	T37.1x1-	T37.1x2-	T37.1x3-	T37.1x4-	T37.1x5-	T37.1x6-
tetradecyl sulfate	T46.8x1-	T46.8x2-	T46.8x3-	T46.8x4-	T46.8x5-	T46.8x6-
thiopental	T41.1x1-	T41.1x2-	T41.1x3-	T41.1x4-	T41.1x5-	T41.1x6-
thiosalicylate	T39.091-	T39.092-	T39.093-	T39.094-	T39.095-	T39.096-
thiosulfate	T50.6x1-	T50.6x2-	T50.6x3-	T50.6x4-	T50.6x5-	T50.6x6-
tolbutamide	T38.3x1-	T38.3x2-	T38.3x3-	T38.3x4-	T38.3x5-	T38.3x6-
tyropanoate	T50.8x1-	T50.8x2-	T50.8x3-	T50.8x4-	T50.8x5-	T50.8x6-
valproate	T42.6x1-	T42.6x2-	T42.6x3-	T42.6x4-	T42.6x5-	T42.6x6-
versenate	T50.6x1-	T50.6x2-	T50.6x3-	T50.6x4-	T50.6x5-	T50.6x6-
Sodium-free salt	T50.901-	T50.902-	T50.903-	T50.904-	T50.905-	T50.906-
Sodium-removing resin	T50.3x1-	T50.3x2-	T50.3x3-	T50.3x4-	T50.3x5-	T50.3x6-
Soft soap	T55.0x1-	T55.0x2-	T55.0x3-	T55.0x4-	—	—
Solanine	T62.2x1-	T62.2x2-	T62.2x3-	T62.2x4-	—	—
berries	T62.1x1-	T62.1x2-	T62.1x3-	T62.1x4-	—	—
Solanum dulcamara	T62.2x1-	T62.2x2-	T62.2x3-	T62.2x4-	—	—
berries	T62.1x1-	T62.1x2-	T62.1x3-	T62.1x4-	—	—
Solapsone	T37.1x1-	T37.1x2-	T37.1x3-	T37.1x4-	T37.1x5-	T37.1x6-
Solar lotion	T49.3x1-	T49.3x2-	T49.3x3-	T49.3x4-	T49.3x5-	T49.3x6-
Solasulfone	T37.1x1-	T37.1x2-	T37.1x3-	T37.1x4-	T37.1x5-	T37.1x6-

Table of Drugs & Chemicals	POISONING				Adverse Effect	Underdosing
	Accidental (Unintentional)	Self-Harm (Intentional)	Assault	Undetermined		
Soldering fluid	T65.891-	T65.892-	T65.893-	T65.894-	—	—
Solid substance	T65.91x-	T65.92x-	T65.93x-	T65.94x-	—	—
specified NEC	T65.891-	T65.892-	T65.893-	T65.894-	—	—
Solvent, industrial NEC	T52.91x-	T52.92x-	T52.93x-	T52.94x-	—	—
naphtha	T52.0x1-	T52.0x2-	T52.0x3-	T52.0x4-	—	—
petroleum	T52.0x1-	T52.0x2-	T52.0x3-	T52.0x4-	—	—
specified NEC	T52.8x1-	T52.8x2-	T52.8x3-	T52.8x4-	—	—
Soma	T42.8x1-	T42.8x2-	T42.8x3-	T42.8x4-	T42.8x5-	T42.8x6-
Somatorelin	T38.891-	T38.892-	T38.893-	T38.894-	T38.895-	T38.896-
Somatostatin	T38.991-	T38.992-	T38.993-	T38.994-	T38.995-	T38.996-
Somatotropin	T38.811-	T38.812-	T38.813-	T38.814-	T38.815-	T38.816-
Somatrem	T38.811-	T38.812-	T38.813-	T38.814-	T38.815-	T38.816-
Somatropin	T38.811-	T38.812-	T38.813-	T38.814-	T38.815-	T38.816-
Sominex	T45.0x1-	T45.0x2-	T45.0x3-	T45.0x4-	T45.0x5-	T45.0x6-
Somnos	T42.6x1-	T42.6x2-	T42.6x3-	T42.6x4-	T42.6x5-	T42.6x6-
Somonal	T42.3x1-	T42.3x2-	T42.3x3-	T42.3x4-	T42.3x5-	T42.3x6-
Soneryl	T42.3x1-	T42.3x2-	T42.3x3-	T42.3x4-	T42.3x5-	T42.3x6-
Soothing syrup	T50.901-	T50.902-	T50.903-	T50.904-	T50.905-	T50.906-
Sopor	T42.6x1-	T42.6x2-	T42.6x3-	T42.6x4-	T42.6x5-	T42.6x6-
Soporific	T42.71x-	T42.72x-	T42.73x-	T42.74x-	T42.75x-	T42.76x-
Soporific drug	T42.71x-	T42.72x-	T42.73x-	T42.74x-	T42.75x-	T42.76x-
specified type NEC	T42.6x1-	T42.6x2-	T42.6x3-	T42.6x4-	T42.6x5-	T42.6x6-
Sorbide nitrate	T46.3x1-	T46.3x2-	T46.3x3-	T46.3x4-	T46.3x5-	T46.3x6-
Sorbitol	T47.4x1-	T47.4x2-	T47.4x3-	T47.4x4-	T47.4x5-	T47.4x6-
Sotalol	T44.7x1-	T44.7x2-	T44.7x3-	T44.7x4-	T44.7x5-	T44.7x6-
Sotradecol	T46.8x1-	T46.8x2-	T46.8x3-	T46.8x4-	T46.8x5-	T46.8x6-
Soysterol	T46.6x1-	T46.6x2-	T46.6x3-	T46.6x4-	T46.6x5-	T46.6x6-
Spacoline	T44.3x1-	T44.3x2-	T44.3x3-	T44.3x4-	T44.3x5-	T44.3x6-
Spanish fly	T49.8x1-	T49.8x2-	T49.8x3-	T49.8x4-	T49.8x5-	T49.8x6-
Sparine	T43.3x1-	T43.3x2-	T43.3x3-	T43.3x4-	T43.3x5-	T43.3x6-
Sparteine	T48.0x1-	T48.0x2-	T48.0x3-	T48.0x4-	T48.0x5-	T48.0x6-
Spasmolytic						
anticholinergics	T44.3x1-	T44.3x2-	T44.3x3-	T44.3x4-	T44.3x5-	T44.3x6-
autonomic	T44.3x1-	T44.3x2-	T44.3x3-	T44.3x4-	T44.3x5-	T44.3x6-
bronchial NEC	T48.6x1-	T48.6x2-	T48.6x3-	T48.6x4-	T48.6x5-	T48.6x6-
quaternary ammonium	T44.3x1-	T44.3x2-	T44.3x3-	T44.3x4-	T44.3x5-	T44.3x6-
skeletal muscle NEC	T48.1x1-	T48.1x2-	T48.1x3-	T48.1x4-	T48.1x5-	T48.1x6-
Spectinomycin	T36.5x1-	T36.5x2-	T36.5x3-	T36.5x4-	T36.5x5-	T36.5x6-
Speed	T43.621-	T43.622-	T43.623-	T43.624-	T43.625-	T43.626-
Spermicide	T49.8x1-	T49.8x2-	T49.8x3-	T49.8x4-	T49.8x5-	T49.8x6-
Spider (bite) (venom)	T63.391-	T63.392-	T63.393-	T63.394-	—	—
antivenin	T50.Z11-	T50.Z12-	T50.Z13-	T50.Z14-	T50.Z15-	T50.Z16-
Spigelia (root)	T37.4x1-	T37.4x2-	T37.4x3-	T37.4x4-	T37.4x5-	T37.4x6-
Spindle inactivator	T50.4x1-	T50.4x2-	T50.4x3-	T50.4x4-	T50.4x5-	T50.4x6-
Spiperone	T43.4x1-	T43.4x2-	T43.4x3-	T43.4x4-	T43.4x5-	T43.4x6-
Spiramycin	T36.3x1-	T36.3x2-	T36.3x3-	T36.3x4-	T36.3x5-	T36.3x6-
Spirapril	T46.4x1-	T46.4x2-	T46.4x3-	T46.4x4-	T46.4x5-	T46.4x6-
Spirilene	T43.591-	T43.592-	T43.593-	T43.594-	T43.595-	T43.596-
Spirit (s) (neutral) NEC	T51.0x1-	T51.0x2-	T51.0x3-	T51.0x4-	—	—
beverage	T51.0x1-	T51.0x2-	T51.0x3-	T51.0x4-	—	—
industrial	T51.0x1-	T51.0x2-	T51.0x3-	T51.0x4-	—	—
mineral	T52.0x1-	T52.0x2-	T52.0x3-	T52.0x4-	—	—
of salt — see Hydrochloric acid						
surgical	T51.0x1-	T51.0x2-	T51.0x3-	T51.0x4-	—	—
Spironolactone	T50.0x1-	T50.0x2-	T50.0x3-	T50.0x4-	T50.0x5-	T50.0x6-
Spiroperidol	T43.4x1-	T43.4x2-	T43.4x3-	T43.4x4-	T43.4x5-	T43.4x6-
Sponge, absorbable (gelatin)	T45.7x1-	T45.7x2-	T45.7x3-	T45.7x4-	T45.7x5-	T45.7x6-
Sporostacin	T49.0x1-	T49.0x2-	T49.0x3-	T49.0x4-	T49.0x5-	T49.0x6-

Table of Drugs & Chemicals	POISONING				Adverse Effect	Underdosing
	Accidental (Unintentional)	Self-Harm (Intentional)	Assault	Undetermined		
Spray (aerosol)	T65.91x-	T65.92x-	T65.93x-	T65.94x-	—	—
cosmetic	T65.891-	T65.892-	T65.893-	T65.894-	—	—
medicinal NEC	T50.901-	T50.902-	T50.903-	T50.904-	T50.905-	T50.906-
pesticides — see Pesticides						
specified content — see specific substance						
Spurge flax	T62.2x1-	T62.2x2-	T62.2x3-	T62.2x4-	—	—
Spurges	T62.2x1-	T62.2x2-	T62.2x3-	T62.2x4-	—	—
Sputum viscosity-lowering drug	T48.4x1-	T48.4x2-	T48.4x3-	T48.4x4-	T48.4x5-	T48.4x6-
Squill	T46.0x1-	T46.0x2-	T46.0x3-	T46.0x4-	T46.0x5-	T46.0x6-
rat poison	T60.4x1-	T60.4x2-	T60.4x3-	T60.4x4-	—	—
Squirting cucumber (cathartic)	T47.2x1-	T47.2x2-	T47.2x3-	T47.2x4-	T47.2x5-	T47.2x6-
Stains	T65.6x1-	T65.6x2-	T65.6x3-	T65.6x4-	—	—
Stannous fluoride	T49.7x1-	T49.7x2-	T49.7x3-	T49.7x4-	T49.7x5-	T49.7x6-
Stanolone	T38.7x1-	T38.7x2-	T38.7x3-	T38.7x4-	T38.7x5-	T38.7x6-
Stanozolol	T38.7x1-	T38.7x2-	T38.7x3-	T38.7x4-	T38.7x5-	T38.7x6-
Staphisagria or stavesacre (pediculicide)	T49.0x1-	T49.0x2-	T49.0x3-	T49.0x4-	T49.0x5-	T49.0x6-
Starch	T50.901-	T50.902-	T50.903-	T50.904-	T50.905-	T50.906-
Stelazine	T43.3x1-	T43.3x2-	T43.3x3-	T43.3x4-	T43.3x5-	T43.3x6-
Stemetil	T43.3x1-	T43.3x2-	T43.3x3-	T43.3x4-	T43.3x5-	T43.3x6-
Stepronin	T48.4x1-	T48.4x2-	T48.4x3-	T48.4x4-	T48.4x5-	T48.4x6-
Sterculia	T47.4x1-	T47.4x2-	T47.4x3-	T47.4x4-	T47.4x5-	T47.4x6-
Sternutator gas	T59.891-	T59.892-	T59.893-	T59.894-	—	—
Steroid	T38.0x1-	T38.0x2-	T38.0x3-	T38.0x4-	T38.0x5-	T38.0x6-
anabolic	T38.7x1-	T38.7x2-	T38.7x3-	T38.7x4-	T38.7x5-	T38.7x6-
androgenic	T38.7x1-	T38.7x2-	T38.7x3-	T38.7x4-	T38.7x5-	T38.7x6-
antineoplastic, hormone	T38.7x1-	T38.7x2-	T38.7x3-	T38.7x4-	T38.7x5-	T38.7x6-
estrogen	T38.5x1-	T38.5x2-	T38.5x3-	T38.5x4-	T38.5x5-	T38.5x6-
ENT agent	T49.6x1-	T49.6x2-	T49.6x3-	T49.6x4-	T49.6x5-	T49.6x6-
ophthalmic preparation	T49.5x1-	T49.5x2-	T49.5x3-	T49.5x4-	T49.5x5-	T49.5x6-
topical NEC	T49.0x1-	T49.0x2-	T49.0x3-	T49.0x4-	T49.0x5-	T49.0x6-
Stibine	T56.891-	T56.892-	T56.893-	T56.894-	—	—
Stibogluconate	T37.3x1-	T37.3x2-	T37.3x3-	T37.3x4-	T37.3x5-	T37.3x6-
Stibophen	T37.4x1-	T37.4x2-	T37.4x3-	T37.4x4-	T37.4x5-	T37.4x6-
Stilbamidine (isetionate)	T37.3x1-	T37.3x2-	T37.3x3-	T37.3x4-	T37.3x5-	T37.3x6-
Stilbestrol	T38.5x1-	T38.5x2-	T38.5x3-	T38.5x4-	T38.5x5-	T38.5x6-
Stilboestrol	T38.5x1-	T38.5x2-	T38.5x3-	T38.5x4-	T38.5x5-	T38.5x6-
Stimulant						
central nervous system — see also Psychostimulant	T43.601-	T43.602-	T43.603-	T43.604-	T43.605-	T43.606-
analeptics	T50.7x1-	T50.7x2-	T50.7x3-	T50.7x4-	T50.7x5-	T50.7x6-
opiate antagonist	T50.7x1-	T50.7x2-	T50.7x3-	T50.7x4-	T50.7x5-	T50.7x6-
psychotherapeutic NEC — see also Psychotherapeutic drug	T43.601-	T43.602-	T43.603-	T43.604-	T43.605-	T43.606-
specified NEC	T43.691-	T43.692-	T43.693-	T43.694-	T43.695-	T43.696-
respiratory	T48.901-	T48.902-	T48.903-	T48.904-	T48.905-	T48.906-
Stone-dissolving drug	T50.901-	T50.902-	T50.903-	T50.904-	T50.905-	T50.906-
Storage battery (cells) (acid)	T54.2x1-	T54.2x2-	T54.2x3-	T54.2x4-	—	—
Stovaine	T41.3x1-	T41.3x2-	T41.3x3-	T41.3x4-	T41.3x5-	T41.3x6-
infiltration (subcutaneous)	T41.3x1-	T41.3x2-	T41.3x3-	T41.3x4-	T41.3x5-	T41.3x6-
nerve block (peripheral) (plexus)	T41.3x1-	T41.3x2-	T41.3x3-	T41.3x4-	T41.3x5-	T41.3x6-
spinal	T41.3x1-	T41.3x2-	T41.3x3-	T41.3x4-	T41.3x5-	T41.3x6-
topical (surface)	T41.3x1-	T41.3x2-	T41.3x3-	T41.3x4-	T41.3x5-	T41.3x6-

Table of Drugs & Chemicals	Poisoning Accidental (Unintentional)	Poisoning Self-Harm (Intentional)	Assault	Undetermined	Adverse Effect	Underdosing
Stovarsal	T37.8x1-	T37.8x2-	T37.8x3-	T37.8x4-	T37.8x5-	T37.8x6-
Stove gas — see Gas, stove						
Stoxil	T49.5x1-	T49.5x2-	T49.5x3-	T49.5x4-	T49.5x5-	T49.5x6-
Stramonium	T48.6x1-	T48.6x2-	T48.6x3-	T48.6x4-	T48.6x5-	T48.6x6-
natural state	T62.2x1-	T62.2x2-	T62.2x3-	T62.2x4-	—	—
Streptodornase	T45.3x1-	T45.3x2-	T45.3x3-	T45.3x4-	T45.3x5-	T45.3x6-
Streptoduocin	T36.5x1-	T36.5x2-	T36.5x3-	T36.5x4-	T36.5x5-	T36.5x6-
Streptokinase	T45.611-	T45.612-	T45.613-	T45.614-	T45.615-	T45.616-
Streptomycin (derivative)	T36.5x1-	T36.5x2-	T36.5x3-	T36.5x4-	T36.5x5-	T36.5x6-
Streptonivicin	T36.5x1-	T36.5x2-	T36.5x3-	T36.5x4-	T36.5x5-	T36.5x6-
Streptovarycin	T36.5x1-	T36.5x2-	T36.5x3-	T36.5x4-	T36.5x5-	T36.5x6-
Streptozocin	T45.1x1-	T45.1x2-	T45.1x3-	T45.1x4-	T45.1x5-	T45.1x6-
Streptozotocin	T45.1x1-	T45.1x2-	T45.1x3-	T45.1x4-	T45.1x5-	T45.1x6-
Stripper (paint) (solvent)	T52.8x1-	T52.8x2-	T52.8x3-	T52.8x4-	—	—
Strobane	T60.1x1-	T60.1x2-	T60.1x3-	T60.1x4-	—	—
Strofantina	T46.0x1-	T46.0x2-	T46.0x3-	T46.0x4-	T46.0x5-	T46.0x6-
Strophanthin (g) (k)	T46.0x1-	T46.0x2-	T46.0x3-	T46.0x4-	T46.0x5-	T46.0x6-
Strophanthus	T46.0x1-	T46.0x2-	T46.0x3-	T46.0x4-	T46.0x5-	T46.0x6-
Strophantin	T46.0x1-	T46.0x2-	T46.0x3-	T46.0x4-	T46.0x5-	T46.0x6-
Strophantin-g	T46.0x1-	T46.0x2-	T46.0x3-	T46.0x4-	T46.0x5-	T46.0x6-
Strychnine (nonmedicinal) (pesticide) (salts)	T65.1x1-	T65.1x2-	T65.1x3-	T65.1x4-	—	—
medicinal	T48.291-	T48.292-	T48.293-	T48.294-	T48.295-	T48.296-
Strychnos (ignatii) — see Strychnine						
Styramate	T42.8x1-	T42.8x2-	T42.8x3-	T42.8x4-	T42.8x5-	T42.8x6-
Styrene	T65.891-	T65.892-	T65.893-	T65.894-		
Succinimide, antiepileptic or anticonvulsant	T42.2x1-	T42.2x2-	T42.2x3-	T42.2x4-	T42.2x5-	T42.2x6-
mercuric — see Mercury						
Succinylcholine	T48.1x1-	T48.1x2-	T48.1x3-	T48.1x4-	T48.1x5-	T48.1x6-
Succinylsulfathiazole	T37.0x1-	T37.0x2-	T37.0x3-	T37.0x4-	T37.0x5-	T37.0x6-
Sucralfate	T47.1x1-	T47.1x2-	T47.1x3-	T47.1x4-	T47.1x5-	T47.1x6-
Sucrose	T50.3x1-	T50.3x2-	T50.3x3-	T50.3x4-	T50.3x5-	T50.3x6-
Sufentanil	T40.4x1-	T40.4x2-	T40.4x3-	T40.4x4-	T40.4x5-	T40.4x6-
Sulbactam	T36.0x1-	T36.0x2-	T36.0x3-	T36.0x4-	T36.0x5-	T36.0x6-
Sulbenicillin	T36.0x1-	T36.0x2-	T36.0x3-	T36.0x4-	T36.0x5-	T36.0x6-
Sulbentine	T49.0x1-	T49.0x2-	T49.0x3-	T49.0x4-	T49.0x5-	T49.0x6-
Sulfacetamide	T49.0x1-	T49.0x2-	T49.0x3-	T49.0x4-	T49.0x5-	T49.0x6-
ophthalmic preparation	T49.5x1-	T49.5x2-	T49.5x3-	T49.5x4-	T49.5x5-	T49.5x6-
Sulfachlorpyridazine	T37.0x1-	T37.0x2-	T37.0x3-	T37.0x4-	T37.0x5-	T37.0x6-
Sulfacitine	T37.0x1-	T37.0x2-	T37.0x3-	T37.0x4-	T37.0x5-	T37.0x6-
Sulfadiasulfone sodium	T37.0x1-	T37.0x2-	T37.0x3-	T37.0x4-	T37.0x5-	T37.0x6-
Sulfadiazine	T37.0x1-	T37.0x2-	T37.0x3-	T37.0x4-	T37.0x5-	T37.0x6-
silver (topical)	T49.0x1-	T49.0x2-	T49.0x3-	T49.0x4-	T49.0x5-	T49.0x6-
Sulfadimethoxine	T37.0x1-	T37.0x2-	T37.0x3-	T37.0x4-	T37.0x5-	T37.0x6-
Sulfadimidine	T37.0x1-	T37.0x2-	T37.0x3-	T37.0x4-	T37.0x5-	T37.0x6-
Sulfadoxine	T37.0x1-	T37.0x2-	T37.0x3-	T37.0x4-	T37.0x5-	T37.0x6-
with pyrimethamine	T37.2x1-	T37.2x2-	T37.2x3-	T37.2x4-	T37.2x5-	T37.2x6-
Sulfaethidole	T37.0x1-	T37.0x2-	T37.0x3-	T37.0x4-	T37.0x5-	T37.0x6-
Sulfafurazole	T37.0x1-	T37.0x2-	T37.0x3-	T37.0x4-	T37.0x5-	T37.0x6-
Sulfaguanidine	T37.0x1-	T37.0x2-	T37.0x3-	T37.0x4-	T37.0x5-	T37.0x6-
Sulfalene	T37.0x1-	T37.0x2-	T37.0x3-	T37.0x4-	T37.0x5-	T37.0x6-
Sulfaloxate	T37.0x1-	T37.0x2-	T37.0x3-	T37.0x4-	T37.0x5-	T37.0x6-
Sulfaloxic acid	T37.0x1-	T37.0x2-	T37.0x3-	T37.0x4-	T37.0x5-	T37.0x6-
Sulfamazone	T39.2x1-	T39.2x2-	T39.2x3-	T39.2x4-	T39.2x5-	T39.2x6-
Sulfamerazine	T37.0x1-	T37.0x2-	T37.0x3-	T37.0x4-	T37.0x5-	T37.0x6-
Sulfameter	T37.0x1-	T37.0x2-	T37.0x3-	T37.0x4-	T37.0x5-	T37.0x6-
Sulfamethazine	T37.0x1-	T37.0x2-	T37.0x3-	T37.0x4-	T37.0x5-	T37.0x6-
Sulfamethizole	T37.0x1-	T37.0x2-	T37.0x3-	T37.0x4-	T37.0x5-	T37.0x6-

Table of Drugs & Chemicals	Poisoning Accidental (Unintentional)	Poisoning Self-Harm (Intentional)	Assault	Undetermined	Adverse Effect	Underdosing
Sulfamethoxazole	T37.0x1-	T37.0x2-	T37.0x3-	T37.0x4-	T37.0x5-	T37.0x6-
with trimethoprim	T36.8x1-	T36.8x2-	T36.8x3-	T36.8x4-	T36.8x5-	T36.8x6-
Sulfamethoxydiazine	T37.0x1-	T37.0x2-	T37.0x3-	T37.0x4-	T37.0x5-	T37.0x6-
Sulfamethoxypyridazine	T37.0x1-	T37.0x2-	T37.0x3-	T37.0x4-	T37.0x5-	T37.0x6-
Sulfamethylthiazole	T37.0x1-	T37.0x2-	T37.0x3-	T37.0x4-	T37.0x5-	T37.0x6-
Sulfametoxydiazine	T37.0x1-	T37.0x2-	T37.0x3-	T37.0x4-	T37.0x5-	T37.0x6-
Sulfamidopyrine	T39.2x1-	T39.2x2-	T39.2x3-	T39.2x4-	T39.2x5-	T39.2x6-
Sulfamonomethoxine	T37.0x1-	T37.0x2-	T37.0x3-	T37.0x4-	T37.0x5-	T37.0x6-
Sulfamoxole	T37.0x1-	T37.0x2-	T37.0x3-	T37.0x4-	T37.0x5-	T37.0x6-
Sulfamylon	T49.0x1-	T49.0x2-	T49.0x3-	T49.0x4-	T49.0x5-	T49.0x6-
Sulfan blue (diagnostic dye)	T50.8x1-	T50.8x2-	T50.8x3-	T50.8x4-	T50.8x5-	T50.8x6-
Sulfanilamide	T37.0x1-	T37.0x2-	T37.0x3-	T37.0x4-	T37.0x5-	T37.0x6-
Sulfanilylguanidine	T37.0x1-	T37.0x2-	T37.0x3-	T37.0x4-	T37.0x5-	T37.0x6-
Sulfaperin	T37.0x1-	T37.0x2-	T37.0x3-	T37.0x4-	T37.0x5-	T37.0x6-
Sulfaphenazole	T37.0x1-	T37.0x2-	T37.0x3-	T37.0x4-	T37.0x5-	T37.0x6-
Sulfaphenylthiazole	T37.0x1-	T37.0x2-	T37.0x3-	T37.0x4-	T37.0x5-	T37.0x6-
Sulfaproxyline	T37.0x1-	T37.0x2-	T37.0x3-	T37.0x4-	T37.0x5-	T37.0x6-
Sulfapyridine	T37.0x1-	T37.0x2-	T37.0x3-	T37.0x4-	T37.0x5-	T37.0x6-
Sulfapyrimidine	T37.0x1-	T37.0x2-	T37.0x3-	T37.0x4-	T37.0x5-	T37.0x6-
Sulfarsphenamine	T37.8x1-	T37.8x2-	T37.8x3-	T37.8x4-	T37.8x5-	T37.8x6-
Sulfasalazine	T37.0x1-	T37.0x2-	T37.0x3-	T37.0x4-	T37.0x5-	T37.0x6-
Sulfasuxidine	T37.0x1-	T37.0x2-	T37.0x3-	T37.0x4-	T37.0x5-	T37.0x6-
Sulfasymazine	T37.0x1-	T37.0x2-	T37.0x3-	T37.0x4-	T37.0x5-	T37.0x6-
Sulfated amylopectin	T47.8x1-	T47.8x2-	T47.8x3-	T47.8x4-	T47.8x5-	T47.8x6-
Sulfathiazole	T37.0x1-	T37.0x2-	T37.0x3-	T37.0x4-	T37.0x5-	T37.0x6-
Sulfatostearate	T49.2x1-	T49.2x2-	T49.2x3-	T49.2x4-	T49.2x5-	T49.2x6-
Sulfinpyrazone	T50.4x1-	T50.4x2-	T50.4x3-	T50.4x4-	T50.4x5-	T50.4x6-
Sulfiram	T49.0x1-	T49.0x2-	T49.0x3-	T49.0x4-	T49.0x5-	T49.0x6-
Sulfisomidine	T37.0x1-	T37.0x2-	T37.0x3-	T37.0x4-	T37.0x5-	T37.0x6-
Sulfisoxazole	T37.0x1-	T37.0x2-	T37.0x3-	T37.0x4-	T37.0x5-	T37.0x6-
ophthalmic preparation	T49.5x1-	T49.5x2-	T49.5x3-	T49.5x4-	T49.5x5-	T49.5x6-
Sulfobromophthalein (sodium)	T50.8x1-	T50.8x2-	T50.8x3-	T50.8x4-	T50.8x5-	T50.8x6-
Sulfobromphthalein	T50.8x1-	T50.8x2-	T50.8x3-	T50.8x4-	T50.8x5-	T50.8x6-
Sulfogaiacol	T48.4x1-	T48.4x2-	T48.4x3-	T48.4x4-	T48.4x5-	T48.4x6-
Sulfomyxin	T36.8x1-	T36.8x2-	T36.8x3-	T36.8x4-	T36.8x5-	T36.8x6-
Sulfonal	T42.6x1-	T42.6x2-	T42.6x3-	T42.6x4-	T42.6x5-	T42.6x6-
Sulfonamide NEC	T37.0x1-	T37.0x2-	T37.0x3-	T37.0x4-	T37.0x5-	T37.0x6-
eye	T49.5x1-	T49.5x2-	T49.5x3-	T49.5x4-	T49.5x5-	T49.5x6-
Sulfonazide	T37.1x1-	T37.1x2-	T37.1x3-	T37.1x4-	T37.1x5-	T37.1x6-
Sulfones	T37.1x1-	T37.1x2-	T37.1x3-	T37.1x4-	T37.1x5-	T37.1x6-
Sulfonethylmethane	T42.6x1-	T42.6x2-	T42.6x3-	T42.6x4-	T42.6x5-	T42.6x6-
Sulfonmethane	T42.6x1-	T42.6x2-	T42.6x3-	T42.6x4-	T42.6x5-	T42.6x6-
Sulfonphthal, sulfonphthol	T50.8x1-	T50.8x2-	T50.8x3-	T50.8x4-	T50.8x5-	T50.8x6-
Sulfonylurea derivatives, oral	T38.3x1-	T38.3x2-	T38.3x3-	T38.3x4-	T38.3x5-	T38.3x6-
Sulforidazine	T43.3x1-	T43.3x2-	T43.3x3-	T43.3x4-	T43.3x5-	T43.3x6-
Sulfoxone	T37.1x1-	T37.1x2-	T37.1x3-	T37.1x4-	T37.1x5-	T37.1x6-
Sulfur, sulfurated, sulfuric, sulfurous, sulfuryl (compounds NEC) (medicinal)	T49.4x1-	T49.4x2-	T49.4x3-	T49.4x4-	T49.4x5-	T49.4x6-
acid	T54.2x1-	T54.2x2-	T54.2x3-	T54.2x4-	—	—
dioxide (gas)	T59.1x1-	T59.1x2-	T59.1x3-	T59.1x4-	—	—
ether — see Ether(s)						
hydrogen	T59.6x1-	T59.6x2-	T59.6x3-	T59.6x4-	—	—
medicinal (keratolytic) (ointment) NEC	T49.4x1-	T49.4x2-	T49.4x3-	T49.4x4-	T49.4x5-	T49.4x6-
ointment	T49.0x1-	T49.0x2-	T49.0x3-	T49.0x4-	T49.0x5-	T49.0x6-
pesticide (vapor)	T60.91x-	T60.92x-	T60.93x-	T60.94x-	—	—
vapor NEC	T59.891-	T59.892-	T59.893-	T59.894-	—	—

DRUGS & CHEMICALS

Table of Drugs & Chemicals	POISONING Accidental (Unintentional)	Self-Harm (Intentional)	Assault	Undetermined	Adverse Effect	Underdosing
Sulfuric acid	T54.2x1-	T54.2x2-	T54.2x3-	T54.2x4-	—	—
Sulglicotide	T47.1x1-	T47.1x2-	T47.1x3-	T47.1x4-	T47.1x5-	T47.1x6-
Sulindac	T39.391-	T39.392-	T39.393-	T39.394-	T39.395-	T39.396-
Sulisatin	T47.2x1-	T47.2x2-	T47.2x3-	T47.2x4-	T47.2x5-	T47.2x6-
Sulisobenzone	T49.3x1-	T49.3x2-	T49.3x3-	T49.3x4-	T49.3x5-	T49.3x6-
Sulkowitch's reagent	T50.8x1-	T50.8x2-	T50.8x3-	T50.8x4-	T50.8x5-	T50.8x6-
Sulmetozine	T44.3x1-	T44.3x2-	T44.3x3-	T44.3x4-	T44.3x5-	T44.3x6-
Suloctidil	T46.7x1-	T46.7x2-	T46.7x3-	T46.7x4-	T46.7x5-	T46.7x6-
Sulph- — see also Sulf-						
Sulphadiazine	T37.0x1-	T37.0x2-	T37.0x3-	T37.0x4-	T37.0x5-	T37.0x6-
Sulphadimethoxine	T37.0x1-	T37.0x2-	T37.0x3-	T37.0x4-	T37.0x5-	T37.0x6-
Sulphadimidine	T37.0x1-	T37.0x2-	T37.0x3-	T37.0x4-	T37.0x5-	T37.0x6-
Sulphadione	T37.1x1-	T37.1x2-	T37.1x3-	T37.1x4-	T37.1x5-	T37.1x6-
Sulphafurazole	T37.0x1-	T37.0x2-	T37.0x3-	T37.0x4-	T37.0x5-	T37.0x6-
Sulphamethizole	T37.0x1-	T37.0x2-	T37.0x3-	T37.0x4-	T37.0x5-	T37.0x6-
Sulphamethoxazole	T37.0x1-	T37.0x2-	T37.0x3-	T37.0x4-	T37.0x5-	T37.0x6-
Sulphan blue	T50.8x1-	T50.8x2-	T50.8x3-	T50.8x4-	T50.8x5-	T50.8x6-
Sulphaphenazole	T37.0x1-	T37.0x2-	T37.0x3-	T37.0x4-	T37.0x5-	T37.0x6-
Sulphapyridine	T37.0x1-	T37.0x2-	T37.0x3-	T37.0x4-	T37.0x5-	T37.0x6-
Sulphasalazine	T37.0x1-	T37.0x2-	T37.0x3-	T37.0x4-	T37.0x5-	T37.0x6-
Sulphinpyrazone	T50.4x1-	T50.4x2-	T50.4x3-	T50.4x4-	T50.4x5-	T50.4x6-
Sulpiride	T43.591-	T43.592-	T43.593-	T43.594-	T43.595-	T43.596-
Sulprostone	T48.0x1-	T48.0x2-	T48.0x3-	T48.0x4-	T48.0x5-	T48.0x6-
Sulpyrine	T39.2x1-	T39.2x2-	T39.2x3-	T39.2x4-	T39.2x5-	T39.2x6-
Sultamicillin	T36.0x1-	T36.0x2-	T36.0x3-	T36.0x4-	T36.0x5-	T36.0x6-
Sulthiame	T42.6x1-	T42.6x2-	T42.6x3-	T42.6x4-	T42.6x5-	T42.6x6-
Sultiame	T42.6x1-	T42.6x2-	T42.6x3-	T42.6x4-	T42.6x5-	T42.6x6-
Sultopride	T43.591-	T43.592-	T43.593-	T43.594-	T43.595-	T43.596-
Sumatriptan	T39.8x1-	T39.8x2-	T39.8x3-	T39.8x4-	T39.8x5-	T39.8x6-
Sunflower seed oil	T46.6x1-	T46.6x2-	T46.6x3-	T46.6x4-	T46.6x5-	T46.6x6-
Superinone	T48.4x1-	T48.4x2-	T48.4x3-	T48.4x4-	T48.4x5-	T48.4x6-
Suprofen	T39.311-	T39.312-	T39.313-	T39.314-	T39.315-	T39.316-
Suramin (sodium)	T37.4x1-	T37.4x2-	T37.4x3-	T37.4x4-	T37.4x5-	T37.4x6-
Surfacaine	T41.3x1-	T41.3x2-	T41.3x3-	T41.3x4-	T41.3x5-	T41.3x6-
Surital	T41.1x1-	T41.1x2-	T41.1x3-	T41.1x4-	T41.1x5-	T41.1x6-
Sutilains	T45.3x1-	T45.3x2-	T45.3x3-	T45.3x4-	T45.3x5-	T45.3x6-
Suxamethonium (chloride)	T48.1x1-	T48.1x2-	T48.1x3-	T48.1x4-	T48.1x5-	T48.1x6-
Suxethonium (chloride)	T48.1x1-	T48.1x2-	T48.1x3-	T48.1x4-	T48.1x5-	T48.1x6-
Suxibuzone	T39.2x1-	T39.2x2-	T39.2x3-	T39.2x4-	T39.2x5-	T39.2x6-
Sweet niter spirit	T46.3x1-	T46.3x2-	T46.3x3-	T46.3x4-	T46.3x5-	T46.3x6-
Sweet oil (birch)	T49.3x1-	T49.3x2-	T49.3x3-	T49.3x4-	T49.3x5-	T49.3x6-
Sweetener	T50.901-	T50.902-	T50.903-	T50.904-	T50.905-	T50.906-
Sym-dichloroethyl ether	T53.6x1-	T53.6x2-	T53.6x3-	T53.6x4-	—	—
Sympatholytic NEC	T44.8x1-	T44.8x2-	T44.8x3-	T44.8x4-	T44.8x5-	T44.8x6-
haloalkylamine	T44.8x1-	T44.8x2-	T44.8x3-	T44.8x4-	T44.8x5-	T44.8x6-
Sympathomimetic NEC	T44.901-	T44.902-	T44.903-	T44.904-	T44.905-	T44.906-
anti-common-cold	T48.5x1-	T48.5x2-	T48.5x3-	T48.5x4-	T48.5x5-	T48.5x6-
bronchodilator	T48.6x1-	T48.6x2-	T48.6x3-	T48.6x4-	T48.6x5-	T48.6x6-
specified NEC	T44.991-	T44.992-	T44.993-	T44.994-	T44.995-	T44.996-
Synagis	T50.B91-	T50.B92-	T50.B93-	T50.B94-	T50.B95-	T50.B96-
Synalar	T49.0x1-	T49.0x2-	T49.0x3-	T49.0x4-	T49.0x5-	T49.0x6-
Synthroid	T38.1x1-	T38.1x2-	T38.1x3-	T38.1x4-	T38.1x5-	T38.1x6-
Syntocinon	T48.0x1-	T48.0x2-	T48.0x3-	T48.0x4-	T48.0x5-	T48.0x6-
Syrosingopine	T46.5x1-	T46.5x2-	T46.5x3-	T46.5x4-	T46.5x5-	T46.5x6-
Systemic drug	T45.91x-	T45.92x-	T45.93x-	T45.94x-	T45.95x-	T45.96x-
specified NEC	T45.8x1-	T45.8x2-	T45.8x3-	T45.8x4-	T45.8x5-	T45.8x6-

Table of Drugs & Chemicals	POISONING Accidental (Unintentional)	Self-Harm (Intentional)	Assault	Undetermined	Adverse Effect	Underdosing
2,4,5-T	T60.3x1-	T60.3x2-	T60.3x3-	T60.3x4-	—	—
Tablets — see also specified substance	T50.901-	T50.902-	T50.903-	T50.904-	T50.905-	T50.906-
Tace	T38.5x1-	T38.5x2-	T38.5x3-	T38.5x4-	T38.5x5-	T38.5x6-
Tacrine	T44.0x1-	T44.0x2-	T44.0x3-	T44.0x4-	T44.0x5-	T44.0x6-
Tadalafil	T46.7x1-	T46.7x2-	T46.7x3-	T46.7x4-	T46.7x5-	T46.7x6-
Talampicillin	T36.0x1-	T36.0x2-	T36.0x3-	T36.0x4-	T36.0x5-	T36.0x6-
Talbutal	T42.3x1-	T42.3x2-	T42.3x3-	T42.3x4-	T42.3x5-	T42.3x6-
Talc powder	T49.3x1-	T49.3x2-	T49.3x3-	T49.3x4-	T49.3x5-	T49.3x6-
Talcum	T49.3x1-	T49.3x2-	T49.3x3-	T49.3x4-	T49.3x5-	T49.3x6-
Taleranol	T38.6x1-	T38.6x2-	T38.6x3-	T38.6x4-	T38.6x5-	T38.6x6-
Tamoxifen	T38.6x1-	T38.6x2-	T38.6x3-	T38.6x4-	T38.6x5-	T38.6x6-
Tamsulosin	T44.6x1-	T44.6x2-	T44.6x3-	T44.6x4-	T44.6x5-	T44.6x6-
Tandearil, tanderil	T39.2x1-	T39.2x2-	T39.2x3-	T39.2x4-	T39.2x5-	T39.2x6-
Tannic acid	T49.2x1-	T49.2x2-	T49.2x3-	T49.2x4-	T49.2x5-	T49.2x6-
medicinal (astringent)	T49.2x1-	T49.2x2-	T49.2x3-	T49.2x4-	T49.2x5-	T49.2x6-
Tannin — see Tannic acid						
Tansy	T62.2x1-	T62.2x2-	T62.2x3-	T62.2x4-	—	—
TAO	T36.3x1-	T36.3x2-	T36.3x3-	T36.3x4-	T36.3x5-	T36.3x6-
Tapazole	T38.2x1-	T38.2x2-	T38.2x3-	T38.2x4-	T38.2x5-	T38.2x6-
Tar NEC	T52.0x1-	T52.0x2-	T52.0x3-	T52.0x4-	—	—
camphor	T60.1x1-	T60.1x2-	T60.1x3-	T60.1x4-	—	—
distillate	T49.1x1-	T49.1x2-	T49.1x3-	T49.1x4-	T49.1x5-	T49.1x6-
fumes	T59.891-	T59.892-	T59.893-	T59.894-	—	—
medicinal	T49.1x1-	T49.1x2-	T49.1x3-	T49.1x4-	T49.1x5-	T49.1x6-
ointment	T49.1x1-	T49.1x2-	T49.1x3-	T49.1x4-	T49.1x5-	T49.1x6-
Taractan	T43.591-	T43.592-	T43.593-	T43.594-	T43.595-	T43.596-
Tarantula (venomous)	T63.321-	T63.322-	T63.323-	T63.324-	—	—
Tartar emetic	T37.8x1-	T37.8x2-	T37.8x3-	T37.8x4-	T37.8x5-	T37.8x6-
Tartaric acid	T65.891-	T65.892-	T65.893-	T65.894-	—	—
Tartrate, laxative	T47.4x1-	T47.4x2-	T47.4x3-	T47.4x4-	T47.4x5-	T47.4x6-
Tartrated antimony (anti-infective)	T37.8x1-	T37.8x2-	T37.8x3-	T37.8x4-	T37.8x5-	T37.8x6-
Tauromustine	T45.1x1-	T45.1x2-	T45.1x3-	T45.1x4-	T45.1x5-	T45.1x6-
TCA — see Trichloroacetic acid						
TCDD	T53.7x1-	T53.7x2-	T53.7x3-	T53.7x4-	—	—
TDI (vapor)	T65.0x1-	T65.0x2-	T65.0x3-	T65.0x4-	—	—
Tear						
gas	T59.3x1-	T59.3x2-	T59.3x3-	T59.3x4-	—	—
solution	T49.5x1-	T49.5x2-	T49.5x3-	T49.5x4-	T49.5x5-	T49.5x6-
Teclothiazide	T50.2x1-	T50.2x2-	T50.2x3-	T50.2x4-	T50.2x5-	T50.2x6-
Teclozan	T37.3x1-	T37.3x2-	T37.3x3-	T37.3x4-	T37.3x5-	T37.3x6-
Tegafur	T45.1x1-	T45.1x2-	T45.1x3-	T45.1x4-	T45.1x5-	T45.1x6-
Tegretol	T42.1x1-	T42.1x2-	T42.1x3-	T42.1x4-	T42.1x5-	T42.1x6-
Teicoplanin	T36.8x1-	T36.8x2-	T36.8x3-	T36.8x4-	T36.8x5-	T36.8x6-
Telepaque	T50.8x1-	T50.8x2-	T50.8x3-	T50.8x4-	T50.8x5-	T50.8x6-
Tellurium	T56.891-	T56.892-	T56.893-	T56.894-	—	—
fumes	T56.891-	T56.892-	T56.893-	T56.894-	—	—
TEM	T45.1x1-	T45.1x2-	T45.1x3-	T45.1x4-	T45.1x5-	T45.1x6-
Temazepam	T42.4x1-	T42.4x2-	T42.4x3-	T42.4x4-	T42.4x5-	T42.4x6-
Temocillin	T36.0x1-	T36.0x2-	T36.0x3-	T36.0x4-	T36.0x5-	T36.0x6-
Tenamfetamine	T43.621-	T43.622-	T43.623-	T43.624-	T43.625-	T43.626-
Teniposide	T45.1x1-	T45.1x2-	T45.1x3-	T45.1x4-	T45.1x5-	T45.1x6-
Tenitramine	T46.3x1-	T46.3x2-	T46.3x3-	T46.3x4-	T46.3x5-	T46.3x6-
Tenoglicin	T48.4x1-	T48.4x2-	T48.4x3-	T48.4x4-	T48.4x5-	T48.4x6-
Tenonitrozole	T37.3x1-	T37.3x2-	T37.3x3-	T37.3x4-	T37.3x5-	T37.3x6-
Tenoxicam	T39.391-	T39.392-	T39.393-	T39.394-	T39.395-	T39.396-
TEPA	T45.1x1-	T45.1x2-	T45.1x3-	T45.1x4-	T45.1x5-	T45.1x6-
TEPP	T60.0x1-	T60.0x2-	T60.0x3-	T60.0x4-	—	—

DRUGS & CHEMICALS

Table of Drugs & Chemicals	POISONING Accidental (Unintentional)	Self-Harm (Intentional)	Assault	Undetermined	Adverse Effect	Underdosing
Teprotide	T46.5x1-	T46.5x2-	T46.5x3-	T46.5x4-	T46.5x5-	T46.5x6-
Terazosin	T44.6x1-	T44.6x2-	T44.6x3-	T44.6x4-	T44.6x5-	T44.6x6-
Terbufos	T60.0x1-	T60.0x2-	T60.0x3-	T60.0x4-	—	—
Terbutaline	T48.6x1-	T48.6x2-	T48.6x3-	T48.6x4-	T48.6x5-	T48.6x6-
Terconazole	T49.0x1-	T49.0x2-	T49.0x3-	T49.0x4-	T49.0x5-	T49.0x6-
Terfenadine	T45.0x1-	T45.0x2-	T45.0x3-	T45.0x4-	T45.0x5-	T45.0x6-
Teriparatide (acetate)	T50.991-	T50.992-	T50.993-	T50.994-	T50.995-	T50.996-
Terizidone	T37.1x1-	T37.1x2-	T37.1x3-	T37.1x4-	T37.1x5-	T37.1x6-
Terlipressin	T38.891-	T38.892-	T38.893-	T38.894-	T38.895-	T38.896-
Terodiline	T46.3x1-	T46.3x2-	T46.3x3-	T46.3x4-	T46.3x5-	T46.3x6-
Teroxalene	T37.4x1-	T37.4x2-	T37.4x3-	T37.4x4-	T37.4x5-	T37.4x6-
Terpin (cis) hydrate	T48.4x1-	T48.4x2-	T48.4x3-	T48.4x4-	T48.4x5-	T48.4x6-
Terramycin	T36.4x1-	T36.4x2-	T36.4x3-	T36.4x4-	T36.4x5-	T36.4x6-
Tertatolol	T44.7x1-	T44.7x2-	T44.7x3-	T44.7x4-	T44.7x5-	T44.7x6-
Tessalon	T48.3x1-	T48.3x2-	T48.3x3-	T48.3x4-	T48.3x5-	T48.3x6-
Testolactone	T38.7x1-	T38.7x2-	T38.7x3-	T38.7x4-	T38.7x5-	T38.7x6-
Testosterone	T38.7x1-	T38.7x2-	T38.7x3-	T38.7x4-	T38.7x5-	T38.7x6-
Tetanus toxoid or vaccine	T50.A91-	T50.A92-	T50.A93-	T50.A94-	T50.A95-	T50.A96-
antitoxin	T50.Z11-	T50.Z12-	T50.Z13-	T50.Z14-	T50.Z15-	T50.Z16-
immune globulin (human)	T50.Z11-	T50.Z12-	T50.Z13-	T50.Z14-	T50.Z15-	T50.Z16-
toxoid	T50.A91-	T50.A92-	T50.A93-	T50.A94-	T50.A95-	T50.A96-
with diphtheria toxoid	T50.A21-	T50.A22-	T50.A23-	T50.A24-	T50.A25-	T50.A26-
with pertussis	T50.A11-	T50.A12-	T50.A13-	T50.A14-	T50.A15-	T50.A16-
Tetrabenazine	T43.591-	T43.592-	T43.593-	T43.594-	T43.595-	T43.596-
Tetracaine	T41.3x1-	T41.3x2-	T41.3x3-	T41.3x4-	T41.3x5-	T41.3x6-
nerve block (peripheral) (plexus)	T41.3x1-	T41.3x2-	T41.3x3-	T41.3x4-	T41.3x5-	T41.3x6-
regional	T41.3x1-	T41.3x2-	T41.3x3-	T41.3x4-	T41.3x5-	T41.3x6-
spinal	T41.3x1-	T41.3x2-	T41.3x3-	T41.3x4-	T41.3x5-	T41.3x6-
Tetrachlorethylene — see Tetrachloroethylene						
Tetrachlormethiazide	T50.2x1-	T50.2x2-	T50.2x3-	T50.2x4-	T50.2x5-	T50.2x6-
2,3,7,8-Tetrachlorodibenzo-p-dioxin	T53.7x1-	T53.7x2-	T53.7x3-	T53.7x4-	—	—
Tetrachloroethane	T53.6x1-	T53.6x2-	T53.6x3-	T53.6x4-	—	—
vapor	T53.6x1-	T53.6x2-	T53.6x3-	T53.6x4-	—	—
paint or varnish	T53.6x1-	T53.6x2-	T53.6x3-	T53.6x4-	—	—
Tetrachloroethylene (liquid)	T53.3x1-	T53.3x2-	T53.3x3-	T53.3x4-	—	—
medicinal	T37.4x1-	T37.4x2-	T37.4x3-	T37.4x4-	T37.4x5-	T37.4x6-
vapor	T53.3x1-	T53.3x2-	T53.3x3-	T53.3x4-		
Tetrachloromethane — see Carbon tetrachloride						
Tetracosactide	T38.811-	T38.812-	T38.813-	T38.814-	T38.815-	T38.816-
Tetracosactrin	T38.811-	T38.812-	T38.813-	T38.814-	T38.815-	T38.816-
Tetracycline	T36.4x1-	T36.4x2-	T36.4x3-	T36.4x4-	T36.4x5-	T36.4x6-
ophthalmic preparation	T49.5x1-	T49.5x2-	T49.5x3-	T49.5x4-	T49.5x5-	T49.5x6-
topical NEC	T49.0x1-	T49.0x2-	T49.0x3-	T49.0x4-	T49.0x5-	T49.0x6-
Tetradifon	T60.8x1-	T60.8x2-	T60.8x3-	T60.8x4-		
Tetradotoxin	T61.771-	T61.772-	T61.773-	T61.774-	—	—
Tetraethyl lead	T56.0x1-	T56.0x2-	T56.0x3-	T56.0x4-	—	—
pyrophosphate	T60.0x1-	T60.0x2-	T60.0x3-	T60.0x4-	—	—
Tetraethylammonium chloride	T44.2x1-	T44.2x2-	T44.2x3-	T44.2x4-	T44.2x5-	T44.2x6-
Tetraethylthiuram disulfide	T50.6x1-	T50.6x2-	T50.6x3-	T50.6x4-	T50.6x5-	T50.6x6-
Tetrahydroaminoacridine	T44.0x1-	T44.0x2-	T44.0x3-	T44.0x4-	T44.0x5-	T44.0x6-
Tetrahydrocannabinol	T40.7x1-	T40.7x2-	T40.7x3-	T40.7x4-	T40.7x5-	T40.7x6-
Tetrahydrofuran	T52.8x1-	T52.8x2-	T52.8x3-	T52.8x4-		
Tetrahydronaphthalene	T52.8x1-	T52.8x2-	T52.8x3-	T52.8x4-		
Tetrahydrozoline	T49.5x1-	T49.5x2-	T49.5x3-	T49.5x4-	T49.5x5-	T49.5x6-

Table of Drugs & Chemicals	POISONING Accidental (Unintentional)	Self-Harm (Intentional)	Assault	Undetermined	Adverse Effect	Underdosing
Tetralin	T52.8x1-	T52.8x2-	T52.8x3-	T52.8x4-	—	—
Tetramethrin	T60.2x1-	T60.2x2-	T60.2x3-	T60.2x4-	—	—
Tetramethylthiuram (disulfide) NEC	T60.3x1-	T60.3x2-	T60.3x3-	T60.3x4-	—	—
medicinal	T49.0x1-	T49.0x2-	T49.0x3-	T49.0x4-	T49.0x5-	T49.0x6-
Tetramisole	T37.4x1-	T37.4x2-	T37.4x3-	T37.4x4-	T37.4x5-	T37.4x6-
Tetranicotinoyl fructose	T46.7x1-	T46.7x2-	T46.7x3-	T46.7x4-	T46.7x5-	T46.7x6-
Tetrazepam	T42.4x1-	T42.4x2-	T42.4x3-	T42.4x4-	T42.4x5-	T42.4x6-
Tetronal	T42.6x1-	T42.6x2-	T42.6x3-	T42.6x4-	T42.6x5-	T42.6x6-
Tetryl	T65.3x1-	T65.3x2-	T65.3x3-	T65.3x4-		
Tetrylammonium chloride	T44.2x1-	T44.2x2-	T44.2x3-	T44.2x4-	T44.2x5-	T44.2x6-
Tetryzoline	T49.5x1-	T49.5x2-	T49.5x3-	T49.5x4-	T49.5x5-	T49.5x6-
Thalidomide	T45.1x1-	T45.1x2-	T45.1x3-	T45.1x4-	T45.1x5-	T45.1x6-
Thallium (compounds) (dust) NEC	T56.811-	T56.812-	T56.813-	T56.814-	—	—
pesticide	T60.4x1-	T60.4x2-	T60.4x3-	T60.4x4-	—	—
THC	T40.7x1-	T40.7x2-	T40.7x3-	T40.7x4-	T40.7x5-	T40.7x6-
Thebacon	T48.3x1-	T48.3x2-	T48.3x3-	T48.3x4-	T48.3x5-	T48.3x6-
Thebaine	T40.2x1-	T40.2x2-	T40.2x3-	T40.2x4-	T40.2x5-	T40.2x6-
Thenoic acid	T49.6x1-	T49.6x2-	T49.6x3-	T49.6x4-	T49.6x5-	T49.6x6-
Thenyldiamine	T45.0x1-	T45.0x2-	T45.0x3-	T45.0x4-	T45.0x5-	T45.0x6-
Theobromine (calcium salicylate)	T48.6x1-	T48.6x2-	T48.6x3-	T48.6x4-	T48.6x5-	T48.6x6-
sodium salicylate	T48.6x1-	T48.6x2-	T48.6x3-	T48.6x4-	T48.6x5-	T48.6x6-
Theophyllamine	T48.6x1-	T48.6x2-	T48.6x3-	T48.6x4-	T48.6x5-	T48.6x6-
Theophylline	T48.6x1-	T48.6x2-	T48.6x3-	T48.6x4-	T48.6x5-	T48.6x6-
aminobenzoic acid	T48.6x1-	T48.6x2-	T48.6x3-	T48.6x4-	T48.6x5-	T48.6x6-
ethylenediamine	T48.6x1-	T48.6x2-	T48.6x3-	T48.6x4-	T48.6x5-	T48.6x6-
piperazine p-amino-benzoate	T48.6x1-	T48.6x2-	T48.6x3-	T48.6x4-	T48.6x5-	T48.6x6-
Thiabendazole	T37.4x1-	T37.4x2-	T37.4x3-	T37.4x4-	T37.4x5-	T37.4x6-
Thialbarbital	T41.1x1-	T41.1x2-	T41.1x3-	T41.1x4-	T41.1x5-	T41.1x6-
Thiamazole	T38.2x1-	T38.2x2-	T38.2x3-	T38.2x4-	T38.2x5-	T38.2x6-
Thiambutosine	T37.1x1-	T37.1x2-	T37.1x3-	T37.1x4-	T37.1x5-	T37.1x6-
Thiamine	T45.2x1-	T45.2x2-	T45.2x3-	T45.2x4-	T45.2x5-	T45.2x6-
Thiamphenicol	T36.2x1-	T36.2x2-	T36.2x3-	T36.2x4-	T36.2x5-	T36.2x6-
Thiamylal	T41.1x1-	T41.1x2-	T41.1x3-	T41.1x4-	T41.1x5-	T41.1x6-
sodium	T41.1x1-	T41.1x2-	T41.1x3-	T41.1x4-	T41.1x5-	T41.1x6-
Thiazesim	T43.291-	T43.292-	T43.293-	T43.294-	T43.295-	T43.296-
Thiazides (diuretics)	T50.2x1-	T50.2x2-	T50.2x3-	T50.2x4-	T50.2x5-	T50.2x6-
Thiazinamium metilsulfate	T43.3x1-	T43.3x2-	T43.3x3-	T43.3x4-	T43.3x5-	T43.3x6-
Thiethylperazine	T43.3x1-	T43.3x2-	T43.3x3-	T43.3x4-	T43.3x5-	T43.3x6-
Thimerosal	T49.0x1-	T49.0x2-	T49.0x3-	T49.0x4-	T49.0x5-	T49.0x6-
ophthalmic preparation	T49.5x1-	T49.5x2-	T49.5x3-	T49.5x4-	T49.5x5-	T49.5x6-
Thioacetazone	T37.1x1-	T37.1x2-	T37.1x3-	T37.1x4-	T37.1x5-	T37.1x6-
with isoniazid	T37.1x1-	T37.1x2-	T37.1x3-	T37.1x4-	T37.1x5-	T37.1x6-
Thiobarbital sodium	T41.1x1-	T41.1x2-	T41.1x3-	T41.1x4-	T41.1x5-	T41.1x6-
Thiobarbiturate anesthetic	T41.1x1-	T41.1x2-	T41.1x3-	T41.1x4-	T41.1x5-	T41.1x6-
Thiobismol	T37.8x1-	T37.8x2-	T37.8x3-	T37.8x4-	T37.8x5-	T37.8x6-
Thiobutabarbital sodium	T41.1x1-	T41.1x2-	T41.1x3-	T41.1x4-	T41.1x5-	T41.1x6-
Thiocarbamate (insecticide)	T60.0x1-	T60.0x2-	T60.0x3-	T60.0x4-	—	—
Thiocarbamide	T38.2x1-	T38.2x2-	T38.2x3-	T38.2x4-	T38.2x5-	T38.2x6-
Thiocarbarsone	T37.8x1-	T37.8x2-	T37.8x3-	T37.8x4-	T37.8x5-	T37.8x6-
Thiocarlide	T37.1x1-	T37.1x2-	T37.1x3-	T37.1x4-	T37.1x5-	T37.1x6-
Thioctamide	T50.991-	T50.992-	T50.993-	T50.994-	T50.995-	T50.996-
Thioctic acid	T50.991-	T50.992-	T50.993-	T50.994-	T50.995-	T50.996-
Thiofos	T60.0x1-	T60.0x2-	T60.0x3-	T60.0x4-	—	—
Thioglycolate	T49.4x1-	T49.4x2-	T49.4x3-	T49.4x4-	T49.4x5-	T49.4x6-
Thioglycolic acid	T65.891-	T65.892-	T65.893-	T65.894-		
Thioguanine	T45.1x1-	T45.1x2-	T45.1x3-	T45.1x4-	T45.1x5-	T45.1x6-
Thiomercaptomerin	T50.2x1-	T50.2x2-	T50.2x3-	T50.2x4-	T50.2x5-	T50.2x6-

Table of Drugs & Chemicals	POISONING Accidental (Unintentional)	POISONING Self-Harm (Intentional)	Assault	Undetermined	Adverse Effect	Underdosing
Thiomerin	T50.2x1-	T50.2x2-	T50.2x3-	T50.2x4-	T50.2x5-	T50.2x6-
Thiomersal	T49.0x1-	T49.0x2-	T49.0x3-	T49.0x4-	T49.0x5-	T49.0x6-
Thionazin	T60.0x1-	T60.0x2-	T60.0x3-	T60.0x4-	—	—
Thiopental (sodium)	T41.1x1-	T41.1x2-	T41.1x3-	T41.1x4-	T41.1x5-	T41.1x6-
Thiopentone (sodium)	T41.1x1-	T41.1x2-	T41.1x3-	T41.1x4-	T41.1x5-	T41.1x6-
Thiopropazate	T43.3x1-	T43.3x2-	T43.3x3-	T43.3x4-	T43.3x5-	T43.3x6-
Thioproperazine	T43.3x1-	T43.3x2-	T43.3x3-	T43.3x4-	T43.3x5-	T43.3x6-
Thioridazine	T43.3x1-	T43.3x2-	T43.3x3-	T43.3x4-	T43.3x5-	T43.3x6-
Thiosinamine	T49.3x1-	T49.3x2-	T49.3x3-	T49.3x4-	T49.3x5-	T49.3x6-
Thiotepa	T45.1x1-	T45.1x2-	T45.1x3-	T45.1x4-	T45.1x5-	T45.1x6-
Thiothixene	T43.4x1-	T43.4x2-	T43.4x3-	T43.4x4-	T43.4x5-	T43.4x6-
Thiouracil (benzyl) (methyl) (propyl)	T38.2x1-	T38.2x2-	T38.2x3-	T38.2x4-	T38.2x5-	T38.2x6-
Thiourea	T38.2x1-	T38.2x2-	T38.2x3-	T38.2x4-	T38.2x5-	T38.2x6-
Thiphenamil	T44.3x1-	T44.3x2-	T44.3x3-	T44.3x4-	T44.3x5-	T44.3x6-
Thiram	T60.3x1-	T60.3x2-	T60.3x3-	T60.3x4-	—	—
medicinal	T49.2x1-	T49.2x2-	T49.2x3-	T49.2x4-	T49.2x5-	T49.2x6-
Thonzylamine (systemic)	T45.0x1-	T45.0x2-	T45.0x3-	T45.0x4-	T45.0x5-	T45.0x6-
mucosal decongestant	T48.5x1-	T48.5x2-	T48.5x3-	T48.5x4-	T48.5x5-	T48.5x6-
Thorazine	T43.3x1-	T43.3x2-	T43.3x3-	T43.3x4-	T43.3x5-	T43.3x6-
Thorium dioxide suspension	T50.8x1-	T50.8x2-	T50.8x3-	T50.8x4-	T50.8x5-	T50.8x6-
Thornapple	T62.2x1-	T62.2x2-	T62.2x3-	T62.2x4-	—	—
Throat drug NEC	T49.6x1-	T49.6x2-	T49.6x3-	T49.6x4-	T49.6x5-	T49.6x6-
Thrombin	T45.7x1-	T45.7x2-	T45.7x3-	T45.7x4-	T45.7x5-	T45.7x6-
Thrombolysin	T45.611-	T45.612-	T45.613-	T45.614-	T45.615-	T45.616-
Thromboplastin	T45.7x1-	T45.7x2-	T45.7x3-	T45.7x4-	T45.7x5-	T45.7x6-
Thurfyl nicotinate	T46.7x1-	T46.7x2-	T46.7x3-	T46.7x4-	T46.7x5-	T46.7x6-
Thymol	T49.0x1-	T49.0x2-	T49.0x3-	T49.0x4-	T49.0x5-	T49.0x6-
Thymopentin	T37.5x1-	T37.5x2-	T37.5x3-	T37.5x4-	T37.5x5-	T37.5x6-
Thymoxamine	T46.7x1-	T46.7x2-	T46.7x3-	T46.7x4-	T46.7x5-	T46.7x6-
Thymus extract	T38.891-	T38.892-	T38.893-	T38.894-	T38.895-	T38.896-
Thyreotrophic hormone	T38.811-	T38.812-	T38.813-	T38.814-	T38.815-	T38.816-
Thyroglobulin	T38.1x1-	T38.1x2-	T38.1x3-	T38.1x4-	T38.1x5-	T38.1x6-
Thyroid (hormone)	T38.1x1-	T38.1x2-	T38.1x3-	T38.1x4-	T38.1x5-	T38.1x6-
Thyrolar	T38.1x1-	T38.1x2-	T38.1x3-	T38.1x4-	T38.1x5-	T38.1x6-
Thyrotrophin	T38.811-	T38.812-	T38.813-	T38.814-	T38.815-	T38.816-
Thyrotropic hormone	T38.811-	T38.812-	T38.813-	T38.814-	T38.815-	T38.816-
Thyroxine	T38.1x1-	T38.1x2-	T38.1x3-	T38.1x4-	T38.1x5-	T38.1x6-
Tiabendazole	T37.4x1-	T37.4x2-	T37.4x3-	T37.4x4-	T37.4x5-	T37.4x6-
Tiamizide	T50.2x1-	T50.2x2-	T50.2x3-	T50.2x4-	T50.2x5-	T50.2x6-
Tianeptine	T43.291-	T43.292-	T43.293-	T43.294-	T43.295-	T43.296-
Tiapamil	T46.1x1-	T46.1x2-	T46.1x3-	T46.1x4-	T46.1x5-	T46.1x6-
Tiapride	T43.591-	T43.592-	T43.593-	T43.594-	T43.595-	T43.596-
Tiaprofenic acid	T39.311-	T39.312-	T39.313-	T39.314-	T39.315-	T39.316-
Tiaramide	T39.8x1-	T39.8x2-	T39.8x3-	T39.8x4-	T39.8x5-	T39.8x6-
Ticarcillin	T36.0x1-	T36.0x2-	T36.0x3-	T36.0x4-	T36.0x5-	T36.0x6-
Ticlatone	T49.0x1-	T49.0x2-	T49.0x3-	T49.0x4-	T49.0x5-	T49.0x6-
Ticlopidine	T45.521-	T45.522-	T45.523-	T45.524-	T45.525-	T45.526-
Ticrynafen	T50.1x1-	T50.1x2-	T50.1x3-	T50.1x4-	T50.1x5-	T50.1x6-
Tidiacic	T50.991-	T50.992-	T50.993-	T50.994-	T50.995-	T50.996-
Tiemonium	T44.3x1-	T44.3x2-	T44.3x3-	T44.3x4-	T44.3x5-	T44.3x6-
iodide	T44.3x1-	T44.3x2-	T44.3x3-	T44.3x4-	T44.3x5-	T44.3x6-
Tienilic acid	T50.1x1-	T50.1x2-	T50.1x3-	T50.1x4-	T50.1x5-	T50.1x6-
Tifenamil	T44.3x1-	T44.3x2-	T44.3x3-	T44.3x4-	T44.3x5-	T44.3x6-
Tigan	T45.0x1-	T45.0x2-	T45.0x3-	T45.0x4-	T45.0x5-	T45.0x6-
Tigloidine	T44.3x1-	T44.3x2-	T44.3x3-	T44.3x4-	T44.3x5-	T44.3x6-
Tilactase	T47.5x1-	T47.5x2-	T47.5x3-	T47.5x4-	T47.5x5-	T47.5x6-
Tiletamine	T41.291-	T41.292-	T41.293-	T41.294-	T41.295-	T41.296-
Tilidine	T40.4x1-	T40.4x2-	T40.4x3-	T40.4x4-	—	—

Table of Drugs & Chemicals	POISONING Accidental (Unintentional)	POISONING Self-Harm (Intentional)	Assault	Undetermined	Adverse Effect	Underdosing
Timepidium bromide	T44.3x1-	T44.3x2-	T44.3x3-	T44.3x4-	T44.3x5-	T44.3x6-
Timiperone	T43.4x1-	T43.4x2-	T43.4x3-	T43.4x4-	T43.4x5-	T43.4x6-
Timolol	T44.7x1-	T44.7x2-	T44.7x3-	T44.7x4-	T44.7x5-	T44.7x6-
Tin (chloride) (dust) (oxide) NEC	T56.6x1-	T56.6x2-	T56.6x3-	T56.6x4-	—	—
anti-infectives	T37.8x1-	T37.8x2-	T37.8x3-	T37.8x4-	T37.8x5-	T37.8x6-
Tincture, iodine — see Iodine						
Tindal	T43.3x1-	T43.3x2-	T43.3x3-	T43.3x4-	T43.3x5-	T43.3x6-
Tinidazole	T37.3x1-	T37.3x2-	T37.3x3-	T37.3x4-	T37.3x5-	T37.3x6-
Tinoridine	T39.8x1-	T39.8x2-	T39.8x3-	T39.8x4-	T39.8x5-	T39.8x6-
Tiocarlide	T37.1x1-	T37.1x2-	T37.1x3-	T37.1x4-	T37.1x5-	T37.1x6-
Tioclomarol	T45.511-	T45.512-	T45.513-	T45.514-	T45.515-	T45.516-
Tioconazole	T49.0x1-	T49.0x2-	T49.0x3-	T49.0x4-	T49.0x5-	T49.0x6-
Tioguanine	T45.1x1-	T45.1x2-	T45.1x3-	T45.1x4-	T45.1x5-	T45.1x6-
Tiopronin	T50.991-	T50.992-	T50.993-	T50.994-	T50.995-	T50.996-
Tiotixene	T43.4x1-	T43.4x2-	T43.4x3-	T43.4x4-	T43.4x5-	T43.4x6-
Tioxolone	T49.4x1-	T49.4x2-	T49.4x3-	T49.4x4-	T49.4x5-	T49.4x6-
Tipepidine	T48.3x1-	T48.3x2-	T48.3x3-	T48.3x4-	T48.3x5-	T48.3x6-
Tiquizium bromide	T44.3x1-	T44.3x2-	T44.3x3-	T44.3x4-	T44.3x5-	T44.3x6-
Tiratricol	T38.1x1-	T38.1x2-	T38.1x3-	T38.1x4-	T38.1x5-	T38.1x6-
Tisopurine	T50.4x1-	T50.4x2-	T50.4x3-	T50.4x4-	T50.4x5-	T50.4x6-
Titanium (compounds) (vapor)	T56.891-	T56.892-	T56.893-	T56.894-	—	—
dioxide	T49.3x1-	T49.3x2-	T49.3x3-	T49.3x4-	T49.3x5-	T49.3x6-
ointment	T49.3x1-	T49.3x2-	T49.3x3-	T49.3x4-	T49.3x5-	T49.3x6-
oxide	T49.3x1-	T49.3x2-	T49.3x3-	T49.3x4-	T49.3x5-	T49.3x6-
tetrachloride	T56.891-	T56.892-	T56.893-	T56.894-	—	—
Titanocene	T56.891-	T56.892-	T56.893-	T56.894-	—	—
Titroid	T38.1x1-	T38.1x2-	T38.1x3-	T38.1x4-	T38.1x5-	T38.1x6-
Tizanidine	T42.8x1-	T42.8x2-	T42.8x3-	T42.8x4-	T42.8x5-	T42.8x6-
TMTD	T60.3x1-	T60.3x2-	T60.3x3-	T60.3x4-	—	—
TNT (fumes)	T65.3x1-	T65.3x2-	T65.3x3-	T65.3x4-	—	—
Toadstool	T62.0x1-	T62.0x2-	T62.0x3-	T62.0x4-	—	—
Tobacco NEC	T65.291-	T65.292-	T65.293-	T65.294-	—	—
cigarettes	T65.221-	T65.222-	T65.223-	T65.224-	—	—
Indian	T62.2x1-	T62.2x2-	T62.2x3-	T62.2x4-	—	—
smoke, second-hand	T65.221-	T65.222-	T65.223-	T65.224-	—	—
Tobramycin	T36.5x1-	T36.5x2-	T36.5x3-	T36.5x4-	T36.5x5-	T36.5x6-
Tocainide	T46.2x1-	T46.2x2-	T46.2x3-	T46.2x4-	T46.2x5-	T46.2x6-
Tocoferol	T45.2x1-	T45.2x2-	T45.2x3-	T45.2x4-	T45.2x5-	T45.2x6-
Tocopherol	T45.2x1-	T45.2x2-	T45.2x3-	T45.2x4-	T45.2x5-	T45.2x6-
acetate	T45.2x1-	T45.2x2-	T45.2x3-	T45.2x4-	T45.2x5-	T45.2x6-
Tocosamine	T48.0x1-	T48.0x2-	T48.0x3-	T48.0x4-	T48.0x5-	T48.0x6-
Todralazine	T46.5x1-	T46.5x2-	T46.5x3-	T46.5x4-	T46.5x5-	T46.5x6-
Tofisopam	T42.4x1-	T42.4x2-	T42.4x3-	T42.4x4-	T42.4x5-	T42.4x6-
Tofranil	T43.011-	T43.012-	T43.013-	T43.014-	T43.015-	T43.016-
Toilet deodorizer	T65.891-	T65.892-	T65.893-	T65.894-	—	—
Tolamolol	T44.7x1-	T44.7x2-	T44.7x3-	T44.7x4-	T44.7x5-	T44.7x6-
Tolazamide	T38.3x1-	T38.3x2-	T38.3x3-	T38.3x4-	T38.3x5-	T38.3x6-
Tolazoline	T46.7x1-	T46.7x2-	T46.7x3-	T46.7x4-	T46.7x5-	T46.7x6-
Tolbutamide (sodium)	T38.3x1-	T38.3x2-	T38.3x3-	T38.3x4-	T38.3x5-	T38.3x6-
Tolciclate	T49.0x1-	T49.0x2-	T49.0x3-	T49.0x4-	T49.0x5-	T49.0x6-
Tolmetin	T39.391-	T39.392-	T39.393-	T39.394-	T39.395-	T39.396-
Tolnaftate	T49.0x1-	T49.0x2-	T49.0x3-	T49.0x4-	T49.0x5-	T49.0x6-
Tolonidine	T46.5x1-	T46.5x2-	T46.5x3-	T46.5x4-	T46.5x5-	T46.5x6-
Toloxatone	T42.6x1-	T42.6x2-	T42.6x3-	T42.6x4-	T42.6x5-	T42.6x6-
Tolperisone	T44.3x1-	T44.3x2-	T44.3x3-	T44.3x4-	T44.3x5-	T44.3x6-
Tolserol	T42.8x1-	T42.8x2-	T42.8x3-	T42.8x4-	T42.8x5-	T42.8x6-

DRUGS & CHEMICALS

Table of Drugs & Chemicals	POISONING Accidental (Unintentional)	POISONING Self-Harm (Intentional)	POISONING Assault	POISONING Undetermined	Adverse Effect	Underdosing
Toluene (liquid)	T52.2x1-	T52.2x2-	T52.2x3-	T52.2x4-	—	—
diisocyanate	T65.0x1-	T65.0x2-	T65.0x3-	T65.0x4-	—	—
Toluidine	T65.891-	T65.892-	T65.893-	T65.894-	—	—
vapor	T59.891-	T59.892-	T59.893-	T59.894-	—	—
Toluol (liquid)	T52.2x1-	T52.2x2-	T52.2x3-	T52.2x4-	—	—
vapor	T52.2x1-	T52.2x2-	T52.2x3-	T52.2x4-	—	—
Toluylenediamine	T65.3x1-	T65.3x2-	T65.3x3-	T65.3x4-	—	—
Tolylene-2,4-diisocyanate	T65.0x1-	T65.0x2-	T65.0x3-	T65.0x4-	—	—
Tonic NEC	T50.901-	T50.902-	T50.903-	T50.904-	T50.905-	T50.906-
Topical action drug NEC	T49.91x-	T49.92x-	T49.93x-	T49.94x-	T49.95x-	T49.96x-
ear, nose or throat	T49.6x1-	T49.6x2-	T49.6x3-	T49.6x4-	T49.6x5-	T49.6x6-
eye	T49.5x1-	T49.5x2-	T49.5x3-	T49.5x4-	T49.5x5-	T49.5x6-
skin	T49.91x-	T49.92x-	T49.93x-	T49.94x-	T49.95x-	T49.96x-
specified NEC	T49.8x1-	T49.8x2-	T49.8x3-	T49.8x4-	T49.8x5-	T49.8x6-
Toquizine	T44.3x1-	T44.3x2-	T44.3x3-	T44.3x4-	T44.3x5-	T44.3x6-
Toremifene	T38.6x1-	T38.6x2-	T38.6x3-	T38.6x4-	T38.6x5-	T38.6x6-
Tosylchloramide sodium	T49.8x1-	T49.8x2-	T49.8x3-	T49.8x4-	T49.8x5-	T49.8x6-
Toxaphene (dust) (spray)	T60.1x1-	T60.1x2-	T60.1x3-	T60.1x4-	—	—
Toxin, diphtheria (Schick Test)	T50.8x1-	T50.8x2-	T50.8x3-	T50.8x4-	T50.8x5-	T50.8x6-
Toxoid						
combined	T50.A21-	T50.A22-	T50.A23-	T50.A24-	T50.A25-	T50.A26-
diphtheria	T50.A91-	T50.A92-	T50.A93-	T50.A94-	T50.A95-	T50.A96-
tetanus	T50.A91-	T50.A92-	T50.A93-	T50.A94-	T50.A95-	T50.A96-
Trace element NEC	T45.8x1-	T45.8x2-	T45.8x3-	T45.8x4-	T45.8x5-	T45.8x6-
Tractor fuel NEC	T52.0x1-	T52.0x2-	T52.0x3-	T52.0x4-	—	—
Tragacanth	T50.991-	T50.992-	T50.993-	T50.994-	T50.995-	T50.996-
Tramadol	T40.4x1-	T40.4x2-	T40.4x3-	T40.4x4-	T40.4x5-	T40.4x6-
Tramazoline	T48.5x1-	T48.5x2-	T48.5x3-	T48.5x4-	T48.5x5-	T48.5x6-
Tranexamic acid	T45.621-	T45.622-	T45.623-	T45.624-	T45.625-	T45.626-
Tranilast	T45.0x1-	T45.0x2-	T45.0x3-	T45.0x4-	T45.0x5-	T45.0x6-
Tranquilizer NEC	T43.501-	T43.502-	T43.503-	T43.504-	T43.505-	T43.506-
with hypnotic or sedative	T42.6x1-	T42.6x2-	T42.6x3-	T42.6x4-	T42.6x5-	T42.6x6-
benzodiazepine NEC	T42.4x1-	T42.4x2-	T42.4x3-	T42.4x4-	T42.4x5-	T42.4x6-
butyrophenone NEC	T43.4x1-	T43.4x2-	T43.4x3-	T43.4x4-	T43.4x5-	T43.4x6-
carbamate	T43.591-	T43.592-	T43.593-	T43.594-	T43.595-	T43.596-
dimethylamine	T43.3x1-	T43.3x2-	T43.3x3-	T43.3x4-	T43.3x5-	T43.3x6-
ethylamine	T43.3x1-	T43.3x2-	T43.3x3-	T43.3x4-	T43.3x5-	T43.3x6-
hydroxyzine	T43.591-	T43.592-	T43.593-	T43.594-	T43.595-	T43.596-
major NEC	T43.501-	T43.502-	T43.503-	T43.504-	T43.505-	T43.506-
penothiazine NEC	T43.3x1-	T43.3x2-	T43.3x3-	T43.3x4-	T43.3x5-	T43.3x6-
phenothiazine-based	T43.3x1-	T43.3x2-	T43.3x3-	T43.3x4-	T43.3x5-	T43.3x6-
piperazine NEC	T43.3x1-	T43.3x2-	T43.3x3-	T43.3x4-	T43.3x5-	T43.3x6-
piperidine	T43.3x1-	T43.3x2-	T43.3x3-	T43.3x4-	T43.3x5-	T43.3x6-
propylamine	T43.3x1-	T43.3x2-	T43.3x3-	T43.3x4-	T43.3x5-	T43.3x6-
specified NEC	T43.591-	T43.592-	T43.593-	T43.594-	T43.595-	T43.596-
thioxanthene NEC	T43.591-	T43.592-	T43.593-	T43.594-	T43.595-	T43.596-
Tranxene	T42.4x1-	T42.4x2-	T42.4x3-	T42.4x4-	T42.4x5-	T42.4x6-
Tranylcypromine	T43.1x1-	T43.1x2-	T43.1x3-	T43.1x4-	T43.1x5-	T43.1x6-
Trapidil	T46.3x1-	T46.3x2-	T46.3x3-	T46.3x4-	T46.3x5-	T46.3x6-
Trasentine	T44.3x1-	T44.3x2-	T44.3x3-	T44.3x4-	T44.3x5-	T44.3x6-
Travert	T50.3x1-	T50.3x2-	T50.3x3-	T50.3x4-	T50.3x5-	T50.3x6-
Trazodone	T43.211-	T43.212-	T43.213-	T43.214-	T43.215-	T43.216-
Trecator	T37.1x1-	T37.1x2-	T37.1x3-	T37.1x4-	T37.1x5-	T37.1x6-
Treosulfan	T45.1x1-	T45.1x2-	T45.1x3-	T45.1x4-	T45.1x5-	T45.1x6-
Tretamine	T45.1x1-	T45.1x2-	T45.1x3-	T45.1x4-	T45.1x5-	T45.1x6-
Tretinoin	T49.0x1-	T49.0x2-	T49.0x3-	T49.0x4-	T49.0x5-	T49.0x6-
Tretoquinol	T48.6x1-	T48.6x2-	T48.6x3-	T48.6x4-	T48.6x5-	T48.6x6-
Triacetin	T49.0x1-	T49.0x2-	T49.0x3-	T49.0x4-	T49.0x5-	T49.0x6-
Triacetoxyanthracene	T49.4x1-	T49.4x2-	T49.4x3-	T49.4x4-	T49.4x5-	T49.4x6-
Triacetyloleandomycin	T36.3x1-	T36.3x2-	T36.3x3-	T36.3x4-	T36.3x5-	T36.3x6-
Triamcinolone	T49.0x1-	T49.0x2-	T49.0x3-	T49.0x4-	T49.0x5-	T49.0x6-
ENT agent	T49.6x1-	T49.6x2-	T49.6x3-	T49.6x4-	T49.6x5-	T49.6x6-
hexacetonide	T49.0x1-	T49.0x2-	T49.0x3-	T49.0x4-	T49.0x5-	T49.0x6-
ophthalmic preparation	T49.5x1-	T49.5x2-	T49.5x3-	T49.5x4-	T49.5x5-	T49.5x6-
topical NEC	T49.0x1-	T49.0x2-	T49.0x3-	T49.0x4-	T49.0x5-	T49.0x6-
Triampyzine	T44.3x1-	T44.3x2-	T44.3x3-	T44.3x4-	T44.3x5-	T44.3x6-
Triamterene	T50.2x1-	T50.2x2-	T50.2x3-	T50.2x4-	T50.2x5-	T50.2x6-
Triazine (herbicide)	T60.3x1-	T60.3x2-	T60.3x3-	T60.3x4-	—	—
Triaziquone	T45.1x1-	T45.1x2-	T45.1x3-	T45.1x4-	T45.1x5-	T45.1x6-
Triazolam	T42.4x1-	T42.4x2-	T42.4x3-	T42.4x4-	T42.4x5-	T42.4x6-
Triazole (herbicide)	T60.3x1-	T60.3x2-	T60.3x3-	T60.3x4-	—	—
Tribenoside	T46.991-	T46.992-	T46.993-	T46.994-	T46.995-	T46.996-
Tribromacetaldehyde	T42.6x1-	T42.6x2-	T42.6x3-	T42.6x4-	T42.6x5-	T42.6x6-
Tribromoethanol, rectal	T41.291-	T41.292-	T41.293-	T41.294-	T41.295-	T41.296-
Tribromomethane	T42.6x1-	T42.6x2-	T42.6x3-	T42.6x4-	T42.6x5-	T42.6x6-
Trichlorethane	T53.2x1-	T53.2x2-	T53.2x3-	T53.2x4-	—	—
Trichlorethylene	T53.2x1-	T53.2x2-	T53.2x3-	T53.2x4-	—	—
Trichlorfon	T60.0x1-	T60.0x2-	T60.0x3-	T60.0x4-	—	—
Trichlormethiazide	T50.2x1-	T50.2x2-	T50.2x3-	T50.2x4-	T50.2x5-	T50.2x6-
Trichlormethine	T45.1x1-	T45.1x2-	T45.1x3-	T45.1x4-	T45.1x5-	T45.1x6-
Trichloroacetic acid, trichloracetic acid	T54.2x1-	T54.2x2-	T54.2x3-	T54.2x4-	—	—
medicinal	T49.4x1-	T49.4x2-	T49.4x3-	T49.4x4-	T49.4x5-	T49.4x6-
Trichloroethane	T53.2x1-	T53.2x2-	T53.2x3-	T53.2x4-	—	—
Trichloroethanol	T42.6x1-	T42.6x2-	T42.6x3-	T42.6x4-	T42.6x5-	T42.6x6-
Trichloroethyl phosphate	T42.6x1-	T42.6x2-	T42.6x3-	T42.6x4-	T42.6x5-	T42.6x6-
Trichloroethylene (liquid) (vapor)	T53.2x1-	T53.2x2-	T53.2x3-	T53.2x4-	—	—
anesthetic (gas)	T41.0x1-	T41.0x2-	T41.0x3-	T41.0x4-	T41.0x5-	T41.0x6-
vapor NEC	T53.2x1-	T53.2x2-	T53.2x3-	T53.2x4-	—	—
Trichlorofluoromethane NEC	T53.5x1-	T53.5x2-	T53.5x3-	T53.5x4-	—	—
Trichloronate	T60.0x1-	T60.0x2-	T60.0x3-	T60.0x4-	—	—
2,4,5-Trichlorophen-oxyacetic acid	T60.3x1-	T60.3x2-	T60.3x3-	T60.3x4-	—	—
Trichloropropane	T53.6x1-	T53.6x2-	T53.6x3-	T53.6x4-	—	—
Trichlorotriethylamine	T45.1x1-	T45.1x2-	T45.1x3-	T45.1x4-	T45.1x5-	T45.1x6-
Trichomonacides NEC	T37.3x1-	T37.3x2-	T37.3x3-	T37.3x4-	T37.3x5-	T37.3x6-
Trichomycin	T36.7x1-	T36.7x2-	T36.7x3-	T36.7x4-	T36.7x5-	T36.7x6-
Triclobisonium chloride	T49.0x1-	T49.0x2-	T49.0x3-	T49.0x4-	T49.0x5-	T49.0x6-
Triclocarban	T49.0x1-	T49.0x2-	T49.0x3-	T49.0x4-	T49.0x5-	T49.0x6-
Triclofos	T42.6x1-	T42.6x2-	T42.6x3-	T42.6x4-	T42.6x5-	T42.6x6-
Triclosan	T49.0x1-	T49.0x2-	T49.0x3-	T49.0x4-	T49.0x5-	T49.0x6-
Tricresyl phosphate	T65.891-	T65.892-	T65.893-	T65.894-	—	—
solvent	T52.91x-	T52.92x-	T52.93x-	T52.94x-	—	—
Tricyclamol chloride	T44.3x1-	T44.3x2-	T44.3x3-	T44.3x4-	T44.3x5-	T44.3x6-
Tridesilon	T49.0x1-	T49.0x2-	T49.0x3-	T49.0x4-	T49.0x5-	T49.0x6-
Tridihexethyl iodide	T44.3x1-	T44.3x2-	T44.3x3-	T44.3x4-	T44.3x5-	T44.3x6-
Tridione	T42.2x1-	T42.2x2-	T42.2x3-	T42.2x4-	T42.2x5-	T42.2x6-
Trientine	T45.8x1-	T45.8x2-	T45.8x3-	T45.8x4-	T45.8x5-	T45.8x6-
Triethanolamine NEC	T54.3x1-	T54.3x2-	T54.3x3-	T54.3x4-	—	—
detergent	T54.3x1-	T54.3x2-	T54.3x3-	T54.3x4-	—	—
trinitrate (biphosphate)	T46.3x1-	T46.3x2-	T46.3x3-	T46.3x4-	T46.3x5-	T46.3x6-
Triethanomelamine	T45.1x1-	T45.1x2-	T45.1x3-	T45.1x4-	T45.1x5-	T45.1x6-
Triethylenemelamine	T45.1x1-	T45.1x2-	T45.1x3-	T45.1x4-	T45.1x5-	T45.1x6-
Triethylenephosphoramide	T45.1x1-	T45.1x2-	T45.1x3-	T45.1x4-	T45.1x5-	T45.1x6-
Triethylenethiophospho-ramide	T45.1x1-	T45.1x2-	T45.1x3-	T45.1x4-	T45.1x5-	T45.1x6-
Trifluoperazine	T43.3x1-	T43.3x2-	T43.3x3-	T43.3x4-	T43.3x5-	T43.3x6-
Trifluoroethyl vinyl ether	T41.0x1-	T41.0x2-	T41.0x3-	T41.0x4-	T41.0x5-	T41.0x6-
Trifluperidol	T43.4x1-	T43.4x2-	T43.4x3-	T43.4x4-	T43.4x5-	T43.4x6-
Triflupromazine	T43.3x1-	T43.3x2-	T43.3x3-	T43.3x4-	T43.3x5-	T43.3x6-

DRUGS & CHEMICALS

Table of Drugs & Chemicals	POISONING Accidental (Unintentional)	POISONING Self-Harm (Intentional)	POISONING Assault	POISONING Undetermined	Adverse Effect	Underdosing
Trifluridine	T37.5x1-	T37.5x2-	T37.5x3-	T37.5x4-	T37.5x5-	T37.5x6-
Triflusal	T45.521-	T45.522-	T45.523-	T45.524-	T45.525-	T45.526-
Trihexyphenidyl	T44.3x1-	T44.3x2-	T44.3x3-	T44.3x4-	T44.3x5-	T44.3x6-
Triiodothyronine	T38.1x1-	T38.1x2-	T38.1x3-	T38.1x4-	T38.1x5-	T38.1x6-
Trilene	T41.0x1-	T41.0x2-	T41.0x3-	T41.0x4-	T41.0x5-	T41.0x6-
Trilostane	T38.991-	T38.992-	T38.993-	T38.994-	T38.995-	T38.996-
Trimebutine	T44.3x1-	T44.3x2-	T44.3x3-	T44.3x4-	T44.3x5-	T44.3x6-
Trimecaine	T41.3x1-	T41.3x2-	T41.3x3-	T41.3x4-	T41.3x5-	T41.3x6-
Trimeprazine (tartrate)	T44.3x1-	T44.3x2-	T44.3x3-	T44.3x4-	T44.3x5-	T44.3x6-
Trimetaphan camsilate	T44.2x1-	T44.2x2-	T44.2x3-	T44.2x4-	T44.2x5-	T44.2x6-
Trimetazidine	T46.7x1-	T46.7x2-	T46.7x3-	T46.7x4-	T46.7x5-	T46.7x6-
Trimethadione	T42.2x1-	T42.2x2-	T42.2x3-	T42.2x4-	T42.2x5-	T42.2x6-
Trimethaphan	T44.2x1-	T44.2x2-	T44.2x3-	T44.2x4-	T44.2x5-	T44.2x6-
Trimethidinium	T44.2x1-	T44.2x2-	T44.2x3-	T44.2x4-	T44.2x5-	T44.2x6-
Trimethobenzamide	T45.0x1-	T45.0x2-	T45.0x3-	T45.0x4-	T45.0x5-	T45.0x6-
Trimethoprim	T37.8x1-	T37.8x2-	T37.8x3-	T37.8x4-	T37.8x5-	T37.8x6-
with sulfamethoxazole	T36.8x1-	T36.8x2-	T36.8x3-	T36.8x4-	T36.8x5-	T36.8x6-
Trimethylcarbinol	T51.3x1-	T51.3x2-	T51.3x3-	T51.3x4-	—	—
Trimethylpsoralen	T49.3x1-	T49.3x2-	T49.3x3-	T49.3x4-	T49.3x5-	T49.3x6-
Trimeton	T45.0x1-	T45.0x2-	T45.0x3-	T45.0x4-	T45.0x5-	T45.0x6-
Trimetrexate	T45.1x1-	T45.1x2-	T45.1x3-	T45.1x4-	T45.1x5-	T45.1x6-
Trimipramine	T43.011-	T43.012-	T43.013-	T43.014-	T43.015-	T43.016-
Trimustine	T45.1x1-	T45.1x2-	T45.1x3-	T45.1x4-	T45.1x5-	T45.1x6-
Trinitrine	T46.3x1-	T46.3x2-	T46.3x3-	T46.3x4-	T46.3x5-	T46.3x6-
Trinitrobenzol	T65.3x1-	T65.3x2-	T65.3x3-	T65.3x4-	—	—
Trinitrophenol	T65.3x1-	T65.3x2-	T65.3x3-	T65.3x4-	—	—
Trinitrotoluene (fumes)	T65.3x1-	T65.3x2-	T65.3x3-	T65.3x4-	—	—
Trional	T42.6x1-	T42.6x2-	T42.6x3-	T42.6x4-	T42.6x5-	T42.6x6-
Triorthocresyl phosphate	T65.891-	T65.892-	T65.893-	T65.894-	—	—
Trioxide of arsenic	T57.0x1-	T57.0x2-	T57.0x3-	T57.0x4-	—	—
Trioxysalen	T49.4x1-	T49.4x2-	T49.4x3-	T49.4x4-	T49.4x5-	T49.4x6-
Tripamide	T50.2x1-	T50.2x2-	T50.2x3-	T50.2x4-	T50.2x5-	T50.2x6-
Triparanol	T46.6x1-	T46.6x2-	T46.6x3-	T46.6x4-	T46.6x5-	T46.6x6-
Tripelennamine	T45.0x1-	T45.0x2-	T45.0x3-	T45.0x4-	T45.0x5-	T45.0x6-
Triperiden	T44.3x1-	T44.3x2-	T44.3x3-	T44.3x4-	T44.3x5-	T44.3x6-
Triperidol	T43.4x1-	T43.4x2-	T43.4x3-	T43.4x4-	T43.4x5-	T43.4x6-
Triphenylphosphate	T65.891-	T65.892-	T65.893-	T65.894-	—	—
Triple						
bromides	T42.6x1-	T42.6x2-	T42.6x3-	T42.6x4-	T42.6x5-	T42.6x6-
carbonate	T47.1x1-	T47.1x2-	T47.1x3-	T47.1x4-	T47.1x5-	T47.1x6-
vaccine						
DPT	T50.A11-	T50.A12-	T50.A13-	T50.A14-	T50.A15-	T50.A16-
including pertussis	T50.A11-	T50.A12-	T50.A13-	T50.A14-	T50.A15-	T50.A16-
MMR	T50.B91-	T50.B92-	T50.B93-	T50.B94-	T50.B95-	T50.B96-
Triprolidine	T45.0x1-	T45.0x2-	T45.0x3-	T45.0x4-	T45.0x5-	T45.0x6-
Trisodium hydrogen edetate	T50.6x1-	T50.6x2-	T50.6x3-	T50.6x4-	T50.6x5-	T50.6x6-
Trisoralen	T49.3x1-	T49.3x2-	T49.3x3-	T49.3x4-	T49.3x5-	T49.3x6-
Trisulfapyrimidines	T37.0x1-	T37.0x2-	T37.0x3-	T37.0x4-	T37.0x5-	T37.0x6-
Trithiozine	T44.3x1-	T44.3x2-	T44.3x3-	T44.3x4-	T44.3x5-	T44.3x6-
Tritiozine	T44.3x1-	T44.3x2-	T44.3x3-	T44.3x4-	T44.3x5-	T44.3x6-
Tritoqualine	T45.0x1-	T45.0x2-	T45.0x3-	T45.0x4-	T45.0x5-	T45.0x6-
Trofosfamide	T45.1x1-	T45.1x2-	T45.1x3-	T45.1x4-	T45.1x5-	T45.1x6-
Troleandomycin	T36.3x1-	T36.3x2-	T36.3x3-	T36.3x4-	T36.3x5-	T36.3x6-
Trolnitrate (phosphate)	T46.3x1-	T46.3x2-	T46.3x3-	T46.3x4-	T46.3x5-	T46.3x6-
Tromantadine	T37.5x1-	T37.5x2-	T37.5x3-	T37.5x4-	T37.5x5-	T37.5x6-
Trometamol	T50.2x1-	T50.2x2-	T50.2x3-	T50.2x4-	T50.2x5-	T50.2x6-
Tromethamine	T50.2x1-	T50.2x2-	T50.2x3-	T50.2x4-	T50.2x5-	T50.2x6-
Tronothane	T41.3x1-	T41.3x2-	T41.3x3-	T41.3x4-	T41.3x5-	T41.3x6-
Tropacine	T44.3x1-	T44.3x2-	T44.3x3-	T44.3x4-	T44.3x5-	T44.3x6-
Tropatepine	T44.3x1-	T44.3x2-	T44.3x3-	T44.3x4-	T44.3x5-	T44.3x6-
Tropicamide	T44.3x1-	T44.3x2-	T44.3x3-	T44.3x4-	T44.3x5-	T44.3x6-
Trospium chloride	T44.3x1-	T44.3x2-	T44.3x3-	T44.3x4-	T44.3x5-	T44.3x6-
Troxerutin	T46.991-	T46.992-	T46.993-	T46.994-	T46.995-	T46.996-
Troxidone	T42.2x1-	T42.2x2-	T42.2x3-	T42.2x4-	T42.2x5-	T42.2x6-
Tryparsamide	T37.3x1-	T37.3x2-	T37.3x3-	T37.3x4-	T37.3x5-	T37.3x6-
Trypsin	T45.3x1-	T45.3x2-	T45.3x3-	T45.3x4-	T45.3x5-	T45.3x6-
Tryptizol	T43.011-	T43.012-	T43.013-	T43.014-	T43.015-	T43.016-
TSH	T38.811-	T38.812-	T38.813-	T38.814-	T38.815-	T38.816-
Tuaminoheptane	T48.5x1-	T48.5x2-	T48.5x3-	T48.5x4-	T48.5x5-	T48.5x6-
Tuberculin, purified protein derivative (PPD)	T50.8x1-	T50.8x2-	T50.8x3-	T50.8x4-	T50.8x5-	T50.8x6-
Tubocurare	T48.1x1-	T48.1x2-	T48.1x3-	T48.1x4-	T48.1x5-	T48.1x6-
Tubocurarine (chloride)	T48.1x1-	T48.1x2-	T48.1x3-	T48.1x4-	T48.1x5-	T48.1x6-
Tulobuterol	T48.6x1-	T48.6x2-	T48.6x3-	T48.6x4-	T48.6x5-	T48.6x6-
Turpentine (spirits of)	T52.8x1-	T52.8x2-	T52.8x3-	T52.8x4-	—	—
vapor	T52.8x1-	T52.8x2-	T52.8x3-	T52.8x4-	—	—
Tybamate	T43.591-	T43.592-	T43.593-	T43.594-	T43.595-	T43.596-
Tyloxapol	T48.4x1-	T48.4x2-	T48.4x3-	T48.4x4-	T48.4x5-	T48.4x6-
Tymazoline	T48.5x1-	T48.5x2-	T48.5x3-	T48.5x4-	T48.5x5-	T48.5x6-
Typhoid-paratyphoid vaccine	T50.A91-	T50.A92-	T50.A93-	T50.A94-	T50.A95-	T50.A96-
Typhus vaccine	T50.A91-	T50.A92-	T50.A93-	T50.A94-	T50.A95-	T50.A96-
Tyropanoate	T50.8x1-	T50.8x2-	T50.8x3-	T50.8x4-	T50.8x5-	T50.8x6-
Tyrothricin	T49.6x1-	T49.6x2-	T49.6x3-	T49.6x4-	T49.6x5-	T49.6x6-
ENT agent	T49.6x1-	T49.6x2-	T49.6x3-	T49.6x4-	T49.6x5-	T49.6x6-
ophthalmic preparation	T49.5x1-	T49.5x2-	T49.5x3-	T49.5x4-	T49.5x5-	T49.5x6-
Ufenamate	T39.391-	T39.392-	T39.393-	T39.394-	T39.395-	T39.396-
Ultraviolet light protectant	T49.3x1-	T49.3x2-	T49.3x3-	T49.3x4-	T49.3x5-	T49.3x6-
Undecenoic acid	T49.0x1-	T49.0x2-	T49.0x3-	T49.0x4-	T49.0x5-	T49.0x6-
Undecoylium	T49.0x1-	T49.0x2-	T49.0x3-	T49.0x4-	T49.0x5-	T49.0x6-
Undecylenic acid (derivatives)	T49.0x1-	T49.0x2-	T49.0x3-	T49.0x4-	T49.0x5-	T49.0x6-
Unna's boot	T49.3x1-	T49.3x2-	T49.3x3-	T49.3x4-	T49.3x5-	T49.3x6-
Unsaturated fatty acid	T46.6x1-	T46.6x2-	T46.6x3-	T46.6x4-	T46.6x5-	T46.6x6-
Uracil mustard	T45.1x1-	T45.1x2-	T45.1x3-	T45.1x4-	T45.1x5-	T45.1x6-
Uramustine	T45.1x1-	T45.1x2-	T45.1x3-	T45.1x4-	T45.1x5-	T45.1x6-
Urapidil	T46.5x1-	T46.5x2-	T46.5x3-	T46.5x4-	T46.5x5-	T46.5x6-
Urari	T48.1x1-	T48.1x2-	T48.1x3-	T48.1x4-	T48.1x5-	T48.1x6-
Urate oxidase	T50.4x1-	T50.4x2-	T50.4x3-	T50.4x4-	T50.4x5-	T50.4x6-
Urea	T47.3x1-	T47.3x2-	T47.3x3-	T47.3x4-	T47.3x5-	T47.3x6-
peroxide	T49.0x1-	T49.0x2-	T49.0x3-	T49.0x4-	T49.0x5-	T49.0x6-
stibamine	T37.4x1-	T37.4x2-	T37.4x3-	T37.4x4-	T37.4x5-	T37.4x6-
topical	T49.8x1-	T49.8x2-	T49.8x3-	T49.8x4-	T49.8x5-	T49.8x6-
Urethane	T45.1x1-	T45.1x2-	T45.1x3-	T45.1x4-	T45.1x5-	T45.1x6-
Urginea (maritima) (scilla) — see Squill						
Uric acid metabolism drug NEC	T50.4x1-	T50.4x2-	T50.4x3-	T50.4x4-	T50.4x5-	T50.4x6-
Uricosuric agent	T50.4x1-	T50.4x2-	T50.4x3-	T50.4x4-	T50.4x5-	T50.4x6-
Urinary anti-infective	T37.8x1-	T37.8x2-	T37.8x3-	T37.8x4-	T37.8x5-	T37.8x6-
Urofollitropin	T38.811-	T38.812-	T38.813-	T38.814-	T38.815-	T38.816-
Urokinase	T45.611-	T45.612-	T45.613-	T45.614-	T45.615-	T45.616-
Urokon	T50.8x1-	T50.8x2-	T50.8x3-	T50.8x4-	T50.8x5-	T50.8x6-
Ursodeoxycholic acid	T50.991-	T50.992-	T50.993-	T50.994-	T50.995-	T50.996-
Ursodiol	T50.991-	T50.992-	T50.993-	T50.994-	T50.995-	T50.996-
Urtica	T62.2x1-	T62.2x2-	T62.2x3-	T62.2x4-	—	—
Utility gas — see Gas, utility						

DRUGS & CHEMICALS

Table of Drugs & Chemicals	Accidental (Unintentional)	Self-Harm (Intentional)	Assault	Undetermined	Adverse Effect	Underdosing
Vaccine NEC	T50.Z91-	T50.Z92-	T50.Z93-	T50.Z94-	T50.Z95-	T50.Z96-
antineoplastic	T50.Z91-	T50.Z92-	T50.Z93-	T50.Z94-	T50.Z95-	T50.Z96-
bacterial NEC	T50.A91-	T50.A92-	T50.A93-	T50.A94-	T50.A95-	T50.A96-
with other bacterial component	T50.A21-	T50.A22-	T50.A23-	T50.A24-	T50.A25-	T50.A26-
pertussis component	T50.A11-	T50.A12-	T50.A13-	T50.A14-	T50.A15-	T50.A16-
viral-rickettsial component	T50.A21-	T50.A22-	T50.A23-	T50.A24-	T50.A25-	T50.A26-
mixed NEC	T50.A21-	T50.A22-	T50.A23-	T50.A24-	T50.A25-	T50.A26-
BCG	T50.A91-	T50.A92-	T50.A93-	T50.A94-	T50.A95-	T50.A96-
cholera	T50.A91-	T50.A92-	T50.A93-	T50.A94-	T50.A95-	T50.A96-
diphtheria	T50.A91-	T50.A92-	T50.A93-	T50.A94-	T50.A95-	T50.A96-
with tetanus	T50.A21-	T50.A22-	T50.A23-	T50.A24-	T50.A25-	T50.A26-
and pertussis	T50.A11-	T50.A12-	T50.A13-	T50.A14-	T50.A15-	T50.A16-
influenza	T50.B91-	T50.B92-	T50.B93-	T50.B94-	T50.B95-	T50.B96-
measles	T50.B91-	T50.B92-	T50.B93-	T50.B94-	T50.B95-	T50.B96-
with mumps and rubella	T50.B91-	T50.B92-	T50.B93-	T50.B94-	T50.B95-	T50.B96-
meningococcal	T50.A91-	T50.A92-	T50.A93-	T50.A94-	T50.A95-	T50.A96-
mumps	T50.B91-	T50.B92-	T50.B93-	T50.B94-	T50.B95-	T50.B96-
paratyphoid	T50.A91-	T50.A92-	T50.A93-	T50.A94-	T50.A95-	T50.A96-
pertussis	T50.A11-	T50.A12-	T50.A13-	T50.A14-	T50.A15-	T50.A16-
with diphtheria	T50.A11-	T50.A12-	T50.A13-	T50.A14-	T50.A15-	T50.A16-
and tetanus	T50.A11-	T50.A12-	T50.A13-	T50.A14-	T50.A15-	T50.A16-
with other component	T50.A11-	T50.A12-	T50.A13-	T50.A14-	T50.A15-	T50.A16-
plague	T50.A91-	T50.A92-	T50.A93-	T50.A94-	T50.A95-	T50.A96-
poliomyelitis	T50.B91-	T50.B92-	T50.B93-	T50.B94-	T50.B95-	T50.B96-
poliovirus	T50.B91-	T50.B92-	T50.B93-	T50.B94-	T50.B95-	T50.B96-
rabies	T50.B91-	T50.B92-	T50.B93-	T50.B94-	T50.B95-	T50.B96-
respiratory syncytial virus	T50.B91-	T50.B92-	T50.B93-	T50.B94-	T50.B95-	T50.B96-
rickettsial NEC	T50.A91-	T50.A92-	T50.A93-	T50.A94-	T50.A95-	T50.A96-
with bacterial component	T50.A21-	T50.A22-	T50.A23-	T50.A24-	T50.A25-	T50.A26-
Rocky Mountain spotted fever	T50.A91-	T50.A92-	T50.A93-	T50.A94-	T50.A95-	T50.A96-
rubella	T50.B91-	T50.B92-	T50.B93-	T50.B94-	T50.B95-	T50.B96-
sabin oral	T50.B91-	T50.B92-	T50.B93-	T50.B94-	T50.B95-	T50.B96-
smallpox	T50.B11-	T50.B12-	T50.B13-	T50.B14-	T50.B15-	T50.B16-
TAB	T50.A91-	T50.A92-	T50.A93-	T50.A94-	T50.A95-	T50.A96-
tetanus	T50.A91-	T50.A92-	T50.A93-	T50.A94-	T50.A95-	T50.A96-
typhoid	T50.A91-	T50.A92-	T50.A93-	T50.A94-	T50.A95-	T50.A96-
typhus	T50.A91-	T50.A92-	T50.A93-	T50.A94-	T50.A95-	T50.A96-
viral NEC	T50.B91-	T50.B92-	T50.B93-	T50.B94-	T50.B95-	T50.B96-
yellow fever	T50.B91-	T50.B92-	T50.B93-	T50.B94-	T50.B95-	T50.B96-
Vaccinia immune globulin	T50.Z11-	T50.Z12-	T50.Z13-	T50.Z14-	T50.Z15-	T50.Z16-
Vaginal contraceptives	T49.8x1-	T49.8x2-	T49.8x3-	T49.8x4-	T49.8x5-	T49.8x6-
Valerian						
root	T42.6x1-	T42.6x2-	T42.6x3-	T42.6x4-	T42.6x5-	T42.6x6-
tincture	T42.6x1-	T42.6x2-	T42.6x3-	T42.6x4-	T42.6x5-	T42.6x6-
Valethamate bromide	T44.3x1-	T44.3x2-	T44.3x3-	T44.3x4-	T44.3x5-	T44.3x6-
Valisone	T49.0x1-	T49.0x2-	T49.0x3-	T49.0x4-	T49.0x5-	T49.0x6-
Valium	T42.4x1-	T42.4x2-	T42.4x3-	T42.4x4-	T42.4x5-	T42.4x6-
Valmid	T42.6x1-	T42.6x2-	T42.6x3-	T42.6x4-	T42.6x5-	T42.6x6-
Valnoctamide	T42.6x1-	T42.6x2-	T42.6x3-	T42.6x4-	T42.6x5-	T42.6x6-
Valproate (sodium)	T42.6x1-	T42.6x2-	T42.6x3-	T42.6x4-	T42.6x5-	T42.6x6-
Valproic acid	T42.6x1-	T42.6x2-	T42.6x3-	T42.6x4-	T42.6x5-	T42.6x6-
Valpromide	T42.6x1-	T42.6x2-	T42.6x3-	T42.6x4-	T42.6x5-	T42.6x6-
Vanadium	T56.891-	T56.892-	T56.893-	T56.894-	—	—
Vancomycin	T36.8x1-	T36.8x2-	T36.8x3-	T36.8x4-	T36.8x5-	T36.8x6-
Vapor — see also Gas	T59.91x-	T59.92x-	T59.93x-	T59.94x-	—	—
kiln (carbon monoxide)	T58.8x1-	T58.8x2-	T58.8x3-	T58.8x4-	—	—
lead — see Lead						
specified source NEC	T59.891-	T59.892-	T59.893-	T59.894-	—	—
Vardenafil	T46.7x1-	T46.7x2-	T46.7x3-	T46.7x4-	T46.7x5-	T46.7x6-

Table of Drugs & Chemicals	Accidental (Unintentional)	Self-Harm (Intentional)	Assault	Undetermined	Adverse Effect	Underdosing
Varicose reduction drug	T46.8x1-	T46.8x2-	T46.8x3-	T46.8x4-	T46.8x5-	T46.8x6-
Varnish	T65.4x1-	T65.4x2-	T65.4x3-	T65.4x4-	—	—
cleaner	T52.91x-	T52.92x-	T52.93x-	T52.94x-	—	—
Vaseline	T49.3x1-	T49.3x2-	T49.3x3-	T49.3x4-	T49.3x5-	T49.3x6-
Vasodilan	T46.7x1-	T46.7x2-	T46.7x3-	T46.7x4-	T46.7x5-	T46.7x6-
Vasodilator						
coronary NEC	T46.3x1-	T46.3x2-	T46.3x3-	T46.3x4-	T46.3x5-	T46.3x6-
peripheral NEC	T46.7x1-	T46.7x2-	T46.7x3-	T46.7x4-	T46.7x5-	T46.7x6-
Vasopressin	T38.891-	T38.892-	T38.893-	T38.894-	T38.895-	T38.896-
Vasopressor drugs	T38.891-	T38.892-	T38.893-	T38.894-	T38.895-	T38.896-
Vecuronium bromide	T48.1x1-	T48.1x2-	T48.1x3-	T48.1x4-	T48.1x5-	T48.1x6-
Vegetable extract, astringent	T49.2x1-	T49.2x2-	T49.2x3-	T49.2x4-	T49.2x5-	T49.2x6-
Venlafaxine	T43.211-	T43.212-	T43.213-	T43.214-	T43.215-	T43.216-
Venom, venomous (bite) (sting)	T63.91x-	T63.92x-	T63.93x-	T63.94x-	—	—
ant	T63.421-	T63.422-	T63.423-	T63.424-	—	—
amphibian NEC	T63.831-	T63.832-	T63.833-	T63.834-	—	—
animal NEC	T63.891-	T63.892-	T63.893-	T63.894-	—	—
arthropod NEC	T63.481-	T63.482-	T63.483-	T63.484-	—	—
bee	T63.441-	T63.442-	T63.443-	T63.444-	—	—
centipede	T63.411-	T63.412-	T63.413-	T63.414-	—	—
fish	T63.591-	T63.592-	T63.593-	T63.594-	—	—
frog	T63.811-	T63.812-	T63.813-	T63.814-	—	—
hornet	T63.451-	T63.452-	T63.453-	T63.454-	—	—
insect NEC	T63.481-	T63.482-	T63.483-	T63.484-	—	—
lizard	T63.121-	T63.122-	T63.123-	T63.124-	—	—
marine						
animals	T63.691-	T63.692-	T63.693-	T63.694-	—	—
bluebottle	T63.611-	T63.612-	T63.613-	T63.614-	—	—
jellyfish NEC	T63.621-	T63.622-	T63.623-	T63.624-	—	—
Portugese Man-o-war	T63.611-	T63.612-	T63.613-	T63.614-	—	—
sea anemone	T63.631-	T63.632-	T63.633-	T63.634-	—	—
specified NEC	T63.691-	T63.692-	T63.693-	T63.694-	—	—
fish	T63.591-	T63.592-	T63.593-	T63.594-	—	—
sting ray	T63.511-	T63.512-	T63.513-	T63.514-	—	—
plants	T63.711-	T63.712-	T63.713-	T63.714-	—	—
millipede (tropical)	T63.411-	T63.412-	T63.413-	T63.414-	—	—
plant NEC	T63.791-	T63.792-	T63.793-	T63.794-	—	—
marine	T63.711-	T63.712-	T63.713-	T63.714-	—	—
reptile	T63.191-	T63.192-	T63.193-	T63.194-	—	—
gila monster	T63.111-	T63.112-	T63.113-	T63.114-	—	—
lizard NEC	T63.121-	T63.122-	T63.123-	T63.124-	—	—
scorpion	T63.2x1-	T63.2x2-	T63.2x3-	T63.2x4-	—	—
snake	T63.001-	T63.002-	T63.003-	T63.004-	—	—
African NEC	T63.081-	T63.082-	T63.083-	T63.084-	—	—
American (North) (South) NEC	T63.061-	T63.062-	T63.063-	T63.064-	—	—
Asian	T63.081-	T63.082-	T63.083-	T63.084-	—	—
Australian	T63.071-	T63.072-	T63.073-	T63.074-	—	—
cobra	T63.041-	T63.042-	T63.043-	T63.044-	—	—
coral snake	T63.021-	T63.022-	T63.023-	T63.024-	—	—
rattlesnake	T63.011-	T63.012-	T63.013-	T63.014-	—	—
specified NEC	T63.091-	T63.092-	T63.093-	T63.094-	—	—
taipan	T63.031-	T63.032-	T63.033-	T63.034-	—	—
specified NEC	T63.891-	T63.892-	T63.893-	T63.894-	—	—
spider	T63.301-	T63.302-	T63.303-	T63.304-	—	—
black widow	T63.311-	T63.312-	T63.313-	T63.314-	—	—
brown recluse	T63.331-	T63.332-	T63.333-	T63.334-	—	—
specified NEC	T63.391-	T63.392-	T63.393-	T63.394-	—	—
tarantula	T63.321-	T63.322-	T63.323-	T63.324-	—	—
sting ray	T63.511-	T63.512-	T63.513-	T63.514-	—	—
toad	T63.821-	T63.822-	T63.823-	T63.824-	—	—
wasp	T63.461-	T63.462-	T63.463-	T63.464-	—	—

DRUGS & CHEMICALS

Table of Drugs & Chemicals	POISONING Accidental (Unintentional)	POISONING Self-Harm (Intentional)	POISONING Assault	POISONING Undeter-mined	Adverse Effect	Underdosing
Venous sclerosing drug NEC	T46.8x1-	T46.8x2-	T46.8x3-	T46.8x4-	T46.8x5-	T46.8x6-
Ventolin — see Albuterol						
Veramon	T42.3x1-	T42.3x2-	T42.3x3-	T42.3x4-	T42.3x5-	T42.3x6-
Verapamil	T46.1x1-	T46.1x2-	T46.1x3-	T46.1x4-	T46.1x5-	T46.1x6-
Veratrine	T46.5x1-	T46.5x2-	T46.5x3-	T46.5x4-	T46.5x5-	T46.5x6-
Veratrum						
album	T62.2x1-	T62.2x2-	T62.2x3-	T62.2x4-	—	—
alkaloids	T46.5x1-	T46.5x2-	T46.5x3-	T46.5x4-	T46.5x5-	T46.5x6-
viride	T62.2x1-	T62.2x2-	T62.2x3-	T62.2x4-	—	—
Verdigris	T60.3x1-	T60.3x2-	T60.3x3-	T60.3x4-	—	—
Veronal	T42.3x1-	T42.3x2-	T42.3x3-	T42.3x4-	T42.3x5-	T42.3x6-
Veroxil	T37.4x1-	T37.4x2-	T37.4x3-	T37.4x4-	T37.4x5-	T37.4x6-
Versenate	T50.6x1-	T50.6x2-	T50.6x3-	T50.6x4-	T50.6x5-	T50.6x6-
Versidyne	T39.8x1-	T39.8x2-	T39.8x3-	T39.8x4-	T39.8x5-	T39.8x6-
Vetrabutine	T48.0x1-	T48.0x2-	T48.0x3-	T48.0x4-	T48.0x5-	T48.0x6-
Vidarabine	T37.5x1-	T37.5x2-	T37.5x3-	T37.5x4-	T37.5x5-	T37.5x6-
Vienna						
green	T57.0x1-	T57.0x2-	T57.0x3-	T57.0x4-	—	—
insecticide	T60.2x1-	T60.2x2-	T60.2x3-	T60.2x4-	—	—
red	T57.0x1-	T57.0x2-	T57.0x3-	T57.0x4-	—	—
pharmaceutical dye	T50.991-	T50.992-	T50.993-	T50.994-	T50.995-	T50.996-
Vigabatrin	T42.6x1-	T42.6x2-	T42.6x3-	T42.6x4-	T42.6x5-	T42.6x6-
Viloxazine	T43.291-	T43.292-	T43.293-	T43.294-	T43.295-	T43.296-
Viminol	T39.8x1-	T39.8x2-	T39.8x3-	T39.8x4-	T39.8x5-	T39.8x6-
Vinbarbital, vinbarbitone	T42.3x1-	T42.3x2-	T42.3x3-	T42.3x4-	T42.3x5-	T42.3x6-
Vinblastine	T45.1x1-	T45.1x2-	T45.1x3-	T45.1x4-	T45.1x5-	T45.1x6-
Vinburnine	T46.7x1-	T46.7x2-	T46.7x3-	T46.7x4-	T46.7x5-	T46.7x6-
Vincamine	T45.1x1-	T45.1x2-	T45.1x3-	T45.1x4-	T45.1x5-	T45.1x6-
Vincristine	T45.1x1-	T45.1x2-	T45.1x3-	T45.1x4-	T45.1x5-	T45.1x6-
Vindesine	T45.1x1-	T45.1x2-	T45.1x3-	T45.1x4-	T45.1x5-	T45.1x6-
Vinesthene, vinethene	T41.0x1-	T41.0x2-	T41.0x3-	T41.0x4-	T41.0x5-	T41.0x6-
Vinorelbine tartrate	T45.1x1-	T45.1x2-	T45.1x3-	T45.1x4-	T45.1x5-	T45.1x6-
Vinpocetine	T46.7x1-	T46.7x2-	T46.7x3-	T46.7x4-	T46.7x5-	T46.7x6-
Vinyl						
acetate	T65.891-	T65.892-	T65.893-	T65.894-	—	—
bital	T42.3x1-	T42.3x2-	T42.3x3-	T42.3x4-	T42.3x5-	T42.3x6-
bromide	T65.891-	T65.892-	T65.893-	T65.894-	—	—
chloride	T59.891-	T59.892-	T59.893-	T59.894-	—	—
ether	T41.0x1-	T41.0x2-	T41.0x3-	T41.0x4-	T41.0x5-	T41.0x6-
Vinylbital	T42.3x1-	T42.3x2-	T42.3x3-	T42.3x4-	T42.3x5-	T42.3x6-
Vinylidene chloride	T65.891-	T65.892-	T65.893-	T65.894-	—	—
Vioform	T37.8x1-	T37.8x2-	T37.8x3-	T37.8x4-	T37.8x5-	T37.8x6-
topical	T49.0x1-	T49.0x2-	T49.0x3-	T49.0x4-	T49.0x5-	T49.0x6-
Viomycin	T36.8x1-	T36.8x2-	T36.8x3-	T36.8x4-	T36.8x5-	T36.8x6-
Viosterol	T45.2x1-	T45.2x2-	T45.2x3-	T45.2x4-	T45.2x5-	T45.2x6-
Viper (venom)	T63.091-	T63.092-	T63.093-	T63.094-	—	—
Viprynium	T37.4x1-	T37.4x2-	T37.4x3-	T37.4x4-	T37.4x5-	T37.4x6-
Viquidil	T46.7x1-	T46.7x2-	T46.7x3-	T46.7x4-	T46.7x5-	T46.7x6-
Viral vaccine NEC	T50.B91-	T50.B92-	T50.B93-	T50.B94-	T50.B95-	T50.B96-
Virginiamycin	T36.8x1-	T36.8x2-	T36.8x3-	T36.8x4-	T36.8x5-	T36.8x6-
Virugon	T37.5x1-	T37.5x2-	T37.5x3-	T37.5x4-	T37.5x5-	T37.5x6-
Viscous agent	T50.901-	T50.902-	T50.903-	T50.904-	T50.905-	T50.906-
Visine	T49.5x1-	T49.5x2-	T49.5x3-	T49.5x4-	T49.5x5-	T49.5x6-
Visnadine	T46.3x1-	T46.3x2-	T46.3x3-	T46.3x4-	T46.3x5-	T46.3x6-

Table of Drugs & Chemicals	POISONING Accidental (Unintentional)	POISONING Self-Harm (Intentional)	POISONING Assault	POISONING Undeter-mined	Adverse Effect	Underdosing
Vitamin NEC	T45.2x1-	T45.2x2-	T45.2x3-	T45.2x4-	T45.2x5-	T45.2x6-
A	T45.2x1-	T45.2x2-	T45.2x3-	T45.2x4-	T45.2x5-	T45.2x6-
B NEC	T45.2x1-	T45.2x2-	T45.2x3-	T45.2x4-	T45.2x5-	T45.2x6-
nicotinic acid	T46.7x1-	T46.7x2-	T46.7x3-	T46.7x4-	T46.7x5-	T46.7x6-
B1	T45.2x1-	T45.2x2-	T45.2x3-	T45.2x4-	T45.2x5-	T45.2x6-
B2	T45.2x1-	T45.2x2-	T45.2x3-	T45.2x4-	T45.2x5-	T45.2x6-
B6	T45.2x1-	T45.2x2-	T45.2x3-	T45.2x4-	T45.2x5-	T45.2x6-
B12	T45.2x1-	T45.2x2-	T45.2x3-	T45.2x4-	T45.2x5-	T45.2x6-
B15	T45.2x1-	T45.2x2-	T45.2x3-	T45.2x4-	T45.2x5-	T45.2x6-
C	T45.2x1-	T45.2x2-	T45.2x3-	T45.2x4-	T45.2x5-	T45.2x6-
D	T45.2x1-	T45.2x2-	T45.2x3-	T45.2x4-	T45.2x5-	T45.2x6-
D2	T45.2x1-	T45.2x2-	T45.2x3-	T45.2x4-	T45.2x5-	T45.2x6-
D3	T45.2x1-	T45.2x2-	T45.2x3-	T45.2x4-	T45.2x5-	T45.2x6-
E	T45.2x1-	T45.2x2-	T45.2x3-	T45.2x4-	T45.2x5-	T45.2x6-
E acetate	T45.2x1-	T45.2x2-	T45.2x3-	T45.2x4-	T45.2x5-	T45.2x6-
hematopoietic	T45.8x1-	T45.8x2-	T45.8x3-	T45.8x4-	T45.8x5-	T45.8x6-
K NEC	T45.7x1-	T45.7x2-	T45.7x3-	T45.7x4-	T45.7x5-	T45.7x6-
K1	T45.7x1-	T45.7x2-	T45.7x3-	T45.7x4-	T45.7x5-	T45.7x6-
K2	T45.7x1-	T45.7x2-	T45.7x3-	T45.7x4-	T45.7x5-	T45.7x6-
PP	T45.2x1-	T45.2x2-	T45.2x3-	T45.2x4-	T45.2x5-	T45.2x6-
ulceroprotectant	T47.1x1-	T47.1x2-	T47.1x3-	T47.1x4-	T47.1x5-	T47.1x6-
Vleminckx's solution	T49.4x1-	T49.4x2-	T49.4x3-	T49.4x4-	T49.4x5-	T49.4x6-
Voltaren — see Diclofenac sodium						
Warfarin	T45.511-	T45.512-	T45.513-	T45.514-	T45.515-	T45.516-
rodenticide	T60.4x1-	T60.4x2-	T60.4x3-	T60.4x4-	—	—
sodium	T60.4x1-	T60.4x2-	T60.4x3-	T60.4x4-	—	—
Wasp (sting)	T63.461-	T63.462-	T63.463-	T63.464-	—	—
Water						
balance drug	T50.3x1-	T50.3x2-	T50.3x3-	T50.3x4-	T50.3x5-	T50.3x6-
distilled	T50.3x1-	T50.3x2-	T50.3x3-	T50.3x4-	T50.3x5-	T50.3x6-
gas — see Gas, water						
incomplete combustion of — see Carbon, monoxide, fuel, utility						
hemlock	T62.2x1-	T62.2x2-	T62.2x3-	T62.2x4-	—	—
moccasin (venom)	T63.061-	T63.062-	T63.063-	T63.064-	—	—
purified	T50.3x1-	T50.3x2-	T50.3x3-	T50.3x4-	T50.3x5-	T50.3x6-
Wax (paraffin) (petroleum)	T52.0x1-	T52.0x2-	T52.0x3-	T52.0x4-	—	—
automobile	T65.891-	T65.892-	T65.893-	T65.894-	—	—
floor	T52.0x1-	T52.0x2-	T52.0x3-	T52.0x4-	—	—
Weed killers NEC	T60.3x1-	T60.3x2-	T60.3x3-	T60.3x4-	—	—
Welldorm	T42.6x1-	T42.6x2-	T42.6x3-	T42.6x4-	T42.6x5-	T42.6x6-
White						
arsenic	T57.0x1-	T57.0x2-	T57.0x3-	T57.0x4-	—	—
hellebore	T62.2x1-	T62.2x2-	T62.2x3-	T62.2x4-	—	—
lotion (keratolytic)	T49.4x1-	T49.4x2-	T49.4x3-	T49.4x4-	T49.4x5-	T49.4x6-
spirit	T52.0x1-	T52.0x2-	T52.0x3-	T52.0x4-	—	—
Whitewash	T65.891-	T65.892-	T65.893-	T65.894-	—	—
Whole blood (human)	T45.8x1-	T45.8x2-	T45.8x3-	T45.8x4-	T45.8x5-	T45.8x6-
Wild						
black cherry	T62.2x1-	T62.2x2-	T62.2x3-	T62.2x4-	—	—
poisonous plants NEC	T62.2x1-	T62.2x2-	T62.2x3-	T62.2x4-	—	—
Window cleaning fluid	T65.891-	T65.892-	T65.893-	T65.894-	—	—
Wintergreen (oil)	T49.3x1-	T49.3x2-	T49.3x3-	T49.3x4-	T49.3x5-	T49.3x6-
Wisterine	T62.2x1-	T62.2x2-	T62.2x3-	T62.2x4-	—	—
Witch hazel	T49.2x1-	T49.2x2-	T49.2x3-	T49.2x4-	T49.2x5-	T49.2x6-
Wood alcohol or spirit	T51.1x1-	T51.1x2-	T51.1x3-	T51.1x4-	—	—
Wool fat (hydrous)	T49.3x1-	T49.3x2-	T49.3x3-	T49.3x4-	T49.3x5-	T49.3x6-
Woorali	T48.1x1-	T48.1x2-	T48.1x3-	T48.1x4-	T48.1x5-	T48.1x6-
Wormseed, American	T37.4x1-	T37.4x2-	T37.4x3-	T37.4x4-	T37.4x5-	T37.4x6-

Table of Drugs & Chemicals	POISONING				Adverse Effect	Underdosing
	Accidental (Unintentional)	Self-Harm (Intentional)	Assault	Undetermined		
Xamoterol	T44.5x1-	T44.5x2-	T44.5x3-	T44.5x4-	T44.5x5-	T44.5x6-
Xanthine diuretics	T50.2x1-	T50.2x2-	T50.2x3-	T50.2x4-	T50.2x5-	T50.2x6-
Xanthinol nicotinate	T46.7x1-	T46.7x2-	T46.7x3-	T46.7x4-	T46.7x5-	T46.7x6-
Xanthotoxin	T49.3x1-	T49.3x2-	T49.3x3-	T49.3x4-	T49.3x5-	T49.3x6-
Xantinol nicotinate	T46.7x1-	T46.7x2-	T46.7x3-	T46.7x4-	T46.7x5-	T46.7x6-
Xantocillin	T36.0x1-	T36.0x2-	T36.0x3-	T36.0x4-	T36.0x5-	T36.0x6-
Xenon (127Xe) (133Xe)	T50.8x1-	T50.8x2-	T50.8x3-	T50.8x4-	T50.8x5-	T50.8x6-
Xenysalate	T49.4x1-	T49.4x2-	T49.4x3-	T49.4x4-	T49.4x5-	T49.4x6-
Xibornol	T37.8x1-	T37.8x2-	T37.8x3-	T37.8x4-	T37.8x5-	T37.8x6-
Xigris	T45.511-	T45.512-	T45.513-	T45.514-	T45.515-	T45.516-
Xipamide	T50.2x1-	T50.2x2-	T50.2x3-	T50.2x4-	T50.2x5-	T50.2x6-
Xylene (vapor)	T52.2x1-	T52.2x2-	T52.2x3-	T52.2x4-	—	—
Xylocaine (infiltration) (topical)	T41.3x1-	T41.3x2-	T41.3x3-	T41.3x4-	T41.3x5-	T41.3x6-
nerve block (peripheral) (plexus)	T41.3x1-	T41.3x2-	T41.3x3-	T41.3x4-	T41.3x5-	T41.3x6-
spinal	T41.3x1-	T41.3x2-	T41.3x3-	T41.3x4-	T41.3x5-	T41.3x6-
Xylol (vapor)	T52.2x1-	T52.2x2-	T52.2x3-	T52.2x4-	—	—
Xylometazoline	T48.5x1-	T48.5x2-	T48.5x3-	T48.5x4-	T48.5x5-	T48.5x6-
Yeast	T45.2x1-	T45.2x2-	T45.2x3-	T45.2x4-	T45.2x5-	T45.2x6-
dried	T45.2x1-	T45.2x2-	T45.2x3-	T45.2x4-	T45.2x5-	T45.2x6-
Yellow						
fever vaccine	T50.B91-	T50.B92-	T50.B93-	T50.B94-	T50.B95-	T50.B96-
jasmine	T62.2x1-	T62.2x2-	T62.2x3-	T62.2x4-		
phenolphthalein	T47.2x1-	T47.2x2-	T47.2x3-	T47.2x4-	T47.2x5-	T47.2x6-
Yew	T62.2x1-	T62.2x2-	T62.2x3-	T62.2x4-		
Yohimbic acid	T40.991-	T40.992-	T40.993-	T40.994-	T40.995-	T40.996-
Zactane	T39.8x1-	T39.8x2-	T39.8x3-	T39.8x4-	T39.8x5-	T39.8x6-
Zalcitabine	T37.5x1-	T37.5x2-	T37.5x3-	T37.5x4-	T37.5x5-	T37.5x6-
Zaroxolyn	T50.2x1-	T50.2x2-	T50.2x3-	T50.2x4-	T50.2x5-	T50.2x6-
Zephiran (topical)	T49.0x1-	T49.0x2-	T49.0x3-	T49.0x4-	T49.0x5-	T49.0x6-
ophthalmic preparation	T49.5x1-	T49.5x2-	T49.5x3-	T49.5x4-	T49.5x5-	T49.5x6-
Zeranol	T38.7x1-	T38.7x2-	T38.7x3-	T38.7x4-	T38.7x5-	T38.7x6-
Zerone	T51.1x1-	T51.1x2-	T51.1x3-	T51.1x4-		
Zidovudine	T37.5x1-	T37.5x2-	T37.5x3-	T37.5x4-	T37.5x5-	T37.5x6-
Zimeldine	T43.221-	T43.222-	T43.223-	T43.224-	T43.225-	T43.226-
Zinc (compounds) (fumes) (vapor) NEC	T56.5x1-	T56.5x2-	T56.5x3-	T56.5x4-	—	—
anti-infectives	T49.0x1-	T49.0x2-	T49.0x3-	T49.0x4-	T49.0x5-	T49.0x6-
antivaricose	T46.8x1-	T46.8x2-	T46.8x3-	T46.8x4-	T46.8x5-	T46.8x6-
bacitracin	T49.0x1-	T49.0x2-	T49.0x3-	T49.0x4-	T49.0x5-	T49.0x6-
chloride (mouthwash)	T49.6x1-	T49.6x2-	T49.6x3-	T49.6x4-	T49.6x5-	T49.6x6-
chromate	T56.5x1-	T56.5x2-	T56.5x3-	T56.5x4-	—	—
gelatin	T49.3x1-	T49.3x2-	T49.3x3-	T49.3x4-	T49.3x5-	T49.3x6-
oxide	T49.3x1-	T49.3x2-	T49.3x3-	T49.3x4-	T49.3x5-	T49.3x6-
plaster	T49.3x1-	T49.3x2-	T49.3x3-	T49.3x4-	T49.3x5-	T49.3x6-
peroxide	T49.0x1-	T49.0x2-	T49.0x3-	T49.0x4-	T49.0x5-	T49.0x6-
pesticides	T56.5x1-	T56.5x2-	T56.5x3-	T56.5x4-	—	—
phosphide	T60.4x1-	T60.4x2-	T60.4x3-	T60.4x4-		
pyrithionate	T49.4x1-	T49.4x2-	T49.4x3-	T49.4x4-	T49.4x5-	T49.4x6-
stearate	T49.3x1-	T49.3x2-	T49.3x3-	T49.3x4-	T49.3x5-	T49.3x6-
sulfate	T49.5x1-	T49.5x2-	T49.5x3-	T49.5x4-	T49.5x5-	T49.5x6-
ENT agent	T49.6x1-	T49.6x2-	T49.6x3-	T49.6x4-	T49.6x5-	T49.6x6-
ophthalmic solution	T49.5x1-	T49.5x2-	T49.5x3-	T49.5x4-	T49.5x5-	T49.5x6-
topical NEC	T49.0x1-	T49.0x2-	T49.0x3-	T49.0x4-	T49.0x5-	T49.0x6-
undecylenate	T49.0x1-	T49.0x2-	T49.0x3-	T49.0x4-	T49.0x5-	T49.0x6-
Zineb	T60.0x1-	T60.0x2-	T60.0x3-	T60.0x4-	—	—
Zinostatin	T45.1x1-	T45.1x2-	T45.1x3-	T45.1x4-	T45.1x5-	T45.1x6-
Zipeprol	T48.3x1-	T48.3x2-	T48.3x3-	T48.3x4-	T48.3x5-	T48.3x6-
Zofenopril	T46.4x1-	T46.4x2-	T46.4x3-	T46.4x4-	T46.4x5-	T46.4x6-
Zolpidem	T42.6x1-	T42.6x2-	T42.6x3-	T42.6x4-	T42.6x5-	T42.6x6-
Zomepirac	T39.391-	T39.392-	T39.393-	T39.394-	T39.395-	T39.396-
Zopiclone	T42.6x1-	T42.6x2-	T42.6x3-	T42.6x4-	T42.6x5-	T42.6x6-
Zorubicin	T45.1x1-	T45.1x2-	T45.1x3-	T45.1x4-	T45.1x5-	T45.1x6-
Zotepine	T43.591-	T43.592-	T43.593-	T43.594-	T43.595-	T43.596-
Zovant	T45.511-	T45.512-	T45.513-	T45.514-	T45.515-	T45.516-
Zoxazolamine	T42.8x1-	T42.8x2-	T42.8x3-	T42.8x4-	T42.8x5-	T42.8x6-
Zuclopenthixol	T43.4x1-	T43.4x2-	T43.4x3-	T43.4x4-	T43.4x5-	T43.4x6-
Zygadenus (venenosus)	T62.2x1-	T62.2x2-	T62.2x3-	T62.2x4-	—	—
Zyprexa	T43.591-	T43.592-	T43.593-	T43.594-	T43.595-	T43.596-

DRUGS & CHEMICALS

Table of Drugs & Chemicals	POISONING				Adverse Effect	Underdosing	Table of Drugs & Chemicals	POISONING				Adverse Effect	Underdosing
	Accidental (Unintentional)	Self-Harm (Intentional)	Assault	Undetermined				Accidental (Unintentional)	Self-Harm (Intentional)	Assault	Undetermined		

A

Abandonment (causing exposure to weather conditions) (with intent to injure or kill) NEC X58

Abuse (adult) (child) (mental) (physical) (sexual) X58

Accident (to) X58
  aircraft (in transit) (powered) — *see also* Accident, transport, aircraft
    due to, caused by cataclysm — *see* Forces of nature, by type
  animal-drawn vehicle — *see* Accident, transport, animal-drawn vehicle occupant
  animal-rider — *see* Accident, transport, animal-rider
  automobile — *see* Accident, transport, car occupant
  bare foot water skier V94.4
  boat, boating — *see also* Accident, watercraft
    striking swimmer
      powered V94.11
      unpowered V94.12
  bus — *see* Accident, transport, bus occupant
  cable car, not on rails V98.0
    on rails — *see* Accident, transport, streetcar occupant
  car — *see* Accident, transport, car occupant
  caused by, due to
    animal NEC W64
    chain hoist W24.0
    cold (excessive) — *see* Exposure, cold
    corrosive liquid, substance — *see* Table of Drugs and Chemicals
    cutting or piercing instrument — *see* Contact, with, by type of instrument
    drive belt W24.0
    electric
      current — *see* Exposure, electric current
      motor (*see also* Contact, with, by type of machine) W31.3
        current (of) W86.8
    environmental factor NEC X58
    explosive material — *see* Explosion
    fire, flames — *see* Exposure, fire
    firearm missile — *see* Discharge, firearm by type
    heat (excessive) — *see* Heat
    hot — *see* Contact, with, hot
    ignition — *see* Ignition
    lifting device W24.0
    lightning — *see* subcategory T75.0
      causing fire — *see* Exposure, fire
    machine, machinery — *see* Contact, with, by type of machine
    natural factor NEC X58
    pulley (block) W24.0
    radiation — *see* Radiation
    steam X13.1
      inhalation X13.0
      pipe X16
    thunderbolt — *see* subcategory T75.0
      causing fire — *see* Exposure, fire
    transmission device W24.1
  coach — *see* Accident, transport, bus occupant
  coal car — *see* Accident, transport, industrial vehicle occupant
  diving — *see also* Fall, into, water
    with
      drowning or submersion — *see* Drowning
  forklift — *see* Accident, transport, industrial vehicle occupant
  heavy transport vehicle NOS — *see* Accident, transport, truck occupant
  ice yacht V98.2

Accident (to) X58 — *continued*
  in
    medical, surgical procedure
      as, or due to misadventure — *see* Misadventure
      causing an abnormal reaction or later complication without mention of misadventure (*see also* Complication of or following, by type of procedure) Y84.9
  land yacht V98.1
  late effect of — *see* W00-X58 with 7th character S
  logging car — *see* Accident, transport, industrial vehicle occupant
  machine, machinery — *see also* Contact, with, by type of machine
    on board watercraft V93.69
      explosion — *see* Explosion, in, watercraft
      fire — *see* Burn, on board watercraft
      powered craft V93.63
        ferry boat V93.61
        fishing boat V93.62
        jetskis V93.63
        liner V93.61
        merchant ship V93.60
        passenger ship V93.61
        sailboat V93.64
  mine tram — *see* Accident, transport, industrial vehicle occupant
  mobility scooter (motorized) — *see* Accident, transport, pedestrian, conveyance, specified type NEC
  motor scooter — *see* Accident, transport, motorcyclist
  motor vehicle NOS (traffic) (*see also* Accident, transport) V89.2
    nontraffic V89.0
    three-wheeled NOS — *see* Accident, transport, three-wheeled motor vehicle occupant
  motorcycle NOS — *see* Accident, transport, motorcyclist
  nonmotor vehicle NOS (nontraffic) (*see also* Accident, transport) V89.1
    traffic NOS V89.3
  nontraffic (victim's mode of transport NOS) V88.9
    collision (between) V88.7
      bus and truck V88.5
      car and:
        bus V88.3
        pickup V88.2
        three-wheeled motor vehicle V88.0
        train V88.6
        truck V88.4
        two-wheeled motor vehicle V88.0
        van V88.2
      specified vehicle NEC and:
        three-wheeled motor vehicle V88.1
        two-wheeled motor vehicle V88.1
    known mode of transport — *see* Accident, transport, by type of vehicle
    noncollision V88.8

Accident (to) X58 — *continued*
  on board watercraft V93.89
    powered craft V93.83
      ferry boat V93.81
      fishing boat V93.82
      jetskis V93.83
      liner V93.81
      merchant ship V93.80
      passenger ship V93.81
    unpowered craft V93.88
      canoe V93.85
      inflatable V93.86
        in tow
          recreational V94.31
          specified NEC V94.32
      kayak V93.85
      sailboat V93.84
      surfboard V93.88
      water skis V93.87
      windsurfer V93.88
  parachutist V97.29
    entangled in object V97.21
    injured on landing V97.22
  pedal cycle — *see* Accident, transport, pedal cyclist
  pedestrian (on foot)
    with
      another pedestrian W51
        with fall W03
          due to ice or snow W00.0
      on pedestrian conveyance NEC V00.09
      roller skater (in-line) V00.01
      skate boarder V00.02
      transport vehicle — *see* Accident, transport
    on pedestrian conveyance — *see* Accident, transport, pedestrian, conveyance
  pickup truck or van — *see* Accident, transport, pickup truck occupant
  quarry truck — *see* Accident, transport, industrial vehicle occupant
  railway vehicle (any) (in motion) — *see* Accident, transport, railway vehicle occupant
    due to cataclysm — *see* Forces of nature, by type
  scooter (non-motorized) — *see* Accident, transport, pedestrian, conveyance, scooter
  sequelae of — *see* W00-X58 with 7th character S
  skateboard — *see* Accident, transport, pedestrian, conveyance, skateboard
  ski(ing) — *see* Accident, transport, pedestrian, conveyance
  lift V98.3
  specified cause NEC X58
  streetcar — *see* Accident, transport, streetcar occupant
  traffic (victim's mode of transport NOS) V87.9
    collision (between) V87.7
      bus and truck V87.5
      car and:
        bus V87.3
        pickup V87.2
        three-wheeled motor vehicle V87.0
        train V87.6
        truck V87.4
        two-wheeled motor vehicle V87.0
        van V87.2
      specified vehicle NEC and:
        three-wheeled motor vehicle V87.1
        two-wheeled motor vehicle V87.1
    known mode of transport — *see* Accident, transport, by type of vehicle
    noncollision V87.8

Accident (to) X58 — *continued*
transport (involving injury to) V99
  18 wheeler — *see* Accident, transport, truck
    occupant
  agricultural vehicle occupant (nontraffic)
    V84.9
    driver V84.5
    hanger-on V84.7
    passenger V84.6
    traffic V84.3
      driver V84.0
      hanger-on V84.2
      passenger V84.1
    while boarding or alighting V84.4
  aircraft NEC V97.89
    military NEC V97.818
      with civlian aircraft V97.810
      civilian injured by V97.811
    occupant injured (in)
      nonpowered craft accident V96.9
        balloon V96.00
          collision V96.03
          crash V96.01
          explosion V96.05
          fire V96.04
          forced landing V96.02
          specified type NEC V96.09
        glider V96.20
          collision V96.23
          crash V96.21
          explosion V96.25
          fire V96.24
          forced landing V96.22
          specified type NEC V96.29
        hang glider V96.10
          collision V96.13
          crash V96.11
          explosion V96.15
          fire V96.14
          forced landing V96.12
          specified type NEC V96.19
        specified craft NEC V96.8
      powered craft accident V95.9
        fixed wing NEC
          commercial V95.30
            collision V95.33
            crash V95.31
            explosion V95.35
            fire V95.34
            forced landing V95.32
            specified type NEC V95.39
          private V95.20
            collision V95.23
            crash V95.21
            explosion V95.25
            fire V95.24
            forced landing V95.22
            specified type NEC V95.29
        glider V95.10
          collision V95.13
          crash V95.11
          explosion V95.15
          fire V95.14
          forced landing V95.12
          specified type NEC V95.19
        helicopter V95.00
          collision V95.03
          crash V95.01
          explosion V95.05
          fire V95.04
          forced landing V95.02
          specified type NEC V95.09

Accident (to) X58 — *continued*
transport (involving injury to) V99—*continued*
  aircraft NEC V97.89 — *continued*
    occupant injured (in) — *continued*
      powered craft accident V95.9 —
        continued
        spacecraft V95.40
          collision V95.43
          crash V95.41
          explosion V95.45
          fire V95.44
          forced landing V95.42
          specified type NEC V95.49
        specified craft NEC V95.8
        ultralight V95.10
          collision V95.13
          crash V95.11
          explosion V95.15
          fire V95.14
          forced landing V95.12
          specified type NEC V95.19
        specified accident NEC V97.0
      while boarding or alighting V97.1
    person (injured by)
      falling from, in or on aircraft V97.0
      machinery on aircraft V97.89
      on ground with aircraft involvement
        V97.39
      rotating propeller V97.32
      struck by object falling from aircraft
        V97.31
      sucked into aircraft jet V97.33
      while boarding or alighting aircraft
        V97.1
  airport (battery-powered) passenger vehicle
    — *see* Accident, transport, industrial
    vehicle occupant
  all-terrain vehicle occupant (nontraffic)
    V86.99
    driver V86.59
    dune buggy — *see* Accident, transport,
      dune buggy occupant
    hanger-on V86.79
    passenger V86.69
    snowmobile — *see* Accident, transport,
      snowmobile occupant
    traffic V86.39
      driver V86.09
      hanger-on V86.29
      passenger V86.19
    while boarding or alighting V86.49
  ambulance occupant (traffic) V86.31
    driver V86.01
    hanger-on V86.21
    nontraffic V86.91
      driver V86.51
      passenger V86.11
    while boarding or alighting V86.41

Accident (to) X58 — *continued*
transport (involving injury to) V99—*continued*
  animal-drawn vehicle occupant (in) V80.929
    collision (with)
      animal V80.12
        being ridden V80.711
      animal-drawn vehicle V80.721
      bus V80.42
      car V80.42
      fixed or stationary object V80.82
      military vehicle V80.920
      nonmotor vehicle V80.791
      pedal cycle V80.22
      pedestrian V80.12
      pickup V80.42
      railway train or vehicle V80.62
      specified motor vehicle NEC V80.52
      streetcar V80.731
      truck V80.42
      two-or three-wheeled motor vehicle
        V80.32
      van V80.42
    noncollision V80.02
    specified circumstance NEC V80.928
  animal-rider V80.919
    collision (with)
      animal V80.11
        being ridden V80.710
      animal-drawn vehicle V80.720
      bus V80.41
      car V80.41
      fixed or stationary object V80.81
      military vehicle V80.910
      nonmotor vehicle V80.790
      pedal cycle V80.21
      pedestrian V80.11
      pickup V80.41
      railway train or vehicle V80.61
      specified motor vehicle NEC V80.51
      streetcar V80.730
      truck V80.41
      two-or three-wheeled motor vehicle
        V80.31
      van V80.41
    noncollision V80.018
      specified as horse rider V80.010
    specified circumstance NEC V80.918
  armored car — *see* Accident, transport, truck
    occupant
  battery-powered truck (baggage) (mail) —
    see Accident, transport, industrial vehicle
    occupant

EXTERNAL CAUSES

Accident (to) X58 — *continued*
  transport (involving injury to) V99—*continued*
  bus occupant V79.9
    collision (with)
      animal (traffic) V70.9
        being ridden (traffic) V76.9
          nontraffic V76.3
            while boarding or alighting V76.4
        nontraffic V70.3
        while boarding or alighting V70.4
      animal-drawn vehicle (traffic) V76.9
        nontraffic V76.3
        while boarding or alighting V76.4
      bus (traffic) V74.9
        nontraffic V74.3
        while boarding or alighting V74.4
      car (traffic) V73.9
        nontraffic V73.3
        while boarding or alighting V73.4
      motor vehicle NOS (traffic) V79.60
        nontraffic V79.20
        specified type NEC (traffic) V79.69
          nontraffic V79.29
      pedal cycle (traffic) V71.9
        nontraffic V71.3
        while boarding or alighting V71.4
      pickup truck (traffic) V73.9
        nontraffic V73.3
        while boarding or alighting V73.4
      railway vehicle (traffic) V75.9
        nontraffic V75.3
        while boarding or alighting V75.4
      specified vehicle NEC (traffic) V76.9
        nontraffic V76.3
        while boarding or alighting V76.4
      stationary object (traffic) V77.9
        nontraffic V77.3
        while boarding or alighting V77.4
      streetcar (traffic) V76.9
        nontraffic V76.3
        while boarding or alighting V76.4
      three wheeled motor vehicle (traffic) V72.9
        nontraffic V72.3
        while boarding or alighting V72.4
      truck (traffic) V74.9
        nontraffic V74.3
        while boarding or alighting V74.4
      two wheeled motor vehicle (traffic) V72.9
        nontraffic V72.3
        while boarding or alighting V72.4
      van (traffic) V73.9
        nontraffic V73.3
        while boarding or alighting V73.4
    driver
      collision (with)
        animal (traffic) V70.5
          being ridden (traffic) V76.5
            nontraffic V76.0
          nontraffic V70.0
        animal-drawn vehicle (traffic) V76.5
          nontraffic V76.0
        bus (traffic) V74.5
          nontraffic V74.0
        car (traffic) V73.5
          nontraffic V73.0
        motor vehicle NOS (traffic) V79.40
          nontraffic V79.00
          specified type NEC (traffic) V79.49
            nontraffic V79.09
        pedal cycle (traffic) V71.5
          nontraffic V71.0
        pickup truck (traffic) V73.5
          nontraffic V73.0
        railway vehicle (traffic) V75.5
          nontraffic V75.0

Accident (to) X58 — *continued*
  transport (involving injury to) V99—*continued*
  bus occupant V79.9 — *continued*
    driver — *continued*
      collision (with) — *continued*
        specified vehicle NEC (traffic) V76.5
          nontraffic V76.0
        stationary object (traffic) V77.5
          nontraffic V77.0
        streetcar (traffic) V76.5
          nontraffic V76.0
        three wheeled motor vehicle (traffic) V72.5
          nontraffic V72.0
        truck (traffic) V74.5
          nontraffic V74.0
        two wheeled motor vehicle (traffic) V72.5
          nontraffic V72.0
        van (traffic) V73.5
          nontraffic V73.0
      noncollision accident (traffic) V78.5
        nontraffic V78.0
    hanger-on
      collision (with)
        animal (traffic) V70.7
          being ridden (traffic) V76.7
            nontraffic V76.2
          nontraffic V70.2
        animal-drawn vehicle (traffic) V76.7
          nontraffic V76.2
        bus (traffic) V74.7
          nontraffic V74.2
        car (traffic) V73.7
          nontraffic V73.2
        pedal cycle (traffic) V71.7
          nontraffic V71.2
        pickup truck (traffic) V73.7
          nontraffic V73.2
        railway vehicle (traffic) V75.7
          nontraffic V75.2
        specified vehicle NEC (traffic) V76.7
          nontraffic V76.2
        stationary object (traffic) V77.7
          nontraffic V77.2
        streetcar (traffic) V76.7
          nontraffic V76.2
        three wheeled motor vehicle (traffic) V72.7
          nontraffic V72.2
        truck (traffic) V74.7
          nontraffic V74.2
        two wheeled motor vehicle (traffic) V72.7
          nontraffic V72.2
        van (traffic) V73.7
          nontraffic V73.2
      noncollision accident (traffic) V78.7
        nontraffic V78.2
      noncollision accident (traffic) V78.9
        nontraffic V78.3
        while boarding or alighting V78.4
      nontraffic V79.3

Accident (to) X58 — *continued*
  transport (involving injury to) V99—*continued*
  bus occupant V79.9 — *continued*
    passenger
      collision (with)
        animal (traffic) V70.6
          being ridden (traffic) V76.6
            nontraffic V76.1
          nontraffic V70.1
        animal-drawn vehicle (traffic) V76.6
          nontraffic V76.1
        bus (traffic) V74.6
          nontraffic V74.1
        car (traffic) V73.6
          nontraffic V73.1
        motor vehicle NOS (traffic) V79.50
          nontraffic V79.10
          specified type NEC (traffic) V79.59
            nontraffic V79.19
        pedal cycle (traffic) V71.6
          nontraffic V71.1
        pickup truck (traffic) V73.6
          nontraffic V73.1
        railway vehicle (traffic) V75.6
          nontraffic V75.1
        specified vehicle NEC (traffic) V76.6
          nontraffic V76.1
        stationary object (traffic) V77.6
          nontraffic V77.1
        streetcar (traffic) V76.6
          nontraffic V76.1
        three wheeled motor vehicle (traffic) V72.6
          nontraffic V72.1
        truck (traffic) V74.6
          nontraffic V74.1
        two wheeled motor vehicle (traffic) V72.6
          nontraffic V72.1
        van (traffic) V73.6
          nontraffic V73.1
      noncollision accident (traffic) V78.6
        nontraffic V78.1
    specified type NEC V79.88
      military vehicle V79.81

EXTERNAL CAUSES

Accident (to) X58 — *continued*
  transport (involving injury to) V99—*continued*
    cable car, not on rails V98.0
      on rails — *see* Accident, transport,
        streetcar occupant
    car occupant V49.9
      ambulance occupant — *see* Accident,
        transport, ambulance occupant
      collision (with)
        animal (traffic) V40.9
          being ridden (traffic) V46.9
            nontraffic V46.3
            while boarding or alighting V46.4
          nontraffic V40.3
          while boarding or alighting V40.4
        animal-drawn vehicle (traffic) V46.9
          nontraffic V46.3
          while boarding or alighting V46.4
        bus (traffic) V44.9
          nontraffic V44.3
          while boarding or alighting V44.4
        car (traffic) V43.92
          nontraffic V43.32
          while boarding or alighting V43.42
        motor vehicle NOS (traffic) V49.60
          nontraffic V49.20
          specified type NEC (traffic) V49.69
            nontraffic V49.29
        pedal cycle (traffic) V41.9
          nontraffic V41.3
          while boarding or alighting V41.4
        pickup truck (traffic) V43.93
          nontraffic V43.33
          while boarding or alighting V43.43
        railway vehicle (traffic) V45.9
          nontraffic V45.3
          while boarding or alighting V45.4
        specified vehicle NEC (traffic) V46.9
          nontraffic V46.3
          while boarding or alighting V46.4
        sport utility vehicle (traffic) V43.91
          nontraffic V43.31
          while boarding or alighting V43.41
        stationary object (traffic) V47.92
          nontraffic V47.32
          while boarding or alighting V47.4
        streetcar (traffic) V46.9
          nontraffic V46.3
          while boarding or alighting V46.4
        three wheeled motor vehicle (traffic)
          V42.9
          nontraffic V42.3
          while boarding or alighting V42.4
        truck (traffic) V44.9
          nontraffic V44.3
          while boarding or alighting V44.4
        two wheeled motor vehicle (traffic)
          V42.9
          nontraffic V42.3
          while boarding or alighting V42.4
        van (traffic) V43.94
          nontraffic V43.34
          while boarding or alighting V43.44

Accident (to) X58 — *continued*
  transport (involving injury to) V99—*continued*
    car occupant V49.9 — *continued*
      driver
        collision (with)
          animal (traffic) V40.5
            being ridden (traffic) V46.5
            nontraffic V46.0
            nontraffic V40.0
          animal-drawn vehicle (traffic) V46.5
            nontraffic V46.0
          bus (traffic) V44.5
            nontraffic V44.0
          car (traffic) V43.52
            nontraffic V43.02
          motor vehicle NOS (traffic) V49.40
            nontraffic V49.00
            specified type NEC (traffic) V49.49
              nontraffic V49.09
          pedal cycle (traffic) V41.5
            nontraffic V41.0
          pickup truck (traffic) V43.53
            nontraffic V43.03
          railway vehicle (traffic) V45.5
            nontraffic V45.0
          specified vehicle NEC (traffic) V46.5
            nontraffic V46.0
          sport utility vehicle (traffic) V43.51
            nontraffic V43.01
          stationary object (traffic) V47.52
            nontraffic V47.02
          streetcar (traffic) V46.5
            nontraffic V46.0
          three wheeled motor vehicle (traffic)
           V42.5
            nontraffic V42.0
          truck (traffic) V44.5
            nontraffic V44.0
          two wheeled motor vehicle (traffic)
           V42.5
            nontraffic V42.0
          van (traffic) V43.54
            nontraffic V43.04
        noncollision accident (traffic) V48.5
        nontraffic V48.0

Accident (to) X58 — *continued*
  transport (involving injury to) V99—*continued*
    car occupant V49.9 — *continued*
      hanger-on
        collision (with)
          animal (traffic) V40.7
            being ridden (traffic) V46.7
            nontraffic V46.2
            nontraffic V40.2
          animal-drawn vehicle (traffic) V46.7
            nontraffic V46.2
          bus (traffic) V44.7
            nontraffic V44.2
          car (traffic) V43.72
            nontraffic V43.22
          pedal cycle (traffic) V41.7
            nontraffic V41.2
          pickup truck (traffic) V43.73
            nontraffic V43.23
          railway vehicle (traffic) V45.7
            nontraffic V45.2
          specified vehicle NEC (traffic) V46.7
            nontraffic V46.2
          sport utility vehicle (traffic) V43.71
            nontraffic V43.21
          stationary object (traffic) V47.7
            nontraffic V47.2
          streetcar (traffic) V46.7
            nontraffic V46.2
          three wheeled motor vehicle (traffic)
           V42.7
            nontraffic V42.2
          truck (traffic) V44.7
            nontraffic V44.2
          two wheeled motor vehicle (traffic)
           V42.7
            nontraffic V42.2
          van (traffic) V43.74
            nontraffic V43.24
        noncollision accident (traffic) V48.7
        nontraffic V48.2
      noncollision accident (traffic) V48.9
        nontraffic V48.3
        while boarding or alighting V48.4
      nontraffic V49.3

Accident (to) X58 — *continued*
  transport (involving injury to) V99—*continued*
    car occupant V49.9 — *continued*
      passenger
        collision (with)
          animal (traffic) V40.6
            being ridden (traffic) V46.6
              nontraffic V46.1
            nontraffic V40.1
          animal-drawn vehicle (traffic) V46.6
            nontraffic V46.1
          bus (traffic) V44.6
            nontraffic V44.1
          car (traffic) V43.62
            nontraffic V43.12
          motor vehicle NOS (traffic) V49.50
            nontraffic V49.10
            specified type NEC (traffic) V49.59
              nontraffic V49.19
          pedal cycle (traffic) V41.6
            nontraffic V41.1
          pickup truck (traffic) V43.63
            nontraffic V43.13
          railway vehicle (traffic) V45.6
            nontraffic V45.1
          specified vehicle NEC (traffic) V46.6
            nontraffic V46.1
          sport utility vehicle (traffic) V43.61
            nontraffic V43.11
          stationary object (traffic) V47.62
            nontraffic V47.12
          streetcar (traffic) V46.6
            nontraffic V46.1
          three wheeled motor vehicle (traffic) V42.6
            nontraffic V42.1
          truck (traffic) V44.6
            nontraffic V44.1
          two wheeled motor vehicle (traffic) V42.6
            nontraffic V42.1
          van (traffic) V43.64
            nontraffic V43.14
        noncollision accident (traffic) V48.6
          nontraffic V48.1
        specified type NEC V49.88
        military vehicle V49.81

Accident (to) X58 — *continued*
  transport (involving injury to) V99—*continued*
    coal car — *see* Accident, transport, industrial vehicle occupant
    construction vehicle occupant (nontraffic) V85.9
      driver V85.5
      hanger-on V85.7
      passenger V85.6
      traffic V85.3
        driver V85.0
        hanger-on V85.2
        passenger V85.1
      while boarding or alighting V85.4
    dirt bike rider — *see* Accident, transport, all-terrain vehicle occupant
    due to cataclysm — *see* Forces of nature, by type
    dune buggy occupant (nontraffic) V86.93
      driver V86.53
      hanger-on V86.73
      passenger V86.63
      traffic V86.33
        driver V86.03
        hanger-on V86.23
        passenger V86.13
      while boarding or alighting V86.43
    forklift — *see* Accident, transport, industrial vehicle occupant
    go cart — *see* Accident, transport, all-terrain vehicle occupant
    golf cart — *see* Accident, transport, all-terrain vehicle occupant
    heavy transport vehicle occupant — *see* Accident, transport, truck occupant
    ice yacht V98.2
    industrial vehicle occupant (nontraffic) V83.9
      driver V83.5
      hanger-on V83.7
      passenger V83.6
      traffic V83.3
        driver V83.0
        hanger-on V83.2
        passenger V83.1
      while boarding or alighting V83.4
    interurban electric car — *see* Accident, transport, streetcar
    land yacht V98.1
    logging car — *see* Accident, transport, industrial vehicle occupant
    military vehicle occupant (traffic) V86.34
      driver V86.04
      hanger-on V86.24
      nontraffic V86.94
        driver V86.54
        hanger-on V86.74
        passenger V86.64
      passenger V86.14
      while boarding or alighting V86.44
    mine tram — *see* Accident, transport, industrial vehicle occupant
    motor vehicle NEC occupant (traffic) V89.2
    motorcoach — *see* Accident, transport, bus occupant

Accident (to) X58 — *continued*
  transport (involving injury to) V99—*continued*
    motorcyclist V29.9
      collision (with)
        animal (traffic) V20.9
          being ridden (traffic) V26.9
            nontraffic V26.2
            while boarding or alighting V26.3
          nontraffic V20.2
          while boarding or alighting V20.3
        animal-drawn vehicle (traffic) V26.9
          nontraffic V26.2
          while boarding or alighting V26.3
        bus (traffic) V24.9
          nontraffic V24.2
          while boarding or alighting V24.3
        car (traffic) V23.9
          nontraffic V23.2
          while boarding or alighting V23.3
        motor vehicle NOS (traffic) V29.60
          nontraffic V29.20
          specified type NEC (traffic) V29.69
            nontraffic V29.29
        pedal cycle (traffic) V21.9
          nontraffic V21.2
          while boarding or alighting V21.3
        pickup truck (traffic) V23.9
          nontraffic V23.2
          while boarding or alighting V23.3
        railway vehicle (traffic) V25.9
          nontraffic V25.2
          while boarding or alighting V25.3
        specified vehicle NEC (traffic) V26.9
          nontraffic V26.2
          while boarding or alighting V26.3
        stationary object (traffic) V27.9
          nontraffic V27.2
          while boarding or alighting V27.3
        streetcar (traffic) V26.9
          nontraffic V26.2
          while boarding or alighting V26.3
        three wheeled motor vehicle (traffic) V22.9
          nontraffic V22.2
          while boarding or alighting V22.3
        truck (traffic) V24.9
          nontraffic V24.2
          while boarding or alighting V24.3
        two wheeled motor vehicle (traffic) V22.9
          nontraffic V22.2
          while boarding or alighting V22.3
        van (traffic) V23.9
          nontraffic V23.2
          while boarding or alighting V23.3

EXTERNAL CAUSES

Accident (to) X58 — *continued*
transport (involving injury to) V99—*continued*
motorcyclist V29.9 — *continued*
driver
collision (with)
animal (traffic) V20.4
being ridden (traffic) V26.4
nontraffic V26.0
nontraffic V20.0
animal-drawn vehicle (traffic) V26.4
nontraffic V26.0
bus (traffic) V24.4
nontraffic V24.0
car (traffic) V23.4
nontraffic V23.0
motor vehicle NOS (traffic) V29.40
nontraffic V29.00
specified type NEC (traffic) V29.49
nontraffic V29.09
pedal cycle (traffic) V21.4
nontraffic V21.0
pickup truck (traffic) V23.4
nontraffic V23.0
railway vehicle (traffic) V25.4
nontraffic V25.0
specified vehicle NEC (traffic) V26.4
nontraffic V26.0
stationary object (traffic) V27.4
nontraffic V27.0
streetcar (traffic) V26.4
nontraffic V26.0
three wheeled motor vehicle (traffic) V22.4
nontraffic V22.0
truck (traffic) V24.4
nontraffic V24.0
two wheeled motor vehicle (traffic) V22.4
nontraffic V22.0
van (traffic) V23.4
nontraffic V23.0
noncollision accident (traffic) V28.4
nontraffic V28.0
noncollision accident (traffic) V28.9
nontraffic V28.2
while boarding or alighting V28.3
nontraffic V29.3

Accident (to) X58 — *continued*
transport (involving injury to) V99—*continued*
motorcyclist V29.9 — *continued*
passenger
collision (with)
animal (traffic) V20.5
being ridden (traffic) V26.5
nontraffic V26.1
nontraffic V20.1
animal-drawn vehicle (traffic) V26.5
nontraffic V26.1
bus (traffic) V24.5
nontraffic V24.1
car (traffic) V23.5
nontraffic V23.1
motor vehicle NOS (traffic) V29.50
nontraffic V29.10
specified type NEC (traffic) V29.59
nontraffic V29.19
pedal cycle (traffic) V21.5
nontraffic V21.1
pickup truck (traffic) V23.5
nontraffic V23.1
railway vehicle (traffic) V25.5
nontraffic V25.1
specified vehicle NEC (traffic) V26.5
nontraffic V26.1
stationary object (traffic) V27.5
nontraffic V27.1
streetcar (traffic) V26.5
nontraffic V26.1
three wheeled motor vehicle (traffic) V22.5
nontraffic V22.1
truck (traffic) V24.5
nontraffic V24.1
two wheeled motor vehicle (traffic) V22.5
nontraffic V22.1
van (traffic) V23.5
nontraffic V23.1
noncollision accident (traffic) V28.5
nontraffic V28.1
specified type NEC V29.88
military vehicle V29.81

Accident (to) X58 — *continued*
transport (involving injury to) V99—*continued*
occupant (of)
aircraft (powered) V95.9
fixed wing
commercial — *see* Accident, transport, aircraft, occupant, powered, fixed wing, commercial
private — *see* Accident, transport, aircraft, occupant, powered, fixed wing, private
nonpowered V96.9
specified NEC V95.8
airport battery-powered vehicle — *see* Accident, transport, industrial vehicle occupant
all-terrain vehicle (ATV) — *see* Accident, transport, all-terrain vehicle occupant
animal-drawn vehicle — *see* Accident, transport, animal-drawn vehicle occupant
automobile — *see* Accident, transport, car occupant
balloon V96.00
battery-powered vehicle — *see* Accident, transport, industrial vehicle occupant
bicycle — *see* Accident, transport, pedal cyclist
motorized — *see* Accident, transport, motorcycle rider
boat NEC — *see* Accident, watercraft
bulldozer — *see* Accident, transport, construction vehicle occupant
bus — *see* Accident, transport, bus occupant
cable car (on rails) — *see also* Accident, transport, streetcar occupant
not on rails V98.0
car — *see also* Accident, transport, car occupant
cable (on rails) — *see also* Accident, transport, streetcar occupant
not on rails V98.0
coach — *see* Accident, transport, bus occupant
coal-car — *see* Accident, transport, industrial vehicle occupant
digger — *see* Accident, transport, construction vehicle occupant
dump truck — *see* Accident, transport, construction vehicle occupant
earth-leveler — *see* Accident, transport, construction vehicle occupant
farm machinery (self-propelled) — *see* Accident, transport, agricultural vehicle occupant
forklift — *see* Accident, transport, industrial vehicle occupant
glider (unpowered) V96.20
hang V96.10
powered (microlight) (ultralight) — *see* Accident, transport, aircraft, occupant, powered, glider
glider (unpowered) NEC V96.20
hang-glider V96.10
harvester — *see* Accident, transport, agricultural vehicle occupant
heavy (transport) vehicle — *see* Accident, transport, truck occupant
helicopter — *see* Accident, transport, aircraft, occupant, helicopter
ice-yacht V98.2
kite (carrying person) V96.8
land-yacht V98.1
logging car — *see* Accident, transport, industrial vehicle occupant

Accident (to) X58 — *continued*
transport (involving injury to) V99—*continued*
occupant (of) — *continued*
mechanical shovel — *see* Accident, transport, construction vehicle occupant
microlight — *see* Accident, transport, aircraft, occupant, powered, glider
minibus — *see* Accident, transport, pickup truck occupant
minivan — *see* Accident, transport, pickup truck occupant
moped — *see* Accident, transport, motorcycle
motor scooter — *see* Accident, transport, motorcycle
motorcycle (with sidecar) — *see* Accident, transport, motorcycle
pedal cycle — *see also* Accident, transport, pedal cyclist
pickup (truck) — *see* Accident, transport, pickup truck occupant
railway (train) (vehicle) (subterranean) (elevated) — *see* Accident, transport, railway vehicle occupant
rickshaw — *see* Accident, transport, pedal cycle
motorized — *see* Accident, transport, three-wheeled motor vehicle
pedal driven — *see* Accident, transport, pedal cyclist
road-roller — *see* Accident, transport, construction vehicle occupant
ship NOS V94.9
ski-lift (chair) (gondola) V98.3
snowmobile — *see* Accident, transport, snowmobile occupant
spacecraft, spaceship — *see* Accident, transport, aircraft, occupant, spacecraft
sport utility vehicle — *see* Accident, transport, pickup truck occupant
streetcar (interurban) (operating on public street or highway) — *see* Accident, transport, streetcar occupant
SUV — *see* Accident, transport, pickup truck occupant
téléférique V98.0
three-wheeled vehicle (motorized) — *see also* Accident, transport, three-wheeled motor vehicle occupant
nonmotorized — *see* Accident, transport, pedal cycle
tractor (farm) (and trailer) — *see* Accident, transport, agricultural vehicle occupant
train — *see* Accident, transport, railway vehicle occupant
tram — *see* Accident, transport, streetcar occupant
in mine or quarry — *see* Accident, transport, industrial vehicle occupant
tricycle — *see* Accident, transport, pedal cycle
motorized — *see* Accident, transport, three-wheeled motor vehicle
trolley — *see* Accident, transport, streetcar occupant
in mine or quarry — *see* Accident, transport, industrial vehicle occupant
tub, in mine or quarry — *see* Accident, transport, industrial vehicle occupant
ultralight — *see* Accident, transport, aircraft, occupant, powered, glider
van — *see* Accident, transport, van occupant

Accident (to) X58 — *continued*
transport (involving injury to) V99—*continued*
occupant (of) — *continued*
vehicle NEC V89.9
heavy transport — *see* Accident, transport, truck occupant
motor (traffic) NEC V89.2
nontraffic NEC V89.0
watercraft NOS V94.9
causing drowning — *see* Drowning, resulting from accident to boat
parachutist V97.29
after accident to aircraft — *see* Accident, transport, aircraft
entangled in object V97.21
injured on landing V97.22
pedal cyclist V19.9
collision (with)
animal (traffic) V10.9
being ridden (traffic) V16.9
nontraffic V16.2
while boarding or alighting V16.3
nontraffic V10.2
while boarding or alighting V10.3
animal-drawn vehicle (traffic) V16.9
nontraffic V16.2
while boarding or alighting V16.3
bus (traffic) V14.9
nontraffic V14.2
while boarding or alighting V14.3
car (traffic) V13.9
nontraffic V13.2
while boarding or alighting V13.3
motor vehicle NOS (traffic) V19.60
nontraffic V19.20
specified type NEC (traffic) V19.69
nontraffic V19.29
pedal cycle (traffic) V11.9
nontraffic V11.2
while boarding or alighting V11.3
pickup truck (traffic) V13.9
nontraffic V13.2
while boarding or alighting V13.3
railway vehicle (traffic) V15.9
nontraffic V15.2
while boarding or alighting V15.3
specified vehicle NEC (traffic) V16.9
nontraffic V16.2
while boarding or alighting V16.3
stationary object (traffic) V17.9
nontraffic V17.2
while boarding or alighting V17.3
streetcar (traffic) V16.9
nontraffic V16.2
while boarding or alighting V16.3
three wheeled motor vehicle (traffic) V12.9
nontraffic V12.2
while boarding or alighting V12.3
truck (traffic) V14.9
nontraffic V14.2
while boarding or alighting V14.3
two wheeled motor vehicle (traffic) V12.9
nontraffic V12.2
while boarding or alighting V12.3
van (traffic) V13.9
nontraffic V13.2
while boarding or alighting V13.3

Accident (to) X58 — *continued*
transport (involving injury to) V99—*continued*
pedal cyclist V19.9 — *continued*
driver
collision (with)
animal (traffic) V10.4
being ridden (traffic) V16.4
nontraffic V16.0
nontraffic V10.0
animal-drawn vehicle (traffic) V16.4
nontraffic V16.0
bus (traffic) V14.4
nontraffic V14.0
car (traffic) V13.4
nontraffic V13.0
motor vehicle NOS (traffic) V19.40
nontraffic V19.00
specified type NEC (traffic) V19.49
nontraffic V19.09
pedal cycle (traffic) V11.4
nontraffic V11.0
pickup truck (traffic) V13.4
nontraffic V13.0
railway vehicle (traffic) V15.4
nontraffic V15.0
specified vehicle NEC (traffic) V16.4
nontraffic V16.0
stationary object (traffic) V17.4
nontraffic V17.0
streetcar (traffic) V16.4
nontraffic V16.0
three wheeled motor vehicle (traffic) V12.4
nontraffic V12.0
truck (traffic) V14.4
nontraffic V14.0
two wheeled motor vehicle (traffic) V12.4
nontraffic V12.0
van (traffic) V13.4
nontraffic V13.0
noncollision accident (traffic) V18.4
nontraffic V18.0
noncollision accident (traffic) V18.9
nontraffic V18.2
while boarding or alighting V18.3
nontraffic V19.3

EXTERNAL CAUSES

EXTERNAL CAUSES

Accident (to) X58 — *continued*
  transport (involving injury to) V99—*continued*
    pedal cyclist V19.9 — *continued*
      passenger
        collision (with)
          animal (traffic) V10.5
            being ridden (traffic) V16.5
              nontraffic V16.1
            nontraffic V10.1
          animal-drawn vehicle (traffic) V16.5
            nontraffic V16.1
          bus (traffic) V14.5
            nontraffic V14.1
          car (traffic) V13.5
            nontraffic V13.1
          motor vehicle NOS (traffic) V19.50
            nontraffic V19.10
            specified type NEC (traffic) V19.59
              nontraffic V19.19
          pedal cycle (traffic) V11.5
            nontraffic V11.1
          pickup truck (traffic) V13.5
            nontraffic V13.1
          railway vehicle (traffic) V15.5
            nontraffic V15.1
          specified vehicle NEC (traffic) V16.5
            nontraffic V16.1
          stationary object (traffic) V17.5
            nontraffic V17.1
          streetcar (traffic) V16.5
            nontraffic V16.1
          three wheeled motor vehicle (traffic)
            V12.5
            nontraffic V12.1
          truck (traffic) V14.5
            nontraffic V14.1
          two wheeled motor vehicle (traffic)
            V12.5
            nontraffic V12.1
          van (traffic) V13.5
            nontraffic V13.1
        noncollision accident (traffic) V18.5
          nontraffic V18.1
      specified type NEC V19.88
      military vehicle V19.81

Accident (to) X58 — *continued*
  transport (involving injury to) V99—*continued*
    pedestrian
      conveyance (occupant) V09.9
        babystroller V00.828
        collision (with) V09.9
          animal being ridden or animal
            drawn vehicle V06.99
            nontraffic V06.09
            traffic V06.19
          bus or heavy transport V04.99
            nontraffic V04.09
            traffic V04.19
          car V03.99
            nontraffic V03.09
            traffic V03.19
          pedal cycle V01.99
            nontraffic V01.09
            traffic V01.19
          pickup truck or van V03.99
            nontraffic V03.09
            traffic V03.19
          railway (train) (vehicle) V05.99
            nontraffic V05.09
            traffic V05.19
          stationary object V00.822
          streetcar V06.99
            nontraffic V06.09
            traffic V06.19
          two-or three-wheeled motor vehicle
            V02.99
            nontraffic V02.09
            traffic V02.19
          vehicle V09.9
            animal-drawn V06.99
              nontraffic V06.09
              traffic V06.19
            motor
              nontraffic V09.00
              traffic V09.20
        fall V00.821
        nontraffic V09.1
          involving motor vehicle NEC
            V09.00
        traffic V09.3
          involving motor vehicle NEC
            V09.20

Accident (to) X58 — *continued*
  transport (involving injury to) V99—*continued*
    pedestrian — *continued*
      conveyance (occupant) V09.9 —
        continued
        flat-bottomed NEC V00.388
        collision (with) V09.9
          animal being ridden or animal
            drawn vehicle V06.99
            nontraffic V06.09
            traffic V06.19
          bus or heavy transport V04.99
            nontraffic V04.09
            traffic V04.19
          car V03.99
            nontraffic V03.09
            traffic V03.19
          pedal cycle V01.99
            nontraffic V01.09
            traffic V01.19
          pickup truck or van V03.99
            nontraffic V03.09
            traffic V03.19
          railway (train) (vehicle) V05.99
            nontraffic V05.09
            traffic V05.19
          stationary object V00.382
          streetcar V06.99
            nontraffic V06.09
            traffic V06.19
          two-or three-wheeled motor vehicle
            V02.99
            nontraffic V02.09
            traffic V02.19
          vehicle V09.9
            animal-drawn V06.99
              nontraffic V06.09
              traffic V06.19
            motor
              nontraffic V09.00
              traffic V09.20
        fall V00.381
        nontraffic V09.1
          involving motor vehicle NEC
            V09.00
        snow
          board — *see* Accident, transport,
            pedestrian, conveyance, snow
            board
          ski — *see* Accident, transport,
            pedestrian, conveyance, skis
            (snow)
        traffic V09.3
          involving motor vehicle NEC
            V09.20

EXTERNAL CAUSES

EXTERNAL CAUSES

EXTERNAL CAUSES

Accident (to) X58 — *continued*
  transport (involving injury to) V99—*continued*
    pedestrian — *continued*
      conveyance (occupant) V09.9 —
        continued
        skis (snow) V00.328
          collision (with) V09.9
            animal being ridden or animal
              drawn vehicle V06.99
              nontraffic V06.09
              traffic V06.19
            bus or heavy transport V04.99
              nontraffic V04.09
              traffic V04.19
            car V03.99
              nontraffic V03.09
              traffic V03.19
            pedal cycle V01.99
              nontraffic V01.09
              traffic V01.19
            pickup truck or van V03.99
              nontraffic V03.09
              traffic V03.19
            railway (train) (vehicle) V05.99
              nontraffic V05.09
              traffic V05.19
            stationary object V00.322
            streetcar V06.99
              nontraffic V06.09
              traffic V06.19
            two-or three-wheeled motor vehicle
              V02.99
              nontraffic V02.09
              traffic V02.19
            vehicle V09.9
              animal-drawn V06.99
                nontraffic V06.09
                traffic V06.19
              motor
                nontraffic V09.00
                traffic V09.20
        fall V00.321
        nontraffic V09.1
          involving motor vehicle NEC
            V09.00
        traffic V09.3
          involving motor vehicle NEC
            V09.20

Accident (to) X58 — *continued*
  transport (involving injury to) V99—*continued*
    pedestrian — *continued*
      conveyance (occupant) V09.9 —
        continued
        sled V00.228
          collision (with) V09.9
            animal being ridden or animal
              drawn vehicle V06.99
              nontraffic V06.09
              traffic V06.19
            bus or heavy transport V04.99
              nontraffic V04.09
              traffic V04.19
            car V03.99
              nontraffic V03.09
              traffic V03.19
            pedal cycle V01.99
              nontraffic V01.09
              traffic V01.19
            pickup truck or van V03.99
              nontraffic V03.09
              traffic V03.19
            railway (train) (vehicle) V05.99
              nontraffic V05.09
              traffic V05.19
            stationary object V00.222
            streetcar V06.99
              nontraffic V06.09
            traffic V06.19
            two-or three-wheeled motor vehicle
              V02.99
              nontraffic V02.09
              traffic V02.19
            vehicle V09.9
             animal-drawn V06.99
              nontraffic V06.09
              traffic V06.19
             motor
              nontraffic V09.00
              traffic V09.20
        fall V00.221
        nontraffic V09.1
          involving motor vehicle NEC
            V09.00
        traffic V09.3
          involving motor vehicle NEC
            V09.20

Accident (to) X58 — *continued*
  transport (involving injury to) V99—*continued*
    pedestrian — *continued*
      conveyance (occupant) V09.9 —
        continued
        snow board V00.318
          collision (with) V09.9
            animal being ridden or animal
              drawn vehicle V06.99
              nontraffic V06.09
              traffic V06.19
            bus or heavy transport V04.99
              nontraffic V04.09
              traffic V04.19
            car V03.99
              nontraffic V03.09
              traffic V03.19
            pedal cycle V01.99
              nontraffic V01.09
              traffic V01.19
            pickup truck or van V03.99
              nontraffic V03.09
              traffic V03.19
            railway (train) (vehicle) V05.99
              nontraffic V05.09
              traffic V05.19
            stationary object V00.312
            streetcar V06.99
              nontraffic V06.09
              traffic V06.19
            two-or three-wheeled motor vehicle
              V02.99
              nontraffic V02.09
              traffic V02.19
            vehicle V09.9
             animal-drawn V06.99
              nontraffic V06.09
              traffic V06.19
             motor
              nontraffic V09.00
              traffic V09.20
        fall V00.311
        nontraffic V09.1
          involving motor vehicle NEC
            V09.00
        traffic V09.3
          involving motor vehicle NEC
            V09.20

EXTERNAL CAUSES

Accident (to) X58 — *continued*
  transport (involving injury to) V99—*continued*
    pedestrian — *continued*
      conveyance (occupant) V09.9 — *continued*
        specified type NEC V00.898
        collision (with) V09.9
          animal being ridden or animal drawn vehicle V06.99
            nontraffic V06.09
            traffic V06.19
          bus or heavy transport V04.99
            nontraffic V04.09
            traffic V04.19
          car V03.99
            nontraffic V03.09
            traffic V03.19
          pedal cycle V01.99
            nontraffic V01.09
            traffic V01.19
          pickup truck or van V03.99
            nontraffic V03.09
            traffic V03.19
          railway (train) (vehicle) V05.99
            nontraffic V05.09
            traffic V05.19
          stationary object V00.892
          streetcar V06.99
            nontraffic V06.09
            traffic V06.19
          two-or three-wheeled motor vehicle V02.99
            nontraffic V02.09
            traffic V02.19
          vehicle V09.9
            animal-drawn V06.99
              nontraffic V06.09
              traffic V06.19
            motor
              nontraffic V09.00
              traffic V09.20
    fall V00.891
    nontraffic V09.1
      involving motor vehicle NEC V09.00
    traffic V09.3
      involving motor vehicle NEC V09.20

Accident (to) X58 — *continued*
  transport (involving injury to) V99—*continued*
    pedestrian — *continued*
      conveyance (occupant) V09.9 — *continued*
        traffic V09.3
          involving motor vehicle V09.20
            military V09.21
          specified type NEC V09.29
      wheelchair (powered) V00.818
        collision (with) V09.9
          animal being ridden or animal drawn vehicle V06.99
            nontraffic V06.09
            traffic V06.19
          bus or heavy transport V04.99
            nontraffic V04.09
            traffic V04.19
          car V03.99
            nontraffic V03.09
            traffic V03.19
          pedal cycle V01.99
            nontraffic V01.09
            traffic V01.19
          pickup truck or van V03.99
            nontraffic V03.09
            traffic V03.19
          railway (train) (vehicle) V05.99
            nontraffic V05.09
            traffic V05.19
          stationary object V00.812
          streetcar V06.99
            nontraffic V06.09
            traffic V06.19
          two-or three-wheeled motor vehicle V02.99
            nontraffic V02.09
            traffic V02.19
          vehicle V09.9
            animal-drawn V06.99
              nontraffic V06.09
              traffic V06.19
            motor
              nontraffic V09.00
              traffic V09.20
        fall V00.811
        nontraffic V09.1
          involving motor vehicle NEC V09.00
        traffic V09.3
          involving motor vehicle NEC V09.20
      wheeled shoe V00.158
        colliding with stationary object V00.152
        fall V00.151

Accident (to) X58 — *continued*
  transport (involving injury to) V99—*continued*
    pedestrian — *continued*
      on foot — *see also* Accident, pedestrian collision (with)
        animal being ridden or animal drawn vehicle V06.90
          nontraffic V06.00
          traffic V06.10
        bus or heavy transport V04.90
          nontraffic V04.00
          traffic V04.10
        car V03.90
          nontraffic V03.00
          traffic V03.10
        pedal cycle V01.90
          nontraffic V01.00
          traffic V01.10
        pickup truck or van V03.90
          nontraffic V03.00
          traffic V03.10
        railway (train) (vehicle) V05.90
          nontraffic V05.00
          traffic V05.10
        streetcar V06.90
          nontraffic V06.00
          traffic V06.10
        two-or three-wheeled motor vehicle V02.90
          nontraffic V02.00
          traffic V02.10
        vehicle V09.9
          animal-drawn V06.90
            nontraffic V06.00
            traffic V06.10
          motor
            nontraffic V09.00
            traffic V09.20
      nontraffic V09.1
        involving motor vehicle V09.00
          military V09.01
          specified type NEC V09.09
      traffic V09.3
        involving motor vehicle V09.20
          military V09.21
          specified type NEC V09.29

Accident (to) X58 — *continued*
transport (involving injury to) V99—*continued*
person NEC (unknown way or
transportation) V99
collision (between)
bus (with)
heavy transport vehicle (traffic) V87.5
nontraffic V88.5
car (with)
bus (traffic) V87.3
nontraffic V88.3
heavy transport vehicle (traffic) V87.4
nontraffic V88.4
nontraffic V88.5
pickup truck or van (traffic) V87.2
nontraffic V88.2
train or railway vehicle (traffic) V87.6
nontraffic V88.6
two-or three-wheeled motor vehicle
(traffic) V87.0
nontraffic V88.0
motor vehicle (traffic) NEC V87.7
nontraffic V88.7
two-or three-wheeled vehicle (with)
(traffic)
motor vehicle NEC V87.1
nontraffic V88.1
nonmotor vehicle (collision) (noncollision)
(traffic) V87.9
nontraffic V88.9

Accident (to) X58 — *continued*
transport (involving injury to) V99—*continued*
pickup truck occupant V59.9
collision (with)
animal (traffic) V50.9
being ridden (traffic) V56.9
nontraffic V56.3
while boarding or alighting V56.4
nontraffic V50.3
while boarding or alighting V50.4
animal-drawn vehicle (traffic) V56.9
nontraffic V56.3
while boarding or alighting V56.4
bus (traffic) V54.9
nontraffic V54.3
while boarding or alighting V54.4
car (traffic) V53.9
nontraffic V53.3
while boarding or alighting V53.4
motor vehicle NOS (traffic) V59.60
nontraffic V59.20
specified type NEC (traffic) V59.69
nontraffic V59.29
pedal cycle (traffic) V51.9
nontraffic V51.3
while boarding or alighting V51.4
pickup truck (traffic) V53.9
nontraffic V53.3
while boarding or alighting V53.4
railway vehicle (traffic) V55.9
nontraffic V55.3
while boarding or alighting V55.4
specified vehicle NEC (traffic) V56.9
nontraffic V56.3
while boarding or alighting V56.4
stationary object (traffic) V57.9
nontraffic V57.3
while boarding or alighting V57.4
streetcar (traffic) V56.9
nontraffic V56.3
while boarding or alighting V56.4
three wheeled motor vehicle (traffic)
V52.9
nontraffic V52.3
while boarding or alighting V52.4
truck (traffic) V54.9
nontraffic V54.3
while boarding or alighting V54.4
two wheeled motor vehicle (traffic)
V52.9
nontraffic V52.3
while boarding or alighting V52.4
van (traffic) V53.9
nontraffic V53.3
while boarding or alighting V53.4

Accident (to) X58 — *continued*
transport (involving injury to) V99—*continued*
pickup truck occupant V59.9 — *continued*
driver
collision (with)
animal (traffic) V50.5
being ridden (traffic) V56.5
nontraffic V56.0
nontraffic V50.0
animal-drawn vehicle (traffic) V56.5
nontraffic V56.0
bus (traffic) V54.5
nontraffic V54.0
car (traffic) V53.5
nontraffic V53.0
motor vehicle NOS (traffic) V59.40
nontraffic V59.00
specified type NEC (traffic) V59.49
nontraffic V59.09
pedal cycle (traffic) V51.5
nontraffic V51.0
pickup truck (traffic) V53.5
nontraffic V53.0
railway vehicle (traffic) V55.5
nontraffic V55.0
specified vehicle NEC (traffic) V56.5
nontraffic V56.0
stationary object (traffic) V57.5
nontraffic V57.0
streetcar (traffic) V56.5
nontraffic V56.0
three wheeled motor vehicle (traffic)
V52.5
nontraffic V52.0
truck (traffic) V54.5
nontraffic V54.0
two wheeled motor vehicle (traffic)
V52.5
nontraffic V52.0
van (traffic) V53.5
nontraffic V53.0
noncollision accident (traffic) V58.5
nontraffic V58.0

EXTERNAL CAUSES

Accident (to) X58 — *continued*
transport (involving injury to) V99—*continued*
  pickup truck occupant V59.9 — *continued*
   hanger-on
    collision (with)
     animal (traffic) V50.7
      being ridden (traffic) V56.7
       nontraffic V56.2
      nontraffic V50.2
     animal-drawn vehicle (traffic) V56.7
      nontraffic V56.2
     bus (traffic) V54.7
      nontraffic V54.2
     car (traffic) V53.7
      nontraffic V53.2
     pedal cycle (traffic) V51.7
      nontraffic V51.2
     pickup truck (traffic) V53.7
      nontraffic V53.2
     railway vehicle (traffic) V55.7
      nontraffic V55.2
     specified vehicle NEC (traffic) V56.7
      nontraffic V56.2
     stationary object (traffic) V57.7
      nontraffic V57.2
     streetcar (traffic) V56.7
      nontraffic V56.2
     three wheeled motor vehicle (traffic) V52.7
      nontraffic V52.2
     truck (traffic) V54.7
      nontraffic V54.2
     two wheeled motor vehicle (traffic) V52.7
      nontraffic V52.2
     van (traffic) V53.7
      nontraffic V53.2
    noncollision accident (traffic) V58.7
     nontraffic V58.2

Accident (to) X58 — *continued*
transport (involving injury to) V99—*continued*
  pickup truck occupant V59.9 — *continued*
   noncollision accident (traffic) V58.9
    nontraffic V58.3
    while boarding or alighting V58.4
   nontraffic V59.3
   passenger
    collision (with)
     animal (traffic) V50.6
      being ridden (traffic) V56.6
       nontraffic V56.1
      nontraffic V50.1
     animal-drawn vehicle (traffic) V56.6
      nontraffic V56.1
     bus (traffic) V54.6
      nontraffic V54.1
     car (traffic) V53.6
      nontraffic V53.1
     motor vehicle NOS (traffic) V59.50
      nontraffic V59.10
      specified type NEC (traffic) V59.59
       nontraffic V59.19
     pedal cycle (traffic) V51.6
      nontraffic V51.1
     pickup truck (traffic) V53.6
      nontraffic V53.1
     railway vehicle (traffic) V55.6
      nontraffic V55.1
     specified vehicle NEC (traffic) V56.6
      nontraffic V56.1
     stationary object (traffic) V57.6
      nontraffic V57.1
     streetcar (traffic) V56.6
      nontraffic V56.1
     three wheeled motor vehicle (traffic) V52.6
      nontraffic V52.1
     truck (traffic) V54.6
      nontraffic V54.1
     two wheeled motor vehicle (traffic) V52.6
      nontraffic V52.1
     van (traffic) V53.6
      nontraffic V53.1
    noncollision accident (traffic) V58.6
     nontraffic V58.1
   specified type NEC V59.88
    military vehicle V59.81

Accident (to) X58 — *continued*
transport (involving injury to) V99—*continued*
  quarry truck — *see* Accident, transport, industrial vehicle occupant
  race car — *see* Accident, transport, motor vehicle NEC occupant
  railway vehicle occupant V81.9
   collision (with) V81.3
    motor vehicle (non-military) (traffic) V81.1
     military V81.83
     nontraffic V81.0
    rolling stock V81.2
    specified object NEC V81.3
   during derailment V81.7
    with antecedent collision — *see* Accident, transport, railway vehicle occupant, collision
   explosion V81.81
   fall (in railway vehicle) V81.5
    during derailment V81.7
     with antecedent collision — *see* Accident, transport, railway vehicle occupant, collision
    from railway vehicle V81.6
     during derailment V81.7
      with antecedent collision — *see* Accident, transport, railway vehicle occupant, collision
    while boarding or alighting V81.4
   fire V81.81
   object falling onto train V81.82
   specified type NEC V81.89
   while boarding or alighting V81.4
  ski lift V98.3
  snowmobile occupant (nontraffic) V86.92
   driver V86.52
   hanger-on V86.72
   passenger V86.62
   traffic V86.32
    driver V86.02
    hanger-on V86.22
    passenger V86.12
   while boarding or alighting V86.42
  specified NEC V98.8
  sport utility vehicle occupant — *see also* Accident, transport, pickup truck occupant

EXTERNAL CAUSES

EXTERNAL CAUSES

Accident (to) X58 — *continued*
transport (involving injury to) V99—*continued*
three-wheeled motor vehicle occupant
  V39.9 — *continued*
  hanger-on
    collision (with)
      animal (traffic) V30.7
        being ridden (traffic) V36.7
          nontraffic V36.2
        nontraffic V30.2
      animal-drawn vehicle (traffic) V36.7
        nontraffic V36.2
      bus (traffic) V34.7
        nontraffic V34.2
      car (traffic) V33.7
        nontraffic V33.2
      pedal cycle (traffic) V31.7
        nontraffic V31.2
      pickup truck (traffic) V33.7
        nontraffic V33.2
      railway vehicle (traffic) V35.7
        nontraffic V35.2
      specified vehicle NEC (traffic) V36.7
        nontraffic V36.2
      stationary object (traffic) V37.7
        nontraffic V37.2
      streetcar (traffic) V36.7
        nontraffic V36.2
      three wheeled motor vehicle (traffic)
        V32.7
        nontraffic V32.2
      truck (traffic) V34.7
        nontraffic V34.2
      two wheeled motor vehicle (traffic)
        V32.7
        nontraffic V32.2
      van (traffic) V33.7
        nontraffic V33.2
    noncollision accident (traffic) V38.7
      nontraffic V38.2

Accident (to) X58 — *continued*
transport (involving injury to) V99—*continued*
three-wheeled motor vehicle occupant
  V39.9 — *continued*
  noncollision accident (traffic) V38.9
    nontraffic V38.3
    while boarding or alighting V38.4
  nontraffic V39.3
  passenger
    collision (with)
      animal (traffic) V30.6
        being ridden (traffic) V36.6
          nontraffic V36.1
        nontraffic V30.1
      animal-drawn vehicle (traffic) V36.6
        nontraffic V36.1
      bus (traffic) V34.6
        nontraffic V34.1
      car (traffic) V33.6
        nontraffic V33.1
      motor vehicle NOS (traffic) V39.50
        nontraffic V39.10
        specified type NEC (traffic) V39.59
          nontraffic V39.19
      pedal cycle (traffic) V31.6
        nontraffic V31.1
      pickup truck (traffic) V33.6
        nontraffic V33.1
      railway vehicle (traffic) V35.6
        nontraffic V35.1
      specified vehicle NEC (traffic) V36.6
        nontraffic V36.1
      stationary object (traffic) V37.6
        nontraffic V37.1
      streetcar (traffic) V36.6
        nontraffic V36.1
      three wheeled motor vehicle (traffic)
        V32.6
        nontraffic V32.1
      truck (traffic) V34.6
        nontraffic V34.1
      two wheeled motor vehicle (traffic)
        V32.6
        nontraffic V32.1
      van (traffic) V33.6
        nontraffic V33.1
    noncollision accident (traffic) V38.6
      nontraffic V38.1
  specified type NEC V39.89
    military vehicle V39.81

Accident (to) X58 — *continued*
transport (involving injury to) V99—*continued*
tractor (farm) (and trailer) — *see* Accident,
  transport, agricultural vehicle occupant
tram — *see* Accident, transport, streetcar
  in mine or quarry — *see* Accident,
  transport, industrial vehicle occupant
trolley — *see* Accident, transport, streetcar
  in mine or quarry — *see* Accident,
  transport, industrial vehicle occupant
truck (heavy) occupant V69.9
  collision (with)
    animal (traffic) V60.9
      being ridden (traffic) V66.9
        nontraffic V66.3
        while boarding or alighting V66.4
      nontraffic V60.3
      while boarding or alighting V60.4
    animal-drawn vehicle (traffic) V66.9
      nontraffic V66.3
      while boarding or alighting V66.4
    bus (traffic) V64.9
      nontraffic V64.3
      while boarding or alighting V64.4
    car (traffic) V63.9
      nontraffic V63.3
      while boarding or alighting V63.4
    motor vehicle NOS (traffic) V69.60
      nontraffic V69.20
      specified type NEC (traffic) V69.69
        nontraffic V69.29
    pedal cycle (traffic) V61.9
      nontraffic V61.3
      while boarding or alighting V61.4
    pickup truck (traffic) V63.9
      nontraffic V63.3
      while boarding or alighting V63.4
    railway vehicle (traffic) V65.9
      nontraffic V65.3
      while boarding or alighting V65.4
    specified vehicle NEC (traffic) V66.9
      nontraffic V66.3
      while boarding or alighting V66.4
    stationary object (traffic) V67.9
      nontraffic V67.3
      while boarding or alighting V67.4
    streetcar (traffic) V66.9
      nontraffic V66.3
      while boarding or alighting V66.4
    three wheeled motor vehicle (traffic)
      V62.9
      nontraffic V62.3
      while boarding or alighting V62.4
    truck (traffic) V64.9
      nontraffic V64.3
      while boarding or alighting V64.4
    two wheeled motor vehicle (traffic)
      V62.9
      nontraffic V62.3
      while boarding or alighting V62.4
    van (traffic) V63.9
      nontraffic V63.3
      while boarding or alighting V63.4

Accident (to) X58 — *continued*
  transport (involving injury to) V99—*continued*
    truck (heavy) occupant V69.9 — *continued*
      driver
        collision (with)
          animal (traffic) V60.5
            being ridden (traffic) V66.5
              nontraffic V66.0
            nontraffic V60.0
          animal-drawn vehicle (traffic) V66.5
            nontraffic V66.0
          bus (traffic) V64.5
            nontraffic V64.0
          car (traffic) V63.5
            nontraffic V63.0
          motor vehicle NOS (traffic) V69.40
            nontraffic V69.00
              specified type NEC (traffic) V69.49
                nontraffic V69.09
          pedal cycle (traffic) V61.5
            nontraffic V61.0
          pickup truck (traffic) V63.5
            nontraffic V63.0
          railway vehicle (traffic) V65.5
            nontraffic V65.0
          specified vehicle NEC (traffic) V66.5
            nontraffic V66.0
          stationary object (traffic) V67.5
            nontraffic V67.0
          streetcar (traffic) V66.5
            nontraffic V66.0
          three wheeled motor vehicle (traffic)
            V62.5
            nontraffic V62.0
          truck (traffic) V64.5
            nontraffic V64.0
          two wheeled motor vehicle (traffic)
            V62.5
            nontraffic V62.0
          van (traffic) V63.5
            nontraffic V63.0
        noncollision accident (traffic) V68.5
          nontraffic V68.0

Accident (to) X58 — *continued*
  transport (involving injury to) V99—*continued*
    truck (heavy) occupant V69.9 — *continued*
      dump — *see* Accident, transport,
        construction vehicle occupant
      hanger-on
        collision (with)
          animal (traffic) V60.7
            being ridden (traffic) V66.7
              nontraffic V66.2
            nontraffic V60.2
          animal-drawn vehicle (traffic) V66.7
            nontraffic V66.2
          bus (traffic) V64.7
            nontraffic V64.2
          car (traffic) V63.7
            nontraffic V63.2
          pedal cycle (traffic) V61.7
            nontraffic V61.2
          pickup truck (traffic) V63.7
            nontraffic V63.2
          railway vehicle (traffic) V65.7
            nontraffic V65.2
          specified vehicle NEC (traffic) V66.7
            nontraffic V66.2
          stationary object (traffic) V67.7
            nontraffic V67.2
          streetcar (traffic) V66.7
            nontraffic V66.2
          three wheeled motor vehicle (traffic)
            V62.7
            nontraffic V62.2
          truck (traffic) V64.7
            nontraffic V64.2
          two wheeled motor vehicle (traffic)
            V62.7
            nontraffic V62.2
          van (traffic) V63.7
            nontraffic V63.2
        noncollision accident (traffic) V68.7
          nontraffic V68.2

Accident (to) X58 — *continued*
  transport (involving injury to) V99—*continued*
    truck (heavy) occupant V69.9 — *continued*
      noncollision accident (traffic) V68.9
        nontraffic V68.3
        while boarding or alighting V68.4
      nontraffic V69.3
      passenger
        collision (with)
          animal (traffic) V60.6
            being ridden (traffic) V66.6
              nontraffic V66.1
            nontraffic V60.1
          animal-drawn vehicle (traffic) V66.6
            nontraffic V66.1
          bus (traffic) V64.6
            nontraffic V64.1
          car (traffic) V63.6
            nontraffic V63.1
          motor vehicle NOS (traffic) V69.50
            nontraffic V69.10
              specified type NEC (traffic) V69.59
                nontraffic V69.19
          pedal cycle (traffic) V61.6
            nontraffic V61.1
          pickup truck (traffic) V63.6
            nontraffic V63.1
          railway vehicle (traffic) V65.6
            nontraffic V65.1
          specified vehicle NEC (traffic) V66.6
            nontraffic V66.1
          stationary object (traffic) V67.6
            nontraffic V67.1
          streetcar (traffic) V66.6
            nontraffic V66.1
          three wheeled motor vehicle (traffic)
            V62.6
            nontraffic V62.1
          truck (traffic) V64.6
            nontraffic V64.1
          two wheeled motor vehicle (traffic)
            V62.6
            nontraffic V62.1
          van (traffic) V63.6
            nontraffic V63.1
        noncollision accident (traffic) V68.6
          nontraffic V68.1
      pickup — *see* Accident, transport, pickup
        truck occupant
      specified type NEC V69.88
        military vehicle V69.81

EXTERNAL CAUSES

EXTERNAL CAUSES

Accident (to) X58 — *continued*
transport (involving injury to) V99—*continued*
van occupant V59.9
  collision (with)
    animal (traffic) V50.9
      being ridden (traffic) V56.9
        nontraffic V56.3
        while boarding or alighting V56.4
      nontraffic V50.3
      while boarding or alighting V50.4
    animal-drawn vehicle (traffic) V56.9
      nontraffic V56.3
      while boarding or alighting V56.4
    bus (traffic) V54.9
      nontraffic V54.3
      while boarding or alighting V54.4
    car (traffic) V53.9
      nontraffic V53.3
      while boarding or alighting V53.4
    motor vehicle NOS (traffic) V59.60
      nontraffic V59.20
      specified type NEC (traffic) V59.69
        nontraffic V59.29
    pedal cycle (traffic) V51.9
      nontraffic V51.3
      while boarding or alighting V51.4
    pickup truck (traffic) V53.9
      nontraffic V53.3
      while boarding or alighting V53.4
    railway vehicle (traffic) V55.9
      nontraffic V55.3
      while boarding or alighting V55.4
    specified vehicle NEC (traffic) V56.9
      nontraffic V56.3
      while boarding or alighting V56.4
    stationary object (traffic) V57.9
      nontraffic V57.3
      while boarding or alighting V57.4
    streetcar (traffic) V56.9
      nontraffic V56.3
      while boarding or alighting V56.4
    three wheeled motor vehicle (traffic)
      V52.9
      nontraffic V52.3
      while boarding or alighting V52.4
    truck (traffic) V54.9
      nontraffic V54.3
      while boarding or alighting V54.4
    two wheeled motor vehicle (traffic)
      V52.9
      nontraffic V52.3
      while boarding or alighting V52.4
    van (traffic) V53.9
      nontraffic V53.3
      while boarding or alighting V53.4

Accident (to) X58 — *continued*
transport (involving injury to) V99—*continued*
van occupant V59.9 — *continued*
  driver
    collision (with)
      animal (traffic) V50.5
        being ridden (traffic) V56.5
          nontraffic V56.0
        nontraffic V50.0
      animal-drawn vehicle (traffic) V56.5
        nontraffic V56.0
      bus (traffic) V54.5
        nontraffic V54.0
      car (traffic) V53.5
        nontraffic V53.0
      motor vehicle NOS (traffic) V59.40
        nontraffic V59.00
        specified type NEC (traffic) V59.49
          nontraffic V59.09
      pedal cycle (traffic) V51.5
        nontraffic V51.0
      pickup truck (traffic) V53.5
        nontraffic V53.0
      railway vehicle (traffic) V55.5
        nontraffic V55.0
      specified vehicle NEC (traffic) V56.5
        nontraffic V56.0
      stationary object (traffic) V57.5
        nontraffic V57.0
      streetcar (traffic) V56.5
        nontraffic V56.0
      three wheeled motor vehicle (traffic)
        V52.5
        nontraffic V52.0
      truck (traffic) V54.5
        nontraffic V54.0
      two wheeled motor vehicle (traffic)
        V52.5
        nontraffic V52.0
      van (traffic) V53.5
        nontraffic V53.0
    noncollision accident (traffic) V58.5
      nontraffic V58.0

Accident (to) X58 — *continued*
transport (involving injury to) V99—*continued*
van occupant V59.9 — *continued*
  hanger-on
    collision (with)
      animal (traffic) V50.7
        being ridden (traffic) V56.7
          nontraffic V56.2
        nontraffic V50.2
      animal-drawn vehicle (traffic) V56.7
        nontraffic V56.2
      bus (traffic) V54.7
        nontraffic V54.2
      car (traffic) V53.7
        nontraffic V53.2
      pedal cycle (traffic) V51.7
        nontraffic V51.2
      pickup truck (traffic) V53.7
        nontraffic V53.2
      railway vehicle (traffic) V55.7
        nontraffic V55.2
      specified vehicle NEC (traffic) V56.7
        nontraffic V56.2
      stationary object (traffic) V57.7
        nontraffic V57.2
      streetcar (traffic) V56.7
        nontraffic V56.2
      three wheeled motor vehicle (traffic)
        V52.7
        nontraffic V52.2
      truck (traffic) V54.7
        nontraffic V54.2
      two wheeled motor vehicle (traffic)
        V52.7
        nontraffic V52.2
      van (traffic) V53.7
        nontraffic V53.2
    noncollision accident (traffic) V58.7
      nontraffic V58.2

EXTERNAL CAUSES

Accident (to) X58 — *continued*
  transport (involving injury to) V99—*continued*
    van occupant V59.9 — *continued*
      noncollision accident (traffic) V58.9
        nontraffic V58.3
        while boarding or alighting V58.4
      nontraffic V59.3
      passenger
        collision (with)
          animal (traffic) V50.6
            being ridden (traffic) V56.6
              nontraffic V56.1
            nontraffic V50.1
          animal-drawn vehicle (traffic) V56.6
            nontraffic V56.1
          bus (traffic) V54.6
            nontraffic V54.1
          car (traffic) V53.6
            nontraffic V53.1
          motor vehicle NOS (traffic) V59.50
            nontraffic V59.10
            specified type NEC (traffic) V59.59
              nontraffic V59.19
          pedal cycle (traffic) V51.6
            nontraffic V51.1
          pickup truck (traffic) V53.6
            nontraffic V53.1
          railway vehicle (traffic) V55.6
            nontraffic V55.1
          specified vehicle NEC (traffic) V56.6
            nontraffic V56.1
          stationary object (traffic) V57.6
            nontraffic V57.1
          streetcar (traffic) V56.6
            nontraffic V56.1
          three wheeled motor vehicle (traffic) V52.6
            nontraffic V52.1
          truck (traffic) V54.6
            nontraffic V54.1
          two wheeled motor vehicle (traffic) V52.6
            nontraffic V52.1
          van (traffic) V53.6
            nontraffic V53.1
        noncollision accident (traffic) V58.6
          nontraffic V58.1
      specified type NEC V59.88
      military vehicle V59.81

Accident (to) X58 — *continued*
  transport (involving injury to) V99—*continued*
    watercraft occupant — *see* Accident, watercraft
    vehicle NEC V89.9
      animal-drawn NEC — *see* Accident, transport, animal-drawn vehicle occupant
      special
        agricultural — *see* Accident, transport, agricultural vehicle occupant
        construction — *see* Accident, transport, construction vehicle occupant
        industrial — *see* Accident, transport, industrial vehicle occupant
        three-wheeled NEC (motorized) — *see* Accident, transport, three-wheeled motor vehicle occupant
  watercraft V94.9
    causing
      drowning — *see* Drowning, due to, accident to, watercraft
      injury NEC V91.89
        crushed between craft and object V91.19
          powered craft V91.13
            ferry boat V91.11
            fishing boat V91.12
            jetskis V91.13
            liner V91.11
            merchant ship V91.10
            passenger ship V91.11
          unpowered craft V91.18
            canoe V91.15
            inflatable V91.16
            kayak V91.15
            sailboat V91.14
            surfboard V91.18
            windsurfer V91.18
        fall on board V91.29
          powered craft V91.23
            ferry boat V91.21
            fishing boat V91.22
            jetskis V91.23
            liner V91.21
            merchant ship V91.20
            passenger ship V91.21
          unpowered craft
            canoe V91.25
            inflatable V91.26
            kayak V91.25
            sailboat V91.24
        fire on board causing burn V91.09
          powered craft V91.03
            ferry boat V91.01
            fishing boat V91.02
            jetskis V91.03
            liner V91.01
            merchant ship V91.00
            passenger ship V91.01
          unpowered craft V91.08
            canoe V91.05
            inflatable V91.06
            kayak V91.05
            sailboat V91.04
            surfboard V91.08
            water skis V91.07
            windsurfer V91.08

Accident (to) X58 — *continued*
  watercraft V94.9 — *continued*
    causing — *continued*
      injury NEC V91.89 — *continued*
        hit by falling object V91.39
          powered craft V91.33
            ferry boat V91.31
            fishing boat V91.32
            jetskis V91.33
            liner V91.31
            merchant ship V91.30
            passenger ship V91.31
          unpowered craft V91.38
            canoe V91.35
            inflatable V91.36
            kayak V91.35
            sailboat V91.34
            surfboard V91.38
            water skis V91.37
            windsurfer V91.38
        specified type NEC V91.89
          powered craft V91.83
            ferry boat V91.81
            fishing boat V91.82
            jetskis V91.83
            liner V91.81
            merchant ship V91.80
            passenger ship V91.81
          unpowered craft V91.88
            canoe V91.85
            inflatable V91.86
            kayak V91.85
            sailboat V91.84
            surfboard V91.88
            water skis V91.87
            windsurfer V91.88
    due to, caused by cataclysm — *see* Forces of nature, by type
    military NEC V94.818
      with civilian watercraft V94.810
      civilian in water injured by V94.811
    nonpowered, struck by
      nonpowered vessel V94.22
      powered vessel V94.21
    specified type NEC V94.89
    striking swimmer
      powered V94.11
      unpowered V94.12

EXTERNAL CAUSES

Acid throwing (assault) Y08.89
Activity (involving) (of victim at time of event)
    Y93.9
  aerobic and step exercise (class) Y93.A3
  alpine skiing Y93.23
  animal care NEC Y93.K9
  arts and handcrafts NEC Y93.D9
  athletics NEC Y93.79
  athletics played as a team or group NEC
    Y93.69
  athletics played individually NEC Y93.59
  baking Y93.G3
  ballet Y93.41
  barbells Y93.B3
  BASE (Building, Antenna, Span, Earth)
    jumping Y93.33
  baseball Y93.64
  basketball Y93.67
  bathing (personal) Y93.E1
  beach volleyball Y93.68
  bike riding Y93.55
  blackout game Y93.85
  boogie boarding Y93.18
  bowling Y93.54
  boxing Y93.71
  brass instrument playing Y93.J4
  building construction Y93.H3
  bungee jumping Y93.34
  calisthenics Y93.A2
  canoeing (in calm and turbulent water) Y93.16
  capture the flag Y93.6A
  cardiorespiratory exercise NEC Y93.A9
  caregiving (providing) NEC Y93.F9
    bathing Y93.F1
    lifting Y93.F2
  cellular
    communication device Y93.C2
    telephone Y93.C2
  challenge course Y93.A5
  cheerleading Y93.45
  choking game Y93.85
  circuit training Y93.A4
  cleaning
    floor Y93.E5
  climbing NEC Y93.39
    mountain Y93.31
    rock Y93.31
    wall Y93.31
  clothing care and maintenance NEC Y93.E9
  combatives Y93.75
  computer
    keyboarding Y93.C1
    technology NEC Y93.C9
  confidence course Y93.A5
  construction (building) Y93.H3
  cooking and baking Y93.G3
  cool down exercises Y93.A2
  cricket Y93.69
  crocheting Y93.D1
  cross country skiing Y93.24
  dancing (all types) Y93.41
  digging
    dirt Y93.H1
  dirt digging Y93.H1
  dishwashing Y93.G1
  diving (platform) (springboard) Y93.12
    underwater Y93.15
  dodge ball Y93.6A
  downhill skiing Y93.23
  drum playing Y93.J2
  dumbbells Y93.B3
  electronic
    devices NEC Y93.C9
      hand held interactive Y93.C2
    game playing (using) (with)
      interactive device Y93.C2
      keyboard or other stationary device
        Y93.C1
  elliptical machine Y93.A1

Activity (involving) (of victim at time of event)
  Y93.9 — *continued*
  exercise(s)
    machines ((primarily) for)
      cardiorespiratory conditioning Y93.A1
      muscle strengthening Y93.B1
    muscle strengthening (non-machine) NEC
      Y93.B9
  external motion NEC Y93.19
    rollercoaster Y93.I1
  fainting game Y93.85
  field hockey Y93.65
  figure skating (pairs) (singles) Y93.21
  flag football Y93.62
  floor mopping and cleaning Y93.E5
  food preparation and clean up Y93.G1
  football (American) NOS Y93.61
    flag Y93.62
    tackle Y93.61
    touch Y93.62
  four square Y93.6A
  free weights Y93.B3
  frisbee (ultimate) Y93.74
  furniture
    building Y93.D3
    finishing Y93.D3
    repair Y93.D3
  game playing (electronic)
    using interactive device Y93.C2
    using keyboard or other stationary device
      Y93.C1
  gardening Y93.H2
  golf Y93.53
  grass drills Y93.A6
  grilling and smoking food Y93.G2
  grooming and shearing an animal Y93.K3
  guerilla drills Y93.A6
  gymnastics (rhythmic) Y93.43
  hand held interactive electronic device Y93.C2
  handball Y93.73
  handcrafts NEC Y93.D9
  hang gliding Y93.35
  hiking (on level or elevated terrain) Y93.01
  hockey (ice) Y93.22
    field Y93.65
  horseback riding Y93.52
  household (interior) maintenance NEC Y93.E9
  ice NEC Y93.29
    dancing Y93.21
    hockey Y93.22
    skating Y93.21
  inline roller skating Y93.51
  ironing Y93.E4
  judo Y93.75
  jumping (off) NEC Y93.39
    BASE (Building, Antenna, Span, Earth)
      Y93.33
    bungee Y93.34
    jacks Y93.A2
    rope Y93.56
  jumping jacks Y93.A2
  jumping rope Y93.56
  karate Y93.75
  kayaking (in calm and turbulent water) Y93.16
  keyboarding (computer) Y93.C1
  kickball Y93.6A
  knitting Y93.D1
  lacrosse Y93.65
  land maintenance NEC Y93.H9
  landscaping Y93.H2
  laundry Y93.E2
  machines (exercise)
    primarily for cardiorespiratory conditioning
      Y93.A1
    primarily for muscle strengthening Y93.B1

Activity (involving) (of victim at time of event)
  Y93.9 — *continued*
  maintenance
    exterior building NEC Y93.H9
    household (interior) NEC Y93.E9
    land Y93.H9
    property Y93.H9
  marching (on level or elevated terrain) Y93.01
  martial arts Y93.75
  microwave oven Y93.G3
  milking an animal Y93.K2
  mopping (floor) Y93.E5
  mountain climbing Y93.31
  muscle strengthening
    exercises (non-machine) NEC Y93.B9
    machines Y93.B1
  musical keyboard (electronic) playing Y93.J1
  nordic skiing Y93.24
  obstacle course Y93.A5
  oven (microwave) Y93.G3
  packing up and unpacking in moving to a new
    residence Y93.E6
  parasailing Y93.19
  pass out game Y93.85
  percussion instrument playing NEC Y93.J2
  personal
    bathing and showering Y93.E1
    hygiene NEC Y93.E8
    showering Y93.E1
  physical games generally associated with
    school recess, summer camp and children
    Y93.6A
  physical training NEC Y93.A9
  piano playing Y93.J1
  pilates Y93.B4
  platform diving Y93.12
  playing musical instrument
    brass instrument Y93.J4
    drum Y93.J2
    musical keyboard (electronic) Y93.J1
    percussion instrument NEC Y93.J2
    piano Y93.J1
    string instrument Y93.J3
    winds instrument Y93.J4
  property maintenance
    exterior NEC Y93.H9
    interior NEC Y93.E9
  pruning (garden and lawn) Y93.H2
  pull-ups Y93.B2
  push-ups Y93.B2
  racquetball Y93.73
  rafting (in calm and turbulent water) Y93.16
  raking (leaves) Y93.H1
  rappelling Y93.32
  refereeing a sports activity Y93.81
  residential relocation Y93.E6
  rhythmic gymnastics Y93.43
  rhythmic movement NEC Y93.49
  riding
    horseback Y93.52
    rollercoaster Y93.I1
  rock climbing Y93.31
  roller skating (inline) Y93.51
  rollercoaster riding Y93.I1
  rough housing and horseplay Y93.83
  rowing (in calm and turbulent water) Y93.16
  rugby Y93.63
  running Y93.02
  SCUBA diving Y93.15
  sewing Y93.D2
  shoveling Y93.H1
    dirt Y93.H1
    snow Y93.H1
  showering (personal) Y93.E1
  sit-ups Y93.B2
  skateboarding Y93.51
  skating (ice) Y93.21
    roller Y93.51

EXTERNAL CAUSES

Activity (involving) (of victim at time of event) Y93.9 — *continued*
  skiing (alpine) (downhill) Y93.23
    cross country Y93.24
    nordic Y93.24
    water Y93.17
  sledding (snow) Y93.23
  sleeping (sleep) Y93.84
  smoking and grilling food Y93.G2
  snorkeling Y93.15
  snow NEC Y93.29
    boarding Y93.23
    shoveling Y93.H1
    sledding Y93.23
    tubing Y93.23
  soccer Y93.66
  softball Y93.64
  specified NEC Y93.89
  spectator at an event Y93.82
  sports NEC Y93.79
    sports played as a team or group NEC Y93.69
    sports played individually NEC Y93.59
  springboard diving Y93.12
  squash Y93.73
  stationary bike Y93.A1
  step (stepping) exercise (class) Y93.A3
  stepper machine Y93.A1
  stove Y93.G3
  string instrument playing Y93.J3
  surfing Y93.18
    wind Y93.18
  swimming Y93.11
  tackle football Y93.61
  tap dancing Y93.41
  tennis Y93.73
  tobogganing Y93.23
  touch football Y93.62
  track and field events (non-running) Y93.57
    running Y93.02
  trampoline Y93.44
  treadmill Y93.A1
  trimming shrubs Y93.H2
  tubing (in calm and turbulent water) Y93.16
    snow Y93.23
  ultimate frisbee Y93.74
  underwater diving Y93.15
  unpacking in moving to a new residence Y93.E6
  use of stove, oven and microwave oven Y93.G3
  vacuuming Y93.E3
  volleyball (beach) (court) Y93.68
  wake boarding Y93.17
  walking (on level or elevated terrain) Y93.01
    an animal Y93.K1
  walking an animal Y93.K1
  wall climbing Y93.31
  warm up and cool down exercises Y93.A2
  water NEC Y93.19
    aerobics Y93.14
    craft NEC Y93.19
    exercise Y93.14
    polo Y93.13
    skiing Y93.17
    sliding Y93.18
    survival training and testing Y93.19
  weeding (garden and lawn) Y93.H2
  wind instrument playing Y93.J4
  windsurfing Y93.18
  wrestling Y93.72
  yoga Y93.42
Adverse effect of drugs — *see* Table of Drugs and Chemicals
Aerosinusitis — *see* Air, pressure
After-effect, late — *see* Sequelae

Air
  blast in war operations — *see* War operations, air blast
  pressure
    change, rapid
      during
        ascent W94.29
          while (in) (surfacing from)
            aircraft W94.23
            deep water diving W94.21
            underground W94.22
        descent W94.39
          in
            aircraft W94.31
            water W94.32
    high, prolonged W94.0
    low, prolonged W94.12
      due to residence or long visit at high altitude W94.11
Alpine sickness W94.11
Altitude sickness W94.11
Anaphylactic shock, anaphylaxis — *see* Table of Drugs and Chemicals
Andes disease W94.11
Arachnidism, arachnoidism X58
Arson (with intent to injure or kill) X97
Asphyxia, asphyxiation
  by
    food (bone) (seed) — *see* categories T17 and T18
    gas — *see also* Table of Drugs and Chemicals legal
      execution — *see* Legal, intervention, gas
      intervention — *see* Legal, intervention, gas
  from
    fire — *see also* Exposure, fire
      in war operations — *see* War operations, fire
    ignition — *see* Ignition
    vomitus T17.81
  in war operations — *see* War operations, restriction of airway
Aspiration
  food (any type) (into respiratory tract) (with asphyxia, obstruction respiratory tract, suffocation) — *see* categories T17 and T18
  foreign body — *see* Foreign body, aspiration
  vomitus (with asphyxia, obstruction respiratory tract, suffocation) T17.81-
Assassination (attempt) — *see* Assault
Assault (homicidal) (by) (in) Y09
  arson X97
  bite (of human being) Y04.1
  bodily force Y04.8
    bite Y04.1
    bumping into Y04.2
    sexual — *see* subcategories T74.0, T76.0
    unarmed fight Y04.0
  bomb X96.9
    antipersonnel X96.0
    fertilizer X96.3
    gasoline X96.1
    letter X96.2
    petrol X96.1
    pipe X96.3
    specified NEC X96.8
  brawl (hand) (fists) (foot) (unarmed) Y04.0
  burning, burns (by fire) NEC X97
    acid Y08.89
    caustic, corrosive substance Y08.89
    chemical from swallowing caustic, corrosive substance — *see* Table of Drugs and Chemicals
    cigarette(s) X97

Assault (homicidal) (by) (in) Y09 — *continued*
  burning, burns (by fire) NEC X97 — *continued*
    hot object X98.9
      fluid NEC X98.2
      household appliance X98.3
      specified NEC X98.8
      steam X98.0
      tap water X98.1
      vapors X98.0
    scalding — *see* Assault, burning
    steam X98.0
    vitriol Y08.89
  caustic, corrosive substance (gas) Y08.89
  crashing of
    aircraft Y08.81
    motor vehicle Y03.8
      pushed in front of Y02.0
      run over Y03.0
      specified NEC Y03.8
  cutting or piercing instrument X99.9
    dagger X99.2
    glass X99.0
    knife X99.1
    specified NEC X99.8
    sword X99.2
  dagger X99.2
  drowning (in) X92.9
    bathtub X92.0
    natural water X92.3
    specified NEC X92.8
    swimming pool X92.1
      following fall X92.2
  dynamite X96.8
  explosive(s) (material) X96.9
  fight (hand) (fists) (foot) (unarmed) Y04.0
    with weapon — *see* Assault, by type of weapon
  fire X97
  firearm X95.9
    airgun X95.01
    handgun X93
    hunting rifle X94.1
    larger X94.9
      specified NEC X94.8
    machine gun X94.2
    shotgun X94.0
    specified NEC X95.8
  from high place Y01
  gunshot (wound) NEC — *see* Assault, firearm, by type
  incendiary device X97
  injury Y09
    to child due to criminal abortion attempt NEC Y08.89
  knife X99.1
  late effect of — *see* X92-Y08 with 7th character S
  placing before moving object NEC Y02.8
    motor vehicle Y02.0
  poisoning — *see* categories T36-T65 with 7th character S
  puncture, any part of body — *see* Assault, cutting or piercing instrument
  pushing
    before moving object NEC Y02.8
      motor vehicle Y02.0
      subway train Y02.1
      train Y02.1
  rape T74.2-
  scalding — *see* Assault, burning
  sequelae of — *see* X92-Y08 with 7th character S
  sexual (by bodily force) T74.2-
  shooting — *see* Assault, firearm
  specified means NEC Y08.89
  stab, any part of body — *see* Assault, cutting or piercing instrument
  steam X98.0

EXTERNAL CAUSES

Assault (homicidal) (by) (in) Y09 — *continued*
  striking against
    other person Y04.2
    sports equipment Y08.09
      baseball bat Y08.02
      hockey stick Y08.01
  struck by
    sports equipment Y08.09
      baseball bat Y08.02
      hockey stick Y08.01
  submersion — *see* Assault, drowning
  violence Y09
  weapon Y09
    blunt Y00
    cutting or piercing — *see* Assault, cutting or
      piercing instrument
    firearm — *see* Assault, firearm
  wound Y09
    cutting — *see* Assault, cutting or piercing
      instrument
    gunshot — *see* Assault, firearm
    knife X99.1
    piercing — *see* Assault, cutting or piercing
      instrument
    puncture — *see* Assault, cutting or piercing
      instrument
    stab — *see* Assault, cutting or piercing
      instrument
Attack by mammals NEC W55.89
Avalanche — *see* Landslide
Aviator's disease — *see* Air, pressure

B

Barotitis, barodontalgia, barosinusitis, barotrauma (otitic) (sinus) — *see* Air, pressure
Battered (baby) (child) (person) (syndrome) X58
Bayonet wound W26.1
  in
    legal intervention — *see* Legal, intervention, sharp object, bayonet
    war operations — *see* War operations, combat
  stated as undetermined whether accidental or intentional Y28.8
  suicide (attempt) X78.2
Bean in nose — *see* categories T17 and T18
Bed set on fire NEC — *see* Exposure, fire, uncontrolled, building, bed
Beheading (by guillotine)
  homicide X99.9
  legal execution — *see* Legal, intervention
Bending, injury in (prolonged) (static) X50.1
Bends — *see* Air, pressure, change
Bite, bitten by
  alligator W58.01
  arthropod (nonvenomous) NEC W57
  bull W55.21
  cat W55.01
  cow W55.21
  crocodile W58.11
  dog W54.0
  goat W55.31
  hoof stock NEC W55.31
  horse W55.11
  human being (accidentally) W50.3
    with intent to injure or kill Y04.1
    as, or caused by, a crowd or human stampede (with fall) W52
    assault Y04.1
    homicide (attempt) Y04.1
    in
      fight Y04.1
  insect (nonvenomous) W57
  lizard (nonvenomous) W59.01
  mammal NEC W55.81
    marine W56.31
  marine animal (nonvenomous) W56.81
  millipede W57
  moray eel W56.51
  mouse W53.01
  person(s) (accidentally) W50.3
    with intent to injure or kill Y04.1
    as, or caused by, a crowd or human stampede (with fall) W52
    assault Y04.1
    homicide (attempt) Y04.1
    in
      fight Y04.1
  pig W55.41
  raccoon W55.51
  rat W53.11
  reptile W59.81
    lizard W59.01
    snake W59.11
    turtle W59.21
    terrestrial W59.81
  rodent W53.81
    mouse W53.01
    rat W53.11
    specified NEC W53.81
    squirrel W53.21
  shark W56.41
  sheep W55.31
  snake (nonvenomous) W59.11
  spider (nonvenomous) W57
  squirrel W53.21

Blast (air) in war operations — *see* War operations, blast
Blizzard X37.2
Blood alcohol level Y90.9
  100-119mg/100ml Y90.5
  120-199mg/100ml Y90.6
  20-39mg/100ml Y90.1
  200-239mg/100ml Y90.7
  40-59mg/100ml Y90.2
  60-79mg/100ml Y90.3
  80-99mg/100ml Y90.4
  less than 20mg/100ml Y90.0
  presence in blood, level not specified Y90.9
Blow X58
  by law-enforcing agent, police (on duty) — *see* Legal, intervention, manhandling
  blunt object — *see* Legal, intervention, blunt object
Blowing up — *see* Explosion
Brawl (hand) (fists) (foot) Y04.0
Breakage (accidental) (part of)
  ladder (causing fall) W11
  scaffolding (causing fall) W12
Broken
  glass, contact with — *see* Contact, with, glass
  power line (causing electric shock) W85
Bumping against, into (accidentally)
  object NEC W22.8
    with fall — *see* Fall, due to, bumping against, object
    caused by crowd or human stampede (with fall) W52
    sports equipment W21.9
  person(s) W51
    with fall W03
      due to ice or snow W00.0
    assault Y04.2
    caused by, a crowd or human stampede (with fall) W52
    homicide (attempt) Y04.2
  sports equipment W21.9
Burn, burned, burning (accidental) (by) (from) (on)
  acid NEC — *see* Table of Drugs and Chemicals
  bed linen — *see* Exposure, fire, uncontrolled, in building, bed
  blowtorch X08.8
    with ignition of clothing NEC X06.2
      nightwear X05
  bonfire, campfire (controlled) — *see also* Exposure, fire, controlled, not in building
    uncontrolled — *see* Exposure, fire, uncontrolled, not in building
  candle X08.8
    with ignition of clothing NEC X06.2
      nightwear X05
  caustic liquid, substance (external) (internal) NEC — *see* Table of Drugs and Chemicals
  chemical (external) (internal) — *see also* Table of Drugs and Chemicals
    in war operations — *see* War operations. fire
  cigar(s) or cigarette(s) X08.8
    with ignition of clothing NEC X06.2
      nightwear X05
  clothes, clothing NEC (from controlled fire) X06.2
    with conflagration — *see* Exposure, fire, uncontrolled, building
    not in building or structure — *see* Exposure, fire, uncontrolled, not in building
  cooker (hot) X15.8
    stated as undetermined whether accidental or intentional Y27.3
    suicide (attempt) X77.3
  electric blanket X16
  engine (hot) X17

EXTERNAL CAUSES

Burn, burned, burning (accidental) (by) (from) (on) — *continued*
fire, flames — *see* Exposure, fire
flare, Very pistol — *see* Discharge, firearm NEC
heat
  from appliance (electrical) (household) X15.8
    cooker X15.8
    hotplate X15.2
    kettle X15.8
    light bulb X15.8
    saucepan X15.3
    skillet X15.3
    stated as undetermined whether accidental or intentional Y27.3
    stove X15.0
    suicide (attempt) X77.3
    toaster X15.1
  in local application or packing during medical or surgical procedure Y63.5
heating
  appliance, radiator or pipe X16
homicide (attempt) — *see* Assault, burning
hot
  air X14.1
  cooker X15.8
  drink X10.0
  engine X17
  fat X10.2
  fluid NEC X12
  food X10.1
  gases X14.1
  heating appliance X16
  household appliance NEC X15.8
  kettle X15.8
  liquid NEC X12
  machinery X17
  metal (molten) (liquid) NEC X18
  object (not producing fire or flames) NEC X19
  oil (cooking) X10.2
  pipe(s) X16
  radiator X16
  saucepan (glass) (metal) X15.3
  stove (kitchen) X15.0
  substance NEC X19
    caustic or corrosive NEC — *see* Table of Drugs and Chemicals
  toaster X15.1
  tool X17
  vapor X13.1
  water (tap) — *see* Contact, with, hot, tap water
hotplate X15.2
  suicide (attempt) X77.3
ignition — *see* Ignition
in war operations — *see* War operations, fire
inflicted by other person X97
  by hot objects, hot vapor, and steam — *see* Assault, burning, hot object
internal, from swallowed caustic, corrosive liquid, substance — *see* Table of Drugs and Chemicals
iron (hot) X15.8
  stated as undetermined whether accidental or intentional Y27.3
  suicide (attempt) X77.3
kettle (hot) X15.8
  stated as undetermined whether accidental or intentional Y27.3
  suicide (attempt) X77.3
lamp (flame) X08.8
  with ignition of clothing NEC X06.2
    nightwear X05
lighter (cigar) (cigarette) X08.8
  with ignition of clothing NEC X06.2
    nightwear X05

Burn, burned, burning (accidental) (by) (from) (on) — *continued*
lightning — *see* subcategory T75.0
  causing fire — *see* Exposure, fire
liquid (boiling) (hot) NEC X12
  stated as undetermined whether accidental or intentional Y27.2
  suicide (attempt) X77.2
local application of externally applied substance in medical or surgical care Y63.5
machinery (hot) X17
matches X08.8
  with ignition of clothing NEC X06.2
    nightwear X05
mattress — *see* Exposure, fire, uncontrolled, building, bed
medicament, externally applied Y63.5
metal (hot) (liquid) (molten) NEC X18
nightwear (nightclothes, nightdress, gown, pajamas, robe) X05
object (hot) NEC X19
on board watercraft
  due to
    accident to watercraft V91.09
      powered craft V91.03
        ferry boat V91.01
        fishing boat V91.02
        jetskis V91.03
        liner V91.01
        merchant ship V91.00
        passenger ship V91.01
      unpowered craft V91.08
        canoe V91.05
        inflatable V91.06
        kayak V91.05
        sailboat V91.04
        surfboard V91.08
        water skis V91.07
        windsurfer V91.08
    fire on board V93.09
      ferry boat V93.01
      fishing boat V93.02
      jetskis V93.03
      liner V93.01
      merchant ship V93.00
      passenger ship V93.01
      powered craft NEC V93.03
      sailboat V93.04
    specified heat source NEC on board V93.19
      ferry boat V93.11
      fishing boat V93.12
      jetskis V93.13
      liner V93.11
      merchant ship V93.10
      passenger ship V93.11
      powered craft NEC V93.13
      sailboat V93.14
pipe (hot) X16
  smoking X08.8
  with ignition of clothing NEC X06.2
    nightwear X05
powder — *see* Powder burn
radiator (hot) X16
saucepan (hot) (glass) (metal) X15.3
  stated as undetermined whether accidental or intentional Y27.3
  suicide (attempt) X77.3
self-inflicted X76
  stated as undetermined whether accidental or intentional Y26
stated as undetermined whether accidental or intentional Y27.0

Burn, burned, burning (accidental) (by) (from) (on) — *continued*
steam X13.1
  pipe X16
    stated as undetermined whether accidental or intentional Y27.8
  stated as undetermined whether accidental or intentional Y27.0
  suicide (attempt) X77.0
stove (hot) (kitchen) X15.0
  stated as undetermined whether accidental or intentional Y27.3
  suicide (attempt) X77.3
substance (hot) NEC X19
  boiling X12
    stated as undetermined whether accidental or intentional Y27.2
    suicide (attempt) X77.2
  molten (metal) X18
suicide (attempt) NEC X76
  hot
    household appliance X77.3
    object X77.9
therapeutic misadventure
  heat in local application or packing during medical or surgical procedure Y63.5
  overdose of radiation Y63.2
toaster (hot) X15.1
  stated as undetermined whether accidental or intentional Y27.3
  suicide (attempt) X77.3
tool (hot) X17
torch, welding X08.8
  with ignition of clothing NEC X06.2
    nightwear X05
trash fire (controlled) — *see* Exposure, fire, controlled, not in building
  uncontrolled — *see* Exposure, fire, uncontrolled, not in building
vapor (hot) X13.1
  stated as undetermined whether accidental or intentional Y27.0
  suicide (attempt) X77.0
Very pistol — *see* Discharge, firearm NEC
Butted by animal W55.82
  bull W55.22
  cow W55.22
  goat W55.32
  horse W55.12
  pig W55.42
  sheep W55.32

EXTERNAL CAUSES

C

Caisson disease — *see* Air, pressure, change
Campfire (exposure to) (controlled) — *see also*
    Exposure, fire, controlled, not in building
  uncontrolled — *see* Exposure, fire,
    uncontrolled, not in building
Capital punishment (any means) — *see*
  Legal, intervention
Car sickness T75.3
Casualty (not due to war) NEC X58
  war — *see* War operations
Cat
  bite W55.01
  scratch W55.03
Cataclysm, cataclysmic (any injury) NEC —
  see Forces of nature
Catching fire — *see* Exposure, fire
Caught
  between
    folding object W23.0
    objects (moving) (stationary and moving)
      W23.0
      and machinery — *see* Contact, with, by
        type of machine
      stationary W23.1
    sliding door and door frame W23.0
  by, in
    machinery (moving parts of) — *see* Contact,
      with, by type of machine
    washing-machine wringer W23.0
    under packing crate (due to losing grip)
      W23.1
Cave-in caused by cataclysmic earth
  surface movement or eruption — *see*
  Landslide
Change(s) in air pressure — *see* Air,
  pressure, change
Choked, choking (on) (any object except food
  or vomitus)
  food (bone) (seed) — *see* categories T17 and
    T18
  vomitus T17.81-
Civil insurrection — *see* War operations
Cloudburst (any injury) X37.8
Cold, exposure to (accidental) (excessive)
  (extreme) (natural) (place) NEC — *see*
  Exposure, cold
Collapse
  building W20.1
    burning (uncontrolled fire) X00.2
  dam or man-made structure (causing earth
    movement) X36.0
  machinery — *see* Contact, with, by type of
    machine
  structure W20.1
    burning (uncontrolled fire) X00.2
Collision (accidental) NEC (*see also* Accident,
  transport) V89.9
  pedestrian W51
    with fall W03
      due to ice or snow W00.0
      involving pedestrian conveyance — *see*
        Accident, transport, pedestrian,
        conveyance
    and
      crowd or human stampede (with fall) W52
      object W22.8
        with fall — *see* Fall, due to, bumping
          against, object
  person(s) — *see* Collision, pedestrian

Collision (accidental) NEC (*see also* Accident,
  transport) V89.9 — *continued*
  transport vehicle NEC V89.9
    and
      avalanche, fallen or not moving — *see*
        Accident, transport
        falling or moving — *see* Landslide
      landslide, fallen or not moving — *see*
        Accident, transport
        falling or moving — *see* Landslide
      due to cataclysm — *see* Forces of nature, by
        type
      intentional, purposeful suicide (attempt) —
        see Suicide, collision
Combustion, spontaneous — *see* Ignition
Complication (delayed) of or following
  (medical or surgical procedure) Y84.9
  with misadventure — *see* Misadventure
  amputation of limb(s) Y83.5
  anastomosis (arteriovenous) (blood vessel)
    (gastrojejunal) (tendon) (natural or
    artificial material) Y83.2
  aspiration (of fluid) Y84.4
    tissue Y84.8
  biopsy Y84.8
  blood
    sampling Y84.7
    transfusion
      procedure Y84.8
  bypass Y83.2
  catheterization (urinary) Y84.6
    cardiac Y84.0
  colostomy Y83.3
  cystostomy Y83.3
  dialysis (kidney) Y84.1
  drug — *see* Table of Drugs and Chemicals
  due to misadventure — *see* Misadventure
  duodenostomy Y83.3
  electroshock therapy Y84.3
  external stoma, creation of Y83.3
  formation of external stoma Y83.3
  gastrostomy Y83.3
  graft Y83.2
  hypothermia (medically-induced) Y84.8
  implant, implantation (of)
    artificial
      internal device (cardiac pacemaker)
        (electrodes in brain) (heart valve
        prosthesis) (orthopedic) Y83.1
      material or tissue (for anastomosis or
        bypass) Y83.2
        with creation of external stoma Y83.3
    natural tissues (for anastomosis or bypass)
      Y83.2
      with creation of external stoma Y83.3
  infusion
    procedure Y84.8
  injection — *see* Table of Drugs and Chemicals
    procedure Y84.8
  insertion of gastric or duodenal sound Y84.5
  insulin-shock therapy Y84.3
  paracentesis (abdominal) (thoracic) (aspirative)
    Y84.4
  procedures other than surgical operation —
    see Complication of or following, by type
    of procedure
  radiological procedure or therapy Y84.2
  removal of organ (partial) (total) NEC Y83.6
  sampling
    blood Y84.7
    fluid NEC Y84.4
    tissue Y84.8
  shock therapy Y84.3

Complication (delayed) of or following
  (medical or surgical procedure) Y84.9 —
  continued
  surgical operation NEC (*see also* Complication
    of or following, by type of operation)
    Y83.9
    reconstructive NEC Y83.4
      with
        anastomosis, bypass or graft Y83.2
        formation of external stoma Y83.3
    specified NEC Y83.8
  transfusion — *see also* Table of Drugs and
    Chemicals
    procedure Y84.8
  transplant, transplantation (heart) (kidney)
    (liver) (whole organ, any) Y83.0
    partial organ Y83.4
  ureterostomy Y83.3
  vaccination — *see also* Table of Drugs and
    Chemicals
    procedure Y84.8
Compression
  divers' squeeze — *see* Air, pressure, change
  trachea by
    food (lodged in esophagus) — *see* categories
      T17 and T18
    vomitus (lodged in esophagus) T17.81-
Conflagration — *see* Exposure, fire,
  uncontrolled
Constriction (external)
  hair W49.01
  jewelry W49.04
  ring W49.04
  rubber band W49.03
  specified item NEC W49.09
  string W49.02
  thread W49.02
Contact (accidental)
  with
    abrasive wheel (metalworking) W31.1
    alligator W58.09
      bite W58.01
      crushing W58.03
      strike W58.02
    amphibian W62.9
      frog W62.0
      toad W62.1
    animal (nonvenomous) NEC W64
      marine W56.89
        bite W56.81
        dolphin — *see* Contact, with, dolphin
        fish NEC — *see* Contact, with, fish
        mammal — *see* Contact, with, mammal,
          marine
        orca — *see* Contact, with, orca
        sea lion — *see* Contact, with, sea lion
        shark — *see* Contact, with, shark
        strike W56.82
    animate mechanical force NEC W64
    arrow W21.89
      not thrown, projected or falling W45.8
    arthropods (nonvenomous) W57
    axe W27.0
    band-saw (industrial) W31.2
    bayonet — *see* Bayonet wound
    bee(s) X58
    bench-saw (industrial) W31.2
    bird W61.99
      bite W61.91
      chicken — *see* Contact, with, chicken
      duck — *see* Contact, with, duck
      goose — *see* Contact, with, goose
      macaw — *see* Contact, with, macaw
      parrot — *see* Contact, with, parrot
      psittacine — *see* Contact, with, psittacine
      strike W61.92
      turkey — *see* Contact, with, turkey
    blender W29.0

Contact (accidental) — *continued*
  with — *continued*
    boiling water X12
      stated as undetermined whether accidental
        or intentional Y27.2
      suicide (attempt) X77.2
    bore, earth-drilling or mining (land)
      (seabed) W31.0
    buffalo — *see* Contact, with, hoof stock NEC
    bull W55.29
      bite W55.21
      gored W55.22
      strike W55.22
    bumper cars W31.81
    camel — *see* Contact, with, hoof stock NEC
    can
      lid W26.8
      opener W27.4
        powered W29.0
    cat W55.09
      bite W55.01
      scratch W55.03
    caterpillar (venomous) X58
    centipede (venomous) X58
    chain
      hoist W24.0
        agricultural operations W30.89
      saw W29.3
    chicken W61.39
      peck W61.33
      strike W61.32
    chisel W27.0
    circular saw W31.2
    cobra X58
    combine (harvester) W30.0
    conveyer belt W24.1
    cooker (hot) X15.8
      stated as undetermined whether accidental
        or intentional Y27.3
      suicide (attempt) X77.3
    coral X58
    cotton gin W31.82
    cow W55.29
      bite W55.21
      strike W55.22
    crane W24.0
      agricultural operations W30.89
    crocodile W58.19
      bite W58.11
      crushing W58.13
      strike W58.12
    dagger W26.1
      stated as undetermined whether accidental
        or intentional Y28.2
      suicide (attempt) X78.2
    dairy equipment W31.82
    dart W21.89
      not thrown, projected or falling W45.8
    deer — *see* Contact, with, hoof stock NEC
    derrick W24.0
      agricultural operations W30.89
        hay W30.2
    dog W54.8
      bite W54.0
      strike W54.1
    dolphin W56.09
      bite W56.01
      strike W56.02
    donkey — *see* Contact, with, hoof stock NEC
    drill (powered) W29.8
      earth (land) (seabed) W31.0
      nonpowered W27.8
    drive belt W24.0
      agricultural operations W30.89
    dry ice — *see* Exposure, cold, man-made
    dryer (clothes) (powered) (spin) W29.2

Contact (accidental) — *continued*
  with — *continued*
    duck W61.69
      bite W61.61
      strike W61.62
    earth(-)
      drilling machine (industrial) W31.0
      scraping machine in stationary use
        W31.83
    edge of stiff paper W26.2
    electric
      beater W29.0
      blanket X16
      fan W29.2
        commercial W31.82
      knife W29.1
      mixer W29.0
    elevator (building) W24.0
      agricultural operations W30.89
        grain W30.3
    engine(s), hot NEC X17
    excavating machine W31.0
    farm machine W30.9
    feces — *see* Contact, with, by type of animal
    fer de lance X58
    fish W56.59
      bite W56.51
      shark — *see* Contact, with, shark
      strike W56.52
    flying horses W31.81
    forging (metalworking) machine W31.1
    fork W27.4
    forklift (truck) W24.0
      agricultural operations W30.89
    frog W62.0
    garden
      cultivator (powered) W29.3
        riding W30.89
      fork W27.1
    gas turbine W31.3
    Gila monster X58
    giraffe — *see* Contact, with, hoof stock NEC
    glass (sharp) (broken) W25
      with subsequent fall W18.02
      assault X99.0
      due to fall — *see* Fall, by type
      stated as undetermined whether accidental
        or intentional Y28.0
      suicide (attempt) X78.0
    goat W55.39
      bite W55.31
      strike W55.32
    goose W61.59
      bite W61.51
      strike W61.52
    hand
      saw W27.0
      tool (not powered) NEC W27.8
        powered W29.8
    harvester W30.0
    hay-derrick W30.2
    heat NEC X19
      from appliance (electrical) (household) —
        see Contact, with, hot, household
        appliance
      heating appliance X16
    heating
      appliance (hot) X16
      pad (electric) X16
    hedge-trimmer (powered) W29.3
    hoe W27.1
    hoist (chain) (shaft) NEC W24.0
      agricultural W30.89
    hoof stock NEC W55.39
      bite W55.31
      strike W55.32
    hornet(s) X58

Contact (accidental) — *continued*
  with — *continued*
    horse W55.19
      bite W55.11
      strike W55.12
    hot
      air X14.1
        inhalation X14.0
      cooker X15.8
      drinks X10.0
      engine X17
      fats X10.2
      fluids NEC X12
        assault X98.2
        suicide (attempt) X77.2
        undetermined whether accidental or
          intentional Y27.2
      food X10.1
      gases X14.1
        inhalation X14.0
      heating appliance X16
      household appliance X15.8
        assault X98.3
        cooker X15.8
        hotplate X15.2
        kettle X15.8
        light bulb X15.8
        object NEC X19
          assault X98.8
          stated as undetermined whether
            accidental or intentional Y27.9
          suicide (attempt) X77.8
        saucepan X15.3
        skillet X15.3
        stated as undetermined whether
          accidental or intentional Y27.3
        stove X15.0
        suicide (attempt) X77.3
        toaster X15.1
      kettle X15.8
      light bulb X15.8
      liquid NEC (*see also* Burn) X12
        drinks X10.0
        stated as undetermined whether
          accidental or intentional Y27.2
        suicide (attempt) X77.2
        tap water X11.8
          stated as undetermined whether
            accidental or intentional Y27.1
          suicide (attempt) X77.1
      machinery X17
      metal (molten) (liquid) NEC X18
      object (not producing fire or flames) NEC
        X19
      oil (cooking) X10.2
      pipe X16
      plate X15.2
      radiator X16
      saucepan (glass) (metal) X15.3
      skillet X15.3
      stove (kitchen) X15.0
      substance NEC X19
      tap-water X11.8
        assault X98.1
        heated on stove X12
          stated as undetermined whether
            accidental or intentional Y27.2
          suicide (attempt) X77.2
        in bathtub X11.0
        running X11.1
        stated as undetermined whether
          accidental or intentional Y27.1
        suicide (attempt) X77.1
      toaster X15.1
      tool X17
      vapors X13.1
        inhalation X13.0

EXTERNAL CAUSES

Contact (accidental) — *continued*
  with — *continued*
    hot — *continued*
      water (tap) X11.8
        boiling X12
          stated as undetermined whether
            accidental or intentional Y27.2
          suicide (attempt) X77.2
        heated on stove X12
          stated as undetermined whether
            accidental or intentional Y27.2
          suicide (attempt) X77.2
        in bathtub X11.0
        running X11.1
        stated as undetermined whether
          accidental or intentional Y27.1
        suicide (attempt) X77.1
    hotplate X15.2
    ice-pick W27.4
    insect (nonvenomous) NEC W57
    kettle (hot) X15.8
    knife W26.0
      assault X99.1
      electric W29.1
      stated as undetermined whether accidental
        or intentional Y28.1
      suicide (attempt) X78.1
    lathe (metalworking) W31.1
      turnings W45.8
      woodworking W31.2
    lawnmower (powered) (ridden) W28
      causing electrocution W86.8
      suicide (attempt) X83.1
      unpowered W27.1
    lift, lifting (devices) W24.0
      agricultural operations W30.89
      shaft W24.0
    liquefied gas — *see* Exposure, cold, man-made
    liquid air, hydrogen, nitrogen — *see*
      Exposure, cold, man-made
    lizard (nonvenomous) W59.09
      bite W59.01
      strike W59.02
    llama — *see* Contact, with, hoof stock NEC
    macaw W61.19
      bite W61.11
      strike W61.12
    machine, machinery W31.9
      abrasive wheel W31.1
      agricultural including animal-powered
        W30.9
      combine harvester W30.0
      grain storage elevator W30.3
      hay derrick W30.2
      power take-off device W30.1
      reaper W30.0
      specified NEC W30.89
      thresher W30.0
      transport vehicle, stationary W30.81
      band saw W31.2
      bench saw W31.2
      circular saw W31.2
      commercial NEC W31.82
      drilling, metal (industrial) W31.1
      earth-drilling W31.0
      earthmoving or scraping W31.89
      excavating W31.89
      forging machine W31.1
      gas turbine W31.3
      hot X17
      internal combustion engine W31.3
      land drill W31.0
      lathe W31.1
      lifting (devices) W24.0
      metal drill W31.1
      metalworking (industrial) W31.1
      milling, metal W31.1

Contact (accidental) — *continued*
  with — *continued*
    machine, machinery W31.9 — *continued*
      mining W31.0
      molding W31.2
      overhead plane W31.2
      power press, metal W31.1
      prime mover W31.3
      printing W31.89
      radial saw W31.2
      recreational W31.81
      roller-coaster W31.81
      rolling mill, metal W31.1
      sander W31.2
      seabed drill W31.0
      shaft
        hoist W31.0
        lift W31.0
      specified NEC W31.89
      spinning W31.89
      steam engine W31.3
      transmission W24.1
      undercutter W31.0
      water driven turbine W31.3
      weaving W31.89
      woodworking or forming (industrial)
        W31.89
    mammal (feces) (urine) W55.89
      bull — *see* Contact, with, bull
      cat — *see* Contact, with, cat
      cow — *see* Contact, with, cow
      goat — *see* Contact, with, goat
      hoof stock — *see* Contact, with, hoof stock
      horse — *see* Contact, with, horse
      marine W56.39
        dolphin — *see* Contact, with, dolphin
        orca — *see* Contact, with, orca
        sea lion — *see* Contact, with, sea lion
        specified NEC W56.39
          bite W56.31
          strike W56.32
      pig — *see* Contact, with, pig
      raccoon — *see* Contact, with, raccoon
      rodent — *see* Contact, with, rodent
      sheep — *see* Contact, with, sheep
      specified NEC W55.89
        bite W55.81
        strike W55.82
    marine
      animal W56.89
        bite W56.81
        dolphin — *see* Contact, with, dolphin
        fish NEC — *see* Contact, with, fish
        mammal — *see* Contact, with, mammal,
          marine
        orca — *see* Contact, with, orca
        sea lion — *see* Contact, with, sea lion
        shark — *see* Contact, with, shark
        strike W56.82
    meat
      grinder (domestic) W29.0
        industrial W31.82
        nonpowered W27.4
      slicer (domestic) W29.0
        industrial W31.82
    merry go round W31.81
    metal, hot (liquid) (molten) NEC X18
    millipede W57
    nail W45.0
      gun W29.4
    needle (sewing) W27.3
      hypodermic W46.0
        contaminated W46.1

Contact (accidental) — *continued*
  with — *continued*
    object (blunt) NEC
      hot NEC X19
      legal intervention — *see* Legal,
        intervention, blunt object
      sharp NEC W45.8
        inflicted by other person NEC W45.8
        stated as
          intentional homicide (attempt) — *see*
            Assault, cutting or piercing
            instrument
          legal intervention — *see* Legal,
            intervention, sharp object
        self-inflicted X78.9
    orca W56.29
      bite W56.21
      strike W56.22
    overhead plane W31.2
    paper (as sharp object) W26.2
    paper-cutter W27.5
    parrot W61.09
      bite W61.01
      strike W61.02
    pig W55.49
      bite W55.41
      strike W55.42
    pipe, hot X16
    pitchfork W27.1
    plane (metal) (wood) W27.0
      overhead W31.2
    plant thorns, spines, sharp leaves or other
      mechanisms W60
    powered
      garden cultivator W29.3
      household appliance, implement, or
        machine W29.8
      saw (industrial) W31.2
        hand W29.8
    printing machine W31.89
    psittacine bird W61.29
      bite W61.21
      macaw — *see* Contact, with, macaw
      parrot — *see* Contact, with, parrot
      strike W61.22
    pulley (block) (transmission) W24.0
      agricultural operations W30.89
    raccoon W55.59
      bite W55.51
      strike W55.52
    radial-saw (industrial) W31.2
    radiator (hot) X16
    rake W27.1
    rattlesnake X58
    reaper W30.0
    reptile W59.89
      lizard — *see* Contact, with, lizard
      snake — *see* Contact, with, snake
      specified NEC W59.89
        bite W59.81
        crushing W59.83
        strike W59.82
      turtle — *see* Contact, with, turtle
    rivet gun (powered) W29.4
    road scraper — *see* Accident, transport,
      construction vehicle
    rodent (feces) (urine) W53.89
      bite W53.81
      mouse W53.09
        bite W53.01
      rat W53.19
        bite W53.11
      specified NEC W53.89
        bite W53.81
      squirrel W53.29
        bite W53.21
    roller coaster W31.81

EXTERNAL CAUSES

Contact (accidental) — *continued*
with — *continued*
  rope NEC W24.0
    agricultural operations W30.89
  saliva — *see* Contact, with, by type of
    animal
  sander W29.8
    industrial W31.2
  saucepan (hot) (glass) (metal) X15.3
  saw W27.0
    band (industrial) W31.2
    bench (industrial) W31.2
    chain W29.3
    hand W27.0
  sawing machine, metal W31.1
  scissors W27.2
  scorpion X58
  screwdriver W27.0
    powered W29.8
  sea
    anemone, cucumber or urchin (spine) X58
    lion W56.19
      bite W56.11
      strike W56.12
  serpent — *see* Contact, with, snake, by type
  sewing-machine (electric) (powered) W29.2
    not powered W27.8
  shaft (hoist) (lift) (transmission) NEC W24.0
    agricultural W30.89
  shark W56.49
    bite W56.41
    strike W56.42
  sharp object(s) W26.9
    specified NEC W26.8
  shears (hand) W27.2
    powered (industrial) W31.1
      domestic W29.2
  sheep W55.39
    bite W55.31
    strike W55.32
  shovel W27.8
    steam — *see* Accident, transport,
      construction vehicle
  snake (nonvenomous) W59.19
    bite W59.11
    crushing W59.13
    strike W59.12
  spade W27.1
  spider (venomous) X58
  spin-drier W29.2
  spinning machine W31.89
  splinter W45.8
  sports equipment W21.9
  staple gun (powered) W29.8
  steam X13.1
    engine W31.3
    inhalation X13.0
    pipe X16
    shovel W31.89
  stove (hot) (kitchen) X15.0
  substance, hot NEC X19
    molten (metal) X18
  sword W26.1
    assault X99.2
    stated as undetermined whether accidental
      or intentional Y28.2
    suicide (attempt) X78.2
  tarantula X58
  thresher W30.0
  tin can lid W26.8
  toad W62.1
  toaster (hot) X15.1

Contact (accidental) — *continued*
with — *continued*
  tool W27.8
    hand (not powered) W27.8
      auger W27.0
      axe W27.0
      can opener W27.4
      chisel W27.0
      fork W27.4
      garden W27.1
      handsaw W27.0
      hoe W27.1
      ice-pick W27.4
      kitchen utensil W27.4
      manual
        lawn mower W27.1
        sewing machine W27.8
      meat grinder W27.4
      needle (sewing) W27.3
        hypodermic W46.0
          contaminated W46.1
      paper cutter W27.5
      pitchfork W27.1
      rake W27.1
      scissors W27.2
      screwdriver W27.0
      specified NEC W27.8
      workbench W27.0
    hot X17
    powered W29.8
      blender W29.0
        commercial W31.82
      can opener W29.0
        commercial W31.82
      chainsaw W29.3
      clothes dryer W29.2
        commercial W31.82
      dishwasher W29.2
        commercial W31.82
      edger W29.3
      electric fan W29.2
        commercial W31.82
      electric knife W29.1
      food processor W29.0
        commercial W31.82
      garbage disposal W29.0
        commercial W31.82
      garden tool W29.3
      hedge trimmer W29.3
      ice maker W29.0
        commercial W31.82
      kitchen appliance W29.0
        commercial W31.82
      lawn mower W28
      meat grinder W29.0
        commercial W31.82
      mixer W29.0
        commercial W31.82
      rototiller W29.3
      sewing machine W29.2
        commercial W31.82
      washing machine W29.2
        commercial W31.82
  transmission device (belt, cable, chain, gear,
    pinion, shaft) W24.1
    agricultural operations W30.89
  turbine (gas) (water-driven) W31.3
  turkey W61.49
    peck W61.43
    strike W61.42
  turtle (nonvenomous) W59.29
    bite W59.21
    strike W59.22
    terrestrial W59.89
      bite W59.81
      crushing W59.83
      strike W59.82

Contact (accidental) — *continued*
with — *continued*
  under-cutter W31.0
  urine — *see* Contact, with, by type of animal
  vehicle
    agricultural use (transport) — *see*
      Accident, transport, agricultural
      vehicle
      not on public highway W30.81
    industrial use (transport) — *see* Accident,
      transport, industrial vehicle
      not on public highway W31.83
    off-road use (transport) — *see* Accident,
      transport, all-terrain or off-road
      vehicle
      not on public highway W31.83
    special construction use (transport) — *see*
      Accident, transport, construction
      vehicle
      not on public highway W31.83
  venomous
    animal X58
    arthropods X58
    lizard X58
    marine animal NEC X58
    marine plant NEC X58
    millipedes (tropical) X58
    plant(s) X58
    snake X58
    spider X58
    viper X58
  washing-machine (powered) W29.2
  wasp X58
  weaving-machine W31.89
  winch W24.0
    agricultural operations W30.89
  wire NEC W24.0
    agricultural operations W30.89
  wood slivers W45.8
  yellow jacket X58
  zebra — *see* Contact, with, hoof stock NEC
  pressure X50.9
  stress X50.9
Coup de soleil X32
Crash
  aircraft (in transit) (powered) V95.9
    balloon V96.01
    fixed wing NEC (private) V95.21
      commercial V95.31
    glider V96.21
      hang V96.11
      powered V95.11
    helicopter V95.01
    in war operations — *see* War operations,
      destruction of aircraft
    microlight V95.11
    nonpowered V96.9
      specified NEC V96.8
    powered NEC V95.8
    stated as
      homicide (attempt) Y08.81
      suicide (attempt) X83.0
    ultralight V95.11
  spacecraft V95.41
  transport vehicle NEC (*see also* Accident,
    transport) V89.9
    homicide (attempt) Y03.8
    motor NEC (traffic) V89.2
      homicide (attempt) Y03.8
      suicide (attempt) — *see* Suicide, collision
Cruelty (mental) (physical) (sexual) X58

EXTERNAL CAUSES

Crushed (accidentally) X58
between objects (moving) (stationary and moving) W23.0
stationary W23.1
by
alligator W58.03
avalanche NEC — *see* Landslide
cave-in W20.0
caused by cataclysmic earth surface movement — *see* Landslide
crocodile W58.13
crowd or human stampede W52
falling
aircraft V97.39
in war operations — *see* War operations, destruction of aircraft
earth, material W20.0
caused by cataclysmic earth surface movement — *see* Landslide
object NEC W20.8
landslide NEC — *see* Landslide
lizard (nonvenomous) W59.09
machinery — *see* Contact, with, by type of machine
reptile NEC W59.89
snake (nonvenomous) W59.13
in
machinery — *see* Contact, with, by type of machine
Cut, cutting (any part of body) (accidental) — *see also* Contact, with, by object or machine
during medical or surgical treatment as misadventure — *see* Index to Diseases and Injuries, Complications
homicide (attempt) — *see* Assault, cutting or piercing instrument
inflicted by other person — *see* Assault, cutting or piercing instrument
legal
execution — *see* Legal, intervention
intervention — *see* Legal, intervention, sharp object
machine NEC (*see also* Contact, with, by type of machine) W31.9
self-inflicted — *see* Suicide, cutting or piercing instrument
suicide (attempt) — *see* Suicide, cutting or piercing instrument
Cyclone (any injury) X37.1

D

Decapitation (accidental circumstances) NEC X58
homicide X99.9
legal execution — *see* Legal, intervention
Dehydration from lack of water X58
Deprivation X58
Derailment (accidental)
railway (rolling stock) (train) (vehicle) (without antecedent collision) V81.7
with antecedent collision — *see* Accident, transport, railway vehicle occupant
streetcar (without antecedent collision) V82.7
with antecedent collision — *see* Accident, transport, streetcar occupant
Descent
parachute (voluntary) (without accident to aircraft) V97.29
due to accident to aircraft — *see* Accident, transport, aircraft
Desertion X58
Destitution X58
Disability, late effect or sequela of injury — *see* Sequelae
Discharge (accidental)
airgun W34.010
assault X95.01
homicide (attempt) X95.01
stated as undetermined whether accidental or intentional Y24.0
suicide (attempt) X74.01
BB gun — *see* Discharge, airgun
firearm (accidental) W34.00
assault X95.9
handgun (pistol) (revolver) W32.0
assault X93
homicide (attempt) X93
legal intervention — *see* Legal, intervention, firearm, handgun
stated as undetermined whether accidental or intentional Y22
suicide (attempt) X72
homicide (attempt) X95.9
hunting rifle W33.02
assault X94.1
homicide (attempt) X94.1
legal intervention
injuring
bystander Y35.032
law enforcement personnel Y35.031
suspect Y35.033
stated as undetermined whether accidental or intentional Y23.1
suicide (attempt) X73.1
larger W33.00
assault X94.9
homicide (attempt) X94.9
hunting rifle — *see* Discharge, firearm, hunting rifle
legal intervention — *see* Legal, intervention, firearm by type of firearm
machine gun — *see* Discharge, firearm, machine gun
shotgun — *see* Discharge, firearm, shotgun
specified NEC W33.09
assault X94.8
homicide (attempt) X94.8
legal intervention
injuring
bystander Y35.092
law enforcement personnel Y35.091
suspect Y35.093
stated as undetermined whether accidental or intentional Y23.8

Discharge (accidental) — *continued*
firearm (accidental) W34.00 — *continued*
larger W33.00 — *continued*
specified NEC W33.09 — *continued*
suicide (attempt) X73.8
stated as undetermined whether accidental or intentional Y23.9
suicide (attempt) X73.9
legal intervention
injuring
bystander Y35.002
law enforcement personnel Y35.001
suspect Y35.03
using rubber bullet
injuring
bystander Y35.042
law enforcement personnel Y35.041
suspect Y35.043
machine gun W33.03
assault X94.2
homicide (attempt) X94.2
legal intervention — *see* Legal, intervention, firearm, machine gun
stated as undetermined whether accidental or intentional Y23.3
suicide (attempt) X73.2
pellet gun — *see* Discharge, airgun
shotgun W33.01
assault X94.0
homicide (attempt) X94.0
legal intervention — *see* Legal, intervention, firearm, specified NEC
stated as undetermined whether accidental or intentional Y23.0
suicide (attempt) X73.0
specified NEC W34.09
assault X95.8
homicide (attempt) X95.8
legal intervention — *see* Legal, intervention, firearm, specified NEC
stated as undetermined whether accidental or intentional Y24.8
suicide (attempt) X74.8
stated as undetermined whether accidental or intentional Y24.9
suicide (attempt) X74.9
Very pistol W34.09
assault X95.8
homicide (attempt) X95.8
stated as undetermined whether accidental or intentional Y24.8
suicide (attempt) X74.8
firework(s) W39
stated as undetermined whether accidental or intentional Y25
gas-operated gun NEC W34.018
airgun — *see* Discharge, airgun
assault X95.09
homicide (attempt) X95.09
paintball gun — *see* Discharge, paintball gun
stated as undetermined whether accidental or intentional Y24.8
suicide (attempt) X74.09
gun NEC — *see also* Discharge, firearm NEC
air — *see* Discharge, airgun
BB — *see* Discharge, airgun
for single hand use — *see* Discharge, firearm, handgun
hand — *see* Discharge, firearm, handgun
machine — *see* Discharge, firearm, machine gun
other specified — *see* Discharge, firearm NEC
paintball — *see* Discharge, paintball gun
pellet — *see* Discharge, airgun
handgun — *see* Discharge, firearm, handgun

Discharge (accidental) — *continued*
  machine gun — *see* Discharge, firearm,
      machine gun
  paintball gun W34.011
    assault X95.02
    homicide (attempt) X95.02
    stated as undetermined whether accidental
        or intentional Y24.8
    suicide (attempt) X74.02
  pistol — *see* Discharge, firearm, handgun
    flare — *see* Discharge, firearm, Very pistol
    pellet — *see* Discharge, airgun
    Very — *see* Discharge, firearm, Very pistol
  revolver — *see* Discharge, firearm, handgun
  rifle (hunting) — *see* Discharge, firearm,
      hunting rifle
  shotgun — *see* Discharge, firearm, shotgun
  spring-operated gun NEC W34.018
    assault X95.09
    homicide (attempt) X95.09
    stated as undetermined whether accidental
        or intentional Y24.8
    suicide (attempt) X74.09

Disease
  Andes W94.11
  aviator's — *see* Air, pressure
  range W94.11

**Diver's disease, palsy, paralysis,
    squeeze** — *see* Air, pressure
Diving (into water) — *see* Accident, diving
Dog bite W54.0
Dragged by transport vehicle NEC (*see also*
    Accident, transport) V09.9
Drinking poison (accidental) — *see* Table of
    Drugs and Chemicals
**Dropped (accidentally) while being
    carried or supported by other person**
    W04

Drowning (accidental) W74
  assault X92.9
  due to
    accident (to)
      machinery — *see* Contact, with, by type of
          machine
      watercraft V90.89
        burning V90.29
          powered V90.23
            fishing boat V90.22
            jetskis V90.23
            merchant ship V90.20
            passenger ship V90.21
          unpowered V90.28
            canoe V90.25
            inflatable V90.26
            kayak V90.25
            sailboat V90.24
            water skis V90.27
        crushed V90.39
          powered V90.33
            fishing boat V90.32
            jetskis V90.33
            merchant ship V90.30
            passenger ship V90.31
          unpowered V90.38
            canoe V90.35
            inflatable V90.36
            kayak V90.35
            sailboat V90.34
            water skis V90.37
        overturning V90.09
          powered V90.03
            fishing boat V90.02
            jetskis V90.03
            merchant ship V90.00
            passenger ship V90.01
          unpowered V90.08
            canoe V90.05
            inflatable V90.06
            kayak V90.05
            sailboat V90.04
        sinking V90.19
          powered V90.13
            fishing boat V90.12
            jetskis V90.13
            merchant ship V90.10
            passenger ship V90.11
          unpowered V90.18
            canoe V90.15
            inflatable V90.16
            kayak V90.15
            sailboat V90.14
        specified type NEC V90.89
          powered V90.83
            fishing boat V90.82
            jetskis V90.83
            merchant ship V90.80
            passenger ship V90.81
          unpowered V90.88
            canoe V90.85
            inflatable V90.86
            kayak V90.85
            sailboat V90.84
            water skis V90.87

Drowning (accidental) W74 — *continued*
  due to — *continued*
    avalanche — *see* Landslide
    cataclysmic
      earth surface movement NEC — *see* Forces
          of nature, earth movement
      storm — *see* Forces of nature, cataclysmic
          storm
    cloudburst X37.8
    cyclone X37.1
    fall overboard (from) V92.09
      powered craft V92.03
        ferry boat V92.01
        fishing boat V92.02
        jetskis V92.03
        liner V92.01
        merchant ship V92.00
        passenger ship V92.01
      resulting from
        accident to watercraft — *see* Drowning,
            due to, accident to, watercraft
        being washed overboard (from) V92.29
          powered craft V92.23
            ferry boat V92.21
            fishing boat V92.22
            jetskis V92.23
            liner V92.21
            merchant ship V92.20
            passenger ship V92.21
          unpowered craft V92.28
            canoe V92.25
            inflatable V92.26
            kayak V92.25
            sailboat V92.24
            surfboard V92.28
            water skis V92.27
            windsurfer V92.28
        motion of watercraft V92.19
          powered craft V92.13
            ferry boat V92.11
            fishing boat V92.12
            jetskis V92.13
            liner V92.11
            merchant ship V92.10
            passenger ship V92.11
          unpowered craft
            canoe V92.15
            inflatable V92.16
            kayak V92.15
            sailboat V92.14
      unpowered craft V92.08
        canoe V92.05
        inflatable V92.06
        kayak V92.05
        sailboat V92.04
        surfboard V92.08
        water skis V92.07
        windsurfer V92.08
    hurricane X37.0
    jumping into water from watercraft (involved
        in accident) — *see also* Drowning, due
        to, accident to, watercraft
      without accident to or on watercraft
          W16.711
    tidal wave NEC — *see* Forces of nature, tidal
        wave
    torrential rain X37.8

EXTERNAL CAUSES

Drowning (accidental) W74 — *continued*
following
  fall
    into
      bathtub W16.211
      bucket W16.221
      fountain — *see* Drowning, following,
        fall, into, water, specified NEC
      quarry — *see* Drowning, following, fall,
        into, water, specified NEC
      reservoir — *see* Drowning, following,
        fall, into, water, specified NEC
      swimming pool W16.011
        stated as undetermined whether
          accidental or intentional Y21.3
        striking
          bottom W16.021
          wall W16.031
        suicide (attempt) X71.2
      water NOS W16.41
        natural (lake) (open sea) (pond) (river)
          (stream) W16.111
          striking
            bottom W16.121
            side W16.131
        specified NEC W16.311
          striking
            bottom W16.321
            wall W16.331
    overboard NEC — *see* Drowning, due to,
      fall overboard
  jump or dive
    from boat W16.711
      striking bottom W16.721
    into
      fountain — *see* Drowning, following,
        jump or dive, into, water, specified
        NEC
      quarry — *see* Drowning, following, jump
        or dive, into, water, specified NEC
      reservoir — *see* Drowning, following,
        jump or dive, into, water, specified
        NEC
      swimming pool W16.511
        striking
          bottom W16.521
          wall W16.531
        suicide (attempt) X71.2
      water NOS W16.91
        natural (lake) (open sea) (pond) (river)
          (stream) W16.611
        specified NEC W16.811
          striking
            bottom W16.821
            wall W16.831
        striking bottom W16.621

Drowning (accidental) W74 — *continued*
homicide (attempt) X92.9
in
  bathtub (accidental) W65
    assault X92.0
    following fall W16.211
      stated as undetermined whether
        accidental or intentional Y21.1
    stated as undetermined whether accidental
      or intentional Y21.0
    suicide (attempt) X71.0
  lake — *see* Drowning, in, natural water
  natural water (lake) (open sea) (pond) (river)
    (stream) W69
    assault X92.3
    following
      dive or jump W16.611
        striking bottom W16.621
      fall W16.111
        striking
          bottom W16.121
          side W16.131
    stated as undetermined whether accidental
      or intentional Y21.4
    suicide (attempt) X71.3
  quarry — *see* Drowning, in, specified place
    NEC
  quenching tank — *see* Drowning, in,
    specified place NEC
  reservoir — *see* Drowning, in, specified
    place NEC
  river — *see* Drowning, in, natural water
  sea — *see* Drowning, in, natural water
  specified place NEC W73
    assault X92.8
    following
      dive or jump W16.811
        striking
          bottom W16.821
          wall W16.831
      fall W16.311
        striking
          bottom W16.321
          wall W16.331
    stated as undetermined whether accidental
      or intentional Y21.8
    suicide (attempt) X71.8
  stream — *see* Drowning, in, natural water
  swimming pool W67
    assault X92.1
      following fall X92.2
    following
      dive or jump W16.511
        striking
          bottom W16.521
          wall W16.531
      fall W16.011
        striking
          bottom W16.021
          wall W16.031
    stated as undetermined whether accidental
      or intentional Y21.2
    following fall Y21.3
    suicide (attempt) X71.1
    following fall X71.2
  war operations — *see* War operations,
    restriction of airway
resulting from accident to watercraft — *see*
  Drowning, due to, accident, watercraft
self-inflicted X71.9
stated as undetermined whether accidental or
  intentional Y21.9
suicide (attempt) X71.9

E

Earth falling (on) W20.0
  caused by cataclysmic earth surface movement
    or eruption — *see* Landslide
Earth (surface) movement NEC — *see*
  Forces of nature, earth movement
Earthquake (any injury) X34
Effect(s) (adverse) of
  air pressure (any) — *see* Air, pressure
  cold, excessive (exposure to) — *see* Exposure,
    cold
  heat (excessive) — *see* Heat
  hot place (weather) — *see* Heat
  insolation X30
  late — *see* Sequelae
  motion — *see* Motion
  nuclear explosion or weapon in war
    operations — *see* War operations, nuclear
    weapon
  radiation — *see* Radiation
  travel — *see* Travel
Electric shock (accidental) (by) (in) — *see*
  Exposure, electric current
Electrocution (accidental) — *see* Exposure,
  electric current
Endotracheal tube wrongly placed
  during anesthetic procedure
Entanglement
  in
    bed linen, causing suffocation — *see*
      category T71
    wheel of pedal cycle V19.88
Entry of foreign body or material — *see*
  Foreign body
Environmental pollution related
  condition — *see* Z57
Execution, legal (any method) — *see* Legal,
  intervention
Exhaustion
  cold — *see* Exposure, cold
  due to excessive exertion (*see also*
    Overexertion) X50.9
  heat — *see* Heat
Explosion (accidental) (of) (with secondary fire)
  W40.9
  acetylene W40.1
  aerosol can W36.1
  air tank (compressed) (in machinery) W36.2
  aircraft (in transit) (powered) NEC V95.9
    balloon V96.05
    fixed wing NEC (private) V95.25
      commercial V95.35
    glider V96.25
      hang V96.15
      powered V95.15
    helicopter V95.05
    in war operations — *see* War operations,
      destruction of aircraft
    microlight V95.15
    nonpowered V96.9
      specified NEC V96.8
    powered NEC V95.8
    stated as
      homicide (attempt) Y03.8
      suicide (attempt) X83.0
    ultralight V95.15
  anesthetic gas in operating room W40.1
  antipersonnel bomb W40.8
    assault X96.0
    homicide (attempt) X96.0
    suicide (attempt) X75
  assault X96.9
  bicycle tire W37.0
  blasting (cap) (materials) W40.0
  boiler (machinery), not on transport vehicle
    W35
    on watercraft — *see* Explosion, in, watercraft

Explosion (accidental) (of) (with secondary fire) W40.9 — *continued*
- butane W40.1
- caused by other person X96.9
- coal gas W40.1
- detonator W40.0
- dump (munitions) W40.8
- dynamite W40.0
  - in
    - assault X96.8
    - homicide (attempt) X96.8
    - legal intervention
      - injuring
        - bystander Y35.112
        - law enforcement personnel Y35.111
        - suspect Y35.113
    - suicide (attempt) X75
- explosive (material) W40.9
  - gas W40.1
  - in blasting operation W40.0
  - specified NEC W40.8
    - in
      - assault X96.8
      - homicide (attempt) X96.8
      - legal intervention
        - injuring
          - bystander Y35.192
          - law enforcement personnel Y35.191
          - suspect Y35.193
      - suicide (attempt) X75
- factory (munitions) W40.8
- fertilizer bomb W40.8
  - assault X96.3
  - homicide (attempt) X96.3
  - suicide (attempt) X75
- fire-damp W40.1
- firearm (parts) NEC W34.19
  - airgun W34.110
  - BB gun W34.110
  - gas, air or spring-operated gun NEC W34.118
  - handgun W32.1
  - hunting rifle W33.12
  - larger firearm W33.10
    - specified NEC W33.19
  - machine gun W33.13
  - paintball gun W34.111
  - pellet gun W34.110
  - shotgun W33.11
  - Very pistol [flare] W34.19
- fireworks W39
- gas (coal) (explosive) W40.1
  - cylinder W36.9
    - aerosol can W36.1
    - air tank W36.2
    - pressurized W36.3
    - specified NEC W36.8
- gasoline (fumes) (tank) not in moving motor vehicle W40.1
  - bomb W40.8
    - assault X96.1
    - homicide (attempt) X96.1
    - suicide (attempt) X75
  - in motor vehicle — *see* Accident, transport, by type of vehicle
- grain store W40.8
- grenade W40.8
  - in
    - assault X96.8
    - homicide (attempt) X96.8
    - legal intervention
      - injuring
        - bystander Y35.192
        - law enforcement personnel Y35.191
        - suspect Y35.193
    - suicide (attempt) X75
- handgun (parts) — *see* Explosion, firearm, hangun (parts)

Explosion (accidental) (of) (with secondary fire) W40.9 — *continued*
- homicide (attempt) X96.9
  - antipersonnel bomb — *see* Explosion, antipersonnel bomb
  - fertilizer bomb — *see* Explosion, fertilizer bomb
  - gasoline bomb — *see* Explosion, gasoline bomb
  - letter bomb — *see* Explosion, letter bomb
  - pipe bomb — *see* Explosion, pipe bomb
  - specified NEC X96.8
- hose, pressurized W37.8
- hot water heater, tank (in machinery) W35
  - on watercraft — *see* Explosion, in, watercraft
- in, on
  - dump W40.8
  - factory W40.8
  - mine (of explosive gases) NEC W40.1
  - watercraft V93.59
    - powered craft V93.53
      - ferry boat V93.51
      - fishing boat V93.52
      - jetskis V93.53
      - liner V93.51
      - merchant ship V93.50
      - passenger ship V93.51
      - sailboat V93.54
- letter bomb W40.8
  - assault X96.2
  - homicide (attempt) X96.2
  - suicide (attempt) X75
- machinery — *see also* Contact, with, by type of machine
  - on board watercraft — *see* Explosion, in, watercraft
  - pressure vessel — *see* Explosion, by type of vessel
- methane W40.1
- mine W40.1
- missile NEC W40.8
- mortar bomb W40.8
  - in
    - assault X96.8
    - homicide (attempt) X96.8
    - legal intervention
      - injuring
        - bystander Y35.192
        - law enforcement personnel Y35.191
        - suspect Y35.193
    - suicide (attempt) X75
- munitions (dump) (factory) W40.8
- pipe, pressurized W37.8
  - bomb W40.8
    - assault X96.4
    - homicide (attempt) X96.4
    - suicide (attempt) X75
- pressure, pressurized
  - cooker W38
  - gas tank (in machinery) W36.3
  - hose W37.8
  - pipe W37.8
  - specified device NEC W38
  - tire W37.8
    - bicycle W37.0
  - vessel (in machinery) W38
- propane W40.1
- self-inflicted X75
- shell (artillery) NEC W40.8
  - during war operations — *see* War operations, explosion
  - in
    - legal intervention
      - injuring
        - bystander Y35.122
        - law enforcement personnel Y35.121
        - suspect Y35.123
  - war — *see* War operations, explosion

Explosion (accidental) (of) (with secondary fire) W40.9 — *continued*
- spacecraft V95.45
- stated as undetermined whether accidental or intentional Y25
- steam or water lines (in machinery) W37.8
- stove W40.9
- suicide (attempt) X75
- tire, pressurized W37.8
  - bicycle W37.0
- undetermined whether accidental or intentional Y25
- vehicle tire NEC W37.8
  - bicycle W37.0
- war operations — *see* War operations, explosion

Exposure (to) X58
- air pressure change — *see* Air, pressure
- cold (accidental) (excessive) (extreme) (natural) (place) X31
  - assault Y08.89
  - due to
    - man-made conditions W93.8
      - dry ice (contact) W93.01
        - inhalation W93.02
      - liquid air (contact) (hydrogen) (nitrogen) W93.11
        - inhalation W93.12
      - refrigeration unit (deep freeze) W93.2
  - suicide (attempt) X83.2
  - weather (conditions) X31
  - homicide (attempt) Y08.89
  - self-inflicted X83.2
- due to abandonment or neglect X58
- electric current W86.8
  - appliance (faulty) W86.8
    - domestic W86.0
  - caused by other person Y08.89
  - conductor (faulty) W86.1
  - control apparatus (faulty) W86.1
  - electric power generating plant, distribution station W86.1
  - electroshock gun — *see* Exposure, electric current, taser
  - high-voltage cable W85
  - homicide (attempt) Y08.89
  - legal execution — *see* Legal, intervention, specified means NEC
  - lightning — *see* subcategory T75.0
  - live rail W86.8
  - misadventure in medical or surgical procedure in electroshock therapy Y63.4
  - motor (electric) (faulty) W86.8
    - domestic W86.0
  - self-inflicted X83.1
  - specified NEC W86.8
    - domestic W86.0
  - stun gun — *see* Exposure, electric current, taser
  - suicide (attempt) X83.1
  - taser W86.8
    - assault Y08.89
    - legal intervention — *see* category Y35
    - self-harm (intentional) X83.8
    - undetermined intent Y33
  - third rail W86.8
  - transformer (faulty) W86.1
  - transmission lines W85
- environmental tobacco smoke X58
- excessive
  - cold — *see* Exposure, cold
  - heat (natural) NEC X30
    - man-made W92
- factor(s) NOS X58
  - environmental NEC X58
  - man-made NEC W99
  - natural NEC — *see* Forces of nature
  - specified NEC X58

EXTERNAL CAUSES

Exposure (to) X58— *continued*
  fire, flames (accidental) X08.8
    assault X97
    campfire — *see* Exposure, fire, controlled,
      not in building
    controlled (in)
      with ignition (of) clothing (*see also* Ignition,
        clothes) X06.2
        nightwear X05
      bonfire — *see* Exposure, fire, controlled,
        not in building
      brazier (in building or structure) — *see also*
        Exposure, fire, controlled, building
        not in building or structure — *see*
          Exposure, fire, controlled, not in
          building
      building or structure X02.0
        with
          fall from building X02.3
          from building X02.5
          injury due to building collapse X02.2
          smoke inhalation X02.1
        hit by object from building X02.4
        specified mode of injury NEC X02.8
      fireplace, furnace or stove — *see*
        Exposure, fire, controlled, building
      not in building or structure X03.0
        with
          fall X03.3
          smoke inhalation X03.1
        hit by object X03.4
        specified mode of injury NEC X03.8
      trash — *see* Exposure, fire, controlled, not
        in building
    fireplace — *see* Exposure, fire, controlled,
      building
    fittings or furniture (in building or structure)
      (uncontrolled) — *see* Exposure, fire,
      uncontrolled, building
    forest (uncontrolled) — *see* Exposure, fire,
      uncontrolled, not in building
    grass (uncontrolled) — *see* Exposure, fire,
      uncontrolled, not in building
    hay (uncontrolled) — *see* Exposure, fire,
      uncontrolled, not in building
    homicide (attempt) X97
    ignition of highly flammable material X04
    in, of, on, starting in
      machinery — *see* Contact, with, by type of
        machine
      motor vehicle (in motion) (*see also*
        Accident, transport, occupant by type
        of vehicle) V87.8
        with collision — *see* Collision
      railway rolling stock, train, vehicle V81.81
        with collision — *see* Accident, transport,
          railway vehicle occupant
      street car (in motion) V82.8
        with collision — *see* Accident, transport,
          streetcar occupant
      transport vehicle NEC — *see also* Accident,
        transport
        with collision — *see* Collision
      war operations — *see also* War operations,
        fire
        from nuclear explosion — *see* War
          operations, nuclear weapons

Exposure (to) X58— *continued*
  fire, flames (accidental) X08.8 — *continued*
    in, of, on, starting in — *continued*
      watercraft (in transit) (not in transit)
        V91.09
      localized — *see* Burn, on board
        watercraft, due to, fire on board
      powered craft V91.03
        ferry boat V91.01
        fishing boat V91.02
        jet skis V91.03
        liner V91.01
        merchant ship V91.00
        passenger ship V91.01
      unpowered craft V91.08
        canoe V91.05
        inflatable V91.06
        kayak V91.05
        sailboat V91.04
        surfboard V91.08
        waterskis V91.07
        windsurfer V91.08
    lumber (uncontrolled) — *see* Exposure, fire,
      uncontrolled, not in building
    mine (uncontrolled) — *see* Exposure, fire,
      uncontrolled, not in building
    prairie (uncontrolled) — *see* Exposure, fire,
      uncontrolled, not in building
    resulting from
      explosion — *see* Explosion
      lightning X08.8
    self-inflicted X76
    specified NEC X08.8
    started by other person X97
    stated as undetermined whether accidental
      or intentional Y26
    stove — *see* Exposure, fire, controlled,
      building
    suicide (attempt) X76
    tunnel (uncontrolled) — *see* Exposure, fire,
      uncontrolled, not in building
    uncontrolled
      in building or structure X00.0
        with
          fall from building X00.3
          injury due to building collapse X00.2
          jump from building X00.5
          smoke inhalation X00.1
        bed X08.00
          due to
            cigarette X08.01
            specified material NEC X08.09
        furniture NEC X08.20
          due to
            cigarette X08.21
            specified material NEC X08.29
        hit by object from building X00.4
        sofa X08.10
          due to
            cigarette X08.11
            specified material NEC X08.19
        specified mode of injury NEC X00.8
      not in building or structure (any) X01.0
        with
          fall X01.3
          smoke inhalation X01.1
        hit by object X01.4
        specified mode of injury NEC X01.8
    undetermined whether accidental or
      intentional Y26
  forces of nature NEC — *see* Forces of nature
  G-forces (abnormal) W49.9
  gravitational forces (abnormal) W49.9
  heat (natural) NEC — *see* Heat
  high-pressure jet (hydraulic) (pneumatic)
    W49.9
  hydraulic jet W49.9
  inanimate mechanical force W49.9

Exposure (to) X58— *continued*
  jet, high-pressure (hydraulic) (pneumatic)
    W49.9
  lightning — *see* subcategory T75.0
    causing fire — *see* Exposure, fire
  mechanical forces NEC W49.9
    animate NEC W64
    inanimate NEC W49.9
  noise W42.9
    supersonic W42.0
  noxious substance — *see* Table of Drugs and
    Chemicals
  pneumatic jet W49.9
  prolonged in deep-freeze unit or refrigerator
    W93.2
  radiation — *see* Radiation
  smoke — *see also* Exposure, fire
    tobacco, second hand Z77.22
  specified factors NEC X58
  sunlight X32
    man-made (sun lamp) W89.8
    tanning bed W89.1
  supersonic waves W42.0
  transmission line(s), electric W85
  vibration W49.9
  waves
    infrasound W49.9
    sound W42.9
    supersonic W42.0
  weather NEC — *see* Forces of nature
External cause status Y99.9
  child assisting in compensated work for family
    Y99.8
  civilian activity done for financial or other
    compensation Y99.0
  civilian activity done for income or pay Y99.0
  family member assisting in compensated work
    for other family member Y99.8
  hobby not done for income Y99.8
  leisure activity Y99.8
  military activity Y99.1
  off-duty activity of military personnel Y99.8
  recreation or sport not for income or while a
    student Y99.8
  specified NEC Y99.8
  student activity Y99.8
  volunteer activity Y99.2

F

Factors, supplemental
alcohol
  blood level
    100-119mg/100ml Y90.5
    120-199mg/100ml Y90.6
    20-39mg/100ml Y90.1
    200-239mg/100ml Y90.7
    240mg/100ml or more Y90.8
    40-59mg/100ml Y90.2
    60-79mg/100ml Y90.3
    80-99mg/100ml Y90.4
    less than 20mg/100ml Y90.0
    presence in blood, level not specified
      Y90.9
    presence in blood, but level not specified
      Y90.9
  environmental-pollution-related condition —
    see Z57
  nosocomial condition Y95
  work-related condition Y99.0

Failure
in suture or ligature during surgical procedure
  Y65.2
mechanical, of instrument or apparatus (any)
  (during any medical or surgical
  procedure) Y65.8
sterile precautions (during medical and
  surgical care) — *see* Misadventure, failure,
  sterile precautions, by type ofprocedure
to
  introduce tube or instrument Y65.4
    endotracheal tube during anesthesia
      Y65.3
  make curve (transport vehicle) NEC — *see*
    Accident, transport
  remove tube or instrument Y65.4

Fall, falling (accidental) W19
building W20.1
  burning (uncontrolled fire) X00.3
down
  embankment W17.81
  escalator W10.0
  hill W17.81
  ladder W11
  ramp W10.2
  stairs, steps W10.9
due to
  bumping against
    object W18.00
      sharp glass W18.02
      specified NEC W18.09
      sports equipment W18.01
    person W03
      due to ice or snow W00.0
      on pedestrian conveyance — *see*
        Accident, transport, pedestrian,
        conveyance
  collision with another person W03
    due to ice or snow W00.0
    involving pedestrian conveyance — *see*
      Accident, transport, pedestrian,
      conveyance
  grocery cart tipping over W17.82
  ice or snow W00.9
    from one level to another W00.2
      on stairs or steps W00.1
    involving pedestrian conveyance — *see*
      Accident, transport, pedestrian,
      conveyance
    on same level W00.0

Fall, falling (accidental) W19 — *continued*
due to — *continued*
  slipping (on moving sidewalk) W01.0
    with subsequent striking against object
      W01.10
      furniture W01.190
      sharp object W01.119
        glass W01.110
        power tool or machine W01.111
        specified NEC W01.118
      specified NEC W01.198
  striking against
    object W18.00
      sharp glass W18.02
      specified NEC W18.09
      sports equipment W18.01
    person W03
      due to ice or snow W00.0
      on pedestrian conveyance — *see*
        Accident, transport, pedestrian,
        conveyance
earth (with asphyxia or suffocation (by
  pressure)) — *see* Earth, falling
from, off, out of
  aircraft NEC (with accident to aircraft NEC)
    V97.0
    while boarding or alighting V97.1
  balcony W13.0
  bed W06
  boat, ship, watercraft NEC (with drowning
    or submersion) — *see* Drowning, due to,
    fall overboard
    with hitting bottom or object V94.0
  bridge W13.1
  building W13.9
    burning (uncontrolled fire) X00.3
  cavity W17.2
  chair W07
  cherry picker W17.89
  cliff W15
  dock W17.4
  embankment W17.81
  escalator W10.0
  flagpole W13.8
  furniture NEC W08
  grocery cart W17.82
  haystack W17.89
  high place NEC W17.89
    stated as undetermined whether accidental
      or intentional Y30
  hole W17.2
  incline W10.2
  ladder W11
  lifting device W17.89
  machine, machinery — *see also* Contact,
    with, by type of machine
    not in operation W17.89
  manhole W17.1
  mobile elevated work platform [MEWP]
    W17.89
  motorized mobility scooter W05.2
  one level to another NEC W17.89
    intentional, purposeful, suicide (attempt)
      X80
    stated as undetermined whether accidental
      or intentional Y30
  pit W17.2
  playground equipment W09.8
    jungle gym W09.2
    slide W09.0
    swing W09.1
  quarry W17.89
  railing W13.9
  ramp W10.2
  roof W13.2
  scaffolding W12
  scooter (nonmotorized) W05.1
    motorized mobility W05.2

Fall, falling (accidental) W19 — *continued*
from, off, out of — *continued*
  sky lift W17.89
  stairs, steps W10.9
    curb W10.1
    due to ice or snow W00.1
    escalator W10.0
    incline W10.2
    ramp W10.2
    sidewalk curb W10.1
    specified NEC W10.8
  stepladder W11
  storm drain W17.1
  streetcar NEC V82.6
    with antecedent collision — *see* Accident,
      transport, streetcar occupant
    while boarding or alighting V82.4
  structure NEC W13.8
    burning (uncontrolled fire) X00.3
  table W08
  toilet W18.11
    with subsequent striking against object
      W18.12
  train NEC V81.6
    during derailment (without antecedent
      collision) V81.7
      with antecedent collision — *see*
        Accident, transport, railway vehicle
        occupant
    while boarding or alighting V81.4
  transport vehicle after collision — *see*
    Accident, transport, by type of vehicle,
    collision
  tree W14
  vehicle (in motion) NEC (*see also* Accident,
    transport) V89.9
    motor NEC (*see also* Accident, transport,
      occupant, by type of vehicle) V87.8
    stationary W17.89
      while boarding or alighting — *see*
        Accident, transport, by type of
        vehicle, while boarding or alighting
  viaduct W13.8
  wall W13.8
  watercraft — *see also* Drowning, due to, fall
    overboard
    with hitting bottom or object V94.0
  well W17.0
  wheelchair, non-moving W05.0
    powered — *see* Accident, transport,
      pedestrian, conveyance occupant,
      specified type NEC
  window W13.4
in, on
  aircraft NEC V97.0
    with accident to aircraft V97.0
    while boarding or alighting V97.1
  bathtub (empty) W18.2
    filled W16.212
      causing drowning W16.211
  escalator W10.0
  incline W10.2
  ladder W11
  machine, machinery — *see* Contact, with, by
    type of machine
  object, edged, pointed or sharp (with cut) —
    see Fall, by type
  playground equipment W09.8
    jungle gym W09.2
    slide W09.0
    swing W09.1
  ramp W10.2
  scaffolding W12
  shower W18.2
    causing drowning W16.211

Forces of nature X39.8 — *continued*
  earthquake X34
  flood (caused by) X38
    dam collapse X36.0
    tidal wave — *see* Forces of nature, tidal wave
  heat (natural) X30
  hurricane X37.0
  landslide X36.1
    causing transport accident — *see* Accident, transport, by type of vehicle
  lightning — *see* subcategory T75.0
    causing fire — *see* Exposure, fire
  mudslide X36.1
    causing transport accident — *see* Accident, transport, by type of vehicle
  radiation (natural) X39.08
    radon X39.01
  radon X39.01
  specified force NEC X39.8
  storm surge X37.0
  structure collapse causing earth movement X36.0
  sunlight X32
  tidal wave X37.41
    due to
      earthquake X37.41
      landslide X37.43
      storm X37.42
      volcanic eruption X37.41
  tornado X37.1
  tsunami X37.41
  twister X37.1
  typhoon X37.0
  volcanic eruption X35
Foreign body
  aspiration — *see* Index to Diseases and Injuries, Foreign body, respiratory tract
  embedded in skin W45
  entering through skin W45.8
    can lid W26.8
    nail W45.0
    paper W26.2
    specified NEC W45.8
    splinter W45.8
Forest fire (exposure to) — *see* Exposure, fire, uncontrolled, not in building
Found injured X58
  from exposure (to) — *see* Exposure
  on
    highway, road(way), street V89.9
    railway right of way V81.9
Fracture (circumstances unknown or unspecified) X58
  due to specified cause NEC X58
Freezing — *see* Exposure, cold
Frostbite X31
  due to man-made conditions — *see* Exposure, cold, man-made
Frozen — *see* Exposure, cold

G

Gored by bull W55.22
Gunshot wound W34.00

H

Hailstones, injured by X39.8
Hanged herself or himself — *see* Hanging, self-inflicted
Hanging (accidental) (*see also* category) T71
  legal execution — *see* Legal, intervention, specified means NEC
Heat (effects of) (excessive) X30
  due to
    man-made conditions W92
      on board watercraft V93.29
        fishing boat V93.22
        merchant ship V93.20
        passenger ship V93.21
        sailboat V93.24
        specified powered craft NEC V93.23
    weather (conditions) X30
  from
    electric heating apparatus causing burning X16
    nuclear explosion in war operations — *see* War operations, nuclear weapons
  inappropriate in local application or packing in medical or surgical procedure Y63.5
Hemorrhage
  delayed following medical or surgical treatment without mention of misadventure — *see* Index to Diseases and Injuries, Complication(s)
  during medical or surgical treatment as misadventure — *see* Index to Diseases and Injuries, Complication(s)
High
  altitude (effects) — *see* Air, pressure, low
  level of radioactivity, effects — *see* Radiation
  pressure (effects) — *see* Air, pressure, high
  temperature, effects — *see* Heat
Hit, hitting (accidental) by — *see* Struck by
Hitting against — *see* Striking against
Homicide (attempt) (justifiable) — *see* Assault
Hot
  place, effects — *see also* Heat
  weather, effects X30
House fire (uncontrolled) — *see* Exposure, fire, uncontrolled, building
Humidity, causing problem X39.8
Hunger X58
Hurricane (any injury) X37.0
Hypobarism, hypobaropathy — *see* Air, pressure, low

EXTERNAL CAUSES

I

EXTERNAL CAUSES

Ictus
caloris — *see also* Heat
solaris X30

Ignition (accidental) (*see also* Exposure, fire)
X08.8
anesthetic gas in operating room W40.1
apparel X06.2
from highly flammable material X04
nightwear X05
bed linen (sheets) (spreads) (pillows) (mattress)
— *see* Exposure, fire, uncontrolled,
building, bed
benzine X04
clothes, clothing NEC (from controlled fire)
X06.2
from
highly flammable material X04
ether X04
in operating room W40.1
explosive material — *see* Explosion
gasoline X04
jewelry (plastic) (any) X06.0
kerosene X04
material
explosive — *see* Explosion
highly flammable with secondary explosion
X04
nightwear X05
paraffin X04
petrol X04

Immersion (accidental) — *see also* Drowning
hand or foot due to cold (excessive) X31

Implantation of quills of porcupine
W55.89

Inanition (from) (hunger) X58
thirst X58

Inappropriate operation performed
correct operation on wrong side or body part
(wrong side) (wrong site) Y65.53
operation intended for another patient done
on wrong patient Y65.52
wrong operation performed on correct patient
Y65.51

Inattention after, at birth (homicidal intent)
(infanticidal intent) X58

Incident, adverse
device
anesthesiology Y70.8
accessory Y70.2
diagnostic Y70.0
miscellaneous Y70.8
monitoring Y70.0
prosthetic Y70.2
rehabilitative Y70.1
surgical Y70.3
therapeutic Y70.1
cardiovascular Y71.8
accessory Y71.2
diagnostic Y71.0
miscellaneous Y71.8
monitoring Y71.0
prosthetic Y71.2
rehabilitative Y71.1
surgical Y71.3
therapeutic Y71.1
gastroenterology Y73.8
accessory Y73.2
diagnostic Y73.0
miscellaneous Y73.8
monitoring Y73.0
prosthetic Y73.2
rehabilitative Y73.1
surgical Y73.3
therapeutic Y73.1

Incident, adverse — *continued*
device — *continued*
general
hospital Y74.8
accessory Y74.2
diagnostic Y74.0
miscellaneous Y74.8
monitoring Y74.0
prosthetic Y74.2
rehabilitative Y74.1
surgical Y74.3
therapeutic Y74.1
surgical Y81.8
accessory Y81.2
diagnostic Y81.0
miscellaneous Y81.8
monitoring Y81.0
prosthetic Y81.2
rehabilitative Y81.1
surgical Y81.3
therapeutic Y81.1
gynecological Y76.8
accessory Y76.2
diagnostic Y76.0
miscellaneous Y76.8
monitoring Y76.0
prosthetic Y76.2
rehabilitative Y76.1
surgical Y76.3
therapeutic Y76.1
medical Y82.9
specified type NEC Y82.8
neurological Y75.8
accessory Y75.2
diagnostic Y75.0
miscellaneous Y75.8
monitoring Y75.0
prosthetic Y75.2
rehabilitative Y75.1
surgical Y75.3
therapeutic Y75.1
obstetrical Y76.8
accessory Y76.2
diagnostic Y76.0
miscellaneous Y76.8
monitoring Y76.0
prosthetic Y76.2
rehabilitative Y76.1
surgical Y76.3
therapeutic Y76.1
ophthalmic Y77.8
accessory Y77.2
diagnostic Y77.0
miscellaneous Y77.8
monitoring Y77.0
prosthetic Y77.2
rehabilitative Y77.1
surgical Y77.3
therapeutic Y77.1
orthopedic Y79.8
accessory Y79.2
diagnostic Y79.0
miscellaneous Y79.8
monitoring Y79.0
prosthetic Y79.2
rehabilitative Y79.1
surgical Y79.3
therapeutic Y79.1
otorhinolaryngological Y72.8
accessory Y72.2
diagnostic Y72.0
miscellaneous Y72.8
monitoring Y72.0
prosthetic Y72.2
rehabilitative Y72.1
surgical Y72.3
therapeutic Y72.1

Incident, adverse — *continued*
device — *continued*
personal use Y74.8
accessory Y74.2
diagnostic Y74.0
miscellaneous Y74.8
monitoring Y74.0
prosthetic Y74.2
rehabilitative Y74.1
surgical Y74.3
therapeutic Y74.1
physical medicine Y80.8
accessory Y80.2
diagnostic Y80.0
miscellaneous Y80.8
monitoring Y80.0
prosthetic Y80.2
rehabilitative Y80.1
surgical Y80.3
therapeutic Y80.1
plastic surgical Y81.8
accessory Y81.2
diagnostic Y81.0
miscellaneous Y81.8
monitoring Y81.0
prosthetic Y81.2
rehabilitative Y81.1
surgical Y81.3
therapeutic Y81.1
radiological Y78.8
accessory Y78.2
diagnostic Y78.0
miscellaneous Y78.8
monitoring Y78.0
prosthetic Y78.2
rehabilitative Y78.1
surgical Y78.3
therapeutic Y78.1
urology Y73.8
accessory Y73.2
diagnostic Y73.0
miscellaneous Y73.8
monitoring Y73.0
prosthetic Y73.2
rehabilitative Y73.1
surgical Y73.3
therapeutic Y73.1

Incineration (accidental) — *see* Exposure, fire
Infanticide — *see* Assault
Infrasound waves (causing injury) W49.9
Ingestion
foreign body (causing injury) (with obstruction)
— *see* Foreign body, alimentary canal
poisonous
plant(s) X58
substance NEC — *see* Table of Drugs and
Chemicals
Inhalation
excessively cold substance, man-made — *see*
Exposure, cold, man-made
food (any type) (into respiratory tract) (with
asphyxia, obstruction respiratory tract,
suffocation) — *see* categories T17 and T18
foreign body — *see* Foreign body, aspiration
gastric contents (with asphyxia, obstruction
respiratory passage, suffocation) T17.81-
hot air or gases X14.0
liquid air, hydrogen, nitrogen W93.12
suicide (attempt) X83.2
steam X13.0
assault X98.0
stated as undetermined whether accidental
or intentional Y27.0
suicide (attempt) X77.0
toxic gas — *see* Table of Drugs and Chemicals
vomitus (with asphyxia, obstruction respiratory
passage, suffocation) T17.81-

EXTERNAL CAUSES

Injury, injured (accidental(ly)) NOS X58
  by, caused by, from
    assault — *see* Assault
    law-enforcing agent, police, in course of
      legal intervention — *see* Legal
      intervention
    suicide (attempt) X83.8
  due to, in
    civil insurrection — *see* War operations
    fight (*see also* Assault, fight) Y04.0
    war operations — *see* War operations
  homicide (*see also* Assault) Y09
  inflicted (by)
    in course of arrest (attempted), suppression
      of disturbance, maintenance of order, by
      law-enforcing agents — *see* Legal
      intervention
    other person
      stated as
        accidental X58
        intentional, homicide (attempt) — *see*
          Assault
        undetermined whether accidental or
          intentional Y33
    purposely (inflicted) by other person(s) — *see*
      Assault
    self-inflicted X83.8
      stated as accidental X58
    specified cause NEC X58
    undetermined whether accidental or intentional
      Y33
Insolation, effects X30
Insufficient nourishment X58
Interruption of respiration (by)
  food (lodged in esophagus) — *see* categories
    T17 and T18
  vomitus (lodged in esophagus) T17.81-
Intervention, legal — *see* Legal intervention
Intoxication
  drug — *see* Table of Drugs and Chemicals
  poison — *see* Table of Drugs and Chemicals

J

Jammed (accidentally)
  between objects (moving) (stationary and
    moving) W23.0
    stationary W23.1
Jumped, jumping
  before moving object NEC X81.8
    motor vehicle X81.0
    subway train X81.1
    train X81.1
    undetermined whether accidental or
      intentional Y31
  from
    boat (into water) voluntarily, without
      accident (to or on boat) W16.712
      with
        accident to or on boat — *see* Accident,
          watercraft
        drowning or submersion W16.711
          suicide (attempt) X71.3
        striking bottom W16.722
          causing drowning W16.721
    building (*see also* Jumped, from, high place)
      W13.9
      burning (uncontrolled fire) X00.5
    high place NEC W17.89
      suicide (attempt) X80
      undetermined whether accidental or
        intentional Y30
    structure (*see also* Jumped, from, high place)
      W13.9
      burning (uncontrolled fire) X00.5
  into water W16.92
    causing drowning W16.91
    from, off watercraft — *see* Jumped, from,
      boat
    in
      natural body W16.612
        causing drowning W16.611
        striking bottom W16.622
          causing drowning W16.621
      specified place NEC W16.812
        causing drowning W16.811
        striking
          bottom W16.822
            causing drowning W16.821
          wall W16.832
            causing drowning W16.831
      swimming pool W16.512
        causing drowning W16.511
        striking
          bottom W16.522
            causing drowning W16.521
          wall W16.532
            causing drowning W16.531
  suicide (attempt) X71.3

K

Kicked by
  animal NEC W55.82
  person(s) (accidentally) W50.1
    with intent to injure or kill Y04.0
    as, or caused by, a crowd or human
      stampede (with fall) W52
    assault Y04.0
    homicide (attempt) Y04.0
    in
      fight Y04.0
      legal intervention
        injuring
          bystander Y35.812
          law enforcement personnel Y35.811
          suspect Y35.813
Kicking
  against
    object W22.8
      sports equipment W21.9
      stationary W22.09
        sports equipment W21.89
    person — *see* Striking against, person
    sports equipment W21.9
  carpet stretcher with knee X50.3
Killed, killing (accidentally) NOS (*see also*
  Injury) X58
  in
    action — *see* War operations
    brawl, fight (hand) (fists) (foot) Y04.0
      by weapon — *see also* Assault
        cutting, piercing — *see* Assault, cutting
          or piercing instrument
        firearm — *see* Discharge, firearm, by
          type, homicide
  self
    stated as
      accident NOS X58
      suicide — *see* Suicide
    undetermined whether accidental or
      intentional Y33
Kneeling (prolonged) (static) X50.1
Knocked down (accidentally) (by) NOS X58
  animal (not being ridden) NEC — *see also*
    Struck by, by type of animal
  crowd or human stampede W52
  person W51
    in brawl, fight Y04.0
  transport vehicle NEC (*see also* Accident,
    transport) V09.9

EXTERNAL CAUSES

L

Laceration NEC — *see* Injury
Lack of
 care (helpless person) (infant) (newborn) X58
 food except as result of abandonment or neglect X58
  due to abandonment or neglect X58
 water except as result of transport accident X58
  due to transport accident — *see* Accident, transport, by type
 helpless person, infant, newborn X58
Landslide (falling on transport vehicle) X36.1
 caused by collapse of man-made structure X36.0
Late effect — *see* Sequelae
Legal
 execution (any method) — *see* Legal, intervention
 intervention (by)
  baton — *see* Legal, intervention, blunt object, baton
  bayonet — *see* Legal, intervention, sharp object, bayonet
  blow — *see* Legal, intervention, manhandling
  blunt object
   baton
    injuring
     bystander Y35.312
     law enforcement personnel Y35.311
     suspect Y35.313
   injuring
    bystander Y35.302
    law enforcement personnel Y35.301
    suspect Y35.303
   specified NEC
    injuring
     bystander Y35.392
     law enforcement personnel Y35.391
     suspect Y35.393
   stave
    injuring
     bystander Y35.392
     law enforcement personnel Y35.391
     suspect Y35.393
  bomb — *see* Legal, intervention, explosive
  cutting or piercing instrument — *see* Legal, intervention, sharp object
  dynamite — *see* Legal, intervention, explosive, dynamite
  explosive(s)
   dynamite
    injuring
     bystander Y35.112
     law enforcement personnel Y35.111
     suspect Y35.113
   grenade
    injuring
     bystander Y35.192
     law enforcement personnel Y35.191
     suspect Y35.193
   injuring
    bystander Y35.102
    law enforcement personnel Y35.101
    suspect Y35.103
   mortar bomb
    injuring
     bystander Y35.192
     law enforcement personnel Y35.191
     suspect Y35.193
   shell
    injuring
     bystander Y35.122
     law enforcement personnel Y35.121
     suspect Y35.123

Legal — *continued*
 intervention (by) — *continued*
  explosive(s) — *continued*
   specified NEC
    injuring
     bystander Y35.192
     law enforcement personnel Y35.191
     suspect Y35.193
  firearm(s) (discharge)
   handgun
    injuring
     bystander Y35.022
     law enforcement personnel Y35.021
     suspect Y35.023
   injuring
    bystander Y35.002
    law enforcement personnel Y35.001
    suspect Y35.003
   machine gun
    injuring
     bystander Y35.012
     law enforcement personnel Y35.011
     suspect Y35.013
   rifle pellet
    injuring
     bystander Y35.032
     law enforcement personnel Y35.031
     suspect Y35.033
   rubber bullet
    injuring
     bystander Y35.042
     law enforcement personnel Y35.041
     suspect Y35.043
   shotgun — *see* Legal, intervention, firearm, specified NEC
   specified NEC
    injuring
     bystander Y35.092
     law enforcement personnel Y35.091
     suspect Y35.093
  gas (asphyxiation) (poisoning)
   injuring
    bystander Y35.202
    law enforcement personnel Y35.201
    suspect Y35.203
   specified NEC
    injuring
     bystander Y35.292
     law enforcement personnel Y35.291
     suspect Y35.293
   tear gas
    injuring
     bystander Y35.212
     law enforcement personnel Y35.211
     suspect Y35.213
  grenade — *see* Legal, intervention, explosive, grenade
  injuring
   bystander Y35.92
   law enforcement personnel Y35.91
   suspect Y35.93
  late effect (of) — *see* with 7th character S Y35
  manhandling
   injuring
    bystander Y35.812
    law enforcement personnel Y35.811
    suspect Y35.813
  sequelae (of) — *see* with 7th character S Y35
  sharp objects
   bayonet
    injuring
     bystander Y35.412
     law enforcement personnel Y35.411
     suspect Y35.413

Legal — *continued*
 intervention (by) — *continued*
  sharp objects — *continued*
   injuring
    bystander Y35.402
    law enforcement personnel Y35.401
    suspect Y35.403
   specified NEC
    injuring
     bystander Y35.492
     law enforcement personnel Y35.491
     suspect Y35.493
  specified means NEC
   injuring
    bystander Y35.892
    law enforcement personnel Y35.891
    suspect Y35.893
  stabbing — *see* Legal, intervention, sharp object
  stave — *see* Legal, intervention, blunt object, stave
  tear gas — *see* Legal, intervention, gas, tear gas
  truncheon — *see* Legal, intervention, blunt object, stave
Lifting — *see* Overexertion
 heavy objects X50.0
 weights X50.0
Lightning (shock) (stroke) (struck by) — *see* subcategory T75.0
 causing fire — *see* Exposure, fire
Loss of control (transport vehicle) NEC — *see* Accident, transport
Lost at sea NOS — *see* Drowning, due to, fall overboard
Low
 pressure (effects) — *see* Air, pressure, low
 temperature (effects) — *see* Exposure, cold
Lying before train, vehicle or other moving object X81.8
 subway train X81.1
 train X81.1
 undetermined whether accidental or intentional Y31
Lynching — *see* Assault

M

Malfunction (mechanism or component) (of)
  firearm W34.10
    airgun W34.110
    BB gun W34.110
    gas, air or spring-operated gun NEC
      W34.118
    handgun W32.1
    hunting rifle W33.12
    larger firearm W33.10
      specified NEC W33.19
    machine gun W33.13
    paintball gun W34.111
    pellet gun W34.110
    shotgun W33.11
    specified NEC W34.19
    Very pistol [flare] W34.19
  handgun — *see* Malfunction, firearm, handgun
Maltreatment — *see* Perpetrator
Mangled (accidentally) NOS X58
Manhandling (in brawl, fight) Y04.0
  legal intervention — *see* Legal, intervention,
    manhandling
Manslaughter (nonaccidental) — *see* Assault
Mauled by animal NEC W55.89
Medical procedure, complication of
  (delayed or as an abnormal reaction without
    mention of misadventure) —*see* Complication
    of or following, by specified type of
    procedure
  due to or as a result of misadventure — *see*
    Misadventure
Melting (due to fire) — *see also* Exposure, fire
  apparel NEC X06.3
  clothes, clothing NEC X06.3
  nightwear X05
  fittings or furniture (burning building)
    (uncontrolled fire) X00.8
  nightwear X05
  plastic jewelry X06.1
Mental cruelty X58
Military operations (injuries to military and
  civilians occuring during peacetime on
  military property and during routine military
  exercises and operations) (by) (from)
  (involving) Y37.90-
  air blast Y37.20-
  aircraft
    destruction — *see* Military operations,
      destruction of aircraft
    airway restriction — *see* Military operations,
      restriction of airways
    asphyxiation — *see* Military operations,
      restriction of airways
  biological weapons Y37.6x-
  blast Y37.20-
  blast fragments Y37.20-
  blast wave Y37.20-
  blast wind Y37.20-
  bomb Y37.20-
    dirty Y37.50-
    gasoline Y37.31-
    incendiary Y37.31-
    petrol Y37.31-
  bullet Y37.43-
    incendiary Y37.32-
    rubber Y37.41-
  chemical weapons Y37.7x-
  combat
    hand to hand (unarmed) combat Y37.44-
    using blunt or piercing object Y37.45-
  conflagration — *see* Military operations, fire
  conventional warfare NEC Y37.49-
  depth-charge Y37.01-

Military operations (injuries to military and
  civilians occuring during peacetime on
  military property and during routine military
  exercises and operations) (by) (from)
  (involving) Y37.90- — *continued*
  destruction of aircraft Y37.10-
    due to
      air to air missile Y37.11-
      collision with other aircraft Y37.12-
      detonation (accidental) of onboard
        munitions and explosives Y37.14-
      enemy fire or explosives Y37.11-
      explosive placed on aircraft Y37.11-
      onboard fire Y37.13-
      rocket propelled grenade [RPG] Y37.11-
      small arms fire Y37.11-
      surface to air missile Y37.11-
    specified NEC Y37.19-
  detonation (accidental) of
    onboard marine weapons Y37.05-
    own munitions or munitions launch device
      Y37.24-
  dirty bomb Y37.50-
  explosion (of) Y37.20-
    aerial bomb Y37.21-
    bomb NOS (*see also* Military operations,
      bomb(s)) Y37.20-
    fragments Y37.20-
    grenade Y37.29-
    guided missile Y37.22-
    improvised explosive device [IED] (person-
      borne) (roadside) (vehicle-borne)
      Y37.23-
    land mine Y37.29-
    marine mine (at sea) (in harbor) Y37.02-
    marine weapon Y37.00-
      specified NEC Y37.09-
    own munitions or munitions launch device
      (accidental) Y37.24-
    sea-based artillery shell Y37.03-
    specified NEC Y37.29-
    torpedo Y37.04-
  fire Y37.30-
    specified NEC Y37.39-
  firearms
    discharge Y37.43-
    pellets Y37.42-
  flamethrower Y37.33-
  fragments (from) (of)
    improvised explosive device [IED] (person-
      borne) (roadside) (vehicle-borne)
      Y37.26-
    munitions Y37.25-
    specified NEC Y37.29-
    weapons Y37.27-
  friendly fire Y37.92-
  hand to hand (unarmed) combat Y37.44-
  hot substances — *see* Military operations, fire
  incendiary bullet Y37.32-
  nuclear weapon (effects of) Y37.50-
    acute radiation exposure Y37.54-
    blast pressure Y37.51-
    direct blast Y37.51-
    direct heat Y37.53-
    fallout exposure Y37.54-
    fireball Y37.53-
    indirect blast (struck or crushed by blast
      debris) (being thrown by blast) Y37.52-
    ionizing radiation (immediate exposure)
      Y37.54-
    nuclear radiation Y37.54-
    radiation
      ionizing (immediate exposure) Y37.54-
      nuclear Y37.54-
      thermal Y37.53-
    secondary effects Y37.54-
    specified NEC Y37.59-
    thermal radiation Y37.53-

Military operations (injuries to military and
  civilians occuring during peacetime on
  military property and during routine military
  exercises and operations) (by) (from)
  (involving) Y37.90- — *continued*
  restriction of air (airway)
    intentional Y37.46-
    unintentional Y37.47-
  rubber bullets Y37.41-
  shrapnel NOS Y37.29-
  suffocation — *see* Military operations,
    restriction of airways
  unconventional warfare NEC Y37.7x-
  underwater blast NOS Y37.00-
  warfare
    conventional NEC Y37.49-
    unconventional NEC Y37.7x-
  weapon of mass destruction [WMD] Y37.91-
  weapons
    biological weapons Y37.6x-
    chemical Y37.7x-
    nuclear (effects of) Y37.50-
      acute radiation exposure Y37.54-
      blast pressure Y37.51-
      direct blast Y37.51-
      direct heat Y37.53-
      fallout exposure Y37.54-
      fireball Y37.53-
      indirect blast (struck or crushed by blast
        debris) (being thrown by blast)
        Y37.52-
      radiation
        ionizing (immediate exposure) Y37.54-
        nuclear Y37.54-
        thermal Y37.53-
      secondary effects Y37.54-
      specified NEC Y37.59-
    of mass destruction [WMD] Y37.91-
**Misadventure(s) to patient(s) during
surgical or medical care** Y69
  contaminated medical or biological substance
    (blood, drug, fluid) Y64.9
    administered (by) NEC Y64.9
    immunization Y64.1
    infusion Y64.0
    injection Y64.1
    specified means NEC Y64.8
    transfusion Y64.0
    vaccination Y64.1
  excessive amount of blood or other fluid
    during transfusion or infusion Y63.0
  failure
    in dosage Y63.9
    electroshock therapy Y63.4
    inappropriate temperature (too hot or too
      cold) in local application and packing
      Y63.5
    infusion
      excessive amount of fluid Y63.0
      incorrect dilution of fluid Y63.1
    insulin-shock therapy Y63.4
    nonadministration of necessary drug or
      biological substance Y63.6
    overdose — *see* Table of Drugs and
      Chemicals
    radiation, in therapy Y63.2
    radiation
      overdose Y63.2
    specified procedure NEC Y63.8
    transfusion
      excessive amount of blood Y63.0
  mechanical, of instrument or apparatus (any)
    (during any procedure) Y65.8
  sterile precautions (during procedure) Y62.9
    aspiration of fluid or tissue (by puncture or
      catheterization, except heart) Y62.6
    biopsy (except needle aspiration) Y62.8
      needle (aspirating) Y62.6
    blood sampling Y62.6

EXTERNAL CAUSES

Misadventure(s) to patient(s) during surgical or medical care Y69 — *continued*
failure — *continued*
    sterile precautions (during procedure) Y62.9 — *continued*
      catheterization Y62.6
        heart Y62.5
      dialysis (kidney) Y62.2
      endoscopic examination Y62.4
      enema Y62.8
      immunization Y62.3
      infusion Y62.1
      injection Y62.3
      needle biopsy Y62.6
      paracentesis (abdominal) (thoracic) Y62.6
      perfusion Y62.2
      puncture (lumbar) Y62.6
      removal of catheter or packing Y62.8
      specified procedure NEC Y62.8
      surgical operation Y62.0
      transfusion Y62.1
      vaccination Y62.3
    suture or ligature during surgical procedure Y65.2
    to introduce or to remove tube or instrument — *see* Failure, to
  hemorrhage — *see* Index to Diseases and Injuries, Complication(s)
  inadvertent exposure of patient to radiation Y63.3
  inappropriate
    operation performed — *see* Inappropriate operation performed
    temperature (too hot or too cold) in local application or packing Y63.5
  infusion (*see also* Misadventure, by type, infusion) Y69
    excessive amount of fluid Y63.0
    incorrect dilution of fluid Y63.1
    wrong fluid Y65.1
  mismatched blood in transfusion Y65.0
  nonadministration of necessary drug or biological substance Y63.6
  overdose — *see* Table of Drugs and Chemicals
  radiation (in therapy)
  perforation — *see* Index to Diseases and Injuries, Complication(s)
  performance of inappropriate operation — *see* Inappropriate operation performed
  puncture — *see* Index to Diseases and Injuries, Complication(s)
  specified type NEC Y65.8
    failure
      suture or ligature during surgical operation Y65.2
      to introduce or to remove tube or instrument — *see* Failure, to
    infusion of wrong fluid Y65.1
    performance of inappropriate operation — *see* Inappropriate operation performed
    transfusion of mismatched blood Y65.0
    wrong
      fluid in infusion Y65.1
      placement of endotracheal tube during anesthetic procedure Y65.3
  transfusion — *see* Misadventure, by type, transfusion
    excessive amount of blood Y63.0
    mismatched blood Y65.0
  wrong
    drug given in error — *see* Table of Drugs and Chemicals
    fluid in infusion Y65.1
    placement of endotracheal tube during anesthetic procedure Y65.3
Mismatched blood in transfusion Y65.0
Motion sickness T75.3
Mountain sickness W94.11
Mudslide (of cataclysmic nature) — *see* Landslide

Murder (attempt) — *see* Assault

N

Nail
  contact with W45.0
    gun W29.4
  embedded in skin W45.0
Neglect (criminal) (homicidal intent) X58
Noise (causing injury) (pollution) W42.9
  supersonic W42.0
Nonadministration (of)
  drug or biological substance (necessary) Y63.6
  surgical and medical care Y66
Nosocomial condition Y95

O

Object
  falling
    from, in, on, hitting
      machinery — *see* Contact, with, by type of machine
  set in motion by
    accidental explosion or rupture of pressure vessel W38
    firearm — *see* Discharge, firearm, by type
    machine(ry) — *see* Contact, with, by type of machine
Overdose (drug) — *see* Table of Drugs and Chemicals
  radiation Y63.2
Overexertion X50.9
  from
    prolonged static or awkward postures X50.1
    repetitive movements X50.3
    specified strenuous movements or postures NEC X50.9
    strenuous movement or load X50.0
Overexposure (accidental) (to)
  cold (*see also* Exposure, cold) X31
    due to man-made conditions — *see* Exposure, cold, man-made
  heat (*see also* Heat) X30
  radiation — *see* Radiation
  radioactivity W88.0
  sun (sunburn) X32
  weather NEC — *see* Forces of nature
  wind NEC — *see* Forces of nature
Overheated — *see* Heat
Overturning (accidental)
  machinery — *see* Contact, with, by type of machine
  transport vehicle NEC (*see also* Accident, transport) V89.9
  watercraft (causing drowning, submersion) — *see also* Drowning, due to, accident to, watercraft, overturning
    causing injury except drowning or submersion — *see* Accident, watercraft, causing, injury NEC

P

Parachute descent (voluntary) (without accident to aircraft) V97.29
  due to accident to aircraft — *see* Accident, transport, aircraft
Pecked by bird W61.99
Perforation during medical or surgical treatment as misadventure — *see* Index to Diseases and Injuries, Complication(s)
Perpetrator, perpetration, of assault, maltreatment and neglect (by) Y07.9
  boyfriend Y07.03
  brother Y07.410
    stepbrother Y07.435
  coach Y07.53
  cousin
    female Y07.491
    male Y07.490
  daycare provider Y07.519
    at-home
      adult care Y07.512
      childcare Y07.510
    care center
      adult care Y07.513
      childcare Y07.511
  family member NEC Y07.499
  father Y07.11
    adoptive Y07.13
    foster Y07.420
    stepfather Y07.430
  foster father Y07.420
  foster mother Y07.421
  girl friend Y07.04
  healthcare provider Y07.529
    mental health Y07.521
    specified NEC Y07.528
  husband Y07.01
  instructor Y07.53
  mother Y07.12
    adoptive Y07.14
    foster Y07.421
    stepmother Y07.433
  nonfamily member Y07.50
    specified NEC Y07.59
  nurse Y07.528
  occupational therapist Y07.528
  partner of parent
    female Y07.434
    male Y07.432
  physical therapist Y07.528
  sister Y07.411
  speech therapist Y07.528
  stepbrother Y07.435
  stepfather Y07.430
  stepmother Y07.433
  stepsister Y07.436
  teacher Y07.53
  wife Y07.02
Piercing — *see* Contact, with, by type of object or machine
Pinched
  between objects (moving) (stationary and moving) W23.0
  stationary W23.1
Pinned under machine(ry) — *see* Contact, with, by type of machine
Place of occurrence Y92.9
  abandoned house Y92.89
  airplane Y92.813
  airport Y92.520
  ambulatory health services establishment NEC Y92.538
  ambulatory surgery center Y92.530
  amusement park Y92.831

Place of occurrence Y92.9 — *continued*
  apartment (co-op) — *see* Place of occurrence, residence, apartment
  assembly hall Y92.29
  bank Y92.510
  barn Y92.71
  baseball field Y92.320
  basketball court Y92.310
  beach Y92.832
  boarding house — *see* Place of occurrence, residence, boarding house
  boat Y92.814
  bowling alley Y92.39
  bridge Y92.89
  building under construction Y92.61
  bus Y92.811
    station Y92.521
  cafe Y92.511
  campsite Y92.833
  campus — *see* Place of occurrence, school
  canal Y92.89
  car Y92.810
  casino Y92.59
  children's home — *see* Place of occurrence, residence, institutional, orphanage
  church Y92.22
  cinema Y92.26
  clubhouse Y92.29
  coal pit Y92.64
  college (community) Y92.214
  condominium — *see* Place of occurrence, residence, apartment
  construction area — *see* Place of occurrence, industrial and construction area
  convalescent home — *see* Place of occurrence, residence, institutional, nursing home
  court-house Y92.240
  cricket ground Y92.328
  cultural building Y92.258
    art gallery Y92.250
    museum Y92.251
    music hall Y92.252
    opera house Y92.253
    specified NEC Y92.258
    theater Y92.254
  dancehall Y92.252
  day nursery Y92.210
  dentist office Y92.531
  derelict house Y92.89
  desert Y92.820
  dock NOS Y92.89
  dockyard Y92.62
  doctor's office Y92.531
  dormitory — *see* Place of occurrence, residence, institutional, school dormitory
  dry dock Y92.62
  factory (building) (premises) Y92.63
  farm (land under cultivation) (outbuildings) Y92.79
    barn Y92.71
    chicken coop Y92.72
    field Y92.73
    hen house Y92.72
    house — *see* Place of occurrence, residence, house
    orchard Y92.74
    specified NEC Y92.79
  football field Y92.321
  forest Y92.821
  freeway Y92.411
  gallery Y92.250
  garage (commercial) Y92.59
    boarding house Y92.044
    military base Y92.135
    mobile home Y92.025
    nursing home Y92.124
    orphanage Y92.114
    private house Y92.015

Place of occurrence Y92.9 — *continued*
  garage (commercial) Y92.59 — *continued*
    reform school Y92.155
  gas station Y92.524
  gasworks Y92.69
  golf course Y92.39
  gravel pit Y92.64
  grocery Y92.512
  gymnasium Y92.39
  handball court Y92.318
  harbor Y92.89
  harness racing course Y92.39
  healthcare provider office Y92.531
  highway (interstate) Y92.411
  hill Y92.828
  hockey rink Y92.330
  home — *see* Place of occurrence, residence
  hospice — *see* Place of occurrence, residence, institutional, nursing home
  hospital Y92.239
    cafeteria Y92.233
    corridor Y92.232
    operating room Y92.234
    patient
      bathroom Y92.231
      room Y92.230
    specified NEC Y92.238
  hotel Y92.59
  house — *see also* Place of occurrence, residence
    abandoned Y92.89
    under construction Y92.61
  industrial and construction area (yard) Y92.69
    building under construction Y92.61
    dock Y92.62
    dry dock Y92.62
    factory Y92.63
    gasworks Y92.69
    mine Y92.64
    oil rig Y92.65
    pit Y92.64
    power station Y92.69
    shipyard Y92.62
    specified NEC Y92.69
    tunnel under construction Y92.69
    workshop Y92.69
  kindergarten Y92.211
  lacrosse field Y92.328
  lake Y92.828
  library Y92.241
  mall Y92.59
  market Y92.512
  marsh Y92.828
  military
    base — *see* Place of occurrence, residence, institutional, military base
    training ground Y92.84
  mine Y92.64
  mosque Y92.22
  motel Y92.59
  motorway (interstate) Y92.411
  mountain Y92.828
  movie-house Y92.26
  museum Y92.251
  music-hall Y92.252
  not applicable Y92.9
  nuclear power station Y92.69
  nursing home — *see* Place of occurrence, residence, institutional, nursing home
  office building Y92.59
  offshore installation Y92.65
  oil rig Y92.65
  old people's home — *see* Place of occurrence, residence, institutional, specified NEC
  opera-house Y92.253
  orphanage — *see* Place of occurrence, residence, institutional, orphanage
  outpatient surgery center Y92.530

EXTERNAL CAUSES

Q

R

Radiation (exposure to)
  arc lamps W89.0
  atomic power plant (malfunction) NEC W88.1
  complication of or abnormal reaction to
    medical radiotherapy Y84.2
  electromagnetic, ionizing W88.0
  gamma rays W88.1
  in
    war operations (from or following nuclear
      explosion) — *see* War operations
  inadvertent exposure of patient (receiving test
    or therapy) Y63.3
  infrared (heaters and lamps) W90.1
    excessive heat from W92
  ionized, ionizing (particles, artificially
    accelerated)
    radioisotopes W88.1
    specified NEC W88.8
    x-rays W88.0
  isotopes, radioactive — *see* Radiation,
    radioactive isotopes
  laser(s) W90.2
    in war operations — *see* War operations
    misadventure in medical care Y63.2
  light sources (man-made visible and ultraviolet)
    W89.9
    natural X32
    specified NEC W89.8
    tanning bed W89.1
    welding light W89.0
  man-made visible light W89.9
    specified NEC W89.8
    tanning bed W89.1
    welding light W89.0
  microwave W90.8
  misadventure in medical or surgical procedure
    Y63.2
  natural NEC X39.08
    radon X39.01
  overdose (in medical or surgical procedure)
    Y63.2
  radar W90.0
  radioactive isotopes (any) W88.1
    atomic power plant malfunction W88.1
    misadventure in medical or surgical
      treatment Y63.2
  radiofrequency W90.0
  radium NEC W88.1
  sun X32
  ultraviolet (light) (man-made) W89.9
    natural X32
    specified NEC W89.8
    tanning bed W89.1
    welding light W89.0
  welding arc, torch, or light W89.0
    excessive heat from W92
  x-rays (hard) (soft) W88.0
Range disease W94.11
Rape (attempted) T74.2-
Rat bite W53.11
Reaching (prolonged) (static) X50.1
Reaction, abnormal to medical
  procedure (*see also* Complication of or
    following, by type of procedure) Y84.9
  with misadventure — *see* Misadventure
  biologicals — *see* Table of Drugs and
    Chemicals
  drugs — *see* Table of Drugs and Chemicals
  vaccine — *see* Table of Drugs and Chemicals

Recoil
  airgun W34.110
  BB gun W34.110
  firearm NEC W34.19
  gas, air or spring-operated gun NEC
    W34.118
  handgun W32.1
  hunting rifle W33.12
  larger firearm W33.10
    specified NEC W33.19
  machine gun W33.13
  paintball gun W34.111
  pellet W34.110
  shotgun W33.11
  Very pistol [flare] W34.19
Reduction in
  atmospheric pressure — *see* Air, pressure,
    change
Rock falling on or hitting (accidentally)
  (person) W20.8
  in cave-in W20.0
Run over (accidentally) (by)
  animal (not being ridden) NEC W55.89
  machinery — *see* Contact, with, by specified
    type of machine
  transport vehicle NEC (*see also* Accident,
    transport) V09.9
    intentional homicide (attempt) Y03.0
    motor NEC V09.20
      intentional homicide (attempt) Y03.0
Running
  before moving object X81.8
    motor vehicle X81.0
Running off, away
  animal (being ridden) (*see also* Accident,
    transport) V80.918
    not being ridden W55.89
  animal-drawn vehicle NEC (*see also* Accident,
    transport) V80.928
  highway, road(way), street
    transport vehicle NEC (*see also* Accident,
    transport) V89.9
Rupture pressurized devices — *see*
  Explosion, by type of device

S

Saturnism — *see* Table of Drugs and
  Chemicals, lead
Scald, scalding (accidental) (by) (from) (in)
  X19
  air (hot) X14.1
  gases (hot) X14.1
  homicide (attempt) — *see* Assault, burning, hot
    object
  inflicted by other person
    stated as intentional, homicide (attempt) —
      see Assault, burning, hot object
  liquid (boiling) (hot) NEC X12
    stated as undetermined whether accidental
      or intentional Y27.2
    suicide (attempt) X77.2
  local application of externally applied
    substance in medical or surgical care
    Y63.5
  metal (molten) (liquid) (hot) NEC X18
  self-inflicted X77.9
  stated as undetermined whether accidental or
    intentional Y27.8
  steam X13.1
    assault X98.0
    stated as undetermined whether accidental
      or intentional Y27.0
    suicide (attempt) X77.0
  suicide (attempt) X77.9
  vapor (hot) X13.1
    assault X98.0
    stated as undetermined whether accidental
      or intentional Y27.0
    suicide (attempt) X77.0
Scratched by
  cat W55.03
  person(s) (accidentally) W50.4
    with intent to injure or kill Y04.0
    as, or caused by, a crowd or human
      stampede (with fall) W52
    assault Y04.0
    homicide (attempt) Y04.0
    in
      fight Y04.0
      legal intervention
        injuring
          bystander Y35.892
          law enforcement personnel Y35.891
          suspect Y35.893
Seasickness T75.3
Self-harm NEC — *see also* External cause by
  type, undetermined whether accidental or
  intentional
  intentional — *see* Suicide
  poisoning NEC — *see* Table of Drugs and
    Chemicals, accident
Self-inflicted (injury) NEC — *see also* External
  cause by type, undetermined whether
  accidental or intentional
  intentional — *see* Suicide
  poisoning NEC — *see* Table of Drugs and
    Chemicals, accident
Sequelae (of)
  accident NEC — *see* W00-X58 with 7th
    character S
  assault (homicidal) (any means) — *see* X92-
    Y08 with 7th character S
  homicide, attempt (any means) — *see* X92-Y08
    with 7th character S
  injury undetermined whether accidentally or
    purposely inflicted — *see* Y21-Y33 with
    7th character S
  intentional self-harm (classifiable to X71-X83)
    — *see* X71-X83 with 7th character S
  legal intervention — *see* with 7th character S
    Y35

EXTERNAL CAUSES

Struck (accidentally) by — *continued*
hockey (ice)
field
puck W21.221
stick W21.211
puck W21.220
stick W21.210
assault Y08.01
landslide — *see* Landslide
law-enforcement agent (on duty) — *see* Legal,
intervention, manhandling
with blunt object — *see* Legal, intervention,
blunt object
lightning — *see* subcategory T75.0
causing fire — *see* Exposure, fire
machine — *see* Contact, with, by type of
machine
mammal NEC W55.89
marine W56.32
marine animal W56.82
missile
firearm — *see* Discharge, firearm by type
in war operations — *see* War operations,
missile
object W22.8
blunt W22.8
assault Y00
suicide (attempt) X79
undetermined whether accidental or
intentional Y29
falling W20.8
from, in, on
building W20.1
burning (uncontrolled fire) X00.4
cataclysmic
earth surface movement NEC — *see*
Landslide
storm — *see* Forces of nature,
cataclysmic storm
cave-in W20.0
earthquake X34
machine (in operation) — *see* Contact,
with, by type of machine
structure W20.1
burning X00.4
transport vehicle (in motion) — *see*
Accident, transport, by type of
vehicle
watercraft V93.49
due to
accident to craft V91.39
powered craft V91.33
ferry boat V91.31
fishing boat V91.32
jetskis V91.33
liner V91.31
merchant ship V91.30
passenger ship V91.31
unpowered craft V91.38
canoe V91.35
inflatable V91.36
kayak V91.35
sailboat V91.34
surfboard V91.38
windsurfer V91.38
powered craft V93.43
ferry boat V93.41
fishing boat V93.42
jetskis V93.43
liner V93.41
merchant ship V93.40
passenger ship V93.41
unpowered craft V93.48
sailboat V93.44
surfboard V93.48
windsurfer V93.48

Struck (accidentally) by — *continued*
object W22.8 — *continued*
moving NEC W20.8
projected W20.8
assault Y00
in sports W21.9
assault Y08.09
ball W21.00
baseball W21.03
basketball W21.05
football W21.01
golf ball W21.04
soccer W21.02
softball W21.07
specified NEC W21.09
volleyball W21.06
bat or racquet
baseball bat W21.11
assault Y08.02
golf club W21.13
assault Y08.09
specified NEC W21.19
assault Y08.09
tennis racquet W21.12
assault Y08.09
hockey (ice)
field
puck W21.221
stick W21.211
puck W21.220
stick W21.210
assault Y08.01
specified NEC W21.89
set in motion by explosion — *see* Explosion
thrown W20.8
assault Y00
in sports W21.9
assault Y08.09
ball W21.00
baseball W21.03
basketball W21.05
football W21.01
golf ball W21.04
soccer W21.02
soft ball W21.07
specified NEC W21.09
volleyball W21.06
bat or racquet
baseball bat W21.11
assault Y08.02
golf club W21.13
assault Y08.09
specified NEC W21.19
assault Y08.09
tennis racquet W21.12
assault Y08.09
hockey (ice)
field
puck W21.221
stick W21.211
puck W21.220
stick W21.210
assault Y08.01
specified NEC W21.89
other person(s) W50.0
with
blunt object W22.8
intentional, homicide (attempt) Y00
sports equipment W21.9
undetermined whether accidental or
intentional Y29
fall W03
due to ice or snow W00.0
as, or caused by, a crowd or human
stampede (with fall) W52
assault Y04.2
homicide (attempt) Y04.2

Struck (accidentally) by — *continued*
other person(s) W50.0 — *continued*
in legal intervention
injuring
bystander Y35.812
law enforcement personnel Y35.811
suspect Y35.813
sports equipment W21.9
police (on duty) — *see* Legal, intervention,
manhandling
with blunt object — *see* Legal, intervention,
blunt object
sports equipment W21.9
assault Y08.09
ball W21.00
baseball W21.03
basketball W21.05
football W21.01
golf ball W21.04
soccer W21.02
soft ball W21.07
specified NEC W21.09
volleyball W21.06
bat or racquet
baseball bat W21.11
assault Y08.02
golf club W21.13
assault Y08.09
specified NEC W21.19
assault Y08.09
tennis racquet W21.12
assault Y08.09
cleats (shoe) W21.31
foot wear NEC W21.39
football helmet W21.81
hockey (ice)
field
puck W21.221
stick W21.211
puck W21.220
stick W21.210
assault Y08.01
skate blades W21.32
specified NEC W21.89
assault Y08.09
thunderbolt — *see* subcategory T75.0
causing fire — *see* Exposure, fire
transport vehicle NEC (*see also* Accident,
transport) V09.9
intentional, homicide (attempt) Y03.0
motor NEC (*see also* Accident, transport)
V09.20
homicide Y03.0
vehicle (transport) NEC — *see* Accident,
transport, by type of vehicle
stationary (falling from jack, hydraulic lift,
ramp) W20.8
Stumbling
over
animal NEC W01.0
with fall W18.09
carpet, rug or (small) object W22.8
with fall W18.09
person W51
with fall W03
due to ice or snow W00.0
without fall W18.40
due to
specified NEC W18.49
stepping from one level to another
W18.43
stepping into hole or opening W18.42
stepping on object W18.41
Submersion (accidental) — *see* Drowning

Suffocation (accidental) (by external means) (by pressure) (mechanical) (*see also* category) T71
  due to, by
    avalanche — *see* Landslide
    explosion — *see* Explosion
    fire — *see* Exposure, fire
    food, any type (aspiration) (ingestion) (inhalation) — *see* categories T17 and T18
    ignition — *see* Ignition
    landslide — *see* Landslide
    machine(ry) — *see* Contact, with, by type of machine
    vomitus (aspiration) (inhalation) T17.81-
  in
    burning building X00.8
Suicide, suicidal (attempted) (by) X83.8
  blunt object X79
  burning, burns X76
    hot object X77.9
      fluid NEC X77.2
      household appliance X77.3
      specified NEC X77.8
      steam X77.0
      tap water X77.1
      vapors X77.0
  caustic substance — *see* Table of Drugs and Chemicals
  cold, extreme X83.2
  collision of motor vehicle with
    motor vehicle X82.0
    specified NEC X82.8
    train X82.1
    tree X82.2
  crashing of aircraft X83.0
  cut (any part of body) X78.9
  cutting or piercing instrument X78.9
    dagger X78.2
    glass X78.0
    knife X78.1
    specified NEC X78.8
    sword X78.2
  drowning (in) X71.9
    bathtub X71.0
    natural water X71.3
    specified NEC X71.8
    swimming pool X71.1
      following fall X71.2
  electrocution X83.1
  explosive(s) (material) X75
  fire, flames X76
  firearm X74.9
    airgun X74.01
    handgun X72
    hunting rifle X73.1
    larger X73.9
      specified NEC X73.8
    machine gun X73.2
    shotgun X73.0
    specified NEC X74.8
  hanging X83.8
  hot object — *see* Suicide, burning, hot object
  jumping
    before moving object X81.8
      motor vehicle X81.0
      subway train X81.1
      train X81.1
    from high place X80
  late effect of attempt — *see* X71-X83 with 7th character S
  lying before moving object, train, vehicle X81.8
  poisoning — *see* Table of Drugs and Chemicals
  puncture (any part of body) — *see* Suicide, cutting or piercing instrument
  scald — *see* Suicide, burning, hot object

Suicide, suicidal (attempted) (by) X83.8 — continued
  sequelae of attempt — *see* X71-X83 with 7th character S
  sharp object (any) — *see* Suicide, cutting or piercing instrument
  shooting — *see* Suicide, firearm
  specified means NEC X83.8
  stab (any part of body) — *see* Suicide, cutting or piercing instrument
  steam, hot vapors X77.0
  strangulation X83.8
  submersion — *see* Suicide, drowning
  suffocation X83.8
  wound NEC X83.8
Sunstroke X32
Supersonic waves (causing injury) W42.0
Surgical procedure, complication of
    (delayed or as an abnormal reaction without mention of misadventure) — *see also* Complication of or following, by type of procedure
  due to or as a result of misadventure — *see* Misadventure
Swallowed, swallowing
  foreign body — *see* Foreign body, alimentary canal
  poison — *see* Table of Drugs and Chemicals
  substance
    caustic or corrosive — *see* Table of Drugs and Chemicals
    poisonous — *see* Table of Drugs and Chemicals

Tackle in sport W03
Terrorism (involving) Y38.80
  biological weapons Y38.6x-
  chemical weapons Y38.7x-
  conflagration Y38.3x-
  drowning and submersion Y38.89-
  explosion Y38.2x-
    destruction of aircraft Y38.1x-
    marine weapons Y38.0x-
  fire Y38.3x-
  firearms Y38.4x-
  hot substances Y38.3x-
  lasers Y38.89-
  nuclear weapons Y38.5x-
  piercing or stabbing instruments Y38.89-
  secondary effects Y38.9x-
  specified method NEC Y38.89-
  suicide bomber Y38.81-
Thirst X58
Threat to breathing
  aspiration — *see* Aspiration
  due to cave-in, falling earth or substance NEC — *see* category T71
Thrown (accidentally)
  against part (any) of or object in transport vehicle (in motion) NEC — *see also* Accident, transport
  from
    high place, homicide (attempt) Y01
    machinery — *see* Contact, with, by type of machine
    transport vehicle NEC (*see also* Accident, transport) V89.9
  off — *see* Thrown, from
Thunderbolt — *see* subcategory T75.0
  causing fire — *see* Exposure, fire
Tidal wave (any injury) NEC — *see* Forces of nature, tidal wave
Took
  overdose (drug) — *see* Table of Drugs and Chemicals
  poison — *see* Table of Drugs and Chemicals
Tornado (any injury) X37.1
Torrential rain (any injury) X37.8
Torture X58
Trampled by animal NEC W55.89
Trapped (accidentally)
  between objects (moving) (stationary and moving) — *see* Caught
  by part (any) of
    motorcycle V29.88
    pedal cycle V19.88
    transport vehicle NEC (*see also* Accident, transport) V89.9
Travel (effects) (sickness) T75.3
Tree falling on or hitting (accidentally) (person) W20.8
Tripping
  over
    animal W01.0
      with fall W01.0
    carpet, rug or (small) object W22.8
      with fall W18.09
    person W51
      with fall W03
        due to ice or snow W00.0
  without fall W18.40
    due to
      specified NEC W18.49
      stepping from one level to another W18.43
      stepping into hole or opening W18.42
      stepping on object W18.41

EXTERNAL CAUSES

Twisted by person(s) (accidentally) W50.2
  with intent to injure or kill Y04.0
  as, or caused by, a crowd or human stampede
    (with fall) W52
  assault Y04.0
  homicide (attempt) Y04.0
  in
    fight Y04.0
    legal intervention — *see* Legal, intervention,
      manhandling
Twisting (prolonged) (static) X50.1

Underdosing of necessary drugs,
  medicaments or biological
  substances Y63.6
Undetermined intent (contact) (exposure)
  automobile collision Y32
  blunt object Y29
  drowning (submersion) (in) Y21.9
    bathtub Y21.0
      after fall Y21.1
    natural water (lake) (ocean) (pond) (river)
      (stream) Y21.4
    specified place NEC Y21.8
    swimming pool Y21.2
      after fall Y21.3
  explosive material Y25
  fall, jump or push from high place Y30
  falling, lying or running before moving object
    Y31
  fire Y26
  firearm discharge Y24.9
    airgun (BB) (pellet) Y24.0
    handgun (pistol) (revolver) Y22
    hunting rifle Y23.1
    larger Y23.9
      hunting rifle Y23.1
      machine gun Y23.3
      military Y23.2
      shotgun Y23.0
      specified type NEC Y23.8
    machine gun Y23.3
    military Y23.2
    shotgun Y23.0
    specified type NEC Y24.8
    Very pistol Y24.8
  hot object Y27.9
    fluid NEC Y27.2
    household appliance Y27.3
    specified object NEC Y27.8
    steam Y27.0
    tap water Y27.1
    vapor Y27.0
  jump, fall or push from high place Y30
  lying, falling or running before moving object
    Y31
  motor vehicle crash Y32
  push, fall or jump from high place Y30
  running, falling or lying before moving object
    Y31
  sharp object Y28.9
    dagger Y28.2
    glass Y28.0
    knife Y28.1
    specified object NEC Y28.8
    sword Y28.2
  smoke Y26
  specified event NEC Y33
Use of hand as hammer X50.3

Vibration (causing injury) W49.9
Victim (of)
  avalanche — *see* Landslide
  earth movements NEC — *see* Forces of nature,
    earth movement
  earthquake X34
  flood — *see* Flood
  landslide — *see* Landslide
  lightning — *see* subcategory T75.0
    causing fire — *see* Exposure, fire
  storm (cataclysmic) NEC — *see* Forces of
    nature, cataclysmic storm
  volcanic eruption X35
Volcanic eruption (any injury) X35
Vomitus, gastric contents in air passages
  (with asphyxia, obstruction or suffocation)
  T17.81-

W

Walked into stationary object (any)
 W22.09
 furniture W22.03
 lamppost W22.02
 wall W22.01
War operations (injuries to military personnel
 and civilians during war, civil insurrection
 and peacekeeping missions) (by) (from)
 (involving) Y36.90
 after cessation of hostilities Y36.89-
 explosion (of)
 bomb placed during war operations
 Y36.82-
 mine placed during war operations
 Y36.81-
 specified NEC Y36.88-
 air blast Y36.20-
 aircraft
 destruction — *see* War operations,
 destruction of aircraft
 airway restriction — *see* War operations,
 restriction of airways
 asphyxiation — *see* War operations, restriction
 of airways
 biological weapons Y36.6x-
 blast Y36.20-
 blast fragments Y36.20-
 blast wave Y36.20-
 blast wind Y36.20-
 bomb Y36.20-
 dirty Y36.50-
 gasoline Y36.31-
 incendiary Y36.31-
 petrol Y36.31-
 bullet Y36.43-
 incendiary Y36.32-
 rubber Y36.41-
 chemical weapons Y36.7x-
 combat
 hand to hand (unarmed) combat Y36.44-
 using blunt or piercing object Y36.45-
 conflagration — *see* War operations, fire
 conventional warfare NEC Y36.49-
 depth-charge Y36.01-
 destruction of aircraft Y36.10-
 due to
 air to air missile Y36.11-
 collision with other aircraft Y36.12-
 detonation (accidental) of onboard
 munitions and explosives Y36.14-
 enemy fire or explosives Y36.11-
 explosive placed on aircraft Y36.11-
 onboard fire Y36.13-
 rocket propelled grenade [RPG] Y36.11-
 small arms fire Y36.11-
 surface to air missile Y36.11-
 specified NEC Y36.19-
 detonation (accidental) of
 onboard marine weapons Y36.05-
 own munitions or munitions launch device
 Y36.24-
 dirty bomb Y36.50-

War operations (injuries to military personnel
 and civilians during war, civil insurrection
 and peacekeeping missions) (by) (from)
 (involving) Y36.90 — *continued*
 explosion (of) Y36.20-
 aerial bomb Y36.21-
 after cessation of hostilities
 bomb placed during war operations
 Y36.82-
 mine placed during war operations
 Y36.81-
 bomb NOS (*see also* War operations,
 bomb(s)) Y36.20-
 fragments Y36.20-
 grenade Y36.29-
 guided missile Y36.22-
 improvised explosive device [IED] (person-
 borne) (roadside) (vehicle-borne)
 Y36.23-
 land mine Y36.29-
 marine mine (at sea) (in harbor) Y36.02-
 marine weapon Y36.00-
 specified NEC Y36.09-
 own munitions or munitions launch device
 (accidental) Y36.24-
 sea-based artillery shell Y36.03-
 specified NEC Y36.29-
 torpedo Y36.04-
 fire Y36.30-
 specified NEC Y36.39-
 firearms
 discharge Y36.43-
 pellets Y36.42-
 flamethrower Y36.33-
 fragments (from) (of)
 improvised explosive device [IED] (person-
 borne) (roadside) (vehicle-borne)
 Y36.26-
 munitions Y36.25-
 specified NEC Y36.29-
 weapons Y36.27-
 friendly fire Y36.92
 hand to hand (unarmed) combat Y36.44-
 hot substances — *see* War operations, fire
 incendiary bullet Y36.32-
 nuclear weapon (effects of) Y36.50-
 acute radiation exposure Y36.54-
 blast pressure Y36.51-
 direct blast Y36.51-
 direct heat Y36.53-
 fallout exposure Y36.54-
 fireball Y36.53-
 indirect blast (struck or crushed by blast
 debris) (being thrown by blast) Y36.52-
 ionizing radiation (immediate exposure)
 Y36.54-
 nuclear radiation Y36.54-
 radiation
 ionizing (immediate exposure) Y36.54-
 nuclear Y36.54-
 thermal Y36.53-
 secondary effects Y36.54-
 specified NEC Y36.59-
 thermal radiation Y36.53-
 restriction of air (airway)
 intentional Y36.46-
 unintentional Y36.47-
 rubber bullets Y36.41-
 shrapnel NOS Y36.29-
 suffocation — *see* War operations, restriction
 of airways
 unconventional warfare NEC Y36.7x-
 underwater blast NOS Y36.00-
 warfare
 conventional NEC Y36.49-
 unconventional NEC Y36.7x-

War operations (injuries to military personnel
 and civilians during war, civil insurrection
 and peacekeeping missions) (by) (from)
 (involving) Y36.90 — *continued*
 weapon of mass destruction [WMD] Y36.91
 weapons
 biological weapons Y36.6x-
 chemical Y36.7x-
 nuclear (effects of) Y36.50-
 acute radiation exposure Y36.54-
 blast pressure Y36.51-
 direct blast Y36.51-
 direct heat Y36.53-
 fallout exposure Y36.54-
 fireball Y36.53-
 radiation
 ionizing (immediate exposure) Y36.54-
 nuclear Y36.54-
 thermal Y36.53-
 secondary effects Y36.54-
 specified NEC Y36.59-
 of mass destruction [WMD] Y36.91
Washed
 away by flood — *see* Flood
 off road by storm (transport vehicle) — *see*
 Forces of nature, cataclysmic storm
Weather exposure NEC — *see* Forces of
 nature
Weightlessness (causing injury) (effects of) (in
 spacecraft, real or simulated) X52
Work related condition Y99.0
Wound (accidental) NEC (*see also* Injury) X58
 battle (*see also* War operations) Y36.90
 gunshot — *see* Discharge, firearm by type
Wreck transport vehicle NEC (*see also*
 Accident, transport) V89.9
Wrong
 device implanted into correct surgical site
 Y65.51
 fluid in infusion Y65.1
 patient, procedure performed on Y65.52
 procedure (operation) on correct patient
 Y65.51

X

Y

Z

EXTERNAL CAUSES

Chapter 1 – Certain infectious and parasitic diseases (A00-B99)

Includes: Diseases generally recognized as communicable or transmissible

Use additional code to identify resistance to antimicrobial drugs (Z16.-)

Excludes 1:   certain localized infections — see body system, related chapters
Excludes ❷: carrier or suspected carrier of infectious disease (Z22-)
infectious and parasitic diseases complicating pregnancy, childbirth and the puerperium (O98.-)
infectious and parasitic diseases specific to the perinatal period (P35-P39)
influenza and other acute respiratory infections (J00-J22)

This chapter contains the following blocks:

A00-A09	Intestinal infectious diseases
A15-A19	Tuberculosis
A20-A28	Certain zoonotic bacterial diseases
A30-A49	Other bacterial diseases
A50-A64	Infections with a predominantly sexual mode of transmission
A65-A69	Other spirochetal diseases
A70-A74	Other diseases caused by chlamydiae
A75-A79	Rickettsioses
A80-A89	Viral and prion infections of the central nervous system
A90-A99	Arthropod-borne viral fevers and viral hemorrhagic fevers
B00-B09	Viral infections characterized by skin and mucous membrane lesions
B10	Other human herpesviruses
B15-B19	Viral hepatitis
B20	Human immunodeficiency virus [HIV] disease
B25-B34	Other viral diseases
B35-B49	Mycoses
B50-B64	Protozoal diseases
B65-B83	Helminthiases
B85-B89	Pediculosis, acariasis and other infestations
B90-B94	Sequelae of infectious and parasitic diseases
B95-B97	Bacterial and viral infectious agents
B99	Other infectious diseases

Chapter-Specific Coding Guidelines

C. Chapter-Specific Coding Guidelines
In addition to general coding guidelines, there are guidelines for specific diagnoses and/or conditions in the classification. Unless otherwise indicated, these guidelines apply to all health care settings. Please refer to Section II for guidelines on the selection of principal diagnosis.

1. Chapter 1: Certain Infectious and Parasitic Diseases (A00-B99)

a. Human Immunodeficiency Virus (HIV) Infections

1) Code only confirmed cases
Code only confirmed cases of HIV infection/illness. This is an exception to the hospital inpatient guideline Section II, H.

In this context, "confirmation" does not require documentation of positive serology or culture for HIV; the provider's diagnostic statement that the patient is HIV positive, or has an HIV-related illness is sufficient.

2) Selection and sequencing of HIV codes

(a) Patient admitted for HIV-related condition
If a patient is admitted for an HIV-related condition, the principal diagnosis should be B20, Human immunodeficiency virus [HIV] disease followed by additional diagnosis codes for all reported HIV-related conditions.

(b) Patient with HIV disease admitted for unrelated condition
If a patient with HIV disease is admitted for an unrelated condition (such as a traumatic injury), the code for the unrelated condition (e.g., the nature of injury code) should be the principal diagnosis. Other diagnoses would be B20 followed by additional diagnosis codes for all reported HIV-related conditions.

(c) Whether the patient is newly diagnosed
Whether the patient is newly diagnosed or has had previous admissions/encounters for HIV conditions is irrelevant to the sequencing decision.

(d) Asymptomatic human immunodeficiency virus
Z21, Asymptomatic human immunodeficiency virus [HIV] infection status, is to be applied when the patient without any documentation of symptoms is listed as being "HIV positive," "known HIV," "HIV test positive," or similar terminology. Do not use this code if the term "AIDS" is used or if the patient is treated for any HIV-related illness or is described as having any condition(s) resulting from his/her HIV positive status; use B20 in these cases.

(e) Patients with inconclusive HIV serology
Patients with inconclusive HIV serology, but no definitive diagnosis or manifestations of the illness, may be assigned code R75, Inconclusive laboratory evidence of human immunodeficiency virus [HIV].

(f) Previously diagnosed HIV-related illness
Patients with any known prior diagnosis of an HIV-related illness should be coded to B20. Once a patient has developed an HIV-related illness, the patient should always be assigned code B20 on every subsequent admission/encounter. Patients previously diagnosed with any HIV illness (B20) should never be assigned to R75 or Z21, Asymptomatic human immunodeficiency virus [HIV] infection status.

(g) HIV Infection in Pregnancy, Childbirth and the Puerperium
During pregnancy, childbirth or the puerperium, a patient admitted (or presenting for a health care encounter) because of an HIV-related illness should receive a principal diagnosis code of O98.7-, Human immunodeficiency [HIV] disease complicating pregnancy, childbirth and the puerperium, followed by B20 and the code(s) for the HIV-related illness(es). Codes from Chapter 15 always take sequencing priority.

Patients with asymptomatic HIV infection status admitted (or presenting for a health care encounter) during pregnancy, childbirth, or the puerperium should receive codes of O98.7- and Z21.

(h) Encounters for testing for HIV
If a patient is being seen to determine his/her HIV status, use code Z11.4, Encounter for screening for human immunodeficiency virus [HIV]. Use additional codes for any associated high risk behavior.

If a patient with signs or symptoms is being seen for HIV testing, code the signs and symptoms. An additional counseling code Z71.7, Human immunodeficiency virus [HIV] counseling, may be used if counseling is provided during the encounter for the test.

When a patient returns to be informed of his/her HIV test results and the test result is negative, use code Z71.7, Human immunodeficiency virus [HIV] counseling.

If the results are positive, see previous guidelines and assign codes as appropriate.

b. Infectious agents as the cause of diseases classified to other chapters
Certain infections are classified in chapters other than Chapter 1 and no organism is identified as part of the infection code. In these instances, it is necessary to use an additional code from Chapter 1 to identify the organism. A code from category B95, Streptococcus, Staphylococcus, and Enterococcus as the cause of diseases classified to other chapters, B96, Other bacterial agents as the cause of diseases classified to other chapters, or B97, Viral agents as the cause of diseases classified to other chapters, is to be used as an additional code to identify the organism. An instructional note will be found at the infection code advising that an additional organism code is required.

c. Infections resistant to antibiotics
Many bacterial infections are resistant to current antibiotics. It is necessary to identify all infections documented as antibiotic resistant. Assign a code from category Z16, Resistance to antimicrobial drugs, following the infection code only if the infection code does not identify drug resistance.

d. Sepsis, Severe Sepsis, and Septic Shock

1) Coding of Sepsis and Severe Sepsis

(a) Sepsis
For a diagnosis of sepsis, assign the appropriate code for the underlying systemic infection. If the type of infection or causal organism is not further specified, assign code A41.9, Sepsis, unspecified organism.

A code from subcategory R65.2, Severe sepsis, should not be assigned unless severe sepsis or an associated acute organ dysfunction is documented.

(i) Negative or inconclusive blood cultures and sepsis
Negative or inconclusive blood cultures do not preclude a diagnosis of sepsis in patients with clinical evidence of the condition, however, the provider should be queried.

(ii) Urosepsis
The term urosepsis is a nonspecific term. It is not to be considered synonymous with sepsis. It has no default code in the Alphabetic Index. Should a provider use this term, he/she must be queried for clarification.

A00-A00

(iii) Sepsis with organ dysfunction

If a patient has sepsis and associated acute organ dysfunction or multiple organ dysfunction (MOD), follow the instructions for coding severe sepsis.

(iv) Acute organ dysfunction that is not clearly associated with the sepsis

If a patient has sepsis and an acute organ dysfunction, but the medical record documentation indicates that the acute organ dysfunction is related to a medical condition other than the sepsis, do not assign a code from subcategory R65.2, Severe sepsis. An acute organ dysfunction must be associated with the sepsis in order to assign the severe sepsis code. If the documentation is not clear as to whether an acute organ dysfunction is related to the sepsis or another medical condition, query the provider.

(b) Severe sepsis

The coding of severe sepsis requires a minimum of 2 codes: first a code for the underlying systemic infection, followed by a code from subcategory R65.2, Severe sepsis. If the causal organism is not documented, assign code A41.9, Sepsis, unspecified organism, for the infection. Additional code(s) for the associated acute organ dysfunction are also required.

Due to the complex nature of severe sepsis, some cases may require querying the provider prior to assignment of the codes.

2) Septic shock

(a) Septic shock

Septic shock generally refers to circulatory failure associated with severe sepsis, and therefore, it represents a type of acute organ dysfunction.

For cases of septic shock, the code for the systemic infection should be sequenced first, followed by code R65.21, Severe sepsis with septic shock or code T81.12, Postprocedural septic shock. Any additional codes for the other acute organ dysfunctions should also be assigned. As noted in the sequencing instructions in the Tabular List, the code for septic shock cannot be assigned as a principal diagnosis.

3) Sequencing of severe sepsis

If severe sepsis is present on admission, and meets the definition of principal diagnosis, the underlying systemic infection should be assigned as principal diagnosis followed by the appropriate code from subcategory R65.2 as required by the sequencing rules in the Tabular List. A code from subcategory R65.2 can never be assigned as a principal diagnosis.

When severe sepsis develops during an encounter (it was not present on admission) the underlying systemic infection and the appropriate code from subcategory R65.2 should be assigned as secondary diagnoses.

Severe sepsis may be present on admission but the diagnosis may not be confirmed until sometime after admission. If the documentation is not clear whether severe sepsis was present on admission, the provider should be queried.

4) Sepsis and severe sepsis with a localized infection

If the reason for admission is both sepsis or severe sepsis and a localized infection, such as pneumonia or cellulitis, a code(s) for the underlying systemic infection should be assigned first and the code for the localized infection should be assigned as a secondary diagnosis. If the patient has severe sepsis, a code from subcategory R65.2 should also be assigned as a secondary diagnosis. If the patient is admitted with a localized infection, such as pneumonia, and sepsis/severe sepsis doesn't develop until after admission, the localized infection should be assigned first, followed by the appropriate sepsis/severe sepsis codes.

5) Sepsis due to a postprocedural infection

(a) Documentation of causal relationship

As with all postprocedural complications, code assignment is based on the provider's documentation of the relationship between the infection and the procedure.

(b) Sepsis due to a postprocedural infection

For such cases, the postprocedural infection code, such as, T80.2, Infections following infusion, transfusion, and therapeutic injection, T81.4, Infection following a procedure, T88.0, Infection following immunization, or O86.0, Infection of obstetric surgical wound, should be coded first, followed by the code for the specific infection. If the patient has severe sepsis the appropriate code from subcategory R65.2 should also be assigned with the additional code(s) for any acute organ dysfunction.

(c) Postprocedural infection and postprocedural septic shock

In cases where a postprocedural infection has occurred and has resulted in severe sepsis the code for the precipitating complication such as code T81.4, Infection following a procedure, or O86.0, Infection of obstetrical surgical wound should be coded first followed by code R65.20, Severe sepsis without septic shock and a code for the systemic infection. A code for the systemic infection should also be assigned.

If a postprocedural infection has resulted in postprocedural septic shock, the code for the precipitating complication such as T81.4, Infection following a procedure, or O86.0, Infection of obstetrical surgical wound should be coded first followed by code T81.12-, Postprocedural septic shock. A code for the systemic infection should also be assigned.

6) Sepsis and severe sepsis associated with a noninfectious process (condition)

In some cases a noninfectious process (condition), such as trauma, may lead to an infection which can result in sepsis or severe sepsis. If sepsis or severe sepsis is documented as associated with a noninfectious condition, such as a burn or serious injury, and this condition meets the definition for principal diagnosis, the code for the noninfectious condition should be sequenced first, followed by the code for the resulting infection. If severe sepsis, is present a code from subcategory R65.2 should also be assigned with any associated organ dysfunction(s) codes. It is not necessary to assign a code from subcategory R65.1, Systemic inflammatory response syndrome (SIRS) of non-infectious origin, for these cases.

If the infection meets the definition of principal diagnosis it should be sequenced before the non-infectious condition. When both the associated non-infectious condition and the infection meet the definition of principal diagnosis either may be assigned as principal diagnosis.

Only one code from category R65, Symptoms and signs specifically associated with systemic inflammation and infection, should be assigned. Therefore, when a non-infectious condition leads to an infection resulting in severe sepsis, assign the appropriate code from subcategory R65.2, Severe sepsis. Do not additionally assign a code from subcategory R65.1, Systemic inflammatory response syndrome (SIRS) of non-infectious origin.

See Section I.C.18. SIRS due to non-infectious process.

7) Sepsis and septic shock complicating abortion, pregnancy, childbirth, and the puerperium

See Section I.C.15. Sepsis and septic shock complicating abortion, pregnancy, childbirth and the puerperium.

8) Newborn sepsis

See Section I.C.16.f. Bacterial sepsis of Newborn.

e. Methicillin Resistant *Staphylococcus aureus* (MRSA) Conditions

1) Selection and sequencing of MRSA codes

(a) Combination codes for MRSA infection

When a patient is diagnosed with an infection that is due to methicillin resistant *Staphylococcus aureus* (MRSA), and that infection has a combination code that includes the causal organism (e.g., sepsis, pneumonia) assign the appropriate combination code for the condition (e.g., code A41.02, Sepsis due to methicillin resistant Staphylococcus aureus or code J15.212, Pneumonia due to methicillin resistant Staphylococcus aureus). Do not assign code B95.62, Methicillin resistant Staphylococcus aureus infection as the cause of the diseases classified elsewhere, as an additional code because the combination code includes the type of infection and the MRSA organism. Do not assign a code from subcategory Z16.11, Resistance to penicillins, as an additional diagnosis.

See Section C.1. for instructions on coding and sequencing of sepsis and severe sepsis.

(b) Other codes for MRSA infection

When there is documentation of a current infection (e.g., wound infection, stitch abscess, urinary tract infection) due to MRSA, and that infection does not have a combination code that includes the causal organism, assign the appropriate code to identify the condition along with code B95.62, Methicillin resistant Staphylococcus aureus infection as the cause of diseases classified elsewhere for the MRSA infection. Do not assign a code from subcategory Z16.11, Resistance to penicillins.

(c) Methicillin susceptible Staphylococcus aureus (MSSA) and MRSA colonization

The condition or state of being colonized or carrying MSSA or MRSA is called colonization or carriage, while an individual person is described as being colonized or being a carrier. Colonization means that MSSA and MSRA is present on or in the body without necessarily causing illness. A positive MRSA colonization test might be documented by the provider as "MRSA screen positive" or "MRSA nasal swab positive".

Assign code Z22.322, Carrier or suspected carrier of methicillin resistant Staphylococcus aureus, for patients documented as having MRSA colonization. Assign code Z22.321, Carrier or suspected carrier of methicillin susceptible Staphylococcus aureus, for patient documented as having MSSA colonization. Colonization is not necessarily indicative of a disease process or as the cause of a specific condition the patient may have unless documented as such by the provider.

(d) MRSA colonization and infection

If a patient is documented as having both MRSA colonization and infection during a hospital admission, code Z22.322, Carrier or suspected carrier of methicillin resistant Staphylococcus aureus, and a code for the MRSA infection may both be assigned.

f.   Zika virus infections
1)   Code only confirmed cases

Code only a confirmed diagnosis of Zika virus (A92.5, Zika virus disease) as documented by the provider. This is an exception to the hospital inpatient guideline Section II, H. In this context, "confirmation" does not require documentation of the type of test performed; the physician's diagnostic statement that the condition is confirmed is sufficient. This code should be assigned regardless of the stated mode of transmission.

If the provider documents "suspected", "possible" or "probable" Zika, do not assign code A92.5. Assign a code(s) explaining the reason for the encounter (such as fever, rash, or joint pain) or Z20.828, Contact with and (suspected) exposure to other viral communicable diseases.

A00-I A00

Intestinal infectious diseases (A00-A09)

A00- <u>Cholera</u> — An acute infectious disease caused by Vibrio cholerae manifested by diarrhea and severe dehydration.

cc**A00.0** **Cholera due to Vibrio cholerae 01, biovar <u>cholerae</u>**
Classical cholera

cc**A00.1** **Cholera due to Vibrio cholerae 01, biovar <u>el tor</u>**
Cholera el tor

cc**A00.9** **Cholera, unspecified**

A01- <u>Typhoid</u> and paratyphoid fevers — An acute infectious disease caused by a Salmonella organism and characterized by acute fever and Peyer's patches in the intestines.

A01.0- <u>Typhoid</u> fever — A form due to infection with Salmonella typhi.
Infection due to Salmonella typhi

cc**A01.00** **Typhoid fever, unspecified**

cc**A01.01** **Typhoid <u>meningitis</u>**

cc**A01.02** **Typhoid fever with <u>heart</u> involvement**
Typhoid endocarditis
Typhoid myocarditis

cc**A01.03** **Typhoid <u>pneumonia</u>**

cc**A01.04** **Typhoid <u>arthritis</u>**

cc**A01.05** **Typhoid <u>osteomyelitis</u>**

cc**A01.09** **Typhoid fever with other complications**

cc**A01.1** **<u>Paratyphoid</u> fever <u>A</u>** — A form due to infection with Salmonella enteritidis paratyphi A.

cc**A01.2** **<u>Paratyphoid</u> fever <u>B</u>** — A form due to infection with Salmonella enteritidis paratyphi B.

cc**A01.3** **<u>Paratyphoid</u> fever <u>C</u>** — A form due to infection with Salmonella enteritidis paratyphi C.

cc**A01.4** **<u>Paratyphoid</u> fever, unspecified**
Infection due to Salmonella paratyphi NOS

A02- <u>Other salmonella</u> infections — Cellular injury due to competitive metabolism after invasion and multiplication of Salmonella organisms.
Includes: Infection or foodborne intoxication due to any Salmonella species other than S. typhi and S. paratyphi

cc**A02.0** **Salmonella <u>enteritis</u>** — Infection of the gastrointestinal tract by Salmonella.
Salmonellosis

mcc**A02.1** **Salmonella <u>sepsis</u>** — A systemic disease caused by persistence of Salmonella and/or their toxins in the blood.

A02.2- <u>Localized</u> salmonella infections

A02.20 **Localized salmonella infection, unspecified**

mcc**A02.21** **Salmonella <u>meningitis</u>**

mcc**A02.22** **Salmonella <u>pneumonia</u>**

cc**A02.23** **Salmonella <u>arthritis</u>**

cc**A02.24** **Salmonella <u>osteomyelitis</u>**

cc**A02.25** **Salmonella <u>pyelonephritis</u>**
Salmonella tubulo-interstitial nephropathy

cc**A02.29** **Salmonella with other localized infection**

cc**A02.8** **Other specified salmonella infections**

cc**A02.9** **Salmonella infection, unspecified**

A03- <u>Shigellosis</u> — An acute infectious disease due to the genus shigella, tribe Salmonelleae, which causes dysentery.

cc**A03.0** **Shigellosis due to Shigella dysenteriae**
Group A shigellosis [Shiga-Kruse dysentery]

A03.1 **Shigellosis due to Shigella flexneri**
Group B shigellosis

A03.2 **Shigellosis due to Shigella boydii**
Group C shigellosis

A03.3 **Shigellosis due to Shigella sonnei**
Group D shigellosis

A03.8 **Other shigellosis**

A03.9 **Shigellosis, unspecified**
Bacillary dysentery NOS

A04- <u>Other bacterial intestinal</u> infections — Escherichia coli – Intestinal infection due to the species Escherichia coli in massive numbers, although common in man's intestinal flora.

Excludes 1: *bacterial foodborne intoxications, NEC (A05.-)*
tuberculous enteritis (A18.32)

cc**A04.0** **Enteropathogenic <u>Escherichia coli</u> infection**

cc**A04.1** **Enterotoxigenic <u>Escherichia coli</u> infection**

cc**A04.2** **Enteroinvasive <u>Escherichia coli</u> infection**

cc**A04.3** **Enterohemorrhagic <u>Escherichia coli</u> infection**

cc**A04.4** **Other intestinal <u>Escherichia coli</u> infections**
Escherichia coli enteritis NOS

cc**A04.5** **Campylobacter enteritis**

cc**A04.6** **Enteritis due to Yersinia enterocolitica**
Excludes 1: *extraintestinal yersiniosis (A28.2)*

cc**A04.7** **Enterocolitis due to Clostridium difficile**
Foodborne intoxication by Clostridium difficile
Pseudomembraneous colitis

cc**A04.8** **Other specified bacterial intestinal infections**

cc**A04.9** **Bacterial intestinal infection, unspecified**
Bacterial enteritis NOS

A05- Other bacterial <u>foodborne</u> intoxications, not elsewhere classified
Excludes 1: *Clostridium difficile foodborne intoxication and infection (A04.7)*
Escherichia coli infection (A04.0-A04.4)
listeriosis (A32.-)
salmonella foodborne intoxication and infection (A02.-)
toxic effect of noxious foodstuffs (T61-T62)

cc**A05.0** **Foodborne staphylococcal intoxication**

cc**A05.1** **Botulism food poisoning** — A form caused by the neurotoxin (Botulin) produced by the growth of Clostridium botulinum in improperly canned or preserved foods.
Botulism NOS
Classical foodborne intoxication due to Clostridium botulinum
Excludes 1: *infant botulism (A48.51)*
wound botulism (A48.52)

cc**A05.2** **Foodborne Clostridium perfringens [Clostridium welchii] intoxication**
Enteritis necroticans
Pig-bel

cc**A05.3** **Foodborne Vibrio parahaemolyticus intoxication**

cc**A05.4** **Foodborne Bacillus cereus intoxication**

cc**A05.5** **Foodborne Vibrio vulnificus intoxication**

cc**A05.8** **Other specified bacterial foodborne intoxications**

A05.9 **Bacterial foodborne intoxication, unspecified**

A06- <u>Amebiasis</u> — The state of being infected with Entamoeba histolytica.
Includes: Infection due to Entamoeba histolytica
Excludes 1: *other protozoal intestinal diseases (A07.-)*
Excludes ❷: *acanthamebiasis (B60.1-)*
Naegleriasis (B60.2)

cc**A06.0** **Acute amebic dysentery**
Acute amebiasis
Intestinal amebiasis NOS

cc**A06.1** **Chronic intestinal amebiasis**

cc**A06.2** **Amebic nondysenteric colitis**

cc**A06.3** **Ameboma of intestine**
Ameboma NOS

mcc**A06.4** **Amebic liver abscess**
Hepatic amebiasis

mcc**A06.5** **Amebic lung abscess**
Amebic abscess of lung (and liver)

mcc**A06.6** **Amebic brain abscess**
Amebic abscess of brain (and liver) (and lung)

A06.7 **Cutaneous amebiasis**

A06.8- **Amebic infection of other sites**

cc**A06.81** **Amebic cystitis**

cc**A06.82** **Other amebic genitourinary infections**
Amebic balanitis
Amebic vesiculitis
Amebic vulvovaginitis

cc **A06.89   Other amebic infections**
Amebic appendicitis
Amebic splenic abscess

A06.9   Amebiasis, unspecified

A07-   Other protozoal intestinal diseases

A07.0   Balantidiasis — Infection of the colon by the protozoa Balantidium coli.
Balantidial dysentery

cc **A07.1   Giardiasis [lambliasis]** — Infection of the small intestine by the species Giardia lamblia.

cc **A07.2   Cryptosporidiosis** — Intestinal infection caused by Cryptosporidium parvum.

cc **A07.3   Isosporiasis**
Infection due to Isospora belli and Isospora hominis
Intestinal coccidiosis
Isosporosis

cc **A07.4   Cyclosporiasis** — Intestinal infection, with severe diarrhea, caused by Cyclospora cayetanensis, associated with eating contaminated raspberries.

cc **A07.8   Other specified protozoal intestinal diseases**
Intestinal microsporidiosis
Intestinal trichomoniasis
Sarcocystosis
Sarcosporidiosis

cc **A07.9   Protozoal intestinal disease, unspecified**
Flagellate diarrhea
Protozoal colitis
Protozoal diarrhea
Protozoal dysentery

A08-   Viral and other specified intestinal infections
Excludes 1:   influenza with involvement of gastrointestinal tract (J09.x3, J10.2, J11.2)

cc **A08.0   Rotaviral enteritis** — Inflammation of the intestine, primarily the small intestine, caused by a group of RNA viruses and often seen in children.

A08.1-   Acute gastroenteropathy due to Norwalk agent and other small round viruses

cc **A08.11   Acute gastroenteropathy due to Norwalk agent** — Inflammation of the intestine, primarily the small intestine, caused by the adenovirus group of disease-causing viruses.
Acute gastroenteropathy due to Norovirus
Acute gastroenteropathy due to Norwalk-like agent

cc **A08.19   Acute gastroenteropathy due to other small round viruses**
Acute gastroenteropathy due to small round virus [SRV] NOS

cc **A08.2   Adenoviral enteritis**

A08.3-   Other viral enteritis

cc **A08.31   Calicivirus enteritis** — Inflammation of the intestine, primarily the small intestine, caused by a subgroup of Picornaviruses.

cc **A08.32   Astrovirus enteritis** — Inflammation of the intestine, primarily the small intestine, caused by the Astrovirus.

cc **A08.39   Other viral enteritis**
Coxsackie virus enteritis — Inflammation of the intestine, primarily the small intestine, caused by the Coxsackie virus from the enterovirus group.
Echovirus enteritis — Inflammation of the intestine, primarily the small intestine, caused by the Echovirus from the enterovirus group.
Enterovirus enteritis NEC
Torovirus enteritis

A08.4   Viral intestinal infection, unspecified
Viral enteritis NOS
Viral gastroenteritis NOS
Viral gastroenteropathy NOS

A08.8   Other specified intestinal infections

A09   Infectious gastroenteritis and colitis, unspecified — Inflammation of the
cc   colon, small intestine, and stomach of an infectious origin.
Infectious colitis NOS
Infectious enteritis NOS
Infectious gastroenteritis NOS
*Excludes 1:   colitis NOS (K52.9)
diarrhea NOS (R19.7)
enteritis NOS (K52.9)
gastroenteritis NOS (K52.9)
noninfective gastroenteritis and colitis, unspecified [K52.9]*

Tuberculosis (A15-A19)

Includes: Infections due to Mycobacterium tuberculosis and Mycobacterium bovis
*Excludes 1:   congenital tuberculosis (P37.0)
nonspecific reaction to test for tuberculosis without active tuberculosis (R76.1-)
pneumoconiosis associated with tuberculosis, any type in A15 (J65)
positive PPD (R76.11)
positive tuberculin skin test without active tuberculosis (R76.11)
sequelae of tuberculosis (B90.-)
silicotuberculosis (J65)*

A15-   Respiratory tuberculosis — An infectious disease caused by Mycobacterium tuberculosis or Mycobacterium bovis and characterized by involvement of respiratory tissues.

cc **A15.0   Tuberculosis of lung**
Tuberculous bronchiectasis
Tuberculous fibrosis of lung
Tuberculous pneumonia
Tuberculous pneumothorax

cc **A15.4   Tuberculosis of intrathoracic lymph nodes**
Tuberculosis of hilar lymph nodes
Tuberculosis of mediastinal lymph nodes
Tuberculosis of tracheobronchial lymph nodes
Excludes 1:   tuberculosis specified as primary (A15.7)

cc **A15.5   Tuberculosis of larynx, trachea and bronchus**
Tuberculosis of bronchus
Tuberculosis of glottis
Tuberculosis of larynx
Tuberculosis of trachea

cc **A15.6   Tuberculous pleurisy**
Tuberculosis of pleura
Tuberculous empyema
Excludes 1:   primary respiratory tuberculosis (A15.7)

cc **A15.7   Primary respiratory tuberculosis**

cc **A15.8   Other respiratory tuberculosis**
Mediastinal tuberculosis
Nasopharyngeal tuberculosis
Tuberculosis of nose
Tuberculosis of sinus [any nasal]

cc **A15.9   Respiratory tuberculosis unspecified**

A17-   Tuberculosis of nervous system — An infectious disease caused by Mycobacterium tuberculosis or Mycobacterium bovis and characterized by involvement of meninges and the nervous system.

MCC **A17.0   Tuberculous meningitis**
Tuberculosis of meninges (cerebral) (spinal)
Tuberculous leptomeningitis
Excludes 1:   tuberculous meningoencephalitis (A17.82)

MCC **A17.1   Meningeal tuberculoma**
Tuberculoma of meninges (cerebral) (spinal)
Excludes ❷: tuberculoma of brain and spinal cord (A17.81)

A17.8-   Other tuberculosis of nervous system

MCC **A17.81   Tuberculoma of brain and spinal cord**
Tuberculous abscess of brain and spinal cord

MCC **A17.82   Tuberculous meningoencephalitis**
Tuberculous myelitis

MCC **A17.83   Tuberculous neuritis**
Tuberculous mononeuropathy

MCC **A17.89   Other tuberculosis of nervous system**
Tuberculous polyneuropathy

cc **A17.9   Tuberculosis of nervous system, unspecified**

A18-   Tuberculosis of other organs

A18.0-   Tuberculosis of bones and joints

cc **A18.01   Tuberculosis of spine**
Pott's disease or curvature of spine
Tuberculous arthritis
Tuberculous osteomyelitis of spine
Tuberculous spondylitis

cc **A18.02   Tuberculous arthritis of other joints**
Tuberculosis of hip (joint)
Tuberculosis of knee (joint)

cc **A18.03   Tuberculosis of other bones**
Tuberculous mastoiditis
Tuberculous osteomyelitis

A 0 6 - A 1 8

cc **A18.09** **Other musculoskeletal tuberculosis**
　　　　Tuberculous myositis
　　　　Tuberculous synovitis
　　　　Tuberculous tenosynovitis

A18.1- **Tuberculosis of <u>genitourinary</u> system** — An infectious disease caused by Mycobacterium tuberculosis or Mycobacterium bovis and characterized by involvement of the genitourinary system.

cc **A18.10** **Tuberculosis of genitourinary system, unspecified**

cc **A18.11** **Tuberculosis of kidney and ureter**

cc **A18.12** **Tuberculosis of bladder**

cc **A18.13** **Tuberculosis of other urinary organs**
　　　　Tuberculous urethritis

cc **A18.14** **Tuberculosis of prostate** — [♂, Age/15-124]

cc **A18.15** **Tuberculosis of other male genital organs** — [♂]

cc **A18.16** **Tuberculosis of cervix** — [♀]

cc **A18.17** **Tuberculous female pelvic inflammatory disease** — [♀]
　　　　Tuberculous endometritis
　　　　Tuberculous oophoritis and salpingitis

cc **A18.18** **Tuberculosis of other female genital organs** — [♀]
　　　　Tuberculous ulceration of vulva

cc **A18.2** **Tuberculous peripheral <u>lymphadenopathy</u>**
　　　　Tuberculous adenitis
　　　Excludes ❷:　*tuberculosis of bronchial and mediastinal lymph nodes (A15.4)*
　　　　　tuberculosis of mesenteric and retroperitoneal lymph nodes (A18.39)
　　　　　tuberculous tracheobronchial adenopathy (A15.4)

A18.3- **Tuberculosis of <u>intestines</u>, peritoneum and mesenteric glands**

MCC **A18.31** **Tuberculous peritonitis**
　　　　Tuberculous ascites

cc **A18.32** **Tuberculous enteritis**
　　　　Tuberculosis of anus and rectum
　　　　Tuberculosis of intestine (large) (small)

cc **A18.39** **Retroperitoneal tuberculosis**
　　　　Tuberculosis of mesenteric glands
　　　　Tuberculosis of retroperitoneal (lymph glands)

cc **A18.4** **Tuberculosis of <u>skin</u> and subcutaneous tissue**
　　　　Erythema induratum, tuberculous
　　　　Lupus excedens
　　　　Lupus vulgaris NOS
　　　　Lupus vulgaris of eyelid
　　　　Scrofuloderma
　　　　Tuberculosis of external ear
　　　Excludes ❷:　*lupus erythematosus (L93.-)*
　　　　　lupus NOS (M32.9)
　　　　　systemic (M32.-)

A18.5- **Tuberculosis of <u>eye</u>**
　　　Excludes ❷:　*lupus vulgaris of eyelid (A18.4)*

cc **A18.50** **Tuberculosis of eye, unspecified**

cc **A18.51** **Tuberculous episcleritis**

cc **A18.52** **Tuberculous keratitis**
　　　　Tuberculous interstitial keratitis
　　　　Tuberculous keratoconjunctivitis (interstitial) (phlyctenular)

cc **A18.53** **Tuberculous chorioretinitis**

cc **A18.54** **Tuberculous iridocyclitis**

cc **A18.59** **Other tuberculosis of eye**
　　　　Tuberculous conjunctivitis

cc **A18.6** **Tuberculosis of (inner) (middle) <u>ear</u>**
　　　　Tuberculous otitis media
　　　Excludes ❷:　*tuberculosis of external ear (A18.4)*
　　　　　tuberculous mastoiditis (A18.03)

cc **A18.7** **Tuberculosis of <u>adrenal</u> glands**
　　　　Tuberculous Addison's disease

A18.8- **Tuberculosis of <u>other specified</u> organs**

cc **A18.81** **Tuberculosis of thyroid gland**

cc **A18.82** **Tuberculosis of other endocrine glands**
　　　　Tuberculosis of pituitary gland
　　　　Tuberculosis of thymus gland

cc **A18.83** **Tuberculosis of digestive tract organs, not elsewhere classified**
　　　Excludes 1:　*tuberculosis of intestine (A18.32)*

cc **A18.84** **Tuberculosis of heart**
　　　　Tuberculous cardiomyopathy
　　　　Tuberculous endocarditis
　　　　Tuberculous myocarditis
　　　　Tuberculous pericarditis

cc **A18.85** **Tuberculosis of spleen**

cc **A18.89** **Tuberculosis of other sites**
　　　　Tuberculosis of muscle
　　　　Tuberculous cerebral arteritis

A19- **<u>Miliary</u> tuberculosis** — An infectious disease caused by Mycobacterium tuberculosis or Mycobacterium bovis and characterized by dissemination of viable tubercle bacilli into the bloodstream with infection throughout the body.
　　　Includes:　Disseminated tuberculosis
　　　　　Generalized tuberculosis
　　　　　Tuberculous polyserositis

MCC **A19.0** **Acute miliary tuberculosis of a single specified site**

MCC **A19.1** **Acute miliary tuberculosis of multiple sites**

MCC **A19.2** **Acute miliary tuberculosis, unspecified**

MCC **A19.8** **Other miliary tuberculosis**

MCC **A19.9** **Miliary tuberculosis, unspecified**

Certain zoonotic bacterial diseases (A20-A28)

A20- **<u>Plague</u>** — A febrile infectious disease caused by Yersinia pestis, characterized by acute fever and chills followed by prostration and commonly marked with delirium, headache, vomiting, and diarrhea. Primarily a disease of rodents, it is transmitted to man by the bite of infected fleas and communicated from patient to patient.
　　　Includes:　Infection due to Yersinia pestis

MCC **A20.0** **Bubonic plague**

MCC **A20.1** **Cellulocutaneous plague**

MCC **A20.2** **Pneumonic plague**

MCC **A20.3** **Plague meningitis**

MCC **A20.7** **Septicemic plague**

MCC **A20.8** **Other forms of plague**
　　　　Abortive plague
　　　　Asymptomatic plague
　　　　Pestis minor

MCC **A20.9** **Plague, unspecified**

A21- **<u>Tularemia</u>** — A febrile infectious disease (resembling plague) caused by Francisella tularensis, and characterized by fever, chills, headache, and myalgia. It is transmitted to man by bites from infected flies, fleas, ticks, and lice.
　　　Includes:　Deer-fly fever
　　　　　Infection due to Francisella tularensis
　　　　　Rabbit fever

cc **A21.0** **Ulceroglandular tularemia**

cc **A21.1** **Oculoglandular tularemia**
　　　　Ophthalmic tularemia

cc **A21.2** **Pulmonary tularemia**

cc **A21.3** **Gastrointestinal tularemia**
　　　　Abdominal tularemia

cc **A21.7** **Generalized tularemia**

cc **A21.8** **Other forms of tularemia**

cc **A21.9** **Tularemia, unspecified**

A22- **<u>Anthrax</u>** — An infectious disease caused by Bacillus anthracis and characterized by ulcerated papules which form black eschars with following necrosis. It is transmitted to man by direct and indirect contact with infected animals and their commerical products.
　　　Includes:　Infection due to Bacillus anthracis

cc **A22.0** **Cutaneous anthrax**
　　　　Malignant carbuncle
　　　　Malignant pustule

MCC **A22.1** **Pulmonary anthrax**
　　　　Inhalation anthrax
　　　　Ragpicker's disease
　　　　Woolsorter's disease

cc **A22.2** **Gastrointestinal anthrax**

MCC **A22.7** **Anthrax sepsis**

cc **A22.8** **Other forms of anthrax**
　　　　Anthrax meningitis

cc **A22.9** **Anthrax, unspecified**

A18 – A22

A23-   **Brucellosis** — An infectious disease caused by Brucella bacterial species, characterized by fever, chills, headache, aches and pains, and weakness.

Includes: Malta fever
Mediterranean fever
Undulant fever

A23.0   **Brucellosis due to Brucella melitensis**

A23.1   **Brucellosis due to Brucella abortus**

A23.2   **Brucellosis due to Brucella suis**

A23.3   **Brucellosis due to Brucella canis**

cc **A23.8**   **Other brucellosis**

cc **A23.9**   **Brucellosis, unspecified**

A24-   **Glanders and melioidosis**

cc **A24.0**   **Glanders** — An infectious disease caused by Pseudomonas mallei and characterized by inflammation of mucous membranes and development of nodules of the skin which break down to ulcers. It is transmitted to man by infected horses.

Infection due to Pseudomonas mallei
Malleus

cc **A24.1**   **Acute and fulminating melioidosis**
Melioidosis pneumonia
Melioidosis sepsis

cc **A24.2**   **Subacute and chronic melioidosis**

cc **A24.3**   **Other melioidosis**

cc **A24.9**   **Melioidosis, unspecified** — An infectious disease caused by Pseudomonas pseudomallei, variously marked by fever, chills, bloodstained sputum, diarrhea, abdominal pain, and in less acute cases granulomatous pneumonia and multiple skin abscess formations.

Infection due to Pseudomonas pseudomallei NOS
Whitmore's disease

A25-   **Rat-bite fevers**

cc **A25.0**   **Spirillosis** — An infectious disease caused by Spirillum minor and characterized by local inflammation at the site of the rat bite, regional lymphadenopathy, macular red-brown rash, and fever of sudden onset.

Sodoku

cc **A25.1**   **Streptobacillosis** — An infectious disease caused by Streptobacillus moniliformis and characterized by sudden onset of fever, erythematous eruption, polyarthritis, adenitis, headache, and vomiting.

Epidemic arthritic erythema
Haverhill fever
Streptobacillary rat-bite fever

cc **A25.9**   **Rat-bite fever, unspecified**

A26-   **Erysipeloid** — An infectious disease caused by Erysipelothrix insidiosa or Erysipelothrix rhusiopathiae and characterized by local inflammation at an abrasion site after contact with infected meat.

A26.0   **Cutaneous erysipeloid**
Erythema migrans

mcc **A26.7**   **Erysipelothrix sepsis**

A26.8   **Other forms of erysipeloid**

A26.9   **Erysipeloid, unspecified**

A27-   **Leptospirosis** — An infectious bacterial disease caused by the genus Leptospira and generally characterized by fever, chills, headache, malaise, and occasionally meningitis, uveitis, hepatitis, and nephritis.

cc **A27.0**   **Leptospirosis icterohemorrhagica** — A form caused by Leptospira icterhaemorrhagiae and characterized by fever, jaundice, myalgia, hemorrhage, anemia, and sometimes vascular collapse.

Leptospiral or spirochetal jaundice (hemorrhagic)
Weil's disease

A27.8-   **Other forms of leptospirosis**

mcc **A27.81**   **Aseptic meningitis in leptospirosis**

cc **A27.89**   **Other forms of leptospirosis**

cc **A27.9**   **Leptospirosis, unspecified**

A28-   **Other zoonotic bacterial diseases, not elsewhere classified**

cc **A28.0**   **Pasteurellosis** — An infectious disease caused by Pasteurella multocida and variously characterized by local infections, respiratory infections, or systemic infections such as meningitis and bacteremia.

cc **A28.1**   **Cat-scratch disease** — An infectious disease caused by Bartonella henselae and characterized by regional lymphadenitis, granulomatous skin reaction at the site of injury from a cat, and mild fever.

Cat-scratch fever

cc **A28.2**   **Extraintestinal yersiniosis**
Excludes 1:   enteritis due to Yersinia enterocolitica (A04.6)
plague (A20.-)

cc **A28.8**   **Other specified zoonotic bacterial diseases, not elsewhere classified**

cc **A28.9**   **Zoonotic bacterial disease, unspecified**

Other bacterial diseases (A30-A49)

A30-   **Leprosy [Hansen's disease]** — A chronic infectious disease caused by Mycobacterium leprae and primarily characterized by granulomatous lesions of the skin, peripheral nerves, and mucous membranes.

Includes: Infection due to Mycobacterium leprae
Excludes 1:   sequelae of leprosy (B92)

cc **A30.0**   **Indeterminate leprosy**
I leprosy

cc **A30.1**   **Tuberculoid leprosy**
TT leprosy

cc **A30.2**   **Borderline tuberculoid leprosy**
BT leprosy

cc **A30.3**   **Borderline leprosy**
BB leprosy

cc **A30.4**   **Borderline lepromatous leprosy**
BL leprosy

cc **A30.5**   **Lepromatous leprosy**
LL leprosy

cc **A30.8**   **Other forms of leprosy**

cc **A30.9**   **Leprosy, unspecified**

A31-   **Infection due to other mycobacteria**
Excludes ❷: leprosy (A30.-)
tuberculosis (A15-A19)

cc **A31.0**   **Pulmonary mycobacterial infection**
Infection due to Mycobacterium avium
Infection due to Mycobacterium intracellulare [Battey bacillus]
Infection due to Mycobacterium kansasii

cc **A31.1**   **Cutaneous mycobacterial infection**
Buruli ulcer
Infection due to Mycobacterium marinum
Infection due to Mycobacterium ulcerans

cc **A31.2**   **Disseminated mycobacterium avium-intracellulare complex (DMAC)**
MAC sepsis

cc **A31.8**   **Other mycobacterial infections**

cc **A31.9**   **Mycobacterial infection, unspecified**
Atypical mycobacterial infection NOS
Mycobacteriosis NOS

A32-   **Listeriosis** — An infectious disease caused by Listeria monocytogenes and characterized by sore throat with glandular swelling, monocytosis, septicemia, conjunctivitis, involvement of the liver, and localized purulent mucous membrane inflammations.

Includes: Listerial foodborne infection
Excludes 1:   neonatal (disseminated) listeriosis (P37.2)

cc **A32.0**   **Cutaneous listeriosis**

A32.1-   **Listerial meningitis and meningoencephalitis**

cc **A32.11**   **Listerial meningitis**

cc **A32.12**   **Listerial meningoencephalitis**

mcc **A32.7**   **Listerial sepsis**

A32.8-   **Other forms of listeriosis**

cc **A32.81**   **Oculoglandular listeriosis**

cc **A32.82**   **Listerial endocarditis**

cc **A32.89**   **Other forms of listeriosis**
Listerial cerebral arteritis

cc **A32.9**   **Listeriosis, unspecified**

A33   **Tetanus neonatorum** — [Age/0]
mcc

A34   **Obstetrical tetanus** — [♀, Age/12-55]
cc

A35   **Other tetanus** — An infectious disease complication of wounds caused by the toxin
mcc   produced by Clostridium tetani and characterized by tonic spasms of the voluntary muscles, hyperreflexia resulting in trismus (lockjaw), severe cases developing generalized convulsions and respiratory distress.

Tetanus NOS
Excludes 1:   obstetrical tetanus (A34)
tetanus neonatorum (A33)

Excludes 1: = NOT CODED HERE! (Do not code both)   **531**   Excludes ❷: = Not Included Here

A36- <u>Diphtheria</u> — An infectious disease caused by Corynebacterium diphtheriae, and characterized by a membrane in the pharynx, sore throat, fever, nausea, vomiting, headache, and chills.

- CC **A36.0** **Pharyngeal diphtheria**
  Diphtheritic membranous angina
  Tonsillar diphtheria

- CC **A36.1** **Nasopharyngeal diphtheria**

- CC **A36.2** **Laryngeal diphtheria**
  Diphtheritic laryngotracheitis

- CC **A36.3** **Cutaneous diphtheria**
  Excludes ❷: erythrasma (L08.1)

- **A36.8-** **Other diphtheria**
  - CC **A36.81** **Diphtheritic cardiomyopathy**
    Diphtheritic myocarditis
  - CC **A36.82** **Diphtheritic radiculomyelitis**
  - CC **A36.83** **Diphtheritic polyneuritis**
  - CC **A36.84** **Diphtheritic tubulo-interstitial nephropathy**
  - CC **A36.85** **Diphtheritic cystitis**
  - CC **A36.86** **Diphtheritic conjunctivitis**
  - CC **A36.89** **Other diphtheritic complications**
    Diphtheritic peritonitis

- CC **A36.9** **Diphtheria, unspecified**

A37- <u>Whooping cough</u> — An infectious disease caused by Bordetella pertussis and characterized by progressive and repetitive paroxysmal coughing, mild systemic complaints, lymphocytosis, and inspiratory whoop.

- **A37.0-** **Whooping cough due to Bordetella pertussis**
  - CC **A37.00** **Whooping cough due to Bordetella pertussis without pneumonia**
  - MCC **A37.01** **Whooping cough due to Bordetella pertussis with pneumonia**

- **A37.1-** **Whooping cough due to Bordetella parapertussis**
  - CC **A37.10** **Whooping cough due to Bordetella parapertussis without pneumonia**
  - MCC **A37.11** **Whooping cough due to Bordetella parapertussis with pneumonia**

- **A37.8-** **Whooping cough due to other Bordetella species**
  - CC **A37.80** **Whooping cough due to other Bordetella species without pneumonia**
  - MCC **A37.81** **Whooping cough due to other Bordetella species with pneumonia**

- **A37.9-** **Whooping cough, unspecified species**
  - CC **A37.90** **Whooping cough, unspecified species without pneumonia**
  - MCC **A37.91** **Whooping cough, unspecified species with pneumonia**

A38- <u>Scarlet fever</u> — An acute febrile infectious disease caused by Group A Streptococcus and characterized by high fever, sore throat, and skin rash.
  Includes: scarlatina
  Excludes ❷: streptococcal sore throat (J02.0)

- CC **A38.0** **Scarlet fever with otitis media**
- CC **A38.1** **Scarlet fever with myocarditis**
- CC **A38.8** **Scarlet fever with other complications**
- CC **A38.9** **Scarlet fever, uncomplicated**
  Scarlet fever, NOS

A39- <u>Meningococcal</u> infection — Infectious diseases caused by Neisseria meningitidis.

- MCC **A39.0** **Meningococcal meningitis** — A form characterized by inflammation of the cerebral and spinal meninges.

- MCC **A39.1** **Waterhouse-Friderichsen syndrome** — The fulminating form characterized by abrupt sudden high fever, chills, myalgias, nausea, vomiting, headache, widespread ecchymotic rash, and buccal mucosa and conjunctival hemorrhages, with cyanosis, hypotension, profound shock, and bilateral adrenal hemorrhages.
  Meningococcal hemorrhagic adrenalitis
  Meningococcic adrenal syndrome

- MCC **A39.2** **Acute meningococcemia**
- MCC **A39.3** **Chronic meningococcemia**
- MCC **A39.4** **Meningococcemia, unspecified**

- **A39.5-** **Meningococcal heart disease**
  - MCC **A39.50** **Meningococcal carditis, unspecified**
  - MCC **A39.51** **Meningococcal endocarditis**
  - MCC **A39.52** **Meningococcal myocarditis**
  - MCC **A39.53** **Meningococcal pericarditis**

- **A39.8-** **Other meningococcal infections**
  - MCC **A39.81** **Meningococcal encephalitis**
  - CC **A39.82** **Meningococcal retrobulbar neuritis**
  - CC **A39.83** **Meningococcal arthritis**
  - CC **A39.84** **Postmeningococcal arthritis**
  - CC **A39.89** **Other meningococcal infections**
    Meningococcal conjunctivitis

- CC **A39.9** **Meningococcal infection, unspecified**
  Meningococcal disease NOS

A40- <u>Streptococcal sepsis</u> — Streptococcal bacteria in the bloodstream marked by high fever, shaking, chills, prostration, and if untreated, hypotension, shock, and death.
  Code first: Postprocedural streptococcal sepsis (T81.4-)
  Streptococcal sepsis during labor (O75.3)
  Streptococcal sepsis following abortion or ectopic or molar pregnancy (O03-O07, O08.0)
  Streptococcal sepsis following immunization (T88.0)
  Streptococcal sepsis following infusion, transfusion or therapeutic injection (T80.2-)
  Excludes 1: neonatal (P36.0-P36.1)
  puerperal sepsis (O85)
  sepsis due to Streptococcus, group D (A41.81)

- MCC **A40.0** **Sepsis due to streptococcus, group A**
- MCC **A40.1** **Sepsis due to streptococcus, group B**
- MCC **A40.3** **Sepsis due to Streptococcus pneumoniae**
  Pneumococcal sepsis
- MCC **A40.8** **Other streptococcal sepsis**
- MCC **A40.9** **Streptococcal sepsis, unspecified**

A41- <u>Other sepsis</u>
 AHA 16:1Q:p32 – Resolving sepsis
 Code first: Postprocedural sepsis (T81.4-)
   Sepsis during labor (O75.3)
   Sepsis following abortion, ectopic or molar pregnancy
     (O03-O07, O08.0)
   Sepsis following immunization (T88.0)
   Sepsis following infusion, transfusion or therapeutic injection
     (T80.2-)
 Excludes 1: *bacteremia NOS (R78.81)*
   neonatal (P36.-)
   puerperal sepsis (O85)
   streptococcal sepsis (A40.-)
 Excludes ❷: *sepsis (due to) (in) actinomycotic (A42.7)*
   sepsis (due to) (in) anthrax (A22.7)
   sepsis (due to) (in) candidal (B37.7)
   sepsis (due to) (in) Erysipelothrix (A26.7)
   sepsis (due to) (in) extraintestinal yersiniosis (A28.2)
   sepsis (due to) (in) gonococcal (A54.86)
   sepsis (due to) (in) herpesviral (B00.7)
   sepsis (due to) (in) listerial (A32.7)
   sepsis (due to) (in) melioidosis (A24.1)
   sepsis (due to) (in) meningococcal (A39.2-A39.4)
   sepsis (due to) (in) plague (A20.7)
   sepsis (due to) (in) tularemia (A21.7)
   toxic shock syndrome (A48.3)

A41.0- Sepsis due to <u>Staphylococcus aureus</u> — Staphylococcus aureus bacteria in the bloodstream marked by high fever, shaking, chills, prostration, and if untreated, hypotension, shock, and death.

MCC**A41.01 <u>Sepsis</u> due to methicillin <u>susceptible</u> Staphylococcus aureus** — A form caused by a form of the bacterium Staphylococcus aureus that is susceptible to antibiotic treatment.
   MSSA sepsis
   Staphylococcus aureus sepsis NOS

MCC**A41.02 <u>Sepsis</u> due to methicillin <u>resistant</u> Staphylococcus aureus** — A form caused by a form of the bacterium Staphylococcus aureus that is resistant to treatment from beta-lactam class antibiotics.

MCC**A41.1 Sepsis due to other specified staphylococcus**
   Coagulase negative staphylococcus sepsis

MCC**A41.2 Sepsis due to unspecified staphylococcus**

MCC**A41.3 Sepsis due to <u>Hemophilus influenzae</u>**

MCC**A41.4 Sepsis due to anaerobes**
   Excludes 1: *gas gangrene (A48.0)*

A41.5- Sepsis due to other Gram-negative organisms

MCC**A41.50 Gram-negative sepsis, unspecified**
   Gram-negative sepsis NOS

MCC**A41.51 Sepsis due to <u>Escherichia coli [E. coli]</u>**

MCC**A41.52 Sepsis due to <u>Pseudomonas</u>**
   Pseudomonas aeroginosa

MCC**A41.53 Sepsis due to <u>Serratia</u>**

MCC**A41.59 Other Gram-negative sepsis**

A41.8- Other specified sepsis

MCC**A41.81 Sepsis due to <u>Enterococcus</u>**

MCC**A41.89 Other specified sepsis**

MCC**A41.9 Sepsis, unspecified organism**
   Septicemia NOS

A42- <u>Actinomycosis</u> — A group of gram-positive infectious diseases classified to the bacterial families Actinomycetaceae and Propionibacteriaceae, often by Actinomyces israelii.
 Excludes 1: *actinomycetoma (B47.1)*

CC**A42.0 Pulmonary actinomycosis**

CC**A42.1 Abdominal actinomycosis**

CC**A42.2 Cervicofacial actinomycosis**

MCC**A42.7 Actinomycotic sepsis**

A42.8- Other forms of actinomycosis

CC**A42.81 Actinomycotic meningitis**

CC**A42.82 Actinomycotic encephalitis**

CC**A42.89 Other forms of actinomycosis**

CC**A42.9 Actinomycosis, unspecified**

A43- <u>Nocardiosis</u> — Infection by bacterium of the genus Nocardia, most commonly Nocardia asteroides or Nocardia brasiliensis.

CC**A43.0 Pulmonary nocardiosis**

CC**A43.1 Cutaneous nocardiosis**

CC**A43.8 Other forms of nocardiosis**

CC**A43.9 Nocardiosis, unspecified**

A44- <u>Bartonellosis</u> — An infectious bacterial disease caused by Bartonella bacilliformis, and characterized by acute febrile hemolytic anemia, and hemangioma-like nodules on the skin.

CC**A44.0 Systemic bartonellosis**
   Oroya fever

CC**A44.1 Cutaneous and mucocutaneous bartonellosis**
   Verruga peruana

CC**A44.8 Other forms of bartonellosis**

CC**A44.9 Bartonellosis, unspecified**

A46 <u>Erysipelas</u> — An infectious contagious disease of the skin and subcutaneous tissue caused by Group A Beta-hemolytic Streptococcus, and characterized by obstructed lymphatics, redness and swelling of the affected areas, and sometimes large tension bullae.
 Excludes 1: *postpartum or puerperal erysipelas (O86.89)*

A48- Other bacterial diseases, not elsewhere classified
 Excludes 1: *actinomycetoma (B47.1)*

MCC**A48.0 Gas gangrene** — An acute infectious disease caused by the genus Clostridium, and characterized by severe, painful histotoxic infection of muscles and subcutaneous tissues which fill with gas and a serosanguineous exudate.
   Clostridial cellulitis
   Clostridial myonecrosis

MCC**A48.1 Legionnaires' disease** — An infectious disease caused by the genus Legionella, usually by Legionella pneumophila and characterized by infection of the respiratory sytem, fever, chills, and cough.

A48.2 Nonpneumonic Legionnaires' disease [Pontiac fever] — A milder form resembling the flu.

MCC**A48.3 Toxic shock syndrome** — An acute infectious bacterial disease caused by Staphylococcus aureus or Group A Streptococcus bacteria, characterized by abrupt onset of high fever, vomiting, diarrhea, sunburn-like rash, and myalgia, followed by hypotension and in severe cases, shock and multi-organ failure.
   Use additional code to identify the organism (B95, B96)
   Excludes 1: *endotoxic shock NOS (R57.8)*
     sepsis NOS (A41.9)

A48.4 Brazilian purpuric fever
   Systemic Hemophilus aegyptius infection

A48.5- Other specified botulism
   Non-foodborne intoxication due to toxins of Clostridium botulinum [C. botulinum]
   Excludes 1: *food poisoning due to toxins of Clostridium botulinum (A05.1)*

CC**A48.51 Infant botulism** — [Age/0-17]

CC**A48.52 Wound botulism**
   Non-foodborne botulism NOS
   Use additional code for associated wound

A48.8 Other specified bacterial diseases

A49- Bacterial <u>infection</u> of <u>unspecified site</u>
 Excludes 1: *bacterial agents as the cause of diseases classified elsewhere (B95-B96)*
   chlamydial infection NOS (A74.9)
   meningococcal infection NOS (A39.9)
   rickettsial infection NOS (A79.9)
   spirochetal infection NOS (A69.9)

A49.0- Staphylococcal infection, unspecified site

A49.01 Methicillin <u>susceptible</u> Staphylococcus aureus <u>infection</u>, unspecified site — An infection caused by a form of the bacterium Staphylococcus aureus that is susceptible to antibiotic treatment.
   Methicillin susceptible Staphylococcus aureus (MSSA) infection
   Staphylococcus aureus infection NOS

A49.02 Methicillin <u>resistant</u> Staphylococcus aureus <u>infection</u>, unspecified site — An infection caused by a form of the bacterium Staphylococcus aureus that is resistant to treatment from beta-lactam class antibiotics.
   Methicillin resistant Staphylococcus aureus (MRSA) infection

A49.1 Streptococcal infection, unspecified site

A49.2 Hemophilus influenzae infection, unspecified site

A49.3 Mycoplasma infection, unspecified site

A49.8 Other bacterial infections of unspecified site

A49.9 Bacterial infection, unspecified
 Excludes 1: *bacteremia NOS (R78.81)*

A41-A49

Infections with a <u>predominantly sexual mode</u> of transmission (A50-A64)

Excludes 1: *human immunodeficiency virus [HIV] disease (B20)*
nonspecific and nongonococcal urethritis (N34.1)
Reiter's disease (M02.3-)

A50- <u>Congenital</u> syphilis — An infectious bacterial disease caused by Treponema pallidum, which is transmitted transplacentally to the fetus from an infected pregnant woman.

A50.0- **Early congenital syphilis, symptomatic** — A form characterized by an enlarged liver and spleen, periostitis and osteochondritis, purulent nasal discharge, and skin lesions and patches on mucous membranes.
>   Any congenital syphilitic condition specified as early or manifest less than two years after birth.

CC **A50.01** **Early congenital syphilitic oculopathy**

CC **A50.02** **Early congenital syphilitic osteochondropathy**

CC **A50.03** **Early congenital syphilitic pharyngitis**
>   Early congenital syphilitic laryngitis

CC **A50.04** **Early congenital syphilitic pneumonia**

CC **A50.05** **Early congenital syphilitic rhinitis**

CC **A50.06** **Early cutaneous congenital syphilis**

CC **A50.07** **Early mucocutaneous congenital syphilis**

CC **A50.08** **Early visceral congenital syphilis**

CC **A50.09** **Other early congenital syphilis, symptomatic**

A50.1 **Early congenital syphilis, latent**
>   Congenital syphilis without clinical manifestations, with positive serological reaction and negative spinal fluid test, less than two years after birth

CC **A50.2** **Early congenital syphilis, unspecified**
>   Congenital syphilis NOS less than two years after birth

A50.3- **Late congenital syphilitic oculopathy**
>   *Excludes 1:* *Hutchinson's triad (A50.53)*

CC **A50.30** **Late congenital syphilitic oculopathy, unspecified**

CC **A50.31** **Late congenital syphilitic interstitial keratitis**

CC **A50.32** **Late congenital syphilitic chorioretinitis**

CC **A50.39** **Other late congenital syphilitic oculopathy**

A50.4- **Late congenital neurosyphilis [juvenile neurosyphilis]**
>   Use additional code to identify any associated mental disorder
>   *Excludes 1:* *Hutchinson's triad (A50.53)*

CC **A50.40** **Late congenital neurosyphilis, unspecified**
>   Juvenile neurosyphilis NOS

MCC **A50.41** **Late congenital syphilitic meningitis**

MCC **A50.42** **Late congenital syphilitic encephalitis**

CC **A50.43** **Late congenital syphilitic polyneuropathy**

CC **A50.44** **Late congenital syphilitic optic nerve atrophy**

CC **A50.45** **Juvenile general paresis**
>   Dementia paralytica juvenilis
>   Juvenile tabetoparetic neurosyphilis

CC **A50.49** **Other late congenital neurosyphilis**
>   Juvenile tabes dorsalis

A50.5- **Other late congenital syphilis, symptomatic**
>   Any congenital syphilitic condition specified as late or manifest two years or more after birth

CC **A50.51** **Clutton's joints**

CC **A50.52** **Hutchinson's teeth**

CC **A50.53** **Hutchinson's triad**

CC **A50.54** **Late congenital cardiovascular syphilis**

CC **A50.55** **Late congenital syphilitic arthropathy**

CC **A50.56** **Late congenital syphilitic osteochondropathy**

CC **A50.57** **Syphilitic saddle nose**

CC **A50.59** **Other late congenital syphilis, symptomatic**

A50.6 **Late congenital syphilis, latent**
>   Congenital syphilis without clinical manifestations, with positive serological reaction and negative spinal fluid test, two years or more after birth

A50.7 **Late congenital syphilis, unspecified**
>   Congenital syphilis NOS two years or more after birth

A50.9 **Congenital syphilis, unspecified**

A51- <u>Early</u> syphilis — The acquired infectious bacterial disease caused by Treponema pallidum.

A51.0 **Primary genital syphilis** — A first stage form characterized by a small, painless open sore or ulcer (called a chancre) on the genitals that heals by itself in 3 to 6 weeks.
>   Syphilitic chancre NOS

A51.1 **Primary anal syphilis** — A first stage form characterized by a small, painless open sore or ulcer (called a chancre) on the anus or rectum that heals by itself in 3 to 6 weeks.

A51.2 **Primary syphilis of other sites** — A first stage form characterized by a small, painless open sore or ulcer (called a chancre) on the mouth, skin, or other areas that heals by itself in 3 to 6 weeks.

A51.3- **Secondary syphilis of skin and mucous membranes** — The second stage of the acquired infectious bacterial disease caused by Treponema pallidum.

CC **A51.31** **Condyloma latum**

CC **A51.32** **Syphilitic alopecia**

CC **A51.39** **Other secondary syphilis of skin**
>   Syphilitic leukoderma
>   Syphilitic mucous patch
>   *Excludes 1:* *late syphilitic leukoderma (A52.79)*

A51.4- **Other secondary syphilis** — The second stage of the acquired infectious bacterial disease caused by Treponema pallidum.

MCC **A51.41** **Secondary syphilitic meningitis**

CC **A51.42** **Secondary syphilitic female pelvic disease** — [♀]

CC **A51.43** **Secondary syphilitic oculopathy**
>   Secondary syphilitic chorioretinitis
>   Secondary syphilitic iridocyclitis, iritis
>   Secondary syphilitic uveitis

CC **A51.44** **Secondary syphilitic nephritis**

CC **A51.45** **Secondary syphilitic hepatitis**

CC **A51.46** **Secondary syphilitic osteopathy**

CC **A51.49** **Other secondary syphilitic conditions**
>   Secondary syphilitic lymphadenopathy
>   Secondary syphilitic myositis

A51.5 **Early syphilis, latent**
>   Syphilis (acquired) without clinical manifestations, with positive serological reaction and negative spinal fluid test, less than two years after infection

A51.9 **Early syphilis, unspecified**

A52- <u>Late</u> syphilis — The third stage of the acquired infectious bacterial disease caused by Treponema pallidum.

A52.0- **Cardiovascular and cerebrovascular syphilis**

CC **A52.00** **Cardiovascular syphilis, unspecified**

CC **A52.01** **Syphilitic aneurysm of aorta**

CC **A52.02** **Syphilitic aortitis**

CC **A52.03** **Syphilitic endocarditis**
>   Syphilitic aortic valve incompetence or stenosis
>   Syphilitic mitral valve stenosis
>   Syphilitic pulmonary valve regurgitation

CC **A52.04** **Syphilitic cerebral arteritis**

CC **A52.05** **Other cerebrovascular syphilis**
>   Syphilitic cerebral aneurysm (ruptured) (non-ruptured)
>   Syphilitic cerebral thrombosis

CC **A52.06** **Other syphilitic heart involvement**
>   Syphilitic coronary artery disease
>   Syphilitic myocarditis
>   Syphilitic pericarditis

CC **A52.09** **Other cardiovascular syphilis**

A52.1- **Symptomatic neurosyphilis**

CC **A52.10** **Symptomatic neurosyphilis, unspecified**

CC **A52.11** **Tabes dorsalis**
>   Locomotor ataxia (progressive)
>   Tabetic neurosyphilis

CC **A52.12** **Other cerebrospinal syphilis**

MCC **A52.13** **Late syphilitic meningitis**

MCC **A52.14** **Late syphilitic encephalitis**

CC **A52.15** **Late syphilitic neuropathy**
>   Late syphilitic acoustic neuritis
>   Late syphilitic optic (nerve) atrophy
>   Late syphilitic polyneuropathy
>   Late syphilitic retrobulbar neuritis

CC **A52.16** **Charcot's arthropathy (tabetic)**

(margin tab) A50-A52

CC **A52.17 General paresis**
Dementia paralytica

CC **A52.19 Other symptomatic neurosyphilis**
Syphilitic parkinsonism

CC **A52.2 Asymptomatic neurosyphilis**

CC **A52.3 Neurosyphilis, unspecified**
Gumma (syphilitic)
Syphilis (late)
Syphiloma

A52.7- Other symptomatic late syphilis

CC **A52.71 Late syphilitic oculopathy**
Late syphilitic chorioretinitis
Late syphilitic episcleritis

CC **A52.72 Syphilis of lung and bronchus**

CC **A52.73 Symptomatic late syphilis of other respiratory organs**

CC **A52.74 Syphilis of liver and other viscera**
Late syphilitic peritonitis

CC **A52.75 Syphilis of kidney and ureter**
Syphilitic glomerular disease

CC **A52.76 Other genitourinary symptomatic late syphilis**
Late syphilitic female pelvic inflammatory disease

CC **A52.77 Syphilis of bone and joint**

CC **A52.78 Syphilis of other musculoskeletal tissue**
Late syphilitic bursitis
Syphilis [stage unspecified] of bursa
Syphilis [stage unspecified] of muscle
Syphilis [stage unspecified] of synovium
Syphilis [stage unspecified] of tendon

CC **A52.79 Other symptomatic late syphilis**
Late syphilitic leukoderma
Syphilis of adrenal gland
Syphilis of pituitary gland
Syphilis of thyroid gland
Syphilitic splenomegaly
Excludes 1:   syphilitic leukoderma (secondary) (A51.39)

A52.8 Late syphilis, latent
Syphilis (acquired) without clinical manifestations, with positive serological reaction and negative spinal fluid test, two years or more after infection

A52.9 Late syphilis, unspecified

A53- Other and unspecified syphilis

A53.0 Latent syphilis, unspecified as early or late
Latent syphilis NOS
Positive serological reaction for syphilis

A53.9 Syphilis, unspecified
Infection due to Treponema pallidum NOS
Syphilis (acquired) NOS
Excludes 1:   syphilis NOS under two years of age (A50.2)

A54- Gonococcal infection — An infectious bacterial disease caused by Neisseria gonorrhoeae and characterized by a purulent, sexually transmitted infection most commonly affecting the urethra and genital organs.

A54.0- Gonococcal infection of lower genitourinary tract without periurethral or accessory gland abscess
Excludes 1:   gonococcal infection with genitourinary gland abscess (A54.1)
gonococcal infection with periurethral abscess (A54.1)

CC **A54.00 Gonococcal infection of lower genitourinary tract, unspecified**

CC **A54.01 Gonococcal cystitis and urethritis, unspecified**

CC **A54.02 Gonococcal vulvovaginitis, unspecified** — [♀]

CC **A54.03 Gonococcal cervicitis, unspecified** — [♀]

CC **A54.09 Other gonococcal infection of lower genitourinary tract**

CC **A54.1 Gonococcal infection of lower genitourinary tract with periurethral and accessory gland abscess**
Gonococcal Bartholin's gland abscess

A54.2- Gonococcal pelviperitonitis and other gonococcal genitourinary infection

CC **A54.21 Gonococcal infection of kidney and ureter**

CC **A54.22 Gonococcal prostatitis** — [♂]

CC **A54.23 Gonococcal infection of other male genital organs** — [♂]
Gonococcal epididymitis
Gonococcal orchitis

CC **A54.24 Gonococcal female pelvic inflammatory disease** — [♀]
Gonococcal pelviperitonitis
Excludes 1:   gonococcal peritonitis (A54.85)

CC **A54.29 Other gonococcal genitourinary infections**

A54.3- Gonococcal infection of eye

CC **A54.30 Gonococcal infection of eye, unspecified**

CC **A54.31 Gonococcal conjunctivitis**
Ophthalmia neonatorum due to gonococcus

CC **A54.32 Gonococcal iridocyclitis**

CC **A54.33 Gonococcal keratitis**

CC **A54.39 Other gonococcal eye infection**
Gonococcal endophthalmia

A54.4- Gonococcal infection of musculoskeletal system

CC **A54.40 Gonococcal infection of musculoskeletal system, unspecified**

CC **A54.41 Gonococcal spondylopathy**

CC **A54.42 Gonococcal arthritis**
Excludes ❷: gonococcal infection of spine (A54.41)

CC **A54.43 Gonococcal osteomyelitis**
Excludes ❷: gonococcal infection of spine (A54.41)

CC **A54.49 Gonococcal infection of other musculoskeletal tissue**
Gonococcal bursitis
Gonococcal myositis
Gonococcal synovitis
Gonococcal tenosynovitis

A54.5 Gonococcal pharyngitis

A54.6 Gonococcal infection of anus and rectum

A54.8- Other gonococcal infections

MCC **A54.81 Gonococcal meningitis**

CC **A54.82 Gonococcal brain abscess**

CC **A54.83 Gonococcal heart infection**
Gonococcal endocarditis
Gonococcal myocarditis
Gonococcal pericarditis

CC **A54.84 Gonococcal pneumonia**

CC **A54.85 Gonococcal peritonitis**
Excludes 1:   gonococcal pelviperitonitis (A54.24)

MCC **A54.86 Gonococcal sepsis**

CC **A54.89 Other gonococcal infections**
Gonococcal keratoderma
Gonococcal lymphadenitis

CC **A54.9 Gonococcal infection, unspecified**

A55 Chlamydial lymphogranuloma (venereum) — An infectious bacterial disease caused by Chlamydia trachomatis and characterized by a painless primary urethral lesion and regional lymphadenopathy which is transmitted sexually.
Climatic or tropical bubo
Durand-Nicolas-Favre disease
Esthiomene
Lymphogranuloma inguinale

A56- Other sexually transmitted chlamydial diseases
Includes: Sexually transmitted diseases due to Chlamydia Trachomatis
Excludes 1:   neonatal chlamydial conjunctivitis (P39.1)
neonatal chlamydial pneumonia (P23.1)
Excludes ❷: chlamydial lymphogranuloma (A55)
conditions classified to A74.-

A56.0- Chlamydial infection of lower genitourinary tract — An infectious bacterial disease caused by Chlamydia trachomatis affecting the lower genitourinary tract.

A56.00 Chlamydial infection of lower genitourinary tract, unspecified

A56.01 Chlamydial cystitis and urethritis

A56.02 Chlamydial vulvovaginitis — [♀]

A56.09 Other chlamydial infection of lower genitourinary tract
Chlamydial cervicitis

A56.1- Chlamydial infection of pelviperitoneum and other genitourinary organs

A56.11 Chlamydial female pelvic inflammatory disease — [♀]

A56.19 Other chlamydial genitourinary infection
Chlamydial epididymitis
Chlamydial orchitis

A56.2 Chlamydial infection of genitourinary tract, unspecified

A
5
2
-
A
5
6

Excludes 1: = NOT CODED HERE! (Do not code both)   *Excludes ❷:* = Not Included Here

A56.3   **Chlamydial infection of anus and rectum**

A56.4   **Chlamydial infection of pharynx**

A56.8   **Sexually transmitted chlamydial infection of other sites**

A57   <u>Chancroid</u> — An infectious, bacterial disease caused by Haemophilus ducreyi and characterized by a painful genital ulceration and diffuse inguinal lymphadenitis that is transmitted sexually.
> Ulcus molle

A58   <u>Granuloma inguinale</u> — An infectious bacterial disease caused by Calymmatobacterium granulomatis and characterized by a mildly painful cutaneous or mucocutaneous genital lesion that is transmitted sexually.
> Donovanosis

A59-   <u>Trichomoniasis</u> — A parasitic disease caused by Trichomonas vaginalis and principally affecting the lower genitourinary tract that is transmitted sexually.
> *Excludes ❷: intestinal trichomoniasis (A07.8)*

   A59.0-   **Urogenital trichomoniasis**

     A59.00   **Urogenital trichomoniasis, unspecified**
> Fluor (vaginalis) due to Trichomonas
> Leukorrhea (vaginalis) due to Trichomonas

     A59.01   **Trichomonal vulvovaginitis** — [♀]

     A59.02   **Trichomonal prostatitis** — [♂]

     A59.03   **Trichomonal cystitis and urethritis**

     A59.09   **Other urogenital trichomoniasis**
> Trichomonas cervicitis

   A59.8   **Trichomoniasis of other sites**

   A59.9   **Trichomoniasis, unspecified**

A60-   <u>Anogenital herpesviral [herpes simplex] infections</u> — Viral infections of the genitourinary tract caused by herpes simplex virus, Type 2, and characterized by herpetic vesicles that is transmitted sexually and may be accompanied by fever, headache, and malaise.

   A60.0-   **Herpesviral infection of genitalia and urogenital tract**

     A60.00   **Herpesviral infection of urogenital system, unspecified**

     A60.01   **Herpesviral infection of penis** — [♂]

     A60.02   **Herpesviral infection of other male genital organs** — [♂]

     A60.03   **Herpesviral cervicitis** — [♀]

     A60.04   **Herpesviral vulvovaginitis** — [♀]
> Herpesviral [herpes simplex] ulceration
> Herpesviral [herpes simplex] vaginitis
> Herpesviral [herpes simplex] vulvitis

     A60.09   **Herpesviral infection of other urogenital tract**

   A60.1   **Herpesviral infection of perianal skin and rectum**

   A60.9   **Anogenital herpesviral infection, unspecified**

A63-   **Other predominantly sexually transmitted diseases, not elsewhere classified**
> *Excludes ❷: molluscum contagiosum (B08.1)*
>   *papilloma of cervix (D26.0)*

   A63.0   **Anogenital (venereal) warts** — An epidermal infectious viral disease caused by a human papillomavirus and characterized by cauliflower-like growths on the external genitals and transmitted mainly through infected genital contact.
> Anogenital warts due to (human) papillomavirus [HPV]
> Condyloma acuminatum

   A63.8   **Other specified predominantly sexually transmitted diseases**

A64   **Unspecified sexually transmitted disease**

Other spirochetal diseases (A65-A69)

> *Excludes ❷: leptospirosis (A27.-)*
>   *syphilis (A50-A53)*

A65   <u>Nonvenereal syphilis</u> — An infectious bacterial disease caused by species of Spirochaeta that are very similar to, but different from, syphilis.
> Bejel — An infectious bacterial disease caused by Treponema pallidium and characterized by a primary oral lesion, rashes, papillomas, and occasionally by laryngitis, pharyngitis, periostitis, generalized lymphadenopathy, and nodular ulcerations.
> Endemic syphilis
> Njovera

A66-   <u>Yaws</u> — An infectious bacterial disease caused by Treponema pertenue and characterized by a primary granulomatous lesion, later crops of granulomatous papules, and ulcerative necrosis of the lesions.
> Includes: Bouba
>   Frambesia (tropica)
>   Pian

   A66.0   **Initial lesions of yaws**
> Chancre of yaws
> Frambesia, initial or primary
> Initial frambesial ulcer
> Mother yaw

   A66.1   **Multiple papillomata and wet crab yaws**
> Frambesioma
> Pianoma
> Plantar or palmar papilloma of yaws

   A66.2   **Other early skin lesions of yaws**
> Cutaneous yaws, less than five years after infection
> Early yaws (cutaneous) (macular) (maculopapular) (micropapular) (papular)
> Frambeside of early yaws

   A66.3   **Hyperkeratosis of yaws**
> Ghoul hand
> Hyperkeratosis, palmar or plantar (early) (late) due to yaws
> Worm-eaten soles

   A66.4   **Gummata and ulcers of yaws**
> Gummatous frambeside
> Nodular late yaws (ulcerated)

   A66.5   **Gangosa**
> Rhinopharyngitis mutilans

   A66.6   **Bone and joint lesions of yaws**
> Yaws ganglion
> Yaws goundou
> Yaws gumma, bone
> Yaws gummatous osteitis or periostitis
> Yaws hydrarthrosis
> Yaws osteitis
> Yaws periostitis (hypertrophic)

   A66.7   **Other manifestations of yaws**
> Juxta-articular nodules of yaws
> Mucosal yaws

   A66.8   **Latent yaws**
> Yaws without clinical manifestations, with positive serology

   A66.9   **Yaws, unspecified**

A67-   <u>Pinta [carate]</u> — An infectious bacterial disease caused by Treponema carateum and characterized by chronic dermatosis with depigmentation.

   A67.0   **Primary lesions of pinta**
> Chancre (primary) of pinta
> Papule (primary) of pinta

   A67.1   **Intermediate lesions of pinta**
> Erythematous plaques of pinta
> Hyperchromic lesions of pinta
> Hyperkeratosis of pinta
> Pintids

   A67.2   **Late lesions of pinta**
> Achromic skin lesions of pinta
> Cicatricial skin lesions of pinta
> Dyschromic skin lesions of pinta

   A67.3   **Mixed lesions of pinta**
> Achromic with hyperchromic skin lesions of pinta [carate]

   A67.9   **Pinta, unspecified**

A68- **Relapsing fevers** — An infectious bacterial disease caused by the genus Borrelia that is characterized by febrile episodes with interim afebrile periods.

    Includes: **Recurrent fever**

    Excludes ❷: *Lyme disease (A69.2-)*

cc **A68.0** **Louse-borne relapsing fever** — A form transmitted to man by the human body louse that is caused by Borrelia recurrentis.

    Relapsing fever due to Borrelia recurrentis

cc **A68.1** **Tick-borne relapsing fever** — A form transmitted to man by ticks.

    Relapsing fever due to any Borrelia species other than Borrelia recurrentis

cc **A68.9** **Relapsing fever, unspecified**

A69- **Other spirochetal infections**

A69.0 **Necrotizing ulcerative stomatitis** — An inflammatory bacterial disease characterized by ulcerative oral lesions with severe pain.

    Cancrum oris
    Fusospirochetal gangrene
    Noma
    Stomatitis gangrenosa

cc **A69.1** **Other Vincent's infections**

    Fusospirochetal pharyngitis
    Necrotizing ulcerative (acute) gingivitis
    Necrotizing ulcerative (acute) gingivostomatitis
    Spirochetal stomatitis
    Trench mouth
    Vincent's angina
    Vincent's gingivitis

A69.2- **Lyme disease** — An infectious bacterial disease that is transmitted by ticks, caused by Borella burgdorferi and characterized by erythematous lesions, arthritis, myalgia, malaise, and other multiple systemic manifestations.

    Erythema chronicum migrans due to Borrelia burgdorferi

cc **A69.20** **Lyme disease, unspecified**

cc **A69.21** **Meningitis due to Lyme disease**

cc **A69.22** **Other neurologic disorders in Lyme disease**

    Cranial neuritis
    Meningoencephalitis
    Polyneuropathy

cc **A69.23** **Arthritis due to Lyme disease**

cc **A69.29** **Other conditions associated with Lyme disease**

    Myopericarditis due to Lyme disease

A69.8 **Other specified spirochetal infections**

A69.9 **Spirochetal infection, unspecified**

Other diseases caused by chlamydiae (A70-A74)

    Excludes 1:   *sexually transmitted chlamydial diseases (A55-A56)*

A70 **Chlamydia psittaci infections** — An infectious bacterial disease caused by
cc Chlamydia psittaci and characterized by sore throat, myalgia, cough, confusion, weakness, fever, hepatosplenomegaly, and headache.

    Ornithosis
    Parrot fever
    Psittacosis

A71- **Trachoma** — An infectious bacterial disease caused by Chlamydia trachomatis and characterized by acute inflammation of the conjunctiva.

    Excludes 1:   *sequelae of trachoma (B94.0)*

A71.0 **Initial stage of trachoma**

    Trachoma dubium

A71.1 **Active stage of trachoma**

    Granular conjunctivitis (trachomatous)
    Trachomatous follicular conjunctivitis
    Trachomatous pannus

A71.9 **Trachoma, unspecified**

A74- **Other diseases caused by chlamydiae**

    Excludes 1:   *neonatal chlamydial conjunctivitis (P39.1)*
              neonatal chlamydial pneumonia (P23.1)
              Reiter's disease (M02.3-)
              sexually transmitted chlamydial diseases (A55-A56)

    Excludes ❷: *chlamydial pneumonia (J16.0)*

A74.0 **Chlamydial conjunctivitis** — An infectious bacterial disease caused by Chlamydia trachomatis affecting the conjunctiva.

    Paratrachoma

A74.8- **Other chlamydial diseases**

A74.81 **Chlamydial peritonitis**

A74.89 **Other chlamydial diseases**

A74.9 **Chlamydial infection, unspecified**

    Chlamydiosis NOS

Rickettsioses (A75-A79)

A75- **Typhus fever**

    Excludes 1:   *rickettsiosis due to Ehrlichia sennetsu (A79.81)*

cc **A75.0** **Epidemic louse-borne typhus fever due to Rickettsia prowazekii** — An infectious bacterial disease caused by Rickettsia prowazekii and characterized by high fever, severe inflammation of the brain, and maculopapular rash, transmitted to man by lice.

    Classical typhus (fever)
    Epidemic (louse-borne) typhus

cc **A75.1** **Recrudescent typhus [Brill's disease]** — A recrudescence of louse-borne (epidemic) typhus occurs when latent infection reactivates with the same symptoms but of lower intensity.

    Brill-Zinsser disease

cc **A75.2** **Typhus fever due to Rickettsia typhi** — An infectious bacterial disease caused by Rickettsia typhi and characterized by fever and a maculopapular rash, transmitted to man by fleas.

    Murine (flea-borne) typhus

cc **A75.3** **Typhus fever due to Rickettsia tsutsugamushi** — An infectious bacterial disease caused by Orientia tsutsugamushi and characterized by fever and a maculopapular rash, transmitted to man by mites.

    Scrub (mite-borne) typhus
    Tsutsugamushi fever

cc **A75.9** **Typhus fever, unspecified**

    Typhus (fever) NOS

A77- **Spotted fever [tick-borne rickettsioses]**

cc **A77.0** **Spotted fever due to Rickettsia rickettsii** — An infectious bacterial disease caused by Rickettsia rickettsii and characterized by fever, skin rash, myalgias, intense headache, and prostration, transmitted to man by ticks.

    Rocky Mountain spotted fever
    Sao Paulo fever

cc **A77.1** **Spotted fever due to Rickettsia conorii** — An infectious bacterial disease caused by Rickettsia conorii and characterized by a primary lesion at the site of tick attachment, a maculopapular exanthem, headache, photophobia, arthralgia, and diffuse myalgia, transmitted to man by ticks.

    African tick typhus
    Boutonneuse fever
    India tick typhus
    Kenya tick typhus
    Marseilles fever
    Mediterranean tick fever

cc **A77.2** **Spotted fever due to Rickettsia siberica**

    North Asian tick fever
    Siberian tick typhus

cc **A77.3** **Spotted fever due to Rickettsia australis**

    Queensland tick typhus

A77.4- **Ehrlichiosis** — An infectious bacterial disease caused by the genus Ehrlichia and characterized by symptoms that may include fever, headache, myalgia, thrombocytopenia, and leukopenia, transmitted to man by ticks.

    Excludes 1:   *Rickettsiosis due to Ehrlichia sennetsu (A79.81)*

cc **A77.40** **Ehrlichiosis, unspecified**

cc **A77.41** **Ehrlichiosis chafeensis [E. chafeensis]**

cc **A77.49** **Other ehrlichiosis**

cc **A77.8** **Other spotted fevers**

cc **A77.9** **Spotted fever, unspecified**

    Tick-borne typhus NOS

A78 **Q fever** — An infectious bacterial disease caused by Coxiella burnetii and characterized
cc by severe headache, sweating, fever, and pneumonia.

    Infection due to Coxiella burnetii
    Nine Mile fever
    Quadrilateral fever

A79- **Other rickettsioses**

cc **A79.0** **Trench fever** — An infectious bacterial disease caused by Rochalimaea quintana and characterized by recurrent febrile episodes, severe headache, profuse sweating, myalgias, a macular rash on the chest and abdomen, and splenomegaly, transmitted to man by lice.

    Quintan fever
    Wolhynian fever

cc **A79.1** **Rickettsialpox due to Rickettsia akari**

    Kew Garden fever
    Vesicular rickettsiosis

A79.8- **Other specified rickettsioses**

cc **A79.81** **Rickettsiosis due to Ehrlichia sennetsu**

cc **A79.89** **Other specified rickettsioses**

cc **A79.9** **Rickettsiosis, unspecified**

    Rickettsial infection NOS

Excludes 1: = NOT CODED HERE! (Do not code both)   **537**   *Excludes ❷:* = Not Included Here

Viral and prion infections of the central nervous system (A80-A89)

Excludes 1:   postpolio syndrome (G14)
              sequelae of poliomyelitis (B91)
              sequelae of viral encephalitis (B94.1)

A80- Acute poliomyelitis — A viral infectious disease caused by the poliovirus, a human enterovirus, and characterized by fever, muscular pain, spasm, and paralysis which may affect the central nervous system and cause permanent muscular deformity.

MCC **A80.0 Acute paralytic poliomyelitis, vaccine-associated**

MCC **A80.1 Acute paralytic poliomyelitis, wild virus, imported**

MCC **A80.2 Acute paralytic poliomyelitis, wild virus, indigenous**

A80.3- Acute paralytic poliomyelitis, other and unspecified

MCC **A80.30 Acute paralytic poliomyelitis, unspecified**

MCC **A80.39 Other acute paralytic poliomyelitis**

A80.4 Acute nonparalytic poliomyelitis

A80.9 Acute poliomyelitis, unspecified

A81- Atypical virus infections of central nervous system
Includes: Diseases of the central nervous system caused by prions
Use additional code to identify:
Dementia with behavioral disturbance (F02.81)
Dementia without behavioral disturbance (F02.80)

A81.0- Creutzfeldt-Jakob disease

CC **A81.00 Creutzfeldt-Jakob disease, unspecified**
Jakob-Creutzfeldt disease, unspecified

CC **A81.01 Variant Creutzfeldt-Jakob disease** — A transmissible spongiform encephalopathy (TSE) causing prominent psychiatric/behavioral symptoms with delayed neurologic signs that results in death and is related to "mad cow disease" (bovine spongiform encephalopathy).
vCJD

CC **A81.09 Other Creutzfeldt-Jakob disease** — A transmissible spongiform encephalopathy (TSE) causing progressive presenile dementia, encephalopathy, and a downhill course resulting in death.
CJD
Familial Creutzfeldt-Jakob disease
Iatrogenic Creutzfeldt-Jakob disease
Sporadic Creutzfeldt-Jakob disease
Subacute spongiform encephalopathy (with dementia)

CC **A81.1 Subacute sclerosing panencephalitis** — A rare viral infectious disease affecting the brain and causing progressive mental deterioration with blindness, profound dementia, and hypothalmic dysfunction in the terminal phase.
Dawson's inclusion body encephalitis
Van Bogaert's sclerosing leukoencephalopathy

CC **A81.2 Progressive multifocal leukoencephalopathy** — A viral infectious disease characterized by demyelination of the cerebral cortex in immunologically compromised patients with symptoms of confusion, disorientation, poor memory, speech and visual disturbances, weakness, and paralysis.
Multifocal leukoencephalopathy NOS

A81.8- Other atypical virus infections of central nervous system

CC **A81.81 Kuru** — A transmissible spongiform encephalopathy (TSE) affecting the central nervous system causing tremors, flaccid paralysis, and death; found in the Fore and neighboring peoples of the mountainous regions of Papua New Guinea who practice ritualistic cannibalism.

CC **A81.82 Gerstmann-Sträussler-Scheinker syndrome** — A prion disease caused by the inheritance of a PrP gene with mutations and characterized by difficulty speaking, unsteadiness, and amyloid plaques.
GSS syndrome

CC **A81.83 Fatal familial insomnia** — A prion disease caused by the inheritance of a PrP gene with mutations and characterized by complete sleeplessness and pathological lesions in the thalamus.
FFI

CC **A81.89 Other atypical virus infections of central nervous system**

CC **A81.9 Atypical virus infection of central nervous system, unspecified**
Prion diseases of the central nervous system NOS

A82- Rabies — An infectious viral disease caused by the rabies virus and characterized by infection of the central nervous system with fever, excitation, convulsions, lacrimation, salivation, paralysis, pharyngeal spasms, coma, and usually death.

CC **A82.0 Sylvatic rabies**

CC **A82.1 Urban rabies**

CC **A82.9 Rabies, unspecified**

A83- Mosquito-borne viral encephalitis — A group of infectious viral diseases characterized by inflammation of the brain and transmitted to man by mosquitoes.
Includes: Mosquito-borne viral meningoencephalitis
Excludes ❷: Venezuelan equine encephalitis (A92.2)
              West Nile fever (A92.3-)
              West Nile virus (A92.3-)

MCC **A83.0 Japanese encephalitis**

MCC **A83.1 Western equine encephalitis**

MCC **A83.2 Eastern equine encephalitis**

MCC **A83.3 St. Louis encephalitis**

MCC **A83.4 Australian encephalitis**
Kunjin virus disease

MCC **A83.5 California encephalitis**
California meningoencephalitis
La Crosse encephalitis

MCC **A83.6 Rocio virus disease**

MCC **A83.8 Other mosquito-borne viral encephalitis**

MCC **A83.9 Mosquito-borne viral encephalitis, unspecified**

A84- Tick-borne viral encephalitis — A group of infectious viral diseases (arbovirus) caused by the genus Flavivirus, and characterized by convulsions, fever, nuchal rigidity, nausea, vomiting, and paralysis in its severe form, and transmitted to man by ticks.
Includes: Tick-borne viral meningoencephalitis

MCC **A84.0 Far Eastern tick-borne encephalitis [Russian spring-summer encephalitis]**

MCC **A84.1 Central European tick-borne encephalitis**

MCC **A84.8 Other tick-borne viral encephalitis**
Louping ill
Powassan virus disease

MCC **A84.9 Tick-borne viral encephalitis, unspecified**

A85- Other viral encephalitis, not elsewhere classified
Includes: Specified viral encephalomyelitis NEC
            Specified viral meningoencephalitis NEC
Excludes 1:   benign myalgic encephalomyelitis (G93.3)
              encephalitis due to cytomegalovirus (B25.8)
              encephalitis due to herpesvirus NEC (B10.0-)
              encephalitis due to herpesvirus [herpes simplex] (B00.4)
              encephalitis due to measles virus (B05.0)
              encephalitis due to mumps virus (B26.2)
              encephalitis due to poliomyelitis virus (A80.-)
              encephalitis due to zoster (B02.0)
              lymphocytic choriomeningitis (A87.2)

CC **A85.0 Enteroviral encephalitis**
Enteroviral encephalomyelitis

CC **A85.1 Adenoviral encephalitis**
Adenoviral meningoencephalitis

MCC **A85.2 Arthropod-borne viral encephalitis, unspecified**
Excludes 1:   West Nile virus with encephalitis (A92.31)

CC **A85.8 Other specified viral encephalitis**
Encephalitis lethargica
Von Economo-Cruchet disease

A86 Unspecified viral encephalitis
CC   Viral encephalomyelitis NOS
     Viral meningoencephalitis NOS

A87- Viral meningitis — A viral infectious inflammation of the meninges caused by Enteroviruses and characterized by malaise, fever, headache, stiff neck, and a relatively shorter benign course than bacterial meningitis.
Excludes 1:   meningitis due to herpesvirus [herpes simplex] (B00.3)
              meningitis due to measles virus (B05.1)
              meningitis due to mumps virus (B26.1)
              meningitis due to poliomyelitis virus (A80.-)
              meningitis due to zoster (B02.1)

CC **A87.0 Enteroviral meningitis**
Coxsackievirus meningitis
Echovirus meningitis

CC **A87.1 Adenoviral meningitis**

CC **A87.2 Lymphocytic choriomeningitis**
Lymphocytic meningoencephalitis

CC **A87.8 Other viral meningitis**

CC **A87.9 Viral meningitis, unspecified**

A88- **Other viral infections of central nervous system, not elsewhere classified**

  Excludes 1:   *viral encephalitis NOS (A86)*
                  viral meningitis NOS (A87.9)

cc **A88.0** **Enteroviral exanthematous fever [Boston exanthem]** — A viral infectious inflammation of the central nervous system caused by Enteroviruses.

A88.1 **Epidemic vertigo**

cc **A88.8** **Other specified viral infections of central nervous system**

A89 **Unspecified viral infection of central nervous system**
cc

Arthropod-borne viral fevers and viral hemorrhagic fevers (A90-A99)

A90 **Dengue fever [classical dengue]** — A mosquito-borne viral disease caused by
cc   the dengue virus that is characterized by fever, headache, severe myalgias, and characteristic rash.

  Excludes 1:   *dengue hemorrhagic fever (A91)*

A91 **Dengue hemorrhagic fever** — A mosquito-borne viral disease caused by
cc   the dengue virus that is characterized by fever, headache, severe myalgias, and characteristic rash that then develops bleeding, low platelet count, and dangerously low blood pressure.

A92- **Other mosquito-borne viral fevers** — Infectious febrile viral diseases transmitted by mosquitoes.

  Excludes 1:   *Ross River disease (B33.1)*

cc **A92.0** **Chikungunya virus disease**
         Chikungunya (hemorrhagic) fever

cc **A92.1** **O'nyong-nyong fever**

cc **A92.2** **Venezuelan equine fever**
         Venezuelan equine encephalitis
         Venezuelan equine encephalomyelitis virus disease

A92.3- **West Nile virus infection** — An infectious disease caused by the genus Flavivirus and characterized by a mild fever and flu-like symptoms and in severe cases, encephalitis. It originated in Africa and was first identified in the United States in 1999.
         West Nile fever

mcc **A92.30** **West Nile virus infection, unspecified**
         West Nile fever NOS
         West Nile fever without complications
         West Nile virus NOS

mcc **A92.31** **West Nile virus infection with encephalitis**
         West Nile encephalitis
         West Nile encephalomyelitis

mcc **A92.32** **West Nile virus infection with other neurologic manifestation**
         Use additional code to specify the neurologic manifestation

mcc **A92.39** **West Nile virus infection with other complications**
         Use additional code to specify the other conditions

cc **A92.4** **Rift Valley fever**

cc **A92.5** **Zika virus disease** — An infectious disease caused by the Zika virus that is characterized by fever, maculopapular rash, joint pain, and conjunctivitis, and infection during pregnancy can cause fetal microcephaly or other birth defects.
         Zika virus fever
         Zika virus infection
         Zika NOS

cc **A92.8** **Other specified mosquito-borne viral fevers**

cc **A92.9** **Mosquito-borne viral fever, unspecified**

A93- **Other arthropod-borne viral fevers, not elsewhere classified**

cc **A93.0** **Oropouche virus disease**
         Oropouche fever

cc **A93.1** **Sandfly fever**
         Pappataci fever
         Phlebotomus fever

cc **A93.2** **Colorado tick fever**

cc **A93.8** **Other specified arthropod-borne viral fevers**
         Piry virus disease
         Vesicular stomatitis virus disease [Indiana fever]

A94 **Unspecified arthropod-borne viral fever**
cc   Arboviral fever NOS
     Arbovirus infection NOS

A95- **Yellow fever** — A mosquito-borne viral disease caused by the genus Flavivirus that is characterized by fever, chills, jaundice, albuminuria, hemorrhage, and renal damage.

cc **A95.0** **Sylvatic yellow fever**
         Jungle yellow fever

cc **A95.1** **Urban yellow fever**

cc **A95.9** **Yellow fever, unspecified**

A96- **Arenaviral hemorrhagic fever** — Hemorrhagic fevers caused by Arenaviruses.

cc **A96.0** **Junin hemorrhagic fever**
         Argentinian hemorrhagic fever

cc **A96.1** **Machupo hemorrhagic fever**
         Bolivian hemorrhagic fever

A96.2 **Lassa fever**

cc **A96.8** **Other arenaviral hemorrhagic fevers**

cc **A96.9** **Arenaviral hemorrhagic fever, unspecified**

A98- **Other viral hemorrhagic fevers, not elsewhere classified**

  Excludes 1:   *chikungunya hemorrhagic fever (A92.0)*
                  dengue hemorrhagic fever (A91)

cc **A98.0** **Crimean-Congo hemorrhagic fever**
         Central Asian hemorrhagic fever

cc **A98.1** **Omsk hemorrhagic fever**

cc **A98.2** **Kyasanur Forest disease**

A98.3 **Marburg virus disease**

A98.4 **Ebola virus disease**

cc **A98.5** **Hemorrhagic fever with renal syndrome**
         Epidemic hemorrhagic fever
         Korean hemorrhagic fever
         Russian hemorrhagic fever
         Hantaan virus disease
         Hantavirus disease with renal manifestations
         Nephropathia epidemica
         Songo fever

         Excludes 1:   *hantavirus (cardio)-pulmonary syndrome (B33.4)*

cc **A98.8** **Other specified viral hemorrhagic fevers**

A99 **Unspecified viral hemorrhagic fever**
cc

Viral infections characterized by skin and mucous membrane lesions (B00-B09)

B00- **Herpesviral [herpes simplex] infections** — A viral infectious disease affecting the skin and mucous membranes caused by the herpes simplex virus, usually Type 1.

  Excludes 1:   *congenital herpesviral infections (P35.2)*
  Excludes ❷: *anogenital herpesviral infection (A60.-)*
                  gammaherpesviral mononucleosis (B27.0-)
                  herpangina (B08.5)

B00.0 **Eczema herpeticum**
         Kaposi's varicelliform eruption

B00.1 **Herpesviral vesicular dermatitis**
         Herpes simplex facialis
         Herpes simplex labialis
         Herpes simplex otitis externa
         Vesicular dermatitis of ear
         Vesicular dermatitis of lip

cc **B00.2** **Herpesviral gingivostomatitis and pharyngotonsillitis**
         Herpesviral pharyngitis

mcc **B00.3** **Herpesviral meningitis**

mcc **B00.4** **Herpesviral encephalitis**
         Herpesviral meningoencephalitis
         Simian B disease

         Excludes 1:   *herpesviral encephalitis due to herpesvirus 6 and 7 (B10.01, B10.09)*
                         non-simplex herpesviral encephalitis (B10.0-)

B00.5- **Herpesviral ocular disease**

cc **B00.50** **Herpesviral ocular disease, unspecified**

cc **B00.51** **Herpesviral iridocyclitis**
         Herpesviral iritis
         Herpesviral uveitis, anterior

cc **B00.52** **Herpesviral keratitis**
         Herpesviral keratoconjunctivitis

cc **B00.53** **Herpesviral conjunctivitis**

cc **B00.59** **Other herpesviral disease of eye**
         Herpesviral dermatitis of eyelid

A 8 8 I B 0 0

MCC **B00.7** **Disseminated** herpesviral disease
Herpesviral sepsis
B00.8- Other forms of herpesviral infections
CC **B00.81** Herpesviral **hepatitis**
MCC **B00.82** Herpes simplex **myelitis**
CC **B00.89** Other herpesviral infection
Herpesviral whitlow
B00.9 Herpesviral infection, unspecified
Herpes simplex infection NOS

B01- **Varicella [chickenpox]** — A highly contagious viral disease caused by Varicella-zoster virus, (the same virus which causes herpes zoster) that is characterized by fever and a rash which progresses rapidly from macules to papules to vesicles to pustules to crusts.
CC **B01.0** Varicella meningitis
B01.1- Varicella encephalitis, myelitis and encephalomyelitis
Postchickenpox encephalitis, myelitis and encephalomyelitis
MCC **B01.11** Varicella encephalitis and encephalomyelitis
Postchickenpox encephalitis and encephalomyelitis
MCC **B01.12** Varicella myelitis
Postchickenpox myelitis
MCC **B01.2** Varicella pneumonia
B01.8- Varicella with other complications
CC **B01.81** Varicella keratitis
CC **B01.89** Other varicella complications
CC **B01.9** Varicella without complication
Varicella NOS

B02- **Zoster [herpes zoster]** — A viral infectious disease caused by Varicella-zoster virus, (the same virus which causes chickenpox) that is characterized by unilateral radicular pain and a vesicular eruption to the surface area of an infected spinal or cerebral sensory ganglion.
Includes: Shingles
Zona
CC **B02.0** Zoster **encephalitis**
Zoster meningoencephalitis
MCC **B02.1** Zoster **meningitis**
B02.2- Zoster with **other nervous** system involvement
CC **B02.21** Postherpetic geniculate ganglionitis
CC **B02.22** Postherpetic trigeminal neuralgia
CC **B02.23** Postherpetic polyneuropathy
MCC **B02.24** Postherpetic myelitis
Herpes zoster myelitis
CC **B02.29** Other postherpetic nervous system involvement
Postherpetic radiculopathy
B02.3- Zoster **ocular** disease
CC **B02.30** Zoster ocular disease, unspecified
CC **B02.31** Zoster conjunctivitis
CC **B02.32** Zoster iridocyclitis
CC **B02.33** Zoster keratitis
Herpes zoster keratoconjunctivitis
CC **B02.34** Zoster scleritis
CC **B02.39** Other herpes zoster eye disease
Zoster blepharitis
CC **B02.7** **Disseminated** zoster
CC **B02.8** Zoster with other complications
Herpes zoster otitis externa
B02.9 Zoster without complications
Zoster NOS

B03 **Smallpox**
CC **Note:** In 1980 the 33rd World Health Assembly declared that smallpox had been eradicated. The classification is maintained for surveillance purposes.

B04 **Monkeypox** — An infectious viral disease caused by the Monkeypox virus that is
CC characterized by fever, rash, respiratory symptoms, and lymphadenopathy.

B05- **Measles** — A contagious viral infection caused by the measles virus, and characterized by fever, conjunctivitis, and a generalized maculopapular eruption.
Includes: Morbilli
Excludes 1: *subacute sclerosing panencephalitis (A81.1)*
MCC **B05.0** Measles complicated by encephalitis
Postmeasles encephalitis
CC **B05.1** Measles complicated by meningitis
Postmeasles meningitis
MCC **B05.2** Measles complicated by pneumonia
Postmeasles pneumonia
B05.3 Measles complicated by otitis media
Postmeasles otitis media
CC **B05.4** Measles with intestinal complications
B05.8- Measles with other complications
CC **B05.81** Measles keratitis and keratoconjunctivitis
CC **B05.89** Other measles complications
B05.9 Measles without complication
Measles NOS

B06- **Rubella [German measles]** — A contagious viral infection caused by the rubella virus, and characterized by a three-day generalized maculapapular rash.
Excludes 1: *congenital rubella (P35.0)*
B06.0- Rubella with neurological complications
CC **B06.00** Rubella with neurological complication, unspecified
MCC **B06.01** Rubella encephalitis
Rubella meningoencephalitis
CC **B06.02** Rubella meningitis
CC **B06.09** Other neurological complications of rubella
B06.8- Rubella with other complications
CC **B06.81** Rubella pneumonia
CC **B06.82** Rubella arthritis
CC **B06.89** Other rubella complications
B06.9 Rubella without complication
Rubella NOS

B07- **Viral warts** — An epidermal infectious viral disease caused by a human papillomavirus, that is characterized by a raised, round papillomatous growth with a horny surface that is most often located on the dorsal aspect of the hands and fingers.
Includes: Verruca simplex
Verruca vulgaris
Viral warts due to human papillomavirus
Excludes 2: *anogenital (venereal) warts (A63.0)*
papilloma of bladder (D41.4)
papilloma of cervix (D26.0)
papilloma larynx (D14.1)
B07.0 Plantar wart — A form characterized by location on the soles of the feet, and lying deep within the epidermis.
Verruca plantaris
B07.8 Other viral warts
Common wart
Flat wart
Verruca plana
B07.9 Viral wart, unspecified

B08- Other viral infections characterized by skin and mucous membrane lesions, not elsewhere classified
Excludes 1: *vesicular stomatitis virus disease (A93.8)*
B08.0- Other orthopoxvirus infections
Excludes 2: *monkeypox (B04)*
B08.01- Cowpox and vaccinia not from vaccine
B08.010 Cowpox — A viral infectious disease of cattle that is caused by the Cowpox virus, which infects man through skin contact and is characterized by vesicopustular lesions on the hands, face, and/or other cutaneous sites.
B08.011 Vaccinia not from vaccine — An infection that results from the accidentally induced vaccinia virus and is not from an intentional medical care vaccination.
Excludes 1: *vaccinia (from vaccination) (generalized) (T88.1)*
B08.02 Orf virus disease
Contagious pustular dermatitis
Ecthyma contagiosum
B08.03 Pseudocowpox [milker's node] — A viral disease characterized by circumscribed nodules on the hands of workers who milk cows infected with cowpox.

B08.04   **Paravaccinia, unspecified**

B08.09   **Other orthopoxvirus infections**
Orthopoxvirus infection NOS

B08.1   **Molluscum contagiosum** — An infectious viral disease caused by a Poxvirus, and characterized by discrete pearly skin papules containing caseous matter.

B08.2-   **Exanthema subitum [sixth disease]** — A sudden, mild viral illness caused by the human herpesvirus that is characterized by a few days of fever, followed by a faint pink rash, usually seen on the trunk.
Roseola infantum

B08.20   **Exanthema subitum [sixth disease], unspecified** — [Age/0-17]
Roseola infantum, unspecified

B08.21   **Exanthema subitum [sixth disease] due to human herpesvirus 6** — [Age/0-17]
Roseola infantum due to human herpesvirus 6

B08.22   **Exanthema subitum [sixth disease] due to human herpesvirus 7** — [Age/0-17]
Roseola infantum due to human herpesvirus 7

CC B08.3   **Erythema infectiosum [fifth disease]** — A contagious viral infectious disease that is caused by Parvovirus B19 and is characterized by a rose-colored macular rash, occurring mainly in children.

B08.4   **Enteroviral vesicular stomatitis with exanthem** — An infectious viral disease caused by Coxsackie A virus, and characterized by vesicular eruption of hands, feet, and mouth. NOTE: Foot and mouth disease (B08.8) is a separate and different infection.
Hand, foot and mouth disease

B08.5   **Enteroviral vesicular pharyngitis**
Herpangina

B08.6-   **Parapoxvirus infections**

B08.60   **Parapoxvirus infection, unspecified**

B08.61   **Bovine stomatitis** — A cutaneous infection in humans caused by contact with cattle infected with bovine papular stomatitis.

B08.62   **Sealpox** — A cutaneous infection in humans caused by contact with seals and sea lions infected with the sealpox virus.

B08.69   **Other parapoxvirus infections**

B08.7-   **Yatapoxvirus infections**

B08.70   **Yatapoxvirus infection, unspecified**

CC B08.71   **Tanapox virus disease** — A viral infection caused by the Tanapox virus that is characterized by fever, headaches, and often itching at the cutaneous lesion sites.

B08.72   **Yaba pox virus disease** — A viral infection caused by the Yaba monkey tumor virus that is characterized by a tumor or nodule containing histiocytes.
Yaba monkey tumor disease

B08.79   **Other yatapoxvirus infections**

B08.8   **Other specified viral infections characterized by skin and mucous membrane lesions**
Enteroviral lymphonodular pharyngitis
Foot-and-mouth disease — An infectious viral disease caused by picornavirus affecting cattle and rarely humans.
Poxvirus NEC

B09   **Unspecified viral infection characterized by skin and mucous membrane lesions**
Viral enanthema NOS
Viral exanthema NOS

Other human herpesviruses (B10)

B10-   **Other human herpesviruses**
Excludes ②: *cytomegalovirus (B25.9)*
Epstein-Barr virus (B27.0-)
herpes NOS (B00.9)
herpes simplex (B00-)
herpes zoster (B02-)
human herpesvirus NOS (B00-)
human herpesvirus 1 and 2 (B00-)
human herpesvirus 3 (B01.-, B02.-)
human herpesvirus 4 (B27.0-)
human herpesvirus 5 (B25-)
varicella (B01-)
zoster (B02-)

B10.0-   **Other human herpesvirus encephalitis** — Inflammation of the brain caused by a human herpesvirus infection.
Excludes ②: *herpes encephalitis NOS (B00.4)*
herpes simplex encephalitis (B00.4)
human herpesvirus encephalitis (B00.4)
simian B herpes virus encephalitis (B00.4)

MCC B10.01   **Human herpesvirus 6 encephalitis**

MCC B10.09   **Other human herpesvirus encephalitis**
Human herpesvirus 7 encephalitis

B10.8-   **Other human herpesvirus infection**

B10.81   **Human herpesvirus 6 infection**

B10.82   **Human herpesvirus 7 infection**

B10.89   **Other human herpesvirus infection**
Human herpesvirus 8 infection
Kaposi's sarcoma-associated herpesvirus infection

Viral hepatitis (B15-B19)

Excludes 1:   *sequelae of viral hepatitis (B94.2)*
Excludes ②: *cytomegaloviral hepatitis (B25.1)*
herpesviral [herpes simplex] hepatitis (B00.81)

B15-   **Acute hepatitis A** — The initial/first stage (within the first 6 months after someone is exposed) of an infection and inflammation of the liver caused by the hepatitis A virus, that is characterized by jaundice, anorexia, nausea, dark urine, pale stool, and vomiting.

MCC B15.0   **Hepatitis A with hepatic coma**

CC B15.9   **Hepatitis A without hepatic coma**
Hepatitis A (acute) (viral) NOS

B16-   **Acute hepatitis B** — The initial/first stage (within the first 6 months after someone is exposed) of an infection and inflammation of the liver caused by the hepatitis B virus, that is characterized by jaundice, urticarial skin lesions, and arthritis.

MCC B16.0   **Acute hepatitis B with delta-agent with hepatic coma**

CC B16.1   **Acute hepatitis B with delta-agent without hepatic coma**

MCC B16.2   **Acute hepatitis B without delta-agent with hepatic coma**

CC B16.9   **Acute hepatitis B without delta-agent and without hepatic coma**
Hepatitis B (acute) (viral) NOS

B17-   **Other acute viral hepatitis** — The initial/first stage (within the first 6 months after someone is exposed) of an infection and inflammation of the liver caused by a hepatitis virus.

CC B17.0   **Acute delta-(super) infection of hepatitis B carrier**

B17.1-   **Acute hepatitis C**

CC B17.10   **Acute hepatitis C without hepatic coma**
Acute hepatitis C NOS

MCC B17.11   **Acute hepatitis C with hepatic coma**

CC B17.2   **Acute hepatitis E**

CC B17.8   **Other specified acute viral hepatitis**
Hepatitis non-A non-B (acute) (viral) NEC

CC B17.9   **Acute viral hepatitis, unspecified**
Acute hepatitis NOS
Acute infectious hepatitis NOS

B08 - B17

B18- __Chronic__ viral hepatitis — The second, long-term illness stage of an infection and inflammation of the liver caused by a hepatitis virus.
    Includes: Carrier of viral hepatitis

CC **B18.0**   **Chronic viral hepatitis B with delta-agent**

CC **B18.1**   **Chronic viral hepatitis B without delta-agent**
         Carrier of viral hepatitis B
         Chronic (viral) hepatitis B

   B18.2   **Chronic viral hepatitis C**
         Carrier of viral hepatitis C

CC **B18.8**   **Other chronic viral hepatitis**
         Carrier of other viral hepatitis

CC **B18.9**   **Chronic viral hepatitis, unspecified**
         Carrier of unspecified viral hepatitis

B19- __Unspecified__ viral hepatitis

MCC **B19.0**   **Unspecified viral hepatitis with hepatic coma**

   B19.1-   **Unspecified viral hepatitis B**

   CC **B19.10**   **Unspecified viral hepatitis B without hepatic coma**
         Unspecified viral hepatitis B NOS

   MCC **B19.11**   **Unspecified viral hepatitis B with hepatic coma**

   B19.2-   **Unspecified viral hepatitis C**

   B19.20   **Unspecified viral hepatitis C without hepatic coma**
         Viral hepatitis C NOS

   MCC **B19.21**   **Unspecified viral hepatitis C with hepatic coma**

CC **B19.9**   **Unspecified viral hepatitis without hepatic coma**
         Viral hepatitis NOS

Human immunodeficiency virus [HIV] disease (B20)

B20   **Human immunodeficiency virus [HIV] disease** — A viral infectious disease
MCC   caused by the human immunodeficiency virus that attacks the immune system causing the body to have trouble fighting off disease.
    Includes: Acquired immune deficiency syndrome [AIDS]
                AIDS-related complex [ARC]
                HIV infection, symptomatic
    Code first Human immunodeficiency virus [HIV] disease complicating pregnancy, childbirth and the puerperium, if applicable (O98.7-)
    Use additional code(s) to identify all manifestations of HIV infection
    Excludes 1:   *asymptomatic human immunodeficiency virus [HIV] infection status (Z21)*
                exposure to HIV virus (Z20.6)
                inconclusive serologic evidence of HIV (R75)

Other viral diseases (B25-B34)

B25- __Cytomegaloviral disease__ — An infectious viral disease caused by the Cytomegalovirus that is characterized by fever and swollen glands.
    Excludes 1:   *congenital cytomegalovirus infection (P35.1)*
                cytomegaloviral mononucleosis (B27.1-)

MCC **B25.0**   **Cytomegaloviral pneumonitis**

CC **B25.1**   **Cytomegaloviral hepatitis**

MCC **B25.2**   **Cytomegaloviral pancreatitis**

CC **B25.8**   **Other cytomegaloviral diseases**
         Cytomegaloviral encephalitis

CC **B25.9**   **Cytomegaloviral disease, unspecified**

B26- __Mumps__ — An infectious viral disease of the paramyxovirus group, and marked most commonly by inflammation of parotid glands.
    Includes: Epidemic parotitis
                Infectious parotitis

CC **B26.0**   **Mumps orchitis** — [♂]

MCC **B26.1**   **Mumps meningitis**

MCC **B26.2**   **Mumps encephalitis**

CC **B26.3**   **Mumps pancreatitis**

   B26.8-   **Mumps with other complications**

   CC **B26.81**   **Mumps hepatitis**

   CC **B26.82**   **Mumps myocarditis**

   CC **B26.83**   **Mumps nephritis**

   CC **B26.84**   **Mumps polyneuropathy**

   CC **B26.85**   **Mumps arthritis**

   CC **B26.89**   **Other mumps complications**

   B26.9   **Mumps without complication**
         Mumps NOS
         Mumps parotitis NOS

B27- __Infectious mononucleosis__
    Includes: Glandular fever
                Monocytic angina
                Pfeiffer's disease

   B27.0-   **Gammaherpesviral mononucleosis** — An infectious viral disease caused by Epstein-Barr virus, that is characterized by inflammation of the pharynx, fever, malaise, lymphadenopathy, and hepatosplenomegaly.
         Mononucleosis due to Epstein-Barr virus

   B27.00   **Gammaherpesviral mononucleosis without complication**

   B27.01   **Gammaherpesviral mononucleosis with polyneuropathy**

   B27.02   **Gammaherpesviral mononucleosis with meningitis**

   B27.09   **Gammaherpesviral mononucleosis with other complications**
         Hepatomegaly in gammaherpesviral mononucleosis

   B27.1-   **Cytomegaloviral mononucleosis** — An infectious viral disease caused by cytomegalovirus that is characterized by inflammation of the pharynx, fever, malaise, lymphadenopathy, and hepatosplenomegaly.

   B27.10   **Cytomegaloviral mononucleosis without complications**

   B27.11   **Cytomegaloviral mononucleosis with polyneuropathy**

   B27.12   **Cytomegaloviral mononucleosis with meningitis**

   B27.19   **Cytomegaloviral mononucleosis with other complication**
         Hepatomegaly in cytomegaloviral mononucleosis

   B27.8-   **Other infectious mononucleosis**

   B27.80   **Other infectious mononucleosis without complication**

   B27.81   **Other infectious mononucleosis with polyneuropathy**

   B27.82   **Other infectious mononucleosis with meningitis**

   B27.89   **Other infectious mononucleosis with other complication**
         Hepatomegaly in other infectious mononucleosis

   B27.9-   **Infectious mononucleosis, unspecified**

   B27.90   **Infectious mononucleosis, unspecified without complication**

   B27.91   **Infectious mononucleosis, unspecified with polyneuropathy**

   B27.92   **Infectious mononucleosis, unspecified with meningitis**

   B27.99   **Infectious mononucleosis, unspecified with other complication**
         Hepatomegaly in unspecified infectious mononucleosis

B30- __Viral conjunctivitis__ — An infectious viral disease usually caused by an Adenovirus that is characterized by inflammation of the conjunctiva.
    Excludes 1:   *herpesviral [herpes simplex] ocular disease (B00.5)*
                ocular zoster (B02.3)

   B30.0   **Keratoconjunctivitis due to adenovirus**
         Epidemic keratoconjunctivitis
         Shipyard eye

   B30.1   **Conjunctivitis due to adenovirus**
         Acute adenoviral follicular conjunctivitis
         Swimming-pool conjunctivitis

   B30.2   **Viral pharyngoconjunctivitis**

   B30.3   **Acute epidemic hemorrhagic conjunctivitis (enteroviral)**
         Conjunctivitis due to coxsackievirus 24
         Conjunctivitis due to enterovirus 70
         Hemorrhagic conjunctivitis (acute) (epidemic)

   B30.8   **Other viral conjunctivitis**
         Newcastle conjunctivitis

   B30.9   **Viral conjunctivitis, unspecified**

B33-   **Other viral diseases, not elsewhere classified**

   B33.0   **Epidemic myalgia** — An infectious viral disease caused by Coxsackie B virus, and characterized by sudden, sharp, paroxysmal chest pain, headache, myalgia, and fever of brief duration.
         Bornholm disease

CC **B33.1**   **Ross River disease**
         Epidemic polyarthritis and exanthema
         Ross River fever

   B33.2-   **Viral carditis** — An infectious viral disease of the heart caused by the Coxsackie virus.
         Coxsackie (virus) carditis

   CC **B33.20**   **Viral carditis, unspecified**

   CC **B33.21**   **Viral endocarditis**

   CC **B33.22**   **Viral myocarditis**

   CC **B33.23**   **Viral pericarditis**

   B33.24   **Viral cardiomyopathy**

Sidebar: B 18 - B 33

B33.3   **Retrovirus infections, not elsewhere classified**
Retrovirus infection NOS

cc **B33.4**   **Hantavirus (cardio)-pulmonary syndrome [HPS] [HCPS]** — An infectious viral disease caused by an RNA virus, that is characterized by fever, cough, muscle aches, headache, lethargy, and shortness-of-breath, which can rapidly deteriorate into acute respiratory failure.
Hantavirus disease with pulmonary manifestations
Sin nombre virus disease
Use additional code to identify any associated acute kidney failure (N17.9)
Excludes 1:   *hantavirus disease with renal manifestations (A98.5)*
hemorrhagic fever with renal manifestations (A98.5)

B33.8   **Other specified viral diseases**
Excludes 1:   *anogenital human papillomavirus infection (A63.0)*
viral warts due to human papillomavirus infection (B07)

B34-   **Viral infection of unspecified site**
Excludes 1:   *anogenital human papillomavirus infection (A63.0)*
cytomegaloviral disease NOS (B25.9)
herpesvirus [herpes simplex] infection NOS (B00.9)
retrovirus infection NOS (B33.3)
viral agents as the cause of diseases classified elsewhere (B97-)
viral warts due to human papillomavirus infection (B07)

B34.0   **Adenovirus infection, unspecified**

B34.1   **Enterovirus infection, unspecified**
Coxsackievirus infection NOS
Echovirus infection NOS

B34.2   **Coronavirus infection, unspecified**
Excludes 1:   *pneumonia due to SARS-associated coronavirus (J12.81)*

cc **B34.3**   **Parvovirus infection, unspecified**

B34.4   **Papovavirus infection, unspecified**

B34.8   **Other viral infections of unspecified site**

B34.9   **Viral infection, unspecified**
Viremia NOS

Mycoses (B35-B49)

Excludes ❷: *hypersensitivity pneumonitis due to organic dust (J67.-)*
mycosis fungoides (C84.0-)

B35-   **Dermatophytosis** — A group of infectious superficial fungal skin diseases caused by a dermatophyte.
Includes: Favus
Infections due to species of Epidermophyton, Micro-sporum and Trichophyton
Tinea, any type except those in B36.-

B35.0   **Tinea barbae and tinea capitis**
Beard ringworm
Kerion
Scalp ringworm
Sycosis, mycotic

B35.1   **Tinea unguium**
Dermatophytic onychia
Dermatophytosis of nail
Onychomycosis
Ringworm of nails

B35.2   **Tinea manuum**
Dermatophytosis of hand
Hand ringworm

B35.3   **Tinea pedis**
Athlete's foot
Dermatophytosis of foot
Foot ringworm

B35.4   **Tinea corporis**
Ringworm of the body

B35.5   **Tinea imbricata**
Tokelau

B35.6   **Tinea cruris**
Dhobi itch
Groin ringworm
Jock itch

B35.8   **Other dermatophytoses**
Disseminated dermatophytosis
Granulomatous dermatophytosis

B35.9   **Dermatophytosis, unspecified**
Ringworm NOS

B36-   **Other superficial mycoses**

B36.0   **Pityriasis versicolor** — A superficial fungal skin disease characterized by discolored, hyperpigmented spots or plaques on the chest and back with a slight scale formation.
Tinea flava
Tinea versicolor

B36.1   **Tinea nigra** — A superficial fungal skin disease characterized by black discoloration of the skin and caused by Cladosporium Wernecki.
Keratomycosis nigricans palmaris
Microsporosis nigra
Pityriasis nigra

B36.2   **White piedra** — A superficial fungal skin disease characterized by white fungal masses on the hair shafts, which may occasionally cause a systemic infection in debilitated patients.
Tinea blanca

B36.3   **Black piedra** — A superficial fungal skin disease characterized by black nodular masses of fungi on the hair shafts.

B36.8   **Other specified superficial mycoses**

B36.9   **Superficial mycosis, unspecified**

B37-   **Candidiasis** — Infectious fungal diseases caused by the genus Candida, and characterized by stubborn infection of the moist areas of the body.
Includes: Candidosis
Moniliasis
Excludes 1:   *neonatal candidiasis (P37.5)*

cc **B37.0**   **Candidal stomatitis** — A form characterized by whitish spots in the mouth, caused by Candida albicans.
Oral thrush

MCC **B37.1**   **Pulmonary candidiasis** — A form characterized by infection of the lung tissues that can develop into pneumonia.
Candidal bronchitis
Candidal pneumonia

B37.2   **Candidiasis of skin and nail**
Candidal onychia
Candidal paronychia
Excludes ❷: *diaper dermatitis (L22)*

B37.3   **Candidiasis of vulva and vagina** — [♀]
Candidal vulvovaginitis
Monilial vulvovaginitis
Vaginal thrush

B37.4-   **Candidiasis of other urogenital sites**
cc **B37.41**   **Candidal cystitis and urethritis**

B37.42   **Candidal balanitis**

cc **B37.49**   **Other urogenital candidiasis**
Candidal pyelonephritis

MCC **B37.5**   **Candidal meningitis**

MCC **B37.6**   **Candidal endocarditis**

MCC **B37.7**   **Candidal sepsis**
AHA 14:2Q:p13 – Sepsis due to non-Candida Albicans
AHA 14:4Q:p46 – Sepsis due to non-Candida Albicans, clarification
Disseminated candidiasis
Systemic candidiasis

B37.8-   **Candidiasis of other sites**
cc **B37.81**   **Candidal esophagitis**

cc **B37.82**   **Candidal enteritis**
Candidal proctitis

cc **B37.83**   **Candidal cheilitis**

cc **B37.84**   **Candidal otitis externa**

cc **B37.89**   **Other sites of candidiasis**
Candidal osteomyelitis

B37.9   **Candidiasis, unspecified**
Thrush NOS

B
3
3
-
B
3
7

B38- __Coccidioidomycosis__ — Infectious fungal diseases caused by Coccidioides immitis, and characterized by respiratory origin of pulmonary disease, and dissemination.

CC **B38.0** **Acute pulmonary coccidioidomycosis**

CC **B38.1** **Chronic pulmonary coccidioidomycosis**

CC **B38.2** **Pulmonary coccidioidomycosis, unspecified**

CC **B38.3** **Cutaneous coccidioidomycosis**

MCC **B38.4** **Coccidioidomycosis meningitis**

CC **B38.7** **Disseminated coccidioidomycosis**
     Generalized coccidioidomycosis

B38.8- **Other forms of coccidioidomycosis**

CC **B38.81** **Prostatic coccidioidomycosis** — [♂]

CC **B38.89** **Other forms of coccidioidomycosis**

CC **B38.9** **Coccidioidomycosis, unspecified**

B39- __Histoplasmosis__ — Infectious fungal diseases caused by the genus Histoplasma.
Code first associated AIDS (B20)
Use additional code for any associated manifestations, such as:
   Eendocarditis (I39)
   Meningitis (G02)
   Pericarditis (I32)
   Retinitits (H32)

MCC **B39.0** **Acute pulmonary histoplasmosis capsulati**

MCC **B39.1** **Chronic pulmonary histoplasmosis capsulati**

MCC **B39.2** **Pulmonary histoplasmosis capsulati, unspecified**

MCC **B39.3** **Disseminated histoplasmosis capsulati**
     Generalized histoplasmosis capsulati

B39.4 **Histoplasmosis capsulati, unspecified**
     American histoplasmosis

B39.5 **Histoplasmosis duboisii**
     African histoplasmosis

B39.9 **Histoplasmosis, unspecified**

B40- __Blastomycosis__ — An infectious fungal disease caused by Blastomyces dermatitidis, and characterized by involvement of the skin, lungs, and other viscera, occurring primarily in North America.
   Excludes 1:   *Brazilian blastomycosis (B41.-)*
                    keloidal blastomycosis (B48.0)

CC **B40.0** **Acute pulmonary blastomycosis**

CC **B40.1** **Chronic pulmonary blastomycosis**

CC **B40.2** **Pulmonary blastomycosis, unspecified**

CC **B40.3** **Cutaneous blastomycosis**

CC **B40.7** **Disseminated blastomycosis**
     Generalized blastomycosis

B40.8- **Other forms of blastomycosis**

CC **B40.81** **Blastomycotic meningoencephalitis**
     Meningomyelitis due to blastomycosis

CC **B40.89** **Other forms of blastomycosis**

CC **B40.9** **Blastomycosis, unspecified**

B41- __Paracoccidioidomycosis__ — An infectious fungal disease caused by Paracoccidioides brasiliensis, and characterized by systemic infection which may affect a few organs to almost all organs.
   Includes: **Brazilian blastomycosis**
                    Lutz' disease

CC **B41.0** **Pulmonary paracoccidioidomycosis**

CC **B41.7** **Disseminated paracoccidioidomycosis**
     Generalized paracoccidioidomycosis

CC **B41.8** **Other forms of paracoccidioidomycosis**

CC **B41.9** **Paracoccidioidomycosis, unspecified**

B42- __Sporotrichosis__ — An infectious fungal disease caused by Sporothrix schenckii, and characterized primarily by suppurating nodules along the lymphatics of the skin and subcutaneous tissue, and occasionally developing into other tissues and organs.

B42.0 **Pulmonary sporotrichosis**

B42.1 **Lymphocutaneous sporotrichosis**

B42.7 **Disseminated sporotrichosis**
     Generalized sporotrichosis

B42.8- **Other forms of sporotrichosis**

B42.81 **Cerebral sporotrichosis**
     Meningitis due to sporotrichosis

B42.82 **Sporotrichosis arthritis**

B42.89 **Other forms of sporotrichosis**

B42.9 **Sporotrichosis, unspecified**

B43- __Chromomycosis__ and __pheomycotic__ abscess — An infectious fungal disease caused by closely related fungal organisms Cladosporium carrionii, Fonsecaea pedrosoi, Fonsecaea compactum, and Phialophora verrucosa, and characterized by chronic granulomatous nodules in the skin and subcutaneous tissue and occasionally multiple subcutaneous pheomycotic cysts and abscesses.

B43.0 **Cutaneous chromomycosis**
     Dermatitis verrucosa

B43.1 **Pheomycotic brain abscess**
     Cerebral chromomycosis

B43.2 **Subcutaneous pheomycotic abscess and cyst**

B43.8 **Other forms of chromomycosis**

B43.9 **Chromomycosis, unspecified**

B44- __Aspergillosis__ — An infectious fungal disease caused by the genus Aspergillus, and characterized by inflammatory granulomatous lesions in the skin, ear, orbit, nasal sinuses, lungs, and occasionally in the bones and meninges.
   Includes: **Aspergilloma**

MCC **B44.0** **Invasive pulmonary aspergillosis**

CC **B44.1** **Other pulmonary aspergillosis**

CC **B44.2** **Tonsillar aspergillosis**

CC **B44.7** **Disseminated aspergillosis**
     Generalized aspergillosis

B44.8- **Other forms of aspergillosis**

CC **B44.81** **Allergic bronchopulmonary aspergillosis**

CC **B44.89** **Other forms of aspergillosis**

CC **B44.9** **Aspergillosis, unspecified**

B45- __Cryptococcosis__ — An infectious fungal disease caused by Cryptococcus neoformans, and characterized by involving the lungs, skin, brain, and meninges.

CC **B45.0** **Pulmonary cryptococcosis**

MCC **B45.1** **Cerebral cryptococcosis**
     Cryptococcal meningitis
     Cryptococcosis meningocerebralis

CC **B45.2** **Cutaneous cryptococcosis**

CC **B45.3** **Osseous cryptococcosis**

CC **B45.7** **Disseminated cryptococcosis**
     Generalized cryptococcosis

CC **B45.8** **Other forms of cryptococcosis**

CC **B45.9** **Cryptococcosis, unspecified**

B46- __Zygomycosis__ — A group of infectious fungal (Zygomycetes) diseases marked by a variety of manifestations depending upon which organism is the infective agent and the body part(s) infected.

MCC **B46.0** **Pulmonary mucormycosis**

MCC **B46.1** **Rhinocerebral mucormycosis**

MCC **B46.2** **Gastrointestinal mucormycosis**

MCC **B46.3** **Cutaneous mucormycosis**
     Subcutaneous mucormycosis

MCC **B46.4** **Disseminated mucormycosis**
     Generalized mucormycosis

MCC **B46.5** **Mucormycosis, unspecified**

MCC **B46.8** **Other zygomycoses**
     Entomophthoromycosis

MCC **B46.9** **Zygomycosis, unspecified**
     Phycomycosis NOS

B47- __Mycetoma__

CC **B47.0** **Eumycetoma** — A fungal disease (Eumycetes) that is characterized by chronic, suppurative, granulomatous subcutaneous tissues and bones with sinus formation.
     Madura foot, mycotic
     Maduromycosis

CC **B47.1** **Actinomycetoma** — An infectious disease caused by actinomycetes that is characterized by chronic, suppurative, granulomatous subcutaneous tissues and bones with sinus formation.

CC **B47.9** **Mycetoma, unspecified**
     Madura foot NOS

**B
3
8
I
B
4
7**

B48- Other mycoses, not elsewhere classified

B48.0 **Lobomycosis** — An infectious fungal disease caused by Loboa loboi that is characterized by slow-growing keloid-like skin tumors.
　　Keloidal blastomycosis
　　Lobo's disease

B48.1 **Rhinosporidiosis** — An infectious fungal disease caused by Rhinosporidium seeberi that is characterized by small tumor-like masses usually in the nose and nasopharynx.

CC B48.2 **Allescheriasis** — An infectious fungal disease caused by Allescheria [Petriellidium] boydii that is characterized by suppurative, granulomatous skin and subcutaneous lesions.
　　Infection due to Pseudallescheria boydii
　　Excludes 1:   eumycetoma (B47.0)

CC B48.3 **Geotrichosis** — A fungal infection caused by Geotrichum candidum that affects the oral cavity and sometimes the lungs.
　　Geotrichum stomatitis

CC B48.4 **Penicillosis** — A fungal infection caused by Penicillium marneffei that affects immunocompromised patients that is characterized by fever, skin lesions, and lymphandenopathy.

CC B48.8 **Other specified mycoses**
　　AHA 14:2Q:p13 – Sepsis due to non-Candida Albicans
　　AHA 14:4Q:p46 – Sepsis due to non-Candida Albicans, clarification
　　Adiaspiromycosis
　　Infection of tissue and organs by Alternaria
　　Infection of tissue and organs by Drechslera
　　Infection of tissue and organs by Fusarium
　　Infection of tissue and organs by saprophytic fungi NEC

B49 Unspecified mycosis
CC　　Fungemia NOS

Protozoal diseases (B50-B64)

Excludes 1:   amebiasis (A06.-)
　　other protozoal intestinal diseases (A07.-)

B50- Plasmodium falciparum malaria — A mosquito-borne parasitic disease caused by Plasmodium falciparum that is characterized by respiratory distress, severe anemia, pulmonary edema, circulatory shock, and organ failure.
　　Includes: Mixed infections of Plasmodium falciparum with any other Plasmodium species

CC B50.0 **Plasmodium falciparum malaria with cerebral complications**
　　Cerebral malaria NOS

CC B50.8 **Other severe and complicated Plasmodium falciparum malaria**
　　Severe or complicated Plasmodium falciparum malaria NOS

MCC B50.9 **Plasmodium falciparum malaria, unspecified**

B51- Plasmodium vivax malaria — A mosquito-borne parasitic disease caused by Plasmodium vivax that is characterized by fever, headache, chills and vomiting, respiratory distress, anemia, and weakness. Clinical relapses may occur weeks to months after the first infection.
　　Includes: Mixed infections of Plasmodium vivax with other Plasmodium species, except Plasmodium falciparum
　　Excludes 1:   Plasmodium vivav with Plasmodium falciparum (B50.-)

CC B51.0 **Plasmodium vivax malaria with rupture of spleen**
CC B51.8 **Plasmodium vivax malaria with other complications**
CC B51.9 **Plasmodium vivax malaria without complication**
　　Plasmodium vivax malaria NOS

B52- Plasmodium malariae malaria — A mosquito-borne parasitic disease caused by Plasmodium malariae that is characterized by fever, headache, chills and vomiting, respiratory distress, anemia, and weakness.
　　Includes: Mixed infections of Plasmodium malariae with other Plasmodium species, except Plasmodium falciparum and Plasmodium vivax
　　Excludes 1:   Plasmodium falciparum (B50.-)
　　　Plasmodium vivax (B51.-)

CC B52.0 **Plasmodium malariae malaria with nephropathy**
CC B52.8 **Plasmodium malariae malaria with other complications**
CC B52.9 **Plasmodium malariae malaria without complication**
　　Plasmodium malariae malaria NOS

B53- Other specified malaria

CC B53.0 **Plasmodium ovale malaria** — A mosquito-borne parasitic disease caused by Plasmodium ovale that is characterized by fever, headache, chills and vomiting, respiratory distress, anemia, and weakness. Clinical relapses may occur weeks to months after the first infection.
　　Excludes 1:   **Plasmodium ovale with Plasmodium falciparum (B50.-)**
　　　Plasmodium ovale with Plasmodium malariae (B52.-)
　　　Plasmodium ovale with Plasmodium vivax (B51.-)

CC B53.1 **Malaria due to simian plasmodia** — A mosquito-borne parasitic disease caused by Plasmodium knowlesi that is characterized by fever, headache, chills and vomiting, respiratory distress, anemia, and weakness.
　　Excludes 1:   **malaria due to simian plasmodia with Plasmodium falciparum (B50.-)**
　　　malaria due to simian plasmodia with Plasmodium malariae (B52.-)
　　　malaria due to simian plasmodia with Plasmodium ovale (B53.0)
　　　malaria due to simian plasmodia with Plasmodium vivax (B51.-)

CC B53.8 **Other malaria, not elsewhere classified**

B54 Unspecified malaria
CC

B55- Leishmaniasis — Parasitic diseases caused by the protozoan genus Leishmaniasis through the bite of sandflies.

CC B55.0 **Visceral leishmaniasis** — Leishmaniasis that is characterized by fever, chills, weight loss, splenomegaly, leukopenia, anemia, and potentially fatal if untreated.
　　Kala-azar
　　Post-kala-azar dermal leishmaniasis

CC B55.1 **Cutaneous leishmaniasis** — Leishmaniasis that is characterized by ulcerated sores with small papules on the edge of the sore.

CC B55.2 **Mucocutaneous leishmaniasis** — Leishmaniasis that is characterized by ulceration of the skin and mucous membranes of the throat and nose.

CC B55.9 **Leishmaniasis, unspecified**

B56- African trypanosomiasis

CC B56.0 **Gambiense trypanosomiasis** — A parasitic disease caused by Trypanosoma brucei gambiense, and characterized by a primary lesion at the tsetse fly bite, fever, lymphadenopathy (especially of posterior neck), and invasion of the central nervous system with somnolence and coma which develops slower than the Rhodesian form.
　　Infection due to Trypanosoma brucei gambiense
　　West African sleeping sickness

CC B56.1 **Rhodesiense trypanosomiasis** — A parasitic disease caused by Trypanosoma brucei rhodesiense that is characterized by a primary lesion at the tsetse fly bite, fever, lymphadenopathy (especially of posterior neck), and invasion of the central nervous system with somnolence and coma which develops more rapidly than the Gambian form.
　　East African sleeping sickness
　　Infection due to Trypanosoma brucei rhodesiense

CC B56.9 **African trypanosomiasis, unspecified**
　　Sleeping sickness NOS

B57- Chagas' disease — A parasitic disease caused by Trypanosoma cruzi that is characterized by primary lesion at the site of entry (skin, conjunctiva), fever, headache, swollen lymph glands, facial and generalized edema, and can progress to involve various organs.
　　Includes: American trypanosomiasis
　　　Infection due to Trypanosoma cruzi

CC B57.0 **Acute Chagas' disease with heart involvement**
　　Acute Chagas' disease with myocarditis

CC B57.1 **Acute Chagas' disease without heart involvement**
　　Acute Chagas' disease NOS

CC B57.2 **Chagas' disease (chronic) with heart involvement**
　　American trypanosomiasis NOS
　　Chagas' disease (chronic) NOS
　　Chagas' disease (chronic) with myocarditis
　　Trypanosomiasis NOS

B57.3- **Chagas' disease (chronic) with digestive system involvement**
CC B57.30 **Chagas' disease with digestive system involvement, unspecified**
CC B57.31 **Megaesophagus in Chagas' disease**
CC B57.32 **Megacolon in Chagas' disease**
CC B57.39 **Other digestive system involvement in Chagas' disease**

B 4 8 – B 5 7

B57.4- **Chagas' disease (chronic) with nervous system involvement**
cc B57.40 **Chagas' disease with nervous system involvement, unspecified**
cc B57.41 **Meningitis in Chagas' disease**
cc B57.42 **Meningoencephalitis in Chagas' disease**
cc B57.49 **Other nervous system involvement in Chagas' disease**
cc B57.5 **Chagas' disease (chronic) with other organ involvement**

B58- <u>**Toxoplasmosis**</u> — A parasitic disease caused by Toxoplasma gondii, and characterized by involvement of various organs.
    Includes: Infection due to Toxoplasma gondii
    Excludes 1: *congenital toxoplasmosis (P37.1)*
  B58.0- **Toxoplasma oculopathy**
   cc B58.00 **Toxoplasma oculopathy, unspecified**
   cc B58.01 **Toxoplasma chorioretinitis**
   cc B58.09 **Other toxoplasma oculopathy**
      Toxoplasma uveitis
 cc B58.1 **Toxoplasma hepatitis**
MCC B58.2 **Toxoplasma meningoencephalitis**
MCC B58.3 **Pulmonary toxoplasmosis**
  B58.8- **Toxoplasmosis with other organ involvement**
   MCC B58.81 **Toxoplasma myocarditis**
   cc B58.82 **Toxoplasma myositis**
   cc B58.83 **Toxoplasma tubulo-interstitial nephropathy**
      Toxoplasma pyelonephritis
   cc B58.89 **Toxoplasmosis with other organ involvement**
 cc B58.9 **Toxoplasmosis, unspecified**

B59 <u>**Pneumocystosis**</u> — A highly contagious interstitial plasma cell pneumonia caused by
MCC Pneumocystis carinii and Pneumocystis jiroveci that is usually seen in immunocompromised patients.
    Pneumonia due to Pneumocystis carinii
    Pneumonia due to Pneumocystis jiroveci

B60- <u>**Other protozoal diseases**</u>, not elsewhere classified
    Excludes 1: *cryptosporidiosis (A07.2)*
        intestinal microsporidiosis (A07.8)
        isosporiasis (A07.3)
 cc B60.0 **Babesiosis** — An infectious parasitic (tick-borne) disease caused by the genus Babesia, and characterized by a malaria-like fever, myalgia, hemolytic anemia, and splenomegaly.
      Piroplasmosis
  B60.1- **Acanthamebiasis** — An infectious parasitic disease caused by the free-living soil and water ameoba Acanthameoba that is characterized by skin ulcers and granulomas, and can progress to infect the meninges.
   cc B60.10 **Acanthamebiasis, unspecified**
   B60.11 **Meningoencephalitis due to Acanthamoeba (culbertsoni)**
   B60.12 **Conjunctivitis due to Acanthamoeba**
   B60.13 **Keratoconjunctivitis due to Acanthamoeba** —
      [Unacceptable PDX]
   cc B60.19 **Other acanthamebic disease**
 cc B60.2 **Naegleriasis** — An infectious parasitic disease caused by the free-living soil and warm water ameoba Naegleria fowleri that is characterized by infection of the nervous system and brain.
     Primary amebic meningoencephalitis
  B60.8 **Other specified protozoal diseases**
     Microsporidiosis

B64 **Unspecified protozoal disease**

Helminthiases (B65-B83)

B65- <u>**Schistosomiasis**</u> [bilharziasis] — A parasitic disease caused by the genus Schistosoma (caused by schistosomes worms) that is characterized by abdominal pain and infection of the gastrointestinal and urinary tracts.
    Includes: Snail fever
 cc B65.0 **Schistosomiasis due to Schistosoma haematobium [urinary schistosomiasis]**
 cc B65.1 **Schistosomiasis due to Schistosoma mansoni [intestinal schistosomiasis]**
 cc B65.2 **Schistosomiasis due to Schistosoma japonicum**
     Asiatic schistosomiasis
 cc B65.3 **Cercarial dermatitis**
     Swimmer's itch

cc B65.8 **Other schistosomiasis**
    Infection due to Schistosoma intercalatum
    Infection due to Schistosoma mattheei
    Infection due to Schistosoma mekongi
cc B65.9 **Schistosomiasis, unspecified**

B66- **Other fluke infections**
 cc B66.0 **Opisthorchiasis** — A parasitic disease caused by Opisthorchis felineus and viverrini that is characterized by liver infestation which, in its severe form, presents hepatomegaly, jaundice, liver abscess, and pancreatitis.
    Infection due to cat liver fluke
    Infection due to Opisthorchis (felineus) (viverrini)
 cc B66.1 **Clonorchiasis** — A parasitic disease caused by Clonorchis (Oristhorchis) sinensis that is characterized by infestation and inflammation of the gallbladder, bile ducts, and liver.
    Chinese liver fluke disease
    Infection due to Clonorchis sinensis
    Oriental liver fluke disease
 cc B66.2 **Dicroceliasis** — A parasitic disease caused by Dicrocoelium dendriticum that is characterized by infection of the bile ducts.
    Infection due to Dicrocoelium dendriticum
    Lancet fluke infection
 cc B66.3 **Fascioliasis** — A parasitic disease caused by the genus Fasciola with symptoms characterized by fever, malaise, urticaria, and nonproductive cough, with large flukes obstructing the biliary tract where they live.
    Infection due to Fasciola gigantica
    Infection due to Fasciola hepatica
    Infection due to Fasciola indica
    Sheep liver fluke disease
 cc B66.4 **Paragonimiasis** — A parasitic disease caused by the genus Paragonimus that is characterized by lung infestation with resulting hemoptysis, fever, and occasionally by pleural conditions, and right heart failure.
    Infection due to Paragonimus species
    Lung fluke disease
    Pulmonary distomiasis
 cc B66.5 **Fasciolopsiasis** — A parasitic disease caused by Fasciolopsis buski that is characterized by abdominal pain, intermittent diarrhea, flatus, and excessive appetite or anorexia.
    Infection due to Fasciolopsis buski
    Intestinal distomiasis
  B66.8 **Other specified fluke infections**
    Echinostomiasis
    Heterophyiasis
    Metagonimiasis
    Nanophyetiasis
    Watsoniasis
  B66.9 **Fluke infection, unspecified**

B67- <u>**Echinococcosis**</u> — A parasitic disease caused by Echinococcus granulosus that is characterized by chronic space-occupying lesions of various organs.
    Includes: Hydatidosis
 cc B67.0 **Echinococcus granulosus infection of liver**
 cc B67.1 **Echinococcus granulosus infection of lung**
 cc B67.2 **Echinococcus granulosus infection of bone**
  B67.3- **Echinococcus granulosus infection, other and multiple sites**
   cc B67.31 **Echinococcus granulosus infection, thyroid gland**
   cc B67.32 **Echinococcus granulosus infection, multiple sites**
   cc B67.39 **Echinococcus granulosus infection, other sites**
 cc B67.4 **Echinococcus granulosus infection, unspecified**
    Dog tapeworm (infection)
 cc B67.5 **Echinococcus multilocularis infection of liver**
  B67.6- **Echinococcus multilocularis infection, other and multiple sites**
   cc B67.61 **Echinococcus multilocularis infection, multiple sites**
   cc B67.69 **Echinococcus multilocularis infection, other sites**
 cc B67.7 **Echinococcus multilocularis infection, unspecified**
 cc B67.8 **Echinococcosis, unspecified, of liver**
  B67.9- **Echinococcosis, other and unspecified**
   cc B67.90 **Echinococcosis, unspecified**
      Echinococcosis NOS
   cc B67.99 **Other echinococcosis**

B57-B67 (side tab)

B68- Taeniasis — A parasitic disease caused by adult intestinal tapeworms growing to 3 to 25 feet (1 to 7.5 m) in length.
    Excludes 1:   cysticercosis (B69.-)

cc **B68.0** **Taenia solium taeniasis**
        Pork tapeworm (infection)

cc **B68.1** **Taenia saginata taeniasis**
        Beef tapeworm (infection)
        Infection due to adult tapeworm Taenia saginata

cc **B68.9** **Taeniasis, unspecified**

B69- Cysticercosis — A parasitic disease caused by the larvae of Taenia solium and characterized by mechanical injury at the larval site which may infest the muscle and often the brain and meninges.
    Includes: Cysticerciasis infection due to larval form of Taenia solium

cc **B69.0** **Cysticercosis of central nervous system**

cc **B69.1** **Cysticercosis of eye**

    B69.8- **Cysticercosis of other sites**

    cc **B69.81** **Myositis in cysticercosis**

    cc **B69.89** **Cysticercosis of other sites**

cc **B69.9** **Cysticercosis, unspecified**

B70- **Diphyllobothriasis and sparganosis**

cc **B70.0** **Diphyllobothriasis** — A parasitic disease caused by Diphyllobothrium latum, characterized by a small intestinal tapeworm of up to 30 feet (9 m) in length, and acquired from eating infected raw or undercooked freshwater fish.
        Diphyllobothrium (adult) (latum) (pacificum) infection
        Fish tapeworm (infection)
    Excludes ❷: larval diphyllobothriasis (B70.1)

cc **B70.1** **Sparganosis** — A parasitic disease caused by the larvae identified below and characterized by invasion of subcutaneous tissue, causing inflammation and fibrosis.
        Infection due to Sparganum (mansoni) (proliferum)
        Infection due to Spirometra larva
        Larval diphyllobothriasis
        Spirometrosis

B71- **Other cestode infections**

cc **B71.0** **Hymenolepiasis** — A parasitic disease caused by Hymenolepis nana and characterized by a 1.6 inch (4 cm) ileal tapeworm which has a lifespan of a few weeks.
        Dwarf tapeworm infection
        Rat tapeworm (infection)

cc **B71.1** **Dipylidiasis**

cc **B71.8** **Other specified cestode infections**
        Coenurosis

    B71.9 **Cestode infection, unspecified**
        Tapeworm (infection) NOS

B72 Dracunculiasis — A parasitic disease caused by the guinea worm that is characterized
cc by development of a worm under the skin causing burning pain at the site.
    Includes: **Guinea worm infection**
        Infection due to Dracunculus medinensis

B73- Onchocerciasis — A parasitic disease caused by Onchocerca volvulus that is characterized by skin nodules, eye lesions, and dermatitis with lymphatic symptoms.
    Includes: **Onchocerca volvulus infection**
        Onchocercosis
        River blindness

    B73.0- **Onchocerciasis with eye disease**

    cc **B73.00** **Onchocerciasis with eye involvement, unspecified**

    cc **B73.01** **Onchocerciasis with endophthalmitis**

    cc **B73.02** **Onchocerciasis with glaucoma**

    cc **B73.09** **Onchocerciasis with other eye involvement**
        Infestation of eyelid due to onchocerciasis

cc **B73.1** **Onchocerciasis without eye disease**

B74- **Filariasis**
    Excludes ❷: onchocerciasis (B73)
           tropical (pulmonary) eosinophilia NOS (J82)

cc **B74.0** **Filariasis due to Wuchereria bancrofti** — A parasitic disease caused by Wuchereria bancrofti that is characterized by frequent attacks of fever, lymphangitis, lymphadenitis, and in the most severe cases elephantiasis.
        Bancroftian elephantiasis
        Bancroftian filariasis

cc **B74.1** **Filariasis due to Brugia malayi** — A parasitic disease caused by Brugia malayi and characterized usually by more acute symptoms than bancroftian filariasis, and in which elephantiasis is more common, but spares the bladder and genitalia.

cc **B74.2** **Filariasis due to Brugia timori** — A parasitic disease caused by Brugia malayi.

cc **B74.3** **Loiasis** — A parasitic disease caused by Loa loa, and characterized by worms 1 to 2 inches (2.5 to 5 cm) in length which move freely in connective tissue giving rise to edematous swelling (Calabar swellings), and frequently infest the conjunctiva with occasional serious complications such as encephalitis.
        Calabar swelling
        Eyeworm disease of Africa
        Loa loa infection

cc **B74.4** **Mansonelliasis** — A parasitic disease caused by Mansonella ozzardi that is characterized by adult worms inhabiting the visceral adipose tissue, and are usually asymptomatic.
        Infection due to Mansonella ozzardi
        Infection due to Mansonella perstans
        Infection due to Mansonella streptocerca

cc **B74.8** **Other filariases**
        Dirofilariasis

cc **B74.9** **Filariasis, unspecified**

B75 Trichinellosis — A parasitic disease caused by Trichinella spiralis, and characterized in
cc the early stages by diarrhea, nausea, colic, and fever, and in the later stages characterized by stiffness, pain, swelling of the muscles, splinter hemorrhages, sweating, and insomnia.
    Includes: **Infection due to Trichinella species**
           Trichiniasis

B76- **Hookworm diseases**
    Includes: **Uncinariasis**

cc **B76.0** **Ancylostomiasis** — A parasitic disease caused by genus Ancylostoma that is characterized by adult worms in the small intestine, causing abdominal pain, diarrhea, malnutrition, and in severe cases anemia.
        Infection due to Ancylostoma species

cc **B76.1** **Necatoriasis** — A parasitic disease caused by Necator americanus that is characterized by adult worms in the small intestine causing abdominal pain, diarrhea, and malnutrition.
        Infection due to Necator americanus

cc **B76.8** **Other hookworm diseases**

cc **B76.9** **Hookworm disease, unspecified**
        Cutaneous larva migrans NOS

B77- Ascariasis — A parasitic disease caused by Ascaris lumbricoides that is characterized by giant intestinal worms and in severe cases by pneumonitis and intestinal blockage.
    Includes: **Ascaridiasis**
           Roundworm infection

cc **B77.0** **Ascariasis with intestinal complications**

    B77.8- **Ascariasis with other complications**

    mcc **B77.81** **Ascariasis pneumonia**

    cc **B77.89** **Ascariasis with other complications**

cc **B77.9** **Ascariasis, unspecified**

B78- Strongyloidiasis — A parasitic disease caused by Strongyloides stercoralis and characterized by roundworm infestation of the small intestine with watery, mucus diarrhea, and migratory larvae infestation of the lungs, rupturing the alveoli.
    Excludes 1:   trichostrongyliasis (B81.2)

cc **B78.0** **Intestinal strongyloidiasis**

    B78.1 **Cutaneous strongyloidiasis**

cc **B78.7** **Disseminated strongyloidiasis**

cc **B78.9** **Strongyloidiasis, unspecified**

B79 Trichuriasis — A parasitic disease caused by Trichuris trichiura, and characterized by
cc whipworm infestation of the large intestine and rectum causing chronic diarrhea, mucus stools, and rectal prolapse.
    Includes: **Trichocephaliasis**
           Whipworm (disease) (infection)

B80 Enterobiasis — A parasitic disease caused by Enterobius vermicularis that is
cc characterized by pinworm infestation of the large intestine causing intense perineal itching in symptomatic patients.
    Includes: **Oxyuriasis**
           Pinworm infection
           Threadworm infection

B81- **Other intestinal helminthiases, not elsewhere classified**
    Excludes 1:   angiostrongyliasis due to Parastrongylus cantonensis (B83.2)

cc **B81.0** **Anisakiasis** — A parasitic disease caused by Ascaris lumbricoides and characterized by giant intestinal worms and in severe cases by pneumonitis and intestinal blockage.
        Infection due to Anisakis larva

cc **B81.1** **Intestinal capillariasis** — A parasitic disease caused by Capillaria philippinensis, and characterized by adult worms infesting the small intestine causing rampant diarrhea, malabsorption, electrolyte imbalance, and in severe cases lead to death.
        Capillariasis NOS
        Infection due to Capillaria philippinensis
    Excludes ❷: hepatic capillariasis (B83.8)

B
6
8
–
B
8
1

---

cc **B81.2** **Trichostrongyliasis** — A parasitic disease caused by the genus Trichostrongylus, and characterized by worms infesting the intestines causing anemia in some patients, but patients usually are infected with other intestinal parasites making symptom differentiation difficult.

cc **B81.3** **Intestinal angiostrongyliasis**
Angiostrongyliasis due to Parastrongylus costaricensis

cc **B81.4** **Mixed intestinal helminthiases**
Infection due to intestinal helminths classified to more than one of the categories B65.0-B81.3 and B81.8
Mixed helminthiasis NOS

cc **B81.8** **Other specified intestinal helminthiases**
Infection due to Oesophagostomum species [esophagostomiasis]
Infection due to Ternidens diminutus [ternidensiasis]

B82- **Unspecified intestinal parasitism**

cc **B82.0** **Intestinal helminthiasis, unspecified**

B82.9 **Intestinal parasitism, unspecified**

B83- **Other helminthiases**
Excludes 1:   capillariasis NOS (B81.1)
Excludes ❷: intestinal capillariasis (B81.1)

B83.0 **Visceral larva migrans** — A parasitic disease caused by the larva of genus Toxocara, and characterized by migrating larvae causing eosinophilia, visceral involvement, and fever.
Toxocariasis

B83.1 **Gnathostomiasis** — A parasitic disease caused by Gnathostoma spinigerum, and characterized by worm infestation causing subcutaneous abscesses.
Wandering swelling

B83.2 **Angiostrongyliasis due to Parastrongylus cantonensis** — A parasitic disease of larval infestation characterized by larval migration to the central nervous system resulting in eosinophilic meningoencephalitis.
Eosinophilic meningoencephalitis due to Parastrongylus cantonensis
Excludes ❷: intestinal angiostrongyliasis (B81.3)

B83.3 **Syngamiasis** — A parasitic disease caused by Syngamus trachea (gapeworm) in humans that is characterized by worm infestation in the trachea, usually found in birds.
Syngamosis

B83.4 **Internal hirudiniasis** — A parasitic infestation of leeches to the mouth, pharynx, or larynx.
Excludes ❷: external hirudiniasis (B88.3)

B83.8 **Other specified helminthiases**
Acanthocephaliasis
Gongylonemiasis
Hepatic capillariasis
Metastrongyliasis
Thelaziasis

B83.9 **Helminthiasis, unspecified**
Worms NOS
Excludes 1:   intestinal helminthiasis NOS (B82.0)

Pediculosis, acariasis and other infestations (B85-B89)

B85- **Pediculosis** and **phthiriasis** — Parasitic diseases caused by lice, and marked by intense itching.

B85.0 **Pediculosis due to Pediculus humanus capitis**
Head-louse infestation

B85.1 **Pediculosis due to Pediculus humanus corporis**
Body-louse infestation

B85.2 **Pediculosis, unspecified**

B85.3 **Phthiriasis**
Infestation by crab-louse
Infestation by Phthirus pubis

B85.4 **Mixed pediculosis and phthiriasis**
Infestation classifiable to more than one of the categories B85.0-B85.3

B86 **Scabies** — A parasitic infestation of the skin by Sarcoptes scabiei, and characterized by nocturnal itching and rash, due to the burrowing under the skin by mites.
Sarcoptic itch

B87- **Myiasis** — A parasitic infestation of the body by fly maggots.
Includes: Infestation by larva of flies

B87.0 **Cutaneous myiasis**
Creeping myiasis

B87.1 **Wound myiasis**
Traumatic myiasis

B87.2 **Ocular myiasis**

B87.3 **Nasopharyngeal myiasis**
Laryngeal myiasis

B87.4 **Aural myiasis**

B87.8- **Myiasis of other sites**

B87.81 **Genitourinary myiasis**

B87.82 **Intestinal myiasis**

B87.89 **Myiasis of other sites**

B87.9 **Myiasis, unspecified**

B88- **Other infestations**

B88.0 **Other acariasis** — Parasitic infestations of mites.
Acarine dermatitis
Dermatitis due to Demodex species
Dermatitis due to Dermanyssus gallinae
Dermatitis due to Liponyssoides sanguineus
Trombiculosis
Excludes ❷: scabies (B86)

B88.1 **Tungiasis [sandflea infestation]** — A skin-burrowing flea which causes intense irritation and, in severe cases, ulceration.

B88.2 **Other arthropod infestations**
Scarabiasis

B88.3 **External hirudiniasis** — A parasitic infestation of leeches to the skin.
Leech infestation NOS
Excludes ❷: internal hirudiniasis (B83.4)

B88.8 **Other specified infestations**
Ichthyoparasitism due to Vandellia cirrhosa
Linguatulosis
Porocephaliasis

B88.9 **Infestation, unspecified**
Infestation (skin) NOS
Infestation by mites NOS
Skin parasites NOS

B89 **Unspecified parasitic disease**

B81-B89 (side tab)

Sequelae of infectious and parasitic diseases (B90-B94)

Note: Categories B90-B94 are to be used to indicate conditions in categories A00-B89 as the cause of sequelae, which are themselves classified elsewhere. The "sequelae" include conditions specified as such; they also include residuals of diseases classifiable to the above categories if there is evidence that the disease itself is no longer present. Codes from these categories are not to be used for chronic infections. Code chronic current infections to active infectious disease as appropriate.

Code first condition resulting from (sequela) the infectious or parasitic disease

B90-   Sequelae of tuberculosis

B90.0   Sequelae of central nervous system tuberculosis

B90.1   Sequelae of genitourinary tuberculosis

B90.2   Sequelae of tuberculosis of bones and joints

B90.8   Sequelae of tuberculosis of other organs
Excludes ❷: sequelae of respiratory tuberculosis (B90.9)

B90.9   Sequelae of respiratory and unspecified tuberculosis
Sequelae of tuberculosis NOS

B91   Sequelae of poliomyelitis
Excludes 1:   postpolio syndrome (G14)

B92   Sequelae of leprosy

B94-   Sequelae of other and unspecified infectious and parasitic diseases

B94.0   Sequelae of trachoma

B94.1   Sequelae of viral encephalitis

B94.2   Sequelae of viral hepatitis

B94.8   Sequelae of other specified infectious and parasitic diseases

B94.9   Sequelae of unspecified infectious and parasitic disease

Bacterial and viral infectious agents (B95-B97)

Note: These categories are provided for use as supplementary or additional codes to identify the infectious agent(s) in diseases classified elsewhere.

B95-   Streptococcus, Staphylococcus, and Enterococcus as the cause of diseases classified elsewhere

B95.0   Streptococcus, group A, as the cause of diseases classified elsewhere

B95.1   Streptococcus, group B, as the cause of diseases classified elsewhere

B95.2   Enterococcus as the cause of diseases classified elsewhere

B95.3   Streptococcus pneumoniae as the cause of diseases classified elsewhere

B95.4   Other streptococcus as the cause of diseases classified elsewhere

B95.5   Unspecified streptococcus as the cause of diseases classified elsewhere

B95.6-   Staphylococcus aureus as the cause of diseases classified elsewhere

B95.61   Methicillin susceptible Staphylococcus aureus infection as the cause of diseases classified elsewhere
Methicillin susceptible Staphylococcus aureus (MSSA) infection as the cause of diseases classified elsewhere
Staphylococcus aureus infection NOS as the cause of diseases classified elsewhere

B95.62   Methicillin resistant Staphylococcus aureus infection as the cause of diseases classified elsewhere
Methicillin resistant Staphylococcus aureus (MRSA) infection as the cause of diseases classified elsewhere

B95.7   Other staphylococcus as the cause of diseases classified elsewhere

B95.8   Unspecified staphylococcus as the cause of diseases classified elsewhere

B96-   Other bacterial agents as the cause of diseases classified elsewhere

B96.0   Mycoplasma pneumoniae [M. pneumoniae] as the cause of diseases classified elsewhere
Pleuro-pneumonia-like-organism [PPLO]

B96.1   Klebsiella pneumoniae [K. pneumoniae] as the cause of diseases classified elsewhere

B96.2-   Escherichia coli [E. coli] as the cause of diseases classified elsewhere

B96.20   Unspecified Escherichia coli [E. coli] as the cause of diseases classified elsewhere
Escherichia coli [E. coli] NOS

B96.21   Shiga toxin-producing Escherichia coli [E. coli] (STEC) O157 as the cause of diseases classified elsewhere
E. coli O157:H- (nonmotile) with confirmation of Shiga toxin
E. coli O157 with confirmation of Shiga toxin when H antigen is unknown, or is not H7
O157:H7 Escherichia coli [E. coli] with or without confirmation of Shiga toxin-production
Shiga toxin-producing Escherichia coli [E. coli] O157:H7 with or without confirmation of Shiga toxin-production
STEC O157:H7 with or without confirmation of Shiga toxin-production

B96.22   Other specified Shiga toxin-producing Escherichia coli [E. coli] (STEC) as the cause of diseases classified elsewhere
Non-O157 Shiga toxin-producing Escherichia coli [E. coli]
Non-O157 Shiga toxin-producing Escherichia coli [E. coli] with known O group

B96.23   Unspecified Shiga toxin-producing Escherichia coli [E. coli] (STEC) as the cause of diseases classified elsewhere
Shiga toxin-producing Escherichia coli [E. coli] with specified O group
STEC NOS

B96.29   Other Escherichia coli [E. coli] as the cause of diseases classified elsewhere
Non-Shiga toxin-producing [E. coli]

B96.3   Hemophilus influenzae [H. influenzae] as the cause of diseases classified elsewhere

B96.4   Proteus (mirabilis) (morganii) as the cause of diseases classified elsewhere

B96.5   Pseudomonas (aeruginosa) (mallei) (pseudomallei) as the cause of diseases classified elsewhere
AHA 15:1Q:p18 – Auricular chondritis due to Pseudomonas aeruginosa

B96.6   Bacteroides fragilis [B. fragilis] as the cause of diseases classified elsewhere

B96.7   Clostridium perfringens [C. perfringens] as the cause of diseases classified elsewhere

B96.8-   Other specified bacterial agents as the cause of diseases classified elsewhere

B96.81   Helicobacter pylori [H. pylori] as the cause of diseases classified elsewhere

B96.82   Vibrio vulnificus as the cause of diseases classified elsewhere

B96.89   Other specified bacterial agents as the cause of diseases classified elsewhere

B97-   Viral agents as the cause of diseases classified elsewhere

B97.0   Adenovirus as the cause of diseases classified elsewhere

B97.1-   Enterovirus as the cause of diseases classified elsewhere

B97.10   Unspecified enterovirus as the cause of diseases classified elsewhere

B97.11   Coxsackievirus as the cause of diseases classified elsewhere

B97.12   Echovirus as the cause of diseases classified elsewhere

B97.19   Other enterovirus as the cause of diseases classified elsewhere

B90 - B97

B97.2- Coronavirus as the cause of diseases classified elsewhere

cc **B97.21** SARS-associated coronavirus as the cause of diseases classified elsewhere

> *Excludes 1:* *pneumonia due to SARS-associated coronavirus (J12.81)*

B97.29 Other coronavirus as the cause of diseases classified elsewhere

B97.3- Retrovirus as the cause of diseases classified elsewhere

> *Excludes 1:* *Human immunodeficiency virus [HIV] disease (B20)*

B97.30 Unspecified retrovirus as the cause of diseases classified elsewhere

B97.31 Lentivirus as the cause of diseases classified elsewhere

B97.32 Oncovirus as the cause of diseases classified elsewhere

cc **B97.33** Human T-cell lymphotrophic virus, type I [HTLV-I] as the cause of diseases classified elsewhere

cc **B97.34** Human T-cell lymphotrophic virus, type II [HTLV-II] as the cause of diseases classified elsewhere

cc **B97.35** Human immunodeficiency virus, type 2 [HIV 2] as the cause of diseases classified elsewhere

B97.39 Other retrovirus as the cause of diseases classified elsewhere

B97.4 Respiratory syncytial virus as the cause of diseases classified elsewhere

B97.5 Reovirus as the cause of diseases classified elsewhere

B97.6 Parvovirus as the cause of diseases classified elsewhere

B97.7 Papillomavirus as the cause of diseases classified elsewhere

B97.8- Other viral agents as the cause of diseases classified elsewhere

B97.81 Human metapneumovirus as the cause of diseases classified elsewhere

B97.89 Other viral agents as the cause of diseases classified elsewhere

Other infectious diseases (B99)

B99- Other and unspecified infectious diseases

B99.8 Other infectious disease

B99.9 Unspecified infectious disease

Chapter 2 – Neoplasms (C00-D49)

Note: **Functional activity**

All neoplasms are classified in this chapter, whether they are functionally active or not. An additional code from Chapter 4 may be used, to identify functional activity associated with any neoplasm.

Morphology [Histology]

Chapter 2 classifies neoplasms primarily by site (topography), with broad groupings for behavior, malignant, in situ, benign, etc. The Table of Neoplasms should be used to identify the correct topography code. In a few cases, such as for malignant melanoma and certain neuroendocrine tumors, the morphology (histologic type) is included in the category and codes.

Primary malignant neoplasms overlapping site boundaries

A primary malignant neoplasm that overlaps two or more contiguous (next to each other) sites should be classified to the subcategory/code .8 ("overlapping lesion"), unless the combination is specifically indexed elsewhere. For multiple neoplasms of the same site that are not contiguous, such as tumors in different quadrants of the same breast, codes for each site should be assigned.

Malignant neoplasm of ectopic tissue

Malignant neoplasms of ectopic tissue are to be coded to the site mentioned, e.g., ectopic pancreatic malignant neoplasms are coded to pancreas, unspecified (C25.9).

This chapter contains the following blocks:

C00-C14	Malignant neoplasm of lip, oral cavity and pharynx
C15-C26	Malignant neoplasm of digestive organs
C30-C39	Malignant neoplasm of respiratory and intrathoracic organs
C40-C41	Malignant neoplasm of bone and articular cartilage
C43-C44	Melanoma and other malignant neoplasms of skin
C45-C49	Malignant neoplasms of mesothelial and soft tissue
C50	Malignant neoplasm of breast
C51-C58	Malignant neoplasm of female genital organs
C60-C63	Malignant neoplasm of male genital organs
C64-C68	Malignant neoplasm of urinary tract
C69-C72	Malignant neoplasm of eye, brain and other parts of central nervous system
C73-C75	Malignant neoplasm of thyroid and other endocrine glands
C7A	Malignant neuroendocrine tumors
C7B	Secondary neuroendocrine tumors
C76-C80	Malignant neoplasms of ill-defined, other secondary and unspecified sites
C81-C96	Malignant neoplasms of lymphoid, hematopoietic and related tissue
D00-D09	In situ neoplasms
D10-D36	Benign neoplasms, except benign neuroendocrine tumors
D3A	Benign neuroendocrine tumors
D37-D48	Neoplasms of uncertain behavior, polycythemia vera and myelodysplastic syndromes
D49	Neoplasms of unspecified behavior

Chapter-Specific Coding Guidelines

C. **Chapter-Specific Coding Guidelines**

In addition to general coding guidelines, there are guidelines for specific diagnoses and/or conditions in the classification. Unless otherwise indicated, these guidelines apply to all health care settings. Please refer to Section II for guidelines on the selection of principal diagnosis.

2. **Chapter 2: Neoplasms (C00-D49)**

General guidelines

Chapter 2 of the ICD-10-CM contains the codes for most benign and all malignant neoplasms. Certain benign neoplasms, such as prostatic adenomas, may be found in the specific body system chapters. To properly code a neoplasm it is necessary to determine from the record if the neoplasm is benign, in-situ, malignant, or of uncertain histologic behavior. If malignant, any secondary (metastatic) sites should also be determined.

Primary malignant neoplasms overlapping site boundaries

A primary malignant neoplasm that overlaps two or more contiguous (next to each other) sites should be classified to the subcategory/code .8 ('overlapping lesion'), unless the combination is specifically indexed elsewhere. For multiple neoplasms of the same site that are not contiguous such as tumors in different quadrants of the same breast, codes for each site should be assigned.

Malignant neoplasm of ectopic tissue

Malignant neoplasms of ectopic tissue are to be coded to the site of origin mentioned, e.g., ectopic pancreatic malignant neoplasms involving the stomach are coded to pancreas, unspecified (C25.9).

The neoplasm table in the Alphabetic Index should be referenced first. However, if the histological term is documented, that term should be referenced first, rather than going immediately to the Neoplasm Table, in order to determine which column in the Neoplasm Table is appropriate. For example, if the documentation indicates "adenoma," refer to the term in the Alphabetic Index to review the entries under this term and the instructional note to "see also neoplasm, by site, benign." The table provides the proper code based on the type of neoplasm and the site. It is important to select the proper column in the table that corresponds to the type of neoplasm. The Tabular List should then be referenced to verify that the correct code has been selected from the table and that a more specific site code does not exist.

See Section I.C.21. Factors influencing health status and contact with health services, Status, for information regarding Z15.0, codes for genetic susceptibility to cancer.

a. **Treatment directed at the malignancy**

If the treatment is directed at the malignancy, designate the malignancy as the principal diagnosis.

The only exception to this guideline is if a patient admission/encounter is solely for the administration of chemotherapy, immunotherapy or radiation therapy, assign the appropriate Z51.– code as the first-listed or principal diagnosis, and the diagnosis or problem for which the service is being performed as a secondary diagnosis.

b. **Treatment of secondary site**

When a patient is admitted because of a primary neoplasm with metastasis and treatment is directed toward the secondary site only, the secondary neoplasm is designated as the principal diagnosis even though the primary malignancy is still present.

c. **Coding and sequencing of complications**

Coding and sequencing of complications associated with the malignancies or with the therapy thereof are subject to the following guidelines:

1) **Anemia associated with malignancy**

When admission/encounter is for management of an anemia associated with the malignancy, and the treatment is only for anemia, the appropriate code for the malignancy is sequenced as the principal or first-listed diagnosis followed by the appropriate code for the anemia (such as code D63.0, Anemia in neoplastic disease).

2) **Anemia associated with chemotherapy, immunotherapy and radiation therapy**

When the admission/encounter is for management of an anemia associated with an adverse effect of the administration of chemotherapy or immunotherapy and the only treatment is for the anemia, the anemia code is sequenced first followed by the appropriate codes for the neoplasm and the adverse effect (T45.1X5, Adverse effect of antineoplastic and immunosuppressive drugs).

When the admission/encounter is for management of an anemia associated with an adverse effect of radiotherapy, the anemia code should be sequenced first, followed by the appropriate neoplasm code and code Y84.2, Radiological procedure and radiotherapy as the cause of abnormal reaction of the patient, or of later complication, without mention of misadventure at the time of the procedure.

3) **Management of dehydration due to the malignancy**

When the admission/encounter is for management of dehydration due to the malignancy and only the dehydration is being treated (intravenous rehydration), the dehydration is sequenced first, followed by the code(s) for the malignancy.

4) **Treatment of a complication resulting from a surgical procedure**

When the admission/encounter is for treatment of a complication resulting from a surgical procedure, designate the complication as the principal or first-listed diagnosis if treatment is directed at resolving the complication.

d. **Primary malignancy previously excised**

When a primary malignancy has been previously excised or eradicated from its site and there is no further treatment directed to that site and there is no evidence of any existing primary malignancy, a code from category Z85, Personal history of malignant neoplasm, should be used to indicate the former site of the malignancy. Any mention of extension, invasion, or metastasis to another site is coded as a secondary malignant neoplasm to that site. The secondary site may be the principal or first-listed with the Z85 code used as a secondary code.

e. **Admissions/Encounters involving chemotherapy, immunotherapy and radiation therapy**

1) **Episode of care involves surgical removal of neoplasm**

When an episode of care involves the surgical removal of a neoplasm, primary or secondary site, followed by adjunct chemotherapy or radiation treatment during the same episode of care, the code for the neoplasm should be assigned as principal or first-listed diagnosis.

C00-C00

2) Patient admission/encounter solely for administration of chemotherapy, immunotherapy and radiation therapy

If a patient admission/encounter is solely for the administration of chemotherapy, immunotherapy or radiation therapy assign code Z51.0, Encounter for antineoplastic radiation therapy, or Z51.11, Encounter for antineoplastic chemotherapy, or Z51.12, Encounter for antineoplastic immunotherapy as the first-listed or principal diagnosis. If a patient receives more than one of these therapies during the same admission more than one of these codes may be assigned, in any sequence.

The malignancy for which the therapy is being administered should be assigned as a secondary diagnosis.

3) Patient admitted for radiation therapy, chemotherapy or immunotherapy and develops complications

When a patient is admitted for the purpose of radiotherapy, immunotherapy or chemotherapy and develops complications such as uncontrolled nausea and vomiting or dehydration, the principal or first-listed diagnosis is Z51.0, Encounter for antineoplastic radiation therapy, or Z51.11, Encounter for antineoplastic chemotherapy, or Z51.12, Encounter for antineoplastic immunotherapy followed by any codes for the complications.

f. Admission/encounter to determine extent of malignancy

When the reason for admission/encounter is to determine the extent of the malignancy, or for a procedure such as paracentesis or thoracentesis, the primary malignancy or appropriate metastatic site is designated as the principal or first-listed diagnosis, even though chemotherapy or radiotherapy is administered.

g. Symptoms, signs, and abnormal findings listed in Chapter 18 associated with neoplasms

Symptoms, signs, and ill-defined conditions listed in Chapter 18 characteristic of, or associated with, an existing primary or secondary site malignancy cannot be used to replace the malignancy as principal or first-listed diagnosis, regardless of the number of admissions or encounters for treatment and care of the neoplasm.

See section I.C.21. Factors influencing health status and contact with health services, Encounter for prophylactic organ removal.

h. Admission/encounter for pain control/management

See Section I.C.6. for information on coding admission/encounter for pain control/management.

i. Malignancy in two or more noncontiguous sites

A patient may have more than one malignant tumor in the same organ. These tumors may represent different primaries or metastatic disease, depending on the site. Should the documentation be unclear, the provider should be queried as to the status of each tumor so that the correct codes can be assigned.

j. Disseminated malignant neoplasm, unspecified

Code C80.0, Disseminated malignant neoplasm, unspecified, is for use only in those cases where the patient has advanced metastatic disease and no known primary or secondary sites are specified. It should not be used in place of assigning codes for the primary site and all known secondary sites.

k. Malignant neoplasm without specification of site

Code C80.1, Malignant (primary) neoplasm, unspecified, equates to Cancer, unspecified. This code should only be used when no determination can be made as to the primary site of a malignancy. This code should rarely be used in the inpatient setting.

l. Sequencing of neoplasm codes

1) Encounter for treatment of primary malignancy

If the reason for the encounter is for treatment of a primary malignancy, assign the malignancy as the principal/first-listed diagnosis. The primary site is to be sequenced first, followed by any metastatic sites.

2) Encounter for treatment of secondary malignancy

When an encounter is for a primary malignancy with metastasis and treatment is directed toward the metastatic (secondary) site(s) only, the metastatic site(s) is designated as the principal/first-listed diagnosis. The primary malignancy is coded as an additional code.

3) Malignant neoplasm in a pregnant patient

When a pregnant woman has a malignant neoplasm, a code from subcategory O9A.1-, Malignant neoplasm complicating pregnancy, childbirth, and the puerperium, should be sequenced first, followed by the appropriate code from Chapter 2 to indicate the type of neoplasm.

4) Encounter for complication associated with a neoplasm

When an encounter is for management of a complication associated with a neoplasm, such as dehydration, and the treatment is only for the complication, the complication is coded first, followed by the appropriate code(s) for the neoplasm.

The exception to this guideline is anemia. When the admission/encounter is for management of an anemia associated with the malignancy, and the treatment is only for anemia, the appropriate code for the malignancy is sequenced as the principal or first-listed diagnosis followed by code D63.0, Anemia in neoplastic disease.

5) Complication from surgical procedure for treatment of a neoplasm

When an encounter is for treatment of a complication resulting from a surgical procedure performed for the treatment of the neoplasm, designate the complication as the principal/first-listed diagnosis. See guideline regarding the coding of a current malignancy versus personal history to determine if the code for the neoplasm should also be assigned.

6) Pathologic fracture due to a neoplasm

When an encounter is for a pathological fracture due to a neoplasm, and the focus of treatment is the fracture, a code from subcategory M84.5, Pathological fracture in neoplastic disease, should be sequenced first, followed by the code for the neoplasm.

If the focus of treatment is the neoplasm with an associated pathological fracture, the neoplasm code should be sequenced first, followed by a code from M84.5 for the pathological fracture.

m. Current malignancy versus personal history of malignancy

When a primary malignancy has been excised but further treatment, such as an additional surgery for the malignancy, radiation therapy or chemotherapy is directed to that site, the primary malignancy code should be used until treatment is completed.

When a primary malignancy has been previously excised or eradicated from its site, there is no further treatment (of the malignancy) directed to that site, and there is no evidence of any existing primary malignancy, a code from category Z85, Personal history of malignant neoplasm, should be used to indicate the former site of the malignancy.

See Section I.C.21. Factors influencing health status and contact with health services, History (of).

n. Leukemia, Multiple Myeloma, and Malignant Plasma Cell Neoplasms in remission versus personal history

The categories for leukemia, and category C90, Multiple myeloma and malignant plasma cell neoplasms, have codes indicating whether or not the leukemia has achieved remission. There are also codes Z85.6, Personal history of leukemia, and Z85.79, Personal history of other malignant neoplasms of lymphoid, hematopoietic and related tissues. If the documentation is unclear, as to whether the leukemia has achieved remission, the provider should be queried.

See Section I.C.21. Factors influencing health status and contact with health services, History (of).

o. Aftercare following surgery for neoplasm

See Section I.C.21. Factors influencing health status and contact with health services, Aftercare.

p. Follow-up care for completed treatment of a malignancy

See Section I.C.21. Factors influencing health status and contact with health services, Follow-up.

q. Prophylactic organ removal for prevention of malignancy

See Section I.C.21. Factors influencing health status and contact with health services, Prophylactic organ removal.

r. Malignant neoplasm associated with transplanted organ

A malignant neoplasm of a transplanted organ should be coded as a transplant complication. Assign first the appropriate code from category T86.-, Complications of transplanted organs and tissue, followed by code C80.2, Malignant neoplasm associated with transplanted organ. Use an additional code for the specific malignancy.

Malignant neoplasms (C00-C96)

Malignant neoplasms, stated or presumed to be primary (of specified sites), and certain specified histologies, except neuroendocrine, and of lymphoid, hematopoietic and related tissue (C00-C75)

Malignant neoplasms of lip, oral cavity and pharynx (C00-C14)

C00-   Malignant neoplasm of lip — Any new and abnormal growth of the lips in which tissue growth is uncontrolled and has the properties of anaplasia, invasion, and metastases.
Use additional code to identify:
    Alcohol abuse and dependence (F10.-)
    History of tobacco dependence (Z87.891)
    Tobacco dependence (F17.-)
    Tobacco use (Z72.0)
Excludes 1:   malignant melanoma of lip (C43.0)
            Merkel cell carcinoma of lip (C4A.0)
            other and unspecified malignant neoplasm of skin of lip
            (C44.0-)
ANATOMY OF THE LIPS — The lips are the highly mobile upper and lower skeletal muscle margins of the anterior wall of the oral cavity.
PHYSIOLOGY OF THE LIPS — The lips have a variety of sensory receptors that are useful in judging the temperature and texture of foods. Their normal reddish color is due to an abundance of blood vessels near their surfaces.

C00.0   Malignant neoplasm of <u>external</u> <u>upper</u> lip
        Malignant neoplasm of lipstick area of upper lip
        Malignant neoplasm of upper lip NOS
        Malignant neoplasm of vermilion border of upper lip

C00.1   Malignant neoplasm of <u>external</u> <u>lower</u> lip
        Malignant neoplasm of lower lip NOS
        Malignant neoplasm of lipstick area of lower lip
        Malignant neoplasm of vermilion border of lower lip

C00.2   Malignant neoplasm of external lip, unspecified
        Malignant neoplasm of vermilion border of lip NOS

C00.3   Malignant neoplasm of <u>upper</u> lip, <u>inner</u> aspect
        Malignant neoplasm of buccal aspect of upper lip
        Malignant neoplasm of frenulum of upper lip
        Malignant neoplasm of mucosa of upper lip
        Malignant neoplasm of oral aspect of upper lip

C00.4   Malignant neoplasm of <u>lower</u> lip, <u>inner</u> aspect
        Malignant neoplasm of buccal aspect of lower lip
        Malignant neoplasm of frenulum of lower lip
        Malignant neoplasm of mucosa of lower lip
        Malignant neoplasm of oral aspect of lower lip

C00.5   Malignant neoplasm of lip, unspecified, inner aspect
        Malignant neoplasm of buccal aspect of lip, unspecified
        Malignant neoplasm of frenulum of lip, unspecified
        Malignant neoplasm of mucosa of lip, unspecified
        Malignant neoplasm of oral aspect of lip, unspecified

C00.6   Malignant neoplasm of <u>commissure</u> of lip, unspecified

C00.8   Malignant neoplasm of <u>overlapping</u> sites of lip

C00.9   Malignant neoplasm of lip, unspecified

C01   Malignant neoplasm of <u>base of tongue</u> — Any new and abnormal growth of the base of the tongue (the posterior third of the tongue which is attached to the floor of the mouth) in which tissue growth is uncontrolled and has the properties of anaplasia, invasion, and metastases.
        Malignant neoplasm of dorsal surface of base of tongue
        Malignant neoplasm of fixed part of tongue NOS
        Malignant neoplasm of posterior third of tongue
    Use additional code to identify:
        Alcohol abuse and dependence (F10.-)
        History of tobacco dependence (Z87.891)
        Tobacco dependence (F17.-)
        Tobacco use (Z72.0)

C02-   Malignant neoplasm of other and unspecified parts of tongue — Any new and abnormal growth of the tongue (other than the base) in which tissue growth is uncontrolled and has the properties of anaplasia, invasion, and metastases.
Use additional code to identify:
    Alcohol abuse and dependence (F10.-)
    History of tobacco dependence (Z87.891)
    Tobacco dependence (F17.-)
    Tobacco use (Z72.0)
ANATOMY OF THE TONGUE —The tongue is the movable, muscular organ on the floor of the mouth. The lingual tonsils are a mass of lymphoid tissue at the root, and the frenulum is the mucous membrane fold which attaches the undersurface of the tongue to the floor of the mouth.
PHYSIOLOGY OF THE TONGUE — The tongue functions primarily as the organ for sense of taste, as well as aiding in the chewing and swallowing of food, and the articulation of sound. The lingual tonsils aid in the elimination of bacteria entering the oral cavity. The frenulum somewhat restricts the movement of the tongue.

TONGUE — SAGITTAL VIEW

C02.0   Malignant neoplasm of <u>dorsal surface</u> of tongue
        Malignant neoplasm of anterior two-thirds of tongue, dorsal surface
    Excludes ❷: malignant neoplasm of dorsal surface of base of tongue (C01)

C02.1   Malignant neoplasm of <u>border</u> of tongue
        Malignant neoplasm of tip of tongue

C02.2   Malignant neoplasm of <u>ventral</u> surface of tongue
        Malignant neoplasm of anterior two-thirds of tongue, ventral surface
        Malignant neoplasm of frenulum linguae

C02.3   Malignant neoplasm of <u>anterior two-thirds</u> of tongue, part unspecified
        Malignant neoplasm of middle third of tongue NOS
        Malignant neoplasm of mobile part of tongue NOS

C02.4   Malignant neoplasm of <u>lingual</u> tonsil — A mass of lymphoid tissue at the root of the tongue.
    Excludes ❷: malignant neoplasm of tonsil NOS (C09.9)

C02.8   Malignant neoplasm of <u>overlapping</u> sites of tongue
        Malignant neoplasm of two or more contiguous sites of tongue

C02.9   Malignant neoplasm of tongue, unspecified

C03-   Malignant neoplasm of <u>gum</u> — Any new and abnormal growth of the gums in which tissue growth is uncontrolled and has the properties of anaplasia, invasion, and metastases.
    **Includes: Malignant neoplasm of alveolar (ridge) mucosa
                Malignant neoplasm of gingiva**
    Use additional code to identify:
        Alcohol abuse and dependence (F10.-)
        History of tobacco dependence (Z87.891)
        Tobacco dependence (F17.-)
        Tobacco use (Z72.0)
Excludes ❷: malignant odontogenic neoplasms (C41.0-C41.1)
ANATOMY OF THE GUMS — The gums (gingiva) are fibrous and mucous membrane tissues which surround the roots of erupted teeth and the crowns of unerupted teeth, and cover the alveolar process of the maxilla and mandible.
PHYSIOLOGY OF THE GUMS — The gums (gingiva) function to help protect and support the roots of the teeth.

C03.0   Malignant neoplasm of <u>upper</u> gum
C03.1   Malignant neoplasm of <u>lower</u> gum
C03.9   Malignant neoplasm of gum, unspecified

C00
-
C03

C04- **Malignant neoplasm of <u>floor of mouth</u>** — Any new and abnormal growth of the floor of the mouth in which tissue growth is uncontrolled and has the properties of anaplasia, invasion, and metastases.
Use additional code to identify:
  Alcohol abuse and dependence (F10.-)
  History of tobacco dependence (Z87.891)
  Tobacco dependence (F17.-)
  Tobacco use (Z72.0)
  ANATOMY OF THE FLOOR OF MOUTH — The floor of mouth is the musculomembranous tissue which forms the inferior wall of the oral cavity.
  PHYSIOLOGY OF THE FLOOR OF MOUTH — The floor of mouth functions to enclose the inferior floor of the oral cavity between the mandibular bodies.

C04.0 **Malignant neoplasm of <u>anterior</u> floor of mouth**
  Malignant neoplasm of anterior to the premolar-canine junction

C04.1 **Malignant neoplasm of <u>lateral</u> floor of mouth**

C04.8 **Malignant neoplasm of <u>overlapping</u> sites of floor of mouth**

C04.9 **Malignant neoplasm of floor of mouth, unspecified**

C05- **Malignant neoplasm of <u>palate</u>** — Any new and abnormal growth of the palate in which tissue growth is uncontrolled and has the properties of anaplasia, invasion, and metastases.
Use additional code to identify:
  Alcohol abuse and dependence (F10.-)
  History of tobacco dependence (Z87.891)
  Tobacco dependence (F17.-)
  Tobacco use (Z72.0)
Excludes 1:   Kaposi's sarcoma of palate (C46.2)

C05.0 **Malignant neoplasm of <u>hard</u> palate** — The palatine process of the maxilla that separates the nasal and oral cavities.

C05.1 **Malignant neoplasm of <u>soft</u> palate** — The muscular extension of the hard palate in the superior-posterior portion of the oral cavity.
  Excludes ❷: malignant neoplasm of nasopharyngeal surface of soft palate (C11.3)

C05.2 **Malignant neoplasm of <u>uvula</u>** — The cone-shaped projection of the soft palate which hangs over the area of the root of the tongue.

C05.8 **Malignant neoplasm of <u>overlapping</u> sites of palate**

C05.9 **Malignant neoplasm of palate, unspecified**
  Malignant neoplasm of roof of mouth

C06- **Malignant neoplasm of <u>other and unspecified parts of mouth</u>** — Any new and abnormal growth of the other and unspecified parts of the mouth in which tissue growth is uncontrolled, and has the properties of anaplasia, invasion and metastases.
Use additional code to identify:
  Alcohol abuse and dependence (F10.-)
  History of tobacco dependence (Z87.891)
  Tobacco dependence (F17.-)
  Tobacco use (Z72.0)
  ANATOMY OF OTHER PARTS OF THE MOUTH — The cheeks are the layers of skin, subcutaneous tissue, and certain muscles which form the lateral walls of the oral cavity. The vestibule is the space which lies between the cheeks or lips and the gingiva and teeth. The hard palate is the superior wall of the oral cavity formed by the palatine processes of the maxilla. The soft palate is the muscular extension of the hard palate in the superior-posterior oral cavity. The uvula is the cone-shaped projection of the soft palate. The retromolar area is the nonspecific area of tissue located behind the third molar teeth.
  PHYSIOLOGY OF OTHER PARTS OF THE MOUTH — The cheeks have certain muscles which are associated with chewing and facial expression. The soft palate contracts to allow swallowing, and prevents food from entering the nasal cavity.

C06.0 **Malignant neoplasm of <u>cheek mucosa</u>** — The mucous membrane of the cheeks.
  Malignant neoplasm of buccal mucosa NOS
  Malignant neoplasm of internal cheek

C06.1 **Malignant neoplasm of <u>vestibule</u> of mouth** — The lining between the cheeks and lips, and the gingiva and teeth.
  Malignant neoplasm of buccal sulcus (upper) (lower)
  Malignant neoplasm of labial sulcus (upper) (lower)

C06.2 **Malignant neoplasm of <u>retromolar area</u>** — The nonspecific area of tissue located behind the third molar.

C06.8- **Malignant neoplasm of overlapping sites of other and unspecified parts of mouth**

C06.80 **Malignant neoplasm of overlapping sites of unspecified parts of mouth**

C06.89 **Malignant neoplasm of overlapping sites of other parts of mouth**
  "Book leaf" neoplasm [ventral surface of tongue and floor of mouth]

C06.9 **Malignant neoplasm of mouth, unspecified**
  Malignant neoplasm of minor salivary gland, unspecified site
  Malignant neoplasm of oral cavity NOS

C07- **Malignant neoplasm of <u>parotid gland</u>** — Any new and abnormal growth of the parotid gland in which tissue growth is uncontrolled and has the properties of anaplasia, invasion, and metastases.
Use additional code to identify:
  Alcohol abuse and dependence (F10.-)
  Exposure to environmental tobacco smoke (Z77.22)
  Exposure to tobacco smoke in the perinatal period (P96.81)
  History of tobacco dependence (Z87.891)
  Occupational exposure to environmental tobacco smoke (Z57.31)
  Tobacco dependence (F17.-)
  Tobacco use (Z72.0)

PAROTID GLAND

C08- **Malignant neoplasm of other and unspecified major salivary glands**
Includes: malignant neoplasm of salivary ducts
Use additional code to identify:
  Alcohol abuse and dependence (F10.-)
  Exposure to environmental tobacco smoke (Z77.22)
  Exposure to tobacco smoke in the perinatal period (P96.81)
  History of tobacco dependence (Z87.891)
  Occupational exposure to environmental tobacco smoke (Z57.31)
  Tobacco dependence (F17.-)
  Tobacco use (Z72.0)
Excludes 1:   malignant neoplasms of specified minor salivary glands which are classified according to their anatomical location
Excludes ❷: malignant neoplasms of minor salivary glands NOS (C06.9)
  malignant neoplasm of parotid gland (C07)
  ANATOMY OF THE MAJOR SALIVARY GLANDS — There are three pairs of major salivary glands. The two parotid glands lie above the mouth, and below and in front of the ears with ducts (Stenson's ducts) which run down through the cheeks and empty into the roof of the mouth opposite of the second molar. The two submandibular (submaxillary) glands lie in the floor of the mouth on the inside surface of the mandible, with ducts (Wharton's ducts) opening beneath the tongue, and with other ducts opening near the frenulum of the tongue. The two sublingual glands lie beneath the tongue, with ducts opening near the frenulum of the tongue. Both sympathetic and parasympathetic nerves stimulate the major salivary glands.
  PHYSIOLOGY OF THE MAJOR SALIVARY GLANDS — The major salivary glands function to secrete saliva which moistens food particles, helps to bind them together, and begins digestion of carbohydrates. Saliva also dissolves various food chemicals so they can be tasted. There are two types of secretory cells. Serous cells produce a watery fluid which contains a digestive enzyme, called amylase. Mucous cells produce a thick stringy liquid that binds food together and acts as a lubricant during swallowing. Sympathetic nerves stimulate the glands to secrete a small quantity of saliva to keep the mouth moist. Parasympathetic nerves stimulate the glands reflexly when the person sees, smells, or even thinks about pleasant food.

SALIVARY GLANDS

C08.0 **Malignant neoplasm of <u>submandibular gland</u>** — Any new and abnormal growth of the submandibular (submaxillary) glands in which tissue growth is uncontrolled and has the properties of anaplasia, invasion, and metastases.
  Malignant neoplasm of submaxillary gland

C08.1 **Malignant neoplasm of <u>sublingual gland</u>** — Any new and abnormal growth of the sublingual glands in which tissue growth is uncontrolled and has the properties of anaplasia, invasion, and metastases.

C08.9   **Malignant neoplasm of major salivary gland, unspecified**
Malignant neoplasm of salivary gland (major) NOS

C09-   **Malignant neoplasm of <u>tonsil</u>** — Any new and abnormal growth of the tonsils (the small, almond-shaped masses of lymphatic tissue on either side of the tongue in the posterior oral cavity) in which tissue growth is uncontrolled and has the properties of anaplasia, invasion, and metastases.
Use additional code to identify:
Alcohol abuse and dependence (F10.-)
Exposure to environmental tobacco smoke (Z77.22)
Exposure to tobacco smoke in the perinatal period (P96.81)
History of tobacco dependence (Z87.891)
Occupational exposure to environmental tobacco smoke (Z57.31)
Tobacco dependence (F17.-)
Tobacco use (Z72.0)
Excludes ❷: *malignant neoplasm of lingual tonsil (C02.4)*
malignant neoplasm of pharyngeal tonsil (C11.1)

C09.0   **Malignant neoplasm of tonsillar <u>fossa</u>** — The depression in which the tonsils are located.

C09.1   **Malignant neoplasm of tonsillar <u>pillar</u> (anterior) (posterior)** — The mucous membrane folds attached to the soft palate.

C09.8   **Malignant neoplasm of <u>overlapping</u> sites of tonsil**

C09.9   **Malignant neoplasm of tonsil, unspecified**
Malignant neoplasm of tonsil NOS
Malignant neoplasm of faucial tonsils
Malignant neoplasm of palatine tonsils

C10-   **Malignant neoplasm of <u>oropharynx</u>** — Any new and abnormal growth of the oropharynx in which tissue growth is uncontrolled and has the properties of anaplasia, invasion, and metastases.
Use additional code to identify:
Alcohol abuse and dependence (F10.-)
Exposure to environmental tobacco smoke (Z77.22)
Exposure to tobacco smoke in the perinatal period (P96.81)
History of tobacco dependence (Z87.891)
Occupational exposure to environmental tobacco smoke (Z57.31)
Tobacco dependence (F17.-)
Tobacco use (Z72.0)
Excludes ❷: *malignant neoplasm of tonsil (C09.-)*
ANATOMY OF THE OROPHARYNX — The tonsils are masses of lymphatic tissue located on either side of the tongue in the posterior oral cavity. The tonsillar fossa is the depression in which the tonsils are located. The tonsillar pillars are the mucous membrane folds attached to the soft palate. The vallecula is the anterior and medial surface of the pharyngoepiglottic fold.
PHYSIOLOGY OF THE OROPHARYNX — The tonsils function to help fight off bacteria by releasing bacteria-consuming phagocytes.

OROPHARYNX

C10.0   **Malignant neoplasm of <u>vallecula</u>** — The depression between the lateral and median glossoepiglottic folds on each side.

C10.1   **Malignant neoplasm of anterior surface of <u>epiglottis</u>** — That portion of the lip-like structure covering the larynx which faces the oral cavity.
Malignant neoplasm of epiglottis, free border [margin]
Malignant neoplasm of glossoepiglottic fold(s)
Excludes ❷: *malignant neoplasm of epiglottis (suprahyoid portion) NOS (C32.1)*

C10.2   **Malignant neoplasm of <u>lateral wall</u> of oropharynx**

C10.3   **Malignant neoplasm of <u>posterior wall</u> of oropharynx**

C10.4   **Malignant neoplasm of <u>branchial cleft</u>** — An area of the lateral part of the neck that is present from the failure of obliteration of the second branchial cleft in embryonic development.
Malignant neoplasm of branchial cyst [site of neoplasm]

C10.8   **Malignant neoplasm of <u>overlapping</u> sites of oropharynx**
Malignant neoplasm of junctional region of oropharynx

C10.9   **Malignant neoplasm of oropharynx, unspecified**

C11-   **Malignant neoplasm of <u>nasopharynx</u>** — Any new and abnormal growth of the nasopharynx in which tissue growth is uncontrolled and has the properties of anaplasia, invasion, and metastases.
Use additional code to identify:
Exposure to environmental tobacco smoke (Z77.22)
Exposure to tobacco smoke in the perinatal period (P96.81)
History of tobacco dependence (Z87.891)
Occupational exposure to environmental tobacco smoke (Z57.31)
Tobacco dependence (F17.-)
Tobacco use (Z72.0)
ANATOMY OF THE NASOPHARYNX — The nasopharynx is the upper portion of the pharynx which lies above the soft palate. The adenoids are the masses of lymphatic tissue in the posterior wall of the nasopharynx.
PHYSIOLOGY OF THE NASOPHARYNX — The nasopharynx functions to connect the nasal cavity with the back of the oral cavity to allow nasal breathing and sinus drainage. The adenoids help in the prevention of bacteria entering the body.

C11.0   **Malignant neoplasm of <u>superior wall</u> of nasopharynx**

NASOPHARYNX

Malignant neoplasm of roof of nasopharynx — The upper limit of the nasopharynx.

C11.1   **Malignant neoplasm of <u>posterior wall</u> of nasopharynx**
Malignant neoplasm of adenoid — A mass of lymphatic tissue in the posterior wall.
Malignant neoplasm of pharyngeal tonsil — Synonym for Adenoid.

C11.2   **Malignant neoplasm of <u>lateral wall</u> of nasopharynx**
Malignant neoplasm of fossa of Rosenmüller — Synonym for Pharyngeal Recess.
Malignant neoplasm of opening of auditory tube — The area where the auditory (Eustachian) tube enters the nasopharynx from the middle ear.
Malignant neoplasm of pharyngeal recess — Slit-like lateral extension in the nasopharyngeal wall.

C11.3   **Malignant neoplasm of <u>anterior wall</u> of nasopharynx**
Malignant neoplasm of floor of nasopharynx
Malignant neoplasm of nasopharyngeal (anterior) (posterior) surface of soft palate
Malignant neoplasm of posterior margin of nasal choana
Malignant neoplasm of posterior margin of nasal septum

C11.8   **Malignant neoplasm of <u>overlapping</u> sites of nasopharynx**

C11.9   **Malignant neoplasm of nasopharynx, unspecified**
Malignant neoplasm of nasopharyngeal wall NOS

C12   **Malignant neoplasm of <u>pyriform sinus</u>** — Any new and abnormal growth of the pyriform sinus (the elongated depression of the hypopharynx lying between the laryngeal opening and the outer wall of the hypopharynx) in which tissue growth is uncontrolled and has the properties of anaplasia, invasion, and metastases.
Malignant neoplasm of pyriform fossa
Use additional code to identify:
Exposure to environmental tobacco smoke (Z77.22)
Exposure to tobacco smoke in the perinatal period (P96.81)
History of tobacco dependence (Z87.891)
Occupational exposure to environmental tobacco smoke (Z57.31)
Tobacco dependence (F17.-)
Tobacco use (Z72.0)

C08 – C12

C13- **Malignant neoplasm of** <u>hypopharynx</u> — Any new and abnormal growth of the hypopharynx in which tissue growth is uncontrolled and has the properties of anaplasia, invasion, and metastases.

Use additional code to identify:
Exposure to environmental tobacco smoke (Z77.22)
Exposure to tobacco smoke in the perinatal period (P96.81)
History of tobacco dependence (Z87.891)
Occupational exposure to environmental tobacco smoke (Z57.31)
Tobacco dependence (F17.-)
Tobacco use (Z72.0)

Excludes ❷: *malignant neoplasm of pyriform sinus (C12)*

ANATOMY OF THE HYPOPHARYNX — The hypopharynx is the cavity which lies from the upper border of the epiglottis to the opening of the larynx and esophagus. The pyriform sinus is the elongated depression of the hypopharynx lying between the laryngeal opening and the outer wall of the hypopharynx. The aryepiglottic fold is the mucous membrane fold on each side of the epiglottis.

PHYSIOLOGY OF THE HYPOPHARYNX — The hypopharynx functions to help in swallowing and breathing.

C13.0 **Malignant neoplasm of** <u>postcricoid region</u> — The lower portion of the hypopharynx.

C13.1 **Malignant neoplasm of** <u>aryepiglottic fold</u>**, hypopharyngeal aspect**
Malignant neoplasm of aryepiglottic fold, marginal zone
Malignant neoplasm of aryepiglottic fold NOS
Malignant neoplasm of interarytenoid fold, marginal zone
Malignant neoplasm of interarytenoid fold NOS
Excludes ❷: *malignant neoplasm of aryepiglottic fold or interarytenoid fold, laryngeal aspect (C32.1)*

C13.2 **Malignant neoplasm of** <u>posterior wall</u> **of hypopharynx**

C13.8 **Malignant neoplasm of** <u>overlapping</u> **sites of hypopharynx**

C13.9 **Malignant neoplasm of hypopharynx, unspecified**
Malignant neoplasm of hypopharyngeal wall NOS

C14- **Malignant neoplasm of other and ill-defined sites in the lip, oral cavity and pharynx**
Use additional code to identify:
Alcohol abuse and dependence (F10.-)
Exposure to environmental tobacco smoke (Z77.22)
Exposure to tobacco smoke in the perinatal period (P96.81)
History of tobacco dependence (Z87.891)
Occupational exposure to environmental tobacco smoke (Z57.31)
Tobacco dependence (F17.-)
Tobacco use (Z72.0)
Excludes 1: *malignant neoplasm of oral cavity NOS (C06.9)*

C14.0 **Malignant neoplasm of pharynx, unspecified**

C14.2 **Malignant neoplasm of Waldeyer's ring** — Any new and abnormal growth of Waldeyer's ring (the ring of lymphoid tissue located in the nasopharynx and oropharynx) in which tissue growth is uncontrolled and has the properties of anaplasia, invasion, and metastases.

C14.8 **Malignant neoplasm of overlapping sites of lip, oral cavity and pharynx**
Primary malignant neoplasm of two or more contiguous sites of lip, oral cavity and pharynx
Excludes 1: *"book leaf" neoplasm [ventral surface of tongue and floor of mouth] (C06.89)*

Malignant neoplasms of digestive organs (C15-C26)

Excludes 1: *Kaposi's sarcoma of gastrointestinal sites (C46.4)*
Excludes ❷: *gastrointestinal stromal tumors (C49.A-)*

C15- **Malignant neoplasm of** <u>esophagus</u> — Any new and abnormal growth of the esophagus in which tissue growth is uncontrolled and has the properties of anaplasia, invasion, and metastases.
Use additional code to identify:
Alcohol abuse and dependence (F10.-)
ANATOMY OF THE ESOPHAGUS — The esophagus, located between the pharynx and stomach, is a collapsible musculomembranous alimentary tract tube about 10 inches (25 cm) long. The esophagus is lined with mucous glands.
PHYSIOLOGY OF THE ESOPHAGUS — The esophagus is the passageway for food from the mouth to the stomach. The mucous glands moisten and lubricate the inner lining to facilitate the passage of food. Situated just above the stomach opening lies the contracted circular muscles which prevent regurgitation.

ESOPHAGUS — ANTERIOR VIEW

ESOPHAGUS — SECTION

cc **C15.3** **Malignant neoplasm of** <u>upper third</u> **of esophagus** — The proximal (upper) approximate one-third of the esophagus above the diaphragm (also known as the cervical esophagus).

cc **C15.4** **Malignant neoplasm of** <u>middle third</u> **of esophagus** — The middle approximate one-third of the esophagus within the diaphragm (also known as the thoracic esophagus).

cc **C15.5** **Malignant neoplasm of** <u>lower third</u> **of esophagus** — The distal (lower) approximate one-third of the esophagus below the diaphragm (also known as the abdominal esophagus).
Excludes 1: *malignant neoplasm of cardio-esophageal junction (C16.0)*

cc **C15.8** **Malignant neoplasm of** <u>overlapping</u> **sites of esophagus**

cc **C15.9** **Malignant neoplasm of esophagus, unspecified**

C16- **Malignant neoplasm of <u>stomach</u>** — Any new and abnormal growth of the stomach in which tissue growth is uncontrolled and has the properties of anaplasia, invasion, and metastases.
Use additional code to identify:
    Alcohol abuse and dependence (F10.-)
Excludes ❷: malignant carcinoid tumor of the stomach (C7A.092)
ANATOMY OF THE STOMACH — The stomach, located in the upper abdomen, is a pouch-like organ of the alimentary tract connecting with the esophagus in the proximal (upper) portion and the duodenum in the distal (lower) portion and is about 10 to 12 inches (25 to 30 cm) long. The cardia lies at the opening of the esophagus at the fundus of the stomach. The fundus is the upper ballooned area of the stomach. The body is the main part of the stomach and is located between the fundus and the pyloric antrum and the duodenum. When empty, the mucous membrane on the interior surface forms longitudinal folds, called rugae. There are three mucosal glands which secrete digestive juices and mucus. These are the gastric glands, which are located throughout the body of the stomach; the cardiac glands, which are found near the esophageal opening; and the pyloric glands, which are located in the pyloric (distal) region. There are three layers of smooth muscle, and a serosal covering of visceral peritoneum. The vagus nerve stimulates the gastric glands. The stomach has a rich arterial blood supply through the celiac artery. The venous blood is drained into the hepatic portal system.

PHYSIOLOGY OF THE STOMACH — The stomach functions to receive food from the esophagus, mixes it with the gastric juice, initiates the digestion of proteins with pepsin, carries on a limited amount of absorption, and moves food into the small intestine by peristaltic muscle action. The gastric glands produce mucous, digestive enzymes (pepsin), hydrochloric acid, and an intrinsic factor, forming the gastric juice. The mucous is thought to help prevent the pepsin and hydrochloric acid from digesting the stomach surface. The stomach may absorb small quantities of water, glucose, certain salts, and alcohol. The parasympathetic vagus nerve stimulates the gastric glands to secrete large amounts of gastric juice which, in turn, releases gastrin, a hormone that causes the gastric glands to increase their secretory activity.

STOMACH

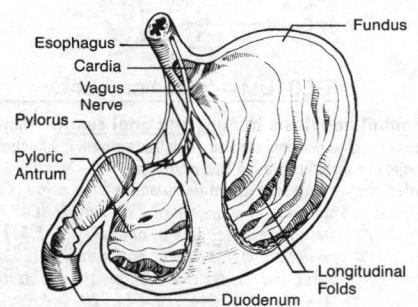

STOMACH — ANTERIOR (CUT-AWAY) VIEW

cc **C16.0** **Malignant neoplasm of <u>cardia</u>** — The opening and junction of the stomach from the esophagus.
    Malignant neoplasm of cardiac orifice
    Malignant neoplasm of cardio-esophageal junction
    Malignant neoplasm of esophagus and stomach
    Malignant neoplasm of gastro-esophageal junction

cc **C16.1** **Malignant neoplasm of <u>fundus</u> of stomach** — The ballooned upper end of the stomach lying above a transverse line drawn from the cardia.

cc **C16.2** **Malignant neoplasm of <u>body</u> of stomach** — The main pouch-like portion.

cc **C16.3** **Malignant neoplasm of <u>pyloric antrum</u>** — That portion between the body and the pylorus.
    Malignant neoplasm of gastric antrum

cc **C16.4** **Malignant neoplasm of <u>pylorus</u>** — The opening between the pyloric antrum and the duodenum.
    Malignant neoplasm of prepylorus
    Malignant neoplasm of pyloric canal

cc **C16.5** **Malignant neoplasm of lesser curvature of stomach, unspecified** — The smaller, innermost curved vertical portion from the esophagus to the duodenum.
    Malignant neoplasm of lesser curvature of stomach, not classifiable to C16.1-C16.4

cc **C16.6** **Malignant neoplasm of greater curvature of stomach, unspecified** — The larger, outermost curved vertical portion from the esophagus to the duodenum.
    Malignant neoplasm of greater curvature of stomach, not classifiable to C16.0-C16.4

cc **C16.8** **Malignant neoplasm of <u>overlapping</u> sites of stomach**

cc **C16.9** **Malignant neoplasm of stomach, unspecified**
    Gastric cancer NOS

C17- **Malignant neoplasm of <u>small intestine</u>** — Any new and abnormal growth of the small intestine, including duodenum, in which tissue growth is uncontrolled and has the properties of anaplasia, invasion, and metastases.
Excludes 1:   malignant carcinoid tumors of the small intestine (C7A.01)
ANATOMY OF THE SMALL INTESTINE — The small intestine is the tubular organ of the alimentary tract between the stomach and large intestine and is about 16 to 20 feet (5 to 6 m) long, and has 3 parts: Duodenum, jejunum, and ileum. The duodenum is the first portion about 10 inches (25 cm) long connected at its proximal end to the stomach. The jejunum is the middle, approximately two-fifths, portion. The ileum is the distal portion which connects with the large intestine. Both the jejunum and ileum are suspended from the posterior abdominal wall by the mesentery.

PHYSIOLOGY OF THE SMALL INTESTINE — The small intestine functions to absorb water and the nutrients produced through digestion. The food is passed through the small intestine by the contraction of its circular smooth muscle layer, called peristalsis. The duodenum releases several enzymes and mixes the pancreatic and bile juices with food from the stomach. The jejunum and ileum continue mixing and absorbing until the remaining substances pass into the large intestine.

SMALL INTESTINE

cc **C17.0** **Malignant neoplasm of <u>duodenum</u>** — The most proximal portion connected with the stomach.

cc **C17.1** **Malignant neoplasm of <u>jejunum</u>** — The middle portion which is larger in diameter than the ileum.

cc **C17.2** **Malignant neoplasm of <u>ileum</u>** — The distal portion connecting with the cecum.
    Excludes 1:   malignant neoplasm of ileocecal valve (C18.0)

cc **C17.3** **<u>Meckel's</u> diverticulum, malignant** — A sacculation or appendage of the ileum, specified as malignant.
    Excludes 1:   Meckel's diverticulum, congenital (Q43.0)

cc **C17.8** **Malignant neoplasm of <u>overlapping</u> sites of small intestine**

cc **C17.9** **Malignant neoplasm of small intestine, unspecified**

C18- **Malignant neoplasm of <u>colon</u>** — Any new and abnormal growth of the large intestine in which tissue growth is uncontrolled and has the properties of anaplasia, invasion, and metastases.

Excludes 1:   *malignant carcinoid tumors of the colon (C7A.02-)*

ANATOMY OF THE COLON — The colon (large intestine) is the tubular organ of the alimentary tract between the small intestine and the rectum, and is about 5 feet (1.5 m) long. The colon has four main segments: Ascending, transverse, descending, and sigmoid. The ascending colon arises from the cecum, the pouch-like structure, and continues upwards where it turns (hepatic flexure) and connects to the transverse colon. The transverse colon extends horizontally and turns (splenic flexure) downward connecting to the descending colon. The descending colon extends downward to the rectum, and is called the sigmoid (flexure) colon where it makes an S-shaped curve over the pelvic brim. The appendix projects downward from the cecum.

PHYSIOLOGY OF THE COLON — The colon (large intestine) functions in a minor capacity to absorb water and electrolytes, and to move by peristalsis, nonabsorbed substances to the rectum for defecation. Many bacteria normally inhabit the colon and serve to further break down substances for colonic absorption.

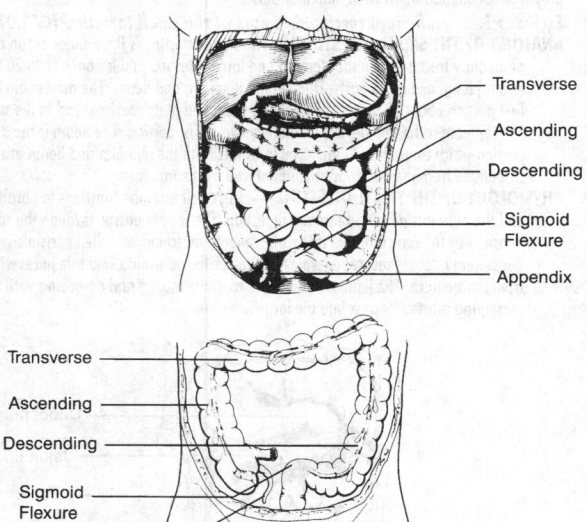

LARGE INTESTINE (COLON)

cc **C18.0** **Malignant neoplasm of <u>cecum</u>** — The dilated pouch at the proximal end of the ascending colon.

    Malignant neoplasm of ileocecal valve — The sphincter muscle valve between the ileum and the colon.

cc **C18.1** **Malignant neoplasm of <u>appendix</u>** — The closed appendage which projects downward from the cecum.

cc **C18.2** **Malignant neoplasm of <u>ascending colon</u>** — That portion which extends upward from the cecum to the transverse colon at the hepatic flexure.

cc **C18.3** **Malignant neoplasm of <u>hepatic flexure</u>** — The bend of the colon where the ascending colon turns to become the transverse colon.

cc **C18.4** **Malignant neoplasm of <u>transverse colon</u>** — That portion which lies horizontally between ascending colon at the hepatic flexure and the descending colon at the splenic flexure.

cc **C18.5** **Malignant neoplasm of <u>splenic flexure</u>** — The bend of the colon where the transverse colon turns downward to become the descending colon.

cc **C18.6** **Malignant neoplasm of <u>descending colon</u>** — That portion which extends downward from the transeverse colon at the splenic flexure to the sigmoid colon.

cc **C18.7** **Malignant neoplasm of <u>sigmoid colon</u>** — That portion of the colon from the descending colon to the rectum, which forms an S-shaped curve over the pelvic brim.

    Malignant neoplasm of sigmoid (flexure)

    Excludes 1:   *malignant neoplasm of rectosigmoid junction (C19)*

cc **C18.8** **Malignant neoplasm of <u>overlapping</u> sites of colon**

cc **C18.9** **Malignant neoplasm of colon, unspecified**

    Malignant neoplasm of large intestine NOS

C19 **Malignant neoplasm of <u>rectosigmoid junction</u>** — Any new and abnormal
cc growth of the rectosigmoid junction in which tissue growth is uncontrolled and has the properties of anaplasia, invasion, and metastases.

    Malignant neoplasm of colon with rectum

    Malignant neoplasm of rectosigmoid (colon)

Excludes 1:   *malignant carcinoid tumors of the colon (C7A.02-)*

C20 **Malignant neoplasm of <u>rectum</u>** — Any new and abnormal growth of the rectum
cc in which tissue growth is uncontrolled and has the properties of anaplasia, invasion, and metastases.

    Malignant neoplasm of rectal ampulla — The dilated portion just proximal to the anus.

Excludes 1:   *malignant carcinoid tumor of the rectum (C7A.026)*

ANATOMY OF THE RECTUM AND ANUS — The rectum is the musculomembranous portion of the alimentary tract between the colon and anus, approximately 5 inches (13 cm) long. The anus is the internal canal from the rectum which ends the alimentary tract at the anal opening. The rectosigmoid junction is that portion of the alimentary tract between the distal end of the sigmoid colon and the proximal end of the rectum.

PHYSIOLOGY OF THE RECTUM AND ANUS — The rectum and anus function to eliminate feces from the alimentary tract. A reflex signal is sent when the rectum fills and urgency to defecate is perceived. The external voluntary muscle is voluntarily relaxed to defecate.

RECTUM

RECTUM — ANTERIOR (CUT-AWAY) VIEW

C21- **Malignant neoplasm of <u>anus and anal canal</u>** — Any new and abnormal growth of the anus and anal canal in which tissue growth is uncontrolled and has the properties of anaplasia, invasion, and metastases.

Excludes ❷: *malignant carcinoid tumors of the colon (C7A.02-)*

    malignant melanoma of anal margin (C43.51)

    malignant melanoma of anal skin (C43.51)

    malignant melanoma of perianal skin (C43.51)

    other and unspecified malignant neoplasm of anal margin (C44.500, C44.510, C44.520, C44.590)

    other and unspecified malignant neoplasm of anal skin (C44.500, C44.510, C44.520, C44.590)

    other and unspecified malignant neoplasm of perianal skin (C44.500, C44.510, C44.520, C44.590)

cc **C21.0** **Malignant neoplasm of anus, unspecified**

cc **C21.1** **Malignant neoplasm of <u>anal canal</u>** — That portion of the alimentary tract between the sigmoid colon and the external opening of the anus.

    Malignant neoplasm of anal sphincter

cc **C21.2** **Malignant neoplasm of <u>cloacogenic zone</u>** — The anorectal region originating from a persistant remnant of the cloacal membrane of the embryo.

cc **C21.8** **Malignant neoplasm of <u>overlapping</u> sites of rectum, anus and anal canal**

    Malignant neoplasm of anorectal junction

    Malignant neoplasm of anorectum

    Primary malignant neoplasm of two or more contiguous sites of rectum, anus and anal canal

---

Excludes 1: = NOT CODED HERE! (Do not code both)   *Excludes ❷:* = Not Included Here

C22- Malignant neoplasm of <u>liver and intrahepatic bile ducts</u> — Any new and abnormal growth of the liver and intrahepatic ducts in which the tissue growth is uncontrolled, and has the properties of anaplasia, invasion and metastases.

Use additional code to identify:
   Alcohol abuse and dependence (F10.-)
   Hepatitis B (B16.-, B18.0-B18.1)
   Hepatitis C (B17.1-, B18.2)

Excludes 1: *malignant neoplasm of biliary tract NOS (C24.9)*
secondary malignant neoplasm of liver and intrahepatic bile duct (C78.7)

ANATOMY OF THE LIVER — The liver is the largest organ in the body, weighing about 3 pounds (1 kg) in the adult. Located in the upper right quadrant of the abdominal cavity, its superior surface lies under the dome of the diaphragm. There are 4 lobes of the liver. The common bile duct is formed by the joining of the hepatic duct, which carries bile from the liver, and the cystic duct, which carries bile from the gallbladder. The common duct then carries the bile into the duodenum through an opening on the duodenal papilla. The hepatic artery furnishes arterial blood for the nourishment of the liver cells. The portal vein carries blood containing products of digestion from the intestinal tract into the liver. Internally, the liver lobules are the functional units of liver substance. Bile is secreted by the liver cells into tiny canals, or canaliculi, and then is emptied into a bile duct.

PHYSIOLOGY OF THE LIVER — One of the regulatory functions of the liver is that of controlling the blood sugar level. The liver is able to both absorb excess sugar and dispense it into the blood. The liver also stores and secretes other essential nutrients. It chemically processes these materials and detoxifies many substances that could be harmful if allowed to accumulate in the body. Its bile salts are necessary for the absorption of vitamin K from the gastrointestinal tract, which in turn, is needed for the production of prothrombin. Another important liver function is that of producing bile. A brownish-yellow fluid, it is secreted continuously by the liver in amounts averaging about 20 fluid ounces (600 ml). per day. Bile contains the bile salts which are very important in the digestion of fat.

LIVER — ANTERIOR VIEW

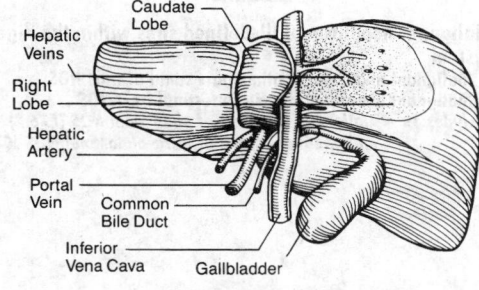

LIVER — POSTERIOR VIEW

cc **C22.0** <u>Liver cell</u> **carcinoma** — A form originating in the liver cells.
   Hepatocellular carcinoma
   Hepatoma

cc **C22.1** <u>Intrahepatic bile duct</u> **carcinoma** — The small channels between the hepatic lobules, which drain into the bile ductules.
   Cholangiocarcinoma
   Excludes 1: *malignant neoplasm of hepatic duct (C24.0)*

cc **C22.2** <u>Hepatoblastoma</u> — A malignant intrahepatic tumor occurring in infants and young children and consisting chiefly of embryonic hepatic tissue.

cc **C22.3** <u>Angiosarcoma</u> of liver
   Kupffer cell sarcoma

cc **C22.4** Other sarcomas of liver

cc **C22.7** Other specified carcinomas of liver

cc **C22.8** Malignant neoplasm of liver, primary, unspecified as to type

cc **C22.9** Malignant neoplasm of liver, not specified as primary or secondary

C23 Malignant neoplasm of <u>gallbladder</u> — Any new and abnormal
cc growth of the gallbladder in which tissue growth is uncontrolled and has the properties of anaplasia, invasion, and metastases.

ANATOMY OF THE GALLBLADDER — The gallbladder is the musculomembranous, pear-shaped bile reservoir located on the undersurface of the liver. The cystic duct is the tubular drain of the gallbladder which merges with the hepatic duct to form the common bile duct. The common bile duct merges with the pancreatic duct in the dilatated area known as the ampulla of Vater. The sphincter of Oddi is the muscle which encircles the bile duct where it enters the duodenum.

PHYSIOLOGY OF THE GALLBLADDER — The gallbladder functions to store and concentrate the bile and release the bile on demand to the small intestine for the digestion of fats. The cystic duct, hepatic duct, and common bile duct convey the bile into the duodenum. The sphincter of Oddi contracts to prevent reflux of intestinal contents back into the bile ducts.

GALLBLADDER

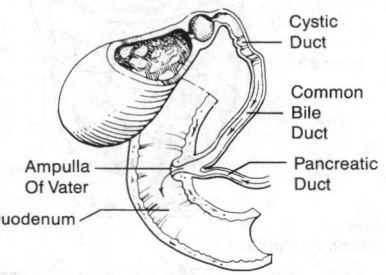

GALLBLADDER — ANTERIOR (CUT-AWAY) VIEW

C24- Malignant neoplasm of other and unspecified parts of biliary tract
   Excludes 1: *malignant neoplasm of intrahepatic bile duct (C22.1)*

cc **C24.0** Malignant neoplasm of <u>extrahepatic bile duct</u> — Any new and abnormal growth in an extrahepatic bile duct (bile ducts which are not within the liver capsule) in which tissue growth is uncontrolled and has the properties of anaplasia, invasion, and metastases.
   Malignant neoplasm of biliary duct or passage NOS
   Malignant neoplasm of common bile duct
   Malignant neoplasm of cystic duct
   Malignant neoplasm of hepatic duct

cc **C24.1** Malignant neoplasm of <u>ampulla of Vater</u> — Any new and abnormal growth of the ampulla of Vater (the dilatation formed by the merger of the pancreatic and common bile ducts just proximal to opening into the duodenum) in which tissue growth is uncontrolled and has the properties of anaplasia, invasion, and metastases.

cc **C24.8** Malignant neoplasm of <u>overlapping</u> sites of biliary tract
   Malignant neoplasm involving both intrahepatic and extrahepatic bile ducts
   Primary malignant neoplasm of two or more contiguous sites of biliary tract

cc **C24.9** Malignant neoplasm of biliary tract, unspecified

C25- **Malignant neoplasm of** <u>pancreas</u> — Any new and abnormal growth of the pancreas and pancreatic ducts in which the tissue growth is uncontrolled and has the properties of anaplasia, invasion, and metastases.
Code also exocrine pancreatic insufficiency (K86.81)
Use additional code to identify:
   Alcohol abuse and dependence (F10.-)
ANATOMY OF THE PANCREAS — The pancreas is a slender organ about 6 to 9 inches (15 to 23 cm) long lying horizontally and located in the abdomen behind and under the stomach. The pancreas is divided into 3 areas. The head, lying in the curve formed by the duodenum; the body, the main portion, lying between the head and tail; and the tail, the most lateral portion blunting up against the spleen. The cells that produce pancreatic juice are called pancreatic acinar cells, and they make up the bulk of the pancreas. These cells are clustered around tiny tubes which drain into the pancreatic duct (duct of Wirsung). This duct connects with the duodenum at the same place where the bile ducts join the duodenum. The second type of pancreatic cells are arranged in groups closely associated with blood vessels, and are called islets of Langerhans. The pancreas arterial blood is supplied via the common hepatic artery, the gastroduodenal artery, the pancreatico-duodenal arches, the splenic artery, and also from the superior mesenteric artery.
PHYSIOLOGY OF THE PANCREAS — The pancreas functions as both an exocrine gland, producing pancreatic juice, and as an endocrine gland, producing the hormones insulin and glucagen. The pancreatic juice contains enzymes capable of digesting carbohydrates, fats, proteins, and nucleic acids, and is produced by the pancreatic acinar cells. This juice is drained into the duodenum. The pancreatic hormones which are produced by the islets of Langerhans cells regulate blood glucose level.

PANCREAS

PANCREAS — ANTERIOR VIEW

CC **C25.0** **Malignant neoplasm of** <u>head</u> **of pancreas** — The medial portion lying in the duodenal curve.

CC **C25.1** **Malignant neoplasm of** <u>body</u> **of pancreas** — The main portion lying horizontally between the head and tail.

CC **C25.2** **Malignant neoplasm of** <u>tail</u> **of pancreas** — The most lateral portion blunting up against the spleen.

CC **C25.3** **Malignant neoplasm of** <u>pancreatic duct</u> — The duct that runs the length of the pancreas emptying the pancreatic juice into the duodenum.

CC **C25.4** **Malignant neoplasm of** <u>endocrine</u> **pancreas** — The cells within the pancreas that produce hormones.
   Malignant neoplasm of islets of Langerhans
   Use additional code to identify any functional activity

CC **C25.7** **Malignant neoplasm of other parts of pancreas**
   Malignant neoplasm of neck of pancreas

CC **C25.8** **Malignant neoplasm of** <u>overlapping</u> **sites of pancreas**

CC **C25.9** **Malignant neoplasm of pancreas, unspecified**

C26- **Malignant neoplasm of other and ill-defined digestive organs**
   Excludes 1:   *malignant neoplasm of peritoneum and retroperitoneum (C48.-)*

C26.0 **Malignant neoplasm of intestinal tract, part unspecified**
   Malignant neoplasm of intestine NOS

C26.1 **Malignant neoplasm of** <u>spleen</u> — Any new and abnormal growth of the spleen in which the tissue growth is uncontrolled and has the properties of anaplasia, invasion, and metastases.
   Excludes 1:   *Hodgkin lymphoma (C81.-)*
               non-Hodgkin lymphoma (C82-C85)
ANATOMY OF THE SPLEEN — The spleen is a gland-like organ, located in the upper abdomen behind the stomach and at the tail of the pancreas, and is about 5 inches (13 cm) in length. The spleen contains both white pulp and red pulp.
PHYSIOLOGY OF THE SPLEEN — The spleen functions as both a large lymph node (white pulp) that filters the blood and produces lymphocytes and monocytes, and as a red blood cell reservoir (red pulp) and disintegrator of worn-out red blood cells. It also plays a role in producing antibodies. Although important, the spleen is not essential to life.

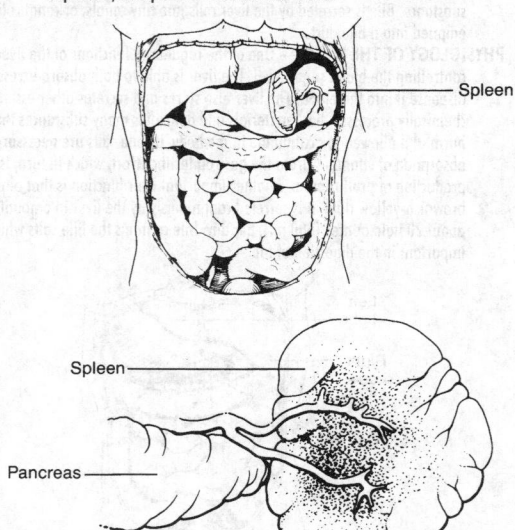

SPLEEN

C26.9 **Malignant neoplasm of ill-defined sites within the digestive system**
   Malignant neoplasm of alimentary canal or tract NOS
   Malignant neoplasm of gastrointestinal tract NOS
   Excludes 1:   *malignant neoplasm of abdominal NOS (C76.2)*
               malignant neoplasm of intra-abdominal NOS (C76.2)

C25-C26

Malignant neoplasms of respiratory and intrathoracic organs (C30-C39)

Includes: Malignant neoplasm of middle ear
Excludes 1: mesothelioma (C45.-)

C30- **Malignant neoplasm of nasal cavity and middle ear**

C30.0 **Malignant neoplasm of <u>nasal cavity</u>** — Any new and abnormal growth of the nasal cavity in which the tissue growth is uncontrolled and has the properties of anaplasia, invasion, and metastases.

    Malignant neoplasm of cartilage of nose
    Malignant neoplasm of nasal concha
    Malignant neoplasm of internal nose
    Malignant neoplasm of septum of nose
    Malignant neoplasm of vestibule of nose

    Excludes 1: *malignant melanoma of skin of nose (C43.31)*
        malignant neoplasm of nasal bone (C41.0)
        malignant neoplasm of nose NOS (C76.0)
        malignant neoplasm of olfactory bulb (C72.2-)
        malignant neoplasm of posterior margin of nasal septum and choana (C11.3)
        malignant neoplasm of turbinates (C41.0)
        other and unspecified malignant neoplasm of skin of nose (C44.301, C44.311, C44.321, C44.391)

ANATOMY OF THE NASAL CAVITIES — The nasal cavity is located between the external nose and the nasopharynx with the nasal bones, and parts of the ethmoid, frontal, sphenoid, vomer, and palatine bones forming the roof, and the maxilla and palatine bones forming the floor.

PHYSIOLOGY OF THE NASAL CAVITIES — The nasal cavity functions to moisten, filter, and warm air as it passes to the lungs. It also contains the sense of smell organ, and helps with speech.

C30.1 **Malignant neoplasm of <u>middle ear</u>** — Any new and abnormal growth of the middle ear in which the tissue growth is uncontrolled and has the properties of anaplasia, invasion, and metastases.

    Malignant neoplasm of antrum tympanicum
    Malignant neoplasm of auditory tube
    Malignant neoplasm of eustachian tube
    Malignant neoplasm of inner ear
    Malignant neoplasm of mastoid air cells
    Malignant neoplasm of tympanic cavity

    Excludes 1: *malignant melanoma of skin of (external) ear (C43.2-)*
        malignant neoplasm of auricular canal (external) (C43.2-,C44.2-)
        malignant neoplasm of bone of ear (meatus) (C41.0)
        malignant neoplasm of cartilage of ear (C49.0)
        other and unspecified malignant neoplasm of skin of (external) ear (C44.2-)

ANATOMY OF THE MIDDLE EAR — The middle ear is the air-filled space behind the tympanic membrane of the external ear which connects the inner ear, mastoid cells, ossicles, and auditory tube. The auditory tube (Eustachian tube) passes between the middle ear and the nasopharynx.

PHYSIOLOGY OF THE MIDDLE EAR — The middle ear transfers, modulates, and amplifies the sound to the inner ear. The auditory tube functions to equalize air pressure within the middle ear to the outside air pressure, and to drain any fluid that may unnaturally accumulate in the middle ear.

EAR

C31- **Malignant neoplasm of accessory <u>sinuses</u>** — Any new and abnormal growth of the accessory sinuses in which the tissue growth is uncontrolled and has the properties of anaplasia, invasion, and metastases.

ANATOMY OF THE ACCESSORY SINUSES — The paired paranasal sinuses (maxillary, ethmoidal, frontal, and sphenoidal) are the bony cavities lined with mucous membranes which communicate with the nasal cavity.

PHYSIOLOGY OF THE ACCESSORY SINUSES — The paranasal cavities function to lighten the bones of the skull, warm air, and give resonance to the voice.

ACCESSORY SINUSES

C31.0 **Malignant neoplasm of <u>maxillary</u> sinus** — The largest of the one of the four paired, air-filled paranasal sinuses located under the eye in the maxillary bone.

    Malignant neoplasm of antrum (Highmore) (maxillary)

C31.1 **Malignant neoplasm of <u>ethmoidal</u> sinus** — One of the four paired, air-filled paranasal sinuses located within the ethmoid bone cavities that lies between the nose and the eyes.

C31.2 **Malignant neoplasm of <u>frontal</u> sinus** — One of the four paired, air-filled paranasal sinuses located above the eye in the frontal bone.

C31.3 **Malignant neoplasm of <u>sphenoid</u> sinus** — One of the four paired, air-filled paranasal sinuses located behind the eyes and nose in the sphenoid bone.

C31.8 **Malignant neoplasm of <u>overlapping</u> sites of accessory sinuses**

C31.9 **Malignant neoplasm of accessory sinus, unspecified**

C32- **Malignant neoplasm of <u>larynx</u>** — Any new and abnormal growth of the larynx in which tissue growth is uncontrolled and has the properties of anaplasia, invasion, and metastases.

Use additional code to identify:
    Alcohol abuse and dependence (F10.-)
    Exposure to environmental tobacco smoke (Z77.22)
    Exposure to tobacco smoke in the perinatal period (P96.81)
    History of tobacco dependence (Z87.891)
    Occupational exposure to environmental tobacco smoke (Z57.31)
    Tobacco dependence (F17.-)
    Tobacco use (Z72.0)

ANATOMY OF THE LARYNX — The larynx is the musculocartilaginous structure, lined with mucous membrane located between the root of the tongue and the trachea. The glottis is the slit-like opening of the larynx formed by the true vocal cords. The supraglottis is that portion of the larynx situated above the glottis. There are nine laryngeal cartilages, three paired and three single.

PHYSIOLOGY OF THE LARYNX — The larynx functions to guard the entrance of the trachea from food and liquids, to control the expulsion of air, and to produce sound. The glottis produces sound, controls pitch, and when closed prevents food from entering the trachea. The supraglottis is an area of the larynx which helps to prevent food and liquid from entering the trachea. The laryngeal cartilages frame and support the larynx and its muscles.

LARYNX

Continued on next page

C30-C32

Continued from previous page

LARYNX — ANTERIOR (CUT-AWAY) VIEW

C32.0 **Malignant neoplasm of <u>glottis</u>** — The true vocal cords formed by the two folds opening into the larynx which produce sound and control pitch.
  Malignant neoplasm of intrinsic larynx
  Malignant neoplasm of laryngeal commissure (anterior) (posterior)
  Malignant neoplasm of vocal cord (true) NOS

C32.1 **Malignant neoplasm of <u>supraglottis</u>** — That portion of the larynx situated above the glottis.
  Malignant neoplasm of aryepiglottic fold or interarytenoid fold, laryngeal aspect
  Malignant neoplasm of epiglottis (suprahyoid portion) NOS
  Malignant neoplasm of extrinsic larynx
  Malignant neoplasm of false vocal cord
  Malignant neoplasm of posterior (laryngeal) surface of epiglottis
  Malignant neoplasm of ventricular bands
  Excludes ❷: *malignant neoplasm of anterior surface of epiglottis (C10.1)*
      malignant neoplasm of aryepiglottic fold or interarytenoid fold, hypopharyngeal aspect (C13.1)
      malignant neoplasm of aryepiglottic fold or interarytenoid fold, marginal zone (C13.1)
      malignant neoplasm of aryepiglottic fold or interarytenoid fold NOS (C13.1)

C32.2 **Malignant neoplasm of <u>subglottis</u>** — That portion of the larynx just below the true vocal cords and above the trachea.

C32.3 **Malignant neoplasm of <u>laryngeal cartilage</u>** — The 9 fibrous connective tissue structures which frame and support the larynx and its muscles.

C32.8 **Malignant neoplasm of <u>overlapping</u> sites of larynx**

C32.9 **Malignant neoplasm of larynx, unspecified**

C33 **Malignant neoplasm of <u>trachea</u>** — Any new and abnormal growth of the trachea
CC in which tissue growth is uncontrolled and has the properties of anaplasia, invasion, and metastases.
  Use additional code to identify:
  Exposure to environmental tobacco smoke (Z77.22)
  Exposure to tobacco smoke in the perinatal period (P96.81)
  History of tobacco dependence (Z87.891)
  Occupational exposure to environmental tobacco smoke (Z57.31)
  Tobacco dependence (F17.-)
  Tobacco use (Z72.0)
  ANATOMY OF THE TRACHEA — The trachea is a cylindrical tube about 1 inch (2.5 cm) in length. It extends downward in front of the esophagus and into the thoracic cavity, where it splits into the right and left bronchi.
  PHYSIOLOGY OF THE TRACHEA — The trachea and bronchi allow for the rapid transport of air to and from the lung tissue.

C34- **Malignant neoplasm of bronchus and lung** — Any new and abnormal growth of the bronchus and lungs in which the tissue growth is uncontrolled and has the properties of anaplasia, invasion, and metastases.
  Use additional code to identify:
  Exposure to environmental tobacco smoke (Z77.22)
  Exposure to tobacco smoke in the perinatal period (P96.81)
  History of tobacco dependence (Z87.891)
  Occupational exposure to environmental tobacco smoke (Z57.31)
  Tobacco dependence (F17.-)
  Tobacco use (Z72.0)
  Excludes 1: *Kaposi's sarcoma of lung (C46.5-)*
      malignant carcinoid tumor of the bronchus and lung (C7A.090)
  ANATOMY OF THE BRONCHUS AND LUNGS — The bronchial tree consists of branched airways leading from the trachea to the microscopic air sacs. The 2 main branches, the right and left bronchi, subdivide into secondary or lobar bronchi which, in turn, branch into finer tubes down to the bronchioles. The lungs are soft, spongy, cone-shaped organs located in the thoracic cavity. The right and left lungs are separated medially by the heart and the mediastinum, and they are enclosed by the diaphragm and the thoracic cage. The right lung is divided into 3 lobes called the upper (superior), middle, and lower (inferior). The left lung is divided into 2 lobes, the upper and lower. The lobes are subdivided into lobules which are composed of bronchioles, alveolar sacs, alveoli, nerves, and associated blood and lymphatic vessels. The alveoli are thin-walled, microscopic air sacs that open only on the side communicating with the inhaled air. Venous blood is pumped from the right ventricle of the heart to the lungs by the right and left pulmonary arteries. (NOTE: Pulmonary arteries carry venous blood, the opposite of the rest of the arteries.) The arterialized blood returns to the left atrium of the heart via the pulmonary veins. (NOTE: Blood vessels with blood flow going to the heart are termed veins.)
  PHYSIOLOGY OF THE BRONCHUS AND LUNGS — The lungs are organs that perform pulmonary ventilation. The alveoli are the microscopic structures responsible for the exchange of oxygen into the blood and carbon dioxide out of the body. Inspiration (inhalation) and expiration (exhalation) are complex central nervous system functions. Two groups of nerve cell bodies in the medulla of the brain compose the inspiratory center and the expiratory center. These 2 centers act reciprocally; that is, when one is stimulated and discharging, the other is inhibited. Both centers discharge nerve impulses to the intercostal muscles. When the inspiration center discharges nerve impulses, the diaphragm moves down and the external intercostal muscles contract, causing inflation. Inflation of the lungs causes stimulation of stretch receptors, which send impulses to the medulla, which in turn stimulates the expiratory center. Two other respiratory centers are contained in the pons which modify and control the medullary centers' activities, and are called the apneustic center and the pneumotaxic center. In addition to the above centers, there is also a chemical reaction which helps to control pulmonary ventilation. The carbon dioxide level in the blood is directly measured by the medulla, and respiration is adjusted accordingly. A decrease in the oxygen level, sensed by nerve endings in the common carotid artery and the aortic arch, will also stimulate a respiratory adjustment, but it does not play a noticeable difference in pulmonary ventilation.

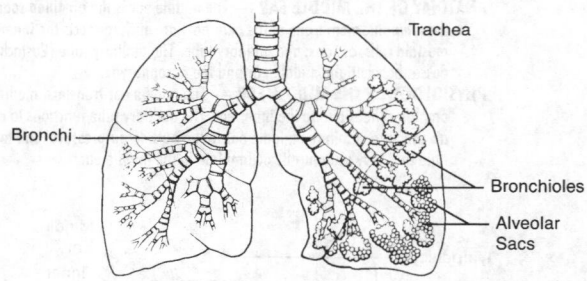

LUNGS — ANTERIOR (CUT-AWAY) VIEW

C34.0- **Malignant neoplasm of <u>main bronchus</u>** — The branched airways leading from the trachea to any one of the 5 lobes of the lung.
    Malignant neoplasm of carina
    Malignant neoplasm of hilus (of lung)

CC **C34.00** **Malignant neoplasm of unspecified main bronchus**

CC **C34.01** **Malignant neoplasm of <u>right</u> main bronchus**

CC **C34.02** **Malignant neoplasm of <u>left</u> main bronchus**

C34.1- **Malignant neoplasm of <u>upper lobe, bronchus or lung</u>** — The two uppermost cone-shaped organs of respiration.

CC **C34.10** **Malignant neoplasm of upper lobe, unspecified bronchus or lung**

CC **C34.11** **Malignant neoplasm of upper lobe, <u>right</u> bronchus or lung**

CC **C34.12** **Malignant neoplasm of upper lobe, <u>left</u> bronchus or lung**

cc C34.2   **Malignant neoplasm of <u>middle lobe, bronchus or lung</u>** — The single cone-shaped organ of respiration located between the upper and lower lobes of the right side.

C34.3-   **Malignant neoplasm of <u>lower lobe, bronchus or lung</u>** — The two lowermost cone-shaped organs of respiration.

    cc C34.30   **Malignant neoplasm of lower lobe, unspecified bronchus or lung**

    cc C34.31   **Malignant neoplasm of lower lobe, <u>right</u> bronchus or lung**

    cc C34.32   **Malignant neoplasm of lower lobe, <u>left</u> bronchus or lung**

C34.8-   **Malignant neoplasm of <u>overlapping sites</u> of bronchus and lung**

    cc C34.80   **Malignant neoplasm of overlapping sites of unspecified bronchus and lung**

    cc C34.81   **Malignant neoplasm of overlapping sites of <u>right</u> bronchus and lung**

    cc C34.82   **Malignant neoplasm of overlapping sites of <u>left</u> bronchus and lung**

C34.9-   **Malignant neoplasm of <u>unspecified part</u> of bronchus or lung**

    cc C34.90   **Malignant neoplasm of unspecified part of unspecified bronchus or lung**

        Lung cancer NOS

    cc C34.91   **Malignant neoplasm of unspecified part of <u>right</u> bronchus or lung**

    cc C34.92   **Malignant neoplasm of unspecified part of <u>left</u> bronchus or lung**

C37   **Malignant neoplasm of <u>thymus</u>** — Any new and abnormal growth of the thymus
cc (the flat bi-lobed organ lying behind the sternum which is large during childhood but shrinks dramatically in the adult, and is composed of lymphoid material, and possibly some hormonal endocrine tissue) in which tissue growth is uncontrolled and has the properties of anaplasia, invasion, and metastases.
  ANATOMY OF THE THYMUS — The thymus is the small, flat bi-lobed organ lying behind the sternum, and composed of lymphoid material.
  PHYSIOLOGY OF THE THYMUS — The thymus functions during childhood by producing lymphocytes and aids in the development of the individual's immunity.
  Excludes 1:   *malignant carcinoid tumor of the thymus (C7A.091)*

C38-   **Malignant neoplasm of heart, mediastinum and pleura** — Any new and abnormal growth of the heart, mediastinum, and pleura in which the tissue growth is uncontrolled and has the properties of anaplasia, invasion, and metastases.
  Excludes 1:   *mesothelioma (C45.-)*
  ANATOMY OF THE HEART, MEDIASTINUM, AND PLEURA — The heart is the 4 chambered, muscular, blood pumping organ behind the mediastinum in the thorax, and is approximately 5.5 inches (14 cm) long and 3.5 inches (9 cm) wide. The heart has 3 layers: The endocardium, myocardium, and pericardium. The endocardium is the interior lining of endothelium. The myocardium is the thick muscular layer. The pericardium is the double-layered serous membrane protecting the heart from friction as it beats. The heart has 4 valves and 4 chambers: The tricuspid valve, mitral valve, aortic valve, the pulmonary valve, right and left atria and right and left ventricles. The mediastinum is the mass of tissue between the sternum and vertebral column which divides the thoracic cavity. The pleura are closed double-layered serous membranous sacs surrounding the lungs. The parietal pleura is the layer which lines the thoracic walls opposite to the visceral pleura. The visceral pleura is the layer which adheres to the lungs and together with the parietal, forms the pleural cavity.
  PHYSIOLOGY OF THE HEART, MEDIASTINUM, AND PLEURA — The heart functions to pump and maintain sufficient pressure of the blood to constantly meet the needs of the body cells. The venous blood is returned from the body via the inferior and superior vena cava to the right atrium where it is pooled momentarily before the tricuspid valve opens and allows the venous blood to enter the right ventricle. The right ventricle then contracts forcing the blood through the pulmonary valve to the lungs. The lungs return the reoxygenated blood to the left atrium where it is pooled momentarily before the mitral valve opens and allows the venous blood to enter the left ventricle. The left ventricle then contracts, forcing the blood through the aortic valve to all the tissues of the body. The pleura functions to prevent friction of the lungs against the thoracic wall during respiration. There is a small amount of serous fluid in the pleural cavity which lubricates the facing membranes.

HEART — ANTERIOR (CUT-AWAY) VIEW

PLEURA

PLEURA — TRANSVERSE SECTION

cc C38.0   **Malignant neoplasm of <u>heart</u>** — The hollow, 4 chambered muscular organ which pumps the blood and maintains circulation.
    Malignant neoplasm of pericardium
    Excludes 1:   *malignant neoplasm of great vessels (C49.3)*

cc C38.1   **Malignant neoplasm of <u>anterior mediastinum</u>** — That portion of the cavity which lies in front, near the chest that contains the heart.

C
3
4
-
C
3
8

Excludes 1: = NOT CODED HERE! (Do not code both)   *Excludes ❷:* = Not Included Here

cc **C38.2 Malignant neoplasm of <u>posterior mediastinum</u>** — That portion of the cavity which lies behind the heart and contains the descending aorta, thoracic duct, the esophagus, and the vagus nerve.

cc **C38.3 Malignant neoplasm of mediastinum, part unspecified**

cc **C38.4 Malignant neoplasm of <u>pleura</u>** — The pleura are closed double-layered serous membranous sacs surrounding the lungs.

cc **C38.8 Malignant neoplasm of <u>overlapping sites</u> of heart, mediastinum and pleura**

C39- Malignant neoplasm of other and ill-defined sites in the respiratory system and intrathoracic organs
Use additional code to identify:
Exposure to environmental tobacco smoke (Z77.22)
Exposure to tobacco smoke in the perinatal period (P96.81)
History of tobacco dependence (Z87.891)
Occupational exposure to environmental tobacco smoke (Z57.31)
Tobacco dependence (F17.-)
Tobacco use (Z72.0)
Excludes 1: *intrathoracic malignant neoplasm NOS (C76.1)*
thoracic malignant neoplasm NOS (C76.1)

C39.0 Malignant neoplasm of upper respiratory tract, part unspecified

C39.9 Malignant neoplasm of lower respiratory tract, part unspecified
Malignant neoplasm of respiratory tract NOS

Malignant neoplasms of bone and articular cartilage (C40-C41)

Includes: Malignant neoplasm of cartilage (articular) (joint)
Malignant neoplasm of periosteum
Excludes 1: *malignant neoplasm of bone marrow NOS (C96.9)*
malignant neoplasm of synovia (C49.-)

C40- Malignant neoplasm of bone and articular cartilage of limbs — Any new and abnormal growth of the bone and articular cartilage of the limbs in which tissue growth is uncontrolled and has the properties of anaplasia, invasion, and metastases. NOTE: For illustrations, see Chapter19.
Use additional code to identify major osseous defect, if applicable (M89.7-)

C40.0- Malignant neoplasm of <u>scapula and long bones of upper limb</u>

cc **C40.00 Malignant neoplasm of scapula and long bones of unspecified upper limb**

cc **C40.01 Malignant neoplasm of scapula and long bones of <u>right</u> upper limb**

cc **C40.02 Malignant neoplasm of scapula and long bones of <u>left</u> upper limb**

C40.1- Malignant neoplasm of <u>short bones of upper limb</u>

cc **C40.10 Malignant neoplasm of <u>short bones of unspecified upper limb</u>**

cc **C40.11 Malignant neoplasm of short bones of <u>right</u> upper limb**

cc **C40.12 Malignant neoplasm of short bones of <u>left</u> upper limb**

C40.2- Malignant neoplasm of <u>long bones of lower limb</u>

cc **C40.20 Malignant neoplasm of long bones of unspecified lower limb**

cc **C40.21 Malignant neoplasm of long bones of <u>right</u> lower limb**

cc **C40.22 Malignant neoplasm of long bones of <u>left</u> lower limb**

C40.3- Malignant neoplasm of <u>short bones of lower limb</u>

cc **C40.30 Malignant neoplasm of short bones of unspecified lower limb**

cc **C40.31 Malignant neoplasm of short bones of <u>right</u> lower limb**

cc **C40.32 Malignant neoplasm of short bones of <u>left</u> lower limb**

C40.8- Malignant neoplasm of <u>overlapping sites</u> of bone and articular cartilage of limb

cc **C40.80 Malignant neoplasm of overlapping sites of bone and articular cartilage of unspecified limb**

cc **C40.81 Malignant neoplasm of overlapping sites of bone and articular cartilage of <u>right</u> limb**

cc **C40.82 Malignant neoplasm of overlapping sites of bone and articular cartilage of <u>left</u> limb**

C40.9- Malignant neoplasm of unspecified bones and articular cartilage of limb

cc **C40.90 Malignant neoplasm of unspecified bones and articular cartilage of unspecified limb**

cc **C40.91 Malignant neoplasm of unspecified bones and articular cartilage of <u>right</u> limb**

cc **C40.92 Malignant neoplasm of unspecified bones and articular cartilage of <u>left</u> limb**

C41- Malignant neoplasm of bone and articular cartilage of other and unspecified sites — Any new and abnormal growth of the bone and articular cartilage other than the limbs in which tissue growth is uncontrolled and has the properties of anaplasia, invasion, and metastases. NOTE: For illustrations, see Chapter19.
Excludes 1: *malignant neoplasm of bones of limbs (C40.-)*
malignant neoplasm of cartilage of ear (C49.0)
malignant neoplasm of cartilage of eyelid (C49.0)
malignant neoplasm of cartilage of larynx (C32.3)
malignant neoplasm of cartilage of limbs (C40.-)
malignant neoplasm of cartilage of nose (C30.0)

cc **C41.0 Malignant neoplasm of <u>bones of skull and face</u>**
Malignant neoplasm of maxilla (superior)
Malignant neoplasm of orbital bone
Excludes ❷: *carcinoma, any type except intraosseous or odontogenic of:*
maxillary sinus (C31.0)
upper jaw (C03.0)
malignant neoplasm of jaw bone (lower) (C41.1)

cc **C41.1 Malignant neoplasm of <u>mandible</u>**
Malignant neoplasm of inferior maxilla
Malignant neoplasm of lower jaw bone
Excludes ❷: *carcinoma, any type except intraosseous or odontogenic of:*
jaw NOS (C03.9)
lower (C03.1)
malignant neoplasm of upper jaw bone (C41.0)

cc **C41.2 Malignant neoplasm of <u>vertebral column</u>**
Excludes 1: *malignant neoplasm of sacrum and coccyx (C41.4)*

cc **C41.3 Malignant neoplasm of <u>ribs, sternum and clavicle</u>**

cc **C41.4 Malignant neoplasm of <u>pelvic bones, sacrum and coccyx</u>**

cc **C41.9 Malignant neoplasm of bone and articular cartilage, unspecified**

Melanoma and other malignant neoplasms of skin (C43-C44)

C43- Malignant <u>melanoma</u> of skin — Any new and abnormal growth of the melanin-pigmented cells in which tissue growth is uncontrolled and has the properties of anaplasia, invasion, and metastases; usually developing from a nevus.
Excludes 1: *melanoma in situ (D03.-)*
Excludes ❷: *malignant melanoma of skin of genital organs (C51-C52, C60.-, C63.-)*
Merkel cell carcinoma (C4A.-)
sites other than skin — code to malignant neoplasm of the site

C43.0 Malignant melanoma of <u>lip</u>
Excludes 1: *malignant neoplasm of vermilion border of lip (C00.0-C00.2)*

C43.1- Malignant melanoma of <u>eyelid, including canthus</u>
C43.10 Malignant melanoma of unspecified eyelid, including canthus
C43.11 Malignant melanoma of <u>right</u> eyelid, including canthus
C43.12 Malignant melanoma of <u>left</u> eyelid, including canthus

C43.2- Malignant melanoma of <u>ear and external auricular canal</u>
C43.20 Malignant melanoma of unspecified ear and external auricular canal
C43.21 Malignant melanoma of <u>right</u> ear and external auricular canal
C43.22 Malignant melanoma of <u>left</u> ear and external auricular canal

C43.3- Malignant melanoma of other and unspecified parts of face
C43.30 Malignant melanoma of unspecified part of face
C43.31 Malignant melanoma of <u>nose</u>
C43.39 Malignant melanoma of other parts of face

C43.4 Malignant melanoma of <u>scalp and neck</u>

C 3 8 - C 4 3

C43.5- Malignant melanoma of <u>trunk</u>
  Excludes ❷: malignant neoplasm of anus NOS (C21.0)
          malignant neoplasm of scrotum (C63.2)

  C43.51 Malignant melanoma of <u>anal skin</u>
    Malignant melanoma of anal margin
    Malignant melanoma of perianal skin

  C43.52 Malignant melanoma of <u>skin of breast</u>

  C43.59 Malignant melanoma of other part of <u>trunk</u>

C43.6- Malignant melanoma of <u>upper limb</u>, including shoulder

  C43.60 Malignant melanoma of unspecified upper limb, including shoulder

  C43.61 Malignant melanoma of <u>right</u> upper limb, including shoulder

  C43.62 Malignant melanoma of <u>left</u> upper limb, including shoulder

C43.7- Malignant melanoma of <u>lower limb</u>, including hip

  C43.70 Malignant melanoma of unspecified lower limb, including hip

  C43.71 Malignant melanoma of <u>right</u> lower limb, including hip

  C43.72 Malignant melanoma of <u>left</u> lower limb, including hip

C43.8 Malignant melanoma of <u>overlapping sites</u> of skin

C43.9 Malignant melanoma of skin, unspecified
  Malignant melanoma of unspecified site of skin
  Melanoma (malignant) NOS

C4A- <u>Merkel cell</u> carcinoma — An aggressive neuroendocrine skin cancer that arises from Merkel cells in the epidermis and is often associated with the Merkel cell polyomavirus (MCV).

C4A.0 Merkel cell carcinoma of <u>lip</u>
  Excludes 1: malignant neoplasm of vermilion border of lip (C00.0-C00.2)

C4A.1- Merkel cell carcinoma of <u>eyelid, including canthus</u>

  C4A.10 Merkel cell carcinoma of unspecified eyelid, including canthus

  C4A.11 Merkel cell carcinoma of <u>right</u> eyelid, including canthus

  C4A.12 Merkel cell carcinoma of <u>left</u> eyelid, including canthus

C4A.2- Merkel cell carcinoma of <u>ear and external auricular canal</u>

  C4A.20 Merkel cell carcinoma of unspecified ear and external auricular canal

  C4A.21 Merkel cell carcinoma of <u>right</u> ear and external auricular canal

  C4A.22 Merkel cell carcinoma of <u>left</u> ear and external auricular canal

C4A.3- Merkel cell carcinoma of other and unspecified parts of face

  C4A.30 Merkel cell carcinoma of unspecified part of face

  C4A.31 Merkel cell carcinoma of <u>nose</u>

  C4A.39 Merkel cell carcinoma of other parts of face

C4A.4 Merkel cell carcinoma of <u>scalp and neck</u>

C4A.5- Merkel cell carcinoma of trunk
  Excludes ❷: malignant neoplasm of anus NOS (C21.0)
          malignant neoplasm of scrotum (C63.2)

  C4A.51 Merkel cell carcinoma of <u>anal skin</u>
    Merkel cell carcinoma of anal margin
    Merkel cell carcinoma of perianal skin

  C4A.52 Merkel cell carcinoma of <u>skin of breast</u>

  C4A.59 Merkel cell carcinoma of other part of trunk

C4A.6- Merkel cell carcinoma of <u>upper limb</u>, including shoulder

  C4A.60 Merkel cell carcinoma of unspecified upper limb, including shoulder

  C4A.61 Merkel cell carcinoma of <u>right</u> upper limb, including shoulder

  C4A.62 Merkel cell carcinoma of <u>left</u> upper limb, including shoulder

C4A.7- Merkel cell carcinoma of <u>lower limb</u>, including hip

  C4A.70 Merkel cell carcinoma of unspecified lower limb, including hip

  C4A.71 Merkel cell carcinoma of <u>right</u> lower limb, including hip

  C4A.72 Merkel cell carcinoma of <u>left</u> lower limb, including hip

C4A.8 Merkel cell carcinoma of <u>overlapping sites</u>

C4A.9 Merkel cell carcinoma, unspecified
  Merkel cell carcinoma of unspecified site
  Merkel cell carcinoma NOS

C44- <u>Other and unspecified malignant</u> neoplasm of <u>skin</u> — Any new and abnormal growth of the skin (basal cell carcinoma arises in the skin's basal cells) (squamous cell carcinoma arises in the skin's squamous cells) that is not classified elsewhere in which tissue growth is uncontrolled and has the properties of anaplasia, invasion, and metastases.
Includes: **Malignant neoplasm of sebaceous glands** — The holocrine glands which secrete a mixture of fatty material and cellular debris onto the hairs and help to keep the skin soft, pliable, and relatively waterproof.
    Malignant neoplasm of sweat glands — The sweat glands of two types; the large apocrine glands of the axilla and perianal tissues that when stimulated by emotion produce sweat with an odor, and the smaller eccrine glands which produce the watery sweat for body cooling after stimulation from a rise in body temperature.
Excludes 1: Kaposi's sarcoma of skin (C46.0)
        malignant melanoma of skin (C43.-)
        malignant neoplasm of skin of genital organs (C51-C52, C60.-, C63.2)
        Merkel cell carcinoma (C4A.-)
ANATOMY OF THE SKIN — The skin is the outer covering of the body, consisting of the epidermis and dermis, and which rests upon the subcutaneous tissue. The epidermis is the outermost layer of the skin which develops keratin, a tough, fibrous waterproof protein, and lacks blood vessels. The dermis is the tough, elastic vascular connective tissue layer of the skin which contains the sebaceous and sweat glands.
PHYSIOLOGY OF THE SKIN — The skin functions to protect the body from invading microorganisms, limits the loss of water from deep tissues, assists in homeostasis, aids in the regulation of body temperature, acts as the sense organ for the cutaneous senses, and is a source of vitamin D when it is exposed to light.

SKIN

C44.0- Other and unspecified malignant neoplasm of skin of <u>lip</u>
  Excludes 1: malignant neoplasm of lip (C00.-)

  C44.00 <u>Unspecified</u> malignant neoplasm of skin of lip

  C44.01 <u>Basal cell</u> carcinoma of skin of lip

  C44.02 <u>Squamous cell</u> carcinoma of skin of lip

  C44.09 <u>Other specified</u> malignant neoplasm of skin of lip

C44.1- Other and unspecified malignant neoplasm of skin of <u>eyelid, including canthus</u>
  Excludes 1: connective tissue of eyelid (C49.0)

  C44.10- <u>Unspecified</u> malignant neoplasm of skin of eyelid, including canthus

    C44.101 Unspecified malignant neoplasm of skin of unspecified eyelid, including canthus

    C44.102 Unspecified malignant neoplasm of skin of <u>right</u> eyelid, including canthus

    C44.109 Unspecified malignant neoplasm of skin of <u>left</u> eyelid, including canthus

  C44.11- <u>Basal cell</u> carcinoma of skin of eyelid, including canthus

    C44.111 Basal cell carcinoma of skin of unspecified eyelid, including canthus

    C44.112 Basal cell carcinoma of skin of <u>right</u> eyelid, including canthus

    C44.119 Basal cell carcinoma of skin of <u>left</u> eyelid, including canthus

  C44.12- <u>Squamous cell</u> carcinoma of skin of eyelid, including canthus

    C44.121 Squamous cell carcinoma of skin of unspecified eyelid, including canthus

    C44.122 Squamous cell carcinoma of skin of <u>right</u> eyelid, including canthus

C
4
3
-
C
4
4

C44.129   Squamous cell carcinoma of skin of <u>left</u> eyelid, including canthus

C44.19-   <u>Other specified</u> malignant neoplasm of skin of eyelid, including canthus

C44.191   Other specified malignant neoplasm of skin of unspecified eyelid, including canthus

C44.192   Other specified malignant neoplasm of skin of <u>right</u> eyelid, including canthus

C44.199   Other specified malignant neoplasm of skin of <u>left</u> eyelid, including canthus

C44.2-   Other and unspecified malignant neoplasm of skin of <u>ear and external auricular canal</u>

    Excludes 1:   connective tissue of ear (C49.0)

C44.20-   <u>Unspecified</u> malignant neoplasm of skin of ear and external auricular canal

C44.201   Unspecified malignant neoplasm of skin of unspecified ear and external auricular canal

C44.202   Unspecified malignant neoplasm of skin of <u>right</u> ear and external auricular canal

C44.209   Unspecified malignant neoplasm of skin of <u>left</u> ear and external auricular canal

C44.21-   <u>Basal cell</u> carcinoma of skin of ear and external auricular canal

C44.211   Basal cell carcinoma of skin of unspecified ear and external auricular canal

C44.212   Basal cell carcinoma of skin of <u>right</u> ear and external auricular canal

C44.219   Basal cell carcinoma of skin of <u>left</u> ear and external auricular canal

C44.22-   <u>Squamous cell</u> carcinoma of skin of ear and external auricular canal

C44.221   Squamous cell carcinoma of skin of unspecified ear and external auricular canal

C44.222   Squamous cell carcinoma of skin of <u>right</u> ear and external auricular canal

C44.229   Squamous cell carcinoma of skin of <u>left</u> ear and external auricular canal

C44.29-   <u>Other specified</u> malignant neoplasm of skin of ear and external auricular canal

C44.291   Other specified malignant neoplasm of skin of unspecified ear and external auricular canal

C44.292   Other specified malignant neoplasm of skin of <u>right</u> ear and external auricular canal

C44.299   Other specified malignant neoplasm of skin of <u>left</u> ear and external auricular canal

C44.3-   Other and unspecified malignant neoplasm of skin of <u>other and unspecified parts of face</u>

C44.30-   <u>Unspecified</u> malignant neoplasm of skin of other and unspecified parts of face

C44.300   Unspecified malignant neoplasm of skin of unspecified part of face

C44.301   Unspecified malignant neoplasm of skin of <u>nose</u>

C44.309   Unspecified malignant neoplasm of skin of <u>other parts</u> of face

C44.31-   <u>Basal cell</u> carcinoma of skin of other and unspecified parts of face

C44.310   Basal cell carcinoma of skin of unspecified parts of face

C44.311   Basal cell carcinoma of skin of <u>nose</u>

C44.319   Basal cell carcinoma of skin of <u>other parts</u> of face

C44.32-   <u>Squamous cell</u> carcinoma of skin of other and unspecified parts of face

C44.320   Squamous cell carcinoma of skin of unspecified parts of face

C44.321   Squamous cell carcinoma of skin of <u>nose</u>

C44.329   Squamous cell carcinoma of skin of <u>other parts</u> of face

C44.39-   <u>Other specified</u> malignant neoplasm of skin of other and unspecified parts of face

C44.390   Other specified malignant neoplasm of skin of unspecified parts of face

C44.391   Other specified malignant neoplasm of skin of <u>nose</u>

C44.399   Other specified malignant neoplasm of skin of <u>other parts</u> of face

C44.4-   Other and unspecified malignant neoplasm of skin of <u>scalp and neck</u>

C44.40   <u>Unspecified</u> malignant neoplasm of skin of scalp and neck

C44.41   <u>Basal cell</u> carcinoma of skin of scalp and neck

C44.42   <u>Squamous cell</u> carcinoma of skin of scalp and neck

C44.49   <u>Other specified</u> malignant neoplasm of skin of scalp and neck

C44.5-   Other and unspecified malignant neoplasm of skin of <u>trunk</u>

    Excludes 1:   anus NOS (C21.0)
              scrotum (C63.2)

C44.50-   <u>Unspecified</u> malignant neoplasm of skin of trunk

C44.500   Unspecified malignant neoplasm of <u>anal skin</u>
    Unspecified malignant neoplasm of anal margin
    Unspecified malignant neoplasm of perianal skin

C44.501   Unspecified malignant neoplasm of skin of <u>breast</u>

C44.509   Unspecified malignant neoplasm of skin of other part of trunk

C44.51-   <u>Basal cell</u> carcinoma of skin of trunk

C44.510   Basal cell carcinoma of <u>anal skin</u>
    Basal cell carcinoma of anal margin
    Basal cell carcinoma of perianal skin

C44.511   Basal cell carcinoma of skin of <u>breast</u>

C44.519   Basal cell carcinoma of skin of other part of trunk

C44.52-   <u>Squamous cell</u> carcinoma of skin of trunk

C44.520   Squamous cell carcinoma of <u>anal skin</u>
    Squamous cell carcinoma of anal margin
    Squamous cell carcinoma of perianal skin

C44.521   Squamous cell carcinoma of skin of <u>breast</u>

C44.529   Squamous cell carcinoma of skin of other part of trunk

C44.59-   <u>Other specified</u> malignant neoplasm of skin of trunk

C44.590   Other specified malignant neoplasm of <u>anal skin</u>
    Other specified malignant neoplasm of anal margin
    Other specified malignant neoplasm of perianal skin

C44.591   Other specified malignant neoplasm of skin of <u>breast</u>

C44.599   Other specified malignant neoplasm of skin of other part of trunk

C44.6-   Other and unspecified malignant neoplasm of skin of <u>upper limb</u>, including shoulder

C44.60-   <u>Unspecified</u> malignant neoplasm of skin of upper limb, including shoulder

C44.601   Unspecified malignant neoplasm of skin of unspecified upper limb, including shoulder

C44.602   Unspecified malignant neoplasm of skin of <u>right</u> upper limb, including shoulder

C44.609   Unspecified malignant neoplasm of skin of <u>left</u> upper limb, including shoulder

C44.61-   <u>Basal cell</u> carcinoma of skin of upper limb, including shoulder

C44.611   Basal cell carcinoma of skin of unspecified upper limb, including shoulder

C44.612   Basal cell carcinoma of skin of <u>right</u> upper limb, including shoulder

C44.619   Basal cell carcinoma of skin of <u>left</u> upper limb, including shoulder

C44.62- <u>Squamous cell</u> carcinoma of skin of upper limb, including shoulder

- **C44.621** Squamous cell carcinoma of skin of unspecified upper limb, including shoulder
- **C44.622** Squamous cell carcinoma of skin of <u>right</u> upper limb, including shoulder
- **C44.629** Squamous cell carcinoma of skin of <u>left</u> upper limb, including shoulder

C44.69- <u>Other specified</u> malignant neoplasm of skin of upper limb, including shoulder

- **C44.691** Other specified malignant neoplasm of skin of unspecified upper limb, including shoulder
- **C44.692** Other specified malignant neoplasm of skin of <u>right</u> upper limb, including shoulder
- **C44.699** Other specified malignant neoplasm of skin of <u>left</u> upper limb, including shoulder

C44.7- Other and unspecified malignant neoplasm of skin of <u>lower limb</u>, including hip

C44.70- <u>Unspecified</u> malignant neoplasm of skin of lower limb, including hip

- **C44.701** Unspecified malignant neoplasm of skin of unspecified lower limb, including hip
- **C44.702** Unspecified malignant neoplasm of skin of <u>right</u> lower limb, including hip
- **C44.709** Unspecified malignant neoplasm of skin of <u>left</u> lower limb, including hip

C44.71- <u>Basal cell</u> carcinoma of skin of lower limb, including hip

- **C44.711** Basal cell carcinoma of skin of unspecified lower limb, including hip
- **C44.712** Basal cell carcinoma of skin of <u>right</u> lower limb, including hip
- **C44.719** Basal cell carcinoma of skin of <u>left</u> lower limb, including hip

C44.72- <u>Squamous cell</u> carcinoma of skin of lower limb, including hip

- **C44.721** Squamous cell carcinoma of skin of unspecified lower limb, including hip
- **C44.722** Squamous cell carcinoma of skin of <u>right</u> lower limb, including hip
- **C44.729** Squamous cell carcinoma of skin of <u>left</u> lower limb, including hip

C44.79- <u>Other specified</u> malignant neoplasm of skin of lower limb, including hip

- **C44.791** Other specified malignant neoplasm of skin of unspecified lower limb, including hip
- **C44.792** Other specified malignant neoplasm of skin of <u>right</u> lower limb, including hip
- **C44.799** Other specified malignant neoplasm of skin of <u>left</u> lower limb, including hip

C44.8- Other and unspecified malignant neoplasm of <u>overlapping sites</u> of skin

- **C44.80** <u>Unspecified</u> malignant neoplasm of overlapping sites of skin
- **C44.81** <u>Basal cell</u> carcinoma of overlapping sites of skin
- **C44.82** <u>Squamous cell</u> carcinoma of overlapping sites of skin
- **C44.89** <u>Other specified</u> malignant neoplasm of overlapping sites of skin

C44.9- Other and unspecified malignant neoplasm of skin, unspecified

- **C44.90** <u>Unspecified</u> malignant neoplasm of skin, unspecified
  Malignant neoplasm of unspecified site of skin
- **C44.91** <u>Basal cell</u> carcinoma of skin, unspecified
- **C44.92** <u>Squamous cell</u> carcinoma of skin, unspecified
- **C44.99** <u>Other specified</u> malignant neoplasm of skin, unspecified

Malignant neoplasms of mesothelial and soft tissue (C45-C49)

C45- <u>Mesothelioma</u> — Any new and abnormal growth of the tissue that lines most of the internal organs (mesothelium) in which tissue growth is uncontrolled and has the properties of anaplasia, invasion, and metastases and is most often associated with asbestos exposure.

cc **C45.0** Mesothelioma of <u>pleura</u>
Excludes 1: other malignant neoplasm of pleura (C38.4)

cc **C45.1** Mesothelioma of <u>peritoneum</u>
Mesothelioma of cul-de-sac
Mesothelioma of mesentery
Mesothelioma of mesocolon
Mesothelioma of omentum
Mesothelioma of peritoneum (parietal) (pelvic)
Excludes 1: other malignant neoplasm of soft tissue of peritoneum (C48.-)

cc **C45.2** Mesothelioma of <u>pericardium</u>
Excludes 1: other malignant neoplasm of pericardium (C38.0)

C45.7 Mesothelioma of other sites

C45.9 Mesothelioma, unspecified

C46- <u>Kaposi's sarcoma</u> — Any new and abnormal growth of cells that line the lymph and blood vessels (endothelium) in which tissue growth is uncontrolled and has the properties of anaplasia and invasion and is often seen in HIV disease and other immunocompromised conditions.
Code first any human immunodeficiency virus [HIV] disease (B20)

cc **C46.0** Kaposi's sarcoma of <u>skin</u>

cc **C46.1** Kaposi's sarcoma of <u>soft tissue</u>
Kaposi's sarcoma of blood vessel
Kaposi's sarcoma of connective tissue
Kaposi's sarcoma of fascia
Kaposi's sarcoma of ligament
Kaposi's sarcoma of lymphatic(s) NEC
Kaposi's sarcoma of muscle
Excludes ❷: Kaposi's sarcoma of lymph glands and nodes (C46.3)

cc **C46.2** Kaposi's sarcoma of <u>palate</u>

cc **C46.3** Kaposi's sarcoma of <u>lymph nodes</u>

cc **C46.4** Kaposi's sarcoma of <u>gastrointestinal</u> sites

C46.5- Kaposi's sarcoma of <u>lung</u>

cc **C46.50** Kaposi's sarcoma of unspecified lung
cc **C46.51** Kaposi's sarcoma of <u>right</u> lung
cc **C46.52** Kaposi's sarcoma of <u>left</u> lung

cc **C46.7** Kaposi's sarcoma of other sites

cc **C46.9** Kaposi's sarcoma, unspecified
Kaposi's sarcoma of unspecified site

C47- Malignant neoplasm of <u>peripheral nerves</u> and <u>autonomic nervous system</u> — Any new and abnormal growth of the peripheral and autonomic nervous system in which tissue growth is uncontrolled and has the properties of anaplasia, invasion, and metastases.
Includes: Malignant neoplasm of sympathetic and parasympathetic nerves and ganglia
Excludes 1: Kaposi's sarcoma of soft tissue (C46.1)

cc **C47.0** Malignant neoplasm of peripheral nerves of head, face and neck
Excludes 1: malignant neoplasm of peripheral nerves of orbit (C69.6-)

C47.1- Malignant neoplasm of peripheral nerves of <u>upper limb</u>, including shoulder

cc **C47.10** Malignant neoplasm of peripheral nerves of unspecified upper limb, including shoulder
cc **C47.11** Malignant neoplasm of peripheral nerves of <u>right</u> upper limb, including shoulder
cc **C47.12** Malignant neoplasm of peripheral nerves of <u>left</u> upper limb, including shoulder

C47.2- Malignant neoplasm of peripheral nerves of <u>lower limb</u>, including hip

cc **C47.20** Malignant neoplasm of peripheral nerves of unspecified lower limb, including hip
cc **C47.21** Malignant neoplasm of peripheral nerves of <u>right</u> lower limb, including hip
cc **C47.22** Malignant neoplasm of peripheral nerves of <u>left</u> lower limb, including hip

C44 - C47

CC **C47.3** **Malignant neoplasm of peripheral nerves of <u>thorax</u>**

CC **C47.4** **Malignant neoplasm of peripheral nerves of <u>abdomen</u>**

CC **C47.5** **Malignant neoplasm of peripheral nerves of <u>pelvis</u>**

CC **C47.6** **Malignant neoplasm of peripheral nerves of trunk, unspecified**
Malignant neoplasm of peripheral nerves of unspecified part of trunk

CC **C47.8** **Malignant neoplasm of <u>overlapping sites</u> of peripheral nerves and autonomic nervous system**

CC **C47.9** **Malignant neoplasm of peripheral nerves and autonomic nervous system, unspecified**
Malignant neoplasm of unspecified site of peripheral nerves and autonomic nervous system

C48- **Malignant neoplasm of retroperitoneum and peritoneum** — Any new and abnormal growth of the retroperitoneum and peritoneum in which tissue growth is uncontrolled and has the properties of anaplasia, invasion, and metastases.
Excludes 1: *Kaposi's sarcoma of connective tissue (C46.1)*
mesothelioma (C45.-)

ANATOMY OF THE RETROPERITONEUM AND PERITONEUM — The retroperitoneum is the space behind the peritoneum and borders the deep muscles of the back which contain the kidneys, adrenals, most of the duodenum, ascending and descending colon, and the pancreas. The peritoneum is the serous membrane which contains most of the abdominal contents, and where it is doubled upon itself it forms supporting structures called ligaments.

PHYSIOLOGY OF THE RETROPERITONEUM AND PERITONEUM —The peritoneum encapsules and protects the abdominal visceral organs allowing them to move slightly without damaging function.

PERITONEUM — (FEMALE) SAGITTAL VIEW

CC **C48.0** **Malignant neoplasm of <u>retroperitoneum</u>** — The space which is behind the peritoneum and borders the deep muscles of the back.

CC **C48.1** **Malignant neoplasm of specified parts of <u>peritoneum</u>**
Malignant neoplasm of cul-de-sac — The area formed by the peritoneal fold behind the uterus and between the rectum and uterus.
Malignant neoplasm of mesentery — The peritoneal fold encircling most of the small bowel and attached to the posterior abdominal wall.
Malignant neoplasm of mesocolon — The peritoneal fold attaching the colon to the posterior abdominal wall.
Malignant neoplasm of omentum — The peritoneal fold attached to the stomach and extending down over the abdominal cavity.
Malignant neoplasm of parietal peritoneum — The serous membrane that lines the abdominal walls and the undersurface of the diaphragm.
Malignant neoplasm of pelvic peritoneum — The serous membrane that lines the pelvic cavity which is continuous with the parietal peritoneum.

CC **C48.2** **Malignant neoplasm of peritoneum, unspecified**

CC **C48.8** **Malignant neoplasm of <u>overlapping sites</u> of retroperitoneum and peritoneum**

C49- **Malignant neoplasm of <u>other connective and soft tissue</u>** — Any new and abnormal growth of the connective and other soft tissue in which tissue growth is uncontrolled and has the properties of anaplasia, invasion invasion, and metastases.
Includes: **Malignant neoplasm of blood vessel** — The musculomembranous tubes of the cardiovascular system that carry blood from the heart to the body cells and back again.
Malignant neoplasm of bursa — A pad-like sac or cavity of connective tissue lined with a synovial membrane which contains a viscid fluid and serves to prevent friction between structures where friction is likely to occur.
Malignant neoplasm of cartilage — The tough but flexible tissue that covers the ends of the bones at a joint and gives shape and support to other body parts.
Malignant neoplasm of fascia — A fibrous membrane which covers, supports, and separates muscles, and lies between the skin and underlying tissue.
Malignant neoplasm of fat — A soft mass of adipose tissue which creates pads between various organs, and serves as an energy reserve for the body.
Malignant neoplasm of ligament, except uterine — A band of fibrous connective tissue that connects bones and cartilages, serving to support and strengthen joints.
Malignant neoplasm of lymphatic vessel — The musculomembranous tubes of the lymphatic system that carry lymph fluid.
Malignant neoplasm of muscle — Groups of tissue made up of cells that contract together to produce movement.
Malignant neoplasm of synovia — The transparent alkaline fluid (synovial fluid) secreted by the synovial membranes into the joints, bursa, and tendons.
Malignant neoplasm of tendon (sheath) — The fibrous connective tissue cords which attach the muscles to bones and other structures.
Excludes 1: *malignant neoplasm of cartilage (of):*
articular (C40-C41)
larynx (C32.3)
nose (C30.0)
malignant neoplasm of connective tissue of breast (C50.-)
Excludes ❷: *Kaposi's sarcoma of soft tissue (C46.1)*
malignant neoplasm of heart (C38.0)
malignant neoplasm of peripheral nerves and autonomic nervous system (C47.-)
malignant neoplasm of peritoneum (C48.2)
malignant neoplasm of retroperitoneum (C48.0)
malignant neoplasm of uterine ligament (C57.3)
mesothelioma (C45.-)

CC **C49.0** **Malignant neoplasm of connective and soft tissue of <u>head, face and neck</u>**
Malignant neoplasm of connective tissue of ear
Malignant neoplasm of connective tissue of eyelid
Excludes 1: *connective tissue of orbit (C69.6-)*

C49.1- **Malignant neoplasm of connective and soft tissue of <u>upper limb</u>, including shoulder**

CC **C49.10** **Malignant neoplasm of connective and soft tissue of unspecified upper limb, including shoulder**

CC **C49.11** **Malignant neoplasm of connective and soft tissue of <u>right</u> upper limb, including shoulder**

CC **C49.12** **Malignant neoplasm of connective and soft tissue of <u>left</u> upper limb, including shoulder**

C49.2- **Malignant neoplasm of connective and soft tissue of <u>lower limb</u>, including hip**

CC **C49.20** **Malignant neoplasm of connective and soft tissue of unspecified lower limb, including hip**

CC **C49.21** **Malignant neoplasm of connective and soft tissue of <u>right</u> lower limb, including hip**

CC **C49.22** **Malignant neoplasm of connective and soft tissue of <u>left</u> lower limb, including hip**

CC **C49.3** **Malignant neoplasm of connective and soft tissue of <u>thorax</u>**
AHA T5:3Q:p19 – Synovial sarcoma, chest
Malignant neoplasm of axilla
Malignant neoplasm of diaphragm
Malignant neoplasm of great vessels
Excludes 1: *malignant neoplasm of breast (C50.-)*
malignant neoplasm of heart (C38.0)
malignant neoplasm of mediastinum (C38.1-C38.3)
malignant neoplasm of thymus (C37)

CC **C49.4** **Malignant neoplasm of connective and soft tissue of <u>abdomen</u>**
Malignant neoplasm of abdominal wall
Malignant neoplasm of hypochondrium

Excludes 1: = NOT CODED HERE! (Do not code both)   **568**   *Excludes ❷:* = Not Included Here

cc **C49.5** **Malignant neoplasm of connective and soft tissue of <u>pelvis</u>**
Malignant neoplasm of buttock
Malignant neoplasm of groin
Malignant neoplasm of perineum

cc **C49.6** **Malignant neoplasm of connective and soft tissue of trunk, unspecified**
Malignant neoplasm of back NOS

cc **C49.8** **Malignant neoplasm of <u>overlapping sites</u> of connective and soft tissue**
Primary malignant neoplasm of two or more contiguous sites of connective and soft tissue

cc **C49.9** **Malignant neoplasm of connective and soft tissue, unspecified**

C49.A- **Gastrointestinal stromal tumor** — A soft tissue sarcoma of the gastrointestinal tract (GIST) originating from interstitial cells of Cajal.

cc **C49.A0** **Gastrointestinal stromal tumor, unspecified site**

cc **C49.A1** **Gastrointestinal stromal tumor of esophagus**

cc **C49.A2** **Gastrointestinal stromal tumor of stomach**

cc **C49.A3** **Gastrointestinal stromal tumor of small intestine**

cc **C49.A4** **Gastrointestinal stromal tumor of large intestine**

cc **C49.A5** **Gastrointestinal stromal tumor of rectum**

cc **C49.A9** **Gastrointestinal stromal tumor of other sites**

Malignant neoplasms of breast (C50)

C50- **Malignant neoplasm of <u>breast</u>** — Any new and abnormal growth of the breast in which tissue growth is uncontrolled and has the properties of anaplasia, invasion, and metastases.
Includes: **Connective tissue of breast**
                Paget's disease of breast
                Paget's disease of nipple
Use additional code to identify estrogen receptor status (Z17.0, Z17.1)
Excludes 1:   skin of breast (C44.501, C44.511, C44.521, C44.591)
ANATOMY OF THE FEMALE BREAST — The female breast is the modified cutaneous glandular prominence overlying the pectoral muscle on the anterior chest, and contains the milk-producing mammary glands. The areola is the circular pigmented area around the nipple. The nipple is the pigmented projection and contains the ends of the mammary ducts.
PHYSIOLOGY OF THE FEMALE BREAST — The female breast functions to secrete nourishing milk for the newborn. During pregnancy, hormones increase the size of the mammary glands, and following delivery, the pituitary gland secretes prolactin, which stimulates the mammary glands to produce milk. The mammary ducts convey the milk to the nipple.

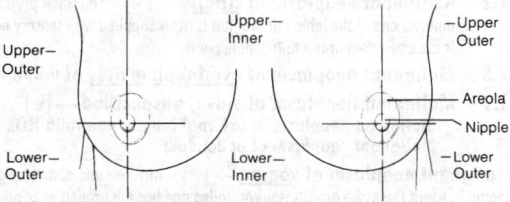

Upper—Inner
Upper—Outer
Upper—Outer
Areola
Nipple
Lower—Outer
Lower—Inner
Lower—Outer
FEMALE BREASTS — ANTERIOR VIEW (QUADRANTS)

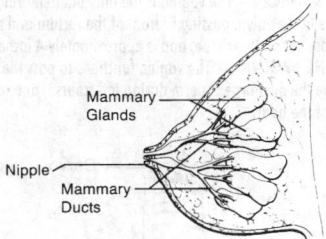

Mammary Glands
Nipple
Mammary Ducts
FEMALE BREAST — SAGITTAL VIEW

C50.0- **Malignant neoplasm of <u>nipple and areola</u>** — Nipple – The projection arising from the approximate center of the areola that contains the ends of the mammary ducts. Areola – The pigmented circular or ellipital area of the approximate center of the breast with the nipple projecting.

     C50.01- **Malignant neoplasm of nipple and areola, <u>female</u>**

         C50.011 **Malignant neoplasm of nipple and areola, <u>right</u> female breast** — [♀]

         C50.012 **Malignant neoplasm of nipple and areola, <u>left</u> female breast** — [♀]

         C50.019 **Malignant neoplasm of nipple and areola, unspecified female breast** — [♀]

     C50.02- **Malignant neoplasm of nipple and areola, <u>male</u>**

         C50.021 **Malignant neoplasm of nipple and areola, <u>right</u> male breast** — [♂]

         C50.022 **Malignant neoplasm of nipple and areola, <u>left</u> male breast** — [♂]

         C50.029 **Malignant neoplasm of nipple and areola, unspecified male breast** — [♂]

C50.1- **Malignant neoplasm of <u>central portion</u> of breast** — The general area that is located behind the areola in the center of breast mass.

     C50.11- **Malignant neoplasm of central portion of breast, <u>female</u>**

         C50.111 **Malignant neoplasm of central portion of <u>right</u> female breast** — [♀]

         C50.112 **Malignant neoplasm of central portion of <u>left</u> female breast** — [♀]

         C50.119 **Malignant neoplasm of central portion of unspecified female breast** — [♀]

     C50.12- **Malignant neoplasm of central portion of breast, <u>male</u>**

         C50.121 **Malignant neoplasm of central portion of <u>right</u> male breast** — [♂]

         C50.122 **Malignant neoplasm of central portion of <u>left</u> male breast** — [♂]

         C50.129 **Malignant neoplasm of central portion of unspecified male breast** — [♂]

C50.2- **Malignant neoplasm of <u>upper-inner quadrant</u> of breast** — That area above the nipple and towards the other breast.

     C50.21- **Malignant neoplasm of upper-inner quadrant of breast, <u>female</u>**

         C50.211 **Malignant neoplasm of upper-inner quadrant of <u>right</u> female breast** — [♀]

         C50.212 **Malignant neoplasm of upper-inner quadrant of <u>left</u> female breast** — [♀]

         C50.219 **Malignant neoplasm of upper-inner quadrant of unspecified female breast** — [♀]

     C50.22- **Malignant neoplasm of upper-inner quadrant of breast, <u>male</u>**

         C50.221 **Malignant neoplasm of upper-inner quadrant of <u>right</u> male breast** — [♂]

         C50.222 **Malignant neoplasm of upper-inner quadrant of <u>left</u> male breast** — [♂]

         C50.229 **Malignant neoplasm of upper-inner quadrant of unspecified male breast** — [♂]

C50.3- **Malignant neoplasm of <u>lower-inner quadrant</u> of breast** — That area below the nipple and towards the other breast.

     C50.31- **Malignant neoplasm of lower-inner quadrant of breast, <u>female</u>**

         C50.311 **Malignant neoplasm of lower-inner quadrant of <u>right</u> female breast** — [♀]

         C50.312 **Malignant neoplasm of lower-inner quadrant of <u>left</u> female breast** — [♀]

         C50.319 **Malignant neoplasm of lower-inner quadrant of unspecified female breast** — [♀]

     C50.32- **Malignant neoplasm of lower-inner quadrant of breast, <u>male</u>**

         C50.321 **Malignant neoplasm of lower-inner quadrant of <u>right</u> male breast** — [♂]

         C50.322 **Malignant neoplasm of lower-inner quadrant of <u>left</u> male breast** — [♂]

         C50.329 **Malignant neoplasm of lower-inner quadrant of unspecified male breast** — [♂]

C50.4- **Malignant neoplasm of <u>upper-outer quadrant</u> of breast** — That area above the nipple and to the side of the body.

     C50.41- **Malignant neoplasm of upper-outer quadrant of breast, <u>female</u>**

         C50.411 **Malignant neoplasm of upper-outer quadrant of <u>right</u> female breast** — [♀]

         C50.412 **Malignant neoplasm of upper-outer quadrant of <u>left</u> female breast** — [♀]

C50.419 Malignant neoplasm of upper-outer quadrant of unspecified female breast — [♀]

C50.42- Malignant neoplasm of upper-outer quadrant of breast, <u>male</u>

    C50.421 Malignant neoplasm of upper-outer quadrant of <u>right</u> male breast — [♂]

    C50.422 Malignant neoplasm of upper-outer quadrant of <u>left</u> male breast — [♂]

    C50.429 Malignant neoplasm of upper-outer quadrant of unspecified male breast — [♂]

C50.5- Malignant neoplasm of <u>lower-outer quadrant</u> of breast — That area below the nipple and to the side of the body.

C50.51- Malignant neoplasm of lower-outer quadrant of breast, <u>female</u>

    C50.511 Malignant neoplasm of lower-outer quadrant of <u>right</u> female breast — [♀]

    C50.512 Malignant neoplasm of lower-outer quadrant of <u>left</u> female breast — [♀]

    C50.519 Malignant neoplasm of lower-outer quadrant of unspecified female breast — [♀]

C50.52- Malignant neoplasm of lower-outer quadrant of breast, <u>male</u>

    C50.521 Malignant neoplasm of lower-outer quadrant of <u>right</u> male breast — [♂]

    C50.522 Malignant neoplasm of lower-outer quadrant of <u>left</u> male breast — [♂]

    C50.529 Malignant neoplasm of lower-outer quadrant of unspecified male breast — [♂]

C50.6- Malignant neoplasm of <u>axillary tail</u> of breast — That area which tapers away from the breast towards the axilla.

C50.61- Malignant neoplasm of axillary tail of breast, <u>female</u>

    C50.611 Malignant neoplasm of axillary tail of <u>right</u> female breast — [♀]

    C50.612 Malignant neoplasm of axillary tail of <u>left</u> female breast — [♀]

    C50.619 Malignant neoplasm of axillary tail of unspecified female breast — [♀]

C50.62- Malignant neoplasm of axillary tail of breast, <u>male</u>

    C50.621 Malignant neoplasm of axillary tail of <u>right</u> male breast — [♂]

    C50.622 Malignant neoplasm of axillary tail of <u>left</u> male breast — [♂]

    C50.629 Malignant neoplasm of axillary tail of unspecified male breast — [♂]

C50.8- Malignant neoplasm of <u>overlapping sites</u> of breast

C50.81- Malignant neoplasm of overlapping sites of breast, <u>female</u>

    C50.811 Malignant neoplasm of overlapping sites of <u>right</u> female breast — [♀]

    C50.812 Malignant neoplasm of overlapping sites of <u>left</u> female breast — [♀]

    C50.819 Malignant neoplasm of overlapping sites of unspecified female breast — [♀]

C50.82- Malignant neoplasm of overlapping sites of breast, <u>male</u>

    C50.821 Malignant neoplasm of overlapping sites of <u>right</u> male breast — [♂]

    C50.822 Malignant neoplasm of overlapping sites of <u>left</u> male breast — [♂]

    C50.829 Malignant neoplasm of overlapping sites of unspecified male breast — [♂]

C50.9- Malignant neoplasm of breast of unspecified site

C50.91- Malignant neoplasm of breast of unspecified site, <u>female</u>

    C50.911 Malignant neoplasm of unspecified site of <u>right</u> female breast — [♀]

    C50.912 Malignant neoplasm of unspecified site of <u>left</u> female breast — [♀]

    C50.919 Malignant neoplasm of unspecified site of unspecified female breast — [♀]

C50.92- Malignant neoplasm of breast of unspecified site, <u>male</u>

    C50.921 Malignant neoplasm of unspecified site of <u>right</u> male breast — [♂]

    C50.922 Malignant neoplasm of unspecified site of <u>left</u> male breast — [♂]

    C50.929 Malignant neoplasm of unspecified site of unspecified male breast — [♂]

Malignant neoplasms of female genital organs (C51-C58)

    Includes: Malignant neoplasm of skin of female genital organs

C51- **Malignant neoplasm of <u>vulva</u>** — Any new and abnormal growth of the vulva in which the tissue growth is uncontrolled and has the properties of anaplasia, invasion, and metastases.

  Excludes 1:   *carcinoma in situ of vulva (D07.1)*

  ANATOMY OF THE VULVA — The vulva is the group of external female genital organs comprising the labia majora, labia minora, clitoris, and vestibular glands.

  PHYSIOLOGY OF THE VULVA — The vulva functions to protect the genital organs at the entrance of the vagina, and aid in sexual stimulation and lubrication during intercourse.

EXTERNAL FEMALE GENITALS

C51.0 **Malignant neoplasm of <u>labium majus</u>** — [♀] — The longitudinal cutaneous folds of skin covering adipose tissue which enclose and protect the other female reproductive organs.

    Malignant neoplasm of Bartholin's [greater vestibular] gland — The mucous-secreting glands on each side of the vaginal orifice.

C51.1 **Malignant neoplasm of <u>labium minus</u>** — [♀] — The longitudinal flaps of skin on both sides of the vaginal opening and located within the labia majora that merge to form a hood-like covering around the clitoris.

C51.2 **Malignant neoplasm of <u>clitoris</u>** — [♀] — The small projection at the anterior end of the labia minora that is richly supplied with sensory nerve fibers and is the equivalent organ to the male penis.

C51.8 **Malignant neoplasm of <u>overlapping sites</u> of vulva** — [♀]

C51.9 **Malignant neoplasm of vulva, unspecified** — [♀]
    Malignant neoplasm of external female genitalia NOS
    Malignant neoplasm of pudendum

C52 **Malignant neoplasm of <u>vagina</u>** — [♀] — Any new and abnormal growth of the vagina in which the tissue growth is uncontrolled and has the properties of anaplasia, invasion, and metastases.

  Excludes 1:   *carcinoma in situ of vagina (D07.2)*

  ANATOMY OF THE VAGINA — The vagina is the musculomembranous tube extending from the uterus to the vulva, passing in front of the rectum and behind the bladder, and attached by loose connective tissue, and is approximately 4 inches (10 cm) in length.

  PHYSIOLOGY OF THE VAGINA — The vagina functions to pass the fetus to birth during delivery, receive the discharged sperm during intercourse, and convey the menstrual discharge out of the body.

VAGINA — CUT-AWAY VIEW

Excludes 1: = NOT CODED HERE! (Do not code both)   **570**   *Excludes ❷:* = Not Included Here

C53- **Malignant neoplasm of cervix uteri** — The lower neck of the uterus which extends downward into the upper portion of the vagina.
    Excludes 1:   *carcinoma in situ of cervix uteri (D06.-)*

C53.0   **Malignant neoplasm of endocervix** — [♀] – The mucous membrane lining of the cervix.

C53.1   **Malignant neoplasm of exocervix** — [♀] – That part of the cervix lined with squamous epithelium extending onto the lip of the cervix.

C53.8   **Malignant neoplasm of overlapping sites of cervix uteri** — [♀]

C53.9   **Malignant neoplasm of cervix uteri, unspecified** — [♀]

C54-   **Malignant neoplasm of corpus uteri** — Any new and abnormal growth of the

UTERUS AND ADNEXA

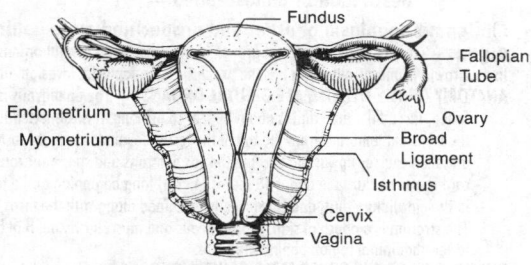

UTERUS AND ADNEXA — CUT-AWAY

body of the uterus in which tissue growth is uncontrolled and has the properties of anaplasia, invasion, and metastases.

ANATOMY OF THE UTERUS — The uterus is the hollow, muscular organ which receives the embryo and is about 2.8 inches (7 cm) in length, and up to 2 inches (5 cm) in width. The cervix is the lower third of the uterus which extends downward into the upper portion of the vagina. The isthmus is the narrowed lower end of the body of the uterus. The body is the bulky upper portion with the dome above the fallopian tube orifices, called the fundus. The endometrium is the mucous membrane interior lining upon the thick muscular myometrium of the body.

PHYSIOLOGY OF THE UTERUS — The uterus functions to receive the embryo, serves as attachment for the placenta, enlarges to allow for the fetus to grow, and rhythmically contracts for delivery of the fetus.

C54.0   **Malignant neoplasm of isthmus uteri** — [♀] – The narrowed part between the body and the cervix.
     Malignant neoplasm of lower uterine segment

C54.1   **Malignant neoplasm of endometrium** — [♀] – The endometrium is the mucous membrane interior lining upon the thick muscular myometrium of the body.

C54.2   **Malignant neoplasm of myometrium** — [♀] – The thick, smooth muscle layer of the uterine walls which is interlaced with connective tissue.

C54.3   **Malignant neoplasm of fundus uteri** — [♀] – The dome-shaped portion above the orifices of the fallopian tubes.

C54.8   **Malignant neoplasm of overlapping sites of corpus uteri** — [♀]

C54.9   **Malignant neoplasm of corpus uteri, unspecified** — [♀]

C55   **Malignant neoplasm of uterus, part unspecified** — [♀]

C56- **Malignant neoplasm of ovary** — Any new and abnormal growth of the ovary (the flat, ovoid paired sexual glands in the female which produce the human reproductive cell, the ova) in which tissue growth is uncontrolled and has the properties of anaplasia, invasion, and metastases.
Use additional code to identify any functional activity
ANATOMY OF THE OVARIES — The ovaries are the paired, flat, ovoid female sexual glands located on each side of the uterus and attached to the broad ligament, and are approximately 1.4 inches (3.5 cm) in length and 0.8 inches (2 cm) in width.
PHYSIOLOGY OF THE OVARIES — The ovaries function to produce the human reproductive cell, and produce sexual hormones.

cc **C56.1**   **Malignant neoplasm of right ovary** — [♀]

cc **C56.2**   **Malignant neoplasm of left ovary** — [♀]

cc **C56.9**   **Malignant neoplasm of unspecified ovary** — [♀]

C57- **Malignant neoplasm of other and unspecified female genital organs** — Any new and abnormal growth of the other uterine adnexa in which tissue growth is uncontrolled and has the properties of anaplasia, invasion, and metastases.

C57.0- **Malignant neoplasm of fallopian tube** — The long, slender tube that extends from the uterus to the area next to the ovary which transfers the ova to the uterus for implantation.
     Malignant neoplasm of oviduct
     Malignant neoplasm of uterine tube

C57.00   **Malignant neoplasm of unspecified fallopian tube** — [♀]

C57.01   **Malignant neoplasm of right fallopian tube** — [♀]

C57.02   **Malignant neoplasm of left fallopian tube** — [♀]

C57.1- **Malignant neoplasm of broad ligament** — The peritoneal fold that supports the uterus on each side.

C57.10   **Malignant neoplasm of unspecified broad ligament** — [♀]

C57.11   **Malignant neoplasm of right broad ligament** — [♀]

C57.12   **Malignant neoplasm of left broad ligament** — [♀]

C57.2- **Malignant neoplasm of round ligament** — The fibromuscular band attached to the uterus, just below the fallopian tube entrance, and to the pelvic wall.

C57.20   **Malignant neoplasm of unspecified round ligament** — [♀]

C57.21   **Malignant neoplasm of right round ligament** — [♀]

C57.22   **Malignant neoplasm of left round ligament** — [♀]

C57.3   **Malignant neoplasm of parametrium** — [♀] – The loose connective tissue between the serous layers of the broad ligaments.
     Malignant neoplasm of uterine ligament NOS

C57.4   **Malignant neoplasm of uterine adnexa, unspecified** — [♀]

C57.7   **Malignant neoplasm of other specified female genital organs** — [♀]
     Malignant neoplasm of wolffian body or duct

C57.8   **Malignant neoplasm of overlapping sites of female genital organs** — [♀]
     Primary malignant neoplasm of two or more contiguous sites of the female genital organs whose point of origin cannot be determined
     Primary tubo-ovarian malignant neoplasm whose point of origin cannot be determined
     Primary utero-ovarian malignant neoplasm whose point of origin cannot be determined

C57.9   **Malignant neoplasm of female genital organ, unspecified** — [♀]
     Malignant neoplasm of female genitourinary tract NOS

C58   **Malignant neoplasm of placenta** — [♀, Age/12-55] – Any new and abnormal growth of the placenta in which tissue growth is uncontrolled and has the properties of anaplasia, invasion, and metastases.
Includes: **Choriocarcinoma NOS**
           Chorionepithelioma NOS
Excludes 1:   *chorioadenoma (destruens) (D39.2)*
           hydatidiform mole NOS (O01.9)
           invasive hydatidiform mole (D39.2)
           male choriocarcinoma NOS (C62.9-)
           malignant hydatidiform mole (D39.2)
ANATOMY OF THE PLACENTA — The placenta is the highly vascular disc-shaped organ within the pregnant uterus which connects with the fetus through the umbilical cord.
PHYSIOLOGY OF THE PLACENTA — The placenta functions to provide the fetus with nourishment, to filter the maternal blood, and, as an endocrine gland, to produce chorionic gonadotrophins, estrogen, and progesterone.

C 5 3 - C 5 8

Malignant neoplasms of male genital organs (C60-C63)

Includes: Malignant neoplasm of skin of male genital organs

C60- **Malignant neoplasm of <u>penis</u>** — Any new and abnormal growth of the penis in which the tissue growth is uncontrolled and has the properties of anaplasia, invasion, and metastases.

ANATOMY OF THE PENIS — The penis is a cylindrical organ which contains the urethra, located at the base of the male perineum. The body (shaft) is composed of 3 columns of erectile tissue, including a pair of dorsally located corpora cavernosa and a single corpus spongiosum below. The corpus spongiosum, through which the urethra extends, is enlarged at its distal end to form a sensitive, cone-shaped glans penis. A loose fold of skin, called the prepuce (foreskin) covers the glans penis, unless removed by circumcision.

PHYSIOLOGY OF THE PENIS — The penis functions as the specialized organ in the male that when erect is inserted into the female vagina for sexual intercourse. It also functions to convey urine and seminal fluid through the urethra to the outside. Erection is obtained by sexual excitement, stimulating parasympathetic nerve impulses causing blood engorgement of the corpora cavernosa and corpus spongiosum.

PENIS — FRONTAL VIEW

C60.0 **Malignant neoplasm of <u>prepuce</u>** — [♂] – The foreskin which covers the glans penis, unless circumcision has been performed.
Malignant neoplasm of foreskin

C60.1 **Malignant neoplasm of <u>glans</u> penis** — [♂] – The cone-shaped distal end of the penis that contains numerous sensory nerve fibers.

C60.2 **Malignant neoplasm of <u>body</u> of penis** — [♂] – The shaft of the penis composed of 3 columns of erectile tissue.
Malignant neoplasm of corpus cavernosum — The pair of dorsally located erectile tissue columns running the length of the penis.

C60.8 **Malignant neoplasm of <u>overlapping sites</u> of penis** — [♂]

C60.9 **Malignant neoplasm of penis, unspecified** — [♂]
Malignant neoplasm of skin of penis NOS

C61 **Malignant neoplasm of <u>prostate</u>** — [♂] – Any new and abnormal growth of the prostate in which tissue growth is uncontrolled and has the properties of anaplasia, invasion, and metastases.
Use additional code to identify:
Hormone sensitivity status (Z19.1-Z19.2)
Rising PSA following treatment for malignant neoplasm of prostate (R97.21)
Excludes 1: *malignant neoplasm of seminal vesicle (C63.7)*
ANATOMY OF THE PROSTATE — The prostate is a walnut-shaped gland which surrounds the bladder neck, and is contracted by smooth muscle with ducts opening into the urethra, and is 1.6 inches (4 cm) across and 1.2 inches (3 cm) thick.
PHYSIOLOGY OF THE PROSTATE — The prostate secretes a thin, milky fluid with an alkaline pH which enhances the motility of sperm cells and neutralizes the acidic pH of the vagina.

C62- **Malignant neoplasm of <u>testis</u>** — Any new and abnormal growth of the testis in which tissue growth is uncontrolled and has the properties of anaplasia, invasion, and metastases.
Use additional code to identify any functional activity
ANATOMY OF THE TESTES — The testes are the ovoid structures in the scrotum, suspended by a spermatic cord, and approximately 2 inches (5 cm) in length and 1.2 inches (3 cm) in diameter. Each testis is enclosed by a tough, white fibrous capsule called the tunica albuginea.
PHYSIOLOGY OF THE TESTES — The testes function to produce sperm cells for human reproduction, and secrete male hormones.

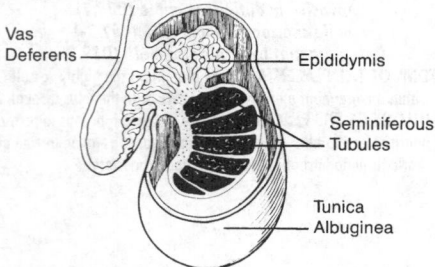

TESTIS — CUT-AWAY

C62.0- **Malignant neoplasm of <u>undescended</u> testis** — A testis which has failed to descend into the scrotum and remains in the inguinal canal.
Malignant neoplasm of ectopic testis
Malignant neoplasm of retained testis

C62.00 **Malignant neoplasm of unspecified undescended testis** — [♂]

C62.01 **Malignant neoplasm of undescended <u>right</u> testis** — [♂]

C62.02 **Malignant neoplasm of undescended <u>left</u> testis** — [♂]

C62.1- **Malignant neoplasm of <u>descended</u> testis** — The normal position of the testis in the scrotum.
Malignant neoplasm of scrotal testis

C62.10 **Malignant neoplasm of unspecified descended testis** — [♂]

C62.11 **Malignant neoplasm of descended <u>right</u> testis** — [♂]

C62.12 **Malignant neoplasm of descended <u>left</u> testis** — [♂]

C62.9- **Malignant neoplasm of testis, <u>unspecified whether descended or undescended</u>**

C62.90 **Malignant neoplasm of unspecified testis, unspecified whether descended or undescended** — [♂]
Malignant neoplasm of testis NOS

C62.91 **Malignant neoplasm of <u>right</u> testis, unspecified whether descended or undescended** — [♂]

C62.92 **Malignant neoplasm of <u>left</u> testis, unspecified whether descended or undescended** — [♂]

C63- **Malignant neoplasm of other and unspecified male genital organs** — Any new and abnormal growth of the other male genital organs in which the tissue growth is uncontrolled and has the properties of anaplasia, invasion, and metastases.
ANATOMY OF THE OTHER MALE GENITAL ORGANS — The epididymis is a tightly coiled, threadlike tube that is about 20 feet (6 m) long. It is connected to ducts within the testis and emerges from the top of the testis, descends along its posterior surface, and then courses upward to become the vas deferans and spermatic cord. The spermatic cord is a muscular tube about 18 inches (45 cm) long beginning at the testis and ending in the ejaculatory duct, and is externally contained along with the testis, in the scrotum. The scrotum is a pouch of skin, subcutaneous and muscular tissue, that hangs from the lower abdominal region behind the penis.
PHYSIOLOGY OF THE OTHER MALE GENITAL ORGANS — The epididymis functions to store and mature sperm cells, and to transport the sperm from the testicular ducts to the spermatic cord. The spermatic cord transports the sperm to the ejaculatory duct. The scrotum protects the testis and spermatic cord by contracting and relaxing the dartos muscle.

MALE GENITAL ORGANS — SAGITTAL VIEW

C63.0- **Malignant neoplasm of <u>epididymis</u>** — The tightly coiled tube attached to each testis where sperm cells mature and are stored.

C63.00 **Malignant neoplasm of unspecified epididymis** — [♂]

C63.01 **Malignant neoplasm of <u>right</u> epididymis** — [♂]

C63.02 **Malignant neoplasm of <u>left</u> epididymis** — [♂]

C63.1- **Malignant neoplasm of <u>spermatic cord</u>** — The muscular tube which transports the sperm from the epididymis to the ejaculatory duct.

C63.10 **Malignant neoplasm of unspecified spermatic cord** — [♂]

C63.11 **Malignant neoplasm of <u>right</u> spermatic cord** — [♂]

C63.12 **Malignant neoplasm of <u>left</u> spermatic cord** — [♂]

C63.2 **Malignant neoplasm of <u>scrotum</u>** — [♂] – The pouch of skin, subcutaneous, and muscular tissue that encloses and protects the testes, and hangs from the trunk behind the penis.
Malignant neoplasm of skin of scrotum — The protective dermal covering of the scrotum.

C63.7 **Malignant neoplasm of other specified male genital organs** — [♂]

      Malignant neoplasm of seminal vesicle — The tube-like glands attached to the vas deferens near the base of the bladder which secrete a slightly alkaline fluid rich in nutrients and prostaglandins.

      Malignant neoplasm of tunica vaginalis — The serous membrane covering the front and sides of the testis and epididymis.

C63.8 **Malignant neoplasm of overlapping sites of male genital organs** — [♂]

      Primary malignant neoplasm of two or more contiguous sites of male genital organs whose point of origin cannot be determined

C63.9 **Malignant neoplasm of male genital organ, unspecified** — [♂]

      Malignant neoplasm of male genitourinary tract NOS

Malignant neoplasms of urinary tract (C64-C68)

C64- **Malignant neoplasm of kidney, except renal pelvis** — Any new and abnormal growth of the kidney in which the tissue growth is uncontrolled and has the properties of anaplasia, invasion, and metastases.

    Excludes 1:   *malignant carcinoid tumor of the kidney (C7A.093)*
                        malignant neoplasm of renal calyces (C65.-)
                        malignant neoplasm of renal pelvis (C65.-)

  ANATOMY OF THE KIDNEYS — The kidneys are reddish-brown, bean-shaped organs about 4.7 inches (12 cm) long, 2.3 inches (6 cm) wide, and 1.2 inches (3 cm) thick, and are located on either side of the vertebral column in the retroperitoneal space. The kidneys are supplied with arterial blood from the renal arteries which branch off from the aorta, and are drained by the renal veins which connect with the inferior vena cava. The renal pelvis is the funnel-shaped urinary collecting system of the kidney at the upper end of a ureter.

  PHYSIOLOGY OF THE KIDNEYS — The kidneys function to remove metabolic wastes from the blood by transferring them into the urine. They also regulate red blood cell production, blood pressure, calcium absorption, and the pH level of the blood.

KIDNEY — ANTERIOR VIEW

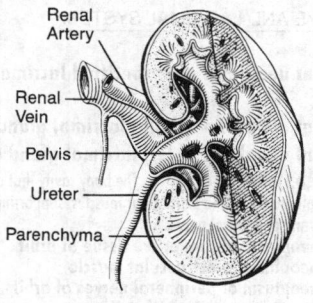

KIDNEY — (CUT AWAY VIEW)

cc **C64.1** **Malignant neoplasm of right kidney, except renal pelvis**
cc **C64.2** **Malignant neoplasm of left kidney, except renal pelvis**
cc **C64.9** **Malignant neoplasm of unspecified kidney, except renal pelvis**

C65- **Malignant neoplasm of renal pelvis** — Any new and abnormal growth of the kidney pelvis in which the tissue growth is uncontrolled and has the properties of anaplasia, invasion, and metastases.

    Includes: **Malignant neoplasm of pelviureteric junction** — The funnel-shaped urine collecting system of the kidneys.

                    Malignant neoplasm of renal calyces — The minor subdivisions of the renal pelvis.

cc **C65.1** **Malignant neoplasm of right renal pelvis**
cc **C65.2** **Malignant neoplasm of left renal pelvis**
cc **C65.9** **Malignant neoplasm of unspecified renal pelvis**

C66- **Malignant neoplasm of ureter** — Any new and abnormal growth of the ureter (the musculomembranous tubes which convey urine from the kidneys to the bladder) in which the tissue growth is uncontrolled and has the properties of anaplasia, invasion, and metastases.

    Excludes 1:   *malignant neoplasm of ureteric orifice of bladder (C67.6)*

cc **C66.1** **Malignant neoplasm of right ureter**
cc **C66.2** **Malignant neoplasm of left ureter**
cc **C66.9** **Malignant neoplasm of unspecified ureter**

C67- **Malignant neoplasm of bladder** — Any new and abnormal growth of the bladder in which the tissue growth is uncontrolled and has the properties of anaplasia, invasion, and metastases.

    AHA 16:1Q:p19 – Malignant neoplasm of neobladder

  ANATOMY OF THE BLADDER — The urinary bladder is a hollow, collapsible musculomembranous organ, and is located within the pelvic cavity, behind the symphysis pubis. In the male, it lies against the rectum, and in the female it lies against the vagina and uterus. When filled it may contain 17 fluid ounces (500 ml) of urine and pushes upward indenting the abdominal cavity. The trigone area is the floor of the bladder formed by three points, the two ureteral orifices and the urethral orifice. The dome is the expandable superior surface of the bladder. The bladder neck is that area surrounding the urethral orifice. The ureteric orifice is that area surrounding the ureteral openings. The urachus in the adult forms the middle umbilical ligament of the bladder.

  PHYSIOLOGY OF THE BLADDER — The urinary bladder functions as a reservoir for the urine produced by the kidneys until the individual expels the urine (micturition). Micturition occurs when the bladder becomes distended with urine and stretch receptor nerves stimulate the micturition center in the sacral spinal cord. Parasympathetic nerve impulses start rhythmically contracting the bladder and the individual senses an urgency to urinate. Following the midbrain decision to urinate, the external urethral

BLADDER

BLADDER — ANTERIOR (CUT-AWAY) VIEW

sphincter is relaxed, and urination begins as the bladder muscle contracts.

C67.0 **Malignant neoplasm of trigone of bladder** — The area of the bladder floor formed by the ureteral orifices and the urethral orifice.

C67.1 **Malignant neoplasm of dome of bladder** — The expandable superior surface of the bladder.

C67.2 **Malignant neoplasm of lateral wall of bladder**

C67.3 **Malignant neoplasm of anterior wall of bladder**

C67.4 **Malignant neoplasm of posterior wall of bladder**

C67.5 **Malignant neoplasm of bladder neck** — The outlet area of bladder surrounding the urethral orifice.

    Malignant neoplasm of internal urethral orifice

C67.6 **Malignant neoplasm of ureteric orifice** — The opening of a ureter into the bladder.

C67.7 **Malignant neoplasm of urachus** — The fetal urinary tract that in the adult forms the middle umbilical ligament of the bladder.

C67.8 **Malignant neoplasm of overlapping sites of bladder**

C67.9 **Malignant neoplasm of bladder, unspecified**

C
6
3
-
C
6
7

C
6
8
I
C
6
9

C68-   Malignant neoplasm of other and unspecified urinary organs
    Excludes 1:   *malignant neoplasm of female genitourinary tract NOS (C57.9)*
                    malignant neoplasm of male genitourinary tract NOS (C63.9)
    cc **C68.0   Malignant neoplasm of <u>urethra</u>** — Any new and abnormal growth of the urethra (the musculomembranous tube which conveys urine from the bladder to the outside at the urethral orifice) in which the tissue growth is uncontrolled and has the properties of anaplasia, invasion, and metastases.
        Excludes 1:   *malignant neoplasm of urethral orifice of bladder (C67.5)*
    cc **C68.1   Malignant neoplasm of <u>paraurethral glands</u>** — Any new and abnormal growth of the paraurethral glands (the small rudimentary glands that open on either side of the posterior portion of the urethral orifice) in which the tissue growth is uncontrolled and has the properties of anaplasia, invasion, and metastases.
    cc **C68.8   Malignant neoplasm of overlapping sites of urinary organs**
        Primary malignant neoplasm of two or more contiguous sites of urinary organs whose point of origin cannot be determined
    cc **C68.9   Malignant neoplasm of urinary organ, unspecified**
        Malignant neoplasm of urinary system NOS

Malignant neoplasms of eye, brain and other parts of central nervous system (C69-C72)

C69-   Malignant neoplasm of <u>eye and adnexa</u> — Any new and abnormal growth of the eye and adnexa in which the tissue growth is uncontrolled and has the properties of anaplasia, invasion, and metastases.
    Excludes 1:   *malignant neoplasm of connective tissue of eyelid (C49.0)*
                    malignant neoplasm of eyelid (skin) (C43.1-, C44.1-)
                    malignant neoplasm of optic nerve (C72.3-)
    ANATOMY OF THE EYES — The eyes are hollow spherical structures about 1 inch (2.5 cm) in diameter, located in and protected by the orbital socket in the skull. The sclera (outer layer) is protective, and its anterior portion, the cornea, is transparent so that it can refract light entering the eye. The crystalline lens is a transparent elastic structure whose shape is controlled by the action of ciliary muscles. The iris is a muscular diaphragm that controls the dilation of the pupil. The ciliary body consists of smooth muscle with suspensory ligaments which hold the lens in place and adjust the focus of the lens. The extraocular muscles attach the eyeball to the orbit by 6 different muscles. The lacrimal glands are located in the upper outer corner of the eyes. The conjunctiva is the delicate mucous membrane which lines the eyelids and covers the exposed surface of the sclera. The retina is the inner layer of the eye, and is continuous with the optic nerve. It contains the visual receptor cells, including the rods and cones. The choroid is the middle layer which contains the dark brown pigment and is the vascular layer. The anterior and posterior chambers contain the watery fluid in the hollow bulk of the eye. The lacrimal duct is located at the inner lower corner of each eye and connects with the nasal cavity.
    PHYSIOLOGY OF THE EYES — The eyes are the primary organ of sight, and are directly connected to the brain through the retina and optic nerve. The lens and cornea refract light waves to focus them on the retina. The retina contains visual receptor cells, called rods and cones. The rods are responsible for colorless vision, like in dim light, and the cones are responsible for color vision through their light-sensitive pigment sets. The iris is constricted or dilated by the ciliary body and allows for varying amounts of light to enter the eye. The extraocular muscles function to rotate the eyeballs to look at desired objects . The lacrimal glands function to keep protective tears on the conjunctiva and cornea. The conjunctiva is the protective mucous membrane covering the eyelids and exposed portion of the sclera. The choroid functions as a vascular blood supply to most eye structures and absorbs excess light through its dark pigment. The lacrimal duct drains the tears from the eyes into the nasal cavities.

EYE — SAGITTAL VIEW

C69.0-   Malignant neoplasm of <u>conjunctiva</u> — The delicate mucous membrane that lines the eyelids and exposed surface of the sclera.
    C69.00   Malignant neoplasm of unspecified conjunctiva
    C69.01   Malignant neoplasm of <u>right</u> conjunctiva
    C69.02   Malignant neoplasm of <u>left</u> conjunctiva

C69.1-   Malignant neoplasm of <u>cornea</u> — The clear, transparent fibrous outer tissue layer of the anterior eyeball including the iris, pupil, and anterior chamber that is continuous with the sclera.
    C69.10   Malignant neoplasm of unspecified cornea
    C69.11   Malignant neoplasm of <u>right</u> cornea
    C69.12   Malignant neoplasm of <u>left</u> cornea
C69.2-   Malignant neoplasm of <u>retina</u> — The innermost layer of the eyeball, consisting of an outer pigmented layer and an inner nervous layer which includes the rods and cones and is continuous with the optic nerve.
    Excludes 1:   *dark area on retina (D49.81)*
                    neoplasm of unspecified behavior of retina and choroid (D49.81)
                    retinal freckle (D49.81)
    C69.20   Malignant neoplasm of unspecified retina
    C69.21   Malignant neoplasm of <u>right</u> retina
    C69.22   Malignant neoplasm of <u>left</u> retina
C69.3-   Malignant neoplasm of <u>choroid</u> — The thin, dark brown pigmented vascular layer between the retina and the sclera that covers the eyeball, except for the anterior light-entering portion.
    C69.30   Malignant neoplasm of unspecified choroid
    C69.31   Malignant neoplasm of <u>right</u> choroid
    C69.32   Malignant neoplasm of <u>left</u> choroid
C69.4-   Malignant neoplasm of <u>ciliary body</u> — The smooth muscle layer which adjusts the iris and lens.
    C69.40   Malignant neoplasm of unspecified ciliary body
    C69.41   Malignant neoplasm of <u>right</u> ciliary body
    C69.42   Malignant neoplasm of <u>left</u> ciliary body
C69.5-   Malignant neoplasm of <u>lacrimal gland and duct</u> — The tear-secreting glands and their ducts that lie at the upper-outer angle of the orbit.
    Malignant neoplasm of lacrimal sac — The dilated upper end of the nasolacrimal duct.
    Malignant neoplasm of nasolacrimal duct — The passage which conveys the tears from the lacrimal sac into the interior nasal meatus.

EYE AND LACRIMAL SYSTEM

    C69.50   Malignant neoplasm of unspecified lacrimal gland and duct
    C69.51   Malignant neoplasm of <u>right</u> lacrimal gland and duct
    C69.52   Malignant neoplasm of <u>left</u> lacrimal gland and duct
C69.6-   Malignant neoplasm of <u>orbit</u> — The bony cavity that contains and protects the eyeball, including the extraocular muscles, supporting and connecting connective tissue, and peripheral nerves.
    Malignant neoplasm of connective tissue of orbit
    Malignant neoplasm of extraocular muscle
    Malignant neoplasm of peripheral nerves of orbit
    Malignant neoplasm of retrobulbar tissue
    Malignant neoplasm of retro-ocular tissue
    Excludes 1:   *malignant neoplasm of orbital bone (C41.0)*
    C69.60   Malignant neoplasm of unspecified orbit
    C69.61   Malignant neoplasm of <u>right</u> orbit
    C69.62   Malignant neoplasm of <u>left</u> orbit
C69.8-   Malignant neoplasm of <u>overlapping sites</u> of eye and adnexa
    C69.80   Malignant neoplasm of overlapping sites of unspecified eye and adnexa
    C69.81   Malignant neoplasm of overlapping sites of <u>right</u> eye and adnexa
    C69.82   Malignant neoplasm of overlapping sites of <u>left</u> eye and adnexa

C69.9- **Malignant neoplasm of unspecified site of eye**
Malignant neoplasm of eyeball

C69.90 **Malignant neoplasm of unspecified site of unspecified eye**

C69.91 **Malignant neoplasm of unspecified site of <u>right</u> eye**

C69.92 **Malignant neoplasm of unspecified site of <u>left</u> eye**

C70- **Malignant neoplasm of <u>meninges</u>** — Any new and abnormal growth of the meninges in which tissue growth is uncontrolled and has the properties of anaplasia, invasion, and metastasis.

cc **C70.0** **Malignant neoplasm of <u>cerebral</u> meninges** — The three protective covering membranes of the brain, consisting of the dura mater (outermost), the arachnoid (middle), and the pia mater (innermost) that are continuous with the spinal meninges.

cc **C70.1** **Malignant neoplasm of <u>spinal</u> meninges** — The three protective covering membranes of the spinal cord which are continuous with the cerebral meninges.

cc **C70.9** **Malignant neoplasm of meninges, unspecified**

C71- **Malignant neoplasm of <u>brain</u>** — Any new and abnormal growth of the brain in which tissue growth is uncontrolled and has the properties of anaplasia, invasion, and metastases.
AHA 14:3Q:p3 – Astrocytoma
Excludes 1: *malignant neoplasm of cranial nerves (C72.2-C72.5)*
retrobulbar malignant neoplasm (C69.6-)
ANATOMY OF THE BRAIN — The brain is the largest and most complex part of the nervous system, and is located in the cranial cavity. The cerebrum is the largest part of the brain, and is divided sagittally (front and back through the center) into 2 hemispheres. The corpus callosum lies below and connects the 2 hemispheres. The thalamus lies below the corpus callosum on either side of the third ventricle. The hypothalamus lies above the brain stem and forms the floor of the third ventricle. The basal ganglia are masses of gray matter located deep within the cerebral hemispheres, including the globus pallidus. The corpus striatum consists of 2 of the basal ganglia, the caudate and lentiform nuclei. The frontal lobe forms the anterior portion of each cerebral hemisphere. The temporal lobes lie below the frontal lobe on the lateral side of each cerebral hemisphere. The parietal lobe forms the superior portion of the cerebrum, lying posterior to the frontal lobe. The occipital lobe forms the posterior portion of each cerebral hemisphere. The ventricles are a series of interconnected cavities of the brain and are continuous with the central canal of the spinal cord, which are filled with the cerebrospinal fluid. The cerebellum is the second largest portion of the brain, located below the occipital lobe and behind the brain stem. The brain stem connects the upper end of the spinal cord with the cerebrum. It contains the pons, cerebral peduncle, medulla oblongata, and midbrain. The tapetum is a layer of fibers from the corpus callosum forming the roof and lateral walls of the lateral ventricles.

PHYSIOLOGY OF THE BRAIN — The cerebrum, including its lobes and cerebral cortex, is concerned with the higher brain functions, such as memory, thought, reasoning, and voluntary muscle control. The basal ganglia function as relay stations for motor impulses. The thalamus functions as a central relay station for sensory impulses. The hypothalamus functions to control homeostasis by regulation of the heart rate, arterial blood pressure, body temperature, body weight, and sleep. The ventricles are filled by continuously replaced cerebrospinal fluid which serves to protect the brain by absorbing shocks and removing any waste substances. It also provides a stable ionic concentration in the central nervous system, which is important for maximum nerve impulse transfers. The cerebellum functions primarily as a reflex center in the coordination of skeletal muscle movements and the maintenance of equilibrium. The pons transmits impulses between the cerebrum and other parts of the nervous system and contains centers that help to regulate the rate and depth of breathing. The medulla oblongata transmits all ascending and descending impulses, and contains several vital and nonvital reflex centers. The midbrain contains reflex centers associated with eye and head movements.

BRAIN — POSTERIOR VIEW

BRAIN — SAGITTAL VIEW

cc **C71.0** **Malignant neoplasm of <u>cerebrum</u>, except lobes and ventricles**
Malignant neoplasm of supratentorial NOS

cc **C71.1** **Malignant neoplasm of <u>frontal lobe</u>** — The anterior portion of the cerebral hemispheres.

cc **C71.2** **Malignant neoplasm of <u>temporal lobe</u>** — The lower lateral portion of the cerebral hemispheres.

cc **C71.3** **Malignant neoplasm of <u>parietal lobe</u>** — The upper central portion of the cerebral hemispheres.

cc **C71.4** **Malignant neoplasm of <u>occipital lobe</u>** — The posterior portion of the cerebral hemispheres.

cc **C71.5** **Malignant neoplasm of <u>cerebral ventricle</u>** — The three cavities within the brain that are filled with cerebrospinal fluid, including the two lateral ventricles and the third ventricle.
Excludes 1: *malignant neoplasm of fourth cerebral ventricle (C71.7)*

cc **C71.6** **Malignant neoplasm of <u>cerebellum</u>** — That part of the brain, below the occipital lobe of the cerebrum and posterior to the brain stem, that functions to control the voluntary muscles and coordination.

cc **C71.7** **Malignant neoplasm of <u>brain stem</u>** — The stem-like portion of the brain connecting the cerebrum with the spinal cord.
Malignant neoplasm of fourth cerebral ventricle — The cavity within the brain that is filled with cerebrospinal fluid and located at the base of the brain surrounding the pons.
Infratentorial malignant neoplasm NOS

cc **C71.8** **Malignant neoplasm of <u>overlapping sites</u> of brain**

cc **C71.9** **Malignant neoplasm of brain, unspecified**

C72- **Malignant neoplasm of spinal cord, cranial nerves and other parts of central nervous system** — Any new and abnormal growth of the spinal cord, cranial nerves, and other parts of the central nervous system in which tissue growth is uncontrolled and has the properties of anaplasia, invasion, and metastases.
Excludes 1: *malignant neoplasm of meninges (C70.-)*
malignant neoplasm of peripheral nerves and autonomic nervous system (C47.-)
ANATOMY OF THE NERVOUS SYSTEM, OTHER THAN THE BRAIN — The cranial nerves are the 12 pairs of nerves arising from the brain stem and cerebrum and serving the various organs of the head. The meninges, both cerebral and spinal are the 3 membranes which completely enclose the brain and spinal cord, and contain the cerebrospinal fluid. The spinal cord is the vertebral canal extension of the central nervous system with most of the body's nerves leaving and entering along its length.
PHYSIOLOGY OF THE NERVOUS SYSTEM, OTHER THAN THE BRAIN — The cranial nerves serve the various specific organs of the head, with some being sensory only (olfactory, optic), others are mostly motor (abducens), while most are of mixed sensory and motor nerves. The meninges function to protect the brain and spinal cord from injury and infection, and contain the cerebrospinal fluid. The spinal cord functions to supply the body with 31 pairs of nerves that branch out to serve all the parts of the body below the neck.

cc **C72.0** **Malignant neoplasm of <u>spinal cord</u>** — That part of the central nervous system found in the vertebral column canal which is continuous with the medulla oblongata.

cc **C72.1** **Malignant neoplasm of <u>cauda equina</u>** — The group of spinal nerve roots that extend from the lower part of the spinal cord.

C72.2- **Malignant neoplasm of <u>olfactory nerve</u>** — The first cranial nerve that receives sensory impulses of smell from the nasal cavity.
Malignant neoplasm of olfactory bulb

cc **C72.20** **Malignant neoplasm of unspecified olfactory nerve**

cc **C72.21** **Malignant neoplasm of <u>right</u> olfactory nerve**

cc **C72.22** **Malignant neoplasm of <u>left</u> olfactory nerve**

C
6
9
-
C
7
2

C72.3- **Malignant neoplasm of <u>optic nerve</u>** — The second cranial nerve that innervates the retina.

cc **C72.30** **Malignant neoplasm of unspecified optic nerve**

cc **C72.31** **Malignant neoplasm of <u>right</u> optic nerve**

cc **C72.32** **Malignant neoplasm of <u>left</u> optic nerve**

C72.4- **Malignant neoplasm of <u>acoustic nerve</u>** — The eighth cranial nerve that innervates the cochlea (the organ of sound input).

cc **C72.40** **Malignant neoplasm of unspecified acoustic nerve**

cc **C72.41** **Malignant neoplasm of <u>right</u> acoustic nerve**

cc **C72.42** **Malignant neoplasm of <u>left</u> acoustic nerve**

C72.5- **Malignant neoplasm of <u>other and unspecified cranial nerves</u>**

cc **C72.50** **Malignant neoplasm of unspecified cranial nerve**
Malignant neoplasm of cranial nerve NOS

cc **C72.59** **Malignant neoplasm of other cranial nerves**

cc **C72.9-** **Malignant neoplasm of central nervous system, unspecified**
Malignant neoplasm of unspecified site of central nervous system
Malignant neoplasm of nervous system NOS

Malignant neoplasms of thyroid and other endocrine glands (C73-C75)

C73 **Malignant neoplasm of <u>thyroid</u> gland** — Any new and abnormal growth of the thyroid gland in which tissue growth is uncontrolled and has the properties of anaplasia, invasion, and metastases.
Use additional code to identify any functional activity
ANATOMY OF THE THYROID — The thyroid gland is the bi-lobed endocrine gland of the front of the neck and joined by a narrow isthmus.
PHYSIOLOGY OF THE THYROID — The thyroid gland produces the hormones (thyroxine and triiodothyronine) which help to regulate the metabolic rate of the body.

THYROID GLAND

THYROID GLAND — ANTERIOR (DETAIL) VIEW

C74- **Malignant neoplasm of <u>adrenal</u> gland** — Any new and abnormal growth of the adrenal gland in which tissue growth is uncontrolled and has the properties of anaplasia, invasion, and metastases.
ANATOMY OF THE ADRENAL GLAND— The adrenal gland is the pyramid-shaped endocrine gland which sits upon the top of each kidney, and is highly vascular.
PHYSIOLOGY OF THE ADRENAL GLAND — The adrenal gland produces several important hormones, among them: Adrenalin, noradrenalin, aldosterone, cortisol, and some sex hormones.

C74.0- **Malignant neoplasm of <u>cortex</u> of adrenal gland** — The bulk of the gland covering the medulla that contains the steroid-producing cells.

cc **C74.00** **Malignant neoplasm of cortex of unspecified adrenal gland**

cc **C74.01** **Malignant neoplasm of cortex of <u>right</u> adrenal gland**

cc **C74.02** **Malignant neoplasm of cortex of <u>left</u> adrenal gland**

C74.1- **Malignant neoplasm of <u>medulla</u> of adrenal gland** — The inner portion of the gland that contains the epinephrine- (adrenaline) and norepinephrine- (noradrenaline) producing cells.

cc **C74.10** **Malignant neoplasm of medulla of unspecified adrenal gland**

cc **C74.11** **Malignant neoplasm of medulla of <u>right</u> adrenal gland**

cc **C74.12** **Malignant neoplasm of medulla of <u>left</u> adrenal gland**

C74.9- **Malignant neoplasm of unspecified part of adrenal gland**

cc **C74.90** **Malignant neoplasm of unspecified part of unspecified adrenal gland**

cc **C74.91** **Malignant neoplasm of unspecified part of <u>right</u> adrenal gland**

cc **C74.92** **Malignant neoplasm of unspecified part of <u>left</u> adrenal gland**

C75- **Malignant neoplasms of other <u>endocrine glands</u> and related structures** — Any new and abnormal growth of the other endocrine glands and related structures in which tissue growth is uncontrolled and has the properties of anaplasia, invasion, and metastases.
Excludes 1: malignant carcinoid tumors (C7A.0-)
malignant neoplasm of adrenal gland (C74.-)
malignant neoplasm of endocrine pancreas (C25.4)
malignant neoplasm of islets of Langerhans (C25.4)
malignant neoplasm of ovary (C56.-)
malignant neoplasm of testis (C62.-)
malignant neoplasm of thymus (C37)
malignant neoplasm of thyroid gland (C73)
malignant neuroendocrine tumors (C7A.-)

ANATOMY OF THE PARATHYROID GLANDS, PITUITARY GLAND, PINEAL GLAND, AND THE CAROTID AND AORTIC BODIES — The parathyroid glands are 4 small glands, 2 on the posterior surface of the thyroid lobes. The pituitary gland is the small endocrine gland located in the sella turcica of the sphenoid bone at the base of the cerebrum, and is about 0.4 inches (1 cm) in diameter. The pineal gland is the small endocrine gland located below the posterior base of the corpus callosum, and attached to the upper portion of the thalamus. The carotid bodies are small neurovascular structures at the carotid bifurcation. The aortic body is the small neurovascular structure located at the aortic arch.
PHYSIOLOGY OF THE PARATHYROID GLANDS, PITUITARY GLAND, PINEAL GLAND, AND THE CAROTID AND AORTIC BODIES — The parathyroid glands secretes one hormone, the parathyroid hormone which causes an increase in the blood calcium level and a decrease in the blood phosphate level. The pituitary gland functions as the central endocrine gland by producing hormones which stimulate many of the other endocrine glands, and has 2 lobes. The anterior lobe (adenohypophysis) produces the growth hormone, prolactin, thyroid-stimulating hormone, follicle-stimulating and luteinizing hormones, and adrenocorticotropic hormone. The posterior lobe (neurohypophysis) secretes the antidiuretic hormone, and oxytocin. The pineal gland produces the hormone melatonin. The aortic body monitors and regulates the reflex respiration.

ENDOCRINE GLANDS

cc **C75.0** **Malignant neoplasm of <u>parathyroid gland</u>** — The four (two on the posterior surface of each thyroid lobe) small endocrine glands which secrete the parathyroid hormone.

cc **C75.1** **Malignant neoplasm of <u>pituitary gland</u>** — The small endocrine gland at the base of the brain which produces many important hormones.

cc **C75.2** **Malignant neoplasm of <u>craniopharyngeal duct</u>** — The duct of embryonic development of the Rathke's pouch (the small colloid-filled cysts and clefts next to the pituitary gland left over from embryonic development).

cc **C75.3** **Malignant neoplasm of <u>pineal gland</u>** — The small endocrine gland below the posterior base of the corpus callosum, which produces the hormone melatonin.

cc **C75.4** **Malignant neoplasm of <u>carotid body</u>** — The small neurovascular structures at the bifurcation of the carotid arteries which monitor the oxygen content of the blood.

cc **C75.5** **Malignant neoplasm of <u>aortic body</u> and other paraganglia** — The aortic body is the small neurovascular structure at the aortic arch which monitors and regulates reflex respiration.

cc **C75.8** **Malignant neoplasm with <u>pluriglandular involvement</u>, unspecified**

cc **C75.9** **Malignant neoplasm of endocrine gland, unspecified**

Malignant neuroendocrine tumors (C7A)

C7A- **Malignant <u>neuroendocrine tumors</u>** — Any new and abnormal growth that arises from endocrine or neuroendocrine cells rather than from where the tumor is located in which the tissue growth is uncontrolled and has the properties of anaplasia, invasion, and metastases (also known as carcinoid tumors, especially when arising in the gastrointestinal tract).
Code also any associated multiple endocrine neoplasia [MEN] syndromes (E31.2-)
Use additional code to identify any associated endocrine syndrome, such as:
  Carcinoid syndrome (E34.0)
Excludes ❷: *malignant pancreatic islet cell tumors (C25.4)*
             Merkel cell carcinoma (C4A.-)

C7A.0- **Malignant <u>carcinoid</u> tumors**

cc **C7A.00** **Malignant carcinoid tumor of unspecified site**

C7A.01- **Malignant carcinoid tumors of the <u>small intestine</u>**

cc **C7A.010** **Malignant carcinoid tumor of the <u>duodenum</u>**

cc **C7A.011** **Malignant carcinoid tumor of the <u>jejunum</u>**

cc **C7A.012** **Malignant carcinoid tumor of the <u>ileum</u>**

cc **C7A.019** **Malignant carcinoid tumor of the small intestine, unspecified portion**

C7A.02- **Malignant carcinoid tumors of the <u>appendix, large intestine, and rectum</u>**

cc **C7A.020** **Malignant carcinoid tumor of the <u>appendix</u>**

cc **C7A.021** **Malignant carcinoid tumor of the <u>cecum</u>**

cc **C7A.022** **Malignant carcinoid tumor of the <u>ascending colon</u>**

cc **C7A.023** **Malignant carcinoid tumor of the <u>transverse colon</u>**

cc **C7A.024** **Malignant carcinoid tumor of the <u>descending colon</u>**

cc **C7A.025** **Malignant carcinoid tumor of the <u>sigmoid colon</u>**

cc **C7A.026** **Malignant carcinoid tumor of the <u>rectum</u>**

cc **C7A.029** **Malignant carcinoid tumor of the large intestine, unspecified portion**
  Malignant carcinoid tumor of the colon NOS

C7A.09- **Malignant <u>carcinoid</u> tumors of other sites**

cc **C7A.090** **Malignant carcinoid tumor of the <u>bronchus and lung</u>**

cc **C7A.091** **Malignant carcinoid tumor of the <u>thymus</u>**

cc **C7A.092** **Malignant carcinoid tumor of the <u>stomach</u>**

cc **C7A.093** **Malignant carcinoid tumor of the <u>kidney</u>**

cc **C7A.094** **Malignant carcinoid tumor of the foregut, unspecified**

cc **C7A.095** **Malignant carcinoid tumor of the midgut, unspecified**

cc **C7A.096** **Malignant carcinoid tumor of the hindgut, unspecified**

cc **C7A.098** **Malignant carcinoid tumors of other sites**

cc **C7A.1** **Malignant <u>poorly differentiated</u> neuroendocrine tumors**
  High grade neuroendocrine carcinoma, any site
  Malignant poorly differentiated neuroendocrine carcinoma, any site
  Malignant poorly differentiated neuroendocrine tumor NOS

cc **C7A.8** **Other malignant neuroendocrine tumors**

Secondary neuroendocrine tumors (C7B)

C7B- **<u>Secondary neuroendocrine</u> tumors** — The migration of malignant neuroendocrine cells from an original (primary) site to other sites in the body.
Use additional code to identify any functional activity

C7B.0- **<u>Secondary carcinoid</u> tumors**

C7B.00 **Secondary carcinoid tumors, unspecified site**

cc **C7B.01** **Secondary carcinoid tumors of <u>distant lymph nodes</u>**

cc **C7B.02** **Secondary carcinoid tumors of <u>liver</u>**

cc **C7B.03** **Secondary carcinoid tumors of <u>bone</u>**

cc **C7B.04** **Secondary carcinoid tumors of <u>peritoneum</u>**
  Mesentary metastasis of carcinoid tumor

cc **C7B.09** **Secondary carcinoid tumors of other sites**

C7B.1 **<u>Secondary Merkel cell</u> carcinoma** — The migration of malignant Merkel cell carcinoma cells from an original (primary) site to other sites in the body.
  Merkel cell carcinoma nodal presentation
  Merkel cell carcinoma visceral metastatic presentation

cc **C7B.8** **Other secondary neuroendocrine tumors**

Malignant neoplasms of ill-defined, other secondary and unspecified sites (C76-C80)

C76- **Malignant neoplasm of other and ill-defined sites** — Any new and abnormal growth of the other and ill-defined sites in which tissue growth is uncontrolled and has the properties of anaplasia, invasion, and metastases.
Excludes 1:   *malignant neoplasm of female genitourinary tract NOS (C57.9)*
             malignant neoplasm of male genitourinary tract NOS (C63.9)
             malignant neoplasm of lymphoid, hematopoietic and related tissue (C81-C96)
             malignant neoplasm of skin (C44.-)
             malignant neoplasm of unspecified site NOS (C80.1)

C76.0 **Malignant neoplasm of head, face and neck**
  Malignant neoplasm of cheek NOS
  Malignant neoplasm of nose NOS

C76.1 **Malignant neoplasm of thorax**
  Intrathoracic malignant neoplasm NOS
  Malignant neoplasm of axilla NOS
  Thoracic malignant neoplasm NOS

C76.2 **Malignant neoplasm of abdomen**

C76.3 **Malignant neoplasm of pelvis**
  Malignant neoplasm of groin NOS
  Malignant neoplasm of sites overlapping systems within the pelvis
  Rectovaginal (septum) malignant neoplasm
  Rectovesical (septum) malignant neoplasm

C76.4- **Malignant neoplasm of <u>upper limb</u>**

C76.40 **Malignant neoplasm of unspecified upper limb**

C76.41 **Malignant neoplasm of <u>right</u> upper limb**

C76.42 **Malignant neoplasm of <u>left</u> upper limb**

C76.5- **Malignant neoplasm of <u>lower limb</u>**

C76.50 **Malignant neoplasm of unspecified lower limb**

C76.51 **Malignant neoplasm of <u>right</u> lower limb**

C76.52 **Malignant neoplasm of <u>left</u> lower limb**

C76.8 **Malignant neoplasm of other specified ill-defined sites**
  Malignant neoplasm of overlapping ill-defined sites

C75 - C76

C77- **Secondary** and unspecified malignant neoplasm of <u>lymph nodes</u> —
The migration of malignant cells from an original (primary) site to any of the lymph nodes.

> Excludes 1: *malignant neoplasm of lymph nodes, specified as primary (C81-C86, C88, C96.-)*
> *mesentary metastasis of carcinoid tumor (C7B.04)*
> *secondary carcinoid tumors of distant lymph nodes (C7B.01)*

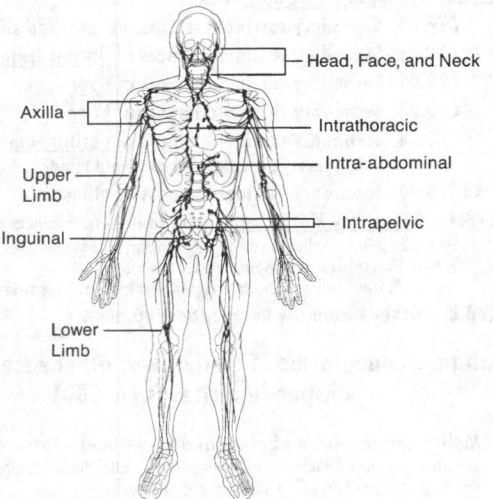

Head, Face, and Neck
Axilla
Intrathoracic
Upper Limb
Intra-abdominal
Inguinal
Intrapelvic
Lower Limb

LYMPH NODES

cc **C77.0** Secondary and unspecified malignant neoplasm of lymph nodes of <u>head, face and neck</u>
Secondary and unspecified malignant neoplasm of supraclavicular lymph nodes

cc **C77.1** Secondary and unspecified malignant neoplasm of <u>intrathoracic</u> lymph nodes

cc **C77.2** Secondary and unspecified malignant neoplasm of <u>intra-abdominal</u> lymph nodes

cc **C77.3** Secondary and unspecified malignant neoplasm of <u>axilla and upper limb</u> lymph nodes
Secondary and unspecified malignant neoplasm of pectoral lymph nodes

cc **C77.4** Secondary and unspecified malignant neoplasm of <u>inguinal and lower limb</u> lymph nodes

cc **C77.5** Secondary and unspecified malignant neoplasm of <u>intrapelvic</u> lymph nodes

cc **C77.8** Secondary and unspecified malignant neoplasm of lymph nodes of multiple regions

cc **C77.9** Secondary and unspecified malignant neoplasm of lymph node, unspecified

C78- **Secondary** malignant neoplasm of <u>respiratory</u> and <u>digestive</u> organs — The migration of malignant cells from an original (primary) site to the tissues of the respiratory and digestive organs.

> Excludes 1: *secondary carcinoid tumors of liver (C7B.02)*
> *secondary carcinoid tumors of peritoneum (C7B.04)*
> Excludes ❷: *lymph node metastases (C77.0)*

C78.0- Secondary malignant neoplasm of <u>lung</u>

cc **C78.00** Secondary malignant neoplasm of unspecified lung

cc **C78.01** Secondary malignant neoplasm of <u>right</u> lung

cc **C78.02** Secondary malignant neoplasm of <u>left</u> lung

cc **C78.1** Secondary malignant neoplasm of <u>mediastinum</u>

cc **C78.2** Secondary malignant neoplasm of <u>pleura</u>

C78.3- Secondary malignant neoplasm of other and unspecified respiratory organs

cc **C78.30** Secondary malignant neoplasm of unspecified respiratory organ

cc **C78.39** Secondary malignant neoplasm of other respiratory organs

cc **C78.4** Secondary malignant neoplasm of <u>small intestine</u>

cc **C78.5** Secondary malignant neoplasm of <u>large intestine and rectum</u>

cc **C78.6** Secondary malignant neoplasm of <u>retroperitoneum and peritoneum</u>

cc **C78.7** Secondary malignant neoplasm of <u>liver and intrahepatic bile duct</u>

C78.8- Secondary malignant neoplasm of other and unspecified digestive organs

cc **C78.80** Secondary malignant neoplasm of unspecified digestive organ

cc **C78.89** Secondary malignant neoplasm of other digestive organs
Code also exocrine pancreatic insufficiency (K86.81)

C79- **Secondary** malignant neoplasm of other and unspecified sites — The migration of malignant cells from an original (primary) site to other tissues.

> Excludes 1: *secondary carcinoid tumors (C7B.-)*
> *secondary neuroendocrine tumors (C7B.-)*
> Excludes ❷: *lymph node metastases (C77.0)*

C79.0- Secondary malignant neoplasm of <u>kidney and renal pelvis</u>

cc **C79.00** Secondary malignant neoplasm of unspecified kidney and renal pelvis

cc **C79.01** Secondary malignant neoplasm of <u>right</u> kidney and renal pelvis

cc **C79.02** Secondary malignant neoplasm of <u>left</u> kidney and renal pelvis

C79.1- Secondary malignant neoplasm of bladder and other and unspecified urinary organs

cc **C79.10** Secondary malignant neoplasm of unspecified urinary organs

cc **C79.11** Secondary malignant neoplasm of <u>bladder</u>

cc **C79.19** Secondary malignant neoplasm of <u>other urinary organs</u>

cc **C79.2** Secondary malignant neoplasm of <u>skin</u>

> Excludes 1: *secondary Merkel cell carcinoma (C7B.1)*

C79.3- Secondary malignant neoplasm of brain and cerebral meninges

cc **C79.31** Secondary malignant neoplasm of <u>brain</u>

cc **C79.32** Secondary malignant neoplasm of <u>cerebral meninges</u>

C79.4- Secondary malignant neoplasm of other and unspecified parts of nervous system

cc **C79.40** Secondary malignant neoplasm of unspecified part of nervous system

cc **C79.49** Secondary malignant neoplasm of other parts of nervous system

C79.5- Secondary malignant neoplasm of bone and bone marrow

> Excludes 1: *secondary carcinoid tumors of bone (C7B.03)*

cc **C79.51** Secondary malignant neoplasm of <u>bone</u>

cc **C79.52** Secondary malignant neoplasm of <u>bone marrow</u>

C79.6- Secondary malignant neoplasm of <u>ovary</u>

cc **C79.60** Secondary malignant neoplasm of unspecified ovary — [♀]

cc **C79.61** Secondary malignant neoplasm of <u>right</u> ovary — [♀]

cc **C79.62** Secondary malignant neoplasm of <u>left</u> ovary — [♀]

C79.7- Secondary malignant neoplasm of <u>adrenal gland</u>

cc **C79.70** Secondary malignant neoplasm of unspecified adrenal gland

cc **C79.71** Secondary malignant neoplasm of <u>right</u> adrenal gland

cc **C79.72** Secondary malignant neoplasm of <u>left</u> adrenal gland

C79.8- Secondary malignant neoplasm of other specified sites

cc **C79.81** Secondary malignant neoplasm of <u>breast</u>

cc **C79.82** Secondary malignant neoplasm of <u>genital organs</u>

cc **C79.89** Secondary malignant neoplasm of other specified sites

cc **C79.9** Secondary malignant neoplasm of unspecified site
Metastatic cancer NOS
Metastatic disease NOS

> Excludes 1: *carcinomatosis NOS (C80.0)*
> *generalized cancer NOS (C80.0)*
> *malignant (primary) neoplasm of unspecified site (C80.1)*

C 7 7 - C 7 9

C80- Malignant neoplasm <u>without specification of site</u> — Any new and abnormal growth of an unspecified site in which the tissue growth has the properties of anaplasia, invasion, and metastases.

> *Excludes 1:   malignant carcinoid tumor of unspecified site (C7A.00)*
> *malignant neoplasm of specified multiple sites — code to each site*

cc **C80.0 <u>Disseminated</u> malignant neoplasm, unspecified**
Carcinomatosis NOS
Generalized cancer, unspecified site (primary) (secondary)
Generalized malignancy, unspecified site (primary) (secondary)

C80.1 Malignant (primary) neoplasm, unspecified
Cancer NOS
Cancer unspecified site (primary)
Carcinoma unspecified site (primary)
Malignancy unspecified site (primary)

> *Excludes 1:   secondary malignant neoplasm of unspecified site (C79.9)*

cc **C80.2 Malignant neoplasm associated with <u>transplanted organ</u>** —
[Unacceptable PDX]
Code first complication of transplanted organ (T86.-)
Use additional code to identify the specific malignancy

Malignant neoplasms of lymphoid, hematopoietic and related tissue (C81-C96)

> *Excludes ❷: Kaposi's sarcoma of lymph nodes (C46.3)*
> *secondary and unspecified neoplasm of lymph nodes (C77.-)*
> *secondary neoplasm of bone marrow (C79.52)*
> *secondary neoplasm of spleen (C78.89)*

C81- <u>Hodgkin lymphoma</u> — A malignant lymphoma (a malignancy that starts in the white blood cells called lymphocytes) of the lymphatic system (lymph, lymph nodes, lymph vessels) characterized by the histologic identification of Reed-Stemberg cells.

> *Excludes 1:   personal history of Hodgkin lymphoma (Z85.71)*

C81.0- <u>Nodular lymphocyte predominant</u> Hodgkin lymphoma — A form marked by large cell variants of Reed-Stemberg cells called popcorn cells.

cc **C81.00 Nodular lymphocyte predominant Hodgkin lymphoma, unspecified site**

cc **C81.01 Nodular lymphocyte predominant Hodgkin lymphoma, lymph nodes of <u>head, face, and neck</u>**

cc **C81.02 Nodular lymphocyte predominant Hodgkin lymphoma, <u>intrathoracic</u> lymph nodes**

cc **C81.03 Nodular lymphocyte predominant Hodgkin lymphoma, <u>intra-abdominal</u> lymph nodes**

cc **C81.04 Nodular lymphocyte predominant Hodgkin lymphoma, lymph nodes of <u>axilla and upper limb</u>**

cc **C81.05 Nodular lymphocyte predominant Hodgkin lymphoma, lymph nodes of <u>inguinal region and lower limb</u>**

cc **C81.06 Nodular lymphocyte predominant Hodgkin lymphoma, <u>intrapelvic</u> lymph nodes**

cc **C81.07 Nodular lymphocyte predominant Hodgkin lymphoma, <u>spleen</u>**

cc **C81.08 Nodular lymphocyte predominant Hodgkin lymphoma, lymph nodes of <u>multiple sites</u>**

cc **C81.09 Nodular lymphocyte predominant Hodgkin lymphoma, <u>extranodal and solid organ sites</u>**

C81.1- <u>Nodular sclerosis</u> Hodgkin lymphoma — A form marked by large tumor nodules with extensive scar tissue and lacunar cells.
Nodular sclerosis classical Hodgkin lymphoma

cc **C81.10 Nodular sclerosis Hodgkin lymphoma, unspecified site**

cc **C81.11 Nodular sclerosis Hodgkin lymphoma, lymph nodes of <u>head, face, and neck</u>**

cc **C81.12 Nodular sclerosis Hodgkin lymphoma, <u>intrathoracic</u> lymph nodes**

cc **C81.13 Nodular sclerosis Hodgkin lymphoma, <u>intra-abdominal</u> lymph nodes**

cc **C81.14 Nodular sclerosis Hodgkin lymphoma, lymph nodes of <u>axilla and upper limb</u>**

cc **C81.15 Nodular sclerosis Hodgkin lymphoma, lymph nodes of <u>inguinal region and lower limb</u>**

cc **C81.16 Nodular sclerosis Hodgkin lymphoma, <u>intrapelvic</u> lymph nodes**

cc **C81.17 Nodular sclerosis Hodgkin lymphoma, <u>spleen</u>**

cc **C81.18 Nodular sclerosis Hodgkin lymphoma, lymph nodes of <u>multiple sites</u>**

cc **C81.19 Nodular sclerosis Hodgkin lymphoma, <u>extranodal and solid organ sites</u>**

C81.2- <u>Mixed cellularity</u> Hodgkin lymphoma — A form marked by many Reed-Stemberg cells and the presence of several other types of cells.
Mixed cellularity classical Hodgkin lymphoma

cc **C81.20 Mixed cellularity Hodgkin lymphoma, unspecified site**

cc **C81.21 Mixed cellularity Hodgkin lymphoma, lymph nodes of <u>head, face, and neck</u>**

cc **C81.22 Mixed cellularity Hodgkin lymphoma, <u>intrathoracic</u> lymph nodes**

cc **C81.23 Mixed cellularity Hodgkin lymphoma, <u>intra-abdominal</u> lymph nodes**

cc **C81.24 Mixed cellularity Hodgkin lymphoma, lymph nodes of <u>axilla and upper limb</u>**

cc **C81.25 Mixed cellularity Hodgkin lymphoma, lymph nodes of <u>inguinal region and lower limb</u>**

cc **C81.26 Mixed cellularity Hodgkin lymphoma, <u>intrapelvic</u> lymph nodes**

cc **C81.27 Mixed cellularity Hodgkin lymphoma, <u>spleen</u>**

cc **C81.28 Mixed cellularity Hodgkin lymphoma, lymph nodes of <u>multiple sites</u>**

cc **C81.29 Mixed cellularity Hodgkin lymphoma, <u>extranodal and solid organ sites</u>**

C81.3- <u>Lymphocyte depleted</u> Hodgkin lymphoma — A form marked by an abundance of Reed-Stemberg cells and few normal cells.
Lymphocyte depleted classical Hodgkin lymphoma

cc **C81.30 Lymphocyte depleted Hodgkin lymphoma, unspecified site**

cc **C81.31 Lymphocyte depleted Hodgkin lymphoma, lymph nodes of <u>head, face, and neck</u>**

cc **C81.32 Lymphocyte depleted Hodgkin lymphoma, <u>intrathoracic</u> lymph nodes**

cc **C81.33 Lymphocyte depleted Hodgkin lymphoma, <u>intra-abdominal</u> lymph nodes**

cc **C81.34 Lymphocyte depleted Hodgkin lymphoma, lymph nodes of <u>axilla and upper limb</u>**

cc **C81.35 Lymphocyte depleted Hodgkin lymphoma, lymph nodes of <u>inguinal region and lower limb</u>**

cc **C81.36 Lymphocyte depleted Hodgkin lymphoma, <u>intrapelvic</u> lymph nodes**

cc **C81.37 Lymphocyte depleted Hodgkin lymphoma, <u>spleen</u>**

cc **C81.38 Lymphocyte depleted Hodgkin lymphoma, lymph nodes of <u>multiple sites</u>**

cc **C81.39 Lymphocyte depleted Hodgkin lymphoma, <u>extranodal and solid organ sites</u>**

C81.4- <u>Lymphocyte-rich</u> Hodgkin lymphoma — A form marked by an abundance of normal-appearing lymphocytes and classic Reed-Stemberg cells.

> *Excludes 1:   nodular lymphocyte predominant Hodgkin lymphoma (C81.0-)*

Lymphocyte-rich classical Hodgkin lymphoma

cc **C81.40 Lymphocyte-rich Hodgkin lymphoma, unspecified site**

cc **C81.41 Lymphocyte-rich Hodgkin lymphoma, lymph nodes of <u>head, face, and neck</u>**

cc **C81.42 Lymphocyte-rich Hodgkin lymphoma, <u>intrathoracic</u> lymph nodes**

cc **C81.43 Lymphocyte-rich Hodgkin lymphoma, <u>intra-abdominal</u> lymph nodes**

cc **C81.44 Lymphocyte-rich Hodgkin lymphoma, lymph nodes of <u>axilla and upper limb</u>**

cc **C81.45 Lymphocyte-rich Hodgkin lymphoma, lymph nodes of <u>inguinal region and lower limb</u>**

cc **C81.46 Lymphocyte-rich Hodgkin lymphoma, <u>intrapelvic</u> lymph nodes**

cc **C81.47 Lymphocyte-rich Hodgkin lymphoma, <u>spleen</u>**

cc **C81.48 Lymphocyte-rich Hodgkin lymphoma, lymph nodes of <u>multiple sites</u>**

cc **C81.49 Lymphocyte-rich Hodgkin lymphoma, <u>extranodal and solid organ sites</u>**

C80
-
C81

C81.7-   Other Hodgkin lymphoma
          Classical Hodgkin lymphoma NOS
          Other classical Hodgkin lymphoma
    cc C81.70   Other Hodgkin lymphoma, unspecified site
    cc C81.71   Other Hodgkin lymphoma, lymph nodes of head, face, and neck
    cc C81.72   Other Hodgkin lymphoma, intrathoracic lymph nodes
    cc C81.73   Other Hodgkin lymphoma, intra-abdominal lymph nodes
    cc C81.74   Other Hodgkin lymphoma, lymph nodes of axilla and upper limb
    cc C81.75   Other Hodgkin lymphoma, lymph nodes of inguinal region and lower limb
    cc C81.76   Other Hodgkin lymphoma, intrapelvic lymph nodes
    cc C81.77   Other Hodgkin lymphoma, spleen
    cc C81.78   Other Hodgkin lymphoma, lymph nodes of multiple sites
    cc C81.79   Other Hodgkin lymphoma, extranodal and solid organ sites

C81.9-   Hodgkin lymphoma, unspecified
    cc C81.90   Hodgkin lymphoma, unspecified, unspecified site
    cc C81.91   Hodgkin lymphoma, unspecified, lymph nodes of head, face, and neck
    cc C81.92   Hodgkin lymphoma, unspecified, intrathoracic lymph nodes
    cc C81.93   Hodgkin lymphoma, unspecified, intra-abdominal lymph nodes
    cc C81.94   Hodgkin lymphoma, unspecified, lymph nodes of axilla and upper limb
    cc C81.95   Hodgkin lymphoma, unspecified, lymph nodes of inguinal region and lower limb
    cc C81.96   Hodgkin lymphoma, unspecified, intrapelvic lymph nodes
    cc C81.97   Hodgkin lymphoma, unspecified, spleen
    cc C81.98   Hodgkin lymphoma, unspecified, lymph nodes of multiple sites
    cc C81.99   Hodgkin lymphoma, unspecified, extranodal and solid organ sites

C82-   Follicular lymphoma — A (non-Hodgkin lymphoma) lymphoma characterized by the histologic identification of certain follicle center B-cell lymphocytes, called centrocytes (small cells) and centroblasts (large cells). Grading of follicular lymphoma is based on various morphological criteria, most commonly by the number of abnormal cells detected under a high-power field microscope.
    Includes: Follicular lymphoma with or without diffuse areas
    Excludes 1:   mature T/NK-cell lymphomas (C84.-)
                   personal history of non-Hodgkin lymphoma (Z85.72)

C82.0-   Follicular lymphoma grade I
    cc C82.00   Follicular lymphoma grade I, unspecified site
    cc C82.01   Follicular lymphoma grade I, lymph nodes of head, face, and neck
    cc C82.02   Follicular lymphoma grade I, intrathoracic lymph nodes
    cc C82.03   Follicular lymphoma grade I, intra-abdominal lymph nodes
    cc C82.04   Follicular lymphoma grade I, lymph nodes of axilla and upper limb
    cc C82.05   Follicular lymphoma grade I, lymph nodes of inguinal region and lower limb
    cc C82.06   Follicular lymphoma grade I, intrapelvic lymph nodes
    cc C82.07   Follicular lymphoma grade I, spleen
    cc C82.08   Follicular lymphoma grade I, lymph nodes of multiple sites
    cc C82.09   Follicular lymphoma grade I, extranodal and solid organ sites

C82.1-   Follicular lymphoma grade II
    cc C82.10   Follicular lymphoma grade II, unspecified site
    cc C82.11   Follicular lymphoma grade II, lymph nodes of head, face, and neck
    cc C82.12   Follicular lymphoma grade II, intrathoracic lymph nodes
    cc C82.13   Follicular lymphoma grade II, intra-abdominal lymph nodes
    cc C82.14   Follicular lymphoma grade II, lymph nodes of axilla and upper limb

    cc C82.15   Follicular lymphoma grade II, lymph nodes of inguinal region and lower limb
    cc C82.16   Follicular lymphoma grade II, intrapelvic lymph nodes
    cc C82.17   Follicular lymphoma grade II, spleen
    cc C82.18   Follicular lymphoma grade II, lymph nodes of multiple sites
    cc C82.19   Follicular lymphoma grade II, extranodal and solid organ sites

C82.2-   Follicular lymphoma grade III, unspecified
    cc C82.20   Follicular lymphoma grade III, unspecified, unspecified site
    cc C82.21   Follicular lymphoma grade III, unspecified, lymph nodes of head, face, and neck
    cc C82.22   Follicular lymphoma grade III, unspecified, intrathoracic lymph nodes
    cc C82.23   Follicular lymphoma grade III, unspecified, intra-abdominal lymph nodes
    cc C82.24   Follicular lymphoma grade III, unspecified, lymph nodes of axilla and upper limb
    cc C82.25   Follicular lymphoma grade III, unspecified, lymph nodes of inguinal region and lower limb
    cc C82.26   Follicular lymphoma grade III, unspecified, intrapelvic lymph nodes
    cc C82.27   Follicular lymphoma grade III, unspecified, spleen
    cc C82.28   Follicular lymphoma grade III, unspecified, lymph nodes of multiple sites
    cc C82.29   Follicular lymphoma grade III, unspecified, extranodal and solid organ sites

C82.3-   Follicular lymphoma grade IIIa
    cc C82.30   Follicular lymphoma grade IIIa, unspecified site
    cc C82.31   Follicular lymphoma grade IIIa, lymph nodes of head, face, and neck
    cc C82.32   Follicular lymphoma grade IIIa, intrathoracic lymph nodes
    cc C82.33   Follicular lymphoma grade IIIa, intra-abdominal lymph nodes
    cc C82.34   Follicular lymphoma grade IIIa, lymph nodes of axilla and upper limb
    cc C82.35   Follicular lymphoma grade IIIa, lymph nodes of inguinal region and lower limb
    cc C82.36   Follicular lymphoma grade IIIa, intrapelvic lymph nodes
    cc C82.37   Follicular lymphoma grade IIIa, spleen
    cc C82.38   Follicular lymphoma grade IIIa, lymph nodes of multiple sites
    cc C82.39   Follicular lymphoma grade IIIa, extranodal and solid organ sites

C82.4-   Follicular lymphoma grade IIIb
    cc C82.40   Follicular lymphoma grade IIIb, unspecified site
    cc C82.41   Follicular lymphoma grade IIIb, lymph nodes of head, face, and neck
    cc C82.42   Follicular lymphoma grade IIIb, intrathoracic lymph nodes
    cc C82.43   Follicular lymphoma grade IIIb, intra-abdominal lymph nodes
    cc C82.44   Follicular lymphoma grade IIIb, lymph nodes of axilla and upper limb
    cc C82.45   Follicular lymphoma grade IIIb, lymph nodes of inguinal region and lower limb
    cc C82.46   Follicular lymphoma grade IIIb, intrapelvic lymph nodes
    cc C82.47   Follicular lymphoma grade IIIb, spleen
    cc C82.48   Follicular lymphoma grade IIIb, lymph nodes of multiple sites
    cc C82.49   Follicular lymphoma grade IIIb, extranodal and solid organ sites

C82.5-   Diffuse follicle center lymphoma
    cc C82.50   Diffuse follicle center lymphoma, unspecified site
    cc C82.51   Diffuse follicle center lymphoma, lymph nodes of head, face, and neck

C
8
1
-
C
8
2

cc **C82.52** Diffuse follicle center lymphoma, <u>intrathoracic</u> lymph nodes

cc **C82.53** Diffuse follicle center lymphoma, <u>intra-abdominal</u> lymph nodes

cc **C82.54** Diffuse follicle center lymphoma, lymph nodes of <u>axilla and upper limb</u>

cc **C82.55** Diffuse follicle center lymphoma, lymph nodes of <u>inguinal region and lower limb</u>

cc **C82.56** Diffuse follicle center lymphoma, <u>intrapelvic</u> lymph nodes

cc **C82.57** Diffuse follicle center lymphoma, <u>spleen</u>

cc **C82.58** Diffuse follicle center lymphoma, lymph nodes of <u>multiple sites</u>

cc **C82.59** Diffuse follicle center lymphoma, <u>extranodal and solid organ sites</u>

C82.6- <u>Cutaneous follicle center</u> lymphoma

cc **C82.60** Cutaneous follicle center lymphoma, unspecified site

cc **C82.61** Cutaneous follicle center lymphoma, lymph nodes of <u>head, face, and neck</u>

cc **C82.62** Cutaneous follicle center lymphoma, <u>intrathoracic</u> lymph nodes

cc **C82.63** Cutaneous follicle center lymphoma, <u>intra-abdominal</u> lymph nodes

cc **C82.64** Cutaneous follicle center lymphoma, lymph nodes of <u>axilla and upper limb</u>

cc **C82.65** Cutaneous follicle center lymphoma, lymph nodes of <u>inguinal region and lower limb</u>

cc **C82.66** Cutaneous follicle center lymphoma, intrapelvic lymph nodes

cc **C82.67** Cutaneous follicle center lymphoma, <u>spleen</u>

cc **C82.68** Cutaneous follicle center lymphoma, lymph nodes of <u>multiple sites</u>

cc **C82.69** Cutaneous follicle center lymphoma, <u>extranodal and solid organ sites</u>

C82.8- <u>Other types</u> of follicular lymphoma

cc **C82.80** Other types of follicular lymphoma, unspecified site

cc **C82.81** Other types of follicular lymphoma, lymph nodes of <u>head, face, and neck</u>

cc **C82.82** Other types of follicular lymphoma, <u>intrathoracic</u> lymph nodes

cc **C82.83** Other types of follicular lymphoma, <u>intra-abdominal</u> lymph nodes

cc **C82.84** Other types of follicular lymphoma, lymph nodes of <u>axilla and upper limb</u>

cc **C82.85** Other types of follicular lymphoma, lymph nodes of <u>inguinal region and lower limb</u>

cc **C82.86** Other types of follicular lymphoma, <u>intrapelvic</u> lymph nodes

cc **C82.87** Other types of follicular lymphoma, <u>spleen</u>

cc **C82.88** Other types of follicular lymphoma, lymph nodes of <u>multiple sites</u>

cc **C82.89** Other types of follicular lymphoma, <u>extranodal and solid organ sites</u>

C82.9- Follicular lymphoma, <u>unspecified</u>

cc **C82.90** Follicular lymphoma, unspecified, unspecified site

cc **C82.91** Follicular lymphoma, unspecified, lymph nodes of <u>head, face, and neck</u>

cc **C82.92** Follicular lymphoma, unspecified, <u>intrathoracic</u> lymph nodes

cc **C82.93** Follicular lymphoma, unspecified, <u>intra-abdominal</u> lymph nodes

cc **C82.94** Follicular lymphoma, unspecified, lymph nodes of <u>axilla and upper limb</u>

cc **C82.95** Follicular lymphoma, unspecified, lymph nodes of <u>inguinal region and lower limb</u>

cc **C82.96** Follicular lymphoma, unspecified, <u>intrapelvic</u> lymph nodes

cc **C82.97** Follicular lymphoma, unspecified, <u>spleen</u>

cc **C82.98** Follicular lymphoma, unspecified, lymph nodes of <u>multiple sites</u>

cc **C82.99** Follicular lymphoma, unspecified, <u>extranodal and solid organ sites</u>

C83- <u>Non-follicular</u> lymphoma — A (non-Hodgkin lymphoma) lymphoma characterized by the histologic identification of malignant B-cell lymphocytes.

Excludes 1: *personal history of non-Hodgkin lymphoma (Z85.72)*

C83.0- <u>Small cell</u> B-cell lymphoma
Lymphoplasmacytic lymphoma
Nodal marginal zone lymphoma
Non-leukemic variant of B-CLL
Splenic marginal zone lymphoma

Excludes 1: *chronic lymphocytic leukemia (C91.1)*
mature T/NK-cell lymphomas (C84.-)
Waldenström macroglobulinemia (C88.0)

cc **C83.00** Small cell B-cell lymphoma, unspecified site

cc **C83.01** Small cell B-cell lymphoma, lymph nodes of <u>head, face, and neck</u>

cc **C83.02** Small cell B-cell lymphoma, <u>intrathoracic</u> lymph nodes

cc **C83.03** Small cell B-cell lymphoma, <u>intra-abdominal</u> lymph nodes

cc **C83.04** Small cell B-cell lymphoma, lymph nodes of <u>axilla and upper limb</u>

cc **C83.05** Small cell B-cell lymphoma, lymph nodes of <u>inguinal region and lower limb</u>

cc **C83.06** Small cell B-cell lymphoma, intrapelvic lymph nodes

cc **C83.07** Small cell B-cell lymphoma, <u>spleen</u>

cc **C83.08** Small cell B-cell lymphoma, lymph nodes of <u>multiple sites</u>

cc **C83.09** Small cell B-cell lymphoma, <u>extranodal and solid organ sites</u>

C83.1- <u>Mantle cell</u> lymphoma
Centrocytic lymphoma
Malignant lymphomatous polyposis

cc **C83.10** Mantle cell lymphoma, unspecified site

cc **C83.11** Mantle cell lymphoma, lymph nodes of <u>head, face, and neck</u>

cc **C83.12** Mantle cell lymphoma, <u>intrathoracic</u> lymph nodes

cc **C83.13** Mantle cell lymphoma, <u>intra-abdominal</u> lymph nodes

cc **C83.14** Mantle cell lymphoma, lymph nodes of <u>axilla and upper limb</u>

cc **C83.15** Mantle cell lymphoma, lymph nodes of <u>inguinal region and lower limb</u>

cc **C83.16** Mantle cell lymphoma, <u>intrapelvic</u> lymph nodes

cc **C83.17** Mantle cell lymphoma, <u>spleen</u>

cc **C83.18** Mantle cell lymphoma, lymph nodes of <u>multiple sites</u>

cc **C83.19** Mantle cell lymphoma, <u>extranodal and solid organ sites</u>

C83.3- <u>Diffuse large B-cell</u> lymphoma
Anaplastic diffuse large B-cell lymphoma
CD30-positive diffuse large B-cell lymphoma
Centroblastic diffuse large B-cell lymphoma
Diffuse large B-cell lymphoma, subtype not specified
Immunoblastic diffuse large B-cell lymphoma
Plasmablastic diffuse large B-cell lymphoma
T-cell rich diffuse large B-cell lymphoma

Excludes 1: *mediastinal (thymic) large B-cell lymphoma (C85.2-)*
mature T/NK-cell lymphomas (C84.-)

cc **C83.30** Diffuse large B-cell lymphoma, unspecified site

cc **C83.31** Diffuse large B-cell lymphoma, lymph nodes of <u>head, face, and neck</u>

cc **C83.32** Diffuse large B-cell lymphoma, <u>intrathoracic</u> lymph nodes

cc **C83.33** Diffuse large B-cell lymphoma, <u>intra-abdominal</u> lymph nodes

cc **C83.34** Diffuse large B-cell lymphoma, lymph nodes of <u>axilla and upper limb</u>

cc **C83.35** Diffuse large B-cell lymphoma, lymph nodes of <u>inguinal region and lower limb</u>

cc **C83.36** Diffuse large B-cell lymphoma, <u>intrapelvic</u> lymph nodes

cc **C83.37** Diffuse large B-cell lymphoma, <u>spleen</u>

cc **C83.38** Diffuse large B-cell lymphoma, lymph nodes of <u>multiple sites</u>

C 8 2 - C 8 3

C83 - C84

cc **C83.39** Diffuse large B-cell lymphoma, <u>extranodal and solid organ sites</u>

C83.5- <u>Lymphoblastic (diffuse) lymphoma</u>
B-precursor lymphoma
Lymphoblastic B-cell lymphoma
Lymphoblastic lymphoma NOS
Lymphoblastic T-cell lymphoma
T-precursor lymphoma

cc **C83.50** Lymphoblastic (diffuse) lymphoma, unspecified site

cc **C83.51** Lymphoblastic (diffuse) lymphoma, lymph nodes of <u>head, face, and neck</u>

cc **C83.52** Lymphoblastic (diffuse) lymphoma, <u>intrathoracic</u> lymph nodes

cc **C83.53** Lymphoblastic (diffuse) lymphoma, <u>intra-abdominal</u> lymph nodes

cc **C83.54** Lymphoblastic (diffuse) lymphoma, lymph nodes of <u>axilla and upper limb</u>

cc **C83.55** Lymphoblastic (diffuse) lymphoma, lymph nodes of <u>inguinal region and lower limb</u>

cc **C83.56** Lymphoblastic (diffuse) lymphoma, <u>intrapelvic</u> lymph nodes

cc **C83.57** Lymphoblastic (diffuse) lymphoma, <u>spleen</u>

cc **C83.58** Lymphoblastic (diffuse) lymphoma, lymph nodes of <u>multiple sites</u>

cc **C83.59** Lymphoblastic (diffuse) lymphoma, <u>extranodal and solid organ sites</u>

C83.7- <u>Burkitt</u> lymphoma
Atypical Burkitt lymphoma
Burkitt-like lymphoma
Excludes 1:   mature B-cell leukemia Burkitt type (C91.A-)

cc **C83.70** Burkitt lymphoma, unspecified site

cc **C83.71** Burkitt lymphoma, lymph nodes of <u>head, face, and neck</u>

cc **C83.72** Burkitt lymphoma, <u>intrathoracic</u> lymph nodes

cc **C83.73** Burkitt lymphoma, <u>intra-abdominal</u> lymph nodes

cc **C83.74** Burkitt lymphoma, lymph nodes of <u>axilla and upper limb</u>

cc **C83.75** Burkitt lymphoma, lymph nodes of <u>inguinal region and lower limb</u>

cc **C83.76** Burkitt lymphoma, <u>intrapelvic</u> lymph nodes

cc **C83.77** Burkitt lymphoma, <u>spleen</u>

cc **C83.78** Burkitt lymphoma, lymph nodes of <u>multiple sites</u>

cc **C83.79** Burkitt lymphoma, <u>extranodal and solid organ sites</u>

C83.8- <u>Other non-follicular</u> lymphoma
Intravascular large B-cell lymphoma
Lymphoid granulomatosis
Primary effusion B-cell lymphoma
Excludes 1:   mediastinal (thymic) large B-cell lymphoma (C85.2-)
T-cell rich B-cell lymphoma (C83.3-)

cc **C83.80** Other non-follicular lymphoma, unspecified site

cc **C83.81** Other non-follicular lymphoma, lymph nodes of <u>head, face, and neck</u>

cc **C83.82** Other non-follicular lymphoma, <u>intrathoracic</u> lymph nodes

cc **C83.83** Other non-follicular lymphoma, <u>intra-abdominal</u> lymph nodes

cc **C83.84** Other non-follicular lymphoma, lymph nodes of <u>axilla and upper limb</u>

cc **C83.85** Other non-follicular lymphoma, lymph nodes of <u>inguinal region and lower limb</u>

cc **C83.86** Other non-follicular lymphoma, <u>intrapelvic</u> lymph nodes

cc **C83.87** Other non-follicular lymphoma, <u>spleen</u>

cc **C83.88** Other non-follicular lymphoma, lymph nodes of <u>multiple sites</u>

cc **C83.89** Other non-follicular lymphoma, <u>extranodal and solid organ sites</u>

C83.9- Non-follicular (diffuse) lymphoma, <u>unspecified</u>

cc **C83.90** Non-follicular (diffuse) lymphoma, unspecified, unspecified site

cc **C83.91** Non-follicular (diffuse) lymphoma, unspecified, lymph nodes of <u>head, face, and neck</u>

cc **C83.92** Non-follicular (diffuse) lymphoma, unspecified, <u>intrathoracic</u> lymph nodes

cc **C83.93** Non-follicular (diffuse) lymphoma, unspecified, <u>intra-abdominal</u> lymph nodes

cc **C83.94** Non-follicular (diffuse) lymphoma, unspecified, lymph nodes of <u>axilla and upper limb</u>

cc **C83.95** Non-follicular (diffuse) lymphoma, unspecified, lymph nodes of <u>inguinal region and lower limb</u>

cc **C83.96** Non-follicular (diffuse) lymphoma, unspecified, <u>intrapelvic</u> lymph nodes

cc **C83.97** Non-follicular (diffuse) lymphoma, unspecified, <u>spleen</u>

cc **C83.98** Non-follicular (diffuse) lymphoma, unspecified, lymph nodes of <u>multiple sites</u>

cc **C83.99** Non-follicular (diffuse) lymphoma, unspecified, <u>extranodal and solid organ sites</u>

C84- <u>Mature T/NK-cell</u> lymphomas — A (non-Hodgkin lymphoma) lymphoma characterized by the histologic identification of malignant T- and NK-cell lymphocytes.
Excludes 1:   personal history of non-Hodgkin lymphoma (Z85.72)

C84.0- <u>Mycosis fungoides</u>
Excludes 1:   peripheral T-cell lymphoma, not classified (C84.4-)

cc **C84.00** Mycosis fungoides, unspecified site

cc **C84.01** Mycosis fungoides, lymph nodes of <u>head, face, and neck</u>

cc **C84.02** Mycosis fungoides, <u>intrathoracic</u> lymph nodes

cc **C84.03** Mycosis fungoides, <u>intra-abdominal</u> lymph nodes

cc **C84.04** Mycosis fungoides, lymph nodes of <u>axilla and upper limb</u>

cc **C84.05** Mycosis fungoides, lymph nodes of <u>inguinal region and lower limb</u>

cc **C84.06** Mycosis fungoides, <u>intrapelvic</u> lymph nodes

cc **C84.07** Mycosis fungoides, <u>spleen</u>

cc **C84.08** Mycosis fungoides, lymph nodes of <u>multiple sites</u>

cc **C84.09** Mycosis fungoides, <u>extranodal and solid organ sites</u>

C84.1- <u>Sézary disease</u>

cc **C84.10** Sézary disease, unspecified site

cc **C84.11** Sézary disease, lymph nodes of <u>head, face, and neck</u>

cc **C84.12** Sézary disease, <u>intrathoracic</u> lymph nodes

cc **C84.13** Sézary disease, <u>intra-abdominal</u> lymph nodes

cc **C84.14** Sézary disease, lymph nodes of <u>axilla and upper limb</u>

cc **C84.15** Sézary disease, lymph nodes of <u>inguinal region and lower limb</u>

cc **C84.16** Sézary disease, <u>intrapelvic</u> lymph nodes

cc **C84.17** Sézary disease, <u>spleen</u>

cc **C84.18** Sézary disease, lymph nodes of <u>multiple sites</u>

cc **C84.19** Sézary disease, <u>extranodal and solid organ sites</u>

C84.4- <u>Peripheral T-cell</u> lymphoma, not classified
Lennert's lymphoma
Lymphoepithelioid lymphoma
Mature T-cell lymphoma, not elsewhere classified

cc **C84.40** Peripheral T-cell lymphoma, not classified, unspecified site

cc **C84.41** Peripheral T-cell lymphoma, not classified, lymph nodes of <u>head, face, and neck</u>

cc **C84.42** Peripheral T-cell lymphoma, not classified, <u>intrathoracic</u> lymph nodes

cc **C84.43** Peripheral T-cell lymphoma, not classified, <u>intra-abdominal</u> lymph nodes

cc **C84.44** Peripheral T-cell lymphoma, not classified, lymph nodes of <u>axilla and upper limb</u>

cc **C84.45** Peripheral T-cell lymphoma, not classified, lymph nodes of <u>inguinal region and lower limb</u>

cc **C84.46** Peripheral T-cell lymphoma, not classified, <u>intrapelvic</u> lymph nodes

cc **C84.47** Peripheral T-cell lymphoma, not classified, <u>spleen</u>

cc **C84.48** Peripheral T-cell lymphoma, not classified, lymph nodes of <u>multiple sites</u>

cc **C84.49** Peripheral T-cell lymphoma, not classified, <u>extranodal and solid organ sites</u>

C84.6- <u>Anaplastic large cell</u> lymphoma, ALK-<u>positive</u>
Anaplastic large cell lymphoma, CD30-positive

cc **C84.60** Anaplastic large cell lymphoma, ALK-positive, **unspecified site**

cc **C84.61** Anaplastic large cell lymphoma, ALK-positive, lymph nodes of <u>head, face, and neck</u>

cc **C84.62** Anaplastic large cell lymphoma, ALK-positive, <u>intrathoracic</u> lymph nodes

cc **C84.63** Anaplastic large cell lymphoma, ALK-positive, <u>intra-abdominal</u> lymph nodes

cc **C84.64** Anaplastic large cell lymphoma, ALK-positive, lymph nodes of <u>axilla and upper limb</u>

cc **C84.65** Anaplastic large cell lymphoma, ALK-positive, lymph nodes of <u>inguinal region and lower limb</u>

cc **C84.66** Anaplastic large cell lymphoma, ALK-positive, <u>intrapelvic</u> lymph nodes

cc **C84.67** Anaplastic large cell lymphoma, ALK-positive, <u>spleen</u>

cc **C84.68** Anaplastic large cell lymphoma, ALK-positive, lymph nodes of <u>multiple sites</u>

cc **C84.69** Anaplastic large cell lymphoma, ALK-positive, <u>extranodal and solid organ sites</u>

C84.7- <u>Anaplastic large cell</u> lymphoma, ALK-<u>negative</u>
Excludes 1: *primary cutaneous CD30-positive T-cell proliferations (C86.6-)*

cc **C84.70** Anaplastic large cell lymphoma, ALK-negative, **unspecified site**

cc **C84.71** Anaplastic large cell lymphoma, ALK-negative, lymph nodes of <u>head, face, and neck</u>

cc **C84.72** Anaplastic large cell lymphoma, ALK-negative, <u>intrathoracic</u> lymph nodes

cc **C84.73** Anaplastic large cell lymphoma, ALK-negative, <u>intra-abdominal</u> lymph nodes

cc **C84.74** Anaplastic large cell lymphoma, ALK-negative, lymph nodes of <u>axilla and upper limb</u>

cc **C84.75** Anaplastic large cell lymphoma, ALK-negative, lymph nodes of <u>inguinal region and lower limb</u>

cc **C84.76** Anaplastic large cell lymphoma, ALK-negative, <u>intrapelvic</u> lymph nodes

cc **C84.77** Anaplastic large cell lymphoma, ALK-negative, <u>spleen</u>

cc **C84.78** Anaplastic large cell lymphoma, ALK-negative, lymph nodes of <u>multiple sites</u>

cc **C84.79** Anaplastic large cell lymphoma, ALK-negative, <u>extranodal and solid organ sites</u>

C84.A- <u>Cutaneous T-cell</u> lymphoma, unspecified

cc **C84.A0** Cutaneous T-cell lymphoma, unspecified, unspecified site

cc **C84.A1** Cutaneous T-cell lymphoma, unspecified lymph nodes of <u>head, face, and neck</u>

cc **C84.A2** Cutaneous T-cell lymphoma, unspecified, <u>intrathoracic</u> lymph nodes

cc **C84.A3** Cutaneous T-cell lymphoma, unspecified, <u>intra-abdominal</u> lymph nodes

cc **C84.A4** Cutaneous T-cell lymphoma, unspecified, lymph nodes of <u>axilla and upper limb</u>

cc **C84.A5** Cutaneous T-cell lymphoma, unspecified, lymph nodes of <u>inguinal region and lower limb</u>

cc **C84.A6** Cutaneous T-cell lymphoma, unspecified, <u>intrapelvic</u> lymph nodes

cc **C84.A7** Cutaneous T-cell lymphoma, unspecified, <u>spleen</u>

cc **C84.A8** Cutaneous T-cell lymphoma, unspecified, lymph nodes of <u>multiple sites</u>

cc **C84.A9** Cutaneous T-cell lymphoma, unspecified, <u>extranodal and solid organ sites</u>

C84.Z- <u>Other mature T/NK-cell</u> lymphomas
Note: If T-cell lineage or involvement is mentioned in conjunction with a specific lymphoma, code to the more specific description.
Excludes 1: *angioimmunoblastic T-cell lymphoma (C86.5)*
blastic NK-cell lymphoma (C86.4)
enteropathy-type T-cell lymphoma (C86.2)
extranodal NK-cell lymphoma, nasal type (C86.0)
hepatosplenic T-cell lymphoma (C86.1)
primary cutaneous CD30-positive T-cell proliferations (C86.6)
subcutaneous panniculitis-like T-cell lymphoma (C86.3)
T-cell leukemia (C91.1-)

cc **C84.Z0** Other mature T/NK-cell lymphomas, unspecified site

cc **C84.Z1** Other mature T/NK-cell lymphomas, lymph nodes of <u>head, face, and neck</u>

cc **C84.Z2** Other mature T/NK-cell lymphomas, <u>intrathoracic</u> lymph nodes

cc **C84.Z3** Other mature T/NK-cell lymphomas, <u>intra-abdominal</u> lymph nodes

cc **C84.Z4** Other mature T/NK-cell lymphomas, lymph nodes of <u>axilla and upper limb</u>

cc **C84.Z5** Other mature T/NK-cell lymphomas, lymph nodes of <u>inguinal region and lower limb</u>

cc **C84.Z6** Other mature T/NK-cell lymphomas, <u>intrapelvic</u> lymph nodes

cc **C84.Z7** Other mature T/NK-cell lymphomas, <u>spleen</u>

cc **C84.Z8** Other mature T/NK-cell lymphomas, lymph nodes of <u>multiple sites</u>

cc **C84.Z9** Other mature T/NK-cell lymphomas, <u>extranodal and solid organ sites</u>

C84.9- Mature T/NK-cell lymphomas, <u>unspecified</u>
NK/T cell lymphoma NOS
Excludes 1: *mature T-cell lymphoma, not elsewhere classified (C84.4-)*

cc **C84.90** Mature T/NK-cell lymphomas, unspecified, unspecified site

cc **C84.91** Mature T/NK-cell lymphomas, unspecified, lymph nodes of <u>head, face, and neck</u>

cc **C84.92** Mature T/NK-cell lymphomas, unspecified, <u>intrathoracic</u> lymph nodes

cc **C84.93** Mature T/NK-cell lymphomas, unspecified, <u>intra-abdominal</u> lymph nodes

cc **C84.94** Mature T/NK-cell lymphomas, unspecified, lymph nodes of <u>axilla and upper limb</u>

cc **C84.95** Mature T/NK-cell lymphomas, unspecified, lymph nodes of <u>inguinal region and lower limb</u>

cc **C84.96** Mature T/NK-cell lymphomas, unspecified, <u>intrapelvic</u> lymph nodes

cc **C84.97** Mature T/NK-cell lymphomas, unspecified, <u>spleen</u>

cc **C84.98** Mature T/NK-cell lymphomas, unspecified, lymph nodes of <u>multiple sites</u>

cc **C84.99** Mature T/NK-cell lymphomas, unspecified, <u>extranodal and solid organ sites</u>

C85- <u>Other specified and unspecified types of non-Hodgkin</u> lymphoma
Excludes 1: *other specified types of T/NK-cell lymphoma (C86.-)*
personal history of non-Hodgkin lymphoma (Z85.72)

C85.1- <u>Unspecified B-cell</u> lymphoma
Note: If B-cell lineage or involvement is mentioned in conjunction with a specific lymphoma, code to the more specific description.

cc **C85.10** Unspecified B-cell lymphoma, unspecified site

cc **C85.11** Unspecified B-cell lymphoma, lymph nodes of <u>head, face, and neck</u>

cc **C85.12** Unspecified B-cell lymphoma, <u>intrathoracic</u> lymph nodes

cc **C85.13** Unspecified B-cell lymphoma, <u>intra-abdominal</u> lymph nodes

cc **C85.14** Unspecified B-cell lymphoma, lymph nodes of <u>axilla and upper limb</u>

cc **C85.15** Unspecified B-cell lymphoma, lymph nodes of <u>inguinal region and lower limb</u>

C 8 4 - C 8 5

cc **C85.16** Unspecified B-cell lymphoma, <u>intrapelvic</u> lymph nodes

cc **C85.17** Unspecified B-cell lymphoma, <u>spleen</u>

cc **C85.18** Unspecified B-cell lymphoma, lymph nodes of <u>multiple sites</u>

cc **C85.19** Unspecified B-cell lymphoma, <u>extranodal and solid organ sites</u>

C85.2- <u>Mediastinal (thymic) large B-cell</u> lymphoma

cc **C85.20** Mediastinal (thymic) large B-cell lymphoma, unspecified site

cc **C85.21** Mediastinal (thymic) large B-cell lymphoma, lymph nodes of <u>head, face, and neck</u>

cc **C85.22** Mediastinal (thymic) large B-cell lymphoma, <u>intrathoracic</u> lymph nodes

cc **C85.23** Mediastinal (thymic) large B-cell lymphoma, <u>intra-abdominal</u> lymph nodes

cc **C85.24** Mediastinal (thymic) large B-cell lymphoma, lymph nodes of <u>axilla and upper limb</u>

cc **C85.25** Mediastinal (thymic) large B-cell lymphoma, lymph nodes of <u>inguinal region and lower limb</u>

cc **C85.26** Mediastinal (thymic) large B-cell lymphoma, <u>intrapelvic</u> lymph nodes

cc **C85.27** Mediastinal (thymic) large B-cell lymphoma, <u>spleen</u>

cc **C85.28** Mediastinal (thymic) large B-cell lymphoma, lymph nodes of <u>multiple sites</u>

cc **C85.29** Mediastinal (thymic) large B-cell lymphoma, <u>extranodal and solid organ sites</u>

C85.8- <u>Other specified types of non-Hodgkin</u> lymphoma

cc **C85.80** Other specified types of non-Hodgkin lymphoma, unspecified site

cc **C85.81** Other specified types of non-Hodgkin lymphoma, lymph nodes of <u>head, face, and neck</u>

cc **C85.82** Other specified types of non-Hodgkin lymphoma, <u>intrathoracic</u> lymph nodes

cc **C85.83** Other specified types of non-Hodgkin lymphoma, <u>intra-abdominal</u> lymph nodes

cc **C85.84** Other specified types of non-Hodgkin lymphoma, lymph nodes of <u>axilla and upper limb</u>

cc **C85.85** Other specified types of non-Hodgkin lymphoma, lymph nodes of <u>inguinal region and lower limb</u>

cc **C85.86** Other specified types of non-Hodgkin lymphoma, <u>intrapelvic</u> lymph nodes

cc **C85.87** Other specified types of non-Hodgkin lymphoma, <u>spleen</u>

cc **C85.88** Other specified types of non-Hodgkin lymphoma, lymph nodes of <u>multiple sites</u>

cc **C85.89** Other specified types of non-Hodgkin lymphoma, <u>extranodal and solid organ sites</u>

C85.9- Non-Hodgkin lymphoma, <u>unspecified</u>
Lymphoma NOS
Malignant lymphoma NOS
Non-Hodgkin lymphoma NOS

cc **C85.90** Non-Hodgkin lymphoma, unspecified, unspecified site

cc **C85.91** Non-Hodgkin lymphoma, unspecified, lymph nodes of <u>head, face, and neck</u>

cc **C85.92** Non-Hodgkin lymphoma, unspecified, <u>intrathoracic</u> lymph nodes

cc **C85.93** Non-Hodgkin lymphoma, unspecified, <u>intra-abdominal</u> lymph nodes

cc **C85.94** Non-Hodgkin lymphoma, unspecified, lymph nodes of <u>axilla and upper limb</u>

cc **C85.95** Non-Hodgkin lymphoma, unspecified, lymph nodes of <u>inguinal region and lower limb</u>

cc **C85.96** Non-Hodgkin lymphoma, unspecified, <u>intrapelvic</u> lymph nodes

cc **C85.97** Non-Hodgkin lymphoma, unspecified, <u>spleen</u>

cc **C85.98** Non-Hodgkin lymphoma, unspecified, lymph nodes of <u>multiple sites</u>

cc **C85.99** Non-Hodgkin lymphoma, unspecified, <u>extranodal and solid organ sites</u>

C86- <u>Other specified types of T/NK-cell</u> lymphoma
Excludes 1:   *anaplastic large cell lymphoma, ALK negative (C84.7-)*
anaplastic large cell lymphoma, ALK positive (C84.6-)
mature T/NK-cell lymphomas (C84.-)
other specified types of non-Hodgkin lymphoma (C85.8-)

cc **C86.0** <u>Extranodal NK/T-cell</u> lymphoma, nasal type

cc **C86.1** <u>Hepatosplenic</u> T-cell lymphoma
Alpha-beta and gamma delta types

cc **C86.2** <u>Enteropathy-type</u> (intestinal) T-cell lymphoma
Enteropathy associated T-cell lymphoma

cc **C86.3** <u>Subcutaneous panniculitis-like</u> T-cell lymphoma

cc **C86.4** <u>Blastic NK-cell</u> lymphoma

cc **C86.5** <u>Angioimmunoblastic</u> T-cell lymphoma
Angioimmunoblastic lymphadenopathy with dysproteinemia (AILD)

cc **C86.6** <u>Primary cutaneous CD30-positive</u> T-cell proliferations
Lymphomatoid papulosis
Primary cutaneous anaplastic large cell lymphoma
Primary cutaneous CD30-positive large T-cell lymphoma

C88- **Malignant immunoproliferative diseases and certain other B-cell lymphomas**
Excludes 1:   *B-cell lymphoma, unspecified (C85.1-)*
personal history of other malignant neoplasms of lymphoid, hematopoietic and related tissues (Z85.79)

cc **C88.0** **Waldenström macroglobulinemia**
Lymphoplasmacytic lymphoma with IgM-production
Macroglobulinemia (idiopathic) (primary)
Excludes 1:   *small cell B-cell lymphoma (C83.0)*

cc **C88.2** **Heavy chain disease**
Franklin disease
Gamma heavy chain disease
Mu heavy chain disease

cc **C88.3** **Immunoproliferative small intestinal disease**
Alpha heavy chain disease
Mediterranean lymphoma

cc **C88.4** **Extranodal marginal zone B-cell lymphoma of mucosa-associated lymphoid tissue [MALT-lymphoma]**
Lymphoma of skin-associated lymphoid tissue [SALT-lymphoma]
Lymphoma of bronchial-associated lymphoid tissue [BALT-lymphoma]
Excludes 1:   *high malignant (diffuse large B-cell) lymphoma (C83.3-)*

cc **C88.8** **Other malignant immunoproliferative diseases**

cc **C88.9** **Malignant immunoproliferative disease, unspecified**
Immunoproliferative disease NOS

C90- **Multiple myeloma and malignant plasma cell neoplasms**
Excludes 1:   *personal history of other malignant neoplasms of lymphoid, hematopoietic and related tissues (Z85.79)*

C90.0- <u>Multiple myeloma</u> — A malignancy affecting plasma cells (a type of white blood cell).
Kahler's disease
Medullary plasmacytoma
Myelomatosis
Plasma cell myeloma
Excludes 1:   *solitary myeloma (C90.3-)*
solitary plasmactyoma (C90.3-)

cc **C90.00** Multiple myeloma <u>not</u> having achieved remission
Multiple myeloma with failed remission
Multiple myeloma NOS

cc **C90.01** Multiple myeloma <u>in remission</u>

cc **C90.02** Multiple myeloma <u>in relapse</u>

C90.1- <u>Plasma cell leukemia</u> — A very aggressive malignancy affecting plasma cells (a type of white blood cell), often evolving from multiple myeloma.
Plasmacytic leukemia

cc **C90.10** Plasma cell leukemia <u>not</u> having achieved remission
Plasma cell leukemia with failed remission
Plasma cell leukemia NOS

cc **C90.11** Plasma cell leukemia <u>in remission</u>

cc **C90.12** Plasma cell leukemia <u>in relapse</u>

C90.2- <u>Extramedullary plasmacytoma</u> — A malignant plasma cell tumor forming a solid mass affecting the soft tissues.

cc **C90.20** Extramedullary plasmacytoma <u>not</u> having achieved remission
Extramedullary plasmacytoma with failed remission
Extramedullary plasmacytoma NOS

cc **C90.21** Extramedullary plasmacytoma <u>in remission</u>

cc **C90.22** Extramedullary plasmacytoma <u>in relapse</u>

C90.3- <u>Solitary plasmacytoma</u> — A malignant plasma cell tumor forming a solid mass affecting the bones.
Localized malignant plasma cell tumor NOS
Plasmacytoma NOS
Solitary myeloma

cc **C90.30** Solitary plasmacytoma <u>not</u> having achieved remission
Solitary plasmacytoma with failed remission
Solitary plasmacytoma NOS

cc **C90.31** Solitary plasmacytoma <u>in remission</u>

cc **C90.32** Solitary plasmacytoma <u>in relapse</u>

C91- <u>Lymphoid leukemia</u> — A malignancy affecting circulating lymphocytes, a type of white blood cell, that originates in the bone marrow.
Excludes 1:   *personal history of leukemia (Z85.6)*

C91.0- <u>Acute lymphoblastic</u> leukemia [ALL]
Note: Code C91.0 should only be used for T-cell and B-cell precursor leukemia

cc **C91.00** Acute lymphoblastic leukemia <u>not</u> having achieved remission
Acute lymphoblastic leukemia with failed remission
Acute lymphoblastic leukemia NOS

cc **C91.01** Acute lymphoblastic leukemia, <u>in remission</u>

cc **C91.02** Acute lymphoblastic leukemia, <u>in relapse</u>

C91.1- <u>Chronic lymphocytic</u> leukemia of B-cell type
Lymphoplasmacytic leukemia
Richter syndrome
Excludes 1:   *lymphoplasmacytic lymphoma (C83.0-)*

cc **C91.10** Chronic lymphocytic leukemia of B-cell type <u>not</u> having achieved remission
Chronic lymphocytic leukemia of B-cell type with failed remission
Chronic lymphocytic leukemia of B-cell type NOS

cc **C91.11** Chronic lymphocytic leukemia of B-cell type <u>in remission</u>

cc **C91.12** Chronic lymphocytic leukemia of B-cell type <u>in relapse</u>

C91.3- <u>Prolymphocytic</u> leukemia of <u>B-cell type</u>

cc **C91.30** Prolymphocytic leukemia of B-cell type <u>not</u> having achieved remission
Prolymphocytic leukemia of B-cell type with failed remission
Prolymphocytic leukemia of B-cell type NOS

cc **C91.31** Prolymphocytic leukemia of B-cell type, <u>in remission</u>

cc **C91.32** Prolymphocytic leukemia of B-cell type, <u>in relapse</u>

C91.4- <u>Hairy cell</u> leukemia
Leukemic reticuloendotheliosis

cc **C91.40** Hairy cell leukemia <u>not</u> having achieved remission
Hairy cell leukemia with failed remission
Hairy cell leukemia NOS

cc **C91.41** Hairy cell leukemia, <u>in remission</u>

cc **C91.42** Hairy cell leukemia, <u>in relapse</u>

C91.5- <u>Adult T-cell</u> lymphoma/leukemia (HTLV-1-associated)
Acute variant of adult T-cell lymphoma/leukemia (HTLV-1-associated)
Chronic variant of adult T-cell lymphoma/leukemia (HTLV-1-associated)
Lymphomatoid variant of adult T-cell lymphoma/leukemia (HTLV-1-associated)
Smouldering variant of adult T-cell lymphoma/leukemia (HTLV-1-associated)

cc **C91.50** Adult T-cell lymphoma/leukemia (HTLV-1-associated) <u>not</u> having achieved remission — [Age/15-124]
Adult T-cell lymphoma/leukemia (HTLV-1-associated) with failed remission
Adult T-cell lymphoma/leukemia (HTLV-1-associated) NOS

cc **C91.51** Adult T-cell lymphoma/leukemia (HTLV-1-associated), <u>in remission</u> — [Age/15-124]

cc **C91.52** Adult T-cell lymphoma/leukemia (HTLV-1-associated), <u>in relapse</u> — [Age/15-124]

C91.6- <u>Prolymphocytic</u> leukemia of <u>T-cell type</u>

cc **C91.60** Prolymphocytic leukemia of T-cell type <u>not</u> having achieved remission
Prolymphocytic leukemia of T-cell type with failed remission
Prolymphocytic leukemia of T-cell type NOS

cc **C91.61** Prolymphocytic leukemia of T-cell type, <u>in remission</u>

cc **C91.62** Prolymphocytic leukemia of T-cell type, <u>in relapse</u>

C91.A- <u>Mature B-cell</u> leukemia <u>Burkitt-type</u>
Excludes 1:   *Burkitt lymphoma (C83.7-)*

cc **C91.A0** Mature B-cell leukemia Burkitt-type <u>not</u> having achieved remission
Mature B-cell leukemia Burkitt-type with failed remission
Mature B-cell leukemia Burkitt-type NOS

cc **C91.A1** Mature B-cell leukemia Burkitt-type, <u>in remission</u>

cc **C91.A2** Mature B-cell leukemia Burkitt-type, <u>in relapse</u>

C91.Z- <u>Other lymphoid</u> leukemia
T-cell large granular lymphocytic leukemia (associated with rheumatoid arthritis)

cc **C91.Z0** Other lymphoid leukemia <u>not</u> having achieved remission
Other lymphoid leukemia with failed remission
Other lymphoid leukemia NOS

cc **C91.Z1** Other lymphoid leukemia, <u>in remission</u>

cc **C91.Z2** Other lymphoid leukemia, <u>in relapse</u>

C91.9- <u>Lymphoid leukemia, unspecified</u>

cc **C91.90** Lymphoid leukemia, unspecified <u>not</u> having achieved remission
Lymphoid leukemia with failed remission
Lymphoid leukemia NOS

cc **C91.91** Lymphoid leukemia, unspecified, <u>in remission</u>

cc **C91.92** Lymphoid leukemia, unspecified, <u>in relapse</u>

C92 <u>Myeloid leukemia</u> — A malignancy affecting white blood cell development in which the bone marrow makes abnormal myeloblasts, red blood cells, and platelets.
Includes: Granulocytic leukemia
Myelogenous leukemia
Excludes 1:   *personal history of leukemia (Z85.6)*

C92.0- <u>Acute myeloblastic</u> leukemia
Acute myeloblastic leukemia, minimal differentiation
Acute myeloblastic leukemia (with maturation)
Acute myeloblastic leukemia 1/ETO
Acute myeloblastic leukemia M0
Acute myeloblastic leukemia M1
Acute myeloblastic leukemia M2
Acute myeloblastic leukemia with t(8;21)
Acute myeloblastic leukemia (without a FAB classification) NOS
Refractory anemia with excess blasts in transformation [RAEB T]
Excludes 1:   *acute exacerbation of chronic myeloid leukemia (C92.10)*
refractory anemia with excess of blasts not in transformation (D46.2-)

cc **C92.00** Acute myeloblastic leukemia, <u>not</u> having achieved remission
Acute myeloblastic leukemia with failed remission
Acute myeloblastic leukemia NOS

cc **C92.01** Acute myeloblastic leukemia, <u>in remission</u>

cc **C92.02** Acute myeloblastic leukemia, <u>in relapse</u>

C92.1- <u>Chronic myeloid leukemia, BCR/ABL-positive</u>
Chronic myelogenous leukemia, Philadelphia chromosome (Ph1) positive
Chronic myelogenous leukemia, t(9;22) (q34;q11)
Chronic myelogenous leukemia with crisis of blast cells
Excludes 1:   *atypical chronic myeloid leukemia BCR/ABL-negative (C92.2-)*
chronic myelomonocytic leukemia (C93.1-)
chronic myeloproliferative disease (D47.1)

cc **C92.10** Chronic myeloid leukemia, BCR/ABL-positive, <u>not</u> having achieved remission
Chronic myeloid leukemia, BCR/ABL-positive with failed remission
Chronic myeloid leukemia, BCR/ABL-positive NOS

cc **C92.11** Chronic myeloid leukemia, BCR/ABL-positive, <u>in remission</u>

cc **C92.12** Chronic myeloid leukemia, BCR/ABL-positive, <u>in relapse</u>

C90 - C92 (margin tab)

C92.2- Atypical chronic myeloid leukemia, BCR/ABL-negative

cc **C92.20** Atypical chronic myeloid leukemia, BCR/ABL-negative, **not** having achieved remission
Atypical chronic myeloid leukemia, BCR/ABL-negative with failed remission
Atypical chronic myeloid leukemia, BCR/ABL-negative NOS

cc **C92.21** Atypical chronic myeloid leukemia, BCR/ABL-negative, **in** remission

cc **C92.22** Atypical chronic myeloid leukemia, BCR/ABL-negative, **in** relapse

C92.3- Myeloid sarcoma
A malignant tumor of immature myeloid cells
Chloroma
Granulocytic sarcoma

cc **C92.30** Myeloid sarcoma, **not** having achieved remission
Myeloid sarcoma with failed remission
Myeloid sarcoma NOS

cc **C92.31** Myeloid sarcoma, **in remission**

cc **C92.32** Myeloid sarcoma, **in relapse**

C92.4- Acute promyelocytic leukemia
AML M3
AML Me with t(15;17) and variants

cc **C92.40** Acute promyelocytic leukemia, **not** having achieved remission
Acute promyelocytic leukemia with failed remission
Acute promyelocytic leukemia NOS

cc **C92.41** Acute promyelocytic leukemia, **in remission**

cc **C92.42** Acute promyelocytic leukemia, **in relapse**

C92.5- Acute myelomonocytic leukemia
AML M4
AML M4 Eo with inv(16) or t(16;16)

cc **C92.50** Acute myelomonocytic leukemia, **not** having achieved remission
Acute myelomonocytic leukemia with failed remission
Acute myelomonocytic leukemia NOS

cc **C92.51** Acute myelomonocytic leukemia, **in remission**

cc **C92.52** Acute myelomonocytic leukemia, **in relapse**

C92.6- Acute myeloid leukemia with 11q23-abnormality
Acute myeloid leukemia with variation of MLL-gene

cc **C92.60** Acute myeloid leukemia with 11q23-abnormality **not** having achieved remission
Acute myeloid leukemia with 11q23-abnormality with failed remission
Acute myeloid leukemia with 11q23-abnormality NOS

cc **C92.61** Acute myeloid leukemia with 11q23-abnormality **in remission**

cc **C92.62** Acute myeloid leukemia with 11q23-abnormality **in relapse**

C92.A- Acute myeloid leukemia with multilineage dysplasia
Acute myeloid leukemia with dysplasia of remaining hematopoesis and/or myelodysplastic disease in its history

cc **C92.A0** Acute myeloid leukemia with multilineage dysplasia, **not** having achieved remission
Acute myeloid leukemia with multilineage dysplasia with failed remission
Acute myeloid leukemia with multilineage dysplasia NOS

cc **C92.A1** Acute myeloid leukemia with multilineage dysplasia, **in remission**

cc **C92.A2** Acute myeloid leukemia with multilineage dysplasia, **in relapse**

C92.Z- Other myeloid leukemia

cc **C92.Z0** Other myeloid leukemia **not** having achieved remission
Myeloid leukemia NEC with failed remission
Myeloid leukemia NEC

cc **C92.Z1** Other myeloid leukemia, **in remission**

cc **C92.Z2** Other myeloid leukemia, **in relapse**

C92.9- Myeloid leukemia, unspecified

cc **C92.90** Myeloid leukemia, unspecified, **not** having achieved remission
Myeloid leukemia, unspecified with failed remission
Myeloid leukemia, unspecified NOS

cc **C92.91** Myeloid leukemia, unspecified **in remission**

cc **C92.92** Myeloid leukemia, unspecified **in relapse**

C93- Monocytic leukemia — A malignancy affecting white blood cell development in which the bone marrow makes an excessive number of monocytes.
Includes: Monocytoid leukemia
Excludes 1:   personal history of leukemia (Z85.6)

C93.0- Acute monoblastic/monocytic leukemia
AML M5
AML M5a
AML M5b

cc **C93.00** Acute monoblastic/monocytic leukemia, **not** having achieved remission
Acute monoblastic/monocytic leukemia with failed remission
Acute monoblastic/monocytic leukemia NOS

cc **C93.01** Acute monoblastic/monocytic leukemia, **in remission**

cc **C93.02** Acute monoblastic/monocytic leukemia, **in relapse**

C93.1- Chronic myelomonocytic leukemia
Chronic monocytic leukemia
CMML-1
CMML-2
CMML with eosinophilia

cc **C93.10** Chronic myelomonocytic leukemia **not** having achieved remission
Chronic myelomonocytic leukemia with failed remission
Chronic myelomonocytic leukemia NOS

cc **C93.11** Chronic myelomonocytic leukemia, **in remission**

cc **C93.12** Chronic myelomonocytic leukemia, **in relapse**

C93.3- Juvenile myelomonocytic leukemia

cc **C93.30** Juvenile myelomonocytic leukemia, **not** having achieved remission — [Age/0-17]
Juvenile myelomonocytic leukemia with failed remission
Juvenile myelomonocytic leukemia NOS

cc **C93.31** Juvenile myelomonocytic leukemia, **in remission** — [Age/0-17]

cc **C93.32** Juvenile myelomonocytic leukemia, **in relapse** — [Age/0-17]

C93.Z- Other monocytic leukemia

cc **C93.Z0** Other monocytic leukemia, **not** having achieved remission
Other monocytic leukemia NOS

cc **C93.Z1** Other monocytic leukemia, **in remission**

cc **C93.Z2** Other monocytic leukemia, **in relapse**

C93.9- Monocytic leukemia, unspecified

cc **C93.90** Monocytic leukemia, unspecified, **not** having achieved remission
Monocytic leukemia, unspecified with failed remission
Monocytic leukemia, unspecified NOS

cc **C93.91** Monocytic leukemia, unspecified **in remission**

cc **C93.92** Monocytic leukemia, unspecified **in relapse**

C94- Other leukemias of specified cell type
Excludes 1:   leukemic reticuloendotheliosis (C91.4-)
myelodysplastic syndromes (D46.-)
personal history of leukemia (Z85.6)
plasma cell leukemia (C90.1-)

C94.0- Acute erythroid leukemia
Acute myeloid leukemia M6(a)(b)
Erythroleukemia

cc **C94.00** Acute erythroid leukemia, **not** having achieved remission
Acute erythroid leukemia with failed remission
Acute erythroid leukemia NOS

cc **C94.01** Acute erythroid leukemia, **in remission**

cc **C94.02** Acute erythroid leukemia, **in relapse**

C94.2- Acute megakaryoblastic leukemia
Acute myeloid leukemia M7
Acute megakaryocytic leukemia

cc **C94.20** Acute megakaryoblastic leukemia **not** having achieved remission
Acute megakaryoblastic leukemia with failed remission
Acute megakaryoblastic leukemia NOS

cc **C94.21** Acute megakaryoblastic leukemia, **in remission**

cc **C94.22** Acute megakaryoblastic leukemia, **in relapse**

C94.3- Mast cell leukemia

cc **C94.30** Mast cell leukemia **not** having achieved remission
Mast cell leukemia with failed remission
Mast cell leukemia NOS

cc **C94.31** Mast cell leukemia, **in remission**

cc **C94.32** Mast cell leukemia, **in relapse**

C
9
2
-
C
9
4

C94.4- <u>Acute panmyelosis</u> with myelofibrosis
   Acute myelofibrosis
   Excludes 1:   myelofibrosis NOS (D75.81)
                    secondary myelofibrosis NOS (D75.81)

cc **C94.40** Acute panmyelosis with myelofibrosis <u>not</u> having
   achieved remission
      Acute myelofibrosis NOS
      Acute panmyelosis with myelofibrosis with failed remission
      Acute panmyelosis NOS

cc **C94.41** Acute panmyelosis with myelofibrosis, <u>in remission</u>

cc **C94.42** Acute panmyelosis with myelofibrosis, <u>in relapse</u>

cc **C94.6** Myelodysplastic disease, not classified
      Myeloproliferative disease, not classified

C94.8- <u>Other specified</u> leukemias
      Aggressive NK-cell leukemia
      Acute basophilic leukemia

cc **C94.80** Other specified leukemias <u>not</u> having achieved remission
      Other specified leukemia with failed remission
      Other specified leukemias NOS

cc **C94.81** Other specified leukemias, <u>in remission</u>

cc **C94.82** Other specified leukemias, <u>in relapse</u>

C95- Leukemia of <u>unspecified cell type</u>
   Excludes 1:   personal history of leukemia (Z85.6)

C95.0- <u>Acute</u> leukemia of unspecified cell type
      Acute bilineal leukemia
      Acute mixed lineage leukemia
      Biphenotypic acute leukemia
      Stem cell leukemia of unclear lineage
   Excludes 1:   acute exacerbation of unspecified chronic leukemia
                    (C95.10)

cc **C95.00** Acute leukemia of unspecified cell type <u>not</u> having
   achieved remission
      Acute leukemia of unspecified cell type with failed remission
      Acute leukemia NOS

cc **C95.01** Acute leukemia of unspecified cell type, <u>in remission</u>

cc **C95.02** Acute leukemia of unspecified cell type, <u>in relapse</u>

C95.1- <u>Chronic</u> leukemia of unspecified cell type

cc **C95.10** Chronic leukemia of unspecified cell type <u>not</u> having
   achieved remission
      Chronic leukemia of unspecified cell type with failed remission
      Chronic leukemia NOS

cc **C95.11** Chronic leukemia of unspecified cell type, <u>in remission</u>

cc **C95.12** Chronic leukemia of unspecified cell type, <u>in relapse</u>

C95.9- Leukemia, <u>unspecified</u>

cc **C95.90** Leukemia, unspecified <u>not</u> having achieved remission
      Leukemia, unspecified with failed remission
      Leukemia NOS

cc **C95.91** Leukemia, unspecified, <u>in remission</u>

cc **C95.92** Leukemia, unspecified, <u>in relapse</u>

C96- Other and unspecified malignant neoplasms of lymphoid,
   hematopoietic and related tissue
   Excludes 1:   personal history of other malignant neoplasms of lymphoid,
                    hematopoietic and related tissues (Z85.79)

cc **C96.0** Multifocal and <u>multisystemic</u> (disseminated) Langerhans-cell
   histiocytosis
      Histiocytosis X, multisystemic
      Letterer-Siwe disease
   Excludes 1:   adult pulmonary Langerhans-cell histiocytosis (J84.82)
                    multifocal and unisystemic Langerhans-cell histiocytosis
                    (C96.5)
                    unifocal Langerhans-cell histiocytosis (C96.6)

cc **C96.2** Malignant <u>mast cell</u> tumor
      Aggressive systemic mastocytosis
      Mast cell sarcoma
   Excludes 1:   indolent mastocytosis (D47.0)
                    mast cell leukemia (C94.30)
                    mastocytosis (congenital) (cutaneous) (Q82.2)

cc **C96.4** Sarcoma of <u>dendritic cells</u> (accessory cells)
      Follicular dendritic cell sarcoma
      Interdigitating dendritic cell sarcoma
      Langerhans cell sarcoma

cc **C96.5** Multifocal and <u>unisystemic</u> Langerhans-cell histiocytosis
      Hand-Schüller-Christian disease
      Histiocytosis X, multifocal
   Excludes 1:   multifocal and multisystemic (disseminated)
                    Langerhans-cell histiocytosis (C96.0)
                    unifocal Langerhans-cell histiocytosis (C96.6)

cc **C96.6** <u>Unifocal</u> Langerhans-cell histiocytosis
      Eosinophilic granuloma
      Histiocytosis X, unifocal
      Histiocytosis X NOS
      Langerhans-cell histiocytosis NOS
   Excludes 1:   multifocal and multisysemic (disseminated) Langerhans-
                    cell histiocytosis (C96.0)
                    multifocal and unisystemic Langerhans-cell histiocytosis
                    (C96.5)

cc **C96.A** Histiocytic sarcoma
      Malignant histiocytosis

cc **C96.Z** Other specified malignant neoplasms of lymphoid,
   hematopoietic and related tissue

cc **C96.9** Malignant neoplasm of lymphoid, hematopoietic and related
   tissue, unspecified

In situ neoplasms (D00-D09)

   Includes: Bowen's disease
                   Erythroplasia
                   Grade III intraepithelial neoplasia
                   Queyrat's erythroplasia

D00- <u>Carcinoma in situ</u> of oral cavity, esophagus and stomach — Malignant
   neoplastic tumor cells that still remain within the epithelium without invasion of the
   basement membrane.
   Excludes 1:   melanoma in situ (D03.-)

D00.0- Carcinoma in situ of <u>lip, oral cavity and pharynx</u>
      Use additional code to identify:
      Exposure to environmental tobacco smoke (Z77.22)
      Exposure to tobacco smoke in the perinatal period (P96.81)
      History of tobacco dependence (Z87.891)
      Occupational exposure to environmental tobacco smoke (Z57.31)
      Tobacco dependence (F17.-)
      Tobacco use (Z72.0)
   Excludes 1:   carcinoma in situ of aryepiglottic fold or interarytenoid fold,
                    laryngeal aspect (D02.0)
                    carcinoma in situ of epiglottis NOS (D02.0)
                    carcinoma in situ of epiglottis suprahyoid portion (D02.0)
                    carcinoma in situ of skin of lip (D03.0, D04.0)

   D00.00 Carcinoma in situ of oral cavity, unspecified site

   D00.01 Carcinoma in situ of <u>labial mucosa and vermilion border</u>

   D00.02 Carcinoma in situ of <u>buccal</u> mucosa

   D00.03 Carcinoma in situ of <u>gingiva</u> and edentulous alveolar
   ridge

   D00.04 Carcinoma in situ of <u>soft</u> palate

   D00.05 Carcinoma in situ of <u>hard</u> palate

   D00.06 Carcinoma in situ of <u>floor</u> of mouth

   D00.07 Carcinoma in situ of <u>tongue</u>

   D00.08 Carcinoma in situ of <u>pharynx</u>
      Carcinoma in situ of aryepiglottic fold NOS
      Carcinoma in situ of hypopharyngeal aspect of aryepiglottic
      fold
      Carcinoma in situ of marginal zone of aryepiglottic fold

D00.1 Carcinoma in situ of <u>esophagus</u>

D00.2 Carcinoma in situ of <u>stomach</u>

D01- <u>Carcinoma in situ</u> of other and unspecified digestive organs
   Excludes 1:   melanoma in situ (D03.-)

D01.0 Carcinoma in situ of <u>colon</u>
   Excludes 1:   carcinoma in situ of rectosigmoid junction (D01.1)

D01.1 Carcinoma in situ of <u>rectosigmoid</u> junction

D01.2 Carcinoma in situ of <u>rectum</u>

D01.3 Carcinoma in situ of <u>anus and anal canal</u>
      Anal intraepithelial neoplasia III [AIN III]
      Severe dysplasia of anus
   Excludes 1:   anal intraepithelial neoplasia I and II [AIN I and AIN II]
                    (K62.82)
                    carcinoma in situ of anal margin (D04.5)
                    carcinoma in situ of anal skin (D04.5)
                    carcinoma in situ of perianal skin (D04.5)

D01.4- Carcinoma in situ of other and unspecified parts of intestine
> *Excludes 1:   carcinoma in situ of ampulla of Vater (D01.5)*

D01.40 Carcinoma in situ of unspecified part of intestine

D01.49 Carcinoma in situ of other parts of intestine

D01.5 Carcinoma in situ of <u>liver, gallbladder and bile ducts</u>
> Carcinoma in situ of ampulla of Vater

D01.7 Carcinoma in situ of other specified digestive organs
> Carcinoma in situ of pancreas

D01.9 Carcinoma in situ of digestive organ, unspecified

D02- <u>Carcinoma in situ</u> of middle ear and respiratory system — Malignant neoplastic tumor cells that still remain within the epithelium without invasion of the basement membrane.
> Use additional code to identify:
> Exposure to environmental tobacco smoke (Z77.22)
> Exposure to tobacco smoke in the perinatal period (P96.81)
> History of tobacco dependence (Z87.891)
> Occupational exposure to environmental tobacco smoke (Z57.31)
> Tobacco dependence (F17.-)
> Tobacco use (Z72.0)
> *Excludes 1:   melanoma in situ (D03.-)*

D02.0 Carcinoma in situ of <u>larynx</u>
> Carcinoma in situ of aryepiglottic fold or interarytenoid fold, laryngeal aspect
> Carcinoma in situ of epiglottis (suprahyoid portion)
> *Excludes 1:   carcinoma in situ of aryepiglottic fold or interarytenoid fold NOS (D00.08)*
> *carcinoma in situ of hypopharyngeal aspect (D00.08)*
> *carcinoma in situ of marginal zone (D00.08)*

D02.1 Carcinoma in situ of <u>trachea</u>

D02.2- Carcinoma in situ of <u>bronchus and lung</u>

D02.20 Carcinoma in situ of unspecified bronchus and lung

D02.21 Carcinoma in situ of <u>right</u> bronchus and lung

D02.22 Carcinoma in situ of <u>left</u> bronchus and lung

D02.3 Carcinoma in situ of other parts of respiratory system
> Carcinoma in situ of accessory sinuses
> Carcinoma in situ of middle ear
> Carcinoma in situ of nasal cavities
> *Excludes 1:   carcinoma in situ of ear (external) (skin) (D04.2-)*
> *carcinoma in situ of nose NOS (D09.8)*
> *carcinoma in situ of skin of nose (D04.3)*

D02.4 Carcinoma in situ of respiratory system, unspecified

D03- <u>Melanoma in situ</u> — Malignant melanoma tumor cells that still remain within the epidermis (the outermost layer of skin) without invasion of the deeper tissue layers.

D03.0 Melanoma in situ of <u>lip</u>

D03.1- Melanoma in situ of <u>eyelid, including canthus</u>

D03.10 Melanoma in situ of unspecified eyelid, including canthus

D03.11 Melanoma in situ of <u>right</u> eyelid, including canthus

D03.12 Melanoma in situ of <u>left</u> eyelid, including canthus

D03.2- Melanoma in situ of ear and external auricular canal

D03.20 Melanoma in situ of unspecified <u>ear and external auricular canal</u>

D03.21 Melanoma in situ of <u>right</u> ear and external auricular canal

D03.22 Melanoma in situ of <u>left</u> ear and external auricular canal

D03.3- Melanoma in situ of other and unspecified parts of face

D03.30 Melanoma in situ of unspecified part of face

D03.39 Melanoma in situ of other parts of face

D03.4 Melanoma in situ of <u>scalp and neck</u>

D03.5- Melanoma in situ of trunk

D03.51 Melanoma in situ of <u>anal skin</u>
> Melanoma in situ of anal margin
> Melanoma in situ of perianal skin

D03.52 Melanoma in situ of <u>breast</u> (skin) (soft tissue)

D03.59 Melanoma in situ of other part of trunk

D03.6- Melanoma in situ of <u>upper limb,</u> including shoulder

D03.60 Melanoma in situ of unspecified upper limb, including shoulder

D03.61 Melanoma in situ of <u>right</u> upper limb, including shoulder

D03.62 Melanoma in situ of <u>left</u> upper limb, including shoulder

D03.7- Melanoma in situ of <u>lower limb</u>, including hip

D03.70 Melanoma in situ of unspecified lower limb, including hip

D03.71 Melanoma in situ of <u>right</u> lower limb, including hip

D03.72 Melanoma in situ of <u>left</u> lower limb, including hip

D03.8 Melanoma in situ of other sites
> Melanoma in situ of scrotum
> *Excludes 1:   carcinoma in situ of scrotum (D07.61)*

D03.9 Melanoma in situ, unspecified

D04- <u>Carcinoma in situ</u> of <u>skin</u> — Malignant neoplastic (non-melanoma) tumor cells that still remain within the epidermis (the outermost layer of skin) without invasion of the deeper tissue layers.
> *Excludes 1:   erythroplasia of Queyrat (penis) NOS (D07.4)*
> *melanoma in situ (D03.-)*

D04.0 Carcinoma in situ of <u>skin</u> of <u>lip</u>
> *Excludes 1:   carcinoma in situ of vermilion border of lip (D00.01)*

D04.1- Carcinoma in situ of <u>skin</u> of <u>eyelid, including canthus</u>

D04.10 Carcinoma in situ of skin of unspecified eyelid, including canthus

D04.11 Carcinoma in situ of skin of <u>right</u> eyelid, including canthus

D04.12 Carcinoma in situ of skin of <u>left</u> eyelid, including canthus

D04.2- Carcinoma in situ of <u>skin</u> of <u>ear and external auricular canal</u>

D04.20 Carcinoma in situ of skin of unspecified ear and external auricular canal

D04.21 Carcinoma in situ of skin of <u>right</u> ear and external auricular canal

D04.22 Carcinoma in situ of skin of <u>left</u> ear and external auricular canal

D04.3- Carcinoma in situ of <u>skin</u> of other and unspecified parts of face

D04.30 Carcinoma in situ of skin of unspecified part of face

D04.39 Carcinoma in situ of skin of other parts of face

D04.4 Carcinoma in situ of <u>skin</u> of <u>scalp and neck</u>

D04.5 Carcinoma in situ of <u>skin</u> of <u>trunk</u>
> Carcinoma in situ of anal margin
> Carcinoma in situ of anal skin
> Carcinoma in situ of perianal skin
> Carcinoma in situ of skin of breast
> *Excludes 1:   carcinoma in situ of anus NOS (D01.3)*
> *carcinoma in situ of scrotum (D07.61)*
> *carcinoma in situ of skin of genital organs (D07.-)*

D04.6- Carcinoma in situ of <u>skin</u> of <u>upper limb</u>, including shoulder

D04.60 Carcinoma in situ of skin of unspecified upper limb, including shoulder

D04.61 Carcinoma in situ of skin of <u>right</u> upper limb, including shoulder

D04.62 Carcinoma in situ of skin of <u>left</u> upper limb, including shoulder

D04.7- Carcinoma in situ of <u>skin</u> of <u>lower limb</u>, including hip

D04.70 Carcinoma in situ of skin of unspecified lower limb, including hip

D04.71 Carcinoma in situ of skin of <u>right</u> lower limb, including hip

D04.72 Carcinoma in situ of skin of <u>left</u> lower limb, including hip

D04.8 Carcinoma in situ of <u>skin</u> of other sites

D04.9 Carcinoma in situ of <u>skin</u>, unspecified

D05- <u>Carcinoma in situ</u> of breast — Malignant neoplastic tumor cells that still remain within the epithelium without invasion of the basement membrane.
> *Excludes 1:   carcinoma in situ of skin of breast (D04.5)*
> *melanoma in situ of breast (skin) (D03.5)*
> *Paget's disease of breast or nipple (C50.-)*

D05.0- <u>Lobular</u> carcinoma in situ of breast

D05.00 Lobular carcinoma in situ of unspecified breast

D05.01 Lobular carcinoma in situ of <u>right</u> breast

D05.02 Lobular carcinoma in situ of <u>left</u> breast

D05.1- <u>Intraductal</u> carcinoma in situ of breast

D05.10 Intraductal carcinoma in situ of unspecified breast

D05.11 Intraductal carcinoma in situ of <u>right</u> breast

D05.12 Intraductal carcinoma in situ of <u>left</u> breast

Excludes 1: = NOT CODED HERE! (Do not code both)   **588**   *Excludes ❷: = Not Included Here*

D 0 1 - D 0 5

D05.8- <u>Other specified type</u> of carcinoma in situ of breast

    D05.80 Other specified type of carcinoma in situ of unspecified breast

    D05.81 Other specified type of carcinoma in situ of <u>right</u> breast

    D05.82 Other specified type of carcinoma in situ of <u>left</u> breast

D05.9- <u>Unspecified</u> type of carcinoma in situ of breast

    D05.90 Unspecified type of carcinoma in situ of unspecified breast

    D05.91 Unspecified type of carcinoma in situ of <u>right</u> breast

    D05.92 Unspecified type of carcinoma in situ of <u>left</u> breast

D06- <u>Carcinoma in situ</u> of cervix uteri — Malignant neoplastic tumor cells that still remain within the surface layer of the cervix without invasion of the basement membrane.
    Includes: Cervical adenocarcinoma in situ
                  Cervical intraepithelial glandular neoplasia
                  Cervical intraepithelial neoplasia III [CIN III]
                  Severe dysplasia of cervix uteri
    Excludes 1:   *cervical intraepithelial neoplasia II [CIN II] (N87.1)*
                  cytologic evidence of malignancy of cervix without histologic confirmation (R87.614)
                  high grade squamous intraepithelial lesion (HGSIL) of cervix (R87.613)
                  melanoma in situ of cervix (D03.5)
                  moderate cervical dysplasia (N87.1)

D06.0 Carcinoma in situ of <u>endocervix</u> — [♀]

D06.1 Carcinoma in situ of <u>exocervix</u> — [♀]

D06.7 Carcinoma in situ of other parts of cervix — [♀]

D06.9 Carcinoma in situ of cervix, unspecified — [♀]

D07- <u>Carcinoma in situ</u> of other and unspecified genital organs — Malignant neoplastic tumor cells that still remain within the surface layer without invasion of the basement membrane.
    Excludes 1:   *melanoma in situ of trunk (D03.5)*

D07.0 Carcinoma in situ of <u>endometrium</u> — [♀]

D07.1 Carcinoma in situ of <u>vulva</u> — [♀]
    Severe dysplasia of vulva
    Vulvar intraepithelial neoplasia III [VIN III]
    Excludes 1:   *moderate dysplasia of vulva (N90.1)*
                  vulvar intraepithelial neoplasia II [VIN II] (N90.1)

D07.2 Carcinoma in situ of <u>vagina</u> — [♀]
    Severe dysplasia of vagina
    Vaginal intraepithelial neoplasia III [VAIN III]
    Excludes 1:   *moderate dysplasia of vagina (N89.1)*
                  vaginal intraepithelial neoplasia II [VIN II] (N89.1)

D07.3- Carcinoma in situ of other and unspecified female genital organs

    D07.30 Carcinoma in situ of unspecified female genital organs — [♀]

    D07.39 Carcinoma in situ of other female genital organs — [♀]

D07.4 Carcinoma in situ of <u>penis</u> — [♂]
    Erythroplasia of Queyrat NOS

D07.5 Carcinoma in situ of <u>prostate</u> — [♂]
    Prostatic intraepithelial neoplasia III (PIN III)
    Severe dysplasia of prostate
    Excludes 1:   *dysplasia (mild) (moderate) of prostate (N42.3-)*
                  prostatic intraepithelial neoplasia II [PIN II] (N42.3-)

D07.6- Carcinoma in situ of other and unspecified male genital organs

    D07.60 Carcinoma in situ of unspecified male genital organs — [♂]

    D07.61 Carcinoma in situ of <u>scrotum</u> — [♂]

    D07.69 Carcinoma in situ of other male genital organs — [♂]

D09- <u>Carcinoma in situ</u> of other and unspecified sites — Malignant neoplastic tumor cells that still remain within the surface layer without invasion of the basement membrane.
    Excludes 1:   *melanoma in situ (D03.-)*

D09.0 Carcinoma in situ of <u>bladder</u>

D09.1- Carcinoma in situ of other and unspecified urinary organs

    D09.10 Carcinoma in situ of unspecified urinary organ

    D09.19 Carcinoma in situ of other urinary organs

D09.2- Carcinoma in situ of <u>eye</u>
    Excludes 1:   *carcinoma in situ of skin of eyelid (D04.1-)*

    D09.20 Carcinoma in situ of unspecified eye

    D09.21 Carcinoma in situ of <u>right</u> eye

D09.22 Carcinoma in situ of <u>left</u> eye

D09.3 Carcinoma in situ of <u>thyroid</u> and other endocrine glands
    Excludes 1:   *carcinoma in situ of endocrine pancreas (D01.7)*
                  carcinoma in situ of ovary (D07.39)
                  carcinoma in situ of testis (D07.69)

D09.8 Carcinoma in situ of other specified sites

D09.9 Carcinoma in situ, unspecified

Benign neoplasms, except benign neuroendocrine tumors (D10-D36)

D10- <u>Benign neoplasm</u> of mouth and pharynx — Any new and abnormal growth in which tumor cells progressively multiply, but lack the properties of invasion and metastases (see Malignant Neoplasm code catgories, by site, for anatomical description).

D10.0 Benign neoplasm of <u>lip</u>
    Benign neoplasm of lip (frenulum) (inner aspect) (mucosa) (vermilion border)
    Excludes 1:   *benign neoplasm of skin of lip (D22.0, D23.0)*

D10.1 Benign neoplasm of <u>tongue</u>
    Benign neoplasm of lingual tonsil

D10.2 Benign neoplasm of <u>floor</u> of mouth

D10.3- Benign neoplasm of other and unspecified parts of mouth

    D10.30 Benign neoplasm of unspecified part of mouth

    D10.39 Benign neoplasm of other parts of mouth
        Benign neoplasm of minor salivary gland NOS
        Excludes 1:   *benign odontogenic neoplasms (D16.4-D16.5)*
                  benign neoplasm of mucosa of lip (D10.0)
                  benign neoplasm of nasopharyngeal surface of soft palate (D10.6)

D10.4 Benign neoplasm of <u>tonsil</u>
    Benign neoplasm of tonsil (faucial) (palatine)
    Excludes 1:   *benign neoplasm of lingual tonsil (D10.1)*
                  benign neoplasm of pharyngeal tonsil (D10.6)
                  benign neoplasm of tonsillar fossa (D10.5)
                  benign neoplasm of tonsillar pillars (D10.5)

D10.5 Benign neoplasm of other parts of oropharynx
    Benign neoplasm of epiglottis, anterior aspect
    Benign neoplasm of tonsillar fossa
    Benign neoplasm of tonsillar pillars
    Benign neoplasm of vallecula
    Excludes 1:   *benign neoplasm of epiglottis NOS (D14.1)*
                  benign neoplasm of epiglottis, suprahyoid portion (D14.1)

D10.6 Benign neoplasm of <u>nasopharynx</u>
    Benign neoplasm of pharyngeal tonsil
    Benign neoplasm of posterior margin of septum and choanae

D10.7 Benign neoplasm of <u>hypopharynx</u>

D10.9 Benign neoplasm of pharynx, unspecified

D11- <u>Benign neoplasm</u> of major salivary glands — Any new and abnormal growth in which tumor cells progressively multiply, but lack the properties of invasion and metastases (see Malignant Neoplasm code catgories, by site, for anatomical description).
    Excludes 1:   *benign neoplasms of specified minor salivary glands which are classified according to their anatomic allocation*
                  benign neoplasms of minor salivary glands NOS (D10.39)

D11.0 Benign neoplasm of <u>parotid</u> gland

D11.7 Benign neoplasm of other major salivary glands
    Benign neoplasm of sublingual salivary gland
    Benign neoplasm of submandibular salivary gland

D11.9 Benign neoplasm of major salivary gland, unspecified

D12- <u>Benign neoplasm</u> of colon, rectum, anus and anal canal — Any new and abnormal growth in which tumor cells progressively multiply, but lack the properties of invasion and metastases (see Malignant Neoplasm code catgories, by site, for anatomical description).
    Excludes 1:   *benign carcinoid tumors of the large intestine, and rectum (D3A.02-)*

D12.0 Benign neoplasm of <u>cecum</u>
    Benign neoplasm of ileocecal valve

D12.1 Benign neoplasm of <u>appendix</u>
    Excludes 1:   *benign carcinoid tumor of the appendix (D3A.020)*

D12.2 Benign neoplasm of <u>ascending colon</u>

D12.3 Benign neoplasm of <u>transverse colon</u>
    Benign neoplasm of hepatic flexure
    Benign neoplasm of splenic flexure

D12.4 Benign neoplasm of <u>descending colon</u>

D12.5 Benign neoplasm of <u>sigmoid colon</u>

D12.6 Benign neoplasm of colon, unspecified
Adenomatosis of colon
Benign neoplasm of large intestine NOS
Polyposis (hereditary) of colon
Excludes 1: *inflammatory polyp of colon (K51.4-)*
polyp of colon NOS (K63.5)

D12.7 Benign neoplasm of <u>rectosigmoid</u> junction

D12.8 Benign neoplasm of <u>rectum</u>
Excludes 1: *benign carcinoid tumor of the rectum (D3A.026)*

D12.9 Benign neoplasm of <u>anus and anal canal</u>
Benign neoplasm of anus NOS
Excludes 1: *benign neoplasm of anal margin (D22.5, D23.5)*
benign neoplasm of anal skin (D22.5, D23.5)
benign neoplasm of perianal skin (D22.5, D23.5)

D13- <u>Benign neoplasm</u> of other and ill-defined parts of digestive system — Any new and abnormal growth in which tumor cells progressively multiply, but lack the properties of invasion and metastases (see Malignant Neoplasm code catgories, by site, for anatomical description).
Excludes 1: *benign stromal tumors of digestive system (D21.4)*

D13.0 Benign neoplasm of <u>esophagus</u>

D13.1 Benign neoplasm of <u>stomach</u>
Excludes 1: *benign carcinoid tumor of the stomach (D3A.092)*

D13.2 Benign neoplasm of <u>duodenum</u>
Excludes 1: *benign carcinoid tumor of the duodenum (D3A.010)*

D13.3- Benign neoplasm of other and unspecified parts of small intestine
Excludes 1: *benign carcinoid tumors of the small intestine(D3A.01-)*
benign neoplasm of ileocecal valve (D12.0)

  D13.30 Benign neoplasm of unspecified part of small intestine

  D13.39 Benign neoplasm of other parts of small intestine

D13.4 Benign neoplasm of <u>liver</u>
Benign neoplasm of intrahepatic bile ducts

D13.5 Benign neoplasm of <u>extrahepatic bile ducts</u>

D13.6 Benign neoplasm of <u>pancreas</u>
Excludes 1: *benign neoplasm of endocrine pancreas (D13.7)*

D13.7 Benign neoplasm of <u>endocrine pancreas</u>
Islet cell tumor
Benign neoplasm of islets of Langerhans
Use additional code to identify any functional activity.

D13.9 Benign neoplasm of ill-defined sites within the digestive system
Benign neoplasm of digestive system NOS
Benign neoplasm of intestine NOS
Benign neoplasm of spleen

D14- <u>Benign neoplasm</u> of middle ear and respiratory system — Any new and abnormal growth in which tumor cells progressively multiply, but lack the properties of invasion and metastases (see Malignant Neoplasm code catgories, by site, for anatomical description).

D14.0 Benign neoplasm of middle ear, nasal cavity and accessory sinuses
Benign neoplasm of cartilage of nose
Excludes 1: *benign neoplasm of auricular canal (external) (D22.2-, D23.2-)*
benign neoplasm of bone of ear (D16.4)
benign neoplasm of bone of nose (D16.4)
benign neoplasm of cartilage of ear (D21.0)
benign neoplasm of ear (external) (skin) (D22.2-, D23.2-)
benign neoplasm of nose NOS (D36.7)
benign neoplasm of skin of nose (D22.39, D23.39)
benign neoplasm of olfactory bulb (D33.3)
benign neoplasm of posterior margin of septum and choanae (D10.6)
polyp of accessory sinus (J33.8)
polyp of ear (middle) (H74.4)
polyp of nasal (cavity) (J33.-)

D14.1 Benign neoplasm of <u>larynx</u>
Adenomatous polyp of larynx
Benign neoplasm of epiglottis (suprahyoid portion)
Excludes 1: *benign neoplasm of epiglottis, anterior aspect (D10.5)*
polyp (nonadenomatous) of vocal cord or larynx (J38.1)

D14.2 Benign neoplasm of <u>trachea</u>

D14.3- Benign neoplasm of <u>bronchus and lung</u>
Excludes 1: *benign carcinoid tumor of the bronchus and lung (D3A.090)*

  D14.30 Benign neoplasm of unspecified bronchus and lung

  D14.31 Benign neoplasm of <u>right</u> bronchus and lung

  D14.32 Benign neoplasm of <u>left</u> bronchus and lung

D14.4 Benign neoplasm of respiratory system, unspecified

D15- <u>Benign neoplasm</u> of other and unspecified intrathoracic organs — Any new and abnormal growth in which tumor cells progressively multiply, but lack the properties of invasion and metastases (see Malignant Neoplasm code catgories, by site, for anatomical description).
Excludes 1: *benign neoplasm of mesothelial tissue (D19.-)*

D15.0 Benign neoplasm of <u>thymus</u>
Excludes 1: *benign carcinoid tumor of the thymus (D3A.091)*

D15.1 Benign neoplasm of <u>heart</u>
Excludes 1: *benign neoplasm of great vessels (D21.3)*

D15.2 Benign neoplasm of <u>mediastinum</u>

D15.7 Benign neoplasm of other specified intrathoracic organs

D15.9 Benign neoplasm of intrathoracic organ, unspecified

D16- <u>Benign neoplasm</u> of bone and articular cartilage — Any new and abnormal growth of in which tumor cells progressively multiply, but lack the properties of invasion and metastases (see Malignant Neoplasm code catgories, by site, for anatomical description).
Excludes 1: *benign neoplasm of connective tissue of ear (D21.0)*
benign neoplasm of connective tissue of eyelid (D21.0)
benign neoplasm of connective tissue of larynx (D14.1)
benign neoplasm of connective tissue of nose (D14.0)
benign neoplasm of synovia (D21.-)

D16.0- Benign neoplasm of <u>scapula and long bones of upper limb</u>

  D16.00 Benign neoplasm of scapula and long bones of unspecified upper limb

  D16.01 Benign neoplasm of scapula and long bones of <u>right</u> upper limb

  D16.02 Benign neoplasm of scapula and long bones of <u>left</u> upper limb

D16.1- Benign neoplasm of <u>short bones of upper limb</u>

  D16.10 Benign neoplasm of short bones of unspecified upper limb

  D16.11 Benign neoplasm of short bones of <u>right</u> upper limb

  D16.12 Benign neoplasm of short bones of <u>left</u> upper limb

D16.2- Benign neoplasm of <u>long bones of lower limb</u>

  D16.20 Benign neoplasm of long bones of unspecified lower limb

  D16.21 Benign neoplasm of long bones of <u>right</u> lower limb

  D16.22 Benign neoplasm of long bones of <u>left</u> lower limb

D16.3- Benign neoplasm of <u>short bones of lower limb</u>

  D16.30 Benign neoplasm of short bones of unspecified lower limb

  D16.31 Benign neoplasm of short bones of <u>right</u> lower limb

  D16.32 Benign neoplasm of short bones of <u>left</u> lower limb

D16.4 Benign neoplasm of <u>bones of skull and face</u>
Benign neoplasm of maxilla (superior)
Benign neoplasm of orbital bone
Keratocyst of maxilla
Keratocystic odontogenic tumor of maxilla
Excludes ❷: *benign neoplasm of lower jaw bone (D16.5)*

D16.5 Benign neoplasm of <u>lower jaw</u> bone
Keratocyst of mandible
Keratocystic odontogenic tumor of mandible

D16.6 Benign neoplasm of <u>vertebral</u> column
Excludes 1: *benign neoplasm of sacrum and coccyx (D16.8)*

D16.7 Benign neoplasm of <u>ribs, sternum and clavicle</u>

D16.8 Benign neoplasm of <u>pelvic bones, sacrum and coccyx</u>

D16.9 Benign neoplasm of bone and articular cartilage, unspecified

D17- <u>Benign lipomatous</u> neoplasm — Any new and abnormal growth of adipose cells (fat) in which tumor cells progressively multiply, but lack the properties of invasion and metastases (see Malignant Neoplasm code catgories, by site, for anatomical description).

D17.0 Benign lipomatous neoplasm of <u>skin</u> and subcutaneous tissue of <u>head, face and neck</u>

D17.1 Benign lipomatous neoplasm of <u>skin</u> and subcutaneous tissue of <u>trunk</u>

D12 - D17

D17.2- Benign lipomatous neoplasm of <u>skin</u> and subcutaneous tissue of <u>limb</u>

D17.20 Benign lipomatous neoplasm of skin and subcutaneous tissue of unspecified limb

D17.21 Benign lipomatous neoplasm of skin and subcutaneous tissue of <u>right</u> arm

D17.22 Benign lipomatous neoplasm of skin and subcutaneous tissue of <u>left</u> arm

D17.23 Benign lipomatous neoplasm of skin and subcutaneous tissue of <u>right</u> leg

D17.24 Benign lipomatous neoplasm of skin and subcutaneous tissue of <u>left</u> leg

D17.3- Benign lipomatous neoplasm of <u>skin</u> and subcutaneous tissue of other and unspecified sites

D17.30 Benign lipomatous neoplasm of skin and subcutaneous tissue of unspecified sites

D17.39 Benign lipomatous neoplasm of skin and subcutaneous tissue of other sites

D17.4 Benign lipomatous neoplasm of <u>intrathoracic organs</u>

D17.5 Benign lipomatous neoplasm of <u>intra-abdominal organs</u>

Excludes 1: *benign lipomatous neoplasm of peritoneum and retroperitoneum (D17.79)*

D17.6 Benign lipomatous neoplasm of <u>spermatic cord</u> — [♂]

D17.7- Benign lipomatous neoplasm of other sites

D17.71 Benign lipomatous neoplasm of <u>kidney</u>

D17.72 Benign lipomatous neoplasm of <u>other genitourinary organ</u>

D17.79 Benign lipomatous neoplasm of <u>other sites</u>
Benign lipomatous neoplasm of peritoneum
Benign lipomatous neoplasm of retroperitoneum

D17.9 Benign lipomatous neoplasm, unspecified
Lipoma NOS

D18- Hemangioma and lymphangioma, any site

Excludes 1: *benign neoplasm of glomus jugulare (D35.6)*
blue or pigmented nevus (D22.-)
nevus NOS (D22.-)
vascular nevus (Q82.5)

D18.0- <u>Hemangioma</u> — Any new and abnormal growth of in which tumor cells of newly formed blood vessels progressively multiply, but lack the properties of invasion and metastases.
Angioma NOS
Cavernous nevus

D18.00 Hemangioma unspecified site

D18.01 Hemangioma of <u>skin</u> and subcutaneous tissue

D18.02 Hemangioma of <u>intracranial</u> structures

D18.03 Hemangioma of <u>intra-abdominal</u> structures

D18.09 Hemangioma of other sites

D18.1 <u>Lymphangioma</u>, any site — Any new and abnormal growth in which tumor cells of newly formed lymph spaces and channels progressively multiply, but lack the properties of invasion and metastases.

D19- <u>Benign neoplasm of mesothelial tissue</u> — Any new and abnormal growth of the tissue that lines most of the internal organs (mesothelium) in which tumor cells progressively multiply, but lack the properties of invasion and metastases (see Malignant Neoplasm code catgories, by site, for anatomical description).

D19.0 Benign neoplasm of mesothelial tissue of <u>pleura</u>

D19.1 Benign neoplasm of mesothelial tissue of <u>peritoneum</u>

D19.7 Benign neoplasm of mesothelial tissue of other sites

D19.9 Benign neoplasm of mesothelial tissue, unspecified
Benign mesothelioma NOS

D20- <u>Benign neoplasm</u> of <u>soft tissue</u> of retroperitoneum and peritoneum — Any new and abnormal growth in which tumor cells progressively multiply, but lack the properties of invasion and metastases (see Malignant Neoplasm code catgories, by site, for anatomical description).

Excludes 1: *benign lipomatous neoplasm of peritoneum and retroperitoneum (D17.79)*
benign neoplasm of mesothelial tissue (D19.-)

D20.0 Benign neoplasm of soft tissue of <u>retroperitoneum</u>

D20.1 Benign neoplasm of soft tissue of <u>peritoneum</u>

D21- <u>Other benign neoplasms</u> of <u>connective</u> and other soft tissue — Any new and abnormal growth in which tumor cells progressively multiply, but lack the properties of invasion and metastases (see Malignant Neoplasm code catgories, by site, for anatomical description).

Includes: Benign neoplasm of blood vessel
Benign neoplasm of bursa
Benign neoplasm of cartilage
Benign neoplasm of fascia
Benign neoplasm of fat
Benign neoplasm of ligament, except uterine
Benign neoplasm of lymphatic channel
Benign neoplasm of muscle
Benign neoplasm of synovia
Benign neoplasm of tendon (sheath)
Benign stromal tumors

Excludes 1: *benign neoplasm of articular cartilage (D16.-)*
benign neoplasm of cartilage of larynx (D14.1)
benign neoplasm of cartilage of nose (D14.0)
benign neoplasm of connective tissue of breast (D24.-)
benign neoplasm of peripheral nerves and autonomic nervous system (D36.1-)
benign neoplasm of peritoneum (D20.1)
benign neoplasm of retroperitoneum (D20.0)
benign neoplasm of uterine ligament, any (D28.2)
benign neoplasm of vascular tissue (D18.-)
hemangioma (D18.0-)
lipomatous neoplasm (D17.-)
lymphangioma (D18.1)
uterine leiomyoma (D25.-)

D21.0 Benign neoplasm of connective and other soft tissue of <u>head, face and neck</u>
Benign neoplasm of connective tissue of ear
Benign neoplasm of connective tissue of eyelid

Excludes 1: *benign neoplasm of connective tissue of orbit (D31.6-)*

D21.1- Benign neoplasm of connective and other soft tissue of <u>upper limb</u>, including shoulder

D21.10 Benign neoplasm of connective and other soft tissue of unspecified upper limb, including shoulder

D21.11 Benign neoplasm of connective and other soft tissue of <u>right</u> upper limb, including shoulder

D21.12 Benign neoplasm of connective and other soft tissue of <u>left</u> upper limb, including shoulder

D21.2- Benign neoplasm of connective and other soft tissue of <u>lower limb</u>, including hip

D21.20 Benign neoplasm of connective and other soft tissue of unspecified lower limb, including hip

D21.21 Benign neoplasm of connective and other soft tissue of <u>right</u> lower limb, including hip

D21.22 Benign neoplasm of connective and other soft tissue of <u>left</u> lower limb, including hip

D21.3 Benign neoplasm of connective and other soft tissue of <u>thorax</u>
Benign neoplasm of axilla
Benign neoplasm of diaphragm
Benign neoplasm of great vessels

Excludes 1: *benign neoplasm of heart (D15.1)*
benign neoplasm of mediastinum (D15.2)
benign neoplasm of thymus (D15.0)

D21.4 Benign neoplasm of connective and other soft tissue of <u>abdomen</u>
Benign stromal tumors of abdomen

D21.5 Benign neoplasm of connective and other soft tissue of <u>pelvis</u>

Excludes 1: *benign neoplasm of any uterine ligament (D28.2)*
uterine leiomyoma (D25.-)

D21.6 Benign neoplasm of connective and other soft tissue of trunk, unspecified
Benign neoplasm of back NOS

D21.9 Benign neoplasm of connective and other soft tissue, unspecified

D17 - D21

D22- <u>Melanocytic nevi</u> — Any new and abnormal growth in which pigment-producing cells (a type of melanocyte) progressively multiply, but lack the properties of invasion and metastases (see Malignant Neoplasm code catgories, by site, for anatomical description).
Includes: Atypical nevus
Blue hairy pigmented nevus
Nevus NOS

D22.0 Melanocytic nevi of <u>lip</u>

D22.1- Melanocytic nevi of <u>eyelid, including canthus</u>

D22.10 Melanocytic nevi of unspecified eyelid, including canthus

D22.11 Melanocytic nevi of <u>right</u> eyelid, including canthus

D22.12 Melanocytic nevi of <u>left</u> eyelid, including canthus

D22.2- Melanocytic nevi of <u>ear and external auricular canal</u>

D22.20 Melanocytic nevi of unspecified ear and external auricular canal

D22.21 Melanocytic nevi of <u>right</u> ear and external auricular canal

D22.22 Melanocytic nevi of <u>left</u> ear and external auricular canal

D22.3- Melanocytic nevi of other and unspecified parts of face

D22.30 Melanocytic nevi of unspecified part of face

D22.39 Melanocytic nevi of other parts of face

D22.4 Melanocytic nevi of <u>scalp and neck</u>

D22.5 Melanocytic nevi of <u>trunk</u>
Melanocytic nevi of anal margin
Melanocytic nevi of anal skin
Melanocytic nevi of perianal skin
Melanocytic nevi of skin of breast

D22.6- Melanocytic nevi of <u>upper limb</u>, including shoulder

D22.60 Melanocytic nevi of unspecified upper limb, including shoulder

D22.61 Melanocytic nevi of <u>right</u> upper limb, including shoulder

D22.62 Melanocytic nevi of <u>left</u> upper limb, including shoulder

D22.7- Melanocytic nevi of <u>lower limb</u>, including hip

D22.70 Melanocytic nevi of unspecified lower limb, including hip

D22.71 Melanocytic nevi of <u>right</u> lower limb, including hip

D22.72 Melanocytic nevi of <u>left</u> lower limb, including hip

D22.9 Melanocytic nevi, unspecified

D23- <u>Other benign neoplasms</u> of skin — Any new and abnormal growth in which skin cells progressively multiply, but lack the properties of invasion and metastases (see Malignant Neoplasm code catgories, by site, for anatomical description).
Includes: Benign neoplasm of hair follicles
Benign neoplasm of sebaceous glands
Benign neoplasm of sweat glands
Excludes 1: *benign lipomatous neoplasms of skin (D17.0-D17.3)*
melanocytic nevi (D22.-)

D23.0 <u>Other</u> benign neoplasm of <u>skin</u> of <u>lip</u>
Excludes 1: *benign neoplasm of vermilion border of lip (D10.0)*

D23.1- <u>Other</u> benign neoplasm of <u>skin</u> of <u>eyelid, including canthus</u>

D23.10 Other benign neoplasm of skin of unspecified eyelid, including canthus

D23.11 Other benign neoplasm of skin of <u>right</u> eyelid, including canthus

D23.12 Other benign neoplasm of skin of <u>left</u> eyelid, including canthus

D23.2- <u>Other</u> benign neoplasm of <u>skin</u> of <u>ear and external auricular canal</u>

D23.20 Other benign neoplasm of skin of unspecified ear and external auricular canal

D23.21 Other benign neoplasm of skin of <u>right</u> ear and external auricular canal

D23.22 Other benign neoplasm of skin of <u>left</u> ear and external auricular canal

D23.3- <u>Other</u> benign neoplasm of <u>skin</u> of other and unspecified parts of face

D23.30 Other benign neoplasm of skin of unspecified part of face

D23.39 Other benign neoplasm of skin of other parts of face

D23.4 <u>Other</u> benign neoplasm of <u>skin</u> of <u>scalp and neck</u>

D23.5 <u>Other</u> benign neoplasm of <u>skin</u> of <u>trunk</u>
Other benign neoplasm of anal margin
Other benign neoplasm of anal skin
Other benign neoplasm of perianal skin
Other benign neoplasm of skin of breast
Excludes 1: *benign neoplasm of anus NOS (D12.9)*

D23.6- <u>Other</u> benign neoplasm of <u>skin</u> of <u>upper limb</u>, including shoulder

D23.60 Other benign neoplasm of skin of unspecified upper limb, including shoulder

D23.61 Other benign neoplasm of skin of <u>right</u> upper limb, including shoulder

D23.62 Other benign neoplasm of skin of <u>left</u> upper limb, including shoulder

D23.7- <u>Other</u> benign neoplasm of <u>skin</u> of <u>lower limb</u>, including hip

D23.70 Other benign neoplasm of skin of unspecified lower limb, including hip

D23.71 Other benign neoplasm of skin of <u>right</u> lower limb, including hip

D23.72 Other benign neoplasm of skin of <u>left</u> lower limb, including hip

D23.9 <u>Other</u> benign neoplasm of <u>skin</u>, unspecified

D24- <u>Benign neoplasm</u> of breast — Any new and abnormal growth in which tumor cells progressively multiply, but lack the properties of invasion and metastases (see Malignant Neoplasm code catgories, by site, for anatomical description).
Includes: Benign neoplasm of connective tissue of breast
Benign neoplasm of soft parts of breast
Fibroadenoma of breast
Excludes ❷: *adenofibrosis of breast (N60.2)*
benign cyst of breast (N60.-)
benign mammary dysplasia (N60.-)
benign neoplasm of skin of breast (D22.5, D23.5)
fibrocystic disease of breast (N60.-)

D24.1 Benign neoplasm of <u>right</u> breast

D24.2 Benign neoplasm of <u>left</u> breast

D24.9 Benign neoplasm of unspecified breast

D25- <u>Leiomyoma</u> of uterus — Any new and abnormal growth in which tumor cells progressively multiply, but lack the properties of invasion and metastases (see Malignant Neoplasm code catgories, by site, for anatomical description).
Includes: Uterine fibroid
Uterine fibromyoma
Uterine myoma

D25.0 <u>Submucous</u> leiomyoma of uterus —[♀]

D25.1 <u>Intramural</u> leiomyoma of uterus —[♀]
Interstitial leiomyoma of uterus

D25.2 <u>Subserosal</u> leiomyoma of uterus —[♀]
Subperitoneal leiomyoma of uterus

D25.9 Leiomyoma of uterus, unspecified —[♀]

D26- <u>Other</u> benign neoplasms of <u>uterus</u> — Any new and abnormal growth in which tumor cells progressively multiply, but lack the properties of invasion and metastases (see Malignant Neoplasm code catgories, by site, for anatomical description).

D26.0 Other benign neoplasm of <u>cervix</u> uteri —[♀]

D26.1 Other benign neoplasm of <u>corpus</u> uteri —[♀]

D26.7 Other benign neoplasm of other parts of uterus —[♀]

D26.9 Other benign neoplasm of uterus, unspecified —[♀]

D27- <u>Benign neoplasm</u> of ovary — Any new and abnormal growth in which tumor cells progressively multiply, but lack the properties of invasion and metastases (see Malignant Neoplasm code catgories, by site, for anatomical description).
Use additional code to identify any functional activity.
Excludes ❷: *corpus albicans cyst (N83.2-)*
corpus luteum cyst (N83.1-)
endometrial cyst (N80.1)
follicular (atretic) cyst (N83.0-)
graafian follicle cyst (N83.0-)
ovarian cyst NEC (N83.2-)
ovarian retention cyst (N83.2-)

D27.0 Benign neoplasm of <u>right</u> ovary —[♀]

D27.1 Benign neoplasm of <u>left</u> ovary —[♀]

D27.9 Benign neoplasm of unspecified ovary —[♀]

D28- <u>Benign neoplasm</u> **of other and unspecified female genital organs** — Any new and abnormal growth in which tumor cells progressively multiply, but lack the properties of invasion and metastases (see Malignant Neoplasm code catgories, by site, for anatomical description).

Includes: Adenomatous polyp
            Benign neoplasm of skin of female genital organs
            Benign teratoma

Excludes 1:   *epoophoron cyst (Q50.5)*
            fimbrial cyst (Q50.4)
            Gartner's duct cyst (Q52.4)
            parovarian cyst (Q50.5)

D28.0   **Benign neoplasm of <u>vulva</u>** — [♀]

D28.1   **Benign neoplasm of <u>vagina</u>** — [♀]

D28.2   **Benign neoplasm of <u>uterine tubes and ligaments</u>** — [♀]
            Benign neoplasm of fallopian tube
            Benign neoplasm of uterine ligament (broad) (round)

D28.7   **Benign neoplasm of other specified female genital organs** — [♀]

D28.9   **Benign neoplasm of female genital organ, unspecified** — [♀]

D29- <u>Benign neoplasm</u> **of male genital organs** — Any new and abnormal growth in which tumor cells progressively multiply, but lack the properties of invasion and metastases (see Malignant Neoplasm code catgories, by site, for anatomical description).

Includes: Benign neoplasm of skin of male genital organs

D29.0   **Benign neoplasm of <u>penis</u>** — [♂]

D29.1   **Benign neoplasm of <u>prostate</u>** — [♂]
            Excludes 1:   *enlarged prostate (N40.-)*

D29.2- **Benign neoplasm of <u>testis</u>**
            Use additional code to identify any functional activity.

   D29.20   **Benign neoplasm of unspecified testis** — [♂]

   D29.21   **Benign neoplasm of <u>right</u> testis** — [♂]

   D29.22   **Benign neoplasm of <u>left</u> testis** — [♂]

D29.3- **Benign neoplasm of <u>epididymis</u>**

   D29.30   **Benign neoplasm of unspecified epididymis** — [♂]

   D29.31   **Benign neoplasm of <u>right</u> epididymis** — [♂]

   D29.32   **Benign neoplasm of <u>left</u> epididymis** — [♂]

D29.4   **Benign neoplasm of <u>scrotum</u>** — [♂]
            Benign neoplasm of skin of scrotum

D29.8   **Benign neoplasm of other specified male genital organs** — [♂]
            Benign neoplasm of seminal vesicle
            Benign neoplasm of spermatic cord
            Benign neoplasm of tunica vaginalis

D29.9   **Benign neoplasm of male genital organ, unspecified** — [♂]

D30- <u>Benign neoplasm</u> **of urinary organs** — Any new and abnormal growth in which tumor cells progressively multiply, but lack the properties of invasion and metastases (see Malignant Neoplasm code catgories, by site, for anatomical description).

D30.0- **Benign neoplasm of <u>kidney</u>**
            Excludes 1:   *benign carcinoid tumor of the kidney (D3A.093)*
            benign neoplasm of renal calyces (D30.1-)
            benign neoplasm of renal pelvis (D30.1-)

   D30.00   **Benign neoplasm of unspecified kidney**

   D30.01   **Benign neoplasm of <u>right</u> kidney**

   D30.02   **Benign neoplasm of <u>left</u> kidney**

D30.1- **Benign neoplasm of <u>renal pelvis</u>**

   D30.10   **Benign neoplasm of unspecified renal pelvis**

   D30.11   **Benign neoplasm of <u>right</u> renal pelvis**

   D30.12   **Benign neoplasm of <u>left</u> renal pelvis**

D30.2- **Benign neoplasm of <u>ureter</u>**
            Excludes 1:   *benign neoplasm of ureteric orifice of bladder (D30.3)*

   D30.20   **Benign neoplasm of unspecified ureter**

   D30.21   **Benign neoplasm of <u>right</u> ureter**

   D30.22   **Benign neoplasm of <u>left</u> ureter**

D30.3   **Benign neoplasm of <u>bladder</u>**
            Benign neoplasm of ureteric orifice of bladder
            Benign neoplasm of urethral orifice of bladder

D30.4   **Benign neoplasm of <u>urethra</u>**
            Excludes 1:   *benign neoplasm of urethral orifice of bladder (D30.3)*

D30.8   **Benign neoplasm of other specified urinary organs**
            Benign neoplasm of paraurethral glands

D30.9   **Benign neoplasm of urinary organ, unspecified**
            Benign neoplasm of urinary system NOS

D31- <u>Benign neoplasm</u> **of eye and adnexa** — Any new and abnormal growth in which tumor cells progressively multiply, but lack the properties of invasion and metastases (see Malignant Neoplasm code catgories, by site, for anatomical description).

Excludes 1:   *benign neoplasm of connective tissue of eyelid (D21.0)*
            benign neoplasm of optic nerve (D33.3)
            benign neoplasm of skin of eyelid (D22.1-, D23.1-)

D31.0- **Benign neoplasm of <u>conjunctiva</u>**

   D31.00   **Benign neoplasm of unspecified conjunctiva**

   D31.01   **Benign neoplasm of <u>right</u> conjunctiva**

   D31.02   **Benign neoplasm of <u>left</u> conjunctiva**

D31.1- **Benign neoplasm of <u>cornea</u>**

   D31.10   **Benign neoplasm of unspecified cornea**

   D31.11   **Benign neoplasm of <u>right</u> cornea**

   D31.12   **Benign neoplasm of <u>left</u> cornea**

D31.2- **Benign neoplasm of <u>retina</u>**
            Excludes 1:   *dark area on retina (D49.81)*
            hemangioma of retina (D49.81)
            neoplasm of unspecified behavior of retina and choroid (D49.81)
            retinal freckle (D49.81)

   D31.20   **Benign neoplasm of unspecified retina**

   D31.21   **Benign neoplasm of <u>right</u> retina**

   D31.22   **Benign neoplasm of <u>left</u> retina**

D31.3- **Benign neoplasm of <u>choroid</u>**

   D31.30   **Benign neoplasm of unspecified choroid**

   D31.31   **Benign neoplasm of <u>right</u> choroid**

   D31.32   **Benign neoplasm of <u>left</u> choroid**

D31.4- **Benign neoplasm of <u>ciliary body</u>**

   D31.40   **Benign neoplasm of unspecified ciliary body**

   D31.41   **Benign neoplasm of <u>right</u> ciliary body**

   D31.42   **Benign neoplasm of <u>left</u> ciliary body**

D31.5- **Benign neoplasm of <u>lacrimal gland and duct</u>**
            Benign neoplasm of lacrimal sac
            Benign neoplasm of nasolacrimal duct

   D31.50   **Benign neoplasm of unspecified lacrimal gland and duct**

   D31.51   **Benign neoplasm of <u>right</u> lacrimal gland and duct**

   D31.52   **Benign neoplasm of <u>left</u> lacrimal gland and duct**

D31.6- **Benign neoplasm of unspecified site of orbit**
            Benign neoplasm of connective tissue of orbit
            Benign neoplasm of extraocular muscle
            Benign neoplasm of peripheral nerves of orbit
            Benign neoplasm of retrobulbar tissue
            Benign neoplasm of retro-ocular tissue
            Excludes 1:   *benign neoplasm of orbital bone (D16.4)*

   D31.60   **Benign neoplasm of unspecified site of unspecified orbit**

   D31.61   **Benign neoplasm of unspecified site of <u>right</u> orbit**

   D31.62   **Benign neoplasm of unspecified site of <u>left</u> orbit**

D31.9- **Benign neoplasm of unspecified part of eye**
            Benign neoplasm of eyeball

   D31.90   **Benign neoplasm of unspecified part of unspecified eye**

   D31.91   **Benign neoplasm of unspecified part of <u>right</u> eye**

   D31.92   **Benign neoplasm of unspecified part of <u>left</u> eye**

D32- <u>Benign neoplasm</u> **of meninges** — Any new and abnormal growth in which tumor cells progressively multiply, but lack the properties of invasion and metastases (see Malignant Neoplasm code catgories, by site, for anatomical description).

D32.0   **Benign neoplasm of <u>cerebral meninges</u>**

D32.1   **Benign neoplasm of <u>spinal meninges</u>**

D32.9   **Benign neoplasm of meninges, unspecified**
            Meningioma NOS

D33- <u>Benign neoplasm</u> of brain and other parts of central nervous system — Any new and abnormal growth in which tumor cells progressively multiply, but lack the properties of invasion and metastases (see Malignant Neoplasm code catgories, by site, for anatomical description).

Excludes 1:   angioma (D18.0-)
           benign neoplasm of meninges (D32.-)
           benign neoplasm of peripheral nerves and autonomic nervous system (D36.1-)
           hemangioma (D18.0-)
           neurofibromatosis (Q85.0-)
           retro-ocular benign neoplasm (D31.6-)

D33.0   Benign neoplasm of <u>brain, supratentorial</u>
     Benign neoplasm of cerebral ventricle
     Benign neoplasm of cerebrum
     Benign neoplasm of frontal lobe
     Benign neoplasm of occipital lobe
     Benign neoplasm of parietal lobe
     Benign neoplasm of temporal lobe
     Excludes 1:   benign neoplasm of fourth ventricle (D33.1)

D33.1   Benign neoplasm of <u>brain, infratentorial</u>
     Benign neoplasm of brain stem
     Benign neoplasm of cerebellum
     Benign neoplasm of fourth ventricle

D33.2   Benign neoplasm of brain, unspecified

D33.3   Benign neoplasm of <u>cranial nerves</u>
     Benign neoplasm of olfactory bulb

D33.4   Benign neoplasm of <u>spinal cord</u>

D33.7   Benign neoplasm of other specified parts of central nervous system

D33.9   Benign neoplasm of central nervous system, unspecified
     Benign neoplasm of nervous system (central) NOS

D34   <u>Benign neoplasm</u> of <u>thyroid</u> gland — Any new and abnormal growth in which tumor cells progressively multiply, but lack the properties of invasion and metastases (see Malignant Neoplasm code catgories, by site, for anatomical description).
Use additional code to identify any functional activity

D35- <u>Benign neoplasm</u> of other and unspecified endocrine glands — Any new and abnormal growth in which tumor cells progressively multiply, but lack the properties of invasion and metastases (see Malignant Neoplasm code catgories, by site, for anatomical description).
Use additional code to identify any functional activity
Excludes 1:   benign neoplasm of endocrine pancreas (D13.7)
           benign neoplasm of ovary (D27.-)
           benign neoplasm of testis (D29.2.-)
           benign neoplasm of thymus (D15.0)

D35.0-   Benign neoplasm of <u>adrenal gland</u>
   D35.00   Benign neoplasm of unspecified adrenal gland
   D35.01   Benign neoplasm of <u>right</u> adrenal gland
   D35.02   Benign neoplasm of <u>left</u> adrenal gland

D35.1   Benign neoplasm of <u>parathyroid gland</u>

D35.2   Benign neoplasm of <u>pituitary gland</u>
     AHA 14:3Q:p22 – Pituitary macroadenoma

D35.3   Benign neoplasm of <u>craniopharyngeal duct</u>

D35.4   Benign neoplasm of <u>pineal gland</u>

D35.5   Benign neoplasm of <u>carotid body</u>

D35.6   Benign neoplasm of <u>aortic body</u> and other <u>paraganglia</u>
     Benign tumor of glomus jugulare

D35.7   Benign neoplasm of other specified <u>endocrine glands</u>

D35.9   Benign neoplasm of endocrine gland, unspecified
     Benign neoplasm of unspecified endocrine gland

D36- <u>Benign neoplasm</u> of other and unspecified sites — Any new and abnormal growth in which tumor cells progressively multiply, but lack the properties of invasion and metastases (see Malignant Neoplasm code catgories, by site, for anatomical description).

D36.0   Benign neoplasm of lymph nodes
     Excludes 1:   lymphangioma (D18.1)

D36.1-   Benign neoplasm of <u>peripheral nerves</u> and <u>autonomic nervous system</u>
     Excludes 1:   benign neoplasm of peripheral nerves of orbit (D31.6-)
                neurofibromatosis (Q85.0-)

   D36.10   Benign neoplasm of peripheral nerves and autonomic nervous system, unspecified
   D36.11   Benign neoplasm of peripheral nerves and autonomic nervous system of <u>face, head, and neck</u>

D36.12   Benign neoplasm of peripheral nerves and autonomic nervous system, <u>upper limb</u>, including shoulder

D36.13   Benign neoplasm of peripheral nerves and autonomic nervous system of <u>lower limb</u>, including hip

D36.14   Benign neoplasm of peripheral nerves and autonomic nervous system of <u>thorax</u>

D36.15   Benign neoplasm of peripheral nerves and autonomic nervous system of <u>abdomen</u>

D36.16   Benign neoplasm of peripheral nerves and autonomic nervous system of <u>pelvis</u>

D36.17   Benign neoplasm of peripheral nerves and autonomic nervous system of trunk, unspecified

D36.7   Benign neoplasm of other specified sites
     Benign neoplasm of nose NOS

D36.9   Benign neoplasm, unspecified site

Benign neuroendocrine tumors (D3A)

D3A- <u>Benign neuroendocrine tumors</u> — Any new and abnormal growth that arises from endocrine or neuroendocrine cells rather than from where the tumor is located in which tumor cells progressively multiply, but lack the properties of invasion and metastases (see Malignant Neoplasm code catgories, by site, for anatomical description).
Use additional code to identify any associated endocrine syndrome, such as: Carcinoid syndrome (E34.0)
Excludes ❷: benign pancreatic islet cell tumors (D13.7)
Code also any associated multiple endocrine neoplasia [MEN] syndromes (E31.2-)

D3A.0-   <u>Benign carcinoid</u> tumors
   D3A.00   <u>Benign carcinoid</u> tumor of unspecified site
       Carcinoid tumor NOS

   D3A.01- <u>Benign carcinoid</u> tumors of the small intestine
     D3A.010   Benign carcinoid tumor of the <u>duodenum</u>
     D3A.011   Benign carcinoid tumor of the <u>jejunum</u>
     D3A.012   Benign carcinoid tumor of the <u>ileum</u>
     D3A.019   Benign carcinoid tumor of the small intestine, unspecified portion

   D3A.02- <u>Benign carcinoid</u> tumors of the appendix, large intestine, and rectum
     D3A.020   Benign carcinoid tumor of the <u>appendix</u>
     D3A.021   Benign carcinoid tumor of the <u>cecum</u>
     D3A.022   Benign carcinoid tumor of the <u>ascending colon</u>
     D3A.023   Benign carcinoid tumor of the <u>transverse colon</u>
     D3A.024   Benign carcinoid tumor of the <u>descending colon</u>
     D3A.025   Benign carcinoid tumor of the <u>sigmoid colon</u>
     D3A.026   Benign carcinoid tumor of the <u>rectum</u>
     D3A.029   Benign carcinoid tumor of the large intestine, unspecified portion
         Benign carcinoid tumor of the colon NOS

   D3A.09- <u>Benign carcinoid</u> tumors of other sites
     D3A.090   Benign carcinoid tumor of the <u>bronchus and lung</u>
     D3A.091   Benign carcinoid tumor of the <u>thymus</u>
     D3A.092   Benign carcinoid tumor of the <u>stomach</u>
     D3A.093   Benign carcinoid tumor of the <u>kidney</u>
     D3A.094   Benign carcinoid tumor of the foregut, unspecified
     D3A.095   Benign carcinoid tumor of the midgut, unspecified
     D3A.096   Benign carcinoid tumor of the hindgut, unspecified
     D3A.098   Benign carcinoid tumors of other sites

D3A.8   <u>Other benign neuroendocrine</u> tumors
     Neuroendocrine tumor NOS

D
3
3
–
D
3
A

Neoplasms of uncertain behavior, polycythemia vera and myelodysplastic syndromes (D37-D48)

Note: Categories D37-D44, and D48 classify by site neoplasms of uncertain behavior, i.e., histologic confirmation whether the neoplasm is malignant or benign cannot be made.

Excludes 1:   neoplasms of unspecified behavior (D49.-)

D37- Neoplasm of <u>uncertain behavior</u> of oral cavity and digestive organs — See Note and Excludes 1 at code block D37-D48.

Excludes 1:   stromal tumors of uncertain behavior of digestive system (D48.1)

D37.0- Neoplasm of uncertain behavior of lip, oral cavity and pharynx

Excludes 1:   neoplasm of uncertain behavior of aryepiglottic fold or interarytenoid fold, laryngeal aspect (D38.0)
neoplasm of uncertain behavior of epiglottis NOS (D38.0)
neoplasm of uncertain behavior of skin of lip (D48.5)
neoplasm of uncertain behavior of suprahyoid portion of epiglottis (D38.0)

D37.01 Neoplasm of uncertain behavior of <u>lip</u>
Neoplasm of uncertain behavior of vermilion border of lip

D37.02 Neoplasm of uncertain behavior of <u>tongue</u>

D37.03- Neoplasm of uncertain behavior of the <u>major</u> salivary glands

D37.030 Neoplasm of uncertain behavior of the <u>parotid</u> salivary glands

D37.031 Neoplasm of uncertain behavior of the <u>sublingual</u> salivary glands

D37.032 Neoplasm of uncertain behavior of the <u>submandibular</u> salivary glands

D37.039 Neoplasm of uncertain behavior of the major salivary glands, unspecified

D37.04 Neoplasm of uncertain behavior of the <u>minor</u> salivary glands
Neoplasm of uncertain behavior of submucosal salivary glands of lip
Neoplasm of uncertain behavior of submucosal salivary glands of cheek
Neoplasm of uncertain behavior of submucosal salivary glands of hard palate
Neoplasm of uncertain behavior of submucosal salivary glands of soft palate

D37.05 Neoplasm of uncertain behavior of <u>pharynx</u>
Neoplasm of uncertain behavior of aryepiglottic fold of pharynx NOS
Neoplasm of uncertain behavior of hypopharyngeal aspect of aryepiglottic fold of pharynx
Neoplasm of uncertain behavior of marginal zone of aryepiglottic fold of pharynx

D37.09 Neoplasm of uncertain behavior of other specified sites of the oral cavity

D37.1 Neoplasm of uncertain behavior of <u>stomach</u>

D37.2 Neoplasm of uncertain behavior of <u>small intestine</u>

D37.3 Neoplasm of uncertain behavior of <u>appendix</u>

D37.4 Neoplasm of uncertain behavior of <u>colon</u>

D37.5 Neoplasm of uncertain behavior of <u>rectum</u>
Neoplasm of uncertain behavior of rectosigmoid junction

D37.6 Neoplasm of uncertain behavior of <u>liver, gallbladder and bile ducts</u>
Neoplasm of uncertain behavior of ampulla of Vater

D37.8 Neoplasm of uncertain behavior of other specified digestive organs
Neoplasm of uncertain behavior of anal canal
Neoplasm of uncertain behavior of anal sphincter
Neoplasm of uncertain behavior of anus NOS
Neoplasm of uncertain behavior of esophagus
Neoplasm of uncertain behavior of intestine NOS
Neoplasm of uncertain behavior of pancreas

Excludes 1:   neoplasm of uncertain behavior of anal margin (D48.5)
neoplasm of uncertain behavior of anal skin (D48.5)
neoplasm of uncertain behavior of perianal skin (D48.5)

D37.9 Neoplasm of uncertain behavior of digestive organ, unspecified

D38- Neoplasm of <u>uncertain behavior</u> of middle ear and respiratory and intrathoracic organs — See Note and Excludes 1 at code block D37-D48.

Excludes 1:   neoplasm of uncertain behavior of heart (D48.7)

D38.0 Neoplasm of uncertain behavior of <u>larynx</u>
Neoplasm of uncertain behavior of aryepiglottic fold or interarytenoid fold, laryngeal aspect
Neoplasm of uncertain behavior of epiglottis (suprahyoid portion)

Excludes 1:   neoplasm of uncertain behavior of aryepiglottic fold or interarytenoid fold NOS (D37.05)
neoplasm of uncertain behavior of hypopharyngeal aspect of aryepiglottic fold (D37.05)
neoplasm of uncertain behavior of marginal zone of aryepiglottic fold (D37.05)

D38.1 Neoplasm of uncertain behavior of <u>trachea, bronchus and lung</u>

D38.2 Neoplasm of uncertain behavior of <u>pleura</u>

D38.3 Neoplasm of uncertain behavior of <u>mediastinum</u>

D38.4 Neoplasm of uncertain behavior of <u>thymus</u>

D38.5 Neoplasm of uncertain behavior of other respiratory organs
Neoplasm of uncertain behavior of accessory sinuses
Neoplasm of uncertain behavior of cartilage of nose
Neoplasm of uncertain behavior of middle ear
Neoplasm of uncertain behavior of nasal cavities

Excludes 1:   neoplasm of uncertain behavior of ear (external) (skin) (D48.5)
neoplasm of uncertain behavior of nose NOS (D48.7)
neoplasm of uncertain behavior of skin of nose (D48.5)

D38.6 Neoplasm of uncertain behavior of respiratory organ, unspecified

D39- Neoplasm of <u>uncertain behavior</u> of female genital organs — See Note and Excludes 1 at code block D37-D48.

D39.0 Neoplasm of uncertain behavior of <u>uterus</u> — [♀]

D39.1- Neoplasm of uncertain behavior of <u>ovary</u>
Use additional code to identify any functional activity.

D39.10 Neoplasm of uncertain behavior of unspecified ovary — [♀]

D39.11 Neoplasm of uncertain behavior of <u>right</u> ovary — [♀]

D39.12 Neoplasm of uncertain behavior of <u>left</u> ovary — [♀]

D39.2 Neoplasm of uncertain behavior of <u>placenta</u> — [♀, Age/12-55]
Chorioadenoma destruens
Invasive hydatidiform mole
Malignant hydatidiform mole

Excludes 1:   hydatidiform mole NOS (O01.9)

D39.8 Neoplasm of uncertain behavior of other specified female genital organs — [♀]
Neoplasm of uncertain behavior of skin of female genital organs

D39.9 Neoplasm of uncertain behavior of female genital organ, unspecified — [♀]

D40- Neoplasm of <u>uncertain behavior</u> of male genital organs — See Note and Excludes 1 at code block D37-D48.

D40.0 Neoplasm of uncertain behavior of <u>prostate</u> — [♂]

D40.1- Neoplasm of uncertain behavior of <u>testis</u>

D40.10 Neoplasm of uncertain behavior of unspecified testis — [♂]

D40.11 Neoplasm of uncertain behavior of <u>right</u> testis — [♂]

D40.12 Neoplasm of uncertain behavior of <u>left</u> testis — [♂]

D40.8 Neoplasm of uncertain behavior of other specified male genital organs — [♂]
Neoplasm of uncertain behavior of skin of male genital organs

D40.9 Neoplasm of uncertain behavior of male genital organ, unspecified — [♂]

D41- Neoplasm of <u>uncertain behavior</u> of urinary organs — See Note and Excludes 1 at code block D37-D48.

D41.0- Neoplasm of uncertain behavior of <u>kidney</u>

Excludes 1:   neoplasm of uncertain behavior of renal pelvis (D41.1-)

D41.00 Neoplasm of uncertain behavior of unspecified kidney

D41.01 Neoplasm of uncertain behavior of <u>right</u> kidney

D41.02 Neoplasm of uncertain behavior of <u>left</u> kidney

D37
–
D41

D41.1- Neoplasm of uncertain behavior of <u>renal pelvis</u>

  D41.10 Neoplasm of uncertain behavior of unspecified renal pelvis

  D41.11 Neoplasm of uncertain behavior of <u>right</u> renal pelvis

  D41.12 Neoplasm of uncertain behavior of <u>left</u> renal pelvis

D41.2- Neoplasm of uncertain behavior of <u>ureter</u>

  D41.20 Neoplasm of uncertain behavior of unspecified ureter

  D41.21 Neoplasm of uncertain behavior of <u>right</u> ureter

  D41.22 Neoplasm of uncertain behavior of <u>left</u> ureter

D41.3 Neoplasm of uncertain behavior of <u>urethra</u>

D41.4 Neoplasm of uncertain behavior of <u>bladder</u>

D41.8 Neoplasm of uncertain behavior of other specified urinary organs

D41.9 Neoplasm of uncertain behavior of unspecified urinary organ

D42- Neoplasm of <u>uncertain behavior</u> of meninges — See Note and Excludes 1 at code block D37-D48.

D42.0 Neoplasm of uncertain behavior of <u>cerebral meninges</u>

D42.1 Neoplasm of uncertain behavior of <u>spinal meninges</u>

D42.9 Neoplasm of uncertain behavior of meninges, unspecified

D43- Neoplasm of <u>uncertain behavior</u> of brain and central nervous system — See Note and Excludes 1 at code block D37-D48.

  Excludes 1:   neoplasm of uncertain behavior of peripheral nerves and autonomic nervous system (D48.2)

D43.0 Neoplasm of uncertain behavior of <u>brain, supratentorial</u>
  Neoplasm of uncertain behavior of cerebral ventricle
  Neoplasm of uncertain behavior of cerebrum
  Neoplasm of uncertain behavior of frontal lobe
  Neoplasm of uncertain behavior of occipital lobe
  Neoplasm of uncertain behavior of parietal lobe
  Neoplasm of uncertain behavior of temporal lobe

  Excludes 1:   neoplasm of uncertain behavior of fourth ventricle (D43.1)

D43.1 Neoplasm of uncertain behavior of <u>brain, infratentorial</u>
  Neoplasm of uncertain behavior of brain stem
  Neoplasm of uncertain behavior of cerebellum
  Neoplasm of uncertain behavior of fourth ventricle

D43.2 Neoplasm of uncertain behavior of brain, unspecified

D43.3 Neoplasm of uncertain behavior of <u>cranial nerves</u>

D43.4 Neoplasm of uncertain behavior of <u>spinal cord</u>

D43.8 Neoplasm of uncertain behavior of other specified parts of central nervous system

D43.9 Neoplasm of uncertain behavior of central nervous system, unspecified
  Neoplasm of uncertain behavior of nervous system (central) NOS

D44- Neoplasm of <u>uncertain behavior</u> of endocrine glands — See Note and Excludes 1 at code block D37-D48.

  Excludes 1:   multiple endocrine adenomatosis (E31.2-)
  multiple endocrine neoplasia (E31.2-)
  neoplasm of uncertain behavior of endocrine pancreas(D37.8)
  neoplasm of uncertain behavior of ovary (D39.1-)
  neoplasm of uncertain behavior of testis (D40.1-)
  neoplasm of uncertain behavior of thymus (D38.4)

D44.0 Neoplasm of uncertain behavior of <u>thyroid gland</u>

D44.1- Neoplasm of uncertain behavior of <u>adrenal gland</u>
  Use additional code to identify any functional activity.

  D44.10 Neoplasm of uncertain behavior of unspecified adrenal gland

  D44.11 Neoplasm of uncertain behavior of <u>right</u> adrenal gland

  D44.12 Neoplasm of uncertain behavior of <u>left</u> adrenal gland

D44.2 Neoplasm of uncertain behavior of <u>parathyroid gland</u>

D44.3 Neoplasm of uncertain behavior of <u>pituitary gland</u>
  Use additional code to identify any functional activity.

D44.4 Neoplasm of uncertain behavior of <u>craniopharyngeal duct</u>

D44.5 Neoplasm of uncertain behavior of <u>pineal gland</u>

D44.6 Neoplasm of uncertain behavior of <u>carotid body</u>

D44.7 Neoplasm of uncertain behavior of <u>aortic body</u> and other <u>paraganglia</u>

D44.9 Neoplasm of uncertain behavior of unspecified endocrine gland

D45 <u>Polycythemia vera</u> — A neoplastic proliferation disorder that is characterized by an abnormally high production and concentration of red blood cells (erythrocytes).

  Excludes 1:   familial polycythemia (D75.0)
  secondary polycythemia (D75.1)

D46- <u>Myelodysplastic syndromes</u> — A neoplastic bone marrow cell production disorder in which immature cells to not develop normally into mature, healthy cells.
  Use additional code for adverse effect, if applicable, to identify drug (T36-T50 with fifth or sixth character 5)

  Excludes 2:   drug-induced aplastic anemia (D61.1)

D46.0 Refractory anemia <u>without</u> ring sideroblasts, so stated
  Refractory anemia without sideroblasts, without excess of blasts

D46.1 Refractory anemia <u>with</u> ring sideroblasts — A form producing too few red blood cells and those cells have too much iron inside the cell.
  RARS

D46.2- Refractory anemia <u>with excess of blasts [RAEB]</u> — A form producing too few red blood cells and a greater than normal number of blast cells.

  D46.20 Refractory anemia with excess of blasts, unspecified
    RAEB NOS

  D46.21 Refractory anemia with excess of <u>blasts 1</u>
    RAEB 1

  CC **D46.22** Refractory anemia with excess of <u>blasts 2</u>
    RAEB 2

D46.A Refractory cytopenia with multilineage dysplasia — A form producing too few of at least two types of blood cells (red blood cells, white blood cells, or platelets).

D46.B Refractory cytopenia with multilineage dysplasia <u>and ring sideroblasts</u> — A form producing too few of at least two types of blood cells (red blood cells, white blood cells, or platelets) and those red blood cells have too much iron inside the cell.
  RCMD RS

CC **D46.C** Myelodysplastic syndrome with isolated del(5q) chromosomal abnormality — A form producing too few red blood cells that is characterized by changes in chromosome 5.
  Myelodysplastic syndrome with 5q deletion
  5q minus syndrome NOS

D46.4 Refractory anemia, unspecified

D46.Z Other myelodysplastic syndromes
  Excludes 1:   chronic myelomonocytic leukemia (C93.1-)

D46.9 Myelodysplastic syndrome, unspecified
  Myelodysplasia NOS

D47- Other neoplasms of <u>uncertain behavior</u> of lymphoid, hematopoietic and related tissue

CC **D47.0** <u>Histiocytic and mast cell tumors</u> of uncertain behavior
  Indolent systemic mastocytosis
  Mast cell tumor NOS
  Mastocytoma NOS

  Excludes 1:   malignant mast cell tumor (C96.2)
  mastocytosis (congenital) (cutaneous) (Q82.2)

CC **D47.1** <u>Chronic myeloproliferative disease</u> — A neoplastic bone marrow cell production disorder in which too many blood cells (red blood cells, white blood cells, or platelets) are produced.
  Chronic neutrophilic leukemia
  Myeloproliferative disease, unspecified

  Excludes 1:   atypical chronic chronic myeloid leukemia BCR/ABL-negative (C92.2-)
  chronic myeloid leukemia BCR/ABL-positive (C92.1-)
  myelofibrosis NOS (D75.81)
  myelophthisic anemia (D61.82)
  myelophthisis (D61.82)
  secondary myelofibrosis NOS (D75.81)

D47.2 <u>Monoclonal gammopathy</u>
  Monoclonal gammopathy of undetermined significance [MGUS]

D47.3 <u>Essential (hemorrhagic) thrombocythemia</u> — A neoplastic bone marrow cell production disorder in which too many platelets are formed.
  Essential thrombocytosis
  Idiopathic hemorrhagic thrombocythemia

D47.4 <u>Osteomyelofibrosis</u>
  Chronic idiopathic myelofibrosis
  Myelofibrosis (idiopathic) (with myeloid metaplasia)
  Myelosclerosis (megakaryocytic) with myeloid metaplasia
  Secondary myelofibrosis in myeloproliferative disease

  Excludes 1:   acute myelofibrosis (C94.4-)

D
4
1
-
D
4
7

D47.Z- Other specified neoplasms of uncertain behavior of lymphoid, hematopoietic and related tissue

cc **D47.Z1** Post-transplant lymphoproliferative disorder (PTLD) —
[Unacceptable PDX]
Code first complications of transplanted organs and tissue (T86.-)

cc **D47.Z2** Castleman disease — A lymphoproliferative disorder with varying clinical features that is characterized by proliferation of morphologically benign lymphocytes.
Code also if applicable human herpesvirus 8 infection (B10.89)
Excludes ❷: Kaposi's sarcoma (C46-)

cc **D47.Z9** Other specified neoplasms of uncertain behavior of lymphoid, hematopoietic and related tissue
Histiocytic tumors of uncertain behavior

cc **D47.9** Neoplasm of uncertain behavior of lymphoid, hematopoietic and related tissue, unspecified
Lymphoproliferative disease NOS

D48- Neoplasm of <u>uncertain behavior</u> of other and unspecified sites — See Note and Excludes 1 at code block D37-D48.
Excludes 1: neurofibromatosis (nonmalignant) (Q85.0-)

D48.0 Neoplasm of uncertain behavior of <u>bone and articular cartilage</u>
Excludes 1: neoplasm of uncertain behavior of cartilage of ear (D48.1)
neoplasm of uncertain behavior of cartilage of larynx (D38.0)
neoplasm of uncertain behavior of cartilage of nose (D38.5)
neoplasm of uncertain behavior of connective tissue of eyelid (D48.1)
neoplasm of uncertain behavior of synovia (D48.1)

D48.1 Neoplasm of uncertain behavior of <u>connective and other soft tissue</u>
Neoplasm of uncertain behavior of connective tissue of ear
Neoplasm of uncertain behavior of connective tissue of eyelid
Stromal tumors of uncertain behavior of digestive system
Excludes 1: neoplasm of uncertain behavior of articular cartilage (D48.0)
neoplasm of uncertain behavior of cartilage of larynx (D38.0)
neoplasm of uncertain behavior of cartilage of nose (D38.5)
neoplasm of uncertain behavior of connective tissue of breast (D48.6-)

D48.2 Neoplasm of uncertain behavior of <u>peripheral nerves and autonomic nervous system</u>
Excludes 1: neoplasm of uncertain behavior of peripheral nerves of orbit (D48.7)

D48.3 Neoplasm of uncertain behavior of <u>retroperitoneum</u>

D48.4 Neoplasm of uncertain behavior of <u>peritoneum</u>

D48.5 Neoplasm of uncertain behavior of <u>skin</u>
Neoplasm of uncertain behavior of anal margin
Neoplasm of uncertain behavior of anal skin
Neoplasm of uncertain behavior of perianal skin
Neoplasm of uncertain behavior of skin of breast
Excludes 1: neoplasm of uncertain behavior of anus NOS (D37.8)
neoplasm of uncertain behavior of skin of genital organs (D39.8, D40.8)
neoplasm of uncertain behavior of vermilion border of lip (D37.0)

D48.6- Neoplasm of uncertain behavior of <u>breast</u>
Neoplasm of uncertain behavior of connective tissue of breast
Cystosarcoma phyllodes
Excludes 1: neoplasm of uncertain behavior of skin of breast (D48.5)

D48.60 Neoplasm of uncertain behavior of unspecified breast

D48.61 Neoplasm of uncertain behavior of <u>right</u> breast

D48.62 Neoplasm of uncertain behavior of <u>left</u> breast

D48.7 Neoplasm of uncertain behavior of other specified sites
Neoplasm of uncertain behavior of eye
Neoplasm of uncertain behavior of heart
Neoplasm of uncertain behavior of peripheral nerves of orbit
Excludes 1: neoplasm of uncertain behavior of connective tissue (D48.1)
neoplasm of uncertain behavior of skin of eyelid (D48.5)

D48.9 Neoplasm of uncertain behavior, unspecified

Neoplasms of unspecified behavior (D49)

D49- Neoplasms of <u>unspecified</u> <u>behavior</u>
Note: Category D49 classifies by site neoplasms of unspecified morphology and behavior. The term "mass", unless otherwise stated, is not to be regarded as a neoplastic growth.
Includes: "Growth" NOS
Neoplasm NOS
New growth NOS
Tumor NOS
Excludes 1: neoplasms of uncertain behavior (D37-D44, D48)

D49.0 Neoplasm of unspecified behavior of <u>digestive system</u>
Excludes 1: neoplasm of unspecified behavior of margin of anus (D49.2)
neoplasm of unspecified behavior of perianal skin (D49.2)
neoplasm of unspecified behavior of skin of anus (D49.2)

D49.1 Neoplasm of unspecified behavior of <u>respiratory system</u>

D49.2 Neoplasm of unspecified behavior of <u>bone, soft tissue, and skin</u>
Excludes 1: neoplasm of unspecified behavior of anal canal (D49.0)
neoplasm of unspecified behavior of anus NOS (D49.0)
neoplasm of unspecified behavior of bone marrow (D49.89)
neoplasm of unspecified behavior of cartilage of larynx (D49.1)
neoplasm of unspecified behavior of cartilage of nose (D49.1)
neoplasm of unspecified behavior of connective tissue of breast (D49.3)
neoplasm of unspecified behavior of skin of genital organs (D49.59)
neoplasm of unspecified behavior of vermilion border of lip (D49.0)

D49.3 Neoplasm of unspecified behavior of <u>breast</u>
Excludes 1: neoplasm of unspecified behavior of skin of breast (D49.2)

D49.4 Neoplasm of unspecified behavior of <u>bladder</u>

D49.5- Neoplasm of unspecified behavior of <u>other genitourinary organs</u>

D49.51- Neoplasm of unspecified behavior of <u>kidney</u>

D49.511 Neoplasm of unspecified behavior of <u>right</u> kidney

D49.512 Neoplasm of unspecified behavior of <u>left</u> kidney

D49.519 Neoplasm of unspecified behavior of <u>unspecified</u> kidney

D49.59 Neoplasm of unspecified behavior of other genitourinary organ

D49.6 Neoplasm of unspecified behavior of <u>brain</u>
Excludes 1: neoplasm of unspecified behavior of cerebral meninges (D49.7)
neoplasm of unspecified behavior of cranial nerves (D49.7)

D49.7 Neoplasm of unspecified behavior of <u>endocrine glands and other parts of nervous system</u>
Excludes 1: neoplasm of unspecified behavior of peripheral, sympathetic, and parasympathetic nerves and ganglia (D49.2)

D49.8- Neoplasm of unspecified behavior of other specified sites
Excludes 1: neoplasm of unspecified behavior of eyelid (skin) (D49.2)
neoplasm of unspecified behavior of eyelid cartilage (D49.2)
neoplasm of unspecified behavior of great vessels (D49.2)
neoplasm of unspecified behavior of optic nerve (D49.7)

D49.81 Neoplasm of unspecified behavior of retina and choroid
Dark area on retina
Retinal freckle

D49.89 Neoplasm of unspecified behavior of other specified sites

D49.9 Neoplasm of unspecified behavior of unspecified site

D
4
9
–
D
4
9

Chapter 3 – Diseases of the blood and blood-forming organs and certain disorders involving the immune mechanism (D50-D89)

Excludes 2: *autoimmune disease (systemic) NOS (M35.9)*
certain conditions originating in the perinatal period (P00-P96)
complications of pregnancy, childbirth and the puerperium (O00-O9A)
congenital malformations, deformations and chromosomal abnormalities (Q00-Q99)
endocrine, nutritional and metabolic diseases (E00-E88)
human immunodeficiency virus [HIV] disease (B20)
injury, poisoning and certain other consequences of external causes (S00-T88)
neoplasms (C00-D49)
symptoms, signs and abnormal clinical and laboratory findings, not elsewhere classified (R00-R94)

This chapter contains the following blocks:

D50-D53	Nutritional anemias
D55-D59	Hemolytic anemias
D60-D64	Aplastic and other anemias and other bone marrow failure syndromes
D65-D69	Coagulation defects, purpura and other hemorrhagic conditions
D70-D77	Other disorders of blood and blood-forming organs
D78	Intraoperative and postprocedural complications of the spleen
D80-D89	Certain disorders involving the immune mechanism

Chapter-Specific Coding Guidelines

C.   Chapter-Specific Coding Guidelines
In addition to general coding guidelines, there are guidelines for specific diagnoses and/or conditions in the classification. Unless otherwise indicated, these guidelines apply to all health care settings. Please refer to Section II for guidelines on the selection of principal diagnosis.

3.   Chapter 3: Disease of the Blood and Blood-forming Organs and Certain Disorders Involving the Immune Mechanism (D50-D89)

Reserved for future guideline expansion

Nutritional anemias (D50-D53)

D50-   Iron deficiency anemia — An abnormal reduction of red blood cells caused by low or absent iron stores.
  Includes: Asiderotic anemia
               Hypochromic anemia

D50.0   Iron deficiency anemia secondary to blood loss (chronic)
       Posthemorrhagic anemia (chronic)
       Excludes 1:   acute posthemorrhagic anemia (D62)
                    congenital anemia from fetal blood loss (P61.3)

D50.1   Sideropenic dysphagia
       Kelly-Paterson syndrome
       Plummer-Vinson syndrome

D50.8   Other iron deficiency anemias
       Iron deficiency anemia due to inadequate dietary iron intake

D50.9   Iron deficiency anemia, unspecified

D51-   Vitamin B12 deficiency anemia — A megaloblastic anemia characterized by decreased levels of vitamin B12 absorption.
    Excludes 1:   vitamin B12 deficiency (E53.8)

D51.0   Vitamin B12 deficiency anemia due to intrinsic factor deficiency
       Addison anemia
       Biermer anemia
       Pernicious (congenital) anemia
       Congenital intrinsic factor deficiency

D51.1   Vitamin B12 deficiency anemia due to selective vitamin B12 malabsorption with proteinuria
       Imerslund (Gräsbeck) syndrome
       Megaloblastic hereditary anemia

D51.2   Transcobalamin II deficiency

D51.3   Other dietary vitamin B12 deficiency anemia
       Vegan anemia

D51.8   Other vitamin B12 deficiency anemias

D51.9   Vitamin B12 deficiency anemia, unspecified

D52-   Folate deficiency anemia — Megaloblastic anemia caused by the lack of folic acid (one of the B vitamins) in the blood.
    Excludes 1:   folate deficiency without anemia (E53.8)

D52.0   Dietary folate deficiency anemia
       Nutritional megaloblastic anemia

D52.1   Drug-induced folate deficiency anemia
       Use additional code for adverse effect, if applicable, to identify drug (T36-T50 with fifth or sixth character 5)

D52.8   Other folate deficiency anemias

D52.9   Folate deficiency anemia, unspecified
       Folic acid deficiency anemia NOS

D53-   Other nutritional anemias
    Includes: Megaloblastic anemia unresponsive to vitamin B12 or folate therapy

D53.0   Protein deficiency anemia — An abnormal reduction of blood cells due to decreased protein intake.
       Amino-acid deficiency anemia
       Orotaciduric anemia
       Excludes 1:   Lesch-Nyhan syndrome (E79.1)

D53.1   Other megaloblastic anemias, not elsewhere classified
       Megaloblastic anemia NOS
       Excludes 1:   Di Guglielmo's disease (C94.0)

D53.2   Scorbutic anemia
       Excludes 1:   scurvy (E54)

D53.8   Other specified nutritional anemias
       Anemia associated with deficiency of copper
       Anemia associated with deficiency of molybdenum
       Anemia associated with deficiency of zinc
       Excludes 1:   nutritional deficiencies without anemia, such as:
                    copper deficiency NOS (E61.0)
                    molybdenum deficiency NOS (E61.5)
                    zinc deficiency NOS (E60)

D53.9   Nutritional anemia, unspecified
       Simple chronic anemia
       Excludes 1:   anemia NOS (D64.9)

Hemolytic anemias (D55-D59)

D55-   Anemia due to enzyme disorders — An abnormal reduction of red blood cells due to the breakdown of red blood cells caused by enzyme disorders.
    Excludes 1:   drug-induced enzyme deficiency anemia (D59.2)

D55.0   Anemia due to glucose-6-phosphate dehydrogenase [G6PD] deficiency — A genetic form caused by a deficiency of the enzyme glucose-6-phosphate dehydrogenase.
       Favism
       G6PD deficiency anemia

D55.1   Anemia due to other disorders of glutathione metabolism
       Anemia (due to) enzyme deficiencies, except G6PD, related to the hexose monophosphate [HMP] shunt pathway
       Anemia (due to) hemolytic nonspherocytic (hereditary), type I

D55.2   Anemia due to disorders of glycolytic enzymes — A genetic form caused by a deficiency of the glycolytic enzymes (hexokinase, pyruvate kinase, triose-phosphate isomerase).
       Hemolytic nonspherocytic (hereditary) anemia, type II
       Hexokinase deficiency anemia
       Pyruvate kinase [PK] deficiency anemia
       Triose-phosphate isomerase deficiency anemia
       Excludes 1:   disorders of glycolysis not associated with anemia (E74.8)

D55.3   Anemia due to disorders of nucleotide metabolism

D55.8   Other anemias due to enzyme disorders

D55.9   Anemia due to enzyme disorder, unspecified

D50-D55

D56- <u>Thalassemia</u> — A group of hereditary hemolytic anemias in which the body makes an abnormal form of hemoglobin that has limited capacity to carry oxygen.

    Excludes 1:   *sickle-cell thalassemia (D57.4-)*

    D56.0   <u>Alpha</u> **thalassemia** — A severe form involving defective alpha hemoglobin chain genes.
        Alpha thalassemia major
        Hemoglobin H Constant Spring
        Hemoglobin H disease
        Hydrops fetalis due to alpha thalassemia
        Severe alpha thalassemia
        Triple gene defect alpha thalassemia
        Use additional code, if applicable, for hydrops fetalis due to alpha thalassemia (P56.99)
        Excludes 1:   *alpha thalassemia trait or minor (D56.3)*
                        asymptomatic alpha thalassemia (D56.3)
                        hydrops fetalis due to isoimmunization (P56.0)
                        hydrops fetalis not due to immune hemolysis (P83.2)

    D56.1   <u>Beta</u> **thalassemia** — A severe form involving defective beta hemoglobin chain genes.
        Beta thalassemia major
        Cooley's anemia
        Homozygous beta thalassemia
        Severe beta thalassemia
        Thalassemia intermedia
        Thalassemia major
        Excludes 1:   *beta thalassemia minor (D56.3)*
                        beta thalassemia trait (D56.3)
                        delta-beta thalassemia (D56.2)
                        hemoglobin E-beta thalassemia (D56.5)
                        sickle-cell beta thalassemia (D57.4-)

    D56.2   <u>Delta-beta</u> **thalassemia** — A form involving defective portions of both beta and delta hemoglobin chain genes.
        Homozygous delta-beta thalassemia
        Excludes 1:   *delta-beta thalassemia minor (D56.3)*
                        delta-beta thalassemia trait (D56.3)

    D56.3   **Thalassemia** <u>minor</u> — A less severe form involving defective hemoglobin chain genes.
        Alpha thalassemia minor
        Alpha thalassemia silent carrier
        Alpha thalassemia trait
        Beta thalassemia minor
        Beta thalassemia trait
        Delta-beta thalassemia minor
        Delta-beta thalassemia trait
        Thalassemia trait NOS
        Excludes 1:   *alpha thalassemia (D56.0)*
                        beta thalassemia (D56.1)
                        delta-beta thalassemia (D56.2)
                        hemoglobin E-beta thalassemia (D56.5)
                        sickle-cell trait (D57.3)

    D56.4   **Hereditary persistence of fetal hemoglobin [HPFH]**

    D56.5   <u>Hemoglobin E-beta</u> **thalassemia** — A beta chain variant hemoglobinopathy characeized by the presence of variant hemoglobin E.
        Excludes 1:   *beta thalassemia (D56.1)*
                        beta thalassemia minor (D56.3)
                        beta thalassemia trait (D56.3)
                        delta-beta thalassemia (D56.2)
                        delta-beta thalassemia trait (D56.3)
                        hemoglobin E disease (D58.2)
                        other hemoglobinopathies (D58.2)
                        sickle-cell beta thalassemia (D57.4-)

    D56.8   **Other thalassemias**
        Dominant thalassemia
        Hemoglobin C thalassemia
        Mixed thalassemia
        Thalassemia with other hemoglobinopathy
        Excludes 1:   *hemoglobin C disease (D58.2)*
                        hemoglobin E disease (D58.2)
                        other hemoglobinopathies (D58.2)
                        sickle-cell anemia (D57.-)
                        sickle-cell thalassemia (D57.4)

    D56.9   **Thalassemia, unspecified**
        Mediterranean anemia (with other hemoglobinopathy)

D57- <u>Sickle-cell</u> **disorders** — A hereditary hemolytic disease characterized by abnormal, shortened-lifespan, crescent-shaped hemoglobin resulting in decreased oxygenation of the tissues.
    Use additional code for any associated fever (R50.81)
    Excludes 1:   *other hemoglobinopathies (D58.-)*

    D57.0-   <u>Hb-SS</u> **disease** <u>with crisis</u> — A form in which the patient has abnormal hemoglobin SS, and is experiencing the painful symptoms and conditions caused by the sickled red blood cells which block the blood flow, resulting in significant loss of oxygenation of the tissues.
        Sickle-cell disease NOS with crisis
        Hb-SS disease with vasoocclusive pain
  MCC **D57.00**   **Hb-SS disease with crisis, unspecified**
  MCC **D57.01**   **Hb-SS disease with acute chest syndrome**
  MCC **D57.02**   **Hb-SS disease with splenic sequestration**

    D57.1   **Sickle-cell disease** <u>without</u> **crisis**
        Hb-SS disease without crisis
        Sickle-cell anemia NOS
        Sickle-cell disease NOS
        Sickle-cell disorder NOS

    D57.2-   **Sickle-cell/**<u>Hb-C</u> **disease** — A form in which the patient has abnormal hemoglobin C.
        Hb-SC disease
        Hb-S/Hb-C disease
    D57.20   **Sickle-cell/Hb-C disease** <u>without</u> **crisis**
    D57.21-   **Sickle-cell/Hb-C disease** <u>with</u> **crisis** — A form in which the patient is experiencing the painful symptoms and conditions caused by the sickled red blood cells which block the blood flow, resulting in significant loss of oxygenation of the tissues.
  MCC **D57.211**   **Sickle-cell/Hb-C disease with acute chest syndrome** — A form involving the chest (lungs) with symptoms that resemble pneumonia.
  MCC **D57.212**   **Sickle-cell/Hb-C disease with splenic sequestration** — A form resulting from the sickled cells pooling in the spleen causing pain, damage to the spleen, and sometimes life-threatening drop in hemoglobin.
  MCC **D57.219**   **Sickle-cell/Hb-C disease with crisis, unspecified**
        Sickle-cell/Hb-C disease with crisis NOS

    D57.3   **Sickle-cell** <u>trait</u> — The usually asymptomatic condition of crescent-shaped hemoglobin S inherited from one of the patient's parents.
        Hb-S trait
        Heterozygous hemoglobin S

    D57.4-   **Sickle-cell** <u>thalassemia</u> — A form in which the patient has both the abnormal hemoglobin S gene and the thalassemia gene.
        Sickle-cell beta thalassemia
        Thalassemia Hb-S disease
    D57.40   **Sickle-cell thalassemia** <u>without</u> **crisis**
        Microdrepanocytosis
        Sickle-cell thalassemia NOS
    D57.41-   **Sickle-cell thalassemia** <u>with crisis</u>
        Sickle-cell thalassemia with vasoocclusive pain
  MCC **D57.411**   **Sickle-cell thalassemia with acute chest syndrome** — A form involving the chest (lungs) with symptoms that resemble pneumonia.
  MCC **D57.412**   **Sickle-cell thalassemia with splenic sequestration** — A form resulting from the sickled cells pooling in the spleen causing pain, damage to the spleen, and sometimes a life-threatening drop in hemoglobin.
  MCC **D57.419**   **Sickle-cell thalassemia with crisis, unspecified**
        Sickle-cell thalassemia with crisis NOS

    D57.8-   <u>Other</u> **sickle-cell disorders**
        Hb-SD disease
        Hb-SE disease
    D57.80   **Other sickle-cell disorders** <u>without</u> **crisis**
    D57.81-   **Other sickle-cell disorders** <u>with</u> **crisis**
  MCC **D57.811**   **Other sickle-cell disorders with acute chest syndrome**
  MCC **D57.812**   **Other sickle-cell disorders with splenic sequestration**
  MCC **D57.819**   **Other sickle-cell disorders with crisis, unspecified**
        Other sickle-cell disorders with crisis NOS

D58- <u>Other hereditary</u> hemolytic anemias
  Excludes 1:   *hemolytic anemia of the newborn (P55.-)*
  D58.0   **Hereditary spherocytosis** — An inherited hemolytic anemia in which erythrocytes assume a spheroid shape that is characterized by hemolysis, jaundice, and splenomegaly.
      Acholuric (familial) jaundice
      Congenital (spherocytic) hemolytic icterus
      Minkowski-Chauffard syndrome

      NORMAL RED BLOOD CELL   SPHEROCYTOSIS, RED BLOOD CELL

  D58.1   **Hereditary elliptocytosis** — A hereditary disorder in which the greater proportion of [BT] erythrocytes are elliptical in shape, and which is characterized by varying degrees of increased red cell destruction and anemia.
      Elliptocytosis (congenital)
      Ovalocytosis (congenital) (hereditary)

  D58.2   **Other hemoglobinopathies**
      Abnormal hemoglobin NOS
      Congenital Heinz body anemia
      Hb-C disease
      Hb-D disease
      Hb-E disease
      Hemoglobinopathy NOS
      Unstable hemoglobin hemolytic disease
      Excludes 1:   *familial polycythemia (D75.0)*
              Hb-M disease (D74.0)
              hemoglobin E-beta thalassemia (D56.5)
              hereditary persistence of fetal hemoglobin [HPFH]
                (D56.4)
              high-altitude polycythemia (D75.1)
              methemoglobinemia (D74.-)
              other hemoglobinopathies with thalassemia (D56.8)

  cc **D58.8**   **Other specified hereditary hemolytic anemias**
      Stomatocytosis

  cc **D58.9**   **Hereditary hemolytic anemia, unspecified**

D59- <u>Acquired</u> hemolytic anemia — An abnormal reduction of red blood cells caused by an increased rate of red blood cell destruction and inability of the bone marrow to compensate, which is due to causes other than hereditary factors.

  cc **D59.0**   **<u>Drug-induced</u> autoimmune hemolytic anemia**
      Use additional code for adverse effect, if applicable, to identify drug (T36-T50 with fifth or sixth character 5)

  cc **D59.1**   **Other autoimmune hemolytic anemias** — Acquired hemolytic anemia characterized by serum antibodies attacking red blood cells that is caused by the adverse chemical reaction of drugs.
      Autoimmune hemolytic disease (cold type) (warm type)
      Chronic cold hemagglutinin disease
      Cold agglutinin disease
      Cold agglutinin hemoglobinuria
      Cold type (secondary) (symptomatic) hemolytic anemia
      Warm type (secondary) (symptomatic) hemolytic anemia
      Excludes 1:   *Evans syndrome (D69.41)*
              hemolytic disease of newborn (P55.-)
              paroxysmal cold hemoglobinuria (D59.6)

  cc **D59.2**   **<u>Drug-induced</u> nonautoimmune hemolytic anemia**
      Drug-induced enzyme deficiency anemia
      Use additional code for adverse effect, if applicable, to identify drug (T36-T50 with fifth or sixth character 5)

  mcc **D59.3**   **Hemolytic-uremic syndrome** — A syndrome characterized by microangiopathic anemia, severe thrombocytopenia, and renal failure.
      Use additional code to identify associated:
      E. coli infection (B96.2-)
      Pneumococcal pneumonia (J13)
      Shigella dysenteriae (A03.9)

  cc **D59.4**   **Other nonautoimmune hemolytic anemias**
      Mechanical hemolytic anemia
      Microangiopathic hemolytic anemia
      Toxic hemolytic anemia

  D59.5   **Paroxysmal nocturnal hemoglobinuria [Marchiafava-Micheli]**
      Excludes 1:   *hemoglobinuria NOS (R82.3)*

  D59.6   **Hemoglobinuria due to hemolysis from other external causes**
      Hemoglobinuria from exertion
      March hemoglobinuria
      Paroxysmal cold hemoglobinuria
      Use additional code (Chapter 20) to identify external cause
      Excludes 1:   *hemoglobinuria NOS (R82.3)*

  D59.8   **Other acquired hemolytic anemias**

  cc **D59.9**   **Acquired hemolytic anemia, unspecified**
      Idiopathic hemolytic anemia, chronic

Aplastic and other anemias and other bone marrow failure syndromes (D60-D64)

D60- <u>Acquired pure red cell aplasia</u> [erythroblastopenia] — A bone marrow disorder characterized by decreased production of red blood cells that is often chronic and associated with underlying disorders such as thymomas and autoimmune diseases.
  Includes: Red cell aplasia (acquired) (adult) (with thymoma)
  Excludes 1:   *congenital red cell aplasia (D61.01)*

  mcc **D60.0**   **<u>Chronic</u> acquired pure red cell aplasia**
  mcc **D60.1**   **<u>Transient</u> acquired pure red cell aplasia**
  mcc **D60.8**   **Other acquired pure red cell aplasias**
  mcc **D60.9**   **Acquired pure red cell aplasia, unspecified**

D61- <u>Other aplastic</u> anemias and other bone marrow failure syndromes
  Excludes 1:   *neutropenia (D70.-)*

  D61.0-   **<u>Constitutional</u> aplastic anemia**
      cc **D61.01**   **Constitutional (pure) red blood cell aplasia** — An inherited, progressive hypoplasia of the bone marrow that is characterized by slow growth, abnormal weakness, deformities, and defects and is unaccompanied by leukopenia and thrombocytopenia.
          Blackfan-Diamond syndrome
          Congenital (pure) red cell aplasia
          Familial hypoplastic anemia
          Primary (pure) red cell aplasia
          Red cell (pure) aplasia of infants
          Excludes 1:   *acquired red cell aplasia (D60.9)*

      cc **D61.09**   **Other constitutional aplastic anemia**
          Fanconi's anemia — An inherited disorder that results in deficiency of all bone marrow elements including red blood cells, white blood cells, and platelets and is characterized by skin pigment changes, musculoskeletal deformities, and short stature.
          Pancytopenia with malformations

  mcc **D61.1**   **<u>Drug-induced</u> aplastic anemia** — Decreased bone marrow production of red blood cells due to the chemical effects of drugs.
      Use additional code for adverse effect, if applicable, to identify drug (T36-T50 with fifth or sixth character 5)

  mcc **D61.2**   **Aplastic anemia <u>due to other external agents</u>**
      Code first, if applicable, toxic effects of substances chiefly nonmedicinal as to source (T51-T65)

  mcc **D61.3**   **<u>Idiopathic</u> aplastic anemia**

  D61.8-   **Other specified aplastic anemias and other bone marrow failure syndromes**

      D61.81- <u>Pancytopenia</u> — A deficiency of all bone marrow elements including red and white blood cells and platelets.
          Excludes 1:   *pancytopenia (due to) (with) aplastic anemia (D61.9)*
                  pancytopenia (due to) (with) bone marrow infiltration (D61.82)
                  pancytopenia (due to) (with) congenital (pure) red cell aplasia (D61.01)
                  pancytopenia (due to) (with) hairy cell leukemia (C91.4-)
                  pancytopenia (due to) (with) human immunodeficiency virus disease (B20.-)
                  pancytopenia (due to) (with) leukoerythroblastic anemia (D61.82)
                  pancytopenia (due to) (with) myeloproliferative disease (D47.1)
          Excludes ❷: *pancytopenia (due to) (with) myelodysplastic syndromes (D46.-)*

          mcc **D61.810**   **Antineoplastic <u>chemotherapy induced</u> pancytopenia**
              Excludes ❷: *aplastic anemia due to antineoplastic chemotherapy (D61.1)*

          mcc **D61.811**   **Other <u>drug-induced</u> pancytopenia**
              Excludes ❷: *aplastic anemia due to drugs (D61.1)*

          cc **D61.818**   **Other pancytopenia**

D 5 8 - D 6 1

cc D61.82 Myelophthisis — A condition of bone marrow failure that results from the destruction of bone marrow precursor cells.
Leukoerythroblastic anemia
Myelophthisic anemia
Panmyelophthisis
Excludes 1: *idiopathic myelofibrosis (D47.1)*
myelofibrosis NOS (D75.81)
myelofibrosis with myeloid metaplasia (D47.4)
primary myelofibrosis (D47.1)
secondary myelofibrosis (D75.81)
Code also the underlying disorder, such as:
Malignant neoplasm of breast (C50.-)
Tuberculosis (A15.-)

MCC D61.89 Other specified aplastic anemias and other bone marrow failure syndromes

cc D61.9 Aplastic anemia, unspecified
Hypoplastic anemia NOS
Medullary hypoplasia

D62 Acute posthemorrhagic anemia — An abnormal reduction of red blood cells due
cc to the voluminous escape of blood from the body, more rapidly than the body can replace it.
Excludes 1: *anemia due to chronic blood loss (D50.0)*
blood loss anemia NOS (D50.0)
congenital anemia from fetal blood loss (P61.3)

D63- Anemia in chronic diseases classified elsewhere

D63.0 Anemia in neoplastic disease — [Not Allowed as PDX]
Code first neoplasm (C00-D49)
Excludes 1: *anemia due to antineoplastic chemotherapy (D64.81)*
aplastic anemia due to antineoplastic chemotherapy (D61.1)

D63.1 Anemia in chronic kidney disease — [Not Allowed as PDX]
Erythropoietin resistant anemia (EPO resistant anemia)
Code first underlying chronic kidney disease (CKD) (N18.-)

D63.8 Anemia in other chronic diseases classified elsewhere —
[Not Allowed as PDX]
Code first underlying disease, such as:
Diphyllobothriasis (B70.0)
Hookworm disease (B76.0-B76.9)
Hypothyroidism (E00.0-E03.9)
Malaria (B50.0-B54)
Symptomatic late syphilis (A52.79)
Tuberculosis (A18.89)

D64- Other anemias
Excludes 1: *refractory anemia (D46.-)*
refractory anemia with excess blasts in transformation [RAEB T] (C92.0-)

D64.0 Hereditary sideroblastic anemia — An abnormal reduction of red blood cells caused by a defect in the final stage of hemesynthesis, and which is marked by hypochromic red blood cells and elevated serum iron.
Sex-linked hypochromic sideroblastic anemia

D64.1 Secondary sideroblastic anemia due to disease —
[Not Allowed as PDX]
Code first underlying disease

D64.2 Secondary sideroblastic anemia due to drugs and toxins
Code first poisoning due to drug or toxin, if applicable (T36-T65 with fifth or sixth character 1-4 or 6)
Use additional code for adverse effect, if applicable, to identify drug (T36-T50 with fifth or sixth character 5)

D64.3 Other sideroblastic anemias
Sideroblastic anemia NOS
Pyridoxine-responsive sideroblastic anemia NEC

D64.4 Congenital dyserythropoietic anemia
Dyshematopoietic anemia (congenital)
Excludes 1: *Blackfan-Diamond syndrome (D61.01)*
Di Guglielmo's disease (C94.0)

D64.8- Other specified anemias

D64.81 Anemia due to antineoplastic chemotherapy
AHA 14:4Q:p22 – Anemia secondary to chemotherapy
Antineoplastic chemotherapy induced anemia
Excludes 1: *aplastic anemia due to antineoplastic chemotherapy (D61.1)*
Excludes ❷: *anemia in neoplastic disease (D63.0)*

D64.89 Other specified anemias
Infantile pseudoleukemia

D64.9 Anemia, unspecified

Coagulation defects, purpura and other hemorrhagic conditions (D65-D69)

D65 Disseminated intravascular coagulation [defibrination syndrome] —
MCC An acquired syndrome characterized by consumption coagulopathy and fibrinolysis.
Afibrinogenemia, acquired
Consumption coagulopathy
Diffuse or disseminated intravascular coagulation [DIC]
Fibrinolytic hemorrhage, acquired
Fibrinolytic purpura
Purpura fulminans
Excludes 1: *disseminated intravascular coagulation (complicating):*
abortion or ectopic or molar pregnancy (O00-O07, O08.1)
in newborn (P60)
pregnancy, childbirth and the puerperium (O45.0, O46.0, O67.0, O72.3)

D66 Hereditary factor VIII deficiency — A hereditary deficiency of Factor VIII,
MCC antihemophilic factor, characterized by recurrent hemarthroses, muscular hematomas, retroperitoneal bleeding, and easy bruising.
Classical hemophilia
Deficiency factor VIII (with functional defect)
Hemophilia NOS
Hemophilia A
Excludes 1: *factor VIII deficiency with vascular defect (D68.0)*

D67 Hereditary factor IX deficiency — A hereditary deficiency of Factor IX, plasma
MCC thromboplastin component factor, characterized by severe joint and soft tissue bleeding.
Christmas disease
Factor IX deficiency (with functional defect)
Hemophilia B
Plasma thromboplastin component [PTC] deficiency

D68- Other coagulation defects
Excludes 1: *abnormal coagulation profile (R79.1)*
coagulation defects complicating abortion or ectopic or molar pregnancy (O00-O07, O08.1)
coagulation defects complicating pregnancy, childbirth and the puerperium (O45.0, O46.0, O67.0, O72.3)

cc D68.0 Von Willebrand's disease — A hereditary disease caused by abnormal blood vessels in association with Factor VIII deficiency, and is characterized by superficial skin and mucous membrane bleeding, and some mild joint bleeding.
Angiohemophilia
Factor VIII deficiency with vascular defect
Vascular hemophilia
Excludes 1: *capillary fragility (hereditary) (D69.8)*
factor VIII deficiency NOS (D66)
factor VIII deficiency with functional defect (D66)

cc D68.1 Hereditary factor XI deficiency — A hereditary deficiency of Factor XI, plasma thromboplastin antecedent factor, characterized by mild mucosal bleeding, bruising, and epistaxis.
Hemophilia C
Plasma thromboplastin antecedent [PTA] deficiency
Rosenthal's disease

cc D68.2 Hereditary deficiency of other clotting factors
AC globulin deficiency
Congenital afibrinogenemia
Deficiency of factor I [fibrinogen]
Deficiency of factor II [prothrombin]
Deficiency of factor V [labile]
Deficiency of factor VII [stable]
Deficiency of factor X [Stuart-Prower]
Deficiency of factor XII [Hageman]
Deficiency of factor XIII [fibrin stabilizing]
Dysfibrinogenemia (congenital)
Hypoproconvertinemia
Owren's disease
Proaccelerin deficiency

D68.3- Hemorrhagic disorder due to circulating anticoagulants
AHA 16:1Q:p14x2 – Duodenal ulcer with hemorrhage due to Coumadin therapy

D68.31- Hemorrhagic disorder due to intrinsic circulating anticoagulants, antibodies, or inhibitors

cc D68.311 Acquired hemophilia — A bleeding disorder from a non-genetic origin that is caused by substances in the blood circulation that delays or prevents normal blood clotting.
Autoimmune hemophilia
Autoimmune inhibitors to clotting factors
Secondary hemophilia

---

cc **D68.312** **Antiphospholipid antibody with hemorrhagic disorder** — A bleeding disorder that is due to the autoimmune production of antibodies against phospholipids (cell membrane component).
Lupus anticoagulant (LAC) with hemorrhagic disorder
Systemic lupus erythematosus [SLE] inhibitor with hemorrhagic disorder
Excludes 1:   *antiphospholipid antibody finding without diagnosis (R76.0)*
antiphospholipid antibody syndrome (D68.61)
antiphospholipid antibody with hypercoagulable state (D68.61)
lupus anticoagulant (LAC) finding without diagnosis (R76.0)
lupus anticoagulant (LAC) with hypercoagulable state (D68.62)
systemic lupus erythematosus [SLE] inhibitor finding without diagnosis (R76.0)
systemic lupus erythematosus [SLE] inhibitor with hypercoagulable state (D68.62)

cc **D68.318** **Other hemorrhagic disorder due to intrinsic circulating anticoagulants, antibodies, or inhibitors**
Antithromboplastinemia
Antithromboplastinogenemia
Hemorrhagic disorder due to intrinsic increase in antithrombin
Hemorrhagic disorder due to intrinsic increase in anti-VIIIa
Hemorrhagic disorder due to intrinsic increase in anti-IXa
Hemorrhagic disorder due to intrinsic increase in anti-XIa

cc **D68.32** **Hemorrhagic disorder due to extrinsic circulating anticoagulants**
AHA 16:1Q:p15 – Hemorrhage due to Prasugrel (Effient®)
Drug-induced hemorrhagic disorder
Hemorrhagic disorder due to increase in anti-IIa
Hemorrhagic disorder due to increase in anti-Xa
Hyperheparinemia
Use additional code for adverse effect, if applicable, to identify drug (T45.515-, T45.525-)

cc **D68.4** **Acquired coagulation factor deficiency** — Decreased production of coagulation factors.
Deficiency of coagulation factor due to liver disease
Deficiency of coagulation factor due to vitamin K deficiency
Excludes 1:   *vitamin K deficiency of newborn (P53)*

D68.5- **Primary thrombophilia** — An inherited condition of an increased tendency to form blood clots (thrombosis), potentially leading to deep vein thrombosis or pulmonary embolism.
Primary hypercoagulable states
Excludes 1:   *antiphospholipid syndrome (D68.61)*
lupus anticoagulant (D68.62)
secondary activated protein C resistance (D68.69)
secondary antiphospholipid antibody syndrome (D68.69)
secondary lupus anticoagulant with hypercoagulable state (D68.69)
secondary systemic lupus erythematosus [SLE] inhibitor with hypercoagulable state (D68.69)
systemic lupus erythematosus [SLE] inhibitor finding without diagnosis (R76.0)
systemic lupus erythematosus [SLE] inhibitor with hemorrhagic disorder (D68.312)
thrombotic thrombocytopenic purpura (M31.1)

cc **D68.51** **Activated protein C resistance** — A form caused by the body's poor response to activated protein C that poses a major risk factor for venous thromboembolism.
Factor V Leiden mutation

cc **D68.52** **Prothrombin gene mutation** — A form that impairs the prothrombin anticoagulant process.

cc **D68.59** **Other primary thrombophilia**
Antithrombin III deficiency
Hypercoagulable state NOS
Primary hypercoagulable state NEC
Primary thrombophilia NEC
Protein C deficiency
Protein S deficiency
Thrombophilia NOS

D68.6- **Other thrombophilia**
Other hypercoagulable states
Excludes 1:   *diffuse or disseminated intravascular coagulation [DIC] (D65)*
heparin induced thrombocytopenia (HIT) (D75.82)
hyperhomocysteinemia (E72.11)

cc **D68.61** **Antiphospholipid syndrome** — An increased tendency to form blood clots (thrombosis) that is due to the autoimmune production of antibodies against phospholipids (cell membrane component).
Anticardiolipin syndrome
Antiphospholipid antibody syndrome
Excludes 1:   *antiphospholipid antibody finding without diagnosis (R76.0)*
antiphospholipid antibody with hemorrhagic disorder (D68.312)
lupus anticoagulant syndrome (D68.62)

cc **D68.62** **Lupus anticoagulant syndrome** — An increased tendency to form blood clots (thrombosis) that is associated with systemic lupus.
Lupus anticoagulant
Presence of systemic lupus erythematosus [SLE] inhibitor
Excludes 1:   *anticardiolipin syndrome (D68.61)*
antiphospholipid syndrome (D68.61)
lupus anticoagulant (LAC) finding without diagnosis (R76.0)
lupus anticoagulant (LAC) with hemorrhagic disorder (D68.312)

cc **D68.69** **Other thrombophilia**
Hypercoagulable states NEC
Secondary hypercoagulable state NOS

cc **D68.8** **Other specified coagulation defects**
Excludes 1:   *hemorrhagic disease of newborn (P53)*

cc **D68.9** **Coagulation defect, unspecified**

D69- **Purpura and other hemorrhagic conditions**
Excludes 1:   *benign hypergammaglobulinemic purpura (D89.0)*
cryoglobulinemic purpura (D89.1)
essential (hemorrhagic) thrombocythemia (D47.3)
hemorrhagic thrombocythemia (D47.3)
purpura fulminans (D65)
thrombotic thrombocytopenic purpura (M31.1)
Waldenström hypergammaglobulinemic purpura (D89.0)

cc **D69.0** **Allergic purpura** — A condition characterized by skin and mucous membrane hemorrhages that is caused by a variety of agents including bacteria, drugs, and food.
Allergic vasculitis
Nonthrombocytopenic hemorrhagic purpura
Nonthrombocytopenic idiopathic purpura
Purpura anaphylactoid
Purpura Henoch(-Schönlein)
Purpura rheumatica
Vascular purpura
Excludes 1:   *thrombocytopenic hemorrhagic purpura (D69.3)*

D69.1 **Qualitative platelet defects** — Blood coagulation disorders caused by platelet cellular abnormalities.
Bernard-Soulier [giant platelet] syndrome
Glanzmann's disease
Grey platelet syndrome
Thromboasthenia (hemorrhagic) (hereditary)
Thrombocytopathy
Excludes 1:   *von Willebrand's disease (D68.0)*

D69.2 **Other nonthrombocytopenic purpura**
Purpura NOS
Purpura simplex — Nonthrombocytopenic purpura which is not associated with vascular or intravascular abnormalities, and marked by persistent bruising.
Senile purpura

cc **D69.3** **Immune thrombocytopenic purpura** — An autoimmune form characterized by development of antibodies to one's own platelets, resulting in destruction of the platelets by phagocytosis.
Hemorrhagic (thrombocytopenic) purpura
Idiopathic thrombocytopenic purpura
Tidal platelet dysgenesis

D69.4- **Other primary thrombocytopenia**
Excludes 1:   *transient neonatal thrombocytopenia (P61.0)*
Wiskott-Aldrich syndrome (D82.0)

cc **D69.41** **Evans syndrome** — An abnormally decreased platelet count with purpural hemorrhages of the skin that is marked by hemolytic anemia of an autoimmune cause.

D 6 8 - D 6 9

CC **D69.42** **Congenital and hereditary thrombocytopenia purpura** — An inherited abnormally decreased platelet count with purpural hemorrhages of the skin.
  Congenital thrombocytopenia
  Hereditary thrombocytopenia
  Code first congenital or hereditary disorder, such as:
  Thrombocytopenia with absent radius (TAR syndrome) (Q87.2)

D69.49 **Other primary thrombocytopenia**
  Megakaryocytic hypoplasia
  Primary thrombocytopenia NOS

D69.5- **Secondary thrombocytopenia** — An abnormally decreased platelet count with purpural hemorrhages of the skin resulting from an underlying disease or an external cause.
  AHA 14:4Q:p22 – Secondary thrombocytopenia
  Excludes 1:   *heparin induced thrombocytopenia (HIT) (D75.82)*
       transient thrombocytopenia of newborn (P61.0)

D69.51 **Posttransfusion purpura** — A form resulting from blood transfusions.
  Posttransfusion purpura from whole blood (fresh) or blood products
  PTP

D69.59 **Other secondary thrombocytopenia**

D69.6 **Thrombocytopenia, unspecified**

D69.8 **Other specified hemorrhagic conditions**
  Capillary fragility (hereditary)
  Vascular pseudohemophilia

D69.9 **Hemorrhagic condition, unspecified**

Other disorders of blood and blood-forming organs (D70-D77)

D70- **Neutropenia** — An abnormally low number of neutrophils in the blood.
  Includes: **Agranulocytosis**
        Decreased absolute neurophile count (ANC)
  Use additional code for any associated:
  Fever (R50.81)
  Mucositis (J34.81, K12.3-, K92.81, N76.81)
  Excludes 1:   *neutropenic splenomegaly (D73.81)*
       transient neonatal neutropenia (P61.5)

D70.0 **Congenital agranulocytosis** — An inherited form characterized by severe neutropenia and frequent, recurrent infections.
  Congenital neutropenia
  Infantile genetic agranulocytosis
  Kostmann's disease

D70.1 **Agranulocytosis secondary to cancer chemotherapy**
  AHA 14:4Q:p22 – Neutropenia secondary to chemotherapy
  Use additional code for adverse effect, if applicable, to identify drug (T45.1x5-)
  Code also underlying neoplasm

D70.2 **Other drug-induced agranulocytosis**
  Use additional code for adverse effect, if applicable, to identify drug (T36-T50 with fifth or sixth character 5)

D70.3 **Neutropenia due to infection**

D70.4 **Cyclic neutropenia** — A form characterized by periodic neutropenia with subsequent infections, followed by peripheral neutrophil recovery.
  Cyclic hematopoiesis
  Periodic neutropenia

D70.8 **Other neutropenia**

D70.9 **Neutropenia, unspecified**

D71 **Functional disorders of polymorphonuclear neutrophils** — Inhibiting disorders of granular leukocytes marked by decreased survival or abnormal pooling.
  Cell membrane receptor complex [CR3] defect
  Chronic (childhood) granulomatous disease
  Congenital dysphagocytosis
  Progressive septic granulomatosis

D72- **Other disorders of white blood cells**
  Excludes 1:   *basophilia (D72.824)*
       immunity disorders (D80-D89)
       neutropenia (D70)
       preleukemia (syndrome) (D46.9)

D72.0 **Genetic anomalies of leukocytes**
  Alder (granulation) (granulocyte) anomaly
  Alder syndrome
  Hereditary leukocytic hypersegmentation
  Hereditary leukocytic hyposegmentation
  Hereditary leukomelanopathy
  May-Hegglin (granulation) (granulocyte) anomaly
  May-Hegglin syndrome
  Pelger-Huët (granulation) (granulocyte) anomaly
  Pelger-Huët syndrome
  Excludes 1:   *Chédiak (-Steinbrinck)-Higashi syndrome (E70.330)*

D72.1 **Eosinophilia** — The abnormal accumulation of eosinophil type granular leukocytes in the blood.
  Allergic eosinophilia
  Hereditary eosinophilia
  Excludes 1:   *Löffler's syndrome (J82)*
       pulmonary eosinophilia (J82)

D72.8- **Other specified disorders of white blood cells**
  Excludes 1:   *leukemia (C91-C95)*

D72.81- **Decreased white blood cell count**
  Excludes 1:   *neutropenia (D70.-)*

D72.810 **Lymphocytopenia** — An abnormally low number of lymphocytes in the blood.
  Decreased lymphocytes

D72.818 **Other decreased white blood cell count**
  Basophilic leukopenia
  Eosinophilic leukopenia
  Monocytopenia
  Other decreased leukocytes
  Plasmacytopenia

D72.819 **Decreased white blood cell count, unspecified**
  Decreased leukocytes, unspecified
  Leukocytopenia, unspecified
  Leukopenia
  Excludes 1:   *malignant leukopenia (D70.9)*

D72.82- **Elevated white blood cell count** — An abnormally high number of white blood cells.
  Excludes 1:   *eosinophilia (D72.1)*

D72.820 **Lymphocytosis (symptomatic)** — An abnormal excess of lymphocytes in the blood.
  Elevated lymphocytes

D72.821 **Monocytosis (symptomatic)** — An abnormal increase in the proportion of monocytes in the blood.
  Excludes 1:   *infectious mononucleosis (B27.-)*

D72.822 **Plasmacytosis** — An abnormal increase of plasma cells in the blood.

D72.823 **Leukemoid reaction** — A severe form of leukocytosis that closely resembles leukemia by morphologic appearance, but is due to a physiologic response to stress, infection, or a disease process.
  Basophilic leukemoid reaction
  Leukemoid reaction NOS
  Lymphocytic leukemoid reaction
  Monocytic leukemoid reaction
  Myelocytic leukemoid reaction
  Neutrophilic leukemoid reaction

D72.824 **Basophilia** — An abnormal increase of basophils in the blood.

D72.825 **Bandemia** — An abnormal excess of immature white blood cells (band cells) that is not due to a confirmed infection.
  Bandemia without diagnosis of specific infection
  Excludes 1:   *confirmed infection — code to infection*
       leukemia (C91.-, C92.-, C93.-, C94.-, C95.-)

D72.828 **Other elevated white blood cell count**

D72.829 **Elevated white blood cell count, unspecified**
  Elevated leukocytes, unspecified
  Leukocytosis, unspecified

D72.89 **Other specified disorders of white blood cells**
  Abnormality of white blood cells NEC

D72.9 **Disorder of white blood cells, unspecified**
  Abnormal leukocyte differential NOS

D 6 9 - D 7 2

D73- Diseases of spleen

D73.0 Hyposplenism — The reduced function of the spleen.
Atrophy of spleen
Excludes 1: *asplenia (congenital) (Q89.01)*
postsurgical absence of spleen (Z90.81)

D73.1 Hypersplenism — Increased function of the spleen resulting in the removal of blood cells too early.
Excludes 1: *neutropenic splenomegaly (D73.81)*
primary splenic neutropenia (D73.81)
splenitis, splenomegaly in late syphilis (A52.79)
splenitis, splenomegaly in tuberculosis (A18.85)
splenomegaly NOS (R16.1)
splenomegaly congenital (Q89.0)

D73.2 Chronic congestive splenomegaly — Enlargement of the spleen often associated with portal hypertension.

D73.3 Abscess of spleen — A localized collection of pus caused by the disintegration of splenic tissue.

D73.4 Cyst of spleen — A fluid-filled sac within the spleen.

D73.5 Infarction of spleen — Ischemic tissue necrosis of the spleen.
Splenic rupture, nontraumatic
Torsion of spleen
Excludes 1: *rupture of spleen due to Plasmodium vivax malaria (B51.0)*
traumatic rupture of spleen (S36.03-)

D73.8- Other diseases of spleen

D73.81 Neutropenic splenomegaly — The enlargement of the spleen that results from the abnormal pooling of granular leukocytes.
Werner-Schultz disease

D73.89 Other diseases of spleen
Fibrosis of spleen NOS
Perisplenitis
Splenitis NOS

D73.9 Disease of spleen, unspecified

D74- Methemoglobinemia — The abnormal presence of methemoglobin in the blood which inhibits normal oxygen combination with iron resulting in cyanosis.

cc **D74.0 Congenital methemoglobinemia**
Congenital NADH-methemoglobin reductase deficiency
Hemoglobin-M [Hb-M] disease
Methemoglobinemia, hereditary

cc **D74.8 Other methemoglobinemias**
Acquired methemoglobinemia (with sulfhemoglobinemia)
Toxic methemoglobinemia

cc **D74.9 Methemoglobinemia, unspecified**

D75- Other and unspecified diseases of blood and blood-forming organs
Excludes ❷: *acute lymphadenitis (L04.-)*
chronic lymphadenitis (I88.1)
enlarged lymph nodes (R59.-)
hypergammaglobulinemia NOS (D89.2)
lymphadenitis NOS (I88.9)
mesenteric lymphadenitis (acute) (chronic) (I88.0)

D75.0 Familial erythrocytosis — A hereditary increase in the total red blood cell mass.
Benign polycythemia
Familial polycythemia
Excludes 1: *hereditary ovalocytosis (D58.1)*

D75.1 Secondary polycythemia — An abnormal increase in the total red blood cell mass caused as a consequence of a disease, or an external cause.
Acquired polycythemia
Emotional polycythemia
Erythrocytosis NOS
Hypoxemic polycythemia
Nephrogenous polycythemia
Polycythemia due to erythropoietin
Polycythemia due to fall in plasma volume
Polycythemia due to high altitude
Polycythemia due to stress
Polycythemia NOS
Relative polycythemia
Excludes 1: *polycythemia neonatorum (P61.1)*
polycythemia vera (D45)

D75.8- Other specified diseases of blood and blood-forming organs

cc **D75.81 Myelofibrosis** — [Not Allowed as PDX] – Replacement of the bone marrow with fibrous tissue that is usually secondary to a disease process.
Myelofibrosis NOS
Secondary myelofibrosis NOS
Code first the underlying disorder, such as:
Malignant neoplasm of breast (C50.-)
Use additional code, if applicable, for associated therapy-related myelodysplastic syndrome (D46.-)
Use additional code for adverse effect, if applicable, to identify drug (T45.1x5-)
Excludes 1: *acute myelofibrosis (C94.4-)*
idiopathic myelofibrosis (D47.1)
leukoerythroblastic anemia (D61.82)
myelofibrosis with myeloid metaplasia (D47.4)
myelophthisic anemia (D61.82)
myelophthisis (D61.82)
primary myelofibrosis (D47.1)

D75.82 Heparin induced thrombocytopenia (HIT)

D75.89 Other specified diseases of blood and blood-forming organs

D75.9 Disease of blood and blood-forming organs, unspecified

D76- Other specified diseases with participation of lymphoreticular and reticulohistiocytic tissue
Excludes 1: *(Abt-) Letterer-Siwe disease (C96.0)*
eosinophilic granuloma (C96.6)
Hand-Schüller-Christian disease (C96.5)
histiocytic medullary reticulosis (C96.9)
histiocytic sarcoma (C96.A)
histiocytosis X, multifocal (C96.5)
histiocytosis X, unifocal (C96.6)
Langerhans-cell histiocytosis, multifocal (C96.5)
Langerhans-cell histiocytosis NOS (C96.6)
Langerhans-cell histiocytosis, unifocal (C96.6)
leukemic reticuloendotheliosis (C91.4-)
lipomelanotic reticulosis (I89.8)
malignant histiocytosis (C96.A)
malignant reticulosis (C86.0)
nonlipid reticuloendotheliosis (C96.0)

cc **D76.1 Hemophagocytic lymphohistiocytosis** — The abnormal activation of lymphocytes and macrophages that destroy healthy blood cells.
Familial hemophagocytic reticulosis
Histiocytoses of mononuclear phagocytes

cc **D76.2 Hemophagocytic syndrome, infection-associated**
Use additional code to identify infectious agent or disease.

cc **D76.3 Other histiocytosis syndromes**
Reticulohistiocytoma (giant-cell)
Sinus histiocytosis with massive lymphadenopathy
Xanthogranuloma

D77 Other disorders of blood and blood-forming organs in diseases classified elsewhere — [Not Allowed as PDX]
Code first underlying disease, such as:
Amyloidosis (E85.-)
Congenital early syphilis (A50.0)
Echinococcosis (B67.0-B67.9)
Malaria (B50.0-B54)
Schistosomiasis [bilharziasis] (B65.0-B65.9)
Vitamin C deficiency (E54)
Excludes 1: *rupture of spleen due to Plasmodium vivax malaria (B51.0)*
splenitis, splenomegaly in late syphilis (A52.79)
splenitis, splenomegaly in tuberculosis (A18.85)

Intraoperative and postprocedural complications of the spleen (D78)

D78- **Intraoperative and postprocedural complications of the** <u>spleen</u>

   D78.0- <u>Intraoperative hemorrhage</u> and hematoma of the spleen complicating a procedure
      Excludes 1:   *intraoperative hemorrhage and hematoma of the spleen due to accidental puncture or laceration during a procedure (D78.1-)*

    cc **D78.01** Intraoperative hemorrhage and hematoma of the spleen complicating a procedure on the spleen

    cc **D78.02** Intraoperative hemorrhage and hematoma of the spleen complicating other procedure

   D78.1- <u>Accidental puncture</u> and laceration of the spleen during a procedure

    cc **D78.11** Accidental puncture and laceration of the spleen during a procedure on the spleen

    cc **D78.12** Accidental puncture and laceration of the spleen during other procedure

   D78.2- <u>Postprocedural hemorrhage</u> of the spleen following a procedure

    cc **D78.21** Postprocedural <u>hemorrhage</u> of the spleen following a procedure on the spleen

    cc **D78.22** Postprocedural <u>hemorrhage</u> of the spleen following other procedure

   D78.3- <u>Postprocedural hematoma and seroma</u> of the spleen following a procedure

    cc **D78.31** Postprocedural <u>hematoma</u> of the spleen following a procedure on the spleen

    cc **D78.32** Postprocedural <u>hematoma</u> of the spleen following other procedure

    cc **D78.33** Postprocedural <u>seroma</u> of the spleen following a procedure on the spleen

    cc **D78.34** Postprocedural <u>seroma</u> of the spleen following other procedure

   D78.8- **Other intraoperative and postprocedural complications of the spleen**
      Use additional code, if applicable, to further specify disorder

    cc **D78.81** Other intraoperative complications of the spleen

    cc **D78.89** Other postprocedural complications of the spleen

Certain disorders involving the immune mechanism (D80-D89)

  Includes: **Defects in the complement system**
      Immunodeficiency disorders, except human immunodeficiency virus [HIV] disease
      Sarcoidosis
  Excludes 1:   *autoimmune disease (systemic) NOS (M35.9)*
      functional disorders of polymorphonuclear neutrophils (D71)
      human immunodeficiency virus [HIV] disease (B20)

D80- **Immunodeficiency with predominantly antibody defects**

  cc **D80.0** <u>Hereditary</u> hypogammaglobulinemia — An inherited immunological deficiency state characterized by abnormally low levels of gammaglobulins.
    Autosomal recessive agammaglobulinemia (Swiss type)
    X-linked agammaglobulinemia [Bruton] (with growth hormone deficiency)

  cc **D80.1** <u>Nonfamilial</u> hypogammaglobulinemia — An immunological deficiency state characterized by abnormally low levels of gammaglobulins.
    Agammaglobulinemia with immunoglobulin-bearing B-lymphocytes
    Common variable agammaglobulinemia [CVAgamma]
    Hypogammaglobulinemia NOS

  cc **D80.2** <u>Selective</u> deficiency of immunoglobulin <u>A [IgA]</u> — An immunological deficiency state characterized by abnormally low levels of IgA class immunoglobins.

  cc **D80.3** <u>Selective</u> deficiency of immunoglobulin <u>G [IgG]</u> subclasses — An immunological deficiency state characterized by abnormally low levels of IgG class immunoglobins.

  cc **D80.4** <u>Selective</u> deficiency of immunoglobulin <u>M [IgM]</u> — An immunological deficiency state characterized by abnormally low levels of IgM class immunoglobins.

  cc **D80.5** <u>Immunodeficiency</u> with increased immunoglobulin <u>M [IgM]</u> — An immunological deficiency state characterized by increased levels of IgM class immunoglobins.

  cc **D80.6** <u>Antibody deficiency</u> with near-normal immunoglobulins or with hyperimmunoglobulinemia

  cc **D80.7** **Transient hypogammaglobulinemia of <u>infancy</u>**

  cc **D80.8** **Other immunodeficiencies with predominantly antibody defects**
    Kappa light chain deficiency

  cc **D80.9** **Immunodeficiency with predominantly antibody defects, unspecified**

D81- **Combined immunodeficiencies** — Immunological deficiency of both humoral and cell-mediated immunity.
    Excludes 1:   *autosomal recessive agammaglobulinemia (Swiss type) (D80.0)*

  cc **D81.0** **Severe combined immunodeficiency [SCID] <u>with reticular dysgenesis</u>**

  cc **D81.1** **Severe combined immunodeficiency [SCID] <u>with low T- and B-cell numbers</u>**

  cc **D81.2** **Severe combined immunodeficiency [SCID] <u>with low or normal B-cell numbers</u>**

  cc **D81.3** <u>Adenosine</u> deaminase [ADA] deficiency

  cc **D81.4** <u>Nezelof's</u> syndrome

  cc **D81.5** <u>Purine</u> nucleoside phosphorylase [PNP] deficiency

  cc **D81.6** **Major histocompatibility complex <u>class I</u> deficiency**
    Bare lymphocyte syndrome

  cc **D81.7** **Major histocompatibility complex <u>class II</u> deficiency**

   D81.8- **Other combined immunodeficiencies**

    D81.81- **Biotin-dependent carboxylase deficiency**
      Multiple carboxylase deficiency
      Excludes 1:   *biotin-dependent carboxylase deficiency due to dietary deficiency of biotin (E53.8)*

      D81.810 **Biotinidase deficiency**

      D81.818 **Other biotin-dependent carboxylase deficiency**
        Holocarboxylase synthetase deficiency
        Other multiple carboxylase deficiency

      D81.819 **Biotin-dependent carboxylase deficiency, unspecified**
        Multiple carboxylase deficiency, unspecified

  cc **D81.89** **Other combined immunodeficiencies**

  cc **D81.9** **Combined immunodeficiency, unspecified**
    Severe combined immunodeficiency disorder [SCID] NOS

D82- **Immunodeficiency** associated with other <u>major defects</u>
    Excludes 1:   *ataxia telangiectasia [Louis-Bar] (G11.3)*

  cc **D82.0** **Wiskott-Aldrich syndrome**
    Immunodeficiency with thrombocytopenia and eczema

  cc **D82.1** **Di George's syndrome**
    Pharyngeal pouch syndrome
    Thymic alymphoplasia
    Thymic aplasia or hypoplasia with immunodeficiency

    D82.2 **Immunodeficiency with short-limbed stature**

    D82.3 **Immunodeficiency following hereditary defective response to Epstein-Barr virus**
    X-linked lymphoproliferative disease

    D82.4 **Hyperimmunoglobulin E [IgE] syndrome**

    D82.8 **Immunodeficiency associated with other specified major defects**

    D82.9 **Immunodeficiency associated with major defect, unspecified**

D83- **Common variable** **immunodeficiency**

  cc **D83.0** **Common variable immunodeficiency with predominant abnormalities of B-cell numbers and function**

  cc **D83.1** **Common variable immunodeficiency with predominant immunoregulatory T-cell disorders**

  cc **D83.2** **Common variable immunodeficiency with autoantibodies to B- or T-cells**

  cc **D83.8** **Other common variable immunodeficiencies**

  cc **D83.9** **Common variable immunodeficiency, unspecified**

Excludes 1: = NOT CODED HERE! (Do not code both)

Excludes ❷: = Not Included Here

D78 – D83 *(side tab)*

D84- Other immunodeficiencies

D84.0 Lymphocyte function antigen-1 [LFA-1] defect

D84.1 Defects in the complement system
C1 esterase inhibitor [C1-INH] deficiency

CC **D84.8 Other specified immunodeficiencies**

CC **D84.9 Immunodeficiency, unspecified**

D86- Sarcoidosis — A chronic, progressive disease of unknown etiology characterized by granulomatous cells collecting into nodule-like masses that may affect any organ or tissue, including the liver, lungs, skin, lymph nodes, spleen, and eyes.

D86.0 Sarcoidosis of lung

D86.1 Sarcoidosis of lymph nodes

D86.2 Sarcoidosis of lung with sarcoidosis of lymph nodes

D86.3 Sarcoidosis of skin

D86.8- Sarcoidosis of other sites

D86.81 Sarcoid meningitis

D86.82 Multiple cranial nerve palsies in sarcoidosis

D86.83 Sarcoid iridocyclitis

D86.84 Sarcoid pyelonephritis
Tubulo-interstitial nephropathy in sarcoidosis

D86.85 Sarcoid myocarditis

D86.86 Sarcoid arthropathy
Polyarthritis in sarcoidosis

D86.87 Sarcoid myositis

D86.89 Sarcoidosis of other sites
Hepatic granuloma
Uveoparotid fever [Heerfordt]

D86.9 Sarcoidosis, unspecified

D89- Other disorders involving the immune mechanism, not elsewhere classified

Excludes 1: *hyperglobulinemia NOS (R77.1)*
monoclonal gammopathy (of undetermined significance) (D47.2)

Excludes ❷: *transplant failure and rejection (T86.-)*

D89.0 Polyclonal hypergammaglobulinemia — The abnormal excess of multiple types of immunoglobulins in the blood.
Benign hypergammaglobulinemic purpura
Polyclonal gammopathy NOS

D89.1 Cryoglobulinemia — The abnormal presence of cryoglobins (certain temperature sensitive proteins) in the blood.
Cryoglobulinemic purpura
Cryoglobulinemic vasculitis
Essential cryoglobulinemia
Idiopathic cryoglobulinemia
Mixed cryoglobulinemia
Primary cryoglobulinemia
Secondary cryoglobulinemia

D89.2 Hypergammaglobulinemia, unspecified

D89.3 Immune reconstitution syndrome
Immune reconstitution inflammatory syndrome [IRIS]
Use additional code for adverse effect, if applicable, to identify drug (T36-T50 with fifth or sixth character 5)

D89.4- Mast cell activation syndrome and related disorders

Excludes 1: *aggressive systemic mastocytosis (C96.2)*
cutaneous mastocytosis (Q82.2)
indolent systemic mastocytosis (D47.0)
malignant mastocytoma (C96.2)
mast cell leukemia (C94.3-)
mastocytoma (D47.0)
systemic mastocytosis associated with a clonal hematologic non-mast cell lineage disease (SM-AHNMD) (D47.0)

D89.40 Mast cell activation, unspecified
Mast cell activation disorder, unspecified
Mast cell activation syndrome, NOS

D89.41 Monoclonal mast cell activation syndrome — A disorder involving hyperresponsive mast cells that is characterized by flushing, pruritis, urticaria, headache, gastrointestinal symptoms, and hypotension.

D89.42 Idiopathic mast cell activation syndrome — A form without an underlying cause.

D89.43 Secondary mast cell activation — A form occurring as an indirect result of another disease or condition.
Secondary mast cell activation syndrome
Code also underlying etiology, if known

D89.49 Other mast cell activation disorder
Other mast cell activation syndrome

D89.8- Other specified disorders involving the immune mechanism, not elsewhere classified

D89.81- Graft-versus-host disease — A condition in which the donor tissue or organ (graft) contains immunogenic cells that attack the recipient's (host) tissue, most often the skin, eyes, blood, liver, and gastrointestinal tract.
Code first underlying cause, such as:
Complications of transplanted organs and tissue (T86.-)
Complications of blood transfusion (T80.89)
Use additional code to identify associated manifestations, such as:
Desquamative dermatitis (L30.8)
Diarrhea (R19.7)
Elevated bilirubin (R17)
Hair loss (L65.9)

CC **D89.810 Acute graft-versus-host disease** —
[Unacceptable PDX] — A form usually appearing within two months of the transplant.

CC **D89.811 Chronic graft-versus-host disease** —
[Unacceptable PDX] — A form usually appearing during the third month of the transplant or later.

CC **D89.812 Acute on chronic graft-versus-host disease** —
[Unacceptable PDX]

CC **D89.813 Graft-versus-host disease, unspecified** —
[Unacceptable PDX]

D89.82 Autoimmune lymphoproliferative syndrome [ALPS] — An inherited disorder of the immune system that is characterized by an excessive accumulation of lymphocytes in the body that often results in anemia, thrombocytopenia, and neutropenia.

D89.89 Other specified disorders involving the immune mechanism, not elsewhere classified

Excludes 1: *human immunodeficiency virus disease (B20)*

D89.9 Disorder involving the immune mechanism, unspecified
AHA 15:3Q:p22 – Immunocompromised state not due to medication or underlying disease
Immune disease NOS

D 8 4 - D 8 9

D89–D89

Chapter 4 – Endocrine, nutritional and metabolic diseases (E00-E89)

Note: All neoplasms, whether functionally active or not, are classified in Chapter 2. Appropriate codes in this chapter (i.e. E05.8, E07.0, E16-E31, E34.-) may be used as additional codes to indicate either functional activity by neoplasms and ectopic endocrine tissue or hyperfunction and hypofunction of endocrine glands associated with neoplasms and other conditions classified elsewhere.

Excludes 1:   transitory endocrine and metabolic disorders specific to newborn (P70-P74)

This chapter contains the following blocks:

E00-E07	Disorders of thyroid gland
E08-E13	Diabetes mellitus
E15-E16	Other disorders of glucose regulation and pancreatic internal secretion
E20-E35	Disorders of other endocrine glands
E36	Intraoperative complications of endocrine system
E40-E46	Malnutrition
E50-E64	Other nutritional deficiencies
E65-E68	Overweight, obesity and other hyperalimentation
E70-E88	Metabolic disorders
E89	Postprocedural endocrine and metabolic complications and disorders, not elsewhere classified

Chapter-Specific Coding Guidelines

C.   Chapter-Specific Coding Guidelines
In addition to general coding guidelines, there are guidelines for specific diagnoses and/or conditions in the classification. Unless otherwise indicated, these guidelines apply to all health care settings. Please refer to Section II for guidelines on the selection of principal diagnosis.

4.   Chapter 4: Endocrine, Nutritional, and Metabolic Diseases (E00-E89)

a.   Diabetes mellitus
The diabetes mellitus codes are combination codes that include the type of diabetes mellitus, the body system affected, and the complications affecting that body system. As many codes within a particular category as are necessary to describe all of the complications of the disease may be used. They should be sequenced based on the reason for a particular encounter. Assign as many codes from categories E08 – E13 as needed to identify all of the associated conditions that the patient has.

1)   Type of diabetes
The age of a patient is not the sole determining factor, though most type 1 diabetics develop the condition before reaching puberty. For this reason type 1 diabetes mellitus is also referred to as juvenile diabetes.

2)   Type of diabetes mellitus not documented
If the type of diabetes mellitus is not documented in the medical record the default is E11.-, Type 2 diabetes mellitus.

3)   Diabetes mellitus and the use of insulin *and oral hypoglycemics*
If the documentation in a medical record does not indicate the type of diabetes but does indicate that the patient uses insulin, code E11, Type 2 diabetes mellitus, should be assigned. Code Z79.4, Long-term (current) use of insulin, or Z79.84, Long term (current) use of oral hypoglycemic drugs, should also be assigned to indicate that the patient uses insulin or hypoglycemic drugs. Code Z79.4 should not be assigned if insulin is given temporarily to bring a type 2 patient's blood sugar under control during an encounter.

4)   Diabetes mellitus in pregnancy and gestational diabetes
See Section I.C.15. Diabetes mellitus in pregnancy.
See Section I.C.15. Gestational (pregnancy induced) diabetes.

5)   Complications due to insulin pump malfunction

(a)   Underdose of insulin due to insulin pump failure
An underdose of insulin due to an insulin pump failure should be assigned to a code from subcategory T85.6, Mechanical complication of other specified internal and external prosthetic devices, implants and grafts, that specifies the type of pump malfunction, as the principal or first-listed code, followed by code T38.3x6-, Underdosing of insulin and oral hypoglycemic [antidiabetic] drugs. Additional codes for the type of diabetes mellitus and any associated complications due to the underdosing should also be assigned.

(b)   Overdose of insulin due to insulin pump failure
The principal or first-listed code for an encounter due to an insulin pump malfunction resulting in an overdose of insulin, should also be T85.6-, Mechanical complication of other specified internal and external prosthetic devices, implants and grafts, followed by code T38.3x1-, Poisoning by insulin and oral hypoglycemic [antidiabetic] drugs, accidental (unintentional).

6)   Secondary diabetes mellitus
Codes under categories E08, Diabetes mellitus due to underlying condition, and E09, Drug or chemical induced diabetes mellitus, and E13, Other specified diabetes mellitus, identify complications/manifestations associated with secondary diabetes mellitus. Secondary diabetes is always caused by another condition or event (e.g., cystic fibrosis, malignant neoplasm of pancreas, pancreatectomy, adverse effect of drug, or poisoning).

(a)   Secondary diabetes mellitus and the use of insulin *or oral hypoglycemic drugs*
For patients who routinely use insulin *or hypoglycemic drugs,* code Z79.4, Long-term (current) use of insulin, *or Z79.84, Long term (current) use of oral hypoglycemic drugs,* should also be assigned. Code Z79.4 should not be assigned if insulin is given temporarily to bring a patient's blood sugar under control during an encounter.

(b)   Assigning and sequencing secondary diabetes codes and its causes
The sequencing of the secondary diabetes codes in relationship to codes for the cause of the diabetes is based on the Tabular List instructions for categories E08, E09 and E13.

(i)   Secondary diabetes mellitus due to pancreatectomy
For postpancreatectomy diabetes mellitus (lack of insulin due to the surgical removal of all or part of the pancreas), assign code E89.1, Postprocedural hypoinsulinemia. Assign a code from category E13 and a code from subcategory Z90.41-, Acquired absence of pancreas, as additional codes.

(ii)   Secondary diabetes due to drugs
Secondary diabetes may be caused by an adverse effect of correctly administered medications, poisoning or sequela of poisoning.

See section I.C.19.e for coding of adverse effects and poisoning, and section I.C.20 for external cause code reporting.

Disorders of thyroid gland (E00-E07)

E00-   Congenital iodine-deficiency syndrome — The fetal developmental failure of the thyroid gland to secrete enough thyroid hormones to maintain the normal metabolic rate (congenital hypothyroidism) that is characterized by arrested physical and mental development, dystrophy of the bones and soft parts, and lowered basal metabolism.
Use additional code (F70-F79) to identify associated intellectual disabilities.
Excludes 1:   subclinical iodine-deficiency hypothyroidism (E02)

E00.0   Congenital iodine-deficiency syndrome, neurological type
Endemic cretinism, neurological type

E00.1   Congenital iodine-deficiency syndrome, myxedematous type
Endemic hypothyroid cretinism
Endemic cretinism, myxedematous type

E00.2   Congenital iodine-deficiency syndrome, mixed type
Endemic cretinism, mixed type

E00.9   Congenital iodine-deficiency syndrome, unspecified
Congenital iodine-deficiency hypothyroidism NOS
Endemic cretinism NOS

E01-   Iodine-deficiency related thyroid disorders and allied conditions
Excludes 1:   congenital iodine-deficiency syndrome (E00.-)
*   subclinical iodine-deficiency hypothyroidism (E02)*

E01.0   Iodine-deficiency related diffuse (endemic) goiter — An enlargement of the thyroid gland with associated swelling in the front part of the neck that is associated with dietary iodine deficiency.

E01.1   Iodine-deficiency related multinodular (endemic) goiter — An enlargement of the thyroid gland with associated swelling in the front part of the neck that is associated with dietary iodine deficiency and characterized by the formation of multiple nodules within the thyroid.
Iodine-deficiency related nodular goiter

E01.2   Iodine-deficiency related (endemic) goiter, unspecified
Endemic goiter NOS

E01.8   Other iodine-deficiency related thyroid disorders and allied conditions
Acquired iodine-deficiency hypothyroidism NOS

E02   Subclinical iodine-deficiency hypothyroidism — A milder form of hypothyroidism that is associated with dietary iodine deficiency.

E03-   Other hypothyroidism
Excludes 1:   iodine-deficiency related hypothyroidism (E00-E02)
*   postprocedural hypothyroidism (E89.0)*

E03.0   Congenital hypothyroidism with diffuse goiter — The failure of the thyroid gland to secrete enough thyroid hormones that is present at birth and causes a general inflammation of the thyroid gland.
Congenital parenchymatous goiter (nontoxic)
Congenital goiter (nontoxic) NOS
Excludes 1:   transitory congenital goiter with normal function (P72.0)

E00 - E03

E03.1 <u>Congenital</u> hypothyroidism <u>without</u> goiter
Aplasia of thyroid (with myxedema)
Congenital atrophy of thyroid
Congenital hypothyroidism NOS

E03.2 Hypothyroidism <u>due to medicaments</u> and other exogenous substances
Code first poisoning due to drug or toxin, if applicable (T36-T65 with fifth or sixth character 1-4 or 6)
Use additional code for adverse effect, if applicable, to identify drug (T36-T50 with fifth or sixth character 5)

E03.3 <u>Postinfectious</u> hypothyroidism

E03.4 <u>Atrophy</u> of thyroid (acquired)
Excludes 1:   congenital atrophy of thyroid (E03.1)

MCC **E03.5** Myxedema <u>coma</u> — A life-threatening form of severe, longstanding hypothyroidism that is characterized by loss of brain function.

E03.8 Other specified hypothyroidism

E03.9 Hypothyroidism, unspecified
Myxedema NOS

E04- Other <u>nontoxic goiter</u>
*Excludes 1:   congenital goiter (NOS) (diffuse) (parenchymatous) (E03.0)
iodine-deficiency related goiter (E00-E02)*

E04.0 Nontoxic <u>diffuse</u> goiter — Hypertrophy of the thyroid with a generalized enlargement of the thyroid gland.
Diffuse (colloid) nontoxic goiter
Simple nontoxic goiter

E04.1 Nontoxic <u>single</u> thyroid nodule — Hypertrophy of the thyroid with the presence of a single nodule.
Colloid nodule (cystic) (thyroid)
Nontoxic uninodular goiter
Thyroid (cystic) nodule NOS

E04.2 Nontoxic <u>multinodular</u> goiter — Hypertrophy of the thyroid with the presence of multiple nodules.
Cystic goiter NOS
Multinodular (cystic) goiter NOS

E04.8 Other specified nontoxic goiter

E04.9 Nontoxic goiter, unspecified
Goiter NOS
Nodular goiter (nontoxic) NOS

E05- <u>Thyrotoxicosis</u> [hyperthyroidism] — The condition of elevated levels of circulating thyroid hormones.
*Excludes 1:   chronic thyroiditis with transient thyrotoxicosis (E06.2)
neonatal thyrotoxicosis (P72.1)*

E05.0- Thyrotoxicosis <u>with diffuse goiter</u> — A form marked by a generalized enlargement of the thyroid gland.
Exophthalmic or toxic goiter NOS
Graves' disease
Toxic diffuse goiter

E05.00 Thyrotoxicosis with diffuse goiter <u>without</u> thyrotoxic crisis or storm

MCC **E05.01** Thyrotoxicosis with diffuse goiter <u>with</u> thyrotoxic crisis or storm — An acute, life-threatening state of excessive release of thyroid hormones that is characterized by a rapid increase in the body's temperature, blood pressure, and heart rate.

E05.1- Thyrotoxicosis with <u>toxic single thyroid nodule</u> — A form marked by the presence of a single nodule.
Thyrotoxicosis with toxic uninodular goiter

E05.10 Thyrotoxicosis with toxic single thyroid nodule <u>without</u> thyrotoxic crisis or storm

MCC **E05.11** Thyrotoxicosis with toxic single thyroid nodule <u>with</u> thyrotoxic crisis or storm — An acute, life-threatening state of excessive release of thyroid hormones that is characterized by a rapid increase in the body's temperature, blood pressure, and heart rate.

E05.2- Thyrotoxicosis with <u>toxic multinodular</u> goiter — A form marked by the presence of multiple nodules.
Toxic nodular goiter NOS

E05.20 Thyrotoxicosis with toxic multinodular goiter <u>without</u> thyrotoxic crisis or storm

MCC **E05.21** Thyrotoxicosis with toxic multinodular goiter <u>with</u> thyrotoxic crisis or storm — An acute, life-threatening state of excessive release of thyroid hormones that is characterized by a rapid increase in the body's temperature, blood pressure, and heart rate.

E05.3- Thyrotoxicosis from <u>ectopic thyroid tissue</u> — A form marked by thyroid-tissue hormones from a thyroid nodule which is not within the thyroid gland.

E05.30 Thyrotoxicosis from ectopic thyroid tissue <u>without</u> thyrotoxic crisis or storm

MCC **E05.31** Thyrotoxicosis from ectopic thyroid tissue <u>with</u> thyrotoxic crisis or storm — An acute, life-threatening state of excessive release of thyroid hormones that is characterized by a rapid increase in the body's temperature, blood pressure, and heart rate.

E05.4- Thyrotoxicosis <u>factitia</u> — A form marked by the ingestion of excessive amounts of exogenous thyroid hormone.

E05.40 Thyrotoxicosis factitia <u>without</u> thyrotoxic crisis or storm

MCC **E05.41** Thyrotoxicosis factitia <u>with</u> thyrotoxic crisis or storm — An acute, life-threatening state of excessive release of thyroid hormones that is characterized by a rapid increase in the body's temperature, blood pressure, and heart rate.

E05.8- Other thyrotoxicosis
Overproduction of thyroid-stimulating hormone

E05.80 Other thyrotoxicosis <u>without</u> thyrotoxic crisis or storm

MCC **E05.81** Other thyrotoxicosis <u>with</u> thyrotoxic crisis or storm — An acute, life-threatening state of excessive release of thyroid hormones that is characterized by a rapid increase in the body's temperature, blood pressure, and heart rate.

E05.9- Thyrotoxicosis, <u>unspecified</u>
Hyperthyroidism NOS

E05.90 Thyrotoxicosis, unspecified <u>without</u> thyrotoxic crisis or storm

MCC **E05.91** Thyrotoxicosis, unspecified <u>with</u> thyrotoxic crisis or storm

E06- <u>Thyroiditis</u> — Inflammation of the thyroid gland.
Excludes 1:   postpartum thyroiditis (O90.5)

CC **E06.0** <u>Acute</u> thyroiditis — A sudden, severe onset of inflammation of the thyroid gland usually caused by a bacterial infection.
Abscess of thyroid
Pyogenic thyroiditis
Suppurative thyroiditis
Use additional code (B95-B97) to identify infectious agent.

E06.1 <u>Subacute</u> thyroiditis — Inflammation of the thyroid marked by the presence of giant cells, granulomas in the gland, and masses of colloid.
de Quervain thyroiditis
Giant-cell thyroiditis
Granulomatous thyroiditis
Nonsuppurative thyroiditis
Viral thyroiditis
Excludes 1:   autoimmune thyroiditis (E06.3)

E06.2 <u>Chronic</u> thyroiditis with transient thyrotoxicosis — A form with brief periods of elevated circulating thyroid hormones.
Excludes 1:   autoimmune thyroiditis (E06.3)

E06.3 <u>Autoimmune</u> thyroiditis — An autoimmune disease of progressive inflammation of the thyroid gland characterized by diffuse lymphocytic infiltration and fibrotic replacement of thyroid tissue.
Hashimoto's thyroiditis
Hashitoxicosis (transient)
Lymphadenoid goiter
Lymphocytic thyroiditis
Struma lymphomatosa

E06.4 <u>Drug-induced</u> thyroiditis
Use additional code for adverse effect, if applicable, to identify drug (T36-T50 with fifth or sixth character 5)

E06.5 Other chronic thyroiditis
Chronic fibrous thyroiditis
Chronic thyroiditis NOS
Ligneous thyroiditis
Riedel thyroiditis

E06.9 Thyroiditis, unspecified

E07- <u>Other disorders</u> of thyroid

E07.0 Hypersecretion of calcitonin — A condition resulting in the body's depletion of calcium and phosphate levels caused by thyrocalcitonin (a thyroid hormone which responds to excessive calcium in the body).
C-cell hyperplasia of thyroid
Hypersecretion of thyrocalcitonin

E07.1 Dyshormogenetic goiter — Thyroid hyperplasia due to enzyme defects in thyroid-hormone synthesis.
Familial dyshormogenetic goiter
Pendred's syndrome
Excludes 1:   transitory congenital goiter with normal function (P72.0)

E07.8- Other specified disorders of thyroid

E07.81 Sick-euthyroid syndrome — A transient alteration in thyroid hormone metabolism (low levels of serum thyroid hormones) caused by a nonthyroidal illness or condition.
Euthyroid sick-syndrome

Excludes 1: = NOT CODED HERE! (Do not code both)   **610**   *Excludes ❷:* = Not Included Here

E03 - E07

E07.89   Other specified disorders of thyroid
Abnormality of thyroid-binding globulin
Hemorrhage of thyroid
Infarction of thyroid

E07.9   Disorder of thyroid, unspecified

Diabetes mellitus (E08-E13)

E08-   Diabetes mellitus due to underlying condition — A complex metabolic syndrome characterized by consistently high blood sugar (glucose) levels, glycosuria, and metabolic effects caused by faulty pancreatic insulin production, thus producing insufficient amounts of insulin that is due to another medical condition.

AHA 13:3Q:p20 — Hyperglycemia together with another diabetes code
AHA 13:3Q:p20 — Uncontrolled type 1 diabetes with ketoacidosis
AHA 16:1Q:p12 — Cause-and-effect condition relationships

Code first the underlying condition, such as:
Congenital rubella (P35.0)
Cushing's syndrome (E24.-)
Cystic fibrosis (E84.-)
Malignant neoplasm (C00-C96)
Malnutrition (E40-E46)
Pancreatitis and other diseases of the pancreas (K85-, K86-)
Use additional code to identify control using:
Insulin (Z79.4)
Oral antidiabetic drugs (Z79.84)
Oral hypoglycemic drugs (Z79.84)

Excludes 1:   drug or chemical induced diabetes mellitus (E09-)
gestational diabetes (O24.4-)
neonatal diabetes mellitus (P70.2)
postpancreatectomy diabetes mellitus (E13-)
postprocedural diabetes mellitus (E13-)
secondary diabetes mellitus NEC (E13-)
type 1 diabetes mellitus (E10-)
type 2 diabetes mellitus (E11-)

E08.0-   Diabetes mellitus due to underlying condition with hyperosmolarity — A form with extremely high blood sugar (glucose) levels and without the presence of ketones.

MCC **E08.00   Diabetes mellitus due to underlying condition with hyperosmolarity without nonketotic hyperglycemic-hyperosmolar coma (NKHHC)** — [Not Allowed as PDX]

MCC **E08.01   Diabetes mellitus due to underlying condition with hyperosmolarity with coma** — [Not Allowed as PDX]

E08.1-   Diabetes mellitus due to underlying condition with ketoacidosis — The potentially life-threatening complication of ketone poisoning caused by very low insulin that forces the body to use fat for fuel. When the fat breaks down, its waste products (acids called ketone bodies) build up in the blood and urine.

MCC **E08.10   Diabetes mellitus due to underlying condition with ketoacidosis without coma** — [Not Allowed as PDX]

MCC **E08.11   Diabetes mellitus due to underlying condition with ketoacidosis with coma** — [Not Allowed as PDX]

E08.2-   Diabetes mellitus due to underlying condition with kidney complications

E08.21   Diabetes mellitus due to underlying condition with diabetic nephropathy — [Not Allowed as PDX] – A progressive kidney disease caused by damage to the blood capillaries of the kidney's glomeruli that is due to the long-term effects of diabetes.
Diabetes mellitus due to underlying condition with intercapillary glomerulosclerosis
Diabetes mellitus due to underlying condition with intracapillary glomerulonephrosis
Diabetes mellitus due to underlying condition with Kimmelstiel-Wilson disease

E08.22   Diabetes mellitus due to underlying condition with diabetic chronic kidney disease — [Not Allowed as PDX]
Use additional code to identify stage of chronic kidney disease (N18.1-N18.6)

E08.29   Diabetes mellitus due to underlying condition with other diabetic kidney complication — [Not Allowed as PDX]
Renal tubular degeneration in diabetes mellitus due to underlying condition

E08.3-   Diabetes mellitus due to underlying condition with ophthalmic complications

E08.31-   Diabetes mellitus due to underlying condition with unspecified diabetic retinopathy — A diabetic complication caused by damage to the blood vessels of the retina.

E08.311   Diabetes mellitus due to underlying condition with unspecified diabetic retinopathy with macular edema — [Not Allowed as PDX]

E08.319   Diabetes mellitus due to underlying condition with unspecified diabetic retinopathy without macular edema — [Not Allowed as PDX]

E08.32-   Diabetes mellitus due to underlying condition with mild nonproliferative diabetic retinopathy
Diabetes mellitus due to underlying condition with nonproliferative diabetic retinopathy NOS

One of the following 7th characters is to be assigned to codes in subcategory E08.32- to designate laterality of the disease:
1   Right eye
2   Left eye
3   Bilateral
9   Unspecified eye

E08.321-   Diabetes mellitus due to underlying condition with mild nonproliferative diabetic retinopathy with macular edema — [Not Allowed as PDX]

E08.329-   Diabetes mellitus due to underlying condition with mild nonproliferative diabetic retinopathy without macular edema — [Not Allowed as PDX]

E08.33-   Diabetes mellitus due to underlying condition with moderate nonproliferative diabetic retinopathy
One of the following 7th characters is to be assigned to codes in subcategory E08.33- to designate laterality of the disease:
1   Right eye
2   Left eye
3   Bilateral
9   Unspecified eye

E08.331-   Diabetes mellitus due to underlying condition with moderate nonproliferative diabetic retinopathy with macular edema — [Not Allowed as PDX]

E08.339-   Diabetes mellitus due to underlying condition with moderate nonproliferative diabetic retinopathy without macular edema — [Not Allowed as PDX]

E08.34-   Diabetes mellitus due to underlying condition with severe nonproliferative diabetic retinopathy
One of the following 7th characters is to be assigned to codes in subcategory E08.34- to designate laterality of the disease:
1   Right eye
2   Left eye
3   Bilateral
9   Unspecified eye

E08.341-   Diabetes mellitus due to underlying condition with severe nonproliferative diabetic retinopathy with macular edema — [Not Allowed as PDX]

E08.349-   Diabetes mellitus due to underlying condition with severe nonproliferative diabetic retinopathy without macular edema — [Not Allowed as PDX]

E08.35-   Diabetes mellitus due to underlying condition with proliferative diabetic retinopathy
One of the following 7th characters is to be assigned to codes in subcategory E08.35- to designate laterality of the disease:
1   Right eye
2   Left eye
3   Bilateral
9   Unspecified eye

E08.351-   Diabetes mellitus due to underlying condition with proliferative diabetic retinopathy with macular edema — [Not Allowed as PDX]

E 07 – E 08

E08.352- Diabetes mellitus due to underlying condition with proliferative diabetic retinopathy <u>with traction retinal detachment involving the macula</u> — [Not Allowed as PDX]

E08.353- Diabetes mellitus due to underlying condition with proliferative diabetic retinopathy with traction retinal detachment <u>not</u> involving the macula — [Not Allowed as PDX]

E08.354- Diabetes mellitus due to underlying condition with proliferative diabetic retinopathy <u>with combined</u> traction retinal detachment and rhegmatogenous retinal detachment — [Not Allowed as PDX]

E08.355- Diabetes mellitus due to underlying condition <u>with stable</u> proliferative diabetic retinopathy — [Not Allowed as PDX]

E08.359- Diabetes mellitus due to underlying condition with proliferative diabetic retinopathy <u>without</u> macular edema — [Not Allowed as PDX]

E08.36 Diabetes mellitus due to underlying condition with diabetic <u>cataract</u> — [Not Allowed as PDX] — The diabetic complication resulting in the clouding of the ocular lens.

E08.37x- Diabetes mellitus due to underlying condition with diabetic macular edema, <u>resolved</u> following treatment — [Not Allowed as PDX]

> **One of the following 7th characters is to be assigned to code E08.37x- to designate laterality of the disease:**
> 1   Right eye
> 2   Left eye
> 3   Bilateral
> 9   Unspecified eye

E08.39 Diabetes mellitus due to underlying condition with other diabetic <u>ophthalmic complication</u> — [Not Allowed as PDX]
Use additional code to identify manifestation, such as:
    Diabetic glaucoma (H40-H42)

E08.4- Diabetes mellitus due to <u>underlying condition</u> with <u>neurological</u> complications

E08.40 Diabetes mellitus due to underlying condition with diabetic <u>neuropathy, unspecified</u> — [Not Allowed as PDX]

E08.41 Diabetes mellitus due to underlying condition with diabetic <u>mononeuropathy</u> — [Not Allowed as PDX] — The diabetic nerve damage complication caused by microvascular damage to nerves in a single location.

E08.42 Diabetes mellitus due to underlying condition with diabetic <u>polyneuropathy</u> — [Not Allowed as PDX] — The diabetic nerve damage complication caused by microvascular damage to multiple nerves in various locations.
    Diabetes mellitus due to underlying condition with diabetic neuralgia

E08.43 Diabetes mellitus due to underlying condition with diabetic <u>autonomic</u> (poly)neuropathy — [Not Allowed as PDX] — The diabetic nerve damage complication caused by microvascular damage to autonomic (internal organs) nerves in various locations.
    AHA 13:4Q:p114 – Diabetic gastroparesis
    Diabetes mellitus due to underlying condition with diabetic gastroparesis

E08.44 Diabetes mellitus due to underlying condition with diabetic <u>amyotrophy</u> — [Not Allowed as PDX] — The diabetic nerve damage complication caused by microvascular damage to the nerves of the hips, buttocks, thighs, or legs and usually on one side of the body.

E08.49 Diabetes mellitus due to underlying condition with other diabetic neurological complication — [Not Allowed as PDX]

E08.5- Diabetes mellitus due to <u>underlying condition</u> with <u>circulatory</u> complications

E08.51 Diabetes mellitus due to underlying condition with <u>diabetic peripheral angiopathy without</u> gangrene — [Not Allowed as PDX] — The diabetic complication causing decay of the lining of peripheral blood vessels.

CC **E08.52** Diabetes mellitus due to underlying condition with <u>diabetic peripheral angiopathy with gangrene</u> — [Not Allowed as PDX]
    Diabetes mellitus due to underlying condition with diabetic gangrene

E08.59 Diabetes mellitus due to underlying condition with other circulatory complications — [Not Allowed as PDX]

E08.6- Diabetes mellitus due to <u>underlying condition</u> with other specified complications

E08.61- Diabetes mellitus due to underlying condition with diabetic <u>arthropathy</u>

E08.610 Diabetes mellitus due to underlying condition with diabetic <u>neuropathic</u> arthropathy — [Not Allowed as PDX] — The diabetic complication of neurovascular damage of joints resulting in loss of sensation and subsequent joint damage.
    Diabetes mellitus due to underlying condition with Charcot's joints

E08.618 Diabetes mellitus due to underlying condition with other diabetic arthropathy — [Not Allowed as PDX]

E08.62- Diabetes mellitus due to underlying condition with <u>skin</u> complications

E08.620 Diabetes mellitus due to underlying condition with diabetic <u>dermatitis</u> — [Not Allowed as PDX] — The diabetic complication of cutaneous damage resulting in various skin conditions (inflammation, infection, lesions).
    Diabetes mellitus due to underlying condition with diabetic necrobiosis lipoidica

E08.621 Diabetes mellitus due to underlying condition with <u>foot ulcer</u> — [Not Allowed as PDX]
Use additional code to identify site of ulcer (L97.4-, L97.5-)

E08.622 Diabetes mellitus due to underlying condition with <u>other skin ulcer</u> — [Not Allowed as PDX]
Use additional code to identify site of ulcer (L97.1-L97.9, L98.41-L98.49)

E08.628 Diabetes mellitus due to underlying condition with other skin complications — [Not Allowed as PDX]

E08.63- Diabetes mellitus due to underlying condition with <u>oral</u> complications

E08.630 Diabetes mellitus due to underlying condition with periodontal disease — [Not Allowed as PDX]

E08.638 Diabetes mellitus due to underlying condition with other oral complications — [Not Allowed as PDX]

E08.64- Diabetes mellitus due to underlying condition with <u>hypoglycemia</u>

MCC **E08.641** Diabetes mellitus due to underlying condition with hypoglycemia <u>with coma</u> — [Not Allowed as PDX]

E08.649 Diabetes mellitus due to underlying condition with hypoglycemia <u>without coma</u> — [Not Allowed as PDX]

E08.65 Diabetes mellitus due to underlying condition with <u>hyperglycemia</u> — [Not Allowed as PDX] — The diabetic condition of having high sugar (glucose) levels in the blood and urine causing excessive thirst and frequent urination.

E08.69 Diabetes mellitus due to underlying condition with <u>other specified</u> complication — [Not Allowed as PDX]
Use additional code to identify complication

E08.8 Diabetes mellitus due to <u>underlying condition</u> with <u>unspecified</u> complications — [Not Allowed as PDX]

E08.9 Diabetes mellitus due to <u>underlying condition</u> <u>without</u> complications — [Not Allowed as PDX]

E08 – E08

E09-   <u>Drug or chemical induced</u> **diabetes mellitus** — A complex metabolic syndrome characterized by consistently high blood sugar (glucose) levels, glycosuria, and metabolic effects caused by faulty pancreatic insulin production, thus producing insufficient amounts of insulin that is due to effect of a drug or chemical.

    AHA 13:3Q:p20 — Hyperglycemia together with another diabetes code

    AHA 13:3Q:p20 — Uncontrolled type 1 diabetes with ketoacidosis

    AHA 16:1Q:p12 — Cause-and-effect condition relationships

    Code first poisoning due to drug or toxin, if applicable (T36-T65 with fifth or sixth character 1-4 or 6)

    Use additional code for adverse effect, if applicable, to identify drug (T36-T50 with fifth or sixth character 5)

    Use additional code to identify control using:

      Insulin (Z79.4)

      Oral antidiabetic drugs (Z79.84)

      Oral hypoglycemic drugs (Z79.84)

    Excludes 1:   *diabetes mellitus due to underlying condition (E08.-)*

               gestational diabetes (O24.4-)

               neonatal diabetes mellitus (P70.2)

               postpancreatectomy diabetes mellitus (E13.-)

               postprocedural diabetes mellitus (E13.-)

               secondary diabetes mellitus NEC (E13.-)

               type 1 diabetes mellitus (E10.-)

               type 2 diabetes mellitus (E11.-)

E09.0-   <u>Drug or chemical induced</u> **diabetes mellitus with** <u>hyperosmolarity</u> — A form with extremely high blood sugar (glucose) levels and without the presence of ketones.

MCC **E09.00**   Drug or chemical induced diabetes mellitus with hyperosmolarity <u>without</u> nonketotic hyperglycemic-hyperosmolar coma (NKHHC)

MCC **E09.01**   Drug or chemical induced diabetes mellitus with hyperosmolarity <u>with coma</u>

E09.1-   <u>Drug or chemical induced</u> **diabetes mellitus with** <u>ketoacidosis</u> — The potentially life-threatening complication of ketone poisoning caused by very low insulin that forces the body to use fat for fuel. When the fat breaks down, its waste products (acids called ketone bodies) build up in the blood and urine.

MCC **E09.10**   Drug or chemical induced diabetes mellitus with ketoacidosis <u>without</u> coma

MCC **E09.11**   Drug or chemical induced diabetes mellitus with ketoacidosis <u>with coma</u>

E09.2-   <u>Drug or chemical induced</u> **diabetes mellitus with** <u>kidney</u> **complications**

   E09.21   Drug or chemical induced diabetes mellitus with diabetic <u>nephropathy</u> — A progressive kidney disease caused by damage to the blood capillaries of the kidney's glomeruli that is due to the long-term effects of diabetes.

      Drug or chemical induced diabetes mellitus with intercapillary glomerulosclerosis

      Drug or chemical induced diabetes mellitus with intracapillary glomerulonephrosis

      Drug or chemical induced diabetes mellitus with Kimmelstiel-Wilson disease

   E09.22   Drug or chemical induced diabetes mellitus with diabetic <u>chronic kidney disease</u>

      Use additional code to identify stage of chronic kidney disease (N18.1-N18.6)

   E09.29   Drug or chemical induced diabetes mellitus with other diabetic kidney complication

      Drug or chemical induced diabetes mellitus with renal tubular degeneration

E09.3-   <u>Drug or chemical induced</u> **diabetes mellitus with** <u>ophthalmic</u> **complications**

   E09.31-   Drug or chemical induced diabetes mellitus with <u>unspecified</u> diabetic retinopathy — A diabetic complication caused by damage to the blood vessels of the retina.

     E09.311   Drug or chemical induced diabetes mellitus with unspecified diabetic retinopathy <u>with macular edema</u>

     E09.319   Drug or chemical induced diabetes mellitus with unspecified diabetic retinopathy <u>without</u> macular edema

E09.32-   Drug or chemical induced diabetes mellitus with <u>mild</u> <u>non</u>proliferative diabetic retinopathy

    Drug or chemical induced diabetes mellitus with nonproliferative diabetic retinopathy NOS

> One of the following 7th characters is to be assigned to codes in subcategory E09.32- to designate laterality of the disease:
> 1   Right eye
> 2   Left eye
> 3   Bilateral
> 9   Unspecified eye

   E09.321-   Drug or chemical induced diabetes mellitus with mild nonproliferative diabetic retinopathy <u>with macular edema</u>

   E09.329-   Drug or chemical induced diabetes mellitus with mild nonproliferative diabetic retinopathy <u>without</u> macular edema

E09.33-   Drug or chemical induced diabetes mellitus with <u>moderate</u> <u>non</u>proliferative diabetic retinopathy

> One of the following 7th characters is to be assigned to codes in subcategory E09.33- to designate laterality of the disease:
> 1   Right eye
> 2   Left eye
> 3   Bilateral
> 9   Unspecified eye

   E09.331-   Drug or chemical induced diabetes mellitus with moderate nonproliferative diabetic retinopathy <u>with macular edema</u>

   E09.339-   Drug or chemical induced diabetes mellitus with moderate nonproliferative diabetic retinopathy <u>without</u> macular edema

E09.34-   Drug or chemical induced diabetes mellitus with <u>severe</u> <u>non</u>proliferative diabetic retinopathy

> One of the following 7th characters is to be assigned to codes in subcategory E09.34- to designate laterality of the disease:
> 1   Right eye
> 2   Left eye
> 3   Bilateral
> 9   Unspecified eye

   E09.341-   Drug or chemical induced diabetes mellitus with severe nonproliferative diabetic retinopathy <u>with macular edema</u>

   E09.349-   Drug or chemical induced diabetes mellitus with severe nonproliferative diabetic retinopathy <u>without</u> macular edema

E09.35-   Drug or chemical induced diabetes mellitus with <u>proliferative</u> diabetic retinopathy

> One of the following 7th characters is to be assigned to codes in subcategory E09.35- to designate laterality of the disease:
> 1   Right eye
> 2   Left eye
> 3   Bilateral
> 9   Unspecified eye

   E09.351-   Drug or chemical induced diabetes mellitus with proliferative diabetic retinopathy <u>with macular edema</u>

   E09.352-   Drug or chemical induced diabetes mellitus with proliferative diabetic retinopathy <u>with traction retinal detachment involving the macula</u> — [Not Allowed as PDX]

   E09.353-   Drug or chemical induced diabetes mellitus with proliferative diabetic retinopathy with traction retinal detachment <u>not</u> involving the macula — [Not Allowed as PDX]

   E09.354-   Drug or chemical induced diabetes mellitus with proliferative diabetic retinopathy <u>with combined</u> traction retinal detachment and rhegmatogenous retinal detachment — [Not Allowed as PDX]

E09.355- Drug or chemical induced diabetes mellitus <u>with</u> <u>stable</u> proliferative diabetic retinopathy —
[Not Allowed as PDX]

E09.359- Drug or chemical induced diabetes mellitus with proliferative diabetic retinopathy <u>without</u> macular edema

E09.36 Drug or chemical induced diabetes mellitus with diabetic <u>cataract</u> — The diabetic complication resulting in the clouding of the ocular lens.

E09.37x- Drug or chemical induced diabetes mellitus with diabetic macular edema, <u>resolved</u> following treatment —
[Not Allowed as PDX]

One of the following 7th characters is to be assigned to code E09.37x- to designate laterality of the disease:
1   Right eye
2   Left eye
3   Bilateral
9   Unspecified eye

E09.39 Drug or chemical induced diabetes mellitus with other diabetic <u>ophthalmic complication</u>
Use additional code to identify manifestation, such as:
Diabetic glaucoma (H40-H42)

E09.4- <u>Drug or chemical induced</u> diabetes mellitus with <u>neurological</u> complications

E09.40 Drug or chemical induced diabetes mellitus with neurological complications with diabetic <u>neuropathy,</u> <u>unspecified</u>

E09.41 Drug or chemical induced diabetes mellitus with neurological complications with diabetic mononeuropathy — The diabetic nerve damage complication caused by microvascular damage to nerves in a single location.

E09.42 Drug or chemical induced diabetes mellitus with neurological complications with diabetic polyneuropathy — The diabetic nerve damage complication caused by microvascular damage to multiple nerves in various locations.
Drug or chemical induced diabetes mellitus with diabetic neuralgia

E09.43 Drug or chemical induced diabetes mellitus with neurological complications with diabetic <u>autonomic</u> (poly)neuropathy — The diabetic nerve damage complication caused by microvascular damage to autonomic (internal organs) nerves in various locations.
AHA 13:4Q:p114 – Diabetic gastroparesis
Drug or chemical induced diabetes mellitus with diabetic gastroparesis

E09.44 Drug or chemical induced diabetes mellitus with neurological complications with diabetic <u>amyotrophy</u> — The diabetic nerve damage complication caused by microvascular damage to the nerves of the hips, buttocks, thighs, or legs and usually on one side of the body.

E09.49 Drug or chemical induced diabetes mellitus with neurological complications with other diabetic neurological complication

E09.5- <u>Drug or chemical induced</u> diabetes mellitus with <u>circulatory</u> complications

E09.51 Drug or chemical induced diabetes mellitus with <u>diabetic</u> <u>peripheral angiopathy without</u> gangrene — The diabetic complication causing decay of the lining of peripheral blood vessels.

CC **E09.52** Drug or chemical induced diabetes mellitus with <u>diabetic</u> <u>peripheral angiopathy with</u> <u>gangrene</u>
Drug or chemical induced diabetes mellitus with diabetic gangrene

E09.59 Drug or chemical induced diabetes mellitus with other circulatory complications

E09.6- <u>Drug or chemical induced</u> diabetes mellitus with other specified complications

E09.61- Drug or chemical induced diabetes mellitus with diabetic <u>arthropathy</u>

E09.610 Drug or chemical induced diabetes mellitus with diabetic <u>neuropathic</u> arthropathy — The diabetic complication of neurovascular damage of joints resulting in loss of sensation and subsequent joint damage.
Drug or chemical induced diabetes mellitus with Charcot's joints

E09.618 Drug or chemical induced diabetes mellitus with other diabetic arthropathy

E09.62- Drug or chemical induced diabetes mellitus with <u>skin</u> complications

E09.620 Drug or chemical induced diabetes mellitus with diabetic <u>dermatitis</u> — The diabetic complication of cutaneous damage resulting in various skin conditions (inflammation, infection, lesions).
Drug or chemical induced diabetes mellitus with diabetic necrobiosis lipoidica

E09.621 Drug or chemical induced diabetes mellitus with <u>foot ulcer</u>
Use additional code to identify site of ulcer (L97.4-, L97.5-)

E09.622 Drug or chemical induced diabetes mellitus with <u>other skin ulcer</u>
Use additional code to identify site of ulcer (L97.1-L97.9, L98.41-L98.49)

E09.628 Drug or chemical induced diabetes mellitus with other skin complications

E09.63- Drug or chemical induced diabetes mellitus with <u>oral</u> complications

E09.630 Drug or chemical induced diabetes mellitus with periodontal disease

E09.638 Drug or chemical induced diabetes mellitus with other oral complications

E09.64- Drug or chemical induced diabetes mellitus with <u>hypoglycemia</u>

MCC **E09.641** Drug or chemical induced diabetes mellitus with hypoglycemia <u>with coma</u>

E09.649 Drug or chemical induced diabetes mellitus with hypoglycemia <u>without</u> coma

E09.65 Drug or chemical induced diabetes mellitus with <u>hyperglycemia</u> — The diabetic condition of having high sugar (glucose) levels in the blood and urine causing excessive thirst and frequent urination.

E09.69 Drug or chemical induced diabetes mellitus with <u>other</u> <u>specified</u> complication
Use additional code to identify complication

E09.8 <u>Drug or chemical induced</u> diabetes mellitus with <u>unspecified</u> complications

E09.9 <u>Drug or chemical induced</u> diabetes mellitus <u>without</u> complications

E10- <u>Type 1 diabetes mellitus</u> — A complex metabolic syndrome characterized by consistently high blood (glucose) sugar, glycosuria, and metabolic effects caused by severely faulty pancreatic insulin production, thus producing little or no insulin.
AHA 13:3Q:p20 — Hyperglycemia together with another diabetes code
AHA 13:3Q:p20 — Uncontrolled type 1 diabetes with ketoacidosis
AHA 16:1Q:p12 – Cause-and-effect condition relationships
Includes: Brittle diabetes (mellitus)
Diabetes (mellitus) due to autoimmune process
Diabetes (mellitus) due to immune mediated pancreatic islet beta-cell destruction
Idiopathic diabetes (mellitus)
Juvenile onset diabetes (mellitus)
Ketosis-prone diabetes (mellitus)
Excludes 1: *diabetes mellitus due to underlying condition (E08.-)*
drug or chemical induced diabetes mellitus (E09.-)
gestational diabetes (O24.4-)
hyperglycemia NOS (R73.9)
neonatal diabetes mellitus (P70.2)
postpancreatectomy diabetes mellitus (E13.-)
postprocedural diabetes mellitus (E13.-)
secondary diabetes mellitus NEC (E13.-)
type 2 diabetes mellitus (E11.-)

E10.1- <u>Type 1</u> diabetes mellitus with <u>ketoacidosis</u> — The potentially life-threatening complication of ketone poisoning caused by very low insulin that forces the body to use fat for fuel. When the fat breaks down, its waste products (acids called ketone bodies) build up in the blood and urine.

MCC **E10.10** <u>Type 1</u> diabetes mellitus with ketoacidosis <u>without</u> coma

MCC **E10.11** <u>Type 1</u> diabetes mellitus with ketoacidosis <u>with</u> coma

E10.2- <u>Type 1</u> diabetes mellitus with <u>kidney</u> complications
E10.21 <u>Type 1</u> diabetes mellitus with diabetic <u>nephropathy</u> — A progressive kidney disease caused by damage to the blood capillaries of the kidney's glomeruli that is due to the long-term effects of diabetes.
Type 1 diabetes mellitus with intercapillary glomerulosclerosis
Type 1 diabetes mellitus with intracapillary glomerulonephrosis
Type 1 diabetes mellitus with Kimmelstiel-Wilson disease
E10.22 <u>Type 1</u> diabetes mellitus with diabetic <u>chronic kidney disease</u>
Use additional code to identify stage of chronic kidney disease (N18.1-N18.6)
E10.29 <u>Type 1</u> diabetes mellitus with other diabetic kidney complication
Type 1 diabetes mellitus with renal tubular degeneration

E10.3- <u>Type 1</u> diabetes mellitus with <u>ophthalmic</u> complications
E10.31- <u>Type 1</u> diabetes mellitus with <u>unspecified</u> diabetic <u>retinopathy</u> — A diabetic complication caused by damage to the blood vessels of the retina.
E10.311 <u>Type 1</u> diabetes mellitus with unspecified diabetic retinopathy <u>with</u> macular edema
E10.319 <u>Type 1</u> diabetes mellitus with unspecified diabetic retinopathy <u>without</u> macular edema
E10.32- <u>Type 1</u> diabetes mellitus with <u>mild</u> <u>non</u>proliferative diabetic retinopathy
Type 1 diabetes mellitus with nonproliferative diabetic retinopathy NOS
One of the following 7th characters is to be assigned to codes in subcategory E10.32- to designate laterality of the disease:
1 Right eye
2 Left eye
3 Bilateral
9 Unspecified eye
E10.321- <u>Type 1</u> diabetes mellitus with mild nonproliferative diabetic retinopathy <u>with macular edema</u>
E10.329- <u>Type 1</u> diabetes mellitus with mild nonproliferative diabetic retinopathy <u>without</u> macular edema

E10.33- <u>Type 1</u> diabetes mellitus with <u>moderate</u> <u>non</u>proliferative diabetic retinopathy
One of the following 7th characters is to be assigned to codes in subcategory E10.33- to designate laterality of the disease:
1 Right eye
2 Left eye
3 Bilateral
9 Unspecified eye
E10.331- <u>Type 1</u> diabetes mellitus with moderate nonproliferative diabetic retinopathy <u>with macular edema</u>
E10.339- <u>Type 1</u> diabetes mellitus with moderate nonproliferative diabetic retinopathy <u>without</u> macular edema
E10.34- <u>Type 1</u> diabetes mellitus with <u>severe</u> <u>non</u>proliferative diabetic retinopathy
One of the following 7th characters is to be assigned to codes in subcategory E10.34- to designate laterality of the disease:
1 Right eye
2 Left eye
3 Bilateral
9 Unspecified eye
E10.341- <u>Type 1</u> diabetes mellitus with severe nonproliferative diabetic retinopathy <u>with macular edema</u>
E10.349- <u>Type 1</u> diabetes mellitus with severe nonproliferative diabetic retinopathy <u>without</u> macular edema
E10.35- <u>Type 1</u> diabetes mellitus with <u>proliferative</u> diabetic retinopathy
One of the following 7th characters is to be assigned to codes in subcategory E10.35- to designate laterality of the disease:
1 Right eye
2 Left eye
3 Bilateral
9 Unspecified eye
E10.351- <u>Type 1</u> diabetes mellitus with proliferative diabetic retinopathy <u>with macular edema</u>
E10.352- <u>Type 1</u> diabetes mellitus with proliferative diabetic retinopathy <u>with traction retinal detachment involving the macula</u> — [Not Allowed as PDX]
E10.353- <u>Type 1</u> diabetes mellitus with proliferative diabetic retinopathy with traction retinal detachment <u>not</u> involving the macula — [Not Allowed as PDX]
E10.354- <u>Type 1</u> diabetes mellitus with proliferative diabetic retinopathy <u>with combined</u> traction retinal detachment and rhegmatogenous retinal detachment — [Not Allowed as PDX]
E10.355- <u>Type 1</u> diabetes mellitus <u>with stable</u> proliferative diabetic retinopathy — [Not Allowed as PDX]
E10.359- <u>Type 1</u> diabetes mellitus with proliferative diabetic retinopathy <u>without</u> macular edema
E10.36 <u>Type 1</u> diabetes mellitus with diabetic <u>cataract</u> — The diabetic complication resulting in the clouding of the ocular lens.
E10.37x- <u>Type 1</u> diabetes mellitus with diabetic macular edema, <u>resolved</u> following treatment — [Not Allowed as PDX]
One of the following 7th characters is to be assigned to code E10.37x- to designate laterality of the disease:
1 Right eye
2 Left eye
3 Bilateral
9 Unspecified eye
E10.39 <u>Type 1</u> diabetes mellitus with other diabetic <u>ophthalmic complication</u>
Use additional code to identify manifestation, such as:
Diabetic glaucoma (H40-H42)

E10.4-   Type 1 diabetes mellitus with neurological complications
    E10.40   Type 1 diabetes mellitus with diabetic neuropathy, unspecified
    E10.41   Type 1 diabetes mellitus with diabetic mononeuropathy — The diabetic nerve damage complication caused by microvascular damage to nerves in a single location.
    E10.42   Type 1 diabetes mellitus with diabetic polyneuropathy — The diabetic nerve damage complication caused by microvascular damage to multiple nerves in various locations.
        Type 1 diabetes mellitus with diabetic neuralgia
    E10.43   Type 1 diabetes mellitus with diabetic autonomic (poly)neuropathy — The diabetic nerve damage complication caused by microvascular damage to autonomic (internal organs) nerves in various locations.
        AHA 13:4Q:p114 – Diabetic gastroparesis
        Type 1 diabetes mellitus with diabetic gastroparesis
    E10.44   Type 1 diabetes mellitus with diabetic amyotrophy — The diabetic nerve damage complication caused by microvascular damage to the nerves of the hips, buttocks, thighs, or legs and usually on one side of the body.
    E10.49   Type 1 diabetes mellitus with other diabetic neurological complication
E10.5-   Type 1 diabetes mellitus with circulatory complications
    E10.51   Type 1 diabetes mellitus with diabetic peripheral angiopathy without gangrene — The diabetic complication causing decay of the lining of peripheral blood vessels.
    CC E10.52   Type 1 diabetes mellitus with diabetic peripheral angiopathy with gangrene
        Type 1 diabetes mellitus with diabetic gangrene
    E10.59   Type 1 diabetes mellitus with other circulatory complications
E10.6-   Type 1 diabetes mellitus with other specified complications
    E10.61-   Type 1 diabetes mellitus with diabetic arthropathy
        E10.610   Type 1 diabetes mellitus with diabetic neuropathic arthropathy — The diabetic complication of neurovascular damage of joints resulting in loss of sensation and subsequent joint damage.
            Type 1 diabetes mellitus with Charcot's joints
        E10.618   Type 1 diabetes mellitus with other diabetic arthropathy
    E10.62-   Type 1 diabetes mellitus with skin complications
        E10.620   Type 1 diabetes mellitus with diabetic dermatitis — The diabetic complication of cutaneous damage resulting in various skin conditions (inflammation, infection, lesions).
            Type 1 diabetes mellitus with diabetic necrobiosis lipoidica
        E10.621   Type 1 diabetes mellitus with foot ulcer
            Use additional code to identify site of ulcer (L97.4-, L97.5-)
        E10.622   Type 1 diabetes mellitus with other skin ulcer
            Use additional code to identify site of ulcer (L97.1-L97.9, L98.41-L98.49)
        E10.628   Type 1 diabetes mellitus with other skin complications
    E10.63-   Type 1 diabetes mellitus with oral complications
        E10.630   Type 1 diabetes mellitus with periodontal disease
        E10.638   Type 1 diabetes mellitus with other oral complications
    E10.64-   Type 1 diabetes mellitus with hypoglycemia
    MCC E10.641   Type 1 diabetes mellitus with hypoglycemia with coma
        E10.649   Type 1 diabetes mellitus with hypoglycemia without coma
    E10.65   Type 1 diabetes mellitus with hyperglycemia — The diabetic condition of having high sugar (glucose) levels in the blood and urine causing excessive thirst and frequent urination.
    E10.69   Type 1 diabetes mellitus with other specified complication
        Use additional code to identify complication
E10.8   Type 1 diabetes mellitus with unspecified complications
E10.9   Type 1 diabetes mellitus without complications

E11-   Type 2 diabetes mellitus — A complex metabolic syndrome characterized by consistently high blood sugar (glucose) levels, glycosuria, and metabolic effects caused by the body's inability to properly use the insulin produced (insulin resistance) and eventually resulting in faulty pancreatic insulin production, thus producing insufficient amounts of insulin.
    AHA 13:3Q:p20 – Hyperglycemia together with another diabetes code
    AHA 13:3Q:p20 – Uncontrolled type 1 diabetes with ketoacidosis
    AHA 16:1Q:p12 – Cause-and-effect condition relationships
    Includes: Diabetes (mellitus) due to insulin secretory defect
            Diabetes NOS
            Insulin resistant diabetes (mellitus)
    Use additional code to identify control using:
      Insulin (Z79.4)
      Oral antidiabetic drugs (Z79.84)
      Oral hypoglycemic drugs (Z79.84)
    Excludes 1:   *diabetes mellitus due to underlying condition (E08.-)*
            drug or chemical induced diabetes mellitus (E09.-)
            gestational diabetes (O24.4-)
            neonatal diabetes mellitus (P70.2)
            postpancreatectomy diabetes mellitus (E13.-)
            postprocedural diabetes mellitus (E13.-)
            secondary diabetes mellitus NEC (E13.-)
            type 1 diabetes mellitus (E10.-)
E11.0-   Type 2 diabetes mellitus with hyperosmolarity — A form with extremely high blood sugar (glucose) levels and without the presence of ketones.
    MCC E11.00   Type 2 diabetes mellitus with hyperosmolarity without nonketotic hyperglycemic-hyperosmolar coma (NKHHC)
    MCC E11.01   Type 2 diabetes mellitus with hyperosmolarity with coma
E11.2-   Type 2 diabetes mellitus with kidney complications
    E11.21   Type 2 diabetes mellitus with diabetic nephropathy — A progressive kidney disease caused by damage to the blood capillaries of the kidney's glomeruli that is due to the long-term effects of diabetes.
        Type 2 diabetes mellitus with intercapillary glomerulosclerosis
        Type 2 diabetes mellitus with intracapillary glomerulonephrosis
        Type 2 diabetes mellitus with Kimmelstiel-Wilson disease
    E11.22   Type 2 diabetes mellitus with diabetic chronic kidney disease
        Use additional code to identify stage of chronic kidney disease (N18.1-N18.6)
    E11.29   Type 2 diabetes mellitus with other diabetic kidney complication
        Type 2 diabetes mellitus with renal tubular degeneration
E11.3-   Type 2 diabetes mellitus with ophthalmic complications
    E11.31-   Type 2 diabetes mellitus with unspecified diabetic retinopathy — A diabetic complication caused by damage to the blood vessels of the retina.
        E11.311   Type 2 diabetes mellitus with unspecified diabetic retinopathy with macular edema
        E11.319   Type 2 diabetes mellitus with unspecified diabetic retinopathy without macular edema
    E11.32-   Type 2 diabetes mellitus with mild nonproliferative diabetic retinopathy
        Type 2 diabetes mellitus with nonproliferative diabetic retinopathy NOS

> **One of the following 7th characters is to be assigned to codes in subcategory E11.32- to designate laterality of the disease:**
> 1   Right eye
> 2   Left eye
> 3   Bilateral
> 9   Unspecified eye

        E11.321-   Type 2 diabetes mellitus with mild nonproliferative diabetic retinopathy with macular edema
        E11.329-   Type 2 diabetes mellitus with mild nonproliferative diabetic retinopathy without macular edema

Side tab: E10-E11

E11.33- <u>Type 2</u> diabetes mellitus with <u>moderate</u> <u>non</u>proliferative diabetic retinopathy

> One of the following 7th characters is to be assigned to codes in subcategory E11.33- to designate laterality of the disease:
> 1 Right eye
> 2 Left eye
> 3 Bilateral
> 9 Unspecified eye

E11.331- <u>Type 2</u> diabetes mellitus with moderate nonproliferative diabetic retinopathy <u>with macular edema</u>

E11.339- <u>Type 2</u> diabetes mellitus with moderate nonproliferative diabetic retinopathy <u>without</u> macular edema

E11.34- <u>Type 2</u> diabetes mellitus with <u>severe</u> <u>non</u>proliferative diabetic retinopathy

> One of the following 7th characters is to be assigned to codes in subcategory E11.34- to designate laterality of the disease:
> 1 Right eye
> 2 Left eye
> 3 Bilateral
> 9 Unspecified eye

E11.341- <u>Type 2</u> diabetes mellitus with severe nonproliferative diabetic retinopathy <u>with macular edema</u>

E11.349- <u>Type 2</u> diabetes mellitus with severe nonproliferative diabetic retinopathy <u>without</u> macular edema

E11.35- <u>Type 2</u> diabetes mellitus with <u>proliferative</u> diabetic retinopathy

> One of the following 7th characters is to be assigned to codes in subcategory E11.35- to designate laterality of the disease:
> 1 Right eye
> 2 Left eye
> 3 Bilateral
> 9 Unspecified eye

E11.351- <u>Type 2</u> diabetes mellitus with proliferative diabetic retinopathy <u>with macular edema</u>

E11.352- <u>Type 2</u> diabetes mellitus with proliferative diabetic retinopathy <u>with traction retinal detachment involving the macula</u> — [Not Allowed as PDX]

E11.353- <u>Type 2</u> diabetes mellitus with proliferative diabetic retinopathy with traction retinal detachment <u>not</u> involving the macula — [Not Allowed as PDX]

E11.354- <u>Type 2</u> diabetes mellitus with proliferative diabetic retinopathy <u>with combined</u> traction retinal detachment and rhegmatogenous retinal detachment — [Not Allowed as PDX]

E11.355- <u>Type 2</u> diabetes mellitus <u>with stable</u> proliferative diabetic retinopathy — [Not Allowed as PDX]

E11.359- <u>Type 2</u> diabetes mellitus with proliferative diabetic retinopathy <u>without</u> macular edema

E11.36 <u>Type 2</u> diabetes mellitus with diabetic <u>cataract</u> — The diabetic complication resulting in the clouding of the ocular lens.

E11.37x- <u>Type 2</u> diabetes mellitus with diabetic macular edema, <u>resolved</u> following treatment — [Not Allowed as PDX]

> One of the following 7th characters is to be assigned to code E11.37x- to designate laterality of the disease:
> 1 Right eye
> 2 Left eye
> 3 Bilateral
> 9 Unspecified eye

E11.39 <u>Type 2</u> diabetes mellitus with other diabetic <u>ophthalmic complication</u>
Use additional code to identify manifestation, such as:
   Diabetic glaucoma (H40-H42)

E11.4- <u>Type 2</u> diabetes mellitus with <u>neurological</u> complications

E11.40 <u>Type 2</u> diabetes mellitus with diabetic <u>neuropathy, unspecified</u>

E11.41 <u>Type 2</u> diabetes mellitus with diabetic <u>mononeuropathy</u> — The diabetic nerve damage complication caused by microvascular damage to nerves in a single location.

E11.42 <u>Type 2</u> diabetes mellitus with diabetic <u>polyneuropathy</u> — The diabetic nerve damage complication caused by microvascular damage to multiple nerves in various locations.
   Type 2 diabetes mellitus with diabetic neuralgia

E11.43 <u>Type 2</u> diabetes mellitus with diabetic <u>autonomic (poly)neuropathy</u> — The diabetic nerve damage complication caused by microvascular damage to autonomic (internal organs) nerves in various locations.
   AHA 13:4Q:p114 – Diabetic gastroparesis
   Type 2 diabetes mellitus with diabetic gastroparesis

E11.44 <u>Type 2</u> diabetes mellitus with diabetic <u>amyotrophy</u> — The diabetic nerve damage complication caused by microvascular damage to the nerves of the hips, buttocks, thighs, or legs and usually on one side of the body.

E11.49 <u>Type 2</u> diabetes mellitus with other diabetic neurological complication

E11.5- <u>Type 2</u> diabetes mellitus with <u>circulatory</u> complications

E11.51 <u>Type 2</u> diabetes mellitus with diabetic <u>peripheral angiopathy without</u> gangrene — The diabetic complication causing decay of the lining of peripheral blood vessels.

cc **E11.52** <u>Type 2</u> diabetes mellitus with diabetic <u>peripheral angiopathy with gangrene</u>
   Type 2 diabetes mellitus with diabetic gangrene

E11.59 <u>Type 2</u> diabetes mellitus with other circulatory complications

E11.6- <u>Type 2</u> diabetes mellitus with <u>other specified</u> complications

E11.61- <u>Type 2</u> diabetes mellitus with diabetic <u>arthropathy</u>

E11.610 <u>Type 2</u> diabetes mellitus with diabetic <u>neuropathic arthropathy</u> — The diabetic complication of neurovascular damage of joints resulting in loss of sensation and subsequent joint damage.
   Type 2 diabetes mellitus with Charcot's joints

E11.618 <u>Type 2</u> diabetes mellitus with other diabetic arthropathy

E11.62- <u>Type 2</u> diabetes mellitus with <u>skin</u> complications

E11.620 <u>Type 2</u> diabetes mellitus with diabetic <u>dermatitis</u> — The diabetic complication of cutaneous damage resulting in various skin conditions (inflammation, infection, lesions).
   Type 2 diabetes mellitus with diabetic necrobiosis lipoidica

E11.621 <u>Type 2</u> diabetes mellitus with <u>foot ulcer</u>
   Use additional code to identify site of ulcer (L97.4-, L97.5-)

E11.622 <u>Type 2</u> diabetes mellitus with <u>other skin ulcer</u>
   Use additional code to identify site of ulcer (L97.1-L97.9, L98.41-L98.49)

E11.628 <u>Type 2</u> diabetes mellitus with other skin complications

E11.63- <u>Type 2</u> diabetes mellitus with <u>oral</u> complications

E11.630 <u>Type 2</u> diabetes mellitus with periodontal disease

E11.638 <u>Type 2</u> diabetes mellitus with other oral complications

E11.64- <u>Type 2</u> diabetes mellitus with <u>hypoglycemia</u>

MCC **E11.641** <u>Type 2</u> diabetes mellitus with hypoglycemia <u>with coma</u>

E11.649 <u>Type 2</u> diabetes mellitus with hypoglycemia <u>without</u> coma
   AHA 15:3Q:p21 – Diabetes mellitus with acute encephalopathy secondary to hypoglycemia

E11.65 <u>Type 2</u> diabetes mellitus with <u>hyperglycemia</u> — The diabetic condition of having high sugar (glucose) levels in the blood and urine causing excessive thirst and frequent urination.

E11.69 <u>Type 2</u> diabetes mellitus with <u>other specified</u> complication
   Use additional code to identify complication

E11.8 <u>Type 2</u> diabetes mellitus with <u>unspecified</u> complications

E11.9 <u>Type 2</u> diabetes mellitus <u>without</u> complications —
   [Questionable Admission]

E11-E11

E13- <u>Other specified</u> diabetes mellitus — A complex metabolic syndrome characterized by consistently high blood sugar (glucose) levels, glycosuria, and metabolic effects caused by faulty pancreatic insulin production, thus producing insufficient amounts of insulin.

    AHA 13:3Q:p20 – Hyperglycemia together with another diabetes code
    AHA 13:3Q:p20 – Uncontrolled type 1 diabetes with ketoacidosis
    AHA 16:1Q:p12 – Cause-and-effect condition relationships

    Includes: Diabetes mellitus due to genetic defects of beta-cell function
              Diabetes mellitus due to genetic defects in insulin action
              Postpancreatectomy diabetes mellitus
              Postprocedural diabetes mellitus
              Secondary diabetes mellitus NEC

    Use additional code to identify control using:
      Insulin (Z79.4)
      Oral antidiabetic drugs (Z79.84)
      Oral hypoglycemic drugs (Z79.84)

    Excludes 1:   *diabetes (mellitus) due to autoimmune process (E10.-)*
              diabetes (mellitus) due to immune mediated pancreatic islet beta-cell destruction (E10.-)
              diabetes mellitus due to underlying condition (E08.-)
              drug or chemical induced diabetes mellitus (E09.-)
              gestational diabetes (O24.4-)
              neonatal diabetes mellitus (P70.2)
              type 1 diabetes mellitus (E10.-)
              type 2 diabetes mellitus (E11.-)

E13.0- <u>Other specified</u> diabetes mellitus with <u>hyperosmolarity</u> — A form with extremely high blood sugar (glucose) levels and without the presence of ketones.

  MCC **E13.00** Other specified diabetes mellitus with hyperosmolarity <u>without</u> nonketotic hyperglycemic-hyperosmolar coma (NKHHC)

  MCC **E13.01** Other specified diabetes mellitus with hyperosmolarity <u>with coma</u>

E13.1- <u>Other specified</u> diabetes mellitus with <u>ketoacidosis</u> — The potentially life-threatening complication of ketone poisoning caused by very low insulin that forces the body to use fat for fuel. When the fat breaks down, its waste products (acids called ketone bodies) build up in the blood and urine.

  MCC **E13.10** Other specified diabetes mellitus with ketoacidosis <u>without</u> coma
      AHA 13:1Q:p26 – Type 2 diabetes mellitus with diabetic ketoacidosis
      AHA 16:2Q:p10 – Unspecified diabetes type with ketoacidosis

  MCC **E13.11** Other specified diabetes mellitus with ketoacidosis <u>with coma</u>

E13.2- Other specified diabetes mellitus with <u>kidney</u> complications

  E13.21 Other specified diabetes mellitus with diabetic <u>nephropathy</u> — A progressive kidney disease caused by damage to the blood capillaries of the kidney's glomeruli that is due to the long-term effects of diabetes.
    Other specified diabetes mellitus with intercapillary glomerulosclerosis
    Other specified diabetes mellitus with intracapillary glomerulonephrosis
    Other specified diabetes mellitus with Kimmelstiel-Wilson disease

  E13.22 Other specified diabetes mellitus with diabetic <u>chronic kidney disease</u>
    Use additional code to identify stage of chronic kidney disease (N18.1-N18.6)

  E13.29 Other specified diabetes mellitus with other diabetic kidney complication
    Other specified diabetes mellitus with renal tubular degeneration

E13.3- <u>Other specified</u> diabetes mellitus with ophthalmic complications

  E13.31- Other specified diabetes mellitus with <u>unspecified diabetic retinopathy</u> — A diabetic complication caused by damage to the blood vessels of the retina.

    E13.311 Other specified diabetes mellitus with unspecified diabetic retinopathy <u>with macular edema</u>

    E13.319 Other specified diabetes mellitus with unspecified diabetic retinopathy <u>without</u> macular edema

E13.32- Other specified diabetes mellitus with <u>mild nonproliferative</u> diabetic retinopathy
  Other specified diabetes mellitus with nonproliferative diabetic retinopathy NOS

  One of the following 7th characters is to be assigned to codes in subcategory E13.32- to designate laterality of the disease:
    1   Right eye
    2   Left eye
    3   Bilateral
    9   Unspecified eye

  E13.321- Other specified diabetes mellitus with mild nonproliferative diabetic retinopathy <u>with macular edema</u>

  E13.329- Other specified diabetes mellitus with mild nonproliferative diabetic retinopathy <u>without</u> macular edema

E13.33- Other specified diabetes mellitus with <u>moderate nonproliferative</u> diabetic retinopathy

  One of the following 7th characters is to be assigned to codes in subcategory E13.33- to designate laterality of the disease:
    1   Right eye
    2   Left eye
    3   Bilateral
    9   Unspecified eye

  E13.331- Other specified diabetes mellitus with moderate nonproliferative diabetic retinopathy <u>with macular edema</u>

  E13.339- Other specified diabetes mellitus with moderate nonproliferative diabetic retinopathy <u>without</u> macular edema

E13.34- Other specified diabetes mellitus with <u>severe nonproliferative</u> diabetic retinopathy

  One of the following 7th characters is to be assigned to codes in subcategory E13.34- to designate laterality of the disease:
    1   Right eye
    2   Left eye
    3   Bilateral
    9   Unspecified eye

  E13.341- Other specified diabetes mellitus with severe nonproliferative diabetic retinopathy <u>with macular edema</u>

  E13.349- Other specified diabetes mellitus with severe nonproliferative diabetic retinopathy <u>without</u> macular edema

E13.35- Other specified diabetes mellitus with <u>proliferative</u> diabetic retinopathy

  One of the following 7th characters is to be assigned to codes in subcategory E13.35- to designate laterality of the disease:
    1   Right eye
    2   Left eye
    3   Bilateral
    9   Unspecified eye

  E13.351- Other specified diabetes mellitus with proliferative diabetic retinopathy <u>with macular edema</u>

  E13.352- Other specified diabetes mellitus with proliferative diabetic retinopathy <u>with traction retinal detachment involving the macula</u> — [Not Allowed as PDX]

  E13.353- Other specified diabetes mellitus with proliferative diabetic retinopathy with traction retinal detachment <u>not</u> involving the macula — [Not Allowed as PDX]

  E13.354- Other specified diabetes mellitus with proliferative diabetic retinopathy <u>with combined</u> traction retinal detachment and rhegmatogenous retinal detachment — [Not Allowed as PDX]

Excludes 1: = NOT CODED HERE! (Do not code both)   **618**   *Excludes ❷:* = Not Included Here

E13.355- Other specified diabetes mellitus <u>with stable</u> proliferative diabetic retinopathy —
[Not Allowed as PDX]

E13.359- Other specified diabetes mellitus with proliferative diabetic retinopathy <u>without</u> macular edema

E13.36 Other specified diabetes mellitus with diabetic <u>cataract</u> — The diabetic complication resulting in the clouding of the ocular lens.

E13.37x- Other specified diabetes mellitus with diabetic macular edema, <u>resolved</u> following treatment — [Not Allowed as PDX]

One of the following 7th characters is to be assigned to code E13.37x- to designate laterality of the disease:
1   Right eye
2   Left eye
3   Bilateral
9   Unspecified eye

E13.39 Other specified diabetes mellitus with other diabetic <u>ophthalmic complication</u>
Use additional code to identify manifestation, such as:
Diabetic glaucoma (H40-H42)

E13.4- <u>Other specified</u> diabetes mellitus with <u>neurological</u> complications

E13.40 Other specified diabetes mellitus with diabetic <u>neuropathy, unspecified</u>

E13.41 Other specified diabetes mellitus with diabetic <u>mononeuropathy</u> — The diabetic nerve damage complication caused by microvascular damage to nerves in a single location.

E13.42 Other specified diabetes mellitus with diabetic <u>polyneuropathy</u> — The diabetic nerve damage complication caused by microvascular damage to multiple nerves in various locations.
Other specified diabetes mellitus with diabetic neuralgia

E13.43 Other specified diabetes mellitus with diabetic <u>autonomic (poly)neuropathy</u> — The diabetic nerve damage complication caused by microvascular damage to autonomic (internal organs) nerves in various locations.
AHA 13:4Q:p114 – Diabetic gastroparesis
Other specified diabetes mellitus with diabetic gastroparesis

E13.44 Other specified diabetes mellitus with diabetic <u>amyotrophy</u> — The diabetic nerve damage complication caused by microvascular damage to the nerves of the hips, buttocks, thighs, or legs and usually on one side of the body.

E13.49 Other specified diabetes mellitus with other diabetic neurological complication

E13.5- <u>Other specified</u> diabetes mellitus with <u>circulatory</u> complications

E13.51 Other specified diabetes mellitus with diabetic <u>peripheral angiopathy without</u> gangrene — The diabetic complication causing decay of the lining of peripheral blood vessels.

CC **E13.52** Other specified diabetes mellitus with diabetic <u>peripheral angiopathy with gangrene</u>
Other specified diabetes mellitus with diabetic gangrene

E13.59 Other specified diabetes mellitus with other circulatory complications

E13.6- <u>Other specified</u> diabetes mellitus with other specified complications

E13.61- Other specified diabetes mellitus with diabetic <u>arthropathy</u>

E13.610 Other specified diabetes mellitus with diabetic <u>neuropathic arthropathy</u> — The diabetic complication of neurovascular damage of joints resulting in loss of sensation and subsequent joint damage.
Other specified diabetes mellitus with Charcot's joints

E13.618 Other specified diabetes mellitus with other diabetic arthropathy

E13.62- Other specified diabetes mellitus with <u>skin</u> complications

E13.620 Other specified diabetes mellitus with diabetic <u>dermatitis</u> — The diabetic complication of cutaneous damage resulting in various skin conditions (inflammation, infection, lesions).
Other specified diabetes mellitus with diabetic necrobiosis lipoidica

E13.621 Other specified diabetes mellitus with <u>foot ulcer</u>
Use additional code to identify site of ulcer (L97.4-, L97.5-)

E13.622 Other specified diabetes mellitus with <u>other skin ulcer</u>
Use additional code to identify site of ulcer (L97.1-L97.9, L98.41-L98.49)

E13.628 Other specified diabetes mellitus with other skin complications

E13.63- Other specified diabetes mellitus with <u>oral</u> complications

E13.630 Other specified diabetes mellitus with periodontal disease

E13.638 Other specified diabetes mellitus with other oral complications

E13.64- Other specified diabetes mellitus with <u>hypoglycemia</u>

MCC **E13.641** Other specified diabetes mellitus with hypoglycemia <u>with coma</u>

E13.649 Other specified diabetes mellitus with hypoglycemia <u>without</u> coma

E13.65 Other specified diabetes mellitus with <u>hyperglycemia</u> — The diabetic condition of having high sugar (glucose) levels in the blood and urine causing excessive thirst and frequent urination.

E13.69 Other specified diabetes mellitus with <u>other specified complication</u>
Use additional code to identify complication

E13.8 <u>Other specified</u> diabetes mellitus with <u>unspecified</u> complications

E13.9 <u>Other specified</u> diabetes mellitus <u>without</u> complications — [Questionable Admission]

Other disorders of glucose regulation and pancreatic internal secretion (E15-E16)

E15 <u>Nondiabetic</u> hypoglycemic coma — Unarousable unconsciousness due to a
CC decreased level of blood glucose.
Includes: Drug-induced insulin coma in nondiabetic
Hyperinsulinism with hypoglycemic coma
Hypoglycemic coma NOS

E16- Other disorders of pancreatic internal secretion

E16.0 <u>Drug-induced hypoglycemia</u> without coma
Use additional code for adverse effect, if applicable, to identify drug (T36-T50 with fifth or sixth character 5)
Excludes 1:   diabetes with hypoglycemia without coma (E09.692)

E16.1 Other hypoglycemia
Functional hyperinsulinism
Functional nonhyperinsulinemic hypoglycemia
Hyperinsulinism NOS
Hyperplasia of pancreatic islet beta cells NOS
Excludes 1:   diabetes with hypoglycemia (E08.649, E10.649, E11.649, E13.649)
hypoglycemia in infant of diabetic mother (P70.1)
neonatal hypoglycemia (P70.4)

E16.2 Hypoglycemia, unspecified
Excludes 1:   diabetes with hypoglycemia (E08.649, E10.649, E11.649, E13.649)

E16.3 Increased secretion of glucagon
Hyperplasia of pancreatic endocrine cells with glucagon excess

E16.4 Increased secretion of gastrin
Hypergastrinemia
Hyperplasia of pancreatic endocrine cells with gastrin excess
Zollinger-Ellison syndrome — A syndrome characterized by gastrin-secreting, pancreatic tumors causing hyperacidity, and ulcers in the stomach and duodenum.

E16.8 Other specified disorders of pancreatic internal secretion
Increased secretion from endocrine pancreas of growth hormone-releasing hormone
Increased secretion from endocrine pancreas of pancreatic polypeptide
Increased secretion from endocrine pancreas of somatostatin
Increased secretion from endocrine pancreas of vasoactive-intestinal polypeptide

E16.9 Disorder of pancreatic internal secretion, unspecified
Islet-cell hyperplasia NOS
Pancreatic endocrine cell hyperplasia NOS

E
1
3
-
E
1
6

Excludes 1: = NOT CODED HERE! (Do not code both)   619   *Excludes* ❷: = Not Included Here

Disorders of other endocrine glands (E20-E35)

Excludes 1:   *galactorrhea (N64.3)*
                  gynecomastia (N62)

E20- Hypoparathyroidism — Abnormal decrease in the function of the parathyroid glands.
Excludes 1:   *Di George's syndrome (D82.1)*
                  postprocedural hypoparathyroidism (E89.2)
                  tetany NOS (R29.0)
                  transitory neonatal hypoparathyroidism (P71.4)

E20.0   Idiopathic hypoparathyroidism

E20.1   Pseudohypoparathyroidism

E20.8   Other hypoparathyroidism

E20.9   Hypoparathyroidism, unspecified
           Parathyroid tetany

E21- Hyperparathyroidism and other disorders of parathyroid gland
Excludes 1:   *adult osteomalacia (M83.-)*
                  ectopic hyperparathyroidism (E34.2)
                  familial hypocalciuric hypercalcemia (E83.52)
                  hungry bone syndrome (E83.81)
                  infantile and juvenile osteomalacia (E55.0)

E21.0   Primary hyperparathyroidism — Abnormally increased activity of the parathyroid glands that secrete too much parathyroid hormone occurring as a result of a parathyroid condition, most commonly an adenoma.
           Hyperplasia of parathyroid
           Osteitis fibrosa cystica generalisata [von Recklinghausen's disease of bone]

E21.1   Secondary hyperparathyroidism, not elsewhere classified
Excludes 1:   *secondary hyperparathyroidism of renal origin (N25.81)*

E21.2   Other hyperparathyroidism
           Tertiary hyperparathyroidism
Excludes 1:   *familial hypocalciuric hypercalcemia (E83.52)*

E21.3   Hyperparathyroidism, unspecified

E21.4   Other specified disorders of parathyroid gland

E21.5   Disorder of parathyroid gland, unspecified

E22- Hyperfunction of pituitary gland
Excludes 1:   *Cushing's syndrome (E24.-)*
                  Nelson's syndrome (E24.1)
                  overproduction of ACTH not associated with Cushing's disease (E27.0)
                  overproduction of pituitary ACTH (E24.0)
                  overproduction of thyroid-stimulating hormone (E05.8-)

E22.0   Acromegaly and pituitary gigantism — ACROMEGALY – A chronic disease of middle-aged persons characterized by elongation and enlargement of bones of the extremities and certain head bones caused by the hypersecretion of the pituitary growth hormone. GIGANTISM – Excessive development of the bones of the hands, feet, and face due to the overproduction of the growth hormone.
           Overproduction of growth hormone
Excludes 1:   *constitutional gigantism (E34.4)*
                  constitutional tall stature (E34.4)
                  increased secretion from endocrine pancreas of growth hormone-releasing hormone (E16.8)

cc **E22.1   Hyperprolactinemia**
           Use additional code for adverse effect, if applicable, to identify drug (T36-T50 with fifth or sixth character 5)

cc **E22.2   Syndrome of inappropriate secretion of antidiuretic hormone**

cc **E22.8   Other hyperfunction of pituitary gland**
           Central precocious puberty

cc **E22.9   Hyperfunction of pituitary gland, unspecified**

E23- Hypofunction and other disorders of the pituitary gland
Includes: The listed conditions whether the disorder is in the pituitary or the hypothalamus
Excludes 1:   *postprocedural hypopituitarism (E89.3)*

cc **E23.0   Hypopituitarism** — Defective or absent function of the entire pituitary gland.
           Fertile eunuch syndrome
           Hypogonadotropic hypogonadism
           Idiopathic growth hormone deficiency
           Isolated deficiency of gonadotropin
           Isolated deficiency of growth hormone
           Isolated deficiency of pituitary hormone
           Kallmann's syndrome
           Lorain-Levi short stature
           Necrosis of pituitary gland (postpartum)
           Panhypopituitarism
           Pituitary cachexia
           Pituitary insufficiency NOS
           Pituitary short stature
           Sheehan's syndrome
           Simmonds' disease

E23.1   Drug-induced hypopituitarism
           Use additional code for adverse effect, if applicable, to identify drug (T36-T50 with fifth or sixth character 5)

cc **E23.2   Diabetes insipidus** — A disorder characterized by excessive water intake and output, which results from inadequate pituitary secretion of antidiuretic hormone (vasopressin).
Excludes 1:   *nephrogenic diabetes insipidus (N25.1)*

E23.3   Hypothalamic dysfunction, not elsewhere classified
Excludes 1:   *Prader-Willi syndrome (Q87.1)*
                  Russell-Silver syndrome (Q87.1)

E23.6   Other disorders of pituitary gland
           Abscess of pituitary
           Adiposogenital dystrophy

E23.7   Disorder of pituitary gland, unspecified

E24- Cushing's syndrome
Excludes 1:   *congenital adrenal hyperplasia (E25.0)*

cc **E24.0   Pituitary-dependent Cushing's disease** — A syndrome resulting from hypersecretion of the adrenal cortex in which there is excessive production of cortisol caused by dysfunction of the pituitary gland upon the adrenal gland that is characterized by adiposity, osteoporosis, amenorrhea, impotence, capillary fragility, edema, and bruisability.
           Overproduction of pituitary ACTH
           Pituitary-dependent hypercorticalism

cc **E24.1   Nelson's syndrome**

cc **E24.2   Drug-induced Cushing's syndrome** — A syndrome resulting from taking too much glucosteroid medicine that is characterized by adiposity, osteoporosis, amenorrhea, impotence, capillary fragility, edema, and bruisability.
           Use additional code for adverse effect, if applicable, to identify drug (T36-T50 with fifth or sixth character 5)

cc **E24.3   Ectopic ACTH syndrome** — A form caused by the production of ACTH by tissue other than the pituitary gland, such as an oat cell carcinoma of the lung.

cc **E24.4   Alcohol-induced pseudo-Cushing's syndrome**

cc **E24.8   Other Cushing's syndrome**

cc **E24.9   Cushing's syndrome, unspecified**

E25- Adrenogenital disorders — Disorders of the genital organs resulting from adrenal dysfunction.
Includes: Adrenogenital syndromes, virilizing or feminizing, whether acquired or due to adrenal hyperplasia consequent on inborn enzyme defects in hormone synthesis
           Female adrenal pseudohermaphroditism
           Female heterosexual precocious pseudopuberty
           Male isosexual precocious pseudopuberty
           Male macrogenitosomia praecox
           Male sexual precocity with adrenal hyperplasia
           Male virilization (female)
Excludes 1:   *indeterminate sex and pseudohermaphroditism (Q56)*
                  chromosomal abnormalities (Q90-Q99)

E25.0   Congenital adrenogenital disorders associated with enzyme deficiency
           Congenital adrenal hyperplasia
           21-Hydroxylase deficiency
           Salt-losing congenital adrenal hyperplasia

E25.8   Other adrenogenital disorders
           Idiopathic adrenogenital disorder
           Use additional code for adverse effect, if applicable, to identify drug (T36-T50 with fifth or sixth character 5)

E25.9   Adrenogenital disorder, unspecified
           Adrenogenital syndrome NOS

E20-E25

E26- **Hyperaldosteronism** — A disease of electrolyte metabolism caused by the excessive secretion of aldosterone, and marked by hypertension, hypocholemia, alkalosis, muscular weakness, polyuria, and polydypsia.

E26.0- **Primary** hyperaldosteronism — A form caused by diseases of the adrenal glands.

E26.01 **Conn's syndrome** — A form due to a tumor of a single adrenal gland.
Code also adrenal adenoma (D35.0-)

E26.02 **Glucocorticoid-remediable aldosteronism** — An inherited form that results from the formation of a hybrid gene.
Familial aldosteronism type I

E26.09 **Other primary hyperaldosteronism**
Primary aldosteronism due to adrenal hyperplasia (bilateral)

E26.1 **Secondary** hyperaldosteronism — A form caused by non-adrenal conditions producing an effect upon the adrenal glands.

E26.8- **Other** hyperaldosteronism

E26.81 **Bartter's syndrome** — An inherited form caused by hyperplasia of the juxtaglomerular cells of the kidney and also marked by hypokalemic alkalosis and short stature.

E26.89 **Other hyperaldosteronism**

E26.9 **Hyperaldosteronism, unspecified**
Aldosteronism NOS
Hyperaldosteronism NOS

E27- **Other disorders of adrenal gland**

CC **E27.0** **Other adrenocortical overactivity**
Overproduction of ACTH, not associated with Cushing's disease
Premature adrenarche
Excludes 1: *Cushing's syndrome (E24.-)*

CC **E27.1** **Primary adrenocortical insufficiency** — A condition of decreased cortisol production that results in a variety of symptoms including malaise, loss of appetite, orthostatic hypotension, weight loss, anemia, pre-renal azotemia, hyperpigmentation, and hyponatremia.
Addison's disease
Autoimmune adrenalitis
Excludes 1: *Addison only phenotype adrenoleukodystrophy (E71.528)*
amyloidosis (E85.-)
tuberculous Addison's disease (A18.7)
Waterhouse-Friderichsen syndrome (A39.1)

CC **E27.2** **Addisonian crisis** — A sudden, severe decrease in adrenal cortex cortisol production causing serious exacerbation of symptoms, notably low blood pressure and dehydration.
Adrenal crisis
Adrenocortical crisis

CC **E27.3** **Drug-induced adrenocortical insufficiency**
Use additional code for adverse effect, if applicable, to identify drug (T36-T50 with fifth or sixth character 5)

E27.4- **Other and unspecified adrenocortical insufficiency**
Excludes 1: *adrenoleukodystrophy [Addison-Schilder] (E71.528)*
Waterhouse-Friderichsen syndrome (A39.1)

CC **E27.40** **Unspecified adrenocortical insufficiency**
Adrenocortical insufficiency NOS
Hypoaldosteronism

CC **E27.49** **Other adrenocortical insufficiency**
Adrenal hemorrhage
Adrenal infarction

CC **E27.5** **Adrenomedullary hyperfunction** — A condition in which the adrenal medulla oversecretes its hormones.
Adrenomedullary hyperplasia
Catecholamine hypersecretion

E27.8 **Other specified disorders of adrenal gland**
Abnormality of cortisol-binding globulin

E27.9 **Disorder of adrenal gland, unspecified**

E28- **Ovarian dysfunction** — Disturbance or impairment of the normal ovarian hormonal function.
Excludes 1: *isolated gonadotropin deficiency (E23.0)*
postprocedural ovarian failure (E89.4-)

E28.0 **Estrogen excess** — [♀]
Use additional code for adverse effect, if applicable, to identify drug (T36-T50 with fifth or sixth character 5)

E28.1 **Androgen excess** — [♀]
Hypersecretion of ovarian androgens
Use additional code for adverse effect, if applicable, to identify drug (T36-T50 with fifth or sixth character 5)

E28.2 **Polycystic ovarian syndrome** — [♀] — An endocrine system disorder involving the ovaries of uncertain origin that is characterized by menstrual disorders, ovarian custs, infertility, increased levels of male hormones, and metabolic effects.
Sclerocystic ovary syndrome
Stein-Leventhal syndrome

E28.3- **Primary ovarian failure** — Abnormal ovarian function due to a disorder within the ovaries themselves.
Excludes 1: *pure gonadal dysgenesis (Q99.1)*
Turner's syndrome (Q96.-)

E28.31- **Premature menopause** — The earlier than normal cessation of menstruation.

E28.310 **Symptomatic premature menopause** — [♀, Age/15-124]
Symptoms such as flushing, sleeplessness, headache, lack of concentration, associated with premature menopause

E28.319 **Asymptomatic premature menopause** — [♀, Age/15-124]
Premature menopause NOS

E28.39 **Other primary ovarian failure** — [♀]
Decreased estrogen
Resistant ovary syndrome

E28.8 **Other ovarian dysfunction** — [♀]
Ovarian hyperfunction NOS
Excludes 1: *postprocedural ovarian failure (E89.4-)*

E28.9 **Ovarian dysfunction, unspecified** — [♀]

E29- **Testicular dysfunction** — Disturbance or impairment of the normal testicular hormonal function.
Excludes 1: *androgen insensitivity syndrome (E34.5-)*
azoospermia or oligospermia NOS (N46.0-N46.1)
isolated gonadotropin deficiency (E23.0)
Klinefelter's syndrome (Q98.0-Q98.1, Q98.4)

E29.0 **Testicular hyperfunction** — [♂] — An abnormal increase in the production of testicular hormones.
Hypersecretion of testicular hormones

E29.1 **Testicular hypofunction** — [♂] — An abnormal decrease in the production of testicular hormones.
Defective biosynthesis of testicular androgen NOS
5-delta-Reductase deficiency (with male pseudohermaphroditism)
Testicular hypogonadism NOS
Use additional code for adverse effect, if applicable, to identify drug (T36-T50 with fifth or sixth character 5)
Excludes 1: *postprocedural testicular hypofunction (E89.5)*

E29.8 **Other testicular dysfunction** — [♂]

E29.9 **Testicular dysfunction, unspecified** — [♂]

E30- **Disorders of puberty, not elsewhere classified**

E30.0 **Delayed puberty** — Development of secondary sexual characteristics after the average period for that development.
Constitutional delay of puberty
Delayed sexual development

E30.1 **Precocious puberty** — [Age/0-17] — Early development of secondary sexual characteristics.
Precocious menstruation
Excludes 1: *Albright (-McCune) (-Sternberg) syndrome (Q78.1)*
central precocious puberty (E22.8)
congenital adrenal hyperplasia (E25.0)
female heterosexual precocious pseudopuberty (E25.-)
male isosexual precocious pseudopuberty (E25.-)

E30.8 **Other disorders of puberty** — [Age/0-17]
Premature thelarche

E30.9 **Disorder of puberty, unspecified**

E31- **Polyglandular dysfunction** — A condition in which mulitple endocrine glands dysfunction sequentially or simultaneously that is due to a common cause.
Excludes 1: *ataxis telangiectasia [Louis-Bar] (G11.3)*
dystrophia myotonica [Steinert] (G71.11)
pseudohypoparathyroidism (E20.1)

E31.0 **Autoimmune polyglandular failure** — A form due to an autoimmune disorder.
Schmidt's syndrome

E31.1 **Polyglandular hyperfunction** — A form in which the dysfunctioning glands produce an increased volume of hormones.
Excludes 1: *multiple endocrine adenomatosis (E31.2-)*
multiple endocrine neoplasia (E31.2-)

E26-E31

E31.2- <u>Multiple endocrine neoplasia [MEN] syndromes</u> — A group of genetically distinct familial diseases involving adenomatous hyperplasia and tumor formation (malignant or benign) in several endocrine glands.
> Multiple endocrine adenomatosis
Code also any associated malignancies and other conditions associated with the syndromes

E31.20 **Multiple endocrine neoplasia [MEN] syndrome, unspecified**
> Multiple endocrine adenomatosis NOS
> Multiple endocrine neoplasia [MEN] syndrome NOS

E31.21 **Multiple endocrine neoplasia [MEN] <u>type I</u>** — A form involving tumors of the parathyroid glands, pancreatic islet cells, and pituitary gland that often results in the development of kidney stones and peptic ulcer disease.
> Wermer's syndrome

E31.22 **Multiple endocrine neoplasia [MEN] <u>type IIA</u>** — A form characterized by medullary carcinoma of the thyroid gland and pheochromocytomas, which usually raises blood pressure, sometimes to severe levels, and hyperparathyroidism.
> Sipple's syndrome

E31.23 **Multiple endocrine neoplasia [MEN] <u>type IIB</u>** — A form with similar features to MEN type IIA, but with the additional distinct feature of mucosal neuromas.

E31.8 **Other polyglandular dysfunction**

E31.9 **Polyglandular dysfunction, unspecified**

E32- **Diseases of <u>thymus</u>**
> *Excludes 1:* *aplasia or hypoplasia of thymus with immunodeficiency (D82.1)*
> *myasthenia gravis (G70.0)*

E32.0 **Persistent <u>hyperplasia</u> of thymus** — A sustained, abnormal increase of thymus cells.
> Hypertrophy of thymus

cc **E32.1** **<u>Abscess</u> of thymus** — A localized collection of pus caused by the disintegration of thymus cells.

E32.8 **Other diseases of thymus**
> *Excludes 1:* *aplasia or hypoplasia with immunodeficiency (D82.1)*
> *thymoma (D15.0)*

E32.9 **Disease of thymus, unspecified**

E34- **<u>Other endocrine disorders</u>**
> *Excludes 1:* *pseudohypoparathyroidism (E20.1)*

cc **E34.0** **Carcinoid syndrome** — A symptom complex caused by catecholamine secretion from carcinoid tumors.
> **Note:** May be used as an additional code to identify functional activity associated with a carcinoid tumor.

E34.1 **Other hypersecretion of intestinal hormones**

E34.2 **Ectopic hormone secretion, not elsewhere classified**
> *Excludes 1:* *ectopic ACTH syndrome (E24.3)*

E34.3 **Short stature due to endocrine disorder** — The condition of being abnormally small in whole body size that is due to an endocrine developmental dysfunction.
> Constitutional short stature
> Laron-type short stature
> *Excludes 1:* *achondroplastic short stature (Q77.4)*
> *hypochondroplastic short stature (Q77.4)*
> *nutritional short stature (E45)*
> *pituitary short stature (E23.0)*
> *progeria (E34.8)*
> *renal short stature (N25.0)*
> *Russell-Silver syndrome (Q87.1)*
> *short-limbed stature with immunodeficiency (D82.2)*
> *short stature in specific dysmorphic syndromes — code to syndrome – see Alphabetical Index*
> *short stature NOS (R62.52)*

E34.4 **Constitutional tall stature** — A condition of excessive growth that is caused by over-production of growth hormone.
> Constitutional gigantism

E34.5- <u>Androgen insensitivity syndrome</u> — A condition in which an individual is chromosomally-male (testes with testicular function), but can develop a wide range of gender characteristics from typical female external genitalia to predominantly male genitalia, that is due to the inability to respond to the male hormones (androgens).

E34.50 **Androgen insensitivity syndrome, unspecified**
> Androgen insensitivity NOS

E34.51 **<u>Complete</u> androgen insensitivity syndrome** — A form in which the individual develops normal female external genitalia including a vagina (but no uterus or ovaries) and has undescended testes.
> Complete androgen insensitivity
> de Quervain syndrome
> Goldberg-Maxwell syndrome

E34.52 **<u>Partial</u> androgen insensitivity syndrome** — A form in which the external genitalia development ranges between underdeveloped male external genitalia to partially-developed female genitalia.
> Partial androgen insensitivity
> Reifenstein syndrome

E34.8 **Other specified endocrine disorders**
> Pineal gland dysfunction
> Progeria
> *Excludes ❷:* *pseudohypoparathyroidism (E20.1)*

E34.9 **Endocrine disorder, unspecified**
> Endocrine disturbance NOS
> Hormone disturbance NOS

E35 **Disorders of endocrine glands in diseases classified elsewhere** — [Not Allowed as PDX]
Code first underlying disease, such as:
> Late congenital syphilis of thymus gland [Dubois disease] (A50.5)
Use additional code, if applicable, to identify:
> Sequelae of tuberculosis of other organs (B90.8)
> *Excludes 1:* *Echinococcus granulosus infection of thyroid gland (B67.3)*
> *meningococcal hemorrhagic adrenalitis (A39.1)*
> *syphilis of endocrine gland (A52.79)*
> *tuberculosis of adrenal gland, except calcification (A18.7)*
> *tuberculosis of endocrine gland NEC (A18.82)*
> *tuberculosis of thyroid gland (A18.81)*
> *Waterhouse-Friderichsen syndrome (A39.1)*

Intraoperative complications of endocrine system (E36)

E36- **<u>Intraoperative complications</u> of endocrine system**
> *Excludes ❷:* *postprocedural endocrine and metabolic complications and disorders, not elsewhere classified (E89.-)*

E36.0- **Intraoperative hemorrhage and hematoma of an endocrine system organ or structure complicating a procedure**
> *Excludes 1:* *intraoperative hemorrhage and hematoma of an endocrine system organ or structure due to accidental puncture or laceration during a procedure (E36.1-)*

cc **E36.01** **Intraoperative hemorrhage and hematoma of an endocrine system organ or structure complicating an endocrine system procedure**

cc **E36.02** **Intraoperative hemorrhage and hematoma of an endocrine system organ or structure complicating other procedure**

E36.1- **<u>Accidental puncture</u> and laceration of an endocrine system organ or structure during a procedure**

cc **E36.11** **Accidental puncture and laceration of an endocrine system organ or structure during an endocrine system procedure**

cc **E36.12** **Accidental puncture and laceration of an endocrine system organ or structure during other procedure**

E36.8 **<u>Other intraoperative complications</u> of endocrine system**
> **Use additional code, if applicable, to further specify disorder**

Malnutrition (E40-E46)

Excludes 1: *intestinal malabsorption (K90.-)*
sequelae of protein-calorie malnutrition (E64.0)
Excludes ②: *nutritional anemias (D50-D53)*
starvation (T73.0)

E40 **Kwashiorkor** — A severe, protein-deficiency type of malnutrition marked by changes in
MCC skin and hair pigment, edema, retarded growth, and pathologic changes in the liver.
Severe malnutrition with nutritional edema with dyspigmentation of skin and hair
Excludes 1: *marasmic kwashiorkor (E42)*

E41 **Nutritional marasmus** — A protein-calorie malnutrition due to a deficiency in calorie
MCC intake that is characterized by severe tissue wasting, loss of subcutaneous fat, and often
dehydration.
Severe malnutrition with marasmus
Excludes 1: *marasmic kwashiorkor (E42)*

E42 **Marasmic kwashiorkor**
MCC **Intermediate form severe protein-calorie malnutrition**
Severe protein-calorie malnutrition with signs of both kwashiorkor and marasmus

E43 **Unspecified severe protein-calorie malnutrition**
MCC **Starvation edema**

E44- **Protein-calorie malnutrition of moderate and mild degree**
CC **E44.0** **Moderate protein-calorie malnutrition**
CC **E44.1** **Mild protein-calorie malnutrition**

E45 **Retarded development following protein-calorie malnutrition** — An
CC abnormally undersized person resulting from malnutrition.
Nutritional short stature
Nutritional stunting
Physical retardation due to malnutrition

E46 **Unspecified protein-calorie malnutrition**
CC **Malnutrition NOS**
Protein-calorie imbalance NOS
Excludes 1: *nutritional deficiency NOS (E63.9)*

Other nutritional deficiencies (E50-E64)

Excludes ②: *nutritional anemias (D50-D53)*

E50- **Vitamin A deficiency** — A nutritional disorder resulting from less than the normal
amount of vitamin A in the diet.
Excludes 1: *sequelae of vitamin A deficiency (E64.1)*

E50.0 **Vitamin A deficiency with conjunctival xerosis** — A form marked by
dryness of the conjunctiva.

E50.1 **Vitamin A deficiency with Bitot's spot and conjunctival
xerosis** — A form marked by dryness of the conjunctiva with foamy gray,
triangular spots on the conjunctiva.
Bitot's spot in the young child

E50.2 **Vitamin A deficiency with corneal xerosis** — A form marked by
dryness of the cornea.

E50.3 **Vitamin A deficiency with corneal ulceration and xerosis** — A
form marked by dryness of the cornea, with local, necrotic corneal tissue defects.

E50.4 **Vitamin A deficiency with keratomalacia** — A form marked by
softening of the cornea.

E50.5 **Vitamin A deficiency with night blindness** — A form marked by the
inability to see at night.

E50.6 **Vitamin A deficiency with xerophthalmic scars of cornea** — A
form marked by opaque regions on the cornea.

E50.7 **Other ocular manifestations of vitamin A deficiency**
Xerophthalmia NOS

E50.8 **Other manifestations of vitamin A deficiency**
Follicular keratosis — A form marked by horny growth of the skin.
Xeroderma — A form marked by dry, rough, discolored, and sometimes scaly
skin.

E50.9 **Vitamin A deficiency, unspecified**
Hypovitaminosis A NOS

E51- **Thiamine deficiency**
Excludes 1: *sequelae of thiamine deficiency (E64.8)*

E51.1- **Beriberi** — A nutritional disorder resulting from less than the normal amount of
thiamine in the diet, which is marked by peripheral neurologic, cerebral, and
cardiovascular abnormalities.

CC **E51.11** **Dry beriberi** — A form affecting the peripheral nervous system.
Beriberi NOS
Beriberi with polyneuropathy

CC **E51.12** **Wet beriberi** — A form affecting the cardiovascular and circulatory
systems.
Beriberi with cardiovascular manifestations
Cardiovascular beriberi
Shoshin disease

CC **E51.2** **Wernicke's encephalopathy** — A condition marked by neurological
symptoms caused by depletion of the vitamin B1 reserves.

CC **E51.8** **Other manifestations of thiamine deficiency**

CC **E51.9** **Thiamine deficiency, unspecified**

E52 **Niacin deficiency [pellagra]** — A nutritional disorder resulting from less than the
normal amount of niacin in the diet.
Niacin (-tryptophan) deficiency
Nicotinamide deficiency
Pellagra (alcoholic)
Excludes 1: *sequelae of niacin deficiency (E64.8)*

E53- **Deficiency of other B group vitamins**
Excludes 1: *sequelae of vitamin B deficiency (E64.8)*

CC **E53.0** **Riboflavin deficiency** — A nutritional disorder resulting from less than the
normal amount of riboflavin (B2) in the diet, which is marked by stomatitis, lip
lesions, seborrhea of the nose, and vascularization of cornea.
Ariboflavinosis
Vitamin B2 deficiency

E53.1 **Pyridoxine deficiency** — A nutritional disorder resulting from less than the
normal amount of vitamin B6 in the diet, which is marked by dermatitis around the
eyes and mouth, neuritis, anorexia, nausea, and vomiting.
Vitamin B6 deficiency
Excludes 1: *pyridoxine-responsive sideroblastic anemia (D64.3)*

E53.8 **Deficiency of other specified B group vitamins**
Biotin deficiency
Cyanocobalamin deficiency
Folate deficiency
Folic acid deficiency
Pantothenic acid deficiency
Vitamin B12 deficiency
Excludes 1: *folate deficiency anemia (D52.-)*
vitamin B12 deficiency anemia (D51.-)

E53.9 **Vitamin B deficiency, unspecified**

E54 **Ascorbic acid deficiency** — A nutritional disorder resulting from less than the
normal amount of vitamin C in the diet, which is marked by lowered resistance to infections,
joint tenderness, and susceptibility to dental disorders.
Deficiency of vitamin C
Scurvy
Excludes 1: *scorbutic anemia (D53.2)*
sequelae of vitamin C deficiency (E64.2)

E55- **Vitamin D deficiency** — A nutritional disorder resulting from less than the normal
amount of vitamin D in the diet, which is marked by bone disorders.
Excludes 1: *adult osteomalacia (M83.-)*
osteoporosis (M80.-)
sequelae of rickets (E64.3)

CC **E55.0** **Rickets, active** — A form marked by inadequate deposition of lime salts in
developing cartilage and newly formed bone causing malformation which is seen
during childhood.
Infantile osteomalacia
Juvenile osteomalacia
Excludes 1: *celiac rickets (K90.0)*
Crohn's rickets (K50.-)
hereditary vitamin D-dependent rickets (E83.32)
inactive rickets (E64.3)
renal rickets (N25.0)
sequelae of rickets (E64.3)
vitamin D-resistant rickets (E83.31)

E55.9 **Vitamin D deficiency, unspecified**
Avitaminosis D — Less than the normal amount of vitamin D in the diet.

E40
I
E55

E56- Other vitamin deficiencies
Excludes 1:   sequelae of other vitamin deficiencies (E64.8)

E56.0 **Deficiency of vitamin E**

E56.1 **Deficiency of vitamin K**
Excludes 1:   deficiency of coagulation factor due to vitamin K deficiency (D68.4)
vitamin K deficiency of newborn (P53)

E56.8 **Deficiency of other vitamins**

E56.9 **Vitamin deficiency, unspecified**

E58 Dietary calcium deficiency
Excludes 1:   disorders of calcium metabolism (E83.5-)
sequelae of calcium deficiency (E64.8)

E59 Dietary selenium deficiency
Keshan disease
Excludes 1:   sequelae of selenium deficiency (E64.8)

E60 Dietary zinc deficiency

E61- Deficiency of other nutrient elements
Use additional code for adverse effect, if applicable, to identify drug   (T36-T50 with fifth or sixth character 5)
Excludes 1:   disorders of mineral metabolism (E83.-)
iodine deficiency related thyroid disorders (E00-E02)
sequelae of malnutrition and other nutritional deficiencies (E64.-)

E61.0 **Copper deficiency**

E61.1 **Iron deficiency**
Excludes 1:   iron deficiency anemia (D50.-)

E61.2 **Magnesium deficiency**

E61.3 **Manganese deficiency**

E61.4 **Chromium deficiency**

E61.5 **Molybdenum deficiency**

E61.6 **Vanadium deficiency**

E61.7 **Deficiency of multiple nutrient elements**

E61.8 **Deficiency of other specified nutrient elements**

E61.9 **Deficiency of nutrient element, unspecified**

E63- Other nutritional deficiencies
Excludes 1:   dehydration (E86.0)
failure to thrive, adult (R62.7)
failure to thrive, child (R62.51)
feeding problems in newborn (P92.-)
sequelae of malnutrition and other nutritional deficiencies (E64.-)

E63.0 **Essential fatty acid [EFA] deficiency**

E63.1 **Imbalance of constituents of food intake**

E63.8 **Other specified nutritional deficiencies**

E63.9 **Nutritional deficiency, unspecified**

E64- Sequelae of malnutrition and other nutritional deficiencies
Note: This category is to be used to indicate conditions in categories E43, E44, E46, E50-E63 as the cause of sequelae, which are themselves classified elsewhere. The "sequelae" include conditions specified as such; they also include the late effects of diseases classifiable to the above categories if the disease itself is no longer present
Code first condition resulting from (sequela) of malnutrition and other nutritional deficiencies

CC **E64.0** **Sequelae of protein-calorie malnutrition**
Excludes ❷: retarded development following protein-calorie malnutrition (E45)

E64.1 **Sequelae of vitamin A deficiency**

E64.2 **Sequelae of vitamin C deficiency**

E64.3 **Sequelae of rickets**

E64.8 **Sequelae of other nutritional deficiencies**

E64.9 **Sequelae of unspecified nutritional deficiency**

Overweight, obesity and other hyperalimentation (E65-E68)

E65 Localized adiposity — An abnormal amount of fat concentrated in one part of the body.
Fat pad — An abnormal amount of fat concentrated into a well-defined circumscribed area.

E66- Overweight and obesity — The abnormally increased body weight for height due to the excess storage of body fat.
Code first obesity complicating pregnancy, childbirth and the puerperium, if applicable (O99.21-)
Use additional code to identify body mass index (BMI), if known (Z68.-)
Excludes 1:   adiposogenital dystrophy (E23.6)
lipomatosis NOS (E88.2)
lipomatosis dolorosa [Dercum] (E88.2)
Prader-Willi syndrome (Q87.1)

E66.0- Obesity due to excess calories — A form caused by the excess intake of food calories that is not due to a medical, genetic, or psychiatric condition, and is not drug-induced.

E66.01 Morbid (severe) obesity due to excess calories — A form usually identified and diagnosed as at least twice a person's ideal weight, 100 pounds over a person's ideal weight, or a body mass index (BMI) that is greater than 40.
Excludes 1:   morbid (severe) obesity with alveolar hypoventilation (E66.2)

E66.09 **Other obesity due to excess calories** — [Questionable Admission]

E66.1 Drug-induced obesity — [Questionable Admission]
Use additional code for adverse effect, if applicable, to identify drug (T36-T50 with fifth or sixth character 5)

CC **E66.2** Morbid (severe) obesity with alveolar hypoventilation — A condition of decreased oxygen levels and elevated carbon dioxide levels that is associated with obesity.
Obesity hypoventilation syndrome (OHS)
Pickwickian syndrome

E66.3 Overweight — The first grade of the overweight/obesity continuum, followed by obesity, morbid obesity, and superobesity, or simply a person's weight (excessive bone and muscle mass) that is in greater proportion to their height.

E66.8 **Other obesity** — [Questionable Admission]

E66.9 **Obesity, unspecified** — [Questionable Admission]
Obesity NOS

E67- Other hyperalimentation — The excessive ingestion or administration of nutrients into the body.
Excludes 1:   hyperalimentation NOS (R63.2)
sequelae of hyperalimentation (E68)

E67.0 **Hypervitaminosis A** — A disorder caused by excessive amounts of vitamin A in the blood, marked by skin pigmentation, pruritis, and loss of hair.

E67.1 **Hypercarotinemia** — An excessive amount of the yellow or red pigment, carotene, in the blood.

E67.2 **Megavitamin-B6 syndrome** — A disorder caused by excessive amounts of vitamin B6 in the blood.

E67.3 **Hypervitaminosis D** — A disorder caused by excessive amounts of vitamin D in the blood, marked by weakness, fatigue, and loss of weight.

E67.8 **Other specified hyperalimentation**

E68 Sequelae of hyperalimentation
Code first condition resulting from (sequela) of hyperalimentation

Metabolic disorders (E70-E88)

Excludes 1:   androgen insensitivity syndrome (E34.5-)
congenital adrenal hyperplasia (E25.0)
Ehlers-Danlos syndrome (Q79.6)
hemolytic anemias attributable to enzyme disorders (D55.-)
Marfan's syndrome (Q87.4)
5-alpha-reductase deficiency (E29.1)

E70- Disorders of aromatic amino-acid metabolism — Abnormalities of a group of chemically similar organic compounds that form the chief structure of proteins.

CC **E70.0** Classical phenylketonuria — An inherited disease caused by the body's failure to oxidize the amino-acid phenylalanine, resulting in tremor, spasticity, convulsions, and mental deficiency.

CC **E70.1** **Other hyperphenylalaninemias**

E70.2- Disorders of tyrosine metabolism
Excludes 1:   transitory tyrosinemia of newborn (P74.5)

CC **E70.20** **Disorder of tyrosine metabolism, unspecified**

CC **E70.21** Tyrosinemia — The abnormal level of tyrosine in the blood.
Hypertyrosinemia

Excludes 1: = NOT CODED HERE! (Do not code both)

Excludes ❷: = Not Included Here

E56 I E70

cc **E70.29   Other disorders of tyrosine metabolism**
　　Alkaptonuria — The abnormal presence of alkapton bodies in the urine.
　　Ochronosis — A disorder characterized by discoloration of certain tissues of the body caused by the deposit of alkapton bodies.

E70.3-   Albinism — A disorder characterized by absence of pigment in the skin, hair, and eyes.

cc **E70.30   Albinism, unspecified**

E70.31- Ocular albinism

cc **E70.310   X-linked ocular albinism**

cc **E70.311   Autosomal recessive ocular albinism**

cc **E70.318   Other ocular albinism**

cc **E70.319   Ocular albinism, unspecified**

E70.32- Oculocutaneous albinism
　　Excludes 1:   Chediak-Higashi syndrome (E70.330)
　　　　　Hermansky-Pudlak syndrome (E70.331)

cc **E70.320   Tyrosinase negative oculocutaneous albinism**
　　Albinism I
　　Oculocutaneous albinism ty-neg

cc **E70.321   Tyrosinase positive oculocutaneous albinism**
　　Albinism II
　　Oculocutaneous albinism ty-pos

cc **E70.328   Other oculocutaneous albinism**
　　Cross syndrome

cc **E70.329   Oculocutaneous albinism, unspecified**

E70.33- Albinism with hematologic abnormality

cc **E70.330   Chediak-Higashi syndrome**

cc **E70.331   Hermansky-Pudlak syndrome**

cc **E70.338   Other albinism with hematologic abnormality**

cc **E70.339   Albinism with hematologic abnormality, unspecified**

cc **E70.39   Other specified albinism**
　　Piebaldism

E70.4-   Disorders of histidine metabolism — Abnormal function of the amino acid, histidine, which is essential for the optimal growth of infants, and breaks down to produce histamine.

cc **E70.40   Disorders of histidine metabolism, unspecified**

cc **E70.41   Histidinemia** — An inherited histidine metabolic defect characterized by excessive amounts of histidine in the blood and urine.

cc **E70.49   Other disorders of histidine metabolism**

cc **E70.5   Disorders of tryptophan metabolism**

cc **E70.8   Other disorders of aromatic amino-acid metabolism**

cc **E70.9   Disorder of aromatic amino-acid metabolism, unspecified**

E71-   Disorders of branched-chain amino-acid metabolism and fatty-acid metabolism — Abnormal function of the amino acids essential for the optimal growth of infants.

cc **E71.0   Maple-syrup-urine disease** — An inherited enzyme defect in the metabolism of branched-chain amino acids.

E71.1-   Other disorders of branched-chain amino-acid metabolism

E71.11- Branched-chain organic acidurias

cc **E71.110   Isovaleric acidemia**

cc **E71.111   3-methylglutaconic aciduria**

cc **E71.118   Other branched-chain organic acidurias**

E71.12- Disorders of propionate metabolism

cc **E71.120   Methylmalonic acidemia**

cc **E71.121   Propionic acidemia**

cc **E71.128   Other disorders of propionate metabolism**

cc **E71.19   Other disorders of branched-chain amino-acid metabolism**
　　Hyperleucine-isoleucinemia
　　Hypervalinemia

cc **E71.2   Disorder of branched-chain amino-acid metabolism, unspecified**

E71.3-   Disorders of fatty-acid metabolism — Conditions resulting from the abnormal fatty acid chemical process that may be characterized by hypoglycemia, coma, muscle weakness, cardiomyopathy, or rhabdomyalgias.
　　Excludes 1:   peroxisomal disorders (E71.5)
　　　　　Refsum's disease (G60.1)
　　　　　Schilder's disease (G37.0)
　　Excludes ❷: carnitine deficiency due to inborn error of metabolism (E71.42)

E71.30   Disorder of fatty-acid metabolism, unspecified

E71.31- Disorders of fatty-acid oxidation

cc **E71.310   Long chain/very long chain acyl CoA dehydrogenase deficiency**
　　LCAD
　　VLCAD

cc **E71.311   Medium chain acyl CoA dehydrogenase deficiency**
　　MCAD

cc **E71.312   Short chain acyl CoA dehydrogenase deficiency**
　　SCAD

cc **E71.313   Glutaric aciduria type II**
　　Glutaric aciduria type II A
　　Glutaric aciduria type II B
　　Glutaric aciduria type II C
　　Excludes 1:   glutaric aciduria (type 1) NOS (E72.3)

cc **E71.314   Muscle carnitine palmitoyltransferase deficiency**

cc **E71.318   Other disorders of fatty-acid oxidation**

cc **E71.32   Disorders of ketone metabolism**

cc **E71.39   Other disorders of fatty-acid metabolism**

E71.4-   Disorders of carnitine metabolism
　　Excludes 1:   muscle carnitine palmitoyltransferase deficiency (E71.314)

E71.40   Disorder of carnitine metabolism, unspecified

E71.41   Primary carnitine deficiency — A condition of lower than normal levels of carnitine concentration in plasma or tissues that is caused by a defect in the carnitine transporter mechanism.

E71.42   Carnitine deficiency due to inborn errors of metabolism — A form caused by metabolic disorders.
　　Code also associated inborn error or metabolism

E71.43   Iatrogenic carnitine deficiency — A form resulting from medical treatment.
　　Carnitine deficiency due to hemodialysis
　　Carnitine deficiency due to valproic acid therapy

E71.44- Other secondary carnitine deficiency

E71.440   Ruvalcaba-Myhre-Smith syndrome

E71.448   Other secondary carnitine deficiency

E71.5-   Peroxisomal disorders — Inherited conditions resulting from the abnormal formation or functioning of the subcellular membrane-bound organelles (peroxisomes) that contain enzymes involved in the metabolism of very long chain fatty acids.
　　Excludes 1:   Schilder's disease (G37.0)

cc **E71.50   Peroxisomal disorder, unspecified**

E71.51- Disorders of peroxisome biogenesis
　　Group 1 peroxisomal disorders
　　Excludes 1:   Refsum's disease (G60.1)

cc **E71.510   Zellweger syndrome** — A genetic peroxisomal leukodystrophy disorder characterized by enlarged liver, lack of muscle tone, mental retardation, and vision disturbances.

cc **E71.511   Neonatal adrenoleukodystrophy** — A form of X-linked adrenoleukodystrophy (see inclusion term below) occurring in the neonatal period.
　　Excludes 1:   X-linked adrenoleukodystrophy (E71.42-)

cc **E71.518   Other disorders of peroxisome biogenesis**

E71.52- X-linked adrenoleukodystrophy — A genetic peroxisomal disorder occurring in childhood that is characterized by mental retardation, spasticity, blindness, and is invariably fatal.

cc **E71.520   Childhood cerebral X-linked adrenoleukodystrophy**

cc **E71.521   Adolescent X-linked adrenoleukodystrophy**

cc **E71.522   Adrenomyeloneuropathy**

cc **E71.528   Other X-linked adrenoleukodystrophy**
　　Addison only phenotype adrenoleukodystrophy
　　Addison-Schilder adrenoleukodystrophy

cc **E71.529   X-linked adrenoleukodystrophy, unspecified type**

cc **E71.53   Other group 2 peroxisomal disorders**

E71.54- Other peroxisomal disorders

cc **E71.540 Rhizomelic chondrodysplasia punctata** — A genetic peroxisomal disorder characterized by shortening of the proximal limbs and joints, round face, high forehead, and a small, upturned nose.

    Excludes 1:   *chondrodysplasia punctata NOS (Q77.3)*

cc **E71.541 Zellweger-like syndrome**

cc **E71.542 Other group 3 peroxisomal disorders**

cc **E71.548 Other peroxisomal disorders**

E72- Other disorders of amino-acid metabolism

    Excludes 1:   *disorders of:*
        aromatic amino-acid metabolism (E70.-)
        branched-chain amino-acid metabolism (E71.0-E71.2)
        fatty-acid metabolism (E71.3)
        gout (M1A.-, M10.-)
        purine and pyrimidine metabolism (E79.-)

E72.0- Disorders of amino-acid transport — Abnormalities of a group of chemically similar organic compounds that form the chief structure of proteins.

    Excludes 1:   *disorders of tryptophan metabolism (E70.5)*

cc **E72.00 Disorders of amino-acid transport, unspecified**

cc **E72.01 Cystinuria** — An inherited, metabolic disorder characterized by large amounts of cystine in the urine resulting in the formation of urinary calculi.

cc **E72.02 Hartnup's disease** — A disorder of the intestinal and renal transport of amino acids, marked by amino acid in the urine, skin rash, and other biochemical abnormalities.

cc **E72.03 Lowe's syndrome**
    Use additional code for associated glaucoma (H42)

cc **E72.04 Cystinosis** — An inherited disease of cystine metabolism resulting in abnormal deposition of cystine in body tissues.
    Fanconi (-de Toni) (-Debré) syndrome with cystinosis
    Excludes 1:   *Fanconi (-de Toni) (-Debré) syndrome without cystinosis (E72.09)*

cc **E72.09 Other disorders of amino-acid transport**
    Fanconi (-de Toni) (-Debré) syndrome, unspecified

E72.1- Disorders of sulfur-bearing amino-acid metabolism — The abnormal function of amino acids containing sulphur compounds.
    Excludes 1:   *cystinosis (E72.04)*
        cystinuria (E72.01)
        transcobalamin II deficiency (D51.2)

cc **E72.10 Disorders of sulfur-bearing amino-acid metabolism, unspecified**

cc **E72.11 Homocystinuria** — The abnormal presence of large amounts of homocystine in the urine caused by an error of sulfur amino acid metabolism due to a deficiency of the liver enzyme cystathionine synthase.
    Cystathionine synthase deficiency

cc **E72.12 Methylenetetrahydrofolate reductase deficiency**

cc **E72.19 Other disorders of sulfur-bearing amino-acid metabolism**
    Cystathioninuria
    Methioninemia
    Sulfite oxidase deficiency

E72.2- Disorders of urea cycle metabolism — Abnormal function of the series of reactions that produce urea, which is important in removing ammonia from the body.
    Excludes 1:   *disorders of ornithine metabolism (E72.4)*

cc **E72.20 Disorder of urea cycle metabolism, unspecified**
    Hyperammonemia
    Excludes 1:   *hyperammonemia-hyperornithinemia-homocitrullinemia syndrome E72.4*
        transient hyperammonemia of newborn (P74.6)

cc **E72.21 Argininemia**

cc **E72.22 Arginosuccinic aciduria**

cc **E72.23 Citrullinemia**

cc **E72.29 Other disorders of urea cycle metabolism**

cc **E72.3 Disorders of lysine and hydroxylysine metabolism** — The abnormal function of lysine and hydroxylysine metabolism.
    Glutaric aciduria NOS
    Glutaric aciduria (type I)
    Hydroxylysinemia
    Hyperlysinemia
    Excludes 1:   *glutaric aciduria type II (E71.313)*
        Refsum's dsease (G60.1)
        Zellweger syndrome (E71.510)

cc **E72.4 Disorders of ornithine metabolism** — The abnormal function of orinthine metabolism.
    Hyperammonemia-Hyperornithinemia-Homocitrullinemia syndrome
    Ornithinemia (types I, II)
    Ornithine transcarbamylase deficiency
    Excludes 1:   *hereditary choroidal dystrophy (H31.2-)*

E72.5- Disorders of glycine metabolism — The abnormal function of glycine metabolism.

cc **E72.50 Disorder of glycine metabolism, unspecified**

cc **E72.51 Non-ketotic hyperglycinemia**

cc **E72.52 Trimethylaminuria**

cc **E72.53 Hyperoxaluria**
    Oxalosis
    Oxaluria

cc **E72.59 Other disorders of glycine metabolism**
    D-glycericacidemia
    Hyperhydroxyprolinemia
    Hyperprolinemia (types I, II)
    Sarcosinemia

cc **E72.8 Other specified disorders of amino-acid metabolism**
    Disorders of beta-amino-acid metabolism
    Disorders of gamma-glutamyl cycle

cc **E72.9 Disorder of amino-acid metabolism, unspecified**

E73- Lactose intolerance — Abnormal decrease or impaired digestion of lactose, a sugar found in milk.

E73.0 Congenital lactase deficiency — An inherited condition of insufficient levels of the enzyme lactase.

E73.1 Secondary lactase deficiency — A condition of insufficient levels of the enzyme lactase that is due to disease conditions, usually of the small intestine.

E73.8 Other lactose intolerance

E73.9 Lactose intolerance, unspecified

E74- Other disorders of carbohydrate metabolism
    Excludes 1:   *diabetes mellitus (E08-E13)*
        hypoglycemia NOS (E16.2)
        increased secretion of glucagon (E16.3)
        mucopolysaccharidosis (E76.0-E76.3)

E74.0- Glycogen storage disease — An inherited metabolic disorder of glycogen storage.

cc **E74.00 Glycogen storage disease, unspecified**

cc **E74.01 von Gierke disease**
    Type I glycogen storage disease

cc **E74.02 Pompe disease**
    Cardiac glycogenosis
    Type II glycogen storage disease

cc **E74.03 Cori disease**
    Forbes disease
    Type III glycogen storage disease

cc **E74.04 McArdle disease**
    Type V glycogen storage disease

cc **E74.09 Other glycogen storage disease**
    Andersen disease
    Hers disease
    Tauri disease
    Glycogen storage disease, types 0, IV, VI-XI
    Liver phosphorylase deficiency
    Muscle phosphofructokinase deficiency

E74.1- Disorders of fructose metabolism — A metabolic disorder of fructose metabolism.
    Excludes 1:   *muscle phosphofructokinase deficiency (E74.09)*

E74.10 Disorder of fructose metabolism, unspecified

E74.11 Essential fructosuria — A benign, hereditary carbohydrate metabolism disorder characterized by fructosemia and fructosuria.
    Fructokinase deficiency

E74.12 Hereditary fructose intolerance — A hereditary disorder involving deficient activity of the hepatic enzyme fructose-1-phosphate aldolase, marked by hypoglycemia in infants' diets.
    Fructosemia

E74.19 Other disorders of fructose metabolism
    Fructose-1, 6-diphosphatase deficiency

E71-E74

E74.2-   **Disorders of galactose metabolism** — A metabolic disorder of galactose metabolism.

cc **E74.20   Disorders of galactose metabolism, unspecified**

cc **E74.21   Galactosemia** — An inherited disorder of galactose metabolism marked by hepatomegaly, cataracts, and mental retardation.

cc **E74.29   Other disorders of galactose metabolism**
Galactokinase deficiency

E74.3-   **Other disorders of intestinal carbohydrate absorption**
Excludes ❷: lactose intolerance (E73.-)

E74.31   Sucrase-isomaltase deficiency

E74.39   Other disorders of intestinal carbohydrate absorption
Disorder of intestinal carbohydrate absorption NOS
Glucose-galactose malabsorption
Sucrase deficiency

cc **E74.4   Disorders of pyruvate metabolism and gluconeogenesis**
Deficiency of phosphoenolpyruvate carboxykinase
Deficiency of pyruvate carboxylase
Deficiency of pyruvate dehydrogenase
Excludes 1:   disorders of pyruvate metabolism and gluconeogenesis with anemia (D55.-)
Leigh's syndrome (G31.82)

cc **E74.8   Other specified disorders of carbohydrate metabolism**
Essential pentosuria
Renal glycosuria

E74.9   Disorder of carbohydrate metabolism, unspecified

E75-   **Disorders of sphingolipid metabolism and other lipid storage disorders** — Inherited disorders characterized by abnormal cellular lipid metabolism.
Excludes 1:   mucolipidosis, types I-III (E77.0-E77.1)
Refsum's disease (G60.1)

E75.0-   **GM2 gangliosidosis** — An inherited abnormal accumulation of GM2 ganglioside in lysosomes.

cc **E75.00   GM2 gangliosidosis, unspecified**

cc **E75.01   Sandhoff disease**

cc **E75.02   Tay-Sachs disease** — A form with hexosaminidase A enzyme deficiency that is characterized by neurodegeneration, difficulty swallowing, and physical developmental disabilities.

cc **E75.09   Other GM2 gangliosidosis**
Adult GM2 gangliosidosis
Juvenile GM2 gangliosidosis

E75.1-   **Other and unspecified gangliosidosis**

cc **E75.10   Unspecified gangliosidosis**
Gangliosidosis NOS

cc **E75.11   Mucolipidosis IV**

cc **E75.19   Other gangliosidosis**
GM1 gangliosidosis
GM3 gangliosidosis

E75.2-   **Other sphingolipidosis** — Inherited lipid storage disorders relating to sphingolipid metabolism.
Excludes 1:   adrenoleukodystrophy [Addison-Schilder] (E71.528)

E75.21   Fabry (-Anderson) disease — A form with a-galactosidase A enzyme deficiency that is characterized by full body and/or limb pain, infarction of organs, and fatigue.

E75.22   Gaucher disease — A form with glococerebrosidase enzyme deficiency that is characterized by bruising, fatigue, anemia, hepatosplenomegaly, and pancytopenia.

cc **E75.23   Krabbe disease** — A form with galactocerebrosidase enzyme deficiency that is characterized by spasticity, neurodegeneration, blindness, and seizures.

E75.24-   **Niemann-Pick disease** — A form with sphingomyelinase enzyme deficiency that is characterized by mental retardation, spasticity, splenomegaly, and thrombocytopenia.

E75.240   Niemann-Pick disease type A

E75.241   Niemann-Pick disease type B

E75.242   Niemann-Pick disease type C

E75.243   Niemann-Pick disease type D

E75.248   Other Niemann-Pick disease

E75.249   Niemann-Pick disease, unspecified

cc **E75.25   Metachromatic leukodystrophy**

cc **E75.29   Other sphingolipidosis**
Farber's syndrome
Sulfatase deficiency
Sulfatide lipidosis

E75.3   Sphingolipidosis, unspecified

cc **E75.4   Neuronal ceroid lipofuscinosis**
Batten disease
Bielschowsky-Jansky disease
Kufs disease
Spielmeyer-Vogt disease

E75.5   Other lipid storage disorders
Cerebrotendinous cholesterosis [van Bogaert-Scherer-Epstein]
Wolman's disease

E75.6   Lipid storage disorder, unspecified

E76-   **Disorders of glycosaminoglycan metabolism** — Inherited diseases of defective glycosaminoglycan metabolism causing abnormal accumulation in the tissues.

E76.0-   **Mucopolysaccharidosis, type I**

cc **E76.01   Hurler's syndrome**

cc **E76.02   Hurler-Scheie syndrome**

cc **E76.03   Scheie's syndrome**

cc E76.1   **Mucopolysaccharidosis, type II**
Hunter's syndrome

E76.2-   **Other mucopolysaccharidoses**

E76.21-   Morquio mucopolysaccharidoses

cc **E76.210   Morquio A mucopolysaccharidoses**
Classic Morquio syndrome
Morquio syndrome A
Mucopolysaccharidosis, type IVA

cc **E76.211   Morquio B mucopolysaccharidoses**
Morquio-like mucopolysaccharidoses
Morquio-like syndrome
Morquio syndrome B
Mucopolysaccharidosis, type IVB

cc **E76.219   Morquio mucopolysaccharidoses, unspecified**
Morquio syndrome
Mucopolysaccharidosis, type IV

cc **E76.22   Sanfilippo mucopolysaccharidoses**
Mucopolysaccharidosis, type III (A) (B) (C) (D)
Sanfilippo A syndrome
Sanfilippo B syndrome
Sanfilippo C syndrome
Sanfilippo D syndrome

cc **E76.29   Other mucopolysaccharidoses**
beta-Glucuronidase deficiency
Maroteaux-Lamy (mild) (severe) syndrome
Mucopolysaccharidosis, types VI, VII

cc **E76.3   Mucopolysaccharidosis, unspecified**

cc **E76.8   Other disorders of glucosaminoglycan metabolism**

cc **E76.9   Glucosaminoglycan metabolism disorder, unspecified**

E77-   **Disorders of glycoprotein metabolism** — Inherited diseases of defective glycoprotein metabolism causing abnormal accumulation in the tissues.

E77.0   Defects in post-translational modification of lysosomal enzymes
Mucolipidosis II [I-cell disease]
Mucolipidosis III [pseudo-Hurler polydystrophy]

E77.1   Defects in glycoprotein degradation
Aspartylglucosaminuria
Fucosidosis
Mannosidosis
Sialidosis [mucolipidosis I]

E77.8   Other disorders of glycoprotein metabolism

E77.9   Disorder of glycoprotein metabolism, unspecified

E78-   **Disorders of lipoprotein metabolism and other lipidemias** — Inherited diseases of defective lipoprotein metabolism causing abnormal accumulation in the tissues, and disorders involving lipids in the blood.
Excludes 1:   sphingolipidosis (E75.0-E75.3)

E78.0-   Pure hypercholesterolemia — A disorder caused by an increase in beta lipoproteins and cholesterol in the plasma.

E78.00   Pure hypercholesterolemia, unspecified
Fredrickson's hyperlipoproteinemia, type IIa
Hyperbetalipoproteinemia
Low-density-lipoprotein-type [LDL] hyperlipoproteinemia

E78.01   Familial hypercholesterolemia — A form caused by genetic mutations involved in LDL-C metabolism.

E
7
4
-
E
7
8

E78.1 Pure hyperglyceridemia — A disorder caused by an increase in triglycerides or pre-beta lipoproteins in the plasma.
  Elevated fasting triglycerides
  Endogenous hyperglyceridemia
  Fredrickson's hyperlipoproteinemia, type IV
  Hyperlipidemia, group B
  Hyperprebetalipoproteinemia
  Very-low-density-lipoprotein-type [VLDL] hyperlipoproteinemia

E78.2 Mixed hyperlipidemia — A disorder caused by an increase of beta lipoproteins and cholesterol, and triglycerides and pre-beta lipoproteins in the plasma.
  Broad- or floating-betalipoproteinemia
  Combined hyperlipidemia NOS
  Elevated cholesterol with elevated triglycerides NEC
  Fredrickson's hyperlipoproteinemia, type IIb or III
  Hyperbetalipoproteinemia with prebetalipoproteinemia
  Hypercholesteremia with endogenous hyperglyceridemia
  Hyperlipidemia, group C
  Tubo-eruptive xanthoma
  Xanthoma tuberosum
  Excludes 1:   cerebrotendinous cholesterosis [van Bogaert-Scherer-Epstein] (E75.5)
  *   familial combined hyperlipidemia (E78.4)*

E78.3 Hyperchylomicronemia — A disorder caused by the presence of large quantities of chylomicrons resulting from an absence or deficiency of the lipoprotein lipase.
  Chylomicron retention disease
  Fredrickson's hyperlipoproteinemia, type I or V
  Hyperlipidemia, group D
  Mixed hyperglyceridemia

E78.4 Other hyperlipidemia
  Familial combined hyperlipidemia

E78.5 Hyperlipidemia, unspecified

E78.6 Lipoprotein deficiency — An abnormal decrease in the blood plasma lipoprotein levels.
  Abetalipoproteinemia
  Depressed HDL cholesterol
  High-density lipoprotein deficiency
  Hypoalphalipoproteinemia
  Hypobetalipoproteinemia (familial)
  Lecithin cholesterol acyltransferase deficiency
  Tangier disease

E78.7- Disorders of bile acid and cholesterol metabolism
  Excludes 1:   Niemann-Pick disease type C (E75.242)

E78.70 Disorder of bile acid and cholesterol metabolism, unspecified

cc **E78.71 Barth syndrome**

cc **E78.72 Smith-Lemli-Opitz syndrome**

E78.79 Other disorders of bile acid and cholesterol metabolism

E78.8- Other disorders of lipoprotein metabolism

E78.81 Lipoid dermatoarthritis

E78.89 Other lipoprotein metabolism disorders

E78.9 Disorder of lipoprotein metabolism, unspecified

E79- Disorders of purine and pyrimidine metabolism — Inherited diseases of defective purine and pyrimidine metabolism causing abnormal accumulation in the tissues.
  Excludes 1:   Ataxia-telangiectasia (Q87.1)
  *   Bloom's syndrome (Q82.8)*
  *   Cockayne's syndrome (Q87.1)*
  *   calculus of kidney (N20.0)*
  *   combined immunodeficiency disorders (D81.-)*
  *   Fanconi's anemia (D61.09)*
  *   gout (M1A.-, M10.-)*
  *   orotaciduric anemia (D53.0)*
  *   progeria (E34.8)*
  *   Werner's syndrome (E34.8)*
  *   xeroderma pigmentosum (Q82.1)*

E79.0 Hyperuricemia without signs of inflammatory arthritis and tophaceous disease
  Asymptomatic hyperuricemia

cc **E79.1 Lesch-Nyhan syndrome**
  HGPRT deficiency

cc **E79.2 Myoadenylate deaminase deficiency**

cc **E79.8 Other disorders of purine and pyrimidine metabolism**
  Hereditary xanthinuria

cc **E79.9 Disorder of purine and pyrimidine metabolism, unspecified**

E80- Disorders of porphyrin and bilirubin metabolism — Inherited diseases of defective porphyrin and bilirubin metabolism causing abnormal accumulation in the tissues.
  Includes: Defects of catalase and peroxidase

cc **E80.0 Hereditary erythropoietic porphyria**
  Congenital erythropoietic porphyria
  Erythropoietic protoporphyria

cc **E80.1 Porphyria cutanea tarda**

E80.2- Other and unspecified porphyria

cc **E80.20 Unspecified porphyria**
  Porphyria NOS

cc **E80.21 Acute intermittent (hepatic) porphyria**

cc **E80.29 Other porphyria**
  Hereditary coproporphyria

cc **E80.3 Defects of catalase and peroxidase**
  Acatalasia [Takahara]

E80.4 Gilbert syndrome

E80.5 Crigler-Najjar syndrome

E80.6 Other disorders of bilirubin metabolism
  Dubin-Johnson syndrome
  Rotor's syndrome

E80.7 Disorder of bilirubin metabolism, unspecified

E83- Disorders of mineral metabolism — Abnormal chemical processing of the organic, life-sustaining chemical process of the nonorganic homogenous solid substances.
  Excludes 1:   dietary mineral deficiency (E58-E61)
  *   parathyroid disorders (E20-E21)*
  *   vitamin D deficiency (E55.-)*

E83.0- Disorders of copper metabolism — Abnormal chemical processing of the metallic element copper, which is essential to several enzyme systems.

E83.00 Disorder of copper metabolism, unspecified

E83.01 Wilson's disease — A hereditary, degenerative syndrome that allows abnormal accumulation of copper in various organs (brain, liver, kidney, and cornea) due to a defect in copper metabolism.
  Code also associated Kayser Fleischer ring (H18.04-)

E83.09 Other disorders of copper metabolism
  Menkes' (kinky hair) (steely hair) disease

E83.1- Disorders of iron metabolism — Abnormal chemical processing of the metallic element iron, which is essential in the formation of hemoglobin.
  Excludes 1:   iron deficiency anemia (D50.-)
  *   sideroblastic anemia (D64.0-D64.3)*

E83.10 Disorder of iron metabolism, unspecified

E83.11- Hemochromatosis — A disease of iron metabolism characterized by excessive iron deposition in tissues, especially the liver, bronze-like pigmentation of the skin, and diabetes mellitus.

E83.110 Hereditary hemochromatosis
  Bronzed diabetes
  Pigmentary cirrhosis (of liver)
  Primary (hereditary) hemochromatosis

E83.111 Hemochromatosis due to repeated red blood cell transfusions
  Iron overload due to repeated red blood cell transfusions
  Transfusion (red blood cell) associated hemochromatosis

E83.118 Other hemochromatosis

E83.119 Hemochromatosis, unspecified

E83.19 Other disorders of iron metabolism
  Use additional code, if applicable, for idiopathic pulmonary hemosiderosis (J84.03)

E83.2 Disorders of zinc metabolism — Abnormal chemical processing of the metallic element zinc, which is essential in the body's general nutrition.
  Acrodermatitis enteropathica

E83.3- Disorders of phosphorus metabolism and phosphatases — Abnormal chemical processing of the nonmetallic element phosphorus, which is essential in energy metabolism, bone minerlization, and for conversion of glycogen to glucose.
  Excludes 1:   adult osteomalacia (M83.-)
  *   osteoporosis (M80.-)*

E83.30 Disorder of phosphorus metabolism, unspecified

E83.31 Familial hypophosphatemia
  Vitamin D-resistant osteomalacia
  Vitamin D-resistant rickets
  Excludes 1:   vitamin D-deficiency rickets (E55.0)

E83.32 **Hereditary vitamin D-dependent rickets (type 1) (type 2)**
25-hydroxyvitamin D 1-alpha-hydroxylase deficiency
Pseudovitamin D deficiency
Vitamin D receptor defect

E83.39 **Other disorders of phosphorus metabolism**
Acid phosphatase deficiency
Hypophosphatasia

E83.4- **Disorders of <u>magnesium metabolism</u>** — Abnormal chemical processing of the metallic element magnesium, which activates certain enzymes to catalyze phosphate ions.

E83.40 **Disorders of magnesium metabolism, unspecified**

E83.41 **Hypermagnesemia**

E83.42 **Hypomagnesemia**

E83.49 **Other disorders of magnesium metabolism**

E83.5- **Disorders of <u>calcium metabolism</u>** — Abnormal chemical processing of the metallic element calcium, which is essential to bone formation, blood coagulation, lactation, and for function of the nerves and muscles.
Excludes 1: *chondrocalcinosis (M11.1-M11.2)*
hungry bone syndrome (E83.81)
hyperparathyroidism (E21.0-E21.3)

E83.50 **Unspecified disorder of calcium metabolism**

E83.51 **Hypocalcemia** — An abnormal decrease of calcium in the blood.

E83.52 **Hypercalcemia** — An excessive amount of calcium in the blood.
Familial hypocalciuric hypercalcemia

E83.59 **Other disorders of calcium metabolism**
Idiopathic hypercalciuria

E83.8- **Other disorders of mineral metabolism**

E83.81 **Hungry bone syndrome** — A hypocalcemic condition that is characterized by the sudden removal of serum calcium from the circulation and deposition into the bones, that is most often due to parathyroidectomy for hyperparathyroidism.

E83.89 **Other disorders of mineral metabolism**

E83.9 **Disorder of mineral metabolism, unspecified**

E84- **Cystic fibrosis** — An inherited disease of infants and children of the exocrine glands, marked by chronic pulmonary disease, frequent lung infections with mucous, pancreas and gastrointestinal dysfucntion, and poor growth in children.
Includes: **Mucoviscidosis**
Code also exocrine pancreatic insufficiency (K86.81)

MCC **E84.0** **Cystic fibrosis with <u>pulmonary</u> manifestations** — A form affecting the respiratory system with chronic obstructive pulmonary disease, frequent lung infections, and/or respiratory failure.
Use additional code to identify any infectious organism present, such as:
Pseudomonas (B96.5)

E84.1- **Cystic fibrosis with <u>intestinal</u> manifestations** — A form affecting the gastrointestinal system with malabsorption, pancreatic insufficiency, and/or organ involvement.

MCC **E84.11** **Meconium ileus in cystic fibrosis** — [Age/0] – An obstruction of the ileum in the newborn due to blocking of the intestine with thick meconium.
Excludes 1: *meconium ileus not due to cystic fibrosis (P76.0)*

CC **E84.19** **Cystic fibrosis with other intestinal manifestations**
Distal intestinal obstruction syndrome

CC **E84.8** **Cystic fibrosis with other manifestations**

CC **E84.9** **Cystic fibrosis, unspecified**

E85- **Amyloidosis** — A metabolic disorder marked by the deposition of an abnormal protein (amyloid - inappropriately folded proteins) in organs and tissues in amounts sufficient to impair normal function.
Excludes 1: *Alzheimer's disease (G30.0-)*

CC **E85.0** **Non-neuropathic heredofamilial amyloidosis** — A hereditary form characterized by regular attacks of inflammation in the lining of the abdominal cavity, chest cavity, skin or joints, along with recurrent high fevers.
Hereditary amyloid nephropathy

CC **E85.1** **Neuropathic heredofamilial amyloidosis** — A hereditary form characterized by paresthesias, sharp pains, and diminished sensitivity to pain.
AHA 12:4Q:p99 – Neuropathic heredofamilial amyloidosis
Amyloid polyneuropathy (Portuguese)

CC **E85.2** **Heredofamilial amyloidosis, unspecified**

CC **E85.3** **Secondary systemic amyloidosis**
Hemodialysis-associated amyloidosis

CC **E85.4** **Organ-limited amyloidosis**
Localized amyloidosis

CC **E85.8** **Other amyloidosis**

CC **E85.9** **Amyloidosis, unspecified**

E86- **Volume depletion** — Abnormally decreased body fluid levels.
Use additional code(s) for any associated disorders of electrolyte and acid-base balance (E87.-)
Excludes 1: *dehydration of newborn (P74.1)*
hypovolemic shock NOS (R57.1)
postprocedural hypovolemic shock (T81.19)
traumatic hypovolemic shock (T79.4)

E86.0 **Dehydration** — The abnormal depletion of the total body water level that is necessary for normal cellular function.
AHA 14:1Q:p7 – Dehydration with hypernatremia/hyponatremia

E86.1 **Hypovolemia** — The abnormal depletion of the blood volume, especially the volume of blood plasma.
Depletion of volume of plasma

E86.9 **Volume depletion, unspecified**

E87- **Other disorders of fluid, electrolyte and acid-base balance**
Excludes 1: *diabetes insipidus (E23.2)*
electrolyte imbalance associated with hyperemesis gravidarum (O21.1)
electrolyte imbalance following ectopic or molar pregnancy (O08.5)
familial periodic paralysis (G72.3)

CC **E87.0** **Hyperosmolality and hypernatremia** — An abnormally increased osmolar/sodium concentration.
AHA 14:1Q:p7 – Dehydration with hypernatremia
Sodium [Na] excess — An abnormally high sodium level in the blood.
Sodium [Na] overload — An abnormally high sodium level in the blood.

CC **E87.1** **Hypo-osmolality and hyponatremia** — An abnormally decreased osmolar/sodium concentration.
AHA 14:1Q:p7 – Dehydration with hyponatremia
Sodium [Na] deficiency — An abnormally low sodium level in the blood.
Excludes 1: *syndrome of inappropriate secretion of antidiuretic hormone (E22.2)*

CC **E87.2** **Acidosis** — The condition of excessive acidity of body fluids, due to the accumulation of acids, or the reduction of base concentration.
Acidosis NOS
Lactic acidosis — A form caused by excessive lactic acid in the body fluids.
Metabolic acidosis — A form resulting from acid increase other than carbonic acid.
Respiratory acidosis — A form resulting from the excess retention of carbon dioxide in the body.
Excludes 1: *diabetic acidosis — see categories E08-E10, E13 with ketoacidosis*

CC **E87.3** **Alkalosis** — The condition of excessive alkalinity (base) of body fluids, due to the accumulation of alkalies or the reduction of acids.
Alkalosis NOS
Metabolic alkalosis — A form resulting from the loss of noncarbonic acids, often from excessive vomiting.
Respiratory alkalosis — A form resulting from the excess loss of carbon dioxide in the body, often from hyperventilation.

CC **E87.4** **Mixed disorder of acid-base balance**

E87.5 **Hyperkalemia** — The abnormally increased potassium level in the blood.
Potassium [K] excess
Potassium [K] overload

E87.6 **Hypokalemia** — The abnormally decreased potassium level in the blood.
Potassium [K] deficiency

E87.7- **Fluid overload** — Abnormally increased body fluid levels.
Excludes 1: *edema NOS (R60.9)*
fluid retention (R60.9)

E87.70 **Fluid overload, unspecified**

E87.71 **Transfusion associated circulatory overload** — The condition of increased body fluid levels due to recent transfusion of blood and/or blood components that is characterized by acute respiratory distress, increased blood pressure, and a positive fluid balance.
Fluid overload due to transfusion (blood) (blood components)
TACO

E87.79 **Other fluid overload**

E87.8 **Other disorders of electrolyte and fluid balance, not elsewhere classified**
Electrolyte imbalance NOS
Hyperchloremia
Hypochloremia

E
8
3
-
E
8
7

E88-   Other and unspecified metabolic disorders
Use additional codes for associated conditions
Excludes 1:   histiocytosis X (chronic) (C96.6)

E88.0-   Disorders of plasma-protein metabolism, not elsewhere classified
Excludes 1:   disorder of lipoprotein metabolism (E78.-)
monoclonal gammopathy (of undetermined significance) (D47.2)
polyclonal hypergammaglobulinemia (D89.0)
Waldenström macroglobulinemia (C88.0)

E88.01   Alpha-1-antitrypsin deficiency — An inherited plasma protein disorder resulting in liver and lung damage.
AAT deficiency

E88.09   Other disorders of plasma-protein metabolism, not elsewhere classified
Bisalbuminemia

E88.1   Lipodystrophy, not elsewhere classified
Lipodystrophy NOS
Excludes 1:   Whipple's disease (K90.81)

E88.2   Lipomatosis, not elsewhere classified
Lipomatosis NOS
Lipomatosis (Check) dolorosa [Dercum]

ᴹᶜᶜ **E88.3   Tumor lysis syndrome** — A group of metabolic conditions that are caused by the byproducts of tumor necrosis and are characterized by hyperkalemia, hyperphosphatemia, hyperuricemia, and hypocalcemia and can lead to acute renal failure.
Tumor lysis syndrome (spontaneous)
Tumor lysis syndrome following antineoplastic drug chemotherapy
Use additional code for adverse effect, if applicable, to identify drug (T45.1X5-)

E88.4-   Mitochondrial metabolism disorders — Inherited conditions resulting from the disturbances/dysfunction of mitochondrial DNA.
Excludes 1:   disorders of pyruvate metabolism (E74.4)
Kearns-Sayre syndrome (H49.81)
Leber's disease (H47.22)
Leigh's encephalopathy (G31.82)
Mitochondrial myopathy, NEC (G71.3)
Reye's syndrome (G93.7)

ᴄᴄ **E88.40   Mitochondrial metabolism disorder, unspecified**

ᴄᴄ **E88.41   MELAS syndrome** — A form characterized by migraine-like attacks, encephalopathy, myopathy, and strokes.
Mitochondrial myopathy, encephalopathy, lactic acidosis and stroke-like episodes

ᴄᴄ **E88.42   MERRF syndrome** — A form characterized by seizure disorder, myoclonus, progressive ataxia, and spasticity, with muscle biopsies that reveal ragged red fibers.
Myoclonic epilepsy associated with ragged-red fibers
Code also progressive myoclonic epilepsy (G40.3-)

ᴄᴄ **E88.49   Other mitochondrial metabolism disorders**

E88.8-   Other specified metabolic disorders

E88.81   Metabolic syndrome — A disorder of energy utilization and storage.
Dysmetabolic syndrome X
Use additional codes for associated manifestations, such as:
Obesity (E66.-)

E88.89   Other specified metabolic disorders
Launois-Bensaude adenolipomatosis
Excludes 1:   adult pulmonary Langerhans cell histiocytosis (J84.82)

E88.9   Metabolic disorder, unspecified

Postprocedural endocrine and metabolic complications and disorders, not elsewhere classified (E89)

E89-   Postprocedural endocrine and metabolic complications and disorders, not elsewhere classified
Excludes ❷: intraoperative complications of endocrine system organ or structure (E36.0-, E36.1-, E36.8)

E89.0   Postprocedural hypothyroidism
Postirradiation hypothyroidism
Postsurgical hypothyroidism

ᴄᴄ **E89.1   Postprocedural hypoinsulinemia**
Postpancreatectomy hyperglycemia
Postsurgical hypoinsulinemia
Use additional code, if applicable, to identify:
Acquired absence of pancreas (Z90.41-)
Diabetes mellitus (postpancreatectomy) (postprocedural) (E13.-)
Insulin use (Z79.4)
Excludes 1:   transient postprocedural hyperglycemia (R73.9)
transient postprocedural hypoglycemia (E16.2)

E89.2   Postprocedural hypoparathyroidism
Parathyroprival tetany

E89.3   Postprocedural hypopituitarism
Postirradiation hypopituitarism

E89.4-   Postprocedural ovarian failure

E89.40   Asymptomatic postprocedural ovarian failure — [♀]
Postprocedural ovarian failure NOS

E89.41   Symptomatic postprocedural ovarian failure — [♀]
Symptoms such as flushing, sleeplessness, headache, lack of concentration, associated with postprocedural menopause

E89.5   Postprocedural testicular hypofunction — [♂]

ᴄᴄ **E89.6   Postprocedural adrenocortical (-medullary) hypofunction**

E89.8-   Other postprocedural endocrine and metabolic complications and disorders

E89.81-   Postprocedural hemorrhage of an endocrine system organ or structure following a procedure

ᴄᴄ **E89.810   Postprocedural hemorrhage of an endocrine system organ or structure following an endocrine system procedure**

ᴄᴄ **E89.811   Postprocedural hemorrhage of an endocrine system organ or structure following other procedure**

E89.82-   Postprocedural hematoma and seroma of an endocrine system organ or structure

ᴄᴄ **E89.820   Postprocedural hematoma of an endocrine system organ or structure following an endocrine system procedure**

ᴄᴄ **E89.821   Postprocedural hematoma of an endocrine system organ or structure following other procedure**

ᴄᴄ **E89.822   Postprocedural seroma of an endocrine system organ or structure following an endocrine system procedure**

ᴄᴄ **E89.823   Postprocedural seroma of an endocrine system organ or structure following other procedure**

ᴄᴄ **E89.89   Other postprocedural endocrine and metabolic complications and disorders**
Use additional code, if applicable, to further specify disorder

E 8 8 – E 8 9

Chapter – 5 Mental, behavioral and neurodevelopmental disorders (F01-F99)

Includes: Disorders of psychological development
Excludes ❷: symptoms, signs and abnormal clinical laboratory findings, not elsewhere classified (R00-R99)

This chapter contains the following blocks:

F01-F09	Mental disorders due to known physiological conditions
F10-F19	Mental and behavioral disorders due to psychoactive substance use
F20-F29	Schizophrenia, schizotypal, delusional, and other non-mood psychotic disorders
F30-F39	Mood [affective] disorders
F40-F48	Anxiety, dissociative, stress-related, somatoform and other nonpsychotic mental disorders
F50-F59	Behavioral syndromes associated with physiological disturbances and physical factors
F60-F69	Disorders of adult personality and behavior
F70-F79	Intellectual disabilities
F80-F89	Pervasive and specific developmental disorders
F90-F98	Behavioral and emotional disorders with onset usually occurring in childhood and adolescence
F99	Unspecified mental disorder

Chapter-Specific Coding Guidelines

C. Chapter-Specific Coding Guidelines
In addition to general coding guidelines, there are guidelines for specific diagnoses and/or conditions in the classification. Unless otherwise indicated, these guidelines apply to all health care settings. Please refer to Section II for guidelines on the selection of principal diagnosis.

5. Chapter 5: Mental and Behavioral Disorders (F01 – F99)

a. Pain disorders related to psychological factors
Assign code F45.41, for pain that is exclusively related to psychological disorders. As indicated by the Excludes1 note under category G89, a code from category G89 should not be assigned with code F45.41.

Code F45.42, Pain disorders with related psychological factors, should be used should be used with a code from category G89, Pain, not elsewhere classified, if there is documentation of a psychological component for a patient with acute or chronic pain.

See Section I.C.6. Pain.

b. Mental and behavioral disorders due to psychoactive substance use

1) In Remission
Selection of codes for "in remission" for categories F10-F19, Mental and behavioral disorders due to psychoactive substance use (categories F10-F19 with -.21) requires the provider's clinical judgment. The appropriate codes for "in remission" are assigned only on the basis of provider documentation (as defined in the Official Guidelines for Coding and Reporting).

2) Psychoactive Substance Use, Abuse And Dependence
When the provider documentation refers to use, abuse and dependence of the same substance (e.g. alcohol, opioid, cannabis, etc.), only one code should be assigned to identify the pattern of use based on the following hierarchy:
- If both use and abuse are documented, assign only the code for abuse
- If both abuse and dependence are documented, assign only the code for dependence
- If use, abuse and dependence are all documented, assign only the code for dependence
- If both use and dependence are documented, assign only the code for dependence

3) Psychoactive Substance Use
As with all other diagnoses, the codes for psychoactive substance use (F10.9-, F11.9-, F12.9-, F13.9-, F14.9-, F15.9-, F16.9-) should only be assigned based on provider documentation and when they meet the definition of a reportable diagnosis (see Section III, Reporting Additional Diagnoses). The codes are to be used only when the psychoactive substance use is associated with a mental or behavioral disorder, and such a relationship is documented by the provider.

Mental disorders due to known physiological conditions (F01-F09)

Note: This block comprises a range of mental disorders grouped together on the basis of their having in common a demonstrable etiology in cerebral disease, brain injury, or other insult leading to cerebral dysfunction. The dysfunction may be primary, as in diseases, injuries, and insults that affect the brain directly and selectively; or secondary, as in systemic diseases and disorders that attack the brain only as one of the multiple organs or systems of the body that are involved.

F01-   Vascular dementia
Vascular dementia as a result of infarction of the brain due to vascular disease, including hypertensive cerebrovascular disease
Includes: Arteriosclerotic dementia
Code first the underlying physiological condition or sequelae of cerebrovascular disease

F01.5-   Vascular dementia

F01.50   Vascular dementia **without** behavioral disturbance —
[Age/15-124]
Major neurocognitive disorder without behavioral disturbance

cc F01.51   Vascular dementia **with** behavioral disturbance —
[Age/15-124]
Major neurocognitive disorder due to vascular disease, with behavioral disturbance
Major neurocognitive disorder with aggressive behavior
Major neurocognitive disorder with combative behavior
Major neurocognitive disorder with violent behavior
Vascular dementia with aggressive behavior
Vascular dementia with combative behavior
Vascular dementia with violent behavior
Use additional code, if applicable, to identify wandering in vasuclar dementia (Z91.83)

F02-   Dementia in other diseases classified elsewhere
Includes: Major neurocognitive disorder in other diseases classified elsewhere
Code first the underlying physiological condition, such as:
Alzheimer's (G30.-)
Cerebral lipidosis (E75.4)
Creutzfeldt-Jakob disease (A81.0-)
Dementia with Lewy bodies (G31.83)
Dementia with Parkinsonism (G31.83)
Epilepsy and recurrent seizures (G40.-)
Frontotemporal dementia (G31.09)
Hepatolenticular degeneration (E83.0)
Human immunodeficiency virus [HIV] disease (B20)
Huntington's disease (G10)
Hypercalcemia (E83.52)
Hypothyroidism, acquired (E00-E03.-)
Intoxications (T36-T65)
Jakob-Creutzfeldt disease (A81.0-)
Multiple sclerosis (G35)
Neurosyphilis (A52.17)
Niacin deficiency [pellagra] (E52)
Parkinson's disease (G20)
Pick's disease (G31.01)
Polyarteritis nodosa (M30.0)
Prion disease (A81.9)
Systemic lupus erythematosus (M32.-)
Traumatic brain injury (S06.-)
Trypanosomiasis (B56.-, B57.-)
Vitamin B deficiency (E53.8)
Excludes ❷: dementia in alcohol and psychoactive substance disorders (F10-F19, with .17, .27, .97)
vascular dementia (F01.5-)

F02.8-   Dementia in other diseases classified elsewhere

F02.80   Dementia in other diseases classified elsewhere **without** behavioral disturbance — [Not Allowed as PDX]
Dementia in other diseases classified elsewhere NOS
Major neurocognitive disorder in other diseases classified elsewhere

cc F02.81   Dementia in other diseases classified elsewhere **with** behavioral disturbance — [Not Allowed as PDX]
Dementia in other diseases classified elsewhere with aggressive behavior
Dementia in other diseases classified elsewhere with combative behavior
Dementia in other diseases classified elsewhere with violent behavior
Major neurocognitive disorder in other diseases classified elsewhere with aggressive behavior
Major neurocognitive disorder in other diseases classified elsewhere with combative behavior
Major neurocognitive disorder in other diseases classified elsewhere with violent behavior
Use additional code, if applicable, to identify wandering in dementia in conditions classified elsewhere (Z91.83)

F01 F02

F03- <u>Unspecified</u> <u>dementia</u>
Presenile dementia NOS
Presenile psychosis NOS
Primary degenerative dementia NOS
Senile dementia NOS
Senile dementia depressed or paranoid type
Senile psychosis NOS
Excludes 1: *senility NOS (R41.81)*
Excludes ❷: *mild memory disturbance due to known physiological condition (F06.8)*
senile dementia with delirium or acute confusional state (F05)

F03.9- Unspecified dementia
F03.90 Unspecified dementia without behavioral disturbance — [Age/15-124]
Dementia NOS

CC **F03.91** Unspecified dementia with behavioral disturbance — [Age/15-124]
Unspecified dementia with aggressive behavior
Unspecified dementia with combative behavior
Unspecified dementia with violent behavior
Use additional code, if applicable, to identify wandering in unspecified dementia (Z91.83)

F04 <u>Amnestic disorder due to known physiological condition</u>
Korsakov's psychosis or syndrome, nonalcoholic
Code first the underlying physiological condition
Excludes 1: *amnesia NOS (R41.3)*
anterograde amnesia (R41.1)
dissociative amnesia (F44.0)
retrograde amnesia (R41.2)
Excludes ❷: *alcohol-induced or unspecified Korsakov's syndrome (F10.26, F10.96)*
Korsakov's syndrome induced by other psychoactive substances (F13.26, F13.96, F19.16, F19.26, F19.96)

F05 <u>Delirium due to known physiological condition</u>
CC
Acute or subacute brain syndrome
Acute or subacute confusional state (nonalcoholic)
Acute or subacute infective psychosis
Acute or subacute organic reaction
Acute or subacute psycho-organic syndrome
Delirium of mixed etiology
Delirium superimposed on dementia
Sundowning
Code first the underlying physiological condition
Excludes 1: *delirium NOS (R41.0)*
Excludes ❷: *delirium tremens alcohol-induced or unspecified (F10.231, F10.921)*

F06- <u>Other mental disorders due to known physiological condition</u>
Includes: Mental disorders due to endocrine disorder
Mental disorders due to exogenous hormone
Mental disorders due to exogenous toxic substance
Mental disorders due to primary cerebral disease
Mental disorders due to somatic illness
Mental disorders due to systemic disease affecting the brain
Code first the underlying physiological condition
Excludes 1: *unspecified dementia (F03)*
Excludes ❷: *delirium due to known physiological condition (F05)*
dementia as classified in F01-F02
other mental disorders associated with alcohol and other psychoactive substances (F10-F19)

CC **F06.0** <u>Psychotic</u> disorder with <u>hallucinations</u> due to known physiological condition
Organic hallucinatory state (nonalcoholic)
Excludes ❷: *hallucinations and perceptual disturbance induced by alcohol and other psychoactive substances (F10-F19 with .151, .251, .951)*
schizophrenia (F20.-)

F06.1 <u>Catatonic</u> disorder due to known physiological condition
Catatonia associated with another mental disorder
Catatonia NOS
Excludes 1: *catatonic stupor (R40.1)*
stupor NOS (R40.1)
Excludes ❷: *catatonic schizophrenia (F20.2)*
dissociative stupor (F44.2)

CC **F06.2** <u>Psychotic</u> disorder with <u>delusions</u> due to known physiological condition
Paranoid and paranoid-hallucinatory organic states
Schizophrenia-like psychosis in epilepsy
Excludes ❷: *alcohol and drug-induced psychotic disorder (F10-F19 with .150, .250, .950)*
brief psychotic disorder (F23)
delusional disorder (F22)
schizophrenia (F20.-)

F06.3- <u>Mood disorder due to known physiological condition</u>
Excludes ❷: *mood disorders due to alcohol and other psychoactive substances (F10-F19 with .14, .24, .94)*
mood disorders, not due to known physiological condition or unspecified (F30-F39)

F06.30 Mood disorder due to known physiological condition, unspecified

F06.31 Mood disorder due to known physiological condition with <u>depressive features</u>

F06.32 Mood disorder due to known physiological condition with <u>major depressive-like</u> episode

F06.33 Mood disorder due to known physiological condition with <u>manic</u> features

F06.34 Mood disorder due to known physiological condition with <u>mixed</u> features

F06.4 <u>Anxiety</u> disorder <u>due to known physiological condition</u>
Excludes ❷: *anxiety disorders due to alcohol and other psychoactive substances (F10-F19 with .180, .280, .980)*
anxiety disorders, not due to known physiological condition or unspecified (F40.-, F41.-)

F06.8 <u>Other specified</u> mental disorders <u>due to known physiological condition</u>
Epileptic psychosis NOS
Organic dissociative disorder
Organic emotionally labile [asthenic] disorder

F07- <u>Personality and behavioral</u> disorders <u>due to known physiological condition</u>
Code first the underlying physiological condition

F07.0 <u>Personality change</u> due to known physiological condition
Frontal lobe syndrome
Limbic epilepsy personality syndrome
Lobotomy syndrome
Organic personality disorder
Organic pseudopsychopathic personality
Organic pseudoretarded personality
Postleucotomy syndrome
Code first underlying physiological condition
Excludes 1: *mild cognitive impairment (G31.84)*
postconcussional syndrome (F07.81)
postencephalitic syndrome (F07.89)
signs and symptoms involving emotional state (R45.-)
Excludes ❷: *specific personality disorder (F60.-)*

F07.8- Other personality and behavioral disorders due to known physiological condition

F07.81 <u>Postconcussional syndrome</u>
Postcontusional syndrome (encephalopathy)
Post-traumatic brain syndrome, nonpsychotic
Use additional code to identify associated post-traumatic headache, if applicable (G44.3-)
Excludes 1: *current concussion (brain) (S06.0-)*
postencephalitic syndrome (F07.89)

F07.89 Other personality and behavioral disorders due to known physiological condition
Postencephalitic syndrome
Right hemispheric organic affective disorder

F07.9 Unspecified personality and behavioral disorder due to known physiological condition
Organic psychosyndrome

F09 <u>Unspecified</u> mental disorder <u>due to known physiological condition</u>
Mental disorder NOS due to known physiological condition
Organic brain syndrome NOS
Organic mental disorder NOS
Organic psychosis NOS
Symptomatic psychosis NOS
Code first the underlying physiological condition
Excludes 1: *psychosis NOS (F29)*

F03-F09 (side tab)

Mental and behavioral disorders due to psychoactive substance use (F10-F19)

F10- **Alcohol related disorders**
Use additional code for blood alcohol level, if applicable (Y90.-)

F10.1- **Alcohol abuse**
Excludes 1: *alcohol dependence (F10.2-)*
alcohol use, unspecified (F10.9-)

F10.10 **Alcohol abuse, uncomplicated**
Alcohol use disorder, mild

F10.12- **Alcohol abuse with intoxication**

F10.120 Alcohol abuse with intoxication, uncomplicated

CC **F10.121** Alcohol abuse with intoxication delirium

F10.129 Alcohol abuse with intoxication, unspecified

CC **F10.14** **Alcohol abuse with alcohol-induced mood disorder**
Alcohol use disorder, mild, with alcohol-induced bipolar or related disorder
Alcohol use disorder, mild, with alcohol-induced depressive disorder

F10.15- **Alcohol abuse with alcohol-induced psychotic disorder**

F10.150 Alcohol abuse with alcohol-induced psychotic disorder with delusions

CC **F10.151** Alcohol abuse with alcohol-induced psychotic disorder with hallucinations

CC **F10.159** Alcohol abuse with alcohol-induced psychotic disorder, unspecified

F10.18- **Alcohol abuse with other alcohol-induced disorders**

CC **F10.180** Alcohol abuse with alcohol-induced anxiety disorder

CC **F10.181** Alcohol abuse with alcohol-induced sexual dysfunction

F10.182 Alcohol abuse with alcohol-induced sleep disorder

CC **F10.188** Alcohol abuse with other alcohol-induced disorder

CC **F10.19** Alcohol abuse with unspecified alcohol-induced disorder

F10.2- **Alcohol dependence**
Excludes 1: *alcohol abuse (F10.1-)*
alcohol use, unspecified (F10.9-)
Excludes ❷: *toxic effect of alcohol (T51.0-)*

F10.20 **Alcohol dependence, uncomplicated**
Alcohol use disorder, moderate
Alcohol use disorder, severe

F10.21 **Alcohol dependence, in remission**

F10.22- **Alcohol dependence with intoxication**
Acute drunkenness (in alcoholism)
Excludes ❷: *alcohol dependence with withdrawal (F10.23-)*

F10.220 **Alcohol dependence with intoxication, uncomplicated**

CC **F10.221** Alcohol dependence with intoxication delirium

F10.229 Alcohol dependence with intoxication, unspecified

F10.23- **Alcohol dependence with withdrawal**
AHA 15:2Q:p15 – Alcohol withdrawal with alcohol abuse
Excludes ❷: *alcohol dependence with intoxication (F10.22-)*

CC **F10.230** **Alcohol dependence with withdrawal, uncomplicated**

CC **F10.231** Alcohol dependence with withdrawal delirium

CC **F10.232** Alcohol dependence with withdrawal with perceptual disturbance

CC **F10.239** Alcohol dependence with withdrawal, unspecified

CC **F10.24** **Alcohol dependence with alcohol-induced mood disorder**
Alcohol use disorder, moderate, with alcohol-induced bipolar or related disorder
Alcohol use disorder, moderate, with alcohol-induced depressive disorder
Alcohol use disorder, severe, with alcohol-induced bipolar or related disorder
Alcohol use disorder, severe, with alcohol-induced depressive disorder

F10.25- **Alcohol dependence with alcohol-induced psychotic disorder**

F10.250 Alcohol dependence with alcohol-induced psychotic disorder with delusions

CC **F10.251** Alcohol dependence with alcohol-induced psychotic disorder with hallucinations

CC **F10.259** Alcohol dependence with alcohol-induced psychotic disorder, unspecified

F10.26 **Alcohol dependence with alcohol-induced persisting amnestic disorder**
Alcohol use disorder, moderate, with alcohol-induced major neurocognitive disorder, amnestic-confabulatory type
Alcohol use disorder, severe, with alcohol-induced major neurocognitive disorder, amnestic-confabulatory type

CC **F10.27** **Alcohol dependence with alcohol-induced persisting dementia**
Alcohol use disorder, moderate, with alcohol-induced major neurocognitive disorder, nonamnestic-confabulatory type
Alcohol use disorder, severe, with alcohol-induced major neurocognitive disorder, nonamnestic-confabulatory type

F10.28- **Alcohol dependence with other alcohol-induced disorders**

CC **F10.280** Alcohol dependence with alcohol-induced anxiety disorder

CC **F10.281** Alcohol dependence with alcohol-induced sexual dysfunction

F10.282 Alcohol dependence with alcohol-induced sleep disorder

CC **F10.288** Alcohol dependence with other alcohol-induced disorder
Alcohol use disorder, moderate, with alcohol-induced mild neurocognitive disorder
Alcohol use disorder, severe, with alcohol-induced mild neurocognitive disorder

CC **F10.29** Alcohol dependence with unspecified alcohol-induced disorder

F10.9- **Alcohol use, unspecified**
Excludes 1: *alcohol abuse (F10.1-)*
alcohol dependence (F10.2-)

F10.92- **Alcohol use, unspecified with intoxication**

F10.920 Alcohol use, unspecified with intoxication, uncomplicated

CC **F10.921** Alcohol use, unspecified with intoxication delirium

F10.929 Alcohol use, unspecified with intoxication, unspecified

CC **F10.94** **Alcohol use, unspecified with alcohol-induced mood disorder**
Alcohol-induced bipolar or related disorder, without use disorder
Alcohol-induced depressive disorder, without use disorder

F10.95- **Alcohol use, unspecified with alcohol-induced psychotic disorder**

F10.950 Alcohol use, unspecified with alcohol-induced psychotic disorder with delusions

CC **F10.951** Alcohol use, unspecified with alcohol-induced psychotic disorder with hallucinations

CC **F10.959** Alcohol use, unspecified with alcohol-induced psychotic disorder, unspecified
Alcohol-induced psychotic disorder, without use disorder

F10.96 **Alcohol use, unspecified with alcohol-induced persisting amnestic disorder**
Alcohol-induced major neurocognitive disorder, amnestic-confabulatory type, without use disorder

F10.97 **Alcohol use, unspecified with alcohol-induced persisting dementia**
Alcohol-induced major neurocognitive disorder, nonamnestic-confabulatory type, without use disorder

F10.98- **Alcohol use, unspecified with other alcohol-induced disorders**

CC **F10.980** Alcohol use, unspecified with alcohol-induced anxiety disorder
Alcohol-induced anxiety disorder, without use disorder

CC **F10.981** Alcohol use, unspecified with alcohol-induced sexual dysfunction
Alcohol-induced sexual dysfunction, without use disorder

F10-F10

cc **F10.982** Alcohol use, unspecified with alcohol-induced <u>sleep</u> disorder
Alcohol-induced sleep disorder, without use disorder

cc **F10.988** Alcohol use, unspecified with other alcohol-induced disorder
Alcohol-induced mild neurocognitive disorder, without use disorder

cc **F10.99** Alcohol use, unspecified with unspecified alcohol-induced disorder

F11- <u>Opioid related disorders</u>

F11.1- Opioid abuse
Excludes 1: *opioid dependence (F11.2-)*
opioid use, unspecified (F11.9-)

F11.10 Opioid abuse, <u>uncomplicated</u>
Opioid use disorder, mild

F11.12- Opioid abuse <u>with intoxication</u>

F11.120 Opioid abuse with intoxication, <u>uncomplicated</u>

cc **F11.121** Opioid abuse with intoxication <u>delirium</u>

F11.122 Opioid abuse with intoxication <u>with perceptual disturbance</u>

F11.129 Opioid abuse with intoxication, <u>unspecified</u>

F11.14 Opioid abuse <u>with</u> opioid-induced <u>mood</u> disorder
Opioid use disorder, mild, with opioid-induced depressive disorder

F11.15- Opioid abuse <u>with</u> opioid-induced <u>psychotic</u> disorder

cc **F11.150** Opioid abuse with opioid-induced psychotic disorder <u>with delusions</u>

cc **F11.151** Opioid abuse with opioid-induced psychotic disorder <u>with hallucinations</u>

F11.159 Opioid abuse with opioid-induced psychotic disorder, unspecified

F11.18- Opioid abuse <u>with</u> <u>other</u> opioid-induced disorder

F11.181 Opioid abuse with opioid-induced <u>sexual dysfunction</u>

F11.182 Opioid abuse with opioid-induced <u>sleep</u> disorder

F11.188 Opioid abuse with other opioid-induced disorder

F11.19 Opioid abuse with unspecified opioid-induced disorder

F11.2- <u>Opioid dependence</u>
Excludes 1: *opioid abuse (F11.1-)*
opioid use, unspecified (F11.9-)
Excludes ❷: *opioid poisoning (T40.0-T40.2-)*

cc **F11.20** Opioid dependence, <u>uncomplicated</u>
Opioid use disorder, moderate
Opioid use disorder, severe

F11.21 Opioid dependence, <u>in remission</u>

F11.22- Opioid dependence <u>with intoxication</u>
Excludes 1: *opioid dependence with withdrawal (F11.23)*

F11.220 Opioid dependence with intoxication, <u>uncomplicated</u>

cc **F11.221** Opioid dependence with intoxication <u>delirium</u>

cc **F11.222** Opioid dependence with intoxication <u>with perceptual disturbance</u>

F11.229 Opioid dependence with intoxication, <u>unspecified</u>

cc **F11.23** Opioid dependence with withdrawal
Excludes 1: *opioid dependence with intoxication (F11.22-)*

F11.24 Opioid dependence <u>with</u> opioid-induced <u>mood</u> disorder
Opioid use disorder, moderate, with opioid-induced depressive disorder

F11.25- Opioid dependence <u>with</u> opioid-induced <u>psychotic</u> disorder

cc **F11.250** Opioid dependence with opioid-induced psychotic disorder <u>with delusions</u>

cc **F11.251** Opioid dependence with opioid-induced psychotic disorder <u>with hallucinations</u>

cc **F11.259** Opioid dependence with opioid-induced psychotic disorder, unspecified

F11.28- Opioid dependence <u>with</u> <u>other</u> opioid-induced disorder

cc **F11.281** Opioid dependence <u>with</u> opioid-induced <u>sexual dysfunction</u>

cc **F11.282** Opioid dependence with opioid-induced <u>sleep</u> disorder

cc **F11.288** Opioid dependence with other opioid-induced disorder

F11.29 Opioid dependence with unspecified opioid-induced disorder

F11.9- <u>Opioid use, unspecified</u>
Excludes 1: *opioid abuse (F11.1-)*
opioid dependence (F11.2-)

F11.90 Opioid use, unspecified, <u>uncomplicated</u>

F11.92- Opioid use, unspecified <u>with intoxication</u>
Excludes 1: *opioid use, unspecified with withdrawal (F11.93)*

F11.920 Opioid use, unspecified with intoxication, <u>uncomplicated</u>

cc **F11.921** Opioid use, unspecified with intoxication <u>delirium</u>
Opioid-induced delirium

F11.922 Opioid use, unspecified with intoxication <u>with perceptual disturbance</u>

F11.929 Opioid use, unspecified with intoxication, unspecified

cc **F11.93** Opioid use, unspecified <u>with withdrawal</u>
Excludes 1: *opioid use, unspecified with intoxication (F11.92-)*

F11.94 Opioid use, unspecified <u>with</u> opioid-induced <u>mood</u> disorder
Opioid-induced depressive disorder, without use disorder

F11.95- Opioid use, unspecified <u>with</u> opioid-induced <u>psychotic</u> disorder

cc **F11.950** Opioid use, unspecified with opioid-induced psychotic disorder <u>with delusions</u>

cc **F11.951** Opioid use, unspecified with opioid-induced psychotic disorder <u>with hallucinations</u>

F11.959 Opioid use, unspecified with opioid-induced psychotic disorder, unspecified

F11.98- Opioid use, unspecified <u>with</u> <u>other</u> specified opioid-induced disorder

F11.981 Opioid use, unspecified <u>with</u> opioid-induced <u>sexual dysfunction</u>
Opioid-induced sexual dysfunction, without use disorder

F11.982 Opioid use, unspecified <u>with</u> opioid-induced <u>sleep</u> disorder
Opioid-induced sleep disorder, without use disorder

F11.988 Opioid use, unspecified <u>with</u> <u>other</u> opioid-induced disorder
Opioid-induced anxiety disorder, without use disorder

F11.99 Opioid use, unspecified with unspecified opioid-induced disorder

F12- <u>Cannabis related disorders</u>
Includes: Marijuana

F12.1- Cannabis <u>abuse</u>
Excludes 1: *cannabis dependence (F12.2-)*
cannabis use, unspecified (F12.9-)

F12.10 Cannabis abuse, <u>uncomplicated</u>
Cannabis use disorder, mild

F12.12- Cannabis abuse <u>with intoxication</u>

F12.120 Cannabis abuse with intoxication, <u>uncomplicated</u>

cc **F12.121** Cannabis abuse with intoxication <u>delirium</u>

F12.122 Cannabis abuse with intoxication <u>with perceptual disturbance</u>

F12.129 Cannabis abuse with intoxication, <u>unspecified</u>

F12.15- Cannabis abuse <u>with psychotic</u> disorder

cc **F12.150** Cannabis abuse with psychotic disorder <u>with delusions</u>

cc **F12.151** Cannabis abuse with psychotic disorder <u>with hallucinations</u>

F12.159 Cannabis abuse with psychotic disorder, unspecified

F12.18- Cannabis abuse <u>with</u> <u>other</u> cannabis-induced disorder

F12.180 Cannabis abuse with cannabis-induced <u>anxiety</u> disorder

F10 - F12

F12.188   Cannabis abuse with other cannabis-induced disorder
Cannabis use disorder, mild, with cannabis-induced sleep disorder

F12.19   Cannabis abuse with unspecified cannabis-induced disorder

F12.2-   Cannabis <u>dependence</u>
Excludes 1:   *cannabis abuse (F12.1-)*
cannabis use, unspecified (F12.9-)
Excludes ❷: *cannabis poisoning (T40.7-)*

F12.20   Cannabis dependence, <u>uncomplicated</u>
Cannabis use disorder, moderate
Cannabis use disorder, severe

F12.21   Cannabis dependence, <u>in remission</u>

F12.22-   Cannabis dependence <u>with intoxication</u>

F12.220   Cannabis dependence with intoxication, <u>uncomplicated</u>

cc**F12.221**   Cannabis dependence with intoxication <u>delirium</u>

F12.222   Cannabis dependence with intoxication <u>with perceptual disturbance</u>

F12.229   Cannabis dependence with intoxication, unspecified

F12.25-   Cannabis dependence <u>with psychotic</u> disorder

cc**F12.250**   Cannabis dependence with psychotic disorder <u>with delusions</u>

cc**F12.251**   Cannabis dependence with psychotic disorder <u>with hallucinations</u>

F12.259   Cannabis dependence with psychotic disorder, unspecified

F12.28-   Cannabis dependence <u>with other</u> cannabis-induced disorder

F12.280   Cannabis dependence with cannabis-induced <u>anxiety</u> disorder

F12.288   Cannabis dependence with other cannabis-induced disorder
Cannabis use disorder, moderate, with cannabis-induced sleep disorder
Cannabis use disorder, severe, with cannabis-induced sleep disorder
Cannabis withdrawal

F12.29   Cannabis dependence with unspecified cannabis-induced disorder

F12.9-   <u>Cannabis use, unspecified</u>
Excludes 1:   *cannabis abuse (F12.1-)*
cannabis dependence (F12.2-)

F12.90   Cannabis use, unspecified, <u>uncomplicated</u>

F12.92-   Cannabis use, unspecified <u>with intoxication</u>

F12.920   Cannabis use, unspecified with intoxication, <u>uncomplicated</u>

cc**F12.921**   Cannabis use, unspecified with intoxication <u>delirium</u>

F12.922   Cannabis use, unspecified with intoxication <u>with perceptual disturbance</u>

F12.929   Cannabis use, unspecified with intoxication, <u>unspecified</u>

F12.95-   Cannabis use, unspecified <u>with psychotic</u> disorder

cc**F12.950**   Cannabis use, unspecified with psychotic disorder <u>with delusions</u>

cc**F12.951**   Cannabis use, unspecified with psychotic disorder <u>with hallucinations</u>

F12.959   Cannabis use, unspecified with psychotic disorder, unspecified
Cannabis-induced psychotic disorder, without use disorder

F12.98-   Cannabis use, unspecified <u>with other</u> cannabis-induced disorder

F12.980   Cannabis use, unspecified with <u>anxiety</u> disorder
Cannabis-induced anxiety disorder, without use disorder

F12.988   Cannabis use, unspecified with other cannabis-induced disorder
Cannabis-induced sleep disorder, without use disorder

F12.99   Cannabis use, unspecified with unspecified cannabis-induced disorder

F13-   <u>Sedative, hypnotic, or anxiolytic related disorders</u>

F13.1-   Sedative, hypnotic or anxiolytic-related <u>abuse</u>
Excludes 1:   *sedative, hypnotic or anxiolytic-related dependence (F13.2-)*
sedative, hypnotic, or anxiolytic use, unspecified (F13.9-)

F13.10   Sedative, hypnotic or anxiolytic abuse, <u>uncomplicated</u>
Sedative, hypnotic, or anxiolytic use disorder, mild

F13.12-   Sedative, hypnotic or anxiolytic abuse <u>with intoxication</u>

F13.120   Sedative, hypnotic or anxiolytic abuse with intoxication, <u>uncomplicated</u>

cc**F13.121**   Sedative, hypnotic or anxiolytic abuse with intoxication <u>delirium</u>

F13.129   Sedative, hypnotic or anxiolytic abuse with intoxication, <u>unspecified</u>

F13.14   Sedative, hypnotic or anxiolytic abuse <u>with</u> sedative, hypnotic or anxiolytic-induced <u>mood</u> disorder
Sedative, hypnotic, or anxiolytic use disorder, mild, with sedative, hypnotic, or anxiolytic-induced bipolar or related disorder
Sedative, hypnotic, or anxiolytic use disorder, mild, with sedative, hypnotic, or anxiolytic-induced depressive disorder

F13.15-   Sedative, hypnotic or anxiolytic abuse <u>with</u> sedative, hypnotic or anxiolytic-induced <u>psychotic</u> disorder

cc**F13.150**   Sedative, hypnotic or anxiolytic abuse with sedative, hypnotic or anxiolytic-induced psychotic disorder <u>with delusions</u>

cc**F13.151**   Sedative, hypnotic or anxiolytic abuse with sedative, hypnotic or anxiolytic-induced psychotic disorder <u>with hallucinations</u>

F13.159   Sedative, hypnotic or anxiolytic abuse with sedative, hypnotic or anxiolytic-induced psychotic disorder, unspecified

F13.18-   Sedative, hypnotic or anxiolytic abuse <u>with other</u> sedative, hypnotic or anxiolytic-induced disorders

F13.180   Sedative, hypnotic or anxiolytic abuse <u>with</u> sedative, hypnotic or anxiolytic-induced <u>anxiety</u> disorder

F13.181   Sedative, hypnotic or anxiolytic abuse <u>with</u> sedative, hypnotic or anxiolytic-induced <u>sexual dysfunction</u>

F13.182   Sedative, hypnotic or anxiolytic abuse <u>with</u> sedative, hypnotic or anxiolytic-induced <u>sleep</u> disorder

F13.188   Sedative, hypnotic or anxiolytic abuse with other sedative, hypnotic or anxiolytic-induced disorder

F13.19   Sedative, hypnotic or anxiolytic abuse with unspecified sedative, hypnotic or anxiolytic-induced disorder

F13.2-   Sedative, hypnotic or anxiolytic-related <u>dependence</u>
Excludes 1:   *sedative, hypnotic or anxiolytic-related abuse (F13.1-)*
sedative, hypnotic, or anxiolytic use, unspecified (F13.9-)
Excludes ❷: *sedative, hypnotic, or anxiolytic poisoning (T42.-)*

cc**F13.20**   Sedative, hypnotic or anxiolytic dependence, <u>uncomplicated</u>

F13.21   Sedative, hypnotic or anxiolytic dependence, <u>in remission</u>

F13.22-   Sedative, hypnotic or anxiolytic dependence <u>with intoxication</u>
Excludes 1:   *sedative, hypnotic or anxiolytic dependence with withdrawal (F13.23-)*

F13.220   Sedative, hypnotic or anxiolytic dependence with intoxication, <u>uncomplicated</u>

cc**F13.221**   Sedative, hypnotic or anxiolytic dependence with intoxication <u>delirium</u>

F13.229   Sedative, hypnotic or anxiolytic dependence with intoxication, <u>unspecified</u>

F
1
2
-
F
1
3

F13.23- Sedative, hypnotic or anxiolytic dependence <u>with</u> <u>withdrawal</u>
Sedative, hypnotic, or anxiolytic use disorder, moderate
Sedative, hypnotic, or anxiolytic use disorder, severe
Excludes 1: sedative, hypnotic or anxiolytic dependence with intoxication (F13.22-)

cc **F13.230** Sedative, hypnotic or anxiolytic dependence with withdrawal, <u>uncomplicated</u>

cc **F13.231** Sedative, hypnotic or anxiolytic dependence <u>with</u> withdrawal <u>delirium</u>

cc **F13.232** Sedative, hypnotic or anxiolytic dependence <u>with</u> withdrawal <u>with perceptual disturbance</u>
Sedative, hypnotic, or anxiolytic withdrawal with perceptual disturbances

cc **F13.239** Sedative, hypnotic or anxiolytic dependence with withdrawal, unspecified
Sedative, hypnotic, or anxiolytic withdrawal without perceptual disturbances

F13.24 Sedative, hypnotic or anxiolytic dependence <u>with</u> sedative, hypnotic or anxiolytic-induced <u>mood</u> disorder
Sedative, hypnotic, or anxiolytic use disorder, moderate, with sedative, hypnotic, or anxiolytic-induced bipolar or related disorder
Sedative, hypnotic, or anxiolytic use disorder, moderate, with sedative, hypnotic, or anxiolytic-induced depressive disorder
Sedative, hypnotic, or anxiolytic use disorder, severe, with sedative, hypnotic, or anxiolytic-induced bipolar or related disorder
Sedative, hypnotic, or anxiolytic use disorder, severe, with sedative, hypnotic, or anxiolytic-induced depressive disorder

F13.25- Sedative, hypnotic or anxiolytic dependence <u>with</u> sedative, hypnotic or anxiolytic-induced <u>psychotic</u> disorder

cc **F13.250** Sedative, hypnotic or anxiolytic dependence with sedative, hypnotic or anxiolytic-induced psychotic disorder <u>with delusions</u>

cc **F13.251** Sedative, hypnotic or anxiolytic dependence with sedative, hypnotic or anxiolytic-induced psychotic disorder <u>with hallucinations</u>

cc **F13.259** Sedative, hypnotic or anxiolytic dependence with sedative, hypnotic or anxiolytic-induced psychotic disorder, <u>unspecified</u>

cc **F13.26** Sedative, hypnotic or anxiolytic dependence <u>with</u> sedative, hypnotic or anxiolytic-induced <u>persisting</u> <u>amnestic</u> disorder

cc **F13.27** Sedative, hypnotic or anxiolytic dependence <u>with</u> sedative, hypnotic or anxiolytic-induced <u>persisting</u> <u>dementia</u>
Sedative, hypnotic, or anxiolytic use disorder, moderate, with sedative, hypnotic, or anxiolytic-induced major neurocognitive disorder
Sedative, hypnotic, or anxiolytic use disorder, severe, with sedative, hypnotic, or anxiolytic-induced major neurocognitive disorder

F13.28- Sedative, hypnotic or anxiolytic dependence <u>with</u> <u>other</u> sedative, hypnotic or anxiolytic-induced disorders

cc **F13.280** Sedative, hypnotic or anxiolytic dependence <u>with</u> sedative, hypnotic or anxiolytic-induced <u>anxiety</u> disorder

cc **F13.281** Sedative, hypnotic or anxiolytic dependence <u>with</u> sedative, hypnotic or anxiolytic-induced <u>sexual</u> <u>dysfunction</u>

cc **F13.282** Sedative, hypnotic or anxiolytic dependence <u>with</u> sedative, hypnotic or anxiolytic-induced <u>sleep</u> disorder

cc **F13.288** Sedative, hypnotic or anxiolytic dependence with other sedative, hypnotic or anxiolytic-induced disorder
Sedative, hypnotic, or anxiolytic use disorder, moderate, with sedative, hypnotic, or anxiolytic-induced mild neurocognitive disorder
Sedative, hypnotic, or anxiolytic use disorder, severe, with sedative, hypnotic, or anxiolytic-induced mild neurocognitive disorder

F13.29 Sedative, hypnotic or anxiolytic dependence with unspecified sedative, hypnotic or anxiolytic-induced disorder

F13.9- <u>Sedative, hypnotic or anxiolytic-related use, unspecified</u>
Excludes 1: sedative, hypnotic or anxiolytic-related abuse (F13.1-)
sedative, hypnotic or anxiolytic-related dependence (F13.2-)

F13.90 Sedative, hypnotic, or anxiolytic use, unspecified, <u>uncomplicated</u>

F13.92- Sedative, hypnotic or anxiolytic use, unspecified <u>with</u> <u>intoxication</u>
Excludes 1: sedative, hypnotic or anxiolytic use, unspecified with withdrawal (F13.93-)

F13.920 Sedative, hypnotic or anxiolytic use, unspecified with intoxication, <u>uncomplicated</u>

cc **F13.921** Sedative, hypnotic or anxiolytic use, unspecified with intoxication <u>delirium</u>
Sedative, hypnotic, or anxiolytic-induced delirium

F13.929 Sedative, hypnotic or anxiolytic use, unspecified with intoxication, <u>unspecified</u>

F13.93- Sedative, hypnotic or anxiolytic use, unspecified <u>with</u> <u>withdrawal</u>
Excludes 1: sedative, hypnotic or anxiolytic use, unspecified with intoxication (F13.92-)

cc **F13.930** Sedative, hypnotic or anxiolytic use, unspecified with withdrawal, <u>uncomplicated</u>

cc **F13.931** Sedative, hypnotic or anxiolytic use, unspecified with withdrawal <u>delirium</u>

cc **F13.932** Sedative, hypnotic or anxiolytic use, unspecified with withdrawal <u>with perceptual disturbances</u>

cc **F13.939** Sedative, hypnotic or anxiolytic use, unspecified with withdrawal, unspecified

F13.94 Sedative, hypnotic or anxiolytic use, unspecified <u>with</u> sedative, hypnotic or anxiolytic-induced <u>mood</u> disorder
Sedative, hypnotic, or anxiolytic-induced bipolar or related disorder, without use disorder
Sedative, hypnotic, or anxiolytic-induced depressive disorder, without use disorder

F13.95- Sedative, hypnotic or anxiolytic use, unspecified <u>with</u> sedative, hypnotic or anxiolytic-induced <u>psychotic</u> disorder

cc **F13.950** Sedative, hypnotic or anxiolytic use, unspecified with sedative, hypnotic or anxiolytic-induced psychotic disorder <u>with delusions</u>

cc **F13.951** Sedative, hypnotic or anxiolytic use, unspecified with sedative, hypnotic or anxiolytic-induced psychotic disorder <u>with hallucinations</u>

F13.959 Sedative, hypnotic or anxiolytic use, unspecified with sedative, hypnotic or anxiolytic-induced psychotic disorder, unspecified
Sedative, hypnotic, or anxiolytic-induced psychotic disorder, without use disorder

F13.96 Sedative, hypnotic or anxiolytic use, unspecified <u>with</u> sedative, hypnotic or anxiolytic-induced <u>persisting</u> <u>amnestic</u> disorder

cc **F13.97** Sedative, hypnotic or anxiolytic use, unspecified <u>with</u> sedative, hypnotic or anxiolytic-induced <u>persisting</u> <u>dementia</u>
Sedative, hypnotic, or anxiolytic-induced major neurocognitive disorder, without use disorder

F13.98- Sedative, hypnotic or anxiolytic use, unspecified <u>with</u> <u>other</u> sedative, hypnotic or anxiolytic-induced disorders

F13.980 Sedative, hypnotic or anxiolytic use, unspecified <u>with</u> sedative, hypnotic or anxiolytic-induced <u>anxiety</u> disorder
Sedative, hypnotic, or anxiolytic-induced anxiety disorder, without use disorder

F13.981 Sedative, hypnotic or anxiolytic use, unspecified <u>with</u> sedative, hypnotic or anxiolytic-induced <u>sexual dysfunction</u>
Sedative, hypnotic, or anxiolytic-induced sexual dysfunction disorder, without use disorder

F13 - F13

F13.982 Sedative, hypnotic or anxiolytic use, unspecified <u>with</u> sedative, hypnotic or anxiolytic-induced <u>sleep</u> disorder
> Sedative, hypnotic, or anxiolytic-induced sleep disorder, without use disorder

F13.988 Sedative, hypnotic or anxiolytic use, unspecified with other sedative, hypnotic or anxiolytic-induced disorder
> Sedative, hypnotic, or anxiolytic-induced mild neurocognitive disorder

F13.99 Sedative, hypnotic or anxiolytic use, unspecified with unspecified sedative, hypnotic or anxiolytic-induced disorder

F14- <u>Cocaine related disorders</u>
Excludes ❷: other stimulant-related disorders (F15.-)

F14.1- Cocaine <u>abuse</u>
Excludes 1: cocaine dependence (F14.2-)
*   cocaine use, unspecified (F14.9-)*

F14.10 Cocaine abuse, <u>uncomplicated</u>
> Cocaine use disorder, mild

F14.12- Cocaine abuse <u>with intoxication</u>

F14.120 Cocaine abuse with intoxication, <u>uncomplicated</u>

cc **F14.121** Cocaine abuse with intoxication <u>with delirium</u>

F14.122 Cocaine abuse with intoxication <u>with perceptual disturbance</u>

F14.129 Cocaine abuse with intoxication, <u>unspecified</u>

F14.14 Cocaine abuse <u>with</u> cocaine-induced <u>mood</u> disorder
> Cocaine use disorder, mild, with cocaine-induced bipolar or related disorder
> Cocaine use disorder, mild, with cocaine-induced depressive disorder

F14.15- Cocaine abuse <u>with</u> cocaine-induced <u>psychotic</u> disorder

cc **F14.150** Cocaine abuse with cocaine-induced psychotic disorder <u>with delusions</u>

cc **F14.151** Cocaine abuse with cocaine-induced psychotic disorder <u>with hallucinations</u>

F14.159 Cocaine abuse with cocaine-induced psychotic disorder, unspecified

F14.18 Cocaine abuse <u>with other</u> cocaine-induced disorder

F14.180 Cocaine abuse <u>with</u> cocaine-induced <u>anxiety</u> disorder

F14.181 Cocaine abuse with cocaine-induced <u>sexual dysfunction</u>

F14.182 Cocaine abuse <u>with</u> cocaine-induced <u>sleep</u> disorder

F14.188 Cocaine abuse with other cocaine-induced disorder
> Cocaine use disorder, mild, with cocaine-induced obsessive-compulsive or related disorder

F14.19 Cocaine abuse with unspecified cocaine-induced disorder

F14.2- Cocaine <u>dependence</u>
Excludes 1: cocaine abuse (F14.1-)
*   cocaine use, unspecified (F14.9-)*
Excludes ❷: cocaine poisoning (T40.5-)

cc **F14.20** Cocaine dependence, <u>uncomplicated</u>
> Cocaine use disorder, moderate
> Cocaine use disorder, severe

F14.21 Cocaine dependence, <u>in remission</u>

F14.22- Cocaine dependence <u>with intoxication</u>
Excludes 1: cocaine dependence with withdrawal (F14.23)

F14.220 Cocaine dependence with intoxication, <u>uncomplicated</u>

cc **F14.221** Cocaine dependence with intoxication <u>delirium</u>

cc **F14.222** Cocaine dependence with intoxication <u>with perceptual disturbance</u>

cc **F14.229** Cocaine dependence with intoxication, <u>unspecified</u>

cc **F14.23** Cocaine dependence <u>with withdrawal</u>
Excludes 1: cocaine dependence with intoxication (F14.22-)

F14.24 Cocaine dependence <u>with</u> cocaine-induced <u>mood</u> disorder
> Cocaine use disorder, moderate, with cocaine-induced bipolar or related disorder
> Cocaine use disorder, moderate, with cocaine-induced depressive disorder
> Cocaine use disorder, severe, with cocaine-induced bipolar or related disorder
> Cocaine use disorder, severe, with cocaine-induced depressive disorder

F14.25- Cocaine dependence <u>with</u> cocaine-induced <u>psychotic</u> disorder

cc **F14.250** Cocaine dependence with cocaine-induced psychotic disorder <u>with delusions</u>

cc **F14.251** Cocaine dependence with cocaine-induced psychotic disorder <u>with hallucinations</u>

cc **F14.259** Cocaine dependence with cocaine-induced psychotic disorder, unspecified

F14.28- Cocaine dependence <u>with other</u> cocaine-induced disorder

cc **F14.280** Cocaine dependence with cocaine-induced <u>anxiety</u> disorder

cc **F14.281** Cocaine dependence with cocaine-induced <u>sexual dysfunction</u>

cc **F14.282** Cocaine dependence with cocaine-induced <u>sleep</u> disorder

cc **F14.288** Cocaine dependence with other cocaine-induced disorder
> Cocaine use disorder, moderate, with cocaine-induced obsessive-compulsive or related disorder
> Cocaine use disorder, severe, with cocaine-induced obsessive-compulsive or related disorder

F14.29 Cocaine dependence with unspecified cocaine-induced disorder

F14.9- Cocaine <u>use, unspecified</u>
Excludes 1: cocaine abuse (F14.1-)
*   cocaine dependence (F14.2-)*

F14.90 Cocaine use, unspecified, <u>uncomplicated</u>

F14.92- Cocaine use, unspecified <u>with intoxication</u>

F14.920 Cocaine use, unspecified with intoxication, <u>uncomplicated</u>

cc **F14.921** Cocaine use, unspecified with intoxication <u>delirium</u>

F14.922 Cocaine use, unspecified with intoxication <u>with perceptual disturbance</u>

F14.929 Cocaine use, unspecified with intoxication, <u>unspecified</u>

F14.94 Cocaine use, unspecified <u>with</u> cocaine-induced <u>mood</u> disorder
> Cocaine-induced bipolar or related disorder, without use disorder
> Cocaine-induced depressive disorder, without use disorder

F14.95- Cocaine use, unspecified <u>with</u> cocaine-induced <u>psychotic</u> disorder

cc **F14.950** Cocaine use, unspecified with cocaine-induced psychotic disorder <u>with delusions</u>

cc **F14.951** Cocaine use, unspecified with cocaine-induced psychotic disorder <u>with hallucinations</u>

F14.959 Cocaine use, unspecified with cocaine-induced psychotic disorder, unspecified
> Cocaine-induced psychotic disorder, without use disorder

F14.98- Cocaine use, unspecified <u>with other</u> specified cocaine-induced disorder

F14.980 Cocaine use, unspecified with cocaine-induced <u>anxiety</u> disorder
> Cocaine-induced anxiety disorder, without use disorder

F14.981 Cocaine use, unspecified with cocaine-induced <u>sexual dysfunction</u>
> Cocaine-induced sexual dysfunction disorder, without use disorder

F14.982 Cocaine use, unspecified with cocaine-induced <u>sleep</u> disorder
> Cocaine-induced sleep disorder, without use disorder

F
1
3
-
F
1
4

F14.988   Cocaine use, unspecified with other cocaine-induced disorder
Cocaine-induced obsessive compulsive or related disorder

F14.99   Cocaine use, unspecified with unspecified cocaine-induced disorder

F15-   <u>Other stimulant related disorders</u>
Includes: Amphetamine-related disorders
Caffeine
Excludes ❷: cocaine-related disorders (F14.-)

F15.1-   Other stimulant <u>abuse</u>
Excludes 1:   other stimulant dependence (F15.2-)
other stimulant use, unspecified (F15.9-)

F15.10   Other stimulant abuse, <u>uncomplicated</u>
Amphetamine type substance use disorder, mild
Other or unspecified stimulant use disorder, mild

F15.12-   Other stimulant abuse <u>with intoxication</u>

F15.120   Other stimulant abuse with intoxication, <u>uncomplicated</u>

CC F15.121   Other stimulant abuse with intoxication <u>delirium</u>

F15.122   Other stimulant abuse with intoxication <u>with perceptual disturbance</u>
Amphetamine or other stimulant use disorder, mild, with amphetamine or other stimulant intoxication, with perceptual disturbances

F15.129   Other stimulant abuse with intoxication, <u>unspecified</u>
Amphetamine or other stimulant use disorder, mild, with amphetamine or other stimulant intoxication, without perceptual disturbances

F15.14   Other stimulant abuse <u>with</u> stimulant-induced <u>mood</u> disorder
Amphetamine or other stimulant use disorder, mild, with amphetamine or other stimulant-induced bipolar or related disorder
Amphetamine or other stimulant use disorder, mild, with amphetamine or other stimulant-induced depressive disorder

F15.15-   Other stimulant abuse <u>with</u> stimulant-induced <u>psychotic</u> disorder

CC F15.150   Other stimulant abuse with stimulant-induced psychotic disorder <u>with delusions</u>

CC F15.151   Other stimulant abuse with stimulant-induced psychotic disorder <u>with hallucinations</u>

F15.159   Other stimulant abuse with stimulant-induced psychotic disorder, unspecified

F15.18-   Other stimulant abuse <u>with</u> <u>other</u> stimulant-induced disorder

F15.180   Other stimulant abuse with stimulant-induced <u>anxiety</u> disorder

F15.181   Other stimulant abuse with stimulant-induced <u>sexual dysfunction</u>

F15.182   Other stimulant abuse with stimulant-induced <u>sleep</u> disorder

F15.188   Other stimulant abuse with other stimulant-induced disorder
Amphetamine or other stimulant use disorder, mild, with amphetamine or other stimulant-induced obsessive-compulsive or related disorder

F15.19   Other stimulant abuse with unspecified stimulant-induced disorder

F15.2-   Other stimulant <u>dependence</u>
Excludes 1:   other stimulant abuse (F15.1-)
other stimulant use, unspecified (F15.9-)

CC F15.20   Other stimulant dependence, <u>uncomplicated</u>
Amphetamine type substance use disorder, moderate
Amphetamine type substance use disorder, severe
Other or unspecified stimulant use disorder, moderate
Other or unspecified stimulant use disorder, severe

F15.21   Other stimulant dependence, <u>in remission</u>

F15.22-   Other stimulant dependence <u>with intoxication</u>
Excludes 1:   other stimulant dependence with withdrawal (F15.23)

F15.220   Other stimulant dependence with intoxication, <u>uncomplicated</u>

CC F15.221   Other stimulant dependence with intoxication <u>delirium</u>

CC F15.222   Other stimulant dependence with intoxication <u>with perceptual disturbance</u>
Amphetamine or other stimulant use disorder, moderate, with amphetamine or other stimulant intoxication, with perceptual disturbances
Amphetamine or other stimulant use disorder, severe, with amphetamine or other stimulant intoxication, with perceptual disturbances

F15.229   Other stimulant dependence with intoxication, <u>unspecified</u>
Amphetamine or other stimulant use disorder, moderate, with amphetamine or other stimulant intoxication, without perceptual disturbances
Amphetamine or other stimulant use disorder, severe, with amphetamine or other stimulant intoxication, without perceptual disturbances

CC F15.23   Other stimulant dependence <u>with withdrawal</u>
Amphetamine or other stimulant withdrawal
Excludes 1:   other stimulant dependence with intoxication (F15.22-)

F15.24   Other stimulant dependence <u>with</u> stimulant-induced <u>mood</u> disorder
Amphetamine or other stimulant use disorder, moderate, with amphetamine or other stimulant-induced bipolar or related disorder
Amphetamine or other stimulant use disorder, moderate, with amphetamine or other stimulant-induced depressive disorder
Amphetamine or other stimulant use disorder, severe, with amphetamine or other stimulant-induced bipolar or related disorder
Amphetamine or other stimulant use disorder, severe, with amphetamine or other stimulant-induced depressive disorder

F15.25-   Other stimulant dependence <u>with</u> stimulant-induced <u>psychotic</u> disorder

CC F15.250   Other stimulant dependence with stimulant-induced psychotic disorder <u>with delusions</u>

CC F15.251   Other stimulant dependence with stimulant-induced psychotic disorder <u>with hallucinations</u>

CC F15.259   Other stimulant dependence with stimulant-induced psychotic disorder, unspecified

F15.28-   Other stimulant dependence <u>with</u> <u>other</u> stimulant-induced disorder

CC F15.280   Other stimulant dependence <u>with</u> stimulant-induced <u>anxiety</u> disorder

CC F15.281   Other stimulant dependence <u>with</u> stimulant-induced <u>sexual dysfunction</u>

CC F15.282   Other stimulant dependence with stimulant-induced <u>sleep</u> disorder

CC F15.288   Other stimulant dependence with other stimulant-induced disorder
Amphetamine or other stimulant use disorder, moderate, with amphetamine or other stimulant-induced obsessive-compulsive or related disorder
Amphetamine or other stimulant use disorder, severe, with amphetamine or other stimulant-induced obsessive-compulsive or related disorder

F15.29   Other stimulant dependence with unspecified stimulant-induced disorder

F15.9-   Other stimulant <u>use, unspecified</u>
Excludes 1:   other stimulant abuse (F15.1-)
other stimulant dependence (F15.2-)

F15.90   Other stimulant use, unspecified, <u>uncomplicated</u>

F15.92- Other stimulant use, unspecified <u>with intoxication</u>
  Excludes 1:   *other stimulant use, unspecified with withdrawal (F15.93)*

  F15.920 Other stimulant use, unspecified with intoxication, <u>uncomplicated</u>

cc **F15.921** Other stimulant use, unspecified with intoxication <u>delirium</u>
    Amphetamine or other stimulant-induced delirium

  F15.922 Other stimulant use, unspecified with intoxication <u>with perceptual disturbance</u>

  F15.929 Other stimulant use, unspecified with intoxication, <u>unspecified</u>
    Caffeine intoxication

cc **F15.93** Other stimulant use, unspecified, <u>with withdrawal</u>
  Caffeine withdrawal
  Excludes 1:   *other stimulant use, unspecified with intoxication (F15.92-)*

F15.94 Other stimulant use, unspecified <u>with</u> stimulant-induced <u>mood</u> disorder
  Amphetamine or other stimulant-induced bipolar or related disorder, without use disorder
  Amphetamine or other stimulant-induced depressive disorder, without use disorder

F15.95- Other stimulant use, unspecified <u>with</u> stimulant-induced <u>psychotic</u> disorder

cc **F15.950** Other stimulant use, unspecified with stimulant-induced psychotic disorder <u>with delusions</u>

cc **F15.951** Other stimulant use, unspecified with stimulant-induced psychotic disorder <u>with hallucinations</u>

  F15.959 Other stimulant use, unspecified with stimulant-induced psychotic disorder, unspecified
    Amphetamine or other stimulant-induced psychotic disorder, without use disorder

F15.98- Other stimulant use, unspecified <u>with</u> <u>other</u> stimulant-induced disorder

  F15.980 Other stimulant use, unspecified with stimulant-induced <u>anxiety</u> disorder
    Amphetamine or other stimulant-induced anxiety disorder, without use disorder
    Caffeine-induced anxiety disorder, without use disorder

  F15.981 Other stimulant use, unspecified with stimulant-induced <u>sexual dysfunction</u>
    Amphetamine or other stimulant-induced sexual dysfunction disorder, without use disorder

  F15.982 Other stimulant use, unspecified with stimulant-induced <u>sleep</u> disorder
    Amphetamine or other stimulant-induced sleep disorder, without use disorder
    Caffeine-induced sleep disorder, without use disorder

  F15.988 Other stimulant use, unspecified with other stimulant-induced disorder
    Amphetamine or other stimulant-induced obsessive-compulsive or related disorder, without use disorder

F15.99 Other stimulant use, unspecified with unspecified stimulant-induced disorder

F16- <u>Hallucinogen related disorders</u>
  Includes: Ecstasy
          PCP
          Phencyclidine

F16.1- Hallucinogen <u>abuse</u>
  Excludes 1:   *hallucinogen dependence (F16.2-)*
              hallucinogen use, unspecified (F16.9-)

F16.10 Hallucinogen abuse, <u>uncomplicated</u>
  Other hallucinogen use disorder, mild
  Phencyclidine use disorder, mild

F16.12- Hallucinogen abuse <u>with intoxication</u>

  F16.120 Hallucinogen abuse with intoxication, <u>uncomplicated</u>

cc **F16.121** Hallucinogen abuse with intoxication with <u>delirium</u>

  F16.122 Hallucinogen abuse with intoxication <u>with perceptual disturbance</u>

  F16.129 Hallucinogen abuse with intoxication, <u>unspecified</u>

F16.14 Hallucinogen abuse <u>with</u> hallucinogen-induced <u>mood</u> disorder
  Other hallucinogen use disorder, mild, with other hallucinogen-induced bipolar or related disorder
  Other hallucinogen use disorder, mild, with other hallucinogen-induced depressive disorder
  Phencyclidine use disorder, mild, with phencyclidine-induced bipolar or related disorder
  Phencyclidine use disorder, mild, with phencyclidine-induced depressive disorder

F16.15- Hallucinogen abuse <u>with</u> hallucinogen-induced <u>psychotic</u> disorder

cc **F16.150** Hallucinogen abuse with hallucinogen-induced psychotic disorder <u>with delusions</u>

cc **F16.151** Hallucinogen abuse with hallucinogen-induced psychotic disorder <u>with hallucinations</u>

  F16.159 Hallucinogen abuse with hallucinogen-induced psychotic disorder, unspecified

F16.18- Hallucinogen abuse <u>with</u> <u>other</u> hallucinogen-induced disorder

  F16.180 Hallucinogen abuse with hallucinogen-induced <u>anxiety</u> disorder

  F16.183 Hallucinogen abuse with hallucinogen <u>persisting perception disorder (flashbacks)</u>

  F16.188 Hallucinogen abuse with other hallucinogen-induced disorder

F16.19 Hallucinogen abuse with unspecified hallucinogen-induced disorder

F16.2- Hallucinogen <u>dependence</u>
  Excludes 1:   *hallucinogen abuse (F16.1-)*
              hallucinogen use, unspecified (F16.9-)

cc **F16.20** Hallucinogen dependence, <u>uncomplicated</u>
  Other hallucinogen use disorder, moderate
  Other hallucinogen use disorder, severe
  Phencyclidine use disorder, moderate
  Phencyclidine use disorder, severe

F16.21 Hallucinogen dependence, <u>in remission</u>

F16.22- Hallucinogen dependence <u>with intoxication</u>

  F16.220 Hallucinogen dependence with intoxication, <u>uncomplicated</u>

cc **F16.221** Hallucinogen dependence with intoxication with <u>delirium</u>

  F16.229 Hallucinogen dependence with intoxication, <u>unspecified</u>

F16.24 Hallucinogen dependence <u>with</u> hallucinogen-induced <u>mood</u> disorder
  Other hallucinogen use disorder, moderate, with other hallucinogen-induced bipolar or related disorder
  Other hallucinogen use disorder, moderate, with other hallucinogen-induced depressive disorder
  Other hallucinogen use disorder, severe, with other hallucinogen-induced bipolar or related disorder
  Other hallucinogen use disorder, severe, with other hallucinogen-induced depressive disorder
  Phencyclidine use disorder, moderate, with phencyclidine-induced bipolar or related disorder
  Phencyclidine use disorder, moderate, with phencyclidine-induced depressive disorder
  Phencyclidine use disorder, severe, with phencyclidine-induced bipolar or related disorder
  Phencyclidine use disorder, severe, with phencyclidine-induced depressive disorder

F16.25- Hallucinogen dependence <u>with</u> hallucinogen-induced <u>psychotic</u> disorder

cc **F16.250** Hallucinogen dependence with hallucinogen-induced psychotic disorder <u>with delusions</u>

cc **F16.251** Hallucinogen dependence with hallucinogen-induced psychotic disorder <u>with hallucinations</u>

cc **F16.259** Hallucinogen dependence with hallucinogen-induced psychotic disorder, unspecified

F16.28- Hallucinogen dependence <u>with</u> <u>other</u> hallucinogen-induced disorder

cc **F16.280** Hallucinogen dependence <u>with</u> hallucinogen-induced <u>anxiety</u> disorder

F15 - F16

cc **F16.283**   Hallucinogen dependence <u>with</u> hallucinogen <u>persisting perception disorder (flashbacks)</u>

cc **F16.288**   Hallucinogen dependence with other hallucinogen-induced disorder

F16.29   Hallucinogen dependence with unspecified hallucinogen-induced disorder

F16.9-   Hallucinogen <u>use, unspecified</u>
> Excludes 1: *hallucinogen abuse (F16.1-)*
> *hallucinogen dependence (F16.2-)*

F16.90   Hallucinogen use, unspecified, <u>uncomplicated</u>

F16.92-   Hallucinogen use, unspecified <u>with intoxication</u>

F16.920   Hallucinogen use, unspecified with intoxication, <u>uncomplicated</u>

cc **F16.921**   Hallucinogen use, unspecified with intoxication with <u>delirium</u>
> Other hallucinogen intoxication delirium

F16.929   Hallucinogen use, unspecified with intoxication, <u>unspecified</u>

F16.94   Hallucinogen use, unspecified <u>with</u> hallucinogen-induced <u>mood</u> disorder
> Other hallucinogen-induced bipolar or related disorder, without use disorder
> Other hallucinogen-induced depressive disorder, without use disorder
> Phencyclidine-induced bipolar or related disorder, without use disorder
> Phencyclidine-induced depressive disorder, without use disorder

F16.95-   Hallucinogen use, unspecified <u>with</u> hallucinogen-induced <u>psychotic</u> disorder

cc **F16.950**   Hallucinogen use, unspecified with hallucinogen-induced psychotic disorder <u>with delusions</u>

cc **F16.951**   Hallucinogen use, unspecified with hallucinogen-induced psychotic disorder <u>with hallucinations</u>

F16.959   Hallucinogen use, unspecified with hallucinogen-induced psychotic disorder, unspecified
> Other hallucinogen-induced psychotic disorder, without use disorder
> Phencyclidine-induced psychotic disorder, without use disorder

F16.98-   Hallucinogen use, unspecified <u>with other</u> specified hallucinogen-induced disorder

F16.980   Hallucinogen use, unspecified with hallucinogen-induced <u>anxiety</u> disorder
> Other hallucinogen-induced anxiety disorder, without use disorder
> Phencyclidine-induced anxiety disorder, without use disorder

F16.983   Hallucinogen use, unspecified <u>with</u> hallucinogen <u>persisting perception disorder (flashbacks)</u>

F16.988   Hallucinogen use, unspecified with other hallucinogen-induced disorder

F16.99   Hallucinogen use, unspecified with unspecified hallucinogen-induced disorder

F17-   <u>Nicotine dependence</u>
> Excludes 1: *history of tobacco dependence (Z87.891)*
> *tobacco use NOS (Z72.0)*
> Excludes 2: *tobacco use (smoking) during pregnancy, childbirth and the puerperium (O99.33-)*
> *toxic effect of nicotine (T65.2-)*

F17.2-   Nicotine <u>dependence</u>
> AHA 13:4Q:p108 – Smoker
> AHA 13:4Q:p108 – Nicotine dependence

F17.20-   Nicotine <u>dependence, unspecified</u>

F17.200   Nicotine dependence, unspecified, <u>uncomplicated</u> — [Unacceptable PDX]
> Tobacco use disorder, mild
> Tobacco use disorder, moderate
> Tobacco use disorder, severe

F17.201   Nicotine dependence, unspecified, <u>in remission</u> — [Unacceptable PDX]

cc **F17.203**   Nicotine dependence unspecified, <u>with withdrawal</u>
> Tobacco withdrawal

F17.208   Nicotine dependence, unspecified, with other nicotine-induced disorders

F17.209   Nicotine dependence, unspecified, with unspecified nicotine-induced disorders

F17.21-   Nicotine dependence, <u>cigarettes</u>
> AHA 13:4Q:p109 – Nicotine dependence and COPD

F17.210   Nicotine dependence, cigarettes, <u>uncomplicated</u> — [Unacceptable PDX]

F17.211   Nicotine dependence, cigarettes, <u>in remission</u> — [Unacceptable PDX]

cc **F17.213**   Nicotine dependence, cigarettes, <u>with withdrawal</u>

F17.218   Nicotine dependence, cigarettes, with other nicotine-induced disorders

F17.219   Nicotine dependence, cigarettes, with unspecified nicotine-induced disorders

F17.22-   Nicotine dependence, <u>chewing tobacco</u>

F17.220   Nicotine dependence, chewing tobacco, <u>uncomplicated</u> — [Unacceptable PDX]

F17.221   Nicotine dependence, chewing tobacco, <u>in remission</u> — [Unacceptable PDX]

cc **F17.223**   Nicotine dependence, chewing tobacco, <u>with withdrawal</u>

F17.228   Nicotine dependence, chewing tobacco, with other nicotine-induced disorders

F17.229   Nicotine dependence, chewing tobacco, with unspecified nicotine-induced disorders

F17.29-   Nicotine dependence, <u>other tobacco product</u>

F17.290   Nicotine dependence, other tobacco product, <u>uncomplicated</u> — [Unacceptable PDX]

F17.291   Nicotine dependence, other tobacco product, <u>in remission</u> — [Unacceptable PDX]

cc **F17.293**   Nicotine dependence, other tobacco product, <u>with withdrawal</u>

F17.298   Nicotine dependence, other tobacco product, with other nicotine-induced disorders

F17.299   Nicotine dependence, other tobacco product, with unspecified nicotine-induced disorders

F18-   <u>Inhalant related disorders</u>
> Includes: Volatile solvents

F18.1-   Inhalant <u>abuse</u>
> Excludes 1: *inhalant dependence (F18.2-)*
> *inhalant use, unspecified (F18.9-)*

F18.10   Inhalant abuse, <u>uncomplicated</u>
> Inhalant use disorder, mild

F18.12-   Inhalant abuse <u>with intoxication</u>

F18.120   Inhalant abuse with intoxication, <u>uncomplicated</u>

cc **F18.121**   Inhalant abuse with intoxication <u>delirium</u>

F18.129   Inhalant abuse with intoxication, <u>unspecified</u>

F18.14   Inhalant abuse <u>with</u> inhalant-induced <u>mood</u> disorder
> Inhalant use disorder, mild, with inhalant-induced depressive disorder

F18.15-   Inhalant abuse <u>with</u> inhalant-induced <u>psychotic</u> disorder

cc **F18.150**   Inhalant abuse with inhalant-induced psychotic disorder <u>with delusions</u>

cc **F18.151**   Inhalant abuse with inhalant-induced psychotic disorder <u>with hallucinations</u>

F18.159   Inhalant abuse with inhalant-induced psychotic disorder, unspecified

cc **F18.17**   Inhalant abuse <u>with</u> inhalant-induced <u>dementia</u>
> Inhalant use disorder, mild, with inhalant-induced major neurocognitive disorder

F18.18-   Inhalant abuse <u>with other</u> inhalant-induced disorders

F18.180   Inhalant abuse with inhalant-induced <u>anxiety</u> disorder

F18.188   Inhalant abuse with other inhalant-induced disorder
> Inhalant use disorder, mild, with inhalant-induced mild neurocognitive disorder

F18.19   Inhalant abuse with unspecified inhalant-induced disorder

F 16 - F 18

F18.2-   Inhalant dependence
Excludes 1:   *inhalant abuse (F18.1-)*
inhalant use, unspecified (F18.9-)

cc **F18.20   Inhalant dependence, uncomplicated**
Inhalant use disorder, moderate
Inhalant use disorder, severe

F18.21   Inhalant dependence, in remission

F18.22- Inhalant dependence with intoxication

F18.220   Inhalant dependence with intoxication, uncomplicated

cc **F18.221   Inhalant dependence with intoxication delirium**

F18.229   Inhalant dependence with intoxication, unspecified

F18.24   Inhalant dependence with inhalant-induced mood disorder
Inhalant use disorder, moderate, with inhalant-induced depressive disorder
Inhalant use disorder, severe, with inhalant-induced depressive disorder

F18.25- Inhalant dependence with inhalant-induced psychotic disorder

cc **F18.250   Inhalant dependence with inhalant-induced psychotic disorder with delusions**

cc **F18.251   Inhalant dependence with inhalant-induced psychotic disorder with hallucinations**

cc **F18.259   Inhalant dependence with inhalant-induced psychotic disorder, unspecified**

cc **F18.27   Inhalant dependence with inhalant-induced dementia**
Inhalant use disorder, moderate, with inhalant-induced major neurocognitive disorder
Inhalant use disorder, severe, with inhalant-induced major neurocognitive disorder

F18.28- Inhalant dependence with other inhalant-induced disorders

cc **F18.280   Inhalant dependence with inhalant-induced anxiety disorder**

cc **F18.288   Inhalant dependence with other inhalant-induced disorder**
Inhalant use disorder, moderate, with inhalant-induced mild neurocognitive disorder
Inhalant use disorder, severe, with inhalant-induced mild neurocognitive disorder

F18.29   Inhalant dependence with unspecified inhalant-induced disorder

F18.9-   Inhalant use, unspecified
Excludes 1:   *inhalant abuse (F18.1-)*
inhalant dependence (F18.2-)

F18.90   Inhalant use, unspecified, uncomplicated

F18.92- Inhalant use, unspecified with intoxication

F18.920   Inhalant use, unspecified with intoxication, uncomplicated

cc **F18.921   Inhalant use, unspecified with intoxication with delirium**

F18.929   Inhalant use, unspecified with intoxication, unspecified

F18.94   Inhalant use, unspecified with inhalant-induced mood disorder
Inhalant-induced depressive disorder

F18.95- Inhalant use, unspecified with inhalant-induced psychotic disorder

cc **F18.950   Inhalant use, unspecified with inhalant-induced psychotic disorder with delusions**

cc **F18.951   Inhalant use, unspecified with inhalant-induced psychotic disorder with hallucinations**

F18.959   Inhalant use, unspecified with inhalant-induced psychotic disorder, unspecified

cc **F18.97   Inhalant use, unspecified with inhalant-induced persisting dementia**
Inhalant-induced major neurocognitive disorder

F18.98- Inhalant use, unspecified with other inhalant-induced disorders

F18.980   Inhalant use, unspecified with inhalant-induced anxiety disorder

F18.988   Inhalant use, unspecified with other inhalant-induced disorder
Inhalant-induced mild neurocognitive disorder

F18.99   Inhalant use, unspecified with unspecified inhalant-induced disorder

F19-   Other psychoactive substance related disorders
Includes: Polysubstance drug use (indiscriminate drug use)

F19.1-   Other psychoactive substance abuse
Excludes 1:   *other psychoactive substance dependence (F19.2-)*
other psychoactive substance use, unspecified (F19.9-)

F19.10   Other psychoactive substance abuse, uncomplicated
Other (or unknown) substance use disorder, mild

F19.12- Other psychoactive substance abuse with intoxication

F19.120   Other psychoactive substance abuse with intoxication, uncomplicated

cc **F19.121   Other psychoactive substance abuse with intoxication delirium**

F19.122   Other psychoactive substance abuse with intoxication with perceptual disturbances

F19.129   Other psychoactive substance abuse with intoxication, unspecified

F19.14   Other psychoactive substance abuse with psychoactive substance-induced mood disorder
Other (or unknown) substance use disorder, mild, with other (or unknown) substance-induced bipolar or related disorder
Other (or unknown) substance use disorder, mild, with other (or unknown) substance-induced depressive disorder

F19.15- Other psychoactive substance abuse with psychoactive substance-induced psychotic disorder

cc **F19.150   Other psychoactive substance abuse with psychoactive substance-induced psychotic disorder with delusions**

cc **F19.151   Other psychoactive substance abuse with psychoactive substance-induced psychotic disorder with hallucinations**

F19.159   Other psychoactive substance abuse with psychoactive substance-induced psychotic disorder, unspecified

F19.16   Other psychoactive substance abuse with psychoactive substance-induced persisting amnestic disorder

cc **F19.17   Other psychoactive substance abuse with psychoactive substance-induced persisting dementia**
Other (or unknown) substance use disorder, mild, with other (or unknown) substance-induced major neurocognitive disorder

F19.18- Other psychoactive substance abuse with other psychoactive substance-induced disorders

F19.180   Other psychoactive substance abuse with psychoactive substance-induced anxiety disorder

F19.181   Other psychoactive substance abuse with psychoactive substance-induced sexual dysfunction

F19.182   Other psychoactive substance abuse with psychoactive substance-induced sleep disorder

F19.188   Other psychoactive substance abuse with other psychoactive substance-induced disorder
Other (or unknown) substance use disorder, mild, with other (or unknown) substance-induced mild neurocognitive disorder
Other (or unknown) substance use disorder, mild, with other (or unknown) substance-induced obsessive-compulsive or related disorder

F19.19   Other psychoactive substance abuse with unspecified psychoactive substance-induced disorder

F19.2-   Other psychoactive substance dependence
Excludes 1:   *other psychoactive substance abuse (F19.1-)*
other psychoactive substance use, unspecified (F19.9-)

cc **F19.20   Other psychoactive substance dependence, uncomplicated**
Other (or unknown) substance use disorder, moderate
Other (or unknown) substance use disorder, severe

F19.21   Other psychoactive substance dependence, in remission

F18 - F19

F19.22- Other psychoactive substance dependence <u>with</u> <u>intoxication</u>
> *Excludes 1:*   *other psychoactive substance dependence with withdrawal (F19.23-)*

   F19.220 Other psychoactive substance dependence with intoxication, <u>uncomplicated</u>

cc **F19.221** Other psychoactive substance dependence with intoxication <u>delirium</u>

cc **F19.222** Other psychoactive substance dependence with intoxication <u>with perceptual disturbance</u>

   F19.229 Other psychoactive substance dependence with intoxication, <u>unspecified</u>

F19.23- Other psychoactive substance dependence <u>with</u> <u>withdrawal</u>
> *Excludes 1:*   *other psychoactive substance dependence with intoxication (F19.22-)*

cc **F19.230** Other psychoactive substance dependence with withdrawal, <u>uncomplicated</u>

cc **F19.231** Other psychoactive substance dependence with withdrawal <u>delirium</u>

cc **F19.232** Other psychoactive substance dependence with withdrawal <u>with perceptual disturbance</u>

cc **F19.239** Other psychoactive substance dependence with withdrawal, <u>unspecified</u>

F19.24 Other psychoactive substance dependence <u>with</u> psychoactive substance-induced <u>mood</u> disorder
> Other (or unknown) substance use disorder, moderate, with other (or unknown) substance-induced bipolar or related disorder
> Other (or unknown) substance use disorder, moderate, with other (or unknown) substance-induced depressive disorder
> Other (or unknown) substance use disorder, severe, with other (or unknown) substance-induced bipolar or related disorder
> Other (or unknown) substance use disorder, severe, with other (or unknown) substance-induced depressive disorder

F19.25- Other psychoactive substance dependence <u>with</u> psychoactive substance-induced <u>psychotic</u> disorder

cc **F19.250** Other psychoactive substance dependence with psychoactive substance-induced psychotic disorder <u>with delusions</u>

cc **F19.251** Other psychoactive substance dependence with psychoactive substance-induced psychotic disorder <u>with hallucinations</u>

cc **F19.259** Other psychoactive substance dependence with psychoactive substance-induced psychotic disorder, unspecified

cc **F19.26** Other psychoactive substance dependence <u>with</u> psychoactive substance-induced <u>persisting amnestic</u> disorder

cc **F19.27** Other psychoactive substance dependence <u>with</u> psychoactive substance-induced <u>persisting dementia</u>
> Other (or unknown) substance use disorder, moderate, with other (or unknown) substance-induced major neurocognitive disorder
> Other (or unknown) substance use disorder, severe, with other (or unknown) substance-induced major neurocognitive disorder

F19.28- Other psychoactive substance dependence <u>with</u> <u>other</u> psychoactive substance-induced disorders

cc **F19.280** Other psychoactive substance dependence with psychoactive substance-induced <u>anxiety</u> disorder

cc **F19.281** Other psychoactive substance dependence with psychoactive substance-induced <u>sexual dysfunction</u>

cc **F19.282** Other psychoactive substance dependence with psychoactive substance-induced <u>sleep</u> disorder

cc **F19.288** Other psychoactive substance dependence with other psychoactive substance-induced disorder
> Other (or unknown) substance use disorder, moderate, with other (or unknown) substance-induced mild neurocognitive disorder
> Other (or unknown) substance use disorder, severe, with other (or unknown) substance-induced mild neurocognitive disorder
> Other (or unknown) substance use disorder, moderate, with other (or unknown) substance-induced obsessive-compulsive or related disorder
> Other (or unknown) substance use disorder, severe, with other (or unknown) substance-induced obsessive-compulsive or related disorder

F19.29 Other psychoactive substance dependence with unspecified psychoactive substance-induced disorder

F19.9- Other psychoactive substance <u>use, unspecified</u>
> *Excludes 1:*   *other psychoactive substance abuse (F19.1-)*
>   *other psychoactive substance dependence (F19.2-)*

F19.90 Other psychoactive substance use, unspecified, <u>uncomplicated</u>

F19.92- Other psychoactive substance use, unspecified <u>with</u> <u>intoxication</u>
> *Excludes 1:*   *other psychoactive substance use, unspecified with withdrawal (F19.93)*

   F19.920 Other psychoactive substance use, unspecified with intoxication, <u>uncomplicated</u>

cc **F19.921** Other psychoactive substance use, unspecified with intoxication <u>with delirium</u>
> Other (or unknown) substance-induced delirium

   F19.922 Other psychoactive substance use, unspecified with intoxication <u>with perceptual disturbance</u>

   F19.929 Other psychoactive substance use, unspecified with intoxication, <u>unspecified</u>

F19.93- Other psychoactive substance use, unspecified <u>with</u> <u>withdrawal</u>
> *Excludes 1:*   *other psychoactive substance use, unspecified with intoxication (F19.92-)*

cc **F19.930** Other psychoactive substance use, unspecified with withdrawal, <u>uncomplicated</u>

cc **F19.931** Other psychoactive substance use, unspecified with withdrawal <u>delirium</u>

cc **F19.932** Other psychoactive substance use, unspecified with withdrawal <u>with perceptual disturbance</u>

cc **F19.939** Other psychoactive substance use, unspecified with withdrawal, <u>unspecified</u>

F19.94 Other psychoactive substance use, unspecified <u>with</u> psychoactive substance-induced <u>mood</u> disorder
> Other (or unknown) substance-induced bipolar or related disorder, without use disorder
> Other (or unknown) substance-induced depressive disorder, without use disorder

F19.95- Other psychoactive substance use, unspecified <u>with</u> psychoactive substance-induced <u>psychotic</u> disorder

cc **F19.950** Other psychoactive substance use, unspecified with psychoactive substance-induced psychotic disorder <u>with delusions</u>

cc **F19.951** Other psychoactive substance use, unspecified with psychoactive substance-induced psychotic disorder <u>with hallucinations</u>

   F19.959 Other psychoactive substance use, unspecified with psychoactive substance-induced psychotic disorder, unspecified
> Other (or unknown) substance-induced psychotic disorder, without use disorder

F19.96 Other psychoactive substance use, unspecified <u>with</u> psychoactive substance-induced <u>persisting amnestic</u> disorder

cc **F19.97** Other psychoactive substance use, unspecified <u>with</u> psychoactive substance-induced <u>persisting dementia</u>
> Other (or unknown) substance-induced major neurocognitive disorder, without use disorder

F 1 9 - F 1 9

F19.98- Other psychoactive substance use, unspecified <u>with</u> <u>other</u> psychoactive substance-induced disorders

    F19.980 Other psychoactive substance use, unspecified <u>with</u> psychoactive substance-induced <u>anxiety</u> disorder
        Other (or unknown) substance-induced anxiety disorder, without use disorder

    F19.981 Other psychoactive substance use, unspecified <u>with</u> psychoactive substance-induced <u>sexual dysfunction</u>
        Other (or unknown) substance-induced sexual dysfunction, without use disorder

    F19.982 Other psychoactive substance use, unspecified <u>with</u> psychoactive substance-induced <u>sleep</u> disorder
        Other (or unknown) substance-induced sleep disorder, without use disorder

    F19.988 Other psychoactive substance use, unspecified with other psychoactive substance-induced disorder
        Other (or unknown) substance-induced mild neurocognitive disorder, without use disorder
        Other (or unknown) substance-induced obsessive-compulsive or related disorder, without use disorder

    F19.99 Other psychoactive substance use, unspecified with unspecified psychoactive substance-induced disorder

Schizophrenia, schizotypal, delusional, and other non-mood psychotic disorders (F20-F29)

F20- <u>Schizophrenia</u>
   Excludes 1: *brief psychotic disorder (F23)*
              cyclic schizophrenia (F25.0)
              mood [affective] disorders with psychotic symptoms (F30.2, F31.2, F31.5, F31.64, F32.3, F33.3)
              schizoaffective disorder (F25.-)
              schizophrenic reaction NOS (F23)
   Excludes 2: *schizophrenic reaction in:*
              alcoholism (F10.15-, F10.25-, F10.95-)
              brain disease (F06.2)
              epilepsy (F06.2)
              psychoactive drug use (F11-F19 with .15, .25, .95)
              schizotypal disorder (F21)

CC **F20.0** Paranoid schizophrenia
    Paraphrenic schizophrenia
   Excludes 1: *involutional paranoid state (F22)*
              paranoia (F22)

CC **F20.1** Disorganized schizophrenia
    Hebephrenic schizophrenia
    Hebephrenia

CC **F20.2** Catatonic schizophrenia
    Schizophrenic catalepsy
    Schizophrenic catatonia
    Schizophrenic flexibilitas cerea
   Excludes 1: *catatonic stupor (R40.1)*

F20.3 Undifferentiated schizophrenia
    Atypical schizophrenia
   Excludes 1: *acute schizophrenia-like psychotic disorder (F23)*
   Excludes 2: *post-schizophrenic depression (F32.89)*

CC **F20.5** Residual schizophrenia
    Restzustand (schizophrenic)
    Schizophrenic residual state

F20.8- Other schizophrenia

  CC **F20.81** Schizophreniform disorder
      Schizophreniform psychosis NOS

  CC **F20.89** Other schizophrenia
      Cenesthopathic schizophrenia
      Simple schizophrenia

F20.9 Schizophrenia, unspecified

F21 <u>Schizotypal</u> disorder
    Borderline schizophrenia
    Latent schizophrenia
    Latent schizophrenic reaction
    Prepsychotic schizophrenia
    Prodromal schizophrenia
    Pseudoneurotic schizophrenia
    Pseudopsychopathic schizophrenia
    Schizotypal personality disorder
   Excludes 2: *Asperger's syndrome (F84.5)*
              schizoid personality disorder (F60.1)

F22 Delusional disorders
    Delusional dysmorphophobia
    Involutional paranoid state
    Paranoia
    Paranoia querulans
    Paranoid psychosis
    Paranoid state
    Paraphrenia (late)
    Sensitiver Beziehungswahn
   Excludes 1: *mood [affective] disorders with psychotic symptoms (F30.2, F31.2, F31.5, F31.64, F32.3, F33.3)*
              paranoid schizophrenia (F20.0)
   Excludes 2: *paranoid personality disorder (F60.0)*
              paranoid psychosis, psychogenic (F23)
              paranoid reaction (F23)

F23 <u>Brief</u> psychotic disorder
CC
    Paranoid reaction
    Psychogenic paranoid psychosis
   Excludes 2: *mood [affective] disorders with psychotic symptoms (F30.2, F31.2, F31.5, F31.64, F32.3, F33.3)*

F24 <u>Shared</u> psychotic disorder
    Folie à deux
    Induced paranoid disorder
    Induced psychotic disorder

F25- <u>Schizoaffective</u> disorders
   Excludes 1: *mood [affective] disorders with psychotic symptoms (F30.2, F31.2, F31.5, F31.64, F32.3, F33.3)*
              schizophrenia (F20.-)

  F25.0 Schizoaffective disorder, <u>bipolar</u> type
      Cyclic schizophrenia
      Schizoaffective disorder, manic type
      Schizoaffective disorder, mixed type
      Schizoaffective psychosis, bipolar type
      Schizophreniform psychosis, manic type

  F25.1 Schizoaffective disorder, <u>depressive</u> type
      Schizoaffective psychosis, depressive type
      Schizophreniform psychosis, depressive type

  F25.8 Other schizoaffective disorders

  F25.9 Schizoaffective disorder, unspecified
      Schizoaffective psychosis NOS

F28 Other psychotic disorder <u>not</u> due to a substance or known physiological condition
    Chronic hallucinatory psychosis

F29 Unspecified psychosis <u>not</u> due to a substance or known physiological condition
    Psychosis NOS
   Excludes 1: *mental disorder NOS (F99)*
              unspecified mental disorder due to known physiological condition (F09)

Mood [affective] disorders (F30-F39)

F30- <u>Manic episode</u>
   Includes: Bipolar disorder, single manic episode
             Mixed affective episode
   Excludes 1: *bipolar disorder (F31.-)*
              major depressive disorder, single episode (F32.-)
              major depressive disorder, recurrent (F33.-)

  F30.1- Manic episode <u>without</u> psychotic symptoms
  CC **F30.10** Manic episode without psychotic symptoms, unspecified
  CC **F30.11** Manic episode without psychotic symptoms, <u>mild</u>
  CC **F30.12** Manic episode without psychotic symptoms, <u>moderate</u>
  CC **F30.13** Manic episode, severe, without psychotic symptoms

  CC **F30.2** Manic episode, severe <u>with psychotic symptoms</u>
      Manic stupor
      Mania with mood-congruent psychotic symptoms
      Mania with mood-incongruent psychotic symptoms

  F30.3 Manic episode in <u>partial</u> remission

  F30.4 Manic episode in <u>full</u> remission

  F30.8 Other manic episodes
      Hypomania

  CC **F30.9** Manic episode, unspecified
      Mania NOS

F19 - F30

F31- Bipolar disorder
Includes: Manic-depressive illness
Manic-depressive psychosis
Manic-depressive reaction
Excludes 1: bipolar disorder, single manic episode (F30.-)
major depressive disorder, single episode (F32.-)
major depressive disorder, recurrent (F33.-)
Excludes ❷: cyclothymia (F34.0)

CC **F31.0 Bipolar disorder, current episode hypomanic**

F31.1- Bipolar disorder, current episode manic without psychotic features

CC **F31.10 Bipolar disorder, current episode manic without psychotic features, unspecified**

CC **F31.11 Bipolar disorder, current episode manic without psychotic features, mild**

CC **F31.12 Bipolar disorder, current episode manic without psychotic features, moderate**

CC **F31.13 Bipolar disorder, current episode manic without psychotic features, severe**

CC **F31.2 Bipolar disorder, current episode manic severe with psychotic features**
Bipolar disorder, current episode manic with mood-congruent psychotic symptoms
Bipolar disorder, current episode manic with mood-incongruent psychotic symptoms

F31.3- Bipolar disorder, current episode depressed, mild or moderate severity

CC **F31.30 Bipolar disorder, current episode depressed, mild or moderate severity, unspecified**

CC **F31.31 Bipolar disorder, current episode depressed, mild**

CC **F31.32 Bipolar disorder, current episode depressed, moderate**

CC **F31.4 Bipolar disorder, current episode depressed, severe, without psychotic features**

CC **F31.5 Bipolar disorder, current episode depressed, severe, with psychotic features**
Bipolar disorder, current episode depressed with mood-incongruent psychotic symptoms
Bipolar disorder, current episode depressed with mood-congruent psychotic symptoms

F31.6- Bipolar disorder, current episode mixed

CC **F31.60 Bipolar disorder, current episode mixed, unspecified**

CC **F31.61 Bipolar disorder, current episode mixed, mild**

CC **F31.62 Bipolar disorder, current episode mixed, moderate**

CC **F31.63 Bipolar disorder, current episode mixed, severe, without psychotic features**

CC **F31.64 Bipolar disorder, current episode mixed, severe, with psychotic features**
Bipolar disorder, current episode mixed with mood-congruent psychotic symptoms
Bipolar disorder, current episode mixed with mood-incongruent psychotic symptoms

F31.7- Bipolar disorder, currently in remission

F31.70 Bipolar disorder, currently in remission, most recent episode unspecified

F31.71 Bipolar disorder, in partial remission, most recent episode hypomanic

F31.72 Bipolar disorder, in full remission, most recent episode hypomanic

F31.73 Bipolar disorder, in partial remission, most recent episode manic

F31.74 Bipolar disorder, in full remission, most recent episode manic

F31.75 Bipolar disorder, in partial remission, most recent episode depressed

F31.76 Bipolar disorder, in full remission, most recent episode depressed

F31.77 Bipolar disorder, in partial remission, most recent episode mixed

F31.78 Bipolar disorder, in full remission, most recent episode mixed

F31.8- Other bipolar disorders

CC **F31.81 Bipolar II disorder**

CC **F31.89 Other bipolar disorder**
Recurrent manic episodes NOS

F31.9 Bipolar disorder, unspecified

F32- Major depressive disorder, single episode
Includes: Single episode of agitated depression
Single episode of depressive reaction
Single episode of major depression
Single episode of psychogenic depression
Single episode of reactive depression
Single episode of vital depression
Excludes 1: bipolar disorder (F31.-)
manic episode (F30.-)
recurrent depressive disorder (F33.-)
Excludes ❷: adjustment disorder (F43.2)

CC **F32.0 Major depressive disorder, single episode, mild**

CC **F32.1 Major depressive disorder, single episode, moderate**

CC **F32.2 Major depressive disorder, single episode, severe without psychotic features**

CC **F32.3 Major depressive disorder, single episode, severe with psychotic features**
Single episode of major depression with mood-congruent psychotic symptoms
Single episode of major depression with mood-incongruent psychotic symptoms
Single episode of major depression with psychotic symptoms
Single episode of psychogenic depressive psychosis
Single episode of psychotic depression
Single episode of reactive depressive psychosis

F32.4 Major depressive disorder, single episode, in partial remission

F32.5 Major depressive disorder, single episode, in full remission

F32.8- Other depressive episodes

F32.81 Premenstrual dysphoric disorder — [♀]
Excludes 1: premenstrual tension syndrome (N94.3)

F32.89 Other specified depressive episodes
Atypical depression
Post-schizophrenic depression
Single episode of "masked" depression NOS

F32.9 Major depressive disorder, single episode, unspecified
AHA 13:4Q:p107 – Chronic depression
Depression NOS
Depressive disorder NOS
Major depression NOS

F33- Major depressive disorder, recurrent
Includes: Recurrent episodes of depressive reaction
Recurrent episodes of endogenous depression
Recurrent episodes of major depression
Recurrent episodes of psychogenic depression
Recurrent episodes of reactive depression
Recurrent episodes of seasonal depressive disorder
Recurrent episodes of vital depression
Excludes 1: bipolar disorder (F31.-)
manic episode (F30.-)

CC **F33.0 Major depressive disorder, recurrent, mild**

CC **F33.1 Major depressive disorder, recurrent, moderate**

CC **F33.2 Major depressive disorder, recurrent severe without psychotic features**

CC **F33.3 Major depressive disorder, recurrent, severe with psychotic symptoms**
Endogenous depression with psychotic symptoms
Recurrent severe episodes of major depression with mood-congruent psychotic symptoms
Recurrent severe episodes of major depression with mood-incongruent psychotic symptoms
Recurrent severe episodes of major depression with psychotic symptoms
Recurrent severe episodes of psychogenic depressive psychosis
Recurrent severe episodes of psychotic depression
Recurrent severe episodes of reactive depressive psychosis

F33.4- Major depressive disorder, recurrent, in remission

CC **F33.40 Major depressive disorder, recurrent, in remission, unspecified**

F33.41 Major depressive disorder, recurrent, in partial remission

F33.42 Major depressive disorder, recurrent, in full remission

F31-F33

Excludes 1: = NOT CODED HERE! (Do not code both) Excludes ❷: = Not Included Here

cc **F33.8**   **Other recurrent depressive disorders**
     Recurrent brief depressive episodes

cc **F33.9**   **Major depressive disorder, recurrent, unspecified**
     Monopolar depression NOS

F34-   Persistent mood [affective] disorders

   F34.0   **Cyclothymic disorder**
     Affective personality disorder
     Cycloid personality
     Cyclothymia
     Cyclothymic personality

   F34.1   **Dysthymic disorder**
     Depressive neurosis
     Depressive personality disorder
     Dysthymia
     Neurotic depression
     Persistent anxiety depression
     Persistent depressive disorder

     Excludes ❷: *anxiety depression (mild or not persistent) (F41.8)*

   F34.8-   **Other persistent mood [affective] disorders**

   cc **F34.81**   **Disruptive mood dysregulation disorder**

   cc **F34.89**   **Other specified persistent mood disorders**

   cc **F34.9**   **Persistent mood [affective] disorder, unspecified**

F39   **Unspecified mood [affective] disorder**
     Affective psychosis NOS

Anxiety, dissociative, stress-related, somatoform and other nonpsychotic mental disorders (F40-F48)

F40-   Phobic anxiety disorders

   F40.0-   Agoraphobia

     F40.00   **Agoraphobia, unspecified**

     F40.01   **Agoraphobia with panic disorder**
       Panic disorder with agoraphobia

       Excludes 1:   *panic disorder without agoraphobia (F41.0)*

     F40.02   **Agoraphobia without panic disorder**

   F40.1-   Social phobias
     Anthropophobia
     Social anxiety disorder of childhood
     Social neurosis

     F40.10   **Social phobia, unspecified**

     F40.11   **Social phobia, generalized**

   F40.2-   Specific (isolated) phobias
     Excludes ❷: *dysmorphophobia (nondelusional) (F45.22)*
               nosophobia (F45.22)

     F40.21-   Animal type phobia

       F40.210   **Arachnophobia**
         Fear of spiders

       F40.218   **Other animal type phobia**

     F40.22-   Natural environment type phobia

       F40.220   **Fear of thunderstorms**

       F40.228   **Other natural environment type phobia**

     F40.23-   Blood, injection, injury type phobia

       F40.230   **Fear of blood**

       F40.231   **Fear of injections and transfusions**

       F40.232   **Fear of other medical care**

       F40.233   **Fear of injury**

     F40.24-   Situational type phobia

       F40.240   **Claustrophobia**

       F40.241   **Acrophobia**

       F40.242   **Fear of bridges**

       F40.243   **Fear of flying**

       F40.248   **Other situational type phobia**

     F40.29-   Other specified phobia

       F40.290   **Androphobia**
         Fear of men

       F40.291   **Gynephobia**
         Fear of women

       F40.298   **Other specified phobia**

   F40.8   **Other phobic anxiety disorders**
     Phobic anxiety disorder of childhood

F40.9   **Phobic anxiety disorder, unspecified**
     Phobia NOS
     Phobic state NOS

F41-   Other anxiety disorders
     Excludes ❷: *anxiety in:*
            acute stress reaction (F43.0)
            transient adjustment reaction (F43.2)
            neurasthenia (F48.8)
            psychophysiologic disorders (F45.-)
            separation anxiety (F93.0)

   F41.0   **Panic disorder [episodic paroxysmal anxiety] without agoraphobia**
     Panic attack
     Panic state

     Excludes 1:   *panic disorder with agoraphobia (F40.01)*

   F41.1   **Generalized anxiety disorder**
     Anxiety neurosis
     Anxiety reaction
     Anxiety state
     Overanxious disorder

     Excludes ❷: *neurasthenia (F48.8)*

   F41.3   **Other mixed anxiety disorders**

   F41.8   **Other specified anxiety disorders**
     Anxiety depression (mild or not persistent)
     Anxiety hysteria
     Mixed anxiety and depressive disorder

   F41.9   **Anxiety disorder, unspecified**
     Anxiety NOS

F42-   Obsessive-compulsive disorder
     Excludes ❷: *obsessive-compulsive personality (disorder) (F60.5)*
            obsessive-compulsive symptoms occurring in depression (F32-F33)
            obsessive-compulsive symptoms occurring in schizophrenia (F20.-)

   F42.2   **Mixed obsessional thoughts and acts**

   F42.3   **Hoarding disorder**

   F42.4   **Excoriation (skin-picking) disorder**

     Excludes 1:   *factitial dermatitis (L98.1)*
            other specified behavioral and emotional disorders with onset usually occurring in early childhood and adolescence (F98.8)

   F42.8   **Other obsessive-compulsive disorder**
     Anancastic neurosis
     Obsessive-compulsive neurosis

   F42.9   **Obsessive-compulsive disorder, unspecified**

F43-   Reaction to severe stress, and adjustment disorders

   F43.0   **Acute stress reaction**
     Acute crisis reaction
     Acute reaction to stress
     Combat and operational stress reaction
     Combat fatigue
     Crisis state
     Psychic shock

   F43.1-   Post-traumatic stress disorder (PTSD)
     Traumatic neurosis

     F43.10   **Post-traumatic stress disorder, unspecified**

     F43.11   **Post-traumatic stress disorder, acute**

     F43.12   **Post-traumatic stress disorder, chronic**

   F43.2-   Adjustment disorders
     Culture shock
     Grief reaction
     Hospitalism in children

     Excludes ❷: *separation anxiety disorder of childhood (F93.0)*

     F43.20   **Adjustment disorder, unspecified**

     F43.21   **Adjustment disorder with depressed mood**
       AHA 14:1Q:p25 – Complicated bereavement

     F43.22   **Adjustment disorder with anxiety**

     F43.23   **Adjustment disorder with mixed anxiety and depressed mood**

     F43.24   **Adjustment disorder with disturbance of conduct**

     F43.25   **Adjustment disorder with mixed disturbance of emotions and conduct**

     F43.29   **Adjustment disorder with other symptoms**

F33 - F43 *(side tab)*

F43.8   Other reactions to severe stress
Other specified trauma and stressor-related disorder

F43.9   Reaction to severe stress, unspecified
Trauma and stressor-related disorder, NOS

F44-   Dissociative and conversion disorders
Includes: Conversion hysteria
Conversion reaction
Hysteria
Hysterical psychosis
Excludes ❷: malingering [conscious simulation] (Z76.5)

F44.0   Dissociative amnesia
Excludes 1:   amnesia NOS (R41.3)
anterograde amnesia (R41.1)
dissociative amnesia with dissociative fugue (F44.1)
retrograde amnesia (R41.2)
Excludes ❷: alcohol-or other psychoactive substance-induced
amnestic disorder (F10, F13, F19 with .26, .96)
amnestic disorder due to known physiological condition
(F04)
postictal amnesia in epilepsy (G40.-)

F44.1   Dissociative fugue
Dissociative amnesia with dissociative fugue
Excludes ❷: postictal fugue in epilepsy (G40.-)

F44.2   Dissociative stupor
Excludes 1:   catatonic stupor (R40.1)
stupor NOS (R40.1)
Excludes ❷: catatonic disorder due to known physiological condition
(F06.1)
depressive stupor (F32, F33)
manic stupor (F30, F31)

F44.4   Conversion disorder with motor symptom or deficit
Dissociative motor disorders
Psychogenic aphonia
Psychogenic dysphonia

F44.5   Conversion disorder with seizures or convulsions
Dissociative convulsions

F44.6   Conversion disorder with sensory symptom or deficit
Dissociative anesthesia and sensory loss
Psychogenic deafness

F44.7   Conversion disorder with mixed symptom presentation

F44.8-   Other dissociative and conversion disorders

F44.81   Dissociative identity disorder
Multiple personality disorder

F44.89   Other dissociative and conversion disorders
Ganser's syndrome
Psychogenic confusion
Psychogenic twilight state
Trance and possession disorders

F44.9   Dissociative and conversion disorder, unspecified
Dissociative disorder NOS

F45-   Somatoform disorders
Excludes ❷: dissociative and conversion disorders (F44.-)
factitious disorders (F68.1-)
hair-plucking (F63.3)
lalling (F80.0)
lisping (F80.0)
malingering [conscious simulation] (Z76.5)
nail-biting (F98.8)
psychological or behavioral factors associated with disorders
or diseases classified elsewhere (F54)
sexual dysfunction, not due to a substance or known
physiological condition (F52.-)
thumb-sucking (F98.8)
tic disorders (in childhood and adolescence) (F95.-)
Tourette's syndrome (F95.2)
trichotillomania (F63.3)

F45.0   Somatization disorder
Briquet's disorder
Multiple psychosomatic disorder

F45.1   Undifferentiated somatoform disorder
Somatic symptom disorder
Undifferentiated psychosomatic disorder

F45.2-   Hypochondriacal disorders
Excludes ❷: delusional dysmorphophobia (F22)
fixed delusions about bodily functions or shape (F22)

F45.20   Hypochondriacal disorder, unspecified

F45.21   Hypochondriasis
Hypochondriacal neurosis
Illness anxiety disorder

F45.22   Body dysmorphic disorder
Dysmorphophobia (nondelusional)
Nosophobia

F45.29   Other hypochondriacal disorders

F45.4-   Pain disorders related to psychological factors
Excludes 1:   pain NOS (R52)

F45.41   Pain disorder exclusively related to psychological factors
Somatoform pain disorder (persistent)

F45.42   Pain disorder with related psychological factors
Code also associated acute or chronic pain (G89.-)

F45.8   Other somatoform disorders
Psychogenic dysmenorrhea
Psychogenic dysphagia, including "globus hystericus"
Psychogenic pruritus
Psychogenic torticollis
Somatoform autonomic dysfunction
Teeth grinding
Excludes 1:   sleep related teeth grinding (G47.63)

F45.9   Somatoform disorder, unspecified
Psychosomatic disorder NOS

F48-   Other nonpsychotic mental disorders

F48.1   Depersonalization-derealization syndrome

F48.2   Pseudobulbar affect
Involuntary emotional expression disorder
Code first underlying cause, if known, such as:
Amyotrophic lateral sclerosis (G12.21)
Multiple sclerosis (G35)
Sequelae of cerebrovascular disease (I69-)
Sequelae of traumatic intracranial injury (S06-)

F48.8   Other specified nonpsychotic mental disorders
Dhat syndrome
Neurasthenia
Occupational neurosis, including writer's cramp
Psychasthenia
Psychasthenic neurosis
Psychogenic syncope

F48.9   Nonpsychotic mental disorder, unspecified
Neurosis NOS

Behavioral syndromes associated with physiological disturbances and physical factors (F50-F59)

F50-   Eating disorders
Excludes 1:   anorexia NOS (R63.0)
feeding difficulties (R63.3)
polyphagia (R63.2)
Excludes ❷: feeding disorder in infancy or childhood (F98.2-)

F50.0-   Anorexia nervosa
Excludes 1:   loss of appetite (R63.0)
psychogenic loss of appetite (F50.89)

cc **F50.00   Anorexia nervosa, unspecified**

cc **F50.01   Anorexia nervosa, restricting type**

cc **F50.02   Anorexia nervosa, binge eating/purging type**
Excludes 1:   bulimia nervosa (F50.2)

cc **F50.2   Bulimia nervosa**
Bulimia NOS
Hyperorexia nervosa
Excludes 1:   anorexia nervosa, binge eating/purging type (F50.02)

F50.8-   Other eating disorders
Excludes ❷: pica of infancy and childhood (F98.3)

F50.81   Binge eating disorder

F50.89   Other specified eating disorder
Pica in adults
Psychogenic loss of appetite

F50.9   Eating disorder, unspecified
Atypical anorexia nervosa
Atypical bulimia nervosa

Excludes 1: = NOT CODED HERE! (Do not code both)   **646**   *Excludes ❷:* = Not Included Here

F
4
3
-
F
5
0

F51- <u>Sleep disorders</u> <u>not</u> due to a substance or known physiological condition

Excludes ❷: organic sleep disorders (G47.-)

F51.0- <u>Insomnia</u> not due to a substance or known physiological condition

Excludes ❷: alcohol related insomnia (F10.182, F10.282, F10.982)
drug-related insomnia (F11.182, F11.282, F11.982, F13.182, F13.282, F13.982, F14.182, F14.282, F14.982, F15.182, F15.282, F15.982, F19.182, F19.282, F19.982)
insomnia NOS (G47.0-)
insomnia due to known physiological condition (G47.0-)
organic insomnia (G47.0-)
sleep deprivation (Z72.820)

F51.01 <u>Primary</u> insomnia
Idiopathic insomnia

F51.02 <u>Adjustment</u> insomnia

F51.03 <u>Paradoxical</u> insomnia

F51.04 <u>Psychophysiologic</u> insomnia

F51.05 Insomnia due to other mental disorder
Code also associated mental disorder

F51.09 Other insomnia not due to a substance or known physiological condition

F51.1- <u>Hypersomnia</u> not due to a substance or known physiological condition

Excludes ❷: alcohol related hypersomnia (F10.182, F10.282, F10.982)
drug-related hypersomnia (F11.182, F11.282, F11.982, F13.182, F13.282, F13.982, F14.182, F14.282, F14.982, F15.182, F15.282, F15.982, F19.182, F19.282, F19.982)
hypersomnia NOS (G47.10)
hypersomnia due to known physiological condition (G47.10)
idiopathic hypersomnia (G47.11, G47.12)
narcolepsy (G47.4-)

F51.11 <u>Primary</u> hypersomnia

F51.12 <u>Insufficient</u> sleep syndrome
Excludes 1:   sleep deprivation (Z72.820)

F51.13 Hypersomnia due to other mental disorder
Code also associated mental disorder

F51.19 Other hypersomnia not due to a substance or known physiological condition

F51.3 Sleepwalking [somnambulism]

F51.4 Sleep terrors [night terrors]

F51.5 Nightmare disorder
Dream anxiety disorder

F51.8 Other sleep disorders not due to a substance or known physiological condition

F51.9 Sleep disorder not due to a substance or known physiological condition, unspecified
Emotional sleep disorder NOS

F52- <u>Sexual dysfunction</u> <u>not</u> due to a substance or known physiological condition

Excludes ❷: Dhat syndrome (F48.8)

F52.0 Hypoactive sexual desire disorder
Lack or loss of sexual desire
Sexual anhedonia
Excludes 1:   decreased libido (R68.82)

F52.1 Sexual aversion disorder
Sexual aversion and lack of sexual enjoyment

F52.2- Sexual arousal disorders
Failure of genital response

F52.21 Male erectile disorder — [♂]
Psychogenic impotence
Excludes 1:   impotence of organic origin (N52.-)
impotence NOS (N52.-)

F52.22 Female sexual arousal disorder — [♀]

F52.3- Orgasmic disorder
Inhibited orgasm
Psychogenic anorgasmy

F52.31 Female orgasmic disorder — [♀]

F52.32 Male orgasmic disorder — [♂]
Delayed ejaculation

F52.4 Premature ejaculation — [♂]

F52.5 Vaginismus not due to a substance or known physiological condition — [♀]
Psychogenic vaginismus
Excludes ❷: vaginismus (due to a known physiological condition) (N94.2)

F52.6 Dyspareunia not due to a substance or known physiological condition — [♀]
Genito-pelvic pain penetration disorder
Psychogenic dyspareunia
Excludes ❷: dyspareunia (due to a known physiological condition) (N94.1-)

F52.8 Other sexual dysfunction not due to a substance or known physiological condition
Excessive sexual drive
Nymphomania
Satyriasis

F52.9 Unspecified sexual dysfunction not due to a substance or known physiological condition — [Unacceptable PDX]
Sexual dysfunction NOS

F53 <u>Puerperal psychosis</u> — [♀, Age/12-55]
Postpartum depression
Excludes 1:   mood disorders with psychotic features (F30.2, F31.2, F31.5, F31.64, F32.3, F33.3)
postpartum dysphoria (O90.6)
psychosis in schizophrenia, schizotypal, delusional, and other psychotic disorders (F20-F29)

F54 Psychological and behavioral factors associated with disorders or diseases classified elsewhere — [Not Allowed as PDX]
Psychological factors affecting physical conditions
Code first the associated physical disorder, such as:
Asthma (J45.-)
Dermatitis (L23-L25)
Gastric ulcer (K25.-)
Mucous colitis (K58.-)
Ulcerative colitis (K51.-)
Urticaria (L50.-)
Excludes ❷: tension-type headache (G44.2)

F55- Abuse of non-psychoactive substances
Excludes ❷: abuse of psychoactive substances (F10-F19)

F55.0 Abuse of antacids

F55.1 Abuse of herbal or folk remedies

F55.2 Abuse of laxatives

F55.3 Abuse of steroids or hormones

F55.4 Abuse of vitamins

F55.8 Abuse of other non-psychoactive substances

F59 Unspecified behavioral syndromes associated with physiological disturbances and physical factors
Psychogenic physiological dysfunction NOS

Disorders of adult personality and behavior (F60-F69)

F60- <u>Specific personality disorders</u>

F60.0 Paranoid personality disorder
Expansive paranoid personality (disorder)
Fanatic personality (disorder)
Querulant personality (disorder)
Paranoid personality (disorder)
Sensitive paranoid personality (disorder)
Excludes ❷: paranoia (F22)
paranoia querulans (F22)
paranoid psychosis (F22)
paranoid schizophrenia (F20.0)
paranoid state (F22)

F60.1 Schizoid personality disorder
Excludes ❷: Asperger's syndrome (F84.5)
delusional disorder (F22)
schizoid disorder of childhood (F84.5)
schizophrenia (F20.-)
schizotypal disorder (F21)

F51-F60

F60.2   Antisocial personality disorder
    Amoral personality (disorder)
    Asocial personality (disorder)
    Dissocial personality disorder
    Psychopathic personality (disorder)
    Sociopathic personality (disorder)
    Excludes 1:   conduct disorders (F91.-)
    Excludes ❷: borderline personality disorder (F60.3)

F60.3   Borderline personality disorder
    Aggressive personality (disorder)
    Emotionally unstable personality disorder
    Explosive personality (disorder)
    Excludes ❷: antisocial personality disorder (F60.2)

F60.4   Histrionic personality disorder
    Hysterical personality (disorder)
    Psychoinfantile personality (disorder)

F60.5   Obsessive-compulsive personality disorder
    Anankastic personality (disorder)
    Compulsive personality (disorder)
    Obsessional personality (disorder)
    Excludes ❷: obsessive-compulsive disorder (F42.-)

F60.6   Avoidant personality disorder
    Anxious personality disorder

F60.7   Dependent personality disorder
    Asthenic personality (disorder)
    Inadequate personality (disorder)
    Passive personality (disorder)

F60.8-   Other specific personality disorders

    F60.81   Narcissistic personality disorder

    F60.89   Other specific personality disorders
        Eccentric personality disorder
        "Haltlose" type personality disorder
        Immature personality disorder
        Passive-aggressive personality disorder
        Psychoneurotic personality disorder
        Self-defeating personality disorder

F60.9   Personality disorder, unspecified
    Character disorder NOS
    Character neurosis NOS
    Pathological personality NOS

F63-   Impulse disorders
    *Excludes ❷: habitual excessive use of alcohol or psychoactive substances
                (F10-F19)
            impulse disorders involving sexual behavior (F65.-)*

F63.0   Pathological gambling
    Compulsive gambling
    Excludes 1:   gambling and betting NOS (Z72.6)
    *Excludes ❷: excessive gambling by manic patients (F30, F31)
            gambling in antisocial personality disorder (F60.2)*

F63.1   Pyromania
    Pathological fire-setting
    *Excludes ❷: fire-setting (by) (in):
                adult with antisocial personality disorder (F60.2)
                alcohol or psychoactive substance intoxication (F10-
                F19)
                conduct disorders (F91.-)
                mental disorders due to known physiological
                condition (F01-F09)
                schizophrenia (F20.-)*

F63.2   Kleptomania
    Pathological stealing
    *Excludes 1:   shoplifting as the reason for observation for suspected
                mental disorder (Z03.8)*
    *Excludes ❷: depressive disorder with stealing (F31-F33)
                stealing due to underlying mental condition-code to
                mental condition
                stealing in mental disorders due to known physiological
                condition (F01-F09)*

F63.3   Trichotillomania
    Hair plucking
    Excludes ❷: other stereotyped movement disorder (F98.4)

F63.8-   Other impulse disorders

    F63.81   Intermittent explosive disorder

    F63.89   Other impulse disorders

F63.9   Impulse disorder, unspecified
    Impulse control disorder NOS

F64-   Gender identity disorders

F64.0   Transsexualism
    Gender identity disorder in adolescence and adulthood
    Gender dysphoria in adolescence and adults

F64.1   Dual role transvestism
    Use additional code to identify sex reassignment status (Z87.890)
    Excludes 1:   gender identity disorder in childhood (F64.2)
    Excludes ❷: fetishistic transvestism (F65.1)

F64.2   Gender identity disorder of childhood — [Age/0-17]
    Gender dysphoria in children
    *Excludes 1:   gender identity disorder in adolescence and adulthood
                (F64.0)*
    Excludes ❷: sexual maturation disorder (F66)

F64.8   Other gender identity disorders

F64.9   Gender identity disorder, unspecified
    Gender-role disorder NOS

F65-   Paraphilias

F65.0   Fetishism

F65.1   Transvestic fetishism
    Fetishistic transvestism

F65.2   Exhibitionism

F65.3   Voyeurism

F65.4   Pedophilia

F65.5-   Sadomasochism

    F65.50   Sadomasochism, unspecified

    F65.51   Sexual masochism

    F65.52   Sexual sadism

F65.8-   Other paraphilias

    F65.81   Frotteurism

    F65.89   Other paraphilias
        Necrophilia

F65.9   Paraphilia, unspecified
    Sexual deviation NOS

F66   Other sexual disorders
    Sexual maturation disorder
    Sexual relationship disorder

F68-   Other disorders of adult personality and behavior

    F68.1-   Factitious disorder
        Compensation neurosis
        Elaboration of physical symptoms for psychological reasons
        Hospital hopper syndrome
        Münchausen's syndrome
        Peregrinating patient
        *Excludes ❷: factitial dermatitis (L98.1)
                    person feigning illness (with obvious motivation)
                    (Z76.5)*

    cc **F68.10   Factitious disorder, unspecified**

        **F68.11   Factitious disorder with predominantly _psychological_
                signs and symptoms**

    cc **F68.12   Factitious disorder with predominantly _physical_ signs and
                symptoms**

        **F68.13   Factitious disorder with _combined_ psychological and
                physical signs and symptoms**

    F68.8   Other specified disorders of adult personality and behavior

F69   Unspecified disorder of adult personality and behavior — [Age/15-124]

Intellectual disabilities (F70-F79)

Code first any associated physical or developmental disorders
    Excludes 1:   borderline intellectual functioning, IQ above 70 to 84 (R41.83)

F70   Mild intellectual disabilities
    IQ level 50-55 to approximately 70
    Mild mental subnormality

F71   Moderate intellectual disabilities
    IQ level 35-40 to 50-55
    Moderate mental subnormality

F72   Severe intellectual disabilities
cc   IQ 20-25 to 35-40
    Severe mental subnormality

F73   Profound intellectual disabilities
cc   IQ level below 20-25
    Profound mental subnormality

Excludes 1: = NOT CODED HERE! (Do not code both)   **648**   *Excludes ❷:* = Not Included Here

F
6
0
-
F
7
3

F78   Other intellectual disabilities

F79   Unspecified intellectual disabilities
     Mental deficiency NOS
     Mental subnormality NOS

Pervasive and specific developmental disorders (F80-F89)

F80-   Specific developmental disorders of speech and language

     F80.0   **Phonological disorder**
         Dyslalia
         Functional speech articulation disorder
         Lalling
         Lisping
         Phonological developmental disorder
         Speech articulation developmental disorder
         Speech-sound disorder

         Excludes 1:   *speech articulation impairment due to aphasia NOS (R47.01)*
                        speech articulation impairment due to apraxia (R48.2)

         Excludes ❷: *speech articulation impairment due to hearing loss (F80.4)*
                        speech articulation impairment due to intellectual disabilities (F70-F79)
                        speech articulation impairment with expressive language developmental disorder (F80.1)
                        speech articulation impairment with mixed receptive expressive language developmental disorder (F80.2)

     F80.1   **Expressive language disorder**
         Developmental dysphasia or aphasia, expressive type
         Excludes 1:   *mixed receptive-expressive language disorder (F80.2)*
                        dysphasia and aphasia NOS (R47.-)
         Excludes ❷: *acquired aphasia with epilepsy [Landau-Kleffner] (G40.80-)*
                        intellectual disabilities (F70-F79)
                        pervasive developmental disorders (F84.-)
                        selective mutism (F94.0)

     F80.2   **Mixed receptive-expressive language disorder**
         Developmental dysphasia or aphasia, receptive type
         Developmental Wernicke's aphasia
         Excludes 1:   *central auditory processing disorder (H93.25)*
                        dysphasia or aphasia NOS (R47.-)
                        expressive language disorder (F80.1)
                        expressive type dysphasia or aphasia (F80.1)
                        word deafness (H93.25)
         Excludes ❷: *acquired aphasia with epilepsy [Landau-Kleffner] (G40.80-)*
                        intellectual disabilities (F70-F79)
                        pervasive developmental disorders (F84.-)
                        selective mutism (F94.0)

     F80.4   **Speech and language development delay due to hearing loss**
         Code also type of hearing loss (H90.-, H91.-)

     F80.8-   Other developmental disorders of speech and language

         F80.81   **Childhood onset fluency disorder**
              Cluttering NOS
              Stuttering NOS
              Excludes 1:   *adult onset fluency disorder (F98.5)*
                            fluency disorder in conditions classified elsewhere (R47.82)
                            fluency disorder (stuttering) following cerebrovascular disease (I69. with final characters -23)

         F80.82   **Social pragmatic communication disorder**
              Excludes 1:   *Asperger's syndrome (F84.5)*
                            autistic disorder (F84.0)

         F80.89   Other developmental disorders of speech and language

     F80.9   **Developmental disorder of speech and language, unspecified**
         Communication disorder NOS
         Language disorder NOS

F81-   Specific developmental disorders of scholastic skills

     F81.0   **Specific reading disorder**
         "Backward reading"
         Developmental dyslexia
         Specific reading retardation
         Excludes 1:   *alexia NOS (R48.0)*
                        dyslexia NOS (R48.0)

     F81.2   **Mathematics disorder**
         Developmental acalculia
         Developmental arithmetical disorder
         Developmental Gerstmann's syndrome
         Excludes 1:   *acalculia NOS (R48.8)*
         Excludes ❷: *arithmetical difficulties associated with a reading disorder (F81.0)*
                        arithmetical difficulties associated with a spelling disorder (F81.81)
                        arithmetical difficulties due to inadequate teaching (Z55.8)

     F81.8-   Other developmental disorders of scholastic skills

         F81.81   **Disorder of written expression**
              Specific spelling disorder

         F81.89   Other developmental disorders of scholastic skills

     F81.9   **Developmental disorder of scholastic skills, unspecified** —
         [Unacceptable PDX]
         Knowledge acquisition disability NOS
         Learning disability NOS
         Learning disorder NOS

F82   Specific developmental disorder of motor function
     Clumsy child syndrome
     Developmental coordination disorder
     Developmental dyspraxia
     Excludes 1:   *abnormalities of gait and mobility (R26.-)*
                    lack of coordination (R27.-)
     Excludes ❷: *lack of coordination secondary to intellectual disabilities (F70-F79)*

F84-   Pervasive developmental disorders
     Use additional code to identify any associated medical condition and intellectual disabilities

     cc **F84.0**   **Autistic disorder**
         Autism spectrum disorder
         Infantile autism
         Infantile psychosis
         Kanner's syndrome
         Excludes 1:   *Asperger's syndrome (F84.5)*

     cc **F84.2**   **Rett's syndrome**
         Excludes 1:   *Asperger's syndrome (F84.5)*
                        autistic disorder (F84.0)
                        other childhood disintegrative disorder (F84.3)

     cc **F84.3**   **Other childhood disintegrative disorder** — [Age/0-17]
         Dementia infantilis
         Disintegrative psychosis
         Heller's syndrome
         Symbiotic psychosis
     Use additional code to identify any associated neurological condition
         Excludes 1:   *Asperger's syndrome (F84.5)*
                        autistic disorder (F84.0)
                        Rett's syndrome (F84.2)

     cc **F84.5**   **Asperger's syndrome**
         Asperger's disorder
         Autistic psychopathy
         Schizoid disorder of childhood

     cc **F84.8**   **Other pervasive developmental disorders**
         Overactive disorder associated with intellectual disabilities and stereotyped movements

     cc **F84.9**   **Pervasive developmental disorder, unspecified**
         Atypical autism

F88   Other disorders of psychological development
     Developmental agnosia
     Global developmental delay
     Other specified neurodevelopmental disorder

F89   Unspecified disorder of psychological development
     Developmental disorder NOS
     Neurodevelopmental disorder NOS

F78 - F89

Behavioral and emotional disorders with onset usually occurring in childhood and adolescence (F90-F98)

Note: Codes within categories F90-F98 may be used regardless of the age of a patient. These disorders generally have onset within the childhood or adolescent years, but may continue throughout life or not be diagnosed until adulthood.

F90- **Attention-deficit hyperactivity disorders**

    Includes: Attention deficit disorder with hyperactivity
                     Attention deficit syndrome with hyperactivity

    Excludes ❷: *anxiety disorders (F40.-, F41.-)*
                         mood [affective] disorders (F30-F39)
                         pervasive developmental disorders (F84.-)
                         schizophrenia (F20.-)

F90.0 Attention-deficit hyperactivity disorder, predominantly <u>inattentive</u> type

F90.1 Attention-deficit hyperactivity disorder, predominantly <u>hyperactive</u> type

F90.2 Attention-deficit hyperactivity disorder, <u>combined</u> type

F90.8 Attention-deficit hyperactivity disorder, other type

F90.9 Attention-deficit hyperactivity disorder, unspecified type
    Attention-deficit hyperactivity disorder of childhood or adolescence NOS
    Attention-deficit hyperactivity disorder NOS

F91- **Conduct disorders**

    Excludes 1:   *antisocial behavior (Z72.81-)*
                  antisocial personality disorder (F60.2)

    Excludes ❷: *conduct problems associated with attention-deficit hyperactivity disorder (F90.-)*
                  mood [affective] disorders (F30-F39)
                  pervasive developmental disorders (F84.-)
                  schizophrenia (F20.-)

F91.0 Conduct disorder <u>confined to family context</u>

F91.1 Conduct disorder, <u>childhood-onset</u> type
    Unsocialized conduct disorder
    Conduct disorder, solitary aggressive type
    Unsocialized aggressive disorder

F91.2 Conduct disorder, <u>adolescent-onset</u> type
    Socialized conduct disorder
    Conduct disorder, group type

F91.3 <u>Oppositional defiant</u> disorder

F91.8 Other conduct disorders
    Other specified conduct disorder
    Other specified disruptive disorder

F91.9 Conduct disorder, unspecified
    Behavioral disorder NOS
    Conduct disorder NOS
    Disruptive behavior disorder NOS
    Disruptive disorder NOS

F93- **Emotional disorders with onset specific to childhood**

F93.0 Separation anxiety disorder of childhood
    Excludes ❷: *mood [affective] disorders (F30-F39)*
                  nonpsychotic mental disorders (F40-F48)
                  phobic anxiety disorder of childhood (F40.8)
                  social phobia (F40.1)

F93.8 Other childhood emotional disorders
    Identity disorder
    Excludes ❷: *gender identity disorder of childhood (F64.2)*

F93.9 Childhood emotional disorder, unspecified

F94- **Disorders of social functioning with onset specific to childhood and adolescence**

F94.0 Selective mutism
    Elective mutism
    Excludes ❷: *pervasive developmental disorders (F84.-)*
                  schizophrenia (F20.-)
                  specific developmental disorders of speech and language (F80.-)
                  transient mutism as part of separation anxiety in young children (F93.0)

F94.1 Reactive attachment disorder of childhood
    Use additional code to identify any associated failure to thrive or growth retardation
    Excludes 1:   *disinhibited attachment disorder of childhood (F94.2)*
                normal variation in pattern of selective attachment
    Excludes ❷: *Asperger's syndrome (F84.5)*
                  maltreatment syndromes (T74.-)
                  sexual or physical abuse in childhood, resulting in psychosocial problems (Z62.81-)

F94.2 Disinhibited attachment disorder of childhood
    Affectionless psychopathy
    Institutional syndrome
    Excludes 1:   *reactive attachment disorder of childhood (F94.1)*
    Excludes ❷: *Asperger's syndrome (F84.5)*
                  attention-deficit hyperactivity disorders (F90.-)
                  hospitalism in children (F43.2-)

F94.8 Other childhood disorders of social functioning

F94.9 Childhood disorder of social functioning, unspecified

F95- **Tic disorder**

F95.0 Transient tic disorder
    Provisional tic disorder

F95.1 Chronic motor or vocal tic disorder

F95.2 Tourette's disorder
    Combined vocal and multiple motor tic disorder [de la Tourette]
    Tourette's syndrome

F95.8 Other tic disorders

F95.9 Tic disorder, unspecified
    Tic NOS

F98- **Other behavioral and emotional disorders with onset usually occurring in childhood and adolescence**
    Excludes ❷: *breath-holding spells (R06.89)*
                  gender identity disorder of childhood (F64.2)
                  Kleine-Levin syndrome (G47.13)
                  obsessive-compulsive disorder (F42.-)
                  sleep disorders not due to a substance or known physiological condition (F51.-)

F98.0 Enuresis <u>not</u> due to a substance or known physiological condition
    Enuresis (primary) (secondary) of nonorganic origin
    Functional enuresis
    Psychogenic enuresis
    Urinary incontinence of nonorganic origin
    Excludes 1:   *enuresis NOS (R32)*

F98.1 Encopresis <u>not</u> due to a substance or known physiological condition
    Functional encopresis
    Incontinence of feces of nonorganic origin
    Psychogenic encopresis
    Use additional code to identify the cause of any coexisting constipation
    Excludes 1:   *encopresis NOS (R15.-)*

F98.2- Other feeding disorders of infancy and childhood
    Excludes 1:   *feeding difficulties (R63.3)*
    Excludes ❷: *anorexia nervosa and other eating disorders (F50.-)*
                  feeding problems of newborn (P92.-)
                  pica of infancy or childhood (F98.3)

F98.21 Rumination disorder of infancy

F98.29 Other feeding disorders of infancy and early childhood

F98.3 Pica of infancy and childhood

F98.4　**Stereotyped movement disorders**
　　　　Stereotype/habit disorder
　　Excludes 1:　abnormal involuntary movements (R25.-)
　　Excludes ❷:　compulsions in obsessive-compulsive disorder (F42.-)
　　　　　　　　hair plucking (F63.3)
　　　　　　　　movement disorders of organic origin (G20-G25)
　　　　　　　　nail-biting (F98.8)
　　　　　　　　nose-picking (F98.8)
　　　　　　　　stereotypies that are part of a broader psychiatric
　　　　　　　　　　condition (F01-F95)
　　　　　　　　thumb-sucking (F98.8)
　　　　　　　　tic disorders (F95.-)
　　　　　　　　trichotillomania (F63.3)

F98.5　**Adult onset fluency disorder**
　　Excludes 1:　childhood onset fluency disorder (F80.81)
　　　　　　　　dysphasia (R47.02)
　　　　　　　　fluency disorder in conditions classified elsewhere
　　　　　　　　　　(R47.82)
　　　　　　　　fluency disorder (stuttering) following cerebrovascular
　　　　　　　　　　disease (I69. with final characters -23)
　　　　　　　　tic disorders (F95.-)

F98.8　**Other specified behavioral and emotional disorders with
　　　　onset usually occurring in childhood and adolescence**
　　　　Excessive masturbation
　　　　Nail-biting
　　　　Nose-picking
　　　　Thumb-sucking

F98.9　**Unspecified behavioral and emotional disorders with onset
　　　　usually occurring in childhood and adolescence**

Unspecified mental disorder (F99)

F99　**Mental disorder, not otherwise specified**
　　　Mental illness NOS
　　Excludes 1:　unspecified mental disorder due to known physiological
　　　　　　　　condition (F09)

F
9
9
–
F
9
9

Chapter 6 – Diseases of the nervous system (G00-G99)

Excludes ❷: certain conditions originating in the perinatal period (P04-P96)
certain infectious and parasitic diseases (A00-B99)
complications of pregnancy, childbirth and the puerperium (O00-O9A)
congenital malformations, deformations, and chromosomal abnormalities (Q00-Q99)
endocrine, nutritional and metabolic diseases (E00-E88)
injury, poisoning and certain other consequences of external causes (S00-T88)
neoplasms (C00-D49)
symptoms, signs and abnormal clinical and laboratory findings, not elsewhere classified (R00-R94)

This chapter contains the following blocks:

G00-G09	Inflammatory diseases of the central nervous system
G10-G14	Systemic atrophies primarily affecting the central nervous system
G20-G26	Extrapyramidal and movement disorders
G30-G32	Other degenerative diseases of the nervous system
G35-G37	Demyelinating diseases of the central nervous system
G40-G47	Episodic and paroxysmal disorders
G50-G59	Nerve, nerve root and plexus disorders
G60-G65	Polyneuropathies and other disorders of the peripheral nervous system
G70-G73	Diseases of myoneural junction and muscle
G80-G83	Cerebral palsy and other paralytic syndromes
G89-G99	Other disorders of the nervous system

Chapter-Specific Coding Guidelines

C.   Chapter-Specific Coding Guidelines

In addition to general coding guidelines, there are guidelines for specific diagnoses and/or conditions in the classification. Unless otherwise indicated, these guidelines apply to all health care settings. Please refer to Section II for guidelines on the selection of principal diagnosis.

6.   Chapter 6: Diseases of Nervous System and Sense Organs (G00-G99)

a.   Dominant/nondominant side

Codes from category G81, Hemiplegia and hemiparesis, and subcategories, G83.1, Monoplegia of lower limb, G83.2, Monoplegia of upper limb, and G83.3, Monoplegia, unspecified, identify whether the dominant or nondominant side is affected. Should the affected side be documented, but not specified as dominant or nondominant, and the classification system does not indicate a default, code selection is as follows:
• For ambidextrous patients, the default should be dominant.
• If the left side is affected, the default is non-dominant.
• If the right side is affected, the default is dominant.

b.   Pain - Category G89

1)   General coding information

Codes in category G89, Pain, not elsewhere classified, may be used in conjunction with codes from other categories and chapters to provide more detail about acute or chronic pain and neoplasm-related pain, unless otherwise indicated below.

If the pain is not specified as acute or chronic, post-thoracotomy, postprocedural, or neoplasm-related, do not assign codes from category G89.

A code from category G89 should not be assigned if the underlying (definitive) diagnosis is known, unless the reason for the encounter is pain control/management and not management of the underlying condition.

When an admission or encounter is for a procedure aimed at treating the underlying condition (e.g., spinal fusion, kyphoplasty), a code for the underlying condition (e.g., vertebral fracture, spinal stenosis) should be assigned as the principal diagnosis. No code from category G89 should be assigned.

(a)   Category G89 Codes as Principal or First-Listed Diagnosis

Category G89 codes are acceptable as principal diagnosis or the first-listed code:
• When pain control or pain management is the reason for the admission/encounter (e.g., a patient with displaced intervertebral disc, nerve impingement and severe back pain presents for injection of steroid into the spinal canal). The underlying cause of the pain should be reported as an additional diagnosis, if known.

• When a patient is admitted for the insertion of a neurostimulator for pain control, assign the appropriate pain code as the principal or first-listed diagnosis. When an admission or encounter is for a procedure aimed at treating the underlying condition and a neurostimulator is inserted for pain control during the same admission/encounter, a code for the underlying condition should be assigned as the principal diagnosis and the appropriate pain code should be assigned as a secondary diagnosis.

(b)   Use of Category G89 Codes in Conjunction with Site Specific Pain Codes

(i)   Assigning Category G89 and Site-Specific Pain Codes

Codes from category G89 may be used in conjunction with codes that identify the site of pain (including codes from chapter 18) if the category G89 code provides additional information. For example, if the code describes the site of the pain, but does not fully describe whether the pain is acute or chronic, then both codes should be assigned.

(ii)   Sequencing of Category G89 Codes with Site-Specific Pain Codes

The sequencing of category G89 codes with site-specific pain codes (including chapter 18 codes), is dependent on the circumstances of the encounter/admission as follows:
• If the encounter is for pain control or pain management, assign the code from category G89 followed by the code identifying the specific site of pain (e.g., encounter for pain management for acute neck pain from trauma is assigned code G89.11, Acute pain due to trauma, followed by code M54.2, Cervicalgia, to identify the site of pain).

• If the encounter is for any other reason except pain control or pain management, and a related definitive diagnosis has not been established (confirmed) by the provider, assign the code for the specific site of pain first, followed by the appropriate code from category G89.

2)   Pain due to devices, implants and grafts
See Section I.C.19. Pain due to medical devices.

3)   Postoperative Pain

The provider's documentation should be used to guide the coding of postoperative pain, as well as *Section III. Reporting Additional Diagnoses and Section IV. Diagnostic Coding and Reporting in the Outpatient Setting.*

The default for post-thoracotomy and other postoperative pain not specified as acute or chronic is the code for the acute form.

Routine or expected postoperative pain immediately after surgery should not be coded.

(a)   Postoperative pain not associated with specific postoperative complication

Postoperative pain not associated with a specific postoperative complication is assigned to the appropriate postoperative pain code in category G89.

(b)   Postoperative pain associated with specific postoperative complication

Postoperative pain associated with a specific postoperative complication (such as painful wire sutures) is assigned to the appropriate code(s) found in Chapter 19, Injury, poisoning, and certain other consequences of external causes. If appropriate, use additional code(s) from category G89 to identify acute or chronic pain (G89.18 or G89.28).

4)   Chronic pain

Chronic pain is classified to subcategory G89.2. There is no time frame defining when pain becomes chronic pain. The provider's documentation should be used to guide use of these codes.

5)   Neoplasm Related Pain

Code G89.3 is assigned to pain documented as being related, associated or due to cancer, primary or secondary malignancy, or tumor. This code is assigned regardless of whether the pain is acute or chronic.

This code may be assigned as the principal or first-listed code when the stated reason for the admission/encounter is documented as pain control/pain management. The underlying neoplasm should be reported as an additional diagnosis.
When the reason for the admission/encounter is management of the neoplasm and the pain associated with the neoplasm is also documented, code G89.3 may be assigned as an additional diagnosis. It is not necessary to assign an additional code for the site of the pain.

See Section I.C.2 for instructions on the sequencing of neoplasms for all other stated reasons for the admission/encounter (except for pain control/pain management).

6)   Chronic pain syndrome

Central pain syndrome (G89.0) and chronic pain syndrome (G89.4) are different than the term "chronic pain," and therefore codes should only be used when the provider has specifically documented this condition.
See Section I.C.5. Pain disorders related to psychological factors.

G00-G99

Inflammatory diseases of the central nervous system (G00-G09)

G00- **Bacterial meningitis, not elsewhere classified** — Bacterial inflammation of the meninges.
    Includes: **Bacterial arachnoiditis** — Bacterial inflammation of the arachnoidea, the delicate membrane between the dura mater and the pia mater.
        Bacterial leptomeningitis — Bacterial inflammation of the pia mater and the arachnoid membranes.
        Bacterial meningitis — Bacterial inflammation of the meninges.
        Bacterial pachymeningitis — Bacterial inflammation of the dura mater.
    Excludes 1:   *bacterial:*
        meningoencephalitis (G04.2)
        meningomyelitis (G04.2)

MCC **G00.0** **Hemophilus meningitis** — A form due to hemophilus microorganisms.
    Meningitis due to Hemophilus influenzae

MCC **G00.1** **Pneumococcal meningitis** — A form due to pneumococcal microorganisms.
    Meningitis due to Streptococcal pneumoniae

MCC **G00.2** **Streptococcal meningitis** — A form due to streptococcal microorganisms.
    Use additional code to further identify organism (B95.0-B95.5)

MCC **G00.3** **Staphylococcal meningitis** — A form due to staphylococcal microorganisms.
    Use additional code to further identify organism (B95.61-B95.8)

MCC **G00.8** **Other bacterial meningitis**
    Meningitis due to Escherichia coli
    Meningitis due to Friedländer's bacillus
    Meningitis due to Klebsiella
    Use additional code to further identify organism (B96.-)

MCC **G00.9** **Bacterial meningitis, unspecified**
    Meningitis due to gram-negative bacteria, unspecified
    Purulent meningitis NOS
    Pyogenic meningitis NOS
    Suppurative meningitis NOS

G01 **Meningitis in bacterial diseases classified elsewhere** —
MCC **[Not Allowed as PDX]**
    Code first underlying disease
    Excludes 1:   *meningitis (in):*
        gonococcal (A54.81)
        leptospirosis (A27.81)
        listeriosis (A32.11)
        Lyme disease (A69.21)
        meningococcal (A39.0)
        neurosyphilis (A52.13)
        tuberculosis (A17.0)
        meningoencephalitis and meningomyelitis in bacterial diseases classified elsewhere (G05)

G02 **Meningitis in other infectious and parasitic diseases classified**
MCC **elsewhere** — **[Not Allowed as PDX]**
    Code first underlying disease, such as:
    African trypanosomiasis (B56-)
    Poliovirus infection (A80-)
    Excludes 1:   *candidal meningitis (B37.5)*
        coccidioidomycosis meningitis (B38.4)
        cryptococcal meningitis (B45.1)
        herpesviral [herpes simplex] meningitis (B00.3)
        infectious mononucleosis complicated by meningitis (B27- with fifth character 2)
        measles complicated by meningitis (B05.1)
        meningoencephalitis and meningomyelitis in other infectious and parasitic diseases classified elsewhere (G05)
        mumps meningitis (B26.1)
        rubella meningitis (B06.02)
        varicella [chickenpox] meningitis (B01.0)
        zoster meningitis (B02.1)

G03- **Meningitis due to other and unspecified causes**
    Includes: **Arachnoiditis NOS**
        Leptomeningitis NOS
        Meningitis NOS
        Pachymeningitis NOS
    Excludes 1:   *meningoencephalitis (G04.-)*
        meningomyelitis (G04.-)

MCC **G03.0** **Nonpyogenic meningitis** — Inflammation of the meninges characterized by the lack of pus in the cerebrospinal fluid.
    Aseptic meningitis
    Nonbacterial meningitis

CC **G03.1** **Chronic meningitis**

CC **G03.2** **Benign recurrent meningitis [Mollaret]**

MCC **G03.8** **Meningitis due to other specified causes**
MCC **G03.9** **Meningitis, unspecified**
    Arachnoiditis (spinal) NOS

G04- **Encephalitis, myelitis and encephalomyelitis**
    Includes: **Acute ascending myelitis** — Inflammation of the spinal cord that is characterized by the progression of myelopathy toward the head.
        Meningoencephalitis — Inflammation of the brain and the meninges that is not of bacterial origin.
        Meningomyelitis — Inflammation of the spinal cord and its membranes that is not of bacterial origin.
    Excludes 1:   *encephalopathy NOS (G93.40)*
    Excludes ❷: *acute transverse myelitis (G37.3-)*
        alcoholic encephalopathy (G31.2)
        benign myalgic encephalomyelitis (G93.3)
        multiple sclerosis (G35)
        subacute necrotizing myelitis (G37.4)
        toxic encephalitis (G92)
        toxic encephalopathy (G92)

G04.0- **Acute disseminated encephalitis and encephalomyelitis (ADEM)**
    Excludes 1:   *acute necrotizing hemorrhagic encephalopathy (G04.3-)*
        other noninfectious acute disseminated encephalomyelitis (noninfectious ADEM) (G04.81)

MCC **G04.00** **Acute disseminated encephalitis and encephalomyelitis, unspecified**

MCC **G04.01** **Postinfectious acute disseminated encephalitis and encephalomyelitis (postinfectious ADEM)** — An inflammatory demyelinating disease of the brain and/or spinal cord following an infection.
    Excludes 1:   *post chickenpox encephalitis (B01.1)*
        post measles encephalitis (B05.0)
        post measles myelitis (B05.1)

MCC **G04.02** **Postimmunization acute disseminated encephalitis, myelitis and encephalomyelitis** — An inflammatory demyelinating disease of the brain and/or spinal cord following an immunization.
    Encephalitis, post immunization
    Encephalomyelitis, post immunization
    Use additional code to identify the vaccine (T50.A-, T50.B-, T50.Z-)

CC **G04.1** **Tropical spastic paraplegia** — A chronic and progressive disease of the nervous system caused by infection with the human T-cell lymphotrophic virus (HTLV-1).

MCC **G04.2** **Bacterial meningoencephalitis and meningomyelitis, not elsewhere classified**

G04.3- **Acute necrotizing hemorrhagic encephalopathy**
    Excludes 1:   *acute disseminated encephalitis and encephalomyelitis (G04.0-)*

MCC **G04.30** **Acute necrotizing hemorrhagic encephalopathy, unspecified**

MCC **G04.31** **Postinfectious acute necrotizing hemorrhagic encephalopathy** — An inflammatory autoimmune demyelinating disease of the brain that destroys white matter following an infection.

MCC **G04.32** **Postimmunization acute necrotizing hemorrhagic encephalopathy** — An inflammatory autoimmune demyelinating disease of the brain that destroys white matter following an immunization.
    Use additional code to identify the vaccine (T50.A-, T50.B-, T50.Z-)

MCC **G04.39** **Other acute necrotizing hemorrhagic encephalopathy**
    Code also underlying etiology, if applicable

G04.8- **Other encephalitis, myelitis and encephalomyelitis**
    Code also any associated seizure (G40.-, R56.9)

MCC **G04.81** **Other encephalitis and encephalomyelitis**
    Noninfectious acute disseminated encephalomyelitis (noninfectious ADEM)

MCC **G04.89** **Other myelitis**

G04.9- **Encephalitis, myelitis and encephalomyelitis, unspecified**

MCC **G04.90** **Encephalitis and encephalomyelitis, unspecified**
    Ventriculitis (cerebral) NOS

MCC **G04.91** **Myelitis, unspecified**

G05- **Encephalitis, myelitis and encephalomyelitis in diseases classified elsewhere**
Code first underlying disease, such as:
Human immunodeficiency virus [HIV] disease (B20)
Poliovirus (A80.-)
Suppurative otitis media (H66.01-H66.4)
Trichinellosis (B75)
Excludes 1:   adenoviral encephalitis, myelitis and encephalomyelitis (A85.1)
congenital toxoplasmosis encephalitis, myelitis and
encephalomyelitis (P37.1)
cytomegaloviral encephalitis, myelitis and encephalomyelitis
(B25.8)
encephalitis, myelitis and encephalomyelitis (in) measles
(B05.0)
encephalitis, myelitis and encephalomyelitis (in) systemic lupus
erythematosus (M32.19)
enteroviral encephalitis, myelitis and encephalomyelitis
(A85.0)
eosinophilic meningoencephalitis (B83.2)
herpesviral [herpes simplex] encephalitis, myelitis and
encephalomyelitis (B00.4)
listerial encephalitis, myelitis and encephalomyelitis (A32.12)
meningococcal encephalitis, myelitis and encephalomyelitis
(A39.81)
mumps encephalitis, myelitis and encephalomyelitis (B26.2)
postchickenpox encephalitis, myelitis and encephalomyelitis
(B01.1-)
rubella encephalitis, myelitis and encephalomyelitis (B06.01)
toxoplasmosis encephalitis, myelitis and encephalomyelitis
(B58.2)
zoster encephalitis, myelitis and encephalomyelitis (B02.0)

MCC **G05.3** **Encephalitis and encephalomyelitis in diseases classified elsewhere** — [Not Allowed as PDX]
Meningoencephalitis in diseases classified elsewhere

MCC **G05.4** **Myelitis in diseases classified elsewhere** — [Not Allowed as PDX]
Meningomyelitis in diseases classified elsewhere

G06- **Intracranial and intraspinal abscess and granuloma**
Use additional code (B95-B97) to identify infectious agent.

MCC **G06.0** **Intracranial abscess and granuloma** — A localized collection of pus caused by the disintegration of tissue in the brain or its membranes that usually occurs as a secondary infection.
Brain [any part] abscess (embolic)
Cerebellar abscess (embolic)
Cerebral abscess (embolic)
Intracranial epidural abscess or granuloma
Intracranial extradural abscess or granuloma
Intracranial subdural abscess or granuloma
Otogenic abscess (embolic)
Excludes 1:   tuberculous intracranial abscess and granuloma
(A17.81)

MCC **G06.1** **Intraspinal abscess and granuloma** — A localized collection of pus caused by the disintegration of tissue in the spinal cord or its membranes that usually occurs as a secondary infection.
Abscess (embolic) of spinal cord [any part]
Intraspinal epidural abscess or granuloma
Intraspinal extradural abscess or granuloma
Intraspinal subdural abscess or granuloma
Excludes 1:   tuberculous intraspinal abscess and granuloma (A17.81)

MCC **G06.2** **Extradural and subdural abscess, unspecified**

G07 **Intracranial and intraspinal abscess and granuloma in diseases**
MCC **classified elsewhere** — [Not Allowed as PDX]
Code first underlying disease, such as:
Schistosomiasis granuloma of brain (B65.-)
Excludes 1:   abscess of brain:
amebic (A06.6)
chromomycotic (B43.1)
gonococcal (A54.82)
tuberculous (A17.81)
tuberculoma of meninges (A17.1)

G08 **Intracranial and intraspinal phlebitis and thrombophlebitis** —
MCC Inflammation, or inflammation with thrombus formation, of the large venous channels which drain the cerebrum, some diploic and meningeal veins into the neck, and from the spinal cord. NOTE: Code G08 refers to phlebitis and thrombophlebitis due to a pus producing microorganism or its poisonous products. See "of nonpyogenic origin" in excludes below.
Septic embolism of intracranial or intraspinal venous sinuses and veins
Septic endophlebitis of intracranial or intraspinal venous sinuses and veins
Septic phlebitis of intracranial or intraspinal venous sinuses and veins
Septic thrombophlebitis of intracranial or intraspinal venous sinuses and veins
Septic thrombosis of intracranial or intraspinal venous sinuses and veins
Excludes 1:   intracranial phlebitis and thrombophlebitis complicating:
abortion, ectopic or molar pregnancy (O00-O07, O08.7)
pregnancy, childbirth and the puerperium (O22.5, O87.3)
nonpyogenic intracranial phlebitis and thrombophlebitis
(I67.6)
Excludes ❷: intracranial phlebitis and thrombophlebitis complicating
nonpyogenic intraspinal phlebitis and thrombophlebitis
(G95.1)

G09 **Sequelae of inflammatory diseases of central nervous system**
Note: Category G09 is to be used to indicate conditions whose primary classification is to G00-G08 as the cause of sequelae, themselves classifiable elsewhere. The "sequelae" include conditions specified as residuals.
Code first condition resulting from (sequela) of inflammatory diseases of central nervous system

Systemic atrophies primarily affecting the central nervous system (G10-G14)

G10 **Huntington's disease** — A hereditary, degenerative disease characterized by
CC involuntary, abrupt, spasmodic, irregular movements of short duration involving the fingers, hands, arms, face, tongue, or head and chronic dementia.
Huntington's chorea
Huntington's dementia

G11- **Hereditary ataxia** — Inherited disorders characterized by slowly progressive incoordination of gait with poor coordination of hands, speech, and eye movements and often developing cerebellar atrophy.
Excludes ❷: cerebral palsy (G80.-)
hereditary and idiopathic neuropathy (G60.-)
metabolic disorders (E70-E88)

CC **G11.0** **Congenital nonprogressive ataxia**

CC **G11.1** **Early-onset cerebellar ataxia**
Early-onset cerebellar ataxia with essential tremor
Early-onset cerebellar ataxia with myoclonus [Hunt's ataxia]
Early-onset cerebellar ataxia with retained tendon reflexes
Friedreich's ataxia (autosomal recessive)
X-linked recessive spinocerebellar ataxia

CC **G11.2** **Late-onset cerebellar ataxia** — [Age/15-124]

CC **G11.3** **Cerebellar ataxia with defective DNA repair**
Ataxia telangiectasia [Louis-Bar]
Excludes ❷: Cockayne's syndrome (Q87.1)
other disorders of purine and pyrimidine metabolism
(E79.-)
xeroderma pigmentosum (Q82.1)

CC **G11.4** **Hereditary spastic paraplegia** — An inherited paraplegia characterized by spasticity of the muscles of the paralyzed part and increased tendon reflexes.

CC **G11.8** **Other hereditary ataxias**

CC **G11.9** **Hereditary ataxia, unspecified**
Hereditary cerebellar ataxia NOS
Hereditary cerebellar degeneration
Hereditary cerebellar disease
Hereditary cerebellar syndrome

G12- **Spinal muscular atrophy and related syndromes** — A wasting of muscle tissues caused by the progressive degeneration of the motor cells of the spinal cord.

CC **G12.0** **Infantile spinal muscular atrophy, type I [Werdnig-Hoffman]** — A hereditary spinal muscular atrophy disease present at birth, caused by the degeneration of the anterior horn cells of the spinal cord and is marked by decreased fetal movements in utero, progressive muscular weakness, hypotonia, complete flaccid paralysis, and death.

G05-G12

cc **G12.1   Other inherited spinal muscular atrophy**
Adult form spinal muscular atrophy
Childhood form, type II spinal muscular atrophy
Distal spinal muscular atrophy
Juvenile form, type III spinal muscular atrophy [Kugelberg-Welander] — Spinal muscular atrophy caused by the degeneration of anterior horn cells of the spinal cord beginning in adolescence and marked by wasting and weakness of the legs and pelvic girdle.
Progressive bulbar palsy of childhood [Fazio-Londe]
Scapuloperoneal form spinal muscular atrophy

G12.2-   Motor neuron disease — Degeneration of the motor neurons of the brain and spinal cord.

cc **G12.20   Motor neuron disease, unspecified**

cc **G12.21   Amyotrophic lateral sclerosis** — [Age/15-124] – A progressive, degenerative disease of the motor neurons in the brain and spinal cord characterized by atrophy and weakness of the muscles innervated by them, and eventually dysphagia, dysarthria, and facial weakness (also called Lou Gehrig's disease).
Progressive spinal muscle atrophy

cc **G12.22   Progressive bulbar palsy** — A type of amyotrophic lateral sclerosis caused by degeneration of the motor neurons of the cranial nerve nuclei, and characterized by progressive weakness and wasting of the pharyngeal muscles, the tongue, the facial muscles, dysarthria, and dysphagia.

cc **G12.29   Other motor neuron disease**
Familial motor neuron disease
Primary lateral sclerosis

cc **G12.8   Other spinal muscular atrophies and related syndromes**

cc **G12.9   Spinal muscular atrophy, unspecified**

G13-   Systemic atrophies primarily affecting central nervous system in diseases classified elsewhere

G13.0   Paraneoplastic neuromyopathy and neuropathy — [Not Allowed as PDX]
Carcinomatous neuromyopathy
Sensorial paraneoplastic neuropathy [Denny Brown]
Code first underlying neoplasm (C00-D49)

G13.1   Other systemic atrophy primarily affecting central nervous system in neoplastic disease — [Not Allowed as PDX]
Paraneoplastic limbic encephalopathy
Code first underlying neoplasm (C00-D49)

G13.2   Systemic atrophy primarily affecting central nervous system in myxedema — [Not Allowed as PDX]
Code first underlying disease, such as:
Hypothyroidism (E03-)
Myxedematous congenital iodine deficiency (E00.1)

G13.8   Systemic atrophy primarily affecting central nervous system in other diseases classified elsewhere — [Not Allowed as PDX]
Code first underlying disease

G14   Postpolio syndrome — A condition presenting long after the acute infection phase (often decades later) characterized by slowly progressive muscle weakness, pain, fatigue, and muscle atrophy.
Includes: Postpolio myelitic syndrome
Excludes 1:   sequelae of poliomyelitis (B91)

Extrapyramidal and movement disorders (G20-G26)

G20   Parkinson's disease — A chronic, degenerative nervous system disease that causes the destruction of dopamine-producing cells and is characterized by a fine, slowly spreading tremor, muscular weakness and rigidity, and a peculiar gait.
Hemiparkinsonism
Idiopathic Parkinsonism or Parkinson's disease
Paralysis agitans
Parkinsonism or Parkinson's disease NOS
Primary Parkinsonism or Parkinson's disease
Excludes 1:   dementia with Parkinsonism (G31.83)

G21-   Secondary parkinsonism — A symptom complex with similar characteristics to Parkinson's disease that is caused as a consequence of other diseases or external agents.
Excludes 1:   dementia with Parkinsonism (G31.83)
Huntington's disease (G10)
Shy-Drager syndrome (G90.3)
syphilitic Parkinsonism (A52.19)

MCC **G21.0   Malignant neuroleptic syndrome** — A condition characterized by multiple symptoms, including hyperthermia and rigidity that is caused by an adverse effect of neuroleptic (antipsychotic) drug therapy.
Use additional code for adverse effect, if applicable, to identify drug (T43.3x5, T43.4x5, T43.505, T43.595)
Excludes 1:   neuroleptic induced parkinsonism (G21.11)

G21.1-   Other drug-induced secondary parkinsonism

cc **G21.11   Neuroleptic induced parkinsonism**
Use additional code for adverse effect, if applicable, to identify drug (T43.3x5, T43.4x5, T43.505, T43.595)
Excludes 1:   malignant neuroleptic syndrome (G21.0)

cc **G21.19   Other drug-induced secondary parkinsonism**
Use additional code for adverse effect, if applicable, to identify drug (T36-T50 with fifth or sixth character 5)

cc **G21.2   Secondary parkinsonism due to other external agents**
Code first (T51-T65) to identify external agent

cc **G21.3   Postencephalitic parkinsonism**

G21.4   Vascular parkinsonism

cc **G21.8   Other secondary parkinsonism**

cc **G21.9   Secondary parkinsonism, unspecified**

G23-   Other degenerative diseases of basal ganglia — Deterioration of the masses of gray matter at the base of the cerebral hemispheres which function to relay motor impulses.
Excludes ❷: multi-system degeneration of the autonomic nervous system (G90.3)

cc **G23.0   Hallervorden-Spatz disease** — A hereditary degeneration of the globus pallidus marked by accumulations of iron pigment, progressive rigidity, choreoathetoid movements, dysarthria, and progressive mental deterioration.
Pigmentary pallidal degeneration

cc **G23.1   Progressive supranuclear ophthalmoplegia [Steele-Richardson-Olszewski]** — A chronic degenerative disease involving the basal ganglia characterized by early paralysis of the eye movements, parkinsonian features, generalized spasticity, progressive dysarthria, and mild dementia.
Progressive supranuclear palsy

cc **G23.2   Striatonigral degeneration** — The degeneration of the striatonigral elements of the basal ganglia characterized by gait imbalance, rigidity, progressive spasticity, and speech which becomes slow and indistinct.

cc **G23.8   Other specified degenerative diseases of basal ganglia**
Calcification of basal ganglia

cc **G23.9   Degenerative disease of basal ganglia, unspecified**

G24-   Dystonia — A movement disorder characterized by involuntary muscle contractions.
Includes: Dyskinesia
Excludes ❷: athetoid cerebral palsy (G80.3)

G24.0-   Drug-induced dystonia — A condition characterized by abnormal postures and muscle spasms that is caused by drugs.
Use additional code for adverse effect, if applicable, to identify drug (T36-T50 with fifth or sixth character 5)

G24.01   Drug-induced subacute dyskinesia
Drug-induced blepharospasm
Drug-induced orofacial dyskinesia
Neuroleptic induced tardive dyskinesia
Tardive dyskinesia

cc **G24.02   Drug-induced acute dystonia**
Acute dystonic reaction to drugs
Neuroleptic induced acute dystonia

cc **G24.09   Other drug-induced dystonia**

G24.1   Genetic torsion dystonia — A hereditary movement disorder characterized by painful contortions of the muscles of the trunk and extremities that produces twisting and repetitive movements and abnormal posture.
Dystonia deformans progressiva
Dystonia musculorum deformans
Familial torsion dystonia
Idiopathic familial dystonia
Idiopathic (torsion) dystonia NOS
(Schwalbe-) Ziehen-Oppenheim disease

cc **G24.2   Idiopathic nonfamilial dystonia** — A form of unknown cause.

G24.3   Spasmodic torticollis — A form causing the head to rotate to one side and pull down toward the chest.
Excludes 1:   congenital torticollis (Q68.0)
hysterical torticollis (F44.4)
ocular torticollis (R29.891)
psychogenic torticollis (F45.8)
torticollis NOS (M43.6)
traumatic recurrent torticollis (S13.4)

G24.4   Idiopathic orofacial dystonia — A form affecting the jaw, lips, and/or tongue.
Orofacial dyskinesia
Excludes 1:   drug induced orofacial dyskinesia (G24.01)

G24.5   Blepharospasm — A form affecting the eyelids which may close for extended periods of time.
Excludes 1:   drug induced blepharospasm (G24.01)

G
1
2
-
G
2
4

cc **G24.8   Other dystonia**
Acquired torsion dystonia NOS

G24.9   Dystonia, unspecified
Dyskinesia NOS

G25- Other extrapyramidal and movement disorders — EXTRAPYRAMIDAL DISEASE — A dysfunction of the nerve fibers which are important in maintenance of equilibrium and muscle tone. MOVEMENT DISORDERS — Varying degrees of inability to voluntarily control muscle action.
Excludes ❷: sleep related movement disorders (G47.6-)

G25.0   Essential tremor — A movement disorder characterized by bilateral, symmetric, involuntary quivering which begins in the fingers and hands.
Familial tremor
Excludes 1:   tremor NOS (R25.1)

G25.1   Drug-induced tremor — A tremor movement disorder caused by effects of drugs.
Use additional code for adverse effect, if applicable, to identify drug (T36-T50 with fifth or sixth character 5)

G25.2   Other specified forms of tremor
Intention tremor

G25.3   Myoclonus — The sudden, involuntary twitching contractions (jerks) of a muscle or a group of muscles.
Drug-induced myoclonus
Palatal myoclonus
Use additional code for adverse effect, if applicable, to identify drug (T36-T50 with fifth or sixth character 5)
Excludes 1:   facial myokymia (G51.4)
myoclonic epilepsy (G40.-)

G25.4   Drug-induced chorea
Use additional code for adverse effect, if applicable, to identify drug (T36-T50 with fifth or sixth character 5)

G25.5   Other chorea
Chorea NOS
Excludes 1:   chorea NOS with heart involvement (I02.0)
Huntington's chorea (G10)
rheumatic chorea (I02.-)
Sydenham's chorea (I02.-)

G25.6- Drug-induced tics and other tics of organic origin

G25.61   Drug-induced tics
Use additional code for adverse effect, if applicable, to identify drug (T36-T50 with fifth or sixth character 5)

G25.69   Other tics of organic origin — Repetitive, spasmodic movements or twitching that occur in an irregular fashion and resemble voluntary movements and are of nonpsychogenic origin.
Excludes 1:   habit spasm (F95.9)
tic NOS (F95.9)
Tourette's syndrome (F95.2)

G25.7- Other and unspecified drug induced movement disorders
Use additional code for adverse effect, if applicable, to identify drug (T36-T50 with fifth or sixth character 5)

G25.70   Drug-induced movement disorder, unspecified

G25.71   Drug-induced akathisia
Drug-induced acathisia
Neuroleptic induced acute akathisia

G25.79   Other drug-induced movement disorders

G25.8- Other specified extrapyramidal and movement disorders

G25.81   Restless legs syndrome — Discomfort deep inside the legs that is relieved by keeping the legs in motion.

cc **G25.82   Stiff-man syndrome** — A condition characterized by progressive painful fluctuating rigidity of the trunk and limb muscles of an unknown origin.

G25.83   Benign shuddering attacks — A neurological phenomenon movement disorder that is usually seen in children and is nonepileptic in origin.

G25.89   Other specified extrapyramidal and movement disorders

cc **G25.9   Extrapyramidal and movement disorder, unspecified**

G26   Extrapyramidal and movement disorders in diseases classified elsewhere — [Not Allowed as PDX]
Code first underlying disease

Other degenerative diseases of the nervous system (G30-G32)

G30- Alzheimer's disease — Diffuse atrophy of the cerebral cortex due to neuronal degeneration and marked by increasing loss of memory, intellectual function, and disturbances in speech.
Includes: Alzheimer's dementia senile and presenile forms
Use additional code to identify:
Delirium, if applicable (F05)
Dementia with behavioral disturbance (F02.81)
Dementia without behavioral disturbance (F02.80)
Excludes 1:   senile degeneration of brain NEC (G31.1)
senile dementia NOS (F03)
senility NOS (R41.81)

G30.0   Alzheimer's disease with <u>early</u> onset

G30.1   Alzheimer's disease with <u>late</u> onset — [Age/15-124]

G30.8   Other Alzheimer's disease

G30.9   Alzheimer's disease, unspecified

G31- Other degenerative diseases of nervous system, not elsewhere classified
Use additional code to identify:
Dementia with behavioral disturbance (F02.81)
Dementia without behavioral disturbance (F02.80)
Excludes ❷: Reye's syndrome (G93.7)

G31.0- Frontotemporal dementia — A neurodegenerative disorder of the frontal and anterior temporal lobes of the brain.

G31.01   Pick's disease — A form marked by severe atrophy of the frontal and temporal lobes that is characterized by symptoms similar to Alzheimer's disease with personality, orientation, and attention span more affected.
Primary progressive aphasia
Progressive isolated aphasia

G31.09   Other frontotemporal dementia
Frontal dementia — A form signifying neuropsychological features localized to the frontal lobes.

G31.1   Senile degeneration of brain, not elsewhere classified
Excludes 1:   Alzheimer's disease (G30.-)
senility NOS (R41.81)

G31.2   Degeneration of nervous system due to alcohol
Alcoholic cerebellar ataxia
Alcoholic cerebellar degeneration
Alcoholic cerebral degeneration
Alcoholic encephalopathy
Dysfunction of the autonomic nervous system due to alcohol
Code also associated alcoholism (F10-)

G31.8- Other specified degenerative diseases of nervous system

cc **G31.81   Alpers disease** — Deterioration of the nerve cells and glia in all layers of the cerebral cortex and marked by symptoms in early infancy of convulsions, dementia, blindness, deafness, and paralysis.
Grey-matter degeneration

cc **G31.82   Leigh's disease** —Deterioration and symmetrical areas of necrosis in the midbrain and pons and substance of the medulla, with involvement of the cerebral hemispheres and cerebellum probably caused by a defect involving tricarboxylic acid cycle, and marked by cerebellar ataxia, hemiparesis, quadriplegia, and in the severe form death.
Subacute necrotizing encephalopathy

G31.83   Dementia with Lewy bodies — A neurodegenerative disorder with Parkinsonian motor features that is characterized by unexplained falls, prominent visual hallucinations, delusions, and gait abnormalities.
Dementia with Parkinsonism
Lewy body dementia
Lewy body disease

G31.84   Mild cognitive impairment, so stated — A mental-functioning disorder in which the patient demonstrates some degree of mental impairment but does not meet the criteria for dementia.
Excludes 1:   age related cognitive decline (R41.81)
altered mental status (R41.82)
cerebral degeneration (G31.9)
change in mental status (R41.82)
cognitive deficits following (sequelae of) cerebral hemorrhage or infarction (I69.01-, I69.11-, I69.21-, I69.31-, I69.81-, I69.91-)
cognitive impairment due to intracranial or head injury (S06.-)
dementia (F01-, F02-, F03)
mild memory disturbance (F06.8)
neurologic neglect syndrome (R41.4)
personality change, nonpsychotic (F68.8)

G 2 4 - G 3 1

G31.85   **Corticobasal degeneration**

G31.89   **Other specified degenerative diseases of nervous system**

G31.9   **Degenerative disease of nervous system, unspecified**

G32-   **Other degenerative disorders of nervous system in diseases classified elsewhere**

cc G32.0   **Subacute combined degeneration of spinal cord in diseases classified elsewhere** — [Not Allowed as PDX]
   Dana-Putnam syndrome
   Sclerosis of spinal cord (combined) (dorsolateral) (posterolateral)
   Code first underlying disease, such as:
   Anemia (D51.9)
   Dietary (D51.3)
   Pernicious (D51.0)
   Vitamin B12 deficiency (E53.8)
   Excludes 1:   syphilitic combined degeneration of spinal cord (A52.11)

G32.8-   **Other specified degenerative disorders of nervous system in diseases classified elsewhere**
   Code first underlying disease, such as:
   Amyloidosis cerebral degeneration (E85.-)
   Cerebral degeneration (due to) hypothyroidism (E00.0-E03.9)
   Cerebral degeneration (due to) neoplasm (C00-D49)
   Cerebral degeneration (due to) vitamin B deficiency, except thiamine (E52-E53-)
   Excludes 1:   superior hemorrhagic polioencephalitis [Wernicke's encephalopathy] (E51.2)

cc G32.81   **Cerebellar ataxia in diseases classified elsewhere** — [Not Allowed as PDX]
   Code first underlying disease, such as:
   Celiac disease (with gluten ataxia) (K90.0)
   Cerebellar ataxia (in) neoplastic disease (paraneoplastic cerebellar degeneration) (C00-D49)
   Non-celiac gluten ataxia (M35.9)
   Excludes 1:   systemic atrophy primarily affecting the central nervous system in alcoholic cerebellar ataxia (G13.2)
   systemic atrophy primarily affecting the central nervous system in myxedema (G13.2)

G32.89   **Other specified degenerative disorders of nervous system in diseases classified elsewhere** — [Not Allowed as PDX]
   Degenerative encephalopathy in diseases classified elsewhere

Demyelinating diseases of the central nervous system (G35-G37)

G35   **Multiple sclerosis** — A demyelinating disease of the white matter of the central nervous system of unknown etiology and characterized by paralysis or paresis of the upper or lower limbs, visual loss, paresthesia, speech disturbances, and occasionally dementia.
   Disseminated multiple sclerosis
   Generalized multiple sclerosis
   Multiple sclerosis NOS
   Multiple sclerosis of brain stem
   Multiple sclerosis of cord

G36-   **Other acute disseminated demyelination** — Destruction of the myelin sheath surrounding nerve fibers of the central nervous system.
   Excludes 1:   postinfectious encephalitis and encephalomyelitis NOS (G04.01)

cc G36.0   **Neuromyelitis optica [Devic]** — A combined demyelination of the optic nerve and the spinal cord that is marked by visual loss and possibly blindness, and flaccid paralysis of the extremities.
   Demyelination in optic neuritis
   Excludes 1:   optic neuritis NOS (H46)

cc G36.1   **Acute and subacute hemorrhagic leukoencephalitis [Hurst]**

cc G36.8   **Other specified acute disseminated demyelination**

cc G36.9   **Acute disseminated demyelination, unspecified**

G37-   **Other demyelinating diseases of central nervous system**

cc G37.0   **Diffuse sclerosis of central nervous system** — Myelinoclastic diffuse sclerosis characterized by mental and neurologic deterioration, intellectual deterioration, increased spasticity, blindness, and deafness.
   Periaxial encephalitis
   Schilder's disease
   Excludes 1:   X linked adrenoleukodystrophy (E71.52-)

cc G37.1   **Central demyelination of corpus callosum** — A degeneration of the corpus callosum of unknown etiology characterized by diffuse signs of cerebral disease, mental symptoms, convulsions, tremors, and other motor disabilities.

cc G37.2   **Central pontine myelinolysis** — A disease caused by the destruction of myelin localized to the base of the pons and characterized by quadriplegia, and facial, glossal, and pharyngeal paralysis with mutism.

cc G37.3   **Acute transverse myelitis in demyelinating disease of central nervous system** — A rapidly developing inflammation of the spinal cord.
   Acute transverse myelitis NOS
   Acute transverse myelopathy
   Excludes 1:   multiple sclerosis (G35)
   neuromyelitis optica [Devic] (G36.0)

MCC G37.4   **Subacute necrotizing myelitis of central nervous system**

cc G37.5   **Concentric sclerosis [Balo] of central nervous system** — A demyelinating disease characterized by concentric areas of demyelination and without recognizable clinical symptoms.

cc G37.8   **Other specified demyelinating diseases of central nervous system**

cc G37.9   **Demyelinating disease of central nervous system, unspecified**

Episodic and paroxysmal disorders (G40-G47)

G40-   **Epilepsy and recurrent seizures** — A neurological disorder of excessive and abnormal brain cell activity that is characterized by a sudden change in how the cells of the brain send electrical signals that causes susceptibility to recurrent seizures. STATUS EPILEPTICUS — An epileptic seizure of greater than five minutes or more than one seizure within a five-minute period without recovery between them.
   Note: The following terms are to be considered equivalent to intractable: pharmacoresistant (pharmacologically resistant), treatment resistant, refractory (medically) and poorly controlled.
   Excludes 1:   conversion disorder with seizures (F44.5)
   convulsions NOS (R56.9)
   post traumatic seizures (R56.1)
   seizure (convulsive) NOS (R56.9)
   seizure of newborn (P90)
   Excludes ❷: hippocampal sclerosis (G93.81)
   mesial temporal sclerosis (G93.81)
   temporal sclerosis (G93.81)
   Todd's paralysis (G83.84)

G40.0-   **Localization-related (focal) (partial) idiopathic epilepsy and epileptic syndromes with seizures of localized onset** — A type that begins in a limited region of the brain that is characterized by a dazed or staring expression.
   Benign childhood epilepsy with centrotemporal EEG spikes
   Childhood epilepsy with occipital EEG paroxysms
   Excludes 1:   adult onset localization-related epilepsy (G40.1-, G40.2-)

G40.00-   **Localization-related (focal) (partial) idiopathic epilepsy and epileptic syndromes with seizures of localized onset, not intractable**
   Localization-related (focal) (partial) idiopathic epilepsy and epileptic syndromes with seizures of localized onset without intractability

cc G40.001   **Localization-related (focal) (partial) idiopathic epilepsy and epileptic syndromes with seizures of localized onset, not intractable, with status epilepticus**

cc G40.009   **Localization-related (focal) (partial) idiopathic epilepsy and epileptic syndromes with seizures of localized onset, not intractable, without status epilepticus**
   Localization-related (focal) (partial) idiopathic epilepsy and epileptic syndromes with seizures of localized onset NOS

G40.01-   **Localization-related (focal) (partial) idiopathic epilepsy and epileptic syndromes with seizures of localized onset, intractable**

cc G40.011   **Localization-related (focal) (partial) idiopathic epilepsy and epileptic syndromes with seizures of localized onset, intractable, with status epilepticus**

cc G40.019   **Localization-related (focal) (partial) idiopathic epilepsy and epileptic syndromes with seizures of localized onset, intractable, without status epilepticus**

G40.1- <u>Localization-related</u> (focal) (partial) symptomatic epilepsy and epileptic syndromes <u>with simple partial seizures</u> — A type that begins in a limited region of the brain and is characterized by uncontrolled shaking, altered emotions, and sensory changes, but without loss of consciousness.
> Attacks without alteration of consciousness
> Epilepsia partialis continua [Kozhevnikof]
> Simple partial seizures developing into secondarily generalized seizures

G40.10- Localization-related (focal) (partial) symptomatic epilepsy and epileptic syndromes with simple partial seizures, <u>not</u> intractable
> Localization-related (focal) (partial) symptomatic epilepsy and epileptic syndromes with simple partial seizures without intractability

CC **G40.101** Localization-related (focal) (partial) symptomatic epilepsy and epileptic syndromes with simple partial seizures, <u>not</u> intractable, <u>with status epilepticus</u>

CC **G40.109** Localization-related (focal) (partial) symptomatic epilepsy and epileptic syndromes with simple partial seizures, <u>not</u> intractable, <u>without</u> status epilepticus
> Localization-related (focal) (partial) symptomatic epilepsy and epileptic syndromes with simple partial seizures NOS

G40.11- Localization-related (focal) (partial) symptomatic epilepsy and epileptic syndromes with simple partial seizures, <u>intractable</u>

CC **G40.111** Localization-related (focal) (partial) symptomatic epilepsy and epileptic syndromes with simple partial seizures, intractable, <u>with status epilepticus</u>

CC **G40.119** Localization-related (focal) (partial) symptomatic epilepsy and epileptic syndromes with simple partial seizures, intractable, <u>without</u> status epilepticus

G40.2- <u>Localization-related</u> (focal) (partial) symptomatic epilepsy and epileptic syndromes <u>with complex partial seizures</u> — A type that begins in a limited region of the brain that is characterized by a dazed or staring expression, repetitious, purposeless movements, and a loss of consciousness.
> Attacks with alteration of consciousness, often with automatisms
> Complex partial seizures developing into secondarily generalized seizures

G40.20- Localization-related (focal) (partial) symptomatic epilepsy and epileptic syndromes with complex partial seizures, <u>not</u> intractable
> Localization-related (focal) (partial) symptomatic epilepsy and epileptic syndromes with complex partial seizures without intractability

CC **G40.201** Localization-related (focal) (partial) symptomatic epilepsy and epileptic syndromes with complex partial seizures, <u>not</u> intractable, <u>with status epilepticus</u>

CC **G40.209** Localization-related (focal) (partial) symptomatic epilepsy and epileptic syndromes with complex partial seizures, <u>not</u> intractable, <u>without</u> status epilepticus
> Localization-related (focal) (partial) symptomatic epilepsy and epileptic syndromes with complex partial seizures NOS

G40.21- Localization-related (focal) (partial) symptomatic epilepsy and epileptic syndromes with complex partial seizures, <u>intractable</u>

CC **G40.211** Localization-related (focal) (partial) symptomatic epilepsy and epileptic syndromes with complex partial seizures, intractable, <u>with status epilepticus</u>

CC **G40.219** Localization-related (focal) (partial) symptomatic epilepsy and epileptic syndromes with complex partial seizures, intractable, <u>without</u> status epilepticus

G40.3- <u>Generalized</u> idiopathic epilepsy and epileptic syndromes — A type characterized by the electrical discharge spread to involve all of the brain, symmetric tonic contraction of all voluntary muscles, decerebrate posturing, followed by clonic violent expiratory contractions with expulsion of saliva, possibly tongue biting, and loss of consciousness.
> Code also MERRF syndrome, if applicable (E88.42)

G40.30- <u>Generalized</u> idiopathic epilepsy and epileptic syndromes, <u>not</u> intractable
> Generalized idiopathic epilepsy and epileptic syndromes without intractability

MCC **G40.301** <u>Generalized</u> idiopathic epilepsy and epileptic syndromes, <u>not</u> intractable, <u>with status epilepticus</u>

G40.309 <u>Generalized</u> idiopathic epilepsy and epileptic syndromes, <u>not</u> intractable, <u>without</u> status epilepticus
> Generalized idiopathic epilepsy and epileptic syndromes NOS

G40.31- <u>Generalized</u> idiopathic epilepsy and epileptic syndromes, <u>intractable</u>

MCC **G40.311** <u>Generalized</u> idiopathic epilepsy and epileptic syndromes, intractable, <u>with status epilepticus</u>

MCC **G40.319** <u>Generalized</u> idiopathic epilepsy and epileptic syndromes, intractable, <u>without</u> status epilepticus

G40.A- <u>Absence epileptic</u> syndrome — A type characterized by staring, brief lapses of awareness and subtle body movements, but without post-seizure confusion, contractions of convulsions, or loss of consciousness.
> Absence epileptic syndrome NOS
> Childhood absence epilepsy [pyknolepsy]
> Juvenile absence epilepsy

G40.A0- Absence epileptic syndrome, <u>not</u> intractable

G40.A01 Absence epileptic syndrome, not intractable, <u>with status epilepticus</u>

G40.A09 Absence epileptic syndrome, not intractable, <u>without</u> status epilepticus

G40.A1- Absence epileptic syndrome, <u>intractable</u>

CC **G40.A11** Absence epileptic syndrome, intractable, <u>with status epilepticus</u>

CC **G40.A19** Absence epileptic syndrome, intractable, <u>without</u> status epilepticus

G40.B- <u>Juvenile myoclonic</u> epilepsy [impulsive petit mal] — A form that manifests itself usually between the ages of 12 and 18.

G40.B0- Juvenile myoclonic epilepsy, <u>not</u> intractable

CC **G40.B01** Juvenile myoclonic epilepsy, not intractable, <u>with status epilepticus</u>

CC **G40.B09** Juvenile myoclonic epilepsy, not intractable, <u>without</u> status epilepticus

G40.B1- Juvenile myoclonic epilepsy, <u>intractable</u>

CC **G40.B11** Juvenile myoclonic epilepsy, intractable, <u>with status epilepticus</u>

CC **G40.B19** Juvenile myoclonic epilepsy, intractable, <u>without</u> status epilepticus

G40.4- <u>Other generalized</u> epilepsy and epileptic syndromes
> Epilepsy with grand mal seizures on awakening
> Epilepsy with myoclonic absences
> Epilepsy with myoclonic-astatic seizures
> Grand mal seizure NOS
> Nonspecific atonic epileptic seizures
> Nonspecific clonic epileptic seizures
> Nonspecific myoclonic epileptic seizures
> Nonspecific tonic epileptic seizures
> Nonspecific tonic-clonic epileptic seizures
> Symptomatic early myoclonic encephalopathy

G40.40- Other <u>generalized</u> epilepsy and epileptic syndromes, <u>not</u> intractable
> Other generalized epilepsy and epileptic syndromes without intractability
> Other generalized epilepsy and epileptic syndromes NOS

G40.401 Other <u>generalized</u> epilepsy and epileptic syndromes, <u>not</u> intractable, <u>with status epilepticus</u>

G40.409 Other <u>generalized</u> epilepsy and epileptic syndromes, <u>not</u> intractable, <u>without</u> status epilepticus

G40 - G40

G40.41- Other <u>generalized</u> epilepsy and epileptic syndromes, <u>intractable</u>

cc G40.411   Other <u>generalized</u> epilepsy and epileptic syndromes, intractable, <u>with status epilepticus</u>

cc G40.419   Other <u>generalized</u> epilepsy and epileptic syndromes, intractable, <u>without</u> status epilepticus

G40.5- Epileptic seizures <u>related to external causes</u>
   Epileptic seizures related to alcohol
   Epileptic seizures related to drugs
   Epileptic seizures related to hormonal changes
   Epileptic seizures related to sleep deprivation
   Epileptic seizures related to stress
   Use additional code for adverse effect, if applicable, to identify drug (T36-T50 with fifth or sixth digit 5)
   Code also, if applicable, associated epilepsy and recurrent seizures (G40-)

G40.50- Epileptic seizures related to external causes, <u>not</u> intractable

cc G40.501   Epileptic seizures related to external causes, <u>not</u> intractable, <u>with status epilepticus</u>

cc G40.509   Epileptic seizures related to external causes, <u>not</u> intractable, <u>without</u> status epilepticus
   Epileptic seizures related to external causes NOS

G40.8- <u>Other epilepsy and recurrent seizures</u>
   Epilepsies and epileptic syndromes undetermined as to whether they are focal or generalized
   Landau-Kleffner syndrome

G40.80- Other epilepsy

cc G40.801   Other epilepsy, <u>not</u> intractable, <u>with status epilepticus</u>
   Other epilepsy without intractability with status epilepticus

cc G40.802   Other epilepsy, <u>not</u> intractable, <u>without</u> status epilepticus
   Other epilepsy NOS
   Other epilepsy without intractability without status epilepticus

cc G40.803   Other epilepsy, <u>intractable</u>, <u>with status epilepticus</u>

cc G40.804   Other epilepsy, <u>intractable</u>, <u>without</u> status epilepticus

G40.81- Lennox-Gastaut syndrome

cc G40.811   Lennox-Gastaut syndrome, <u>not</u> intractable, <u>with status epilepticus</u>

cc G40.812   Lennox-Gastaut syndrome, <u>not</u> intractable, <u>without</u> status epilepticus

cc G40.813   Lennox-Gastaut syndrome, <u>intractable</u>, <u>with status epilepticus</u>

cc G40.814   Lennox-Gastaut syndrome, <u>intractable</u>, <u>without</u> status epilepticus

G40.82- Epileptic spasms — A type characterized by brief, sudden spasms of the flexor muscles of the neck, trunk, and limbs manifesting during the first year of life.
   Infantile spasms
   Salaam attacks
   West's syndrome

cc G40.821   Epileptic spasms, <u>not</u> intractable, <u>with status epilepticus</u>

cc G40.822   Epileptic spasms, <u>not</u> intractable, <u>without</u> status epilepticus

cc G40.823   Epileptic spasms, <u>intractable</u>, <u>with status epilepticus</u>

cc G40.824   Epileptic spasms, <u>intractable</u>, <u>without</u> status epilepticus

cc G40.89 Other seizures
   Excludes 1:   post traumatic seizures (R56.1)
               recurrent seizures NOS (G40.909)
               seizure NOS (R56.9)

G40.9- <u>Epilepsy, unspecified</u>

G40.90- Epilepsy, unspecified, <u>not</u> intractable
   Epilepsy, unspecified, without intractability

G40.901   Epilepsy, unspecified, <u>not</u> intractable, <u>with status epilepticus</u>

G40.909   Epilepsy, unspecified, <u>not</u> intractable, <u>without</u> status epilepticus
   Epilepsy NOS
   Epileptic convulsions NOS
   Epileptic fits NOS
   Epileptic seizures NOS
   Recurrent seizures NOS
   Seizure disorder NOS

G40.91- Epilepsy, unspecified, <u>intractable</u>
   Intractable seizure disorder NOS

cc G40.911   Epilepsy, unspecified, intractable, <u>with status epilepticus</u>

cc G40.919   Epilepsy, unspecified, intractable, <u>without</u> status epilepticus

G43- <u>Migraine</u> — A neurological primary headache disorder that is characterized by episodic attacks of headache and associated symptoms.
   Note: The following terms are to be considered equivalent to intractable: pharmacoresistant (pharmacologically resistant), treatment resistant, refractory (medically) and poorly controlled.
   Use additional code for adverse effect, if applicable, to identify drug (T36-T50 with fifth or sixth character 5)
   Excludes 1:   *headache NOS (R51)*
               lower half migraine (G44.00)
   Excludes ❷: *headache syndromes (G44.-)*

G43.0- <u>Migraine without aura</u> — A form characterized by moderate to severe headaches lasting 4-72 hours with varying symptoms including nausea and/or vomiting, photophobia, and phonophobia.
   Common migraine
   Excludes 1:   *chronic migraine without aura (G43.7-)*

G43.00- Migraine without aura, <u>not</u> intractable
   Migraine without aura without mention of refractory migraine

G43.001   Migraine without aura, <u>not</u> intractable, <u>with status migrainosus</u> — A form lasting more than 72 hours.

G43.009   Migraine without aura, <u>not</u> intractable, <u>without</u> status migrainosus
   Migraine without aura NOS

G43.01- Migraine without aura, <u>intractable</u> — INTRACTABLE – Provider stated, and/or see Note at G43-.
   Migraine without aura with refractory migraine

G43.011   Migraine without aura, intractable, <u>with status migrainosus</u> — A form lasting more than 72 hours.

G43.019   Migraine without aura, intractable, <u>without</u> status migrainosus

G43.1- <u>Migraine with aura</u> — A form characterized by moderate to severe headaches with preceding or accompanying visual (most common), sensory, motor, and/or speech aura with the features of "migraine without aura" usually following the aura symptoms.
   Basilar migraine
   Classical migraine
   Migraine equivalents
   Migraine preceded or accompanied by transient focal neurological phenomena
   Migraine triggered seizures
   Migraine with acute-onset aura
   Migraine with aura without headache (migraine equivalents)
   Migraine with prolonged aura
   Migraine with typical aura
   Retinal migraine
   Code also any associated seizure (G40.-, R56.9)
   Excludes 1:   *persistent migraine aura (G43.5-, G43.6-)*

G43.10- Migraine with aura, <u>not</u> intractable
   Migraine with aura without mention of refractory migraine

G43.101   Migraine with aura, <u>not</u> intractable, <u>with status migrainosus</u> — A form lasting more than 72 hours.

G43.109   Migraine with aura, <u>not</u> intractable, <u>without</u> status migrainosus
   Migraine with aura NOS

G43.11- Migraine with aura, <u>intractable</u> — INTRACTABLE – Provider stated, and/or see Note at G43-.
   Migraine with aura with refractory migraine

G43.111   Migraine with aura, intractable, <u>with status migrainosus</u> — A form lasting more than 72 hours.

G43.119   Migraine with aura, intractable, <u>without</u> status migrainosus

G 4 0 - G 4 3

G43.4- <u>Hemiplegic</u> migraine — A form characterized by recurrent headaches with aura and temporary, unilateral hemiparesis or hemiplegia.
Familial migraine
Sporadic migraine

G43.40- Hemiplegic migraine, <u>not</u> intractable
Hemiplegic migraine without refractory migraine

G43.401   Hemiplegic migraine, <u>not</u> intractable, <u>with</u> status migrainosus — A form lasting more than 72 hours.

G43.409   Hemiplegic migraine, <u>not</u> intractable, <u>without</u> status migrainosus
Hemiplegic migraine NOS

G43.41- Hemiplegic migraine, <u>intractable</u> — INTRACTABLE – Provider stated, and/or see Note at G43-.
Hemiplegic migraine with refractory migraine

G43.411   Hemiplegic migraine, intractable, <u>with</u> status migrainosus — A form lasting more than 72 hours.

G43.419   Hemiplegic migraine, intractable, <u>without</u> status migrainosus

G43.5- <u>Persistent</u> migraine aura <u>without</u> cerebral infarction — A form characterized by aura symptoms that persist for more than two weeks and are without radiographic evidence of infarction.

G43.50- Persistent migraine aura without cerebral infarction, <u>not</u> intractable
Persistent migraine aura without cerebral infarction, without refractory migraine

G43.501   Persistent migraine aura without cerebral infarction, not intractable, <u>with</u> status migrainosus — A form lasting more than 72 hours.

G43.509   Persistent migraine aura without cerebral infarction, not intractable, <u>without</u> status migrainosus
Persistent migraine aura NOS

G43.51- Persistent migraine aura without cerebral infarction, <u>intractable</u> — INTRACTABLE – Provider stated, and/or see Note at G43-.
Persistent migraine aura without cerebral infarction, with refractory migraine

G43.511   Persistent migraine aura without cerebral infarction, intractable, <u>with status migrainosus</u> — A form lasting more than 72 hours.

G43.519   Persistent migraine aura without cerebral infarction, intractable, <u>without</u> status migrainosus

G43.6- <u>Persistent</u> migraine aura <u>with cerebral infarction</u> — A form characterized by aura symptoms that are not reversible within seven days and/or are associated with radiographic evidence of infarction.
Code also the type of cerebral infarction (I63.-)

G43.60- Persistent migraine aura with cerebral infarction, <u>not</u> intractable
Persistent migraine aura with cerebral infarction, without refractory migraine

CC **G43.601   Persistent migraine aura with cerebral infarction, <u>not</u> intractable, <u>with</u> status migrainosus** — A form lasting more than 72 hours.

CC **G43.609   Persistent migraine aura with cerebral infarction, <u>not</u> intractable, <u>without</u> status migrainosus**

G43.61- Persistent migraine aura with cerebral infarction, <u>intractable</u> — INTRACTABLE – Provider stated, and/or see Note at G43-.
Persistent migraine aura with cerebral infarction, with refractory migraine

CC **G43.611   Persistent migraine aura with cerebral infarction, intractable, <u>with status migrainosus</u>** — A form lasting more than 72 hours.

CC **G43.619   Persistent migraine aura with cerebral infarction, intractable, <u>without</u> status migrainosus**

G43.7   <u>Chronic</u> migraine <u>without aura</u> — A form marked by headache occurring 15 or more days per month for more than three months and is not the result of medication overuse.
Transformed migraine
Excludes 1:   migraine without aura (G43.0-)

G43.70- Chronic migraine without aura, <u>not</u> intractable
Chronic migraine without aura, without refractory migraine

G43.701   Chronic migraine without aura, <u>not</u> intractable, <u>with status migrainosus</u> — A form lasting more than 72 hours.

G43.709   Chronic migraine without aura, <u>not</u> intractable, <u>without</u> status migrainosus
Chronic migraine without aura NOS

G43.71- Chronic migraine without aura, <u>intractable</u> — INTRACTABLE – Provider stated, and/or see Note at G43-.
Chronic migraine without aura, with refractory migraine

G43.711   Chronic migraine without aura, intractable, <u>with</u> status migrainosus — A form lasting more than 72 hours.

G43.719   Chronic migraine without aura, intractable, <u>without</u> status migrainosus

G43.A- <u>Cyclical vomiting</u> — A form marked by intense nausea and vomiting that lasts from one hour to days and is without headache.

G43.A0   Cyclical vomiting, <u>not</u> intractable
Cyclical vomiting, without refractory migraine

G43.A1   Cyclical vomiting, <u>intractable</u> — INTRACTABLE – Provider stated, and/or see Note at G43-.
Cyclical vomiting, with refractory migraine

G43.B- <u>Ophthalmoplegic</u> migraine — A form marked by severe headache and pain usually surrounding the eyeball that is often associated with eye muscle weakness.

G43.B0   Ophthalmoplegic migraine, <u>not</u> intractable
Ophthalmoplegic migraine, without refractory migraine

G43.B1   Ophthalmoplegic migraine, <u>intractable</u> — INTRACTABLE – Provider stated, and/or see Note at G43-.
Ophthalmoplegic migraine, with refractory migraine

G43.C- <u>Periodic headache syndromes in child or adult</u> — Other forms that affect children, adolescents, or adults with varying symptoms including abdominal pain and vertigo.

G43.C0   Periodic headache syndromes in child or adult, <u>not</u> intractable
Periodic headache syndromes in child or adult, without refractory migraine

G43.C1   Periodic headache syndromes in child or adult, <u>intractable</u> — INTRACTABLE – Provider stated, and/or see Note at G43-.
Periodic headache syndromes in child or adult, with refractory migraine

G43.D- <u>Abdominal</u> migraine — A form marked by abdominal pain, nausea, and vomiting that is usually seen in children.

G43.D0   Abdominal migraine, <u>not</u> intractable
Abdominal migraine, without refractory migraine

G43.D1   Abdominal migraine, <u>intractable</u> — INTRACTABLE – Provider stated, and/or see Note at G43-.
Abdominal migraine, with refractory migraine

G43.8-   <u>Other</u> migraine

G43.80- Other migraine, <u>not</u> intractable
Other migraine, without refractory migraine

G43.801   Other migraine, <u>not</u> intractable, <u>with status migrainosus</u> — A form lasting more than 72 hours.

G43.809   Other migraine, <u>not</u> intractable, <u>without</u> status migrainosus

G43.81- Other migraine, <u>intractable</u> — INTRACTABLE – Provider stated, and/or see Note at G43-.
Other migraine, with refractory migraine

G43.811   Other migraine, intractable, <u>with status migrainosus</u> — A form lasting more than 72 hours.

G43.819   Other migraine, intractable, <u>without</u> status migrainosus

G43.82- Menstrual migraine, <u>not</u> intractable — A form characterized by being associated with the menstrual cycle.
Menstrual headache, not intractable
Menstrual migraine, without refractory migraine
Menstrually related migraine, not intractable
Pre-menstrual headache, not intractable
Pre-menstrual migraine, not intractable
Pure menstrual migraine, not intractable
Code also associated premenstrual tension syndrome (N94.3)

G43.821   Menstrual migraine, <u>not</u> intractable, <u>with status migrainosus</u> — [♀] – A form lasting more than 72 hours.

G43.829   Menstrual migraine, <u>not</u> intractable, <u>without</u> status migrainosus — [♀]
Menstrual migraine NOS

G43.83- **Menstrual migraine, <u>intractable</u>** — A form characterized by being associated with the menstrual cycle. INTRACTABLE – Provider stated, and/or see Note at G43-.
  Menstrual headache, intractable
  Menstrual migraine, with refractory migraine
  Menstrually related migraine, intractable
  Pre-menstrual headache, intractable
  Pre-menstrual migraine, intractable
  Pure menstrual migraine, intractable
  Code also associated premenstrual tension syndrome (N94.3)

  G43.831 **Menstrual migraine, <u>intractable</u>, <u>with status</u> <u>migrainosus</u>** — [♀] – A form lasting more than 72 hours.

  G43.839 **Menstrual migraine, <u>intractable</u>, <u>without</u> status migrainosus** — [♀]

G43.9- **Migraine, <u>unspecified</u>**

  G43.90- **Migraine, unspecified, <u>not</u> intractable**
    Migraine, unspecified, without refractory migraine

  G43.901 **Migraine, unspecified, <u>not</u> intractable, <u>with status</u> <u>migrainosus</u>** — A form lasting more than 72 hours.
    Status migrainosus NOS

  G43.909 **Migraine, unspecified, <u>not</u> intractable, <u>without</u> status migrainosus**
    Migraine NOS

  G43.91- **Migraine, unspecified, <u>intractable</u>** — INTRACTABLE – Provider stated, and/or see Note at G43-.
    Migraine, unspecified, with refractory migraine

  G43.911 **Migraine, unspecified, intractable, <u>with status</u> <u>migrainosus</u>** — A form lasting more than 72 hours.

  G43.919 **Migraine, unspecified, intractable, <u>without</u> status migrainosus**

G44- **Other headache syndromes**
  Excludes 1:   *headache NOS (R51)*
  Excludes ❷: *atypical facial pain (G50.1)*
           headache due to lumbar puncture (G97.1)
           migraines (G43.-)
           trigeminal neuralgia (G50.0)

  G44.0- **Cluster headaches and other trigeminal autonomic cephalgias (TAC)** — CLUSTER HEADACHE – A neurological primary headache disorder that is characterized by extremely painful, unilateral headaches that typically occur at the same time of day for several weeks until the "cluster" period is over. TRIGEMINAL AUTONOMIC CEPHALGIAS – A group of primary headaches that involves the activation of the trigeminal-autonomic reflex.

    G44.00- **<u>Cluster headache syndrome, unspecified</u>**
      Ciliary neuralgia
      Cluster headache NOS
      Histamine cephalgia
      Lower half migraine
      Migrainous neuralgia

    G44.001 **Cluster headache syndrome, unspecified, <u>intractable</u>** — INTRACTABLE – Provider stated (also review Note at G43-).

    G44.009 **Cluster headache syndrome, unspecified, <u>not</u> intractable**
      Cluster headache syndrome NOS

  G44.01- **<u>Episodic</u> cluster headache** — A form that is characterized by cycles of headaches (commonly one to several per day for several weeks) followed by a pain-free interval of months to years.

    G44.011 **Episodic cluster headache, <u>intractable</u>** — INTRACTABLE – Provider stated (also review Note at G43-).

    G44.019 **Episodic cluster headache, <u>not</u> intractable**
      Episodic cluster headache NOS

  G44.02- **<u>Chronic</u> cluster headache** — A form that is characterized by cycles of headaches without sustained periods of remission.

    G44.021 **Chronic cluster headache, <u>intractable</u>** — INTRACTABLE – Provider stated (also review Note at G43-).

    G44.029 **Chronic cluster headache, <u>not</u> intractable**
      Chronic cluster headache NOS

G44.03- **<u>Episodic paroxysmal hemicrania</u>** — A type of primary headache that is characterized by throbbing, claw-like, or boring pain usually on one side of the face, has a duration of minutes to less than one hour, occurs multiple times per day, and has sustained periods of remission.
  Paroxysmal hemicrania NOS

  G44.031 **Episodic paroxysmal hemicrania, <u>intractable</u>** — INTRACTABLE – Provider stated (also review Note at G43-).

  G44.039 **Episodic paroxysmal hemicrania, <u>not</u> intractable**
    Episodic paroxysmal hemicrania NOS

G44.04- **<u>Chronic paroxysmal hemicrania</u>** — A type of primary headache that is characterized by throbbing, claw-like, or boring pain usually on one side of the face, has a duration of minutes to less than one hour, occurs multiple times per day, and does not have sustained periods of remission.

  G44.041 **Chronic paroxysmal hemicrania, <u>intractable</u>** — INTRACTABLE – Provider stated (also review Note at G43-).

  G44.049 **Chronic paroxysmal hemicrania, <u>not</u> intractable**
    Chronic paroxysmal hemicrania NOS

G44.05- **Short lasting unilateral <u>neuralgiform headache</u> with conjunctival injection and tearing (SUNCT)** — A type of primary headache that is characterized by a very short duration (less than a minute), occurs very frequently (many times per hour), watery eyes, and bloodshot eyes that are caused by the dilation of blood vessels.

  G44.051 **Short lasting unilateral neuralgiform headache with conjunctival injection and tearing (SUNCT), <u>intractable</u>** — INTRACTABLE – Provider stated (also review Note at G43-).

  G44.059 **Short lasting unilateral neuralgiform headache with conjunctival injection and tearing (SUNCT), <u>not</u> intractable**
    Short lasting unilateral neuralgiform headache with conjunctival injection and tearing (SUNCT) NOS

G44.09- **Other <u>trigeminal autonomic cephalgias</u> (TAC)**

  G44.091 **Other trigeminal autonomic cephalgias (TAC), <u>intractable</u>** — INTRACTABLE – Provider stated (also review Note at G43-).

  G44.099 **Other trigeminal autonomic cephalgias (TAC), <u>not</u> intractable**

G44.1 **<u>Vascular headache, not elsewhere classified</u>**
  Excludes ❷: *cluster headache (G44.0)*
           complicated headache syndromes (G44.5-)
           drug-induced headache (G44.4-)
           migraine (G43-)
           other specified headache syndromes (G44.8-)
           post-traumatic headache (G44.3-)
           tension-type headache (G44.2-)

G44.2- **<u>Tension-type</u> headache** — A common type of primary headache characterized by a mild to moderate pain, tightness in the muscles of the head, and tenderness of the head muscles and is not associated with a psychological condition.

  G44.20- **Tension-type headache, <u>unspecified</u>**

    G44.201 **Tension-type headache, unspecified, <u>intractable</u>** — INTRACTABLE – Provider stated (also review Note at G43-).

    G44.209 **Tension-type headache, unspecified, <u>not</u> intractable**
      Tension headache NOS

  G44.21- **<u>Episodic</u> tension-type headache** — A form that occurs less than several times a month (approximately 15 or less).

    G44.211 **Episodic tension-type headache, <u>intractable</u>** — INTRACTABLE – Provider stated (also review Note at G43-).

    G44.219 **Episodic tension-type headache, <u>not</u> intractable**
      Episodic tension-type headache NOS

  G44.22- **<u>Chronic</u> tension-type headache** — A form that occurs more than several times a month (approximately 15 or more).

    G44.221 **Chronic tension-type headache, <u>intractable</u>** — INTRACTABLE – Provider stated (also review Note at G43-).

    G44.229 **Chronic tension-type headache, <u>not</u> intractable**
      Chronic tension-type headache NOS

G44.3- **<u>Post-traumatic</u> headache** — A type of headache that is the result of a head injury and that usually starts within two weeks post injury.

  G44.30- **Post-traumatic headache, <u>unspecified</u>**

    G44.301 **Post-traumatic headache, unspecified, <u>intractable</u>** — INTRACTABLE – Provider stated (also review Note at G43-).

G 4 3 - G 4 4

G44.309 Post-traumatic headache, unspecified, <u>not</u> intractable
Post-traumatic headache NOS

G44.31- <u>Acute</u> post-traumatic headache — A form that goes away by the third month.

G44.311 Acute post-traumatic headache, <u>intractable</u> — INTRACTABLE – Provider stated (also review Note at G43-).

G44.319 Acute post-traumatic headache, <u>not</u> intractable
Acute post-traumatic headache NOS

G44.32- <u>Chronic</u> post-traumatic headache — A form that continues beyond the third month.

G44.321 Chronic post-traumatic headache, <u>intractable</u> — INTRACTABLE – Provider stated (also review Note at G43-).

G44.329 Chronic post-traumatic headache, <u>not</u> intractable
Chronic post-traumatic headache NOS

G44.4- <u>Drug-induced</u> headache, not elsewhere classified
Medication overuse headache — A type of headache that is the result of excessive use of medication (often medication used for headaches) which resolves after the medication is withdrawn.
Use additional code for adverse effect, if applicable, to identify drug (T36-T50 with fifth or sixth character 5)

G44.40 Drug-induced headache, not elsewhere classified, <u>not</u> intractable

G44.41 Drug-induced headache, not elsewhere classified, <u>intractable</u> — INTRACTABLE – Provider stated (also review Note at G43-).

G44.5- Complicated headache syndromes

G44.51 Hemicrania continua — A type of primary headache that is characterized by unilateral, daily, and continuous headaches that are without pain-free periods and respond to therapeutic doses of indomethacin.

G44.52 New daily persistent headache (NDPH) — A type of primary headache that is characterized by daily and unremitting pain that continues for more than three months and is bilateral in location.

G44.53 Primary thunderclap headache — A type of primary headache that is characterized by very sudden onset (usually less than one minute) and very severe pain that is not due to an underlying pathology like cerebral hemorrhage.

G44.59 Other complicated headache syndrome

G44.8- Other specified headache syndromes

G44.81 Hypnic headache — A type of primary headache that is characterized by onset during sleep ("alarm clock" headache), begins after the age of 50, and is short-lived (typically 30 minutes).

G44.82 Headache associated with sexual activity — A type of primary headache that is characterized by a dull, bilateral ache during sexual activity and increases with sexual excitement.
Orgasmic headache
Preorgasmic headache

G44.83 Primary cough headache — A type of primary headache that is characterized by onset due to coughing and usually lasts less than 30 minutes.

G44.84 Primary exertional headache — A type of primary headache that is characterized by onset due to physical exertion and may last from minutes to two days.

G44.85 Primary stabbing headache — A type of primary headache that is characterized by sharp, jabbing-like pains in the orbit, temple, and parietal areas that recurs at irregular intervals from one to many per day.

G44.89 Other headache syndrome

G45- <u>Transient cerebral ischemic attacks</u> and related syndromes — An episode of neurologic dysfunction caused by temporary decreased blood flow to the brain, spinal cord, or retina and without residual effects or infarction.
Excludes 1:   *neonatal cerebral ischemia (P91.0)*
                transient retinal artery occlusion (H34.0-)

cc **G45.0** Vertebro-basilar artery syndrome — A form originating in the vertebral and basilar arteries.

cc **G45.1** Carotid artery syndrome (hemispheric) — A form originating in a carotid artery that usually affects one hemisphere of the brain that is often caused by anatomical compression of a carotid artery while turning the head to one side for a brief to extended period of time.

cc **G45.2** Multiple and bilateral precerebral artery syndromes

cc **G45.3** Amaurosis fugax — A form characterized by transient visual loss in one eye.

G45.4 Transient global amnesia — A neurologic condition characterized by an acute, temporary loss of short-term memory.
Excludes 1:   *amnesia NOS (R41.3)*

cc **G45.8** Other transient cerebral ischemic attacks and related syndromes

cc **G45.9** Transient cerebral ischemic attack, unspecified
Spasm of cerebral artery
TIA
Transient cerebral ischemia NOS

G46- <u>Vascular syndromes of brain in cerebrovascular diseases</u> — The symptomatic conditions resulting from a cerebrovascular disease (occlusion, sclerosis, etc.) to a particular artery and the part of the brain it supplies.
Code first underlying cerebrovascular disease (I60-I69)

cc **G46.0** Middle cerebral artery syndrome

cc **G46.1** Anterior cerebral artery syndrome

cc **G46.2** Posterior cerebral artery syndrome

G46.3 Brain stem stroke syndrome
Benedikt syndrome
Claude syndrome
Foville syndrome
Millard-Gubler syndrome
Wallenberg syndrome
Weber syndrome

G46.4 Cerebellar stroke syndrome

G46.5 Pure motor lacunar syndrome

G46.6 Pure sensory lacunar syndrome

G46.7 Other lacunar syndromes

G46.8 Other vascular syndromes of brain in cerebrovascular diseases

G47- <u>Sleep disorders</u> — A condition that affects or disrupts the natural sleep pattern.
Excludes ❷: *nightmares (F51.5)*
            nonorganic sleep disorders (F51.-)
            sleep terrors (F51.4)
            sleepwalking (F51.3)

G47.0- <u>Insomnia</u> — A condition that disrupts the natural sleep pattern that is characterized by poor quality sleep, difficulty falling asleep, difficulty staying asleep, waking up too early, and multiple spontaneous awakenings.
Excludes ❷: *alcohol related insomnia (F10.182, F10.282, F10.982)*
            drug-related insomnia F11.182, F11.282, F11.982, F13.182, F13.282, F13.982, F14.182, F14.282, F14.982, F15.182, F15.282, F15.982, F19.182, F19.282, F19.982
            idiopathic insomnia (F51.01)
            insomnia due to a mental disorder (F51.05)
            insomnia not due to a substance or known physiological condition (F51.0-)
            nonorganic insomnia (F51.0-)
            primary insomnia (F51.01)
            sleep apnea (G47.3-)

G47.00 Insomnia, unspecified
Insomnia NOS

G47.01 Insomnia due to medical condition
Code also associated medical condition

G47.09 Other insomnia

G47.1- <u>Hypersomnia</u> — A condition of excessive daytime sleepiness that is not relieved by naps or prolonged sleep periods and often results in difficulty waking up, long nighttime sleeping, decreased energy, confusion, disorientation, and poor motor coordination.
Excludes ❷: *alcohol-related hypersomnia (F10.182, F10.282, F10.982)*
            drug-related hypersomnia F11.182, F11.282, F11.982, F13.182, F13.282, F13.982, F14.182, F14.282, F14.982, F15.182, F15.282, F15.982, F19.182, F19.282, F19.982
            hypersomnia due to a mental disorder (F51.13)
            hypersomnia not due to a substance or known physiological condition (F51.1-)
            primary hypersomnia (F51.11)
            sleep apnea (G47.3-)

G47.10 Hypersomnia, unspecified
Hypersomnia NOS

G47.11 <u>Idiopathic</u> hypersomnia <u>with long sleep time</u>
Idiopathic hypersomnia NOS

G47.12 <u>Idiopathic</u> hypersomnia <u>without</u> long sleep time

G47.13 Recurrent hypersomnia — A form that lasts for days to weeks at a time and occurs several times a year.
Kleine-Levin syndrome
Menstrual related hypersomnia

G47.14 Hypersomnia due to medical condition
Code also associated medical condition

G47.19 Other hypersomnia

G 4 4 - G 4 7

G47.2- <u>Circadian rhythm</u> sleep disorders — A condition that affects or disrupts the normal 24-hour sleep-wake pattern.
Disorders of the sleep wake schedule
Inversion of nyctohemeral rhythm
Inversion of sleep rhythm

G47.20 Circadian rhythm sleep disorder, unspecified type
Sleep wake schedule disorder NOS

G47.21 Circadian rhythm sleep disorder, <u>delayed</u> sleep phase type — A form in which the patient goes to bed later than desired and rises later than desired.
Delayed sleep phase syndrome

G47.22 Circadian rhythm sleep disorder, <u>advanced</u> sleep phase type — A form in which the patient goes to bed earlier than desired and rises earlier than desired.

G47.23 Circadian rhythm sleep disorder, <u>irregular</u> sleep wake type — A form in which the patient has difficulty establishing a natural sleep-wake pattern.
Irregular sleep-wake pattern

G47.24 Circadian rhythm sleep disorder, <u>free</u> running type — A form occurring in patients who are not synchronized to the normal 24-hour day due to absence of environmental cues (e.g., blind persons).

G47.25 Circadian rhythm sleep disorder, <u>jet lag</u> type — A form characterized by difficulty adjusting to rapid travel over several time zones that results in lack of alertness and sleepiness.

G47.26 Circadian rhythm sleep disorder, <u>shift work</u> type — A form characterized by difficulty adjusting to night-shift work or varying shift-work schedules.

G47.27 Circadian rhythm sleep disorder in conditions classified elsewhere — [Not Allowed as PDX]
Code first underlying condition

G47.29 Other circadian rhythm sleep disorder

G47.3- <u>Sleep apnea</u> — The periodic cessation of breathing during sleep that is not classified elsewhere (see Excludes 1 below).
Code also any associated underlying condition
Excludes 1: *apnea NOS (R06.81)*
Cheyne-Stokes breathing (R06.3)
pickwickian syndrome (E66.2)
sleep apnea of newborn (P28.3)

G47.30 Sleep apnea, unspecified
Sleep apnea NOS

G47.31 <u>Primary</u> central sleep apnea — A form associated with a lack of sufficient neural impulses to the respiratory system.

G47.32 <u>High altitude</u> periodic breathing — A normal phenomenon form that occurs at higher altitudes and is characterized by brief apneic periods (3 to 10 seconds), but is not associated with altitude illness.

G47.33 <u>Obstructive</u> sleep apnea (adult) (pediatric) — A form that is due to structural abnormalities in the back of the throat that briefly collapses and blocks the airway.
Excludes 1: *obstructive sleep apnea of newborn (P28.3)*

G47.34 <u>Idiopathic</u> sleep related nonobstructive alveolar hypoventilation — A condition of insufficient ventilation during sleep that causes deficient oxygenation of the blood, but is not due to an obstructive airway condition.
Sleep related hypoxia

G47.35 <u>Congenital</u> central alveolar hypoventilation syndrome — A condition of insufficient ventilation during sleep that causes deficient oxygenation of the blood that has been determined as congenital in origin. (Note: see Excludes above)

G47.36 Sleep related hypoventilation in conditions classified elsewhere — [Not Allowed as PDX]
Sleep related hypoxemia in conditions classified elsewhere
Code first underlying condition

G47.37 Central sleep apnea <u>in conditions classified elsewhere</u> — [Not Allowed as PDX]
Code first underlying condition

G47.39 Other sleep apnea

G47.4- Narcolepsy and cataplexy

G47.41- Narcolepsy — A neurological disorder of chronic recurrent attacks of drowsiness and sleep during the daytime.

G47.411 Narcolepsy <u>with</u> cataplexy — A form with the sudden, brief loss of muscle control triggered by strong emotion or emotional response.

G47.419 Narcolepsy <u>without</u> cataplexy
Narcolepsy NOS

G47.42- Narcolepsy in conditions classified elsewhere
Code first underlying condition

G47.421 Narcolepsy in conditions classified elsewhere <u>with cataplexy</u> — [Not Allowed as PDX]

G47.429 Narcolepsy in conditions classified elsewhere <u>without</u> cataplexy — [Not Allowed as PDX]

G47.5- Parasomnia — The condition of abnormal behavioral or physiological events associated with sleep and sleep stages.
Excludes 1: *alcohol induced parasomnia (F10.182, F10.282, F10.982)*
drug induced parasomnia (F11.182, F11.282, F11.982, F13.182, F13.282, F13.982, F14.182, F14.282, F14.982, F15.182, F15.282, F15.982, F19.182, F19.282, F19.982)
parasomnia not due to a substance or known physiological condition (F51.8)

G47.50 Parasomnia, unspecified
Parasomnia NOS

G47.51 Confusional arousals — A form that may begin with yelling or crying and violently moving around in bed, in which the sleeper seems to be alert and upset after awakening.

G47.52 REM sleep behavior disorder — A form that occurs during the rapid eye movement state of sleep, in which the sleeper acts out his or her dream.

G47.53 Recurrent isolated sleep paralysis — A form with the sensation of feeling paralyzed upon awakening.

G47.54 Parasomnia in conditions classified elsewhere — [Not Allowed as PDX]
Code first underlying condition

G47.59 Other parasomnia

G47.6- Sleep related movement disorders — The condition of involuntary movement occurring during sleep.
Excludes ❷: *restless legs syndrome (G25.81)*

G47.61 Periodic limb movement disorder — A form characterized by the repetitive, brief involuntary movement of the limbs (usually legs) during sleep that occurs between non-movement periods.
Periodic limb movement disorder

G47.62 Sleep related leg cramps — A form involving the painful contraction of the leg muscles.

G47.63 Sleep related bruxism — A form involving the grinding of the teeth during sleep.
Excludes 1: *psychogenic bruxism (F45.8)*

G47.69 Other sleep related movement disorders

G47.8 Other sleep disorders

G47.9 Sleep disorder, unspecified
Sleep disorder NOS

Nerve, nerve root and plexus disorders (G50-G59)

Excludes 1: *current traumatic nerve, nerve root and plexus disorders — see Injury, nerve by body region*
neuralgia NOS (M79.2)
neuritis NOS (M79.2)
peripheral neuritis in pregnancy (O26.82-)
radiculitis NOS (M54.1-)

G50- Disorders of <u>trigeminal nerve</u>
Includes: Disorders of 5th cranial nerve

G50.0 Trigeminal neuralgia — A sudden, severe, excruciating episodic pain in the area supplied by the trigeminal nerve.
Syndrome of paroxysmal facial pain
Tic douloureux

G50.1 Atypical facial pain

G50.8 Other disorders of trigeminal nerve

G50.9 Disorder of trigeminal nerve, unspecified

G51- <u>Facial nerve</u> disorders
Includes: Disorders of 7th cranial nerve

G51.0 Bell's palsy — Facial paralysis caused by a lesion of the facial nerve and marked by characteristic distortion of the face.
Facial palsy

G51.1 Geniculate ganglionitis — Inflammation of the geniculate ganglion characterized by severe, sharp pain occurring in the region of the external ear.
Excludes 1: *postherpetic geniculate ganglionitis (B02.21)*

G 4 7 - G 5 1

G51.2   **Melkersson's syndrome** — A hereditary facial palsy characterized by facial swelling and occasionally fissured tongue.
     Melkersson-Rosenthal syndrome

G51.3   **Clonic hemifacial spasm**

G51.4   **Facial myokymia**

G51.8   **Other disorders of facial nerve**

G51.9   **Disorder of facial nerve, unspecified**

G52-   **Disorders of other cranial nerves**
    Excludes ❷: *disorders of acoustic [8th] nerve (H93.3)*
            disorders of optic [2nd] nerve (H46, H47.0)
            paralytic strabismus due to nerve palsy (H49.0-H49.2)

G52.0   **Disorders of olfactory nerve**
     Disorders of 1st cranial nerve

G52.1   **Disorders of glossopharyngeal nerve**
     Disorder of 9th cranial nerve
     Glossopharyngeal neuralgia — Pharyngeal spasms of pain in the sensory distribution of the ninth cranial nerve.

G52.2   **Disorders of vagus nerve**
     Disorders of pneumogastric [10th] nerve

G52.3   **Disorders of hypoglossal nerve**
     Disorders of 12th cranial nerve

G52.7   **Disorders of multiple cranial nerves**
     Polyneuritis cranialis — Inflammation of two or more of the cranial nerves at the same time.

G52.8   **Disorders of other specified cranial nerves**

G52.9   **Cranial nerve disorder, unspecified**

G53   **Cranial nerve disorders in diseases classified elsewhere** — [Not Allowed as PDX]
    Code first underlying disease, such as:
     Neoplasm (C00-D49)
    Excludes 1:   *multiple cranial nerve palsy in sarcoidosis (D86.82)*
            multiple cranial nerve palsy in syphilis (A52.15)
            postherpetic geniculate ganglionitis (B02.21)
            postherpetic trigeminal neuralgia (B02.22)

G54-   **Nerve root and plexus disorders**
    Excludes 1:   *current traumatic nerve root and plexus disorders — see nerve injury by body region*
            intervertebral disc disorders (M50-M51)
            neuralgia or neuritis NOS (M79.2)
            neuritis or radiculitis brachial NOS (M54.13)
            neuritis or radiculitis lumbar NOS (M54.16)
            neuritis or radiculitis lumbosacral NOS (M54.17)
            neuritis or radiculitis thoracic NOS (M54.14)
            radiculitis NOS (M54.10)
            radiculopathy NOS (M54.10)
            spondylosis (M47.-)

G54.0   **Brachial plexus disorders**
     Thoracic outlet syndrome — Compression of the brachial plexus nerve trunks characterized by numbness and tingling of the hand, weakness and wasting of the small muscles of the hand, and painful paresthesias.

G54.1   **Lumbosacral plexus disorders**

G54.2   **Cervical root disorders, not elsewhere classified**

G54.3   **Thoracic root disorders, not elsewhere classified** — [Unacceptable PDX]

G54.4   **Lumbosacral root disorders, not elsewhere classified**

G54.5   **Neuralgic amyotrophy** — Pain across the shoulder and upper arm, with atrophy and paralysis of the muscles of the shoulder girdle.
     Parsonage-Aldren-Turner syndrome
     Shoulder-girdle neuritis
    Excludes 1:   *neuralgic amyotrophy in diabetes mellitus (E08-E13 with .44)*

G54.6   **Phantom limb syndrome with pain** — The sensation that pain exists in the amputated part of the limb due to stimulation of those transsected nerve ends which normally innervate the distal part of that limb.

G54.7   **Phantom limb syndrome without pain** — The sensation that the limb exists in the amputated part of the limb.
     Phantom limb syndrome NOS

G54.8   **Other nerve root and plexus disorders**

G54.9   **Nerve root and plexus disorder, unspecified**

G55   **Nerve root and plexus compressions** <u>in diseases classified elsewhere</u> — [Not Allowed as PDX]
    Code first underlying disease, such as:
     Neoplasm (C00-D49)
    Excludes 1:   *nerve root compression (due to) (in) ankylosing spondylitis (M45.-)*
            nerve root compression (due to) (in) dorsopathies (M53.-, M54.-)
            nerve root compression (due to) (in) intervertebral disc disorders (M50.1.-, M51.1.-)
            nerve root compression (due to) (in) spondylopathies (M46.-, M48.-)

G56-   **Mononeuropathies of** <u>upper</u> **limb**
    Excludes 1:   *current traumatic nerve disorder — see nerve injury by body region*

G56.0-   <u>**Carpal tunnel**</u> **syndrome** — Fluctuating numbness, paresthesias, and pain in the hand due to compression of the median nerve at the wrist.

    G56.00   **Carpal tunnel syndrome, unspecified upper limb**

    G56.01   **Carpal tunnel syndrome, <u>right</u> upper limb**

    G56.02   **Carpal tunnel syndrome, <u>left</u> upper limb**

    G56.03   **Carpal tunnel syndrome, <u>bilateral</u> upper limbs**

G56.1-   <u>**Other lesions**</u> **of median nerve**

    G56.10   **Other lesions of median nerve, unspecified upper limb**

    G56.11   **Other lesions of median nerve, <u>right</u> upper limb**

    G56.12   **Other lesions of median nerve, <u>left</u> upper limb**

    G56.13   **Other lesions of median nerve, <u>bilateral</u> upper limbs**

G56.2-   **Lesion of <u>ulnar nerve</u>** — Pain, numbness, and weakness of the hand and forearm caused by injury or compression of the ulnar nerve at the elbow.
     Tardy ulnar nerve palsy

    G56.20   **Lesion of ulnar nerve, unspecified upper limb**

    G56.21   **Lesion of ulnar nerve, <u>right</u> upper limb**

    G56.22   **Lesion of ulnar nerve, <u>left</u> upper limb**

    G56.23   **Lesion of ulnar nerve, <u>bilateral</u> upper limbs**

G56.3-   **Lesion of <u>radial nerve</u>** — Wrist drop, paralysis of the extension of the elbow, weakness of elbow flexion, and paralysis of the extension of the fingers, thumb, and wrist due to a lesion of the radial nerve.

    G56.30   **Lesion of radial nerve, unspecified upper limb**

    G56.31   **Lesion of radial nerve, <u>right</u> upper limb**

    G56.32   **Lesion of radial nerve, <u>left</u> upper limb**

    G56.33   **Lesion of radial nerve, <u>bilateral</u> upper limbs**

G56.4-   <u>**Causalgia**</u> **of <u>upper</u> limb** — A condition characterized by intense burning pain of the upper limb with skin sensitivity, discoloration, and increased localized temperature that is most likely due to peripheral nerve damage.
     Complex regional pain syndrome II of upper limb — A form identified as following a distinct nerve injury.
    Excludes 1:   *complex regional pain syndrome I of lower limb (G90.52-)*
            complex regional pain syndrome I of upper limb (G90.51-)
            complex regional pain syndrome II of lower limb (G57.7-)
            reflex sympathetic dystrophy of lower limb (G90.52-)
            reflex sympathetic dystrophy of upper limb (G90.51-)

    G56.40   **Causalgia of unspecified upper limb**

    G56.41   **Causalgia of <u>right</u> upper limb**

    G56.42   **Causalgia of <u>left</u> upper limb**

    G56.43   **Causalgia of <u>bilateral</u> upper limbs**

G56.8-   <u>**Other specified**</u> **mononeuropathies of <u>upper</u> limb**
     Interdigital neuroma of upper limb

    G56.80   **Other specified mononeuropathies of unspecified upper limb**

    G56.81   **Other specified mononeuropathies of <u>right</u> upper limb**

    G56.82   **Other specified mononeuropathies of <u>left</u> upper limb**

    G56.83   **Other specified mononeuropathies of <u>bilateral</u> upper limbs**

G56.9-   <u>**Unspecified mono**</u>**neuropathy of <u>upper</u> limb**

    G56.90   **Unspecified mononeuropathy of unspecified upper limb**

    G56.91   **Unspecified mononeuropathy of <u>right</u> upper limb**

    G56.92   **Unspecified mononeuropathy of <u>left</u> upper limb**

    G56.93   **Unspecified mononeuropathy of <u>bilateral</u> upper limbs**

G51 - G56

G57- **Mononeuropathies of lower limb**
  Excludes 1:   current traumatic nerve disorder — see nerve injury by body region

G57.0- **Lesion of sciatic nerve**
  Excludes 1:   sciatica NOS (M54.3-)
  Excludes ❷: sciatica attributed to intervertebral disc disorder (M51.1.-)
  G57.00 **Lesion of sciatic nerve, unspecified lower limb**
  G57.01 **Lesion of sciatic nerve, right lower limb**
  G57.02 **Lesion of sciatic nerve, left lower limb**
  G57.03 **Lesion of sciatic nerve, bilateral lower limbs**

G57.1- **Meralgia paresthetica** — Compression of the femoral cutaneous nerve at the inguinal ligament characterized by paresthesia, pain, and numbness of the outer surface of the thigh.
    Lateral cutaneous nerve of thigh syndrome
  G57.10 **Meralgia paresthetica, unspecified lower limb**
  G57.11 **Meralgia paresthetica, right lower limb**
  G57.12 **Meralgia paresthetica, left lower limb**
  G57.13 **Meralgia paresthetica, bilateral lower limbs**

G57.2- **Lesion of femoral nerve**
  G57.20 **Lesion of femoral nerve, unspecified lower limb**
  G57.21 **Lesion of femoral nerve, right lower limb**
  G57.22 **Lesion of femoral nerve, left lower limb**
  G57.23 **Lesion of femoral nerve, bilateral lower limbs**

G57.3- **Lesion of lateral popliteal nerve**
    Peroneal nerve palsy
  G57.30 **Lesion of lateral popliteal nerve, unspecified lower limb**
  G57.31 **Lesion of lateral popliteal nerve, right lower limb**
  G57.32 **Lesion of lateral popliteal nerve, left lower limb**
  G57.33 **Lesion of lateral popliteal nerve, bilateral lower limbs**

G57.4- **Lesion of medial popliteal nerve**
  G57.40 **Lesion of medial popliteal nerve, unspecified lower limb**
  G57.41 **Lesion of medial popliteal nerve, right lower limb**
  G57.42 **Lesion of medial popliteal nerve, left lower limb**
  G57.43 **Lesion of medial popliteal nerve, bilateral lower limbs**

G57.5- **Tarsal tunnel syndrome** — Compression of the posterior tibial nerve characterized by pain, numbness, and tingling of the sole of the foot.
  G57.50 **Tarsal tunnel syndrome, unspecified lower limb**
  G57.51 **Tarsal tunnel syndrome, right lower limb**
  G57.52 **Tarsal tunnel syndrome, left lower limb**
  G57.53 **Tarsal tunnel syndrome, bilateral lower limbs**

G57.6- **Lesion of plantar nerve**
    Morton's metatarsalgia — Episodic pain, or traumatic nodular mass of nerve tissue in the region of the third and fourth metatarsals of the foot.
  G57.60 **Lesion of plantar nerve, unspecified lower limb**
  G57.61 **Lesion of plantar nerve, right lower limb**
  G57.62 **Lesion of plantar nerve, left lower limb**
  G57.63 **Lesion of plantar nerve, bilateral lower limbs**

G57.7- **Causalgia of lower limb** — A condition characterized by intense burning pain of the lower limb with skin sensitivity, discoloration, and increased localized temperature that is most likely due to peripheral nerve damage.
    Complex regional pain syndrome II of lower limb
  Excludes 1:   complex regional pain syndrome I of lower limb (G90.52-)
                complex regional pain syndrome I of upper limb (G90.51-)
                complex regional pain syndrome II of upper limb (G56.4-)
                reflex sympathetic dystrophy of lower limb (G90.52-)
                reflex sympathetic dystrophy of upper limb (G90.51-)
  G57.70 **Causalgia of unspecified lower limb**
  G57.71 **Causalgia of right lower limb**
  G57.72 **Causalgia of left lower limb**
  G57.73 **Causalgia of bilateral lower limbs**

G57.8- **Other specified mononeuropathies of lower limb**
    Interdigital neuroma of lower limb
  G57.80 **Other specified mononeuropathies of unspecified lower limb**
  G57.81 **Other specified mononeuropathies of right lower limb**
  G57.82 **Other specified mononeuropathies of left lower limb**
  G57.83 **Other specified mononeuropathies of bilateral lower limbs**

G57.9- **Unspecified mononeuropathy of lower limb**
  G57.90 **Unspecified mononeuropathy of unspecified lower limb**
  G57.91 **Unspecified mononeuropathy of right lower limb**
  G57.92 **Unspecified mononeuropathy of left lower limb**
  G57.93 **Unspecified mononeuropathy of bilateral lower limbs**

G58- **Other mononeuropathies**
  G58.0   **Intercostal neuropathy**
  G58.7   **Mononeuritis multiplex**
  G58.8   **Other specified mononeuropathies**
  G58.9   **Mononeuropathy, unspecified**

G59 **Mononeuropathy in diseases classified elsewhere** — [Not Allowed as PDX]
  Code first underlying disease
  Excludes 1:   diabetic mononeuropathy (E08-E13 with .41)
                syphilitic nerve paralysis (A52.19)
                syphilitic neuritis (A52.15)
                tuberculous mononeuropathy (A17.83)

Polyneuropathies and other disorders of the peripheral nervous system (G60-G65)

  Excludes 1:   neuralgia NOS (M79.2)
                neuritis NOS (M79.2)
                peripheral neuritis in pregnancy (O26.82-)
                radiculitis NOS (M54.10)

G60- **Hereditary and idiopathic neuropathy** — A peripheral nerve disease that is genetically transmitted or is of unknown origin.
  G60.0   **Hereditary motor and sensory neuropathy** — An inherited neuropathy characterized by lightning pains, hyperkeratosis feet, painless ulcers, severe distal sensory loss, and muscle wasting.
    Charcot-Marie-Tooth disease
    Déjérine-Sottas disease
    Hereditary motor and sensory neuropathy, types I-IV
    Hypertrophic neuropathy of infancy
    Peroneal muscular atrophy (axonal type) (hypertrophic type)
    Roussy-Levy syndrome
  CC G60.1 **Refsum's disease** — An inherited defect of acid metabolism characterized by chronic polyneuritis, retinitis pigmentosa, and mild ataxia.
    Infantile Refsum disease
  G60.2   **Neuropathy in association with hereditary ataxia**
  G60.3   **Idiopathic progressive neuropathy** — A condition of increasingly persistent disease of the peripheral nerves of undetermined origin.
  G60.8   **Other hereditary and idiopathic neuropathies**
    Dominantly inherited sensory neuropathy
    Morvan's disease
    Nelaton's syndrome
    Recessively inherited sensory neuropathy
  G60.9   **Hereditary and idiopathic neuropathy, unspecified**

G61- **Inflammatory polyneuropathy** — Disease of the nervous system caused by inflammation and cellular damage.
  CC G61.0 **Guillain-Barre syndrome** — An acute progressive ascending motor neuron paralysis of unknown etiology (most likely autoimmune) characterized by paresthesia, flaccid paralysis, spreading from the legs towards the head, and in some cases respiratory paralysis.
    AHA 14:2Q:p4 – Acute inflammatory demyelinating polyneuropathy
    Acute (post-)infective polyneuritis
    Miller Fisher Syndrome
  G61.1   **Serum neuropathy**
    Use additional code for adverse effect, if applicable, to identify serum (T50-)
  G61.8- **Other inflammatory polyneuropathies**
  CC G61.81 **Chronic inflammatory demyelinating polyneuritis** — A slowly progressive sensorimotor condition characterized by symmetrical weakness and paresthesias.
  G61.82 **Multifocal motor neuropathy**
    MMN

(side tab) G 57 - G 61

G61.89 Other inflammatory polyneuropathies

G61.9 Inflammatory polyneuropathy, unspecified

G62- Other and unspecified polyneuropathies

G62.0 Drug-induced polyneuropathy — Damage of multiple peripheral nerves due to the cellular damaging effects of drugs.
Use additional code for adverse effect, if applicable, to identify drug (T36-T50 with fifth or sixth character 5)

G62.1 Alcoholic polyneuropathy — Damage of the peripheral nerves due to the cellular destructive effects of excess alcohol.

G62.2 Polyneuropathy due to other toxic agents
Code first (T51-T65) to identify toxic agent

G62.8- Other specified polyneuropathies

cc **G62.81 Critical illness polyneuropathy** — A functional disturbance or damage of the peripheral nervous system that is associated with sepsis, multi-organ failure, and SIRS.
    Acute motor neuropathy

G62.82 Radiation-induced polyneuropathy
Use additional external cause code (W88-W90, X39.0-) to identify cause

G62.89 Other specified polyneuropathies
    AHA 16:2Q:p11 – Anti-MAG peripheral neuropathy

G62.9 Polyneuropathy, unspecified
    Neuropathy NOS

G63 Polyneuropathy in diseases classified elsewhere — [Not Allowed as PDX]
    AHA 12:4Q:p99 – Polyneuropathy
Code first underlying disease, such as:
    Amyloidosis (E85.-)
    Endocrine disease, except diabetes (E00-E07, E15-E16, E20-E34)
    Metabolic diseases (E70-E88)
    Neoplasm (C00-D49)
    Nutritional deficiency (E40-E64)

Excludes 1:   *polyneuropathy (in):*
      diabetes mellitus (E08-E13 with .42)
      diphtheria (A36.83)
      infectious mononucleosis (B27.0-B27.9 with 1)
      Lyme disease (A69.22)
      mumps (B26.84)
      postherpetic (B02.23)
      rheumatoid arthritis (M05.33)
      scleroderma (M34.83)
      systemic lupus erythematosus (M32.19)

G64 Other disorders of peripheral nervous system
    Disorder of peripheral nervous system NOS

G65- Sequelae of inflammatory and toxic polyneuropathies
Code first condition resulting from (sequela) of inflammatory and toxic polyneuropathies

G65.0 Sequelae of Guillain-Barré syndrome

G65.1 Sequelae of other inflammatory polyneuropathy

G65.2 Sequelae of toxic polyneuropathy

Diseases of myoneural junction and muscle (G70-G73)

G70- Myasthenia gravis and other myoneural disorders
Excludes 1:   *botulism (A05.1, A48.51-A48.52)*
      transient neonatal myasthenia gravis (P94.0)

G70.0- Myasthenia gravis — An autoimmune condition characterized by progressive muscular weakness on exertion followed by recovery of strength after a period of rest.

G70.00 Myasthenia gravis without (acute) exacerbation
    Myasthenia gravis NOS

MCC **G70.01 Myasthenia gravis with (acute) exacerbation** — A relatively sudden, severe onset of difficulty breathing caused by significant weakness of the muscles that control breathing.
    Myasthenia gravis in crisis

G70.1 Toxic myoneural disorders — Disorders of the muscles and nerves caused by the cellular damaging effect of toxic substances.
Code first (T51-T65) to identify toxic agent

G70.2 Congenital and developmental myasthenia

G70.8- Other specified myoneural disorders

cc **G70.80 Lambert-Eaton syndrome, unspecified** — An autoimmune, neuromuscular junction disorder that is characterized by muscle weakness, difficulty swallowing, dry mouth, and vision changes.
    Lambert-Eaton syndrome NOS

cc **G70.81 Lambert-Eaton syndrome in disease classified elsewhere** — [Not Allowed as PDX]
Code first underlying disease
Excludes 1:   *Lambert-Eaton syndrome in neoplastic disease (G73.1)*

G70.89 Other specified myoneural disorders

G70.9 Myoneural disorder, unspecified

G71- Primary disorders of muscles
Excludes ❷: *arthrogryposis multiplex congenita (Q74.3)*
      metabolic disorders (E70-E88)
      myositis (M60.-)

cc **G71.0 Muscular dystrophy** — A group of inherited muscular dystrophies characterized by progressive muscular weakness and degeneration of muscle fibers.
    Autosomal recessive, childhood type, muscular dystrophy resembling Duchenne or Becker muscular dystrophy
    Benign [Becker] muscular dystrophy
    Benign scapuloperoneal muscular dystrophy with early contractures [Emery-Dreifuss]
    Congenital muscular dystrophy NOS
    Congenital muscular dystrophy with specific morphological abnormalities of the muscle fiber
    Distal muscular dystrophy
    Facioscapulohumeral muscular dystrophy
    Limb-girdle muscular dystrophy
    Ocular muscular dystrophy
    Oculopharyngeal muscular dystrophy
    Scapuloperoneal muscular dystrophy
    Severe [Duchenne] muscular dystrophy

G71.1- Myotonic disorders — Disorders characterized by sustained contraction of muscles with decreased ability of muscular relaxation.

G71.11 Myotonic muscular dystrophy — An inherited disorder of the muscles that is characterized by progressive muscular weakness and wasting, cataracts, heart conduction defects, and endocrine changes.
    Dystrophia myotonica [Steinert]
    Myotonia atrophica
    Myotonic dystrophy
    Proximal myotonic myopathy (PROMM)
    Steinert disease

G71.12 Myotonia congenita — An inherited disorder of the muscles that usually begins in childhood and is characterized by very stiff muscles of the hands, legs, and eyelids and associated muscular hypertrophy.
    Acetazolamide responsive myotonia congenita
    Dominant myotonia congenita [Thomsen disease]
    Myotonia levior
    Recessive myotonia congenita [Becker disease]

G71.13 Myotonic chondrodystrophy — An inherited disorder of the muscles with onset at or soon after birth that is characterized by a more severe form of myotonia, muscular hypertrophy, and multiple skeletal deformities.
    Chondrodystrophic myotonia
    Congenital myotonic chondrodystrophy
    Schwartz-Jampel disease

G71.14 Drug-induced myotonia
Use additional code for adverse effect, if applicable, to identify drug (T36-T50 with fifth or sixth character 5)

G71.19 Other specified myotonic disorders
    Myotonia fluctuans
    Myotonia permanens
    Neuromyotonia [Isaacs]
    Paramyotonia congenita (of von Eulenburg)
    Pseudomyotonia
    Symptomatic myotonia

cc **G71.2 Congenital myopathies** — An inherited group of rare disorders characterized by slowly progressive or nonprogressive myopathy.
    Central core disease
    Fiber-type disproportion
    Minicore disease
    Multicore disease
    Myotubular (centronuclear) myopathy
    Nemaline myopathy
Excludes 1:   *arthrogryposis multiplex congenita (Q74.3)*

G71.3 Mitochondrial myopathy, not elsewhere classified
Excludes 1:   *Kearns-Sayre syndrome (H49.81)*
      Leber's disease (H47.21)
      Leigh's encephalopathy (G31.82)
      mitochondrial metabolism disorders (E88.4.-)
      Reye's syndrome (G93.7)

G71.8 Other primary disorders of muscles

G71.9 Primary disorder of muscle, unspecified
    Hereditary myopathy NOS

G61-G71

G72- Other and unspecified myopathies

Excludes 1: arthrogryposis multiplex congenita (Q74.3)
dermatopolymyositis (M33.-)
ischemic infarction of muscle (M62.2-)
myositis (M60.-)
polymyositis (M33.2.-)

cc **G72.0 Drug-induced myopathy**
Use additional code for adverse effect, if applicable, to identify drug (T36-T50 with fifth or sixth character 5)

cc **G72.1 Alcoholic myopathy**
Use additional code to identify alcoholism (F10.-)

cc **G72.2 Myopathy due to other toxic agents**
Code first (T51-T65) to identify toxic agent

G72.3 Periodic paralysis — An inherited disorder of the voluntary muscles that is characterized by sudden attacks of weakness and paralysis.
Familial periodic paralysis
Hyperkalemic periodic paralysis (familial)
Hypokalemic periodic paralysis (familial)
Myotonic periodic paralysis (familial)
Normokalemic paralysis (familial)
Potassium sensitive periodic paralysis
Excludes 1: paramyotonia congenita (of von Eulenburg) (G71.19)

G72.4- Inflammatory and immune myopathies, not elsewhere classified

G72.41 Inclusion body myositis [IBM] — An inflammatory muscle disease that is characterized by slowly progressive weakness that leads to balance problems, impaired finger gripping, and dysphagia.

G72.49 Other inflammatory and immune myopathies, not elsewhere classified
Inflammatory myopathy NOS

G72.8- Other specified myopathies

cc **G72.81 Critical illness myopathy** — A functional disturbance or damage to the neuromuscular system that is associated with sepsis, multi-organ failure, and SIRS.
Acute necrotizing myopathy
Acute quadriplegic myopathy
Intensive care (ICU) myopathy
Myopathy of critical illness

G72.89 Other specified myopathies

G72.9 Myopathy, unspecified

G73- Disorders of myoneural junction and muscle in diseases classified elsewhere

cc **G73.1 Lambert-Eaton syndrome in neoplastic disease** —
[Unacceptable PDX] [Not Allowed as PDX]
Code first underlying neoplasm (C00-D49)
Excludes 1: Lambert-Eaton syndrome not associated with neoplasm (G70.80-G70.81)

cc **G73.3 Myasthenic syndromes in other diseases classified elsewhere** — [Not Allowed as PDX]
Code first underlying, such as:
Neoplasm (C00-D49)
Thyrotoxicosis (E05.-)

G73.7 Myopathy in diseases classified elsewhere — [Not Allowed as PDX]
Code first underlying disease, such as:
Glycogen storage disease (E74.0)
Hyperparathyroidism (E21.0, E21.3)
Hypoparathyroidism (E20.-)
Lipid storage disorders (E75.-)
Excludes 1: myopathy in:
rheumatoid arthritis (M05.32)
sarcoidosis (D86.87)
scleroderma (M34.82)
sicca syndrome [Sjögren] (M35.03)
systemic lupus erythematosus (M32.19)

Cerebral palsy and other paralytic syndromes (G80-G83)

G80- Cerebral palsy — A nonprogressive, brain damaging disturbance of the prenatal or perinatal period characterized by persistent, qualitative motor dysfunction, paralysis, and in severe cases mental retardation.
Excludes 1: hereditary spastic paraplegia (G11.4)

MCC **G80.0 Spastic quadriplegic cerebral palsy** — A form characterized by paralysis of all four limbs.
Congenital spastic paralysis (cerebral)

cc **G80.1 Spastic diplegic cerebral palsy** — The most common form due to bilateral damage of the corticospinal tracts and characterized by lower limb paralysis showing the typical "scissor" gait and is associated with prematurity.
Spastic cerebral palsy NOS

cc **G80.2 Spastic hemiplegic cerebral palsy** — A form resulting from damage to the sensorimotor cortex that controls one side of the body and characterized by hemiparesis, growth arrest of the affected limbs, sensory deficits, and occasionally a seizure disorder which is usually associated with head trauma and is present at birth.

cc **G80.3 Athetoid cerebral palsy** — A form damaging the basal ganglia that is characterized by uncontrolled movements of the trunk and extremities.
Double athetosis (syndrome)
Dyskinetic cerebral palsy
Dystonic cerebral palsy
Vogt disease

G80.4 Ataxic cerebral palsy — A rare form that is characterized by movements that are not smooth and appear jerky.

G80.8 Other cerebral palsy
Mixed cerebral palsy syndromes

G80.9 Cerebral palsy, unspecified
Cerebral palsy NOS

G81- Hemiplegia and hemiparesis — Paralysis of one side of the body.
AHA 14:1Q:p23 – Hemiplegia
AHA 15:1Q:p25 – Left sided (nondominant) weakness
Note: This category is to be used only when hemiplegia (complete) (incomplete) is reported without further specification, or is stated to be old or longstanding but of unspecified cause. The category is also for use in multiple coding to identify these types of hemiplegia resulting from any cause.
Excludes 1: congenital cerebral palsy (G80.-)
hemiplegia and hemiparesis due to sequela of cerebrovascular disease (I69.05-, I69.15-, I69.25-, I69.35-, I69.85-, I69.95-)

G81.0- Flaccid hemiplegia — Paralysis of one side of the body with loss of tone of the muscles of the paralyzed part and absence of tendon reflexes.
cc **G81.00 Flaccid hemiplegia affecting unspecified side**
cc **G81.01 Flaccid hemiplegia affecting right dominant side**
cc **G81.02 Flaccid hemiplegia affecting left dominant side**
cc **G81.03 Flaccid hemiplegia affecting right nondominant side**
cc **G81.04 Flaccid hemiplegia affecting left nondominant side**

G81.1- Spastic hemiplegia — Paralysis of one side of the body marked by spasticity of the muscles of the paralyzed part and increased tendon reflexes.
cc **G81.10 Spastic hemiplegia affecting unspecified side**
cc **G81.11 Spastic hemiplegia affecting right dominant side**
cc **G81.12 Spastic hemiplegia affecting left dominant side**
cc **G81.13 Spastic hemiplegia affecting right nondominant side**
cc **G81.14 Spastic hemiplegia affecting left nondominant side**

G81.9- Hemiplegia, unspecified
cc **G81.90 Hemiplegia, unspecified affecting unspecified side**
cc **G81.91 Hemiplegia, unspecified affecting right dominant side**
cc **G81.92 Hemiplegia, unspecified affecting left dominant side**
cc **G81.93 Hemiplegia, unspecified affecting right nondominant side**
cc **G81.94 Hemiplegia, unspecified affecting left nondominant side**

G
7
2
-
G
8
1

G82- Paraplegia (paraparesis) and quadriplegia (quadriparesis)
Note: This category is to be used only when the listed conditions are reported without further specification, or are stated to be old or longstanding but of unspecified cause. The category is also for use in multiple coding to identify these conditions resulting from any cause.
Excludes 1:   *congenital cerebral palsy (G80.-)*
           functional quadriplegia (R53.2)
           hysterical paralysis (F44.4)

G82.2- Paraplegia — Loss or impairment of function of the legs and lower part of the body.
      Paralysis of both lower limbs NOS
      Paraparesis (lower) NOS
      Paraplegia (lower) NOS

CC **G82.20 Paraplegia, unspecified**
CC **G82.21 Paraplegia, complete**
CC **G82.22 Paraplegia, incomplete**

G82.5- Quadriplegia — Loss or impairment of motor function of all four limbs.
MCC **G82.50 Quadriplegia, unspecified**
MCC **G82.51 Quadriplegia, C1-C4 complete**
MCC **G82.52 Quadriplegia, C1-C4 incomplete**
MCC **G82.53 Quadriplegia, C5-C7 complete**
MCC **G82.54 Quadriplegia, C5-C7 incomplete**

G83- Other paralytic syndromes
Note: This category is to be used only when the listed conditions are reported without further specification, or are stated to be old or longstanding but of unspecified cause. The category is also for use in multiple coding to identify these conditions resulting from any cause.
Includes: Paralysis (complete) (incomplete), except as in G80-G82

CC **G83.0 Diplegia of upper limbs** — Loss or impairment of function of the upper limbs.
      Diplegia (upper)
      Paralysis of both upper limbs

G83.1- Monoplegia of lower limb — Loss or impairment of function of one of the lower limbs.
      Paralysis of lower limb
Excludes 1:   *monoplegia of lower limbs due to sequela of cerebrovascular disease (I69.04-, I69.14-, I69.24-, I69.34-, I69.84-, I69.94-)*

G83.10 Monoplegia of lower limb affecting unspecified side
G83.11 Monoplegia of lower limb affecting right dominant side
G83.12 Monoplegia of lower limb affecting left dominant side
G83.13 Monoplegia of lower limb affecting right nondominant side
G83.14 Monoplegia of lower limb affecting left nondominant side

G83.2- Monoplegia of upper limb — Loss or impairment of function of one of the upper limbs.
      Paralysis of upper limb
Excludes 1:   *monoplegia of upper limbs due to sequela of cerebrovascular disease (I69.03-, I69.13-, I69.23-, I69.33-, I69.83-, I69.93-)*

G83.20 Monoplegia of upper limb affecting unspecified side
G83.21 Monoplegia of upper limb affecting right dominant side
G83.22 Monoplegia of upper limb affecting left dominant side
G83.23 Monoplegia of upper limb affecting right nondominant side
G83.24 Monoplegia of upper limb affecting left nondominant side

G83.3- Monoplegia, unspecified
G83.30 Monoplegia, unspecified affecting unspecified side
G83.31 Monoplegia, unspecified affecting right dominant side
G83.32 Monoplegia, unspecified affecting left dominant side
G83.33 Monoplegia, unspecified affecting right nondominant side
G83.34 Monoplegia, unspecified affecting left nondominant side

CC **G83.4 Cauda equina syndrome** — Compression of the spinal nerve roots marked by areflexic paralysis, paresthesia, and dull aching pains of the perineum, bladder, and sacrum.
      Neurogenic bladder due to cauda equina syndrome — Dysfunction of the urinary bladder due to cauda equina syndrome.
Excludes 1:   *cord bladder NOS (G95.89)*
           neurogenic bladder NOS (N31.9)

MCC **G83.5 Locked-in state** — A condition marked by a severe, nonreactive paralysis while remaining conscious.

G83.8- Other specified paralytic syndromes
Excludes 1:   *paralytic syndromes due to current spinal cord injury-code to spinal cord injury (S14, S24, S34)*

G83.81 Brown-Séquard syndrome
G83.82 Anterior cord syndrome
G83.83 Posterior cord syndrome
G83.84 Todd's paralysis (postepileptic)
G83.89 Other specified paralytic syndromes
G83.9 Paralytic syndrome, unspecified

Other disorders of the nervous system (G89-G99)

G89- Pain, not elsewhere classified
Code also related psychological factors associated with pain (F45.42)
Excludes 1:   *generalized pain NOS (R52)*
           pain disorders exclusively related to psychological factors (F45.41)
           pain NOS (R52)
Excludes 2:   *atypical face pain (G50.1)*
           headache syndromes (G44.-)
           localized pain, unspecified type — code to pain by site, such as:
              abdomen pain (R10.-)
              back pain (M54.9)
              breast pain (N64.4)
              chest pain (R07.1-R07.9)
              ear pain (H92.0-)
              eye pain (H57.1)
              headache (R51)
              joint pain (M25.5-)
              limb pain (M79.6-)
              lumbar region pain (M54.5)
              painful urination (R30.9)
              pelvic and perineal pain (R10.2)
              shoulder pain (M25.51-)
              spine pain (M54.-)
              throat pain (R07.0)
              tongue pain (K14.6)
              tooth pain (K08.8)
           migraines (G43.-)
           myalgia (M79.1)
           pain from prosthetic devices, implants, and grafts (T82.84, T83.84, T84.84, T85.84-)
           phantom limb syndrome with pain (G54.6)
           renal colic (N23)
           vulvar vestibulitis (N94.810)
           vulvodynia (N94.81-)

G89.0 Central pain syndrome — Pain caused by damage to the central nervous system.
      Déjérine-Roussy syndrome
      Myelopathic pain syndrome
      Thalamic pain syndrome (hyperesthetic)

G89.1- Acute pain, not elsewhere classified
G89.11 Acute pain due to trauma
G89.12 Acute post-thoracotomy pain
      Post-thoracotomy pain NOS
G89.18 Other acute postprocedural pain
      Postoperative pain NOS
      Postprocedural pain NOS

G89.2- Chronic pain, not elsewhere classified
Excludes 1:   *causalgia, lower limb (G57.7-)*
           causalgia, upper limb (G56.4-)
           central pain syndrome (G89.0)
           chronic pain syndrome (G89.4)
           complex regional pain syndrome II, lower limb (G57.7-)
           complex regional pain syndrome II, upper limb (G56.4-)
           neoplasm related chronic pain (G89.3)
           reflex sympathetic dystrophy (G90.5-)

G89.21 Chronic pain due to trauma
G89.22 Chronic post-thoracotomy pain
G89.28 Other chronic postprocedural pain
      Other chronic postoperative pain
G89.29 Other chronic pain

G
8
2
-
G
8
9

G89.3   <u>Neoplasm</u> related pain (acute) (chronic)
    Cancer associated pain
    Pain due to malignancy (primary) (secondary)
    Tumor associated pain

G89.4   <u>Chronic pain syndrome</u>
    Chronic pain associated with significant psychosocial dysfunction

G90- Disorders of autonomic nervous system
    Excludes 1:   *dysfunction of the autonomic nervous system due to alcohol (G31.2)*

G90.0- Idiopathic peripheral autonomic neuropathy
    G90.01 **Carotid sinus syncope** — A temporary loss of consciousness due to the overactivity of the carotid sinus reflex.
        Carotid sinus syndrome

    G90.09 Other idiopathic peripheral autonomic neuropathy
        Idiopathic peripheral autonomic neuropathy NOS

G90.1   Familial dysautonomia [Riley-Day]

G90.2   Horner's syndrome
    Bernard(-Horner) syndrome
    Cervical sympathetic dystrophy or paralysis

CC **G90.3**   Multi-system degeneration of the autonomic nervous system
    Neurogenic orthostatic hypotension [Shy-Drager]
    Excludes 1:   *orthostatic hypotension NOS (I95.1)*

G90.4   **Autonomic dysreflexia** — A condition of the spinal cord sympathetic nervous system signals resulting in hypertension, vasoconstriction, bradycardia, blurred vision, and sweating.
    Use additional code to identify the cause, such as:
        Fecal impaction (K56.41)
        Pressure ulcer (pressure area) (L89.-)
        Urinary tract infection (N39.0)

G90.5- **Complex regional pain syndrome I (CRPS I)** — A condition most often affecting one of the limbs of the sympathetic nervous system marked by burning pain, sweating, hyperesthesia, and skin atrophy most likely caused as a result of an injury to nerves or blood vessels.
    Reflex sympathetic dystrophy
    Excludes 1:   *causalgia of lower limb (G57.7-)*
                  causalgia of upper limb (G56.4-)
                  complex regional pain syndrome II of lower limb (G57.7-)
                  complex regional pain syndrome II of upper limb (G56.4-)

    CC **G90.50** Complex regional pain syndrome I, unspecified

    G90.51- Complex regional pain syndrome I of <u>upper</u> limb
        CC **G90.511** Complex regional pain syndrome I of <u>right</u> upper limb
        CC **G90.512** Complex regional pain syndrome I of <u>left</u> upper limb
        CC **G90.513** Complex regional pain syndrome I of upper limb, <u>bilateral</u>
        CC **G90.519** Complex regional pain syndrome I of <u>unspecified</u> upper limb

    G90.52- Complex regional pain syndrome I of <u>lower</u> limb
        CC **G90.521** Complex regional pain syndrome I of <u>right</u> lower limb
        CC **G90.522** Complex regional pain syndrome I of <u>left</u> lower limb
        CC **G90.523** Complex regional pain syndrome I of lower limb, <u>bilateral</u>
        CC **G90.529** Complex regional pain syndrome I of <u>unspecified</u> lower limb

    CC **G90.59** Complex regional pain syndrome I of other specified site

G90.8   Other disorders of autonomic nervous system

G90.9   Disorder of the autonomic nervous system, unspecified

G91- <u>Hydrocephalus</u> — An abnormal accumulation of cerebrospinal fluid.
    Includes: Acquired hydrocephalus
    Excludes 1:   *Arnold-Chiari syndrome with hydrocephalus (Q07.-)*
                  congenital hydrocephalus (Q03.-)
                  spina bifida with hydrocephalus (Q05.-)

CC **G91.0**   <u>Communicating</u> hydrocephalus — An abnormal accumulation of cerebrospinal fluid that is secondary to a disease process.
    Secondary normal pressure hydrocephalus

CC **G91.1**   <u>Obstructive</u> hydrocephalus — An abnormal accumulation of cerebrospinal fluid that develops as a result of a blockage in the normal circulation of cerebrospinal fluid within the brain.

CC **G91.2**   <u>(Idiopathic) normal pressure</u> hydrocephalus — An abnormal accumulation of cerebrospinal fluid that is characterized by dementia, urinary incontinence, and gait disturbance and is without a known cause.
    Normal pressure hydrocephalus NOS

CC **G91.3**   <u>Post-traumatic</u> hydrocephalus, unspecified

G91.4   Hydrocephalus <u>in diseases classified elsewhere</u> —
    [Not Allowed as PDX]
    AHA 14:3Q:p3 – Hydrocephalus in disease classified elsewhere
    Code first underlying condition, such as:
        Congenital syphilis (A50.4-)
        Neoplasm (C00-D49)
    Excludes 1:   *hydrocephalus due to congenital toxoplasmosis (P37.1)*

CC **G91.8**   Other hydrocephalus

CC **G91.9**   Hydrocephalus, unspecified

G92   **Toxic encephalopathy** — A degenerative condition of the brain caused by the toxic
MCC   effect of certain substances.
    Toxic encephalitis
    Toxic metabolic encephalopathy
    Code first (T51-T65) to identify toxic agent

G93- Other disorders of brain
    G93.0   **Cerebral cysts** — An encapsulated fluid-filled cyst of the brain and meninges.
        Arachnoid cyst
        Porencephalic cyst, acquired
        Excludes 1:   *acquired periventricular cysts of newborn (P91.1)*
                      congenital cerebral cysts (Q04.6)

    CC **G93.1**   **Anoxic brain damage, not elsewhere classified** — Cellular brain tissue injury due to the absence or lack of oxygen.
        Excludes 1:   *cerebral anoxia due to anesthesia during labor and delivery (O74.3)*
                      cerebral anoxia due to anesthesia during the puerperium (O89.2)
                      neonatal anoxia (P84)

    G93.2   **Benign intracranial hypertension** — Cerebral edema resulting in raised intracranial pressure with headache, nausea, vomiting, and occasional sixth nerve palsy.
        Excludes 1:   *hypertensive encephalopathy (I67.4)*

    G93.3   **Postviral fatigue syndrome** — The abnormal lack or loss of strength after recovery from a viral infection.
        Benign myalgic encephalomyelitis
        Excludes 1:   *chronic fatigue syndrome NOS (R53.82)*

    G93.4- Other and unspecified encephalopathy
        Excludes 1:   *alcoholic encephalopathy (G31.2)*
                      encephalopathy in diseases classified elsewhere (G94)
                      hypertensive encephalopathy (I67.4)
                      toxic (metabolic) encephalopathy (G92)

    MCC **G93.40** Encephalopathy, unspecified

    MCC **G93.41** Metabolic encephalopathy — A generalized cerebral dysfunction due to metabolic disorders.
        AHA 15:3Q:p21 – Diabetes mellitus with acute encephalopathy secondary to hypoglycemia
        Septic encephalopathy

    MCC **G93.49** Other encephalopathy
        Encephalopathy NEC

    MCC **G93.5**   **Compression of brain** — Pressure on the brain usually due to space-occupying diseases.
        Arnold-Chiari type 1 compression of brain
        Compression of brain (stem)
        Herniation of brain (stem)
        Excludes 1:   *diffuse traumatic compression of brain (S06.2-)*
                      focal traumatic compression of brain (S06.3-)

    MCC **G93.6**   **Cerebral edema** — An excessive accumulation of fluid in the brain substance.
        Excludes 1:   *cerebral edema due to birth injury (P11.0)*
                      traumatic cerebral edema (S06.1-)

G89 - G93

Excludes 1: = NOT CODED HERE! (Do not code both)   *Excludes 2:* = Not Included Here

MCC **G93.7** **Reye's syndrome** — [Age/0-17] — An acute encephalopathy in children usually following certain infections and marked by fatty degeneration of the liver, rapid development of brain swelling, hepatomegaly, and seizures.
Code first (T39.0-), if salicylates-induced

G93.8- **Other specified disorders of brain**

G93.81 **Temporal sclerosis** — The condition of loss of neurons and scarring of the temporal lobe that is usually due to brain injuries or diseases and results in seizure activity.
Hippocampal sclerosis
Mesial temporal sclerosis

MCC **G93.82** **Brain death** — The condition of complete and irreversible cessation of all brain function and activity.

G93.89 **Other specified disorders of brain**
Postradiation encephalopathy

G93.9 **Disorder of brain, unspecified**

G94 **Other disorders of brain in diseases classified elsewhere** —
[Not Allowed as PDX]
Code first underlying disease
Excludes 1: *encephalopathy in congenital syphilis (A50.49)*
encephalopathy in influenza (J09.X9, J10.81, J11.81)
encephalopathy in syphilis (A52.19)
hydrocephalus in diseases classified elsewhere (G91.4)

G95- **Other and unspecified diseases of spinal cord**
Excludes ❷: *myelitis (G04.-)*

CC **G95.0** **Syringomyelia and syringobulbia** — SYRINGOMYELIA – A destructive spinal cord condition resulting in cavity formation and characterized by weakness and wasting of the small muscles of the hand, with accompanying loss of pain sensation. SYRINGOBULBIA – A destructive cavitary disorder of the brainstem characterized by weakness and wasting of the tongue, dysphagia, dysarthria, and general loss of sensation to the face.

G95.1- **Vascular myelopathies** — Functional disorders of the spinal cord caused by vascular hemorrhagic conditions.
Excludes ❷: *intraspinal phlebitis and thrombophlebitis, except non-pyogenic (G08)*

MCC **G95.11** **Acute infarction of spinal cord (embolic) (nonembolic)** — Obstructive ischemic tissue necrosis of the spinal cord.
Anoxia of spinal cord
Arterial thrombosis of spinal cord

MCC **G95.19** **Other vascular myelopathies**
Edema of spinal cord
Hematomyelia
Nonpyogenic intraspinal phlebitis and thrombophlebitis
Subacute necrotic myelopathy

G95.2- **Other and unspecified cord compression**

CC **G95.20** **Unspecified cord compression**

CC **G95.29** **Other cord compression**

G95.8- **Other specified diseases of spinal cord**
Excludes 1: *neurogenic bladder NOS (N31.9)*
neurogenic bladder due to cauda equina syndrome (G83.4)
neuromuscular dysfunction of bladder without spinal cord lesion (N31.-)

CC **G95.81** **Conus medullaris syndrome**

CC **G95.89** **Other specified diseases of spinal cord**
Cord bladder NOS
Drug-induced myelopathy
Radiation-induced myelopathy
Excludes 1: *myelopathy NOS (G95.9)*

CC **G95.9** **Disease of spinal cord, unspecified**
Myelopathy NOS

G96- **Other disorders of central nervous system**

CC **G96.0** **Cerebrospinal fluid leak**
Excludes 1: *cerebrospinal fluid leak from spinal puncture (G97.0)*

G96.1- **Disorders of meninges, not elsewhere classified**

CC **G96.11** **Dural tear**
AHA 14:4Q:p24 – Durotomy secondary to previous epidural injections
Excludes 1: *accidental puncture or laceration of dura during a procedure (G97.41)*

G96.12 **Meningeal adhesions (cerebral) (spinal)**

G96.19 **Other disorders of meninges, not elsewhere classified**

G96.8 **Other specified disorders of central nervous system**

G96.9 **Disorder of central nervous system, unspecified**

G97- **Intraoperative and postprocedural complications** and disorders of nervous system, not elsewhere classified
Excludes ❷: *intraoperative and postprocedural cerebrovascular infarction (I97.81-, I97.82-)*

CC **G97.0** **Cerebrospinal fluid leak from spinal puncture**

G97.1 **Other reaction to spinal and lumbar puncture**
Headache due to lumbar puncture

CC **G97.2** **Intracranial hypotension following ventricular shunting**

G97.3- **Intraoperative hemorrhage and hematoma** of a nervous system organ or structure complicating a procedure
Excludes 1: *intraoperative hemorrhage and hematoma of a nervous system organ or structure due to accidental puncture and laceration during a procedure (G97.4-)*

CC **G97.31** **Intraoperative hemorrhage and hematoma of a nervous system organ or structure complicating a nervous system procedure**

CC **G97.32** **Intraoperative hemorrhage and hematoma of a nervous system organ or structure complicating other procedure**

G97.4- **Accidental puncture and laceration** of a nervous system organ or structure during a procedure

CC **G97.41** **Accidental puncture or laceration of dura during a procedure**
Incidental (inadvertent) durotomy

CC **G97.48** **Accidental puncture and laceration of other nervous system organ or structure during a nervous system procedure**

CC **G97.49** **Accidental puncture and laceration of other nervous system organ or structure during other procedure**

G97.5- **Postprocedural hemorrhage** of a nervous system organ or structure following a procedure

CC **G97.51** **Postprocedural hemorrhage** of a nervous system organ or structure following a nervous system procedure

CC **G97.52** **Postprocedural hemorrhage** of a nervous system organ or structure following other procedure

G97.6- **Postprocedural hematoma and seroma** of a nervous system organ or structure following a procedure

CC **G97.61** **Postprocedural hematoma** of a nervous system organ or structure following a nervous system procedure

CC **G97.62** **Postprocedural hematoma** of a nervous system organ or structure following other procedure

CC **G97.63** **Postprocedural seroma** of a nervous system organ or structure following a nervous system procedure

CC **G97.64** **Postprocedural seroma** of a nervous system organ or structure following other procedure

G97.8- **Other intraoperative and postprocedural complications and disorders of nervous system**
Use additional code to further specify disorder

CC **G97.81** **Other intraoperative complications of nervous system**

CC **G97.82** **Other postprocedural complications and disorders of nervous system**

G98- **Other disorders of nervous system not elsewhere classified**
Includes: Nervous system disorder NOS

G98.0 **Neurogenic arthritis, not elsewhere classified**
Nonsyphilitic neurogenic arthropathy NEC
Nonsyphilitic neurogenic spondylopathy NEC
Excludes 1: *spondylopathy (in):*
syringomyelia and syringobulbia (G95.0)
tabes dorsalis (A52.11)

G98.8 **Other disorders of nervous system**
Nervous system disorder NOS

G
9
3
–
G
9
8

G99- Other disorders of nervous system in diseases classified elsewhere

CC **G99.0 Autonomic neuropathy in diseases classified elsewhere** —
[Not Allowed as PDX]
Code first underlying disease, such as:
Amyloidosis (E85.-)
Gout (M1A.-, M10.-)
Hyperthyroidism (E05.-)
Excludes 1: diabetic autonomic neuropathy (E08-E14 with .43)

CC **G99.2 Myelopathy in diseases classified elsewhere** —
[Not Allowed as PDX]
Code first underlying disease, such as:
Neoplasm (C00-D49)
Excludes 1: myelopathy in:
intervertebral disease (M50.0-, M51.0-)
spondylosis (M47.0-, M47.1-)

G99.8 Other specified disorders of nervous system in diseases classified elsewhere — [Not Allowed as PDX]
Code first underlying disorder, such as:
Amyloidosis (E85.-)
Avitaminosis (E56.9)
Excludes 1: nervous system involvement in:
cysticercosis (B69.0)
rubella (B06.0-)
syphilis (A52.1-)

Chapter 7 – Diseases of the eye and adnexa (H00-H59)

Note: Use an external cause code following the code for the eye condition, if applicable, to identify the cause of the eye condition

Excludes ❷: certain conditions originating in the perinatal period (P04-P96)

certain infectious and parasitic diseases (A00-B99)

complications of pregnancy, childbirth and the puerperium (O00-O9A)

congenital malformations, deformations, and chromosomal abnormalities (Q00-Q99)

diabetes mellitus related eye conditions (E09.3-, E10.3-, E11.3-, E13.3-)

endocrine, nutritional and metabolic diseases (E00-E88)

injury (trauma) of eye and orbit (S05.-)

injury, poisoning and certain other consequences of external causes (S00-T88)

neoplasms (C00-D49)

symptoms, signs and abnormal clinical and laboratory findings, not elsewhere classified (R00-R94)

syphilis related eye disorders (A50.01, A50.3-, A51.43, A52.71)

This chapter contains the following blocks:

H00-H05	Disorders of eyelid, lacrimal system and orbit
H10-H11	Disorders of conjunctiva
H15-H22	Disorders of sclera, cornea, iris and ciliary body
H25-H28	Disorders of lens
H30-H36	Disorders of choroid and retina
H40-H42	Glaucoma
H43-H44	Disorders of vitreous body and globe
H46-H47	Disorders of optic nerve and visual pathways
H49-H52	Disorders of ocular muscles, binocular movement, accommodation and refraction
H53-H54	Visual disturbances and blindness
H55-H57	Other disorders of eye and adnexa
H59	Intraoperative and postprocedural complications and disorders of eye and adnexa, not elsewhere classified

Chapter-Specific Coding Guidelines

C. Chapter-Specific Coding Guidelines

In addition to general coding guidelines, there are guidelines for specific diagnoses and/or conditions in the classification. Unless otherwise indicated, these guidelines apply to all health care settings. Please refer to Section II for guidelines on the selection of principal diagnosis.

7. Chapter 7: Diseases of Eye and Adnexa (H00-H59)

a. Glaucoma

1) Assigning Glaucoma Codes

Assign as many codes from category H40, Glaucoma, as needed to identify the type of glaucoma, the affected eye, and the glaucoma stage.

2) Bilateral glaucoma with same type and stage

When a patient has bilateral glaucoma and both eyes are documented as being the same type and stage, and there is a code for bilateral glaucoma, report only the code for the type of glaucoma, bilateral, with the seventh character for the stage.

When a patient has bilateral glaucoma and both eyes are documented as being the same type and stage, and the classification does not provide a code for bilateral glaucoma (i.e. subcategories H40.10, H40.11 and H40.20) report only one code for the type of glaucoma with the appropriate seventh character for the stage.

3) Bilateral glaucoma stage with different types or stages

When a patient has bilateral glaucoma and each eye is documented as having a different type or stage, and the classification distinguishes laterality, assign the appropriate code for each eye rather than the code for bilateral glaucoma.

When a patient has bilateral glaucoma and each eye is documented as having a different type, and the classification does not distinguish laterality (i.e. subcategories H40.10, H40.11 and H40.20), assign one code for each type of glaucoma with the appropriate seventh character for the stage.

When a patient has bilateral glaucoma and each eye is documented as having the same type, but different stage, and the classification does not distinguish laterality (i.e. subcategories H40.10, H40.11 and H40.20), assign a code for the type of glaucoma for each eye with the seventh character for the specific glaucoma stage documented for each eye.

4) Patient admitted with glaucoma and stage evolves during the admission

If a patient is admitted with glaucoma and the stage progresses during the admission, assign the code for highest stage documented.

5) Indeterminate stage glaucoma

Assignment of the seventh character "4" for "indeterminate stage" should be based on the clinical documentation. The seventh character "4" is used for glaucomas whose stage cannot be clinically determined. This seventh character should not be confused with the seventh character "0", unspecified, which should be assigned when there is no documentation regarding the stage of the glaucoma.

Disorders of eyelid, lacrimal system and orbit (H00-H05)

Excludes ❷: open wound of eyelid (S01.1-)
superficial injury of eyelid (S00.1-, S00.2-)

H00- Hordeolum and chalazion

H00.0- Hordeolum (externum) (internum) of eyelid

H00.01- Hordeolum externum — Purulent inflammation of the sebaceous glands of the external eyelid surface, most often caused by Staphylococcus.
Hordeolum NOS
Stye

H00.011	Hordeolum externum **right upper** eyelid
H00.012	Hordeolum externum **right lower** eyelid
H00.013	Hordeolum externum **right** eye, **unspecified** eyelid
H00.014	Hordeolum externum **left upper** eyelid
H00.015	Hordeolum externum **left lower** eyelid
H00.016	Hordeolum externum **left** eye, **unspecified** eyelid
H00.019	Hordeolum externum **unspecified** eye, **unspecified** eyelid

H00.02- Hordeolum internum — Purulent inflammation of the sebaceous glands of the internal eyelid surface, most often caused by Staphylococcus.
Infection of meibomian gland — A form affecting the meibomian glands of the conjunctiva of the eyelids.

H00.021	Hordeolum internum **right upper** eyelid
H00.022	Hordeolum internum **right lower** eyelid
H00.023	Hordeolum internum **right** eye, **unspecified** eyelid
H00.024	Hordeolum internum **left upper** eyelid
H00.025	Hordeolum internum **left lower** eyelid
H00.026	Hordeolum internum **left** eye, **unspecified** eyelid
H00.029	Hordeolum internum **unspecified** eye, **unspecified** eyelid

H00.03- Abscess of eyelid — A localized collection of pus caused by the disintegration of eyelid tissues.
Furuncle of eyelid — An acute circumscribed inflammation of the subcutaneous tissue of the eyelid.

H00.031	Abscess of **right upper** eyelid
H00.032	Abscess of **right lower** eyelid
H00.033	Abscess of eyelid **right** eye, **unspecified** eyelid
H00.034	Abscess of **left upper** eyelid
H00.035	Abscess of **left lower** eyelid
H00.036	Abscess of eyelid **left** eye, **unspecified** eyelid
H00.039	Abscess of eyelid **unspecified** eye, **unspecified** eyelid

H00.1- Chalazion — Chronic inflammation of a meibomian gland with formation of a granulomatous mass.
Meibomian (gland) cyst
Excludes ❷: infected meibomian gland (H00.02-)

H00.11	Chalazion **right upper** eyelid
H00.12	Chalazion **right lower** eyelid
H00.13	Chalazion **right** eye, **unspecified** eyelid
H00.14	Chalazion **left upper** eyelid
H00.15	Chalazion **left lower** eyelid
H00.16	Chalazion **left** eye, **unspecified** eyelid
H00.19	Chalazion **unspecified** eye, **unspecified** eyelid

H01- Other inflammation of eyelid

H01.0- Blepharitis — Inflammation of edges of the eyelids involving hair follicles and glands.
Excludes 1: blepharoconjunctivitis (H10.5-)

H01.00- Unspecified blepharitis

H01.001	Unspecified blepharitis **right upper** eyelid
H01.002	Unspecified blepharitis **right lower** eyelid
H01.003	Unspecified blepharitis **right** eye, **unspecified** eyelid

H0 0 - H0 1

H01.004   Unspecified blepharitis <u>left</u> <u>upper</u> eyelid
H01.005   Unspecified blepharitis <u>left</u> <u>lower</u> eyelid
H01.006   Unspecified blepharitis <u>left</u> eye, <u>unspecified</u> eyelid
H01.009   Unspecified blepharitis <u>unspecified</u> eye, <u>unspecified</u> eyelid

H01.01- <u>Ulcerative</u> blepharitis — A form characterized by an eating away of a localized eyelid area.

H01.011   Ulcerative blepharitis <u>right</u> <u>upper</u> eyelid
H01.012   Ulcerative blepharitis <u>right</u> <u>lower</u> eyelid
H01.013   Ulcerative blepharitis <u>right</u> eye, <u>unspecified</u> eyelid
H01.014   Ulcerative blepharitis <u>left</u> <u>upper</u> eyelid
H01.015   Ulcerative blepharitis <u>left</u> <u>lower</u> eyelid
H01.016   Ulcerative blepharitis <u>left</u> eye, <u>unspecified</u> eyelid
H01.019   Ulcerative blepharitis <u>unspecified</u> eye, <u>unspecified</u> eyelid

H01.02- <u>Squamous</u> blepharitis — A form characterized by the development of scales.

H01.021   Squamous blepharitis <u>right</u> <u>upper</u> eyelid
H01.022   Squamous blepharitis <u>right</u> <u>lower</u> eyelid
H01.023   Squamous blepharitis <u>right</u> eye, <u>unspecified</u> eyelid
H01.024   Squamous blepharitis <u>left</u> <u>upper</u> eyelid
H01.025   Squamous blepharitis <u>left</u> <u>lower</u> eyelid
H01.026   Squamous blepharitis <u>left</u> eye, <u>unspecified</u> eyelid
H01.029   Squamous blepharitis <u>unspecified</u> eye, <u>unspecified</u> eyelid

H01.1- <u>Noninfectious dermatoses</u> of eyelid

H01.11- <u>Allergic dermatitis</u> of eyelid — An inflammatory reaction caused by an allergen.
      Contact dermatitis of eyelid

H01.111   Allergic dermatitis of <u>right</u> <u>upper</u> eyelid
H01.112   Allergic dermatitis of <u>right</u> <u>lower</u> eyelid
H01.113   Allergic dermatitis of <u>right</u> eye, <u>unspecified</u> eyelid
H01.114   Allergic dermatitis of <u>left</u> <u>upper</u> eyelid
H01.115   Allergic dermatitis of <u>left</u> <u>lower</u> eyelid
H01.116   Allergic dermatitis of <u>left</u> eye, <u>unspecified</u> eyelid
H01.119   Allergic dermatitis of <u>unspecified</u> eye, <u>unspecified</u> eyelid

H01.12- <u>Discoid lupus erythematosus</u> of eyelid — A superficial inflammation of the eyelids with red macules.

H01.121   Discoid lupus erythematosus of <u>right</u> <u>upper</u> eyelid
H01.122   Discoid lupus erythematosus of <u>right</u> <u>lower</u> eyelid
H01.123   Discoid lupus erythematosus of <u>right</u> eye, <u>unspecified</u> eyelid
H01.124   Discoid lupus erythematosus of <u>left</u> <u>upper</u> eyelid
H01.125   Discoid lupus erythematosus of <u>left</u> <u>lower</u> eyelid
H01.126   Discoid lupus erythematosus of <u>left</u> eye, <u>unspecified</u> eyelid
H01.129   Discoid lupus erythematosus of <u>unspecified</u> eye, <u>unspecified</u> eyelid

H01.13- <u>Eczematous dermatitis</u> of eyelid — An inflammatory reaction involving the eyelids.

H01.131   Eczematous dermatitis of <u>right</u> <u>upper</u> eyelid
H01.132   Eczematous dermatitis of <u>right</u> <u>lower</u> eyelid
H01.133   Eczematous dermatitis of <u>right</u> eye, <u>unspecified</u> eyelid
H01.134   Eczematous dermatitis of <u>left</u> <u>upper</u> eyelid
H01.135   Eczematous dermatitis of <u>left</u> <u>lower</u> eyelid
H01.136   Eczematous dermatitis of <u>left</u> eye, <u>unspecified</u> eyelid
H01.139   Eczematous dermatitis of <u>unspecified</u> eye, <u>unspecified</u> eyelid

H01.14- <u>Xeroderma</u> of eyelid — Dryness and roughness of the eyelid skin.

H01.141   Xeroderma of <u>right</u> <u>upper</u> eyelid
H01.142   Xeroderma of <u>right</u> <u>lower</u> eyelid
H01.143   Xeroderma of <u>right</u> eye, <u>unspecified</u> eyelid
H01.144   Xeroderma of <u>left</u> <u>upper</u> eyelid

H01.145   Xeroderma of <u>left</u> <u>lower</u> eyelid
H01.146   Xeroderma of <u>left</u> eye, <u>unspecified</u> eyelid
H01.149   Xeroderma of <u>unspecified</u> eye, <u>unspecified</u> eyelid

H01.8   Other specified inflammations of eyelid
H01.9   Unspecified inflammation of eyelid
      Inflammation of eyelid NOS

H02-   Other disorders of eyelid
   Excludes 1:   congenital malformations of eyelid (Q10.0-Q10.3)

H02.0-   <u>Entropion</u> and trichiasis of eyelid — The turning inward of the eyelid edge.

H02.00- <u>Unspecified</u> entropion of eyelid

H02.001   Unspecified entropion of <u>right</u> <u>upper</u> eyelid
H02.002   Unspecified entropion of <u>right</u> <u>lower</u> eyelid
H02.003   Unspecified entropion of <u>right</u> eye, <u>unspecified</u> eyelid
H02.004   Unspecified entropion of <u>left</u> <u>upper</u> eyelid
H02.005   Unspecified entropion of <u>left</u> <u>lower</u> eyelid
H02.006   Unspecified entropion of <u>left</u> eye, <u>unspecified</u> eyelid
H02.009   Unspecified entropion of <u>unspecified</u> eye, <u>unspecified</u> eyelid

H02.01- <u>Cicatricial</u> entropion of eyelid — A form caused by contraction of conjunctival scar tissue.

H02.011   Cicatricial entropion of <u>right</u> <u>upper</u> eyelid
H02.012   Cicatricial entropion of <u>right</u> <u>lower</u> eyelid
H02.013   Cicatricial entropion of <u>right</u> eye, <u>unspecified</u> eyelid
H02.014   Cicatricial entropion of <u>left</u> <u>upper</u> eyelid
H02.015   Cicatricial entropion of <u>left</u> <u>lower</u> eyelid
H02.016   Cicatricial entropion of <u>left</u> eye, <u>unspecified</u> eyelid
H02.019   Cicatricial entropion of <u>unspecified</u> eye, <u>unspecified</u> eyelid

H02.02- <u>Mechanical</u> entropion of eyelid — A form caused by external forces.

H02.021   Mechanical entropion of <u>right</u> <u>upper</u> eyelid
H02.022   Mechanical entropion of <u>right</u> <u>lower</u> eyelid
H02.023   Mechanical entropion of <u>right</u> eye, <u>unspecified</u> eyelid
H02.024   Mechanical entropion of <u>left</u> <u>upper</u> eyelid
H02.025   Mechanical entropion of <u>left</u> <u>lower</u> eyelid
H02.026   Mechanical entropion of <u>left</u> eye, <u>unspecified</u> eyelid
H02.029   Mechanical entropion of <u>unspecified</u> eye, <u>unspecified</u> eyelid

H02.03- <u>Senile</u> entropion of eyelid — A form caused by loss of tone of the obicularis oculi muscle.

H02.031   Senile entropion of <u>right</u> <u>upper</u> eyelid — [Age/15-124]
H02.032   Senile entropion of <u>right</u> <u>lower</u> eyelid — [Age/15-124]
H02.033   Senile entropion of <u>right</u> eye, <u>unspecified</u> eyelid — [Age/15-124]
H02.034   Senile entropion of <u>left</u> <u>upper</u> eyelid — [Age/15-124]
H02.035   Senile entropion of <u>left</u> <u>lower</u> eyelid — [Age/15-124]
H02.036   Senile entropion of <u>left</u> eye, <u>unspecified</u> eyelid — [Age/15-124]
H02.039   Senile entropion of <u>unspecified</u> eye, <u>unspecified</u> eyelid — [Age/15-124]

H02.04- <u>Spastic</u> entropion of eyelid — A form caused by tonic spasm of the obicularis oculi muscle.

H02.041   Spastic entropion of <u>right</u> <u>upper</u> eyelid
H02.042   Spastic entropion of <u>right</u> <u>lower</u> eyelid
H02.043   Spastic entropion of <u>right</u> eye, <u>unspecified</u> eyelid
H02.044   Spastic entropion of <u>left</u> <u>upper</u> eyelid
H02.045   Spastic entropion of <u>left</u> <u>lower</u> eyelid
H02.046   Spastic entropion of <u>left</u> eye, <u>unspecified</u> eyelid
H02.049   Spastic entropion of <u>unspecified</u> eye, <u>unspecified</u> eyelid

H 0 1 - H 0 2

H02.05- **Trichiasis without entropian** — The inward inversion of the eyelashes which rub against the cornea.

H02.051	Trichiasis without entropian <u>right</u> <u>upper</u> eyelid
H02.052	Trichiasis without entropian <u>right</u> <u>lower</u> eyelid
H02.053	Trichiasis without entropian <u>right</u> eye, <u>unspecified</u> eyelid
H02.054	Trichiasis without entropian <u>left</u> <u>upper</u> eyelid
H02.055	Trichiasis without entropian <u>left</u> <u>lower</u> eyelid
H02.056	Trichiasis without entropian <u>left</u> eye, <u>unspecified</u> eyelid
H02.059	Trichiasis without entropian <u>unspecified</u> eye, <u>unspecified</u> eyelid

H02.1- **Ectropion** of eyelid — The turning outward of the eyelid edge.

H02.10- **Unspecified** ectropion of eyelid

H02.101	Unspecified ectropion of <u>right</u> <u>upper</u> eyelid
H02.102	Unspecified ectropion of <u>right</u> <u>lower</u> eyelid
H02.103	Unspecified ectropion of <u>right</u> eye, <u>unspecified</u> eyelid
H02.104	Unspecified ectropion of <u>left</u> <u>upper</u> eyelid
H02.105	Unspecified ectropion of <u>left</u> <u>lower</u> eyelid
H02.106	Unspecified ectropion of <u>left</u> eye, <u>unspecified</u> eyelid
H02.109	Unspecified ectropion of <u>unspecified</u> eye, <u>unspecified</u> eyelid

H02.11- **Cicatricial** ectropion of eyelid — A form caused by contraction of conjunctival scar tissue.

H02.111	Cicatricial ectropion of <u>right</u> <u>upper</u> eyelid
H02.112	Cicatricial ectropion of <u>right</u> <u>lower</u> eyelid
H02.113	Cicatricial ectropion of <u>right</u> eye, <u>unspecified</u> eyelid
H02.114	Cicatricial ectropion of <u>left</u> <u>upper</u> eyelid
H02.115	Cicatricial ectropion of <u>left</u> <u>lower</u> eyelid
H02.116	Cicatricial ectropion of <u>left</u> eye, <u>unspecified</u> eyelid
H02.119	Cicatricial ectropion of <u>unspecified</u> eye, <u>unspecified</u> eyelid

H02.12- **Mechanical** ectropion of eyelid — A form caused by external forces.

H02.121	Mechanical ectropion of <u>right</u> <u>upper</u> eyelid
H02.122	Mechanical ectropion of <u>right</u> <u>lower</u> eyelid
H02.123	Mechanical ectropion of <u>right</u> eye, <u>unspecified</u> eyelid
H02.124	Mechanical ectropion of <u>left</u> <u>upper</u> eyelid
H02.125	Mechanical ectropion of <u>left</u> <u>lower</u> eyelid
H02.126	Mechanical ectropion of <u>left</u> eye, <u>unspecified</u> eyelid
H02.129	Mechanical ectropion of <u>unspecified</u> eye, <u>unspecified</u> eyelid

H02.13- **Senile** ectropion of eyelid — A form caused by loss of tone of the obicularis oculi muscle.

H02.131	Senile ectropion of <u>right</u> <u>upper</u> eyelid — [Age/15-124]
H02.132	Senile ectropion of <u>right</u> <u>lower</u> eyelid — [Age/15-124]
H02.133	Senile ectropion of <u>right</u> eye, <u>unspecified</u> eyelid — [Age/15-124]
H02.134	Senile ectropion of <u>left</u> <u>upper</u> eyelid — [Age/15-124]
H02.135	Senile ectropion of <u>left</u> <u>lower</u> eyelid — [Age/15-124]
H02.136	Senile ectropion of <u>left</u> eye, <u>unspecified</u> eyelid — [Age/15-124]
H02.139	Senile ectropion of <u>unspecified</u> eye, <u>unspecified</u> eyelid — [Age/15-124]

H02.14- **Spastic** ectropion of eyelid — A form caused by tonic spasm of the obicularis oculi muscle.

H02.141	Spastic ectropion of <u>right</u> <u>upper</u> eyelid
H02.142	Spastic ectropion of <u>right</u> <u>lower</u> eyelid
H02.143	Spastic ectropion of <u>right</u> eye, <u>unspecified</u> eyelid
H02.144	Spastic ectropion of <u>left</u> <u>upper</u> eyelid
H02.145	Spastic ectropion of <u>left</u> <u>lower</u> eyelid
H02.146	Spastic ectropion of <u>left</u> eye, <u>unspecified</u> eyelid
H02.149	Spastic ectropion of <u>unspecified</u> eye, <u>unspecified</u> eyelid

H02.2- **Lagophthalmos** — Incomplete closure of the eyelids.

H02.20- **Unspecified** lagophthalmos

H02.201	Unspecified lagophthalmos <u>right</u> <u>upper</u> eyelid
H02.202	Unspecified lagophthalmos <u>right</u> <u>lower</u> eyelid
H02.203	Unspecified lagophthalmos <u>right</u> eye, <u>unspecified</u> eyelid
H02.204	Unspecified lagophthalmos <u>left</u> <u>upper</u> eyelid
H02.205	Unspecified lagophthalmos <u>left</u> <u>lower</u> eyelid
H02.206	Unspecified lagophthalmos <u>left</u> eye, <u>unspecified</u> eyelid
H02.209	Unspecified lagophthalmos <u>unspecified</u> eye, <u>unspecified</u> eyelid

H02.21- **Cicatricial** lagophthalmos — A form caused by contraction of an eyelid scar.

H02.211	Cicatricial lagophthalmos <u>right</u> <u>upper</u> eyelid
H02.212	Cicatricial lagophthalmos <u>right</u> <u>lower</u> eyelid
H02.213	Cicatricial lagophthalmos <u>right</u> eye, <u>unspecified</u> eyelid
H02.214	Cicatricial lagophthalmos <u>left</u> <u>upper</u> eyelid
H02.215	Cicatricial lagophthalmos <u>left</u> <u>lower</u> eyelid
H02.216	Cicatricial lagophthalmos <u>left</u> eye, <u>unspecified</u> eyelid
H02.219	Cicatricial lagophthalmos <u>unspecified</u> eye, <u>unspecified</u> eyelid

H02.22- **Mechanical** lagophthalmos — A form caused by external forces.

H02.221	Mechanical lagophthalmos <u>right</u> <u>upper</u> eyelid
H02.222	Mechanical lagophthalmos <u>right</u> <u>lower</u> eyelid
H02.223	Mechanical lagophthalmos <u>right</u> eye, <u>unspecified</u> eyelid
H02.224	Mechanical lagophthalmos <u>left</u> <u>upper</u> eyelid
H02.225	Mechanical lagophthalmos <u>left</u> <u>lower</u> eyelid
H02.226	Mechanical lagophthalmos <u>left</u> eye, <u>unspecified</u> eyelid
H02.229	Mechanical lagophthalmos <u>unspecified</u> eye, <u>unspecified</u> eyelid

H02.23- **Paralytic** lagophthalmos — A form caused by impairment of the facial nerve.

H02.231	Paralytic lagophthalmos <u>right</u> <u>upper</u> eyelid
H02.232	Paralytic lagophthalmos <u>right</u> <u>lower</u> eyelid
H02.233	Paralytic lagophthalmos <u>right</u> eye, <u>unspecified</u> eyelid
H02.234	Paralytic lagophthalmos <u>left</u> <u>upper</u> eyelid
H02.235	Paralytic lagophthalmos <u>left</u> <u>lower</u> eyelid
H02.236	Paralytic lagophthalmos <u>left</u> eye, <u>unspecified</u> eyelid
H02.239	Paralytic lagophthalmos <u>unspecified</u> eye, <u>unspecified</u> eyelid

H02.3- **Blepharochalasis** — Hypertrophy with loss of elasticity of the upper eyelids resulting in drooping.
   Pseudoptosis — Apparent ptosis of an eyelid resulting from a fold of skin or fat.

H02.30	Blepharochalasis <u>unspecified</u> eye, <u>unspecified</u> eyelid
H02.31	Blepharochalasis <u>right</u> <u>upper</u> eyelid
H02.32	Blepharochalasis <u>right</u> <u>lower</u> eyelid
H02.33	Blepharochalasis <u>right</u> eye, <u>unspecified</u> eyelid
H02.34	Blepharochalasis <u>left</u> <u>upper</u> eyelid
H02.35	Blepharochalasis <u>left</u> <u>lower</u> eyelid
H02.36	Blepharochalasis <u>left</u> eye, <u>unspecified</u> eyelid

H02.4- **Ptosis** of eyelid — Prolapse or drooping of the upper eyelid.

H02.40- **Unspecified** ptosis of eyelid

H02.401	Unspecified ptosis of <u>right</u> eyelid
H02.402	Unspecified ptosis of <u>left</u> eyelid
H02.403	Unspecified ptosis of <u>bilateral</u> eyelids
H02.409	Unspecified ptosis of <u>unspecified</u> eyelid

H02.41- **Mechanical** ptosis of eyelid — A form caused by external forces.

H02.411	Mechanical ptosis of <u>right</u> eyelid
H02.412	Mechanical ptosis of <u>left</u> eyelid

H02 - H02

H02.413   Mechanical ptosis of <u>bilateral</u> eyelids

H02.419   Mechanical ptosis of <u>unspecified</u> eyelid

H02.42- <u>Myogenic</u> ptosis of eyelid — A form caused by impairment of the ocular muscles.

H02.421   Myogenic ptosis of <u>right</u> eyelid

H02.422   Myogenic ptosis of <u>left</u> eyelid

H02.423   Myogenic ptosis of <u>bilateral</u> eyelids

H02.429   Myogenic ptosis of <u>unspecified</u> eyelid

H02.43- <u>Paralytic</u> ptosis of eyelid — A form caused by severe impairment of the third nerve.

Neurogenic ptosis of eyelid

H02.431   Paralytic ptosis of <u>right</u> eyelid

H02.432   Paralytic ptosis of <u>left</u> eyelid

H02.433   Paralytic ptosis of <u>bilateral</u> eyelids

H02.439   Paralytic ptosis <u>unspecified</u> eyelid

H02.5-   Other disorders affecting eyelid function

Excludes ❷: blepharospasm (G24.5)
organic tic (G25.69)
psychogenic tic (F95.-)

H02.51- <u>Abnormal innervation syndrome</u> — Conditions due to crossed or fused ocular nerves.

H02.511   Abnormal innervation syndrome <u>right</u> <u>upper</u> eyelid

H02.512   Abnormal innervation syndrome <u>right</u> <u>lower</u> eyelid

H02.513   Abnormal innervation syndrome <u>right</u> eye, <u>unspecified</u> eyelid

H02.514   Abnormal innervation syndrome <u>left</u> <u>upper</u> eyelid

H02.515   Abnormal innervation syndrome <u>left</u> <u>lower</u> eyelid

H02.516   Abnormal innervation syndrome <u>left</u> eye, <u>unspecified</u> eyelid

H02.519   Abnormal innervation syndrome <u>unspecified</u> eye, <u>unspecified</u> eyelid

H02.52- <u>Blepharophimosis</u> — Decreased width of the opening of the eyelids.

Ankyloblepharon — The abnormal adhesion of the ciliary body edges to the eyelid.

H02.521   Blepharophimosis <u>right</u> <u>upper</u> eyelid

H02.522   Blepharophimosis <u>right</u> <u>lower</u> eyelid

H02.523   Blepharophimosis <u>right</u> eye, <u>unspecified</u> eyelid

H02.524   Blepharophimosis <u>left</u> <u>upper</u> eyelid

H02.525   Blepharophimosis <u>left</u> <u>lower</u> eyelid

H02.526   Blepharophimosis <u>left</u> eye, <u>unspecified</u> eyelid

H02.529   Blepharophimosis <u>unspecified</u> eye, <u>unspecified</u> lid

H02.53- <u>Eyelid retraction</u> — The drawing-back of an eyelid.

Eyelid lag

H02.531   Eyelid retraction <u>right</u> <u>upper</u> eyelid

H02.532   Eyelid retraction <u>right</u> <u>lower</u> eyelid

H02.533   Eyelid retraction <u>right</u> eye, <u>unspecified</u> eyelid

H02.534   Eyelid retraction <u>left</u> <u>upper</u> eyelid

H02.535   Eyelid retraction <u>left</u> <u>lower</u> eyelid

H02.536   Eyelid retraction <u>left</u> eye, <u>unspecified</u> eyelid

H02.539   Eyelid retraction <u>unspecified</u> eye, <u>unspecified</u> lid

H02.59- Other disorders affecting eyelid function

Deficient blink reflex — Impairment of the normal blink reflex.

Sensory disorders — Abnormal conditions of eyelid function due to dysfunctional sensory stimulation.

H02.6-   <u>Xanthelasma</u> of eyelid — A fat deposit under the skin of the eyelid and usually toward the inner canthus.

H02.60   Xanthelasma of <u>unspecified</u> eye, <u>unspecified</u> eyelid

H02.61   Xanthelasma of <u>right</u> <u>upper</u> eyelid

H02.62   Xanthelasma of <u>right</u> <u>lower</u> eyelid

H02.63   Xanthelasma of <u>right</u> eye, <u>unspecified</u> eyelid

H02.64   Xanthelasma of <u>left</u> <u>upper</u> eyelid

H02.65   Xanthelasma of <u>left</u> <u>lower</u> eyelid

H02.66   Xanthelasma of <u>left</u> eye, <u>unspecified</u> eyelid

H02.7-   Other and unspecified degenerative disorders of eyelid and periocular area

H02.70   Unspecified degenerative disorders of eyelid and periocular area

H02.71- <u>Chloasma</u> of eyelid and periocular area — Abnormal eyelid pigmentation with yellowish-brown spots or patches.

Dyspigmentation of eyelid — Abnormal eyelid pigmentation.

Hyperpigmentation of eyelid — The abnormal excessive pigmentation of an eyelid.

H02.711   Chloasma of <u>right</u> <u>upper</u> eyelid and periocular area

H02.712   Chloasma of <u>right</u> <u>lower</u> eyelid and periocular area

H02.713   Chloasma of <u>right</u> eye, <u>unspecified</u> eyelid and periocular area

H02.714   Chloasma of <u>left</u> <u>upper</u> eyelid and periocular area

H02.715   Chloasma of <u>left</u> <u>lower</u> eyelid and periocular area

H02.716   Chloasma of <u>left</u> eye, <u>unspecified</u> eyelid and periocular area

H02.719   Chloasma of <u>unspecified</u> eye, <u>unspecified</u> eyelid and periocular area

H02.72- <u>Madarosis</u> of eyelid and periocular area — The abnormal loss of eyelashes.

Hypotrichosis of eyelid — The abnormal reduction or lack of eyelid hair.

H02.721   Madarosis of <u>right</u> <u>upper</u> eyelid and periocular area

H02.722   Madarosis of <u>right</u> <u>lower</u> eyelid and periocular area

H02.723   Madarosis of <u>right</u> eye, <u>unspecified</u> eyelid and periocular area

H02.724   Madarosis of <u>left</u> <u>upper</u> eyelid and periocular area

H02.725   Madarosis of <u>left</u> <u>lower</u> eyelid and periocular area

H02.726   Madarosis of <u>left</u> eye, <u>unspecified</u> eyelid and periocular area

H02.729   Madarosis of <u>unspecified</u> eye, <u>unspecified</u> eyelid and periocular area

H02.73- <u>Vitiligo</u> of eyelid and periocular area — A form marked by destruction of melanocytes.

Hypopigmentation of eyelid — The abnormal lack of pigmentation of an eyelid.

H02.731   Vitiligo of <u>right</u> <u>upper</u> eyelid and periocular area

H02.732   Vitiligo of <u>right</u> <u>lower</u> eyelid and periocular area

H02.733   Vitiligo of <u>right</u> eye, <u>unspecified</u> eyelid and periocular area

H02.734   Vitiligo of <u>left</u> <u>upper</u> eyelid and periocular area

H02.735   Vitiligo of <u>left</u> <u>lower</u> eyelid and periocular area

H02.736   Vitiligo of <u>left</u> eye, <u>unspecified</u> eyelid and periocular area

H02.739   Vitiligo of <u>unspecified</u> eye, <u>unspecified</u> eyelid and periocular area

H02.79   Other degenerative disorders of eyelid and periocular area

H02.8-   Other specified disorders of <u>eyelid</u>

H02.81- <u>Retained foreign body in eyelid</u> — The continued presence of foreign material in an eyelid.

Use additional code to identify the type of retained foreign body (Z18.-)

Excludes 1:   laceration of eyelid with foreign body (S01.12-)
retained intraocular foreign body (H44.6-, H44.7-)
superficial foreign body of eyelid and periocular area (S00.25-)

H02.811   Retained foreign body in <u>right</u> <u>upper</u> eyelid

H02.812   Retained foreign body in <u>right</u> <u>lower</u> eyelid

H02.813   Retained foreign body in <u>right</u> eye, <u>unspecified</u> eyelid

H02.814   Retained foreign body in <u>left</u> <u>upper</u> eyelid

H02.815   Retained foreign body in <u>left</u> <u>lower</u> eyelid

H02.816   Retained foreign body in <u>left</u> eye, <u>unspecified</u> eyelid

H02.819   Retained foreign body in <u>unspecified</u> eye, <u>unspecified</u> eyelid

H02.82- <u>Cysts</u> of eyelid — An encapsulated, fluid-filled sac of an eyelid.

Sebaceous cyst of eyelid — A cyst of a sebaceous gland.

H02.821   Cysts of <u>right</u> <u>upper</u> eyelid

H02.822   Cysts of <u>right</u> <u>lower</u> eyelid

H02-H02

H02.823   Cysts of <u>right</u> eye, <u>unspecified</u> eyelid
H02.824   Cysts of <u>left</u> <u>upper</u> eyelid
H02.825   Cysts of <u>left</u> <u>lower</u> eyelid
H02.826   Cysts of <u>left</u> eye, <u>unspecified</u> eyelid
H02.829   Cysts of <u>unspecified</u> eye, <u>unspecified</u> eyelid

H02.83- <u>Dermatochalasis</u> of eyelid — Excess and lax skin of the eyelids.

H02.831   Dermatochalasis of <u>right</u> <u>upper</u> eyelid
H02.832   Dermatochalasis of <u>right</u> <u>lower</u> eyelid
H02.833   Dermatochalasis of <u>right</u> eye, <u>unspecified</u> eyelid
H02.834   Dermatochalasis of <u>left</u> <u>upper</u> eyelid
H02.835   Dermatochalasis of <u>left</u> <u>lower</u> eyelid
H02.836   Dermatochalasis of <u>left</u> eye, <u>unspecified</u> eyelid
H02.839   Dermatochalasis of <u>unspecified</u> eye, <u>unspecified</u> eyelid

H02.84- <u>Edema</u> of eyelid — The abnormal accumulation of intercellular fluid of an eyelid.
  Hyperemia of eyelid — The abnormal congestion of blood of an eyelid.

H02.841   Edema of <u>right</u> <u>upper</u> eyelid
H02.842   Edema of <u>right</u> <u>lower</u> eyelid
H02.843   Edema of <u>right</u> eye, <u>unspecified</u> eyelid
H02.844   Edema of <u>left</u> <u>upper</u> eyelid
H02.845   Edema of <u>left</u> <u>lower</u> eyelid
H02.846   Edema of <u>left</u> eye, <u>unspecified</u> eyelid
H02.849   Edema of <u>unspecified</u> eye, <u>unspecified</u> eyelid

H02.85- <u>Elephantiasis</u> of eyelid — The massive hypertrophy of eyelid tissues.

H02.851   Elephantiasis of <u>right</u> <u>upper</u> eyelid
H02.852   Elephantiasis of <u>right</u> <u>lower</u> eyelid
H02.853   Elephantiasis of <u>right</u> eye, <u>unspecified</u> eyelid
H02.854   Elephantiasis of <u>left</u> <u>upper</u> eyelid
H02.855   Elephantiasis of <u>left</u> <u>lower</u> eyelid
H02.856   Elephantiasis of <u>left</u> eye, <u>unspecified</u> eyelid
H02.859   Elephantiasis of <u>unspecified</u> eye, <u>unspecified</u> eyelid

H02.86- <u>Hypertrichosis</u> of eyelid — The excessive growth of eyelid hair.

H02.861   Hypertrichosis of <u>right</u> <u>upper</u> eyelid
H02.862   Hypertrichosis of <u>right</u> <u>lower</u> eyelid
H02.863   Hypertrichosis of <u>right</u> eye, <u>unspecified</u> eyelid
H02.864   Hypertrichosis of <u>left</u> <u>upper</u> eyelid
H02.865   Hypertrichosis of <u>left</u> <u>lower</u> eyelid
H02.866   Hypertrichosis of <u>left</u> eye, <u>unspecified</u> eyelid
H02.869   Hypertrichosis of <u>unspecified</u> eye, <u>unspecified</u> eyelid

H02.87- <u>Vascular anomalies</u> of eyelid — Abnormal conditions of the eyelid blood vessels.

H02.871   Vascular anomalies of <u>right</u> <u>upper</u> eyelid
H02.872   Vascular anomalies of <u>right</u> <u>lower</u> eyelid
H02.873   Vascular anomalies of <u>right</u> eye, <u>unspecified</u> eyelid
H02.874   Vascular anomalies of <u>left</u> <u>upper</u> eyelid
H02.875   Vascular anomalies of <u>left</u> <u>lower</u> eyelid
H02.876   Vascular anomalies of <u>left</u> eye, <u>unspecified</u> eyelid
H02.879   Vascular anomalies of <u>unspecified</u> eye, <u>unspecified</u> eyelid

H02.89   Other specified disorders of eyelid
  Hemorrhage of eyelid — Bleeding from the eyelids.

H02.9   Unspecified disorder of eyelid
  Disorder of eyelid NOS

H04- Disorders of <u>lacrimal system</u>
  Excludes 1:   congenital malformations of lacrimal system (Q10.4-Q10.6)

H04.0- <u>Dacryoadenitis</u> — Inflammation of a lacrimal gland.

H04.00- <u>Unspecified</u> dacryoadenitis

H04.001   Unspecified dacryoadenitis, <u>right</u> lacrimal gland
H04.002   Unspecified dacryoadenitis, <u>left</u> lacrimal gland
H04.003   Unspecified dacryoadenitis, <u>bilateral</u> lacrimal glands

H04.009   Unspecified dacryoadenitis, <u>unspecified</u> lacrimal gland

H04.01- <u>Acute</u> dacryoadenitis — A form characterized by sudden, severe onset.

H04.011   Acute dacryoadenitis, <u>right</u> lacrimal gland
H04.012   Acute dacryoadenitis, <u>left</u> lacrimal gland
H04.013   Acute dacryoadenitis, <u>bilateral</u> lacrimal glands
H04.019   Acute dacryoadenitis, <u>unspecified</u> lacrimal gland

H04.02- <u>Chronic</u> dacryoadenitis — A form characterized by slow development and persistence over a long period of time.

H04.021   Chronic dacryoadenitis, <u>right</u> lacrimal gland
H04.022   Chronic dacryoadenitis, <u>left</u> lacrimal gland
H04.023   Chronic dacryoadenitis, <u>bilateral</u> lacrimal gland
H04.029   Chronic dacryoadenitis, <u>unspecified</u> lacrimal gland

H04.03- <u>Chronic enlargement</u> of lacrimal gland — A form characterized by continued increased size.

H04.031   Chronic enlargement of <u>right</u> lacrimal gland
H04.032   Chronic enlargement of <u>left</u> lacrimal gland
H04.033   Chronic enlargement of <u>bilateral</u> lacrimal glands
H04.039   Chronic enlargement of <u>unspecified</u> lacrimal gland

H04.1- Other disorders of <u>lacrimal gland</u>

H04.11- <u>Dacryops</u> — The constant flow of tears.

H04.111   Dacryops of <u>right</u> lacrimal gland
H04.112   Dacryops of <u>left</u> lacrimal gland
H04.113   Dacryops of <u>bilateral</u> lacrimal glands
H04.119   Dacryops of <u>unspecified</u> lacrimal gland

H04.12- <u>Dry eye</u> syndrome — The abnormal decrease of tear production.
  Tear film insufficiency, NOS

H04.121   Dry eye syndrome of <u>right</u> lacrimal gland
H04.122   Dry eye syndrome of <u>left</u> lacrimal gland
H04.123   Dry eye syndrome of <u>bilateral</u> lacrimal glands
H04.129   Dry eye syndrome of <u>unspecified</u> lacrimal gland

H04.13- <u>Lacrimal cyst</u> — Encapsulated, fluid-filled sacs of a lacrimal gland.
  Lacrimal cystic degeneration

H04.131   Lacrimal cyst, <u>right</u> lacrimal gland
H04.132   Lacrimal cyst, <u>left</u> lacrimal gland
H04.133   Lacrimal cyst, <u>bilateral</u> lacrimal glands
H04.139   Lacrimal cyst, <u>unspecified</u> lacrimal gland

H04.14- <u>Primary</u> lacrimal <u>gland atrophy</u> — The wasting-away of a lacrimal gland resulting from a lacrimal disorder.

H04.141   Primary lacrimal gland atrophy, <u>right</u> lacrimal gland
H04.142   Primary lacrimal gland atrophy, <u>left</u> lacrimal gland
H04.143   Primary lacrimal gland atrophy, <u>bilateral</u> lacrimal glands
H04.149   Primary lacrimal gland atrophy, <u>unspecified</u> lacrimal gland

H04.15- <u>Secondary</u> lacrimal <u>gland atrophy</u>

H04.151   Secondary lacrimal gland atrophy, <u>right</u> lacrimal gland
H04.152   Secondary lacrimal gland atrophy, <u>left</u> lacrimal gland
H04.153   Secondary lacrimal gland atrophy, <u>bilateral</u> lacrimal glands
H04.159   Secondary lacrimal gland atrophy, <u>unspecified</u> lacrimal gland

H04.16- <u>Lacrimal gland dislocation</u> — The wasting-away of a lacrimal gland resulting from another ocular disease.

H04.161   Lacrimal gland dislocation, <u>right</u> lacrimal gland
H04.162   Lacrimal gland dislocation, <u>left</u> lacrimal gland
H04.163   Lacrimal gland dislocation, <u>bilateral</u> lacrimal glands
H04.169   Lacrimal gland dislocation, <u>unspecified</u> lacrimal gland

H04.19   Other specified disorders of lacrimal gland

H04.2- <u>Epiphora</u> — The overflow of tears down the cheek.

H04.20- <u>Unspecified</u> epiphora

H02 - H04

H04.201   Unspecified epiphora, <u>right</u> lacrimal gland

H04.202   Unspecified epiphora, <u>left</u> lacrimal gland

H04.203   Unspecified epiphora, <u>bilateral</u> lacrimal glands

H04.209   Unspecified epiphora, <u>unspecified</u> lacrimal gland

H04.21- Epiphora due to <u>excess lacrimation</u> — A form caused by excessive tear production.

H04.211   Epiphora due to excess lacrimation, <u>right</u> lacrimal gland

H04.212   Epiphora due to excess lacrimation, <u>left</u> lacrimal gland

H04.213   Epiphora due to excess lacrimation, <u>bilateral</u> lacrimal glands

H04.219   Epiphora due to excess lacrimation, <u>unspecified</u> lacrimal gland

H04.22- Epiphora due to <u>insufficient drainage</u> — A form resulting from blocked drainage.

H04.221   Epiphora due to insufficient drainage, <u>right</u> lacrimal gland

H04.222   Epiphora due to insufficient drainage, <u>left</u> lacrimal gland

H04.223   Epiphora due to insufficient drainage, <u>bilateral</u> lacrimal glands

H04.229   Epiphora due to insufficient drainage, <u>unspecified</u> lacrimal gland

H04.3-   <u>Acute</u> and unspecified <u>inflammation of lacrimal passages</u>
> Excludes 1:   neonatal dacryocystitis (P39.1)

H04.30- Unspecified <u>dacryocystitis</u>

H04.301   Unspecified dacryocystitis of <u>right</u> lacrimal passage

H04.302   Unspecified dacryocystitis of <u>left</u> lacrimal passage

H04.303   Unspecified dacryocystitis of <u>bilateral</u> lacrimal passages

H04.309   Unspecified dacryocystitis of <u>unspecified</u> lacrimal passage

H04.31- <u>Phlegmonous dacryocystitis</u> — Inflammation of the connective tissue of a lacrimal sac.

H04.311   Phlegmonous dacryocystitis of <u>right</u> lacrimal passage

H04.312   Phlegmonous dacryocystitis of <u>left</u> lacrimal passage

H04.313   Phlegmonous dacryocystitis of <u>bilateral</u> lacrimal passages

H04.319   Phlegmonous dacryocystitis of <u>unspecified</u> lacrimal passage

H04.32- <u>Acute</u> dacryocystitis — The sudden, severe onset of inflammation of a lacrimal sac.
> **Acute dacryopericystitis** — A form affecting the tissues surrounding a lacrimal sac.

H04.321   Acute dacryocystitis of <u>right</u> lacrimal passage

H04.322   Acute dacryocystitis of <u>left</u> lacrimal passage

H04.323   Acute dacryocystitis of <u>bilateral</u> lacrimal passages

H04.329   Acute dacryocystitis of <u>unspecified</u> lacrimal passage

H04.33- <u>Acute lacrimal canaliculitis</u> — The sudden, severe onset of inflammation of the short passage between the lacrimal lake and the lacrimal sac.

H04.331   Acute lacrimal canaliculitis of <u>right</u> lacrimal passage

H04.332   Acute lacrimal canaliculitis of <u>left</u> lacrimal passage

H04.333   Acute lacrimal canaliculitis of <u>bilateral</u> lacrimal passages

H04.339   Acute lacrimal canaliculitis of <u>unspecified</u> lacrimal passage

H04.4-   <u>Chronic</u> inflammation of lacrimal passages

H04.41- <u>Chronic dacryocystitis</u> — Inflammation of a lacrimal sac that develops slowly and persists over a long period of time.

H04.411   Chronic dacryocystitis of <u>right</u> lacrimal passage

H04.412   Chronic dacryocystitis of <u>left</u> lacrimal passage

H04.413   Chronic dacryocystitis of <u>bilateral</u> lacrimal passages

H04.419   Chronic dacryocystitis of <u>unspecified</u> lacrimal passage

H04.42- Chronic lacrimal <u>canaliculitis</u> — Inflammation of the short passage between the lacrimal lake and the lacrimal sac that develops slowly and persists over a long period of time.

H04.421   Chronic lacrimal canaliculitis of <u>right</u> lacrimal passage

H04.422   Chronic lacrimal canaliculitis of <u>left</u> lacrimal passage

H04.423   Chronic lacrimal canaliculitis of <u>bilateral</u> lacrimal passages

H04.429   Chronic lacrimal canaliculitis of <u>unspecified</u> lacrimal passage

H04.43- Chronic lacrimal <u>mucocele</u> — Dilatation with mucous secretion of the lacrimal passages.

H04.431   Chronic lacrimal mucocele of <u>right</u> lacrimal passage

H04.432   Chronic lacrimal mucocele of <u>left</u> lacrimal passage

H04.433   Chronic lacrimal mucocele of <u>bilateral</u> lacrimal passages

H04.439   Chronic lacrimal mucocele of <u>unspecified</u> lacrimal passage

H04.5-   <u>Stenosis and insufficiency</u> of lacrimal passages

H04.51- <u>Dacryolith</u> — An abnormal concretion within the lacrimal passages.

H04.511   Dacryolith of <u>right</u> lacrimal passage

H04.512   Dacryolith of <u>left</u> lacrimal passage

H04.513   Dacryolith of <u>bilateral</u> lacrimal passages

H04.519   Dacryolith of <u>unspecified</u> lacrimal passage

H04.52- <u>Eversion</u> of lacrimal <u>punctum</u> — The turning outward of the eyelid lacrimal opening.

H04.521   Eversion of <u>right</u> lacrimal punctum

H04.522   Eversion of <u>left</u> lacrimal punctum

H04.523   Eversion of <u>bilateral</u> lacrimal punctum

H04.529   Eversion of <u>unspecified</u> lacrimal punctum

H04.53- <u>Neonatal obstruction</u> of <u>nasolacrimal duct</u> — The blockage of the nasal tear-draining duct that specifically develops after birth and is not due to a fetal distortion of the duct.
> Excludes 1:   congenital stenosis and stricture of lacrimal duct (Q10.5)

H04.531   Neonatal obstruction of <u>right</u> nasolacrimal duct — [Age/0]

H04.532   Neonatal obstruction of <u>left</u> nasolacrimal duct — [Age/0]

H04.533   Neonatal obstruction of <u>bilateral</u> nasolacrimal duct — [Age/0]

H04.539   Neonatal obstruction of <u>unspecified</u> nasolacrimal duct — [Age/0]

H04.54- <u>Stenosis</u> of lacrimal <u>canaliculi</u> — The narrowing of the passage between the punctum and the lacrimal sac.

H04.541   Stenosis of <u>right</u> lacrimal canaliculi

H04.542   Stenosis of <u>left</u> lacrimal canaliculi

H04.543   Stenosis of <u>bilateral</u> lacrimal canaliculi

H04.549   Stenosis of <u>unspecified</u> lacrimal canaliculi

H04.55- <u>Acquired stenosis</u> of <u>nasolacrimal duct</u> — The narrowing of the nasal tear-draining duct.

H04.551   Acquired stenosis of <u>right</u> nasolacrimal duct

H04.552   Acquired stenosis of <u>left</u> nasolacrimal duct

H04.553   Acquired stenosis of <u>bilateral</u> nasolacrimal duct

H04.559   Acquired stenosis of <u>unspecified</u> nasolacrimal duct

H04.56- <u>Stenosis</u> of lacrimal <u>punctum</u> — The narrowing of the eyelid lacrimal opening.

H04.561   Stenosis of <u>right</u> lacrimal punctum

H04.562   Stenosis of <u>left</u> lacrimal punctum

H04.563   Stenosis of <u>bilateral</u> lacrimal punctum

H04.569   Stenosis of <u>unspecified</u> lacrimal punctum

H04.57- <u>Stenosis</u> of lacrimal <u>sac</u> — The narrowing of the lacrimal sac.

H04.571   Stenosis of <u>right</u> lacrimal sac

H04.572   Stenosis of <u>left</u> lacrimal sac

H04.573   Stenosis of <u>bilateral</u> lacrimal sac
H04.579   Stenosis of <u>unspecified</u> lacrimal sac
H04.6-   Other changes of lacrimal passages
  H04.61- Lacrimal <u>fistula</u> — An abnormal passage of the lacrimal passages.
    H04.611   Lacrimal fistula <u>right</u> lacrimal passage
    H04.612   Lacrimal fistula <u>left</u> lacrimal passage
    H04.613   Lacrimal fistula <u>bilateral</u> lacrimal passages
    H04.619   Lacrimal fistula <u>unspecified</u> lacrimal passage
  H04.69   Other changes of lacrimal passages
H04.8-   Other disorders of lacrimal system
  H04.81- <u>Granuloma</u> of lacrimal passages — The formation of granular tissue within a lacrimal passage.
    H04.811   Granuloma of <u>right</u> lacrimal passage
    H04.812   Granuloma of <u>left</u> lacrimal passage
    H04.813   Granuloma of <u>bilateral</u> lacrimal passages
    H04.819   Granuloma of <u>unspecified</u> lacrimal passage
  H04.89   Other disorders of lacrimal system
H04.9   Disorder of lacrimal system, unspecified

H05-   Disorders of <u>orbit</u>
  Excludes 1:   congenital malformation of orbit (Q10.7)
  H05.0-   <u>Acute inflammation</u> of orbit — The sudden, severe onset of inflammation of the cavity that contains the eyeball.
    H05.00   <u>Unspecified</u> acute inflammation of orbit
    H05.01- <u>Cellulitis</u> of orbit — A form marked by the inflammation of the cellular tissue.
      Abscess of orbit — A form marked by the localized collection of pus caused by the disintegration of orbital tissues.
      cc H05.011   Cellulitis of <u>right</u> orbit
      cc H05.012   Cellulitis of <u>left</u> orbit
      cc H05.013   Cellulitis of <u>bilateral</u> orbits
      cc H05.019   Cellulitis of <u>unspecified</u> orbit
    H05.02- <u>Osteomyelitis</u> of orbit — A form characterized by inflammation of the orbital bone and bone marrow.
      cc H05.021   Osteomyelitis of <u>right</u> orbit
      cc H05.022   Osteomyelitis of <u>left</u> orbit
      cc H05.023   Osteomyelitis of <u>bilateral</u> orbits
      cc H05.029   Osteomyelitis of <u>unspecified</u> orbit
    H05.03- <u>Periostitis</u> of orbit — A form characterized by inflammation of the orbital periosteum.
      cc H05.031   Periostitis of <u>right</u> orbit
      cc H05.032   Periostitis of <u>left</u> orbit
      cc H05.033   Periostitis of <u>bilateral</u> orbits
      cc H05.039   Periostitis of <u>unspecified</u> orbit
    H05.04- <u>Tenonitis</u> of orbit — A form characterized by inflammation of the orbital tendons.
      H05.041   Tenonitis of <u>right</u> orbit
      H05.042   Tenonitis of <u>left</u> orbit
      H05.043   Tenonitis of <u>bilateral</u> orbits
      H05.049   Tenonitis of <u>unspecified</u> orbit
  H05.1-   <u>Chronic inflammatory disorders of orbit</u> — Inflammatory disorders of the cavity that contains the eyeball which develop slowly and persist over a long period of time.
    H05.10   <u>Unspecified</u> chronic inflammatory disorders of orbit
    H05.11- <u>Granuloma</u> of orbit — A form characterized by the formation of granular tissue.
      Pseudotumor (inflammatory) of orbit — A form marked by a mass of granular and fibrous inflammatory tissue.
      H05.111   Granuloma of <u>right</u> orbit
      H05.112   Granuloma of <u>left</u> orbit
      H05.113   Granuloma of <u>bilateral</u> orbits
      H05.119   Granuloma of <u>unspecified</u> orbit
    H05.12- Orbital <u>myositis</u> — A form characterized by inflammation of the orbital muscles.
      H05.121   Orbital myositis, <u>right</u> orbit
      H05.122   Orbital myositis, <u>left</u> orbit
      H05.123   Orbital myositis, <u>bilateral</u>
      H05.129   Orbital myositis, <u>unspecified</u> orbit

H05.2-   <u>Exophthalmic conditions</u> — The abnormal protrusion of the eyeball.
  H05.20   Unspecified exophthalmos
  H05.21- <u>Displacement</u> (lateral) of <u>globe</u> — A form characterized by the movement of the eyeball towards the side.
    H05.211   Displacement (lateral) of globe, <u>right</u> eye
    H05.212   Displacement (lateral) of globe, <u>left</u> eye
    H05.213   Displacement (lateral) of globe, <u>bilateral</u>
    H05.219   Displacement (lateral) of globe, <u>unspecified</u> eye
  H05.22- <u>Edema</u> of orbit — A form characterized by the localized accumulation of intercellular orbital fluid.
    Orbital congestion
    H05.221   Edema of <u>right</u> orbit
    H05.222   Edema of <u>left</u> orbit
    H05.223   Edema of <u>bilateral</u> orbit
    H05.229   Edema of <u>unspecified</u> orbit
  H05.23- <u>Hemorrhage</u> of orbit — A form characterized by bleeding from the orbit.
    H05.231   Hemorrhage of <u>right</u> orbit
    H05.232   Hemorrhage of <u>left</u> orbit
    H05.233   Hemorrhage of <u>bilateral</u> orbit
    H05.239   Hemorrhage of <u>unspecified</u> orbit
  H05.24- <u>Constant</u> exophthalmos — A form characterized by continued protrusion.
    H05.241   Constant exophthalmos, <u>right</u> eye
    H05.242   Constant exophthalmos, <u>left</u> eye
    H05.243   Constant exophthalmos, <u>bilateral</u>
    H05.249   Constant exophthalmos, <u>unspecified</u> eye
  H05.25- <u>Intermittent</u> exophthalmos — A form characterized by the occurrence of protrusion at separated intervals.
    H05.251   Intermittent exophthalmos, <u>right</u> eye
    H05.252   Intermittent exophthalmos, <u>left</u> eye
    H05.253   Intermittent exophthalmos, <u>bilateral</u>
    H05.259   Intermittent exophthalmos, <u>unspecified</u> eye
  H05.26- <u>Pulsating</u> exophthalmos — A form characterized by slight forward movement associated with vascular blood flow.
    H05.261   Pulsating exophthalmos, <u>right</u> eye
    H05.262   Pulsating exophthalmos, <u>left</u> eye
    H05.263   Pulsating exophthalmos, <u>bilateral</u>
    H05.269   Pulsating exophthalmos, <u>unspecified</u> eye
H05.3-   <u>Deformity</u> of <u>orbit</u> — The abnormal distortion of the normal orbital shape.
  Excludes 1:   congenital deformity of orbit (Q10.7)
              hypertelorism (Q75.2)
  H05.30   <u>Unspecified</u> deformity of orbit
  H05.31- <u>Atrophy</u> of orbit — A form resulting from the abnormal wasting-away of the orbital tissues.
    H05.311   Atrophy of <u>right</u> orbit
    H05.312   Atrophy of <u>left</u> orbit
    H05.313   Atrophy of <u>bilateral</u> orbit
    H05.319   Atrophy of <u>unspecified</u> orbit
  H05.32- Deformity of orbit <u>due to bone disease</u>
    Code also associated bone disease
    H05.321   Deformity of <u>right</u> orbit due to bone disease
    H05.322   Deformity of <u>left</u> orbit due to bone disease
    H05.323   Deformity of <u>bilateral</u> orbits due to bone disease
    H05.329   Deformity of <u>unspecified</u> orbit due to bone disease
  H05.33- Deformity of orbit <u>due to trauma or surgery</u>
    H05.331   Deformity of <u>right</u> orbit due to trauma or surgery
    H05.332   Deformity of <u>left</u> orbit due to trauma or surgery
    H05.333   Deformity of <u>bilateral</u> orbits due to trauma or surgery
    H05.339   Deformity of <u>unspecified</u> orbit due to trauma or surgery
  H05.34- <u>Enlargement</u> of orbit — A form resulting from the abnormal increase in the size of the orbital tissues.
    H05.341   Enlargement of <u>right</u> orbit
    H05.342   Enlargement of <u>left</u> orbit

H04 | H05

H05.343 Enlargement of <u>bilateral</u> orbits

H05.349 Enlargement of <u>unspecified</u> orbit

H05.35- <u>Exostosis</u> of orbit — A form characterized by an abnormal bony growth the of the orbit.

H05.351 Exostosis of <u>right</u> orbit

H05.352 Exostosis of <u>left</u> orbit

H05.353 Exostosis of <u>bilateral</u> orbits

H05.359 Exostosis of <u>unspecified</u> orbit

H05.4- <u>Enophthalmos</u> — A backward displacement of the eyeball into the orbit.

H05.40- <u>Unspecified</u> enophthalmos

H05.401 Unspecified enophthalmos, <u>right</u> eye

H05.402 Unspecified enophthalmos, <u>left</u> eye

H05.403 Unspecified enophthalmos, <u>bilateral</u>

H05.409 Unspecified enophthalmos, <u>unspecified</u> eye

H05.41- Enophthalmos <u>due to atrophy</u> of orbital tissue — A form resulting from the wasting-away of orbital tissues.

H05.411 Enophthalmos due to atrophy of orbital tissue, <u>right</u> eye

H05.412 Enophthalmos due to atrophy of orbital tissue, <u>left</u> eye

H05.413 Enophthalmos due to atrophy of orbital tissue, <u>bilateral</u>

H05.419 Enophthalmos due to atrophy of orbital tissue, <u>unspecified</u> eye

H05.42- Enophthalmos <u>due to trauma or surgery</u>

H05.421 Enophthalmos due to trauma or surgery, <u>right</u> eye

H05.422 Enophthalmos due to trauma or surgery, <u>left</u> eye

H05.423 Enophthalmos due to trauma or surgery, <u>bilateral</u>

H05.429 Enophthalmos due to trauma or surgery, <u>unspecified</u> eye

H05.5- <u>Retained (old) foreign body</u> following penetrating wound of <u>orbit</u> — The continued presence of foreign material within the orbit.
Retrobulbar foreign body
Use additional code to identify the type of retained foreign body (Z18.-)
Excludes 1:   *current penetrating wound of orbit (S05.4-)*
Excludes ❷: *retained foreign body of eyelid (H02.81-)*
                retained intraocular foreign body (H44.6-, H44.7-)

H05.50 Retained (old) foreign body following penetrating wound of <u>unspecified</u> orbit

H05.51 Retained (old) foreign body following penetrating wound of <u>right</u> orbit

H05.52 Retained (old) foreign body following penetrating wound of <u>left</u> orbit

H05.53 Retained (old) foreign body following penetrating wound of <u>bilateral</u> orbits

H05.8- <u>Other</u> disorders of <u>orbit</u>

H05.81- <u>Cyst</u> of orbit — An encapsulated, fluid-filled sac of the orbit.
Encephalocele of orbit

H05.811 Cyst of <u>right</u> orbit

H05.812 Cyst of <u>left</u> orbit

H05.813 Cyst of <u>bilateral</u> orbits

H05.819 Cyst of <u>unspecified</u> orbit

H05.82- <u>Myopathy</u> of extraocular muscles — Abnormal disorders and conditions of the extraocular muscles.

H05.821 Myopathy of extraocular muscles, <u>right</u> orbit

H05.822 Myopathy of extraocular muscles, <u>left</u> orbit

H05.823 Myopathy of extraocular muscles, <u>bilateral</u>

H05.829 Myopathy of extraocular muscles, <u>unspecified</u> orbit

H05.89 Other disorders of orbit

H05.9 Unspecified disorder of orbit

Disorders of conjunctiva (H10-H11)

H10- <u>Conjunctivitis</u> — Inflammation of the conjunctiva.
Excludes 1:   *keratoconjunctivitis (H16.2-)*

H10.0- <u>Mucopurulent</u> conjunctivitis — A form characterized by mucous membrane pus formation.

H10.01- <u>Acute follicular</u> conjunctivitis — A form characterized by dense localized infiltrations of lymphoid tissue.

H10.011 Acute follicular conjunctivitis, <u>right</u> eye

H10.012 Acute follicular conjunctivitis, <u>left</u> eye

H10.013 Acute follicular conjunctivitis, <u>bilateral</u>

H10.019 Acute follicular conjunctivitis, <u>unspecified</u> eye

H10.02- <u>Other mucopurulent</u> conjunctivitis

H10.021 Other mucopurulent conjunctivitis, <u>right</u> eye

H10.022 Other mucopurulent conjunctivitis, <u>left</u> eye

H10.023 Other mucopurulent conjunctivitis, <u>bilateral</u>

H10.029 Other mucopurulent conjunctivitis, <u>unspecified</u> eye

H10.1- <u>Acute atopic</u> conjunctivitis — A form caused by an allergen.
Acute papillary conjunctivitis

H10.10 Acute atopic conjunctivitis, <u>unspecified</u> eye

H10.11 Acute atopic conjunctivitis, <u>right</u> eye

H10.12 Acute atopic conjunctivitis, <u>left</u> eye

H10.13 Acute atopic conjunctivitis, <u>bilateral</u>

H10.2- <u>Other acute</u> conjunctivitis

H10.21- <u>Acute toxic</u> conjunctivitis — A form caused by an external irritant (smoke, smog, cleaning chemical vapors, etc.), but not causing a burn, corrosion, or other injury to the conjunctival tissue.
Acute chemical conjunctivitis
Code first (T51-T65) to identify chemical and intent
Excludes 1:   *burn and corrosion of eye and adnexa (T26.-)*

H10.211 Acute toxic conjunctivitis, <u>right</u> eye

H10.212 Acute toxic conjunctivitis, <u>left</u> eye

H10.213 Acute toxic conjunctivitis, <u>bilateral</u>

H10.219 Acute toxic conjunctivitis, <u>unspecified</u> eye

H10.22- <u>Pseudomembranous</u> conjunctivitis — A form characterized by fibrous exudates which form a false membrane.

H10.221 Pseudomembranous conjunctivitis, <u>right</u> eye

H10.222 Pseudomembranous conjunctivitis, <u>left</u> eye

H10.223 Pseudomembranous conjunctivitis, <u>bilateral</u>

H10.229 Pseudomembranous conjunctivitis, <u>unspecified</u> eye

H10.23- <u>Serous</u> conjunctivitis, except viral — A form characterized by a watery discharge that is not viral in origin.
Excludes 1:   *viral conjunctivitis (B30.-)*

H10.231 Serous conjunctivitis, except viral, <u>right</u> eye

H10.232 Serous conjunctivitis, except viral, <u>left</u> eye

H10.233 Serous conjunctivitis, except viral, <u>bilateral</u>

H10.239 Serous conjunctivitis, except viral, <u>unspecified</u> eye

H10.3- <u>Unspecified acute</u> conjunctivitis
Excludes 1:   *ophthalmia neonatorum NOS (P39.1)*

H10.30 Unspecified acute conjunctivitis, <u>unspecified</u> eye

H10.31 Unspecified acute conjunctivitis, <u>right</u> eye

H10.32 Unspecified acute conjunctivitis, <u>left</u> eye

H10.33 Unspecified acute conjunctivitis, <u>bilateral</u>

H10.4- <u>Chronic</u> conjunctivitis — Inflammation of the conjunctiva that develops slowly and persists over a long period of time.

H10.40- <u>Unspecified</u> chronic conjunctivitis

H10.401 Unspecified chronic conjunctivitis, <u>right</u> eye

H10.402 Unspecified chronic conjunctivitis, <u>left</u> eye

H10.403 Unspecified chronic conjunctivitis, <u>bilateral</u>

H10.409 Unspecified chronic conjunctivitis, <u>unspecified</u> eye

H10.41- Chronic <u>giant papillary</u> conjunctivitis — A form that is characterized by groups of papillary inflammatory cells and caused by wearing of contact lenses.

H10.411 Chronic giant papillary conjunctivitis, <u>right</u> eye

H10.412 Chronic giant papillary conjunctivitis, <u>left</u> eye

H10.413 Chronic giant papillary conjunctivitis, <u>bilateral</u>

H10.419 Chronic giant papillary conjunctivitis, <u>unspecified</u> eye

H10.42- <u>Simple</u> chronic conjunctivitis — A form resulting from mild continuous acute symptoms.

H10.421 Simple chronic conjunctivitis, <u>right</u> eye

H10.422 Simple chronic conjunctivitis, <u>left</u> eye

H10.423 Simple chronic conjunctivitis, <u>bilateral</u>

H05-H10

H10.429   Simple chronic conjunctivitis, <u>unspecified</u> eye

H10.43- Chronic <u>follicular</u> conjunctivitis — A form characterized by dense localized infiltrations of lymphoid tissue.

    H10.431   Chronic follicular conjunctivitis, <u>right</u> eye

    H10.432   Chronic follicular conjunctivitis, <u>left</u> eye

    H10.433   Chronic follicular conjunctivitis, <u>bilateral</u>

    H10.439   Chronic follicular conjunctivitis, <u>unspecified</u> eye

H10.44   <u>Vernal</u> conjunctivitis — A form characterized by onset during the spring and summer months.

    Excludes 1:   vernal keratoconjunctivitis with limbar and corneal involvement (H16.26-)

H10.45   <u>Other chronic allergic</u> conjunctivitis

H10.5- <u>Blepharoconjunctivitis</u> — Inflammation of the eyelids and conjunctiva.

H10.50- <u>Unspecified</u> blepharoconjunctivitis

    H10.501   Unspecified blepharoconjunctivitis, <u>right</u> eye

    H10.502   Unspecified blepharoconjunctivitis, <u>left</u> eye

    H10.503   Unspecified blepharoconjunctivitis, <u>bilateral</u>

    H10.509   Unspecified blepharoconjunctivitis, <u>unspecified</u> eye

H10.51- <u>Ligneous</u> conjunctivitis — A form characterized by pseudomembranous lesions developing on the tarsal conjunctiva.

    H10.511   Ligneous conjunctivitis, <u>right</u> eye

    H10.512   Ligneous conjunctivitis, <u>left</u> eye

    H10.513   Ligneous conjunctivitis, <u>bilateral</u>

    H10.519   Ligneous conjunctivitis, <u>unspecified</u> eye

H10.52- <u>Angular</u> blepharoconjunctivitis — A form affecting the canthal area.

    H10.521   Angular blepharoconjunctivitis, <u>right</u> eye

    H10.522   Angular blepharoconjunctivitis, <u>left</u> eye

    H10.523   Angular blepharoconjunctivitis, <u>bilateral</u>

    H10.529   Angular blepharoconjunctivitis, <u>unspecified</u> eye

H10.53- <u>Contact</u> blepharoconjunctivitis — A form caused by various substances.

    H10.531   Contact blepharoconjunctivitis, <u>right</u> eye

    H10.532   Contact blepharoconjunctivitis, <u>left</u> eye

    H10.533   Contact blepharoconjunctivitis, <u>bilateral</u>

    H10.539   Contact blepharoconjunctivitis, <u>unspecified</u> eye

H10.8- Other conjunctivitis

H10.81- <u>Pingueculitis</u> — An inflammatory disorder of the pingueculae (yellowish, slightly raised, lipid-like deposits on the conjunctiva) characterized by acute inflammation, vascularized conjunctiva, redness, and irritation.

    Excludes 1:   pinguecula (H11.15-)

    H10.811   Pingueculitis, <u>right</u> eye

    H10.812   Pingueculitis, <u>left</u> eye

    H10.813   Pingueculitis, <u>bilateral</u>

    H10.819   Pingueculitis, <u>unspecified</u> eye

H10.89   Other conjunctivitis

H10.9   Unspecified conjunctivitis

H11- <u>Other disorders of conjunctiva</u>

    Excludes 1:   keratoconjunctivitis (H16.2-)

H11.0- <u>Pterygium of eye</u> — A triangular-shaped thickening of the conjunctiva extending from the inner canthus over the cornea towards the pupil.

    Excludes 1:   pseudopterygium (H11.81-)

PTERYGIUM — RIGHT EYE

H11.00- <u>Unspecified</u> pterygium of eye

    H11.001   Unspecified pterygium of <u>right</u> eye

    H11.002   Unspecified pterygium of <u>left</u> eye

    H11.003   Unspecified pterygium of eye, <u>bilateral</u>

H11.009   Unspecified pterygium of <u>unspecified</u> eye

H11.01- <u>Amyloid</u> pterygium — A form with amyloid deposition in blood vessel walls.

    H11.011   Amyloid pterygium of <u>right</u> eye

    H11.012   Amyloid pterygium of <u>left</u> eye

    H11.013   Amyloid pterygium of eye, <u>bilateral</u>

    H11.019   Amyloid pterygium of <u>unspecified</u> eye

H11.02- <u>Central</u> pterygium of eye — A form which encroaches on the center of the cornea.

    H11.021   Central pterygium of <u>right</u> eye

    H11.022   Central pterygium of <u>left</u> eye

    H11.023   Central pterygium of eye, <u>bilateral</u>

    H11.029   Central pterygium of <u>unspecified</u> eye

H11.03- <u>Double</u> pterygium of eye — Bilateral pterygiums occurring at the same time.

    H11.031   Double pterygium of <u>right</u> eye

    H11.032   Double pterygium of <u>left</u> eye

    H11.033   Double pterygium of eye, <u>bilateral</u>

    H11.039   Double pterygium of <u>unspecified</u> eye

H11.04- <u>Peripheral</u> pterygium of eye, <u>stationary</u> — A stage in which the head of the pterygium remains permanently attached to the same point on the cornea.

    H11.041   Peripheral pterygium, stationary, <u>right</u> eye

    H11.042   Peripheral pterygium, stationary, <u>left</u> eye

    H11.043   Peripheral pterygium, stationary, <u>bilateral</u>

    H11.049   Peripheral pterygium, stationary, <u>unspecified</u> eye

H11.05- <u>Peripheral</u> pterygium of eye, <u>progressive</u> — A stage in which the growth extends toward the center of the cornea.

    H11.051   Peripheral pterygium, progressive, <u>right</u> eye

    H11.052   Peripheral pterygium, progressive, <u>left</u> eye

    H11.053   Peripheral pterygium, progressive, <u>bilateral</u>

    H11.059   Peripheral pterygium, progressive, <u>unspecified</u> eye

H11.06- <u>Recurrent</u> pterygium of eye — A form which returns after the initial condition has healed.

    H11.061   Recurrent pterygium of <u>right</u> eye

    H11.062   Recurrent pterygium of <u>left</u> eye

    H11.063   Recurrent pterygium of eye, <u>bilateral</u>

    H11.069   Recurrent pterygium of <u>unspecified</u> eye

H11.1- Conjunctival degenerations and deposits

    Excludes ❷: pseudopterygium (H11.81)

H11.10   Unspecified conjunctival degenerations

H11.11- <u>Conjunctival deposits</u> — Extraneous inorganic matter collected on the conjunctiva.

    H11.111   Conjunctival deposits, <u>right</u> eye

    H11.112   Conjunctival deposits, <u>left</u> eye

    H11.113   Conjunctival deposits, <u>bilateral</u>

    H11.119   Conjunctival deposits, <u>unspecified</u> eye

H11.12- Conjunctival <u>concretions</u> — A condition marked by a hardening of the conjunctiva.

    H11.121   Conjunctival concretions, <u>right</u> eye

    H11.122   Conjunctival concretions, <u>left</u> eye

    H11.123   Conjunctival concretions, <u>bilateral</u>

    H11.129   Conjunctival concretions, <u>unspecified</u> eye

H11.13- Conjunctival <u>pigmentations</u> — The pigmental discoloration of the conjunctiva.

    Conjunctival argyrosis [argyria] — A poisoning of the conjunctiva by silver, or a silver salt, causing a permanent ash gray discolorization.

    H11.131   Conjunctival pigmentations, <u>right</u> eye

    H11.132   Conjunctival pigmentations, <u>left</u> eye

    H11.133   Conjunctival pigmentations, <u>bilateral</u>

    H11.139   Conjunctival pigmentations, <u>unspecified</u> eye

H11.14- Conjunctival <u>xerosis</u>, <u>unspecified</u> — An abnormal dryness of the conjunctiva.

    Excludes 1:   xerosis of conjunctiva due to vitamin A deficiency (E50.0, E50.1)

    H11.141   Conjunctival xerosis, <u>unspecified</u>, <u>right</u> eye

    H11.142   Conjunctival xerosis, <u>unspecified</u>, <u>left</u> eye

H10 - H11

H11.143 Conjunctival xerosis, <u>unspecified</u>, <u>bilateral</u>
H11.149 Conjunctival xerosis, <u>unspecified</u>, <u>unspecified</u> eye
H11.15- <u>Pinguecula</u> — A yellowish thickening of the conjunctiva on the inner and outer margins of the cornea.
　　Excludes 1: pingueculitis (H10.81-)
H11.151 Pinguecula, <u>right</u> eye
H11.152 Pinguecula, <u>left</u> eye
H11.153 Pinguecula, <u>bilateral</u>
H11.159 Pinguecula, <u>unspecified</u> eye
H11.2- <u>Conjunctival scars</u> — The dense healing tissue of the conjunctiva.
H11.21- Conjunctival <u>adhesions and strands (localized)</u> — The formation of fibrous tissue of the conjunctiva.
H11.211 Conjunctival adhesions and strands (localized), <u>right</u> eye
H11.212 Conjunctival adhesions and strands (localized), <u>left</u> eye
H11.213 Conjunctival adhesions and strands (localized), <u>bilateral</u>
H11.219 Conjunctival adhesions and strands (localized), <u>unspecified</u> eye
H11.22- Conjunctival <u>granuloma</u> — The formation of granulation tissue of the conjunctiva.
H11.221 Conjunctival granuloma, <u>right</u> eye
H11.222 Conjunctival granuloma, <u>left</u> eye
H11.223 Conjunctival granuloma, <u>bilateral</u>
H11.229 Conjunctival granuloma, <u>unspecified</u>
H11.23- <u>Symblepharon</u> — The adhesion of the eyelid conjunctiva and the eyeball following an injury.
H11.231 Symblepharon, <u>right</u> eye
H11.232 Symblepharon, <u>left</u> eye
H11.233 Symblepharon, <u>bilateral</u>
H11.239 Symblepharon, <u>unspecified</u> eye
H11.24- <u>Scarring</u> of conjunctiva — The dense post wound-healing tissue of the conjunctiva.
H11.241 Scarring of conjunctiva, <u>right</u> eye
H11.242 Scarring of conjunctiva, <u>left</u> eye
H11.243 Scarring of conjunctiva, <u>bilateral</u>
H11.249 Scarring of conjunctiva, <u>unspecified</u> eye
H11.3- Conjunctival <u>hemorrhage</u> — Bleeding from the conjunctiva.
　　Subconjunctival hemorrhage
H11.30 Conjunctival hemorrhage, <u>unspecified</u> eye
H11.31 Conjunctival hemorrhage, <u>right</u> eye
H11.32 Conjunctival hemorrhage, <u>left</u> eye
H11.33 Conjunctival hemorrhage, <u>bilateral</u>
H11.4- <u>Other conjunctival vascular</u> disorders and cysts
H11.41- <u>Vascular abnormalities</u> of conjunctiva
　　Conjunctival aneurysm — The dilatation of a conjunctival artery.
H11.411 Vascular abnormalities of conjunctiva, <u>right</u> eye
H11.412 Vascular abnormalities of conjunctiva, <u>left</u> eye
H11.413 Vascular abnormalities of conjunctiva, <u>bilateral</u>
H11.419 Vascular abnormalities of conjunctiva, <u>unspecified</u> eye
H11.42- Conjunctival <u>edema</u> — The excessive amount of fluid within the conjunctiva.
H11.421 Conjunctival edema, <u>right</u> eye
H11.422 Conjunctival edema, <u>left</u> eye
H11.423 Conjunctival edema, <u>bilateral</u>
H11.429 Conjunctival edema, <u>unspecified</u> eye
H11.43- Conjunctival <u>hyperemia</u> — The abnormal excessive amount of blood in the conjunctiva.
H11.431 Conjunctival hyperemia, <u>right</u> eye
H11.432 Conjunctival hyperemia, <u>left</u> eye
H11.433 Conjunctival hyperemia, <u>bilateral</u>
H11.439 Conjunctival hyperemia, <u>unspecified</u> eye

H11.44- Conjunctival <u>cysts</u> — An encapsulated, fluid-filled sac of the conjunctiva.
H11.441 Conjunctival cysts, <u>right</u> eye
H11.442 Conjunctival cysts, <u>left</u> eye
H11.443 Conjunctival cysts, <u>bilateral</u>
H11.449 Conjunctival cysts, <u>unspecified</u> eye
H11.8- <u>Other specified disorders of conjunctiva</u>
H11.81- <u>Pseudopterygium</u> of conjunctiva — A scar on the conjunctiva that is usually firmly attached to the underlying tissue.
H11.811 Pseudopterygium of conjunctiva, <u>right</u> eye
H11.812 Pseudopterygium of conjunctiva, <u>left</u> eye
H11.813 Pseudopterygium of conjunctiva, <u>bilateral</u>
H11.819 Pseudopterygium of conjunctiva, <u>unspecified</u> eye
H11.82- <u>Conjunctivochalasis</u> — The formation of redundant conjunctival tissue which overlies the lower eyelid margin.
H11.821 Conjunctivochalasis, <u>right</u> eye
H11.822 Conjunctivochalasis, <u>left</u> eye
H11.823 Conjunctivochalasis, <u>bilateral</u>
H11.829 Conjunctivochalasis, <u>unspecified</u> eye
H11.89 Other specified disorders of conjunctiva
H11.9 Unspecified disorder of conjunctiva

Disorders of sclera, cornea, iris and ciliary body (H15-H22)

H15- <u>Disorders of sclera</u>
H15.0- <u>Scleritis</u> — Inflammation of the sclera.
H15.00- <u>Unspecified</u> scleritis
H15.001 Unspecified scleritis, <u>right</u> eye
H15.002 Unspecified scleritis, <u>left</u> eye
H15.003 Unspecified scleritis, <u>bilateral</u>
H15.009 Unspecified scleritis, <u>unspecified</u> eye
H15.01- <u>Anterior</u> scleritis — A form characterized by affecting that portion towards the front of the eye, including the corneal margins.
H15.011 Anterior scleritis, <u>right</u> eye
H15.012 Anterior scleritis, <u>left</u> eye
H15.013 Anterior scleritis, <u>bilateral</u>
H15.019 Anterior scleritis, <u>unspecified</u> eye
H15.02- <u>Brawny</u> scleritis — A form characterized by thickening of the corneal margins.
H15.021 Brawny scleritis, <u>right</u> eye
H15.022 Brawny scleritis, <u>left</u> eye
H15.023 Brawny scleritis, <u>bilateral</u>
H15.029 Brawny scleritis, <u>unspecified</u> eye
H15.03- <u>Posterior</u> scleritis — A form characterized by involvement of the underlying retina and choroid.
　　Sclerotenonitis
H15.031 Posterior scleritis, <u>right</u> eye
H15.032 Posterior scleritis, <u>left</u> eye
H15.033 Posterior scleritis, <u>bilateral</u>
H15.039 Posterior scleritis, <u>unspecified</u> eye
H15.04- <u>Scleritis with corneal involvement</u> — A form characterized by an inflammatory reaction in the cornea.
H15.041 Scleritis with corneal involvement, <u>right</u> eye
H15.042 Scleritis with corneal involvement, <u>left</u> eye
H15.043 Scleritis with corneal involvement, <u>bilateral</u>
H15.049 Scleritis with corneal involvement, <u>unspecified</u> eye
H15.05- <u>Scleromalacia perforans</u> — A form characterized by degeneration and softening that is often seen in patients with rheumatoid arthritis.
H15.051 Scleromalacia perforans, <u>right</u> eye
H15.052 Scleromalacia perforans, <u>left</u> eye
H15.053 Scleromalacia perforans, <u>bilateral</u>
H15.059 Scleromalacia perforans, <u>unspecified</u> eye
H15.09- <u>Other</u> scleritis
　　Scleral abscess — A localized collection of pus, caused by the disintegration of scleral tissue.
H15.091 Other scleritis, <u>right</u> eye
H15.092 Other scleritis, <u>left</u> eye

H11-H15

H15.093   Other scleritis, **bilateral**
H15.099   Other scleritis, **unspecified** eye

H15.1- — **Episcleritis** — Inflammation of the loose connective tissue of the sclera.

H15.10- **Unspecified** episcleritis

H15.101   Unspecified episcleritis, **right** eye
H15.102   Unspecified episcleritis, **left** eye
H15.103   Unspecified episcleritis, **bilateral**
H15.109   Unspecified episcleritis, **unspecified** eye

H15.11- Episcleritis **periodica fugax** — A form characterized by the sudden accumulation of blood which lasts a short time.

H15.111   Episcleritis periodica fugax, **right** eye
H15.112   Episcleritis periodica fugax, **left** eye
H15.113   Episcleritis periodica fugax, **bilateral**
H15.119   Episcleritis periodica fugax, **unspecified** eye

H15.12- **Nodular** episcleritis — A form characterized by the formation of nodules.

H15.121   Nodular episcleritis, **right** eye
H15.122   Nodular episcleritis, **left** eye
H15.123   Nodular episcleritis, **bilateral**
H15.129   Nodular episcleritis, **unspecified** eye

H15.8- **Other disorders** of sclera

Excludes ❷: blue sclera (Q13.5)
                   degenerative myopia (H44.2-)

H15.81- **Equatorial staphyloma** — A form characterized by bulging at the equatorial region of the eye.

H15.811   Equatorial staphyloma, **right** eye
H15.812   Equatorial staphyloma, **left** eye
H15.813   Equatorial staphyloma, **bilateral**
H15.819   Equatorial staphyloma, **unspecified** eye

H15.82- **Localized anterior staphyloma** — A form characterized by protrusion in the anterior part of the eye.

H15.821   Localized anterior staphyloma, **right** eye
H15.822   Localized anterior staphyloma, **left** eye
H15.823   Localized anterior staphyloma, **bilateral**
H15.829   Localized anterior staphyloma, **unspecified** eye

H15.83- **Staphyloma posticum** — A form characterized by the backward bulging of the sclera.

H15.831   Staphyloma posticum, **right** eye
H15.832   Staphyloma posticum, **left** eye
H15.833   Staphyloma posticum, **bilateral**
H15.839   Staphyloma posticum, **unspecified** eye

H15.84- Scleral **ectasia** — The abnormal protrusion of the sclera and cornea.

H15.841   Scleral ectasia, **right** eye
H15.842   Scleral ectasia, **left** eye
H15.843   Scleral ectasia, **bilateral**
H15.849   Scleral ectasia, **unspecified** eye

H15.85- **Ring staphyloma** — A form characterized by bulging in a ring-like shape.

H15.851   Ring staphyloma, **right** eye
H15.852   Ring staphyloma, **left** eye
H15.853   Ring staphyloma, **bilateral**
H15.859   Ring staphyloma, **unspecified** eye

H15.89 Other disorders of sclera

H15.9 Unspecified disorder of sclera

H16- **Keratitis** — Inflammation of the cornea.

H16.0- **Corneal ulcer** — The abnormal erosion of the corneal tissue.

H16.00- **Unspecified** corneal ulcer

H16.001   Unspecified corneal ulcer, **right** eye
H16.002   Unspecified corneal ulcer, **left** eye
H16.003   Unspecified corneal ulcer, **bilateral**
H16.009   Unspecified corneal ulcer, **unspecified** eye

H16.01- **Central** corneal ulcer — A form situated in the central area of the cornea.

H16.011   Central corneal ulcer, **right** eye
H16.012   Central corneal ulcer, **left** eye

H16.013   Central corneal ulcer, **bilateral**
H16.019   Central corneal ulcer, **unspecified** eye

H16.02- **Ring** corneal ulcer — A form marked by the development of connected peripheral ulcers.

H16.021   Ring corneal ulcer, **right** eye
H16.022   Ring corneal ulcer, **left** eye
H16.023   Ring corneal ulcer, **bilateral**
H16.029   Ring corneal ulcer, **unspecified** eye

H16.03- Corneal ulcer **with hypopyon** — A form associated with pus in the anterior chamber.

H16.031   Corneal ulcer with hypopyon, **right** eye
H16.032   Corneal ulcer with hypopyon, **left** eye
H16.033   Corneal ulcer with hypopyon, **bilateral**
H16.039   Corneal ulcer with hypopyon, **unspecified** eye

H16.04- **Marginal** corneal ulcer — A form situated in the lateral margins of the cornea.

H16.041   Marginal corneal ulcer, **right** eye
H16.042   Marginal corneal ulcer, **left** eye
H16.043   Marginal corneal ulcer, **bilateral**
H16.049   Marginal corneal ulcer, **unspecified** eye

H16.05- **Mooren's** corneal ulcer — A form of a marginal, pus-forming ulcer usually seen in elderly patients.

H16.051   Mooren's corneal ulcer, **right** eye
H16.052   Mooren's corneal ulcer, **left** eye
H16.053   Mooren's corneal ulcer, **bilateral**
H16.059   Mooren's corneal ulcer, **unspecified** eye

H16.06- **Mycotic** corneal ulcer — A form caused by a fungus.

H16.061   Mycotic corneal ulcer, **right** eye
H16.062   Mycotic corneal ulcer, **left** eye
H16.063   Mycotic corneal ulcer, **bilateral**
H16.069   Mycotic corneal ulcer, **unspecified** eye

H16.07- **Perforated** corneal ulcer — A form involving the entire thickness of the cornea.

H16.071   Perforated corneal ulcer, **right** eye
H16.072   Perforated corneal ulcer, **left** eye
H16.073   Perforated corneal ulcer, **bilateral**
H16.079   Perforated corneal ulcer, **unspecified** eye

H16.1- Other and **unspecified** superficial keratitis without **conjunctivitis** — Direct inflammation of the corneal epithelium, without associated conjunctivitis.

H16.10- **Unspecified superficial** keratitis

H16.101   Unspecified superficial keratitis, **right** eye
H16.102   Unspecified superficial keratitis, **left** eye
H16.103   Unspecified superficial keratitis, **bilateral**
H16.109   Unspecified superficial keratitis, **unspecified** eye

H16.11- **Macular** keratitis — A form characterized by circumscribed opacity of the cornea.

Areolar keratitis — A form marked by small, circular spots.
Nummular keratitis — A form marked by circular corneal deposits.
Stellate keratitis — A form marked by star-shaped opacities.
Striate keratitis — A form marked by lines of opacity on the cornea.

H16.111   Macular keratitis, **right** eye
H16.112   Macular keratitis, **left** eye
H16.113   Macular keratitis, **bilateral**
H16.119   Macular keratitis, **unspecified** eye

H16.12- **Filamentary** keratitis — A form characterized by twisted filaments of mucoid material on the surface of the cornea.

H16.121   Filamentary keratitis, **right** eye
H16.122   Filamentary keratitis, **left** eye
H16.123   Filamentary keratitis, **bilateral**
H16.129   Filamentary keratitis, **unspecified** eye

H16.13- **Photokeratitis** — A form characterized by fluorescein-positive infiltrates.

Snow blindness — A form resulting from intensified, reflected sunlight off of snow.
Welders keratitis — A form resulting from ultraviolet light from welding torches.

H16.131   Photokeratitis, **right** eye
H16.132   Photokeratitis, **left** eye

H
1
5
-
H
1
6

Excludes 1: = NOT CODED HERE! (Do not code both)   **683**   *Excludes* ❷: = Not Included Here

H16.133   Photokeratitis, **bilateral**

H16.139   Photokeratitis, **unspecified** eye

H16.14-   **Punctate** keratitis — A form characterized by the formation of cellular and fibrous deposits on the cornea.

H16.141   Punctate keratitis, **right** eye

H16.142   Punctate keratitis, **left** eye

H16.143   Punctate keratitis, **bilateral**

H16.149   Punctate keratitis, **unspecified** eye

H16.2-   **Keratoconjunctivitis** — Inflammation of the cornea and conjunctiva.

H16.20-   **Unspecified** keratoconjunctivitis
Superficial keratitis with conjunctivitis NOS

H16.201   Unspecified keratoconjunctivitis, **right** eye

H16.202   Unspecified keratoconjunctivitis, **left** eye

H16.203   Unspecified keratoconjunctivitis, **bilateral**

H16.209   Unspecified keratoconjunctivitis, **unspecified** eye

H16.21-   **Exposure** keratoconjunctivitis — A form characterized by air exposure with drying of the conjunctiva and cornea.

H16.211   Exposure keratoconjunctivitis, **right** eye

H16.212   Exposure keratoconjunctivitis, **left** eye

H16.213   Exposure keratoconjunctivitis, **bilateral**

H16.219   Exposure keratoconjunctivitis, **unspecified** eye

H16.22-   Keratoconjunctivitis **sicca, not specified as Sjögren's** — A form characterized by conjunctival blood congestion, lacrimal drying, and thickening of the cornea.
   Excludes 1:   *Sjögren's syndrome (M35.01)*

H16.221   Keratoconjunctivitis sicca, not specified as Sjögren's, **right** eye

H16.222   Keratoconjunctivitis sicca, not specified as Sjögren's, **left** eye

H16.223   Keratoconjunctivitis sicca, not specified as Sjögren's, **bilateral**

H16.229   Keratoconjunctivitis sicca, not specified as Sjögren's, **unspecified** eye

H16.23-   **Neurotrophic** keratoconjunctivitis — A form of neurogenic origin.

H16.231   Neurotrophic keratoconjunctivitis, **right** eye

H16.232   Neurotrophic keratoconjunctivitis, **left** eye

H16.233   Neurotrophic keratoconjunctivitis, **bilateral**

H16.239   Neurotrophic keratoconjunctivitis, **unspecified** eye

H16.24-   **Ophthalmia nodosa** — Inflammation of the conjunctiva produced by caterpillar hairs.

H16.241   Ophthalmia nodosa, **right** eye

H16.242   Ophthalmia nodosa, **left** eye

H16.243   Ophthalmia nodosa, **bilateral**

H16.249   Ophthalmia nodosa, **unspecified** eye

H16.25-   **Phlyctenular** keratoconjunctivitis — A form characterized by small, gray, circumscribed lesions of the corneal limbus.

H16.251   Phlyctenular keratoconjunctivitis, **right** eye

H16.252   Phlyctenular keratoconjunctivitis, **left** eye

H16.253   Phlyctenular keratoconjunctivitis, **bilateral**

H16.259   Phlyctenular keratoconjunctivitis, **unspecified** eye

H16.26-   **Vernal** keratoconjunctivitis, **with limbar and corneal involvement** — A form characterized by onset during the spring and summer months.
   Excludes 1:   *vernal conjunctivitis without limbar and corneal involvement (H10.44)*

H16.261   Vernal keratoconjunctivitis, with limbar and corneal involvement, **right** eye

H16.262   Vernal keratoconjunctivitis, with limbar and corneal involvement, **left** eye

H16.263   Vernal keratoconjunctivitis, with limbar and corneal involvement, **bilateral**

H16.269   Vernal keratoconjunctivitis, with limbar and corneal involvement, **unspecified** eye

H16.29-   **Other** keratoconjunctivitis

H16.291   Other keratoconjunctivitis, **right** eye

H16.292   Other keratoconjunctivitis, **left** eye

H16.293   Other keratoconjunctivitis, **bilateral**

H16.299   Other keratoconjunctivitis, **unspecified** eye

H16.3-   **Interstitial and deep** keratitis — Inflammation of the cornea with deposits deep in the layers of the cornea resulting in a ground-glass appearance.

H16.30-   **Unspecified interstitial** keratitis

H16.301   Unspecified interstitial keratitis, **right** eye

H16.302   Unspecified interstitial keratitis, **left** eye

H16.303   Unspecified interstitial keratitis, **bilateral**

H16.309   Unspecified interstitial keratitis, **unspecified** eye

H16.31-   **Corneal abscess** — A localized collection of pus, caused by the disintegration of corneal tissues.

H16.311   Corneal abscess, **right** eye

H16.312   Corneal abscess, **left** eye

H16.313   Corneal abscess, **bilateral**

H16.319   Corneal abscess, **unspecified** eye

H16.32-   **Diffuse interstitial** keratitis — A form characterized by general involvement of the cornea.
Cogan's syndrome

H16.321   Diffuse interstitial keratitis, **right** eye

H16.322   Diffuse interstitial keratitis, **left** eye

H16.323   Diffuse interstitial keratitis, **bilateral**

H16.329   Diffuse interstitial keratitis, **unspecified** eye

H16.33-   **Sclerosing** keratitis — A form marked by deep opacity and associated with inflammation of the sclera.

H16.331   Sclerosing keratitis, **right** eye

H16.332   Sclerosing keratitis, **left** eye

H16.333   Sclerosing keratitis, **bilateral**

H16.339   Sclerosing keratitis, **unspecified** eye

H16.39-   **Other interstitial** and deep keratitis

H16.391   Other interstitial and deep keratitis, **right** eye

H16.392   Other interstitial and deep keratitis, **left** eye

H16.393   Other interstitial and deep keratitis, **bilateral**

H16.399   Other interstitial and deep keratitis, **unspecified** eye

H16.4-   **Corneal neovascularization** — The abnormal formation of new blood vessels.

H16.40-   **Unspecified** corneal neovascularization

H16.401   Unspecified corneal neovascularization, **right** eye

H16.402   Unspecified corneal neovascularization, **left** eye

H16.403   Unspecified corneal neovascularization, **bilateral**

H16.409   Unspecified corneal neovascularization, **unspecified** eye

H16.41-   **Ghost vessels (corneal)** — The presence of corneal blood vessels which have no blood flow.

H16.411   Ghost vessels (corneal), **right** eye

H16.412   Ghost vessels (corneal), **left** eye

H16.413   Ghost vessels (corneal), **bilateral**

H16.419   Ghost vessels (corneal), **unspecified** eye

H16.42-   **Pannus (corneal)** — The superficial vascularization of the cornea with infiltration of granulation tissue.

H16.421   Pannus (corneal), **right** eye

H16.422   Pannus (corneal), **left** eye

H16.423   Pannus (corneal), **bilateral**

H16.429   Pannus (corneal), **unspecified** eye

H16.43-   **Localized vascularization** of cornea — The formation of corneal blood vessels in a circumscribed area.

H16.431   Localized vascularization of cornea, **right** eye

H16.432   Localized vascularization of cornea, **left** eye

H16.433   Localized vascularization of cornea, **bilateral**

H16.439   Localized vascularization of cornea, **unspecified** eye

H16.44-   **Deep vascularization** of cornea — The abnormal formation of blood vessels in the deep corneal layers.

H16.441   Deep vascularization of cornea, **right** eye

H16.442   Deep vascularization of cornea, **left** eye

H16.443   Deep vascularization of cornea, **bilateral**

H16.449   Deep vascularization of cornea, **unspecified** eye

H16-H16

H16.8   Other keratitis — [Unacceptable PDX]

H16.9   Unspecified keratitis

H17-   <u>Corneal scars and opacities</u> — The dense post-healing tissue of the cornea, and the inability to pass light through the cornea.

H17.0-   <u>Adherent leukoma</u> — A form adhering to the iris.

   H17.00   Adherent leukoma, <u>unspecified</u> eye

   H17.01   Adherent leukoma, <u>right</u> eye

   H17.02   Adherent leukoma, <u>left</u> eye

   H17.03   Adherent leukoma, <u>bilateral</u>

H17.1-   <u>Central corneal opacity</u> — A form affecting the center of the cornea.

   H17.10   Central corneal opacity, <u>unspecified</u> eye

   H17.11   Central corneal opacity, <u>right</u> eye

   H17.12   Central corneal opacity, <u>left</u> eye

   H17.13   Central corneal opacity, <u>bilateral</u>

H17.8-   Other corneal scars and opacities

   H17.81-   <u>Minor opacity</u> of cornea — A form which is not severe enough to interfere with vision.

     Corneal nebula — A form which can only be seen by oblique illumination.

     H17.811   Minor opacity of cornea, <u>right</u> eye

     H17.812   Minor opacity of cornea, <u>left</u> eye

     H17.813   Minor opacity of cornea, <u>bilateral</u>

     H17.819   Minor opacity of cornea, <u>unspecified</u> eye

   H17.82-   <u>Peripheral opacity</u> of cornea — A form affecting the noncentral margins of the cornea.

     H17.821   Peripheral opacity of cornea, <u>right</u> eye

     H17.822   Peripheral opacity of cornea, <u>left</u> eye

     H17.823   Peripheral opacity of cornea, <u>bilateral</u>

     H17.829   Peripheral opacity of cornea, <u>unspecified</u> eye

   H17.89   Other corneal scars and opacities

H17.9   Unspecified corneal scar and opacity

H18-   <u>Other disorders of cornea</u>

H18.0-   Corneal pigmentations and deposits

   H18.00-   <u>Unspecified corneal deposit</u>

     H18.001   Unspecified corneal deposit, <u>right</u> eye

     H18.002   Unspecified corneal deposit, <u>left</u> eye

     H18.003   Unspecified corneal deposit, <u>bilateral</u>

     H18.009   Unspecified corneal deposit, <u>unspecified</u> eye

   H18.01-   <u>Anterior corneal pigmentations</u> — The deposition of colored matter in the outer layer of the cornea.

     Staehli's line — A horizontal brown mark on the cornea that is seen in aged persons.

     H18.011   Anterior corneal pigmentations, <u>right</u> eye

     H18.012   Anterior corneal pigmentations, <u>left</u> eye

     H18.013   Anterior corneal pigmentations, <u>bilateral</u>

     H18.019   Anterior corneal pigmentations, <u>unspecified</u> eye

   H18.02-   <u>Argentous corneal deposits</u> — Silver corneal deposits.

     H18.021   Argentous corneal deposits, <u>right</u> eye

     H18.022   Argentous corneal deposits, <u>left</u> eye

     H18.023   Argentous corneal deposits, <u>bilateral</u>

     H18.029   Argentous corneal deposits, <u>unspecified</u> eye

   H18.03-   <u>Corneal deposits in metabolic disorders</u>

     Code also associated metabolic disorder

     H18.031   Corneal deposits in metabolic disorders, <u>right</u> eye

     H18.032   Corneal deposits in metabolic disorders, <u>left</u> eye

     H18.033   Corneal deposits in metabolic disorders, <u>bilateral</u>

     H18.039   Corneal deposits in metabolic disorders, <u>unspecified</u> eye

   H18.04-   <u>Kayser-Fleischer ring</u> — A dark pigmented ring at the outer margin of the cornea.

     Code also associated Wilson's disease (E83.01)

     H18.041   Kayser-Fleischer ring, <u>right</u> eye

     H18.042   Kayser-Fleischer ring, <u>left</u> eye

     H18.043   Kayser-Fleischer ring, <u>bilateral</u>

     H18.049   Kayser-Fleischer ring, <u>unspecified</u> eye

   H18.05-   <u>Posterior corneal pigmentations</u> — The deposition of colored matter in the innermost layer of the cornea.

     Krukenberg's spindle — A vertical spindle-shaped, brownish-red opacity on the posterior surface of the cornea.

     H18.051   Posterior corneal pigmentations, <u>right</u> eye

     H18.052   Posterior corneal pigmentations, <u>left</u> eye

     H18.053   Posterior corneal pigmentations, <u>bilateral</u>

     H18.059   Posterior corneal pigmentations, <u>unspecified</u> eye

   H18.06-   <u>Stromal corneal pigmentations</u> — The deposition of colored matter in the main layers of the cornea.

     Hematocornea — The presence of hematin deposits within the corneal layers.

     H18.061   Stromal corneal pigmentations, <u>right</u> eye

     H18.062   Stromal corneal pigmentations, <u>left</u> eye

     H18.063   Stromal corneal pigmentations, <u>bilateral</u>

     H18.069   Stromal corneal pigmentations, <u>unspecified</u> eye

H18.1-   <u>Bullous keratopathy</u> — A form contained in a small sac of tissue.

   H18.10   Bullous keratopathy, <u>unspecified</u> eye

   H18.11   Bullous keratopathy, <u>right</u> eye

   H18.12   Bullous keratopathy, <u>left</u> eye

   H18.13   Bullous keratopathy, <u>bilateral</u>

H18.2-   Other and unspecified <u>corneal edema</u> — Excessive fluid in the cornea.

   H18.20   <u>Unspecified corneal edema</u>

   H18.21-   Corneal edema <u>secondary to contact lens</u> — A form caused by the irritating effects of contact lenses.

     Excludes ❷: *other corneal disorders due to contact lens (H18.82-)*

     H18.211   Corneal edema secondary to contact lens, <u>right</u> eye

     H18.212   Corneal edema secondary to contact lens, <u>left</u> eye

     H18.213   Corneal edema secondary to contact lens, <u>bilateral</u>

     H18.219   Corneal edema secondary to contact lens, <u>unspecified</u> eye

   H18.22-   <u>Idiopathic</u> corneal edema — A form which is not associated with another disease.

     H18.221   Idiopathic corneal edema, <u>right</u> eye

     H18.222   Idiopathic corneal edema, <u>left</u> eye

     H18.223   Idiopathic corneal edema, <u>bilateral</u>

     H18.229   Idiopathic corneal edema, <u>unspecified</u> eye

   H18.23-   <u>Secondary</u> corneal edema — A form resulting from a disease or ocular injury.

     H18.231   Secondary corneal edema, <u>right</u> eye

     H18.232   Secondary corneal edema, <u>left</u> eye

     H18.233   Secondary corneal edema, <u>bilateral</u>

     H18.239   Secondary corneal edema, <u>unspecified</u> eye

H18.3-   <u>Changes of corneal membranes</u> — A change in the normal formation of the corneal membranes.

   H18.30   <u>Unspecified</u> corneal membrane change

   H18.31-   <u>Folds and rupture in Bowman's membrane</u> — A form affecting the second-most outer corneal layer.

     H18.311   Folds and rupture in Bowman's membrane, <u>right</u> eye

     H18.312   Folds and rupture in Bowman's membrane, <u>left</u> eye

     H18.313   Folds and rupture in Bowman's membrane, <u>bilateral</u>

     H18.319   Folds and rupture in Bowman's membrane, <u>unspecified</u> eye

   H18.32-   <u>Folds in Descemet's membrane</u> — A doubling upon itself of the second-most inner corneal layer.

     H18.321   Folds in Descemet's membrane, <u>right</u> eye

     H18.322   Folds in Descemet's membrane, <u>left</u> eye

     H18.323   Folds in Descemet's membrane, <u>bilateral</u>

     H18.329   Folds in Descemet's membrane, <u>unspecified</u> eye

   H18.33-   <u>Rupture in Descemet's membrane</u> — A forcible tearing of the second-most inner corneal layer.

     H18.331   Rupture in Descemet's membrane, <u>right</u> eye

     H18.332   Rupture in Descemet's membrane, <u>left</u> eye

     H18.333   Rupture in Descemet's membrane, <u>bilateral</u>

H16 – H18

H18.339   Rupture in Descemet's membrane, <u>unspecified</u> eye

H18.4-   <u>Corneal degeneration</u> — Deterioration or loss of function of the corneal tissues.
> *Excludes 1:   Mooren's ulcer (H16.0-)*
> *recurrent erosion of cornea (H18.83-)*

H18.40   <u>Unspecified</u> corneal degeneration

H18.41-   <u>Arcus senilis</u> — Lipoid degeneration resulting in a gray-white ring on the cornea occurring with advancing age.
> **Senile corneal changes** — Corneal deteriorations occurring in advancing age.

H18.411   Arcus senilis, <u>right</u> eye
H18.412   Arcus senilis, <u>left</u> eye
H18.413   Arcus senilis, <u>bilateral</u>
H18.419   Arcus senilis, <u>unspecified</u> eye

H18.42-   <u>Band keratopathy</u> — Band-like superficial gray-white flecks on the cornea.

H18.421   Band keratopathy, <u>right</u> eye
H18.422   Band keratopathy, <u>left</u> eye
H18.423   Band keratopathy, <u>bilateral</u>
H18.429   Band keratopathy, <u>unspecified</u> eye

H18.43   Other calcerous corneal degeneration

H18.44-   <u>Keratomalacia</u> — Softening of the cornea.
> *Excludes 1:   keratomalacia due to vitamin A deficiency (E50.4)*

H18.441   Keratomalacia, <u>right</u> eye
H18.442   Keratomalacia, <u>left</u> eye
H18.443   Keratomalacia, <u>bilateral</u>
H18.449   Keratomalacia, <u>unspecified</u> eye

H18.45-   Nodular corneal degeneration — Nodular-like hypertrophy of the cornea.

H18.451   Nodular corneal degeneration, <u>right</u> eye
H18.452   Nodular corneal degeneration, <u>left</u> eye
H18.453   Nodular corneal degeneration, <u>bilateral</u>
H18.459   Nodular corneal degeneration, <u>unspecified</u> eye

H18.46-   <u>Peripheral</u> corneal degeneration — Deterioration of the edges of the cornea.

H18.461   Peripheral corneal degeneration, <u>right</u> eye
H18.462   Peripheral corneal degeneration, <u>left</u> eye
H18.463   Peripheral corneal degeneration, <u>bilateral</u>
H18.469   Peripheral corneal degeneration, <u>unspecified</u> eye

H18.49   Other corneal degeneration

H18.5-   <u>Hereditary corneal dystrophies</u> — An inherited corneal disorder of cellular abnormality.

H18.50   Unspecified hereditary corneal dystrophies

H18.51   Endothelial corneal dystrophy — A form affecting the innermost layer of the cornea.
> **Fuchs' dystrophy**

H18.52   Epithelial (juvenile) corneal dystrophy — A form affecting the epithelial layer occurring early in life.

H18.53   Granular corneal dystrophy — A form characterized by the presence of small opacities in the superficial layers of the cornea occurring during the first decade of life.

H18.54   Lattice corneal dystrophy — A form affecting the corneal lattice.

H18.55   Macular corneal dystrophy — A form affecting the corneal macula.

H18.59   Other hereditary corneal dystrophies

H18.6-   Keratoconus — A conical protrusion of the center of the cornea without inflammation.

H18.60-   Keratoconus, <u>unspecified</u>

H18.601   Keratoconus, unspecified, <u>right</u> eye
H18.602   Keratoconus, unspecified, <u>left</u> eye
H18.603   Keratoconus, unspecified, <u>bilateral</u>
H18.609   Keratoconus, unspecified, <u>unspecified</u> eye

H18.61-   Keratoconus, <u>stable</u> — A form marked by slow, persistent progression.

H18.611   Keratoconus, stable, <u>right</u> eye
H18.612   Keratoconus, stable, <u>left</u> eye
H18.613   Keratoconus, stable, <u>bilateral</u>
H18.619   Keratoconus, stable, <u>unspecified</u> eye

H18.62-   Keratoconus, <u>unstable</u> — A form marked by rapid progression.
> **Acute hydrops** — A form marked by sudden, severe onset.

H18.621   Keratoconus, unstable, <u>right</u> eye
H18.622   Keratoconus, unstable, <u>left</u> eye
H18.623   Keratoconus, unstable, <u>bilateral</u>
H18.629   Keratoconus, unstable, <u>unspecified</u> eye

H18.7-   <u>Other and unspecified corneal deformities</u>
> *Excludes 1:   congenital malformations of cornea (Q13.3-Q13.4)*

H18.70   Unspecified corneal deformity

H18.71-   Corneal <u>ectasia</u> — The protrusion of a thinned, scarred cornea.

H18.711   Corneal ectasia, <u>right</u> eye
H18.712   Corneal ectasia, <u>left</u> eye
H18.713   Corneal ectasia, <u>bilateral</u>
H18.719   Corneal ectasia, <u>unspecified</u> eye

H18.72-   Corneal <u>staphyloma</u> — The protrusion of the cornea.

H18.721   Corneal staphyloma, <u>right</u> eye
H18.722   Corneal staphyloma, <u>left</u> eye
H18.723   Corneal staphyloma, <u>bilateral</u>
H18.729   Corneal staphyloma, <u>unspecified</u> eye

H18.73-   <u>Descemetocele</u> — Herniation of the Descemet membrane.

H18.731   Descemetocele, <u>right</u> eye
H18.732   Descemetocele, <u>left</u> eye
H18.733   Descemetocele, <u>bilateral</u>
H18.739   Descemetocele, <u>unspecified</u> eye

H18.79-   <u>Other</u> corneal deformities

H18.791   Other corneal deformities, <u>right</u> eye
H18.792   Other corneal deformities, <u>left</u> eye
H18.793   Other corneal deformities, <u>bilateral</u>
H18.799   Other corneal deformities, <u>unspecified</u> eye

H18.8-   Other specified disorders of cornea

H18.81-   <u>Anesthesia and hypoesthesia</u> of cornea — Decreased sensitivity of the cornea.

H18.811   Anesthesia and hypoesthesia of cornea, <u>right</u> eye
H18.812   Anesthesia and hypoesthesia of cornea, <u>left</u> eye
H18.813   Anesthesia and hypoesthesia of cornea, <u>bilateral</u>
H18.819   Anesthesia and hypoesthesia of cornea, <u>unspecified</u> eye

H18.82-   Corneal disorder due to contact lens — A form caused by the irritating effects of contact lenses.
> *Excludes ❷: corneal edema due to contact lens (H18.21-)*

H18.821   Corneal disorder due to contact lens, <u>right</u> eye
H18.822   Corneal disorder due to contact lens, <u>left</u> eye
H18.823   Corneal disorder due to contact lens, <u>bilateral</u>
H18.829   Corneal disorder due to contact lens, <u>unspecified</u> eye

H18.83-   <u>Recurrent erosion</u> of cornea — The failure of the epithelial layer to fuse with the basement mambrane seen in recurring corneal ulcers.

H18.831   Recurrent erosion of cornea, <u>right</u> eye
H18.832   Recurrent erosion of cornea, <u>left</u> eye
H18.833   Recurrent erosion of cornea, <u>bilateral</u>
H18.839   Recurrent erosion of cornea, <u>unspecified</u> eye

H18.89-   <u>Other specified</u> disorders of cornea

H18.891   Other specified disorders of cornea, <u>right</u> eye
H18.892   Other specified disorders of cornea, <u>left</u> eye
H18.893   Other specified disorders of cornea, <u>bilateral</u>
H18.899   Other specified disorders of cornea, <u>unspecified</u> eye

H18.9   Unspecified disorder of cornea

H
1
8
-
H
1
8

H20-   <u>Iridocyclitis</u> — Inflammation of the iris and the ciliary body.

  H20.0-   <u>Acute and subacute</u> **iridocyclitis** — A sudden, severe onset of inflammation of the iris and the ciliary body.

    <u>Acute anterior uveitis</u> — A sudden, severe onset of inflammation of the iris and ciliary body.

    <u>Acute cyclitis</u> — A sudden, severe onset of inflammation of the ciliary body.

    <u>Acute iritis</u> — A sudden, severe onset of inflammation of the iris.

    <u>Subacute anterior uveitis</u> — A relatively sudden, severe onset of inflammation of the iris and ciliary body.

    <u>Subacute cyclitis</u> — A relatively sudden, severe onset of inflammation of the ciliary body.

    <u>Subacute iritis</u> — A relatively sudden, severe onset of inflammation of the iris.

    Excludes 1:   *iridocyclitis, iritis, uveitis (due to) (in) diabetes mellitus (E08-E13 with .39)*

      iridocyclitis, iritis, uveitis (due to) (in) diphtheria (A36.89)

      iridocyclitis, iritis, uveitis (due to) (in) gonococcal (A54.32)

      iridocyclitis, iritis, uveitis (due to) (in) herpes (simplex) (B00.51)

      iridocyclitis, iritis, uveitis (due to) (in) herpes zoster (B02.32)

      iridocyclitis, iritis, uveitis (due to) (in) late congenital syphilis (A50.39)

      iridocyclitis, iritis, uveitis (due to) (in) late syphilis (A52.71)

      iridocyclitis, iritis, uveitis (due to) (in) sarcoidosis (D86.83)

      iridocyclitis, iritis, uveitis (due to) (in) syphilis (A51.43)

      iridocyclitis, iritis, uveitis (due to) (in) toxoplasmosis (B58.09)

      iridocyclitis, iritis, uveitis (due to) (in) tuberculosis (A18.54)

  CC **H20.00**   <u>Unspecified</u> acute and subacute iridocyclitis

  H20.01-   <u>Primary</u> **iridocyclitis** — A form characterized by the infection originating within the iris and ciliary body.

    CC **H20.011**   Primary iridocyclitis, <u>right</u> eye

    CC **H20.012**   Primary iridocyclitis, <u>left</u> eye

    CC **H20.013**   Primary iridocyclitis, <u>bilateral</u>

    CC **H20.019**   Primary iridocyclitis, <u>unspecified</u> eye

  H20.02-   <u>Recurrent acute</u> **iridocyclitis** — A form characterized by the return of infection after it has healed.

    CC **H20.021**   Recurrent acute iridocyclitis, <u>right</u> eye

    CC **H20.022**   Recurrent acute iridocyclitis, <u>left</u> eye

    CC **H20.023**   Recurrent acute iridocyclitis, <u>bilateral</u>

    CC **H20.029**   Recurrent acute iridocyclitis, <u>unspecified</u> eye

  H20.03-   <u>Secondary infectious</u> **iridocyclitis** — A form characterized by the infection spreading from other ocular or periocular tissues.

    CC **H20.031**   Secondary infectious iridocyclitis, <u>right</u> eye

    CC **H20.032**   Secondary infectious iridocyclitis, <u>left</u> eye

    CC **H20.033**   Secondary infectious iridocyclitis, <u>bilateral</u>

    CC **H20.039**   Secondary infectious iridocyclitis, <u>unspecified</u> eye

  H20.04-   <u>Secondary non</u>infectious **iridocyclitis** — A form characterized by an inflammatory reaction from other ocular or periocular infections.

    H20.041   Secondary noninfectious iridocyclitis, <u>right</u> eye

    H20.042   Secondary noninfectious iridocyclitis, <u>left</u> eye

    H20.043   Secondary noninfectious iridocyclitis, <u>bilateral</u>

    H20.049   Secondary noninfectious iridocyclitis, <u>unspecified</u> eye

  H20.05-   <u>Hypopyon</u> — An abnormal accumulation of pus in the anterior chamber of the eye.

    H20.051   Hypopyon, <u>right</u> eye

    H20.052   Hypopyon, <u>left</u> eye

    H20.053   Hypopyon, <u>bilateral</u>

    H20.059   Hypopyon, <u>unspecified</u> eye

  H20.1-   <u>Chronic</u> **iridocyclitis** — Inflammation of the iris and ciliary body which develops slowly and persists over a long period of time.

    Use additional code for any associated cataract (H26.21-)

    Excludes ❷: *posterior cyclitis (H30.2-)*

  H20.10   Chronic iridocyclitis, <u>unspecified</u> eye

  H20.11   Chronic iridocyclitis, <u>right</u> eye

  H20.12   Chronic iridocyclitis, <u>left</u> eye

H20.13   Chronic iridocyclitis, <u>bilateral</u>

  H20.2-   <u>Lens-induced</u> **iridocyclitis** — A form characterized by secondary inflammatory reactions due to disorders of the lens.

  H20.20   Lens-induced iridocyclitis, <u>unspecified</u> eye

  H20.21   Lens-induced iridocyclitis, <u>right</u> eye

  H20.22   Lens-induced iridocyclitis, <u>left</u> eye

  H20.23   Lens-induced iridocyclitis, <u>bilateral</u>

  H20.8-   Other iridocyclitis

    Excludes ❷: *glaucomatocyclitis crises (H40.4-)*

      posterior cyclitis (H30.2-)

      sympathetic uveitis (H44.13-)

  H20.81-   <u>Fuchs' heterochromic</u> **cyclitis** — A form characterized by lightening of the iris color and a few keratic deposits on the cornea.

    H20.811   Fuchs' heterochromic cyclitis, <u>right</u> eye

    H20.812   Fuchs' heterochromic cyclitis, <u>left</u> eye

    H20.813   Fuchs' heterochromic cyclitis, <u>bilateral</u>

    H20.819   Fuchs' heterochromic cyclitis, <u>unspecified</u> eye

  H20.82-   <u>Vogt-Koyanagi syndrome</u> — A syndrome characterized by chronic iridocyclitis, exudative choroiditis, and patchy depigmentation of the skin and hair.

    H20.821   Vogt-Koyanagi syndrome, <u>right</u> eye

    H20.822   Vogt-Koyanagi syndrome, <u>left</u> eye

    H20.823   Vogt-Koyanagi syndrome, <u>bilateral</u>

    H20.829   Vogt-Koyanagi syndrome, <u>unspecified</u> eye

 CC **H20.9**   Unspecified iridocyclitis

    Uveitis NOS

H21-   <u>Other disorders of iris and ciliary body</u>

  Excludes ❷: *sympathetic uveitis (H44.1-)*

  H21.0-   <u>Hyphema</u> — Hemorrhage within the anterior chamber of the eye.

    Excludes 1:   *traumatic hyphema (S05.1-)*

  H21.00   Hyphema, <u>unspecified</u> eye

  H21.01   Hyphema, <u>right</u> eye

  H21.02   Hyphema, <u>left</u> eye

  H21.03   Hyphema, <u>bilateral</u>

  H21.1-   <u>Other vascular disorders</u> of iris and ciliary body

    <u>Neovascularization of iris or ciliary body</u> — The formation of new abnormal blood vessels of the iris and ciliary body.

    <u>Rubeosis iridis</u> — An abnormal condition characterized by the new formation of vessels and connective tissue on the surface of the iris.

    Rubeosis of iris

  H21.1x-   <u>Other vascular disorders</u> of iris and ciliary body

    H21.1x1   Other vascular disorders of iris and ciliary body, <u>right</u> eye

    H21.1x2   Other vascular disorders of iris and ciliary body, <u>left</u> eye

    H21.1x3   Other vascular disorders of iris and ciliary body, <u>bilateral</u>

    H21.1x9   Other vascular disorders of iris and ciliary body, <u>unspecified</u> eye

  H21.2-   Degeneration of iris and ciliary body — Deteriorations of the iris and ciliary body.

  H21.21-   <u>Degeneration of chamber angle</u> — Loss of the normal ciliary body chamber angle.

    H21.211   Degeneration of chamber angle, <u>right</u> eye

    H21.212   Degeneration of chamber angle, <u>left</u> eye

    H21.213   Degeneration of chamber angle, <u>bilateral</u>

    H21.219   Degeneration of chamber angle, <u>unspecified</u> eye

  H21.22-   <u>Degeneration of ciliary body</u> — Deterioration of the ciliary body tissues.

    H21.221   Degeneration of ciliary body, <u>right</u> eye

    H21.222   Degeneration of ciliary body, <u>left</u> eye

    H21.223   Degeneration of ciliary body, <u>bilateral</u>

    H21.229   Degeneration of ciliary body, <u>unspecified</u> eye

  H21.23-   <u>Degeneration of iris (pigmentary)</u> — Abnormal deterioration of the iris pigment.

    <u>Translucency of iris</u> — A form marked by enough loss of pigment to allow light to pass through.

    H21.231   Degeneration of iris (pigmentary), <u>right</u> eye

    H21.232   Degeneration of iris (pigmentary), <u>left</u> eye

---

H21.233   Degeneration of iris (pigmentary), <u>bilateral</u>
H21.239   Degeneration of iris (pigmentary), <u>unspecified</u> eye
H21.24- <u>Degeneration of pupillary margin</u> — Deterioration of the inner edge of the iris, surrounding the pupil.
    H21.241   Degeneration of pupillary margin, <u>right</u> eye
    H21.242   Degeneration of pupillary margin, <u>left</u> eye
    H21.243   Degeneration of pupillary margin, <u>bilateral</u>
    H21.249   Degeneration of pupillary margin, <u>unspecified</u> eye
H21.25- <u>Iridoschisis</u> — Splitting of the iris into two layers.
    H21.251   Iridoschisis, <u>right</u> eye
    H21.252   Iridoschisis, <u>left</u> eye
    H21.253   Iridoschisis, <u>bilateral</u>
    H21.259   Iridoschisis, <u>unspecified</u> eye
H21.26- <u>Iris atrophy</u> (essential) (progressive) — The wasting-away of the iris.
    H21.261   Iris atrophy (essential) (progressive), <u>right</u> eye
    H21.262   Iris atrophy (essential) (progressive), <u>left</u> eye
    H21.263   Iris atrophy (essential) (progressive), <u>bilateral</u>
    H21.269   Iris atrophy (essential) (progressive), <u>unspecified</u> eye
H21.27- <u>Miotic pupillary cyst</u> — Serous filled sacs upon the pupillary margin of the iris.
    H21.271   Miotic pupillary cyst, <u>right</u> eye
    H21.272   Miotic pupillary cyst, <u>left</u> eye
    H21.273   Miotic pupillary cyst, <u>bilateral</u>
    H21.279   Miotic pupillary cyst, <u>unspecified</u> eye
H21.29 Other iris atrophy
H21.3- <u>Cyst of iris, ciliary body and anterior chamber</u> — Encapsulated, fluid-filled sacs of the iris, ciliary body, and anterior chamber.
    Excludes ❷: miotic pupillary cyst (H21.27-)
H21.30- <u>Idiopathic</u> cysts of iris, ciliary body or anterior chamber — A form characterized by unknown etiology.
    Cyst of iris, ciliary body or anterior chamber NOS
    H21.301   Idiopathic cysts of iris, ciliary body or anterior chamber, <u>right</u> eye
    H21.302   Idiopathic cysts of iris, ciliary body or anterior chamber, <u>left</u> eye
    H21.303   Idiopathic cysts of iris, ciliary body or anterior chamber, <u>bilateral</u>
    H21.309   Idiopathic cysts of iris, ciliary body or anterior chamber, <u>unspecified</u> eye
H21.31- <u>Exudative</u> cysts of iris or anterior chamber — A form characterized by cellular debris within the cysts.
    H21.311   Exudative cysts of iris or anterior chamber, <u>right</u> eye
    H21.312   Exudative cysts of iris or anterior chamber, <u>left</u> eye
    H21.313   Exudative cysts of iris or anterior chamber, <u>bilateral</u>
    H21.319   Exudative cysts of iris or anterior chamber, <u>unspecified</u> eye
H21.32- <u>Implantation</u> cysts of iris, ciliary body or anterior chamber — A form characterized by down-growth of epithelium.
    H21.321   Implantation cysts of iris, ciliary body or anterior chamber, <u>right</u> eye
    H21.322   Implantation cysts of iris, ciliary body or anterior chamber, <u>left</u> eye
    H21.323   Implantation cysts of iris, ciliary body or anterior chamber, <u>bilateral</u>
    H21.329   Implantation cysts of iris, ciliary body or anterior chamber, <u>unspecified</u> eye
H21.33- <u>Parasitic</u> cyst of iris, ciliary body or anterior chamber — A form characterized by infestation by a parasite.
    cc H21.331   Parasitic cyst of iris, ciliary body or anterior chamber, <u>right</u> eye
    cc H21.332   Parasitic cyst of iris, ciliary body or anterior chamber, <u>left</u> eye
    cc H21.333   Parasitic cyst of iris, ciliary body or anterior chamber, <u>bilateral</u>

cc **H21.339**   Parasitic cyst of iris, ciliary body or anterior chamber, <u>unspecified</u> eye
H21.34- <u>Primary cyst of pars plana</u> — A form characterized by development associated with ciliary body disorder of the ciliary ring.
    H21.341   Primary cyst of pars plana, <u>right</u> eye
    H21.342   Primary cyst of pars plana, <u>left</u> eye
    H21.343   Primary cyst of pars plana, <u>bilateral</u>
    H21.349   Primary cyst of pars plana, <u>unspecified</u> eye
H21.35- <u>Exudative cyst of pars plana</u> — A form characterized by cellular debris within the cysts of the ciliary ring.
    H21.351   Exudative cyst of pars plana, <u>right</u> eye
    H21.352   Exudative cyst of pars plana, <u>left</u> eye
    H21.353   Exudative cyst of pars plana, <u>bilateral</u>
    H21.359   Exudative cyst of pars plana, <u>unspecified</u> eye
H21.4- <u>Pupillary membranes</u> — Abnormal pupillary membrane formation.
    Iris bombé — The condition in which the iris is bowed forward with aqueous humor behind it.
    Pupillary occlusion — Complete closure of the pupillary opening.
    Pupillary seclusion — Complete covering of the iris and pupillary opening by the formation of a membrane.
    Excludes 1: congenital pupillary membranes (Q13.8)
H21.40 Pupillary membranes, <u>unspecified</u> eye
H21.41 Pupillary membranes, <u>right</u> eye
H21.42 Pupillary membranes, <u>left</u> eye
H21.43 Pupillary membranes, <u>bilateral</u>
H21.5- Other and unspecified adhesions and disruptions of iris and ciliary body
    Excludes 1: corectopia (Q13.2)
H21.50- <u>Unspecified adhesions of iris</u>
    Synechia (iris) NOS
    H21.501   Unspecified adhesions of iris, <u>right</u> eye
    H21.502   Unspecified adhesions of iris, <u>left</u> eye
    H21.503   Unspecified adhesions of iris, <u>bilateral</u>
    H21.509   Unspecified adhesions of iris and ciliary body, <u>unspecified</u> eye
H21.51- <u>Anterior synechiae (iris)</u> — Adherence of the iris to the cornea.
    H21.511   Anterior synechiae (iris), <u>right</u> eye
    H21.512   Anterior synechiae (iris), <u>left</u> eye
    H21.513   Anterior synechiae (iris), <u>bilateral</u>
    H21.519   Anterior synechiae (iris), <u>unspecified</u> eye
H21.52- <u>Goniosynechiae</u> — Adherence of the iris to the cornea at the angle of the anterior chamber.
    H21.521   Goniosynechiae, <u>right</u> eye
    H21.522   Goniosynechiae, <u>left</u> eye
    H21.523   Goniosynechiae, <u>bilateral</u>
    H21.529   Goniosynechiae, <u>unspecified</u> eye
H21.53- <u>Iridodialysis</u> — The separation or loosening of the iris from its attachment.
    H21.531   Iridodialysis, <u>right</u> eye
    H21.532   Iridodialysis, <u>left</u> eye
    H21.533   Iridodialysis, <u>bilateral</u>
    H21.539   Iridodialysis, <u>unspecified</u> eye
H21.54- <u>Posterior synechiae (iris)</u> — Adherence of the iris to the lens.
    H21.541   Posterior synechiae (iris), <u>right</u> eye
    H21.542   Posterior synechiae (iris), <u>left</u> eye
    H21.543   Posterior synechiae (iris), <u>bilateral</u>
    H21.549   Posterior synechiae (iris), <u>unspecified</u> eye
H21.55- <u>Recession of chamber angle</u> — The drawing-back of the angle of the anterior chamber.
    H21.551   Recession of chamber angle, <u>right</u> eye
    H21.552   Recession of chamber angle, <u>left</u> eye
    H21.553   Recession of chamber angle, <u>bilateral</u>
    H21.559   Recession of chamber angle, <u>unspecified</u> eye

H21 – H21

H21.56- Pupillary abnormalities
     Deformed pupil — A physically impaired pupil.
     Ectopic pupil — Displacement of the pupil.
     Rupture of sphincter, pupil — The forcible tearing of the pupil.
     Excludes 1:   *congenital deformity of pupil (Q13.2-)*

    H21.561   **Pupillary abnormality, right eye**

    H21.562   **Pupillary abnormality, left eye**

    H21.563   **Pupillary abnormality, bilateral**

    H21.569   **Pupillary abnormality, unspecified eye**

H21.8-   **Other specified disorders of iris and ciliary body**

    H21.81   **Floppy iris syndrome** — A potentially complicating condition, usually caused by a history of taking alpha-blockers, in which the iris does not stay properly dilated during cataract surgery.
      Intraoperative floppy iris syndrome (IFIS)
      Use additional code for adverse effect, if applicable, to identify drug (T36-T50 with fifth or sixth character 5)

    H21.82   **Plateau iris syndrome (post-iridectomy) (postprocedural)** — The abnormal anatomical condition of angle crowding that may lead to acute angle-closure glaucoma.

    H21.89   **Other specified disorders of iris and ciliary body**

H21.9   **Unspecified disorder of iris and ciliary body**

H22   **Disorders of iris and ciliary body in diseases classified elsewhere** —
[Not Allowed as PDX]
Code first underlying disease, such as:
   Gout (M1A.-, M10.-)
   Leprosy (A30.-)
   Parasitic disease (B89)

Disorders of lens (H25-H28)

H25-   **Age-related cataract** — The opacity (inability to pass light through) of the crystalline lens of the eye with onset later in life.
    AHA 16:1Q:p32 – Bilateral cataracts with separate surgical encounters
    Senile cataract
    Excludes ❷: *capsular glaucoma with pseudoexfoliation of lens (H40.1-)*

H25.0-   **Age-related incipient cataract** — A form characterized by localized areas of opacity.

    H25.01-   **Cortical age-related cataract** — A form characterized by the opacity situated in the cortical layers of the lens.

      H25.011   **Cortical age-related cataract, right eye** — [Age/15-124]

      H25.012   **Cortical age-related cataract, left eye** — [Age/15-124]

      H25.013   **Cortical age-related cataract, bilateral** — [Age/15-124]

      H25.019   **Cortical age-related cataract, unspecified eye** — [Age/15-124]

    H25.03-   **Anterior subcapsular polar age-related cataract** — A form characterized by the opacity situated beneath the front, center portion of the capsule of the lens.

      H25.031   **Anterior subcapsular polar age-related cataract, right eye** — [Age/15-124]

      H25.032   **Anterior subcapsular polar age-related cataract, left eye** — [Age/15-124]

      H25.033   **Anterior subcapsular polar age-related cataract, bilateral** — [Age/15-124]

      H25.039   **Anterior subcapsular polar age-related cataract, unspecified eye** — [Age/15-124]

    H25.04-   **Posterior subcapsular polar age-related cataract** — A form characterized by the opacity situated beneath the back, center portion of the capsule of the lens.

      H25.041   **Posterior subcapsular polar age-related cataract, right eye** — [Age/15-124]

      H25.042   **Posterior subcapsular polar age-related cataract, left eye** — [Age/15-124]

      H25.043   **Posterior subcapsular polar age-related cataract, bilateral** — [Age/15-124]

      H25.049   **Posterior subcapsular polar age-related cataract, unspecified eye** — [Age/15-124]

    H25.09-   **Other age-related incipient cataract**
      Coronary age-related cataract — A form marked by club-like opacities, with clear edges and center.
      Punctate age-related cataract — A form marked by dot-like opacities.
      Water clefts

      H25.091   **Other age-related incipient cataract, right eye** — [Age/15-124]

      H25.092   **Other age-related incipient cataract, left eye** — [Age/15-124]

      H25.093   **Other age-related incipient cataract, bilateral** — [Age/15-124]

      H25.099   **Other age-related incipient cataract, unspecified eye** — [Age/15-124]

H25.1-   **Age-related nuclear cataract** — A form characterized by hardening opacity of the center of the lens.
     Cataracta brunescens — A form marked by brown discoloration.
     Nuclear sclerosis cataract — A form characterized by hardening opacity of the center of the lens.

    H25.10   **Age-related nuclear cataract, unspecified eye** — [Age/15-124]

    H25.11   **Age-related nuclear cataract, right eye** — [Age/15-124]

    H25.12   **Age-related nuclear cataract, left eye** — [Age/15-124]

    H25.13   **Age-related nuclear cataract, bilateral** — [Age/15-124]

H25.2-   **Age-related cataract, morgagnian type** — A form characterized by a shrunken, soft, wrinkled, opaque lens.
     Age-related hypermature cataract

    H25.20   **Age-related cataract, morgagnian type, unspecified eye** — [Age/15-124]

    H25.21   **Age-related cataract, morgagnian type, right eye** — [Age/15-124]

    H25.22   **Age-related cataract, morgagnian type, left eye** — [Age/15-124]

    H25.23   **Age-related cataract, morgagnian type, bilateral** — [Age/15-124]

H25.8-   **Other age-related cataract**

    H25.81-   **Combined forms of age-related cataract**

      H25.811   **Combined forms of age-related cataract, right eye** — [Age/15-124]

      H25.812   **Combined forms of age-related cataract, left eye** — [Age/15-124]

      H25.813   **Combined forms of age-related cataract, bilateral** — [Age/15-124]

      H25.819   **Combined forms of age-related cataract, unspecified eye** — [Age/15-124]

    H25.89   **Other age-related cataract** — [Age/15-124]

H25.9   **Unspecified age-related cataract** — [Age/15-124]

H26-   **Other cataract**
    Excludes 1:   *congenital cataract (Q12.0)*

H26.0-   **Infantile and juvenile cataract** — The opacity (inability to pass light through) of the crystalline lens of the eye characterized by onset early in life.

    H26.00-   **Unspecified infantile and juvenile cataract**

      H26.001   **Unspecified infantile and juvenile cataract, right eye** — [Age/0-17]

      H26.002   **Unspecified infantile and juvenile cataract, left eye** — [Age/0-17]

      H26.003   **Unspecified infantile and juvenile cataract, bilateral** — [Age/0-17]

      H26.009   **Unspecified infantile and juvenile cataract, unspecified eye** — [Age/0-17]

    H26.01-   **Infantile and juvenile cortical, lamellar, or zonular cataract** — A form characterized by the opacity affecting only the middle layers of the lens.

      H26.011   **Infantile and juvenile cortical, lamellar, or zonular cataract, right eye** — [Age/0-17]

      H26.012   **Infantile and juvenile cortical, lamellar, or zonular cataract, left eye** — [Age/0-17]

      H26.013   **Infantile and juvenile cortical, lamellar, or zonular cataract, bilateral** — [Age/0-17]

H21 - H26

H26.019 Infantile and juvenile cortical, lamellar, or zonular cataract, <u>unspecified</u> eye — [Age/0-17]

H26.03- Infantile and juvenile <u>nuclear</u> cataract — A form characterized by the opacity affecting the center of the lens.

H26.031 Infantile and juvenile nuclear cataract, <u>right</u> eye — [Age/0-17]

H26.032 Infantile and juvenile nuclear cataract, <u>left</u> eye — [Age/0-17]

H26.033 Infantile and juvenile nuclear cataract, <u>bilateral</u> — [Age/0-17]

H26.039 Infantile and juvenile nuclear cataract, <u>unspecified</u> eye — [Age/0-17]

H26.04- <u>Anterior</u> subcapsular polar infantile and juvenile cataract — A form characterized by the opacity situated beneath the front, center portion of the capsule of the lens.

H26.041 Anterior subcapsular polar infantile and juvenile cataract, <u>right</u> eye — [Age/0-17]

H26.042 Anterior subcapsular polar infantile and juvenile cataract, <u>left</u> eye — [Age/0-17]

H26.043 Anterior subcapsular polar infantile and juvenile cataract, <u>bilateral</u> — [Age/0-17]

H26.049 Anterior subcapsular polar infantile and juvenile cataract, <u>unspecified</u> eye — [Age/0-17]

H26.05- <u>Posterior</u> subcapsular polar infantile and juvenile cataract — A form characterized by the opacity situated beneath the back, center portion of the capsule of the lens.

H26.051 Posterior subcapsular polar infantile and juvenile cataract, <u>right</u> eye — [Age/0-17]

H26.052 Posterior subcapsular polar infantile and juvenile cataract, <u>left</u> eye — [Age/0-17]

H26.053 Posterior subcapsular polar infantile and juvenile cataract, <u>bilateral</u> — [Age/0-17]

H26.059 Posterior subcapsular polar infantile and juvenile cataract, <u>unspecified</u> eye — [Age/0-17]

H26.06- <u>Combined</u> forms of infantile and juvenile cataract

H26.061 Combined forms of infantile and juvenile cataract, <u>right</u> eye — [Age/0-17]

H26.062 Combined forms of infantile and juvenile cataract, <u>left</u> eye — [Age/0-17]

H26.063 Combined forms of infantile and juvenile cataract, <u>bilateral</u> — [Age/0-17]

H26.069 Combined forms of infantile and juvenile cataract, <u>unspecified</u> eye — [Age/0-17]

H26.09 Other infantile and juvenile cataract — [Age/0-17]

H26.1- <u>Traumatic</u> cataract — The opacity (inability to pass light through) of the crystalline lens of the eye due to an external injury.
Use additional code (Chapter 20) to identify external cause

H26.10- <u>Unspecified</u> traumatic cataract

H26.101 Unspecified traumatic cataract, <u>right</u> eye

H26.102 Unspecified traumatic cataract, <u>left</u> eye

H26.103 Unspecified traumatic cataract, <u>bilateral</u>

H26.109 Unspecified traumatic cataract, <u>unspecified</u> eye

H26.11- <u>Localized</u> traumatic opacities — A form characterized by opacities appearing in small circumscribed areas.

H26.111 Localized traumatic opacities, <u>right</u> eye

H26.112 Localized traumatic opacities, <u>left</u> eye

H26.113 Localized traumatic opacities, <u>bilateral</u>

H26.119 Localized traumatic opacities, <u>unspecified</u> eye

H26.12- <u>Partially resolved</u> traumatic cataract — A form characterized by partial clearing of the opacity.

H26.121 Partially resolved traumatic cataract, <u>right</u> eye

H26.122 Partially resolved traumatic cataract, <u>left</u> eye

H26.123 Partially resolved traumatic cataract, <u>bilateral</u>

H26.129 Partially resolved traumatic cataract, <u>unspecified</u> eye

H26.13- <u>Total</u> traumatic cataract — A form characterized by complete opacity.

H26.131 Total traumatic cataract, <u>right</u> eye

H26.132 Total traumatic cataract, <u>left</u> eye

H26.133 Total traumatic cataract, <u>bilateral</u>

H26.139 Total traumatic cataract, <u>unspecified</u> eye

H26.2- <u>Complicated</u> cataract

H26.20 <u>Unspecified</u> complicated cataract
Cataracta complicata NOS

H26.21- Cataract <u>with neovascularization</u> — A form characterized by the formation of new abnormal blood vessels.
Code also associated condition, such as:
Chronic iridocyclitis (H20.1-)

H26.211 Cataract with neovascularization, <u>right</u> eye

H26.212 Cataract with neovascularization, <u>left</u> eye

H26.213 Cataract with neovascularization, <u>bilateral</u>

H26.219 Cataract with neovascularization, <u>unspecified</u> eye

H26.22- Cataract <u>secondary to ocular disorders</u> (degenerative) (inflammatory) — The opacity (inability to pass light through) of the crystalline lens of the eye due to ocular disorders and diseases.
Code also associated ocular disorder

H26.221 Cataract secondary to ocular disorders (degenerative) (inflammatory), <u>right</u> eye

H26.222 Cataract secondary to ocular disorders (degenerative) (inflammatory), <u>left</u> eye

H26.223 Cataract secondary to ocular disorders (degenerative) (inflammatory), <u>bilateral</u>

H26.229 Cataract secondary to ocular disorders (degenerative) (inflammatory), <u>unspecified</u> eye

H26.23- <u>Glaucomatous flecks</u> (subcapsular)
Code first underlying glaucoma (H40-H42)

H26.231 Glaucomatous flecks (subcapsular), <u>right</u> eye

H26.232 Glaucomatous flecks (subcapsular), <u>left</u> eye

H26.233 Glaucomatous flecks (subcapsular), <u>bilateral</u>

H26.239 Glaucomatous flecks (subcapsular), <u>unspecified</u> eye

H26.3- <u>Drug-induced</u> cataract
Toxic cataract
Use additional code for adverse effect, if applicable, to identify drug (T36-T50 with fifth or sixth character 5)

H26.30 Drug-induced cataract, <u>unspecified</u> eye

H26.31 Drug-induced cataract, <u>right</u> eye

H26.32 Drug-induced cataract, <u>left</u> eye

H26.33 Drug-induced cataract, <u>bilateral</u>

H26.4- <u>Secondary</u> cataract

H26.40 <u>Unspecified</u> secondary cataract

H26.41- <u>Soemmering's ring</u> — A recurrent doughnut-shaped opacity occurring after cataract surgery.

H26.411 Soemmering's ring, <u>right</u> eye

H26.412 Soemmering's ring, <u>left</u> eye

H26.413 Soemmering's ring, <u>bilateral</u>

H26.419 Soemmering's ring, <u>unspecified</u> eye

H26.49- <u>Other</u> secondary cataract

H26.491 Other secondary cataract, <u>right</u> eye

H26.492 Other secondary cataract, <u>left</u> eye

H26.493 Other secondary cataract, <u>bilateral</u>

H26.499 Other secondary cataract, <u>unspecified</u> eye

H26.8 Other specified cataract

H26.9 Unspecified cataract

H27- Other disorders of lens
Excludes 1: congenital lens malformations (Q12.-)
mechanical complications of intraocular lens implant (T85.2)
pseudophakia (Z96.1)

H27.0- <u>Aphakia</u> — Absence of the crystalline lens of the eye.
Acquired absence of lens
Acquired aphakia
Aphakia due to trauma
Excludes 1: cataract extraction status (Z98.4-)
congenital absence of lens (Q12.3)
congenital aphakia (Q12.3)

H27.00 Aphakia, <u>unspecified</u> eye

H27.01 Aphakia, <u>right</u> eye

H27.02 Aphakia, <u>left</u> eye

H27.03 Aphakia, <u>bilateral</u>

H26-H27

H27.1- Dislocation of lens — Dislocation of the crystalline lens of the eye.

H27.10 Unspecified dislocation of lens

H27.11- Subluxation of lens — Partial dislocation of the crystalline lens of the eye.

H27.111 Subluxation of lens, right eye

H27.112 Subluxation of lens, left eye

H27.113 Subluxation of lens, bilateral

H27.119 Subluxation of lens, unspecified eye

H27.12- Anterior dislocation of lens — The movement forward of the crystalline lens of the eye from its normal position.

H27.121 Anterior dislocation of lens, right eye

H27.122 Anterior dislocation of lens, left eye

H27.123 Anterior dislocation of lens, bilateral

H27.129 Anterior dislocation of lens, unspecified eye

H27.13- Posterior dislocation of lens — The movement backward of the crystalline lens of the eye from its normal position.

H27.131 Posterior dislocation of lens, right eye

H27.132 Posterior dislocation of lens, left eye

H27.133 Posterior dislocation of lens, bilateral

H27.139 Posterior dislocation of lens, unspecified eye

H27.8 Other specified disorders of lens

H27.9 Unspecified disorder of lens

H28 Cataract in diseases classified elsewhere — [Not Allowed as PDX]
Code first underlying disease, such as:
Hypoparathyroidism (E20.-)
Myotonia (G71.1-)
Myxedema (E03.-)
Protein-calorie malnutrition (E40-E46)
Excludes 1: cataract in diabetes mellitus (E08.36, E09.36, E10.36, E11.36, E13.36)

Disorders of choroid and retina (H30-H36)

H30- Chorioretinal inflammation — Inflammation of the retina and/or choroid.

H30.0- Focal chorioretinal inflammation — Inflammation of the central retina and/or choroid.
Focal chorioretinitis
Focal choroiditis
Focal retinitis
Focal retinochoroiditis

H30.00- Unspecified focal chorioretinal inflammation
Focal chorioretinitis NOS
Focal choroiditis NOS
Focal retinitis NOS
Focal retinochoroiditis NOS

H30.001 Unspecified focal chorioretinal inflammation, right eye

H30.002 Unspecified focal chorioretinal inflammation, left eye

H30.003 Unspecified focal chorioretinal inflammation, bilateral

H30.009 Unspecified focal chorioretinal inflammation, unspecified eye

H30.01- Focal chorioretinal inflammation, juxtapapillary

H30.011 Focal chorioretinal inflammation, juxtapapillary, right eye

H30.012 Focal chorioretinal inflammation, juxtapapillary, left eye

H30.013 Focal chorioretinal inflammation, juxtapapillary, bilateral

H30.019 Focal chorioretinal inflammation, juxtapapillary, unspecified eye

H30.02- Focal chorioretinal inflammation of posterior pole

H30.021 Focal chorioretinal inflammation of posterior pole, right eye

H30.022 Focal chorioretinal inflammation of posterior pole, left eye

H30.023 Focal chorioretinal inflammation of posterior pole, bilateral

H30.029 Focal chorioretinal inflammation of posterior pole, unspecified eye

H30.03- Focal chorioretinal inflammation, peripheral

H30.031 Focal chorioretinal inflammation, peripheral, right eye

H30.032 Focal chorioretinal inflammation, peripheral, left eye

H30.033 Focal chorioretinal inflammation, peripheral, bilateral

H30.039 Focal chorioretinal inflammation, peripheral, unspecified eye

H30.04- Focal chorioretinal inflammation, macular or paramacular

H30.041 Focal chorioretinal inflammation, macular or paramacular, right eye

H30.042 Focal chorioretinal inflammation, macular or paramacular, left eye

H30.043 Focal chorioretinal inflammation, macular or paramacular, bilateral

H30.049 Focal chorioretinal inflammation, macular or paramacular, unspecified eye

H30.1- Disseminated chorioretinal inflammation — Inflammation of multiple sites throughout the retina and choroid.
Disseminated chorioretinitis
Disseminated choroiditis
Disseminated retinitis
Disseminated retinochoroiditis
Excludes ❷: exudative retinopathy (H35.02-)

H30.10- Unspecified disseminated chorioretinal inflammation
Disseminated chorioretinitis NOS
Disseminated choroiditis NOS
Disseminated retinitis NOS
Disseminated retinochoroiditis NOS

CC **H30.101** Unspecified disseminated chorioretinal inflammation, right eye

CC **H30.102** Unspecified disseminated chorioretinal inflammation, left eye

CC **H30.103** Unspecified disseminated chorioretinal inflammation, bilateral

CC **H30.109** Unspecified disseminated chorioretinal inflammation, unspecified eye

H30.11- Disseminated chorioretinal inflammation of posterior pole

CC **H30.111** Disseminated chorioretinal inflammation of posterior pole, right eye

CC **H30.112** Disseminated chorioretinal inflammation of posterior pole, left eye

CC **H30.113** Disseminated chorioretinal inflammation of posterior pole, bilateral

CC **H30.119** Disseminated chorioretinal inflammation of posterior pole, unspecified eye

H30.12- Disseminated chorioretinal inflammation, peripheral

CC **H30.121** Disseminated chorioretinal inflammation, peripheral right eye

CC **H30.122** Disseminated chorioretinal inflammation, peripheral, left eye

CC **H30.123** Disseminated chorioretinal inflammation, peripheral, bilateral

CC **H30.129** Disseminated chorioretinal inflammation, peripheral, unspecified eye

H30.13- Disseminated chorioretinal inflammation, generalized

CC **H30.131** Disseminated chorioretinal inflammation, generalized, right eye

CC **H30.132** Disseminated chorioretinal inflammation, generalized, left eye

CC **H30.133** Disseminated chorioretinal inflammation, generalized, bilateral

CC **H30.139** Disseminated chorioretinal inflammation, generalized, unspecified eye

H30.14- Acute posterior multifocal placoid pigment epitheliopathy

CC **H30.141** Acute posterior multifocal placoid pigment epitheliopathy, right eye cc **H30.142** Acute posterior multifocal placoid pigment epitheliopathy, <u>left</u> eye

cc **H30.143** Acute posterior multifocal placoid pigment epitheliopathy, <u>bilateral</u>

cc **H30.149** Acute posterior multifocal placoid pigment epitheliopathy, <u>unspecified</u> eye

H30.2- <u>Posterior cyclitis</u> — Specific inflammation of the peripheral retina characterized by "snowbanks" of inflammatory cells.
　　　Pars planitis

H30.20 Posterior cyclitis, <u>unspecified</u> eye

H30.21 Posterior cyclitis, <u>right</u> eye

H30.22 Posterior cyclitis, <u>left</u> eye

H30.23 Posterior cyclitis, <u>bilateral</u>

H30.8- <u>Other</u> chorioretinal inflammations

H30.81- <u>Harada's disease</u> — Inflammation of the choroid and retina associated with uveomeningitis.

H30.811 Harada's disease, <u>right</u> eye

H30.812 Harada's disease, <u>left</u> eye

H30.813 Harada's disease, <u>bilateral</u>

H30.819 Harada's disease, <u>unspecified</u> eye

H30.89- <u>Other</u> chorioretinal inflammations

cc **H30.891** Other chorioretinal inflammations, <u>right</u> eye

cc **H30.892** Other chorioretinal inflammations, <u>left</u> eye

cc **H30.893** Other chorioretinal inflammations, <u>bilateral</u>

cc **H30.899** Other chorioretinal inflammations, <u>unspecified</u> eye

H30.9- <u>Unspecified</u> chorioretinal inflammation
　　　Chorioretinitis NOS
　　　Choroiditis NOS
　　　Neuroretinitis NOS
　　　Retinitis NOS
　　　Retinochoroiditis NOS

cc **H30.90** Unspecified chorioretinal inflammation, <u>unspecified</u> eye

cc **H30.91** Unspecified chorioretinal inflammation, <u>right</u> eye

cc **H30.92** Unspecified chorioretinal inflammation, <u>left</u> eye

cc **H30.93** Unspecified chorioretinal inflammation, <u>bilateral</u>

H31- <u>Other disorders of choroid</u>

H31.0- <u>Chorioretinal scars</u> — Dense, wound-healing tissue of the choroid and retina.

　　　Excludes ❷: postsurgical chorioretinal scars (H59.81-)

H31.00- <u>Unspecified</u> chorioretinal scars

H31.001 Unspecified chorioretinal scars, <u>right</u> eye

H31.002 Unspecified chorioretinal scars, <u>left</u> eye

H31.003 Unspecified chorioretinal scars, <u>bilateral</u>

H31.009 Unspecified chorioretinal scars, <u>unspecified</u> eye

H31.01- <u>Macula scars</u> of posterior pole (postinflammatory) (post-traumatic) — A form affecting the macula.

　　　Excludes 1: postprocedural chorioretinal scar (H59.81-)

H31.011 Macula scars of posterior pole (postinflammatory) (post-traumatic), <u>right</u> eye

H31.012 Macula scars of posterior pole (postinflammatory) (post-traumatic), <u>left</u> eye

H31.013 Macula scars of posterior pole (postinflammatory) (post-traumatic), <u>bilateral</u>

H31.019 Macula scars of posterior pole (postinflammatory) (post-traumatic), <u>unspecified</u> eye

H31.02- <u>Solar retinopathy</u> — A form due to solar radiation affecting the macula.

H31.021 Solar retinopathy, <u>right</u> eye

H31.022 Solar retinopathy, <u>left</u> eye

H31.023 Solar retinopathy, <u>bilateral</u>

H31.029 Solar retinopathy, <u>unspecified</u> eye

H31.09- <u>Other</u> chorioretinal scars

H31.091 Other chorioretinal scars, <u>right</u> eye

H31.092 Other chorioretinal scars, <u>left</u> eye

H31.093 Other chorioretinal scars, <u>bilateral</u>

H31.099 Other chorioretinal scars, <u>unspecified</u> eye

H31.1- <u>Choroidal degeneration</u> — Deterioration of the choroid tissue.

　　　Excludes ❷: angioid streaks of macula (H35.33)

H31.10- <u>Unspecified</u> choroidal degeneration
　　　Choroidal sclerosis NOS

H31.101 Choroidal degeneration, unspecified, <u>right</u> eye

H31.102 Choroidal degeneration, unspecified, <u>left</u> eye

H31.103 Choroidal degeneration, unspecified, <u>bilateral</u>

H31.109 Choroidal degeneration, unspecified, <u>unspecified</u> eye

H31.11- <u>Age-related choroidal atrophy</u> — A form characterized by wasting-away of the choroid occurring in advancing age.

H31.111 Age-related choroidal atrophy, <u>right</u> eye — [Age/15-124]

H31.112 Age-related choroidal atrophy, <u>left</u> eye — [Age/15-124]

H31.113 Age-related choroidal atrophy, <u>bilateral</u> — [Age/15-124]

H31.119 Age-related choroidal atrophy, <u>unspecified</u> eye — [Age/15-124]

H31.12- <u>Diffuse secondary atrophy</u> of choroid — A form due to systemic diseases and affecting the whole of the choroid.

H31.121 Diffuse secondary atrophy of choroid, <u>right</u> eye

H31.122 Diffuse secondary atrophy of choroid, <u>left</u> eye

H31.123 Diffuse secondary atrophy of choroid, <u>bilateral</u>

H31.129 Diffuse secondary atrophy of choroid, <u>unspecified</u> eye

H31.2- <u>Hereditary choroidal dystrophy</u> — Inherited dystrophic and atrophic deteriorations of the choroid.

　　　Excludes ❷: hyperornithinemia (E72.4)
　　　　　　　　ornithinemia (E72.4)

H31.20 Hereditary choroidal dystrophy, unspecified

H31.21 Choroideremia — A form characterized by primary choroidal degeneration with night blindness.

H31.22 Choroidal dystrophy (central areolar) (generalized) (peripapillary) — A form affecting the central portion of the choroid capillaries.

H31.23 Gyrate atrophy, choroid — A form affecting the whole of the choroid blood vessels.

H31.29 Other hereditary choroidal dystrophy

H31.3- <u>Choroidal hemorrhage and rupture</u> — The escape of blood and forcible tearing of a blood vessel wall.

H31.30- <u>Unspecified</u> choroidal hemorrhage

H31.301 Unspecified choroidal hemorrhage, <u>right</u> eye

H31.302 Unspecified choroidal hemorrhage, <u>left</u> eye

H31.303 Unspecified choroidal hemorrhage, <u>bilateral</u>

H31.309 Unspecified choroidal hemorrhage, <u>unspecified</u> eye

H31.31- <u>Expulsive</u> choroidal hemorrhage — A form characterized by expulsion of blood into the choroid and retinal tissues.

H31.311 Expulsive choroidal hemorrhage, <u>right</u> eye

H31.312 Expulsive choroidal hemorrhage, <u>left</u> eye

H31.313 Expulsive choroidal hemorrhage, <u>bilateral</u>

H31.319 Expulsive choroidal hemorrhage, <u>unspecified</u> eye

H31.32- Choroidal <u>rupture</u> — The forcible tearing of a choroid blood vessel.

cc **H31.321** Choroidal rupture, <u>right</u> eye

cc **H31.322** Choroidal rupture, <u>left</u> eye

cc **H31.323** Choroidal rupture, <u>bilateral</u>

cc **H31.329** Choroidal rupture, <u>unspecified</u> eye

H31.4- Choroidal <u>detachment</u> — The separation of the choroid layers.

H31.40- <u>Unspecified</u> choroidal detachment

cc **H31.401** Unspecified choroidal detachment, <u>right</u> eye

cc **H31.402** Unspecified choroidal detachment, <u>left</u> eye

cc **H31.403** Unspecified choroidal detachment, <u>bilateral</u>

cc **H31.409** Unspecified choroidal detachment, <u>unspecified</u> eye

H31.41- <u>Hemorrhagic</u> choroidal detachment — A form characterized by blood within the separation.

cc **H31.411** Hemorrhagic choroidal detachment, <u>right</u> eye

cc **H31.412** Hemorrhagic choroidal detachment, <u>left</u> eye

H
3
0
–
H
3
1

cc **H31.413** **Hemorrhagic choroidal detachment, bilateral**

cc **H31.419** **Hemorrhagic choroidal detachment, unspecified eye**

H31.42- **Serous choroidal detachment** — A form characterized by fluid within the separation.

cc **H31.421** **Serous choroidal detachment, right eye**

cc **H31.422** **Serous choroidal detachment, left eye**

cc **H31.423** **Serous choroidal detachment, bilateral**

cc **H31.429** **Serous choroidal detachment, unspecified eye**

H31.8 **Other specified disorders of choroid**

H31.9 **Unspecified disorder of choroid**

H32 **Chorioretinal disorders in diseases classified elsewhere** —
[Not Allowed as PDX]
Code first underlying disease, such as:
   Congenital toxoplasmosis (P37.1)
   Histoplasmosis (B39.-)
   Leprosy (A30.-)
Excludes 1:   chorioretinitis (in):
               toxoplasmosis (acquired) (B58.01)
               tuberculosis (A18.53)

H33- **Retinal detachments and breaks** — The separation of the retinal layer from the pigment epithelium, and the break in continuity of the retinal layer.
   Excludes 1:   detachment of retinal pigment epithelium (H35.72-, H35.73-)

H33.0- **Retinal detachment with retinal break**
   Rhegmatogenous retinal detachment
   Excludes 1:   serous retinal detachment (without retinal break) (H33.2-)

H33.00- **Unspecified retinal detachment with retinal break**

H33.001 **Unspecified retinal detachment with retinal break, right eye**

H33.002 **Unspecified retinal detachment with retinal break, left eye**

H33.003 **Unspecified retinal detachment with retinal break, bilateral**

H33.009 **Unspecified retinal detachment with retinal break, unspecified eye**

H33.01- **Retinal detachment with single break** — A form characterized by one current retinal break.

H33.011 **Retinal detachment with single break, right eye**

H33.012 **Retinal detachment with single break, left eye**

H33.013 **Retinal detachment with single break, bilateral**

H33.019 **Retinal detachment with single break, unspecified eye**

H33.02- **Retinal detachment with multiple breaks** — A form characterized by two or more current retinal breaks.

H33.021 **Retinal detachment with multiple breaks, right eye**

H33.022 **Retinal detachment with multiple breaks, left eye**

H33.023 **Retinal detachment with multiple breaks, bilateral**

H33.029 **Retinal detachment with multiple breaks, unspecified eye**

H33.03- **Retinal detachment with giant retinal tear** — A form characterized by a relatively large current break (tear).

H33.031 **Retinal detachment with giant retinal tear, right eye**

H33.032 **Retinal detachment with giant retinal tear, left eye**

H33.033 **Retinal detachment with giant retinal tear, bilateral**

H33.039 **Retinal detachment with giant retinal tear, unspecified eye**

H33.04- **Retinal detachment with retinal dialysis** — A form characterized by a demonstrable current break at the ora serrata.

H33.041 **Retinal detachment with retinal dialysis, right eye**

H33.042 **Retinal detachment with retinal dialysis, left eye**

H33.043 **Retinal detachment with retinal dialysis, bilateral**

H33.049 **Retinal detachment with retinal dialysis, unspecified eye**

H33.05- **Total retinal detachment** — A form characterized by a current complete, or almost complete, separation of the retinal layer.

H33.051 **Total retinal detachment, right eye**

H33.052 **Total retinal detachment, left eye**

H33.053 **Total retinal detachment, bilateral**

H33.059 **Total retinal detachment, unspecified eye**

H33.1- **Retinoschisis and retinal cysts** — Splitting of the retinal layers, and fluid-filled sacs of the retina.
   Excludes 1:   congenital retinoschisis (Q14.1)
                  microcystoid degeneration of retina (H35.42-)

H33.10- **Unspecified retinoschisis**

H33.101 **Unspecified retinoschisis, right eye**

H33.102 **Unspecified retinoschisis, left eye**

H33.103 **Unspecified retinoschisis, bilateral**

H33.109 **Unspecified retinoschisis, unspecified eye**

H33.11- **Cyst of ora serrata** — A form characterized by fluid-filled sacs in the serrated junction between the retina and the ciliary body.

H33.111 **Cyst of ora serrata, right eye**

H33.112 **Cyst of ora serrata, left eye**

H33.113 **Cyst of ora serrata, bilateral**

H33.119 **Cyst of ora serrata, unspecified eye**

H33.12- **Parasitic cyst of retina** — A form characterized by infestation of a parasite.

cc **H33.121** **Parasitic cyst of retina, right eye**

cc **H33.122** **Parasitic cyst of retina, left eye**

cc **H33.123** **Parasitic cyst of retina, bilateral**

cc **H33.129** **Parasitic cyst of retina, unspecified eye**

H33.19- **Other retinoschisis and retinal cysts**
   Pseudocyst of retina — A dilated space of the retina.

H33.191 **Other retinoschisis and retinal cysts, right eye**

H33.192 **Other retinoschisis and retinal cysts, left eye**

H33.193 **Other retinoschisis and retinal cysts, bilateral**

H33.199 **Other retinoschisis and retinal cysts, unspecified eye**

H33.2- **Serous retinal detachment** — The separation of the retinal layers from the pigment epithelium with serous fluid.
   Retinal detachment NOS
   Retinal detachment without retinal break
   Excludes 1:   central serous chorioretinopathy (H35.71-)

cc **H33.20** **Serous retinal detachment, unspecified eye**

cc **H33.21** **Serous retinal detachment, right eye**

cc **H33.22** **Serous retinal detachment, left eye**

cc **H33.23** **Serous retinal detachment, bilateral**

H33.3- **Retinal breaks without detachment** — A break, tear, or hole without separation of retinal layers.
   Excludes 1:   chorioretinal scars after surgery for detachment (H59.81-)
                  peripheral retinal degeneration without break (H35.4-)

H33.30- **Unspecified retinal break**

H33.301 **Unspecified retinal break, right eye**

H33.302 **Unspecified retinal break, left eye**

H33.303 **Unspecified retinal break, bilateral**

H33.309 **Unspecified retinal break, unspecified eye**

H33.31- **Horseshoe tear of retina without detachment** — A form characterized by a horseshoe-shaped tear of the retinal layer.
   Operculum of retina without detachment — A form marked by the retinal tear completely free of the retinal surface.

H33.311 **Horseshoe tear of retina without detachment, right eye**

H33.312 **Horseshoe tear of retina without detachment, left eye**

H33.313 **Horseshoe tear of retina without detachment, bilateral**

H33.319 **Horseshoe tear of retina without detachment, unspecified eye**

H33.32- **Round hole of retina without detachment** — A form characterized by a round-shaped atrophic hole through the retinal layer.

H33.321 **Round hole, right eye**

H33.322 **Round hole, left eye**

H33.323 **Round hole, bilateral**

H33.329 **Round hole, unspecified eye**

H3 1 - H3 3

H33.33- <u>Multiple defects</u> of retina without detachment — A form characterized by two or more breaks, tears, or holes.

H33.331 Multiple defects of retina without detachment, <u>right</u> eye

H33.332 Multiple defects of retina without detachment, <u>left</u> eye

H33.333 Multiple defects of retina without detachment, <u>bilateral</u>

H33.339 Multiple defects of retina without detachment, <u>unspecified</u> eye

H33.4- <u>Traction</u> detachment of retina — The separation of the retinal layer at its attachment due to the pulling force of the vitreous on the retina.
Proliferative vitreo-retinopathy with retinal detachment

cc **H33.40** Traction detachment of retina, <u>unspecified</u> eye

cc **H33.41** Traction detachment of retina, <u>right</u> eye

cc **H33.42** Traction detachment of retina, <u>left</u> eye

cc **H33.43** Traction detachment of retina, <u>bilateral</u>

cc **H33.8** Other retinal detachments

H34- <u>Retinal vascular occlusions</u> — The obstruction of blood flow to and from the retina.
Excludes 1:   amaurosis fugax (G45.3)

H34.0- <u>Transient retinal artery occlusion</u> — Temporary blockage of a retinal arterial branch.

cc **H34.00** Transient retinal artery occlusion, <u>unspecified</u> eye

cc **H34.01** Transient retinal artery occlusion, <u>right</u> eye

cc **H34.02** Transient retinal artery occlusion, <u>left</u> eye

cc **H34.03** Transient retinal artery occlusion, <u>bilateral</u>

H34.1- <u>Central retinal artery occlusion</u> — Blockage of the central retinal artery resulting in sudden and complete, or almost complete, loss of vision.

cc **H34.10** Central retinal artery occlusion, <u>unspecified</u> eye

cc **H34.11** Central retinal artery occlusion, <u>right</u> eye

cc **H34.12** Central retinal artery occlusion, <u>left</u> eye

cc **H34.13** Central retinal artery occlusion, <u>bilateral</u>

H34.2- Other retinal artery occlusions

H34.21- <u>Partial retinal artery</u> occlusion — Incomplete blockage of the retinal artery and its branches.
Hollenhorst's plaque — Erythromatous emboli deposits in the retinal arterioles.
Retinal microembolism — A blood clot of a very minute size in a retinal artery.

cc **H34.211** Partial retinal artery occlusion, <u>right</u> eye

cc **H34.212** Partial retinal artery occlusion, <u>left</u> eye

cc **H34.213** Partial retinal artery occlusion, <u>bilateral</u>

cc **H34.219** Partial retinal artery occlusion, <u>unspecified</u> eye

H34.23- <u>Retinal artery branch</u> occlusion — Blockage of a retinal arterial branch resulting in sudden partial loss of vision.

cc **H34.231** Retinal artery branch occlusion, <u>right</u> eye

cc **H34.232** Retinal artery branch occlusion, <u>left</u> eye

cc **H34.233** Retinal artery branch occlusion, <u>bilateral</u>

cc **H34.239** Retinal artery branch occlusion, <u>unspecified</u> eye

H34.8- Other retinal vascular occlusions

H34.81- <u>Central retinal vein</u> occlusion — Blockage of the central retinal vein leading to increased intraocular pressure and retinal hemorrhages.

One of the following 7th characters is to be assigned to codes in subcategory H34.81- to designate the severity of the occlusion:
0   With macular edema
1   With retinal neovascularization
2   Stable
Old retinal vein occlusion

cc-0-2 **H34.811-** Central retinal vein occlusion, <u>right</u> eye

cc-0-2 **H34.812-** Central retinal vein occlusion, <u>left</u> eye

cc-0-2 **H34.813-** Central retinal vein occlusion, <u>bilateral</u>

cc-0-2 **H34.819-** Central retinal vein occlusion, <u>unspecified</u> eye

H34.82- <u>Venous engorgement</u> — The abnormal accumulation of venous blood in the retinal veins.
Incipient retinal vein occlusion — A form marked by the beginning of blockage.
Partial retinal vein occlusion — A form marked by incomplete blockage.

H34.821 Venous engorgement, <u>right</u> eye

H34.822 Venous engorgement, <u>left</u> eye

H34.823 Venous engorgement, <u>bilateral</u>

H34.829 Venous engorgement, <u>unspecified</u> eye

H34.83- <u>Tributary (branch) retinal vein occlusion</u> — Blockage of a tortuous retinal vein branch which may cause retinal hemorrhage.

One of the following 7th characters is to be assigned to codes in subcategory H34.83- to designate the severity of the occlusion:
0   With macular edema
1   With retinal neovascularization
2   Stable
Old tributary (branch) retinal vein occlusion

H34.831- Tributary (branch) retinal vein occlusion, <u>right</u> eye

H34.832- Tributary (branch) retinal vein occlusion, <u>left</u> eye

H34.833- Tributary (branch) retinal vein occlusion, <u>bilateral</u>

H34.839- Tributary (branch) retinal vein occlusion, <u>unspecified</u> eye

cc **H34.9** Unspecified retinal vascular occlusion

H35- <u>Other retinal disorders</u>
Excludes ❷: diabetic retinal disorders (E08.311- E08.359, E09.311- E09.359, E10.311- E10.359, E11.311- E11.359, E13.311- E13.359)

H35.0- <u>Background retinopathy</u> and retinal vascular changes — A disease of the retinal capillaries that is caused by some condition other than diabetes.
Code also any associated hypertension (I10.)

H35.00 <u>Unspecified</u> background retinopathy

H35.01- <u>Changes in retinal vascular appearance</u> — New, abnormal vascular development.
Retinal vascular sheathing — The white-line appearance of thickened retinal arterial walls.

H35.011 Changes in retinal vascular appearance, <u>right</u> eye

H35.012 Changes in retinal vascular appearance, <u>left</u> eye

H35.013 Changes in retinal vascular appearance, <u>bilateral</u>

H35.019 Changes in retinal vascular appearance, <u>unspecified</u> eye

H35.02- <u>Exudative retinopathy</u> — A disease of the retinal capillaries characterized by masses of white or yellowish exudate which deposit on the posterior part of the fundus oculi.
Coats retinopathy

H35.021 Exudative retinopathy, <u>right</u> eye

H35.022 Exudative retinopathy, <u>left</u> eye

H35.023 Exudative retinopathy, <u>bilateral</u>

H35.029 Exudative retinopathy, <u>unspecified</u> eye

H35.03- <u>Hypertensive</u> retinopathy — A disease of the retinal capillaries due to the effects of hypertension.

H35.031 Hypertensive retinopathy, <u>right</u> eye

H35.032 Hypertensive retinopathy, <u>left</u> eye

H35.033 Hypertensive retinopathy, <u>bilateral</u>

H35.039 Hypertensive retinopathy, <u>unspecified</u> eye

H35.04- <u>Retinal micro-aneurysms</u>, unspecified — The presence of small dilated arterial sacs.

H35.041 Retinal micro-aneurysms, unspecified, <u>right</u> eye

H35.042 Retinal micro-aneurysms, unspecified, <u>left</u> eye

H35.043 Retinal micro-aneurysms, unspecified, <u>bilateral</u>

H35.049 Retinal micro-aneurysms, unspecified, <u>unspecified</u> eye

H35.05- <u>Retinal neovascularization</u>, unspecified — The abnormal development of new retinal blood vessels.

H35.051 Retinal neovascularization, unspecified, <u>right</u> eye

H35.052 Retinal neovascularization, unspecified, <u>left</u> eye

H35.053 Retinal neovascularization, unspecified, <u>bilateral</u>

H35.059 Retinal neovascularization, unspecified, <u>unspecified</u> eye

H35.06- <u>Retinal vasculitis</u> — Inflammation of the retinal blood vessels.
Eales disease — A disease characterized by recurrent hemorrhages into the retina and vitreous.
Retinal perivasculitis — Inflammation of the retinal perivascular sheaths.

H35.061 Retinal vasculitis, <u>right</u> eye

H33-H35

H35.062   Retinal vasculitis, <u>left</u> eye
H35.063   Retinal vasculitis, <u>bilateral</u>
H35.069   Retinal vasculitis, <u>unspecified</u> eye
H35.07- <u>Retinal telangiectasis</u> — The abnormal dilatation of a group of retinal capillaries.
H35.071   Retinal telangiectasis, <u>right</u> eye
H35.072   Retinal telangiectasis, <u>left</u> eye
H35.073   Retinal telangiectasis, <u>bilateral</u>
H35.079   Retinal telangiectasis, <u>unspecified</u> eye
H35.09   Other intraretinal microvascular abnormalities
Retinal varices — Enlarged, tortuous retinal capillary vessels.
H35.1-   <u>Retinopathy of prematurity</u> — A developmental disorder of premature infants in which the normal development of the retinal vasculature is arrested and results in fibrovascular proliferation.
H35.10- Retinopathy of prematurity, <u>unspecified</u>
Retinopathy of prematurity NOS
H35.101   Retinopathy of prematurity, unspecified, <u>right</u> eye
H35.102   Retinopathy of prematurity, unspecified, <u>left</u> eye
H35.103   Retinopathy of prematurity, unspecified, <u>bilateral</u>
H35.109   Retinopathy of prematurity, unspecified, <u>unspecified</u> eye
H35.11- Retinopathy of prematurity, <u>stage 0</u> — The mildest form with no identifiable line of demarcation.
H35.111   Retinopathy of prematurity, stage 0, <u>right</u> eye
H35.112   Retinopathy of prematurity, stage 0, <u>left</u> eye
H35.113   Retinopathy of prematurity, stage 0, <u>bilateral</u>
H35.119   Retinopathy of prematurity, stage 0, <u>unspecified</u> eye
H35.12- Retinopathy of prematurity, <u>stage 1</u> — Blood vessel growth is mildly abnormal and a line of demarcation develops.
H35.121   Retinopathy of prematurity, stage 1, <u>right</u> eye
H35.122   Retinopathy of prematurity, stage 1, <u>left</u> eye
H35.123   Retinopathy of prematurity, stage 1, <u>bilateral</u>
H35.129   Retinopathy of prematurity, stage 1, <u>unspecified</u> eye
H35.13- Retinopathy of prematurity, <u>stage 2</u> — Blood vessel growth is moderately abnormal and the line becomes a ridge.
H35.131   Retinopathy of prematurity, stage 2, <u>right</u> eye
H35.132   Retinopathy of prematurity, stage 2, <u>left</u> eye
H35.133   Retinopathy of prematurity, stage 2, <u>bilateral</u>
H35.139   Retinopathy of prematurity, stage 2, <u>unspecified</u> eye
H35.14- Retinopathy of prematurity, <u>stage 3</u> — Blood vessel growth is severely abnormal and extra-retinal vascular proliferation occurs.
H35.141   Retinopathy of prematurity, stage 3, <u>right</u> eye
H35.142   Retinopathy of prematurity, stage 3, <u>left</u> eye
H35.143   Retinopathy of prematurity, stage 3, <u>bilateral</u>
H35.149   Retinopathy of prematurity, stage 3, <u>unspecified</u> eye
H35.15- Retinopathy of prematurity, <u>stage 4</u> — Blood vessel growth is severely abnormal and there is a partially detached retina.
H35.151   Retinopathy of prematurity, stage 4, <u>right</u> eye
H35.152   Retinopathy of prematurity, stage 4, <u>left</u> eye
H35.153   Retinopathy of prematurity, stage 4, <u>bilateral</u>
H35.159   Retinopathy of prematurity, stage 4, <u>unspecified</u> eye
H35.16- Retinopathy of prematurity, <u>stage 5</u> — There is a total retinal detachment.
H35.161   Retinopathy of prematurity, stage 5, <u>right</u> eye
H35.162   Retinopathy of prematurity, stage 5, <u>left</u> eye
H35.163   Retinopathy of prematurity, stage 5, <u>bilateral</u>
H35.169   Retinopathy of prematurity, stage 5, <u>unspecified</u> eye
H35.17- <u>Retrolental fibroplasia</u> — A condition in which the retina is already scarred.
H35.171   Retrolental fibroplasia, <u>right</u> eye
H35.172   Retrolental fibroplasia, <u>left</u> eye

H35.173   Retrolental fibroplasia, <u>bilateral</u>
H35.179   Retrolental fibroplasia, <u>unspecified</u> eye
H35.2-   <u>Other non-diabetic proliferative retinopathy</u>
Proliferative vitreo-retinopathy
Excludes 1:   proliferative vitreo-retinopathy with retinal detachment (H33.4-)
H35.20   Other non-diabetic proliferative retinopathy, <u>unspecified</u> eye
H35.21   Other non-diabetic proliferative retinopathy, <u>right</u> eye
H35.22   Other non-diabetic proliferative retinopathy, <u>left</u> eye
H35.23   Other non-diabetic proliferative retinopathy, <u>bilateral</u>
H35.3-   Degeneration of macula and posterior pole — Deterioration of the yellow pigmented point of sharpest vision of the retina.
H35.30   Unspecified macular degeneration — [Age/15-124]
Age-related macular degeneration
H35.31- Nonexudative age-related macular degeneration — A form characterized by progressive cellular destruction and the lack of cellular debris.
Atrophic age-related macular degeneration
Dry age-related macular degeneration
One of the following 7th characters is to be assigned to codes in subcategory H35.31- to designate the stage of the disease:
0   Stage unspecified
1   Early dry stage
2   Intermediate dry stage
3   Advanced atrophic without subfoveal involvement
Advanced dry stage
4   Advanced atrophic with subfoveal involvement
H35.311-   Nonexudative age-related macular degeneration, <u>right</u> eye — [Age/15-124]
H35.312-   Nonexudative age-related macular degeneration, <u>left</u> eye — [Age/15-124]
H35.313-   Nonexudative age-related macular degeneration, <u>bilateral</u> — [Age/15-124]
H35.319-   Nonexudative age-related macular degeneration, <u>unspecified</u> eye — [Age/15-124]
H35.32- Exudative age-related macular degeneration — A form characterized by progressive cellular destruction and cellular debris.
Wet age-related macular degeneration
One of the following 7th characters is to be assigned to codes in subcategory H35.32- to designate the stage of the disease:
0   Stage unspecified
1   With active choroidal neovascularization
2   With inactive choroidal neovascularization
With involuted or regressed neovascularization
3   With inactive scar
H35.321-   Exudative age-related macular degeneration, <u>right</u> eye — [Age/15-124]
H35.322-   Exudative age-related macular degeneration, <u>left</u> eye — [Age/15-124]
H35.323-   Exudative age-related macular degeneration, <u>bilateral</u> — [Age/15-124]
H35.329-   Exudative age-related macular degeneration, <u>unspecified</u> eye — [Age/15-124]
H35.33   Angioid streaks of macula — A form characterized by dark brown pigmented streaks which anastomose and may be mistaken for blood vessels.
H35.34- <u>Macular cyst, hole, or pseudohole</u> — A form characterized by a membrane break of the macula.
H35.341   Macular cyst, hole, or pseudohole, <u>right</u> eye
H35.342   Macular cyst, hole, or pseudohole, <u>left</u> eye
H35.343   Macular cyst, hole, or pseudohole, <u>bilateral</u>
H35.349   Macular cyst, hole, or pseudohole, <u>unspecified</u> eye
H35.35- <u>Cystoid macular degeneration</u> — A form characterized by appearance of cyst-like macular and foveal cavities.
Excludes 1:   cystoid macular edema following cataract surgery (H59.03-)
H35.351   Cystoid macular degeneration, <u>right</u> eye
H35.352   Cystoid macular degeneration, <u>left</u> eye
H35.353   Cystoid macular degeneration, <u>bilateral</u>

H35.359 Cystoid macular degeneration, <u>unspecified</u> eye

H35.36- <u>Drusen (degenerative) of macula</u> — Hyaline excrescences of the Bruch's membrane of the choroid.

H35.361 Drusen (degenerative) of macula, <u>right</u> eye

H35.362 Drusen (degenerative) of macula, <u>left</u> eye

H35.363 Drusen (degenerative) of macula, <u>bilateral</u>

H35.369 Drusen (degenerative) of macula, <u>unspecified</u> eye

H35.37- <u>Puckering of macula</u> — A form characterized by wrinkling of the macular surface.

H35.371 Puckering of macula, <u>right</u> eye

H35.372 Puckering of macula, <u>left</u> eye

H35.373 Puckering of macula, <u>bilateral</u>

H35.379 Puckering of macula, <u>unspecified</u> eye

H35.38- <u>Toxic maculopathy</u> — A form caused by the effects of toxic substances.
Code first poisoning due to drug or toxin, if applicable (T36-T65 with fifth or sixth character 1-4 or 6)
Use additional code for adverse effect, if applicable, to identify drug (T36-T50 with fifth or sixth character 5)

H35.381 Toxic maculopathy, <u>right</u> eye

H35.382 Toxic maculopathy, <u>left</u> eye

H35.383 Toxic maculopathy, <u>bilateral</u>

H35.389 Toxic maculopathy, <u>unspecified</u> eye

H35.4- <u>Peripheral retinal degeneration</u> — Deterioration of the retina other than the macula.
Excludes 1: *hereditary retinal degeneration (dystrophy) (H35.5-)*
peripheral retinal degeneration with retinal break (H33.3-)

H35.40 <u>Unspecified</u> peripheral retinal degeneration

H35.41- <u>Lattice</u> degeneration of retina — A form characterized by atrophy of the retinal lattice.
Palisade degeneration of retina

H35.411 Lattice degeneration of retina, <u>right</u> eye

H35.412 Lattice degeneration of retina, <u>left</u> eye

H35.413 Lattice degeneration of retina, <u>bilateral</u>

H35.419 Lattice degeneration of retina, <u>unspecified</u> eye

H35.42- <u>Microcystoid</u> degeneration of retina — A form characterized by atrophic small cysts occurring in advancing age.

H35.421 Microcystoid degeneration of retina, <u>right</u> eye

H35.422 Microcystoid degeneration of retina, <u>left</u> eye

H35.423 Microcystoid degeneration of retina, <u>bilateral</u>

H35.429 Microcystoid degeneration of retina, <u>unspecified</u> eye

H35.43- <u>Paving stone</u> degeneration of retina — A form characterized by the paving stone appearance of the retina.

H35.431 Paving stone degeneration of retina, <u>right</u> eye

H35.432 Paving stone degeneration of retina, <u>left</u> eye

H35.433 Paving stone degeneration of retina, <u>bilateral</u>

H35.439 Paving stone degeneration of retina, <u>unspecified</u> eye

H35.44- Age-related reticular degeneration of retina — A form characterized by an atrophic net-like appearance.

H35.441 Age-related reticular degeneration of retina, <u>right</u> eye — [Age/15-124]

H35.442 Age-related reticular degeneration of retina, <u>left</u> eye — [Age/15-124]

H35.443 Age-related reticular degeneration of retina, <u>bilateral</u> — [Age/15-124]

H35.449 Age-related reticular degeneration of retina, <u>unspecified</u> eye — [Age/15-124]

H35.45- <u>Secondary pigmentary</u> degeneration — A form characterized by pigmentary changes due to nonocular diseases.

H35.451 Secondary pigmentary degeneration, <u>right</u> eye

H35.452 Secondary pigmentary degeneration, <u>left</u> eye

H35.453 Secondary pigmentary degeneration, <u>bilateral</u>

H35.459 Secondary pigmentary degeneration, <u>unspecified</u> eye

H35.46- <u>Secondary vitreoretinal</u> degeneration — A form characterized by destruction of vitreoretinal tissue due to nonocular diseases.

H35.461 Secondary vitreoretinal degeneration, <u>right</u> eye

H35.462 Secondary vitreoretinal degeneration, <u>left</u> eye

H35.463 Secondary vitreoretinal degeneration, <u>bilateral</u>

H35.469 Secondary vitreoretinal degeneration, <u>unspecified</u> eye

H35.5- **Hereditary retinal dystrophy** — Inherited dystrophic and atrophic retinal deteriorations.
Excludes 1: *dystrophies primarily involving Bruch's membrane (H31.1-)*

H35.50 Unspecified hereditary retinal dystrophy

H35.51 Vitreoretinal dystrophy — A form characterized by cystoid structure changes of the central retina.

H35.52 Pigmentary retinal dystrophy — A form characterized by retinal pigmentary atrophy.
Albipunctate retinal dystrophy
Retinitis pigmentosa
Tapetoretinal dystrophy

H35.53 Other dystrophies primarily involving the sensory retina
Stargardt's disease — A form marked by whitish foveal flecks and progressive foveal atrophy.

H35.54 Dystrophies primarily involving the retinal pigment epithelium
Vitelliform retinal dystrophy — A form marked by orange-yellow foveal disc.

H35.6- <u>Retinal hemorrhage</u> — The escape of blood into the retina.

H35.60 Retinal hemorrhage, <u>unspecified</u> eye

H35.61 Retinal hemorrhage, <u>right</u> eye

H35.62 Retinal hemorrhage, <u>left</u> eye

H35.63 Retinal hemorrhage, <u>bilateral</u>

H35.7- <u>Separation of retinal layers</u> — The abnormal separation of the pigment epithelium from the choroid.
Excludes 1: *retinal detachment (serous) (H33.2-)*
rhegmatogenous retinal detachment (H33.0-)

cc **H35.70** Unspecified separation of retinal layers

H35.71- <u>Central serous chorioretinopathy</u> — A form characterized by serous fluid separation in the center of the retina.

H35.711 Central serous chorioretinopathy, <u>right</u> eye

H35.712 Central serous chorioretinopathy, <u>left</u> eye

H35.713 Central serous chorioretinopathy, <u>bilateral</u>

H35.719 Central serous chorioretinopathy, <u>unspecified</u> eye

H35.72- <u>Serous</u> detachment of retinal pigment epithelium — The separation of the retinal pigment epithelium from the choroid by serous fluid.

cc **H35.721** Serous detachment of retinal pigment epithelium, <u>right</u> eye

cc **H35.722** Serous detachment of retinal pigment epithelium, <u>left</u> eye

cc **H35.723** Serous detachment of retinal pigment epithelium, <u>bilateral</u>

cc **H35.729** Serous detachment of retinal pigment epithelium, <u>unspecified</u> eye

H35.73- <u>Hemorrhagic</u> detachment of retinal pigment epithelium — The separation of the retinal pigment epithelium from the choroid by the escape of blood into that separation.

cc **H35.731** Hemorrhagic detachment of retinal pigment epithelium, <u>right</u> eye

cc **H35.732** Hemorrhagic detachment of retinal pigment epithelium, <u>left</u> eye

cc **H35.733** Hemorrhagic detachment of retinal pigment epithelium, <u>bilateral</u>

cc **H35.739** Hemorrhagic detachment of retinal pigment epithelium, <u>unspecified</u> eye

H35.8- **Other specified retinal disorders**
Excludes ❷: *retinal hemorrhage (H35.6-)*

H35.81 Retinal edema — The accumulation of intercellular fluid.
Retinal cotton wool spots — The white or gray fluid opacities in the retina composed of cytoid bodies.

cc **H35.82** Retinal ischemia — Deficiency of blood supply to the retina.

H35.89 Other specified retinal disorders

H35 - H35

H35.9   Unspecified retinal disorder

H36   Retinal disorders in diseases classified elsewhere — [Not Allowed as PDX]
Code first underlying disease, such as:
Lipid storage disorders (E75.-)
Sickle-cell disorders (D57.-)
*Excludes 1:   arteriosclerotic retinopathy (H35.0-)
diabetic retinopathy (E08.3-, E09.3-, E10.3-, E11.3-, E13.3-)*

Glaucoma (H40-H42)

H40-   Glaucoma — An abnormal increase in intraocular pressure.
*Excludes 1:   absolute glaucoma (H44.51-)
congenital glaucoma (Q15.0)
traumatic glaucoma due to birth injury (P15.3)*

H40.0-   Glaucoma suspect — A relatively low increase in intraocular pressure which does not meet all the criteria for the formal diagnosis of glaucoma.

H40.00-   Preglaucoma, unspecified

H40.001   Preglaucoma, unspecified, right eye

H40.002   Preglaucoma, unspecified, left eye

H40.003   Preglaucoma, unspecified, bilateral

H40.009   Preglaucoma, unspecified, unspecified eye

H40.01-   Open angle with borderline findings, low risk — A form with the angle of the anterior chamber open.
Open angle, low risk

H40.011   Open angle with borderline findings, low risk, right eye

H40.012   Open angle with borderline findings, low risk, left eye

H40.013   Open angle with borderline findings, low risk, bilateral

H40.019   Open angle with borderline findings, low risk, unspecified eye

H40.02-   Open angle with borderline findings, high risk — A form with the angle of the anterior chamber open.
Open angle, high risk

H40.021   Open angle with borderline findings, high risk, right eye

H40.022   Open angle with borderline findings, high risk, left eye

H40.023   Open angle with borderline findings, high risk, bilateral

H40.029   Open angle with borderline findings, high risk, unspecified eye

H40.03-   Anatomical narrow angle — A form characterized by the finding of a narrowed angle of the anterior chamber.
Primary angle closure suspect

H40.031   Anatomical narrow angle, right eye

H40.032   Anatomical narrow angle, left eye

H40.033   Anatomical narrow angle, bilateral

H40.039   Anatomical narrow angle, unspecified eye

H40.04-   Steroid responder

H40.041   Steroid responder, right eye

H40.042   Steroid responder, left eye

H40.043   Steroid responder, bilateral

H40.049   Steroid responder, unspecified eye

H40.05-   Ocular hypertension — A form characterized by increased ocular blood pressure.

H40.051   Ocular hypertension, right eye

H40.052   Ocular hypertension, left eye

H40.053   Ocular hypertension, bilateral

H40.059   Ocular hypertension, unspecified eye

H40.06-   Primary angle closure without glaucoma damage — An abnormal increase in intraocular pressure with the angle of the anterior chamber narrowed and without pre-existing ocular disease.

H40.061   Primary angle closure without glaucoma damage, right eye

H40.062   Primary angle closure without glaucoma damage, left eye

H40.063   Primary angle closure without glaucoma damage, bilateral

H40.069   Primary angle closure without glaucoma damage, unspecified eye

H40.1-   Open-angle glaucoma — An abnormal increase in intraocular pressure with the angle of the anterior chamber open.

H40.10x-   Unspecified open-angle glaucoma
One of the following 7th characters is to be assigned to code H40.10x- to designate the stage of glaucoma:
0   Stage unspecified
1   Mild stage
2   Moderate stage
3   Severe stage
4   Indeterminate stage

H40.11-   Primary open-angle glaucoma — A form without a pre-existing ocular disease.
Chronic simple glaucoma
One of the following 7th characters is to be assigned to each code in subcategory H40.11- to designate the stage of glaucoma:
0   Stage unspecified
1   Mild stage
2   Moderate stage
3   Severe stage
4   Indeterminate stage

H40.111-   Primary open-angle glaucoma, right eye

H40.112-   Primary open-angle glaucoma, left eye

H40.113-   Primary open-angle glaucoma, bilateral

H40.119-   Primary open-angle glaucoma, unspecified eye

H40.12-   Low-tension glaucoma — A form marked by a relatively low increased intraocular pressure.
One of the following 7th characters is to be assigned to code H40.12- to designate the stage of glaucoma:
0   Stage unspecified
1   Mild stage
2   Moderate stage
3   Severe stage
4   Indeterminate stage

H40.121-   Low-tension glaucoma, right eye — [Unacceptable PDX]

H40.122-   Low-tension glaucoma, left eye — [Unacceptable PDX]

H40.123-   Low-tension glaucoma, bilateral — [Unacceptable PDX]

H40.129-   Low-tension glaucoma, unspecified eye — [Unacceptable PDX]

H40.13-   Pigmentary glaucoma — A form marked by an abnormal amount of pigment in the anterior chamber.
One of the following 7th characters is to be assigned to code H40.13- to designate the stage of glaucoma:
0   Stage unspecified
1   Mild stage
2   Moderate stage
3   Severe stage
4   Indeterminate stage

H40.131-   Pigmentary glaucoma, right eye — [Unacceptable PDX]

H40.132-   Pigmentary glaucoma, left eye — [Unacceptable PDX]

H40.133-   Pigmentary glaucoma, bilateral — [Unacceptable PDX]

H40.139-   Pigmentary glaucoma, unspecified eye — [Unacceptable PDX]

H40.14-   Capsular glaucoma with pseudoexfoliation of lens — A form marked by the presence of flakes or clumps of proteinaceous substance within the eye.
One of the following 7th characters is to be assigned to code H40.14- to designate the stage of glaucoma:
0   Stage unspecified
1   Mild stage
2   Moderate stage
3   Severe stage
4   Indeterminate stage

H40.141-   Capsular glaucoma with pseudoexfoliation of lens, right eye

H40.142-   Capsular glaucoma with pseudoexfoliation of lens, left eye

H40.143-   Capsular glaucoma with pseudoexfoliation of lens, bilateral

H 3 5 - H 4 0

H40.149- Capsular glaucoma with pseudoexfoliation of lens, <u>unspecified</u> eye

H40.15- <u>Residual stage</u> of open-angle glaucoma

H40.151 Residual stage of open-angle glaucoma, <u>right</u> eye — [Unacceptable PDX]

H40.152 Residual stage of open-angle glaucoma, <u>left</u> eye — [Unacceptable PDX]

H40.153 Residual stage of open-angle glaucoma, <u>bilateral</u> — [Unacceptable PDX]

H40.159 Residual stage of open-angle glaucoma, <u>unspecified</u> eye — [Unacceptable PDX]

H40.2- <u>Primary angle-closure glaucoma</u> — An abnormal increase in intraocular pressure with the angle of the anterior chamber narrowed and without pre-existing ocular disease.

Excludes 1:   *aqueous misdirection (H40.83-)*
              malignant glaucoma (H40.83-)

H40.20x- <u>Unspecified</u> primary angle-closure glaucoma

One of the following 7th characters is to be assigned to code H40.20x- to designate the stage of glaucoma:
  0   Stage unspecified
  1   Mild stage
  2   Moderate stage
  3   Severe stage
  4   Indeterminate stage

H40.21- <u>Acute</u> angle-closure glaucoma — A form marked by sudden, severe onset.
Acute angle-closure glaucoma attack
Acute angle-closure glaucoma crisis

CC **H40.211** Acute angle-closure glaucoma, <u>right</u> eye

CC **H40.212** Acute angle-closure glaucoma, <u>left</u> eye

CC **H40.213** Acute angle-closure glaucoma, <u>bilateral</u>

CC **H40.219** Acute angle-closure glaucoma, <u>unspecified</u> eye

H40.22- <u>Chronic</u> angle-closure glaucoma — A form marked by slow development, and persistence over a long period of time, often unnoticed.
Chronic primary angle-closure glaucoma

One of the following 7th characters is to be assigned to code H40.22- to designate the stage of glaucoma:
  0   Stage unspecified
  1   Mild stage
  2   Moderate stage
  3   Severe stage
  4   Indeterminate stage

H40.221- Chronic angle-closure glaucoma, <u>right</u> eye

H40.222- Chronic angle-closure glaucoma, <u>left</u> eye

H40.223- Chronic angle-closure glaucoma, <u>bilateral</u>

H40.229- Chronic angle-closure glaucoma, <u>unspecified</u> eye

H40.23- <u>Intermittent</u> angle-closure glaucoma — A form occurring at separated intervals.

H40.231 Intermittent angle-closure glaucoma, <u>right</u> eye

H40.232 Intermittent angle-closure glaucoma, <u>left</u> eye

H40.233 Intermittent angle-closure glaucoma, <u>bilateral</u>

H40.239 Intermittent angle-closure glaucoma, <u>unspecified</u> eye

H40.24- <u>Residual stage</u> of angle-closure glaucoma

H40.241 Residual stage of angle-closure glaucoma, <u>right</u> eye

H40.242 Residual stage of angle-closure glaucoma, <u>left</u> eye

H40.243 Residual stage of angle-closure glaucoma, <u>bilateral</u>

H40.249 Residual stage of angle-closure glaucoma, <u>unspecified</u> eye

H40.3- Glaucoma <u>secondary to eye trauma</u>
Code also underlying condition
One of the following 7th characters is to be assigned to code H40.3- to designate the stage of glaucoma:
  0   Stage unspecified
  1   Mild stage
  2   Moderate stage
  3   Severe stage
  4   Indeterminate stage

H40.30x- Glaucoma secondary to eye trauma, <u>unspecified</u> eye

H40.31x- Glaucoma secondary to eye trauma, <u>right</u> eye

H40.32x- Glaucoma secondary to eye trauma, <u>left</u> eye

H40.33x- Glaucoma secondary to eye trauma, <u>bilateral</u>

H40.4- Glaucoma <u>secondary to eye inflammation</u>
Code also underlying condition
One of the following 7th characters is to be assigned to code H40.4- to designate the stage of glaucoma:
  0   Stage unspecified
  1   Mild stage
  2   Moderate stage
  3   Severe stage
  4   Indeterminate stage

H40.40x- Glaucoma secondary to eye inflammation, <u>unspecified</u> eye

H40.41x- Glaucoma secondary to eye inflammation, <u>right</u> eye

H40.42x- Glaucoma secondary to eye inflammation, <u>left</u> eye

H40.43x- Glaucoma secondary to eye inflammation, <u>bilateral</u>

H40.5- Glaucoma <u>secondary to other eye disorders</u>
Code also underlying eye disorder
One of the following 7th characters is to be assigned to code H40.5- to designate the stage of glaucoma:
  0   Stage unspecified
  1   Mild stage
  2   Moderate stage
  3   Severe stage
  4   Indeterminate stage

H40.50x- Glaucoma secondary to other eye disorders, <u>unspecified</u> eye

H40.51x- Glaucoma secondary to other eye disorders, <u>right</u> eye

H40.52x- Glaucoma secondary to other eye disorders, <u>left</u> eye

H40.53x- Glaucoma secondary to other eye disorders, <u>bilateral</u>

H40.6- Glaucoma <u>secondary to drugs</u>
Use additional code for adverse effect, if applicable, to identify drug (T36-T50 with fifth or sixth character 5)
One of the following 7th characters is to be assigned to code H40.6- to designate the stage of glaucoma:
  0   Stage unspecified
  1   Mild stage
  2   Moderate stage
  3   Severe stage
  4   Indeterminate stage

H40.60x- Glaucoma secondary to drugs, <u>unspecified</u> eye

H40.61x- Glaucoma secondary to drugs, <u>right</u> eye

H40.62x- Glaucoma secondary to drugs, <u>left</u> eye

H40.63x- Glaucoma secondary to drugs, <u>bilateral</u>

H40.8- <u>Other</u> glaucoma

H40.81- Glaucoma <u>with increased episcleral venous pressure</u> — A form due to increased venous pressure of the scleral vessels.

H40.811 Glaucoma with increased episcleral venous pressure, <u>right</u> eye

H40.812 Glaucoma with increased episcleral venous pressure, <u>left</u> eye

H40.813 Glaucoma with increased episcleral venous pressure, <u>bilateral</u>

H40.819 Glaucoma with increased episcleral venous pressure, <u>unspecified</u> eye

H40.82- <u>Hypersecretion</u> glaucoma — A form due to increased production of aqueous.

H40.821 Hypersecretion glaucoma, <u>right</u> eye

H40.822 Hypersecretion glaucoma, <u>left</u> eye

H40 - H40

H40.823   Hypersecretion glaucoma, _bilateral_

H40.829   Hypersecretion glaucoma, _unspecified_ eye

H40.83- _Aqueous misdirection_ — An abnormal increase in intraocular pressure caused by the flow of aqueous back into the central cavity of eye, rather than forward.

   Malignant glaucoma

H40.831   Aqueous misdirection, _right_ eye

H40.832   Aqueous misdirection, _left_ eye

H40.833   Aqueous misdirection, _bilateral_

H40.839   Aqueous misdirection, _unspecified_ eye

H40.89   Other specified glaucoma

H40.9   Unspecified glaucoma

H42   Glaucoma _in diseases classified elsewhere_ — [Not Allowed as PDX]
   Code first underlying condition, such as:
      Amyloidosis (E85.-)
      Aniridia (Q13.1)
      Lowe's syndrome (E72.03)
      Reiger's anomaly (Q13.81)
      Specified metabolic disorder (E70-E88)
   Excludes 1:   glaucoma (in) onchocerciasis (B73.02)
      glaucoma (in) syphilis (A52.71)
      glaucoma (in) tuberculous (A18.59)
   Excludes ❷: glaucoma (in) diabetes mellitus (E08.39, E09.39, E10.39, E11.39, E13.39)

Disorders of vitreous body and globe (H43-H44)

H43-   _Disorders of vitreous body_

H43.0-   Vitreous _prolapse_ — The downward displacement of the vitreous body.
   Excludes 1:   vitreous syndrome following cataract surgery (H59.0-)
      traumatic vitreous prolapse (S05.2-)

H43.00   Vitreous prolapse, _unspecified_ eye

H43.01   Vitreous prolapse, _right_ eye

H43.02   Vitreous prolapse, _left_ eye

H43.03   Vitreous prolapse, _bilateral_

H43.1-   Vitreous _hemorrhage_ — The abnormal escape of blood into the vitreous.

H43.10   Vitreous hemorrhage, _unspecified_ eye

H43.11   Vitreous hemorrhage, _right_ eye

H43.12   Vitreous hemorrhage, _left_ eye

H43.13   Vitreous hemorrhage, _bilateral_

H43.2-   _Crystalline deposits_ in vitreous body — The deposition of angular solids within the vitreous.

H43.20   Crystalline deposits in vitreous body, _unspecified_ eye

H43.21   Crystalline deposits in vitreous body, _right_ eye

H43.22   Crystalline deposits in vitreous body, _left_ eye

H43.23   Crystalline deposits in vitreous body, _bilateral_

H43.3-   Other vitreous opacities

H43.31- _Vitreous membranes and strands_ — The formation of abnormal vitreous membranes or strands of tissue.

H43.311   Vitreous membranes and strands, _right_ eye

H43.312   Vitreous membranes and strands, _left_ eye

H43.313   Vitreous membranes and strands, _bilateral_

H43.319   Vitreous membranes and strands, _unspecified_ eye

H43.39- _Other_ vitreous _opacities_
   Vitreous floaters — Small particles of proteins or cells which float in the vitreous body.

H43.391   Other vitreous opacities, _right_ eye

H43.392   Other vitreous opacities, _left_ eye

H43.393   Other vitreous opacities, _bilateral_

H43.399   Other vitreous opacities, _unspecified_ eye

H43.8-   Other disorders of vitreous body
   Excludes 1:   proliferative vitreo-retinopathy with retinal detachment (H33.4-)
   Excludes ❷: vitreous abscess (H44.02-)

H43.81- _Vitreous degeneration_ — Deterioration of vitreous and its functional ability.
   Vitreous detachment — A form marked by separation of lining membrane from the retina.

H43.811   Vitreous degeneration, _right_ eye

H43.812   Vitreous degeneration, _left_ eye

H43.813   Vitreous degeneration, _bilateral_

H43.819   Vitreous degeneration, _unspecified_ eye

H43.82- _Vitreomacular adhesion_ — The abnormal persistent attachment of the membrane separating the vitreous gel and the macula (which normally separates during the aging process) that may result in retinal deformity or damage and cause visual impairment.
   Vitreomacular traction

H43.821   Vitreomacular adhesion, _right_ eye — [Age/15-124]

H43.822   Vitreomacular adhesion, _left_ eye — [Age/15-124]

H43.823   Vitreomacular adhesion, _bilateral_ — [Age/15-124]

H43.829   Vitreomacular adhesion, _unspecified_ eye — [Age/15-124]

H43.89   Other disorders of vitreous body

H43.9   Unspecified disorder of vitreous body

H44-   _Disorders of globe_
   Includes: Disorders affecting multiple structures of eye

H44.0-   _Purulent endophthalmitis_ — A pus-producing inflammation of the ocular cavities.
   Use additional code to identify organism
   Excludes 1:   bleb associated endophthalmitis (H59.4-)

H44.00- _Unspecified_ purulent endophthalmitis

cc **H44.001   Unspecified purulent endophthalmitis, _right_ eye**

cc **H44.002   Unspecified purulent endophthalmitis, _left_ eye**

cc **H44.003   Unspecified purulent endophthalmitis, _bilateral_**

cc **H44.009   Unspecified purulent endophthalmitis, _unspecified_ eye**

H44.01- _Panophthalmitis_ (acute) — Inflammation of all of the structures or tissues of the eye.

cc **H44.011   Panophthalmitis (acute), _right_ eye**

cc **H44.012   Panophthalmitis (acute), _left_ eye**

cc **H44.013   Panophthalmitis (acute), _bilateral_**

cc **H44.019   Panophthalmitis (acute), _unspecified_ eye**

H44.02- _Vitreous abscess_ (chronic) — A localized collection of pus caused by the disintegration of vitreous tissues.

cc **H44.021   Vitreous abscess (chronic), _right_ eye**

cc **H44.022   Vitreous abscess (chronic), _left_ eye**

cc **H44.023   Vitreous abscess (chronic), _bilateral_**

cc **H44.029   Vitreous abscess (chronic), _unspecified_ eye**

H44.1-   _Other_ endophthalmitis
   Excludes 1:   bleb associated endophthalmitis (H59.4-)
   Excludes ❷: ophthalmia nodosa (H16.2-)

H44.11- _Panuveitis_ — Inflammation of the entire uveal tract.

cc **H44.111   Panuveitis, _right_ eye**

cc **H44.112   Panuveitis, _left_ eye**

cc **H44.113   Panuveitis, _bilateral_**

cc **H44.119   Panuveitis, _unspecified_ eye**

H44.12- _Parasitic endophthalmitis_, unspecified

cc **H44.121   Parasitic endophthalmitis, unspecified, _right_ eye**

cc **H44.122   Parasitic endophthalmitis, unspecified, _left_ eye**

cc **H44.123   Parasitic endophthalmitis, unspecified, _bilateral_**

cc **H44.129   Parasitic endophthalmitis, unspecified, _unspecified_ eye**

H44.13- _Sympathetic uveitis_ — Granulomatous inflammation of the uveal tract.

cc **H44.131   Sympathetic uveitis, _right_ eye**

cc **H44.132   Sympathetic uveitis, _left_ eye**

cc **H44.133   Sympathetic uveitis, _bilateral_**

cc **H44.139   Sympathetic uveitis, _unspecified_ eye**

cc **H44.19   Other endophthalmitis**

H44.2-   _Degenerative myopia_ — Progressive nearsightedness leading to retinal detachment and blindness.
   Malignant myopia

H44.20   Degenerative myopia, _unspecified_ eye

H44.21   Degenerative myopia, _right_ eye

H44.22   Degenerative myopia, _left_ eye

H44.23   Degenerative myopia, _bilateral_

H44.3-   Other and unspecified degenerative disorders of globe

H44.30   Unspecified degenerative disorder of globe

H44.31- _Chalcosis_ — The abnormal presence of copper in the globe.

H40 | H44

H44.311 Chalcosis, __right__ eye
H44.312 Chalcosis, __left__ eye
H44.313 Chalcosis, __bilateral__
H44.319 Chalcosis, __unspecified__ eye

H44.32- __Siderosis__ of eye — The abnormal deposit of iron in the conjunctiva marked by a rust-brown or yellowish discoloration.
H44.321 Siderosis of eye, __right__ eye
H44.322 Siderosis of eye, __left__ eye
H44.323 Siderosis of eye, __bilateral__
H44.329 Siderosis of eye, __unspecified__ eye

H44.39- __Other__ degenerative disorders of globe
H44.391 Other degenerative disorders of globe, __right__ eye
H44.392 Other degenerative disorders of globe, __left__ eye
H44.393 Other degenerative disorders of globe, __bilateral__
H44.399 Other degenerative disorders of globe, __unspecified__ eye

H44.4- __Hypotony__ of eye — Low intraocular pressure.
H44.40 __Unspecified__ hypotony of eye
H44.41- __Flat anterior chamber__ hypotony of eye — A condition characterized by loss of intraocular fluid within the anterior chamber resulting in compression of the chamber from surrounding tissues.
H44.411 Flat anterior chamber hypotony of __right__ eye
H44.412 Flat anterior chamber hypotony of __left__ eye
H44.413 Flat anterior chamber hypotony of eye, __bilateral__
H44.419 Flat anterior chamber hypotony of __unspecified__ eye

H44.42- Hypotony of eye __due to ocular fistula__ — An abnormal passage for the intraocular cavities resulting in decreased intraocular pressure.
H44.421 Hypotony of __right__ eye due to ocular fistula
H44.422 Hypotony of __left__ eye due to ocular fistula
H44.423 Hypotony of eye due to ocular fistula, __bilateral__
H44.429 Hypotony of __unspecified__ eye due to ocular fistula

H44.43- Hypotony of eye __due to other ocular disorders__
H44.431 Hypotony of eye due to other ocular disorders, __right__ eye
H44.432 Hypotony of eye due to other ocular disorders, __left__ eye
H44.433 Hypotony of eye due to other ocular disorders, __bilateral__
H44.439 Hypotony of eye due to other ocular disorders, __unspecified__ eye

H44.44- __Primary__ hypotony of eye — Low intraocular pressure without a determinate cause.
H44.441 Primary hypotony of __right__ eye
H44.442 Primary hypotony of __left__ eye
H44.443 Primary hypotony of eye, __bilateral__
H44.449 Primary hypotony of __unspecified__ eye

H44.5- __Degenerated conditions of globe__
H44.50 __Unspecified__ degenerated conditions of globe
H44.51- __Absolute glaucoma__ — The final stage of glaucoma characterized by pain in the eye and blindness.
H44.511 Absolute glaucoma, __right__ eye
H44.512 Absolute glaucoma, __left__ eye
H44.513 Absolute glaucoma, __bilateral__
H44.519 Absolute glaucoma, __unspecified__ eye

H44.52- __Atrophy__ of globe — A wasting-away of the globe tissues.
Phthisis bulbi
H44.521 Atrophy of globe, __right__ eye
H44.522 Atrophy of globe, __left__ eye
H44.523 Atrophy of globe, __bilateral__
H44.529 Atrophy of globe, __unspecified__ eye

H44.53- __Leucocoria__ — A reflection from the pupil due to the presence of a whitish mass in the pupillary area of the eye.
H44.531 Leucocoria, __right__ eye
H44.532 Leucocoria, __left__ eye
H44.533 Leucocoria, __bilateral__
H44.539 Leucocoria, __unspecified__ eye

H44.6- __Retained (old) intraocular foreign body, magnetic__ — The existing, noncurrent presence of a nonocular tissue particle that contains iron (or other magnetic elements), and is located within the intraocular tissues.
Use additional code to identify magnetic foreign body (Z18.11)
Excludes 1: *current intraocular foreign body (S05.-)*
Excludes ❷: *retained foreign body in eyelid (H02.81-)*
retained (old) foreign body following penetrating wound of orbit (H05.5-)
retained (old) intraocular foreign body, nonmagnetic (H44.7-)

H44.60- __Unspecified__ retained (old) intraocular foreign body, __magnetic__
H44.601 Unspecified retained (old) intraocular foreign body, magnetic, __right__ eye
H44.602 Unspecified retained (old) intraocular foreign body, magnetic, __left__ eye
H44.603 Unspecified retained (old) intraocular foreign body, magnetic, __bilateral__
H44.609 Unspecified retained (old) intraocular foreign body, magnetic, __unspecified__ eye

H44.61- Retained (old) __magnetic__ foreign body __in anterior chamber__
H44.611 Retained (old) magnetic foreign body in anterior chamber, __right__ eye
H44.612 Retained (old) magnetic foreign body in anterior chamber, __left__ eye
H44.613 Retained (old) magnetic foreign body in anterior chamber, __bilateral__
H44.619 Retained (old) magnetic foreign body in anterior chamber, __unspecified__ eye

H44.62- Retained (old) __magnetic__ foreign body __in iris or ciliary body__
H44.621 Retained (old) magnetic foreign body in iris or ciliary body, __right__ eye
H44.622 Retained (old) magnetic foreign body in iris or ciliary body, __left__ eye
H44.623 Retained (old) magnetic foreign body in iris or ciliary body, __bilateral__
H44.629 Retained (old) magnetic foreign body in iris or ciliary body, __unspecified__ eye

H44.63- Retained (old) __magnetic__ foreign body __in lens__
H44.631 Retained (old) magnetic foreign body in lens, __right__ eye
H44.632 Retained (old) magnetic foreign body in lens, __left__ eye
H44.633 Retained (old) magnetic foreign body in lens, __bilateral__
H44.639 Retained (old) magnetic foreign body in lens, __unspecified__ eye

H44.64- Retained (old) __magnetic__ foreign body __in posterior wall of globe__
H44.641 Retained (old) magnetic foreign body in posterior wall of globe, __right__ eye
H44.642 Retained (old) magnetic foreign body in posterior wall of globe, __left__ eye
H44.643 Retained (old) magnetic foreign body in posterior wall of globe, __bilateral__
H44.649 Retained (old) magnetic foreign body in posterior wall of globe, __unspecified__ eye

H44.65- Retained (old) __magnetic__ foreign body __in vitreous body__
H44.651 Retained (old) magnetic foreign body in vitreous body, __right__ eye
H44.652 Retained (old) magnetic foreign body in vitreous body, __left__ eye
H44.653 Retained (old) magnetic foreign body in vitreous body, __bilateral__
H44.659 Retained (old) magnetic foreign body in vitreous body, __unspecified__ eye

H44 - H44

H44.69- Retained (old) intraocular foreign body, <u>magnetic, in other or multiple sites</u>

H44.691 Retained (old) intraocular foreign body, magnetic, in other or multiple sites, <u>right</u> eye

H44.692 Retained (old) intraocular foreign body, magnetic, in other or multiple sites, <u>left</u> eye

H44.693 Retained (old) intraocular foreign body, magnetic, in other or multiple sites, <u>bilateral</u>

H44.699 Retained (old) intraocular foreign body, magnetic, in other or multiple sites, <u>unspecified</u> eye

H44.7- <u>Retained (old) intraocular foreign body, nonmagnetic</u> — The existing, noncurrent presence of a nonocular tissue particle or mass that contains no iron (or other magnetic elements), and is located within the intraocular tissues.
Use additional code to identify nonmagnetic foreign body (Z18.01-Z18.10, Z18.12, Z18.2-Z18.9)

Excludes 1:   *current intraocular foreign body (S05.-)*
Excludes ❷: *retained foreign body in eyelid (H02.81-)*
          retained (old) foreign body following penetrating wound of orbit (H05.5-)
          retained (old) intraocular foreign body, magnetic (H44.6-)

H44.70- <u>Unspecified</u> retained (old) intraocular foreign body, <u>nonmagnetic</u>

H44.701 Unspecified retained (old) intraocular foreign body, nonmagnetic, <u>right</u> eye

H44.702 Unspecified retained (old) intraocular foreign body, nonmagnetic, <u>left</u> eye

H44.703 Unspecified retained (old) intraocular foreign body, nonmagnetic, <u>bilateral</u>

H44.709 Unspecified retained (old) intraocular foreign body, nonmagnetic, <u>unspecified</u> eye
Retained (old) intraocular foreign body NOS

H44.71- Retained (<u>nonmagnetic</u>) (old) foreign body <u>in anterior chamber</u>

H44.711 Retained (nonmagnetic) (old) foreign body in anterior chamber, <u>right</u> eye

H44.712 Retained (nonmagnetic) (old) foreign body in anterior chamber, <u>left</u> eye

H44.713 Retained (nonmagnetic) (old) foreign body in anterior chamber, <u>bilateral</u>

H44.719 Retained (nonmagnetic) (old) foreign body in anterior chamber, <u>unspecified</u> eye

H44.72- Retained (<u>nonmagnetic</u>) (old) foreign body <u>in iris or ciliary body</u>

H44.721 Retained (nonmagnetic) (old) foreign body in iris or ciliary body, <u>right</u> eye

H44.722 Retained (nonmagnetic) (old) foreign body in iris or ciliary body, <u>left</u> eye

H44.723 Retained (nonmagnetic) (old) foreign body in iris or ciliary body, <u>bilateral</u>

H44.729 Retained (nonmagnetic) (old) foreign body in iris or ciliary body, <u>unspecified</u> eye

H44.73- Retained (<u>nonmagnetic</u>) (old) foreign body <u>in lens</u>

H44.731 Retained (nonmagnetic) (old) foreign body in lens, <u>right</u> eye

H44.732 Retained (nonmagnetic) (old) foreign body in lens, <u>left</u> eye

H44.733 Retained (nonmagnetic) (old) foreign body in lens, <u>bilateral</u>

H44.739 Retained (nonmagnetic) (old) foreign body in lens, <u>unspecified</u> eye

H44.74- Retained (<u>nonmagnetic</u>) (old) foreign body <u>in posterior wall of globe</u>

H44.741 Retained (nonmagnetic) (old) foreign body in posterior wall of globe, <u>right</u> eye

H44.742 Retained (nonmagnetic) (old) foreign body in posterior wall of globe, <u>left</u> eye

H44.743 Retained (nonmagnetic) (old) foreign body in posterior wall of globe, <u>bilateral</u>

H44.749 Retained (nonmagnetic) (old) foreign body in posterior wall of globe, <u>unspecified</u> eye

H44.75- Retained (<u>nonmagnetic</u>) (old) foreign body <u>in vitreous body</u>

H44.751 Retained (nonmagnetic) (old) foreign body in vitreous body, <u>right</u> eye

H44.752 Retained (nonmagnetic) (old) foreign body in vitreous body, <u>left</u> eye

H44.753 Retained (nonmagnetic) (old) foreign body in vitreous body, <u>bilateral</u>

H44.759 Retained (nonmagnetic) (old) foreign body in vitreous body, <u>unspecified</u> eye

H44.79- Retained (old) intraocular foreign body, <u>nonmagnetic, in other or multiple sites</u>

H44.791 Retained (old) intraocular foreign body, nonmagnetic, in other or multiple sites, <u>right</u> eye

H44.792 Retained (old) intraocular foreign body, nonmagnetic, in other or multiple sites, <u>left</u> eye

H44.793 Retained (old) intraocular foreign body, nonmagnetic, in other or multiple sites, <u>bilateral</u>

H44.799 Retained (old) intraocular foreign body, nonmagnetic, in other or multiple sites, <u>unspecified</u> eye

H44.8- Other disorders of globe

H44.81- <u>Hemophthalmos</u> — Diffusion of blood into the eyeball.

H44.811 Hemophthalmos, <u>right</u> eye

H44.812 Hemophthalmos, <u>left</u> eye

H44.813 Hemophthalmos, <u>bilateral</u>

H44.819 Hemophthalmos, <u>unspecified</u> eye

H44.82- <u>Luxation</u> of globe — The abnormal dislocation or displacement of the globe and its tissues.

H44.821 Luxation of globe, <u>right</u> eye

H44.822 Luxation of globe, <u>left</u> eye

H44.823 Luxation of globe, <u>bilateral</u>

H44.829 Luxation of globe, <u>unspecified</u> eye

H44.89 Other disorders of globe

H44.9 Unspecified disorder of globe

Disorders of optic nerve and visual pathways (H46-H47)

H46- <u>Optic neuritis</u> — Inflammation of the optic nerve within the eyeball.
Excludes ❷: *ischemic optic neuropathy (H47.01-)*
          neuromyelitis optica [Devic] (G36.0)

H46.0- <u>Optic papillitis</u> — Inflammation of the optic disc.

cc **H46.00** Optic papillitis, <u>unspecified</u> eye

cc **H46.01** Optic papillitis, <u>right</u> eye

cc **H46.02** Optic papillitis, <u>left</u> eye

cc **H46.03** Optic papillitis, <u>bilateral</u>

H46.1- <u>Retrobulbar neuritis</u> — The sudden, severe onset of inflammation of that portion of the optic nerve which is behind the eyeball.
Retrobulbar neuritis NOS
Excludes 1:   *syphilitic retrobulbar neuritis (A52.15)*

cc **H46.10** Retrobulbar neuritis, <u>unspecified</u> eye

cc **H46.11** Retrobulbar neuritis, <u>right</u> eye

cc **H46.12** Retrobulbar neuritis, <u>left</u> eye

cc **H46.13** Retrobulbar neuritis, <u>bilateral</u>

H46.2 Nutritional optic neuropathy — A disorder of the optic nerve due to a defect in nutrition.

H46.3 Toxic optic neuropathy — A disorder of the optic nerve due to the toxic effect of substances.
Code first (T51-T65) to identify cause

cc **H46.8** Other optic neuritis

cc **H46.9** Unspecified optic neuritis

H47- Other disorders of optic [2nd] nerve and visual pathways

H47.0- Disorders of optic nerve, not elsewhere classified

H47.01- <u>Ischemic optic neuropathy</u> — A disorder of the optic nerve due to a deficient blood supply.

H47.011 Ischemic optic neuropathy, <u>right</u> eye

H47.012 Ischemic optic neuropathy, <u>left</u> eye

H47.013 Ischemic optic neuropathy, <u>bilateral</u>

H44-H47

H47.019   Ischemic optic neuropathy, <u>unspecified</u> eye

H47.02- <u>Hemorrhage</u> in optic nerve sheath — The escape of blood within the covering of the optic nerve.

H47.021   Hemorrhage in optic nerve sheath, <u>right</u> eye

H47.022   Hemorrhage in optic nerve sheath, <u>left</u> eye

H47.023   Hemorrhage in optic nerve sheath, <u>bilateral</u>

H47.029   Hemorrhage in optic nerve sheath, <u>unspecified</u> eye

H47.03- Optic nerve <u>hypoplasia</u> — The congenital condition of underdevelopment of one or both optic nerves that results in varying degrees of vision loss.

H47.031   Optic nerve hypoplasia, <u>right</u> eye

H47.032   Optic nerve hypoplasia, <u>left</u> eye

H47.033   Optic nerve hypoplasia, <u>bilateral</u>

H47.039   Optic nerve hypoplasia, <u>unspecified</u> eye

H47.09- <u>Other disorders of optic nerve, not elsewhere classified</u>
Compression of optic nerve — The forced pressure upon the optic nerve.

H47.091   Other disorders of optic nerve, not elsewhere classified, <u>right</u> eye

H47.092   Other disorders of optic nerve, not elsewhere classified, <u>left</u> eye

H47.093   Other disorders of optic nerve, not elsewhere classified, <u>bilateral</u>

H47.099   Other disorders of optic nerve, not elsewhere classified, <u>unspecified</u> eye

H47.1- <u>Papilledema</u> — The abnormal accumulation of intercellular fluid of the optic nerve within the eyeball.

cc **H47.10   Unspecified papilledema**

cc **H47.11   Papilledema associated with increased intracranial pressure**

H47.12   Papilledema associated with decreased ocular pressure

H47.13   Papilledema associated with retinal disorder

H47.14- <u>Foster-Kennedy syndrome</u> — A form associated with optic neuritis and optic atrophy.

H47.141   Foster-Kennedy syndrome, <u>right</u> eye

H47.142   Foster-Kennedy syndrome, <u>left</u> eye

H47.143   Foster-Kennedy syndrome, <u>bilateral</u>

H47.149   Foster-Kennedy syndrome, <u>unspecified</u> eye

H47.2- <u>Optic atrophy</u> — The abnormal wasting-away of the optic nerve within the eyeball.

H47.20   <u>Unspecified</u> optic atrophy

H47.21- <u>Primary</u> optic atrophy — A form resulting from a condition of the optic nerve.

H47.211   Primary optic atrophy, <u>right</u> eye

H47.212   Primary optic atrophy, <u>left</u> eye

H47.213   Primary optic atrophy, <u>bilateral</u>

H47.219   Primary optic atrophy, <u>unspecified</u> eye

H47.22   <u>Hereditary</u> optic atrophy — A form inherited from one's parents.
Leber's optic atrophy — A form marked by progressive optic atrophy, with onset usually in males in their twenties.

H47.23- <u>Glaucomatous</u> optic atrophy — A form resulting from the continuous effects of glaucoma upon the optic disc.

H47.231   Glaucomatous optic atrophy, <u>right</u> eye

H47.232   Glaucomatous optic atrophy, <u>left</u> eye

H47.233   Glaucomatous optic atrophy, <u>bilateral</u>

H47.239   Glaucomatous optic atrophy, <u>unspecified</u> eye

H47.29- <u>Other</u> optic atrophy
Temporal pallor of optic disc — A form affecting only a portion of the optic disc.

H47.291   Other optic atrophy, <u>right</u> eye

H47.292   Other optic atrophy, <u>left</u> eye

H47.293   Other optic atrophy, <u>bilateral</u>

H47.299   Other optic atrophy, <u>unspecified</u> eye

H47.3- <u>Other disorders of optic disc</u>

H47.31- <u>Coloboma</u> of optic disc — A defect of the optic disc resulting from a failure of the fetal fissure to close.

H47.311   Coloboma of optic disc, <u>right</u> eye

H47.312   Coloboma of optic disc, <u>left</u> eye

H47.313   Coloboma of optic disc, <u>bilateral</u>

H47.319   Coloboma of optic disc, <u>unspecified</u> eye

H47.32- <u>Drusen</u> of optic disc — The whitish, hyaline lesions of the optic disc.

H47.321   Drusen of optic disc, <u>right</u> eye

H47.322   Drusen of optic disc, <u>left</u> eye

H47.323   Drusen of optic disc, <u>bilateral</u>

H47.329   Drusen of optic disc, <u>unspecified</u> eye

H47.33- <u>Pseudopapilledema</u> of optic disc — The abnormal elevation of the optic disc.

H47.331   Pseudopapilledema of optic disc, <u>right</u> eye

H47.332   Pseudopapilledema of optic disc, <u>left</u> eye

H47.333   Pseudopapilledema of optic disc, <u>bilateral</u>

H47.339   Pseudopapilledema of optic disc, <u>unspecified</u> eye

H47.39- <u>Other</u> disorders of optic disc

H47.391   Other disorders of optic disc, <u>right</u> eye

H47.392   Other disorders of optic disc, <u>left</u> eye

H47.393   Other disorders of optic disc, <u>bilateral</u>

H47.399   Other disorders of optic disc, <u>unspecified</u> eye

H47.4- <u>Disorders of optic chiasm</u> — Conditions resulting from effects upon the crossing of the optic nerves.
Code also underlying condition

cc **H47.41   Disorders of optic chiasm in (due to) inflammatory disorders**

cc **H47.42   Disorders of optic chiasm in (due to) neoplasm**

cc **H47.43   Disorders of optic chiasm in (due to) vascular disorders**

cc **H47.49   Disorders of optic chiasm in (due to) other disorders**

H47.5- <u>Disorders of other visual pathways</u> — Conditions resulting from disturbances of the optic nerve other than the optic chiasm.
Disorders of optic tracts, geniculate nuclei and optic radiations
Code also underlying condition

H47.51- Disorders of visual pathways <u>in (due to) inflammatory disorders</u>

cc **H47.511   Disorders of visual pathways in (due to) inflammatory disorders, <u>right</u> side**

cc **H47.512   Disorders of visual pathways in (due to) inflammatory disorders, <u>left</u> side**

cc **H47.519   Disorders of visual pathways in (due to) inflammatory disorders, <u>unspecified</u> side**

H47.52- Disorders of visual pathways <u>in (due to) neoplasm</u>

cc **H47.521   Disorders of visual pathways in (due to) neoplasm, <u>right</u> side**

cc **H47.522   Disorders of visual pathways in (due to) neoplasm, <u>left</u> side**

cc **H47.529   Disorders of visual pathways in (due to) neoplasm, <u>unspecified</u> side**

H47.53- Disorders of visual pathways <u>in (due to) vascular disorders</u>

cc **H47.531   Disorders of visual pathways in (due to) vascular disorders, <u>right</u> side**

cc **H47.532   Disorders of visual pathways in (due to) vascular disorders, <u>left</u> side**

cc **H47.539   Disorders of visual pathways in (due to) vascular disorders, <u>unspecified</u> side**

H47.6- <u>Disorders of visual cortex</u> — Conditions resulting from disturbances of the visual centers of the brain.
Code also underlying condition
Excludes 1:   injury to visual cortex S04.04

H47.61- <u>Cortical blindness</u> — Blindness resulting from a lesion of the visual area of the cerebral cortex.

H47.611   Cortical blindness, <u>right</u> side of brain

H47.612   Cortical blindness, <u>left</u> side of brain

H47.619   Cortical blindness, <u>unspecified</u> side of brain

H47.62- Disorders of visual cortex <u>in (due to) inflammatory disorders</u>

cc **H47.621   Disorders of visual cortex in (due to) inflammatory disorders, <u>right</u> side of brain**

cc **H47.622   Disorders of visual cortex in (due to) inflammatory disorders, <u>left</u> side of brain**

H47-H47

CC **H47.629** Disorders of visual cortex in (due to) inflammatory disorders, <u>unspecified</u> side of brain

H47.63- Disorders of visual cortex <u>in (due to) neoplasm</u>

CC **H47.631** Disorders of visual cortex in (due to) neoplasm, <u>right</u> side of brain

CC **H47.632** Disorders of visual cortex in (due to) neoplasm, <u>left</u> side of brain

CC **H47.639** Disorders of visual cortex in (due to) neoplasm, <u>unspecified</u> side of brain

H47.64- Disorders of visual cortex <u>in (due to) vascular disorders</u>

CC **H47.641** Disorders of visual cortex in (due to) vascular disorders, <u>right</u> side of brain

CC **H47.642** Disorders of visual cortex in (due to) vascular disorders, <u>left</u> side of brain

CC **H47.649** Disorders of visual cortex in (due to) vascular disorders, <u>unspecified</u> side of brain

H47.9   Unspecified disorder of visual pathways

Disorders of ocular muscles, binocular movement, accommodation and refraction (H49-H52)

Excludes ❷: nystagmus and other irregular eye movements (H55)

H49- <u>Paralytic strabismus</u> — Deviation due to paralysis of an extraocular muscle.

Excludes ❷: internal ophthalmoplegia (H52.51-)
internuclear ophthalmoplegia (H51.2-)
progressive supranuclear ophthalmoplegia (G23.1)

H49.0- <u>Third</u> [oculomotor] nerve palsy

H49.00 Third [oculomotor] nerve palsy, <u>unspecified</u> eye

H49.01 Third [oculomotor] nerve palsy, <u>right</u> eye

H49.02 Third [oculomotor] nerve palsy, <u>left</u> eye

H49.03 Third [oculomotor] nerve palsy, <u>bilateral</u>

H49.1- <u>Fourth</u> [trochlear] nerve palsy

H49.10 Fourth [trochlear] nerve palsy, <u>unspecified</u> eye

H49.11 Fourth [trochlear] nerve palsy, <u>right</u> eye

H49.12 Fourth [trochlear] nerve palsy, <u>left</u> eye

H49.13 Fourth [trochlear] nerve palsy, <u>bilateral</u>

H49.2- <u>Sixth</u> [abducent] nerve palsy

H49.20 Sixth [abducent] nerve palsy, <u>unspecified</u> eye

H49.21 Sixth [abducent] nerve palsy, <u>right</u> eye

H49.22 Sixth [abducent] nerve palsy, <u>left</u> eye

H49.23 Sixth [abducent] nerve palsy, <u>bilateral</u>

H49.3- <u>Total</u> (external) ophthalmoplegia — Paralysis of the external and internal ocular muscles.

H49.30 Total (external) ophthalmoplegia, <u>unspecified</u> eye

H49.31 Total (external) ophthalmoplegia, <u>right</u> eye

H49.32 Total (external) ophthalmoplegia, <u>left</u> eye

H49.33 Total (external) ophthalmoplegia, <u>bilateral</u>

H49.4- <u>Progressive</u> external ophthalmoplegia — Paralysis which progresses from one extraocular muscle to another.

Excludes 1: Kearns-Sayre syndrome (H49.81-)

H49.40 Progressive external ophthalmoplegia, <u>unspecified</u> eye

H49.41 Progressive external ophthalmoplegia, <u>right</u> eye

H49.42 Progressive external ophthalmoplegia, <u>left</u> eye

H49.43 Progressive external ophthalmoplegia, <u>bilateral</u>

H49.8- Other paralytic strabismus

H49.81- <u>Kearns-Sayre syndrome</u> — A rare neuromuscular disorder that is characterized by paralysis which progresses from one extraocular muscle to another and is associated with pigmentary retinopathy.

Progressive external ophthalmoplegia with pigmentary retinopathy

Use additional code for other manifestation, such as: Heart block (I45.9)

CC **H49.811** Kearns-Sayre syndrome, <u>right</u> eye

CC **H49.812** Kearns-Sayre syndrome, <u>left</u> eye

CC **H49.813** Kearns-Sayre syndrome, <u>bilateral</u>

CC **H49.819** Kearns-Sayre syndrome, <u>unspecified</u> eye

H49.88- <u>Other</u> paralytic strabismus — Paralysis of the external ocular muscles.

External ophthalmoplegia NOS

H49.881 Other paralytic strabismus, <u>right</u> eye

H49.882 Other paralytic strabismus, <u>left</u> eye

H49.883 Other paralytic strabismus, <u>bilateral</u>

H49.889 Other paralytic strabismus, <u>unspecified</u> eye

H49.9   Unspecified paralytic strabismus

H50- Other strabismus

H50.0- <u>Esotropia</u> — The turning inward of the eyes.

Convergent concomitant strabismus — Esotropia due to faulty insertion of eye muscles.

Excludes 1: intermittent esotropia (H50.31-, H50.32)

H50.00 <u>Unspecified</u> esotropia

H50.01- <u>Monocular</u> esotropia — A form characterized by affecting only one eye.

H50.011 Monocular esotropia, <u>right</u> eye

H50.012 Monocular esotropia, <u>left</u> eye

H50.02- Monocular esotropia <u>with A pattern</u>

H50.021 Monocular esotropia with A pattern, <u>right</u> eye

H50.022 Monocular esotropia with A pattern, <u>left</u> eye

H50.03- Monocular esotropia <u>with V pattern</u>

H50.031 Monocular esotropia with V pattern, <u>right</u> eye

H50.032 Monocular esotropia with V pattern, <u>left</u> eye

H50.04- Monocular esotropia <u>with other noncomitancies</u>

H50.041 Monocular esotropia with other noncomitancies, <u>right</u> eye

H50.042 Monocular esotropia with other noncomitancies, <u>left</u> eye

H50.05 Alternating esotropia — A form characterized by affecting each eye alternately.

H50.06 Alternating esotropia with A pattern

H50.07 Alternating esotropia with V pattern

H50.08 Alternating esotropia with other noncomitancies

H50.1- <u>Exotropia</u> — The turning outward of the eyes.

Divergent concomitant strabismus

Excludes 1: intermittent exotropia (H50.33-, H50.34)

H50.10 <u>Unspecified</u> exotropia

H50.11- <u>Monocular</u> exotropia — A form characterized by affecting only one eye.

H50.111 Monocular exotropia, <u>right</u> eye

H50.112 Monocular exotropia, <u>left</u> eye

H50.12- Monocular exotropia <u>with A pattern</u>

H50.121 Monocular exotropia with A pattern, <u>right</u> eye

H50.122 Monocular exotropia with A pattern, <u>left</u> eye

H50.13- Monocular exotropia <u>with V pattern</u>

H50.131 Monocular exotropia with V pattern, <u>right</u> eye

H50.132 Monocular exotropia with V pattern, <u>left</u> eye

H50.14- Monocular exotropia <u>with other noncomitancies</u>

H50.141 Monocular exotropia with other noncomitancies, <u>right</u> eye

H50.142 Monocular exotropia with other noncomitancies, <u>left</u> eye

H50.15 Alternating exotropia — A form characterized by affecting each eye alternately.

H50.16 Alternating exotropia with A pattern

H50.17 Alternating exotropia with V pattern

H50.18 Alternating exotropia with other noncomitancies

H50.2- <u>Vertical strabismus</u> — Upward deviation of an eye.

Hypertropia

H50.21 Vertical strabismus, <u>right</u> eye

H50.22 Vertical strabismus, <u>left</u> eye

H50.3- <u>Intermittent heterotropia</u> — Deviation of the eyes that occurs at intervals.

H50.30 <u>Unspecified</u> intermittent heterotropia

H50.31- Intermittent <u>monocular</u> esotropia — Inward deviation of one eye occurring at intervals.

H50.311 Intermittent monocular esotropia, <u>right</u> eye

H47-H50

H50.312   Intermittent monocular esotropia, <u>left</u> eye

H50.32   **Intermittent alternating esotropia** — Inward deviation of alternating eyes occurring at intervals.

H50.33-   **Intermittent <u>monocular</u> <u>exotropia</u>** — Outward deviation of one eye occurring at intervals.

H50.331   Intermittent monocular exotropia, <u>right</u> eye

H50.332   Intermittent monocular exotropia, <u>left</u> eye

H50.34   **Intermittent alternating <u>exotropia</u>** — Outward deviation of alternating eyes occurring at intervals.

H50.4-   **Other and unspecified heterotropia**

H50.40   **Unspecified heterotropia**

H50.41-   **<u>Cyclotropia</u>** — Rotational deviation of an eye.

H50.411   **Cyclotropia, right eye**

H50.412   **Cyclotropia, left eye**

H50.42   **Monofixation syndrome** — The mild deviation of an eye, which does not cause diplopia.

H50.43   **Accommodative component in esotropia**

H50.5-   **Heterophoria** — Deviation after visual alignment.

H50.50   **Unspecified heterophoria**

H50.51   **Esophoria** — A form characterized by turning inward.

H50.52   **Exophoria** — A form characterized by turning outward.

H50.53   **Vertical heterophoria** — A form characterized by turning upward.

H50.54   **Cyclophoria** — A form characterized by rotational turning.

H50.55   **Alternating heterophoria** — A form characterized by affecting each eye alternately.

H50.6-   **Mechanical strabismus** — Deviation due to external forces.

H50.60   **Mechanical strabismus, unspecified**

H50.61-   **Brown's sheath syndrome** — A form affecting the extraocular tendon sheaths.

H50.611   **Brown's sheath syndrome, <u>right</u> eye**

H50.612   **Brown's sheath syndrome, <u>left</u> eye**

H50.69   **Other mechanical strabismus**
  Strabismus due to adhesions
  Traumatic limitation of duction of eye muscle

H50.8-   **Other specified strabismus**

H50.81-   **Duane's syndrome** — An inherited syndrome characterized by limitation of abduction and deficient convergence.

H50.811   **Duane's syndrome, <u>right</u> eye**

H50.812   **Duane's syndrome, <u>left</u> eye**

H50.89   **Other specified strabismus**

H50.9   **Unspecified strabismus**

H51-   **Other disorders of binocular movement**

H51.0   **Palsy (spasm) of conjugate gaze**

H51.1-   **Convergence insufficiency and excess**

H51.11   **Convergence insufficiency** — Impairment of convergence.

H51.12   **Convergence excess** — Overcompensation of convergence.

H51.2-   **<u>Internuclear ophthalmoplegia</u>** — Paralysis of extraocular muscles due to a lesion between the nuclei of the motor nerves of the eye.

H51.20   **Internuclear ophthalmoplegia, <u>unspecified</u> eye**

H51.21   **Internuclear ophthalmoplegia, <u>right</u> eye**

H51.22   **Internuclear ophthalmoplegia, <u>left</u> eye**

H51.23   **Internuclear ophthalmoplegia, <u>bilateral</u>**

H51.8   **Other specified disorders of binocular movement**

H51.9   **Unspecified disorder of binocular movement**

H52-   **Disorders of refraction and accommodation** — REFRACTION — The deflection or change of direction of light as it passes through the lens. ACCOMMODATION — The adjustment in the shape and curvature of the lens when looking far away and near.

H52.0-   **<u>Hypermetropia</u>** — An error of refraction in which the focal point is behind the retina causing near objects to be out of focus (farsightedness).

H52.00   **Hypermetropia, <u>unspecified</u> eye**

H52.01   **Hypermetropia, <u>right</u> eye**

H52.02   **Hypermetropia, <u>left</u> eye**

H52.03   **Hypermetropia, <u>bilateral</u>**

H52.1-   **<u>Myopia</u>** — An error of refraction in which the focal point is in front of the retina causing objects far away not to be in focus (nearsightedness).
  Excludes 1:   *degenerative myopia (H44.2-)*

H52.10   **Myopia, <u>unspecified</u> eye**

H52.11   **Myopia, <u>right</u> eye**

H52.12   **Myopia, <u>left</u> eye**

H52.13   **Myopia, <u>bilateral</u>**

H52.2-   **<u>Astigmatism</u>** — An error in refraction in which light is not sharply focused to a point on the retina, but to a diffuse area of the retina.

H52.20-   **<u>Unspecified</u> astigmatism**

H52.201   **Unspecified astigmatism, <u>right</u> eye**

H52.202   **Unspecified astigmatism, <u>left</u> eye**

H52.203   **Unspecified astigmatism, <u>bilateral</u>**

H52.209   **Unspecified astigmatism, <u>unspecified</u> eye**

H52.21-   **<u>Irregular</u> astigmatism** — A form in which the diffuse focus is different from one meridian to the other.

H52.211   **Irregular astigmatism, <u>right</u> eye**

H52.212   **Irregular astigmatism, <u>left</u> eye**

H52.213   **Irregular astigmatism, <u>bilateral</u>**

H52.219   **Irregular astigmatism, <u>unspecified</u> eye**

H52.22-   **<u>Regular</u> astigmatism** — A form in which the diffuse focus is uniform from one meridian to the other.

H52.221   **Regular astigmatism, <u>right</u> eye**

H52.222   **Regular astigmatism, <u>left</u> eye**

H52.223   **Regular astigmatism, <u>bilateral</u>**

H52.229   **Regular astigmatism, <u>unspecified</u> eye**

H52.3-   **Anisometropia and aniseikonia**

H52.31   **Anisometropia** — A condition in which refractive power of the eyes is unequal.

H52.32   **Aniseikonia** — A condition in which the size and shape of the ocular image of one differs from that of the other.

H52.4   **Presbyopia** — A defect of vision in advancing age involving loss of accommodation or recession of near points, due to a loss of elasticity of the crystalline lens.

H52.5-   **<u>Disorders of accommodation</u>** — The adjustment in the shape and curvature of the lens when looking far away and near.

H52.51-   **<u>Internal ophthalmoplegia</u> (complete) (total)** — Paralysis of the internal ocular muscles.

H52.511   **Internal ophthalmoplegia (complete) (total), <u>right</u> eye**

H52.512   **Internal ophthalmoplegia (complete) (total), <u>left</u> eye**

H52.513   **Internal ophthalmoplegia (complete) (total), <u>bilateral</u>**

H52.519   **Internal ophthalmoplegia (complete) (total), <u>unspecified</u> eye**

H52.52-   **<u>Paresis of accommodation</u>** — A loss of accommodation due to a partial or complete paralysis of the ciliary muscle and lens.

H52.521   **Paresis of accommodation, <u>right</u> eye**

H52.522   **Paresis of accommodation, <u>left</u> eye**

H52.523   **Paresis of accommodation, <u>bilateral</u>**

H52.529   **Paresis of accommodation, <u>unspecified</u> eye**

H52.53-   **<u>Spasm</u> of accommodation** — A sudden, involuntary contraction of the ciliary muscles producing excess of accommodation for near objects.

H52.531   **Spasm of accommodation, <u>right</u> eye**

H52.532   **Spasm of accommodation, <u>left</u> eye**

H52.533   **Spasm of accommodation, <u>bilateral</u>**

H52.539   **Spasm of accommodation, <u>unspecified</u> eye**

H52.6   **Other disorders of refraction**

H52.7   **Unspecified disorder of refraction**

Excludes 1: = NOT CODED HERE! (Do not code both)   *Excludes ❷:* = Not Included Here

Visual disturbances and blindness (H53-H54)

H53- Visual disturbances — Impairment of the sense of sight.

H53.0- Amblyopia ex anopsia — Decreased visual acuity (reduction in clarity or sharpness of vision).

> Excludes 1: amblyopia due to vitamin A deficiency (E50.5)

H53.00- Unspecified amblyopia

H53.001 Unspecified amblyopia, right eye

H53.002 Unspecified amblyopia, left eye

H53.003 Unspecified amblyopia, bilateral

H53.009 Unspecified amblyopia, unspecified eye

H53.01- Deprivation amblyopia — A form due to absence of light stimuli.

H53.011 Deprivation amblyopia, right eye

H53.012 Deprivation amblyopia, left eye

H53.013 Deprivation amblyopia, bilateral

H53.019 Deprivation amblyopia, unspecified eye

H53.02- Refractive amblyopia — A form due to the deflection of light.

H53.021 Refractive amblyopia, right eye

H53.022 Refractive amblyopia, left eye

H53.023 Refractive amblyopia, bilateral

H53.029 Refractive amblyopia, unspecified eye

H53.03- Strabismic amblyopia — A form due to suppression of vision in one eye to avoid diplopia.

> Excludes 1: strabismus (H50.-)

H53.031 Strabismic amblyopia, right eye

H53.032 Strabismic amblyopia, left eye

H53.033 Strabismic amblyopia, bilateral

H53.039 Strabismic amblyopia, unspecified eye

H53.04- Amblyopia suspect — Identified significant risk of amblyopia, but without certainty of diagnosis.

H53.041 Amblyopia suspect, right eye

H53.042 Amblyopia suspect, left eye

H53.043 Amblyopia suspect, bilateral

H53.049 Amblyopia suspect, unspecified eye

H53.1- Subjective visual disturbances — Impairment and distortion of sight as perceived by the patient.

> Excludes 1: subjective visual disturbances due to vitamin A deficiency (E50.5)
> visual hallucinations (R44.1)

H53.10 Unspecified subjective visual disturbances

H53.11 Day blindness — Diminished vision in bright light.
   Hemeralopia

H53.12- Transient visual loss — The temporary, complete loss of sight.
   Scintillating scotoma — Diminished vision with a luminous wall-like appearance.

> Excludes 1: amaurosis fugax (G45.3-)
> transient retinal artery occlusion (H34.0-)

CC **H53.121 Transient visual loss, right eye**

CC **H53.122 Transient visual loss, left eye**

CC **H53.123 Transient visual loss, bilateral**

CC **H53.129 Transient visual loss, unspecified eye**

H53.13- Sudden visual loss — The immediate, complete loss of sight.

CC **H53.131 Sudden visual loss, right eye**

CC **H53.132 Sudden visual loss, left eye**

CC **H53.133 Sudden visual loss, bilateral**

CC **H53.139 Sudden visual loss, unspecified eye**

H53.14- Visual discomfort — Uneasiness and lack of comfort of the eyes.
   Asthenopia — Weakness or tiring of the eyes accompanied by pain, headache, and dimness of vision.
   Photophobia — An unusual intolerance of light.

H53.141 Visual discomfort, right eye

H53.142 Visual discomfort, left eye

H53.143 Visual discomfort, bilateral

H53.149 Visual discomfort, unspecified

H53.15 Visual distortions of shape and size
   Metamorphopsia — Visual distortion of an object's size and shape.

H53.16 Psychophysical visual disturbances — Impairment of sight due to emotional stimuli.

H53.19 Other subjective visual disturbances
   Visual halos — The perception of a halo of light around an object.

H53.2 Diplopia — The perception of two images of the same object.
   Double vision

H53.3- Other and unspecified disorders of binocular vision

H53.30 Unspecified disorder of binocular vision

H53.31 Abnormal retinal correspondence

H53.32 Fusion with defective stereopsis

H53.33 Simultaneous visual perception without fusion

H53.34 Suppression of binocular vision

H53.4- Visual field defects

H53.40 Unspecified visual field defects

H53.41- Scotoma involving central area — Diminished vision at the center of the sighted object.
   Central scotoma

H53.411 Scotoma involving central area, right eye

H53.412 Scotoma involving central area, left eye

H53.413 Scotoma involving central area, bilateral

H53.419 Scotoma involving central area, unspecified eye

H53.42- Scotoma of blind spot area — Diminished vision at some area other than the center of the sighted object.
   Enlarged blind spot

H53.421 Scotoma of blind spot area, right eye

H53.422 Scotoma of blind spot area, left eye

H53.423 Scotoma of blind spot area, bilateral

H53.429 Scotoma of blind spot area, unspecified eye

H53.43- Sector or arcuate defects — An arc-shaped diminished vision area of the sighted object.
   Arcuate scotoma
   Bjerrum scotoma

H53.431 Sector or arcuate defects, right eye

H53.432 Sector or arcuate defects, left eye

H53.433 Sector or arcuate defects, bilateral

H53.439 Sector or arcuate defects, unspecified eye

H53.45- Other localized visual field defect — Diminished vision within the visual field.
   Peripheral visual field defect
   Ring scotoma NOS
   Scotoma NOS

H53.451 Other localized visual field defect, right eye

H53.452 Other localized visual field defect, left eye

H53.453 Other localized visual field defect, bilateral

H53.459 Other localized visual field defect, unspecified eye

H53.46- Homonymous bilateral field defects — Defective vision affecting the right and left halves of the eyes' visual field.
   Homonymous hemianopia
   Homonymous hemianopsia
   Quadrant anopia
   Quadrant anopsia

H53.461 Homonymous bilateral field defects, right side

H53.462 Homonymous bilateral field defects, left side

H53.469 Homonymous bilateral field defects, unspecified side
   Homonymous bilateral field defects NOS

H53.47 Heteronymous bilateral field defects — Defective vision affecting the nasal or temporal halves of the eyes' visual field.
   Heteronymous hemianop(s)ia

H53.48- Generalized contraction of visual field

H53.481 Generalized contraction of visual field, right eye

H53.482 Generalized contraction of visual field, left eye

H53.483 Generalized contraction of visual field, bilateral

H53.489 Generalized contraction of visual field, unspecified eye

H53.5- Color vision deficiencies — Impairment of color perception.
   Color blindness

> Excludes 2: day blindness (H53.11)

H53.50 Unspecified color vision deficiencies
   Color blindness NOS

H53.51 Achromatopsia — Inability to differentiate colors.

H53 - H53

Excludes 1: = NOT CODED HERE! (Do not code both)   **705**   Excludes 2: = Not Included Here

H53.52 Acquired color vision deficiency — A form developed after birth and not hereditary.

H53.53 Deuteranomaly — A form characterized by sensory loss of red-green colors without shortened spectrum.
   Deuteranopia

H53.54 Protanomaly — A form characterized by sensory loss of red-green colors with shortened spectrum.
   Protanopia

H53.55 Tritanomaly — A form characterized by sensory loss of blue and yellow colors.
   Tritanopia

H53.59 Other color vision deficiencies

H53.6- Night blindness — Impairment of vision at night or in dim light.
   Excludes 1: *night blindness due to vitamin A deficiency (E50.5)*

H53.60 Unspecified night blindness

H53.61 Abnormal dark adaptation curve — The abnormally slow adjustment from light to darkness.

H53.62 Acquired night blindness — A form developed after birth and not hereditary.

H53.63 Congenital night blindness — A form present at birth.

H53.69 Other night blindness

H53.7- Vision sensitivity deficiencies

H53.71 Glare sensitivity

H53.72 Impaired contrast sensitivity

H53.8 Other visual disturbances

H53.9 Unspecified visual disturbance

H54- Blindness and low vision
   Note: For definition of visual impairment categories see table below
   Code first any associated underlying cause of the blindness
   Excludes 1: *amaurosis fugax (G45.3)*

H54.0 Blindness, both eyes
   Visual impairment categories 3, 4, 5 in both eyes.

H54.1- Blindness, one eye, low vision other eye
   Visual impairment categories 3, 4, 5 in one eye, with categories 1 or 2 in the other eye

H54.10 Blindness, one eye, low vision other eye, unspecified eyes

H54.11 Blindness, right eye, low vision left eye

H54.12 Blindness, left eye, low vision right eye

H54.2 Low vision, both eyes
   Visual impairment categories 1 or 2 in both eyes.

H54.3 Unqualified visual loss, both eyes
   Visual impairment category 9 in both eyes.

H54.4- Blindness, one eye
   Visual impairment categories 3, 4, 5 in one eye [normal vision in other eye]

H54.40 Blindness, one eye, unspecified eye

H54.41 Blindness, right eye, normal vision left eye

H54.42 Blindness, left eye, normal vision right eye

H54.5- Low vision, one eye
   Visual impairment categories 1 or 2 in one eye [normal vision in other eye]

H54.50 Low vision, one eye, unspecified eye

H54.51 Low vision, right eye, normal vision left eye

H54.52 Low vision, left eye, normal vision right eye

H54.6- Unqualified visual loss, one eye
   Visual impairment category 9 in one eye [normal vision in other eye]

H54.60 Unqualified visual loss, one eye, unspecified

H54.61 Unqualified visual loss, right eye, normal vision left eye

H54.62 Unqualified visual loss, left eye, normal vision right eye

H54.7 Unspecified visual loss — [Unacceptable PDX]
   Visual impairment category 9 NOS

H54.8 Legal blindness, as defined in USA
   Blindness NOS according to USA definition
   Excludes 1: *legal blindness with specification of impairment level (H54.0-H54.7)*
   Note: The table below gives a classification of severity of visual impairment recommended by a WHO Study Group on the Prevention of Blindness, Geneva, 6-10 November 1972.
   The term "low vision" in category H54 comprises categories 1 and 2 of the table, the term "blindness" categories 3, 4 and 5, and the term "unqualified visual loss" category 9.
   If the extent of the visual field is taken into account, patients with a field no greater than 10 but greater than 5 around central fixation should be placed in category 3 and patients with a field no greater than 5 around central fixation should be placed in category 4, even if the central acuity is not impaired.

Category of Visual Impairment	Visual Acuity With Best Possible Correction	
	Maximum less than:	Minimum equal to or better than:
1	6/18 3/10 (0.3) 20/70	6/60 1/10 (0.1) 20/200
2	6/60 1/10 (0.1) 20/200	3/60 1/20 (0.5) 20/400
3	3/60 1/20 (0.05) 20/400	1/60 (finger counting at one meter) 1/50 (0.02) 5/300 (20/1200)
4	1/60 (finger counting at one meter) 1/50 (0.02) 5/300	Light perception
5	No light perception	—
9	Undetermined or unspecified	—

Other disorders of eye and adnexa (H55-H57)

H55- Nystagmus and other irregular eye movements

H55.0- Nystagmus — Constant, involuntary eyeball movements.

H55.00 Unspecified nystagmus

H55.01 Congenital nystagmus — A form characterized by presence at birth.

H55.02 Latent nystagmus — A form characterized by occurring only when one eye is covered.

H55.03 Visual deprivation nystagmus — A form characterized by occurring after being in a light-free environment.

H55.04 Dissociated nystagmus — A form characterized by dissimilar movements of both eyes.

H55.09 Other forms of nystagmus

H55.8- Other irregular eye movements

H55.81 Saccadic eye movements

H55.89 Other irregular eye movements

H57- Other disorders of eye and adnexa

H57.0- Anomalies of pupillary function

H57.00 Unspecified anomaly of pupillary function

H57.01 Argyll Robertson pupil, atypical — The absence of the pupillary light reflex, but no decrease in the power of accommodation.
   Excludes 1: *syphilitic Argyll Robertson pupil (A52.19)*

H57.02 Anisocoria — Inequality of the size of pupils (the open circular area formed by the iris).

H57.03 Miosis — The continued, abnormal contraction of the pupil.

H57.04 Mydriasis — The continued, abnormal dilation of the pupil.

H57.05- Tonic pupil — A condition which responds in a slow and delayed manner.

H57.051 Tonic pupil, right eye

H57.052 Tonic pupil, left eye

H57.053 Tonic pupil, bilateral

H57.059 Tonic pupil, unspecified eye

H57.09 Other anomalies of pupillary function

H57.1- Ocular pain

H57.10 Ocular pain, unspecified eye

H57.11 Ocular pain, right eye

H57.12 Ocular pain, left eye

H53 - H57

H57.13   Ocular pain, <u>bilateral</u>
H57.8   Other specified disorders of eye and adnexa
H57.9   Unspecified disorder of eye and adnexa — [Unacceptable PDX]

Intraoperative and postprocedural complications and disorders of eye and adnexa, not elsewhere classified (H59)

H59-   Intraoperative and postprocedural complications and disorders of eye and adnexa, not elsewhere classified

Excludes 1:   *mechanical complication of intraocular lens (T85.2)*
mechanical complication of other ocular prosthetic devices, implants and grafts (T85.3)
pseudophakia (Z96.1)
secondary cataracts (H26.4-)

H59.0-   Disorders of the eye <u>following cataract surgery</u>

H59.01- <u>Keratopathy (bullous aphakic)</u> following cataract surgery
Vitreal corneal syndrome
Vitreous (touch) syndrome

cc H59.011   Keratopathy (bullous aphakic) following cataract surgery, <u>right</u> eye

cc H59.012   Keratopathy (bullous aphakic) following cataract surgery, <u>left</u> eye

cc H59.013   Keratopathy (bullous aphakic) following cataract surgery, <u>bilateral</u>

cc H59.019   Keratopathy (bullous aphakic) following cataract surgery, <u>unspecified</u> eye

H59.02- <u>Cataract (lens) fragments in eye</u> following cataract surgery

H59.021   Cataract (lens) fragments in eye following cataract surgery, <u>right</u> eye

H59.022   Cataract (lens) fragments in eye following cataract surgery, <u>left</u> eye

H59.023   Cataract (lens) fragments in eye following cataract surgery, <u>bilateral</u>

H59.029   Cataract (lens) fragments in eye following cataract surgery, <u>unspecified</u> eye

H59.03- <u>Cystoid macular edema</u> following cataract surgery

cc H59.031   Cystoid macular edema following cataract surgery, <u>right</u> eye

cc H59.032   Cystoid macular edema following cataract surgery, <u>left</u> eye

cc H59.033   Cystoid macular edema following cataract surgery, <u>bilateral</u>

cc H59.039   Cystoid macular edema following cataract surgery, <u>unspecified</u> eye

H59.09- <u>Other disorders of the eye</u> following cataract surgery

cc H59.091   Other disorders of the <u>right</u> eye following cataract surgery

cc H59.092   Other disorders of the <u>left</u> eye following cataract surgery

cc H59.093   Other disorders of the eye following cataract surgery, <u>bilateral</u>

cc H59.099   Other disorders of <u>unspecified</u> eye following cataract surgery

H59.1-   <u>Intraoperative hemorrhage and hematoma of eye and adnexa complicating a procedure</u>

Excludes 1:   *intraoperative hemorrhage and hematoma of eye and adnexa due to accidental puncture or laceration during a procedure (H59.2-)*

H59.11- <u>Intraoperative hemorrhage and hematoma</u> of eye and adnexa complicating <u>an ophthalmic procedure</u>

cc H59.111   Intraoperative hemorrhage and hematoma of <u>right</u> eye and adnexa complicating an ophthalmic procedure

cc H59.112   Intraoperative hemorrhage and hematoma of <u>left</u> eye and adnexa complicating an ophthalmic procedure

cc H59.113   Intraoperative hemorrhage and hematoma of eye and adnexa complicating an ophthalmic procedure, <u>bilateral</u>

cc H59.119   Intraoperative hemorrhage and hematoma of <u>unspecified</u> eye and adnexa complicating an ophthalmic procedure

H59.12- <u>Intraoperative hemorrhage and hematoma</u> of eye and adnexa complicating <u>other procedure</u>

cc H59.121   Intraoperative hemorrhage and hematoma of <u>right</u> eye and adnexa complicating other procedure

cc H59.122   Intraoperative hemorrhage and hematoma of <u>left</u> eye and adnexa complicating other procedure

cc H59.123   Intraoperative hemorrhage and hematoma of eye and adnexa complicating other procedure, <u>bilateral</u>

cc H59.129   Intraoperative hemorrhage and hematoma of <u>unspecified</u> eye and adnexa complicating other procedure

H59.2-   <u>Accidental puncture and laceration</u> of eye and adnexa during a procedure

H59.21- Accidental puncture and laceration of eye and adnexa during an <u>ophthalmic procedure</u>

cc H59.211   Accidental puncture and laceration of <u>right</u> eye and adnexa during an ophthalmic procedure

cc H59.212   Accidental puncture and laceration of <u>left</u> eye and adnexa during an ophthalmic procedure

cc H59.213   Accidental puncture and laceration of eye and adnexa during an ophthalmic procedure, <u>bilateral</u>

cc H59.219   Accidental puncture and laceration of <u>unspecified</u> eye and adnexa during an ophthalmic procedure

H59.22- Accidental puncture and laceration of eye and adnexa during <u>other procedure</u>

cc H59.221   Accidental puncture and laceration of <u>right</u> eye and adnexa during other procedure

cc H59.222   Accidental puncture and laceration of <u>left</u> eye and adnexa during other procedure

cc H59.223   Accidental puncture and laceration of eye and adnexa during other procedure, <u>bilateral</u>

cc H59.229   Accidental puncture and laceration of <u>unspecified</u> eye and adnexa during other procedure

H59.3-   <u>Postprocedural hemorrhage, hematoma and seroma</u> of eye and adnexa following a procedure

H59.31- Postprocedural <u>hemorrhage</u> of eye and adnexa following an <u>ophthalmic procedure</u>

cc H59.311   Postprocedural hemorrhage of <u>right</u> eye and adnexa following an ophthalmic procedure

cc H59.312   Postprocedural hemorrhage of <u>left</u> eye and adnexa following an ophthalmic procedure

cc H59.313   Postprocedural hemorrhage of eye and adnexa following an ophthalmic procedure, <u>bilateral</u>

cc H59.319   Postprocedural hemorrhage of <u>unspecified</u> eye and adnexa following an ophthalmic procedure

H59.32- Postprocedural <u>hemorrhage</u> of eye and adnexa following <u>other procedure</u>

cc H59.321   Postprocedural hemorrhage of <u>right</u> eye and adnexa following other procedure

cc H59.322   Postprocedural hemorrhage of <u>left</u> eye and adnexa following other procedure

cc H59.323   Postprocedural hemorrhage of eye and adnexa following other procedure, <u>bilateral</u>

cc H59.329   Postprocedural hemorrhage of <u>unspecified</u> eye and adnexa following other procedure

H59.33- Postprocedural <u>hematoma</u> of eye and adnexa following an <u>ophthalmic procedure</u>

cc H59.331   Postprocedural hematoma of <u>right</u> eye and adnexa following an ophthalmic procedure

cc H59.332   Postprocedural hematoma of <u>left</u> eye and adnexa following an ophthalmic procedure

cc H59.333   Postprocedural hematoma of eye and adnexa following an ophthalmic procedure, <u>bilateral</u>

cc H59.339   Postprocedural hematoma of <u>unspecified</u> eye and adnexa following an ophthalmic procedure

H59.34- Postprocedural <u>hematoma</u> of eye and adnexa following <u>other procedure</u>

- CC H59.341 Postprocedural hematoma of <u>right</u> eye and adnexa following other procedure
- CC H59.342 Postprocedural hematoma of <u>left</u> eye and adnexa following other procedure
- CC H59.343 Postprocedural hematoma of eye and adnexa following other procedure, <u>bilateral</u>
- CC H59.349 Postprocedural hematoma of <u>unspecified</u> eye and adnexa following other procedure

H59.35- Postprocedural <u>seroma</u> of eye and adnexa following an <u>ophthalmic procedure</u>

- CC H59.351 Postprocedural seroma of <u>right</u> eye and adnexa following an ophthalmic procedure
- CC H59.352 Postprocedural seroma of <u>left</u> eye and adnexa following an ophthalmic procedure
- CC H59.353 Postprocedural seroma of eye and adnexa following an ophthalmic procedure, <u>bilateral</u>
- CC H59.359 Postprocedural seroma of <u>unspecified</u> eye and adnexa following an ophthalmic procedure

H59.36- Postprocedural <u>seroma</u> of eye and adnexa following <u>other procedure</u>

- CC H59.361 Postprocedural seroma of <u>right</u> eye and adnexa following other procedure
- CC H59.362 Postprocedural seroma of <u>left</u> eye and adnexa following other procedure
- CC H59.363 Postprocedural seroma of eye and adnexa following other procedure, <u>bilateral</u>
- CC H59.369 Postprocedural seroma of <u>unspecified</u> eye and adnexa following other procedure

H59.4- Inflammation (infection) of postprocedural bleb
  Postprocedural blebitis
  Excludes 1:   filtering (vitreous) bleb after glaucoma surgery status (Z98.83)

- H59.40 Inflammation (infection) of postprocedural bleb, unspecified
- H59.41 Inflammation (infection) of postprocedural bleb, stage 1
- H59.42 Inflammation (infection) of postprocedural bleb, stage 2
- H59.43 Inflammation (infection) of postprocedural bleb, stage 3
  Bleb endophthalmitis

H59.8- Other intraoperative and postprocedural complications and disorders of eye and adnexa, not elsewhere classified

H59.81- <u>Chorioretinal scars after surgery for detachment</u>

- CC H59.811 Chorioretinal scars after surgery for detachment, <u>right</u> eye
- CC H59.812 Chorioretinal scars after surgery for detachment, <u>left</u> eye
- CC H59.813 Chorioretinal scars after surgery for detachment, <u>bilateral</u>
- CC H59.819 Chorioretinal scars after surgery for detachment, <u>unspecified</u> eye

- CC H59.88 Other intraoperative complications of eye and adnexa, not elsewhere classified
- CC H59.89 Other postprocedural complications and disorders of eye and adnexa, not elsewhere classified

H59 - H59

Chapter 8 – Diseases of the ear and mastoid process (H60-H95)

Note: Use an external cause code following the code for the ear condition, if applicable, to identify the cause of the ear condition

Excludes ❷: *certain conditions originating in the perinatal period (P04-P96)*
certain infectious and parasitic diseases (A00-B99)
complications of pregnancy, childbirth and the puerperium (O00-O9A)
congenital malformations, deformations and chromosomal abnormalities (Q00-Q99)
endocrine, nutritional and metabolic diseases (E00-E88)
injury, poisoning and certain other consequences of external causes (S00-T88)
neoplasms (C00-D49)
symptoms, signs and abnormal clinical and laboratory findings, not elsewhere classified (R00-R94)

This chapter contains the following blocks:
H60-H62   Diseases of external ear
H65-H75   Diseases of middle ear and mastoid
H80-H83   Diseases of inner ear
H90-H94   Other disorders of ear
H95   Intraoperative and postprocedural complications and disorders of ear and mastoid process, not elsewhere classified

Chapter-Specific Coding Guidelines

C.   Chapter-Specific Coding Guidelines
In addition to general coding guidelines, there are guidelines for specific diagnoses and/or conditions in the classification. Unless otherwise indicated, these guidelines apply to all health care settings. Please refer to Section II for guidelines on the selection of principal diagnosis.

8. Chapter 8: Diseases of Ear and Mastoid Process (H60-H95)

Reserved for future guideline expansion

Diseases of external ear (H60-H62)

H60- Otitis externa — Inflammation of the external ear.
H60.0- Abscess of external ear — A localized collection of pus caused by the disintegration of external ear tissue.
Boil of external ear
Carbuncle of auricle or external auditory canal — A necrotizing infection of the external ear and subcutaneous tissue composed of a cluster of boils (furuncles), with multiple formed or incipient draining sinuses.
Furuncle of external ear — A painful infectious nodule formed in the skin by circumscribed inflammation of the corium and subcutaneous tissue.
H60.00 Abscess of external ear, <u>unspecified</u> ear
H60.01 Abscess of <u>right</u> external ear
H60.02 Abscess of <u>left</u> external ear
H60.03 Abscess of external ear, <u>bilateral</u>
H60.1- Cellulitis of external ear — Cellular tissue inflammation of the external ear.
Cellulitis of auricle
Cellulitis of external auditory canal
H60.10 Cellulitis of external ear, <u>unspecified</u> ear
H60.11 Cellulitis of <u>right</u> external ear
H60.12 Cellulitis of <u>left</u> external ear
H60.13 Cellulitis of external ear, <u>bilateral</u>
H60.2- Malignant otitis externa — An extremely severe, necrotic bacterial inflammation of the external ear, often caused by Pseudomonas aeruginosa.
cc H60.20 Malignant otitis externa, <u>unspecified</u> ear
cc H60.21 Malignant otitis externa, <u>right</u> ear
cc H60.22 Malignant otitis externa, <u>left</u> ear
cc H60.23 Malignant otitis externa, <u>bilateral</u>
H60.3- Other infective otitis externa — Inflammation of the external ear caused by invasion of microorganisms.
H60.31- Diffuse otitis externa — A form which affects most of the external ear, including the external auditory canal.
H60.311 Diffuse otitis externa, <u>right</u> ear
H60.312 Diffuse otitis externa, <u>left</u> ear
H60.313 Diffuse otitis externa, <u>bilateral</u>

H60.319 Diffuse otitis externa, <u>unspecified</u> ear
H60.32- Hemorrhagic otitis externa — A form marked by escape of blood at the infected areas.
H60.321 Hemorrhagic otitis externa, <u>right</u> ear
H60.322 Hemorrhagic otitis externa, <u>left</u> ear
H60.323 Hemorrhagic otitis externa, <u>bilateral</u>
H60.329 Hemorrhagic otitis externa, <u>unspecified</u> ear
H60.33- Swimmer's ear — The sudden, severe onset of bacterial inflammation of the external ear, seen in warm humid weather and commonly precipitated by swimming.
H60.331 Swimmer's ear, <u>right</u> ear
H60.332 Swimmer's ear, <u>left</u> ear
H60.333 Swimmer's ear, <u>bilateral</u>
H60.339 Swimmer's ear, <u>unspecified</u> ear
H60.39- Other infective otitis externa
H60.391 Other infective otitis externa, <u>right</u> ear
H60.392 Other infective otitis externa, <u>left</u> ear
H60.393 Other infective otitis externa, <u>bilateral</u>
H60.399 Other infective otitis externa, <u>unspecified</u> ear
H60.4- Cholesteatoma of external ear — A cyst-like mass containing keratin debris and epithelial cells of the external ear.
Keratosis obturans of external ear (canal)
Excludes ❷: *cholesteatoma of middle ear (H71.-)*
recurrent cholesteatoma of postmastoidectomy cavity (H95.0-)
H60.40 Cholesteatoma of external ear, <u>unspecified</u> ear
H60.41 Cholesteatoma of <u>right</u> external ear
H60.42 Cholesteatoma of <u>left</u> external ear
H60.43 Cholesteatoma of external ear, <u>bilateral</u>
H60.5- Acute noninfective otitis externa — The sudden, severe onset of inflammation of the external ear that is not caused by invasion of microorganisms.
H60.50- Unspecified acute noninfective otitis externa
Acute otitis externa NOS
H60.501 Unspecified acute noninfective otitis externa, <u>right</u> ear
H60.502 Unspecified acute noninfective otitis externa, <u>left</u> ear
H60.503 Unspecified acute noninfective otitis externa, <u>bilateral</u>
H60.509 Unspecified acute noninfective otitis externa, <u>unspecified</u> ear
H60.51- Acute actinic otitis externa — A form caused by the photochemical effects of sunlight and other high-intensity light.
H60.511 Acute actinic otitis externa, <u>right</u> ear
H60.512 Acute actinic otitis externa, <u>left</u> ear
H60.513 Acute actinic otitis externa, <u>bilateral</u>
H60.519 Acute actinic otitis externa, <u>unspecified</u> ear
H60.52- Acute chemical otitis externa — A form caused by the effects of chemical substances.
H60.521 Acute chemical otitis externa, <u>right</u> ear
H60.522 Acute chemical otitis externa, <u>left</u> ear
H60.523 Acute chemical otitis externa, <u>bilateral</u>
H60.529 Acute chemical otitis externa, <u>unspecified</u> ear
H60.53- Acute contact otitis externa — A form caused by the irritating effects of a substance in direct contact with the ear.
H60.531 Acute contact otitis externa, <u>right</u> ear
H60.532 Acute contact otitis externa, <u>left</u> ear
H60.533 Acute contact otitis externa, <u>bilateral</u>
H60.539 Acute contact otitis externa, <u>unspecified</u> ear
H60.54- Acute eczematoid otitis externa — A form resembling eczema.
H60.541 Acute eczematoid otitis externa, <u>right</u> ear
H60.542 Acute eczematoid otitis externa, <u>left</u> ear
H60.543 Acute eczematoid otitis externa, <u>bilateral</u>
H60.549 Acute eczematoid otitis externa, <u>unspecified</u> ear
H60.55- Acute reactive otitis externa
H60.551 Acute reactive otitis externa, <u>right</u> ear
H60.552 Acute reactive otitis externa, <u>left</u> ear

H60 - H60

H60.553   Acute reactive otitis externa, <u>bilateral</u>

H60.559   Acute reactive otitis externa, <u>unspecified</u> ear

H60.59-   <u>Other noninfective acute</u> otitis externa

    H60.591   Other noninfective acute otitis externa, <u>right</u> ear

    H60.592   Other noninfective acute otitis externa, <u>left</u> ear

    H60.593   Other noninfective acute otitis externa, <u>bilateral</u>

    H60.599   Other noninfective acute otitis externa, <u>unspecified</u> ear

H60.6-   <u>Unspecified chronic</u> otitis externa — Inflammation of the external ear that is not caused by the invasion of microorganisms that develops slowly and persists over a long period of time.

    H60.60   Unspecified chronic otitis externa, <u>unspecified</u> ear

    H60.61   Unspecified chronic otitis externa, <u>right</u> ear

    H60.62   Unspecified chronic otitis externa, <u>left</u> ear

    H60.63   Unspecified chronic otitis externa, <u>bilateral</u>

H60.8-   <u>Other</u> otitis externa

H60.8x-   <u>Other</u> otitis externa

    H60.8x1   Other otitis externa, <u>right</u> ear

    H60.8x2   Other otitis externa, <u>left</u> ear

    H60.8x3   Other otitis externa, <u>bilateral</u>

    H60.8x9   Other otitis externa, <u>unspecified</u> ear

H60.9-   <u>Unspecified</u> otitis externa

    H60.90   Unspecified otitis externa, <u>unspecified</u> ear

    H60.91   Unspecified otitis externa, <u>right</u> ear

    H60.92   Unspecified otitis externa, <u>left</u> ear

    H60.93   Unspecified otitis externa, <u>bilateral</u>

H61-   <u>Other disorders of external ear</u> — Disorders of that portion to the outside of the tympanic membrane.

H61.0-   <u>Chondritis and perichondritis</u> of external ear — The inflammation/infection of the fibrous connective tissue that covers the cartilage of the external ear.

    AHA 15:1Q:p18 – Auricular chondritis due to Pseudomonas aeruginosa

    Chondrodermatitis nodularis chronica helicis

    Perichondritis of auricle

    Perichondritis of pinna

H61.00-   <u>Unspecified</u> perichondritis of external ear

    H61.001   Unspecified perichondritis of <u>right</u> external ear

    H61.002   Unspecified perichondritis of <u>left</u> external ear

    H61.003   Unspecified perichondritis of external ear, <u>bilateral</u>

    H61.009   Unspecified perichondritis of external ear, <u>unspecified</u> ear

H61.01-   <u>Acute perichondritis</u> of external ear — The sudden, severe inflammation/infection of the fibrous connective tissue that covers the cartilage of the external ear.

    H61.011   Acute perichondritis of <u>right</u> external ear

    H61.012   Acute perichondritis of <u>left</u> external ear

    H61.013   Acute perichondritis of external ear, <u>bilateral</u>

    H61.019   Acute perichondritis of external ear, <u>unspecified</u> ear

H61.02-   Chronic perichondritis of external ear — The inflammation/infection of the fibrous connective tissue that covers the cartilage of the external ear that is marked by slow development and persists over a long period of time.

    H61.021   Chronic perichondritis of <u>right</u> external ear

    H61.022   Chronic perichondritis of <u>left</u> external ear

    H61.023   Chronic perichondritis of external ear, <u>bilateral</u>

    H61.029   Chronic perichondritis of external ear, <u>unspecified</u> ear

H61.03-   <u>Chondritis</u> of external ear — The inflammation/infection of the cartilage of the ear.

    Chondritis of auricle

    Chondritis of pinna

    H61.031   Chondritis of <u>right</u> external ear

    H61.032   Chondritis of <u>left</u> external ear

    H61.033   Chondritis of external ear, <u>bilateral</u>

    H61.039   Chondritis of external ear, <u>unspecified</u> ear

---

H61.1-   Noninfective disorders of pinna

    Excludes ❷: *cauliflower ear (M95.1-)*

              gouty tophi of ear (M1A.-)

H61.10-   <u>Unspecified noninfective disorders</u> of pinna

    Disorder of pinna NOS

    H61.101   Unspecified noninfective disorders of pinna, <u>right</u> ear

    H61.102   Unspecified noninfective disorders of pinna, <u>left</u> ear

    H61.103   Unspecified noninfective disorders of pinna, <u>bilateral</u>

    H61.109   Unspecified noninfective disorders of pinna, <u>unspecified</u> ear

H61.11-   <u>Acquired deformity</u> of pinna — A distortion of that portion of the external ear lying outside of the head which is not congenital.

    Acquired deformity of auricle

    Excludes ❷: *cauliflower ear (M95.1-)*

    H61.111   Acquired deformity of pinna, <u>right</u> ear

    H61.112   Acquired deformity of pinna, <u>left</u> ear

    H61.113   Acquired deformity of pinna, <u>bilateral</u>

    H61.119   Acquired deformity of pinna, <u>unspecified</u> ear

H61.12-   <u>Hematoma</u> of pinna — The localized collection of blood within the tissues of that portion of the ear which lies outside of the head.

    Hematoma of auricle

    H61.121   Hematoma of pinna, <u>right</u> ear

    H61.122   Hematoma of pinna, <u>left</u> ear

    H61.123   Hematoma of pinna, <u>bilateral</u>

    H61.129   Hematoma of pinna, <u>unspecified</u> ear

H61.19-   <u>Other noninfective disorders</u> of pinna

    H61.191   Noninfective disorders of pinna, <u>right</u> ear

    H61.192   Noninfective disorders of pinna, <u>left</u> ear

    H61.193   Noninfective disorders of pinna, <u>bilateral</u>

    H61.199   Noninfective disorders of pinna, <u>unspecified</u> ear

H61.2-   <u>Impacted cerumen</u> — The lodged or wedged accumulation of the wax-like secretion in the external auditory canal.

    Wax in ear

    H61.20   Impacted cerumen, <u>unspecified</u> ear — [Questionable Admission]

    H61.21   Impacted cerumen, <u>right</u> ear — [Questionable Admission]

    H61.22   Impacted cerumen, <u>left</u> ear — [Questionable Admission]

    H61.23   Impacted cerumen, <u>bilateral</u> — [Questionable Admission]

H61.3-   <u>Acquired stenosis</u> of external ear canal — The abnormal narrowing of the external auditory canal which is not inherited.

    Collapse of external ear canal

    Excludes 1:   *postprocedural stenosis of external ear canal (H95.81-)*

H61.30-   Acquired stenosis of external ear canal, <u>unspecified</u>

    H61.301   Acquired stenosis of <u>right</u> external ear canal, unspecified

    H61.302   Acquired stenosis of <u>left</u> external ear canal, unspecified

    H61.303   Acquired stenosis of external ear canal, unspecified, <u>bilateral</u>

    H61.309   Acquired stenosis of external ear canal, unspecified, <u>unspecified</u> ear

H61.31-   <u>Acquired stenosis</u> of external ear canal <u>secondary to trauma</u> — A form due to external physical injury.

    H61.311   Acquired stenosis of <u>right</u> external ear canal secondary to trauma

    H61.312   Acquired stenosis of <u>left</u> external ear canal secondary to trauma

    H61.313   Acquired stenosis of external ear canal secondary to trauma, <u>bilateral</u>

    H61.319   Acquired stenosis of external ear canal secondary to trauma, <u>unspecified</u> ear

H61.32-   <u>Acquired stenosis</u> of external ear canal <u>secondary to inflammation and infection</u> — A form resulting from the enlarging effects of inflammation/infection.

    H61.321   Acquired stenosis of <u>right</u> external ear canal secondary to inflammation and infection

---

H 60 - H 61 (side tab)

H61.322 Acquired stenosis of <u>left</u> external ear canal secondary to inflammation and infection

H61.323 Acquired stenosis of external ear canal secondary to inflammation and infection, <u>bilateral</u>

H61.329 Acquired stenosis of external ear canal secondary to inflammation and infection, <u>unspecified</u> ear

H61.39- Other acquired stenosis of external ear canal

H61.391 Other acquired stenosis of <u>right</u> external ear canal

H61.392 Other acquired stenosis of <u>left</u> external ear canal

H61.393 Other acquired stenosis of external ear canal, <u>bilateral</u>

H61.399 Other acquired stenosis of external ear canal, <u>unspecified</u> ear

H61.8- Other specified disorders of external ear

H61.81- <u>Exostosis</u> of external canal — A benign bony growth projecting from the external ear canal.

H61.811 Exostosis of <u>right</u> external canal

H61.812 Exostosis of <u>left</u> external canal

H61.813 Exostosis of external canal, <u>bilateral</u>

H61.819 Exostosis of external canal, <u>unspecified</u> ear

H61.89- <u>Other specified disorders</u> of external ear

H61.891 Other specified disorders of <u>right</u> external ear

H61.892 Other specified disorders of <u>left</u> external ear

H61.893 Other specified disorders of external ear, <u>bilateral</u>

H61.899 Other specified disorders of external ear, <u>unspecified</u> ear

H61.9- Disorder of external ear, unspecified

H61.90 Disorder of external ear, unspecified, <u>unspecified</u> ear

H61.91 Disorder of <u>right</u> external ear, unspecified

H61.92 Disorder of <u>left</u> external ear, unspecified

H61.93 Disorder of external ear, unspecified, <u>bilateral</u>

H62- Disorders of external ear <u>in diseases classified elsewhere</u>

H62.4- Otitis externa <u>in other diseases classified elsewhere</u>
Code first underlying disease, such as:
  Erysipelas (A46)
  Impetigo (L01.0)
Excludes 1:   otitis externa (in):
  candidiasis (B37.84)
  herpes viral [herpes simplex] (B00.1)
  herpes zoster (B02.8)

H62.40 Otitis externa in other diseases classified elsewhere, <u>unspecified</u> ear — [Not Allowed as PDX]

H62.41 Otitis externa in other diseases classified elsewhere, <u>right</u> ear — [Not Allowed as PDX]

H62.42 Otitis externa in other diseases classified elsewhere, <u>left</u> ear — [Not Allowed as PDX]

H62.43 Otitis externa in other diseases classified elsewhere, <u>bilateral</u> — [Not Allowed as PDX]

H62.8- Other disorders of external ear <u>in diseases classified elsewhere</u>
Code first underlying disease, such as:
  Gout (M1A.-, M10.-)

H62.8x- Other disorders of external ear in diseases classified elsewhere

H62.8x1 Other disorders of <u>right</u> external ear in diseases classified elsewhere — [Not Allowed as PDX]

H62.8x2 Other disorders of <u>left</u> external ear in diseases classified elsewhere — [Not Allowed as PDX]

H62.8x3 Other disorders of external ear in diseases classified elsewhere, <u>bilateral</u> — [Not Allowed as PDX]

H62.8x9 Other disorders of external ear in diseases classified elsewhere, <u>unspecified</u> ear — [Not Allowed as PDX]

Diseases of middle ear and mastoid (H65-H75)

H65- <u>Nonsuppurative</u> <u>otitis media</u> — The inflammation of the middle ear, without pus formation.
Includes: Nonsuppurative otitis media with myringitis
Use additional code for any associated perforated tympanic membrane (H72.-)
Use additional code to identify:
  Exposure to environmental tobacco smoke (Z77.22)
  Exposure to tobacco smoke in the perinatal period (P96.81)
  History of tobacco dependence (Z87.891)
  Occupational exposure to environmental tobacco smoke (Z57.31)
  Tobacco dependence (F17.-)
  Tobacco use (Z72.0)

H65.0- <u>Acute serous</u> otitis media — The sudden, severe onset of inflammation of the middle ear that is characterized by serous exudation, without pus formation.
  Acute and subacute secretory otitis

H65.00 Acute serous otitis media, <u>unspecified</u> ear

H65.01 Acute serous otitis media, <u>right</u> ear

H65.02 Acute serous otitis media, <u>left</u> ear

H65.03 Acute serous otitis media, <u>bilateral</u>

H65.04 Acute serous otitis media, recurrent, <u>right</u> ear

H65.05 Acute serous otitis media, recurrent, <u>left</u> ear

H65.06 Acute serous otitis media, recurrent, <u>bilateral</u>

H65.07 Acute serous otitis media, recurrent, <u>unspecified</u> ear

H65.1- <u>Other acute</u> nonsuppurative otitis media
Excludes 1:   otitic barotrauma (T70.0)
  otitis media (acute) NOS (H66.9)

H65.11- Acute and subacute <u>allergic</u> otitis media (mucoid) (sanguinous) (serous) — The sudden, severe onset of inflammation of the middle ear that is caused by an allergic reaction.

H65.111 Acute and subacute allergic otitis media (mucoid) (sanguinous) (serous), <u>right</u> ear

H65.112 Acute and subacute allergic otitis media (mucoid) (sanguinous) (serous), <u>left</u> ear

H65.113 Acute and subacute allergic otitis media (mucoid) (sanguinous) (serous), <u>bilateral</u>

H65.114 Acute and subacute allergic otitis media (mucoid) (sanguinous) (serous), recurrent, <u>right</u> ear

H65.115 Acute and subacute allergic otitis media (mucoid) (sanguinous) (serous), recurrent, <u>left</u> ear

H65.116 Acute and subacute allergic otitis media (mucoid) (sanguinous) (serous), recurrent, <u>bilateral</u>

H65.117 Acute and subacute allergic otitis media (mucoid) (sanguinous) (serous), recurrent, <u>unspecified</u> ear

H65.119 Acute and subacute allergic otitis media (mucoid) (sanguinous) (serous), <u>unspecified</u> ear

H65.19- <u>Other acute</u> nonsuppurative otitis media
  Acute and subacute mucoid otitis media
  Acute and subacute nonsuppurative otitis media NOS
  Acute and subacute sanguinous otitis media
  Acute and subacute seromucinous otitis media

H65.191 Other acute nonsuppurative otitis media, <u>right</u> ear

H65.192 Other acute nonsuppurative otitis media, <u>left</u> ear

H65.193 Other acute nonsuppurative otitis media, <u>bilateral</u>

H65.194 Other acute nonsuppurative otitis media, recurrent, <u>right</u> ear

H65.195 Other acute nonsuppurative otitis media, recurrent, <u>left</u> ear

H65.196 Other acute nonsuppurative otitis media, recurrent, <u>bilateral</u>

H65.197 Other acute nonsuppurative otitis media recurrent, <u>unspecified</u> ear

H65.199 Other acute nonsuppurative otitis media, <u>unspecified</u> ear

H65.2- <u>Chronic serous</u> otitis media — Inflammation of the middle ear that develops slowly and persists over a long period of time, without pus formation.
  Chronic tubotympanal catarrh

H65.20 Chronic serous otitis media, <u>unspecified</u> ear

H65.21 Chronic serous otitis media, <u>right</u> ear

H65.22 Chronic serous otitis media, <u>left</u> ear

H65.23 Chronic serous otitis media, <u>bilateral</u>

H61 - H65

H65.3- **Chronic mucoid** otitis media — A form characterized by mucus-like substance in the middle ear, without pus formation.
  Chronic mucinous otitis media
  Chronic secretory otitis media
  Chronic transudative otitis media
  Glue ear
  Excludes 1:   *adhesive middle ear disease (H74.1)*

  H65.30 Chronic mucoid otitis media, **unspecified** ear
  H65.31 Chronic mucoid otitis media, **right** ear
  H65.32 Chronic mucoid otitis media, **left** ear
  H65.33 Chronic mucoid otitis media, **bilateral**

H65.4- **Other chronic nonsuppurative** otitis media

  H65.41- **Chronic allergic** otitis media — A form caused by an allergic reaction.
    H65.411 Chronic allergic otitis media, **right** ear
    H65.412 Chronic allergic otitis media, **left** ear
    H65.413 Chronic allergic otitis media, **bilateral**
    H65.419 Chronic allergic otitis media, **unspecified** ear

  H65.49- **Other chronic** nonsuppurative otitis media
    Chronic exudative otitis media
    Chronic nonsuppurative otitis media NOS
    Chronic otitis media with effusion (nonpurulent)
    Chronic seromucinous otitis media
    H65.491 Other chronic nonsuppurative otitis media, **right** ear
    H65.492 Other chronic nonsuppurative otitis media, **left** ear
    H65.493 Other chronic nonsuppurative otitis media, **bilateral**
    H65.499 Other chronic nonsuppurative otitis media, **unspecified** ear

H65.9- **Unspecified nonsuppurative** otitis media
  Allergic otitis media NOS
  Catarrhal otitis media NOS
  Exudative otitis media NOS
  Mucoid otitis media NOS
  Otitis media with effusion (nonpurulent) NOS
  Secretory otitis media NOS
  Seromucinous otitis media NOS
  Serous otitis media NOS
  Transudative otitis media NOS
  H65.90 Unspecified nonsuppurative otitis media, **unspecified** ear
  H65.91 Unspecified nonsuppurative otitis media, **right** ear
  H65.92 Unspecified nonsuppurative otitis media, **left** ear
  H65.93 Unspecified nonsuppurative otitis media, **bilateral**

H66- **Suppurative and unspecified** otitis media — The inflammation of the middle ear, with pus formation.
  Includes: Suppurative and unspecified otitis media with myringitis
  Use additional code to identify:
  Exposure to environmental tobacco smoke (Z77.22)
  Exposure to tobacco smoke in the perinatal period (P96.81)
  History of tobacco dependence (Z87.891)
  Occupational exposure to environmental tobacco smoke (Z57.31)
  Tobacco dependence (F17.-)
  Tobacco use (Z72.0)

H66.0- **Acute suppurative** otitis media — The sudden, severe onset of inflammation of the middle ear; with pus formation.

  H66.00- Acute suppurative otitis media **without** spontaneous rupture of ear drum
    H66.001 Acute suppurative otitis media without spontaneous rupture of ear drum, **right** ear
    H66.002 Acute suppurative otitis media without spontaneous rupture of ear drum, **left** ear
    H66.003 Acute suppurative otitis media without spontaneous rupture of ear drum, **bilateral**
    H66.004 Acute suppurative otitis media without spontaneous rupture of ear drum, **recurrent, right** ear
    H66.005 Acute suppurative otitis media without spontaneous rupture of ear drum, **recurrent, left** ear
    H66.006 Acute suppurative otitis media without spontaneous rupture of ear drum, **recurrent, bilateral**

    H66.007 Acute suppurative otitis media without spontaneous rupture of ear drum, **recurrent, unspecified** ear
    H66.009 Acute suppurative otitis media without spontaneous rupture of ear drum, **unspecified** ear

  H66.01- Acute suppurative otitis media **with spontaneous rupture of ear drum** — A form marked by the nontraumatic tearing open of the ear drum.
    H66.011 Acute suppurative otitis media with spontaneous rupture of ear drum, **right** ear
    H66.012 Acute suppurative otitis media with spontaneous rupture of ear drum, **left** ear
    H66.013 Acute suppurative otitis media with spontaneous rupture of ear drum, **bilateral**
    H66.014 Acute suppurative otitis media with spontaneous rupture of ear drum, **recurrent, right** ear
    H66.015 Acute suppurative otitis media with spontaneous rupture of ear drum, **recurrent, left** ear
    H66.016 Acute suppurative otitis media with spontaneous rupture of ear drum, **recurrent, bilateral**
    H66.017 Acute suppurative otitis media with spontaneous rupture of ear drum, **recurrent, unspecified** ear
    H66.019 Acute suppurative otitis media with spontaneous rupture of ear drum, **unspecified** ear

H66.1- **Chronic tubotympanic** suppurative otitis media — Inflammation of the tympanic cavity of the middle ear that develops slowly and persists over a long period of time, with pus formation.
  Benign chronic suppurative otitis media
  Chronic tubotympanic disease
  Use additional code for any associated perforated tympanic membrane (H72.-)
  H66.10 Chronic tubotympanic suppurative otitis media, **unspecified**
  H66.11 Chronic tubotympanic suppurative otitis media, **right** ear
  H66.12 Chronic tubotympanic suppurative otitis media, **left** ear
  H66.13 Chronic tubotympanic suppurative otitis media, **bilateral**

H66.2- **Chronic atticoantral** suppurative otitis media — Inflammation of the upper portion of the middle ear that develops slowly and persists over a long period of time, with pus formation that drains through a perforation of the tympanic membrane.
  Chronic atticoantral disease
  Use additional code for any associated perforated tympanic membrane (H72.-)
  H66.20 Chronic atticoantral suppurative otitis media, **unspecified** ear
  H66.21 Chronic atticoantral suppurative otitis media, **right** ear
  H66.22 Chronic atticoantral suppurative otitis media, **left** ear
  H66.23 Chronic atticoantral suppurative otitis media, **bilateral**

H66.3- **Other chronic** suppurative otitis media
  Chronic suppurative otitis media NOS
  Use additional code for any associated perforated tympanic membrane (H72.-)
  Excludes 1:   *tuberculous otitis media (A18.6)*

  H66.3x- **Other chronic** suppurative otitis media
    H66.3x1 Other chronic suppurative otitis media, **right** ear
    H66.3x2 Other chronic suppurative otitis media, **left** ear
    H66.3x3 Other chronic suppurative otitis media, **bilateral**
    H66.3x9 Other chronic suppurative otitis media, **unspecified** ear

H66.4- **Suppurative** otitis media, **unspecified**
  Purulent otitis media NOS
  Use additional code for any associated perforated tympanic membrane (H72.-)
  H66.40 Suppurative otitis media, unspecified, **unspecified** ear
  H66.41 Suppurative otitis media, unspecified, **right** ear
  H66.42 Suppurative otitis media, unspecified, **left** ear
  H66.43 Suppurative otitis media, unspecified, **bilateral**

H66.9- Otitis media, <u>unspecified</u>
     Otitis media NOS
     Acute otitis media NOS
     Chronic otitis media NOS
     Use additional code for any associated perforated tympanic membrane (H72.-)

    H66.90 Otitis media, unspecified, <u>unspecified</u> ear
    H66.91 Otitis media, unspecified, <u>right</u> ear
    H66.92 Otitis media, unspecified, <u>left</u> ear
    H66.93 Otitis media, unspecified, <u>bilateral</u>

H67- Otitis media <u>in diseases classified elsewhere</u>
    Code first underlying disease, such as:
    Viral disease NEC (B00-B34)
    Use additional code for any associated perforated tympanic membrane (H72.-)

    Excludes 1:   *otitis media in:*
         influenza (J09.X9, J10.83, J11.83)
         measles (B05.3)
         scarlet fever (A38.0)
         tuberculosis (A18.6)

    H67.1 Otitis media in diseases classified elsewhere, <u>right</u> ear — [Not Allowed as PDX]
    H67.2 Otitis media in diseases classified elsewhere, <u>left</u> ear — [Not Allowed as PDX]
    H67.3 Otitis media in diseases classified elsewhere, <u>bilateral</u> — [Not Allowed as PDX]
    H67.9 Otitis media in diseases classified elsewhere, <u>unspecified</u> ear — [Not Allowed as PDX]

H68- Eustachian salpingitis and obstruction
    H68.0- <u>Eustachian salpingitis</u> — Inflammation of the Eustachian (auditory) tube.
      H68.00- <u>Unspecified</u> Eustachian salpingitis
        H68.001 Unspecified Eustachian salpingitis, <u>right</u> ear
        H68.002 Unspecified Eustachian salpingitis, <u>left</u> ear
        H68.003 Unspecified Eustachian salpingitis, <u>bilateral</u>
        H68.009 Unspecified Eustachian salpingitis, <u>unspecified</u> ear
      H68.01- <u>Acute</u> Eustachian salpingitis — A form marked by sudden, severe onset.
        H68.011 Acute Eustachian salpingitis, <u>right</u> ear
        H68.012 Acute Eustachian salpingitis, <u>left</u> ear
        H68.013 Acute Eustachian salpingitis, <u>bilateral</u>
        H68.019 Acute Eustachian salpingitis, <u>unspecified</u> ear
      H68.02- <u>Chronic</u> Eustachian salpingitis — A form marked by slow development and persistence over a long period of time.
        H68.021 Chronic Eustachian salpingitis, <u>right</u> ear
        H68.022 Chronic Eustachian salpingitis, <u>left</u> ear
        H68.023 Chronic Eustachian salpingitis, <u>bilateral</u>
        H68.029 Chronic Eustachian salpingitis, <u>unspecified</u> ear
    H68.1- <u>Obstruction</u> of Eustachian tube — Blockage of the Eustachian (auditory) tube.
      Stenosis of Eustachian tube — A reduction in the lumen of the Eustachian (auditory) tube.
      Stricture of Eustachian tube — A narrowing of the lumen of the Eustachian (auditory) tube.
      H68.10- <u>Unspecified</u> obstruction of Eustachian tube
        H68.101 Unspecified obstruction of Eustachian tube, <u>right</u> ear
        H68.102 Unspecified obstruction of Eustachian tube, <u>left</u> ear
        H68.103 Unspecified obstruction of Eustachian tube, <u>bilateral</u>
        H68.109 Unspecified obstruction of Eustachian tube, <u>unspecified</u> ear
      H68.11- <u>Osseous</u> obstruction of Eustachian tube — A form marked by bony overgrowth.
        H68.111 Osseous obstruction of Eustachian tube, <u>right</u> ear
        H68.112 Osseous obstruction of Eustachian tube, <u>left</u> ear
        H68.113 Osseous obstruction of Eustachian tube, <u>bilateral</u>
        H68.119 Osseous obstruction of Eustachian tube, <u>unspecified</u> ear

H68.12- <u>Intrinsic cartilagenous</u> obstruction of Eustachian tube — A form marked by overgrowth of the Eustachian tube cartilage.
    H68.121 Intrinsic cartilagenous obstruction of Eustachian tube, <u>right</u> ear
    H68.122 Intrinsic cartilagenous obstruction of Eustachian tube, <u>left</u> ear
    H68.123 Intrinsic cartilagenous obstruction of Eustachian tube, <u>bilateral</u>
    H68.129 Intrinsic cartilagenous obstruction of Eustachian tube, <u>unspecified</u> ear
H68.13- <u>Extrinsic cartilagenous</u> obstruction of Eustachian tube — A form marked by overgrowth of the cartilage surrounding the Eustachian tube.
    Compression of Eustachian tube
    H68.131 Extrinsic cartilagenous obstruction of Eustachian tube, <u>right</u> ear
    H68.132 Extrinsic cartilagenous obstruction of Eustachian tube, <u>left</u> ear
    H68.133 Extrinsic cartilagenous obstruction of Eustachian tube, <u>bilateral</u>
    H68.139 Extrinsic cartilagenous obstruction of Eustachian tube, <u>unspecified</u> ear

H69- Other and unspecified disorders of Eustachian tube
    H69.0- <u>Patulous</u> Eustachian tube — An abnormally wide, distended Eustachian (auditory) tube.
      H69.00 Patulous Eustachian tube, <u>unspecified</u> ear
      H69.01 Patulous Eustachian tube, <u>right</u> ear
      H69.02 Patulous Eustachian tube, <u>left</u> ear
      H69.03 Patulous Eustachian tube, <u>bilateral</u>
    H69.8- <u>Other specified</u> disorders of Eustachian tube
      H69.80 Other specified disorders of Eustachian tube, <u>unspecified</u> ear
      H69.81 Other specified disorders of Eustachian tube, <u>right</u> ear
      H69.82 Other specified disorders of Eustachian tube, <u>left</u> ear
      H69.83 Other specified disorders of Eustachian tube, <u>bilateral</u>
    H69.9- <u>Unspecified</u> Eustachian tube disorder
      H69.90 Unspecified Eustachian tube disorder, <u>unspecified</u> ear
      H69.91 Unspecified Eustachian tube disorder, <u>right</u> ear
      H69.92 Unspecified Eustachian tube disorder, <u>left</u> ear
      H69.93 Unspecified Eustachian tube disorder, <u>bilateral</u>

H70- Mastoiditis and related conditions
    H70.0- <u>Acute mastoiditis</u> — The sudden, severe onset of inflammation of the mastoid antrum (air cells) of the mastoid process of the temporal bone.
      Abscess of mastoid — A localized collection of pus caused by the disintegration of the mastoid antrum cells.
      Empyema of mastoid — The accumulation of pus within the mastoid antrum.
    H70.00- Acute mastoiditis <u>without</u> complications — A form without complications.
      CC **H70.001 Acute mastoiditis without complications, <u>right</u> ear**
      CC **H70.002 Acute mastoiditis without complications, <u>left</u> ear**
      CC **H70.003 Acute mastoiditis without complications, <u>bilateral</u>**
      CC **H70.009 Acute mastoiditis without complications, <u>unspecified</u> ear**
    H70.01- <u>Subperiosteal abscess</u> of mastoid — A localized collection of pus caused by the disintegration of mastoid antrum cells beneath the periosteum layer.
      CC **H70.011 Subperiosteal abscess of mastoid, <u>right</u> ear**
      CC **H70.012 Subperiosteal abscess of mastoid, <u>left</u> ear**
      CC **H70.013 Subperiosteal abscess of mastoid, <u>bilateral</u>**
      CC **H70.019 Subperiosteal abscess of mastoid, <u>unspecified</u> ear**
    H70.09- Acute mastoiditis <u>with other complications</u>
      CC **H70.091 Acute mastoiditis with other complications, <u>right</u> ear**
      CC **H70.092 Acute mastoiditis with other complications, <u>left</u> ear**
      CC **H70.093 Acute mastoiditis with other complications, <u>bilateral</u>**
      CC **H70.099 Acute mastoiditis with other complications, <u>unspecified</u> ear**

H 6 6 – H 7 0

H70.1- <u>Chronic mastoiditis</u> — Inflammation of the mastoid antrum (air cells) of the mastoid process of the temporal bone which develops slowly and persists over a long period of time.
    Caries of mastoid — The decay of the mastoid bony substance.
    Fistula of mastoid — An abnormal passage of the mastoid.
    Excludes 1:   *tuberculous mastoiditis (A18.03)*

  H70.10   Chronic mastoiditis, <u>unspecified</u> ear
  H70.11   Chronic mastoiditis, <u>right</u> ear
  H70.12   Chronic mastoiditis, <u>left</u> ear
  H70.13   Chronic mastoiditis, <u>bilateral</u>

H70.2- <u>Petrositis</u> — Inflammation of the petrous region of the temporal bone.
    Inflammation of petrous bone

  H70.20- <u>Unspecified</u> petrositis
    H70.201   Unspecified petrositis, <u>right</u> ear
    H70.202   Unspecified petrositis, <u>left</u> ear
    H70.203   Unspecified petrositis, <u>bilateral</u>
    H70.209   Unspecified petrositis, <u>unspecified</u> ear

  H70.21- <u>Acute</u> petrositis — A form characterized by sudden, severe onset.
    H70.211   Acute petrositis, <u>right</u> ear
    H70.212   Acute petrositis, <u>left</u> ear
    H70.213   Acute petrositis, <u>bilateral</u>
    H70.219   Acute petrositis, <u>unspecified</u> ear

  H70.22- <u>Chronic</u> petrositis — A form characterized by slow development and persistence over a long period of time.
    H70.221   Chronic petrositis, <u>right</u> ear
    H70.222   Chronic petrositis, <u>left</u> ear
    H70.223   Chronic petrositis, <u>bilateral</u>
    H70.229   Chronic petrositis, <u>unspecified</u> ear

H70.8- <u>Other mastoiditis and related conditions</u>
    Excludes 1:   *preauricular sinus and cyst (Q18.1)*
                 sinus, fistula, and cyst of branchial cleft (Q18.0)

  H70.81- <u>Postauricular fistula</u> — An abnormal passage just behind the mastoid cavity.
    H70.811   Postauricular fistula, <u>right</u> ear
    H70.812   Postauricular fistula, <u>left</u> ear
    H70.813   Postauricular fistula, <u>bilateral</u>
    H70.819   Postauricular fistula, <u>unspecified</u> ear

  H70.89- <u>Other mastoiditis and related conditions</u>
    H70.891   Other mastoiditis and related conditions, <u>right</u> ear
    H70.892   Other mastoiditis and related conditions, <u>left</u> ear
    H70.893   Other mastoiditis and related conditions, <u>bilateral</u>
    H70.899   Other mastoiditis and related conditions, <u>unspecified</u> ear

H70.9- <u>Unspecified mastoiditis</u>
  H70.90   Unspecified mastoiditis, <u>unspecified</u> ear
  H70.91   Unspecified mastoiditis, <u>right</u> ear
  H70.92   Unspecified mastoiditis, <u>left</u> ear
  H70.93   Unspecified mastoiditis, <u>bilateral</u>

H71- <u>Cholesteatoma of middle ear</u> — A cyst-like sac filled with keratin debris of the middle ear.
    Excludes ❷: *cholesteatoma of external ear (H60.4-)*
                 recurrent cholesteatoma of postmastoidectomy cavity (H95.0-)

H71.0- <u>Cholesteatoma of attic</u> — A form located in the upper portion of the middle ear.
  H71.00   Cholesteatoma of attic, <u>unspecified</u> ear
  H71.01   Cholesteatoma of attic, <u>right</u> ear
  H71.02   Cholesteatoma of attic, <u>left</u> ear
  H71.03   Cholesteatoma of attic, <u>bilateral</u>

H71.1- <u>Cholesteatoma of tympanum</u> — A form adjacent to the tympanic membrane.
  H71.10   Cholesteatoma of tympanum, <u>unspecified</u> ear
  H71.11   Cholesteatoma of tympanum, <u>right</u> ear
  H71.12   Cholesteatoma of tympanum, <u>left</u> ear
  H71.13   Cholesteatoma of tympanum, <u>bilateral</u>

H71.2- <u>Cholesteatoma of mastoid</u> — A form located in the mastoid antrum.
  H71.20   Cholesteatoma of mastoid, <u>unspecified</u> ear
  H71.21   Cholesteatoma of mastoid, <u>right</u> ear

H71.22   Cholesteatoma of mastoid, <u>left</u> ear
H71.23   Cholesteatoma of mastoid, <u>bilateral</u>

H71.3- <u>Diffuse cholesteatosis</u> — A form marked by the presence of cholesteatoma formation throughout the middle ear.
  H71.30   Diffuse cholesteatosis, <u>unspecified</u> ear
  H71.31   Diffuse cholesteatosis, <u>right</u> ear
  H71.32   Diffuse cholesteatosis, <u>left</u> ear
  H71.33   Diffuse cholesteatosis, <u>bilateral</u>

H71.9- <u>Unspecified</u> cholesteatoma
  H71.90   Unspecified cholesteatoma, <u>unspecified</u> ear
  H71.91   Unspecified cholesteatoma, <u>right</u> ear
  H71.92   Unspecified cholesteatoma, <u>left</u> ear
  H71.93   Unspecified cholesteatoma, <u>bilateral</u>

H72- <u>Perforation of tympanic membrane</u> — The tearing open of a hole in the tympanic membrane (ear drum).
    Includes: **Persistent post-traumatic perforation of ear drum** — A form which persists over a long period of time after healing by primary intent.
                 Postinflammatory perforation of ear drum — A form which occurs as a sequelae to an inflammatory reaction of the ear drum.
    Code first any associated otitis media (H65.-, H66.1-, H66.2-, H66.3-, H66.4-, H66.9-, H67.-)
    Excludes 1:   *acute suppurative otitis media with rupture of the tympanic membrane (H66.01-)*
                 traumatic rupture of ear drum (S09.2-)

H72.0- <u>Central</u> perforation of tympanic membrane — A form in which the hole is in the approximate center of the tympanic membrane.
  H72.00   Central perforation of tympanic membrane, <u>unspecified</u> ear
  H72.01   Central perforation of tympanic membrane, <u>right</u> ear
  H72.02   Central perforation of tympanic membrane, <u>left</u> ear
  H72.03   Central perforation of tympanic membrane, <u>bilateral</u>

H72.1- <u>Attic</u> perforation of tympanic membrane — A form in which the hole is to the uppermost margin of the tympanic membrane.
    Perforation of pars flaccida
  H72.10   Attic perforation of tympanic membrane, <u>unspecified</u> ear
  H72.11   Attic perforation of tympanic membrane, <u>right</u> ear
  H72.12   Attic perforation of tympanic membrane, <u>left</u> ear
  H72.13   Attic perforation of tympanic membrane, <u>bilateral</u>

H72.2- <u>Other marginal perforations of tympanic membrane</u>
  H72.2x- <u>Other marginal perforations</u> of tympanic membrane
    H72.2x1   Other marginal perforations of tympanic membrane, <u>right</u> ear
    H72.2x2   Other marginal perforations of tympanic membrane, <u>left</u> ear
    H72.2x3   Other marginal perforations of tympanic membrane, <u>bilateral</u>
    H72.2x9   Other marginal perforations of tympanic membrane, <u>unspecified</u> ear

H72.8- <u>Other perforations of tympanic membrane</u>
  H72.81- <u>Multiple</u> perforations of tympanic membrane
    H72.811   Multiple perforations of tympanic membrane, <u>right</u> ear
    H72.812   Multiple perforations of tympanic membrane, <u>left</u> ear
    H72.813   Multiple perforations of tympanic membrane, <u>bilateral</u>
    H72.819   Multiple perforations of tympanic membrane, <u>unspecified</u> ear

  H72.82- <u>Total</u> perforations of tympanic membrane — A form in which the entire tympanic membrane is obliterated.
    H72.821   Total perforations of tympanic membrane, <u>right</u> ear
    H72.822   Total perforations of tympanic membrane, <u>left</u> ear
    H72.823   Total perforations of tympanic membrane, <u>bilateral</u>
    H72.829   Total perforations of tympanic membrane, <u>unspecified</u> ear

H72.9- <u>Unspecified</u> perforation of tympanic membrane
  H72.90   Unspecified perforation of tympanic membrane, <u>unspecified</u> ear

H70 - H72

H72.91 Unspecified perforation of tympanic membrane, <u>right</u> ear
H72.92 Unspecified perforation of tympanic membrane, <u>left</u> ear
H72.93 Unspecified perforation of tympanic membrane, <u>bilateral</u>

H73- Other disorders of tympanic membrane
H73.0- <u>Acute myringitis</u> — The sudden, severe onset of inflammation of the ear drum.
  Excludes 1:   acute myringitis with otitis media (H65, H66)
  H73.00- <u>Unspecified</u> acute myringitis
     Acute tympanitis NOS
     H73.001 Acute myringitis, <u>right</u> ear
     H73.002 Acute myringitis, <u>left</u> ear
     H73.003 Acute myringitis, <u>bilateral</u>
     H73.009 Acute myringitis, <u>unspecified</u> ear
  H73.01- <u>Bullous</u> myringitis — A form marked by serous or hemorrhagic blebs.
     H73.011 Bullous myringitis, <u>right</u> ear
     H73.012 Bullous myringitis, <u>left</u> ear
     H73.013 Bullous myringitis, <u>bilateral</u>
     H73.019 Bullous myringitis, <u>unspecified</u> ear
  H73.09- <u>Other</u> acute myringitis
     H73.091 Other acute myringitis, <u>right</u> ear
     H73.092 Other acute myringitis, <u>left</u> ear
     H73.093 Other acute myringitis, <u>bilateral</u>
     H73.099 Other acute myringitis, <u>unspecified</u> ear
H73.1- <u>Chronic myringitis</u> — Inflammation of the ear drum that develops slowly and persists over a long period of time.
     Chronic tympanitis
  Excludes 1:   chronic myringitis with otitis media (H65, H66)
  H73.10 Chronic myringitis, <u>unspecified</u> ear
  H73.11 Chronic myringitis, <u>right</u> ear
  H73.12 Chronic myringitis, <u>left</u> ear
  H73.13 Chronic myringitis, <u>bilateral</u>
H73.2- <u>Unspecified myringitis</u>
  H73.20 Unspecified myringitis, <u>unspecified</u> ear
  H73.21 Unspecified myringitis, <u>right</u> ear
  H73.22 Unspecified myringitis, <u>left</u> ear
  H73.23 Unspecified myringitis, <u>bilateral</u>
H73.8- Other specified disorders of tympanic membrane
  H73.81- <u>Atrophic flaccid tympanic membrane</u> — A wasting-away of the tympanic membrane with deterioration in the tone of the membrane.
     H73.811 Atrophic flaccid tympanic membrane, <u>right</u> ear
     H73.812 Atrophic flaccid tympanic membrane, <u>left</u> ear
     H73.813 Atrophic flaccid tympanic membrane, <u>bilateral</u>
     H73.819 Atrophic flaccid tympanic membrane, <u>unspecified</u> ear
  H73.82- <u>Atrophic nonflaccid tympanic membrane</u> — A wasting-away of the tympanic membrane without loss of tone of the membrane.
     H73.821 Atrophic nonflaccid tympanic membrane, <u>right</u> ear
     H73.822 Atrophic nonflaccid tympanic membrane, <u>left</u> ear
     H73.823 Atrophic nonflaccid tympanic membrane, <u>bilateral</u>
     H73.829 Atrophic nonflaccid tympanic membrane, <u>unspecified</u> ear
  H73.89- <u>Other specified</u> disorders of tympanic membrane
     H73.891 Other specified disorders of tympanic membrane, <u>right</u> ear
     H73.892 Other specified disorders of tympanic membrane, <u>left</u> ear
     H73.893 Other specified disorders of tympanic membrane, <u>bilateral</u>
     H73.899 Other specified disorders of tympanic membrane, <u>unspecified</u> ear
H73.9- <u>Unspecified disorder of tympanic membrane</u>
  H73.90 Unspecified disorder of tympanic membrane, <u>unspecified</u> ear
  H73.91 Unspecified disorder of tympanic membrane, <u>right</u> ear
  H73.92 Unspecified disorder of tympanic membrane, <u>left</u> ear
  H73.93 Unspecified disorder of tympanic membrane, <u>bilateral</u>

H74- Other disorders of middle ear mastoid
  Excludes ❷: mastoiditis (H70.-)
H74.0- <u>Tympanosclerosis</u> — The formation and infiltration of hard fibrous tissue in the middle ear.
  H74.01 Tympanosclerosis, <u>right</u> ear
  H74.02 Tympanosclerosis, <u>left</u> ear
  H74.03 Tympanosclerosis, <u>bilateral</u>
  H74.09 Tympanosclerosis, <u>unspecified</u> ear
H74.1- <u>Adhesive middle ear disease</u> — The abnormal adherence together of the middle ear structures by fibrous tissue which restricts their function.
     Adhesive otitis
  Excludes 1:   glue ear (H65.3-)
  H74.11 Adhesive <u>right</u> middle ear disease
  H74.12 Adhesive <u>left</u> middle ear disease
  H74.13 Adhesive middle ear disease, <u>bilateral</u>
  H74.19 Adhesive middle ear disease, <u>unspecified</u> ear
H74.2- <u>Discontinuity and dislocation of ear ossicles</u> — The displacement of ear ossicles from their normal positions.
  H74.20 Discontinuity and dislocation of ear ossicles, <u>unspecified</u> ear
  H74.21 Discontinuity and dislocation of <u>right</u> ear ossicles
  H74.22 Discontinuity and dislocation of <u>left</u> ear ossicles
  H74.23 Discontinuity and dislocation of ear ossicles, <u>bilateral</u>
H74.3- Other acquired abnormalities of ear ossicles
  H74.31- <u>Ankylosis</u> of ear ossicles — The abnormal fixation of the middle ear ossicles.
     H74.311 Ankylosis of ear ossicles, <u>right</u> ear
     H74.312 Ankylosis of ear ossicles, <u>left</u> ear
     H74.313 Ankylosis of ear ossicles, <u>bilateral</u>
     H74.319 Ankylosis of ear ossicles, <u>unspecified</u> ear
  H74.32- <u>Partial loss</u> of ear ossicles — The deterioration or partial destruction of ear ossicles.
     H74.321 Partial loss of ear ossicles, <u>right</u> ear
     H74.322 Partial loss of ear ossicles, <u>left</u> ear
     H74.323 Partial loss of ear ossicles, <u>bilateral</u>
     H74.329 Partial loss of ear ossicles, <u>unspecified</u> ear
  H74.39- <u>Other acquired abnormalities</u> of ear ossicles
     H74.391 Other acquired abnormalities of <u>right</u> ear ossicles
     H74.392 Other acquired abnormalities of <u>left</u> ear ossicles
     H74.393 Other acquired abnormalities of ear ossicles, <u>bilateral</u>
     H74.399 Other acquired abnormalities of ear ossicles, <u>unspecified</u> ear
H74.4- <u>Polyp</u> of middle ear — A protruding growth of the middle ear.
  H74.40 Polyp of middle ear, <u>unspecified</u> ear
  H74.41 Polyp of <u>right</u> middle ear
  H74.42 Polyp of <u>left</u> middle ear
  H74.43 Polyp of middle ear, <u>bilateral</u>
H74.8- <u>Other specified disorders of middle ear and mastoid</u>
  H74.8x- Other specified disorders of middle ear and mastoid
     H74.8x1 Other specified disorders of <u>right</u> middle ear and mastoid
     H74.8x2 Other specified disorders of <u>left</u> middle ear and mastoid
     H74.8x3 Other specified disorders of middle ear and mastoid, <u>bilateral</u>
     H74.8x9 Other specified disorders of middle ear and mastoid, <u>unspecified</u> ear
H74.9- <u>Unspecified disorder of middle ear and mastoid</u>
  H74.90 Unspecified disorder of middle ear and mastoid, <u>unspecified</u> ear
  H74.91 Unspecified disorder of <u>right</u> middle ear and mastoid
  H74.92 Unspecified disorder of <u>left</u> middle ear and mastoid
  H74.93 Unspecified disorder of middle ear and mastoid, <u>bilateral</u>

H72 – H74

H75- Other disorders of middle ear and mastoid <u>in diseases classified elsewhere</u>
    Code first underlying disease

H75.0- Mastoiditis <u>in infectious and parasitic diseases classified elsewhere</u>
      Excludes 1:   mastoiditis (in):
                syphilis (A52.77)
                tuberculosis (A18.03)

H75.00 Mastoiditis in infectious and parasitic diseases classified elsewhere, <u>unspecified</u> ear — [Not Allowed as PDX]

H75.01 Mastoiditis in infectious and parasitic diseases classified elsewhere, <u>right</u> ear — [Not Allowed as PDX]

H75.02 Mastoiditis in infectious and parasitic diseases classified elsewhere, <u>left</u> ear — [Not Allowed as PDX]

H75.03 Mastoiditis in infectious and parasitic diseases classified elsewhere, <u>bilateral</u> — [Not Allowed as PDX]

H75.8- Other specified disorders of middle ear and mastoid <u>in diseases classified elsewhere</u>

H75.80 Other specified disorders of middle ear and mastoid in diseases classified elsewhere, <u>unspecified</u> ear — [Not Allowed as PDX]

H75.81 Other specified disorders of <u>right</u> middle ear and mastoid in diseases classified elsewhere — [Not Allowed as PDX]

H75.82 Other specified disorders of <u>left</u> middle ear and mastoid in diseases classified elsewhere — [Not Allowed as PDX]

H75.83 Other specified disorders of middle ear and mastoid in diseases classified elsewhere, <u>bilateral</u> — [Not Allowed as PDX]

Diseases of inner ear (H80-H83)

H80- <u>Otosclerosis</u> — The abnormal formation of spongy bone in the labyrinth of the ear.
    Includes: Otospongiosis

H80.0- Otosclerosis involving <u>oval window</u>, <u>non</u>obliterative

H80.00 Otosclerosis involving oval window, <u>non</u>obliterative, <u>unspecified</u> ear

H80.01 Otosclerosis involving oval window, <u>non</u>obliterative, <u>right</u> ear

H80.02 Otosclerosis involving oval window, <u>non</u>obliterative, <u>left</u> ear

H80.03 Otosclerosis involving oval window, <u>non</u>obliterative, <u>bilateral</u>

H80.1- Otosclerosis involving <u>oval window</u>, <u>obliterative</u> — A form resulting in complete replacement of the oval window by the spongy bone.

H80.10 Otosclerosis involving oval window, <u>obliterative</u>, <u>unspecified</u> ear

H80.11 Otosclerosis involving oval window, <u>obliterative</u>, <u>right</u> ear

H80.12 Otosclerosis involving oval window, <u>obliterative</u>, <u>left</u> ear

H80.13 Otosclerosis involving oval window, <u>obliterative</u>, <u>bilateral</u>

H80.2- <u>Cochlear</u> otosclerosis — A form affecting the cochlea of the inner ear.
      Otosclerosis involving otic capsule — A form involving the enclosing skeletal portion of the inner ear.
      Otosclerosis involving round window — A form affecting the round window of the inner ear.

H80.20 Cochlear otosclerosis, <u>unspecified</u> ear

H80.21 Cochlear otosclerosis, <u>right</u> ear

H80.22 Cochlear otosclerosis, <u>left</u> ear

H80.23 Cochlear otosclerosis, <u>bilateral</u>

H80.8- <u>Other</u> otosclerosis

H80.80 Other otosclerosis, <u>unspecified</u> ear

H80.81 Other otosclerosis, <u>right</u> ear

H80.82 Other otosclerosis, <u>left</u> ear

H80.83 Other otosclerosis, <u>bilateral</u>

H80.9- <u>Unspecified</u> otosclerosis

H80.90 Unspecified otosclerosis, <u>unspecified</u> ear

H80.91 Unspecified otosclerosis, <u>right</u> ear

H80.92 Unspecified otosclerosis, <u>left</u> ear

H80.93 Unspecified otosclerosis, <u>bilateral</u>

H81- Disorders of vestibular function
      Excludes 1:   epidemic vertigo (A88.1)
                vertigo NOS (R42)

H81.0- <u>Ménière's disease</u> — A disease of the inner ear characterized by deafness, ringing of the ears, dizziness, and a sensation of fullness or pressure in the ears.
      Labyrinthine hydrops
      Ménière's syndrome or vertigo

H81.01 Ménière's disease, <u>right</u> ear

H81.02 Ménière's disease, <u>left</u> ear

H81.03 Ménière's disease, <u>bilateral</u>

H81.09 Ménière's disease, <u>unspecified</u> ear

H81.1- <u>Benign paroxysmal vertigo</u> — An illusion of the external world moving due to disturbances of the vestibular centers or pathways in the central nervous system associated with a specific position of the head.

H81.10 Benign paroxysmal vertigo, <u>unspecified</u> ear

H81.11 Benign paroxysmal vertigo, <u>right</u> ear

H81.12 Benign paroxysmal vertigo, <u>left</u> ear

H81.13 Benign paroxysmal vertigo, <u>bilateral</u>

H81.2- <u>Vestibular neuronitis</u> — An illusion of the external world moving due to disturbances of the vestibular centers or pathways in the central nervous system due to inflammation of the vestibular nerves.

H81.20 Vestibular neuronitis, <u>unspecified</u> ear

H81.21 Vestibular neuronitis, <u>right</u> ear

H81.22 Vestibular neuronitis, <u>left</u> ear

H81.23 Vestibular neuronitis, <u>bilateral</u>

H81.3- <u>Other</u> peripheral vertigo — An illusion of the external world moving due to disturbances of the vestibular centers or pathways in the central nervous system.

H81.31- <u>Aural vertigo</u> — A form due to pressure of cerumen on the ear drum.

H81.311 Aural vertigo, <u>right</u> ear

H81.312 Aural vertigo, <u>left</u> ear

H81.313 Aural vertigo, <u>bilateral</u>

H81.319 Aural vertigo, <u>unspecified</u> ear

H81.39- <u>Other peripheral vertigo</u>
      Lermoyez' syndrome
      Otogenic vertigo
      Peripheral vertigo NOS

H81.391 Other peripheral vertigo, <u>right</u> ear

H81.392 Other peripheral vertigo, <u>left</u> ear

H81.393 Other peripheral vertigo, <u>bilateral</u>

H81.399 Other peripheral vertigo, <u>unspecified</u> ear

H81.4- Vertigo of <u>central origin</u> — The illusion of true (rotational) vertigo due to a disease of the central nervous system.
      Central positional nystagmus

H81.41 Vertigo of central origin, <u>right</u> ear

H81.42 Vertigo of central origin, <u>left</u> ear

H81.43 Vertigo of central origin, <u>bilateral</u>

H81.49 Vertigo of central origin, <u>unspecified</u> ear

H81.8- Other disorders of vestibular function

H81.8x- <u>Other disorders of vestibular function</u>

H81.8x1 Other disorders of vestibular function, <u>right</u> ear

H81.8x2 Other disorders of vestibular function, <u>left</u> ear

H81.8x3 Other disorders of vestibular function, <u>bilateral</u>

H81.8x9 Other disorders of vestibular function, <u>unspecified</u> ear

H81.9- <u>Unspecified</u> disorder of vestibular function
      Vertiginous syndrome NOS

H81.90 Unspecified disorder of vestibular function, <u>unspecified</u> ear

H81.91 Unspecified disorder of vestibular function, <u>right</u> ear

H81.92 Unspecified disorder of vestibular function, <u>left</u> ear

H81.93 Unspecified disorder of vestibular function, <u>bilateral</u>

H82- Vertiginous syndromes <u>in diseases classified elsewhere</u>
    Code first underlying disease
      Excludes 1:   epidemic vertigo (A88.1)

H82.1 Vertiginous syndromes in diseases classified elsewhere, <u>right</u> ear — [Not Allowed as PDX]

H82.2 Vertiginous syndromes in diseases classified elsewhere, <u>left</u> ear — [Not Allowed as PDX]

H 7 5 - H 8 2

H82.3 Vertiginous syndromes in diseases classified elsewhere, <u>bilateral</u> — [Not Allowed as PDX]

H82.9 Vertiginous syndromes in diseases classified elsewhere, <u>unspecified</u> ear — [Not Allowed as PDX]

H83- Other diseases of inner ear

H83.0- <u>Labyrinthitis</u> — Inflammation of the inner ear labyrinth.

H83.01 Labyrinthitis, <u>right</u> ear

H83.02 Labyrinthitis, <u>left</u> ear

H83.03 Labyrinthitis, <u>bilateral</u>

H83.09 Labyrinthitis, <u>unspecified</u> ear

H83.1- <u>Labyrinthine fistula</u> — An abnormal passage communicating with the labyrinth.

H83.11 Labyrinthine fistula, <u>right</u> ear

H83.12 Labyrinthine fistula, <u>left</u> ear

H83.13 Labyrinthine fistula, <u>bilateral</u>

H83.19 Labyrinthine fistula, <u>unspecified</u> ear

H83.2- <u>Labyrinthine dysfunction</u> — An abnormal impairment of function of the inner ear.
Labyrinthine hypersensitivity
Labyrinthine hypofunction
Labyrinthine loss of function

H83.2x- <u>Labyrinthine dysfunction</u>

H83.2x1 Labyrinthine dysfunction, <u>right</u> ear

H83.2x2 Labyrinthine dysfunction, <u>left</u> ear

H83.2x3 Labyrinthine dysfunction, <u>bilateral</u>

H83.2x9 Labyrinthine dysfunction, <u>unspecified</u> ear

H83.3- Noise effects on inner ear
Acoustic trauma of inner ear
Noise-induced hearing loss of inner ear

H83.3x- <u>Noise effects on inner ear</u>

H83.3x1 Noise effects on <u>right</u> inner ear

H83.3x2 Noise effects on <u>left</u> inner ear

H83.3x3 Noise effects on inner ear, <u>bilateral</u>

H83.3x9 Noise effects on inner ear, <u>unspecified</u> ear

H83.8- Other specified diseases of inner ear

H83.8x- <u>Other specified</u> diseases of inner ear

H83.8x1 Other specified diseases of <u>right</u> inner ear

H83.8x2 Other specified diseases of <u>left</u> inner ear

H83.8x3 Other specified diseases of inner ear, <u>bilateral</u>

H83.8x9 Other specified diseases of inner ear, <u>unspecified</u> ear

H83.9- <u>Unspecified</u> disease of inner ear

H83.90 Unspecified disease of inner ear, <u>unspecified</u> ear

H83.91 Unspecified disease of <u>right</u> inner ear

H83.92 Unspecified disease of <u>left</u> inner ear

H83.93 Unspecified disease of inner ear, <u>bilateral</u>

Other disorders of ear (H90-H94)

H90- Conductive and sensorineural hearing loss — CONDUCTIVE HEARING LOSS — The decreased ability to perceive sounds due to a defect of the sound conducting apparatus of the ear. SENSORINEURAL HEARING LOSS — The decreased ability to perceive sounds due to a defect in the sensory mechanism of the ear or nerves.
Excludes 1:   deaf nonspeaking NEC (H91.3)
deafness NOS (H91.9-)
hearing loss NOS (H91.9-)
noise-induced hearing loss (H83.3-)
ototoxic hearing loss (H91.0-)
sudden (idiopathic) hearing loss (H91.2-)
AHA 15:2Q:p7x2 – Mixed hearing loss, bilateral

H90.0 <u>Conductive</u> hearing loss, <u>bilateral</u>

H90.1- <u>Conductive</u> hearing loss, <u>unilateral</u> with unrestricted hearing on the contralateral side

H90.11 Conductive hearing loss, unilateral, <u>right</u> ear, with unrestricted hearing on the contralateral side

H90.12 Conductive hearing loss, unilateral, <u>left</u> ear, with unrestricted hearing on the contralateral side

H90.2 <u>Conductive</u> hearing loss, <u>unspecified</u>
Conductive deafness NOS

H90.3 <u>Sensorineural</u> hearing loss, <u>bilateral</u>

H90.4- <u>Sensorineural</u> hearing loss, <u>unilateral</u> with unrestricted hearing on the contralateral side

H90.41 Sensorineural hearing loss, unilateral, <u>right</u> ear, with unrestricted hearing on the contralateral side

H90.42 Sensorineural hearing loss, unilateral, <u>left</u> ear, with unrestricted hearing on the contralateral side

H90.5 Unspecified <u>sensorineural</u> hearing loss
Central hearing loss NOS
Congenital deafness NOS
Neural hearing loss NOS
Perceptive hearing loss NOS
Sensorineural deafness NOS
Sensory hearing loss NOS
Excludes 1:   abnormal auditory perception (H93.2-)
psychogenic deafness (F44.6)

H90.6 <u>Mixed</u> conductive and sensorineural hearing loss, <u>bilateral</u>

H90.7- <u>Mixed</u> conductive and sensorineural hearing loss, <u>unilateral</u> with unrestricted hearing on the contralateral side

H90.71 Mixed conductive and sensorineural hearing loss, unilateral, <u>right</u> ear, with unrestricted hearing on the contralateral side

H90.72 Mixed conductive and sensorineural hearing loss, unilateral, <u>left</u> ear, with unrestricted hearing on the contralateral side

H90.8 Mixed conductive and sensorineural hearing loss, <u>unspecified</u>

H90.A- Conductive and sensorineural hearing loss <u>with restricted hearing on the contralateral side</u>

H90.A1- <u>Conductive</u> hearing loss, unilateral, with restricted hearing on the contralateral side

H90.A11 Conductive hearing loss, unilateral, <u>right</u> ear, with restricted hearing on the contralateral side

H90.A12 Conductive hearing loss, unilateral, <u>left</u> ear, with restricted hearing on the contralateral side

H90.A2- <u>Sensorineural</u> hearing loss, unilateral, with restricted hearing on the contralateral side

H90.A21 Sensorineural hearing loss, unilateral, <u>right</u> ear, with restricted hearing on the contralateral side

H90.A22 Sensorineural hearing loss, unilateral, <u>left</u> ear, with restricted hearing on the contralateral side

H90.A3- <u>Mixed</u> conductive and sensorineural hearing loss, unilateral, with restricted hearing on the contralateral side

H90.A31 Mixed conductive and sensorineural hearing loss, unilateral, <u>right</u> ear, with restricted hearing on the contralateral side

H90.A32 Mixed conductive and sensorineural hearing loss, unilateral, <u>left</u> ear, with restricted hearing on the contralateral side

H91- <u>Other and unspecified hearing loss</u>
Excludes 1:   abnormal auditory perception (H93.2-)
hearing loss as classified in H90.-
impacted cerumen (H61.2-)
noise-induced hearing loss (H83.3-)
psychogenic deafness (F44.6)
transient ischemic deafness (H93.01-)

H91.0- <u>Ototoxic hearing loss</u> — The decreased ability to perceive sounds due to a drug, toxin, or other external substance.
Code first poisoning due to drug or toxin, if applicable (T36-T65 with fifth or sixth character 1-4 or 6)
Use additional code for adverse effect, if applicable, to identify drug (T36-T50 with fift or sixth character 5)

H91.01 Ototoxic hearing loss, <u>right</u> ear

H91.02 Ototoxic hearing loss, <u>left</u> ear

H91.03 Ototoxic hearing loss, <u>bilateral</u>

H91.09 Ototoxic hearing loss, <u>unspecified</u> ear

H91.1- <u>Presbycusis</u> — Progressive loss of hearing ability due to the normal aging process.
Presbyacusia

H91.10 Presbycusis, <u>unspecified</u> ear

H91.11 Presbycusis, <u>right</u> ear

H91.12 Presbycusis, <u>left</u> ear

H91.13 Presbycusis, <u>bilateral</u>

H82 - H91

H91.2- Sudden idiopathic hearing loss — The sudden decreased ability to perceive sounds due to an unknown cause.

    Sudden hearing loss NOS

  H91.20 Sudden idiopathic hearing loss, unspecified ear

  H91.21 Sudden idiopathic hearing loss, right ear

  H91.22 Sudden idiopathic hearing loss, left ear

  H91.23 Sudden idiopathic hearing loss, bilateral

H91.3 Deaf nonspeaking, not elsewhere classified

H91.8- Other specified hearing loss

  H91.8x- Other specified hearing loss

    H91.8x1 Other specified hearing loss, right ear

    H91.8x2 Other specified hearing loss, left ear

    H91.8x3 Other specified hearing loss, bilateral

    H91.8x9 Other specified hearing loss, unspecified ear

H91.9- Unspecified hearing loss

    Deafness NOS

    High frequency deafness

    Low frequency deafness

  H91.90 Unspecified hearing loss, unspecified ear

  H91.91 Unspecified hearing loss, right ear

  H91.92 Unspecified hearing loss, left ear

  H91.93 Unspecified hearing loss, bilateral

H92- Otalgia and effusion of ear

  H92.0- Otalgia — Pain in the ear.

    H92.01 Otalgia, right ear

    H92.02 Otalgia, left ear

    H92.03 Otalgia, bilateral

    H92.09 Otalgia, unspecified ear

  H92.1- Otorrhea — Inflammation of the ear with purulent discharge.

    Excludes 1: *leakage of cerebrospinal fluid through ear (G96.0)*

    H92.10 Otorrhea, unspecified ear

    H92.11 Otorrhea, right ear

    H92.12 Otorrhea, left ear

    H92.13 Otorrhea, bilateral

  H92.2- Otorrhagia — The abnormal discharge of blood from the ear.

    Excludes 1: *traumatic otorrhagia — code to injury*

    H92.20 Otorrhagia, unspecified ear

    H92.21 Otorrhagia, right ear

    H92.22 Otorrhagia, left ear

    H92.23 Otorrhagia, bilateral

H93- Other disorders of ear, not elsewhere classified

  H93.0- Degenerative and vascular disorders of ear

    Excludes 1: *presbycusis (H91.1)*

    H93.01- Transient ischemic deafness — A temporary loss of hearing ability due to decreased blood flow to the ear.

      H93.011 Transient ischemic deafness, right ear

      H93.012 Transient ischemic deafness, left ear

      H93.013 Transient ischemic deafness, bilateral

      H93.019 Transient ischemic deafness, unspecified ear

    H93.09- Unspecified degenerative and vascular disorders of ear

      H93.091 Unspecified degenerative and vascular disorders of right ear

      H93.092 Unspecified degenerative and vascular disorders of left ear

      H93.093 Unspecified degenerative and vascular disorders of ear, bilateral

      H93.099 Unspecified degenerative and vascular disorders of unspecified ear

  H93.1- Tinnitus — A ringing, buzzing, or clicking noise in the ear.

  H93.11 Tinnitus, right ear

  H93.12 Tinnitus, left ear

  H93.13 Tinnitus, bilateral

  H93.19 Tinnitus, unspecified ear

H93.A- Pulsatile tinnitus — A beating or pulsing sound in the ear that is synchronous with the heartbeat.

  H93.A1 Pulsatile tinnitus, right ear

  H93.A2 Pulsatile tinnitus, left ear

  H93.A3 Pulsatile tinnitus, bilateral

  H93.A9 Pulsatile tinnitus, unspecified ear

H93.2- Other abnormal auditory perceptions

  Excludes 2: *auditory hallucinations (R44.0)*

  H93.21- Auditory recruitment — An abnormal increase in the perceived intensity of a sound out of proportion to the actual increase in the sound level.

    H93.211 Auditory recruitment, right ear

    H93.212 Auditory recruitment, left ear

    H93.213 Auditory recruitment, bilateral

    H93.219 Auditory recruitment, unspecified ear

  H93.22- Diplacusis — An abnormal perception of pitch characterized by hearing two tones for every sound produced.

    H93.221 Diplacusis, right ear

    H93.222 Diplacusis, left ear

    H93.223 Diplacusis, bilateral

    H93.229 Diplacusis, unspecified ear

  H93.23- Hyperacusis — The abnormal sensitivity to sound.

    H93.231 Hyperacusis, right ear

    H93.232 Hyperacusis, left ear

    H93.233 Hyperacusis, bilateral

    H93.239 Hyperacusis, unspecified ear

  H93.24- Temporary auditory threshold shift — A condition of temporary decreased auditory sensitivity to accommodate a higher decible environment.

    H93.241 Temporary auditory threshold shift, right ear

    H93.242 Temporary auditory threshold shift, left ear

    H93.243 Temporary auditory threshold shift, bilateral

    H93.249 Temporary auditory threshold shift, unspecified ear

  H93.25 Central auditory processing disorder — A disorder characterized by difficulty in the processing of auditory frequency, intensity, and temporal information in the central nervous system.

    Congenital auditory imperception

    Word deafness

  Excludes 1: *mixed receptive-expressive language disorder (F80.2)*

  H93.29- Other abnormal auditory perceptions

    H93.291 Other abnormal auditory perceptions, right ear

    H93.292 Other abnormal auditory perceptions, left ear

    H93.293 Other abnormal auditory perceptions, bilateral

    H93.299 Other abnormal auditory perceptions, unspecified ear

H93.3- Disorders of acoustic nerve

    Disorder of 8th cranial nerve

  Excludes 1: *acoustic neuroma (D33.3)*

          syphilitic acoustic neuritis (A52.15)

  H93.3x- Disorders of acoustic nerve — Dysfunction of the acoustic nerve.

    H93.3x1 Disorders of right acoustic nerve

    H93.3x2 Disorders of left acoustic nerve

    H93.3x3 Disorders of bilateral acoustic nerves

    H93.3x9 Disorders of unspecified acoustic nerve

H93.8- Other specified disorders of ear

  H93.8x- Other specified disorders of ear

    H93.8x1 Other specified disorders of right ear

    H93.8x2 Other specified disorders of left ear

    H93.8x3 Other specified disorders of ear, bilateral

    H93.8x9 Other specified disorders of ear, unspecified ear

H93.9- Unspecified disorder of ear

  H93.90 Unspecified disorder of ear, unspecified ear — [Unacceptable PDX]

  H93.91 Unspecified disorder of right ear — [Unacceptable PDX]

  H93.92 Unspecified disorder of left ear — [Unacceptable PDX]

  H93.93 Unspecified disorder of ear, bilateral — [Unacceptable PDX]

H91-H93

H94- Other disorders of ear <u>in diseases classified elsewhere</u>

H94.0- Acoustic neuritis <u>in infectious and parasitic diseases classified elsewhere</u>
Code first underlying disease, such as:
  Parasitic disease (B65-B89)
  Excludes 1: *acoustic neuritis (in):*
              herpes zoster (B02.29)
              syphilis (A52.15)

H94.00 Acoustic neuritis in infectious and parasitic diseases classified elsewhere, <u>unspecified</u> ear — [Not Allowed as PDX]

H94.01 Acoustic neuritis in infectious and parasitic diseases classified elsewhere, <u>right</u> ear — [Not Allowed as PDX]

H94.02 Acoustic neuritis in infectious and parasitic diseases classified elsewhere, <u>left</u> ear — [Not Allowed as PDX]

H94.03 Acoustic neuritis in infectious and parasitic diseases classified elsewhere, <u>bilateral</u> — [Not Allowed as PDX]

H94.8- Other specified disorders of ear <u>in diseases classified elsewhere</u>
Code first underlying disease, such as:
  Congenital syphilis (A50.0)
  Excludes 1: *aural myiasis (B87.4)*
              syphilitic labyrinthitis (A52.79)

H94.80 Other specified disorders of ear in diseases classified elsewhere, <u>unspecified</u> ear — [Not Allowed as PDX]

H94.81 Other specified disorders of <u>right</u> ear in diseases classified elsewhere — [Not Allowed as PDX]

H94.82 Other specified disorders of <u>left</u> ear in diseases classified elsewhere — [Not Allowed as PDX]

H94.83 Other specified disorders of ear in diseases classified elsewhere, <u>bilateral</u> — [Not Allowed as PDX]

Intraoperative and postprocedural complications and disorders of ear and mastoid process, not elsewhere classified (H95)

H95- <u>Intraoperative and postprocedural complications</u> and disorders of ear and mastoid process, not elsewhere classified

H95.0- <u>Recurrent cholesteatoma of postmastoidectomy cavity</u>

H95.00 Recurrent cholesteatoma of postmastoidectomy cavity, <u>unspecified</u> ear

H95.01 Recurrent cholesteatoma of postmastoidectomy cavity, <u>right</u> ear

H95.02 Recurrent cholesteatoma of postmastoidectomy cavity, <u>left</u> ear

H95.03 Recurrent cholesteatoma of postmastoidectomy cavity, <u>bilateral</u> ears

H95.1- <u>Other</u> disorders of ear and mastoid process <u>following mastoidectomy</u>

H95.11- Chronic inflammation of postmastoidectomy cavity

H95.111 Chronic inflammation of postmastoidectomy cavity, <u>right</u> ear

H95.112 Chronic inflammation of postmastoidectomy cavity, <u>left</u> ear

H95.113 Chronic inflammation of postmastoidectomy cavity, <u>bilateral</u> ears

H95.119 Chronic inflammation of postmastoidectomy cavity, <u>unspecified</u> ear

H95.12- <u>Granulation</u> of <u>postmastoidectomy cavity</u>

H95.121 Granulation of postmastoidectomy cavity, <u>right</u> ear

H95.122 Granulation of postmastoidectomy cavity, <u>left</u> ear

H95.123 Granulation of postmastoidectomy cavity, <u>bilateral</u> ears

H95.129 Granulation of postmastoidectomy cavity, <u>unspecified</u> ear

H95.13- <u>Mucosal cyst</u> of <u>postmastoidectomy cavity</u>

H95.131 Mucosal cyst of postmastoidectomy cavity, <u>right</u> ear

H95.132 Mucosal cyst of postmastoidectomy cavity, <u>left</u> ear

H95.133 Mucosal cyst of postmastoidectomy cavity, <u>bilateral</u> ears

H95.139 Mucosal cyst of postmastoidectomy cavity, <u>unspecified</u> ear

H95.19- <u>Other</u> disorders <u>following mastoidectomy</u>

H95.191 Other disorders following mastoidectomy, <u>right</u> ear

H95.192 Other disorders following mastoidectomy, <u>left</u> ear

H95.193 Other disorders following mastoidectomy, <u>bilateral</u> ears

H95.199 Other disorders following mastoidectomy, <u>unspecified</u> ear

H95.2- <u>Intraoperative hemorrhage and hematoma</u> of ear and mastoid process complicating a procedure
  Excludes 1: *intraoperative hemorrhage and hematoma of ear and mastoid process due to accidental puncture or laceration during a procedure (H95.3-)*

CC **H95.21** Intraoperative hemorrhage and hematoma of ear and mastoid process complicating a <u>procedure on the ear and mastoid process</u>

CC **H95.22** Intraoperative hemorrhage and hematoma of ear and mastoid process complicating <u>other procedure</u>

H95.3- <u>Accidental puncture and laceration</u> of ear and mastoid process during a procedure

CC **H95.31** Accidental puncture and laceration of the ear and mastoid process during a <u>procedure on the ear and mastoid process</u>

CC **H95.32** Accidental puncture and laceration of the ear and mastoid process during <u>other procedure</u>

H95.4- <u>Postprocedural</u> <u>hemorrhage</u> of ear and mastoid process following a procedure

CC **H95.41** Postprocedural hemorrhage of ear and mastoid process following a <u>procedure on the ear and mastoid process</u>

CC **H95.42** Postprocedural hemorrhage of ear and mastoid process following <u>other procedure</u>

H95.5- <u>Postprocedural</u> <u>hematoma and seroma</u> of ear and mastoid process following a procedure

CC **H95.51** Postprocedural <u>hematoma</u> of ear and mastoid process following a <u>procedure on the ear and mastoid process</u>

CC **H95.52** Postprocedural <u>hematoma</u> of ear and mastoid process following <u>other procedure</u>

CC **H95.53** Postprocedural <u>seroma</u> of ear and mastoid process following a <u>procedure on the ear and mastoid process</u>

CC **H95.54** Postprocedural <u>seroma</u> of ear and mastoid process following <u>other procedure</u>

H95.8- Other intraoperative and postprocedural complications and disorders of the ear and mastoid process, not elsewhere classified
  Excludes ❷: *postprocedural complications and disorders following mastoidectomy (H95.0-, H95.1-)*

H95.81- <u>Postprocedural stenosis</u> of external ear canal

CC **H95.811** Postprocedural stenosis of <u>right</u> external ear canal

CC **H95.812** Postprocedural stenosis of <u>left</u> external ear canal

CC **H95.813** Postprocedural stenosis of external ear canal, <u>bilateral</u>

CC **H95.819** Postprocedural stenosis of <u>unspecified</u> external ear canal

CC **H95.88** Other intraoperative complications and disorders of the ear and mastoid process, no telsewhere classified
  Use additional code, if applicable, to further specify disorder

CC **H95.89** Other postprocedural complications and disorders of the ear and mastoid process, not elsewhere classified
  Use additional code, if applicable, to further specify disorder

H
9
4
I
H
9
5

H
9
5
-
H
9
5

Chapter 9 – Diseases of the circulatory system (I00-I99)

Excludes ❷: *certain conditions originating in the perinatal period*
(P04-P96)
certain infectious and parasitic diseases (A00-B99)
complications of pregnancy, childbirth and the puerperium
(O00-O9A)
congenital malformations, deformations, and chromosomal
abnormalities (Q00-Q99)
endocrine, nutritional and metabolic diseases (E00-E88)
injury, poisoning and certain other consequences of external
causes (S00-T88)
neoplasms (C00-D49)
symptoms, signs and abnormal clinical and laboratory findings,
not elsewhere classified (R00-R94)
systemic connective tissue disorders (M30-M36)
transient cerebral ischemic attacks and related syndromes
(G45-)

This chapter contains the following blocks:

I00-I02	**Acute rheumatic fever**
I05-I09	**Chronic rheumatic heart diseases**
I10-I16	**Hypertensive diseases**
I20-I25	**Ischemic heart diseases**
I26-I28	**Pulmonary heart disease and diseases of pulmonary circulation**
I30-I52	**Other forms of heart disease**
I60-I69	**Cerebrovascular diseases**
I70-I79	**Diseases of arteries, arterioles and capillaries**
I80-I89	**Diseases of veins, lymphatic vessels and lymph nodes, not elsewhere classified**
I95-I99	**Other and unspecified disorders of the circulatory system**

Chapter-Specific Coding Guidelines

C. Chapter-Specific Coding Guidelines

In addition to general coding guidelines, there are guidelines for specific diagnoses and/or conditions in the classification. Unless otherwise indicated, these guidelines apply to all health care settings. Please refer to Section II for guidelines on the selection of principal diagnosis.

9. Chapter 9: Diseases of Circulatory System (I00-I99)

a. Hypertension

The classification presumes a causal relationship between hypertension and heart involvement and between hypertension and kidney involvement, as the two conditions are linked by the term "with" in the Alphabetic Index. These conditions should be coded as related even in the absence of provider documentation explicitly linking them, unless the documentation clearly states the conditions are unrelated.

For hypertension and conditions not specifically linked by relational terms such as "with," "associated with" or "due to" in the classification, provider documentaton must link the conditions in order to code them as related.

1) Hypertension with Heart Disease

Hypertension with heart conditions classified to I50.- or I51.4-I51.9, are assigned to, a code from category I11, Hypertensive heart disease, when a causal relationship is stated (due to hypertension) or implied (hypertensive). Use an additional code from category I50, Heart failure, to identify the type of heart failure in those patients with heart failure.

The same heart conditions (I50.-, I51.4-I51.9) with hypertension, ~~but without a stated causal relationship,~~ are coded separately if the provider has specifically documented a different cause. Sequence according to the circumstances of the admission/encounter.

2) Hypertensive Chronic Kidney Disease

Assign codes from category I12, Hypertensive chronic kidney disease, when both hypertension and a condition classifiable to category N18, Chronic kidney disease (CKD), are present. ~~Unlike hypertension with heart disease, ICD-10-CM presumes a cause- and-effect relationship and classifies chronic kidney disease with hypertension as hypertensive chronic kidney disease.~~ CKD should not be coded as hypertensive if the physician has specifically documented a different cause.

The appropriate code from category N18 should be used as a secondary code with a code from category I12 to identify the stage of chronic kidney disease.

See Section I.C.14. Chronic kidney disease.

If a patient has hypertensive chronic kidney disease and acute renal failure, an additional code for the acute renal failure is required.

3) Hypertensive Heart and Chronic Kidney Disease

Assign codes from combination category I13, Hypertensive heart and chronic kidney disease, when ~~both hypertensive kidney disease and hypertensive heart disease are stated in the diagnosis~~ there is hypertension with both heart and kidney involvement. ~~Assume a relationship between the hypertension and the chronic kidney disease, whether or not the condition is so designated.~~ If heart failure is present, assign an additional code from category I50 to identify the type of heart failure.

The appropriate code from category N18, Chronic kidney disease, should be used as a secondary code with a code from category I13 to identify the stage of chronic kidney disease.

See Section I.C.14. Chronic kidney disease.

The codes in category I13, Hypertensive heart and chronic kidney disease, are combination codes that include hypertension, heart disease and chronic kidney disease. The Includes note at I13 specifies that the conditions included at I11 and I12 are included together in I13. If apatient has hypertension, heart disease and chronic kidney disease then a code from I13 should be used, not individual codes for hypertension, heart disease and chronic kidney disease, or codes from I11 or I12.

For patients with both acute renal failure and chronic kidney disease, an additional code for acute renal failure is required.

4) Hypertensive Cerebrovascular Disease

For hypertensive cerebrovascular disease, first assign the appropriate code from categories I60-I69, followed by the appropriate hypertension code.

5) Hypertensive Retinopathy

Subcategory H35.0, Background retinopathy and retinal vascular changes, should be used with a code from category I10-I15, Hypertensive disease to include the systemic hypertension. The sequencing is based on the reason for the encounter.

6) Hypertension, Secondary

Secondary hypertension is due to an underlying condition. Two codes are required: one to identify the underlying etiology and one from category I15 to identify the hypertension. Sequencing of codes is determined by the reason for admission/encounter.

7) Hypertension, Transient

Assign code R03.0, Elevated blood pressure reading without diagnosis of hypertension, unless patient has an established diagnosis of hypertension. Assign code O13.-, Gestational [pregnancy-induced] hypertension without significant proteinuria, or O14.-, Pre-eclampsia, for transient hypertension of pregnancy.

8) Hypertension, Controlled

This diagnostic statement usually refers to an existing state of hypertension under control by therapy. Assign the appropriate code from categories I10-I15, Hypertensive diseases.

9) Hypertension, Uncontrolled

Uncontrolled hypertension may refer to untreated hypertension or hypertension not responding to current therapeutic regimen. In either case, assign the appropriate code from categories I10-I15, Hypertensive diseases.

10) Hypertensive Crisis

Assign a code from category I16, Hypertensive crisis, for documented hypertensive urgency, hypertensive emergency or unspecified hypertensive crisis. Code also any identified hypertensive disease (I10-I15). The sequencing is based on the reason for the encounter.

b. Atherosclerotic Coronary Artery Disease and Angina

ICD-10-CM has combination codes for atherosclerotic heart disease with angina pectoris. The subcategories for these codes are I25.11, Atherosclerotic heart disease of native coronary artery with angina pectoris and I25.7, Atherosclerosis of coronary artery bypass graft(s) and coronary artery of transplanted heart with angina pectoris.

When using one of these combination codes it is not necessary to use an additional code for angina pectoris. A causal relationship can be assumed in a patient with both atherosclerosis and angina pectoris, unless the documentation indicates the angina is due to something other than the atherosclerosis.

If a patient with coronary artery disease is admitted due to an acute myocardial infarction (AMI), the AMI should be sequenced before the coronary artery disease.

See Section I.C.9. Acute myocardial infarction (AMI).

c. Intraoperative and Postprocedural Cerebrovascular Accident

Medical record documentation should clearly specify the cause-and-effect relationship between the medical intervention and the cerebrovascular accident in order to assign a code for intraoperative or postprocedural cerebrovascular accident.

I00 - I00

Proper code assignment depends on whether it was an infarction or hemorrhage and whether it occurred intraoperatively or postoperatively. If it was a cerebral hemorrhage, code assignment depends on the type of procedure performed.

d. Sequelae of Cerebrovascular Disease

1) Category I69, Sequelae of Cerebrovascular disease

Category I69 is used to indicate conditions classifiable to categories I60-I67 as the causes of sequela (neurologic deficits), themselves classified elsewhere. These "late effects" include neurologic deficits that persist after initial onset of conditions classifiable to categories I60-I67. The neurologic deficits caused by cerebrovascular disease may be present from the onset or may arise at any time after the onset of the condition classifiable to categories I60-I67.

Codes from category I69, Sequelae of cerebrovascular disease, that specify hemiplegia, hemiparesis and monoplegia identify whether the dominant or nondominant side is affected. Should the affected side be documented, but not specified as dominant or nondominant, and the classification system does not indicate a default, code selection is as follows:
- For ambidextrous patients, the default should be dominant.
- If the left side is affected, the default is nondominant.
- If the right side is affected, the default is dominant.

2) Codes from category I69 with codes from I60-I67

Codes from category I69 may be assigned on a health care record with codes from I60-I67, if the patient has a current cerebrovascular disease and deficits from an old cerebrovascular disease.

3) Codes from category I69 and Personal history of transient ischemic attack (TIA) and cerebral infarction (Z86.73)

Codes from category I69 should not be assigned if the patient does not have neurologic deficits.

See Section I.C.21.c4. History (of) for use of personal history codes.

e. Acute myocardial infarction (AMI)

1) ST elevation myocardial infarction (STEMI) and non ST elevation myocardial infarction (NSTEMI)

The ICD-10-CM codes for acute myocardial infarction (AMI) identify the site, such as anterolateral wall or true posterior wall. Subcategories I21.0-I21.2 and code I21.3 are used for ST elevation myocardial infarction (STEMI). Code I21.4, Non-ST elevation (NSTEMI) myocardial infarction, is used for non ST elevation myocardial infarction (NSTEMI) and nontransmural MIs.

If NSTEMI evolves to STEMI, assign the STEMI code. If STEMI converts to NSTEMI due to thrombolytic therapy, it is still coded as STEMI.

For encounters occurring while the myocardial infarction is equal to, or less than, four weeks old, including transfers to another acute setting or a postacute setting, and ~~the patient requires continued care for~~ the myocardial infarction meets the definition for "other diagnoses" (see Section III, Reporting Additional Diagnoses), codes from category I21 may continue to be reported. For encounters after the 4 week time frame and the   patient is still receiving care related to the myocardial infarction, the appropriate aftercare code should be assigned, rather than a code from category I21. For old or healed myocardial infarctions not requiring further care, code I25.2, Old myocardial infarction, may be assigned.

2) Acute myocardial infarction, unspecified

Code I21.3, ST elevation (STEMI) myocardial infarction of unspecified site, is the default for the unspecified acute myocardial infarction. If only STEMI or transmural MI without the site is documented, assign code I21.3.

3) AMI documented as nontransmural or subendocardial but site provided

If an AMI is documented as nontransmural or subendocardial, but the site is provided, it is still coded as a subendocardial AMI.

See Section I.C.21.3 for information on coding status post administration of tPA in a different facility within the last 24 hours.

4) Subsequent acute myocardial infarction

A code from category I22, Subsequent ST elevation (STEMI) and non ST elevation (NSTEMI) myocardial infarction, is to be used when a patient who has suffered an AMI has a new AMI within the 4 week time frame of the initial AMI. A code from category I22 must be used in conjunction with a code from category I21. The sequencing of the I22 and I21 codes depends on the circumstances of the encounter.

Acute rheumatic fever (I00-I02)

I00 Rheumatic fever <u>without</u> heart involvement — A systemic inflammatory disease, with a severe onset, occurring as a delayed sequela of group A beta-hemolytic Streptococcus characterized by connective tissue inflammation, especially the blood vessels and joints.

Includes: Arthritis, rheumatic, acute or subacute
Excludes 1:   rheumatic fever with heart involvement (I01.0 - I01.9)

I01- Rheumatic fever <u>with</u> heart involvement — A systemic inflammatory disease, with a severe onset, as a delayed sequela of group A beta-hemolytic Streptococcus characterized by connective tissue inflammation, specifically the heart, and of blood vessels and joints.

Excludes 1:   chronic diseases of rheumatic origin (I05-I09) unless rheumatic fever is also present or there is evidence of reactivation or activity of the rheumatic process

cc I01.0 Acute rheumatic pericarditis — A form characterized by inflammation of the outer fibrous and serous protective layers of the heart.
  Any condition in I00 with pericarditis
  Rheumatic pericarditis (acute)
Excludes 1:   acute pericarditis not specified as rheumatic (I30.-)

cc I01.1 Acute rheumatic endocarditis — A form characterized by inflammation of the inner serous lining membrane of the heart, including the valves of the heart.
  Any condition in I00 with endocarditis or valvulitis
  Acute rheumatic valvulitis

cc I01.2 Acute rheumatic myocarditis — A form characterized by inflammation of the cardiac muscle.
  Any condition in I00 with myocarditis

cc I01.8 Other acute rheumatic heart disease
  Any condition in I00 with other or multiple types of heart involvement
  Acute rheumatic pancarditis — A form marked by inflammation of the pericardium and endocardium.

cc I01.9 Acute rheumatic heart disease, unspecified
  Any condition in I00 with unspecified type of heart involvement
  Rheumatic carditis, acute
  Rheumatic heart disease, active or acute

I02- Rheumatic <u>chorea</u> — Abrupt, involuntary, purposeless movements, muscular weakness, and emotional lability associated with rheumatic fever.
Includes: Sydenham's chorea
Excludes 1:   chorea NOS (G25.5)
                  Huntington's chorea (G10)

cc I02.0 Rheumatic chorea with heart involvement — A form marked by association with cardiac inflammation.
  Chorea NOS with heart involvement
  Rheumatic chorea with heart involvement of any type classifiable under I01.-

cc I02.9 Rheumatic chorea without heart involvement
  Rheumatic chorea NOS

Chronic rheumatic heart diseases (I05-I09)

I05- Rheumatic <u>mitral valve diseases</u> — Persistent, degenerative, rheumatic inflammatory lesions of the mitral valve.
Includes: Conditions classifiable to both I05.0 and I05.2-I05.9, whether specified as rheumatic or not
Excludes 1:   mitral valve disease specified as nonrheumatic (I34.-)
                  mitral valve disease with aortic and/or tricuspid valve involvement (I08.-)

I05.0 Rheumatic mitral stenosis — A form characterized by reduction in the mitral valve orifice size.
  Mitral (valve) obstruction (rheumatic) — A form marked by blockage of the mitral valve orifice.

I05.1 Rheumatic mitral insufficiency — A form characterized by the inadequate function of the mitral valve.
  Rheumatic mitral incompetence — A form marked by inadequate function of the mitral valve.
  Rheumatic mitral regurgitation — A form marked by backflow of blood through the mitral valve.
Excludes 1:   mitral insufficiency not specified as rheumatic (I34.0)

I05.2 Rheumatic mitral stenosis <u>with insufficiency</u> — A form characterized by both reduction in the mitral valve orifice size and inadequate function and/or backflow of blood through the mitral valve.
  Rheumatic mitral stenosis with incompetence or regurgitation

I05.8 Other rheumatic mitral valve diseases
  Rheumatic mitral (valve) failure — A form characterized by the inability of the mitral valve to perform normally.

Excludes 1: = NOT CODED HERE! (Do not code both)   **722**   *Excludes ❷:* = Not Included Here

I05.9   Rheumatic mitral valve disease, unspecified
Rheumatic mitral (valve) disorder (chronic) NOS

I06-   Rheumatic aortic valve diseases — Persistent, degenerative, rheumatic inflammatory lesions of the aortic valve.
Excludes 1:   aortic valve disease not specified as rheumatic (I35.-)
aortic valve disease with mitral and/or tricuspid valve involvement (I08.-)

I06.0   Rheumatic aortic stenosis — A form characterized by reduction in the aortic valve orifice size.
Rheumatic aortic (valve) obstruction — A form marked by blockage of the aortic valve orifice size.

I06.1   Rheumatic aortic insufficiency — A form characterized by both reduction in the aortic valve orifice size and inadequate function.
Rheumatic aortic incompetence — A form marked by inadequate function of the aortic valve.
Rheumatic aortic regurgitation — A form marked by backflow of blood through the aortic valve.

I06.2   Rheumatic aortic stenosis with insufficiency — A form characterized by both reduction in the aortic valve orifice size and inadequate function and/or backflow of blood through the aortic valve.
Rheumatic aortic stenosis with incompetence or regurgitation

I06.8   Other rheumatic aortic valve diseases

I06.9   Rheumatic aortic valve disease, unspecified
Rheumatic aortic (valve) disease NOS

I07-   Rheumatic tricuspid valve diseases — Persistent, degenerative, rheumatic inflammatory lesions of the tricuspid valve.
Includes: Rheumatic tricuspid valve diseases specified as rheumatic or unspecified
Excludes 1:   tricuspid valve disease specified as nonrheumatic (I36.-)
tricuspid valve disease with aortic and/or mitral valve involvement (I08.-)

I07.0   Rheumatic tricuspid stenosis — A form characterized by reduction in the tricuspid valve orifice size.
Tricuspid (valve) stenosis (rheumatic)

I07.1   Rheumatic tricuspid insufficiency — A form characterized by the inadequate function of the tricuspid valve.
Tricuspid (valve) insufficiency (rheumatic)

I07.2   Rheumatic tricuspid stenosis and insufficiency — A form characterized by both reduction in the tricuspid valve orifice size and inadequate function and/or backflow of blood through the tricuspid valve.

I07.8   Other rheumatic tricuspid valve diseases

I07.9   Rheumatic tricuspid valve disease, unspecified
Rheumatic tricuspid valve disorder NOS

I08-   Multiple valve diseases — Persistent, degenerative, rheumatic inflammatory lesions of two or more heart valves.
Includes: Multiple valve diseases specified as rheumatic or unspecified
Excludes 1:   endocarditis, valve unspecified (I38)
multiple valve disease specified a nonrheumatic (I34.-, I35.-, I36.-, I37.-, I38.-, Q22.-, Q23.-, Q24.8-)
rheumatic valve disease NOS (I09.1)

I08.0   Rheumatic disorders of both mitral and aortic valves
Involvement of both mitral and aortic valves specified as rheumatic or unspecified

I08.1   Rheumatic disorders of both mitral and tricuspid valves

I08.2   Rheumatic disorders of both aortic and tricuspid valves

I08.3   Combined rheumatic disorders of mitral, aortic and tricuspid valves

I08.8   Other rheumatic multiple valve diseases

I08.9   Rheumatic multiple valve disease, unspecified

I09-   Other rheumatic heart diseases
cc **I09.0   Rheumatic myocarditis** — Persistent, degenerative, rheumatic inflammatory lesions of the myocardium.
Excludes 1:   myocarditis not specified as rheumatic (I51.4)

I09.1   Rheumatic diseases of endocardium, valve unspecified
Rheumatic endocarditis (chronic)
Rheumatic valvulitis (chronic)
Excludes 1:   endocarditis, valve unspecified (I38)

cc **I09.2   Chronic rheumatic pericarditis** — Persistent, degenerative, rheumatic inflammatory lesions of the outer fibrous and serous protective layers of the heart.
Adherent pericardium, rheumatic — A rheumatic degenerative condition characterized by increased friction and stickiness of the pericardium layers.
Chronic rheumatic mediastinopericarditis — A rheumatic, degenerative, adhesive inflammation of the pericardium extending to the mediastinum.
Chronic rheumatic myopericarditis — A rheumatic, degenerative inflammatory condition of the myocardium and pericardium.
Excludes 1:   chronic pericarditis not specified as rheumatic (I31.-)

I09.8-   Other specified rheumatic heart diseases
cc **I09.81   Rheumatic heart failure** — A rheumatic condition resulting in markedly decreased cardiac output and marked by venocapillary congestion, hypertension, and edema.
Use additional code to identify type of heart failure (I50.-)

I09.89   Other specified rheumatic heart diseases
Rheumatic disease of pulmonary valve — Persistent, degenerative, rheumatic inflammatory lesions of the pulmonary valve.

I09.9   Rheumatic heart disease, unspecified
Rheumatic carditis
Excludes 1:   rheumatoid carditis (M05.31)

Hypertensive diseases (I10-I16)

Use additional code to identify:
Exposure to environmental tobacco smoke (Z77.22)
History of tobacco dependence (Z87.891)
Occupational exposure to environmental tobacco smoke (Z57.31)
Tobacco dependence (F17.-)
Tobacco use (Z72.0)
Excludes 1:   neonatal hypertension (P29.2)
primary pulmonary hypertension (I27.0)
Excludes ❷: hypertensive disease complicating pregnancy, childbirth and the puerperium (O10-O11, O13-O16)

I10   Essential (primary) hypertension — [Questionable Admission] – Persistently high arterial blood pressure, measuring above 140 mm Hg systolic and 90 mm Hg diastolic, and without a discoverable organic cause.
Includes: High blood pressure
Hypertension (arterial) (benign) (essential) (malignant) (primary) (systemic)
Excludes 1:   hypertensive disease complicating pregnancy, childbirth and the puerperium (O10-O11, O13-O16)
Excludes ❷: essential (primary) hypertension involving vessels of brain (I60-I69)
essential (primary) hypertension involving vessels of eye (H35.0-)

I11-   Hypertensive heart disease — Heart function abnormality resulting from hypertension.
Includes: Any condition in I51.4-I51.9 due to hypertension

I11.0   Hypertensive heart disease with heart failure — A form resulting in the decreased ability of the heart to pump enough blood to meet the needs of the body's tissues.
Hypertensive heart failure
Use additional code to identify type of heart failure (I50.-)

I11.9   Hypertensive heart disease without heart failure
Hypertensive heart disease NOS

I12-   Hypertensive chronic kidney disease — Kidney damage and malfunction (usually parenchymal ischemia) that is associated with or resulting from hypertension.
Includes: Any condition in N18 and N26 due to hypertension
Arteriosclerosis of kidney — Thickening and loss of elasticity of the arterioles of the kidney.
Arteriosclerotic nephritis (chronic) (interstitial) — Inflammation of the kidney due to arteriolar ischemia.
Hypertensive nephropathy — Functional disease of the kidney due to hypertension.
Nephrosclerosis — Inflammation of the kidney due to arteriolar ischemia.
Excludes 1:   hypertension due to kidney disease (I15.0, I15.1)
renovascular hypertension (I15.0)
secondary hypertension (I15.-)
Excludes ❷: acute kidney failure (N17.-)

cc **I12.0   Hypertensive chronic kidney disease with stage 5 chronic kidney disease or end stage renal disease**
Use additional code to identify the stage of chronic kidney disease (N18.5, N18.6)

I12.9   Hypertensive chronic kidney disease with stage 1 through stage 4 chronic kidney disease, or unspecified chronic kidney disease
Hypertensive chronic kidney disease NOS
Hypertensive renal disease NOS
Use additional code to identify the stage of chronic kidney disease (N18.1-N18.4, N18.9)

I05 - I12

I13- **Hypertensive** <u>heart and chronic kidney</u> **disease** — Kidney damage with heart and kidney functional abnormalities resulting from hypertension.
  Includes: Any condition in I11.- with any condition in I12.-
        Cardiorenal disease
        Cardiovascular renal disease — A form marked by hypertensive disease of the heart, blood vessels, and kidneys.

CC **I13.0** **Hypertensive heart and chronic kidney disease** <u>with heart failure</u> **and** <u>stage 1 through stage 4</u> **chronic kidney disease, or unspecified chronic kidney disease**
    Use additional code to identify type of heart failure (I50.-)
    Use additional code to identify stage of chronic kidney disease (N18.1-N18.4, N18.9)

I13.1- **Hypertensive heart and chronic kidney disease** <u>without</u> **heart failure**

  I13.10 **Hypertensive heart and chronic kidney disease without heart failure,** <u>with stage 1 through stage 4</u> **chronic kidney disease, or unspecified chronic kidney disease**
      Hypertensive heart disease and hypertensive chronic kidney disease NOS
      Use additional code to identify the stage of chronic kidney disease (N18.1-N18.4, N18.9)

  CC **I13.11** **Hypertensive heart and chronic kidney disease without heart failure,** <u>with stage 5</u> **chronic kidney disease, or end stage renal disease**
      Use additional code to identify the stage of chronic kidney disease (N18.5, N18.6)

CC **I13.2** **Hypertensive heart and chronic kidney disease** <u>with heart failure</u> **and** <u>with stage 5</u> **chronic kidney disease, or end stage renal disease**
    Use additional code to identify type of heart failure (I50.-)
    Use additional code to identify the stage of chronic kidney disease (N18.5, N18.6)

I15- <u>Secondary</u> **hypertension** — Elevated arterial blood pressure due to various primary diseases.
  Code also underlying condition
  Excludes 1: *postprocedural hypertension (I97.3)*
  Excludes ❷: *secondary hypertension involving vessels of brain (I60-I69)*
        secondary hypertension involving vessels of eye (H35.0-)
  I15.0 **Renovascular hypertension** — A form caused by primary renal disease.
  I15.1 **Hypertension secondary to other renal disorders**
  I15.2 **Hypertension secondary to endocrine disorders**
  I15.8 **Other secondary hypertension**
  I15.9 **Secondary hypertension, unspecified**

I16- **Hypertensive crisis** — The rapid elevation of blood pressure that is high enough to cause organ damage.
  Code also any identified hypertensive disease (I10-I15)
  I16.0 **Hypertensive urgency** — The rapid elevation of blood pressure without associated progressive organ dysfunction.
  CC **I16.1** **Hypertensive emergency** — The rapid elevation of blood pressure that can lead to impending or progressive organ dysfunction.
  CC **I16.9** **Hypertensive crisis, unspecified**

Ischemic heart diseases (I20-I25)

Use additional code to identify presence of hypertension (I10-I16)

I20- <u>Angina pectoris</u> — Severe, squeezing or pressure-like thoracic pain that is caused by reduced oxygenation of the cardiac muscle and often brought on by some form of exertion or stress.
  Use additional code to identify:
    Exposure to environmental tobacco smoke (Z77.22)
    History of tobacco dependence (Z87.891)
    Occupational exposure to environmental tobacco smoke (Z57.31)
    Tobacco dependence (F17.-)
    Tobacco use (Z72.0)
  Excludes 1: *angina pectoris with atherosclerotic heart disease of native coronary arteries (I25.1-)*
        atherosclerosis of coronary artery bypass graft(s) and coronary artery of transplanted heart with angina pectoris (I25.7-)
        postinfarction angina (I23.7)

CC **I20.0** <u>Unstable</u> **angina** — Angina which is increased in frequency and duration, provoked with less than usual stimuli, occurs with abrupt onset (often while resting), and/or usual relief (rest and/or medication) does not help relieve it.
      Accelerated angina
      Crescendo angina
      De novo effort angina
      Intermediate coronary syndrome
      Preinfarction syndrome
      Worsening effort angina

CC **I20.1** **Angina pectoris** <u>with documented spasm</u> — A form with attacks associated with ST-segment elevations on EKG that often occur during rest.
      Angiospastic angina
      Prinzmetal angina
      Spasm-induced angina
      Variant angina

I20.8 <u>Other forms</u> **of angina pectoris**
      Angina equivalent
      Angina of effort
      Coronary slow flow syndrome
      Stable angina
      Stenocardia
    Use additioal code(s) for symptoms associated with angina equivalent

I20.9 **Angina pectoris,** <u>unspecified</u>
      Angina NOS
      Anginal syndrome
      Cardiac angina
      Ischemic chest pain

I21- **ST elevation (STEMI) and non-ST elevation (NSTEMI)** <u>myocardial infarction</u> — A severe, sudden onset of myocardial necrosis due to obstruction of the coronary artery blood flow to an area of heart muscle.
  AHA 12:4Q:p102 – Two STEMI myocardial infarctions a week apart in hospital
  AHA 12:4Q:p103 – Two STEMI myocardial infarctions a week apart after discharge
  AHA 13:1Q:p25 – Four-week time frame of the initial acute myocardial infarction
  Includes: **Cardiac infarction**
      Coronary (artery) embolism — An obstructing blood clot in the coronary arteries.
      Coronary (artery) occlusion — An obstruction of a coronary artery by thrombosis or as a result of a spasm.
      Coronary (artery) rupture — Forcible tearing of a coronary artery.
      Coronary (artery) thrombosis — The formation or presence of an aggregation of blood factors, primarily platelets and fibrin forming a blood clot.
      Infarction of heart, myocardium, or ventricle
      Myocardial infarction specified as acute or with a stated duration of 4 weeks (28 days) or less from onset
  Use additional code, if applicable, to identify:
    Exposure to environmental tobacco smoke (Z77.22)
    History of tobacco dependence (Z87.891)
    Occupational exposure to environmental tobacco smoke (Z57.31)
    Status post administration of tPA (rtPA) in a different facility within the last 24 hours prior to admission to current facility (Z92.82)
    Tobacco dependence (F17.-)
    Tobacco use (Z72.0)
  Excludes ❷: *old myocardial infarction (I25.2)*
        postmyocardial infarction syndrome (I24.1)
        subsequent myocardial infarction (I22.-)

I21.0- <u>ST elevation (STEMI)</u> **myocardial infarction of** <u>anterior wall</u> — Infarction of the front portion of the heart that is defined by an ST segment elevation on EKG indicating a relatively large area of heart muscle is affected.

MCC **I21.01** **ST elevation (STEMI) myocardial infarction involving** <u>left main</u> **coronary artery** — A form identifying the obstruction in the left main coronary artery.

MCC **I21.02** **ST elevation (STEMI) myocardial infarction involving** <u>left anterior descending</u> **coronary artery** — A form identifying the obstruction in the left anterior descending coronary artery.
      ST elevation (STEMI) myocardial infarction involving diagonal coronary artery

MCC **I21.09** **ST elevation (STEMI) myocardial infarction involving** <u>other coronary artery</u> **of anterior wall**
      Acute transmural myocardial infarction of anterior wall — TRANSMURAL — A form involving the entire thickness of the heart muscle.
      Anteroapical transmural (Q wave) infarction (acute)
      Anterolateral transmural (Q wave) infarction (acute)
      Anteroseptal transmural (Q wave) infarction (acute)
      Transmural (Q wave) infarction (acute) (of) anterior (wall) NOS

I21.1- <u>ST elevation (STEMI)</u> **myocardial infarction of** <u>inferior wall</u> — Infarction of the lower portion of the heart that is defined by an ST segment elevation on EKG indicating a relatively large area of heart muscle is affected.

MCC **I21.11** **ST elevation (STEMI) myocardial infarction involving** <u>right coronary</u> **artery** — A form identifying the obstruction in the right coronary artery.
      Inferoposterior transmural (Q wave) infarction (acute) — TRANSMURAL — A form involving the entire thickness of the heart muscle.

Excludes 1: = NOT CODED HERE! (Do not code both)   **724**   *Excludes ❷:* = Not Included Here

I13-I21

MCC **I21.19** **ST elevation (STEMI)** myocardial infarction involving **other coronary** artery of inferior wall
> **Acute transmural myocardial infarction of inferior wall** — TRANSMURAL – A form involving the entire thickness of the heart muscle.
> **Inferolateral transmural (Q wave) infarction (acute)**
> **Transmural (Q wave) infarction (acute) (of) diaphragmatic wall**
> **Transmural (Q wave) infarction (acute) (of) inferior (wall) NOS**
> *Excludes ❷: ST elevation (STEMI) myocardial infarction involving left circumflex coronary artery (I21.21)*

I21.2- **ST elevation (STEMI)** myocardial infarction of **other sites** — Infarction of the heart that is defined by an ST segment elevation on EKG indicating a relatively large area of heart muscle is affected.

MCC **I21.21** **ST elevation (STEMI)** myocardial infarction involving **left circumflex** coronary artery — A form identifying the obstruction in the left circumflex coronary artery.
> **ST elevation (STEMI) myocardial infarction involving oblique marginal coronary artery**

MCC **I21.29** **ST elevation (STEMI)** myocardial infarction involving **other sites**
> **Acute transmural myocardial infarction of other sites** — TRANSMURAL – A form involving the entire thickness of the heart muscle.
> **Apical-lateral transmural (Q wave) infarction (acute)**
> **Basal-lateral transmural (Q wave) infarction (acute)**
> **High lateral transmural (Q wave) infarction (acute)**
> **Lateral (wall) NOS transmural (Q wave) infarction (acute)**
> **Posterior (true) transmural (Q wave) infarction (acute)**
> **Posterobasal transmural (Q wave) infarction (acute)**
> **Posterolateral transmural (Q wave) infarction (acute)**
> **Posteroseptal transmural (Q wave) infarction (acute)**
> **Septal transmural (Q wave) infarction (acute) NOS**

MCC **I21.3** **ST elevation (STEMI)** myocardial infarction of **unspecified site** — Infarction of an unspecified area of the heart that is defined by an ST segment elevation on EKG indicating a relatively large area of heart muscle is affected.
> **Acute transmural myocardial infarction of unspecified site**
> **Myocardial infarction (acute) NOS**
> **Transmural (Q wave) myocardial infarction NOS**

MCC **I21.4** **Non-ST elevation (NSTEMI)** myocardial infarction — Infarction of the heart that is defined by NOT having an ST segment elevation on EKG and by a positive blood test for troponin (a protein released when the heart muscle is damaged) indicating a relatively small area of heart muscle is affected.
> **Acute subendocardial myocardial infarction**
> **Non-Q wave myocardial infarction NOS**
> **Nontransmural myocardial infarction NOS**

I22- **Subsequent** ST elevation (STEMI) and non-ST elevation (NSTEMI) **myocardial infarction** — See Includes Note below.
> **AHA 12:4Q:p102 – Two STEMI myocardial infarctions a week apart in hospital**
> **AHA 12:4Q:p103 – Two STEMI myocardial infarctions a week apart after discharge**
> **AHA 13:1Q:p25 – Four-week time frame of the initial acute myocardial infarction**

> Includes: **Acute myocardial infarction occurring within four weeks (28 days) of a previous acute myocardial infarction, regardless of site**
> **Cardiac infarction**
> **Coronary (artery) embolism** — An obstructing blood clot in the coronary arteries.
> **Coronary (artery) occlusion** — An obstruction of a coronary artery by thrombosis or as a result of a spasm.
> **Coronary (artery) rupture** — Forcible tearing of a coronary artery.
> **Coronary (artery) thrombosis** — The formation or presence of an aggregation of blood factors, primarily platelets and fibrin forming a blood clot.
> **Infarction of heart, myocardium, or ventricle**
> **Recurrent myocardial infarction**
> **Reinfarction of myocardium**
> **Rupture of heart, myocardium, or ventricle**

Use additional code, if applicable, to identify:
> **Exposure to environmental tobacco smoke (Z77.22)**
> **History of tobacco dependence (Z87.891)**
> **Occupational exposure to environmental tobacco smoke (Z57.31)**
> **Status post administration of tPA (rtPA) in a different facility within the last 24 hours prior to admission to current facility (Z92.82)**
> **Tobacco dependence (F17.-)**
> **Tobacco use (Z72.0)**

MCC **I22.0** **Subsequent** **ST elevation (STEMI)** myocardial infarction of **anterior wall** — Infarction of the front portion of the heart that occurs within 4 weeks of a previous infarction that is defined by an ST segment elevation on EKG indicating a relatively large area of heart muscle is affected.
> **Subsequent acute transmural myocardial infarction of anterior wall** — TRANSMURAL – A form involving the entire thickness of the heart muscle.
> **Subsequent transmural (Q wave) infarction (acute) (of) anterior (wall) NOS**
> **Subsequent anteroapical transmural (Q wave) infarction (acute)**
> **Subsequent anterolateral transmural (Q wave) infarction (acute)**
> **Subsequent anteroseptal transmural (Q wave) infarction (acute)**

MCC **I22.1** **Subsequent** **ST elevation (STEMI)** myocardial infarction of **inferior wall** — Infarction of the lower portion of the heart that occurs within 4 weeks of a previous infarction that is defined by an ST segment elevation on EKG indicating a relatively large area of heart muscle is affected.
> **Subsequent acute transmural myocardial infarction of inferior wall** — TRANSMURAL – A form involving the entire thickness of the heart muscle.
> **Subsequent transmural (Q wave) infarction (acute) (of) diaphragmatic wall**
> **Subsequent transmural (Q wave) infarction (acute) (of) inferior (wall) NOS**
> **Subsequent inferolateral transmural (Q wave) infarction (acute)**
> **Subsequent inferoposterior transmural (Q wave) infarction (acute)**

MCC **I22.2** **Subsequent** **non-ST elevation (NSTEMI)** myocardial infarction — Infarction of the heart that occurs within 4 weeks of a previous infarction that is defined by NOT having an ST segment elevation on EKG and by a positive blood test for troponin (a protein released when the heart muscle is damaged) indicating a relatively small area of heart muscle is affected.
> **Subsequent acute subendocardial myocardial infarction**
> **Subsequent non-Q wave myocardial infarction NOS**
> **Subsequent nontransmural myocardial infarction NOS**

MCC **I22.8** **Subsequent** **ST elevation (STEMI)** myocardial infarction of **other sites** — Infarction of the heart that occurs within 4 weeks of a previous infarction that is defined by an ST segment elevation on EKG indicating a relatively large area of heart muscle is affected.
> **Subsequent acute transmural myocardial infarction of other sites** — TRANSMURAL – A form involving the entire thickness of the heart muscle.
> **Subsequent apical-lateral transmural (Q wave) myocardial infarction (acute)**
> **Subsequent basal-lateral transmural (Q wave) myocardial infarction (acute)**
> **Subsequent high lateral transmural (Q wave) myocardial infarction (acute)**
> **Subsequent transmural (Q wave) myocardial infarction (acute) (of) lateral (wall) NOS**
> **Subsequent posterior (true)transmural (Q wave) myocardial infarction (acute)**
> **Subsequent posterobasal transmural (Q wave) myocardial infarction (acute)**
> **Subsequent posterolateral transmural (Q wave) myocardial infarction (acute)**
> **Subsequent posteroseptal transmural (Q wave) myocardial infarction (acute)**
> **Subsequent septal NOS transmural (Q wave) myocardial infarction (acute)**

MCC **I22.9** **Subsequent** **ST elevation (STEMI)** myocardial infarction of **unspecified site** — Infarction of an unspecified area the heart that occurs within 4 weeks of a previous infarction that is defined by an ST segment elevation on EKG indicating a relatively large area of heart muscle is affected.
> **Subsequent acute myocardial infarction of unspecified site**
> **Subsequent myocardial infarction (acute) NOS**

I23- **Certain current complications following** ST elevation (STEMI) and non-ST elevation (NSTEMI) **myocardial infarction (within the 28 day period)**

CC **I23.0** **Hemopericardium** as current complication following acute myocardial infarction — [Age/15-124] – The abnormal presence of effused blood in the pericardial cavity.
> *Excludes 1:   hemopericardium not specified as current complication following acute myocardial infarction (I31.2)*

CC **I23.1** **Atrial septal defect** as current complication following acute myocardial infarction — [Age/15-124] – A break or opening in the atrial septum (wall).
> *Excludes 1:   acquired atrial septal defect not specified as current complication following acute myocardial infarction (I51.0)*

I
2
1
-
I
2
3

CC **I23.2** <u>**Ventricular septal defect**</u> **as current complication following acute myocardial infarction** — [Age/15-124] – A break or opening in the ventricular septum (wall).
   Excludes 1:   *acquired ventricular septal defect not specified as current complication following acute myocardial infarction (I51.0)*

CC **I23.3** <u>**Rupture of cardiac wall**</u> **without hemopericardium as current complication following acute myocardial infarction** — [Age/15-124] – A tear of the heart muscle.

MCC **I23.4** <u>**Rupture of chordae tendineae**</u> **as current complication following acute myocardial infarction** – A forcible tearing of the strong, cord-like attachments of the heart valves to the papillary muscles.
   Excludes 1:   *rupture of chordae tendineae not specified as current complication following acute myocardial infarction (I51.1)*

MCC **I23.5** <u>**Rupture of papillary muscle**</u> **as current complication following acute myocardial infarction** – A forcible tearing of the conical intraventricular muscles attached to the chordae tendineae and heart wall.
   Excludes 1:   *rupture of papillary muscle not specified as current complication following acute myocardial infarction (I51.2)*

CC **I23.6** <u>**Thrombosis of atrium, auricular appendage, and ventricle**</u> **as current complications following acute myocardial infarction** — [Age/15-124] – The formation or presence of an aggregation of blood factors, primarily platelets and fibrin forming a blood clot.
   Excludes 1:   *thrombosis of atrium, auricular appendage, and ventricle not specified as current complication following acute myocardial infarction (I51.3)*

CC **I23.7** <u>**Postinfarction angina**</u> — [Age/15-124] – Angina occurring from a few hours and up to 30 days following an acute myocardial infarction.
   AHA 15:2Q:p16 – Postinfarction angina

CC **I23.8** <u>**Other current complications**</u> **following acute myocardial infarction** — [Age/15-124]

I24- <u>**Other acute**</u> **ischemic heart diseases**
   Excludes 1:   *angina pectoris (I20.-)*
                 transient myocardial ischemia in newborn (P29.4)

CC **I24.0** <u>**Acute coronary thrombosis**</u> <u>**not**</u> **resulting in myocardial infarction**
   Acute coronary (artery) (vein) embolism not resulting in myocardial infarction
   Acute coronary (artery) (vein) occlusion not resulting in myocardial infarction
   Acute coronary (artery) (vein) thromboembolism not resulting in myocardial infarction
   Excludes 1:   *atherosclerotic heart disease (I25.1-)*

CC **I24.1** <u>**Dressler's syndrome**</u> — Pericarditis with fever, leukocytosis, and pleurisy, occurring after an acute myocardial infarction.
   Postmyocardial infarction syndrome
   Excludes 1:   *postinfarction angina (I23.7)*

CC **I24.8** **Other forms of acute ischemic heart disease**

CC **I24.9** **Acute ischemic heart disease, unspecified**
   Excludes 1:   *ischemic heart disease (chronic) NOS (I25.9)*

I25- <u>**Chronic**</u> **ischemic heart disease**
   Use additional code to identify:
   Chronic total occlusion of coronary artery (I25.82)
   Exposure to environmental tobacco smoke (Z77.22)
   History of tobacco dependence (Z87.891)
   Occupational exposure to environmental tobacco smoke (Z57.31)
   Tobacco dependence (F17.-)
   Tobacco use (Z72.0)

I25.1- <u>**Atherosclerotic heart disease**</u> <u>**of native**</u> **coronary artery** —
Coronary artery narrowing caused by deposition of plaque-forming cholesterol and other lipids within the lumen of those arteries.
   Atherosclerotic cardiovascular disease
   Coronary (artery) atheroma
   Coronary (artery) atherosclerosis
   Coronary (artery) disease
   Coronary (artery) sclerosis
   Use additional code, if applicable, to identify:
   Coronary atherosclerosis due to calcified coronary lesion (I25.84)
   Coronary atherosclerosis due to lipid rich plaque (I25.83)
   Excludes ❷: *atheroembolism (I75.-)*
                 atherosclerosis of coronary artery bypass graft(s) and transplanted heart (I25.7-)

I25.10 **Atherosclerotic heart disease of native coronary artery** <u>**without**</u> **angina pectoris** — [Age/15-124]
   Atherosclerotic heart disease NOS

I25.11- **Atherosclerotic heart disease of native coronary artery** <u>**with angina pectoris**</u> — A form with severe, squeezing or pressure-like thoracic pain that is caused by reduced oxygenation of the cardiac muscle and often brought on by some form of exertion or stress.
   AHA 15:2Q:p16 – Postinfarction angina with atherosclerosis

CC **I25.110** **Atherosclerotic heart disease of native coronary artery with** <u>**unstable**</u> **angina pectoris** — [Age/15-124]
   Excludes 1:   *unstable angina without atherosclerotic heart disease (I20.0)*

I25.111 **Atherosclerotic heart disease of native coronary artery with angina pectoris** <u>**with documented spasm**</u> — [Age/15-124]
   Excludes 1:   *angina pectoris with documented spasm without atherosclerotic heart disease (I20.1)*

I25.118 **Atherosclerotic heart disease of native coronary artery with** <u>**other forms**</u> **of angina pectoris** — [Age/15-124]
   Excludes 1:   *other forms of angina pectoris without atherosclerotic heart disease (I20.8)*

I25.119 **Atherosclerotic heart disease of native coronary artery with** <u>**unspecified**</u> **angina pectoris** — [Age/15-124]
   Atherosclerotic heart disease with angina NOS
   Atherosclerotic heart disease with ischemic chest pain
   Excludes 1:   *unspecified angina pectoris without atherosclerotic heart disease (I20.9)*

I25.2 <u>**Old**</u> **myocardial infarction** — A known past myocardial infarction, not presenting any symptoms during the current episode of care.
   Healed myocardial infarction
   Past myocardial infarction diagnosed by ECG or other investigation, but currently presenting no symptoms

CC **I25.3** <u>**Aneurysm**</u> **of heart** — An abnormal enlargement and thinning of a portion of the heart wall.
   Mural aneurysm
   Ventricular aneurysm

I25.4- **Coronary artery aneurysm and dissection**

I25.41 **Coronary artery aneurysm** — An abnormal enlargement and thinning of a portion of a coronary artery wall.
   Coronary arteriovenous fistula, acquired
   Excludes 1:   *congenital coronary (artery) aneurysm (Q24.5)*

MCC **I25.42** **Coronary artery dissection** — The splitting of the coronary artery wall that allows blood to flow within the wall layers.

I25.5 **Ischemic cardiomyopathy** — A weakened, dilated, and enlarged heart muscle that is caused by the decreased blood supply.
   Excludes ❷: *coronary atherosclerosis (I25.1-, I25.7-)*

I25.6 **Silent myocardial ischemia** — Decreased blood supply to the heart muscle that isn't producing any symptoms.

I25.7- <u>**Atherosclerosis**</u> **of coronary artery bypass graft(s) and coronary artery of transplanted heart** <u>**with angina pectoris**</u>
   Use additional code, if applicable, to identify:
   Coronary atherosclerosis due to calcified coronary lesion (I25.84)
   Coronary atherosclerosis due to lipid rich plaque (I25.83)
   Excludes 1:   *atherosclerosis of bypass graft(s) of transplanted heart without angina pectoris (I25.812)*
                 atherosclerosis of coronary artery bypass graft(s) without angina pectoris (I25.810)
                 atherosclerosis of native coronary artery of transplanted heart without angina pectoris (I25.811)
                 embolism or thrombus of coronary artery bypass graft(s) (T82.8-)

I25.70- **Atherosclerosis of** <u>**coronary artery bypass graft(s), unspecified, with angina pectoris**</u> — Narrowing of a coronary artery bypass graft caused by deposition of plaque-forming cholesterol and other lipids within the lumen of those arteries and severe, squeezing or pressure-like thoracic pain that is caused by reduced oxygenation of the cardiac muscle and often brought on by some form of exertion or stress.

CC **I25.700** **Atherosclerosis of coronary artery bypass graft(s), unspecified,** <u>**with unstable**</u> **angina pectoris** — [Age/15-124]
   Excludes 1:   *unstable angina pectoris without atherosclerosis of coronary artery bypass graft (I20.0)*

I 2 3 - I 2 5

I25.701 Atherosclerosis of coronary artery bypass graft(s), unspecified, with angina pectoris <u>with documented spasm</u> — [Age/15-124]
Excludes 1:   *angina pectoris with documented spasm without atherosclerosis of coronary artery bypass graft (I20.1)*

I25.708 Atherosclerosis of coronary artery bypass graft(s), unspecified, <u>with other forms</u> of angina pectoris — [Age/15-124]
Excludes 1:   *other forms of angina pectoris without atherosclerosis of coronary artery bypass graft (I20.8)*

I25.709 Atherosclerosis of coronary artery bypass graft(s), unspecified, <u>with unspecified</u> angina pectoris — [Age/15-124]
Excludes 1:   *unspecified angina pectoris without atherosclerosis of coronary artery bypass graft (I20.9)*

I25.71- Atherosclerosis of <u>autologous vein coronary artery bypass graft(s)</u> <u>with angina pectoris</u>

cc **I25.710** Atherosclerosis of autologous <u>vein</u> coronary artery bypass graft(s) <u>with unstable</u> angina pectoris — [Age/15-124]
Excludes 1:   *unstable angina without atherosclerosis of autologous vein coronary artery bypass graft(s) (I20.0)*

cc **I25.711** Atherosclerosis of autologous <u>vein</u> coronary artery bypass graft(s) with angina pectoris <u>with documented spasm</u> — [Age/15-124]
Excludes 1:   *angina pectoris with documented spasm without atherosclerosis of autologous vein coronary artery bypass graft(s) (I20.1)*

cc **I25.718** Atherosclerosis of autologous <u>vein</u> coronary artery bypass graft(s) <u>with other forms</u> of angina pectoris — [Age/15-124]
Excludes 1:   *other forms of angina pectoris without atherosclerosis of autologous vein coronary artery bypass graft(s) (I20.8)*

cc **I25.719** Atherosclerosis of autologous <u>vein</u> coronary artery bypass graft(s) <u>with unspecified</u> angina pectoris — [Age/15-124]
Excludes 1:   *unspecified angina pectoris without atherosclerosis of autologous vein coronary artery bypass graft(s) (I20.9)*

I25.72- Atherosclerosis of autologous <u>artery</u> coronary artery bypass graft(s) <u>with angina pectoris</u>
Atherosclerosis of internal mammary artery graft with angina pectoris

cc **I25.720** Atherosclerosis of autologous <u>artery</u> coronary artery bypass graft(s) <u>with unstable</u> angina pectoris — [Age/15-124]
Excludes 1:   *unstable angina without atherosclerosis of autologous artery coronary artery bypass graft(s) (I20.0)*

cc **I25.721** Atherosclerosis of autologous <u>artery</u> coronary artery bypass graft(s) with angina pectoris <u>with documented spasm</u> — [Age/15-124]
Excludes 1:   *angina pectoris with documented spasm without atherosclerosis of autologous artery coronary artery bypass graft(s) (I20.1)*

cc **I25.728** Atherosclerosis of autologous <u>artery</u> coronary artery bypass graft(s) <u>with other forms</u> of angina pectoris — [Age/15-124]
Excludes 1:   *other forms of angina pectoris without atherosclerosis of autologous artery coronary artery bypass graft(s) (I20.8)*

cc **I25.729** Atherosclerosis of autologous <u>artery</u> coronary artery bypass graft(s) <u>with unspecified</u> angina pectoris — [Age/15-124]
Excludes 1:   *unspecified angina pectoris without atherosclerosis of autologous artery coronary artery bypass graft(s) (I20.9)*

I25.73- Atherosclerosis of <u>nonautologous biological</u> coronary artery bypass graft(s) <u>with angina pectoris</u>

cc **I25.730** Atherosclerosis of <u>nonautologous biological</u> coronary artery bypass graft(s) <u>with unstable</u> angina pectoris — [Age/15-124]
Excludes 1:   *unstable angina without atherosclerosis of nonautologous biological coronary artery bypass graft(s) (I20.0)*

cc **I25.731** Atherosclerosis of <u>nonautologous biological</u> coronary artery bypass graft(s) with angina pectoris <u>with documented spasm</u> — [Age/15-124]
Excludes 1:   *angina pectoris with documented spasm without atherosclerosis of nonautologous biological coronary artery bypass graft(s) (I20.1)*

cc **I25.738** Atherosclerosis of <u>nonautologous biological</u> coronary artery bypass graft(s) <u>with other forms</u> of angina pectoris — [Age/15-124]
Excludes 1:   *other forms of angina pectoris without atherosclerosis of nonautologous biological coronary artery bypass graft(s) (I20.8)*

cc **I25.739** Atherosclerosis of <u>nonautologous biological</u> coronary artery bypass graft(s) <u>with unspecified</u> angina pectoris — [Age/15-124]
Excludes 1:   *unspecified angina pectoris without atherosclerosis of nonautologous biological coronary artery bypass graft(s) (I20.9)*

I25.75- Atherosclerosis of <u>native coronary artery of transplanted heart with angina pectoris</u> — Narrowing of a native coronary artery of a transplanted heart caused by deposition of plaque-forming cholesterol and other lipids within the lumen of those arteries and severe, squeezing or pressure-like thoracic pain that is caused by reduced oxygenation of the cardiac muscle and often brought on by some form of exertion or stress.
Excludes 1:   *atherosclerosis of native coronary artery of transplanted heart without angina pectoris (I25.811)*

cc **I25.750** Atherosclerosis of native coronary artery of transplanted heart <u>with unstable</u> angina

cc **I25.751** Atherosclerosis of native coronary artery of transplanted heart with angina pectoris <u>with documented spasm</u>

cc **I25.758** Atherosclerosis of native coronary artery of transplanted heart <u>with other forms</u> of angina pectoris

cc **I25.759** Atherosclerosis of native coronary artery of transplanted heart <u>with unspecified</u> angina pectoris

I25.76- Atherosclerosis of <u>bypass graft</u> of coronary artery of <u>transplanted heart with angina pectoris</u> — Narrowing of a coronary artery bypass graft of a transplanted heart caused by deposition of plaque-forming cholesterol and other lipids within the lumen of those arteries and severe, squeezing or pressure-like thoracic pain that is caused by reduced oxygenation of the cardiac muscle and often brought on by some form of exertion or stress.
Excludes 1:   *atherosclerosis of bypass graft of coronary artery of transplanted heart without angina pectoris (I25.812)*

cc **I25.760** Atherosclerosis of bypass graft of coronary artery of transplanted heart <u>with unstable angina</u> — [Age/15-124]

cc **I25.761** Atherosclerosis of bypass graft of coronary artery of transplanted heart with angina pectoris <u>with documented spasm</u> — [Age/15-124]

cc **I25.768** Atherosclerosis of bypass graft of coronary artery of transplanted heart <u>with other forms</u> of angina pectoris — [Age/15-124]

cc **I25.769** Atherosclerosis of bypass graft of coronary artery of transplanted heart <u>with unspecified</u> angina pectoris — [Age/15-124]

I25 - I25

I25.79- Atherosclerosis of <u>other</u> coronary artery bypass graft(s) <u>with angina pectoris</u>

cc **I25.790** Atherosclerosis of other coronary artery bypass graft(s) <u>with unstable</u> angina pectoris — [Age/15-124]
>   *Excludes 1:*   unstable angina without atherosclerosis of other coronary artery bypassgraft(s) (I20.0)

cc **I25.791** Atherosclerosis of other coronary artery bypass graft(s) with angina pectoris <u>with documented spasm</u> — [Age/15-124]
>   *Excludes 1:*   angina pectoris with documented spasm without atherosclerosis of other coronary artery bypass graft(s) (I20.1)

cc **I25.798** Atherosclerosis of other coronary artery bypass graft(s) <u>with other forms</u> of angina pectoris — [Age/15-124]
>   *Excludes 1:*   other forms of angina pectoris without atherosclerosis of other coronary artery bypass graft(s) (I20.8)

cc **I25.799** Atherosclerosis of other coronary artery bypass graft(s) <u>with unspecified</u> angina pectoris — [Age/15-124]
>   *Excludes 1:*   unspecified angina pectoris without atherosclerosis of other coronary artery bypass graft(s) (I20.9)

I25.8- Other forms of chronic ischemic heart disease

I25.81- <u>Atherosclerosis of other coronary vessels</u> <u>without</u> angina pectoris — Coronary artery narrowing caused by deposition of plaque-forming cholesterol and other lipids within the lumen of those arteries without the symptoms of angina pectoris.
Use additional code, if applicable, to identify:
Coronary atherosclerosis due to calcified coronary lesion (I25.84)
Coronary atherosclerosis due to lipid rich plaque (I25.83)
>   *Excludes 1:*   atherosclerotic heart disease of native coronary artery without angina pectoris (I25.10)

cc **I25.810** Atherosclerosis of <u>coronary artery bypass graft(s)</u> <u>without</u> angina pectoris — [Age/15-124] — A form occurring in a coronary artery bypass graft.
Atherosclerosis of coronary artery bypass graft NOS
>   *Excludes 1:*   atherosclerosis of coronary bypass graft(s) with angina pectoris (I25.70-I25.73-, I25.79-)

cc **I25.811** Atherosclerosis of <u>native coronary artery of transplanted heart</u> <u>without</u> angina pectoris — A form occurring in a native coronary artery of a transplanted heart.
Atherosclerosis of native coronary artery of transplanted heart NOS
>   *Excludes 1:*   atherosclerosis of native coronary artery of transplanted heart with angina pectoris (I25.75-)

cc **I25.812** Atherosclerosis of <u>bypass graft of coronary artery of transplanted heart</u> <u>without</u> angina pectoris — [Age/15-124] — A form occurring in a coronary artery bypass graft of a transplanted heart.
Atherosclerosis of bypass graft of transplanted heart NOS
>   *Excludes 1:*   atherosclerosis of bypass graft of transplanted heart with angina pectoris (I25.76)

I25.82 <u>Chronic total occlusion of coronary artery</u> — [Unacceptable PDX] — A complete blockage of a coronary artery without an acute occlusion that has been present for an extended duration.
Complete occlusion of coronary artery
Total occlusion of coronary artery
Code first coronary atherosclerosis (I25.1-, I25.7-, I25.81-)
>   *Excludes 1:*   acute coronary occlusion with myocardial infarction (I21.-, I22.-)
>   acute coronary occlusion without myocardial infarction (I24.0)

I25.83 Coronary atherosclerosis <u>due to lipid rich plaque</u> — [Age/15-124] [Unacceptable PDX] — The identification of a coronary artery plaque that contains a greater than usual percentage of lipid material and results in a higher propensity to rupture than more fibrotic plaques.
Code first coronary atherosclerosis (I25.1-, I25.7-, I25.81-)

I25.84 Coronary atherosclerosis <u>due to calcified coronary lesion</u> — [Unacceptable PDX] — The identification of a calcified coronary artery lesion that results in a higher propensity to rupture than more fibrotic plaques.
Coronary atherosclerosis due to severely calcified coronary lesion
Code first coronary atherosclerosis (I25.1-, I25.7-, I25.81-)

I25.89 Other forms of chronic ischemic heart disease

I25.9 Chronic ischemic heart disease, unspecified
Ischemic heart disease (chronic) NOS

Pulmonary heart disease and diseases of pulmonary circulation (I26-I28)

I26- Pulmonary embolism — The closure of a pulmonary artery or one of its branches by a blood clot that traveled through the bloodstream to the lungs.
Includes: Pulmonary (acute) (artery) (vein) infarction
Pulmonary (acute) (artery) (vein) thromboembolism
Pulmonary (acute) (artery) (vein) thrombosis
>   *Excludes ❷:*   chronic pulmonary embolism (I27.82)
>   personal history of pulmonary embolism (Z86.711)
>   pulmonary embolism complicating abortion, ectopic or molar pregnancy (O00-O07, O08.2)
>   pulmonary embolism complicating pregnancy, childbirth and the puerperium (O88.-)
>   pulmonary embolism due to complications of surgical and medical care (T80.0, T81.7-, T82.8-)
>   pulmonary embolism due to trauma (T79.0, T79.1)
>   septic (non-pulmonary) arterial embolism (I76)

I26.0- Pulmonary embolism <u>with acute cor pulmonale</u> — A relatively severe sudden onset of right heart decreased efficiency due to pulmonary hypertension caused by a pulmonary embolism.

MCC **I26.01** <u>Septic</u> pulmonary embolism with acute cor pulmonale — [Unacceptable PDX] — A form due to a localized collection of pus and bacteria that travels through the venous system to the heart and then continues into the pulmonary arterial system, where it lodges in a pulmonary vessel.
Code first underlying infection

MCC **I26.02** <u>Saddle</u> embolus of pulmonary artery with acute cor pulmonale — A form characterized by a large embolism that straddles the bifurcation of the main pulmonary artery.

MCC **I26.09** <u>Other</u> pulmonary embolism with acute cor pulmonale
AHA 14:4Q:p21 – Pulmonary hypertension with acute cor pulmonale
Acute cor pulmonale NOS

I26.9- Pulmonary embolism <u>without</u> acute cor pulmonale

MCC **I26.90** <u>Septic</u> pulmonary embolism without acute cor pulmonale — [Unacceptable PDX]
Code first underlying infection

MCC **I26.92** <u>Saddle</u> embolus of pulmonary artery without acute cor pulmonale

MCC **I26.99** <u>Other</u> pulmonary embolism without acute cor pulmonale
Acute pulmonary embolism NOS
Pulmonary embolism NOS

I27- Other pulmonary heart diseases

cc **I27.0** Primary pulmonary hypertension — Persistently high arterial blood pressure within the pulmonary circulation that is due to an organic cause.
>   *Excludes 1:*   pulmonary hypertension NOS (I27.2)
>   secondary pulmonary hypertension (I27.2)

cc **I27.1** Kyphoscoliotic heart disease — Pulmonary hypertension due to severe hypoventilation that is caused by kyphoscoliosis (backward and lateral curvature of the spinal column).

I27.2 Other secondary pulmonary hypertension
AHA 14:4Q:p21 – Pulmonary hypertension
Pulmonary hypertension NOS
Code also associated underlying condition

I27.8- Other specified pulmonary heart diseases

I27.81 Cor pulmonale (chronic) — Persistent pulmonary hypertension secondary to disease of the blood vessels of the lung.
AHA 14:4Q:p21 – Cor pulmonale
Cor pulmonale NOS
>   *Excludes 1:*   acute cor pulmonale (I26.0-)

cc **I27.82 Chronic pulmonary embolism** — A pulmonary vascular congestion condition characterized by the restriction or closure of the pulmonary artery or one of its branches by a blood clot(s) that persists over a long period of time.
Use additional code, if applicable, for associated long-term (current) use of anticoagulants (Z79.01)
Excludes 1:   personal history of pulmonary embolism (Z86.711)

I27.89 Other specified pulmonary heart diseases
Eisenmenger's complex
Eisenmenger's syndrome
Excludes 1:   Eisenmenger's defect (Q21.8)

I27.9 Pulmonary heart disease, unspecified
Chronic cardiopulmonary disease

I28- Other diseases of pulmonary vessels

cc **I28.0 Arteriovenous fistula of pulmonary vessels** — An abnormal communication between a pulmonary artery and vein.
Excludes 1:   congenital arteriovenous fistula (Q25.72)

cc **I28.1 Aneurysm of pulmonary artery** — A dilated sac in the wall of a pulmonary artery.
Excludes 1:   congenital aneurysm (Q25.79)
congenital arteriovenous aneurysm (Q25.72)

I28.8 Other diseases of pulmonary vessels
Pulmonary arteritis — Inflammation of a pulmonary arterial wall.
Pulmonary endarteritis — Inflammation of the innermost lining of a pulmonary artery.
Rupture of pulmonary vessels — The forcible tearing of a pulmonary blood vessel wall.
Stenosis of pulmonary vessels — The narrowing of the lumen of a pulmonary blood vessel.
Stricture of pulmonary vessels — The decrease in caliber of a pulmonary blood vessel.

I28.9 Disease of pulmonary vessels, unspecified

Other forms of heart disease (I30-I52)

I30- Acute pericarditis — Inflammation of the outer fibrous and serous protective layers of the heart that is marked by a short and relatively severe course.
Includes: Acute mediastinopericarditis — A form marked by association with inflammation of the mediastinum.
Acute myopericarditis — A form marked by association with inflammation of the myocardium.
Acute pericardial effusion — The abnormal increase of pericardial fluids caused by the overproduction of fluid due to a disease affecting the pericardium.
Acute pleuropericarditis — A form marked by association with inflammation of the pleura.
Acute pneumopericarditis — A form marked by association with inflammation of the lung.
Excludes 1:   Dressler's syndrome (I24.1)
rheumatic pericarditis (acute) (I01.0)

cc **I30.0 Acute nonspecific idiopathic pericarditis** — Acute pericarditis of an unknown cause.

cc **I30.1 Infective pericarditis** — A form caused by microorganisms.
Pneumococcal pericarditis — A form caused by pneumococcal microorganisms.
Pneumopyopericardium — A form marked by pus formation involving the pericardium and the lung.
Purulent pericarditis — A form marked by pus formation, indicating a bacterial infection.
Pyopericarditis — A form marked by pus formation within the pericardium.
Pyopericardium — A form marked by pus formation within the pericardium.
Pyopneumopericardium — A form marked by pus formation involving the pericardium and the lung.
Staphylococcal pericarditis — A form caused by staphylococcal microorganisms.
Streptococcal pericarditis — A form caused by streptococcal microorganisms.
Suppurative pericarditis — A form marked by the production of pus.
Viral pericarditis — A form caused by a virus.
Use additional code (B95-B97) to identify infectious agent

cc **I30.8 Other forms of acute pericarditis**

cc **I30.9 Acute pericarditis, unspecified**

I31- Other diseases of pericardium
Excludes 1:   diseases of pericardium specified as rheumatic (I09.2)
postcardiotomy syndrome (I97.0)
traumatic injury to pericardium (S26.-)

cc **I31.0 Chronic adhesive pericarditis** — The condition of dense, fibrous tissue between the parietal and visceral layers of the pericardium.
Accretio cordis
Adherent pericardium
Adhesive mediastinopericarditis

cc **I31.1 Chronic constrictive pericarditis** — Inflammation of the pericardium characterized by thickening and loss of elasticity.
Concretio cordis
Pericardial calcification

cc **I31.2 Hemopericardium, not elsewhere classified** — The abnormal presence of effused blood in the pericardial cavity that is not due to trauma or a complication of a myocardial infarction.
Excludes 1:   hemopericardium as current complication following acute myocardial infarction (I23.0)

cc **I31.3 Pericardial effusion (noninflammatory)** — The abnormal presence of excessive fluid in the pericardial cavity.
Chylopericardium — A form with chylous fluid.
Excludes 1:   acute pericardial effusion (I30.9)

cc **I31.4 Cardiac tamponade** — [Unacceptable PDX] — The abnormal accumulation of fluid in the pericardium causing increased pressure on the heart so that ventricular filling is impaired and cardiac output is decreased.
Code first underlying cause

cc **I31.8 Other specified diseases of pericardium**
Epicardial plaques
Focal pericardial adhesions

cc **I31.9 Disease of pericardium, unspecified**
Pericarditis (chronic) NOS

I32 Pericarditis in diseases classified elsewhere — [Not Allowed as PDX]
cc **Code first underlying disease**
Excludes 1:   pericarditis (in):
coxsackie (virus) (B33.23)
gonococcal (A54.83)
meningococcal (A39.53)
rheumatoid (arthritis) (M05.31)
syphilitic (A52.06)
systemic lupus erythematosus (M32.12)
tuberculosis (A18.84)

I33- Acute and subacute endocarditis — Inflammation of the endocardium, including the valves, with a sudden, severe onset or a more gradual and subtle development.
Excludes 1:   acute rheumatic endocarditis (I01.1)
endocarditis NOS (I38)

mcc **I33.0 Acute and subacute infective endocarditis** — Inflammation of the endocardium, including the valves, caused by a bacterial or fungal infection, and presenting with sudden, severe onset or a more gradual and subtle development.
Bacterial endocarditis (acute) (subacute)
Infective endocarditis (acute) (subacute) NOS
Endocarditis lenta (acute) (subacute)
Malignant endocarditis (acute) (subacute)
Purulent endocarditis (acute) (subacute)
Septic endocarditis (acute) (subacute)
Ulcerative endocarditis (acute) (subacute)
Vegetative endocarditis (acute) (subacute)
Use additional code (B95-B97) to identify infectious agent

mcc **I33.9 Acute and subacute endocarditis, unspecified**
Acute endocarditis NOS
Acute myoendocarditis NOS
Acute periendocarditis NOS
Subacute endocarditis NOS
Subacute myoendocarditis NOS
Subacute periendocarditis NOS

I34- Nonrheumatic mitral valve disorders — Impaired function of the mitral valve that is not due to rheumatic fever.
Excludes 1:   mitral valve disease (I05.9)
mitral valve failure (I05.8)
mitral valve stenosis (I05.0)
mitral valve disorder of unspecified cause with diseases of aortic and/or tricuspid valve(s) (I08.-)
mitral valve disorder of unspecified cause with mitral stenosis or obstruction (I05.0)
mitral valve disorder specified as congenital (Q23.2, Q23.3)
mitral valve disorder specified as rheumatic (I05.-)

I34.0 Nonrheumatic mitral (valve) insufficiency — Inadequate function of the mitral valve.
Nonrheumatic mitral (valve) incompetence NOS — Synonym for Insufficiency.
Nonrheumatic mitral (valve) regurgitation NOS — The backflow of blood through the mitral valve.

I34.1 Nonrheumatic mitral (valve) prolapse — A form in which the valve leaflets do not close smoothly and evenly.
Floppy nonrheumatic mitral valve syndrome
Excludes 1:   Marfan's syndrome (Q87.4-)

I34.2 Nonrheumatic mitral (valve) stenosis — Reduction in the mitral valve orifice size.

I27-I34

I34.8   **Other nonrheumatic mitral valve disorders**

I34.9   **Nonrheumatic mitral valve disorder, unspecified**

I35-   <u>Nonrheumatic aortic valve disorders</u> — Impaired function of the aortic valve that is not due to rheumatic fever.

     Excludes 1:   *aortic valve disorder of unspecified cause but with diseases of mitral and/or tricuspid valve(s) (I08.-)*
             aortic valve disorder specified as congenital (Q23.0, Q23.1)
             aortic valve disorder specified as rheumatic (I06.-)
             hypertrophic subaortic stenosis (I42.1)

I35.0   **Nonrheumatic aortic (valve) stenosis** — Reduction in the aortic valve orifice size.

I35.1   **Nonrheumatic aortic (valve) insufficiency** — Inadequate function of the aortic valve.
       Nonrheumatic aortic (valve) incompetence NOS — Synonym for Insufficiency.
       Nonrheumatic aortic (valve) regurgitation NOS — The backflow of blood through the aortic valve.

I35.2   **Nonrheumatic aortic (valve) stenosis with insufficiency** — Reduction in the aortic valve orifice size with dysfunction of the aortic valve.

I35.8   **Other nonrheumatic aortic valve disorders**

I35.9   **Nonrheumatic aortic valve disorder, unspecified**

I36-   <u>Nonrheumatic tricuspid valve disorders</u> — Impaired function of the tricuspid valve that is not due to rheumatic fever.

     Excludes 1:   *tricuspid valve disorders of unspecified cause (I07.-)*
             tricuspid valve disorders specified as congenital (Q22.4, Q22.8, Q22.9)
             tricuspid valve disorders specified as rheumatic (I07.-)
             tricuspid valve disorders with aortic and/or mitral valve involvement (I08.-)

I36.0   **Nonrheumatic tricuspid (valve) stenosis** — Reduction in the tricuspid valve orifice size.

I36.1   **Nonrheumatic tricuspid (valve) insufficiency** — Inadequate function of the tricuspid valve.
       Nonrheumatic tricuspid (valve) incompetence — Synonym for Insufficiency.
       Nonrheumatic tricuspid (valve) regurgitation — The backflow of blood through the tricuspid valve.

I36.2   **Nonrheumatic tricuspid (valve) stenosis with insufficiency** — Reduction in the tricuspid valve orifice size with inadequate function of the tricuspid valve.

I36.8   **Other nonrheumatic tricuspid valve disorders**

I36.9   **Nonrheumatic tricuspid valve disorder, unspecified**

I37-   <u>Nonrheumatic pulmonary valve disorders</u> — Impaired function of the pulmonary valve that is not due to rheumatic fever.

     Excludes 1:   *pulmonary valve disorder specified as congenital (Q22.1, Q22.2, Q22.3)*
             pulmonary valve disorder specified as rheumatic (I09.89)

I37.0   **Nonrheumatic pulmonary valve stenosis** — Reduction in the pulmonary valve orifice size.

I37.1   **Nonrheumatic pulmonary valve insufficiency** — Inadequate function of the pulmonary valve.
       Nonrheumatic pulmonary valve incompetence — Synonym for Insufficiency.
       Nonrheumatic pulmonary valve regurgitation

I37.2   **Nonrheumatic pulmonary valve stenosis with insufficiency** — Reduction in the pulmonary valve orifice size with inadequate function of the tricuspid valve.

I37.8   **Other nonrheumatic pulmonary valve disorders**

I37.9   **Nonrheumatic pulmonary valve disorder, unspecified**

I38   **Endocarditis, valve unspecified**
CC
     Includes: **Endocarditis (chronic) NOS**
             Valvular incompetence NOS
             Valvular insufficiency NOS
             Valvular regurgitation NOS
             Valvular stenosis NOS
             Valvulitis (chronic) NOS
     Excludes 1:   *congenital insufficiency of cardiac valve NOS (Q24.8)*
             congenital stenosis of cardiac valve NOS (Q24.8)
             endocardial fibroelastosis (I42.4)
             endocarditis specified as rheumatic (I09.1)

I39   **Endocarditis and heart valve disorders** <u>in diseases classified</u>
CC   <u>elsewhere</u> — [Not Allowed as PDX]
     Code first underlying disease, such as:
       Q fever (A78)
     Excludes 1:   *endocardial involvement in:*
             candidiasis (B37.6)
             gonococcal infection (A54.83)
             Libman-Sacks disease (M32.11)
             listerosis (A32.82)
             meningococcal infection (A39.51)
             rheumatoid arthritis (M05.31)
             syphilis (A52.03)
             tuberculosis (A18.84)
             typhoid fever (A01.02)

I40-   <u>Acute myocarditis</u> — Inflammation of the myocardium with a sudden, severe onset.
     Includes: **Subacute myocarditis** — A form with a more gradual and subtle development.
     Excludes 1:   *acute rheumatic myocarditis (I01.2)*

MCC **I40.0**   **Infective myocarditis** — Inflammation of the myocardium caused by bacterial microorganisms.
       Septic myocarditis
       Use additional code (B95-B97) to identify infectious agent

MCC **I40.1**   **Isolated myocarditis** — Inflammation of the myocardium chiefly affecting the interstitial fibrous tissue and of an unknown etiology.
       Fiedler's myocarditis
       Giant cell myocarditis
       Idiopathic myocarditis

MCC **I40.8**   **Other acute myocarditis**

MCC **I40.9**   **Acute myocarditis, unspecified**

I41   **Myocarditis** <u>in diseases classified elsewhere</u> — [Not Allowed as PDX]
MCC   **Code first underlying disease, such as:**
       Typhus (A75.0-A75.9)
     Excludes 1:   *myocarditis (in):*
             Chagas' disease (chronic) (B57.2)
             acute (B57.0)
             coxsackie (virus) infection (B33.22)
             diphtheritic (A36.81)
             gonococcal (A54.83)
             influenzal (J09.X9, J10.82, J11.82)
             meningococcal (A39.52)
             mumps (B26.82)
             rheumatoid arthritis (M05.31)
             sarcoid (D86.85)
             syphilis (A52.06)
             toxoplasmosis (B58.81)
             tuberculous (A18.84)

I42-   <u>Cardiomyopathy</u> — A disease of the heart muscle, usually of an unknown cause.
     Includes: **Myocardiopathy**
     Code first pre-existing cardiomyopathy complicating pregnancy and puerperium (O99.4)
     Excludes ❷: *ischemic cardiomyopathy (I25.5)*
             peripartum cardiomyopathy (O90.3)
             ventricular hypertrophy (I51.7)

CC **I42.0**   **Dilated cardiomyopathy** — The weakening and enlargement (dilation) of the left ventricular wall that leads to insufficient pumping function.
       Congestive cardiomyopathy

CC **I42.1**   **Obstructive hypertrophic cardiomyopathy** — A disease of unknown cause characterized by asymmetric hypertrophy of the left ventricle wall with variable obstruction of the left ventricle outflow tract.
       Hypertrophic subaortic stenosis (idiopathic)

CC **I42.2**   **Other hypertrophic cardiomyopathy** — Hypertrophy of the left ventricle wall.
       Nonobstructive hypertrophic cardiomyopathy

CC **I42.3**   **Endomyocardial (eosinophilic) disease** — A restrictive form left ventricular dysfunction associated with eosinophilia and fibrous tissue of the myocardium.
       Endomyocardial (tropical) fibrosis
       Löffler's endocarditis

CC **I42.4**   **Endocardial fibroelastosis** — A condition characterized by hypertrophy of the left ventricle wall caused by increased fibroelastic tissue production, often with increased ventricular capacity.
       Congenital cardiomyopathy
       Elastomyofibrosis

CC **I42.5**   **Other restrictive cardiomyopathy** — A form which progressively restricts the contractions of the ventricles.
       Constrictive cardiomyopathy NOS

I34 - I42

cc **I42.6** **Alcoholic cardiomyopathy** — A disease of the heart muscle tissue due to the adverse chemical effects of excessive alcohol.
> Code also presence of alcoholism (F10.-)

cc **I42.7** **Cardiomyopathy** <u>due to drug and external agent</u>
> Code first poisoning due to drug or toxin, if applicable (T36-T65 with fifth or sixth character 1-4 or 6)
> Use additional code for adverse effect, if applicable, to identify drug (T36-T50 with fifth or sixth character 5)

cc **I42.8** **Other cardiomyopathies**

cc **I42.9** **Cardiomyopathy, unspecified**
> **Cardiomyopathy (primary) (secondary) NOS**

I43 **Cardiomyopathy** <u>in diseases classified elsewhere</u> — [Not Allowed as PDX]
cc Code first underlying disease, such as:
> Amyloidosis (E85.-)
> Glycogen storage disease (E74.0)
> Gout (M10.0-)
> Thyrotoxicosis (E05.0-E05.9-)
> *Excludes 1:*   *cardiomyopathy (in):*
>> *coxsackie (virus) (B33.24)*
>> *diphtheria (A36.81)*
>> *sarcoidosis (D86.85)*
>> *tuberculosis (A18.84)*

I44- <u>Atrioventricular</u> and left bundle-branch block

I44.0 **Atrioventricular block, <u>first</u> degree** — Impairment of conduction at the atrioventricular node which is prolonged, but the heart makes all of its beats.

I44.1 **Atrioventricular block, <u>second</u> degree** — Impairment of conduction at the atrioventricular node with partial progressive block and intermittent dropped beats.
> **Atrioventricular block, type I and II**
> **Möbitz block block, type I and II**
> **Second degree block, type I and II**
> **Wenckebach's block**

cc **I44.2** **Atrioventricular block, <u>complete</u>** — Impairment of conduction at the atrioventricular node when no impulses are conducted.
> **Complete heart block NOS**
> **Third degree block**

I44.3- **Other and unspecified atrioventricular block**
> **Atrioventricular block NOS**

I44.30 <u>Unspecified</u> **atrioventricular block**

I44.39 <u>Other</u> **atrioventricular block**

I44.4 <u>Left anterior</u> **fascicular block** — [Questionable Admission] – Conduction impairment of the left anterior superior branch of the left bundle of His.

I44.5 <u>Left posterior</u> **fascicular block** — [Questionable Admission] – Conduction impairment of the left posterior inferior branch of the left bundle of His.

I44.6- **Other and unspecified fascicular block**

I44.60 <u>Unspecified</u> **fascicular block** — [Questionable Admission]
> **Left bundle-branch hemiblock NOS**

I44.69 <u>Other</u> **fascicular block** — [Questionable Admission]

I44.7 **Left bundle-branch block, <u>unspecified</u>** — [Questionable Admission]

I45- **Other conduction disorders**

I45.0 <u>Right fascicular</u> **block** — [Questionable Admission] – Conduction impairment of the right branch of the bundle of His.

I45.1- **Other and unspecified right bundle-branch block**

I45.10 **Unspecified right bundle-branch block** — [Questionable Admission]
> **Right bundle-branch block NOS**

I45.19 **Other right bundle-branch block** — [Questionable Admission]

cc **I45.2** **Bifascicular block** — Conduction impairment of the right branch and the left branch of the bundle of His.

cc **I45.3** **Trifascicular block** — Conduction impairment of all three branches of the bundle of His.

I45.4 **Nonspecific intraventricular block**
> **Bundle-branch block NOS**

I45.5 **Other specified heart block**
> **Sinoatrial block** — Partial or complete conduction impairment of the sinoatrial node.
> **Sinoauricular block**
> *Excludes 1:*   *heart block NOS (I45.9)*

I45.6 **Pre-excitation syndrome** — A conductive cardiac disease that is characterized by the association of paroxysmal tachycardia and premature ventricular impulses.
> **Accelerated atrioventricular conduction**
> **Accessory atrioventricular conduction**
> **Anomalous atrioventricular excitation**
> **Lown-Ganong-Levine syndrome**
> **Pre-excitation atrioventricular conduction**
> **Wolff-Parkinson-White syndrome**

I45.8- **Other specified conduction disorders**

I45.81 **Long QT syndrome** — A disorder (often hereditary) of the heart's electrical rhythm that is characterized by arrhythmia, syncope, dizziness, and sudden death.

cc **I45.89** **Other specified conduction disorders**
> **AHA 13:2Q:p31 – Short QT syndrome**
> **Atrioventricular [AV] dissociation**
> **Interference dissociation**
> **Isorhythmic dissociation**
> **Nonparoxysmal AV nodal tachycardia**

I45.9 **Conduction disorder, unspecified**
> **Heart block NOS**
> **Stokes-Adams syndrome** — A syndrome characterized by heart block and attacks of sudden loss of consciousness.

I46- <u>Cardiac arrest</u> — The sudden cessation (stopping) of cardiac function, with disappearance of arterial blood pressure.
> *Excludes 1:*   *cardiogenic shock (R57.0)*

MCC **I46.2** **Cardiac arrest due to underlying <u>cardiac</u> condition**
> Code first underlying cardiac condition

MCC **I46.8** **Cardiac arrest due to <u>other</u> underlying condition**
> Code first underlying condition

MCC **I46.9** **Cardiac arrest, cause <u>unspecified</u>**

I47- <u>Paroxysmal tachycardia</u> — A condition marked by attacks of rapid action of the heart having sudden onset and cessation.
> Code first tachycardia complicating:
> Abortion or ectopic or molar pregnancy (O00-O07, O08.8)
> Obstetric surgery and procedures (O75.4)
> *Excludes 1:*   *sinoauricular tachycardia NOS (R00.0)*
>> *sinus [sinusal] tachycardia NOS (R00.0)*
>> *tachycardia NOS (R00.0)*

cc **I47.0** **Re-entry ventricular arrhythmia**

cc **I47.1** <u>Supraventricular</u> **tachycardia** — An abnormally rapid atrial rhythm, usually in excess of 160 beats per minute resulting in decreased cardiac output.
> **Atrial (paroxysmal) tachycardia**
> **Atrioventricular [AV] (paroxysmal) tachycardia**
> **Atrioventricular re-entrant (nodal) tachycardia [AVNRT] [AVRT]**
> **Junctional (paroxysmal) tachycardia**
> **Nodal (paroxysmal) tachycardia**

cc **I47.2** **Ventricular tachycardia** — An abnormally rapid ventricular rhythm with aberrant ventricular excitation, usually in excess of 100 beats per minute, which is generated within the ventricle and is most commonly associated with atrioventricular dissociation.
> **AHA 13:3Q:p23 – Catecholaminergic polymorphic ventricular tachycardia (CPVT)**

I47.9 **Paroxysmal tachycardia, unspecified**
> **Bouveret (-Hoffman) syndrome**

I48- <u>Atrial</u> **fibrillation and flutter**

I48.0 <u>Paroxysmal</u> **atrial <u>fibrillation</u>** — Atrial arrhythmia characterized by rapid, randomized contractions of the atria causing an irregular and often rapid ventricular rate that are classified as recurrent episodes that stops on its own in less than 7 days.

cc **I48.1** <u>Persistent</u> **atrial <u>fibrillation</u>** — Atrial arrhythmia characterized by rapid, randomized contractions of the atria causing an irregular and often rapid ventricular rate that are classified as recurrent episodes that lasts more than 7 days.

I48.2 <u>Chronic</u> **atrial <u>fibrillation</u>** — Atrial arrhythmia characterized by rapid, randomized contractions of the atria causing an irregular and often rapid ventricular rate that is classified as an ongoing long-term episode.
> **Permanent atrial fibrillation**

cc **I48.3** <u>Typical</u> **atrial <u>flutter</u>** — A condition of cardiac arrhythmia in which the atrial contractions are rapid (200-300 per minute range). The ventricles are unable to respond to each atrial impulse, so that a partial block usually is present.
> **Type I atrial flutter**

cc **I48.4** <u>Atypical</u> **atrial <u>flutter</u>** — A condition of cardiac arrhythmia in which the atrial contractions are very rapid (300-400 per minute range). The ventricles are unable to respond to each atrial impulse, so that a partial block usually is present.
> **Type II atrial flutter**

**I
4
2
-
I
4
8**

I48.9- <u>Unspecified</u> atrial fibrillation and atrial flutter

    I48.91 Unspecified atrial <u>fibrillation</u>

cc **I48.92** Unspecified atrial <u>flutter</u>

I49- Other cardiac arrhythmias
    Code first cardiac arrhythmia complicating:
        Abortion or ectopic or molar pregnancy (O00-O07, O08.8)
        Obstetric surgery and procedures (O75.4)
    Excludes 1:   *bradycardia NOS (R00.1)*
                 neonatal dysrhythmia (P29.1-)
                 sinoatrial bradycardia (R00.1)
                 sinus bradycardia (R00.1)
                 vagal bradycardia (R00.1)

  I49.0- <u>Ventricular</u> fibrillation and flutter

mcc **I49.01** Ventricular fibrillation — An arrhythmia characterized by quivering of the ventricle due to rapid repetitive excitation of myocardial fibers without coordinated contraction of the ventricle that results in the loss of the heart pumping and collapse of cardiac output and blood pressure.

mcc **I49.02** Ventricular flutter — A possible transition stage between ventricular tachycardia and ventricular fibrillation with the EKG showing rapid, uniform, and virtually regular oscillations, 180 or more per minute.

  I49.1 Atrial premature depolarization — An early appearing cardiac beat originating in an atria.
        Atrial premature beats

cc **I49.2** Junctional premature depolarization — An early appearing cardiac beat originating in the atrioventricular node.

  I49.3 Ventricular premature depolarization — An early appearing cardiac beat originating in the Purkinje fibers of the ventricles.

  I49.4- Other and unspecified premature depolarization

    I49.40 Unspecified premature depolarization
        Premature beats NOS

    I49.49 Other premature depolarization
        Ectopic beats — A heart beat originating at some point other than a sinus node.
        Extrasystoles — A premature contraction of the heart that is independent of the normal rhythm and arises in response to an impulse in some part of the heart other than the sinoatrial node.
        Extrasystolic arrhythmias
        Premature contractions

  I49.5 Sick sinus syndrome — Cardiac arrhythmia characterized by severe sinus bradycardia alone, sinus bradycardia alternating with tachycardia, or sinus bradycardia with atrioventricular block.
        Tachycardia-bradycardia syndrome

  I49.8 Other specified cardiac arrhythmias
        Coronary sinus rhythm disorder
        Ectopic rhythm disorder
        Nodal rhythm disorder

  I49.9 Cardiac arrhythmia, unspecified
        Arrhythmia (cardiac) NOS

I50- <u>Heart failure</u> — The decreased ability of the heart to pump enough blood to meet the needs of the body's tissues.
    AHA 14:1Q:p25 – Diastolic or systolic heart failure
    AHA 14:4Q:p21 – Decompensated right heart failure
    AHA 16:1Q:p10 – Diastolic or systolic heart failure (HFpEF, HFrEF)
    Code first:
        Heart failure complicating abortion or ectopic or molar pregnancy (O00-O07, O08.8)
        Heart failure due to hypertension (I11.0)
        Heart failure due to hypertension with chronic kidney disease (I13.-)
        Heart failure following surgery (I97.13-)
        Obstetric surgery and procedures (O75.4)
        Rheumatic heart failure (I09.81)
    Excludes 1:   *neonatal cardiac failure (P29.0)*
    Excludes ❷: *cardiac arrest (I46.-)*

cc **I50.1** Left ventricular failure — A condition of decreased cardiac output of the left ventricle.
        Cardiac asthma
        Edema of lung with heart disease NOS
        Edema of lung with heart failure
        Left heart failure
        Pulmonary edema with heart disease NOS
        Pulmonary edema with heart failure
    Excludes 1:   *edema of lung without heart disease or heart failure (J81.-)*
             pulmonary edema without heart disease or failure (J81.-)

I50.2- <u>Systolic</u> (congestive) heart failure — A form caused by the left ventricle's inability to contract with enough force to pump adequate amounts of blood through the body that is characterized by excessive fluid retention, congestion in the lungs, and swelling of the legs and ankles.
    Excludes 1:   *combined systolic (congestive) and diastolic (congestive) heart failure (I50.4-)*

cc **I50.20** <u>Unspecified</u> systolic (congestive) heart failure

mcc **I50.21** <u>Acute</u> systolic (congestive) heart failure — A form marked by a sudden, severe onset.

cc **I50.22** <u>Chronic</u> systolic (congestive) heart failure — A form that persists over a long period of time.

mcc **I50.23** <u>Acute on chronic</u> systolic (congestive) heart failure — A form that persists over a long period of time and has a sudden, severe exacerbation of the condition.
        AHA 13:2Q:p33 – Decompensated systolic heart failure

I50.3- <u>Diastolic</u> (congestive) heart failure — A form caused by the left ventricle's inability to relax properly and fill with blood as a result of stiffening of the heart muscle that is characterized by excessive fluid retention, congestion in the lungs, and swelling of the legs and ankles.
    Excludes 1:   *combined systolic (congestive) and diastolic (congestive) heart failure (I50.4-)*

cc **I50.30** <u>Unspecified</u> diastolic (congestive) heart failure

mcc **I50.31** <u>Acute</u> diastolic (congestive) heart failure — A form marked by a sudden, severe onset.

cc **I50.32** <u>Chronic</u> diastolic (congestive) heart failure — A form that persists over a long period of time.

mcc **I50.33** <u>Acute on chronic</u> diastolic (congestive) heart failure — A form that persists over a long period of time and has a sudden, severe exacerbation of the condition.

I50.4- <u>Combined</u> systolic (congestive) and diastolic (congestive) heart failure — A form in which the left ventricle's inability to contract and relax are both present.

cc **I50.40** <u>Unspecified</u> combined systolic (congestive) and diastolic (congestive) heart failure

mcc **I50.41** <u>Acute</u> combined systolic (congestive) and diastolic (congestive) heart failure — A form marked by a sudden, severe onset.

cc **I50.42** <u>Chronic</u> combined systolic (congestive) and diastolic (congestive) heart failure — A form that persists over a long period of time.

mcc **I50.43** <u>Acute on chronic</u> combined systolic (congestive) and diastolic (congestive) heart failure — A form that persists over a long period of time and has a sudden, severe exacerbation of the condition.

I50.9 Heart failure, <u>unspecified</u>
        Biventricular (heart) failure NOS
        Cardiac, heart or myocardial failure NOS
        Congestive heart disease
        Congestive heart failure NOS
        Right ventricular failure (secondary to left heart failure)
    Excludes ❷: *fluid overload (E87.70)*

I51- Complications and ill-defined descriptions of heart disease
    Excludes 1:   *any condition in I51.4-I51.9 due to hypertension (I11.-)*
             any condition in I51.4-I51.9 due to hypertension and chronic kidney disease (I13.-)
             heart disease specified as rheumatic (I00-I09)

cc **I51.0** Cardiac septal defect, acquired — [Age/15-124]
        Acquired septal atrial defect (old)
        Acquired septal auricular defect (old)
        Acquired septal ventricular defect (old)
    Excludes 1:   *cardiac septal defect as current complication following acute myocardial infarction (I23.1, I23.2)*

mcc **I51.1** Rupture of chordae tendineae, not elsewhere classified — A forcible tearing of the strong, cord-like attachments of the heart valves to the papillary muscles.
    Excludes 1:   *rupture of chordae tendineae as current complication following acute myocardial infarction (I23.4)*

mcc **I51.2** Rupture of papillary muscle, not elsewhere classified — A forcible tearing of the conical intraventricular muscles attached to the chordae tendineae and heart wall.
    Excludes 1:   *rupture of papillary muscle as current complication following acute myocardial infarction (I23.5)*

I 48 - I 51

I51.3   Intracardiac thrombosis, not elsewhere classified
AHA 13:1Q:p24 – Left atrial appendage thrombus
Apical thrombosis (old)
Atrial thrombosis (old)
Auricular thrombosis (old)
Mural thrombosis (old)
Ventricular thrombosis (old)
*Excludes 1:   intracardiac thrombosis as current complication
following acute myocardial infarction (I23.6)*

I51.4   Myocarditis, unspecified — Inflammation of the heart muscle.
Chronic (interstitial) myocarditis
Myocardial fibrosis
Myocarditis NOS
Excludes 1:   acute or subacute myocarditis (I40.-)

I51.5   Myocardial degeneration — Deterioration of the heart muscle tissue.
Fatty degeneration of heart or myocardium
Myocardial disease
Senile degeneration of heart or myocardium

I51.7   Cardiomegaly — The abnormal enlargement of the heart.
Cardiac dilatation
Cardiac hypertrophy
Ventricular dilatation

I51.8-   Other ill-defined heart diseases
cc **I51.81 Takotsubo syndrome** — A reversible left ventricular dysfunction in
patients without coronary disease that is precipitated by emotional or
physiological stress.
Reversible left ventricular dysfunction following sudden
emotional stress
Stress induced cardiomyopathy
Takotsubo cardiomyopathy
Transient left ventricular apical ballooning syndrome

I51.89 Other ill-defined heart diseases
Carditis (acute) (chronic)
Pancarditis (acute) (chronic)

I51.9   Heart disease, unspecified

I52   Other heart disorders in diseases classified elsewhere —
[Not Allowed as PDX]
Code first underlying disease, such as:
Congenital syphilis (A50.5)
Mucopolysaccharidosis (E76.3)
Schistosomiasis (B65.0-B65.9)
Excludes 1:   heart disease (in):
gonococcal infection (A54.83)
meningococcal infection (A39.50)
rheumatoid arthritis (M05.31)
syphilis (A52.06)

Cerebrovascular diseases (I60-I69)

Use additional code to identify presence of:
Alcohol abuse and dependence (F10.-)
Exposure to environmental tobacco smoke (Z77.22)
History of tobacco dependence (Z87.891)
Hypertension (I10-I15)
Occupational exposure to environmental tobacco smoke (Z57.31)
Tobacco dependence (F17.-)
Tobacco use (Z72.0)
*Excludes 1:   transient cerebral ischemic attacks and related syndromes
(G45.-)*
traumatic intracranial hemorrhage (S06.-)

I60-   Nontraumatic subarachnoid hemorrhage — A hemorrhage into the
subarachnoid (beneath the arachnoid layer of cerebral meninges) space.
Includes: Ruptured cerebral aneurysm
Excludes 1:   syphilitic ruptured cerebral aneurysm (A52.05)
Excludes ❷: sequelae of subarachnoid hemorrhage (I69.0-)

**I60.0-   Nontraumatic subarachnoid hemorrhage from carotid siphon
and bifurcation**
mcc **I60.00 Nontraumatic subarachnoid hemorrhage from unspecified
carotid siphon and bifurcation**
mcc **I60.01 Nontraumatic subarachnoid hemorrhage from right
carotid siphon and bifurcation**
mcc **I60.02 Nontraumatic subarachnoid hemorrhage from left carotid
siphon and bifurcation**
**I60.1-   Nontraumatic subarachnoid hemorrhage from middle cerebral
artery**
mcc **I60.10 Nontraumatic subarachnoid hemorrhage from unspecified
middle cerebral artery**

mcc **I60.11 Nontraumatic subarachnoid hemorrhage from right
middle cerebral artery**
mcc **I60.12 Nontraumatic subarachnoid hemorrhage from left middle
cerebral artery**
mcc **I60.2   Nontraumatic subarachnoid hemorrhage from anterior
communicating artery**
**I60.3-   Nontraumatic subarachnoid hemorrhage from posterior
communicating artery**
mcc **I60.30 Nontraumatic subarachnoid hemorrhage from unspecified
posterior communicating artery**
mcc **I60.31 Nontraumatic subarachnoid hemorrhage from right
posterior communicating artery**
mcc **I60.32 Nontraumatic subarachnoid hemorrhage from left
posterior communicating artery**
mcc **I60.4   Nontraumatic subarachnoid hemorrhage from basilar artery**
I60.5-   Nontraumatic subarachnoid hemorrhage from vertebral artery
mcc **I60.50 Nontraumatic subarachnoid hemorrhage from unspecified
vertebral artery**
mcc **I60.51 Nontraumatic subarachnoid hemorrhage from right
vertebral artery**
mcc **I60.52 Nontraumatic subarachnoid hemorrhage from left
vertebral artery**
mcc **I60.6   Nontraumatic subarachnoid hemorrhage from other
intracranial arteries**
mcc **I60.7   Nontraumatic subarachnoid hemorrhage from unspecified
intracranial artery**
Ruptured (congenital) berry aneurysm
Ruptured (congenital) cerebral aneurysm
Subarachnoid hemorrhage (nontraumatic) from cerebral artery NOS
Subarachnoid hemorrhage (nontraumatic) from communicating
artery NOS
Excludes 1:   berry aneurysm, nonruptured (I67.1)
mcc **I60.8   Other nontraumatic subarachnoid hemorrhage**
Meningeal hemorrhage
Rupture of cerebral arteriovenous malformation
mcc **I60.9   Nontraumatic subarachnoid hemorrhage, unspecified**

I61-   Nontraumatic intracerebral hemorrhage — A hemorrhage within the brain.
Excludes ❷: sequelae of intracerebral hemorrhage (I69.1-)
mcc **I61.0   Nontraumatic intracerebral hemorrhage in hemisphere,
subcortical** — A hemorrhage beneath the cerebral cortex.
Deep intracerebral hemorrhage (nontraumatic)
mcc **I61.1   Nontraumatic intracerebral hemorrhage in hemisphere,
cortical** — A hemorrhage in the cerebral cortex.
Cerebral lobe hemorrhage (nontraumatic)
Superficial intracerebral hemorrhage (nontraumatic)
mcc **I61.2   Nontraumatic intracerebral hemorrhage in hemisphere,
unspecified**
mcc **I61.3   Nontraumatic intracerebral hemorrhage in brain stem** — A
hemorrhage in the brain stem.
mcc **I61.4   Nontraumatic intracerebral hemorrhage in cerebellum** — A
hemorrhage in the cerebellum.
mcc **I61.5   Nontraumatic intracerebral hemorrhage, intraventricular** — A
hemorrhage into the ventricles of the brain.
mcc **I61.6   Nontraumatic intracerebral hemorrhage, multiple localized** —
A form marked by separate, distinct sites.
mcc **I61.8   Other nontraumatic intracerebral hemorrhage**
mcc **I61.9   Nontraumatic intracerebral hemorrhage, unspecified**

I62-   Other and unspecified nontraumatic intracranial hemorrhage
Excludes ❷: sequelae of intracranial hemorrhage (I69.2)
I62.0-   Nontraumatic subdural hemorrhage — A hemorrhage below the dura
layer of meninges but does not involve the brain, but can compress on the brain.
mcc **I62.00 Nontraumatic subdural hemorrhage, unspecified**
mcc **I62.01 Nontraumatic acute subdural hemorrhage** — A form with a
sudden, severe onset.
mcc **I62.02 Nontraumatic subacute subdural hemorrhage** — A form that
develops over several days.
mcc **I62.03 Nontraumatic chronic subdural hemorrhage** — A form that
develops over several weeks.

I
5
1
-
I
6
2

MCC **I62.1** **Nontraumatic extradural hemorrhage** — A hemorrhage between the skull and meninges which does not involve the brain.
    Nontraumatic epidural hemorrhage — A hemorrhage situated upon or outside the dura (the outermost layer of cerebral meninges).

CC **I62.9** **Nontraumatic intracranial hemorrhage, unspecified**

I63- **Cerebral infarction** — Local cerebral tissue ischemia that produces a neurological brain impairment.
    Includes: Occlusion and stenosis of cerebral and precerebral arteries, resulting in cerebral infarction
    Use additional code, if applicable, to identify status post administration of tPA (rtPA) in a different facility within the last 24 hours prior to admission to current facility (Z92.82)
    Use additional code, if known, to indicate National Institutes of Health Stroke Scale (NIHSS) score (R29.7)
    Excludes ❷: *sequelae of cerebral infarction (I69.3-)*

I63.0- **Cerebral infarction due to thrombosis of precerebral arteries** — A form marked by an abnormal aggregation of blood factors causing inadequate blood flow of the branched arteries before they anatomically branch into the brain.

MCC **I63.00** **Cerebral infarction due to thrombosis of unspecified precerebral artery**

I63.01- **Cerebral infarction due to thrombosis of vertebral artery**

MCC **I63.011** **Cerebral infarction due to thrombosis of right vertebral artery**

MCC **I63.012** **Cerebral infarction due to thrombosis of left vertebral artery**

MCC **I63.013** **Cerebral infarction due to thrombosis of bilateral vertebral arteries**

MCC **I63.019** **Cerebral infarction due to thrombosis of unspecified vertebral artery**

MCC **I63.02** **Cerebral infarction due to thrombosis of basilar artery**

I63.03- **Cerebral infarction due to thrombosis of carotid artery**

MCC **I63.031** **Cerebral infarction due to thrombosis of right carotid artery**

MCC **I63.032** **Cerebral infarction due to thrombosis of left carotid artery**

MCC **I63.033** **Cerebral infarction due to thrombosis of bilateral carotid arteries**

MCC **I63.039** **Cerebral infarction due to thrombosis of unspecified carotid artery**

MCC **I63.09** **Cerebral infarction due to thrombosis of other precerebral artery**

I63.1- **Cerebral infarction due to embolism of precerebral arteries** — A form marked by obstruction caused by a blood clot or foreign substances of the branched arteries before they anatomically branch into the brain.

MCC **I63.10** **Cerebral infarction due to embolism of unspecified precerebral artery**

I63.11- **Cerebral infarction due to embolism of vertebral artery**

MCC **I63.111** **Cerebral infarction due to embolism of right vertebral artery**

MCC **I63.112** **Cerebral infarction due to embolism of left vertebral artery**

MCC **I63.113** **Cerebral infarction due to embolism of bilateral vertebral arteries**

MCC **I63.119** **Cerebral infarction due to embolism of unspecified vertebral artery**

MCC **I63.12** **Cerebral infarction due to embolism of basilar artery**

I63.13- **Cerebral infarction due to embolism of carotid artery**

MCC **I63.131** **Cerebral infarction due to embolism of right carotid artery**

MCC **I63.132** **Cerebral infarction due to embolism of left carotid artery**

MCC **I63.133** **Cerebral infarction due to embolism of bilateral carotid arteries**

MCC **I63.139** **Cerebral infarction due to embolism of unspecified carotid artery**

MCC **I63.19** **Cerebral infarction due to embolism of other precerebral artery**

I63.2- **Cerebral infarction due to unspecified occlusion or stenosis of precerebral arteries**

MCC **I63.20** **Cerebral infarction due to unspecified occlusion or stenosis of unspecified precerebral arteries**

I63.21- **Cerebral infarction due to unspecified occlusion or stenosis of vertebral arteries**

MCC **I63.211** **Cerebral infarction due to unspecified occlusion or stenosis of right vertebral arteries**

MCC **I63.212** **Cerebral infarction due to unspecified occlusion or stenosis of left vertebral arteries**

MCC **I63.213** **Cerebral infarction due to unspecified occlusion or stenosis of bilateral vertebral arteries**

MCC **I63.219** **Cerebral infarction due to unspecified occlusion or stenosis of unspecified vertebral arteries**

MCC **I63.22** **Cerebral infarction due to unspecified occlusion or stenosis of basilar arteries**

I63.23- **Cerebral infarction due to unspecified occlusion or stenosis of carotid arteries**

MCC **I63.231** **Cerebral infarction due to unspecified occlusion or stenosis of right carotid arteries**

MCC **I63.232** **Cerebral infarction due to unspecified occlusion or stenosis of left carotid arteries**

MCC **I63.233** **Cerebral infarction due to unspecified occlusion or stenosis of bilateral carotid arteries**

MCC **I63.239** **Cerebral infarction due to unspecified occlusion or stenosis of unspecified carotid arteries**

MCC **I63.29** **Cerebral infarction due to unspecified occlusion or stenosis of other precerebral arteries**

I63.3- **Cerebral infarction due to thrombosis of cerebral arteries** — A form marked by an abnormal aggregation of blood factors causing inadequate blood flow of the arteries within the brain.

MCC **I63.30** **Cerebral infarction due to thrombosis of unspecified cerebral artery**

I63.31- **Cerebral infarction due to thrombosis of middle cerebral artery**

MCC **I63.311** **Cerebral infarction due to thrombosis of right middle cerebral artery**

MCC **I63.312** **Cerebral infarction due to thrombosis of left middle cerebral artery**

MCC **I63.313** **Cerebral infarction due to thrombosis of bilateral middle cerebral arteries**

MCC **I63.319** **Cerebral infarction due to thrombosis of unspecified middle cerebral artery**

I63.32- **Cerebral infarction due to thrombosis of anterior cerebral artery**

MCC **I63.321** **Cerebral infarction due to thrombosis of right anterior cerebral artery**

MCC **I63.322** **Cerebral infarction due to thrombosis of left anterior cerebral artery**

MCC **I63.323** **Cerebral infarction due to thrombosis of bilateral anterior arteries**

MCC **I63.329** **Cerebral infarction due to thrombosis of unspecified anterior cerebral artery**

I63.33- **Cerebral infarction due to thrombosis of posterior cerebral artery**

MCC **I63.331** **Cerebral infarction due to thrombosis of right posterior cerebral artery**

MCC **I63.332** **Cerebral infarction due to thrombosis of left posterior cerebral artery**

MCC **I63.333** **Cerebral infarction due to thrombosis of bilateral posterior arteries**

MCC **I63.339** **Cerebral infarction due to thrombosis of unspecified posterior cerebral artery**

I63.34- **Cerebral infarction due to thrombosis of cerebellar artery**

MCC **I63.341** **Cerebral infarction due to thrombosis of right cerebellar artery**

MCC **I63.342** **Cerebral infarction due to thrombosis of left cerebellar artery**

MCC **I63.343** Cerebral infarction due to <u>thrombosis</u> of <u>bilateral</u> cerebellar arteries

MCC **I63.349** Cerebral infarction due to <u>thrombosis</u> of <u>unspecified</u> cerebellar artery

MCC **I63.39** Cerebral infarction due to <u>thrombosis</u> of other <u>cerebral</u> artery

I63.4- Cerebral infarction due to <u>embolism</u> of <u>cerebral</u> arteries — A form marked by obstruction caused by a blood clot or foreign substances of the arteries within the brain.

MCC **I63.40** Cerebral infarction due to <u>embolism</u> of <u>unspecified</u> cerebral artery

I63.41- Cerebral infarction due to <u>embolism</u> of <u>middle</u> cerebral artery

MCC **I63.411** Cerebral infarction due to <u>embolism</u> of <u>right</u> middle cerebral artery

MCC **I63.412** Cerebral infarction due to <u>embolism</u> of <u>left</u> middle cerebral artery

MCC **I63.413** Cerebral infarction due to <u>embolism</u> of <u>bilateral</u> middle cerebral arteries

MCC **I63.419** Cerebral infarction due to <u>embolism</u> of <u>unspecified</u> middle cerebral artery

I63.42- Cerebral infarction due to <u>embolism</u> of <u>anterior</u> cerebral artery

MCC **I63.421** Cerebral infarction due to <u>embolism</u> of <u>right</u> anterior cerebral artery

MCC **I63.422** Cerebral infarction due to <u>embolism</u> of <u>left</u> anterior cerebral artery

MCC **I63.423** Cerebral infarction due to <u>embolism</u> of <u>bilateral</u> anterior cerebral arteries

MCC **I63.429** Cerebral infarction due to <u>embolism</u> of <u>unspecified</u> anterior cerebral artery

I63.43- Cerebral infarction due to <u>embolism</u> of <u>posterior</u> cerebral artery

MCC **I63.431** Cerebral infarction due to <u>embolism</u> of <u>right</u> posterior cerebral artery

MCC **I63.432** Cerebral infarction due to <u>embolism</u> of <u>left</u> posterior cerebral artery

MCC **I63.433** Cerebral infarction due to <u>embolism</u> of <u>bilateral</u> posterior cerebral arteries

MCC **I63.439** Cerebral infarction due to <u>embolism</u> of <u>unspecified</u> posterior cerebral artery

I63.44- Cerebral infarction due to <u>embolism</u> of <u>cerebellar</u> artery

MCC **I63.441** Cerebral infarction due to <u>embolism</u> of <u>right</u> cerebellar artery

MCC **I63.442** Cerebral infarction due to <u>embolism</u> of <u>left</u> cerebellar artery

MCC **I63.443** Cerebral infarction due to <u>embolism</u> of <u>bilateral</u> cerebellar arteries

MCC **I63.449** Cerebral infarction due to <u>embolism</u> of <u>unspecified</u> cerebellar artery

MCC **I63.49** Cerebral infarction due to <u>embolism</u> of <u>other cerebral</u> artery

I63.5- Cerebral infarction due to <u>unspecified occlusion or stenosis of cerebral arteries</u>

MCC **I63.50** Cerebral infarction due to <u>unspecified</u> occlusion or stenosis of unspecified cerebral artery

I63.51- Cerebral infarction due to <u>unspecified</u> occlusion or stenosis of <u>middle</u> cerebral artery

MCC **I63.511** Cerebral infarction due to <u>unspecified</u> occlusion or stenosis of <u>right</u> middle cerebral artery

MCC **I63.512** Cerebral infarction due to <u>unspecified</u> occlusion or stenosis of <u>left</u> middle cerebral artery

MCC **I63.513** Cerebral infarction due to <u>unspecified</u> occlusion or stenosis of <u>bilateral</u> middle arteries

MCC **I63.519** Cerebral infarction due to <u>unspecified</u> occlusion or stenosis of <u>unspecified</u> middle cerebral artery

I63.52- Cerebral infarction due to <u>unspecified</u> occlusion or stenosis of <u>anterior</u> cerebral artery

MCC **I63.521** Cerebral infarction due to <u>unspecified</u> occlusion or stenosis of <u>right</u> anterior cerebral artery

MCC **I63.522** Cerebral infarction due to <u>unspecified</u> occlusion or stenosis of <u>left</u> anterior cerebral artery

MCC **I63.523** Cerebral infarction due to <u>unspecified</u> occlusion or stenosis of <u>bilateral</u> anterior arteries

MCC **I63.529** Cerebral infarction due to <u>unspecified</u> occlusion or stenosis of <u>unspecified</u> anterior cerebral artery

I63.53- Cerebral infarction due to <u>unspecified</u> occlusion or stenosis of <u>posterior</u> cerebral artery

MCC **I63.531** Cerebral infarction due to <u>unspecified</u> occlusion or stenosis of <u>right</u> posterior cerebral artery

MCC **I63.532** Cerebral infarction due to <u>unspecified</u> occlusion or stenosis of <u>left</u> posterior cerebral artery

MCC **I63.533** Cerebral infarction due to <u>unspecified</u> occlusion or stenosis of <u>bilateral</u> posterior arteries

MCC **I63.539** Cerebral infarction due to <u>unspecified</u> occlusion or stenosis of <u>unspecified</u> posterior cerebral artery

I63.54- Cerebral infarction due to <u>unspecified</u> occlusion or stenosis of <u>cerebellar</u> artery

MCC **I63.541** Cerebral infarction due to <u>unspecified</u> occlusion or stenosis of <u>right</u> cerebellar artery

MCC **I63.542** Cerebral infarction due to <u>unspecified</u> occlusion or stenosis of <u>left</u> cerebellar artery

MCC **I63.543** Cerebral infarction due to <u>unspecified</u> occlusion or stenosis of <u>bilateral</u> cerebellar arteries

MCC **I63.549** Cerebral infarction due to <u>unspecified</u> occlusion or stenosis of <u>unspecified</u> cerebellar artery

MCC **I63.59** Cerebral infarction due to <u>unspecified</u> occlusion or stenosis of <u>other cerebral</u> artery

MCC **I63.6** Cerebral infarction due to <u>cerebral venous thrombosis,</u> nonpyogenic

MCC **I63.8** <u>Other</u> cerebral infarction

MCC **I63.9** Cerebral infarction, <u>unspecified</u>
   AHA 15:1Q:p25 – Cerebral infarction
   Stroke NOS

I65- <u>Occlusion and stenosis</u> of <u>precerebral</u> arteries, <u>not resulting in cerebral infarction</u> — Decreased blood flow conditions of the branched arteries before they anatomically branch into the brain.
   Includes: **Embolism of precerebral artery** — Obstruction caused by foreign substances or a blood clot.
   Narrowing of precerebral artery — Inadequate blood flow due to decreased lumenal patency.
   Obstruction (complete) (partial) of precerebral artery — Blockage by any means.
   Thrombosis of precerebral artery — An abnormal aggregation of blood factors causing inadequate blood flow.
   Excludes 1: *insufficiency, NOS, of precerebral artery (G45.-)*
   insufficiency of precerebral arteries causing cerebral infarction (I63.0-I63.2)

I65.0- <u>Occlusion and stenosis</u> of <u>vertebral</u> artery
   I65.01 Occlusion and stenosis of <u>right</u> vertebral artery
   I65.02 Occlusion and stenosis of <u>left</u> vertebral artery
   I65.03 Occlusion and stenosis of <u>bilateral</u> vertebral arteries
   I65.09 Occlusion and stenosis of <u>unspecified</u> vertebral artery

I65.1 <u>Occlusion and stenosis</u> of <u>basilar</u> artery

I65.2- <u>Occlusion and stenosis</u> of <u>carotid</u> artery
   I65.21 Occlusion and stenosis of <u>right</u> carotid artery
   I65.22 Occlusion and stenosis of <u>left</u> carotid artery
   I65.23 Occlusion and stenosis of <u>bilateral</u> carotid arteries
   I65.29 Occlusion and stenosis of <u>unspecified</u> carotid artery

I65.8 <u>Occlusion and stenosis</u> of <u>other</u> precerebral arteries

I65.9 <u>Occlusion and stenosis</u> of <u>unspecified</u> precerebral artery
   Occlusion and stenosis of precerebral artery NOS

I 63 - I 65

I66- **Occlusion and stenosis** of **cerebral** arteries, **not resulting in cerebral infarction** — Blocked blood flow of the arteries within brain.
Includes: **Embolism of cerebral artery** — Obstruction caused by foreign substances or a blood clot.
Narrowing of cerebral artery — Inadequate blood flow due to decreased lumenal patency.
Obstruction (complete) (partial) of cerebral artery — Blockage by any means.
Thrombosis of cerebral artery — An abnormal aggregation of blood factors causing inadequate blood flow.
Excludes 1: *occlusion and stenosis of cerebral artery causing cerebral infarction (I63.3-I63.5)*

I66.0- **Occlusion and stenosis** of **middle cerebral** artery
I66.01 Occlusion and stenosis of **right** middle cerebral artery
I66.02 Occlusion and stenosis of **left** middle cerebral artery
I66.03 Occlusion and stenosis of **bilateral** middle cerebral arteries
I66.09 Occlusion and stenosis of **unspecified** middle cerebral artery

I66.1- **Occlusion and stenosis** of **anterior cerebral** artery
I66.11 Occlusion and stenosis of **right** anterior cerebral artery
I66.12 Occlusion and stenosis of **left** anterior cerebral artery
I66.13 Occlusion and stenosis of **bilateral** anterior cerebral arteries
I66.19 Occlusion and stenosis of **unspecified** anterior cerebral artery

I66.2- **Occlusion and stenosis** of **posterior cerebral** artery
I66.21 Occlusion and stenosis of **right** posterior cerebral artery
I66.22 Occlusion and stenosis of **left** posterior cerebral artery
I66.23 Occlusion and stenosis of **bilateral** posterior cerebral arteries
I66.29 Occlusion and stenosis of **unspecified** posterior cerebral artery

I66.3 **Occlusion and stenosis** of **cerebellar** arteries
I66.8 **Occlusion and stenosis** of **other cerebral** arteries
Occlusion and stenosis of perforating arteries
I66.9 **Occlusion and stenosis** of **unspecified cerebral** artery

I67- **Other cerebrovascular diseases**
Excludes ❷: *sequelae of the listed conditions (I69.8)*

MCC **I67.0** **Dissection of cerebral arteries, nonruptured** — The tearing of the lining of a cerebral artery.
Excludes 1: *ruptured cerebral arteries (I60.7)*

I67.1 **Cerebral aneurysm, nonruptured** — A sac formed by the dilatation of a cerebral arterial wall, in which the arterial wall has not torn open.
Cerebral aneurysm NOS
Cerebral arteriovenous fistula, acquired
Internal carotid artery aneurysm, intracranial portion
Internal carotid artery aneurysm, NOS
Excludes 1: *congenital cerebral aneurysm, nonruptured (Q28.-)*
ruptured cerebral aneurysm (I60.7)

I67.2 **Cerebral atherosclerosis** — [Age/15-124] — Narrowing of the cerebral an/or the precerebral arteries caused by deposition of plaque-forming cholesterol and other lipids within the lumen of those arteries.
Atheroma of cerebral and precerebral arteries

CC **I67.3** **Progressive vascular leukoencephalopathy**
Binswanger's disease

CC **I67.4** **Hypertensive encephalopathy** — A degenerative condition of the brain resulting from severe hypertension.

CC **I67.5** **Moyamoya disease** — The arterial graphic appearance of a filmy network of small vessels (resembling a puff of smoke) replacing the normal vascular pattern at the termination of the internal carotid artery; seen in patients with sudden cerebrovascular insufficiency.

CC **I67.6** **Nonpyogenic thrombosis of intracranial venous system** — An abnormal aggregation of blood factors causing obstruction of the intracranial venous sinus that is not formed by pus-producing organisms.
Nonpyogenic thrombosis of cerebral vein
Nonpyogenic thrombosis of intracranial venous sinus
Excludes 1: *nonpyogenic thrombosis of intracranial venous system causing infarction (I63.6)*

CC **I67.7** **Cerebral arteritis, not elsewhere classified**
Granulomatous angiitis of the nervous system
Excludes 1: *allergic granulomatous angiitis (M30.1)*

I67.8- **Other specified cerebrovascular diseases**
CC **I67.81** **Acute cerebrovascular insufficiency** — Inadequate function of the cerebrovascular system, but not diagnostic of transient cerebral ischemia or stroke.
Acute cerebrovascular insufficiency unspecified as to location or reversibility

CC **I67.82** **Cerebral ischemia** — Prolonged, persistent deficiency of blood supply to the brain.
Chronic cerebral ischemia

MCC **I67.83** **Posterior reversible encephalopathy syndrome** — A syndrome characterized by headache, visual disturbance, and seizures that is often due to hypertension.
PRES

I67.84- **Cerebral vasospasm and vasoconstriction**
CC **I67.841** **Reversible cerebrovascular vasoconstriction syndrome** — A cerebrovascular disorder associated with arterial dilation and constriction that is characterized by thunderclap headaches and sometime seizures.
Call-Fleming syndrome
Code first underlying condition, if applicable, such as eclampsia (O15.00-O15.9)

CC **I67.848** **Other cerebral vasospasm and vasoconstriction**

CC **I67.89** **Other cerebrovascular disease**

I67.9 **Cerebrovascular disease, unspecified**

I68- **Cerebrovascular disorders** **in diseases classified elsewhere**
I68.0 **Cerebral amyloid angiopathy** — [Not Allowed as PDX]
Code first underlying amyloidosis (E85.-)

CC **I68.2** **Cerebral arteritis in other diseases classified elsewhere** — [Not Allowed as PDX]
Code first underlying disease
Excludes 1: *cerebral arteritis (in):*
listerosis (A32.89)
systemic lupus erythematosus (M32.19)
syphilis (A52.04)
tuberculosis (A18.89)

I68.8 **Other cerebrovascular disorders in diseases classified elsewhere** — [Not Allowed as PDX]
Code first underlying disease
Excludes 1: *syphilitic cerebral aneurysm (A52.05)*

I69- **Sequelae** of cerebrovascular disease
AHA 12:4Q:p106 – Affected side not specified (dominant and nondominant)
Note: Category I69 is to be used to indicate conditions in I60-I67 as the cause of sequelae. The "sequelae" include conditions specified as such or as residuals which may occur at any time after the onset of the causal condition.
Excludes 1: *personal history of cerebral infarction without residual deficit (Z86.73)*
personal history of prolonged reversible ischemic neurologic deficit (PRIND) (Z86.73)
personal history of reversible ischemic neurologcial deficit (RIND) (Z86.73)
sequelae of traumatic intracranial injury (S06.-)
transient ischemic attack (TIA) (G45.9)

I69.0- **Sequelae** of nontraumatic **subarachnoid** hemorrhage
I69.00 **Unspecified** sequelae of nontraumatic **subarachnoid** hemorrhage
I69.01- **Cognitive** deficits following nontraumatic **subarachnoid** hemorrhage
I69.010 **Attention and concentration** deficit following nontraumatic subarachnoid hemorrhage
I69.011 **Memory** deficit following nontraumatic subarachnoid hemorrhage
I69.012 **Visuospatial deficit and spatial neglect** following nontraumatic subarachnoid hemorrhage
I69.013 **Psychomotor** deficit following nontraumatic subarachnoid hemorrhage
I69.014 **Frontal lobe and executive function** deficit following nontraumatic subarachnoid hemorrhage
I69.015 **Cognitive social or emotional** deficit following nontraumatic subarachnoid hemorrhage

I 6 6 - I 6 9

I69.018 Other symptoms and signs involving cognitive functions following nontraumatic subarachnoid hemorrhage

I69.019 Unspecified symptoms and signs involving cognitive functions following nontraumatic subarachnoid hemorrhage

I69.02- Speech and language deficits following nontraumatic subarachnoid hemorrhage

I69.020 Aphasia following nontraumatic subarachnoid hemorrhage

I69.021 Dysphasia following nontraumatic subarachnoid hemorrhage

I69.022 Dysarthria following nontraumatic subarachnoid hemorrhage

I69.023 Fluency disorder following nontraumatic subarachnoid hemorrhage
　Stuttering following nontraumatic subarachnoid hemorrhage

I69.028 Other speech and language deficits following nontraumatic subarachnoid hemorrhage

I69.03- Monoplegia of upper limb following nontraumatic subarachnoid hemorrhage

I69.031 Monoplegia of upper limb following nontraumatic subarachnoid hemorrhage affecting right dominant side

I69.032 Monoplegia of upper limb following nontraumatic subarachnoid hemorrhage affecting left dominant side

I69.033 Monoplegia of upper limb following nontraumatic subarachnoid hemorrhage affecting right non-dominant side

I69.034 Monoplegia of upper limb following nontraumatic subarachnoid hemorrhage affecting left non-dominant side

I69.039 Monoplegia of upper limb following nontraumatic subarachnoid hemorrhage affecting unspecified side

I69.04- Monoplegia of lower limb following nontraumatic subarachnoid hemorrhage

I69.041 Monoplegia of lower limb following nontraumatic subarachnoid hemorrhage affecting right dominant side

I69.042 Monoplegia of lower limb following nontraumatic subarachnoid hemorrhage affecting left dominant side

I69.043 Monoplegia of lower limb following nontraumatic subarachnoid hemorrhage affecting right non-dominant side

I69.044 Monoplegia of lower limb following nontraumatic subarachnoid hemorrhage affecting left non-dominant side

I69.049 Monoplegia of lower limb following nontraumatic subarachnoid hemorrhage affecting unspecified side

I69.05- Hemiplegia and hemiparesis following nontraumatic subarachnoid hemorrhage

CC I69.051 Hemiplegia and hemiparesis following nontraumatic subarachnoid hemorrhage affecting right dominant side

CC I69.052 Hemiplegia and hemiparesis following nontraumatic subarachnoid hemorrhage affecting left dominant side

CC I69.053 Hemiplegia and hemiparesis following nontraumatic subarachnoid hemorrhage affecting right non-dominant side

CC I69.054 Hemiplegia and hemiparesis following nontraumatic subarachnoid hemorrhage affecting left non-dominant side

CC I69.059 Hemiplegia and hemiparesis following nontraumatic subarachnoid hemorrhage affecting unspecified side

I69.06- Other paralytic syndrome following nontraumatic subarachnoid hemorrhage
Use additional code to identify type of paralytic syndrome, such as:
　Locked-in state (G83.5)
　Quadriplegia (G82.5-)
Excludes 1: hemiplegia/hemiparesis following nontraumatic subarachnoid hemorrhage (I69.05-)
　monoplegia of lower limb following nontraumatic subarachnoid hemorrhage (I69.04-)
　monoplegia of upper limb following nontraumatic subarachnoid hemorrhage (I69.03-)

I69.061 Other paralytic syndrome following nontraumatic subarachnoid hemorrhage affecting right dominant side

I69.062 Other paralytic syndrome following nontraumatic subarachnoid hemorrhage affecting left dominant side

I69.063 Other paralytic syndrome following nontraumatic subarachnoid hemorrhage affecting right non-dominant side

I69.064 Other paralytic syndrome following nontraumatic subarachnoid hemorrhage affecting left non-dominant side

I69.065 Other paralytic syndrome following nontraumatic subarachnoid hemorrhage, bilateral

I69.069 Other paralytic syndrome following nontraumatic subarachnoid hemorrhage affecting unspecified side

I69.09- Other sequelae of nontraumatic subarachnoid hemorrhage

I69.090 Apraxia following nontraumatic subarachnoid hemorrhage

I69.091 Dysphagia following nontraumatic subarachnoid hemorrhage
Use additional code to identify the type of dysphagia, if known (R13.1-)

I69.092 Facial weakness following nontraumatic subarachnoid hemorrhage
　Facial droop following nontraumatic subarachnoid hemorrhage

I69.093 Ataxia following nontraumatic subarachnoid hemorrhage

I69.098 Other sequelae following nontraumatic subarachnoid hemorrhage
　Alterations of sensation following nontraumatic subarachnoid hemorrhage
　Disturbance of vision following nontraumatic subarachnoid hemorrhage
Use additional code to identify the sequelae

I69.1- Sequelae of nontraumatic intracerebral hemorrhage

I69.10 Unspecified sequelae of nontraumatic intracerebral hemorrhage

I69.11- Cognitive deficits following nontraumatic intracerebral hemorrhage

I69.110 Attention and concentration deficit following nontraumatic intracerebral hemorrhage

I69.111 Memory deficit following nontraumatic intracerebral hemorrhage

I69.112 Visuospatial deficit and spatial neglect following nontraumatic intracerebral hemorrhage

I69.113 Psychomotor deficit following nontraumatic intracerebral hemorrhage

I69.114 Frontal lobe and executive function deficit following nontraumatic intracerebral hemorrhage

I69.115 Cognitive social or emotional deficit following nontraumatic intracerebral hemorrhage

I69.118 Other symptoms and signs involving cognitive functions following nontraumatic intracerebral hemorrhage

I69 - I69

I69.119 <u>Unspecified symptoms and signs</u> involving cognitive functions following nontraumatic <u>intracerebral</u> hemorrhage

I69.12- <u>Speech and language</u> deficits following nontraumatic <u>intracerebral</u> hemorrhage

I69.120 <u>Aphasia</u> following nontraumatic <u>intracerebral</u> hemorrhage

I69.121 <u>Dysphasia</u> following nontraumatic <u>intracerebral</u> hemorrhage

I69.122 <u>Dysarthria</u> following nontraumatic <u>intracerebral</u> hemorrhage

I69.123 <u>Fluency disorder</u> following nontraumatic <u>intracerebral</u> hemorrhage
Stuttering following nontraumatic intracerebral hemorrhage

I69.128 <u>Other speech and language</u> deficits following nontraumatic <u>intracerebral</u> hemorrhage

I69.13- <u>Monoplegia</u> of <u>upper limb</u> following nontraumatic <u>intracerebral</u> hemorrhage

I69.131 Monoplegia of upper limb following nontraumatic <u>intracerebral</u> hemorrhage affecting <u>right</u> dominant side

I69.132 Monoplegia of upper limb following nontraumatic <u>intracerebral</u> hemorrhage affecting <u>left</u> dominant side

I69.133 Monoplegia of upper limb following nontraumatic <u>intracerebral</u> hemorrhage affecting <u>right non-</u>dominant side

I69.134 Monoplegia of upper limb following nontraumatic <u>intracerebral</u> hemorrhage affecting <u>left non-</u>dominant side

I69.139 Monoplegia of upper limb following nontraumatic <u>intracerebral</u> hemorrhage affecting <u>unspecified</u> side

I69.14- <u>Monoplegia</u> of <u>lower limb</u> following nontraumatic <u>intracerebral</u> hemorrhage

I69.141 Monoplegia of lower limb following nontraumatic <u>intracerebral</u> hemorrhage affecting <u>right</u> dominant side

I69.142 Monoplegia of lower limb following nontraumatic <u>intracerebral</u> hemorrhage affecting <u>left</u> dominant side

I69.143 Monoplegia of lower limb following nontraumatic <u>intracerebral</u> hemorrhage affecting <u>right non-</u>dominant side

I69.144 Monoplegia of lower limb following nontraumatic <u>intracerebral</u> hemorrhage affecting <u>left non-</u>dominant side

I69.149 Monoplegia of lower limb following nontraumatic <u>intracerebral</u> hemorrhage affecting <u>unspecified</u> side

I69.15- <u>Hemiplegia and hemiparesis</u> following nontraumatic <u>intracerebral</u> hemorrhage

cc **I69.151** <u>Hemiplegia and hemiparesis</u> following nontraumatic <u>intracerebral</u> hemorrhage affecting <u>right</u> dominant side

cc **I69.152** <u>Hemiplegia and hemiparesis</u> following nontraumatic <u>intracerebral</u> hemorrhage affecting <u>left</u> dominant side

cc **I69.153** <u>Hemiplegia and hemiparesis</u> following nontraumatic <u>intracerebral</u> hemorrhage affecting <u>right non-</u>dominant side

cc **I69.154** <u>Hemiplegia and hemiparesis</u> following nontraumatic <u>intracerebral</u> hemorrhage affecting <u>left non-</u>dominant side

cc **I69.159** <u>Hemiplegia and hemiparesis</u> following nontraumatic <u>intracerebral</u> hemorrhage affecting <u>unspecified side</u>

I69.16- <u>Other paralytic</u> syndrome following nontraumatic <u>intracerebral</u> hemorrhage
Use additional code to identify type of paralytic syndrome, such as:
Locked-in state (G83.5)
Quadriplegia (G82.5-)
Excludes 1:   hemiplegia/hemiparesis following nontraumatic intracerebral hemorrhage (I69.15-)
monoplegia of lower limb following nontraumatic intracerebral hemorrhage (I69.14-)
monoplegia of upper limb following nontraumatic intracerebral hemorrhage (I69.13-)

I69.161 Other paralytic syndrome following nontraumatic <u>intracerebral</u> hemorrhage affecting <u>right</u> dominant side

I69.162 Other paralytic syndrome following nontraumatic <u>intracerebral</u> hemorrhage affecting <u>left</u> dominant side

I69.163 Other paralytic syndrome following nontraumatic <u>intracerebral</u> hemorrhage affecting <u>right non-</u>dominant side

I69.164 Other paralytic syndrome following nontraumatic <u>intracerebral</u> hemorrhage affecting <u>left non-</u>dominant side

I69.165 Other paralytic syndrome following nontraumatic <u>intracerebral</u> hemorrhage, <u>bilateral</u>

I69.169 Other paralytic syndrome following nontraumatic intracerebral hemorrhage affecting <u>unspecified side</u>

I69.19- <u>Other sequelae</u> of nontraumatic <u>intracerebral</u> hemorrhage

I69.190 <u>Apraxia</u> following nontraumatic <u>intracerebral</u> hemorrhage

I69.191 <u>Dysphagia</u> following nontraumatic <u>intracerebral</u> hemorrhage
Use additional code to identify the type of dysphagia, if known (R13.1-)

I69.192 <u>Facial weakness</u> following nontraumatic <u>intracerebral</u> hemorrhage
Facial droop following nontraumatic intracerebral hemorrhage

I69.193 <u>Ataxia</u> following nontraumatic <u>intracerebral</u> hemorrhage

I69.198 <u>Other sequelae</u> of nontraumatic <u>intracerebral</u> hemorrhage
Alteration of sensations following nontraumatic intracerebral hemorrhage
Disturbance of vision following nontraumatic intracerebral hemorrhage
Use additional code to identify the sequelae

I69.2- <u>Sequelae</u> of other nontraumatic <u>intracranial</u> hemorrhage

I69.20 <u>Unspecified</u> sequelae of other nontraumatic <u>intracranial</u> hemorrhage

I69.21- <u>Cognitive</u> deficits following other nontraumatic <u>intracranial</u> hemorrhage

I69.210 <u>Attention and concentration</u> deficit following other nontraumatic <u>intracranial</u> hemorrhage

I69.211 <u>Memory</u> deficit following other nontraumatic <u>intracranial</u> hemorrhage

I69.212 <u>Visuospatial deficit and spatial neglect</u> following other nontraumatic <u>intracranial</u> hemorrhage

I69.213 <u>Psychomotor</u> deficit following other nontraumatic <u>intracranial</u> hemorrhage

I69.214 <u>Frontal lobe and executive function</u> deficit following other nontraumatic <u>intracranial</u> hemorrhage

I69.215 <u>Cognitive social or emotional</u> deficit following other nontraumatic <u>intracranial</u> hemorrhage

I69.218 <u>Other symptoms and signs</u> involving cognitive functions following other nontraumatic <u>intracranial</u> hemorrhage

I69.219 **Unspecified symptoms and signs** involving cognitive functions following other nontraumatic <u>intracranial</u> hemorrhage

I69.22- **Speech and language** deficits following other nontraumatic <u>intracranial</u> hemorrhage

I69.220 **Aphasia** following other nontraumatic <u>intracranial</u> hemorrhage

I69.221 **Dysphasia** following other nontraumatic <u>intracranial</u> hemorrhage

I69.222 **Dysarthria** following other nontraumatic <u>intracranial</u> hemorrhage

I69.223 **Fluency disorder** following other nontraumatic <u>intracranial</u> hemorrhage
Stuttering following other nontraumatic intracranial hemorrhage

I69.228 **Other speech and language** deficits following other nontraumatic <u>intracranial</u> hemorrhage

I69.23- **Monoplegia** of <u>upper limb</u> following other nontraumatic <u>intracranial</u> hemorrhage

I69.231 Monoplegia of upper limb following other nontraumatic <u>intracranial</u> hemorrhage affecting <u>right</u> dominant side

I69.232 Monoplegia of upper limb following other nontraumatic <u>intracranial</u> hemorrhage affecting <u>left</u> dominant side

I69.233 Monoplegia of upper limb following other nontraumatic <u>intracranial</u> hemorrhage affecting <u>right</u> <u>non</u>-dominant side

I69.234 Monoplegia of upper limb following other nontraumatic <u>intracranial</u> hemorrhage affecting <u>left</u> <u>non</u>-dominant side

I69.239 Monoplegia of upper limb following other nontraumatic <u>intracranial</u> hemorrhage affecting <u>unspecified side</u>

I69.24- **Monoplegia** of <u>lower limb</u> following other nontraumatic <u>intracranial</u> hemorrhage

I69.241 Monoplegia of lower limb following other nontraumatic <u>intracranial</u> hemorrhage affecting <u>right</u> dominant side

I69.242 Monoplegia of lower limb following other nontraumatic <u>intracranial</u> hemorrhage affecting <u>left</u> dominant side

I69.243 Monoplegia of lower limb following other nontraumatic <u>intracranial</u> hemorrhage affecting <u>right</u> <u>non</u>-dominant side

I69.244 Monoplegia of lower limb following other nontraumatic <u>intracranial</u> hemorrhage affecting <u>left</u> <u>non</u>-dominant side

I69.249 Monoplegia of lower limb following other nontraumatic <u>intracranial</u> hemorrhage affecting <u>unspecified side</u>

I69.25- **Hemiplegia and hemiparesis** following other nontraumatic <u>intracranial</u> hemorrhage

cc **I69.251** **Hemiplegia and hemiparesis** following other nontraumatic <u>intracranial</u> hemorrhage affecting <u>right</u> dominant side

cc **I69.252** **Hemiplegia and hemiparesis** following other nontraumatic <u>intracranial</u> hemorrhage affecting <u>left</u> dominant side

cc **I69.253** **Hemiplegia and hemiparesis** following other nontraumatic <u>intracranial</u> hemorrhage affecting <u>right</u> <u>non</u>-dominant side

cc **I69.254** **Hemiplegia and hemiparesis** following other nontraumatic <u>intracranial</u> hemorrhage affecting <u>left</u> <u>non</u>-dominant side

cc **I69.259** **Hemiplegia and hemiparesis** following other nontraumatic <u>intracranial</u> hemorrhage affecting <u>unspecified side</u>

I69.26- **Other paralytic** syndrome following other nontraumatic <u>intracranial</u> hemorrhage
Use additional code to identify type of paralytic syndrome, such as:
   Locked-in state (G83.5)
   Quadriplegia (G82.5-)
   Excludes 1:   *hemiplegia/hemiparesis following other nontraumatic intracranial hemorrhage (I69.25-)*
       monoplegia of lower limb following other nontraumatic intracranial hemorrhage (I69.24-)
       monoplegia of upper limb following other nontraumatic intracranial hemorrhage (I69.23-)

I69.261 Other paralytic syndrome following other nontraumatic <u>intracranial</u> hemorrhage affecting <u>right</u> dominant side

I69.262 Other paralytic syndrome following other nontraumatic <u>intracranial</u> hemorrhage affecting <u>left</u> dominant side

I69.263 Other paralytic syndrome following other nontraumatic <u>intracranial</u> hemorrhage affecting <u>right</u> <u>non</u>-dominant side

I69.264 Other paralytic syndrome following other nontraumatic <u>intracranial</u> hemorrhage affecting <u>left</u> <u>non</u>-dominant side

I69.265 Other paralytic syndrome following other nontraumatic <u>intracranial</u> hemorrhage, <u>bilateral</u>

I69.269 Other paralytic syndrome following other nontraumatic <u>intracranial</u> hemorrhage affecting <u>unspecified side</u>

I69.29- **Other sequelae** of other nontraumatic <u>intracranial</u> hemorrhage

I69.290 **Apraxia** following other nontraumatic <u>intracranial</u> hemorrhage

I69.291 **Dysphagia** following other nontraumatic <u>intracranial</u> hemorrhage
Use additional code to identify the type of dysphagia, if known (R13.1-)

I69.292 **Facial weakness** following other nontraumatic <u>intracranial</u> hemorrhage
Facial droop following other nontraumatic intracranial hemorrhage

I69.293 **Ataxia** following other nontraumatic <u>intracranial</u> hemorrhage

I69.298 **Other sequelae** of other nontraumatic <u>intracranial</u> hemorrhage
Alteration of sensation following other nontraumatic intracranial hemorrhage
Disturbance of vision following other nontraumatic intracranial hemorrhage
Use additional code to identify the sequelae

I69.3- **Sequelae** of <u>cerebral infarction</u>
AHA 13:4Q:p127 – Admission to rehabilitation facility following an acute stroke
AHA 13:4Q:p128 – Residual aphasia and hemiplegia following acute cerebral infarction
AHA 15:1Q:p25 – Hemiplegia/hemiparesis of an old CVA
Sequelae of stroke NOS

I69.30 **Unspecified** sequelae of cerebral <u>infarction</u>

I69.31- **Cognitive** deficits following cerebral <u>infarction</u>

I69.310 **Attention and concentration** deficit following cerebral <u>infarction</u>

I69.311 **Memory** deficit following cerebral <u>infarction</u>

I69.312 **Visuospatial deficit and spatial neglect** following cerebral <u>infarction</u>

I69.313 **Psychomotor** deficit following cerebral <u>infarction</u>

I69.314 **Frontal lobe and executive function** deficit following cerebral <u>infarction</u>

I69.315 **Cognitive social or emotional** deficit following cerebral <u>infarction</u>

I 69 - I 69

I69.318 <u>Other symptoms and signs</u> involving cognitive functions following cerebral <u>infarction</u>

I69.319 <u>Unspecified symptoms and signs</u> involving cognitive functions following cerebral <u>infarction</u>

I69.32- <u>Speech and language</u> deficits following cerebral infarction

I69.320 <u>Aphasia</u> following cerebral <u>infarction</u>

I69.321 <u>Dysphasia</u> following cerebral <u>infarction</u>

I69.322 <u>Dysarthria</u> following cerebral <u>infarction</u>

I69.323 <u>Fluency disorder</u> following cerebral <u>infarction</u>
Stuttering following cerebral infarction

I69.328 <u>Other speech and language</u> deficits following cerebral <u>infarction</u>

I69.33- <u>Monoplegia</u> of <u>upper limb</u> following cerebral infarction

I69.331 Monoplegia of upper limb following cerebral <u>infarction</u> affecting <u>right</u> dominant side

I69.332 Monoplegia of upper limb following cerebral <u>infarction</u> affecting <u>left</u> dominant side

I69.333 Monoplegia of upper limb following cerebral <u>infarction</u> affecting <u>right</u> <u>non-dominant</u> side

I69.334 Monoplegia of upper limb following cerebral <u>infarction</u> affecting <u>left</u> <u>non-dominant</u> side

I69.339 Monoplegia of upper limb following cerebral <u>infarction</u> affecting <u>unspecified side</u>

I69.34- <u>Monoplegia</u> of <u>lower limb</u> following cerebral <u>infarction</u>

I69.341 Monoplegia of lower limb following cerebral <u>infarction</u> affecting <u>right</u> dominant side

I69.342 Monoplegia of lower limb following cerebral <u>infarction</u> affecting <u>left</u> dominant side

I69.343 Monoplegia of lower limb following cerebral <u>infarction</u> affecting <u>right</u> <u>non-dominant</u> side

I69.344 Monoplegia of lower limb following cerebral <u>infarction</u> affecting <u>left</u> <u>non-dominant</u> side

I69.349 Monoplegia of lower limb following cerebral <u>infarction</u> affecting <u>unspecified side</u>

I69.35- <u>Hemiplegia and hemiparesis</u> following cerebral <u>infarction</u>

cc **I69.351** <u>Hemiplegia and hemiparesis</u> following cerebral <u>infarction</u> affecting <u>right</u> dominant side

cc **I69.352** <u>Hemiplegia and hemiparesis</u> following cerebral <u>infarction</u> affecting <u>left</u> dominant side

cc **I69.353** <u>Hemiplegia and hemiparesis</u> following cerebral <u>infarction</u> affecting <u>right</u> <u>non-dominant</u> side

cc **I69.354** <u>Hemiplegia and hemiparesis</u> following cerebral <u>infarction</u> affecting <u>left</u> <u>non-dominant</u> side

cc **I69.359** <u>Hemiplegia and hemiparesis</u> following cerebral <u>infarction</u> affecting <u>unspecified side</u>

I69.36- <u>Other paralytic</u> syndrome following cerebral <u>infarction</u>
Use additional code to identify type of paralytic syndrome, such as:
Locked-in state (G83.5)
Quadriplegia (G82.5-)
Excludes 1: *hemiplegia/hemiparesis following cerebral infarction (I69.35-)*
monoplegia of lower limb following cerebral infarction (I69.34-)
monoplegia of upper limb following cerebral infarction (I69.33-)

I69.361 Other paralytic syndrome following cerebral <u>infarction</u> affecting <u>right</u> dominant side

I69.362 Other paralytic syndrome following cerebral <u>infarction</u> affecting <u>left</u> dominant side

I69.363 Other paralytic syndrome following cerebral <u>infarction</u> affecting <u>right</u> <u>non-dominant</u> side

I69.364 Other paralytic syndrome following cerebral <u>infarction</u> affecting <u>left</u> <u>non-dominant</u> side

I69.365 Other paralytic syndrome following cerebral <u>infarction</u>, <u>bilateral</u>

I69.369 Other paralytic syndrome following cerebral <u>infarction</u> affecting <u>unspecified side</u>

I69.39- <u>Other sequelae</u> of cerebral <u>infarction</u>

I69.390 <u>Apraxia</u> following cerebral <u>infarction</u>

I69.391 <u>Dysphagia</u> following cerebral <u>infarction</u>
Use additional code to identify the type of dysphagia, if known (R13.1-)

I69.392 <u>Facial weakness</u> following cerebral <u>infarction</u>
Facial droop following cerebral infarction

I69.393 <u>Ataxia</u> following cerebral <u>infarction</u>

I69.398 <u>Other sequelae</u> of cerebral <u>infarction</u>
Alteration of sensation following cerebral infarction
Disturbance of vision following cerebral infarction
Use additional code to identify the sequelae

I69.8- <u>Sequelae</u> of <u>other cerebrovascular diseases</u>
Excludes 1: *sequelae of traumatic intracranial injury (S06.-)*

I69.80 <u>Unspecified</u> sequelae of <u>other</u> cerebrovascular disease

I69.81- <u>Cognitive</u> deficits following <u>other</u> cerebrovascular disease

I69.810 <u>Attention and concentration</u> deficit following <u>other</u> cerebrovascular disease

I69.811 <u>Memory</u> deficit following <u>other</u> cerebrovascular disease

I69.812 <u>Visuospatial deficit and spatial neglect</u> following <u>other</u> cerebrovascular disease

I69.813 <u>Psychomotor</u> deficit following <u>other</u> cerebrovascular disease

I69.814 <u>Frontal lobe and executive function</u> deficit following <u>other</u> cerebrovascular disease

I69.815 <u>Cognitive social or emotional</u> deficit following <u>other</u> cerebrovascular disease

I69.818 <u>Other symptoms and signs</u> involving cognitive functions following <u>other</u> cerebrovascular disease

I69.819 <u>Unspecified symptoms and signs</u> involving cognitive functions following <u>other</u> cerebrovascular disease

I69.82- <u>Speech and language</u> deficits following <u>other</u> cerebrovascular disease

I69.820 <u>Aphasia</u> following <u>other</u> cerebrovascular disease

I69.821 <u>Dysphasia</u> following <u>other</u> cerebrovascular disease

I69.822 <u>Dysarthria</u> following <u>other</u> cerebrovascular disease

I69.823 <u>Fluency disorder</u> following <u>other</u> cerebrovascular disease
Stuttering following other cerebrovascular disease

I69.828 <u>Other speech and language</u> deficits following <u>other</u> cerebrovascular disease

I69.83- <u>Monoplegia</u> of <u>upper limb</u> following <u>other</u> cerebrovascular disease

I69.831 Monoplegia of upper limb following <u>other</u> cerebrovascular disease affecting <u>right</u> dominant side

I69.832 Monoplegia of upper limb following <u>other</u> cerebrovascular disease affecting <u>left</u> dominant side

I69.833 Monoplegia of upper limb following <u>other</u> cerebrovascular disease affecting <u>right</u> <u>non-dominant</u> side

I69.834 Monoplegia of upper limb following <u>other</u> cerebrovascular disease affecting <u>left</u> <u>non-dominant</u> side

I69.839 Monoplegia of upper limb following <u>other</u> cerebrovascular disease affecting <u>unspecified side</u>

I69.84- <u>Monoplegia</u> of <u>lower limb</u> following <u>other</u> cerebrovascular disease

I69.841 Monoplegia of lower limb following <u>other</u> cerebrovascular disease affecting <u>right</u> dominant side

I69.842 Monoplegia of lower limb following <u>other</u> cerebrovascular disease affecting <u>left</u> dominant side

I69.843 Monoplegia of lower limb following <u>other</u> cerebrovascular disease affecting <u>right</u> <u>non-dominant</u> side

I69 - I69

I69.844   Monoplegia of lower limb following other cerebrovascular disease affecting left non-dominant side

I69.849   Monoplegia of lower limb following other cerebrovascular disease affecting unspecified side

I69.85-   Hemiplegia and hemiparesis following other cerebrovascular disease

CC I69.851   Hemiplegia and hemiparesis following other cerebrovascular disease affecting right dominant side

CC I69.852   Hemiplegia and hemiparesis following other cerebrovascular disease affecting left dominant side

CC I69.853   Hemiplegia and hemiparesis following other cerebrovascular disease affecting right non-dominant side

CC I69.854   Hemiplegia and hemiparesis following other cerebrovascular disease affecting left non-dominant side

CC I69.859   Hemiplegia and hemiparesis following other cerebrovascular disease affecting unspecified side

I69.86-   Other paralytic syndrome following other cerebrovascular disease

Use additional code to identify type of paralytic syndrome, such as:
   Locked-in state (G83.5)
   Quadriplegia (G82.5-)
   Excludes 1:   hemiplegia/hemiparesis following other cerebrovascular disease (I69.85-)
      monoplegia of lower limb following other cerebrovascular disease (I69.84-)
      monoplegia of upper limb following other cerebrovascular disease (I69.83-)

I69.861   Other paralytic syndrome following other cerebrovascular disease affecting right dominant side

I69.862   Other paralytic syndrome following other cerebrovascular disease affecting left dominant side

I69.863   Other paralytic syndrome following other cerebrovascular disease affecting right non-dominant side

I69.864   Other paralytic syndrome following other cerebrovascular disease affecting left non-dominant side

I69.865   Other paralytic syndrome following other cerebrovascular disease, bilateral

I69.869   Other paralytic syndrome following other cerebrovascular disease affecting unspecified side

I69.89-   Other sequelae of other cerebrovascular disease

I69.890   Apraxia following other cerebrovascular disease

I69.891   Dysphagia following other cerebrovascular disease
Use additional code to identify the type of dysphagia, if known (R13.1-)

I69.892   Facial weakness following other cerebrovascular disease
      Facial droop following other cerebrovascular disease

I69.893   Ataxia following other cerebrovascular disease

I69.898   Other sequelae of other cerebrovascular disease
      Alteration of sensation following other cerebrovascular disease
      Disturbance of vision following other cerebrovascular disease
Use additional code to identify the sequelae

I69.9-   Sequelae of unspecified cerebrovascular diseases
   Excludes 1:   sequelae of stroke (I69.3)
      sequelae of traumatic intracranial injury (S06.-)

I69.90   Unspecified sequelae of unspecified cerebrovascular disease

I69.91-   Cognitive deficits following unspecified cerebrovascular disease

I69.910   Attention and concentration deficit following unspecified cerebrovascular disease

I69.911   Memory deficit following unspecified cerebrovascular disease

I69.912   Visuospatial deficit and spatial neglect following unspecified cerebrovascular disease

I69.913   Psychomotor deficit following unspecified cerebrovascular disease

I69.914   Frontal lobe and executive function deficit following unspecified cerebrovascular disease

I69.915   Cognitive social or emotional deficit following unspecified cerebrovascular disease

I69.918   Other symptoms and signs involving cognitive functions following unspecified cerebrovascular disease

I69.919   Unspecified symptoms and signs involving cognitive functions following unspecified cerebrovascular disease

I69.92-   Speech and language deficits following unspecified cerebrovascular disease

I69.920   Aphasia following unspecified cerebrovascular disease

I69.921   Dysphasia following unspecified cerebrovascular disease

I69.922   Dysarthria following unspecified cerebrovascular disease

I69.923   Fluency disorder following unspecified cerebrovascular disease
      Stuttering following unspecified cerebrovascular disease

I69.928   Other speech and language deficits following unspecified cerebrovascular disease

I69.93-   Monoplegia of upper limb following unspecified cerebrovascular disease

I69.931   Monoplegia of upper limb following unspecified cerebrovascular disease affecting right dominant side

I69.932   Monoplegia of upper limb following unspecified cerebrovascular disease affecting left dominant side

I69.933   Monoplegia of upper limb following unspecified cerebrovascular disease affecting right non-dominant side

I69.934   Monoplegia of upper limb following unspecified cerebrovascular disease affecting left non-dominant side

I69.939   Monoplegia of upper limb following unspecified cerebrovascular disease affecting unspecified side

I69.94-   Monoplegia of lower limb following unspecified cerebrovascular disease

I69.941   Monoplegia of lower limb following unspecified cerebrovascular disease affecting right dominant side

I69.942   Monoplegia of lower limb following unspecified cerebrovascular disease affecting left dominant side

I69.943   Monoplegia of lower limb following unspecified cerebrovascular disease affecting right non-dominant side

I69.944   Monoplegia of lower limb following unspecified cerebrovascular disease affecting left non-dominant side

I69.949   Monoplegia of lower limb following unspecified cerebrovascular disease affecting unspecified side

I69.95-   Hemiplegia and hemiparesis following unspecified cerebrovascular disease

CC I69.951   Hemiplegia and hemiparesis following unspecified cerebrovascular disease affecting right dominant side

CC I69.952   Hemiplegia and hemiparesis following unspecified cerebrovascular disease affecting left dominant side

I
6
9
-
I
6
9

CC **I69.953** **Hemiplegia and hemiparesis** following <u>unspecified</u> cerebrovascular disease affecting <u>right</u> <u>non-dominant</u> side

CC **I69.954** **Hemiplegia and hemiparesis** following <u>unspecified</u> cerebrovascular disease affecting <u>left</u> <u>non-dominant</u> side

CC **I69.959** **Hemiplegia and hemiparesis** following <u>unspecified</u> cerebrovascular disease affecting <u>unspecified side</u>

I69.96- <u>Other paralytic</u> syndrome following <u>unspecified</u> cerebrovascular disease
Use additional code to identify type of paralytic syndrome, such as:
  Locked-in state (G83.5)
  Quadriplegia (G82.5-)
Excludes 1: *hemiplegia/hemiparesis following unspecified cerebrovascular disease (I69.95-)*
  monoplegia of lower limb following unspecified cerebrovascular disease (I69.94-)
  monoplegia of upper limb following unspecified cerebrovascular disease (I69.93-)

I69.961 **Other paralytic syndrome following <u>unspecified</u> cerebrovascular disease affecting <u>right</u> dominant side**

I69.962 **Other paralytic syndrome following <u>unspecified</u> cerebrovascular disease affecting <u>left</u> dominant side**

I69.963 **Other paralytic syndrome following <u>unspecified</u> cerebrovascular disease affecting <u>right</u> <u>non-dominant</u> side**

I69.964 **Other paralytic syndrome following <u>unspecified</u> cerebrovascular disease affecting <u>left</u> <u>non-dominant</u> side**

I69.965 **Other paralytic syndrome following <u>unspecified</u> cerebrovascular disease, <u>bilateral</u>**

I69.969 **Other paralytic syndrome following <u>unspecified</u> cerebrovascular disease affecting <u>unspecified side</u>**

I69.99- <u>Other sequelae</u> of <u>unspecified</u> cerebrovascular disease

I69.990 **<u>Apraxia</u> following <u>unspecified</u> cerebrovascular disease**

I69.991 **<u>Dysphagia</u> following <u>unspecified</u> cerebrovascular disease**
Use additional code to identify the type of dysphagia, if known (R13.1-)

I69.992 **<u>Facial weakness</u> following <u>unspecified</u> cerebrovascular disease**
Facial droop following unspecified cerebrovascular disease

I69.993 **<u>Ataxia</u> following <u>unspecified</u> cerebrovascular disease**

I69.998 **<u>Other sequelae</u> following <u>unspecified</u> cerebrovascular disease**
Alteration in sensation following unspecified cerebrovascular disease
Disturbance of vision following unspecified cerebrovascular disease
Use additional code to identify the sequelae

Diseases of arteries, arterioles and capillaries (I70-I79)

I70- **Atherosclerosis** — Narrowing of an arterial wall caused by deposition of plaque-forming cholesterol and other lipids within the lumen.
Includes: **Arteriolosclerosis** — Thickening, hardening, and loss of elasticity of the arteriole walls.
  Arterial degeneration — Deterioration and decrease in normal function of an artery.
  Arteriosclerosis — Thickening, hardening, and loss of elasticity of the arterial walls which in its severe form may cause complete obliteration of the lumen of the artery.
  Arteriosclerotic vascular disease — Thickening, hardening, and loss of elasticity of the arterial vascular system.
  Arteriovascular degeneration — Deterioration and decrease in normal function of an artery.
  Atheroma — The plaque of degenerated, thickened arterial intima with deposits of cholesterol and lipid material.
  Endarteritis deformans or obliterans — Inflammation of the inner lining of an artery resulting from fatty degeneration, lime salt deposits, and with narrowed or obliterated lumen.
  Senile arteritis — Prolonged inflammation of an artery.
  Senile endarteritis — Prolonged inflammation of the innermost lining of an artery.
  Vascular degeneration — Deterioration and decrease in normal function of an artery.
Use additional code to identify:
  Exposure to environmental tobacco smoke (Z77.22)
  History of tobacco dependence (Z87.891)
  Occupational exposure to environmental tobacco smoke (Z57.31)
  Tobacco dependence (F17.-)
  Tobacco use (Z72.0)
Excludes ❷: *arteriosclerotic cardiovascular disease (I25.1-)*
  arteriosclerotic heart disease (I25.1-)
  atheroembolism (I75.-)
  cerebral atherosclerosis (I67.2)
  coronary atherosclerosis (I25.1-)
  mesenteric atherosclerosis (K55.1)
  precerebral atherosclerosis (I67.2)
  primary pulmonary atherosclerosis (I27.0)

I70.0 **Atherosclerosis of aorta** — [Age/15-124]

I70.1 **Atherosclerosis of renal artery** — [Age/15-124]
Goldblatt's kidney
Excludes ❷: *atherosclerosis of renal arterioles (I12.-)*

I70.2- **Atherosclerosis of <u>native arteries of the extremities</u>**
Mönckeberg's (medial) sclerosis
Use additional code, if applicable, to identify chronic total occlusion of artery of extremity (I70.92)
Excludes ❷: *atherosclerosis of bypass graft of extremities (I70.30-I70.79)*

I70.20- <u>Unspecified</u> atherosclerosis of <u>native</u> arteries of extremities

I70.201 **<u>Unspecified</u> atherosclerosis of <u>native</u> arteries of extremities, <u>right</u> leg** — [Age/15-124]

I70.202 **<u>Unspecified</u> atherosclerosis of <u>native</u> arteries of extremities, <u>left</u> leg** — [Age/15-124]

I70.203 **<u>Unspecified</u> atherosclerosis of <u>native</u> arteries of extremities, <u>bilateral legs</u>** — [Age/15-124]

I70.208 **<u>Unspecified</u> atherosclerosis of <u>native</u> arteries of extremities, <u>other extremity</u>** — [Age/15-124]

I70.209 **<u>Unspecified</u> atherosclerosis of <u>native</u> arteries of extremities, <u>unspecified extremity</u>** — [Age/15-124]

I70.21- **Atherosclerosis of <u>native</u> arteries of extremities <u>with intermittent claudication</u>**

I70.211 **Atherosclerosis of <u>native</u> arteries of extremities <u>with intermittent claudication</u>, <u>right</u> leg** — [Age/15-124]

I70.212 **Atherosclerosis of <u>native</u> arteries of extremities <u>with intermittent claudication</u>, <u>left</u> leg** — [Age/15-124]

I70.213 **Atherosclerosis of <u>native</u> arteries of extremities <u>with intermittent claudication</u>, <u>bilateral</u> legs** — [Age/15-124]

I70.218 **Atherosclerosis of <u>native</u> arteries of extremities <u>with intermittent claudication</u>, <u>other extremity</u>** — [Age/15-124]

I70.219 **Atherosclerosis of <u>native</u> arteries of extremities <u>with intermittent claudication</u>, <u>unspecified extremity</u>** — [Age/15-124]

I 69 - I 70

I70.22- **Atherosclerosis of <u>native</u> arteries of extremities <u>with rest pain</u>**
Includes: Any condition classifiable to I70.21-

    I70.221 **Atherosclerosis of <u>native</u> arteries of extremities <u>with rest pain</u>, <u>right</u> leg** — [Age/15-124]

    I70.222 **Atherosclerosis of <u>native</u> arteries of extremities <u>with rest pain</u>, <u>left</u> leg** — [Age/15-124]

    I70.223 **Atherosclerosis of <u>native</u> arteries of extremities <u>with rest pain</u>, <u>bilateral</u> legs** — [Age/15-124]

    I70.228 **Atherosclerosis of <u>native</u> arteries of extremities <u>with rest pain</u>, <u>other extremity</u>** — [Age/15-124]

    I70.229 **Atherosclerosis of native arteries of extremities <u>with rest pain</u>, <u>unspecified extremity</u>** — [Age/15-124]

I70.23- **Atherosclerosis of <u>native</u> arteries of <u>right</u> leg <u>with ulceration</u>**
Includes: Any condition classifiable to I70.211 and I70.221
Use additional code to identify severity of ulcer (L97.-)

    I70.231 **Atherosclerosis of <u>native</u> arteries of <u>right</u> leg <u>with ulceration</u> of <u>thigh</u>** — [Age/15-124]

    I70.232 **Atherosclerosis of <u>native</u> arteries of <u>right</u> leg <u>with ulceration</u> of <u>calf</u>** — [Age/15-124]

    I70.233 **Atherosclerosis of <u>native</u> arteries of <u>right</u> leg <u>with ulceration</u> of <u>ankle</u>** — [Age/15-124]

    I70.234 **Atherosclerosis of <u>native</u> arteries of <u>right</u> leg <u>with ulceration</u> of <u>heel and midfoot</u>** — [Age/15-124]
        Atherosclerosis of native arteries of right leg with ulceration of plantar surface of midfoot

    I70.235 **Atherosclerosis of <u>native</u> arteries of <u>right</u> leg <u>with ulceration</u> of <u>other part of foot</u>** — [Age/15-124]
        Atherosclerosis of native arteries of right leg extremities with ulceration of toe

    I70.238 **Atherosclerosis of <u>native</u> arteries of <u>right</u> leg <u>with ulceration</u> of other part of <u>lower right leg</u>** — [Age/15-124]

    I70.239 **Atherosclerosis of <u>native</u> arteries of <u>right</u> leg <u>with ulceration</u> of <u>unspecified site</u>** — [Age/15-124]

I70.24- **Atherosclerosis of <u>native</u> arteries of <u>left</u> leg <u>with ulceration</u>**
Includes: Any condition classifiable to I70.212 and I70.222
Use additional code to identify severity of ulcer (L97.-)

    I70.241 **Atherosclerosis of <u>native</u> arteries of <u>left</u> leg <u>with ulceration</u> of <u>thigh</u>** — [Age/15-124]

    I70.242 **Atherosclerosis of <u>native</u> arteries of <u>left</u> leg <u>with ulceration</u> of <u>calf</u>** — [Age/15-124]

    I70.243 **Atherosclerosis of <u>native</u> arteries of <u>left</u> leg <u>with ulceration</u> of <u>ankle</u>** — [Age/15-124]

    I70.244 **Atherosclerosis of <u>native</u> arteries of <u>left</u> leg <u>with ulceration</u> of <u>heel and midfoot</u>** — [Age/15-124]
        Atherosclerosis of native arteries of left leg with ulceration of plantar surface of midfoot

    I70.245 **Atherosclerosis of <u>native</u> arteries of <u>left</u> leg <u>with ulceration</u> of <u>other part of foot</u>** — [Age/15-124]
        Atherosclerosis of native arteries of left leg extremities with ulceration of toe

    I70.248 **Atherosclerosis of <u>native</u> arteries of <u>left</u> leg <u>with ulceration</u> of other part of <u>lower left leg</u>** — [Age/15-124]

    I70.249 **Atherosclerosis of <u>native</u> arteries of <u>left</u> leg <u>with ulceration</u> of <u>unspecified site</u>** — [Age/15-124]

I70.25 **Atherosclerosis of <u>native</u> arteries of <u>other extremities with ulceration</u>** — [Age/15-124]
Includes: Any condition classifiable to I70.218 and I70.228
Use additional code to identify the severity of the ulcer (L98.49-)

I70.26- **Atherosclerosis of <u>native</u> arteries of extremities <u>with gangrene</u>**
Includes: Any condition classifiable to I70.21-, I70.22-, I70.23-, I70.24-, and I70.25-
Use additional code to identify the severity of any ulcer (L97.-, L98.49-), if applicable

  cc I70.261 **Atherosclerosis of <u>native</u> arteries of extremities <u>with gangrene</u>, <u>right</u> leg** — [Age/15-124]

  cc I70.262 **Atherosclerosis of <u>native</u> arteries of extremities <u>with gangrene</u>, <u>left</u> leg** — [Age/15-124]

  cc I70.263 **Atherosclerosis of <u>native</u> arteries of extremities <u>with gangrene</u>, <u>bilateral</u> legs** — [Age/15-124]

  cc I70.268 **Atherosclerosis of <u>native</u> arteries of extremities <u>with gangrene</u>, <u>other extremity</u>** — [Age/15-124]

  cc I70.269 **Atherosclerosis of <u>native</u> arteries of extremities <u>with gangrene</u>, <u>unspecified extremity</u>** — [Age/15-124]

I70.29- **<u>Other</u> atherosclerosis of <u>native</u> arteries of extremities**

    I70.291 **<u>Other</u> atherosclerosis of <u>native</u> arteries of extremities, <u>right</u> leg** — [Age/15-124]

    I70.292 **<u>Other</u> atherosclerosis of <u>native</u> arteries of extremities, <u>left</u> leg** — [Age/15-124]

    I70.293 **<u>Other</u> atherosclerosis of <u>native</u> arteries of extremities, <u>bilateral</u> legs** — [Age/15-124]

    I70.298 **<u>Other</u> atherosclerosis of <u>native</u> arteries of extremities, <u>other extremity</u>** — [Age/15-124]

    I70.299 **<u>Other</u> atherosclerosis of <u>native</u> arteries of extremities, <u>unspecified extremity</u>** — [Age/15-124]

I70.3- **Atherosclerosis of <u>unspecified type of bypass graft(s)</u> of the extremities**
Use additional code, if applicable, to identify chronic total occlusion of artery of extremity (I70.92)
Excludes 1:   *embolism or thrombus of bypass graft(s) of extremities (T82.8-)*

I70.30- **<u>Unspecified</u> atherosclerosis of <u>unspecified type of bypass graft(s)</u> of the extremities**

    I70.301 **<u>Unspecified</u> atherosclerosis of unspecified type of bypass <u>graft(s)</u> of the extremities, <u>right</u> leg** — [Age/15-124]

    I70.302 **<u>Unspecified</u> atherosclerosis of unspecified type of bypass <u>graft(s)</u> of the extremities, <u>left</u> leg** — [Age/15-124]

    I70.303 **<u>Unspecified</u> atherosclerosis of unspecified type of bypass <u>graft(s)</u> of the extremities, <u>bilateral</u> legs** — [Age/15-124]

    I70.308 **<u>Unspecified</u> atherosclerosis of unspecified type of bypass <u>graft(s)</u> of the extremities, <u>other extremity</u>** — [Age/15-124]

    I70.309 **<u>Unspecified</u> atherosclerosis of unspecified type of bypass <u>graft(s)</u> of the extremities, <u>unspecified extremity</u>** — [Age/15-124]

I70.31- **Atherosclerosis of <u>unspecified type of bypass graft(s)</u> of the extremities <u>with intermittent claudication</u>**

    I70.311 **Atherosclerosis of unspecified type of bypass <u>graft(s)</u> of the extremities <u>with intermittent claudication</u>, <u>right</u> leg** — [Age/15-124]

    I70.312 **Atherosclerosis of unspecified type of bypass <u>graft(s)</u> of the extremities <u>with intermittent claudication</u>, <u>left</u> leg** — [Age/15-124]

    I70.313 **Atherosclerosis of unspecified type of bypass <u>graft(s)</u> of the extremities <u>with intermittent claudication</u>, <u>bilateral</u> legs** — [Age/15-124]

    I70.318 **Atherosclerosis of unspecified type of bypass graft(s) of the extremities <u>with intermittent claudication</u>, <u>other extremity</u>** — [Age/15-124]

    I70.319 **Atherosclerosis of unspecified type of bypass graft(s) of the extremities <u>with intermittent claudication</u>, <u>unspecified extremity</u>** — [Age/15-124]

I70.32- **Atherosclerosis of <u>unspecified type of bypass graft(s)</u> of the extremities <u>with rest pain</u>**
Includes: Any condition classifiable to I70.31-

    I70.321 **Atherosclerosis of unspecified type of bypass <u>graft(s)</u> of the extremities <u>with rest pain</u>, <u>right</u> leg** — [Age/15-124]

    I70.322 **Atherosclerosis of unspecified type of bypass <u>graft(s)</u> of the extremities <u>with rest pain</u>, <u>left</u> leg** — [Age/15-124]

I70 - I70

I70.323 Atherosclerosis of unspecified type of bypass graft(s) of the extremities with rest pain, bilateral legs — [Age/15-124]

I70.328 Atherosclerosis of unspecified type of bypass graft(s) of the extremities with rest pain, other extremity — [Age/15-124]

I70.329 Atherosclerosis of unspecified type of bypass graft(s) of the extremities with rest pain, unspecified extremity — [Age/15-124]

I70.33- Atherosclerosis of unspecified type of bypass graft(s) of the right leg with ulceration
Includes: Any condition classifiable to I70.311 and I70.321
Use additional code to identify severity of ulcer (L97.-)

cc I70.331 Atherosclerosis of unspecified type of bypass graft(s) of the right leg with ulceration of thigh — [Age/15-124]

cc I70.332 Atherosclerosis of unspecified type of bypass graft(s) of the right leg with ulceration of calf — [Age/15-124]

cc I70.333 Atherosclerosis of unspecified type of bypass graft(s) of the right leg with ulceration of ankle — [Age/15-124]

cc I70.334 Atherosclerosis of unspecified type of bypass graft(s) of the right leg with ulceration of heel and midfoot — [Age/15-124]
    Atherosclerosis of unspecified type of bypass graft(s) of right leg with ulceration of plantar surface of midfoot

I70.335 Atherosclerosis of unspecified type of bypass graft(s) of the right leg with ulceration of other part of foot — [Age/15-124]
    Atherosclerosis of unspecified type of bypass graft(s) of the right leg with ulceration of toe

cc I70.338 Atherosclerosis of unspecified type of bypass graft(s) of the right leg with ulceration of other part of lower leg — [Age/15-124]

cc I70.339 Atherosclerosis of unspecified type of bypass graft(s) of the right leg with ulceration of unspecified site — [Age/15-124]

I70.34- Atherosclerosis of unspecified type of bypass graft(s) of the left leg with ulceration
Includes: Any condition classifiable to I70.312 and I70.322
Use additional code to identify severity of ulcer (L97.-)

cc I70.341 Atherosclerosis of unspecified type of bypass graft(s) of the left leg with ulceration of thigh — [Age/15-124]

cc I70.342 Atherosclerosis of unspecified type of bypass graft(s) of the left leg with ulceration of calf — [Age/15-124]

cc I70.343 Atherosclerosis of unspecified type of bypass graft(s) of the left leg with ulceration of ankle — [Age/15-124]

cc I70.344 Atherosclerosis of unspecified type of bypass graft(s) of the left leg with ulceration of heel and midfoot — [Age/15-124]
    Atherosclerosis of unspecified type of bypass graft(s) of left leg with ulceration of plantar surface of midfoot

I70.345 Atherosclerosis of unspecified type of bypass graft(s) of the left leg with ulceration of other part of foot — [Age/15-124]
    Atherosclerosis of unspecified type of bypass graft(s) of the left leg with ulceration of toe

cc I70.348 Atherosclerosis of unspecified type of bypass graft(s) of the left leg with ulceration of other part of lower leg — [Age/15-124]

cc I70.349 Atherosclerosis of unspecified type of bypass graft(s) of the left leg with ulceration of unspecified site — [Age/15-124]

I70.35 Atherosclerosis of unspecified type of bypass graft(s) of other extremity with ulceration — [Age/15-124]
Includes: Any condition classifiable to I70.318 and I70.328
Use additional code to identify severity of ulcer (L98.49-)

I70.36- Atherosclerosis of unspecified type of bypass graft(s) of the extremities with gangrene
Includes: Any condition classifiable to I70.31-, I70.32-, I70.33-, I70.34-, I70.35
Use additional code to identify the severity of any ulcer (L97.-, L98.49-), if applicable

cc I70.361 Atherosclerosis of unspecified type of bypass graft(s) of the extremities with gangrene, right leg — [Age/15-124]

cc I70.362 Atherosclerosis of unspecified type of bypass graft(s) of the extremities with gangrene, left leg — [Age/15-124]

cc I70.363 Atherosclerosis of unspecified type of bypass graft(s) of the extremities with gangrene, bilateral legs — [Age/15-124]

cc I70.368 Atherosclerosis of unspecified type of bypass graft(s) of the extremities with gangrene, other extremity — [Age/15-124]

cc I70.369 Atherosclerosis of unspecified type of bypass graft(s) of the extremities with gangrene, unspecified extremity — [Age/15-124]

I70.39- Other atherosclerosis of unspecified type of bypass graft(s) of the extremities

I70.391 Other atherosclerosis of unspecified type of bypass graft(s) of the extremities, right leg — [Age/15-124]

I70.392 Other atherosclerosis of unspecified type of bypass graft(s) of the extremities, left leg — [Age/15-124]

I70.393 Other atherosclerosis of unspecified type of bypass graft(s) of the extremities, bilateral legs — [Age/15-124]

I70.398 Other atherosclerosis of unspecified type of bypass graft(s) of the extremities, other extremity — [Age/15-124]

I70.399 Other atherosclerosis of unspecified type of bypass graft(s) of the extremities, unspecified extremity — [Age/15-124]

I70.4- Atherosclerosis of autologous vein bypass graft(s) of the extremities
Use additional code, if applicable, to identify chronic total occlusion of artery of extremity (I70.92)

I70.40- Unspecified atherosclerosis of autologous vein bypass graft(s) of the extremities

I70.401 Unspecified atherosclerosis of autologous vein bypass graft(s) of the extremities, right leg — [Age/15-124]

I70.402 Unspecified atherosclerosis of autologous vein bypass graft(s) of the extremities, left leg — [Age/15-124]

I70.403 Unspecified atherosclerosis of autologous vein bypass graft(s) of the extremities, bilateral legs — [Age/15-124]

I70.408 Unspecified atherosclerosis of autologous vein bypass graft(s) of the extremities, other extremity — [Age/15-124]

I70.409 Unspecified atherosclerosis of autologous vein bypass graft(s) of the extremities, unspecified extremity — [Age/15-124]

I70.41- Atherosclerosis of autologous vein bypass graft(s) of the extremities with intermittent claudication

I70.411 Atherosclerosis of autologous vein bypass graft(s) of the extremities with intermittent claudication, right leg — [Age/15-124]

I70.412 Atherosclerosis of autologous vein bypass graft(s) of the extremities with intermittent claudication, left leg — [Age/15-124]

I70.413 Atherosclerosis of autologous vein bypass graft(s) of the extremities with intermittent claudication, bilateral legs — [Age/15-124]

I70.418 Atherosclerosis of autologous vein bypass graft(s) of the extremities with intermittent claudication, other extremity — [Age/15-124]

I70-I70

I70.419   Atherosclerosis of autologous <u>vein</u> bypass graft(s) of the extremities <u>with intermittent claudication</u>, <u>unspecified extremity</u> — [Age/15-124]

I70.42-   Atherosclerosis of autologous <u>vein</u> bypass graft(s) of the extremities <u>with rest pain</u>
Includes: Any condition classifiable to I70.41-

I70.421   Atherosclerosis of autologous vein bypass graft(s) of the extremities <u>with rest pain</u>, <u>right</u> leg — [Age/15-124]

I70.422   Atherosclerosis of autologous <u>vein</u> bypass graft(s) of the extremities <u>with rest pain</u>, <u>left</u> leg — [Age/15-124]

I70.423   Atherosclerosis of autologous vein bypass graft(s) of the extremities <u>with rest pain</u>, <u>bilateral</u> legs — [Age/15-124]

I70.428   Atherosclerosis of autologous <u>vein</u> bypass graft(s) of the extremities <u>with rest pain</u>, <u>other extremity</u> — [Age/15-124]

I70.429   Atherosclerosis of autologous <u>vein</u> bypass graft(s) of the extremities <u>with rest pain</u>, <u>unspecified extremity</u> — [Age/15-124]

I70.43-   Atherosclerosis of autologous vein bypass graft(s) of the <u>right</u> leg <u>with ulceration</u>
Includes: Any condition classifiable to I70.411 and I70.421
Use additional code to identify severity of ulcer (L97.-)

cc **I70.431**   Atherosclerosis of autologous <u>vein</u> bypass graft(s) of the <u>right</u> leg <u>with ulceration</u> of <u>thigh</u> — [Age/15-124]

cc **I70.432**   Atherosclerosis of autologous <u>vein</u> bypass graft(s) of the <u>right</u> leg <u>with ulceration</u> of <u>calf</u> — [Age/15-124]

cc **I70.433**   Atherosclerosis of autologous <u>vein</u> bypass graft(s) of the <u>right</u> leg <u>with ulceration</u> of <u>ankle</u> — [Age/15-124]

cc **I70.434**   Atherosclerosis of autologous vein bypass graft(s) of the <u>right</u> leg <u>with ulceration</u> of <u>heel and midfoot</u> — [Age/15-124]
Atherosclerosis of autologous vein bypass graft(s) of right leg with ulceration of plantar surface of midfoot

I70.435   Atherosclerosis of autologous <u>vein</u> bypass graft(s) of the <u>right</u> leg <u>with ulceration</u> of <u>other part of foot</u> — [Age/15-124]
Atherosclerosis of autologous vein bypass graft(s) of right leg with ulceration of toe

cc **I70.438**   Atherosclerosis of autologous <u>vein</u> bypass graft(s) of the <u>right</u> leg with ulceration of <u>other part of lower leg</u> — [Age/15-124]

cc **I70.439**   Atherosclerosis of autologous <u>vein</u> bypass graft(s) of the <u>right</u> leg <u>with ulceration</u> of <u>unspecified site</u> — [Age/15-124]

I70.44-   Atherosclerosis of autologous <u>vein</u> bypass graft(s) of the <u>left</u> leg <u>with ulceration</u>
Includes: Any condition classifiable to I70.412 and I70.422
Use additional code to identify severity of ulcer (L97.-)

cc **I70.441**   Atherosclerosis of autologous <u>vein</u> bypass graft(s) of the <u>left</u> leg <u>with ulceration</u> of <u>thigh</u> — [Age/15-124]

cc **I70.442**   Atherosclerosis of autologous <u>vein</u> bypass graft(s) of the <u>left</u> leg <u>with ulceration</u> of <u>calf</u> — [Age/15-124]

cc **I70.443**   Atherosclerosis of autologous <u>vein</u> bypass graft(s) of the <u>left</u> leg <u>with ulceration</u> of <u>ankle</u> — [Age/15-124]

cc **I70.444**   Atherosclerosis of autologous <u>vein</u> bypass graft(s) of the <u>left</u> leg <u>with ulceration</u> of <u>heel and midfoot</u> — [Age/15-124]
Atherosclerosis of autologous vein bypass graft(s) of left leg with ulceration of plantar surface of midfoot

I70.445   Atherosclerosis of autologous <u>vein</u> bypass graft(s) of the <u>left</u> leg <u>with ulceration</u> of <u>other part of foot</u> — [Age/15-124]
Atherosclerosis of autologous vein bypass graft(s) of left leg with ulceration of toe

cc **I70.448**   Atherosclerosis of autologous <u>vein</u> bypass graft(s) of the <u>left</u> leg <u>with ulceration</u> of <u>other part of lower leg</u> — [Age/15-124]

cc **I70.449**   Atherosclerosis of autologous <u>vein</u> bypass graft(s) of the <u>left</u> leg <u>with ulceration</u> of <u>unspecified site</u> — [Age/15-124]

I70.45   Atherosclerosis of autologous <u>vein</u> bypass graft(s) of <u>other extremity</u> <u>with ulceration</u> — [Age/15-124]
Includes: Any condition classifiable to I70.418, I70.428, and I70.438
Use additional code to identify severity of ulcer (L98.49)

I70.46-   Atherosclerosis of autologous <u>vein</u> bypass graft(s) of the extremities <u>with gangrene</u>
Includes: Any condition classifiable to I70.41-, I70.42-, and I70.43-, I70.44-, I70.45
Use additional code to identify the severity of any ulcer (L97.-, L98.49-), if applicable

cc **I70.461**   Atherosclerosis of autologous <u>vein</u> bypass graft(s) of the extremities <u>with gangrene</u>, <u>right</u> leg — [Age/15-124]

cc **I70.462**   Atherosclerosis of autologous <u>vein</u> bypass graft(s) of the extremities <u>with gangrene</u>, <u>left</u> leg — [Age/15-124]

cc **I70.463**   Atherosclerosis of autologous <u>vein</u> bypass graft(s) of the extremities <u>with gangrene</u>, <u>bilateral</u> legs — [Age/15-124]

cc **I70.468**   Atherosclerosis of autologous <u>vein</u> bypass graft(s) of the extremities <u>with gangrene</u>, <u>other extremity</u> — [Age/15-124]

cc **I70.469**   Atherosclerosis of autologous <u>vein</u> bypass graft(s) of the extremities <u>with gangrene</u>, <u>unspecified extremity</u> — [Age/15-124]

I70.49-   <u>Other</u> atherosclerosis of autologous <u>vein</u> bypass graft(s) of the extremities

I70.491   <u>Other</u> atherosclerosis of autologous <u>vein</u> bypass graft(s) of the extremities, <u>right</u> leg — [Age/15-124]

I70.492   <u>Other</u> atherosclerosis of autologous <u>vein</u> bypass graft(s) of the extremities, <u>left</u> leg — [Age/15-124]

I70.493   <u>Other</u> atherosclerosis of autologous <u>vein</u> bypass graft(s) of the extremities, bilateral legs — [Age/15-124]

I70.498   <u>Other</u> atherosclerosis of autologous <u>vein</u> bypass graft(s) of the extremities, other extremity — [Age/15-124]

I70.499   <u>Other</u> atherosclerosis of autologous <u>vein</u> bypass graft(s) of the extremities, unspecified extremity — [Age/15-124]

I70.5-   Atherosclerosis of nonautologous <u>biological</u> bypass graft(s) of the extremities
Use additional code, if applicable, to identify chronic total occlusion of artery of extremity (I70.92)

I70.50-   <u>Unspecified</u> atherosclerosis of nonautologous <u>biological</u> bypass graft(s) of the extremities

I70.501   <u>Unspecified</u> atherosclerosis of nonautologous <u>biological</u> bypass graft(s) of the extremities, <u>right</u> leg — [Age/15-124]

I70.502   <u>Unspecified</u> atherosclerosis of nonautologous <u>biological</u> bypass graft(s) of the extremities, <u>left</u> leg — [Age/15-124]

I70.503   <u>Unspecified</u> atherosclerosis of nonautologous <u>biological</u> bypass graft(s) of the extremities, <u>bilateral</u> legs — [Age/15-124]

I70.508   <u>Unspecified</u> atherosclerosis of nonautologous <u>biological</u> bypass graft(s) of the extremities, <u>other extremity</u> — [Age/15-124]

I70.509   <u>Unspecified</u> atherosclerosis of nonautologous <u>biological</u> bypass graft(s) of the extremities, <u>unspecified extremity</u> — [Age/15-124]

I70 - I70

I70.51- Atherosclerosis of nonautologous <u>biological</u> bypass graft(s) of the extremities <u>with intermittent claudication</u>

I70.511 Atherosclerosis of nonautologous <u>biological</u> bypass graft(s) of the extremities <u>with intermittent claudication, right</u> leg — [Age/15-124]

I70.512 Atherosclerosis of nonautologous <u>biological</u> bypass graft(s) of the extremities <u>with intermittent claudication, left</u> leg — [Age/15-124]

I70.513 Atherosclerosis of nonautologous <u>biological</u> bypass graft(s) of the extremities <u>with intermittent claudication, bilateral</u> legs — [Age/15-124]

I70.518 Atherosclerosis of nonautologous <u>biological</u> bypass graft(s) of the extremities <u>with intermittent claudication, other extremity</u> — [Age/15-124]

I70.519 Atherosclerosis of nonautologous <u>biological</u> bypass graft(s) of the extremities <u>with intermittent claudication, unspecified extremity</u> — [Age/15-124]

I70.52- Atherosclerosis of nonautologous <u>biological</u> bypass graft(s) of the extremities <u>with rest pain</u>
Includes: Any condition classifiable to I70.51-

I70.521 Atherosclerosis of nonautologous <u>biological</u> bypass graft(s) of the extremities <u>with rest pain, right</u> leg — [Age/15-124]

I70.522 Atherosclerosis of nonautologous <u>biological</u> bypass graft(s) of the extremities <u>with rest pain, left</u> leg — [Age/15-124]

I70.523 Atherosclerosis of nonautologous <u>biological</u> bypass graft(s) of the extremities <u>with rest pain, bilateral</u> legs — [Age/15-124]

I70.528 Atherosclerosis of nonautologous <u>biological</u> bypass graft(s) of the extremities <u>with rest pain, other extremity</u> — [Age/15-124]

I70.529 Atherosclerosis of nonautologous <u>biological</u> bypass graft(s) of the extremities <u>with rest pain, unspecified extremity</u> — [Age/15-124]

I70.53- Atherosclerosis of nonautologous <u>biological</u> bypass graft(s) of the <u>right leg with ulceration</u>
Includes: Any condition classifiable to I70.511 and I70.521
Use additional code to identify severity of ulcer (L97.-)

CC **I70.531** Atherosclerosis of nonautologous <u>biological</u> bypass graft(s) of the <u>right</u> leg <u>with ulceration</u> of <u>thigh</u> — [Age/15-124]

CC **I70.532** Atherosclerosis of nonautologous <u>biological</u> bypass graft(s) of the <u>right</u> leg <u>with ulceration</u> of <u>calf</u> — [Age/15-124]

CC **I70.533** Atherosclerosis of nonautologous <u>biological</u> bypass graft(s) of the <u>right</u> leg <u>with ulceration</u> of <u>ankle</u> — [Age/15-124]

CC **I70.534** Atherosclerosis of nonautologous <u>biological</u> bypass graft(s) of the <u>right</u> leg <u>with ulceration</u> of <u>heel and midfoot</u> — [Age/15-124]
Atherosclerosis of nonautologous biological bypass graft(s) of right leg with ulceration of plantar surface of midfoot

I70.535 Atherosclerosis of nonautologous <u>biological</u> bypass graft(s) of the <u>right</u> leg <u>with ulceration</u> of <u>other part of foot</u> — [Age/15-124]
Atherosclerosis of nonautologous biological bypass graft(s) of the right leg with ulceration of toe

CC **I70.538** Atherosclerosis of nonautologous <u>biological</u> bypass graft(s) of the <u>right</u> leg <u>with ulceration</u> of <u>other part of lower leg</u> — [Age/15-124]

CC **I70.539** Atherosclerosis of nonautologous <u>biological</u> bypass graft(s) of the <u>right</u> leg <u>with ulceration</u> of <u>unspecified site</u> — [Age/15-124]

I70.54- Atherosclerosis of nonautologous <u>biological</u> bypass graft(s) of the <u>left leg with ulceration</u>
Includes: Any condition classifiable to I70.512 and I70.522
Use additional code to identify severity of ulcer (L97.-)

CC **I70.541** Atherosclerosis of nonautologous <u>biological</u> bypass graft(s) of the <u>left</u> leg <u>with ulceration</u> of <u>thigh</u> — [Age/15-124]

CC **I70.542** Atherosclerosis of nonautologous <u>biological</u> bypass graft(s) of the <u>left</u> leg <u>with ulceration</u> of <u>calf</u> — [Age/15-124]

CC **I70.543** Atherosclerosis of nonautologous <u>biological</u> bypass graft(s) of the <u>left</u> leg <u>with ulceration</u> of <u>ankle</u> — [Age/15-124]

CC **I70.544** Atherosclerosis of nonautologous <u>biological</u> bypass graft(s) of the <u>left</u> leg <u>with ulceration</u> of <u>heel and midfoot</u> — [Age/15-124]
Atherosclerosis of nonautologous biological bypass graft(s) of left leg with ulceration of plantar surface of midfoot

I70.545 Atherosclerosis of nonautologous <u>biological</u> bypass graft(s) of the <u>left</u> leg <u>with ulceration</u> of <u>other part of foot</u> — [Age/15-124]
Atherosclerosis of nonautologous biological bypass graft(s) of the left leg with ulceration of toe

CC **I70.548** Atherosclerosis of nonautologous <u>biological</u> bypass graft(s) of the <u>left</u> leg <u>with ulceration</u> of <u>other part of lower leg</u> — [Age/15-124]

CC **I70.549** Atherosclerosis of nonautologous <u>biological</u> bypass graft(s) of the <u>left</u> leg <u>with ulceration</u> of <u>unspecified site</u> — [Age/15-124]

I70.55 Atherosclerosis of nonautologous <u>biological</u> bypass graft(s) of <u>other extremity with ulceration</u> — [Age/15-124]
Includes: Any condition classifiable to I70.518, I70.528, and I70.538
Use additional code to identify severity of ulcer (L98.49)

I70.56- Atherosclerosis of nonautologous <u>biological</u> bypass graft(s) of the extremities <u>with gangrene</u>
Includes: Any condition classifiable to I70.51-, I70.52-, and I70.53-, I70.54-, I70.55
Use additional code to identify the severity of any ulcer (L97.-, L98.49-), if applicable

CC **I70.561** Atherosclerosis of nonautologous <u>biological</u> bypass graft(s) of the extremities <u>with gangrene, right</u> leg — [Age/15-124]

CC **I70.562** Atherosclerosis of nonautologous <u>biological</u> bypass graft(s) of the extremities <u>with gangrene, left</u> leg — [Age/15-124]

CC **I70.563** Atherosclerosis of nonautologous <u>biological</u> bypass graft(s) of the extremities <u>with gangrene, bilateral</u> legs — [Age/15-124]

CC **I70.568** Atherosclerosis of nonautologous <u>biological</u> bypass graft(s) of the extremities <u>with gangrene, other extremity</u> — [Age/15-124]

CC **I70.569** Atherosclerosis of nonautologous <u>biological</u> bypass graft(s) of the extremities <u>with gangrene, unspecified extremity</u> — [Age/15-124]

I70.59- <u>Other</u> atherosclerosis of nonautologous <u>biological</u> bypass graft(s) of the extremities

I70.591 <u>Other</u> atherosclerosis of nonautologous <u>biological</u> bypass graft(s) of the extremities, <u>right</u> leg — [Age/15-124]

I70.592 <u>Other</u> atherosclerosis of nonautologous <u>biological</u> bypass graft(s) of the extremities, <u>left</u> leg — [Age/15-124]

I70.593 <u>Other</u> atherosclerosis of nonautologous <u>biological</u> bypass graft(s) of the extremities, <u>bilateral</u> legs — [Age/15-124]

I70.598 <u>Other</u> atherosclerosis of nonautologous <u>biological</u> bypass graft(s) of the extremities, <u>other</u> extremity — [Age/15-124]

I70.599 <u>Other</u> atherosclerosis of nonautologous <u>biological</u> bypass graft(s) of the extremities, <u>unspecified</u> extremity — [Age/15-124]

I70.6- Atherosclerosis of <u>nonbiological</u> bypass graft(s) of the extremities
> Use additional code, if applicable, to identify chronic total occlusion of artery of extremity (I70.92)

I70.60- <u>Unspecified</u> atherosclerosis of <u>nonbiological</u> bypass graft(s) of the extremities

I70.601 <u>Unspecified</u> atherosclerosis of <u>nonbiological</u> bypass graft(s) of the extremities, <u>right</u> leg — [Age/15-124]

I70.602 <u>Unspecified</u> atherosclerosis of <u>nonbiological</u> bypass graft(s) of the extremities, <u>left</u> leg — [Age/15-124]

I70.603 <u>Unspecified</u> atherosclerosis of <u>nonbiological</u> bypass graft(s) of the extremities, <u>bilateral</u> legs — [Age/15-124]

I70.608 <u>Unspecified</u> atherosclerosis of <u>nonbiological</u> bypass graft(s) of the extremities, <u>other</u> extremity — [Age/15-124]

I70.609 <u>Unspecified</u> atherosclerosis of <u>nonbiological</u> bypass graft(s) of the extremities, <u>unspecified</u> extremity — [Age/15-124]

I70.61- Atherosclerosis of <u>nonbiological</u> bypass graft(s) of the extremities <u>with intermittent claudication</u>

I70.611 Atherosclerosis of <u>nonbiological</u> bypass graft(s) of the extremities <u>with intermittent claudication</u>, <u>right</u> leg — [Age/15-124]

I70.612 Atherosclerosis of <u>nonbiological</u> bypass graft(s) of the extremities <u>with intermittent claudication</u>, <u>left</u> leg — [Age/15-124]

I70.613 Atherosclerosis of <u>nonbiological</u> bypass graft(s) of the extremities <u>with intermittent claudication</u>, <u>bilateral</u> legs — [Age/15-124]

I70.618 Atherosclerosis of <u>nonbiological</u> bypass graft(s) of the extremities <u>with intermittent claudication</u>, <u>other extremity</u> — [Age/15-124]

I70.619 Atherosclerosis of <u>nonbiological</u> bypass graft(s) of the extremities <u>with intermittent claudication</u>, <u>unspecified extremity</u> — [Age/15-124]

I70.62- Atherosclerosis of <u>nonbiological</u> bypass graft(s) of the extremities <u>with rest pain</u>
> Includes: Any condition classifiable to I70.61-

I70.621 Atherosclerosis of <u>nonbiological</u> bypass graft(s) of the extremities <u>with rest pain</u>, <u>right</u> leg — [Age/15-124]

I70.622 Atherosclerosis of <u>nonbiological</u> bypass graft(s) of the extremities <u>with rest pain</u>, <u>left</u> leg — [Age/15-124]

I70.623 Atherosclerosis of <u>nonbiological</u> bypass graft(s) of the extremities <u>with rest pain</u>, <u>bilateral</u> legs — [Age/15-124]

I70.628 Atherosclerosis of <u>nonbiological</u> bypass graft(s) of the extremities <u>with rest pain</u>, <u>other extremity</u> — [Age/15-124]

I70.629 Atherosclerosis of <u>nonbiological</u> bypass graft(s) of the extremities <u>with rest pain</u>, <u>unspecified extremity</u> — [Age/15-124]

I70.63- Atherosclerosis of <u>nonbiological</u> bypass graft(s) of the <u>right</u> leg <u>with ulceration</u>
> Includes: Any condition classifiable to I70.611 and I70.621
> Use additional code to identify severity of ulcer (L97.-)

cc I70.631 Atherosclerosis of <u>nonbiological</u> bypass graft(s) of the <u>right</u> leg <u>with ulceration</u> of <u>thigh</u> — [Age/15-124]

cc I70.632 Atherosclerosis of <u>nonbiological</u> bypass graft(s) of the <u>right</u> leg <u>with ulceration</u> of <u>calf</u> — [Age/15-124]

cc I70.633 Atherosclerosis of <u>nonbiological</u> bypass graft(s) of the <u>right</u> leg <u>with ulceration</u> of <u>ankle</u> — [Age/15-124]

cc I70.634 Atherosclerosis of <u>nonbiological</u> bypass graft(s) of the <u>right</u> leg <u>with ulceration</u> of <u>heel and midfoot</u> — [Age/15-124]
> Atherosclerosis of nonbiological bypass graft(s) of right leg with ulceration of plantar surface of midfoot

I70.635 Atherosclerosis of <u>nonbiological</u> bypass graft(s) of the <u>right</u> leg <u>with ulceration</u> of <u>other part of foot</u> — [Age/15-124]
> Atherosclerosis of nonbiological bypass graft(s) of the right leg with ulceration of toe

cc I70.638 Atherosclerosis of <u>nonbiological</u> bypass graft(s) of the <u>right</u> leg <u>with ulceration</u> of <u>other part of lower leg</u> — [Age/15-124]

cc I70.639 Atherosclerosis of <u>nonbiological</u> bypass graft(s) of the <u>right</u> leg <u>with ulceration</u> of <u>unspecified site</u> — [Age/15-124]

I70.64- Atherosclerosis of <u>nonbiological</u> bypass graft(s) of the <u>left</u> leg <u>with ulceration</u>
> Includes: Any condition classifiable to I70.612 and I70.622
> Use additional code to identify severity of ulcer (L97.-)

cc I70.641 Atherosclerosis of <u>nonbiological</u> bypass graft(s) of the <u>left</u> leg <u>with ulceration</u> of <u>thigh</u> — [Age/15-124]

cc I70.642 Atherosclerosis of <u>nonbiological</u> bypass graft(s) of the <u>left</u> leg <u>with ulceration</u> of <u>calf</u> — [Age/15-124]

cc I70.643 Atherosclerosis of <u>nonbiological</u> bypass graft(s) of the <u>left</u> leg <u>with ulceration</u> of <u>ankle</u> — [Age/15-124]

cc I70.644 Atherosclerosis of <u>nonbiological</u> bypass graft(s) of the <u>left</u> leg <u>with ulceration</u> of <u>heel and midfoot</u> — [Age/15-124]
> Atherosclerosis of nonbiological bypass graft(s) of left leg with ulceration of plantar surface of midfoot

I70.645 Atherosclerosis of <u>nonbiological</u> bypass graft(s) of the <u>left</u> leg <u>with ulceration</u> of <u>other part of foot</u> — [Age/15-124]
> Atherosclerosis of nonbiological bypass graft(s) of the left leg with ulceration of toe

cc I70.648 Atherosclerosis of <u>nonbiological</u> bypass graft(s) of the <u>left</u> leg <u>with ulceration</u> of <u>other part of lower leg</u> — [Age/15-124]

cc I70.649 Atherosclerosis of <u>nonbiological</u> bypass graft(s) of the <u>left</u> leg <u>with ulceration</u> of <u>unspecified site</u> — [Age/15-124]

I70.65 Atherosclerosis of <u>nonbiological</u> bypass graft(s) of <u>other extremity</u> <u>with ulceration</u> — [Age/15-124]
> Includes: Any condition classifiable to I70.618 and I70.628
> Use additional code to identify severity of ulcer (L98.49)

I70.66- Atherosclerosis of <u>nonbiological</u> bypass graft(s) of the extremities <u>with gangrene</u>
> Includes: Any condition classifiable to I70.61-, I70.62-, I70.63-, I70.64-, I70.65
> Use additional code to identify the severity of any ulcer (L97.-, L98.49-), if applicable

cc I70.661 Atherosclerosis of <u>nonbiological</u> bypass graft(s) of the extremities <u>with gangrene</u>, <u>right</u> leg — [Age/15-124]

cc I70.662 Atherosclerosis of <u>nonbiological</u> bypass graft(s) of the extremities <u>with gangrene</u>, <u>left</u> leg — [Age/15-124]

cc I70.663 Atherosclerosis of <u>nonbiological</u> bypass graft(s) of the extremities <u>with gangrene</u>, <u>bilateral</u> legs — [Age/15-124]

cc I70.668 Atherosclerosis of <u>nonbiological</u> bypass graft(s) of the extremities <u>with gangrene</u>, <u>other extremity</u> — [Age/15-124]

cc I70.669 Atherosclerosis of <u>nonbiological</u> bypass graft(s) of the extremities <u>with gangrene</u>, <u>unspecified extremity</u> — [Age/15-124]

I70.69- <u>Other</u> atherosclerosis of <u>nonbiological</u> bypass graft(s) of the extremities

I70.691 <u>Other</u> atherosclerosis of <u>nonbiological</u> bypass graft(s) of the extremities, <u>right</u> leg — [Age/15-124]

I70.692 <u>Other</u> atherosclerosis of <u>nonbiological</u> bypass graft(s) of the extremities, <u>left</u> leg — [Age/15-124]

I70.693 <u>Other</u> atherosclerosis of <u>nonbiological</u> bypass graft(s) of the extremities, <u>bilateral</u> legs — [Age/15-124]

I70 - I70

I70.698   <u>Other</u> atherosclerosis of <u>nonbiological</u> bypass graft(s) of the extremities, <u>other extremity</u> — [Age/15-124]

I70.699   <u>Other</u> atherosclerosis of <u>nonbiological</u> bypass graft(s) of the extremities, <u>unspecified extremity</u> — [Age/15-124]

I70.7- Atherosclerosis of <u>other</u> type of bypass graft(s) of the extremities
Use additional code, if applicable, to identify chronic total occlusion of artery of extremity (I70.92)

I70.70- <u>Unspecified</u> atherosclerosis of <u>other</u> type of bypass graft(s) of the extremities

I70.701   <u>Unspecified</u> atherosclerosis of <u>other</u> type of bypass graft(s) of the extremities, <u>right</u> leg — [Age/15-124]

I70.702   <u>Unspecified</u> atherosclerosis of <u>other</u> type of bypass graft(s) of the extremities, <u>left</u> leg — [Age/15-124]

I70.703   <u>Unspecified</u> atherosclerosis of <u>other</u> type of bypass graft(s) of the extremities, <u>bilateral</u> legs — [Age/15-124]

I70.708   <u>Unspecified</u> atherosclerosis of <u>other</u> type of bypass graft(s) of the extremities, <u>other extremity</u> — [Age/15-124]

I70.709   <u>Unspecified</u> atherosclerosis of <u>other</u> type of bypass graft(s) of the extremities, <u>unspecified extremity</u> — [Age/15-124]

I70.71- Atherosclerosis of <u>other</u> type of bypass graft(s) of the extremities <u>with intermittent claudication</u>

I70.711   Atherosclerosis of <u>other</u> type of bypass graft(s) of the extremities <u>with intermittent claudication</u>, <u>right</u> leg — [Age/15-124]

I70.712   Atherosclerosis of <u>other</u> type of bypass graft(s) of the extremities <u>with intermittent claudication</u>, <u>left</u> leg — [Age/15-124]

I70.713   Atherosclerosis of <u>other</u> type of bypass graft(s) of the extremities <u>with intermittent claudication</u>, <u>bilateral</u> legs — [Age/15-124]

I70.718   Atherosclerosis of <u>other</u> type of bypass graft(s) of the extremities <u>with intermittent claudication</u>, <u>other extremity</u> — [Age/15-124]

I70.719   Atherosclerosis of <u>other</u> type of bypass graft(s) of the extremities <u>with intermittent claudication</u>, <u>unspecified extremity</u> — [Age/15-124]

I70.72- Atherosclerosis of <u>other</u> type of bypass graft(s) of the extremities <u>with rest pain</u>
Includes: Any condition classifiable to I70.71-

I70.721   Atherosclerosis of <u>other</u> type of bypass graft(s) of the extremities <u>with rest pain</u>, <u>right</u> leg — [Age/15-124]

I70.722   Atherosclerosis of <u>other</u> type of bypass graft(s) of the extremities <u>with rest pain</u>, <u>left</u> leg — [Age/15-124]

I70.723   Atherosclerosis of <u>other</u> type of bypass graft(s) of the extremities <u>with rest pain</u>, <u>bilateral</u> legs — [Age/15-124]

I70.728   Atherosclerosis of <u>other</u> type of bypass graft(s) of the extremities <u>with rest pain</u>, <u>other extremity</u> — [Age/15-124]

I70.729   Atherosclerosis of <u>other</u> type of bypass graft(s) of the extremities <u>with rest pain</u>, <u>unspecified extremity</u> — [Age/15-124]

I70.73- Atherosclerosis of <u>other</u> type of bypass graft(s) of the <u>right</u> leg <u>with ulceration</u>
Includes: Any condition classifiable to I70.711 and I70.721
Use additional code to identify severity of ulcer (L97.-)

cc I70.731   Atherosclerosis of <u>other</u> type of bypass graft(s) of the <u>right</u> leg <u>with ulceration</u> of <u>thigh</u> — [Age/15-124]

cc I70.732   Atherosclerosis of <u>other</u> type of bypass graft(s) of the <u>right</u> leg <u>with ulceration</u> of <u>calf</u> — [Age/15-124]

cc I70.733   Atherosclerosis of <u>other</u> type of bypass graft(s) of the <u>right</u> leg <u>with ulceration</u> of <u>ankle</u> — [Age/15-124]

cc I70.734   Atherosclerosis of <u>other</u> type of bypass graft(s) of the <u>right</u> leg <u>with ulceration</u> of <u>heel and midfoot</u> — [Age/15-124]
Atherosclerosis of other type of bypass graft(s) of right leg with ulceration of plantar surface of midfoot

I70.735   Atherosclerosis of <u>other</u> type of bypass graft(s) of the <u>right</u> leg <u>with ulceration</u> of <u>other part of foot</u> — [Age/15-124]
Atherosclerosis of other type of bypass graft(s) of right leg with ulceration of toe

cc I70.738   Atherosclerosis of <u>other</u> type of bypass graft(s) of the <u>right</u> leg <u>with ulceration</u> of <u>other part of lower leg</u> — [Age/15-124]

cc I70.739   Atherosclerosis of <u>other</u> type of bypass graft(s) of the <u>right</u> leg <u>with ulceration</u> of <u>unspecified site</u> — [Age/15-124]

I70.74- Atherosclerosis of <u>other</u> type of bypass graft(s) of the <u>left</u> leg <u>with ulceration</u>
Includes: Any condition classifiable to I70.712 and I70.722
Use additional code to identify severity of ulcer (L97.-)

cc I70.741   Atherosclerosis of <u>other</u> type of bypass graft(s) of the <u>left</u> leg <u>with ulceration</u> of <u>thigh</u> — [Age/15-124]

cc I70.742   Atherosclerosis of <u>other</u> type of bypass graft(s) of the <u>left</u> leg <u>with ulceration</u> of <u>calf</u> — [Age/15-124]

cc I70.743   Atherosclerosis of <u>other</u> type of bypass graft(s) of the <u>left</u> leg <u>with ulceration</u> of <u>ankle</u> — [Age/15-124]

cc I70.744   Atherosclerosis of <u>other</u> type of bypass graft(s) of the <u>left</u> leg <u>with ulceration</u> of <u>heel and midfoot</u> — [Age/15-124]
Atherosclerosis of other type of bypass graft(s) of left leg with ulceration of plantar surface of midfoot

I70.745   Atherosclerosis of <u>other</u> type of bypass graft(s) of the <u>left</u> leg <u>with ulceration</u> of <u>other part of foot</u> — [Age/15-124]
Atherosclerosis of other type of bypass graft(s) of left leg with ulceration of toe

cc I70.748   Atherosclerosis of <u>other</u> type of bypass graft(s) of the <u>left</u> leg <u>with ulceration</u> of <u>other part of lower leg</u> — [Age/15-124]

cc I70.749   Atherosclerosis of <u>other</u> type of bypass graft(s) of the <u>left</u> leg <u>with ulceration</u> of <u>unspecified site</u> — [Age/15-124]

I70.75   Atherosclerosis of <u>other</u> type of bypass graft(s) <u>of other extremity with ulceration</u> — [Age/15-124]
Includes: Any condition classifiable to I70.718 and I70.728
Use additional code to identify severity of ulcer (L98.49)

I70.76- Atherosclerosis of <u>other</u> type of bypass graft(s) of the extremities <u>with gangrene</u>
Includes: Any condition classifiable to I70.71-, I70.72-, I70.73-, I70.74-, I70.75
Use additional code to identify the severity of any ulcer (L97.-, L98.49-), if applicable

cc I70.761   Atherosclerosis of <u>other</u> type of bypass graft(s) of the extremities <u>with gangrene</u>, <u>right</u> leg — [Age/15-124]

cc I70.762   Atherosclerosis of <u>other</u> type of bypass graft(s) of the extremities <u>with gangrene</u>, <u>left</u> leg — [Age/15-124]

cc I70.763   Atherosclerosis of <u>other</u> type of bypass graft(s) of the extremities <u>with gangrene</u>, <u>bilateral</u> legs — [Age/15-124]

cc I70.768   Atherosclerosis of <u>other</u> type of bypass graft(s) of the extremities <u>with gangrene</u>, <u>other extremity</u> — [Age/15-124]

cc I70.769   Atherosclerosis of <u>other</u> type of bypass graft(s) of the extremities <u>with gangrene</u>, <u>unspecified extremity</u> — [Age/15-124]

I70.79- <u>Other</u> atherosclerosis of <u>other</u> type of bypass graft(s) of the extremities

I70.791   <u>Other</u> atherosclerosis of <u>other</u> type of bypass graft(s) of the extremities, <u>right</u> leg — [Age/15-124]

I70.792   <u>Other</u> atherosclerosis of <u>other</u> type of bypass graft(s) of the extremities, <u>left</u> leg — [Age/15-124]

I70.793 **Other** atherosclerosis of **other type of bypass graft(s) of the extremities, bilateral legs** — [Age/15-124]

I70.798 **Other** atherosclerosis of **other type of bypass graft(s) of the extremities, other extremity** — [Age/15-124]

I70.799 **Other** atherosclerosis of **other type of bypass graft(s) of the extremities, unspecified extremity** — [Age/15-124]

I70.8 **Atherosclerosis of other arteries** — [Age/15-124]

I70.9- **Other and unspecified atherosclerosis**

I70.90 **Unspecified atherosclerosis** — [Age/15-124]

I70.91 **Generalized atherosclerosis** — [Age/15-124]

cc **I70.92** **Chronic total occlusion of artery of the extremities** — [Age/15-124] [Unacceptable PDX]
Complete occlusion of artery of the extremities
Total occlusion of artery of the extremities
Code first atherosclerosis of arteries of the extremities (I70.2-, I70.3-, I70.4-, I70.5-, I70.6-, I70.7-)

I71- **Aortic aneurysm and dissection** — AORTIC ANEURYSM – A sac formed by the dilatation of the aortic wall. AORTIC DISSECTION – A longitudinal splitting of the aortic arterial wall.

Excludes 1: *aortic ectasia (I77.81-)*
syphilitic aortic aneurysm (A52.01)
traumatic aortic aneurysm (S25.09, S35.09)

Dilatation of Arterial Wall

ARTERIAL ANEURYSM

Dissected Aortic Wall

DISSECTING AORTIC ANEURYSM

I71.0- **Dissection of aorta** — A longitudinal splitting of the aortic arterial wall.

MCC **I71.00** **Dissection of unspecified site of aorta**

MCC **I71.01** **Dissection of thoracic aorta**

MCC **I71.02** **Dissection of abdominal aorta**

MCC **I71.03** **Dissection of thoracoabdominal aorta**

MCC **I71.1** **Thoracic aortic aneurysm, ruptured** — A form in the thoracic aorta in which the wall ruptures and results in a massive hemorrhage.

I71.2 **Thoracic aortic aneurysm, without rupture**

MCC **I71.3** **Abdominal aortic aneurysm, ruptured** — A form in the abdominal aorta in which the wall ruptures, resulting in massive hemorrhage.

I71.4 **Abdominal aortic aneurysm, without rupture**

MCC **I71.5** **Thoracoabdominal aortic aneurysm, ruptured** — A form in the thoracic and abdominal aorta in which the wall ruptures, resulting in massive hemorrhage.

I71.6 **Thoracoabdominal aortic aneurysm, without rupture**

MCC **I71.8** **Aortic aneurysm of unspecified site, ruptured**
Rupture of aorta NOS

I71.9 **Aortic aneurysm of unspecified site, without rupture**
Aneurysm of aorta
Dilatation of aorta
Hyaline necrosis of aorta

I72- **Other aneurysm** — A sac formed by the dilatation of an arterial wall.
Includes: **Aneurysm (cirsoid) (false) (ruptured)** — CIRSOID – A form in which the blood vessels become dilated, lengthened, and tortuous. FALSE – A form in which the entire wall is injured and the blood is contained by the surrounding tissues, with eventual formation of a sac communicating with the artery. RUPTURED – A form in which the arterial wall ruptures resulting in massive hemorrhage.

Excludes ❷: *acquired aneurysm (I77.0)*
aneurysm (of) aorta (I71-)
aneurysm (of) arteriovenous NOS (Q27.3-)
carotid artery dissection (I77.71)
cerebral (nonruptured) aneurysm (I67.1)
coronary aneurysm (I25.4)
coronary artery dissection (I25.42)
dissection of artery NEC (I77.79)
dissection of precerebral artery, congenital (nonruptured) (Q28.1)
heart aneurysm (I25.3)
iliac artery dissection (I77.72)
pulmonary artery aneurysm (I28.1)
renal artery dissection (I77.73)
retinal aneurysm (H35.0)
ruptured cerebral aneurysm (I60.7)
varicose aneurysm (I77.0)
vertebral artery dissection (I77.74)

I72.0 **Aneurysm of carotid artery** — A form affecting the carotid arteries which supply blood to the brain and head.
Aneurysm of common carotid artery
Aneurysm of external carotid artery
Aneurysm of internal carotid artery, extracranial portion
Excludes 1: *aneurysm of internal carotid artery, intracranial portion (I67.1)*
aneurysm of internal carotid artery NOS (I67.1)

I72.1 **Aneurysm of artery of upper extremity**

I72.2 **Aneurysm of renal artery**

I72.3 **Aneurysm of iliac artery**

I72.4 **Aneurysm of artery of lower extremity**

I72.5 **Aneurysm of other precerebral arteries**
Aneurysm of basilar artery (trunk)
Excludes ❷: *aneurysm of carotid artery (I72.0)*
aneurysm of vertebral artery (I72.6)
dissection of carotid artery (I77.71)
dissection of other precerebral arteries (I77.75)
dissection of vertebral artery (I77.74)

I72.6 **Aneurysm of vertebral artery**
Excludes ❷: *dissection of vertebral artery (I77.74)*

I72.8 **Aneurysm of other specified arteries**

I72.9 **Aneurysm of unspecified site**

I73- **Other peripheral vascular diseases**
Excludes ❷: *chilblains (T69.1)*
frostbite (T33-T34)
immersion hand or foot (T69.0-)
spasm of cerebral artery (G45.9)

I73.0- **Raynaud's syndrome** — Paroxysmal digital cyanosis of an undetermined primary cause.
Raynaud's disease
Raynaud's phenomenon (secondary) — Paroxysmal digital cyanosis followed by redness of the skin of the digits which is precipitated by cold or emotional upset, and may be due to a number of regional or systemic disorders.

I73.00 **Raynaud's syndrome without gangrene**

cc **I73.01** **Raynaud's syndrome with gangrene** — A form with the death of tissue.

I73.1 **Thromboangiitis obliterans [Buerger's disease]** — Inflammatory occlusions of the more distal arteries, resulting in circulatory insufficiency of the toes and fingers, and thrombosis of superficial veins and is most commonly seen in young men who smoke.

I73.8- **Other specified peripheral vascular diseases**
Excludes 1: *diabetic (peripheral) angiopathy (E08-E13 with .51-.52)*
I73.81 **Erythromelalgia** — A rare condition of paroxysmal vasodilation with intense burning pain (most frequently in the extremities), severe redness, and increased temperature.

I70 - I73

I73.89 **Other specified peripheral vascular diseases**
    Acrocyanosis — Arteriolar vasoconstriction combined with dilatation of the subpapillary venous plexus of the skin resulting in symmetric coldness and cyanotic discoloration of the skin of the hands and feet.
    Erythrocyanosis — Bluish-red discoloration on the legs and thighs associated with cyanosis.
    Simple acroparesthesia [Schultze's type] — Tingling, numbness, and stiffness of the extremities of the simple form which tends to end in acrocyanosis.
    Vasomotor acroparesthesia [Nothnagel's type] — Tingling, numbness, and stiffness in the extremities of the vasomotor or angiospastic form.

I73.9 **Peripheral vascular disease, unspecified**
    Intermittent claudication — Pain, tension, and weakness while walking until it becomes impossible to continue.
    Peripheral angiopathy NOS
    Spasm of artery — A sudden, involuntary contraction of an arterial wall.
    Excludes 1:   *atherosclerosis of the extremities (I70.2- – I70.7-)*

I74- **Arterial <u>embolism and thrombosis</u>** — EMBOLISM — A blood clot or other substance blocking an artery. THROMBOSIS — An abnormal aggregation of blood factors causing an arterial obstruction.
    Includes: **Embolic infarction** — A localized necrosis of tissue resulting from an arterial embolism.
        Embolic occlusion — Blockage of an artery by an embolus.
        Thrombotic infarction — A localized necrosis of tissue resulting from a thrombotic occlusion.
        Thrombotic occlusion — Blockage of an artery by a thrombosis.
    Code first embolism and thrombosis complicating abortion or ectopic or molar pregnancy (O00-O07, O08.2)
    Code first embolism and thrombosis complicating pregnancy, childbirth and the puerperium (O88.-)
    Excludes ❷: *atheroembolism (I75.-)*
        basilar embolism and thrombosis (I63.0-I63.2, I65.1)
        carotid embolism and thrombosis (I63.0-I63.2, I65.2)
        cerebral embolism and thrombosis (I63.3-I63.5, I66.-)
        coronary embolism and thrombosis (I21-I25)
        mesenteric embolism and thrombosis (K55.0-)
        ophthalmic embolism and thrombosis (H34-)
        precerebral embolism and thrombosis NOS (I63.0-I63.2, I65.9)
        pulmonary embolism and thrombosis (I26-)
        renal embolism and thrombosis (N28.0)
        retinal embolism and thrombosis (H34-)
        septic embolism and thrombosis (I76)
        vertebral embolism and thrombosis (I63.0-I63.2, I65.0)

I74.0- **Embolism and thrombosis of <u>abdominal aorta</u>**
MCC I74.01 **<u>Saddle</u> embolism abdominal aorta** — A form characterized by a large embolism that straddles the bifurcation of the abdominal aorta.

CC I74.09 **Other arterial embolism and thrombosis of abdominal aorta**
    Aortic bifurcation syndrome
    Aortoiliac obstruction — A form affecting the abdominal aorta and the iliac arteries.
    Leriche's syndrome — A syndrome caused by obstruction of the terminal aorta characterized by muscle fatigue in the legs, absence of pulsation in the femoral arteries, and coldness of the lower extremities.

I74.1- **Embolism and thrombosis of other and unspecified parts of aorta**
CC I74.10 **Embolism and thrombosis of unspecified parts of aorta**
CC I74.11 **Embolism and thrombosis of <u>thoracic</u> aorta**
CC I74.19 **Embolism and thrombosis of other parts of aorta**
CC I74.2 **Embolism and thrombosis of arteries of the <u>upper</u> extremities**
CC I74.3 **Embolism and thrombosis of arteries of the <u>lower</u> extremities**
CC I74.4 **Embolism and thrombosis of arteries of extremities, unspecified**
    Peripheral arterial embolism NOS
CC I74.5 **Embolism and thrombosis of <u>iliac</u> artery**
CC I74.8 **Embolism and thrombosis of other arteries**
CC I74.9 **Embolism and thrombosis of unspecified artery**

I75- **<u>Atheroembolism</u>** — The blockage of a terminal artery caused by the lodging of atheromatous (fatty) plaque debris in a terminal artery branch.
    Includes: **Atherothrombotic microembolism**
        Cholesterol embolism

I75.0- **Atheroembolism of <u>extremities</u>**
I75.01- **Atheroembolism of <u>upper</u> extremity**
CC I75.011 **Atheroembolism of <u>right</u> upper extremity**
CC I75.012 **Atheroembolism of <u>left</u> upper extremity**

CC I75.013 **Atheroembolism of <u>bilateral</u> upper extremities**
CC I75.019 **Atheroembolism of <u>unspecified</u> upper extremity**
I75.02- **Atheroembolism of <u>lower</u> extremity**
CC I75.021 **Atheroembolism of <u>right</u> lower extremity**
CC I75.022 **Atheroembolism of <u>left</u> lower extremity**
CC I75.023 **Atheroembolism of <u>bilateral</u> lower extremities**
CC I75.029 **Atheroembolism of <u>unspecified</u> lower extremity**
I75.8- **Atheroembolism of other sites**
CC I75.81 **Atheroembolism of <u>kidney</u>**
    Use additional code for any associated acute kidney failure and chronic kidney disease (N17.-, N18.-)
CC I75.89 **Atheroembolism of <u>other site</u>**

I76 **<u>Septic</u> arterial embolism** — [Unacceptable PDX] — A localized collection of pus and bacteria that often originates in the heart or lungs and then travels through the systemic arterial system where it lodges in small vessels throughout the body, often in the brain, retina, and digits.
CC
    Code first underlying infection, such as:
      Infective endocarditis (I33.0)
      Lung abscess (J85.-)
    Use additional code to identify the site of the embolism (I74.-)
    Excludes ❷: *septic pulmonary embolism (I26.01, I26.90)*

I77- **Other disorders of arteries and arterioles**
    Excludes ❷: *collagen (vascular) diseases (M30-M36)*
        hypersensitivity angiitis (M31.0)
        pulmonary artery (I28.-)

I77.0 **Arteriovenous fistula, acquired** — An abnormal communication between an artery and a vein.
    Aneurysmal varix
    Arteriovenous aneurysm, acquired
    Excludes 1:   *arteriovenous aneurysm NOS (Q27.3-)*
        presence of arteriovenous shunt (fistula) for dialysis (Z99.2)
        traumatic — see injury of blood vessel by body region
    Excludes ❷: *cerebral (I67.1)*
        coronary (I25.4)

I77.1 **Stricture of artery** — Decrease in caliber of an artery.
    Narrowing of artery

CC I77.2 **Rupture of artery** — A forcible tearing of the arterial wall.
    Erosion of artery — A wasting-away of the arterial wall.
    Fistula of artery — An abnormal communication of an artery with another organ or tissue area.
    Ulcer of artery — An eating-away of the arterial wall.
    Excludes 1:   *traumatic rupture of artery — see injury of blood vessel by body region*

I77.3 **Arterial fibromuscular dysplasia** — The abnormal multiplication or increase in the number of normal cells and the normal arrangement of the fibromuscular layers of an artery.
    Fibromuscular hyperplasia (of) carotid artery
    Fibromuscular hyperplasia (of) renal artery
CC I77.4 **Celiac artery compression syndrome** — Recurrent abdominal pain caused by the compression of the celiac artery by the median arcuate ligament of the diaphragm.

CC I77.5 **Necrosis of artery** — Death of the arterial wall tissue.

I77.6 **Arteritis, unspecified**
    Aortitis NOS
    Endarteritis NOS
    Excludes 1:   *arteritis or endarteritis:*
        aortic arch (M31.4)
        cerebral NEC (I67.7)
        coronary (I25.89)
        deformans (I70.-)
        giant cell (M31.5., M31.6)
        obliterans (I70.-)
        senile (I70.-)

I77.7- **Other arterial dissection** — The splitting of an arterial wall that allows blood to flow within the wall layers.
    Excludes ❷: *dissection of aorta (I71.0-)*
        dissection of coronary artery (I25.42)

MCC I77.70 **Dissection of unspecified artery**
MCC I77.71 **Dissection of carotid artery**
MCC I77.72 **Dissection of iliac artery**
MCC I77.73 **Dissection of renal artery**
MCC I77.74 **Dissection of vertebral artery**
    Excludes ❷: *aneurysm of vertebral artery (I72.6)*

Excludes 1: = NOT CODED HERE! (Do not code both)   **750**   *Excludes ❷:* = Not Included Here

I73 - I77

MCC **I77.75 Dissection of other precerebral arteries**
Dissection of basilar artery (trunk)
Excludes ❷: *aneurysm of carotid artery (I72.0)*
aneurysm of other precerebral arteries (I72.5)
aneurysm of vertebral artery (I72.6)
dissection of carotid artery (I77.71)
dissection of vertebral artery (I77.74)

MCC **I77.76 Dissection of artery of upper extremity**

MCC **I77.77 Dissection of artery of lower extremitiy**

MCC **I77.79 Dissection of other specified artery**

I77.8- Other specified disorders of arteries and arterioles

I77.81- Aortic ectasia — The abnormal widening of the aortic wall that is not diagnostic of an aneurysm.
Ectasis aorta
Excludes 1:   *aortic aneurysm and dissection (I71.0-)*

I77.810 Thoracic aortic ectasia

I77.811 Abdominal aortic ectasia

I77.812 Thoracoabdominal aortic ectasia

I77.819 Aortic ectasia, unspecified site

I77.89 Other specified disorders of arteries and arterioles

I77.9 Disorder of arteries and arterioles, unspecified

I78- Diseases of capillaries

I78.0 Hereditary hemorrhagic telangiectasia — A hereditary disorder characterized by multiple telangiectatic lesions on the face, mouth, nose, and hand in association with epistaxis or gastrointestinal bleeding.
Rendu-Osler-Weber disease

I78.1 Nevus, non-neoplastic — Hypertrophy of the skin capillaries characterized by a reddish swelling or patch on the skin.
Araneus nevus
Senile nevus
Spider nevus
Stellar nevus
Excludes 1:   *nevus NOS (D22.-)*
vascular NOS (Q82.5)
Excludes ❷: *blue nevus (D22.-)*
flammeus nevus (Q82.5)
hairy nevus (D22.-)
melanocytic nevus (D22.-)
pigmented nevus (D22.-)
portwine nevus (Q82.5)
sanguineous nevus (Q82.5)
strawberry nevus (Q82.5)
verrucous nevus (Q82.5)

I78.8 Other diseases of capillaries

I78.9 Disease of capillaries, unspecified

I79- Disorders of arteries, arterioles and capillaries in diseases classified elsewhere

I79.0 Aneurysm of aorta in diseases classified elsewhere — [Not Allowed as PDX]
Code first underlying disease
Excludes 1:   *syphilitic aneurysm (A52.01)*

I79.1 Aortitis in diseases classified elsewhere — [Not Allowed as PDX]
Code first underlying disease
Excludes 1:   *syphilitic aortitis (A52.02)*

I79.8 Other disorders of arteries, arterioles and capillaries in diseases classified elsewhere — [Not Allowed as PDX]
Code first underlying disease, such as:
Amyloidosis (E85.-)
Excludes 1:   *diabetic (peripheral) angiopathy (E08-E13 with .51-.52)*
syphilitic endarteritis (A52.09)
tuberculous endarteritis (A18.89)

Diseases of veins, lymphatic vessels and lymph nodes, not elsewhere classified (I80-I89)

I80- Phlebitis and thrombophlebitis — PHLEBITIS – Inflammation of a vein attended by edema, stiffness, and pain at the site of inflammation. THROMBOPHLEBITIS – A partial or complete occlusion of a vein by a thrombus, with secondary inflammatory reaction in the wall of the vein.
Includes: **Endophlebitis** — Inflammation of the innermost lining of a vein.
Inflammation, vein — Tissue reaction to a venous condition or injury.
Periphlebitis — Inflammation of the external coat of the vein and the surrounding tissue.
Suppurative phlebitis — Pus-producing inflammation of a vein.
Code first phlebitis and thrombophlebitis complicating abortion, ectopic or molar pregnancy (O00-O07, O08.7)
Code first phlebitis and thrombophlebitis complicating pregnancy, childbirth and the puerperium (O22-, O87-)
Excludes 1:   *venous embolism and thrombosis of lower extremities (I82.4-, I82.5-, I82.81-)*

I80.0- Phlebitis and thrombophlebitis of superficial vessels of lower extremities
Phlebitis and thrombophlebitis of femoropopliteal vein

I80.00 Phlebitis and thrombophlebitis of superficial vessels of unspecified lower extremity

I80.01 Phlebitis and thrombophlebitis of superficial vessels of right lower extremity

I80.02 Phlebitis and thrombophlebitis of superficial vessels of left lower extremity

I80.03 Phlebitis and thrombophlebitis of superficial vessels of lower extremities, bilateral

I80.1- Phlebitis and thrombophlebitis of femoral vein

CC **I80.10 Phlebitis and thrombophlebitis of unspecified femoral vein**

CC **I80.11 Phlebitis and thrombophlebitis of right femoral vein**

CC **I80.12 Phlebitis and thrombophlebitis of left femoral vein**

CC **I80.13 Phlebitis and thrombophlebitis of femoral vein, bilateral**

I80.2- Phlebitis and thrombophlebitis of other and unspecified deep vessels of lower extremities

I80.20- Phlebitis and thrombophlebitis of unspecified deep vessels of lower extremities

CC **I80.201 Phlebitis and thrombophlebitis of unspecified deep vessels of right lower extremity**

CC **I80.202 Phlebitis and thrombophlebitis of unspecified deep vessels of left lower extremity**

CC **I80.203 Phlebitis and thrombophlebitis of unspecified deep vessels of lower extremities, bilateral**

CC **I80.209 Phlebitis and thrombophlebitis of unspecified deep vessels of unspecified lower extremity**

I80.21- Phlebitis and thrombophlebitis of iliac vein

CC **I80.211 Phlebitis and thrombophlebitis of right iliac vein**

CC **I80.212 Phlebitis and thrombophlebitis of left iliac vein**

CC **I80.213 Phlebitis and thrombophlebitis of iliac vein, bilateral**

CC **I80.219 Phlebitis and thrombophlebitis of unspecified iliac vein**

I80.22- Phlebitis and thrombophlebitis of popliteal vein

CC **I80.221 Phlebitis and thrombophlebitis of right popliteal vein**

CC **I80.222 Phlebitis and thrombophlebitis of left popliteal vein**

CC **I80.223 Phlebitis and thrombophlebitis of popliteal vein, bilateral**

CC **I80.229 Phlebitis and thrombophlebitis of unspecified popliteal vein**

I80.23- Phlebitis and thrombophlebitis of tibial vein

CC **I80.231 Phlebitis and thrombophlebitis of right tibial vein**

CC **I80.232 Phlebitis and thrombophlebitis of left tibial vein**

CC **I80.233 Phlebitis and thrombophlebitis of tibial vein, bilateral**

CC **I80.239 Phlebitis and thrombophlebitis of unspecified tibial vein**

I77-I80

I80.29- Phlebitis and thrombophlebitis of <u>other deep</u> vessels of <u>lower</u> extremities

CC **I80.291** Phlebitis and thrombophlebitis of <u>other deep</u> vessels of <u>right lower</u> extremity

CC **I80.292** Phlebitis and thrombophlebitis of <u>other deep</u> vessels of <u>left lower</u> extremity

CC **I80.293** Phlebitis and thrombophlebitis of <u>other deep</u> vessels of <u>lower</u> extremity, <u>bilateral</u>

CC **I80.299** Phlebitis and thrombophlebitis of <u>other deep</u> vessels of <u>unspecified lower</u> extremity

I80.3 Phlebitis and thrombophlebitis of lower extremities, unspecified

I80.8 Phlebitis and thrombophlebitis of other sites

I80.9 Phlebitis and thrombophlebitis of unspecified site

I81 Portal vein thrombosis — An abnormal clotting aggregation of platelets and fibrin
MCC in the portal vein causing obstruction.

Portal (vein) obstruction — Blocking or clogging of the portal vein due to a thrombus.

Excludes ❷: *hepatic vein thrombosis (I82.0)*
phlebitis of portal vein (K75.1)

Portal Vein

Renal Vein

VENOUS EMBOLISM   PORTAL VEIN THROMBOSIS

I82- Other venous embolism and thrombosis — EMBOLISM — The blocking of a vein by a blood clot, or other substance, which has been brought to the site of obstruction by the blood flow. THROMBOSIS — An abnormal aggregation of blood factors causing an obstruction of a vein that remains in place at the site where it formed. ACUTE — A current episode with the sudden onset of symptoms. CHRONIC — A form that is not diagnosed as an acute episode (but often has had a previous acute episode) that is now being treated for the existing, non-acute condition.

Code first venous embolism and thrombosis complicating:
Abortion, ectopic or molar pregnancy (O00-O07, O08.7)
Pregnancy, childbirth and the puerperium (O22-, O87-)

Excludes ❷: *venous embolism and thrombosis (of):*
cerebral (I63.6, I67.6)
coronary (I21-I25)
intracranial and intraspinal, septic or NOS (G08)
intracranial, nonpyogenic (I67.6)
intraspinal, nonpyogenic (G95.1)
mesenteric (K55.0-)
portal (I81)
pulmonary (I26.-)

MCC **I82.0** Budd-Chiari syndrome — The symptomatic obstruction or occlusion of the hepatic veins (usually of unknown origin) causing enlargement and tenderness of the liver.

Hepatic vein thrombosis — Formation of a thrombus in the hepatic vein causing obstruction.

CC **I82.1** Thrombophlebitis migrans — A recurring phlebitis affecting superficial peripheral veins and sometimes major and visceral veins.

I82.2- Embolism and thrombosis of vena cava and other thoracic veins

I82.21- Embolism and thrombosis of <u>superior</u> vena cava

CC **I82.210** <u>Acute</u> embolism and thrombosis of superior vena cava

Embolism and thrombosis of superior vena cava NOS

CC **I82.211** <u>Chronic</u> embolism and thrombosis of superior vena cava

I82.22- Embolism and thrombosis of <u>inferior</u> vena cava

MCC **I82.220** <u>Acute</u> embolism and thrombosis of inferior vena cava

Embolism and thrombosis of inferior vena cava NOS

MCC **I82.221** <u>Chronic</u> embolism and thrombosis of inferior vena cava

I82.29- Embolism and thrombosis of <u>other thoracic</u> veins

Embolism and thrombosis of brachiocephalic (innominate) vein

CC **I82.290** <u>Acute</u> embolism and thrombosis of other thoracic veins

CC **I82.291** <u>Chronic</u> embolism and thrombosis of other thoracic veins

CC **I82.3** Embolism and thrombosis of renal vein

I82.4- <u>Acute</u> embolism and thrombosis of <u>deep veins</u> of <u>lower extremity</u>

I82.40- Acute embolism and thrombosis of <u>unspecified deep</u> veins of lower extremity

Deep vein thrombosis NOS
DVT NOS

Excludes 1: *acute embolism and thrombosis of unspecified deep veins of distal lower extremity (I82.4Z-) acute embolism and thrombosis of unspecified deep veins of proximal lower extremity (I82.4Y-)*

CC **I82.401** Acute embolism and thrombosis of <u>unspecified deep</u> veins of <u>right</u> lower extremity

CC **I82.402** Acute embolism and thrombosis of <u>unspecified deep</u> veins of <u>left</u> lower extremity

CC **I82.403** Acute embolism and thrombosis of <u>unspecified deep</u> veins of lower extremity, <u>bilateral</u>

CC **I82.409** Acute embolism and thrombosis of <u>unspecified deep</u> veins of <u>unspecified</u> lower extremity

I82.41- Acute embolism and thrombosis of <u>femoral</u> vein

CC **I82.411** Acute embolism and thrombosis of <u>right femoral</u> vein

CC **I82.412** Acute embolism and thrombosis of <u>left femoral</u> vein

CC **I82.413** Acute embolism and thrombosis of <u>femoral</u> vein, <u>bilateral</u>

CC **I82.419** Acute embolism and thrombosis of <u>unspecified femoral</u> vein

I82.42- Acute embolism and thrombosis of <u>iliac</u> vein

CC **I82.421** Acute embolism and thrombosis of <u>right iliac</u> vein

CC **I82.422** Acute embolism and thrombosis of <u>left iliac</u> vein

CC **I82.423** Acute embolism and thrombosis of <u>iliac</u> vein, <u>bilateral</u>

CC **I82.429** Acute embolism and thrombosis of <u>unspecified iliac</u> vein

I82.43- Acute embolism and thrombosis of <u>popliteal</u> vein

CC **I82.431** Acute embolism and thrombosis of <u>right popliteal</u> vein

CC **I82.432** Acute embolism and thrombosis of <u>left popliteal</u> vein

CC **I82.433** Acute embolism and thrombosis of <u>popliteal</u> vein, <u>bilateral</u>

CC **I82.439** Acute embolism and thrombosis of <u>unspecified popliteal</u> vein

I82.44- Acute embolism and thrombosis of <u>tibial</u> vein

CC **I82.441** Acute embolism and thrombosis of <u>right tibial</u> vein

CC **I82.442** Acute embolism and thrombosis of <u>left tibial</u> vein

CC **I82.443** Acute embolism and thrombosis of <u>tibial</u> vein, <u>bilateral</u>

CC **I82.449** Acute embolism and thrombosis of <u>unspecified tibial</u> vein

I82.49- Acute embolism and thrombosis of <u>other specified</u> deep vein of lower extremity

CC **I82.491** Acute embolism and thrombosis of <u>other specified</u> deep vein of <u>right</u> lower extremity

CC **I82.492** Acute embolism and thrombosis of <u>other specified</u> deep vein of <u>left</u> lower extremity

CC **I82.493** Acute embolism and thrombosis of <u>other specified</u> deep vein of lower extremity, <u>bilateral</u>

CC **I82.499** Acute embolism and thrombosis of <u>other specified</u> deep vein of <u>unspecified</u> lower extremity

I 80 - I 82

I82.4Y- Acute embolism and thrombosis of <u>unspecified</u> deep veins of <u>proximal</u> lower extremity
Acute embolism and thrombosis of deep vein of thigh NOS
Acute embolism and thrombosis of deep vein of upper leg NOS

cc **I82.4Y1** Acute embolism and thrombosis of <u>unspecified</u> deep veins of <u>right proximal</u> lower extremity

cc **I82.4Y2** Acute embolism and thrombosis of <u>unspecified</u> deep veins of <u>left proximal</u> lower extremity

cc **I82.4Y3** Acute embolism and thrombosis of <u>unspecified</u> deep veins of <u>proximal</u> lower extremity, <u>bilateral</u>

cc **I82.4Y9** Acute embolism and thrombosis of <u>unspecified</u> deep veins of <u>unspecified proximal</u> lower extremity

I82.4Z- Acute embolism and thrombosis of <u>unspecified</u> deep veins of <u>distal</u> lower extremity
Acute embolism and thrombosis of deep vein of calf NOS
Acute embolism and thrombosis of deep vein of lower leg NOS

cc **I82.4Z1** Acute embolism and thrombosis of <u>unspecified</u> deep veins of <u>right distal</u> lower extremity

cc **I82.4Z2** Acute embolism and thrombosis of <u>unspecified</u> deep veins of <u>left distal</u> lower extremity

cc **I82.4Z3** Acute embolism and thrombosis of <u>unspecified</u> deep veins of <u>distal</u> lower extremity, <u>bilateral</u>

cc **I82.4Z9** Acute embolism and thrombosis of <u>unspecified</u> deep veins of <u>unspecified distal</u> lower extremity

I82.5- <u>Chronic</u> embolism and thrombosis of deep veins of lower extremity
Use additional code, if applicable, for associated long-term (current) use of anticoagulants (Z79.01)
Excludes 1:   personal history of venous embolism and thrombosis (Z86.718)

I82.50- <u>Chronic</u> embolism and thrombosis of <u>unspecified</u> <u>deep</u> veins of lower extremity
Excludes 1:   chronic embolism and thrombosis of unspecified deep veins of distal lower extremity (I82.5Z-)
chronic embolism and thrombosis of unspecified deep veins of proximal lower extremity (I82.5Y-)

cc **I82.501** <u>Chronic</u> embolism and thrombosis of <u>unspecified</u> <u>deep</u> veins of <u>right</u> lower extremity

cc **I82.502** <u>Chronic</u> embolism and thrombosis of <u>unspecified</u> <u>deep</u> veins of <u>left</u> lower extremity

cc **I82.503** <u>Chronic</u> embolism and thrombosis of <u>unspecified</u> <u>deep</u> veins of lower extremity, <u>bilateral</u>

cc **I82.509** <u>Chronic</u> embolism and thrombosis of <u>unspecified</u> <u>deep</u> veins of <u>unspecified</u> lower extremity

I82.51- <u>Chronic</u> embolism and thrombosis of <u>femoral</u> vein

cc **I82.511** <u>Chronic</u> embolism and thrombosis of <u>right femoral</u> vein

cc **I82.512** <u>Chronic</u> embolism and thrombosis of <u>left femoral</u> vein

cc **I82.513** <u>Chronic</u> embolism and thrombosis of <u>femoral</u> vein, <u>bilateral</u>

cc **I82.519** <u>Chronic</u> embolism and thrombosis of <u>unspecified</u> <u>femoral</u> vein

I82.52- <u>Chronic</u> embolism and thrombosis of <u>iliac</u> vein

cc **I82.521** <u>Chronic</u> embolism and thrombosis of <u>right iliac</u> vein

cc **I82.522** <u>Chronic</u> embolism and thrombosis of <u>left iliac</u> vein

cc **I82.523** <u>Chronic</u> embolism and thrombosis of <u>iliac</u> vein, <u>bilateral</u>

cc **I82.529** <u>Chronic</u> embolism and thrombosis of <u>unspecified</u> <u>iliac</u> vein

I82.53- <u>Chronic</u> embolism and thrombosis of <u>popliteal</u> vein

cc **I82.531** <u>Chronic</u> embolism and thrombosis of <u>right popliteal</u> vein

cc **I82.532** <u>Chronic</u> embolism and thrombosis of <u>left popliteal</u> vein

cc **I82.533** <u>Chronic</u> embolism and thrombosis of <u>popliteal</u> vein, <u>bilateral</u>

cc **I82.539** <u>Chronic</u> embolism and thrombosis of <u>unspecified</u> <u>popliteal</u> vein

I82.54- <u>Chronic</u> embolism and thrombosis of <u>tibial</u> vein

cc **I82.541** <u>Chronic</u> embolism and thrombosis of <u>right tibial</u> vein

cc **I82.542** <u>Chronic</u> embolism and thrombosis of <u>left tibial</u> vein

cc **I82.543** <u>Chronic</u> embolism and thrombosis of <u>tibial</u> vein, <u>bilateral</u>

cc **I82.549** <u>Chronic</u> embolism and thrombosis of <u>unspecified</u> <u>tibial</u> vein

I82.59- <u>Chronic</u> embolism and thrombosis of <u>other specified</u> deep vein of lower extremity

cc **I82.591** <u>Chronic</u> embolism and thrombosis of <u>other specified</u> deep vein of <u>right</u> lower extremity

cc **I82.592** <u>Chronic</u> embolism and thrombosis of <u>other specified</u> deep vein of <u>left</u> lower extremity

cc **I82.593** <u>Chronic</u> embolism and thrombosis of <u>other specified</u> deep vein of lower extremity, <u>bilateral</u>

cc **I82.599** <u>Chronic</u> embolism and thrombosis of <u>other specified</u> deep vein of <u>unspecified</u> lower extremity

I82.5Y- <u>Chronic</u> embolism and thrombosis of <u>unspecified deep</u> veins of <u>proximal</u> lower extremity
Chronic embolism and thrombosis of deep veins of thigh NOS
Chronic embolism and thrombosis of deep veins of upper leg NOS

cc **I82.5Y1** <u>Chronic</u> embolism and thrombosis of <u>unspecified</u> deep veins of <u>right proximal</u> lower extremity

cc **I82.5Y2** <u>Chronic</u> embolism and thrombosis of <u>unspecified</u> deep veins of <u>left proximal</u> lower extremity

cc **I82.5Y3** <u>Chronic</u> embolism and thrombosis of <u>unspecified</u> deep veins of <u>proximal</u> lower extremity, <u>bilateral</u>

cc **I82.5Y9** <u>Chronic</u> embolism and thrombosis of <u>unspecified</u> deep veins of <u>unspecified proximal</u> lower extremity

I82.5Z- <u>Chronic</u> embolism and thrombosis of <u>unspecified deep</u> veins of <u>distal</u> lower extremity
Chronic embolism and thrombosis of deep veins of calf NOS
Chronic embolism and thrombosis of deep veins of lower leg NOS

cc **I82.5Z1** <u>Chronic</u> embolism and thrombosis of <u>unspecified</u> deep veins of <u>right distal</u> lower extremity

cc **I82.5Z2** <u>Chronic</u> embolism and thrombosis of <u>unspecified</u> deep veins of <u>left distal</u> lower extremity

cc **I82.5Z3** <u>Chronic</u> embolism and thrombosis of <u>unspecified</u> deep veins of <u>distal</u> lower extremity, bilateral

cc **I82.5Z9** <u>Chronic</u> embolism and thrombosis of <u>unspecified</u> deep veins of unspecified <u>distal</u> lower extremity

I82.6- <u>Acute</u> embolism and thrombosis of <u>veins</u> of <u>upper extremity</u>

I82.60- <u>Acute</u> embolism and thrombosis of <u>unspecified</u> veins of <u>upper</u> extremity

cc **I82.601** Acute embolism and thrombosis of <u>unspecified</u> veins of <u>right</u> upper extremity

cc **I82.602** Acute embolism and thrombosis of <u>unspecified</u> veins of <u>left</u> upper extremity

cc **I82.603** Acute embolism and thrombosis of <u>unspecified</u> veins of upper extremity, <u>bilateral</u>

cc **I82.609** Acute embolism and thrombosis of <u>unspecified</u> veins of <u>unspecified</u> upper extremity

I82.61- Acute embolism and thrombosis of <u>superficial</u> veins of <u>upper</u> extremity
Acute embolism and thrombosis of antecubital vein
Acute embolism and thrombosis of basilic vein
Acute embolism and thrombosis of cephalic vein

cc **I82.611** Acute embolism and thrombosis of <u>superficial</u> veins of <u>right</u> upper extremity

cc **I82.612** Acute embolism and thrombosis of <u>superficial</u> veins of <u>left</u> upper extremity

cc **I82.613** Acute embolism and thrombosis of <u>superficial</u> veins of upper extremity, <u>bilateral</u>

cc **I82.619** Acute embolism and thrombosis of <u>superficial</u> veins of <u>unspecified</u> upper extremity

I82.62- Acute embolism and thrombosis of <u>deep</u> veins of <u>upper</u> extremity
> Acute embolism and thrombosis of brachial vein
> Acute embolism and thrombosis of radial vein
> Acute embolism and thrombosis of ulnar vein

cc **I82.621 Acute embolism and thrombosis of <u>deep</u> veins of <u>right</u> upper extremity**

cc **I82.622 Acute embolism and thrombosis of <u>deep</u> veins of <u>left</u> upper extremity**

cc **I82.623 Acute embolism and thrombosis of <u>deep</u> veins of upper extremity, <u>bilateral</u>**

cc **I82.629 Acute embolism and thrombosis of <u>deep</u> veins of <u>unspecified</u> upper extremity**

I82.7- <u>Chronic</u> embolism and thrombosis of veins of <u>upper</u> extremity
> Use additional code, if applicable, for associated long-term (current) use of anticoagulants (Z79.01)
> *Excludes 1:* *personal history of venous embolism and thrombosis (Z86.718)*

I82.70- <u>Chronic</u> embolism and thrombosis of <u>unspecified</u> veins of <u>upper</u> extremity

cc **I82.701 <u>Chronic</u> embolism and thrombosis of <u>unspecified</u> veins of <u>right</u> upper extremity**

cc **I82.702 <u>Chronic</u> embolism and thrombosis of <u>unspecified</u> veins of <u>left</u> upper extremity**

cc **I82.703 <u>Chronic</u> embolism and thrombosis of <u>unspecified</u> veins of upper extremity, <u>bilateral</u>**

cc **I82.709 <u>Chronic</u> embolism and thrombosis of <u>unspecified</u> veins of <u>unspecified</u> upper extremity**

I82.71- <u>Chronic</u> embolism and thrombosis of <u>superficial</u> veins of <u>upper</u> extremity
> Chronic embolism and thrombosis of antecubital vein
> Chronic embolism and thrombosis of basilic vein
> Chronic embolism and thrombosis of cephalic vein

cc **I82.711 <u>Chronic</u> embolism and thrombosis of <u>superficial</u> veins of <u>right</u> upper extremity**

cc **I82.712 <u>Chronic</u> embolism and thrombosis of <u>superficial</u> veins of <u>left</u> upper extremity**

cc **I82.713 <u>Chronic</u> embolism and thrombosis of <u>superficial</u> veins of upper extremity, <u>bilateral</u>**

cc **I82.719 <u>Chronic</u> embolism and thrombosis of <u>superficial</u> veins of <u>unspecified</u> upper extremity**

I82.72- <u>Chronic</u> embolism and thrombosis of <u>deep</u> veins of <u>upper</u> extremity
> Chronic embolism and thrombosis of brachial vein
> Chronic embolism and thrombosis of radial vein
> Chronic embolism and thrombosis of ulnar vein

cc **I82.721 <u>Chronic</u> embolism and thrombosis of <u>deep</u> veins of <u>right</u> upper extremity**

cc **I82.722 <u>Chronic</u> embolism and thrombosis of <u>deep</u> veins of <u>left</u> upper extremity**

cc **I82.723 <u>Chronic</u> embolism and thrombosis of <u>deep</u> veins of upper extremity, <u>bilateral</u>**

cc **I82.729 Chronic embolism and thrombosis of <u>deep</u> veins of <u>unspecified</u> upper extremity**

I82.A- Embolism and thrombosis of axillary vein

I82.A1- <u>Acute</u> embolism and thrombosis of <u>axillary</u> vein

cc **I82.A11 Acute embolism and thrombosis of <u>right</u> <u>axillary</u> vein**

cc **I82.A12 Acute embolism and thrombosis of <u>left</u> <u>axillary</u> vein**

cc **I82.A13 Acute embolism and thrombosis of <u>axillary</u> vein, <u>bilateral</u>**

cc **I82.A19 Acute embolism and thrombosis of <u>unspecified</u> <u>axillary</u> vein**

I82.A2- <u>Chronic</u> embolism and thrombosis of <u>axillary</u> vein

cc **I82.A21 <u>Chronic</u> embolism and thrombosis of <u>right</u> <u>axillary</u> vein**

cc **I82.A22 <u>Chronic</u> embolism and thrombosis of <u>left</u> <u>axillary</u> vein**

cc **I82.A23 <u>Chronic</u> embolism and thrombosis of <u>axillary</u> vein, <u>bilateral</u>**

cc **I82.A29 <u>Chronic</u> embolism and thrombosis of <u>unspecified</u> <u>axillary</u> vein**

I82.B- Embolism and thrombosis of <u>subclavian</u> vein

I82.B1- <u>Acute</u> embolism and thrombosis of <u>subclavian</u> vein

cc **I82.B11 Acute embolism and thrombosis of <u>right</u> <u>subclavian</u> vein**

cc **I82.B12 Acute embolism and thrombosis of <u>left</u> <u>subclavian</u> vein**

cc **I82.B13 Acute embolism and thrombosis of <u>subclavian</u> vein, <u>bilateral</u>**

cc **I82.B19 Acute embolism and thrombosis of <u>unspecified</u> <u>subclavian</u> vein**

I82.B2- <u>Chronic</u> embolism and thrombosis of <u>subclavian</u> vein

cc **I82.B21 <u>Chronic</u> embolism and thrombosis of <u>right</u> <u>subclavian</u> vein**

cc **I82.B22 <u>Chronic</u> embolism and thrombosis of <u>left</u> <u>subclavian</u> vein**

cc **I82.B23 <u>Chronic</u> embolism and thrombosis of <u>subclavian</u> vein, <u>bilateral</u>**

cc **I82.B29 <u>Chronic</u> embolism and thrombosis of <u>unspecified</u> <u>subclavian</u> vein**

I82.C- Embolism and thrombosis of <u>internal jugular</u> vein

I82.C1- <u>Acute</u> embolism and thrombosis of <u>internal jugular</u> vein

cc **I82.C11 Acute embolism and thrombosis of <u>right</u> <u>internal jugular</u> vein**

cc **I82.C12 Acute embolism and thrombosis of <u>left</u> <u>internal jugular</u> vein**

cc **I82.C13 Acute embolism and thrombosis of <u>internal jugular</u> vein, <u>bilateral</u>**

cc **I82.C19 Acute embolism and thrombosis of <u>unspecified</u> <u>internal jugular</u> vein**

I82.C2- <u>Chronic</u> embolism and thrombosis of <u>internal jugular</u> vein

cc **I82.C21 <u>Chronic</u> embolism and thrombosis of <u>right</u> <u>internal jugular</u> vein**

cc **I82.C22 <u>Chronic</u> embolism and thrombosis of <u>left</u> <u>internal jugular</u> vein**

cc **I82.C23 <u>Chronic</u> embolism and thrombosis of <u>internal jugular</u> vein, <u>bilateral</u>**

cc **I82.C29 <u>Chronic</u> embolism and thrombosis of <u>unspecified</u> <u>internal jugular</u> vein**

I82.8- Embolism and thrombosis of <u>other specified veins</u>
> Use additional code, if applicable, for associated long-term (current) use of anticoagulants (Z79.01)

I82.81- Embolism and thrombosis of <u>superficial</u> veins of <u>lower</u> extremities
> Embolism and thrombosis of saphenous vein (greater) (lesser)

cc **I82.811 Embolism and thrombosis of <u>superficial</u> veins of <u>right</u> lower extremities**

cc **I82.812 Embolism and thrombosis of <u>superficial</u> veins of <u>left</u> lower extremities**

cc **I82.813 Embolism and thrombosis of <u>superficial</u> veins of lower extremities, <u>bilateral</u>**

cc **I82.819 Embolism and thrombosis of <u>superficial</u> veins of <u>unspecified</u> lower extremities**

I82.89- Embolism and thrombosis of <u>other specified veins</u>

cc **I82.890 <u>Acute</u> embolism and thrombosis of other specified veins**

cc **I82.891 <u>Chronic</u> embolism and thrombosis of other specified veins**

I82.9- Embolism and thrombosis of <u>unspecified</u> vein

cc **I82.90 <u>Acute</u> embolism and thrombosis of unspecified vein**
> Embolism of vein NOS
> Thrombosis (vein) NOS

cc **I82.91 <u>Chronic</u> embolism and thrombosis of unspecified vein**

Excludes 1: = NOT CODED HERE! (Do not code both)   **754**   *Excludes ❷:* = Not Included Here

I83- <u>Varicose veins</u> of <u>lower</u> extremities — Dilatated, tortuous superficial veins of the legs.

> Excludes 1:   *varicose veins complicating pregnancy (O22.0-)*
> *varicose veins complicating the puerperium (O87.4)*

I83.0- <u>Varicose veins</u> of <u>lower extremities</u> <u>with ulcer</u> — A form characterized by the sloughing of inflammatory necrotic tissue at the varicose vein site.

> Use additional code to identify severity of ulcer (L97.-)

I83.00- Varicose veins of <u>unspecified</u> lower extremity with ulcer

I83.001   Varicose veins of <u>unspecified</u> lower extremity <u>with ulcer</u> of <u>thigh</u> — [Age/15-124]

I83.002   Varicose veins of <u>unspecified</u> lower extremity <u>with ulcer</u> of <u>calf</u> — [Age/15-124]

I83.003   Varicose veins of <u>unspecified</u> lower extremity <u>with ulcer</u> of <u>ankle</u> — [Age/15-124]

I83.004   Varicose veins of <u>unspecified</u> lower extremity <u>with ulcer</u> of <u>heel and midfoot</u> — [Age/15-124]
> Varicose veins of unspecified lower extremity with ulcer of plantar surface of midfoot

I83.005   Varicose veins of <u>unspecified</u> lower extremity <u>with ulcer</u> <u>other part of foot</u> — [Age/15-124]
> Varicose veins of unspecified lower extremity with ulcer of toe

I83.008   Varicose veins of unspecified lower extremity with <u>ulcer</u> <u>other part of lower leg</u> — [Age/15-124]

I83.009   Varicose veins of <u>unspecified</u> lower extremity <u>with ulcer</u> of <u>unspecified site</u> — [Age/15-124]

I83.01- Varicose veins of <u>right</u> lower extremity <u>with ulcer</u>

I83.011   Varicose veins of <u>right</u> lower extremity <u>with ulcer</u> of <u>thigh</u> — [Age/15-124]

I83.012   Varicose veins of <u>right</u> lower extremity <u>with ulcer</u> of <u>calf</u> — [Age/15-124]

I83.013   Varicose veins of <u>right</u> lower extremity <u>with ulcer</u> of <u>ankle</u> — [Age/15-124]

I83.014   Varicose veins of <u>right</u> lower extremity <u>with ulcer</u> of <u>heel and midfoot</u> — [Age/15-124]
> Varicose veins of right lower extremity with ulcer of plantar surface of midfoot

I83.015   Varicose veins of <u>right</u> lower extremity <u>with ulcer</u> <u>other part of foot</u> — [Age/15-124]
> Varicose veins of right lower extremity with ulcer of toe

I83.018   Varicose veins of <u>right</u> lower extremity <u>with ulcer</u> <u>other part of lower leg</u> — [Age/15-124]

I83.019   Varicose veins of <u>right</u> lower extremity <u>with ulcer</u> of <u>unspecified site</u> — [Age/15-124]

I83.02- Varicose veins of <u>left</u> lower extremity <u>with ulcer</u>

I83.021   Varicose veins of <u>left</u> lower extremity <u>with ulcer</u> of <u>thigh</u> — [Age/15-124]

I83.022   Varicose veins of <u>left</u> lower extremity <u>with ulcer</u> of <u>calf</u> — [Age/15-124]

I83.023   Varicose veins of <u>left</u> lower extremity <u>with ulcer</u> of <u>ankle</u> — [Age/15-124]

I83.024   Varicose veins of <u>left</u> lower extremity <u>with ulcer</u> of <u>heel and midfoot</u> — [Age/15-124]
> Varicose veins of left lower extremity with ulcer of plantar surface of midfoot

I83.025   Varicose veins of <u>left</u> lower extremity <u>with ulcer</u> <u>other part of foot</u> — [Age/15-124]
> Varicose veins of left lower extremity with ulcer of toe

I83.028   Varicose veins of <u>left</u> lower extremity <u>with ulcer</u> <u>other part of lower leg</u> — [Age/15-124]

I83.029   Varicose veins of <u>left</u> lower extremity <u>with ulcer</u> of <u>unspecified site</u> — [Age/15-124]

I83.1- <u>Varicose veins</u> of <u>lower extremities with inflammation</u> — A form characterized by massive tissue reaction and swelling.

I83.10   Varicose veins of <u>unspecified</u> lower extremity <u>with inflammation</u> — [Age/15-124]

I83.11   Varicose veins of <u>right</u> lower extremity <u>with inflammation</u> — [Age/15-124]

I83.12   Varicose veins of <u>left</u> lower extremity <u>with inflammation</u> — [Age/15-124]

I83.2- <u>Varicose veins</u> of <u>lower extremities</u> <u>with both ulcer and inflammation</u> — A form characterized by the sloughing of inflammatory necrotic tissue at the varicose vein site and inflammatory massive tissue reaction and swelling.

> Use additional code to identify severity of ulcer (L97.-)

I83.20- Varicose veins of <u>unspecified</u> lower extremity <u>with both ulcer and inflammation</u>

cc **I83.201**   Varicose veins of <u>unspecified</u> lower extremity <u>with both ulcer</u> of <u>thigh</u> and <u>inflammation</u> — [Age/15-124]

cc **I83.202**   Varicose veins of <u>unspecified</u> lower extremity <u>with both ulcer</u> of <u>calf</u> and <u>inflammation</u> — [Age/15-124]

cc **I83.203**   Varicose veins of <u>unspecified</u> lower extremity <u>with both ulcer</u> of <u>ankle</u> and <u>inflammation</u> — [Age/15-124]

cc **I83.204**   Varicose veins of <u>unspecified</u> lower extremity <u>with both ulcer</u> of <u>heel and midfoot</u> and <u>inflammation</u> — [Age/15-124]
> Varicose veins of unspecified lower extremity with both ulcer of plantar surface of midfoot and inflammation

cc **I83.205**   Varicose veins of <u>unspecified</u> lower extremity <u>with both ulcer</u> <u>other part of foot</u> and <u>inflammation</u> — [Age/15-124]
> Varicose veins of unspecified lower extremity with both ulcer of toe and inflammation

cc **I83.208**   Varicose veins of <u>unspecified</u> lower extremity <u>with both ulcer</u> of <u>other part of lower extremity</u> and <u>inflammation</u> — [Age/15-124]

cc **I83.209**   Varicose veins of unspecified lower extremity <u>with both ulcer</u> of <u>unspecified site</u> and <u>inflammation</u> — [Age/15-124]

I83.21- Varicose veins of <u>right</u> lower extremity <u>with both ulcer and inflammation</u>

cc **I83.211**   Varicose veins of <u>right</u> lower extremity <u>with both ulcer</u> of <u>thigh</u> and <u>inflammation</u> — [Age/15-124]

cc **I83.212**   Varicose veins of <u>right</u> lower extremity <u>with both ulcer</u> of <u>calf</u> and <u>inflammation</u> — [Age/15-124]

cc **I83.213**   Varicose veins of <u>right</u> lower extremity <u>with both ulcer</u> of <u>ankle</u> and <u>inflammation</u> — [Age/15-124]

cc **I83.214**   Varicose veins of <u>right</u> lower extremity <u>with both ulcer</u> of <u>heel and midfoot</u> and <u>inflammation</u> — [Age/15-124]
> Varicose veins of right lower extremity with both ulcer of plantar surface of midfoot and inflammation

cc **I83.215**   Varicose veins of <u>right</u> lower extremity <u>with both ulcer</u> <u>other part of foot</u> and <u>inflammation</u> — [Age/15-124]
> Varicose veins of right lower extremity with both ulcer of toe and inflammation

cc **I83.218**   Varicose veins of <u>right</u> lower extremity <u>with both ulcer</u> of <u>other part of lower extremity</u> and <u>inflammation</u> — [Age/15-124]

cc **I83.219**   Varicose veins of <u>right</u> lower extremity <u>with both ulcer</u> of <u>unspecified site</u> and <u>inflammation</u> — [Age/15-124]

I83.22- Varicose veins of <u>left</u> lower extremity <u>with both ulcer and inflammation</u>

cc **I83.221**   Varicose veins of <u>left</u> lower extremity <u>with both ulcer</u> of <u>thigh</u> and <u>inflammation</u> — [Age/15-124]

cc **I83.222**   Varicose veins of <u>left</u> lower extremity <u>with both ulcer</u> of <u>calf</u> and <u>inflammation</u> — [Age/15-124]

cc **I83.223**   Varicose veins of <u>left</u> lower extremity <u>with both ulcer</u> of <u>ankle</u> and <u>inflammation</u> — [Age/15-124]

cc **I83.224**   Varicose veins of <u>left</u> lower extremity <u>with both ulcer</u> of <u>heel and midfoot</u> and <u>inflammation</u> — [Age/15-124]
> Varicose veins of left lower extremity with both ulcer of plantar surface of midfoot and inflammation

cc **I83.225**   Varicose veins of <u>left</u> lower extremity <u>with both ulcer</u> <u>other part of foot</u> and <u>inflammation</u> — [Age/15-124]
> Varicose veins of left lower extremity with both ulcer of toe and inflammation

I83 - I83

CC **I83.228** **Varicose veins of left lower extremity with both ulcer of other part of lower extremity and inflammation** — [Age/15-124]

CC **I83.229** **Varicose veins of left lower extremity with both ulcer of unspecified site and inflammation** — [Age/15-124]

I83.8- **Varicose veins of lower extremities with other complications**
  I83.81- Varicose veins of lower extremities with pain
    I83.811 **Varicose veins of right lower extremities with pain** — [Age/15-124]
    I83.812 **Varicose veins of left lower extremities with pain** — [Age/15-124]
    I83.813 **Varicose veins of bilateral lower extremities with pain** — [Age/15-124]
    I83.819 **Varicose veins of unspecified lower extremities with pain** — [Age/15-124]
  I83.89- Varicose veins of lower extremities with other complications
    Varicose veins of lower extremities with edema — The accumulation of fluid in the intercellular spaces.
    Varicose veins of lower extremities with swelling — The temporary enlargement of the tissues of a lower limb.
    I83.891 **Varicose veins of right lower extremities with other complications** — [Age/15-124]
    I83.892 **Varicose veins of left lower extremities with other complications** — [Age/15-124]
    I83.893 **Varicose veins of bilateral lower extremities with other complications** — [Age/15-124]
    I83.899 **Varicose veins of unspecified lower extremities with other complications** — [Age/15-124]

I83.9- **Asymptomatic varicose veins of lower extremities**
  Phlebectasia of lower extremities
  Varicose veins of lower extremities
  Varix of lower extremities
  I83.90 **Asymptomatic varicose veins of unspecified lower extremity** — [Age/15-124]
    Varicose veins NOS
  I83.91 **Asymptomatic varicose veins of right lower extremity** — [Age/15-124]
  I83.92 **Asymptomatic varicose veins of left lower extremity** — [Age/15-124]
  I83.93 **Asymptomatic varicose veins of bilateral lower extremities** — [Age/15-124]

I85- **Esophageal varices**
Use additional code to identify:
Alcohol abuse and dependence (F10.-)
I85.0- **Esophageal varices** — Dilatated, tortuous esophageal veins.
  Idiopathic esophageal varices — A form without an identifiable cause.
  Primary esophageal varices — A form arising within the esophageal vein tissue that is not due to another condition or disease.
CC **I85.00** **Esophageal varices without bleeding**
  Esophageal varices NOS
MCC **I85.01** **Esophageal varices with bleeding** — Dilatated, tortuous esophageal veins with escape of blood.
I85.1- **Secondary esophageal varices** — A form due to another condition or disease.
  Esophageal varices secondary to alcoholic liver disease
  Esophageal varices secondary to cirrhosis of liver
  Esophageal varices secondary to schistosomiasis
  Esophageal varices secondary to toxic liver disease
  Code first underlying disease
CC **I85.10** **Secondary esophageal varices without bleeding**
MCC **I85.11** **Secondary esophageal varices with bleeding**

I86- **Varicose veins of other sites**
Excludes 1: varicose veins of unspecified site (I83.9-)
Excludes 2: retinal varices (H35.0-)
I86.0 **Sublingual varices** — Dilatated, tortuous veins under the tongue.
I86.1 **Scrotal varices** — [♂] – Dilatated, tortuous veins within the scrotum.
  Varicocele — A condition of dilatated, tortuous veins of the testicles and epididymides.
I86.2 **Pelvic varices** — Dilatated, tortuous veins within the pelvic cavity.

I86.3 **Vulval varices** — [♀] – Dilatated, tortuous veins of the vulva.
Excludes 1: vulval varices complicating childbirth and the puerperium (O87.8)
  vulval varices complicating pregnancy (O22.1-)
I86.4 **Gastric varices** — Dilatated, tortuous stomach veins.
I86.8 **Varicose veins of other specified sites** — [Age/15-124]
  Varicose ulcer of nasal septum

I87- **Other disorders of veins**
I87.0- **Postthrombotic syndrome** — Conditions resulting from the destructive effects of thrombosis, including increased pressure in the deep and superficial veins, destruction of the valves of the deep veins, and obliteration in severe cases.
  Chronic venous hypertension due to deep vein thrombosis
  Postphlebitic syndrome
Excludes 1: chronic venous hypertension without deep vein thrombosis (I87.3-)
  I87.00- **Postthrombotic syndrome without complications**
    Asymptomatic Postthrombotic syndrome
    I87.001 **Postthrombotic syndrome without complications of right lower extremity**
    I87.002 **Postthrombotic syndrome without complications of left lower extremity**
    I87.003 **Postthrombotic syndrome without complications of bilateral lower extremity**
    I87.009 **Postthrombotic syndrome without complications of unspecified extremity**
      Postthrombotic syndrome NOS
  I87.01- **Postthrombotic syndrome with ulcer** — A form with necrotic tissue sites.
    Use additional code to specify site and severity of ulcer (L97.-)
  CC **I87.011** **Postthrombotic syndrome with ulcer of right lower extremity**
  CC **I87.012** **Postthrombotic syndrome with ulcer of left lower extremity**
  CC **I87.013** **Postthrombotic syndrome with ulcer of bilateral lower extremity**
  CC **I87.019** **Postthrombotic syndrome with ulcer of unspecified lower extremity**
  I87.02- **Postthrombotic syndrome with inflammation** — A form characterized by massive tissue infusion and swelling.
    I87.021 **Postthrombotic syndrome with inflammation of right lower extremity**
    I87.022 **Postthrombotic syndrome with inflammation of left lower extremity**
    I87.023 **Postthrombotic syndrome with inflammation of bilateral lower extremity**
    I87.029 **Postthrombotic syndrome with inflammation of unspecified lower extremity**
  I87.03- **Postthrombotic syndrome with ulcer and inflammation** — A form with necrotic tissue sites and massive tissue infusion and swelling.
    Use additional code to specify site and severity of ulcer (L97.-)
  CC **I87.031** **Postthrombotic syndrome with ulcer and inflammation of right lower extremity**
  CC **I87.032** **Postthrombotic syndrome with ulcer and inflammation of left lower extremity**
  CC **I87.033** **Postthrombotic syndrome with ulcer and inflammation of bilateral lower extremity**
  CC **I87.039** **Postthrombotic syndrome with ulcer and inflammation of unspecified lower extremity**
  I87.09- **Postthrombotic syndrome with other complications**
    I87.091 **Postthrombotic syndrome with other complications of right lower extremity**
    I87.092 **Postthrombotic syndrome with other complications of left lower extremity**
    I87.093 **Postthrombotic syndrome with other complications of bilateral lower extremity**
    I87.099 **Postthrombotic syndrome with other complications of unspecified lower extremity**

CC I87.1 **Compression of vein** — The collapsing walls of a vein due to excessive external pressure around the vein.
    Stricture of vein — Narrowing of the vein's lumen.
    Vena cava syndrome (inferior) (superior) — Compression of the vena cava (usually superior) resulting in edema of the face, neck, and upper arm.
    Excludes ❷: compression of pulmonary vein (I28.8)

I87.2 **Venous insufficiency (chronic) (peripheral)** — Impairment of the venous return, often due to defective venous valves.
    Stasis dermatitis — Eczema and edema of the legs due to varicose veins.
    Excludes 1: stasis dermatitis with varicose veins of lower extremities (I83.1-, I83.2-)

I87.3- **Chronic venous hypertension (idiopathic)** — Increased venous blood pressure in the deep and superficial veins that is not due to deep vein thrombosis.
    Stasis edema
    Excludes 1: chronic venous hypertension due to deep vein thrombosis (I87.0-)
    varicose veins of lower extremities (I83.-)

I87.30- **Chronic venous hypertension (idiopathic) without complications**
    Asymptomatic chronic venous hypertension (idiopathic)

I87.301 **Chronic venous hypertension (idiopathic) without complications of right lower extremity**

I87.302 **Chronic venous hypertension (idiopathic) without complications of left lower extremity**

I87.303 **Chronic venous hypertension (idiopathic) without complications of bilateral lower extremity**

I87.309 **Chronic venous hypertension (idiopathic) without complications of unspecified lower extremity**
    Chronic venous hypertension NOS

I87.31- **Chronic venous hypertension (idiopathic) with ulcer** — A form with necrotic tissue sites.
    Use additional code to specify site and severity of ulcer (L97.-)

CC I87.311 **Chronic venous hypertension (idiopathic) with ulcer of right lower extremity**

CC I87.312 **Chronic venous hypertension (idiopathic) with ulcer of left lower extremity**

CC I87.313 **Chronic venous hypertension (idiopathic) with ulcer of bilateral lower extremity**

CC I87.319 **Chronic venous hypertension (idiopathic) with ulcer of unspecified lower extremity**

I87.32- **Chronic venous hypertension (idiopathic) with inflammation** — A form characterized by massive tissue infusion and swelling.

I87.321 **Chronic venous hypertension (idiopathic) with inflammation of right lower extremity**

I87.322 **Chronic venous hypertension (idiopathic) with inflammation of left lower extremity**

I87.323 **Chronic venous hypertension (idiopathic) with inflammation of bilateral lower extremity**

I87.329 **Chronic venous hypertension (idiopathic) with inflammation of unspecified lower extremity**

I87.33- **Chronic venous hypertension (idiopathic) with ulcer and inflammation** — A form with necrotic tissue sites and massive tissue infusion and swelling.
    Use additional code to specify site and severity of ulcer (L97.-)

CC I87.331 **Chronic venous hypertension (idiopathic) with ulcer and inflammation of right lower extremity**

CC I87.332 **Chronic venous hypertension (idiopathic) with ulcer and inflammation of left lower extremity**

CC I87.333 **Chronic venous hypertension (idiopathic) with ulcer and inflammation of bilateral lower extremity**

CC I87.339 **Chronic venous hypertension (idiopathic) with ulcer and inflammation of unspecified lower extremity**

I87.39- **Chronic venous hypertension (idiopathic) with other complications**

I87.391 **Chronic venous hypertension (idiopathic) with other complications of right lower extremity**

I87.392 **Chronic venous hypertension (idiopathic) with other complications of left lower extremity**

I87.393 **Chronic venous hypertension (idiopathic) with other complications of bilateral lower extremity**

I87.399 **Chronic venous hypertension (idiopathic) with other complications of unspecified lower extremity**

I87.8 **Other specified disorders of veins**
    Phlebosclerosis
    Venofibrosis

I87.9 **Disorder of vein, unspecified**

I88- **Nonspecific lymphadenitis** — Inflammation of lymph tissue causing mild swelling, pain, and tenderness.
    Excludes 1: acute lymphadenitis, except mesenteric (L04.-)
    enlarged lymph nodes NOS (R59.-)
    human immunodeficiency virus [HIV] disease resulting in generalized lymphadenopathy (B20)

I88.0 **Nonspecific mesenteric lymphadenitis** — A form affecting the mesenteric (abdominal cavity) lymph nodes.
    Mesenteric lymphadenitis (acute) (chronic)

I88.1 **Chronic lymphadenitis, except mesenteric** — A form that develops and persists over a relatively long period of time.
    Adenitis
    Lymphadenitis

I88.8 **Other nonspecific lymphadenitis**

I88.9 **Nonspecific lymphadenitis, unspecified**
    Lymphadenitis NOS

I89- **Other noninfective disorders of lymphatic vessels and lymph nodes**
    Excludes 1: chylocele, tunica vaginalis (nonfilarial) NOS (N50.89)
    enlarged lymph nodes NOS (R59.-)
    filarial chylocele (B74.-)
    hereditary lymphedema (Q82.0)

I89.0 **Lymphedema, not elsewhere classified** — Accumulation of interstitial fluid of the lymphatic system.
    Elephantiasis (nonfilarial) NOS — Edema and enlargement of an area due to lymphatic obstruction.
    Lymphangiectasis — Dilatation of the lymphatic vessels.
    Obliteration, lymphatic vessel — The complete destruction of a lymphatic vessel.
    Praecox lymphedema — Puffiness and swelling of the lower limbs seen in girls at or near puberty.
    Secondary lymphedema — Accumulation of interstitial fluid due to secondary obstruction of the lymphatic system.
    Excludes 1: postmastectomy lymphedema (I97.2)

I89.1 **Lymphangitis** — Inflammation of the lymph vessels.
    Chronic lymphangitis
    Lymphangitis NOS
    Subacute lymphangitis
    Excludes 1: acute lymphangitis (L03.-)

I89.8 **Other specified noninfective disorders of lymphatic vessels and lymph nodes**
    Chylocele (nonfilarial) — Severe, massive edema encapsulated by a sac.
    Chylous ascites — The abnormal presence of chyle (triglycerides suspended in water) in the peritoneal cavity.
    Chylous cyst — An abnormal mesenteric sac filled with chyle.
    Lipomelanotic reticulosis — Lymph node hyperplasia of the reticular cells.
    Lymph node or vessel fistula — An abnormal passage of chyle from a lymph duct.
    Lymph node or vessel infarction — A localized area of necrosis due to the massive accumulation of chyle.
    Lymph node or vessel rupture — A forcible tearing of the thoracic duct leaving chyle.

I89.9 **Noninfective disorder of lymphatic vessels and lymph nodes, unspecified**
    Disease of lymphatic vessels NOS

I87 - I89

Other and unspecified disorders of the circulatory system (I95-I99)

I95- <u>Hypotension</u> — Abnormally low blood pressure.
    Excludes 1:   *cardiovascular collapse (R57.9)*
                maternal hypotension syndrome (O26.5-)
                nonspecific low blood pressure reading NOS (R03.1)

  I95.0   **Idiopathic hypotension** — A form of unknown etiology.

  I95.1   **Orthostatic hypotension** — Syncope, or near syncope, due to abnormally low blood pressure when the person stands up.
      Hypotension, postural
      Excludes 1:   *neurogenic orthostatic hypotension [Shy-Drager] (G90.3)*
                  orthostatic hypotension due to drugs (I95.2)

  I95.2   **Hypotension** <u>due to drugs</u>
      Orthostatic hypotension due to drugs
      Use additional code for adverse effect, if applicable, to identify drug (T36-T50 with fifth or sixth character 5)

  I95.3   **Hypotension** <u>of hemodialysis</u> — A form occurring during, or as a result of, hemodialysis.
      Intra-dialytic hypotension

  I95.8-   **Other hypotension**

    I95.81   **Postprocedural hypotension** — A form occurring postoperatively.

    I95.89   **Other hypotension**
        Chronic hypotension

  I95.9   **Hypotension, unspecified**

I96   **Gangrene,** <u>not elsewhere classified</u> — The death of tissue that is usually due to
cc   a loss of vascular supply.
    AHA 13:2Q:p34 – Warfarin induced skin necrosis
    Gangrenous cellulitis
    Excludes 1:   *gangrene in atherosclerosis of native arteries of the extremities (I70.26)*
                gangrene in diabetes mellitus (E08-E13 with .52)
                gangrene in hernia (K40.1, K40.4, K41.1, K41.4, K42.1, K43.1-, K44.1, K45.1, K46.1)
                gangrene in other peripheral vascular diseases (I73-)
                gangrene of certain specified sites — see Alphabetical Index
                gas gangrene (A48.0)
                pyoderma gangrenosum (L88)

I97-   <u>Intraoperative and postprocedural complications</u> and disorders of circulatory system, not elsewhere classified
    Excludes 2:   *postprocedural shock (T81.1-)*

  I97.0   **Postcardiotomy syndrome**

  I97.1-   **Other postprocedural cardiac functional disturbances**
      Excludes 2:   *acute pulmonary insufficiency following thoracic surgery (J95.1)*
                  intraoperative cardiac functional disturbances (I97.7-)

    I97.11-   **Postprocedural cardiac insufficiency**

    cc I97.110   **Postprocedural cardiac insufficiency following cardiac surgery**

    cc I97.111   **Postprocedural cardiac insufficiency following other surgery**

    I97.12-   **Postprocedural cardiac arrest**

    cc I97.120   **Postprocedural cardiac arrest following cardiac surgery**

    cc I97.121   **Postprocedural cardiac arrest following other surgery**

    I97.13-   **Postprocedural heart failure**
      Use additional code to identify the heart failure (I50.-)

    cc I97.130   **Postprocedural heart failure following cardiac surgery**

    cc I97.131   **Postprocedural heart failure following other surgery**

    I97.19-   **Other postprocedural cardiac functional disturbances**
      Use additional code, if applicable, to further specify disorder

    cc I97.190   **Other postprocedural cardiac functional disturbances following cardiac surgery**

    cc I97.191   **Other postprocedural cardiac functional disturbances following other surgery**

  I97.2   **Postmastectomy lymphedema syndrome** — [Age/15-124] — Edema of arm (same side as mastectomy) due to obliteration of lymph nodes and channels from the surgical procedure.
      Elephantiasis due to mastectomy
      Obliteration of lymphatic vessels

  I97.3   **Postprocedural hypertension** — Elevated blood pressure occurring postoperatively.

  I97.4-   <u>Intraoperative hemorrhage and hematoma</u> of a circulatory system organ or structure complicating a procedure
      Excludes 1:   *intraoperative hemorrhage and hematoma of a circulatory system organ or structure due to accidental puncture and laceration during a procedure (I97.5-)*
      Excludes 2:   *intraoperative cerebrovascular hemorrhage complicating a procedure (G97.3-)*

    I97.41-   **Intraoperative hemorrhage and hematoma of a circulatory system organ or structure complicating a circulatory system procedure**

    cc I97.410   **Intraoperative hemorrhage and hematoma of a circulatory system organ or structure** <u>complicating a cardiac catheterization</u>

    cc I97.411   **Intraoperative hemorrhage and hematoma of a circulatory system organ or structure** <u>complicating a cardiac bypass</u>

    cc I97.418   **Intraoperative hemorrhage and hematoma of a circulatory system organ or structure** <u>complicating other circulatory system procedure</u>

    cc I97.42   **Intraoperative hemorrhage and hematoma of a circulatory system organ or structure** <u>complicating other procedure</u>

  I97.5-   <u>Accidental puncture and laceration</u> of a circulatory system organ or structure during a procedure
      Excludes 2:   *accidental puncture and laceration of brain during a procedure (G97.4-)*

    cc I97.51   **Accidental puncture and laceration of a circulatory system organ or structure during a** <u>circulatory system procedure</u>

    cc I97.52   **Accidental puncture and laceration of a circulatory system organ or structure during** <u>other procedure</u>

  I97.6-   <u>Postprocedural hemorrhage, hematoma and seroma</u> of a circulatory system organ or structure following a procedure
      Excludes 2:   *postprocedural cerebrovascular hemorrhage complicating a procedure (G97.5-)*

    I97.61-   **Postprocedural** <u>hemorrhage</u> **of a circulatory system organ or structure following a circulatory system procedure**

    cc I97.610   **Postprocedural** <u>hemorrhage</u> **of a circulatory system organ or structure following a** <u>cardiac catheterization</u>

    cc I97.611   **Postprocedural** <u>hemorrhage</u> **of a circulatory system organ or structure following** <u>cardiac bypass</u>

    cc I97.618   **Postprocedural** <u>hemorrhage</u> **of a circulatory system organ or structure following** <u>other circulatory system procedure</u>

    I97.62-   <u>Postprocedural hemorrhage, hematoma and seroma</u> **of a circulatory system organ or structure** <u>following other procedure</u>

    cc I97.620   **Postprocedural** <u>hemorrhage</u> **of a circulatory system organ or structure following** <u>other procedure</u>

    cc I97.621   **Postprocedural** <u>hematoma</u> **of a circulatory system organ or structure following** <u>other procedure</u>

    cc I97.622   **Postprocedural** <u>seroma</u> **of a circulatory system organ or structure following** <u>other procedure</u>

I95-I97

I97.63- <u>Postprocedural hematoma</u> of a circulatory system organ or structure <u>following a circulatory system procedure</u>

cc I97.630   Postprocedural <u>hematoma</u> of a circulatory system organ or structure following a <u>cardiac catheterization</u>

cc I97.631   Postprocedural <u>hematoma</u> of a circulatory system organ or structure following <u>cardiac bypass</u>

cc I97.638   Postprocedural <u>hematoma</u> of a circulatory system organ or structure following <u>other circulatory system procedure</u>

I97.64- <u>Postprocedural seroma</u> of a circulatory system organ or structure <u>following a circulatory system procedure</u>

cc I97.640   Postprocedural <u>seroma</u> of a circulatory system organ or structure following a <u>cardiac catheterization</u>

cc I97.641   Postprocedural <u>seroma</u> of a circulatory system organ or structure following <u>cardiac bypass</u>

cc I97.648   Postprocedural <u>seroma</u> of a circulatory system organ or structure following <u>other circulatory system procedure</u>

I97.7-   **Intraoperative cardiac functional disturbances**
        Excludes ❷: acute pulmonary insufficiency following thoracic surgery (J95.1)
                     postprocedural cardiac functional disturbances (I97.1-)

I97.71- **Intraoperative cardiac arrest**

cc I97.710   Intraoperative cardiac arrest during <u>cardiac</u> surgery

cc I97.711   Intraoperative cardiac arrest during <u>other</u> surgery

I97.79- **Other intraoperative cardiac functional disturbances**
        Use additional code, if applicable, to further specify disorder

cc I97.790   Other intraoperative cardiac functional disturbances during <u>cardiac</u> surgery

cc I97.791   Other intraoperative cardiac functional disturbances during <u>other</u> surgery

I97.8-   **Other intraoperative and postprocedural complications and disorders of the circulatory system, not elsewhere classified**
        Use additional code, if applicable, to further specify disorder

I97.81- **Intraoperative cerebrovascular infarction**

cc I97.810   Intraoperative cerebrovascular infarction during <u>cardiac</u> surgery

cc I97.811   Intraoperative cerebrovascular infarction during <u>other</u> surgery

I97.82- **Postprocedural cerebrovascular infarction**

cc I97.820   Postprocedural cerebrovascular infarction following <u>cardiac</u> surgery

cc I97.821   Postprocedural cerebrovascular infarction following <u>other</u> surgery

cc I97.88 Other intraoperative complications of the circulatory system, <u>not elsewhere classified</u>

cc I97.89 Other postprocedural complications and disorders of the circulatory system, not elsewhere classified

I99- **Other and unspecified disorders of circulatory system**

I99.8   **Other disorder of circulatory system**

I99.9   **Unspecified disorder of circulatory system**

I
9
9
-
I
9
9

Chapter 10 – Diseases of the respiratory system (J00-J99)

Note: When a respiratory condition is described as occurring in more than one site and is not specifically indexed, it should be classified to the lower anatomic site (e.g. tracheobronchitis to bronchitis in J40).
Use additional code, where applicable, to identify:
Exposure to environmental tobacco smoke (Z77.22)
Exposure to tobacco smoke in the perinatal period (P96.81)
History of tobacco dependence (Z87.891)
Occupational exposure to environmental tobacco smoke (Z57.31)
Tobacco dependence (F17.-)
Tobacco use (Z72.0)

Excludes ❷: *certain conditions originating in the perinatal period (P04-P96)*
certain infectious and parasitic diseases (A00-B99)
complications of pregnancy, childbirth and the puerperium (O00-O9A)
congenital malformations, deformations and chromosomal abnormalities (Q00-Q99)
endocrine, nutritional and metabolic diseases (E00-E88)
injury, poisoning and certain other consequences of external causes (S00-T88)
neoplasms (C00-D49)
smoke inhalation (T59.81-)
symptoms, signs and abnormal clinical and laboratory findings, not elsewhere classified (R00-R94)

This chapter contains the following blocks:

J00-J06	Acute upper respiratory infections
J09-J18	Influenza and pneumonia
J20-J22	Other acute lower respiratory infections
J30-J39	Other diseases of upper respiratory tract
J40-J47	Chronic lower respiratory diseases
J60-J70	Lung diseases due to external agents
J80-J84	Other respiratory diseases principally affecting the interstitium
J85-J86	Suppurative and necrotic conditions of the lower respiratory tract
J90-J94	Other diseases of the pleura
J95	Intraoperative and postprocedural complications and disorders of respiratory system, not elsewhere classified
J96-J99	Other diseases of the respiratory system

Chapter-Specific Coding Guidelines

C.   Chapter-Specific Coding Guidelines
In addition to general coding guidelines, there are guidelines for specific diagnoses and/or conditions in the classification. Unless otherwise indicated, these guidelines apply to all health care settings. Please refer to Section II for guidelines on the selection of principal diagnosis.

10.   Chapter 10: Diseases of the Respiratory System (J00-J99)

a.   Chronic Obstructive Pulmonary Disease [COPD] and Asthma

1)   Acute exacerbation of chronic obstructive bronchitis and asthma
The codes in categories J44 and J45 distinguish between uncomplicated cases and those in acute exacerbation. An acute exacerbation is a worsening or a decompensation of a chronic condition. An acute exacerbation is not equivalent to an infection superimposed on a chronic condition, though an exacerbation may be triggered by an infection.

b.   Acute Respiratory Failure

1)   Acute respiratory failure as principal diagnosis
A code from subcategory J96.0, Acute respiratory failure, or subcategory J96.2, Acute and chronic respiratory failure, may be assigned as a principal diagnosis when it is the condition established after study to be chiefly responsible for occasioning the admission to the hospital, and the selection is supported by the Alphabetic Index and Tabular List. However, chapter-specific coding guidelines (such as obstetrics, poisoning, HIV, newborn) that provide sequencing direction take precedence.

2)   Acute respiratory failure as secondary diagnosis
Respiratory failure may be listed as a secondary diagnosis if it occurs after admission, or if it is present on admission, but does not meet the definition of principal diagnosis.

3)   Sequencing of acute respiratory failure and another acute condition
When a patient is admitted with respiratory failure and another acute condition, (e.g., myocardial infarction, cerebrovascular accident, aspiration pneumonia), the principal diagnosis will not be the same in every situation. This applies whether the other acute condition is a respiratory or nonrespiratory condition. Selection of the principal diagnosis will be dependent on the circumstances of admission. If both the respiratory failure and the other acute condition are equally responsible for occasioning the admission to the hospital, and there are no chapter-specific sequencing rules, the guideline regarding two or more diagnoses that equally meet the definition for principal diagnosis (*Section II, C.*) may be applied in these situations.

If the documentation is not clear as to whether acute respiratory failure and another condition are equally responsible for occasioning the admission, query the provider for clarification.

c.   Influenza due to certain identified influenza viruses
Code only confirmed cases of influenza due to certain identified influenza viruses (category J09), and due to other identified influenza virus (category J10). This is an exception to the hospital inpatient guideline Section II, H. (Uncertain Diagnosis).

In this context, "confirmation" does not require documentation of positive laboratory testing specific for avian or other novel influenza A or other identified influenza virus. However, coding should be based on the provider's diagnostic statement that the patient has avian influenza, or other novel influenza A, for category J09, or has another particular identified strain of influenza, such as H1N1 or H3N2, but not identified as novel or variant, for category J10.

If the provider records "suspected" or "possible" or "probable" avian influenza, or novel influenza, or other identified influenza, then the appropriate influenza code from category J11, Influenza due to unidentified influenza virus, should be assigned. A code from category J09, Influenza due to certain identified influenza viruses, should not be assigned nor should a code from category J10, Influenza due to other identified influenza virus.

d.   Ventilator associated Pneumonia

1)   Documentation of Ventilator associated Pneumonia
As with all procedural or postprocedural complications, code assignment is based on the provider's documentation of the relationship between the condition and the procedure.

Code J95.851, Ventilator associated pneumonia, should be assigned only when the provider has documented ventilator associated pneumonia (VAP). An additional code to identify the organism (e.g., Pseudomonas aeruginosa, code B96.5) should also be assigned. Do not assign an additional code from categories J12-J18 to identify the type of pneumonia.

Code J95.851 should not be assigned for cases where the patient has pneumonia and is on a mechanical ventilator and the provider has not specifically stated that the pneumonia is ventilator-associated pneumonia. If the documentation is unclear as to whether the patient has a pneumonia that is a complication attributable to the mechanical ventilator, query the provider.

2)   Ventilator associated Pneumonia Develops after Admission
A patient may be admitted with one type of pneumonia (e.g., code J13, Pneumonia due to Streptococcus pneumonia) and subsequently develop VAP. In this instance, the principal diagnosis would be the appropriate code from categories J12-J18 for the pneumonia diagnosed at the time of admission. Code J95.851, Ventilator associated pneumonia, would be assigned as an additional diagnosis when the provider has also documented the presence of ventilator associated pneumonia.

Acute upper respiratory infections (J00-J06)

Excludes 1:   chronic obstructive pulmonary disease with acute lower respiratory infection (J44.0)
influenza virus with other respiratory manifestations (J09.x2, J10.1, J11.1)

J00   Acute nasopharyngitis [common cold] — A sudden severe onset of mucous membrane inflammation of the nasopharynx that is marked by nasal congestion, continuous watery discharge, and malaise.
Acute rhinitis
Coryza (acute)
Infective nasopharyngitis NOS
Infective rhinitis
Nasal catarrh, acute
Nasopharyngitis NOS
Excludes 1:   acute pharyngitis (J02.-)
acute sore throat NOS (J02.9)
pharyngitis NOS (J02.9)
rhinitis NOS (J31.0)
sore throat NOS (J02.9)
Excludes ❷: allergic rhinitis (J30.1-J30.9)
chronic pharyngitis (J31.2)
chronic rhinitis (J31.0)
chronic sore throat (J31.2)
nasopharyngitis, chronic (J31.1)
vasomotor rhinitis (J30.0)

J00 - J00

J01- **Acute sinusitis** — A sudden, severe onset of inflammation of the paranasal sinuses.
Includes: **Acute abscess of sinus** — A form marked by a localized collection of pus caused by the disintegration of sinus mucous membrane tissue.
Acute empyema of sinus — A form marked by an accumulation of pus within the sinus cavities.
Acute infection of sinus — A form caused by microorganisms.
Acute inflammation of sinus — A sudden, severe onset of inflammation of the paranasal sinuses.
Acute suppuration of sinus — A form marked by a pus-producing inflammation of the sinuses.
Use additional code (B95-B97) to identify infectious agent
Excludes 1: *sinusitis NOS (J32.9)*
Excludes ❷: *chronic sinusitis (J32.0-J32.8)*

J01.0- **Acute maxillary sinusitis** — A form affecting one of the paranasal sinuses, located in the body of the maxilla.
Acute antritis — A sudden, severe inflammation of the maxillary antrum.

J01.00 **Acute maxillary sinusitis, unspecified**

J01.01 **Acute recurrent maxillary sinusitis**

J01.1- **Acute frontal sinusitis** — A form affecting one of the paired paranasal sinuses, located in the frontal bone.

J01.10 **Acute frontal sinusitis, unspecified**

J01.11 **Acute recurrent frontal sinusitis**

J01.2- **Acute ethmoidal sinusitis** — A form affecting one of the grouped paranasal sinuses, located in the ethmoid bone.

J01.20 **Acute ethmoidal sinusitis, unspecified**

J01.21 **Acute recurrent ethmoidal sinusitis**

J01.3- **Acute sphenoidal sinusitis** — A form affecting one of the paired paranasal sinuses, located in the anterior part of the body of the sphenoid bone.

J01.30 **Acute sphenoidal sinusitis, unspecified**

J01.31 **Acute recurrent sphenoidal sinusitis**

J01.4- **Acute pansinusitis** — A sudden, severe inflammation involving all of the paranasal sinuses.

J01.40 **Acute pansinusitis, unspecified**

J01.41 **Acute recurrent pansinusitis**

J01.8- **Other acute sinusitis**

J01.80 **Other acute sinusitis**
Acute sinusitis involving more than one sinus but not pansinusitis

J01.81 **Other acute recurrent sinusitis**
Acute recurrent sinusitis involving more than one sinus but not pansinusitis

J01.9- **Acute sinusitis, unspecified**

J01.90 **Acute sinusitis, unspecified**

J01.91 **Acute recurrent sinusitis, unspecified**

J02- **Acute pharyngitis** — A sudden, severe inflammation of the pharynx.
Includes: **Acute sore throat** — A common term referring to acute pharyngitis.
Excludes 1: *acute laryngopharyngitis (J06.0)*
peritonsillar abscess (J36)
pharyngeal abscess (J39.1)
retropharyngeal abscess (J39.0)
Excludes ❷: *chronic pharyngitis (J31.2)*

J02.0 **Streptococcal pharyngitis** — An infectious disease caused by Streptococcus pyogenes, and characterized by severe sore throat, fever, vomiting, headache, and malaise.
Septic pharyngitis
Streptococcal sore throat
Excludes ❷: *scarlet fever (A38.-)*

J02.8 **Acute pharyngitis due to other specified organisms**
Use additional code (B95-B97) to identify infectious agent
Excludes 1: *acute pharyngitis due to coxsackie virus (B08.5)*
acute pharyngitis due to gonococcus (A54.5)
acute pharyngitis due to herpes [simplex] virus (B00.2)
acute pharyngitis due to infectious mononucleosis (B27.-)
enteroviral vesicular pharyngitis (B08.5)

J02.9 **Acute pharyngitis, unspecified**
Gangrenous pharyngitis (acute) — A form characterized by gangrenous patches.
Infective pharyngitis (acute) NOS
Pharyngitis (acute) NOS
Sore throat (acute) NOS
Suppurative pharyngitis (acute) — A form characterized by the production of pus.
Ulcerative pharyngitis (acute) — A form characterized by ulcers covered by a yellow, membrane-like deposit in the pharynx, with fever, pain, and prostration.

J03- **Acute tonsillitis** — A sudden, severe onset of inflammation of the tonsils, in which the tonsils are red and swollen.
Excludes 1: *acute sore throat (J02.-)*
hypertrophy of tonsils (J35.1)
peritonsillar abscess (J36)
sore throat NOS (J02.9)
streptococcal sore throat (J02.0)
Excludes ❷: *chronic tonsillitis (J35.0)*

J03.0- **Streptococcal tonsillitis** — A form caused by streptococcal microorganisms.

J03.00 **Acute streptococcal tonsillitis, unspecified**

J03.01 **Acute recurrent streptococcal tonsillitis**

J03.8- **Acute tonsillitis due to other specified organisms**
Use additional code (B95-B97) to identify infectious agent.
Excludes 1: *diphtheritic tonsillitis (A36.0)*
herpesviral pharyngotonsillitis (B00.2)
streptococcal tonsillitis (J03.0)
tuberculous tonsillitis (A15.8)
Vincent's tonsillitis (A69.1)

J03.80 **Acute tonsillitis due to other specified organisms**

J03.81 **Acute recurrent tonsillitis due to other specified organisms**

J03.9- **Acute tonsillitis, unspecified**
Follicular tonsillitis (acute) — A form characterized by affecting the crypts.
Gangrenous tonsillitis (acute) — A form characterized by gangrenous patches.
Infective tonsillitis (acute)
Tonsillitis (acute) NOS
Ulcerative tonsillitis (acute) — A form characterized by the eating-away and disintegration of the tonsil tissue.

J03.90 **Acute tonsillitis, unspecified**

J03.91 **Acute recurrent tonsillitis, unspecified**

J04- **Acute laryngitis and tracheitis** — A sudden, severe onset of inflammation of the larynx and/or trachea.
Use additional code (B95-B97) to identify infectious agent.
Excludes 1: *acute obstructive laryngitis [croup] and epiglottitis (J05.-)*
Excludes ❷: *laryngismus (stridulus) (J38.5)*

J04.0 **Acute laryngitis** — A sudden, severe onset of inflammation of the larynx.
Edematous laryngitis (acute) — A form characterized by abnormally large amounts of intercellular fluid of the laryngeal tissues.
Laryngitis (acute) NOS
Subglottic laryngitis (acute)
Suppurative laryngitis (acute) — A form caused by the production of pus.
Ulcerative laryngitis (acute) — A form characterized by the eating-away of laryngeal tissue.
Excludes 1: *acute obstructive laryngitis (J05.0)*
Excludes ❷: *chronic laryngitis (J37.0)*

J04.1- **Acute tracheitis** — A sudden, severe onset of inflammation of the trachea.
Acute viral tracheitis — A form caused by viral microorganisms.
Catarrhal tracheitis (acute) — A form caused by severe inflammation of the mucous membranes.
Tracheitis (acute) NOS
Excludes ❷: *chronic tracheitis (J42)*

J04.10 **Acute tracheitis without obstruction**

MCC **J04.11** **Acute tracheitis with obstruction** — A form marked by blockage of the airflow.

J04.2 **Acute laryngotracheitis** — A sudden, severe onset of inflammation of the larynx and trachea.
Laryngotracheitis NOS
Tracheitis (acute) with laryngitis (acute)
Excludes 1: *acute obstructive laryngotracheitis (J05.0)*
Excludes ❷: *chronic laryngotracheitis (J37.1)*

J04.3- **Supraglottitis, unspecified** — A form affecting the tissues just above the vocal cords.

J04.30 **Supraglottitis, unspecified, without obstruction**

MCC **J04.31** **Supraglottitis, unspecified, with obstruction** — A form marked by blockage of the airflow.

J05- **Acute obstructive laryngitis [croup] and epiglottitis**
Use additional code (B95-B97) to identify infectious agent.

J05.0 **Acute obstructive laryngitis [croup]** — A sudden, severe onset of obstruction of the larynx in infants and young children characterized by resonant barking cough, laryngeal spasm, difficult breathing, and hoarseness, usually due to an upper respiratory infection.
Obstructive laryngitis (acute) NOS
Obstructive laryngotracheitis NOS

J05.1-   **Acute <u>epiglottitis</u>** — A sudden, severe onset of inflammation of the flap of tissue at the opening to the larynx.

    Excludes ❷: *epiglottitis, chronic (J37.0)*

cc **J05.10**   **Acute epiglottitis <u>without</u> obstruction**
    Epiglottitis NOS

mcc **J05.11**   **Acute epiglottitis <u>with obstruction</u>** — A form marked by blockage of the airflow.

J06-   **Acute upper respiratory infections of multiple and unspecified sites**

    Excludes 1: *acute respiratory infection NOS (J22)*
                   streptococcal pharyngitis (J02.0)

J06.0   **Acute laryngopharyngitis** — A sudden, severe onset of inflammation of the larynx and pharynx.

J06.9   **Acute upper respiratory infection, unspecified**
    Upper respiratory disease, acute
    Upper respiratory infection NOS

Influenza and pneumonia (J09-J18)

    Excludes ❷: *allergic or eosinophilic pneumonia (J82)*
                  aspiration pneumonia NOS (J69.0)
                  congenital pneumonia (P23.9)
                  lipid pneumonia (J69.1)
                  meconium pneumonia (P24.01)
                  neonatal aspiration pneumonia (P24.-)
                  pneumonia due to solids and liquids (J69.-)
                  rheumatic pneumonia (I00)
                  ventilator associated pneumonia (J95.851)

J09-   **Influenza due to certain identified influenza viruses** — Infection of the respiratory tract by certain influenza viruses.

    Excludes 1: *influenza due to other identified influenza virus (J10-)*
                  influenza due to unidentified influenza virus (J11-)
                  seasonal influenza due to other identified influenza virus (J10-)
                  seasonal influenza due to unidentified influenza virus (J11-)

J09.x-   **Influenza due to <u>identified novel influenza A virus</u>** — Infection of the respiratory tract by novel influenza A viruses.
    Avian influenza
    Bird influenza
    Influenza A/H5N1
    Influenza of other animal origin, not bird or swine
    Swine influenza virus (viruses that normally cause infections in pigs)

mcc **J09.x1**   **Influenza due to identified novel influenza A virus <u>with pneumonia</u>** — A form marked by the concurring presence of inflammation of the lungs with exudate-filled air spaces.
    Code also, if applicable, associated:
    Lung abscess (J85.1)
    Other specified type of pneumonia

J09.x2   **Influenza due to identified novel influenza A virus <u>with other respiratory</u> manifestations** — A form marked by fever, chills, malaise, cough, coryza, muscle aches, and prostration which may involve the upper respiratory organs.
    Influenza due to identified novel influenza A virus NOS
    Influenza due to identified novel influenza A virus with laryngitis
    Influenza due to identified novel influenza A virus with pharyngitis
    Influenza due to identified novel influenza A virus with upper respiratory symptoms
    Use additional code, if applicable, for associated:
    Pleural effusion (J91.8)
    Sinusitis (J01.-)

J09.x3   **Influenza due to identified novel influenza A virus <u>with gastrointestinal manifestations</u>** — A form marked by infection of the gastrointestinal tract.
    Influenza due to identified novel influenza A virus gastroenteritis

    Excludes 1: *"intestinal flu" [viral gastroenteritis] (A08-)*

J09.x9   **Influenza due to identified novel influenza A virus <u>with</u> other manifestations**
    Influenza due to identified novel influenza A virus with encephalopathy
    Influenza due to identified novel influenza A virus with myocarditis
    Influenza due to identified novel influenza A virus with otitis media
    Use additional code to identify manifestation

J10-   **Influenza due to <u>other identified influenza</u> virus** — Infection of the respiratory tract by other (non novel influenza A viruses) influenza viruses.

    Excludes 1: *influenza due to avian influenza virus (J09.x-)*
                  influenza due to swine flu (J09.x-)
                  influenza due to unidentified influenza virus (J11-)

J10.0-   **Influenza due to <u>other</u> identified influenza virus <u>with pneumonia</u>** — A form marked by the concurring presence of inflammation of the lungs with exudate-filled air spaces.
    Code also associated lung abscess, if applicable (J85.1)

mcc **J10.00**   **Influenza due to <u>other</u> identified influenza virus <u>with unspecified type of pneumonia</u>**

mcc **J10.01**   **Influenza due to <u>other</u> identified influenza virus <u>with the same other identified influenza virus pneumonia</u>**

mcc **J10.08**   **Influenza due to <u>other</u> identified influenza virus <u>with other specified pneumonia</u>**
    Code also other specified type of pneumonia

J10.1   **Influenza due to <u>other</u> identified influenza virus <u>with other respiratory</u> manifestations** — A form marked by fever, chills, malaise, cough, coryza, muscle aches, and prostration which may involve the upper respiratory organs.
    Influenza due to other identified influenza virus NOS
    Influenza due to other identified influenza virus with laryngitis
    Influenza due to other identified influenza virus with pharyngitis
    Influenza due to other identified influenza virus with upper respiratory symptoms
    Use additional code for associated pleural effusion, if applicable (J91.8)
    Use additional code for associated sinusitis, if applicable (J01.-)

J10.2   **Influenza due to <u>other</u> identified influenza virus <u>with gastrointestinal manifestations</u>** — A form marked by infection of the gastrointestinal tract.
    Influenza due to other identified influenza virus gastroenteritis

    Excludes 1: *"intestinal flu" [viral gastroenteritis] (A08.-)*

J10.8-   **Influenza due to <u>other</u> identified influenza virus <u>with other manifestations</u>**

J10.81   **Influenza due to <u>other</u> identified influenza virus <u>with encephalopathy</u>**

J10.82   **Influenza due to <u>other</u> identified influenza virus <u>with myocarditis</u>**

J10.83   **Influenza due to <u>other</u> identified influenza virus <u>with otitis media</u>**
    Use additional code for any associated perforated tympanic membrane (H72.-)

J10.89   **Influenza due to <u>other</u> identified influenza virus <u>with other manifestations</u>**
    Use additional codes to identify the manifestations

J11-   **Influenza due to <u>unidentified influenza virus</u>**

J11.0-   **Influenza due to <u>unidentified</u> influenza virus with pneumonia** — A form marked by the concurring presence of inflammation of the lungs with exudate-filled air spaces.
    Code also associated lung abscess, if applicable (J85.1)

mcc **J11.00**   **Influenza due to <u>unidentified</u> influenza virus <u>with unspecified type of pneumonia</u>**
    Influenza with pneumonia NOS

mcc **J11.08**   **Influenza due to <u>unidentified</u> influenza virus <u>with specified pneumonia</u>**
    Code also other specified type of pneumonia

J11.1   **Influenza due to <u>unidentified</u> influenza virus <u>with other respiratory</u> manifestations** — A form marked by fever, chills, malaise, cough, coryza, muscle aches, and prostration which may involve the upper respiratory organs.
    Influenza NOS
    Influenzal laryngitis NOS
    Influenzal pharyngitis NOS
    Influenza with upper respiratory symptoms NOS
    Use additional code for associated pleural effusion, if applicable (J91.8)
    Use additional code for associated sinusitis, if applicable (J01.-)

J11.2   **Influenza due to <u>unidentified</u> influenza virus <u>with gastrointestinal manifestations</u>** — A form marked by infection of the gastrointestinal tract.
    Influenza gastroenteritis NOS

    Excludes 1: *"intestinal flu" [viral gastroenteritis] (A08.-)*

J 0 5 - J 1 1

Excludes 1: = NOT CODED HERE! (Do not code both)

Excludes ❷: = Not Included Here

J11.8- **Influenza due to <u>unidentified</u> influenza virus <u>with other manifestations</u>**

    J11.81 **Influenza due to <u>unidentified</u> influenza virus <u>with encephalopathy</u>**
        Influenzal encephalopathy NOS

    J11.82 **Influenza due to <u>unidentified</u> influenza virus <u>with myocarditis</u>**
        Influenzal myocarditis NOS

    J11.83 **Influenza due to <u>unidentified</u> influenza virus <u>with otitis media</u>**
        Influenzal otitis media NOS
        Use additional code for any associated perforated tympanic membrane (H72.-)

    J11.89 **Influenza due to <u>unidentified</u> influenza virus <u>with other manifestations</u>**
        Use additional codes to identify the manifestations

J12- **Viral pneumonia, <u>not elsewhere classified</u>** — Inflammation of the lung with exudate-filled air spaces caused by viral microorganisms.
    Includes: Bronchopneumonia due to viruses other than influenza viruses
    Code first associated influenza, if applicable (J09.x1, J10.0-, J11.0-)
    Code also associated abscess, if applicable (J85.1)
    Excludes 1:   *aspiration pneumonia due to anesthesia during labor and delivery (O74.0)*
        aspiration pneumonia due to anesthesia during pregnancy (O29)
        aspiration pneumonia due to anesthesia during puerperium (O89.0)
        aspiration pneumonia due to solids and liquids (J69.-)
        aspiration pneumonia NOS (J69.0)
        congenital pneumonia (P23.0)
        congenital rubella pneumonitis (P35.0)
        interstitial pneumonia NOS (J84.9)
        lipid pneumonia (J69.1)
        neonatal aspiration pneumonia (P24.-)

MCC **J12.0** **Adenoviral pneumonia** — A form caused by the group of adenovirus microorganisms.

MCC **J12.1** **Respiratory syncytial virus pneumonia** — A form caused by the group of respiratory syncytial virus (RSV) microorganisms.

MCC **J12.2** **Parainfluenza virus pneumonia** — A form caused by the group of parainfluenzal viral (HPIVs) microorganisms.

MCC **J12.3** **Human metapneumovirus pneumonia** — A form caused by the group of human metapneumovirus (hMPV) microorganisms.

    J12.8- **Other viral pneumonia**

   MCC **J12.81** **Pneumonia due to SARS-associated coronavirus** — A form caused by the group of SARS-associated coronavirus (SARS-CoV) microorganisms.
        Severe acute respiratory syndrome NOS

   MCC **J12.89** **Other viral pneumonia**

MCC **J12.9** **Viral pneumonia, unspecified**

J13 **Pneumonia due to Streptococcus pneumoniae** — Inflammation of the lungs
MCC with exudate-filled air spaces caused by Streptococcal pneumoconiae microorganisms.
    Bronchopneumonia due to S. pneumoniae
    Code first associated influenza, if applicable (J09.x1, J10.0-, J11.0-)
    Code also associated abscess, if applicable (J85.1)
    Excludes 1:   *congenital pneumonia due to S. pneumoniae (P23.6)*
        lobar pneumonia, unspecified organism (J18.1)
        pneumonia due to other streptococci (J15.3-J15.4)

J14 **Pneumonia due to Hemophilus influenzae** — A form caused by the
MCC microorganism Hemophilus influenzae, usually seen with chronic bronchopulmonary disease but may occur rarely as a primary infection.
    Bronchopneumonia due to H. influenzae
    Code first associated influenza, if applicable (J09.x1, J10.0-, J11.0-)
    Code also associated abscess, if applicable (J85.1)
    Excludes 1:   *congenital pneumonia due to H. influenzae (P23.6)*

J15- **Bacterial pneumonia, <u>not elsewhere classified</u>**
    Includes: Bronchopneumonia due to bacteria other than S. pneumoniae and H. influenzae
    Code first associated influenza, if applicable (J09.x1, J10.0-, J11.0-)
    Code also associated abscess, if applicable (J85.1)
    Excludes 1:   *chlamydial pneumonia (J16.0)*
        congenital pneumonia (P23.-)
        Legionnaires' disease (A48.1)
        spirochetal pneumonia (A69.8)

MCC **J15.0** **Pneumonia due to Klebsiella pneumoniae** — A form caused by the microorganism Klebsiella pneumoniae and characterized by massive mucoid inflammatory exudates in the lung.

MCC **J15.1** **Pneumonia due to Pseudomonas** — A form caused by the pseudomonas microorganisms, including Pseudomonas aeruginosa.

    J15.2- **Pneumonia due to staphylococcus** — A form caused by staphylococcal microorganisms, many strains of which are antibiotic resistant.

   MCC **J15.20** **Pneumonia due to staphylococcus, unspecified**

    J15.21- **Pneumonia due to Staphylococcus aureus**

   MCC **J15.211** **Pneumonia due to methicillin susceptible Staphylococcus aureus** — A form caused by a form of the bacterium Staphylococcus aureus that is susceptible to antibiotic treatment.
        MSSA pneumonia
        Pneumonia due to Staphylococcus aureus NOS

   MCC **J15.212** **Pneumonia due to methicillin resistant Staphylococcus aureus** — A form caused by a form of the bacterium Staphylococcus aureus that is resistant to treatment from beta-lactam class antibiotics.

   MCC **J15.29** **Pneumonia due to other staphylococcus**

MCC **J15.3** **Pneumonia due to streptococcus, group B** — A form caused by Streptococcus agalactiae.

MCC **J15.4** **Pneumonia due to other streptococci**
    Excludes 1:   *pneumonia due to streptococcus, group B (J15.3)*
        pneumonia due to Streptococcus pneumoniae (J13)

MCC **J15.5** **Pneumonia due to Escherichia coli** — A form caused by Escherichia coli, normally present in intestinal flora, but pathogenic in the lungs.

MCC **J15.6** **Pneumonia due to other aerobic Gram-negative bacteria**
    Pneumonia due to Serratia marcescens — A form caused by the species Serratia marcescens.

MCC **J15.7** **Pneumonia due to Mycoplasma pneumoniae** — The most common form of primary atypical pneumonia caused by the microorganism Mycoplasma pneumoniae.

MCC **J15.8** **Pneumonia due to other specified bacteria**

MCC **J15.9** **Unspecified bacterial pneumonia**
    Pneumonia due to gram-positive bacteria

J16- **Pneumonia due to other infectious organisms, <u>not elsewhere classified</u>**
    Code first associated influenza, if applicable (J09.x1, J10.0-, J11.0-)
    Code also associated abscess, if applicable (J85.1)
    Excludes 1:   *congenital pneumonia (P23.-)*
        ornithosis (A70)
        pneumocystosis (B59)
        pneumonia NOS (J18.9)

MCC **J16.0** **Chlamydial pneumonia** — A form caused by the chlamydial gram-negative bacteria.

MCC **J16.8** **Pneumonia due to other specified infectious organisms**

J11-J16 (side tab)

Excludes 1: = NOT CODED HERE! (Do not code both)   **764**   *Excludes ❷: =* Not Included Here

J17 **Pneumonia** <u>in diseases classified elsewhere</u> — [Not Allowed as PDX]
MCC   Code first underlying disease, such as:
    Q fever (A78)
    Rheumatic fever (I00)
    Schistosomiasis (B65.0-B65.9)
    Excludes 1:   *candidial pneumonia (B37.1)*
            chlamydial pneumonia (J16.0)
            gonorrheal pneumonia (A54.84)
            histoplasmosis pneumonia (B39.0-B39.2)
            measles pneumonia (B05.2)
            nocardiosis pneumonia (A43.0)
            pneumocystosis (B59)
            pneumonia due to Pneumocystis carinii (B59)
            pneumonia due to Pneumocystis jiroveci (B59)
            pneumonia in actinomycosis (A42.0)
            pneumonia in anthrax (A22.1)
            pneumonia in ascariasis (B77.81)
            pneumonia in aspergillosis (B44.0-B44.1)
            pneumonia in coccidioidomycosis (B38.0-B38.2)
            pneumonia in cytomegalovirus disease (B25.0)
            pneumonia in toxoplasmosis (B58.3)
            rubella pneumonia (B06.81)
            salmonella pneumonia (A02.22)
            spirochetal infection NEC with pneumonia (A69.8)
            tularemia pneumonia (A21.2)
            typhoid fever with pneumonia (A01.03)
            varicella pneumonia (B01.2)
            whooping cough with pneumonia (A37 with fifth-character 1)

J18- **Pneumonia,** <u>unspecified organism</u>
    AHA 14:3Q:p4 – SIRS secondary to pneumonia
    Code first associated influenza, if applicable (J09.x1, J10.0-, J11.0-)
    Excludes 1: *abscess of lung with pneumonia (J85.1)*
           aspiration pneumonia due to anesthesia during labor and delivery (O74.0)
           aspiration pneumonia due to anesthesia during pregnancy (O29)
           aspiration pneumonia due to anesthesia during puerperium (O89.0)
           aspiration pneumonia due to solids and liquids (J69.-)
           aspiration pneumonia NOS (J69.0)
           congenital pneumonia (P23.0)
           drug-induced interstitial lung disorder (J70.2-J70.4)
           interstitial pneumonia NOS (J84.9)
           lipid pneumonia (J69.1)
           neonatal aspiration pneumonia (P24.-)
           pneumonitis due to external agents (J67-J70)
           pneumonitis due to fumes and vapors (J68.0)
           usual interstitial pneumonia (J84.17)

MCC **J18.0** **Bronchopneumonia, unspecified organism** — Inflammation of the lungs which usually begins in the terminal bronchioles and causes the air spaces to become filled with exudates.
    Excludes 1: *hypostatic bronchopneumonia (J18.2)*
           lipid pneumonia (J69.1)
    Excludes ❷: *acute bronchiolitis (J21.-)*
           chronic bronchiolitis (J44.9)

MCC **J18.1** **Lobar pneumonia, unspecified organism**

CC **J18.2** **Hypostatic pneumonia, unspecified organism**
    Hypostatic bronchopneumonia
    Passive pneumonia

MCC **J18.8** **Other pneumonia, unspecified organism**

MCC **J18.9** **Pneumonia, unspecified organism**

Other acute lower respiratory infections (J20-J22)

    Excludes ❷: *chronic obstructive pulmonary disease with acute lower respiratory infection (J44.0)*

J20- **Acute bronchitis** — A sudden, severe onset of inflammation of the bronchi.
    Includes: **Acute and subacute bronchitis (with) bronchospasm** — A form marked by spasmodic contraction (tightening) of the muscles in the walls of the bronchioles.
        Acute and subacute bronchitis (with) tracheitis
        Acute and subacute bronchitis (with) tracheobronchitis, acute
        Acute and subacute fibrinous bronchitis
        Acute and subacute membranous bronchitis
        Acute and subacute purulent bronchitis
        Acute and subacute septic bronchitis
    Excludes 1: *bronchitis NOS (J40)*
           tracheobronchitis NOS (J40)
    Excludes ❷: *acute bronchitis with bronchiectasis (J47.0)*
           acute bronchitis with chronic obstructive asthma (J44.0)
           acute bronchitis with chronic obstructive pulmonary disease (J44.0)
           allergic bronchitis NOS (J45.909-)
           bronchitis due to chemicals, fumes and vapors (J68.0)
           chronic bronchitis NOS (J42)
           chronic mucopurulent bronchitis (J41.1)
           chronic obstructive bronchitis (J44.-)
           chronic obstructive tracheobronchitis (J44.-)
           chronic simple bronchitis (J41.0)
           chronic tracheobronchitis (J42)

J20.0 **Acute bronchitis due to Mycoplasma pneumoniae**
J20.1 **Acute bronchitis due to Hemophilus influenzae**
J20.2 **Acute bronchitis due to streptococcus**
J20.3 **Acute bronchitis due to coxsackievirus**
J20.4 **Acute bronchitis due to parainfluenza virus**
J20.5 **Acute bronchitis due to respiratory syncytial virus**
J20.6 **Acute bronchitis due to rhinovirus**
J20.7 **Acute bronchitis due to echovirus**
J20.8 **Acute bronchitis due to other specified organisms**
J20.9 **Acute bronchitis, unspecified**

J21- **Acute bronchiolitis** — A sudden, severe onset of inflammation of the bronchioles (the fine, small bronchial tubes).
    Includes: **Acute bronchiolitis with bronchospasm** — A form marked by spasmodic contraction (tightening) of the muscles in the walls of the bronchioles.
    Excludes ❷: *respiratory bronchiolitis interstitial lung disease (J84.115)*

CC **J21.0** **Acute bronchiolitis due to respiratory syncytial virus**
CC **J21.1** **Acute bronchiolitis due to human metapneumovirus**
CC **J21.8** **Acute bronchiolitis due to other specified organisms**
CC **J21.9** **Acute bronchiolitis, unspecified**
    Bronchiolitis (acute)
    Excludes 1: *chronic bronchiolitis (J44-)*

J22 **Unspecified acute lower respiratory infection**
    Acute (lower) respiratory (tract) infection NOS
    Excludes 1: *upper respiratory infection (acute) (J06.9)*

Other diseases of upper respiratory tract (J30-J39)

J30- **Vasomotor and allergic rhinitis** — ALLERGIC RHINITIS – Inflammation of the mucous membrane of the nose due to hypersensitivity of a particular allergen.
    Includes: **Spasmodic rhinorrhea**
    Excludes 1: *allergic rhinitis with asthma (bronchial) (J45.909)*
           rhinitis NOS (J31.0)

J30.0 **Vasomotor rhinitis** — A non-allergic form without a known cause.
J30.1 **Allergic rhinitis due to pollens** — A form caused by the allergen pollen (the microspores of flowering plants).
    Allergy NOS due to pollen
    Hay fever
    Pollinosis
J30.2 **Other seasonal allergic rhinitis**
J30.5 **Allergic rhinitis due to food** — A form due to food allergens.
J30.8- **Other allergic rhinitis**
    J30.81 **Allergic rhinitis due to animal (cat) (dog) hair and dander** — A form due to the old skin and hair cells of animals.
    J30.89 **Other allergic rhinitis**
        Perennial allergic rhinitis

J
1
7
-
J
3
0

J30.9 **Allergic rhinitis, unspecified**

J31- **Chronic rhinitis, nasopharyngitis and pharyngitis**
Use additional code to identify:
Exposure to environmental tobacco smoke (Z77.22)
Exposure to tobacco smoke in the perinatal period (P96.81)
History of tobacco dependence (Z87.891)
Occupational exposure to environmental tobacco smoke (Z57.31)
Tobacco dependence (F17.-)
Tobacco use (Z72.0)

J31.0 **Chronic rhinitis** — Inflammation of the nasal mucous membrane which persists over a long period of time.
Atrophic rhinitis (chronic) — A form marked by wasting of the mucous membrane and glands.
Granulomatous rhinitis (chronic) — A form marked by the formation of granulomas.
Hypertrophic rhinitis (chronic) — A form in which the mucous membrane swells and thickens.
Obstructive rhinitis (chronic) — A form in which the mucous membrane swells sufficiently to obstruct the airflow.
Ozena
Purulent rhinitis (chronic) — A form marked by production of pus.
Rhinitis (chronic) NOS
Ulcerative rhinitis (chronic) — A form marked by the eating-away of the nasal mucous membrane.
Excludes 1: allergic rhinitis (J30.1-J30.9)
vasomotor rhinitis (J30.0)

J31.1 **Chronic nasopharyngitis** — Inflammation of the nasal and pharyngeal mucous membranes which develops slowly and persists over a long period of time.
Excludes ❷: acute nasopharyngitis (J00)

J31.2 **Chronic pharyngitis** — Inflammation of the pharynx persisting over a long period of time.
Chronic sore throat
Atrophic pharyngitis (chronic)
Granular pharyngitis (chronic)
Hypertrophic pharyngitis (chronic)
Excludes ❷: acute pharyngitis (J02.9)

J32- **Chronic sinusitis** — Inflammation of one or more of the nasal sinuses which persists over a long period of time.
Includes: **Sinus abscess** — The localized collection of pus within a sinus which persists over a long period of time.
Sinus empyema — The accumulation of pus within a sinus cavity over a long period of time.
Sinus infection
Sinus suppuration — A form characterized by the production of pus.
Use additional code to identify:
Exposure to environmental tobacco smoke (Z77.22)
Exposure to tobacco smoke in the perinatal period (P96.81)
History of tobacco dependence (Z87.891)
Infectious agent (B95-B97)
Occupational exposure to environmental tobacco smoke (Z57.31)
Tobacco dependence (F17-)
Tobacco use (Z72.0)
Excludes ❷: acute sinusitis (J01-)

J32.0 **Chronic maxillary sinusitis** — A form affecting one of the paired maxillary sinuses.
Antritis (chronic) — A form affecting the maxillary antrum.
Maxillary sinusitis NOS

J32.1 **Chronic frontal sinusitis** — A form affecting one of the paired frontal sinuses.
Frontal sinusitis NOS

J32.2 **Chronic ethmoidal sinusitis** — A form affecting one of the paired groups of ethmoidal sinuses.
Ethmoidal sinusitis NOS
Excludes 1: Woakes' ethmoiditis (J33.1)

J32.3 **Chronic sphenoidal sinusitis** — A form affecting one of the paired sphenoidal sinuses.
Sphenoidal sinusitis NOS

J32.4 **Chronic pansinusitis** — A form affecting two or more of the sinuses at the same time.
Pansinusitis NOS

J32.8 **Other chronic sinusitis**
Sinusitis (chronic) involving more than one sinus but not pansinusitis

J32.9 **Chronic sinusitis, unspecified**
Sinusitis (chronic) NOS

J33- **Nasal polyp** — A protruding growth from the nasal mucous membrane.
Use additional code to identify:
Exposure to environmental tobacco smoke (Z77.22)
Exposure to tobacco smoke in the perinatal period (P96.81)
History of tobacco dependence (Z87.891)
Occupational exposure to environmental tobacco smoke (Z57.31)
Tobacco dependence (F17.-)
Tobacco use (Z72.0)
Excludes 1: adenomatous polyps (D14.0)

J33.0 **Polyp of nasal cavity** — A protruding mucous membrane growth within the nose.
Choanal polyp
Nasopharyngeal polyp

J33.1 **Polypoid sinus degeneration** — Deterioration of the nasal sinus mucous membrane due to polypoid growth.
Woakes' syndrome or ethmoiditis

J33.8 **Other polyp of sinus**
Accessory polyp of sinus — A mucous membrane growth of one of the accessory sinuses.
Ethmoidal polyp of sinus — A mucous membrane growth of the ethmoidal sinus.
Maxillary polyp of sinus — A mucous membrane growth of the maxillary sinus.
Sphenoidal polyp of sinus — A mucous membrane growth of the sphenoidal sinus.

J33.9 **Nasal polyp, unspecified**

J34- **Other and unspecified disorders of nose and nasal sinuses**
Excludes ❷: varicose ulcer of nasal septum (I86.8)

J34.0 **Abscess, furuncle and carbuncle of nose** — A localized collection of purulent fluid caused by the disintegration of nasal tissue.
Cellulitis of nose — Cellular tissue inflammation of the nose.
Necrosis of nose — The localized death of nasal tissue cells.
Ulceration of nose — An eating-away of the nasal tissue.

J34.1 **Cyst and mucocele of nose and nasal sinus** — The abnormal dilatation of a sinus cavity with accumulated mucous secretion.

J34.2 **Deviated nasal septum** — An abnormality of the nasoseptal cartilage characterized by a turning away from the midline to either side.
Deflection or deviation of septum (nasal) (acquired)
Excludes 1: congenital deviated nasal septum (Q67.4)

J34.3 **Hypertrophy of nasal turbinates** — An enlargement of the turbinate bones of the nasal cavity and their lining membranes.

J34.8- **Other specified disorders of nose and nasal sinuses**
J34.81 **Nasal mucositis (ulcerative)** — Inflammation and/or ulcerative sores of the nasal mucosal surfaces.
Code also type of associated therapy, such as:
Antineoplastic and immunosuppressive drugs (T45.1x-)
Radiological procedure and radiotherapy (Y84.2)
Excludes ❷: gastrointestinal mucositis (ulcerative) (K92.81)
mucositis (ulcerative) of vagina and vulva (N76.81)
oral mucositis (ulcerative) (K12.3-)

J34.89 **Other specified disorders of nose and nasal sinuses**
Perforation of nasal septum NOS
Rhinolith — A nasal stone or concretion.

J34.9 **Unspecified disorder of nose and nasal sinuses**

J35- **Chronic diseases of tonsils and adenoids**
Use additional code to identify:
Exposure to environmental tobacco smoke (Z77.22)
Exposure to tobacco smoke in the perinatal period (P96.81)
History of tobacco dependence (Z87.891)
Occupational exposure to environmental tobacco smoke (Z57.31)
Tobacco dependence (F17.-)
Tobacco use (Z72.0)

J35.0- **Chronic tonsillitis and adenoiditis** — Inflammation of the palatine tonsils and/or the adenoids that persists over a long period of time.
Excludes ❷: acute tonsillitis (J03.-)

J35.01 **Chronic tonsillitis** — A form affecting the palatine tonsils.

J35.02 **Chronic adenoiditis** — A form affecting the adenoids.

J35.03 **Chronic tonsillitis and adenoiditis** — A form affecting both the palatine tonsils and the adenoids.

J35.1 **Hypertrophy of tonsils** — The abnormal enlargement of the tonsils.
Enlargement of tonsils
Excludes 1: hypertrophy of tonsils with tonsillitis (J35.0-)

J35.2 **Hypertrophy of adenoids** — The abnormal enlargement of the adenoids.
Enlargement of adenoids
Excludes 1: hypertrophy of adenoids with adenoiditis (J35.0-)

J30 - J35

J35.3   **Hypertrophy of tonsils with hypertrophy of adenoids**
 Excludes 1:   *hypertrophy of tonsils and adenoids with tonsillitis and adenoiditis (J35.03)*

J35.8   **Other chronic diseases of tonsils and adenoids**
 Adenoid vegetations — A fungus-like growth of lymphoid tissue in the nasopharynx.
 Amygdalolith — A chalky, hard mass within a tonsil.
 Calculus, tonsil — A hard mass within a tonsil.
 Cicatrix of tonsil (and adenoid) — The new healing tissue of tonsils and/or adenoids.
 Tonsillar tag — A small appendage of tonsillar tissue.
 Ulcer of tonsil — An eating-away of the tonsillar tissue.

J35.9   **Chronic disease of tonsils and adenoids, unspecified**
 Disease (chronic) of tonsils and adenoids NOS

J36   **Peritonsillar abscess** — A localized collection of pus caused by the disintegration of
CC   the connective tissue of the tonsil capsule.
 Includes: **Abscess of tonsil** — A localized collection of pus caused by the disintegration of tonsillar lymphoid tissue.
 Peritonsillar cellulitis
 Quinsy
 Use additional code (B95-B97) to identify infectious agent
 Excludes 1:   *acute tonsillitis (J03.-)*
 chronic tonsillitis (J35.0)
 retropharyngeal abscess (J39.0)
 tonsillitis NOS (J03.9-)

J37-   **Chronic laryngitis and laryngotracheitis** — Inflammation of the larynx and/or larynx and trachea which develops slowly and persists over a long period of time.
 Use additional code to identify:
 Exposure to environmental tobacco smoke (Z77.22)
 Exposure to tobacco smoke in the perinatal period (P96.81)
 History of tobacco dependence (Z87.891)
 Infectious agent (B95-B97)
 Occupational exposure to environmental tobacco smoke (Z57.31)
 Tobacco dependence (F17.-)
 Tobacco use (Z72.0)

J37.0   **Chronic laryngitis** — Inflammation of the larynx which develops slowly and persists over a long period of time.
 Catarrhal laryngitis — A form marked by atrophy of the mucous membrane.
 Hypertrophic laryngitis — A form marked by the thickening and swelling of the mucous membrane.
 Sicca laryngitis — A form marked by glue-like secretions.
 Excludes ❷: *acute laryngitis (J04.0)*
 obstructive (acute) laryngitis (J05.0)

J37.1   **Chronic laryngotracheitis** — Inflammation of the larynx and trachea which develops slowly and persists over a long period of time.
 Laryngitis, chronic, with tracheitis (chronic)
 Tracheitis, chronic, with laryngitis
 Excludes 1:   *chronic tracheitis (J42)*
 Excludes ❷: *acute laryngotracheitis (J04.2)*
 acute tracheitis (J04.1)

J38-   **Diseases of vocal cords and larynx, not elsewhere classified**
 Use additional code to identify:
 Exposure to environmental tobacco smoke (Z77.22)
 Exposure to tobacco smoke in the perinatal period (P96.81)
 History of tobacco dependence (Z87.891)
 Occupational exposure to environmental tobacco smoke (Z57.31)
 Tobacco dependence (F17.-)
 Tobacco use (Z72.0)
 Excludes 1:   *congenital laryngeal stridor (P28.89)*
 obstructive laryngitis (acute) (J05.0)
 postprocedural subglottic stenosis (J95.5)
 stridor (R06.1)
 ulcerative laryngitis (J04.0)

J38.0-   **Paralysis of vocal cords and larynx** — Loss of motor function of the vocal cords or larynx.
 Laryngoplegia — Paralysis of the larynx.
 Paralysis of glottis — A loss of motor function of the vocal apparatus of the larynx.

J38.00   **Paralysis of vocal cords and larynx, unspecified**

J38.01   **Paralysis of vocal cords and larynx, unilateral**

J38.02   **Paralysis of vocal cords and larynx, bilateral**

J38.1   **Polyp of vocal cord and larynx** — A mucous membrane protruding growth of the vocal cords or larynx.
 Excludes 1:   *adenomatous polyps (D14.1)*

J38.2   **Nodules of vocal cords** — Small, white nodules occurring on the vocal cords.
 Chorditis (fibrinous) (nodosa) (tuberosa)
 Singer's nodes
 Teacher's nodes

J38.3   **Other diseases of vocal cords**
 Abscess of vocal cords — A localized collection of pus caused by the disintegration of the vocal cord tissue.
 Cellulitis of vocal cords — Inflammation of the cellular tissue of the vocal cords.
 Granuloma of vocal cords — The formation of a granuloma on the vocal cords.
 Leukokeratosis of vocal cords
 Leukoplakia of vocal cords — White, thickened patches of the mucous membrane lining of the vocal cords.

J38.4   **Edema of larynx** — The accumulation of intercellular fluid of the laryngeal tissues.
 Edema (of) glottis — The accumulation of intercellular fluid of the vocal apparatus.
 Subglottic edema — The accumulation of intercellular fluid of the tissues below the vocal cord apparatus.
 Supraglottic edema — The accumulation of intercellular fluid in the tissues above the vocal apparatus.
 Excludes 1:   *acute obstructive laryngitis [croup] (J05.0)*
 edematous laryngitis (J04.0)

J38.5   **Laryngeal spasm** — A sudden, violent involuntary contraction of the laryngeal muscles.
 Laryngismus (stridulus)

J38.6   **Stenosis of larynx** — The abnormal reduction in the laryngeal orifice size.

J38.7   **Other diseases of larynx**
 Abscess of larynx — A localized collection of pus caused by the disintegration of laryngeal tissue.
 Cellulitis of larynx — Inflammation of the cellular tissue of the larynx.
 Disease of larynx NOS
 Necrosis of larynx — The death of a localized group of laryngeal cells.
 Pachyderma of larynx — Localized, warty epithelial thickenings on the larynx.
 Perichondritis of larynx — Inflammation of the dense connective tissue around the laryngeal cartilages.
 Ulcer of larynx — An eating-away of the laryngeal tissue.

J39-   **Other diseases of upper respiratory tract**
 Excludes 1:   *acute respiratory infection NOS (J22)*
 acute upper respiratory infection (J06.9)
 upper respiratory inflammation due to chemicals, gases, fumes or vapors (J68.2)

CC **J39.0**   **Retropharyngeal and parapharyngeal abscess** — A localized collection of pus caused by the disintegration of the fascial tissue between the pharyngeal wall and the prevertebral fascia or the connective tissue within the pharynx.
 Peripharyngeal abscess
 Excludes 1:   *peritonsillar abscess (J36)*

CC **J39.1**   **Other abscess of pharynx**
 Cellulitis of pharynx — Inflammation of the cellular pharyngeal tissue.
 Nasopharyngeal abscess — A localized collection of pus caused by the disintegration of the nasopharyngeal tissue.

J39.2   **Other diseases of pharynx**
 Cyst of pharynx — A fluid-filled sac of the pharynx.
 Edema of pharynx — The abnormal accumulation of intercellular fluid of the pharynx.
 Excludes ❷: *chronic pharyngitis (J31.2)*
 ulcerative pharyngitis (J02.9)

J39.3   **Upper respiratory tract hypersensitivity reaction, site unspecified**
 Excludes 1:   *hypersensitivity reaction of upper respiratory tract, such as:*
 extrinsic allergic alveolitis (J67.9)
 pneumoconiosis (J60-J67.9)

J39.8   **Other specified diseases of upper respiratory tract**

J39.9   **Disease of upper respiratory tract, unspecified**

J
3
5
-
J
3
9

Chronic lower respiratory diseases (J40-J47)

Excludes 1:   *bronchitis due to chemicals, gases, fumes and vapors (J68.0)*
Excludes ❷*:*   *cystic fibrosis (E84-)*

J40   Bronchitis, <u>not specified as acute or chronic</u>
    Bronchitis NOS
    Bronchitis with tracheitis NOS
    Catarrhal bronchitis
    Tracheobronchitis NOS
    Use additional code to identify:
    Exposure to environmental tobacco smoke (Z77.22)
    Exposure to tobacco smoke in the perinatal period (P96.81)
    History of tobacco dependence (Z87.891)
    Occupational exposure to environmental tobacco smoke (Z57.31)
    Tobacco dependence (F17-)
    Tobacco use (Z72.0)
    Excludes 1:   *acute bronchitis (J20.-)*
           allergic bronchitis NOS (J45.909-)
           asthmatic bronchitis NOS (J45.9-)
           bronchitis due to chemicals, gases, fumes and vapors (J68.0)

J41-   Simple and mucopurulent chronic bronchitis
    Use additional code to identify:
    Exposure to environmental tobacco smoke (Z77.22)
    Exposure to tobacco smoke in the perinatal period (P96.81)
    History of tobacco dependence (Z87.891)
    Occupational exposure to environmental tobacco smoke (Z57.31)
    Tobacco dependence (F17-)
    Tobacco use (Z72.0)
    Excludes 1:   *chronic bronchitis NOS (J42)*
           chronic obstructive bronchitis (J44-)

    J41.0   Simple chronic bronchitis — A form marked by mild, persistent symptoms of coughing and expectoration.

    J41.1   Mucopurulent chronic bronchitis — A form marked by persistent, significant mucopurulent discharge.

    J41.8   Mixed simple and mucopurulent chronic bronchitis

J42   Unspecified chronic bronchitis
    Chronic bronchitis NOS
    Chronic tracheitis
    Chronic tracheobronchitis
    Use additional code to identify:
    Exposure to environmental tobacco smoke (Z77.22)
    Exposure to tobacco smoke in the perinatal period (P96.81)
    History of tobacco dependence (Z87.891)
    Occupational exposure to environmental tobacco smoke (Z57.31)
    Tobacco dependence (F17-)
    Tobacco use (Z72.0)
    Excludes 1:   *chronic asthmatic bronchitis (J44-)*
           chronic bronchitis with airways obstruction (J44-)
           chronic emphysematous bronchitis (J44-)
           chronic obstructive pulmonary disease NOS (J44.9)
           simple and mucopurulent chronic bronchitis (J41-)

J43-   Emphysema — The abnormal increase in the size of the air spaces distal to the terminal bronchioles with destructive changes.
    Use additional code to identify:
    Exposure to environmental tobacco smoke (Z77.22)
    History of tobacco dependence (Z87.891)
    Occupational exposure to environmental tobacco smoke (Z57.31)
    Tobacco dependence (F17-)
    Tobacco use (Z72.0)
    Excludes 1:   *compensatory emphysema (J98.3)*
           emphysema due to inhalation of chemicals, gases, fumes or
             vapors (J68.4)
           emphysema with chronic (obstructive) bronchitis (J44-)
           emphysematous (obstructive) bronchitis (J44-)
           interstitial emphysema (J98.2)
           mediastinal emphysema (J98.2)
           neonatal interstitial emphysema (P25.0)
           surgical (subcutaneous) emphysema (T81.82)
           traumatic subcutaneous emphysema (T79.7)

    J43.0   Unilateral pulmonary emphysema [MacLeod's syndrome] — A form with greater translucency over one lung.
        Swyer-James syndrome
        Unilateral emphysema
        Unilateral hyperlucent lung
        Unilateral pulmonary artery functional hypoplasia
        Unilateral transparency of lung

    J43.1   Panlobular emphysema — A form marked by generalized areas of destructive dilatations.
        Panacinar emphysema

    J43.2   Centrilobular emphysema — A form marked by localized areas of destructive dilatations.

    J43.8   Other emphysema

    J43.9   Emphysema, unspecified
        Bullous emphysema (lung) (pulmonary) — A form marked by large blebs.
        Emphysema (lung) (pulmonary) NOS
        Emphysematous bleb — A form characterized by single or multiple large cystic alveolar dilatations of the air spaces.
        Vesicular emphysema (lung) (pulmonary)

J44-   <u>Other chronic obstructive pulmonary disease</u> — A disease of decreased ability of the lungs to perform ventilation due to diffuse obstruction of the pulmonary system.
    AHA 13:4Q:p109 – Nicotine dependence and COPD
    AHA 13:4Q:p129 – Chronic hypoxic respiratory failure and COPD
    Includes: Asthma with chronic obstructive pulmonary disease
               Chronic asthmatic (obstructive) bronchitis
               Chronic bronchitis with airways obstruction
               Chronic bronchitis with emphysema
               Chronic emphysematous bronchitis
               Chronic obstructive asthma
               Chronic obstructive bronchitis
               Chronic obstructive tracheobronchitis
    Use additional code to identify:
    Exposure to environmental tobacco smoke (Z77.22)
    History of tobacco dependence (Z87.891)
    Occupational exposure to environmental tobacco smoke (Z57.31)
    Tobacco dependence (F17-)
    Tobacco use (Z72.0)
    Code also type of asthma, if applicable (J45.-)
    Excludes 1:   *bronchiectasis (J47-)*
           chronic bronchitis NOS (J42)
           chronic simple and mucopurulent bronchitis (J41-)
           chronic tracheitis (J42)
           chronic tracheobronchitis (J42)
           emphysema without chronic bronchitis (J43-)
    Excludes ❷*:*   *lung diseases due to external agents (J60-J70)*

cc **J44.0   Chronic obstructive pulmonary disease <u>with acute lower respiratory infection</u>**
        Use additional code to identify the infection

cc **J44.1   Chronic obstructive pulmonary disease <u>with (acute) exacerbation</u>** — A form characterized by a sudden, severe increase in severity.
        Decompensated COPD
        Decompensated COPD with (acute) exacerbation
        Excludes ❷*:*   *chronic obstructive pulmonary disease [COPD] with*
                    acute bronchitis (J44.0)

    J44.9   Chronic obstructive pulmonary disease, unspecified
        Chronic obstructive airway disease NOS
        Chronic obstructive lung disease NOS

J45-   <u>Asthma</u> — A chronic inflammatory disorder of the airways which results in narrowing of the airways and is characterized by difficult and labored breathing with coughing and wheezing.
    AHA 12:4Q:p99 – Acute exacerbation of asthma and status asthmaticus
        together
    Includes: Allergic (predominantly) asthma
               Allergic bronchitis NOS
               Allergic rhinitis with asthma
               Atopic asthma
               Extrinsic allergic asthma
               Hay fever with asthma
               Idiosyncratic asthma
               Intrinsic nonallergic asthma
               Nonallergic asthma
    Use additional code to identify:
    Exposure to environmental tobacco smoke (Z77.22)
    Exposure to tobacco smoke in the perinatal period (P96.81)
    History of tobacco dependence (Z87.891)
    Occupational exposure to environmental tobacco smoke (Z57.31)
    Tobacco dependence (F17.-)
    Tobacco use (Z72.0)
    Excludes 1:   *detergent asthma (J69.8)*
           eosinophilic asthma (J82)
           lung diseases due to external agents (J60-J70)
           miner's asthma (J60)
           wheezing NOS (R06.2)
           wood asthma (J67.8)
    Excludes ❷*:*   *asthma with chronic obstructive pulmonary disease (J44.9)*
           chronic asthmatic (obstructive) bronchitis (J44.9)
           chronic obstructive asthma (J44.9)

    J45.2-   Mild intermittent asthma — A severity of symptoms frequency classification of two or fewer episodes per week.

        J45.20   Mild intermittent asthma, uncomplicated
            Mild intermittent asthma NOS

J 4 0 - J 4 5

cc**J45.21** **Mild intermittent asthma with (acute) exacerbation** — A form characterized by a sudden, severe increase in severity.

cc**J45.22** **Mild intermittent asthma with status asthmaticus** — A continuous, obstructive asthmatic state unrelieved after initial therapy measures.

J45.3- **Mild persistent asthma** — A severity of symptoms frequency classification of two or more episodes per week.

J45.30 **Mild persistent asthma, uncomplicated**
    Mild persistent asthma NOS

cc**J45.31** **Mild persistent asthma with (acute) exacerbation** — A form characterized by a sudden, severe increase in severity.

cc**J45.32** **Mild persistent asthma with status asthmaticus** — A continuous, obstructive asthmatic state unrelieved after initial therapy measures.

J45.4- **Moderate persistent asthma** — A severity of symptoms frequency classification of daily episodes.

J45.40 **Moderate persistent asthma, uncomplicated**
    Moderate persistent asthma NOS

cc**J45.41** **Moderate persistent asthma with (acute) exacerbation** — A form characterized by a sudden, severe increase in severity.

cc**J45.42** **Moderate persistent asthma with status asthmaticus** — A continuous, obstructive asthmatic state unrelieved after initial therapy measures.

J45.5- **Severe persistent asthma** — A severity of symptoms frequency classification of continuous episodes.

J45.50 **Severe persistent asthma, uncomplicated**
    Severe persistent asthma NOS

cc**J45.51** **Severe persistent asthma with (acute) exacerbation** — A form characterized by a sudden, severe increase in severity.

cc**J45.52** **Severe persistent asthma with status asthmaticus** — A continuous, obstructive asthmatic state unrelieved after initial therapy measures.

J45.9- **Other and unspecified asthma**

J45.90- **Unspecified asthma**
    Asthmatic bronchitis NOS
    Childhood asthma NOS
    Late onset asthma

cc**J45.901** **Unspecified asthma with (acute) exacerbation** — A form characterized by a sudden, severe increase in severity.

cc**J45.902** **Unspecified asthma with status asthmaticus** — A continuous, obstructive asthmatic state unrelieved after initial therapy measures.

J45.909 **Unspecified asthma, uncomplicated**
    Asthma NOS

J45.99- **Other asthma**

J45.990 **Exercise induced bronchospasm** — A form causing difficulty exhaling air that is triggered by exercise or strenuous activity.

J45.991 **Cough variant asthma** — A form in which coughing is the patient's only symptom.

J45.998 **Other asthma**

J47- **Bronchiectasis** — Persistent dilatation of the bronchi with coughing, foul-smelling breath, and mucopurulent expectoration.
Includes: Bronchiolectasis
Use additional code to identify:
    Exposure to environmental tobacco smoke (Z77.22)
    Exposure to tobacco smoke in the perinatal period (P96.81)
    History of tobacco dependence (Z87.891)
    Occupational exposure to environmental tobacco smoke (Z57.31)
    Tobacco dependence (F17-)
    Tobacco use (Z72.0)
Excludes 1:   congenital bronchiectasis (Q33.4)
                 tuberculous bronchiectasis (current disease) (A15.0)

cc**J47.0** **Bronchiectasis with acute lower respiratory infection**
    Bronchiectasis with acute bronchitis
    Use additional code to identify the infection

cc**J47.1** **Bronchiectasis with (acute) exacerbation** — A form characterized by a sudden, severe increase in severity.

J47.9 **Bronchiectasis, uncomplicated**
    Bronchiectasis NOS

Lung diseases due to external agents (J60-J70)

Excludes ❷: asthma (J45-)
                 malignant neoplasm of bronchus and lung (C34-)

J60 **Coalworker's pneumoconiosis** — [Age/15-124] – Destructive deposition of substantial amounts of coal dust particles in the lungs.
    Anthracosilicosis
    Anthracosis
    Black lung disease
    Coalworker's lung
Excludes 1:   coalworker pneumoconiosis with tuberculosis, any type in A15 (J65)

J61 **Pneumoconiosis due to asbestos and other mineral fibers** — [Age/15-124] – Destructive deposition of magnesium and calcium silicate in the lung tissues.
    Asbestosis
Excludes 1:   pleural plaque with asbestosis (J92.0)
                 pneumoconiosis with tuberculosis, any type in A15 (J65)

J62- **Pneumoconiosis due to dust containing silica**
Includes: Silicotic fibrosis (massive) of lung
Excludes 1:   pneumoconiosis with tuberculosis, any type in A15 (J65)

J62.0 **Pneumoconiosis due to talc dust** — Destructive deposition of magnesium silicate in the lung tissues.

J62.8 **Pneumoconiosis due to other dust containing silica** — Destructive deposition of silicon dioxide in the lung tissues.
    Silicosis NOS

J63- **Pneumoconiosis due to other inorganic dusts**
Excludes 1:   pneumoconiosis with tuberculosis, any type in A15 (J65)

J63.0 **Aluminosis (of lung)** — Destructive deposition of aluminum particles in the lung tissues.

J63.1 **Bauxite fibrosis (of lung)** — Destructive deposition of bauxite fumes containing fine particles of alumina and silica which lead to extreme pulmonary emphysema.

J63.2 **Berylliosis** — Destructive deposition of beryllium salts or dust in the lung tissues characterized by the formation of granulomas.

J63.3 **Graphite fibrosis (of lung)** — Fibrotic, destructive deposition of mineralized carbon in the lung tissues.

J63.4 **Siderosis** — Destructive deposition of iron particles in the lung tissue.

J63.5 **Stannosis** — Destructive deposition of tin oxide in the lung tissues.

J63.6 **Pneumoconiosis due to other specified inorganic dusts**

J64 **Unspecified pneumoconiosis**
Excludes 1:   pneumonoconiosis with tuberculosis, any type in A15 (J65)

J65 **Pneumoconiosis associated with tuberculosis**
    Any condition in J60-J64 with tuberculosis, any type in A15
    Silicotuberculosis

J66- **Airway disease due to specific organic dust**
Excludes ❷: allergic alveolitis (J67.-)
                 asbestosis (J61)
                 bagassosis (J67.1)
                 farmer's lung (J67.0)
                 hypersensitivity pneumonitis due to organic dust (J67.-)
                 reactive airways dysfunction syndrome (J68.3)

J66.0 **Byssinosis** — A disease of the lung tissues caused by the inhalation of cotton dust.
    Airway disease due to cotton dust

J66.1 **Flax-dressers' disease** — A disease of the lung tissue caused by the inhalation of flax plant particles.

J66.2 **Cannabinosis** — A disease of the lung caused by the inhalation of cannabis smoke.

J66.8 **Airway disease due to other specific organic dusts**

J67- **Hypersensitivity pneumonitis due to organic dust**
Includes: Allergic alveolitis and pneumonitis due to inhaled organic dust and particles of fungal, actinomycetic or other origin
Excludes 1:   pneumonitis due to inhalation of chemicals, gases, fumes or vapors (J68.0)

J67.0 **Farmer's lung** — A form of hypersensitivity alveolitis caused by exposure to moldy hay that has fermented.
    Harvester's lung
    Haymaker's lung
    Moldy hay disease

J45-J67

J67.1 **Bagassosis** — A form of hypersensitivity pneumonitis due to inhalation of bagasse dust; the moldy, dusty fibrous waste of sugar cane after removal of the sugar-containing sap.
> **Bagasse disease**
> **Bagasse pneumonitis**

J67.2 **Bird fancier's lung** — A condition marked by cough, shortness of breath, fever, and chills caused by bird's excreta and seen in persons with extensive exposure to birds.
> **Budgerigar fancier's disease or lung** — A form due to extensive exposure to an Australian parakeet (Budgerigar).
> **Pigeon fancier's disease or lung** — A form due to extensive exposure to pigeons.

J67.3 **Suberosis** — Pneumoconiosis due to inhalation and tissue reaction to cork dust.
> **Corkhandler's disease or lung**
> **Corkworker's disease or lung**

J67.4 **Maltworker's lung** — A form of hypersensitivity alveolitis caused by working with germinated malt.
> **Alveolitis due to Aspergillus clavatus** — A hypersensitivity from the organism Aspergillus clavatus.

J67.5 **Mushroom-worker's lung** — A form of hypersensitivity alveolitis caused by work involving the cultivating of mushrooms.

J67.6 **Maple-bark-stripper's lung** — A form of hypersensitivity alveolitis caused by work involving the stripping of bark from maple trees.
> **Alveolitis due to Cryptostroma corticale** — A form of hypersensitivity alveolitis caused by Cryptostroma corticale, a fungi which grows under the bark of certain trees.
> **Cryptostromosis**

CC **J67.7** **Air conditioner and humidifier lung**
> **Allergic alveolitis due to fungal, thermophilic actinomycetes and other organisms growing in ventilation [air conditioning] systems**

CC **J67.8** **Hypersensitivity pneumonitis due to other organic dusts**
> **Cheese-washer's lung** — A hypersensitivity lung disease caused by fungus released during cheese production.
> **Coffee-worker's lung** — A hypersensitivity lung disease caused by work involving coffee bean processing dust.
> **Fish-meal worker's lung** — A hypersensitivity lung disease caused by work involving the production of fish meal.
> **Furrier's lung** — A hypersensitivity lung disease caused by work involving furs.
> **Sequoiosis** — A hypersensitivity lung disease caused by sawdust.

CC **J67.9** **Hypersensitivity pneumonitis due to unspecified organic dust**
> **Allergic alveolitis (extrinsic) NOS**
> **Hypersensitivity pneumonitis NOS**

J68- **Respiratory conditions due to inhalation of chemicals, gases, fumes and vapors** — Inflammation and other respiratory conditions due to the adverse effects of gaseous fumes and vapors.
> **Code first (T51-T65) to identify cause**
> **Use additional code to identify associated respiratory conditions, such as:**
> **Acute respiratory failure (J96.0-)**

CC **J68.0** **Bronchitis and pneumonitis due to chemicals, gases, fumes and vapors** — Inflammation of the bronchi and/or lungs due to the adverse effects of gaseous fumes and vapors.
> **Chemical bronchitis (acute)**

MCC **J68.1** **Pulmonary edema due to chemicals, gases, fumes and vapors** — A sudden, severe onset of an excessive amount of intercellular fluid due to the effects of gaseous fumes and vapors.
> **Chemical pulmonary edema (acute) (chronic)**
> *Excludes 1:* *pulmonary edema (acute) (chronic) NOS (J81-)*

J68.2 **Upper respiratory inflammation due to chemicals, gases, fumes and vapors, not elsewhere classified**

J68.3 **Other acute and subacute respiratory conditions due to chemicals, gases, fumes and vapors**
> **Reactive airways dysfunction syndrome**

J68.4 **Chronic respiratory conditions due to chemicals, fumes and vapors**
> **Emphysema (diffuse) (chronic) due to inhalation of chemicals, gases, fumes and vapors** — The prolonged, persistent increase in the size of the air spaces distal to the terminal bronchioles due to inhalation of chemical fumes and vapors.
> **Obliterative bronchiolitis (chronic) (subacute) due to inhalation of chemicals, gases, fumes and vapors** — The destructive inflammation of the bronchi and bronchioles due to inhalation of chemical fumes and vapors.
> **Pulmonary fibrosis (chronic) due to inhalation of chemicals, gases, fumes and vapors** — The prolonged, persistent development of fibrous tissue of the lung due to inhalation of chemical fumes and vapors.
> *Excludes 1:* *chronic pulmonary edema due to chemicals, gases, fumes and vapors (J68.1)*

J68.8 **Other respiratory conditions due to chemicals, gases, fumes and vapors**

J68.9 **Unspecified respiratory condition due to chemicals, gases, fumes and vapors**

J69- **Pneumonitis due to solids and liquids** — Inflammation of the lungs caused by the inhalation of solid and/or liquid matter.
> *Excludes 1:* *neonatal aspiration syndromes (P24-)*
> *postprocedural pneumonitis (J95.4)*

MCC **J69.0** **Pneumonitis due to inhalation of food and vomit**
> **Aspiration pneumonia NOS**
> **Aspiration pneumonia (due to) food (regurgitated)**
> **Aspiration pneumonia (due to) gastric secretions**
> **Aspiration pneumonia (due to) milk**
> **Aspiration pneumonia (due to) vomit**
> **Code also any associated foreign body in respiratory tract (T17-)**
> *Excludes 1:* *chemical pneumonitis due to anesthesia (J95.4)*
> *obstetric aspiration pneumonia (O74.0)*

MCC **J69.1** **Pneumonitis due to inhalation of oils and essences**
> **Exogenous lipoid pneumonia**
> **Lipid pneumonia NOS**
> **Code first (T51-T65) to identify substance**
> *Excludes 1:* *endogenous lipoid pneumonia (J84.89)*

MCC **J69.8** **Pneumonitis due to inhalation of other solids and liquids**
> **Pneumonitis due to aspiration of blood**
> **Pneumonitis due to aspiration of detergent**
> **Code first (T51-T65) to identify substance**

J70- **Respiratory conditions due to other external agents**

CC **J70.0** **Acute pulmonary manifestations due to radiation** —
> Inflammation of the lungs due to the adverse effects of radiation.
> **Radiation pneumonitis**
> **Use additional code (W88-W90, X39.0-) to identify the external cause**

CC **J70.1** **Chronic and other pulmonary manifestations due to radiation**
> **Fibrosis of lung following radiation** — The fibrotic tissue reaction of the lung which develops slowly over a period of time and is caused by the adverse effects of radiation.
> **Use additional code (W88-W90, X39.0-) to identify the external cause**

J70.2 **Acute drug-induced interstitial lung disorders**
> **Use additional code for adverse effect, if applicable, to identify drug (T36-T50 with fifth or sixth character 5)**
> *Excludes 1:* *interstitial pneumonia NOS (J84.9)*
> *lymphoid interstitial pneumonia (J84.2)*

J70.3 **Chronic drug-induced interstitial lung disorders**
> **Use additional code for adverse effect, if applicable, to identify drug (T36-T50 with fifth or sixth character 5)**
> *Excludes 1:* *interstitial pneumonia NOS (J84.9)*
> *lymphoid interstitial pneumonia (J84.2)*

J70.4 **Drug-induced interstitial lung disorders, unspecified**
> **Use additional code for adverse effect, if applicable, to identify drug (T36-T50 with fifth or sixth character 5)**
> *Excludes 1:* *interstitial pneumonia NOS (J84.9)*
> *lymphoid interstitial pneumonia (J84.2)*

J70.5 **Respiratory conditions due to smoke inhalation**
> AHA 13:4Q:p121 – Acute respiratory failure due to smoke inhalation
> **Smoke inhalation NOS**
> *Excludes 1:* *smoke inhalation due to chemicals, gases, fumes and vapors (J68.9)*

J70.8 **Respiratory conditions due to other specified external agents**
> **Code first (T51-T65) to identify the external agent**

J70.9 **Respiratory conditions due to unspecified external agent**
> **Code first (T51-T65) to identify the external agent**

J67-J70

Other respiratory diseases principally affecting the interstitium (J80-J84)

J80 **Acute respiratory distress syndrome** — A syndrome characterized by damage to
CC the pulmonary capillary endothelium, alveolar hemorrhage, and interstitial edema following severe shock, trauma, or major thoracic surgery.
    Acute respiratory distress syndrome in adult or child
    Adult hyaline membrane disease
    Excludes 1:   *respiratory distress syndrome in newborn (perinatal) (P22.0)*

J81- **Pulmonary edema** — The severe, sudden accumulation of intercellular fluid of the lungs not due to heart disease.
    Use additional code to identify:
    Exposure to environmental tobacco smoke (Z77.22)
    History of tobacco dependence (Z87.891)
    Occupational exposure to environmental tobacco smoke (Z57.31)
    Tobacco dependence (F17-)
    Tobacco use (Z72.0)
    Excludes 1:   *chemical (acute) pulmonary edema (J68.1)*
        hypostatic pneumonia (J18.2)
        passive pneumonia (J18.2)
        pulmonary edema due to external agents (J60-J70)
        pulmonary edema with heart disease NOS (I50.1)
        pulmonary edema with heart failure (I50.1)

MCC J81.0   <u>**Acute**</u> **pulmonary edema** — A sudden, severe onset.
    Acute edema of lung

CC J81.1   <u>**Chronic**</u> **pulmonary edema** — A form that persists over a long period of time.
    Pulmonary congestion (chronic) (passive)
    Pulmonary edema NOS

J82 **Pulmonary eosinophilia, not elsewhere classified** — The abnormal
CC infiltration of the pulmonary tissues by eosinophils.
    Allergic pneumonia
    Eosinophilic asthma
    Eosinophilic pneumonia
    Löffler's pneumonia
    Tropical (pulmonary) eosinophilia NOS
    Excludes 1:   *pulmonary eosinophilia due to aspergillosis (B44-)*
        pulmonary eosinophilia due to drugs (J70.2-J70.4)
        pulmonary eosinophilia due to specified parasitic infection (B50-B83)
        pulmonary eosinophilia due to systemic connective tissue disorders (M30-M36)
        pulmonary infiltrate NOS (R91.8)

J84- **Other interstitial pulmonary diseases**
    Excludes 1:   *drug-induced interstitial lung disorders (J70.2-J70.4)*
        interstitial emphysema (J98.2)
        lung diseases due to external agents (J60-J70)

J84.0- **Alveolar and parieto-alveolar conditions**

CC J84.01   **Alveolar proteinosis** — The abnormal filling of the distal alveoli with proteinaceous material which prevents ventilation of the affected areas.

CC J84.02   **Pulmonary alveolar microlithiasis** — The abnormal deposition of minute calculi in the alveoli of the lungs.

CC J84.03   **Idiopathic pulmonary hemosiderosis** — [Not Allowed as PDX] — The abnormal deposition of iron pigment in the lung tissue.
    Essential brown induration of lung
    Code first underlying disease, such as:
    Disorders of iron metabolism (E83.1-)
    Excludes 1:   *acute idiopathic pulmonary hemorrhage in infants [AIPHI] (R04.81)*

CC J84.09   **Other alveolar and parieto-alveolar conditions**

J84.1- **Other interstitial pulmonary diseases with fibrosis**
    Excludes 1:   *pulmonary fibrosis (chronic) due to inhalation of chemicals, gases, fumes or vapors (J68.4)*
        pulmonary fibrosis (chronic) following radiation (J70.1)

J84.10   **Pulmonary fibrosis, unspecified** — The progressive fibrous tissue replacement of the pulmonary alveolar walls leading to difficult or labored breathing.
    Capillary fibrosis of lung
    Cirrhosis of lung (chronic) NOS
    Fibrosis of lung (atrophic) (chronic) (confluent) (massive) (perialveolar) (peribronchial) NOS
    Induration of lung (chronic) NOS
    Postinflammatory pulmonary fibrosis — Progressive fibrosis of the pulmonary alveolar walls with difficult breathing following inflammatory reaction within the lung tissue.

J84.11- **Idiopathic interstitial pneumonia** — The abnormal accumulation of damaged (e.g., fibrotic, inflammatory, plasma) cells in the space between the air sacs (alveoli) of the lungs that is not due to a known underlying cause and is primarily differentiated by histological appearance.
    Excludes 1:   *lymphoid interstitial pneumonia (J84.2)*
        pneumocystis pneumonia (B59)

J84.111   **Idiopathic interstitial pneumonia, not otherwise specified**

J84.112   **Idiopathic pulmonary fibrosis** — A progressive fibrotic lung disease that is limited to the lungs with the histological appearance of usual interstitial pneumonia (UIP).
    Cryptogenic fibrosing alveolitis
    Idiopathic fibrosing alveolitis

J84.113   **Idiopathic non-specific interstitial pneumonitis** — A form marked by the histological appearance of diffuse inflammation with some degree of interstitial fibrosis.
    Excludes 1:   *non-specific interstitial pneumonia NOS, or due to known underlying cause (J84.89)*

CC J84.114   **Acute interstitial pneumonitis** — A rapidly progressive, severe form with the histological appearance of organizing diffuse alveolar damage and without an identifiable underlying etiology.
    Hamman-Rich syndrome
    Excludes 1:   *pneumocystis pneumonia (B59)*

J84.115   **Respiratory bronchiolitis interstitial lung disease** — A form marked by the patchy accumulation of macrophages in the peribronchiolar alveolar spaces and associated with the pathologic lesion of respiratory bronchiolitis with bronchiolocentric distribution.

CC J84.116   **Cryptogenic organizing pneumonia** — A form marked by the proliferation of granulation tissue within small airways and alveolar ducts with the histological appearance of organizing pneumonia.
    Excludes 1:   *organizing pneumonia NOS, or due to known underlying cause (J84.89)*

CC J84.117   **Desquamative interstitial pneumonia** — A form marked by the accumulation of macrophages in the alveoli that affects the lungs in a diffuse manner.

J84.17   **Other interstitial pulmonary diseases with fibrosis in diseases classified elsewhere** — [Not Allowed as PDX]
    Interstitial pneumonia (nonspecific) (usual) due to collagen vascular disease
    Interstitial pneumonia (nonspecific) (usual) in diseases classified elsewhere
    Organizing pneumonia due to collagen vascular disease
    Organizing pneumonia in diseases classified elsewhere
    Code first underlying disease, such as:
    Progressive systemic sclerosis (M34.0)
    Rheumatoid arthritis (M05.00-M06.9)
    Systemic lupus erythematosis (M32.0-M32.9)

CC J84.2   **Lymphoid interstitial pneumonia** — A form marked by lymphocytic and plasma cells in the interstitial spaces.
    Lymphoid interstitial pneumonitis

J84.8- **Other specified interstitial pulmonary diseases**
    Excludes 1:   *exogenous lipoid pneumonia (J69.1)*
        unspecified lipoid pneumonia (J69.1)

MCC J84.81   **Lymphangioleiomyomatosis** — [♀] — An obstructive lung disorder that affects women that is caused by the proliferation of smooth muscle cells surrounding the small airways and alveoli, and by cystic destruction of the lung tissue.
    Lymphangiomyomatosis

CC J84.82   **Adult pulmonary Langerhans cell histiocytosis** — [Age/15-124] — An interstitial lung disorder that is characterized by focal Langerhans' cell granulomas that invade and destroy distal bronchioles.
    Adult PLCH

MCC J84.83   **Surfactant mutations of the lung** — A severe form that decreases lung elasticity and results in alveolar collapse that is caused by a genetic abnormailty of the lung surfactant protein.

J84.84- **Other interstitial lung diseases of childhood**

MCC J84.841   **Neuroendocrine cell hyperplasia of infancy** — A form characterized by rapid breathing with the histological appearance of hyperplasia of neuroendocrine celss in the bronchioles.

MCC J84.842   **Pulmonary interstitial glycogenosis** — A form marked by glycogen in the alveolar insterstitial spaces.

MCC J84.843   **Alveolar capillary dysplasia with vein misalignment** — A developmental lung disorder characterized by abnormal development of the alveolar capillary vascular system.

MCC J84.848   **Other interstitial lung diseases of childhood**

J80-J84

J84.89   **Other specified interstitial pulmonary diseases**
    Endogenous lipoid pneumonia — A pneumonia-like reaction of the lung tissue due to the aspiration of oils and fat tissues from the patient's own body.
    Interstitial pneumonitis
    Non-specific interstitial pneumonitis NOS
    Organizing pneumonia NOS
    Code first, if applicable:
      Poisoning due to drug or toxin (T51-T65 with fifth or sixth character to indicate intent), for toxic pneumonopathy
      Underlying cause of pneumonopathy, if known
    Use additional code, for adverse effect, to identify drug (T36-T50 with fifth or sixth character 5), if drug-induced
    Excludes 1:   *cryptogenic organizing pneumonia (J84.116)*
        idiopathic non-specific interstitial pneumonitis (J84.113)
        lipoid pneumonia, exogenous or unspecified (J69.1)
        lymphoid interstitial pneumonia (J84.2)

cc **J84.9**   **Interstitial pulmonary disease, unspecified**
    Interstitial pneumonia NOS

Suppurative and necrotic conditions of the lower respiratory tract (J85-J86)

J85-   **Abscess of lung and mediastinum**
    Use additional code (B95-B97) to identify infectious agent

mcc **J85.0**   **Gangrene and necrosis of lung** — The death of lung tissue cells.

mcc **J85.1**   **Abscess of lung with pneumonia** — A localized collection of pus caused by the disintegration of lung tissue with inflammation of the lung.
    Code also the type of pneumonia

mcc **J85.2**   **Abscess of lung without pneumonia** — A localized collection of pus caused by the disintegration of lung tissue.
    Abscess of lung NOS

mcc **J85.3**   **Abscess of mediastinum** — A localized collection of pus caused by the disintegration of mediastinal tissues.

J86-   **Pyothorax** — The accumulation of pus within the thoracic cavity.
    Use additional code (B95-B97) to identify infectious agent
    Excludes 1:   *abscess of lung (J85.-)*
        pyothorax due to tuberculosis (A15.6)

mcc **J86.0**   **Pyothorax with fistula** — A form associated with an abnormal passage of the thoracic cavity.
    Any condition classifiable to J86.9 with fistula
    Bronchocutaneous fistula — A form characterized by an abnormal passage between the bronchial region and the skin.
    Bronchopleural fistula — A form characterized by an abnormal passage from the bronchial area to the pleura.
    Hepatopleural fistula — A form characterized by an abnormal passage between the liver and the pleura.
    Mediastinal fistula — A form characterized by an abnormal passage of the mediastinum.
    Pleural fistula — A form characterized by an abnormal passage of the pleura.
    Thoracic fistula — A form characterized by an abnormal passage of the thoracic cavity.

mcc **J86.9**   **Pyothorax without fistula**
    Abscess of pleura — An abnormal localized accumulation of pus in the pleural cavity.
    Abscess of thorax — An abnormal accumulation of pus within the thoracic cavity.
    Empyema (chest) (lung) (pleura) — An abnormal localized accumulation of pus within the thoracic cavity.
    Fibrinopurulent pleurisy — Inflammation of the pleura characterized by a localized collection of pus which contains fibrin.
    Purulent pleurisy — Inflammation of the pleura with a localized collection of pus.
    Pyopneumothorax — The abnormal massive collection of pus and air or gas in the pleural cavity.
    Septic pleurisy — Inflammation of the pleura with a localized collection of pus caused by the decomposition of microorganisms.
    Seropurulent pleurisy — Inflammation of the pleura with a localized collection of pus and serous fluid.
    Suppurative pleurisy — Inflammation of the pleura with a localized collection of pus and serous fluid.

Other diseases of the pleura (J90-J94)

J90   **Pleural effusion, <u>not elsewhere classified</u>** — Inflammation of the pleura with
cc   an abnormal accumulation of pleural fluid in the pleural space.
    Encysted pleurisy — A form characterized by adhesions that localize the pleural effusion.
    Pleural effusion NOS
    Pleurisy with effusion (exudative) (serous)
    Excludes 1:   *chylous (pleural) effusion (J94.0)*
        malignant pleural effusion (J91.0))
        pleurisy NOS (R09.1)
        tuberculous pleural effusion (A15.6)

J91-   **Pleural effusion <u>in conditions classified elsewhere</u>**
    Excludes ❷: *pleural effusion in heart failure (I50.-)*
        pleural effusion in systemic lupus erythematosus (M32.13)

cc **J91.0**   **Malignant pleural effusion** — [Not Allowed as PDX] — The presence of malignant cells in the pleural fluid.
    Code first underlying neoplasm

cc **J91.8**   **Pleural effusion in other conditions classified elsewhere** —
    [Not Allowed as PDX]
    AHA 15:2Q:p15 – Pleural effusion in congestive heart failure patients
    Code first underlying disease, such as:
    Filariasis (B74.0-B74.9)
    Influenza (J09.x2, J10.1, J11.1)

J92-   **Pleural plaque** — The fibrous thickening of the pleura.
    Includes: **Pleural thickening**

J92.0   **Pleural plaque <u>with presence of asbestos</u>**

J92.9   **Pleural plaque <u>without</u> asbestos**
    Pleural plaque NOS

J93-   **Pneumothorax and air leak** — The abnormal accumulation or presence of air or gas in the pleural space.
    Excludes 1:   *congenital or perinatal pneumothorax (P25.1)*
        postprocedural air leak (J95.812)
        postprocedural pneumothorax (J95.811)
        traumatic pneumothorax (S27.0)
        tuberculous (current disease) pneumothorax (A15.-)
        pyopneumothorax (J86-)

mcc **J93.0**   **Spontaneous <u>tension</u> pneumothorax** — A severe form of unknown cause in which a significant portion of the lung collapses and results in compression on the chest structures, including the major blood vessels, trachea, and heart.

J93.1-   **Other <u>spontaneous</u> pneumothorax**

cc **J93.11**   **<u>Primary</u> spontaneous pneumothorax** — A form of unknown cause that causes a partial collapse of the lung.

cc **J93.12**   **<u>Secondary</u> spontaneous pneumothorax** —
    [Unacceptable PDX] — A form due to another disease condition that causes a partial collapse of the lung.
    Code first underlying condition, such as:
    Catamenial pneumothorax due to endometriosis (N80.8)
    Cystic fibrosis (E84-)
    Eosinophilic pneumonia (J82)
    Lymphangioleiomyomatosis (J84.81)
    Malignant neoplasm of bronchus amd lung (C34-)
    Marfan's syndrome (Q87.4)
    Pneumonia due to Pneumocystis carinii (B59)
    Secondary malignant neoplasm of lung (C78.0-)
    Spontaneous rupture of the esophagus (K22.3)

J93.8-   **Other pneumothorax and air leak**

cc **J93.81**   **<u>Chronic</u> pneumothorax** — A form marked by slow development, or persistence, over a period of time that causes a partial collapse of the lung.

cc **J93.82**   **Other <u>air leak</u>** — A form marked by the persistent escape of air from the lung into the pleural space without causing a partial collapse of the lung.
    Persistent air leak

cc **J93.83**   **Other pneumothorax**
    Acute pneumothorax — A form marked by sudden, severe onset that causes a partial collapse of the lung.
    Spontaneous pneumothorax NOS

cc **J93.9**   **Pneumothorax, unspecified**
    Pneumothorax NOS

J 84 - J 93

J94- Other pleural conditions

Excludes 1: *pleurisy NOS (R09.1)*
traumatic hemopneumothorax (S27.2)
traumatic hemothorax (S27.1)
tuberculous pleural conditions (current disease) (A15.-)

cc **J94.0** **Chylous effusion** — An abnormal accumulation of chyle in the pleural space.
Chyliform effusion

J94.1 **Fibrothorax** — An abnormal accumulation of fibrosis in the pleural space.

cc **J94.2** **Hemothorax** — An abnormal accumulation of effused blood in the pleural space.
Hemopneumothorax — An abnormal accumulation of effused blood and air in the pleural space.

cc **J94.8** **Other specified pleural conditions**
Hydropneumothorax — An abnormal accumulation of watery fluid and air in the pleural space.
Hydrothorax — An abnormal accumulation of watery fluid in the pleural space.

J94.9 **Pleural condition, unspecified**

Intraoperative and postprocedural complications and disorders of respiratory system, not elsewhere classified (J95)

J95- **Intraoperative and postprocedural complications** and disorders of respiratory system, not elsewhere classified

Excludes ❷: *aspiration pneumonia (J69.-)*
emphysema (subcutaneous) resulting from a procedure (T81.82)
hypostatic pneumonia (J18.2)
pulmonary manifestations due to radiation (J70.0-J70.1)

J95.0- Tracheostomy complications

cc **J95.00** **Unspecified tracheostomy complication**

cc **J95.01** **Hemorrhage from tracheostomy stoma**

cc **J95.02** **Infection of tracheostomy stoma**
Use additional code to identify type of infection, such as:
Cellulitis of neck (L03.8)
Sepsis (A40, A41.-)

cc **J95.03** **Malfunction of tracheostomy stoma**
Mechanical complication of tracheostomy stoma
Obstruction of tracheostomy airway
Tracheal stenosis due to tracheostomy

cc **J95.04** **Tracheo-esophageal fistula following tracheostomy**

cc **J95.09** **Other tracheostomy complication**

MCC **J95.1** **Acute pulmonary insufficiency following thoracic surgery**

Excludes ❷: *functional disturbances following cardiac surgery (I97.0, I97.1-)*

MCC **J95.2** **Acute pulmonary insufficiency following nonthoracic surgery**

Excludes ❷: *functional disturbances following cardiac surgery (I97.0, I97.1-)*

MCC **J95.3** **Chronic pulmonary insufficiency following surgery**

Excludes ❷: *functional disturbances following cardiac surgery (I97.0, I97.1-)*

cc **J95.4** **Chemical pneumonitis due to anesthesia**
Mendelson's syndrome
Postprocedural aspiration pneumonia
Use additional code for adverse effect, if applicable, to identify drug (T41- with fifth or sixth character 5)

Excludes 1: *aspiration pneumonitis due to anesthesia complicating labor and delivery (O74.0)*
aspiration pneumonitis due to anesthesia complicating pregnancy (O29)
aspiration pneumonitis due to anesthesia complicating the puerperium (O89.01)

cc **J95.5** **Postprocedural subglottic stenosis**

J95.6- Intraoperative hemorrhage and hematoma of a respiratory system organ or structure complicating a procedure

Excludes 1: *intraoperative hemorrhage and hematoma of a respiratory system organ or structure due to accidental puncture and laceration during procedure (J95.7-)*

cc **J95.61** **Intraoperative hemorrhage and hematoma of a respiratory system organ or structure complicating a respiratory system procedure**

cc **J95.62** **Intraoperative hemorrhage and hematoma of a respiratory system organ or structure complicating other procedure**

J95.7- Accidental puncture and laceration of a respiratory system organ or structure during a procedure

Excludes ❷: *postprocedural pneumothorax (J95.811)*

cc **J95.71** **Accidental puncture and laceration of a respiratory system organ or structure during a respiratory system procedure**

cc **J95.72** **Accidental puncture and laceration of a respiratory system organ or structure during other procedure**

J95.8- Other intraoperative and postprocedural complications and disorders of respiratory system, not elsewhere classified

J95.81- Postprocedural pneumothorax and air leak

cc **J95.811** **Postprocedural pneumothorax**

cc **J95.812** **Postprocedural air leak**

J95.82- Postprocedural respiratory failure

Excludes 1: *respiratory failure in other conditions (J96-)*

MCC **J95.821** **Acute postprocedural respiratory failure**
Postprocedural respiratory failure NOS

MCC **J95.822** **Acute and chronic postprocedural respiratory failure**

J95.83- Postprocedural hemorrhage of a respiratory system organ or structure following a procedure

cc **J95.830** **Postprocedural hemorrhage of a respiratory system organ or structure following a respiratory system procedure**

cc **J95.831** **Postprocedural hemorrhage of a respiratory system organ or structure following other procedure**

cc **J95.84** **Transfusion-related acute lung injury (TRALI)** — A pulmonary disorder occurring 1-6 hours post transfusion that is characterized by pulmonary distress, bilateral noncardiogenic pulmonary edema, hypotension, fever, and hypoxemia.

J95.85- Complication of respirator [ventilator]

cc **J95.850** **Mechanical complication of respirator**

Excludes 1: *encounter for respirator [ventilator] dependence during power failure (Z99.12)*

cc **J95.851** **Ventilator associated pneumonia**
Ventilator associated pneumonitis
Use additional code to identify the organism, if known (B95-, B96-, B97-)

Excludes 1: *ventilator lung in newborn (P27.8)*

cc **J95.859** **Other complication of respirator [ventilator]**

J95.86- Postprocedural hematoma and seroma of a respiratory system organ or structure following a procedure

cc **J95.860** **Postprocedural hematoma of a respiratory system organ or structure following a respiratory system procedure**

cc **J95.861** **Postprocedural hematoma of a respiratory system organ or structure following other procedure**

cc **J95.862** **Postprocedural seroma of a respiratory system organ or structure following a respiratory system procedure**

cc **J95.863** **Postprocedural seroma of a respiratory system organ or structure following other procedure**

cc **J95.88** **Other intraoperative complications of respiratory system, not elsewhere classified**

cc **J95.89** **Other postprocedural complications and disorders of respiratory system, not elsewhere classified**
Use additional code to identify disorder, such as:
Aspiration pneumonia (J69.-)
Bacterial or viral pneumonia (J12-J18)

Excludes ❷: *acute pulmonary insufficiency following thoracic surgery (J95.1)*
postprocedural subglottic stenosis (J95.5)

J94 - J95

Other diseases of the respiratory system (J96-J99)

J96- **Respiratory failure, <u>not elsewhere classified</u>**
    Excludes 1:   acute respiratory distress syndrome (J80)
                cardiorespiratory failure (R09.2)
                newborn respiratory distress syndrome (P22.0)
                postprocedural respiratory failure (J95.82-)
                respiratory arrest (R09.2)
                respiratory arrest of newborn (P28.81)
                respiratory failure of newborn (P28.5)

  J96.0- **<u>Acute respiratory failure</u>** — A sudden, severe onset of decreased pulmonary function due to an abnormally low arterial oxygen level or an abnormally high arterial carbon dioxide level.
      AHA 13:4Q:p121 – Acute respiratory failure due to smoke inhalation

  MCC **J96.00** **Acute respiratory failure, <u>unspecified</u> whether with hypoxia or hypercapnia**

  MCC **J96.01** **Acute respiratory failure <u>with hypoxia</u>** — Insufficient level of oxygen reaching the tissues.

  MCC **J96.02** **Acute respiratory failure <u>with hypercapnia</u>** — Abnormally high arterial carbon dioxide level.

  J96.1- **<u>Chronic</u> respiratory failure**
      AHA 13:4Q:p129 – Chronic hypoxic respiratory failure and COPD

  CC **J96.10** **Chronic respiratory failure, <u>unspecified</u> whether with hypoxia or hypercapnia**

  CC **J96.11** **Chronic respiratory failure <u>with hypoxia</u>** — Insufficient level of oxygen reaching the tissues.

  CC **J96.12** **Chronic respiratory failure <u>with hypercapnia</u>** — Abnormally high arterial carbon dioxide level.

  J96.2- **<u>Acute and chronic</u> respiratory failure**
      Acute on chronic respiratory failure

  MCC **J96.20** **Acute and chronic respiratory failure, <u>unspecified</u> whether with hypoxia or hypercapnia**

  MCC **J96.21** **Acute and chronic respiratory failure <u>with hypoxia</u>** — Insufficient level of oxygen reaching the tissues.

  MCC **J96.22** **Acute and chronic respiratory failure <u>with hypercapnia</u>** — Abnormally high arterial carbon dioxide level.

  J96.9- **Respiratory failure, <u>unspecified</u>**

  MCC **J96.90** **Respiratory failure, unspecified, <u>unspecified</u> whether with hypoxia or hypercapnia**

  MCC **J96.91** **Respiratory failure, unspecified <u>with hypoxia</u>** — Insufficient level of oxygen reaching the tissues.

  MCC **J96.92** **Respiratory failure, unspecified <u>with hypercapnia</u>** — Abnormally high arterial carbon dioxide level.

J98- **Other respiratory disorders**
    Use additional code to identify:
    Exposure to environmental tobacco smoke (Z77.22)
    Exposure to tobacco smoke in the perinatal period (P96.81)
    History of tobacco dependence (Z87.891)
    Occupational exposure to environmental tobacco smoke (Z57.31)
    Tobacco dependence (F17.-)
    Tobacco use (Z72.0)
    Excludes 1:   newborn apnea (P28.4)
                newborn sleep apnea (P28.3)
    Excludes 2:   apnea NOS (R06.81)
                sleep apnea (G47.3-)

  J98.0- **Diseases of bronchus, <u>not elsewhere classified</u>**

    J98.01 **Acute bronchospasm** — The sudden, severe onset of narrowing of the bronchial airways.
        Excludes 1:   acute bronchiolitis with bronchospasm (J21.-)
                 acute bronchitis with bronchospasm (J20.-)
                 asthma (J45.-)
                 exercise induced bronchospasm (J45.990)

    J98.09 **Other diseases of bronchus, not elsewhere classified**
        Broncholithiasis — The abnormal presence of calculi within the bronchial branches.
        Calcification of bronchus — The abnormal deposition of calcium salts in the bronchial tissues.
        Stenosis of bronchus — The abnormal reduction in the size of the bronchial airways.
        Tracheobronchial collapse — The abnormal reduction in the size of the bronchial or tracheal lumens.
        Tracheobronchial dyskinesia
        Ulcer of bronchus — A tissue-destroying sore of the bronchial tissues.

J98.1- **Pulmonary collapse** — An acute, airless state of all or part of a lung.
    Excludes 1:   therapeutic collapse of lung status (Z98.3)

  CC **J98.11** **Atelectasis** — The airless collapse (alveolar deflation) of part or all of a lung.
      Excludes 1:   newborn atelectasis
                 tuberculous atelectasis (current disease) (A15)

  CC **J98.19** **Other pulmonary collapse**

J98.2 **Interstitial emphysema** — The abnormal presence of air in the peribronchial and interstitial tissues of the lungs.
    Mediastinal emphysema — The abnormal presence of air in the mediastinal tissues.
    Excludes 1:   emphysema NOS (J43.9)
                emphysema in newborn (P25.0)
                surgical emphysema (subcutaneous) (T81.82)
                traumatic subcutaneous emphysema (T79.7)

J98.3 **Compensatory emphysema** — Excessive inhalation of lung tissue following a morbid lung tissue condition.

J98.4 **Other disorders of lung**
    Calcification of lung — The abnormal deposition of calcium salts within the pulmonary tissue.
    Cystic lung disease (acquired) — The abnormal presence of cystic air spaces.
    Lung disease NOS
    Pulmolithiasis — The abnormal presence of calculi within the pulmonary system.
    Excludes 1:   acute interstitial pneumonitis (J84.114)
                pulmonary insufficiency following surgery (J95.1-J95.2)

J98.5- **Diseases of mediastinum, <u>not elsewhere classified</u>**
    Excludes 2:   abscess of mediastinum (J85.3)

  MCC **J98.51** **Mediastinitis** — Inflammation of the mediastinum.
      Code first underlying condition, if applicable, such as postoperative mediastinitis (T81.-)

  MCC **J98.59** **Other diseases of mediastinum, not elsewhere classified**
      Fibrosis of mediastinum — The abnormal presence of fibrous tissue within the mediastinum.
      Hernia of mediastinum — The abnormal protrusion of the mediastinum into other parts of the thoracic cavity.
      Retraction of mediastinum — The abnormal drawing-back of the normal mediastinal area.

J98.6 **Disorders of diaphragm**
    Diaphragmatitis — Inflammation of the diaphragm.
    Paralysis of diaphragm — The abnormal loss or impairment of the motor function of the diaphragm.
    Relaxation of diaphragm — The abnormal decrease in the diaphragm tension.
    Excludes 1:   congenital malformation of diaphragm NEC (Q79.1)
                congenital diaphragmatic hernia (Q79.0)
    Excludes 2:   diaphragmatic hernia (K44.-)

J98.8 **Other specified respiratory disorders**

J98.9 **Respiratory disorder, unspecified**
    Respiratory disease (chronic) NOS

J99 **Respiratory disorders <u>in diseases classified elsewhere</u>** —
    [Not Allowed as PDX]
    Code first underlying disease, such as:
    Amyloidosis (E85.-)
    Ankylosing spondylitis (M45)
    Congenital syphilis (A50.5)
    Cryoglobulinemia (D89.1)
    Early congenital syphilis (A50.0)
    Schistosomiasis (B65.0-B65.9)
    Excludes 1:   respiratory disorders in:
                 amebiasis (A06.5)
                 blastomycosis (B40.0-B40.2)
                 candidiasis (B37.1)
                 coccidioidomycosis (B38.0-B38.2)
                 cystic fibrosis with pulmonary manifestations (E84.0)
                 dermatomyositis (M33.01, M33.11)
                 histoplasmosis (B39.0-B39.2)
                 late syphilis (A52.72, A52.73)
                 polymyositis (M33.21)
                 sicca syndrome (M35.02)
                 systemic lupus erythematosus (M32.13)
                 systemic sclerosis (M34.81)
                 Wegener's granulomatosis (M31.30-M31.31)

J
9
6
-
J
9
9

Chapter 11 – Diseases of the digestive system (K00-K95)

Excludes ❷: certain conditions originating in the perinatal period
(P04-P96)
certain infectious and parasitic diseases (A00-B99)
complications of pregnancy, childbirth and the puerperium
(O00-O9A)
congenital malformations, deformations and chromosomal
abnormalities (Q00-Q99)
endocrine, nutritional and metabolic diseases (E00-E88)
injury, poisoning and certain other consequences of external
causes (S00-T88)
neoplasms (C00-D49)
symptoms, signs and abnormal clinical and laboratory findings,
not elsewhere classified (R00-R94)

This chapter contains the following blocks:

K00-K14	Diseases of oral cavity and salivary glands
K20-K31	Diseases of esophagus, stomach and duodenum
K35-K38	Diseases of appendix
K40-K46	Hernia
K50-K52	Noninfective enteritis and colitis
K55-K64	Other diseases of intestines
K65-K68	Diseases of peritoneum and retroperitoneum
K70-K77	Diseases of liver
K80-K87	Disorders of gallbladder, biliary tract and pancreas
K90-K95	Other diseases of the digestive system

Chapter-Specific Coding Guidelines

C. Chapter-Specific Coding Guidelines
In addition to general coding guidelines, there are guidelines for specific diagnoses and/or conditions in the classification. Unless otherwise indicated, these guidelines apply to all health care settings. Please refer to Section II for guidelines on the selection of principal diagnosis.

11. Chapter 11: Diseases of the Digestive System (K00-K94)

Reserved for future guideline expansion

Diseases of oral cavity and salivary glands (K00-K14)

K00- Disorders of tooth development and eruption
Excludes ❷: embedded and impacted teeth (K01.-)

K00.0   Anodontia — Congenital absence of all or some of the teeth.
Hypodontia — Congenital absence of some of the teeth.
Oligodontia — The presence of less than the normal number of teeth, some of them being congenitally absent.
Excludes 1: acquired absence of teeth (K08.1-)

K00.1   Supernumerary teeth — An excess number of teeth.
Distomolar — Any tooth found distal to a third molar.
Fourth molar — A supernumerary molar distal to the third molar.
Mesiodens — A small supernumerary tooth situated palatally between the maxillary central incisor.
Paramolar — A supernumerary tooth appearing adjacent to a molar.
Supplementary teeth — Additional teeth.
Excludes ❷: supernumerary roots (K00.2)

K00.2   Abnormalities of size and form of teeth
Concrescence of teeth — The union of the roots of 2 approximating teeth by a deposit of cementum.
Dens evaginatus — The eruption of teeth before calcification is complete.
Dens in dente — A malformed tooth resulting from invagination of the crown before it is calcified.
Dens invaginatus — Synonym for Dens In Dente.
Enamel pearls — Tiny globules of enamel, firmly adherent to a tooth.
Fusion of teeth — The abnormal coherence of 2 or more teeth.
Gemination of teeth — The division of a tooth bud which results in the formation of 2 teeth, or of a double crown formed on a single root with a single pulp canal.
Macrodontia — An abnormal increase in the size of the teeth.
Microdontia — An abnormal smallness of the size of the teeth.
Peg-shaped [conical] teeth — Malformed teeth, with a characteristic peg-shaped appearance.
Supernumerary roots — An excess number of roots.
Taurodontism — An elongated variation in molar teeth form.
Tuberculum paramolare — A small nodule of tooth close to a molar.
Excludes 1: abnormalities of teeth due to congenital syphilis (A50.5)
tuberculum Carabelli, which is regarded as a normal variation and should not be coded

K00.3   Mottled teeth — A patchy discoloration of the teeth.
Dental fluorosis — A mottled discoloration of the enamel of the teeth resulting from ingestion of excessive amounts of fluorine during tooth development.
Mottling of enamel — A patchy or spotting of discoloration of the enamel.
Nonfluoride enamel opacities — An abnormal discoloration of the enamel by a nonfluoride cause.
Excludes ❷: deposits [accretions] on teeth (K03.6)

K00.4   Disturbances in tooth formation
Aplasia and hypoplasia of cementum — The lack or incomplete development of the bone-like connective tissue covering the root of a tooth.
Dilaceration of tooth — Developmental injury to a tooth characterized by a crease or band at the junction of the crown or root, or by tortuous roots with abnormal curvatures.
Enamel hypoplasia (neonatal) (postnatal) (prenatal) — Incomplete or defective development of the enamel of the teeth.
Regional odontodysplasia — The abnormal development of a group of teeth.
Turner's tooth — A permanent tooth enamel hypoplasia resulting from the spread of infection.
Excludes 1: Hutchinson's teeth and mulberry molars in congenital syphilis (A50.5)
Excludes ❷: mottled teeth (K00.3)

K00.5   Hereditary disturbances in tooth structure, not elsewhere classified
Amelogenesis imperfecta — An inherited condition resulting in defective development of the enamel of the teeth which is brown in color.
Dentinal dysplasia — An inherited condition affecting both the primary and secondary dentition, in which the teeth have short, distorted roots.
Dentinogenesis imperfecta — An inherited condition characterized by defective formation and calcification of the dentin, giving the teeth a brown or blue opalescent appearance.
Odontogenesis imperfecta — Synonym for Dentinogenesis, Imperfecta.
Shell teeth — An inherited condition in which the enamel appears essentially normal, the dentin is extremely thin, and the pulp chamber is enlarged.

K00.6   Disturbances in tooth eruption
Dentia praecox — A primary tooth that erupts during the neonatal period.
Natal tooth — A prematurely erupted deciduous tooth, visible in the jaw at birth.
Neonatal tooth — A primary tooth that erupts during the neonatal period.
Premature eruption of tooth — Appearance of a tooth before the proper time.
Premature shedding of primary [deciduous] tooth — The early loss of primary teeth before the proper time.
Prenatal teeth — Synonym for Natal Tooth.
Retained [persistent] primary tooth — The abnormal retention of primary teeth beyond the normal time.
Excludes ❷: embedded and impacted teeth (K01-)

K00.7   Teething syndrome — The uncomfortable symptoms associated with the process of erupting teeth.

K00.8   Other disorders of tooth development
Color changes during tooth formation
Intrinsic staining of teeth NOS
Excludes ❷: posteruptive color changes (K03.7)

K00.9   Disorder of tooth development, unspecified
Disorder of odontogenesis NOS

K01- Embedded and impacted teeth
Excludes 1: abnormal position of fully erupted teeth (M26.3-)

K01.0   Embedded teeth — An unerupted tooth, usually one completely covered by bone.

K01.1   Impacted teeth — A tooth so placed in the jaw that it is unable to erupt.

K02- Dental caries — The progressive decalcification of the hard, inorganic portion of a tooth caused by the action of microorganisms and followed by disintegration of the soft, organic portion.
Includes: Caries of dentine
Dental cavities
Early childhood caries
Pre-eruptive caries
Recurrent caries (dentino enamel junction) (enamel) (to the pulp)
Tooth decay

K02.3   Arrested dental caries — A form marked by the cessation of the decaying process.
Arrested coronal and root caries

K02.5- Dental caries on pit and fissure surface
Dental caries on chewing surface of tooth

K02.51   Dental caries on pit and fissure surface limited to enamel — A form involving the very hard, white substance that covers the dentin and forms the crown of a tooth.
White spot lesions [initial caries] on pit and fissure surface of tooth

K
0
0
–
K
0
2

K02.52 Dental caries on pit and fissure surface penetrating into dentin — A form involving the primary, hard tooth substance which surrounds the root and is covered by enamel.
  Primary dental caries, cervical origin

K02.53 Dental caries on pit and fissure surface penetrating into pulp — A form involving the organic, viable center portion of a tooth.

K02.6- Dental caries on smooth surface

K02.61 Dental caries on smooth surface limited to enamel — A form involving the very hard, white substance that covers the dentin and forms the crown of a tooth.
  White spot lesions [initial caries] on smooth surface of tooth

K02.62 Dental caries on smooth surface penetrating into dentin — A form involving the primary, hard tooth substance which surrounds the root and is covered by enamel.

K02.63 Dental caries on smooth surface penetrating into pulp — A form involving the very hard, white substance that covers the dentin and forms the crown of a tooth.

K02.7 Dental root caries — A form involving the dental roots.

K02.9 Dental caries, unspecified

K03- Other diseases of hard tissues of teeth
  Excludes ❷: *bruxism (F45.8)*
  dental caries (K02.-)
  teeth-grinding NOS (F45.8)

K03.0 Excessive attrition of teeth — The abnormal wearing-away of the teeth in the course of normal use.
  Approximal wear of teeth
  Occlusal wear of teeth

K03.1 Abrasion of teeth — The mechanical or chemical friction process which wears away the substance of the teeth.
  Dentifrice abrasion of teeth
  Habitual abrasion of teeth
  Occupational abrasion of teeth
  Ritual abrasion of teeth
  Traditional abrasion of teeth
  Wedge defect NOS

K03.2 Erosion of teeth — The disintegration of tooth substance on surfaces free from attrition by mastication.
  Erosion of teeth due to diet
  Erosion of teeth due to drugs and medicaments
  Erosion of teeth due to persistent vomiting
  Erosion of teeth NOS
  Idiopathic erosion of teeth
  Occupational erosion of teeth

K03.3 Pathological resorption of teeth — The removal of enamel and other calcific portions of a tooth as a result of a pathological process.
  Internal granuloma of pulp
  Resorption of teeth (external)

K03.4 Hypercementosis — The abnormal, excessive growth of tooth cementum.
  Cementation hyperplasia — The excessive proliferation of normal cementum cells in normal arrangement leading to an overall increase in size.

K03.5 Ankylosis of teeth — The abnormal fusion of the root cementum with the adjacent alveolar bone.

K03.6 Deposits [accretions] on teeth — The abnormal addition of material growing on the teeth.
  Betel deposits [accretions] on teeth
  Black deposits [accretions] on teeth
  Extrinsic staining of teeth NOS
  Green deposits [accretions] on teeth
  Materia alba deposits [accretions] on teeth
  Orange deposits [accretions] on teeth
  Staining of teeth NOS
  Subgingival dental calculus
  Supragingival dental calculus
  Tobacco deposits [accretions] on teeth

K03.7 Posteruptive color changes of dental hard tissues — The abnormal discoloration of the teeth after they have broken out of the alveolar tissues.
  Excludes ❷: *deposits [accretions] on teeth (K03.6)*

K03.8- Other specified diseases of hard tissues of teeth

K03.81 Cracked tooth — The abnormal cracking or breaking of a tooth that is not due to trauma.
  Excludes 1: *asymptomatic craze lines in enamel — omit code*
  broken or fractured tooth due to trauma (S02.5)

K03.89 Other specified diseases of hard tissues of teeth

K03.9 Disease of hard tissues of teeth, unspecified

K04- Diseases of pulp and periapical tissues

K04.0- Pulpitis — Inflammation of the soft, neurovascular portion of the center of a tooth.
  Acute pulpitis — A form marked by sudden, severe onset.
  Chronic (hyperplastic) (ulcerative) pulpitis — A form marked by slow, progressive development.

CC **K04.01 Reversible pulpitis** — A form that can be restored.

CC **K04.02 Irreversible pulpitis** — A form with irreversible damage.

K04.1 Necrosis of pulp — The death of pulp tissue.
  Pulpal gangrene — The death of pulp tissue due to deficient or absent blood supply.

K04.2 Pulp degeneration — The deterioration of the pulp tissue and its function.
  Denticles — A relatively large, calcified growth within the pulp.
  Pulpal calcifications — Synonym for Denticles.
  Pulpal stones — Synonym for Denticles.

K04.3 Abnormal hard tissue formation in pulp — The abnormal replacement of the pulp tissue with hard tissue such as dentin.
  Secondary or irregular dentine

CC **K04.4 Acute apical periodontitis of pulpal origin** — A sudden, severe onset of inflammation of the dental periosteum, alveolar bone, and adjacent gingiva, originating from the pulp tissue.
  Acute apical periodontitis NOS
  Excludes 1: *acute periodontitis (K05.2-)*

K04.5 Chronic apical periodontitis — A progressive, slowly developing inflammation of the dental periosteum, alveolar bone, and adjacent gingiva.
  Apical or periapical granuloma — The abnormal formation of granulomas in the periapical tissues.
  Apical periodontitis NOS
  Excludes 1: *chronic periodontitis (K05.3-)*

K04.6 Periapical abscess with sinus — A localized collection of pus caused by the disintegration of the dental periosteum, alveolar bone, and adjacent gingiva, with a draining sinus outside of the area of inflammation.
  Dental abscess with sinus
  Dentoalveolar abscess with sinus

K04.7 Periapical abscess without sinus — A localized collection of pus caused by the disintegration of the dental periosteum, alveolar bone, and adjacent gingiva, without the formation of a draining sinus.
  Dental abscess without sinus
  Dentoalveolar abscess without sinus
  Periapical abscess without sinus

K04.8 Radicular cyst — An epithelium-lined sac at the apex of a tooth.
  Apical (periodontal) cyst
  Periapical cyst
  Residual radicular cyst
  Excludes ❷: *lateral periodontal cyst (K09.0)*

K04.9- Other and unspecified diseases of pulp and periapical tissues

K04.90 Unspecified diseases of pulp and periapical tissues

K04.99 Other diseases of pulp and periapical tissues

K05- Gingivitis and periodontal diseases
  Use additional code to identify:
  Alcohol abuse and dependence (F10.-)
  Exposure to environmental tobacco smoke (Z77.22)
  Exposure to tobacco smoke in the perinatal period (P96.81)
  History of tobacco dependence (Z87.891)
  Occupational exposure to environmental tobacco smoke (Z57.31)
  Tobacco dependence (F17.-)
  Tobacco use (Z72.0)

K05.0- Acute gingivitis — A sudden, severe onset of inflammation of the gums.
  Excludes 1: *acute necrotizing ulcerative gingivitis (A69.1)*
  herpesviral [herpes simplex] gingivostomatitis (B00.2)

K05.00 Acute gingivitis, <u>plaque</u> induced — A form that is due to the presence of plaque.
  Acute gingivitis NOS
  Plaque-induced gingival disease

K05.01 Acute gingivitis, <u>non</u>-plaque induced — A form that is due to conditions other than the presence of plaque.

K 0 2 - K 0 5

K05.1- **Chronic gingivitis** — Inflammation of the gums which develops slowly and persists over a long period of time.
  Desquamative gingivitis (chronic) — A form marked by the shedding of the gingival surface epithelium.
  Gingivitis (chronic) NOS
  Hyperplastic gingivitis (chronic) — A form marked by the abnormal increase in the size and arrangement of normal gingival cells.
  Pregnancy associated gingivitis
  Simple marginal gingivitis (chronic) — A form marked by engorgement of the gingiva with blood and edema.
  Ulcerative gingivitis (chronic) — A form marked by the eating-away of the gingival tissue.

  Code first, if applicable, diseases of the digestive system complicating pregnancy (O99.61-)

K05.10 **Chronic gingivitis, <u>plaque</u> induced** — A form that is due to the presence of plaque.
  Chronic gingivitis NOS
  Gingivitis NOS

K05.11 **Chronic gingivitis, <u>non-plaque</u> induced** — A form that is due to conditions other than the presence of plaque.

K05.2- **<u>Aggressive periodontitis</u>** — A sudden, severe onset of inflammation of the supporting structure tissues of the teeth, including the gingival and alveolar bone.
  Acute pericoronitis — A form marked by the inflammation of the gingiva surrounding the crown of a partially erupted tooth, including the cementum, alveolar bone, and gingiva.

  Excludes 1:   *acute apical periodontitis (K04.4)*
                periapical abscess (K04.7)
                periapical abscess with sinus (K04.6)

K05.20 **Aggressive periodontitis, <u>unspecified</u>**

K05.21- **Aggressive periodontitis, <u>localized</u>** — A progressive inflammation with periodontal damage of the supporting structures of the teeth that is usually confined to the permanent first molars and incisors.
  Periodontal abscess — A localized collection of pus caused by the disintegration of the supporting structure tissues of the teeth.

  K05.211 **Aggressive periodontitis, localized, <u>slight</u>**
  K05.212 **Aggressive periodontitis, localized, <u>moderate</u>**
  K05.213 **Aggressive periodontitis, localized, <u>severe</u>**
  K05.219 **Aggressive periodontitis, localized, <u>unspecified</u> severity**

K05.22- **Aggressive periodontitis, <u>generalized</u>** — A progressive inflammation with periodontal damage of the supporting structures of the teeth that affects at least 3 permanent teeth other than the permanent first molars and incisors.

  K05.221 **Aggressive periodontitis, generalized, <u>slight</u>**
  K05.222 **Aggressive periodontitis, generalized, <u>moderate</u>**
  K05.223 **Aggressive periodontitis, generalized, <u>severe</u>**
  K05.229 **Aggressive periodontitis, generalized, <u>unspecified</u> severity**

K05.3- **<u>Chronic periodontitis</u>** — Inflammation of the supporting tissues of the teeth including the cementum, alveolar bone, and gingiva, which develops slowly and persists over a long period of time.
  Chronic pericoronitis — A form marked by the inflammation of the gingiva surrounding the crown of a partially erupted tooth.
  Complex periodontitis — See Chronic Periodontitis above.
  Periodontitis NOS
  Simplex periodontitis — A form due to a variety of local irritants.

  Excludes 1:   *chronic apical periodontitis (K04.5)*

K05.30 **Chronic periodontitis, <u>unspecified</u>**

K05.31- **Chronic periodontitis, <u>localized</u>** — A form affecting the permanent first molars and incisors.

  K05.311 **Chronic periodontitis, localized, <u>slight</u>**
  K05.312 **Chronic periodontitis, localized, <u>moderate</u>**
  K05.313 **Chronic periodontitis, localized, <u>severe</u>**
  K05.319 **Chronic periodontitis, localized, <u>unspecified</u> severity**

K05.32- **Chronic periodontitis, <u>generalized</u>** — A form affecting at least 3 permanent teeth other than the permanent first molars and incisors.

  K05.321 **Chronic periodontitis, generalized, <u>slight</u>**
  K05.322 **Chronic periodontitis, generalized, <u>moderate</u>**
  K05.323 **Chronic periodontitis, generalized, <u>severe</u>**
  K05.329 **Chronic periodontitis, generalized, <u>unspecified</u> severity**

K05.4 **Periodontosis** — The noninflammatory degenerative destruction of the periodontal tissues.
  Juvenile periodontosis

K05.5 **Other periodontal diseases**
  Combined periodontic-endodontic lesion
  Narrow gingival width (of periodontal soft tissue)
  Excludes ❷: *leukoplakia of gingiva (K13.21)*

K05.6 **Periodontal disease, unspecified**

K06- **Other disorders of gingiva and edentulous alveolar ridge**
  Excludes ❷: *acute gingivitis (K05.0)*
                atrophy of edentulous alveolar ridge (K08.2)
                chronic gingivitis (K05.1)
                gingivitis NOS (K05.1)

K06.0 **Gingival recession** — The abnormal receding of the gingival margin from the neck of a tooth.
  Gingival recession (generalized) (localized) (postinfective) (postprocedural)

K06.1 **Gingival enlargement** — The abnormal hypertrophy of the gums.
  Gingival fibromatosis — An inherited condition characterized by hypertrophy of the gums prior to the time of eruption of the teeth.

K06.2 **Gingival and edentulous alveolar ridge lesions associated with trauma**
  Irritative hyperplasia of edentulous ridge [denture hyperplasia]
  Use additional code (Chapter 20) to identify external cause or denture status (Z97.2)

K06.3 **Horizontal alveolar bone loss**

K06.8 **Other specified disorders of gingiva and edentulous alveolar ridge**
  Fibrous epulis — A fibrous tumor originating in the periosteum of the lower jaw and gingiva.
  Flabby alveolar ridge
  Giant cell epulis — A fibrous tumor originating in the periosteum of the lower jaw and gingiva.
  Peripheral giant cell granuloma of gingiva — A pedunculated lesion of the gingiva or alveolar ridge.
  Pyogenic granuloma of gingiva
  Vertical ridge deficiency
  Excludes ❷: *gingival cyst (K09.0)*

K06.9 **Disorder of gingiva and edentulous alveolar ridge, unspecified**

K08- **Other disorders of teeth and supporting structures**
  Excludes ❷: *dentofacial anomalies [including malocclusion] (M26.-)*
                disorders of jaw (M27.-)

K08.0 **Exfoliation of teeth due to systemic causes** — The deterioration and loss of teeth due to systemic diseases which affect the development and support of the teeth.
  Code also underlying systemic condition

K08.1- **<u>Complete loss</u> of teeth** — The acquired absence of some or all of the natural teeth.
  Acquired loss of teeth, complete
  Excludes 1:   *congenital absence of teeth (K00.0)*
                exfoliation of teeth due to systemic causes (K08.0)
                partial loss of teeth (K08.4-)

K08.10- **Complete loss of teeth, <u>unspecified</u> cause**
  K08.101 **Complete loss of teeth, unspecified cause, class I**
  K08.102 **Complete loss of teeth, unspecified cause, class II**
  K08.103 **Complete loss of teeth, unspecified cause, class III**
  K08.104 **Complete loss of teeth, unspecified cause, class IV**
  K08.109 **Complete loss of teeth, unspecified cause, unspecified class**
          Edentulism NOS

K08.11- **Complete loss of teeth <u>due to trauma</u>** — Loss due to physical injury.
  K08.111 **Complete loss of teeth due to trauma, class I**
  K08.112 **Complete loss of teeth due to trauma, class II**
  K08.113 **Complete loss of teeth due to trauma, class III**
  K08.114 **Complete loss of teeth due to trauma, class IV**
  K08.119 **Complete loss of teeth due to trauma, unspecified class**

K08.12- **Complete loss of teeth <u>due to periodontal diseases</u>** — Loss due to a diseased condition of the teeth supporting structures.
  K08.121 **Complete loss of teeth due to periodontal diseases, class I**
  K08.122 **Complete loss of teeth due to periodontal diseases, class II**

K05 – K08

K08.123 Complete loss of teeth due to periodontal diseases, class III

K08.124 Complete loss of teeth due to periodontal diseases, class IV

K08.129 Complete loss of teeth due to periodontal diseases, unspecified class

K08.13- Complete loss of teeth <u>due to caries</u> — Loss due to cavities.

K08.131 Complete loss of teeth due to caries, class I

K08.132 Complete loss of teeth due to caries, class II

K08.133 Complete loss of teeth due to caries, class III

K08.134 Complete loss of teeth due to caries, class IV

K08.139 Complete loss of teeth due to caries, unspecified class

K08.19- Complete loss of teeth <u>due to other</u> specified cause

K08.191 Complete loss of teeth due to other specified cause, class I

K08.192 Complete loss of teeth due to other specified cause, class II

K08.193 Complete loss of teeth due to other specified cause, class III

K08.194 Complete loss of teeth due to other specified cause, class IV

K08.199 Complete loss of teeth due to other specified cause, unspecified class

K08.2- **Atrophy of edentulous alveolar ridge** — A wasting-away of a toothless alveolar ridge.

K08.20 **Unspecified atrophy of edentulous alveolar ridge**
Atrophy of the mandible NOS
Atrophy of the maxilla NOS

K08.21 **Minimal atrophy of the mandible**
Minimal atrophy of the edentulous mandible

K08.22 **Moderate atrophy of the mandible**
Moderate atrophy of the edentulous mandible

K08.23 **Severe atrophy of the mandible**
Severe atrophy of the edentulous mandible

K08.24 **Minimal atrophy of maxilla**
Minimal atrophy of the edentulous maxilla

K08.25 **Moderate atrophy of the maxilla**
Moderate atrophy of the edentulous maxilla

K08.26 **Severe atrophy of the maxilla**
Severe atrophy of the edentulous maxilla

K08.3 **Retained dental root** — A retained dental root fragment still present after loss of the rest of the tooth.

K08.4- <u>Partial loss</u> of teeth — The acquired absence of some of the natural teeth.
Acquired loss of teeth, partial
Excludes 1: *complete loss of teeth (K08.1-)*
congenital absence of teeth (K00.0)
Excludes ❷: *exfoliation of teeth due to systemic causes (K08.0)*

K08.40- Partial loss of teeth, <u>unspecified</u> cause

K08.401 Partial loss of teeth, unspecified cause, class I

K08.402 Partial loss of teeth, unspecified cause, class II

K08.403 Partial loss of teeth, unspecified cause, class III

K08.404 Partial loss of teeth, unspecified cause, class IV

K08.409 Partial loss of teeth, unspecified cause, unspecified class
Tooth extraction status NOS

K08.41- Partial loss of teeth <u>due to trauma</u> — Loss due to physical injury.

K08.411 Partial loss of teeth due to trauma, class I

K08.412 Partial loss of teeth due to trauma, class II

K08.413 Partial loss of teeth due to trauma, class III

K08.414 Partial loss of teeth due to trauma, class IV

K08.419 Partial loss of teeth due to trauma, unspecified class

K08.42- Partial loss of teeth <u>due to periodontal diseases</u> — Loss due to a diseased condition of the teeth supporting structures.

K08.421 Partial loss of teeth due to periodontal diseases, class I

K08.422 Partial loss of teeth due to periodontal diseases, class II

K08.423 Partial loss of teeth due to periodontal diseases, class III

K08.424 Partial loss of teeth due to periodontal diseases, class IV

K08.429 Partial loss of teeth due to periodontal diseases, unspecified class

K08.43- Partial loss of teeth <u>due to caries</u> — Loss due to cavities.

K08.431 Partial loss of teeth due to caries, class I

K08.432 Partial loss of teeth due to caries, class II

K08.433 Partial loss of teeth due to caries, class III

K08.434 Partial loss of teeth due to caries, class IV

K08.439 Partial loss of teeth due to caries, unspecified class

K08.49- Partial loss of teeth <u>due to other</u> specified cause

K08.491 Partial loss of teeth due to other specified cause, class I

K08.492 Partial loss of teeth due to other specified cause, class II

K08.493 Partial loss of teeth due to other specified cause, class III

K08.494 Partial loss of teeth due to other specified cause, class IV

K08.499 Partial loss of teeth due to other specified cause, unspecified class

K08.5- **Unsatisfactory restoration of tooth**
Defective bridge, crown, filling
Defective dental restoration
Excludes 1: *dental restoration status (Z98.811)*
Excludes ❷: *endosseous dental implant failure (M27.6-)*
unsatisfactory endodontic treatment (M27.5-)

K08.50 **Unsatisfactory restoration of tooth, unspecified**
Defective dental restoration NOS

K08.51 **Open restoration margins of tooth**
Dental restoration failure of marginal integrity
Open margin on tooth restoration
Poor gingival margin to tooth restoration

K08.52 **Unrepairable overhanging of dental restorative materials**
Overhanging of tooth restoration

K08.53- **Fractured dental restorative material**
Excludes 1: *cracked tooth (K03.81)*
traumatic fracture of tooth (S02.5)

K08.530 **Fractured dental restorative material <u>without</u> loss of material**

K08.531 **Fractured dental restorative material <u>with loss of material</u>**

K08.539 **Fractured dental restorative material, <u>unspecified</u>**

K08.54 **Contour of existing restoration of tooth biologically incompatible with oral health**
Dental restoration failure of periodontal anatomical integrity
Unacceptable contours of existing restoration of tooth
Unacceptable morphology of existing restoration of tooth

K08.55 **Allergy to existing dental restorative material**
Use additional code to identify the specific type of allergy

K08.56 **Poor aesthetic of existing restoration of tooth**
Dental restoration aesthetically inadequate or displeasing

K08.59 **Other unsatisfactory restoration of tooth**
Other defective dental restoration

K08.8- **Other specified disorders of teeth and supporting structures**

K08.81 **Primary occlusal trauma**

K08.82 **Secondary occlusal trauma**

K08.89 **Other specified disorders of teeth and supporting structures**
Enlargement of alveolar ridge NOS
Insufficient anatomic crown height
Insufficient clinical crown length
Irregular alveolar process
Toothache NOS

K08.9 **Disorder of teeth and supporting structures, unspecified**

K
0
8
-
K
0
8

K09- Cysts of oral region, not elsewhere classified
Includes: Lesions showing histological features both of aneurysmal cyst
and of another fibro-osseous lesion
Excludes ❷: cysts of jaw (M27.0-, M27.4-)
radicular cyst (K04.8)

K09.0 Developmental odontogenic cysts — A cyst of the odontogenic
epithelium of the jaws.
Dentigerous cyst
Eruption cyst
Follicular cyst
Gingival cyst
Lateral periodontal cyst
Primordial cyst
Excludes ❷: keratocysts (D16.4, D16.5)
odontogenic keratocystic tumors (D16.4, D16.5)

K09.1 Developmental (nonodontogenic) cysts of oral region
Cyst (of) incisive canal
Cyst (of) palatine of papilla
Globulomaxillary cyst
Median palatal cyst
Nasoalveolar cyst
Nasolabial cyst
Nasopalatine duct cyst

K09.8 Other cysts of oral region, not elsewhere classified
Dermoid cyst
Epidermoid cyst
Lymphoepithelial cyst
Epstein's pearl

K09.9 Cyst of oral region, unspecified

K11- Diseases of salivary glands
Use additional code to identify:
Alcohol abuse and dependence (F10.-)
Exposure to environmental tobacco smoke (Z77.22)
Exposure to tobacco smoke in the perinatal period (P96.81)
History of tobacco dependence (Z87.891)
Occupational exposure to environmental tobacco smoke (Z57.31)
Tobacco dependence (F17.-)
Tobacco use (Z72.0)

K11.0 Atrophy of salivary gland — A wasting-away of the salivary gland tissue.

K11.1 Hypertrophy of salivary gland — The abnormal enlargement of the
salivary glands and their tissues.

K11.2- Sialoadenitis — Inflammation of a salivary gland.
Parotitis
Excludes 1:   epidemic parotitis (B26.-)
mumps (B26.-)
uveoparotid fever [Heerfordt] (D86.89)

K11.20 Sialoadenitis, unspecified

K11.21 Acute sialoadenitis — A form marked by sudden, severe onset.
Excludes 1:   acute recurrent sialoadenitis (K11.22)

K11.22 Acute <u>recurrent</u> sialoadenitis — A form marked by sudden, severe
onset following a previous episode.

K11.23 Chronic sialoadenitis — A form marked by slow, persistent progression.

cc **K11.3 Abscess of salivary gland** — A localized collection of pus caused by the
disintegration of salivary gland tissues.

cc **K11.4 Fistula of salivary gland** — An abnormal passage of a salivary gland.
Excludes 1:   congenital fistula of salivary gland (Q38.4)

K11.5 Sialolithiasis — The abnormal presence of a salivary calculi.
Calculus of salivary gland or duct
Stone of salivary gland or duct

K11.6 Mucocele of salivary gland — A mucous cyst of a salivary gland.
Mucous extravasation cyst of salivary gland — An encapsulated sac
containing blood of a salivary gland.
Mucous retention cyst of salivary gland — An encapsulated sac
containing glandular secretions of a salivary gland.
Ranula — A cystic tumor of a salivary gland.

K11.7 Disturbances of salivary secretion
Hypoptyalism — The abnormally decreased secretion of saliva.
Ptyalism — The abnormally excessive secretion of saliva.
Xerostomia — Dryness of the mouth caused by the decrease of normal salivary
secretion.
Excludes ❷: dry mouth NOS (R68.2)

K11.8 Other diseases of salivary glands
Benign lymphoepithelial lesion of salivary gland
Mikulicz' disease
Necrotizing sialometaplasia
Sialectasia
Stenosis of salivary duct
Stricture of salivary duct
Excludes 1:   sicca syndrome [Sjögren] (M35.0-)

K11.9 Disease of salivary gland, unspecified
Sialoadenopathy NOS

K12- Stomatitis and related lesions — Inflammation and/or ulcerative sores of the oral
mucosal surfaces.
Use additional code to identify:
Alcohol abuse and dependence (F10.-)
Exposure to environmental tobacco smoke (Z77.22)
Exposure to tobacco smoke in the perinatal period (P96.81)
History of tobacco dependence (Z87.891)
Occupational exposure to environmental tobacco smoke (Z57.31)
Tobacco dependence (F17.-)
Tobacco use (Z72.0)
Excludes 1:   cancrum oris (A69.0)
cheilitis (K13.0)
gangrenous stomatitis (A69.0)
herpesviral [herpes simplex] gingivostomatitis (B00.2)
noma (A69.0)

K12.0 Recurrent oral aphthae — Small ulcers on the mucous membrane of the
mouth.
Aphthous stomatitis (major) (minor)
Bednar's aphthae
Periadenitis mucosa necrotica recurrens
Recurrent aphthous ulcer
Stomatitis herpetiformis

K12.1 Other forms of stomatitis
Stomatitis NOS
Denture stomatitis
Ulcerative stomatitis
Vesicular stomatitis
Excludes 1:   acute necrotizing ulcerative stomatitis (A69.1)
Vincent's stomatitis (A69.1)

cc **K12.2 Cellulitis and abscess of mouth** — CELLULITIS – Inflammation of the
oral cellular tissue. ABSCESS – A localized collection of pus, caused by the
disintegration of oral tissue.
Cellulitis of mouth (floor)
Submandibular abscess
Excludes ❷: abscess of salivary gland (K11.3)
abscess of tongue (K14.0)
periapical abscess (K04.6-K04.7)
periodontal abscess (K05.21)
peritonsillar abscess (J36)

K12.3- <u>Oral mucositis (ulcerative)</u> — The eating-away of the oral mucosa.
Mucositis (oral) (oropharyneal)
Excludes ❷: gastrointestinal mucositis (ulcerative) (K92.81)
mucositis (ulcerative) of vagina and vulva (N76.81)
nasal mucositis (ulcerative) (J34.81)

K12.30 Oral mucositis (ulcerative), <u>unspecified</u>

K12.31 Oral mucositis (ulcerative) <u>due to antineoplastic therapy</u>
Use additional code for adverse effect, if applicable, to identify
antineoplastic and immunosuppressive drugs (T45.1x5)
Use additional code for other antineoplastic therapy, such as:
Radiological procedure and radiotherapy (Y84.2)

K12.32 Oral mucositis (ulcerative) <u>due to other drugs</u>
Use additional code for adverse effect, if applicable, to identify
drug (T36-T50 with fifth or sixth character 5)

K12.33 Oral mucositis (ulcerative) <u>due to radiation</u>
Use additional external cause code (W88-W90, X39.0-) to
identify cause

K12.39 Other oral mucositis (ulcerative)
Viral oral mucositis (ulcerative)

K
0
9
-
K
1
2

K13-   Other diseases of lip and oral mucosa
    Includes: Epithelial disturbances of tongue
    Use additional code to identify:
      Alcohol abuse and dependence (F10.-)
      Exposure to environmental tobacco smoke (Z77.22)
      Exposure to tobacco smoke in the perinatal period (P96.81)
      History of tobacco dependence (Z87.891)
      Occupational exposure to environmental tobacco smoke (Z57.31)
      Tobacco dependence (F17.-)
      Tobacco use (Z72.0)
    Excludes ❷: certain disorders of gingiva and edentulous alveolar ridge
              (K05-K06)
              cysts of oral region (K09.-)
              diseases of tongue (K14.-)
              stomatitis and related lesions (K12.-)

K13.0   Diseases of lips
      Abscess of lips — A localized collection of pus caused by the disintegration of the tissues of the lips.
      Angular cheilitis — Superficial erosions and fissuring at the angles of the mouth.
      Cellulitis of lips — Superficial erosions and fissuring of the lips.
      Cheilitis NOS
      Cheilodynia — Pain in the lips.
      Cheilosis — The abnormal fissuring and dry scaling of the vermilion surface of the lips and the angles of the mouth.
      Exfoliative cheilitis — Persistent peeling, dryness, and flaking of the lips.
      Fistula of lips — An abnormal passage of the lip tissue.
      Glandular cheilitis — Inflammation of the minor salivary glands of the lower lip.
      Hypertrophy of lips — An abnormal enlargement of the lips.
      Perlèche NEC — See Angular Cheilitis above.
      Excludes 1:   ariboflavinosis (E53.0)
              cheilitis due to radiation-related disorders (L55-L59)
              congenital fistula of lips (Q38.0)
              congenital hypertrophy of lips (Q18.6)
              Perlèche due to candidiasis (B37.83)
              Perlèche due to riboflavin deficiency (E53.0)

K13.1   Cheek and lip biting — Habitual biting of the lip and oral mucosa that is usually seen in children with emotional issues.

K13.2-   Leukoplakia and other disturbances of oral epithelium, including tongue
      Excludes 1:   carcinoma in situ of oral epithelium (D00.0-)
              hairy leukoplakia (K13.3)

    K13.21   Leukoplakia of oral mucosa, including tongue — Thick, whitish patches which develop upon the mucous membrane of the oral mucosa.
        Leukokeratosis of oral mucosa
        Leukoplakia of gingiva, lips, tongue
      Excludes 1:   hairy leukoplakia (K13.3)
              leukokeratosis nicotina palati (K13.24)

    K13.22   Minimal keratinized residual ridge mucosa
        Minimal keratinization of alveolar ridge mucosa

    K13.23   Excessive keratinized residual ridge mucosa
        Excessive keratinization of alveolar ridge mucosa

    K13.24   Leukokeratosis nicotina palati — The formation of whitish patches on the tongue due to the effects of cigarette smoking.
        Smoker's palate

    K13.29   Other disturbances of oral epithelium, including tongue
        Erythroplakia of mouth or tongue
        Focal epithelial hyperplasia of mouth or tongue
        Leukoedema of mouth or tongue
        Other oral epithelium disturbances

K13.3   Hairy leukoplakia — Whitish patches of the oral mucosa with a fuzzy appearance that are due to the Epstein-Barr virus and more often seen in immunocompromised pateints.

K13.4   Granuloma and granuloma-like lesions of oral mucosa — An oral mucosal granular growth.
      Eosinophilic granuloma — Oral mucosal cystic lesions containing lipid and eosinophils.
      Granuloma pyogenicum — An oral mucosal granular growth with the formation of pus.
      Verrucous xanthoma — A wart-like growth of the oral mucosa.

K13.5   Oral submucous fibrosis — The formation of fibrous tissue in the oral tissue layers below the mucous membrane.
      Submucous fibrosis of tongue

K13.6   Irritative hyperplasia of oral mucosa — The abnormal increase in the number of normal cells caused by irritative effects.
      Excludes ❷: irritative hyperplasia of edentulous ridge [denture hyperplasia] (K06.2)

K13.7-   Other and unspecified lesions of oral mucosa
    K13.70   Unspecified lesions of oral mucosa
    K13.79   Other lesions of oral mucosa
        Focal oral mucinosis

K14-   Diseases of tongue
    Use additional code to identify:
      Alcohol abuse and dependence (F10.-)
      Exposure to environmental tobacco smoke (Z77.22)
      History of tobacco dependence (Z87.891)
      Occupational exposure to environmental tobacco smoke (Z57.31)
      Tobacco dependence (F17.-)
      Tobacco use (Z72.0)
    Excludes ❷: erythroplakia (K13.29)
              focal epithelial hyperplasia (K13.29)
              leukedema of tongue (K13.29)
              leukoplakia of tongue (K13.21)
              hairy leukoplakia (K13.3)
              macroglossia (congenital) (Q38.2)
              submucous fibrosis of tongue (K13.5)

K14.0   Glossitis — Inflammation of the tongue.
      Abscess of tongue — A localized collection of pus caused by the disintegration of glossal tissue.
      Ulceration (traumatic) of tongue — A localized eating-away of glossal tissue.
      Excludes 1:   atrophic glossitis (K14.4)

K14.1   Geographic tongue — A condition characterized by white or yellowish plaque on the tongue gradually denuding to red patches with thickened white borders.
      Benign migratory glossitis
      Glossitis areata exfoliativa

K14.2   Median rhomboid glossitis — A congenital anomaly of the tongue characterized by reddish patches on the midline surface of the tongue.

K14.3   Hypertrophy of tongue papillae — Enlargement of the dorsal surface taste bud structures.
      Black hairy tongue — A form marked by the presence of a brown, fur-like patch on the dorsal surface of the tongue.
      Coated tongue — A form marked by a whitish or yellowish layer on the dorsal surface consisting of cellular debris.
      Hypertrophy of foliate papillae — A form affecting the parallel mucosal folds on the margins of the tongue at the junction of its body and root.
      Lingua villosa nigra — Synonym for Black Hairy Tongue.

K14.4   Atrophy of tongue papillae — A wasting-away of the dorsal surface taste bud structures.
      Atrophic glossitis

K14.5   Plicated tongue — A disease characterized by cracks and divisions in the dorsal surface of the tongue.
      Fissured tongue
      Furrowed tongue
      Scrotal tongue
      Excludes 1:   fissured tongue, congenital (Q38.3)

K14.6   Glossodynia — A painful tongue.
      Glossopyrosis — A burning sensation in the tongue.
      Painful tongue

K14.8   Other diseases of tongue
      Atrophy of tongue — An abnormal wasting-away of the glossal tissue.
      Crenated tongue — The abnormal notching of the surface of the tongue.
      Enlargement of tongue — The abnormal increase in the size of the tongue.
      Glossocele — The abnormal swelling and/or protrusion of the tongue.
      Glossoptosis — The downward displacement of the tongue.
      Hypertrophy of tongue — The abnormal overgrowth of the tongue.

K14.9   Disease of tongue, unspecified
      Glossopathy NOS

K
1
3
-
K
1
4

Excludes 1: = NOT CODED HERE! (Do not code both)

Excludes ❷: = Not Included Here

Diseases of esophagus, stomach and duodenum (K20-K31)

Excludes ❷: hiatus hernia (K44.-)

K20- Esophagitis — Inflammation of the esophagus.
   Use additional code to identify:
      Alcohol abuse and dependence (F10.-)
   Excludes 1:   erosion of esophagus (K22.1-)
                  esophagitis with gastro-esophageal reflux disease (K21.0)
                  reflux esophagitis (K21.0)
                  ulcerative esophagitis (K22.1-)
   Excludes ❷: eosinophilic gastritis or gastroenteritis (K52.81)

K20.0 Eosinophilic esophagitis — A condition involving eosinophil accumulation in the tissues lining the esophagus and characterized by severe inflammation that affects the ability to swallow.

K20.8 Other esophagitis
   Abscess of esophagus — A localized collection of pus in the esophagus formed by the disintegration of tissues.

K20.9 Esophagitis, unspecified
   Esophagitis NOS

K21- Gastro-esophageal reflux disease — A disease caused by a reflux of acid and pepsin from the stomach.
   AHA 16:1Q:p18 — Laryngopharyngeal reflux disease
   Excludes 1:   newborn esophageal reflux (P78.83)

K21.0 Gastro-esophageal reflux disease with esophagitis — A form with inflammation of the esophagus.
   Reflux esophagitis

K21.9 Gastro-esophageal reflux disease without esophagitis
   Esophageal reflux NOS

K22- Other diseases of esophagus
   Excludes ❷: esophageal varices (I85.-)

K22.0 Achalasia of cardia — Failure to relax the smooth muscle fibers of the esophagogastric sphincter due to degeneration of the ganglion cells in the wall of the esophagus.
   Achalasia NOS
   Cardiospasm
   Excludes 1:   congenital cardiospasm (Q39.5)

K22.1- Ulcer of esophagus — An open sore of the lining of the esophagus.
   Barrett's ulcer — See Ulcer of Esophagus above.
   Erosion of esophagus — The eating-away of the lining of the esophagus.
   Fungal ulcer of esophagus — A form caused by necrotic fungal infection.
   Peptic ulcer of esophagus — A form caused by the action of the acid gastric juice.
   Ulcer of esophagus due to ingestion of chemicals
   Ulcer of esophagus due to ingestion of drugs and medicaments
   Ulcerative esophagitis — See Ulcer of Esophagus above.
   Code first poisoning due to drug or toxin, if applicable (T36-T65 with fifth or sixth character 1-4 or 6)
   Use additional code for adverse effect, if applicable, to identify drug (T36-T50 with fifth or sixth character 5)
   Excludes 1:   Barrett's esophagus (K22.7-)

CC **K22.10 Ulcer of esophagus without bleeding**
   Ulcer of esophagus NOS

MCC **K22.11 Ulcer of esophagus with bleeding** — A form with the escape of blood from the ulcer site.
   Excludes ❷: bleeding esophageal varices (I85.01, I85.11)

K22.2 Esophageal obstruction — Blocking or clogging of the esophagus.
   Compression of esophagus — External pressure on the esophagus causing narrowing of the esophageal lumen.
   Constriction of esophagus — The narrowing of the esophagus.
   Stenosis of esophagus — The decrease in caliber of the esophagus.
   Stricture of esophagus — The narrowing of the esophagus.
   Excludes 1:   congenital stenosis or stricture of esophagus (Q39.3)

MCC **K22.3 Perforation of esophagus** — A hole or opening through the esophageal wall.
   Rupture of esophagus — Forcible tearing or disruption through the esophageal wall.
   Excludes 1:   traumatic perforation of (thoracic) esophagus (S27.8-)

K22.4 Dyskinesia of esophagus — Impairment of the muscular control of the esophagus.
   Corkscrew esophagus — Esophageal spasm giving the appearance of a corkscrew.
   Diffuse esophageal spasm — The strong, painful, incoordinated, nonpropulsive contractions of the esophagus.
   Spasm of esophagus — The painful contractions of the esophagus.
   Excludes 1:   cardiospasm (K22.0)

K22.5 Diverticulum of esophagus, acquired — A defect in the esophagus creating a herniated sac or pouch of tissue.
   Esophageal pouch, acquired — A pocket-like space or sac in the esophagus.
   Excludes 1:   diverticulum of esophagus (congenital) (Q39.6)

MCC **K22.6 Gastro-esophageal laceration-hemorrhage syndrome** — The slit-like bleeding lacerations of the esophagogastric junction following several days of severe vomiting.
   Mallory-Weiss syndrome

K22.7- Barrett's esophagus — A metaplastic disorder of the lining of the lower esophagus caused by gastroesophageal reflux damage to the esophageal mucosa that is characterized by esophageal lining cells changing from squamous cells to goblet cells (usually found in the small intestine).
   Barrett's disease
   Barrett's syndrome
   Excludes 1:   Barrett's ulcer (K22.1)
                  malignant neoplasm of esophagus (C15.-)

K22.70 Barrett's esophagus without dysplasia
   Barrett's esophagus NOS

K22.71- Barrett's esophagus with dysplasia — A form with the development and presence of abnormal, potentially cancerous cells.

K22.710 Barrett's esophagus with low grade dysplasia

K22.711 Barrett's esophagus with high grade dysplasia

K22.719 Barrett's esophagus with dysplasia, unspecified

K22.8 Other specified diseases of esophagus
   Hemorrhage of esophagus NOS
   Excludes ❷: esophageal varices (I85.-)
                  Paterson-Kelly syndrome (D50.1)

K22.9 Disease of esophagus, unspecified

K23 Disorders of esophagus in diseases classified elsewhere —
   [Not Allowed as PDX]
   Code first underlying disease, such as:
      Congenital syphilis (A50.5)
   Excludes 1:   late syphilis (A52.79)
                  megaesophagus due to Chagas' disease (B57.31)
                  tuberculosis (A18.83)

K25- Gastric ulcer — An inflammatory, necrotic, sloughing defect (open sore) in the gastric mucosa.
   Includes: Erosion (acute) of stomach
                    Pylorus ulcer (peptic) — A form located in the pyloric antrum of the stomach.
                    Stomach ulcer (peptic) — A form located in any portion of the stomach.
   Use additional code to identify:
      Alcohol abuse and dependence (F10.-)
   Excludes 1:   acute gastritis (K29.0-)
                  peptic ulcer NOS (K27.-)

Erosive Gastric Ulcer

GASTRIC ULCER

MCC **K25.0 Acute gastric ulcer with hemorrhage** — A form marked by sudden, severe onset with hemorrhage at the site of the ulcer.

MCC **K25.1 Acute gastric ulcer with perforation** — A form marked by sudden, severe onset with the creation of a hole through the stomach wall into the abdominal cavity.

MCC **K25.2 Acute gastric ulcer with both hemorrhage and perforation** — A form marked by sudden, severe onset with hemorrhage and a hole through the stomach wall into the abdominal cavity.

CC **K25.3 Acute gastric ulcer without hemorrhage or perforation**

MCC **K25.4 Chronic or unspecified gastric ulcer with hemorrhage** — A form marked by slow, persistent progression with hemorrhage at the site of the ulcer.

MCC **K25.5 Chronic or unspecified gastric ulcer with perforation** — A form marked by slow, persistent progression with the creation of a hole through the stomach wall into the abdominal cavity.

MCC **K25.6 Chronic or unspecified gastric ulcer with both hemorrhage and perforation** — A form marked by slow, persistent progression with hemorrhage and a hole through the stomach wall into the abdominal cavity.

K25.7 Chronic gastric ulcer without hemorrhage or perforation

K20 - K25

Excludes 1: = NOT CODED HERE! (Do not code both)   Excludes ❷: = Not Included Here

K25.9   Gastric ulcer, <u>unspecified as acute or chronic</u>, without hemorrhage or perforation

K26-   <u>Duodenal ulcer</u> — An inflammatory, necrotic sloughing defect (open sore) in the duodenal mucosa.
   Includes: Duodenum ulcer (peptic)
              Erosion (acute) of duodenum
              Postpyloric ulcer (peptic)
   Use additional code to identify:
     Alcohol abuse and dependence (F10.-)
   Excludes 1:   peptic ulcer NOS (K27.-)

MCC **K26.0   <u>Acute</u> duodenal ulcer with hemorrhage** — A form marked by sudden, severe onset with hemorrhage at the site of the ulcer.

MCC **K26.1   <u>Acute</u> duodenal ulcer with perforation** — A form marked by sudden, severe onset with the creation of a hole through the duodenal wall into the abdominal cavity.

MCC **K26.2   <u>Acute</u> duodenal ulcer with both hemorrhage and perforation** — A form marked by sudden, severe onset with hemorrhage and a hole through the duodenal wall into the abdominal cavity.

CC **K26.3   <u>Acute</u> duodenal ulcer without hemorrhage or perforation**

MCC **K26.4   Chronic or unspecified duodenal ulcer with hemorrhage** — A form marked by slow, persistent progression with hemorrhage at the site of the ulcer.
        AHA 16:1Q:p14 – Duodenal ulcer with hemorrhage due to Coumadin therapy

MCC **K26.5   Chronic or unspecified duodenal ulcer with perforation** — A form marked by slow, persistent progression with the creation of a hole through the duodenal wall into the abdominal cavity.

MCC **K26.6   Chronic or unspecified duodenal ulcer with both hemorrhage and perforation** — A form marked by slow, persistent progression with hemorrhage and a hole through the duodenal wall into the abdominal cavity.

K26.7   Chronic duodenal ulcer without hemorrhage or perforation

K26.9   Duodenal ulcer, <u>unspecified as acute or chronic</u>, without hemorrhage or perforation

K27-   <u>Peptic ulcer</u>, site unspecified — An inflammatory, necrotic, sloughing defect (open sore) in an unspecified site of the gastroduodenal mucosa.
   Includes: Gastroduodenal ulcer NOS
              Peptic ulcer NOS
   Use additional code to identify:
     Alcohol abuse and dependence (F10.-)
   Excludes 1:   peptic ulcer of newborn (P78.82)

MCC **K27.0   <u>Acute</u> peptic ulcer, site unspecified, with hemorrhage** — A form marked by sudden, severe onset with hemorrhage at the site of the ulcer.

MCC **K27.1   <u>Acute</u> peptic ulcer, site unspecified, with perforation** — A form marked by sudden, severe onset with the creation of a hole through the site wall into the abdominal cavity.

MCC **K27.2   <u>Acute</u> peptic ulcer, site unspecified, with both hemorrhage and perforation** — A form marked by sudden, severe onset with hemorrhage and a hole through the site wall into the abdominal cavity.

CC **K27.3   <u>Acute</u> peptic ulcer, site unspecified, without hemorrhage or perforation**

MCC **K27.4   Chronic or unspecified peptic ulcer, site unspecified, with hemorrhage** — A form marked by slow, persistent progression with hemorrhage at the site of the ulcer.

MCC **K27.5   Chronic or unspecified peptic ulcer, site unspecified, with perforation** — A form marked by slow, persistent progression with hemorrhage and a hole through the site wall into the abdominal cavity.

MCC **K27.6   Chronic or unspecified peptic ulcer, site unspecified, with both hemorrhage and perforation** — A form marked by slow, persistent progression with hemorrhage and a hole through the site wall into the abdominal cavity.

K27.7   Chronic peptic ulcer, site unspecified, without hemorrhage or perforation

K27.9   Peptic ulcer, site unspecified, <u>unspecified as acute or chronic</u>, without hemorrhage or perforation

K28-   <u>Gastrojejunal ulcer</u> — An inflammatory, necrotic, sloughing defect (open sore) of the stomach and jejunum anastomotic site.
   Includes: Anastomotic ulcer (peptic) or erosion
              Gastrocolic ulcer (peptic) or erosion
              Gastrointestinal ulcer (peptic) or erosion
              Gastrojejunal ulcer (peptic) or erosion
              Jejunal ulcer (peptic) or erosion
              Marginal ulcer (peptic) or erosion
              Stomal ulcer (peptic) or erosion
   Use additional code to identify:
     Alcohol abuse and dependence (F10.-)
   Excludes 1:   primary ulcer of small intestine (K63.3)

MCC **K28.0   <u>Acute</u> gastrojejunal ulcer with hemorrhage** — A form marked by sudden, severe onset with hemorrhage at the site of the ulcer.

MCC **K28.1   <u>Acute</u> gastrojejunal ulcer with perforation** — A form marked by sudden, severe onset with the creation of a hole through the site wall into the abdominal cavity.

MCC **K28.2   <u>Acute</u> gastrojejunal ulcer with both hemorrhage and perforation** — A form marked by sudden, severe onset with hemorrhage and a hole through the site wall into the abdominal cavity.

CC **K28.3   <u>Acute</u> gastrojejunal ulcer without hemorrhage or perforation**

MCC **K28.4   Chronic or unspecified gastrojejunal ulcer with hemorrhage** — A form marked by slow, persistent progression with hemorrhage at the site of the ulcer.

MCC **K28.5   Chronic or unspecified gastrojejunal ulcer with perforation** — A form marked by slow, persistent progression with the creation of a hole through the site wall into the abdominal cavity.

MCC **K28.6   Chronic or unspecified gastrojejunal ulcer with both hemorrhage and perforation** — A form marked by slow, persistent progression with hemorrhage and a hole through the site wall into the abdominal cavity.

K28.7   Chronic gastrojejunal ulcer without hemorrhage or perforation

K28.9   Gastrojejunal ulcer, <u>unspecified as acute or chronic</u>, without hemorrhage or perforation

K29-   Gastritis and duodenitis
   Excludes 1:   eosinophilic gastritis or gastroenteritis (K52.81)
              Zollinger-Ellison syndrome (E16.4)

K29.0-   <u>Acute gastritis</u> — The sudden, severe onset of inflammation of the stomach.
   Use additional code to identify:
     Alcohol abuse and dependence (F10.-)
   Excludes 1:   erosion (acute) of stomach (K25.-)

K29.00   Acute gastritis <u>without</u> bleeding

MCC **K29.01   Acute gastritis <u>with bleeding</u>**

K29.2-   <u>Alcoholic</u> gastritis — Inflammation of the stomach resulting from the overconsumption of alcoholic beverages.
   Use additional code to identify:
     Alcohol abuse and dependence (F10.-)

K29.20   Alcoholic gastritis <u>without</u> bleeding

MCC **K29.21   Alcoholic gastritis <u>with bleeding</u>**

K29.3-   <u>Chronic superficial</u> gastritis — Inflammation of the innermost layer of the stomach mucosa that persists over a period of time.

K29.30   Chronic superficial gastritis <u>without</u> bleeding

MCC **K29.31   Chronic superficial gastritis <u>with bleeding</u>**

K29.4-   <u>Chronic atrophic</u> gastritis — Gastritis which persists over a period of time resulting in a wasting-away of the stomach.
        Gastric atrophy

K29.40   Chronic atrophic gastritis <u>without</u> bleeding

MCC **K29.41   Chronic atrophic gastritis <u>with bleeding</u>**

K29.5-   <u>Unspecified chronic</u> gastritis
        Chronic antral gastritis
        Chronic fundal gastritis

K29.50   Unspecified chronic gastritis <u>without</u> bleeding

MCC **K29.51   Unspecified chronic gastritis <u>with bleeding</u>**

K29.6-   <u>Other</u> gastritis
        Giant hypertrophic gastritis — A form marked by gross hypertrophy of the stomach lining.
        Granulomatous gastritis — A form marked by granulomatous inflammation.
        Ménétrier's disease — See Giant Hypertrophic Gastritis above.

K29.60   Other gastritis <u>without</u> bleeding

MCC **K29.61   Other gastritis <u>with bleeding</u>**

K25-K29

K29.7- **Gastritis, unspecified**

   K29.70 **Gastritis, unspecified, without bleeding**

MCC K29.71 **Gastritis, unspecified, with bleeding**

K29.8- **Duodenitis** — Inflammation of the duodenum.

   K29.80 **Duodenitis without bleeding**

MCC K29.81 **Duodenitis with bleeding**

K29.9- **Gastroduodenitis, unspecified**

   K29.90 **Gastroduodenitis, unspecified, without bleeding**

MCC K29.91 **Gastroduodenitis, unspecified, with bleeding**

K30 Functional dyspepsia — The impairment of the power or function of digestion.
  Indigestion — The abnormal decrease of the stomach to break down food into absorbable substances.
    Excludes 1:   *dyspepsia NOS (R10.13)*
              heartburn (R12)
              nervous dyspepsia (F45.8)
              neurotic dyspepsia (F45.8)
              psychogenic dyspepsia (F45.8)

K31- Other diseases of stomach and duodenum
  Includes: **Functional disorders of stomach**
    Excludes ❷: *diabetic gastroparesis (E08.43, E09.43, E10.43, E11.43, E13.43)*
              diverticulum of duodenum (K57.00-K57.13)

CC **K31.0 Acute dilatation of stomach** — The abnormal enlargement of the stomach.
    Acute distention of stomach

CC **K31.1 Adult hypertrophic pyloric stenosis** — [Age/15-124] — Obstruction of the pyloric opening of the stomach into the duodenum associated with the abnormal increase in the size of the pyloric cells.
    Pyloric stenosis NOS
    Excludes 1: *congenital or infantile pyloric stenosis (Q40.0)*

PYLORIC STENOSIS

K31.2 Hourglass stricture and stenosis of stomach — A decrease in caliber at the middle of the stomach forming an hourglass appearance of the stomach.
    Excludes 1: *congenital hourglass stomach (Q40.2)*
             hourglass contraction of stomach (K31.89)

K31.3 Pylorospasm, not elsewhere classified — The sudden, involuntary contraction of the pyloric muscles of the stomach.
    Excludes 1: *congenital or infantile pylorospasm (Q40.0)*
             neurotic pylorospasm (F45.8)
             psychogenic pylorospasm (F45.8)

HOURGLASS STRICTURE OF STOMACH

K31.4 Gastric diverticulum — A protruding pouch of mucous membrane through a defect in the muscular wall of the stomach.
    Excludes 1: *congenital diverticulum of stomach (Q40.2)*

CC **K31.5 Obstruction of duodenum**
    Constriction of duodenum — A narrowing of the duodenum due to a loss in elasticity of the duodenal muscular walls.
    Duodenal ileus (chronic) — Obstruction and blockage of the duodenum which develops slowly and persists over a period of time.
    Stenosis of duodenum — A reduction in the size of the duodenal lumen.
    Stricture of duodenum — A decrease in caliber of the duodenal lumen.
    Volvulus of duodenum — Obstruction of the duodenum due to a knotting or twisting of the duodenum.
    Excludes 1: *congenital stenosis of duodenum (Q41.0)*

CC **K31.6 Fistula of stomach and duodenum** — An abnormal passage leading from the stomach or duodenum.
    Gastrocolic fistula — An abnormal passage between the stomach and the intestine.
    Gastrojejunocolic fistula — An abnormal passage between the stomach and the jejunum.

K31.7 Polyp of stomach and duodenum — A mucous membrane protruding growth.
    Excludes 1: *adenomatous polyp of stomach (D13.1)*

K31.8- Other specified diseases of stomach and duodenum
  K31.81- Angiodysplasia of stomach and duodenum — The presence of small vascular abnormalities of the stomach or duodenum.

  MCC **K31.811 Angiodysplasia of stomach and duodenum with bleeding**

     K31.819 Angiodysplasia of stomach and duodenum without bleeding
           Angiodysplasia of stomach and duodenum NOS

MCC **K31.82 Dieulafoy lesion (hemorrhagic) of stomach and duodenum** — A severe, often recurrent, hemorrhage from a pinpoint, non-ulcerated arterial lesion of the stomach or duodenum.
    Excludes ❷: *Dieulafoy lesion of intestine (K63.81)*

K31.83 Achlorhydria — The decreased, or absent, production of hydrochloric stomach acid.

K31.84 Gastroparesis — The condition of paralysis, or impaired contraction capacity of the stomach resulting in defective gastric emptying.
    AHA 13:4Q:p114 – Diabetic gastroparesis
    Gastroparalysis
    Code first undrlying disease, if known, such as:
      Anorexia nervosa (F50.0-)
      Diabetes mellitus (E08.43, E09.43, E10.43, E11.43, E13.43)
      Scleroderma (M34-)

K31.89 Other diseases of stomach and duodenum

K31.9 Disease of stomach and duodenum, unspecified

Diseases of appendix (K35-K38)

K35- Acute appendicitis — The sudden, severe onset of inflammation of the appendix.

MCC **K35.2 Acute appendicitis with generalized peritonitis** — A form resulting in the general inflammation of the lining membrane of the peritoneum.
    Appendicitis (acute) with generalized (diffuse) peritonitis following rupture or perforation of appendix
    Perforated appendix NOS
    Ruptured appendix NOS

MCC **K35.3 Acute appendicitis with localized peritonitis** — A form resulting in the localized inflammation of the lining membrane of the peritoneum.
    Acute appendicitis with or without perforation or rupture with localized peritonitis
    Acute appendicitis with or without perforation or rupture with peritonitis NOS
    Acute appendicitis with peritoneal abscess — A form marked by the localized collection of pus caused by the disintegration of peritoneal tissue.

K35.8- Other and unspecified acute appendicitis

CC **K35.80 Unspecified acute appendicitis**
    Acute appendicitis NOS
    Acute appendicitis without (localized) (generalized) peritonitis

CC **K35.89 Other acute appendicitis**

K36 Other appendicitis
  Chronic appendicitis — Inflammation of the appendix which develops slowly and persists over a long period of time.
  Recurrent appendicitis — Inflammation of the appendix which returns periodically.

K37 Unspecified appendicitis
    Excludes 1: *unspecified appendicitis with peritonitis (K35.2-K35.3)*

K38- Other diseases of appendix

K38.0 Hyperplasia of appendix

K38.1 Appendicular concretions — The presence of hardened tissue within the appendix.
    Fecalith of appendix — An appendiceal concretion formed around a center of fecal matter.
    Stercolith of appendix — Synonym for Fecalith of Appendix.

K38.2 Diverticulum of appendix — A pouch of mucous membrane which protrudes through the appendiceal muscular wall.

K38.3 Fistula of appendix — An abnormal passage leading outside of the appendix.

K29-K38

K38.8 **Other specified diseases of appendix**
Intussusception of appendix — The inward prolapse of the appendix into the intestine.

K38.9 **Disease of appendix, unspecified**

Hernia (K40-K46)

Note: Hernia with both gangrene and obstruction is classified to hernia with gangrene.
Includes: Acquired hernia
Congenital [except diaphragmatic or hiatus] hernia
Recurrent hernia

K40- **Inguinal hernia** — Protrusion of the intestine through the inguinal opening.
Includes: Bubonocele — See Indirect Inguinal Hernia below.
Direct inguinal hernia — Protrusion occurs directly through the abdominal wall.
Double inguinal hernia — Bilateral inguinal hernias.
Indirect inguinal hernia — Protrusion occurs through the internal inguinal ring into the inguinal canal.
Inguinal hernia NOS
Oblique inguinal hernia
Scrotal hernia — An inguinal hernia in which the herniated intestine descends into the scrotum.

K40.0- **Bilateral inguinal hernia, with obstruction, without gangrene** — A bilateral form marked by blockage of that portion of the alimentary tract, but without necrosis.
Inguinal hernia (bilateral) causing obstruction without gangrene
Incarcerated inguinal hernia (bilateral) without gangrene
Irreducible inguinal hernia (bilateral) without gangrene
Strangulated inguinal hernia (bilateral) without gangrene

CC **K40.00** **Bilateral inguinal hernia, with obstruction, without gangrene, not specified as recurrent**
Bilateral inguinal hernia, with obstruction, without gangrene NOS

CC **K40.01** **Bilateral inguinal hernia, with obstruction, without gangrene, recurrent**

K40.1- **Bilateral inguinal hernia, with gangrene** — A bilateral form marked by necrosis of the protruded segment due to deficient blood supply.

MCC **K40.10** **Bilateral inguinal hernia, with gangrene, not specified as recurrent**
Bilateral inguinal hernia, with gangrene NOS

MCC **K40.11** **Bilateral inguinal hernia, with gangrene, recurrent**

K40.2- **Bilateral inguinal hernia, without obstruction or gangrene**

K40.20 **Bilateral inguinal hernia, without obstruction or gangrene, not specified as recurrent**
Bilateral inguinal hernia NOS

K40.21 **Bilateral inguinal hernia, without obstruction or gangrene, recurrent**

K40.3- **Unilateral inguinal hernia, with obstruction, without gangrene** — A form marked by blockage of that portion of the alimentary tract, but without necrosis.
Inguinal hernia (unilateral) causing obstruction without gangrene
Incarcerated inguinal hernia (unilateral) without gangrene
Irreducible inguinal hernia (unilateral) without gangrene
Strangulated inguinal hernia (unilateral) without gangrene

CC **K40.30** **Unilateral inguinal hernia, with obstruction, without gangrene, not specified as recurrent**
Inguinal hernia, with obstruction NOS
Unilateral inguinal hernia, with obstruction, without gangrene NOS

CC **K40.31** **Unilateral inguinal hernia, with obstruction, without gangrene, recurrent**

K40.4- **Unilateral inguinal hernia, with gangrene** — A form marked by necrosis of the protruded segment due to deficient blood supply.

MCC **K40.40** **Unilateral inguinal hernia, with gangrene, not specified as recurrent**
Inguinal hernia with gangrene NOS
Unilateral inguinal hernia with gangrene NOS

MCC **K40.41** **Unilateral inguinal hernia, with gangrene, recurrent**

K40.9- **Unilateral inguinal hernia, without obstruction or gangrene**

K40.90 **Unilateral inguinal hernia, without obstruction or gangrene, not specified as recurrent**
Inguinal hernia NOS
Unilateral inguinal hernia NOS

K40.91 **Unilateral inguinal hernia, without obstruction or gangrene, recurrent**

K41- **Femoral hernia** — Protrusion of an abdominal organ through a defect in the femoral ring.

K41.0- **Bilateral femoral hernia, with obstruction, without gangrene** — A bilateral form marked by blockage of that portion of the alimentary tract, but without necrosis.
Femoral hernia (bilateral) causing obstruction, without gangrene
Incarcerated femoral hernia (bilateral), without gangrene
Irreducible femoral hernia (bilateral), without gangrene
Strangulated femoral hernia (bilateral), without gangrene

CC **K41.00** **Bilateral femoral hernia, with obstruction, without gangrene, not specified as recurrent**
Bilateral femoral hernia, with obstruction, without gangrene NOS

CC **K41.01** **Bilateral femoral hernia, with obstruction, without gangrene, recurrent**

K41.1- **Bilateral femoral hernia, with gangrene** — A bilateral form marked by necrosis of the protruded segment due to deficient blood supply.

MCC **K41.10** **Bilateral femoral hernia, with gangrene, not specified as recurrent**
Bilateral femoral hernia, with gangrene NOS

MCC **K41.11** **Bilateral femoral hernia, with gangrene, recurrent**

K41.2- **Bilateral femoral hernia, without obstruction or gangrene**

K41.20 **Bilateral femoral hernia, without obstruction or gangrene, not specified as recurrent**
Bilateral femoral hernia NOS

K41.21 **Bilateral femoral hernia, without obstruction or gangrene, recurrent**

K41.3- **Unilateral femoral hernia, with obstruction, without gangrene** — A form marked by blockage of that portion of the alimentary tract, but without necrosis.
Femoral hernia (unilateral) causing obstruction, without gangrene
Incarcerated femoral hernia (unilateral), without gangrene
Irreducible femoral hernia (unilateral), without gangrene
Strangulated femoral hernia (unilateral), without gangrene

CC **K41.30** **Unilateral femoral hernia, with obstruction, without gangrene, not specified as recurrent**
Femoral hernia, with obstruction NOS
Unilateral femoral hernia, with obstruction NOS

CC **K41.31** **Unilateral femoral hernia, with obstruction, without gangrene, recurrent**

K41.4- **Unilateral femoral hernia, with gangrene** — A form marked by necrosis of the protruded segment due to deficient blood supply.

MCC **K41.40** **Unilateral femoral hernia, with gangrene, not specified as recurrent**
Femoral hernia, with gangrene NOS
Unilateral femoral hernia, with gangrene NOS

MCC **K41.41** **Unilateral femoral hernia, with gangrene, recurrent**

K41.9- **Unilateral femoral hernia, without obstruction or gangrene**

K41.90 **Unilateral femoral hernia, without obstruction or gangrene, not specified as recurrent**
Femoral hernia NOS
Unilateral femoral hernia NOS

K41.91 **Unilateral femoral hernia, without obstruction or gangrene, recurrent**

K42- **Umbilical hernia** — Protrusion of the intestine through the umbilicus.
Includes: Paraumbilical hernia
Excludes 1: omphalocele (Q79.2)

CC **K42.0** **Umbilical hernia with obstruction, without gangrene** — A form marked by blockage of that portion of the alimentary tract, but without necrosis.
Umbilical hernia causing obstruction, without gangrene
Incarcerated umbilical hernia, without gangrene
Irreducible umbilical hernia, without gangrene
Strangulated umbilical hernia, without gangrene

MCC **K42.1** **Umbilical hernia with gangrene** — A form marked by necrosis of the protruded segment due to deficient blood supply.
Gangrenous umbilical hernia

K42.9 **Umbilical hernia without obstruction or gangrene**
Umbilical hernia NOS

K38 - K42

K43- Ventral hernia — Protrusion of an abdominal organ through a defect in the abdominal wall.

CC **K43.0   Incisional hernia with obstruction, without gangrene** — A form resulting from an incision in the abdominal wall with blockage of that organ's function, but without necrosis.
> Incarcerated incisional hernia, without gangrene
> Incisional hernia causing obstruction, without gangrene
> Irreducible incisional hernia, without gangrene
> Strangulated incisional hernia, without gangrene

MCC **K43.1   Incisional hernia with gangrene** — A form resulting from an incision in the abdominal wall with necrosis.
> Gangrenous incisional hernia

K43.2   Incisional hernia without obstruction, or gangrene
> Incisional hernia NOS

CC **K43.3   Parastomal hernia with obstruction, without gangrene** — A form occurring at a stomal site in the abdominal wall with blockage of that organ's function, but without necrosis.
> Incarcerated parastomal hernia, without gangrene
> Irreducible parastomal hernia, without gangrene
> Parastomal hernia causing obstruction, without gangrene
> Strangulated parastomal hernia, without gangrene

MCC **K43.4   Parastomal hernia with gangrene** — A form occurring at a stomal site in the abdominal wall with necrosis.
> Gangrenous parastomal hernia

K43.5   Parastomal hernia without obstruction, or gangrene
> Parastomal hernia NOS

CC **K43.6   Other and unspecified ventral hernia with obstruction, without gangrene**
> Epigastric hernia, without gangrene
> Hypogastric hernia causing obstruction, without gangrene
> Incarcerated epigastric hernia, without gangrene
> Incarcerated hypogastric hernia, without gangrene
> Incarcerated midline hernia, without gangrene
> Incarcerated spigelian hernia, without gangrene
> Incarcerated subxiphoid hernia, without gangrene
> Irreducible epigastric hernia, without gangrene
> Irreducible hypogastric hernia, without gangrene
> Irreducible midline hernia, without gangrene
> Irreducible spigelian hernia, without gangrene
> Irreducible subxiphoid hernia, without gangrene
> Midline hernia causing obstruction, without gangrene
> Spigelian hernia causing obstruction, without gangrene
> Strangulated epigastric hernia, without gangrene
> Strangulated hypogastric hernia, without gangrene
> Strangulated midline hernia, without gangrene
> Strangulated spigelian hernia, without gangrene
> Strangulated subxiphoid hernia, without gangrene
> Subxiphoid hernia causing obstruction, without gangrene

MCC **K43.7   Other and unspecified ventral hernia with gangrene**
> Any condition listed under K43.6 specified as gangenous

K43.9   Ventral hernia without obstruction or gangrene
> Epigastric hernia
> Ventral hernia NOS

K44- Diaphragmatic hernia — Protrusion of an organ through the diaphragm.
> Includes: Hiatus hernia (esophageal) (sliding)
> Paraesophageal hernia
> *Excludes 1:   congenital diaphragmatic hernia (Q79.0)*
> *congenital hiatus hernia (Q40.1)*

CC **K44.0   Diaphragmatic hernia with obstruction, without gangrene** — Protrusion of an organ through the diaphragm with blockage of that organ's function, but without necrosis.
> Diaphragmatic hernia causing obstruction
> Incarcerated diaphragmatic hernia
> Irreducible diaphragmatic hernia
> Strangulated diaphragmatic hernia

MCC **K44.1   Diaphragmatic hernia with gangrene** — Protrusion of an organ through a defect in the diaphragm which has resulted in the necrosis of the herniated organ due to a deficient blood supply.
> Gangrenous diaphragmatic hernia

K44.9   Diaphragmatic hernia without obstruction or gangrene
> Diaphragmatic hernia NOS

K45- Other abdominal hernia
> Includes: Abdominal hernia, specified site NEC
> Lumbar hernia
> Obturator hernia
> Pudendal hernia
> Retroperitoneal hernia
> Sciatic hernia

CC **K45.0   Other specified abdominal hernia with obstruction, without gangrene**
> Other specified abdominal hernia causing obstruction
> Other specified incarcerated abdominal hernia
> Other specified irreducible abdominal hernia
> Other specified strangulated abdominal hernia

MCC **K45.1   Other specified abdominal hernia with gangrene**
> Any condition listed under K45 specified as gangrenous

K45.8   Other specified abdominal hernia without obstruction or gangrene

K46- Unspecified abdominal hernia
> Includes: Enterocele
> Epiplocele
> Hernia NOS
> Interstitial hernia
> Intestinal hernia
> Intra-abdominal hernia
> *Excludes 1:   vaginal enterocele (N81.5)*

CC **K46.0   Unspecified abdominal hernia with obstruction, without gangrene**
> Unspecified abdominal hernia causing obstruction
> Unspecified incarcerated abdominal hernia
> Unspecified irreducible abdominal hernia
> Unspecified strangulated abdominal hernia

MCC **K46.1   Unspecified abdominal hernia with gangrene**
> Any condition listed under K46 specified as gangrenous

K46.9   Unspecified abdominal hernia without obstruction or gangrene
> Abdominal hernia NOS

Noninfective enteritis and colitis (K50-K52)

> Includes: Noninfective inflammatory bowel disease
> *Excludes 1:   irritable bowel syndrome (K58.-)*
> *megacolon (K59.3-)*

K50- Crohn's disease [regional enteritis] — A chronic, granulomatous, inflammatory disease characterized by thickening of intestinal walls, low-grade fever, lymphoid hyperplasia, nonspecific granulomas, and mesenteric lymphadenitis.
> AHA 12:4Q:p104 — Crohn's disease of small intestine with abscess
> Includes: Granulomatous enteritis
> Use additional code to identify manifestations, such as:
> Pyoderma gangrenosum (L88)
> *Excludes 1:   ulcerative colitis (K51.-)*

K50.0- Crohn's disease of small intestine — A chronic, granulomatous, inflammatory disease characterized by thickening of the small intestinal walls, low-grade fever, lymphoid hyperplasia, nonspecific granulomas, and mesenteric lymphadenitis.
> Crohn's disease [regional enteritis] of duodenum — A form affecting the duodenum.
> Crohn's disease [regional enteritis] of ileum — A form affecting the ileum.
> Crohn's disease [regional enteritis] of jejunum — A form affecting the jejunum.
> Regional ileitis
> Terminal ileitis
> *Excludes 1:   Crohn's disease of both small and large intestine (K50.8-)*

CC **K50.00 Crohn's disease of small intestine without complications**

K50.01- Crohn's disease of small intestine with complications

CC **K50.011   Crohn's disease of small intestine with rectal bleeding** — A form with the escape of blood from the rectum.

CC **K50.012   Crohn's disease of small intestine with intestinal obstruction** — A form with blockage of the intestine.

CC **K50.013   Crohn's disease of small intestine with fistula** — A form with a communicating passage from the small intestine.

CC **K50.014   Crohn's disease of small intestine with abscess** — A form with a localized collection of pus.

CC **K50.018   Crohn's disease of small intestine with other complication**

K
4
3
–
K
5
0

cc **K50.019** **Crohn's disease of small intestine with <u>unspecified</u> complications**

K50.1- **Crohn's disease of <u>large intestine</u>** — A chronic, granulomatous, inflammatory disease characterized by thickening of the large intestinal walls, low-grade fever, lymphoid hyperplasia, nonspecific granulomas, and mesenteric lymphadenitis.

    Crohn's disease [regional enteritis] of colon
    Crohn's disease [regional enteritis] of large bowel
    Crohn's disease [regional enteritis] of rectum
    Granulomatous colitis
    Regional colitis

    Excludes 1:   *Crohn's disease of both small and large intestine (K50.8-)*

cc **K50.10** **Crohn's disease of large intestine <u>without</u> complications**

K50.11- **Crohn's disease of large intestine <u>with</u> complications**

cc **K50.111** **Crohn's disease of large intestine with <u>rectal bleeding</u>** — A form with the escape of blood from the rectum.

cc **K50.112** **Crohn's disease of large intestine with <u>intestinal obstruction</u>** — A form with blockage of the intestine.

cc **K50.113** **Crohn's disease of large intestine with <u>fistula</u>** — A form with a communicating passage from the large intestine.

cc **K50.114** **Crohn's disease of large intestine with <u>abscess</u>** — A form with a localized collection of pus.

cc **K50.118** **Crohn's disease of large intestine with <u>other</u> complication**

cc **K50.119** **Crohn's disease of large intestine with <u>unspecified</u> complications**

K50.8- **Crohn's disease of <u>both small and large intestine</u>** — A chronic, granulomatous, inflammatory disease characterized by thickening of the small and large intestinal walls, low-grade fever, lymphoid hyperplasia, nonspecific granulomas, and mesenteric lymphadenitis.

cc **K50.80** **Crohn's disease of both small and large intestine <u>without</u> complications**

K50.81- **Crohn's disease of both small and large intestine <u>with</u> complications**

cc **K50.811** **Crohn's disease of both small and large intestine with <u>rectal bleeding</u>** — A form with the escape of blood from the rectum.

cc **K50.812** **Crohn's disease of both small and large intestine with <u>intestinal obstruction</u>** — A form with blockage of the intestine.

cc **K50.813** **Crohn's disease of both small and large intestine with <u>fistula</u>** — A form with a communicating passage from the small and/or large intestine.

cc **K50.814** **Crohn's disease of both small and large intestine with <u>abscess</u>** — A form with a localized collection of pus.

cc **K50.818** **Crohn's disease of both small and large intestine with <u>other</u> complication**

cc **K50.819** **Crohn's disease of both small and large intestine with <u>unspecified</u> complications**

K50.9- **Crohn's disease, <u>unspecified</u>**

cc **K50.90** **Crohn's disease, unspecified, <u>without</u> complications**
    Crohn's disease NOS
    Regional enteritis NOS

K50.91- **Crohn's disease, unspecified, <u>with</u> complications**

cc **K50.911** **Crohn's disease, unspecified, with <u>rectal bleeding</u>** — A form with the escape of blood from the rectum.

cc **K50.912** **Crohn's disease, unspecified, with <u>intestinal obstruction</u>** — A form with blockage of the intestine.

cc **K50.913** **Crohn's disease, unspecified, with <u>fistula</u>** — A form with a communicating passage from the small and/or large intestine.

cc **K50.914** **Crohn's disease, unspecified, with <u>abscess</u>** — A form with a localized collection of pus.

cc **K50.918** **Crohn's disease, unspecified, with other complication**

cc **K50.919** **Crohn's disease, unspecified, with <u>unspecified</u> complications**

K51- **<u>Ulcerative colitis</u>** — A chronic, recurrent, inflammatory, and ulcerative disease of the intestine that is characterized by bloody diarrhea, lower abdominal cramps, abdominal tenderness, and fever.

Use additional code to identify manifestations, such as:
    Pyoderma gangrenosum (L88)

    Excludes 1:   *Crohn's disease [regional enteritis] (K50.-)*

K51.0- **Ulcerative <u>(chronic) pancolitis</u>** — A chronic, recurrent, inflammatory, and ulcerative disease of the small and large intestine and rectum that is characterized by bloody diarrhea, lower abdominal cramps, abdominal tenderness, and fever.

    Backwash ileitis

cc **K51.00** **Ulcerative (chronic) pancolitis <u>without</u> complications**
    Ulcerative (chronic) pancolitis NOS

K51.01- **Ulcerative (chronic) pancolitis <u>with</u> complications**

cc **K51.011** **Ulcerative (chronic) pancolitis with <u>rectal bleeding</u>** — A form with the escape of blood from the rectum.

cc **K51.012** **Ulcerative (chronic) pancolitis with <u>intestinal obstruction</u>** — A form with blockage of the intestine.

cc **K51.013** **Ulcerative (chronic) pancolitis with <u>fistula</u>** — A form with a communicating passage from the intestine and/or rectum.

cc **K51.014** **Ulcerative (chronic) pancolitis with <u>abscess</u>** — A form with a localized collection of pus.

cc **K51.018** **Ulcerative (chronic) pancolitis with <u>other</u> complication**

cc **K51.019** **Ulcerative (chronic) pancolitis with <u>unspecified</u> complications**

K51.2- **Ulcerative <u>(chronic) proctitis</u>** — A chronic, recurrent, inflammatory, and ulcerative disease of the rectum that is characterized by bloody diarrhea, lower abdominal cramps, abdominal tenderness, and fever.

cc **K51.20** **Ulcerative (chronic) proctitis <u>without</u> complications**
    Ulcerative (chronic) proctitis NOS

K51.21- **Ulcerative (chronic) proctitis <u>with</u> complications**

cc **K51.211** **Ulcerative (chronic) proctitis with <u>rectal bleeding</u>** — A form with the escape of blood from the rectum.

cc **K51.212** **Ulcerative (chronic) proctitis with <u>intestinal obstruction</u>** — A form with blockage of the intestine.

cc **K51.213** **Ulcerative (chronic) proctitis with <u>fistula</u>** — A form with a communicating passage from the rectum.

cc **K51.214** **Ulcerative (chronic) proctitis with <u>abscess</u>** — A form with a localized collection of pus.

cc **K51.218** **Ulcerative (chronic) proctitis with <u>other</u> complication**

cc **K51.219** **Ulcerative (chronic) proctitis with <u>unspecified</u> complications**

K51.3- **Ulcerative <u>(chronic) rectosigmoiditis</u>** — A chronic, recurrent, inflammatory, and ulcerative disease of the sigmoid colon and rectum that is characterized by bloody diarrhea, lower abdominal cramps, abdominal tenderness, and fever.

cc **K51.30** **Ulcerative (chronic) rectosigmoiditis <u>without</u> complications**
    Ulcerative (chronic) rectosigmoiditis NOS

K51.31- **Ulcerative (chronic) rectosigmoiditis <u>with</u> complications**

cc **K51.311** **Ulcerative (chronic) rectosigmoiditis with <u>rectal bleeding</u>** — A form with the escape of blood from the rectum.

cc **K51.312** **Ulcerative (chronic) rectosigmoiditis with <u>intestinal obstruction</u>** — A form with blockage of the intestine.

cc **K51.313** **Ulcerative (chronic) rectosigmoiditis with <u>fistula</u>** — A form with a communicating passage from the sigmoid colon and/or rectum.

cc **K51.314** **Ulcerative (chronic) rectosigmoiditis with <u>abscess</u>** — A form with a localized collection of pus.

cc **K51.318** **Ulcerative (chronic) rectosigmoiditis with <u>other</u> complication**

cc **K51.319** **Ulcerative (chronic) rectosigmoiditis with <u>unspecified</u> complications**

K51.4- **<u>Inflammatory polyps of colon</u>** — A form with inflamed, protruding polyps.

    Excludes 1:   *adenomatous polyp of colon (D12.6)*
        polyposis of colon (D12.6)
        polyps of colon NOS (K63.5)

cc **K51.40** **Inflammatory polyps of colon <u>without</u> complications**
    Inflammatory polyps of colon NOS

K 5 0 - K 5 1

K51.41- Inflammatory polyps of colon <u>with</u> complications

cc **K51.411 Inflammatory polyps of colon with <u>rectal bleeding</u>** — A form with the escape of blood from the rectum.

cc **K51.412 Inflammatory polyps of colon with <u>intestinal obstruction</u>** — A form with blockage of the intestine.

cc **K51.413 Inflammatory polyps of colon with <u>fistula</u>** — A form with a communicating passage from the intestine.

cc **K51.414 Inflammatory polyps of colon with <u>abscess</u>** — A form with a localized collection of pus.

cc **K51.418 Inflammatory polyps of colon with <u>other</u> complication**

cc **K51.419 Inflammatory polyps of colon with <u>unspecified</u> complications**

K51.5- <u>Left sided colitis</u> — A chronic, recurrent, inflammatory, and ulcerative disease of the transverse and sigmoid colon that is characterized by bloody diarrhea, lower abdominal cramps, abdominal tenderness, and fever.

   Left hemicolitis

cc **K51.50 Left sided colitis <u>without</u> complications**
   Left sided colitis NOS

K51.51- Left sided colitis <u>with</u> complications

cc **K51.511 Left sided colitis with <u>rectal bleeding</u>** — A form with the escape of blood from the rectum.

cc **K51.512 Left sided colitis with <u>intestinal obstruction</u>** — A form with blockage of the intestine.

cc **K51.513 Left sided colitis with <u>fistula</u>** — A form with a communicating passage from the transverse and/or sigmoid colon.

cc **K51.514 Left sided colitis with <u>abscess</u>** — A form with a localized collection of pus.

cc **K51.518 Left sided colitis with <u>other</u> complication**

cc **K51.519 Left sided colitis with <u>unspecified</u> complications**

K51.8- <u>Other ulcerative colitis</u>

cc **K51.80 Other ulcerative colitis <u>without</u> complications**

K51.81- Other ulcerative colitis <u>with</u> complications

cc **K51.811 Other ulcerative colitis with <u>rectal bleeding</u>** — A form with the escape of blood from the rectum.

cc **K51.812 Other ulcerative colitis with <u>intestinal obstruction</u>** — A form with blockage of the intestine.

cc **K51.813 Other ulcerative colitis with <u>fistula</u>** — A form with a communicating passage from the intestine.

cc **K51.814 Other ulcerative colitis with <u>abscess</u>** — A form with a localized collection of pus.

cc **K51.818 Other ulcerative colitis with <u>other</u> complication**

cc **K51.819 Other ulcerative colitis with <u>unspecified</u> complications**

K51.9- <u>Ulcerative colitis, unspecified</u>

cc **K51.90 Ulcerative colitis, unspecified, <u>without</u> complications**

K51.91- Ulcerative colitis, unspecified, <u>with</u> complications

cc **K51.911 Ulcerative colitis, unspecified with <u>rectal bleeding</u>** — A form with the escape of blood from the rectum.

cc **K51.912 Ulcerative colitis, unspecified with <u>intestinal obstruction</u>** — A form with blockage of the intestine.

cc **K51.913 Ulcerative colitis, unspecified with <u>fistula</u>** — A form with a communicating passage from the intestine.

cc **K51.914 Ulcerative colitis, unspecified with <u>abscess</u>** — A form with a localized collection of pus.

cc **K51.918 Ulcerative colitis, unspecified with <u>other</u> complication**

cc **K51.919 Ulcerative colitis, unspecified with <u>unspecified</u> complications**

K52- Other and unspecified noninfective gastroenteritis and colitis

cc **K52.0 Gastroenteritis and colitis due to radiation** — Inflammation of the stomach and small intestine and/or colon due to the adverse effects of radiation.

cc **K52.1 Toxic gastroenteritis and colitis** — Inflammation of the stomach and small intestine and/or colon due to the chemically poisoning effects of toxic substances.
   Drug-induced gastroenteritis and colitis — A form due to drugs.
   Code first (T51-T65) to identify toxic agent
   Use additional code for adverse effect, if applicable, to identify drug (T36-T50 with fifth or sixth character 5)

K52.2- Allergic and dietetic gastroenteritis and colitis — Inflammation of the stomach and small intestine and/or colon due to effects of an allergen.
   Food hypersensitivity gastroenteritis or colitis
   Use additional code to identify type of food allergy (Z91.01-, Z91.02-)
   Excludes ❷: allergic eosinophilic colitis (K52.82)
   *   allergic eosinophilic esophagitis (K20.0)*
   *   allergic eosinophilic gastritis (K52.81)*
   *   allergic eosinophilic gastroenteritis (K52.81)*
   *   food protein-induced proctocolitis (K52.82)*

K52.21 Food protein-induced enterocolitis syndrome
   Use additional code for hypovolemic shock, if present (R57.1)

K52.22 Food protein-induced enteropathy

K52.29 Other allergic and dietetic gastroenteritis and colitis
   Food hypersensitivity gastroenteritis or colitis
   Immediate gastrointestinal hypersensitivity

K52.3 Indeterminate colitis
   Colonic inflammatory bowel disease unclassified (IBDU)
   Excludes 1:   unspecified colitis (K52.9)

K52.8- Other specified noninfective gastroenteritis and colitis

K52.81 Eosinophilic gastritis or gastroenteritis — A condition involving eosinophil accumulation in the tissues lining the stomach and intestines that is characterized by inflammation, vomiting, and severe abdominal pain.
   Eosinophilic enteritis
   Excludes ❷: eosinophilic esophagitis (K20.0)

K52.82 Eosinophilic colitis — A condition involving eosinophil accumulation in the tissues lining the large intestine that is characterized by inflammation, abdominal pain, diarrhea, and/or blood in the stool.
   Allergic proctocolitis
   Food-induced eosinophilic proctocolitis
   Food protein-induced proctocolitis
   Milk protein-induced proctocolitis

K52.83- Microscopic colitis — An inflammatory intestinal condition that is characterized by chronic nonbloody watery diarrhea with a normal appearing colon on colonoscopy, but some inflammatory changes on biopsy.

K52.831 Collagenous colitis

K52.832 Lymphocytic colitis

K52.838 Other microscopic colitis

K52.839 Microscopic colitis, unspecified

K52.89 Other specified noninfective gastroenteritis and colitis

K52.9 Noninfective gastroenteritis and colitis, unspecified
   Colitis NOS
   Enteritis NOS
   Gastroenteritis NOS
   Ileitis NOS
   Jejunitis NOS
   Sigmoiditis NOS
   Excludes 1:   diarrhea NOS (R19.7)
   *   functional diarrhea (K59.1)*
   *   infectious gastroenteritis and colitis NOS (A09)*
   *   neonatal diarrhea (noninfective) (P78.3)*
   *   psychogenic diarrhea (F45.8)*

K 5 1 - K 5 2

Other diseases of intestines (K55-K64)

K55- **Vascular disorders** of intestine — The condition of an inadequate, functional decrease of blood flow to the intestine.

    Excludes 1:   *necrotizing enterocolitis of newborn (P77.-)*

    K55.0- **Acute vascular disorders of intestine** — The sudden, severe onset of an inadequate, functional decrease of blood flow to the intestine.

        Infarction of appendices epiploicae — Ischemic necrosis of the intestinal, peritoneum-covered tabs of adipose tissue.

        Mesenteric (artery) (vein) embolism — The sudden blocking of the mesenteric artery by a blood clot or foreign material.

        Mesenteric (artery) (vein) infarction — Localized tissue necrosis of the mesentery resulting from obstruction of circulation in that area.

        Mesenteric (artery) (vein) thrombosis — The abnormal formation of a clot in a mesenteric artery or arteriole.

      K55.01- Acute (reversible) **ischemia** of **small intestine** — The sudden, severe onset of inflammation of the small intestine due to and associated with a deficiency of blood supply.

    MCC **K55.011** **Focal (segmental) acute (reversible) ischemia of small intestine**

    MCC **K55.012** **Diffuse acute (reversible) ischemia of small intestine**

    MCC **K55.019** **Acute (reversible) ischemia of small intestine, extent unspecified**

      K55.02- Acute **infarction** of **small intestine** — Ischemic necrosis of the small intestine due to obstruction of the circulation to that area.

        Gangrene of small intestine
        Necrosis of small intestine

    MCC **K55.021** **Focal (segmental) acute infarction of small intestine**

    MCC **K55.022** **Diffuse acute infarction of small intestine**

    MCC **K55.029** **Acute infarction of small intestine, extent unspecified**

      K55.03- Acute (reversible) **ischemia** of **large intestine** — The sudden, severe onset of inflammation of the large intestine due to and associated with a deficiency of blood supply.

        Acute fulminant ischemic colitis
        Subacute ischemic colitis

    MCC **K55.031** **Focal (segmental) acute (reversible) ischemia of large intestine**

    MCC **K55.032** **Diffuse acute (reversible) ischemia of large intestine**

    MCC **K55.039** **Acute (reversible) ischemia of large intestine, extent unspecified**

      K55.04- Acute **infarction** of **large intestine** — Ischemic necrosis of the large intestine due to obstruction of the circulation to that area.

        Gangrene of large intestine
        Necrosis of large intestine

    MCC **K55.041** **Focal (segmental) acute infarction of large intestine**

    MCC **K55.042** **Diffuse acute infarction of large intestine**

    MCC **K55.049** **Acute infarction of large intestine, extent unspecified**

      K55.05- Acute (reversible) **ischemia** of intestine, **part unspecified**

    MCC **K55.051** **Focal (segmental) acute (reversible) ischemia of intestine, part unspecified**

    MCC **K55.052** **Diffuse acute (reversible) ischemia of intestine, part unspecified**

    MCC **K55.059** **Acute (reversible) ischemia of intestine, part and extent unspecified**

      K55.06- Acute **infarction** of intestine, part **unspecified**

        Acute intestinal infarction
        Gangrene of intestine
        Necrosis of intestine

    MCC **K55.061** **Focal (segmental) acute infarction of intestine, part unspecified**

    MCC **K55.062** **Diffuse acute infarction of intestine, part unspecified**

    MCC **K55.069** **Acute infarction of intestine, part and extent unspecified**

CC **K55.1** **Chronic** vascular disorders of intestine — Inadequate, functional decrease of blood flow to the intestine which develops slowly and persists over a long period of time.

    Chronic ischemic colitis — Inflammation of the large intestine and associated with a deficiency of blood supply which develops slowly and persists over a long period of time.

    Chronic ischemic enteritis — Inflammation of the small intestine and associated with a deficiency of blood supply which develops slowly and persists over a long period of time.

    Chronic ischemic enterocolitis — Inflammation of the small and large intestine and associated with a deficiency of blood supply which develops slowly and persists over a long period of time.

    Ischemic stricture of intestine — The abnormal deficiency of blood supply to a localized area of the intestine resulting in contracture of the intestinal smooth muscles.

    Mesenteric atherosclerosis — The narrowing of the mesenteric arteries.

    Mesenteric vascular insufficiency — Abdominal pain after eating due to a deficiency of blood supply to the smooth muscle of the intestine.

K55.2- **Angiodysplasia** of colon — The presence of small, vascular abnormalities of the intestines.

    K55.20 Angiodysplasia of colon **without** hemorrhage

    MCC **K55.21** Angiodysplasia of colon **with hemorrhage**

K55.3- **Necrotizing enterocolitis** — A gastrointestinal disorder involving infection and inflammation that results in weakening and destruction of the intestinal tissues.

    Excludes 1:   *necrotizing enterocolitis of newborn (P77.-)*

    Excludes ❷: *necrotizing enterocolitis due to Clostridium difficile (A04.7)*

    MCC **K55.30** **Necrotizing enterocolitis, unspecified**
        Necrotizing enterocolitis, NOS

    MCC **K55.31** **Stage 1 necrotizing enterocolitis**
        Necrotizing enterocolitis without pneumatosis, without perforation

    MCC **K55.32** **Stage 2 necrotizing enterocolitis**
        Necrotizing enterocolitis with pneumatosis, without perforation

    MCC **K55.33** **Stage 3 necrotizing enterocolitis**
        Necrotizing enterocolitis with perforation
        Necrotizing enterocolitis with pneumatosis and perforation

CC **K55.8** **Other vascular disorders of intestine**

CC **K55.9** **Vascular disorder of intestine, unspecified**
    Ischemic colitis
    Ischemic enteritis
    Ischemic enterocolitis

K56- **Paralytic ileus and intestinal obstruction without hernia**

    Excludes 1:   *congenital stricture or stenosis of intestine (Q41-Q42)*
         cystic fibrosis with meconium ileus (E84.11)
         ischemic stricture of intestine (K55.1)
         meconium ileus NOS (P76.0)
         neonatal intestinal obstructions classifiable to P76.-
         obstruction of duodenum (K31.5)
         postprocedural intestinal obstruction (K91.3)
         stenosis of anus or rectum (K62.4)
         intestinal obstruction with hernia (K40-K46)

CC **K56.0** **Paralytic ileus** — The neurogenic impairment of peristalsis.
    Paralysis of bowel
    Paralysis of colon
    Paralysis of intestine
    Excludes 1:   *gallstone ileus (K56.3)*
         ileus NOS (K56.7)
         obstructive ileus NOS (K56.69)

CC **K56.1** **Intussusception** — The prolapse (invagination, telescoping, sliding into) of one part of the intestine to an immediate adjacent part.
    Intussusception or invagination of bowel
    Intussusception or invagination of colon
    Intussusception or invagination of intestine
    Intussusception or invagination of rectum
    Excludes ❷: *intussusception of appendix (K38.8)*

MCC **K56.2** **Volvulus** — An intestinal obstruction due to a knotting or twisting of the intestine.
    Strangulation of colon or intestine
    Torsion of colon or intestine
    Twist of colon or intestine
    Excludes ❷: *volvulus of duodenum (K31.5)*

CC **K56.3** **Gallstone ileus** — An acute ileal obstruction due to the wedging or lodging of a gallstone in the small intestine.
    Obstruction of intestine by gallstone

K
5
5
-
K
5
6

K56.4- Other impaction of intestine

K56.41 Fecal impaction — An obstruction of the intestine due to the wedging or lodging of a fecal mass.
> Excludes 1:   constipation (K59.0-)
> incomplete defecation (R15.0)

cc **K56.49 Other impaction of intestine**

cc **K56.5 Intestinal adhesions [bands] with obstruction (postprocedural) (postinfection)** — The blockage of the intestine resulting from the constricting effects of intestinal or peritoneal adhesions.
> Abdominal hernia due to adhesions with obstruction
> Peritoneal adhesions [bands] with intestinal obstruction (postprocedural) (postinfection)

K56.6- Other and unspecified intestinal obstruction

cc **K56.60 Unspecified intestinal obstruction**
> Intestinal obstruction NOS
> Excludes 1:   intestinal obstruction due to specified condition – code to condition

cc **K56.69 Other intestinal obstruction**
> Enterostenosis NOS
> Obstructive ileus NOS
> Occlusion of colon or intestine NOS
> Stenosis of colon or intestine NOS
> Stricture of colon or intestine NOS
> Excludes 1:   intestinal obstruction due to specified condition – code to condition

cc **K56.7 Ileus, unspecified**
> Excludes 1:   obstructive ileus (K56.69)

K57- Diverticular disease of intestine — A small mucosal pouch or sac (diverticula) which herniates through a defect in the muscular layer of the intestine. DIVERTICULOSIS – The presence of small mucosal pouches or sacs (diverticula) which herniate through defects in the muscular layer of the intestine. DIVERTICULITIS – Inflammation and/or infection of the diverticula, and if ruptured form abscesses.
> Excludes 1:   congenital diverticulum of intestine (Q43.8)
> Meckel's diverticulum (Q43.0)
> Excludes ❷: diverticulum of appendix (K38.2)

K57.0- Diverticulitis of small intestine with perforation and abscess — A form affecting the small intestine with ruptured diverticula and abscess formation.
> Diverticulitis of small intestine with peritonitis
> Excludes 1:   diverticulitis of both small and large intestine with perforation and abscess (K57.4-)

cc **K57.00 Diverticulitis of small intestine with perforation and abscess without bleeding**

mcc **K57.01 Diverticulitis of small intestine with perforation and abscess with bleeding** — A form with the escape of blood.

K57.1- Diverticular disease of small intestine without perforation or abscess
> Excludes 1:   diverticular disease of both small and large intestine without perforation or abscess (K57.5-)

K57.10 Diverticulosis of small intestine without perforation or abscess without bleeding
> Diverticular disease of small intestine NOS

mcc **K57.11 Diverticulosis of small intestine without perforation or abscess with bleeding** — A form with the escape of blood.

cc **K57.12 Diverticulitis of small intestine without perforation or abscess without bleeding**

mcc **K57.13 Diverticulitis of small intestine without perforation or abscess with bleeding** — A form with the escape of blood.

K57.2- Diverticulitis of large intestine with perforation and abscess — A form affecting the large intestine with ruptured diverticula and abscess formation.
> Diverticulitis of colon with peritonitis
> Excludes 1:   diverticulitis of both small and large intestine with perforation and abscess (K57.4-)

cc **K57.20 Diverticulitis of large intestine with perforation and abscess without bleeding**

mcc **K57.21 Diverticulitis of large intestine with perforation and abscess with bleeding** — A form with the escape of blood.

K57.3- Diverticular disease of large intestine without perforation or abscess
> Excludes 1:   diverticular disease of both small and large intestine without perforation or abscess (K57.5-)

K57.30 Diverticulosis of large intestine without perforation or abscess without bleeding
> Diverticular disease of colon NOS

mcc **K57.31 Diverticulosis of large intestine without perforation or abscess with bleeding** — A form with the escape of blood.

cc **K57.32 Diverticulitis of large intestine without perforation or abscess without bleeding**

mcc **K57.33 Diverticulitis of large intestine without perforation or abscess with bleeding** — A form with the escape of blood.

K57.4- Diverticulitis of both small and large intestine with perforation and abscess — A form affecting the small and large intestine with ruptured diverticula and abscess formation.
> Diverticulitis of both small and large intestine with peritonitis

cc **K57.40 Diverticulitis of both small and large intestine with perforation and abscess without bleeding**

mcc **K57.41 Diverticulitis of both small and large intestine with perforation and abscess with bleeding** — A form with the escape of blood.

K57.5- Diverticular disease of both small and large intestine without perforation or abscess

K57.50 Diverticulosis of both small and large intestine without perforation or abscess without bleeding
> Diverticular disease of both small and large intestine NOS

mcc **K57.51 Diverticulosis of both small and large intestine without perforation or abscess with bleeding** — A form with the escape of blood.

cc **K57.52 Diverticulitis of both small and large intestine without perforation or abscess without bleeding**

mcc **K57.53 Diverticulitis of both small and large intestine without perforation or abscess with bleeding** — A form with the escape of blood.

K57.8- Diverticulitis of intestine, part unspecified, with perforation and abscess — A form affecting the intestine with ruptured diverticula and abscess formation.
> Diverticulitis of intestine NOS with peritonitis

cc **K57.80 Diverticulitis of intestine, part unspecified, with perforation and abscess without bleeding**

mcc **K57.81 Diverticulitis of intestine, part unspecified, with perforation and abscess with bleeding** — A form with the escape of blood.

K57.9- Diverticular disease of intestine, part unspecified, without perforation or abscess

K57.90 Diverticulosis of intestine, part unspecified, without perforation or abscess without bleeding
> Diverticular disease of intestine NOS

mcc **K57.91 Diverticulosis of intestine, part unspecified, without perforation or abscess with bleeding** — A form with the escape of blood.

cc **K57.92 Diverticulitis of intestine, part unspecified, without perforation or abscess without bleeding**

mcc **K57.93 Diverticulitis of intestine, part unspecified, without perforation or abscess with bleeding** — A form with the escape of blood.

K58- Irritable bowel syndrome — A noninflammatory functional disorder of the intestine characterized by abdominal pain, diarrhea, constipation, passage of mucus, and/or bloating.
> Includes: Irritable colon
> Spastic colon

K58.0 Irritable bowel syndrome with diarrhea

K58.1 Irritable bowel syndrome with constipation

K58.2 Mixed irritable bowel syndrome

K58.8 Other irritable bowel syndrome

K58.9 Irritable bowel syndrome without diarrhea
> Irritable bowel syndrome NOS

K56 - K58

K59- **Other functional intestinal disorders**
   Excludes 1:   *change in bowel habit NOS (R19.4)*
                  intestinal malabsorption (K90.-)
                  psychogenic intestinal disorders (F45.8)
   Excludes ❷: *functional disorders of stomach (K31.-)*

  K59.0- **Constipation** — Difficult and infrequent defecation.
        Use additional code for adverse effect, if applicable, to identify drug (T36-T50 with fifth or sixth character 5)
      Excludes 1:   *fecal impaction (K56.41)*
                 incomplete defecation (R15.0)

    K59.00 **Constipation, unspecified**
    K59.01 <u>Slow transit</u> **constipation** — A form marked by a delay in the movement of fecal material throughout the colon secondary to smooth muscle dysfunction.
    K59.02 <u>Outlet dysfunction</u> **constipation** — A form marked by dysfunction of the pelvic floor muscles during defecation.
    K59.03 <u>Drug-induced</u> **constipation** — A form due to a drug that alters the nerve input to the gastrointestinal tract.
        Use additional code for adverse effect, if applicable, to identify drug (T36-T50 with fifth or sixth character 5)
    K59.04 <u>Chronic idiopathic</u> **constipation** — A form of unknown cause that is marked by its continued presence over a considerable period of time, usually more than 3 months.
        Functional constipation
    K59.09 **Other constipation**
        Chronic constipation

  K59.1 **Functional diarrhea** — The abnormal frequency and liquidity of feces due to a dysfunction of the gastrointestinal tract.
      Excludes 1:   *diarrhea NOS (R19.7)*
                 irritable bowel syndrome with diarrhea (K58.0)

  cc **K59.2** **Neurogenic bowel, not elsewhere classified** — The neurologic disruption of normal defecation most commonly seen in patients with spinal cord dysfunction.

  K59.3- **Megacolon, not elsewhere classified** — An abnormally large or dilated colon.
        Dilatation of colon — The abnormal stretching of the colon beyond its normal dimensions.
        Code first, if applicable, (T51-T65) to identify toxic agent
      Excludes 1:   *congenital megacolon (aganglionic) (Q43.1)*
                 megacolon (due to) (in) Chagas' disease (B57.32)
                 megacolon (due to) (in) Clostridium difficile (A04.7)
                 megacolon (due to) (in) Hirschsprung's disease (Q43.1)

    cc **K59.31** **Toxic megacolon** — The significant dilatation of the colon with associated severe symptoms including fever, tachycardia, leukocytosis, and/or anemia.

    cc **K59.39** **Other megacolon**
        Megacolon NOS

  K59.4 **Anal spasm** — A sudden, transitory constriction of the anal canal.
        Proctalgia fugax — Spasmodic pain high in the rectum.

  K59.8 **Other specified functional intestinal disorders**
        Atony of colon — The lack of normal tone or strength of the colon.
        Pseudo-obstruction (acute) (chronic) of intestine

  K59.9 **Functional intestinal disorder, unspecified**

K60- **Fissure and fistula of anal and rectal regions**
   Excludes 1:   *fissure and fistula of anal and rectal regions with abscess or cellulitis (K61.-)*
   Excludes ❷: *anal sphincter tear (healed) (nontraumatic) (old) (K62.81)*

  K60.0 **Acute anal fissure** — A sudden onset of a linear, ulcerative division of anal epithelium.
  K60.1 **Chronic anal fissure** — A persistent linear, ulcerative division of anal epithelium.
  K60.2 **Anal fissure, unspecified**
  K60.3 **Anal fistula** — An abnormal passage from the anal canal.
  K60.4 **Rectal fistula** — An abnormal passage from the rectum.
        Fistula of rectum to skin — An abnormal passage from the rectum, usually rectal crypts, to the skin.
      Excludes 1:   *rectovaginal fistula (N82.3)*
                 vesicorectal fistual (N32.1)
  K60.5 **Anorectal fistula** — An abnormal passage between the anus and the rectum.

K61- **Abscess of anal and rectal regions**
   Includes: **Abscess of anal and rectal regions**
                Cellulitis of anal and rectal regions

  cc **K61.0** **Anal abscess** — A localized collection of pus caused by the disintegration of the anal tissues.
        Perianal abscess — A form located immediately beneath the skin adjacent to the anal canal.
      Excludes 1:   *intrasphincteric abscess (K61.4)*

  cc **K61.1** **Rectal abscess** — A localized collection of pus caused by the disintegration of the rectal tissues.
        AHA 12:4Q:p104 – Rectal abscess with Crohn's disease of small intestine
        Perirectal abscess — Purulent inflammation of the tissue immediately surrounding the rectum.
      Excludes 1:   *ischiorectal abscess (K61.3)*

  cc **K61.2** **Anorectal abscess** — A form localized to the anus and the rectum.
  cc **K61.3** **Ischiorectal abscess** — A form localized to the ischium and the rectum.
        Abscess of ischiorectal fossa
  cc **K61.4** **Intrasphincteric abscess** — A form localized to the space between the interior and external anal sphincters.

K62- **Other diseases of anus and rectum**
   Includes: **Anal canal**
   Excludes ❷: *colostomy and enterostomy malfunction (K94.0-, K94.1-)*
                 fecal incontinence (R15.-)
                 hemorrhoids (K64-)

  K62.0 **Anal polyp** — A protruding mucous membrane growth of the anus.
  K62.1 **Rectal polyp** — A protruding mucous membrane growth of the rectum.
      Excludes 1:   *adenomatous polyp (D12.8)*
  K62.2 **Anal prolapse** — The abnormal protrusion of the anal mucosa through the anal opening.
        Prolapse of anal canal
  K62.3 **Rectal prolapse** — The abnormal protrusion of the rectal mucosa through the anus.
        Prolapse of rectal mucosa
  K62.4 **Stenosis of anus and rectum** — The abnormal decrease in caliber of the rectal and/or anal canal.
        Stricture of anus (sphincter) — The abnormal decrease in the ability of the anal sphincter muscle to relax.
  cc **K62.5** **Hemorrhage of anus and rectum** — The escape of blood from the anus and/or rectum.
      Excludes 1:   *gastrointestinal bleeding NOS (K92.2)*
                 melena (K92.1)
                 neonatal rectal hemorrhage (P54.2)
  cc **K62.6** **Ulcer of anus and rectum** — The abnormal eating-away of anal and/or rectal tissue.
        Solitary ulcer of anus and rectum
        Stercoral ulcer of anus and rectum
      Excludes 1:   *fissure and fistula of anus and rectum (K60-)*
                 ulcerative colitis (K51-)
  K62.7 **Radiation proctitis** — Inflammation of the anus and/or rectum due to the effects of radiation.
        Use additional code to identify the type of radiation (W90-)
  K62.8- **Other specified diseases of anus and rectum**
      Excludes ❷: *ulcerative proctitis (K51.2)*
    K62.81 **Anal sphincter tear (healed) (nontraumatic) (old)** — The presence of a forceful disruption of the anal sphincter tissues that is not due to acute trauma.
        Tear of anus, nontraumatic
        Use additional code for any associated fecal incontinence (R15.-)
      Excludes ❷: *anal fissure (K60.-)*
                 anal sphincter tear (healed) (old) complicating delivery (O34.7-)
                 traumatic tear of anal sphincter (S31.831)

    K62.82 **Dysplasia of anus** — The abnormal shape and/or size of anal cells.
        Anal intraepithelial neoplasia I and II (AIN I and II) (histologically confirmed)
        Dysplasia of anus NOS
        Mild and moderate dysplasia of anus (histologically confirmed)
      Excludes 1:   *abnormal results from anal cytologic examination without histologic confirmation (R85.61-)*
                 anal intraepithelial neoplasia III (D01.3)
                 carcinoma in situ of anus (D01.3)
                 HGSIL of anus (R85.613)
                 severe dysplasia of anus (D01.3)

K 5 9 - K 6 2

K62.89   Other specified diseases of anus and rectum
> Proctitis NOS
> Use additional code for any associated fecal incontinence (R15.-)

K62.9   Disease of anus and rectum, unspecified

K63-   Other diseases of intestine

CC **K63.0   Abscess of intestine** — A localized collection of pus caused by the disintegration of intestinal tissue.
> Excludes 1:   abscess of intestine with Crohn's disease (K50.014, K50.114, K50.814, K50.914)
> abscess of intestine with diverticular disease (K57.0, K57.2, K57.4, K57.8)
> abscess of intestine with ulcerative colitis (K51.014, K51.214, K51.314, K51.414, K51.514, K51.814, K51.914)
> Excludes ❷: abscess of anal and rectal regions (K61-)
> abscess of appendix (K35.3)

MCC **K63.1   Perforation of intestine (nontraumatic)** — The tearing open of an intestinal wall.
> Perforation (nontraumatic) of rectum
> Excludes 1:   perforation (nontraumatic) of duodenum (K26.-)
> perforation (nontraumatic) of intestine with diverticular disease (K57.0, K57.2, K57.4, K57.8)
> Excludes ❷: perforation (nontraumatic) of appendix (K35.2, K35.3)

CC **K63.2   Fistula of intestine** — The abnormal passage of the intestine.
> Excludes 1:   fistula of duodenum (K31.6)
> fistula of intestine with Crohn's disease (K50.013, K50.113, K50.813, K50.913)
> fistula of intestine with ulcerative colitis (K51.013, K51.213, K51.313, K51.413, K51.513, K51.813, K51.913)
> Excludes ❷: fistula of anal and rectal regions (K60.-)
> fistula of appendix (K38.3)
> intestinal-genital fistula, female (N82.2-N82.4)
> vesicointestinal fistula (N32.1)

CC **K63.3   Ulcer of intestine** — The localized eating-away of intestinal tissue.
> Primary ulcer of small intestine
> Excludes 1:   duodenal ulcer (K26-)
> gastrointestinal ulcer (K28-)
> gastrojejunal ulcer (K28-)
> jejunal ulcer (K28-)
> peptic ulcer, site unspecified (K27-)
> ulcer of intestine with perforation (K63.1)
> ulcer of anus or rectum (K62.6)
> ulcerative colitis (K51-)

K63.4   Enteroptosis — The downward displacement of the intestine in the abdominal cavity.

K63.5   Polyp of colon — A protruding mucous membrane growth of the large intestine.
> AHA 15:2Q:p14 – Hyperplastic colon polyp
> Excludes 1:   adenomatous polyp of colon (D12.6)
> inflammatory polyp of colon (K51.4-)
> polyposis of colon (D12.6)

K63.8-   Other specified diseases of intestine

MCC **K63.81   Dieulafoy lesion of intestine** — A severe, often recurrent, hemorrhage from a pinpoint, non-ulcerated arterial lesion of the intestine.
> Excludes ❷: Dieulafoy lesion of stomach and duodenum (K31.82)

K63.89   Other specified diseases of intestine

K63.9   Disease of intestine, unspecified

K64-   Hemorrhoids and perianal venous thrombosis — HEMORRHOIDS – A varicose dilatation of one of the veins of the hemorrhoidal plexus.
> Includes: Piles
> Excludes 1:   hemorrhoids complicating childbirth and the puerperium (O87.2)
> hemorrhoids complicating pregnancy (O22.4)

K64.0   First degree hemorrhoids
> Grade/stage I hemorrhoids
> Hemorrhoids (bleeding) without prolapse outside of anal canal

K64.1   Second degree hemorrhoids
> Grade/stage II hemorrhoids
> Hemorrhoids (bleeding) that prolapse with straining, but retract spontaneously

K64.2   Third degree hemorrhoids
> Grade/stage III hemorrhoids
> Hemorrhoids (bleeding) that prolapse with straining and require manual replacement back inside anal canal

K64.3   Fourth degree hemorrhoids
> Grade/stage IV hemorrhoids
> Hemorrhoids (bleeding) with prolapsed tissue that cannot be manually replaced

K64.4   Residual hemorrhoidal skin tags — Small, hemorrhoidal tissue walls remaining after primary treatment.
> External hemorrhoids NOS
> Skin tags of anus

K64.5   Perianal venous thrombosis
> External hemorrhoids with thrombosis
> Perianal hematoma
> Thrombosed hemorrhoids NOS

K64.8   Other hemorrhoids
> Internal hemorrhoids, without mention of degree
> Prolapsed hemorrhoids, degree not specified

K64.9   Unspecified hemorrhoids
> Hemorrhoids (bleeding) NOS
> Hemorrhoids (bleeding) without mention of degree

Diseases of peritoneum and retroperitoneum (K65-K68)

K65-   Peritonitis — Inflammation of the peritoneum.
> AHA 13:2Q:p31 – Epiploic appendagitis
> Use additional code (B95-B97), to identify infectious agent
> Excludes 1:   acute appendicitis with generalized peritonitis (K35.2)
> aseptic peritonitis (T81.6)
> benign paroxysmal peritonitis (E85.0)
> chemical peritonitis (T81.6)
> diverticulitis of both small and large intestine with peritonitis (K57.4-)
> diverticulitis of colon with peritonitis (K57.2-)
> diverticulitis of intestine, NOS, with peritonitis (K57.8-)
> diverticulitis of small intestine with peritonitis (K57.0-)
> gonococcal peritonitis (A54.85)
> neonatal peritonitis (P78.0-P78.1)
> pelvic peritonitis, female (N73.3-N73.5)
> periodic familial peritonitis (E85.0)
> peritonitis due to talc or other foreign substance (T81.6)
> peritonitis in chlamydia (A74.81)
> peritonitis in diphtheria (A36.89)
> peritonitis in syphilis (late) (A52.74)
> peritonitis in tuberculosis (A18.31)
> peritonitis with or following abortion or ectopic or molar pregnancy (O00-O07, O08.0)
> peritonitis with or following appendicitis (K35-)
> peritonitis with or following diverticular disease of intestine (K57-)
> puerperal peritonitis (O85)
> retroperitoneal infections (K68-)

MCC **K65.0   Generalized (acute) peritonitis** — A form that has spread to most of the peritoneal tissues.
> Pelvic peritonitis (acute), male
> Subphrenic peritonitis (acute)
> Suppurative peritonitis (acute)

MCC **K65.1   Peritoneal abscess** — A form characterized by the localized collection of pus.
> Abdominopelvic abscess
> Abscess (of) omentum
> Abscess (of) peritoneum
> Mesenteric abscess
> Retrocecal abscess
> Subdiaphragmatic abscess
> Subhepatic abscess
> Subphrenic abscess

MCC **K65.2   Spontaneous bacterial peritonitis** — A form characterized by the lack of an identifiable source of infection that is often associated with ascites and cirrhosis.
> Excludes 1:   bacterial peritonitis NOS (K65.9)

MCC **K65.3   Choleperitonitis** — A peritoneal inflammatory reaction resulting from the escape of bile into the peritoneum.
> Peritonitis due to bile

CC **K65.4   Sclerosing mesenteritis** — A mesenteric inflammatory condition that is characterized by fat necrosis, inflammation, and fibrosis.
> Fat necrosis of peritoneum
> (Idiopathic) sclerosing mesenteric fibrosis
> Mesenteric lipodystrophy
> Mesenteric panniculitis
> Retractile mesenteritis

MCC **K65.8   Other peritonitis**
> Chronic proliferative peritonitis
> Peritonitis due to urine

K62 - K65

MCC **K65.9   Peritonitis, unspecified**
        Bacterial peritonitis NOS

K66-   Other disorders of peritoneum
    Excludes ❷: ascites (R18.-)
                peritoneal effusion (chronic) (R18.8)

    K66.0   Peritoneal adhesions (postprocedural) (postinfection) — The formation of fibrous bands within the peritoneum which abnormally restrict the function of the adhered organs.
        AHA 14:1Q:p3 – Peritoneal adhesions
        Adhesions (of) abdominal (wall)
        Adhesions (of) diaphragm
        Adhesions (of) intestine
        Adhesions (of) male pelvis
        Adhesions (of) omentum
        Adhesions (of) stomach
        Adhesive bands
        Mesenteric adhesions
        Excludes 1:   female pelvic adhesions [bands] (N73.6)
                   peritoneal adhesions with intestinal obstruction (K56.5)

MCC **K66.1   Hemoperitoneum** — The abnormal escape of blood into the peritoneum.
        Excludes 1:   traumatic hemoperitoneum (S36.8-)

    K66.8   Other specified disorders of peritoneum

    K66.9   Disorder of peritoneum, unspecified

K67-   Disorders of peritoneum in infectious diseases classified
MCC   **elsewhere** — [Not Allowed as PDX]
    Code first underlying disease, such as :
    Congenital syphilis (A50.0)
    Helminthiasis (B65.0-B83.9)
    Excludes 1:   peritonitis in chlamydia (A74.81)
                peritonitis in diphtheria (A36.89)
                peritonitis in gonococcal (A54.85)
                peritonitis in syphilis (late) (A52.74)
                peritonitis in tuberculosis (A18.31)

K68-   Disorders of retroperitoneum
    K68.1-   Retroperitoneal abscess — The microorganism invasion of the tissues between the parietal peritoneum and the posterior abdominal wall that contains the kidneys, adrenal glands, ureters, and major abdominal vessels.

    CC **K68.11   Postprocedural retroperitoneal abscess** — A form occurring following a procedure.

    MCC **K68.12   Psoas muscle abscess** — The localized collection of pus of the psoas muscle.

    MCC **K68.19   Other retroperitoneal abscess**

MCC **K68.9   Other disorders of retroperitoneum**

Diseases of liver (K70-K77)

Excludes 1:   jaundice NOS (R17)
Excludes ❷: hemochromatosis (E83.11-)
                Reye's syndrome (G93.7)
                viral hepatitis (B15-B19)
                Wilson's disease (E83.0)

K70-   Alcoholic liver disease
    Use additional code to identify:
    Alcohol abuse and dependence (F10.-)

    K70.0   Alcoholic fatty liver — [Age/15-124] – The abnormal accumulation of fat in the liver in persons with excessive chronic alcoholism.

    K70.1-   Alcoholic hepatitis — The sudden, severe onset of inflammation of the liver resulting from necrosis due to alcohol abuse.

        K70.10   Alcoholic hepatitis _without_ ascites — [Age/15-124]

        K70.11   Alcoholic hepatitis _with ascites_ — [Age/15-124] – The abnormal accumulation of fluid in the abdominal cavity.

    K70.2   Alcoholic fibrosis and sclerosis of liver — [Age/15-124] – The degeneration of liver tissue with fibrosis due to chronic excessive exposure to alcohol as a hepatotoxin.

    K70.3-   Alcoholic cirrhosis of liver — The degeneration of liver tissue with scarring due to chronic excessive exposure to alcohol as a hepatotoxin.
        Alcoholic cirrhosis NOS

        K70.30   Alcoholic cirrhosis of liver _without_ ascites — [Age/15-124]

        K70.31   Alcoholic cirrhosis of liver _with ascites_ — [Age/15-124] – The abnormal accumulation of fluid in the abdominal cavity.

    K70.4-   Alcoholic hepatic failure — Complete, or almost complete, loss of function of the liver due to chronic excessive exposure to alcohol as a hepatotoxin.
        Acute alcoholic hepatic failure
        Alcoholic hepatic failure NOS
        Chronic alcoholic hepatic failure
        Subacute alcoholic hepatic failure

        K70.40   Alcoholic hepatic failure _without_ coma — [Age/15-124]

    MCC **K70.41   Alcoholic hepatic failure _with coma_** — [Age/15-124] – A form with loss of consciousness.

    K70.9   Alcoholic liver disease, unspecified — [Age/15-124]

K71-   Toxic liver disease — The degeneration of liver tissue due to a toxic substance other than alcohol.
    Includes: Drug-induced idiosyncratic (unpredictable) liver disease
                Drug-induced toxic (predictable) liver disease
    Code first poisoning due to drug or toxin, if applicable (T36-T65 with fifth or sixth character 1-4 or 6)
    Use additional code for adverse effect, if applicable, to identify drug (T36-T50 with fifth or sixth character 5)
    Excludes ❷: alcoholic liver disease (K70.-)
                Budd-Chiari syndrome (I82.0)

    K71.0   Toxic liver disease with cholestasis — Damage to the liver that prevents the production and/or flow of bile from the liver.
        Cholestasis with hepatocyte injury
        "Pure" cholestasis

    K71.1-   Toxic liver disease with hepatic necrosis — The severe onset of liver dysfunction and localized tissue death of the hepatic tissues.
        Hepatic failure (acute) (chronic) due to drugs

        K71.10   Toxic liver disease with hepatic necrosis, _without_ coma

    MCC **K71.11   Toxic liver disease with hepatic necrosis, _with coma_** — A form with loss of consciousness.

    K71.2   Toxic liver disease with acute hepatitis — The sudden, severe onset of an inflammatory reaction of the hepatic tissues.

    K71.3   Toxic liver disease with chronic persistent hepatitis — An inflammatory reaction of the liver which is usually benign and characterized by little or no "piece-meal necrosis" of the liver cells.

    K71.4   Toxic liver disease with chronic lobular hepatitis — A form affecting a lobe of the liver.

    K71.5-   Toxic liver disease with chronic active hepatitis — An inflammatory reaction of the liver which persists for more than six months' duration.
        Toxic liver disease with lupoid hepatitis

        K71.50   Toxic liver disease with chronic active hepatitis _without_ ascites

        K71.51   Toxic liver disease with chronic active hepatitis _with ascites_ — The abnormal accumulation of fluid in the abdominal cavity.

    K71.6   Toxic liver disease with hepatitis, not elsewhere classified

    K71.7   Toxic liver disease with fibrosis and cirrhosis of liver — Degeneration of the liver tissue with fibrosis.

    K71.8   Toxic liver disease with other disorders of liver
        Toxic liver disease with focal nodular hyperplasia
        Toxic liver disease with hepatic granulomas
        Toxic liver disease with peliosis hepatis
        Toxic liver disease with veno-occlusive disease of liver

    K71.9   Toxic liver disease, unspecified

K72-   Hepatic failure, not elsewhere classified
    AHA 16:2Q:p35 – Hepatic failure with coma
    Includes: Fulminant hepatitis NEC, with hepatic failure
                Hepatic encephalopathy NOS
                Liver (cell) necrosis with hepatic failure
                Malignant hepatitis NEC, with hepatic failure
                Yellow liver atrophy or dystrophy
    Excludes 1:   alcoholic hepatic failure (K70.4)
                hepatic failure with toxic liver disease (K71.1-)
                icterus of newborn (P55-P59)
                postprocedural hepatic failure (K91.82)
    Excludes ❷: hepatic failure complicating abortion or ectopic or molar pregnancy (O00-O07, O08.8)
                hepatic failure complicating pregnancy, childbirth and the puerperium (O26.6-)
                viral hepatitis with hepatic coma (B15-B19)

    K72.0-   _Acute and subacute_ hepatic failure — Complete, or almost complete, loss of function of the liver.
        AHA 14:2Q:p13 – Shock liver
        AHA 15:2Q:p17 – Acute nonviral hepatitis
        Acute non-viral hepatitis NOS

    MCC **K72.00   Acute and subacute hepatic failure _without_ coma**

K
6
5
-
K
7
2

MCC **K72.01 Acute and subacute hepatic failure with coma** — A form with loss of consciousness.

K72.1- Chronic hepatic failure — The significantly ongoing loss of function of the liver.

K72.10 Chronic hepatic failure without coma

MCC **K72.11 Chronic hepatic failure with coma** — A form with loss of consciousness.

K72.9- Hepatic failure, unspecified

K72.90 Hepatic failure, unspecified without coma

MCC **K72.91 Hepatic failure, unspecified with coma** — A form with loss of consciousness.
Hepatic coma NOS

K73- Chronic hepatitis, not elsewhere classified
Excludes 1:   alcoholic hepatitis (chronic) (K70.1-)
drug-induced hepatitis (chronic) (K71.-)
granulomatous hepatitis (chronic) NEC (K75.3)
reactive, nonspecific hepatitis (chronic) (K75.2)
viral hepatitis (chronic) (B15-B19)

K73.0 Chronic persistent hepatitis, not elsewhere classified
K73.1 Chronic lobular hepatitis, not elsewhere classified
K73.2 Chronic active hepatitis, not elsewhere classified
K73.8 Other chronic hepatitis, not elsewhere classified
K73.9 Chronic hepatitis, unspecified

K74- Fibrosis and cirrhosis of liver
Code also, if applicable, viral hepatitis (acute) (chronic) (B15-B19)
Excludes 1:   alcoholic cirrhosis (of liver) (K70.3)
alcoholic fibrosis of liver (K70.2)
cardiac sclerosis of liver (K76.1)
cirrhosis (of liver) with toxic liver disease (K71.7)
congenital cirrhosis (of liver) (P78.81)
pigmentary cirrhosis (of liver) (E83.110)

K74.0 Hepatic fibrosis — Degeneration of the liver tissue with fibrosis.
K74.1 Hepatic sclerosis — Degeneration of the liver tissue with replacement by connective tissue.
K74.2 Hepatic fibrosis with hepatic sclerosis — Degeneration of the liver tissue with fibrosis and replacement by connective tissue.
K74.3 Primary biliary cirrhosis — Cirrhosis of the liver due to obstruction or infection of the major extrahepatic or intrahepatic bile ducts.
Chronic nonsuppurative destructive cholangitis
K74.4 Secondary biliary cirrhosis — Cirrhosis of the liver due to obstruction or infection of the major extrahepatic or intrahepatic bile ducts that is caused by another disease or condition.

K74.6- Other and unspecified cirrhosis of liver
K74.60 Unspecified cirrhosis of liver
Cirrhosis (of liver) NOS
K74.69 Other cirrhosis of liver — Degeneration of the liver tissue with fibrosis and inflammation.
Cryptogenic cirrhosis (of liver)
Macronodular cirrhosis (of liver)
Micronodular cirrhosis (of liver)
Mixed type cirrhosis (of liver)
Portal cirrhosis (of liver)
Postnecrotic cirrhosis (of liver)

K75- Other inflammatory liver diseases
Excludes ❷: toxic liver disease (K71.-)

MCC **K75.0 Abscess of liver** — A localized collection of pus caused by the disintegration of hepatic tissue.
Cholangitic hepatic abscess
Hematogenic hepatic abscess
Hepatic abscess NOS
Lymphogenic hepatic abscess
Pylephlebitic hepatic abscess
Excludes 1:   amebic liver abscess (A06.4)
cholangitis without liver abscess (K83.0)
pylephlebitis without liver abscess (K75.1)
Excludes ❷: acute or subacute hepatitis NOS (B17.9)
acute or subacute non-viral hepatitis NOS (K72.0)
chronic hepatitis NEC (K73.8)

MCC **K75.1 Phlebitis of portal vein** — Inflammation of the portal vein.
Pylephlebitis
Excludes 1:   pylephlebitic liver abscess (K75.0)

K75.2 Nonspecific reactive hepatitis
Excludes 1:   acute or subacute hepatitis (K72.0-)
chronic hepatitis NEC (K73.-)
viral hepatitis (B15-B19)

K75.3 Granulomatous hepatitis, not elsewhere classified
Excludes 1:   acute or subacute hepatitis (K72.0-)
chronic hepatitis NEC (K73.-)
viral hepatitis (B15-B19)

K75.4 Autoimmune hepatitis — An autoimmune disease (the body's immune system attacks itself) that is characterized by hepatocellular inflammation and necrosis which tends to progress to cirrhosis.
Lupoid hepatitis NEC

K75.8- Other specified inflammatory liver diseases
K75.81 Nonalcoholic steatohepatitis (NASH) — Inflammation of the liver caused by the buildup of fat in the liver, but is not associated with alcohol consumption.
K75.89 Other specified inflammatory liver diseases
K75.9 Inflammatory liver disease, unspecified
Hepatitis NOS
Excludes 1:   acute or subacute hepatitis (K72.0-)
chronic hepatitis NEC (K73.-)
viral hepatitis (B15-B19)

K76- Other diseases of liver
Excludes ❷: alcoholic liver disease (K70.-)
amyloid degeneration of liver (E85.-)
cystic disease of liver (congenital) (Q44.6)
hepatic vein thrombosis (I82.0)
hepatomegaly NOS (R16.0)
pigmentary cirrhosis (of liver) (E83.110)
portal vein thrombosis (I81)
toxic liver disease (K71.-)

K76.0 Fatty (change of) liver, not elsewhere classified — The abnormal accumulation of fat in the liver.
Nonalcoholic fatty liver disease (NAFLD)
Excludes 1:   nonalcoholic steatohepatitis (NASH) (K75.81)

K76.1 Chronic passive congestion of liver — The excessive accumulation of escaped blood in the liver tissues.
Cardiac cirrhosis
Cardiac sclerosis

MCC **K76.2 Central hemorrhagic necrosis of liver**
Excludes 1:   liver necrosis with hepatic failure (K72-)

MCC **K76.3 Infarction of liver** — A localized area of necrosis due to obstruction of circulation to that area.

K76.4 Peliosis hepatis — A vascular condition of the liver that is characterized by multiple blood-filled cystic cavities.
Hepatic angiomatosis

K76.5 Hepatic veno-occlusive disease — A syndrome characterized by hepatomegaly due to obstruction of the small veins of the liver (hepatic venules and hepatic sinusoids) that is most often seen in post stem cell and post chemotherapy patients (also called Sinusoidal Obstruction Syndrome (SOS)).
Excludes 1:   Budd-Chiari syndrome (I82.0)

CC **K76.6 Portal hypertension** — An abnormally increased blood pressure in the portal venous system; a frequent complication of cirrhosis of the liver.
Use additional code for any associated complications, such as:
Portal hypertensive gastropathy (K31.89)

MCC **K76.7 Hepatorenal syndrome** — Renal failure associated with acute or chronic liver disease.
Excludes 1:   hepatorenal syndrome following labor and delivery (O90.4)
postprocedural hepatorenal syndrome (K91.83)

K76.8- Other specified diseases of liver
K76.81 Hepatopulmonary syndrome — [Unacceptable PDX] – A complication of liver disease that affects the lungs and is characterized by low blood oxygen levels and shortness of breath.
Code first underlying disease, such as:
Alcoholic cirrhosis of liver (K70.3-)
Cirrhosis of liver without mention of alcohol (K74.6-)
K76.89 Other specified diseases of liver
Cyst (simple) of liver — The presence of a fluid-filled sac of the liver.
Focal nodular hyperplasia of liver — The presence of benign vascular growth nodules of the liver.
Hepatoptosis — The abnormal downward displacement of the liver.
K76.9 Liver disease, unspecified

K72 - K76

K77 Liver disorders in diseases classified elsewhere — [Not Allowed as PDX]

CC   Code first underlying disease, such as:
    Amyloidosis (E85.-)
    Congenital syphilis (A50.0, A50.5)
    Congenital toxoplasmosis (P37.1)
    Schistosomiasis (B65.0-B65.9)

    Excludes 1:   alcoholic hepatitis (K70.1-)
              alcoholic liver disease (K70.-)
              cytomegaloviral hepatitis (B25.1)
              herpesviral [herpes simplex] hepatitis (B00.81)
              infectious mononucleosis with liver disease (B27.0-B27.9
                with .9)
              mumps hepatitis (B26.81)
              sarcoidosis with liver disease (D86.89)
              secondary syphilis with liver disease (A51.45)
              syphilis (late) with liver disease (A52.74)
              toxoplasmosis (acquired) hepatitis (B58.1)
              tuberculosis with liver disease (A18.83)

Disorders of gallbladder, biliary tract and pancreas (K80-K87)

K80- **Cholelithiasis** — The formation and presence of gallbladder calculi.
    Excludes 1:   retained cholelithiasis following cholecystectomy (K91.86)

K80.0- **Calculus of gallbladder with acute cholecystitis** — The presence of one or more gallstones associated with the severe, sudden onset of gallbladder inflammation.
    Any condition listed in K80.2 with acute cholecystitis

CC **K80.00** **Calculus of gallbladder with acute cholecystitis without obstruction**

CC **K80.01** **Calculus of gallbladder with acute cholecystitis with obstruction** — The blockage of a part of the biliary system.

K80.1- **Calculus of gallbladder with other cholecystitis** — The presence of one or more gallstones with inflammation of the gallbladder of a chronic or unspecified intensity.

CC **K80.10** **Calculus of gallbladder with chronic cholecystitis without obstruction**
    Cholelithiasis with cholecystitis NOS

CC **K80.11** **Calculus of gallbladder with chronic cholecystitis with obstruction** — The blockage of a part of the biliary system.

CC **K80.12** **Calculus of gallbladder with acute and chronic cholecystitis without obstruction**

CC **K80.13** **Calculus of gallbladder with acute and chronic cholecystitis with obstruction** — The blockage of a part of the biliary system.

CC **K80.18** **Calculus of gallbladder with other cholecystitis without obstruction**

CC **K80.19** **Calculus of gallbladder with other cholecystitis with obstruction** — The blockage of a part of the biliary system.

K80.2- **Calculus of gallbladder without cholecystitis** — The presence of one or more gallstones without associated inflammation of the gallbladder.
    Cholecystolithiasis without cholecystitis
    Cholelithiasis (without cholecystitis)
    Colic (recurrent) of gallbladder (without cholecystitis)
    Gallstone (impacted) of cystic duct (without cholecystitis)
    Gallstone (impacted) of gallbladder (without cholecystitis)

K80.20 **Calculus of gallbladder without cholecystitis without obstruction**

CC **K80.21** **Calculus of gallbladder without cholecystitis with obstruction** — The blockage of a part of the biliary system.

K80.3- **Calculus of bile duct with cholangitis** — The presence of one or more gallstones in the bile duct with inflammation of the bile duct.
    Any condition listed in K80.5 with cholangitis

CC **K80.30** **Calculus of bile duct with cholangitis, unspecified, without obstruction**

CC **K80.31** **Calculus of bile duct with cholangitis, unspecified, with obstruction** — The blockage of a part of the biliary system.

CC **K80.32** **Calculus of bile duct with acute cholangitis without obstruction**

CC **K80.33** **Calculus of bile duct with acute cholangitis with obstruction** — The blockage of a part of the biliary system.

CC **K80.34** **Calculus of bile duct with chronic cholangitis without obstruction**

CC **K80.35** **Calculus of bile duct with chronic cholangitis with obstruction** — The blockage of a part of the biliary system.

CC **K80.36** **Calculus of bile duct with acute and chronic cholangitis without obstruction**

CC **K80.37** **Calculus of bile duct with acute and chronic cholangitis with obstruction** — The blockage of a part of the biliary system.

K80.4- **Calculus of bile duct with cholecystitis** — The presence of one or more gallstones in the bile duct with gallbladder inflammation.
    Any condition listed in K80.5 with cholecystitis (with cholangitis)

CC **K80.40** **Calculus of bile duct with cholecystitis, unspecified, without obstruction**

CC **K80.41** **Calculus of bile duct with cholecystitis, unspecified, with obstruction** — The blockage of a part of the biliary system.

CC **K80.42** **Calculus of bile duct with acute cholecystitis without obstruction**

CC **K80.43** **Calculus of bile duct with acute cholecystitis with obstruction** — The blockage of a part of the biliary system.

CC **K80.44** **Calculus of bile duct with chronic cholecystitis without obstruction**

CC **K80.45** **Calculus of bile duct with chronic cholecystitis with obstruction** — The blockage of a part of the biliary system.

CC **K80.46** **Calculus of bile duct with acute and chronic cholecystitis without obstruction**

CC **K80.47** **Calculus of bile duct with acute and chronic cholecystitis with obstruction** — The blockage of a part of the biliary system.

K80.5- **Calculus of bile duct without cholangitis or cholecystitis** — The presence of one or more gallstones in the bile duct.
    Choledocholithiasis (without cholangitis or cholecystitis)
    Gallstone (impacted) of bile duct NOS (without cholangitis or cholecystitis)
    Gallstone (impacted) of common duct (without cholangitis or cholecystitis)
    Gallstone (impacted) of hepatic duct (without cholangitis or cholecystitis)
    Hepatic cholelithiasis (without cholangitis or cholecystitis)
    Hepatic colic (recurrent) (without cholangitis or cholecystitis)

K80.50 **Calculus of bile duct without cholangitis or cholecystitis without obstruction**

CC **K80.51** **Calculus of bile duct without cholangitis or cholecystitis with obstruction** — The blockage of a part of the biliary system.

K80.6- **Calculus of gallbladder and bile duct with cholecystitis** — The presence of one or more gallstones in the gallbladder and bile duct with gallbladder inflammation.

CC **K80.60** **Calculus of gallbladder and bile duct with cholecystitis, unspecified, without obstruction**

CC **K80.61** **Calculus of gallbladder and bile duct with cholecystitis, unspecified, with obstruction** — The blockage of a part of the biliary system.

CC **K80.62** **Calculus of gallbladder and bile duct with acute cholecystitis without obstruction**

CC **K80.63** **Calculus of gallbladder and bile duct with acute cholecystitis with obstruction** — The blockage of a part of the biliary system.

CC **K80.64** **Calculus of gallbladder and bile duct with chronic cholecystitis without obstruction**

CC **K80.65** **Calculus of gallbladder and bile duct with chronic cholecystitis with obstruction** — The blockage of a part of the biliary system.

CC **K80.66** **Calculus of gallbladder and bile duct with acute and chronic cholecystitis without obstruction**

MCC **K80.67** **Calculus of gallbladder and bile duct with acute and chronic cholecystitis with obstruction** — The blockage of a part of the biliary system.

K80.7- **Calculus of gallbladder and bile duct without cholecystitis** — The presence of one or more gallstones in the gallbladder and bile duct.

K80.70 **Calculus of gallbladder and bile duct without cholecystitis without obstruction**

CC **K80.71** **Calculus of gallbladder and bile duct without cholecystitis with obstruction** — The blockage of a part of the biliary system.

K80.8- **Other cholelithiasis**

K80.80 **Other cholelithiasis without obstruction**

K 7 7 - K 8 0

cc **K80.81** **Other cholelithiasis with obstruction** — The blockage of a part of the biliary system.

K81- Cholecystitis

Excludes 1:   *cholecystitis with cholelithiasis (K80.-)*

cc **K81.0** **Acute cholecystitis** — The sudden, severe onset of inflammation of the gallbladder.

    Abscess of gallbladder — A localized collection of pus caused by the disintegration of gallbladder tissues.

    Angiocholecystitis — A form associated with an unusually vascular formation of the gallbladder.

    Emphysematous (acute) cholecystitis — A form caused by gas-producing organisms.

    Empyema of gallbladder — A form marked by the accumulation of pus within the gallbladder.

    Gangrene of gallbladder — A form marked by the death of gallbladder tissue due to decreased vascular supply.

    Gangrenous cholecystitis — A form marked by the death of gallbladder tissue due to decreased vascular supply.

    Suppurative cholecystitis — A form marked by the production of pus.

K81.1 **Chronic cholecystitis** — Inflammation of the gallbladder presenting with mild symptoms over a long period of time.

cc **K81.2** **Acute cholecystitis with chronic cholecystitis** — Inflammation of the gallbladder with both persistent and severe, sudden onset.

K81.9 **Cholecystitis, unspecified**

K82- Other diseases of gallbladder

Excludes 1:   *nonvisualization of gallbladder (R93.2)*
                 postcholecystectomy syndrome (K91.5)

cc **K82.0** **Obstruction of gallbladder** — The blockage of draining bile from the gallbladder.

    Occlusion of cystic duct or gallbladder without cholelithiasis
    Stenosis of cystic duct or gallbladder without cholelithiasis
    Stricture of cystic duct or gallbladder without cholelithiasis

    Excludes 1:   *obstruction of gallbladder with cholelithiasis (K80.-)*

cc **K82.1** **Hydrops of gallbladder** — The abnormal accumulation of serous fluid within the gallbladder.

    Mucocele of gallbladder — The abnormal dilatation of the gallbladder with accumulated mucus secretion.

mcc **K82.2** **Perforation of gallbladder** — The forcible tearing of the gallbladder wall.

    Rupture of cystic duct or gallbladder — The tearing-open of the cystic duct or gallbladder walls.

cc **K82.3** **Fistula of gallbladder** — An abnormal passage of the gallbladder.

    Cholecystocolic fistula — An abnormal passage communicating the gallbladder with the intestine.

    Cholecystoduodenal fistula — An abnormal passage communicating the gallbladder with the duodenum.

K82.4 **Cholesterolosis of gallbladder** — The abnormal deposition of cholesterol in the gallbladder tissues.

    Strawberry gallbladder — The abnormal condition of cholesterol deposition in the gallbladder resulting in a strawberry-like appearance.

    Excludes 1:   *cholesterolosis of gallbladder with cholecystitis (K81-)*
                      cholesterolosis of gallbladder with cholelithiasis (K80-)

K82.8 **Other specified diseases of gallbladder**

    Adhesions of cystic duct or gallbladder — The formation of fibrous bands of tissue of the gallbladder or cystic duct.

    Atrophy of cystic duct or gallbladder — The abnormal wasting-away of the gallbladder or cystic duct.

    Cyst of cystic duct or gallbladder — The abnormal accumulation of fluid contained in a sac of the gallbladder or cystic duct.

    Dyskinesia of cystic duct or gallbladder — The abnormal function of the filling and emptying mechanism of the gallbladder or cystic duct.

    Hypertrophy of cystic duct or gallbladder — The abnormal enlargement of constituent cells of the gallbladder or cystic duct.

    Nonfunctioning of cystic duct or gallbladder — The absence of normal gallbladder or cystic duct function.

    Ulcer of cystic duct or gallbladder — An eating-away of a localized area of the gallbladder or cystic duct.

K82.9 **Disease of gallbladder, unspecified**

K83- Other diseases of biliary tract

Excludes 1:   *postcholecystectomy syndrome (K91.5)*
Excludes ❷: *conditions involving the gallbladder (K81-K82)*
                 conditions involving the cystic duct (K81-K82)

cc **K83.0** **Cholangitis** — Inflammation of a bile duct.

    Ascending cholangitis — A form affecting the upper bile ducts.

    Cholangitis NOS

    Primary cholangitis — A form resulting from direct invasion.

    Recurrent cholangitis — A form marked by the return of symptoms after a remission.

    Sclerosing cholangitis — A form marked by the hardening of the bile duct walls.

    Secondary cholangitis — A form caused by the effects of a systemic disease or toxin.

    Stenosing cholangitis — A form marked by a decrease in caliber of the bile duct's lumen.

    Suppurative cholangitis — A form marked by the production of pus.

    Excludes 1:   *cholangitic liver abscess (K75.0)*
                     cholangitis with choledocholithiasis (K80.3-, K80.4-)
                     chronic nonsuppurative destructive cholangitis (K74.3)

mcc **K83.1** **Obstruction of bile duct** — The blockage of a bile duct.

    AHA 16:1Q:p18 – Biliary obstruction from neoplasm

    Occlusion of bile duct without cholelithiasis — The blockage of a bile duct.

    Stenosis of bile duct without cholelithiasis — The abnormal reduction in the size of a bile duct lumen.

    Stricture of bile duct without cholelithiasis — The decrease in caliber of a bile duct lumen.

    Excludes 1:   *congenital obstruction of bile duct (Q44.3)*
                     obstruction of bile duct with cholelithiasis (K80.-)

mcc **K83.2** **Perforation of bile duct** — The tearing-open of a bile duct wall.

    Rupture of bile duct

cc **K83.3** **Fistula of bile duct** — An abnormal passage communicating from a bile duct.

    Choledochoduodenal fistula — An abnormal passage communicating a bile duct with the duodenum.

K83.4 **Spasm of sphincter of Oddi** — The abnormal function of the muscle fibers encircling the common bile duct as it enters the duodenum.

K83.5 **Biliary cyst** — An encapsulated, fluid-filled sac of a bile duct.

K83.8 **Other specified diseases of biliary tract**

    Adhesions of biliary tract — The formation of fibrous tissue bands affecting a bile duct.

    Atrophy of biliary tract — The abnormal wasting-away of bile duct tissues.

    Hypertrophy of biliary tract — The abnormal enlargement of the constituent cells of a bile duct.

    Ulcer of biliary tract — An abnormal eating-away of a localized area of a bile duct.

K83.9 **Disease of biliary tract, unspecified**

K85- Acute pancreatitis — The sudden, severe onset of inflammation of the pancreas.

  Includes: **Acute (recurrent) pancreatitis** — Multiple episodes of sudden, severe onset of inflammation of the pancreas.

             Subacute pancreatitis — A form marked by slightly milder onset and severity.

K85.0- **Idiopathic acute pancreatitis** — The sudden, severe onset of inflammation of the pancreas without a known cause.

mcc **K85.00** **Idiopathic acute pancreatitis without necrosis or infection**

mcc **K85.01** **Idiopathic acute pancreatitis with uninfected necrosis**

mcc **K85.02** **Idiopathic acute pancreatitis with infected necrosis**

K85.1- **Biliary acute pancreatitis** — The sudden, severe onset of inflammation of the pancreas due to a disease or condition in the biliary system.

    Gallstone pancreatitis — The sudden, severe onset of inflammation of the pancreas due to effects of gallstones.

mcc **K85.10** **Biliary acute pancreatitis without necrosis or infection**

mcc **K85.11** **Biliary acute pancreatitis with uninfected necrosis**

mcc **K85.12** **Biliary acute pancreatitis with infected necrosis**

K85.2- **Alcohol-induced acute pancreatitis** — The sudden, severe onset of inflammation of the pancreas due to the effects of alcohol.

    Excludes ❷: *alcohol-induced chronic pancreatitis (K86.0)*

mcc **K85.20** **Alcohol-induced acute pancreatitis without necrosis or infection**

mcc **K85.21** **Alcohol-induced acute pancreatitis with uninfected necrosis**

mcc **K85.22** **Alcohol-induced acute pancreatitis with infected necrosis**

K80 - K85

K85.3- <u>Drug-induced</u> acute pancreatitis — The sudden, severe onset of inflammation of the pancreas due to the effects of drugs.
Use additional code for adverse effect, if applicable, to identify drug (T36-T50 with fifth or sixth character 5)
Use additional code to identify drug abuse and dependence (F11.- – F17.-)

MCC **K85.30** Drug-induced acute pancreatitis <u>without</u> necrosis or infection

MCC **K85.31** Drug-induced acute pancreatitis <u>with uninfected necrosis</u>

MCC **K85.32** Drug-induced acute pancreatitis <u>with infected necrosis</u>

K85.8- <u>Other</u> acute pancreatitis

MCC **K85.80** Other acute pancreatitis <u>without</u> necrosis or infection

MCC **K85.81** Other acute pancreatitis <u>with uninfected necrosis</u>

MCC **K85.82** Other acute pancreatitis <u>with infected necrosis</u>

K85.9- Acute pancreatitis, <u>unspecified</u>
Pancreatitis NOS

MCC **K85.90** Acute pancreatitis <u>without</u> necrosis or infection, unspecified

MCC **K85.91** Acute pancreatitis <u>with uninfected necrosis</u>, unspecified

MCC **K85.92** Acute pancreatitis <u>with infected necrosis</u>, unspecified

K86- **Other diseases of pancreas**
Excludes ❷: *fibrocystic disease of pancreas (E84-)*
islet cell tumor (of pancreas) (D13.7)
pancreatic steatorrhea (K90.3)

CC **K86.0** **Alcohol-induced chronic pancreatitis** — Inflammation of the pancreas which persists over a long period of time that results in the loss of exocrine and endocrine function due to the effects of alcohol.
Code also exocrine pancreatic insufficiency (K86.81)
Use additional code to identify:
Alcohol abuse and dependence (F10-)
Excludes ❷: *alcohol induced acute pancreatitis (K85.2-)*

CC **K86.1** **Other chronic pancreatitis**
Chronic pancreatitis NOS
Infectious chronic pancreatitis — Inflammation of the pancreas which persists over a long period of time that results in the loss of exocrine and endocrine function due to invading microorganisms.
Recurrent chronic pancreatitis — Inflammation of the pancreas which persists over a long period of time that results in the loss of exocrine and endocrine function that recurs but is not diagnostic of acute pancreatitis.
Relapsing chronic pancreatitis — Inflammation of the pancreas which persists over a long period of time that results in the loss of exocrine and endocrine function that recurs but is not diagnostic of acute pancreatitis.
Code also exocrine pancreatic insufficiency (K86.81)

CC **K86.2** **Cyst of pancreas** — The abnormal presence of a fluid-filled sac in the pancreas.

CC **K86.3** **Pseudocyst of pancreas** — The abnormal presence of a pancreatic juice-filled sac in the abdomen.

K86.8- **Other specified diseases of pancreas**

K86.81 **Exocrine pancreatic insufficiency** — The inadequate production of pancreatic enzymes resulting in maldigestion, malabsorption, and nutrient deficiencies.

K86.89 **Other specified diseases of pancreas**
Aseptic pancreatic necrosis, unrelated to acute pancreatitis — The localized death of pancreatic tissue cells which is not associated with invading microorganisms.
Atrophy of pancreas — An abnormal wasting-away of the pancreas.
Calculus of pancreas — An abnormal concretion within the pancreas.
Cirrhosis of pancreas — The loss of normal microscopic tissue formation.
Fibrosis of pancreas — The abnormal formation of fibrous tissue which replaces the pancreatic tissue.
Pancreatic fat necrosis, unrelated to acute pancreatitis — The localized death of pancreatic tissue due to the splitting of neutral fats into fatty acids and glycerol.
Pancreatic infantilism — A condition affecting normal growth caused by defective pancreatic function.
Pancreatic necrosis NOS, unrelated to acute pancreatitis

K86.9 **Disease of pancreas, unspecified**

K87 **Disorders of gallbladder, biliary tract and pancreas <u>in diseases classified elsewhere</u>** — [Not Allowed as PDX]
Code first underlying disease
Excludes 1: *cytomegaloviral pancreatitis(B25.2)*
mumps pancreatitis (B26.3)
syphilitic gallbladder (A52.74)
syphilitic pancreas (A52.74)
tuberculosis of gallbladder (A18.83)
tuberculosis of pancreas (A18.83)

Other diseases of the digestive system (K90-K95)

K90- **Intestinal malabsorption** — Inadequate absorption of nutrients from the intestinal tract.
Excludes 1: *intestinal malabsorption following gastrointestinal surgery (K91.2)*

K90.0 **Celiac disease** — Inadequate absorption of nutrients from the intestinal tract precipitated by ingestion of gluten-containing (a protein of wheat) foods, and characterized by the degeneration of intestinal cells and fatty stools.
Celiac disease with steatorrhea
Gluten-sensitive enteropathy
Nontropical sprue
Code also exocrine pancreatic insufficiency (K86.81)
Use additional code for associated disorders including:
Dermatitis herpetiformis (L13.0)
Gluten ataxia (G32.81)

CC **K90.1** **Tropical sprue** — Inadequate absorption of nutrients from the intestinal tract occurring in the tropics and associated with anemia due to folic acid deficiency.
Sprue NOS
Tropical steatorrhea

CC **K90.2** **Blind loop syndrome, not elsewhere classified** — Inadequate intestinal absorption due to changes in the anatomy of the small intestine.
Blind loop syndrome NOS
Excludes 1: *congenital blind loop syndrome (Q43.8)*
postsurgical blind loop syndrome (K91.2)

CC **K90.3** **Pancreatic steatorrhea** — The excessive amount of fat in the feces, of pancreatic origin.

K90.4- **Other malabsorption due to intolerance**
Excludes ❷: *gluten-sensitive enteropathy (K90.0)*
lactose intolerance (E73.-)

CC **K90.41** **Non-celiac gluten sensitivity** — The condition of difficulty tolerating the ingestion of gluten-containing (a protein of wheat) foods that produce gastrointestinal symptoms, headaches, "foggy mind," joint pain, and chronic fatigue, but is not diagnostic of celiac disease.
Gluten-sensitivity NOS
Non-celiac gluten-sensitive enteropathy

CC **K90.49** **Malabsorption due to intolerance, not elsewhere classified**
Malabsorption due to intolerance to carbohydrate
Malabsorption due to intolerance to fat
Malabsorption due to intolerance to protein
Malabsorption due to intolerance to starch

K90.8- **Other intestinal malabsorption**

CC **K90.81** **Whipple's disease** — A disease caused by infection with Tropheryma whipplei that is characterized by "foamy" appearing enlarged mesenteric lymph nodes, malabsorption, progressive debility, and articular abnormalities.

CC **K90.89** **Other intestinal malabsorption**

CC **K90.9** **Intestinal malabsorption, unspecified**

K91- **<u>Intraoperative and postprocedural complications</u> and disorders of digestive system, not elsewhere classified**
Excludes ❷: *complications of artificial opening of digestive system (K94-)*
complications of bariatric procedures (K95-)
gastrojejunal ulcer (K28-)
postprocedural (radiation) retroperitoneal abscess (K68.11)
radiation colitis (K52.0)
radiation gastroenteritis (K52.0)
radiation proctitis (K62.7)

K91.0 **Vomiting following gastrointestinal surgery** — The forcible expulsion of the stomach contents through the mouth following gastrointestinal surgery.

K91.1 **Postgastric surgery syndromes**
Dumping syndrome — A symptom complex marked by nausea, weakness, sweating, tachycardia, vomiting, diarrhea, and syncope that occurs after ingestion of food by postgastrectomy or gastrojejunostomy patients.
Postgastrectomy syndrome — Synonym for Dumping Syndrome.
Postvagotomy syndrome — A form of dumping syndrome following a vagotomy.

CC **K91.2** **Postsurgical malabsorption, not elsewhere classified**
Postsurgical blind loop syndrome — Inadequate intestinal absorption following a surgical procedure.
Excludes 1: *malabsorption osteomalacia in adults (M83.2)*
malabsorption osteoporosis, postsurgical (M80.8-, M81.8)

CC **K91.3** **Postprocedural intestinal obstruction** — The blockage of the intestine following a surgical procedure.

K91.5 **Postcholecystectomy syndrome** — A syndrome characterized by abdominal pain or jaundice following a cholecystectomy.

K91.6- <u>Intraoperative hemorrhage and hematoma</u> of a digestive system organ or structure complicating a procedure
    Excludes 1:   *intraoperative hemorrhage and hematoma of a digestive system organ or structure due to accidental puncture and laceration during a procedure (K91.7-)*

CC **K91.61** Intraoperative hemorrhage and hematoma of a digestive system organ or structure complicating a <u>digestive system procedure</u>

CC **K91.62** Intraoperative hemorrhage and hematoma of a digestive system organ or structure complicating <u>other procedure</u>

K91.7- <u>Accidental puncture and laceration</u> of a digestive system organ or structure during a procedure

CC **K91.71** Accidental puncture and laceration of a digestive system organ or structure during a <u>digestive system procedure</u>

CC **K91.72** Accidental puncture and laceration of a digestive system organ or structure during <u>other procedure</u>

K91.8- Other intraoperative and postprocedural complications and disorders of digestive system

CC **K91.81** Other intraoperative complications of digestive system

CC **K91.82** Postprocedural hepatic failure

CC **K91.83** Postprocedural hepatorenal syndrome

K91.84- <u>Postprocedural hemorrhage</u> of a digestive system organ or structure following a procedure

CC **K91.840** Postprocedural hemorrhage of a digestive system organ or structure following a <u>digestive system procedure</u>

CC **K91.841** Postprocedural hemorrhage of a digestive system organ or structure following <u>other procedure</u>

K91.85- Complications of intestinal pouch — The abnormal function or condition of a surgically created intestinal pouch.

CC **K91.850** **Pouchitis** — Inflammation of the surgically created pouch with symptoms that may include diarrhea, bloody stool, urgency, incontinence, abdominal pain, and fever.
        Inflammation of internal ileoanal pouch

CC **K91.858** **Other complications of intestinal pouch**

CC **K91.86** Retained cholelithiasis following cholecystectomy

K91.87- <u>Postprocedural hematoma and seroma</u> of a digestive system organ or structure following a procedure

CC **K91.870** Postprocedural <u>hematoma</u> of a digestive system organ or structure following a <u>digestive system procedure</u>

CC **K91.871** Postprocedural <u>hematoma</u> of a digestive system organ or structure following <u>other procedure</u>

CC **K91.872** Postprocedural <u>seroma</u> of a digestive system organ or structure following a <u>digestive system procedure</u>

CC **K91.873** Postprocedural <u>seroma</u> of a digestive system organ or structure following <u>other procedure</u>

CC **K91.89** Other postprocedural complications and disorders of digestive system
    Use additional code, if applicable, to further specify disorder
    Excludes ❷: *postprocedural retroperitoneal abscess (K68.11)*

K92- **Other diseases of digestive system**
    Excludes 1:   *neonatal gastrointestinal hemorrhage (P54.0-P54.3)*

CC **K92.0** **Hematemesis** — The abnormal presence of blood in the vomitus.

CC **K92.1** **Melena** — Black, tarry-colored feces due to the abnormal escape of blood into the fecal material.
    Excludes 1:   *occult blood in feces (R19.5)*

CC **K92.2** **Gastrointestinal hemorrhage, unspecified** — The abnormal escape of blood from the gastrointestinal tract.
    Gastric hemorrhage NOS
    Intestinal hemorrhage NOS
    Excludes 1:   *acute hemorrhagic gastritis (K29.01)*
               hemorrhage of anus and rectum (K62.5)
               angiodysplasia of stomach with hemorrhage (K31.811)
               diverticular disease with hemorrhage (K57.-)
               gastritis and duodenitis with hemorrhage (K29.-)
               peptic ulcer with hemorrhage (K25-K28)

K92.8- **Other specified diseases of the digestive system**

CC **K92.81** **Gastrointestinal mucositis (ulcerative)** — Inflammation and/or ulcerative sores of the gastrointestinal mucosal surfaces.
    Code also type of associated therapy, such as:
      Antineoplastic and immunosuppressive drugs (T45.1x-)
      Radiological procedure and radiotherapy (Y84.2)
    Excludes ❷: *mucositis (ulcerative) of vagina and vulva (N76.81)*
               nasal mucositis (ulcerative) (J34.81)
               oral mucositis (ulcerative) (K12.3-)

K92.89 Other specified diseases of the digestive system

K92.9 Disease of digestive system, unspecified

K94- **Complications of artificial openings of the digestive system**

K94.0- <u>Colostomy</u> complications — The abnormal function or condition of a colostomy.

K94.00 **Colostomy complication, unspecified**

CC **K94.01** Colostomy hemorrhage — A form with the abnormal escape of blood.

CC **K94.02** Colostomy infection — A form characterized by cellular inflammation that is caused by microorganisms.
    Use additional code to specify type of infection, such as:
      Cellulitis of abdominal wall (L03.311)
      Sepsis (A40.-, A41.-)

CC **K94.03** Colostomy malfunction — The abnormal, or cessation of, function of a colostomy.
    Mechanical complication of colostomy

CC **K94.09** **Other complications of colostomy**

K94.1- <u>Enterostomy</u> complications — The abnormal function or condition of an enterostomy.

K94.10 **Enterostomy complication, unspecified**

CC **K94.11** Enterostomy hemorrhage — A form with the abnormal escape of blood.

CC **K94.12** Enterostomy infection — A form characterized by cellular inflammation that is caused by microorganisms.
    Use additional code to specify type of infection, such as:
      Cellulitis of abdominal wall (L03.311)
      Sepsis (A40.-, A41.-)

CC **K94.13** Enterostomy malfunction — The abnormal, or cessation of, function of an enterostomy.
    Mechanical complication of enterostomy

CC **K94.19** **Other complications of enterostomy**

K94.2- <u>Gastrostomy</u> complications — The abnormal function or condition of a gastrostomy.

K94.20 **Gastrostomy complication, unspecified**

K94.21 Gastrostomy hemorrhage — A form with the abnormal escape of blood.

CC **K94.22** Gastrostomy infection — A form characterized by cellular inflammation that is caused by microorganisms.
    Use additional code to specify type of infection, such as:
      Cellulitis of abdominal wall (L03.311)
      Sepsis (A40.-, A41.-)

CC **K94.23** Gastrostomy malfunction — The abnormal, or cessation of, function of a gastrostomy.
    Mechanical complication of gastrostomy

K94.29 **Other complications of gastrostomy**

K94.3- <u>Esophagostomy</u> complications — The abnormal function or condition of an esophagostomy.

CC **K94.30** **Esophagostomy complications, unspecified**

CC **K94.31** Esophagostomy hemorrhage — A form with the abnormal escape of blood.

CC **K94.32** Esophagostomy infection — A form characterized by cellular inflammation that is caused by microorganisms.
    Use additional code to identify the infection

CC **K94.33** Esophagostomy malfunction — The abnormal, or cessation of, function of an esophagostomy.
    Mechanical complication of esophagostomy

CC **K94.39** **Other complications of esophagostomy**

K91-K94 (side tab)

K95   Complications of bariatric procedures

K95.0-   Complications of gastric band procedure

cc **K95.01   Infection due to gastric band procedure** — A form characterized by cellular inflammation that is caused by microorganisms.
Use additional code to specify type of infection or organism, such as:
Bacterial and viral infectious agents (B95.-, B96.-)
Cellulitis of abdominal wall (L03.311)
Sepsis (A40-, A41-)

cc **K95.09   Other complications of gastric band procedure**
Use additional code, if applicable, to further specify complication

K95.8-   Complications of other bariatric procedure

Excludes 1:   *complications of gastric band surgery (K95.0-)*

cc **K95.81   Infection due to other bariatric procedure** — A form characterized by cellular inflammation that is caused by microorganisms.
Use additional code to specify type of infection or organism, such as:
Bacterial and viral infectious agents (B95.-, B96.-)
Cellulitis of abdominal wall (L03.311)
Sepsis (A04-, A41-)

cc **K95.89   Other complications of other bariatric procedure**
Use additional code, if applicable, to further specify complication

Chapter 12 – Diseases of the skin and subcutaneous tissue (L00-L99)

Excludes ❷: *certain conditions originating in the perinatal period (P04-P96)*
certain infectious and parasitic diseases (A00-B99)
complications of pregnancy, childbirth and the puerperium (O00-O9A)
congenital malformations, deformations, and chromosomal abnormalities (Q00-Q99)
endocrine, nutritional and metabolic diseases (E00-E88)
lipomelanotic reticulosis (I89.8)
neoplasms (C00-D49)
symptoms, signs and abnormal clinical and laboratory findings, not elsewhere classified (R00-R94)
systemic connective tissue disorders (M30-M36)
viral warts (B07-)

This chapter contains the following blocks:

L00-L08	Infections of the skin and subcutaneous tissue
L10-L14	Bullous disorders
L20-L30	Dermatitis and eczema
L40-L45	Papulosquamous disorders
L49-L54	Urticaria and erythema
L55-L59	Radiation-related disorders of the skin and subcutaneous tissue
L60-L75	Disorders of skin appendages
L76	Intraoperative and postprocedural complications of skin and subcutaneous tissue
L80-L99	Other disorders of the skin and subcutaneous tissue

Chapter-Specific Coding Guidelines

C.   Chapter-Specific Coding Guidelines
In addition to general coding guidelines, there are guidelines for specific diagnoses and/or conditions in the classification. Unless otherwise indicated, these guidelines apply to all health care settings. Please refer to Section II for guidelines on the selection of principal diagnosis.

12.   Chapter 12: Diseases of the Skin and Subcutaneous Tissue (L00-L99)

a.   Pressure ulcer stage codes

1)   Pressure ulcer stages
Codes from category L89, Pressure ulcer, ~~are combination codes that~~ identify the site of the pressure ulcer as well as the stage of the ulcer.

The ICD-10-CM classifies pressure ulcer stages based on severity, which is designated by stages 1-4, unspecified stage and unstageable.

Assign as many codes from category L89 as needed to identify all the pressure ulcers the patient has, if applicable.

2)   Unstageable pressure ulcers
Assignment of the code for unstageable pressure ulcer (L89.--0) should be based on the clinical documentation. These codes are used for pressure ulcers whose stage cannot be clinically determined (e.g., the ulcer is covered by eschar or has been treated with a skin or muscle graft) and pressure ulcers that are documented as deep tissue injury but not documented as due to trauma. This code should not be confused with the codes for unspecified stage (L89.--9). When there is no documentation regarding the stage of the pressure ulcer, assign the appropriate code for unspecified stage (L89.--9).

3)   Documented pressure ulcer stage
Assignment of the pressure ulcer stage code should be guided by clinical documentation of the stage or documentation of the terms found in the Alphabetic Index. For clinical terms describing the stage that are not found in the Alphabetic Index, and there is no documentation of the stage, the provider should be queried.

4)   Patients admitted with pressure ulcers documented as healed
No code is assigned if the documentation states that the pressure ulcer is completely healed.

5)   Patients admitted with pressure ulcers documented as healing
Pressure ulcers described as healing should be assigned the appropriate pressure ulcer stage code based on the documentation in the medical record. If the documentation does not provide information about the stage of the healing pressure ulcer, assign the appropriate code for unspecified stage.

If the documentation is unclear as to whether the patient has a current (new) pressure ulcer or if the patient is being treated for a healing pressure ulcer, query the provider.

For ulcers that were present on admission but healed at the time of discharge, assign the code for the site and stage of the pressure ulcer at the time of admission.

6)   Patient admitted with pressure ulcer evolving into another stage during the admission
If a patient is admitted with a pressure ulcer at one stage and it progresses to a higher stage, ~~assign the code for the highest stage reported for that site~~ two separate codes should be assigned: one code for the site and stage of the ulcer on admission and a second code for the same ulcer site and the highest stage reported during the stay.

Infections of the skin and subcutaneous tissue (L00-L08)

Use additional code (B95-B97) to identify infectious agent
Excludes ❷: *hordeolum (H00.0)*
infective dermatitis (L30.3)
local infections of skin classified in Chapter 1
lupus panniculitis (L93.2)
panniculitis NOS (M79.3)
panniculitis of neck and back (M54.0-)
Perlèche NOS (K13.0)
Perlèche due to candidiasis (B37.0)
Perlèche due to riboflavin deficiency (E53.0)
pyogenic granuloma (L98.0)
relapsing panniculitis [Weber-Christian] (M35.6)
viral warts (B07.-)
zoster (B02.-)

L00   Staphylococcal scalded skin syndrome — A blistering skin disease caused by a toxin produced from a Staphylococcus bacterial infection.
   Ritter's disease
   Use additional code to identify percentage of skin exfoliation (L49.-)
   Excludes 1:   *bullous impetigo (L01.03)*
   pemphigus neonatorum (L01.03)
   toxic epidermal necrolysis [Lyell] (L51.2)

L01-   Impetigo
   Excludes 1:   *impetigo herpetiformis (L40.1)*

   L01.0-   Impetigo — A contagious skin infection characterized by vesicles and pustules that rupture and form a yellow crust, usually caused by Streptococcus.
      Impetigo contagiosa
      Impetigo vulgaris

      L01.00   Impetigo, unspecified
         Impetigo NOS

      L01.01   Non-bullous impetigo — A form caused by Staphylococcus or Streptococcus that is usually caused by a break in the skin and smaller blisters.

      L01.02   Bockhart's impetigo — A form marked by inflammation of the hair follicles with pus formation.
         Impetigo follicularis
         Perifolliculitis NOS
         Superficial pustular perifolliculitis

      L01.03   Bullous impetigo — A form caused by Staphylococcus that occurs in infants and children and forms larger blisters.
         Impetigo neonatorum
         Pemphigus neonatorum

      L01.09   Other impetigo
         Ulcerative impetigo — A form with an open sore.

   L01.1   Impetiginization of other dermatoses

L02-   Cutaneous abscess, furuncle and carbuncle — ABSCESS – A localized collection of pus caused by the disintegration of skin tissue. CARBUNCLE – A necrotizing infection of the skin and subcutaneous tissue composed of a cluster of boils (furuncles), with multiple formed or incipient draining sinuses. FURUNCLE (BOIL) – A painful nodule formed in the skin characterized by circumscribed inflammation of the corium and subcutaneous tissue.
   Use additional code to identify organism (B95-B96)
   Excludes ❷: *abscess of anus and rectal regions (K61.-)*
   abscess of female genital organs (external) (N76.4)
   abscess of male genital organs (external) (N48.2, N49.-)

   L02.0-   Cutaneous abscess, furuncle and carbuncle of <u>face</u>
      Excludes ❷: *abscess of ear, external (H60.0)*
      abscess of eyelid (H00.0)
      abscess of head [any part, except face] (L02.8)
      abscess of lacrimal gland (H04.0)
      abscess of lacrimal passages (H04.3)
      abscess of mouth (K12.2)
      abscess of nose (J34.0)
      abscess of orbit (H05.0)
      submandibular abscess (K12.2)

   CC **L02.01   Cutaneous <u>abscess</u> of face**

L00 - L02 (side tab)

L02.02 <u>Furuncle</u> of face
    Boil of face
    Folliculitis of face

L02.03 <u>Carbuncle</u> of face

L02.1- Cutaneous abscess, furuncle and carbuncle of <u>neck</u>

  cc **L02.11** Cutaneous <u>abscess</u> of neck

  L02.12 <u>Furuncle</u> of neck
      Boil of neck
      Folliculitis of neck

  L02.13 <u>Carbuncle</u> of neck

L02.2- Cutaneous abscess, furuncle and carbuncle of <u>trunk</u>
    Excludes 1:   *non-newborn omphalitis (L08.82)*
                   omphalitis of newborn (P38.-)
    Excludes ❷: *abscess of breast (N61.1)*
                   abscess of buttocks (L02.3)
                   abscess of female external genital organs (N76.4)
                   abscess of male external genital organs (N48.2, N49.-)
                   abscess of hip (L02.4)

  L02.21- Cutaneous <u>abscess</u> of trunk

    cc **L02.211** Cutaneous abscess of <u>abdominal wall</u>

    cc **L02.212** Cutaneous abscess of <u>back</u> [any part, except buttock]

    cc **L02.213** Cutaneous abscess of <u>chest wall</u>

    cc **L02.214** Cutaneous abscess of <u>groin</u>

    cc **L02.215** Cutaneous abscess of <u>perineum</u>

    cc **L02.216** Cutaneous abscess of <u>umbilicus</u>

    cc **L02.219** Cutaneous abscess of trunk, <u>unspecified</u>

  L02.22- <u>Furuncle</u> of trunk
      Boil of trunk
      Folliculitis of trunk

    L02.221 Furuncle of <u>abdominal wall</u>

    L02.222 Furuncle of <u>back</u> [any part, except buttock]

    L02.223 Furuncle of <u>chest wall</u>

    L02.224 Furuncle of <u>groin</u>

    L02.225 Furuncle of <u>perineum</u>

    L02.226 Furuncle of umbilicus

    L02.229 Furuncle of trunk, <u>unspecified</u>

  L02.23- <u>Carbuncle</u> of trunk

    L02.231 Carbuncle of <u>abdominal wall</u>

    L02.232 Carbuncle of <u>back</u> [any part, except buttock]

    L02.233 Carbuncle of <u>chest wall</u>

    L02.234 Carbuncle of <u>groin</u>

    L02.235 Carbuncle of <u>perineum</u>

    L02.236 Carbuncle of <u>umbilicus</u>

    L02.239 Carbuncle of trunk, <u>unspecified</u>

L02.3- Cutaneous abscess, furuncle and carbuncle of <u>buttock</u>
    Excludes 1:   *pilonidal cyst with abscess (L05.01)*

  cc **L02.31** Cutaneous <u>abscess</u> of buttock
      Cutaneous abscess of gluteal region

  L02.32 <u>Furuncle</u> of buttock
      Boil of buttock
      Folliculitis of buttock
      Furuncle of gluteal region

  L02.33 <u>Carbuncle</u> of buttock
      Carbuncle of gluteal region

L02.4- Cutaneous abscess, furuncle and carbuncle of <u>limb</u>
    Excludes ❷: *cutaneous abscess, furuncle and carbuncle of groin*
                   (L02.214, L02.224, L02.234)
                   cutaneous abscess, furuncle and carbuncle of hand
                   (L02.5-)
                   cutaneous abscess, furuncle and carbuncle of foot
                   (L02.6-)

  L02.41- Cutaneous <u>abscess</u> of limb

    cc **L02.411** Cutaneous abscess of <u>right</u> <u>axilla</u>

    cc **L02.412** Cutaneous abscess of <u>left</u> <u>axilla</u>

    cc **L02.413** Cutaneous abscess of <u>right</u> <u>upper</u> limb

    cc **L02.414** Cutaneous abscess of <u>left</u> <u>upper</u> limb

    cc **L02.415** Cutaneous abscess of <u>right</u> <u>lower</u> limb

    cc **L02.416** Cutaneous abscess of <u>left</u> <u>lower</u> limb

    cc **L02.419** Cutaneous abscess of limb, <u>unspecified</u>

L02.42- <u>Furuncle</u> of limb
      Boil of limb
      Folliculitis of limb

  L02.421 Furuncle of <u>right</u> <u>axilla</u>

  L02.422 Furuncle of <u>left</u> <u>axilla</u>

  L02.423 Furuncle of <u>right</u> <u>upper</u> limb

  L02.424 Furuncle of <u>left</u> <u>upper</u> limb

  L02.425 Furuncle of <u>right</u> <u>lower</u> limb

  L02.426 Furuncle of <u>left</u> <u>lower</u> limb

  L02.429 Furuncle of limb, <u>unspecified</u>

L02.43- <u>Carbuncle</u> of limb

  L02.431 Carbuncle of <u>right</u> <u>axilla</u>

  L02.432 Carbuncle of <u>left</u> <u>axilla</u>

  L02.433 Carbuncle of <u>right</u> <u>upper</u> limb

  L02.434 Carbuncle of <u>left</u> <u>upper</u> limb

  L02.435 Carbuncle of <u>right</u> <u>lower</u> limb

  L02.436 Carbuncle of <u>left</u> <u>lower</u> limb

  L02.439 Carbuncle of limb, <u>unspecified</u>

L02.5- Cutaneous abscess, furuncle and carbuncle of <u>hand</u>

  L02.51- Cutaneous <u>abscess</u> of hand

    cc **L02.511** Cutaneous abscess of <u>right</u> hand

    cc **L02.512** Cutaneous abscess of <u>left</u> hand

    cc **L02.519** Cutaneous abscess of <u>unspecified</u> hand

  L02.52- <u>Furuncle</u> hand
      Boil of hand
      Folliculitis of hand

    L02.521 Furuncle <u>right</u> hand

    L02.522 Furuncle <u>left</u> hand

    L02.529 Furuncle <u>unspecified</u> hand

  L02.53- <u>Carbuncle</u> of hand

    L02.531 Carbuncle of <u>right</u> hand

    L02.532 Carbuncle of <u>left</u> hand

    L02.539 Carbuncle of <u>unspecified</u> hand

L02.6- Cutaneous abscess, furuncle and carbuncle of <u>foot</u>

  L02.61- Cutaneous <u>abscess</u> of foot

    cc **L02.611** Cutaneous abscess of <u>right</u> foot

    cc **L02.612** Cutaneous abscess of <u>left</u> foot

    cc **L02.619** Cutaneous abscess of <u>unspecified</u> foot

  L02.62- <u>Furuncle</u> of foot
      Boil of foot
      Folliculitis of foot

    L02.621 Furuncle of <u>right</u> foot

    L02.622 Furuncle of <u>left</u> foot

    L02.629 Furuncle of <u>unspecified</u> foot

  L02.63- <u>Carbuncle</u> of foot

    L02.631 Carbuncle of <u>right</u> foot

    L02.632 Carbuncle of <u>left</u> foot

    L02.639 Carbuncle of <u>unspecified</u> foot

L02.8- Cutaneous abscess, furuncle and carbuncle of <u>other sites</u>

  L02.81- Cutaneous <u>abscess</u> of other sites

    cc **L02.811** Cutaneous abscess of <u>head</u> [any part, except face]

    cc **L02.818** Cutaneous abscess of <u>other</u> sites

  L02.82- <u>Furuncle</u> of other sites
      Boil of other sites
      Folliculitis of other sites

    L02.821 Furuncle of <u>head</u> [any part, except face]

    L02.828 Furuncle of <u>other</u> sites

  L02.83- <u>Carbuncle</u> of other sites

    L02.831 Carbuncle of <u>head</u> [any part, except face]

    L02.838 Carbuncle of <u>other</u> sites

L02.9- Cutaneous abscess, furuncle and carbuncle, <u>unspecified</u>

  cc **L02.91** Cutaneous <u>abscess</u>, unspecified

  L02.92 <u>Furuncle</u>, unspecified
      Boil NOS
      Furunculosis NOS

  L02.93 <u>Carbuncle</u>, unspecified

L02
-
L02

L03- <u>Cellulitis and acute lymphangitis</u> — CELLULITIS – Cellular tissue inflammation.
ACUTE LYMPHANGITIS – The sudden, severe onset of inflammation of a lymphatic vessel.
Excludes ❷: cellulitis of anal and rectal region (K61.-)
cellulitis of external auditory canal (H60.1)
cellulitis of eyelid (H00.0)
cellulitis of female external genital organs (N76.4)
cellulitis of lacrimal apparatus (H04.3)
cellulitis of male external genital organs (N48.2, N49.-)
cellulitis of mouth (K12.2)
cellulitis of nose (J34.0)
eosinophilic cellulitis [Wells] (L98.3)
febrile neutrophilic dermatosis [Sweet] (L98.2)
lymphangitis (chronic) (subacute) (I89.1)

L03.0- **Cellulitis and acute lymphangitis of finger and toe**
Infection of nail
Onychia — Inflammation of the nail matrix, resulting in the shedding of the nail.
Paronychia — Inflammation of the folds of tissue surrounding the fingernail.
Perionychia — Inflammation of the folds of tissue surrounding the fingernail.

L03.01- <u>Cellulitis</u> of <u>finger</u>
Felon
Whitlow
Excludes 1:   herpetic whitlow (B00.89)
L03.011 **Cellulitis of <u>right</u> finger**
L03.012 **Cellulitis of <u>left</u> finger**
L03.019 **Cellulitis of <u>unspecified</u> finger**
L03.02- **Acute <u>lymphangitis</u> of <u>finger</u>**
Hangnail with lymphangitis of finger
L03.021 **Acute lymphangitis of <u>right</u> finger**
L03.022 **Acute lymphangitis of <u>left</u> finger**
L03.029 **Acute lymphangitis of <u>unspecified</u> finger**
L03.03- <u>Cellulitis</u> of <u>toe</u>
L03.031 **Cellulitis of <u>right</u> toe**
L03.032 **Cellulitis of <u>left</u> toe**
L03.039 **Cellulitis of <u>unspecified</u> toe**
L03.04- **Acute <u>lymphangitis</u> of <u>toe</u>**
Hangnail with lymphangitis of toe
L03.041 **Acute lymphangitis of <u>right</u> toe**
L03.042 **Acute lymphangitis of <u>left</u> toe**
L03.049 **Acute lymphangitis of <u>unspecified</u> toe**
L03.1- **Cellulitis and acute lymphangitis of other parts of limb**
L03.11- <u>Cellulitis</u> of other parts of <u>limb</u>
Excludes ❷: cellulitis of fingers (L03.01-)
cellulitis of toes (L03.03-)
groin (L03.314)
cc **L03.111** **Cellulitis of <u>right</u> <u>axilla</u>**
cc **L03.112** **Cellulitis of <u>left</u> <u>axilla</u>**
cc **L03.113** **Cellulitis of <u>right</u> <u>upper</u> limb**
cc **L03.114** **Cellulitis of <u>left</u> <u>upper</u> limb**
cc **L03.115** **Cellulitis of <u>right</u> <u>lower</u> limb**
cc **L03.116** **Cellulitis of <u>left</u> <u>lower</u> limb**
cc **L03.119** **Cellulitis of <u>unspecified</u> part of limb**
L03.12- **Acute <u>lymphangitis</u> of other parts of <u>limb</u>**
Excludes ❷: acute lymphangitis of fingers (L03.2-)
acute lymphangitis of toes (L03.04-)
acute lymphangitis of groin (L03.324)
cc **L03.121** **Acute lymphangitis of <u>right</u> <u>axilla</u>**
cc **L03.122** **Acute lymphangitis of <u>left</u> <u>axilla</u>**
cc **L03.123** **Acute lymphangitis of <u>right</u> <u>upper</u> limb**
cc **L03.124** **Acute lymphangitis of <u>left</u> <u>upper</u> limb**
cc **L03.125** **Acute lymphangitis of <u>right</u> <u>lower</u> limb**
cc **L03.126** **Acute lymphangitis of <u>left</u> <u>lower</u> limb**
cc **L03.129** **Acute lymphangitis of <u>unspecified</u> part of limb**

L03.2- **Cellulitis and acute lymphangitis of face and neck**
L03.21- **Cellulitis and acute lymphangitis of face**
cc **L03.211** <u>Cellulitis</u> of <u>face</u>
Excludes ❷: abscess of orbit (H05.01-)
cellulitis of ear (H60.1-)
cellulitis of eyelid (H00.0-)
cellulitis of head (L03.81)
cellulitis of lacrimal apparatus (H04.3)
cellulitis of lip (K13.0)
cellulitis of mouth (K12.2)
cellulitis of nose (internal) (J34.0)
cellulitis of orbit (H05.01-)
cellulitis of scalp (L03.81)
cc **L03.212** **Acute <u>lymphangitis</u> of <u>face</u>**
cc **L03.213** **Periorbital cellulitis**
Preseptal cellulitis
L03.22- **Cellulitis and acute lymphangitis of neck**
cc **L03.221** <u>Cellulitis</u> of <u>neck</u>
cc **L03.222** **Acute <u>lymphangitis</u> of <u>neck</u>**
L03.3- **Cellulitis and acute lymphangitis of trunk**
L03.31- <u>Cellulitis</u> of <u>trunk</u>
Excludes ❷: cellulitis of anal and rectal regions (K61.-)
cellulitis of breast NOS (N61.0)
cellulitis of female external genital organs (N76.4)
cellulitis of male external genital organs (N48.2, N49.-)
omphalitis of newborn (P38.-)
puerperal cellulitis of breast (O91.2)
cc **L03.311** **Cellulitis of <u>abdominal wall</u>**
Excludes ❷: cellulitis of umbilicus (L03.316)
cellulitis of groin (L03.314)
cc **L03.312** **Cellulitis of <u>back</u> [any part except buttock]**
cc **L03.313** **Cellulitis of <u>chest wall</u>**
cc **L03.314** **Cellulitis of <u>groin</u>**
cc **L03.315** **Cellulitis of <u>perineum</u>**
cc **L03.316** **Cellulitis of <u>umbilicus</u>**
cc **L03.317** **Cellulitis of <u>buttock</u>**
cc **L03.319** **Cellulitis of trunk, <u>unspecified</u>**
L03.32- **Acute <u>lymphangitis</u> of <u>trunk</u>**
cc **L03.321** **Acute lymphangitis of <u>abdominal wall</u>**
cc **L03.322** **Acute lymphangitis of <u>back</u> [any part except buttock]**
cc **L03.323** **Acute lymphangitis of <u>chest wall</u>**
cc **L03.324** **Acute lymphangitis of <u>groin</u>**
cc **L03.325** **Acute lymphangitis of <u>perineum</u>**
cc **L03.326** **Acute lymphangitis of <u>umbilicus</u>**
cc **L03.327** **Acute lymphangitis of <u>buttock</u>**
cc **L03.329** **Acute lymphangitis of trunk, <u>unspecified</u>**
L03.8- **Cellulitis and acute lymphangitis of other sites**
L03.81- **Cellulitis of other sites**
cc **L03.811** <u>Cellulitis</u> of <u>head</u> [any part, except face]
Cellulitis of scalp
Excludes ❷: cellulitis of face (L03.211)
cc **L03.818** <u>Cellulitis</u> of <u>other</u> sites
L03.89- **Acute lymphangitis of other sites**
cc **L03.891** **Acute <u>lymphangitis</u> of <u>head</u> [any part, except face]**
cc **L03.898** **Acute <u>lymphangitis</u> of <u>other</u> sites**
L03.9- **Cellulitis and acute lymphangitis, unspecified**
cc **L03.90** **Cellulitis, <u>unspecified</u>**
cc **L03.91** **Acute lymphangitis, <u>unspecified</u>**
Excludes 1:   lymphangitis NOS (I89.1)

L
0
3
–
L
0
3

L04- **Acute lymphadenitis** — The sudden, severe onset of infectious inflammation of the lymph glands or nodes.
    Includes: Abscess (acute) of lymph nodes, except mesenteric
        Acute lymphadenitis, except mesenteric
    Excludes 1: *chronic or subacute lymphadenitis, except mesenteric (I88.1)*
        enlarged lymph nodes (R59.-)
        human immunodeficiency virus [HIV] disease resulting in
          generalized lymphadenopathy (B20)
        lymphadenitis NOS (I88.9)
        nonspecific mesenteric lymphadenitis (I88.0)

L04.0 **Acute lymphadenitis of face, head and neck**

L04.1 **Acute lymphadenitis of trunk**

L04.2 **Acute lymphadenitis of upper limb**
    Acute lymphadenitis of axilla
    Acute lymphadenitis of shoulder

L04.3 **Acute lymphadenitis of lower limb**
    Acute lymphadenitis of hip
    Excludes ❷: acute lymphadenitis of groin (L04.1)

L04.8 **Acute lymphadenitis of other sites**

L04.9 **Acute lymphadenitis, unspecified**

L05- **Pilonidal cyst and sinus** — A hair-containing sacrococcygeal dermoid cyst or sinus that often opens at a postanal dimple.

L05.0- **Pilonidal cyst and sinus with abscess** — A form with a localized collection of pus.

  CC **L05.01** **Pilonidal cyst <u>with abscess</u>**
    Pilonidal abscess
    Pilonidal dimple with abscess
    Postanal dimple with abscess
    Excludes ❷: congenital sacral dimple (Q82.6)
        parasacral dimple (Q82.6)

  CC **L05.02** **Pilonidal sinus <u>with abscess</u>**
    Coccygeal fistula with abscess
    Coccygeal sinus with abscess
    Pilonidal fistula with abscess

L05.9- **Pilonidal cyst and sinus without abscess**

  L05.91 **Pilonidal cyst <u>without</u> abscess**
    Pilonidal dimple
    Postanal dimple
    Pilonidal cyst NOS
    Excludes ❷: congenital sacral dimple (Q82.6)
        parasacral dimple (Q82.6)

  L05.92 **Pilonidal sinus <u>without</u> abscess**
    Coccygeal fistula
    Coccygeal sinus without abscess
    Pilonidal fistula

L08- **Other local infections of skin and subcutaneous tissue**

L08.0 **Pyoderma** — A nonspecific purulent skin infection.
    Dermatitis gangrenosa — A form characterized by unique skin lesions, and often associated with an underlying systemic disease.
    Purulent dermatitis — Inflammation of the skin with pus.
    Septic dermatitis — Inflammation of the skin with decomposition of microorganisms.
    Suppurative dermatitis — Inflammation of the skin with production of pus.
    Excludes 1: pyoderma gangrenosum (L88)
        pyoderma vegetans (L08.81)

  CC **L08.1** **Erythrasma** — A chronic bacterial skin infection caused by Corynebacterium minutissimum that occurs primarily in the folds of the skin.

L08.8- **Other specified local infections of the skin and subcutaneous tissue**

  L08.81 **Pyoderma vegetans** — A purulent skin infection that is characterized by large verrucous plaques and elevated borders with an unknown cause.
    Excludes 1: pyoderma gangrenosum (L88)
        pyoderma NOS (L08.0)

  L08.82 **Omphalitis not of newborn** — Infection of the umbilical stump.
    Excludes 1: omphalitis of newborn (P38.-)

  L08.89 **Other specified local infections of the skin and subcutaneous tissue**

L08.9 **Local infection of the skin and subcutaneous tissue, unspecified**

Bullous disorders (L10-L14)

    Excludes 1: *benign familial pemphigus [Hailey-Hailey] (Q82.8)*
        staphylococcal scalded skin syndrome (L00)
        toxic epidermal necrolysis [Lyell] (L51.2)

L10- **Pemphigus** — A group of distinctive autoimmune diseases marked by successive crops of bullae.
    Excludes 1: pemphigus neonatorum (L01.03)

  CC **L10.0** **Pemphigus vulgaris** — A form manifested by suprabasal, intraepidermal bullae of the skin and mucous membranes with sores often in the mouth.

  CC **L10.1** **Pemphigus vegetans** — A mild, pustular variant of pemphigus.

  CC **L10.2** **Pemphigus foliaceous** — A form characterized by generalized vesicular and scaling skin eruption.

  CC **L10.3** **Brazilian pemphigus [fogo selvagem]** — A form endemic to some South American countries that is transmitted by an insect.

  CC **L10.4** **Pemphigus erythematosus** — Chronic pemphigus characterized by lesions limited to the face and chest, and resembling those of disseminated lupus erythematosus.
    Senear-Usher syndrome

  CC **L10.5** **Drug-induced pemphigus**
    Use additional code for adverse effect, if applicable, to identify drug (T36-T50 with fifth or sixth character 5)

L10.8- **Other pemphigus**

  CC **L10.81** **Paraneoplastic pemphigus** — A form characterized by painful sores in the mouth, lips, and esophagus that is a complication of cancer, usually a lymphoma.

  CC **L10.89** **Other pemphigus**

  CC **L10.9** **Pemphigus, unspecified**

L11- **Other acantholytic disorders**

L11.0 **Acquired keratosis follicularis**
    Excludes 1: keratosis follicularis (congenital) [Darier-White] (Q82.8)

L11.1 **Transient acantholytic dermatosis [Grover]**

L11.8 **Other specified acantholytic disorders**

L11.9 **Acantholytic disorder, unspecified**

L12- **Pemphigoid** — A group of bullous connective tissue autoimmune skin diseases that are similar but clearly distinguishable from those of the pemphigus group.
    Excludes 1: herpes gestationis (O26.4-)
        impetigo herpetiformis (L40.1)

  CC **L12.0** **Bullous pemphigoid** — A chronic, generalized bullous eruption that usually occurs in elderly adults, but rarely the mouth.

L12.1 **Cicatricial pemphigoid** — A form affecting mucous membranes, but not the skin.
    Benign mucous membrane pemphigoid

L12.2 **Chronic bullous disease of childhood** — [Age/0-17]
    Juvenile dermatitis herpetiformis

L12.3- **Acquired epidermolysis bullosa**
    Excludes 1: epidermolysis bullosa (congenital) (Q81.-)

  CC **L12.30** **Acquired epidermolysis bullosa, unspecified**

  CC **L12.31** **Epidermolysis bullosa due to drug**
    Use additional code for adverse effect, if applicable, to identify drug (T36-T50 with fifth or sixth character 5)

  CC **L12.35** **Other acquired epidermolysis bullosa**

  CC **L12.8** **Other pemphigoid**

  CC **L12.9** **Pemphigoid, unspecified**

L13- **Other bullous disorders**

L13.0 **Dermatitis herpetiformis** — A chronic dermatitis characterized by grouped, symmetrical erythematous, papular, vesicular eczematous, or bullous lesions that occur in successive crops in varied combinations and accompanied by burning and itching.
    Duhring's disease
    Hydroa herpetiformis
    Excludes 1: juvenile dermatitis herpetiformis (L12.2)
        senile dermatitis herpetiformis (L12.0)

L13.1 **Subcorneal pustular dermatitis** — A chronic, pustular disease that is characterized by a relapsing course with sterile, pustular blebs and chiefly affecting women in middle life.
    Sneddon-Wilkinson disease

L13.8 **Other specified bullous disorders**

L13.9 **Bullous disorder, unspecified**

Excludes 1: = NOT CODED HERE! (Do not code both)
        802   *Excludes ❷:* = Not Included Here

L 0 4 – L 1 3

L14 Bullous disorders <u>in diseases classified elsewhere</u> —
[Not Allowed as PDX]
Code first underlying disease

Dermatitis and eczema (L20-L30)

Note: In this block the terms dermatitis and eczema are used synonymously and interchangeably.

Excludes ❷: chronic (childhood) granulomatous disease (D71)
dermatitis gangrenosa (L08.0)
dermatitis herpetiformis (L13.0)
dry skin dermatitis (L85.3)
factitial dermatitis (L98.1)
perioral dermatitis (L71.0)
radiation-related disorders of the skin and subcutaneous tissue (L55-L59)
stasis dermatitis (I87.2)

L20- <u>Atopic dermatitis</u> — A chronic skin disease of unknown etiology that is characterized by dry and itchy skin, and rash on the face, inside of the elbows, and behind the knees.

L20.0 Besnier's prurigo

L20.8- Other atopic dermatitis
Excludes ❷: circumscribed neurodermatitis (L28.0)

L20.81 Atopic neurodermatitis
Diffuse neurodermatitis

L20.82 Flexural eczema

L20.83 Infantile (acute) (chronic) eczema — [Age/0-17]

L20.84 Intrinsic (allergic) eczema

L20.89 Other atopic dermatitis

L20.9 Atopic dermatitis, unspecified

L21- Seborrheic dermatitis — A chronic inflammatory skin disease of unknown etiology that is characterized by scaly, stubborn dandruff, and itchy and red skin.
Excludes ❷: infective dermatitis (L30.3)
seborrheic keratosis (L82.-)

L21.0 Seborrhea capitis — [Age/0-17]
Cradle cap

L21.1 Seborrheic infantile dermatitis — [Age/0-17]

L21.8 Other seborrheic dermatitis

L21.9 Seborrheic dermatitis, unspecified
Seborrhea NOS

L22 Diaper dermatitis — A cutaneous reaction in an infant (or one who wears a diaper) that is localized to the areas ordinarily covered by, and in contact with, the diaper.
Diaper erythema
Diaper rash
Psoriasiform diaper rash

L23- <u>Allergic contact dermatitis</u> — An acute, allergic response inflammation of the skin caused by contact with various substances to which a delayed hypersensitivity has been acquired.
Excludes 1: allergy NOS (T78.40)
contact dermatitis NOS (L25.9)
dermatitis NOS (L30.9)
Excludes ❷: dermatitis due to substances taken internally (L27.-)
dermatitis of eyelid (H01.1-)
diaper dermatitis (L22)
eczema of external ear (H60.5-)
irritant contact dermatitis (L24.-)
perioral dermatitis (L71.0)
radiation-related disorders of the skin and subcutaneous tissue (L55-L59)

L23.0 Allergic contact dermatitis due to <u>metals</u>
Allergic contact dermatitis due to chromium
Allergic contact dermatitis due to nickel

L23.1 Allergic contact dermatitis due to <u>adhesives</u>

L23.2 Allergic contact dermatitis due to <u>cosmetics</u>

L23.3 Allergic contact dermatitis due to <u>drugs in contact with skin</u>
Use additional code for adverse effect, if applicable, to identify drug (T36-T50 with fifth or sixth character 5)
Excludes ❷: dermatitis due to ingested drugs and medicaments (L27.0-L27.1)

L23.4 Allergic contact dermatitis due to <u>dyes</u>

L23.5 Allergic contact dermatitis due to <u>other chemical products</u>
Allergic contact dermatitis due to cement
Allergic contact dermatitis due to insecticide
Allergic contact dermatitis due to plastic
Allergic contact dermatitis due to rubber

L23.6 Allergic contact dermatitis due to <u>food in contact with the skin</u>
Excludes ❷: dermatitis due to ingested food (L27.2)

L23.7 Allergic contact dermatitis due to <u>plants, except food</u>
Excludes ❷: allergy NOS due to pollen (J30.1)

L23.8- Allergic contact dermatitis due to other agents

L23.81 Allergic contact dermatitis due to <u>animal (cat) (dog) dander</u>
Allergic contact dermatitis due to animal (cat) (dog) hair

L23.89 Allergic contact dermatitis due to <u>other</u> agents

L23.9 Allergic contact dermatitis, <u>unspecified</u> cause
Allergic contact eczema NOS

L24- <u>Irritant</u> contact dermatitis — An acute inflammation of the skin caused by contact with various substances.
Excludes 1: allergy NOS (T78.40)
contact dermatitis NOS (L25.9)
dermatitis NOS (L30.9)
Excludes ❷: allergic contact dermatitis (L23.-)
dermatitis due to substances taken internally (L27.-)
dermatitis of eyelid (H01.1-)
diaper dermatitis (L22)
eczema of external ear (H60.5-)
perioral dermatitis (L71.0)
radiation-related disorders of the skin and subcutaneous tissue (L55-L59)

L24.0 Irritant contact dermatitis due to <u>detergents</u>

L24.1 Irritant contact dermatitis due to <u>oils and greases</u>

L24.2 Irritant contact dermatitis due to <u>solvents</u>
Irritant contact dermatitis due to chlorocompound
Irritant contact dermatitis due to cyclohexane
Irritant contact dermatitis due to ester
Irritant contact dermatitis due to glycol
Irritant contact dermatitis due to hydrocarbon
Irritant contact dermatitis due to ketone

L24.3 Irritant contact dermatitis due to <u>cosmetics</u>

L24.4 Irritant contact dermatitis due to <u>drugs in contact with skin</u>
Use additional code for adverse effect, if applicable, to identify drug (T36-T50 with fifth or sixth character 5)

L24.5 Irritant contact dermatitis due to <u>other chemical products</u>
Irritant contact dermatitis due to cement
Irritant contact dermatitis due to insecticide
Irritant contact dermatitis due to plastic
Irritant contact dermatitis due to rubber

L24.6 Irritant contact dermatitis due to <u>food in contact with skin</u>
Excludes ❷: dermatitis due to ingested food (L27.2)

L24.7 Irritant contact dermatitis due to <u>plants, except food</u>
Excludes ❷: allergy NOS to pollen (J30.1)

L24.8- Irritant contact dermatitis due to other agents

L24.81 Irritant contact dermatitis due to <u>metals</u>
Irritant contact dermatitis due to chromium
Irritant contact dermatitis due to nickel

L24.89 Irritant contact dermatitis due to <u>other agents</u>
Irritant contact dermatitis due to dyes

L24.9 Irritant contact dermatitis, <u>unspecified</u> cause
Irritant contact eczema NOS

L25- <u>Unspecified</u> contact dermatitis
Excludes 1: allergic contact dermatitis (L23.-)
allergy NOS (T78.40)
dermatitis NOS (L30.9)
irritant contact dermatitis (L24.-)
Excludes ❷: dermatitis due to ingested substances (L27.-)
dermatitis of eyelid (H01.1-)
eczema of external ear (H60.5-)
perioral dermatitis (L71.0)
radiation-related disorders of the skin and subcutaneous tissue (L55-L59)

L25.0 Unspecified contact dermatitis due to <u>cosmetics</u>

L25.1 Unspecified contact dermatitis due to <u>drugs in contact with skin</u>
Use additional code for adverse effect, if applicable, to identify drug (T36-T50 with fifth or sixth character 5)
Excludes ❷: dermatitis due to ingested drugs and medicaments (L27.0-L27.1)

L25.2 Unspecified contact dermatitis due to <u>dyes</u>

L25.3   Unspecified contact dermatitis due to <u>other chemical products</u>
Unspecified contact dermatitis due to cement
Unspecified contact dermatitis due to insecticide

L25.4   Unspecified contact dermatitis due to <u>food in contact with skin</u>
Excludes ❷: dermatitis due to ingested food (L27.2)

L25.5   Unspecified contact dermatitis due to <u>plants, except food</u>
Excludes 1:   nettle rash (L50.9)
Excludes ❷: allergy NOS due to pollen (J30.1)

L25.8   Unspecified contact dermatitis due to <u>other</u> agents

L25.9   Unspecified contact dermatitis, <u>unspecified</u> cause
Contact dermatitis (occupational) NOS
Contact eczema (occupational) NOS

L26   Exfoliative dermatitis — An inflammatory skin disease that is characterized by excessive shedding or peeling of the nonviable outer layer of the skin caused by excessive growth of the basal layer of the skin.
Hebra's pityriasis
Excludes 1:   Ritter's disease (L00)

L27-   Dermatitis <u>due to substances taken internally</u> — Inflammation of the skin due to substances taken internally.
Excludes 1:   allergy NOS (T78.40)
Excludes ❷: adverse food reaction, except dermatitis (T78.0-T78.1)
contact dermatitis (L23-L25)
drug photoallergic response (L56.1)
drug phototoxic response (L56.0)
urticaria (L50.-)

L27.0   <u>Generalized</u> skin eruption due to drugs and medicaments taken internally
Use additional code for adverse effect, if applicable, to identify drug (T36-T50 with fifth or sixth character 5)

L27.1   <u>Localized</u> skin eruption due to drugs and medicaments taken internally
Use additional code for adverse effect, if applicable, to identify drug (T36-T50 with fifth or sixth character 5)

L27.2   Dermatitis due to ingested <u>food</u>
Excludes ❷: dermatitis due to food in contact with skin (L23.6, L24.6, L25.4)

L27.8   Dermatitis due to <u>other</u> substances taken internally

L27.9   Dermatitis due to <u>unspecified</u> substance taken internally

L28-   Lichen simplex chronicus and prurigo

L28.0   Lichen simplex chronicus — A skin disorder that is characterized by chronic itching and scratching, by the self-perpetuating scratch-itch cycle.
Circumscribed neurodermatitis
Lichen NOS

L28.1   Prurigo nodularis — A form of neurodermatitis with discrete, firm, rough-surfaced, intensely itchy nodules occurring on extensor surfaces of the extremities.

L28.2   Other prurigo
Prurigo NOS
Prurigo Hebra
Prurigo mitis
Urticaria papulosa

L29-   Pruritus
Excludes 1:   neurotic excoriation (L98.1)
psychogenic pruritus (F45.8)

L29.0   Pruritus ani — The intense, chronic itching of the anal region.

L29.1   Pruritus scroti — [♂] – The intense, chronic itching of the scrotal region.

L29.2   Pruritus vulvae — [♀] – The intense, chronic itching of the vulvar region.

L29.3   Anogenital pruritus, unspecified

L29.8   Other pruritus

L29.9   Pruritus, unspecified
Itch NOS

L30-   <u>Other and unspecified</u> dermatitis
Excludes ❷: contact dermatitis (L23-L25)
dry skin dermatitis (L85.3)
small plaque parapsoriasis (L41.3)
stasis dermatitis (I87.2)

L30.0   Nummular dermatitis — A skin eruption condition characterized by distinct, coin-shaped (nummular) sores.

L30.1   Dyshidrosis [pompholyx] — A skin eruption condition characterized by vesicular eruption on the palms and soles, and is accompanied by intense itching.

L30.2   Cutaneous autosensitization — A skin eruption condition characterized by widespread eruption from a distant local focus.
Candidid [levurid]
Dermatophytid
Eczematid

L30.3   Infective dermatitis
Infectious eczematoid dermatitis

L30.4   Erythema intertrigo — A superficial inflammatory skin disease characterized by macerated, erythematous patches on opposing skin surfaces, such as under pendulous breasts.

L30.5   Pityriasis alba — A common skin disorder characterized by hypopigmented, round to oval scaling patches on the face, neck, and shoulders.

L30.8   Other specified dermatitis

L30.9   Dermatitis, unspecified
Eczema NOS

Papulosquamous disorders (L40-L45)

L40-   Psoriasis

L40.0   Psoriasis vulgaris — A chronic, recurrent inflammatory skin disease characterized by rounded, circumscribed, erythematous, dry scaling patches that are covered by silvery-white lamellated scales.
Nummular psoriasis
Plaque psoriasis

L40.1   Generalized pustular psoriasis — A form marked by pus-filled blisters.
Impetigo herpetiformis
Von Zumbusch's disease

L40.2   Acrodermatitis continua

L40.3   Pustulosis palmaris et plantaris — A form marked by pus-filled blisters of the fingers and toes.

L40.4   Guttate psoriasis — A form marked by teardrop shaped lesions.

L40.5-   Arthropathic psoriasis — Psoriasis associated with arthritis, especially of the distal interphalangeal joints.

L40.50   Arthropathic psoriasis, unspecified

L40.51   Distal interphalangeal psoriatic arthropathy

L40.52   Psoriatic arthritis mutilans

L40.53   Psoriatic spondylitis

L40.54   Psoriatic juvenile arthropathy

L40.59   Other psoriatic arthropathy

L40.8   Other psoriasis
Flexural psoriasis

L40.9   Psoriasis, unspecified

L41-   Parapsoriasis — A group of maculopapular, scaly erythrodermas of slow development.
Excludes 1:   poikiloderma vasculare atrophicans (L94.5)

L41.0   Pityriasis lichenoides et varioliformis acuta — A form marked by a polymorphous eruption composed of macules, papules, and occasional vesicles.
Mucha-Habermann disease

L41.1   Pityriasis lichenoides chronica — A form marked by erythematous, yellowish, scaly macules.

L41.3   Small plaque parapsoriasis

L41.4   Large plaque parapsoriasis

L41.5   Retiform parapsoriasis

L41.8   Other parapsoriasis

L41.9   Parapsoriasis, unspecified

L42   Pityriasis rosea — A mild inflammatory exanthem characterized by salmon-colored papular and macular lesions that are usually seen parallel to the lines of cleavage of the skin.

L43-   Lichen planus — An inflammatory skin disease characterized by wide, flat, itchy papules that have a distinctive sheen and occur in circumscribed patches.
Excludes 1:   lichen planopilaris (L66.1)

L43.0   Hypertrophic lichen planus

L43.1   Bullous lichen planus

L43.2   Lichenoid drug reaction
Use additional code for adverse effect, if applicable, to identify drug (T36-T50 with fifth or sixth character 5)

L43.3   Subacute (active) lichen planus
Lichen planus tropicus

L43.8   Other lichen planus

L43.9   Lichen planus, unspecified

L44- **Other papulosquamous disorders**

L44.0 **Pityriasis rubra pilaris** — A rare, chronic inflammatory skin disease characterized by small follicular papules, and disseminated yellowish-pink scaling patches.

L44.1 **Lichen nitidus** — A rare skin disease characterized by numerous, pinhead-size, flat, glistening discrete papules.

L44.2 **Lichen striatus** — A skin disorder characterized by linear lichenoid papules, usually occurring in young children.

L44.3 **Lichen ruber moniliformis**

L44.4 **Infantile papular acrodermatitis [Gianotti-Crosti]** — [Age/0-17]

L44.8 **Other specified papulosquamous disorders**

L44.9 **Papulosquamous disorder, unspecified**

L45 **Papulosquamous disorders in diseases classified elsewhere** — [Not Allowed as PDX]
Code first underlying disease

Urticaria and erythema (L49-L54)

Excludes 1: Lyme disease (A69.2-)
rosacea (L71.-)

L49- **Exfoliation due to erythematous conditions according to extent of body surface involved**
Code first erythematous condition causing exfoliation, such as:
Ritter's disease (L00)
(Staphylococcal) scalded skin syndrom (L00)
Stevens-Johnson syndrome (L51.1)
Stevens-Johnson syndrome-toxic epidermal necrolysis overlap syndrome (L51.3)
Toxic epidermal necrolysis (L51.2)

L49.0 **Exfoliation due to erythematous condition involving less than 10 percent of body surface** — [Unacceptable PDX]
Exfoliation due to erythematous condition NOS

L49.1 **Exfoliation due to erythematous condition involving 10-19 percent of body surface** — [Unacceptable PDX]

L49.2 **Exfoliation due to erythematous condition involving 20-29 percent of body surface** — [Unacceptable PDX]

cc **L49.3** **Exfoliation due to erythematous condition involving 30-39 percent of body surface** — [Unacceptable PDX]

cc **L49.4** **Exfoliation due to erythematous condition involving 40-49 percent of body surface** — [Unacceptable PDX]

cc **L49.5** **Exfoliation due to erythematous condition involving 50-59 percent of body surface** — [Unacceptable PDX]

cc **L49.6** **Exfoliation due to erythematous condition involving 60-69 percent of body surface** — [Unacceptable PDX]

cc **L49.7** **Exfoliation due to erythematous condition involving 70-79 percent of body surface** — [Unacceptable PDX]

cc **L49.8** **Exfoliation due to erythematous condition involving 80-89 percent of body surface** — [Unacceptable PDX]

cc **L49.9** **Exfoliation due to erythematous condition involving 90 or more percent of body surface** — [Unacceptable PDX]

L50- **Urticaria** — A vascular reaction of the skin characterized by elevated wheals, welts, or reddened patches and associated with severe itching or stinging.

Excludes 1: allergic contact dermatitis (L23-)
angioneurotic edema (T78.3)
giant urticaria (T78.3)
hereditary angio-edema (D84.1)
Quincke's edema (T78.3)
serum urticaria (T80.6-)
solar urticaria (L56.3)
urticaria neonatorum (P83.8)
urticaria papulosa (L28.2)
urticaria pigmentosa (Q82.2)

L50.0 **Allergic urticaria** — A form due to a hypersensitive reaction to an allergen.

L50.1 **Idiopathic urticaria** — A form of unknown origin.

L50.2 **Urticaria due to cold and heat** — A form due to the exposure effects of cold or heat.

Excludes 2: familial cold urticaria (M04.2)

L50.3 **Dermatographic urticaria** — A form due to the skin's hypersensitivity to the minor trauma of daily life that is characterized by raised and inflamed skin where the object disrupted the skin.

L50.4 **Vibratory urticaria** — A form occurring after contact with vibratory equipment.

L50.5 **Cholinergic urticaria** — A form produced by the action of internal acetylcholine or mast cells that are released in increased amounts during emotional stress or increased environmental heat.

L50.6 **Contact urticaria** — A form due to contact with an item or substance.

L50.8 **Other urticaria**
Chronic urticaria — A form that persists and recurs over a long period of time.
Recurrent periodic urticaria

L50.9 **Urticaria, unspecified**

L51- **Erythema multiforme** — An inflammatory skin disease characterized by a variety of skin eruptions including rashes, red welts, and/or purple or blistered areas that is often due to a herpes virus or response to medications or illness.
Use additional code for adverse effect, if applicable, to identify drug (T36-T50 with fifth or sixth character 5)
Use additional code to identify associated manifestations, such as:
Arthropathy associated with dermatological disorders (M14.8-)
Conjunctival edema (H11.42)
Conjunctivitis (H10.22-)
Corneal scars and opacities (H17-)
Corneal ulcer (H16.0-)
Edema of eyelid (H02.84)
Inflammation of eyelid (H01.8)
Keratoconjunctivitis sicca (H16.22-)
Mechanical lagophthalmos (H02.22-)
Stomatitis (K12-)
Symblepharon (H11.23-)
Use additional code to identify percentage of skin exfoliation (L49.-)

Excludes 1: staphylococcal scalded skin syndrome (L00)
Ritter's disease (L00)

L51.0 **Nonbullous erythema multiforme**

cc **L51.1** **Stevens-Johnson syndrome** — A form within the same spectrum as toxic epidermal necrolysis that is characterized by severe, extensive skin lesions, involvement of the mucous membranes, and generally involves less than 10% of the body surface.

cc **L51.2** **Toxic epidermal necrolysis [Lyell]** — A form within the same spectrum as Stevens-Johnson syndrome that is characterized by severe, extensive skin lesions, involvement of the mucous membranes with multiple large blisters, and generally involves more than 30% of the body surface.

cc **L51.3** **Stevens-Johnson syndrome-toxic epidermal necrolysis overlap syndrome** — A form within the same spectrum as toxic epidermal necrolysis that is characterized by severe, extensive skin lesions, involvement of the mucous membranes, and generally involves 10% to 30% of the body surface.
SJS-TEN overlap syndrome

L51.8 **Other erythema multiforme**

L51.9 **Erythema multiforme, unspecified**
Erythema iris — A form marked by the formation of concentric rings, producing a target-like appearance.
Erythema multiforme major NOS — A form marked by typical target-like rashes or raised, edematous papules with involvement of one or more mucous membranes but not diagnostic of Stevens-Johnson syndrome or toxic epidermal necrolysis.
Erythema multiforme minor NOS — A form marked by typical target-like rashes or raised, edematous papules.
Herpes iris — A form marked by vesicular lesions.

L52 **Erythema nodosum** — An acute skin disease characterized by tender, red nodules that are due to exudation of blood and serum.

Excludes 1: tuberculous erythema nodosum (A18.4)

L53- **Other erythematous conditions**
Excludes 1: erythema ab igne (L59.0)
erythema due to external agents in contact with skin (L23-L25)
erythema intertrigo (L30.4)

cc **L53.0** **Toxic erythema** — A generalized, diffuse erythematous eruption that is due to a drug or toxin.
Code first poisoning due to drug or toxin, if applicable (T36-T65 with fifth or sixth character 1-4 or 6)
Use additional code for adverse effect, if applicable, to identify drug (T36-T50 with fifth or sixth character 5)
Excludes 1: neonatal erythema toxicum (P83.1)

cc **L53.1** **Erythema annulare centrifugum**

cc **L53.2** **Erythema marginatum**

cc **L53.3** **Other chronic figurate erythema**

L53.8 **Other specified erythematous conditions**

L53.9 **Erythematous condition, unspecified**
Erythema NOS
Erythroderma NOS

Excludes 1: = NOT CODED HERE! (Do not code both)   Excludes 2: = Not Included Here

L54 **Erythema in diseases classified elsewhere** — [Not Allowed as PDX]
Code first underlying disease

Radiation-related disorders of the skin and subcutaneous tissue (L55-L59)

L55- **Sunburn** — An injury to the skin following excessive exposure to the ultraviolet rays of sunlight.

   L55.0 **Sunburn of first degree** — A form affecting the outer layer (epidermis) of the skin causing redness, tenderness, and mild pain.

   L55.1 **Sunburn of second degree** — A form affecting the outer layer (epidermis) and a portion of the inner layer (dermis) of the skin causing blisters.

   L55.2 **Sunburn of third degree** — A form affecting the full-thickness of the skin (epidermis and dermis) and often the underlying subcutaneous tissues.

   L55.9 **Sunburn, unspecified**

L56- **Other acute skin changes due to ultraviolet radiation** — An injury to the skin following excessive exposure to ultraviolet rays (sunlight).
Use additional code to identify the source of the ultraviolet radiation (W89, X32)

   L56.0 **Drug phototoxic response** — A form caused by a nonimmunologic type of photosensitivity.
Use additional code for adverse effect, if applicable, to identify drug (T36-T50 with fifth or sixth character 5)

   L56.1 **Drug photoallergic response** — A form caused by an immunologic type of photosensitivity.
Use additional code for adverse effect, if applicable, to identify drug (T36-T50 with fifth or sixth character 5)

   L56.2 **Photocontact dermatitis [berloque dermatitis]** — A form aggravated by oil found in perfumes and colognes.

   L56.3 **Solar urticaria** — A form causing acute inflammation of the skin.

   L56.4 **Polymorphous light eruption** — A form characterized by skin lesions.

   L56.5 **Disseminated superficial actinic porokeratosis (DSAP)** — An autosomal dominantly inherited skin disorder induced by ultraviolet light causing dry patches on the arms and legs.

   L56.8 **Other specified acute skin changes due to ultraviolet radiation**

   L56.9 **Acute skin change due to ultraviolet radiation, unspecified**

L57- **Skin changes due to chronic exposure to nonionizing radiation**
Use additional code to identify the source of the ultraviolet radiation (W89, X32)

   L57.0 **Actinic keratosis** — A premalignant skin lesion characterized by sharply outlined, reddened growth that is caused by excessive exposure to the sun.
Keratosis NOS
Senile keratosis
Solar keratosis

   L57.1 **Actinic reticuloid** — A photosensitivity dermatitis that is characterized by itchy, red, inflamed skin that resembles reticulosis on biopsy.

   L57.2 **Cutis rhomboidalis nuchae**

   L57.3 **Poikiloderma of Civatte**

   L57.4 **Cutis laxa senilis**
Elastosis senilis

   L57.5 **Actinic granuloma**

   L57.8 **Other skin changes due to chronic exposure to nonionizing radiation**
Farmer's skin
Sailor's skin
Solar dermatitis

   L57.9 **Skin changes due to chronic exposure to nonionizing radiation, unspecified**

L58- **Radiodermatitis** — Damage to the skin from ionizing radiation.
Use additional code to identify the source of the radiation (W88, W90)

   L58.0 **Acute radiodermatitis**

   L58.1 **Chronic radiodermatitis**

   L58.9 **Radiodermatitis, unspecified**

L59- **Other disorders of skin and subcutaneous tissue related to radiation**

   L59.0 **Erythema ab igne [dermatitis ab igne]** — Localized areas of erythema and/or hyperpigmentation caused by repeated exposure to infrared (heat) radiation.

   L59.8 **Other specified disorders of the skin and subcutaneous tissue related to radiation**

   L59.9 **Disorder of the skin and subcutaneous tissue related to radiation, unspecified**

Disorders of skin appendages (L60-L75)

Excludes 1: congenital malformations of integument (Q84.-)

L60- **Nail disorders**
Excludes ❷: clubbing of nails (R68.3)
onychia and paronychia (L03.0-)

   L60.0 **Ingrowing nail** — The inward growing of the nail into the soft tissues.

   L60.1 **Onycholysis** — The loosening of the nails from their nailbeds.

   L60.2 **Onychogryphosis** — An abnormal overgrowth of the nails with an inward curvature.

   L60.3 **Nail dystrophy** — Abnormal changes in nail texture, structure, or color.

   L60.4 **Beau's lines** — Ridges or indentations in the nail plate.

   L60.5 **Yellow nail syndrome** — Yellow coloring of the nails due to an underlying disease, usually lyphedema.

   L60.8 **Other nail disorders**

   L60.9 **Nail disorder, unspecified**

L62 **Nail disorders in diseases classified elsewhere** — [Not Allowed as PDX]
Code first underlying disease, such as:
Pachydermoperiostosis (M89.4-)

L63- **Alopecia areata** — An abnormal autoimmune loss of hair in sharply defined patches usually on the beard or scalp.

   L63.0 **Alopecia (capitis) totalis** — A form losing all the hair on the scalp.

   L63.1 **Alopecia universalis** — A form losing all the hair on the body, including pubic hair.

   L63.2 **Ophiasis** — A form marked by involvement of the temporal and occipital margins of the scalp in a continuous band.

   L63.8 **Other alopecia areata**

   L63.9 **Alopecia areata, unspecified**

L64- **Androgenic alopecia** — The loss of hair on the scalp caused by diminished hair follicles.
Includes: Male-pattern baldness

   L64.0 **Drug-induced androgenic alopecia**
Use additional code for adverse effect, if applicable, to identify drug (T36-T50 with fifth or sixth character 5)

   L64.8 **Other androgenic alopecia**

   L64.9 **Androgenic alopecia, unspecified**

L65- **Other nonscarring hair loss**
Use additional code for adverse effect, if applicable, to identify drug (T36-T50 with fifth or sixth character 5)
Excludes 1: trichotillomania (F63.3)

   L65.0 **Telogen effluvium**

   L65.1 **Anagen effluvium**

   L65.2 **Alopecia mucinosa**

   L65.8 **Other specified nonscarring hair loss**

   L65.9 **Nonscarring hair loss, unspecified**
Alopecia NOS

L66- **Cicatricial alopecia [scarring hair loss]**

   L66.0 **Pseudopelade**

   L66.1 **Lichen planopilaris**
Follicular lichen planus

   L66.2 **Folliculitis decalvans**

   L66.3 **Perifolliculitis capitis abscedens**

   L66.4 **Folliculitis ulerythematosa reticulata**

   L66.8 **Other cicatricial alopecia**
AHA 15:1Q:p19 – Cicatricial alopecia due to second degree burns

   L66.9 **Cicatricial alopecia, unspecified**

L67- **Hair color and hair shaft abnormalities**
Excludes 1: monilethrix (Q84.1)
pili annulati (Q84.1)
telogen effluvium (L65.0)

   L67.0 **Trichorrhexis nodosa**

   L67.1 **Variations in hair color**
Canities
Greyness, hair (premature)
Heterochromia of hair
Poliosis circumscripta, acquired
Poliosis NOS

**L
5
4
-
L
6
7**

L67.8   Other hair color and hair shaft abnormalities
   Fragilitas crinium

L67.9   Hair color and hair shaft abnormality, unspecified

L68-   Hypertrichosis — The excessive growth or coverage of hair.
   Includes: Excess hair
   Excludes 1:   congenital hypertrichosis (Q84.2)
                  persistent lanugo (Q84.2)

L68.0   Hirsutism

L68.1   Acquired hypertrichosis lanuginosa

L68.2   Localized hypertrichosis

L68.3   Polytrichia

L68.8   Other hypertrichosis

L68.9   Hypertrichosis, unspecified

L70-   Acne — An inflammatory pilosebaceous disease.
   Excludes 2:   acne keloid (L73.0)

L70.0   Acne vulgaris — A form characterized by comedones, papules, pustules, cysts, and nodules occurring chiefly on the face, neck, upper trunk, and upper arms.

L70.1   Acne conglobata — A form characterized by numerous comedones, pus, and cyst and sinus formation with severe scarring.

L70.2   Acne varioliformis — A form characterized by superficial, brownish-red papulopustules occurring on the forehead and scalp.
   Acne necrotica miliaris

L70.3   Acne tropica — A severe form occurring in the tropics.

L70.4   Infantile acne — [Age/0-17] — A form presenting in the first year of life.

L70.5   Acné excoriée — Hyperpigmentation of healed acne sites that have been exacerbated by the individual applying pressure.
   Acné excoriée des jeunes filles
   Picker's acne

L70.8   Other acne

L70.9   Acne, unspecified

L71-   Rosacea — A chronic inflammatory disease of the capillary-rich areas of the face that is characterized by erythema, pustules, and telangiectasia.
   Use additional code for adverse effect, if applicable, to identify drug (T36-T50 with fifth or sixth character 5)

L71.0   Perioral dermatitis — A papular, sometimes pustular eruption of the area surrounding the mouth, and occurring almost exclusively in women between the ages of 20 and 35.

L71.1   Rhinophyma — A form of rosacea marked by nodular swelling, redness, sebaceous hyperplasia, and congestion of the distal portion of the nose.

L71.8   Other rosacea

L71.9   Rosacea, unspecified

L72-   Follicular cysts of skin and subcutaneous tissue

L72.0   Epidermal cyst — An encapsulated keratin-filled sac of the epidermis that has implanted into the dermis.

L72.1-   Pilar and trichodermal cyst

L72.11   Pilar cyst — An encapsulated keratin-filled sac of the epidermis that is derived from the outer root sheath of a hair follicle.

L72.12   Trichodermal cyst — Pilar cyst(s) that grow extensively and rapidly, multiplying into a tumor-like mass.
   Trichilemmal (proliferating) cyst

L72.2   Steatocystoma multiplex — A skin disorder characterized by the development of multiple cysts.

L72.3   Sebaceous cyst — An encapsulated, keratin and sebum-filled sac of a pilosebaceous unit.
   Excludes 2:   pilar cyst (L72.11)
                  trichilemmal (proliferating) cyst (L72.12)

L72.8   Other follicular cysts of the skin and subcutaneous tissue

L72.9   Follicular cyst of the skin and subcutaneous tissue, unspecified

L73-   Other follicular disorders

L73.0   Acne keloid — A keloid-like scar from a follicular-based pustule.

L73.1   Pseudofolliculitis barbae — An inflammatory skin condition of shaved hair (usually facial) in which the hair curls back into the skin causing a foreign body like reaction.

L73.2   Hidradenitis suppurativa — Inflammation of the apocrine sweat glands with secondary infection marked by abscessed cutaneous nodules and sinus formation.

L73.8   Other specified follicular disorders
   Sycosis barbae

L73.9   Follicular disorder, unspecified

L74-   Eccrine sweat disorders
   Excludes 2:   generalized hyperhidrosis (R61)

L74.0   Miliaria rubra — A condition caused by the obstruction of the sweat ducts that is characterized by discrete, pruritic, erythematous papulovesicles.

L74.1   Miliaria crystallina

L74.2   Miliaria profunda
   Miliaria tropicalis

L74.3   Miliaria, unspecified

L74.4   Anhidrosis — The diminished or complete absence of sweat secretion.
   Hypohidrosis

L74.5-   Focal hyperhidrosis — Excessive sweating involving one or more specific locations on the body.

L74.51-   Primary focal hyperhidrosis — A form not related to an underlying condition.

L74.510   Primary focal hyperhidrosis, axilla

L74.511   Primary focal hyperhidrosis, face

L74.512   Primary focal hyperhidrosis, palms

L74.513   Primary focal hyperhidrosis, soles

L74.519   Primary focal hyperhidrosis, unspecified

L74.52   Secondary focal hyperhidrosis — A form due to an underlying condition or medical treatment.
   Frey's syndrome — A form characterized by warmth and sweating in the face due to eating certain foods and often associated as a consequence of parotid gland damage.

L74.8   Other eccrine sweat disorders

L74.9   Eccrine sweat disorder, unspecified
   Sweat gland disorder NOS

L75-   Apocrine sweat disorders
   Excludes 1:   dyshidrosis (L30.1)
                  hidradenitis suppurativa (L73.2)

L75.0   Bromhidrosis — Foul-smelling sweat due to the decomposition of microorganisms of the apocrine sweat glands.

L75.1   Chromhidrosis — The abnormal coloration of sweat.

L75.2   Apocrine miliaria — A skin disease characterized by conical, flesh-colored, or grayish, intensely pruritic, discrete follicular papules.
   Fox-Fordyce disease

L75.8   Other apocrine sweat disorders

L75.9   Apocrine sweat disorder, unspecified

Intraoperative and postprocedural complications of skin and subcutaneous tissue (L76)

L76-   Intraoperative and postprocedural complications of skin and subcutaneous tissue

L76.0-   Intraoperative hemorrhage and hematoma of skin and subcutaneous tissue complicating a procedure
   Excludes 1:   intraoperative hemorrhage and hematoma of skin and subcutaneous tissue due to accidental puncture and laceration during a procedure (L76.1-)

cc **L76.01   Intraoperative hemorrhage and hematoma of skin and subcutaneous tissue complicating a dermatologic procedure**

cc **L76.02   Intraoperative hemorrhage and hematoma of skin and subcutaneous tissue complicating other procedure**

L76.1-   Accidental puncture and laceration of skin and subcutaneous tissue during a procedure

cc **L76.11   Accidental puncture and laceration of skin and subcutaneous tissue during a dermatologic procedure**

cc **L76.12   Accidental puncture and laceration of skin and subcutaneous tissue during other procedure**

L76.2-   Postprocedural hemorrhage of skin and subcutaneous tissue following a procedure

cc **L76.21   Postprocedural hemorrhage of skin and subcutaneous tissue following a dermatologic procedure**

cc **L76.22   Postprocedural hemorrhage of skin and subcutaneous tissue following other procedure**

L 6 7 - L 7 6

L76.3-   <u>Postprocedural hematoma and seroma</u> of skin and subcutaneous tissue following a procedure

cc **L76.31**   Postprocedural <u>hematoma</u> of skin and subcutaneous tissue following a <u>dermatologic procedure</u>

cc **L76.32**   Postprocedural <u>hematoma</u> of skin and subcutaneous tissue following <u>other procedure</u>

cc **L76.33**   Postprocedural <u>seroma</u> of skin and subcutaneous tissue following a <u>dermatologic procedure</u>

cc **L76.34**   Postprocedural <u>seroma</u> of skin and subcutaneous tissue following <u>other procedure</u>

L76.8-   Other intraoperative and postprocedural complications of skin and subcutaneous tissue
Use additional code, if applicable, to further specify disorder

L76.81   Other intraoperative complications of skin and subcutaneous tissue

L76.82   Other postprocedural complications of skin and subcutaneous tissue

Other disorders of the skin and subcutaneous tissue (L80-L99)

L80   **Vitiligo** — An epidermal pigment cell destructive disorder of an unknown etiology marked by paper-white macules and patches and usually affecting the skin over bony prominences.
*Excludes ❷: vitiligo of eyelids (H02.73-)
                vitiligo of vulva (N90.89)*

L81-   Other disorders of pigmentation
*Excludes 1:   birthmark NOS (Q82.5)
               Peutz-Jeghers syndrome (Q85.8)*
Excludes ❷: nevus — see Alphabetical Index

L81.0   Postinflammatory hyperpigmentation

L81.1   Chloasma

L81.2   Freckles

L81.3   Café au lait spots

L81.4   Other melanin hyperpigmentation
Lentigo

L81.5   Leukoderma, not elsewhere classified

L81.6   Other disorders of diminished melanin formation

L81.7   Pigmented purpuric dermatosis
Angioma serpiginosum

L81.8   Other specified disorders of pigmentation
Iron pigmentation
Tattoo pigmentation

L81.9   Disorder of pigmentation, unspecified

L82-   **Seborrheic keratosis** — A benign skin tumor of epidermal origin that forms numerous yellow or brown raised lesions.
Includes: Basal cell papilloma
            Dermatosis papulosa nigra
            Leser-Trélat disease
Excludes ❷: seborrheic dermatitis (L21.-)

L82.0   **Inflamed seborrheic keratosis** — A form marked by symptomatic inflammation of the lesion.

L82.1   Other seborrheic keratosis
Seborrheic keratosis NOS

L83   **Acanthosis nigricans** — A hypertrophic skin disease characterized by hyperpigmentation and papillary hypertrophy of the body fold regions.
Confluent and reticulated papillomatosis

L84   **Corns and callosities** — CORN — The inward thickening of the outer layer of the skin caused by friction and pressure. CALLOSITIES — The localized thickening of the skin caused by abnormal friction or pressure.
Callus
Clavus

L85-   Other epidermal thickening
Excludes ❷: hypertrophic disorders of the skin (L91.-)

L85.0   **Acquired ichthyosis** — A generalized skin disorder marked by dryness, roughness, and scaliness that is due to hypertrophy of the outer layer of the skin.
Excludes 1:   congenital ichthyosis (Q80.-)

L85.1   **Acquired keratosis [keratoderma] palmaris et plantaris** — A hypertrophic skin disorder marked by thickening of the outer layer of the skin of the palms and soles.
Excludes 1:   inherited keratosis palmaris et plantaris (Q82.8)

L85.2   Keratosis punctata (palmaris et plantaris)

L85.3   Xerosis cutis
Dry skin dermatitis

L85.8   Other specified epidermal thickening
Cutaneous horn

L85.9   Epidermal thickening, unspecified

L86   Keratoderma in diseases classified elsewhere — [Not Allowed as PDX]
Code first underlying disease, such as:
    Reiter's disease (M02.3-)
*Excludes 1:   gonococcal keratoderma (A54.89)
               gonococcal keratosis (A54.89)
               keratoderma due to vitamin A deficiency (E50.8)
               keratosis due to vitamin A deficiency (E50.8)
               xeroderma due to vitamin A deficiency (E50.8)*

L87-   Transepidermal elimination disorders
Excludes 1:   granuloma annulare (perforating) (L92.0)

L87.0   Keratosis follicularis et parafollicularis in cutem penetrans — A hypertrophic, follicular skin disease characterized by keratotic pegs of the hair follicles and eccrine ducts that extend down into the corium.
Kyrle disease
Hyperkeratosis follicularis penetrans

L87.1   Reactive perforating collagenosis

L87.2   Elastosis perforans serpiginosa — A hypertrophic skin disorder marked by loss of the normal elasticity of the skin.

L87.8   Other transepidermal elimination disorders

L87.9   Transepidermal elimination disorder, unspecified

L88   Pyoderma gangrenosum — A fungating, pedunculated growth of the skin in which
cc   the granulations consist of masses of pyogenic organisms.
Phagedenic pyoderma
Excludes 1:   dermatitis gangrenosa (L08.0)

L89-   <u>Pressure ulcer</u> — A localized, inflammatory, necrotic skin defect that develops slowly and persists over a period of time that is caused by prolonged pressure at the site.
Includes: Bed sore
            Decubitus ulcer
            Plaster ulcer
            Pressure area
            Pressure sore
Code first any associated gangrene (I96)
*Excludes ❷: decubitus (trophic) ulcer of cervix (uteri) (N86)
               diabetic ulcers (E08.621, E08.622, E09.621, E09.622, E10.621, E10.622, E11.621, E11.622, E13.621, E13.622)
               non-pressure chronic ulcer of skin (L97.-)
               skin infections (L00-L08)
               varicose ulcer (I83.0, I83.2)*

L89.0-   <u>Pressure ulcer</u> of elbow

L89.00-   Pressure ulcer of <u>unspecified elbow</u>

L89.000   Pressure ulcer of <u>unspecified</u> elbow, unstageable

L89.001   Pressure ulcer of <u>unspecified</u> elbow, stage 1
Healing pressure ulcer of unspecified elbow, stage 1
Pressure pre-ulcer skin changes limited to persistent focal edema, unspecified elbow

L89.002   Pressure ulcer of <u>unspecified</u> elbow, stage 2
Healing pressure ulcer of unspecified elbow, stage 2
Pressure ulcer with abrasion, blister, partial thickness skin loss involving epidermis and/or dermis, unspecified elbow

mcc **L89.003**   Pressure ulcer of <u>unspecified</u> elbow, stage 3
Healing pressure ulcer of unspecified elbow, stage 3
Pressure ulcer with full thickness skin loss involving damage or necrosis of subcutaneous tissue, unspecified elbow

mcc **L89.004**   Pressure ulcer of <u>unspecified</u> elbow, stage 4
Healing pressure ulcer of unspecified elbow, stage 4
Pressure ulcer with necrosis of soft tissues through to underlying muscle, tendon, or bone, unspecified elbow

L89.009   Pressure ulcer of <u>unspecified</u> elbow, unspecified stage
Healing pressure ulcer of elbow NOS
Healing pressure ulcer of unspecified elbow, unspecified stage

L89.01- Pressure ulcer of <u>right elbow</u>

L89.010   Pressure ulcer of <u>right elbow</u>, unstageable

L89.011   Pressure ulcer of <u>right elbow</u>, stage 1
Healing pressure ulcer of right elbow, stage 1
Pressure pre-ulcer skin changes limited to persistent focal edema, right elbow

L89.012   Pressure ulcer of <u>right elbow</u>, stage 2
Healing pressure ulcer of right elbow, stage 2
Pressure ulcer with abrasion, blister, partial thickness skin loss involving epidermis and/or dermis, right elbow

MCC L89.013   Pressure ulcer of <u>right elbow</u>, stage 3
Healing pressure ulcer of right elbow, stage 3
Pressure ulcer with full thickness skin loss involving damage or necrosis of subcutaneous tissue, right elbow

MCC L89.014   Pressure ulcer of <u>right elbow</u>, stage 4
Healing pressure ulcer of right elbow, stage 4
Pressure ulcer with necrosis of soft tissues through to underlying muscle, tendon, or bone, right elbow

L89.019   Pressure ulcer of <u>right elbow</u>, unspecified stage
Healing pressure right of elbow NOS
Healing pressure ulcer of unspecified elbow, unspecified stage

L89.02- Pressure ulcer of <u>left elbow</u>

L89.020   Pressure ulcer of <u>left elbow</u>, unstageable

L89.021   Pressure ulcer of <u>left elbow</u>, stage 1
Healing pressure ulcer of left elbow, stage 1
Pressure pre-ulcer skin changes limited to persistent focal edema, left elbow

L89.022   Pressure ulcer of <u>left elbow</u>, stage 2
Healing pressure ulcer of left elbow, stage 2
Pressure ulcer with abrasion, blister, partial thickness skin loss involving epidermis and/or dermis, left elbow

MCC L89.023   Pressure ulcer of <u>left elbow</u>, stage 3
Healing pressure ulcer of left elbow, stage 3
Pressure ulcer with full thickness skin loss involving damage or necrosis of subcutaneous tissue, left elbow

MCC L89.024   Pressure ulcer of <u>left elbow</u>, stage 4
Healing pressure ulcer of left elbow, stage 4
Pressure ulcer with necrosis of soft tissues through to underlying muscle, tendon, or bone, left elbow

L89.029   Pressure ulcer of <u>left elbow</u>, unspecified stage
Healing pressure ulcer of left of elbow NOS
Healing pressure ulcer of unspecified elbow, unspecified stage

L89.1- <u>Pressure ulcer</u> of back

L89.10- Pressure ulcer of <u>unspecified</u> part of <u>back</u>

L89.100   Pressure ulcer of <u>unspecified</u> part of <u>back</u>, unstageable

L89.101   Pressure ulcer of <u>unspecified</u> part of <u>back</u>, stage 1
Healing pressure ulcer of unspecified part of back, stage 1
Pressure pre-ulcer skin changes limited to persistent focal edema, unspecified part of back

L89.102   Pressure ulcer of <u>unspecified</u> part of <u>back</u>, stage 2
Healing pressure ulcer of unspecified part of back, stage 2
Pressure ulcer with abrasion, blister, partial thickness skin loss involving epidermis and/or dermis, unspecified part of back

MCC L89.103   Pressure ulcer of <u>unspecified</u> part of <u>back</u>, stage 3
Healing pressure ulcer of unspecified part of back, stage 3
Pressure ulcer with full thickness skin loss involving damage or necrosis of subcutaneous tissue, unspecified part of back

MCC L89.104   Pressure ulcer of <u>unspecified</u> part of <u>back</u>, stage 4
Healing pressure ulcer of unspecified part of back, stage 4
Pressure ulcer with necrosis of soft tissues through to underlying muscle, tendon, or bone, unspecified part of back

L89.109   Pressure ulcer of <u>unspecified</u> part of <u>back</u>, unspecified stage
Healing pressure ulcer of unspecified part of back NOS
Healing pressure ulcer of unspecified part of back, unspecified stage

L89.11- Pressure ulcer of <u>right upper back</u>
Pressure ulcer of right shoulder blade

L89.110   Pressure ulcer of <u>right upper back</u>, unstageable

L89.111   Pressure ulcer of <u>right upper back</u>, stage 1
Healing pressure ulcer of right upper back, stage 1
Pressure pre-ulcer skin changes limited to persistent focal edema, right upper back

L89.112   Pressure ulcer of <u>right upper back</u>, stage 2
Healing pressure ulcer of right upper back, stage 2
Pressure ulcer with abrasion, blister, partial thickness skin loss involving epidermis and/or dermis, right upper back

MCC L89.113   Pressure ulcer of <u>right upper back</u>, stage 3
Healing pressure ulcer of right upper back, stage 3
Pressure ulcer with full thickness skin loss involving damage or necrosis of subcutaneous tissue, right upper back

MCC L89.114   Pressure ulcer of <u>right upper back</u>, stage 4
Healing pressure ulcer of right upper back, stage 4
Pressure ulcer with necrosis of soft tissues through to underlying muscle, tendon, or bone, right upper back

L89.119   Pressure ulcer of <u>right upper back</u>, unspecified stage
Healing pressure ulcer of right upper back NOS
Healing pressure ulcer of right upper back, unspecified stage

L89.12- Pressure ulcer of <u>left upper back</u>
Pressure ulcer of left shoulder blade

L89.120   Pressure ulcer of <u>left upper back</u>, unstageable

L89.121   Pressure ulcer of <u>left upper back</u>, stage 1
Healing pressure ulcer of left upper back, stage 1
Pressure pre-ulcer skin changes limited to persistent focal edema, left upper back

L89.122   Pressure ulcer of <u>left upper back</u>, stage 2
Healing pressure ulcer of left upper back, stage 2
Pressure ulcer with abrasion, blister, partial thickness skin loss involving epidermis and/or dermis, left upper back

MCC L89.123   Pressure ulcer of <u>left upper back</u>, stage 3
Healing pressure ulcer of left upper back, stage 3
Pressure ulcer with full thickness skin loss involving damage or necrosis of subcutaneous tissue, left upper back

MCC L89.124   Pressure ulcer of <u>left upper back</u>, stage 4
Healing pressure ulcer of left upper back, stage 4
Pressure ulcer with necrosis of soft tissues through to underlying muscle, tendon, or bone, left upper back

L89.129   Pressure ulcer of <u>left upper back</u>, unspecified stage
Healing pressure ulcer of left upper back NOS
Healing pressure ulcer of left upper back, unspecified stage

L89.13- Pressure ulcer of <u>right lower back</u>

L89.130   Pressure ulcer of <u>right lower back</u>, unstageable

L89.131   Pressure ulcer of <u>right lower back</u>, stage 1
Healing pressure ulcer of right lower back, stage 1
Pressure pre-ulcer skin changes limited to persistent focal edema, right lower back

L89.132   Pressure ulcer of <u>right lower back</u>, stage 2
Healing pressure ulcer of right lower back, stage 2
Pressure ulcer with abrasion, blister, partial thickness skin loss involving epidermis and/or dermis, right lower back

MCC L89.133   Pressure ulcer of <u>right lower back</u>, stage 3
Healing pressure ulcer of right lower back, stage 3
Pressure ulcer with full thickness skin loss involving damage or necrosis of subcutaneous tissue, right lower back

MCC L89.134   Pressure ulcer of <u>right lower back</u>, stage 4
Healing pressure ulcer of right lower back, stage 4
Pressure ulcer with necrosis of soft tissues through to underlying muscle, tendon, or bone, right lower back

L89.139   Pressure ulcer of <u>right lower back</u>, unspecified stage
Healing pressure ulcer of right lower back NOS
Healing pressure ulcer of right lower back, unspecified stage

L89 - L89

L89.14- Pressure ulcer of <u>left lower back</u>

    L89.140 Pressure ulcer of <u>left lower back</u>, unstageable

    L89.141 Pressure ulcer of <u>left lower back</u>, stage 1
        Healing pressure ulcer of left lower back, stage 1
        Pressure pre-ulcer skin changes limited to persistent focal edema, left lower back

    L89.142 Pressure ulcer of <u>left lower back</u>, stage 2
        Healing pressure ulcer of left lower back, stage 2
        Pressure ulcer with abrasion, blister, partial thickness skin loss involving epidermis and/or dermis, left lower back

    MCC L89.143 Pressure ulcer of <u>left lower back</u>, stage 3
        Healing pressure ulcer of left lower back, stage 3
        Pressure ulcer with full thickness skin loss involving damage or necrosis of subcutaneous tissue, left lower back

    MCC L89.144 Pressure ulcer of <u>left lower back</u>, stage 4
        Healing pressure ulcer of left lower back, stage 4
        Pressure ulcer with necrosis of soft tissues through to underlying muscle, tendon, or bone, left lower back

    L89.149 Pressure ulcer of <u>left lower back</u>, unspecified stage
        Healing pressure ulcer of left lower back NOS
        Healing pressure ulcer of left lower back, unspecified stage

L89.15- Pressure ulcer of <u>sacral</u> region
    Pressure ulcer of coccyx
    Pressure ulcer of tailbone

    L89.150 Pressure ulcer of <u>sacral</u> region, unstageable

    L89.151 Pressure ulcer of <u>sacral</u> region, stage 1
        Healing pressure ulcer of sacral region, stage 1
        Pressure pre-ulcer skin changes limited to persistent focal edema, sacral region

    L89.152 Pressure ulcer of <u>sacral</u> region, stage 2
        Healing pressure ulcer of sacral region, stage 2
        Pressure ulcer with abrasion, blister, partial thickness skin loss involving epidermis and/or dermis, sacral region

    MCC L89.153 Pressure ulcer of <u>sacral</u> region, stage 3
        Healing pressure ulcer of sacral region, stage 3
        Pressure ulcer with full thickness skin loss involving damage or necrosis of subcutaneous tissue, sacral region

    MCC L89.154 Pressure ulcer of <u>sacral</u> region, stage 4
        Healing pressure ulcer of sacral region, stage 4
        Pressure ulcer with necrosis of soft tissues through to underlying muscle, tendon, or bone, sacral region

    L89.159 Pressure ulcer of <u>sacral</u> region, unspecified stage
        Healing pressure ulcer of sacral region NOS
        Healing pressure ulcer of sacral region, unspecified stage

L89.2- <u>Pressure ulcer</u> of hip

L89.20- Pressure ulcer of <u>unspecified hip</u>

    L89.200 Pressure ulcer of <u>unspecified hip</u>, unstageable

    L89.201 Pressure ulcer of <u>unspecified hip</u>, stage 1
        Healing pressure ulcer of unspecified hip back, stage 1
        Pressure pre-ulcer skin changes limited to persistent focal edema, unspecified hip

    L89.202 Pressure ulcer of <u>unspecified hip</u>, stage 2
        Healing pressure ulcer of unspecified hip, stage 2
        Pressure ulcer with abrasion, blister, partial thickness skin loss involving epidermis and/or dermis, unspecified hip

    MCC L89.203 Pressure ulcer of <u>unspecified hip</u>, stage 3
        Healing pressure ulcer of unspecified hip, stage 3
        Pressure ulcer with full thickness skin loss involving damage or necrosis of subcutaneous tissue, unspecified hip

    MCC L89.204 Pressure ulcer of <u>unspecified hip</u>, stage 4
        Healing pressure ulcer of unspecified hip, stage 4
        Pressure ulcer with necrosis of soft tissues through to underlying muscle, tendon, or bone, unspecified hip

    L89.209 Pressure ulcer of <u>unspecified hip</u>, unspecified stage
        Healing pressure ulcer of unspecified hip NOS
        Healing pressure ulcer of unspecified hip, unspecified stage

L89.21- Pressure ulcer of <u>right hip</u>

    L89.210 Pressure ulcer of <u>right hip</u>, unstageable

    L89.211 Pressure ulcer of <u>right hip</u>, stage 1
        Healing pressure ulcer of right hip back, stage 1
        Pressure pre-ulcer skin changes limited to persistent focal edema, right hip

    L89.212 Pressure ulcer of <u>right hip</u>, stage 2
        Healing pressure ulcer of right hip, stage 2
        Pressure ulcer with abrasion, blister, partial thickness skin loss involving epidermis and/or dermis, right hip

    MCC L89.213 Pressure ulcer of <u>right hip</u>, stage 3
        Healing pressure ulcer of right hip, stage 3
        Pressure ulcer with full thickness skin loss involving damage or necrosis of subcutaneous tissue, right hip

    MCC L89.214 Pressure ulcer of <u>right hip</u>, stage 4
        Healing pressure ulcer of right hip, stage 4
        Pressure ulcer with necrosis of soft tissues through to underlying muscle, tendon, or bone, right hip

    L89.219 Pressure ulcer of <u>right hip</u>, unspecified stage
        Healing pressure ulcer of right hip NOS
        Healing pressure ulcer of right hip, unspecified stage

L89.22- Pressure ulcer of <u>left hip</u>

    L89.220 Pressure ulcer of <u>left hip</u>, unstageable

    L89.221 Pressure ulcer of <u>left hip</u>, stage 1
        Healing pressure ulcer of left hip back, stage 1
        Pressure pre-ulcer skin changes limited to persistent focal edema, left hip

    L89.222 Pressure ulcer of <u>left hip</u>, stage 2
        Healing pressure ulcer of left hip, stage 2
        Pressure ulcer with abrasion, blister, partial thickness skin loss involving epidermis and/or dermis, left hip

    MCC L89.223 Pressure ulcer of <u>left hip</u>, stage 3
        Healing pressure ulcer of left hip, stage 3
        Pressure ulcer with full thickness skin loss involving damage or necrosis of subcutaneous tissue, left hip

    MCC L89.224 Pressure ulcer of <u>left hip</u>, stage 4
        Healing pressure ulcer of left hip, stage 4
        Pressure ulcer with necrosis of soft tissues through to underlying muscle, tendon, or bone, left hip

    L89.229 Pressure ulcer of <u>left hip</u>, unspecified stage
        Healing pressure ulcer of left hip NOS
        Healing pressure ulcer of left hip, unspecified stage

L89.3- <u>Pressure ulcer</u> of buttock

L89.30- Pressure ulcer of <u>unspecified buttock</u>

    L89.300 Pressure ulcer of <u>unspecified buttock</u>, unstageable

    L89.301 Pressure ulcer of <u>unspecified buttock</u>, stage 1
        Healing pressure ulcer of unspecified buttock, stage 1
        Pressure pre-ulcer skin changes limited to persistent focal edema, unspecified buttock

    L89.302 Pressure ulcer of <u>unspecified buttock</u>, stage 2
        Healing pressure ulcer of unspecified buttock, stage 2
        Pressure ulcer with abrasion, blister, partial thickness skin loss involving epidermis and/or dermis, unspecified buttock

    MCC L89.303 Pressure ulcer of <u>unspecified buttock</u>, stage 3
        Healing pressure ulcer of unspecified buttock, stage 3
        Pressure ulcer with full thickness skin loss involving damage or necrosis of subcutaneous tissue, unspecified buttock

    MCC L89.304 Pressure ulcer of <u>unspecified buttock</u>, stage 4
        Healing pressure ulcer of unspecified buttock, stage 4
        Pressure ulcer with necrosis of soft tissues through to underlying muscle, tendon, or bone, unspecified buttock

    L89.309 Pressure ulcer of <u>unspecified buttock</u>, unspecified stage
        Healing pressure ulcer of unspecified buttock NOS
        Healing pressure ulcer of unspecified buttock, unspecified stage

L89.31- Pressure ulcer of <u>right buttock</u>

    L89.310 Pressure ulcer of <u>right buttock</u>, unstageable

    L89.311 Pressure ulcer of <u>right buttock</u>, stage 1
        Healing pressure ulcer of right buttock, stage 1
        Pressure pre-ulcer skin changes limited to persistent focal edema, right buttock

L89 - L89

L89.312 Pressure ulcer of <u>right buttock</u>, stage 2
Healing pressure ulcer of right buttock, stage 2
Pressure ulcer with abrasion, blister, partial thickness skin loss involving epidermis and/or dermis, right buttock

MCC L89.313 Pressure ulcer of <u>right buttock</u>, stage 3
Healing pressure ulcer of right buttock, stage 3
Pressure ulcer with full thickness skin loss involving damage or necrosis of subcutaneous tissue, right buttock

MCC L89.314 Pressure ulcer of <u>right buttock</u>, stage 4
Healing pressure ulcer of right buttock, stage 4
Pressure ulcer with necrosis of soft tissues through to underlying muscle, tendon, or bone, right buttock

L89.319 Pressure ulcer of <u>right buttock</u>, unspecified stage
Healing pressure ulcer of right buttock NOS
Healing pressure ulcer of right buttock, unspecified stage

L89.32- Pressure ulcer of <u>left buttock</u>

L89.320 Pressure ulcer of <u>left buttock</u>, unstageable

L89.321 Pressure ulcer of <u>left buttock</u>, stage 1
Healing pressure ulcer of left buttock, stage 1
Pressure pre-ulcer skin changes limited to persistent focal edema, left buttock

L89.322 Pressure ulcer of <u>left buttock</u>, stage 2
Healing pressure ulcer of left buttock, stage 2
Pressure ulcer with abrasion, blister, partial thickness skin loss involving epidermis and/or dermis, left buttock

MCC L89.323 Pressure ulcer of <u>left buttock</u>, stage 3
Healing pressure ulcer of left buttock, stage 3
Pressure ulcer with full thickness skin loss involving damage or necrosis of subcutaneous tissue, left buttock

MCC L89.324 Pressure ulcer of <u>left buttock</u>, stage 4
Healing pressure ulcer of left buttock, stage 4
Pressure ulcer with necrosis of soft tissues through to underlying muscle, tendon, or bone, left buttock

L89.329 Pressure ulcer of <u>left buttock</u>, unspecified stage
Healing pressure ulcer of left buttock NOS
Healing pressure ulcer of left buttock, unspecified stage

L89.4- <u>Pressure ulcer</u> of contiguous site of back, buttock and hip

L89.40 Pressure ulcer of <u>contiguous site of back, buttock and hip</u>, unspecified stage
Healing pressure ulcer of contiguous site of back, buttock and hip NOS
Healing pressure ulcer of contiguous site of back, buttock and hip, unspecified stage

L89.41 Pressure ulcer of <u>contiguous site of back, buttock and hip</u>, stage 1
Healing pressure ulcer of contiguous site of back, buttock and hip, stage 1
Pressure pre-ulcer skin changes limited to persistent focal edema, contiguous site of back, buttock and hip

L89.42 Pressure ulcer of <u>contiguous site of back, buttock and hip</u>, stage 2
Healing pressure ulcer of contiguous site of back, buttock and hip, stage 2
Pressure ulcer with abrasion, blister, partial thickness skin loss involving epidermis and/or dermis, contiguous site of back, buttock and hip

MCC L89.43 Pressure ulcer of <u>contiguous site of back, buttock and hip</u>, stage 3
Healing pressure ulcer of contiguous site of back, buttock and hip, stage 3
Pressure ulcer with full thickness skin loss involving damage or necrosis of subcutaneous tissue, contiguous site of back, buttock and hip

MCC L89.44 Pressure ulcer of <u>contiguous site of back, buttock and hip</u>, stage 4
Healing pressure ulcer of contiguous site of back, buttock and hip, stage 4
Pressure ulcer with necrosis of soft tissues through to underlying muscle, tendon, or bone, contiguous site of back, buttock and hip

L89.45 Pressure ulcer of <u>contiguous site of back, buttock and hip</u>, unstageable

L89.5- <u>Pressure ulcer</u> of ankle

L89.50- Pressure ulcer of <u>unspecified ankle</u>

L89.500 Pressure ulcer of <u>unspecified ankle</u>, unstageable

L89.501 Pressure ulcer of <u>unspecified ankle</u>, stage 1
Healing pressure ulcer of unspecified ankle, stage 1
Pressure pre-ulcer skin changes limited to persistent focal edema, unspecified ankle

L89.502 Pressure ulcer of <u>unspecified ankle</u>, stage 2
Healing pressure ulcer of unspecified ankle, stage 2
Pressure ulcer with abrasion, blister, partial thickness skin loss involving epidermis and/or dermis, unspecified ankle

MCC L89.503 Pressure ulcer of <u>unspecified ankle</u>, stage 3
Healing pressure ulcer of unspecified ankle, stage 3
Pressure ulcer with full thickness skin loss involving damage or necrosis of subcutaneous tissue, unspecified ankle

MCC L89.504 Pressure ulcer of <u>unspecified ankle</u>, stage 4
Healing pressure ulcer of unspecified ankle, stage 4
Pressure ulcer with necrosis of soft tissues through to underlying muscle, tendon, or bone, unspecified ankle

L89.509 Pressure ulcer of <u>unspecified ankle</u>, unspecified stage
Healing pressure ulcer of unspecified ankle NOS
Healing pressure ulcer of unspecified ankle, unspecified stage

L89.51- Pressure ulcer of <u>right ankle</u>

L89.510 Pressure ulcer of <u>right ankle</u>, unstageable

L89.511 Pressure ulcer of <u>right ankle</u>, stage 1
Healing pressure ulcer of right ankle, stage 1
Pressure pre-ulcer skin changes limited to persistent focal edema, right ankle

L89.512 Pressure ulcer of <u>right ankle</u>, stage 2
Healing pressure ulcer of right ankle, stage 2
Pressure ulcer with abrasion, blister, partial thickness skin loss involving epidermis and/or dermis, right ankle

MCC L89.513 Pressure ulcer of <u>right ankle</u>, stage 3
Healing pressure ulcer of right ankle, stage 3
Pressure ulcer with full thickness skin loss involving damage or necrosis of subcutaneous tissue, right ankle

MCC L89.514 Pressure ulcer of <u>right ankle</u>, stage 4
Healing pressure ulcer of right ankle, stage 4
Pressure ulcer with necrosis of soft tissues through to underlying muscle, tendon, or bone, right ankle

L89.519 Pressure ulcer of <u>right ankle</u>, unspecified stage
Healing pressure ulcer of right ankle NOS
Healing pressure ulcer of right ankle, unspecified stage

L89.52- Pressure ulcer of <u>left ankle</u>

L89.520 Pressure ulcer of <u>left ankle</u>, unstageable

L89.521 Pressure ulcer of <u>left ankle</u>, stage 1
Healing pressure ulcer of left ankle, stage 1
Pressure pre-ulcer skin changes limited to persistent focal edema, left ankle

L89.522 Pressure ulcer of <u>left ankle</u>, stage 2
Healing pressure ulcer of left ankle, stage 2
Pressure ulcer with abrasion, blister, partial thickness skin loss involving epidermis and/or dermis, left ankle

MCC L89.523 Pressure ulcer of <u>left ankle</u>, stage 3
Healing pressure ulcer of left ankle, stage 3
Pressure ulcer with full thickness skin loss involving damage or necrosis of subcutaneous tissue, left ankle

MCC L89.524 Pressure ulcer of <u>left ankle</u>, stage 4
Healing pressure ulcer of left ankle, stage 4
Pressure ulcer with necrosis of soft tissues through to underlying muscle, tendon, or bone, left ankle

L89.529 Pressure ulcer of <u>left ankle</u>, unspecified stage
Healing pressure ulcer of left ankle NOS
Healing pressure ulcer of left ankle, unspecified stage

L89 - L89

L89.6-   <u>Pressure ulcer</u> of heel

   L89.60- Pressure ulcer of <u>unspecified</u> <u>heel</u>

   L89.600   Pressure ulcer of <u>unspecified</u> <u>heel</u>, unstageable

   L89.601   Pressure ulcer of <u>unspecified</u> <u>heel</u>, stage 1
   Healing pressure ulcer of unspecified heel, stage 1
   Pressure pre-ulcer skin changes limited to persistent focal edema, unspecified heel

   L89.602   Pressure ulcer of <u>unspecified</u> <u>heel</u>, stage 2
   Healing pressure ulcer of unspecified heel, stage 2
   Pressure ulcer with abrasion, blister, partial thickness skin loss involving epidermis and/or dermis, unspecified heel

   MCC **L89.603**   Pressure ulcer of <u>unspecified</u> <u>heel</u>, stage 3
   Healing pressure ulcer of unspecified heel, stage 3
   Pressure ulcer with full thickness skin loss involving damage or necrosis of subcutaneous tissue, unspecified heel

   MCC **L89.604**   Pressure ulcer of <u>unspecified</u> <u>heel</u>, stage 4
   Healing pressure ulcer of unspecified heel, stage 4
   Pressure ulcer with necrosis of soft tissues through to underlying muscle, tendon, or bone, unspecified heel

   L89.609   Pressure ulcer of <u>unspecified</u> <u>heel</u>, unspecified stage
   Healing pressure ulcer of unspecified heel NOS
   Healing pressure ulcer of unspecified heel, unspecified stage

   L89.61- Pressure ulcer of <u>right heel</u>

   L89.610   Pressure ulcer of <u>right heel</u>, unstageable

   L89.611   Pressure ulcer of <u>right heel</u>, stage 1
   Healing pressure ulcer of right heel, stage 1
   Pressure pre-ulcer skin changes limited to persistent focal edema, right heel

   L89.612   Pressure ulcer of <u>right heel</u>, stage 2
   Healing pressure ulcer of right heel, stage 2
   Pressure ulcer with abrasion, blister, partial thickness skin loss involving epidermis and/or dermis, right heel

   MCC **L89.613**   Pressure ulcer of <u>right heel</u>, stage 3
   Healing pressure ulcer of right heel, stage 3
   Pressure ulcer with full thickness skin loss involving damage or necrosis of subcutaneous tissue, right heel

   MCC **L89.614**   Pressure ulcer of <u>right heel</u>, stage 4
   Healing pressure ulcer of right heel, stage 4
   Pressure ulcer with necrosis of soft tissues through to underlying muscle, tendon, or bone, right heel

   L89.619   Pressure ulcer of <u>right heel</u>, unspecified stage
   Healing pressure ulcer of right heel NOS
   Healing pressure ulcer of unspecified heel, right stage

   L89.62- Pressure ulcer of <u>left heel</u>

   L89.620   Pressure ulcer of <u>left heel</u>, unstageable

   L89.621   Pressure ulcer of <u>left heel</u>, stage 1
   Healing pressure ulcer of left heel, stage 1
   Pressure pre-ulcer skin changes limited to persistent focal edema, left heel

   L89.622   Pressure ulcer of <u>left heel</u>, stage 2
   Healing pressure ulcer of left heel, stage 2
   Pressure ulcer with abrasion, blister, partial thickness skin loss involving epidermis and/or dermis, left heel

   MCC **L89.623**   Pressure ulcer of <u>left heel</u>, stage 3
   Healing pressure ulcer of left heel, stage 3
   Pressure ulcer with full thickness skin loss involving damage or necrosis of subcutaneous tissue, left heel

   MCC **L89.624**   Pressure ulcer of <u>left heel</u>, stage 4
   Healing pressure ulcer of left heel, stage 4
   Pressure ulcer with necrosis of soft tissues through to underlying muscle, tendon, or bone, left heel

   L89.629   Pressure ulcer of <u>left heel</u>, unspecified stage
   Healing pressure ulcer of left heel NOS
   Healing pressure ulcer of left heel, unspecified stage

L89.8-   <u>Pressure ulcer</u> of other site

   L89.81- Pressure ulcer of <u>head</u>
   Pressure ulcer of face

   L89.810   Pressure ulcer of <u>head</u>, unstageable

   L89.811   Pressure ulcer of <u>head</u>, stage 1
   Healing pressure ulcer of head, stage 1
   Pressure pre-ulcer skin changes limited to persistent focal edema, head

   L89.812   Pressure ulcer of <u>head</u>, stage 2
   Healing pressure ulcer of head, stage 2
   Pressure ulcer with abrasion, blister, partial thickness skin loss involving epidermis and/or dermis, head

   MCC **L89.813**   Pressure ulcer of <u>head</u>, stage 3
   Healing pressure ulcer of head, stage 3
   Pressure ulcer with full thickness skin loss involving damage or necrosis of subcutaneous tissue, head

   MCC **L89.814**   Pressure ulcer of <u>head</u>, stage 4
   Healing pressure ulcer of head, stage 4
   Pressure ulcer with necrosis of soft tissues through to underlying muscle, tendon, or bone, head

   L89.819   Pressure ulcer of <u>head</u>, unspecified stage
   Healing pressure ulcer of head NOS
   Healing pressure ulcer of head, unspecified stage

   L89.89- Pressure ulcer of other site

   L89.890   Pressure ulcer of <u>other</u> site, unstageable

   L89.891   Pressure ulcer of <u>other</u> site, stage 1
   Healing pressure ulcer of other site, stage 1
   Pressure pre-ulcer skin changes limited to persistent focal edema, other site

   L89.892   Pressure ulcer of <u>other</u> site, stage 2
   Healing pressure ulcer of other site, stage 2
   Pressure ulcer with abrasion, blister, partial thickness skin loss involving epidermis and/or dermis, other site

   MCC **L89.893**   Pressure ulcer of <u>other</u> site, stage 3
   Healing pressure ulcer of other site, stage 3
   Pressure ulcer with full thickness skin loss involving damage or necrosis of subcutaneous tissue, other site

   MCC **L89.894**   Pressure ulcer of <u>other</u> site, stage 4
   Healing pressure ulcer of other site, stage 4
   Pressure ulcer with necrosis of soft tissues through to underlying muscle, tendon, or bone, other site

   L89.899   Pressure ulcer of <u>other</u> site, unspecified stage
   Healing pressure ulcer of other site NOS
   Healing pressure ulcer of other site, unspecified stage

L89.9-   <u>Pressure ulcer</u> of unspecified site

   L89.90   Pressure ulcer of <u>unspecified site</u>, unspecified stage
   Healing pressure ulcer of unspecified site NOS
   Healing pressure ulcer of unspecified site, unspecified stage

   L89.91   Pressure ulcer of <u>unspecified site</u>, stage 1
   Healing pressure ulcer of unspecified site, stage 1
   Pressure pre-ulcer skin changes limited to persistent focal edema, unspecified site

   L89.92   Pressure ulcer of <u>unspecified site</u>, stage 2
   Healing pressure ulcer of unspecified site, stage 2
   Pressure ulcer with abrasion, blister, partial thickness skin loss involving epidermis and/or dermis, unspecified site

   MCC **L89.93**   Pressure ulcer of <u>unspecified site</u>, stage 3
   Healing pressure ulcer of unspecified site, stage 3
   Pressure ulcer with full thickness skin loss involving damage or necrosis of subcutaneous tissue, unspecified site

   MCC **L89.94**   Pressure ulcer of <u>unspecified site</u>, stage 4
   Healing pressure ulcer of unspecified site, stage 4
   Pressure ulcer with necrosis of soft tissues through to underlying muscle, tendon, or bone, unspecified site

   L89.95   Pressure ulcer of <u>unspecified site</u>, unstageable

L 8 9 – L 8 9

L90-   Atrophic disorders of skin — Skin diseases characterized by wasting-away of the skin tissue.

L90.0   Lichen sclerosus et atrophicus
> Excludes ❷: lichen sclerosus of external female genital organs (N90.4)
> lichen sclerosus of external male genital organs (N48.0)

L90.1   Anetoderma of Schweninger-Buzzi

L90.2   Anetoderma of Jadassohn-Pellizzari

L90.3   Atrophoderma of Pasini and Pierini

L90.4   Acrodermatitis chronica atrophicans

L90.5   Scar conditions and fibrosis of skin
> AHA 15:1Q:p19 – Skin contracture due to third degree burns
> Adherent scar (skin)
> Cicatrix
> Disfigurement of skin due to scar
> Fibrosis of skin NOS
> Scar NOS
> Excludes ❷: hypertrophic scar (L91.0)
> keloid scar (L91.0)

L90.6   Striae atrophicae

L90.8   Other atrophic disorders of skin

L90.9   Atrophic disorder of skin, unspecified

L91-   Hypertrophic disorders of skin

L91.0   Hypertrophic scar — A firm, elevated, irregularly-shaped growth of the skin due to excessive amounts of collagen in the skin during healing of a wound. It may also appear without a history of trauma.
> Keloid
> Keloid scar
> Excludes ❷: acne keloid (L73.0)
> scar NOS (L90.5)

L91.8   Other hypertrophic disorders of the skin

L91.9   Hypertrophic disorder of the skin, unspecified

L92-   Granulomatous disorders of skin and subcutaneous tissue — Skin diseases characterized by the development of granulomatous tissue.
> Excludes ❷: actinic granuloma (L57.5)

L92.0   Granuloma annulare
> Perforating granuloma annulare

L92.1   Necrobiosis lipoidica, not elsewhere classified
> Excludes 1:   necrobiosis lipoidica associated with diabetes mellitus (E08-E13 with .620)

L92.2   Granuloma faciale [eosinophilic granuloma of skin]

L92.3   Foreign body granuloma of the skin and subcutaneous tissue
> Use additional code to identify the type of retained foreign body (Z18.-)

L92.8   Other granulomatous disorders of the skin and subcutaneous tissue

L92.9   Granulomatous disorder of the skin and subcutaneous tissue, unspecified

L93-   Lupus erythematosus — A superficial autimmune skin disorder characterized by inflammation, red macules, adherent scales, and patulous follicles that fall off, leaving scars.
> Use additional code for adverse effect, if applicable, to identify drug (T36-T50 with fifth or sixth character 5)
> Excludes 1:   lupus exedens (A18.4)
> lupus vulgaris (A18.4)
> scleroderma (M34.-)
> systemic lupus erythematosus (M32.-)

L93.0   Discoid lupus erythematosus — A form primarily affecting the face, ears, and scalp.
> Lupus erythematosus NOS

L93.1   Subacute cutaneous lupus erythematosus — A form primarily affecting women that is characterized by scaly annular lesions and plaques.

L93.2   Other local lupus erythematosus
> Lupus erythematosus profundus
> Lupus panniculitis — A form marked by subcutaneous nodules.

L94-   Other localized connective tissue disorders
> Excludes 1:   systemic connective tissue disorders (M30-M36)

L94.0   Localized scleroderma [morphea] — A chronic, atrophic skin disease characterized by replacement of localized areas of the skin and subcutaneous tissues with constricting connective tissue.
> Circumscribed scleroderma

L94.1   Linear scleroderma — A form marked by a line of thickened skin that affects the muscle and bone below it, often causing the arm or leg to not grow at the same pace as the other.
> En coup de sabre lesion

L94.2   Calcinosis cutis — The abnormal deposition of calcium salts forming nodules in the skin.

L94.3   Sclerodactyly — A chronic, atrophic skin disease characterized by replacement of localized areas of the skin and subcutaneous tissues with constricting connective tissue.

L94.4   Gottron's papules — A connective tissue disease that is characterized by inflammation of the skin and often the underlying muscles.

L94.5   Poikiloderma vasculare atrophicans — A skin disorder characterized by mottled dispigmentation, telangiectasia, and atrophy.

L94.6   Ainhum — The growth of constricting fibrous tissue around the base of a toe that eventually leads to loss of the digit.

L94.8   Other specified localized connective tissue disorders

L94.9   Localized connective tissue disorder, unspecified

L95-   Vasculitis limited to skin, not elsewhere classified
> Excludes 1:   angioma serpiginosum (L81.7)
> Henoch(-Schönlein) purpura (D69.0)
> hypersensitivity angiitis (M31.0)
> lupus panniculitis (L93.2)
> panniculitis NOS (M79.3)
> panniculitis of neck and back (M54.0-)
> polyarteritis nodosa (M30.0)
> relapsing panniculitis (M35.6)
> rheumatoid vasculitis (M05.2)
> serum sickness (T80.6-)
> urticaria (L50-)
> Wegener's granulomatosis (M31.3-)

L95.0   Livedoid vasculitis — A chronic skin and vascular disorder characterized by painful purple marks and ulcers of the lower extremities.
> Atrophie blanche (en plaque)

L95.1   Erythema elevatum diutinum — A chronic skin and vascular disorder characterized by red, purple, brown, or yellow nodules of the extremities.

L95.8   Other vasculitis limited to the skin

L95.9   Vasculitis limited to the skin, unspecified

L97-   Non-pressure chronic ulcer of lower limb, not elsewhere classified — A localized, inflammatory, necrotic skin defect of the lower extermity that develops slowly and persists over a period of time and is NOT caused by prolonged pressure at the site.
> Includes: Chronic ulcer of skin of lower limb NOS
> Non-healing ulcer of skin
> Non-infected sinus of skin
> Trophic ulcer NOS
> Tropical ulcer NOS
> Ulcer of skin of lower limb NOS
> Code first any associated underlying condition, such as:
> Any associated gangrene (I96)
> Atherosclerosis of the lower extremities (I70.23-, I70.24-, I70.33-, I70.34-, I70.43-, I70.44-, I70.53-, I70.54-, I70.63-, I70.64-, I70.73-, I70.74-)
> Chronic venous hypertension (I87.31-, I87.33-)
> Diabetic ulcers (E08.621, E08.622, E09.621, E09.622, E10.621, E10.622, E11.621, E11.622, E13.621, E13.622)
> Postphlebitic syndrome (I87.01-, I87.03-)
> Postthrombotic syndrome (I87.01-, I87.03-)
> Varicose ulcer (I83.0-, I83.2-)
> Excludes ❷: pressure ulcer (pressure area) (L89.-)
> skin infections (L00-L08)
> specific infections classified to A00-B99

L97.1-   Non-pressure chronic ulcer of thigh

L97.10-   Non-pressure chronic ulcer of unspecified thigh

cc **L97.101   Non-pressure chronic ulcer of unspecified thigh limited to breakdown of skin**

cc **L97.102   Non-pressure chronic ulcer of unspecified thigh with fat layer exposed**

cc **L97.103   Non-pressure chronic ulcer of unspecified thigh with necrosis of muscle**

cc **L97.104   Non-pressure chronic ulcer of unspecified thigh with necrosis of bone**

cc **L97.109   Non-pressure chronic ulcer of unspecified thigh with unspecified severity**

L97.11-   Non-pressure chronic ulcer of right thigh

cc **L97.111   Non-pressure chronic ulcer of right thigh limited to breakdown of skin**

cc **L97.112   Non-pressure chronic ulcer of right thigh with fat layer exposed**

L90 – L97

cc **L97.113** **Non-pressure chronic ulcer of <u>right</u> thigh <u>with</u> <u>necrosis of muscle</u>**

cc **L97.114** **Non-pressure chronic ulcer of <u>right</u> thigh <u>with</u> <u>necrosis of bone</u>**

cc **L97.119** **Non-pressure chronic ulcer of <u>right</u> thigh with <u>unspecified</u> severity**

L97.12- **Non-pressure chronic ulcer of <u>left</u> thigh**

cc **L97.121** **Non-pressure chronic ulcer of <u>left</u> thigh limited to <u>breakdown of skin</u>**

cc **L97.122** **Non-pressure chronic ulcer of <u>left</u> thigh <u>with fat</u> <u>layer exposed</u>**

cc **L97.123** **Non-pressure chronic ulcer of <u>left</u> thigh <u>with</u> <u>necrosis of muscle</u>**

cc **L97.124** **Non-pressure chronic ulcer of <u>left</u> thigh <u>with</u> <u>necrosis of bone</u>**

cc **L97.129** **Non-pressure chronic ulcer of <u>left</u> thigh with <u>unspecified</u> severity**

L97.2- **<u>Non-pressure chronic ulcer</u> of calf**

L97.20- **Non-pressure chronic ulcer of <u>unspecified calf</u>**

cc **L97.201** **Non-pressure chronic ulcer of <u>unspecified</u> calf limited to <u>breakdown of skin</u>**

cc **L97.202** **Non-pressure chronic ulcer of <u>unspecified</u> calf <u>with</u> <u>fat layer exposed</u>**

cc **L97.203** **Non-pressure chronic ulcer of <u>unspecified</u> calf <u>with</u> <u>necrosis of muscle</u>**

cc **L97.204** **Non-pressure chronic ulcer of <u>unspecified</u> calf <u>with</u> <u>necrosis of bone</u>**

cc **L97.209** **Non-pressure chronic ulcer of <u>unspecified</u> calf with <u>unspecified</u> severity**

L97.21- **Non-pressure chronic ulcer of <u>right</u> calf**

cc **L97.211** **Non-pressure chronic ulcer of <u>right</u> calf limited to <u>breakdown of skin</u>**

cc **L97.212** **Non-pressure chronic ulcer of <u>right</u> calf <u>with fat</u> <u>layer exposed</u>**

cc **L97.213** **Non-pressure chronic ulcer of <u>right</u> calf <u>with</u> <u>necrosis of muscle</u>**

cc **L97.214** **Non-pressure chronic ulcer of <u>right</u> calf <u>with</u> <u>necrosis of bone</u>**

cc **L97.219** **Non-pressure chronic ulcer of <u>right</u> calf with <u>unspecified</u> severity**

L97.22- **Non-pressure chronic ulcer of <u>left</u> calf**

cc **L97.221** **Non-pressure chronic ulcer of <u>left</u> calf limited to <u>breakdown of skin</u>**

cc **L97.222** **Non-pressure chronic ulcer of <u>left</u> calf <u>with fat</u> <u>layer exposed</u>**

cc **L97.223** **Non-pressure chronic ulcer of <u>left</u> calf <u>with necrosis</u> of muscle**

cc **L97.224** **Non-pressure chronic ulcer of <u>left</u> calf <u>with necrosis</u> of bone**

cc **L97.229** **Non-pressure chronic ulcer of <u>left</u> calf with <u>unspecified</u> severity**

L97.3- **<u>Non-pressure chronic ulcer</u> of ankle**

L97.30- **Non-pressure chronic ulcer of <u>unspecified ankle</u>**

cc **L97.301** **Non-pressure chronic ulcer of <u>unspecified</u> ankle limited to <u>breakdown of skin</u>**

cc **L97.302** **Non-pressure chronic ulcer of <u>unspecified</u> ankle <u>with fat layer exposed</u>**

cc **L97.303** **Non-pressure chronic ulcer of <u>unspecified</u> ankle <u>with necrosis of muscle</u>**

cc **L97.304** **Non-pressure chronic ulcer of <u>unspecified</u> ankle <u>with necrosis of bone</u>**

cc **L97.309** **Non-pressure chronic ulcer of <u>unspecified</u> ankle with <u>unspecified</u> severity**

L97.31- **Non-pressure chronic ulcer of <u>right</u> ankle**

cc **L97.311** **Non-pressure chronic ulcer of <u>right</u> ankle limited to <u>breakdown of skin</u>**

cc **L97.312** **Non-pressure chronic ulcer of <u>right</u> ankle <u>with fat</u> <u>layer exposed</u>**

cc **L97.313** **Non-pressure chronic ulcer of <u>right</u> ankle <u>with</u> <u>necrosis of muscle</u>**

cc **L97.314** **Non-pressure chronic ulcer of <u>right</u> ankle <u>with</u> <u>necrosis of bone</u>**

cc **L97.319** **Non-pressure chronic ulcer of <u>right</u> ankle with <u>unspecified</u> severity**

L97.32- **Non-pressure chronic ulcer of <u>left ankle</u>**

cc **L97.321** **Non-pressure chronic ulcer of <u>left</u> ankle limited to <u>breakdown of skin</u>**

cc **L97.322** **Non-pressure chronic ulcer of <u>left</u> ankle <u>with fat</u> <u>layer exposed</u>**

cc **L97.323** **Non-pressure chronic ulcer of <u>left</u> ankle <u>with</u> <u>necrosis of muscle</u>**

cc **L97.324** **Non-pressure chronic ulcer of <u>left</u> ankle <u>with</u> <u>necrosis of bone</u>**

cc **L97.329** **Non-pressure chronic ulcer of <u>left</u> ankle with <u>unspecified</u> severity**

L97.4- **<u>Non-pressure chronic ulcer</u> of heel and midfoot**
Non-pressure chronic ulcer of plantar surface of midfoot

L97.40- **Non-pressure chronic ulcer of <u>unspecified heel and</u> <u>midfoot</u>**

cc **L97.401** **Non-pressure chronic ulcer of <u>unspecified</u> heel and midfoot limited to <u>breakdown of skin</u>**

cc **L97.402** **Non-pressure chronic ulcer of <u>unspecified</u> heel and midfoot <u>with fat layer exposed</u>**

cc **L97.403** **Non-pressure chronic ulcer of <u>unspecified</u> heel and midfoot <u>with necrosis of muscle</u>**

cc **L97.404** **Non-pressure chronic ulcer of <u>unspecified</u> heel and midfoot <u>with necrosis of bone</u>**

cc **L97.409** **Non-pressure chronic ulcer of unspecified heel and midfoot with <u>unspecified</u> severity**

L97.41- **Non-pressure chronic ulcer of <u>right heel and midfoot</u>**

cc **L97.411** **Non-pressure chronic ulcer of <u>right</u> heel and midfoot limited to <u>breakdown of skin</u>**

cc **L97.412** **Non-pressure chronic ulcer of <u>right</u> heel and midfoot <u>with fat layer exposed</u>**

cc **L97.413** **Non-pressure chronic ulcer of <u>right</u> heel and midfoot <u>with necrosis of muscle</u>**

cc **L97.414** **Non-pressure chronic ulcer of <u>right</u> heel and midfoot <u>with necrosis of bone</u>**

cc **L97.419** **Non-pressure chronic ulcer of <u>right</u> heel and midfoot with <u>unspecified</u> severity**

L97.42- **Non-pressure chronic ulcer of <u>left heel and midfoot</u>**

cc **L97.421** **Non-pressure chronic ulcer of <u>left</u> heel and midfoot limited to <u>breakdown of skin</u>**

cc **L97.422** **Non-pressure chronic ulcer of <u>left</u> heel and midfoot <u>with fat layer exposed</u>**

cc **L97.423** **Non-pressure chronic ulcer of <u>left</u> heel and midfoot <u>with necrosis of muscle</u>**

cc **L97.424** **Non-pressure chronic ulcer of <u>left</u> heel and midfoot <u>with necrosis of bone</u>**

cc **L97.429** **Non-pressure chronic ulcer of <u>left</u> heel and midfoot with <u>unspecified</u> severity**

L97.5- **<u>Non-pressure chronic ulcer</u> of other part of foot**
Non-pressure chronic ulcer of toe

L97.50- **Non-pressure chronic ulcer of <u>other part of unspecified</u> <u>foot</u>**

L97.501 **Non-pressure chronic ulcer of <u>other part of</u> <u>unspecified foot</u> limited to <u>breakdown of skin</u>**

L97.502 **Non-pressure chronic ulcer of <u>other part of</u> <u>unspecified foot</u> <u>with fat layer exposed</u>**

L97.503 **Non-pressure chronic ulcer of <u>other part of</u> <u>unspecified foot</u> <u>with necrosis of muscle</u>**

L97.504 **Non-pressure chronic ulcer of <u>other part of</u> <u>unspecified foot</u> <u>with necrosis of bone</u>**

L97.509 **Non-pressure chronic ulcer of <u>other part of</u> <u>unspecified foot</u> with <u>unspecified</u> severity**

L97.51- Non-pressure chronic ulcer of <u>other part</u> of <u>right</u> <u>foot</u>

L97.511 Non-pressure chronic ulcer of <u>other part</u> of <u>right</u> foot limited to <u>breakdown of skin</u>

L97.512 Non-pressure chronic ulcer of <u>other part</u> of <u>right</u> foot <u>with fat layer exposed</u>

L97.513 Non-pressure chronic ulcer of <u>other part</u> of <u>right</u> foot <u>with necrosis of muscle</u>

L97.514 Non-pressure chronic ulcer of <u>other part</u> of <u>right</u> foot <u>with necrosis of bone</u>

L97.519 Non-pressure chronic ulcer of <u>other part</u> of <u>right</u> foot with <u>unspecified</u> severity

L97.52- Non-pressure chronic ulcer of other part of left <u>foot</u>

L97.521 Non-pressure chronic ulcer of <u>other part</u> of <u>left</u> foot limited to <u>breakdown of skin</u>

L97.522 Non-pressure chronic ulcer of <u>other part</u> of <u>left</u> foot <u>with fat layer exposed</u>

L97.523 Non-pressure chronic ulcer of <u>other part</u> of <u>left</u> foot <u>with necrosis of muscle</u>

L97.524 Non-pressure chronic ulcer of <u>other part</u> of <u>left</u> foot <u>with necrosis of bone</u>

L97.529 Non-pressure chronic ulcer of <u>other part</u> of <u>left</u> foot with <u>unspecified</u> severity

L97.8- <u>Non-pressure chronic ulcer</u> of other part of lower leg

L97.80 Non-pressure chronic ulcer of <u>other part of unspecified lower leg</u>

cc **L97.801** Non-pressure chronic ulcer of other part of unspecified <u>lower leg</u> limited to <u>breakdown of skin</u>

cc **L97.802** Non-pressure chronic ulcer of other part of unspecified <u>lower leg</u> <u>with fat layer exposed</u>

cc **L97.803** Non-pressure chronic ulcer of other part of unspecified <u>lower leg</u> <u>with necrosis of muscle</u>

cc **L97.804** Non-pressure chronic ulcer of other part of unspecified <u>lower leg</u> <u>with necrosis of bone</u>

cc **L97.809** Non-pressure chronic ulcer of other part of unspecified <u>lower leg</u> with <u>unspecified</u> severity

L97.81- Non-pressure chronic ulcer of <u>other part of right lower leg</u>

cc **L97.811** Non-pressure chronic ulcer of other part of <u>right</u> lower leg limited to <u>breakdown of skin</u>

cc **L97.812** Non-pressure chronic ulcer of other part of <u>right</u> lower leg <u>with fat layer exposed</u>

cc **L97.813** Non-pressure chronic ulcer of other part of <u>right</u> lower leg <u>with necrosis of muscle</u>

cc **L97.814** Non-pressure chronic ulcer of other part of <u>right</u> lower leg <u>with necrosis of bone</u>

cc **L97.819** Non-pressure chronic ulcer of other part of <u>right</u> lower leg with <u>unspecified</u> severity

L97.82- Non-pressure chronic ulcer of <u>other part of left</u> lower leg

cc **L97.821** Non-pressure chronic ulcer of other part of <u>left</u> lower leg limited to <u>breakdown of skin</u>

cc **L97.822** Non-pressure chronic ulcer of other part of <u>left</u> lower leg <u>with fat layer exposed</u>

cc **L97.823** Non-pressure chronic ulcer of other part of <u>left</u> lower leg <u>with necrosis of muscle</u>

cc **L97.824** Non-pressure chronic ulcer of other part of <u>left</u> lower leg <u>with necrosis of bone</u>

cc **L97.829** Non-pressure chronic ulcer of other part of <u>left</u> lower leg with <u>unspecified</u> severity

L97.9- <u>Non-pressure chronic ulcer</u> of <u>unspecified part of lower leg</u>

L97.90- Non-pressure chronic ulcer of <u>unspecified part of unspecified lower leg</u>

cc **L97.901** Non-pressure chronic ulcer of unspecified part of <u>unspecified</u> lower leg limited to <u>breakdown of skin</u>

cc **L97.902** Non-pressure chronic ulcer of unspecified part of <u>unspecified</u> lower leg <u>with fat layer exposed</u>

cc **L97.903** Non-pressure chronic ulcer of unspecified part of <u>unspecified</u> lower leg <u>with necrosis of muscle</u>

cc **L97.904** Non-pressure chronic ulcer of unspecified part of <u>unspecified</u> lower leg <u>with necrosis of bone</u>

cc **L97.909** Non-pressure chronic ulcer of unspecified part of <u>unspecified</u> lower leg with <u>unspecified</u> severity

L97.91- Non-pressure chronic ulcer of <u>unspecified part of right</u> lower leg

cc **L97.911** Non-pressure chronic ulcer of unspecified part of <u>right</u> lower leg limited to <u>breakdown of skin</u>

cc **L97.912** Non-pressure chronic ulcer of unspecified part of <u>right</u> lower leg <u>with fat layer exposed</u>

cc **L97.913** Non-pressure chronic ulcer of unspecified part of <u>right</u> lower leg <u>with necrosis of muscle</u>

cc **L97.914** Non-pressure chronic ulcer of unspecified part of <u>right</u> lower leg <u>with necrosis of bone</u>

cc **L97.919** Non-pressure chronic ulcer of unspecified part of <u>right</u> lower leg with <u>unspecified</u> severity

L97.92- Non-pressure chronic ulcer of <u>unspecified part of left</u> lower leg

cc **L97.921** Non-pressure chronic ulcer of unspecified part of <u>left</u> lower leg limited to <u>breakdown of skin</u>

cc **L97.922** Non-pressure chronic ulcer of unspecified part of <u>left</u> lower leg <u>with fat layer exposed</u>

cc **L97.923** Non-pressure chronic ulcer of unspecified part of <u>left</u> lower leg <u>with necrosis of muscle</u>

cc **L97.924** Non-pressure chronic ulcer of unspecified part of <u>left</u> lower leg <u>with necrosis of bone</u>

cc **L97.929** Non-pressure chronic ulcer of unspecified part of <u>left</u> lower leg with <u>unspecified</u> severity

L98- Other disorders of skin and subcutaneous tissue, <u>not elsewhere classified</u>

L98.0 Pyogenic granuloma — A fungating, pedunculated growth of the skin in which the granulations consist of masses of pyogenic organisms.
Excludes ❷: pyogenic granuloma of gingiva (K06.8)
pyogenic granuloma of maxillary alveolar ridge (K04.5)
pyogenic granuloma of oral mucosa (K13.4)

L98.1 Factitial dermatitis — Self-inflicted skin lesions.
Neurotic excoriation
Excludes 1: excoriation (skin-picking) disorder (F42.4)

L98.2 Febrile neutrophilic dermatosis [Sweet] — A reactive skin disorder characterized by tender papules that develop into plaques and fever.

cc **L98.3** Eosinophilic cellulitis [Wells] — A granulomatous skin disorder characterized by tender cellulitis-like plaques and eosinophils in the dermis.

L98.4- <u>Non-pressure chronic ulcer of skin, not elsewhere classified</u> — A localized, inflammatory, necrotic skin defect that develops slowly and persists over a period of time that is NOT of the lower extermity and that is NOT caused by prolonged pressure at the site.
Chronic ulcer of skin NOS
Tropical ulcer NOS
Ulcer of skin NOS
Excludes ❷: pressure ulcer (pressure area) (L89.-)
gangrene (I96)
skin infections (L00-L08)
specific infections classified to A00-B99
ulcer of lower limb NEC (L97.-)
varicose ulcer (I83.0-I82.2)

L98.41- Non-pressure chronic ulcer of <u>buttock</u>

L98.411 Non-pressure chronic ulcer of buttock limited to <u>breakdown of skin</u>

L98.412 Non-pressure chronic ulcer of buttock <u>with fat layer exposed</u>

L98.413 Non-pressure chronic ulcer of buttock <u>with necrosis of muscle</u>

L98.414 Non-pressure chronic ulcer of buttock <u>with necrosis of bone</u>

L98.419 Non-pressure chronic ulcer of buttock with <u>unspecified</u> severity

L97 L98

L98.42- Non-pressure chronic ulcer of <u>back</u>

    L98.421 Non-pressure chronic ulcer of back limited to <u>breakdown of skin</u>

    L98.422 Non-pressure chronic ulcer of back <u>with fat layer exposed</u>

    L98.423 Non-pressure chronic ulcer of back <u>with necrosis of muscle</u>

    L98.424 Non-pressure chronic ulcer of back <u>with necrosis of bone</u>

    L98.429 Non-pressure chronic ulcer of back with <u>unspecified</u> severity

L98.49- Non-pressure chronic ulcer of skin of <u>other sites</u>
Non-pressure chronic ulcer of skin NOS

    L98.491 Non-pressure chronic ulcer of skin of <u>other sites</u> limited to <u>breakdown of skin</u>

    L98.492 Non-pressure chronic ulcer of skin of <u>other sites</u> <u>with fat layer exposed</u>

    L98.493 Non-pressure chronic ulcer of skin of <u>other sites</u> <u>with necrosis of muscle</u>

    L98.494 Non-pressure chronic ulcer of skin of <u>other sites</u> <u>with necrosis of bone</u>

    L98.499 Non-pressure chronic ulcer of skin of <u>other sites</u> with <u>unspecified</u> severity

L98.5 Mucinosis of the skin — A skin disorder characterized by the abnormal accumulation of mucin in the skin.
Focal mucinosis
Lichen myxedematosus
Reticular erythematous mucinosis
Excludes 1: focal oral mucinosis (K13.79)
    myxedema (E03.9)

L98.6 Other infiltrative disorders of the skin and subcutaneous tissue
Excludes 1: hyalinosis cutis et mucosae (E78.89)

L98.7 Excessive and redundant skin and subcutaneous tissue
Loose or sagging skin following bariatric surgery weight loss
Loose or sagging skin following dietary weight loss
Loose or sagging skin, NOS
Excludes ❷: acquired excess or redundant skin of eyelid (H02.3-)
    congenital excess or redundant skin of eyelid (Q10.3)
    skin changes due to chronic exposure to nonionizing radiation (L57.-)

L98.8 Other specified disorders of the skin and subcutaneous tissue
AHA 13:2Q:p32 – Acrokeratosis paraneoplastica

L98.9 Disorder of the skin and subcutaneous tissue, unspecified

L99 Other disorders of skin and subcutaneous tissue <u>in diseases classified elsewhere</u> — [Not Allowed as PDX]
Code first underlying disease, such as:
Amyloidosis (E85.-)
Excludes 1: skin disorders in diabetes (E08-E13 with .62)
    skin disorders in gonorrhea (A54.89)
    skin disorders in syphilis (A51.31, A52.79)

L98 - L99

Chapter 13 – Diseases of the musculoskeletal system and connective tissue (M00-M99)

Note: Use an external cause code following the code for the musculoskeletal condition, if applicable, to identify the cause of the musculoskeletal condition

Excludes ❷: *arthropathic psoriasis (L40.5-)*
certain conditions originating in the perinatal period (P04-P96)
certain infectious and parasitic diseases (A00-B99)
compartment syndrome (traumatic) (T79.A-)
complications of pregnancy, childbirth and the puerperium (O00-O9A)
congenital malformations, deformations, and chromosomal abnormalities (Q00-Q99)
endocrine, nutritional and metabolic diseases (E00-E88)
injury, poisoning and certain other consequences of external causes (S00-T88)
neoplasms (C00-D49)
symptoms, signs and abnormal clinical and laboratory findings, not elsewhere classified (R00-R94)

This chapter contains the following blocks:

M00-M02	Infectious arthropathies
M04	Autoinflammatory syndromes
M05-M14	Inflammatory polyarthropathies
M15-M19	Osteoarthritis
M20-M25	Other joint disorders
M26-M27	Dentofacial anomalies [including malocclusion] and other disorders of jaw
M30-M36	Systemic connective tissue disorders
M40-M43	Deforming dorsopathies
M45-M49	Spondylopathies
M50-M54	Other dorsopathies
M60-M63	Disorders of muscles
M65-M67	Disorders of synovium and tendon
M70-M79	Other soft tissue disorders
M80-M85	Disorders of bone density and structure
M86-M90	Other osteopathies
M91-M94	Chondropathies
M95	Other disorders of the musculoskeletal system and connective tissue
M96	Intraoperative and postprocedural complications and disorders of musculoskeletal system, not elsewhere classified
M97	Periprosthetic fracture around internal prosthetic joint
M99	Biomechanical lesions, not elsewhere classified

Chapter-Specific Coding Guidelines

C. Chapter-Specific Coding Guidelines

In addition to general coding guidelines, there are guidelines for specific diagnoses and/or conditions in the classification. Unless otherwise indicated, these guidelines apply to all health care settings. Please refer to Section II for guidelines on the selection of principal diagnosis.

13. Chapter 13: Diseases of the Musculoskeletal System and Connective Tissue (M00-M99)

a. Site and laterality

Most of the codes within Chapter 13 have site and laterality designations. The site represents the bone, joint or the muscle involved. For some conditions where more than one bone, joint or muscle is usually involved, such as osteoarthritis, there is a "multiple sites" code available. For categories where no multiple site code is provided and more than one bone, joint or muscle is involved, multiple codes should be used to indicate the different sites involved.

1) Bone versus joint

For certain conditions, the bone may be affected at the upper or lower end, (e.g., avascular necrosis of bone, M87, Osteoporosis, M80, M81). Though the portion of the bone affected may be at the joint, the site designation will be the bone, not the joint.

b. Acute traumatic versus chronic or recurrent musculoskeletal conditions

Many musculoskeletal conditions are a result of previous injury or trauma to a site, or are recurrent conditions. Bone, joint or muscle conditions that are the result of a healed injury are usually found in chapter 13. Recurrent bone, joint or muscle conditions are also usually found in chapter 13. Any current, acute injury should be coded to the appropriate injury code from chapter 19. Chronic or recurrent conditions should generally be coded with a code from chapter 13. If it is difficult to determine from the documentation in the record which code is best to describe a condition, query the provider.

c. Coding of Pathologic Fractures

7th character A is for use as long as the patient is receiving active treatment for the fracture. ~~Examples of active treatment are: surgical treatment, emergency department encounter, evaluation and continuing treatment by the same or a different physician.~~ While the patient may be seen by a new or different provider over the course of treatment for a pathological fracture, assignment of the 7th character is based on whether the patient is undergoing active treatment and not whether the provider is seeing the patient for the first time.

7th character D is to be used for encounters after the patient has completed active treatment. The other 7th characters, listed under each subcategory in the Tabular List, are to be used for subsequent encounters for routine care of fractures during the healing and recovery phase as well as treatment of problems associated with the healing, such as malunions, nonunions, and sequelae.

Care for complications of surgical treatment for fracture repairs during the healing or recovery phase should be coded with the appropriate complication codes.

See Section I.C.19. Coding of traumatic fractures.

d. Osteoporosis

Osteoporosis is a systemic condition, meaning that all bones of the musculoskeletal system are affected. Therefore, site is not a component of the codes under category M81, Osteoporosis without current pathological fracture. The site codes under category M80, Osteoporosis with current pathological fracture, identify the site of the fracture, not the osteoporosis.

1) Osteoporosis without pathological fracture

Category M81, Osteoporosis without current pathological fracture, is for use for patients with osteoporosis who do not currently have a pathologic fracture due to the osteoporosis, even if they have had a fracture in the past. For patients with a history of osteoporosis fractures, status code Z87.310, Personal history of (healed) osteoporosis fracture, should follow the code from M81.

2) Osteoporosis with current pathological fracture

Category M80, Osteoporosis with current pathological fracture, is for patients who have a current pathologic fracture at the time of an encounter. The codes under M80 identify the site of the fracture. A code from category M80, not a traumatic fracture code, should be used for any patient with known osteoporosis who suffers a fracture, even if the patient had a minor fall or trauma, if that fall or trauma would not usually break a normal, healthy bone.

Arthropathies (M00-M25)

Includes: Disorders affecting predominantly peripheral (limb) joints

Infectious arthropathies (M00-M02)

Note: This block comprises arthropathies due to microbiological agents. Distinction is made between the following types of etiological relationship:
  a) direct infection of joint, where organisms invade synovial tissue and microbial antigen is present in the joint;
  b) indirect infection, which may be of two types: a reactive arthropathy, where microbial infection of the body is established but neither organisms nor antigens can be identified in the joint, and a postinfective arthropathy, where microbial antigen is present but recovery of an organism is inconstant and evidence of local multiplication is lacking.

M00- Pyogenic arthritis — An acute inflammation within the joint with pus formation that is due to infection by microorganisms.

M00.0- Staphylococcal arthritis and polyarthritis — A form caused by staphylococcal microorganisms.
  Use additional code (B95.61-B95.8) to identify bacterial agent
  Excludes ❷: infection and inflammatory reaction due to internal joint prosthesis (T84.5-)

cc **M00.00 Staphylococcal arthritis, unspecified joint**

M00.01- Staphylococcal arthritis, shoulder
  cc **M00.011 Staphylococcal arthritis, right shoulder**
  cc **M00.012 Staphylococcal arthritis, left shoulder**
  cc **M00.019 Staphylococcal arthritis, unspecified shoulder**

M00.02- Staphylococcal arthritis, elbow
  cc **M00.021 Staphylococcal arthritis, right elbow**
  cc **M00.022 Staphylococcal arthritis, left elbow**
  cc **M00.029 Staphylococcal arthritis, unspecified elbow**

M00.03- Staphylococcal arthritis, wrist
  Staphylococcal arthritis of carpal bones
  cc **M00.031 Staphylococcal arthritis, right wrist**

M 0 0 - M 0 0

cc M00.032 Staphylococcal arthritis, <u>left</u> wrist

cc M00.039 Staphylococcal arthritis, <u>unspecified</u> wrist

M00.04- Staphylococcal arthritis, <u>hand</u>
Staphylococcal arthritis of metacarpus and phalanges

cc M00.041 Staphylococcal arthritis, <u>right</u> hand

cc M00.042 Staphylococcal arthritis, <u>left</u> hand

cc M00.049 Staphylococcal arthritis, <u>unspecified</u> hand

M00.05- Staphylococcal arthritis, <u>hip</u>

cc M00.051 Staphylococcal arthritis, <u>right</u> hip

cc M00.052 Staphylococcal arthritis, <u>left</u> hip

cc M00.059 Staphylococcal arthritis, <u>unspecified</u> hip

M00.06- Staphylococcal arthritis, <u>knee</u>

cc M00.061 Staphylococcal arthritis, <u>right</u> knee

cc M00.062 Staphylococcal arthritis, <u>left</u> knee

cc M00.069 Staphylococcal arthritis, <u>unspecified</u> knee

M00.07- Staphylococcal arthritis, <u>ankle and foot</u>
Staphylococcal arthritis, tarsus, metatarsus and phalanges

cc M00.071 Staphylococcal arthritis, <u>right</u> ankle and foot

cc M00.072 Staphylococcal arthritis, <u>left</u> ankle and foot

cc M00.079 Staphylococcal arthritis, <u>unspecified</u> ankle and foot

cc M00.08 Staphylococcal arthritis, <u>vertebrae</u>

cc M00.09 Staphylococcal <u>polyarthritis</u>

M00.1- <u>Pneumococcal</u> arthritis and polyarthritis — A form caused by pneumococcal microorganisms.

cc M00.10 Pneumococcal arthritis, <u>unspecified</u> joint

M00.11- Pneumococcal arthritis, <u>shoulder</u>

cc M00.111 Pneumococcal arthritis, <u>right</u> shoulder

cc M00.112 Pneumococcal arthritis, <u>left</u> shoulder

cc M00.119 Pneumococcal arthritis, <u>unspecified</u> shoulder

M00.12- Pneumococcal arthritis, <u>elbow</u>

cc M00.121 Pneumococcal arthritis, <u>right</u> elbow

cc M00.122 Pneumococcal arthritis, <u>left</u> elbow

cc M00.129 Pneumococcal arthritis, <u>unspecified</u> elbow

M00.13- Pneumococcal arthritis, <u>wrist</u>
Pneumococcal arthritis of carpal bones

cc M00.131 Pneumococcal arthritis, <u>right</u> wrist

cc M00.132 Pneumococcal arthritis, <u>left</u> wrist

cc M00.139 Pneumococcal arthritis, <u>unspecified</u> wrist

M00.14- Pneumococcal arthritis, <u>hand</u>
Pneumococcal arthritis of metacarpus and phalanges

cc M00.141 Pneumococcal arthritis, <u>right</u> hand

cc M00.142 Pneumococcal arthritis, <u>left</u> hand

cc M00.149 Pneumococcal arthritis, <u>unspecified</u> hand

M00.15- Pneumococcal arthritis, <u>hip</u>

cc M00.151 Pneumococcal arthritis, <u>right</u> hip

cc M00.152 Pneumococcal arthritis, <u>left</u> hip

cc M00.159 Pneumococcal arthritis, <u>unspecified</u> hip

M00.16- Pneumococcal arthritis, <u>knee</u>

cc M00.161 Pneumococcal arthritis, <u>right</u> knee

cc M00.162 Pneumococcal arthritis, <u>left</u> knee

cc M00.169 Pneumococcal arthritis, <u>unspecified</u> knee

M00.17- Pneumococcal arthritis, <u>ankle and foot</u>
Pneumococcal arthritis, tarsus, metatarsus and phalanges

cc M00.171 Pneumococcal arthritis, <u>right</u> ankle and foot

cc M00.172 Pneumococcal arthritis, <u>left</u> ankle and foot

cc M00.179 Pneumococcal arthritis, <u>unspecified</u> ankle and foot

cc M00.18 Pneumococcal arthritis, <u>vertebrae</u>

cc M00.19 Pneumococcal <u>polyarthritis</u>

M00.2- <u>Other streptococcal</u> arthritis and polyarthritis — A form caused by streptococcal microorganisms.
Use additional code (B95.0-B95.2, B95.4-B95.5) to identify bacterial agent

cc M00.20 Other streptococcal arthritis, <u>unspecified</u> joint

M00.21- Other streptococcal arthritis, <u>shoulder</u>

cc M00.211 Other streptococcal arthritis, <u>right</u> shoulder

cc M00.212 Other streptococcal arthritis, <u>left</u> shoulder

cc M00.219 Other streptococcal arthritis, <u>unspecified</u> shoulder

M00.22- Other streptococcal arthritis, <u>elbow</u>

cc M00.221 Other streptococcal arthritis, <u>right</u> elbow

cc M00.222 Other streptococcal arthritis, <u>left</u> elbow

cc M00.229 Other streptococcal arthritis, <u>unspecified</u> elbow

M00.23- Other streptococcal arthritis, <u>wrist</u>
Other streptococcal arthritis of carpal bones

cc M00.231 Other streptococcal arthritis, <u>right</u> wrist

cc M00.232 Other streptococcal arthritis, <u>left</u> wrist

cc M00.239 Other streptococcal arthritis, <u>unspecified</u> wrist

M00.24- Other streptococcal arthritis, <u>hand</u>
Other streptococcal arthritis metacarpus and phalanges

cc M00.241 Other streptococcal arthritis, <u>right</u> hand

cc M00.242 Other streptococcal arthritis, <u>left</u> hand

cc M00.249 Other streptococcal arthritis, <u>unspecified</u> hand

M00.25- Other streptococcal arthritis, <u>hip</u>

cc M00.251 Other streptococcal arthritis, <u>right</u> hip

cc M00.252 Other streptococcal arthritis, <u>left</u> hip

cc M00.259 Other streptococcal arthritis, <u>unspecified</u> hip

M00.26- Other streptococcal arthritis, <u>knee</u>

cc M00.261 Other streptococcal arthritis, <u>right</u> knee

cc M00.262 Other streptococcal arthritis, <u>left</u> knee

cc M00.269 Other streptococcal arthritis, <u>unspecified</u> knee

M00.27- Other streptococcal arthritis, <u>ankle and foot</u>
Other streptococcal arthritis, tarsus, metatarsus and phalanges

cc M00.271 Other streptococcal arthritis, <u>right</u> ankle and foot

cc M00.272 Other streptococcal arthritis, <u>left</u> ankle and foot

cc M00.279 Other streptococcal arthritis, <u>unspecified</u> ankle and foot

cc M00.28 Other streptococcal arthritis, <u>vertebrae</u>

cc M00.29 Other streptococcal <u>polyarthritis</u>

M00.8- Arthritis and polyarthritis <u>due to other bacteria</u>
Use additional code (B96) to identify bacteria

cc M00.80 Arthritis due to other bacteria, <u>unspecified</u> joint

M00.81- Arthritis due to other bacteria, <u>shoulder</u>

cc M00.811 Arthritis due to other bacteria, <u>right</u> shoulder

cc M00.812 Arthritis due to other bacteria, <u>left</u> shoulder

cc M00.819 Arthritis due to other bacteria, <u>unspecified</u> shoulder

M00.82- Arthritis due to other bacteria, <u>elbow</u>

cc M00.821 Arthritis due to other bacteria, <u>right</u> elbow

cc M00.822 Arthritis due to other bacteria, <u>left</u> elbow

cc M00.829 Arthritis due to other bacteria, <u>unspecified</u> elbow

M00.83- Arthritis due to other bacteria, <u>wrist</u>
Arthritis due to other bacteria, carpal bones

cc M00.831 Arthritis due to other bacteria, <u>right</u> wrist

cc M00.832 Arthritis due to other bacteria, <u>left</u> wrist

cc M00.839 Arthritis due to other bacteria, <u>unspecified</u> wrist

M00.84- Arthritis due to other bacteria, <u>hand</u>
Arthritis due to other bacteria, metacarpus and phalanges

cc M00.841 Arthritis due to other bacteria, <u>right</u> hand

cc M00.842 Arthritis due to other bacteria, <u>left</u> hand

cc M00.849 Arthritis due to other bacteria, <u>unspecified</u> hand

M00.85- Arthritis due to other bacteria, <u>hip</u>

cc M00.851 Arthritis due to other bacteria, <u>right</u> hip

cc M00.852 Arthritis due to other bacteria, <u>left</u> hip

cc M00.859 Arthritis due to other bacteria, <u>unspecified</u> hip

M00.86- Arthritis due to other bacteria, <u>knee</u>

cc M00.861 Arthritis due to other bacteria, <u>right</u> knee

cc M00.862 Arthritis due to other bacteria, <u>left</u> knee

cc M00.869 Arthritis due to other bacteria, <u>unspecified</u> knee

M00.87- Arthritis due to other bacteria, <u>ankle and foot</u>
Arthritis due to other bacteria, tarsus, metatarsus, and phalanges

cc M00.871 Arthritis due to other bacteria, <u>right</u> ankle and foot

cc M00.872 Arthritis due to other bacteria, <u>left</u> ankle and foot

M 0 0 – M 0 0

cc **M00.879** Arthritis due to other bacteria, <u>unspecified</u> ankle and foot

cc **M00.88** Arthritis due to other bacteria, <u>vertebrae</u>

cc **M00.89** <u>Polyarthritis</u> due to other bacteria

cc **M00.9** Pyogenic arthritis, <u>unspecified</u>
  Infective arthritis NOS

M01- Direct infections of joint <u>in infectious and parasitic diseases classified elsewhere</u> — An acute inflammation within the joint caused by the infectious or parasitic organism in an underlying disease.
  Code first underlying disease, such as:
    Leprosy [Hansen's disease] (A30.-)
    Mycoses (B35-B49)
    O'nyong-nyong fever (A92.1)
    Paratyphoid fever (A01.1-A01.4)
  Excludes 1:   arthropathy in Lyme disease (A69.23)
    gonococcal arthritis (A54.42)
    meningococcal arthritis (A39.83)
    mumps arthritis (B26.85)
    postinfective arthropathy (M02.-)
    postmeningococcal arthritis (A39.84)
    reactive arthritis (M02.3-)
    rubella arthritis (B06.82)
    sarcoidosis arthritis (D86.86)
    typhoid fever arthritis (A01.04)
    tuberculosis arthritis (A18.01-A18.02)

M01.x- Direct infection of joint in infectious and parasitic diseases classified elsewhere

cc **M01.x0** Direct infection of <u>unspecified</u> joint in infectious and parasitic diseases classified elsewhere — [Not Allowed as PDX]

M01.x1- Direct infection of <u>shoulder</u> joint in infectious and parasitic diseases classified elsewhere

cc **M01.x11** Direct infection of <u>right</u> shoulder in infectious and parasitic diseases classified elsewhere — [Not Allowed as PDX]

cc **M01.x12** Direct infection of <u>left</u> shoulder in infectious and parasitic diseases classified elsewhere — [Not Allowed as PDX]

cc **M01.x19** Direct infection of <u>unspecified</u> shoulder in infectious and parasitic diseases classified elsewhere — [Not Allowed as PDX]

M01.x2- Direct infection of <u>elbow</u> in infectious and parasitic diseases classified elsewhere

cc **M01.x21** Direct infection of <u>right</u> elbow in infectious and parasitic diseases classified elsewhere — [Not Allowed as PDX]

cc **M01.x22** Direct infection of <u>left</u> elbow in infectious and parasitic diseases classified elsewhere — [Not Allowed as PDX]

cc **M01.x29** Direct infection of <u>unspecified</u> elbow in infectious and parasitic diseases classified elsewhere — [Not Allowed as PDX]

M01.x3- Direct infection of <u>wrist</u> in infectious and parasitic diseases classified elsewhere
  Direct infection of carpal bones in infectious and parasitic diseases classified elsewhere

cc **M01.x31** Direct infection of <u>right</u> wrist in infectious and parasitic diseases classified elsewhere — [Not Allowed as PDX]

cc **M01.x32** Direct infection of <u>left</u> wrist in infectious and parasitic diseases classified elsewhere — [Not Allowed as PDX]

cc **M01.x39** Direct infection of <u>unspecified</u> wrist in infectious and parasitic diseases classified elsewhere — [Not Allowed as PDX]

M01.x4- Direct infection of <u>hand</u> in infectious and parasitic diseases classified elsewhere
  Direct infection of metacarpus and phalanges in infectious and parasitic diseases classified elsewhere

cc **M01.x41** Direct infection of <u>right</u> hand in infectious and parasitic diseases classified elsewhere — [Not Allowed as PDX]

cc **M01.x42** Direct infection of <u>left</u> hand in infectious and parasitic diseases classified elsewhere — [Not Allowed as PDX]

cc **M01.x49** Direct infection of <u>unspecified</u> hand in infectious and parasitic diseases classified elsewhere — [Not Allowed as PDX]

M01.x5- Direct infection of <u>hip</u> in infectious and parasitic diseases classified elsewhere

cc **M01.x51** Direct infection of <u>right</u> hip in infectious and parasitic diseases classified elsewhere — [Not Allowed as PDX]

cc **M01.x52** Direct infection of <u>left</u> hip in infectious and parasitic diseases classified elsewhere — [Not Allowed as PDX]

cc **M01.x59** Direct infection of <u>unspecified</u> hip in infectious and parasitic diseases classified elsewhere — [Not Allowed as PDX]

M01.x6- Direct infection of <u>knee</u> in infectious and parasitic diseases classified elsewhere

cc **M01.x61** Direct infection of <u>right</u> knee in infectious and parasitic diseases classified elsewhere — [Not Allowed as PDX]

cc **M01.x62** Direct infection of <u>left</u> knee in infectious and parasitic diseases classified elsewhere — [Not Allowed as PDX]

cc **M01.x69** Direct infection of <u>unspecified</u> knee in infectious and parasitic diseases classified elsewhere — [Not Allowed as PDX]

M01.x7- Direct infection of <u>ankle and foot</u> in infectious and parasitic diseases classified elsewhere
  Direct infection of tarsus, metatarsus and phalanges in infectious and parasitic diseases classified elsewhere

cc **M01.x71** Direct infection of <u>right</u> ankle and foot in infectious and parasitic diseases classified elsewhere — [Not Allowed as PDX]

cc **M01.x72** Direct infection of <u>left</u> ankle and foot in infectious and parasitic diseases classified elsewhere — [Not Allowed as PDX]

cc **M01.x79** Direct infection of <u>unspecified</u> ankle and foot in infectious and parasitic diseases classified elsewhere — [Not Allowed as PDX]

cc **M01.x8** Direct infection of <u>vertebrae</u> in infectious and parasitic diseases classified elsewhere — [Not Allowed as PDX]

cc **M01.x9** Direct infection of <u>multiple joints</u> in infectious and parasitic diseases classified elsewhere — [Not Allowed as PDX]

M02- <u>Postinfective and reactive arthropathies</u> — Inflammation of the joint following an infection or as a reactive response to an infection elsewhere in the body.
  Code first underlying disease, such as:
    Congenital syphilis [Clutton's joints] (A50.5)
    Enteritis due to Yersinia enterocolitica (A04.6)
    Infective endocarditis (I33.0)
    Viral hepatitis (B15-B19)
  Excludes 1:   Behçet's disease (M35.2)
    direct infections of joint in infectious and parasitic diseases classified elsewhere (M01.-)
    postmeningococcal arthritis (A39.84)
    mumps arthritis (B26.85)
    rubella arthritis (B06.82)
    syphilis arthritis (late) (A52.77)
    rheumatic fever (I00)
    tabetic arthropathy [Charcot's] (A52.16)

M02.0- Arthropathy <u>following intestinal bypass</u> — A form following an intestinal bypass surgery.

M02.00 Arthropathy following intestinal bypass, <u>unspecified</u> site

M02.01- Arthropathy following intestinal bypass, <u>shoulder</u>

M02.011 Arthropathy following intestinal bypass, <u>right</u> shoulder

M02.012 Arthropathy following intestinal bypass, <u>left</u> shoulder

M02.019 Arthropathy following intestinal bypass, <u>unspecified</u> shoulder

M02.02- Arthropathy following intestinal bypass, <u>elbow</u>
   M02.021 Arthropathy following intestinal bypass, <u>right</u> elbow
   M02.022 Arthropathy following intestinal bypass, <u>left</u> elbow
   M02.029 Arthropathy following intestinal bypass, <u>unspecified</u> elbow
M02.03- Arthropathy following intestinal bypass, <u>wrist</u>
    Arthropathy following intestinal bypass, carpal bones
   M02.031 Arthropathy following intestinal bypass, <u>right</u> wrist
   M02.032 Arthropathy following intestinal bypass, <u>left</u> wrist
   M02.039 Arthropathy following intestinal bypass, <u>unspecified</u> wrist
M02.04- Arthropathy following intestinal bypass, <u>hand</u>
    Arthropathy following intestinal bypass, metacarpals and phalanges
   M02.041 Arthropathy following intestinal bypass, <u>right</u> hand
   M02.042 Arthropathy following intestinal bypass, <u>left</u> hand
   M02.049 Arthropathy following intestinal bypass, <u>unspecified</u> hand
M02.05- Arthropathy following intestinal bypass, <u>hip</u>
   M02.051 Arthropathy following intestinal bypass, <u>right</u> hip
   M02.052 Arthropathy following intestinal bypass, <u>left</u> hip
   M02.059 Arthropathy following intestinal bypass, <u>unspecified</u> hip
M02.06- Arthropathy following intestinal bypass, <u>knee</u>
   M02.061 Arthropathy following intestinal bypass, <u>right</u> knee
   M02.062 Arthropathy following intestinal bypass, <u>left</u> knee
   M02.069 Arthropathy following intestinal bypass, <u>unspecified</u> knee
M02.07- Arthropathy following intestinal bypass, <u>ankle and foot</u>
    Arthropathy following intestinal bypass, tarsus, metatarsus and phalanges
   M02.071 Arthropathy following intestinal bypass, <u>right</u> ankle and foot
   M02.072 Arthropathy following intestinal bypass, <u>left</u> ankle and foot
   M02.079 Arthropathy following intestinal bypass, <u>unspecified</u> ankle and foot
M02.08 Arthropathy following intestinal bypass, <u>vertebrae</u>
M02.09 Arthropathy following intestinal bypass, <u>multiple sites</u>
M02.1- <u>Postdysenteric</u> arthropathy — A form following a dysentery infection.
cc M02.10 Postdysenteric arthropathy, <u>unspecified</u> site
M02.11- Postdysenteric arthropathy, <u>shoulder</u>
  cc M02.111 Postdysenteric arthropathy, <u>right</u> shoulder
  cc M02.112 Postdysenteric arthropathy, <u>left</u> shoulder
  cc M02.119 Postdysenteric arthropathy, <u>unspecified</u> shoulder
M02.12- Postdysenteric arthropathy, <u>elbow</u>
  cc M02.121 Postdysenteric arthropathy, <u>right</u> elbow
  cc M02.122 Postdysenteric arthropathy, <u>left</u> elbow
  cc M02.129 Postdysenteric arthropathy, <u>unspecified</u> elbow
M02.13- Postdysenteric arthropathy, <u>wrist</u>
    Postdysenteric arthropathy, carpal bones
  cc M02.131 Postdysenteric arthropathy, <u>right</u> wrist
  cc M02.132 Postdysenteric arthropathy, <u>left</u> wrist
  cc M02.139 Postdysenteric arthropathy, <u>unspecified</u> wrist
M02.14- Postdysenteric arthropathy, <u>hand</u>
    Postdysenteric arthropathy, metacarpus and phalanges
  cc M02.141 Postdysenteric arthropathy, <u>right</u> hand
  cc M02.142 Postdysenteric arthropathy, <u>left</u> hand
  cc M02.149 Postdysenteric arthropathy, <u>unspecified</u> hand
M02.15- Postdysenteric arthropathy, <u>hip</u>
  cc M02.151 Postdysenteric arthropathy, <u>right</u> hip
  cc M02.152 Postdysenteric arthropathy, <u>left</u> hip
  cc M02.159 Postdysenteric arthropathy, <u>unspecified</u> hip
M02.16- Postdysenteric arthropathy, <u>knee</u>
  cc M02.161 Postdysenteric arthropathy, <u>right</u> knee
  cc M02.162 Postdysenteric arthropathy, <u>left</u> knee

cc M02.169 Postdysenteric arthropathy, <u>unspecified</u> knee
M02.17- Postdysenteric arthropathy, <u>ankle and foot</u>
    Postdysenteric arthropathy, tarsus, metatarsus and phalanges
  cc M02.171 Postdysenteric arthropathy, <u>right</u> ankle and foot
  cc M02.172 Postdysenteric arthropathy, <u>left</u> ankle and foot
  cc M02.179 Postdysenteric arthropathy, <u>unspecified</u> ankle and foot
cc M02.18 Postdysenteric arthropathy, <u>vertebrae</u>
cc M02.19 Postdysenteric arthropathy, <u>multiple sites</u>
M02.2- <u>Postimmunization</u> arthropathy — A form following an immunization.
M02.20 Postimmunization arthropathy, <u>unspecified</u> site
M02.21- Postimmunization arthropathy, <u>shoulder</u>
   M02.211 Postimmunization arthropathy, <u>right</u> shoulder
   M02.212 Postimmunization arthropathy, <u>left</u> shoulder
   M02.219 Postimmunization arthropathy, <u>unspecified</u> shoulder
M02.22- Postimmunization arthropathy, <u>elbow</u>
   M02.221 Postimmunization arthropathy, <u>right</u> elbow
   M02.222 Postimmunization arthropathy, <u>left</u> elbow
   M02.229 Postimmunization arthropathy, <u>unspecified</u> elbow
M02.23- Postimmunization arthropathy, <u>wrist</u>
    Postimmunization arthropathy, carpal bones
   M02.231 Postimmunization arthropathy, <u>right</u> wrist
   M02.232 Postimmunization arthropathy, <u>left</u> wrist
   M02.239 Postimmunization arthropathy, <u>unspecified</u> wrist
M02.24- Postimmunization arthropathy, <u>hand</u>
    Postimmunization arthropathy, metacarpus and phalanges
   M02.241 Postimmunization arthropathy, <u>right</u> hand
   M02.242 Postimmunization arthropathy, <u>left</u> hand
   M02.249 Postimmunization arthropathy, <u>unspecified</u> hand
M02.25- Postimmunization arthropathy, <u>hip</u>
   M02.251 Postimmunization arthropathy, <u>right</u> hip
   M02.252 Postimmunization arthropathy, <u>left</u> hip
   M02.259 Postimmunization arthropathy, <u>unspecified</u> hip
M02.26- Postimmunization arthropathy, <u>knee</u>
   M02.261 Postimmunization arthropathy, <u>right</u> knee
   M02.262 Postimmunization arthropathy, <u>left</u> knee
   M02.269 Postimmunization arthropathy, <u>unspecified</u> knee
M02.27- Postimmunization arthropathy, <u>ankle and foot</u>
    Postimmunization arthropathy, tarsus, metatarsus and phalanges
   M02.271 Postimmunization arthropathy, <u>right</u> ankle and foot
   M02.272 Postimmunization arthropathy, <u>left</u> ankle and foot
   M02.279 Postimmunization arthropathy, <u>unspecified</u> ankle and foot
M02.28 Postimmunization arthropathy, <u>vertebrae</u>
M02.29 Postimmunization arthropathy, <u>multiple sites</u>
M02.3- <u>Reiter's disease</u> — An autoimmune form that is characterized by inflammation of the large joints, eyes, and genitals or urinary tract.
    Reactive arthritis
cc M02.30 Reiter's disease, <u>unspecified</u> site
M02.31- Reiter's disease, <u>shoulder</u>
  cc M02.311 Reiter's disease, <u>right</u> shoulder
  cc M02.312 Reiter's disease, <u>left</u> shoulder
  cc M02.319 Reiter's disease, <u>unspecified</u> shoulder
M02.32- Reiter's disease, <u>elbow</u>
  cc M02.321 Reiter's disease, <u>right</u> elbow
  cc M02.322 Reiter's disease, <u>left</u> elbow
  cc M02.329 Reiter's disease, <u>unspecified</u> elbow
M02.33- Reiter's disease, <u>wrist</u>
    Reiter's disease, carpal bones
  cc M02.331 Reiter's disease, <u>right</u> wrist
  cc M02.332 Reiter's disease, <u>left</u> wrist
  cc M02.339 Reiter's disease, <u>unspecified</u> wrist

M 0 2 - M 0 2

M02.34- Reiter's disease, <u>hand</u>
     Reiter's disease, metacarpus and phalanges
   cc M02.341   Reiter's disease, <u>right</u> hand
   cc M02.342   Reiter's disease, <u>left</u> hand
   cc M02.349   Reiter's disease, <u>unspecified</u> hand
M02.35- Reiter's disease, <u>hip</u>
   cc M02.351   Reiter's disease, <u>right</u> hip
   cc M02.352   Reiter's disease, <u>left</u> hip
   cc M02.359   Reiter's disease, <u>unspecified</u> hip
M02.36- Reiter's disease, <u>knee</u>
   cc M02.361   Reiter's disease, <u>right</u> knee
   cc M02.362   Reiter's disease, <u>left</u> knee
   cc M02.369   Reiter's disease, <u>unspecified</u> knee
M02.37- Reiter's disease, <u>ankle and foot</u>
     Reiter's disease, tarsus, metatarsus and phalanges
   cc M02.371   Reiter's disease, <u>right</u> ankle and foot
   cc M02.372   Reiter's disease, <u>left</u> ankle and foot
   cc M02.379   Reiter's disease, <u>unspecified</u> ankle and foot
  cc M02.38 Reiter's disease, <u>vertebrae</u>
  cc M02.39 Reiter's disease, <u>multiple sites</u>
M02.8- <u>Other reactive</u> arthropathies
  cc M02.80 Other reactive arthropathies, <u>unspecified</u> site —
      [Not Allowed as PDX]
M02.81- Other reactive arthropathies, <u>shoulder</u>
   cc M02.811   Other reactive arthropathies, <u>right</u> shoulder —
      [Not Allowed as PDX]
   cc M02.812   Other reactive arthropathies, <u>left</u> shoulder —
      [Not Allowed as PDX]
   cc M02.819   Other reactive arthropathies, <u>unspecified</u>
      shoulder — [Not Allowed as PDX]
M02.82- Other reactive arthropathies, <u>elbow</u>
   cc M02.821   Other reactive arthropathies, <u>right</u> elbow —
      [Not Allowed as PDX]
   cc M02.822   Other reactive arthropathies, <u>left</u> elbow —
      [Not Allowed as PDX]
   cc M02.829   Other reactive arthropathies, <u>unspecified</u> elbow —
      [Not Allowed as PDX]
M02.83- Other reactive arthropathies, <u>wrist</u>
     Other reactive arthropathies, carpal bones
   cc M02.831   Other reactive arthropathies, <u>right</u> wrist —
      [Not Allowed as PDX]
   cc M02.832   Other reactive arthropathies, <u>left</u> wrist —
      [Not Allowed as PDX]
   cc M02.839   Other reactive arthropathies, <u>unspecified</u> wrist —
      [Not Allowed as PDX]
M02.84- Other reactive arthropathies, <u>hand</u>
     Other reactive arthropathies, metacarpus and phalanges
   cc M02.841   Other reactive arthropathies, <u>right</u> hand —
      [Not Allowed as PDX]
   cc M02.842   Other reactive arthropathies, <u>left</u> hand —
      [Not Allowed as PDX]
   cc M02.849   Other reactive arthropathies, <u>unspecified</u> hand —
      [Not Allowed as PDX]
M02.85- Other reactive arthropathies, <u>hip</u>
   cc M02.851   Other reactive arthropathies, <u>right</u> hip —
      [Not Allowed as PDX]
   cc M02.852   Other reactive arthropathies, <u>left</u> hip —
      [Not Allowed as PDX]
   cc M02.859   Other reactive arthropathies, <u>unspecified</u> hip —
      [Not Allowed as PDX]
M02.86- Other reactive arthropathies, <u>knee</u>
   cc M02.861   Other reactive arthropathies, <u>right</u> knee —
      [Not Allowed as PDX]
   cc M02.862   Other reactive arthropathies, <u>left</u> knee —
      [Not Allowed as PDX]
   cc M02.869   Other reactive arthropathies, <u>unspecified</u> knee —
      [Not Allowed as PDX]

M02.87- Other reactive arthropathies, <u>ankle and foot</u>
     Other reactive arthropathies, tarsus, metatarsus and
     phalanges
   cc M02.871   Other reactive arthropathies, <u>right</u> ankle and
      foot — [Not Allowed as PDX]
   cc M02.872   Other reactive arthropathies, <u>left</u> ankle and foot —
      [Not Allowed as PDX]
   cc M02.879   Other reactive arthropathies, <u>unspecified</u> ankle
      and foot — [Not Allowed as PDX]
  cc M02.88 Other reactive arthropathies, <u>vertebrae</u> —
      [Not Allowed as PDX]
  cc M02.89 Other reactive arthropathies, <u>multiple sites</u> —
      [Not Allowed as PDX]
M02.9   Reactive arthropathy, <u>unspecified</u> — [Not Allowed as PDX]

Autoinflammatory syndromes (M04)

M04- <u>Autoinflammatory syndromes</u> — Disorders involving regulation of the immune system that are caused by genetic mutations and are generally characterized by recurrent systemic inflammation, fever, rashes, arthritis, ophthalmic inflammation, headaches, and lymphadenopathy, and some may lead to secondary amyloidosis.
   Excludes ❷: *Crohn's disease (K50.-)*

M04.1   **Periodic fever syndromes** — A form involving recurrent fever episodes.
     Familial Mediterranean fever — A form caused by the mutation of the MEFV gene that is characterized by brief episodes of fever, arthritis, rash on the lower legs, and in some cases pleuritis and peritonitis.
     Hyperimmunoglobin D syndrome — A form caused by the mutation of the MVK gene that is characterized by episodes of fever, cervical lymphadenopathy, diffuse rash, headache, arthritis, and abdominal pain.
     Mevalonate kinase deficiency — A form caused by the mutation of the MVK gene that is characterized by episodes of fever, enlarged spleen, diffuse rash, central nervous system conditions, arthritis, and abdominal pain.
     Tumor necrosis factor receptor associated periodic syndrome [TRAPS] — A form caused by the mutation of the TNFRSF1A gene that is characterized by episodes of fever, migrating rash with deep pain under the rash, periorbital edema, myalgia, arthritis, and abdominal and chest pain.

M04.2   **Cryopyrin-associated periodic syndromes** — A form caused by the mutation of the NLRP3 gene that is characterized by recurrent episodes of fever, urticarial rash, arthralgias, non-infectious conjunctivitis, and headaches.
     Chronic infantile neurological, cutaneous and articular syndrome [CINCA] — A severe form characterized by an ever-present rash, aseptic meningitis, and papilledema.
     Familial cold autoinflammatory syndrome — A milder form triggered by cold exposure.
     Familial cold urticaria — A milder form triggered by cold exposure.
     Muckle-Wells syndrome — A more severe form with more frequent and prolonged episodes and may include headaches from aseptic meningitis.
     Neonatal onset multisystemic inflammatory disorder [NOMID] — A severe form characterized by an ever-present rash, aseptic meningitis, and papilledema.

M04.8   **Other autoinflammatory syndromes**
     Blau syndrome — A form caused by the mutation of the NOD2 gene that is characterized by daily intermittent fevers, rash, granulomatosis, arthritis, and uveitis.
     Deficiency of interleukin 1 receptor antagonist [DIRA] — A form caused by the mutation of the IR1RN gene that is characterized by a severe pustular rash, osteitis, and joint swelling.
     Majeed syndrome — A form caused by the mutation of the LPIN2 gene that is characterized by high fevers, chronic recurrent multifocal osteomyelitis, inflammatory dermatosis, and dyserythropoietic anemia.
     Periodic fever, aphthous stomatitis, pharyngitis, and adenopathy syndrome [PFAPA] — A form caused by the mutation of an unknown gene that is characterized by periodic fever, aphthous stomatitis, pharyngitis, and adenopathy.
     Pyogenic arthritis, pyoderma gangrenosum, and acne syndrome [PAPA] — A form caused by the mutation of the PSTPIP1 gene that is characterized by periodic non-infectious pyogenic arthritis, pyoderma gangrenosum, and cystic acne.

M04.9   **Autoinflammatory syndrome, unspecified**

Inflammatory polyarthropathies (M05-M14)

M05- <u>Rheumatoid arthritis with rheumatoid factor</u> — A chronic, systemic autoimmune inflammatory disease characterized by inflammation of the joint structures with resultant crippling deformities that may affect organs throughout the body with the presence of the rheumatoid factor autoantibody in the blood.

Excludes 1: *juvenile rheumatoid arthritis (M08-)*
rheumatic fever (I00)
rheumatoid arthritis of spine (M45-)

M05.0- <u>Felty's syndrome</u> — A form with an enlarged spleen, abnormally low white blood cell count, and repeated infections.

Rheumatoid arthritis with splenoadenomegaly and leukopenia

M05.00 Felty's syndrome, <u>unspecified</u> site

M05.01- Felty's syndrome, <u>shoulder</u>

    M05.011 Felty's syndrome, <u>right</u> shoulder

    M05.012 Felty's syndrome, <u>left</u> shoulder

    M05.019 Felty's syndrome, <u>unspecified</u> shoulder

M05.02- Felty's syndrome, <u>elbow</u>

    M05.021 Felty's syndrome, <u>right</u> elbow

    M05.022 Felty's syndrome, <u>left</u> elbow

    M05.029 Felty's syndrome, <u>unspecified</u> elbow

M05.03- Felty's syndrome, <u>wrist</u>

    Felty's syndrome, carpal bones

    M05.031 Felty's syndrome, <u>right</u> wrist

    M05.032 Felty's syndrome, <u>left</u> wrist

    M05.039 Felty's syndrome, <u>unspecified</u> wrist

M05.04- Felty's syndrome, <u>hand</u>

    Felty's syndrome, metacarpus and phalanges

    M05.041 Felty's syndrome, <u>right</u> hand

    M05.042 Felty's syndrome, <u>left</u> hand

    M05.049 Felty's syndrome, <u>unspecified</u> hand

M05.05- Felty's syndrome, <u>hip</u>

    M05.051 Felty's syndrome, <u>right</u> hip

    M05.052 Felty's syndrome, <u>left</u> hip

    M05.059 Felty's syndrome, <u>unspecified</u> hip

M05.06- Felty's syndrome, <u>knee</u>

    M05.061 Felty's syndrome, <u>right</u> knee

    M05.062 Felty's syndrome, <u>left</u> knee

    M05.069 Felty's syndrome, <u>unspecified</u> knee

M05.07- Felty's syndrome, <u>ankle and foot</u>

    Felty's syndrome, tarsus, metatarsus and phalanges

    M05.071 Felty's syndrome, <u>right</u> ankle and foot

    M05.072 Felty's syndrome, <u>left</u> ankle and foot

    M05.079 Felty's syndrome, <u>unspecified</u> ankle and foot

M05.09 Felty's syndrome, <u>multiple sites</u>

M05.1- Rheumatoid <u>lung disease</u> <u>with</u> rheumatoid <u>arthritis</u> — A form with pulmonary disorders that may include bronchiolitis, pleural effusion, nodules, and interstitial lung disease.

M05.10 Rheumatoid lung disease with rheumatoid arthritis of <u>unspecified</u> site

M05.11- Rheumatoid lung disease with rheumatoid arthritis of <u>shoulder</u>

    M05.111 Rheumatoid lung disease with rheumatoid arthritis of <u>right</u> shoulder

    M05.112 Rheumatoid lung disease with rheumatoid arthritis of <u>left</u> shoulder

    M05.119 Rheumatoid lung disease with rheumatoid arthritis of <u>unspecified</u> shoulder

M05.12- Rheumatoid lung disease with rheumatoid arthritis of <u>elbow</u>

    M05.121 Rheumatoid lung disease with rheumatoid arthritis of <u>right</u> elbow

    M05.122 Rheumatoid lung disease with rheumatoid arthritis of <u>left</u> elbow

    M05.129 Rheumatoid lung disease with rheumatoid arthritis of <u>unspecified</u> elbow

M05.13- Rheumatoid lung disease with rheumatoid arthritis of <u>wrist</u>

    Rheumatoid lung disease with rheumatoid arthritis, carpal bones

    M05.131 Rheumatoid lung disease with rheumatoid arthritis of <u>right</u> wrist

    M05.132 Rheumatoid lung disease with rheumatoid arthritis of <u>left</u> wrist

    M05.139 Rheumatoid lung disease with rheumatoid arthritis of <u>unspecified</u> wrist

M05.14- Rheumatoid lung disease with rheumatoid arthritis of <u>hand</u>

    Rheumatoid lung disease with rheumatoid arthritis, metacarpus and phalanges

    M05.141 Rheumatoid lung disease with rheumatoid arthritis of <u>right</u> hand

    M05.142 Rheumatoid lung disease with rheumatoid arthritis of <u>left</u> hand

    M05.149 Rheumatoid lung disease with rheumatoid arthritis of <u>unspecified</u> hand

M05.15- Rheumatoid lung disease with rheumatoid arthritis of <u>hip</u>

    M05.151 Rheumatoid lung disease with rheumatoid arthritis of <u>right</u> hip

    M05.152 Rheumatoid lung disease with rheumatoid arthritis of <u>left</u> hip

    M05.159 Rheumatoid lung disease with rheumatoid arthritis of <u>unspecified</u> hip

M05.16- Rheumatoid lung disease with rheumatoid arthritis of <u>knee</u>

    M05.161 Rheumatoid lung disease with rheumatoid arthritis of <u>right</u> knee

    M05.162 Rheumatoid lung disease with rheumatoid arthritis of <u>left</u> knee

    M05.169 Rheumatoid lung disease with rheumatoid arthritis of <u>unspecified</u> knee

M05.17- Rheumatoid lung disease with rheumatoid arthritis of <u>ankle and foot</u>

    Rheumatoid lung disease with rheumatoid arthritis, tarsus, metatarsus and phalanges

    M05.171 Rheumatoid lung disease with rheumatoid arthritis of <u>right</u> ankle and foot

    M05.172 Rheumatoid lung disease with rheumatoid arthritis of <u>left</u> ankle and foot

    M05.179 Rheumatoid lung disease with rheumatoid arthritis of <u>unspecified</u> ankle and foot

M05.19 Rheumatoid lung disease with rheumatoid arthritis of <u>multiple sites</u>

M05.2- Rheumatoid <u>vasculitis</u> <u>with</u> rheumatoid <u>arthritis</u> — A form with vascular disorders involving inflammation of the medium and small arteries throughout the body causing rashes, numbness, tingling, and/or loss of sensation.

M05.20 Rheumatoid vasculitis with rheumatoid arthritis of <u>unspecified</u> site

M05.21- Rheumatoid vasculitis with rheumatoid arthritis of <u>shoulder</u>

    M05.211 Rheumatoid vasculitis with rheumatoid arthritis of <u>right</u> shoulder

    M05.212 Rheumatoid vasculitis with rheumatoid arthritis of <u>left</u> shoulder

    M05.219 Rheumatoid vasculitis with rheumatoid arthritis of <u>unspecified</u> shoulder

M05.22- Rheumatoid vasculitis with rheumatoid arthritis of <u>elbow</u>

    M05.221 Rheumatoid vasculitis with rheumatoid arthritis of <u>right</u> elbow

    M05.222 Rheumatoid vasculitis with rheumatoid arthritis of <u>left</u> elbow

    M05.229 Rheumatoid vasculitis with rheumatoid arthritis of <u>unspecified</u> elbow

M05 - M05

M05.23- Rheumatoid vasculitis with rheumatoid arthritis of <u>wrist</u>
Rheumatoid vasculitis with rheumatoid arthritis, carpal bones

  M05.231 Rheumatoid vasculitis with rheumatoid arthritis of <u>right</u> wrist

  M05.232 Rheumatoid vasculitis with rheumatoid arthritis of <u>left</u> wrist

  M05.239 Rheumatoid vasculitis with rheumatoid arthritis of <u>unspecified</u> wrist

M05.24- Rheumatoid vasculitis with rheumatoid arthritis of <u>hand</u>
Rheumatoid vasculitis with rheumatoid arthritis, metacarpus and phalanges

  M05.241 Rheumatoid vasculitis with rheumatoid arthritis of <u>right</u> hand

  M05.242 Rheumatoid vasculitis with rheumatoid arthritis of <u>left</u> hand

  M05.249 Rheumatoid vasculitis with rheumatoid arthritis of <u>unspecified</u> hand

M05.25- Rheumatoid vasculitis with rheumatoid arthritis of <u>hip</u>

  M05.251 Rheumatoid vasculitis with rheumatoid arthritis of <u>right</u> hip

  M05.252 Rheumatoid vasculitis with rheumatoid arthritis of <u>left</u> hip

  M05.259 Rheumatoid vasculitis with rheumatoid arthritis of <u>unspecified</u> hip

M05.26- Rheumatoid vasculitis with rheumatoid arthritis of <u>knee</u>

  M05.261 Rheumatoid vasculitis with rheumatoid arthritis of <u>right</u> knee

  M05.262 Rheumatoid vasculitis with rheumatoid arthritis of <u>left</u> knee

  M05.269 Rheumatoid vasculitis with rheumatoid arthritis of <u>unspecified</u> knee

M05.27- Rheumatoid vasculitis with rheumatoid arthritis of <u>ankle and foot</u>
Rheumatoid vasculitis with rheumatoid arthritis, tarsus, metatarsus and phalanges

  M05.271 Rheumatoid vasculitis with rheumatoid arthritis of <u>right</u> ankle and foot

  M05.272 Rheumatoid vasculitis with rheumatoid arthritis of <u>left</u> ankle and foot

  M05.279 Rheumatoid vasculitis with rheumatoid arthritis of <u>unspecified</u> ankle and foot

M05.29 Rheumatoid vasculitis with rheumatoid arthritis of <u>multiple sites</u>

M05.3- Rheumatoid <u>heart</u> disease <u>with</u> rheumatoid <u>arthritis</u> — A form with heart disorders.
Rheumatoid carditis
Rheumatoid endocarditis
Rheumatoid myocarditis
Rheumatoid pericarditis

M05.30 Rheumatoid heart disease with rheumatoid arthritis of <u>unspecified</u> site

M05.31- Rheumatoid heart disease with rheumatoid arthritis of <u>shoulder</u>

  M05.311 Rheumatoid heart disease with rheumatoid arthritis of <u>right</u> shoulder

  M05.312 Rheumatoid heart disease with rheumatoid arthritis of <u>left</u> shoulder

  M05.319 Rheumatoid heart disease with rheumatoid arthritis of <u>unspecified</u> shoulder

M05.32- Rheumatoid heart disease with rheumatoid arthritis of <u>elbow</u>

  M05.321 Rheumatoid heart disease with rheumatoid arthritis of <u>right</u> elbow

  M05.322 Rheumatoid heart disease with rheumatoid arthritis of <u>left</u> elbow

  M05.329 Rheumatoid heart disease with rheumatoid arthritis of <u>unspecified</u> elbow

M05.33- Rheumatoid heart disease with rheumatoid arthritis of <u>wrist</u>
Rheumatoid heart disease with rheumatoid arthritis, carpal bones

  M05.331 Rheumatoid heart disease with rheumatoid arthritis of <u>right</u> wrist

  M05.332 Rheumatoid heart disease with rheumatoid arthritis of <u>left</u> wrist

  M05.339 Rheumatoid heart disease with rheumatoid arthritis of <u>unspecified</u> wrist

M05.34- Rheumatoid heart disease with rheumatoid arthritis of <u>hand</u>
Rheumatoid heart disease with rheumatoid arthritis, metacarpus and phalanges

  M05.341 Rheumatoid heart disease with rheumatoid arthritis of <u>right</u> hand

  M05.342 Rheumatoid heart disease with rheumatoid arthritis of <u>left</u> hand

  M05.349 Rheumatoid heart disease with rheumatoid arthritis of <u>unspecified</u> hand

M05.35- Rheumatoid heart disease with rheumatoid arthritis of <u>hip</u>

  M05.351 Rheumatoid heart disease with rheumatoid arthritis of <u>right</u> hip

  M05.352 Rheumatoid heart disease with rheumatoid arthritis of <u>left</u> hip

  M05.359 Rheumatoid heart disease with rheumatoid arthritis of <u>unspecified</u> hip

M05.36- Rheumatoid heart disease with rheumatoid arthritis of <u>knee</u>

  M05.361 Rheumatoid heart disease with rheumatoid arthritis of <u>right</u> knee

  M05.362 Rheumatoid heart disease with rheumatoid arthritis of <u>left</u> knee

  M05.369 Rheumatoid heart disease with rheumatoid arthritis of <u>unspecified</u> knee

M05.37- Rheumatoid heart disease with rheumatoid arthritis of <u>ankle and foot</u>
Rheumatoid heart disease with rheumatoid arthritis, tarsus, metatarsus and phalanges

  M05.371 Rheumatoid heart disease with rheumatoid arthritis of <u>right</u> ankle and foot

  M05.372 Rheumatoid heart disease with rheumatoid arthritis of <u>left</u> ankle and foot

  M05.379 Rheumatoid heart disease with rheumatoid arthritis of <u>unspecified</u> ankle and foot

M05.39 Rheumatoid heart disease with rheumatoid arthritis of <u>multiple sites</u>

M05.4- Rheumatoid <u>myopathy</u> <u>with</u> rheumatoid <u>arthritis</u> — A form involving the muscles causing inflammation and weakness.

cc **M05.40** Rheumatoid myopathy with rheumatoid arthritis of <u>unspecified</u> site

M05.41- Rheumatoid myopathy with rheumatoid arthritis of <u>shoulder</u>

  cc **M05.411** Rheumatoid myopathy with rheumatoid arthritis of <u>right</u> shoulder

  cc **M05.412** Rheumatoid myopathy with rheumatoid arthritis of <u>left</u> shoulder

  cc **M05.419** Rheumatoid myopathy with rheumatoid arthritis of <u>unspecified</u> shoulder

M05.42- Rheumatoid myopathy with rheumatoid arthritis of <u>elbow</u>

  cc **M05.421** Rheumatoid myopathy with rheumatoid arthritis of <u>right</u> elbow

  cc **M05.422** Rheumatoid myopathy with rheumatoid arthritis of <u>left</u> elbow

  cc **M05.429** Rheumatoid myopathy with rheumatoid arthritis of <u>unspecified</u> elbow

M05 – M05

M05.43- Rheumatoid myopathy with rheumatoid arthritis of <u>wrist</u>
Rheumatoid myopathy with rheumatoid arthritis, carpal bones

cc **M05.431** Rheumatoid myopathy with rheumatoid arthritis of <u>right</u> wrist

cc **M05.432** Rheumatoid myopathy with rheumatoid arthritis of <u>left</u> wrist

cc **M05.439** Rheumatoid myopathy with rheumatoid arthritis of <u>unspecified</u> wrist

M05.44- Rheumatoid myopathy with rheumatoid arthritis of <u>hand</u>
Rheumatoid myopathy with rheumatoid arthritis, metacarpus and phalanges

cc **M05.441** Rheumatoid myopathy with rheumatoid arthritis of <u>right</u> hand

cc **M05.442** Rheumatoid myopathy with rheumatoid arthritis of <u>left</u> hand

cc **M05.449** Rheumatoid myopathy with rheumatoid arthritis of <u>unspecified</u> hand

M05.45- Rheumatoid myopathy with rheumatoid arthritis of <u>hip</u>

cc **M05.451** Rheumatoid myopathy with rheumatoid arthritis of <u>right</u> hip

cc **M05.452** Rheumatoid myopathy with rheumatoid arthritis of <u>left</u> hip

cc **M05.459** Rheumatoid myopathy with rheumatoid arthritis of <u>unspecified</u> hip

M05.46- Rheumatoid myopathy with rheumatoid arthritis of <u>knee</u>

cc **M05.461** Rheumatoid myopathy with rheumatoid arthritis of <u>right</u> knee

cc **M05.462** Rheumatoid myopathy with rheumatoid arthritis of <u>left</u> knee

cc **M05.469** Rheumatoid myopathy with rheumatoid arthritis of <u>unspecified</u> knee

M05.47- Rheumatoid myopathy with rheumatoid arthritis of <u>ankle and foot</u>
Rheumatoid myopathy with rheumatoid arthritis, tarsus, metatarsus and phalanges

cc **M05.471** Rheumatoid myopathy with rheumatoid arthritis of <u>right</u> ankle and foot

cc **M05.472** Rheumatoid myopathy with rheumatoid arthritis of <u>left</u> ankle and foot

cc **M05.479** Rheumatoid myopathy with rheumatoid arthritis of <u>unspecified</u> ankle and foot

cc **M05.49** Rheumatoid myopathy with rheumatoid arthritis of <u>multiple sites</u>

M05.5- Rheumatoid <u>polyneuropathy</u> <u>with</u> rheumatoid <u>arthritis</u> — A form affecting the peripheral nervous system causing inflammation, damage to the nerves, and pain.

M05.50 Rheumatoid polyneuropathy with rheumatoid arthritis of <u>unspecified</u> site

M05.51- Rheumatoid polyneuropathy with rheumatoid arthritis of <u>shoulder</u>

M05.511 Rheumatoid polyneuropathy with rheumatoid arthritis of <u>right</u> shoulder

M05.512 Rheumatoid polyneuropathy with rheumatoid arthritis of <u>left</u> shoulder

M05.519 Rheumatoid polyneuropathy with rheumatoid arthritis of <u>unspecified</u> shoulder

M05.52- Rheumatoid polyneuropathy with rheumatoid arthritis of <u>elbow</u>

M05.521 Rheumatoid polyneuropathy with rheumatoid arthritis of <u>right</u> elbow

M05.522 Rheumatoid polyneuropathy with rheumatoid arthritis of <u>left</u> elbow

M05.529 Rheumatoid polyneuropathy with rheumatoid arthritis of <u>unspecified</u> elbow

M05.53- Rheumatoid polyneuropathy with rheumatoid arthritis of <u>wrist</u>
Rheumatoid polyneuropathy with rheumatoid arthritis, carpal bones

M05.531 Rheumatoid polyneuropathy with rheumatoid arthritis of <u>right</u> wrist

M05.532 Rheumatoid polyneuropathy with rheumatoid arthritis of <u>left</u> wrist

M05.539 Rheumatoid polyneuropathy with rheumatoid arthritis of <u>unspecified</u> wrist

M05.54- Rheumatoid polyneuropathy with rheumatoid arthritis of <u>hand</u>
Rheumatoid polyneuropathy with rheumatoid arthritis, metacarpus and phalanges

M05.541 Rheumatoid polyneuropathy with rheumatoid arthritis of <u>right</u> hand

M05.542 Rheumatoid polyneuropathy with rheumatoid arthritis of <u>left</u> hand

M05.549 Rheumatoid polyneuropathy with rheumatoid arthritis of <u>unspecified</u> hand

M05.55- Rheumatoid polyneuropathy with rheumatoid arthritis of <u>hip</u>

M05.551 Rheumatoid polyneuropathy with rheumatoid arthritis of <u>right</u> hip

M05.552 Rheumatoid polyneuropathy with rheumatoid arthritis of <u>left</u> hip

M05.559 Rheumatoid polyneuropathy with rheumatoid arthritis of <u>unspecified</u> hip

M05.56- Rheumatoid polyneuropathy with rheumatoid arthritis of <u>knee</u>

M05.561 Rheumatoid polyneuropathy with rheumatoid arthritis of <u>right</u> knee

M05.562 Rheumatoid polyneuropathy with rheumatoid arthritis of <u>left</u> knee

M05.569 Rheumatoid polyneuropathy with rheumatoid arthritis of <u>unspecified</u> knee

M05.57- Rheumatoid polyneuropathy with rheumatoid arthritis of <u>ankle and foot</u>
Rheumatoid polyneuropathy with rheumatoid arthritis, tarsus, metatarsus and phalanges

M05.571 Rheumatoid polyneuropathy with rheumatoid arthritis of <u>right</u> ankle and foot

M05.572 Rheumatoid polyneuropathy with rheumatoid arthritis of <u>left</u> ankle and foot

M05.579 Rheumatoid polyneuropathy with rheumatoid arthritis of <u>unspecified</u> ankle and foot

M05.59 Rheumatoid polyneuropathy with rheumatoid arthritis of <u>multiple sites</u>

M05.6- Rheumatoid <u>arthritis</u> <u>with</u> involvement of <u>other organs and systems</u>

M05.60 Rheumatoid arthritis of <u>unspecified</u> site with involvement of other organs and systems

M05.61- Rheumatoid arthritis of <u>shoulder</u> with involvement of other organs and systems

M05.611 Rheumatoid arthritis of <u>right</u> shoulder with involvement of other organs and systems

M05.612 Rheumatoid arthritis of <u>left</u> shoulder with involvement of other organs and systems

M05.619 Rheumatoid arthritis of <u>unspecified</u> shoulder with involvement of other organs and systems

M05.62- Rheumatoid arthritis of <u>elbow</u> with involvement of other organs and systems

M05.621 Rheumatoid arthritis of <u>right</u> elbow with involvement of other organs and systems

M05.622 Rheumatoid arthritis of <u>left</u> elbow with involvement of other organs and systems

M05.629 Rheumatoid arthritis of <u>unspecified</u> elbow with involvement of other organs and systems

M05-M05

M05.63- Rheumatoid arthritis of <u>wrist</u> with involvement of other organs and systems
>> Rheumatoid arthritis of carpal bones with involvement of other organs and systems

> **M05.631** Rheumatoid arthritis of <u>right</u> wrist with involvement of other organs and systems

> **M05.632** Rheumatoid arthritis of <u>left</u> wrist with involvement of other organs and systems

> **M05.639** Rheumatoid arthritis of <u>unspecified</u> wrist with involvement of other organs and systems

M05.64- Rheumatoid arthritis of <u>hand</u> with involvement of other organs and systems
>> Rheumatoid arthritis of metacarpus and phalanges with involvement of other organs and systems

> **M05.641** Rheumatoid arthritis of <u>right</u> hand with involvement of other organs and systems

> **M05.642** Rheumatoid arthritis of <u>left</u> hand with involvement of other organs and systems

> **M05.649** Rheumatoid arthritis of <u>unspecified</u> hand with involvement of other organs and systems

M05.65- Rheumatoid arthritis of <u>hip</u> with involvement of other organs and systems

> **M05.651** Rheumatoid arthritis of <u>right</u> hip with involvement of other organs and systems

> **M05.652** Rheumatoid arthritis of <u>left</u> hip with involvement of other organs and systems

> **M05.659** Rheumatoid arthritis of <u>unspecified</u> hip with involvement of other organs and systems

M05.66- Rheumatoid arthritis of <u>knee</u> with involvement of other organs and systems

> **M05.661** Rheumatoid arthritis of <u>right</u> knee with involvement of other organs and systems

> **M05.662** Rheumatoid arthritis of <u>left</u> knee with involvement of other organs and systems

> **M05.669** Rheumatoid arthritis of <u>unspecified</u> knee with involvement of other organs and systems

M05.67- Rheumatoid arthritis of <u>ankle and foot</u> with involvement of other organs and systems
>> Rheumatoid arthritis of tarsus, metatarsus and phalanges with involvement of other organs and systems

> **M05.671** Rheumatoid arthritis of <u>right</u> ankle and foot with involvement of other organs and systems

> **M05.672** Rheumatoid arthritis of <u>left</u> ankle and foot with involvement of other organs and systems

> **M05.679** Rheumatoid arthritis of <u>unspecified</u> ankle and foot with involvement of other organs and systems

M05.69 Rheumatoid arthritis of <u>multiple sites</u> with involvement of other organs and systems

M05.7- Rheumatoid <u>arthritis with</u> rheumatoid <u>factor without</u> organ or systems involvement — A form without the known involvement of other organs or tissues.

M05.70 Rheumatoid arthritis with rheumatoid factor of <u>unspecified</u> site without organ or systems involvement

M05.71- Rheumatoid arthritis with rheumatoid factor of <u>shoulder</u> without organ or systems involvement

> **M05.711** Rheumatoid arthritis with rheumatoid factor of <u>right</u> shoulder without organ or systems involvement

> **M05.712** Rheumatoid arthritis with rheumatoid factor of <u>left</u> shoulder without organ or systems involvement

> **M05.719** Rheumatoid arthritis with rheumatoid factor of <u>unspecified</u> shoulder without organ or systems involvement

M05.72- Rheumatoid arthritis with rheumatoid factor of <u>elbow</u> without organ or systems involvement

> **M05.721** Rheumatoid arthritis with rheumatoid factor of <u>right</u> elbow without organ or systems involvement

> **M05.722** Rheumatoid arthritis with rheumatoid factor of <u>left</u> elbow without organ or systems involvement

> **M05.729** Rheumatoid arthritis with rheumatoid factor of <u>unspecified</u> elbow without organ or systems involvement

M05.73- Rheumatoid arthritis with rheumatoid factor of <u>wrist</u> without organ or systems involvement

> **M05.731** Rheumatoid arthritis with rheumatoid factor of <u>right</u> wrist without organ or systems involvement

> **M05.732** Rheumatoid arthritis with rheumatoid factor of <u>left</u> wrist without organ or systems involvement

> **M05.739** Rheumatoid arthritis with rheumatoid factor of <u>unspecified</u> wrist without organ or systems involvement

M05.74- Rheumatoid arthritis with rheumatoid factor of <u>hand</u> without organ or systems involvement

> **M05.741** Rheumatoid arthritis with rheumatoid factor of <u>right</u> hand without organ or systems involvement

> **M05.742** Rheumatoid arthritis with rheumatoid factor of <u>left</u> hand without organ or systems involvement

> **M05.749** Rheumatoid arthritis with rheumatoid factor of <u>unspecified</u> hand without organ or systems involvement

M05.75- Rheumatoid arthritis with rheumatoid factor of <u>hip</u> without organ or systems involvement

> **M05.751** Rheumatoid arthritis with rheumatoid factor of <u>right</u> hip without organ or systems involvement

> **M05.752** Rheumatoid arthritis with rheumatoid factor of <u>left</u> hip without organ or systems involvement

> **M05.759** Rheumatoid arthritis with rheumatoid factor of <u>unspecified</u> hip without organ or systems involvement

M05.76- Rheumatoid arthritis with rheumatoid factor of <u>knee</u> without organ or systems involvement

> **M05.761** Rheumatoid arthritis with rheumatoid factor of <u>right</u> knee without organ or systems involvement

> **M05.762** Rheumatoid arthritis with rheumatoid factor of <u>left</u> knee without organ or systems involvement

> **M05.769** Rheumatoid arthritis with rheumatoid factor of <u>unspecified</u> knee without organ or systems involvement

M05.77- Rheumatoid arthritis with rheumatoid factor of <u>ankle and foot</u> without organ or systems involvement

> **M05.771** Rheumatoid arthritis with rheumatoid factor of <u>right</u> ankle and foot without organ or systems involvement

> **M05.772** Rheumatoid arthritis with rheumatoid factor of <u>left</u> ankle and foot without organ or systems involvement

> **M05.779** Rheumatoid arthritis with rheumatoid factor of <u>unspecified</u> ankle and foot without organ or systems involvement

M05.79 Rheumatoid arthritis with rheumatoid factor of <u>multiple sites</u> without organ or systems involvement

M05.8- <u>Other</u> rheumatoid arthritis <u>with</u> rheumatoid <u>factor</u>

M05.80 Other rheumatoid arthritis with rheumatoid factor of <u>unspecified</u> site

M05.81- Other rheumatoid arthritis with rheumatoid factor of <u>shoulder</u>

> **M05.811** Other rheumatoid arthritis with rheumatoid factor of <u>right</u> shoulder

> **M05.812** Other rheumatoid arthritis with rheumatoid factor of <u>left</u> shoulder

> **M05.819** Other rheumatoid arthritis with rheumatoid factor of <u>unspecified</u> shoulder

M05 | M05

M05.82- Other rheumatoid arthritis with rheumatoid factor of <u>elbow</u>

    M05.821   Other rheumatoid arthritis with rheumatoid factor of <u>right</u> elbow

    M05.822   Other rheumatoid arthritis with rheumatoid factor of <u>left</u> elbow

    M05.829   Other rheumatoid arthritis with rheumatoid factor of <u>unspecified</u> elbow

M05.83- Other rheumatoid arthritis with rheumatoid factor of <u>wrist</u>

    M05.831   Other rheumatoid arthritis with rheumatoid factor of <u>right</u> wrist

    M05.832   Other rheumatoid arthritis with rheumatoid factor of <u>left</u> wrist

    M05.839   Other rheumatoid arthritis with rheumatoid factor of <u>unspecified</u> wrist

M05.84- Other rheumatoid arthritis with rheumatoid factor of <u>hand</u>

    M05.841   Other rheumatoid arthritis with rheumatoid factor of <u>right</u> hand

    M05.842   Other rheumatoid arthritis with rheumatoid factor of <u>left</u> hand

    M05.849   Other rheumatoid arthritis with rheumatoid factor of <u>unspecified</u> hand

M05.85- Other rheumatoid arthritis with rheumatoid factor of <u>hip</u>

    M05.851   Other rheumatoid arthritis with rheumatoid factor of <u>right</u> hip

    M05.852   Other rheumatoid arthritis with rheumatoid factor of <u>left</u> hip

    M05.859   Other rheumatoid arthritis with rheumatoid factor of <u>unspecified</u> hip

M05.86- Other rheumatoid arthritis with rheumatoid factor of <u>knee</u>

    M05.861   Other rheumatoid arthritis with rheumatoid factor of <u>right</u> knee

    M05.862   Other rheumatoid arthritis with rheumatoid factor of <u>left</u> knee

    M05.869   Other rheumatoid arthritis with rheumatoid factor of <u>unspecified</u> knee

M05.87- Other rheumatoid arthritis with rheumatoid factor of <u>ankle and foot</u>

    M05.871   Other rheumatoid arthritis with rheumatoid factor of <u>right</u> ankle and foot

    M05.872   Other rheumatoid arthritis with rheumatoid factor of <u>left</u> ankle and foot

    M05.879   Other rheumatoid arthritis with rheumatoid factor of <u>unspecified</u> ankle and foot

M05.89   Other rheumatoid arthritis with rheumatoid factor of <u>multiple sites</u>

M05.9   Rheumatoid arthritis with rheumatoid factor, <u>unspecified</u>

M06-   <u>Other rheumatoid arthritis</u>

M06.0-   Rheumatoid <u>arthritis</u> <u>without</u> rheumatoid <u>factor</u> — A chronic, systemic autoimmune inflammatory disease characterized by inflammation of the joint structures with resultant crippling deformities that may affect organs throughout the body WITHOUT the presence of the rheumatoid factor autoantibody in the blood.

    M06.00   Rheumatoid arthritis without rheumatoid factor, <u>unspecified</u> site

M06.01- Rheumatoid arthritis without rheumatoid factor, <u>shoulder</u>

    M06.011   Rheumatoid arthritis without rheumatoid factor, <u>right</u> shoulder

    M06.012   Rheumatoid arthritis without rheumatoid factor, <u>left</u> shoulder

    M06.019   Rheumatoid arthritis without rheumatoid factor, <u>unspecified</u> shoulder

M06.02- Rheumatoid arthritis without rheumatoid factor, <u>elbow</u>

    M06.021   Rheumatoid arthritis without rheumatoid factor, <u>right</u> elbow

    M06.022   Rheumatoid arthritis without rheumatoid factor, <u>left</u> elbow

    M06.029   Rheumatoid arthritis without rheumatoid factor, <u>unspecified</u> elbow

M06.03- Rheumatoid arthritis without rheumatoid factor, <u>wrist</u>

    M06.031   Rheumatoid arthritis without rheumatoid factor, <u>right</u> wrist

    M06.032   Rheumatoid arthritis without rheumatoid factor, <u>left</u> wrist

    M06.039   Rheumatoid arthritis without rheumatoid factor, <u>unspecified</u> wrist

M06.04- Rheumatoid arthritis without rheumatoid factor, <u>hand</u>

    M06.041   Rheumatoid arthritis without rheumatoid factor, <u>right</u> hand

    M06.042   Rheumatoid arthritis without rheumatoid factor, <u>left</u> hand

    M06.049   Rheumatoid arthritis without rheumatoid factor, <u>unspecified</u> hand

M06.05- Rheumatoid arthritis without rheumatoid factor, <u>hip</u>

    M06.051   Rheumatoid arthritis without rheumatoid factor, <u>right</u> hip

    M06.052   Rheumatoid arthritis without rheumatoid factor, <u>left</u> hip

    M06.059   Rheumatoid arthritis without rheumatoid factor, <u>unspecified</u> hip

M06.06- Rheumatoid arthritis without rheumatoid factor, <u>knee</u>

    M06.061   Rheumatoid arthritis without rheumatoid factor, <u>right</u> knee

    M06.062   Rheumatoid arthritis without rheumatoid factor, <u>left</u> knee

    M06.069   Rheumatoid arthritis without rheumatoid factor, <u>unspecified</u> knee

M06.07- Rheumatoid arthritis without rheumatoid factor, <u>ankle and foot</u>

    M06.071   Rheumatoid arthritis without rheumatoid factor, <u>right</u> ankle and foot

    M06.072   Rheumatoid arthritis without rheumatoid factor, <u>left</u> ankle and foot

    M06.079   Rheumatoid arthritis without rheumatoid factor, <u>unspecified</u> ankle and foot

M06.08   Rheumatoid arthritis without rheumatoid factor, <u>vertebrae</u>

M06.09   Rheumatoid arthritis without rheumatoid factor, <u>multiple sites</u>

M06.1   Adult-onset Still's disease — [Age/15-124] — A form characterized by high fevers, salmon-colored rash, and joint pain.

    Excludes 1:   Still's disease NOS (M08.2-)

M06.2-   <u>Rheumatoid bursitis</u> — A form characterized by inflammation of the bursae and tendons.

M06.20   Rheumatoid bursitis, <u>unspecified</u> site

M06.21- Rheumatoid bursitis, <u>shoulder</u>

    M06.211   Rheumatoid bursitis, <u>right</u> shoulder

    M06.212   Rheumatoid bursitis, <u>left</u> shoulder

    M06.219   Rheumatoid bursitis, <u>unspecified</u> shoulder

M06.22- Rheumatoid bursitis, <u>elbow</u>

    M06.221   Rheumatoid bursitis, <u>right</u> elbow

    M06.222   Rheumatoid bursitis, <u>left</u> elbow

    M06.229   Rheumatoid bursitis, <u>unspecified</u> elbow

M06.23- Rheumatoid bursitis, <u>wrist</u>

    M06.231   Rheumatoid bursitis, <u>right</u> wrist

    M06.232   Rheumatoid bursitis, <u>left</u> wrist

    M06.239   Rheumatoid bursitis, <u>unspecified</u> wrist

M05 - M06 (side tab)

M06.24- Rheumatoid bursitis, <u>hand</u>
    M06.241 Rheumatoid bursitis, <u>right</u> hand
    M06.242 Rheumatoid bursitis, <u>left</u> hand
    M06.249 Rheumatoid bursitis, <u>unspecified</u> hand
M06.25- Rheumatoid bursitis, <u>hip</u>
    M06.251 Rheumatoid bursitis, <u>right</u> hip
    M06.252 Rheumatoid bursitis, <u>left</u> hip
    M06.259 Rheumatoid bursitis, <u>unspecified</u> hip
M06.26- Rheumatoid bursitis, <u>knee</u>
    M06.261 Rheumatoid bursitis, <u>right</u> knee
    M06.262 Rheumatoid bursitis, <u>left</u> knee
    M06.269 Rheumatoid bursitis, <u>unspecified</u> knee
M06.27- Rheumatoid bursitis, <u>ankle and foot</u>
    M06.271 Rheumatoid bursitis, <u>right</u> ankle and foot
    M06.272 Rheumatoid bursitis, <u>left</u> ankle and foot
    M06.279 Rheumatoid bursitis, <u>unspecified</u> ankle and foot
M06.28 Rheumatoid bursitis, <u>vertebrae</u>
M06.29 Rheumatoid bursitis, <u>multiple sites</u>
M06.3- <u>Rheumatoid nodule</u> — A form characterized by soft tissue masses that are usually found in the subcutaneous tissue of the hands and arms.
M06.30 Rheumatoid nodule, <u>unspecified</u> site
M06.31- Rheumatoid nodule, <u>shoulder</u>
    M06.311 Rheumatoid nodule, <u>right</u> shoulder
    M06.312 Rheumatoid nodule, <u>left</u> shoulder
    M06.319 Rheumatoid nodule, <u>unspecified</u> shoulder
M06.32- Rheumatoid nodule, <u>elbow</u>
    M06.321 Rheumatoid nodule, <u>right</u> elbow
    M06.322 Rheumatoid nodule, <u>left</u> elbow
    M06.329 Rheumatoid nodule, <u>unspecified</u> elbow
M06.33- Rheumatoid nodule, <u>wrist</u>
    M06.331 Rheumatoid nodule, <u>right</u> wrist
    M06.332 Rheumatoid nodule, <u>left</u> wrist
    M06.339 Rheumatoid nodule, <u>unspecified</u> wrist
M06.34 Rheumatoid nodule, <u>hand</u>
    M06.341 Rheumatoid nodule, <u>right</u> hand
    M06.342 Rheumatoid nodule, <u>left</u> hand
    M06.349 Rheumatoid nodule, <u>unspecified</u> hand
M06.35- Rheumatoid nodule, <u>hip</u>
    M06.351 Rheumatoid nodule, <u>right</u> hip
    M06.352 Rheumatoid nodule, <u>left</u> hip
    M06.359 Rheumatoid nodule, <u>unspecified</u> hip
M06.36- Rheumatoid nodule, <u>knee</u>
    M06.361 Rheumatoid nodule, <u>right</u> knee
    M06.362 Rheumatoid nodule, <u>left</u> knee
    M06.369 Rheumatoid nodule, <u>unspecified</u> knee
M06.37- Rheumatoid nodule, <u>ankle and foot</u>
    M06.371 Rheumatoid nodule, <u>right</u> ankle and foot
    M06.372 Rheumatoid nodule, <u>left</u> ankle and foot
    M06.379 Rheumatoid nodule, <u>unspecified</u> ankle and foot
M06.38 Rheumatoid nodule, <u>vertebrae</u>
M06.39 Rheumatoid nodule, <u>multiple sites</u>
M06.4 Inflammatory polyarthropathy — A form affecting many joints and often symmetrically.
    Excludes 1:   *polyarthritis NOS (M13.0)*
M06.8- <u>Other specified</u> rheumatoid arthritis
M06.80 Other specified rheumatoid arthritis, <u>unspecified</u> site
M06.81- Other specified rheumatoid arthritis, <u>shoulder</u>
    M06.811 Other specified rheumatoid arthritis, <u>right</u> shoulder
    M06.812 Other specified rheumatoid arthritis, <u>left</u> shoulder
    M06.819 Other specified rheumatoid arthritis, <u>unspecified</u> shoulder

M06.82- Other specified rheumatoid arthritis, <u>elbow</u>
    M06.821 Other specified rheumatoid arthritis, <u>right</u> elbow
    M06.822 Other specified rheumatoid arthritis, <u>left</u> elbow
    M06.829 Other specified rheumatoid arthritis, <u>unspecified</u> elbow
M06.83- Other specified rheumatoid arthritis, <u>wrist</u>
    M06.831 Other specified rheumatoid arthritis, <u>right</u> wrist
    M06.832 Other specified rheumatoid arthritis, <u>left</u> wrist
    M06.839 Other specified rheumatoid arthritis, <u>unspecified</u> wrist
M06.84- Other specified rheumatoid arthritis, <u>hand</u>
    M06.841 Other specified rheumatoid arthritis, <u>right</u> hand
    M06.842 Other specified rheumatoid arthritis, <u>left</u> hand
    M06.849 Other specified rheumatoid arthritis, <u>unspecified</u> hand
M06.85- Other specified rheumatoid arthritis, <u>hip</u>
    M06.851 Other specified rheumatoid arthritis, <u>right</u> hip
    M06.852 Other specified rheumatoid arthritis, <u>left</u> hip
    M06.859 Other specified rheumatoid arthritis, <u>unspecified</u> hip
M06.86- Other specified rheumatoid arthritis, <u>knee</u>
    M06.861 Other specified rheumatoid arthritis, <u>right</u> knee
    M06.862 Other specified rheumatoid arthritis, <u>left</u> knee
    M06.869 Other specified rheumatoid arthritis, <u>unspecified</u> knee
M06.87- Other specified rheumatoid arthritis, <u>ankle and foot</u>
    M06.871 Other specified rheumatoid arthritis, <u>right</u> ankle and foot
    M06.872 Other specified rheumatoid arthritis, <u>left</u> ankle and foot
    M06.879 Other specified rheumatoid arthritis, <u>unspecified</u> ankle and foot
M06.88 Other specified rheumatoid arthritis, <u>vertebrae</u>
M06.89 Other specified rheumatoid arthritis, <u>multiple sites</u>
M06.9 Rheumatoid arthritis, <u>unspecified</u>
M07- Enteropathic arthropathies — An inflammatory joint disease that is linked with gastrointestinal pathology.
    Code also associated enteropathy, such as:
      Regional enteritis [Crohn's disease] (K50.-)
      Ulcerative colitis (K51.-)
    Excludes 1:   *psoriatic arthropathies (L40.5-)*
M07.6- Enteropathic arthropathies
M07.60 Enteropathic arthropathies, <u>unspecified</u> site
M07.61- Enteropathic arthropathies, <u>shoulder</u>
    M07.611 Enteropathic arthropathies, <u>right</u> shoulder
    M07.612 Enteropathic arthropathies, <u>left</u> shoulder
    M07.619 Enteropathic arthropathies, <u>unspecified</u> shoulder
M07.62- Enteropathic arthropathies, <u>elbow</u>
    M07.621 Enteropathic arthropathies, <u>right</u> elbow
    M07.622 Enteropathic arthropathies, <u>left</u> elbow
    M07.629 Enteropathic arthropathies, <u>unspecified</u> elbow
M07.63- Enteropathic arthropathies, <u>wrist</u>
    M07.631 Enteropathic arthropathies, <u>right</u> wrist
    M07.632 Enteropathic arthropathies, <u>left</u> wrist
    M07.639 Enteropathic arthropathies, <u>unspecified</u> wrist
M07.64- Enteropathic arthropathies, <u>hand</u>
    M07.641 Enteropathic arthropathies, <u>right</u> hand
    M07.642 Enteropathic arthropathies, <u>left</u> hand
    M07.649 Enteropathic arthropathies, <u>unspecified</u> hand
M07.65- Enteropathic arthropathies, <u>hip</u>
    M07.651 Enteropathic arthropathies, <u>right</u> hip
    M07.652 Enteropathic arthropathies, <u>left</u> hip
    M07.659 Enteropathic arthropathies, <u>unspecified</u> hip

M06-M07

M07.66- Enteropathic arthropathies, <u>knee</u>

   M07.661 Enteropathic arthropathies, <u>right</u> knee

   M07.662 Enteropathic arthropathies, <u>left</u> knee

   M07.669 Enteropathic arthropathies, <u>unspecified</u> knee

M07.67- Enteropathic arthropathies, <u>ankle and foot</u>

   M07.671 Enteropathic arthropathies, <u>right</u> ankle and foot

   M07.672 Enteropathic arthropathies, <u>left</u> ankle and foot

   M07.679 Enteropathic arthropathies, <u>unspecified</u> ankle and foot

M07.68 Enteropathic arthropathies, <u>vertebrae</u>

M07.69 Enteropathic arthropathies, <u>multiple sites</u>

M08- <u>Juvenile arthritis</u> — An autoimmune or inflammatory disease of the synovium of the joints that presents prior to 16-17 years of age that is usually characterized by joint swelling, joint pain, and redness and warmth over the affected joints.

   Code also any associated underlying condition, such as:

     Regional enteritis [Crohn's disease] (K50.-)

     Ulcerative colitis (K51.-)

   Excludes 1:   *arthropathy in Whipple's disease (M14.8)*

                Felty's syndrome (M05.0)

                juvenile dermatomyositis (M33.0-)

                psoriatic juvenile arthropathy (L40.54)

M08.0- <u>Unspecified</u> juvenile rheumatoid arthritis — A form specified as juvenile rheumatoid arthritis with or without the identification of the rheumatoid factor in the blood.

     Juvenile rheumatoid arthritis with or without rheumatoid factor

  M08.00 Unspecified juvenile rheumatoid arthritis of <u>unspecified</u> site

  M08.01- Unspecified juvenile rheumatoid arthritis, <u>shoulder</u>

   M08.011 Unspecified juvenile rheumatoid arthritis, <u>right</u> shoulder

   M08.012 Unspecified juvenile rheumatoid arthritis, <u>left</u> shoulder

   M08.019 Unspecified juvenile rheumatoid arthritis, <u>unspecified</u> shoulder

  M08.02- Unspecified juvenile rheumatoid arthritis of <u>elbow</u>

   M08.021 Unspecified juvenile rheumatoid arthritis, <u>right</u> elbow

   M08.022 Unspecified juvenile rheumatoid arthritis, <u>left</u> elbow

   M08.029 Unspecified juvenile rheumatoid arthritis, <u>unspecified</u> elbow

  M08.03- Unspecified juvenile rheumatoid arthritis, <u>wrist</u>

   M08.031 Unspecified juvenile rheumatoid arthritis, <u>right</u> wrist

   M08.032 Unspecified juvenile rheumatoid arthritis, <u>left</u> wrist

   M08.039 Unspecified juvenile rheumatoid arthritis, <u>unspecified</u> wrist

  M08.04- Unspecified juvenile rheumatoid arthritis, <u>hand</u>

   M08.041 Unspecified juvenile rheumatoid arthritis, <u>right</u> hand

   M08.042 Unspecified juvenile rheumatoid arthritis, <u>left</u> hand

   M08.049 Unspecified juvenile rheumatoid arthritis, <u>unspecified</u> hand

  M08.05- Unspecified juvenile rheumatoid arthritis, <u>hip</u>

   M08.051 Unspecified juvenile rheumatoid arthritis, <u>right</u> hip

   M08.052 Unspecified juvenile rheumatoid arthritis, <u>left</u> hip

   M08.059 Unspecified juvenile rheumatoid arthritis, <u>unspecified</u> hip

  M08.06- Unspecified juvenile rheumatoid arthritis, <u>knee</u>

   M08.061 Unspecified juvenile rheumatoid arthritis, <u>right</u> knee

   M08.062 Unspecified juvenile rheumatoid arthritis, <u>left</u> knee

   M08.069 Unspecified juvenile rheumatoid arthritis, <u>unspecified</u> knee

  M08.07- Unspecified juvenile rheumatoid arthritis, <u>ankle and foot</u>

   M08.071 Unspecified juvenile rheumatoid arthritis, <u>right</u> ankle and foot

   M08.072 Unspecified juvenile rheumatoid arthritis, <u>left</u> ankle and foot

   M08.079 Unspecified juvenile rheumatoid arthritis, <u>unspecified</u> ankle and foot

  M08.08 Unspecified juvenile rheumatoid arthritis, <u>vertebrae</u>

  M08.09 Unspecified juvenile rheumatoid arthritis, <u>multiple sites</u>

M08.1 Juvenile ankylosing spondylitis — A form affecting the vertebral joints and the muscles, tendons, and ligaments of the spine that cause the stiffening of the spine.

   Excludes 1:   *ankylosing spondylitis in adults (M45.0-)*

M08.2- Juvenile rheumatoid arthritis <u>with systemic onset</u> — A juvenile idiopathic arthritis that is characterized by fever and rash in addition to the inflammation of the joints.

    Still's disease NOS

   Excludes 1:   *adult-onset Still's disease (M06.1-)*

  M08.20 Juvenile rheumatoid arthritis with systemic onset, <u>unspecified</u> site

  M08.21- Juvenile rheumatoid arthritis with systemic onset, <u>shoulder</u>

   M08.211 Juvenile rheumatoid arthritis with systemic onset, <u>right</u> shoulder

   M08.212 Juvenile rheumatoid arthritis with systemic onset, <u>left</u> shoulder

   M08.219 Juvenile rheumatoid arthritis with systemic onset, <u>unspecified</u> shoulder

  M08.22- Juvenile rheumatoid arthritis with systemic onset, <u>elbow</u>

   M08.221 Juvenile rheumatoid arthritis with systemic onset, <u>right</u> elbow

   M08.222 Juvenile rheumatoid arthritis with systemic onset, <u>left</u> elbow

   M08.229 Juvenile rheumatoid arthritis with systemic onset, <u>unspecified</u> elbow

  M08.23- Juvenile rheumatoid arthritis with systemic onset, <u>wrist</u>

   M08.231 Juvenile rheumatoid arthritis with systemic onset, <u>right</u> wrist

   M08.232 Juvenile rheumatoid arthritis with systemic onset, <u>left</u> wrist

   M08.239 Juvenile rheumatoid arthritis with systemic onset, <u>unspecified</u> wrist

  M08.24- Juvenile rheumatoid arthritis with systemic onset, <u>hand</u>

   M08.241 Juvenile rheumatoid arthritis with systemic onset, <u>right</u> hand

   M08.242 Juvenile rheumatoid arthritis with systemic onset, <u>left</u> hand

   M08.249 Juvenile rheumatoid arthritis with systemic onset, <u>unspecified</u> hand

  M08.25- Juvenile rheumatoid arthritis with systemic onset, <u>hip</u>

   M08.251 Juvenile rheumatoid arthritis with systemic onset, <u>right</u> hip

   M08.252 Juvenile rheumatoid arthritis with systemic onset, <u>left</u> hip

   M08.259 Juvenile rheumatoid arthritis with systemic onset, <u>unspecified</u> hip

  M08.26- Juvenile rheumatoid arthritis with systemic onset, <u>knee</u>

   M08.261 Juvenile rheumatoid arthritis with systemic onset, <u>right</u> knee

   M08.262 Juvenile rheumatoid arthritis with systemic onset, <u>left</u> knee

   M08.269 Juvenile rheumatoid arthritis with systemic onset, <u>unspecified</u> knee

  M08.27- Juvenile rheumatoid arthritis with systemic onset, <u>ankle and foot</u>

   M08.271 Juvenile rheumatoid arthritis with systemic onset, <u>right</u> ankle and foot

   M08.272 Juvenile rheumatoid arthritis with systemic onset, <u>left</u> ankle and foot

   M08.279 Juvenile rheumatoid arthritis with systemic onset, <u>unspecified</u> ankle and foot

  M08.28 Juvenile rheumatoid arthritis with systemic onset, <u>vertebrae</u>

M08.29 Juvenile rheumatoid arthritis with systemic onset, <u>multiple sites</u>

M08.3   Juvenile rheumatoid polyarthritis (seronegative) — An autoimmune disorder form that is characterized by inflammation of 5 or more joints with soreness, swelling, and stiffness and without the identification of the rheumatoid factor in the blood.

M08.4-   <u>Pauciarticular</u> juvenile rheumatoid arthritis — An autoimmune disorder form that is characterized by inflammation of 4 or less joints with soreness, swelling, and stiffness and usually with the identification of the rheumatoid factor in the blood.

M08.40 Pauciarticular juvenile rheumatoid arthritis, <u>unspecified</u> site

M08.41- Pauciarticular juvenile rheumatoid arthritis, <u>shoulder</u>
- **M08.411   Pauciarticular juvenile rheumatoid arthritis, <u>right</u> shoulder**
- **M08.412   Pauciarticular juvenile rheumatoid arthritis, <u>left</u> shoulder**
- **M08.419   Pauciarticular juvenile rheumatoid arthritis, <u>unspecified</u> shoulder**

M08.42- Pauciarticular juvenile rheumatoid arthritis, <u>elbow</u>
- **M08.421   Pauciarticular juvenile rheumatoid arthritis, <u>right</u> elbow**
- **M08.422   Pauciarticular juvenile rheumatoid arthritis, <u>left</u> elbow**
- **M08.429   Pauciarticular juvenile rheumatoid arthritis, <u>unspecified</u> elbow**

M08.43- Pauciarticular juvenile rheumatoid arthritis, <u>wrist</u>
- **M08.431   Pauciarticular juvenile rheumatoid arthritis, <u>right</u> wrist**
- **M08.432   Pauciarticular juvenile rheumatoid arthritis, <u>left</u> wrist**
- **M08.439   Pauciarticular juvenile rheumatoid arthritis, <u>unspecified</u> wrist**

M08.44- Pauciarticular juvenile rheumatoid arthritis, <u>hand</u>
- **M08.441   Pauciarticular juvenile rheumatoid arthritis, <u>right</u> hand**
- **M08.442   Pauciarticular juvenile rheumatoid arthritis, <u>left</u> hand**
- **M08.449   Pauciarticular juvenile rheumatoid arthritis, <u>unspecified</u> hand**

M08.45- Pauciarticular juvenile rheumatoid arthritis, <u>hip</u>
- **M08.451   Pauciarticular juvenile rheumatoid arthritis, <u>right</u> hip**
- **M08.452   Pauciarticular juvenile rheumatoid arthritis, <u>left</u> hip**
- **M08.459   Pauciarticular juvenile rheumatoid arthritis, <u>unspecified</u> hip**

M08.46- Pauciarticular juvenile rheumatoid arthritis, <u>knee</u>
- **M08.461   Pauciarticular juvenile rheumatoid arthritis, <u>right</u> knee**
- **M08.462   Pauciarticular juvenile rheumatoid arthritis, <u>left</u> knee**
- **M08.469   Pauciarticular juvenile rheumatoid arthritis, <u>unspecified</u> knee**

M08.47- Pauciarticular juvenile rheumatoid arthritis, <u>ankle and foot</u>
- **M08.471   Pauciarticular juvenile rheumatoid arthritis, <u>right</u> ankle and foot**
- **M08.472   Pauciarticular juvenile rheumatoid arthritis, <u>left</u> ankle and foot**
- **M08.479   Pauciarticular juvenile rheumatoid arthritis, <u>unspecified</u> ankle and foot**

M08.48 Pauciarticular juvenile rheumatoid arthritis, vertebrae

M08.8-   <u>Other</u> juvenile arthritis

M08.80 Other juvenile arthritis, <u>unspecified</u> site

M08.81- Other juvenile arthritis, <u>shoulder</u>
- **M08.811   Other juvenile arthritis, <u>right</u> shoulder**
- **M08.812   Other juvenile arthritis, <u>left</u> shoulder**
- **M08.819   Other juvenile arthritis, <u>unspecified</u> shoulder**

M08.82- Other juvenile arthritis, <u>elbow</u>
- **M08.821   Other juvenile arthritis, <u>right</u> elbow**
- **M08.822   Other juvenile arthritis, <u>left</u> elbow**
- **M08.829   Other juvenile arthritis, <u>unspecified</u> elbow**

M08.83- Other juvenile arthritis, <u>wrist</u>
- **M08.831   Other juvenile arthritis, <u>right</u> wrist**
- **M08.832   Other juvenile arthritis, <u>left</u> wrist**
- **M08.839   Other juvenile arthritis, <u>unspecified</u> wrist**

M08.84- Other juvenile arthritis, <u>hand</u>
- **M08.841   Other juvenile arthritis, <u>right</u> hand**
- **M08.842   Other juvenile arthritis, <u>left</u> hand**
- **M08.849   Other juvenile arthritis, <u>unspecified</u> hand**

M08.85- Other juvenile arthritis, <u>hip</u>
- **M08.851   Other juvenile arthritis, <u>right</u> hip**
- **M08.852   Other juvenile arthritis, <u>left</u> hip**
- **M08.859   Other juvenile arthritis, <u>unspecified</u> hip**

M08.86- Other juvenile arthritis, <u>knee</u>
- **M08.861   Other juvenile arthritis, <u>right</u> knee**
- **M08.862   Other juvenile arthritis, <u>left</u> knee**
- **M08.869   Other juvenile arthritis, <u>unspecified</u> knee**

M08.87- Other juvenile arthritis, <u>ankle and foot</u>
- **M08.871   Other juvenile arthritis, <u>right</u> ankle and foot**
- **M08.872   Other juvenile arthritis, <u>left</u> ankle and foot**
- **M08.879   Other juvenile arthritis, <u>unspecified</u> ankle and foot**

M08.88 Other juvenile arthritis, <u>other specified site</u>
Other juvenile arthritis, vertebrae

M08.89 Other juvenile arthritis, <u>multiple sites</u>

M08.9-   Juvenile arthritis, <u>unspecified</u>
Excludes 1:   *juvenile rheumatoid arthritis, unspecified (M08.0-)*

M08.90 Juvenile arthritis, unspecified, <u>unspecified</u> site

M08.91- Juvenile arthritis, unspecified, <u>shoulder</u>
- **M08.911   Juvenile arthritis, unspecified, <u>right</u> shoulder**
- **M08.912   Juvenile arthritis, unspecified, <u>left</u> shoulder**
- **M08.919   Juvenile arthritis, unspecified, <u>unspecified</u> shoulder**

M08.92- Juvenile arthritis, unspecified, <u>elbow</u>
- **M08.921   Juvenile arthritis, unspecified, <u>right</u> elbow**
- **M08.922   Juvenile arthritis, unspecified, <u>left</u> elbow**
- **M08.929   Juvenile arthritis, unspecified, <u>unspecified</u> elbow**

M08.93- Juvenile arthritis, unspecified, <u>wrist</u>
- **M08.931   Juvenile arthritis, unspecified, <u>right</u> wrist**
- **M08.932   Juvenile arthritis, unspecified, <u>left</u> wrist**
- **M08.939   Juvenile arthritis, unspecified, <u>unspecified</u> wrist**

M08.94- Juvenile arthritis, unspecified, <u>hand</u>
- **M08.941   Juvenile arthritis, unspecified, <u>right</u> hand**
- **M08.942   Juvenile arthritis, unspecified, <u>left</u> hand**
- **M08.949   Juvenile arthritis, unspecified, <u>unspecified</u> hand**

M08.95- Juvenile arthritis, unspecified, <u>hip</u>
- **M08.951   Juvenile arthritis, unspecified, <u>right</u> hip**
- **M08.952   Juvenile arthritis, unspecified, <u>left</u> hip**
- **M08.959   Juvenile arthritis, unspecified, <u>unspecified</u> hip**

M08.96- Juvenile arthritis, unspecified, <u>knee</u>
- **M08.961   Juvenile arthritis, unspecified, <u>right</u> knee**
- **M08.962   Juvenile arthritis, unspecified, <u>left</u> knee**
- **M08.969   Juvenile arthritis, unspecified, <u>unspecified</u> knee**

M08.97- Juvenile arthritis, unspecified, <u>ankle and foot</u>
- **M08.971   Juvenile arthritis, unspecified, <u>right</u> ankle and foot**
- **M08.972   Juvenile arthritis, unspecified, <u>left</u> ankle and foot**
- **M08.979   Juvenile arthritis, unspecified, <u>unspecified</u> ankle and foot**

M08.98 Juvenile arthritis, unspecified, <u>vertebrae</u>

M08.99 Juvenile arthritis, unspecified, <u>multiple sites</u>

M08-M08

M1A- **Chronic gout** — A form of arthritis that is characterized by the deposition of urate crystals in and around the joints that causes inflammation and degenerative changes that persists over a long period of time with repeated episodes of soreness and aching.

Use additional code to identify:
Autonomic neuropathy in diseases classified elsewhere (G99.0)
Calculus of urinary tract in diseases classified elsewhere (N22)
Cardiomyopathy in diseases classified elsewhere (I43)
Disorders of external ear in diseases classified elsewhere (H61.1-, H62.8-)
Disorders of iris and ciliary body in diseases classified elsewhere (H22)
Glomerular disorders in diseases classified elsewhere (N08)

Excludes 1: gout NOS (M10.-)
Excludes ➋: acute gout (M10.-)

The appropriate 7th character is to be added to each code from category M1A:
0 **Without** tophus (tophi)
1 **With tophus (tophi)** — The appearance of enlarged joints due to nodular monosodium urate crystal deposits.

M1A.0- **Idiopathic chronic gout** — A form that is of a primary cause (versus due to another condition or disease) or unknown cause.
Chronic gouty bursitis
Primary chronic gout

M1A.00x- Idiopathic chronic gout, <u>unspecified</u> site
M1A.01- Idiopathic chronic gout, <u>shoulder</u>
M1A.011- Idiopathic chronic gout, <u>right</u> shoulder
M1A.012- Idiopathic chronic gout, <u>left</u> shoulder
M1A.019- Idiopathic chronic gout, <u>unspecified</u> shoulder
M1A.02- Idiopathic chronic gout, <u>elbow</u>
M1A.021- Idiopathic chronic gout, <u>right</u> elbow
M1A.022- Idiopathic chronic gout, <u>left</u> elbow
M1A.029- Idiopathic chronic gout, <u>unspecified</u> elbow
M1A.03- Idiopathic chronic gout, <u>wrist</u>
M1A.031- Idiopathic chronic gout, <u>right</u> wrist
M1A.032- Idiopathic chronic gout, <u>left</u> wrist
M1A.039- Idiopathic chronic gout, <u>unspecified</u> wrist
M1A.04- Idiopathic chronic gout, <u>hand</u>
M1A.041- Idiopathic chronic gout, <u>right</u> hand
M1A.042- Idiopathic chronic gout, <u>left</u> hand
M1A.049- Idiopathic chronic gout, <u>unspecified</u> hand
M1A.05- Idiopathic chronic gout, <u>hip</u>
M1A.051- Idiopathic chronic gout, <u>right</u> hip
M1A.052- Idiopathic chronic gout, <u>left</u> hip
M1A.059- Idiopathic chronic gout, <u>unspecified</u> hip
M1A.06- Idiopathic chronic gout, <u>knee</u>
M1A.061- Idiopathic chronic gout, <u>right</u> knee
M1A.062- Idiopathic chronic gout, <u>left</u> knee
M1A.069- Idiopathic chronic gout, <u>unspecified</u> knee
M1A.07- Idiopathic chronic gout, <u>ankle and foot</u>
M1A.071- Idiopathic chronic gout, <u>right</u> ankle and foot
M1A.072- Idiopathic chronic gout, <u>left</u> ankle and foot
M1A.079- Idiopathic chronic gout, <u>unspecified</u> ankle and foot
M1A.08x- Idiopathic chronic gout, <u>vertebrae</u>
M1A.09x- Idiopathic chronic gout, <u>multiple sites</u>

M1A.1- **Lead-induced** chronic gout — A form that is due to the toxic effects of lead and its compounds.
Code first toxic effects of lead and its compounds (T56.0-)

M1A.10x- Lead-induced chronic gout, <u>unspecified</u> site
M1A.11- Lead-induced chronic gout, <u>shoulder</u>
M1A.111- Lead-induced chronic gout, <u>right</u> shoulder
M1A.112- Lead-induced chronic gout, <u>left</u> shoulder
M1A.119- Lead-induced chronic gout, <u>unspecified</u> shoulder
M1A.12- Lead-induced chronic gout, <u>elbow</u>
M1A.121- Lead-induced chronic gout, <u>right</u> elbow
M1A.122- Lead-induced chronic gout, <u>left</u> elbow
M1A.129- Lead-induced chronic gout, <u>unspecified</u> elbow
M1A.13- Lead-induced chronic gout, <u>wrist</u>
M1A.131- Lead-induced chronic gout, <u>right</u> wrist
M1A.132- Lead-induced chronic gout, <u>left</u> wrist
M1A.139- Lead-induced chronic gout, <u>unspecified</u> wrist

M1A.14- Lead-induced chronic gout, <u>hand</u>
M1A.141- Lead-induced chronic gout, <u>right</u> hand
M1A.142- Lead-induced chronic gout, <u>left</u> hand
M1A.149- Lead-induced chronic gout, <u>unspecified</u> hand
M1A.15- Lead-induced chronic gout, <u>hip</u>
M1A.151- Lead-induced chronic gout, <u>right</u> hip
M1A.152- Lead-induced chronic gout, <u>left</u> hip
M1A.159- Lead-induced chronic gout, <u>unspecified</u> hip
M1A.16- Lead-induced chronic gout, <u>knee</u>
M1A.161- Lead-induced chronic gout, <u>right</u> knee
M1A.162- Lead-induced chronic gout, <u>left</u> knee
M1A.169- Lead-induced chronic gout, <u>unspecified</u> knee
M1A.17- Lead-induced chronic gout, <u>ankle and foot</u>
M1A.171- Lead-induced chronic gout, <u>right</u> ankle and foot
M1A.172- Lead-induced chronic gout, <u>left</u> ankle and foot
M1A.179- Lead-induced chronic gout, <u>unspecified</u> ankle and foot
M1A.18x- Lead-induced chronic gout, <u>vertebrae</u>
M1A.19x- Lead-induced chronic gout, <u>multiple sites</u>

M1A.2- **Drug-induced** chronic gout — A form that is due to medications and their effects.
Use additional code for adverse effect, if applicable, to identify drug (T36-T50 with fifth or sixth character 5)

M1A.20x- Drug-induced chronic gout, <u>unspecified</u> site
M1A.21- Drug-induced chronic gout, <u>shoulder</u>
M1A.211- Drug-induced chronic gout, <u>right</u> shoulder
M1A.212- Drug-induced chronic gout, <u>left</u> shoulder
M1A.219- Drug-induced chronic gout, <u>unspecified</u> shoulder
M1A.22- Drug-induced chronic gout, <u>elbow</u>
M1A.221- Drug-induced chronic gout, <u>right</u> elbow
M1A.222- Drug-induced chronic gout, <u>left</u> elbow
M1A.229- Drug-induced chronic gout, <u>unspecified</u> elbow
M1A.23- Drug-induced chronic gout, <u>wrist</u>
M1A.231- Drug-induced chronic gout, <u>right</u> wrist
M1A.232- Drug-induced chronic gout, <u>left</u> wrist
M1A.239- Drug-induced chronic gout, <u>unspecified</u> wrist
M1A.24- Drug-induced chronic gout, <u>hand</u>
M1A.241- Drug-induced chronic gout, <u>right</u> hand
M1A.242- Drug-induced chronic gout, <u>left</u> hand
M1A.249- Drug-induced chronic gout, <u>unspecified</u> hand
M1A.25- Drug-induced chronic gout, <u>hip</u>
M1A.251- Drug-induced chronic gout, <u>right</u> hip
M1A.252- Drug-induced chronic gout, <u>left</u> hip
M1A.259- Drug-induced chronic gout, <u>unspecified</u> hip
M1A.26- Drug-induced chronic gout, <u>knee</u>
M1A.261- Drug-induced chronic gout, <u>right</u> knee
M1A.262- Drug-induced chronic gout, <u>left</u> knee
M1A.269- Drug-induced chronic gout, <u>unspecified</u> knee
M1A.27- Drug-induced chronic gout, <u>ankle and foot</u>
M1A.271- Drug-induced chronic gout, <u>right</u> ankle and foot
M1A.272- Drug-induced chronic gout, <u>left</u> ankle and foot
M1A.279- Drug-induced chronic gout, <u>unspecified</u> ankle and foot
M1A.28x- Drug-induced chronic gout, <u>vertebrae</u>
M1A.29x- Drug-induced chronic gout, <u>multiple sites</u>

M1A.3- Chronic gout <u>due to renal impairment</u> — A form that is due to the decreased function of the kidney resulting in inadequate removal of uric acid from the blood.
Code first associated renal disease

M1A.30x- Chronic gout due to renal impairment, <u>unspecified</u> site
M1A.31- Chronic gout due to renal impairment, <u>shoulder</u>
M1A.311- Chronic gout due to renal impairment, <u>right</u> shoulder
M1A.312- Chronic gout due to renal impairment, <u>left</u> shoulder

M1A.319- Chronic gout due to renal impairment, <u>unspecified</u> shoulder

M1A.32- Chronic gout due to renal impairment, <u>elbow</u>
- **M1A.321-** Chronic gout due to renal impairment, <u>right</u> elbow
- **M1A.322-** Chronic gout due to renal impairment, <u>left</u> elbow
- **M1A.329-** Chronic gout due to renal impairment, <u>unspecified</u> elbow

M1A.33- Chronic gout due to renal impairment, <u>wrist</u>
- **M1A.331-** Chronic gout due to renal impairment, <u>right</u> wrist
- **M1A.332-** Chronic gout due to renal impairment, <u>left</u> wrist
- **M1A.339-** Chronic gout due to renal impairment, <u>unspecified</u> wrist

M1A.34- Chronic gout due to renal impairment, <u>hand</u>
- **M1A.341-** Chronic gout due to renal impairment, <u>right</u> hand
- **M1A.342-** Chronic gout due to renal impairment, <u>left</u> hand
- **M1A.349-** Chronic gout due to renal impairment, <u>unspecified</u> hand

M1A.35- Chronic gout due to renal impairment, <u>hip</u>
- **M1A.351-** Chronic gout due to renal impairment, <u>right</u> hip
- **M1A.352-** Chronic gout due to renal impairment, <u>left</u> hip
- **M1A.359-** Chronic gout due to renal impairment, <u>unspecified</u> hip

M1A.36- Chronic gout due to renal impairment, <u>knee</u>
- **M1A.361-** Chronic gout due to renal impairment, <u>right</u> knee
- **M1A.362-** Chronic gout due to renal impairment, <u>left</u> knee
- **M1A.369-** Chronic gout due to renal impairment, <u>unspecified</u> knee

M1A.37- Chronic gout due to renal impairment, <u>ankle and foot</u>
- **M1A.371-** Chronic gout due to renal impairment, <u>right</u> ankle and foot
- **M1A.372-** Chronic gout due to renal impairment, <u>left</u> ankle and foot
- **M1A.379-** Chronic gout due to renal impairment, <u>unspecified</u> ankle and foot

M1A.38x- Chronic gout due to renal impairment, <u>vertebrae</u>
M1A.39x- Chronic gout due to renal impairment, <u>multiple sites</u>

M1A.4- <u>Other secondary</u> chronic gout
    Code first associated condition

M1A.40x- Other secondary chronic gout, <u>unspecified</u> site

M1A.41- Other secondary chronic gout, <u>shoulder</u>
- **M1A.411-** Other secondary chronic gout, <u>right</u> shoulder
- **M1A.412-** Other secondary chronic gout, <u>left</u> shoulder
- **M1A.419-** Other secondary chronic gout, <u>unspecified</u> shoulder

M1A.42- Other secondary chronic gout, <u>elbow</u>
- **M1A.421-** Other secondary chronic gout, <u>right</u> elbow
- **M1A.422-** Other secondary chronic gout, <u>left</u> elbow
- **M1A.429-** Other secondary chronic gout, <u>unspecified</u> elbow

M1A.43- Other secondary chronic gout, <u>wrist</u>
- **M1A.431-** Other secondary chronic gout, <u>right</u> wrist
- **M1A.432-** Other secondary chronic gout, <u>left</u> wrist
- **M1A.439-** Other secondary chronic gout, <u>unspecified</u> wrist

M1A.44- Other secondary chronic gout, <u>hand</u>
- **M1A.441-** Other secondary chronic gout, <u>right</u> hand
- **M1A.442-** Other secondary chronic gout, <u>left</u> hand
- **M1A.449-** Other secondary chronic gout, <u>unspecified</u> hand

M1A.45- Other secondary chronic gout, <u>hip</u>
- **M1A.451-** Other secondary chronic gout, <u>right</u> hip
- **M1A.452-** Other secondary chronic gout, <u>left</u> hip
- **M1A.459-** Other secondary chronic gout, <u>unspecified</u> hip

M1A.46- Other secondary chronic gout, <u>knee</u>
- **M1A.461-** Other secondary chronic gout, <u>right</u> knee
- **M1A.462-** Other secondary chronic gout, <u>left</u> knee
- **M1A.469-** Other secondary chronic gout, <u>unspecified</u> knee

M1A.47- Other secondary chronic gout, <u>ankle and foot</u>
- **M1A.471-** Other secondary chronic gout, <u>right</u> ankle and foot
- **M1A.472-** Other secondary chronic gout, <u>left</u> ankle and foot
- **M1A.479-** Other secondary chronic gout, <u>unspecified</u> ankle and foot

M1A.48x- Other secondary chronic gout, <u>vertebrae</u>
M1A.49x- Other secondary chronic gout, <u>multiple sites</u>

M1A.9xx- Chronic gout, <u>unspecified</u>

M10- <u>Gout</u> — A form of arthritis that is characterized by the deposition of urate crystals in and around the joints that causes inflammation and degenerative changes that presents as a sudden, severe onset of sharp pain, swelling, redness, and tenderness of the affected joint.
  <u>Acute</u> gout
  Gout <u>attack</u>
  Gout <u>flare</u>
  Gout <u>NOS</u>
  Podagra — A form affecting the big toe.
  Use additional code to identify:
    Autonomic neuropathy in diseases classified elsewhere (G99.0)
    Calculus of urinary tract in diseases classified elsewhere (N22)
    Cardiomyopathy in diseases classified elsewhere (I43)
    Disorders of external ear in diseases classified elsewhere (H61.1-, H62.8-)
    Disorders of iris and ciliary body in diseases classified elsewhere (H22)
    Glomerular disorders in diseases classified elsewhere (N08)
  Excludes ❷: chronic gout (M1A.-)

M10.0- <u>Idiopathic gout</u> — A form that is of a primary cause (versus due to another condition or disease) or unknown cause.
    Gouty bursitis
    Primary gout

M10.00 Idiopathic gout, <u>unspecified</u> site
M10.01- Idiopathic gout, <u>shoulder</u>
- **M10.011** Idiopathic gout, <u>right</u> shoulder
- **M10.012** Idiopathic gout, <u>left</u> shoulder
- **M10.019** Idiopathic gout, <u>unspecified</u> shoulder

M10.02- Idiopathic gout, <u>elbow</u>
- **M10.021** Idiopathic gout, <u>right</u> elbow
- **M10.022** Idiopathic gout, <u>left</u> elbow
- **M10.029** Idiopathic gout, <u>unspecified</u> elbow

M10.03- Idiopathic gout, <u>wrist</u>
- **M10.031** Idiopathic gout, <u>right</u> wrist
- **M10.032** Idiopathic gout, <u>left</u> wrist
- **M10.039** Idiopathic gout, <u>unspecified</u> wrist

M10.04- Idiopathic gout, <u>hand</u>
- **M10.041** Idiopathic gout, <u>right</u> hand
- **M10.042** Idiopathic gout, <u>left</u> hand
- **M10.049** Idiopathic gout, <u>unspecified</u> hand

M10.05- Idiopathic gout, <u>hip</u>
- **M10.051** Idiopathic gout, <u>right</u> hip
- **M10.052** Idiopathic gout, <u>left</u> hip
- **M10.059** Idiopathic gout, <u>unspecified</u> hip

M10.06- Idiopathic gout, <u>knee</u>
- **M10.061** Idiopathic gout, <u>right</u> knee
- **M10.062** Idiopathic gout, <u>left</u> knee
- **M10.069** Idiopathic gout, <u>unspecified</u> knee

M10.07- Idiopathic gout, <u>ankle and foot</u>
- **M10.071** Idiopathic gout, <u>right</u> ankle and foot
- **M10.072** Idiopathic gout, <u>left</u> ankle and foot
- **M10.079** Idiopathic gout, <u>unspecified</u> ankle and foot

M10.08 Idiopathic gout, <u>vertebrae</u>
M10.09 Idiopathic gout, <u>multiple sites</u>

M10.1- <u>Lead-induced</u> gout — A form that is due to the toxic effects of lead and its compounds.
    Code first toxic effects of lead and its compounds (T56.0-)

M10.10 Lead-induced gout, <u>unspecified</u> site
M10.11- Lead-induced gout, <u>shoulder</u>
- **M10.111** Lead-induced gout, <u>right</u> shoulder
- **M10.112** Lead-induced gout, <u>left</u> shoulder
- **M10.119** Lead-induced gout, <u>unspecified</u> shoulder

M1A - M10

M10.12- Lead-induced gout, <u>elbow</u>
   M10.121 Lead-induced gout, <u>right</u> elbow
   M10.122 Lead-induced gout, <u>left</u> elbow
   M10.129 Lead-induced gout, <u>unspecified</u> elbow

M10.13- Lead-induced gout, <u>wrist</u>
   M10.131 Lead-induced gout, <u>right</u> wrist
   M10.132 Lead-induced gout, <u>left</u> wrist
   M10.139 Lead-induced gout, <u>unspecified</u> wrist

M10.14- Lead-induced gout, <u>hand</u>
   M10.141 Lead-induced gout, <u>right</u> hand
   M10.142 Lead-induced gout, <u>left</u> hand
   M10.149 Lead-induced gout, <u>unspecified</u> hand

M10.15- Lead-induced gout, <u>hip</u>
   M10.151 Lead-induced gout, <u>right</u> hip
   M10.152 Lead-induced gout, <u>left</u> hip
   M10.159 Lead-induced gout, <u>unspecified</u> hip

M10.16- Lead-induced gout, <u>knee</u>
   M10.161 Lead-induced gout, <u>right</u> knee
   M10.162 Lead-induced gout, <u>left</u> knee
   M10.169 Lead-induced gout, <u>unspecified</u> knee

M10.17- Lead-induced gout, <u>ankle and foot</u>
   M10.171 Lead-induced gout, <u>right</u> ankle and foot
   M10.172 Lead-induced gout, <u>left</u> ankle and foot
   M10.179 Lead-induced gout, <u>unspecified</u> ankle and foot

M10.18 Lead-induced gout, <u>vertebrae</u>
M10.19 Lead-induced gout, <u>multiple sites</u>

M10.2- <u>Drug-induced</u> gout — A form that is due to medications and their effects.
Use additional code for adverse effect, if applicable, to identify drug
(T36-T50 with fifth or sixth character 5)

M10.20 Drug-induced gout, <u>unspecified</u> site

M10.21- Drug-induced gout, <u>shoulder</u>
   M10.211 Drug-induced gout, <u>right</u> shoulder
   M10.212 Drug-induced gout, <u>left</u> shoulder
   M10.219 Drug-induced gout, <u>unspecified</u> shoulder

M10.22- Drug-induced gout, <u>elbow</u>
   M10.221 Drug-induced gout, <u>right</u> elbow
   M10.222 Drug-induced gout, <u>left</u> elbow
   M10.229 Drug-induced gout, <u>unspecified</u> elbow

M10.23- Drug-induced gout, <u>wrist</u>
   M10.231 Drug-induced gout, <u>right</u> wrist
   M10.232 Drug-induced gout, <u>left</u> wrist
   M10.239 Drug-induced gout, <u>unspecified</u> wrist

M10.24- Drug-induced gout, <u>hand</u>
   M10.241 Drug-induced gout, <u>right</u> hand
   M10.242 Drug-induced gout, <u>left</u> hand
   M10.249 Drug-induced gout, <u>unspecified</u> hand

M10.25- Drug-induced gout, <u>hip</u>
   M10.251 Drug-induced gout, <u>right</u> hip
   M10.252 Drug-induced gout, <u>left</u> hip
   M10.259 Drug-induced gout, <u>unspecified</u> hip

M10.26- Drug-induced gout, <u>knee</u>
   M10.261 Drug-induced gout, <u>right</u> knee
   M10.262 Drug-induced gout, <u>left</u> knee
   M10.269 Drug-induced gout, <u>unspecified</u> knee

M10.27- Drug-induced gout, <u>ankle and foot</u>
   M10.271 Drug-induced gout, <u>right</u> ankle and foot
   M10.272 Drug-induced gout, <u>left</u> ankle and foot
   M10.279 Drug-induced gout, <u>unspecified</u> ankle and foot

M10.28 Drug-induced gout, <u>vertebrae</u>
M10.29 Drug-induced gout, <u>multiple sites</u>

M10.3- Gout <u>due to renal impairment</u> — A form that is due to the decreased
function of the kidney resulting in inadequate removal of uric acid from the blood.
Code first associated renal disease

M10.30 Gout due to renal impairment, <u>unspecified</u> site

M10.31- Gout due to renal impairment, <u>shoulder</u>
   M10.311 Gout due to renal impairment, <u>right</u> shoulder
   M10.312 Gout due to renal impairment, <u>left</u> shoulder
   M10.319 Gout due to renal impairment, <u>unspecified</u> shoulder

M10.32- Gout due to renal impairment, <u>elbow</u>
   M10.321 Gout due to renal impairment, <u>right</u> elbow
   M10.322 Gout due to renal impairment, <u>left</u> elbow
   M10.329 Gout due to renal impairment, <u>unspecified</u> elbow

M10.33- Gout due to renal impairment, <u>wrist</u>
   M10.331 Gout due to renal impairment, <u>right</u> wrist
   M10.332 Gout due to renal impairment, <u>left</u> wrist
   M10.339 Gout due to renal impairment, <u>unspecified</u> wrist

M10.34- Gout due to renal impairment, <u>hand</u>
   M10.341 Gout due to renal impairment, <u>right</u> hand
   M10.342 Gout due to renal impairment, <u>left</u> hand
   M10.349 Gout due to renal impairment, <u>unspecified</u> hand

M10.35- Gout due to renal impairment, <u>hip</u>
   M10.351 Gout due to renal impairment, <u>right</u> hip
   M10.352 Gout due to renal impairment, <u>left</u> hip
   M10.359 Gout due to renal impairment, <u>unspecified</u> hip

M10.36- Gout due to renal impairment, <u>knee</u>
   M10.361 Gout due to renal impairment, <u>right</u> knee
   M10.362 Gout due to renal impairment, <u>left</u> knee
   M10.369 Gout due to renal impairment, <u>unspecified</u> knee

M10.37- Gout due to renal impairment, <u>ankle and foot</u>
   M10.371 Gout due to renal impairment, <u>right</u> ankle and foot
   M10.372 Gout due to renal impairment, <u>left</u> ankle and foot
   M10.379 Gout due to renal impairment, <u>unspecified</u> ankle and foot

M10.38 Gout due to renal impairment, <u>vertebrae</u>
M10.39 Gout due to renal impairment, <u>multiple sites</u>

M10.4- <u>Other secondary</u> gout
Code first associated condition

M10.40 Other secondary gout, <u>unspecified</u> site

M10.41- Other secondary gout, <u>shoulder</u>
   M10.411 Other secondary gout, <u>right</u> shoulder
   M10.412 Other secondary gout, <u>left</u> shoulder
   M10.419 Other secondary gout, <u>unspecified</u> shoulder

M10.42- Other secondary gout, <u>elbow</u>
   M10.421 Other secondary gout, <u>right</u> elbow
   M10.422 Other secondary gout, <u>left</u> elbow
   M10.429 Other secondary gout, <u>unspecified</u> elbow

M10.43- Other secondary gout, <u>wrist</u>
   M10.431 Other secondary gout, <u>right</u> wrist
   M10.432 Other secondary gout, <u>left</u> wrist
   M10.439 Other secondary gout, <u>unspecified</u> wrist

M10.44- Other secondary gout, <u>hand</u>
   M10.441 Other secondary gout, <u>right</u> hand
   M10.442 Other secondary gout, <u>left</u> hand
   M10.449 Other secondary gout, <u>unspecified</u> hand

M10.45- Other secondary gout, <u>hip</u>
   M10.451 Other secondary gout, <u>right</u> hip
   M10.452 Other secondary gout, <u>left</u> hip
   M10.459 Other secondary gout, <u>unspecified</u> hip

M10.46- Other secondary gout, <u>knee</u>
   M10.461 Other secondary gout, <u>right</u> knee
   M10.462 Other secondary gout, <u>left</u> knee
   M10.469 Other secondary gout, <u>unspecified</u> knee

M10 - M10

Excludes 1: = NOT CODED HERE! (Do not code both)
Excludes ❷: = Not Included Here

M10.47- Other secondary gout, <u>ankle and foot</u>
   M10.471 Other secondary gout, <u>right</u> ankle and foot
   M10.472 Other secondary gout, <u>left</u> ankle and foot
   M10.479 Other secondary gout, <u>unspecified</u> ankle and foot
M10.48 Other secondary gout, <u>vertebrae</u>
M10.49 Other secondary gout, <u>multiple sites</u>
M10.9 Gout, <u>unspecified</u>
   Gout NOS

M11- <u>Other crystal arthropathies</u> — A group of joint diseases characterized by the deposition of crystals in the joints.
  M11.0- <u>Hydroxyapatite deposition</u> disease — A form caused the deposition of hydroxyapatite crystals in the joints.
   M11.00 Hydroxyapatite deposition disease, <u>unspecified</u> site
   M11.01- Hydroxyapatite deposition disease, <u>shoulder</u>
    M11.011 Hydroxyapatite deposition disease, <u>right</u> shoulder
    M11.012 Hydroxyapatite deposition disease, <u>left</u> shoulder
    M11.019 Hydroxyapatite deposition disease, <u>unspecified</u> shoulder
   M11.02- Hydroxyapatite deposition disease, <u>elbow</u>
    M11.021 Hydroxyapatite deposition disease, <u>right</u> elbow
    M11.022 Hydroxyapatite deposition disease, <u>left</u> elbow
    M11.029 Hydroxyapatite deposition disease, <u>unspecified</u> elbow
   M11.03- Hydroxyapatite deposition disease, <u>wrist</u>
    M11.031 Hydroxyapatite deposition disease, <u>right</u> wrist
    M11.032 Hydroxyapatite deposition disease, <u>left</u> wrist
    M11.039 Hydroxyapatite deposition disease, <u>unspecified</u> wrist
   M11.04- Hydroxyapatite deposition disease, <u>hand</u>
    M11.041 Hydroxyapatite deposition disease, <u>right</u> hand
    M11.042 Hydroxyapatite deposition disease, <u>left</u> hand
    M11.049 Hydroxyapatite deposition disease, <u>unspecified</u> hand
   M11.05- Hydroxyapatite deposition disease, <u>hip</u>
    M11.051 Hydroxyapatite deposition disease, <u>right</u> hip
    M11.052 Hydroxyapatite deposition disease, <u>left</u> hip
    M11.059 Hydroxyapatite deposition disease, <u>unspecified</u> hip
   M11.06- Hydroxyapatite deposition disease, <u>knee</u>
    M11.061 Hydroxyapatite deposition disease, <u>right</u> knee
    M11.062 Hydroxyapatite deposition disease, <u>left</u> knee
    M11.069 Hydroxyapatite deposition disease, <u>unspecified</u> knee
   M11.07- Hydroxyapatite deposition disease, <u>ankle and foot</u>
    M11.071 Hydroxyapatite deposition disease, <u>right</u> ankle and foot
    M11.072 Hydroxyapatite deposition disease, <u>left</u> ankle and foot
    M11.079 Hydroxyapatite deposition disease, <u>unspecified</u> ankle and foot
   M11.08 Hydroxyapatite deposition disease, <u>vertebrae</u>
   M11.09 Hydroxyapatite deposition disease, <u>multiple sites</u>
  M11.1- <u>Familial chondrocalcinosis</u> — A form caused the deposition of calcium pyrophosphate dihydrate crystals in the joints.
   M11.10 Familial chondrocalcinosis, <u>unspecified</u> site
   M11.11- Familial chondrocalcinosis, <u>shoulder</u>
    M11.111 Familial chondrocalcinosis, <u>right</u> shoulder
    M11.112 Familial chondrocalcinosis, <u>left</u> shoulder
    M11.119 Familial chondrocalcinosis, <u>unspecified</u> shoulder
   M11.12- Familial chondrocalcinosis, <u>elbow</u>
    M11.121 Familial chondrocalcinosis, <u>right</u> elbow
    M11.122 Familial chondrocalcinosis, <u>left</u> elbow
    M11.129 Familial chondrocalcinosis, <u>unspecified</u> elbow
   M11.13- Familial chondrocalcinosis, <u>wrist</u>
    M11.131 Familial chondrocalcinosis, <u>right</u> wrist
    M11.132 Familial chondrocalcinosis, <u>left</u> wrist
    M11.139 Familial chondrocalcinosis, <u>unspecified</u> wrist

M11.14- Familial chondrocalcinosis, <u>hand</u>
   M11.141 Familial chondrocalcinosis, <u>right</u> hand
   M11.142 Familial chondrocalcinosis, <u>left</u> hand
   M11.149 Familial chondrocalcinosis, <u>unspecified</u> hand
M11.15- Familial chondrocalcinosis, <u>hip</u>
   M11.151 Familial chondrocalcinosis, <u>right</u> hip
   M11.152 Familial chondrocalcinosis, <u>left</u> hip
   M11.159 Familial chondrocalcinosis, <u>unspecified</u> hip
M11.16- Familial chondrocalcinosis, <u>knee</u>
   M11.161 Familial chondrocalcinosis, <u>right</u> knee
   M11.162 Familial chondrocalcinosis, <u>left</u> knee
   M11.169 Familial chondrocalcinosis, <u>unspecified</u> knee
M11.17- Familial chondrocalcinosis, <u>ankle and foot</u>
   M11.171 Familial chondrocalcinosis, <u>right</u> ankle and foot
   M11.172 Familial chondrocalcinosis, <u>left</u> ankle and foot
   M11.179 Familial chondrocalcinosis, <u>unspecified</u> ankle and foot
M11.18 Familial chondrocalcinosis, <u>vertebrae</u>
M11.19 Familial chondrocalcinosis, <u>multiple sites</u>
M11.2- <u>Other chondrocalcinosis</u> — A chronic inherited form caused by the deposition of calcium pyrophosphate dihydrate crystals in the joints.
   Chondrocalcinosis NOS
M11.20 Other chondrocalcinosis, <u>unspecified</u> site
M11.21- Other chondrocalcinosis, <u>shoulder</u>
   M11.211 Other chondrocalcinosis, <u>right</u> shoulder
   M11.212 Other chondrocalcinosis, <u>left</u> shoulder
   M11.219 Other chondrocalcinosis, <u>unspecified</u> shoulder
M11.22- Other chondrocalcinosis, <u>elbow</u>
   M11.221 Other chondrocalcinosis, <u>right</u> elbow
   M11.222 Other chondrocalcinosis, <u>left</u> elbow
   M11.229 Other chondrocalcinosis, <u>unspecified</u> elbow
M11.23- Other chondrocalcinosis, <u>wrist</u>
   M11.231 Other chondrocalcinosis, <u>right</u> wrist
   M11.232 Other chondrocalcinosis, <u>left</u> wrist
   M11.239 Other chondrocalcinosis, <u>unspecified</u> wrist
M11.24- Other chondrocalcinosis, <u>hand</u>
   M11.241 Other chondrocalcinosis, <u>right</u> hand
   M11.242 Other chondrocalcinosis, <u>left</u> hand
   M11.249 Other chondrocalcinosis, <u>unspecified</u> hand
M11.25- Other chondrocalcinosis, <u>hip</u>
   M11.251 Other chondrocalcinosis, <u>right</u> hip
   M11.252 Other chondrocalcinosis, <u>left</u> hip
   M11.259 Other chondrocalcinosis, <u>unspecified</u> hip
M11.26- Other chondrocalcinosis, <u>knee</u>
   M11.261 Other chondrocalcinosis, <u>right</u> knee
   M11.262 Other chondrocalcinosis, <u>left</u> knee
   M11.269 Other chondrocalcinosis, <u>unspecified</u> knee
M11.27- Other chondrocalcinosis, <u>ankle and foot</u>
   M11.271 Other chondrocalcinosis, <u>right</u> ankle and foot
   M11.272 Other chondrocalcinosis, <u>left</u> ankle and foot
   M11.279 Other chondrocalcinosis, <u>unspecified</u> ankle and foot
M11.28 Other chondrocalcinosis, <u>vertebrae</u>
M11.29 Other chondrocalcinosis, <u>multiple sites</u>
M11.8- <u>Other specified crystal</u> arthropathies
M11.80 Other specified crystal arthropathies, <u>unspecified</u> site
M11.81- Other specified crystal arthropathies, <u>shoulder</u>
   M11.811 Other specified crystal arthropathies, <u>right</u> shoulder
   M11.812 Other specified crystal arthropathies, <u>left</u> shoulder
   M11.819 Other specified crystal arthropathies, <u>unspecified</u> shoulder

M10-M11

M11.82-Other specified crystal arthropathies, <u>elbow</u>

   M11.821 Other specified crystal arthropathies, <u>right</u> elbow

   M11.822 Other specified crystal arthropathies, <u>left</u> elbow

   M11.829 Other specified crystal arthropathies, <u>unspecified</u> elbow

M11.83-Other specified crystal arthropathies, <u>wrist</u>

   M11.831 Other specified crystal arthropathies, <u>right</u> wrist

   M11.832 Other specified crystal arthropathies, <u>left</u> wrist

   M11.839 Other specified crystal arthropathies, <u>unspecified</u> wrist

M11.84-Other specified crystal arthropathies, <u>hand</u>

   M11.841 Other specified crystal arthropathies, <u>right</u> hand

   M11.842 Other specified crystal arthropathies, <u>left</u> hand

   M11.849 Other specified crystal arthropathies, <u>unspecified</u> hand

M11.85-Other specified crystal arthropathies, <u>hip</u>

   M11.851 Other specified crystal arthropathies, <u>right</u> hip

   M11.852 Other specified crystal arthropathies, <u>left</u> hip

   M11.859 Other specified crystal arthropathies, <u>unspecified</u> hip

M11.86-Other specified crystal arthropathies, <u>knee</u>

   M11.861 Other specified crystal arthropathies, <u>right</u> knee

   M11.862 Other specified crystal arthropathies, <u>left</u> knee

   M11.869 Other specified crystal arthropathies, <u>unspecified</u> knee

M11.87-Other specified crystal arthropathies, <u>ankle and foot</u>

   M11.871 Other specified crystal arthropathies, <u>right</u> ankle and foot

   M11.872 Other specified crystal arthropathies, <u>left</u> ankle and foot

   M11.879 Other specified crystal arthropathies, <u>unspecified</u> ankle and foot

  M11.88 Other specified crystal arthropathies, <u>vertebrae</u>

  M11.89 Other specified crystal arthropathies, <u>multiple sites</u>

 M11.9 Crystal arthropathy, <u>unspecified</u>

M12- <u>Other and unspecified</u> arthropathy

   Excludes 1:   *arthrosis (M15-M19)*
                   cricoarytenoid arthropathy (J38.7)

  M12.0- <u>Chronic postrheumatic arthropathy [Jaccoud]</u> — Chronic inflammation of the joints that follows patients with previous rheumatoid arthritis attacks and the rheumatoid factor is not present in the blood.

   M12.00 Chronic postrheumatic arthropathy [Jaccoud], <u>unspecified</u> site

  M12.01-Chronic postrheumatic arthropathy [Jaccoud], <u>shoulder</u>

   M12.011 Chronic postrheumatic arthropathy [Jaccoud], <u>right</u> shoulder

   M12.012 Chronic postrheumatic arthropathy [Jaccoud], <u>left</u> shoulder

   M12.019 Chronic postrheumatic arthropathy [Jaccoud], <u>unspecified</u> shoulder

  M12.02-Chronic postrheumatic arthropathy [Jaccoud], <u>elbow</u>

   M12.021 Chronic postrheumatic arthropathy [Jaccoud], <u>right</u> elbow

   M12.022 Chronic postrheumatic arthropathy [Jaccoud], <u>left</u> elbow

   M12.029 Chronic postrheumatic arthropathy [Jaccoud], <u>unspecified</u> elbow

  M12.03-Chronic postrheumatic arthropathy [Jaccoud], <u>wrist</u>

   M12.031 Chronic postrheumatic arthropathy [Jaccoud], <u>right</u> wrist

   M12.032 Chronic postrheumatic arthropathy [Jaccoud], <u>left</u> wrist

   M12.039 Chronic postrheumatic arthropathy [Jaccoud], <u>unspecified</u> wrist

M12.04-Chronic postrheumatic arthropathy [Jaccoud], <u>hand</u>

   M12.041 Chronic postrheumatic arthropathy [Jaccoud], <u>right</u> hand

   M12.042 Chronic postrheumatic arthropathy [Jaccoud], <u>left</u> hand

   M12.049 Chronic postrheumatic arthropathy [Jaccoud], <u>unspecified</u> hand

M12.05-Chronic postrheumatic arthropathy [Jaccoud], <u>hip</u>

   M12.051 Chronic postrheumatic arthropathy [Jaccoud], <u>right</u> hip

   M12.052 Chronic postrheumatic arthropathy [Jaccoud], <u>left</u> hip

   M12.059 Chronic postrheumatic arthropathy [Jaccoud], <u>unspecified</u> hip

M12.06-Chronic postrheumatic arthropathy [Jaccoud], <u>knee</u>

   M12.061 Chronic postrheumatic arthropathy [Jaccoud], <u>right</u> knee

   M12.062 Chronic postrheumatic arthropathy [Jaccoud], <u>left</u> knee

   M12.069 Chronic postrheumatic arthropathy [Jaccoud], <u>unspecified</u> knee

M12.07-Chronic postrheumatic arthropathy [Jaccoud], <u>ankle and foot</u>

   M12.071 Chronic postrheumatic arthropathy [Jaccoud], <u>right</u> ankle and foot

   M12.072 Chronic postrheumatic arthropathy [Jaccoud], <u>left</u> ankle and foot

   M12.079 Chronic postrheumatic arthropathy [Jaccoud], <u>unspecified</u> ankle and foot

  M12.08 Chronic postrheumatic arthropathy [Jaccoud], <u>other specified site</u>

      Chronic postrheumatic arthropathy [Jaccoud], vertebrae

  M12.09 Chronic postrheumatic arthropathy [Jaccoud], <u>multiple sites</u>

  M12.1- <u>Kaschin-Beck</u> disease — A chronic osteochondropathy that is characterized by joint pain, stiffness, shortened limb length, and enlarged joints of the fingers that is found primarily in southern China and surrounding areas.

      Osteochondroarthrosis deformans endemica

  M12.10 Kaschin-Beck disease, <u>unspecified</u> site

  M12.11-Kaschin-Beck disease, <u>shoulder</u>

   M12.111 Kaschin-Beck disease, <u>right</u> shoulder

   M12.112 Kaschin-Beck disease, <u>left</u> shoulder

   M12.119 Kaschin-Beck disease, <u>unspecified</u> shoulder

  M12.12-Kaschin-Beck disease, <u>elbow</u>

   M12.121 Kaschin-Beck disease, <u>right</u> elbow

   M12.122 Kaschin-Beck disease, <u>left</u> elbow

   M12.129 Kaschin-Beck disease, <u>unspecified</u> elbow

  M12.13-Kaschin-Beck disease, <u>wrist</u>

   M12.131 Kaschin-Beck disease, <u>right</u> wrist

   M12.132 Kaschin-Beck disease, <u>left</u> wrist

   M12.139 Kaschin-Beck disease, <u>unspecified</u> wrist

  M12.14-Kaschin-Beck disease, <u>hand</u>

   M12.141 Kaschin-Beck disease, <u>right</u> hand

   M12.142 Kaschin-Beck disease, <u>left</u> hand

   M12.149 Kaschin-Beck disease, <u>unspecified</u> hand

  M12.15-Kaschin-Beck disease, <u>hip</u>

   M12.151 Kaschin-Beck disease, <u>right</u> hip

   M12.152 Kaschin-Beck disease, <u>left</u> hip

   M12.159 Kaschin-Beck disease, <u>unspecified</u> hip

  M12.16-Kaschin-Beck disease, <u>knee</u>

   M12.161 Kaschin-Beck disease, <u>right</u> knee

   M12.162 Kaschin-Beck disease, <u>left</u> knee

   M12.169 Kaschin-Beck disease, <u>unspecified</u> knee

M 1 1 - M 1 2

M12.17- Kaschin-Beck disease, <u>ankle and foot</u>
    M12.171 Kaschin-Beck disease, <u>right</u> ankle and foot
    M12.172 Kaschin-Beck disease, <u>left</u> ankle and foot
    M12.179 Kaschin-Beck disease, <u>unspecified</u> ankle and foot
  M12.18 Kaschin-Beck disease, <u>vertebrae</u>
  M12.19 Kaschin-Beck disease, <u>multiple sites</u>
M12.2- <u>Villonodular synovitis (pigmented)</u> — A chronic synovial joint disorder that is characterized by nodular lesions.
  M12.20 Villonodular synovitis (pigmented), <u>unspecified</u> site
  M12.21- Villonodular synovitis (pigmented), <u>shoulder</u>
    M12.211 Villonodular synovitis (pigmented), <u>right</u> shoulder
    M12.212 Villonodular synovitis (pigmented), <u>left</u> shoulder
    M12.219 Villonodular synovitis (pigmented), <u>unspecified</u> shoulder
  M12.22- Villonodular synovitis (pigmented), <u>elbow</u>
    M12.221 Villonodular synovitis (pigmented), <u>right</u> elbow
    M12.222 Villonodular synovitis (pigmented), <u>left</u> elbow
    M12.229 Villonodular synovitis (pigmented), <u>unspecified</u> elbow
  M12.23- Villonodular synovitis (pigmented), <u>wrist</u>
    M12.231 Villonodular synovitis (pigmented), <u>right</u> wrist
    M12.232 Villonodular synovitis (pigmented), <u>left</u> wrist
    M12.239 Villonodular synovitis (pigmented), <u>unspecified</u> wrist
  M12.24- Villonodular synovitis (pigmented), <u>hand</u>
    M12.241 Villonodular synovitis (pigmented), <u>right</u> hand
    M12.242 Villonodular synovitis (pigmented), <u>left</u> hand
    M12.249 Villonodular synovitis (pigmented), <u>unspecified</u> hand
  M12.25- Villonodular synovitis (pigmented), <u>hip</u>
    M12.251 Villonodular synovitis (pigmented), <u>right</u> hip
    M12.252 Villonodular synovitis (pigmented), <u>left</u> hip
    M12.259 Villonodular synovitis (pigmented), <u>unspecified</u> hip
  M12.26- Villonodular synovitis (pigmented), <u>knee</u>
    M12.261 Villonodular synovitis (pigmented), <u>right</u> knee
    M12.262 Villonodular synovitis (pigmented), <u>left</u> knee
    M12.269 Villonodular synovitis (pigmented), <u>unspecified</u> knee
  M12.27- Villonodular synovitis (pigmented), <u>ankle and foot</u>
    M12.271 Villonodular synovitis (pigmented), <u>right</u> ankle and foot
    M12.272 Villonodular synovitis (pigmented), <u>left</u> ankle and foot
    M12.279 Villonodular synovitis (pigmented), <u>unspecified</u> ankle and foot
  M12.28 Villonodular synovitis (pigmented), <u>other specified site</u>
    Villonodular synovitis (pigmented), vertebrae
  M12.29 Villonodular synovitis (pigmented), <u>multiple sites</u>
M12.3- <u>Palindromic rheumatism</u> — A chronic arthropathy that is characterized by sudden attacks of acute pain, swelling, and stiffness that come and go but do not show signs of permanent damage to the joints.
  M12.30 Palindromic rheumatism, <u>unspecified</u> site
  M12.31- Palindromic rheumatism, <u>shoulder</u>
    M12.311 Palindromic rheumatism, <u>right</u> shoulder
    M12.312 Palindromic rheumatism, <u>left</u> shoulder
    M12.319 Palindromic rheumatism, <u>unspecified</u> shoulder
  M12.32- Palindromic rheumatism, <u>elbow</u>
    M12.321 Palindromic rheumatism, <u>right</u> elbow
    M12.322 Palindromic rheumatism, <u>left</u> elbow
    M12.329 Palindromic rheumatism, <u>unspecified</u> elbow
  M12.33- Palindromic rheumatism, <u>wrist</u>
    M12.331 Palindromic rheumatism, <u>right</u> wrist
    M12.332 Palindromic rheumatism, <u>left</u> wrist
    M12.339 Palindromic rheumatism, <u>unspecified</u> wrist
  M12.34- Palindromic rheumatism, <u>hand</u>
    M12.341 Palindromic rheumatism, <u>right</u> hand

    M12.342 Palindromic rheumatism, <u>left</u> hand
    M12.349 Palindromic rheumatism, <u>unspecified</u> hand
  M12.35- Palindromic rheumatism, <u>hip</u>
    M12.351 Palindromic rheumatism, <u>right</u> hip
    M12.352 Palindromic rheumatism, <u>left</u> hip
    M12.359 Palindromic rheumatism, <u>unspecified</u> hip
  M12.36- Palindromic rheumatism, <u>knee</u>
    M12.361 Palindromic rheumatism, <u>right</u> knee
    M12.362 Palindromic rheumatism, <u>left</u> knee
    M12.369 Palindromic rheumatism, <u>unspecified</u> knee
  M12.37- Palindromic rheumatism, <u>ankle and foot</u>
    M12.371 Palindromic rheumatism, <u>right</u> ankle and foot
    M12.372 Palindromic rheumatism, <u>left</u> ankle and foot
    M12.379 Palindromic rheumatism, <u>unspecified</u> ankle and foot
  M12.38 Palindromic rheumatism, <u>other specified site</u>
    Palindromic rheumatism, vertebrae
  M12.39 Palindromic rheumatism, <u>multiple sites</u>
M12.4- <u>Intermittent hydrarthrosis</u> — A rare arthropathy that usually affects women that is characterized by symmetric joint effusions of the knees and often occurring around the menses period.
  M12.40 Intermittent hydrarthrosis, <u>unspecified</u> site
  M12.41- Intermittent hydrarthrosis, <u>shoulder</u>
    M12.411 Intermittent hydrarthrosis, <u>right</u> shoulder
    M12.412 Intermittent hydrarthrosis, <u>left</u> shoulder
    M12.419 Intermittent hydrarthrosis, <u>unspecified</u> shoulder
  M12.42- Intermittent hydrarthrosis, <u>elbow</u>
    M12.421 Intermittent hydrarthrosis, <u>right</u> elbow
    M12.422 Intermittent hydrarthrosis, <u>left</u> elbow
    M12.429 Intermittent hydrarthrosis, <u>unspecified</u> elbow
  M12.43- Intermittent hydrarthrosis, <u>wrist</u>
    M12.431 Intermittent hydrarthrosis, <u>right</u> wrist
    M12.432 Intermittent hydrarthrosis, <u>left</u> wrist
    M12.439 Intermittent hydrarthrosis, <u>unspecified</u> wrist
  M12.44- Intermittent hydrarthrosis, <u>hand</u>
    M12.441 Intermittent hydrarthrosis, <u>right</u> hand
    M12.442 Intermittent hydrarthrosis, <u>left</u> hand
    M12.449 Intermittent hydrarthrosis, <u>unspecified</u> hand
  M12.45- Intermittent hydrarthrosis, <u>hip</u>
    M12.451 Intermittent hydrarthrosis, <u>right</u> hip
    M12.452 Intermittent hydrarthrosis, <u>left</u> hip
    M12.459 Intermittent hydrarthrosis, <u>unspecified</u> hip
  M12.46- Intermittent hydrarthrosis, <u>knee</u>
    M12.461 Intermittent hydrarthrosis, <u>right</u> knee
    M12.462 Intermittent hydrarthrosis, <u>left</u> knee
    M12.469 Intermittent hydrarthrosis, <u>unspecified</u> knee
  M12.47- Intermittent hydrarthrosis, <u>ankle and foot</u>
    M12.471 Intermittent hydrarthrosis, <u>right</u> ankle and foot
    M12.472 Intermittent hydrarthrosis, <u>left</u> ankle and foot
    M12.479 Intermittent hydrarthrosis, <u>unspecified</u> ankle and foot
  M12.48 Intermittent hydrarthrosis, <u>other site</u>
  M12.49 Intermittent hydrarthrosis, <u>multiple sites</u>
M12.5- <u>Traumatic arthropathy</u> — An arthropathy that is due to a traumatic injury to a joint.
  AHA 15:1Q:p17 – Traumatic arthritis of hip secondary to femur fracture
  Excludes 1:   current injury — see Alphabetic Index
        post-traumatic osteoarthritis of first carpometacarpal joint (M18.2-M18.3)
        post-traumatic osteoarthritis of hip (M16.4-M16.5)
        post-traumatic osteoarthritis of knee (M17.2-M17.3)
        post-traumatic osteoarthritis NOS (M19.1-)
        post-traumatic osteoarthritis of other single joints (M19.1-)
  M12.50 Traumatic arthropathy, <u>unspecified</u> site

M12 - M12

M12.51-Traumatic arthropathy, shoulder
- M12.511   Traumatic arthropathy, right shoulder
- M12.512   Traumatic arthropathy, left shoulder
- M12.519   Traumatic arthropathy, unspecified shoulder

M12.52-Traumatic arthropathy, elbow
- M12.521   Traumatic arthropathy, right elbow
- M12.522   Traumatic arthropathy, left elbow
- M12.529   Traumatic arthropathy, unspecified elbow

M12.53-Traumatic arthropathy, wrist
- M12.531   Traumatic arthropathy, right wrist
- M12.532   Traumatic arthropathy, left wrist
- M12.539   Traumatic arthropathy, unspecified wrist

M12.54-Traumatic arthropathy, hand
- M12.541   Traumatic arthropathy, right hand
- M12.542   Traumatic arthropathy, left hand
- M12.549   Traumatic arthropathy, unspecified hand

M12.55-Traumatic arthropathy, hip
- M12.551   Traumatic arthropathy, right hip
- M12.552   Traumatic arthropathy, left hip
- M12.559   Traumatic arthropathy, unspecified hip

M12.56-Traumatic arthropathy, knee
- M12.561   Traumatic arthropathy, right knee
- M12.562   Traumatic arthropathy, left knee
- M12.569   Traumatic arthropathy, unspecified knee

M12.57-Traumatic arthropathy, ankle and foot
- M12.571   Traumatic arthropathy, right ankle and foot
- M12.572   Traumatic arthropathy, left ankle and foot
- M12.579   Traumatic arthropathy, unspecified ankle and foot

M12.58   Traumatic arthropathy, other specified site
  Traumatic arthropathy, vertebrae

M12.59   Traumatic arthropathy, multiple sites

M12.8-   Other specific arthropathies, not elsewhere classified
  Transient arthropathy

M12.80   Other specific arthropathies, not elsewhere classified, unspecified site

M12.81-Other specific arthropathies, not elsewhere classified, shoulder
- M12.811   Other specific arthropathies, not elsewhere classified, right shoulder
- M12.812   Other specific arthropathies, not elsewhere classified, left shoulder
- M12.819   Other specific arthropathies, not elsewhere classified, unspecified shoulder

M12.82-Other specific arthropathies, not elsewhere classified, elbow
- M12.821   Other specific arthropathies, not elsewhere classified, right elbow
- M12.822   Other specific arthropathies, not elsewhere classified, left elbow
- M12.829   Other specific arthropathies, not elsewhere classified, unspecified elbow

M12.83-Other specific arthropathies, not elsewhere classified, wrist
- M12.831   Other specific arthropathies, not elsewhere classified, right wrist
- M12.832   Other specific arthropathies, not elsewhere classified, left wrist
- M12.839   Other specific arthropathies, not elsewhere classified, unspecified wrist

M12.84-Other specific arthropathies, not elsewhere classified, hand
- M12.841   Other specific arthropathies, not elsewhere classified, right hand
- M12.842   Other specific arthropathies, not elsewhere classified, left hand
- M12.849   Other specific arthropathies, not elsewhere classified, unspecified hand

M12.85-Other specific arthropathies, not elsewhere classified, hip
- M12.851   Other specific arthropathies, not elsewhere classified, right hip
- M12.852   Other specific arthropathies, not elsewhere classified, left hip
- M12.859   Other specific arthropathies, not elsewhere classified, unspecified hip

M12.86-Other specific arthropathies, not elsewhere classified, knee
- M12.861   Other specific arthropathies, not elsewhere classified, right knee
- M12.862   Other specific arthropathies, not elsewhere classified, left knee
- M12.869   Other specific arthropathies, not elsewhere classified, unspecified knee

M12.87-Other specific arthropathies, not elsewhere classified, ankle and foot
- M12.871   Other specific arthropathies, not elsewhere classified, right ankle and foot
- M12.872   Other specific arthropathies, not elsewhere classified, left ankle and foot
- M12.879   Other specific arthropathies, not elsewhere classified, unspecified ankle and foot

M12.88   Other specific arthropathies, not elsewhere classified, other specified site
  Other specific arthropathies, not elsewhere classified, vertebrae

M12.89   Other specific arthropathies, not elsewhere classified, multiple sites

M12.9   Arthropathy, unspecified

M13-   Other arthritis
  Excludes 1:   *arthrosis (M15-M19)*
              osteoarthritis (M15-M19)

M13.0   Polyarthritis, unspecified — A form affecting multiple joints and of an unknown cause.

M13.1-   Monoarthritis, not elsewhere classified — A form affecting a single joint and of an unknown cause.
- **M13.10   Monoarthritis, not elsewhere classified, unspecified site**
- **M13.11-Monoarthritis, not elsewhere classified, shoulder**
  - M13.111   Monoarthritis, not elsewhere classified, right shoulder
  - M13.112   Monoarthritis, not elsewhere classified, left shoulder
  - M13.119   Monoarthritis, not elsewhere classified, unspecified shoulder
- **M13.12-Monoarthritis, not elsewhere classified, elbow**
  - M13.121   Monoarthritis, not elsewhere classified, right elbow
  - M13.122   Monoarthritis, not elsewhere classified, left elbow
  - M13.129   Monoarthritis, not elsewhere classified, unspecified elbow
- **M13.13-Monoarthritis, not elsewhere classified, wrist**
  - M13.131   Monoarthritis, not elsewhere classified, right wrist
  - M13.132   Monoarthritis, not elsewhere classified, left wrist
  - M13.139   Monoarthritis, not elsewhere classified, unspecified wrist
- **M13.14-Monoarthritis, not elsewhere classified, hand**
  - M13.141   Monoarthritis, not elsewhere classified, right hand
  - M13.142   Monoarthritis, not elsewhere classified, left hand
  - M13.149   Monoarthritis, not elsewhere classified, unspecified hand
- **M13.15-Monoarthritis, not elsewhere classified, hip**
  - M13.151   Monoarthritis, not elsewhere classified, right hip
  - M13.152   Monoarthritis, not elsewhere classified, left hip
  - M13.159   Monoarthritis, not elsewhere classified, unspecified hip
- **M13.16-Monoarthritis, not elsewhere classified, knee**
  - M13.161   Monoarthritis, not elsewhere classified, right knee

M12-M13

M13.162   Monoarthritis, not elsewhere classified, <u>left</u> knee
M13.169   Monoarthritis, not elsewhere classified, <u>unspecified</u> knee
M13.17- Monoarthritis, not elsewhere classified, <u>ankle and foot</u>
M13.171   Monoarthritis, not elsewhere classified, <u>right</u> ankle and foot
M13.172   Monoarthritis, not elsewhere classified, <u>left</u> ankle and foot
M13.179   Monoarthritis, not elsewhere classified, <u>unspecified</u> ankle and foot
M13.8- <u>Other specified arthritis</u>
    Allergic arthritis — Inflammation of a joint(s) that is due to an allergen.
    Excludes 1:   osteoarthritis (M15-M19)
M13.80 Other specified arthritis, <u>unspecified</u> site
M13.81- Other specified arthritis, <u>shoulder</u>
M13.811   Other specified arthritis, <u>right</u> shoulder
M13.812   Other specified arthritis, <u>left</u> shoulder
M13.819   Other specified arthritis, <u>unspecified</u> shoulder
M13.82- Other specified arthritis, <u>elbow</u>
M13.821   Other specified arthritis, <u>right</u> elbow
M13.822   Other specified arthritis, <u>left</u> elbow
M13.829   Other specified arthritis, <u>unspecified</u> elbow
M13.83- Other specified arthritis, <u>wrist</u>
M13.831   Other specified arthritis, <u>right</u> wrist
M13.832   Other specified arthritis, <u>left</u> wrist
M13.839   Other specified arthritis, <u>unspecified</u> wrist
M13.84- Other specified arthritis, <u>hand</u>
M13.841   Other specified arthritis, <u>right</u> hand
M13.842   Other specified arthritis, <u>left</u> hand
M13.849   Other specified arthritis, <u>unspecified</u> hand
M13.85- Other specified arthritis, <u>hip</u>
M13.851   Other specified arthritis, <u>right</u> hip
M13.852   Other specified arthritis, <u>left</u> hip
M13.859   Other specified arthritis, <u>unspecified</u> hip
M13.86- Other specified arthritis, <u>knee</u>
M13.861   Other specified arthritis, <u>right</u> knee
M13.862   Other specified arthritis, <u>left</u> knee
M13.869   Other specified arthritis, <u>unspecified</u> knee
M13.87- Other specified arthritis, <u>ankle and foot</u>
M13.871   Other specified arthritis, <u>right</u> ankle and foot
M13.872   Other specified arthritis, <u>left</u> ankle and foot
M13.879   Other specified arthritis, <u>unspecified</u> ankle and foot
M13.88 Other specified arthritis, <u>other site</u>
M13.89 Other specified arthritis, <u>multiple sites</u>
M14- Arthropathies <u>in other diseases classified elsewhere</u>
    Excludes 1:   arthropathy in:
        diabetes mellitus (E08-E13 with .61-)
        hematological disorders (M36.2-M36.3)
        hypersensitivity reactions (M36.4)
        neoplastic disease (M36.1)
        neurosyphillis (A52.16)
        sarcoidosis (D86.86)
        enteropathic arthropathies (M07.-)
        juvenile psoriatic arthropathy (L40.54)
        lipoid dermatoarthritis (E78.81)
M14.6- <u>Charcot's joint</u> — An arthropathy that is characterized by decreased sensation at the site (usually a weight bearing joint) that leads to bony abnormalities, deformity, and ulceration.
    Neuropathic arthropathy
    Excludes 1:   Charcot's joint in diabetes mellitus (E08-E13 with .610)
        Charcot's joint in tabes dorsalis (A52.16)
M14.60 Charcot's joint, <u>unspecified</u> site
M14.61- Charcot's joint, <u>shoulder</u>
M14.611   Charcot's joint, <u>right</u> shoulder
M14.612   Charcot's joint, <u>left</u> shoulder
M14.619   Charcot's joint, <u>unspecified</u> shoulder

M14.62- Charcot's joint, <u>elbow</u>
M14.621   Charcot's joint, <u>right</u> elbow
M14.622   Charcot's joint, <u>left</u> elbow
M14.629   Charcot's joint, <u>unspecified</u> elbow
M14.63- Charcot's joint, <u>wrist</u>
M14.631   Charcot's joint, <u>right</u> wrist
M14.632   Charcot's joint, <u>left</u> wrist
M14.639   Charcot's joint, <u>unspecified</u> wrist
M14.64- Charcot's joint, <u>hand</u>
M14.641   Charcot's joint, <u>right</u> hand
M14.642   Charcot's joint, <u>left</u> hand
M14.649   Charcot's joint, <u>unspecified</u> hand
M14.65- Charcot's joint, <u>hip</u>
M14.651   Charcot's joint, <u>right</u> hip
M14.652   Charcot's joint, <u>left</u> hip
M14.659   Charcot's joint, <u>unspecified</u> hip
M14.66- Charcot's joint, <u>knee</u>
M14.661   Charcot's joint, <u>right</u> knee
M14.662   Charcot's joint, <u>left</u> knee
M14.669   Charcot's joint, <u>unspecified</u> knee
M14.67- Charcot's joint, <u>ankle and foot</u>
M14.671   Charcot's joint, <u>right</u> ankle and foot
M14.672   Charcot's joint, <u>left</u> ankle and foot
M14.679   Charcot's joint, <u>unspecified</u> ankle and foot
M14.68 Charcot's joint, <u>vertebrae</u>
M14.69 Charcot's joint, <u>multiple sites</u>
M14.8- Arthropathies <u>in other specified diseases classified elsewhere</u>
    Code first underlying disease, such as:
        Amyloidosis (E85.-)
        Erythema multiforme (L51-)
        Erythema nodosum (L52)
        Hemochromatosis (E83.11-)
        Hyperparathyroidism (E21-)
        Hypothyroidism (E00-E03)
        Sickle-cell disorders (D57-)
        Thyrotoxicosis [hyperthyroidism] (E05-)
        Whipple's disease (K90.81)
M14.80 Arthropathies in other specified diseases classified elsewhere, <u>unspecified</u> site — [Not Allowed as PDX]
M14.81- Arthropathies in other specified diseases classified elsewhere, <u>shoulder</u>
M14.811   Arthropathies in other specified diseases classified elsewhere, <u>right</u> shoulder — [Not Allowed as PDX]
M14.812   Arthropathies in other specified diseases classified elsewhere, <u>left</u> shoulder — [Not Allowed as PDX]
M14.819   Arthropathies in other specified diseases classified elsewhere, <u>unspecified</u> shoulder — [Not Allowed as PDX]
M14.82- Arthropathies in other specified diseases classified elsewhere, <u>elbow</u>
M14.821   Arthropathies in other specified diseases classified elsewhere, <u>right</u> elbow — [Not Allowed as PDX]
M14.822   Arthropathies in other specified diseases classified elsewhere, <u>left</u> elbow — [Not Allowed as PDX]
M14.829   Arthropathies in other specified diseases classified elsewhere, <u>unspecified</u> elbow — [Not Allowed as PDX]
M14.83- Arthropathies in other specified diseases classified elsewhere, <u>wrist</u>
M14.831   Arthropathies in other specified diseases classified elsewhere, <u>right</u> wrist — [Not Allowed as PDX]
M14.832   Arthropathies in other specified diseases classified elsewhere, <u>left</u> wrist — [Not Allowed as PDX]
M14.839   Arthropathies in other specified diseases classified elsewhere, <u>unspecified</u> wrist — [Not Allowed as PDX]
M14.84- Arthropathies in other specified diseases classified elsewhere, <u>hand</u>
M14.841   Arthropathies in other specified diseases classified elsewhere, <u>right</u> hand — [Not Allowed as PDX]
M14.842   Arthropathies in other specified diseases classified elsewhere, <u>left</u> hand — [Not Allowed as PDX]

M13 - M14

M14.849 Arthropathies in other specified diseases classified elsewhere, <u>unspecified</u> hand — [Not Allowed as PDX]

M14.85- Arthropathies in other specified diseases classified elsewhere, <u>hip</u>

M14.851 Arthropathies in other specified diseases classified elsewhere, <u>right</u> hip — [Not Allowed as PDX]

M14.852 Arthropathies in other specified diseases classified elsewhere, <u>left</u> hip — [Not Allowed as PDX]

M14.859 Arthropathies in other specified diseases classified elsewhere, <u>unspecified</u> hip — [Not Allowed as PDX]

M14.86- Arthropathies in other specified diseases classified elsewhere, <u>knee</u>

M14.861 Arthropathies in other specified diseases classified elsewhere, <u>right</u> knee — [Not Allowed as PDX]

M14.862 Arthropathies in other specified diseases classified elsewhere, <u>left</u> knee — [Not Allowed as PDX]

M14.869 Arthropathies in other specified diseases classified elsewhere, <u>unspecified</u> knee — [Not Allowed as PDX]

M14.87- Arthropathies in other specified diseases classified elsewhere, <u>ankle and foot</u>

M14.871 Arthropathies in other specified diseases classified elsewhere, <u>right</u> ankle and foot — [Not Allowed as PDX]

M14.872 Arthropathies in other specified diseases classified elsewhere, <u>left</u> ankle and foot — [Not Allowed as PDX]

M14.879 Arthropathies in other specified diseases classified elsewhere, <u>unspecified</u> ankle and foot — [Not Allowed as PDX]

M14.88 Arthropathies in other specified diseases classified elsewhere, <u>vertebrae</u> — [Not Allowed as PDX]

M14.89 Arthropathies in other specified diseases classified elsewhere, <u>multiple sites</u> — [Not Allowed as PDX]

Osteoarthritis (M15-M19)

Excludes ❷: osteoarthritis of spine (M47.-)

M15- <u>Polyosteoarthritis</u> — A degenerative inflammation of the joints that is caused by the breakdown, weardown, or erosion of the joint cartilage and results in damage to the underlying bone.

Includes: Arthritis of multiple sites

Excludes 1:   bilateral involvement of single joint (M16-M19)

M15.0 Primary generalized (osteo)arthritis — A form occurring without any known secondary cause.

M15.1 Heberden's nodes (with arthropathy) — A form marked by the formation of hard nodules in the distal interphalangeal joints of the fingers and toes.

Interphalangeal distal osteoarthritis

M15.2 Bouchard's nodes (with arthropathy) — A form marked by the formation of hard or gelatinous nodules in the proximal interphalangeal joints of the fingers and toes.

Juxtaphalangeal distal osteoarthritis

M15.3 Secondary multiple arthritis — A form caused by another underlying disease or condition.

Post-traumatic polyosteoarthritis

M15.4 Erosive (osteo)arthritis — A form marked by "saw-tooth" deformities of the interphalangeal joints of the hand.

M15.8 Other polyosteoarthritis

M15.9 Polyosteoarthritis, <u>unspecified</u>

Generalized osteoarthritis NOS

M16- <u>Osteoarthritis</u> of <u>hip</u>

M16.0 <u>Bilateral</u> <u>primary</u> osteoarthritis of hip

M16.1- <u>Unilateral</u> <u>primary</u> osteoarthritis of hip

Primary osteoarthritis of hip NOS

M16.10 Unilateral primary osteoarthritis, <u>unspecified</u> hip

M16.11 Unilateral primary osteoarthritis, <u>right</u> hip

M16.12 Unilateral primary osteoarthritis, <u>left</u> hip

M16.2 <u>Bilateral</u> osteoarthritis <u>resulting from hip dysplasia</u>

M16.3- <u>Unilateral</u> osteoarthritis <u>resulting from hip dysplasia</u>

Dysplastic osteoarthritis of hip NOS

M16.30 Unilateral osteoarthritis resulting from hip dysplasia, <u>unspecified</u> hip

M16.31 Unilateral osteoarthritis resulting from hip dysplasia, <u>right</u> hip

M16.32 Unilateral osteoarthritis resulting from hip dysplasia, <u>left</u> hip

M16.4 <u>Bilateral</u> <u>post-traumatic</u> osteoarthritis of hip

M16.5- <u>Unilateral</u> <u>post-traumatic</u> osteoarthritis of hip

Post-traumatic osteoarthritis of hip NOS

M16.50 Unilateral post-traumatic osteoarthritis, <u>unspecified</u> hip

M16.51 Unilateral post-traumatic osteoarthritis, <u>right</u> hip

M16.52 Unilateral post-traumatic osteoarthritis, <u>left</u> hip

M16.6 <u>Other</u> <u>bilateral</u> secondary osteoarthritis of hip

M16.7 <u>Other</u> <u>unilateral</u> secondary osteoarthritis of hip

Secondary osteoarthritis of hip NOS

M16.9 Osteoarthritis of hip, <u>unspecified</u>

M17- <u>Osteoarthritis</u> of <u>knee</u>

M17.0 <u>Bilateral</u> <u>primary</u> osteoarthritis of knee

M17.1- <u>Unilateral</u> <u>primary</u> osteoarthritis of knee

Primary osteoarthritis of knee NOS

M17.10 Unilateral primary osteoarthritis, <u>unspecified</u> knee

M17.11 Unilateral primary osteoarthritis, <u>right</u> knee

M17.12 Unilateral primary osteoarthritis, <u>left</u> knee

M17.2 <u>Bilateral</u> <u>post-traumatic</u> osteoarthritis of knee

M17.3- <u>Unilateral</u> <u>post-traumatic</u> osteoarthritis of knee

Post-traumatic osteoarthritis of knee NOS

M17.30 Unilateral post-traumatic osteoarthritis, <u>unspecified</u> knee

M17.31 Unilateral post-traumatic osteoarthritis, <u>right</u> knee

M17.32 Unilateral post-traumatic osteoarthritis, <u>left</u> knee

M17.4 <u>Other</u> <u>bilateral</u> secondary osteoarthritis of knee

M17.5 <u>Other</u> <u>unilateral</u> secondary osteoarthritis of knee

Secondary osteoarthritis of knee NOS

M17.9 Osteoarthritis of knee, <u>unspecified</u>

M18- <u>Osteoarthritis</u> of <u>first carpometacarpal</u> joint

M18.0 <u>Bilateral</u> <u>primary</u> osteoarthritis of first carpometacarpal joints

M18.1- <u>Unilateral</u> <u>primary</u> osteoarthritis of first carpometacarpal joint

Primary osteoarthritis of first carpometacarpal joint NOS

M18.10 Unilateral primary osteoarthritis of first carpometacarpal joint, <u>unspecified</u> hand

M18.11 Unilateral primary osteoarthritis of first carpometacarpal joint, <u>right</u> hand

M18.12 Unilateral primary osteoarthritis of first carpometacarpal joint, <u>left</u> hand

M18.2 <u>Bilateral</u> <u>post-traumatic</u> osteoarthritis of first carpometacarpal joints

M18.3- <u>Unilateral</u> <u>post-traumatic</u> osteoarthritis of first carpometacarpal joint

Post-traumatic osteoarthritis of first carpometacarpal joint NOS

M18.30 Unilateral post-traumatic osteoarthritis of first carpometacarpal joint, <u>unspecified</u> hand

M18.31 Unilateral post-traumatic osteoarthritis of first carpometacarpal joint, <u>right</u> hand

M18.32 Unilateral post-traumatic osteoarthritis of first carpometacarpal joint, <u>left</u> hand

M18.4 <u>Other</u> <u>bilateral</u> secondary osteoarthritis of first carpometacarpal joints

M18.5- <u>Other</u> <u>unilateral</u> secondary osteoarthritis of first carpometacarpal joint

Secondary osteoarthritis of first carpometacarpal joint NOS

M18.50 Other unilateral secondary osteoarthritis of first carpometacarpal joint, <u>unspecified</u> hand

M18.51 Other unilateral secondary osteoarthritis of first carpometacarpal joint, <u>right</u> hand

M18.52 Other unilateral secondary osteoarthritis of first carpometacarpal joint, <u>left</u> hand

M18.9 Osteoarthritis of first carpometacarpal joint, <u>unspecified</u>

M14-M18

M19 Other and unspecified osteoarthritis
  Excludes 1:   polyarthritis (M15.-)
  Excludes ❷: arthrosis of spine (M47.-)
            hallux rigidus (M20.2)
            osteoarthritis of spine (M47.-)

M19.0- Primary osteoarthritis of other joints
  M19.01- Primary osteoarthritis, shoulder
    M19.011 Primary osteoarthritis, right shoulder
    M19.012 Primary osteoarthritis, left shoulder
    M19.019 Primary osteoarthritis, unspecified shoulder
  M19.02- Primary osteoarthritis, elbow
    M19.021 Primary osteoarthritis, right elbow
    M19.022 Primary osteoarthritis, left elbow
    M19.029 Primary osteoarthritis, unspecified elbow
  M19.03- Primary osteoarthritis, wrist
    M19.031 Primary osteoarthritis, right wrist
    M19.032 Primary osteoarthritis, left wrist
    M19.039 Primary osteoarthritis, unspecified wrist
  M19.04- Primary osteoarthritis, hand
    Excludes ❷: primary osteoarthritis of first carpometacarpal
              joint (M18.0-, M18.1-)
    M19.041 Primary osteoarthritis, right hand
    M19.042 Primary osteoarthritis, left hand
    M19.049 Primary osteoarthritis, unspecified hand
  M19.07- Primary osteoarthritis ankle and foot
    M19.071 Primary osteoarthritis, right ankle and foot
    M19.072 Primary osteoarthritis, left ankle and foot
    M19.079 Primary osteoarthritis, unspecified ankle and foot

M19.1- Post-traumatic osteoarthritis of other joints
  M19.11- Post-traumatic osteoarthritis, shoulder
    M19.111 Post-traumatic osteoarthritis, right shoulder
    M19.112 Post-traumatic osteoarthritis, left shoulder
    M19.119 Post-traumatic osteoarthritis, unspecified shoulder
  M19.12- Post-traumatic osteoarthritis, elbow
    M19.121 Post-traumatic osteoarthritis, right elbow
    M19.122 Post-traumatic osteoarthritis, left elbow
    M19.129 Post-traumatic osteoarthritis, unspecified elbow
  M19.13- Post-traumatic osteoarthritis, wrist
    M19.131 Post-traumatic osteoarthritis, right wrist
    M19.132 Post-traumatic osteoarthritis, left wrist
    M19.139 Post-traumatic osteoarthritis, unspecified wrist
  M19.14- Post-traumatic osteoarthritis, hand
    Excludes ❷: post-traumatic osteoarthritis of first
              carpometacarpal joint (M18.2-, M18.3-)
    M19.141 Post-traumatic osteoarthritis, right hand
    M19.142 Post-traumatic osteoarthritis, left hand
    M19.149 Post-traumatic osteoarthritis, unspecified hand
  M19.17- Post-traumatic osteoarthritis, ankle and foot
    M19.171 Post-traumatic osteoarthritis, right ankle and foot
    M19.172 Post-traumatic osteoarthritis, left ankle and foot
    M19.179 Post-traumatic osteoarthritis, unspecified ankle
            and foot

M19.2- Secondary osteoarthritis of other joints
  M19.21- Secondary osteoarthritis, shoulder
    M19.211 Secondary osteoarthritis, right shoulder
    M19.212 Secondary osteoarthritis, left shoulder
    M19.219 Secondary osteoarthritis, unspecified shoulder
  M19.22- Secondary osteoarthritis, elbow
    M19.221 Secondary osteoarthritis, right elbow
    M19.222 Secondary osteoarthritis, left elbow
    M19.229 Secondary osteoarthritis, unspecified elbow
  M19.23- Secondary osteoarthritis, wrist
    M19.231 Secondary osteoarthritis, right wrist
    M19.232 Secondary osteoarthritis, left wrist
    M19.239 Secondary osteoarthritis, unspecified wrist

  M19.24- Secondary osteoarthritis, hand
    M19.241 Secondary osteoarthritis, right hand
    M19.242 Secondary osteoarthritis, left hand
    M19.249 Secondary osteoarthritis, unspecified hand
  M19.27- Secondary osteoarthritis, ankle and foot
    M19.271 Secondary osteoarthritis, right ankle and foot
    M19.272 Secondary osteoarthritis, left ankle and foot
    M19.279 Secondary osteoarthritis, unspecified ankle and
            foot

M19.9- Osteoarthritis, unspecified site
  M19.90 Unspecified osteoarthritis, unspecified site
      Arthrosis NOS
      Arthritis NOS
      Osteoarthritis NOS
  M19.91 Primary osteoarthritis, unspecified site
      Primary osteoarthritis NOS
  M19.92 Post-traumatic osteoarthritis, unspecified site
      Post-traumatic osteoarthritis NOS
  M19.93 Secondary osteoarthritis, unspecified site
      Secondary osteoarthritis NOS

Other joint disorders (M20-M25)

  Excludes ❷: joints of the spine (M40-M54)
M20- Acquired deformities of fingers and toes — The deviation of the normal anatomical structure and alignment of the fingers and toes.
  Excludes 1:   acquired absence of fingers and toes (Z89.-)
            congenital absence of fingers and toes (Q71.3-, Q72.3-)
            congenital deformities and malformations of fingers and toes
            (Q66.-, Q68-Q70, Q74.-)
M20.0- Deformity of finger(s)
  Excludes 1:   clubbing of fingers (R68.3)
            palmar fascial fibromatosis [Dupuytren] (M72.0)
            trigger finger (M65.3)
  M20.00- Unspecified deformity of finger(s)
    M20.001 Unspecified deformity of right finger(s)
    M20.002 Unspecified deformity of left finger(s)
    M20.009 Unspecified deformity of unspecified finger(s)
  M20.01- Mallet finger — The permanent flexion of a distal phalanx.
    M20.011 Mallet finger of right finger(s)
    M20.012 Mallet finger of left finger(s)
    M20.019 Mallet finger of unspecified finger(s)
  M20.02- Boutonnière deformity — Flexion of the proximal phalanx and hyperextension of the distal joint.
    M20.021 Boutonnière deformity of right finger(s)
    M20.022 Boutonnière deformity of left finger(s)
    M20.029 Boutonnière deformity of unspecified finger(s)
  M20.03- Swan-neck deformity — Hyperextended proximal interphalangeal joint and flexion of the distal interphalangeal joint.
    M20.031 Swan-neck deformity of right finger(s)
    M20.032 Swan-neck deformity of left finger(s)
    M20.039 Swan-neck deformity of unspecified finger(s)
  M20.09- Other deformity of finger(s)
    M20.091 Other deformity of right finger(s)
    M20.092 Other deformity of left finger(s)
    M20.099 Other deformity of finger(s), unspecified finger(s)
M20.1- Hallux valgus (acquired) — Angulation of the great toe towards other toes of that foot.
  Excludes ❷: bunion (M21.6-)
  M20.10 Hallux valgus (acquired), unspecified foot
  M20.11 Hallux valgus (acquired), right foot
  M20.12 Hallux valgus (acquired), left foot
M20.2- Hallux rigidus — Painful restriction of joint motion of the great toe.
  M20.20 Hallux rigidus, unspecified foot
  M20.21 Hallux rigidus, right foot
  M20.22 Hallux rigidus, left foot

M19 - M20

M20.3- **Hallux varus (acquired)** — Angulation of the great toe away from the other toes of that foot.

   M20.30 Hallux varus (acquired), **unspecified** foot
   M20.31 Hallux varus (acquired), **right** foot
   M20.32 Hallux varus (acquired), **left** foot

M20.4- **Other hammer toe(s) (acquired)** — The claw-like deformity of a toe, other than a great toe.

   M20.40 Other hammer toe(s) (acquired), **unspecified** foot
   M20.41 Other hammer toe(s) (acquired), **right** foot
   M20.42 Other hammer toe(s) (acquired), **left** foot

M20.5- **Other deformities of toe(s) (acquired)**

   M20.5x- Other deformities of toe(s) (acquired)
      M20.5x1 Other deformities of toe(s) (acquired), **right** foot
      M20.5x2 Other deformities of toe(s) (acquired), **left** foot
      M20.5x9 Other deformities of toe(s) (acquired), **unspecified** foot

M20.6- **Acquired** deformities of toe(s), **unspecified**

   M20.60 Acquired deformities of toe(s), **unspecified**, **unspecified** foot
   M20.61 Acquired deformities of toe(s), **unspecified**, **right** foot
   M20.62 Acquired deformities of toe(s), **unspecified**, **left** foot

M21- **Other acquired deformities of limbs** — The deviation of the normal anatomical structure and alignment of the limbs, except of the fingers and toes.

   Excludes 1:   *acquired absence of limb (Z89.-)*
                congenital absence of limbs (Q71-Q73)
                congenital deformities and malformations of limbs (Q65-Q66, Q68-Q74)
   Excludes ❷: *acquired deformities of fingers or toes (M20.-)*
                coxa plana (M91.2)

M21.0- **Valgus** deformity, **not elsewhere classified** — Angulation away from the body.
   Excludes 1:   *metatarsus valgus (Q66.6)*
                talipes calcaneovalgus (Q66.4)

   M21.00 Valgus deformity, not elsewhere classified, **unspecified** site
   M21.02- Valgus deformity, not elsewhere classified, **elbow**
      Cubitus valgus — Angulation of the forearm away from the body.
      M21.021 Valgus deformity, not elsewhere classified, **right** elbow
      M21.022 Valgus deformity, not elsewhere classified, **left** elbow
      M21.029 Valgus deformity, not elsewhere classified, **unspecified** elbow
   M21.05- Valgus deformity, not elsewhere classified, **hip**
      M21.051 Valgus deformity, not elsewhere classified, **right** hip
      M21.052 Valgus deformity, not elsewhere classified, **left** hip
      M21.059 Valgus deformity, not elsewhere classified, **unspecified** hip
   M21.06- Valgus deformity, not elsewhere classified, **knee**
      Genu valgum — The deformity in which the knees are close together.
      Knock knee
      M21.061 Valgus deformity, not elsewhere classified, **right** knee
      M21.062 Valgus deformity, not elsewhere classified, **left** knee
      M21.069 Valgus deformity, not elsewhere classified, **unspecified** knee
   M21.07- Valgus deformity, not elsewhere classified, **ankle**
      M21.071 Valgus deformity, not elsewhere classified, **right** ankle
      M21.072 Valgus deformity, not elsewhere classified, **left** ankle
      M21.079 Valgus deformity, not elsewhere classified, **unspecified** ankle

M21.1- **Varus** deformity, **not elsewhere classified** — Angulation towards the body.
   Excludes 1:   *metatarsus varus (Q66.22)*
                tibia vara (M92.5)

   M21.10 Varus deformity, not elsewhere classified, **unspecified** site
   M21.12- Varus deformity, not elsewhere classified, **elbow**
      Cubitus varus, elbow — Angulation of the forearm towards the body.
      M21.121 Varus deformity, not elsewhere classified, **right** elbow
      M21.122 Varus deformity, not elsewhere classified, **left** elbow
      M21.129 Varus deformity, not elsewhere classified, **unspecified** elbow
   M21.15- Varus deformity, not elsewhere classified, **hip**
      M21.151 Varus deformity, not elsewhere classified, **right** hip
      M21.152 Varus deformity, not elsewhere classified, **left** hip
      M21.159 Varus deformity, not elsewhere classified, **unspecified** hip
   M21.16- Varus deformity, not elsewhere classified, **knee**
      Bow leg
      Genu varum — The deformity in which the knees are more separated.
      M21.161 Varus deformity, not elsewhere classified, **right** knee
      M21.162 Varus deformity, not elsewhere classified, **left** knee
      M21.169 Varus deformity, not elsewhere classified, **unspecified** knee
   M21.17- Varus deformity, not elsewhere classified, **ankle**
      M21.171 Varus deformity, not elsewhere classified, **right** ankle
      M21.172 Varus deformity, not elsewhere classified, **left** ankle
      M21.179 Varus deformity, not elsewhere classified, **unspecified** ankle

M21.2- **Flexion deformity** — The inability to straighten the joint to its normal range of motion postion.

   M21.20 Flexion deformity, **unspecified** site
   M21.21- Flexion deformity, **shoulder**
      M21.211 Flexion deformity, **right** shoulder
      M21.212 Flexion deformity, **left** shoulder
      M21.219 Flexion deformity, **unspecified** shoulder
   M21.22- Flexion deformity, **elbow**
      M21.221 Flexion deformity, **right** elbow
      M21.222 Flexion deformity, **left** elbow
      M21.229 Flexion deformity, **unspecified** elbow
   M21.23- Flexion deformity, **wrist**
      M21.231 Flexion deformity, **right** wrist
      M21.232 Flexion deformity, **left** wrist
      M21.239 Flexion deformity, **unspecified** wrist
   M21.24- Flexion deformity, **finger joints**
      M21.241 Flexion deformity, **right** finger joints
      M21.242 Flexion deformity, **left** finger joints
      M21.249 Flexion deformity, **unspecified** finger joints
   M21.25- Flexion deformity, **hip**
      M21.251 Flexion deformity, **right** hip
      M21.252 Flexion deformity, **left** hip
      M21.259 Flexion deformity, **unspecified** hip
   M21.26- Flexion deformity, **knee**
      M21.261 Flexion deformity, **right** knee
      M21.262 Flexion deformity, **left** knee
      M21.269 Flexion deformity, **unspecified** knee
   M21.27- Flexion deformity, **ankle and toes**
      M21.271 Flexion deformity, **right** ankle and toes
      M21.272 Flexion deformity, **left** ankle and toes
      M21.279 Flexion deformity, **unspecified** ankle and toes

M20 - M21

M21.3- Wrist or foot drop (acquired)

M21.33- Wrist drop (acquired) — Paralysis of the extensor muscles with a dropping deformity of the hand.

M21.331 Wrist drop, right wrist

M21.332 Wrist drop, left wrist

M21.339 Wrist drop, unspecified wrist

M21.37- Foot drop (acquired) — Paralysis of the extensor muscles with a dropping deformity of the foot.

M21.371 Foot drop, right foot

M21.372 Foot drop, left foot

M21.379 Foot drop, unspecified foot

M21.4- Flat foot [pes planus] (acquired) — The flattened-out arch of a foot.

Excludes 1:   congenital pes planus (Q66.5-)

M21.40 Flat foot [pes planus] (acquired), unspecified foot

M21.41 Flat foot [pes planus] (acquired), right foot

M21.42 Flat foot [pes planus] (acquired), left foot

M21.5- Acquired clawhand, clubhand, clawfoot and clubfoot

Excludes 1:   clubfoot, not specified as acquired (Q66.89)

M21.51- Acquired clawhand — A deformity with extension of the 4th and 5th metacarpophalangeal joints with flexion of the 4th and 5th fingers that is caused by damage to the ulnar nerve.

M21.511 Acquired clawhand, right hand

M21.512 Acquired clawhand, left hand

M21.519 Acquired clawhand, unspecified hand

M21.52- Acquired clubhand — A twisting deformity of the hand.

M21.521 Acquired clubhand, right hand

M21.522 Acquired clubhand, left hand

M21.529 Acquired clubhand, unspecified hand

M21.53- Acquired clawfoot — The increased arch of the foot with deformity of the toes.

M21.531 Acquired clawfoot, right foot

M21.532 Acquired clawfoot, left foot

M21.539 Acquired clawfoot, unspecified foot

M21.54- Acquired clubfoot — The turning inward of the heel with turning upward of the inner edge of the foot.

M21.541 Acquired clubfoot, right foot

M21.542 Acquired clubfoot, left foot

M21.549 Acquired clubfoot, unspecified foot

M21.6- Other acquired deformities of foot

Excludes ❷: deformities of toe (acquired) (M20.1-M20.6-)

M21.61- Bunion — Hypertrophy/edema/bursitis of the medial eminence of the first metatarsal head.

M21.611 Bunion of right foot

M21.612 Bunion of left foot

M21.619 Bunion of unspecified foot

M21.62- Bunionette — Hypertrophy/edema/bursitis of the lateral condyle of the fifth metatarsal head.

M21.621 Bunionette of right foot

M21.622 Bunionette of left foot

M21.629 Bunionette of unspecified foot

M21.6x- Other acquired deformities of foot

M21.6x1 Other acquired deformities of right foot

M21.6x2 Other acquired deformities of left foot

M21.6x9 Other acquired deformities of unspecified foot

M21.7- Unequal limb length (acquired)

Note: The site used should correspond to the shorter limb

M21.70 Unequal limb length (acquired), unspecified site

M21.72- Unequal limb length (acquired), humerus

M21.721 Unequal limb length (acquired), right humerus

M21.722 Unequal limb length (acquired), left humerus

M21.729 Unequal limb length (acquired), unspecified humerus

M21.73- Unequal limb length (acquired), ulna and radius

M21.731 Unequal limb length (acquired), right ulna

M21.732 Unequal limb length (acquired), left ulna

M21.733 Unequal limb length (acquired), right radius

M21.734 Unequal limb length (acquired), left radius

M21.739 Unequal limb length (acquired), unspecified ulna and radius

M21.75- Unequal limb length (acquired), femur

M21.751 Unequal limb length (acquired), right femur

M21.752 Unequal limb length (acquired), left femur

M21.759 Unequal limb length (acquired), unspecified femur

M21.76- Unequal limb length (acquired), tibia and fibula

M21.761 Unequal limb length (acquired), right tibia

M21.762 Unequal limb length (acquired), left tibia

M21.763 Unequal limb length (acquired), right fibula

M21.764 Unequal limb length (acquired), left fibula

M21.769 Unequal limb length (acquired), unspecified tibia and fibula

M21.8- Other specified acquired deformities of limbs

Excludes ❷: coxa plana (M91.2)

M21.80 Other specified acquired deformities of unspecified limb

M21.82- Other specified acquired deformities of upper arm

M21.821 Other specified acquired deformities of right upper arm

M21.822 Other specified acquired deformities of left upper arm

M21.829 Other specified acquired deformities of unspecified upper arm

M21.83- Other specified acquired deformities of forearm

M21.831 Other specified acquired deformities of right forearm

M21.832 Other specified acquired deformities of left forearm

M21.839 Other specified acquired deformities of unspecified forearm

M21.85- Other specified acquired deformities of thigh

M21.851 Other specified acquired deformities of right thigh

M21.852 Other specified acquired deformities of left thigh

M21.859 Other specified acquired deformities of unspecified thigh

M21.86- Other specified acquired deformities of lower leg

M21.861 Other specified acquired deformities of right lower leg

M21.862 Other specified acquired deformities of left lower leg

M21.869 Other specified acquired deformities of unspecified lower leg

M21.9- Unspecified acquired deformity of limb and hand

M21.90 Unspecified acquired deformity of unspecified limb

M21.92- Unspecified acquired deformity of upper arm

M21.921 Unspecified acquired deformity of right upper arm

M21.922 Unspecified acquired deformity of left upper arm

M21.929 Unspecified acquired deformity of unspecified upper arm

M21.93- Unspecified acquired deformity of forearm

M21.931 Unspecified acquired deformity of right forearm

M21.932 Unspecified acquired deformity of left forearm

M21.939 Unspecified acquired deformity of unspecified forearm

M21.94- Unspecified acquired deformity of hand

M21.941 Unspecified acquired deformity of hand, right hand

M21.942 Unspecified acquired deformity of hand, left hand

M21.949 Unspecified acquired deformity of hand, unspecified hand

M21.95- Unspecified acquired deformity of thigh

M21.951 Unspecified acquired deformity of right thigh

M21.952 Unspecified acquired deformity of left thigh

M21.959 Unspecified acquired deformity of unspecified thigh

M21 - M21 - M21

M21.96- Unspecified acquired deformity of <u>lower leg</u>
  M21.961 Unspecified acquired deformity of <u>right</u> lower leg
  M21.962 Unspecified acquired deformity of <u>left</u> lower leg
  M21.969 Unspecified acquired deformity of <u>unspecified</u> lower leg

M22- Disorder of <u>patella</u>
  Excludes 1: traumatic dislocation of patella (S83.0-)
  M22.0- <u>Recurrent dislocation</u> of patella — The current dislocation of the patella that is due to previous tissue damage or defect, but is not due to a current traumatic event.
    M22.00 Recurrent dislocation of patella, <u>unspecified</u> knee
    M22.01 Recurrent dislocation of patella, <u>right</u> knee
    M22.02 Recurrent dislocation of patella, <u>left</u> knee
  M22.1- <u>Recurrent subluxation</u> of patella — Partial dislocation of the patella.
    Incomplete dislocation of patella
    M22.10 Recurrent subluxation of patella, <u>unspecified</u> knee
    M22.11 Recurrent subluxation of patella, <u>right</u> knee
    M22.12 Recurrent subluxation of patella, <u>left</u> knee
  M22.2- Patellofemoral disorders
    M22.2x- <u>Patellofemoral disorders</u>
      M22.2x1 Patellofemoral disorders, <u>right</u> knee
      M22.2x2 Patellofemoral disorders, <u>left</u> knee
      M22.2x9 Patellofemoral disorders, <u>unspecified</u> knee
  M22.3- Other derangements of patella
    M22.3x- <u>Other derangements</u> of patella
      M22.3x1 Other derangements of patella, <u>right</u> knee
      M22.3x2 Other derangements of patella, <u>left</u> knee
      M22.3x9 Other derangements of patella, <u>unspecified</u> knee
  M22.4- <u>Chondromalacia</u> patellae — The softening of the patellar cartilage tissue.
    M22.40 Chondromalacia patellae, <u>unspecified</u> knee
    M22.41 Chondromalacia patellae, <u>right</u> knee
    M22.42 Chondromalacia patellae, <u>left</u> knee
  M22.8- Other disorders of patella
    M22.8x- <u>Other disorders</u> of patella
      M22.8x1 Other disorders of patella, <u>right</u> knee
      M22.8x2 Other disorders of patella, <u>left</u> knee
      M22.8x9 Other disorders of patella, <u>unspecified</u> knee
  M22.9- <u>Unspecified disorder</u> of patella
    M22.90 Unspecified disorder of patella, <u>unspecified</u> knee
    M22.91 Unspecified disorder of patella, <u>right</u> knee
    M22.92 Unspecified disorder of patella, <u>left</u> knee

M23- <u>Internal derangement</u> of <u>knee</u> — The instability disorders of the knee joint ligaments and menisci due to the malfunctioning disarrangement of the knee joint structures that is due to a previous direct trauma or an injury (wearing) of repetitive use, but not the result of an acute trauma.
  Excludes 1: ankylosis (M24.66)
    current injury — see injury of knee and lower leg (S80-S89)
    deformity of knee (M21.-)
    osteochondritis dissecans (M93.2)
    recurrent dislocation or subluxation of joints (M24.4)
    recurrent dislocation or subluxation of patella (M22.0-M22.1)
  M23.0- <u>Cystic meniscus</u>
    M23.00- Cystic meniscus, <u>unspecified meniscus</u>
      Cystic meniscus, unspecified lateral meniscus
      Cystic meniscus, unspecified medial meniscus
      M23.000 Cystic meniscus, <u>unspecified</u> <u>lateral</u> meniscus, <u>right</u> knee
      M23.001 Cystic meniscus, <u>unspecified</u> <u>lateral</u> meniscus, <u>left</u> knee
      M23.002 Cystic meniscus, <u>unspecified</u> <u>lateral</u> meniscus, <u>unspecified</u> knee
      M23.003 Cystic meniscus, <u>unspecified</u> <u>medial</u> meniscus, <u>right</u> knee
      M23.004 Cystic meniscus, <u>unspecified</u> <u>medial</u> meniscus, <u>left</u> knee
      M23.005 Cystic meniscus, <u>unspecified</u> <u>medial</u> meniscus, <u>unspecified</u> knee

M23.006 Cystic meniscus, <u>unspecified</u> meniscus, <u>right</u> knee
M23.007 Cystic meniscus, <u>unspecified</u> meniscus, <u>left</u> knee
M23.009 Cystic meniscus, <u>unspecified</u> meniscus, <u>unspecified</u> knee
  M23.01- Cystic meniscus, <u>anterior horn</u> of <u>medial</u> meniscus
    M23.011 Cystic meniscus, anterior horn of medial meniscus, <u>right</u> knee
    M23.012 Cystic meniscus, anterior horn of medial meniscus, <u>left</u> knee
    M23.019 Cystic meniscus, anterior horn of medial meniscus, <u>unspecified</u> knee
  M23.02- Cystic meniscus, <u>posterior horn</u> of <u>medial</u> meniscus
    M23.021 Cystic meniscus, posterior horn of medial meniscus, <u>right</u> knee
    M23.022 Cystic meniscus, posterior horn of medial meniscus, <u>left</u> knee
    M23.029 Cystic meniscus, posterior horn of medial meniscus, <u>unspecified</u> knee
  M23.03- Cystic meniscus, <u>other medial meniscus</u>
    M23.031 Cystic meniscus, other medial meniscus, <u>right</u> knee
    M23.032 Cystic meniscus, other medial meniscus, <u>left</u> knee
    M23.039 Cystic meniscus, other medial meniscus, <u>unspecified</u> knee
  M23.04- Cystic meniscus, <u>anterior horn</u> of <u>lateral</u> meniscus
    M23.041 Cystic meniscus, anterior horn of lateral meniscus, <u>right</u> knee
    M23.042 Cystic meniscus, anterior horn of lateral meniscus, <u>left</u> knee
    M23.049 Cystic meniscus, anterior horn of lateral meniscus, <u>unspecified</u> knee
  M23.05- Cystic meniscus, <u>posterior horn</u> of <u>lateral</u> meniscus
    M23.051 Cystic meniscus, posterior horn of lateral meniscus, <u>right</u> knee
    M23.052 Cystic meniscus, posterior horn of lateral meniscus, <u>left</u> knee
    M23.059 Cystic meniscus, posterior horn of lateral meniscus, <u>unspecified</u> knee
  M23.06- Cystic meniscus, <u>other lateral</u> meniscus
    M23.061 Cystic meniscus, other lateral meniscus, <u>right</u> knee
    M23.062 Cystic meniscus, other lateral meniscus, <u>left</u> knee
    M23.069 Cystic meniscus, other lateral meniscus, <u>unspecified</u> knee
M23.2- Derangement of meniscus <u>due to old tear or injury</u>
  Old bucket-handle tear
  M23.20- Derangement of <u>unspecified</u> meniscus due to old tear or injury
    Derangement of unspecified lateral meniscus due to old tear or injury
    Derangement of unspecified medial meniscus due to old tear or injury
    M23.200 Derangement of <u>unspecified</u> <u>lateral</u> meniscus due to old tear or injury, <u>right</u> knee
    M23.201 Derangement of <u>unspecified</u> <u>lateral</u> meniscus due to old tear or injury, <u>left</u> knee
    M23.202 Derangement of <u>unspecified</u> <u>lateral</u> meniscus due to old tear or injury, <u>unspecified</u> knee
    M23.203 Derangement of <u>unspecified</u> <u>medial</u> meniscus due to old tear or injury, <u>right</u> knee
    M23.204 Derangement of <u>unspecified</u> <u>medial</u> meniscus due to old tear or injury, <u>left</u> knee
    M23.205 Derangement of <u>unspecified</u> <u>medial</u> meniscus due to old tear or injury, <u>unspecified</u> knee
    M23.206 Derangement of <u>unspecified</u> meniscus due to old tear or injury, <u>right</u> knee
    M23.207 Derangement of <u>unspecified</u> meniscus due to old tear or injury, <u>left</u> knee
    M23.209 Derangement of <u>unspecified</u> meniscus due to old tear or injury, <u>unspecified</u> knee

M23.21- Derangement of <u>anterior horn</u> of medial meniscus due to old tear or injury

    M23.211 Derangement of anterior horn of medial meniscus due to old tear or injury, <u>right</u> knee

    M23.212 Derangement of anterior horn of medial meniscus due to old tear or injury, <u>left</u> knee

    M23.219 Derangement of anterior horn of medial meniscus due to old tear or injury, <u>unspecified</u> knee

M23.22- Derangement of <u>posterior horn</u> of <u>medial</u> meniscus due to old tear or injury

    M23.221 Derangement of posterior horn of medial meniscus due to old tear or injury, <u>right</u> knee

    M23.222 Derangement of posterior horn of medial meniscus due to old tear or injury, <u>left</u> knee

    M23.229 Derangement of posterior horn of medial meniscus due to old tear or injury, <u>unspecified</u> knee

M23.23- Derangement of other medial meniscus due to old tear or injury

    M23.231 Derangement of other medial meniscus due to old tear or injury, <u>right</u> knee

    M23.232 Derangement of other medial meniscus due to old tear or injury, <u>left</u> knee

    M23.239 Derangement of other medial meniscus due to old tear or injury, <u>unspecified</u> knee

M23.24- Derangement of <u>anterior horn</u> of <u>lateral</u> meniscus due to old tear or injury

    M23.241 Derangement of anterior horn of lateral meniscus due to old tear or injury, <u>right</u> knee

    M23.242 Derangement of anterior horn of lateral meniscus due to old tear or injury, <u>left</u> knee

    M23.249 Derangement of anterior horn of lateral meniscus due to old tear or injury, <u>unspecified</u> knee

M23.25- Derangement of <u>posterior horn</u> of <u>lateral</u> meniscus due to old tear or injury

    M23.251 Derangement of posterior horn of lateral meniscus due to old tear or injury, <u>right</u> knee

    M23.252 Derangement of posterior horn of lateral meniscus due to old tear or injury, <u>left</u> knee

    M23.259 Derangement of posterior horn of lateral meniscus due to old tear or injury, <u>unspecified</u> knee

M23.26- Derangement of <u>other lateral</u> meniscus due to old tear or injury

    M23.261 Derangement of other lateral meniscus due to old tear or injury, <u>right</u> knee

    M23.262 Derangement of other lateral meniscus due to old tear or injury, <u>left</u> knee

    M23.269 Derangement of other lateral meniscus due to old tear or injury, <u>unspecified</u> knee

M23.3- <u>Other meniscus derangements</u>
    Degenerate meniscus
    Detached meniscus
    Retained meniscus

M23.30- Other meniscus derangements, <u>unspecified</u> meniscus
    Other meniscus derangements, unspecified lateral meniscus
    Other meniscus derangements, unspecified medial meniscus

    M23.300 Other meniscus derangements, <u>unspecified lateral</u> meniscus, <u>right</u> knee

    M23.301 Other meniscus derangements, <u>unspecified lateral</u> meniscus, <u>left</u> knee

    M23.302 Other meniscus derangements, <u>unspecified lateral</u> meniscus, <u>unspecified</u> knee

    M23.303 Other meniscus derangements, <u>unspecified medial</u> meniscus, <u>right</u> knee

    M23.304 Other meniscus derangements, <u>unspecified medial</u> meniscus, <u>left</u> knee

    M23.305 Other meniscus derangements, <u>unspecified medial</u> meniscus, <u>unspecified</u> knee

    M23.306 Other meniscus derangements, <u>unspecified</u> meniscus, <u>right</u> knee

    M23.307 Other meniscus derangements, <u>unspecified</u> meniscus, <u>left</u> knee

    M23.309 Other meniscus derangements, <u>unspecified</u> meniscus, <u>unspecified</u> knee

M23.31- Other meniscus derangements, <u>anterior horn</u> of <u>medial</u> meniscus

    M23.311 Other meniscus derangements, anterior horn of medial meniscus, <u>right</u> knee

    M23.312 Other meniscus derangements, anterior horn of medial meniscus, <u>left</u> knee

    M23.319 Other meniscus derangements, anterior horn of medial meniscus, <u>unspecified</u> knee

M23.32- Other meniscus derangements, <u>posterior horn</u> of <u>medial</u> meniscus

    M23.321 Other meniscus derangements, posterior horn of medial meniscus, <u>right</u> knee

    M23.322 Other meniscus derangements, posterior horn of medial meniscus, <u>left</u> knee

    M23.329 Other meniscus derangements, posterior horn of medial meniscus, <u>unspecified</u> knee

M23.33- Other meniscus derangements, <u>other medial</u> meniscus

    M23.331 Other meniscus derangements, other medial meniscus, <u>right</u> knee

    M23.332 Other meniscus derangements, other medial meniscus, <u>left</u> knee

    M23.339 Other meniscus derangements, other medial meniscus, <u>unspecified</u> knee

M23.34- Other meniscus derangements, <u>anterior horn</u> of <u>lateral</u> meniscus

    M23.341 Other meniscus derangements, anterior horn of lateral meniscus, <u>right</u> knee

    M23.342 Other meniscus derangements, anterior horn of lateral meniscus, <u>left</u> knee

    M23.349 Other meniscus derangements, anterior horn of lateral meniscus, <u>unspecified</u> knee

M23.35- Other meniscus derangements, posterior horn of <u>lateral</u> meniscus

    M23.351 Other meniscus derangements, posterior horn of lateral meniscus, <u>right</u> knee

    M23.352 Other meniscus derangements, posterior horn of lateral meniscus, <u>left</u> knee

    M23.359 Other meniscus derangements, posterior horn of lateral meniscus, <u>unspecified</u> knee

M23.36- Other meniscus derangements, <u>other lateral</u> meniscus

    M23.361 Other meniscus derangements, other lateral meniscus, <u>right</u> knee

    M23.362 Other meniscus derangements, other lateral meniscus, <u>left</u> knee

    M23.369 Other meniscus derangements, other lateral meniscus, <u>unspecified</u> knee

M23.4- <u>Loose body</u> in <u>knee</u> — The presence of nonattached pieces of joint tissue in the knee joint.

    M23.40 Loose body in knee, <u>unspecified</u> knee

    M23.41 Loose body in knee, <u>right</u> knee

    M23.42 Loose body in knee, <u>left</u> knee

M23.5- <u>Chronic instability</u> of <u>knee</u>

    M23.50 Chronic instability of knee, <u>unspecified</u> knee

    M23.51 Chronic instability of knee, <u>right</u> knee

    M23.52 Chronic instability of knee, <u>left</u> knee

M23.6- <u>Other spontaneous disruption of ligament(s)</u> of <u>knee</u>

    M23.60- Other spontaneous disruption of <u>unspecified</u> <u>ligament</u> of knee

        M23.601 Other spontaneous disruption of <u>unspecified</u> ligament of <u>right</u> knee

        M23.602 Other spontaneous disruption of <u>unspecified</u> ligament of <u>left</u> knee

        M23.609 Other spontaneous disruption of <u>unspecified</u> ligament of <u>unspecified</u> knee

M23
-
M23

M23.61- Other spontaneous disruption of <u>anterior cruciate ligament</u> of knee
- **M23.611** Other spontaneous disruption of anterior cruciate ligament of <u>right</u> knee
- **M23.612** Other spontaneous disruption of anterior cruciate ligament of <u>left</u> knee
- **M23.619** Other spontaneous disruption of anterior cruciate ligament of <u>unspecified</u> knee

M23.62- Other spontaneous disruption of <u>posterior cruciate ligament</u> of knee
- **M23.621** Other spontaneous disruption of posterior cruciate ligament of <u>right</u> knee
- **M23.622** Other spontaneous disruption of posterior cruciate ligament of <u>left</u> knee
- **M23.629** Other spontaneous disruption of posterior cruciate ligament of <u>unspecified</u> knee

M23.63- Other spontaneous disruption of <u>medial collateral ligament</u> of knee
- **M23.631** Other spontaneous disruption of medial collateral ligament of <u>right</u> knee
- **M23.632** Other spontaneous disruption of medial collateral ligament of <u>left</u> knee
- **M23.639** Other spontaneous disruption of medial collateral ligament of <u>unspecified</u> knee

M23.64- Other spontaneous disruption of <u>lateral collateral ligament</u> of knee
- **M23.641** Other spontaneous disruption of lateral collateral ligament of <u>right</u> knee
- **M23.642** Other spontaneous disruption of lateral collateral ligament of <u>left</u> knee
- **M23.649** Other spontaneous disruption of lateral collateral ligament of <u>unspecified</u> knee

M23.67- Other spontaneous disruption of <u>capsular ligament</u> of knee
- **M23.671** Other spontaneous disruption of capsular ligament of <u>right</u> knee
- **M23.672** Other spontaneous disruption of capsular ligament of <u>left</u> knee
- **M23.679** Other spontaneous disruption of capsular ligament of <u>unspecified</u> knee

M23.8- Other internal derangements of knee
  Laxity of ligament of knee
  Snapping knee
M23.8x- <u>Other internal derangements</u> of knee
- **M23.8x1** Other internal derangements of <u>right</u> knee
- **M23.8x2** Other internal derangements of <u>left</u> knee
- **M23.8x9** Other internal derangements of <u>unspecified</u> knee

M23.9- <u>Unspecified</u> internal derangement of knee
- **M23.90** Unspecified internal derangement of <u>unspecified</u> knee
- **M23.91** Unspecified internal derangement of <u>right</u> knee
- **M23.92** Unspecified internal derangement of <u>left</u> knee

M24- Other specific joint derangements
  Excludes 1:   *current injury — see injury of joint by body region*
  Excludes ❷: *ganglion (M67.4)*
        snapping knee (M23.8-)
        temporomandibular joint disorders (M26.6-)

M24.0- <u>Loose body in joint</u> — The presence of nonattached pieces of joint tissue in the joint.
  Excludes ❷: loose body in knee (M23.4)
- **M24.00** Loose body in <u>unspecified</u> joint
- **M24.01-** Loose body in <u>shoulder</u>
  - **M24.011** Loose body in <u>right</u> shoulder
  - **M24.012** Loose body in <u>left</u> shoulder
  - **M24.019** Loose body in <u>unspecified</u> shoulder
- **M24.02-** Loose body in <u>elbow</u>
  - **M24.021** Loose body in <u>right</u> elbow
  - **M24.022** Loose body in <u>left</u> elbow
  - **M24.029** Loose body in <u>unspecified</u> elbow

M24.03- Loose body in <u>wrist</u>
- **M24.031** Loose body in <u>right</u> wrist
- **M24.032** Loose body in <u>left</u> wrist
- **M24.039** Loose body in <u>unspecified</u> wrist

M24.04- Loose body in <u>finger</u> joints
- **M24.041** Loose body in <u>right</u> finger joint(s)
- **M24.042** Loose body in <u>left</u> finger joint(s)
- **M24.049** Loose body in <u>unspecified</u> finger joint(s)

M24.05- Loose body in <u>hip</u>
- **M24.051** Loose body in <u>right</u> hip
- **M24.052** Loose body in <u>left</u> hip
- **M24.059** Loose body in <u>unspecified</u> hip

M24.07- Loose body in <u>ankle and toe</u> joints
- **M24.071** Loose body in <u>right</u> ankle
- **M24.072** Loose body in <u>left</u> ankle
- **M24.073** Loose body in <u>unspecified</u> ankle
- **M24.074** Loose body in <u>right</u> toe joint(s)
- **M24.075** Loose body in <u>left</u> toe joint(s)
- **M24.076** Loose body in <u>unspecified</u> toe joints

M24.08 Loose body, <u>other site</u>

M24.1- <u>Other articular cartilage disorders</u>
  Excludes ❷: chondrocalcinosis (M11.1, M11.2-)
        internal derangement of knee (M23.-)
        metastatic calcification (E83.5)
        ochronosis (E70.2)

M24.10 Other articular cartilage disorders, <u>unspecified</u> site
M24.11- Other articular cartilage disorders, <u>shoulder</u>
- **M24.111** Other articular cartilage disorders, <u>right</u> shoulder
- **M24.112** Other articular cartilage disorders, <u>left</u> shoulder
- **M24.119** Other articular cartilage disorders, <u>unspecified</u> shoulder

M24.12- Other articular cartilage disorders, <u>elbow</u>
- **M24.121** Other articular cartilage disorders, <u>right</u> elbow
- **M24.122** Other articular cartilage disorders, <u>left</u> elbow
- **M24.129** Other articular cartilage disorders, <u>unspecified</u> elbow

M24.13- Other articular cartilage disorders, <u>wrist</u>
- **M24.131** Other articular cartilage disorders, <u>right</u> wrist
- **M24.132** Other articular cartilage disorders, <u>left</u> wrist
- **M24.139** Other articular cartilage disorders, <u>unspecified</u> wrist

M24.14- Other articular cartilage disorders, <u>hand</u>
- **M24.141** Other articular cartilage disorders, <u>right</u> hand
- **M24.142** Other articular cartilage disorders, <u>left</u> hand
- **M24.149** Other articular cartilage disorders, <u>unspecified</u> hand

M24.15- Other articular cartilage disorders, <u>hip</u>
- **M24.151** Other articular cartilage disorders, <u>right</u> hip
- **M24.152** Other articular cartilage disorders, <u>left</u> hip
- **M24.159** Other articular cartilage disorders, <u>unspecified</u> hip

M24.17- Other articular cartilage disorders, <u>ankle and foot</u>
- **M24.171** Other articular cartilage disorders, <u>right</u> ankle
- **M24.172** Other articular cartilage disorders, <u>left</u> ankle
- **M24.173** Other articular cartilage disorders, <u>unspecified</u> ankle
- **M24.174** Other articular cartilage disorders, <u>right</u> foot
- **M24.175** Other articular cartilage disorders, <u>left</u> foot
- **M24.176** Other articular cartilage disorders, <u>unspecified</u> foot

M24.2- <u>Disorder of ligament</u>
  Instability secondary to old ligament injury
  Ligamentous laxity NOS
  Excludes 1:   familial ligamentous laxity (M35.7)
  Excludes ❷: internal derangement of knee (M23.5-M23.89)

M24.20 Disorder of ligament, <u>unspecified</u> site
M24.21- Disorder of ligament, <u>shoulder</u>
- **M24.211** Disorder of ligament, <u>right</u> shoulder
- **M24.212** Disorder of ligament, <u>left</u> shoulder

M24.219   Disorder of ligament, <u>unspecified</u> shoulder
M24.22- Disorder of ligament, <u>elbow</u>
   M24.221   Disorder of ligament, <u>right</u> elbow
   M24.222   Disorder of ligament, <u>left</u> elbow
   M24.229   Disorder of ligament, <u>unspecified</u> elbow
M24.23- Disorder of ligament, <u>wrist</u>
   M24.231   Disorder of ligament, <u>right</u> wrist
   M24.232   Disorder of ligament, <u>left</u> wrist
   M24.239   Disorder of ligament, <u>unspecified</u> wrist
M24.24- Disorder of ligament, <u>hand</u>
   M24.241   Disorder of ligament, <u>right</u> hand
   M24.242   Disorder of ligament, <u>left</u> hand
   M24.249   Disorder of ligament, <u>unspecified</u> hand
M24.25- Disorder of ligament, <u>hip</u>
   M24.251   Disorder of ligament, <u>right</u> hip
   M24.252   Disorder of ligament, <u>left</u> hip
   M24.259   Disorder of ligament, <u>unspecified</u> hip
M24.27- Disorder of ligament, <u>ankle and foot</u>
   M24.271   Disorder of ligament, <u>right</u> ankle
   M24.272   Disorder of ligament, <u>left</u> ankle
   M24.273   Disorder of ligament, <u>unspecified</u> ankle
   M24.274   Disorder of ligament, <u>right</u> foot
   M24.275   Disorder of ligament, <u>left</u> foot
   M24.276   Disorder of ligament, <u>unspecified</u> foot
M24.28 Disorder of ligament, <u>vertebrae</u>
M24.3- <u>Pathological dislocation of joint</u>, <u>not elsewhere classified</u> —
The dislocation of a joint that is due to the effects of a disease process.
   Excludes 1:   *congenital dislocation or displacement of joint — see*
            congenital malformations and deformations of the
            musculoskeletal system (Q65-Q79)
           current injury — see injury of joints and ligaments by
            body region
           recurrent dislocation of joint (M24.4-)
M24.30 Pathological dislocation of <u>unspecified</u> joint, not
elsewhere classified
M24.31- Pathological dislocation of <u>shoulder</u>, not elsewhere
classified
   M24.311   Pathological dislocation of <u>right</u> shoulder, not
elsewhere classified
   M24.312   Pathological dislocation of <u>left</u> shoulder, not
elsewhere classified
   M24.319   Pathological dislocation of <u>unspecified</u> shoulder,
not elsewhere classified
M24.32- Pathological dislocation of <u>elbow</u>, not elsewhere
classified
   M24.321   Pathological dislocation of <u>right</u> elbow, not
elsewhere classified
   M24.322   Pathological dislocation of <u>left</u> elbow, not
elsewhere classified
   M24.329   Pathological dislocation of <u>unspecified</u> elbow, not
elsewhere classified
M24.33- Pathological dislocation of <u>wrist</u>, not elsewhere classified
   M24.331   Pathological dislocation of <u>right</u> wrist, not
elsewhere classified
   M24.332   Pathological dislocation of <u>left</u> wrist, not elsewhere
classified
   M24.339   Pathological dislocation of <u>unspecified</u> wrist, not
elsewhere classified
M24.34- Pathological dislocation of <u>hand</u>, not elsewhere classified
   M24.341   Pathological dislocation of <u>right</u> hand, not
elsewhere classified
   M24.342   Pathological dislocation of <u>left</u> hand, not
elsewhere classified
   M24.349   Pathological dislocation of <u>unspecified</u> hand, not
elsewhere classified
M24.35- Pathological dislocation of <u>hip</u>, not elsewhere classified
   M24.351   Pathological dislocation of <u>right</u> hip, not elsewhere
classified

M24.352   Pathological dislocation of <u>left</u> hip, not elsewhere
classified
M24.359   Pathological dislocation of <u>unspecified</u> hip, not
elsewhere classified
M24.36- Pathological dislocation of <u>knee</u>, not elsewhere classified
   M24.361   Pathological dislocation of <u>right</u> knee, not
elsewhere classified
   M24.362   Pathological dislocation of <u>left</u> knee, not elsewhere
classified
   M24.369   Pathological dislocation of <u>unspecified</u> knee, not
elsewhere classified
M24.37- Pathological dislocation of <u>ankle and foot</u>, not elsewhere
classified
   M24.371   Pathological dislocation of <u>right</u> ankle, not
elsewhere classified
   M24.372   Pathological dislocation of <u>left</u> ankle, not
elsewhere classified
   M24.373   Pathological dislocation of <u>unspecified</u> ankle, not
elsewhere classified
   M24.374   Pathological dislocation of <u>right</u> foot, not
elsewhere classified
   M24.375   Pathological dislocation of <u>left</u> foot, not elsewhere
classified
   M24.376   Pathological dislocation of <u>unspecified</u> foot, not
elsewhere classified
M24.4- <u>Recurrent</u> <u>dislocation</u> of joint — The redislocation of a joint following a
period of proper location.
   Recurrent subluxation of joint
   Excludes ❷: *recurrent dislocation of patella (M22.0-M22.1)*
           recurrent vertebral dislocation (M43.3-, M43.4, M43.5-)
M24.40 Recurrent dislocation, <u>unspecified</u> joint
M24.41- Recurrent dislocation, <u>shoulder</u>
   M24.411   Recurrent dislocation, <u>right</u> shoulder
   M24.412   Recurrent dislocation, <u>left</u> shoulder
   M24.419   Recurrent dislocation, <u>unspecified</u> shoulder
M24.42- Recurrent dislocation, <u>elbow</u>
   M24.421   Recurrent dislocation, <u>right</u> elbow
   M24.422   Recurrent dislocation, <u>left</u> elbow
   M24.429   Recurrent dislocation, <u>unspecified</u> elbow
M24.43- Recurrent dislocation, <u>wrist</u>
   M24.431   Recurrent dislocation, <u>right</u> wrist
   M24.432   Recurrent dislocation, <u>left</u> wrist
   M24.439   Recurrent dislocation, <u>unspecified</u> wrist
M24.44- Recurrent dislocation, <u>hand and finger(s)</u>
   M24.441   Recurrent dislocation, <u>right</u> hand
   M24.442   Recurrent dislocation, <u>left</u> hand
   M24.443   Recurrent dislocation, <u>unspecified</u> hand
   M24.444   Recurrent dislocation, <u>right</u> finger
   M24.445   Recurrent dislocation, <u>left</u> finger
   M24.446   Recurrent dislocation, <u>unspecified</u> finger
M24.45- Recurrent dislocation, <u>hip</u>
   M24.451   Recurrent dislocation, <u>right</u> hip
   M24.452   Recurrent dislocation, <u>left</u> hip
   M24.459   Recurrent dislocation, <u>unspecified</u> hip
M24.46- Recurrent dislocation, <u>knee</u>
   M24.461   Recurrent dislocation, <u>right</u> knee
   M24.462   Recurrent dislocation, <u>left</u> knee
   M24.469   Recurrent dislocation, <u>unspecified</u> knee
M24.47- Recurrent dislocation, <u>ankle, foot and toes</u>
   M24.471   Recurrent dislocation, <u>right</u> ankle
   M24.472   Recurrent dislocation, <u>left</u> ankle
   M24.473   Recurrent dislocation, <u>unspecified</u> ankle
   M24.474   Recurrent dislocation, <u>right</u> foot
   M24.475   Recurrent dislocation, <u>left</u> foot
   M24.476   Recurrent dislocation, <u>unspecified</u> foot
   M24.477   Recurrent dislocation, <u>right</u> toe(s)

M24
–
M24

M24.478   Recurrent dislocation, <u>left</u> toe(s)

M24.479   Recurrent dislocation, <u>unspecified</u> toe(s)

M24.5-   <u>Contracture</u> of joint — The condition of decreased flexibility of a joint.

     Excludes 1:   *contracture of muscle without contracture of joint (M62.4-)*

             contracture of tendon (sheath) without contracture of joint (M62.4-)

             Dupuytren's contracture (M72.0)

     Excludes ❷: *acquired deformities of limbs (M20-M21)*

   M24.50   Contracture, <u>unspecified</u> joint

   M24.51- Contracture, <u>shoulder</u>

     M24.511   Contracture, <u>right</u> shoulder

     M24.512   Contracture, <u>left</u> shoulder

     M24.519   Contracture, <u>unspecified</u> shoulder

   M24.52- Contracture, <u>elbow</u>

     M24.521   Contracture, <u>right</u> elbow

     M24.522   Contracture, <u>left</u> elbow

     M24.529   Contracture, <u>unspecified</u> elbow

   M24.53- Contracture, <u>wrist</u>

     M24.531   Contracture, <u>right</u> wrist

     M24.532   Contracture, <u>left</u> wrist

     M24.539   Contracture, <u>unspecified</u> wrist

   M24.54- Contracture, <u>hand</u>

     M24.541   Contracture, <u>right</u> hand

     M24.542   Contracture, <u>left</u> hand

     M24.549   Contracture, <u>unspecified</u> hand

   M24.55- Contracture, <u>hip</u>

     M24.551   Contracture, <u>right</u> hip

     M24.552   Contracture, <u>left</u> hip

     M24.559   Contracture, <u>unspecified</u> hip

   M24.56- Contracture, <u>knee</u>

     M24.561   Contracture, <u>right</u> knee

     M24.562   Contracture, <u>left</u> knee

     M24.569   Contracture, <u>unspecified</u> knee

   M24.57- Contracture, <u>ankle and foot</u>

     M24.571   Contracture, <u>right</u> ankle

     M24.572   Contracture, <u>left</u> ankle

     M24.573   Contracture, <u>unspecified</u> ankle

     M24.574   Contracture, <u>right</u> foot

     M24.575   Contracture, <u>left</u> foot

     M24.576   Contracture, <u>unspecified</u> foot

M24.6-   <u>Ankylosis</u> of joint — The condition of significant stiffness or immobility of a joint.

     Excludes 1:   *stiffness of joint without ankylosis (M25.6-)*

     Excludes ❷: *spine (M43.2-)*

   M24.60   Ankylosis, <u>unspecified</u> joint

   M24.61- Ankylosis, <u>shoulder</u>

     M24.611   Ankylosis, <u>right</u> shoulder

     M24.612   Ankylosis, <u>left</u> shoulder

     M24.619   Ankylosis, <u>unspecified</u> shoulder

   M24.62- Ankylosis, <u>elbow</u>

     M24.621   Ankylosis, <u>right</u> elbow

     M24.622   Ankylosis, <u>left</u> elbow

     M24.629   Ankylosis, <u>unspecified</u> elbow

   M24.63- Ankylosis, <u>wrist</u>

     M24.631   Ankylosis, <u>right</u> wrist

     M24.632   Ankylosis, <u>left</u> wrist

     M24.639   Ankylosis, <u>unspecified</u> wrist

   M24.64- Ankylosis, <u>hand</u>

     M24.641   Ankylosis, <u>right</u> hand

     M24.642   Ankylosis, <u>left</u> hand

     M24.649   Ankylosis, <u>unspecified</u> hand

   M24.65- Ankylosis, <u>hip</u>

     M24.651   Ankylosis, <u>right</u> hip

     M24.652   Ankylosis, <u>left</u> hip

     M24.659   Ankylosis, <u>unspecified</u> hip

   M24.66- Ankylosis, <u>knee</u>

     M24.661   Ankylosis, <u>right</u> knee

     M24.662   Ankylosis, <u>left</u> knee

     M24.669   Ankylosis, <u>unspecified</u> knee

   M24.67- Ankylosis, <u>ankle and foot</u>

     M24.671   Ankylosis, <u>right</u> ankle

     M24.672   Ankylosis, <u>left</u> ankle

     M24.673   Ankylosis, <u>unspecified</u> ankle

     M24.674   Ankylosis, <u>right</u> foot

     M24.675   Ankylosis, <u>left</u> foot

     M24.676   Ankylosis, <u>unspecified</u> foot

M24.7   Protrusio acetabuli

M24.8-   <u>Other specific</u> joint derangements, <u>not elsewhere classified</u>

     Excludes ❷: *iliotibial band syndrome (M76.3)*

   M24.80   Other specific joint derangements of <u>unspecified</u> joint, not elsewhere classified

   M24.81- Other specific joint derangements of <u>shoulder</u>, not elsewhere classified

     M24.811   Other specific joint derangements of <u>right</u> shoulder, not elsewhere classified

     M24.812   Other specific joint derangements of <u>left</u> shoulder, not elsewhere classified

     M24.819   Other specific joint derangements of <u>unspecified</u> shoulder, not elsewhere classified

   M24.82- Other specific joint derangements of <u>elbow</u>, not elsewhere classified

     M24.821   Other specific joint derangements of <u>right</u> elbow, not elsewhere classified

     M24.822   Other specific joint derangements of <u>left</u> elbow, not elsewhere classified

     M24.829   Other specific joint derangements of <u>unspecified</u> elbow, not elsewhere classified

   M24.83- Other specific joint derangements of wrist, not elsewhere classified

     M24.831   Other specific joint derangements of <u>right</u> wrist, not elsewhere classified

     M24.832   Other specific joint derangements of <u>left</u> wrist, not elsewhere classified

     M24.839   Other specific joint derangements of <u>unspecified</u> wrist, not elsewhere classified

   M24.84- Other specific joint derangements of <u>hand</u>, not elsewhere classified

     M24.841   Other specific joint derangements of <u>right</u> hand, not elsewhere classified

     M24.842   Other specific joint derangements of <u>left</u> hand, not elsewhere classified

     M24.849   Other specific joint derangements of <u>unspecified</u> hand, not elsewhere classified

   M24.85- Other specific joint derangements of <u>hip</u>, not elsewhere classified

     Irritable hip

     M24.851   Other specific joint derangements of <u>right</u> hip, not elsewhere classified

     M24.852   Other specific joint derangements of <u>left</u> hip, not elsewhere classified

     M24.859   Other specific joint derangements of <u>unspecified</u> hip, not elsewhere classified

   M24.87- Other specific joint derangements of <u>ankle and foot</u>, not elsewhere classified

     M24.871   Other specific joint derangements of <u>right</u> ankle, not elsewhere classified

     M24.872   Other specific joint derangements of <u>left</u> ankle, not elsewhere classified

     M24.873   Other specific joint derangements of <u>unspecified</u> ankle, not elsewhere classified

     M24.874   Other specific joint derangements of <u>right</u> foot, not elsewhere classified

M24.875   Other specific joint derangements **left** foot, not elsewhere classified

M24.876   Other specific joint derangements of **unspecified** foot, not elsewhere classified

M24.9   Joint derangement, <u>unspecified</u>

M25-   <u>Other joint disorder</u>, <u>not elsewhere classified</u>
　　Excludes ❷: abnormality of gait and mobility (R26.-)
　　　　　　　acquired deformities of limb (M20-M21)
　　　　　　　calcification of bursa (M71.4-)
　　　　　　　calcification of shoulder (joint) (M75.3)
　　　　　　　calcification of tendon (M65.2-)
　　　　　　　difficulty in walking (R26.2)
　　　　　　　temporomandibular joint disorder (M26.6-)

M25.0-   <u>Hemarthrosis</u> — The abnormal presence of free blood in a joint.
　　Excludes 1:   current injury — see injury of joint by body region
　　　　　　　hemophilic arthropathy (M36.2)

cc **M25.00 Hemarthrosis, <u>unspecified</u> joint**
M25.01-Hemarthrosis, <u>shoulder</u>
cc **M25.011   Hemarthrosis, <u>right</u> shoulder**
cc **M25.012   Hemarthrosis, <u>left</u> shoulder**
cc **M25.019   Hemarthrosis, <u>unspecified</u> shoulder**
M25.02-Hemarthrosis, <u>elbow</u>
cc **M25.021   Hemarthrosis, <u>right</u> elbow**
cc **M25.022   Hemarthrosis, <u>left</u> elbow**
cc **M25.029   Hemarthrosis, <u>unspecified</u> elbow**
M25.03-Hemarthrosis, <u>wrist</u>
cc **M25.031   Hemarthrosis, <u>right</u> wrist**
cc **M25.032   Hemarthrosis, <u>left</u> wrist**
cc **M25.039   Hemarthrosis, <u>unspecified</u> wrist**
M25.04-Hemarthrosis, <u>hand</u>
cc **M25.041   Hemarthrosis, <u>right</u> hand**
cc **M25.042   Hemarthrosis, <u>left</u> hand**
cc **M25.049   Hemarthrosis, <u>unspecified</u> hand**
M25.05-Hemarthrosis, <u>hip</u>
cc **M25.051   Hemarthrosis, <u>right</u> hip**
cc **M25.052   Hemarthrosis, <u>left</u> hip**
cc **M25.059   Hemarthrosis, <u>unspecified</u> hip**
M25.06-Hemarthrosis, <u>knee</u>
cc **M25.061   Hemarthrosis, <u>right</u> knee**
cc **M25.062   Hemarthrosis, <u>left</u> knee**
cc **M25.069   Hemarthrosis, <u>unspecified</u> knee**
M25.07-Hemarthrosis, <u>ankle and foot</u>
cc **M25.071   Hemarthrosis, <u>right</u> ankle**
cc **M25.072   Hemarthrosis, <u>left</u> ankle**
cc **M25.073   Hemarthrosis, <u>unspecified</u> ankle**
cc **M25.074   Hemarthrosis, <u>right</u> foot**
cc **M25.075   Hemarthrosis, <u>left</u> foot**
cc **M25.076   Hemarthrosis, <u>unspecified</u> foot**
cc **M25.08 Hemarthrosis, <u>other specified site</u>**
　　　　Hemarthrosis, vertebrae

M25.1-   <u>Fistula of joint</u> — The presence of an abnormal communicating passage of a joint.
M25.10 Fistula, <u>unspecified</u> joint
M25.11-Fistula, <u>shoulder</u>
M25.111   Fistula, <u>right</u> shoulder
M25.112   Fistula, <u>left</u> shoulder
M25.119   Fistula, <u>unspecified</u> shoulder
M25.12-Fistula, <u>elbow</u>
M25.121   Fistula, <u>right</u> elbow
M25.122   Fistula, <u>left</u> elbow
M25.129   Fistula, <u>unspecified</u> elbow
M25.13-Fistula, wrist
M25.131   Fistula, <u>right</u> wrist
M25.132   Fistula, <u>left</u> wrist
M25.139   Fistula, <u>unspecified</u> wrist
M25.14-Fistula, <u>hand</u>
M25.141   Fistula, <u>right</u> hand

M25.142   Fistula, <u>left</u> hand
M25.149   Fistula, <u>unspecified</u> hand
M25.15-Fistula, <u>hip</u>
M25.151   Fistula, <u>right</u> hip
M25.152   Fistula, <u>left</u> hip
M25.159   Fistula, <u>unspecified</u> hip
M25.16-Fistula, <u>knee</u>
M25.161   Fistula, <u>right</u> knee
M25.162   Fistula, <u>left</u> knee
M25.169   Fistula, <u>unspecified</u> knee
M25.17-Fistula, <u>ankle and foot</u>
M25.171   Fistula, <u>right</u> ankle
M25.172   Fistula, <u>left</u> ankle
M25.173   Fistula, <u>unspecified</u> ankle
M25.174   Fistula, <u>right</u> foot
M25.175   Fistula, <u>left</u> foot
M25.176   Fistula, <u>unspecified</u> foot
M25.18 Fistula, <u>other specified site</u>
　　　　Fistula, vertebrae

M25.2-   <u>Flail joint</u> — The condition of abnormal mobility of a joint.
M25.20 Flail joint, <u>unspecified</u> joint
M25.21-Flail joint, <u>shoulder</u>
M25.211   Flail joint, <u>right</u> shoulder
M25.212   Flail joint, <u>left</u> shoulder
M25.219   Flail joint, <u>unspecified</u> shoulder
M25.22-Flail joint, <u>elbow</u>
M25.221   Flail joint, <u>right</u> elbow
M25.222   Flail joint, <u>left</u> elbow
M25.229   Flail joint, <u>unspecified</u> elbow
M25.23-Flail joint, <u>wrist</u>
M25.231   Flail joint, <u>right</u> wrist
M25.232   Flail joint, <u>left</u> wrist
M25.239   Flail joint, <u>unspecified</u> wrist
M25.24-Flail joint, <u>hand</u>
M25.241   Flail joint, <u>right</u> hand
M25.242   Flail joint, <u>left</u> hand
M25.249   Flail joint, <u>unspecified</u> hand
M25.25-Flail joint, <u>hip</u>
M25.251   Flail joint, <u>right</u> hip
M25.252   Flail joint, <u>left</u> hip
M25.259   Flail joint, <u>unspecified</u> hip
M25.26-Flail joint, <u>knee</u>
M25.261   Flail joint, <u>right</u> knee
M25.262   Flail joint, <u>left</u> knee
M25.269   Flail joint, <u>unspecified</u> knee
M25.27-Flail joint, <u>ankle and foot</u>
M25.271   Flail joint, <u>right</u> ankle and foot
M25.272   Flail joint, <u>left</u> ankle and foot
M25.279   Flail joint, <u>unspecified</u> ankle and foot
M25.28 Flail joint, <u>other site</u>

M25.3-   <u>Other instability</u> of joint
　　Excludes 1:   instability of joint secondary to old ligament injury
　　　　　　　(M24.2-)
　　　　　　　instability of joint secondary to removal of joint
　　　　　　　prosthesis (M96.8-)
　　Excludes ❷: spinal instabilities (M53.2-)
M25.30 Other instability, <u>unspecified</u> joint
M25.31-Other instability, <u>shoulder</u>
M25.311   Other instability, <u>right</u> shoulder
M25.312   Other instability, <u>left</u> shoulder
M25.319   Other instability, <u>unspecified</u> shoulder
M25.32-Other instability, <u>elbow</u>
M25.321   Other instability, <u>right</u> elbow
M25.322   Other instability, <u>left</u> elbow
M25.329   Other instability, <u>unspecified</u> elbow

M25.33- Other instability, <u>wrist</u>
    M25.331 Other instability, <u>right</u> wrist
    M25.332 Other instability, <u>left</u> wrist
    M25.339 Other instability, <u>unspecified</u> wrist
M25.34- Other instability, <u>hand</u>
    M25.341 Other instability, <u>right</u> hand
    M25.342 Other instability, <u>left</u> hand
    M25.349 Other instability, <u>unspecified</u> hand
M25.35- Other instability, <u>hip</u>
    M25.351 Other instability, <u>right</u> hip
    M25.352 Other instability, <u>left</u> hip
    M25.359 Other instability, <u>unspecified</u> hip
M25.36- Other instability, <u>knee</u>
    M25.361 Other instability, <u>right</u> knee
    M25.362 Other instability, <u>left</u> knee
    M25.369 Other instability, <u>unspecified</u> knee
M25.37- Other instability, <u>ankle and foot</u>
    M25.371 Other instability, <u>right</u> ankle
    M25.372 Other instability, <u>left</u> ankle
    M25.373 Other instability, <u>unspecified</u> ankle
    M25.374 Other instability, <u>right</u> foot
    M25.375 Other instability, <u>left</u> foot
    M25.376 Other instability, <u>unspecified</u> foot
M25.4- <u>Effusion of joint</u> — The abnormal increased amount of fluid in a joint.
    Excludes 1: *hydrarthrosis in yaws (A66.6)*
                   intermittent hydrarthrosis (M12.4-)
                   other infective (teno)synovitis (M65.1-)
  M25.40 Effusion, <u>unspecified</u> joint
M25.41- Effusion, <u>shoulder</u>
    M25.411 Effusion, <u>right</u> shoulder
    M25.412 Effusion, <u>left</u> shoulder
    M25.419 Effusion, <u>unspecified</u> shoulder
M25.42- Effusion, <u>elbow</u>
    M25.421 Effusion, <u>right</u> elbow
    M25.422 Effusion, <u>left</u> elbow
    M25.429 Effusion, <u>unspecified</u> elbow
M25.43- Effusion, <u>wrist</u>
    M25.431 Effusion, <u>right</u> wrist
    M25.432 Effusion, <u>left</u> wrist
    M25.439 Effusion, <u>unspecified</u> wrist
M25.44- Effusion, <u>hand</u>
    M25.441 Effusion, <u>right</u> hand
    M25.442 Effusion, <u>left</u> hand
    M25.449 Effusion, <u>unspecified</u> hand
M25.45- Effusion, <u>hip</u>
    M25.451 Effusion, <u>right</u> hip
    M25.452 Effusion, <u>left</u> hip
    M25.459 Effusion, <u>unspecified</u> hip
M25.46- Effusion, <u>knee</u>
    M25.461 Effusion, <u>right</u> knee
    M25.462 Effusion, <u>left</u> knee
    M25.469 Effusion, <u>unspecified</u> knee
M25.47- Effusion, <u>ankle and foot</u>
    M25.471 Effusion, <u>right</u> ankle
    M25.472 Effusion, <u>left</u> ankle
    M25.473 Effusion, <u>unspecified</u> ankle
    M25.474 Effusion, <u>right</u> foot
    M25.475 Effusion, <u>left</u> foot
    M25.476 Effusion, <u>unspecified</u> foot
M25.48 Effusion, <u>other site</u>

M25.5- <u>Pain in joint</u> — The condition of discomfort of a joint.
    Excludes ❷: *pain in hand (M79.64-)*
                   pain in fingers (M79.64-)
                   pain in foot (M79.67-)
                   pain in limb (M79.6-)
                   pain in toes (M79.67-)
  M25.50 Pain in <u>unspecified</u> joint
M25.51- Pain in <u>shoulder</u>
    M25.511 Pain in <u>right</u> shoulder
    M25.512 Pain in <u>left</u> shoulder
    M25.519 Pain in <u>unspecified</u> shoulder
M25.52- Pain in <u>elbow</u>
    M25.521 Pain in <u>right</u> elbow
    M25.522 Pain in <u>left</u> elbow
    M25.529 Pain in <u>unspecified</u> elbow
M25.53- Pain in <u>wrist</u>
    M25.531 Pain in <u>right</u> wrist
    M25.532 Pain in <u>left</u> wrist
    M25.539 Pain in <u>unspecified</u> wrist
M25.54- Pain in <u>joints of hand</u>
    M25.541 Pain in joints of hand of <u>right</u> hand
    M25.542 Pain in joints of hand of <u>left</u> hand
    M25.559 Pain in joints of hand of <u>unspecified</u> hand
               Pain in joints of hand NOS
M25.55- Pain in <u>hip</u>
    M25.551 Pain in <u>right</u> hip
    M25.552 Pain in <u>left</u> hip
    M25.559 Pain in <u>unspecified</u> hip
M25.56- Pain in <u>knee</u>
    M25.561 Pain in <u>right</u> knee
    M25.562 Pain in <u>left</u> knee
    M25.569 Pain in <u>unspecified</u> knee
M25.57- Pain in <u>ankle and joints of foot</u>
    M25.571 Pain in <u>right</u> ankle and joints of right foot
    M25.572 Pain in <u>left</u> ankle and joints of left foot
    M25.579 Pain in <u>unspecified</u> ankle and joints of unspecified foot
M25.6- <u>Stiffness of joint, not elsewhere classified</u>
    Excludes 1: *ankylosis of joint (M24.6-)*
                   contracture of joint (M24.5-)
  M25.60 Stiffness of <u>unspecified</u> joint, not elsewhere classified
M25.61- Stiffness of <u>shoulder</u>, not elsewhere classified
    M25.611 Stiffness of <u>right</u> shoulder, not elsewhere classified
    M25.612 Stiffness of <u>left</u> shoulder, not elsewhere classified
    M25.619 Stiffness of <u>unspecified</u> shoulder, not elsewhere classified
M25.62- Stiffness of <u>elbow</u>, not elsewhere classified
    M25.621 Stiffness of <u>right</u> elbow, not elsewhere classified
    M25.622 Stiffness of <u>left</u> elbow, not elsewhere classified
    M25.629 Stiffness of <u>unspecified</u> elbow, not elsewhere classified
M25.63- Stiffness of <u>wrist</u>, not elsewhere classified
    M25.631 Stiffness of <u>right</u> wrist, not elsewhere classified
    M25.632 Stiffness of <u>left</u> wrist, not elsewhere classified
    M25.639 Stiffness of <u>unspecified</u> wrist, not elsewhere classified
M25.64- Stiffness of <u>hand</u>, not elsewhere classified
    M25.641 Stiffness of <u>right</u> hand, not elsewhere classified
    M25.642 Stiffness of <u>left</u> hand, not elsewhere classified
    M25.649 Stiffness of <u>unspecified</u> hand, not elsewhere classified
M25.65- Stiffness of <u>hip</u>, not elsewhere classified
    M25.651 Stiffness of <u>right</u> hip, not elsewhere classified
    M25.652 Stiffness of <u>left</u> hip, not elsewhere classified
    M25.659 Stiffness of <u>unspecified</u> hip, not elsewhere classified

M25 – M25

M25.66-Stiffness of <u>knee</u>, not elsewhere classified
  M25.661 Stiffness of <u>right</u> knee, not elsewhere classified
  M25.662 Stiffness of <u>left</u> knee, not elsewhere classified
  M25.669 Stiffness of <u>unspecified</u> knee, not elsewhere classified
M25.67-Stiffness of <u>ankle and foot</u>, not elsewhere classified
  M25.671 Stiffness of <u>right</u> ankle, not elsewhere classified
  M25.672 Stiffness of <u>left</u> ankle, not elsewhere classified
  M25.673 Stiffness of <u>unspecified</u> ankle, not elsewhere classified
  M25.674 Stiffness of <u>right</u> foot, not elsewhere classified
  M25.675 Stiffness of <u>left</u> foot, not elsewhere classified
  M25.676 Stiffness of <u>unspecified</u> foot, not elsewhere classified
M25.7- <u>Osteophyte</u> — The bony tissue growth along the margins of a joint.
  M25.70 Osteophyte, <u>unspecified</u> joint
  M25.71-Osteophyte, <u>shoulder</u>
    M25.711 Osteophyte, <u>right</u> shoulder
    M25.712 Osteophyte, <u>left</u> shoulder
    M25.719 Osteophyte, <u>unspecified</u> shoulder
  M25.72-Osteophyte, <u>elbow</u>
    M25.721 Osteophyte, <u>right</u> elbow
    M25.722 Osteophyte, <u>left</u> elbow
    M25.729 Osteophyte, <u>unspecified</u> elbow
  M25.73-Osteophyte, <u>wrist</u>
    M25.731 Osteophyte, <u>right</u> wrist
    M25.732 Osteophyte, <u>left</u> wrist
    M25.739 Osteophyte, <u>unspecified</u> wrist
  M25.74-Osteophyte, <u>hand</u>
    M25.741 Osteophyte, <u>right</u> hand
    M25.742 Osteophyte, <u>left</u> hand
    M25.749 Osteophyte, <u>unspecified</u> hand
  M25.75-Osteophyte, <u>hip</u>
    M25.751 Osteophyte, <u>right</u> hip
    M25.752 Osteophyte, <u>left</u> hip
    M25.759 Osteophyte, <u>unspecified</u> hip
  M25.76-Osteophyte, <u>knee</u>
    M25.761 Osteophyte, <u>right</u> knee
    M25.762 Osteophyte, <u>left</u> knee
    M25.769 Osteophyte, <u>unspecified</u> knee
  M25.77-Osteophyte, <u>ankle and foot</u>
    M25.771 Osteophyte, <u>right</u> ankle
    M25.772 Osteophyte, <u>left</u> ankle
    M25.773 Osteophyte, <u>unspecified</u> ankle
    M25.774 Osteophyte, <u>right</u> foot
    M25.775 Osteophyte, <u>left</u> foot
    M25.776 Osteophyte, <u>unspecified</u> foot
  M25.78 Osteophyte, <u>vertebrae</u>
M25.8- <u>Other specified</u> joint disorders
  AHA 14:4Q:p25 – Femoroacetabular impingement
  M25.80 Other specified joint disorders, <u>unspecified</u> joint
  M25.81-Other specified joint disorders, <u>shoulder</u>
    M25.811 Other specified joint disorders, <u>right</u> shoulder
    M25.812 Other specified joint disorders, <u>left</u> shoulder
    M25.819 Other specified joint disorders, <u>unspecified</u> shoulder
  M25.82-Other specified joint disorders, <u>elbow</u>
    M25.821 Other specified joint disorders, <u>right</u> elbow
    M25.822 Other specified joint disorders, <u>left</u> elbow
    M25.829 Other specified joint disorders, <u>unspecified</u> elbow
  M25.83-Other specified joint disorders, <u>wrist</u>
    M25.831 Other specified joint disorders, <u>right</u> wrist
    M25.832 Other specified joint disorders, <u>left</u> wrist
    M25.839 Other specified joint disorders, <u>unspecified</u> wrist

M25.84-Other specified joint disorders, <u>hand</u>
  M25.841 Other specified joint disorders, <u>right</u> hand
  M25.842 Other specified joint disorders, <u>left</u> hand
  M25.849 Other specified joint disorders, <u>unspecified</u> hand
M25.85-Other specified joint disorders, <u>hip</u>
  M25.851 Other specified joint disorders, <u>right</u> hip
  M25.852 Other specified joint disorders, <u>left</u> hip
  M25.859 Other specified joint disorders, <u>unspecified</u> hip
M25.86-Other specified joint disorders, <u>knee</u>
  M25.861 Other specified joint disorders, <u>right</u> knee
  M25.862 Other specified joint disorders, <u>left</u> knee
  M25.869 Other specified joint disorders, <u>unspecified</u> knee
M25.87-Other specified joint disorders, <u>ankle and foot</u>
  M25.871 Other specified joint disorders, <u>right</u> ankle and foot
  M25.872 Other specified joint disorders, <u>left</u> ankle and foot
  M25.879 Other specified joint disorders, <u>unspecified</u> ankle and foot
M25.9 Joint disorder, <u>unspecified</u>

Dentofacial anomalies [including malocclusion] and other disorders of jaw (M26-M27)

Excludes 1: *hemifacial atrophy or hypertrophy (Q67.4)*
  unilateral condylar hyperplasia or hypoplasia (M27.8)

M26- <u>Dentofacial anomalies</u> [including malocclusion]
M26.0- <u>Major</u> anomalies of jaw size — The functionally significant deviation of normal jaw size.
  Excludes 1: *acromegaly (E22.0)*
    Robin's syndrome (Q87.0)
  M26.00 Unspecified anomaly of jaw size
  M26.01 Maxillary hyperplasia — The abnormal, developmental enlargement of the upper jaw bone (maxilla).
  M26.02 Maxillary hypoplasia — The abnormal, developmental smallness of the upper jaw bone (maxilla).
    AHA 14:3Q:p23 – Maxillary hypoplasia
  M26.03 Mandibular hyperplasia — The abnormal, developmental enlargement of the lower jaw bone (mandible).
  M26.04 Mandibular hypoplasia — The abnormal, developmental smallness of the lower jaw bone (mandible).
  M26.05 Macrogenia — The abnormal, developmental enlargement of the chin (mandible).
  M26.06 Microgenia — The abnormal, developmental smallness of the chin (mandible).
  M26.07 Excessive tuberosity of jaw — The abnormal presence of excessive bone and/or soft tissue of the jaw.
    Entire maxillary tuberosity
  M26.09 Other specified anomalies of jaw size
M26.1- Anomalies of <u>jaw-cranial base</u> relationship — The functionally significant deviation of the anatomical location of the jaw in relation to the skull.
  M26.10 Unspecified anomaly of jaw-cranial base relationship
  M26.11 Maxillary asymmetry — The dissimilar position of the upper jaw to the skull.
  M26.12 Other jaw asymmetry
  M26.19 Other specified anomalies of jaw-cranial base relationship
M26.2- Anomalies of <u>dental arch</u> relationship — The malposition of the teeth and alveolar process creating a functionally significant abnormality of the dental arch.
  M26.20 Unspecified anomaly of dental arch relationship
  M26.21-Malocclusion, Angle's class
    M26.211 Malocclusion, Angle's class I
      Neutro-occlusion
    M26.212 Malocclusion, Angle's class II
      Disto-occlusion Division I
      Disto-occlusion Division II
    M26.213 Malocclusion, Angle's class III
      Mesio-occlusion
    M26.219 Malocclusion, Angle's class, unspecified

M25-M26

M26.22- <u>Open occlusal</u> relationship

    M26.220 **Open anterior occlusal relationship**
        Anterior openbite

    M26.221 **Open posterior occlusal relationship**
        Posterior openbite

M26.23 <u>Excessive horizontal overlap</u>
    Excessive horizontal overjet

M26.24 <u>Reverse articulation</u>
    Crossbite (anterior) (posterior)

M26.25 **Anomalies of interarch distance**

M26.29 **Other anomalies of dental arch relationship**
    Midline deviation of dental arch
    Overbite (excessive) deep
    Overbite (excessive) horizontal
    Overbite (excessive) vertical
    Posterior lingual occlusion of mandibular teeth

M26.3- **Anomalies of** <u>tooth position</u> **of fully erupted tooth or teeth**
    Excludes ❷: embedded and impacted teeth (K01.-)

M26.30 **Unspecified anomaly of tooth position of fully erupted tooth or teeth**
    Abnormal spacing of fully erupted tooth or teeth NOS
    Displacement of fully erupted tooth or teeth NOS
    Transposition of fully erupted tooth or teeth NOS

M26.31 **Crowding of fully erupted teeth**

M26.32 **Excessive spacing of fully erupted teeth**
    Diastema of fully erupted tooth or teeth NOS

M26.33 **Horizontal displacement of fully erupted tooth or teeth**
    Tipped tooth or teeth
    Tipping of fully erupted tooth

M26.34 **Vertical displacement of fully erupted tooth or teeth**
    Extruded tooth
    Infraeruption of tooth or teeth
    Supraeruption of tooth or teeth

M26.35 **Rotation of fully erupted tooth or teeth**

M26.36 **Insufficient interocclusal distance of fully erupted teeth (ridge)**
    Lack of adequate intermaxillary vertical dimension of fully erupted teeth

M26.37 **Excessive interocclusal distance of fully erupted teeth**
    Excessive intermaxillary vertical dimension of fully erupted teeth
    Loss of occlusal vertical dimension of fully erupted teeth

M26.39 **Other anomalies of tooth position of fully erupted tooth or teeth**

M26.4 **Malocclusion, unspecified**

M26.5- **Dentofacial** <u>functional abnormalities</u>
    Excludes 1: bruxism (F45.8)
              teeth-grinding NOS (F45.8)

M26.50 **Dentofacial functional abnormalities, unspecified**

M26.51 **Abnormal jaw closure**

M26.52 **Limited mandibular range of motion**

M26.53 **Deviation in opening and closing of the mandible**

M26.54 **Insufficient anterior guidance**
    Insufficient anterior occlusal guidance

M26.55 **Centric occlusion maximum intercuspation discrepancy**
    Excludes 1: centric occlusion NOS (M26.59)

M26.56 **Non-working side interference**
    Balancing side interference

M26.57 **Lack of posterior occlusal support**

M26.59 **Other dentofacial functional abnormalities**
    Centric occlusion (of teeth) NOS
    Malocclusion due to abnormal swallowing
    Malocclusion due to mouth breathing
    Malocclusion due to tongue, lip or finger habits

M26.6- <u>Temporomandibular joint disorders</u> — The abnormal function of the temporomandibular joint.
    Excludes ❷: current temporomandibular joint dislocation (S03.0)
              current temporomandibular joint sprain (S03.4)

M26.60- **Temporomandibular joint disorder,** <u>unspecified</u>

    M26.601 <u>Right</u> **temporomandibular joint disorder, unspecified**

    M26.602 <u>Left</u> **temporomandibular joint disorder, unspecified**

    M26.603 **Bilateral temporomandibular joint disorder, unspecified**

    M26.609 **Unspecified temporomandibular joint disorder,** <u>unspecified side</u>
        Temporomandibular joint disorder NOS

M26.61- <u>Adhesions and ankylosis</u> **of temporomandibular joint** — The immobility and/or fixation of the temporomandibular joint.

    M26.611 **Adhesions and ankylosis of** <u>right</u> **temporomandibular joint**

    M26.612 **Adhesions and ankylosis of** <u>left</u> **temporomandibular joint**

    M26.613 **Adhesions and ankylosis of** <u>bilateral</u> **temporomandibular joint**

    M26.619 **Adhesions and ankylosis of temporomandibular joint,** <u>unspecified side</u>

M26.62- <u>Arthralgia</u> **of temporomandibular joint** — A condition characterized by discomfort and pain of the temporomandibular joint.

    M26.621 **Arthralgia of** <u>right</u> **temporomandibular joint**

    M26.622 **Arthralgia of** <u>left</u> **temporomandibular joint**

    M26.623 **Arthralgia of** <u>bilateral</u> **temporomandibular joint**

    M26.629 **Arthralgia of temporomandibular joint,** <u>unspecified side</u>

M26.63- <u>Articular disc disorder</u> **of temporomandibular joint** — Dysfunction of the temporomandibular joint caused by the deterioration of the temporomandibular articular disc.

    M26.631 **Articular disc disorder of** <u>right</u> **temporomandibular joint**

    M26.632 **Articular disc disorder of** <u>left</u> **temporomandibular joint**

    M26.633 **Articular disc disorder of** <u>bilateral</u> **temporomandibular joint**

    M26.639 **Articular disc disorder of temporomandibular joint,** <u>unspecified side</u>

M26.69 **Other specified disorders of temporomandibular joint**

M26.7- <u>Dental alveolar</u> **anomalies**

M26.70 **Unspecified alveolar anomaly**

M26.71 **Alveolar maxillary hyperplasia** — The abnormal developmental enlargement of the upper jaw alveolar process cavities.

M26.72 **Alveolar mandibular hyperplasia** — The abnormal developmental enlargement of the lower jaw alveolar process cavities.

M26.73 **Alveolar maxillary hypoplasia** — The abnormal developmental smallness of the upper jaw alveolar process cavities.

M26.74 **Alveolar mandibular hypoplasia** — The abnormal developmental smallness of the lower jaw alveolar process cavities.

M26.79 **Other specified alveolar anomalies**

M26.8- <u>Other</u> **dentofacial anomalies**

M26.81 **Anterior soft tissue impingement**
    Anterior soft tissue impingement on teeth

M26.82 **Posterior soft tissue impingement**
    Posterior soft tissue impingement on teeth

M26.89 **Other dentofacial anomalies**

M26.9 **Dentofacial anomaly,** <u>unspecified</u>

M27- **Other diseases of jaws**

M27.0 **Developmental disorders of jaws**
    Latent bone cyst of jaw
    Stafne's cyst
    Torus mandibularis
    Torus palatinus

M27.1 **Giant cell granuloma, central** — An abnormal, benign reparative reaction to an injury of the jaw characterized by the proliferation of numerous fibroplastic giant cells.
    Giant cell granuloma NOS
    Excludes 1: peripheral giant cell granuloma (K06.8)

M26
-
M27

M27.2   **Inflammatory conditions of jaws**
     Osteitis of jaw(s)
     Osteomyelitis (neonatal) jaw(s)
     Osteoradionecrosis jaw(s)
     Periostitis jaw(s)
     Sequestrum of jaw bone
     Use additional code (W88-W90, X39.0) to identify radiation, if radiation-induced
     Excludes ❷: *osteonecrosis of jaw due to drug (M87.180)*

M27.3   **Alveolitis of jaws** — Inflammation of the bony cavities or sockets of the mandible and maxilla.
     Alveolar osteitis
     Dry socket — A form resulting from exposure of the bone after tooth extraction.

M27.4-   **Other and unspecified cysts of jaw**
     Excludes 1:   *cysts of oral region (K09.-)*
         latent bone cyst of jaw (M27.0)
         Stafne's cyst (M27.0)

    M27.40   **Unspecified cyst of jaw**
       Cyst of jaw NOS

    M27.49   **Other cysts of jaw**
       Aneurysmal cyst of jaw — The bulging of the jaw cortex resembling an arterial aneurysm in shape.
       Hemorrhagic cyst of jaw — A cyst of the jaw caused by the escape of blood within a jaw bone.
       Traumatic cyst of jaw — A cyst of the jaw resulting from trauma to the jaw bone.

M27.5-   **Periradicular pathology associated with previous endodontic treatment**

    M27.51   **Perforation of root canal space due to endodontic treatment**

    M27.52   **Endodontic overfill**

    M27.53   **Endodontic underfill**

    M27.59   **Other periradicular pathology associated with previous endodontic treatment**

M27.6-   **Endosseous dental implant failure**

    M27.61   **Osseointegration failure of dental implant**
       Hemorrhagic complications of dental implant placement
       Iatrogenic osseointegration failure of dental implant
       Osseointegration failure of dental implant due to complications of systemic disease
       Osseointegration failure of dental implant due to poor bone quality
       Pre-integration failure of dental implant NOS
       Pre-osseointegration failure of dental implant

    M27.62   **Post-osseointegration biological failure of dental implant**
       Failure of dental implant due to lack of attached gingiva
       Failure of dental implant due to occlusal trauma (caused by poor prosthetic design)
       Failure of dental implant due to parafunctional habits
       Failure of dental implant due to periodontal infection (peri-implantitis)
       Failure of dental implant due to poor oral hygiene
       Iatrogenic post-osseointegration failure of dental implant
       Post-osseointegration failure of dental implant due to complications of systemic disease

    M27.63   **Post-osseointegration mechanical failure of dental implant**
       Failure of dental prosthesis causing loss of dental implant
       Fracture of dental implant
       Excludes ❷: *cracked tooth (K03.81)*
           fractured dental restorative material with loss of material (K08.531)
           fractured dental restorative material without loss of material (K08.530)
           fractured tooth (S02.5)

    M27.69   **Other endosseous dental implant failure**
       Dental implant failure NOS

M27.8   **Other specified diseases of jaws**
     Cherubism
     Exostosis
     Fibrous dysplasia
     Unilateral condylar hyperplasia
     Unilateral condylar hypoplasia
     Excludes 1:   *jaw pain (R68.84)*

M27.9   **Disease of jaws, unspecified**

Systemic connective tissue disorders (M30-M36)

Includes: Autoimmune disease NOS
            Collagen (vascular) disease NOS
            Systemic autoimmune disease
            Systemic collagen (vascular) disease
   Excludes 1:   *autoimmune disease, single organ or single cell-type — code to relevant condition category*

M30-   **Polyarteritis nodosa and related conditions**
     Excludes 1:   *microscopic polyarteritis (M31.7)*

   CC   **M30.0**   **Polyarteritis nodosa** — A systemic vasculitis that is characterized by acute necrotizing inflammation of the small- to medium-sized arteries and microaneurysm formation.

   CC   **M30.1**   **Polyarteritis with lung involvement [Churg-Strauss]** — A form involving the pulmonary circulation.
       Allergic granulomatous angiitis

   CC   **M30.2**   **Juvenile polyarteritis** — A form affecting infants and young children that often has a neurologic component.

   CC   **M30.3**   **Mucocutaneous lymph node syndrome [Kawasaki]** — A form marked by tender lymph nodes and skin and mucous membrane inflammation that usually affects young children.

   CC   **M30.8**   **Other conditions related to polyarteritis nodosa**
       Polyangiitis overlap syndrome

M31-   **Other necrotizing vasculopathies**

   CC   **M31.0**   **Hypersensitivity angiitis** — A group of necrotizing inflammatory diseases affecting primarily the small blood vessels and characterized by palpable purpura.
       Goodpasture's syndrome — Severe, acute glomerulonephritis accompanied by diffuse hemorrhagic inflammation of the lungs.

   MCC   **M31.1**   **Thrombotic microangiopathy** — The formation of thrombi in the arterioles and capillaries.
       Thrombotic thrombocytopenic purpura — Thrombotic microangiopathy associated with thrombocytopenia, hemolytic anemia, azotemia, and fever.

   CC   **M31.2**   **Lethal midline granuloma** — A necrotizing tumor-like granuloma which results in destruction of the mid-face and invariably in death.

     M31.3-   **Wegener's granulomatosis** — Focal necrotizing arteriolitis, and granulomatous lesions of the respiratory tract with widespread inflammation of all of the organs of the body.
       Necrotizing respiratory granulomatosis

     CC   **M31.30**   **Wegener's granulomatosis without renal involvement**
       Wegener's granulomatosis NOS

     CC   **M31.31**   **Wegener's granulomatosis with renal involvement**

   CC   **M31.4**   **Aortic arch syndrome [Takayasu]** — An occlusive polyarteritis of unknown cause usually affecting the branches of the aortic arch.

     M31.5   **Giant cell arteritis with polymyalgia rheumatica**

     M31.6   **Other giant cell arteritis** — Chronic inflammation of the large arteries, usually the temporal, occipital, or ophthalmic arteries, accompanied by the presence of giant cells which cause thickening of the intima with narrowing and eventual occlusion of the lumen.

   CC   **M31.7**   **Microscopic polyangiitis** — A form of polyarteritis nodosa affecting the smallest vessels.
       Microscopic polyarteritis
       Excludes 1:   *polyarteritis nodosa (M30.0)*

   CC   **M31.8**   **Other specified necrotizing vasculopathies**
       Hypocomplementemic vasculitis
       Septic vasculitis

   CC   **M31.9**   **Necrotizing vasculopathy, unspecified**

M32-   **Systemic lupus erythematosus (SLE)** — An inflammatory autoimmune disorder of the connective tissue that is characterized by rash, joint pain, leukopenia, fever, malaise, and in severe cases organ involvement.
     Excludes 1:   *lupus erythematosus (discoid) (NOS) (L93.0)*

     M32.0   **Drug-induced systemic lupus erythematosus**
       Use additional code for adverse effect, if applicable, to identify drug (T36-T50 with fifth or sixth character 5)

     M32.1-   **Systemic lupus erythematosus with organ or system involvement**

       M32.10   **Systemic lupus erythematosus, organ or system involvement unspecified**

    CC   **M32.11**   **Endocarditis in systemic lupus erythematosus**
       Libman-Sacks disease

    CC   **M32.12**   **Pericarditis in systemic lupus erythematosus**
       Lupus pericarditis

       M32.13   **Lung involvement in systemic lupus erythematosus**
       Pleural effusion due to systemic lupus erythematosus

M 2 7 I M 3 2

M32.14 <u>Glomerular</u> disease in systemic lupus erythematosus
> AHA 13:4Q:p125 – Lupus complicated by lupus nephritis
>> Lupus renal disease NOS

M32.15 <u>Tubulo-interstitial nephropathy</u> in systemic lupus erythematosus

M32.19 <u>Other</u> organ or system involvement in systemic lupus erythematosus

M32.8 Other forms of systemic lupus erythematosus

M32.9 Systemic lupus erythematosus, unspecified
> SLE NOS
> Systemic lupus erythematosus NOS
> Systemic lupus erythematosus without organ involvement

M33- <u>Dermatopolymyositis</u> — A connective tissue disease characterized by inflammation of the skin, edema, and inflammation of the muscles.

M33.0- <u>Juvenile</u> dermatopolymyositis

cc **M33.00** Juvenile dermatopolymyositis, organ involvement <u>unspecified</u>

cc **M33.01** Juvenile dermatopolymyositis <u>with respiratory involvement</u>

cc **M33.02** Juvenile dermatopolymyositis <u>with myopathy</u>

cc **M33.09** Juvenile dermatopolymyositis <u>with other organ involvement</u>

M33.1- <u>Other</u> dermatopolymyositis

cc **M33.10** Other dermatopolymyositis, organ involvement <u>unspecified</u>

cc **M33.11** Other dermatopolymyositis <u>with respiratory involvement</u>

cc **M33.12** Other dermatopolymyositis <u>with myopathy</u>

cc **M33.19** Other dermatopolymyositis <u>with other organ involvement</u>

M33.2- <u>Polymyositis</u> — A connective tissue disease characterized by inflammation and degeneration of the muscles, edema, and without skin changes.

cc **M33.20** Polymyositis, organ involvement <u>unspecified</u>

cc **M33.21** Polymyositis <u>with respiratory involvement</u>

cc **M33.22** Polymyositis <u>with myopathy</u>

cc **M33.29** Polymyositis <u>with other organ involvement</u>

M33.9- <u>Dermatopolymyositis, unspecified</u>

cc **M33.90** Dermatopolymyositis, unspecified, organ involvement unspecified

cc **M33.91** Dermatopolymyositis, unspecified <u>with respiratory involvement</u>

cc **M33.92** Dermatopolymyositis, unspecified <u>with myopathy</u>

cc **M33.99** Dermatopolymyositis, unspecified <u>with other organ involvement</u>

M34- Systemic sclerosis [scleroderma] — A chronic disease characterized by diffuse fibrous hardening of the skin and internal organs, loss of elasticity, and deposition of melanin in the basal cells.
> *Excludes 1:*   *circumscribed scleroderma (L94.0)*
>>   *neonatal scleroderma (P83.8)*

M34.0 Progressive systemic sclerosis

M34.1 CR(E)ST syndrome
> Combination of calcinosis, Raynaud's phenomenon, esophageal dysfunction, sclerodactyly, telangiectasia

M34.2 Systemic sclerosis induced by drug and chemical
> Code first poisoning due to drug or toxin, if applicable (T36-T65 with fifth or sixth character 1-4 or 6)
> Use additional code for adverse effect, if applicable, to identify drug (T36-T50 with fifth or sixth character 5)

M34.8- Other forms of systemic sclerosis

cc **M34.81** Systemic sclerosis <u>with lung involvement</u>

cc **M34.82** Systemic sclerosis <u>with myopathy</u>

M34.83 Systemic sclerosis <u>with polyneuropathy</u>

M34.89 Other systemic sclerosis

M34.9 Systemic sclerosis, unspecified

M35- Other systemic involvement of connective tissue
> *Excludes 1:*   *reactive perforating collagenosis (L87.1)*

M35.0- <u>Sicca syndrome</u> [Sjögren] — An autoimmune disorder characterized by drying of the mucous membranes and eyes, enlargement of the parotid glands, and chronic polyarthritis.

M35.00 Sicca syndrome, <u>unspecified</u>

M35.01 Sicca syndrome <u>with keratoconjunctivitis</u>

M35.02 Sicca syndrome <u>with lung involvement</u>

cc **M35.03** Sicca syndrome <u>with myopathy</u>

M35.04 Sicca syndrome <u>with tubulo-interstitial nephropathy</u>
> Renal tubular acidosis in sicca syndrome

M35.09 Sicca syndrome <u>with other organ involvement</u>

cc **M35.1** Other overlap syndromes
> Mixed connective tissue disease
> *Excludes 1:*   *polyangiitis overlap syndrome (M30.8)*

cc **M35.2** Behçet's disease — An autoinflammatory disorder that is characterized by oral ulcers, genital ulcers, and uveitis.

M35.3 Polymyalgia rheumatica — An inflammatory disease characterized by pain and stiffness of the shoulder, upper arms, hips, and neck and elevated erythrocyte sedimentation rate.
> *Excludes 1:*   *polymyalgia rheumatica with giant cell arteritis (M31.5)*

M35.4 Diffuse (eosinophilic) fasciitis — An inflammatory disease affecting the fascia that is usually limited to the arms and legs.

cc **M35.5** Multifocal fibrosclerosis

M35.6 Relapsing panniculitis [Weber-Christian] — Inflammation of the subcutaneous fat with associated relapsing fever.
> *Excludes 1:*   *lupus panniculitis (L93.2)*
>>   *panniculitis NOS (M79.3-)*

M35.7 Hypermobility syndrome — Joints that can move beyond the normal range of motion.
> Familial ligamentous laxity
> *Excludes 1:*   *Ehlers-Danlos syndrome (Q79.6)*
>>   *ligamentous laxity, NOS (M24.2-)*

cc **M35.8** Other specified systemic involvement of connective tissue

M35.9 Systemic involvement of connective tissue, unspecified
> Autoimmune disease (systemic) NOS
> Collagen (vascular) disease NOS

M36- Systemic disorders of connective tissue in diseases classified elsewhere
> *Excludes ❷:*   *arthropathies in diseases classified elsewhere (M14.-)*

cc **M36.0** Dermato(poly)myositis in neoplastic disease — [Not Allowed as PDX]
> Code first underlying neoplasm (C00-D49)

M36.1 Arthropathy in neoplastic disease — [Not Allowed as PDX]
> Code first underlying neoplasm, such as:
>> Leukemia (C91-C95)
>> Malignant histiocytosis (C96.A)
>> Multiple myeloma (C90.0)

M36.2 Hemophilic arthropathy — [Not Allowed as PDX]
> Hemarthrosis in hemophilic arthropathy
> Code first underlying disease, such as:
>> Factor VIII deficiency (D66)
>>> With vascular defect (D68.0)
>> Factor IX deficiency (D67)
>> Hemophilia (classical) (D66)
>> Hemophilia B (D67)
>> Hemophilia C (D68.1)

M36.3 Arthropathy in other blood disorders — [Not Allowed as PDX]

M36.4 Arthropathy in hypersensitivity reactions classified elsewhere — [Not Allowed as PDX]
> Code first underlying disease, such as:
>> Henoch (-Schönlein) purpura (D69.0)
>> Serum sickness (T80.6-)

M36.8 Systemic disorders of connective tissue <u>in other diseases classified elsewhere</u> — [Not Allowed as PDX]
> Code first underlying disease, such as:
>> Alkaptonuria (E70.2)
>> Hypogammaglobulinemia (D80.-)
>> Ochronosis (E70.2)

Dorsopathies (M40-M54)

Deforming dorsopathies (M40-M43)

M40- <u>Kyphosis and lordosis</u>
> *Excludes 1:*   *congenital kyphosis and lordosis (Q76.4)*
>>   *kyphoscoliosis (M41.-)*
>>   *postprocedural kyphosis and lordosis (M96.-)*

M40.0- <u>Postural kyphosis</u> — The increased convexity of the spinal position that is due to improper posture.
> *Excludes 1:*   *osteochondrosis of spine (M42.-)*

M40.00 Postural kyphosis, site <u>unspecified</u>

M40.03 Postural kyphosis, <u>cervicothoracic</u> region

M40.04   Postural kyphosis, <u>thoracic</u> region

M40.05   Postural kyphosis, <u>thoracolumbar</u> region

M40.1-   <u>Other secondary</u> kyphosis

M40.10   Other secondary kyphosis, site <u>unspecified</u>

M40.12   Other secondary kyphosis, <u>cervical</u> region

M40.13   Other secondary kyphosis, <u>cervicothoracic</u> region

M40.14   Other secondary kyphosis, <u>thoracic</u> region

M40.15   Other secondary kyphosis, <u>thoracolumbar</u> region

M40.2-   Other and unspecified kyphosis

M40.20- <u>Unspecified</u> kyphosis

M40.202   Unspecified kyphosis, cervical region

M40.203   Unspecified kyphosis, <u>cervicothoracic</u> region

M40.204   Unspecified kyphosis, <u>thoracic</u> region

M40.205   Unspecified kyphosis, <u>thoracolumbar</u> region

M40.209   Unspecified kyphosis, <u>site unspecified</u>

M40.29- <u>Other</u> kyphosis

M40.292   Other kyphosis, <u>cervical</u> region

M40.293   Other kyphosis, <u>cervicothoracic</u> region

M40.294   Other kyphosis, <u>thoracic</u> region

M40.295   Other kyphosis, <u>thoracolumbar</u> region

M40.299   Other kyphosis, site <u>unspecified</u>

M40.3-   Flatback syndrome — The abnormal alignment of the spine in which the spine appears flat versus naturally curved.

M40.30   Flatback syndrome, <u>site unspecified</u>

M40.35   Flatback syndrome, <u>thoracolumbar</u> region

M40.36   Flatback syndrome, <u>lumbar</u> region

M40.37   Flatback syndrome, <u>lumbosacral</u> region

M40.4-   <u>Postural</u> lordosis — The increased concavity of the spinal position that is due to improper posture.

      Acquired lordosis

M40.40   Postural lordosis, <u>site unspecified</u>

M40.45   Postural lordosis, <u>thoracolumbar</u> region

M40.46   Postural lordosis, <u>lumbar</u> region

M40.47   Postural lordosis, <u>lumbosacral</u> region

M40.5-   Lordosis, <u>unspecified</u>

M40.50   Lordosis, unspecified, site <u>unspecified</u>

M40.55   Lordosis, unspecified, <u>thoracolumbar</u> region

M40.56   Lordosis, unspecified, <u>lumbar</u> region

M40.57   Lordosis, unspecified, <u>lumbosacral</u> region

M41-   Scoliosis — The lateral curvature of the spine.

   Includes: **Kyphoscoliosis** — The backward and lateral curvature of the spine.

   Excludes 1:   *congenital scoliosis NOS (Q67.5)*

         congenital scoliosis due to bony malformation (Q76.3)

         postural congenital scoliosis (Q67.5)

         kyphoscoliotic heart disease (I27.1)

         postprocedural scoliosis (M96.-)

M41.0-   <u>Infantile idiopathic</u> scoliosis — A form usually diagnosed before the age of 3 and with an unknown cause.

M41.00   Infantile idiopathic scoliosis, <u>site unspecified</u>

M41.02   Infantile idiopathic scoliosis, <u>cervical</u> region

M41.03   Infantile idiopathic scoliosis, <u>cervicothoracic</u> region

M41.04   Infantile idiopathic scoliosis, <u>thoracic</u> region

M41.05   Infantile idiopathic scoliosis, <u>thoracolumbar</u> region

M41.06   Infantile idiopathic scoliosis, <u>lumbar</u> region

M41.07   Infantile idiopathic scoliosis, <u>lumbosacral</u> region

M41.08   Infantile idiopathic scoliosis, <u>sacral and sacrococcygeal</u> region

M41.1-   Juvenile and adolescent idiopathic scoliosis

M41.11- <u>Juvenile idiopathic</u> scoliosis — A form usually diagnosed between the ages of 4 and 10 and with an unknown cause.

M41.112   Juvenile idiopathic scoliosis, <u>cervical</u> region

M41.113   Juvenile idiopathic scoliosis, <u>cervicothoracic</u> region

M41.114   Juvenile idiopathic scoliosis, <u>thoracic</u> region

M41.115   Juvenile idiopathic scoliosis, <u>thoracolumbar</u> region

M41.116   Juvenile idiopathic scoliosis, <u>lumbar</u> region

M41.117   Juvenile idiopathic scoliosis, <u>lumbosacral</u> region

M41.119   Juvenile idiopathic scoliosis, <u>site unspecified</u>

M41.12- <u>Adolescent</u> scoliosis — A form usually diagnosed between the ages of 10 and 18 and with an unknown cause.

M41.122   Adolescent idiopathic scoliosis, <u>cervical</u> region

M41.123   Adolescent idiopathic scoliosis, <u>cervicothoracic</u> region

M41.124   Adolescent idiopathic scoliosis, <u>thoracic</u> region

M41.125   Adolescent idiopathic scoliosis, <u>thoracolumbar</u> region

M41.126   Adolescent idiopathic scoliosis, <u>lumbar</u> region

M41.127   Adolescent idiopathic scoliosis, <u>lumbosacral</u> region

M41.129   Adolescent idiopathic scoliosis, <u>site unspecified</u>

M41.2-   <u>Other idiopathic</u> scoliosis

M41.20   Other idiopathic scoliosis, <u>site unspecified</u>

M41.22   Other idiopathic scoliosis, <u>cervical</u> region

M41.23   Other idiopathic scoliosis, <u>cervicothoracic</u> region

M41.24   Other idiopathic scoliosis, <u>thoracic</u> region

M41.25   Other idiopathic scoliosis, <u>thoracolumbar</u> region

M41.26   Other idiopathic scoliosis, <u>lumbar</u> region

M41.27   Other idiopathic scoliosis, <u>lumbosacral</u> region

M41.3-   Thoracogenic scoliosis — A form due to disease or operative trauma to the thoracic cage.

M41.30   Thoracogenic scoliosis, <u>site unspecified</u>

M41.34   Thoracogenic scoliosis, <u>thoracic</u> region

M41.35   Thoracogenic scoliosis, <u>thoracolumbar</u> region

M41.4-   <u>Neuromuscular</u> scoliosis — A form due to a neurologic or muscular disease.

      Scoliosis secondary to cerebral palsy, Friedreich's ataxia, poliomyelitis and other neuromuscular disorders

      Code also underlying condition

M41.40   Neuromuscular scoliosis, <u>site unspecified</u>

M41.41   Neuromuscular scoliosis, <u>occipito-atlanto-axial</u> region

M41.42   Neuromuscular scoliosis, <u>cervical</u> region

M41.43   Neuromuscular scoliosis, <u>cervicothoracic</u> region

M41.44   Neuromuscular scoliosis, <u>thoracic</u> region

M41.45   Neuromuscular scoliosis, <u>thoracolumbar</u> region

M41.46   Neuromuscular scoliosis, <u>lumbar</u> region

M41.47   Neuromuscular scoliosis, <u>lumbosacral</u> region

M41.5-   <u>Other secondary</u> scoliosis

M41.50   Other secondary scoliosis, <u>site unspecified</u>

M41.52   Other secondary scoliosis, <u>cervical</u> region

M41.53   Other secondary scoliosis, <u>cervicothoracic</u> region

M41.54   Other secondary scoliosis, <u>thoracic</u> region

M41.55   Other secondary scoliosis, <u>thoracolumbar</u> region

M41.56   Other secondary scoliosis, <u>lumbar</u> region

M41.57   Other secondary scoliosis, <u>lumbosacral</u> region

M41.8-   <u>Other forms</u> of scoliosis

M41.80   Other forms of scoliosis, <u>site unspecified</u>

M41.82   Other forms of scoliosis, <u>cervical</u> region

M41.83   Other forms of scoliosis, <u>cervicothoracic</u> region

M41.84   Other forms of scoliosis, <u>thoracic</u> region

M41.85   Other forms of scoliosis, <u>thoracolumbar</u> region

M41.86   Other forms of scoliosis, <u>lumbar</u> region

M41.87   Other forms of scoliosis, <u>lumbosacral</u> region

M41.9   Scoliosis, unspecified

M42-   <u>Spinal osteochondrosis</u> — Diseases affecting both the bone and cartilage of the spine.

M42.0-   <u>Juvenile</u> osteochondrosis of spine — A developmental disease of the vertebral bone-growth centers characterized by degeneration and recalcification of the vertebrae with resultant deformity of the spine.

      Calvé's disease

      Scheuermann's disease

   Excludes 1:   *postural kyphosis (M40.0)*

M42.00   Juvenile osteochondrosis of spine, <u>site unspecified</u>

M42.01   Juvenile osteochondrosis of spine, <u>occipito-atlanto-axial</u> region

M42.02   Juvenile osteochondrosis of spine, <u>cervical</u> region

M42.03 Juvenile osteochondrosis of spine, <u>cervicothoracic</u> region

M42.04 Juvenile osteochondrosis of spine, <u>thoracic</u> region

M42.05 Juvenile osteochondrosis of spine, <u>thoracolumbar</u> region

M42.06 Juvenile osteochondrosis of spine, <u>lumbar</u> region

M42.07 Juvenile osteochondrosis of spine, <u>lumbosacral</u> region

M42.08 Juvenile osteochondrosis of spine, <u>sacral and sacrococcygeal</u> region

M42.09 Juvenile osteochondrosis of spine, <u>multiple sites</u> in spine

M42.1- <u>Adult</u> **osteochondrosis of spine** — Degeneration and recalcification of the vertebrae in adults.

M42.10 Adult osteochondrosis of spine, <u>site unspecified</u> — [Age/15-124]

M42.11 Adult osteochondrosis of spine, <u>occipito-atlanto-axial</u> region — [Age/15-124]

M42.12 Adult osteochondrosis of spine, <u>cervical</u> region — [Age/15-124]

M42.13 Adult osteochondrosis of spine, <u>cervicothoracic</u> region — [Age/15-124]

M42.14 Adult osteochondrosis of spine, <u>thoracic</u> region — [Age/15-124]

M42.15 Adult osteochondrosis of spine, <u>thoracolumbar</u> region — [Age/15-124]

M42.16 Adult osteochondrosis of spine, <u>lumbar</u> region — [Age/15-124]

M42.17 Adult osteochondrosis of spine, <u>lumbosacral</u> region — [Age/15-124]

M42.18 Adult osteochondrosis of spine, <u>sacral and sacrococcygeal</u> region — [Age/15-124]

M42.19 Adult osteochondrosis of spine, <u>multiple sites</u> in spine — [Age/15-124]

M42.9 Spinal osteochondrosis, unspecified

M43- <u>Other deforming dorsopathies</u>

Excludes 1: *congenital spondylolysis and spondylolisthesis (Q76.2)*
hemivertebra (Q76.3-Q76.4)
Klippel-Feil syndrome (Q76.1)
lumbarization and sacralization (Q76.4)
platyspondylisis (Q76.4)
spina bifida occulta (Q76.0)
spinal curvature in osteoporosis (M80.-)
spinal curvature in Paget's disease of bone [osteitis deformans] (M88.-)

M43.0- <u>Spondylolysis</u> — A defect in the connection between vertebrae.

Excludes 1: *congenital spondylolysis (Q76.2)*
spondylolisthesis (M43.1)

M43.00 Spondylolysis, <u>site unspecified</u>

M43.01 Spondylolysis, <u>occipito-atlanto-axial</u> region

M43.02 Spondylolysis, <u>cervical</u> region

M43.03 Spondylolysis, <u>cervicothoracic</u> region

M43.04 Spondylolysis, <u>thoracic</u> region

M43.05 Spondylolysis, <u>thoracolumbar</u> region

M43.06 Spondylolysis, <u>lumbar</u> region

M43.07 Spondylolysis, <u>lumbosacral</u> region

M43.08 Spondylolysis, <u>sacral and sacrococcygeal</u> region

M43.09 Spondylolysis, <u>multiple sites</u> in spine

M43.1- <u>Spondylolisthesis</u> — The forward displacement of a vertebra.

Excludes 1: *acute traumatic of lumbosacral region (S33.1)*
acute traumatic of sites other than lumbosacral — code to Fracture, vertebra, by region
congenital spondylolisthesis (Q76.2)

M43.10 Spondylolisthesis, <u>site unspecified</u>

M43.11 Spondylolisthesis, <u>occipito-atlanto-axial</u> region

M43.12 Spondylolisthesis, <u>cervical</u> region

M43.13 Spondylolisthesis, <u>cervicothoracic</u> region

M43.14 Spondylolisthesis, <u>thoracic</u> region

M43.15 Spondylolisthesis, <u>thoracolumbar</u> region

M43.16 Spondylolisthesis, <u>lumbar</u> region

M43.17 Spondylolisthesis, <u>lumbosacral</u> region

M43.18 Spondylolisthesis, <u>sacral and sacrococcygeal</u> region

M43.19 Spondylolisthesis, <u>multiple sites</u> in spine

M43.2- <u>Fusion of spine</u> — Inflammation of the spinal joints that causes the vertebrae to fuse together.

Ankylosis of spinal joint

Excludes 1: *ankylosing spondylitis (M45.0-)*
congenital fusion of spine (Q76.4)

Excludes ❷: *arthrodesis status (Z98.1)*
pseudoarthrosis after fusion or arthrodesis (M96.0)

M43.20 Fusion of spine, <u>site unspecified</u>

M43.21 Fusion of spine, <u>occipito-atlanto-axial</u> region

M43.22 Fusion of spine, <u>cervical</u> region

M43.23 Fusion of spine, <u>cervicothoracic</u> region

M43.24 Fusion of spine, <u>thoracic</u> region

M43.25 Fusion of spine, <u>thoracolumbar</u> region

M43.26 Fusion of spine, <u>lumbar</u> region

M43.27 Fusion of spine, <u>lumbosacral</u> region

M43.28 Fusion of spine, <u>sacral and sacrococcygeal</u> region

M43.3 Recurrent atlantoaxial dislocation with myelopathy

M43.4 Other recurrent atlantoaxial dislocation

M43.5- Other recurrent vertebral dislocation

Excludes 1: *biomechanical lesions NEC (M99.-)*

M43.5x- <u>Other recurrent vertebral dislocation</u>

M43.5x2 Other recurrent vertebral dislocation, <u>cervical</u> region

M43.5x3 Other recurrent vertebral dislocation, <u>cervicothoracic</u> region

M43.5x4 Other recurrent vertebral dislocation, <u>thoracic</u> region

M43.5x5 Other recurrent vertebral dislocation, <u>thoracolumbar</u> region

M43.5x6 Other recurrent vertebral dislocation, <u>lumbar</u> region

M43.5x7 Other recurrent vertebral dislocation, <u>lumbosacral</u> region

M43.5x8 Other recurrent vertebral dislocation, <u>sacral and sacrococcygeal</u> region

M43.5x9 Other recurrent vertebral dislocation, <u>site unspecified</u>

M43.6 Torticollis — The contracted state of the neck muscles causing the characteristic head tilt.

Excludes 1: *congenital (sternomastoid) torticollis (Q68.0)*
current injury — see Injury, of spine, by body region
ocular torticollis (R29.891)
psychogenic torticollis (F45.8)
spasmodic torticollis (G24.3)
torticollis due to birth injury (P15.2)

M43.8- Other specified deforming dorsopathies

Excludes ❷: *kyphosis and lordosis (M40.-)*
scoliosis (M41.-)

M43.8x- <u>Other specified deforming dorsopathies</u>

M43.8x1 Other specified deforming dorsopathies, <u>occipito-atlanto-axial</u> region

M43.8x2 Other specified deforming dorsopathies, <u>cervical</u> region

M43.8x3 Other specified deforming dorsopathies, <u>cervicothoracic</u> region

M43.8x4 Other specified deforming dorsopathies, <u>thoracic</u> region

M43.8x5 Other specified deforming dorsopathies, <u>thoracolumbar</u> region

M43.8x6 Other specified deforming dorsopathies, <u>lumbar</u> region

M43.8x7 Other specified deforming dorsopathies, <u>lumbosacral</u> region

M43.8x8 Other specified deforming dorsopathies, <u>sacral and sacrococcygeal</u> region

M43.8x9 Other specified deforming dorsopathies, <u>site unspecified</u>

M43.9 Deforming dorsopathy, unspecified

Curvature of spine NOS

M
4
2
-
M
4
3

Spondylopathies (M45-M49)

M45- **Ankylosing spondylitis** — Inflammation of the spinal joints that causes the spine to become stiff and inflexible.
    Rheumatoid arthritis of spine — A form of rheumatoid arthritis that affects the vertebrae and marked by immobility, pain, and calcification.
    Excludes 1:   *arthropathy in Reiter's disease (M02.3-)*
                    juvenile (ankylosing) spondylitis (M08.1)
    Excludes ❷: *Behçet's disease (M35.2)*

  M45.0   Ankylosing spondylitis of <u>multiple sites</u> in spine
  M45.1   Ankylosing spondylitis of <u>occipito-atlanto-axial</u> region
  M45.2   Ankylosing spondylitis of <u>cervical</u> region
  M45.3   Ankylosing spondylitis of <u>cervicothoracic</u> region
  M45.4   Ankylosing spondylitis of <u>thoracic</u> region
  M45.5   Ankylosing spondylitis of <u>thoracolumbar</u> region
  M45.6   Ankylosing spondylitis of <u>lumbar</u> region
  M45.7   Ankylosing spondylitis of <u>lumbosacral</u> region
  M45.8   Ankylosing spondylitis <u>sacral and sacrococcygeal</u> region
  M45.9   Ankylosing spondylitis of <u>unspecified</u> sites in spine

M46- Other inflammatory spondylopathies
  M46.0-   <u>Spinal enthesopathy</u> — A disorder of the spinal ligamentous or muscular attachments.
          Disorder of ligamentous or muscular attachments of spine
    M46.00   Spinal enthesopathy, <u>site unspecified</u>
    M46.01   Spinal enthesopathy, <u>occipito-atlanto-axial</u> region
    M46.02   Spinal enthesopathy, <u>cervical</u> region
    M46.03   Spinal enthesopathy, <u>cervicothoracic</u> region
    M46.04   Spinal enthesopathy, <u>thoracic</u> region
    M46.05   Spinal enthesopathy, <u>thoracolumbar</u> region
    M46.06   Spinal enthesopathy, <u>lumbar</u> region
    M46.07   Spinal enthesopathy, <u>lumbosacral</u> region
    M46.08   Spinal enthesopathy, <u>sacral and sacrococcygeal</u> region
    M46.09   Spinal enthesopathy, <u>multiple sites</u> in spine
  M46.1   Sacroiliitis, not elsewhere classified
  M46.2-   <u>Osteomyelitis</u> of vertebra — Inflammation of the vertebrae caused by microorganisms.
    CC **M46.20**   Osteomyelitis of vertebra, <u>site unspecified</u>
    CC **M46.21**   Osteomyelitis of vertebra, <u>occipito-atlanto-axial</u> region
    CC **M46.22**   Osteomyelitis of vertebra, <u>cervical</u> region
    CC **M46.23**   Osteomyelitis of vertebra, <u>cervicothoracic</u> region
    CC **M46.24**   Osteomyelitis of vertebra, <u>thoracic</u> region
    CC **M46.25**   Osteomyelitis of vertebra, <u>thoracolumbar</u> region
    CC **M46.26**   Osteomyelitis of vertebra, <u>lumbar</u> region
    CC **M46.27**   Osteomyelitis of vertebra, <u>lumbosacral</u> region
    CC **M46.28**   Osteomyelitis of vertebra, <u>sacral and sacrococcygeal</u> region
  M46.3-   <u>Infection of intervertebral disc (pyogenic)</u> — Inflammation of an intervertebral disc with pus formation that is due to infection by microorganisms.
          Use additional code (B95-B97) to identify infectious agent
    CC **M46.30**   Infection of intervertebral disc (pyogenic), <u>site unspecified</u>
    CC **M46.31**   Infection of intervertebral disc (pyogenic), <u>occipito-atlanto-axial</u> region
    CC **M46.32**   Infection of intervertebral disc (pyogenic), <u>cervical</u> region
    CC **M46.33**   Infection of intervertebral disc (pyogenic), <u>cervicothoracic</u> region
    CC **M46.34**   Infection of intervertebral disc (pyogenic), <u>thoracic</u> region
    CC **M46.35**   Infection of intervertebral disc (pyogenic), <u>thoracolumbar</u> region
    CC **M46.36**   Infection of intervertebral disc (pyogenic), <u>lumbar</u> region
    CC **M46.37**   Infection of intervertebral disc (pyogenic), <u>lumbosacral</u> region
    CC **M46.38**   Infection of intervertebral disc (pyogenic), <u>sacral and sacrococcygeal</u> region
    CC **M46.39**   Infection of intervertebral disc (pyogenic), <u>multiple sites</u> in spine

M46.4-   <u>Discitis</u>, unspecified
  M46.40   Discitis, unspecified, <u>site unspecified</u>
  M46.41   Discitis, unspecified, <u>occipito-atlanto-axial</u> region
  M46.42   Discitis, unspecified, <u>cervical</u> region
  M46.43   Discitis, unspecified, <u>cervicothoracic</u> region
  M46.44   Discitis, unspecified, <u>thoracic</u> region
  M46.45   Discitis, unspecified, <u>thoracolumbar</u> region
  M46.46   Discitis, unspecified, <u>lumbar</u> region
  M46.47   Discitis, unspecified, <u>lumbosacral</u> region
  M46.48   Discitis, unspecified, <u>sacral and sacrococcygeal</u> region
  M46.49   Discitis, unspecified, <u>multiple sites</u> in spine

M46.5-   <u>Other infective</u> spondylopathies
  M46.50   Other infective spondylopathies, <u>site unspecified</u>
  M46.51   Other infective spondylopathies, <u>occipito-atlanto-axial</u> region
  M46.52   Other infective spondylopathies, <u>cervical</u> region
  M46.53   Other infective spondylopathies, <u>cervicothoracic</u> region
  M46.54   Other infective spondylopathies, <u>thoracic</u> region
  M46.55   Other infective spondylopathies, <u>thoracolumbar</u> region
  M46.56   Other infective spondylopathies, <u>lumbar</u> region
  M46.57   Other infective spondylopathies, <u>lumbosacral</u> region
  M46.58   Other infective spondylopathies, <u>sacral and sacrococcygeal</u> region
  M46.59   Other infective spondylopathies, <u>multiple sites</u> in spine

M46.8-   <u>Other specified inflammatory</u> spondylopathies
  M46.80   Other specified inflammatory spondylopathies, <u>site unspecified</u>
  M46.81   Other specified inflammatory spondylopathies, <u>occipito-atlanto-axial</u> region
  M46.82   Other specified inflammatory spondylopathies, <u>cervical</u> region
  M46.83   Other specified inflammatory spondylopathies, <u>cervicothoracic</u> region
  M46.84   Other specified inflammatory spondylopathies, <u>thoracic</u> region
  M46.85   Other specified inflammatory spondylopathies, <u>thoracolumbar</u> region
  M46.86   Other specified inflammatory spondylopathies, <u>lumbar</u> region
  M46.87   Other specified inflammatory spondylopathies, <u>lumbosacral</u> region
  M46.88   Other specified inflammatory spondylopathies, <u>sacral and sacrococcygeal</u> region
  M46.89   Other specified inflammatory spondylopathies, <u>multiple sites</u> in spine

M46.9-   <u>Unspecified</u> inflammatory spondylopathy
  M46.90   Unspecified inflammatory spondylopathy, <u>site unspecified</u>
  M46.91   Unspecified inflammatory spondylopathy, <u>occipito-atlanto-axial</u> region
  M46.92   Unspecified inflammatory spondylopathy, <u>cervical</u> region
  M46.93   Unspecified inflammatory spondylopathy, <u>cervicothoracic</u> region
  M46.94   Unspecified inflammatory spondylopathy, <u>thoracic</u> region
  M46.95   Unspecified inflammatory spondylopathy, <u>thoracolumbar</u> region
  M46.96   Unspecified inflammatory spondylopathy, <u>lumbar</u> region
  M46.97   Unspecified inflammatory spondylopathy, <u>lumbosacral</u> region
  M46.98   Unspecified inflammatory spondylopathy, <u>sacral and sacrococcygeal</u> region
  M46.99   Unspecified inflammatory spondylopathy, <u>multiple sites</u> in spine

M45 - M46

M47- Spondylosis — Degenerative joint disease of the spine.
   Includes: Arthrosis or osteoarthritis of spine
                Degeneration of facet joints

M47.0- Anterior spinal and vertebral artery compression syndromes

M47.01- Anterior spinal artery compression syndromes — A form resulting in the restriction of blood flow through the anterior spinal artery.

cc **M47.011 Anterior spinal artery compression syndromes, occipito-atlanto-axial region**

cc **M47.012 Anterior spinal artery compression syndromes, cervical region**

cc **M47.013 Anterior spinal artery compression syndromes, cervicothoracic region**

cc **M47.014 Anterior spinal artery compression syndromes, thoracic region**

cc **M47.015 Anterior spinal artery compression syndromes, thoracolumbar region**

cc **M47.016 Anterior spinal artery compression syndromes, lumbar region**

cc **M47.019 Anterior spinal artery compression syndromes, site unspecified**

M47.02- Vertebral artery compression syndromes — A form resulting in the restriction of blood flow through the vertebral artery.

cc **M47.021 Vertebral artery compression syndromes, occipito-atlanto-axial region**

cc **M47.022 Vertebral artery compression syndromes, cervical region**

cc **M47.029 Vertebral artery compression syndromes, site unspecified**

M47.1- Other spondylosis with myelopathy — Degenerative joint disease of the spine that results in a disorder of the spinal cord.
   Spondylogenic compression of spinal cord
   Excludes 1:   vertebral subluxation (M43.3-M43.59)

cc **M47.10 Other spondylosis with myelopathy, site unspecified**

cc **M47.11 Other spondylosis with myelopathy, occipito-atlanto-axial region**

cc **M47.12 Other spondylosis with myelopathy, cervical region**

cc **M47.13 Other spondylosis with myelopathy, cervicothoracic region**

cc **M47.14 Other spondylosis with myelopathy, thoracic region**

cc **M47.15 Other spondylosis with myelopathy, thoracolumbar region**

cc **M47.16 Other spondylosis with myelopathy, lumbar region**

M47.2- Other spondylosis with radiculopathy

M47.20 Other spondylosis with radiculopathy, site unspecified

M47.21 Other spondylosis with radiculopathy, occipito-atlanto-axial region

M47.22 Other spondylosis with radiculopathy, cervical region

M47.23 Other spondylosis with radiculopathy, cervicothoracic region

M47.24 Other spondylosis with radiculopathy, thoracic region

M47.25 Other spondylosis with radiculopathy, thoracolumbar region

M47.26 Other spondylosis with radiculopathy, lumbar region

M47.27 Other spondylosis with radiculopathy, lumbosacral region

M47.28 Other spondylosis with radiculopathy, sacral and sacrococcygeal region

M47.8- Other spondylosis

M47.81- Spondylosis without myelopathy or radiculopathy

M47.811 Spondylosis without myelopathy or radiculopathy, occipito-atlanto-axial region

M47.812 Spondylosis without myelopathy or radiculopathy, cervical region

M47.813 Spondylosis without myelopathy or radiculopathy, cervicothoracic region

M47.814 Spondylosis without myelopathy or radiculopathy, thoracic region

M47.815 Spondylosis without myelopathy or radiculopathy, thoracolumbar region

M47.816 Spondylosis without myelopathy or radiculopathy, lumbar region

M47.817 Spondylosis without myelopathy or radiculopathy, lumbosacral region

M47.818 Spondylosis without myelopathy or radiculopathy, sacral and sacrococcygeal region

M47.819 Spondylosis without myelopathy or radiculopathy, site unspecified

M47.89- Other spondylosis

M47.891 Other spondylosis, occipito-atlanto-axial region

M47.892 Other spondylosis, cervical region

M47.893 Other spondylosis, cervicothoracic region

M47.894 Other spondylosis, thoracic region

M47.895 Other spondylosis, thoracolumbar region

M47.896 Other spondylosis, lumbar region

M47.897 Other spondylosis, lumbosacral region

M47.898 Other spondylosis, sacral and sacrococcygeal region

M47.899 Other spondylosis, site unspecified

M47.9 Spondylosis, unspecified

M48- Other spondylopathies

M48.0- Spinal stenosis — The narrowing of the spinal column with compression of the spinal nerve roots.
   Caudal stenosis

M48.00 Spinal stenosis, site unspecified

M48.01 Spinal stenosis, occipito-atlanto-axial region

M48.02 Spinal stenosis, cervical region

M48.03 Spinal stenosis, cervicothoracic region

M48.04 Spinal stenosis, thoracic region

M48.05 Spinal stenosis, thoracolumbar region

M48.06 Spinal stenosis, lumbar region

M48.07 Spinal stenosis, lumbosacral region

M48.08 Spinal stenosis, sacral and sacrococcygeal region

M48.1- Ankylosing hyperostosis [Forestier] — The spinal arthropathy that is characterized by ossification of the ligaments and connective tissue of the spine.
   Diffuse idiopathic skeletal hyperostosis [DISH]

M48.10 Ankylosing hyperostosis [Forestier], site unspecified

M48.11 Ankylosing hyperostosis [Forestier], occipito-atlanto-axial region

M48.12 Ankylosing hyperostosis [Forestier], cervical region

M48.13 Ankylosing hyperostosis [Forestier], cervicothoracic region

M48.14 Ankylosing hyperostosis [Forestier], thoracic region

M48.15 Ankylosing hyperostosis [Forestier], thoracolumbar region

M48.16 Ankylosing hyperostosis [Forestier], lumbar region

M48.17 Ankylosing hyperostosis [Forestier], lumbosacral region

M48.18 Ankylosing hyperostosis [Forestier], sacral and sacrococcygeal region

M48.19 Ankylosing hyperostosis [Forestier], multiple sites in spine

M48.2- Kissing spine — A disorder in which the spinal processes of adjacent vertebrae are in contact.

M48.20 Kissing spine, site unspecified

M48.21 Kissing spine, occipito-atlanto-axial region

M48.22 Kissing spine, cervical region

M48.23 Kissing spine, cervicothoracic region

M48.24 Kissing spine, thoracic region

M48.25 Kissing spine, thoracolumbar region

M48.26 Kissing spine, lumbar region

M48.27 Kissing spine, lumbosacral region

M48.3- Traumatic spondylopathy — A disorder of the spine as a result of trauma.

cc **M48.30 Traumatic spondylopathy, site unspecified**

cc **M48.31 Traumatic spondylopathy, occipito-atlanto-axial region**

cc **M48.32 Traumatic spondylopathy, cervical region**

cc **M48.33 Traumatic spondylopathy, cervicothoracic region**

cc **M48.34 Traumatic spondylopathy, thoracic region**

cc **M48.35 Traumatic spondylopathy, thoracolumbar region**

cc **M48.36 Traumatic spondylopathy, lumbar region**

cc **M48.37 Traumatic spondylopathy, lumbosacral region**

M
4
7
-
M
4
8

CC **M48.38** Traumatic spondylopathy, <u>sacral and sacrococcygeal</u> region

M48.4- <u>Fatigue fracture</u> of <u>vertebra</u> — A break of a diseased or weakened bone by a minor injury that would otherwise not break a healthy bone.
  Stress fracture of vertebra
  Excludes 1: *pathological fracture NOS (M84.4-)*
      pathological fracture of vertebra due to neoplasm (M84.58)
      pathological fracture of vertebra due to other diagnosis (M84.68)
      pathological fracture of vertebra due to osteoporosis (M80-)
      traumatic fracture of vertebrae (S12.0-S12.3-, S22.0-, S32.0-)

The appropriate 7th character is to be added to each code from subcategory M48.4:
  A **Initial encounter for fracture**
  D **Subsequent encounter for fracture with routine healing**
  G **Subsequent encounter for fracture with delayed healing**
  S **Sequela of fracture**

M48.40x- Fatigue fracture of vertebra, <u>site unspecified</u>
M48.41x- Fatigue fracture of vertebra, <u>occipito-atlanto-axial</u> region
M48.42x- Fatigue fracture of vertebra, <u>cervical</u> region
M48.43x- Fatigue fracture of vertebra, <u>cervicothoracic</u> region
M48.44x- Fatigue fracture of vertebra, <u>thoracic</u> region
M48.45x- Fatigue fracture of vertebra, <u>thoracolumbar</u> region
M48.46x- Fatigue fracture of vertebra, <u>lumbar</u> region
M48.47x- Fatigue fracture of vertebra, <u>lumbosacral</u> region
M48.48x- Fatigue fracture of vertebra, <u>sacral and sacrococcygeal</u> region

M48.5- <u>Collapsed vertebra</u>, <u>not elsewhere classified</u>
  Collapsed vertebra NOS
  Compression fracture of vertebra NOS
  Wedging of vertebra NOS
  Excludes 1: *current injury — see Injury of spine, by body region*
      fatigue fracture of vertebra (M48.4)
      pathological fracture of vertebra due to neoplasm (M84.58)
      pathological fracture of vertebra due to other diagnosis (M84.68)
      pathological fracture of vertebra due to osteoporosis (M80.-)
      pathological fracture NOS (M84.4-)
      stress fracture of vertebra (M48.4-)
      traumatic fracture of vertebra (S12.-, S22.-, S32.-)

The appropriate 7th character is to be added to each code from subcategory M48.5:
  A **Initial encounter for fracture**
  D **Subsequent encounter for fracture with routine healing**
  G **Subsequent encounter for fracture with delayed healing**
  S **Sequela of fracture**

CC-A **M48.50x-** Collapsed vertebra, not elsewhere classified, <u>site unspecified</u>
CC-A **M48.51x-** Collapsed vertebra, not elsewhere classified, <u>occipito-atlanto-axial</u> region
CC-A **M48.52x-** Collapsed vertebra, not elsewhere classified, <u>cervical</u> region
CC-A **M48.53x-** Collapsed vertebra, not elsewhere classified, <u>cervicothoracic</u> region
CC-A **M48.54x-** Collapsed vertebra, not elsewhere classified, <u>thoracic</u> region
CC-A **M48.55x-** Collapsed vertebra, not elsewhere classified, <u>thoracolumbar</u> region
CC-A **M48.56x-** Collapsed vertebra, not elsewhere classified, <u>lumbar</u> region
CC-A **M48.57x-** Collapsed vertebra, not elsewhere classified, <u>lumbosacral</u> region
CC-A **M48.58x-** Collapsed vertebra, not elsewhere classified, <u>sacral and sacrococcygeal</u> region

M48.8- Other specified spondylopathies
  Ossification of posterior longitudinal ligament
  M48.8x- <u>Other specified spondylopathies</u>
    M48.8x1 Other specified spondylopathies, <u>occipito-atlanto-axial</u> region
    M48.8x2 Other specified spondylopathies, <u>cervical</u> region
    M48.8x3 Other specified spondylopathies, <u>cervicothoracic</u> region
    M48.8x4 Other specified spondylopathies, <u>thoracic</u> region
    M48.8x5 Other specified spondylopathies, <u>thoracolumbar</u> region
    M48.8x6 Other specified spondylopathies, <u>lumbar</u> region
    M48.8x7 Other specified spondylopathies, <u>lumbosacral</u> region
    M48.8x8 Other specified spondylopathies, <u>sacral and sacrococcygeal</u> region
    M48.8x9 Other specified spondylopathies, <u>site unspecified</u>
  M48.9 Spondylopathy, <u>unspecified</u>

M49- Spondylopathies <u>in diseases classified elsewhere</u>
  Includes: Curvature of spine in diseases classified elsewhere
      Deformity of spine in diseases classified elsewhere
      Kyphosis in diseases classified elsewhere
      Scoliosis in diseases classified elsewhere
      Spondylopathy in diseases classified elsewhere
  Code first underlying disease, such as:
      Brucellosis (A23.-)
      Charcot-Marie-Tooth disease (G60.0)
      Enterobacterial infections (A01-A04)
      Osteitis fibrosa cystica (E21.0)
  Excludes 1: *curvature of spine in tuberculosis [Pott's] (A18.01)*
      enteropathic arthropathies (M07.-)
      gonococcal spondylitis (A54.41)
      neuropathic spondylopathy in syringomyelia (G95.0)
      neuropathic spondylopathy in tabes dorsalis (A52.11)
      neuropathic [tabes dorsalis] spondylitis (A52.11)
      nonsyphilitic neuropathic spondylopathy NEC (G98.0)
      spondylitis in syphilis (acquired) (A52.77)
      tuberculosis spondylitis (A18.01)
      typhoid fever spondylitis (A01.05)

M49.8- <u>Spondylopathy</u> <u>in diseases classified elsewhere</u>
  M49.80 Spondylopathy in diseases classified elsewhere, <u>site unspecified</u> — [Not Allowed as PDX]
  M49.81 Spondylopathy in diseases classified elsewhere, <u>occipito-atlanto-axial</u> region — [Not Allowed as PDX]
  M49.82 Spondylopathy in diseases classified elsewhere, <u>cervical</u> region — [Not Allowed as PDX]
  M49.83 Spondylopathy in diseases classified elsewhere, <u>cervicothoracic</u> region — [Not Allowed as PDX]
  M49.84 Spondylopathy in diseases classified elsewhere, <u>thoracic</u> region — [Not Allowed as PDX]
  M49.85 Spondylopathy in diseases classified elsewhere, <u>thoracolumbar</u> region — [Not Allowed as PDX]
  M49.86 Spondylopathy in diseases classified elsewhere, <u>lumbar</u> region — [Not Allowed as PDX]
  M49.87 Spondylopathy in diseases classified elsewhere, <u>lumbosacral</u> region — [Not Allowed as PDX]
  M49.88 Spondylopathy in diseases classified elsewhere, <u>sacral and sacrococcygeal</u> region — [Not Allowed as PDX]
  M49.89 Spondylopathy in diseases classified elsewhere, <u>multiple sites</u> in spine — [Not Allowed as PDX]

Other dorsopathies (M50-M54)

Excludes 1: *current injury — see injury of spine by body region*
    discitis NOS (M46.4-)

M50- <u>Cervical disc disorders</u> — The abnormal condition of a cervical disc.
  AHA 16:1Q:p17 – Code to the most superior level of disorder
  Note: Code to the most superior level of disorder
  Includes: Cervicothoracic disc disorders with cervicalgia
      Cervicothoracic disc disorders
  M50.0- Cervical disc disorder <u>with myelopathy</u> — A form that results in a disorder of the spinal cord.
    CC **M50.00** Cervical disc disorder with myelopathy, <u>unspecified cervical</u> region

M48-M50

cc **M50.01 Cervical disc disorder with myelopathy, <u>high cervical</u> region**
   C2-C3 disc disorder with myelopathy
   C3-C4 disc disorder with myelopathy

M50.02-Cervical disc disorder with myelopathy, <u>mid-cervical</u> region

cc **M50.020 Cervical disc disorder with myelopathy, mid-cervical region, <u>unspecified level</u>**

cc **M50.021 Cervical disc disorder at <u>C4-C5 level</u> with myelopathy**
   C4-C5 disc disorder with myelopathy

cc **M50.022 Cervical disc disorder at <u>C5-C6 level</u> with myelopathy**
   C5-C6 disc disorder with myelopathy

cc **M50.023 Cervical disc disorder at <u>C6-C7 level</u> with myelopathy**
   C6-C7 disc disorder with myelopathy

cc **M50.03 Cervical disc disorder with myelopathy, <u>cervicothoracic</u> region**
   C7-T1 disc disorder with myelopathy

M50.1- Cervical disc disorder <u>with radiculopathy</u> — A form with injury (compression and/or inflammation) to the spinal nerve root.
   Excludes ❷: brachial radiculitis NOS (M54.13)

M50.10 Cervical disc disorder with radiculopathy, <u>unspecified cervical</u> region

M50.11 Cervical disc disorder with radiculopathy, <u>high cervical</u> region
   C2-C3 disc disorder with radiculopathy
   C3 radiculopathy due to disc disorder
   C3-C4 disc disorder with radiculopathy
   C4 radiculopathy due to disc disorder

M50.12-Cervical disc disorder with radiculopathy, <u>mid-cervical</u> region

M50.120 Mid-cervical disc disorder, <u>unspecified</u>

M50.121 Cervical disc disorder at <u>C4-C5 level</u> with radiculopathy
   C4-C5 disc disorder with radiculopathy
   C5 radiculopathy due to disc disorder

M50.122 Cervical disc disorder at <u>C5-C6 level</u> with radiculopathy
   C5-C6 disc disorder with radiculopathy
   C6 radiculopathy due to disc disorder

M50.123 Cervical disc disorder at <u>C6-C7 level</u> with radiculopathy
   C6-C7 disc disorder with radiculopathy
   C7 radiculopathy due to disc disorder

M50.13 Cervical disc disorder with radiculopathy, <u>cervicothoracic</u> region
   C7-T1 disc disorder with radiculopathy
   C8 radiculopathy due to disc disorder

M50.2- <u>Other cervical</u> disc displacement — The dislocation of a cervical intervertebral disc.

M50.20 Other cervical disc displacement, <u>unspecified cervical</u> region

M50.21 Other cervical disc displacement, <u>high cervical</u> region
   Other C2-C3 cervical disc displacement
   Other C3-C4 cervical disc displacement

M50.22-Other cervical disc displacement, <u>mid-cervical</u> region

M50.220 Other cervical disc displacement, mid-cervical region, <u>unspecified level</u>

M50.221 Other cervical disc displacement at <u>C4-C5 level</u>
   Other C4-C5 cervical disc displacement

M50.222 Other cervical disc displacement at <u>C5-C6 level</u>
   Other C5-C6 cervical disc displacement

M50.223 Other cervical disc displacement at <u>C6-C7 level</u>
   Other C6-C7 cervical disc displacement

M50.23 Other cervical disc displacement, <u>cervicothoracic</u> region
   Other C7-T1 cervical disc displacement

M50.3- <u>Other cervical</u> disc degeneration — The deterioration of a cervical intervertebral disc.

M50.30 Other cervical disc degeneration, <u>unspecified cervical</u> region

M50.31 Other cervical disc degeneration, <u>high cervical</u> region
   Other C2-C3 cervical disc degeneration
   Other C3-C4 cervical disc degeneration

M50.32-Other cervical disc degeneration, <u>mid-cervical</u> region

M50.320 Other cervical disc degeneration, mid-cervical region, <u>unspecified level</u>

M50.321 Other cervical disc degeneration at <u>C4-C5 level</u>
   Other C4-C5 cervical disc degeneration

M50.322 Other cervical disc degeneration at <u>C5-C6 level</u>
   Other C5-C6 cervical disc degeneration

M50.323 Other cervical disc degeneration at <u>C6-C7 level</u>
   Other C6-C7 cervical disc degeneration

M50.33 Other cervical disc degeneration, <u>cervicothoracic</u> region
   Other C7-T1 cervical disc degeneration

M50.8- <u>Other cervical disc disorders</u>

M50.80 Other cervical disc disorders, <u>unspecified cervical</u> region

M50.81 Other cervical disc disorders, <u>high cervical</u> region
   Other C2-C3 cervical disc disorders
   Other C3-C4 cervical disc disorders

M50.82-Other cervical disc disorders, <u>mid-cervical</u> region

M50.820 Other cervical disc disorders, mid-cervical region, <u>unspecified level</u>

M50.821 Other cervical disc disorders at <u>C4-C5 level</u>
   Other C4-C5 cervical disc disorders

M50.822 Other cervical disc disorders at <u>C5-C6 level</u>
   Other C5-C6 cervical disc disorders

M50.823 Other cervical disc disorders at <u>C6-C7 level</u>
   Other C6-C7 cervical disc disorders

M50.83 Other cervical disc disorders, <u>cervicothoracic</u> region
   Other C7-T1 cervical disc disorders

M50.9- Cervical disc disorder, <u>unspecified</u>

M50.90 Cervical disc disorder, unspecified, <u>unspecified cervical</u> region

M50.91 Cervical disc disorder, unspecified, <u>high cervical</u> region
   C2-C3 cervical disc disorder, unspecified
   C3-C4 cervical disc disorder, unspecified

M50.92-Cervical disc disorder, unspecified, <u>mid-cervical</u> region

M50.920 Unspecified cervical disc disorder, mid-cervical region, <u>unspecified level</u>

M50.921 Unspecified cervical disc disorder at <u>C4-C5 level</u>
   Unspecified C4-C5 cervical disc disorder

M50.922 Unspecified cervical disc disorder at <u>C5-C6 level</u>
   Unspecified C5-C6 cervical disc disorder

M50.923 Unspecified cervical disc disorder at <u>C6-C7 level</u>
   Unspecified C6-C7 cervical disc disorder

M50.93 Cervical disc disorder, unspecified, <u>cervicothoracic</u> region
   C7-T1 cervical disc disorder, unspecified

M51- <u>Thoracic, thoracolumbar, and lumbosacral intervertebral disc disorders</u> — The abnormal condition of a thoracic, thoracolumbar, or lumbosacral disc.
   Excludes ❷: cervical and cervicothoracic disc disorders (M50.-)
   sacral and sacrococcygeal disorders (M53.3)

M51.0- Thoracic, thoracolumbar and lumbosacral intervertebral disc disorders <u>with myelopathy</u> — A form that results in a disorder of the spinal cord.

cc **M51.04 Intervertebral disc disorders with myelopathy, <u>thoracic</u> region**

cc **M51.05 Intervertebral disc disorders with myelopathy, <u>thoracolumbar</u> region**

cc **M51.06 Intervertebral disc disorders with myelopathy, <u>lumbar</u> region**

M51.1- Thoracic, thoracolumbar and lumbosacral intervertebral disc disorders <u>with radiculopathy</u> — A form with injury (compression and/or inflammation) to the spinal nerve root.
   Sciatica due to intervertebral disc disorder
   Excludes 1:   lumbar radiculitis NOS (M54.16)
   sciatica NOS (M54.3)

M51.14 Intervertebral disc disorders with radiculopathy, <u>thoracic</u> region

M51.15 Intervertebral disc disorders with radiculopathy, <u>thoracolumbar</u> region

M 50 - M 51

M51.16 Intervertebral disc disorders with radiculopathy, <u>lumbar</u> region

M51.17 Intervertebral disc disorders with radiculopathy, <u>lumbosacral</u> region

M51.2- <u>Other</u> thoracic, thoracolumbar and lumbosacral intervertebral disc <u>displacement</u> — The dislocation of a thoracic, thoracolumbar, or lumbosacral intervertebral disc.
   Lumbago due to displacement of intervertebral disc

M51.24 Other intervertebral disc displacement, <u>thoracic</u> region

M51.25 Other intervertebral disc displacement, <u>thoracolumbar</u> region

M51.26 Other intervertebral disc displacement, <u>lumbar</u> region

M51.27 Other intervertebral disc displacement, <u>lumbosacral</u> region

M51.3- <u>Other</u> thoracic, thoracolumbar and lumbosacral intervertebral disc <u>degeneration</u> — The deterioration of a thoracic, thoracolumbar, or lumbosacral intervertebral disc.

M51.34 Other intervertebral disc degeneration, <u>thoracic</u> region

M51.35 Other intervertebral disc degeneration, <u>thoracolumbar</u> region

M51.36 Other intervertebral disc degeneration, <u>lumbar</u> region

M51.37 Other intervertebral disc degeneration, <u>lumbosacral</u> region

M51.4- <u>Schmorl's nodes</u> — A bony defect of a spinal vertebra.

M51.44 Schmorl's nodes, <u>thoracic</u> region

M51.45 Schmorl's nodes, <u>thoracolumbar</u> region

M51.46 Schmorl's nodes, <u>lumbar</u> region

M51.47 Schmorl's nodes, <u>lumbosacral</u> region

M51.8- <u>Other</u> thoracic, thoracolumbar and lumbosacral intervertebral disc <u>disorders</u>

M51.84 Other intervertebral disc disorders, <u>thoracic</u> region

M51.85 Other intervertebral disc disorders, <u>thoracolumbar</u> region

M51.86 Other intervertebral disc disorders, <u>lumbar</u> region

M51.87 Other intervertebral disc disorders, <u>lumbosacral</u> region

M51.9 <u>Unspecified</u> thoracic, thoracolumbar and lumbosacral intervertebral disc disorder

M53- <u>Other</u> and <u>unspecified</u> dorsopathies, <u>not elsewhere classified</u>

M53.0 Cervicocranial syndrome — The neurological dysfunction of the upper portion of the cervical spinal cord and associated nerve roots that is caused by misalignment of the cervical vertebrae and characterized by dizziness, headache, tinnitis, and sinus or ear pain.
   Posterior cervical sympathetic syndrome

M53.1 Cervicobrachial syndrome — The neurological dysfunction of the lower portion of the cervical spinal cord and associated nerve roots that is characterized by neck pain with numbness and tingling, and pain down the arm.
   Excludes ❷: cervical disc disorder (M50.-)
        thoracic outlet syndrome (G54.0)

M53.2- Spinal instabilities — The abnormal excessive movement of the spinal vertebrae.
M53.2x- <u>Spinal instabilities</u>

M53.2x1 Spinal instabilities, <u>occipito-atlanto-axial</u> region
M53.2x2 Spinal instabilities, <u>cervical</u> region
M53.2x3 Spinal instabilities, <u>cervicothoracic</u> region
M53.2x4 Spinal instabilities, <u>thoracic</u> region
M53.2x5 Spinal instabilities, <u>thoracolumbar</u> region
M53.2x6 Spinal instabilities, <u>lumbar</u> region
M53.2x7 Spinal instabilities, <u>lumbosacral</u> region
M53.2x8 Spinal instabilities, <u>sacral and sacrococcygeal</u> region
M53.2x9 Spinal instabilities, <u>site unspecified</u>

M53.3 Sacrococcygeal disorders, not elsewhere classified
   Coccygodynia

M53.8- <u>Other specified dorsopathies</u>
M53.80 Other specified dorsopathies, <u>site unspecified</u>
M53.81 Other specified dorsopathies, <u>occipito-atlanto-axial</u> region
M53.82 Other specified dorsopathies, <u>cervical</u> region
M53.83 Other specified dorsopathies, <u>cervicothoracic</u> region

M53.84 Other specified dorsopathies, <u>thoracic</u> region
M53.85 Other specified dorsopathies, <u>thoracolumbar</u> region
M53.86 Other specified dorsopathies, <u>lumbar</u> region
M53.87 Other specified dorsopathies, <u>lumbosacral</u> region
M53.88 Other specified dorsopathies, <u>sacral and sacrococcygeal</u> region

M53.9 Dorsopathy, <u>unspecified</u>

M54- <u>Dorsalgia</u> — Back pain.
   Excludes 1: psychogenic dorsalgia (F45.41)

M54.0- <u>Panniculitis affecting regions of neck and back</u> — Inflammation of the subcutaneous fat of the sacral or back region.
   Excludes 1: lupus panniculitis (L93.2)
        panniculitis NOS (M79.3)
        relapsing [Weber-Christian] panniculitis (M35.6)

M54.00 Panniculitis affecting regions of neck and back, site <u>unspecified</u>
M54.01 Panniculitis affecting regions of neck and back, <u>occipito-atlanto-axial</u> region
M54.02 Panniculitis affecting regions of neck and back, <u>cervical</u> region
M54.03 Panniculitis affecting regions of neck and back, cervicothoracic region
M54.04 Panniculitis affecting regions of neck and back, <u>thoracic</u> region
M54.05 Panniculitis affecting regions of neck and back, <u>thoracolumbar</u> region
M54.06 Panniculitis affecting regions of neck and back, <u>lumbar</u> region
M54.07 Panniculitis affecting regions of neck and back, <u>lumbosacral</u> region
M54.08 Panniculitis affecting regions of neck and back, <u>sacral and sacrococcygeal</u> region
M54.09 Panniculitis affecting regions, neck and back, <u>multiple sites</u> in spine

M54.1- <u>Radiculopathy</u> — Irritation, compression, or inflammation of a spinal nerve root.
   Brachial neuritis or radiculitis NOS
   Lumbar neuritis or radiculitis NOS
   Lumbosacral neuritis or radiculitis NOS
   Thoracic neuritis or radiculitis NOS
   Radiculitis NOS
   Excludes 1: neuralgia and neuritis NOS (M79.2)
        radiculopathy with cervical disc disorder (M50.1)
        radiculopathy with lumbar and other intervertebral disc disorder (M51.1-)
        radiculopathy with spondylosis (M47.2-)

M54.10 Radiculopathy, <u>site unspecified</u>
M54.11 Radiculopathy, <u>occipito-atlanto-axial</u> region
M54.12 Radiculopathy, <u>cervical</u> region
M54.13 Radiculopathy, <u>cervicothoracic</u> region
M54.14 Radiculopathy, <u>thoracic</u> region
M54.15 Radiculopathy, <u>thoracolumbar</u> region
M54.16 Radiculopathy, <u>lumbar</u> region
M54.17 Radiculopathy, <u>lumbosacral</u> region
M54.18 Radiculopathy, <u>sacral and sacrococcygeal</u> region

M54.2 Cervicalgia — Neck pain.
   Excludes 1: cervicalgia due to intervertebral cervical disc disorder (M50.-)

M54.3- <u>Sciatica</u> — Sciatic nerve pain radiating to the buttock and leg.
   Excludes 1: lesion of sciatic nerve (G57.0)
        sciatica due to intervertebral disc disorder (M51.1-)
        sciatica with lumbago (M54.4-)

M54.30 Sciatica, <u>unspecified</u> side
M54.31 Sciatica, <u>right</u> side
M54.32 Sciatica, <u>left</u> side

M54.4- <u>Lumbago with sciatica</u> — Pain in the lumbar region with sciatic nerve pain radiating to the buttock and leg.
   Excludes 1: lumbago with sciatica due to intervertebral disc disorder (M51.1-)

M54.40 Lumbago with sciatica, <u>unspecified</u> side
M54.41 Lumbago with sciatica, <u>right</u> side

M51 – M54

M54.42 Lumbago with sciatica, _left_ side

M54.5 Low back pain — Pain in the lumbar region.
  Loin pain
  Lumbago NOS
  Excludes 1:   *low back strain (S39.012)*
                    lumbago due to intervertebral disc displacement
                    (M51.2-)
                    lumbago with sciatica (M54.4-)

M54.6 Pain in thoracic spine
  Excludes 1:   *pain in thoracic spine due to intervertebral disc*
                    disorder (M51.-)

M54.8- Other dorsalgia
  Excludes 1:   *dorsalgia in thoracic region (M54.6)*
                    low back pain (M54.5)

  M54.81 Occipital neuralgia — A neck and back of the head pain disorder with
    the pain sometimes radiating to the face or side of the face.

  M54.89 Other dorsalgia

M54.9 Dorsalgia, unspecified
  Backache NOS
  Back pain NOS

Soft tissue disorders (M60-M79)

Disorders of muscles (M60-M63)

Excludes 1:   *dermatopolymyositis (M33-)*
                  muscular dystrophies and myopathies (G71-G72)
                  myopathy in amyloidosis (E85.-)
                  myopathy in polyarteritis nodosa (M30.0)
                  myopathy in rheumatoid arthritis (M05.32)
                  myopathy in scleroderma (M34.-)
                  myopathy in Sjögren's syndrome (M35.03)
                  myopathy in systemic lupus erythematosus (M32.-)

M60- Myositis — Inflammation of the muscles.
  Excludes ❷: *inclusion body myositis [IBM] (G72.41)*

  M60.0- Infective myositis — A form caused by microorganisms.
    Tropical pyomyositis
    Use additional code (B95-B97) to identify infectious agent

    M60.00-Infective myositis, _unspecified_ site
    cc **M60.000   Infective myositis, unspecified _right_ _arm_**
                    Infective myositis, right upper limb NOS
    cc **M60.001   Infective myositis, unspecified _left_ _arm_**
                    Infective myositis, left upper limb NOS
    cc **M60.002   Infective myositis, unspecified _arm_**
                    Infective myositis, upper limb NOS
    cc **M60.003   Infective myositis, unspecified _right_ _leg_**
                    Infective myositis, right lower limb NOS
    cc **M60.004   Infective myositis, unspecified _left_ _leg_**
                    Infective myositis, left lower limb NOS
    cc **M60.005   Infective myositis, unspecified _leg_**
                    Infective myositis, lower limb NOS
    cc **M60.009   Infective myositis, unspecified _site_**

    M60.01-Infective myositis, _shoulder_
    cc **M60.011   Infective myositis, _right_ shoulder**
    cc **M60.012   Infective myositis, _left_ shoulder**
    cc **M60.019   Infective myositis, _unspecified_ shoulder**

    M60.02-Infective myositis, _upper arm_
    cc **M60.021   Infective myositis, _right_ upper arm**
    cc **M60.022   Infective myositis, _left_ upper arm**
    cc **M60.029   Infective myositis, _unspecified_ upper arm**

    M60.03-Infective myositis, _forearm_
    cc **M60.031   Infective myositis, _right_ forearm**
    cc **M60.032   Infective myositis, _left_ forearm**
    cc **M60.039   Infective myositis, _unspecified_ forearm**

    M60.04-Infective myositis, _hand and fingers_
    cc **M60.041   Infective myositis, _right_ hand**
    cc **M60.042   Infective myositis, _left_ hand**
    cc **M60.043   Infective myositis, _unspecified_ hand**
    cc **M60.044   Infective myositis, _right_ finger(s)**
    cc **M60.045   Infective myositis, _left_ finger(s)**
    cc **M60.046   Infective myositis, _unspecified_ finger(s)**

M60.05-Infective myositis, _thigh_
cc **M60.051   Infective myositis, _right_ thigh**
cc **M60.052   Infective myositis, _left_ thigh**
cc **M60.059   Infective myositis, _unspecified_ thigh**

M60.06-Infective myositis, _lower leg_
cc **M60.061   Infective myositis, _right_ lower leg**
cc **M60.062   Infective myositis, _left_ lower leg**
cc **M60.069   Infective myositis, _unspecified_ lower leg**

M60.07-Infective myositis, _ankle, foot and toes_
cc **M60.070   Infective myositis, _right_ ankle**
cc **M60.071   Infective myositis, _left_ ankle**
cc **M60.072   Infective myositis, _unspecified_ ankle**
cc **M60.073   Infective myositis, _right_ foot**
cc **M60.074   Infective myositis, _left_ foot**
cc **M60.075   Infective myositis, _unspecified_ foot**
cc **M60.076   Infective myositis, _right_ toe(s)**
cc **M60.077   Infective myositis, _left_ toe(s)**
cc **M60.078   Infective myositis, _unspecified_ toe(s)**

cc **M60.08 Infective myositis, _other_ site**
cc **M60.09 Infective myositis, _multiple sites_**

M60.1- Interstitial myositis — A form with fibrous degeneration of muscle tissue.
  M60.10 Interstitial myositis of _unspecified_ _site_

  M60.11-Interstitial myositis, _shoulder_
    M60.111   Interstitial myositis, _right_ shoulder
    M60.112   Interstitial myositis, _left_ shoulder
    M60.119   Interstitial myositis, _unspecified_ shoulder

  M60.12-Interstitial myositis, _upper arm_
    M60.121   Interstitial myositis, _right_ upper arm
    M60.122   Interstitial myositis, _left_ upper arm
    M60.129   Interstitial myositis, _unspecified_ upper arm

  M60.13-Interstitial myositis, _forearm_
    M60.131   Interstitial myositis, _right_ forearm
    M60.132   Interstitial myositis, _left_ forearm
    M60.139   Interstitial myositis, _unspecified_ forearm

  M60.14-Interstitial myositis, _hand_
    M60.141   Interstitial myositis, _right_ hand
    M60.142   Interstitial myositis, _left_ hand
    M60.149   Interstitial myositis, _unspecified_ hand

  M60.15-Interstitial myositis, _thigh_
    M60.151   Interstitial myositis, _right_ thigh
    M60.152   Interstitial myositis, _left_ thigh
    M60.159   Interstitial myositis, _unspecified_ thigh

  M60.16-Interstitial myositis, _lower leg_
    M60.161   Interstitial myositis, _right_ lower leg
    M60.162   Interstitial myositis, _left_ lower leg
    M60.169   Interstitial myositis, _unspecified_ lower leg

  M60.17-Interstitial myositis, _ankle and foot_
    M60.171   Interstitial myositis, _right_ ankle and foot
    M60.172   Interstitial myositis, _left_ ankle and foot
    M60.179   Interstitial myositis, _unspecified_ ankle and foot

  M60.18 Interstitial myositis, _other_ site
  M60.19 Interstitial myositis, _multiple sites_

M60.2- Foreign body granuloma of soft tissue, _not elsewhere_
  classified — The formation of a tumor-like mass of fibroblast tissue with a
  foreign body reaction.
    Use additional code to identify the type of retained foreign body
    (Z18.-)
    Excludes 1:   *foreign body granuloma of skin and subcutaneous*
                      tissue (L92.3)

  **M60.20 Foreign body granuloma of soft tissue, not elsewhere
    classified, _unspecified_ _site_**

  **M60.21-Foreign body granuloma of soft tissue, not elsewhere
    classified, _shoulder_**

    **M60.211   Foreign body granuloma of soft tissue, not
      elsewhere classified, _right_ shoulder**

M60.212   Foreign body granuloma of soft tissue, not elsewhere classified, **left** shoulder
M60.219   Foreign body granuloma of soft tissue, not elsewhere classified, **unspecified** shoulder
M60.22- Foreign body granuloma of soft tissue, not elsewhere classified, **upper arm**
M60.221   Foreign body granuloma of soft tissue, not elsewhere classified, **right** upper arm
M60.222   Foreign body granuloma of soft tissue, not elsewhere classified, **left** upper arm
M60.229   Foreign body granuloma of soft tissue, not elsewhere classified, **unspecified** upper arm
M60.23- Foreign body granuloma of soft tissue, not elsewhere classified, **forearm**
M60.231   Foreign body granuloma of soft tissue, not elsewhere classified, **right** forearm
M60.232   Foreign body granuloma of soft tissue, not elsewhere classified, **left** forearm
M60.239   Foreign body granuloma of soft tissue, not elsewhere classified, **unspecified** forearm
M60.24- Foreign body granuloma of soft tissue, not elsewhere classified, **hand**
M60.241   Foreign body granuloma of soft tissue, not elsewhere classified, **right** hand
M60.242   Foreign body granuloma of soft tissue, not elsewhere classified, **left** hand
M60.249   Foreign body granuloma of soft tissue, not elsewhere classified, **unspecified** hand
M60.25- Foreign body granuloma of soft tissue, not elsewhere classified, **thigh**
M60.251   Foreign body granuloma of soft tissue, not elsewhere classified, **right** thigh
M60.252   Foreign body granuloma of soft tissue, not elsewhere classified, **left** thigh
M60.259   Foreign body granuloma of soft tissue, not elsewhere classified, **unspecified** thigh
M60.26- Foreign body granuloma of soft tissue, not elsewhere classified, **lower leg**
M60.261   Foreign body granuloma of soft tissue, not elsewhere classified, **right** lower leg
M60.262   Foreign body granuloma of soft tissue, not elsewhere classified, **left** lower leg
M60.269   Foreign body granuloma of soft tissue, not elsewhere classified, **unspecified** lower leg
M60.27- Foreign body granuloma of soft tissue, not elsewhere classified, **ankle and foot**
M60.271   Foreign body granuloma of soft tissue, not elsewhere classified, **right** ankle and foot
M60.272   Foreign body granuloma of soft tissue, not elsewhere classified, **left** ankle and foot
M60.279   Foreign body granuloma of soft tissue, not elsewhere classified, **unspecified** ankle and foot
M60.28   Foreign body granuloma of soft tissue, not elsewhere classified, **other site**
M60.8- **Other myositis**
M60.80   Other myositis, **unspecified site**
M60.81- Other myositis **shoulder**
M60.811   Other myositis, **right** shoulder
M60.812   Other myositis, **left** shoulder
M60.819   Other myositis, **unspecified** shoulder
M60.82- Other myositis, **upper arm**
M60.821   Other myositis, **right** upper arm
M60.822   Other myositis, **left** upper arm
M60.829   Other myositis, **unspecified** upper arm
M60.83- Other myositis, **forearm**
M60.831   Other myositis, **right** forearm
M60.832   Other myositis, **left** forearm
M60.839   Other myositis, **unspecified** forearm

M60.84- Other myositis, **hand**
M60.841   Other myositis, **right** hand
M60.842   Other myositis, **left** hand
M60.849   Other myositis, **unspecified** hand
M60.85- Other myositis, **thigh**
M60.851   Other myositis, **right** thigh
M60.852   Other myositis, **left** thigh
M60.859   Other myositis, **unspecified** thigh
M60.86- Other myositis, **lower leg**
M60.861   Other myositis, **right** lower leg
M60.862   Other myositis, **left** lower leg
M60.869   Other myositis, **unspecified** lower leg
M60.87- Other myositis, **ankle and foot**
M60.871   Other myositis, **right** ankle and foot
M60.872   Other myositis, **left** ankle and foot
M60.879   Other myositis, **unspecified** ankle and foot
M60.88   Other myositis, **other site**
M60.89   Other myositis, **multiple sites**
M60.9   Myositis, **unspecified**
M61- **Calcification and ossification of muscle** — The deposition of calcium, or the conversion into bony tissue, of the muscle.
M61.0- **Myositis ossificans traumatica** — The conversion of traumatized muscular tissue into bony tissue.
M61.00   Myositis ossificans traumatica, **unspecified site**
M61.01- Myositis ossificans traumatica, **shoulder**
M61.011   Myositis ossificans traumatica, **right** shoulder
M61.012   Myositis ossificans traumatica, **left** shoulder
M61.019   Myositis ossificans traumatica, **unspecified** shoulder
M61.02- Myositis ossificans traumatica, **upper arm**
M61.021   Myositis ossificans traumatica, **right** upper arm
M61.022   Myositis ossificans traumatica, **left** upper arm
M61.029   Myositis ossificans traumatica, **unspecified** upper arm
M61.03- Myositis ossificans traumatica, **forearm**
M61.031   Myositis ossificans traumatica, **right** forearm
M61.032   Myositis ossificans traumatica, **left** forearm
M61.039   Myositis ossificans traumatica, **unspecified** forearm
M61.04- Myositis ossificans traumatica, **hand**
M61.041   Myositis ossificans traumatica, **right** hand
M61.042   Myositis ossificans traumatica, **left** hand
M61.049   Myositis ossificans traumatica, **unspecified** hand
M61.05- Myositis ossificans traumatica, **thigh**
M61.051   Myositis ossificans traumatica, **right** thigh
M61.052   Myositis ossificans traumatica, **left** thigh
M61.059   Myositis ossificans traumatica, **unspecified** thigh
M61.06- Myositis ossificans traumatica, **lower leg**
M61.061   Myositis ossificans traumatica, **right** lower leg
M61.062   Myositis ossificans traumatica, **left** lower leg
M61.069   Myositis ossificans traumatica, **unspecified** lower leg
M61.07- Myositis ossificans traumatica, **ankle and foot**
M61.071   Myositis ossificans traumatica, **right** ankle and foot
M61.072   Myositis ossificans traumatica, **left** ankle and foot
M61.079   Myositis ossificans traumatica, **unspecified** ankle and foot
M61.08   Myositis ossificans traumatica, **other site**
M61.09   Myositis ossificans traumatica, **multiple sites**
M61.1- **Myositis ossificans progressiva** — A chronic, progressive conversion of muscle tissue to bony tissue that begins early in life.
Fibrodysplasia ossificans progressiva
M61.10   Myositis ossificans progressiva, **unspecified site**
M61.11- Myositis ossificans progressiva, **shoulder**
M61.111   Myositis ossificans progressiva, **right** shoulder
M61.112   Myositis ossificans progressiva, **left** shoulder

M61.119   Myositis ossificans progressiva, <u>unspecified</u> shoulder
M61.12- Myositis ossificans progressiva, <u>upper arm</u>
   M61.121   Myositis ossificans progressiva, <u>right</u> upper arm
   M61.122   Myositis ossificans progressiva, <u>left</u> upper arm
   M61.129   Myositis ossificans progressiva, <u>unspecified</u> arm
M61.13- Myositis ossificans progressiva, <u>forearm</u>
   M61.131   Myositis ossificans progressiva, <u>right</u> forearm
   M61.132   Myositis ossificans progressiva, <u>left</u> forearm
   M61.139   Myositis ossificans progressiva, <u>unspecified</u> forearm
M61.14- Myositis ossificans progressiva, <u>hand and finger(s)</u>
   M61.141   Myositis ossificans progressiva, <u>right</u> hand
   M61.142   Myositis ossificans progressiva, <u>left</u> hand
   M61.143   Myositis ossificans progressiva, <u>unspecified</u> hand
   M61.144   Myositis ossificans progressiva, <u>right</u> finger(s)
   M61.145   Myositis ossificans progressiva, <u>left</u> finger(s)
   M61.146   Myositis ossificans progressiva, <u>unspecified</u> finger(s)
M61.15- Myositis ossificans progressiva, <u>thigh</u>
   M61.151   Myositis ossificans progressiva, <u>right</u> thigh
   M61.152   Myositis ossificans progressiva, <u>left</u> thigh
   M61.159   Myositis ossificans progressiva, <u>unspecified</u> thigh
M61.16- Myositis ossificans progressiva, <u>lower leg</u>
   M61.161   Myositis ossificans progressiva, <u>right</u> lower leg
   M61.162   Myositis ossificans progressiva, <u>left</u> lower leg
   M61.169   Myositis ossificans progressiva, <u>unspecified</u> lower leg
M61.17- Myositis ossificans progressiva, <u>ankle, foot and toe(s)</u>
   M61.171   Myositis ossificans progressiva, <u>right</u> ankle
   M61.172   Myositis ossificans progressiva, <u>left</u> ankle
   M61.173   Myositis ossificans progressiva, <u>unspecified</u> ankle
   M61.174   Myositis ossificans progressiva, <u>right</u> foot
   M61.175   Myositis ossificans progressiva, <u>left</u> foot
   M61.176   Myositis ossificans progressiva, <u>unspecified</u> foot
   M61.177   Myositis ossificans progressiva, <u>right</u> toe(s)
   M61.178   Myositis ossificans progressiva, <u>left</u> toe(s)
   M61.179   Myositis ossificans progressiva, <u>unspecified</u> toe(s)
M61.18 Myositis ossificans progressiva, <u>other site</u>
M61.19 Myositis ossificans progressiva, <u>multiple sites</u>
M61.2- <u>Paralytic calcification and ossification of muscle</u>
   Myositis ossificans associated with quadriplegia or paraplegia
M61.20 Paralytic calcification and ossification of muscle, <u>unspecified site</u>
M61.21- Paralytic calcification and ossification of muscle, <u>shoulder</u>
   M61.211   Paralytic calcification and ossification of muscle, <u>right</u> shoulder
   M61.212   Paralytic calcification and ossification of muscle, <u>left</u> shoulder
   M61.219   Paralytic calcification and ossification of muscle, <u>unspecified</u> shoulder
M61.22- Paralytic calcification and ossification of muscle, <u>upper arm</u>
   M61.221   Paralytic calcification and ossification of muscle, <u>right</u> upper arm
   M61.222   Paralytic calcification and ossification of muscle, <u>left</u> upper arm
   M61.229   Paralytic calcification and ossification of muscle, <u>unspecified</u> upper arm
M61.23- Paralytic calcification and ossification of muscle, <u>forearm</u>
   M61.231   Paralytic calcification and ossification of muscle, <u>right</u> forearm
   M61.232   Paralytic calcification and ossification of muscle, <u>left</u> forearm
   M61.239   Paralytic calcification and ossification of muscle, <u>unspecified</u> forearm

M61.24- Paralytic calcification and ossification of muscle, <u>hand</u>
   M61.241   Paralytic calcification and ossification of muscle, <u>right</u> hand
   M61.242   Paralytic calcification and ossification of muscle, <u>left</u> hand
   M61.249   Paralytic calcification and ossification of muscle, <u>unspecified</u> hand
M61.25- Paralytic calcification and ossification of muscle, <u>thigh</u>
   M61.251   Paralytic calcification and ossification of muscle, <u>right</u> thigh
   M61.252   Paralytic calcification and ossification of muscle, <u>left</u> thigh
   M61.259   Paralytic calcification and ossification of muscle, <u>unspecified</u> thigh
M61.26- Paralytic calcification and ossification of muscle, <u>lower leg</u>
   M61.261   Paralytic calcification and ossification of muscle, <u>right</u> lower leg
   M61.262   Paralytic calcification and ossification of muscle, <u>left</u> lower leg
   M61.269   Paralytic calcification and ossification of muscle, <u>unspecified</u> lower leg
M61.27- Paralytic calcification and ossification of muscle, <u>ankle and foot</u>
   M61.271   Paralytic calcification and ossification of muscle, <u>right</u> ankle and foot
   M61.272   Paralytic calcification and ossification of muscle, <u>left</u> ankle and foot
   M61.279   Paralytic calcification and ossification of muscle, <u>unspecified</u> ankle and foot
M61.28 Paralytic calcification and ossification of muscle, <u>other site</u>
M61.29 Paralytic calcification and ossification of muscle, <u>multiple sites</u>
M61.3- Calcification and ossification of muscles associated <u>with burns</u>
   Myositis ossificans associated with burns
M61.30 Calcification and ossification of muscles associated with burns, <u>unspecified site</u>
M61.31- Calcification and ossification of muscles associated with burns, <u>shoulder</u>
   M61.311   Calcification and ossification of muscles associated with burns, <u>right</u> shoulder
   M61.312   Calcification and ossification of muscles associated with burns, <u>left</u> shoulder
   M61.319   Calcification and ossification of muscles associated with burns, <u>unspecified</u> shoulder
M61.32- Calcification and ossification of muscles associated with burns, <u>upper arm</u>
   M61.321   Calcification and ossification of muscles associated with burns, <u>right</u> upper arm
   M61.322   Calcification and ossification of muscles associated with burns, <u>left</u> upper arm
   M61.329   Calcification and ossification of muscles associated with burns, <u>unspecified</u> upper arm
M61.33- Calcification and ossification of muscles associated with burns, <u>forearm</u>
   M61.331   Calcification and ossification of muscles associated with burns, <u>right</u> forearm
   M61.332   Calcification and ossification of muscles associated with burns, <u>left</u> forearm
   M61.339   Calcification and ossification of muscles associated with burns, <u>unspecified</u> forearm
M61.34- Calcification and ossification of muscles associated with burns, <u>hand</u>
   M61.341   Calcification and ossification of muscles associated with burns, <u>right</u> hand
   M61.342   Calcification and ossification of muscles associated with burns, <u>left</u> hand

M61

M61-M61

M61.349 Calcification and ossification of muscles associated with burns, <u>unspecified</u> hand

M61.35- Calcification and ossification of muscles associated with burns, <u>thigh</u>

M61.351 Calcification and ossification of muscles associated with burns, <u>right</u> thigh

M61.352 Calcification and ossification of muscles associated with burns, <u>left</u> thigh

M61.359 Calcification and ossification of muscles associated with burns, <u>unspecified</u> thigh

M61.36- Calcification and ossification of muscles associated with burns, <u>lower leg</u>

M61.361 Calcification and ossification of muscles associated with burns, <u>right</u> lower leg

M61.362 Calcification and ossification of muscles associated with burns, <u>left</u> lower leg

M61.369 Calcification and ossification of muscles associated with burns, <u>unspecified</u> lower leg

M61.37- Calcification and ossification of muscles associated with burns, <u>ankle and foot</u>

M61.371 Calcification and ossification of muscles associated with burns, <u>right</u> ankle and foot

M61.372 Calcification and ossification of muscles associated with burns, <u>left</u> ankle and foot

M61.379 Calcification and ossification of muscles associated with burns, <u>unspecified</u> ankle and foot

M61.38 Calcification and ossification of muscles associated with burns, <u>other site</u>

M61.39 Calcification and ossification of muscles associated with burns, <u>multiple sites</u>

M61.4- <u>Other calcification</u> of muscle
Excludes 1:   *calcific tendinitis NOS (M65.2-)*
        calcific tendinitis of shoulder (M75.3)

M61.40 Other calcification of muscle, <u>unspecified site</u>

M61.41- Other calcification of muscle, <u>shoulder</u>

M61.411 Other calcification of muscle, <u>right</u> shoulder

M61.412 Other calcification of muscle, <u>left</u> shoulder

M61.419 Other calcification of muscle, <u>unspecified</u> shoulder

M61.42- Other calcification of muscle, <u>upper arm</u>

M61.421 Other calcification of muscle, <u>right</u> upper arm

M61.422 Other calcification of muscle, <u>left</u> upper arm

M61.429 Other calcification of muscle, <u>unspecified</u> upper arm

M61.43- Other calcification of muscle, <u>forearm</u>

M61.431 Other calcification of muscle, <u>right</u> forearm

M61.432 Other calcification of muscle, <u>left</u> forearm

M61.439 Other calcification of muscle, <u>unspecified</u> forearm

M61.44- Other calcification of muscle, <u>hand</u>

M61.441 Other calcification of muscle, <u>right</u> hand

M61.442 Other calcification of muscle, <u>left</u> hand

M61.449 Other calcification of muscle, <u>unspecified</u> hand

M61.45- Other calcification of muscle, <u>thigh</u>

M61.451 Other calcification of muscle, <u>right</u> thigh

M61.452 Other calcification of muscle, <u>left</u> thigh

M61.459 Other calcification of muscle, <u>unspecified</u> thigh

M61.46- Other calcification of muscle, <u>lower leg</u>

M61.461 Other calcification of muscle, <u>right</u> lower leg

M61.462 Other calcification of muscle, <u>left</u> lower leg

M61.469 Other calcification of muscle, <u>unspecified</u> lower leg

M61.47- Other calcification of muscle, ankle and foot

M61.471 Other calcification of muscle, <u>right</u> ankle and foot

M61.472 Other calcification of muscle, <u>left</u> ankle and foot

M61.479 Other calcification of muscle, <u>unspecified</u> ankle and foot

M61.48 Other calcification of muscle, other site

M61.49 Other calcification of muscle, <u>multiple sites</u>

M61.5- <u>Other ossification</u> of muscle

M61.50 Other ossification of muscle, <u>unspecified site</u>

M61.51- Other ossification of muscle, <u>shoulder</u>

M61.511 Other ossification of muscle, <u>right</u> shoulder

M61.512 Other ossification of muscle, <u>left</u> shoulder

M61.519 Other ossification of muscle, <u>unspecified</u> shoulder

M61.52- Other ossification of muscle, <u>upper arm</u>

M61.521 Other ossification of muscle, <u>right</u> upper arm

M61.522 Other ossification of muscle, <u>left</u> upper arm

M61.529 Other ossification of muscle, <u>unspecified</u> upper arm

M61.53- Other ossification of muscle, <u>forearm</u>

M61.531 Other ossification of muscle, <u>right</u> forearm

M61.532 Other ossification of muscle, <u>left</u> forearm

M61.539 Other ossification of muscle, <u>unspecified</u> forearm

M61.54- Other ossification of muscle, <u>hand</u>

M61.541 Other ossification of muscle, <u>right</u> hand

M61.542 Other ossification of muscle, <u>left</u> hand

M61.549 Other ossification of muscle, <u>unspecified</u> hand

M61.55- Other ossification of muscle, <u>thigh</u>

M61.551 Other ossification of muscle, <u>right</u> thigh

M61.552 Other ossification of muscle, <u>left</u> thigh

M61.559 Other ossification of muscle, <u>unspecified</u> thigh

M61.56- Other ossification of muscle, <u>lower leg</u>

M61.561 Other ossification of muscle, <u>right</u> lower leg

M61.562 Other ossification of muscle, <u>left</u> lower leg

M61.569 Other ossification of muscle, <u>unspecified</u> lower leg

M61.57- Other ossification of muscle, <u>ankle and foot</u>

M61.571 Other ossification of muscle, <u>right</u> ankle and foot

M61.572 Other ossification of muscle, <u>left</u> ankle and foot

M61.579 Other ossification of muscle, <u>unspecified</u> ankle and foot

M61.58 Other ossification of muscle, <u>other site</u>

M61.59 Other ossification of muscle, <u>multiple sites</u>

M61.9 Calcification and ossification of muscle, <u>unspecified</u>

M62- Other disorders of muscle
Excludes 1:   *alcoholic myopathy (G72.1)*
        cramp and spasm (R25.2)
        drug-induced myopathy (G72.0)
        myalgia (M79.1)
        stiff-man syndrome (G25.82)
Excludes ❷: *nontraumatic hematoma of muscle (M79.81)*

M62.0- <u>Separation of muscle (nontraumatic)</u> — The nontraumatic disruption of a muscle attachment or groups of muscles from each other.
    Diastasis of muscle
Excludes 1:   *diastasis recti complicating pregnancy, labor and delivery (O71.8)*
        traumatic separation of muscle — see strain of muscle by body region

M62.00 Separation of muscle (nontraumatic), <u>unspecified site</u>

M62.01- Separation of muscle (nontraumatic), <u>shoulder</u>

M62.011 Separation of muscle (nontraumatic), <u>right</u> shoulder

M62.012 Separation of muscle (nontraumatic), <u>left</u> shoulder

M62.019 Separation of muscle (nontraumatic), <u>unspecified</u> shoulder

M62.02- Separation of muscle (nontraumatic), <u>upper arm</u>

M62.021 Separation of muscle (nontraumatic), <u>right</u> upper arm

M62.022 Separation of muscle (nontraumatic), <u>left</u> upper arm

M62.029 Separation of muscle (nontraumatic), <u>unspecified</u> upper arm

M62.03- Separation of muscle (nontraumatic), <u>forearm</u>

M62.031 Separation of muscle (nontraumatic), <u>right</u> forearm

M62.032 Separation of muscle (nontraumatic), <u>left</u> forearm

M62.039 Separation of muscle (nontraumatic), <u>unspecified</u> forearm

M61 - M62

M62.04- Separation of muscle (nontraumatic), <u>hand</u>

    M62.041   Separation of muscle (nontraumatic), <u>right</u> hand

    M62.042   Separation of muscle (nontraumatic), <u>left</u> hand

    M62.049   Separation of muscle (nontraumatic), <u>unspecified</u> hand

M62.05- Separation of muscle (nontraumatic), <u>thigh</u>

    M62.051   Separation of muscle (nontraumatic), <u>right</u> thigh

    M62.052   Separation of muscle (nontraumatic), <u>left</u> thigh

    M62.059   Separation of muscle (nontraumatic), <u>unspecified</u> thigh

M62.06- Separation of muscle (nontraumatic), <u>lower leg</u>

    M62.061   Separation of muscle (nontraumatic), <u>right</u> lower leg

    M62.062   Separation of muscle (nontraumatic), <u>left</u> lower leg

    M62.069   Separation of muscle (nontraumatic), <u>unspecified</u> lower leg

M62.07- Separation of muscle (nontraumatic), <u>ankle and foot</u>

    M62.071   Separation of muscle (nontraumatic), <u>right</u> ankle and foot

    M62.072   Separation of muscle (nontraumatic), <u>left</u> ankle and foot

    M62.079   Separation of muscle (nontraumatic), <u>unspecified</u> ankle and foot

M62.08 Separation of muscle (nontraumatic), <u>other site</u>

M62.1- <u>Other rupture</u> of muscle (nontraumatic) — The nontraumatic disruption of a muscle tissue.

    Excludes 1:   *traumatic rupture of muscle — see strain of muscle by body region*

    Excludes ❷: *rupture of tendon (M66.-)*

M62.10 Other rupture of muscle (nontraumatic), <u>unspecified</u> <u>site</u>

M62.11- Other rupture of muscle (nontraumatic), <u>shoulder</u>

    M62.111   Other rupture of muscle (nontraumatic), <u>right</u> shoulder

    M62.112   Other rupture of muscle (nontraumatic), <u>left</u> shoulder

    M62.119   Other rupture of muscle (nontraumatic), <u>unspecified</u> shoulder

M62.12- Other rupture of muscle (nontraumatic), <u>upper arm</u>

    M62.121   Other rupture of muscle (nontraumatic), <u>right</u> upper arm

    M62.122   Other rupture of muscle (nontraumatic), <u>left</u> upper arm

    M62.129   Other rupture of muscle (nontraumatic), <u>unspecified</u> upper arm

M62.13- Other rupture of muscle (nontraumatic), <u>forearm</u>

    M62.131   Other rupture of muscle (nontraumatic), <u>right</u> forearm

    M62.132   Other rupture of muscle (nontraumatic), <u>left</u> forearm

    M62.139   Other rupture of muscle (nontraumatic), <u>unspecified</u> forearm

M62.14- Other rupture of muscle (nontraumatic), <u>hand</u>

    M62.141   Other rupture of muscle (nontraumatic), <u>right</u> hand

    M62.142   Other rupture of muscle (nontraumatic), <u>left</u> hand

    M62.149   Other rupture of muscle (nontraumatic), <u>unspecified</u> hand

M62.15- Other rupture of muscle (nontraumatic), <u>thigh</u>

    M62.151   Other rupture of muscle (nontraumatic), <u>right</u> thigh

    M62.152   Other rupture of muscle (nontraumatic), <u>left</u> thigh

    M62.159   Other rupture of muscle (nontraumatic), <u>unspecified</u> thigh

M62.16- Other rupture of muscle (nontraumatic), <u>lower leg</u>

    M62.161   Other rupture of muscle (nontraumatic), <u>right</u> lower leg

    M62.162   Other rupture of muscle (nontraumatic), <u>left</u> lower leg

    M62.169   Other rupture of muscle (nontraumatic), <u>unspecified</u> lower leg

M62.17- Other rupture of muscle (nontraumatic), <u>ankle and foot</u>

    M62.171   Other rupture of muscle (nontraumatic), <u>right</u> ankle and foot

    M62.172   Other rupture of muscle (nontraumatic), <u>left</u> ankle and foot

    M62.179   Other rupture of muscle (nontraumatic), <u>unspecified</u> ankle and foot

M62.18 Other rupture of muscle (nontraumatic), <u>other site</u>

M62.2- <u>Nontraumatic ischemic infarction</u> of muscle — The nontraumatic localized area of muscle necrosis due to obstruction of circulation to that muscle.

    Excludes 1:   *compartment syndrome (traumatic) (T79.A-)*

                    nontraumatic compartment syndrome (M79.A-)

                    traumatic ischemia of muscle (T79.6)

                    rhabdomyolysis (M62.82)

                    Volkmann's ischemic contracture (T79.6)

M62.20 Nontraumatic ischemic infarction of muscle, <u>unspecified site</u>

M62.21- Nontraumatic ischemic infarction of muscle, <u>shoulder</u>

    M62.211   Nontraumatic ischemic infarction of muscle, <u>right</u> shoulder

    M62.212   Nontraumatic ischemic infarction of muscle, <u>left</u> shoulder

    M62.219   Nontraumatic ischemic infarction of muscle, <u>unspecified</u> shoulder

M62.22- Nontraumatic ischemic infarction of muscle, <u>upper arm</u>

    M62.221   Nontraumatic ischemic infarction of muscle, <u>right</u> upper arm

    M62.222   Nontraumatic ischemic infarction of muscle, <u>left</u> upper arm

    M62.229   Nontraumatic ischemic infarction of muscle, <u>unspecified</u> upper arm

M62.23- Nontraumatic ischemic infarction of muscle, <u>forearm</u>

    M62.231   Nontraumatic ischemic infarction of muscle, <u>right</u> forearm

    M62.232   Nontraumatic ischemic infarction of muscle, <u>left</u> forearm

    M62.239   Nontraumatic ischemic infarction of muscle, <u>unspecified</u> forearm

M62.24- Nontraumatic ischemic infarction of muscle, <u>hand</u>

    M62.241   Nontraumatic ischemic infarction of muscle, <u>right</u> hand

    M62.242   Nontraumatic ischemic infarction of muscle, <u>left</u> hand

    M62.249   Nontraumatic ischemic infarction of muscle, <u>unspecified</u> hand

M62.25- Nontraumatic ischemic infarction of muscle, <u>thigh</u>

    M62.251   Nontraumatic ischemic infarction of muscle, <u>right</u> thigh

    M62.252   Nontraumatic ischemic infarction of muscle, <u>left</u> thigh

    M62.259   Nontraumatic ischemic infarction of muscle, <u>unspecified</u> thigh

M62.26- Nontraumatic ischemic infarction of muscle, <u>lower leg</u>

    M62.261   Nontraumatic ischemic infarction of muscle, <u>right</u> lower leg

    M62.262   Nontraumatic ischemic infarction of muscle, <u>left</u> lower leg

    M62.269   Nontraumatic ischemic infarction of muscle, <u>unspecified</u> lower leg

M62.27- Nontraumatic ischemic infarction of muscle, <u>ankle and foot</u>

    M62.271   Nontraumatic ischemic infarction of muscle, <u>right</u> ankle and foot

    M62.272   Nontraumatic ischemic infarction of muscle, <u>left</u> ankle and foot

    M62.279   Nontraumatic ischemic infarction of muscle, <u>unspecified</u> ankle and foot

M62.28 Nontraumatic ischemic infarction of muscle, <u>other site</u>

M62.3 **Immobility syndrome (paraplegic)** — The condition of muscular dysfunction caused by prolonged immobility and disuse of the muscles.

M62.4- <u>Contracture</u> of muscle — The abnormal tightening of a muscle.
  Contracture of tendon (sheath)
  Excludes 1:   contracture of joint (M24.5-)
M62.40 Contracture of muscle, <u>unspecified</u> <u>site</u>
M62.41- Contracture of muscle, <u>shoulder</u>
 M62.411 Contracture of muscle, <u>right</u> shoulder
 M62.412 Contracture of muscle, <u>left</u> shoulder
 M62.419 Contracture of muscle, <u>unspecified</u> shoulder
M62.42- Contracture of muscle, <u>upper arm</u>
 M62.421 Contracture of muscle, <u>right</u> upper arm
 M62.422 Contracture of muscle, <u>left</u> upper arm
 M62.429 Contracture of muscle, <u>unspecified</u> upper arm
M62.43- Contracture of muscle, <u>forearm</u>
 M62.431 Contracture of muscle, <u>right</u> forearm
 M62.432 Contracture of muscle, <u>left</u> forearm
 M62.439 Contracture of muscle, <u>unspecified</u> forearm
M62.44- Contracture of muscle, <u>hand</u>
 M62.441 Contracture of muscle, <u>right</u> hand
 M62.442 Contracture of muscle, <u>left</u> hand
 M62.449 Contracture of muscle, <u>unspecified</u> hand
M62.45- Contracture of muscle, <u>thigh</u>
 M62.451 Contracture of muscle, <u>right</u> thigh
 M62.452 Contracture of muscle, <u>left</u> thigh
 M62.459 Contracture of muscle, <u>unspecified</u> thigh
M62.46- Contracture of muscle, <u>lower leg</u>
 M62.461 Contracture of muscle, <u>right</u> lower leg
 M62.462 Contracture of muscle, <u>left</u> lower leg
 M62.469 Contracture of muscle, <u>unspecified</u> lower leg
M62.47- Contracture of muscle, <u>ankle and foot</u>
 M62.471 Contracture of muscle, <u>right</u> ankle and foot
 M62.472 Contracture of muscle, <u>left</u> ankle and foot
 M62.479 Contracture of muscle, <u>unspecified</u> ankle and foot
M62.48 Contracture of muscle, <u>other site</u>
M62.49 Contracture of muscle, <u>multiple sites</u>

M62.5- <u>Muscle wasting and atrophy, not elsewhere classified</u> — MUSCLE WASTING — The disintegration of the muscle cells. MUSCLE ATROPHY — The abnormal decrease in muscle mass.
  Disuse atrophy NEC
 Excludes 1:   neuralgic amyotrophy (G54.5)
     progressive muscular atrophy (G12.29)
     sarcopenia (M62.84)
 Excludes ❷: pelvic muscle wasting (N81.84)
M62.50 Muscle wasting and atrophy, not elsewhere classified, <u>unspecified site</u>
M62.51- Muscle wasting and atrophy, not elsewhere classified, <u>shoulder</u>
 M62.511 Muscle wasting and atrophy, not elsewhere classified, <u>right</u> shoulder
 M62.512 Muscle wasting and atrophy, not elsewhere classified, <u>left</u> shoulder
 M62.519 Muscle wasting and atrophy, not elsewhere classified, <u>unspecified</u> shoulder
M62.52- Muscle wasting and atrophy, not elsewhere classified, <u>upper arm</u>
 M62.521 Muscle wasting and atrophy, not elsewhere classified, <u>right</u> upper arm
 M62.522 Muscle wasting and atrophy, not elsewhere classified, <u>left</u> upper arm
 M62.529 Muscle wasting and atrophy, not elsewhere classified, <u>unspecified</u> upper arm
M62.53- Muscle wasting and atrophy, not elsewhere classified, <u>forearm</u>
 M62.531 Muscle wasting and atrophy, not elsewhere classified, <u>right</u> forearm

M62.532 Muscle wasting and atrophy, not elsewhere classified, <u>left</u> forearm
M62.539 Muscle wasting and atrophy, not elsewhere classified, <u>unspecified</u> forearm
M62.54- Muscle wasting and atrophy, not elsewhere classified, <u>hand</u>
 M62.541 Muscle wasting and atrophy, not elsewhere classified, <u>right</u> hand
 M62.542 Muscle wasting and atrophy, not elsewhere classified, <u>left</u> hand
 M62.549 Muscle wasting and atrophy, not elsewhere classified, <u>unspecified</u> hand
M62.55- Muscle wasting and atrophy, not elsewhere classified, <u>thigh</u>
 M62.551 Muscle wasting and atrophy, not elsewhere classified, <u>right</u> thigh
 M62.552 Muscle wasting and atrophy, not elsewhere classified, <u>left</u> thigh
 M62.559 Muscle wasting and atrophy, not elsewhere classified, <u>unspecified</u> thigh
M62.56- Muscle wasting and atrophy, not elsewhere classified, <u>lower leg</u>
 M62.561 Muscle wasting and atrophy, not elsewhere classified, <u>right</u> lower leg
 M62.562 Muscle wasting and atrophy, not elsewhere classified, <u>left</u> lower leg
 M62.569 Muscle wasting and atrophy, not elsewhere classified, <u>unspecified</u> lower leg
M62.57- Muscle wasting and atrophy, not elsewhere classified, <u>ankle and foot</u>
 M62.571 Muscle wasting and atrophy, not elsewhere classified, <u>right</u> ankle and foot
 M62.572 Muscle wasting and atrophy, not elsewhere classified, <u>left</u> ankle and foot
 M62.579 Muscle wasting and atrophy, not elsewhere classified, <u>unspecified</u> ankle and foot
M62.58 Muscle wasting and atrophy, not elsewhere classified, <u>other site</u>
M62.59 Muscle wasting and atrophy, not elsewhere classified, <u>multiple sites</u>

M62.8- Other specified disorders of muscle
 Excludes ❷: nontraumatic hematoma of muscle (M79.81)
M62.81 Muscle weakness (generalized) — A decrease in a patient's normal muscle strength.
 Excludes 1:   muscle weakness in sarcopenia (M62.84)
CC **M62.82** Rhabdomyolysis — A condition characterized by the destruction of skeletal muscle that releases potentially toxic muscle cell components into the circulation.
 Excludes 1:   traumatic rhabdomyolysis (T79.6)
M62.83- Muscle spasm — The sudden involuntary contraction of a muscle.
 M62.830 Muscle spasm of back
 M62.831 Muscle spasm of calf
  Charley-horse
 M62.838 Other muscle spasm
M62.84 Sarcopenia
 Age-related sarcopenia
 Code first underlying disease, if applicable, such as:
  Disorders of myoneural junction and muscle disease in diseases classified elsewhere (G73.-)
  Other and unspecified myopathies (G72.-)
  Primary disorders of muscles (G71.-)
M62.89 Other specified disorders of muscle
 Muscle (sheath) hernia
M62.9 Disorder of muscle, unspecified

M62 | M62

M63- **Disorders of muscle in diseases classified elsewhere**
Code first underlying disease, such as:
Leprosy (A30.-)
Neoplasm (C49.-, C79.89, D21.-, D48.1)
Schistosomiasis (B65.-)
Trichinellosis (B75)
Excludes 1: myopathy in cysticercosis (B69.81)
myopathy in endocrine diseases (G73.7)
myopathy in metabolic diseases (G73.7)
myopathy in sarcoidosis (D86.87)
myopathy in secondary syphilis (A51.49)
myopathy in syphilis (late) (A52.78)
myopathy in toxoplasmosis (B58.82)
myopathy in tuberculosis (A18.09)

M63.8- **Disorders of muscle in diseases classified elsewhere**

M63.80 **Disorders of muscle in diseases classified elsewhere, unspecified site** — [Not Allowed as PDX]

M63.81- **Disorders of muscle in diseases classified elsewhere, shoulder**

M63.811 **Disorders of muscle in diseases classified elsewhere, right shoulder** — [Not Allowed as PDX]

M63.812 **Disorders of muscle in diseases classified elsewhere, left shoulder** — [Not Allowed as PDX]

M63.819 **Disorders of muscle in diseases classified elsewhere, unspecified shoulder** — [Not Allowed as PDX]

M63.82- **Disorders of muscle in diseases classified elsewhere, upper arm**

M63.821 **Disorders of muscle in diseases classified elsewhere, right upper arm** — [Not Allowed as PDX]

M63.822 **Disorders of muscle in diseases classified elsewhere, left upper arm** — [Not Allowed as PDX]

M63.829 **Disorders of muscle in diseases classified elsewhere, unspecified upper arm** — [Not Allowed as PDX]

M63.83- **Disorders of muscle in diseases classified elsewhere, forearm**

M63.831 **Disorders of muscle in diseases classified elsewhere, right forearm** — [Not Allowed as PDX]

M63.832 **Disorders of muscle in diseases classified elsewhere, left forearm** — [Not Allowed as PDX]

M63.839 **Disorders of muscle in diseases classified elsewhere, unspecified forearm** — [Not Allowed as PDX]

M63.84- **Disorders of muscle in diseases classified elsewhere, hand**

M63.841 **Disorders of muscle in diseases classified elsewhere, right hand** — [Not Allowed as PDX]

M63.842 **Disorders of muscle in diseases classified elsewhere, left hand** — [Not Allowed as PDX]

M63.849 **Disorders of muscle in diseases classified elsewhere, unspecified hand** — [Not Allowed as PDX]

M63.85- **Disorders of muscle in diseases classified elsewhere, thigh**

M63.851 **Disorders of muscle in diseases classified elsewhere, right thigh** — [Not Allowed as PDX]

M63.852 **Disorders of muscle in diseases classified elsewhere, left thigh** — [Not Allowed as PDX]

M63.859 **Disorders of muscle in diseases classified elsewhere, unspecified thigh** — [Not Allowed as PDX]

M63.86- **Disorders of muscle in diseases classified elsewhere, lower leg**

M63.861 **Disorders of muscle in diseases classified elsewhere, right lower leg** — [Not Allowed as PDX]

M63.862 **Disorders of muscle in diseases classified elsewhere, left lower leg** — [Not Allowed as PDX]

M63.869 **Disorders of muscle in diseases classified elsewhere, unspecified lower leg** — [Not Allowed as PDX]

M63.87- **Disorders of muscle in diseases classified elsewhere, ankle and foot**

M63.871 **Disorders of muscle in diseases classified elsewhere, right ankle and foot** — [Not Allowed as PDX]

M63.872 **Disorders of muscle in diseases classified elsewhere, left ankle and foot** — [Not Allowed as PDX]

M63.879 **Disorders of muscle in diseases classified elsewhere, unspecified ankle and foot** — [Not Allowed as PDX]

M63.88 **Disorders of muscle in diseases classified elsewhere, other site** — [Not Allowed as PDX]

M63.89 **Disorders of muscle in diseases classified elsewhere, multiple sites** — [Not Allowed as PDX]

Disorders of synovium and tendon (M65-M67)

M65- **Synovitis and tenosynovitis** — Inflammation of the synovial membrane or tendon sheath.
Excludes 1: chronic crepitant synovitis of hand and wrist (M70.0-)
current injury — see injury of ligament or tendon by body region
soft tissue disorders related to use, overuse and pressure (M70.-)

M65.0- **Abscess of tendon sheath** — A localized collection of pus caused by the disintegration of a tendon sheath.
Use additional code (B95-B96) to identify bacterial agent.

M65.00 **Abscess of tendon sheath, unspecified site**

M65.01- **Abscess of tendon sheath, shoulder**

M65.011 Abscess of tendon sheath, right shoulder
M65.012 Abscess of tendon sheath, left shoulder
M65.019 Abscess of tendon sheath, unspecified shoulder

M65.02- **Abscess of tendon sheath, upper arm**

M65.021 Abscess of tendon sheath, right upper arm
M65.022 Abscess of tendon sheath, left upper arm
M65.029 Abscess of tendon sheath, unspecified upper arm

M65.03- **Abscess of tendon sheath, forearm**

M65.031 Abscess of tendon sheath, right forearm
M65.032 Abscess of tendon sheath, left forearm
M65.039 Abscess of tendon sheath, unspecified forearm

M65.04- **Abscess of tendon sheath, hand**

M65.041 Abscess of tendon sheath, right hand
M65.042 Abscess of tendon sheath, left hand
M65.049 Abscess of tendon sheath, unspecified hand

M65.05- **Abscess of tendon sheath, thigh**

M65.051 Abscess of tendon sheath, right thigh
M65.052 Abscess of tendon sheath, left thigh
M65.059 Abscess of tendon sheath, unspecified thigh

M65.06- **Abscess of tendon sheath, lower leg**

M65.061 Abscess of tendon sheath, right lower leg
M65.062 Abscess of tendon sheath, left lower leg
M65.069 Abscess of tendon sheath, unspecified lower leg

M65.07- **Abscess of tendon sheath, ankle and foot**

M65.071 Abscess of tendon sheath, right ankle and foot
M65.072 Abscess of tendon sheath, left ankle and foot
M65.079 Abscess of tendon sheath, unspecified ankle and foot

M65.08 **Abscess of tendon sheath, other site**

M65.1- **Other infective (teno)synovitis**

M65.10 **Other infective (teno)synovitis, unspecified site**

M65.11- **Other infective (teno)synovitis, shoulder**

M65.111 Other infective (teno)synovitis, right shoulder
M65.112 Other infective (teno)synovitis, left shoulder
M65.119 Other infective (teno)synovitis, unspecified shoulder

M65.12- **Other infective (teno)synovitis, elbow**

M65.121 Other infective (teno)synovitis, right elbow
M65.122 Other infective (teno)synovitis, left elbow
M65.129 Other infective (teno)synovitis, unspecified elbow

M65.13- **Other infective (teno)synovitis, wrist**

M65.131 Other infective (teno)synovitis, right wrist
M65.132 Other infective (teno)synovitis, left wrist

M63-M65

M65.139   Other infective (teno)synovitis, <u>unspecified</u> wrist
M65.14- Other infective (teno)synovitis, <u>hand</u>
   M65.141   Other infective (teno)synovitis, <u>right</u> hand
   M65.142   Other infective (teno)synovitis, <u>left</u> hand
   M65.149   Other infective (teno)synovitis, <u>unspecified</u> hand
M65.15- Other infective (teno)synovitis, <u>hip</u>
   M65.151   Other infective (teno)synovitis, <u>right</u> hip
   M65.152   Other infective (teno)synovitis, <u>left</u> hip
   M65.159   Other infective (teno)synovitis, <u>unspecified</u> hip
M65.16- Other infective (teno)synovitis, <u>knee</u>
   M65.161   Other infective (teno)synovitis, <u>right</u> knee
   M65.162   Other infective (teno)synovitis, <u>left</u> knee
   M65.169   Other infective (teno)synovitis, <u>unspecified</u> knee
M65.17- Other infective (teno)synovitis, <u>ankle and foot</u>
   M65.171   Other infective (teno)synovitis, <u>right</u> ankle and foot
   M65.172   Other infective (teno)synovitis, <u>left</u> ankle and foot
   M65.179   Other infective (teno)synovitis, <u>unspecified</u> ankle and foot
M65.18   Other infective (teno)synovitis, <u>other site</u>
M65.19   Other infective (teno)synovitis, <u>multiple sites</u>
M65.2-   <u>Calcific tendinitis</u> — The deposition of calcium and its salts in a tendon.
   Excludes 1:   *tendinitis as classified in M75-M77*
                calcified tendinitis of shoulder (M75.3)
M65.20   Calcific tendinitis, <u>unspecified site</u>
M65.22- Calcific tendinitis, <u>upper arm</u>
   M65.221   Calcific tendinitis, <u>right</u> upper arm
   M65.222   Calcific tendinitis, <u>left</u> upper arm
   M65.229   Calcific tendinitis, <u>unspecified</u> upper arm
M65.23- Calcific tendinitis, <u>forearm</u>
   M65.231   Calcific tendinitis, <u>right</u> forearm
   M65.232   Calcific tendinitis, <u>left</u> forearm
   M65.239   Calcific tendinitis, <u>unspecified</u> forearm
M65.24- Calcific tendinitis, <u>hand</u>
   M65.241   Calcific tendinitis, <u>right</u> hand
   M65.242   Calcific tendinitis, <u>left</u> hand
   M65.249   Calcific tendinitis, <u>unspecified</u> hand
M65.25- Calcific tendinitis, <u>thigh</u>
   M65.251   Calcific tendinitis, <u>right</u> thigh
   M65.252   Calcific tendinitis, <u>left</u> thigh
   M65.259   Calcific tendinitis, <u>unspecified</u> thigh
M65.26- Calcific tendinitis, <u>lower leg</u>
   M65.261   Calcific tendinitis, <u>right</u> lower leg
   M65.262   Calcific tendinitis, <u>left</u> lower leg
   M65.269   Calcific tendinitis, <u>unspecified</u> lower leg
M65.27- Calcific tendinitis, <u>ankle and foot</u>
   M65.271   Calcific tendinitis, <u>right</u> ankle and foot
   M65.272   Calcific tendinitis, <u>left</u> ankle and foot
   M65.279   Calcific tendinitis, <u>unspecified</u> ankle and foot
M65.28   Calcific tendinitis, <u>other site</u>
M65.29   Calcific tendinitis, <u>multiple sites</u>
M65.3-   <u>Trigger finger</u> — The temporary arrest of flexion or extension of a finger with subsequent snapping into place.
      Nodular tendinous disease
M65.30   Trigger finger, <u>unspecified</u> finger
M65.31- Trigger <u>thumb</u>
   M65.311   Trigger thumb, <u>right</u> thumb
   M65.312   Trigger thumb, <u>left</u> thumb
   M65.319   Trigger thumb, <u>unspecified</u> thumb
M65.32- Trigger finger, <u>index</u> finger
   M65.321   Trigger finger, <u>right</u> index finger
   M65.322   Trigger finger, <u>left</u> index finger
   M65.329   Trigger finger, <u>unspecified</u> index finger
M65.33- Trigger finger, <u>middle</u> finger
   M65.331   Trigger finger, <u>right</u> middle finger
   M65.332   Trigger finger, <u>left</u> middle finger

M65.339   Trigger finger, <u>unspecified</u> middle finger
M65.34- Trigger finger, <u>ring</u> finger
   M65.341   Trigger finger, <u>right</u> ring finger
   M65.342   Trigger finger, <u>left</u> ring finger
   M65.349   Trigger finger, <u>unspecified</u> ring finger
M65.35- Trigger finger, <u>little</u> finger
   M65.351   Trigger finger, <u>right</u> little finger
   M65.352   Trigger finger, <u>left</u> little finger
   M65.359   Trigger finger, <u>unspecified</u> little finger
M65.4   **Radial styloid tenosynovitis [de Quervain]** — Inflammation of the radial styloid tendon sheath.
M65.8-   <u>Other synovitis and tenosynovitis</u>
M65.80   Other synovitis and tenosynovitis, <u>unspecified</u> site
M65.81- Other synovitis and tenosynovitis, <u>shoulder</u>
   M65.811   Other synovitis and tenosynovitis, <u>right</u> shoulder
   M65.812   Other synovitis and tenosynovitis, <u>left</u> shoulder
   M65.819   Other synovitis and tenosynovitis, <u>unspecified</u> shoulder
M65.82- Other synovitis and tenosynovitis, <u>upper arm</u>
   M65.821   Other synovitis and tenosynovitis, <u>right</u> upper arm
   M65.822   Other synovitis and tenosynovitis, <u>left</u> upper arm
   M65.829   Other synovitis and tenosynovitis, <u>unspecified</u> upper arm
M65.83- Other synovitis and tenosynovitis, <u>forearm</u>
   M65.831   Other synovitis and tenosynovitis, <u>right</u> forearm
   M65.832   Other synovitis and tenosynovitis, <u>left</u> forearm
   M65.839   Other synovitis and tenosynovitis, <u>unspecified</u> forearm
M65.84- Other synovitis and tenosynovitis, <u>hand</u>
   M65.841   Other synovitis and tenosynovitis, <u>right</u> hand
   M65.842   Other synovitis and tenosynovitis, <u>left</u> hand
   M65.849   Other synovitis and tenosynovitis, <u>unspecified</u> hand
M65.85- Other synovitis and tenosynovitis, <u>thigh</u>
   M65.851   Other synovitis and tenosynovitis, <u>right</u> thigh
   M65.852   Other synovitis and tenosynovitis, <u>left</u> thigh
   M65.859   Other synovitis and tenosynovitis, <u>unspecified</u> thigh
M65.86- Other synovitis and tenosynovitis, <u>lower leg</u>
   M65.861   Other synovitis and tenosynovitis, <u>right</u> lower leg
   M65.862   Other synovitis and tenosynovitis, <u>left</u> lower leg
   M65.869   Other synovitis and tenosynovitis, <u>unspecified</u> lower leg
M65.87- Other synovitis and tenosynovitis, <u>ankle and foot</u>
   M65.871   Other synovitis and tenosynovitis, <u>right</u> ankle and foot
   M65.872   Other synovitis and tenosynovitis, <u>left</u> ankle and foot
   M65.879   Other synovitis and tenosynovitis, <u>unspecified</u> ankle and foot
M65.88   Other synovitis and tenosynovitis, <u>other site</u>
M65.89   Other synovitis and tenosynovitis, multiple sites
M65.9   Synovitis and tenosynovitis, <u>unspecified</u>
M66-   <u>Spontaneous rupture of synovium and tendon</u>
   Includes: Rupture that occurs when a normal force is applied to tissues that are inferred to have less than normal strength
   Excludes ❷: *rotator cuff syndrome (M75.1-)*
           rupture where an abnormal force is applied to normal tissue — see injury of tendon by body region
M66.0   **Rupture of popliteal cyst** — An accumulation of effused synovial fluid behind the knee that has ruptured.
M66.1-   **Rupture of <u>synovium</u>** — An accumulation of effused synovial fluid that has ruptured.
      Rupture of synovial cyst
   Excludes ❷: *rupture of popliteal cyst (M66.0)*
M66.10   Rupture of synovium, <u>unspecified</u> joint
M66.11- Rupture of synovium, <u>shoulder</u>
   M66.111   Rupture of synovium, <u>right</u> shoulder
   M66.112   Rupture of synovium, <u>left</u> shoulder

M 6 5 ▪ M 6 6

M66.119 Rupture of synovium, <u>unspecified</u> shoulder

M66.12- Rupture of synovium, <u>elbow</u>

M66.121 Rupture of synovium, <u>right</u> elbow

M66.122 Rupture of synovium, <u>left</u> elbow

M66.129 Rupture of synovium, <u>unspecified</u> elbow

M66.13- Rupture of synovium, <u>wrist</u>

M66.131 Rupture of synovium, <u>right</u> wrist

M66.132 Rupture of synovium, <u>left</u> wrist

M66.139 Rupture of synovium, <u>unspecified</u> wrist

M66.14- Rupture of synovium, <u>hand and fingers</u>

M66.141 Rupture of synovium, <u>right</u> hand

M66.142 Rupture of synovium, <u>left</u> hand

M66.143 Rupture of synovium, <u>unspecified</u> hand

M66.144 Rupture of synovium, <u>right</u> finger(s)

M66.145 Rupture of synovium, <u>left</u> finger(s)

M66.146 Rupture of synovium, <u>unspecified</u> finger(s)

M66.15- Rupture of synovium, <u>hip</u>

M66.151 Rupture of synovium, <u>right</u> hip

M66.152 Rupture of synovium, <u>left</u> hip

M66.159 Rupture of synovium, <u>unspecified</u> hip

M66.17- Rupture of synovium, <u>ankle, foot and toes</u>

M66.171 Rupture of synovium, <u>right</u> ankle

M66.172 Rupture of synovium, <u>left</u> ankle

M66.173 Rupture of synovium, <u>unspecified</u> ankle

M66.174 Rupture of synovium, <u>right</u> foot

M66.175 Rupture of synovium, <u>left</u> foot

M66.176 Rupture of synovium, <u>unspecified</u> foot

M66.177 Rupture of synovium, <u>right</u> toe(s)

M66.178 Rupture of synovium, <u>left</u> toe(s)

M66.179 Rupture of synovium, <u>unspecified</u> toe(s)

M66.18 Rupture of synovium, <u>other site</u>

M66.2- Spontaneous rupture of <u>extensor</u> tendons

M66.20 Spontaneous rupture of extensor tendons, <u>unspecified site</u>

M66.21- Spontaneous rupture of extensor tendons, <u>shoulder</u>

M66.211 Spontaneous rupture of extensor tendons, <u>right</u> shoulder

M66.212 Spontaneous rupture of extensor tendons, <u>left</u> shoulder

M66.219 Spontaneous rupture of extensor tendons, <u>unspecified</u> shoulder

M66.22- Spontaneous rupture of extensor tendons, <u>upper arm</u>

M66.221 Spontaneous rupture of extensor tendons, <u>right</u> upper arm

M66.222 Spontaneous rupture of extensor tendons, <u>left</u> upper arm

M66.229 Spontaneous rupture of extensor tendons, <u>unspecified</u> upper arm

M66.23- Spontaneous rupture of extensor tendons, <u>forearm</u>

M66.231 Spontaneous rupture of extensor tendons, <u>right</u> forearm

M66.232 Spontaneous rupture of extensor tendons, <u>left</u> forearm

M66.239 Spontaneous rupture of extensor tendons, <u>unspecified</u> forearm

M66.24- Spontaneous rupture of extensor tendons, <u>hand</u>

M66.241 Spontaneous rupture of extensor tendons, <u>right</u> hand

M66.242 Spontaneous rupture of extensor tendons, <u>left</u> hand

M66.249 Spontaneous rupture of extensor tendons, <u>unspecified</u> hand

M66.25- Spontaneous rupture of extensor tendons, <u>thigh</u>

M66.251 Spontaneous rupture of extensor tendons, <u>right</u> thigh

M66.252 Spontaneous rupture of extensor tendons, <u>left</u> thigh

M66.259 Spontaneous rupture of extensor tendons, <u>unspecified</u> thigh

M66.26- Spontaneous rupture of extensor tendons, <u>lower leg</u>

M66.261 Spontaneous rupture of extensor tendons, <u>right</u> lower leg

M66.262 Spontaneous rupture of extensor tendons, <u>left</u> lower leg

M66.269 Spontaneous rupture of extensor tendons, <u>unspecified</u> lower leg

M66.27- Spontaneous rupture of extensor tendons, <u>ankle and foot</u>

M66.271 Spontaneous rupture of extensor tendons, <u>right</u> ankle and foot

M66.272 Spontaneous rupture of extensor tendons, <u>left</u> ankle and foot

M66.279 Spontaneous rupture of extensor tendons, <u>unspecified</u> ankle and foot

M66.28 Spontaneous rupture of extensor tendons, <u>other site</u>

M66.29 Spontaneous rupture of extensor tendons, <u>multiple sites</u>

M66.3- Spontaneous rupture of <u>flexor</u> tendons

M66.30 Spontaneous rupture of flexor tendons, <u>unspecified</u> site

M66.31- Spontaneous rupture of flexor tendons, <u>shoulder</u>

M66.311 Spontaneous rupture of flexor tendons, <u>right</u> shoulder

M66.312 Spontaneous rupture of flexor tendons, <u>left</u> shoulder

M66.319 Spontaneous rupture of flexor tendons, <u>unspecified</u> shoulder

M66.32- Spontaneous rupture of flexor tendons, <u>upper arm</u>

M66.321 Spontaneous rupture of flexor tendons, <u>right</u> upper arm

M66.322 Spontaneous rupture of flexor tendons, <u>left</u> upper arm

M66.329 Spontaneous rupture of flexor tendons, <u>unspecified</u> upper arm

M66.33- Spontaneous rupture of flexor tendons, <u>forearm</u>

M66.331 Spontaneous rupture of flexor tendons, <u>right</u> forearm

M66.332 Spontaneous rupture of flexor tendons, <u>left</u> forearm

M66.339 Spontaneous rupture of flexor tendons, <u>unspecified</u> forearm

M66.34- Spontaneous rupture of flexor tendons, <u>hand</u>

M66.341 Spontaneous rupture of flexor tendons, <u>right</u> hand

M66.342 Spontaneous rupture of flexor tendons, <u>left</u> hand

M66.349 Spontaneous rupture of flexor tendons, <u>unspecified</u> hand

M66.35- Spontaneous rupture of flexor tendons, <u>thigh</u>

M66.351 Spontaneous rupture of flexor tendons, <u>right</u> thigh

M66.352 Spontaneous rupture of flexor tendons, <u>left</u> thigh

M66.359 Spontaneous rupture of flexor tendons, <u>unspecified</u> thigh

M66.36- Spontaneous rupture of flexor tendons, <u>lower leg</u>

M66.361 Spontaneous rupture of flexor tendons, <u>right</u> lower leg

M66.362 Spontaneous rupture of flexor tendons, <u>left</u> lower leg

M66.369 Spontaneous rupture of flexor tendons, <u>unspecified</u> lower leg

M66.37- Spontaneous rupture of flexor tendons, <u>ankle and foot</u>

M66.371 Spontaneous rupture of flexor tendons, <u>right</u> ankle and foot

M66.372 Spontaneous rupture of flexor tendons, <u>left</u> ankle and foot

M66.379 Spontaneous rupture of flexor tendons, <u>unspecified</u> ankle and foot

M66.38 Spontaneous rupture of flexor tendons, <u>other site</u>

M66.39 Spontaneous rupture of flexor tendons, <u>multiple sites</u>

M66.8- Spontaneous rupture of <u>other</u> tendons

M66.80 Spontaneous rupture of other tendons, <u>unspecified</u> site

M66.81- Spontaneous rupture of other tendons, <u>shoulder</u>

M
6
6
I
M
6
6

M66.811   Spontaneous rupture of other tendons, <u>right</u> shoulder

M66.812   Spontaneous rupture of other tendons, <u>left</u> shoulder

M66.819   Spontaneous rupture of other tendons, <u>unspecified</u> shoulder

M66.82- Spontaneous rupture of other tendons, <u>upper arm</u>

M66.821   Spontaneous rupture of other tendons, <u>right</u> upper arm

M66.822   Spontaneous rupture of other tendons, <u>left</u> upper arm

M66.829   Spontaneous rupture of other tendons, <u>unspecified</u> upper arm

M66.83- Spontaneous rupture of other tendons, <u>forearm</u>

M66.831   Spontaneous rupture of other tendons, <u>right</u> forearm

M66.832   Spontaneous rupture of other tendons, <u>left</u> forearm

M66.839   Spontaneous rupture of other tendons, <u>unspecified</u> forearm

M66.84- Spontaneous rupture of other tendons, <u>hand</u>

M66.841   Spontaneous rupture of other tendons, <u>right</u> hand

M66.842   Spontaneous rupture of other tendons, <u>left</u> hand

M66.849   Spontaneous rupture of other tendons, <u>unspecified</u> hand

M66.85- Spontaneous rupture of other tendons, <u>thigh</u>

M66.851   Spontaneous rupture of other tendons, <u>right</u> thigh

M66.852   Spontaneous rupture of other tendons, <u>left</u> thigh

M66.859   Spontaneous rupture of other tendons, <u>unspecified</u> thigh

M66.86- Spontaneous rupture of other tendons, <u>lower leg</u>

M66.861   Spontaneous rupture of other tendons, <u>right</u> lower leg

M66.862   Spontaneous rupture of other tendons, <u>left</u> lower leg

M66.869   Spontaneous rupture of other tendons, <u>unspecified</u> lower leg

M66.87- Spontaneous rupture of other tendons, <u>ankle and foot</u>

M66.871   Spontaneous rupture of other tendons, <u>right</u> ankle and foot

M66.872   Spontaneous rupture of other tendons, <u>left</u> ankle and foot

M66.879   Spontaneous rupture of other tendons, <u>unspecified</u> ankle and foot

M66.88   Spontaneous rupture of other tendons, <u>other</u>

M66.89   Spontaneous rupture of other tendons, <u>multiple sites</u>

M66.9   Spontaneous rupture of <u>unspecified</u> tendon
Rupture at musculotendinous junction, nontraumatic

M67-   <u>Other disorders</u> of synovium and tendon
Excludes 1:   palmar fascial fibromatosis [Dupuytren] (M72.0)
tendinitis NOS (M77.9-)
xanthomatosis localized to tendons (E78.2)

M67.0-   <u>Short Achilles tendon (acquired)</u> — The abnormally reduced length of the Achilles tendon.

M67.00   Short Achilles tendon (acquired), <u>unspecified</u> ankle

M67.01   Short Achilles tendon (acquired), <u>right</u> ankle

M67.02   Short Achilles tendon (acquired), <u>left</u> ankle

M67.2-   <u>Synovial hypertrophy</u>, <u>not elsewhere classified</u>
Excludes 1:   villonodular synovitis (pigmented) (M12.2-)

M67.20   Synovial hypertrophy, not elsewhere classified, <u>unspecified</u> site

M67.21- Synovial hypertrophy, not elsewhere classified, <u>shoulder</u>

M67.211   Synovial hypertrophy, not elsewhere classified, <u>right</u> shoulder

M67.212   Synovial hypertrophy, not elsewhere classified, <u>left</u> shoulder

M67.219   Synovial hypertrophy, not elsewhere classified, <u>unspecified</u> shoulder

M67.22- Synovial hypertrophy, not elsewhere classified, <u>upper arm</u>

M67.221   Synovial hypertrophy, not elsewhere classified, <u>right</u> upper arm

M67.222   Synovial hypertrophy, not elsewhere classified, <u>left</u> upper arm

M67.229   Synovial hypertrophy, not elsewhere classified, <u>unspecified</u> upper arm

M67.23- Synovial hypertrophy, not elsewhere classified, <u>forearm</u>

M67.231   Synovial hypertrophy, not elsewhere classified, <u>right</u> forearm

M67.232   Synovial hypertrophy, not elsewhere classified, <u>left</u> forearm

M67.239   Synovial hypertrophy, not elsewhere classified, <u>unspecified</u> forearm

M67.24- Synovial hypertrophy, not elsewhere classified, <u>hand</u>

M67.241   Synovial hypertrophy, not elsewhere classified, <u>right</u> hand

M67.242   Synovial hypertrophy, not elsewhere classified, <u>left</u> hand

M67.249   Synovial hypertrophy, not elsewhere classified, <u>unspecified</u> hand

M67.25- Synovial hypertrophy, not elsewhere classified, <u>thigh</u>

M67.251   Synovial hypertrophy, not elsewhere classified, <u>right</u> thigh

M67.252   Synovial hypertrophy, not elsewhere classified, <u>left</u> thigh

M67.259   Synovial hypertrophy, not elsewhere classified, <u>unspecified</u> thigh

M67.26- Synovial hypertrophy, not elsewhere classified, <u>lower leg</u>

M67.261   Synovial hypertrophy, not elsewhere classified, <u>right</u> lower leg

M67.262   Synovial hypertrophy, not elsewhere classified, <u>left</u> lower leg

M67.269   Synovial hypertrophy, not elsewhere classified, <u>unspecified</u> lower leg

M67.27- Synovial hypertrophy, not elsewhere classified, <u>ankle and foot</u>

M67.271   Synovial hypertrophy, not elsewhere classified, <u>right</u> ankle and foot

M67.272   Synovial hypertrophy, not elsewhere classified, <u>left</u> ankle and foot

M67.279   Synovial hypertrophy, not elsewhere classified, <u>unspecified</u> ankle and foot

M67.28   Synovial hypertrophy, not elsewhere classified, <u>other site</u>

M67.29   Synovial hypertrophy, not elsewhere classified, <u>multiple sites</u>

M67.3-   <u>Transient</u> synovitis — Inflammation of the synovial membrane that only lasts a few days or weeks, has no known cause (traumatic or medical), and most often affects children.
Toxic synovitis
Excludes 1:   palindromic rheumatism (M12.3-)

M67.30   Transient synovitis, <u>unspecified</u> <u>site</u>

M67.31- Transient synovitis, <u>shoulder</u>

M67.311   Transient synovitis, <u>right</u> shoulder

M67.312   Transient synovitis, <u>left</u> shoulder

M67.319   Transient synovitis, <u>unspecified</u> shoulder

M67.32- Transient synovitis, <u>elbow</u>

M67.321   Transient synovitis, <u>right</u> elbow

M67.322   Transient synovitis, <u>left</u> elbow

M67.329   Transient synovitis, <u>unspecified</u> elbow

M67.33- Transient synovitis, <u>wrist</u>

M67.331   Transient synovitis, <u>right</u> wrist

M67.332   Transient synovitis, <u>left</u> wrist

M67.339   Transient synovitis, <u>unspecified</u> wrist

M67.34- Transient synovitis, <u>hand</u>

M67.341   Transient synovitis, <u>right</u> hand

M67.342   Transient synovitis, <u>left</u> hand

M67.349   Transient synovitis, <u>unspecified</u> hand

M 6 6 - M 6 7

M67.35- Transient synovitis, <u>hip</u>
    M67.351 Transient synovitis, <u>right</u> hip
    M67.352 Transient synovitis, <u>left</u> hip
    M67.359 Transient synovitis, <u>unspecified</u> hip
M67.36- Transient synovitis, <u>knee</u>
    M67.361 Transient synovitis, <u>right</u> knee
    M67.362 Transient synovitis, <u>left</u> knee
    M67.369 Transient synovitis, <u>unspecified</u> knee
M67.37- Transient synovitis, <u>ankle and foot</u>
    M67.371 Transient synovitis, <u>right</u> ankle and foot
    M67.372 Transient synovitis, <u>left</u> ankle and foot
    M67.379 Transient synovitis, <u>unspecified</u> ankle and foot
M67.38 Transient synovitis, <u>other site</u>
M67.39 Transient synovitis, <u>multiple sites</u>

M67.4- <u>Ganglion</u> — A cystic tumor of joint tissue or a tendon sheath.
    Ganglion of joint or tendon (sheath)
    Excludes 1:   *ganglion in yaws (A66.6)*
    Excludes ❷: *cyst of bursa (M71.2-M71.3)*
              cyst of synovium (M71.2-M71.3)
M67.40 Ganglion, <u>unspecified site</u>
M67.41- Ganglion, <u>shoulder</u>
    M67.411 Ganglion, <u>right</u> shoulder
    M67.412 Ganglion, <u>left</u> shoulder
    M67.419 Ganglion, <u>unspecified</u> shoulder
M67.42- Ganglion, <u>elbow</u>
    M67.421 Ganglion, <u>right</u> elbow
    M67.422 Ganglion, <u>left</u> elbow
    M67.429 Ganglion, <u>unspecified</u> elbow
M67.43- Ganglion, <u>wrist</u>
    M67.431 Ganglion, <u>right</u> wrist
    M67.432 Ganglion, <u>left</u> wrist
    M67.439 Ganglion, <u>unspecified</u> wrist
M67.44- Ganglion, <u>hand</u>
    M67.441 Ganglion, <u>right</u> hand
    M67.442 Ganglion, <u>left</u> hand
    M67.449 Ganglion, <u>unspecified</u> hand
M67.45- Ganglion, <u>hip</u>
    M67.451 Ganglion, <u>right</u> hip
    M67.452 Ganglion, <u>left</u> hip
    M67.459 Ganglion, <u>unspecified</u> hip
M67.46- Ganglion, <u>knee</u>
    M67.461 Ganglion, <u>right</u> knee
    M67.462 Ganglion, <u>left</u> knee
    M67.469 Ganglion, <u>unspecified</u> knee
M67.47- Ganglion, <u>ankle and foot</u>
    M67.471 Ganglion, <u>right</u> ankle and foot
    M67.472 Ganglion, <u>left</u> ankle and foot
    M67.479 Ganglion, <u>unspecified</u> ankle and foot
M67.48 Ganglion, <u>other site</u>
M67.49 Ganglion, <u>multiple sites</u>

M67.5- <u>Plica syndrome</u> — An inflammatory disorder of the remnants of synovial tissue characterized by swelling, a clicking sensation, and weakness.
    Plica knee
M67.50 Plica syndrome, <u>unspecified</u> knee
M67.51 Plica syndrome, <u>right</u> knee
M67.52 Plica syndrome, <u>left</u> knee

M67.8- <u>Other specified</u> disorders of synovium and tendon
M67.80 Other specified disorders of synovium and tendon, <u>unspecified site</u>
M67.81- Other specified disorders of synovium and tendon, <u>shoulder</u>
    M67.811 Other specified disorders of synovium, <u>right</u> shoulder
    M67.812 Other specified disorders of synovium, <u>left</u> shoulder

    M67.813 Other specified disorders of tendon, <u>right</u> shoulder
    M67.814 Other specified disorders of tendon, <u>left</u> shoulder
    M67.819 Other specified disorders of synovium and tendon, <u>unspecified</u> shoulder
M67.82- Other specified disorders of synovium and tendon, <u>elbow</u>
    M67.821 Other specified disorders of synovium, <u>right</u> elbow
    M67.822 Other specified disorders of synovium, <u>left</u> elbow
    M67.823 Other specified disorders of tendon, <u>right</u> elbow
    M67.824 Other specified disorders of tendon, <u>left</u> elbow
    M67.829 Other specified disorders of synovium and tendon, <u>unspecified</u> elbow
M67.83- Other specified disorders of synovium and tendon, <u>wrist</u>
    M67.831 Other specified disorders of synovium, <u>right</u> wrist
    M67.832 Other specified disorders of synovium, <u>left</u> wrist
    M67.833 Other specified disorders of tendon, <u>right</u> wrist
    M67.834 Other specified disorders of tendon, <u>left</u> wrist
    M67.839 Other specified disorders of synovium and tendon, <u>unspecified</u> forearm
M67.84- Other specified disorders of synovium and tendon, <u>hand</u>
    M67.841 Other specified disorders of synovium, <u>right</u> hand
    M67.842 Other specified disorders of synovium, <u>left</u> hand
    M67.843 Other specified disorders of tendon, <u>right</u> hand
    M67.844 Other specified disorders of tendon, <u>left</u> hand
    M67.849 Other specified disorders of synovium and tendon, <u>unspecified</u> hand
M67.85- Other specified disorders of synovium and tendon, <u>hip</u>
    M67.851 Other specified disorders of synovium, <u>right</u> hip
    M67.852 Other specified disorders of synovium, <u>left</u> hip
    M67.853 Other specified disorders of tendon, <u>right</u> hip
    M67.854 Other specified disorders of tendon, <u>left</u> hip
    M67.859 Other specified disorders of synovium and tendon, <u>unspecified</u> hip
M67.86- Other specified disorders of synovium and tendon, <u>knee</u>
    M67.861 Other specified disorders of synovium, <u>right</u> knee
    M67.862 Other specified disorders of synovium, <u>left</u> knee
    M67.863 Other specified disorders of tendon, <u>right</u> knee
    M67.864 Other specified disorders of tendon, <u>left</u> knee
    M67.869 Other specified disorders of synovium and tendon, <u>unspecified</u> knee
M67.87- Other specified disorders of synovium and tendon, <u>ankle and foot</u>
    M67.871 Other specified disorders of synovium, <u>right</u> ankle and foot
    M67.872 Other specified disorders of synovium, <u>left</u> ankle and foot
    M67.873 Other specified disorders of tendon, <u>right</u> ankle and foot
    M67.874 Other specified disorders of tendon, <u>left</u> ankle and foot
    M67.879 Other specified disorders of synovium and tendon, <u>unspecified</u> ankle and foot
M67.88 Other specified disorders of synovium and tendon, <u>other site</u>
M67.89 Other specified disorders of synovium and tendon, <u>multiple sites</u>
M67.9- <u>Unspecified disorder</u> of synovium and tendon
M67.90 Unspecified disorder of synovium and tendon, <u>unspecified site</u>
M67.91- Unspecified disorder of synovium and tendon, <u>shoulder</u>
    M67.911 Unspecified disorder of synovium and tendon, <u>right</u> shoulder
    M67.912 Unspecified disorder of synovium and tendon, <u>left</u> shoulder
    M67.919 Unspecified disorder of synovium and tendon, <u>unspecified</u> shoulder

M 6 7 - M 6 7

Excludes 1: = NOT CODED HERE! (Do not code both)   *Excludes ❷:* = Not Included Here

M67.92- Unspecified disorder of synovium and tendon, <u>upper arm</u>
    M67.921   Unspecified disorder of synovium and tendon, <u>right</u> upper arm
    M67.922   Unspecified disorder of synovium and tendon, <u>left</u> upper arm
    M67.929   Unspecified disorder of synovium and tendon, <u>unspecified</u> upper arm
M67.93- Unspecified disorder of synovium and tendon, <u>forearm</u>
    M67.931   Unspecified disorder of synovium and tendon, <u>right</u> forearm
    M67.932   Unspecified disorder of synovium and tendon, <u>left</u> forearm
    M67.939   Unspecified disorder of synovium and tendon, <u>unspecified</u> forearm
M67.94- Unspecified disorder of synovium and tendon, <u>hand</u>
    M67.941   Unspecified disorder of synovium and tendon, <u>right</u> hand
    M67.942   Unspecified disorder of synovium and tendon, <u>left</u> hand
    M67.949   Unspecified disorder of synovium and tendon, <u>unspecified</u> hand
M67.95- Unspecified disorder of synovium and tendon, <u>thigh</u>
    M67.951   Unspecified disorder of synovium and tendon, <u>right</u> thigh
    M67.952   Unspecified disorder of synovium and tendon, <u>left</u> thigh
    M67.959   Unspecified disorder of synovium and tendon, <u>unspecified</u> thigh
M67.96- Unspecified disorder of synovium and tendon, <u>lower leg</u>
    M67.961   Unspecified disorder of synovium and tendon, <u>right</u> lower leg
    M67.962   Unspecified disorder of synovium and tendon, <u>left</u> lower leg
    M67.969   Unspecified disorder of synovium and tendon, <u>unspecified</u> lower leg
M67.97- Unspecified disorder of synovium and tendon, <u>ankle and foot</u>
    M67.971   Unspecified disorder of synovium and tendon, <u>right</u> ankle and foot
    M67.972   Unspecified disorder of synovium and tendon, <u>left</u> ankle and foot
    M67.979   Unspecified disorder of synovium and tendon, <u>unspecified</u> ankle and foot
M67.98   Unspecified disorder of synovium and tendon, <u>other site</u>
M67.99   Unspecified disorder of synovium and tendon, <u>multiple sites</u>

Other soft tissue disorders (M70-M79)

M70-   <u>Soft tissue disorders related to use, overuse and pressure</u> —
Inflammation and/or irritation of the soft tissues (synovial membranes, bursae, muscles, tendons) due to use (usual or unusual), overuse, and/or pressure.
Includes: Soft tissue disorders of occupational origin
Use additional external cause code to identify activity causing disorder (Y93.-)
Excludes 1:   *bursitis NOS (M71.9-)*
Excludes ❷: *bursitis of shoulder (M75.5)*
                enthesopathies (M76-M77)
                pressure ulcer (pressure area) (L89.-)

M70.0-   <u>Crepitant synovitis</u> (acute) (chronic) of hand and wrist
    M70.03- Crepitant synovitis (acute) (chronic), <u>wrist</u>
       M70.031   Crepitant synovitis (acute) (chronic), <u>right</u> wrist
       M70.032   Crepitant synovitis (acute) (chronic), <u>left</u> wrist
       M70.039   Crepitant synovitis (acute) (chronic), <u>unspecified</u> wrist
    M70.04- Crepitant synovitis (acute) (chronic), <u>hand</u>
       M70.041   Crepitant synovitis (acute) (chronic), <u>right</u> hand
       M70.042   Crepitant synovitis (acute) (chronic), <u>left</u> hand
       M70.049   Crepitant synovitis (acute) (chronic), <u>unspecified</u> hand

M70.1-   <u>Bursitis</u> of hand
    M70.10   Bursitis, <u>unspecified</u> hand
    M70.11   Bursitis, <u>right</u> hand
    M70.12   Bursitis, <u>left</u> hand
M70.2-   <u>Olecranon</u> bursitis
    M70.20   Olecranon bursitis, <u>unspecified</u> elbow
    M70.21   Olecranon bursitis, <u>right</u> elbow
    M70.22   Olecranon bursitis, <u>left</u> elbow
M70.3-   <u>Other</u> bursitis of <u>elbow</u>
    M70.30   Other bursitis of elbow, <u>unspecified</u> elbow
    M70.31   Other bursitis of elbow, <u>right</u> elbow
    M70.32   Other bursitis of elbow, <u>left</u> elbow
M70.4-   <u>Prepatellar</u> bursitis
    M70.40   Prepatellar bursitis, <u>unspecified</u> knee
    M70.41   Prepatellar bursitis, <u>right</u> knee
    M70.42   Prepatellar bursitis, <u>left</u> knee
M70.5-   <u>Other</u> bursitis of <u>knee</u>
    M70.50   Other bursitis of knee, <u>unspecified</u> knee
    M70.51   Other bursitis of knee, <u>right</u> knee
    M70.52   Other bursitis of knee, <u>left</u> knee
M70.6-   <u>Trochanteric</u> bursitis
       Trochanteric tendinitis
    M70.60   Trochanteric bursitis, <u>unspecified</u> hip
    M70.61   Trochanteric bursitis, <u>right</u> hip
    M70.62   Trochanteric bursitis, <u>left</u> hip
M70.7-   Other bursitis of <u>hip</u>
       Ischial bursitis
    M70.70   Other bursitis of hip, <u>unspecified</u> hip
    M70.71   Other bursitis of hip, <u>right</u> hip
    M70.72   Other bursitis of hip, <u>left</u> hip
M70.8-   <u>Other soft tissue disorders</u> related to use, overuse and pressure
    M70.80   Other soft tissue disorders related to use, overuse and pressure of <u>unspecified</u> site
    M70.81- Other soft tissue disorders related to use, overuse and pressure of <u>shoulder</u>
       M70.811   Other soft tissue disorders related to use, overuse and pressure, <u>right</u> shoulder
       M70.812   Other soft tissue disorders related to use, overuse and pressure, <u>left</u> shoulder
       M70.819   Other soft tissue disorders related to use, overuse and pressure, <u>unspecified</u> shoulder
    M70.82- Other soft tissue disorders related to use, overuse and pressure of <u>upper arm</u>
       M70.821   Other soft tissue disorders related to use, overuse and pressure, <u>right</u> upper arm
       M70.822   Other soft tissue disorders related to use, overuse and pressure, <u>left</u> upper arm
       M70.829   Other soft tissue disorders related to use, overuse and pressure, <u>unspecified</u> upper arms
    M70.83- Other soft tissue disorders related to use, overuse and pressure of <u>forearm</u>
       M70.831   Other soft tissue disorders related to use, overuse and pressure, <u>right</u> forearm
       M70.832   Other soft tissue disorders related to use, overuse and pressure, <u>left</u> forearm
       M70.839   Other soft tissue disorders related to use, overuse and pressure, <u>unspecified</u> forearm
    M70.84- Other soft tissue disorders related to use, overuse and pressure of <u>hand</u>
       M70.841   Other soft tissue disorders related to use, overuse and pressure, <u>right</u> hand
       M70.842   Other soft tissue disorders related to use, overuse and pressure, <u>left</u> hand
       M70.849   Other soft tissue disorders related to use, overuse and pressure, <u>unspecified</u> hand

M70.85- Other soft tissue disorders related to use, overuse and pressure of <u>thigh</u>

    M70.851 Other soft tissue disorders related to use, overuse and pressure, <u>right</u> thigh

    M70.852 Other soft tissue disorders related to use, overuse and pressure, <u>left</u> thigh

    M70.859 Other soft tissue disorders related to use, overuse and pressure, <u>unspecified</u> thigh

M70.86 Other soft tissue disorders related to use, overuse and pressure <u>lower leg</u>

    M70.861 Other soft tissue disorders related to use, overuse and pressure, <u>right</u> lower leg

    M70.862 Other soft tissue disorders related to use, overuse and pressure, <u>left</u> lower leg

    M70.869 Other soft tissue disorders related to use, overuse and pressure, <u>unspecified</u> leg

M70.87- Other soft tissue disorders related to use, overuse and pressure of <u>ankle and foot</u>

    M70.871 Other soft tissue disorders related to use, overuse and pressure, <u>right</u> ankle and foot

    M70.872 Other soft tissue disorders related to use, overuse and pressure, <u>left</u> ankle and foot

    M70.879 Other soft tissue disorders related to use, overuse and pressure, <u>unspecified</u> ankle and foot

M70.88 Other soft tissue disorders related to use, overuse and pressure <u>other site</u>

M70.89 Other soft tissue disorders related to use, overuse and pressure <u>multiple sites</u>

M70.9- <u>Unspecified</u> soft tissue disorder related to use, overuse and pressure

    M70.90 Unspecified soft tissue disorder related to use, overuse and pressure of <u>unspecified</u> <u>site</u>

    M70.91- Unspecified soft tissue disorder related to use, overuse and pressure of <u>shoulder</u>

        M70.911 Unspecified soft tissue disorder related to use, overuse and pressure, <u>right</u> shoulder

        M70.912 Unspecified soft tissue disorder related to use, overuse and pressure, <u>left</u> shoulder

        M70.919 Unspecified soft tissue disorder related to use, overuse and pressure, <u>unspecified</u> shoulder

    M70.92- Unspecified soft tissue disorder related to use, overuse and pressure of <u>upper arm</u>

        M70.921 Unspecified soft tissue disorder related to use, overuse and pressure, <u>right</u> upperarm

        M70.922 Unspecified soft tissue disorder related to use, overuse and pressure, <u>left</u> upperarm

        M70.929 Unspecified soft tissue disorder related to use, overuse and pressure, <u>unspecified</u> upper arm

    M70.93- Unspecified soft tissue disorder related to use, overuse and pressure of <u>forearm</u>

        M70.931 Unspecified soft tissue disorder related to use, overuse and pressure, <u>right</u> forearm

        M70.932 Unspecified soft tissue disorder related to use, overuse and pressure, <u>left</u> forearm

        M70.939 Unspecified soft tissue disorder related to use, overuse and pressure, <u>unspecified</u> forearm

    M70.94- Unspecified soft tissue disorder related to use, overuse and pressure of <u>hand</u>

        M70.941 Unspecified soft tissue disorder related to use, overuse and pressure, <u>right</u> hand

        M70.942 Unspecified soft tissue disorder related to use, overuse and pressure, <u>left</u> hand

        M70.949 Unspecified soft tissue disorder related to use, overuse and pressure, <u>unspecified</u> hand

    M70.95- Unspecified soft tissue disorder related to use, overuse and pressure of <u>thigh</u>

        M70.951 Unspecified soft tissue disorder related to use, overuse and pressure, <u>right</u> thigh

        M70.952 Unspecified soft tissue disorder related to use, overuse and pressure, <u>left</u> thigh

        M70.959 Unspecified soft tissue disorder related to use, overuse and pressure, <u>unspecified</u> thigh

    M70.96- Unspecified soft tissue disorder related to use, overuse and pressure <u>lower leg</u>

        M70.961 Unspecified soft tissue disorder related to use, overuse and pressure, <u>right</u> lower leg

        M70.962 Unspecified soft tissue disorder related to use, overuse and pressure, <u>left</u> lower leg

        M70.969 Unspecified soft tissue disorder related to use, overuse and pressure, <u>unspecified</u> lower leg

    M70.97- Unspecified soft tissue disorder related to use, overuse and pressure of <u>ankle and foot</u>

        M70.971 Unspecified soft tissue disorder related to use, overuse and pressure, <u>right</u> ankle and foot

        M70.972 Unspecified soft tissue disorder related to use, overuse and pressure, <u>left</u> ankle and foot

        M70.979 Unspecified soft tissue disorder related to use, overuse and pressure, <u>unspecified</u> ankle and foot

    M70.98 Unspecified soft tissue disorder related to use, overuse and pressure <u>other</u>

    M70.99 Unspecified soft tissue disorder related to use, overuse and pressure <u>multiple sites</u>

M71- Other bursopathies

    Excludes 1:   bunion (M20.1)

                    bursitis related to use, overuse or pressure (M70.-)

                    enthesopathies (M76-M77)

    M71.0- <u>Abscess of bursa</u> — A localized collection of pus caused by the disintegration of bursal tissue.

    Use additional code (B95.-, B96.-) to identify causative organism

    M71.00 Abscess of bursa, <u>unspecified</u> site

    M71.01- Abscess of bursa, <u>shoulder</u>

        M71.011 Abscess of bursa, <u>right</u> shoulder

        M71.012 Abscess of bursa, <u>left</u> shoulder

        M71.019 Abscess of bursa, <u>unspecified</u> shoulder

    M71.02- Abscess of bursa, <u>elbow</u>

        M71.021 Abscess of bursa, <u>right</u> elbow

        M71.022 Abscess of bursa, <u>left</u> elbow

        M71.029 Abscess of bursa, <u>unspecified</u> elbow

    M71.03- Abscess of bursa, <u>wrist</u>

        M71.031 Abscess of bursa, <u>right</u> wrist

        M71.032 Abscess of bursa, <u>left</u> wrist

        M71.039 Abscess of bursa, <u>unspecified</u> wrist

    M71.04- Abscess of bursa, <u>hand</u>

        M71.041 Abscess of bursa, <u>right</u> hand

        M71.042 Abscess of bursa, <u>left</u> hand

        M71.049 Abscess of bursa, <u>unspecified</u> hand

    M71.05- Abscess of bursa, <u>hip</u>

        M71.051 Abscess of bursa, <u>right</u> hip

        M71.052 Abscess of bursa, <u>left</u> hip

        M71.059 Abscess of bursa, <u>unspecified</u> hip

    M71.06- Abscess of bursa, <u>knee</u>

        M71.061 Abscess of bursa, <u>right</u> knee

        M71.062 Abscess of bursa, <u>left</u> knee

        M71.069 Abscess of bursa, <u>unspecified</u> knee

    M71.07- Abscess of bursa, <u>ankle and foot</u>

        M71.071 Abscess of bursa, <u>right</u> ankle and foot

        M71.072 Abscess of bursa, <u>left</u> ankle and foot

        M71.079 Abscess of bursa, <u>unspecified</u> ankle and foot

    M71.08 Abscess of bursa, other site

    M71.09 Abscess of bursa, <u>multiple sites</u>

    M71.1- <u>Other infective</u> bursitis

    Use additional code (B95.-, B96.-) to identify causative organism

    M71.10 Other infective bursitis, <u>unspecified</u> <u>site</u>

    M71.11- Other infective bursitis, <u>shoulder</u>

M70 - M71

M71.111   Other infective bursitis, <u>right</u> shoulder
M71.112   Other infective bursitis, <u>left</u> shoulder
M71.119   Other infective bursitis, <u>unspecified</u> shoulder
M71.12- Other infective bursitis, <u>elbow</u>
    M71.121   Other infective bursitis, <u>right</u> elbow
    M71.122   Other infective bursitis, <u>left</u> elbow
    M71.129   Other infective bursitis, <u>unspecified</u> elbow
M71.13- Other infective bursitis, <u>wrist</u>
    M71.131   Other infective bursitis, <u>right</u> wrist
    M71.132   Other infective bursitis, <u>left</u> wrist
    M71.139   Other infective bursitis, <u>unspecified</u> wrist
M71.14- Other infective bursitis, <u>hand</u>
    M71.141   Other infective bursitis, <u>right</u> hand
    M71.142   Other infective bursitis, <u>left</u> hand
    M71.149   Other infective bursitis, <u>unspecified</u> hand
M71.15- Other infective bursitis, <u>hip</u>
    M71.151   Other infective bursitis, <u>right</u> hip
    M71.152   Other infective bursitis, <u>left</u> hip
    M71.159   Other infective bursitis, <u>unspecified</u> hip
M71.16- Other infective bursitis, <u>knee</u>
    M71.161   Other infective bursitis, <u>right</u> knee
    M71.162   Other infective bursitis, <u>left</u> knee
    M71.169   Other infective bursitis, <u>unspecified</u> knee
M71.17- Other infective bursitis, <u>ankle and foot</u>
    M71.171   Other infective bursitis, <u>right</u> ankle and foot
    M71.172   Other infective bursitis, <u>left</u> ankle and foot
    M71.179   Other infective bursitis, <u>unspecified</u> ankle and foot
M71.18 Other infective bursitis, other site
M71.19 Other infective bursitis, <u>multiple sites</u>
M71.2- <u>Synovial cyst of popliteal space [Baker]</u> — An accumulation of effused synovial fluid behind the knee that is contained by a membrane.
    Excludes 1:   *synovial cyst of popliteal space with rupture (M66.0)*
M71.20 Synovial cyst of popliteal space [Baker], <u>unspecified</u> knee
M71.21 Synovial cyst of popliteal space [Baker], <u>right</u> knee
M71.22 Synovial cyst of popliteal space [Baker], <u>left</u> knee
M71.3- <u>Other bursal cyst</u> — An accumulation of effused synovial fluid that is contained by a membrane.
    Synovial cyst NOS
    Excludes 1:   *synovial cyst with rupture (M66.1-)*
M71.30 Other bursal cyst, <u>unspecified site</u>
M71.31- Other bursal cyst, <u>shoulder</u>
    M71.311   Other bursal cyst, <u>right</u> shoulder
    M71.312   Other bursal cyst, <u>left</u> shoulder
    M71.319   Other bursal cyst, <u>unspecified</u> shoulder
M71.32- Other bursal cyst, <u>elbow</u>
    M71.321   Other bursal cyst, <u>right</u> elbow
    M71.322   Other bursal cyst, <u>left</u> elbow
    M71.329   Other bursal cyst, <u>unspecified</u> elbow
M71.33- Other bursal cyst, <u>wrist</u>
    M71.331   Other bursal cyst, <u>right</u> wrist
    M71.332   Other bursal cyst, <u>left</u> wrist
    M71.339   Other bursal cyst, <u>unspecified</u> wrist
M71.34- Other bursal cyst, <u>hand</u>
    M71.341   Other bursal cyst, <u>right</u> hand
    M71.342   Other bursal cyst, <u>left</u> hand
    M71.349   Other bursal cyst, <u>unspecified</u> hand
M71.35- Other bursal cyst, <u>hip</u>
    M71.351   Other bursal cyst, <u>right</u> hip
    M71.352   Other bursal cyst, <u>left</u> hip
    M71.359   Other bursal cyst, <u>unspecified</u> hip
M71.37- Other bursal cyst, <u>ankle and foot</u>
    M71.371   Other bursal cyst, <u>right</u> ankle and foot
    M71.372   Other bursal cyst, <u>left</u> ankle and foot
    M71.379   Other bursal cyst, <u>unspecified</u> ankle and foot
M71.38 Other bursal cyst, <u>other site</u>

M71.39 Other bursal cyst, <u>multiple sites</u>
M71.4- <u>Calcium deposit</u> in bursa — The deposition of calcium and its salts in the bursae.
    Excludes ❷: *calcium deposit in bursa of shoulder (M75.3)*
M71.40 Calcium deposit in bursa, <u>unspecified</u> <u>site</u>
M71.42- Calcium deposit in bursa, <u>elbow</u>
    M71.421   Calcium deposit in bursa, <u>right</u> elbow
    M71.422   Calcium deposit in bursa, <u>left</u> elbow
    M71.429   Calcium deposit in bursa, <u>unspecified</u> elbow
M71.43- Calcium deposit in bursa, wrist
    M71.431   Calcium deposit in bursa, <u>right</u> wrist
    M71.432   Calcium deposit in bursa, <u>left</u> wrist
    M71.439   Calcium deposit in bursa, <u>unspecified</u> wrist
M71.44- Calcium deposit in bursa, hand
    M71.441   Calcium deposit in bursa, <u>right</u> hand
    M71.442   Calcium deposit in bursa, <u>left</u> hand
    M71.449   Calcium deposit in bursa, <u>unspecified</u> hand
M71.45- Calcium deposit in bursa, <u>hip</u>
    M71.451   Calcium deposit in bursa, <u>right</u> hip
    M71.452   Calcium deposit in bursa, <u>left</u> hip
    M71.459   Calcium deposit in bursa, <u>unspecified</u> hip
M71.46- Calcium deposit in bursa, <u>knee</u>
    M71.461   Calcium deposit in bursa, <u>right</u> knee
    M71.462   Calcium deposit in bursa, <u>left</u> knee
    M71.469   Calcium deposit in bursa, <u>unspecified</u> knee
M71.47- Calcium deposit in bursa, <u>ankle and foot</u>
    M71.471   Calcium deposit in bursa, <u>right</u> ankle and foot
    M71.472   Calcium deposit in bursa, <u>left</u> ankle and foot
    M71.479   Calcium deposit in bursa, <u>unspecified</u> ankle and foot
M71.48 Calcium deposit in bursa, <u>other site</u>
M71.49 Calcium deposit in bursa, <u>multiple sites</u>
M71.5- <u>Other</u> bursitis, <u>not elsewhere classified</u>
    Excludes 1:   *bursitis NOS (M71.9-)*
    Excludes ❷: *bursitis of shoulder (M75.5)*
                bursitis of tibial collateral [Pellegrini-Stieda] (M76.4-)
M71.50 Other bursitis, not elsewhere classified, <u>unspecified site</u>
M71.52- Other bursitis, not elsewhere classified, <u>elbow</u>
    M71.521   Other bursitis, not elsewhere classified, <u>right</u> elbow
    M71.522   Other bursitis, not elsewhere classified, <u>left</u> elbow
    M71.529   Other bursitis, not elsewhere classified, <u>unspecified</u> elbow
M71.53- Other bursitis, not elsewhere classified, <u>wrist</u>
    M71.531   Other bursitis, not elsewhere classified, <u>right</u> wrist
    M71.532   Other bursitis, not elsewhere classified, <u>left</u> wrist
    M71.539   Other bursitis, not elsewhere classified, <u>unspecified</u> wrist
M71.54- Other bursitis, not elsewhere classified, <u>hand</u>
    M71.541   Other bursitis, not elsewhere classified, <u>right</u> hand
    M71.542   Other bursitis, not elsewhere classified, <u>left</u> hand
    M71.549   Other bursitis, not elsewhere classified, <u>unspecified</u> hand
M71.55- Other bursitis, not elsewhere classified, <u>hip</u>
    M71.551   Other bursitis, not elsewhere classified, <u>right</u> hip
    M71.552   Other bursitis, not elsewhere classified, <u>left</u> hip
    M71.559   Other bursitis, not elsewhere classified, <u>unspecified</u> hip
M71.56- Other bursitis, not elsewhere classified, <u>knee</u>
    M71.561   Other bursitis, not elsewhere classified, <u>right</u> knee
    M71.562   Other bursitis, not elsewhere classified, <u>left</u> knee
    M71.569   Other bursitis, not elsewhere classified, <u>unspecified</u> knee
M71.57- Other bursitis, not elsewhere classified, <u>ankle and foot</u>
    M71.571   Other bursitis, not elsewhere classified, <u>right</u> ankle and foot

M71.572 Other bursitis, not elsewhere classified, <u>left</u> ankle and foot

M71.579 Other bursitis, not elsewhere classified, <u>unspecified</u> ankle and foot

M71.58 Other bursitis, not elsewhere classified, <u>other site</u>

M71.8- <u>Other specified bursopathies</u>

M71.80 Other specified bursopathies, <u>unspecified site</u>

M71.81- Other specified bursopathies, <u>shoulder</u>

M71.811 Other specified bursopathies, <u>right</u> shoulder

M71.812 Other specified bursopathies, <u>left</u> shoulder

M71.819 Other specified bursopathies, <u>unspecified</u> shoulder

M71.82- Other specified bursopathies, <u>elbow</u>

M71.821 Other specified bursopathies, <u>right</u> elbow

M71.822 Other specified bursopathies, <u>left</u> elbow

M71.829 Other specified bursopathies, <u>unspecified</u> elbow

M71.83- Other specified bursopathies, <u>wrist</u>

M71.831 Other specified bursopathies, <u>right</u> wrist

M71.832 Other specified bursopathies, <u>left</u> wrist

M71.839 Other specified bursopathies, <u>unspecified</u> wrist

M71.84- Other specified bursopathies, <u>hand</u>

M71.841 Other specified bursopathies, <u>right</u> hand

M71.842 Other specified bursopathies, <u>left</u> hand

M71.849 Other specified bursopathies, <u>unspecified</u> hand

M71.85- Other specified bursopathies, <u>hip</u>

M71.851 Other specified bursopathies, <u>right</u> hip

M71.852 Other specified bursopathies, <u>left</u> hip

M71.859 Other specified bursopathies, <u>unspecified</u> hip

M71.86- Other specified bursopathies, <u>knee</u>

M71.861 Other specified bursopathies, <u>right</u> knee

M71.862 Other specified bursopathies, <u>left</u> knee

M71.869 Other specified bursopathies, <u>unspecified</u> knee

M71.87- Other specified bursopathies, <u>ankle and foot</u>

M71.871 Other specified bursopathies, <u>right</u> ankle and foot

M71.872 Other specified bursopathies, <u>left</u> ankle and foot

M71.879 Other specified bursopathies, <u>unspecified</u> ankle and foot

M71.88 Other specified bursopathies, <u>other site</u>

M71.89 Other specified bursopathies, <u>multiple sites</u>

M71.9 Bursopathy, <u>unspecified</u>
Bursitis NOS

M72- Fibroblastic disorders

Excludes ❷: retroperitoneal fibromatosis (D48.3)

M72.0 **Palmar fascial fibromatosis [Dupuytren]** — [Age/15-124] — The formation of a fibrous nodule in the palmar fascia.

M72.1 **Knuckle pads** — The formation of nodular fibrous masses on the knuckles of the hands.

M72.2 **Plantar fascial fibromatosis** — The formation of a fibrous nodule in the plantar fascia.
Plantar fasciitis — Inflammation of the plantar fascia.

M72.4 **Pseudosarcomatous fibromatosis** — A sarcoma-like appearing proliferation of fibroblasts in the subcutaneous tissue.
Nodular fasciitis — The formation of nodular fibrous masses of the fascia.

MCC M72.6 **Necrotizing fasciitis** — A fulminating infection of the fascia characterized by cellulitis and thrombosis of the subcutaneous vessels and gangrene of the underlying tissue.
Use additional code (B95.-, B96.-) to identify causative organism

M72.8 **Other fibroblastic disorders**
Abscess of fascia — A localized collection of pus caused by the disintegration of fascial tissue.
Fasciitis NEC
Other infective fasciitis
Use additional code to (B95.-, B96.-) identify causative organism
Excludes 1: diffuse (eosinophilic) fasciitis (M35.4)
necrotizing fasciitis (M72.6)
nodular fasciitis (M72.4)
perirenal fasciitis NOS (N13.5)
perirenal fasciitis with infection (N13.6)
plantar fasciitis (M72.2)

M72.9 Fibroblastic disorder, unspecified
Fasciitis NOS
Fibromatosis NOS

M75- <u>Shoulder lesions</u>

Excludes ❷: shoulder-hand syndrome (M89.0-)

M75.0- <u>Adhesive capsulitis</u> of shoulder — The adhesive inflammation of the shoulder joint capsule with progressive stiffness.
AHA 15:2Q:p23 Frozen shoulder
Frozen shoulder
Periarthritis of shoulder

M75.00 Adhesive capsulitis of <u>unspecified</u> shoulder

M75.01 Adhesive capsulitis of <u>right</u> shoulder

M75.02 Adhesive capsulitis of <u>left</u> shoulder

M75.1- <u>Rotator cuff tear or rupture</u>, <u>not specified as traumatic</u> — The non-traumatic injury of the tendons and/or muscles of the shoulder that hold the humeral head in the shallow glenohumeral joint socket.
Rotator cuff syndrome
Supraspinatus syndrome
Supraspinatus tear or rupture, not specified as traumatic
Excludes 1: tear of rotator cuff, traumatic (S46.01-)

M75.10- <u>Unspecified</u> rotator cuff tear or rupture, not specified as traumatic

M75.100 Unspecified rotator cuff tear or rupture of <u>unspecified</u> shoulder, not specified as traumatic

M75.101 Unspecified rotator cuff tear or rupture of <u>right</u> shoulder, not specified as traumatic

M75.102 Unspecified rotator cuff tear or rupture of <u>left</u> shoulder, not specified as traumatic

M75.11- <u>Incomplete</u> rotator cuff tear or rupture, not specified as traumatic — A form where the tendon(s) have a partial tear but remain intact.

M75.110 Incomplete rotator cuff tear or rupture of <u>unspecified</u> shoulder, not specified as traumatic

M75.111 Incomplete rotator cuff tear or rupture of <u>right</u> shoulder, not specified as traumatic

M75.112 Incomplete rotator cuff tear or rupture of <u>left</u> shoulder, not specified as traumatic

M75.12- <u>Complete</u> rotator cuff tear or rupture, not specified as traumatic — A form where the tendon(s) have a full-thickness tear and often become detached.

M75.120 Complete rotator cuff tear or rupture of <u>unspecified</u> shoulder, not specified as traumatic

M75.121 Complete rotator cuff tear or rupture of <u>right</u> shoulder, not specified as traumatic

M75.122 Complete rotator cuff tear or rupture of <u>left</u> shoulder, not specified as traumatic

M75.2- <u>Bicipital</u> tendinitis — Inflammation of the long head of the biceps tendon.

M75.20 Bicipital tendinitis, <u>unspecified</u> shoulder

M75.21 Bicipital tendinitis, <u>right</u> shoulder

M75.22 Bicipital tendinitis, <u>left</u> shoulder

M75.3- <u>Calcific</u> tendinitis of shoulder — The deposition of calcium in the inflamed tendons of the shoulder.
Calcified bursa of shoulder

M75.30 Calcific tendinitis of <u>unspecified</u> shoulder

M75.31 Calcific tendinitis of <u>right</u> shoulder

M75.32 Calcific tendinitis of <u>left</u> shoulder

M75.4- <u>Impingement syndrome</u> of shoulder — The downward compression of the bursa and/or tendons of the shoulder from the acromion process.

M75.40 Impingement syndrome of <u>unspecified</u> shoulder

M75.41 Impingement syndrome of <u>right</u> shoulder

M75.42 Impingement syndrome of <u>left</u> shoulder

M75.5- <u>Bursitis</u> of shoulder — Inflammation of the shoulder bursa.

M75.50 Bursitis of <u>unspecified</u> shoulder

M75.51 Bursitis of <u>right</u> shoulder

M75.52 Bursitis of <u>left</u> shoulder

M75.8- <u>Other</u> shoulder lesions

M75.80 Other shoulder lesions, <u>unspecified</u> shoulder

M75.81 Other shoulder lesions, <u>right</u> shoulder

M75.82 Other shoulder lesions, <u>left</u> shoulder

M
7
1
-
M
7
5

M75.9- Shoulder lesion, <u>unspecified</u>

    M75.90 Shoulder lesion, unspecified, <u>unspecified</u> shoulder

    M75.91 Shoulder lesion, unspecified, <u>right</u> shoulder

    M75.92 Shoulder lesion, unspecified, <u>left</u> shoulder

M76- Enthesopathies, lower limb, excluding foot

    Excludes ❷: *bursitis due to use, overuse and pressure (M70-)*
                   enthesopathies of ankle and foot (M77.5-)

  M76.0- <u>Gluteal</u> tendinitis — Inflammation of the tendons that attach the gluteal muscles to the femur.

    M76.00 Gluteal tendinitis, <u>unspecified</u> hip

    M76.01 Gluteal tendinitis, <u>right</u> hip

    M76.02 Gluteal tendinitis, <u>left</u> hip

  M76.1- <u>Psoas</u> tendinitis — Inflammation of the iliopsoas tendons.

    M76.10 Psoas tendinitis, <u>unspecified</u> hip

    M76.11 Psoas tendinitis, <u>right</u> hip

    M76.12 Psoas tendinitis, <u>left</u> hip

  M76.2- <u>Iliac crest spur</u> — A mass of bony tissue projecting from the iliac crest.

    M76.20 Iliac crest spur, <u>unspecified</u> hip

    M76.21 Iliac crest spur, <u>right</u> hip

    M76.22 Iliac crest spur, <u>left</u> hip

  M76.3- <u>Iliotibial band syndrome</u> — Inflammation of the iliotibial fascia band of the upper leg and knee.

    M76.30 Iliotibial band syndrome, <u>unspecified</u> leg

    M76.31 Iliotibial band syndrome, <u>right</u> leg

    M76.32 Iliotibial band syndrome, <u>left</u> leg

  M76.4- <u>Tibial collateral bursitis [Pellegrini-Stieda]</u> — Inflammation of the bursa over the tibial collateral ligament.

    M76.40 Tibial collateral bursitis [Pellegrini-Stieda], <u>unspecified</u> leg

    M76.41 Tibial collateral bursitis [Pellegrini-Stieda], <u>right</u> leg

    M76.42 Tibial collateral bursitis [Pellegrini-Stieda], <u>left</u> leg

  M76.5- <u>Patellar</u> tendinitis — Inflammation of the patellar tendon.

    M76.50 Patellar tendinitis, <u>unspecified</u> knee

    M76.51 Patellar tendinitis, <u>right</u> knee

    M76.52 Patellar tendinitis, <u>left</u> knee

  M76.6- <u>Achilles</u> tendinitis — Inflammation of the Achilles tendon.

    Achilles bursitis — Inflammation of the Achilles bursa.

    M76.60 Achilles tendinitis, <u>unspecified</u> leg

    M76.61 Achilles tendinitis, <u>right</u> leg

    M76.62 Achilles tendinitis, <u>left</u> leg

  M76.7- <u>Peroneal</u> tendinitis — Inflammation of the peroneal tendon.

    M76.70 Peroneal tendinitis, <u>unspecified</u> leg

    M76.71 Peroneal tendinitis, <u>right</u> leg

    M76.72 Peroneal tendinitis, <u>left</u> leg

  M76.8- <u>Other specified</u> enthesopathies of lower limb, excluding foot

    M76.81-<u>Anterior tibial syndrome</u>

      M76.811 Anterior tibial syndrome, <u>right</u> leg

      M76.812 Anterior tibial syndrome, <u>left</u> leg

      M76.819 Anterior tibial syndrome, <u>unspecified</u> leg

    M76.82-<u>Posterior tibial tendinitis</u>

      M76.821 Posterior tibial tendinitis, <u>right</u> leg

      M76.822 Posterior tibial tendinitis, <u>left</u> leg

      M76.829 Posterior tibial tendinitis, <u>unspecified</u> leg

    M76.89-Other specified enthesopathies of <u>lower limb</u>, excluding foot

      M76.891 Other specified enthesopathies of <u>right</u> lower limb, excluding foot

      M76.892 Other specified enthesopathies of <u>left</u> lower limb, excluding foot

      M76.899 Other specified enthesopathies of <u>unspecified</u> lower limb, excluding foot

  M76.9 Unspecified enthesopathy, lower limb, excluding foot

M77- Other enthesopathies

  Excludes 1:   *bursitis NOS (M71.9-)*

  Excludes ❷: *bursitis due to use, overuse and pressure (M70.-)*
                 osteophyte (M25.7)
                 spinal enthesopathy (M46.0-)

  M77.0- <u>Medial</u> epicondylitis — Inflammation of the medial epicondyle of the humerus and its surrounding tissue.

    M77.00 Medial epicondylitis, <u>unspecified</u> elbow

    M77.01 Medial epicondylitis, <u>right</u> elbow

    M77.02 Medial epicondylitis, <u>left</u> elbow

  M77.1- <u>Lateral</u> epicondylitis — Inflammation of the lateral epicondyle of the humerus and its surrounding tissue.

    Tennis elbow

    M77.10 Lateral epicondylitis, <u>unspecified</u> elbow

    M77.11 Lateral epicondylitis, <u>right</u> elbow

    M77.12 Lateral epicondylitis, <u>left</u> elbow

  M77.2- <u>Periarthritis</u> of <u>wrist</u> — Inflammation of the tissue surrounding the wrist joint.

    M77.20 Periarthritis, <u>unspecified</u> wrist

    M77.21 Periarthritis, <u>right</u> wrist

    M77.22 Periarthritis, <u>left</u> wrist

  M77.3- <u>Calcaneal spur</u> — A bony tissue projection on the calcaneous.

    M77.30 Calcaneal spur, <u>unspecified</u> foot

    M77.31 Calcaneal spur, <u>right</u> foot

    M77.32 Calcaneal spur, <u>left</u> foot

  M77.4- <u>Metatarsalgia</u>

    Excludes 1:   *Morton's metatarsalgia (G57.6)*

    M77.40 Metatarsalgia, <u>unspecified</u> foot

    M77.41 Metatarsalgia, <u>right</u> foot

    M77.42 Metatarsalgia, <u>left</u> foot

  M77.5- <u>Other</u> enthesopathy of foot

    M77.50 Other enthesopathy of <u>unspecified</u> foot

    M77.51 Other enthesopathy of <u>right</u> foot

    M77.52 Other enthesopathy of <u>left</u> foot

  M77.8 Other enthesopathies, not elsewhere classified

  M77.9 Enthesopathy, unspecified

    Bone spur NOS
    Capsulitis NOS
    Periarthritis NOS
    Tendinitis NOS

M79- Other and unspecified soft tissue disorders, <u>not elsewhere classified</u>

  Excludes 1:   *psychogenic rheumatism (F45.8)*
                 soft tissue pain, psychogenic (F45.41)

  M79.0 Rheumatism, unspecified — A connective tissue disease marked by inflammation, degeneration, and metabolic changes.

    Excludes 1:   *fibromyalgia (M79.7)*
                 palindromic rheumatism (M12.3-)

  M79.1 Myalgia — Pain or inflammation of the muscles.

    Myofascial pain syndrome

    Excludes 1:   *fibromyalgia (M79.7)*
                 myositis (M60.-)

  M79.2 Neuralgia and neuritis, unspecified — Pain or inflammation of the nerves or nerve roots.

    Excludes 1:   *brachial radiculitis NOS (M54.1)*
                 lumbosacral radiculitis NOS (M54.1)
                 mononeuropathies (G56-G58)
                 radiculitis NOS (M54.1)
                 sciatica (M54.3-M54.4)

  M79.3 Panniculitis, unspecified — Inflammation of the subcutaneous fat.

    Excludes 1:   *lupus panniculitis (L93.2)*
                 neck and back panniculitis (M54.0-)
                 relapsing [Weber-Christian] panniculitis (M35.6)

  M79.4 Hypertrophy of (infrapatellar) fat pad — The enlargement of the fat pad of the knee.

  M79.5 Residual foreign body in soft tissue — The retention of a foreign body in the soft tissue following healing of the primary injury.

    Excludes 1:   *foreign body granuloma of skin and subcutaneous tissue (L92.3)*
                 foreign body granuloma of soft tissue (M60.2-)

M75-M79 (side tab)

M79.6- Pain in limb, hand, foot, fingers and toes
   Excludes ❷: pain in joint (M25.5-)

  M79.60- Pain in limb, <u>unspecified</u>
    M79.601 Pain in <u>right</u> arm
       Pain in right upper limb NOS
    M79.602 Pain in <u>left</u> arm
       Pain in left upper limb NOS
    M79.603 Pain in arm, <u>unspecified</u>
       Pain in upper limb NOS
    M79.604 Pain in <u>right</u> leg
       Pain in right lower limb NOS
    M79.605 Pain in <u>left</u> leg
       Pain in left lower limb NOS
    M79.606 Pain in leg, <u>unspecified</u>
       Pain in lower limb NOS
    M79.609 Pain in <u>unspecified</u> limb
       Pain in limb NOS

  M79.62- Pain in <u>upper arm</u>
       Pain in axillary region
    M79.621 Pain in <u>right</u> upper arm
    M79.622 Pain in <u>left</u> upper arm
    M79.629 Pain in <u>unspecified</u> upper arm

  M79.63- Pain in <u>forearm</u>
    M79.631 Pain in <u>right</u> forearm
    M79.632 Pain in <u>left</u> forearm
    M79.639 Pain in <u>unspecified</u> forearm

  M79.64- Pain in <u>hand and fingers</u>
    M79.641 Pain in <u>right</u> hand
    M79.642 Pain in <u>left</u> hand
    M79.643 Pain in <u>unspecified</u> hand
    M79.644 Pain in <u>right</u> finger(s)
    M79.645 Pain in <u>left</u> finger(s)
    M79.646 Pain in <u>unspecified</u> finger(s)

  M79.65- Pain in <u>thigh</u>
    M79.651 Pain in <u>right</u> thigh
    M79.652 Pain in <u>left</u> thigh
    M79.659 Pain in <u>unspecified</u> thigh

  M79.66- Pain in <u>lower leg</u>
    M79.661 Pain in <u>right</u> lower leg
    M79.662 Pain in <u>left</u> lower leg
    M79.669 Pain in <u>unspecified</u> lower leg

  M79.67- Pain in <u>foot and toes</u>
    M79.671 Pain in <u>right</u> foot
    M79.672 Pain in <u>left</u> foot
    M79.673 Pain in <u>unspecified</u> foot
    M79.674 Pain in <u>right</u> toe(s)
    M79.675 Pain in <u>left</u> toe(s)
    M79.676 Pain in <u>unspecified</u> toe(s)

M79.7 Fibromyalgia — A condition of widespread pain of the soft tissues and muscles that is characterized by muscle pain, fatigue, sleep, and hypersensitivity to localized pressure.
    Fibromyositis
    Fibrositis
    Myofibrositis

M79.A- <u>Nontraumatic compartment syndrome</u> — An abnormal condition characterized by increased pressure within a closed tissue space containing muscles and nerves that compromises circulation and may lead to tissue necrosis.
  Code first, if applicable, associated postprocedural complication
  Excludes 1: compartment syndrome NOS (T79.A-)
             fibromyalgia (M79.7)
             nontraumatic ischemic infarction of muscle (M62.2-)
             traumatic compartment syndrome (T79.A-)

  M79.A1- Nontraumatic compartment syndrome of <u>upper extremity</u>
       Nontraumatic compartment syndrome of shoulder, arm, forearm, wrist, hand, and fingers
    cc **M79.A11 Nontraumatic compartment syndrome of <u>right</u> upper extremity**

cc **M79.A12 Nontraumatic compartment syndrome of <u>left</u> upper extremity**
cc **M79.A19 Nontraumatic compartment syndrome of <u>unspecified</u> upper extremity**

  M79.A2- Nontraumatic compartment syndrome of <u>lower extremity</u>
       Nontraumatic compartment syndrome of hip, buttock, thigh, leg, foot, and toes
    cc **M79.A21 Nontraumatic compartment syndrome of <u>right</u> lower extremity**
    cc **M79.A22 Nontraumatic compartment syndrome of <u>left</u> lower extremity**
    cc **M79.A29 Nontraumatic compartment syndrome of <u>unspecified</u> lower extremity**

  cc **M79.A3 Nontraumatic compartment syndrome of <u>abdomen</u>**
  cc **M79.A9 Nontraumatic compartment syndrome of <u>other sites</u>**

M79.8- Other specified soft tissue disorders
  M79.81 Nontraumatic hematoma of soft tissue — A localized swelling mass of clotted blood within a soft tissue site that is not due to an identified injury.
       Nontraumatic hematoma of muscle
       Nontraumatic seroma of muscle and soft tissue
  M79.89 Other specified soft tissue disorders
       Polyalgia — Pain in several of the soft tissues at the same time.

M79.9 Soft tissue disorder, unspecified

Osteopathies and chondropathies (M80-M94)

Disorders of bone density and structure (M80-M85)

M80- <u>Osteoporosis with current pathological fracture</u> — A break of a diseased or weakened bone by a minor injury that would not otherwise break a healthy bone due to a degenerative bone disease of increased porosity of the bone with resultant softening.
  Includes: Osteoporosis with current fragility fracture
  Use additional code to identify major osseous defect, if applicable (M89.7-)
  Excludes 1: collapsed vertebra NOS (M48.5)
             pathological fracture NOS (M84.4)
             wedging of vertebra NOS (M48.5)
  Excludes ❷: personal history of (healed) osteoporosis fracture (Z87.310)

The appropriate 7th character is to be added to each code from category M80:
  A Initial encounter for fracture
  D Subsequent encounter for fracture with routine healing
  G Subsequent encounter for fracture with delayed healing
  K Subsequent encounter for fracture with nonunion
  P Subsequent encounter for fracture with malunion
  S Sequela

M80.0- <u>Age-related</u> osteoporosis <u>with current pathological fracture</u>
       Involutional osteoporosis with current pathological fracture
       Osteoporosis NOS with current pathological fracture
       Postmenopausal osteoporosis with current pathological fracture
       Senile osteoporosis with current pathological fracture

CC-A,K,P **M80.00x- Age-related osteoporosis with current pathological fracture, <u>unspecified site</u> [Age/15-124]**

  M80.01- Age-related osteoporosis with current pathological fracture, <u>shoulder</u>
  CC-A,K,P **M80.011- Age-related osteoporosis with current pathological fracture, <u>right</u> shoulder** — [Age/15-124]
  CC-A,K,P **M80.012- Age-related osteoporosis with current pathological fracture, <u>left</u> shoulder** — [Age/15-124]
  CC-A,K,P **M80.019- Age-related osteoporosis with current pathological fracture, <u>unspecified</u> shoulder** — [Age/15-124]

  M80.02- Age-related osteoporosis with current pathological fracture, <u>humerus</u>
  CC-A,K,P **M80.021- Age-related osteoporosis with current pathological fracture, <u>right</u> humerus** — [Age/15-124]
  CC-A,K,P **M80.022- Age-related osteoporosis with current pathological fracture, <u>left</u> humerus** — [Age/15-124]
  CC-A,K,P **M80.029- Age-related osteoporosis with current pathological fracture, <u>unspecified</u> humerus** — [Age/15-124]

M79 - M80 (side tab)

M80.03- Age-related osteoporosis with current pathological fracture, <u>forearm</u>
   Age-related osteoporosis with current pathological fracture of wrist

CC-A,K,P **M80.031-** Age-related osteoporosis with current pathological fracture, <u>right</u> forearm — [Age/15-124]

CC-A,K,P **M80.032-** Age-related osteoporosis with current pathological fracture, <u>left</u> forearm — [Age/15-124]

CC-A,K,P **M80.039-** Age-related osteoporosis with current pathological fracture, <u>unspecified</u> forearm — [Age/15-124]

M80.04- Age-related osteoporosis with current pathological fracture, <u>hand</u>

CC-A,K,P **M80.041-** Age-related osteoporosis with current pathological fracture, <u>right</u> hand — [Age/15-124]

CC-A,K,P **M80.042-** Age-related osteoporosis with current pathological fracture, <u>left</u> hand — [Age/15-124]

CC-A,K,P **M80.049-** Age-related osteoporosis with current pathological fracture, <u>unspecified</u> hand — [Age/15-124]

M80.05- Age-related osteoporosis with current pathological fracture, <u>femur</u>
   Age-related osteoporosis with current pathological fracture of hip

CC-A,K,P **M80.051-** Age-related osteoporosis with current pathological fracture, <u>right</u> femur — [Age/15-124]

CC-A,K,P **M80.052-** Age-related osteoporosis with current pathological fracture, <u>left</u> femur — [Age/15-124]

CC-A,K,P **M80.059-** Age-related osteoporosis with current pathological fracture, <u>unspecified</u> femur — [Age/15-124]

M80.06- Age-related osteoporosis with current pathological fracture, <u>lower leg</u>

CC-A,K,P **M80.061-** Age-related osteoporosis with current pathological fracture, <u>right</u> lower leg — [Age/15-124]

CC-A,K,P **M80.062-** Age-related osteoporosis with current pathological fracture, <u>left</u> lower leg — [Age/15-124]

CC-A,K,P **M80.069-** Age-related osteoporosis with current pathological fracture, <u>unspecified</u> lower leg — [Age/15-124]

M80.07- Age-related osteoporosis with current pathological fracture, <u>ankle and foot</u>

CC-A,K,P **M80.071-** Age-related osteoporosis with current pathological fracture, <u>right</u> ankle and foot — [Age/15-124]

CC-A,K,P **M80.072-** Age-related osteoporosis with current pathological fracture, <u>left</u> ankle and foot — [Age/15-124]

CC-A,K,P **M80.079-** Age-related osteoporosis with current pathological fracture, <u>unspecified</u> ankle and foot — [Age/15-124]

CC-A,K,P **M80.08x-** Age-related osteoporosis with current pathological fracture, <u>vertebra(e)</u> — [Age/15-124]

M80.8- <u>Other</u> osteoporosis <u>with current pathological fracture</u>
   Drug-induced osteoporosis with current pathological fracture
   Idiopathic osteoporosis with current pathological fracture
   Osteoporosis of disuse with current pathological fracture
   Postoophorectomy osteoporosis with current pathological fracture
   Postsurgical malabsorption osteoporosis with current pathological fracture
   Post-traumatic osteoporosis with current pathological fracture
   Use additional code for adverse effect, if applicable, to identify drug (T36-T50 with fifth or sixth character 5)

CC-A,K,P **M80.80x-** Other osteoporosis with current pathological fracture, <u>unspecified</u> site

M80.81- Other osteoporosis with pathological fracture, <u>shoulder</u>

CC-A,K,P **M80.811-** Other osteoporosis with current pathological fracture, <u>right</u> shoulder

CC-A,K,P **M80.812-** Other osteoporosis with current pathological fracture, <u>left</u> shoulder

CC-A,K,P **M80.819-** Other osteoporosis with current pathological fracture, <u>unspecified</u> shoulder

M80.82- Other osteoporosis with current pathological fracture, <u>humerus</u>

CC-A,K,P **M80.821-** Other osteoporosis with current pathological fracture, <u>right</u> humerus

CC-A,K,P **M80.822-** Other osteoporosis with current pathological fracture, <u>left</u> humerus

CC-A,K,P **M80.829-** Other osteoporosis with current pathological fracture, <u>unspecified</u> humerus

M80.83- Other osteoporosis with current pathological fracture, <u>forearm</u>
   Other osteoporosis with current pathological fracture of wrist

CC-A,K,P **M80.831-** Other osteoporosis with current pathological fracture, <u>right</u> forearm

CC-A,K,P **M80.832-** Other osteoporosis with current pathological fracture, <u>left</u> forearm

CC-A,K,P **M80.839-** Other osteoporosis with current pathological fracture, <u>unspecified</u> forearm

M80.84- Other osteoporosis with current pathological fracture, <u>hand</u>

CC-A,K,P **M80.841-** Other osteoporosis with current pathological fracture, <u>right</u> hand

CC-A,K,P **M80.842-** Other osteoporosis with current pathological fracture, <u>left</u> hand

CC-A,K,P **M80.849-** Other osteoporosis with current pathological fracture, <u>unspecified</u> hand

M80.85- Other osteoporosis with current pathological fracture, <u>femur</u>
   Other osteoporosis with current pathological fracture of hip

CC-A,K,P **M80.851-** Other osteoporosis with current pathological fracture, <u>right</u> femur

CC-A,K,P **M80.852-** Other osteoporosis with current pathological fracture, <u>left</u> femur

CC-A,K,P **M80.859-** Other osteoporosis with current pathological fracture, <u>unspecified</u> femur

M80.86- Other osteoporosis with current pathological fracture, <u>lower leg</u>

CC-A,K,P **M80.861-** Other osteoporosis with current pathological fracture, <u>right</u> lower leg

CC-A,K,P **M80.862-** Other osteoporosis with current pathological fracture, <u>left</u> lower leg

CC-A,K,P **M80.869-** Other osteoporosis with current pathological fracture, <u>unspecified</u> lower leg

M80.87- Other osteoporosis with current pathological fracture, <u>ankle and foot</u>

CC-A,K,P **M80.871-** Other osteoporosis with current pathological fracture, <u>right</u> ankle and foot

CC-A,K,P **M80.872-** Other osteoporosis with current pathological fracture, <u>left</u> ankle and foot

CC-A,K,P **M80.879-** Other osteoporosis with current pathological fracture, <u>unspecified</u> ankle and foot

CC-A,K,P **M80.88x-** Other osteoporosis with current pathological fracture, vertebra(e)

M81- Osteoporosis <u>without</u> current pathological fracture — A degenerative bone disorder due to bone loss and characterized by porosity, softening, decreased bone strength, and susceptibility to relatively minor force fractures.
   Use additional code to identify:
      Major osseous defect, if applicable (M89.7-)
      Personal history of (healed) osteoporosis fracture, if applicable (Z87.310)
   Excludes 1:   *osteoporosis with current pathological fracture (M80.-)*
         Sudeck's atrophy (M89.0)

M81.0 <u>Age-related</u> osteoporosis without current pathological fracture — [Age/15-124]
   Involutional osteoporosis without current pathological fracture
   Osteoporosis NOS
   Postmenopausal osteoporosis without current pathological fracture
   Senile osteoporosis without current pathological fracture

M81.6 <u>Localized</u> osteoporosis [Lequesne]
   Excludes 1:   *Sudeck's atrophy (M89.0)*

M80 - M81

M81.8 <u>Other</u> osteoporosis without current pathological fracture
Drug-induced osteoporosis without current pathological fracture
Idiopathic osteoporosis without current pathological fracture
Osteoporosis of disuse without current pathological fracture
Postoophorectomy osteoporosis without current pathological fracture
Postsurgical malabsorption osteoporosis without current pathological fracture
Post-traumatic osteoporosis without current pathological fracture
Use additional code for adverse effect, if applicable, to identify drug (T36-T50 with fifth or sixth character 5)

M83- <u>Adult osteomalacia</u> — Softening of the bone.
Excludes 1: *infantile and juvenile osteomalacia (E55.0)*
renal osteodystrophy (N25.0)
rickets (active) (E55.0)
rickets (active) sequelae (E64.3)
vitamin D-resistant osteomalacia (E83.3)
vitamin D-resistant rickets (active) (E83.3)

M83.0 **Puerperal osteomalacia** — [♀, Age/12-55] — A form following pregnancy.

M83.1 **Senile osteomalacia** — [Age/15-124] — A form that is age-related.

M83.2 **Adult osteomalacia due to malabsorption** — [Age/15-124] — A form due to the body's decreased ability to absorb nutrients.
Postsurgical malabsorption osteomalacia in adults

M83.3 **Adult osteomalacia due to malnutrition** — [Age/15-124] — A form due to the decreased intake of nutrients.

M83.4 **Aluminum bone disease** — A form due to aluminum toxicity.

M83.5 **Other drug-induced osteomalacia in adults** — [Age/15-124]
Use additional code for adverse effect, if applicable, to identify drug (T36-T50 with fifth or sixth character 5)

M83.8 **Other adult osteomalacia** — [Age/15-124]

M83.9 **Adult osteomalacia, unspecified** — [Age/15-124]

M84- **Disorder of continuity of bone**
Excludes ❷: *traumatic fracture of bone-see fracture, by site*

M84.3- <u>Stress fracture</u> — A fracture that is due to multiple/repetitive stress forces as opposed to an isolated acute traumatic injury event.
Fatigue fracture
March fracture
Stress fracture NOS
Stress reaction
Use additional external cause code(s) to identify the cause of the stress fracture
Excludes 1: *pathological fracture NOS (M84.4.-)*
pathological fracture due to osteoporosis (M80.-)
traumatic fracture (S12.-, S22.-, S32.-, S42.-, S52.-, S62.-, S72.-, S82.-, S92.-)
Excludes ❷: *personal history of (healed) stress (fatigue) fracture (Z87.312)*
stress fracture of vertebra (M48.4-)

The appropriate 7th character is to be added to each code from subcategory M84.3:
A Initial encounter for fracture
D Subsequent encounter for fracture with routine healing
G Subsequent encounter for fracture with delayed healing
K Subsequent encounter for fracture with nonunion
P Subsequent encounter for fracture with malunion
S Sequela

CC-K,P **M84.30x-** Stress fracture, <u>unspecified</u> <u>site</u>
M84.31- Stress fracture, <u>shoulder</u>
CC-K,P **M84.311-** Stress fracture, <u>right</u> shoulder
CC-K,P **M84.312-** Stress fracture, <u>left</u> shoulder
CC-K,P **M84.319-** Stress fracture, <u>unspecified</u> shoulder
M84.32- Stress fracture, <u>humerus</u>
CC-K,P **M84.321-** Stress fracture, <u>right</u> humerus
CC-K,P **M84.322-** Stress fracture, <u>left</u> humerus
CC-K,P **M84.329-** Stress fracture, <u>unspecified</u> humerus
M84.33- Stress fracture, <u>ulna and radius</u>
CC-K,P **M84.331-** Stress fracture, <u>right</u> ulna
CC-K,P **M84.332-** Stress fracture, <u>left</u> ulna
CC-K,P **M84.333-** Stress fracture, <u>right</u> radius
CC-K,P **M84.334-** Stress fracture, <u>left</u> radius
CC-K,P **M84.339-** Stress fracture, <u>unspecified</u> ulna and radius
M84.34- Stress fracture, <u>hand and fingers</u>
CC-K,P **M84.341-** Stress fracture, <u>right</u> hand

CC-K,P **M84.342-** Stress fracture, <u>left</u> hand
CC-K,P **M84.343-** Stress fracture, <u>unspecified</u> hand
CC-K,P **M84.344-** Stress fracture, <u>right</u> finger(s)
CC-K,P **M84.345-** Stress fracture, <u>left</u> finger(s)
CC-K,P **M84.346-** Stress fracture, <u>unspecified</u> finger(s)
M84.35- Stress fracture, <u>pelvis and femur</u>
Stress fracture, hip
CC-K,P **M84.350-** Stress fracture, pelvis
CC-K,P **M84.351-** Stress fracture, <u>right</u> femur
CC-K,P **M84.352-** Stress fracture, <u>left</u> femur
CC-K,P **M84.353-** Stress fracture, <u>unspecified</u> femur
CC-K,P **M84.359-** Stress fracture, hip, <u>unspecified</u>
M84.36- Stress fracture, <u>tibia and fibula</u>
CC-K,P **M84.361-** Stress fracture, <u>right</u> tibia
CC-K,P **M84.362-** Stress fracture, <u>left</u> tibia
CC-K,P **M84.363-** Stress fracture, <u>right</u> fibula
CC-K,P **M84.364-** Stress fracture, <u>left</u> fibula
CC-K,P **M84.369-** Stress fracture, <u>unspecified</u> tibia and fibula
M84.37- Stress fracture, <u>ankle, foot and toes</u>
CC-K,P **M84.371-** Stress fracture, <u>right</u> ankle
CC-K,P **M84.372-** Stress fracture, <u>left</u> ankle
CC-K,P **M84.373-** Stress fracture, <u>unspecified</u> ankle
CC-K,P **M84.374-** Stress fracture, <u>right</u> foot
CC-K,P **M84.375-** Stress fracture, <u>left</u> foot
CC-K,P **M84.376-** Stress fracture, <u>unspecified</u> foot
CC-K,P **M84.377-** Stress fracture, <u>right</u> toe(s)
CC-K,P **M84.378-** Stress fracture, <u>left</u> toe(s)
CC-K,P **M84.379-** Stress fracture, <u>unspecified</u> toe(s)
CC-K,P **M84.38x-** Stress fracture, <u>other site</u>
Excludes ❷: *stress fracture of vertebra (M48.4-)*

M84.4- <u>Pathological fracture</u>, <u>not elsewhere classified</u> — A break of a diseased or weakened bone by a minor injury that would not otherwise break a healthy bone and that is NOT due to osteoporosis.
Chronic fracture
Pathological fracture NOS
Excludes 1: *collapsed vertebra NEC (M48.5)*
pathological fracture in neoplastic disease (M84.5-)
pathological fracture in osteoporosis (M80.-)
pathological fracture in other disease (M84.6-)
stress fracture (M84.3-)
traumatic fracture (S12.-, S22.-, S32.-, S42.-, S52.-, S62.-, S72.-, S82.-, S92.-)
Excludes ❷: *personal history of (healed) pathological fracture (Z87.311)*

The appropriate 7th character is to be added to each code from subcategory M84.4:
A Initial encounter for fracture
D Subsequent encounter for fracture with routine healing
G Subsequent encounter for fracture with delayed healing
K Subsequent encounter for fracture with nonunion
P Subsequent encounter for fracture with malunion
S Sequela

CC-A,K,P **M84.40x-** Pathological fracture, <u>unspecified</u> <u>site</u>
M84.41- Pathological fracture, <u>shoulder</u>
CC-A,K,P **M84.411-** Pathological fracture, <u>right</u> shoulder
CC-A,K,P **M84.412-** Pathological fracture, <u>left</u> shoulder
CC-A,K,P **M84.419-** Pathological fracture, <u>unspecified</u> shoulder
M84.42- Pathological fracture, <u>humerus</u>
CC-A,K,P **M84.421-** Pathological fracture, <u>right</u> humerus
CC-A,K,P **M84.422-** Pathological fracture, <u>left</u> humerus
CC-A,K,P **M84.429-** Pathological fracture, <u>unspecified</u> humerus
M84.43- Pathological fracture, <u>ulna and radius</u>
CC-A,K,P **M84.431-** Pathological fracture, <u>right</u> ulna
CC-A,K,P **M84.432-** Pathological fracture, <u>left</u> ulna
CC-A,K,P **M84.433-** Pathological fracture, <u>right</u> radius
CC-A,K,P **M84.434-** Pathological fracture, <u>left</u> radius
CC-A,K,P **M84.439-** Pathological fracture, <u>unspecified</u> ulna and radius
M84.44- Pathological fracture, <u>hand and fingers</u>
CC-A,K,P **M84.441-** Pathological fracture, <u>right</u> hand

M
8
1
–
M
8
4

CC-A,K,P **M84.442-** Pathological fracture, <u>left</u> hand

CC-A,K,P **M84.443-** Pathological fracture, <u>unspecified</u> hand

CC-A,K,P **M84.444-** Pathological fracture, <u>right</u> finger(s)

CC-A,K,P **M84.445-** Pathological fracture, <u>left</u> finger(s)

CC-A,K,P **M84.446-** Pathological fracture, <u>unspecified</u> finger(s)

M84.45- Pathological fracture, <u>femur and pelvis</u>

CC-A,K,P **M84.451-** Pathological fracture, <u>right</u> femur

CC-A,K,P **M84.452-** Pathological fracture, <u>left</u> femur

CC-A,K,P **M84.453-** Pathological fracture, <u>unspecified</u> femur

CC-A,K,P **M84.454-** Pathological fracture, pelvis

CC-A,K,P **M84.459-** Pathological fracture, hip, <u>unspecified</u>

M84.46- Pathological fracture, <u>tibia and fibula</u>

CC-A,K,P **M84.461-** Pathological fracture, <u>right</u> tibia

CC-A,K,P **M84.462-** Pathological fracture, <u>left</u> tibia

CC-A,K,P **M84.463-** Pathological fracture, <u>right</u> fibula

CC-A,K,P **M84.464-** Pathological fracture, <u>left</u> fibula

CC-A,K,P **M84.469-** Pathological fracture, <u>unspecified</u> tibia and fibula

M84.47- Pathological fracture, <u>ankle, foot and toes</u>

CC-A,K,P **M84.471-** Pathological fracture, <u>right</u> ankle

CC-A,K,P **M84.472-** Pathological fracture, <u>left</u> ankle

CC-A,K,P **M84.473-** Pathological fracture, <u>unspecified</u> ankle

CC-A,K,P **M84.474-** Pathological fracture, <u>right</u> foot

CC-A,K,P **M84.475-** Pathological fracture, <u>left</u> foot

CC-A,K,P **M84.476-** Pathological fracture, <u>unspecified</u> foot

CC-A,K,P **M84.477-** Pathological fracture, <u>right</u> toe(s)

CC-A,K,P **M84.478-** Pathological fracture, <u>left</u> toe(s)

CC-A,K,P **M84.479-** Pathological fracture, <u>unspecified</u> toe(s)

CC-A,K,P **M84.48x-** Pathological fracture, <u>other site</u>

M84.5- Pathological fracture <u>in neoplastic disease</u>
Code also underlying neoplasm

The appropriate 7th character is to be added to each code from subcategory M84.5:
  A   Initial encounter for fracture
  D   Subsequent encounter for fracture with routine healing
  G   Subsequent encounter for fracture with delayed healing
  K   Subsequent encounter for fracture with nonunion
  P   Subsequent encounter for fracture with malunion
  S   Sequela

CC-A,K,P **M84.50x-** Pathological fracture in neoplastic disease, <u>unspecified site</u>

M84.51- Pathological fracture in neoplastic disease, <u>shoulder</u>

CC-A,K,P **M84.511-** Pathological fracture in neoplastic disease, <u>right</u> shoulder

CC-A,K,P **M84.512-** Pathological fracture in neoplastic disease, <u>left</u> shoulder

CC-A,K,P **M84.519-** Pathological fracture in neoplastic disease, <u>unspecified</u> shoulder

M84.52- Pathological fracture in neoplastic disease, <u>humerus</u>

CC-A,K,P **M84.521-** Pathological fracture in neoplastic disease, <u>right</u> humerus

CC-A,K,P **M84.522-** Pathological fracture in neoplastic disease, <u>left</u> humerus

CC-A,K,P **M84.529-** Pathological fracture in neoplastic disease, <u>unspecified</u> humerus

M84.53- Pathological fracture in neoplastic disease, <u>ulna and radius</u>

CC-A,K,P **M84.531-** Pathological fracture in neoplastic disease, <u>right</u> ulna

CC-A,K,P **M84.532-** Pathological fracture in neoplastic disease, <u>left</u> ulna

CC-A,K,P **M84.533-** Pathological fracture in neoplastic disease, <u>right</u> radius

CC-A,K,P **M84.534-** Pathological fracture in neoplastic disease, <u>left</u> radius

CC-A,K,P **M84.539-** Pathological fracture in neoplastic disease, <u>unspecified</u> ulna and radius

M84.54- Pathological fracture in neoplastic disease, <u>hand</u>

CC-A,K,P **M84.541-** Pathological fracture in neoplastic disease, <u>right</u> hand

CC-A,K,P **M84.542-** Pathological fracture in neoplastic disease, <u>left</u> hand

CC-A,K,P **M84.549-** Pathological fracture in neoplastic disease, <u>unspecified</u> hand

M84.55- Pathological fracture in neoplastic disease, <u>pelvis and femur</u>

CC-A,K,P **M84.550-** Pathological fracture in neoplastic disease, pelvis

CC-A,K,P **M84.551-** Pathological fracture in neoplastic disease, <u>right</u> femur

CC-A,K,P **M84.552-** Pathological fracture in neoplastic disease, <u>left</u> femur

CC-A,K,P **M84.553-** Pathological fracture in neoplastic disease, <u>unspecified</u> femur

CC-A,K,P **M84.559-** Pathological fracture in neoplastic disease, hip, <u>unspecified</u>

M84.56- Pathological fracture in neoplastic disease, <u>tibia and fibula</u>

CC-A,K,P **M84.561-** Pathological fracture in neoplastic disease, <u>right</u> tibia

CC-A,K,P **M84.562-** Pathological fracture in neoplastic disease, <u>left</u> tibia

CC-A,K,P **M84.563-** Pathological fracture in neoplastic disease, <u>right</u> fibula

CC-A,K,P **M84.564-** Pathological fracture in neoplastic disease, <u>left</u> fibula

CC-A,K,P **M84.569-** Pathological fracture in neoplastic disease, <u>unspecified</u> tibia and fibula

M84.57- Pathological fracture in neoplastic disease, <u>ankle and foot</u>

CC-A,K,P **M84.571-** Pathological fracture in neoplastic disease, <u>right</u> ankle

CC-A,K,P **M84.572-** Pathological fracture in neoplastic disease, <u>left</u> ankle

CC-A,K,P **M84.573-** Pathological fracture in neoplastic disease, <u>unspecified</u> ankle

CC-A,K,P **M84.574-** Pathological fracture in neoplastic disease, <u>right</u> foot

CC-A,K,P **M84.575-** Pathological fracture in neoplastic disease, <u>left</u> foot

CC-A,K,P **M84.576-** Pathological fracture in neoplastic disease, <u>unspecified</u> foot

CC-A,K,P **M84.58x-** Pathological fracture in neoplastic disease, <u>other specified site</u>
Pathological fracture in neoplastic disease, vertebrae

M84.6- Pathological fracture <u>in other disease</u>
Code also underlying condition
Excludes 1:   *pathological fracture in osteoporosis (M80.-)*

The appropriate 7th character is to be added to each code from subcategory M84.6:
  A   Initial encounter for fracture
  D   Subsequent encounter for fracture with routine healing
  G   Subsequent encounter for fracture with delayed healing
  K   Subsequent encounter for fracture with nonunion
  P   Subsequent encounter for fracture with malunion
  S   Sequela

CC-A,K,P **M84.60x-** Pathological fracture in other disease, <u>unspecified</u> <u>site</u>

M84.61- Pathological fracture in other disease, <u>shoulder</u>

CC-A,K,P **M84.611-** Pathological fracture in other disease, <u>right</u> shoulder

CC-A,K,P **M84.612-** Pathological fracture in other disease, <u>left</u> shoulder

CC-A,K,P **M84.619-** Pathological fracture in other disease, <u>unspecified</u> shoulder

M84.62- Pathological fracture in other disease, <u>humerus</u>

CC-A,K,P **M84.621-** Pathological fracture in other disease, <u>right</u> humerus

CC-A,K,P **M84.622-** Pathological fracture in other disease, <u>left</u> humerus

M84-M84

CC-A,K,P **M84.629-** Pathological fracture in other disease, <u>unspecified</u> humerus

M84.63- Pathological fracture in other disease, <u>ulna and radius</u>

CC-A,K,P **M84.631-** Pathological fracture in other disease, <u>right</u> ulna

CC-A,K,P **M84.632-** Pathological fracture in other disease, <u>left</u> ulna

CC-A,K,P **M84.633-** Pathological fracture in other disease, <u>right</u> radius

CC-A,K,P **M84.634-** Pathological fracture in other disease, <u>left</u> radius

CC-A,K,P **M84.639-** Pathological fracture in other disease, <u>unspecified</u> ulna and radius

M84.64- Pathological fracture in other disease, <u>hand</u>

CC-A,K,P **M84.641-** Pathological fracture in other disease, <u>right</u> hand

CC-A,K,P **M84.642-** Pathological fracture in other disease, <u>left</u> hand

CC-A,K,P **M84.649-** Pathological fracture in other disease, <u>unspecified</u> hand

M84.65- Pathological fracture in other disease, <u>pelvis and femur</u>

CC-A,K,P **M84.650-** Pathological fracture in other disease, pelvis

CC-A,K,P **M84.651-** Pathological fracture in other disease, <u>right</u> femur

CC-A,K,P **M84.652-** Pathological fracture in other disease, <u>left</u> femur

CC-A,K,P **M84.653-** Pathological fracture in other disease, <u>unspecified</u> femur

CC-A,K,P **M84.659-** Pathological fracture in other disease, hip, <u>unspecified</u>

M84.66- Pathological fracture in other disease, <u>tibia and fibula</u>

CC-A,K,P **M84.661-** Pathological fracture in other disease, <u>right</u> tibia

CC-A,K,P **M84.662-** Pathological fracture in other disease, <u>left</u> tibia

CC-A,K,P **M84.663-** Pathological fracture in other disease, <u>right</u> fibula

CC-A,K,P **M84.664-** Pathological fracture in other disease, <u>left</u> fibula

CC-A,K,P **M84.669-** Pathological fracture in other disease, <u>unspecified</u> tibia and fibula

M84.67 Pathological fracture in other disease, ankle and foot

CC-A,K,P **M84.671-** Pathological fracture in other disease, <u>right</u> ankle

CC-A,K,P **M84.672-** Pathological fracture in other disease, <u>left</u> ankle

CC-A,K,P **M84.673-** Pathological fracture in other disease, <u>unspecified</u> ankle

CC-A,K,P **M84.674-** Pathological fracture in other disease, <u>right</u> foot

CC-A,K,P **M84.675-** Pathological fracture in other disease, <u>left</u> foot

CC-A,K,P **M84.676-** Pathological fracture in other disease, <u>unspecified</u> foot

CC-A,K,P **M84.68x-** Pathological fracture in other disease, <u>other site</u>

M84.7- Nontraumatic fracture, not elsewhere classified

M84.75-<u>Atypical femoral</u> fracture

> The appropriate 7th character is to be added to each code from M84.75:
> **A** Initial encounter for fracture
> **D** Subsequent encounter for fracture with routine healing
> **G** Subsequent encounter for fracture with delayed healing
> **K** Subsequent encounter for fracture with nonunion
> **P** Subsequent encounter for fracture with malunion
> **S** Sequela

CC-A,K,P **M84.750-** Atypical femoral fracture, <u>unspecified</u>

CC-A,K,P **M84.751-** <u>Incomplete</u> atypical femoral fracture, <u>right</u> leg

CC-A,K,P **M84.752-** <u>Incomplete</u> atypical femoral fracture, <u>left</u> leg

CC-A,K,P **M84.753-** <u>Incomplete</u> atypical femoral fracture, <u>unspecified</u> leg

CC-A,K,P **M84.754-** <u>Complete</u> transverse atypical femoral fracture, <u>right</u> leg

CC-A,K,P **M84.755-** <u>Complete</u> transverse atypical femoral fracture, <u>left</u> leg

CC-A,K,P **M84.756-** <u>Complete</u> transverse atypical femoral fracture, <u>unspecified</u> leg

CC-A,K,P **M84.757-** <u>Complete</u> oblique atypical femoral fracture, <u>right</u>

CC-A,K,P **M84.758-** <u>Complete</u> oblique atypical femoral fracture, <u>left</u> leg

CC-A,K,P **M84.759-** <u>Complete</u> oblique atypical femoral fracture, <u>unspecified</u> leg

M84.8- <u>Other disorders of continuity of bone</u>

M84.80 Other disorders of continuity of bone, <u>unspecified</u> <u>site</u>

M84.81- Other disorders of continuity of bone, <u>shoulder</u>

M84.811 Other disorders of continuity of bone, <u>right</u> shoulder

M84.812 Other disorders of continuity of bone, <u>left</u> shoulder

M84.819 Other disorders of continuity of bone, <u>unspecified</u> shoulder

M84.82- Other disorders of continuity of bone, <u>humerus</u>

M84.821 Other disorders of continuity of bone, <u>right</u> humerus

M84.822 Other disorders of continuity of bone, <u>left</u> humerus

M84.829 Other disorders of continuity of bone, <u>unspecified</u> humerus

M84.83- Other disorders of continuity of bone, <u>ulna and radius</u>

M84.831 Other disorders of continuity of bone, <u>right</u> ulna

M84.832 Other disorders of continuity of bone, <u>left</u> ulna

M84.833 Other disorders of continuity of bone, <u>right</u> radius

M84.834 Other disorders of continuity of bone, <u>left</u> radius

M84.839 Other disorders of continuity of bone, <u>unspecified</u> ulna and radius

M84.84- Other disorders of continuity of bone, <u>hand</u>

M84.841 Other disorders of continuity of bone, <u>right</u> hand

M84.842 Other disorders of continuity of bone, <u>left</u> hand

M84.849 Other disorders of continuity of bone, <u>unspecified</u> hand

M84.85- Other disorders of continuity of bone, <u>pelvic region and thigh</u>

M84.851 Other disorders of continuity of bone, <u>right</u> pelvic region and thigh

M84.852 Other disorders of continuity of bone, <u>left</u> pelvic region and thigh

M84.859 Other disorders of continuity of bone, <u>unspecified</u> pelvic region and thigh

M84.86- Other disorders of continuity of bone, <u>tibia and fibula</u>

M84.861 Other disorders of continuity of bone, <u>right</u> tibia

M84.862 Other disorders of continuity of bone, <u>left</u> tibia

M84.863 Other disorders of continuity of bone, <u>right</u> fibula

M84.864 Other disorders of continuity of bone, <u>left</u> fibula

M84.869 Other disorders of continuity of bone, <u>unspecified</u> tibia and fibula

M84.87- Other disorders of continuity of bone, <u>ankle and foot</u>

M84.871 Other disorders of continuity of bone, <u>right</u> ankle and foot

M84.872 Other disorders of continuity of bone, <u>left</u> ankle and foot

M84.879 Other disorders of continuity of bone, <u>unspecified</u> ankle and foot

M84.88 Other disorders of continuity of bone, <u>other site</u>

M84.9 Disorder of continuity of bone, <u>unspecified</u>

M85- <u>Other disorders of bone density and structure</u>

Excludes 1:   osteogenesis imperfecta (Q78.0)
osteopetrosis (Q78.2)
osteopoikilosis (Q78.8)
polyostotic fibrous dysplasia (Q78.1)

M85.0- <u>Fibrous dysplasia (monostotic)</u> — The replacement the bone marrow with fibrous tissue that is limited to a single bone.
Excludes ❷: fibrous dysplasia of jaw (M27.8)

M85.00 Fibrous dysplasia (monostotic), <u>unspecified</u> <u>site</u>

M85.01- Fibrous dysplasia (monostotic), <u>shoulder</u>

M85.011 Fibrous dysplasia (monostotic), <u>right</u> shoulder

M85.012 Fibrous dysplasia (monostotic), <u>left</u> shoulder

M85.019 Fibrous dysplasia (monostotic), <u>unspecified</u> shoulder

M85.02- Fibrous dysplasia (monostotic), <u>upper arm</u>

M85.021 Fibrous dysplasia (monostotic), <u>right</u> upper arm

M85.022 Fibrous dysplasia (monostotic), <u>left</u> upper arm

M85.029   Fibrous dysplasia (monostotic), <u>unspecified</u> upper arm

M85.03- Fibrous dysplasia (monostotic), <u>forearm</u>
- M85.031   Fibrous dysplasia (monostotic), <u>right</u> forearm
- M85.032   Fibrous dysplasia (monostotic), <u>left</u> forearm
- M85.039   Fibrous dysplasia (monostotic), <u>unspecified</u> forearm

M85.04- Fibrous dysplasia (monostotic), <u>hand</u>
- M85.041   Fibrous dysplasia (monostotic), <u>right</u> hand
- M85.042   Fibrous dysplasia (monostotic), <u>left</u> hand
- M85.049   Fibrous dysplasia (monostotic), <u>unspecified</u> hand

M85.05- Fibrous dysplasia (monostotic), <u>thigh</u>
- M85.051   Fibrous dysplasia (monostotic), <u>right</u> thigh
- M85.052   Fibrous dysplasia (monostotic), <u>left</u> thigh
- M85.059   Fibrous dysplasia (monostotic), <u>unspecified</u> thigh

M85.06- Fibrous dysplasia (monostotic), <u>lower leg</u>
- M85.061   Fibrous dysplasia (monostotic), <u>right</u> lower leg
- M85.062   Fibrous dysplasia (monostotic), <u>left</u> lower leg
- M85.069   Fibrous dysplasia (monostotic), <u>unspecified</u> lower leg

M85.07 Fibrous dysplasia (monostotic), <u>ankle and foot</u>
- M85.071   Fibrous dysplasia (monostotic), <u>right</u> ankle and foot
- M85.072   Fibrous dysplasia (monostotic), <u>left</u> ankle and foot
- M85.079   Fibrous dysplasia (monostotic), <u>unspecified</u> ankle and foot

M85.08 Fibrous dysplasia (monostotic), <u>other site</u>
M85.09 Fibrous dysplasia (monostotic), <u>multiple sites</u>

M85.1- <u>Skeletal fluorosis</u> — A bone disease marked by excessive fluoride accumulation in the bones.

M85.10 Skeletal fluorosis, <u>unspecified</u> <u>site</u>
M85.11- Skeletal fluorosis, <u>shoulder</u>
- M85.111   Skeletal fluorosis, <u>right</u> shoulder
- M85.112   Skeletal fluorosis, <u>left</u> shoulder
- M85.119   Skeletal fluorosis, <u>unspecified</u> shoulder

M85.12- Skeletal fluorosis, <u>upper arm</u>
- M85.121   Skeletal fluorosis, <u>right</u> upper arm
- M85.122   Skeletal fluorosis, <u>left</u> upper arm
- M85.129   Skeletal fluorosis, <u>unspecified</u> upper arm

M85.13- Skeletal fluorosis, <u>forearm</u>
- M85.131   Skeletal fluorosis, <u>right</u> forearm
- M85.132   Skeletal fluorosis, <u>left</u> forearm
- M85.139   Skeletal fluorosis, <u>unspecified</u> forearm

M85.14- Skeletal fluorosis, <u>hand</u>
- M85.141   Skeletal fluorosis, <u>right</u> hand
- M85.142   Skeletal fluorosis, <u>left</u> hand
- M85.149   Skeletal fluorosis, <u>unspecified</u> hand

M85.15- Skeletal fluorosis, <u>thigh</u>
- M85.151   Skeletal fluorosis, <u>right</u> thigh
- M85.152   Skeletal fluorosis, <u>left</u> thigh
- M85.159   Skeletal fluorosis, <u>unspecified</u> thigh

M85.16- Skeletal fluorosis, <u>lower leg</u>
- M85.161   Skeletal fluorosis, <u>right</u> lower leg
- M85.162   Skeletal fluorosis, <u>left</u> lower leg
- M85.169   Skeletal fluorosis, <u>unspecified</u> lower leg

M85.17- Skeletal fluorosis, <u>ankle and foot</u>
- M85.171   Skeletal fluorosis, <u>right</u> ankle and foot
- M85.172   Skeletal fluorosis, <u>left</u> ankle and foot
- M85.179   Skeletal fluorosis, <u>unspecified</u> ankle and foot

M85.18 Skeletal fluorosis, <u>other site</u>
M85.19 Skeletal fluorosis, <u>multiple sites</u>

M85.2 Hyperostosis of skull — The abnormal formation of new bone on the inner side of the cranial bones.

M85.3- <u>Osteitis condensans</u> — Inflammation of the bone with the marrow cavity filled with osseous tissue.

M85.30 Osteitis condensans, <u>unspecified</u> <u>site</u>
M85.31- Osteitis condensans, shoulder
- M85.311   Osteitis condensans, <u>right</u> shoulder
- M85.312   Osteitis condensans, <u>left</u> shoulder
- M85.319   Osteitis condensans, <u>unspecified</u> shoulder

M85.32- Osteitis condensans, <u>upper arm</u>
- M85.321   Osteitis condensans, <u>right</u> upper arm
- M85.322   Osteitis condensans, <u>left</u> upper arm
- M85.329   Osteitis condensans, <u>unspecified</u> upper arm

M85.33- Osteitis condensans, <u>forearm</u>
- M85.331   Osteitis condensans, <u>right</u> forearm
- M85.332   Osteitis condensans, <u>left</u> forearm
- M85.339   Osteitis condensans, <u>unspecified</u> forearm

M85.34- Osteitis condensans, <u>hand</u>
- M85.341   Osteitis condensans, <u>right</u> hand
- M85.342   Osteitis condensans, <u>left</u> hand
- M85.349   Osteitis condensans, <u>unspecified</u> hand

M85.35- Osteitis condensans, <u>thigh</u>
- M85.351   Osteitis condensans, <u>right</u> thigh
- M85.352   Osteitis condensans, <u>left</u> thigh
- M85.359   Osteitis condensans, <u>unspecified</u> thigh

M85.36- Osteitis condensans, <u>lower leg</u>
- M85.361   Osteitis condensans, <u>right</u> lower leg
- M85.362   Osteitis condensans, <u>left</u> lower leg
- M85.369   Osteitis condensans, <u>unspecified</u> lower leg

M85.37- Osteitis condensans, <u>ankle and foot</u>
- M85.371   Osteitis condensans, <u>right</u> ankle and foot
- M85.372   Osteitis condensans, <u>left</u> ankle and foot
- M85.379   Osteitis condensans, <u>unspecified</u> ankle and foot

M85.38 Osteitis condensans, <u>other site</u>
M85.39 Osteitis condensans, <u>multiple sites</u>

M85.4- <u>Solitary bone cyst</u> — An encapsulated space within bone tissue usually occurring in the metaphyses of long bones of children and adolescents.
    Excludes ❷: *solitary cyst of jaw (M27.4)*

M85.40 Solitary bone cyst, <u>unspecified</u> <u>site</u>
M85.41- Solitary bone cyst, <u>shoulder</u>
- M85.411   Solitary bone cyst, <u>right</u> shoulder
- M85.412   Solitary bone cyst, <u>left</u> shoulder
- M85.419   Solitary bone cyst, <u>unspecified</u> shoulder

M85.42- Solitary bone cyst, <u>humerus</u>
- M85.421   Solitary bone cyst, <u>right</u> humerus
- M85.422   Solitary bone cyst, <u>left</u> humerus
- M85.429   Solitary bone cyst, <u>unspecified</u> humerus

M85.43- Solitary bone cyst, <u>ulna and radius</u>
- M85.431   Solitary bone cyst, <u>right</u> ulna and radius
- M85.432   Solitary bone cyst, <u>left</u> ulna and radius
- M85.439   Solitary bone cyst, <u>unspecified</u> ulna and radius

M85.44- Solitary bone cyst, <u>hand</u>
- M85.441   Solitary bone cyst, <u>right</u> hand
- M85.442   Solitary bone cyst, <u>left</u> hand
- M85.449   Solitary bone cyst, <u>unspecified</u> hand

M85.45- Solitary bone cyst, <u>pelvis</u>
- M85.451   Solitary bone cyst, <u>right</u> pelvis
- M85.452   Solitary bone cyst, <u>left</u> pelvis
- M85.459   Solitary bone cyst, <u>unspecified</u> pelvis

M85.46- Solitary bone cyst, <u>tibia and fibula</u>
- M85.461   Solitary bone cyst, <u>right</u> tibia and fibula
- M85.462   Solitary bone cyst, <u>left</u> tibia and fibula
- M85.469   Solitary bone cyst, <u>unspecified</u> tibia and fibula

M85.47- Solitary bone cyst, <u>ankle and foot</u>
- M85.471   Solitary bone cyst, <u>right</u> ankle and foot
- M85.472   Solitary bone cyst, <u>left</u> ankle and foot
- M85.479   Solitary bone cyst, <u>unspecified</u> ankle and foot

M 8 5 - M 8 5

M85.48 Solitary bone cyst, <u>other site</u>

M85.5- Aneurysmal bone cyst — A form producing a bulge in the bone cortex and appearing similar to an aneurysm.
    Excludes ❷: aneurysmal cyst of jaw (M27.4)

M85.50 Aneurysmal bone cyst, <u>unspecified</u> <u>site</u>

M85.51-Aneurysmal bone cyst, <u>shoulder</u>
  M85.511 Aneurysmal bone cyst, <u>right</u> shoulder
  M85.512 Aneurysmal bone cyst, <u>left</u> shoulder
  M85.519 Aneurysmal bone cyst, <u>unspecified</u> shoulder

M85.52-Aneurysmal bone cyst, <u>upper arm</u>
  M85.521 Aneurysmal bone cyst, <u>right</u> upper arm
  M85.522 Aneurysmal bone cyst, <u>left</u> upper arm
  M85.529 Aneurysmal bone cyst, <u>unspecified</u> upper arm

M85.53-Aneurysmal bone cyst, <u>forearm</u>
  M85.531 Aneurysmal bone cyst, <u>right</u> forearm
  M85.532 Aneurysmal bone cyst, <u>left</u> forearm
  M85.539 Aneurysmal bone cyst, <u>unspecified</u> forearm

M85.54-Aneurysmal bone cyst, <u>hand</u>
  M85.541 Aneurysmal bone cyst, <u>right</u> hand
  M85.542 Aneurysmal bone cyst, <u>left</u> hand
  M85.549 Aneurysmal bone cyst, <u>unspecified</u> hand

M85.55-Aneurysmal bone cyst, <u>thigh</u>
  M85.551 Aneurysmal bone cyst, <u>right</u> thigh
  M85.552 Aneurysmal bone cyst, <u>left</u> thigh
  M85.559 Aneurysmal bone cyst, <u>unspecified</u> thigh

M85.56-Aneurysmal bone cyst, <u>lower leg</u>
  M85.561 Aneurysmal bone cyst, <u>right</u> lower leg
  M85.562 Aneurysmal bone cyst, <u>left</u> lower leg
  M85.569 Aneurysmal bone cyst, <u>unspecified</u> lower leg

M85.57-Aneurysmal bone cyst, <u>ankle and foot</u>
  M85.571 Aneurysmal bone cyst, <u>right</u> ankle and foot
  M85.572 Aneurysmal bone cyst, <u>left</u> ankle and foot
  M85.579 Aneurysmal bone cyst, <u>unspecified</u> ankle and foot

M85.58 Aneurysmal bone cyst, <u>other site</u>

M85.59 Aneurysmal bone cyst, <u>multiple sites</u>

M85.6- <u>Other cyst</u> of bone
    Excludes 1: cyst of jaw NEC (M27.4)
       osteitis fibrosa cystica generalisata [von Recklinghausen's disease of bone] (E21.0)

M85.60 Other cyst of bone, <u>unspecified</u> site

M85.61-Other cyst of bone, <u>shoulder</u>
  M85.611 Other cyst of bone, <u>right</u> shoulder
  M85.612 Other cyst of bone, <u>left</u> shoulder
  M85.619 Other cyst of bone, <u>unspecified</u> shoulder

M85.62-Other cyst of bone, <u>upper arm</u>
  M85.621 Other cyst of bone, <u>right</u> upper arm
  M85.622 Other cyst of bone, <u>left</u> upper arm
  M85.629 Other cyst of bone, <u>unspecified</u> upper arm

M85.63-Other cyst of bone, <u>forearm</u>
  M85.631 Other cyst of bone, <u>right</u> forearm
  M85.632 Other cyst of bone, <u>left</u> forearm
  M85.639 Other cyst of bone, <u>unspecified</u> forearm

M85.64-Other cyst of bone, <u>hand</u>
  M85.641 Other cyst of bone, <u>right</u> hand
  M85.642 Other cyst of bone, <u>left</u> hand
  M85.649 Other cyst of bone, <u>unspecified</u> hand

M85.65-Other cyst of bone, <u>thigh</u>
  M85.651 Other cyst of bone, <u>right</u> thigh
  M85.652 Other cyst of bone, <u>left</u> thigh
  M85.659 Other cyst of bone, <u>unspecified</u> thigh

M85.66-Other cyst of bone, <u>lower leg</u>
  M85.661 Other cyst of bone, <u>right</u> lower leg
  M85.662 Other cyst of bone, <u>left</u> lower leg
  M85.669 Other cyst of bone, <u>unspecified</u> lower leg

M85.67-Other cyst of bone, <u>ankle and foot</u>
  M85.671 Other cyst of bone, <u>right</u> ankle and foot
  M85.672 Other cyst of bone, <u>left</u> ankle and foot
  M85.679 Other cyst of bone, <u>unspecified</u> ankle and foot

M85.68 Other cyst of bone, <u>other site</u>

M85.69 Other cyst of bone, <u>multiple sites</u>

M85.8- <u>Other specified</u> disorders of bone density and structure
    Hyperostosis of bones, except skull
    Osteosclerosis, acquired
    Excludes 1: diffuse idiopathic skeletal hyperostosis [DISH] (M48.1)
       osteosclerosis congenita (Q77.4)
       osteosclerosis fragilitas (generalista) (Q78.2)
       osteosclerosis myelofibrosis (D75.81)

M85.80 Other specified disorders of bone density and structure, <u>unspecified</u> <u>site</u>

M85.81-Other specified disorders of bone density and structure, <u>shoulder</u>
  M85.811 Other specified disorders of bone density and structure, <u>right</u> shoulder
  M85.812 Other specified disorders of bone density and structure, <u>left</u> shoulder
  M85.819 Other specified disorders of bone density and structure, <u>unspecified</u> shoulder

M85.82-Other specified disorders of bone density and structure, <u>upper arm</u>
  M85.821 Other specified disorders of bone density and structure, <u>right</u> upper arm
  M85.822 Other specified disorders of bone density and structure, <u>left</u> upper arm
  M85.829 Other specified disorders of bone density and structure, <u>unspecified</u> upper arm

M85.83-Other specified disorders of bone density and structure, <u>forearm</u>
  M85.831 Other specified disorders of bone density and structure, <u>right</u> forearm
  M85.832 Other specified disorders of bone density and structure, <u>left</u> forearm
  M85.839 Other specified disorders of bone density and structure, <u>unspecified</u> forearm

M85.84-Other specified disorders of bone density and structure, <u>hand</u>
  M85.841 Other specified disorders of bone density and structure, <u>right</u> hand
  M85.842 Other specified disorders of bone density and structure, <u>left</u> hand
  M85.849 Other specified disorders of bone density and structure, <u>unspecified</u> hand

M85.85-Other specified disorders of bone density and structure, <u>thigh</u>
  M85.851 Other specified disorders of bone density and structure, <u>right</u> thigh
  M85.852 Other specified disorders of bone density and structure, <u>left</u> thigh
  M85.859 Other specified disorders of bone density and structure, <u>unspecified</u> thigh

M85.86-Other specified disorders of bone density and structure, <u>lower leg</u>
  M85.861 Other specified disorders of bone density and structure, <u>right</u> lower leg
  M85.862 Other specified disorders of bone density and structure, <u>left</u> lower leg
  M85.869 Other specified disorders of bone density and structure, <u>unspecified</u> lower leg

M85.87-Other specified disorders of bone density and structure, <u>ankle and foot</u>
  M85.871 Other specified disorders of bone density and structure, <u>right</u> ankle and foot
  M85.872 Other specified disorders of bone density and structure, <u>left</u> ankle and foot

M85.879   Other specified disorders of bone density and structure, <u>unspecified</u> ankle and foot

M85.88   Other specified disorders of bone density and structure, <u>other site</u>

M85.89   Other specified disorders of bone density and structure, <u>multiple sites</u>

M85.9   Disorder of bone density and structure, <u>unspecified</u>

Other osteopathies (M86-M90)

Excludes 1:   *postprocedural osteopathies (M96.-)*

M86-   <u>Osteomyelitis</u> — Inflammation of the bone or bone marrow.
Use additional code (B95-B97) to identify infectious agent
Use additional code to identify major osseous defect, if applicable (M89.7-)
Excludes 1:   *osteomyelitis due to:*
            echinococcus (B67.2)
            gonococcus (A54.43)
            salmonella (A02.24)
Excludes ❷: *ostemyelitis of:*
            orbit (H05.0-)
            petrous bone (H70.2-)
            vertebra (M46.2-)

M86.0-   <u>Acute hematogenous</u> osteomyelitis — The sudden, severe onset of inflammation of the bone caused by microorganisms that invade through the bloodstream.

cc **M86.00** Acute hematogenous osteomyelitis, <u>unspecified</u> site

M86.01- Acute hematogenous osteomyelitis, <u>shoulder</u>

cc **M86.011**   Acute hematogenous osteomyelitis, <u>right</u> shoulder

cc **M86.012**   Acute hematogenous osteomyelitis, <u>left</u> shoulder

cc **M86.019**   Acute hematogenous osteomyelitis, <u>unspecified</u> shoulder

M86.02- Acute hematogenous osteomyelitis, <u>humerus</u>

cc **M86.021**   Acute hematogenous osteomyelitis, <u>right</u> humerus

cc **M86.022**   Acute hematogenous osteomyelitis, <u>left</u> humerus

cc **M86.029**   Acute hematogenous osteomyelitis, <u>unspecified</u> humerus

M86.03- Acute hematogenous osteomyelitis, <u>radius and ulna</u>

cc **M86.031**   Acute hematogenous osteomyelitis, <u>right</u> radius and ulna

cc **M86.032**   Acute hematogenous osteomyelitis, <u>left</u> radius and ulna

cc **M86.039**   Acute hematogenous osteomyelitis, <u>unspecified</u> radius and ulna

M86.04- Acute hematogenous osteomyelitis, <u>hand</u>

cc **M86.041**   Acute hematogenous osteomyelitis, <u>right</u> hand

cc **M86.042**   Acute hematogenous osteomyelitis, <u>left</u> hand

cc **M86.049**   Acute hematogenous osteomyelitis, <u>unspecified</u> hand

M86.05- Acute hematogenous osteomyelitis, <u>femur</u>

cc **M86.051**   Acute hematogenous osteomyelitis, <u>right</u> femur

cc **M86.052**   Acute hematogenous osteomyelitis, <u>left</u> femur

cc **M86.059**   Acute hematogenous osteomyelitis, <u>unspecified</u> femur

M86.06- Acute hematogenous osteomyelitis, <u>tibia and fibula</u>

cc **M86.061**   Acute hematogenous osteomyelitis, <u>right</u> tibia and fibula

cc **M86.062**   Acute hematogenous osteomyelitis, <u>left</u> tibia and fibula

cc **M86.069**   Acute hematogenous osteomyelitis, <u>unspecified</u> tibia and fibula

M86.07- Acute hematogenous osteomyelitis, <u>ankle and foot</u>

cc **M86.071**   Acute hematogenous osteomyelitis, <u>right</u> ankle and foot

cc **M86.072**   Acute hematogenous osteomyelitis, <u>left</u> ankle and foot

cc **M86.079**   Acute hematogenous osteomyelitis, <u>unspecified</u> ankle and foot

cc **M86.08** Acute hematogenous osteomyelitis, <u>other sites</u>

cc **M86.09** Acute hematogenous osteomyelitis, <u>multiple sites</u>

M86.1-   <u>Other acute</u> osteomyelitis

cc **M86.10** Other acute osteomyelitis, <u>unspecified</u> <u>site</u>

M86.11- Other acute osteomyelitis, <u>shoulder</u>

cc **M86.111**   Other acute osteomyelitis, <u>right</u> shoulder

cc **M86.112**   Other acute osteomyelitis, <u>left</u> shoulder

cc **M86.119**   Other acute osteomyelitis, <u>unspecified</u> shoulder

M86.12- Other acute osteomyelitis, <u>humerus</u>

cc **M86.121**   Other acute osteomyelitis, <u>right</u> humerus

cc **M86.122**   Other acute osteomyelitis, <u>left</u> humerus

cc **M86.129**   Other acute osteomyelitis, <u>unspecified</u> humerus

M86.13- Other acute osteomyelitis, <u>radius and ulna</u>

cc **M86.131**   Other acute osteomyelitis, <u>right</u> radius and ulna

cc **M86.132**   Other acute osteomyelitis, <u>left</u> radius and ulna

cc **M86.139**   Other acute osteomyelitis, <u>unspecified</u> radius and ulna

M86.14- Other acute osteomyelitis, <u>hand</u>

cc **M86.141**   Other acute osteomyelitis, <u>right</u> hand

cc **M86.142**   Other acute osteomyelitis, <u>left</u> hand

cc **M86.149**   Other acute osteomyelitis, <u>unspecified</u> hand

M86.15- Other acute osteomyelitis, <u>femur</u>

cc **M86.151**   Other acute osteomyelitis, <u>right</u> femur

cc **M86.152**   Other acute osteomyelitis, <u>left</u> femur

cc **M86.159**   Other acute osteomyelitis, <u>unspecified</u> femur

M86.16- Other acute osteomyelitis, <u>tibia and fibula</u>

cc **M86.161**   Other acute osteomyelitis, <u>right</u> tibia and fibula

cc **M86.162**   Other acute osteomyelitis, <u>left</u> tibia and fibula

cc **M86.169**   Other acute osteomyelitis, <u>unspecified</u> tibia and fibula

M86.17- Other acute osteomyelitis, <u>ankle and foot</u>

cc **M86.171**   Other acute osteomyelitis, <u>right</u> ankle and foot

cc **M86.172**   Other acute osteomyelitis, <u>left</u> ankle and foot

cc **M86.179**   Other acute osteomyelitis, <u>unspecified</u> ankle and foot

cc **M86.18** Other acute osteomyelitis, <u>other site</u>

cc **M86.19** Other acute osteomyelitis, <u>multiple sites</u>

M86.2-   <u>Subacute</u> osteomyelitis

cc **M86.20** Subacute osteomyelitis, <u>unspecified</u> site

M86.21- Subacute osteomyelitis, <u>shoulder</u>

cc **M86.211**   Subacute osteomyelitis, <u>right</u> shoulder

cc **M86.212**   Subacute osteomyelitis, <u>left</u> shoulder

cc **M86.219**   Subacute osteomyelitis, <u>unspecified</u> shoulder

M86.22- Subacute osteomyelitis, <u>humerus</u>

cc **M86.221**   Subacute osteomyelitis, <u>right</u> humerus

cc **M86.222**   Subacute osteomyelitis, <u>left</u> humerus

cc **M86.229**   Subacute osteomyelitis, <u>unspecified</u> humerus

M86.23- Subacute osteomyelitis, <u>radius and ulna</u>

cc **M86.231**   Subacute osteomyelitis, <u>right</u> radius and ulna

cc **M86.232**   Subacute osteomyelitis, <u>left</u> radius and ulna

cc **M86.239**   Subacute osteomyelitis, <u>unspecified</u> radius and ulna

M86.24- Subacute osteomyelitis, <u>hand</u>

cc **M86.241**   Subacute osteomyelitis, <u>right</u> hand

cc **M86.242**   Subacute osteomyelitis, <u>left</u> hand

cc **M86.249**   Subacute osteomyelitis, <u>unspecified</u> hand

M86.25- Subacute osteomyelitis, <u>femur</u>

cc **M86.251**   Subacute osteomyelitis, <u>right</u> femur

cc **M86.252**   Subacute osteomyelitis, <u>left</u> femur

cc **M86.259**   Subacute osteomyelitis, <u>unspecified</u> femur

M86.26- Subacute osteomyelitis, <u>tibia and fibula</u>

cc **M86.261**   Subacute osteomyelitis, <u>right</u> tibia and fibula

cc **M86.262**   Subacute osteomyelitis, <u>left</u> tibia and fibula

cc **M86.269**   Subacute osteomyelitis, <u>unspecified</u> tibia and fibula

M86.27- Subacute osteomyelitis, <u>ankle and foot</u>

cc **M86.271**   Subacute osteomyelitis, <u>right</u> ankle and foot cc **M86.272** Subacute osteomyelitis, <u>left</u> ankle and foot

cc **M86.279** Subacute osteomyelitis, <u>unspecified</u> ankle and foot

cc **M86.28** Subacute osteomyelitis, <u>other site</u>

cc **M86.29** Subacute osteomyelitis, <u>multiple sites</u>

M86.3- <u>Chronic multifocal</u> osteomyelitis — An autoinflammatory recurrent disease of the bone that is characterized by inflammation, bone lesions, periodic fevers, and bone pain.

cc **M86.30** Chronic multifocal osteomyelitis, <u>unspecified site</u>

M86.31- Chronic multifocal osteomyelitis, <u>shoulder</u>

cc **M86.311** Chronic multifocal osteomyelitis, <u>right</u> shoulder

cc **M86.312** Chronic multifocal osteomyelitis, <u>left</u> shoulder

cc **M86.319** Chronic multifocal osteomyelitis, <u>unspecified</u> shoulder

M86.32- Chronic multifocal osteomyelitis, <u>humerus</u>

cc **M86.321** Chronic multifocal osteomyelitis, <u>right</u> humerus

cc **M86.322** Chronic multifocal osteomyelitis, <u>left</u> humerus

cc **M86.329** Chronic multifocal osteomyelitis, <u>unspecified</u> humerus

M86.33- Chronic multifocal osteomyelitis, <u>radius and ulna</u>

cc **M86.331** Chronic multifocal osteomyelitis, <u>right</u> radius and ulna

cc **M86.332** Chronic multifocal osteomyelitis, <u>left</u> radius and ulna

cc **M86.339** Chronic multifocal osteomyelitis, <u>unspecified</u> radius and ulna

M86.34- Chronic multifocal osteomyelitis, <u>hand</u>

cc **M86.341** Chronic multifocal osteomyelitis, <u>right</u> hand

cc **M86.342** Chronic multifocal osteomyelitis, <u>left</u> hand

cc **M86.349** Chronic multifocal osteomyelitis, <u>unspecified</u> hand

M86.35- Chronic multifocal osteomyelitis, <u>femur</u>

cc **M86.351** Chronic multifocal osteomyelitis, <u>right</u> femur

cc **M86.352** Chronic multifocal osteomyelitis, <u>left</u> femur

cc **M86.359** Chronic multifocal osteomyelitis, <u>unspecified</u> femur

M86.36- Chronic multifocal osteomyelitis, <u>tibia and fibula</u>

cc **M86.361** Chronic multifocal osteomyelitis, <u>right</u> tibia and fibula

cc **M86.362** Chronic multifocal osteomyelitis, <u>left</u> tibia and fibula

cc **M86.369** Chronic multifocal osteomyelitis, <u>unspecified</u> tibia and fibula

M86.37- Chronic multifocal osteomyelitis, <u>ankle and foot</u>

cc **M86.371** Chronic multifocal osteomyelitis, <u>right</u> ankle and foot

cc **M86.372** Chronic multifocal osteomyelitis, <u>left</u> ankle and foot

cc **M86.379** Chronic multifocal osteomyelitis, <u>unspecified</u> ankle and foot

cc **M86.38** Chronic multifocal osteomyelitis, <u>other site</u>

cc **M86.39** Chronic multifocal osteomyelitis, <u>multiple sites</u>

M86.4- <u>Chronic</u> osteomyelitis <u>with draining sinus</u> — Inflammation of the bone caused by microorganisms that develops slowly and persists over a long period of time and creates a suppuration passage to the skin or other tissues.

cc **M86.40** Chronic osteomyelitis with draining sinus, <u>unspecified site</u>

M86.41- Chronic osteomyelitis with draining sinus, <u>shoulder</u>

cc **M86.411** Chronic osteomyelitis with draining sinus, <u>right</u> shoulder

cc **M86.412** Chronic osteomyelitis with draining sinus, <u>left</u> shoulder

cc **M86.419** Chronic osteomyelitis with draining sinus, <u>unspecified</u> shoulder

M86.42- Chronic osteomyelitis with draining sinus, <u>humerus</u>

cc **M86.421** Chronic osteomyelitis with draining sinus, <u>right</u> humerus

cc **M86.422** Chronic osteomyelitis with draining sinus, <u>left</u> humerus

cc **M86.429** Chronic osteomyelitis with draining sinus, <u>unspecified</u> humerus

M86.43- Chronic osteomyelitis with draining sinus, <u>radius and ulna</u>

cc **M86.431** Chronic osteomyelitis with draining sinus, <u>right</u> radius and ulna

cc **M86.432** Chronic osteomyelitis with draining sinus, <u>left</u> radius and ulna

cc **M86.439** Chronic osteomyelitis with draining sinus, <u>unspecified</u> radius and ulna

M86.44- Chronic osteomyelitis with draining sinus, <u>hand</u>

cc **M86.441** Chronic osteomyelitis with draining sinus, <u>right</u> hand

cc **M86.442** Chronic osteomyelitis with draining sinus, <u>left</u> hand

cc **M86.449** Chronic osteomyelitis with draining sinus, <u>unspecified</u> hand

M86.45- Chronic osteomyelitis with draining sinus, <u>femur</u>

cc **M86.451** Chronic osteomyelitis with draining sinus, <u>right</u> femur

cc **M86.452** Chronic osteomyelitis with draining sinus, <u>left</u> femur

cc **M86.459** Chronic osteomyelitis with draining sinus, <u>unspecified</u> femur

M86.46- Chronic osteomyelitis with draining sinus, <u>tibia and fibula</u>

cc **M86.461** Chronic osteomyelitis with draining sinus, <u>right</u> tibia and fibula

cc **M86.462** Chronic osteomyelitis with draining sinus, <u>left</u> tibia and fibula

cc **M86.469** Chronic osteomyelitis with draining sinus, <u>unspecified</u> tibia and fibula

M86.47- Chronic osteomyelitis with draining sinus, <u>ankle and foot</u>

cc **M86.471** Chronic osteomyelitis with draining sinus, <u>right</u> ankle and foot

cc **M86.472** Chronic osteomyelitis with draining sinus, <u>left</u> ankle and foot

cc **M86.479** Chronic osteomyelitis with draining sinus, <u>unspecified</u> ankle and foot

cc **M86.48** Chronic osteomyelitis with draining sinus, <u>other site</u>

cc **M86.49** Chronic osteomyelitis with draining sinus, <u>multiple sites</u>

M86.5- <u>Other chronic hematogenous</u> osteomyelitis — Inflammation of the bone caused by microorganisms that invade through the bloodstream and that develops slowly and persists over a long period of time.

cc **M86.50** Other chronic hematogenous osteomyelitis, <u>unspecified site</u>

M86.51- Other chronic hematogenous osteomyelitis, <u>shoulder</u>

cc **M86.511** Other chronic hematogenous osteomyelitis, <u>right</u> shoulder

cc **M86.512** Other chronic hematogenous osteomyelitis, <u>left</u> shoulder

cc **M86.519** Other chronic hematogenous osteomyelitis, <u>unspecified</u> shoulder

M86.52- Other chronic hematogenous osteomyelitis, <u>humerus</u>

cc **M86.521** Other chronic hematogenous osteomyelitis, <u>right</u> humerus

cc **M86.522** Other chronic hematogenous osteomyelitis, <u>left</u> humerus

cc **M86.529** Other chronic hematogenous osteomyelitis, <u>unspecified</u> humerus

M86.53- Other chronic hematogenous osteomyelitis, <u>radius and ulna</u>

cc **M86.531** Other chronic hematogenous osteomyelitis, <u>right</u> radius and ulna

cc **M86.532** Other chronic hematogenous osteomyelitis, <u>left</u> radius and ulna

cc **M86.539** Other chronic hematogenous osteomyelitis, <u>unspecified</u> radius and ulna

M86.54- Other chronic hematogenous osteomyelitis, <u>hand</u>

cc **M86.541** Other chronic hematogenous osteomyelitis, <u>right</u> hand

M86 — M86

cc **M86.542** Other chronic hematogenous osteomyelitis, <u>left</u> hand

cc **M86.549** Other chronic hematogenous osteomyelitis, <u>unspecified</u> hand

M86.55- Other chronic hematogenous osteomyelitis, <u>femur</u>

cc **M86.551** Other chronic hematogenous osteomyelitis, <u>right</u> femur

cc **M86.552** Other chronic hematogenous osteomyelitis, <u>left</u> femur

cc **M86.559** Other chronic hematogenous osteomyelitis, <u>unspecified</u> femur

M86.56- Other chronic hematogenous osteomyelitis, <u>tibia and fibula</u>

cc **M86.561** Other chronic hematogenous osteomyelitis, <u>right</u> tibia and fibula

cc **M86.562** Other chronic hematogenous osteomyelitis, <u>left</u> tibia and fibula

cc **M86.569** Other chronic hematogenous osteomyelitis, <u>unspecified</u> tibia and fibula

M86.57- Other chronic hematogenous osteomyelitis, <u>ankle and foot</u>

cc **M86.571** Other chronic hematogenous osteomyelitis, <u>right</u> ankle and foot

cc **M86.572** Other chronic hematogenous osteomyelitis, <u>left</u> ankle and foot

cc **M86.579** Other chronic hematogenous osteomyelitis, <u>unspecified</u> ankle and foot

cc **M86.58** Other chronic hematogenous osteomyelitis, <u>other site</u>

cc **M86.59** Other chronic hematogenous osteomyelitis, <u>multiple sites</u>

M86.6- <u>Other chronic</u> osteomyelitis

cc **M86.60** Other chronic osteomyelitis, <u>unspecified</u> site

M86.61- Other chronic osteomyelitis, <u>shoulder</u>

cc **M86.611** Other chronic osteomyelitis, <u>right</u> shoulder

cc **M86.612** Other chronic osteomyelitis, <u>left</u> shoulder

cc **M86.619** Other chronic osteomyelitis, <u>unspecified</u> shoulder

M86.62- Other chronic osteomyelitis, <u>humerus</u>

cc **M86.621** Other chronic osteomyelitis, <u>right</u> humerus

cc **M86.622** Other chronic osteomyelitis, <u>left</u> humerus

cc **M86.629** Other chronic osteomyelitis, <u>unspecified</u> humerus

M86.63- Other chronic osteomyelitis, <u>radius and ulna</u>

cc **M86.631** Other chronic osteomyelitis, <u>right</u> radius and ulna

cc **M86.632** Other chronic osteomyelitis, <u>left</u> radius and ulna

cc **M86.639** Other chronic osteomyelitis, <u>unspecified</u> radius and ulna

M86.64- Other chronic osteomyelitis, <u>hand</u>

cc **M86.641** Other chronic osteomyelitis, <u>right</u> hand

cc **M86.642** Other chronic osteomyelitis, <u>left</u> hand

cc **M86.649** Other chronic osteomyelitis, <u>unspecified</u> hand

M86.65- Other chronic osteomyelitis, <u>thigh</u>

cc **M86.651** Other chronic osteomyelitis, <u>right</u> thigh

cc **M86.652** Other chronic osteomyelitis, <u>left</u> thigh

cc **M86.659** Other chronic osteomyelitis, <u>unspecified</u> thigh

M86.66- Other chronic osteomyelitis, <u>tibia and fibula</u>

cc **M86.661** Other chronic osteomyelitis, <u>right</u> tibia and fibula

cc **M86.662** Other chronic osteomyelitis, <u>left</u> tibia and fibula

cc **M86.669** Other chronic osteomyelitis, <u>unspecified</u> tibia and fibula

M86.67- Other chronic osteomyelitis, <u>ankle and foot</u>

cc **M86.671** Other chronic osteomyelitis, <u>right</u> ankle and foot

cc **M86.672** Other chronic osteomyelitis, <u>left</u> ankle and foot

cc **M86.679** Other chronic osteomyelitis, <u>unspecified</u> ankle and foot

cc **M86.68** Other chronic osteomyelitis, <u>other site</u>

cc **M86.69** Other chronic osteomyelitis, <u>multiple sites</u>

M86.8- Other osteomyelitis

   Brodie's abscess — A localized necrosis of bone.

M86.8x- <u>Other</u> osteomyelitis

cc **M86.8x0** Other osteomyelitis, multiple sites

cc **M86.8x1** Other osteomyelitis, shoulder

cc **M86.8x2** Other osteomyelitis, upper arm

cc **M86.8x3** Other osteomyelitis, forearm

cc **M86.8x4** Other osteomyelitis, hand

cc **M86.8x5** Other osteomyelitis, thigh

cc **M86.8x6** Other osteomyelitis, lower leg

cc **M86.8x7** Other osteomyelitis, ankle and foot

cc **M86.8x8** Other osteomyelitis, other site

cc **M86.8x9** Other osteomyelitis, unspecified sites

cc **M86.9** Osteomyelitis, <u>unspecified</u>

   Infection of bone NOS

   Periostitis without osteomyelitis

M87- <u>Osteonecrosis</u> — The condition of progressive sclerosis and death of bone tissue that is due to decreased blood flow to the bone.

   Includes: Avascular necrosis of bone

   Use additional code to identify major osseous defect, if applicable (M89.7-)

   Excludes 1:   *juvenile osteonecrosis (M91-M92)*

         osteochondropathies (M90-M93)

M87.0- <u>Idiopathic aseptic necrosis of bone</u> — A form of unknown etiology.

cc **M87.00** Idiopathic aseptic necrosis of <u>unspecified</u> bone

M87.01- Idiopathic aseptic necrosis of <u>shoulder</u>

   Idiopathic aseptic necrosis of clavicle and scapula

cc **M87.011** Idiopathic aseptic necrosis of <u>right</u> shoulder

cc **M87.012** Idiopathic aseptic necrosis of <u>left</u> shoulder

cc **M87.019** Idiopathic aseptic necrosis of <u>unspecified</u> shoulder

M87.02- Idiopathic aseptic necrosis of <u>humerus</u>

cc **M87.021** Idiopathic aseptic necrosis of <u>right</u> humerus

cc **M87.022** Idiopathic aseptic necrosis of <u>left</u> humerus

cc **M87.029** Idiopathic aseptic necrosis of <u>unspecified</u> humerus

M87.03- Idiopathic aseptic necrosis of <u>radius, ulna and carpus</u>

cc **M87.031** Idiopathic aseptic necrosis of <u>right</u> radius

cc **M87.032** Idiopathic aseptic necrosis of <u>left</u> radius

cc **M87.033** Idiopathic aseptic necrosis of <u>unspecified</u> radius

cc **M87.034** Idiopathic aseptic necrosis of <u>right</u> ulna

cc **M87.035** Idiopathic aseptic necrosis of <u>left</u> ulna

cc **M87.036** Idiopathic aseptic necrosis of <u>unspecified</u> ulna

cc **M87.037** Idiopathic aseptic necrosis of <u>right</u> carpus

cc **M87.038** Idiopathic aseptic necrosis of <u>left</u> carpus

cc **M87.039** Idiopathic aseptic necrosis of <u>unspecified</u> carpus

M87.04- Idiopathic aseptic necrosis of <u>hand and fingers</u>

   Idiopathic aseptic necrosis of metacarpals and phalanges of hands

cc **M87.041** Idiopathic aseptic necrosis of <u>right</u> hand

cc **M87.042** Idiopathic aseptic necrosis of <u>left</u> hand

cc **M87.043** Idiopathic aseptic necrosis of <u>unspecified</u> hand

cc **M87.044** Idiopathic aseptic necrosis of <u>right</u> finger(s)

cc **M87.045** Idiopathic aseptic necrosis of <u>left</u> finger(s)

cc **M87.046** Idiopathic aseptic necrosis of <u>unspecified</u> finger(s)

M87.05- Idiopathic aseptic necrosis of <u>pelvis and femur</u>

cc **M87.050** Idiopathic aseptic necrosis of pelvis

cc **M87.051** Idiopathic aseptic necrosis of <u>right</u> femur

cc **M87.052** Idiopathic aseptic necrosis of <u>left</u> femur

cc **M87.059** Idiopathic aseptic necrosis of <u>unspecified</u> femur

   Idiopathic aseptic necrosis of hip NOS

M87.06- Idiopathic aseptic necrosis of <u>tibia and fibula</u>

cc **M87.061** Idiopathic aseptic necrosis of <u>right</u> tibia

cc **M87.062** Idiopathic aseptic necrosis of <u>left</u> tibia

cc **M87.063** Idiopathic aseptic necrosis of <u>unspecified</u> tibia

cc **M87.064** Idiopathic aseptic necrosis of <u>right</u> fibula

cc **M87.065** Idiopathic aseptic necrosis of <u>left</u> fibula

cc **M87.066** Idiopathic aseptic necrosis of <u>unspecified</u> fibula

M 8 6 - M 8 7

M87.07-Idiopathic aseptic necrosis of ankle, foot and toes
Idiopathic aseptic necrosis of metatarsus, tarsus, and phalanges of toes
- cc M87.071 Idiopathic aseptic necrosis of right ankle
- cc M87.072 Idiopathic aseptic necrosis of left ankle
- cc M87.073 Idiopathic aseptic necrosis of unspecified ankle
- cc M87.074 Idiopathic aseptic necrosis of right foot
- cc M87.075 Idiopathic aseptic necrosis of left foot
- cc M87.076 Idiopathic aseptic necrosis of unspecified foot
- cc M87.077 Idiopathic aseptic necrosis of right toe(s)
- cc M87.078 Idiopathic aseptic necrosis of left toe(s)
- cc M87.079 Idiopathic aseptic necrosis of unspecified toe(s)
- cc M87.08 Idiopathic aseptic necrosis of bone, other site
- cc M87.09 Idiopathic aseptic necrosis of bone, multiple sites

M87.1- Osteonecrosis due to drugs
Use additional code for adverse effect, if applicable, to identify drug (T36-T50 with fifth or sixth character 5)
- cc M87.10 Osteonecrosis due to drugs, unspecified bone

M87.11-Osteonecrosis due to drugs, shoulder
- cc M87.111 Osteonecrosis due to drugs, right shoulder
- cc M87.112 Osteonecrosis due to drugs, left shoulder
- cc M87.119 Osteonecrosis due to drugs, unspecified shoulder

M87.12-Osteonecrosis due to drugs, humerus
- cc M87.121 Osteonecrosis due to drugs, right humerus
- cc M87.122 Osteonecrosis due to drugs, left humerus
- cc M87.129 Osteonecrosis due to drugs, unspecified humerus

M87.13-Osteonecrosis due to drugs of radius, ulna and carpus
- cc M87.131 Osteonecrosis due to drugs of right radius
- cc M87.132 Osteonecrosis due to drugs of left radius
- cc M87.133 Osteonecrosis due to drugs of unspecified radius
- cc M87.134 Osteonecrosis due to drugs of right ulna
- cc M87.135 Osteonecrosis due to drugs of left ulna
- cc M87.136 Osteonecrosis due to drugs of unspecified ulna
- cc M87.137 Osteonecrosis due to drugs of right carpus
- cc M87.138 Osteonecrosis due to drugs of left carpus
- cc M87.139 Osteonecrosis due to drugs of unspecified carpus

M87.14-Osteonecrosis due to drugs, hand and fingers
- cc M87.141 Osteonecrosis due to drugs, right hand
- cc M87.142 Osteonecrosis due to drugs, left hand
- cc M87.143 Osteonecrosis due to drugs, unspecified hand
- cc M87.144 Osteonecrosis due to drugs, right finger(s)
- cc M87.145 Osteonecrosis due to drugs, left finger(s)
- cc M87.146 Osteonecrosis due to drugs, unspecified finger(s)

M87.15-Osteonecrosis due to drugs, pelvis and femur
- cc M87.150 Osteonecrosis due to drugs, pelvis
- cc M87.151 Osteonecrosis due to drugs, right femur
- cc M87.152 Osteonecrosis due to drugs, left femur
- cc M87.159 Osteonecrosis due to drugs, unspecified femur

M87.16-Osteonecrosis due to drugs, tibia and fibula
- cc M87.161 Osteonecrosis due to drugs, right tibia
- cc M87.162 Osteonecrosis due to drugs, left tibia
- cc M87.163 Osteonecrosis due to drugs, unspecified tibia
- cc M87.164 Osteonecrosis due to drugs, right fibula
- cc M87.165 Osteonecrosis due to drugs, left fibula
- cc M87.166 Osteonecrosis due to drugs, unspecified fibula

M87.17-Osteonecrosis due to drugs, ankle, foot and toes
- cc M87.171 Osteonecrosis due to drugs, right ankle
- cc M87.172 Osteonecrosis due to drugs, left ankle
- cc M87.173 Osteonecrosis due to drugs, unspecified ankle
- cc M87.174 Osteonecrosis due to drugs, right foot
- cc M87.175 Osteonecrosis due to drugs, left foot
- cc M87.176 Osteonecrosis due to drugs, unspecified foot
- cc M87.177 Osteonecrosis due to drugs, right toe(s)
- cc M87.178 Osteonecrosis due to drugs, left toe(s)
- cc M87.179 Osteonecrosis due to drugs, unspecified toe(s)

M87.18-Osteonecrosis due to drugs, other site
- cc M87.180 Osteonecrosis due to drugs, jaw
- cc M87.188 Osteonecrosis due to drugs, other site
- cc M87.19 Osteonecrosis due to drugs, multiple sites

M87.2- Osteonecrosis due to previous trauma
- cc M87.20 Osteonecrosis due to previous trauma, unspecified bone

M87.21-Osteonecrosis due to previous trauma, shoulder
- cc M87.211 Osteonecrosis due to previous trauma, right shoulder
- cc M87.212 Osteonecrosis due to previous trauma, left shoulder
- cc M87.219 Osteonecrosis due to previous trauma, unspecified shoulder

M87.22-Osteonecrosis due to previous trauma, humerus
- cc M87.221 Osteonecrosis due to previous trauma, right humerus
- cc M87.222 Osteonecrosis due to previous trauma, left humerus
- cc M87.229 Osteonecrosis due to previous trauma, unspecified humerus

M87.23-Osteonecrosis due to previous trauma of radius, ulna and carpus
- cc M87.231 Osteonecrosis due to previous trauma of right radius
- cc M87.232 Osteonecrosis due to previous trauma of left radius
- cc M87.233 Osteonecrosis due to previous trauma of unspecified radius
- cc M87.234 Osteonecrosis due to previous trauma of right ulna
- cc M87.235 Osteonecrosis due to previous trauma of left ulna
- cc M87.236 Osteonecrosis due to previous trauma of unspecified ulna
- cc M87.237 Osteonecrosis due to previous trauma of right carpus
- cc M87.238 Osteonecrosis due to previous trauma of left carpus
- cc M87.239 Osteonecrosis due to previous trauma of unspecified carpus

M87.24-Osteonecrosis due to previous trauma, hand and fingers
- cc M87.241 Osteonecrosis due to previous trauma, right hand
- cc M87.242 Osteonecrosis due to previous trauma, left hand
- cc M87.243 Osteonecrosis due to previous trauma, unspecified hand
- cc M87.244 Osteonecrosis due to previous trauma, right finger(s)
- cc M87.245 Osteonecrosis due to previous trauma, left finger(s)
- cc M87.246 Osteonecrosis due to previous trauma, unspecified finger(s)

M87.25-Osteonecrosis due to previous trauma, pelvis and femur
- cc M87.250 Osteonecrosis due to previous trauma, pelvis
- cc M87.251 Osteonecrosis due to previous trauma, right femur
- cc M87.252 Osteonecrosis due to previous trauma, left femur
- cc M87.256 Osteonecrosis due to previous trauma, unspecified femur

M87.26-Osteonecrosis due to previous trauma, tibia and fibula
- cc M87.261 Osteonecrosis due to previous trauma, right tibia
- cc M87.262 Osteonecrosis due to previous trauma, left tibia
- cc M87.263 Osteonecrosis due to previous trauma, unspecified tibia
- cc M87.264 Osteonecrosis due to previous trauma, right fibula
- cc M87.265 Osteonecrosis due to previous trauma, left fibula
- cc M87.266 Osteonecrosis due to previous trauma, unspecified fibula

M87.27-Osteonecrosis due to previous trauma, ankle, foot and toes
- cc M87.271 Osteonecrosis due to previous trauma, right ankle
- cc M87.272 Osteonecrosis due to previous trauma, left ankle
- cc M87.273 Osteonecrosis due to previous trauma, unspecified ankle
- cc M87.274 Osteonecrosis due to previous trauma, right foot

cc **M87.275** Osteonecrosis due to previous trauma, <u>left</u> foot

cc **M87.276** Osteonecrosis due to previous trauma, <u>unspecified</u> foot

cc **M87.277** Osteonecrosis due to previous trauma, <u>right</u> toe(s)

cc **M87.278** Osteonecrosis due to previous trauma, <u>left</u> toe(s)

cc **M87.279** Osteonecrosis due to previous trauma, <u>unspecified</u> toe(s)

cc **M87.28** Osteonecrosis due to previous trauma, <u>other site</u>

cc **M87.29** Osteonecrosis due to previous trauma, <u>multiple sites</u>

M87.3- <u>Other secondary</u> osteonecrosis

cc **M87.30** Other secondary osteonecrosis, <u>unspecified</u> <u>bone</u>

M87.31- Other secondary osteonecrosis, <u>shoulder</u>

cc **M87.311** Other secondary osteonecrosis, <u>right</u> shoulder

cc **M87.312** Other secondary osteonecrosis, <u>left</u> shoulder

cc **M87.319** Other secondary osteonecrosis, <u>unspecified</u> shoulder

M87.32- Other secondary osteonecrosis, <u>humerus</u>

cc **M87.321** Other secondary osteonecrosis, <u>right</u> humerus

cc **M87.322** Other secondary osteonecrosis, <u>left</u> humerus

cc **M87.329** Other secondary osteonecrosis, <u>unspecified</u> humerus

M87.33- Other secondary osteonecrosis of <u>radius, ulna and carpus</u>

cc **M87.331** Other secondary osteonecrosis of <u>right</u> radius

cc **M87.332** Other secondary osteonecrosis of <u>left</u> radius

cc **M87.333** Other secondary osteonecrosis of <u>unspecified</u> radius

cc **M87.334** Other secondary osteonecrosis of <u>right</u> ulna

cc **M87.335** Other secondary osteonecrosis of <u>left</u> ulna

cc **M87.336** Other secondary osteonecrosis of <u>unspecified</u> ulna

cc **M87.337** Other secondary osteonecrosis of <u>right</u> carpus

cc **M87.338** Other secondary osteonecrosis of <u>left</u> carpus

cc **M87.339** Other secondary osteonecrosis of <u>unspecified</u> carpus

M87.34- Other secondary osteonecrosis, <u>hand and fingers</u>

cc **M87.341** Other secondary osteonecrosis, <u>right</u> hand

cc **M87.342** Other secondary osteonecrosis, <u>left</u> hand

cc **M87.343** Other secondary osteonecrosis, <u>unspecified</u> hand

cc **M87.344** Other secondary osteonecrosis, <u>right</u> finger(s)

cc **M87.345** Other secondary osteonecrosis, <u>left</u> finger(s)

cc **M87.346** Other secondary osteonecrosis, <u>unspecified</u> finger(s)

M87.35- Other secondary osteonecrosis, <u>pelvis and femur</u>

cc **M87.350** Other secondary osteonecrosis, pelvis

cc **M87.351** Other secondary osteonecrosis, <u>right</u> femur

cc **M87.352** Other secondary osteonecrosis, <u>left</u> femur

cc **M87.353** Other secondary osteonecrosis, <u>unspecified</u> femur

M87.36- Other secondary osteonecrosis, <u>tibia and fibula</u>

cc **M87.361** Other secondary osteonecrosis, <u>right</u> tibia

cc **M87.362** Other secondary osteonecrosis, <u>left</u> tibia

cc **M87.363** Other secondary osteonecrosis, <u>unspecified</u> tibia

cc **M87.364** Other secondary osteonecrosis, <u>right</u> fibula

cc **M87.365** Other secondary osteonecrosis, <u>left</u> fibula

cc **M87.366** Other secondary osteonecrosis, <u>unspecified</u> fibula

M87.37- Other secondary osteonecrosis, <u>ankle and foot</u>

cc **M87.371** Other secondary osteonecrosis, <u>right</u> ankle

cc **M87.372** Other secondary osteonecrosis, <u>left</u> ankle

cc **M87.373** Other secondary osteonecrosis, <u>unspecified</u> ankle

cc **M87.374** Other secondary osteonecrosis, <u>right</u> foot

cc **M87.375** Other secondary osteonecrosis, <u>left</u> foot

cc **M87.376** Other secondary osteonecrosis, <u>unspecified</u> foot

cc **M87.377** Other secondary osteonecrosis, <u>right</u> toe(s)

cc **M87.378** Other secondary osteonecrosis, <u>left</u> toe(s)

cc **M87.379** Other secondary osteonecrosis, <u>unspecified</u> toe(s)

cc **M87.38** Other secondary osteonecrosis, <u>other site</u>

cc **M87.39** Other secondary osteonecrosis, <u>multiple sites</u>

M87.8- <u>Other</u> osteonecrosis

cc **M87.80** Other osteonecrosis, <u>unspecified</u> <u>bone</u>

M87.81- Other osteonecrosis, <u>shoulder</u>

cc **M87.811** Other osteonecrosis, <u>right</u> shoulder

cc **M87.812** Other osteonecrosis, <u>left</u> shoulder

cc **M87.819** Other osteonecrosis, <u>unspecified</u> shoulder

M87.82- Other osteonecrosis, <u>humerus</u>

cc **M87.821** Other osteonecrosis, <u>right</u> humerus

cc **M87.822** Other osteonecrosis, <u>left</u> humerus

cc **M87.829** Other osteonecrosis, <u>unspecified</u> humerus

M87.83- Other osteonecrosis of <u>radius, ulna and carpus</u>

cc **M87.831** Other osteonecrosis of <u>right</u> radius

cc **M87.832** Other osteonecrosis of <u>left</u> radius

cc **M87.833** Other osteonecrosis of <u>unspecified</u> radius

cc **M87.834** Other osteonecrosis of <u>right</u> ulna

cc **M87.835** Other osteonecrosis of <u>left</u> ulna

cc **M87.836** Other osteonecrosis of <u>unspecified</u> ulna

cc **M87.837** Other osteonecrosis of <u>right</u> carpus

cc **M87.838** Other osteonecrosis of <u>left</u> carpus

cc **M87.839** Other osteonecrosis of <u>unspecified</u> carpus

M87.84- Other osteonecrosis, <u>hand and fingers</u>

cc **M87.841** Other osteonecrosis, <u>right</u> hand

cc **M87.842** Other osteonecrosis, <u>left</u> hand

cc **M87.843** Other osteonecrosis, <u>unspecified</u> hand

cc **M87.844** Other osteonecrosis, <u>right</u> finger(s)

cc **M87.845** Other osteonecrosis, <u>left</u> finger(s)

cc **M87.849** Other osteonecrosis, <u>unspecified</u> finger(s)

M87.85- Other osteonecrosis, <u>pelvis and femur</u>

cc **M87.850** Other osteonecrosis, pelvis

cc **M87.851** Other osteonecrosis, <u>right</u> femur

cc **M87.852** Other osteonecrosis, <u>left</u> femur

cc **M87.859** Other osteonecrosis, <u>unspecified</u> femur

M87.86- Other osteonecrosis, <u>tibia and fibula</u>

cc **M87.861** Other osteonecrosis, <u>right</u> tibia

cc **M87.862** Other osteonecrosis, <u>left</u> tibia

cc **M87.863** Other osteonecrosis, <u>unspecified</u> tibia

cc **M87.864** Other osteonecrosis, <u>right</u> fibula

cc **M87.865** Other osteonecrosis, <u>left</u> fibula

cc **M87.869** Other osteonecrosis, <u>unspecified</u> fibula

M87.87- Other osteonecrosis, <u>ankle, foot and toes</u>

cc **M87.871** Other osteonecrosis, <u>right</u> ankle

cc **M87.872** Other osteonecrosis, <u>left</u> ankle

cc **M87.873** Other osteonecrosis, <u>unspecified</u> ankle

cc **M87.874** Other osteonecrosis, <u>right</u> foot

cc **M87.875** Other osteonecrosis, <u>left</u> foot

cc **M87.876** Other osteonecrosis, <u>unspecified</u> foot

cc **M87.877** Other osteonecrosis, <u>right</u> toe(s)

cc **M87.878** Other osteonecrosis, <u>left</u> toe(s)

cc **M87.879** Other osteonecrosis, <u>unspecified</u> toe(s)

cc **M87.88** Other osteonecrosis, <u>other site</u>

cc **M87.89** Other osteonecrosis, <u>multiple sites</u>

cc **M87.9** Osteonecrosis, <u>unspecified</u>
Necrosis of bone NOS

M88- <u>Osteitis deformans [Paget's disease of bone]</u> — Inflammation of the bone with softening and deformity, especially bowing of the long bones.

Excludes 1: *osteitis deformans in neoplastic disease (M90.6)*

M88.0 Osteitis deformans of <u>skull</u>

M88.1 Osteitis deformans of <u>vertebrae</u>

M88.8- Osteitis deformans of <u>other bones</u>

M88.81- Osteitis deformans of <u>shoulder</u>

M88.811 Osteitis deformans of <u>right</u> shoulder

M88.812 Osteitis deformans of <u>left</u> shoulder

M88.819 Osteitis deformans of <u>unspecified</u> shoulder

M 8 7 – M 8 8

Excludes 1: = NOT CODED HERE! (Do not code both)   Excludes ❷: = Not Included Here

M88.82- Osteitis deformans of <u>upper arm</u>
    M88.821 Osteitis deformans of <u>right</u> upper arm
    M88.822 Osteitis deformans of <u>left</u> upper arm
    M88.829 Osteitis deformans of <u>unspecified</u> upper arm
M88.83- Osteitis deformans of <u>forearm</u>
    M88.831 Osteitis deformans of <u>right</u> forearm
    M88.832 Osteitis deformans of <u>left</u> forearm
    M88.839 Osteitis deformans of <u>unspecified</u> forearm
M88.84- Osteitis deformans of <u>hand</u>
    M88.841 Osteitis deformans of <u>right</u> hand
    M88.842 Osteitis deformans of <u>left</u> hand
    M88.849 Osteitis deformans of <u>unspecified</u> hand
M88.85- Osteitis deformans of <u>thigh</u>
    M88.851 Osteitis deformans of <u>right</u> thigh
    M88.852 Osteitis deformans of <u>left</u> thigh
    M88.859 Osteitis deformans of <u>unspecified</u> thigh
M88.86- Osteitis deformans of <u>lower leg</u>
    M88.861 Osteitis deformans of <u>right</u> lower leg
    M88.862 Osteitis deformans of <u>left</u> lower leg
    M88.869 Osteitis deformans of <u>unspecified</u> lower leg
M88.87- Osteitis deformans of <u>ankle and foot</u>
    M88.871 Osteitis deformans of <u>right</u> ankle and foot
    M88.872 Osteitis deformans of <u>left</u> ankle and foot
    M88.879 Osteitis deformans of <u>unspecified</u> ankle and foot
M88.88 Osteitis deformans of <u>other bones</u>
    Excludes ❷: osteitis deformans of skull (M88.0)
              osteitis deformans of vertebrae (M88.1)
M88.89 Osteitis deformans of <u>multiple sites</u>
M88.9   Osteitis deformans of <u>unspecified</u> bone
M89- Other disorders of bone
  M89.0- <u>Algoneurodystrophy</u> — Bone deterioration that is due to damage of the supplying nerve.
      Shoulder-hand syndrome
      Sudeck's atrophy
    Excludes 1:   causalgia, lower limb (G57.7-)
              causalgia, upper limb (G56.4-)
              complex regional pain syndrome II, lower limb (G57.7-)
              complex regional pain syndrome II, upper limb (G56.4-)
              reflex sympathetic dystrophy (G90.5-)
  M89.00 Algoneurodystrophy, <u>unspecified</u> <u>site</u>
  M89.01- Algoneurodystrophy, <u>shoulder</u>
    M89.011 Algoneurodystrophy, <u>right</u> shoulder
    M89.012 Algoneurodystrophy, <u>left</u> shoulder
    M89.019 Algoneurodystrophy, <u>unspecified</u> shoulder
  M89.02- Algoneurodystrophy, <u>upper arm</u>
    M89.021 Algoneurodystrophy, <u>right</u> upper arm
    M89.022 Algoneurodystrophy, <u>left</u> upper arm
    M89.029 Algoneurodystrophy, <u>unspecified</u> upper arm
  M89.03- Algoneurodystrophy, <u>forearm</u>
    M89.031 Algoneurodystrophy, <u>right</u> forearm
    M89.032 Algoneurodystrophy, <u>left</u> forearm
    M89.039 Algoneurodystrophy, <u>unspecified</u> forearm
  M89.04- Algoneurodystrophy, <u>hand</u>
    M89.041 Algoneurodystrophy, <u>right</u> hand
    M89.042 Algoneurodystrophy, <u>left</u> hand
    M89.049 Algoneurodystrophy, <u>unspecified</u> hand
  M89.05- Algoneurodystrophy, <u>thigh</u>
    M89.051 Algoneurodystrophy, <u>right</u> thigh
    M89.052 Algoneurodystrophy, <u>left</u> thigh
    M89.059 Algoneurodystrophy, <u>unspecified</u> thigh
  M89.06- Algoneurodystrophy, <u>lower leg</u>
    M89.061 Algoneurodystrophy, <u>right</u> lower leg
    M89.062 Algoneurodystrophy, <u>left</u> lower leg
    M89.069 Algoneurodystrophy, <u>unspecified</u> lower leg
  M89.07- Algoneurodystrophy, <u>ankle and foot</u>
    M89.071 Algoneurodystrophy, <u>right</u> ankle and foot

    M89.072 Algoneurodystrophy, <u>left</u> ankle and foot
    M89.079 Algoneurodystrophy, <u>unspecified</u> ankle and foot
  M89.08 Algoneurodystrophy, <u>other site</u>
  M89.09 Algoneurodystrophy, <u>multiple sites</u>
M89.1- <u>Physeal arrest</u> — The cessation of the normal epiphyseal bone growth.
    Arrest of growth plate
    Epiphyseal arrest
    Growth plate arrest
  M89.12- Physeal arrest, <u>humerus</u>
    M89.121 <u>Complete</u> physeal arrest, <u>right</u> proximal humerus
    M89.122 <u>Complete</u> physeal arrest, <u>left</u> proximal humerus
    M89.123 Partial physeal arrest, <u>right</u> proximal humerus
    M89.124 Partial physeal arrest, <u>left</u> proximal humerus
    M89.125 <u>Complete</u> physeal arrest, <u>right</u> distal humerus
    M89.126 <u>Complete</u> physeal arrest, <u>left</u> distal humerus
    M89.127 Partial physeal arrest, <u>right</u> distal humerus
    M89.128 Partial physeal arrest, <u>left</u> distal humerus
    M89.129 Physeal arrest, humerus, <u>unspecified</u>
  M89.13- Physeal arrest, <u>forearm</u>
    M89.131 <u>Complete</u> physeal arrest, <u>right</u> distal radius
    M89.132 <u>Complete</u> physeal arrest, <u>left</u> distal radius
    M89.133 Partial physeal arrest, <u>right</u> distal radius
    M89.134 Partial physeal arrest, <u>left</u> distal radius
    M89.138 Other physeal arrest of forearm
    M89.139 Physeal arrest, forearm, <u>unspecified</u>
  M89.15- Physeal arrest, <u>femur</u>
    M89.151 <u>Complete</u> physeal arrest, <u>right</u> proximal femur
    M89.152 <u>Complete</u> physeal arrest, <u>left</u> proximal femur
    M89.153 Partial physeal arrest, <u>right</u> proximal femur
    M89.154 Partial physeal arrest, <u>left</u> proximal femur
    M89.155 <u>Complete</u> physeal arrest, <u>right</u> distal femur
    M89.156 <u>Complete</u> physeal arrest, <u>left</u> distal femur
    M89.157 Partial physeal arrest, <u>right</u> distal femur
    M89.158 Partial physeal arrest, <u>left</u> distal femur
    M89.159 Physeal arrest, femur, <u>unspecified</u>
  M89.16- Physeal arrest, <u>lower leg</u>
    M89.160 <u>Complete</u> physeal arrest, <u>right</u> proximal tibia
    M89.161 <u>Complete</u> physeal arrest, <u>left</u> proximal tibia
    M89.162 Partial physeal arrest, <u>right</u> proximal tibia
    M89.163 Partial physeal arrest, <u>left</u> proximal tibia
    M89.164 <u>Complete</u> physeal arrest, <u>right</u> distal tibia
    M89.165 <u>Complete</u> physeal arrest, <u>left</u> distal tibia
    M89.166 Partial physeal arrest, <u>right</u> distal tibia
    M89.167 Partial physeal arrest, <u>left</u> distal tibia
    M89.168 Other physeal arrest of lower leg
    M89.169 Physeal arrest, lower leg, <u>unspecified</u>
  M89.18 Physeal arrest, other site
M89.2- <u>Other disorders of bone development and growth</u>
  M89.20 Other disorders of bone development and growth, <u>unspecified site</u>
  M89.21- Other disorders of bone development and growth, <u>shoulder</u>
    M89.211 Other disorders of bone development and growth, <u>right</u> shoulder
    M89.212 Other disorders of bone development and growth, <u>left</u> shoulder
    M89.219 Other disorders of bone development and growth, <u>unspecified</u> shoulder
  M89.22- Other disorders of bone development and growth, <u>humerus</u>
    M89.221 Other disorders of bone development and growth, <u>right</u> humerus
    M89.222 Other disorders of bone development and growth, <u>left</u> humerus
    M89.229 Other disorders of bone development and growth, <u>unspecified</u> humerus

M88 – M89

M89.23- Other disorders of bone development and growth, <u>ulna and radius</u>

    M89.231 Other disorders of bone development and growth, <u>right</u> ulna

    M89.232 Other disorders of bone development and growth, <u>left</u> ulna

    M89.233 Other disorders of bone development and growth, <u>right</u> radius

    M89.234 Other disorders of bone development and growth, <u>left</u> radius

    M89.239 Other disorders of bone development and growth, <u>unspecified</u> ulna and radius

M89.24- Other disorders of bone development and growth, <u>hand</u>

    M89.241 Other disorders of bone development and growth, <u>right</u> hand

    M89.242 Other disorders of bone development and growth, <u>left</u> hand

    M89.249 Other disorders of bone development and growth, <u>unspecified</u> hand

M89.25- Other disorders of bone development and growth, <u>femur</u>

    M89.251 Other disorders of bone development and growth, <u>right</u> femur

    M89.252 Other disorders of bone development and growth, <u>left</u> femur

    M89.259 Other disorders of bone development and growth, <u>unspecified</u> femur

M89.26- Other disorders of bone development and growth, <u>tibia and fibula</u>

    M89.261 Other disorders of bone development and growth, <u>right</u> tibia

    M89.262 Other disorders of bone development and growth, <u>left</u> tibia

    M89.263 Other disorders of bone development and growth, <u>right</u> fibula

    M89.264 Other disorders of bone development and growth, <u>left</u> fibula

    M89.269 Other disorders of bone development and growth, <u>unspecified</u> lower leg

M89.27- Other disorders of bone development and growth, <u>ankle and foot</u>

    M89.271 Other disorders of bone development and growth, <u>right</u> ankle and foot

    M89.272 Other disorders of bone development and growth, <u>left</u> ankle and foot

    M89.279 Other disorders of bone development and growth, <u>unspecified</u> ankle and foot

M89.28 Other disorders of bone development and growth, <u>other site</u>

M89.29 Other disorders of bone development and growth, <u>multiple sites</u>

M89.3- <u>Hypertrophy</u> of bone — Enlargement of a bone.

M89.30 Hypertrophy of bone, <u>unspecified site</u>

M89.31- Hypertrophy of bone, <u>shoulder</u>

    M89.311 Hypertrophy of bone, <u>right</u> shoulder

    M89.312 Hypertrophy of bone, <u>left</u> shoulder

    M89.319 Hypertrophy of bone, <u>unspecified</u> shoulder

M89.32- Hypertrophy of bone, <u>humerus</u>

    M89.321 Hypertrophy of bone, <u>right</u> humerus

    M89.322 Hypertrophy of bone, <u>left</u> humerus

    M89.329 Hypertrophy of bone, <u>unspecified</u> humerus

M89.33- Hypertrophy of bone, <u>ulna and radius</u>

    M89.331 Hypertrophy of bone, <u>right</u> ulna

    M89.332 Hypertrophy of bone, <u>left</u> ulna

    M89.333 Hypertrophy of bone, <u>right</u> radius

    M89.334 Hypertrophy of bone, <u>left</u> radius

    M89.339 Hypertrophy of bone, <u>unspecified</u> ulna and radius

M89.34- Hypertrophy of bone, <u>hand</u>

    M89.341 Hypertrophy of bone, <u>right</u> hand

    M89.342 Hypertrophy of bone, <u>left</u> hand

    M89.349 Hypertrophy of bone, <u>unspecified</u> hand

M89.35- Hypertrophy of bone, <u>femur</u>

    M89.351 Hypertrophy of bone, <u>right</u> femur

    M89.352 Hypertrophy of bone, <u>left</u> femur

    M89.359 Hypertrophy of bone, <u>unspecified</u> femur

M89.36- Hypertrophy of bone, <u>tibia and fibula</u>

    M89.361 Hypertrophy of bone, <u>right</u> tibia

    M89.362 Hypertrophy of bone, <u>left</u> tibia

    M89.363 Hypertrophy of bone, <u>right</u> fibula

    M89.364 Hypertrophy of bone, <u>left</u> fibula

    M89.369 Hypertrophy of bone, <u>unspecified</u> tibia and fibula

M89.37- Hypertrophy of bone, <u>ankle and foot</u>

    M89.371 Hypertrophy of bone, <u>right</u> ankle and foot

    M89.372 Hypertrophy of bone, <u>left</u> ankle and foot

    M89.379 Hypertrophy of bone, <u>unspecified</u> ankle and foot

M89.38 Hypertrophy of bone, <u>other site</u>

M89.39 Hypertrophy of bone, <u>multiple sites</u>

M89.4- <u>Other hypertrophic</u> osteoarthropathy
    Marie-Bamberger disease — Inflammation and enlargement of the distal fingers and toes that is due to pulmonary disorders.
    Pachydermoperiostosis

M89.40 Other hypertrophic osteoarthropathy, <u>unspecified site</u>

M89.41- Other hypertrophic osteoarthropathy, <u>shoulder</u>

    M89.411 Other hypertrophic osteoarthropathy, <u>right</u> shoulder

    M89.412 Other hypertrophic osteoarthropathy, <u>left</u> shoulder

    M89.419 Other hypertrophic osteoarthropathy, <u>unspecified</u> shoulder

M89.42- Other hypertrophic osteoarthropathy, <u>upper arm</u>

    M89.421 Other hypertrophic osteoarthropathy, <u>right</u> upper arm

    M89.422 Other hypertrophic osteoarthropathy, <u>left</u> upper arm

    M89.429 Other hypertrophic osteoarthropathy, <u>unspecified</u> upper arm

M89.43- Other hypertrophic osteoarthropathy, <u>forearm</u>

    M89.431 Other hypertrophic osteoarthropathy, <u>right</u> forearm

    M89.432 Other hypertrophic osteoarthropathy, <u>left</u> forearm

    M89.439 Other hypertrophic osteoarthropathy, <u>unspecified</u> forearm

M89.44- Other hypertrophic osteoarthropathy, <u>hand</u>

    M89.441 Other hypertrophic osteoarthropathy, <u>right</u> hand

    M89.442 Other hypertrophic osteoarthropathy, <u>left</u> hand

    M89.449 Other hypertrophic osteoarthropathy, <u>unspecified</u> hand

M89.45- Other hypertrophic osteoarthropathy, <u>thigh</u>

    M89.451 Other hypertrophic osteoarthropathy, <u>right</u> thigh

    M89.452 Other hypertrophic osteoarthropathy, <u>left</u> thigh

    M89.459 Other hypertrophic osteoarthropathy, <u>unspecified</u> thigh

M89.46- Other hypertrophic osteoarthropathy, <u>lower leg</u>

    M89.461 Other hypertrophic osteoarthropathy, <u>right</u> lower leg

    M89.462 Other hypertrophic osteoarthropathy, <u>left</u> lower leg

    M89.469 Other hypertrophic osteoarthropathy, <u>unspecified</u> lower leg

M89.47- Other hypertrophic osteoarthropathy, <u>ankle and foot</u>

    M89.471 Other hypertrophic osteoarthropathy, <u>right</u> ankle and foot

    M89.472 Other hypertrophic osteoarthropathy, <u>left</u> ankle and foot

    M89.479 Other hypertrophic osteoarthropathy, <u>unspecified</u> ankle and foot

M89.48 Other hypertrophic osteoarthropathy, <u>other site</u>

M89.49 Other hypertrophic osteoarthropathy, <u>multiple sites</u>

M89.5- <u>Osteolysis</u> — Resorption of bone.
   Use additional code to identify major osseous defect, if applicable (M89.7-)
   Excludes ❷: periprosthetic osteolysis of internal prosthetic joint (T84.05-)

M89.50 Osteolysis, <u>unspecified</u> site
M89.51- Osteolysis, <u>shoulder</u>
   M89.511 Osteolysis, <u>right</u> shoulder
   M89.512 Osteolysis, <u>left</u> shoulder
   M89.519 Osteolysis, <u>unspecified</u> shoulder
M89.52- Osteolysis, <u>upper arm</u>
   M89.521 Osteolysis, <u>right</u> upper arm
   M89.522 Osteolysis, <u>left</u> upper arm
   M89.529 Osteolysis, <u>unspecified</u> upper arm
M89.53- Osteolysis, <u>forearm</u>
   M89.531 Osteolysis, <u>right</u> forearm
   M89.532 Osteolysis, <u>left</u> forearm
   M89.539 Osteolysis, <u>unspecified</u> forearm
M89.54- Osteolysis, <u>hand</u>
   M89.541 Osteolysis, <u>right</u> hand
   M89.542 Osteolysis, <u>left</u> hand
   M89.549 Osteolysis, <u>unspecified</u> hand
M89.55- Osteolysis, <u>thigh</u>
   M89.551 Osteolysis, <u>right</u> thigh
   M89.552 Osteolysis, <u>left</u> thigh
   M89.559 Osteolysis, <u>unspecified</u> thigh
M89.56- Osteolysis, <u>lower leg</u>
   M89.561 Osteolysis, <u>right</u> lower leg
   M89.562 Osteolysis, <u>left</u> lower leg
   M89.569 Osteolysis, <u>unspecified</u> lower leg
M89.57- Osteolysis, <u>ankle and foot</u>
   M89.571 Osteolysis, <u>right</u> ankle and foot
   M89.572 Osteolysis, <u>left</u> ankle and foot
   M89.579 Osteolysis, <u>unspecified</u> ankle and foot
M89.58 Osteolysis, <u>other site</u>
M89.59 Osteolysis, <u>multiple sites</u>

M89.6- <u>Osteopathy after poliomyelitis</u>
   Use additional code (B91) to identify previous poliomyelitis
   Excludes 1: postpolio syndrome (G14)

M89.60 Osteopathy after poliomyelitis, <u>unspecified</u> site
M89.61- Osteopathy after poliomyelitis, <u>shoulder</u>
   M89.611 Osteopathy after poliomyelitis, <u>right</u> shoulder
   M89.612 Osteopathy after poliomyelitis, <u>left</u> shoulder
   M89.619 Osteopathy after poliomyelitis, <u>unspecified</u> shoulder
M89.62- Osteopathy after poliomyelitis, <u>upper arm</u>
   M89.621 Osteopathy after poliomyelitis, <u>right</u> upper arm
   M89.622 Osteopathy after poliomyelitis, <u>left</u> upper arm
   M89.629 Osteopathy after poliomyelitis, <u>unspecified</u> upper arm
M89.63- Osteopathy after poliomyelitis, <u>forearm</u>
   M89.631 Osteopathy after poliomyelitis, <u>right</u> forearm
   M89.632 Osteopathy after poliomyelitis, <u>left</u> forearm
   M89.639 Osteopathy after poliomyelitis, <u>unspecified</u> forearm
M89.64- Osteopathy after poliomyelitis, <u>hand</u>
   M89.641 Osteopathy after poliomyelitis, <u>right</u> hand
   M89.642 Osteopathy after poliomyelitis, <u>left</u> hand
   M89.649 Osteopathy after poliomyelitis, <u>unspecified</u> hand
M89.65- Osteopathy after poliomyelitis, <u>thigh</u>
   M89.651 Osteopathy after poliomyelitis, <u>right</u> thigh
   M89.652 Osteopathy after poliomyelitis, <u>left</u> thigh
   M89.659 Osteopathy after poliomyelitis, <u>unspecified</u> thigh
M89.66- Osteopathy after poliomyelitis, <u>lower leg</u>
   M89.661 Osteopathy after poliomyelitis, <u>right</u> lower leg

M89.662 Osteopathy after poliomyelitis, <u>left</u> lower leg
   M89.669 Osteopathy after poliomyelitis, <u>unspecified</u> lower leg
M89.67- Osteopathy after poliomyelitis, <u>ankle and foot</u>
   M89.671 Osteopathy after poliomyelitis, <u>right</u> ankle and foot
   M89.672 Osteopathy after poliomyelitis, <u>left</u> ankle and foot
   M89.679 Osteopathy after poliomyelitis, <u>unspecified</u> ankle and foot
M89.68 Osteopathy after poliomyelitis, <u>other site</u>
M89.69 Osteopathy after poliomyelitis, <u>multiple sites</u>

M89.7- <u>Major osseous defect</u> — A condition of extensive, localized bone loss that has important implications regarding future diagnosis and restoration options.
   Code first underlying disease, if known, such as:
      Aseptic necrosis of bone (M87.-)
      Malignant neoplasm of bone (C40.-)
      Osteolysis (M89.5)
      Osteomyelitis (M86.-)
      Osteonecrosis (M87.-)
      Osteoporosis (M80.-, M81.-)
      Periprosthetic osteolysis (T84.05-)

M89.70 Major osseous defect, <u>unspecified</u> site
M89.71- Major osseous defect, <u>shoulder</u> region
   Major osseous defect clavicle or scapula
   M89.711 Major osseous defect, <u>right</u> shoulder region
   M89.712 Major osseous defect, <u>left</u> shoulder region
   M89.719 Major osseous defect, <u>unspecified</u> shoulder region
M89.72- Major osseous defect, <u>humerus</u>
   M89.721 Major osseous defect, <u>right</u> humerus
   M89.722 Major osseous defect, <u>left</u> humerus
   M89.729 Major osseous defect, <u>unspecified</u> humerus
M89.73- Major osseous defect, <u>forearm</u>
   Major osseous defect of radius and ulna
   M89.731 Major osseous defect, <u>right</u> forearm
   M89.732 Major osseous defect, <u>left</u> forearm
   M89.739 Major osseous defect, <u>unspecified</u> forearm
M89.74- Major osseous defect, <u>hand</u>
   Major osseous defect of carpus, fingers, metacarpus
   M89.741 Major osseous defect, <u>right</u> hand
   M89.742 Major osseous defect, <u>left</u> hand
   M89.749 Major osseous defect, <u>unspecified</u> hand
M89.75- Major osseous defect, <u>pelvic region and thigh</u>
   Major osseous defect of femur and pelvis
   M89.751 Major osseous defect, <u>right</u> pelvic region and thigh
   M89.752 Major osseous defect, <u>left</u> pelvic region and thigh
   M89.759 Major osseous defect, <u>unspecified</u> pelvic region and thigh
M89.76- Major osseous defect, <u>lower leg</u>
   Major osseous defect of fibula and tibia
   M89.761 Major osseous defect, <u>right</u> lower leg
   M89.762 Major osseous defect, <u>left</u> lower leg
   M89.769 Major osseous defect, <u>unspecified</u> lower leg
M89.77- Major osseous defect, <u>ankle and foot</u>
   Major osseous defect of metatarsus, tarsus, toes
   M89.771 Major osseous defect, <u>right</u> ankle and foot
   M89.772 Major osseous defect, <u>left</u> ankle and foot
   M89.779 Major osseous defect, <u>unspecified</u> ankle and foot
M89.78 Major osseous defect, <u>other site</u>
M89.79 Major osseous defect, <u>multiple sites</u>

M89.8- <u>Other specified</u> disorders of bone
   Infantile cortical hyperostoses
   Post-traumatic subperiosteal ossification
M89.8x- Other specified disorders of bone
   M89.8x0 Other specified disorders of bone, multiple sites
   M89.8x1 Other specified disorders of bone, shoulder
   M89.8x2 Other specified disorders of bone, upper arm
   M89.8x3 Other specified disorders of bone, forearm
   M89.8x4 Other specified disorders of bone, hand

M89
-
M89

M89.8x5   Other specified disorders of bone, thigh
M89.8x6   Other specified disorders of bone, lower leg
M89.8x7   Other specified disorders of bone, ankle and foot
M89.8x8   Other specified disorders of bone, other site
M89.8x9   Other specified disorders of bone, unspecified site
M89.9   Disorder of bone, unspecified

M90-   Osteopathies in diseases classified elsewhere
    Excludes 1:   osteochondritis, osteomyelitis, and osteopathy (in):
        cryptococcosis (B45.3)
        diabetes mellitus (E08-E13 with .69-)
        gonococcal (A54.43)
        neurogenic syphilis (A52.11)
        renal osteodystrophy (N25.0)
        salmonellosis (A02.24)
        secondary syphilis (A51.46)
        syphilis (late) (A52.77)

M90.5-   Osteonecrosis in diseases classified elsewhere
    Code first underlying disease, such as:
        Caisson disease (T70.3)
        Hemoglobinopathy (D50-D64)
cc M90.50   Osteonecrosis in diseases classified elsewhere, unspecified site — [Not Allowed as PDX]
M90.51- Osteonecrosis in diseases classified elsewhere, shoulder
    cc M90.511   Osteonecrosis in diseases classified elsewhere, right shoulder — [Not Allowed as PDX]
    cc M90.512   Osteonecrosis in diseases classified elsewhere, left shoulder — [Not Allowed as PDX]
    cc M90.519   Osteonecrosis in diseases classified elsewhere, unspecified shoulder — [Not Allowed as PDX]
M90.52- Osteonecrosis in diseases classified elsewhere, upper arm
    cc M90.521   Osteonecrosis in diseases classified elsewhere, right upper arm — [Not Allowed as PDX]
    cc M90.522   Osteonecrosis in diseases classified elsewhere, left upper arm — [Not Allowed as PDX]
    cc M90.529   Osteonecrosis in diseases classified elsewhere, unspecified upper arm — [Not Allowed as PDX]
M90.53- Osteonecrosis in diseases classified elsewhere, forearm
    cc M90.531   Osteonecrosis in diseases classified elsewhere, right forearm — [Not Allowed as PDX]
    cc M90.532   Osteonecrosis in diseases classified elsewhere, left forearm — [Not Allowed as PDX]
    cc M90.539   Osteonecrosis in diseases classified elsewhere, unspecified forearm — [Not Allowed as PDX]
M90.54- Osteonecrosis in diseases classified elsewhere, hand
    cc M90.541   Osteonecrosis in diseases classified elsewhere, right hand — [Not Allowed as PDX]
    cc M90.542   Osteonecrosis in diseases classified elsewhere, left hand — [Not Allowed as PDX]
    cc M90.549   Osteonecrosis in diseases classified elsewhere, unspecified hand — [Not Allowed as PDX]
M90.55- Osteonecrosis in diseases classified elsewhere, thigh
    cc M90.551   Osteonecrosis in diseases classified elsewhere, right thigh — [Not Allowed as PDX]
    cc M90.552   Osteonecrosis in diseases classified elsewhere, left thigh — [Not Allowed as PDX]
    cc M90.559   Osteonecrosis in diseases classified elsewhere, unspecified thigh — [Not Allowed as PDX]
M90.56- Osteonecrosis in diseases classified elsewhere, lower leg
    cc M90.561   Osteonecrosis in diseases classified elsewhere, right lower leg — [Not Allowed as PDX]
    cc M90.562   Osteonecrosis in diseases classified elsewhere, left lower leg — [Not Allowed as PDX]
    cc M90.569   Osteonecrosis in diseases classified elsewhere, unspecified lower leg — [Not Allowed as PDX]
M90.57- Osteonecrosis in diseases classified elsewhere, ankle and foot
    cc M90.571   Osteonecrosis in diseases classified elsewhere, right ankle and foot — [Not Allowed as PDX]
    cc M90.572   Osteonecrosis in diseases classified elsewhere, left ankle and foot — [Not Allowed as PDX]

cc M90.579   Osteonecrosis in diseases classified elsewhere, unspecified ankle and foot — [Not Allowed as PDX]
cc M90.58   Osteonecrosis in diseases classified elsewhere, other site — [Not Allowed as PDX]
cc M90.59   Osteonecrosis in diseases classified elsewhere, multiple sites — [Not Allowed as PDX]

M90.6-   Osteitis deformans in neoplastic diseases
    Osteitis deformans in malignant neoplasm of bone
    Code first the neoplasm (C40.-, C41.-)
    Excludes 1:   osteitis deformans [Paget's disease of bone] (M88.-)
M90.60   Osteitis deformans in neoplastic diseases, unspecified site — [Not Allowed as PDX]
M90.61- Osteitis deformans in neoplastic diseases, shoulder
    M90.611   Osteitis deformans in neoplastic diseases, right shoulder — [Not Allowed as PDX]
    M90.612   Osteitis deformans in neoplastic diseases, left shoulder — [Not Allowed as PDX]
    M90.619   Osteitis deformans in neoplastic diseases, unspecified shoulder — [Not Allowed as PDX]
M90.62- Osteitis deformans in neoplastic diseases, upper arm
    M90.621   Osteitis deformans in neoplastic diseases, right upper arm — [Not Allowed as PDX]
    M90.622   Osteitis deformans in neoplastic diseases, left upper arm — [Not Allowed as PDX]
    M90.629   Osteitis deformans in neoplastic diseases, unspecified upper arm — [Not Allowed as PDX]
M90.63- Osteitis deformans in neoplastic diseases, forearm
    M90.631   Osteitis deformans in neoplastic diseases, right forearm — [Not Allowed as PDX]
    M90.632   Osteitis deformans in neoplastic diseases, left forearm — [Not Allowed as PDX]
    M90.639   Osteitis deformans in neoplastic diseases, unspecified forearm — [Not Allowed as PDX]
M90.64- Osteitis deformans in neoplastic diseases, hand
    M90.641   Osteitis deformans in neoplastic diseases, right hand — [Not Allowed as PDX]
    M90.642   Osteitis deformans in neoplastic diseases, left hand — [Not Allowed as PDX]
    M90.649   Osteitis deformans in neoplastic diseases, unspecified hand — [Not Allowed as PDX]
M90.65- Osteitis deformans in neoplastic diseases, thigh
    M90.651   Osteitis deformans in neoplastic diseases, right thigh — [Not Allowed as PDX]
    M90.652   Osteitis deformans in neoplastic diseases, left thigh — [Not Allowed as PDX]
    M90.659   Osteitis deformans in neoplastic diseases, unspecified thigh — [Not Allowed as PDX]
M90.66- Osteitis deformans in neoplastic diseases, lower leg
    M90.661   Osteitis deformans in neoplastic diseases, right lower leg — [Not Allowed as PDX]
    M90.662   Osteitis deformans in neoplastic diseases, left lower leg — [Not Allowed as PDX]
    M90.669   Osteitis deformans in neoplastic diseases, unspecified lower leg — [Not Allowed as PDX]
M90.67- Osteitis deformans in neoplastic diseases, ankle and foot
    M90.671   Osteitis deformans in neoplastic diseases, right ankle and foot — [Not Allowed as PDX]
    M90.672   Osteitis deformans in neoplastic diseases, left ankle and foot — [Not Allowed as PDX]
    M90.679   Osteitis deformans in neoplastic diseases, unspecified ankle and foot — [Not Allowed as PDX]
M90.68   Osteitis deformans in neoplastic diseases, other site — [Not Allowed as PDX]
M90.69   Osteitis deformans in neoplastic diseases, multiple sites — [Not Allowed as PDX]

M89-M90

M90.8- Osteopathy in diseases classified elsewhere
Code first underlying disease, such as:
Rickets (E55.0)
Vitamin-D-resistant rickets (E83.3)

M90.80 Osteopathy in diseases classified elsewhere, unspecified site — [Not Allowed as PDX]

M90.81- Osteopathy in diseases classified elsewhere, shoulder

M90.811 Osteopathy in diseases classified elsewhere, right shoulder — [Not Allowed as PDX]

M90.812 Osteopathy in diseases classified elsewhere, left shoulder — [Not Allowed as PDX]

M90.819 Osteopathy in diseases classified elsewhere, unspecified shoulder — [Not Allowed as PDX]

M90.82- Osteopathy in diseases classified elsewhere, upper arm

M90.821 Osteopathy in diseases classified elsewhere, right upper arm — [Not Allowed as PDX]

M90.822 Osteopathy in diseases classified elsewhere, left upper arm — [Not Allowed as PDX]

M90.829 Osteopathy in diseases classified elsewhere, unspecified upper arm — [Not Allowed as PDX]

M90.83- Osteopathy in diseases classified elsewhere, forearm

M90.831 Osteopathy in diseases classified elsewhere, right forearm — [Not Allowed as PDX]

M90.832 Osteopathy in diseases classified elsewhere, left forearm — [Not Allowed as PDX]

M90.839 Osteopathy in diseases classified elsewhere, unspecified forearm — [Not Allowed as PDX]

M90.84- Osteopathy in diseases classified elsewhere, hand

M90.841 Osteopathy in diseases classified elsewhere, right hand — [Not Allowed as PDX]

M90.842 Osteopathy in diseases classified elsewhere, left hand — [Not Allowed as PDX]

M90.849 Osteopathy in diseases classified elsewhere, unspecified hand — [Not Allowed as PDX]

M90.85- Osteopathy in diseases classified elsewhere, thigh

M90.851 Osteopathy in diseases classified elsewhere, right thigh — [Not Allowed as PDX]

M90.852 Osteopathy in diseases classified elsewhere, left thigh — [Not Allowed as PDX]

M90.859 Osteopathy in diseases classified elsewhere, unspecified thigh — [Not Allowed as PDX]

M90.86- Osteopathy in diseases classified elsewhere, lower leg

M90.861 Osteopathy in diseases classified elsewhere, right lower leg — [Not Allowed as PDX]

M90.862 Osteopathy in diseases classified elsewhere, left lower leg — [Not Allowed as PDX]

M90.869 Osteopathy in diseases classified elsewhere, unspecified lower leg — [Not Allowed as PDX]

M90.87- Osteopathy in diseases classified elsewhere, ankle and foot

M90.871 Osteopathy in diseases classified elsewhere, right ankle and foot — [Not Allowed as PDX]

M90.872 Osteopathy in diseases classified elsewhere, left ankle and foot — [Not Allowed as PDX]

M90.879 Osteopathy in diseases classified elsewhere, unspecified ankle and foot — [Not Allowed as PDX]

M90.88 Osteopathy in diseases classified elsewhere, other site — [Not Allowed as PDX]

M90.89 Osteopathy in diseases classified elsewhere, multiple sites — [Not Allowed as PDX]

Chondropathies (M91-M94)

Excludes 1: *postprocedural chondropathies (M96.-)*

M91- Juvenile osteochondrosis of hip and pelvis — A developmental disease of the hip and pelvis bone-growth centers characterized by degeneration and recalcification of the hip or pelvis with resultant deformity.

Excludes 1: *slipped upper femoral epiphysis (nontraumatic) (M93.0)*

M91.0 Juvenile osteochondrosis of pelvis
Osteochondrosis (juvenile) of acetabulum
Osteochondrosis (juvenile) of iliac crest [Buchanan]
Osteochondrosis (juvenile) of ischiopubic synchondrosis [van Neck]
Osteochondrosis (juvenile) of symphysis pubis [Pierson]

M91.1- Juvenile osteochondrosis of head of femur [Legg-Calvé-Perthes]

M91.10 Juvenile osteochondrosis of head of femur [Legg-Calvé-Perthes], unspecified leg

M91.11 Juvenile osteochondrosis of head of femur [Legg-Calvé-Perthes], right leg

M91.12 Juvenile osteochondrosis of head of femur [Legg-Calvé-Perthes], left leg

M91.2- Coxa plana
Hip deformity due to previous juvenile osteochondrosis

M91.20 Coxa plana, unspecified hip

M91.21 Coxa plana, right hip

M91.22 Coxa plana, left hip

M91.3- Pseudocoxalgia

M91.30 Pseudocoxalgia, unspecified hip

M91.31 Pseudocoxalgia, right hip

M91.32 Pseudocoxalgia, left hip

M91.4- Coxa magna

M91.40 Coxa magna, unspecified hip

M91.41 Coxa magna, right hip

M91.42 Coxa magna, left hip

M91.8- Other juvenile osteochondrosis of hip and pelvis
Juvenile osteochondrosis after reduction of congenital dislocation of hip

M91.80 Other juvenile osteochondrosis of hip and pelvis, unspecified leg

M91.81 Other juvenile osteochondrosis of hip and pelvis, right leg

M91.82 Other juvenile osteochondrosis of hip and pelvis, left leg

M91.9- Juvenile osteochondrosis of hip and pelvis, unspecified

M91.90 Juvenile osteochondrosis of hip and pelvis, unspecified, unspecified leg

M91.91 Juvenile osteochondrosis of hip and pelvis, unspecified, right leg

M91.92 Juvenile osteochondrosis of hip and pelvis, unspecified, left leg

M92- Other juvenile osteochondrosis

M92.0- Juvenile osteochondrosis of humerus
Osteochondrosis (juvenile) of capitulum of humerus [Panner]
Osteochondrosis (juvenile) of head of humerus [Haas]

M92.00 Juvenile osteochondrosis of humerus, unspecified arm

M92.01 Juvenile osteochondrosis of humerus, right arm

M92.02 Juvenile osteochondrosis of humerus, left arm

M92.1- Juvenile osteochondrosis of radius and ulna
Osteochondrosis (juvenile) of lower ulna [Burns]
Osteochondrosis (juvenile) of radial head [Brailsford]

M92.10 Juvenile osteochondrosis of radius and ulna, unspecified arm

M92.11 Juvenile osteochondrosis of radius and ulna, right arm

M92.12 Juvenile osteochondrosis of radius and ulna, left arm

M92.2- Juvenile osteochondrosis, hand

M92.20- Unspecified juvenile osteochondrosis, hand

M92.201 Unspecified juvenile osteochondrosis, right hand

M92.202 Unspecified juvenile osteochondrosis, left hand

M92.209 Unspecified juvenile osteochondrosis, unspecified hand

M92.21- Osteochondrosis (juvenile) of carpal lunate [Kienböck]

   M92.211 Osteochondrosis (juvenile) of carpal lunate [Kienböck], right hand

   M92.212 Osteochondrosis (juvenile) of carpal lunate [Kienböck], left hand

   M92.219 Osteochondrosis (juvenile) of carpal lunate [Kienböck], unspecified hand

M92.22- Osteochondrosis (juvenile) of metacarpal heads [Mauclaire]

   M92.221 Osteochondrosis (juvenile) of metacarpal heads [Mauclaire], right hand

   M92.222 Osteochondrosis (juvenile) of metacarpal heads [Mauclaire], left hand

   M92.229 Osteochondrosis (juvenile) of metacarpal heads [Mauclaire], unspecified hand

M92.29- Other juvenile osteochondrosis, hand

   M92.291 Other juvenile osteochondrosis, right hand

   M92.292 Other juvenile osteochondrosis, left hand

   M92.299 Other juvenile osteochondrosis, unspecified hand

M92.3- Other juvenile osteochondrosis, upper limb

  M92.30 Other juvenile osteochondrosis, unspecified upper limb

  M92.31 Other juvenile osteochondrosis, right upper limb

  M92.32 Other juvenile osteochondrosis, left upper limb

M92.4- Juvenile osteochondrosis of patella
    Osteochondrosis (juvenile) of primary patellar center [Köhler]
    Osteochondrosis (juvenile) of secondary patellar centre [Sinding Larsen]

  M92.40 Juvenile osteochondrosis of patella, unspecified knee

  M92.41 Juvenile osteochondrosis of patella, right knee

  M92.42 Juvenile osteochondrosis of patella, left knee

M92.5- Juvenile osteochondrosis of tibia and fibula
    Osteochondrosis (juvenile) of proximal tibia [Blount]
    Osteochondrosis (juvenile) of tibial tubercle [Osgood-Schlatter]
    Tibia vara

  M92.50 Juvenile osteochondrosis of tibia and fibula, unspecified leg

  M92.51 Juvenile osteochondrosis of tibia and fibula, right leg

  M92.52 Juvenile osteochondrosis of tibia and fibula, left leg

M92.6- Juvenile osteochondrosis of tarsus
    Osteochondrosis (juvenile) of calcaneum [Sever]
    Osteochondrosis (juvenile) of os tibiale externum [Haglund]
    Osteochondrosis (juvenile) of talus [Diaz]
    Osteochondrosis (juvenile) of tarsal navicular [Köhler]

  M92.60 Juvenile osteochondrosis of tarsus, unspecified ankle

  M92.61 Juvenile osteochondrosis of tarsus, right ankle

  M92.62 Juvenile osteochondrosis of tarsus, left ankle

M92.7- Juvenile osteochondrosis of metatarsus
    Osteochondrosis (juvenile) of fifth metatarsus [Iselin]
    Osteochondrosis (juvenile) of second metatarsus [Freiberg]

  M92.70 Juvenile osteochondrosis of metatarsus, unspecified foot

  M92.71 Juvenile osteochondrosis of metatarsus, right foot

  M92.72 Juvenile osteochondrosis of metatarsus, left foot

M92.8 Other specified juvenile osteochondrosis
    Calcaneal apophysitis

M92.9 Juvenile osteochondrosis, unspecified
    Juvenile apophysitis NOS
    Juvenile epiphysitis NOS
    Juvenile osteochondritis NOS
    Juvenile osteochondrosis NOS

M93- Other osteochondropathies
    Excludes ❷: osteochondrosis of spine (M42.-)

M93.0- Slipped upper femoral epiphysis (nontraumatic) — The partial dislocation of the hip that is not due to trauma.
    Use additional code for associated chondrolysis (M94.3)

  M93.00- Unspecified slipped upper femoral epiphysis (nontraumatic)

   M93.001 Unspecified slipped upper femoral epiphysis (nontraumatic), right hip

   M93.002 Unspecified slipped upper femoral epiphysis (nontraumatic), left hip

   M93.003 Unspecified slipped upper femoral epiphysis (nontraumatic), unspecified hip

  M93.01- Acute slipped upper femoral epiphysis (nontraumatic)

   M93.011 Acute slipped upper femoral epiphysis (nontraumatic), right hip

   M93.012 Acute slipped upper femoral epiphysis (nontraumatic), left hip

   M93.013 Acute slipped upper femoral epiphysis (nontraumatic), unspecified hip

  M93.02- Chronic slipped upper femoral epiphysis (nontraumatic)

   M93.021 Chronic slipped upper femoral epiphysis (nontraumatic), right hip

   M93.022 Chronic slipped upper femoral epiphysis (nontraumatic), left hip

   M93.023 Chronic slipped upper femoral epiphysis (nontraumatic), unspecified hip

  M93.03- Acute on chronic slipped upper femoral epiphysis (nontraumatic)

   M93.031 Acute on chronic slipped upper femoral epiphysis (nontraumatic), right hip

   M93.032 Acute on chronic slipped upper femoral epiphysis (nontraumatic), left hip

   M93.033 Acute on chronic slipped upper femoral epiphysis (nontraumatic), unspecified hip

M93.1 Kienböck's disease of adults — [Age/15-124] — Degeneration and recalcification of the bones in adults.
    Adult osteochondrosis of carpal lunates

M93.2- Osteochondritis dissecans — Inflammation of both the bone and cartilage with fragmenting pieces of cartilage into the joint.

  M93.20 Osteochondritis dissecans of unspecified site

  M93.21- Osteochondritis dissecans of shoulder

   M93.211 Osteochondritis dissecans, right shoulder

   M93.212 Osteochondritis dissecans, left shoulder

   M93.219 Osteochondritis dissecans, unspecified shoulder

  M93.22- Osteochondritis dissecans of elbow

   M93.221 Osteochondritis dissecans, right elbow

   M93.222 Osteochondritis dissecans, left elbow

   M93.229 Osteochondritis dissecans, unspecified elbow

  M93.23- Osteochondritis dissecans of wrist

   M93.231 Osteochondritis dissecans, right wrist

   M93.232 Osteochondritis dissecans, left wrist

   M93.239 Osteochondritis dissecans, unspecified wrist

  M93.24- Osteochondritis dissecans of joints of hand

   M93.241 Osteochondritis dissecans, joints of right hand

   M93.242 Osteochondritis dissecans, joints of left hand

   M93.249 Osteochondritis dissecans, joints of unspecified hand

  M93.25- Osteochondritis dissecans of hip

   M93.251 Osteochondritis dissecans, right hip

   M93.252 Osteochondritis dissecans, left hip

   M93.259 Osteochondritis dissecans, unspecified hip

  M93.26- Osteochondritis dissecans knee

   M93.261 Osteochondritis dissecans, right knee

   M93.262 Osteochondritis dissecans, left knee

   M93.269 Osteochondritis dissecans, unspecified knee

  M93.27- Osteochondritis dissecans of ankle and joints of foot

   M93.271 Osteochondritis dissecans, right ankle and joints of right foot

   M93.272 Osteochondritis dissecans, left ankle and joints of left foot

   M93.279 Osteochondritis dissecans, unspecified ankle and joints of foot

  M93.28 Osteochondritis dissecans other site

  M93.29 Osteochondritis dissecans multiple sites

M93.8- Other specified osteochondropathies

  M93.80 Other specified osteochondropathies of unspecified site

M92
I
M93

M93.81- Other specified osteochondropathies of <u>shoulder</u>
  M93.811   Other specified osteochondropathies, <u>right</u> shoulder
  M93.812   Other specified osteochondropathies, <u>left</u> shoulder
  M93.819   Other specified osteochondropathies, <u>unspecified</u> shoulder
M93.82- Other specified osteochondropathies of <u>upper arm</u>
  M93.821   Other specified osteochondropathies, <u>right</u> upper arm
  M93.822   Other specified osteochondropathies, <u>left</u> upper arm
  M93.829   Other specified osteochondropathies, <u>unspecified</u> upper arm
M93.83- Other specified osteochondropathies of <u>forearm</u>
  M93.831   Other specified osteochondropathies, <u>right</u> forearm
  M93.832   Other specified osteochondropathies, <u>left</u> forearm
  M93.839   Other specified osteochondropathies, <u>unspecified</u> forearm
M93.84- Other specified osteochondropathies of <u>hand</u>
  M93.841   Other specified osteochondropathies, <u>right</u> hand
  M93.842   Other specified osteochondropathies, <u>left</u> hand
  M93.849   Other specified osteochondropathies, <u>unspecified</u> hand
M93.85- Other specified osteochondropathies of <u>thigh</u>
  M93.851   Other specified osteochondropathies, <u>right</u> thigh
  M93.852   Other specified osteochondropathies, <u>left</u> thigh
  M93.859   Other specified osteochondropathies, <u>unspecified</u> thigh
M93.86- Other specified osteochondropathies <u>lower leg</u>
  M93.861   Other specified osteochondropathies, <u>right</u> lower leg
  M93.862   Other specified osteochondropathies, <u>left</u> lower leg
  M93.869   Other specified osteochondropathies, <u>unspecified</u> lower leg
M93.87- Other specified osteochondropathies of <u>ankle and foot</u>
  M93.871   Other specified osteochondropathies, <u>right</u> ankle and foot
  M93.872   Other specified osteochondropathies, <u>left</u> ankle and foot
  M93.879   Other specified osteochondropathies, <u>unspecified</u> ankle and foot
M93.88   Other specified osteochondropathies <u>other</u>
M93.89   Other specified osteochondropathies <u>multiple sites</u>
M93.9- Osteochondropathy, <u>unspecified</u>
  Apophysitis NOS
  Epiphysitis NOS
  Osteochondritis NOS
  Osteochondrosis NOS
  M93.90   Osteochondropathy, unspecified of <u>unspecified site</u>
  M93.91- Osteochondropathy, unspecified of <u>shoulder</u>
    M93.911   Osteochondropathy, unspecified, <u>right</u> shoulder
    M93.912   Osteochondropathy, unspecified, <u>left</u> shoulder
    M93.919   Osteochondropathy, unspecified, <u>unspecified</u> shoulder
  M93.92- Osteochondropathy, unspecified of <u>upper arm</u>
    M93.921   Osteochondropathy, unspecified, <u>right</u> upper arm
    M93.922   Osteochondropathy, unspecified, <u>left</u> upper arm
    M93.929   Osteochondropathy, unspecified, <u>unspecified</u> upper arm
  M93.93- Osteochondropathy, unspecified of <u>forearm</u>
    M93.931   Osteochondropathy, unspecified, <u>right</u> forearm
    M93.932   Osteochondropathy, unspecified, <u>left</u> forearm
    M93.939   Osteochondropathy, unspecified, <u>unspecified</u> forearm
  M93.94- Osteochondropathy, unspecified of <u>hand</u>
    M93.941   Osteochondropathy, unspecified, <u>right</u> hand
    M93.942   Osteochondropathy, unspecified, <u>left</u> hand

M93.949   Osteochondropathy, unspecified, <u>unspecified</u> hand
M93.95- Osteochondropathy, unspecified of <u>thigh</u>
  M93.951   Osteochondropathy, unspecified, <u>right</u> thigh
  M93.952   Osteochondropathy, unspecified, <u>left</u> thigh
  M93.959   Osteochondropathy, unspecified, <u>unspecified</u> thigh
M93.96- Osteochondropathy, unspecified <u>lower leg</u>
  M93.961   Osteochondropathy, unspecified, <u>right</u> lower leg
  M93.962   Osteochondropathy, unspecified, <u>left</u> lower leg
  M93.969   Osteochondropathy, unspecified, <u>unspecified</u> lower leg
M93.97- Osteochondropathy, unspecified of <u>ankle and foot</u>
  M93.971   Osteochondropathy, unspecified, <u>right</u> ankle and foot
  M93.972   Osteochondropathy, unspecified, <u>left</u> ankle and foot
  M93.979   Osteochondropathy, unspecified, <u>unspecified</u> ankle and foot
M93.98   Osteochondropathy, unspecified <u>other</u>
M93.99   Osteochondropathy, unspecified <u>multiple sites</u>

M94- <u>Other disorders of cartilage</u>
  M94.0   **Chondrocostal junction syndrome [Tietze]** — Inflammation of the costal cartilages of the ribs with chest pain similar to coronary artery disease.
    Costochondritis
  M94.1   **Relapsing polychondritis** — Inflammation and degeneration of various cartilaginous structures.
  M94.2- <u>Chondromalacia</u> — The softening of the articular cartilage.
    Excludes 1:   chondromalacia patellae (M22.4)
    M94.20   Chondromalacia, <u>unspecified site</u>
    M94.21- Chondromalacia, <u>shoulder</u>
      M94.211   Chondromalacia, <u>right</u> shoulder
      M94.212   Chondromalacia, <u>left</u> shoulder
      M94.219   Chondromalacia, <u>unspecified</u> shoulder
    M94.22- Chondromalacia, <u>elbow</u>
      M94.221   Chondromalacia, <u>right</u> elbow
      M94.222   Chondromalacia, <u>left</u> elbow
      M94.229   Chondromalacia, <u>unspecified</u> elbow
    M94.23- Chondromalacia, <u>wrist</u>
      M94.231   Chondromalacia, <u>right</u> wrist
      M94.232   Chondromalacia, <u>left</u> wrist
      M94.239   Chondromalacia, <u>unspecified</u> wrist
    M94.24- Chondromalacia, joints of <u>hand</u>
      M94.241   Chondromalacia, joints of <u>right</u> hand
      M94.242   Chondromalacia, joints of <u>left</u> hand
      M94.249   Chondromalacia, joints of <u>unspecified</u> hand
    M94.25- Chondromalacia, <u>hip</u>
      M94.251   Chondromalacia, <u>right</u> hip
      M94.252   Chondromalacia, <u>left</u> hip
      M94.259   Chondromalacia, <u>unspecified</u> hip
    M94.26- Chondromalacia, <u>knee</u>
      M94.261   Chondromalacia, <u>right</u> knee
      M94.262   Chondromalacia, <u>left</u> knee
      M94.269   Chondromalacia, <u>unspecified</u> knee
    M94.27- Chondromalacia, <u>ankle and joints of foot</u>
      M94.271   Chondromalacia, <u>right</u> ankle and joints of <u>right</u> foot
      M94.272   Chondromalacia, <u>left</u> ankle and joints of <u>left</u> foot
      M94.279   Chondromalacia, <u>unspecified</u> ankle and joints of foot
    M94.28   Chondromalacia, <u>other site</u>
    M94.29   Chondromalacia, <u>multiple sites</u>

M94.3- <u>Chondrolysis</u> — Resorption of cartilage.
  Code first any associated slipped upper femoral epiphysis (nontraumatic) (M93.0-)

  M94.35- Chondrolysis, <u>hip</u>

    M94.351 Chondrolysis, <u>right</u> hip

    M94.352 Chondrolysis, <u>left</u> hip

    M94.359 Chondrolysis, <u>unspecified</u> hip

M94.8- Other specified disorders of cartilage

  M94.8x- <u>Other specified disorders of cartilage</u>

    M94.8x0 Other specified disorders of cartilage, multiple sites

    M94.8x1 Other specified disorders of cartilage, shoulder

    M94.8x2 Other specified disorders of cartilage, upper arm

    M94.8x3 Other specified disorders of cartilage, forearm

    M94.8x4 Other specified disorders of cartilage, hand

    M94.8x5 Other specified disorders of cartilage, thigh

    M94.8x6 Other specified disorders of cartilage, lower leg

    M94.8x7 Other specified disorders of cartilage, ankle and foot

    M94.8x8 Other specified disorders of cartilage, other site

    M94.8x9 Other specified disorders of cartilage, unspecified sites

M94.9 Disorder of cartilage, <u>unspecified</u>

Other disorders of the musculoskeletal system and connective tissue (M95)

M95- Other acquired deformities of musculoskeletal system and connective tissue
  Excludes ❷: *acquired absence of limbs and organs (Z89-Z90)*
    acquired deformities of limbs (M20-M21)
    congenital malformations and deformations of the musculoskeletal system (Q65-Q79)
    deforming dorsopathies (M40-M43)
    dentofacial anomalies [including malocclusion] (M26.-)
    postprocedural musculoskeletal disorders (M96.-)

M95.0 Acquired deformity of nose
  Excludes ❷: *deviated nasal septum (J34.2)*

M95.1- <u>Cauliflower ear</u> — Formation of fibrous tissue at the site of damaged cartilage of the ear.
  Excludes ❷: *other acquired deformities of ear (H61.1)*

  M95.10 Cauliflower ear, <u>unspecified</u> ear

  M95.11 Cauliflower ear, <u>right</u> ear

  M95.12 Cauliflower ear, <u>left</u> ear

M95.2 Other acquired deformity of <u>head</u>

M95.3 Acquired deformity of <u>neck</u>

M95.4 Acquired deformity of <u>chest and rib</u>
  AHA 14:4Q:p26 – Rib deformity associated with congenital scoliosis

M95.5 Acquired deformity of <u>pelvis</u>
  Excludes 1: *maternal care for known or suspected disproportion (O33.-)*

M95.8 Other specified acquired deformities of musculoskeletal system

M95.9 Acquired deformity of musculoskeletal system, <u>unspecified</u>

Intraoperative and postprocedural complications and disorders of musculoskeletal system, not elsewhere classified (M96)

M96- <u>Intraoperative and postprocedural complications</u> and disorders of musculoskeletal system, not elsewhere classified
  Excludes ❷: *arthropathy following intestinal bypass (M02.0-)*
    complications of internal orthopedic prosthetic devices, implants and grafts (T84.-)
    disorders associated with osteoporosis (M80)
    periprosthetic fracture around internal prosthetic joint (M97.-)
    presence of functional implants and other devices (Z96-Z97)

cc M96.0 Pseudarthrosis after fusion or arthrodesis

M96.1 Postlaminectomy syndrome, not elsewhere classified

M96.2 Postradiation kyphosis

M96.3 Postlaminectomy kyphosis

M96.4 Postsurgical lordosis

M96.5 Postradiation scoliosis

M96.6- <u>Fracture of bone following insertion of orthopedic implant, joint prosthesis, or bone plate</u>
  Intraoperative fracture of bone during insertion of orthopedic implant, joint prosthesis, or bone plate
  Excludes ❷: *complication of internal orthopedic devices, implants or grafts (T84.-)*

  M96.62- Fracture of <u>humerus</u> following insertion of orthopedic implant, joint prosthesis, or bone plate

    cc M96.621 Fracture of humerus following insertion of orthopedic implant, joint prosthesis, or bone plate, <u>right</u> arm

    cc M96.622 Fracture of humerus following insertion of orthopedic implant, joint prosthesis, or bone plate, <u>left</u> arm

    cc M96.629 Fracture of humerus following insertion of orthopedic implant, joint prosthesis, or bone plate, <u>unspecified</u> arm

  M96.63- Fracture of <u>radius or ulna</u> following insertion of orthopedic implant, joint prosthesis, or bone plate

    cc M96.631 Fracture of radius or ulna following insertion of orthopedic implant, joint prosthesis, or bone plate, <u>right</u> arm

    cc M96.632 Fracture of radius or ulna following insertion of orthopedic implant, joint prosthesis, or bone plate, <u>left</u> arm

    cc M96.639 Fracture of radius or ulna following insertion of orthopedic implant, joint prosthesis, or bone plate, <u>unspecified</u> arm

  cc M96.65 Fracture of <u>pelvis</u> following insertion of orthopedic implant, joint prosthesis, or bone plate

  M96.66- Fracture of <u>femur</u> following insertion of orthopedic implant, joint prosthesis, or bone plate

    cc M96.661 Fracture of femur following insertion of orthopedic implant, joint prosthesis, or bone plate, <u>right</u> leg

    cc M96.662 Fracture of femur following insertion of orthopedic implant, joint prosthesis, or bone plate, <u>left</u> leg

    cc M96.669 Fracture of femur following insertion of orthopedic implant, joint prosthesis, or bone plate, <u>unspecified</u> leg

  M96.67- Fracture of <u>tibia or fibula</u> following insertion of orthopedic implant, joint prosthesis, or bone plate

    cc M96.671 Fracture of tibia or fibula following insertion of orthopedic implant, joint prosthesis, or bone plate, <u>right</u> leg

    cc M96.672 Fracture of tibia or fibula following insertion of orthopedic implant, joint prosthesis, or bone plate, <u>left</u> leg

    cc M96.679 Fracture of tibia or fibula following insertion of orthopedic implant, joint prosthesis, or bone plate, <u>unspecified</u> leg

  cc M96.69 Fracture of <u>other bone</u> following insertion of orthopedic implant, joint prosthesis, or bone plate

M94 - M96

M96.8- <u>Other</u> intraoperative and postprocedural complications and disorders of musculoskeletal system, not elsewhere classified

M96.81- <u>Intraoperative hemorrhage and hematoma</u> of a musculoskeletal structure complicating a procedure

> Excludes 1: intraoperative hemorrhage and hematoma of a musculoskeletal structure due to accidental puncture and laceration during a procedure (M96.82-)

cc **M96.810** Intraoperative hemorrhage and hematoma of a musculoskeletal structure complicating a <u>musculoskeletal system procedure</u>

cc **M96.811** Intraoperative hemorrhage and hematoma of a musculoskeletal structure complicating <u>other procedure</u>

M96.82- <u>Accidental puncture and laceration</u> of a musculoskeletal structure during a procedure

cc **M96.820** Accidental puncture and laceration of a musculoskeletal structure during a <u>musculoskeletal system procedure</u>

cc **M96.821** Accidental puncture and laceration of a musculoskeletal structure during <u>other procedure</u>

M96.83- <u>Postprocedural hemorrhage</u> of a musculoskeletal structure following a procedure

cc **M96.830** Postprocedural <u>hemorrhage</u> of a musculoskeletal structure following a <u>musculoskeletal system procedure</u>

cc **M96.831** Postprocedural <u>hemorrhage</u> of a musculoskeletal structure following <u>other procedure</u>

M96.84- <u>Postprocedural hematoma and seroma</u> of a musculoskeletal structure following a procedure

cc **M96.840** Postprocedural <u>hematoma</u> of a musculoskeletal structure following a <u>musculoskeletal system procedure</u>

cc **M96.841** Postprocedural <u>hematoma</u> of a musculoskeletal structure following <u>other procedure</u>

cc **M96.842** Postprocedural <u>seroma</u> of a musculoskeletal structure following a <u>musculoskeletal system procedure</u>

cc **M96.843** Postprocedural <u>seroma</u> of a musculoskeletal structure following <u>other procedure</u>

cc **M96.89** Other intraoperative and postprocedural complications and disorders of the musculoskeletal system
> Instability of joint secondary to removal of joint prosthesis
> Use additional code, if applicable, to further specify disorder

Periprosthetic fracture around internal prosthetic joint (M97)

M97- <u>Periprosthetic</u> fracture around internal prosthetic joint
> Excludes ❷: breakage (fracture) of prosthetic joint (T84.01-)
> fracture of bone following insertion of orthopedic implant, joint prosthesis or bone plate (M96.6-)

> The appropriate 7th character is to be added to each code from category M97:
> A   Initial encounter
> D   Subsequent encounter
> S   Sequela

M97.0- Periprosthetic fracture around internal prosthetic <u>hip</u> joint

cc-a **M97.01x-** Periprosthetic fracture around internal prosthetic <u>right</u> hip joint

cc-a **M97.02x-** Periprosthetic fracture around internal prosthetic <u>left</u> hip joint

M97.1- Periprosthetic fracture around internal prosthetic <u>knee</u> joint

cc-a **M97.11x-** Periprosthetic fracture around internal prosthetic <u>right</u> knee joint

cc-a **M97.12x-** Periprosthetic fracture around internal prosthetic <u>left</u> knee joint

M97.2- Periprosthetic fracture around internal prosthetic <u>ankle</u> joint

cc-a **M97.21x-** Periprosthetic fracture around internal prosthetic <u>right</u> ankle joint

cc-a **M97.22x-** Periprosthetic fracture around internal prosthetic <u>left</u> ankle joint

M97.3- Periprosthetic fracture around internal prosthetic <u>shoulder</u> joint

cc-a **M97.31x-** Periprosthetic fracture around internal prosthetic <u>right</u> shoulder joint

cc-a **M97.32x-** Periprosthetic fracture around internal prosthetic <u>left</u> shoulder joint

M97.4- Periprosthetic fracture around internal prosthetic <u>elbow</u> joint

cc-a **M97.41x-** Periprosthetic fracture around internal prosthetic <u>right</u> elbow joint

cc-a **M97.42x-** Periprosthetic fracture around internal prosthetic <u>left</u> elbow joint

cc-a **M97.8xx-** Periprosthetic fracture around <u>other</u> internal prosthetic joint
> Periprosthetic fracture around internal prosthetic finger joint
> Periprosthetic fracture around internal prosthetic spinal joint
> Periprosthetic fracture around internal prosthetic toe joint
> Periprosthetic fracture around internal prosthetic wrist joint
> Use additional code to identify the joint (Z96.6-)

cc-a **M97.9xx-** Periprosthetic fracture around <u>unspecified</u> internal prosthetic joint

Biomechanical lesions, not elsewhere classified (M99)

M99- Biomechanical lesions, <u>not elsewhere classified</u>
    Note: **This category should not be used if the condition can be classified elsewhere.**

M99.0- <u>Segmental and somatic dysfunction</u>
    M99.00 Segmental and somatic dysfunction of head region
    M99.01 Segmental and somatic dysfunction of cervical region
    M99.02 Segmental and somatic dysfunction of thoracic region
    M99.03 Segmental and somatic dysfunction of lumbar region
    M99.04 Segmental and somatic dysfunction of sacral region
    M99.05 Segmental and somatic dysfunction of pelvic region
    M99.06 Segmental and somatic dysfunction of lower extremity
    M99.07 Segmental and somatic dysfunction of upper extremity
    M99.08 Segmental and somatic dysfunction of rib cage
    M99.09 Segmental and somatic dysfunction of abdomen and other regions

M99.1- <u>Subluxation complex (vertebral)</u>
    cc M99.10 Subluxation complex (vertebral) of head region
    cc M99.11 Subluxation complex (vertebral) of cervical region
    M99.12 Subluxation complex (vertebral) of thoracic region
    M99.13 Subluxation complex (vertebral) of lumbar region
    M99.14 Subluxation complex (vertebral) of sacral region
    M99.15 Subluxation complex (vertebral) of pelvic region
    M99.16 Subluxation complex (vertebral) of lower extremity
    M99.17 Subluxation complex (vertebral) of upper extremity
    cc M99.18 Subluxation complex (vertebral) of rib cage
    M99.19 Subluxation complex (vertebral) of abdomen and other regions

M99.2- <u>Subluxation stenosis</u> of neural canal
    M99.20 Subluxation stenosis of neural canal of head region
    M99.21 Subluxation stenosis of neural canal of cervical region
    M99.22 Subluxation stenosis of neural canal of thoracic region
    M99.23 Subluxation stenosis of neural canal of lumbar region
    M99.24 Subluxation stenosis of neural canal of sacral region
    M99.25 Subluxation stenosis of neural canal of pelvic region
    M99.26 Subluxation stenosis of neural canal of lower extremity
    M99.27 Subluxation stenosis of neural canal of upper extremity
    M99.28 Subluxation stenosis of neural canal of rib cage
    M99.29 Subluxation stenosis of neural canal of abdomen and other regions

M99.3- <u>Osseous stenosis</u> of neural canal
    M99.30 Osseous stenosis of neural canal of head region
    M99.31 Osseous stenosis of neural canal of cervical region
    M99.32 Osseous stenosis of neural canal of thoracic region
    M99.33 Osseous stenosis of neural canal of lumbar region
    M99.34 Osseous stenosis of neural canal of sacral region
    M99.35 Osseous stenosis of neural canal of pelvic region
    M99.36 Osseous stenosis of neural canal of lower extremity
    M99.37 Osseous stenosis of neural canal of upper extremity
    M99.38 Osseous stenosis of neural canal of rib cage
    M99.39 Osseous stenosis of neural canal of abdomen and other regions

M99.4- <u>Connective tissue stenosis</u> of neural canal
    M99.40 Connective tissue stenosis of neural canal of head region
    M99.41 Connective tissue stenosis of neural canal of cervical region
    M99.42 Connective tissue stenosis of neural canal of thoracic region
    M99.43 Connective tissue stenosis of neural canal of lumbar region
    M99.44 Connective tissue stenosis of neural canal of sacral region
    M99.45 Connective tissue stenosis of neural canal of pelvic region
    M99.46 Connective tissue stenosis of neural canal of lower extremity
    M99.47 Connective tissue stenosis of neural canal of upper extremity
    M99.48 Connective tissue stenosis of neural canal of rib cage
    M99.49 Connective tissue stenosis of neural canal of abdomen and other regions

M99.5- <u>Intervertebral disc stenosis</u> of neural canal
    M99.50 Intervertebral disc stenosis of neural canal of head region
    M99.51 Intervertebral disc stenosis of neural canal of cervical region
    M99.52 Intervertebral disc stenosis of neural canal of thoracic region
    M99.53 Intervertebral disc stenosis of neural canal of lumbar region
    M99.54 Intervertebral disc stenosis of neural canal of sacral region
    M99.55 Intervertebral disc stenosis of neural canal of pelvic region
    M99.56 Intervertebral disc stenosis of neural canal of lower extremity
    M99.57 Intervertebral disc stenosis of neural canal of upper extremity
    M99.58 Intervertebral disc stenosis of neural canal of rib cage
    M99.59 Intervertebral disc stenosis of neural canal of abdomen and other regions

M99.6- <u>Osseous and subluxation stenosis</u> of intervertebral foramina
    M99.60 Osseous and subluxation stenosis of intervertebral foramina of head region
    M99.61 Osseous and subluxation stenosis of intervertebral foramina of cervical region
    M99.62 Osseous and subluxation stenosis of intervertebral foramina of thoracic region
    M99.63 Osseous and subluxation stenosis of intervertebral foramina of lumbar region
    M99.64 Osseous and subluxation stenosis of intervertebral foramina of sacral region
    M99.65 Osseous and subluxation stenosis of intervertebral foramina of pelvic region
    M99.66 Osseous and subluxation stenosis of intervertebral foramina of lower extremity
    M99.67 Osseous and subluxation stenosis of intervertebral foramina of upper extremity
    M99.68 Osseous and subluxation stenosis of intervertebral foramina of rib cage
    M99.69 Osseous and subluxation stenosis of intervertebral foramina of abdomen and other regions

M 9 9 | M 9 9

M99.7- **Connective tissue and disc stenosis** of intervertebral foramina

M99.70 Connective tissue and disc stenosis of intervertebral foramina of head region

M99.71 Connective tissue and disc stenosis of intervertebral foramina of cervical region

M99.72 Connective tissue and disc stenosis of intervertebral foramina of thoracic region

M99.73 Connective tissue and disc stenosis of intervertebral foramina of lumbar region

M99.74 Connective tissue and disc stenosis of intervertebral foramina of sacral region

M99.75 Connective tissue and disc stenosis of intervertebral foramina of pelvic region

M99.76 Connective tissue and disc stenosis of intervertebral foramina of lower extremity

M99.77 Connective tissue and disc stenosis of intervertebral foramina of upper extremity

M99.78 Connective tissue and disc stenosis of intervertebral foramina of rib cage

M99.79 Connective tissue and disc stenosis of intervertebral foramina of abdomen and other regions

M99.8- **Other** biomechanical lesions

M99.80 Other biomechanical lesions of head region

M99.81 Other biomechanical lesions of cervical region

M99.82 Other biomechanical lesions of thoracic region

M99.83 Other biomechanical lesions of lumbar region

M99.84 Other biomechanical lesions of sacral region

M99.85 Other biomechanical lesions of pelvic region

M99.86 Other biomechanical lesions of lower extremity

M99.87 Other biomechanical lesions of upper extremity

M99.88 Other biomechanical lesions of rib cage

M99.89 Other biomechanical lesions of abdomen and other regions

M99.9 **Biomechanical lesion, unspecified**

Chapter 14 – Diseases of the genitourinary system (N00-N99)

Excludes ❷: certain conditions originating in the perinatal period (P04-P96)
certain infectious and parasitic diseases (A00-B99)
complications of pregnancy, childbirth and the puerperium (O00-O9A)
congenital malformations, deformations and chromosomal abnormalities (Q00-Q99)
endocrine, nutritional and metabolic diseases (E00-E88)
injury, poisoning and certain other consequences of external causes (S00-T88)
neoplasms (C00-D49)
symptoms, signs and abnormal clinical and laboratory findings, not elsewhere classified (R00-R94)

This chapter contains the following blocks:

N00-N08	Glomerular diseases
N10-N16	Renal tubulo-interstitial diseases
N17-N19	Acute kidney failure and chronic kidney disease
N20-N23	Urolithiasis
N25-N29	Other disorders of kidney and ureter
N30-N39	Other diseases of the urinary system
N40-N53	Diseases of male genital organs
N60-N65	Disorders of breast
N70-N77	Inflammatory diseases of female pelvic organs
N80-N98	Noninflammatory disorders of female genital tract
N99	Intraoperative and postprocedural complications and disorders of genitourinary system, not elsewhere classified

Chapter-Specific Coding Guidelines

C. Chapter-Specific Coding Guidelines
In addition to general coding guidelines, there are guidelines for specific diagnoses and/or conditions in the classification. Unless otherwise indicated, these guidelines apply to all health care settings. Please refer to Section II for guidelines on the selection of principal diagnosis.

14. Chapter 14: Diseases of Genitourinary System (N00-N99)

a. Chronic kidney disease

1) Stages of chronic kidney disease (CKD)
The ICD-10-CM classifies CKD based on severity. The severity of CKD is designated by stages 1-5. Stage 2, code N18.2, equates to mild CKD; stage 3, code N18.3, equates to moderate CKD; and stage 4, code N18.4, equates to severe CKD. Code N18.6, End stage renal disease (ESRD), is assigned when the provider has documented end-stage-renal disease (ESRD).

If both a stage of CKD and ESRD are documented, assign code N18.6 only.

2) Chronic kidney disease and kidney transplant status
Patients who have undergone kidney transplant may still have some form of chronic kidney disease (CKD) because the kidney transplant may not fully restore kidney function. Therefore, the presence of CKD alone does not constitute a transplant complication. Assign the appropriate N18 code for the patient's stage of CKD and code Z94.0, Kidney transplant status. If a transplant complication such as failure or rejection or other transplant complication is documented, see section I.C.19.g for information on coding complications of a kidney transplant. If the documentation is unclear as to whether the patient has a complication of the transplant, query the provider.

3) Chronic kidney disease with other conditions
Patients with CKD may also suffer from other serious conditions, most commonly diabetes mellitus and hypertension. The sequencing of the CKD code in relationship to codes for other contributing conditions is based on the conventions in the Tabular List.

See I.C.9. Hypertensive chronic kidney disease.
See I.C.19. Chronic kidney disease and kidney transplant complications.

Glomerular diseases (N00-N08)

Excludes 1: hypertensive chronic kidney disease (I12.-)
Code also any associated kidney failure (N17-N19).

N00- **Acute nephritic syndrome** — The sudden, sever onset of inflammation of the glomeruli of the kidney of various causes including following a streptococcal infection of the throat or skin.
Includes: Acute glomerular disease
Acute glomerulonephritis — The sudden, severe onset of inflammation and proliferation of the glomeruli of the kidney that is characterized by hematuria, proteinuria, and red blood cell casts.
Acute nephritis — The sudden, severe onset of inflammation of the kidney.
Excludes 1: acute tubulo-interstitial nephritis (N10)
nephritic syndrome NOS (N05.-)

MCC **N00.0** Acute nephritic syndrome <u>with</u> minor glomerular abnormality
Acute nephritic syndrome with minimal change lesion

MCC **N00.1** Acute nephritic syndrome <u>with</u> focal and segmental glomerular lesions
Acute nephritic syndrome with focal and segmental hyalinosis
Acute nephritic syndrome with focal and segmental sclerosis
Acute nephritic syndrome with focal glomerulonephritis

MCC **N00.2** Acute nephritic syndrome <u>with</u> diffuse membranous glomerulonephritis

MCC **N00.3** Acute nephritic syndrome <u>with</u> diffuse mesangial proliferative glomerulonephritis

MCC **N00.4** Acute nephritic syndrome <u>with</u> diffuse endocapillary proliferative glomerulonephritis

MCC **N00.5** Acute nephritic syndrome <u>with</u> diffuse mesangiocapillary glomerulonephritis
Acute nephritic syndrome with membranoproliferative glomerulonephritis, types 1 and 3, or NOS

MCC **N00.6** Acute nephritic syndrome <u>with</u> dense deposit disease
Acute nephritic syndrome with membranoproliferative glomerulonephritis, type 2

MCC **N00.7** Acute nephritic syndrome <u>with</u> diffuse crescentic glomerulonephritis
Acute nephritic syndrome with extracapillary glomerulonephritis

MCC **N00.8** Acute nephritic syndrome <u>with</u> other morphologic changes
Acute nephritic syndrome with proliferative glomerulonephritis NOS

MCC **N00.9** Acute nephritic syndrome with unspecified morphologic changes

N01- **Rapidly progressive nephritic syndrome** — A form characterized by a rapid downhill course, rapid decrease in the glomerular filtration rate, and glomerular crescent formation.
Includes: Rapidly progressive glomerular disease
Rapidly progressive glomerulonephritis
Rapidly progressive nephritis
Excludes 1: nephritic syndrome NOS (N05.-)

MCC **N01.0** Rapidly progressive nephritic syndrome <u>with</u> minor glomerular abnormality
Rapidly progressive nephritic syndrome with minimal change lesion

MCC **N01.1** Rapidly progressive nephritic syndrome <u>with</u> focal and segmental glomerular lesions
Rapidly progressive nephritic syndrome with focal and segmental hyalinosis
Rapidly progressive nephritic syndrome with focal and segmental sclerosis
Rapidly progressive nephritic syndrome with focal glomerulonephritis

MCC **N01.2** Rapidly progressive nephritic syndrome <u>with</u> diffuse membranous glomerulonephritis

MCC **N01.3** Rapidly progressive nephritic syndrome <u>with</u> diffuse mesangial proliferative glomerulonephritis

MCC **N01.4** Rapidly progressive nephritic syndrome <u>with</u> diffuse endocapillary proliferative glomerulonephritis

MCC **N01.5** Rapidly progressive nephritic syndrome <u>with</u> diffuse mesangiocapillary glomerulonephritis
Rapidly progressive nephritic syndrome with membranoproliferative glomerulonephritis, types 1 and 3, or NOS

MCC **N01.6** Rapidly progressive nephritic syndrome <u>with</u> dense deposit disease
Rapidly progressive nephritic syndrome with membranoproliferative glomerulonephritis, type 2

MCC **N01.7** **Rapidly progressive nephritic syndrome with diffuse crescentic glomerulonephritis**
Rapidly progressive nephritic syndrome with extracapillary glomerulonephritis

MCC **N01.8** **Rapidly progressive nephritic syndrome with other morphologic changes**
Rapidly progressive nephritic syndrome with proliferative glomerulonephritis NOS

MCC **N01.9** **Rapidly progressive nephritic syndrome with unspecified morphologic changes**

N02- **Recurrent and persistent hematuria**
Excludes 1: acute cystitis with hematuria (N30.01)
hematuria NOS (R31.9)
hematuria not associated with specified morphologic lesions (R31.-)

CC **N02.0** **Recurrent and persistent hematuria with minor glomerular abnormality**
Recurrent and persistent hematuria with minimal change lesion

CC **N02.1** **Recurrent and persistent hematuria with focal and segmental glomerular lesions**
Recurrent and persistent hematuria with focal and segmental hyalinosis
Recurrent and persistent hematuria with focal and segmental sclerosis
Recurrent and persistent hematuria with focal glomerulonephritis

CC **N02.2** **Recurrent and persistent hematuria with diffuse membranous glomerulonephritis**

CC **N02.3** **Recurrent and persistent hematuria with diffuse mesangial proliferative glomerulonephritis**

CC **N02.4** **Recurrent and persistent hematuria with diffuse endocapillary proliferative glomerulonephritis**

CC **N02.5** **Recurrent and persistent hematuria with diffuse mesangiocapillary glomerulonephritis**
Recurrent and persistent hematuria with membranoproliferative glomerulonephritis, types 1 and 3, or NOS

CC **N02.6** **Recurrent and persistent hematuria with dense deposit disease**
Recurrent and persistent hematuria with membranoproliferative glomerulonephritis, type 2

CC **N02.7** **Recurrent and persistent hematuria with diffuse crescentic glomerulonephritis**
Recurrent and persistent hematuria with extracapillary glomerulonephritis

CC **N02.8** **Recurrent and persistent hematuria with other morphologic changes**
Recurrent and persistent hematuria with proliferative glomerulonephritis NOS

CC **N02.9** **Recurrent and persistent hematuria with unspecified morphologic changes**

N03- **Chronic nephritic syndrome** — A form that persists over a long period of time.
Includes: Chronic glomerular disease
Chronic glomerulonephritis
Chronic nephritis
Excludes 1: chronic tubulo-interstitial nephritis (N11.-)
diffuse sclerosing glomerulonephritis (N05.8-)
nephritic syndrome NOS (N05.-)

CC **N03.0** **Chronic nephritic syndrome with minor glomerular abnormality**
Chronic nephritic syndrome with minimal change lesion

CC **N03.1** **Chronic nephritic syndrome with focal and segmental glomerular lesions**
Chronic nephritic syndrome with focal and segmental hyalinosis
Chronic nephritic syndrome with focal and segmental sclerosis
Chronic nephritic syndrome with focal glomerulonephritis

CC **N03.2** **Chronic nephritic syndrome with diffuse membranous glomerulonephritis**

CC **N03.3** **Chronic nephritic syndrome with diffuse mesangial proliferative glomerulonephritis**

CC **N03.4** **Chronic nephritic syndrome with diffuse endocapillary proliferative glomerulonephritis**

CC **N03.5** **Chronic nephritic syndrome with diffuse mesangiocapillary glomerulonephritis**
Chronic nephritic syndrome with membranoproliferative glomerulonephritis, types 1 and 3, or NOS

CC **N03.6** **Chronic nephritic syndrome with dense deposit disease**
Chronic nephritic syndrome with membranoproliferative glomerulonephritis, type 2

CC **N03.7** **Chronic nephritic syndrome with diffuse crescentic glomerulonephritis**
Chronic nephritic syndrome with extracapillary glomerulonephritis

CC **N03.8** **Chronic nephritic syndrome with other morphologic changes**
Chronic nephritic syndrome with proliferative glomerulonephritis NOS

CC **N03.9** **Chronic nephritic syndrome with unspecified morphologic changes**

N04- **Nephrotic syndrome** — A kidney disease syndrome characterized by massive edema, marked proteinuria, hypoalbuminemia, and hyperlipidemia.
Includes: Congenital nephrotic syndrome
Lipoid nephrosis

CC **N04.0** **Nephrotic syndrome with minor glomerular abnormality**
Nephrotic syndrome with minimal change lesion

CC **N04.1** **Nephrotic syndrome with focal and segmental glomerular lesions**
Nephrotic syndrome with focal and segmental hyalinosis
Nephrotic syndrome with focal and segmental sclerosis
Nephrotic syndrome with focal glomerulonephritis

CC **N04.2** **Nephrotic syndrome with diffuse membranous glomerulonephritis**

CC **N04.3** **Nephrotic syndrome with diffuse mesangial proliferative glomerulonephritis**

CC **N04.4** **Nephrotic syndrome with diffuse endocapillary proliferative glomerulonephritis**

CC **N04.5** **Nephrotic syndrome with diffuse mesangiocapillary glomerulonephritis**
Nephrotic syndrome with membranoproliferative glomerulonephritis, types 1 and 3, or NOS

CC **N04.6** **Nephrotic syndrome with dense deposit disease**
Nephrotic syndrome with membranoproliferative glomerulonephritis, type 2

CC **N04.7** **Nephrotic syndrome with diffuse crescentic glomerulonephritis**
Nephrotic syndrome with extracapillary glomerulonephritis

CC **N04.8** **Nephrotic syndrome with other morphologic changes**
Nephrotic syndrome with proliferative glomerulonephritis NOS

CC **N04.9** **Nephrotic syndrome with unspecified morphologic changes**

N05- **Unspecified nephritic syndrome**
Includes: Glomerular disease NOS
Glomerulonephritis NOS
Nephritis NOS
Nephropathy NOS and renal disease NOS with morphological lesion specified in .0-.8
Excludes 1: nephropathy NOS with no stated morphological lesion (N28.9)
renal disease NOS with no stated morphological lesion (N28.9)
tubulo-interstitial nephritis NOS (N12)

N05.0 **Unspecified nephritic syndrome with minor glomerular abnormality**
Unspecified nephritic syndrome with minimal change lesion

N05.1 **Unspecified nephritic syndrome with focal and segmental glomerular lesions**
Unspecified nephritic syndrome with focal and segmental hyalinosis
Unspecified nephritic syndrome with focal and segmental sclerosis
Unspecified nephritic syndrome with focal glomerulonephritis

CC **N05.2** **Unspecified nephritic syndrome with diffuse membranous glomerulonephritis**

CC **N05.3** **Unspecified nephritic syndrome with diffuse mesangial proliferative glomerulonephritis**

CC **N05.4** **Unspecified nephritic syndrome with diffuse endocapillary proliferative glomerulonephritis**

CC **N05.5** **Unspecified nephritic syndrome with diffuse mesangiocapillary glomerulonephritis**
Unspecified nephritic syndrome with membranoproliferative glomerulonephritis, types 1 and 3, or NOS

N05.6 **Unspecified nephritic syndrome with dense deposit disease**
Unspecified nephritic syndrome with membranoproliferative glomerulonephritis, type 2

N05.7 **Unspecified nephritic syndrome with diffuse crescentic glomerulonephritis**
Unspecified nephritic syndrome with extracapillary glomerulonephritis

N01-N05

N05.8 Unspecified nephritic syndrome <u>with</u> other morphologic changes
Unspecified nephritic syndrome with proliferative glomerulonephritis NOS

N05.9 Unspecified nephritic syndrome <u>with</u> unspecified morphologic changes

N06- <u>Isolated proteinuria with specified morphological lesion</u>
Excludes 1:   proteinuria not associated with specific morphologic lesions (R80.0)

N06.0 Isolated proteinuria <u>with</u> minor glomerular abnormality
Isolated proteinuria with minimal change lesion

N06.1 Isolated proteinuria <u>with</u> focal and segmental glomerular lesions
Isolated proteinuria with focal and segmental hyalinosis
Isolated proteinuria with focal and segmental sclerosis
Isolated proteinuria with focal glomerulonephritis

cc N06.2 Isolated proteinuria <u>with</u> <u>diffuse</u> membranous glomerulonephritis

cc N06.3 Isolated proteinuria <u>with</u> <u>diffuse</u> mesangial proliferative glomerulonephritis

cc N06.4 Isolated proteinuria <u>with</u> <u>diffuse</u> endocapillary proliferative glomerulonephritis

cc N06.5 Isolated proteinuria <u>with</u> <u>diffuse</u> mesangiocapillary glomerulonephritis
Isolated proteinuria with membranoproliferative glomerulonephritis, types 1 and 3, or NOS

N06.6 Isolated proteinuria <u>with</u> dense deposit disease
Isolated proteinuria with membranoproliferative glomerulonephritis, type 2

N06.7 Isolated proteinuria <u>with</u> <u>diffuse</u> crescentic glomerulonephritis
Isolated proteinuria with extracapillary glomerulonephritis

N06.8 Isolated proteinuria <u>with</u> other morphologic lesion
Isolated proteinuria with proliferative glomerulonephritis NOS

N06.9 Isolated proteinuria <u>with</u> unspecified morphologic lesion

N07- <u>Hereditary nephropathy, not elsewhere classified</u>
Excludes ❷: Alport's syndrome (Q87.81-)
hereditary amyloid nephropathy (E85.-)
nail patella syndrome (Q87.2)
non-neuropathic heredofamilial amyloidosis (E85.-)

N07.0 Hereditary nephropathy, not elsewhere classified <u>with</u> minor glomerular abnormality
Hereditary nephropathy, not elsewhere classified with minimal change lesion

N07.1 Hereditary nephropathy, not elsewhere classified <u>with</u> focal and segmental glomerular lesions
Hereditary nephropathy, not elsewhere classified with focal and segmental hyalinosis
Hereditary nephropathy, not elsewhere classified with focal and segmental sclerosis
Hereditary nephropathy, not elsewhere classified with focal glomerulonephritis

cc N07.2 Hereditary nephropathy, not elsewhere classified <u>with</u> <u>diffuse</u> membranous glomerulonephritis

cc N07.3 Hereditary nephropathy, not elsewhere classified <u>with</u> <u>diffuse</u> mesangial proliferative glomerulonephritis

cc N07.4 Hereditary nephropathy, not elsewhere classified <u>with</u> <u>diffuse</u> endocapillary proliferative glomerulonephritis

cc N07.5 Hereditary nephropathy, not elsewhere classified <u>with</u> <u>diffuse</u> mesangiocapillary glomerulonephritis
Hereditary nephropathy, not elsewhere classified with membranoproliferative glomerulonephritis, types 1 and 3, or NOS

N07.6 Hereditary nephropathy, not elsewhere classified <u>with</u> dense deposit disease
Hereditary nephropathy, not elsewhere classified with membranoproliferative glomerulonephritis, type 2

N07.7 Hereditary nephropathy, not elsewhere classified <u>with</u> <u>diffuse</u> crescentic glomerulonephritis
Hereditary nephropathy, not elsewhere classified with extracapillary glomerulonephritis

N07.8 Hereditary nephropathy, not elsewhere classified <u>with</u> other morphologic lesions
Hereditary nephropathy, not elsewhere classified with proliferative glomerulonephritis NOS

N07.9 Hereditary nephropathy, not elsewhere classified <u>with</u> unspecified morphologic lesions

N08 Glomerular disorders <u>in diseases classified elsewhere</u> —
[Not Allowed as PDX]
Glomerulonephritis
Nephritis
Nephropathy
Code first underlying disease, such as:
Amyloidosis (E85.-)
Congenital syphilis (A50.5)
Cryoglobulinemia (D89.1)
Disseminated intravascular coagulation (D65)
Gout (M1A.-, M10.-)
Microscopic polyangiitis (M31.7)
Multiple myeloma (C90.0-)
Sepsis (A40.0-A41.9)
Sickle-cell disease (D57.0-D57.8)
Excludes 1:   glomerulonephritis, nephritis and nephropathy (in):
antiglomerular basement membrane disease (M31.0)
diabetes (E08-E13 with .21)
gonococcal (A54.21)
Goodpasture's syndrome (M31.0)
hemolytic-uremic syndrome (D59.3)
lupus (M32.14)
mumps (B26.83)
syphilis (A52.75)
systemic lupus erythematosus (M32.14)
Wegener's granulomatosis (M31.31)
pyelonephritis in diseases classified elsewhere (N16)
renal tubulo-interstitial disorders classified elsewhere (N16)

Renal tubulo-interstitial diseases (N10-N16)

Includes: Pyelonephritis
Excludes 1:   pyeloureteritis cystica (N28.85)

N10 <u>Acute</u> tubulo-interstitial nephritis — Inflammation of the kidney tissue between
cc the tubules (interstitial) that has a sudden, severe onset.
Acute infectious interstitial nephritis
Acute pyelitis
Acute tubulo-interstitial nephritis
Hemoglobin nephrosis
Myoglobin nephrosis
Use additional code (B95-B97), to identify infectious agent.

N11- <u>Chronic</u> tubulo-interstitial nephritis — Inflammation and fibrosis of the kidney
tissue between the tubules (interstitial) that persists over a long period of time.
Includes: Chronic infectious interstitial nephritis
Chronic pyelitis
Chronic pyelonephritis
Use additional code (B95-B97), to identify infectious agent.

N11.0 Nonobstructive reflux-associated chronic pyelonephritis
Pyelonephritis (chronic) associated with (vesicoureteral) reflux
Excludes 1:   vesicoureteral reflux NOS (N13.70)

cc N11.1 Chronic obstructive pyelonephritis
Pyelonephritis (chronic) associated with anomaly of pelviureteric junction
Pyelonephritis (chronic) associated with anomaly of pyeloureteric junction
Pyelonephritis (chronic) associated with crossing of vessel
Pyelonephritis (chronic) associated with kinking of ureter
Pyelonephritis (chronic) associated with obstruction of ureter
Pyelonephritis (chronic) associated with stricture of pelviureteric junction
Pyelonephritis (chronic) associated with stricture of ureter
Excludes 1:   calculous pyelonephritis (N20.9)
obstructive uropathy (N13.-)

cc N11.8 Other chronic tubulo-interstitial nephritis
Nonobstructive chronic pyelonephritis NOS

cc N11.9 Chronic tubulo-interstitial nephritis, unspecified
Chronic interstitial nephritis NOS
Chronic pyelitis NOS
Chronic pyelonephritis NOS

N12 Tubulo-interstitial nephritis, <u>not specified as acute or chronic</u>
cc Interstitial nephritis NOS
Pyelitis NOS
Pyelonephritis NOS
Excludes 1:   calculous pyelonephritis (N20.9)

N05
-
N12

N13- **Obstructive and reflux uropathy** — HYDRONEPHROSIS —The abnormal accumulation of urine in the renal pelvis due to obstruction of the renal outflow.
*Excludes ❷: calculus of kidney and ureter without hydronephrosis (N20.-)
congenital obstructive defects of renal pelvis and ureter (Q62.0-Q62.3)
hydronephrosis with ureteropelvic junction obstruction (Q62.1)
obstructive pyelonephritis (N11.1)*

CC **N13.0** **Hydronephrosis with ureteropelvic obstruction**
Hydronephrosis due to acquired occlusion of ureteropelvic junction
Excludes ❷: hydronephrosis with ureteropelvic junction obstruction due to calculus (N13.2)

CC **N13.1** **Hydronephrosis with ureteral stricture, not elsewhere classified**
Excludes 1: hydronephrosis with ureteral stricture with infection (N13.6)

CC **N13.2** **Hydronephrosis with renal and ureteral calculous obstruction**
Excludes 1: hydronephrosis with renal and ureteral calculous obstruction with infection (N13.6)

N13.3- **Other and unspecified hydronephrosis**
Excludes 1: hydronephrosis with infection (N13.6)

CC **N13.30** **Unspecified hydronephrosis**

CC **N13.39** **Other hydronephrosis**

CC **N13.4** **Hydroureter** — Distention of a ureter with fluid due to obstruction.
*Excludes 1: congenital hydroureter (Q62.3-)
hydroureter with infection (N13.6)
vesicoureteral-reflux with hydroureter (N13.73-)*

N13.5 **Crossing vessel and stricture of ureter without hydronephrosis** — The decrease in the usual ureteral lumen diameter that is often due to external forces (compression by blood vessels, abnormal growths).
Kinking and stricture of ureter without hydronephrosis
Excludes 1: crossing vessel and stricture of ureter without hydronephrosis with infection (N13.6)

Tubular Muscular Constriction   Kidney

URETERAL CONSTRICTION

CC **N13.6** **Pyonephrosis** — The abnormal accumulation of pus in the renal pelvis due to obstruction of the renal outflow.
Conditions in N13.0-N13.5 with infection
Obstructive uropathy with infection
Use additional code (B95-B97), to identify infectious agent

N13.7- **Vesicoureteral-reflux** — The abnormal backward flow of urine from the bladder into the ureters and kidneys.
Excludes 1: reflux-associated pyelonephritis (N11.0)

N13.70 **Vesicoureteral-reflux, unspecified**
Vesicoureteral-reflux NOS

N13.71 **Vesicoureteral-reflux without reflux nephropathy**

N13.72- **Vesicoureteral-reflux with reflux nephropathy without hydroureter**

N13.721 **Vesicoureteral-reflux with reflux nephropathy without hydroureter, unilateral**

N13.722 **Vesicoureteral-reflux with reflux nephropathy without hydroureter, bilateral**

N13.729 **Vesicoureteral-reflux with reflux nephropathy without hydroureter, unspecified**

N13.73- **Vesicoureteral-reflux with reflux nephropathy with hydroureter**

N13.731 **Vesicoureteral-reflux with reflux nephropathy with hydroureter, unilateral**

N13.732 **Vesicoureteral-reflux with reflux nephropathy with hydroureter, bilateral**

N13.739 **Vesicoureteral-reflux with reflux nephropathy with hydroureter, unspecified**

CC **N13.8** **Other obstructive and reflux uropathy**
Urinary tract obstruction due to specified cause
Code first, if applicable, any causal condition, such as:
Enlarged prostate (N40.1)

N13.9 **Obstructive and reflux uropathy, unspecified**
Urinary tract obstruction NOS

N14- **Drug- and heavy-metal-induced tubulo-interstitial and tubular conditions**
Code first poisoning due to drug or toxin, if applicable (T36-T65 with fifth or sixth character 1-4 or 6)
Use additional code for adverse effect, if applicable, to identify drug (T36-T50 with fifth or sixth character 5)

N14.0 **Analgesic nephropathy** — A form caused by the effects of long term analgesic medication use.

N14.1 **Nephropathy induced by other drugs, medicaments and biological substances**

N14.2 **Nephropathy induced by unspecified drug, medicament or biological substance**

N14.3 **Nephropathy induced by heavy metals**

N14.4 **Toxic nephropathy, not elsewhere classified**

N15- **Other renal tubulo-interstitial diseases**

N15.0 **Balkan nephropathy** — A form of chronic tubulointerstitial disease that is commonly seen in southeastern Europe and marked by urothelial atypia.
Balkan endemic nephropathy

MCC **N15.1** **Renal and perinephric abscess**

N15.8 **Other specified renal tubulo-interstitial diseases**

N15.9 **Renal tubulo-interstitial disease, unspecified**
Infection of kidney NOS
Excludes 1: urinary tract infection NOS (N39.0)

N16 **Renal tubulo-interstitial disorders in diseases classified elsewhere** — [Not Allowed as PDX]
Pyelonephritis
Tubulo-interstitial nephritis
Code first underlying disease, such as:
Brucellosis (A23.0-A23.9)
Cryoglobulinemia (D89.1)
Glycogen storage disease (E74.0)
Leukemia (C91-C95)
Lymphoma (C81.0-C85.9, C96.0-C96.9)
Multiple myeloma (C90.0-)
Sepsis (A40.0-A41.9)
Wilson's disease (E83.0)
*Excludes 1: diphtheritic pyelonephritis and tubulo-interstitial nephritis (A36.84)
pyelonephritis and tubulo-interstitial nephritis in candidiasis (B37.49)
pyelonephritis and tubulo-interstitial nephritis in cystinosis (E72.0)
pyelonephritis and tubulo-interstitial nephritis in salmonella infection (A02.25)
pyelonephritis and tubulo-interstitial nephritis in sarcoidosis (D86.84)
pyelonephritis and tubulo-interstitial nephritis in sicca syndrome [Sjogren's] (M35.04)
pyelonephritis and tubulo-interstitial nephritis in systemic lupus erythematosus (M32.15)
pyelonephritis and tubulo-interstitial nephritis in toxoplasmosis (B58.83)
renal tubular degeneration in diabetes (E08-E13 with .29)
syphilitic pyelonephritis and tubulo-interstitial nephritis (A52.75)*

N 1 3 - N 1 6

Acute kidney failure and chronic kidney disease (N17-N19)

Excludes ❷:　congenital renal failure (P96.0)
　　drug- and heavy-metal-induced tubulo-interstitial and tubular
　　　conditions (N14.-)
　　extrarenal uremia (R39.2)
　　hemolytic-uremic syndrome (D59.3)
　　hepatorenal syndrome (K76.7)
　　postpartum hepatorenal syndrome (O90.4)
　　posttraumatic renal failure (T79.5)
　　prerenal uremia (R39.2)
　　renal failure complicating abortion or ectopic or molar
　　　pregnancy (O00-O07, O08.4)
　　renal failure following labor and delivery (O90.4)
　　renal failure postprocedural (N99.0)

N17-　**Acute** kidney failure — The sudden, severe onset of inadequate kidney function.
　　Code also associated underlying condition
　　Excludes 1:　posttraumatic renal failure (T79.5)

MCC N17.0　Acute kidney failure <u>with tubular necrosis</u> — A form characterized by the destruction of renal tubules.
　　Acute tubular necrosis
　　Renal tubular necrosis
　　Tubular necrosis NOS

MCC N17.1　Acute kidney failure <u>with acute cortical necrosis</u> — A form characterized by the destruction of the renal cortex.
　　Acute cortical necrosis
　　Cortical necrosis NOS
　　Renal cortical necrosis

MCC N17.2　Acute kidney failure <u>with medullary necrosis</u> — A form characterized by the destruction of the renal medulla.
　　Medullary [papillary] necrosis NOS
　　Acute medullary [papillary] necrosis
　　Renal medullary [papillary] necrosis

CC N17.8　<u>Other</u> acute kidney failure

CC N17.9　Acute kidney failure, <u>unspecified</u>
　　Acute kidney injury (nontraumatic)
　　Excludes ❷:　traumatic kidney injury (S37.0-)

N18-　<u>Chronic</u> kidney disease (CKD) — Kidney damage marked by the persistent and usually progressive reduction in the glomerular filtration rate and albuminuria. The stages of chronic kidney disease listed below are based on the level of kidney function (glomerular filtration rate).
　　Code first any associated:
　　　Diabetic chronic kidney disease (E08.22, E09.22, E10.22, E11.22, E13.22)
　　　Hypertensive chronic kidney disease (I12.-, I13.-)
　　Use additional code to identify kidney transplant status, if applicable,
　　　(Z94.0)

N18.1　Chronic kidney disease, stage 1

N18.2　Chronic kidney disease, stage 2 (mild)

N18.3　Chronic kidney disease, stage 3 (moderate)

CC N18.4　Chronic kidney disease, stage 4 (severe)
　　AHA 13:1Q:p24 – Kidney transplant failure with stage IV chronic kidney disease

CC N18.5　Chronic kidney disease, stage 5
　　Excludes 1:　chronic kidney disease, stage 5 requiring chronic dialysis (N18.6)

MCC N18.6　<u>End stage renal disease</u> — A severe form requiring dialysis or kidney transplantation.
　　AHA 13:4Q:p124 – Encounter for hemodialysis
　　AHA 13:4Q:p125 – End stage renal disease
　　Chronic kidney disease requiring chronic dialysis
　　Use additional code to identify dialysis status (Z99.2)

N18.9　Chronic kidney disease, <u>unspecified</u>
　　Chronic renal disease
　　Chronic renal failure NOS
　　Chronic renal insufficiency
　　Chronic uremia

N19　<u>Unspecified</u> kidney failure
　　Uremia NOS
　　Excludes 1:　acute kidney failure (N17.-)
　　　chronic kidney disease (N18.-)
　　　chronic uremia (N18.9)
　　　extrarenal uremia (R39.2)
　　　prerenal uremia (R39.2)
　　　renal insufficiency (acute) (N28.9)
　　　uremia of newborn (P96.0)

Urolithiasis (N20-N23)

N20-　Calculus of kidney and ureter
　　Calculous pyelonephritis
　　Excludes 1:　nephrocalcinosis (E83.5)
　　　that with hydronephrosis (N13.2)

N20.0　Calculus of kidney — An abnormal concretion occurring within the kidney.
　　Nephrolithiasis NOS
　　Renal calculus
　　Renal stone
　　Staghorn calculus
　　Stone in kidney

CC N20.1　Calculus of ureter — An abnormal concretion occurring within the ureter.
　　Ureteric stone

CC N20.2　Calculus of kidney with calculus of ureter

N20.9　Urinary calculus, unspecified

N21-　Calculus of lower urinary tract
　　Includes:　Calculus of lower urinary tract with cystitis and urethritis

N21.0　Calculus in bladder — An abnormal concretion occurring within the bladder.
　　Calculus in diverticulum of bladder
　　Urinary bladder stone
　　Excludes ❷:　staghorn calculus (N20.0)

N21.1　Calculus in urethra — An abnormal concretion occurring within the urethra.
　　Excludes ❷:　calculus of prostate (N42.0)

N21.8　Other lower urinary tract calculus

N21.9　Calculus of lower urinary tract, unspecified
　　Excludes 1:　calculus of urinary tract NOS (N20.9)

N22　Calculus of urinary tract <u>in diseases classified elsewhere</u> —
　　[Not Allowed as PDX]
　　Code first underlying disease, such as:
　　　Gout (M1A.-, M10.-)
　　　Schistosomiasis (B65.0-B65.9)

N23　Unspecified renal colic

Other disorders of kidney and ureter (N25-N29)

Excludes ❷:　disorders of kidney and ureter with urolithiasis (N20-N23)

N25-　Disorders resulting from impaired renal tubular function
　　Excludes 1:　metabolic disorders classifiable to E70-E88

N25.0　Renal osteodystrophy — Various developmental bone formation disorders caused by the hypocalcemic, hyperphosphatemic effects of renal disease.
　　Azotemic osteodystrophy
　　Phosphate-losing tubular disorders
　　Renal rickets
　　Renal short stature

CC N25.1　Nephrogenic diabetes insipidus — Failure of the renal tubules to reabsorb water and with failure to respond to excessive production of antidiuretic hormone.
　　Excludes 1:　diabetes insipidus NOS (E23.2)

N25.8-　Other disorders resulting from impaired renal tubular function

CC N25.81　Secondary hyperparathyroidism of renal origin — A form of hyperparathyroidism due to a renal disease that lowers the serum calcium levels and results in the overstimulation of the parathyroid glands.
　　Excludes 1:　secondary hyperparathyroidism, non-renal (E21.1)

N25.89　Other disorders resulting from impaired renal tubular function
　　Hypokalemic nephropathy — Dysfunction of the kidney associated with low potassium blood levels.
　　Lightwood-Albright syndrome
　　Renal tubular acidosis NOS

N25.9　Disorder resulting from impaired renal tubular function, unspecified

N26-　Unspecified contracted kidney — The abnormal reduction in size of the kidney.
　　Excludes 1:　contracted kidney due to hypertension (I12.-)
　　　diffuse sclerosing glomerulonephritis (N05.8.-)
　　　hypertensive nephrosclerosis (arteriolar) (arteriosclerotic)
　　　　(I12.-)
　　　small kidney of unknown cause (N27.-)

N26.1　Atrophy of kidney (terminal) — The abnormal wasting-away of the kidney.

N26.2　Page kidney — External compression of the kidney (often by a hematoma) causing decreased blood flow to the kidney that results in hypertension.

N26.9　Renal sclerosis, unspecified

Excludes 1: = NOT CODED HERE! (Do not code both)　　　**903**　　　Excludes ❷: = Not Included Here

N27- Small kidney of unknown cause — The abnormally diminished size of the kidney, of an unknown origin.
  Includes: Oligonephronia
  N27.0 Small kidney, <u>unilateral</u>
  N27.1 Small kidney, <u>bilateral</u>
  N27.9 Small kidney, <u>unspecified</u>

N28- Other disorders of kidney and ureter, not elsewhere classified
  CC **N28.0 Ischemia and infarction of kidney**
    Renal artery embolism — Blockage of the renal artery due to a clot of blood.
    Renal artery obstruction — Blockage of the renal artery.
    Renal artery occlusion — Narrowing, or complete closure, of the renal artery.
    Renal artery thrombosis — An abnormal aggregation of blood factors causing a renal artery obstruction.
    Renal infarct — Obstructive ischemic tissue necrosis of the kidney.
    Excludes 1: *atherosclerosis of renal artery (extrarenal part) (I70.1)*
        congenital stenosis of renal artery (Q27.1)
        Goldblatt's kidney (I70.1)
  N28.1 Cyst of kidney, acquired — A closed sac or pouch in a kidney, with a definite wall that contains fluid or semisolid material.
    Cyst (multiple) (solitary) of kidney, acquired
    Excludes 1: *cystic kidney disease (congenital) (Q61.-)*
  N28.8- Other specified disorders of kidney and ureter
    Excludes 1: *hydroureter (N13.4)*
        ureteric stricture with hydronephrosis (N13.1)
        ureteric stricture without hydronephrosis (N13.5)
    N28.81 Hypertrophy of kidney — Abnormal enlargement of a kidney.
    N28.82 Megaloureter — The abnormal enlargment of the lumen of a ureter.
    N28.83 Nephroptosis — Downward displacement of a kidney.
    CC **N28.84 Pyelitis cystica** — Inflammation of the kidney pelvis with the formation of multiple submucosal cysts.
    CC **N28.85 Pyeloureteritis cystica** — Inflammation of the kidney pelvis and ureter with the formation of multiple submucosal cysts.
    CC **N28.86 Ureteritis cystica** — Inflammation of the ureters with formation of multiple submucosal cysts.
    N28.89 Other specified disorders of kidney and ureter
  N28.9 Disorder of kidney and ureter, unspecified
    Nephropathy NOS
    Renal disease (acute) NOS
    Renal insufficiency (acute)
    Excludes 1: *chronic renal insufficiency (N18.9)*
        unspecified nephritic syndrome (N05.-)

N29 Other disorders of kidney and ureter <u>in diseases classified elsewhere</u> — [Not Allowed as PDX]
  Code first underlying disease, such as:
    Amyloidosis (E85.-)
    Nephrocalcinosis (E83.5)
    Schistosomiasis (B65.0-B65.9)
  Excludes 1: *disorders of kidney and ureter in:*
        cystinosis (E72.0)
        gonorrhea (A54.21)
        syphilis (A52.75)
        tuberculosis (A18.11)

Other diseases of the urinary system (N30-N39)

  Excludes 1: *urinary infection (complicating):*
        abortion or ectopic or molar pregnancy (O00-O07, O08.8)
        pregnancy, childbirth and the puerperium (O23.-, O75.3, O86.2-)

N30- <u>Cystitis</u> — Inflammation of the bladder.
  Use additional code to identify infectious agent (B95-B97)
  Excludes 1: *prostatocystitis (N41.3)*
  N30.0- <u>Acute</u> cystitis — A severe, sudden onset of inflammation of the bladder.
    Excludes 1: *irradiation cystitis (N30.4-)*
        trigonitis (N30.3-)
  CC **N30.00 Acute cystitis <u>without</u> hematuria**
  CC **N30.01 Acute cystitis <u>with</u> hematuria** — Blood in the urine.
  N30.1- <u>Interstitial</u> cystitis (chronic) — A persistent inflammatory lesion involving the entire thickness of the bladder, seen most often in women.
    N30.10 Interstitial cystitis (chronic) <u>without</u> hematuria
    N30.11 Interstitial cystitis (chronic) <u>with hematuria</u> — Blood in the urine.

N30.2- Other chronic cystitis
  N30.20 Other chronic cystitis <u>without</u> hematuria
  N30.21 Other chronic cystitis <u>with hematuria</u> — Blood in the urine.
N30.3- <u>Trigonitis</u> — Inflammation or localized hyperemia of the trigone area of the bladder.
    Urethrotrigonitis — Inflammation of the urethra and bladder trigone area.
  N30.30 Trigonitis <u>without</u> hematuria
  N30.31 Trigonitis <u>with hematuria</u> — Blood in the urine.
N30.4- <u>Irradiation</u> cystitis — Inflammation of the bladder due to the effects of radiation.
  CC **N30.40 Irradiation cystitis <u>without</u> hematuria**
  CC **N30.41 Irradiation cystitis <u>with hematuria</u>** — Blood in the urine.
N30.8- <u>Other</u> cystitis
    Abscess of bladder — A localized collection of pus caused by the disintegration of bladder tissues.
  N30.80 Other cystitis <u>without</u> hematuria
  N30.81 Other cystitis <u>with hematuria</u> — Blood in the urine.
N30.9- Cystitis, <u>unspecified</u>
  N30.90 Cystitis, unspecified <u>without</u> hematuria
  N30.91 Cystitis, unspecified <u>with hematuria</u> — Blood in the urine.

N31- Neuromuscular dysfunction of bladder, <u>not elsewhere classified</u>
  Use additional code to identify any associated urinary incontinence (N39.3-N39.4-)
  Excludes 1: *cord bladder NOS (G95.89)*
        neurogenic bladder due to cauda equina syndrome (G83.4)
        neuromuscular dysfunction due to spinal cord lesion (G95.89)
  N31.0 Uninhibited neuropathic bladder, not elsewhere classified
  N31.1 Reflex neuropathic bladder, not elsewhere classified
  N31.2 Flaccid neuropathic bladder, not elsewhere classified
    Atonic (motor) (sensory) neuropathic bladder
    Autonomous neuropathic bladder
    Nonreflex neuropathic bladder
  N31.8 Other neuromuscular dysfunction of bladder
  N31.9 Neuromuscular dysfunction of bladder, unspecified
    Neurogenic bladder dysfunction NOS

N32- Other disorders of bladder
  Excludes ❷: *calculus of bladder (N21.0)*
        cystocele (N81.1-)
        hernia or prolapse of bladder, female (N81.1-)
  N32.0 Bladder-neck obstruction — Blockage of the urethral opening of the bladder.
    Bladder-neck stenosis (acquired)
    Excludes 1: *congenital bladder-neck obstruction (Q64.3-)*
  CC **N32.1 Vesicointestinal fistula** — An abnormal passage between the bladder and the intestine.
    Vesicorectal fistula — An abnormal passage between the bladder and the rectum.

VESICOENTERIC FISTULA

VESICORECTAL FISTULA

N2 7 - N3 2

CC **N32.2   Vesical fistula, not elsewhere classified**
Excludes 1:   fistula between bladder and female genital tract (N82.0-N82.1)

N32.3   Diverticulum of bladder — A pouch created by the herniation of bladder-lining mucous membrane through a defect in the bladder muscular wall.
*Excludes 1:   congenital diverticulum of bladder (Q64.6)
diverticulitis of bladder (N30.8-)*

N32.8-   Other specified disorders of bladder

N32.81   Overactive bladder — A condition of abnormal bladder muscle contraction causing symptoms of urinary frequency, urgency, and/or urge incontinence.
Detrusor muscle hyperactivity
Excludes 1:   frequent urination due to specified bladder condition — code to condition

N32.89   Other specified disorders of bladder
Bladder hemorrhage — The abnormal escape of blood from the bladder tissues.
Bladder hypertrophy — The abnormal enlargement of constituent bladder tissue.
Calcified bladder — The abnormal deposition of calcium in the bladder tissues.
Contracted bladder — The abnormal tightening and drawing inward of the bladder tissues.

N32.9   Bladder disorder, unspecified

N33   Bladder disorders in diseases classified elsewhere —
[Not Allowed as PDX]
Code first underlying disease, such as:
Schistosomiasis (B65.0-B65.9)
*Excludes 1:   bladder disorder in syphilis (A52.76)
bladder disorder in tuberculosis (A18.12)
candidal cystitis (B37.41)
chlamydial cystitis (A56.01)
cystitis in gonorrhea (A54.01)
cystitis in neurogenic bladder (N31.-)
diphtheritic cystitis (A36.85)
syphilitic cystitis (A52.76)
trichomonal cystitis (A59.03)*

N34-   Urethritis and urethral syndrome
Use additional code (B95-B97), to identify infectious agent
*Excludes ❷: Reiter's disease (M02.3-)
urethritis in diseases with a predominantly sexual mode of transmission (A50-A64)
urethrotrigonitis (N30.3-)*

CC **N34.0   Urethral abscess** — A localized collection of pus caused by the disintegration of the urethral tissue.
Abscess (of) Cowper's gland
Abscess (of) Littré's gland
Abscess (of) urethral (gland)
Periurethral abscess
Excludes 1:   urethral caruncle (N36.2)

N34.1   Nonspecific urethritis — Inflammation of the urethra.
Nongonococcal urethritis
Nonvenereal urethritis

N34.2   Other urethritis
Meatitis, urethral — Inflammation of the external urethral opening.
Postmenopausal urethritis
Ulcer of urethra (meatus)
Urethritis NOS

N34.3   Urethral syndrome, unspecified

N35-   Urethral stricture — A decrease in the diameter of the urethral lumen.
*Excludes 1:   congenital urethral stricture (Q64.3-)
postprocedural urethral stricture (N99.1-)*

N35.0-   Post-traumatic urethral stricture
Urethral stricture due to injury
Excludes 1:   postprocedural urethral stricture (N99.1-)

N35.01-   Post-traumatic urethral stricture, male

N35.010   Post-traumatic urethral stricture, male, meatal — [♂]

N35.011   Post-traumatic bulbous urethral stricture

N35.012   Post-traumatic membranous urethral stricture

N35.013   Post-traumatic anterior urethral stricture

N35.014   Post-traumatic urethral stricture, male, unspecified — [♂]

N35.02-   Post-traumatic urethral stricture, female

N35.021   Urethral stricture due to childbirth — [♀]

N35.028   Other post-traumatic urethral stricture, female — [♀]

N35.1-   Postinfective urethral stricture, not elsewhere classified
*Excludes 1:   urethral stricture associated with schistosomiasis (B65.-, N29)
gonococcal urethral stricture (A54.01)
syphilitic urethral stricture (A52.76)*

N35.11-   Postinfective urethral stricture, not elsewhere classified, male

N35.111   Postinfective urethral stricture, not elsewhere classified, male, meatal — [♂]

N35.112   Postinfective bulbous urethral stricture, not elsewhere classified

N35.113   Postinfective membranous urethral stricture, not elsewhere classified

N35.114   Postinfective anterior urethral stricture, not elsewhere classified

N35.119   Postinfective urethral stricture, not elsewhere classified, male, unspecified — [♂]

N35.12   Postinfective urethral stricture, not elsewhere classified, female — [♀]

N35.8   Other urethral stricture
Excludes 1:   postprocedural urethral stricture (N99.1-)

N35.9   Urethral stricture, unspecified

N36-   Other disorders of urethra

CC **N36.0   Urethral fistula** — An abnormal passage involving the urethra.
Urethroperineal fistula
Urethrorectal fistula
Urinary fistula NOS
*Excludes 1:   urethroscrotal fistula (N50.89)
urethrovaginal fistula (N82.1)
urethrovesicovaginal fistula (N82.1)*

N36.1   Urethral diverticulum — A circumscribed pouch or sac of mucous membrane lining through a defect in the muscular layer.

Defect in Muscular Wall
Bladder
Urethra

URETHRAL DIVERTICULUM

N36.2   Urethral caruncle — A small fleshy projection of the urethra.

N36.4-   Urethral functional and muscular disorders
Use additional code to identify associated urinary stress incontinence (N39.3)

N36.41   Hypermobility of urethra — The abnormal displacement of the urethra due to anatomical changes that may lead to urine leakage.

N36.42   Intrinsic sphincter deficiency (ISD) — Weakening of the urethral spincter musculature.

N36.43   Combined hypermobility of urethra and intrinsic sphincter deficiency

N36.44   Muscular disorders of urethra
Bladder sphincter dyssynergy

N36.5   Urethral false passage — The presence of non-urethral passage that transports urine.

N36.8   Other specified disorders of urethra
*Excludes 1:   congenital urethrocele (Q64.7)
female urethrocele (N81.0)*

N36.9   Urethral disorder, unspecified

N32–N36

N37 Urethral disorders <u>in diseases classified elsewhere</u> —
[Not Allowed as PDX]
Code first underlying disease
Excludes 1: urethritis (in):
candidal infection (B37.41)
chlamydial (A56.01)
gonorrhea (A54.01)
syphilis (A52.76)
trichomonal infection (A59.03)
tuberculosis (A18.13)

N39- Other disorders of urinary system
Excludes ❷: hematuria NOS (R31.-)
recurrent or persistent hematuria (N02.-)
recurrent or persistent hematuria with specified morphological
lesion (N02.-)
proteinuria NOS (R80.-)

CC **N39.0** Urinary tract infection, site not specified — The abnormal presence
of microorganisms in the urine indicating an infection of the urinary tract.
Use additional code (B95-B97), to identify infectious agent.
Excludes 1: candidiasis of urinary tract (B37.4-)
neonatal urinary tract infection (P39.3)
urinary tract infection of specified site, such as:
cystitis (N30.-)
urethritis (N34.-)

N39.3 Stress incontinence (female) (male) — The involuntary passage of
urine during physical exertion or activity, laughing, coughing, or sneezing.
Code also any associated overactive bladder (N32.81)
Excludes 1: mixed incontinence (N39.46)

N39.4- Other specified urinary incontinence — The involuntary passage of
urine.
Code also any associated overactive bladder (N32.81)
Excludes 1: enuresis NOS (R32)
functional urinary incontinence (R39.81)
urinary incontinence associated with cognitive
impairment (R39.81)
urinary incontinence NOS (R32)
urinary incontinence of nonorganic origin (F98.0)

N39.41 Urge incontinence — A form associated with a strong, sudden desire to
void.
Excludes 1: mixed incontinence (N39.46)

N39.42 Incontinence without sensory awareness — A form without
warning.
Insensible (urinary) incontinence

N39.43 Post-void dribbling — A form following emptying of the bladder.

N39.44 Nocturnal enuresis — A form while asleep due to a delay in
maturation of the mechanism of inhibition.

N39.45 Continuous leakage — A form with continuous passage of urine in
small amounts.

N39.46 Mixed incontinence
Urge and stress incontinence

N39.49- Other specified urinary incontinence

N39.490 Overflow incontinence — A form in which the bladder is
overfilled and leaks a small amount of urine continuously, and does
not completely empty even after voiding.

N39.491 Coital incontinence — A form occurring during sexual
intercourse or orgasm.

N39.492 Postural (urinary) incontinence — A form occurring as a
result of change of body position.

N39.498 Other specified urinary incontinence
Reflex incontinence — A form in which the micturition reflex
is interrupted.
Total incontinence — A form in which control is lost.

N39.8 Other specified disorders of urinary system

N39.9 Disorder of urinary system, unspecified

Diseases of male genital organs (N40-N53)

N40- <u>Benign prostatic hyperplasia</u> — The abnormal proliferation and/or growth of
prostate cellular tissues.
Includes: Adenofibromatous hypertrophy of prostate
Benign hypertrophy of the prostate
Benign prostatic hypertrophy
BPH
Enlarged prostate
Nodular prostate
Polyp of prostate
Excludes 1: benign neoplasms of prostate (adenoma, benign)
(fibroadenoma) (fibroma) (myoma) (D29.1)
Excludes ❷: malignant neoplasm of prostate (C61)

N40.0 Benign prostatic hyperplasia <u>without</u> lower urinary tract
symptoms — [♂, Age/15-124]
Enlarged prostate NOS
Enlarged prostate without LUTS

N40.1 Benign prostatic hyperplasia <u>with lower urinary tract</u>
<u>symptoms</u> — [♂, Age/15-124]
Enlarged prostate with LUTS
Use additional code for associated symptoms, when specified:
Incomplete bladder emptying (R39.14)
Nocturia (R35.1)
Straining on urination (R39.16)
Urinary frequency (R35.0)
Urinary hesitancy (R39.11)
Urinary incontinence (N39.4-)
Urinary obstruction (N13.8)
Urinary retention (R33.8)
Urinary urgency (R39.15)
Weak urinary stream (R39.12)

N40.2 Nodular prostate <u>without</u> lower urinary tract symptoms —
[♂, Age/15-124] — A form with the presence of nodule(s).
Nodular prostate without LUTS

N40.3 Nodular prostate <u>with lower urinary tract symptoms</u> —
[♂, Age/15-124]
Use additional code for associated symptoms, when specified:
Incomplete bladder emptying (R39.14)
Nocturia (R35.1)
Straining on urination (R39.16)
Urinary frequency (R35.0)
Urinary hesitancy (R39.11)
Urinary incontinence (N39.4-)
Urinary obstruction (N13.8)
Urinary retention (R33.8)
Urinary urgency (R39.15)
Weak urinary stream (R39.12)

N41- <u>Inflammatory</u> diseases of prostate
Use additional code (B95-B97), to identify infectious agent

CC **N41.0** <u>Acute</u> prostatitis — [♂, Age/15-124] — The sudden, severe onset of
inflammation of the prostate.

N41.1 <u>Chronic</u> prostatitis — [♂, Age/15-124] — Inflammation of the prostate which
develops slowly and persists over a long period of time.

CC **N41.2** Abscess of prostate — [♂, Age/15-124] — A localized collection of pus
caused by the disintegration of prostatic tissue.

N41.3 Prostatocystitis — [♂, Age/15-124] — Inflammation of the prostate gland
and bladder.

N41.4 Granulomatous prostatitis — [♂, Age/15-124] — Inflammation of the
prostate with the formation of granular tissue.

N41.8 Other inflammatory diseases of prostate — [♂, Age/15-124]

N41.9 Inflammatory disease of prostate, unspecified — [♂, Age/15-124]
Prostatitis NOS

N42- Other and unspecified disorders of prostate

N42.0 Calculus of prostate — [♂, Age/15-124] — A concretion within the prostate
gland.
Prostatic stone

N42.1 Congestion and hemorrhage of prostate — [♂, Age/15-124] — An
abnormal accumulation or escape of blood within the prostate.
Excludes 1: enlarged prostate (N40.-)
hematuria (R31.-)
hyperplasia of prostate (N40.-)
inflammatory diseases of prostate (N41.-)

N42.3- **Dysplasia of prostate** — The abnormal shape and/or size of prostatic cells.

N42.30 **Unspecified dysplasia of prostate** — [♂]

N42.31 **Prostatic intraepithelial neoplasia** — [♂]
PIN
Prostatic intraepithelial neoplasia I (PIN I)
Prostatic intraepithelial neoplasia II (PIN II)
Excludes 1: *prostatic intraepithelial neoplasia III (PIN III)*
(D07.5)

N42.32 **Atypical small acinar proliferation of prostate** — [♂]

N42.39 **Other dysplasia of prostate** — [♂]

N42.8- **Other specified disorders of prostate**

N42.81 **Prostatodynia syndrome** — [♂, Age/15-124]
Painful prostate syndrome

N42.82 **Prostatosis syndrome** — [♂, Age/15-124]

N42.83 **Cyst of prostate** — [♂, Age/15-124] — An encapsulated, fluid-filled sac of the prostate.

N42.89 **Other specified disorders of prostate** — [♂, Age/15-124]

N42.9 **Disorder of prostate, unspecified** — [♂, Age/15-124]

N43- **Hydrocele and spermatocele**
Includes: **Hydrocele of spermatic cord, testis or tunica vaginalis**
Excludes 1: *congenital hydrocele (P83.5)*

N43.0 **Encysted hydrocele** — [♂] — The abnormal accumulation of serous fluid which occurs outside the cavity of the tunica vaginalis testes.

CC **N43.1** **Infected hydrocele** — [♂] — The abnormal accumulation of serous fluid within the scrotum marked by the invasion of microorganisms.
Use additional code (B95-B97), to identify infectious agent

N43.2 **Other hydrocele** — [♂]

N43.3 **Hydrocele, unspecified** — [♂]

N43.4- **Spermatocele of epididymis** – A cystic mass of the epididymis containing spermatozoa.
Spermatic cyst

N43.40 **Spermatocele of epididymis, unspecified** — [♂]

N43.41 **Spermatocele of epididymis, single** — [♂]

N43.42 **Spermatocele of epididymis, multiple** — [♂]

N44- **Noninflammatory disorders of testis**

N44.0- **Torsion of testis** — The abnormal twisting of a testis within the scrotum.

CC **N44.00** **Torsion of testis, unspecified** — [♂]

CC **N44.01** **Extravaginal torsion of spermatic cord** — [♂] — A form in which the spermatic cord is twisted, proximal to the attachments of the tunica vaginalis.

CC **N44.02** **Intravaginal torsion of spermatic cord** — [♂] — A form in which the spermatic cord is twisted, within the tunica vaginalis.
Torsion of spermatic cord NOS

CC **N44.03** **Torsion of appendix testis** — [♂] — The abnormal twisting of the remnant of the embryologic müllerian duct.

CC **N44.04** **Torsion of appendix epididymis** — [♂] — The abnormal twisting of the remnant of the mesonephros.

N44.1 **Cyst of tunica albuginea testis** — [♂] — An encapsulated, fluid-filled sac of the tunica albuginea.

N44.2 **Benign cyst of testis** — [♂] — An encapsulated, fluid-filled sac of the testis.

N44.8 **Other noninflammatory disorders of the testis** — [♂]

N45- **Orchitis and epididymitis**
Use additional code (B95-B97), to identify infectious agent.

N45.1 **Epididymitis** — [♂] — Inflammation of the epididymis.

N45.2 **Orchitis** — [♂] — Inflammation of the testis.

N45.3 **Epididymo-orchitis** — [♂] — Inflammation of the epididymis and testis.

CC **N45.4** **Abscess of epididymis or testis** — [♂] — A localized collection of pus caused by the disintegration of tissue.

N46- **Male infertility** — The inability or diminished ability of the male to produce offspring.
Excludes 1: *vasectomy status (Z98.52)*

N46.0- **Azoospermia** — The absence of spermatozoa in the semen.
Absolute male infertility
Male infertility due to germinal (cell) aplasia
Male infertility due to spermatogenic arrest (complete)

N46.01 **Organic azoospermia** — [♂, Age/15-124] — A form caused by the diseases or conditions of the sperm-producing testes.
Azoospermia NOS

N46.02- **Azoospermia due to extratesticular causes**
Code also associated cause

N46.021 **Azoospermia due to drug therapy** — [♂, Age/15-124]

N46.022 **Azoospermia due to infection** — [♂, Age/15-124]

N46.023 **Azoospermia due to obstruction of efferent ducts** — [♂, Age/15-124]

N46.024 **Azoospermia due to radiation** — [♂, Age/15-124]

N46.025 **Azoospermia due to systemic disease** — [♂, Age/15-124]

N46.029 **Azoospermia due to other extratesticular causes** — [♂, Age/15-124]

N46.1- **Oligospermia** — The diminished amount of spermatozoa in the seminal fluid.
Male infertility due to germinal cell desquamation
Male infertility due to hypospermatogenesis
Male infertility due to incomplete spermatogenic arrest

N46.11 **Organic oligospermia** — [♂, Age/15-124] — A form caused by the diseases or conditions of the sperm-producing testes.
Oligospermia NOS

N46.12- **Oligospermia due to extratesticular causes**
Code also associated cause

N46.121 **Oligospermia due to drug therapy** — [♂, Age/15-124]

N46.122 **Oligospermia due to infection** — [♂, Age/15-124]

N46.123 **Oligospermia due to obstruction of efferent ducts** — [♂, Age/15-124]

N46.124 **Oligospermia due to radiation** — [♂, Age/15-124]

N46.125 **Oligospermia due to systemic disease** — [♂, Age/15-124]

N46.129 **Oligospermia due to other extratesticular causes** — [♂, Age/15-124]

N46.8 **Other male infertility** — [♂, Age/15-124]

N46.9 **Male infertility, unspecified** — [♂, Age/15-124]

N47- **Disorders of prepuce**

N47.0 **Adherent prepuce, newborn** — [♂, Age/0]

N47.1 **Phimosis** — [♂] — The inability to draw the foreskin back from over the glans.

N47.2 **Paraphimosis** — [♂] — The condition in which the retracted foreskin cannot be pulled back into its normal position causing constriction.

N47.3 **Deficient foreskin** — [♂]

N47.4 **Benign cyst of prepuce** — [♂] — An encapsulated, fluid-filled sac of the prepuce.

N47.5 **Adhesions of prepuce and glans penis** — [♂] — The formation of fibrous bands of the prepuce and/or glans penis.

N47.6 **Balanoposthitis** — [♂] — Inflammation of the glans penis and prepuce.
Use additional code (B95-B97), to identify infectious agent
Excludes 1: *balanitis (N48.1)*

N47.7 **Other inflammatory diseases of prepuce** — [♂]
Use additional code (B95-B97), to identify infectious agent

N47.8 **Other disorders of prepuce** — [♂]

N48- **Other disorders of penis**

N48.0 **Leukoplakia of penis** — [♂] — A disease characterized by the shriveled, white, and glossy appearance of the glans penis with the meatus stenosed.
Balanitis xerotica obliterans
Kraurosis of penis
Lichen sclerosus of external male genital organs
Excludes 1: *carcinoma in situ of penis (D07.4)*

N48.1 **Balanitis** — [♂] — Inflammation of the glans penis.
Use additional code (B95-B97), to identify infectious agent
Excludes 1: *amebic balanitis (A06.8)*
balanitis xerotica obliterans (N48.0)
candidal balanitis (B37.42)
gonococcal balanitis (A54.23)
herpesviral [herpes simplex] balanitis (A60.01)

N48.2- **Other inflammatory disorders of penis**
Use additional code (B95-B97), to identify infectious agent.
Excludes 1: *balanitis (N48.1)*
balanitis xerotica obliterans (N48.0)
balanoposthitis (N47.6)

N48.21 **Abscess of corpus cavernosum and penis** — [♂] – A localized collection of pus caused by the disintegration of corpus cavernosum and/or penile tissue.

N48.22 **Cellulitis of corpus cavernosum and penis** — [♂]

N42 - N48

N48.29 Other inflammatory disorders of penis — [♂]

N48.3- Priapism — An abnormal, persistent erection of the penis which is accompanied by pain and tenderness.
  Painful erection
  Code first underlying cause

CC **N48.30 Priapism, unspecified** — [♂]

CC **N48.31 Priapism due to trauma** — [♂]

CC **N48.32 Priapism due to disease classified elsewhere** — [♂]
  [Not Allowed as PDX]

CC **N48.33 Priapism, drug-induced** — [♂]

CC **N48.39 Other priapism** — [♂]

N48.5 Ulcer of penis — [♂] – The eating-away of penile tissue.

N48.6 Induration penis plastica — [♂] – The abnormal curvature of the penis caused by fibrous tissue that results in painful erection.
  Peyronie's disease
  Plastic induration of penis

N48.8- Other specified disorders of penis

N48.81 Thrombosis of superficial vein of penis — [♂] – An abnormal aggregation of blood factors causing an obstruction of the superficial vein of the penis.

N48.82 Acquired torsion of penis — [♂]
  Acquired torsion of penis NOS
  Excludes 1: *congenital torsion of penis (Q55.63)*

N48.83 Acquired buried penis — [♂] – The condition of the penis being hidden underneath the skin.
  Excludes 1: *congenital hidden penis (Q55.64)*

N48.89 Other specified disorders of penis — [♂]

N48.9 Disorder of penis, unspecified — [♂]

N49- Inflammatory disorders of male genital organs, not elsewhere classified
  Use additional code (B95-B97), to identify infectious agent
  Excludes 1: *inflammation of penis (N48.1, N48.2-)*
    orchitis and epididymitis (N45.-)

N49.0 Inflammatory disorders of seminal vesicle — [♂]
  Vesiculitis NOS

N49.1 Inflammatory disorders of spermatic cord, tunica vaginalis and vas deferens — [♂]
  Vasitis

N49.2 Inflammatory disorders of scrotum — [♂]

N49.3 Fournier gangrene — [♂]

N49.8 Inflammatory disorders of other specified male genital organs — [♂]
  Inflammation of multiple sites in male genital organs

N49.9 Inflammatory disorder of unspecified male genital organ — [♂]
  Abscess of unspecified male genital organ
  Boil of unspecified male genital organ
  Carbuncle of unspecified male genital organ
  Cellulitis of unspecified male genital organ

N50- Other and unspecified disorders of male genital organs
  Excludes ❷: *torsion of testis (N44.0-)*

N50.0 Atrophy of testis — [♂] – The abnormal wasting away of the testis.

N50.1 Vascular disorders of male genital organs — [♂]
  Hematocele, NOS, of male genital organs
  Hemorrhage of male genital organs
  Thrombosis of male genital organs

N50.3 Cyst of epididymis — [♂] – An encapsulated, fluid-filled sac of the epididymis.

N50.8- Other specified disorders of male genital organs

N50.81- Testicular pain

N50.811- Right testicular pain — [♂]

N50.812- Left testicular pain — [♂]

N50.819- Testicular pain, unspecified — [♂]

N50.82 Scrotal pain — [♂]

N50.89 Other specified disorders of male genital organs — [♂]
  Atrophy of scrotum, seminal vesicle, spermatic cord, tunica vaginalis and vas deferens
  Chylocele, tunica vaginalis (nonfilarial) NOS
  Edema of scrotum, seminal vesicle, spermatic cord, tunica vaginalis and vas deferens
  Hypertrophy of scrotum, seminal vesicle, spermatic cord, tunica vaginalis and vas deferens
  Stricture of spermatic cord, tunica vaginalis, and vas deferens
  Ulcer of scrotum, seminal vesicle, spermatic cord, testis, tunica vaginalis and vas deferens
  Urethroscrotal fistula

N50.9 Disorder of male genital organs, unspecified — [♂]

N51 Disorders of male genital organs in diseases classified elsewhere — [♂] [Not Allowed as PDX]
  Code first underlying disease, such as:
    Filariasis (B74.0-B74.9)
  Excludes 1: *amebic balanitis (A06.8)*
    candidal balanitis (B37.42)
    gonococcal balanitis (A54.23)
    gonococcal prostatitis (A54.22)
    herpesviral [herpes simplex] balanitis (A60.01)
    trichomonal prostatitis (A59.02)
    tuberculous prostatitis (A18.14)

N52- Male erectile dysfunction — Inability to achieve or maintain erection of the penis, caused by an anatomical condition.
  Excludes 1: *psychogenic impotence (F52.21)*

N52.0- Vasculogenic erectile dysfunction — A form of vascular origin.

N52.01 Erectile dysfunction due to arterial insufficiency — [♂, Age/15-124]

N52.02 Corporo-venous occlusive erectile dysfunction — [♂, Age/15-124]

N52.03 Combined arterial insufficiency and corporo-venous occlusive erectile dysfunction — [♂, Age/15-124]

N52.1 Erectile dysfunction due to diseases classified elsewhere — [♂, Age/15-124] [Not Allowed as PDX]
  Code first underlying disease

N52.2 Drug-induced erectile dysfunction — [♂, Age/15-124]

N52.3- Postprocedural erectile dysfunction

N52.31 Erectile dysfunction following radical prostatectomy — [♂, Age/15-124]

N52.32 Erectile dysfunction following radical cystectomy — [♂, Age/15-124]

N52.33 Erectile dysfunction following urethral surgery — [♂, Age/15-124]

N52.34 Erectile dysfunction following simple prostatectomy — [♂, Age/15-124]

N52.35 Erectile dysfunction following radiation therapy — [♂, Age/15-124]

N52.36 Erectile dysfunction following interstitial seed therapy — [♂, Age/15-124]

N52.37 Erectile dysfunction following prostate ablative therapy — [♂, Age/15-124]
  Erectile dysfunction following cryotherapy
  Erectile dysfunction following other prostate ablative therapies
  Erectile dysfunction following ultrasound ablative therapies

N52.39 Other and unspecified postprocedural erectile dysfunction — [♂, Age/15-124]

N52.8 Other male erectile dysfunction — [♂, Age/15-124]

N52.9 Male erectile dysfunction, unspecified — [♂, Age/15-124]
  Impotence NOS

N
4
8
-
N
5
2

N53-   Other male sexual dysfunction
   Excludes 1:   *psychogenic sexual dysfunction (F52.-)*

   N53.1-   Ejaculatory dysfunction — The abnormal release of the ejaculate.
      Excludes 1:   *premature ejaculation (F52.4)*

      N53.11   Retarded ejaculation — [♂] – A form that is slow to occur.
      N53.12   Painful ejaculation — [♂] – A form that causes pain.
      N53.13   Anejaculatory orgasm — [♂] – A male orgasm that occurs with ejaculation.
      N53.14   Retrograde ejaculation — [♂] – A condition in which the ejaculate is released into the bladder instead of through the urethra.
      N53.19   Other ejaculatory dysfunction — [♂]
            Ejaculatory dysfunction NOS

   N53.8   Other male sexual dysfunction — [♂]
   N53.9   Unspecified male sexual dysfunction — [♂]

Disorders of breast (N60-N65)

   Excludes 1:   *disorders of breast associated with childbirth (O91-O92)*

N60-   Benign mammary dysplasia — Abnormal development of breast tissue.
   Includes: Fibrocystic mastopathy

   N60.0-   Solitary cyst of breast — A single, encapsulated, fluid-filled sac of the breast.
            Cyst of breast
      N60.01   Solitary cyst of right breast
      N60.02   Solitary cyst of left breast
      N60.09   Solitary cyst of unspecified breast

   N60.1-   Diffuse cystic mastopathy — A disease of the breast characterized by nodular cyst formation, tenderness, fluctuation of size, and ductal epithelial hyperplasia.
            Cystic breast
            Fibrocystic disease of breast
      Excludes 1:   *diffuse cystic mastopathy with epithelial proliferation (N60.3-)*
      N60.11   Diffuse cystic mastopathy of right breast — [Age/15-124]
      N60.12   Diffuse cystic mastopathy of left breast — [Age/15-124]
      N60.19   Diffuse cystic mastopathy of unspecified breast — [Age/15-124]

   N60.2-   Fibroadenosis of breast — A non-neoplastic nodular breast condition with fibrous tissue formation.
            Adenofibrosis of breast
      Excludes ❷: *fibroadenoma of breast (D24.-)*
      N60.21   Fibroadenosis of right breast
      N60.22   Fibroadenosis of left breast
      N60.29   Fibroadenosis of unspecified breast

   N60.3-   Fibrosclerosis of breast — Fibrosis and sclerosis of the breast.
            Cystic mastopathy with epithelial proliferation
      N60.31   Fibrosclerosis of right breast
      N60.32   Fibrosclerosis of left breast
      N60.39   Fibrosclerosis of unspecified breast

   N60.4-   Mammary duct ectasia — A disease characterized by dilatation of the mammary gland ducts, intraductal inflammation, and interstitial inflammatory reaction.
      N60.41   Mammary duct ectasia of right breast
      N60.42   Mammary duct ectasia of left breast
      N60.49   Mammary duct ectasia of unspecified breast

   N60.8-   Other benign mammary dysplasias
      N60.81   Other benign mammary dysplasias of right breast
      N60.82   Other benign mammary dysplasias of left breast
      N60.89   Other benign mammary dysplasias of unspecified breast

   N60.9-   Unspecified benign mammary dysplasia
      N60.91   Unspecified benign mammary dysplasia of right breast
      N60.92   Unspecified benign mammary dysplasia of left breast
      N60.99   Unspecified benign mammary dysplasia of unspecified breast

N61-   Inflammatory disorders of breast
   Excludes 1:   *inflammatory carcinoma of breast (C50.9)*
            inflammatory disorder of breast associated with childbirth (O91.-)
            neonatal infective mastitis (P39.0)
            thrombophlebitis of breast [Mondor's disease] (I80.8)

   N61.0   Mastitis without abscess — Inflammation of the breast.
            Cellulitis (acute) (nonpuerperal) (subacute) of breast NOS
            Cellulitis (acute) (nonpuerperal) (subacute) of nipple NOS
            Infective mastitis (acute) (nonpuerperal) (subacute) — Inflammation of the breast due to the invasion and multiplication of microorganisms.
            Mastitis (acute) (nonpuerperal) (subacute) NOS

   N61.1   Abscess of the breast and nipple — A localized collection of pus caused by the disintegration of mammary or areola tissue.
            Abscess (acute) (chronic) (nonpuerperal) of areola
            Abscess (acute) (chronic) (nonpuerperal) of breast
            Carbuncle of breast — A necrotizing infection of the breast composed of a cluster of boils.
            Mastitis with abscess

N62   Hypertrophy of breast — The abnormal enlargement of the breast.
         Gynecomastia — An abnormally large mammary gland in the male which may sometimes secrete milk.
         Hypertrophy of breast NOS
         Massive pubertal hypertrophy of breast
   Excludes 1:   *breast engorgement of newborn (P83.4)*
            disproportion of reconstructed breast (N65.1)

N63   Unspecified lump in breast
         Nodule(s) NOS in breast

N64-   Other disorders of breast
   Excludes ❷: *mechanical complication of breast prosthesis and implant (T85.4-)*

   N64.0   Fissure and fistula of nipple — A crack-like sore of the nipple.
   N64.1   Fat necrosis of breast — [Unacceptable PDX] – Necrosis of the fatty tissue of the breast.
            Fat necrosis (segmental) of breast
            Code first breast necrosis due to breast graft (T85.898)
   N64.2   Atrophy of breast — The abnormal wasting-away of the breast.
   N64.3   Galactorrhea not associated with childbirth — The abnormal flow of milk from the breasts.
   N64.4   Mastodynia — Pain and discomfort of the breast.
   N64.5-   Other signs and symptoms in breast
      Excludes ❷: *abnormal findings on diagnostic imaging of breast (R92.-)*
      N64.51   Induration of breast — The abnormal hardening of the breast tissue.
      N64.52   Nipple discharge — The abnormal drainage of fluid from the nipple.
            Excludes 1:   *abnormal findings in nipple discharge (R89.-)*
      N64.53   Retraction of nipple — The drawing-back of the nipple.
      N64.59   Other signs and symptoms in breast
   N64.8-   Other specified disorders of breast
      N64.81   Ptosis of breast — [Age/15-124] – The condition of sagging or drooping of the breast.
            Excludes 1:   *ptosis of native breast in relation to reconstructed breast (N65.1)*
      N64.82   Hypoplasia of breast — [Age/15-124] – The condition of postpubertal underdevelopment of the breast.
            Micromastia
            Excludes 1:   *congenital absence of breast (Q83.0)*
                     hypoplasia of native breast in relation to reconstructed breast (N65.1)
      N64.89   Other specified disorders of breast
            Galactocele — A breast mass caused by the occlusion of a milk duct and containing a milk-like liquid.
            Subinvolution of breast (postlactational) — The failure of the breast to return to normal size after enlargement.
   N64.9   Disorder of breast, unspecified

N65-   Deformity and disproportion of reconstructed breast
   N65.0   Deformity of reconstructed breast — [Age/15-124] – The condition of a displeasing shape of the reconstructed breast.
            Contour irregularity in reconstructed breast
            Excess tissue in reconstructed breast
            Misshapen reconstructed breast
   N65.1   Disproportion of reconstructed breast — [Age/15-124] – The condition of a displeasing balance of proportion of the reconstructed breast to the other breast.
            Breast asymmetry between native breast and reconstructed breast
            Disproportion between native breast and reconstructed breast

N53 – N65

Inflammatory diseases of female pelvic organs (N70-N77)

Excludes 1: *inflammatory diseases of female pelvic organs complicating:*
abortion or ectopic or molar pregnancy (O00-O07, O08.0)
pregnancy, childbirth and the puerperium (O23.-, O75.3,
O85, O86.-)

N70- **Salpingitis and oophoritis** — Inflammation of the fallopian tube and the ovary.
Includes: **Abscess (of) fallopian tube** — A localized collection of pus caused by the disintegration of fallopian tube tissue.
Abscess (of) ovary — A localized collection of pus caused by the disintegration of ovarian tissue.
Pyosalpinx — The presence of pus within the fallopian tube.
Salpingo-oophoritis — Inflammation of the fallopian tube and ovary.
Tubo-ovarian abscess — A localized collection of pus caused by the disintegration of tubal and ovarian tissues.
Tubo-ovarian inflammatory disease — Inflammation of the fallopian tube and ovary.
Use additional code (B95-B97), to identify infectious agent
Excludes 1: *gonococcal infection (A54.24)*
tuberculous infection (A18.17)

N70.0- **Acute salpingitis and oophoritis** — The sudden, severe onset of inflammation of the fallopian tube and the ovary.
cc **N70.01** Acute salpingitis — [♀]
cc **N70.02** Acute oophoritis — [♀]
cc **N70.03** Acute salpingitis and oophoritis — [♀]

N70.1- **Chronic salpingitis and oophoritis** — Inflammation of the fallopian tube and ovary that develops slowly and persists over a long period of time.
Hydrosalpinx
N70.11 Chronic salpingitis — [♀]
N70.12 Chronic oophoritis — [♀]
N70.13 Chronic salpingitis and oophoritis — [♀]

N70.9- **Salpingitis and oophoritis, unspecified**
N70.91 Salpingitis, unspecified — [♀]
N70.92 Oophoritis, unspecified — [♀]
N70.93 Salpingitis and oophoritis, unspecified — [♀]

N71- **Inflammatory disease of uterus, except cervix** — Inflammation of the uterus.
Includes: **Endo (myo) metritis** — Inflammation of the mucous membrane lining of the uterus.
Metritis — Inflammation of the uterus.
Myometritis — Inflammation of the muscular wall of the uterus.
Pyometra — The abnormal accumulation of pus within the uterine cavity.
Uterine abscess — A localized collection of pus caused by the disintegration of uterine tissues.
Use additional code (B95-B97), to identify infectious agent
Excludes 1: *hyperplastic endometritis (N85.0-)*
infection of uterus following delivery (O85, O86.-)

cc **N71.0** **Acute inflammatory disease of uterus** — [♀] — The sudden, severe onset.
N71.1 **Chronic inflammatory disease of uterus** — [♀] — Develops slowly and persists over a long period of time.
N71.9 Inflammatory disease of uterus, unspecified — [♀]

N72 **Inflammatory disease of cervix uteri** — [♀] — Inflammation of the neck of the uterus.
Includes: **Cervicitis** (with or without erosion or ectropion)
Endocervicitis (with or without erosion or ectropion)
Exocervicitis (with or without erosion or ectropion)
Use additional code (B95-B97), to identify infectious agent
Excludes 1: *erosion and ectropion of cervix without cervicitis (N86)*

N73- **Other female pelvic inflammatory diseases**
Use additional code (B95-B97), to identify infectious agent
cc **N73.0** **Acute parametritis and pelvic cellulitis** — [♀] — The sudden, severe onset of inflammation of the cellular tissue adjacent to the uterus, and inflammation of the cellular tissue in the pelvic cavity.
Abscess of broad ligament
Abscess of parametrium
Pelvic cellulitis, female
N73.1 **Chronic parametritis and pelvic cellulitis** — [♀] — Inflammation of the cellular tissue adjacent to the uterus, and pelvic cellular tissue that develops slowly and persists over a long period of time.
Any condition in N73.0 specified as chronic
Excludes 1: *tuberculous parametritis and pelvic cellulitis (A18.17)*
N73.2 **Unspecified parametritis and pelvic cellulitis** — [♀]
Any condition in N73.0 unspecified whether acute or chronic
mcc **N73.3** **Female acute pelvic peritonitis** — [♀] — The sudden, severe onset of inflammation of the pelvic cavity cellular tissue.

cc **N73.4** **Female chronic pelvic peritonitis** — [♀] — Inflammation of the pelvic cavity cellular tissue in the female that develops slowly and persists over a long period of time.
Excludes 1: *tuberculous pelvic (female) peritonitis (A18.17)*
N73.5 **Female pelvic peritonitis, unspecified** — [♀]
N73.6 **Female pelvic peritoneal adhesions (postinfective)** — [♀] — The formation of fibrotic adhesive bands within the female pelvic peritoneum.
AHA 14:1Q:p3 – Peritoneal adhesions
Excludes ❷: *postprocedural pelvic peritoneal adhesions (N99.4)*
N73.8 Other specified female pelvic inflammatory diseases — [♀]
N73.9 Female pelvic inflammatory disease, unspecified — [♀]
Female pelvic infection or inflammation NOS

N74 **Female pelvic inflammatory disorders in diseases classified elsewhere** — [♀] [Not Allowed as PDX]
Code first underlying disease
Excludes 1: *chlamydial cervicitis (A56.02)*
chlamydial pelvic inflammatory disease (A56.11)
gonococcal cervicitis (A54.03)
gonococcal pelvic inflammatory disease (A54.24)
herpesviral [herpes simplex] cervicitis (A60.03)
herpesviral [herpes simplex] pelvic inflammatory disease (A60.09)
syphilitic cervicitis (A52.76)
syphilitic pelvic inflammatory disease (A52.76)
trichomonal cervicitis (A59.09)
tuberculous cervicitis (A18.16)
tuberculous pelvic inflammatory disease (A18.17)

N75- **Diseases of Bartholin's gland**
N75.0 **Cyst of Bartholin's gland** — [♀] — An encapsulated, fluid-filled sac of the small glands on either side of the vaginal orifice.
cc **N75.1** **Abscess of Bartholin's gland** — [♀] — A localized collection of pus caused by the disintegration of Bartholin's gland tissue.
N75.8 Other diseases of Bartholin's gland — [♀]
Bartholinitis
N75.9 Disease of Bartholin's gland, unspecified — [♀]

N76- **Other inflammation of vagina and vulva**
Use additional code (B95-B97), to identify infectious agent
Excludes ❷: *senile (atrophic) vaginitis (N95.2)*
vulvar vestibulitis (N94.810)
N76.0 **Acute vaginitis** — [♀] — The sudden, severe onset of inflammation of the vagina.
Acute vulvovaginitis
Vaginitis NOS
Vulvovaginitis NOS
N76.1 **Subacute and chronic vaginitis** — [♀] — Inflammation of the vagina that develops slower than an acute infection and persists over a long period of time.
Chronic vulvovaginitis
Subacute vulvovaginitis
N76.2 **Acute vulvitis** — [♀] — The sudden, severe onset of inflammation of the vulva.
Vulvitis NOS
N76.3 **Subacute and chronic vulvitis** — [♀] — Inflammation of the vulva that develops slower than an acute infection and persists over a long period of time.
cc **N76.4** **Abscess of vulva** — [♀] — A localized collection of pus caused by the disintegration of vulva tissue.
Furuncle of vulva — An inflammatory subcutaneous nodule of the vulva.
N76.5 **Ulceration of vagina** — [♀] — The localized eating-away of vaginal tissue.
N76.6 **Ulceration of vulva** — [♀] — The localized eating-away of vulvar tissue.
N76.8- **Other specified inflammation of vagina and vulva**
cc **N76.81** **Mucositis (ulcerative) of vagina and vulva** — [♀] — Inflammation and/or ulcerative sores of the mucous membranes of the vagina and/or vulva.
Code also type of associated therapy, such as:
Antineoplastic and immunosuppressive drugs (T45.1x-)
Radiological procedure and radiotherapy (Y84.2)
Excludes ❷: *gastrointestinal mucositis (ulcerative) (K92.81)*
nasal mucositis (ulcerative) (J34.81)
oral mucositis (ulcerative) (K12.3-)
N76.89 Other specified inflammation of vagina and vulva — [♀]

N77- Vulvovaginal ulceration and inflammation <u>in diseases classified elsewhere</u>

N77.0 Ulceration of vulva in diseases classified elsewhere — [♀] [Not Allowed as PDX]
Code first underlying disease, such as:
Behçet's disease (M35.2)
Excludes 1:   ulceration of vulva in gonococcal infection (A54.02)
ulceration of vulva in herpesviral [herpes simplex] infection (A60.04)
ulceration of vulva in syphilis (A51.0)
ulceration of vulva in tuberculosis (A18.18)

N77.1 Vaginitis, vulvitis and vulvovaginitis in diseases classified elsewhere — [♀] [Not Allowed as PDX]
Code first underlying disease, such as:
Pinworm (B80)
Excludes 1:   candidal vulvovaginitis (B37.3)
chlamydial vulvovaginitis (A56.02)
gonococcal vulvovaginitis (A54.02)
herpesviral [herpes simplex] vulvovaginitis (A60.04)
trichomonal vulvovaginitis (A59.01)
tuberculous vulvovaginitis (A18.18)
vulvovaginitis in early syphilis (A51.0)
vulvovaginitis in late syphilis (A52.76)

Noninflammatory disorders of female genital tract (N80-N98)

N80- <u>Endometriosis</u> — A condition of endometrial tissue growth outside of the uterus.

N80.0 Endometriosis of uterus — [♀] – A form affecting the endometrium of the uterus.
Adenomyosis — A form characterized by in-growth of the endometrium into the uterine muscle layer.
Excludes 1:   stromal endometriosis (D39.0)

N80.1 Endometriosis of ovary — [♀] – A form affecting the ovary.

N80.2 Endometriosis of fallopian tube — [♀] – A form affecting the fallopian tube.

N80.3 Endometriosis of pelvic peritoneum — [♀] – A form affecting the pelvic peritoneum.

N80.4 Endometriosis of rectovaginal septum and vagina — [♀] – A form affecting the tissue between the rectum and the vagina.

N80.5 Endometriosis of intestine — [♀] – A form affecting the intestine.

N80.6 Endometriosis in cutaneous scar — [♀] – A form appearing in the scar healing tissue of the skin.

N80.8 Other endometriosis — [♀]

N80.9 Endometriosis, unspecified — [♀]

N81- <u>Female genital prolapse</u>
Excludes 1:   genital prolapse complicating pregnancy, labor or delivery (O34.5-)
prolapse and hernia of ovary and fallopian tube (N83.4-)
prolapse of vaginal vault after hysterectomy (N99.3)

N81.0 Urethrocele — [♀] – A hernia of the urethral wall that protrudes into the vagina.
Excludes 1:   urethrocele with cystocele (N81.1-)
urethrocele with prolapse of uterus (N81.2-N81.4)

N81.1- Cystocele — A hernia of the bladder that protrudes into the vagina.
Cystocele with urethrocele
Cystourethrocele — A hernia of the bladder and bladder neck/upper urethra that protrudes into the vagina.
Excludes 1:   cystocele with prolapse of uterus (N81.2-N81.4)

N81.10 Cystocele, unspecified — [♀]
Prolapse of (anterior) vaginal wall NOS

N81.11 Cystocele, midline — [♀] – A hernia of the bladder that protrudes into the vagina due to damage to the central portion of the pubocervical fascia.

N81.12 Cystocele, lateral — [♀] – A hernia of the bladder that protrudes into the vagina due to disruption of the lateral vaginal attachments to the arcus tendineus.
Paravaginal cystocele

N81.2 Incomplete uterovaginal prolapse — [♀] – The downward displacement of the uterus and vaginal walls in which the uterus descends into the introitus.
First degree uterine prolapse — A form with protrusion past the cervical os.
Prolapse of cervix NOS
Second degree uterine prolapse — A form with protrusion into the vaginal orifice.
Excludes 1:   cervical stump prolaspe (N81.85)

N81.3 Complete uterovaginal prolapse — [♀] – The downward displacement of the uterus and vaginal walls in which the uterus descends and protrudes beyond the introitus.
Procidentia (uteri) NOS
Third degree uterine prolapse — A form with protrusion beyond the vaginal orifice.

N81.4 Uterovaginal prolapse, unspecified — [♀]
Prolapse of uterus NOS

N81.5 Vaginal enterocele — [♀] – A herniation of the intestine into the rectal vaginal pouch
Excludes 1:   enterocele with prolapse of uterus (N81.2-N81.4)

N81.6 Rectocele — [♀] – A hernia of the anterior wall of the rectum that protrudes into the vagina.
Prolapse of posterior vaginal wall
Use additional code for any associated fecal incontinence, if applicable (R15.-)
Excludes ❷: perineocele (N81.81)
rectal prolapse (K62.3)
rectocele with prolapse of uterus (N81.2-N81.4)

N81.8- Other female genital prolapse

N81.81 Perineocele — [♀] – A hernia between the rectum and vagina that protrudes into the vagina

N81.82 Incompetence or weakening of pubocervical tissue — [♀]

N81.83 Incompetence or weakening of rectovaginal tissue — [♀]

N81.84 Pelvic muscle wasting — [♀]
Disuse atrophy of pelvic muscles and anal sphincter

N81.85 Cervical stump prolapse — [♀] – The downward displacement of the posthysterectomy cervical stump.

N81.89 Other female genital prolapse — [♀]
Deficient perineum
Old laceration of muscles of pelvic floor — Lacerations of pelvic floor muscles which have healed per primam.

N81.9 Female genital prolapse, unspecified — [♀]

N82- Fistulae involving female genital tract
Excludes 1:   vesicointestinal fistulae (N32.1)

CC **N82.0 Vesicovaginal fistula** — [♀] – An abnormal passage communicating the bladder with the vagina.

CC **N82.1 Other female urinary-genital tract fistulae** — [♀]
Cervicovesical fistula — An abnormal passage communicating the cervix with the bladder.
Ureterovaginal fistula — An abnormal passage communicating the ureter with the vagina.
Urethrovaginal fistula — An abnormal passage communicating the urethra with the vagina.
Uteroureteric fistula — An abnormal passage communicating a ureter with the uterus.
Uterovesical fistula — An abnormal passage communicating the uterus with the bladder.

CC **N82.2 Fistula of vagina to small intestine** — [♀] – An abnormal passage communicating the samll intestine with the vagina.

CC **N82.3 Fistula of vagina to large intestine** — [♀] – An abnormal passage communicating the large intestine with the vagina.
Rectovaginal fistula

CC **N82.4 Other female intestinal-genital tract fistulae** — [♀]
Intestinouterine fistula — An abnormal passage communicating the intestine with the vagina.

CC **N82.5 Female genital tract-skin fistulae** — [♀] – An abnormal passage communicating the female genital tract with the skin.
Uterus to abdominal wall fistula — An abnormal passage communicating the uterus with the abdominal wall.
Vaginoperineal fistula — An abnormal passage communicating the vagina with the perineum.

CC **N82.8 Other female genital tract fistulae** — [♀]

CC **N82.9 Female genital tract fistula, unspecified** — [♀]

N83- Noninflammatory disorders of ovary, fallopian tube and broad ligament
Excludes ❷: hydrosalpinx (N70.1-)

N83.0- <u>Follicular cyst of ovary</u> — An encapsulated, enlarged graafian follicle filled with accumulated transudate.
Cyst of graafian follicle
Hemorrhagic follicular cyst (of ovary)

N83.00 Follicular cyst of ovary, <u>unspecified</u> side — [♀]

N83.01 Follicular cyst of <u>right</u> ovary — [♀]

N83.02 Follicular cyst of <u>left</u> ovary — [♀]

N83.1- <u>Corpus luteum</u> cyst — An encapsulated, enlarged serous-filled corpus luteum, or a localized swelling of clotted blood within a corpus luteum.
> **Hemorrhagic corpus luteum cyst** — The escape of blood from, or forcible tearing of the wall of a corpus luteum cyst.

N83.10 Corpus luteum cyst of ovary, <u>unspecified</u> side — [♀]

N83.11 Corpus luteum cyst of <u>right</u> ovary — [♀]

N83.12 Corpus luteum cyst of <u>left</u> ovary — [♀]

N83.2- Other and unspecified ovarian cysts
> *Excludes 1:*   developmental ovarian cyst (Q50.1)
> neoplastic ovarian cyst (D27.-)
> polycystic ovarian syndrome (E28.2)
> Stein-Leventhal syndrome (E28.2)

N83.20- <u>Unspecified</u> ovarian cysts

N83.201 Unspecified ovarian cyst, <u>right</u> side — [♀]

N83.202 Unspecified ovarian cyst, <u>left</u> side — [♀]

N83.209 Unspecified ovarian cyst, <u>unspecified</u> side — [♀]
> Ovarian cyst, NOS

N83.29- <u>Other</u> ovarian cysts
> Retention cyst of ovary
> Simple cyst of ovary

N83.291 Other ovarian cyst, <u>right</u> side — [♀]

N83.292 Other ovarian cyst, <u>left</u> side — [♀]

N83.299 Other ovarian cyst, <u>unspecified</u> side — [♀]

N83.3- <u>Acquired atrophy</u> of ovary and fallopian tube

N83.31- Acquired atrophy of <u>ovary</u> — An abnormal wasting-away of an ovary.

N83.311 Acquired atrophy of <u>right</u> ovary — [♀]

N83.312 Acquired atrophy of <u>left</u> ovary — [♀]

N83.319 Acquired atrophy of ovary, <u>unspecified</u> side — [♀]
> Acquired atrophy of ovary, NOS

N83.32- Acquired atrophy of <u>fallopian tube</u> — An abnormal wasting-away of a fallopian tube.

N83.321 Acquired atrophy of <u>right</u> fallopian tube — [♀]

N83.322 Acquired atrophy of <u>left</u> fallopian tube — [♀]

N83.329 Acquired atrophy of fallopian tube, <u>unspecified</u> side — [♀]
> Acquired atrophy of fallopian tube, NOS

N83.33- Acquired atrophy of <u>ovary and fallopian tube</u> — An abnormal wasting-away of an ovary and a fallopian tube.

N83.331 Acquired atrophy of <u>right</u> ovary and fallopian tube — [♀]

N83.332 Acquired atrophy of <u>left</u> ovary and fallopian tube — [♀]

N83.339 Acquired atrophy of ovary and fallopian tube, <u>unspecified</u> side — [♀]
> Acquired atrophy of ovary and fallopian tube, NOS

N83.4- <u>Prolapse and hernia</u> of ovary and fallopian tube — An abnormal protrusion or displacement from the normal position of an ovary or fallopian tube.

N83.40 Prolapse and hernia of ovary and fallopian tube, <u>unspecified</u> side — [♀]
> Prolapse and hernia of ovary and fallopian tube, NOS

N83.41 Prolapse and hernia of <u>right</u> ovary and fallopian tube — [♀]

N83.42 Prolapse and hernia of <u>left</u> ovary and fallopian tube — [♀]

N83.5- <u>Torsion</u> of ovary, ovarian pedicle and fallopian tube
> Torsion of accessory tube

N83.51- Torsion of <u>ovary and ovarian pedicle</u> — The abnormal twisting of an ovary and/or an ovarian pedicle.

CC **N83.511** Torsion of <u>right</u> ovary and ovarian pedicle — [♀]

CC **N83.512** Torsion of <u>left</u> ovary and ovarian pedicle — [♀]

CC **N83.519** Torsion of ovary and ovarian pedicle, <u>unspecified</u> side — [♀]
> Torsion of ovary and ovarian pedicle, NOS

N83.52- Torsion of <u>fallopian tube</u> — The abnormal twisting of a fallopian tube.
> **Torsion of hydatid of Morgagni** — The abnormal twisting of a cyst-like remnant of the oviduct.

CC **N83.521** Torsion of <u>right</u> fallopian tube — [♀]

CC **N83.522** Torsion of <u>left</u> fallopian tube — [♀]

CC **N83.529** Torsion of fallopian tube, <u>unspecified</u> side — [♀]
> Torsion of fallopian tube, NOS

CC **N83.53** Torsion of ovary, ovarian pedicle and fallopian tube — [♀] — The abnormal twisting of an ovary, ovarian pedicle and fallopian tube.

N83.6 Hematosalpinx — [♀] — The abnormally retained menstrual fluid in a fallopian tube.
> *Excludes 1:*   hematosalpinx (with) (in):
> hematocolpos (N89.7)
> hematometra (N85.7)
> tubal pregnancy (O00.1-)

N83.7 Hematoma of broad ligament — [♀] — A localized swelling mass of clotted blood in the broad ligament, caused by a break in a blood vessel.

N83.8 Other noninflammatory disorders of ovary, fallopian tube and broad ligament — [♀]
> **Broad ligament laceration syndrome [Allen-Masters]** — A forceful disruption of the broad ligament.

N83.9 Noninflammatory disorder of ovary, fallopian tube and broad ligament, unspecified — [♀]

N84- Polyp of female genital tract
> *Excludes 1:*   adenomatous polyp (D28.-)
> placental polyp (O90.89)

N84.0 Polyp of corpus uteri — [♀] — A protruding mucous membrane growth of that portion of the uterus above the isthmus and below the fallopian tube orifices.
> **Polyp of endometrium** — A sessile benign projecting mass on the endometrium.
> Polyp of uterus NOS
> *Excludes 1:*   polypoid endometrial hyperplasia (N85.0-)

N84.1 Polyp of cervix uteri — [♀] — A protruding mucous membrane growth of the cervix.
> **Mucous polyp of cervix**

N84.2 Polyp of vagina — [♀] — A protruding mucous membrane growth of the vagina.

N84.3 Polyp of vulva — [♀] — A protruding mucous membrane growth of the labia and vulva.
> **Polyp of labia**

N84.8 Polyp of other parts of female genital tract — [♀]

N84.9 Polyp of female genital tract, unspecified — [♀]

N85- Other noninflammatory disorders of uterus, except cervix
> *Excludes 1:*   endometriosis (N80.-)
> inflammatory diseases of uterus (N71.-)
> noninflammatory disorders of cervix, except malposition (N86-N88)
> polyp of corpus uteri (N84.0)
> uterine prolapse (N81.-)

N85.0- Endometrial hyperplasia — The abnormal overgrowth of the endometrium.

N85.00 Endometrial hyperplasia, unspecified — [♀]
> **Hyperplasia (adenomatous) (cystic) (glandular) of endometrium**
> **Hyperplastic endometritis** — The abnormal overgrowth of an inflamed endometrium.

N85.01 Benign endometrial hyperplasia — [♀] — A form caused by the hormonal effects of unopposed estrogens.
> **Endometrial hyperplasia (complex) (simple) without atypia**

N85.02 Endometrial intraepithelial neoplasia [EIN] — [♀] — A form indicating an emergent neoplastic precancerous lesion.
> **Endometrial hyperplasia with atypia**
> *Excludes 1:*   malignant neoplasm of endometrium (with endometrial intraepithelial neoplasia [EIN]) (C54.1)

N85.2 Hypertrophy of uterus — [♀] — The abnormal enlargement of the uterus.
> **Bulky or enlarged uterus**
> *Excludes 1:*   puerperal hypertrophy of uterus (O90.89)

N85.3 Subinvolution of uterus — [♀] — A diffuse, symmetrical uterine enlargement with failure to return to its normal size and position.
> *Excludes 1:*   puerperal subinvolution of uterus (O90.89)

N85.4 Malposition of uterus — [♀] — The abnormal position of the uterus.
> **Anteversion of uterus** — The abnormal forward displacement of the uterus.
> **Retroflexion of uterus** — The abnormal bending backward of the uterus at the cervix.
> **Retroversion of uterus** — The abnormal displacement of the uterus backward, including the cervix.
> *Excludes 1:*   malposition of uterus complicating pregnancy, labor or delivery (O34.5-, O65.5)

Excludes 1: = NOT CODED HERE! (Do not code both)   **912**   *Excludes ❷:* = Not Included Here

N85.5 **Inversion of uterus** — [♀] – The abnormal, persistent turning inside out of the uterus.
> Excludes 1:   *current obstetric trauma (O71.2)*
>   *postpartum inversion of uterus (O71.2)*

N85.6 **Intrauterine synechiae** — [♀] – The abnormal adherence and adhesions of the uterus.

N85.7 **Hematometra** — [♀] – The abnormal accumulation of blood within the uterus.
> **Hematosalpinx with hematometra**
> Excludes 1:   *hematometra with hematocolpos (N89.7)*

N85.8 **Other specified noninflammatory disorders of uterus** — [♀]
> **Atrophy of uterus, acquired** — An abnormal wasting-away of the uterus.
> **Fibrosis of uterus NOS**

N85.9 **Noninflammatory disorder of uterus, unspecified** — [♀]
> **Disorder of uterus NOS**

N86 **Erosion and ectropion of cervix uteri** — [♀]
> **Decubitus (trophic) ulcer of cervix** — The abnormal, localized eating-away of cervical tissue.
> **Eversion of cervix** — The abnormal turning inside out of the cervix.
> Excludes 1:   *erosion and ectropion of cervix with cervicitis (N72)*

N87- **Dysplasia of cervix uteri** — The cellular deviation of the cervical epithelium.
> Excludes 1:   *abnormal results from cervical cytologic examination without*
>   *histologic confirmation (R87.61-)*
>   *carcinoma in situ of cervix uteri (D06.-)*
>   *cervical intraepithelial neoplasia III [CIN III] (D06.-)*
>   *HGSIL of cervix (R87.613)*
>   *severe dysplasia of cervix uteri (D06.-)*

N87.0 **Mild cervical dysplasia** — [♀]
> **Cervical intraepithelial neoplasia I [CIN I]**

N87.1 **Moderate cervical dysplasia** — [♀]
> **Cervical intraepithelial neoplasia II [CIN II]**

N87.9 **Dysplasia of cervix uteri, unspecified** — [♀]
> **Anaplasia of cervix**
> **Cervical atypism**
> **Cervical dysplasia NOS**

N88- **Other noninflammatory disorders of cervix uteri**
> Excludes ❷: *inflammatory disease of cervix (N72)*
>   *polyp of cervix (N84.1)*

N88.0 **Leukoplakia of cervix uteri** — [♀] – The abnormal development of white, thickened patches of the mucous membrane of the cervix.

N88.1 **Old laceration of cervix uteri** — [♀] – The presence of a healed lacerated wound of the cervix.
> **Adhesions of cervix**
> Excludes 1:   *current obstetric trauma (O71.3)*

N88.2 **Stricture and stenosis of cervix uteri** — [♀] – An abnormal narrowing of the cervical opening.
> Excludes 1:   *stricture and stenosis of cervix uteri complicating labor*
>   *(O65.5)*

N88.3 **Incompetence of cervix uteri** — [♀] – The abnormal widening of the cervical opening due to inadequate function.
> **Investigation and management of (suspected) cervical**
> **incompetence in a nonpregnant woman**
> Excludes 1:   *cervical incompetence complicating pregnancy*
>   *(O34.3-)*

N88.4 **Hypertrophic elongation of cervix uteri** — [♀] – The abnormal increased length of the cervix into the vagina due to enlargement of the cervical tissues.

N88.8 **Other specified noninflammatory disorders of cervix uteri** — [♀]
> Excludes 1:   *current obstetric trauma (O71.3)*

N88.9 **Noninflammatory disorder of cervix uteri, unspecified** — [♀]

N89- **Other noninflammatory disorders of vagina**
> Excludes 1:   *abnormal results from vaginal cytologic examination without*
>   *histologic confirmation (R87.62-)*
>   *carcinoma in situ of vagina (D07.2)*
>   *HGSIL of vagina (R87.623)*
>   *inflammation of vagina (N76.-)*
>   *senile (atrophic) vaginitis (N95.2)*
>   *severe dysplasia of vagina (D07.2)*
>   *trichomonal leukorrhea (A59.00)*
>   *vaginal intraepithelial neoplasia [VAIN], grade III (D07.2)*

N89.0 **Mild vaginal dysplasia** — [♀] – The abnormal development of vaginal cellular tissue.
> **Vaginal intraepithelial neoplasia [VAIN], grade I**

N89.1 **Moderate vaginal dysplasia** — [♀] – The abnormal development of vaginal cellular tissue.
> **Vaginal intraepithelial neoplasia [VAIN], grade II**

N89.3 **Dysplasia of vagina, unspecified** — [♀]

N89.4 **Leukoplakia of vagina** — [♀] – The abnormal development of white, thickened patches on the mucous membrane of the vagina.

N89.5 **Stricture and atresia of vagina** — [♀] – The abnormal narrowing, or complete blockage of the vagina.
> **Vaginal adhesions** — The abnormal development of fibrotic tissue in the vagina.
> **Vaginal stenosis** — An abnormal decrease in caliber of the vaginal canal.
> Excludes 1:   *congenital atresia or stricture (Q52.4)*
>   *postprocedural adhesions of vagina (N99.2)*

N89.6 **Tight hymenal ring** — [♀] – An abnormally thick, or impenetrable membranous fold of the vaginal orifice.
> **Rigid hymen**
> **Tight introitus**
> Excludes 1:   *imperforate hymen (Q52.3)*

N89.7 **Hematocolpos** — [♀] – The abnormal filling of the vagina with menstrual blood.
> **Hematocolpos with hematometra or hematosalpinx**

N89.8 **Other specified noninflammatory disorders of vagina** — [♀]
> **Leukorrhea NOS**
> **Old vaginal laceration** — The presence of a healed vaginal laceration.
> **Pessary ulcer of vagina**
> Excludes 1:   *current obstetric trauma (O70.-, O71.4, O71.7-*
>   *O71.8)*
>   *old laceration involving muscles of pelvic floor (N81.8)*

N89.9 **Noninflammatory disorder of vagina, unspecified** — [♀]

N90- **Other noninflammatory disorders of vulva and perineum**
> Excludes 1:   *anogenital (venereal) warts (A63.0)*
>   *carcinoma in situ of vulva (D07.1)*
>   *condyloma acuminatum (A63.0)*
>   *current obstetric trauma (O70.-, O71.7-O71.8)*
>   *inflammation of vulva (N76.-)*
>   *severe dysplasia of vulva (D07.1)*
>   *vulvar intraepithelial neoplasm III [VIN III] (D07.1)*

N90.0 **Mild vulvar dysplasia** — [♀] – The abnormal development of vulvar cellular tissue.
> **Vulvar intrepithelial neoplasia [VIN], grade I**

N90.1 **Moderate vulvar dysplasia** — [♀] – The abnormal development of vulvar cellular tissue.
> **Vulvar intraepithelial neoplasia [VIN], grade II**

N90.3 **Dysplasia of vulva, unspecified** — [♀]

N90.4 **Leukoplakia of vulva** — [♀] – A vulvar dystrophic condition characterized by the development of white, thickened patches.
> **Dystrophy of vulva** — Abnormal hypertrophic cellular changes of the vulva.
> **Kraurosis of vulva** — A vulvar dystrophic condition characterized by a dry, shriveled vulva with leukoplakic patches and intense itching.
> **Lichen sclerosus of external female genital organs**

N90.5 **Atrophy of vulva** — [♀] – An abnormal wasting-away of the vulva.
> **Stenosis of vulva**

N90.6- **Hypertrophy of vulva** — An abnormal enlargement of the vulva.

N90.60 **Unspecified hypertrophy of vulva** — [♀]
> **Unspecified hypertrophy of labia**

N90.61 **Childhood asymmetric labium majus enlargement** — [♀, Age/0-17] – An abnormal enlargement of one side of the vulva due to excessive tissue growth and occurring during pre- and early puberty.
> **CALME**

N90.69 **Other specified hypertrophy of vulva** — [♀]
> **Other specified hypertrophy of labia**

N90.7 **Vulvar cyst** — [♀] – An encapsulated, fluid-filled sac of the vulva.

N85 – N90

N90.8- **Other specified noninflammatory disorders of vulva and perineum**

N90.81- **Female genital mutilation status** — The condition of having the female genitalia removed, in all or part, as a cultural practice performed in Africa, the Middle East, and part of Asia.
Female genital cutting status

N90.810 **Female genital mutilation status, unspecified** — [♀]
Female genital cutting status, unspecified
Female genital mutilation status NOS

N90.811 **Female genital mutilation Type I status** — [♀]
Clitorectomy status
Female genital cutting Type I status

N90.812 **Female genital mutilation Type II status** — [♀]
Clitorectomy with excision of labia minora status
Female genital cutting Type II status

N90.813 **Female genital mutilation Type III status** — [♀]
Female genital cutting Type III status
Infibulation status

N90.818 **Other female genital mutilation status** — [♀]
Female genital cutting Type IV status
Female genital mutilation Type IV status
Other female genital cutting status

N90.89 **Other specified noninflammatory disorders of vulva and perineum** — [♀]
Adhesions of vulva
Hypertrophy of clitoris

N90.9 **Noninflammatory disorder of vulva and perineum, unspecified** — [♀]

N91- **Absent, scanty and rare menstruation**
Excludes 1:   ovarian dysfunction (E28.-)

N91.0 **Primary amenorrhea** — [♀] — The absence of menstruation prior to age 16 years.

N91.1 **Secondary amenorrhea** — [♀] — The absence of menstruation for a period of 6 months or greater.

N91.2 **Amenorrhea, unspecified** — [♀]

N91.3 **Primary oligomenorrhea** — [♀] — The decreased frequency of menstruation.

N91.4 **Secondary oligomenorrhea** — [♀] — The decreased frequency of menstruation that is due to another disease or condition.

N91.5 **Oligomenorrhea, unspecified** — [♀]
Hypomenorrhea NOS

N92- **Excessive, frequent and irregular menstruation**
Excludes 1:   postmenopausal bleeding (N95.0)
precocious puberty (menstruation) (E30.1)

N92.0 **Excessive and frequent menstruation with regular cycle** — [♀] — The abnormal increase or increased number of cycles of menstruation.
Heavy periods NOS — The increased volume of menstrual flow.
Menorrhagia NOS — The excessive uterine bleeding occurring at the regular intervals of menstruation.
Polymenorrhea — Abnormally frequent menstruation.

N92.1 **Excessive and frequent menstruation with irregular cycle** — [♀] — A menstrual cycle which is different than the average four-week interval.
Irregular intermenstrual bleeding — Nonmenstrual uterine bleeding unrelated to menstrual cycle.
Irregular, shortened intervals between menstrual bleeding
Menometrorrhagia
Metrorrhagia

N92.2 **Excessive menstruation at puberty** — [♀, Age/0-17]
Excessive bleeding associated with onset of menstrual periods
Pubertal menorrhagia
Puberty bleeding

N92.3 **Ovulation bleeding** — [♀] — Uterine bleeding associated with ovulation.
Regular intermenstrual bleeding

N92.4 **Excessive bleeding in the premenopausal period** — [♀]
Climacteric menorrhagia or metrorrhagia
Menopausal menorrhagia or metrorrhagia
Preclimacteric menorrhagia or metrorrhagia
Premenopausal menorrhagia or metrorrhagia

N92.5 **Other specified irregular menstruation** — [♀]

N92.6 **Irregular menstruation, unspecified** — [♀]
Irregular bleeding NOS
Irregular periods NOS
Excludes 1:   irregular menstruation with:
lengthened intervals or scanty bleeding (N91.3-N91.5)
shortened intervals or excessive bleeding (N92.1)

N93- **Other abnormal uterine and vaginal bleeding**
Excludes 1:   neonatal vaginal hemorrhage (P54.6)
precocious puberty (menstruation) (E30.1)
pseudomenses (P54.6)

N93.0 **Postcoital and contact bleeding** — [♀] — Abnormal bleeding following sexual intercourse.

N93.1 **Pre-pubertal vaginal bleeding** — [♀, Age/0-17] — Abnormal pre-pubertal vaginal bleeding of an unknown cause, including not due to menstruation.

N93.8 **Other specified abnormal uterine and vaginal bleeding** — [♀]
Dysfunctional or functional uterine or vaginal bleeding NOS

N93.9 **Abnormal uterine and vaginal bleeding, unspecified** — [♀]

N94- **Pain and other conditions associated with female genital organs and menstrual cycle**

N94.0 **Mittelschmerz** — [♀] — Abdominal pain occurring at the time of ovulation.

N94.1- **Dyspareunia** — The occurrence of pain during sexual intercourse.
Excludes 1:   psychogenic dyspareunia (F52.6)

N94.10 **Unspecified dyspareunia** — [♀]

N94.11 **Superficial (introital) dyspareunia** — [♀] — A form occurring on vaginal entry.

N94.12 **Deep dyspareunia** — [♀] — A form occurring with mid or upper vaginal penetration.

N94.19 **Other specified dyspareunia** — [♀]

N94.2 **Vaginismus** — [♀] — The painful spasm of the muscles surrounding the vagina.
Excludes 1:   psychogenic vaginismus (F52.5)

N94.3 **Premenstrual tension syndrome** — [♀] — A syndrome of various symptoms occurring in the days preceding menstruation marked by emotional instability, irritability, insomnia, and headache.
Premenstrual dysphoric disorder — A severe form of premenstrual tension syndrome that significantly disrupts a woman's day-to-day activities.
Code also associated menstrual migraine (G43.82-, G43.83-)
Excludes 1:   premenstrual dysphoric disorder (F32.81)

N94.4 **Primary dysmenorrhea** — [♀] — The excessively painful uterine cramps that accompany menstruation.

N94.5 **Secondary dysmenorrhea** — [♀] — A form that is associated with another medical conditon.

N94.6 **Dysmenorrhea, unspecified** — [♀]
Excludes 1:   psychogenic dysmenorrhea (F45.8)

N94.8- **Other specified conditions associated with female genital organs and menstrual cycle**

N94.81- **Vulvodynia** — The condition of persistent pain in the vulva that is characterized by burning, soreness, itching, rawness, and painful intercourse.

N94.810 **Vulvar vestibulitis** — [♀] — A form marked by pain with symptoms generally limited to the vaginal opening that results in painful vaginal entry (tampons or intercourse) and/or pain associated with sitting or wearing tight clothing.

N94.818 **Other vulvodynia** — [♀]

N94.819 **Vulvodynia, unspecified** — [♀]
Vulvodynia NOS

N94.89 **Other specified conditions associated with female genital organs and menstrual cycle** — [♀]

N94.9 **Unspecified condition associated with female genital organs and menstrual cycle** — [♀]

N95- Menopausal and other perimenopausal disorders
Menopausal and other perimenopausal disorders due to naturally occurring (age-related) menopause and perimenopause

Excludes 1:   *excessive bleeding in the premenopausal period (N92.4)*
menopausal and perimenopausal disorders due to artificial or premature menopause (E89.4-, E28.31-)
premature menopause (E28.31-)

Excludes ❷: *postmenopausal osteoporosis (M81.0-)*
postmenopausal osteoporosis with current pathological fracture (M80.0-)
postmenopausal urethritis (N34.2)

N95.0 Postmenopausal bleeding — [♀] – Abnormal bleeding following menopause.

N95.1 Menopausal and female climacteric states — [♀]
Symptoms such as flushing, sleeplessness, headache, lack of concentration, associated with natural (age-related) menopause
Use additional code for associated symptoms

Excludes 1:   *asymptomatic menopausal state (Z78.0)*
symptoms associated with artificial menopause (E89.41)
symptoms associated with premature menopause (E28.310)

N95.2 Postmenopausal atrophic vaginitis — [♀] – The wasting-away of the vaginal tissues associated with the cessation of menstruation.
Senile (atrophic) vaginitis

N95.8 Other specified menopausal and perimenopausal disorders — [♀]

N95.9 Unspecified menopausal and perimenopausal disorder — [♀]

N96 Recurrent pregnancy loss — [♀]
Investigation or care in a nonpregnant woman with history of recurrent pregnancy loss

Excludes 1:   *recurrent pregancy loss with current pregnancy (O26.2-)*

N97- Female infertility — Inability, or diminished ability, of a female to produce offspring.
Includes: Inability to achieve a pregnancy
Sterility, female NOS

Excludes 1:   *female infertility associated with:*
hypopituitarism (E23.0)
Stein-Leventhal syndrome (E28.2)

Excludes ❷: *incompetence of cervix uteri (N88.3)*

N97.0 Female infertility associated with anovulation — [♀] – A form characterized by absence of ovulation.

N97.1 Female infertility of tubal origin — [♀] – A form resulting from dysfunctional fallopian tube conditions.
Female infertility associated with congenital anomaly of tube
Female infertility due to tubal block
Female infertility due to tubal occlusion
Female infertility due to tubal stenosis

N97.2 Female infertility of uterine origin — [♀] – A form resulting from dysfunctional uterine conditions.
Female infertility associated with congenital anomaly of uterus
Female infertility due to nonimplantation of ovum

N97.8 Female infertility of other origin — [♀]

N97.9 Female infertility, unspecified — [♀]

N98- Complications associated with artificial fertilization

cc **N98.0 Infection associated with artificial insemination** — [♀]

cc **N98.1 Hyperstimulation of ovaries** — [♀]
Hyperstimulation of ovaries NOS
Hyperstimulation of ovaries associated with induced ovulation

cc **N98.2 Complications of attempted introduction of fertilized ovum following in vitro fertilization** — [♀]

cc **N98.3 Complications of attempted introduction of embryo in embryo transfer** — [♀]

cc **N98.8 Other complications associated with artificial fertilization** — [♀]

cc **N98.9 Complication associated with artificial fertilization, unspecified** — [♀]

Intraoperative and postprocedural complications and disorders of genitourinary system, not elsewhere classified (N99)

N99- Intraoperative and postprocedural complications and disorders of genitourinary system, not elsewhere classified

Excludes ❷: *irradiation cystitis (N30.4-)*
postoophorectomy osteoporosis with current pathological fracture (M80.8-)
postoophorectomy osteoporosis without current pathological fracture (M81.8)

N99.0 Postprocedural (acute) (chronic) kidney failure
Use additional code to type of kidney disease

N99.1- Postprocedural urethral stricture
Postcatheterization urethral stricture

N99.11- Postprocedural urethral stricture, male

N99.110 Postprocedural urethral stricture, male, meatal — [♂]

N99.111 Postprocedural bulbous urethral stricture — [♂]

N99.112 Postprocedural membranous urethral stricture — [♂]

N99.113 Postprocedural anterior bulbous urethral stricture — [♂]

N99.114 Postprocedural urethral stricture, male, unspecified — [♂]

N99.115 Postprocedural fossa navicularis urethral stricture

N99.12 Postprocedural urethral stricture, female — [♀]

N99.2 Postprocedural adhesions of vagina — [♀]

N99.3 Prolapse of vaginal vault after hysterectomy — [♀]

N99.4 Postprocedural pelvic peritoneal adhesions

Excludes ❷: *pelvic peritoneal adhesions NOS (N73.6)*
postinfective pelvic peritoneal adhesions (N73.6)

N99.5- Complications of stoma of urinary tract

Excludes ❷: *mechanical complication of urinary catheter (T83.0-)*

N99.51- Complication of cystostomy

cc **N99.510 Cystostomy hemorrhage**

cc **N99.511 Cystostomy infection**

cc **N99.512 Cystostomy malfunction**

cc **N99.518 Other cystostomy complication**

N99.52- Complication of incontinent external stoma of urinary tract

N99.520 Hemorrhage of incontinent external stoma of urinary tract

N99.521 Infection of incontinent external stoma of urinary tract

N99.522 Malfunction of incontinent external stoma of urinary tract

N99.523 Herniation of incontinent stoma of urinary tract

N99.524 Stenosis of incontinent stoma of urinary tract

N99.528 Other complication of incontinent external stoma of urinary tract

N99.53- Complication of continent stoma of urinary tract

N99.530 Hemorrhage of continent stoma of urinary tract

N99.531 Infection of continent stoma of urinary tract

N99.532 Malfunction of continent stoma of urinary tract

N99.533 Herniation of continent stoma of urinary tract

N99.534 Stenosis of continent stoma of urinary tract

N99.538 Other complication of continent stoma of urinary tract

N99.6- **Intraoperative hemorrhage and hematoma** of a genitourinary system organ or structure complicating a procedure
　　Excludes 1: *intraoperative hemorrhage and hematoma of a genitourinary system organ or structure due to accidental puncture or laceration during a procedure (N99.7-)*

cc N99.61 **Intraoperative hemorrhage and hematoma of a genitourinary system organ or structure complicating a genitourinary system procedure**

cc N99.62 **Intraoperative hemorrhage and hematoma of a genitourinary system organ or structure complicating other procedure**

N99.7- **Accidental puncture and laceration of a genitourinary system organ or structure during a procedure**

cc N99.71 **Accidental puncture and laceration of a genitourinary system organ or structure during a genitourinary system procedure**

cc N99.72 **Accidental puncture and laceration of a genitourinary system organ or structure during other procedure**

N99.8- **Other intraoperative and postprocedural complications and disorders of genitourinary system**

N99.81 **Other intraoperative complications of genitourinary system**

N99.82- **Postprocedural hemorrhage** of a genitourinary system organ or structure following a procedure

cc N99.820 **Postprocedural hemorrhage of a genitourinary system organ or structure following a genitourinary system procedure**

cc N99.821 **Postprocedural hemorrhage of a genitourinary system organ or structure following other procedure**

N99.83 **Residual ovary syndrome** — [♀]

N99.84- **Postprocedural hematoma and seroma** of a genitourinary system organ or structure following a procedure

cc N99.840 **Postprocedural hematoma of a genitourinary system organ or structure following a genitourinary system procedure**

cc N99.841 **Postprocedural hematoma of a genitourinary system organ or structure following other procedure**

cc N99.842 **Postprocedural seroma of a genitourinary system organ or structure following a genitourinary system procedure**

cc N99.843 **Postprocedural seroma of a genitourinary system organ or structure following other procedure**

N99.89 **Other postprocedural complications and disorders of genitourinary system**

Chapter 15 – Pregnancy, childbirth and the puerperium (O00-O9A)

Note: CODES FROM THIS CHAPTER ARE FOR USE ONLY ON MATERNAL RECORDS, NEVER ON NEWBORN RECORDS. Codes from this chapter are for use for conditions related to or aggravated by the pregnancy, childbirth, or by the puerperium (maternal causes or obstetric causes)

Use additional code from category Z3A, Weeks of gestation, to identify the specific week of the pregnancy, if known.

Trimesters are counted from the first day of the last menstrual period. They are defined as follows:

1st trimester- less than 14 weeks 0 days
2nd trimester- 14 weeks 0 days to less than 28 weeks 0 days
3rd trimester- 28 weeks 0 days until delivery

Excludes 1: supervision of normal pregnancy (Z34.-)
Excludes ❷: mental and behavioral disorders associated with the puerperium (F53)
        obstetrical tetanus (A34)
        postpartum necrosis of pituitary gland (E23.0)
        puerperal osteomalacia (M83.0)

This chapter contains the following blocks:

O00-O08	Pregnancy with abortive outcome
O09	Supervision of high risk pregnancy
O10-O16	Edema, proteinuria and hypertensive disorders in pregnancy, childbirth and the puerperium
O20-O29	Other maternal disorders predominantly related to pregnancy
O30-O48	Maternal care related to the fetus and amniotic cavity and possible delivery problems
O60-O77	Complications of labor and delivery
O80-O82	Encounter for delivery
O85-O92	Complications predominantly related to the puerperium
O94-O9A	Other obstetric conditions, not elsewhere classified

Chapter-Specific Coding Guidelines

C. Chapter-Specific Coding Guidelines

In addition to general coding guidelines, there are guidelines for specific diagnoses and/or conditions in the classification. Unless otherwise indicated, these guidelines apply to all health care settings. Please refer to Section II for guidelines on the selection of principal diagnosis.

15. Chapter 15: Pregnancy, Childbirth, and the Puerperium (O00-O9A)

a. General Rules for Obstetric Cases

1) Codes from chapter 15 and sequencing priority

Obstetric cases require codes from chapter 15, codes in the range O00-O9A, Pregnancy, Childbirth, and the Puerperium. Chapter 15 codes have sequencing priority over codes from other chapters. Additional codes from other chapters may be used in conjunction with chapter 15 codes to further specify conditions. Should the provider document that the pregnancy is incidental to the encounter, then code Z33.1, Pregnant state, incidental, should be used in place of any chapter 15 codes. It is the provider's responsibility to state that the condition being treated is not affecting the pregnancy.

2) Chapter 15 codes used only on the maternal record

Chapter 15 codes are to be used only on the maternal record, never on the record of the newborn.

3) Final character for trimester

The majority of codes in Chapter 15 have a final character indicating the trimester of pregnancy. The timeframes for the trimesters are indicated at the beginning of the chapter. If trimester is not a component of a code it is because the condition always occurs in a specific trimester, or the concept of trimester of pregnancy is not applicable. Certain codes have characters for only certain trimesters because the condition does not occur in all trimesters, but it may occur in more than just one.

Assignment of the final character for trimester should be based on the provider's documentation of the trimester (or number of weeks) for the current admission/encounter. This applies to the assignment of trimester for pre-existing conditions as well as those that develop during or are due to the pregnancy. The provider's documentation of the number of weeks may be used to assign the appropriate code identifying the trimester.

Whenever delivery occurs during the current admission, and there is an "in childbirth" option for the obstetric complication being coded, the "in childbirth" code should be assigned.

4) Selection of trimester for inpatient admissions that encompass more than one trimesters

In instances when a patient is admitted to a hospital for complications of pregnancy during one trimester and remains in the hospital into a subsequent trimester, the trimester character for the antepartum complication code should be assigned on the basis of the trimester when the complication developed, not the trimester of the discharge. If the condition developed prior to the current admission/encounter or represents a pre-existing condition, the trimester character for the trimester at the time of the admission/encounter should be assigned.

5) Unspecified trimester

Each category that includes codes for trimester has a code for "unspecified trimester." The "unspecified trimester" code should rarely be used, such as when the documentation in the record is insufficient to determine the trimester and it is not possible to obtain clarification.

6) 7th character for Fetus Identification

Where applicable, a 7th character is to be assigned for certain categories (O31, O32, O33.3 - O33.6, O35, O36, O40, O41, O60.1, O60.2, O64, and O69) to identify the fetus for which the complication code applies.

Assign 7th character "0":
  • For single gestations
  • When the documentation in the record is insufficient to determine the fetus affected and it is not possible to obtain clarification.
  • When it is not possible to clinically determine which fetus is affected.

b. Selection of OB Principal or First-listed Diagnosis

1) Routine outpatient prenatal visits

For routine outpatient prenatal visits when no complications are present, a code from category Z34, Encounter for supervision of normal pregnancy, should be used as the first-listed diagnosis. These codes should not be used in conjunction with chapter 15 codes.

2) *Supervision of High-Risk Pregnancy*

Codes from category O09, Supervision of high-risk pregnancy, are intended for use only during the prenatal period. For complications during the labor or delivery episode as a result of a high-risk pregnancy, assign the applicable complication codes from Chapter 15. If there are no complications during the labor and delivery episode, assign code O80, Encounter for full-term uncomplicated delivery.

For routine prenatal outpatient visits for patients with high-risk pregnancies, a code from category O09, Supervision of high-risk pregnancy, should be used as the first-listed diagnosis. Secondary chapter 15 codes may be used in conjunction with these codes if appropriate.

3) Episodes when no delivery occurs

In episodes when no delivery occurs, the principal diagnosis should correspond to the principal complication of the pregnancy which necessitated the encounter. Should more than one complication exist, all of which are treated or monitored, any of the complications codes may be sequenced first.

4) When a delivery occurs

~~When a delivery occurs, the principal diagnosis should correspond to the main circumstances or complication of the delivery.~~ When an obstetric patient is admitted and delivers during that admission, the condition that prompted the admission should be sequenced as the principal diagnosis. If multiple conditions prompted the admission, sequence the one most related to the delivery as the principal diagnosis. A code for any complication of the delivery should be assigned as an additional diagnosis. In cases of cesarean delivery, ~~the selection of the principal diagnosis should be the condition established after study that was responsible for the patient's admission.~~ If the patient was admitted with a condition that resulted in the performance of a cesarean procedure, that condition should be selected as the principal diagnosis. If the reason for the admission/~~encounter~~ was unrelated to the condition resulting in the cesarean delivery, the condition related to the reason for the admission/~~encounter~~ should be selected as the principal diagnosis.

5) Outcome of delivery

A code from category Z37, Outcome of delivery, should be included on every maternal record when a delivery has occurred. These codes are not to be used on subsequent records or on the newborn record.

c. Pre-existing conditions versus conditions due to the pregnancy

Certain categories in Chapter 15 distinguish between conditions of the mother that existed prior to pregnancy (pre-existing) and those that are a direct result of pregnancy. When assigning codes from Chapter 15, it is important to assess if a condition was pre-existing prior to pregnancy or developed during or due to the pregnancy in order to assign the correct code.

O00-O9A

Categories that do not distinguish between pre-existing and pregnancy-related conditions may be used for either. It is acceptable to use codes specifically for the puerperium with codes complicating pregnancy and childbirth if a condition arises postpartum during the delivery encounter.

d. Pre-existing hypertension in pregnancy
Category O10, Pre-existing hypertension complicating pregnancy, childbirth and the puerperium, includes codes for hypertensive heart and hypertensive chronic kidney disease. When assigning one of the O10 codes that includes hypertensive heart disease or hypertensive chronic kidney disease, it is necessary to add a secondary code from the appropriate hypertension category to specify the type of heart failure or chronic kidney disease.

See Section I.C.9. Hypertension.

e. Fetal Conditions Affecting the Management of the Mother

1) Codes from categories O35 and O36
Codes from categories O35, Maternal care for known or suspected fetal abnormality and damage, and O36, Maternal care for other fetal problems, are assigned only when the fetal condition is actually responsible for modifying the management of the mother, i.e., by requiring diagnostic studies, additional observation, special care, or termination of pregnancy. The fact that the fetal condition exists does not justify assigning a code from this series to the mother's record.

2) In utero surgery
In cases when surgery is performed on the fetus, a diagnosis code from category O35, Maternal care for known or suspected fetal abnormality and damage, should be assigned identifying the fetal condition. Assign the appropriate procedure code for the procedure performed.

No code from Chapter 16, the perinatal codes, should be used on the mother's record to identify fetal conditions. Surgery performed in utero on a fetus is still to be coded as an obstetric encounter.

f. HIV Infection in Pregnancy, Childbirth and the Puerperium
During pregnancy, childbirth or the puerperium, a patient admitted because of an HIV-related illness should receive a principal diagnosis from subcategory O98.7-, Human immunodeficiency [HIV] disease complicating pregnancy, childbirth and the puerperium, followed by the code(s) for the HIV-related illness(es).

Patients with asymptomatic HIV infection status admitted during pregnancy, childbirth, or the puerperium should receive codes of O98.7- and Z21, Asymptomatic human immunodeficiency virus [HIV] infection status.

g. Diabetes mellitus in pregnancy
Diabetes mellitus is a significant complicating factor in pregnancy. Pregnant women who are diabetic should be assigned a code from category O24, Diabetes mellitus in pregnancy, childbirth, and the puerperium, first, followed by the appropriate diabetes code(s) (E08-E13) from Chapter 4.

h. Long-term use of insulin *and oral hypoglycemics*
Code Z79.4, Long-term (current) use of insulin, or code Z79.84, Long-term (current) use of oral hypoglycemic drugs, should also be assigned if the diabetes mellitus is being treated with insulin or oral medications. If the patient is treated with both oral medications and insulin, only the code for insulin-controlled should be assigned.

i. Gestational (pregnancy induced) diabetes
Gestational (pregnancy induced) diabetes can occur during the second and third trimester of pregnancy in women who were not diabetic prior to pregnancy. Gestational diabetes can cause complications in the pregnancy similar to those of pre-existing diabetes mellitus. It also puts the woman at greater risk of developing diabetes after the pregnancy. Codes for gestational diabetes are in subcategory O24.4, Gestational diabetes mellitus. No other code from category O24, Diabetes mellitus in pregnancy, childbirth, and the puerperium, should be used with a code from O24.4.

The codes under subcategory O24.4 include diet controlled, and insulin controlled, and controlled by oral hypoglycemic drugs. If a patient with gestational diabetes is treated with both diet and insulin, only the code for insulin-controlled is required. If a patient with gestational diabetes is treated with both diet and oral hypoglycemic medications, only the code for "controlled by oral hypoglycemic drugs" is required. Code Z79.4, Long-term (current) use of insulin or code Z79.84, Long-term (current) use of oral hypoglycemic drugs, should not be assigned with codes from subcategory O24.4.

An abnormal glucose tolerance in pregnancy is assigned a code from subcategory O99.81, Abnormal glucose complicating pregnancy, childbirth, and the puerperium.

j. Sepsis and septic shock complicating abortion, pregnancy, childbirth and the puerperium
When assigning a chapter 15 code for sepsis complicating abortion, pregnancy, childbirth, and the puerperium, a code for the specific type of infection should be assigned as an additional diagnosis. If severe sepsis is present, a code from subcategory R65.2, Severe sepsis, and code(s) for associated organ dysfunction(s) should also be assigned as additional diagnoses.

k. Puerperal sepsis
Code O85, Puerperal sepsis, should be assigned with a secondary code to identify the causal organism (e.g., for a bacterial infection, assign a code from category B95-B96, Bacterial infections in conditions classified elsewhere). A code from category A40, Strepto-coccal sepsis, or A41, Other sepsis, should not be used for puerperal sepsis. If applicable, use additional codes to identify severe sepsis (R65.2-) and any associated acute organ dysfunction.

l. Alcohol and tobacco use during pregnancy, childbirth and the puerperium

1) Alcohol use during pregnancy, childbirth and the puerperium
Codes under subcategory O99.31, Alcohol use complicating pregnancy, childbirth, and the puerperium, should be assigned for any pregnancy case when a mother uses alcohol during the pregnancy or postpartum. A secondary code from category F10, Alcohol related disorders, should also be assigned to identify manifestations of the alcohol use.

2) Tobacco use during pregnancy, childbirth and the puerperium
Codes under subcategory O99.33, Smoking (tobacco) complicating pregnancy, childbirth, and the puerperium, should be assigned for any pregnancy case when a mother uses any type of tobacco product during the pregnancy or postpartum. A secondary code from category F17, Nicotine dependence, Tobacco use, should also be assigned to identify the type of nicotine dependence.

m. Poisoning, toxic effects, adverse effects and underdosing in a pregnant patient
A code from subcategory O9A.2, Injury, poisoning and certain other consequences of external causes complicating pregnancy, childbirth, and the puerperium, should be sequenced first, followed by the appropriate injury, poisoning, toxic effect, adverse effect or underdosing code, and then the additional code(s) that specifies the condition caused by the poisoning, toxic effect, adverse effect or underdosing.

See Section I.C.19. Adverse effects, poisoning, underdosing and toxic effects.

n. Normal Delivery, Code O80

1) Encounter for full term uncomplicated delivery
Code O80 should be assigned when a woman is admitted for a full-term normal delivery and delivers a single, healthy infant without any complications antepartum, during the delivery, or postpartum during the delivery episode. Code O80 is always a principal diagnosis. It is not to be used if any other code from chapter 15 is needed to describe a current complication of the antenatal, delivery, or perinatal period. Additional codes from other chapters may be used with code O80 if they are not related to or are in any way complicating the pregnancy.

2) Uncomplicated delivery with resolved antepartum complication
Code O80 may be used if the patient had a complication at some point during the pregnancy, but the complication is not present at the time of the admission for delivery.

3) Outcome of delivery for O80
Z37.0, Single live birth, is the only outcome of delivery code appropriate for use with O80.

o. The Peripartum and Postpartum Periods

1) Peripartum and Postpartum periods
The postpartum period begins immediately after delivery and continues for six weeks following delivery. The peripartum period is defined as the last month of pregnancy to five months postpartum.

2) Peripartum and postpartum complication
A postpartum complication is any complication occurring within the six-week period.

3) Pregnancy-related complications after 6 week period
Chapter 15 codes may also be used to describe pregnancy-related complications after the peripartum or postpartum period if the provider documents that a condition is pregnancy related.

4) Admission for routine postpartum care following delivery outside hospital
When the mother delivers outside the hospital prior to admission and is admitted for routine postpartum care and no complications are noted, code Z39.0, Encounter for care and examination of mother immediately after delivery, should be assigned as the principal diagnosis.

O00-O9A

5) Pregnancy associated cardiomyopathy

Pregnancy associated cardiomyopathy, code O90.3, is unique in that it may be diagnosed in the third trimester of pregnancy but may continue to progress months after delivery. For this reason, it is referred to as peripartum cardiomyopathy. Code O90.3 is only for use when the cardiomyopathy develops as a result of pregnancy in a woman who did not have pre-existing heart disease.

p. Code O94, Sequelae of complication of pregnancy, childbirth, and the puerperium

1) Code O94

Code O94, Sequelae of complication of pregnancy, childbirth, and the puerperium, is for use in those cases when an initial complication of a pregnancy develops a sequelae requiring care or treatment at a future date.

2) After the initial postpartum period

This code may be used at any time after the initial postpartum period.

3) Sequencing of Code O94

This code, like all sequela codes, is to be sequenced following the code describing the sequelae of the complication.

q. Termination of Pregnancy and Spontaneous abortions

1) Abortion with Liveborn Fetus

When an attempted termination of pregnancy results in a liveborn fetus, assign code Z33.2, Encounter for elective termination of pregnancy and a code from category Z37, Outcome of Delivery.

2) Retained Products of Conception following an abortion

Subsequent encounters for retained products of conception following a spontaneous abortion or elective termination of pregnancy are assigned the appropriate code from category O03, Spontaneous abortion, or codes O07.4, Failed attempted termination of pregnancy without complication and Z33.2, Encounter for elective termination of pregnancy. This advice is appropriate even when the patient was discharged previously with a discharge diagnosis of complete abortion.

3) Complications leading to abortion

Codes from Chapter 15 may be used as additional codes to identify any documented complications of the pregnancy in conjunction with codes in categories in O07 and O08.

r. Abuse in a pregnant patient

For suspected or confirmed cases of abuse of a pregnant patient, a code(s) from subcategories O9A.3, Physical abuse complicating pregnancy, childbirth, and the puerperium, O9A.4, Sexual abuse complicating pregnancy, childbirth, and the puerperium, and O9A.5, Psychological abuse complicating pregnancy, childbirth, and the puerperium, should be sequenced first, followed by the appropriate codes (if applicable) to identify any associated current injury due to physical abuse, sexual abuse, and the perpetrator of abuse.

See Section I.C.19.f. Adult and child abuse, neglect and other maltreatment.

Pregnancy with abortive outcome (O00-O08)

Excludes 1:   *continuing pregnancy in multiple gestation after abortion of one fetus or more (O31.1-, O31.3-)*

O00- Ectopic pregnancy — The development of a fertilized ovum outside of the uterus.
   Includes: **Ruptured ectopic pregnancy** — A breaking open of a fertilized ovum that lies outside of the uterus.
   Use additional code from category O08 to identify any associated complication

O00.0- Abdominal pregnancy — The development of a fertilized ovum within the abdominal cavity.
     Excludes 1:   *maternal care for viable fetus in abdominal pregnancy (O36.7-)*

cc **O00.00 Abdominal pregnancy without intrauterine pregnancy** — [♀, Age/12-55]
     Abdominal pregnancy NOS

cc **O00.01 Abdominal pregnancy with intrauterine pregnancy** — [♀, Age/12-55]

O00.1- Tubal pregnancy — The development of a fertilized ovum within the fallopian tube.
     Fallopian pregnancy
     Rupture of (fallopian) tube due to pregnancy — The forcible tearing of a fallopian tube wall due to a tubal pregnancy.
     Tubal abortion — The expulsion of a tubal pregnancy through the open end (abdominal) of a fallopian tube.

cc **O00.10 Tubal pregnancy without intrauterine pregnancy** — [♀, Age/12-55]
     Tubal pregnancy NOS

cc **O00.11 Tubal pregnancy with intrauterine pregnancy** — [♀, Age/12-55]

O00.2- Ovarian pregnancy — The development of a fertilized ovum within an ovary.

cc **O00.20 Ovarian pregnancy without intrauterine pregnancy** — [♀, Age/12-55]
     Ovarian pregnancy NOS

cc **O00.21 Ovarian pregnancy with intrauterine pregnancy** — [♀, Age/12-55]

O00.8- Other ectopic pregnancy
     Cervical pregnancy — The development of a fertilized ovum within the cervical canal.
     Cornual pregnancy — The development of a fertilized ovum within one of the horns of a bicornate uterus.
     Intraligamentous pregnancy — The development of a fertilized ovum within the broad ligament.
     Mural pregnancy — The development of a fertilized ovum within a fallopian tube uterine orifice.

cc **O00.80 Other ectopic pregnancy without intrauterine pregnancy** — [♀, Age/12-55]
     Other ectopic pregnancy NOS

cc **O00.81 Other ectopic pregnancy with intrauterine pregnancy** — [♀, Age/12-55]

O00.9- Ectopic pregnancy, unspecified

cc **O00.90 Unspecified ectopic pregnancy without intrauterine pregnancy** — [♀, Age/12-55]
     Ectopic pregnancy NOS

cc **O00.91 Unspecified ectopic pregnancy with intrauterine pregnancy** — [♀, Age/12-55]

O01- Hydatidiform mole — An abnormal pregnancy characterized by the cystic degeneration of the chorionic villi, with the appearance of a grape-like mass.
   Use additional code from category O08 to identify any associated complication
     Excludes 1:   *chorioadenoma (destruens) (D39.2)*
                             malignant hydatidiform mole (D39.2)

O01.0 Classical hydatidiform mole — [♀, Age/12-55]
     Complete hydatidiform mole

O01.1 Incomplete and partial hydatidiform mole — [♀, Age/12-55]

O01.9 Hydatidiform mole, unspecified — [♀, Age/12-55]
     Trophoblastic disease NOS
     Vesicular mole NOS

O00-O01

O02- Other abnormal products of conception
  Use additional code from category O08 to identify any associated
  complication
  Excludes 1:   papyraceous fetus (O31.0-)

O02.0 Blighted ovum and nonhydatidiform mole — [♀, Age/12-55] – A
  fertilized ovum that fails to develop.
      Carneous mole
      Fleshy mole
      Intrauterine mole NOS
      Molar pregnancy NEC
      Pathological ovum

O02.1 Missed abortion — [♀, Age/12-55]
      Early fetal death, before completion of 20 weeks of gestation, with
      retention of dead fetus
  Excludes 1:   failed induced abortion (O07-)
                fetal death (intrauterine) (late) (O36.4)
                missed abortion with blighted ovum (O02.0)
                missed abortion with hydatidiform mole (O01-)
                missed abortion with nonhydatidiform (O02.0)
                missed abortion with other abnormal products of
                  conception (O02.8-)
                missed delivery (O36.4)
                stillbirth (P95)

O02.8- Other specified abnormal products of conception
  Excludes 1:   abnormal products of conception with blighted ovum
                  (O02.0)
                abnormal products of conception with hydatidiform
                  mole (O01.-)
                abnormal products of conception with nonhydatidiform
                  mole (O02.0)

  **O02.81 Inappropriate change in quantitative human chorionic
    gonadotropin (hCG) in early pregnancy** — [♀, Age/12-55]
        Biochemical pregnancy
        Chemical pregnancy
        Inappropriate level of quantitative human chorionic
          gonadotropin (hCG) for gestational age in early
          pregnancy

  O02.89 Other specified abnormal products of conception —
      [♀, Age/12-55]

O02.9 Abnormal product of conception, unspecified — [♀, Age/12-55]

O03- Spontaneous abortion — The premature expulsion of the fetus that occurs naturally
and without an apparent cause.
  **Note: Incomplete abortion includes retained products of conception
    following spontaneous abortion**
  Includes: Miscarriage

cc **O03.0 Genital tract and pelvic infection following incomplete
    spontaneous abortion** — [♀, Age/12-55]
      Endometritis following incomplete spontaneous abortion
      Oophoritis following incomplete spontaneous abortion
      Parametritis following incomplete spontaneous abortion
      Pelvic peritonitis following incomplete spontaneous abortion
      Salpingitis following incomplete spontaneous abortion
      Salpingo-oophoritis following incomplete spontaneous abortion
  Excludes 1:   sepsis following incomplete spontaneous abortion
                  (O03.37)
                urinary tract infection following incomplete
                  spontaneous abortion (O03.38)

**O03.1 Delayed or excessive hemorrhage following incomplete
    spontaneous abortion** — [♀, Age/12-55]
      Afibrinogenemia following incomplete spontaneous abortion
      Defibrination syndrome following incomplete spontaneous
        abortion
      Hemolysis following incomplete spontaneous abortion
      Intravascular coagulation following incomplete spontaneous
        abortion

MCC **O03.2 Embolism following incomplete spontaneous abortion** —
      [♀, Age/12-55]
      Air embolism following incomplete spontaneous abortion
      Amniotic fluid embolism following incomplete spontaneous
        abortion
      Blood-clot embolism following incomplete spontaneous abortion
      Embolism NOS following incomplete spontaneous abortion
      Fat embolism following incomplete spontaneous abortion
      Pulmonary embolism following incomplete spontaneous abortion
      Pyemic embolism following incomplete spontaneous abortion
      Septic or septicopyemic embolism following incomplete
        spontaneous abortion
      Soap embolism following incomplete spontaneous abortion

**O03.3- Other and unspecified complications following incomplete
  spontaneous abortion**

cc **O03.30 Unspecified complication following incomplete
    spontaneous abortion** — [♀, Age/12-55]

MCC **O03.31 Shock following incomplete spontaneous abortion** —
      [♀, Age/12-55]
      Circulatory collapse following incomplete spontaneous
        abortion
      Shock (postprocedural) following incomplete spontaneous
        abortion
  Excludes 1:   shock due to infection following incomplete
                  spontaneous abortion (O03.37)

MCC **O03.32 Renal failure following incomplete spontaneous
    abortion** — [♀, Age/12-55]
      Kidney failure (acute) following incomplete spontaneous
        abortion
      Oliguria following incomplete spontaneous abortion
      Renal shutdown following incomplete spontaneous abortion
      Renal tubular necrosis following incomplete spontaneous
        abortion
      Uremia following incomplete spontaneous abortion

cc **O03.33 Metabolic disorder following incomplete spontaneous
    abortion** — [♀, Age/12-55]

cc **O03.34 Damage to pelvic organs following incomplete
    spontaneous abortion** — [♀, Age/12-55]
      Laceration, perforation, tear or chemical damage of bladder
        following incomplete spontaneous abortion
      Laceration, perforation, tear or chemical damage of bowel
        following incomplete spontaneous abortion
      Laceration, perforation, tear or chemical damage of broad
        ligament following incomplete spontaneous abortion
      Laceration, perforation, tear or chemical damage of cervix
        following incomplete spontaneous abortion
      Laceration, perforation, tear or chemical damage of
        periurethral tissue following incomplete spontaneous
        abortion
      Laceration, perforation, tear or chemical damage of uterus
        following incomplete spontaneous abortion
      Laceration, perforation, tear or chemical damage of vagina
        following incomplete spontaneous abortion

cc **O03.35 Other venous complications following incomplete
    spontaneous abortion** — [♀, Age/12-55]

cc **O03.36 Cardiac arrest following incomplete spontaneous
    abortion** — [♀, Age/12-55]

cc **O03.37 Sepsis following incomplete spontaneous abortion** —
      [♀, Age/12-55]
      Use additional code to identify infectious agent (B95-B97)
      Use additional code to identify severe sepsis, if applicable
        (R65.2-)
  Excludes 1:   septic or septicopyemic embolism following
                  incomplete spontaneous abortion (O03.2)

cc **O03.38 Urinary tract infection following incomplete spontaneous
    abortion** — [♀, Age/12-55]
      Cystitis following incomplete spontaneous abortion

cc **O03.39 Incomplete spontaneous abortion with other
    complications** — [♀, Age/12-55]

O03.4 Incomplete spontaneous abortion without complication —
      [♀, Age/12-55]

cc **O03.5 Genital tract and pelvic infection following complete or
    unspecified spontaneous abortion** — [♀, Age/12-55]
      Endometritis following complete or unspecified spontaneous
        abortion
      Oophoritis following complete or unspecified spontaneous abortion
      Parametritis following complete or unspecified spontaneous
        abortion
      Pelvic peritonitis following complete or unspecified spontaneous
        abortion
      Salpingitis following complete or unspecified spontaneous abortion
      Salpingo-oophoritis following complete or unspecified
        spontaneous abortion
  Excludes 1:   sepsis following complete or unspecified spontaneous
                  abortion (O03.87)
                urinary tract infection following complete or
                  unspecified spontaneous abortion (O03.88)

O 0 2 - O 0 3

O03.6 **Delayed or excessive hemorrhage following complete or unspecified** spontaneous abortion — [♀, Age/12-55]
  Afibrinogenemia following complete or unspecified spontaneous abortion
  Defibrination syndrome following complete or unspecified spontaneous abortion
  Hemolysis following complete or unspecified spontaneous abortion
  Intravascular coagulation following complete or unspecified spontaneous abortion

cc O03.7 **Embolism following complete or unspecified** spontaneous abortion — [♀, Age/12-55]
  Air embolism following complete or unspecified spontaneous abortion
  Amniotic fluid embolism following complete or unspecified spontaneous abortion
  Blood-clot embolism following complete or unspecified spontaneous abortion
  Embolism NOS following complete or unspecified spontaneous abortion
  Fat embolism following complete or unspecified spontaneous abortion
  Pulmonary embolism following complete or unspecified spontaneous abortion
  Pyemic embolism following complete or unspecified spontaneous abortion
  Septic or septicopyemic embolism following complete or unspecified spontaneous abortion
  Soap embolism following complete or unspecified spontaneous abortion

O03.8- **Other and unspecified complications following complete or unspecified** spontaneous abortion

cc O03.80 **Unspecified complication following complete or unspecified** spontaneous abortion — [♀, Age/12-55]

MCC O03.81 **Shock following complete or unspecified** spontaneous abortion — [♀, Age/12-55]
  Circulatory collapse following complete or unspecified spontaneous abortion
  Shock (postprocedural) following complete or unspecified spontaneous abortion
  Excludes 1: *shock due to infection following complete or unspecified spontaneous abortion (O03.87)*

MCC O03.82 **Renal failure following complete or unspecified** spontaneous abortion — [♀, Age/12-55]
  Kidney failure (acute) following complete or unspecified spontaneous abortion
  Oliguria following complete or unspecified spontaneous abortion
  Renal shutdown following complete or unspecified spontaneous abortion
  Renal tubular necrosis following complete or unspecified spontaneous abortion
  Uremia following complete or unspecified spontaneous abortion

cc O03.83 **Metabolic disorder following complete or unspecified** spontaneous abortion — [♀, Age/12-55]

cc O03.84 **Damage to pelvic organs following complete or unspecified** spontaneous abortion — [♀, Age/12-55]
  Laceration, perforation, tear or chemical damage of bladder following complete or unspecified spontaneous abortion
  Laceration, perforation, tear or chemical damage of bowel following complete or unspecified spontaneous abortion
  Laceration, perforation, tear or chemical damage of broad ligament following complete or unspecified spontaneous abortion
  Laceration, perforation, tear or chemical damage of cervix following complete or unspecified spontaneous abortion
  Laceration, perforation, tear or chemical damage of periurethral tissue following complete or unspecified spontaneous abortion
  Laceration, perforation, tear or chemical damage of uterus following complete or unspecified spontaneous abortion
  Laceration, perforation, tear or chemical damage of vagina following complete or unspecified spontaneous abortion

cc O03.85 **Other venous complications following complete or unspecified** spontaneous abortion — [♀, Age/12-55]

cc O03.86 **Cardiac arrest following complete or unspecified** spontaneous abortion — [♀, Age/12-55]

cc O03.87 **Sepsis following complete or unspecified** spontaneous abortion — [♀, Age/12-55]
  Use additional code to identify infectious agent (B95-B97)
  Use additional code to identify severe sepsis, if applicable (R65.2-)
  Excludes 1: *septic or septicopyemic embolism following complete or unspecified spontaneousabortion (O03.7)*

cc O03.88 **Urinary tract infection following complete or unspecified** spontaneous abortion — [♀, Age/12-55]
  Cystitis following complete or unspecified spontaneous abortion

cc O03.89 **Complete or unspecified** spontaneous abortion **with other complications** — [♀, Age/12-55]

O03.9 **Complete or unspecified** spontaneous abortion **without complication** — [♀, Age/12-55]
  Miscarriage NOS
  Spontaneous abortion NOS

O04- **Complications following (induced) termination of pregnancy** — The expulsion of the fetus that is brought on intentionally by authorized medical professionals.
  Includes: Complications following (induced) termination of pregnancy
  Excludes 1: *encounter for elective termination of pregnancy, uncomplicated (Z33.2)*
  failed attempted termination of pregnancy (O07.-)

cc O04.5 **Genital tract and pelvic infection following (induced) termination** of pregnancy — [♀, Age/12-55]
  Endometritis following (induced) termination of pregnancy
  Oophoritis following (induced) termination of pregnancy
  Parametritis following (induced) termination of pregnancy
  Pelvic peritonitis following (induced) termination of pregnancy
  Salpingitis following (induced) termination of pregnancy
  Salpingo-oophoritis following (induced) termination of pregnancy
  Excludes 1: *sepsis following (induced) termination of pregnancy (O04.87)*
  urinary tract infection following (induced) termination of pregnancy (O04.88)

O04.6 **Delayed or excessive hemorrhage following (induced) termination** of pregnancy — [♀, Age/12-55]
  Afibrinogenemia following (induced) termination of pregnancy
  Defibrination syndrome following (induced) termination of pregnancy
  Hemolysis following (induced) termination of pregnancy
  Intravascular coagulation following (induced) termination of pregnancy

MCC O04.7 **Embolism following (induced) termination** of pregnancy — [♀, Age/12-55]
  Air embolism following (induced) termination of pregnancy
  Amniotic fluid embolism following (induced) termination of pregnancy
  Blood-clot embolism following (induced) termination of pregnancy
  Embolism NOS following (induced) termination of pregnancy
  Fat embolism following (induced) termination of pregnancy
  Pulmonary embolism following (induced) termination of pregnancy
  Pyemic embolism following (induced) termination of pregnancy
  Septic or septicopyemic embolism following (induced) termination of pregnancy
  Soap embolism following (induced) termination of pregnancy

O04.8- **(Induced) termination of pregnancy with other and unspecified complications**

cc O04.80 **(Induced) termination of pregnancy with unspecified complications** — [♀, Age/12-55]

MCC O04.81 **Shock following (induced) termination of pregnancy** — [♀, Age/12-55]
  Circulatory collapse following (induced) termination of pregnancy
  Shock (postprocedural) following (induced) termination of pregnancy
  Excludes 1: *shock due to infection following (induced) termination of pregnancy (O04.87)*

MCC O04.82 **Renal failure following (induced) termination of pregnancy** — [♀, Age/12-55]
  Kidney failure (acute) following (induced) termination of pregnancy
  Oliguria following (induced) termination of pregnancy
  Renal shutdown following (induced) termination of pregnancy
  Renal tubular necrosis following (induced) termination of pregnancy
  Uremia following (induced) termination of pregnancy

O03 - O04

cc **O04.83** Metabolic disorder following (induced) termination of pregnancy — [♀, Age/12-55]

cc **O04.84** Damage to pelvic organs following (induced) termination of pregnancy — [♀, Age/12-55]
  Laceration, perforation, tear or chemical damage of bladder following (induced) termination of pregnancy
  Laceration, perforation, tear or chemical damage of bowel following (induced) termination of pregnancy
  Laceration, perforation, tear or chemical damage of broad ligament following (induced) termination of pregnancy
  Laceration, perforation, tear or chemical damage of cervix following (induced) termination of pregnancy
  Laceration, perforation, tear or chemical damage of periurethral tissue following (induced) termination of pregnancy
  Laceration, perforation, tear or chemical damage of uterus following (induced) termination of pregnancy
  Laceration, perforation, tear or chemical damage of vagina following (induced) termination of pregnancy

cc **O04.85** Other venous complications following (induced) termination of pregnancy — [♀, Age/12-55]

cc **O04.86** Cardiac arrest following (induced) termination of pregnancy — [♀, Age/12-55]

cc **O04.87** Sepsis following (induced) termination of pregnancy — [♀, Age/12-55]
  Use additional code to identify infectious agent (B95-B97)
  Use additional code to identify severe sepsis, if applicable (R65.2-)
  Excludes 1:   *septic or septicopyemic embolism following (induced) termination of pregnancy (O04.7)*

cc **O04.88** Urinary tract infection following (induced) termination of pregnancy — [♀, Age/12-55]
  Cystitis following (induced) termination of pregnancy

cc **O04.89** (Induced) termination of pregnancy with other complications — [♀, Age/12-55]

O07- Failed attempted termination of pregnancy — The inability of authorized medical professionals to induce the expulsion of the fetus.
  Includes: Failure of attempted induction of termination of pregnancy
              Incomplete elective abortion
  Excludes 1:   *incomplete spontaneous abortion (O03.0-)*

cc **O07.0** Genital tract and pelvic infection following failed attempted termination of pregnancy — [♀, Age/12-55]
  Endometritis following failed attempted termination of pregnancy
  Oophoritis following failed attempted termination of pregnancy
  Parametritis following failed attempted termination of pregnancy
  Pelvic peritonitis following failed attempted termination of pregnancy
  Salpingitis following failed attempted termination of pregnancy
  Salpingo-oophoritis following failed attempted termination of pregnancy
  Excludes 1:   *sepsis following failed attempted termination of pregnancy (O07.37)*
              urinary tract infection following failed attempted termination of pregnancy (O07.38)

cc **O07.1** Delayed or excessive hemorrhage following failed attempted termination of pregnancy — [♀, Age/12-55]
  Afibrinogenemia following failed attempted termination of pregnancy
  Defibrination syndrome following failed attempted termination of pregnancy
  Hemolysis following failed attempted termination of pregnancy
  Intravascular coagulation following failed attempted termination of pregnancy

MCC **O07.2** Embolism following failed attempted termination of pregnancy — [♀, Age/12-55]
  Air embolism following failed attempted termination of pregnancy
  Amniotic fluid embolism following failed attempted termination of pregnancy
  Blood-clot embolism following failed attempted termination of pregnancy
  Embolism NOS following failed attempted termination of pregnancy
  Fat embolism following failed attempted termination of pregnancy
  Pulmonary embolism following failed attempted termination of pregnancy
  Pyemic embolism following failed attempted termination of pregnancy
  Septic or septicopyemic embolism following failed attempted termination of pregnancy
  Soap embolism following failed attempted termination of pregnancy

O07.3- Failed attempted termination of pregnancy with other and unspecified complications

cc **O07.30** Failed attempted termination of pregnancy with unspecified complications — [♀, Age/12-55]

MCC **O07.31** Shock following failed attempted termination of pregnancy — [♀, Age/12-55]
  Circulatory collapse following failed attempted termination of pregnancy
  Shock (postprocedural) following failed attempted termination of pregnancy
  Excludes 1:   *shock due to infection following failed attempted termination of pregnancy (O07.37)*

MCC **O07.32** Renal failure following failed attempted termination of pregnancy — [♀, Age/12-55]
  Kidney failure (acute) following failed attempted termination of pregnancy
  Oliguria following failed attempted termination of pregnancy
  Renal shutdown following failed attempted termination of pregnancy
  Renal tubular necrosis following failed attempted termination of pregnancy
  Uremia following failed attempted termination of pregnancy

cc **O07.33** Metabolic disorder following failed attempted termination of pregnancy — [♀, Age/12-55]

cc **O07.34** Damage to pelvic organs following failed attempted termination of pregnancy — [♀, Age/12-55]
  Laceration, perforation, tear or chemical damage of bladder following failed attempted termination of pregnancy
  Laceration, perforation, tear or chemical damage of bowel following failed attempted termination of pregnancy
  Laceration, perforation, tear or chemical damage of broad ligament following failed attempted termination of pregnancy
  Laceration, perforation, tear or chemical damage of cervix following failed attempted termination of pregnancy
  Laceration, perforation, tear or chemical damage of periurethral tissue following failed attempted termination of pregnancy
  Laceration, perforation, tear or chemical damage of uterus following failed attempted termination of pregnancy
  Laceration, perforation, tear or chemical damage of vagina following failed attempted termination of pregnancy

cc **O07.35** Other venous complications following failed attempted termination of pregnancy — [♀, Age/12-55]

cc **O07.36** Cardiac arrest following failed attempted termination of pregnancy — [♀, Age/12-55]

cc **O07.37** Sepsis following failed attempted termination of pregnancy — [♀, Age/12-55]
  Use additional code (B95-B97), to identify infectious agent
  Use additional code (R65.2-) to identify severe sepsis, if applicable
  Excludes 1:   *septic or septicopyemic embolism following failed attempted termination of pregnancy (O07.2)*

cc **O07.38** Urinary tract infection following failed attempted termination of pregnancy — [♀, Age/12-55]
  Cystitis following failed attempted termination of pregnancy

cc **O07.39** Failed attempted termination of pregnancy with other complications — [♀, Age/12-55]

O07.4 Failed attempted termination of pregnancy without complication — [♀, Age/12-55]

O08- Complications following ectopic and molar pregnancy
  This category is for use with categories O00-O02 to identify any associated complications

cc **O08.0** Genital tract and pelvic infection following ectopic and molar pregnancy — [♀, Age/12-55]
  Endometritis following ectopic and molar pregnancy
  Oophoritis following ectopic and molar pregnancy
  Parametritis following ectopic and molar pregnancy
  Pelvic peritonitis following ectopic and molar pregnancy
  Salpingitis following ectopic and molar pregnancy
  Salpingo-oophoritis following ectopic and molar pregnancy
  Excludes 1:   *sepsis following ectopic and molar pregnancy (O08.82)*
              urinary tract infection (O08.83)

O04-O08

cc **O08.1** <u>Delayed or excessive hemorrhage following ectopic</u> and molar pregnancy — [♀, Age/12-55]
  Afibrinogenemia following ectopic and molar pregnancy
  Defibrination syndrome following ectopic and molar pregnancy
  Hemolysis following ectopic and molar pregnancy
  Intravascular coagulation following ectopic and molar pregnancy
  Excludes 1:   delayed or excessive hemorrhage due to incomplete abortion (O03.1)

MCC **O08.2** <u>Embolism following ectopic</u> and molar pregnancy — [♀, Age/12-55]
  Air embolism following ectopic and molar pregnancy
  Amniotic fluid embolism following ectopic and molar pregnancy
  Blood-clot embolism following ectopic and molar pregnancy
  Embolism NOS following ectopic and molar pregnancy
  Fat embolism following ectopic and molar pregnancy
  Pulmonary embolism following ectopic and molar pregnancy
  Pyemic embolism following ectopic and molar pregnancy
  Septic or septicopyemic embolism following ectopic and molar pregnancy
  Soap embolism following ectopic and molar pregnancy

MCC **O08.3** <u>Shock following ectopic</u> and molar pregnancy — [♀, Age/12-55]
  Circulatory collapse following ectopic and molar pregnancy
  Shock (postprocedural) following ectopic and molar pregnancy
  Excludes 1:   shock due to infection following ectopic and molar pregnancy (O08.82)

MCC **O08.4** <u>Renal failure following ectopic</u> and molar pregnancy — [♀, Age/12-55]
  Kidney failure (acute) following ectopic and molar pregnancy
  Oliguria following ectopic and molar pregnancy
  Renal shutdown following ectopic and molar pregnancy
  Renal tubular necrosis following ectopic and molar pregnancy
  Uremia following ectopic and molar pregnancy

cc **O08.5** <u>Metabolic disorders following</u> an <u>ectopic</u> and molar pregnancy — [♀, Age/12-55]

cc **O08.6** <u>Damage to pelvic organs and tissues following</u> an <u>ectopic</u> and molar pregnancy — [♀, Age/12-55]
  Laceration, perforation, tear or chemical damage of bladder following an ectopic and molar pregnancy
  Laceration, perforation, tear or chemical damage of bowel following an ectopic and molar pregnancy
  Laceration, perforation, tear or chemical damage of broad ligament following an ectopic and molar pregnancy
  Laceration, perforation, tear or chemical damage of cervix following an ectopic and molar pregnancy
  Laceration, perforation, tear or chemical damage of periurethral tissue following an ectopic and molar pregnancy
  Laceration, perforation, tear or chemical damage of uterus following an ectopic and molar pregnancy
  Laceration, perforation, tear or chemical damage of vagina following an ectopic and molar pregnancy

cc **O08.7** Other venous complications following an <u>ectopic</u> and molar pregnancy — [♀, Age/12-55]

O08.8- <u>Other</u> complications following an <u>ectopic</u> and molar pregnancy

cc **O08.81** <u>Cardiac arrest following</u> an <u>ectopic</u> and molar pregnancy — [♀, Age/12-55]

cc **O08.82** <u>Sepsis following ectopic</u> and molar pregnancy — [♀, Age/12-55]
  Use additional code (B95-B97), to identify infectious agent
  Use additional code (R65.2-) to identify severe sepsis, if applicable
  Excludes 1:   septic or septicopyemic embolism following ectopic and molar pregnancy (O08.2)

cc **O08.83** <u>Urinary tract infection following</u> an <u>ectopic</u> and molar pregnancy — [♀, Age/12-55]
  Cystitis following an ectopic and molar pregnancy

cc **O08.89** <u>Other</u> complications following an <u>ectopic</u> and molar pregnancy — [♀, Age/12-55]

cc **O08.9** <u>Unspecified</u> complication following an <u>ectopic</u> and molar pregnancy — [♀, Age/12-55]

Supervision of high risk pregnancy (O09)

O09- <u>Supervision of high risk pregnancy</u> — Conditions (medical and lifestyle) that are present before pregnancy, or present during pregnancy, that prompt providers to provide special monitoring and/or care during the pregnancy.

O09.0- Supervision of pregnancy <u>with history of infertility</u>

O09.00 Supervision of pregnancy with history of infertility, <u>unspecified</u> trimester — [♀, Age/12-55] [Unacceptable PDX]

O09.01 Supervision of pregnancy with history of infertility, <u>first</u> trimester — [♀, Age/12-55] [Unacceptable PDX]

O09.02 Supervision of pregnancy with history of infertility, <u>second</u> trimester — [♀, Age/12-55] [Unacceptable PDX]

O09.03 Supervision of pregnancy with history of infertility, <u>third</u> trimester — [♀, Age/12-55] [Unacceptable PDX]

O09.1- Supervision of pregnancy <u>with history of ectopic pregnancy</u>

O09.10 Supervision of pregnancy with history of ectopic pregnancy, <u>unspecified</u> trimester — [♀, Age/12-55] [Unacceptable PDX]

O09.11 Supervision of pregnancy with history of ectopic pregnancy, <u>first</u> trimester — [♀, Age/12-55] [Unacceptable PDX]

O09.12 Supervision of pregnancy with history of ectopic pregnancy, <u>second</u> trimester — [♀, Age/12-55] [Unacceptable PDX]

O09.13 Supervision of pregnancy with history of ectopic pregnancy, <u>third</u> trimester — [♀, Age/12-55] [Unacceptable PDX]

O09.A- Supervision of pregnancy <u>with history of molar pregnancy</u>

O09.A0 Supervision of pregnancy with history of molar pregnancy, <u>unspecified</u> trimester — [♀, Age/12-55] [Unacceptable PDX]

O09.A1 Supervision of pregnancy with history of molar pregnancy, <u>first</u> trimester — [♀, Age/12-55] [Unacceptable PDX]

O09.A2 Supervision of pregnancy with history of molar pregnancy, <u>second</u> trimester — [♀, Age/12-55] [Unacceptable PDX]

O09.A3 Supervision of pregnancy with history of molar pregnancy, <u>third</u> trimester — [♀, Age/12-55] [Unacceptable PDX]

O09.2- Supervision of pregnancy <u>with other poor reproductive or obstetric history</u>
  Excludes ❷: pregnancy care for patient with history of recurrent pregnancy loss (O26.2-)

O09.21- Supervision of pregnancy <u>with history of pre-term labor</u>

O09.211 Supervision of pregnancy with history of pre-term labor, <u>first</u> trimester — [♀, Age/12-55] [Unacceptable PDX]

O09.212 Supervision of pregnancy with history of pre-term labor, <u>second</u> trimester — [♀, Age/12-55] [Unacceptable PDX]

O09.213 Supervision of pregnancy with history of pre-term labor, <u>third</u> trimester — [♀, Age/12-55] [Unacceptable PDX]

O09.219 Supervision of pregnancy with history of pre-term labor, unspecified trimester — [♀, Age/12-55] [Unacceptable PDX]

O09.29- Supervision of pregnancy <u>with other poor reproductive or obstetric history</u>
  Supervision of pregnancy with history of neonatal death
  Supervision of pregnancy with history of stillbirth

O09.291 Supervision of pregnancy with other poor reproductive or obstetric history, <u>first</u> trimester — [♀, Age/12-55] [Unacceptable PDX]

O09.292 Supervision of pregnancy with other poor reproductive or obstetric history, <u>second</u> trimester — [♀, Age/12-55] [Unacceptable PDX]

O09.293 Supervision of pregnancy with other poor reproductive or obstetric history, <u>third</u> trimester — [♀, Age/12-55] [Unacceptable PDX]

O09.299 Supervision of pregnancy with other poor reproductive or obstetric history, <u>unspecified</u> trimester — [♀, Age/12-55] [Unacceptable PDX]

O08 - O09

O09.3- Supervision of pregnancy <u>with insufficient antenatal care</u>
Supervision of concealed pregnancy
Supervision of hidden pregnancy

O09.30 Supervision of pregnancy with insufficient antenatal care, <u>unspecified</u> trimester — [♀, Age/12-55] [Unacceptable PDX]

O09.31 Supervision of pregnancy with insufficient antenatal care, <u>first</u> trimester — [♀, Age/12-55] [Unacceptable PDX]

O09.32 Supervision of pregnancy with insufficient antenatal care, <u>second</u> trimester — [♀, Age/12-55] [Unacceptable PDX]

O09.33 Supervision of pregnancy with insufficient antenatal care, <u>third</u> trimester — [♀, Age/12-55] [Unacceptable PDX]

O09.4- Supervision of pregnancy <u>with grand multiparity</u>

O09.40 Supervision of pregnancy with grand multiparity, <u>unspecified</u> trimester — [♀, Age/12-55] [Unacceptable PDX]

O09.41 Supervision of pregnancy with grand multiparity, <u>first</u> trimester — [♀, Age/12-55] [Unacceptable PDX]

O09.42 Supervision of pregnancy with grand multiparity, <u>second</u> trimester — [♀, Age/12-55] [Unacceptable PDX]

O09.43 Supervision of pregnancy with grand multiparity, <u>third</u> trimester — [♀, Age/12-55] [Unacceptable PDX]

O09.5- Supervision of elderly primigravida and multigravida
Pregnancy for a female 35 years and older at expected date of delivery

O09.51- <u>Supervision of elderly primigravida</u>

O09.511 Supervision of elderly primigravida, <u>first</u> trimester — [♀, Age/12-55] [Unacceptable PDX]

O09.512 Supervision of elderly primigravida, <u>second</u> trimester — [♀, Age/12-55] [Unacceptable PDX]

O09.513 Supervision of elderly primigravida, <u>third</u> trimester — [♀, Age/12-55] [Unacceptable PDX]

O09.519 Supervision of elderly primigravida, <u>unspecified</u> trimester — [♀, Age/12-55] [Unacceptable PDX]

O09.52- <u>Supervision of elderly multigravida</u>

O09.521 Supervision of elderly multigravida, <u>first</u> trimester — [♀, Age/12-55] [Unacceptable PDX]

O09.522 Supervision of elderly multigravida, <u>second</u> trimester — [♀, Age/12-55] [Unacceptable PDX]

O09.523 Supervision of elderly multigravida, <u>third</u> trimester — [♀, Age/12-55] [Unacceptable PDX]

O09.529 Supervision of elderly multigravida, <u>unspecified</u> trimester — [♀, Age/12-55] [Unacceptable PDX]

O09.6- Supervision of young primigravida and multigravida
Supervision of pregnancy for a female less than 16 years old at expected date of delivery

O09.61- <u>Supervision of young primigravida</u>

O09.611 Supervision of young primigravida, <u>first</u> trimester — [♀, Age/12-55] [Unacceptable PDX]

O09.612 Supervision of young primigravida, <u>second</u> trimester — [♀, Age/12-55] [Unacceptable PDX]

O09.613 Supervision of young primigravida, <u>third</u> trimester — [♀, Age/12-55] [Unacceptable PDX]

O09.619 Supervision of young primigravida, <u>unspecified</u> trimester — [♀, Age/12-55] [Unacceptable PDX]

O09.62- <u>Supervision of young multigravida</u>

O09.621 Supervision of young multigravida, <u>first</u> trimester — [♀, Age/12-55] [Unacceptable PDX]

O09.622 Supervision of young multigravida, <u>second</u> trimester — [♀, Age/12-55] [Unacceptable PDX]

O09.623 Supervision of young multigravida, <u>third</u> trimester — [♀, Age/12-55] [Unacceptable PDX]

O09.629 Supervision of young multigravida, <u>unspecified</u> trimester — [♀, Age/12-55] [Unacceptable PDX]

O09.7- <u>Supervision of high risk pregnancy due to social problems</u>

O09.70 Supervision of high risk pregnancy due to social problems, <u>unspecified</u> trimester — [♀, Age/12-55] [Unacceptable PDX]

O09.71 Supervision of high risk pregnancy due to social problems, <u>first</u> trimester — [♀, Age/12-55] [Unacceptable PDX]

O09.72 Supervision of high risk pregnancy due to social problems, <u>second</u> trimester — [♀, Age/12-55] [Unacceptable PDX]

O09.73 Supervision of high risk pregnancy due to social problems, <u>third</u> trimester — [♀, Age/12-55] [Unacceptable PDX]

O09.8- Supervision of other high risk pregnancies

O09.81- Supervision of pregnancy <u>resulting from assisted reproductive technology</u>
Supervision of pregnancy resulting from in-vitro fertilization
Excludes ❷: gestational carrier status (Z33.3)

O09.811 Supervision of pregnancy resulting from assisted reproductive technology, <u>first</u> trimester — [♀, Age/12-55] [Unacceptable PDX]

O09.812 Supervision of pregnancy resulting from assisted reproductive technology, <u>second</u> trimester — [♀, Age/12-55] [Unacceptable PDX]

O09.813 Supervision of pregnancy resulting from assisted reproductive technology, <u>third</u> trimester — [♀, Age/12-55] [Unacceptable PDX]

O09.819 Supervision of pregnancy resulting from assisted reproductive technology, <u>unspecified</u> trimester — [♀, Age/12-55] [Unacceptable PDX]

O09.82- Supervision of pregnancy <u>with history of in utero procedure during previous pregnancy</u>

O09.821 Supervision of pregnancy with history of in utero procedure during previous pregnancy, <u>first</u> trimester — [♀, Age/12-55] [Unacceptable PDX]

O09.822 Supervision of pregnancy with history of in utero procedure during previous pregnancy, <u>second</u> trimester — [♀, Age/12-55] [Unacceptable PDX]

O09.823 Supervision of pregnancy with history of in utero procedure during previous pregnancy, <u>third</u> trimester — [♀, Age/12-55] [Unacceptable PDX]

O09.829 Supervision of pregnancy with history of in utero procedure during previous pregnancy, <u>unspecified</u> trimester — [♀, Age/12-55] [Unacceptable PDX]

Excludes 1: supervision of pregnancy affected by in utero procedure during current pregnancy (O35.7)

O09.89- Supervision of other high risk pregnancies

O09.891 Supervision of other high risk pregnancies, <u>first</u> trimester — [♀, Age/12-55] [Unacceptable PDX]

O09.892 Supervision of other high risk pregnancies, <u>second</u> trimester — [♀, Age/12-55] [Unacceptable PDX]

O09.893 Supervision of other high risk pregnancies, <u>third</u> trimester — [♀, Age/12-55] [Unacceptable PDX]

O09.899 Supervision of other high risk pregnancies, <u>unspecified</u> trimester — [♀, Age/12-55] [Unacceptable PDX]

O09.9- Supervision of high risk pregnancy, <u>unspecified</u>

O09.90 Supervision of high risk pregnancy, unspecified, <u>unspecified</u> trimester — [♀, Age/12-55] [Unacceptable PDX]

O09.91 Supervision of high risk pregnancy, unspecified, <u>first</u> trimester — [♀, Age/12-55] [Unacceptable PDX]

O09.92 Supervision of high risk pregnancy, unspecified, <u>second</u> trimester — [♀, Age/12-55] [Unacceptable PDX]

O09.93 Supervision of high risk pregnancy, unspecified, <u>third</u> trimester — [♀, Age/12-55] [Unacceptable PDX]

Edema, proteinuria and hypertensive disorders in pregnancy, childbirth and the puerperium (O10-O16)

O10- <u>Pre-existing hypertension</u> **complicating pregnancy, childbirth and the puerperium** — Persistently high arterial blood pressure.
  Includes: Pre-existing hypertension with pre-existing proteinuria complicating pregnancy, childbirth and the puerperium
  Excludes ❷: pre-existing hypertension with superimposed pre-eclampsia complicating pregnancy, childbirth and the puerperium (O11.-)

O10.0- **Pre-existing** <u>essential</u> **hypertension complicating pregnancy, childbirth and the puerperium** — Persistently high arterial blood pressure of a relatively mild degree.
    Any condition in I10 specified as a reason for obstetric care during pregnancy, childbirth or the puerperium

  O10.01-   **Pre-existing essential hypertension** <u>complicating pregnancy,</u>
    cc **O10.011** **Pre-existing essential hypertension complicating pregnancy, <u>first</u> trimester** — [♀, Age/12-55]
    cc **O10.012** **Pre-existing essential hypertension complicating pregnancy, <u>second</u> trimester** — [♀, Age/12-55]
    cc **O10.013** **Pre-existing essential hypertension complicating pregnancy, <u>third</u> trimester** — [♀, Age/12-55]
    O10.019 **Pre-existing essential hypertension complicating pregnancy, <u>unspecified</u> trimester** — [♀, Age/12-55]

  cc **O10.02** **Pre-existing essential hypertension** <u>complicating childbirth</u> — [♀, Age/12-55]

  O10.03 **Pre-existing essential hypertension** <u>complicating the puerperium</u> — [♀, Age/12-55]

O10.1- **Pre-existing** <u>hypertensive heart disease</u> **complicating pregnancy, childbirth and the puerperium** — Persistently high arterial blood pressure resulting in functional cardiac abnormalities.
    Any condition in I11 specified as a reason for obstetric care during pregnancy, childbirth or the puerperium
  Use additional code from I11 to identify the type of hypertensive heart disease

  O10.11-   **Pre-existing hypertensive heart disease** <u>complicating pregnancy</u>
    O10.111 **Pre-existing hypertensive heart disease complicating pregnancy, <u>first</u> trimester** — [♀, Age/12-55]
    O10.112 **Pre-existing hypertensive heart disease complicating pregnancy, <u>second</u> trimester** — [♀, Age/12-55]
    O10.113 **Pre-existing hypertensive heart disease complicating pregnancy, <u>third</u> trimester** — [♀, Age/12-55]
    O10.119 **Pre-existing hypertensive heart disease complicating pregnancy, <u>unspecified</u> trimester** — [♀, Age/12-55]

  O10.12 **Pre-existing hypertensive heart disease** <u>complicating childbirth</u> — [♀, Age/12-55]

  O10.13 **Pre-existing hypertensive heart disease** <u>complicating the puerperium</u> — [♀, Age/12-55]

O10.2- **Pre-existing** <u>hypertensive chronic kidney disease</u> **complicating pregnancy, childbirth and the puerperium** — Persistently high arterial blood pressure resulting in functional kidney abnormalities.
    Any condition in I12 specified as a reason for obstetric care during pregnancy, childbirth or the puerperium
  Use additional code from I12 to identify the type of hypertensive chronic kidney disease

  O10.21-   **Pre-existing hypertensive chronic kidney disease complicating pregnancy**
    O10.211 **Pre-existing hypertensive chronic kidney disease complicating pregnancy, <u>first</u> trimester** — [♀, Age/12-55]
    O10.212 **Pre-existing hypertensive chronic kidney disease complicating pregnancy, <u>second</u> trimester** — [♀, Age/12-55]
    O10.213 **Pre-existing hypertensive chronic kidney disease complicating pregnancy, <u>third</u> trimester** — [♀, Age/12-55]

  O10.219 **Pre-existing hypertensive chronic kidney disease complicating pregnancy, <u>unspecified</u> trimester** — [♀, Age/12-55]

  O10.22 **Pre-existing hypertensive chronic kidney disease** <u>complicating childbirth</u> — [♀, Age/12-55]

  O10.23 **Pre-existing hypertensive chronic kidney disease** <u>complicating the puerperium</u> — [♀, Age/12-55]

O10.3- **Pre-existing** <u>hypertensive heart and chronic kidney disease</u> **complicating pregnancy, childbirth and the puerperium** — Persistently high arterial blood pressure resulting in heart and kidney functional abnormalities.
    Any condition in I13 specified as a reason for obstetric care during pregnancy, childbirth and the puerperium
  Use additional code from I13 to identify the type of hypertensive heart and chronic kidney disease

  O10.31-   **Pre-existing hypertensive heart and chronic kidney disease** <u>complicating pregnancy</u>
    O10.311 **Pre-existing hypertensive heart and chronic kidney disease complicating pregnancy, <u>first</u> trimester** — [♀, Age/12-55]
    O10.312 **Pre-existing hypertensive heart and chronic kidney disease complicating pregnancy, <u>second</u> trimester** — [♀, Age/12-55]
    O10.313 **Pre-existing hypertensive heart and chronic kidney disease complicating pregnancy, <u>third</u> trimester** — [♀, Age/12-55]
    O10.319 **Pre-existing hypertensive heart and chronic kidney disease complicating pregnancy, <u>unspecified</u> trimester** — [♀, Age/12-55]

  O10.32 **Pre-existing hypertensive heart and chronic kidney disease** <u>complicating childbirth</u> — [♀, Age/12-55]

  O10.33 **Pre-existing hypertensive heart and chronic kidney disease** <u>complicating the puerperium</u> — [♀, Age/12-55]

O10.4- **Pre-existing** <u>secondary</u> **hypertension complicating pregnancy, childbirth and the puerperium** — Persistently high arterial blood pressure resulting in functional cardiac abnormalities.
    Any condition in I15 specified as a reason for obstetric care during pregnancy, childbirth or the puerperium
  Use additional code from I15 to identify the type of secondary hypertension

  O10.41-   **Pre-existing secondary hypertension** <u>complicating pregnancy</u>
    cc **O10.411** **Pre-existing secondary hypertension complicating pregnancy, <u>first</u> trimester** — [♀, Age/12-55]
    cc **O10.412** **Pre-existing secondary hypertension complicating pregnancy, <u>second</u> trimester** — [♀, Age/12-55]
    cc **O10.413** **Pre-existing secondary hypertension complicating pregnancy, <u>third</u> trimester** — [♀, Age/12-55]
    O10.419 **Pre-existing secondary hypertension complicating pregnancy, <u>unspecified</u> trimester** — [♀, Age/12-55]

  MCC **O10.42** **Pre-existing secondary hypertension** <u>complicating childbirth</u> — [♀, Age/12-55]

  cc **O10.43** **Pre-existing secondary hypertension** <u>complicating the puerperium</u> — [♀, Age/12-55]

O10.9- <u>Unspecified</u> **pre-existing** <u>hypertension</u> **complicating pregnancy, childbirth and the puerperium**

  O10.91-   **Unspecified pre-existing hypertension** <u>complicating pregnancy</u>
    cc **O10.911** **Unspecified pre-existing hypertension complicating pregnancy, <u>first</u> trimester** — [♀, Age/12-55]
    cc **O10.912** **Unspecified pre-existing hypertension complicating pregnancy, <u>second</u> trimester** — [♀, Age/12-55]
    cc **O10.913** **Unspecified pre-existing hypertension complicating pregnancy, <u>third</u> trimester** — [♀, Age/12-55]
    O10.919 **Unspecified pre-existing hypertension complicating pregnancy, <u>unspecified</u> trimester** — [♀, Age/12-55]

  cc **O10.92** **Unspecified pre-existing hypertension** <u>complicating childbirth</u> — [♀, Age/12-55]

  O10.93 **Unspecified pre-existing hypertension** <u>complicating the puerperium</u> — [♀, Age/12-55]

O
1
0
-
O
1
0

O11- Pre-existing hypertension <u>with pre-eclampsia</u>
> Includes: Conditions in O10 complicated by pre-eclampsia
> Pre-eclampsia superimposed pre-existing hypertension
> Use additional code from O10 to identify the type of hypertension

MCC **O11.1   Pre-existing hypertension with pre-eclampsia, <u>first</u> trimester** — [♀, Age/12-55]

MCC **O11.2   Pre-existing hypertension with pre-eclampsia, <u>second</u> trimester** — [♀, Age/12-55]

MCC **O11.3   Pre-existing hypertension with pre-eclampsia, <u>third</u> trimester** — [♀, Age/12-55]

O11.4   Pre-existing hypertension with pre-eclampsia, <u>complicating childbirth</u> — [♀, Age/12-55]

O11.5   Pre-existing hypertension with pre-eclampsia, <u>complicating the puerperium</u> — [♀, Age/12-55]

O11.9   Pre-existing hypertension with pre-eclampsia, <u>unspecified</u> trimester — [♀, Age/12-55]

O12- Gestational [pregnancy-induced] edema and proteinuria <u>without</u> hypertension

O12.0- <u>Gestational edema</u> — The excessive accumulation of interstitial fluid and venous congestion of the legs that occurs during pregnancy without hypertension.

O12.00 Gestational edema, <u>unspecified</u> trimester — [♀, Age/12-55]

O12.01 Gestational edema, <u>first</u> trimester — [♀, Age/12-55]

O12.02 Gestational edema, <u>second</u> trimester — [♀, Age/12-55]

O12.03 Gestational edema, <u>third</u> trimester — [♀, Age/12-55]

O12.04 Gestational edema, <u>complicating childbirth</u> — [♀, Age/12-55]

O12.05 Gestational edema, <u>complicating the puerperium</u> — [♀, Age/12-55]

O12.1- <u>Gestational proteinuria</u> — The abnormal volume of proteins in the urine that occurs during pregnancy without hypertension.

O12.10 Gestational proteinuria, <u>unspecified</u> trimester — [♀, Age/12-55]

CC **O12.11 Gestational proteinuria, <u>first</u> trimester** — [♀, Age/12-55]

CC **O12.12 Gestational proteinuria, <u>second</u> trimester** — [♀, Age/12-55]

CC **O12.13 Gestational proteinuria, <u>third</u> trimester** — [♀, Age/12-55]

O12.14 Gestational proteinuria, <u>complicating childbirth</u> — [♀, Age/12-55]

O12.15 Gestational proteinuria, <u>complicating the puerperium</u> — [♀, Age/12-55]

O12.2- <u>Gestational edema with proteinuria</u> — The excessive accumulation of interstitial fluid and venous congestion of the legs and the abnormal volume of proteins in the urine that occurs during pregnancy without hypertension.

O12.20 Gestational edema with proteinuria, <u>unspecified</u> trimester — [♀, Age/12-55]

CC **O12.21 Gestational edema with proteinuria, <u>first</u> trimester** — [♀, Age/12-55]

CC **O12.22 Gestational edema with proteinuria, <u>second</u> trimester** — [♀, Age/12-55]

CC **O12.23 Gestational edema with proteinuria, <u>third</u> trimester** — [♀, Age/12-55]

O12.24 Gestational edema with proteinuria, <u>complicating childbirth</u> — [♀, Age/12-55]

O12.25 Gestational edema with proteinuria, <u>complicating the puerperium</u> — [♀, Age/12-55]

O13- Gestational [pregnancy-induced] hypertension <u>without</u> significant proteinuria — Temporary elevated arterial blood pressure noted during pregnancy.
> AHA 16:1Q:p5 – Gestational hypertension
> Includes: Gestational hypertension NOS
> Transient hypertension of pregnancy

O13.1   Gestational [pregnancy-induced] hypertension without significant proteinuria, <u>first</u> trimester — [♀, Age/12-55]

O13.2   Gestational [pregnancy-induced] hypertension without significant proteinuria, <u>second</u> trimester — [♀, Age/12-55]

O13.3   Gestational [pregnancy-induced] hypertension without significant proteinuria, <u>third</u> trimester — [♀, Age/12-55]

O13.4   Gestational [pregnancy-induced] hypertension without significant proteinuria, <u>complicating childbirth</u> — [♀, Age/12-55]

O13.5   Gestational [pregnancy-induced] hypertension without significant proteinuria, <u>complicating the puerperium</u> — [♀, Age/12-55]

O13.9   Gestational [pregnancy-induced] hypertension without significant proteinuria, <u>unspecified</u> trimester — [♀, Age/12-55]

O14- <u>Pre-eclampsia</u> — A pregnancy-induced hypertensive condition characterized by a large volume of proteins in the urine and edema.
> *Excludes 1:   pre-existing hypertension with pre-eclampsia (O11)*

O14.0- <u>Mild to moderate</u> pre-eclampsia

O14.00 Mild to moderate pre-eclampsia, <u>unspecified</u> trimester — [♀, Age/12-55]

CC **O14.02 Mild to moderate pre-eclampsia, <u>second</u> trimester** — [♀, Age/12-55]

CC **O14.03 Mild to moderate pre-eclampsia, <u>third</u> trimester** — [♀, Age/12-55]

O14.04 Mild to moderate pre-eclampsia, <u>complicating childbirth</u> — [♀, Age/12-55]

O14.05 Mild to moderate pre-eclampsia, <u>complicating the puerperium</u> — [♀, Age/12-55]

O14.1- <u>Severe</u> pre-eclampsia
> *Excludes 1:   HELLP syndrome (O14.2-)*

O14.10 Severe pre-eclampsia, <u>unspecified</u> trimester — [♀, Age/12-55]

MCC **O14.12 Severe pre-eclampsia, <u>second</u> trimester** — [♀, Age/12-55]

MCC **O14.13 Severe pre-eclampsia, <u>third</u> trimester** — [♀, Age/12-55]

O14.14 Severe pre-eclampsia, <u>complicating childbirth</u> — [♀, Age/12-55]

O14.15 Severe pre-eclampsia, <u>complicating the puerperium</u> — [♀, Age/12-55]

O14.2- <u>HELLP syndrome</u>
> Severe pre-eclampsia with hemolysis, elevated liver enzymes and low platelet count (HELLP)

O14.20 HELLP syndrome (HELLP), <u>unspecified</u> trimester — [♀, Age/12-55]

MCC **O14.22 HELLP syndrome (HELLP), <u>second</u> trimester** — [♀, Age/12-55]

MCC **O14.23 HELLP syndrome (HELLP), <u>third</u> trimester** — [♀, Age/12-55]

O14.24 HELLP syndrome, <u>complicating childbirth</u> — [♀, Age/12-55]

O14.25 HELLP syndrome, <u>complicating the puerperium</u> — [♀, Age/12-55]

O14.9- <u>Unspecified</u> pre-eclampsia

O14.90 Unspecified pre-eclampsia, <u>unspecified</u> trimester — [♀, Age/12-55]

CC **O14.92 Unspecified pre-eclampsia, <u>second</u> trimester** — [♀, Age/12-55]

CC **O14.93 Unspecified pre-eclampsia, <u>third</u> trimester** — [♀, Age/12-55]

O14.94 Unspecified pre-eclampsia, <u>complicating childbirth</u> — [♀, Age/12-55]

O14.95 Unspecified pre-eclampsia, <u>complicating the puerperium</u> — [♀, Age/12-55]

O15- <u>Eclampsia</u> — The onset of seizures in a women with pre-eclapmsia or pre-existing hypertension conditions.
> Includes: Convulsions following conditions in O10-O14 and O16

O15.0- Eclampsia <u>complicating pregnancy</u>

O15.00 Eclampsia complicating pregnancy, unspecified trimester — [♀, Age/12-55]

MCC **O15.02 Eclampsia complicating pregnancy, <u>second</u> trimester** — [♀, Age/12-55]

MCC **O15.03 Eclampsia complicating pregnancy, <u>third</u> trimester** — [♀, Age/12-55]

MCC **O15.1   Eclampsia <u>complicating labor</u>** — [♀, Age/12-55]

MCC **O15.2   Eclampsia <u>complicating the puerperium</u>** — [♀, Age/12-55]

O15.9   Eclampsia, <u>unspecified</u> as to time period — [♀, Age/12-55]
> Eclampsia NOS

O16- <u>Unspecified</u> maternal hypertension

CC **O16.1   Unspecified maternal hypertension, <u>first</u> trimester** — [♀, Age/12-55]

CC **O16.2   Unspecified maternal hypertension, <u>second</u> trimester** — [♀, Age/12-55]

CC **O16.3   Unspecified maternal hypertension, <u>third</u> trimester** — [♀, Age/12-55]

O 1 1 - O 1 6

O16.4 Unspecified maternal hypertension, <u>complicating childbirth</u> — [♀, Age/12-55]

O16.5 Unspecified maternal hypertension, <u>complicating the puerperium</u> — [♀, Age/12-55]

O16.9 Unspecified maternal hypertension, <u>unspecified</u> trimester — [♀, Age/12-55]

Other maternal disorders predominantly related to pregnancy (O20-O29)

Excludes ❷: *maternal care related to the fetus and amniotic cavity and possible delivery problems (O30-O48)*
maternal diseases classifiable elsewhere but complicating pregnancy, labor and delivery, and the puerperium (O98-O99)

O20- Hemorrhage in early pregnancy
  Includes: Hemorrhage before completion of 20 weeks gestation
  Excludes 1: pregnancy with abortive outcome (O00-O08)

cc **O20.0 Threatened abortion** — [♀, Age/12-55]
    Hemorrhage specified as due to threatened abortion

O20.8 Other hemorrhage in early pregnancy — [♀, Age/12-55]

cc **O20.9 Hemorrhage in early pregnancy, unspecified** — [♀, Age/12-55]

O21- Excessive vomiting in pregnancy

O21.0 Mild hyperemesis gravidarum — [♀, Age/12-55]
    Hyperemesis gravidarum, mild or unspecified, starting before the end of the 20th week of gestation

O21.1 Hyperemesis gravidarum <u>with metabolic disturbance</u> — [♀, Age/12-55]
    Hyperemesis gravidarum, starting before the end of the 20th week of gestation, with metabolic disturbance such as carbohydrate depletion
    Hyperemesis gravidarum, starting before the end of the 20th week of gestation, with metabolic disturbance such as dehydration
    Hyperemesis gravidarum, starting before the end of the 20th week of gestation, with metabolic disturbance such as electrolyte imbalance

O21.2 Late vomiting of pregnancy — [♀, Age/12-55]
    Excessive vomiting starting after 20 completed weeks of gestation

O21.8 Other vomiting complicating pregnancy — [♀, Age/12-55]
    Vomiting due to diseases classified elsewhere, complicating pregnancy
    Use additional code, to identify cause.

O21.9 Vomiting of pregnancy, unspecified — [♀, Age/12-55]

O22- Venous complications and hemorrhoids <u>in pregnancy</u>
  Excludes 1: venous complications of:
    abortion NOS (O03.9)
    ectopic or molar pregnancy (O08.7)
    failed attempted abortion (O07.35)
    induced abortion (O04.85)
    spontaneous abortion (O03.89)
  Excludes ❷: *obstetric pulmonary embolism (O88-)*
    venous complications and hemorrhoids of childbirth and the puerperium (O87-)

O22.0- <u>Varicose veins of lower extremity</u> in pregnancy — Dilated, tortuous leg veins presenting symptoms during pregnancy.
    Varicose veins NOS in pregnancy

O22.00 Varicose veins of lower extremity in pregnancy, <u>unspecified</u> trimester — [♀, Age/12-55]

O22.01 Varicose veins of lower extremity in pregnancy, <u>first</u> trimester — [♀, Age/12-55]

O22.02 Varicose veins of lower extremity in pregnancy, <u>second</u> trimester — [♀, Age/12-55]

O22.03 Varicose veins of lower extremity in pregnancy, <u>third</u> trimester — [♀, Age/12-55]

O22.1- <u>Genital varices</u> in pregnancy — Dilated, tortuous genital veins presenting symptoms during pregnancy.
    Perineal varices in pregnancy
    Vaginal varices in pregnancy
    Vulval varices in pregnancy

O22.10 Genital varices in pregnancy, <u>unspecified</u> trimester — [♀, Age/12-55]

O22.11 Genital varices in pregnancy, <u>first</u> trimester — [♀, Age/12-55]

O22.12 Genital varices in pregnancy, <u>second</u> trimester — [♀, Age/12-55]

O22.13 Genital varices in pregnancy, <u>third</u> trimester — [♀, Age/12-55]

O22.2- <u>Superficial thrombophlebitis</u> in pregnancy — Inflammation of a superficial vein with thrombus formation during pregnancy.
    Phlebitis in pregnancy NOS
    Thrombophlebitis of legs in pregnancy
    Thrombosis in pregnancy NOS
    Use additional code to identify the superficial thrombophlebitis (I80.0-)

cc **O22.20 Superficial thrombophlebitis in pregnancy, <u>unspecified</u> trimester** — [♀, Age/12-55]

cc **O22.21 Superficial thrombophlebitis in pregnancy, <u>first</u> trimester** — [♀, Age/12-55]

cc **O22.22 Superficial thrombophlebitis in pregnancy, <u>second</u> trimester** — [♀, Age/12-55]

cc **O22.23 Superficial thrombophlebitis in pregnancy, <u>third</u> trimester** — [♀, Age/12-55]

O22.3- <u>Deep phlebothrombosis</u> in pregnancy — Inflammation of a deep vein with thrombus formation during pregnancy.
    Deep vein thrombosis, antepartum
    Use additional code to identify the deep vein thrombosis (I82.4-, I82.5-, I82.62-. I82.72-)
    Use additional code, if applicable, for associated long-term (current) use of anticoagulants (Z79.01)

cc **O22.30 Deep phlebothrombosis in pregnancy, <u>unspecified</u> trimester** — [♀, Age/12-55]

MCC **O22.31 Deep phlebothrombosis in pregnancy, <u>first</u> trimester** — [♀, Age/12-55]

MCC **O22.32 Deep phlebothrombosis in pregnancy, <u>second</u> trimester** — [♀, Age/12-55]

MCC **O22.33 Deep phlebothrombosis in pregnancy, <u>third</u> trimester** — [♀, Age/12-55]

O22.4- <u>Hemorrhoids</u> in pregnancy — The varicose dilatation of a vein of the hemorrhoidal plexus during pregnancy.

cc **O22.40 Hemorrhoids in pregnancy, <u>unspecified</u> trimester** — [♀, Age/12-55]

cc **O22.41 Hemorrhoids in pregnancy, <u>first</u> trimester** — [♀, Age/12-55]

cc **O22.42 Hemorrhoids in pregnancy, <u>second</u> trimester** — [♀, Age/12-55]

cc **O22.43 Hemorrhoids in pregnancy, <u>third</u> trimester** — [♀, Age/12-55]

O22.5- <u>Cerebral venous thrombosis</u> in pregnancy — The formation of a thrombus in a cerebral vessel during pregnancy.
    Cerebrovenous sinus thrombosis in pregnancy

cc **O22.50 Cerebral venous thrombosis in pregnancy, <u>unspecified</u> trimester** — [♀, Age/12-55]

cc **O22.51 Cerebral venous thrombosis in pregnancy, <u>first</u> trimester** — [♀, Age/12-55]

cc **O22.52 Cerebral venous thrombosis in pregnancy, <u>second</u> trimester** — [♀, Age/12-55]

cc **O22.53 Cerebral venous thrombosis in pregnancy, <u>third</u> trimester** — [♀, Age/12-55]

O22.8- <u>Other venous complications</u> in pregnancy
  O22.8x-Other venous complications in pregnancy

cc **O22.8x1 Other venous complications in pregnancy, <u>first</u> trimester** — [♀, Age/12-55]

cc **O22.8x2 Other venous complications in pregnancy, <u>second</u> trimester** — [♀, Age/12-55]

cc **O22.8x3 Other venous complications in pregnancy, <u>third</u> trimester** — [♀, Age/12-55]

cc **O22.8x9 Other venous complications in pregnancy, <u>unspecified</u> trimester** — [♀, Age/12-55]

O22.9- Venous complication in pregnancy, <u>unspecified</u>
    Gestational phlebitis NOS
    Gestational phlebopathy NOS
    Gestational thrombosis NOS

cc **O22.90 Venous complication in pregnancy, unspecified, <u>unspecified</u> trimester** — [♀, Age/12-55]

O22.91 Venous complication in pregnancy, unspecified, <u>first</u> trimester — [♀, Age/12-55]

O16 - O22

O22.92 Venous complication in pregnancy, unspecified, <u>second</u> trimester — [♀, Age/12-55]

O22.93 Venous complication in pregnancy, unspecified, <u>third</u> trimester — [♀, Age/12-55]

O23- <u>Infections of genitourinary tract</u> in pregnancy
Use additional code to identify organism (B95-, B96-)
Excludes ❷: gonococcal infections complicating pregnancy, childbirth and the puerperium (O98.2)
infections with a predominantly sexual mode of transmission NOS complicating pregnancy, childbirth and the puerperium (O98.3)
syphilis complicating pregnancy, childbirth and the puerperium (O98.1)
tuberculosis of genitourinary system complicating pregnancy, childbirth and the puerperium (O98.0)
venereal disease NOS complicating pregnancy, childbirth and the puerperium (O98.3)

O23.0- <u>Infections of kidney</u> in pregnancy
Pyelonephritis in pregnancy

O23.00 Infections of kidney in pregnancy, <u>unspecified</u> trimester — [♀, Age/12-55]

cc **O23.01 Infections of kidney in pregnancy, <u>first</u> trimester** — [♀, Age/12-55]

cc **O23.02 Infections of kidney in pregnancy, <u>second</u> trimester** — [♀, Age/12-55]

cc **O23.03 Infections of kidney in pregnancy, <u>third</u> trimester** — [♀, Age/12-55]

O23.1- <u>Infections of bladder</u> in pregnancy

O23.10 Infections of bladder in pregnancy, <u>unspecified</u> trimester — [♀, Age/12-55]

cc **O23.11 Infections of bladder in pregnancy, <u>first</u> trimester** — [♀, Age/12-55]

cc **O23.12 Infections of bladder in pregnancy, <u>second</u> trimester** — [♀, Age/12-55]

cc **O23.13 Infections of bladder in pregnancy, <u>third</u> trimester** — [♀, Age/12-55]

O23.2- <u>Infections of urethra</u> in pregnancy

O23.20 Infections of urethra in pregnancy, <u>unspecified</u> trimester — [♀, Age/12-55]

cc **O23.21 Infections of urethra in pregnancy, <u>first</u> trimester** — [♀, Age/12-55]

cc **O23.22 Infections of urethra in pregnancy, <u>second</u> trimester** — [♀, Age/12-55]

cc **O23.23 Infections of urethra in pregnancy, <u>third</u> trimester** — [♀, Age/12-55]

O23.3- <u>Infections of other parts of urinary tract</u> in pregnancy

O23.30 Infections of other parts of urinary tract in pregnancy, <u>unspecified</u> trimester — [♀, Age/12-55]

cc **O23.31 Infections of other parts of urinary tract in pregnancy, <u>first</u> trimester** — [♀, Age/12-55]

cc **O23.32 Infections of other parts of urinary tract in pregnancy, <u>second</u> trimester** — [♀, Age/12-55]

cc **O23.33 Infections of other parts of urinary tract in pregnancy, <u>third</u> trimester** — [♀, Age/12-55]

O23.4- <u>Unspecified</u> infection of urinary tract in pregnancy

O23.40 Unspecified infection of urinary tract in pregnancy, <u>unspecified</u> trimester — [♀, Age/12-55]

cc **O23.41 Unspecified infection of urinary tract in pregnancy, <u>first</u> trimester** — [♀, Age/12-55]

cc **O23.42 Unspecified infection of urinary tract in pregnancy, <u>second</u> trimester** — [♀, Age/12-55]

cc **O23.43 Unspecified infection of urinary tract in pregnancy, <u>third</u> trimester** — [♀, Age/12-55]

O23.5- <u>Infections of the genital tract</u> in pregnancy

O23.51-   Infection of <u>cervix</u> in pregnancy

cc **O23.511 Infections of cervix in pregnancy, <u>first</u> trimester** — [♀, Age/12-55]

cc **O23.512 Infections of cervix in pregnancy, <u>second</u> trimester** — [♀, Age/12-55]

cc **O23.513 Infections of cervix in pregnancy, <u>third</u> trimester** — [♀, Age/12-55]

O23.519 Infections of cervix in pregnancy, <u>unspecified</u> trimester — [♀, Age/12-55]

O23.52- <u>Salpingo-oophoritis</u> in pregnancy
Oophoritis in pregnancy
Salpingitis in pregnancy

cc **O23.521 Salpingo-oophoritis in pregnancy, <u>first</u> trimester** — [♀, Age/12-55]

cc **O23.522 Salpingo-oophoritis in pregnancy, <u>second</u> trimester** — [♀, Age/12-55]

cc **O23.523 Salpingo-oophoritis in pregnancy, <u>third</u> trimester** — [♀, Age/12-55]

O23.529 Salpingo-oophoritis in pregnancy, <u>unspecified</u> trimester — [♀, Age/12-55]

O23.59- Infection of <u>other part of genital tract</u> in pregnancy

cc **O23.591 Infection of other part of genital tract in pregnancy, <u>first</u> trimester** — [♀, Age/12-55]

cc **O23.592 Infection of other part of genital tract in pregnancy, <u>second</u> trimester** — [♀, Age/12-55]

cc **O23.593 Infection of other part of genital tract in pregnancy, <u>third</u> trimester** — [♀, Age/12-55]

O23.599 Infection of other part of genital tract in pregnancy, <u>unspecified</u> trimester — [♀, Age/12-55]

O23.9- <u>Unspecified</u> genitourinary tract infection in pregnancy
Genitourinary tract infection in pregnancy NOS

O23.90 Unspecified genitourinary tract infection in pregnancy, <u>unspecified</u> trimester — [♀, Age/12-55]

cc **O23.91 Unspecified genitourinary tract infection in pregnancy, <u>first</u> trimester** — [♀, Age/12-55]

cc **O23.92 Unspecified genitourinary tract infection in pregnancy, <u>second</u> trimester** — [♀, Age/12-55]

cc **O23.93 Unspecified genitourinary tract infection in pregnancy, <u>third</u> trimester** — [♀, Age/12-55]

O24- <u>Diabetes mellitus</u> in pregnancy, childbirth, and the puerperium

O24.0- <u>Pre-existing type 1 diabetes mellitus</u>, in pregnancy, childbirth and the puerperium
Juvenile onset diabetes mellitus, in pregnancy, childbirth and the puerperium
Ketosis-prone diabetes mellitus in pregnancy, childbirth and the puerperium
Use additional code from category E10 to further identify any manifestations

O24.01-   Pre-existing <u>type 1</u> diabetes mellitus, <u>in pregnancy</u>

cc **O24.011 Pre-existing type 1 diabetes mellitus, in pregnancy, <u>first</u> trimester** — [♀, Age/12-55]

cc **O24.012 Pre-existing type 1 diabetes mellitus, in pregnancy, <u>second</u> trimester** — [♀, Age/12-55]

cc **O24.013 Pre-existing type 1 diabetes mellitus, in pregnancy, <u>third</u> trimester** — [♀, Age/12-55]

cc **O24.019 Pre-existing type 1 diabetes mellitus, in pregnancy, <u>unspecified</u> trimester** — [♀, Age/12-55]

mcc **O24.02 Pre-existing <u>type 1</u> diabetes mellitus, <u>in childbirth</u>** — [♀, Age/12-55]

cc **O24.03 Pre-existing <u>type 1</u> diabetes mellitus, <u>in the puerperium</u>** — [♀, Age/12-55]

O24.1- Pre-existing <u>type 2</u> diabetes mellitus in pregnancy, childbirth and the puerperium
Insulin-resistant diabetes mellitus in pregnancy, childbirth and the puerperium
Use additional code (for):
From category E11 to further identify any manifestations
Long-term (current) use of insulin (Z79.4)

O24.11-   Pre-existing <u>type 2</u> diabetes mellitus, <u>in pregnancy</u>

cc **O24.111 Pre-existing type 2 diabetes mellitus, in pregnancy, <u>first</u> trimester** — [♀, Age/12-55]

cc **O24.112 Pre-existing type 2 diabetes mellitus, in pregnancy, <u>second</u> trimester** — [♀, Age/12-55]

cc **O24.113 Pre-existing type 2 diabetes mellitus, in pregnancy, <u>third</u> trimester** — [♀, Age/12-55]

O
2
2
-
O
2
4

CC **O24.119 Pre-existing type 2 diabetes mellitus, in pregnancy, unspecified** trimester — [♀, Age/12-55]

MCC **O24.12 Pre-existing type 2 diabetes mellitus, in childbirth** — [♀, Age/12-55]

CC **O24.13 Pre-existing type 2 diabetes mellitus, in the puerperium** — [♀, Age/12-55]

O24.3- Unspecified pre-existing diabetes mellitus in pregnancy, childbirth and the puerperium
Use additional code (for):
From category E11 to further identify any manifestation
Long-term (current) use of insulin (Z79.4)

O24.31- Unspecified pre-existing diabetes mellitus in pregnancy

CC **O24.311 Unspecified pre-existing diabetes mellitus in pregnancy, first** trimester — [♀, Age/12-55]

CC **O24.312 Unspecified pre-existing diabetes mellitus in pregnancy, second** trimester — [♀, Age/12-55]

CC **O24.313 Unspecified pre-existing diabetes mellitus in pregnancy, third** trimester — [♀, Age/12-55]

CC **O24.319 Unspecified pre-existing diabetes mellitus in pregnancy, unspecified** trimester — [♀, Age/12-55]

MCC **O24.32 Unspecified pre-existing diabetes mellitus in childbirth** — [♀, Age/12-55]

CC **O24.33 Unspecified pre-existing diabetes mellitus in the puerperium** — [♀, Age/12-55]

O24.4- Gestational diabetes mellitus
AHA 16:1Q:p5 – Delivery complicated by gestational diabetes
Diabetes mellitus arising in pregnancy
Gestational diabetes mellitus NOS

O24.41- Gestational diabetes mellitus in pregnancy

O24.410 Gestational diabetes mellitus in pregnancy, diet controlled — [♀, Age/12-55]

O24.414 Gestational diabetes mellitus in pregnancy, insulin controlled — [♀, Age/12-55]

O24.415 Gestational diabetes mellitus in pregnancy, controlled by oral hypoglycemic drugs — [♀, Age/12-55]
Gestational diabetes mellitus in pregnancy, controlled by oral antidiabetic drugs

O24.419 Gestational diabetes mellitus in pregnancy, unspecified control — [♀, Age/12-55]
AHA 15:4Q:p34 – Oral medication control of gestational diabetes

O24.42- Gestational diabetes mellitus in childbirth

O24.420 Gestational diabetes mellitus in childbirth, diet controlled — [♀, Age/12-55]

O24.424 Gestational diabetes mellitus in childbirth, insulin controlled — [♀, Age/12-55]

O24.425 Gestational diabetes mellitus in childbirth, controlled by oral hypoglycemic drugs — [♀, Age/12-55]
Gestational diabetes mellitus in childbirth, controlled by oral antidiabetic drugs

O24.429 Gestational diabetes mellitus in childbirth, unspecified control — [♀, Age/12-55]

O24.43- Gestational diabetes mellitus in the puerperium

O24.430 Gestational diabetes mellitus in the puerperium, diet controlled — [♀, Age/12-55]

O24.434 Gestational diabetes mellitus in the puerperium, insulin controlled — [♀, Age/12-55]

O24.435 Gestational diabetes mellitus in puerperium, controlled by oral hypoglycemic drugs — [♀, Age/12-55]
Gestational diabetes mellitus in puerperium, controlled by oral antidiabetic drugs

O24.439 Gestational diabetes mellitus in the puerperium, unspecified control — [♀, Age/12-55]

O24.8- Other pre-existing diabetes mellitus in pregnancy, childbirth and the puerperium
Use additional code (for):
From categories E08, E09 and E13 to further identify any manifestation
Long-term (current) use of insulin (Z79.4)

O24.81- Other pre-existing diabetes mellitus in pregnancy

CC **O24.811 Other pre-existing diabetes mellitus in pregnancy, first** trimester — [♀, Age/12-55]

CC **O24.812 Other pre-existing diabetes mellitus in pregnancy, second** trimester — [♀, Age/12-55]

CC **O24.813 Other pre-existing diabetes mellitus in pregnancy, third** trimester — [♀, Age/12-55]

CC **O24.819 Other pre-existing diabetes mellitus in pregnancy, unspecified** trimester — [♀, Age/12-55]

MCC **O24.82 Other pre-existing diabetes mellitus in childbirth** — [♀, Age/12-55]

CC **O24.83 Other pre-existing diabetes mellitus in the puerperium** — [♀, Age/12-55]

O24.9- Unspecified diabetes mellitus in pregnancy, childbirth and the puerperium
Use additional code for long-term (current) use of insulin (Z79.4)

O24.91- Unspecified diabetes mellitus in pregnancy

CC **O24.911 Unspecified diabetes mellitus in pregnancy, first** trimester — [♀, Age/12-55]

CC **O24.912 Unspecified diabetes mellitus in pregnancy, second** trimester — [♀, Age/12-55]

CC **O24.913 Unspecified diabetes mellitus in pregnancy, third** trimester — [♀, Age/12-55]

CC **O24.919 Unspecified diabetes mellitus in pregnancy, unspecified** trimester — [♀, Age/12-55]

O24.92 Unspecified diabetes mellitus in childbirth — [♀, Age/12-55]

CC **O24.93 Unspecified diabetes mellitus in the puerperium** — [♀, Age/12-55]

O25- Malnutrition in pregnancy, childbirth and the puerperium

O25.1- Malnutrition in pregnancy — The inadequate intake of nutrients during pregnancy.

O25.10 Malnutrition in pregnancy, unspecified trimester — [♀, Age/12-55]

O25.11 Malnutrition in pregnancy, first trimester — [♀, Age/12-55]

O25.12 Malnutrition in pregnancy, second trimester — [♀, Age/12-55]

O25.13 Malnutrition in pregnancy, third trimester — [♀, Age/12-55]

O25.2 Malnutrition in childbirth — [♀, Age/12-55]

O25.3 Malnutrition in the puerperium — [♀, Age/12-55]

O26- Maternal care for other conditions predominantly related to pregnancy

O26.0- Excessive weight gain in pregnancy
Excludes 2: gestational edema (O12.0, O12.2)

O26.00 Excessive weight gain in pregnancy, unspecified trimester — [♀, Age/12-55]

O26.01 Excessive weight gain in pregnancy, first trimester — [♀, Age/12-55]

O26.02 Excessive weight gain in pregnancy, second trimester — [♀, Age/12-55]

O26.03 Excessive weight gain in pregnancy, third trimester — [♀, Age/12-55]

O26.1- Low weight gain in pregnancy

O26.10 Low weight gain in pregnancy, unspecified trimester — [♀, Age/12-55]

O26.11 Low weight gain in pregnancy, first trimester — [♀, Age/12-55]

O26.12 Low weight gain in pregnancy, second trimester — [♀, Age/12-55]

O26.13 Low weight gain in pregnancy, third trimester — [♀, Age/12-55]

O26.2- Pregnancy care for patient with recurrent pregnancy loss

O26.20 Pregnancy care for patient with recurrent pregnancy loss, unspecified trimester — [♀, Age/12-55]

O24 - O26

O26.21 Pregnancy care for patient with recurrent pregnancy loss, first trimester — [♀, Age/12-55]

O26.22 Pregnancy care for patient with recurrent pregnancy loss, second trimester — [♀, Age/12-55]

O26.23 Pregnancy care for patient with recurrent pregnancy loss, third trimester — [♀, Age/12-55]

O26.3- Retained intrauterine contraceptive device in pregnancy

O26.30 Retained intrauterine contraceptive device in pregnancy, unspecified trimester — [♀, Age/12-55]

O26.31 Retained intrauterine contraceptive device in pregnancy, first trimester — [♀, Age/12-55]

O26.32 Retained intrauterine contraceptive device in pregnancy, second trimester — [♀, Age/12-55]

O26.33 Retained intrauterine contraceptive device in pregnancy, third trimester — [♀, Age/12-55]

O26.4- Herpes gestationis — A form of dermatitis herpetiformis that occurs during pregnancy that clears upon delivery.

O26.40 Herpes gestationis, unspecified trimester — [♀, Age/12-55]

O26.41 Herpes gestationis, first trimester — [♀, Age/12-55]

O26.42 Herpes gestationis, second trimester — [♀, Age/12-55]

O26.43 Herpes gestationis, third trimester — [♀, Age/12-55]

O26.5- Maternal hypotension syndrome — Abnormally low blood pressure during pregnancy.
    Supine hypotensive syndrome

O26.50 Maternal hypotension syndrome, unspecified trimester — [♀, Age/12-55]

O26.51 Maternal hypotension syndrome, first trimester — [♀, Age/12-55]

O26.52 Maternal hypotension syndrome, second trimester — [♀, Age/12-55]

O26.53 Maternal hypotension syndrome, third trimester — [♀, Age/12-55]

O26.6- Liver and biliary tract disorders in pregnancy, childbirth and the puerperium
Use additional code to identify the specific disorder
Excludes ❷: hepatorenal syndrome following labor and delivery (O90.4)

O26.61- Liver and biliary tract disorders in pregnancy

CC **O26.611 Liver and biliary tract disorders in pregnancy, first trimester** — [♀, Age/12-55]

CC **O26.612 Liver and biliary tract disorders in pregnancy, second trimester** — [♀, Age/12-55]

CC **O26.613 Liver and biliary tract disorders in pregnancy, third trimester** — [♀, Age/12-55]

O26.619 Liver and biliary tract disorders in pregnancy, unspecified trimester — [♀, Age/12-55]

CC **O26.62 Liver and biliary tract disorders in childbirth** — [♀, Age/12-55]

O26.63 Liver and biliary tract disorders in the puerperium — [♀, Age/12-55]

O26.7- Subluxation of symphysis (pubis) in pregnancy, childbirth and the puerperium — The abnormal displacement or movement of the symphysis pubis during pregnancy.
Excludes 1: traumatic separation of symphysis (pubis) during childbirth (O71.6)

O26.71- Subluxation of symphysis (pubis) in pregnancy

O26.711 Subluxation of symphysis (pubis) in pregnancy, first trimester — [♀, Age/12-55]

O26.712 Subluxation of symphysis (pubis) in pregnancy, second trimester — [♀, Age/12-55]

O26.713 Subluxation of symphysis (pubis) in pregnancy, third trimester — [♀, Age/12-55]

O26.719 Subluxation of symphysis (pubis) in pregnancy, unspecified trimester — [♀, Age/12-55]

O26.72 Subluxation of symphysis (pubis) in childbirth — [♀, Age/12-55]

O26.73 Subluxation of symphysis (pubis) in the puerperium — [♀, Age/12-55]

O26.8- Other specified pregnancy related conditions

O26.81- Pregnancy related exhaustion and fatigue

O26.811 Pregnancy related exhaustion and fatigue, first trimester — [♀, Age/12-55]

O26.812 Pregnancy related exhaustion and fatigue, second trimester — [♀, Age/12-55]

O26.813 Pregnancy related exhaustion and fatigue, third trimester — [♀, Age/12-55]

O26.819 Pregnancy related exhaustion and fatigue, unspecified trimester — [♀, Age/12-55]

O26.82- Pregnancy related peripheral neuritis

O26.821 Pregnancy related peripheral neuritis, first trimester — [♀, Age/12-55]

O26.822 Pregnancy related peripheral neuritis, second trimester — [♀, Age/12-55]

O26.823 Pregnancy related peripheral neuritis, third trimester — [♀, Age/12-55]

O26.829 Pregnancy related peripheral neuritis, unspecified trimester — [♀, Age/12-55]

O26.83- Pregnancy related renal disease
Use additional code to identify the specific disorder

CC **O26.831 Pregnancy related renal disease, first trimester** — [♀, Age/12-55]

CC **O26.832 Pregnancy related renal disease, second trimester** — [♀, Age/12-55]

CC **O26.833 Pregnancy related renal disease, third trimester** — [♀, Age/12-55]

O26.839 Pregnancy related renal disease, unspecified trimester — [♀, Age/12-55]

O26.84- Uterine size-date discrepancy complicating pregnancy
Excludes 1: encounter for suspected problem with fetal growth ruled out (Z03.74)

O26.841 Uterine size-date discrepancy, first trimester — [♀, Age/12-55]

O26.842 Uterine size-date discrepancy, second trimester — [♀, Age/12-55]

O26.843 Uterine size-date discrepancy, third trimester — [♀, Age/12-55]

O26.849 Uterine size-date discrepancy, unspecified trimester — [♀, Age/12-55]

O26.85- Spotting complicating pregnancy — The presence of light vaginal bleeding during pregnancy.

O26.851 Spotting complicating pregnancy, first trimester — [♀, Age/12-55]

O26.852 Spotting complicating pregnancy, second trimester — [♀, Age/12-55]

O26.853 Spotting complicating pregnancy, third trimester — [♀, Age/12-55]

O26.859 Spotting complicating pregnancy, unspecified trimester — [♀, Age/12-55]

O26.86 Pruritic urticarial papules and plaques of pregnancy (PUPPP) — [♀, Age/12-55]
    Polymorphic eruption of pregnancy

O26.87- Cervical shortening — The premature effacing and dilation of the cervix during pregnancy.
Excludes 1: encounter for suspected cervical shortening ruled out (Z03.75)

CC **O26.872 Cervical shortening, second trimester** — [♀, Age/12-55]

CC **O26.873 Cervical shortening, third trimester** — [♀, Age/12-55]

CC **O26.879 Cervical shortening, unspecified trimester** — [♀, Age/12-55]

O26.89- Other specified pregnancy related conditions

O26.891 Other specified pregnancy related conditions, first trimester — [♀, Age/12-55]

O26.892 Other specified pregnancy related conditions, second trimester — [♀, Age/12-55]

O26.893 **Other specified pregnancy related conditions, <u>third</u> trimester** — [♀, Age/12-55]
  AHA 15:3Q:p40 – Prophylactic Rhogam

O26.899 **Other specified pregnancy related conditions, <u>unspecified</u> trimester** — [♀, Age/12-55]

O26.9- **Pregnancy related conditions, <u>unspecified</u>**

O26.90 **Pregnancy related conditions, unspecified, <u>unspecified</u> trimester** — [♀, Age/12-55]

O26.91 **Pregnancy related conditions, unspecified, <u>first</u> trimester** — [♀, Age/12-55]

O26.92 **Pregnancy related conditions, unspecified, <u>second</u> trimester** — [♀, Age/12-55]

O26.93 **Pregnancy related conditions, unspecified, <u>third</u> trimester** — [♀, Age/12-55]

O28- **<u>Abnormal findings</u> on antenatal screening of mother**
  Excludes 1:   diagnostic findings classified elsewhere — see Alphabetical Index

O28.0 **Abnormal hematological finding on antenatal screening of mother** — [♀, Age/12-55]

O28.1 **Abnormal biochemical finding on antenatal screening of mother** — [♀, Age/12-55]

O28.2 **Abnormal cytological finding on antenatal screening of mother** — [♀, Age/12-55]

O28.3 **Abnormal ultrasonic finding on antenatal screening of mother** — [♀, Age/12-55]

O28.4 **Abnormal radiological finding on antenatal screening of mother** — [♀, Age/12-55]

O28.5 **Abnormal chromosomal and genetic finding on antenatal screening of mother** — [♀, Age/12-55]

O28.8 **Other abnormal findings on antenatal screening of mother** — [♀, Age/12-55]

O28.9 **Unspecified abnormal findings on antenatal screening of mother** — [♀, Age/12-55]

O29- **<u>Complications of anesthesia during pregnancy</u>**
  Includes: Maternal complications arising from the administration of a general, regional or local anesthetic, analgesic or other sedation during pregnancy
  Use additional code, if necessary, to identify the complication
  *Excludes ❷: complications of anesthesia during labor and delivery (O74.-)
             complicatios of anesthesia during the puerperium (O89.-)*

O29.0- **<u>Pulmonary complications</u> of anesthesia during pregnancy**

O29.01- **<u>Aspiration pneumonitis</u> due to anesthesia during pregnancy**
  Inhalation of stomach contents or secretions NOS due to anesthesia during pregnancy
  Mendelson's syndrome due to anesthesia during pregnancy

O29.011 **Aspiration pneumonitis due to anesthesia during pregnancy, <u>first</u> trimester** — [♀, Age/12-55]

O29.012 **Aspiration pneumonitis due to anesthesia during pregnancy, <u>second</u> trimester** — [♀, Age/12-55]

O29.013 **Aspiration pneumonitis due to anesthesia during pregnancy, <u>third</u> trimester** — [♀, Age/12-55]

O29.019 **Aspiration pneumonitis due to anesthesia during pregnancy, <u>unspecified</u> trimester** — [♀, Age/12-55]

O29.02- **<u>Pressure collapse of lung</u> due to anesthesia during pregnancy**

O29.021 **Pressure collapse of lung due to anesthesia during pregnancy, <u>first</u> trimester** — [♀, Age/12-55]

O29.022 **Pressure collapse of lung due to anesthesia during pregnancy, <u>second</u> trimester** — [♀, Age/12-55]

O29.023 **Pressure collapse of lung due to anesthesia during pregnancy, <u>third</u> trimester** — [♀, Age/12-55]

O29.029 **Pressure collapse of lung due to anesthesia during pregnancy, <u>unspecified</u> trimester** — [♀, Age/12-55]

O29.09- **<u>Other pulmonary</u> complications of anesthesia during pregnancy**

O29.091 **Other pulmonary complications of anesthesia during pregnancy, <u>first</u> trimester** — [♀, Age/12-55]

O29.092 **Other pulmonary complications of anesthesia during pregnancy, <u>second</u> trimester** — [♀, Age/12-55]

O29.093 **Other pulmonary complications of anesthesia during pregnancy, <u>third</u> trimester** — [♀, Age/12-55]

O29.099 **Other pulmonary complications of anesthesia during pregnancy, <u>unspecified</u> trimester** — [♀, Age/12-55]

O29.1- **<u>Cardiac complications</u> of anesthesia during pregnancy**

O29.11- **<u>Cardiac arrest</u> due to anesthesia during pregnancy**

O29.111 **Cardiac arrest due to anesthesia during pregnancy, <u>first</u> trimester** — [♀, Age/12-55]

O29.112 **Cardiac arrest due to anesthesia during pregnancy, <u>second</u> trimester** — [♀, Age/12-55]

O29.113 **Cardiac arrest due to anesthesia during pregnancy, <u>third</u> trimester** — [♀, Age/12-55]

O29.119 **Cardiac arrest due to anesthesia during pregnancy, <u>unspecified</u> trimester** — [♀, Age/12-55]

O29.12- **<u>Cardiac failure</u> due to anesthesia during pregnancy**

O29.121 **Cardiac failure due to anesthesia during pregnancy, <u>first</u> trimester** — [♀, Age/12-55]

O29.122 **Cardiac failure due to anesthesia during pregnancy, <u>second</u> trimester** — [♀, Age/12-55]

O29.123 **Cardiac failure due to anesthesia during pregnancy, <u>third</u> trimester** — [♀, Age/12-55]

O29.129 **Cardiac failure due to anesthesia during pregnancy, <u>unspecified</u> trimester** — [♀, Age/12-55]

O29.19- **<u>Other cardiac complications</u> of anesthesia during pregnancy**

O29.191 **Other cardiac complications of anesthesia during pregnancy, <u>first</u> trimester** — [♀, Age/12-55]

O29.192 **Other cardiac complications of anesthesia during pregnancy, <u>second</u> trimester** — [♀, Age/12-55]

O29.193 **Other cardiac complications of anesthesia during pregnancy, <u>third</u> trimester** — [♀, Age/12-55]

O29.199 **Other cardiac complications of anesthesia during pregnancy, <u>unspecified</u> trimester** — [♀, Age/12-55]

O29.2- **<u>Central nervous system complications</u> of anesthesia during pregnancy**

O29.21- **<u>Cerebral anoxia</u> due to anesthesia during pregnancy**

O29.211 **Cerebral anoxia due to anesthesia during pregnancy, <u>first</u> trimester** — [♀, Age/12-55]

O29.212 **Cerebral anoxia due to anesthesia during pregnancy, <u>second</u> trimester** — [♀, Age/12-55]

O29.213 **Cerebral anoxia due to anesthesia during pregnancy, <u>third</u> trimester** — [♀, Age/12-55]

O29.219 **Cerebral anoxia due to anesthesia during pregnancy, <u>unspecified</u> trimester** — [♀, Age/12-55]

O29.29- **<u>Other central nervous system complications</u> of anesthesia during pregnancy**

O29.291 **Other central nervous system complications of anesthesia during pregnancy, <u>first</u> trimester** — [♀, Age/12-55]

O29.292 **Other central nervous system complications of anesthesia during pregnancy, <u>second</u> trimester** — [♀, Age/12-55]

O29.293 **Other central nervous system complications of anesthesia during pregnancy, <u>third</u> trimester** — [♀, Age/12-55]

O29.299 **Other central nervous system complications of anesthesia during pregnancy, <u>unspecified</u> trimester** — [♀, Age/12-55]

O29.3- **<u>Toxic reaction to local anesthesia</u> during pregnancy**

O29.3x- **Toxic reaction to local anesthesia during pregnancy**

O29.3x1 **Toxic reaction to local anesthesia during pregnancy, <u>first</u> trimester** — [♀, Age/12-55]

O29.3x2 **Toxic reaction to local anesthesia during pregnancy, <u>second</u> trimester** — [♀, Age/12-55]

O29.3x3 **Toxic reaction to local anesthesia during pregnancy, <u>third</u> trimester** — [♀, Age/12-55]

O29.3x9 **Toxic reaction to local anesthesia during pregnancy, <u>unspecified</u> trimester** — [♀, Age/12-55]

O
2
6
-
O
2
9

O29.4- <u>Spinal and epidural anesthesia induced headache</u> during pregnancy

O29.40 Spinal and epidural anesthesia induced headache during pregnancy, <u>unspecified</u> trimester — [♀, Age/12-55]

O29.41 Spinal and epidural anesthesia induced headache during pregnancy, <u>first</u> trimester — [♀, Age/12-55]

O29.42 Spinal and epidural anesthesia induced headache during pregnancy, <u>second</u> trimester — [♀, Age/12-55]

O29.43 Spinal and epidural anesthesia induced headache during pregnancy, <u>third</u> trimester — [♀, Age/12-55]

O29.5- <u>Other complications of spinal and epidural anesthesia</u> during pregnancy

  O29.5x- Other complications of spinal and epidural anesthesia during pregnancy

    O29.5x1 Other complications of spinal and epidural anesthesia during pregnancy, <u>first</u> trimester — [♀, Age/12-55]

    O29.5x2 Other complications of spinal and epidural anesthesia during pregnancy, <u>second</u> trimester — [♀, Age/12-55]

    O29.5x3 Other complications of spinal and epidural anesthesia during pregnancy, <u>third</u> trimester — [♀, Age/12-55]

    O29.5x9 Other complications of spinal and epidural anesthesia during pregnancy, <u>unspecified</u> trimester — [♀, Age/12-55]

O29.6- <u>Failed or difficult intubation for anesthesia</u> during pregnancy

O29.60 Failed or difficult intubation for anesthesia during pregnancy, <u>unspecified</u> trimester — [♀, Age/12-55]

O29.61 Failed or difficult intubation for anesthesia during pregnancy, <u>first</u> trimester — [♀, Age/12-55]

O29.62 Failed or difficult intubation for anesthesia during pregnancy, <u>second</u> trimester — [♀, Age/12-55]

O29.63 Failed or difficult intubation for anesthesia during pregnancy, <u>third</u> trimester — [♀, Age/12-55]

O29.8- <u>Other complications of anesthesia</u> during pregnancy

  O29.8x- Other complications of anesthesia during pregnancy

    O29.8x1 Other complications of anesthesia during pregnancy, <u>first</u> trimester — [♀, Age/12-55]

    O29.8x2 Other complications of anesthesia during pregnancy, <u>second</u> trimester — [♀, Age/12-55]

    O29.8x3 Other complications of anesthesia during pregnancy, <u>third</u> trimester — [♀, Age/12-55]

    O29.8x9 Other complications of anesthesia during pregnancy, <u>unspecified</u> trimester — [♀, Age/12-55]

O29.9- <u>Unspecified</u> complication of anesthesia during pregnancy

O29.90 Unspecified complication of anesthesia during pregnancy, <u>unspecified</u> trimester — [♀, Age/12-55]

O29.91 Unspecified complication of anesthesia during pregnancy, <u>first</u> trimester — [♀, Age/12-55]

O29.92 Unspecified complication of anesthesia during pregnancy, <u>second</u> trimester — [♀, Age/12-55]

O29.93 Unspecified complication of anesthesia during pregnancy, <u>third</u> trimester — [♀, Age/12-55]

Maternal care related to the fetus and amniotic cavity and possible delivery problems (O30-O48)

O30- <u>Multiple gestation</u> — The presence of more than one developing fetus within the uterus.
Code also any complications specific to multiple gestation

O30.0- <u>Twin</u> pregnancy — The presence of two fetuses.

  O30.00- Twin pregnancy, <u>unspecified number</u> of placenta and <u>unspecified number</u> of amniotic sacs

    O30.001 Twin pregnancy, unspecified number of placenta and unspecified number of amniotic sacs, <u>first</u> trimester — [♀, Age/12-55]

    O30.002 Twin pregnancy, unspecified number of placenta and unspecified number of amniotic sacs, <u>second</u> trimester — [♀, Age/12-55]

    O30.003 Twin pregnancy, unspecified number of placenta and unspecified number of amniotic sacs, <u>third</u> trimester — [♀, Age/12-55]

    O30.009 Twin pregnancy, unspecified number of placenta and unspecified number of amniotic sacs, <u>unspecified</u> trimester — [♀, Age/12-55]

  O30.01- Twin pregnancy, <u>monochorionic/monoamniotic</u>
Twin pregnancy, one placenta, one amniotic sac
Excludes 1: conjoined twins (O30.02-)

    O30.011 Twin pregnancy, monochorionic/monoamniotic, <u>first</u> trimester — [♀, Age/12-55]

    O30.012 Twin pregnancy, monochorionic/monoamniotic, <u>second</u> trimester — [♀, Age/12-55]

    O30.013 Twin pregnancy, monochorionic/monoamniotic, <u>third</u> trimester — [♀, Age/12-55]

    O30.019 Twin pregnancy, monochorionic/monoamniotic, <u>unspecified</u> trimester — [♀, Age/12-55]

  O30.02- <u>Conjoined</u> twin pregnancy

    O30.021 Conjoined twin pregnancy, <u>first</u> trimester — [♀, Age/12-55]

    O30.022 Conjoined twin pregnancy, <u>second</u> trimester — [♀, Age/12-55]

    O30.023 Conjoined twin pregnancy, <u>third</u> trimester — [♀, Age/12-55]

    O30.029 Conjoined twin pregnancy, <u>unspecified</u> trimester — [♀, Age/12-55]

  O30.03- Twin pregnancy, <u>monochorionic/diamniotic</u>
Twin pregnancy, one placenta, two amniotic sacs

    O30.031 Twin pregnancy, monochorionic/diamniotic, <u>first</u> trimester — [♀, Age/12-55]

    O30.032 Twin pregnancy, monochorionic/diamniotic, <u>second</u> trimester — [♀, Age/12-55]

    O30.033 Twin pregnancy, monochorionic/diamniotic, <u>third</u> trimester — [♀, Age/12-55]

    O30.039 Twin pregnancy, monochorionic/diamniotic, <u>unspecified</u> trimester — [♀, Age/12-55]

  O30.04- Twin pregnancy, <u>dichorionic/diamniotic</u>
Twin pregnancy, two placentae, two amniotic sacs

    O30.041 Twin pregnancy, dichorionic/diamniotic, <u>first</u> trimester — [♀, Age/12-55]

    O30.042 Twin pregnancy, dichorionic/diamniotic, <u>second</u> trimester — [♀, Age/12-55]

    O30.043 Twin pregnancy, dichorionic/diamniotic, <u>third</u> trimester — [♀, Age/12-55]

    O30.049 Twin pregnancy, dichorionic/diamniotic, <u>unspecified</u> trimester — [♀, Age/12-55]

  O30.09- Twin pregnancy, <u>unable to determine number</u> of placenta and number of amniotic sacs

    O30.091 Twin pregnancy, unable to determine number of placenta and number of amniotic sacs, <u>first</u> trimester — [♀, Age/12-55]

    O30.092 Twin pregnancy, unable to determine number of placenta and number of amniotic sacs, <u>second</u> trimester — [♀, Age/12-55]

    O30.093 Twin pregnancy, unable to determine number of placenta and number of amniotic sacs, <u>third</u> trimester — [♀, Age/12-55]

    O30.099 Twin pregnancy, unable to determine number of placenta and number of amniotic sacs, <u>unspecified</u> trimester — [♀, Age/12-55]

O
2
9
-
0
3
0

O30.1- **Triplet** pregnancy — The presence of three fetuses.
    AHA 16:2Q:p8 – Triamniotic trichorionic triplet pregnancy

O30.10-   Triplet pregnancy, <u>unspecified number</u> of placenta and <u>unspecified number</u> of amniotic sacs

cc **O30.101** Triplet pregnancy, unspecified number of placenta and unspecified number of amniotic sacs, <u>first</u> trimester — [♀, Age/12-55]

cc **O30.102** Triplet pregnancy, unspecified number of placenta and unspecified number of amniotic sacs, <u>second</u> trimester — [♀, Age/12-55]

cc **O30.103** Triplet pregnancy, unspecified number of placenta and unspecified number of amniotic sacs, <u>third</u> trimester — [♀, Age/12-55]

O30.109 Triplet pregnancy, unspecified number of placenta and unspecified number of amniotic sacs, <u>unspecified</u> trimester — [♀, Age/12-55]

O30.11-   Triplet pregnancy <u>with two or more</u> <u>monochorionic</u> fetuses

cc **O30.111** Triplet pregnancy with two or more monochorionic fetuses, <u>first</u> trimester — [♀, Age/12-55]

cc **O30.112** Triplet pregnancy with two or more monochorionic fetuses, <u>second</u> trimester — [♀, Age/12-55]

cc **O30.113** Triplet pregnancy with two or more monochorionic fetuses, <u>third</u> trimester — [♀, Age/12-55]

O30.119 Triplet pregnancy with two or more monochorionic fetuses, <u>unspecified</u> trimester — [♀, Age/12-55]

O30.12-   Triplet pregnancy <u>with two or more monoamniotic</u> fetuses

cc **O30.121** Triplet pregnancy with two or more monoamniotic fetuses, <u>first</u> trimester — [♀, Age/12-55]

cc **O30.122** Triplet pregnancy with two or more monoamniotic fetuses, <u>second</u> trimester — [♀, Age/12-55]

cc **O30.123** Triplet pregnancy with two or more monoamniotic fetuses, <u>third</u> trimester — [♀, Age/12-55]

O30.129 Triplet pregnancy with two or more monoamniotic fetuses, <u>unspecified</u> trimester — [♀, Age/12-55]

O30.19-   Triplet pregnancy, <u>unable to determine number</u> of placenta and number of amniotic sacs

cc **O30.191** Triplet pregnancy, unable to determine number of placenta and number of amniotic sacs, <u>first</u> trimester — [♀, Age/12-55]

cc **O30.192** Triplet pregnancy, unable to determine number of placenta and number of amniotic sacs, <u>second</u> trimester — [♀, Age/12-55]

cc **O30.193** Triplet pregnancy, unable to determine number of placenta and number of amniotic sacs, <u>third</u> trimester — [♀, Age/12-55]

O30.199 Triplet pregnancy, unable to determine number of placenta and number of amniotic sacs, <u>unspecified</u> trimester — [♀, Age/12-55]

O30.2- <u>Quadruplet</u> pregnancy — The presence of four fetuses.

O30.20-   Quadruplet pregnancy, <u>unspecified number</u> of placenta and <u>unspecified number</u> of amnioticsacs

cc **O30.201** Quadruplet pregnancy, unspecified number of placenta and unspecified number of amniotic sacs, <u>first</u> trimester — [♀, Age/12-55]

cc **O30.202** Quadruplet pregnancy, unspecified number of placenta and unspecified number of amniotic sacs, <u>second</u> trimester — [♀, Age/12-55]

cc **O30.203** Quadruplet pregnancy, unspecified number of placenta and unspecified number of amniotic sacs, <u>third</u> trimester — [♀, Age/12-55]

O30.209 Quadruplet pregnancy, unspecified number of placenta and unspecified number of amniotic sacs, <u>unspecified</u> trimester — [♀, Age/12-55]

O30.21-   Quadruplet pregnancy <u>with two or more</u> <u>monochorionic</u> fetuses

cc **O30.211** Quadruplet pregnancy with two or more monochorionic fetuses, <u>first</u> trimester — [♀, Age/12-55]

cc **O30.212** Quadruplet pregnancy with two or more monochorionic fetuses, <u>second</u> trimester — [♀, Age/12-55]

cc **O30.213** Quadruplet pregnancy with two or more monochorionic fetuses, <u>third</u> trimester — [♀, Age/12-55]

O30.219 Quadruplet pregnancy with two or more monochorionic fetuses, <u>unspecified</u> trimester — [♀, Age/12-55]

O30.22-   Quadruplet pregnancy <u>with two or more</u> <u>monoamniotic</u> fetuses

cc **O30.221** Quadruplet pregnancy with two or more monoamniotic fetuses, <u>first</u> trimester — [♀, Age/12-55]

cc **O30.222** Quadruplet pregnancy with two or more monoamniotic fetuses, <u>second</u> trimester — [♀, Age/12-55]

cc **O30.223** Quadruplet pregnancy with two or more monoamniotic fetuses, <u>third</u> trimester — [♀, Age/12-55]

O30.229 Quadruplet pregnancy with two or more monoamniotic fetuses, <u>unspecified</u> trimester — [♀, Age/12-55]

O30.29-   Quadruplet pregnancy, <u>unable to determine number</u> of placenta and number of amniotic sacs

cc **O30.291** Quadruplet pregnancy, unable to determine number of placenta and number of amniotic sacs, <u>first</u> trimester — [♀, Age/12-55]

cc **O30.292** Quadruplet pregnancy, unable to determine number of placenta and number of amniotic sacs, <u>second</u> trimester — [♀, Age/12-55]

cc **O30.293** Quadruplet pregnancy, unable to determine number of placenta and number of amniotic sacs, <u>third</u> trimester — [♀, Age/12-55]

O30.299 Quadruplet pregnancy, unable to determine number of placenta and number of amniotic sacs, <u>unspecified</u> trimester — [♀, Age/12-55]

O30.8- <u>Other specified</u> multiple gestation
    Multiple gestation pregnancy greater then quadruplets

O30.80-   Other specified multiple gestation, <u>unspecified number</u> of placenta and <u>unspecified number</u> of amniotic sacs

cc **O30.801** Other specified multiple gestation, unspecified number of placenta and unspecified number of amniotic sacs, <u>first</u> trimester — [♀, Age/12-55]

cc **O30.802** Other specified multiple gestation, unspecified number of placenta and unspecified number of amniotic sacs, <u>second</u> trimester — [♀, Age/12-55]

cc **O30.803** Other specified multiple gestation, unspecified number of placenta and unspecified number of amniotic sacs, <u>third</u> trimester — [♀, Age/12-55]

O30.809 Other specified multiple gestation, unspecified number of placenta and unspecified number of amniotic sacs, <u>unspecified</u> trimester — [♀, Age/12-55]

O30 - O30

O30.81-   Other specified multiple gestation <u>with two or more monochorionic</u> fetuses

cc **O30.811**   Other specified multiple gestation with two or more monochorionic fetuses, <u>first</u> trimester — [♀, Age/12-55]

cc **O30.812**   Other specified multiple gestation with two or more monochorionic fetuses, <u>second</u> trimester — [♀, Age/12-55]

cc **O30.813**   Other specified multiple gestation with two or more monochorionic fetuses, <u>third</u> trimester — [♀, Age/12-55]

O30.819   Other specified multiple gestation with two or more monochorionic fetuses, <u>unspecified</u> trimester — [♀, Age/12-55]

O30.82-   Other specified multiple gestation <u>with two or more monoamniotic</u> fetuses

cc **O30.821**   Other specified multiple gestation with two or more monoamniotic fetuses, <u>first</u> trimester — [♀, Age/12-55]

cc **O30.822**   Other specified multiple gestation with two or more monoamniotic fetuses, <u>second</u> trimester — [♀, Age/12-55]

cc **O30.823**   Other specified multiple gestation with two or more monoamniotic fetuses, <u>third</u> trimester — [♀, Age/12-55]

O30.829   Other specified multiple gestation with two or more monoamniotic fetuses, <u>unspecified</u> trimester — [♀, Age/12-55]

O30.89-   Other specified multiple gestation, <u>unable to determine number</u> of placenta and number of amniotic sacs

cc **O30.891**   Other specified multiple gestation, unable to determine number of placenta and number of amniotic sacs, <u>first</u> trimester — [♀, Age/12-55]

cc **O30.892**   Other specified multiple gestation, unable to determine number of placenta and number of amniotic sacs, <u>second</u> trimester — [♀, Age/12-55]

cc **O30.893**   Other specified multiple gestation, unable to determine number of placenta and number of amniotic sacs, <u>third</u> trimester — [♀, Age/12-55]

O30.899   Other specified multiple gestation, unable to determine number of placenta and number of amniotic sacs, <u>unspecified</u> trimester — [♀, Age/12-55]

O30.9- Multiple gestation, <u>unspecified</u>
    Multiple pregnancy NOS

O30.90 Multiple gestation, unspecified, <u>unspecified</u> trimester — [♀, Age/12-55]

O30.91 Multiple gestation, unspecified, <u>first</u> trimester — [♀, Age/12-55]

O30.92 Multiple gestation, unspecified, <u>second</u> trimester — [♀, Age/12-55]

O30.93 Multiple gestation, unspecified, <u>third</u> trimester — [♀, Age/12-55]

O31- <u>Complications specific to multiple gestation</u>
    AHA 12:4Q:p107 – Fetus A and B same as fetus 1 and 2
    Excludes ❷: *delayed delivery of second twin, triplet, etc. (O63.2)*
                  malpresentation of one fetus or more (O32.9)
                   placental transfusion syndromes (O43.0-)

One of the following 7th characters is to be assigned to each code under category O31. 7th character 0 is for single gestations and multiple gestations where the fetus is unspecified. 7th characters 1 through 9 are for cases of multiple gestations to identify the fetus for which the code applies. The appropriate code from category O30, Multiple gestation, must also be assigned when assigning a code from category O31 that has a 7th character of 1 through 9.

  0   Not applicable or unspecified
  1   Fetus 1
  2   Fetus 2
  3   Fetus 3
  4   Fetus 4
  5   Fetus 5
  9   Other fetus

O31.0- <u>Papyraceous fetus</u> — The dead fetus that is pressed flat by the development of the living twin.
    Fetus compressus

O31.00x- Papyraceous fetus, <u>unspecified</u> trimester — [♀, Age/12-55]

O31.01x- Papyraceous fetus, <u>first</u> trimester — [♀, Age/12-55]

O31.02x- Papyraceous fetus, <u>second</u> trimester — [♀, Age/12-55]

O31.03x- Papyraceous fetus, <u>third</u> trimester — [♀, Age/12-55]

O31.1- <u>Continuing pregnancy after spontaneous abortion</u> of one fetus or more

O31.10x- Continuing pregnancy after spontaneous abortion of one fetus or more, <u>unspecified</u> trimester — [♀, Age/12-55]

O31.11x- Continuing pregnancy after spontaneous abortion of one fetus or more, <u>first</u> trimester — [♀, Age/12-55]

O31.12x- Continuing pregnancy after spontaneous abortion of one fetus or more, <u>second</u> trimester — [♀, Age/12-55]

O31.13x- Continuing pregnancy after spontaneous abortion of one fetus or more, <u>third</u> trimester — [♀, Age/12-55]

O31.2- <u>Continuing pregnancy after intrauterine death</u> of one fetus or more

O31.20x- Continuing pregnancy after intrauterine death of one fetus or more, <u>unspecified</u> trimester — [♀, Age/12-55]

O31.21x- Continuing pregnancy after intrauterine death of one fetus or more, <u>first</u> trimester — [♀, Age/12-55]

O31.22x- Continuing pregnancy after intrauterine death of one fetus or more, <u>second</u> trimester — [♀, Age/12-55]

O31.23x- Continuing pregnancy after intrauterine death of one fetus or more, <u>third</u> trimester — [♀, Age/12-55]

O31.3- Continuing pregnancy <u>after elective fetal reduction</u> of one fetus or more
    Continuing pregnancy after selective termination of one fetus or more

O31.30x- Continuing pregnancy after elective fetal reduction of one fetus or more, <u>unspecified</u> trimester — [♀, Age/12-55]

O31.31x- Continuing pregnancy after elective fetal reduction of one fetus or more, <u>first</u> trimester — [♀, Age/12-55]

O31.32x- Continuing pregnancy after elective fetal reduction of one fetus or more, <u>second</u> trimester — [♀, Age/12-55]

O31.33x- Continuing pregnancy after elective fetal reduction of one fetus or more, <u>third</u> trimester — [♀, Age/12-55]

O31.8- Other complications specific to multiple gestation

O31.8x-   <u>Other complications specific to multiple gestation</u>

CC-0-9 **O31.8x1-** Other complications specific to multiple gestation, <u>first</u> trimester — [♀, Age/12-55]

CC-0-9 **O31.8x2-** Other complications specific to multiple gestation, <u>second</u> trimester — [♀, Age/12-55]

CC-0-9 **O31.8x3-** Other complications specific to multiple gestation, <u>third</u> trimester — [♀, Age/12-55]

O31.8x9- Other complications specific to multiple gestation, <u>unspecified</u> trimester — [♀, Age/12-55]

O 3 0 - O 3 1

O32- **Maternal care for malpresentation of fetus**
AHA 12:4Q:p107 – Fetus A and B same as fetus 1 and 2
Includes: The listed conditions as a reason for observation, hospitalization
             or other obstetric care of the mother, or for cesarean
             delivery before onset of labor
Excludes 1:   malpresentation of fetus with obstructed labor (O64.-)

One of the following 7th characters is to be assigned to each code
under category O32. 7th character 0 is for single gestations and
multiple gestations where the fetus is unspecified. 7th
characters 1 through 9 are for cases of multiple gestations to
identify the fetus for which the code applies. The appropriate
code from category O30, Multiple gestation, must also be
assigned when assigning a code from category O32 that has a
7th character of 1 through 9.
0   Not applicable or unspecified
1   Fetus 1
2   Fetus 2
3   Fetus 3
4   Fetus 4
5   Fetus 5
9   Other fetus

O32.0xx- **Maternal care for** <u>unstable lie</u> — [♀, Age/12-55] – A fetal position
which is changes repeatedly.

O32.1xx- **Maternal care for** <u>breech presentation</u> — [♀, Age/12-55] –
Presentation of the buttocks in the birth canal during labor.
Maternal care for buttocks presentation
Maternal care for complete breech
Maternal care for frank breech
Excludes 1:   footling presentation (O32.8)
*   incomplete breech (O32.8)*

BREECH PRESENTATION

O32.2xx- **Maternal care for** <u>transverse and oblique lie</u> —
[♀, Age/12-55] – Presentation of the body (trunk) in the birth canal during
labor.
Maternal care for oblique presentation
Maternal care for transverse presentation

TRANSVERSE LIE

O32.3xx- **Maternal care for** <u>face, brow and chin presentation</u> —
[♀, Age/12-55] – Presentation of the fetal face, brow (forehead), or chin
(mentum) in the birth canal during labor.

FACE/BROW PRESENTATION

O32.4xx- **Maternal care for** <u>high head at term</u> — [♀, Age/12-55] – The
situation of the fetus at term with its head in a cephalic position, but not
presenting into the pelvic brim.
Maternal care for failure of head to enter pelvic brim

O32.6xx- **Maternal care for** <u>compound presentation</u> — [♀, Age/12-55] –
Presentation of the fetus with a prolapsed arm or leg alongside the head or
alongside a breech.

O32.8xx- **Maternal care for** <u>other</u> **malpresentation of fetus** —
[♀, Age/12-55]
Maternal care for footling presentation — Presentation of one or
both feet in the birth canal during labor.
Maternal care for incomplete breech — Breech presentation with only
one of the legs bent at the knees in the birth canal during labor.

O32.9xx- **Maternal care for malpresentation of fetus,** <u>unspecified</u> —
[♀, Age/12-55]

O33- **Maternal care** <u>for disproportion</u> — The relative difference in size between the
fetal head and the pelvis.
AHA 12:4Q:p107 – Fetus A and B same as fetus 1 and 2
Includes: The listed conditions as a reason for observation, hospitalization
             or other obstetric care of the mother, or for cesarean
             delivery before onset of labor
Excludes 1:   disproportion with obstructed labor (O65-O66)

CC **O33.0** **Maternal care for disproportion due to** <u>deformity of maternal
pelvic bones</u> — [♀, Age/12-55]
Maternal care for disproportion due to pelvic deformity causing
disproportion NOS

O33.1 **Maternal care for disproportion due to** <u>generally contracted
pelvis</u> — [♀, Age/12-55] – A pelvic opening that is reduced more than 2 cm in
diameter.
Maternal care for disproportion due to contracted pelvis NOS
causing disproportion

O33.2 **Maternal care for disproportion due to** <u>inlet contraction of
pelvis</u> — [♀, Age/12-55] – The reduced upper opening of the pelvis.
Maternal care for disproportion due to inlet contraction (pelvis)
causing disproportion

O33.3xx- **Maternal care for disproportion due to** <u>outlet contraction of
pelvis</u> — [♀, Age/12-55] – The reduced lower opening of the pelvis.
Maternal care for disproportion due to mid-cavity contraction
(pelvis)
Maternal care for disproportion due to outlet contraction (pelvis)

One of the following 7th characters is to be assigned to
code O33.3. 7th character 0 is for single gestations
and multiple gestations where the fetus is unspecified.
7th characters 1 through 9 are for cases of multiple
gestations to identify the fetus for which the code
applies. The appropriate code from category O30,
Multiple gestation, must also be assigned when
assigning code O33.3 with a 7th character of 1 through
9.
0   Not applicable or unspecified
1   Fetus 1
2   Fetus 2
3   Fetus 3
4   Fetus 4
5   Fetus 5
9   Other fetus

O33.4xx- **Maternal care for disproportion of** <u>mixed maternal and
fetal origin</u> — [♀, Age/12-55]
One of the following 7th characters is to be assigned to
code O33.4. 7th character 0 is for single gestations
and multiple gestations where the fetus is unspecified.
7th characters 1 through 9 are for cases of multiple
gestations to identify the fetus for which the code
applies. The appropriate code from category O30,
Multiple gestation, must also be assigned when
assigning code O33.4 with a 7th character of 1 through
9.
0   Not applicable or unspecified
1   Fetus 1
2   Fetus 2
3   Fetus 3
4   Fetus 4
5   Fetus 5
9   Other fetus

O
3
2
|
O
3
3

O33.5xx- **Maternal care for disproportion due to <u>unusually large fetus</u>** — [♀, Age/12-55] – A larger than average fetus that is too large for the normal maternal pelvis.

Maternal care for disproportion due to disproportion of fetal origin with normally formed fetus

Maternal care for disproportion due to fetal disproportion NOS

One of the following 7th characters is to be assigned to code O33.5. 7th character 0 is for single gestations and multiple gestations where the fetus is unspecified. 7th characters 1 through 9 are for cases of multiple gestations to identify the fetus for which the code applies. The appropriate code from category O30, Multiple gestation, must also be assigned when assigning code O33.5 with a 7th character of 1 through 9.

0   Not applicable or unspecified
1   Fetus 1
2   Fetus 2
3   Fetus 3
4   Fetus 4
5   Fetus 5
9   Other fetus

O33.6xx- **Maternal care for disproportion due to <u>hydrocephalic fetus</u>** — [♀, Age/12-55] – The abnormal massive accumulation of fluid within the fetal cranial vault.

One of the following 7th characters is to be assigned to code O33.6. 7th character 0 is for single gestations and multiple gestations where the fetus is unspecified. 7th characters 1 through 9 are for cases of multiple gestations to identify the fetus for which the code applies. The appropriate code from category O30, Multiple gestation, must also be assigned when assigning code O33.6 with a 7th character of 1 through 9.

0   Not applicable or unspecified
1   Fetus 1
2   Fetus 2
3   Fetus 3
4   Fetus 4
5   Fetus 5
9   Other fetus

O33.7xx- **Maternal care for disproportion due to other <u>fetal deformities</u>** — [♀, Age/12-55]

Maternal care for disproportion due to fetal ascites
Maternal care for disproportion due to fetal hydrops
Maternal care for disproportion due to fetal meningomyelocele
Maternal care for disproportion due to fetal sacral teratoma
Maternal care for disproportion due to fetal tumor

Excludes 1: obstructed labor due to other fetal deformities (O66.3)

One of the following 7th characters is to be assigned to code O33.7. 7th character 0 is for single gestations and multiple gestations where the fetus is unspecified. 7th characters 1 through 9 are for cases of multiple gestations to identify the fetus for which the code applies. The appropriate code from category O30, Multiple gestation, must also be assigned when assigning code O33.7 with a 7th character of 1 through 9.

0   Not applicable or unspecified
1   Fetus 1
2   Fetus 2
3   Fetus 3
4   Fetus 4
5   Fetus 5
9   Other fetus

O33.8 **Maternal care for disproportion of <u>other</u> origin** — [♀, Age/12-55]

O33.9 **Maternal care for disproportion, <u>unspecified</u>** — [♀, Age/12-55]

Maternal care for disproportion due to cephalopelvic disproportion NOS
Maternal care for disproportion due to fetopelvic disproportion NOS

O34- **Maternal care for <u>abnormality of pelvic organs</u>**
Includes: The listed conditions as a reason for hospitalization or other obstetric care of the mother, or for cesarean delivery before onset of labor
Code first any associated obstructed labor (O65.5)
Use additional code for specific condition

O34.0- **Maternal care for <u>congenital malformation of uterus</u>** — Maternal uterine conditions that have been present since birth.
Maternal care for double uterus
Maternal care for uterus bicornis

O34.00 **Maternal care for unspecified congenital malformation of uterus, <u>unspecified</u> trimester** — [♀, Age/12-55]

O34.01 **Maternal care for unspecified congenital malformation of uterus, <u>first</u> trimester** — [♀, Age/12-55]

O34.02 **Maternal care for unspecified congenital malformation of uterus, <u>second</u> trimester** — [♀, Age/12-55]

O34.03 **Maternal care for unspecified congenital malformation of uterus, <u>third</u> trimester** — [♀, Age/12-55]

O34.1- **Maternal care for <u>benign tumor of corpus uteri</u>** — Abnormal growths of the uterus.
Excludes ❷: maternal care for benign tumor of cervix (O34.4-)
maternal care for malignant neoplasm of uterus (O9A.1-)

O34.10 **Maternal care for benign tumor of corpus uteri, <u>unspecified</u> trimester** — [♀, Age/12-55]

O34.11 **Maternal care for benign tumor of corpus uteri, <u>first</u> trimester** — [♀, Age/12-55]

O34.12 **Maternal care for benign tumor of corpus uteri, <u>second</u> trimester** — [♀, Age/12-55]

O34.13 **Maternal care for benign tumor of corpus uteri, <u>third</u> trimester** — [♀, Age/12-55]

O34.2- **Maternal care due to uterine scar from previous surgery**

O34.21- **Maternal care for <u>scar from previous cesarean delivery</u>**

O34.211 **Maternal care for <u>low transverse</u> scar from previous cesarean delivery** — [♀, Age/12-55]

O34.212 **Maternal care for <u>vertical</u> scar from previous cesarean delivery** — [♀, Age/12-55]
Maternal care for classical scar from previous cesarean delivery

O34.219 **Maternal care for <u>unspecified</u> type scar from previous cesarean delivery** — [♀, Age/12-55]

O34.29 **Maternal care due to <u>uterine scar from other previous surgery</u>** — [♀, Age/12-55]
Maternal care due to uterine scar from other transmural uterine incision

O34.3- **Maternal care for <u>cervical incompetence</u>** — The abnormal dilation of the cervix before the onset of labor, usually during the second trimester.
Maternal care for cerclage with or without cervical incompetence
Maternal care for Shirodkar suture with or without cervical incompetence

O34.30 **Maternal care for cervical incompetence, <u>unspecified</u> trimester** — [♀, Age/12-55]

MCC **O34.31** **Maternal care for cervical incompetence, <u>first</u> trimester** — [♀, Age/12-55]

MCC **O34.32** **Maternal care for cervical incompetence, <u>second</u> trimester** — [♀, Age/12-55]

MCC **O34.33** **Maternal care for cervical incompetence, <u>third</u> trimester** — [♀, Age/12-55]

O34.4- **Maternal care for other abnormalities of cervix**

O34.40 **Maternal care for other abnormalities of cervix, <u>unspecified</u> trimester** — [♀, Age/12-55]

O34.41 **Maternal care for other abnormalities of cervix, <u>first</u> trimester** — [♀, Age/12-55]

O34.42 **Maternal care for other abnormalities of cervix, <u>second</u> trimester** — [♀, Age/12-55]

O34.43 **Maternal care for other abnormalities of cervix, <u>third</u> trimester** — [♀, Age/12-55]

O33-O34

O34.5- Maternal care for other abnormalities of gravid uterus

O34.51-   Maternal care for <u>incarceration of gravid uterus</u> — The abnormal confinement of the uterus.

O34.511 **Maternal care for incarceration of gravid uterus, <u>first</u> trimester** — [♀, Age/12-55]

O34.512 **Maternal care for incarceration of gravid uterus, <u>second</u> trimester** — [♀, Age/12-55]

O34.513 **Maternal care for incarceration of gravid uterus, <u>third</u> trimester** — [♀, Age/12-55]

O34.519 **Maternal care for incarceration of gravid uterus, <u>unspecified</u> trimester** — [♀, Age/12-55]

O34.52-   Maternal care for <u>prolapse of gravid uterus</u> — The downward displacement of the gravid uterus.

O34.521 **Maternal care for prolapse of gravid uterus, <u>first</u> trimester** — [♀, Age/12-55]

O34.522 **Maternal care for prolapse of gravid uterus, <u>second</u> trimester** — [♀, Age/12-55]

O34.523 **Maternal care for prolapse of gravid uterus, <u>third</u> trimester** — [♀, Age/12-55]

O34.529 **Maternal care for prolapse of gravid uterus, <u>unspecified</u> trimester** — [♀, Age/12-55]

O34.53-   Maternal care for <u>retroversion of gravid uterus</u> — The abnormal turning backwards of the uterus.

O34.531 **Maternal care for retroversion of gravid uterus, <u>first</u> trimester** — [♀, Age/12-55]

O34.532 **Maternal care for retroversion of gravid uterus, <u>second</u> trimester** — [♀, Age/12-55]

O34.533 **Maternal care for retroversion of gravid uterus, <u>third</u> trimester** — [♀, Age/12-55]

O34.539 **Maternal care for retroversion of gravid uterus, <u>unspecified</u> trimester** — [♀, Age/12-55]

O34.59-   Maternal care for <u>other</u> abnormalities of gravid uterus

O34.591 **Maternal care for other abnormalities of gravid uterus, <u>first</u> trimester** — [♀, Age/12-55]

O34.592 **Maternal care for other abnormalities of gravid uterus, <u>second</u> trimester** — [♀, Age/12-55]

O34.593 **Maternal care for other abnormalities of gravid uterus, <u>third</u> trimester** — [♀, Age/12-55]

O34.599 **Maternal care for other abnormalities of gravid uterus, <u>unspecified</u> trimester** — [♀, Age/12-55]

O34.6- Maternal care for <u>abnormality of vagina</u>

Excludes ❷: maternal care for vaginal varices in pregnancy (O22.1-)

O34.60 **Maternal care for abnormality of vagina, <u>unspecified</u> trimester** — [♀, Age/12-55]

O34.61 **Maternal care for abnormality of vagina, <u>first</u> trimester** — [♀, Age/12-55]

O34.62 **Maternal care for abnormality of vagina, <u>second</u> trimester** — [♀, Age/12-55]

O34.63 **Maternal care for abnormality of vagina, <u>third</u> trimester** — [♀, Age/12-55]

O34.7- Maternal care for <u>abnormality of vulva and perineum</u>

Excludes ❷: maternal care for perineal and vulval varices in pregnancy (O22.1-)

O34.70 **Maternal care for abnormality of vulva and perineum, <u>unspecified</u> trimester** — [♀, Age/12-55]

O34.71 **Maternal care for abnormality of vulva and perineum, <u>first</u> trimester** — [♀, Age/12-55]

O34.72 **Maternal care for abnormality of vulva and perineum, <u>second</u> trimester** — [♀, Age/12-55]

O34.73 **Maternal care for abnormality of vulva and perineum, <u>third</u> trimester** — [♀, Age/12-55]

O34.8- Maternal care for <u>other</u> abnormalities of <u>pelvic organs</u>

O34.80 **Maternal care for other abnormalities of pelvic organs, <u>unspecified</u> trimester** — [♀, Age/12-55]

O34.81 **Maternal care for other abnormalities of pelvic organs, <u>first</u> trimester** — [♀, Age/12-55]

O34.82 **Maternal care for other abnormalities of pelvic organs, <u>second</u> trimester** — [♀, Age/12-55]

O34.83 **Maternal care for other abnormalities of pelvic organs, <u>third</u> trimester** — [♀, Age/12-55]

O34.9- Maternal care for abnormality of pelvic organ, <u>unspecified</u>

O34.90 **Maternal care for abnormality of pelvic organ, unspecified, <u>unspecified</u> trimester** — [♀, Age/12-55]

O34.91 **Maternal care for abnormality of pelvic organ, unspecified, <u>first</u> trimester** — [♀, Age/12-55]

O34.92 **Maternal care for abnormality of pelvic organ, unspecified, <u>second</u> trimester** — [♀, Age/12-55]

O34.93 **Maternal care for abnormality of pelvic organ, unspecified, <u>third</u> trimester** — [♀, Age/12-55]

O35- Maternal care for <u>known or suspected fetal abnormality and damage</u>

AHA 12:4Q:p107 – Fetus A and B same as fetus 1 and 2

Includes: The listed conditions in the fetus as a reason for hospitalization or other obstetric care to the mother, or for termination of pregnancy

Code also any associated maternal condition

Excludes 1:   encounter for suspected maternal and fetal conditions ruled out (Z03.7-)

One of the following 7th characters is to be assigned to each code under category O35. 7th character 0 is for single gestations and multiple gestations where the fetus is unspecified. 7th characters 1 through 9 are for cases of multiple gestations to identify the fetus for which the code applies. The appropriate code from category O30, Multiple gestation, must also be assigned when assigning a code from category O35 that has a 7th character of 1 through 9.

0   Not applicable or unspecified
1   Fetus 1
2   Fetus 2
3   Fetus 3
4   Fetus 4
5   Fetus 5
9   Other fetus

O35.0xx- Maternal care for (suspected) <u>central nervous system malformation in fetus</u> — [♀, Age/12-55]
Maternal care for fetal anencephaly
Maternal care for fetal hydrocephalus
Maternal care for fetal spina bifida
Excludes ❷: chromosomal abnormality in fetus (O35.1)

O35.1xx- Maternal care for (suspected) <u>chromosomal abnormality in fetus</u> — [♀, Age/12-55]

O35.2xx- Maternal care for (suspected) <u>hereditary disease in fetus</u> — [♀, Age/12-55]
Excludes ❷: chromosomal abnormality in fetus (O35.1)

O35.3xx- Maternal care for (suspected) <u>damage to fetus from viral disease in mother</u> — [♀, Age/12-55]
Maternal care for damage to fetus from maternal cytomegalovirus infection
Maternal care for damage to fetus from maternal rubella

O35.4xx- Maternal care for (suspected) damage to fetus <u>from alcohol</u> — [♀, Age/12-55]

O35.5xx- Maternal care for (suspected) damage to fetus <u>by drugs</u> — [♀, Age/12-55]
Maternal care for damage to fetus from drug addiction

O35.6xx- Maternal care for (suspected) damage to fetus <u>by radiation</u> — [♀, Age/12-55]

O35.7xx- Maternal care for (suspected) damage to fetus <u>by other medical procedures</u> — [♀, Age/12-55]
Maternal care for damage to fetus by amniocentesis
Maternal care for damage to fetus by biopsy procedures
Maternal care for damage to fetus by hematological investigation
Maternal care for damage to fetus by intrauterine contraceptive device
Maternal care for damage to fetus by intrauterine surgery

O35.8xx- Maternal care for <u>other</u> (suspected) fetal abnormality and damage — [♀, Age/12-55]
Maternal care for damage to fetus from maternal listeriosis
Maternal care for damage to fetus from maternal toxoplasmosis

O35.9xx- Maternal care for (suspected) fetal abnormality and damage, <u>unspecified</u> — [♀, Age/12-55]

O36- Maternal care <u>for other fetal problems</u>
AHA 12:4Q:p107 – Fetus A and B same as fetus 1 and 2
Includes: The listed conditions in the fetus as a reason for hospitalization or other obstetric care of the mother, or for termination of pregnancy
Excludes 1:   encounter for suspected maternal and fetal conditions ruled out (Z03.7-)
              placental transfusion syndromes (O43.0-)
Excludes ❷: labor and delivery complicated by fetal stress (O77.-)

One of the following 7th characters is to be assigned to each code under category O36. 7th character 0 is for single gestations and multiple gestations where the fetus is unspecified. 7th characters 1 through 9 are for cases of multiple gestations to identify the fetus for which the code applies. The appropriate code from category O30, Multiple gestation, must also be assigned when assigning a code from category O36 that has a 7th character of 1 through 9.
  0   Not applicable or unspecified
  1   Fetus 1
  2   Fetus 2
  3   Fetus 3
  4   Fetus 4
  5   Fetus 5
  9   Other fetus

O36.0- Maternal care for rhesus isoimmunization — The development of Rh-negative agglutinins in an Rh-negative mother in response to the development of Rh-positive fetal agglutinins.
    Maternal care for Rh incompatibility (with hydrops fetalis)

O36.01-   Maternal care for <u>anti-D [Rh] antibodies</u>
                AHA 14:4Q:p17x2 – Maternal care for anti-D [RH] antibodies

CC-0-9 **O36.011-** Maternal care for anti-D [Rh] antibodies, <u>first</u> trimester — [♀, Age/12-55]

CC-0-9 **O36.012-** Maternal care for anti-D [Rh] antibodies, <u>second</u> trimester — [♀, Age/12-55]

CC-0-9 **O36.013-** Maternal care for anti-D [Rh] antibodies, <u>third</u> trimester — [♀, Age/12-55]

O36.019- Maternal care for anti-D [Rh] antibodies, <u>unspecified</u> trimester — [♀, Age/12-55]

O36.09-   Maternal care for other <u>rhesus isoimmunization</u>

CC-0-9 **O36.091-** Maternal care for other rhesus isoimmunization, <u>first</u> trimester — [♀, Age/12-55]

CC-0-9 **O36.092-** Maternal care for other rhesus isoimmunization, <u>second</u> trimester — [♀, Age/12-55]

CC-0-9 **O36.093-** Maternal care for other rhesus isoimmunization, <u>third</u> trimester — [♀, Age/12-55]

O36.099- Maternal care for other rhesus <u>isoimmunization, unspecified</u> trimester — [♀, Age/12-55]

O36.1- Maternal care for other isoimmunization — The development of agglutinins due to a blood-group incompatibility.
    Maternal care for ABO isoimmunization

O36.11-   Maternal care for <u>Anti-A sensitization</u>
                Maternal care for isoimmunization NOS (with hydrops fetalis)

O36.111- Maternal care for Anti-A sensitization, <u>first</u> trimester — [♀, Age/12-55]

O36.112- Maternal care for Anti-A sensitization, <u>second</u> trimester — [♀, Age/12-55]

O36.113- Maternal care for Anti-A sensitization, <u>third</u> trimester — [♀, Age/12-55]

O36.119- Maternal care for Anti-A sensitization, <u>unspecified</u> trimester — [♀, Age/12-55]

O36.19-   Maternal care for <u>other isoimmunization</u>
                Maternal care for Anti-B sensitization

O36.191- Maternal care for other isoimmunization, <u>first</u> trimester — [♀, Age/12-55]

O36.192- Maternal care for other isoimmunization, <u>second</u> trimester — [♀, Age/12-55]

O36.193- Maternal care for other isoimmunization, <u>third</u> trimester — [♀, Age/12-55]

O36.199- Maternal care for other isoimmunization, <u>unspecified</u> trimester — [♀, Age/12-55]

O36.2- Maternal care for <u>hydrops fetalis</u> — The presence of whole body edema of the fetus.
    Maternal care for hydrops fetalis NOS
    Maternal care for hydrops fetalis not associated with isoimmunization
    Excludes 1:   hydrops fetalis associated with ABO isoimmunization (O36.1-)
                  hydrops fetalis associated with rhesus isoimmunization (O36.0-)

O36.20x- Maternal care for hydrops fetalis, <u>unspecified</u> trimester — [♀, Age/12-55]

O36.21x- Maternal care for hydrops fetalis, <u>first</u> trimester — [♀, Age/12-55]

O36.22x- Maternal care for hydrops fetalis, <u>second</u> trimester — [♀, Age/12-55]

O36.23x- Maternal care for hydrops fetalis, <u>third</u> trimester — [♀, Age/12-55]

O36.4xx- Maternal care for intrauterine death — [♀, Age/12-55]
CC-0-9   Maternal care for intrauterine fetal death NOS
            Maternal care for intrauterine fetal death after completion of 20 weeks of gestation
            Maternal care for late fetal death
            Maternal care for missed delivery
    Excludes 1:   missed abortion (O02.1)
                  stillbirth (P95)

O36.5- Maternal care for known or suspected <u>poor fetal growth</u> — The abnormally low fetal weight/size in comparison to gestational age.

O36.51-   Maternal care for known or suspected <u>placental insufficiency</u>

O36.511- Maternal care for known or suspected placental insufficiency, <u>first</u> trimester — [♀, Age/12-55]

O36.512- Maternal care for known or suspected placental insufficiency, <u>second</u> trimester — [♀, Age/12-55]

O36.513- Maternal care for known or suspected placental insufficiency, <u>third</u> trimester — [♀, Age/12-55]

O36.519- Maternal care for known or suspected placental insufficiency, <u>unspecified</u> trimester — [♀, Age/12-55]

O36.59-   Maternal care for <u>other</u> known or suspected poor fetal growth
                Maternal care for known or suspected light-for-dates NOS
                Maternal care for known or suspected small-for-dates NOS

O36.591- Maternal care for other known or suspected poor fetal growth, <u>first</u> trimester — [♀, Age/12-55]

O36.592- Maternal care for other known or suspected poor fetal growth, <u>second</u> trimester — [♀, Age/12-55]

O36.593- Maternal care for other known or suspected poor fetal growth, <u>third</u> trimester — [♀, Age/12-55]

O36.599- Maternal care for other known or suspected poor fetal growth, <u>unspecified</u> trimester — [♀, Age/12-55]

O36.6- Maternal care for <u>excessive fetal growth</u> — The abnormally high fetal weight/size in comparison to gestational age.
    Maternal care for known or suspected large-for-dates

O36.60x- Maternal care for excessive fetal growth, <u>unspecified</u> trimester — [♀, Age/12-55]

O36.61x- Maternal care for excessive fetal growth, <u>first</u> trimester — [♀, Age/12-55]

O36.62x- Maternal care for excessive fetal growth, <u>second</u> trimester — [♀, Age/12-55]

O36.63x- Maternal care for excessive fetal growth, <u>third</u> trimester — [♀, Age/12-55]

O36.7- Maternal care for <u>viable fetus in abdominal</u> pregnancy

O36.70x- Maternal care for viable fetus in abdominal pregnancy, <u>unspecified</u> trimester — [♀, Age/12-55]

O36.71x- Maternal care for viable fetus in abdominal pregnancy, <u>first</u> trimester — [♀, Age/12-55]

O36.72x- Maternal care for viable fetus in abdominal pregnancy, <u>second</u> trimester — [♀, Age/12-55]

O36.73x- Maternal care for viable fetus in abdominal pregnancy, <u>third</u> trimester — [♀, Age/12-55]

O35-O36 (side tab)

O36.8- Maternal care for other specified fetal problems

O36.80x- Pregnancy with <u>inconclusive fetal viability</u> — [♀, Age/12-55] [Unacceptable PDX]
Encounter to determine fetal viability of pregnancy

O36.81- <u>Decreased fetal movements</u>

O36.812- Decreased fetal movements, <u>second</u> trimester — [♀, Age/12-55]

O36.813- Decreased fetal movements, <u>third</u> trimester — [♀, Age/12-55]

O36.819- Decreased fetal movements, <u>unspecified</u> trimester — [♀, Age/12-55]

O36.82- <u>Fetal anemia and thrombocytopenia</u>

O36.821- Fetal anemia and thrombocytopenia, <u>first</u> trimester — [♀, Age/12-55]

O36.822- Fetal anemia and thrombocytopenia, <u>second</u> trimester — [♀, Age/12-55]

O36.823- Fetal anemia and thrombocytopenia, <u>third</u> trimester — [♀, Age/12-55]

O36.829- Fetal anemia and thrombocytopenia, <u>unspecified</u> trimester — [♀, Age/12-55]

O36.89- Maternal care for <u>other specified</u> fetal problems

O36.891- Maternal care for other specified fetal problems, <u>first</u> trimester — [♀, Age/12-55]

O36.892- Maternal care for other specified fetal problems, <u>second</u> trimester — [♀, Age/12-55]

O36.893- Maternal care for other specified fetal problems, <u>third</u> trimester — [♀, Age/12-55]

O36.899- Maternal care for other specified fetal problems, <u>unspecified</u> trimester — [♀, Age/12-55]

O36.9- Maternal care for fetal problem, <u>unspecified</u>

O36.90x- Maternal care for fetal problem, unspecified, <u>unspecified</u> trimester — [♀, Age/12-55]

O36.91x- Maternal care for fetal problem, unspecified, <u>first</u> trimester — [♀, Age/12-55]

O36.92x- Maternal care for fetal problem, unspecified, <u>second</u> trimester — [♀, Age/12-55]

O36.93x- Maternal care for fetal problem, unspecified, <u>third</u> trimester — [♀, Age/12-55]

O40- <u>Polyhydramnios</u> — The excessive amount of amniotic fluid.
AHA 12:4Q:p107 – Fetus A and B same as fetus 1 and 2
AHA 16:1Q:p4 – Polyhydramnios and laceration
Includes: Hydramnios
Excludes 1:   *encounter for suspected maternal and fetal conditions ruled out (Z03.7-)*

One of the following 7th characters is to be assigned to each code under category O40. 7th character 0 is for single gestations and multiple gestations where the fetus is unspecified. 7th characters 1 through 9 are for cases of multiple gestations to identify the fetus for which the code applies. The appropriate code from category O30, Multiple gestation, must also be assigned when assigning a code from category O40 that has a 7th character of 1 through 9.
0   Not applicable or unspecified
1   Fetus 1
2   Fetus 2
3   Fetus 3
4   Fetus 4
5   Fetus 5
9   Other fetus

O40.1xx- Polyhydramnios, <u>first</u> trimester — [♀, Age/12-55]

O40.2xx- Polyhydramnios, <u>second</u> trimester — [♀, Age/12-55]

O40.3xx- Polyhydramnios, <u>third</u> trimester — [♀, Age/12-55]

O40.9xx- Polyhydramnios, <u>unspecified</u> trimester — [♀, Age/12-55]

O41- Other disorders of amniotic fluid and membranes
AHA 12:4Q:p107 – Fetus A and B same as fetus 1 and 2
Excludes 1:   *encounter for suspected maternal and fetal conditions ruled out (Z03.7-)*

One of the following 7th characters is to be assigned to each code under category O41. 7th character 0 is for single gestations and multiple gestations where the fetus is unspecified. 7th characters 1 through 9 are for cases of multiple gestations to identify the fetus for which the code applies. The appropriate code from category O30, Multiple gestation, must also be assigned when assigning a code from category O41 that has a 7th character of 1 through 9.
0   Not applicable or unspecified
1   Fetus 1
2   Fetus 2
3   Fetus 3
4   Fetus 4
5   Fetus 5
9   Other fetus

O41.0- <u>Oligohydramnios</u> — The abnormally low amount of amniotic fluid. Oligohydramnios without rupture of membranes

O41.00x- Oligohydramnios, <u>unspecified</u> trimester — [♀, Age/12-55]

CC-0-9 **O41.01x-** Oligohydramnios, <u>first</u> trimester — [♀, Age/12-55]

CC-0-9 **O41.02x-** Oligohydramnios, <u>second</u> trimester — [♀, Age/12-55]

CC-0-9 **O41.03x-** Oligohydramnios, <u>third</u> trimester — [♀, Age/12-55]

O41.1- Infection of amniotic sac and membranes — Invasion of microorganisms of the amniotic cavity.

O41.10- <u>Infection of amniotic sac and membranes, unspecified</u>

MCC-0-9 **O41.101-** Infection of amniotic sac and membranes, unspecified, <u>first</u> trimester — [♀, Age/12-55]

MCC-0-9 **O41.102-** Infection of amniotic sac and membranes, unspecified, <u>second</u> trimester — [♀, Age/12-55]

MCC-0-9 **O41.103-** Infection of amniotic sac and membranes, unspecified, <u>third</u> trimester — [♀, Age/12-55]

O41.109- Infection of amniotic sac and membranes, unspecified, <u>unspecified</u> trimester — [♀, Age/12-55]

O41.12- <u>Chorioamnionitis</u> — Inflammation of the fetal amniotic membranes caused by microorganisms.

MCC-0-9 **O41.121-** Chorioamnionitis, <u>first</u> trimester — [♀, Age/12-55]

MCC-0-9 **O41.122-** Chorioamnionitis, <u>second</u> trimester — [♀, Age/12-55]

MCC-0-9 **O41.123-** Chorioamnionitis, <u>third</u> trimester — [♀, Age/12-55]

O41.129- Chorioamnionitis, <u>unspecified</u> trimester — [♀, Age/12-55]

O41.14- <u>Placentitis</u> — Inflammation of the placenta caused by microorganisms.

MCC-0-9 **O41.141-** Placentitis, <u>first</u> trimester — [♀, Age/12-55]

MCC-0-9 **O41.142-** Placentitis, <u>second</u> trimester — [♀, Age/12-55]

MCC-0-9 **O41.143-** Placentitis, <u>third</u> trimester — [♀, Age/12-55]

O41.149- Placentitis, <u>unspecified</u> trimester — [♀, Age/12-55]

O41.8- Other specified disorders of amniotic fluid and membranes

O41.8x- <u>Other specified</u> disorders of amniotic fluid and membranes

O41.8x1- Other specified disorders of amniotic fluid and membranes, <u>first</u> trimester — [♀, Age/12-55]

O41.8x2- Other specified disorders of amniotic fluid and membranes, <u>second</u> trimester — [♀, Age/12-55]

O41.8x3- Other specified disorders of amniotic fluid and membranes, <u>third</u> trimester — [♀, Age/12-55]

O41.8x9- Other specified disorders of amniotic fluid and membranes, <u>unspecified</u> trimester — [♀, Age/12-55]

O41.9- Disorder of amniotic fluid and membranes, <u>unspecified</u>

O41.90x- Disorder of amniotic fluid and membranes, unspecified, <u>unspecified</u> trimester — [♀, Age/12-55]

O41.91x- Disorder of amniotic fluid and membranes, unspecified, <u>first</u> trimester — [♀, Age/12-55]

O41.92x- Disorder of amniotic fluid and membranes, unspecified, <u>second</u> trimester — [♀, Age/12-55]

O 3 6 - O 4 1

O41.93x- Disorder of amniotic fluid and membranes, unspecified, third trimester — [♀, Age/12-55]

O42- Premature rupture of membranes — The rupture or tear of the amniotic sac prior to the onset of labor.
AHA 16:1Q:p3,5 – Premature rupture of membranes and laceration

O42.0- Premature rupture of membranes, onset of labor within 24 hours of rupture

O42.00 Premature rupture of membranes, onset of labor within 24 hours of rupture, unspecified weeks of gestation — [♀, Age/12-55]

O42.01- Preterm premature rupture of membranes, onset of labor within 24 hours of rupture
Premature rupture of membranes before 37 completed weeks of gestation

O42.011 Preterm premature rupture of membranes, onset of labor within 24 hours of rupture, first trimester — [♀, Age/12-55]

O42.012 Preterm premature rupture of membranes, onset of labor within 24 hours of rupture, second trimester — [♀, Age/12-55]

O42.013 Preterm premature rupture of membranes, onset of labor within 24 hours of rupture, third trimester — [♀, Age/12-55]

O42.019 Preterm premature rupture of membranes, onset of labor within 24 hours of rupture, unspecified trimester — [♀, Age/12-55]

O42.02 Full-term premature rupture of membranes, onset of labor within 24 hours of rupture — [♀, Age/12-55]
Premature rupture of membranes at or after 37 completed weeks of gestation, onset of labor within 24 hours of rupture

O42.1- Premature rupture of membranes, onset of labor more than 24 hours following rupture

O42.10 Premature rupture of membranes, onset of labor more than 24 hours following rupture, unspecified weeks of gestation — [♀, Age/12-55]

O42.11- Preterm premature rupture of membranes, onset of labor more than 24 hours following rupture
Premature rupture of membranes before 37 completed weeks of gestation

O42.111 Preterm premature rupture of membranes, onset of labor more than 24 hours following rupture, first trimester — [♀, Age/12-55]

O42.112 Preterm premature rupture of membranes, onset of labor more than 24 hours following rupture, second trimester — [♀, Age/12-55]

O42.113 Preterm premature rupture of membranes, onset of labor more than 24 hours following rupture, third trimester — [♀, Age/12-55]

O42.119 Preterm premature rupture of membranes, onset of labor more than 24 hours following rupture, unspecified trimester — [♀, Age/12-55]

O42.12 Full-term premature rupture of membranes, onset of labor more than 24 hours following rupture — [♀, Age/12-55]
Premature rupture of membranes at or after 37 completed weeks of gestation, onset of labor more than 24 hours following rupture

O42.9- Premature rupture of membranes, unspecified as to length of time between rupture and onset of labor

O42.90 Premature rupture of membranes, unspecified as to length of time between rupture and onset of labor, unspecified weeks of gestation — [♀, Age/12-55]

O42.91- Preterm premature rupture of membranes, unspecified as to length of time between rupture and onset of labor
Premature rupture of membranes before 37 completed weeks of gestation

O42.911 Preterm premature rupture of membranes, unspecified as to length of time between rupture and onset of labor, first trimester — [♀, Age/12-55]

O42.912 Preterm premature rupture of membranes, unspecified as to length of time between rupture and onset of labor, second trimester — [♀, Age/12-55]

O42.913 Preterm premature rupture of membranes, unspecified as to length of time between rupture and onset of labor, third trimester — [♀, Age/12-55]

O42.919 Preterm premature rupture of membranes, unspecified as to length of time between rupture and onset of labor, unspecified trimester — [♀, Age/12-55]

O42.92 Full-term premature rupture of membranes, unspecified as to length of time between rupture and onset of labor — [♀, Age/12-55]
Premature rupture of membranes at or after 37 completed weeks of gestation, unspecified as to length of time between rupture and onset of labor

O43- Placental disorders
Excludes ❷: *maternal care for poor fetal growth due to placental insufficiency (O36.5-)*
placenta previa (O44.-)
placental polyp (O90.89)
placentitis (O41.14-)
premature separation of placenta [abruptio placentae] (O45.-)

O43.0- Placental transfusion syndromes — The abnormal flow of blood to the fetus.

O43.01- Fetomaternal placental transfusion syndrome— The abnormal flow of fetal blood cells to the mother through a defect in the placental membranes.
Maternofetal placental transfusion syndrome

O43.011 Fetomaternal placental transfusion syndrome, first trimester — [♀, Age/12-55]

O43.012 Fetomaternal placental transfusion syndrome, second trimester — [♀, Age/12-55]

O43.013 Fetomaternal placental transfusion syndrome, third trimester — [♀, Age/12-55]

O43.019 Fetomaternal placental transfusion syndrome, unspecified trimester — [♀, Age/12-55]

O43.02- Fetus-to-fetus placental transfusion syndrome — The disproportionate flow of blood to one fetus versus the other.

O43.021 Fetus-to-fetus placental transfusion syndrome, first trimester — [♀, Age/12-55]

O43.022 Fetus-to-fetus placental transfusion syndrome, second trimester — [♀, Age/12-55]

O43.023 Fetus-to-fetus placental transfusion syndrome, third trimester — [♀, Age/12-55]

O43.029 Fetus-to-fetus placental transfusion syndrome, unspecified trimester — [♀, Age/12-55]

O43.1- Malformation of placenta — The abnormal development of the placenta.

O43.10- Malformation of placenta, unspecified
Abnormal placenta NOS

O43.101 Malformation of placenta, unspecified, first trimester — [♀, Age/12-55]

O43.102 Malformation of placenta, unspecified, second trimester — [♀, Age/12-55]

O43.103 Malformation of placenta, unspecified, third trimester — [♀, Age/12-55]

O43.109 Malformation of placenta, unspecified, unspecified trimester — [♀, Age/12-55]

O43.11- Circumvallate placenta — A condition in which the layers of the placenta fold into an abnormal position.

O43.111 Circumvallate placenta, first trimester — [♀, Age/12-55]

O43.112 Circumvallate placenta, second trimester — [♀, Age/12-55]

O43.113 Circumvallate placenta, third trimester — [♀, Age/12-55]

O43.119 Circumvallate placenta, unspecified trimester — [♀, Age/12-55]

O43.12-   Velamentous insertion of umbilical cord — The abnormal insertion of the umbilical cord in the placenta.

O43.121   Velamentous insertion of umbilical cord, first trimester — [♀, Age/12-55]

O43.122   Velamentous insertion of umbilical cord, second trimester — [♀, Age/12-55]

O43.123   Velamentous insertion of umbilical cord, third trimester — [♀, Age/12-55]

O43.129   Velamentous insertion of umbilical cord, unspecified trimester — [♀, Age/12-55]

O43.19-   Other malformation of placenta

O43.191   Other malformation of placenta, first trimester — [♀, Age/12-55]

O43.192   Other malformation of placenta, second trimester — [♀, Age/12-55]

O43.193   Other malformation of placenta, third trimester — [♀, Age/12-55]

O43.199   Other malformation of placenta, unspecified trimester — [♀, Age/12-55]

O43.2- Morbidly adherent placenta
Code also associated third stage postpartum hemorrhage, if applicable (O72.0)
Excludes 1:   retained placenta (O73.-)

O43.21-   Placenta accreta — The abnormally deep attachment of the placenta onto the myometrium instead of the endometrium of pregnancy (decidua).

O43.211   Placenta accreta, first trimester — [♀, Age/12-55]

O43.212   Placenta accreta, second trimester — [♀, Age/12-55]

O43.213   Placenta accreta, third trimester — [♀, Age/12-55]

O43.219   Placenta accreta, unspecified trimester — [♀, Age/12-55]

O43.22-   Placenta increta — The abnormally deep attachment of the placenta into the myometrium.

O43.221   Placenta increta, first trimester — [♀, Age/12-55]

O43.222   Placenta increta, second trimester — [♀, Age/12-55]

O43.223   Placenta increta, third trimester — [♀, Age/12-55]

O43.229   Placenta increta, unspecified trimester — [♀, Age/12-55]

O43.23-   Placenta percreta — The abnormally deep attachment of the placenta and through the myometrium.

O43.231   Placenta percreta, first trimester — [♀, Age/12-55]

O43.232   Placenta percreta, second trimester — [♀, Age/12-55]

O43.233   Placenta percreta, third trimester — [♀, Age/12-55]

O43.239   Placenta percreta, unspecified trimester — [♀, Age/12-55]

O43.8- Other placental disorders

O43.81-   Placental infarction — Ischemic placental tissue necrosis due to obstruction of a placental vessel.

O43.811   Placental infarction, first trimester — [♀, Age/12-55]

O43.812   Placental infarction, second trimester — [♀, Age/12-55]

O43.813   Placental infarction, third trimester — [♀, Age/12-55]

O43.819   Placental infarction, unspecified trimester — [♀, Age/12-55]

O43.89-   Other placental disorders
Placental dysfunction

O43.891   Other placental disorders, first trimester — [♀, Age/12-55]

O43.892   Other placental disorders, second trimester — [♀, Age/12-55]

O43.893   Other placental disorders, third trimester — [♀, Age/12-55]

O43.899   Other placental disorders, unspecified trimester — [♀, Age/12-55]

O43.9- Unspecified placental disorder

O43.90 Unspecified placental disorder, unspecified trimester — [♀, Age/12-55]

O43.91 Unspecified placental disorder, first trimester — [♀, Age/12-55]

O43.92 Unspecified placental disorder, second trimester — [♀, Age/12-55]

O43.93 Unspecified placental disorder, third trimester — [♀, Age/12-55]

O44- Placenta previa — The implantation of the placenta in the lower uterine segment.

O44.0-   Complete placenta previa NOS or without hemorrhage
Placenta previa NOS

O44.00 Complete placenta previa NOS or without hemorrhage, unspecified trimester — [♀, Age/12-55]

cc **O44.01 Complete placenta previa NOS or without hemorrhage, first trimester** — [♀, Age/12-55]

cc **O44.02 Complete placenta previa NOS or without hemorrhage, second trimester** — [♀, Age/12-55]

cc **O44.03 Complete placenta previa NOS or without hemorrhage, third trimester** — [♀, Age/12-55]

O44.1-   Complete placenta previa with hemorrhage
Excludes 1:   labor and delivery complicated by hemorrhage from vasa previa (O69.4)

O44.10 Complete placenta previa with hemorrhage, unspecified trimester — [♀, Age/12-55]

mcc **O44.11 Complete placenta previa with hemorrhage, first trimester** — [♀, Age/12-55]

mcc **O44.12 Complete placenta previa with hemorrhage, second trimester** — [♀, Age/12-55]

mcc **O44.13 Complete placenta previa with hemorrhage, third trimester** — [♀, Age/12-55]

O44.2-   Partial placenta previa without hemorrhage
Marginal placenta previa, NOS or without hemorrhage

O44.20 Partial placenta previa NOS or without hemorrhage, unspecified trimester — [♀, Age/12-55]

cc **O44.21 Partial placenta previa NOS or without hemorrhage, first trimester** — [♀, Age/12-55]

cc **O44.22 Partial placenta previa NOS or without hemorrhage, second trimester** — [♀, Age/12-55]

cc **O44.23 Partial placenta previa NOS or without hemorrhage, third trimester** — [♀, Age/12-55]

O44.3-   Partial placenta previa with hemorrhage
Marginal placenta previa with hemorrhage

O44.30 Partial placenta previa with hemorrhage, unspecified trimester — [♀, Age/12-55]

mcc **O44.31 Partial placenta previa with hemorrhage, first trimester** — [♀, Age/12-55]

mcc **O44.32 Partial placenta previa with hemorrhage, second trimester** — [♀, Age/12-55]

mcc **O44.33 Partial placenta previa with hemorrhage, third trimester** — [♀, Age/12-55]

O44.4-   Low lying placenta NOS or without hemorrhage
Low implantation of placenta NOS or without hemorrhage

O44.40 Low lying placenta NOS or without hemorrhage, unspecified trimester — [♀, Age/12-55]

cc **O44.41 Low lying placenta NOS or without hemorrhage, first trimester** — [♀, Age/12-55]

cc **O44.42 Low lying placenta NOS or without hemorrhage, second trimester** — [♀, Age/12-55]

cc **O44.43 Low lying placenta NOS or without hemorrhage, third trimester** — [♀, Age/12-55]

O44.5-   Low lying placenta with hemorrhage
Low implantation of placenta with hemorrhage

O44.50 Low lying placenta with hemorrhage, unspecified trimester — [♀, Age/12-55]

mcc **O44.51 Low lying placenta with hemorrhage, first trimester** — [♀, Age/12-55]

mcc **O44.52 Low lying placenta with hemorrhage, second trimester** — [♀, Age/12-55]

mcc **O44.53 Low lying placenta with hemorrhage, third trimester** — [♀, Age/12-55]

O43 | O44

O45- <u>Premature separation of placenta [abruptio placentae]</u> — The premature detachment of the placenta from the uterus.

O45.0- Premature separation of placenta <u>with coagulation defect</u>

O45.00- Premature separation of placenta with coagulation defect, <u>unspecified</u>

MCC **O45.001** Premature separation of placenta with coagulation defect, unspecified, <u>first</u> trimester — [♀, Age/12-55]

MCC **O45.002** Premature separation of placenta with coagulation defect, unspecified, <u>second</u> trimester — [♀, Age/12-55]

MCC **O45.003** Premature separation of placenta with coagulation defect, unspecified, <u>third</u> trimester — [♀, Age/12-55]

O45.009 Premature separation of placenta with coagulation defect, unspecified, <u>unspecified</u> trimester — [♀, Age/12-55]

O45.01- Premature separation of placenta <u>with afibrinogenemia</u> — A form caused by the decreased ability of the blood to coagulate due to the decrease or absence of fibrinogen in the blood plasma.
Premature separation of placenta with hypofibrinogenemia

MCC **O45.011** Premature separation of placenta with afibrinogenemia, <u>first</u> trimester — [♀, Age/12-55]

MCC **O45.012** Premature separation of placenta with afibrinogenemia, <u>second</u> trimester — [♀, Age/12-55]

MCC **O45.013** Premature separation of placenta with afibrinogenemia, <u>third</u> trimester — [♀, Age/12-55]

O45.019 Premature separation of placenta with afibrinogenemia, <u>unspecified</u> trimester — [♀, Age/12-55]

O45.02- Premature separation of placenta <u>with disseminated intravascular coagulation</u> — The condition of abnormal blood clotting and compromised blood flow.

MCC **O45.021** Premature separation of placenta with disseminated intravascular coagulation, <u>first</u> trimester — [♀, Age/12-55]

MCC **O45.022** Premature separation of placenta with disseminated intravascular coagulation, <u>second</u> trimester — [♀, Age/12-55]

MCC **O45.023** Premature separation of placenta with disseminated intravascular coagulation, <u>third</u> trimester — [♀, Age/12-55]

O45.029 Premature separation of placenta with disseminated intravascular coagulation, <u>unspecified</u> trimester — [♀, Age/12-55]

O45.09- Premature separation of placenta <u>with other coagulation defect</u>

MCC **O45.091** Premature separation of placenta with other coagulation defect, <u>first</u> trimester — [♀, Age/12-55]

MCC **O45.092** Premature separation of placenta with other coagulation defect, <u>second</u> trimester — [♀, Age/12-55]

MCC **O45.093** Premature separation of placenta with other coagulation defect, <u>third</u> trimester — [♀, Age/12-55]

O45.099 Premature separation of placenta with other coagulation defect, <u>unspecified</u> trimester — [♀, Age/12-55]

O45.8- Other premature separation of placenta

O45.8x-<u>Other</u> premature separation of placenta

MCC **O45.8x1** Other premature separation of placenta, <u>first</u> trimester — [♀, Age/12-55]

MCC **O45.8x2** Other premature separation of placenta, <u>second</u> trimester — [♀, Age/12-55]

MCC **O45.8x3** Other premature separation of placenta, <u>third</u> trimester — [♀, Age/12-55]

O45.8x9 Other premature separation of placenta, <u>unspecified</u> trimester — [♀, Age/12-55]

O45.9- Premature separation of placenta, <u>unspecified</u>
Abruptio placentae NOS

O45.90 Premature separation of placenta, unspecified, <u>unspecified</u> trimester — [♀, Age/12-55]

MCC **O45.91** Premature separation of placenta, unspecified, <u>first</u> trimester — [♀, Age/12-55]

MCC **O45.92** Premature separation of placenta, unspecified, <u>second</u> trimester — [♀, Age/12-55]

MCC **O45.93** Premature separation of placenta, unspecified, <u>third</u> trimester — [♀, Age/12-55]

O46- <u>Antepartum hemorrhage, not elsewhere classified</u>
Excludes 1: hemorrhage in early pregnancy (O20.-)
intrapartum hemorrhage NEC (O67.-)
placenta previa (O44.-)
premature separation of placenta [abruptio placentae] (O45.-)

O46.0- Antepartum hemorrhage with coagulation defect — Bloody uterine discharge due to impairment of the blood to normally coagulate.

O46.00- Antepartum hemorrhage <u>with coagulation defect, unspecified</u>

MCC **O46.001** Antepartum hemorrhage with coagulation defect, unspecified, <u>first</u> trimester — [♀, Age/12-55]

MCC **O46.002** Antepartum hemorrhage with coagulation defect, unspecified, <u>second</u> trimester — [♀, Age/12-55]

MCC **O46.003** Antepartum hemorrhage with coagulation defect, unspecified, <u>third</u> trimester — [♀, Age/12-55]

O46.009 Antepartum hemorrhage with coagulation defect, unspecified, <u>unspecified</u> trimester — [♀, Age/12-55]

O46.01- Antepartum hemorrhage <u>with afibrinogenemia</u> — A form caused by the decreased ability of the blood to coagulate due to the decrease or absence of fibrinogen in the blood plasma.
Antepartum hemorrhage with hypofibrinogenemia

MCC **O46.011** Antepartum hemorrhage with afibrinogenemia, <u>first</u> trimester — [♀, Age/12-55]

MCC **O46.012** Antepartum hemorrhage with afibrinogenemia, <u>second</u> trimester — [♀, Age/12-55]

MCC **O46.013** Antepartum hemorrhage with afibrinogenemia, <u>third</u> trimester — [♀, Age/12-55]

O46.019 Antepartum hemorrhage with afibrinogenemia, <u>unspecified</u> trimester — [♀, Age/12-55]

O46.02- Antepartum hemorrhage <u>with disseminated intravascular coagulation</u> — The condition of abnormal blood clotting and compromised blood flow.

MCC **O46.021** Antepartum hemorrhage with disseminated intravascular coagulation, <u>first</u> trimester — [♀, Age/12-55]

MCC **O46.022** Antepartum hemorrhage with disseminated intravascular coagulation, <u>second</u> trimester — [♀, Age/12-55]

MCC **O46.023** Antepartum hemorrhage with disseminated intravascular coagulation, <u>third</u> trimester — [♀, Age/12-55]

O46.029 Antepartum hemorrhage with disseminated intravascular coagulation, <u>unspecified</u> trimester — [♀, Age/12-55]

O46.09- Antepartum hemorrhage <u>with other coagulation defect</u>

MCC **O46.091** Antepartum hemorrhage with other coagulation defect, <u>first</u> trimester — [♀, Age/12-55]

MCC **O46.092** Antepartum hemorrhage with other coagulation defect, <u>second</u> trimester — [♀, Age/12-55]

MCC **O46.093** Antepartum hemorrhage with other coagulation defect, <u>third</u> trimester — [♀, Age/12-55]

O46.099 Antepartum hemorrhage with other coagulation defect, <u>unspecified</u> trimester — [♀, Age/12-55]

O46.8- Other antepartum hemorrhage

O46.8x-<u>Other antepartum hemorrhage</u>

O46.8x1 Other antepartum hemorrhage, <u>first</u> trimester — [♀, Age/12-55]

O46.8x2 Other antepartum hemorrhage, <u>second</u> trimester — [♀, Age/12-55]

O46.8x3 Other antepartum hemorrhage, <u>third</u> trimester — [♀, Age/12-55]

O46.8x9 Other antepartum hemorrhage, unspecified trimester — [♀, Age/12-55]

O45 - O46

O46.9- Antepartum hemorrhage, <u>unspecified</u>

    O46.90 Antepartum hemorrhage, unspecified, <u>unspecified</u> trimester — [♀, Age/12-55]

    O46.91 Antepartum hemorrhage, unspecified, <u>first</u> trimester — [♀, Age/12-55]

    O46.92 Antepartum hemorrhage, unspecified, <u>second</u> trimester — [♀, Age/12-55]

    O46.93 Antepartum hemorrhage, unspecified, <u>third</u> trimester — [♀, Age/12-55]

O47- <u>False labor</u> — Labor symptoms occurring before the actual onset of labor.
    Includes: Braxton Hicks contractions
                    Threatened labor
    Excludes 1:   *preterm labor (O60.-)*

    O47.0- False labor before 37 completed weeks of gestation

        O47.00 False labor before 37 completed weeks of gestation, <u>unspecified</u> trimester — [♀, Age/12-55]

    cc **O47.02** False labor before 37 completed weeks of gestation, <u>second</u> trimester — [♀, Age/12-55]

    cc **O47.03** False labor before 37 completed weeks of gestation, <u>third</u> trimester — [♀, Age/12-55]

  cc **O47.1**   False labor at or after 37 completed weeks of gestation — [♀, Age/12-55]

    O47.9   False labor, unspecified — [♀, Age/12-55]

O48- <u>Late pregnancy</u>

    O48.0   Post-term pregnancy — [♀, Age/12-55]
           AHA 16:1Q:p5 – Delivery complicated by post-term pregnancy
           Pregnancy over 40 completed weeks to 42 completed weeks gestation

    O48.1   Prolonged pregnancy — [♀, Age/12-55]
           Pregnancy which has advanced beyond 42 completed weeks gestation

Complications of labor and delivery (O60-O77)

O60- <u>Preterm labor</u>
    AHA 12:4Q:p107 – Fetus A and B same as fetus 1 and 2
    Includes: Onset (spontaneous) of labor before 37 completed weeks of gestation
    Excludes 1:   *false labor (O47.0-)*
                      threatened labor NOS (O47.0-)

    O60.0- Preterm labor <u>without</u> delivery — The onset of labor before the pregnancy has reached term, and without delivery.

        O60.00 Preterm labor without delivery, <u>unspecified</u> trimester — [♀, Age/12-55]

    MCC **O60.02** Preterm labor without delivery, <u>second</u> trimester — [♀, Age/12-55]

    MCC **O60.03** Preterm labor without delivery, <u>third</u> trimester — [♀, Age/12-55]

    O60.1- Preterm labor <u>with preterm delivery</u> — The onset of labor before the pregnancy has reached term, and with delivery before term.
          AHA 16:2Q:p10 – Twin pregnancy, preterm delivery

        One of the following 7th characters is to be assigned to each code under subcategory O60.1. 7th character 0 is for single gestations and multiple gestations where the fetus is unspecified. 7th characters 1 through 9 are for cases of multiple gestations to identify the fetus for which the code applies. The appropriate code from category O30, Multiple gestation, must also be assigned when assigning a code from subcategory O60.1 that has a 7th character of 1 through 9.
        0   Not applicable or unspecified
        1   Fetus 1
        2   Fetus 2
        3   Fetus 3
        4   Fetus 4
        5   Fetus 5
        9   Other fetus

  CC-0-9 **O60.10x-** Preterm labor with preterm delivery, <u>unspecified</u> trimester — [♀, Age/12-55]
           Preterm labor with delivery NOS

  MCC-0-9 **O60.12x-** Preterm labor <u>second</u> trimester with preterm delivery <u>second</u> trimester — [♀, Age/12-55]

  MCC-0-9 **O60.13x-** Preterm labor <u>second</u> trimester with preterm delivery <u>third</u> trimester — [♀, Age/12-55]

  MCC-0-9 **O60.14x-** Preterm labor <u>third</u> trimester with preterm delivery <u>third</u> trimester — [♀, Age/12-55]

    O60.2- <u>Term delivery with preterm labor</u> — The onset of labor before the pregnancy has reached term, and with delivery at term.

        One of the following 7th characters is to be assigned to each code under subcategory O60.2. 7th character 0 is for single gestations and multiple gestations where the fetus is unspecified. 7th characters 1 through 9 are for cases of multiple gestations to identify the fetus for which the code applies. The appropriate code from category O30, Multiple gestation, must also be assigned when assigning a code from subcategory O60.2 that has a 7th character of 1 through 9.
        0   Not applicable or unspecified
        1   Fetus 1
        2   Fetus 2
        3   Fetus 3
        4   Fetus 4
        5   Fetus 5
        9   Other fetus

  CC-0-9 **O60.20x-** Term delivery with preterm labor, <u>unspecified</u> trimester — [♀, Age/12-55]

  MCC-0-9 **O60.22x-** Term delivery with preterm labor, <u>second</u> trimester — [♀, Age/12-55]

  MCC-0-9 **O60.23x-** Term delivery with preterm labor, <u>third</u> trimester — [♀, Age/12-55]

O61- <u>Failed induction of labor</u>

    O61.0   Failed medical induction of labor — [♀, Age/12-55] – Failure of induction of labor by medical methods, such as oxytocic drugs.
           Failed induction (of labor) by oxytocin
           Failed induction (of labor) by prostaglandins

    O61.1- Failed instrumental induction of labor — [♀, Age/12-55] – Failure of induction of labor by surgical or other instrumental methods.
           Failed mechanical induction (of labor)
           Failed surgical induction (of labor)

    O61.8   Other failed induction of labor — [♀, Age/12-55]

    O61.9   Failed induction of labor, unspecified — [♀, Age/12-55]

O62- <u>Abnormalities of forces of labor</u>

    O62.0   Primary inadequate contractions — [♀, Age/12-55] – Dysfunction and weakness of uterine contractions during the first stage of labor.
           Failure of cervical dilatation
           Primary hypotonic uterine dysfunction
           Uterine inertia during latent phase of labor

    O62.1   Secondary uterine inertia — [♀, Age/12-55] – Dysfunction and weakness of uterine contractions during the second stage of labor.
           Arrested active phase of labor
           Secondary hypotonic uterine dysfunction

    O62.2   Other uterine inertia — [♀, Age/12-55]
           Atony of uterus without hemorrhage — The loss of normal uterine muscle tone, without any associated hemorrhage.
           Atony of uterus NOS
           Desultory labor — Random uterine contractions.
           Hypotonic uterine dysfunction NOS
           Irregular labor — Varying intensity of uterine contractions.
           Poor contractions — Weak uterine contractions.
           Slow slope active phase of labor — Less than the normal intensity of contractions and progression of labor.
           Uterine inertia NOS
    Excludes 1:   *atony of uterus with hemorrhage (postpartum) (O72.1)*
                    postpartum atony of uterus without hemorrhage (O75.89)

    O62.3   Precipitate labor — [♀, Age/12-55] – Frequent, intense contractions with rapid delivery.

O46 - O62

O62.4 Hypertonic, incoordinate, and prolonged uterine contractions — [♀, Age/12-55] – The increased resting tone and uncoordinated, or abnormally long uterine contractions.

Cervical spasm — The abnormally intense contraction of the cervix.
Contraction ring dystocia — The ring-like circular muscle contraction of the uterus.
Dyscoordinate labor — Uncoordinated uterine contractions.
Hour-glass contraction of uterus — The ring-like circular muscle contraction of the uterus.
Hypertonic uterine dysfunction — The increased resting tone of the uterus.
Incoordinate uterine action — Uncoordinated uterine contractions.
Tetanic contractions — The abnormal sustained contraction of the uterus.
Uterine dystocia NOS
Uterine spasm — The abnormally intense contraction of the uterus.
Excludes 1:   dystocia (fetal) (maternal) NOS (O66.9)

O62.8 Other abnormalities of forces of labor — [♀, Age/12-55]

O62.9 Abnormality of forces of labor, unspecified — [♀, Age/12-55]

O63- Long labor — Labor prolonged beyond the normal length of time, generally considered more than 18 hours.

O63.0 Prolonged first stage (of labor) — [♀, Age/12-55]

O63.1 Prolonged second stage (of labor) — [♀, Age/12-55]

O63.2 Delayed delivery of second twin, triplet, etc. — [♀, Age/12-55]

CC **O63.9 Long labor, unspecified** — [♀, Age/12-55]
Prolonged labor NOS

O64- Obstructed labor due to malposition and malpresentation of fetus
AHA 12:4Q:p107 – Fetus A and B same as fetus 1 and 2

One of the following 7th characters is to be assigned to each code under category O64. 7th character 0 is for single gestations and multiple gestations where the fetus is unspecified. 7th characters 1 through 9 are for cases of multiple gestations to identify the fetus for which the code applies. The appropriate code from category O30, Multiple gestation, must also be assigned when assigning a code from category O64 that has a 7th character of 1 through 9.
0   Not applicable or unspecified
1   Fetus 1
2   Fetus 2
3   Fetus 3
4   Fetus 4
5   Fetus 5
9   Other fetus

O64.0xx- Obstructed labor due to incomplete rotation of fetal head — [♀, Age/12-55]
Deep transverse arrest
Obstructed labor due to persistent occipitoiliac (position)
Obstructed labor due to persistent occipitoposterior (position)
Obstructed labor due to persistent occipitosacral (position)
Obstructed labor due to persistent occipitotransverse (position)

O64.1xx- Obstructed labor due to breech presentation — [♀, Age/12-55]
Obstructed labor due to buttocks presentation
Obstructed labor due to complete breech presentation
Obstructed labor due to frank breech presentation

O64.2xx- Obstructed labor due to face presentation — [♀, Age/12-55]
Obstructed labor due to chin presentation

O64.3xx- Obstructed labor due to brow presentation — [♀, Age/12-55]

O64.4xx- Obstructed labor due to shoulder presentation — [♀, Age/12-55]
Prolapsed arm
Excludes 1:   impacted shoulders (O66.0)
*   shoulder dystocia (O66.0)*

O64.5xx- Obstructed labor due to compound presentation — [♀, Age/12-55]

O64.8xx- Obstructed labor due to other malposition and malpresentation — [♀, Age/12-55]
Obstructed labor due to footling presentation
Obstructed labor due to incomplete breech presentation

O64.9xx- Obstructed labor due to malposition and malpresentation, unspecified — [♀, Age/12-55]

O65- Obstructed labor due to maternal pelvic abnormality

O65.0 Obstructed labor due to deformed pelvis — [♀, Age/12-55]

O65.1 Obstructed labor due to generally contracted pelvis — [♀, Age/12-55] – A pelvic opening that is reduced more than 2 cm in diameter.

O65.2 Obstructed labor due to pelvic inlet contraction — [♀, Age/12-55] – The reduced upper opening of the pelvis.

O65.3 Obstructed labor due to pelvic outlet and mid-cavity contraction — [♀, Age/12-55] – The reduced lower opening of the pelvis.

O65.4 Obstructed labor due to fetopelvic disproportion, unspecified — [♀, Age/12-55]
Excludes 1:   dystocia due to abnormality of fetus (O66.2-O66.3)

O65.5 Obstructed labor due to abnormality of maternal pelvic organs — [♀, Age/12-55]
Obstructed labor due to conditions listed in O34.-
Use additional code to identify abnormality of pelvic organs O34.-

O65.8 Obstructed labor due to other maternal pelvic abnormalities — [♀, Age/12-55]

O65.9 Obstructed labor due to maternal pelvic abnormality, unspecified — [♀, Age/12-55]

O66- Other obstructed labor

O66.0 Obstructed labor due to shoulder dystocia — [♀, Age/12-55] – Obstructed labor due to impaction of the shoulders at the pelvic brim.
Impacted shoulders

O66.1 Obstructed labor due to locked twins — [♀, Age/12-55] – Obstructed labor due to entwined necks of twins.

O66.2 Obstructed labor due to unusually large fetus — [♀, Age/12-55]

O66.3 Obstructed labor due to other abnormalities of fetus — [♀, Age/12-55]
Dystocia due to fetal ascites
Dystocia due to fetal hydrops
Dystocia due to fetal meningomyelocele
Dystocia due to fetal sacral teratoma
Dystocia due to fetal tumor
Dystocia due to hydrocephalic fetus
Use additional code to identify cause of obstruction

O66.4- Failed trial of labor

O66.40 Failed trial of labor, unspecified — [♀, Age/12-55]

O66.41 Failed attempted vaginal birth after previous cesarean delivery — [♀, Age/12-55]
Code first rupture of uterus, if applicable (O71.0-, O71.1)

O66.5 Attempted application of vacuum extractor and forceps — [♀, Age/12-55]
Attempted application of vacuum or forceps, with subsequent delivery by forceps or cesarean delivery

O66.6 Obstructed labor due to other multiple fetuses — [♀, Age/12-55]

O66.8 Other specified obstructed labor — [♀, Age/12-55]
Use additional code to identify cause of obstruction

O66.9 Obstructed labor, unspecified — [♀, Age/12-55]
Dystocia NOS
Fetal dystocia NOS
Maternal dystocia NOS

O67- Labor and delivery complicated by intrapartum hemorrhage, not elsewhere classified
Excludes 1:   antepartum hemorrhage NEC (O46.-)
*   placenta previa (O44.-)*
*   premature separation of placenta [abruptio placentae] (O45.-)*
Excludes ❷: postpartum hemorrhage (O72.-)

MCC **O67.0 Intrapartum hemorrhage with coagulation defect** — [♀, Age/12-55]
Intrapartum hemorrhage (excessive) associated with afibrinogenemia
Intrapartum hemorrhage (excessive) associated with disseminated intravascular coagulation
Intrapartum hemorrhage (excessive) associated with hyperfibrinolysis
Intrapartum hemorrhage (excessive) associated with hypofibrinogenemia

O67.8 Other intrapartum hemorrhage — [♀, Age/12-55]
Excessive intrapartum hemorrhage

O67.9 Intrapartum hemorrhage, unspecified — [♀, Age/12-55]

O62 - O67 (side tab)

O68 **Labor and delivery complicated by abnormality of fetal acid-base**
cc **balance** — [♀, Age/12-55]
    Fetal acidemia complicating labor and delivery
    Fetal acidosis complicating labor and delivery
    Fetal alkalosis complicating labor and delivery
    Fetal metabolic acidemia complicating labor and delivery
    Excludes 1:   *fetal stress NOS (O77.9)*
              labor and delivery complicated by electrocardiographic
                  evidence of fetal stress (O77.8)
              labor and delivery complicated by ultrasonic evidence of fetal
                  stress (O77.8)
    Excludes ❷: *abnormality in fetal heart rate or rhythm (O76)*
              labor and delivery complicated by meconium in amniotic fluid
                  (O77.0)

O69- **Labor and delivery complicated by umbilical cord complications**
    AHA 12:4Q:p107 – Fetus A and B same as fetus 1 and 2

One of the following 7th characters is to be assigned to each code under category O69. 7th character 0 is for single gestations and multiple gestations where the fetus is unspecified. 7th characters 1 through 9 are for cases of multiple gestations to identify the fetus for which the code applies. The appropriate code from category O30, Multiple gestation, must also be assigned when assigning a code from category O69 that has a 7th character of 1 through 9.
    0   Not applicable or unspecified
    1   Fetus 1
    2   Fetus 2
    3   Fetus 3
    4   Fetus 4
    5   Fetus 5
    9   Other fetus

O69.0xx- **Labor and delivery complicated by prolapse of cord** — [♀, Age/12-55] – The abnormal presentation of the umbilical cord in the vagina.

O69.1xx- **Labor and delivery complicated by cord around neck, with compression** — [♀, Age/12-55] – The abnormal presence of the umbilical cord wrapped around the fetal neck, with constricting tension on the neck.
    Excludes 1:   *labor and delivery complicated by cord around neck, without compression (O69.81)*

O69.2xx- **Labor and delivery complicated by other cord entanglement, with compression** — [♀, Age/12-55] – Umbilical cord entanglement with the fetus, other than wrapped around the neck, and with constricting tension to the affected part.
    Labor and delivery complicated by compression of cord NOS
    Labor and delivery complicated by entanglement of cords of twins in monoamniotic sac
    Labor and delivery complicated by knot in cord
    Excludes 1:   *labor and delivery complicated by other cord entanglement, without compression (O69.82)*

O69.3xx- **Labor and delivery complicated by short cord** — [♀, Age/12-55] – The abnormally small length of the umbilical cord.

O69.4xx- **Labor and delivery complicated by vasa previa** — [♀, Age/12-55] – The abnormal presentation of the umbilical vessels in front of the fetal head.
    Labor and delivery complicated by hemorrhage from vasa previa

O69.5xx- **Labor and delivery complicated by vascular lesion of cord** — [♀, Age/12-55] – Damage to or medical condition of the umbilical cord vessels.
    Labor and delivery complicated by cord bruising
    Labor and delivery complicated by cord hematoma
    Labor and delivery complicated by thrombosis of umbilical vessels

O69.8- **Labor and delivery complicated by other cord complications**
    O69.81x- **Labor and delivery complicated by cord around neck, without compression** — [♀, Age/12-55]
    O69.82x- **Labor and delivery complicated by other cord entanglement, without compression** — [♀, Age/12-55]
    O69.89x- **Labor and delivery complicated by other cord complications** — [♀, Age/12-55]

O69.9xx- **Labor and delivery complicated by cord complication, unspecified** — [♀, Age/12-55]

O70- **Perineal laceration during delivery**
    AHA 16:1Q:p6-8 – Perineal lacerations
    AHA 16:1Q:p4 – Polyhydramnios and laceration
    AHA 16:1Q:p3,5 – Premature rupture of membranes and laceration
    Includes: Episiotomy extended by laceration — The tearing continuance of the surgical incision of the vulvar orifice.
    Excludes 1:   *obstetric high vaginal laceration alone (O71.4)*

O70.0 **First degree perineal laceration during delivery** — [♀, Age/12-55] – A tear of the superficial layers of the perineal organs.
    Perineal laceration, rupture or tear involving fourchette during delivery
    Perineal laceration, rupture or tear involving labia during delivery
    Perineal laceration, rupture or tear involving skin during delivery
    Perineal laceration, rupture or tear involving vagina during delivery
    Perineal laceration, rupture or tear involving vulva during delivery
    Slight perineal laceration, rupture or tear during delivery

O70.1 **Second degree perineal laceration during delivery** — [♀, Age/12-55] – A tear of the inner and muscular layers of the perineal organs.
    AHA 16:2Q:p34 – Second degree perineal laceration
    Perineal laceration, rupture or tear during delivery as in O70.0, also involving pelvic floor
    Perineal laceration, rupture or tear during delivery as in O70.0, also involving perineal muscles
    Perineal laceration, rupture or tear during delivery as in O70.0, also involving vaginal muscles
    Excludes 1:   *perineal laceration involving anal sphincter (O70.2)*

O70.2- **Third degree perineal laceration during delivery** — A tear of the tissues between the vaginal and perineal muscular layers and the rectal mucosa/sphincter.
    Perineal laceration, rupture or tear during delivery as in O70.1, also involving anal sphincter
    Perineal laceration, rupture or tear during delivery as in O70.1, also involving rectovaginal septum
    Perineal laceration, rupture or tear during delivery as in O70.1, also involving sphincter NOS
    Excludes 1:   *anal sphincter tear during delivery without third degree perineal laceration (O70.4)*
              perineal laceration involving anal or rectal mucosa (O70.3)

cc **O70.20** **Third degree perineal laceration during delivery, unspecified** — [♀, Age/12-55]

cc **O70.21** **Third degree perineal laceration during delivery, IIIa** — [♀, Age/12-55]
    Third degree perineal laceration during delivery with less than 50% of external anal sphincter (EAS) thickness torn

cc **O70.22** **Third degree perineal laceration during delivery, IIIb** — [♀, Age/12-55]
    Third degree perineal laceration during delivery with more than 50% of external anal sphincter (EAS) thickness torn

cc **O70.23** **Third degree perineal laceration during delivery, IIIc** — [♀, Age/12-55]
    Third degree perineal laceration during delivery with both external anal sphincter (EAS) and internal anal sphincter (IAS) torn

cc **O70.3** **Fourth degree perineal laceration during delivery** — [♀, Age/12-55] – A tear that extends into the anal and rectal mucosa.
    Perineal laceration, rupture or tear during delivery as in O70.2, also involving anal mucosa
    Perineal laceration, rupture or tear during delivery as in O70.2, also involving rectal mucosa

cc **O70.4** **Anal sphincter tear complicating delivery, not associated with third degree laceration** — [♀, Age/12-55]
    Excludes 1:   *anal sphincter tear with third degree perineal laceration (O70.2)*

O70.9 **Perineal laceration during delivery, unspecified** — [♀, Age/12-55]

O71- **Other obstetric trauma**
    Includes: Obstetric damage from instruments

O71.0- **Rupture of uterus (spontaneous) before onset of labor** — The tearing-open of the uterus wall, before the onset of labor.
    Excludes 1:   *disruption of (current) cesarean delivery wound (O90.0)*
              laceration of uterus, NEC (O71.81)

    O71.00 **Rupture of uterus before onset of labor, unspecified trimester** — [♀, Age/12-55]

mcc **O71.02** **Rupture of uterus before onset of labor, second trimester** — [♀, Age/12-55]

O68 - O71

MCC **O71.03 Rupture of uterus before onset of labor, <u>third</u> trimester** — [♀, Age/12-55]

MCC **O71.1 Rupture of uterus <u>during labor</u>** — [♀, Age/12-55] — The tearing-open of the uterus wall, during and after labor.
    Rupture of uterus not stated as occurring before onset of labor
    Excludes 1:   *disruption of cesarean delivery wound (O90.0)*
                 laceration of uterus, NEC (O71.81)

cc **O71.2 Postpartum inversion of uterus** — [♀, Age/12-55] — The turning inside out of the uterus.

cc **O71.3 Obstetric laceration of cervix** — [♀, Age/12-55] — A tear of the cervix.
    Annular detachment of cervix

cc **O71.4 Obstetric high vaginal laceration alone** — [♀, Age/12-55] — Laceration of vaginal wall or sulcus without mention of perineal laceration.
    Laceration of vaginal wall without perineal laceration
    Excludes 1:   *obstetric high vaginal laceration with perineal laceration (O70.-)*

cc **O71.5 Other obstetric injury to pelvic organs** — [♀, Age/12-55]
    AHA 14:4Q:p18 – Periurethral laceration during delivery
    AHA 16:1Q:p4 – Periurethral laceration during delivery
    Obstetric injury to bladder — Traumatic damage to the bladder.
    Obstetric injury to urethra — Traumatic damage to the urethra.
    Excludes ❷: *obstetric periurethral trauma (O71.82)*

cc **O71.6 Obstetric damage to pelvic joints and ligaments** — [♀, Age/12-55]
    Obstetric avulsion of inner symphyseal cartilage — The tearing detachment of the cartilage of the symphysis pubis.
    Obstetric damage to coccyx — Injury to the small bone at the end of the sacrum.
    Obstetric traumatic separation of symphysis (pubis) — The separating detachment of the symphysis pubis.

cc **O71.7 Obstetric hematoma of pelvis** — [♀, Age/12-55] — A localized swelling mass of clotted blood caused by a break in a blood vessel.
    Obstetric hematoma of perineum
    Obstetric hematoma of vagina
    Obstetric hematoma of vulva

O71.8- Other specified obstetric trauma
    O71.81 Laceration of uterus, not elsewhere classified — [♀, Age/12-55]
    O71.82 Other specified trauma to perineum and vulva — [♀, Age/12-55]
        AHA 14:4Q:p18 – Periurethral laceration during delivery
        Obstetric periurethral trauma
    O71.89 Other specified obstetric trauma — [♀, Age/12-55]

O71.9 Obstetric trauma, unspecified — [♀, Age/12-55]

O72- <u>Postpartum hemorrhage</u>
    Includes: Hemorrhage after delivery of fetus or infant

cc **O72.0 Third-stage hemorrhage** — [♀, Age/12-55]
    Hemorrhage associated with retained, trapped or adherent placenta
    Retained placenta NOS
    Code also type of adherent placenta (O43.2-)

cc **O72.1 Other immediate postpartum hemorrhage** — [♀, Age/12-55]
    AHA 16:1Q:p4 – Uterine atony with hemorrhage
    Hemorrhage following delivery of placenta
    Postpartum hemorrhage (atonic) NOS
    Uterine atony with hemorrhage
    Excludes 1:   *uterine atony NOS (O62.2)*
                 uterine atony without hemorrhage (O62.2)
                 postpartum atony of uterus without hemorrhage (O75.89)

cc **O72.2 Delayed and secondary postpartum hemorrhage** — [♀, Age/12-55]
    Hemorrhage associated with retained portions of placenta or membranes after the first 24 hours following delivery of placenta
    Retained products of conception NOS, following delivery

O72.3 Postpartum coagulation defects — [♀, Age/12-55]
    Postpartum afibrinogenemia
    Postpartum fibrinolysis

O73- <u>Retained placenta and membranes, without</u> hemorrhage
    Excludes 1:   *placenta accreta (O43.21-)*
                 placenta increta (O43.22-)
                 placenta percreta (O43.23-)

O73.0 Retained placenta without hemorrhage — [♀, Age/12-55]
    Adherent placenta, without hemorrhage
    Trapped placenta without hemorrhage

O73.1 Retained portions of placenta and membranes, without hemorrhage — [♀, Age/12-55]
    Retained products of conception following delivery, without hemorrhage

O74- <u>Complications of anesthesia during labor and delivery</u>
    Includes: Maternal complications arising from the administration of a general, regional or local anesthetic, analgesic or other sedation during labor and delivery
    Use additional code, if applicable, to identify specific complication

O74.0 <u>Aspiration pneumonitis</u> due to anesthesia during labor and delivery — [♀, Age/12-55]
    Inhalation of stomach contents or secretions NOS due to anesthesia during labor and delivery
    Mendelson's syndrome due to anesthesia during labor and delivery

O74.1 Other pulmonary complications of anesthesia during labor and delivery — [♀, Age/12-55]

O74.2 <u>Cardiac complications</u> of anesthesia during labor and delivery — [♀, Age/12-55]

O74.3 <u>Central nervous system</u> complications of anesthesia during labor and delivery — [♀, Age/12-55]

O74.4 Toxic reaction to local anesthesia during labor and delivery — [♀, Age/12-55]

O74.5 <u>Spinal and epidural anesthesia-induced headache</u> during labor and delivery — [♀, Age/12-55]

O74.6 <u>Other complications of spinal and epidural anesthesia</u> during labor and delivery — [♀, Age/12-55]

O74.7 <u>Failed or difficult intubation for anesthesia</u> during labor and delivery — [♀, Age/12-55]

O74.8 <u>Other</u> complications of anesthesia during labor and delivery — [♀, Age/12-55]

O74.9 Complication of anesthesia during labor and delivery, <u>unspecified</u> — [♀, Age/12-55]

O75- Other complications of labor and delivery, <u>not elsewhere classified</u>
    Excludes ❷: *puerperal (postpartum) infection (O86.-)*
                 puerperal (postpartum) sepsis (O85)

O75.0 Maternal distress during labor and delivery — [♀, Age/12-55]

MCC **O75.1 Shock during or following labor and delivery** — [♀, Age/12-55]
    Obstetric shock following labor and delivery

cc **O75.2 Pyrexia during labor, not elsewhere classified** — [♀, Age/12-55]

MCC **O75.3 Other infection during labor** — [♀, Age/12-55]
    Sepsis during labor
    Use additional code (B95-B97), to identify infectious agent

O75.4 Other complications of obstetric surgery and procedures — [♀, Age/12-55]
    Cardiac arrest following obstetric surgery or procedures
    Cardiac failure following obstetric surgery or procedures
    Cerebral anoxia following obstetric surgery or procedures
    Pulmonary edema following obstetric surgery or procedures
    Use additional code to identify specific complication
    Excludes ❷: *complications of anesthesia during labor and delivery (O74.-)*
                 disruption of obstetrical (surgical) wound (O90.0-O90.1)
                 hematoma of obstetrical (surgical) wound (O90.2)
                 infection of obstetrical (surgical) wound (O86.0)

O75.5 Delayed delivery after artificial rupture of membranes — [♀, Age/12-55]

O75.8- Other specified complications of labor and delivery
    O75.81 Maternal exhaustion complicating labor and delivery — [♀, Age/12-55]
    O75.82 Onset (spontaneous) of labor after 37 completed weeks of gestation but before 39 completed weeks of gestation, with delivery by (planned) cesarean section — [♀, Age/12-55]
        Delivery by (planned) cesarean section occurring after 37 completed weeks of gestation but before 39 completed weeks gestation due to (spontaneous) onset of labor
        Code first to specify reason for planned cesarean section, such as:
            Cephalopelvic disproportion (normally formed fetus) (O33.9)
            Previous cesarean delivery (O34.21)
    O75.89 Other specified complications of labor and delivery — [♀, Age/12-55]

O75.9 Complication of labor and delivery, unspecified — [♀, Age/12-55]

O71-O75

Excludes 1: = NOT CODED HERE! (Do not code both)

Excludes ❷: = Not Included Here

O76   <u>Abnormality in fetal heart rate</u> and rhythm complicating labor and delivery — [♀, Age/12-55]

    AHA 13:4Q:p118 – Meconium amniotic fluid and fetal decelerations
     Depressed fetal heart rate tones complicating labor and delivery
     Fetal bradycardia complicating labor and delivery
     Fetal heart rate decelerations complicating labor and delivery
     Fetal heart rate irregularity complicating labor and delivery
     Fetal heart rate abnormal variability complicating labor and delivery
     Fetal tachycardia complicating labor and delivery
     Non-reassuring fetal heart rate or rhythm complicating labor and delivery

    Excludes 1:   *fetal stress NOS (O77.9)*
              labor and delivery complicated by electrocardiographic evidence of fetal stress (O77.8)
              labor and delivery complicated by ultrasonic evidence of fetal stress (O77.8)

    Excludes ❷: *fetal metabolic acidemia (O68)*
              other fetal stress (O77.0-O77.1)

O77-   <u>Other fetal stress</u> complicating labor and delivery

   O77.0   **Labor and delivery complicated by meconium in amniotic fluid** — [♀, Age/12-55] – The unusual presence of fetal bowel meconium in the amniotic fluid.

     AHA 13:4Q:p117 – Delivery complicated by meconium in amniotic fluid

     AHA 13:4Q:p118 – Meconium amniotic fluid and fetal decelerations

   O77.1   **Fetal stress in labor or delivery due to drug administration** — [♀, Age/12-55]

   O77.8   **Labor and delivery complicated by other evidence of fetal stress** — [♀, Age/12-55]
     Labor and delivery complicated by electrocardiographic evidence of fetal stress
     Labor and delivery complicated by ultrasonic evidence of fetal stress

     Excludes 1:   *abnormality of fetal acid-base balance (O68)*
               abnormality in fetal heart rate or rhythm (O76)
               fetal metabolic acidemia (O68)

   O77.9   **Labor and delivery complicated by fetal stress, unspecified** — [♀, Age/12-55]

     Excludes 1:   *abnormality of fetal acid-base balance (O68)*
               abnormality in fetal heart rate or rhythm (O76)
               fetal metabolic acidemia (O68)

Encounter for delivery (O80-O82)

O80   **Encounter for full-term uncomplicated delivery** — [♀, Age/12-55]

    AHA 14:2Q:p9 – Uncomplicated delivery with Pitocin to augment active labor
    Delivery requiring minimal or no assistance, with or without episiotomy, without fetal manipulation [e.g., rotation version] or instrumentation [forceps] of a spontaneous, cephalic, vaginal, full-term, single, live-born infant. This code is for use as a single diagnosis code and is not to be used with any other code from chapter 15.
    Use additional code to indicate outcome of delivery (Z37.0)

O82   **Encounter for cesarean delivery without indication** — [♀, Age/12-55]
    Use additional code to indicate outcome of delivery (Z37.0)

Complications predominantly related to the puerperium (O85-O92)

    Excludes ❷: *mental and behavioral disorders associated with the puerperium (F53)*
               obstetrical tetanus (A34)
               puerperal osteomalacia (M83.0)

O85   **Puerperal sepsis** — [♀, Age/12-55] – Postpartum infection of the bloodstream, including the toxins produced.
MCC
    Postpartum sepsis
    Puerperal peritonitis
    Puerperal pyemia
    Use additional code (B95-B97), to identify infectious agent
    Use additional code (R65.2-) to identify severe sepsis, if applicable

    Excludes 1:   *fever of unknown origin following delivery (O86.4)*
               genital tract infection following delivery (O86.1-)
               obstetric pyemic and septic embolism (O88.3-)
               puerperal septic thrombophlebitis (O86.81)
               urinary tract infection following delivery (O86.2-)
    Excludes ❷: *sepsis during labor (O75.3)*

O86-   <u>Other puerperal infections</u>
    Use additional code (B95-B97), to identify infectious agent
    Excludes ❷: *infection during labor (O75.3)*
               obstetrical tetanus (A34)

   O86.0   **Infection of <u>obstetric surgical wound</u>** — [♀, Age/12-55]
     Infected cesarean delivery wound following delivery
     Infected perineal repair following delivery

   O86.1-   Other infection of <u>genital tract</u> following delivery

    cc   **O86.11 Cervicitis following delivery** — [♀, Age/12-55]

    cc   **O86.12 Endometritis following delivery** — [♀, Age/12-55]

    cc   **O86.13 Vaginitis following delivery** — [♀, Age/12-55]

    cc   **O86.19 Other infection of genital tract following delivery** — [♀, Age/12-55]

   O86.2-   <u>Urinary tract</u> infection following delivery

    cc   **O86.20 Urinary tract infection following delivery, unspecified** — [♀, Age/12-55]
      Puerperal urinary tract infection NOS

    cc   **O86.21 Infection of kidney following delivery** — [♀, Age/12-55]

    cc   **O86.22 Infection of bladder following delivery** — [♀, Age/12-55]
      Infection of urethra following delivery

    cc   **O86.29 Other urinary tract infection following delivery** — [♀, Age/12-55]

   cc   **O86.4**   **<u>Pyrexia</u> of unknown origin following delivery** — [♀, Age/12-55]
     Puerperal infection NOS following delivery
     Puerperal pyrexia NOS following delivery

     Excludes ❷: *pyrexia during labor (O75.2)*

   O86.8-   <u>Other</u> specified puerperal infections

    MCC   **O86.81 Puerperal septic thrombophlebitis** — [♀, Age/12-55]

    MCC   **O86.89 Other specified puerperal infections** — [♀, Age/12-55]

O87-   <u>Venous complications and hemorrhoids</u> in the puerperium
    Includes: Venous complications in labor, delivery and the puerperium
    Excludes ❷: *obstetric embolism (O88-)*
               puerperal septic thrombophlebitis (O86.81)
               venous complications in pregnancy (O22-)

   cc   **O87.0**   **<u>Superficial thrombophlebitis</u> in the puerperium** — [♀, Age/12-55] – Inflammation of a superficial vein with thrombus formation following delivery.
     Puerperal phlebitis NOS
     Puerperal thrombosis NOS

   MCC   **O87.1**   **<u>Deep phlebothrombosis</u> in the puerperium** — [♀, Age/12-55] – Inflammation of a deep vein with thrombus following delivery.
     Deep vein thrombosis, postpartum
     Pelvic thrombophlebitis, postpartum
     Use additional code to identify the deep vein thrombosis (I82.4-, I82.5-, I82.62-, I82.72-)
     Use additional code, if applicable, for associated long-term (current) use of anticoagulants (Z79.01)

   cc   **O87.2**   **<u>Hemorrhoids</u> in the puerperium** — [♀, Age/12-55] – A varicose dilatation of a vein of the hemorrhoidal plexus following delivery.

   cc   **O87.3**   **<u>Cerebral venous thrombosis</u> in the puerperium** — [♀, Age/12-55] – Formation of a thrombus in a cerebral vessel following delivery.
     Cerebrovenous sinus thrombosis in the puerperium

   O87.4   **<u>Varicose veins</u> of lower extremity in the puerperium** — [♀, Age/12-55] – Dilated, tortuous leg veins presenting symptoms following delivery.

   cc   **O87.8**   **Other venous complications in the puerperium** — [♀, Age/12-55]
     Genital varices in the puerperium — Dilated, tortuous vulvar and perineal veins following delivery.

   O87.9   **Venous complication in the puerperium, unspecified** — [♀, Age/12-55]
     Puerperal phlebopathy NOS

O88-   <u>Obstetric embolism</u>
    Excludes 1:   *embolism complicating abortion NOS (O03.2)*
              embolism complicating ectopic or molar pregnancy (O08.2)
              embolism complicating failed attempted abortion (O07.2)
              embolism complicating induced abortion (O04.7)
              embolism complicating spontaneous abortion (O03.2, O03.7)

   O88.0-   **Obstetric <u>air</u> embolism** — The blockage of an artery with an embolism of air or bubbles of nitrogen.

    O88.01-   **Obstetric air embolism <u>in pregnancy</u>**

     MCC   **O88.011 Air embolism in pregnancy, <u>first</u> trimester** — [♀, Age/12-55]

O
7
6
-
O
8
8

MCC **O88.012** **Air embolism in pregnancy, <u>second</u> trimester** — [♀, Age/12-55]

MCC **O88.013** **Air embolism in pregnancy, <u>third</u> trimester** — [♀, Age/12-55]

O88.019 **Air embolism in pregnancy, <u>unspecified</u> trimester** — [♀, Age/12-55]

MCC **O88.02** **Air embolism <u>in childbirth</u>** — [♀, Age/12-55]

MCC **O88.03** **Air embolism <u>in the puerperium</u>** — [♀, Age/12-55]

O88.1- **Amniotic <u>fluid</u> embolism** — The blockage of an artery with an embolism composed of amniotic fluid.
    Anaphylactoid syndrome in pregnancy

O88.11- **Amniotic fluid embolism <u>in pregnancy</u>**

MCC **O88.111** **Amniotic fluid embolism in pregnancy, <u>first</u> trimester** — [♀, Age/12-55]

MCC **O88.112** **Amniotic fluid embolism in pregnancy, <u>second</u> trimester** — [♀, Age/12-55]

MCC **O88.113** **Amniotic fluid embolism in pregnancy, <u>third</u> trimester** — [♀, Age/12-55]

O88.119 **Amniotic fluid embolism in pregnancy, <u>unspecified</u> trimester** — [♀, Age/12-55]

MCC **O88.12** **Amniotic fluid embolism <u>in childbirth</u>** — [♀, Age/12-55]

MCC **O88.13** **Amniotic fluid embolism <u>in the puerperium</u>** — [♀, Age/12-55]

O88.2- **Obstetric <u>thromboembolism</u>** — The blockage of an artery with an embolism composed of clotted blood.

O88.21- **Thromboembolism <u>in pregnancy</u>**
    Obstetric (pulmonary) embolism NOS

MCC **O88.211** **Thromboembolism in pregnancy, <u>first</u> trimester** — [♀, Age/12-55]

MCC **O88.212** **Thromboembolism in pregnancy, <u>second</u> trimester** — [♀, Age/12-55]

MCC **O88.213** **Thromboembolism in pregnancy, <u>third</u> trimester** — [♀, Age/12-55]

O88.219 **Thromboembolism in pregnancy, <u>unspecified</u> trimester** — [♀, Age/12-55]

MCC **O88.22** **Thromboembolism <u>in childbirth</u>** — [♀, Age/12-55]

MCC **O88.23** **Thromboembolism <u>in the puerperium</u>** — [♀, Age/12-55]
    Puerperal (pulmonary) embolism NOS — The blockage of a pulmonary artery with an embolism composed of clotted blood.

O88.3- **Obstetric pyemic and septic embolism**

O88.31- **<u>Pyemic and septic embolism in pregnancy</u>** — The blockage of an artery with an embolism composed of pus or septic debris.

MCC **O88.311** **Pyemic and septic embolism in pregnancy, <u>first</u> trimester** — [♀, Age/12-55]

MCC **O88.312** **Pyemic and septic embolism in pregnancy, <u>second</u> trimester** — [♀, Age/12-55]

MCC **O88.313** **Pyemic and septic embolism in pregnancy, <u>third</u> trimester** — [♀, Age/12-55]

CC **O88.319** **Pyemic and septic embolism in pregnancy, <u>unspecified</u> trimester** — [♀, Age/12-55]

MCC **O88.32** **Pyemic and septic embolism <u>in childbirth</u>** — [♀, Age/12-55]

MCC **O88.33** **Pyemic and septic embolism <u>in the puerperium</u>** — [♀, Age/12-55]

O88.8- **Other obstetric embolism**
    Obstetric fat embolism

O88.81- **<u>Other</u> embolism <u>in pregnancy</u>**

MCC **O88.811** **Other embolism in pregnancy, <u>first</u> trimester** — [♀, Age/12-55]

MCC **O88.812** **Other embolism in pregnancy, <u>second</u> trimester** — [♀, Age/12-55]

MCC **O88.813** **Other embolism in pregnancy, <u>third</u> trimester** — [♀, Age/12-55]

O88.819 **Other embolism in pregnancy, <u>unspecified</u> trimester** — [♀, Age/12-55]

MCC **O88.82** **Other embolism <u>in childbirth</u>** — [♀, Age/12-55]

MCC **O88.83** **Other embolism <u>in the puerperium</u>** — [♀, Age/12-55]

O89- **<u>Complications of anesthesia during the puerperium</u>**
  Includes: Maternal complications arising from the administration of a general, regional or local anesthetic, analgesic or other sedation during the puerperium
  Use additional code, if applicable, to identify specific complication

O89.0- **<u>Pulmonary complications</u> of anesthesia during the puerperium**

O89.01 **Aspiration pneumonitis due to anesthesia during the puerperium** — [♀, Age/12-55]
    Inhalation of stomach contents or secretions NOS due to anesthesia during the puerperium
    Mendelson's syndrome due to anesthesia during the puerperium

O89.09 **Other pulmonary complications of anesthesia during the puerperium** — [♀, Age/12-55]

O89.1 **<u>Cardiac</u> complications of anesthesia during the puerperium** — [♀, Age/12-55]

O89.2 **<u>Central nervous system</u> complications of anesthesia during the puerperium** — [♀, Age/12-55]

O89.3 **<u>Toxic reaction</u> to local anesthesia during the puerperium** — [♀, Age/12-55]

O89.4 **<u>Spinal and epidural anesthesia-induced headache</u> during the puerperium** — [♀, Age/12-55]

O89.5 **<u>Other complications of spinal and epidural anesthesia</u> during the puerperium** — [♀, Age/12-55]

O89.6 **<u>Failed or difficult intubation</u> for anesthesia during the puerperium** — [♀, Age/12-55]

O89.8 **<u>Other</u> complications of anesthesia during the puerperium** — [♀, Age/12-55]

O89.9 **Complication of anesthesia during the puerperium, <u>unspecified</u>** — [♀, Age/12-55]

O90- **Complications of the puerperium, <u>not elsewhere classified</u>**

O90.0 **Disruption of cesarean delivery wound** — [♀, Age/12-55] — The separation of the surgical incision layers.
    Dehiscence of cesarean delivery wound
  Excludes 1: *rupture of uterus (spontaneous) before onset of labor (O71.0-)*
           rupture of uterus during labor (O71.1)

O90.1 **Disruption of perineal obstetric wound** — [♀, Age/12-55] — The separation of the surgical layers of a perineal wound.
    Disruption of wound of episiotomy
    Disruption of wound of perineal laceration
    Secondary perineal tear

O90.2 **Hematoma of obstetric wound** — [♀, Age/12-55] — A localized swelling mass of blood of a cesarean section or perineal wound.

MCC **O90.3** **Peripartum cardiomyopathy** — [♀, Age/12-55] — A condition of cardiac enlargement and congestive heart failure that develops late in pregnancy or in the months following delivery in women without pre-existing heart disease.
    Conditions in I42.- arising during pregnancy and the puerperium
  Excludes 1: *pre-existing heart disease complicating pregnancy and the puerperium (O99.4-)*

MCC **O90.4** **Postpartum acute kidney failure** — [♀, Age/12-55]
    Hepatorenal syndrome following labor and delivery

O90.5 **Postpartum thyroiditis** — [♀, Age/12-55]

O90.6 **Postpartum mood disturbance** — [♀, Age/12-55]
    Postpartum blues
    Postpartum dysphoria
    Postpartum sadness
  Excludes 1: *postpartum depression (F53)*
           puerperal psychosis (F53)

O90.8- **Other complications of the puerperium, <u>not elsewhere classified</u>**

O90.81 **Anemia of the puerperium** — [♀, Age/12-55]
    Postpartum anemia NOS
  Excludes 1: *pre-existing anemia complicating the puerperium (O99.03)*

O90.89 **Other complications of the puerperium, not elsewhere classified** — [♀, Age/12-55]
    Placental polyp

O90.9 **Complication of the puerperium, unspecified** — [♀, Age/12-55]

O
8
8
-
O
9
0

Excludes 1: = NOT CODED HERE! (Do not code both)   **948**   *Excludes ❷:* = Not Included Here

O91- **Infections of breast** associated with pregnancy, the puerperium and lactation
Use additional code to identify infection

O91.0- **Infection of nipple** associated with pregnancy, the puerperium and lactation — Cellular injury of the nipple due to invasion of microorganisms.

O91.01- **Infection of nipple** associated with pregnancy
Gestational abscess of nipple

O91.011 Infection of nipple associated with pregnancy, **first** trimester — [♀, Age/12-55]

O91.012 Infection of nipple associated with pregnancy, **second** trimester — [♀, Age/12-55]

O91.013 Infection of nipple associated with pregnancy, **third** trimester — [♀, Age/12-55]

O91.019 Infection of nipple associated with pregnancy, **unspecified** trimester — [♀, Age/12-55]

O91.02 Infection of nipple associated with the puerperium — [♀, Age/12-55]
Puerperal abscess of nipple

O91.03 Infection of nipple associated with lactation — [♀, Age/12-55]
Abscess of nipple associated with lactation

O91.1- **Abscess of breast** associated with pregnancy, the puerperium and lactation — A localized collection of pus caused by the disintegration of breast tissue.

O91.11- **Abscess of breast** associated with pregnancy
Gestational mammary abscess
Gestational purulent mastitis
Gestational subareolar abscess

O91.111 Abscess of breast associated with pregnancy, **first** trimester — [♀, Age/12-55]

O91.112 Abscess of breast associated with pregnancy, **second** trimester — [♀, Age/12-55]

O91.113 Abscess of breast associated with pregnancy, **third** trimester — [♀, Age/12-55]

O91.119 Abscess of breast associated with pregnancy, **unspecified** trimester — [♀, Age/12-55]

O91.12 Abscess of breast associated with the puerperium — [♀, Age/12-55]
Puerperal mammary abscess
Puerperal purulent mastitis
Puerperal subareolar abscess

O91.13 Abscess of breast associated with lactation — [♀, Age/12-55]
Mammary abscess associated with lactation
Purulent mastitis associated with lactation
Subareolar abscess associated with lactation

O91.2- **Nonpurulent mastitis** associated with pregnancy, the puerperium and lactation — Inflammation of the breast without the presence or formation of pus.

O91.21- **Nonpurulent mastitis** associated with pregnancy
Gestational interstitial mastitis
Gestational lymphangitis of breast
Gestational mastitis NOS
Gestational parenchymatous mastitis

O91.211 Nonpurulent mastitis associated with pregnancy, **first** trimester — [♀, Age/12-55]

O91.212 Nonpurulent mastitis associated with pregnancy, **second** trimester — [♀, Age/12-55]

O91.213 Nonpurulent mastitis associated with pregnancy, **third** trimester — [♀, Age/12-55]

O91.219 Nonpurulent mastitis associated with pregnancy, **unspecified** trimester — [♀, Age/12-55]

O91.22 Nonpurulent mastitis associated with the puerperium — [♀, Age/12-55]
Puerperal interstitial mastitis
Puerperal lymphangitis of breast
Puerperal mastitis NOS
Puerperal parenchymatous mastitis

O91.23 Nonpurulent mastitis associated with lactation — [♀, Age/12-55]
Interstitial mastitis associated with lactation
Lymphangitis of breast associated with lactation
Mastitis NOS associated with lactation
Parenchymatous mastitis associated with lactation

O92- **Other disorders of breast** and disorders of lactation associated with pregnancy and the puerperium

O92.0- **Retracted nipple** associated with pregnancy, the puerperium, and lactation — A condition in which the nipple is drawn back from its normal position.

O92.01- **Retracted nipple** associated with pregnancy

O92.011 Retracted nipple associated with pregnancy, **first** trimester — [♀, Age/12-55]

O92.012 Retracted nipple associated with pregnancy, **second** trimester — [♀, Age/12-55]

O92.013 Retracted nipple associated with pregnancy, **third** trimester — [♀, Age/12-55]

O92.019 Retracted nipple associated with pregnancy, **unspecified** trimester — [♀, Age/12-55]

O92.02 Retracted nipple associated **with the puerperium** — [♀, Age/12-55]

O92.03 Retracted nipple associated **with lactation** — [♀, Age/12-55]

O92.1- **Cracked nipple** associated with pregnancy, the puerperium, and lactation — A condition in which the nipple is split or partially fissured.
Fissure of nipple, gestational or puerperal

O92.11- **Cracked nipple** associated with pregnancy

O92.111 Cracked nipple associated with pregnancy, **first** trimester — [♀, Age/12-55]

O92.112 Cracked nipple associated with pregnancy, **second** trimester — [♀, Age/12-55]

O92.113 Cracked nipple associated with pregnancy, **third** trimester — [♀, Age/12-55]

O92.119 Cracked nipple associated with pregnancy, **unspecified** trimester — [♀, Age/12-55]

O92.12 Cracked nipple associated **with the puerperium** — [♀, Age/12-55]

O92.13 Cracked nipple associated **with lactation** — [♀, Age/12-55]

O92.2- **Other** and unspecified disorders of breast associated with pregnancy and the puerperium

O92.20 Unspecified disorder of breast associated with pregnancy and the puerperium — [♀, Age/12-55]

O92.29 Other disorders of breast associated with pregnancy and the puerperium — [♀, Age/12-55]

O92.3 Agalactia — [♀, Age/12-55] — Absence or failure of the secretion of milk.
Primary agalactia
Excludes 1:   *elective agalactia (O92.5)*
              secondary agalactia (O92.5)
              therapeutic agalactia (O92.5)

O92.4 Hypogalactia — [♀, Age/12-55] — The abnormally low volume of the secretion of milk.

O92.5 Suppressed lactation — [♀, Age/12-55] — The sudden stoppage of milk secretion.
Elective agalactia
Secondary agalactia
Therapeutic agalactia
Excludes 1:   *primary agalactia (O92.3)*

O92.6 Galactorrhea — [♀, Age/12-55] — Persistent secretion of milk, irrespective of nursing.

O92.7- **Other and unspecified disorders of lactation**

O92.70 Unspecified disorders of lactation — [♀, Age/12-55]

O92.79 Other disorders of lactation — [♀, Age/12-55]
Puerperal galactocele — The cystic enlargement of a mammary gland containing milk.

Other obstetric conditions, not elsewhere classified (O94-O9A)

O94 **Sequelae** of complication of pregnancy, childbirth, and the puerperium — [♀, Age/12-55]
Note: This category is to be used to indicate conditions in O00-O77-, O85-O94 and O98-O9A- as the cause of late effects. The sequelae include conditions specified as such, or as late effects, which may occur at any time after the puerperium.
Code first condition resulting from (sequela) of complication of pregnancy, childbirth, and the puerperium

O91-O94

O98- **Maternal infectious and parasitic diseases classifiable elsewhere but complicating pregnancy, childbirth and the puerperium**

Includes: The listed conditions when complicating the pregnant state, when aggravated by the pregnancy, or as a reason for obstetric care

Use additional code (Chapter 1), to identify specific infectious or parasitic disease

Excludes ❷: herpes gestationis (O26.4-)
    infectious carrier state (O99.82-, O99.83-)
    obstetrical tetanus (A34)
    puerperal infection (O86.-)
    puerperal sepsis (O85)
    when the reason for maternal care is that the disease is known or suspected to have affected the fetus (O35-O36)

O98.0- **Tuberculosis complicating pregnancy, childbirth and the puerperium**
    Conditions in A15-A19

O98.01-   **Tuberculosis complicating pregnancy**

cc **O98.011** **Tuberculosis complicating pregnancy, first trimester** — [♀, Age/12-55]

cc **O98.012** **Tuberculosis complicating pregnancy, second trimester** — [♀, Age/12-55]

cc **O98.013** **Tuberculosis complicating pregnancy, third trimester** — [♀, Age/12-55]

O98.019 **Tuberculosis complicating pregnancy, unspecified trimester** — [♀, Age/12-55]

cc **O98.02** **Tuberculosis complicating childbirth** — [♀, Age/12-55]

cc **O98.03** **Tuberculosis complicating the puerperium** — [♀, Age/12-55]

O98.1- **Syphilis complicating pregnancy, childbirth and the puerperium**
    Conditions in A50-A53

O98.11-   **Syphilis complicating pregnancy**

cc **O98.111** **Syphilis complicating pregnancy, first trimester** — [♀, Age/12-55]

cc **O98.112** **Syphilis complicating pregnancy, second trimester** — [♀, Age/12-55]

cc **O98.113** **Syphilis complicating pregnancy, third trimester** — [♀, Age/12-55]

O98.119 **Syphilis complicating pregnancy, unspecified trimester** — [♀, Age/12-55]

cc **O98.12** **Syphilis complicating childbirth** — [♀, Age/12-55]

cc **O98.13** **Syphilis complicating the puerperium** — [♀, Age/12-55]

O98.2- **Gonorrhea complicating pregnancy, childbirth and the puerperium**
    Conditions in A54.-

O98.21-   **Gonorrhea complicating pregnancy**

cc **O98.211** **Gonorrhea complicating pregnancy, first trimester** — [♀, Age/12-55]

cc **O98.212** **Gonorrhea complicating pregnancy, second trimester** — [♀, Age/12-55]

cc **O98.213** **Gonorrhea complicating pregnancy, third trimester** — [♀, Age/12-55]

O98.219 **Gonorrhea complicating pregnancy, unspecified trimester** — [♀, Age/12-55]

cc **O98.22** **Gonorrhea complicating childbirth** — [♀, Age/12-55]

cc **O98.23** **Gonorrhea complicating the puerperium** — [♀, Age/12-55]

O98.3- **Other infections with a predominantly sexual mode of transmission complicating pregnancy, childbirth and the puerperium**
    Conditions in A55-A64

O98.31-   **Other infections with a predominantly sexual mode of transmission complicating pregnancy**

cc **O98.311** **Other infections with a predominantly sexual mode of transmission complicating pregnancy, first trimester** — [♀, Age/12-55]

cc **O98.312** **Other infections with a predominantly sexual mode of transmission complicating pregnancy, second trimester** — [♀, Age/12-55]

cc **O98.313** **Other infections with a predominantly sexual mode of transmission complicating pregnancy, third trimester** — [♀, Age/12-55]

cc **O98.319** **Other infections with a predominantly sexual mode of transmission complicating pregnancy, unspecified trimester** — [♀, Age/12-55]

cc **O98.32** **Other infections with a predominantly sexual mode of transmission complicating childbirth** — [♀, Age/12-55]

cc **O98.33** **Other infections with a predominantly sexual mode of transmission complicating the puerperium** — [♀, Age/12-55]

O98.4- **Viral hepatitis complicating pregnancy, childbirth and the puerperium**
    Conditions in B15-B19

O98.41-   **Viral hepatitis complicating pregnancy**

cc **O98.411** **Viral hepatitis complicating pregnancy, first trimester** — [♀, Age/12-55]

cc **O98.412** **Viral hepatitis complicating pregnancy, second trimester** — [♀, Age/12-55]

cc **O98.413** **Viral hepatitis complicating pregnancy, third trimester** — [♀, Age/12-55]

O98.419 **Viral hepatitis complicating pregnancy, unspecified trimester** — [♀, Age/12-55]

cc **O98.42** **Viral hepatitis complicating childbirth** — [♀, Age/12-55]

cc **O98.43** **Viral hepatitis complicating the puerperium** — [♀, Age/12-55]

O98.5- **Other viral diseases complicating pregnancy, childbirth and the puerperium**
    Conditions in A80-B09, B25-B34, R87.81-, R87.82-

Excludes 1:   human immunodeficiency virus [HIV] disease complicating pregnancy, childbirth and the puerperium (O98.7-)

O98.51-   **Other viral diseases complicating pregnancy**

cc **O98.511** **Other viral diseases complicating pregnancy, first trimester** — [♀, Age/12-55]

cc **O98.512** **Other viral diseases complicating pregnancy, second trimester** — [♀, Age/12-55]

cc **O98.513** **Other viral diseases complicating pregnancy, third trimester** — [♀, Age/12-55]

O98.519 **Other viral diseases complicating pregnancy, unspecified trimester** — [♀, Age/12-55]

cc **O98.52** **Other viral diseases complicating childbirth** — [♀, Age/12-55]

cc **O98.53** **Other viral diseases complicating the puerperium** — [♀, Age/12-55]

O98.6- **Protozoal diseases complicating pregnancy, childbirth and the puerperium**
    Conditions in B50-B64

O98.61-   **Protozoal diseases complicating pregnancy**

cc **O98.611** **Protozoal diseases complicating pregnancy, first trimester** — [♀, Age/12-55]

cc **O98.612** **Protozoal diseases complicating pregnancy, second trimester** — [♀, Age/12-55]

cc **O98.613** **Protozoal diseases complicating pregnancy, third trimester** — [♀, Age/12-55]

O98.619 **Protozoal diseases complicating pregnancy, unspecified trimester** — [♀, Age/12-55]

cc **O98.62** **Protozoal diseases complicating childbirth** — [♀, Age/12-55]

cc **O98.63** **Protozoal diseases complicating the puerperium** — [♀, Age/12-55]

O98.7- **Human immunodeficiency virus [HIV] disease complicating pregnancy, childbirth and the puerperium**
    Use additional code to identify the type of HIV disease:
    Acquired immune deficiency syndrome (AIDS) (B20)
    Asymptomatic HIV status (Z21)
    HIV positive NOS (Z21)
    Symptomatic HIV disease (B20)

O98.71-   **Human immunodeficiency virus [HIV] disease complicating pregnancy**

cc **O98.711** **Human immunodeficiency virus [HIV] disease complicating pregnancy, first trimester** — [♀, Age/12-55]

Excludes 1: = NOT CODED HERE! (Do not code both)   **950**   Excludes ❷: = Not Included Here

cc **O98.712 Human immunodeficiency virus [HIV] disease complicating pregnancy, <u>second</u> trimester** — [♀, Age/12-55]

cc **O98.713 Human immunodeficiency virus [HIV] disease complicating pregnancy, <u>third</u> trimester** — [♀, Age/12-55]

O98.719 Human immunodeficiency virus [HIV] disease complicating pregnancy, <u>unspecified</u> trimester — [♀, Age/12-55]

cc **O98.72 Human immunodeficiency virus [HIV] disease complicating <u>childbirth</u>** — [♀, Age/12-55]

cc **O98.73 Human immunodeficiency virus [HIV] disease complicating <u>the puerperium</u>** — [♀, Age/12-55]

O98.8- <u>Other</u> maternal infectious and parasitic diseases complicating pregnancy, childbirth and the puerperium

O98.81- Other maternal infectious and parasitic diseases complicating <u>pregnancy</u>

cc **O98.811 Other maternal infectious and parasitic diseases complicating pregnancy, <u>first</u> trimester** — [♀, Age/12-55]

cc **O98.812 Other maternal infectious and parasitic diseases complicating pregnancy, <u>second</u> trimester** — [♀, Age/12-55]

cc **O98.813 Other maternal infectious and parasitic diseases complicating pregnancy, <u>third</u> trimester** — [♀, Age/12-55]

O98.819 Other maternal infectious and parasitic diseases complicating pregnancy, <u>unspecified</u> trimester — [♀, Age/12-55]

cc **O98.82 Other maternal infectious and parasitic diseases complicating <u>childbirth</u>** — [♀, Age/12-55]

cc **O98.83 Other maternal infectious and parasitic diseases complicating <u>the puerperium</u>** — [♀, Age/12-55]

O98.9- <u>Unspecified</u> maternal infectious and parasitic disease complicating pregnancy, childbirth and the puerperium

O98.91- Unspecified maternal infectious and parasitic disease complicating <u>pregnancy</u>

cc **O98.911 Unspecified maternal infectious and parasitic disease complicating pregnancy, <u>first</u> trimester** — [♀, Age/12-55]

cc **O98.912 Unspecified maternal infectious and parasitic disease complicating pregnancy, <u>second</u> trimester** — [♀, Age/12-55]

cc **O98.913 Unspecified maternal infectious and parasitic disease complicating pregnancy, <u>third</u> trimester** — [♀, Age/12-55]

O98.919 Unspecified maternal infectious and parasitic disease complicating pregnancy, <u>unspecified</u> trimester — [♀, Age/12-55]

cc **O98.92 Unspecified maternal infectious and parasitic disease complicating <u>childbirth</u>** — [♀, Age/12-55]

cc **O98.93 Unspecified maternal infectious and parasitic disease complicating <u>the puerperium</u>** — [♀, Age/12-55]

O99- <u>Other maternal diseases classifiable elsewhere</u> but complicating pregnancy, childbirth and the puerperium
Includes: Conditions which complicate the pregnant state, are aggravated by the pregnancy or are a main reason for obstetric care
Use additional code to identify specific condition
Excludes ❷: when the reason for maternal care is that the condition is known or suspected to have affected the fetus (O35-O36)

O99.0- <u>Anemia</u> complicating pregnancy, childbirth and the puerperium
AHA 16:1Q:p4 – Pregnancy complicated by anemia
Conditions in D50-D64
Excludes 1: anemia arising in the puerperium (O90.81)
postpartum anemia NOS (O90.81)

O99.01- Anemia complicating <u>pregnancy</u>

O99.011 Anemia complicating pregnancy, <u>first</u> trimester — [♀, Age/12-55]

O99.012 Anemia complicating pregnancy, <u>second</u> trimester — [♀, Age/12-55]

O99.013 Anemia complicating pregnancy, <u>third</u> trimester — [♀, Age/12-55]

O99.019 Anemia complicating pregnancy, <u>unspecified</u> trimester — [♀, Age/12-55]

O99.02 Anemia complicating <u>childbirth</u> — [♀, Age/12-55]

O99.03 Anemia complicating <u>the puerperium</u> — [♀, Age/12-55]
Excludes 1: postpartum anemia not pre-existing prior to delivery (O90.81)

O99.1- <u>Other diseases of the blood and blood-forming organs and certain disorders involving the immune mechanism</u> complicating pregnancy, childbirth and the puerperium
Conditions in D65-D89
Excludes ❷: hemorrhage with coagulation defects (O45.-, O46.0-, O67.0, O72.3)

O99.11- Other diseases of the blood and blood-forming organs and certain disorders involving the immune mechanism complicating <u>pregnancy</u>

cc **O99.111 Other diseases of the blood and blood-forming organs and certain disorders involving the immune mechanism complicating pregnancy, <u>first</u> trimester** — [♀, Age/12-55]

cc **O99.112 Other diseases of the blood and blood-forming organs and certain disorders involving the immune mechanism complicating pregnancy, <u>second</u> trimester** — [♀, Age/12-55]

cc **O99.113 Other diseases of the blood and blood-forming organs and certain disorders involving the immune mechanism complicating pregnancy, <u>third</u> trimester** — [♀, Age/12-55]

cc **O99.119 Other diseases of the blood and blood-forming organs and certain disorders involving the immune mechanism complicating pregnancy, <u>unspecified</u> trimester** — [♀, Age/12-55]

cc **O99.12 Other diseases of the blood and blood-forming organs and certain disorders involving the immune mechanism complicating <u>childbirth</u>** — [♀, Age/12-55]

cc **O99.13 Other diseases of the blood and blood-forming organs and certain disorders involving the immune mechanism complicating <u>the puerperium</u>** — [♀, Age/12-55]

O99.2- <u>Endocrine, nutritional and metabolic diseases</u> complicating pregnancy, childbirth and the puerperium
Conditions in E00-E88
Excludes ❷: diabetes mellitus (O24.-)
malnutrition (O25.-)
postpartum thyroiditis (O90.5)

O99.21- <u>Obesity</u> complicating pregnancy, childbirth, and the puerperium
Use additional code to identify the type of obesity (E66.-)

O99.210 Obesity complicating <u>pregnancy</u>, <u>unspecified</u> trimester — [♀, Age/12-55]

O99.211 Obesity complicating <u>pregnancy</u>, <u>first</u> trimester — [♀, Age/12-55]

O99.212 Obesity complicating <u>pregnancy</u>, <u>second</u> trimester — [♀, Age/12-55]

O99.213 Obesity complicating <u>pregnancy</u>, <u>third</u> trimester — [♀, Age/12-55]

O99.214 Obesity complicating <u>childbirth</u> — [♀, Age/12-55]

O99.215 Obesity complicating <u>the puerperium</u> — [♀, Age/12-55]

O99.28- <u>Other</u> endocrine, nutritional and metabolic diseases complicating pregnancy, childbirth and the puerperium

O99.280 Endocrine, nutritional and metabolic diseases complicating <u>pregnancy</u>, <u>unspecified</u> trimester — [♀, Age/12-55]

O99.281 Endocrine, nutritional and metabolic diseases complicating <u>pregnancy</u>, <u>first</u> trimester — [♀, Age/12-55]

O 9 8 - O 9 9

O99.282 **Endocrine, nutritional and metabolic diseases complicating** <u>pregnancy</u>, <u>second</u> trimester — [♀, Age/12-55]

O99.283 **Endocrine, nutritional and metabolic diseases complicating** <u>pregnancy</u>, <u>third</u> trimester — [♀, Age/12-55]

O99.284 **Endocrine, nutritional and metabolic diseases complicating** <u>childbirth</u> — [♀, Age/12-55]

O99.285 **Endocrine, nutritional and metabolic diseases complicating** <u>the puerperium</u> — [♀, Age/12-55]

O99.3- <u>**Mental disorders and diseases of the nervous system**</u> complicating pregnancy, childbirth and the puerperium

O99.31- <u>**Alcohol use**</u> complicating pregnancy, childbirth, and the puerperium
Use additional code(s) from F10 to identify manifestations of the alcohol use

O99.310 **Alcohol use complicating** <u>pregnancy</u>, <u>unspecified</u> trimester — [♀, Age/12-55]

O99.311 **Alcohol use complicating** <u>pregnancy</u>, <u>first</u> trimester — [♀, Age/12-55]

O99.312 **Alcohol use complicating** <u>pregnancy</u>, <u>second</u> trimester — [♀, Age/12-55]

O99.313 **Alcohol use complicating** <u>pregnancy</u>, <u>third</u> trimester — [♀, Age/12-55]

O99.314 **Alcohol use complicating** <u>childbirth</u> — [♀, Age/12-55]

O99.315 **Alcohol use complicating** <u>the puerperium</u> — [♀, Age/12-55]

O99.32- <u>**Drug use**</u> complicating pregnancy, childbirth, and the puerperium
Use additional code(s) from F11-F16 and F18-F19 to identify manifestations of the drug use

O99.320 **Drug use complicating** <u>pregnancy</u>, <u>unspecified</u> trimester — [♀, Age/12-55]

cc O99.321 **Drug use complicating** <u>pregnancy</u>, <u>first</u> trimester — [♀, Age/12-55]

cc O99.322 **Drug use complicating** <u>pregnancy</u>, <u>second</u> trimester — [♀, Age/12-55]

cc O99.323 **Drug use complicating** <u>pregnancy</u>, <u>third</u> trimester — [♀, Age/12-55]

cc O99.324 **Drug use complicating** <u>childbirth</u> — [♀, Age/12-55]

cc O99.325 **Drug use complicating** <u>the puerperium</u> — [♀, Age/12-55]

O99.33- <u>**Tobacco use disorder**</u> complicating pregnancy, childbirth, and the puerperium
Smoking complicating pregnancy, childbirth, and the puerperium
Use additional code from category F17 to identify type of tobacco nicotine dependence

O99.330 **Smoking (tobacco) complicating** <u>pregnancy</u>, <u>unspecified</u> trimester — [♀, Age/12-55]

O99.331 **Smoking (tobacco) complicating** <u>pregnancy</u>, <u>first</u> trimester — [♀, Age/12-55]

O99.332 **Smoking (tobacco) complicating** <u>pregnancy</u>, <u>second</u> trimester — [♀, Age/12-55]

O99.333 **Smoking (tobacco) complicating** <u>pregnancy</u>, <u>third</u> trimester — [♀, Age/12-55]

O99.334 **Smoking (tobacco) complicating** <u>childbirth</u> — [♀, Age/12-55]

O99.335 **Smoking (tobacco) complicating** <u>the puerperium</u> — [♀, Age/12-55]

O99.34- <u>**Other mental disorders**</u> complicating pregnancy, childbirth, and the puerperium
Conditions in F01-F09 and F20-F99
Excludes ❷: *postpartum mood disturbance (O90.6)*
postnatal psychosis (F53)
puerperal psychosis (F53)

O99.340 **Other mental disorders complicating** <u>pregnancy</u>, <u>unspecified</u> trimester — [♀, Age/12-55]

O99.341 **Other mental disorders complicating** <u>pregnancy</u>, <u>first</u> trimester — [♀, Age/12-55]

O99.342 **Other mental disorders complicating** <u>pregnancy</u>, <u>second</u> trimester — [♀, Age/12-55]

O99.343 **Other mental disorders complicating** <u>pregnancy</u>, <u>third</u> trimester — [♀, Age/12-55]

O99.344 **Other mental disorders complicating** <u>childbirth</u> — [♀, Age/12-55]

O99.345 **Other mental disorders complicating** <u>the puerperium</u> — [♀, Age/12-55]

O99.35- <u>**Diseases of the nervous system**</u> complicating pregnancy, childbirth, and the puerperium
Conditions in G00-G99
Excludes ❷: *pregnancy related peripheral neuritis (O26.8-)*

O99.350 **Diseases of the nervous system complicating** <u>pregnancy</u>, <u>unspecified</u> trimester — [♀, Age/12-55]

O99.351 **Diseases of the nervous system complicating** <u>pregnancy</u>, <u>first</u> trimester — [♀, Age/12-55]

O99.352 **Diseases of the nervous system complicating** <u>pregnancy</u>, <u>second</u> trimester — [♀, Age/12-55]

O99.353 **Diseases of the nervous system complicating** <u>pregnancy</u>, <u>third</u> trimester — [♀, Age/12-55]

cc O99.354 **Diseases of the nervous system complicating** <u>childbirth</u> — [♀, Age/12-55]

cc O99.355 **Diseases of the nervous system complicating** <u>the puerperium</u> — [♀, Age/12-55]

O99.4- <u>**Diseases of the circulatory system**</u> complicating pregnancy, childbirth and the puerperium
AHA 16:2Q:p8 – Preexisting pulmonary hypertension complicating pregnancy
Conditions in I00-I99
Excludes 1: *peripartum cardiomyopathy (O90.3)*
Excludes ❷: *hypertensive disorders (O10-O16)*
obstetric embolism (O88.-)
venous complications and cerebrovenous sinus thrombosis in labor, childbirth and the puerperium (O87-)
venous complications and cerebrovenous sinus thrombosis in pregnancy (O22-)

O99.41- **Diseases of the circulatory system complicating** <u>pregnancy</u>

cc O99.411 **Diseases of the circulatory system complicating pregnancy,** <u>first</u> trimester — [♀, Age/12-55]

cc O99.412 **Diseases of the circulatory system complicating pregnancy,** <u>second</u> trimester — [♀, Age/12-55]

cc O99.413 **Diseases of the circulatory system complicating pregnancy,** <u>third</u> trimester — [♀, Age/12-55]

O99.419 **Diseases of the circulatory system complicating pregnancy,** <u>unspecified</u> trimester — [♀, Age/12-55]

MCC O99.42 **Diseases of the circulatory system complicating** <u>childbirth</u> — [♀, Age/12-55]

cc O99.43 **Diseases of the circulatory system complicating** <u>the puerperium</u> — [♀, Age/12-55]

O99.5- <u>**Diseases of the respiratory system**</u> complicating pregnancy, childbirth and the puerperium
Conditions in J00-J99

O99.51- **Diseases of the respiratory system complicating** <u>pregnancy</u>

O99.511 **Diseases of the respiratory system complicating pregnancy,** <u>first</u> trimester — [♀, Age/12-55]

O99.512 **Diseases of the respiratory system complicating pregnancy,** <u>second</u> trimester — [♀, Age/12-55]

O99.513 **Diseases of the respiratory system complicating pregnancy,** <u>third</u> trimester — [♀, Age/12-55]

O99.519 **Diseases of the respiratory system complicating pregnancy,** <u>unspecified</u> trimester — [♀, Age/12-55]

O99.52 **Diseases of the respiratory system complicating** <u>childbirth</u> — [♀, Age/12-55]

O99.53 **Diseases of the respiratory system complicating** <u>the puerperium</u> — [♀, Age/12-55]

O99 I O99

O99.6- **Diseases of the digestive system** complicating pregnancy, childbirth and the puerperium
   AHA 16:1Q:p4 – Pregnancy complicated by gallstones
   Conditions in K00-K93
   Excludes ❷: hemorrhoids in pregnancy (O22.4-)
   liver and biliary tract disorders in pregnancy, childbirth and the puerperium (O26.6-)

O99.61-   Diseases of the digestive system complicating **pregnancy**

O99.611 Diseases of the digestive system complicating pregnancy, **first** trimester — [♀, Age/12-55]

O99.612 Diseases of the digestive system complicating pregnancy, **second** trimester — [♀, Age/12-55]

O99.613 Diseases of the digestive system complicating pregnancy, **third** trimester — [♀, Age/12-55]

O99.619 Diseases of the digestive system complicating pregnancy, **unspecified** trimester — [♀, Age/12-55]

O99.62 Diseases of the digestive system complicating **childbirth** — [♀, Age/12-55]

O99.63 Diseases of the digestive system complicating **the puerperium** — [♀, Age/12-55]

O99.7- **Diseases of the skin and subcutaneous tissue** complicating pregnancy, childbirth and the puerperium
   Conditions in L00-L99
   Excludes ❷: herpes gestationis (O26.4)
   pruritic urticarial papules and plaques of pregnancy (PUPPP) (O26.86)

O99.71-   Diseases of the skin and subcutaneous tissue complicating **pregnancy**

O99.711 Diseases of the skin and subcutaneous tissue complicating pregnancy, **first** trimester — [♀, Age/12-55]

O99.712 Diseases of the skin and subcutaneous tissue complicating pregnancy, **second** trimester — [♀, Age/12-55]

O99.713 Diseases of the skin and subcutaneous tissue complicating pregnancy, **third** trimester — [♀, Age/12-55]

O99.719 Diseases of the skin and subcutaneous tissue complicating pregnancy, **unspecified** trimester — [♀, Age/12-55]

O99.72 Diseases of the skin and subcutaneous tissue complicating **childbirth** — [♀, Age/12-55]

O99.73 Diseases of the skin and subcutaneous tissue complicating **the puerperium** — [♀, Age/12-55]

O99.8- **Other specified diseases and conditions** complicating pregnancy, childbirth and the puerperium
   Conditions in D00-D48, H00-H95, M00-N99, and Q00-Q99
   Use additional code to identify condition
   Excludes ❷: genitourinary infections in pregnancy (O23-)
   infection of genitourinary tract following delivery (O86.1-O86.3)
   malignant neoplasm complicating pregnancy, childbirth and the puerperium (O9A.1-)
   maternal care for known or suspected abnormality of maternal pelvic organs (O34-)
   postpartum acute kidney failure (O90.4)
   traumatic injuries in pregnancy (O9A.2-)

O99.81-   **Abnormal glucose** complicating pregnancy, childbirth and the puerperium
   Excludes 1:   gestational diabetes (O24.4-)

O99.810 Abnormal glucose complicating **pregnancy** — [♀, Age/12-55]

O99.814 Abnormal glucose complicating **childbirth** — [♀, Age/12-55]

O99.815 Abnormal glucose complicating **the puerperium** — [♀, Age/12-55]

O99.82-   **Streptococcus B carrier state** complicating pregnancy, childbirth and the puerperium
   Excludes 1:   carrier of streptococcus group B (GBS) in a nonpregnant woman (Z22.330)

O99.820 Streptococcus B carrier state complicating **pregnancy** — [♀, Age/12-55] [Unacceptable PDX]

O99.824 Streptococcus B carrier state complicating **childbirth** — [♀, Age/12-55]

O99.825 Streptococcus B carrier state complicating **the puerperium** — [♀, Age/12-55] [Unacceptable PDX]

O99.83-   **Other infection carrier state** complicating pregnancy, childbirth and the puerperium
   Use additional code to identify the carrier state (Z22.-)

cc **O99.830** Other infection carrier state complicating **pregnancy** — [♀, Age/12-55]

cc **O99.834** Other infection carrier state complicating **childbirth** — [♀, Age/12-55]

cc **O99.835** Other infection carrier state complicating **the puerperium** — [♀, Age/12-55]

O99.84-   **Bariatric surgery status** complicating pregnancy, childbirth and the puerperium
   Gastric banding status complicating pregnancy, childbirth and the puerperium
   Gastric bypass status for obesity complicating pregnancy, childbirth and the puerperium
   Obesity surgery status complicating pregnancy, childbirth and the puerperium

O99.840 Bariatric surgery status complicating **pregnancy, unspecified** trimester — [♀, Age/12-55]

O99.841 Bariatric surgery status complicating **pregnancy, first** trimester — [♀, Age/12-55]

O99.842 Bariatric surgery status complicating **pregnancy, second** trimester — [♀, Age/12-55]

O99.843 Bariatric surgery status complicating **pregnancy, third** trimester — [♀, Age/12-55]

O99.844 Bariatric surgery status complicating **childbirth** — [♀, Age/12-55]

O99.845 Bariatric surgery status complicating **the puerperium** — [♀, Age/12-55]

O99.89 **Other specified** diseases and conditions complicating pregnancy, childbirth and the puerperium — [♀, Age/12-55]

O9A- **Maternal malignant neoplasms, traumatic injuries and abuse classifiable elsewhere but complicating pregnancy, childbirth and the puerperium**

O9A.1- **Malignant neoplasm** complicating pregnancy, childbirth and the puerperium
   Conditions in C00-C96
   Use additional code to identify neoplasm
   Excludes ❷: maternal care for benign tumor of corpus uteri (O34.1-)
   maternal care for benign tumor of cervix (O34.4-)

O9A.11-   Malignant neoplasm complicating **pregnancy**

O9A.111 Malignant neoplasm complicating pregnancy, **first** trimester — [♀, Age/12-55]

O9A.112 Malignant neoplasm complicating pregnancy, **second** trimester — [♀, Age/12-55]

O9A.113 Malignant neoplasm complicating pregnancy, **third** trimester — [♀, Age/12-55]

O9A.119 Malignant neoplasm complicating pregnancy, **unspecified** trimester — [♀, Age/12-55]

O9A.12 Malignant neoplasm complicating **childbirth** — [♀, Age/12-55]

O9A.13 Malignant neoplasm complicating **the puerperium** — [♀, Age/12-55]
   AHA 15:3Q:p19 – Malignant neoplasm complicating puerperium

O99 I O9A

O9A.2- Injury, poisoning and certain other consequences of external causes complicating pregnancy, childbirth and the puerperium
    Conditions in S00-T88, except T74 and T76
Use additional code(s) to identify the injury or poisoning
Excludes ❷: physical, sexual and psychological abuse complicating pregnancy, childbirth and the puerperium (O9A.3-, O9A.4-, O9A.5-)

O9A.21-   Injury, poisoning and certain other consequences of external causes complicating pregnancy

O9A.211 Injury, poisoning and certain other consequences of external causes complicating pregnancy, first trimester — [♀, Age/12-55]

O9A.212 Injury, poisoning and certain other consequences of external causes complicating pregnancy, second trimester — [♀, Age/12-55]

O9A.213 Injury, poisoning and certain other consequences of external causes complicating pregnancy, third trimester — [♀, Age/12-55]

O9A.219 Injury, poisoning and certain other consequences of external causes complicating pregnancy, unspecified trimester — [♀, Age/12-55]

O9A.22 Injury, poisoning and certain other consequences of external causes complicating childbirth — [♀, Age/12-55]

O9A.23 Injury, poisoning and certain other consequences of external causes complicating the puerperium — [♀, Age/12-55]

O9A.3- Physical abuse complicating pregnancy, childbirth and the puerperium
    Conditions in T74.11 or T76.11
Use additional code (if applicable):
    To identify any associated current injury due to physical abuse
    To identify the perpetrator of abuse (Y07.-)
Excludes ❷: sexual abuse complicating pregnancy, childbirth and the puerperium (O9A.4-)

O9A.31- Physical abuse complicating pregnancy

O9A.311 Physical abuse complicating pregnancy, first trimester — [♀, Age/12-55]

O9A.312 Physical abuse complicating pregnancy, second trimester — [♀, Age/12-55]

O9A.313 Physical abuse complicating pregnancy, third trimester — [♀, Age/12-55]

O9A.319 Physical abuse complicating pregnancy, unspecified trimester — [♀, Age/12-55]

O9A.32 Physical abuse complicating childbirth — [♀, Age/12-55]

O9A.33 Physical abuse complicating the puerperium — [♀, Age/12-55]

O9A.4- Sexual abuse complicating pregnancy, childbirth and the puerperium
    Conditions in T74.21 or T76.21
Use additional code (if applicable):
    To identify any associated current injury due to sexual abuse
    To identify the perpetrator of abuse (Y07.-)

O9A.41- Sexual abuse complicating pregnancy

O9A.411 Sexual abuse complicating pregnancy, first trimester — [♀, Age/12-55]

O9A.412 Sexual abuse complicating pregnancy, second trimester — [♀, Age/12-55]

O9A.413 Sexual abuse complicating pregnancy, third trimester — [♀, Age/12-55]

O9A.419 Sexual abuse complicating pregnancy, unspecified trimester — [♀, Age/12-55]

O9A.42 Sexual abuse complicating childbirth — [♀, Age/12-55]

O9A.43 Sexual abuse complicating the puerperium — [♀, Age/12-55]

O9A.5- Psychological abuse complicating pregnancy, childbirth and the puerperium
    Conditions in T74.31 or T76.31
Use additional code to identify the perpetrator of abuse (Y07.-)

O9A.51- Psychological abuse complicating pregnancy

O9A.511 Psychological abuse complicating pregnancy, first trimester — [♀, Age/12-55]

O9A.512 Psychological abuse complicating pregnancy, second trimester — [♀, Age/12-55]

O9A.513 Psychological abuse complicating pregnancy, third trimester — [♀, Age/12-55]

O9A.519 Psychological abuse complicating pregnancy, unspecified trimester — [♀, Age/12-55]

O9A.52 Psychological abuse complicating childbirth — [♀, Age/12-55]

O9A.53 Psychological abuse complicating the puerperium — [♀, Age/12-55]

Chapter 16 – Certain conditions originating in the perinatal period (P00-P96)

Note: Codes from this chapter are for use on newborn records only, never on maternal records

Includes: Conditions that have their origin in the fetal or perinatal period (before birth through the first 28 days after birth) even if morbidity occurs later

Excludes ❷: congenital malformations, deformations and chromosomal abnormalities (Q00-Q99)
endocrine, nutritional and metabolic diseases (E00-E88)
injury, poisoning and certain other consequences of external causes (S00-T88)
neoplasms (C00-D49)
tetanus neonatorum (A33)

This chapter contains the following blocks:

P00-P04	Newborn affected by maternal factors and by complications of pregnancy, labor, and delivery
P05-P08	Disorders of newborn related to length of gestation and fetal growth
P09	Abnormal findings on neonatal screening
P10-P15	Birth trauma
P19-P29	Respiratory and cardiovascular disorders specific to the perinatal period
P35-P39	Infections specific to the perinatal period
P50-P61	Hemorrhagic and hematological disorders of newborn
P70-P74	Transitory endocrine and metabolic disorders specific to newborn
P76-P78	Digestive system disorders of newborn
P80-P83	Conditions involving the integument and temperature regulation of newborn
P84	Other problems with newborn
P90-P96	Other disorders originating in the perinatal period

Chapter-Specific Coding Guidelines

C. Chapter-Specific Coding Guidelines
In addition to general coding guidelines, there are guidelines for specific diagnoses and/or conditions in the classification. Unless otherwise indicated, these guidelines apply to all health care settings. Please refer to Section II for guidelines on the selection of principal diagnosis.

16. Chapter 16: Certain Conditions Originating in the Perinatal Period (P00-P96)
For coding and reporting purposes the perinatal period is defined as before birth through the 28th day following birth. The following guidelines are provided for reporting purposes

a. General Perinatal Rules

1) Use of Chapter 16 Codes
Codes in this chapter are never for use on the maternal record.

Codes from Chapter 15, the obstetric chapter, are never permitted on the newborn record. Chapter 16 codes may be used throughout the life of the patient if the condition is still present.

2) Principal Diagnosis for Birth Record
When coding the birth episode in a newborn record, assign a code from category Z38, Liveborn infants according to place of birth and type of delivery, as the principal diagnosis. A code from category Z38 is assigned only once, to a newborn at the time of birth. If a newborn is transferred to another institution, a code from category Z38 should not be used at the receiving hospital.

A code from category Z38 is used only on the newborn record, not on the mother's record.

3) Use of Codes from other Chapters with Codes from Chapter 16
Codes from other chapters may be used with codes from chapter 16 if the codes from the other chapters provide more specific detail. Codes for signs and symptoms may be assigned when a definitive diagnosis has not been established. If the reason for the encounter is a perinatal condition, the code from chapter 16 should be sequenced first.

4) Use of Chapter 16 Codes after the Perinatal Period
Should a condition originate in the perinatal period, and continue throughout the life of the patient, the perinatal code should continue to be used regardless of the patient's age.

5) Birth process or community acquired conditions
If a newborn has a condition that may be either due to the birth process or community acquired and the documentation does not indicate which it is, the default is due to the birth process and the code from Chapter 16 should be used. If the condition is community-acquired, a code from Chapter 16 should not be assigned.

6) Code all clinically significant conditions
All clinically significant conditions noted on routine newborn examination should be coded. A condition is clinically significant if it requires:
- clinical evaluation; or
- therapeutic treatment; or
- diagnostic procedures; or
- extended length of hospital stay; or
- increased nursing care and/or monitoring; or
- has implications for future health care needs

Note: The perinatal guidelines listed above are the same as the general coding guidelines for "additional diagnoses", except for the final point regarding implications for future health care needs. Codes should be assigned for conditions that have been specified by the provider as having implications for future health care needs.

b. Observation and Evaluation of Newborns for Suspected Conditions not Found
~~Reserved for future expansion~~

1) Assign a code from category Z05, Observation and evaluation of newborns and infants for suspected conditions ruled out, to identify those instances when a healthy newborn is evaluated for a suspected condition that is determined after study not to be present. Do not use a code from category Z05 when the patient has identified signs or symptoms of a suspected problem; in such cases code the sign or symptom.

2) A code from category Z05 may also be assigned as a principal or first-listed code for readmissions or encounters when the code from category Z38 code no longer applies. Codes from category Z05 are for use only for healthy newborns and infants for which no condition after study is found to be present.

3) Z05 on a birth record
A code from category Z05 is to be used as a secondary code after the code from category Z38, Liveborn infants according to place of birth and type of delivery.

c. Coding Additional Perinatal Diagnoses

1) Assigning codes for conditions that require treatment
Assign codes for conditions that require treatment or further investigation, prolong the length of stay, or require resource utilization.

2) Codes for conditions specified as having implications for future health care needs
Assign codes for conditions that have been specified by the provider as having implications for future health care needs.

Note: This guideline should not be used for adult patients.

d. Prematurity and Fetal Growth Retardation
Providers utilize different criteria in determining prematurity. A code for prematurity should not be assigned unless it is documented. Assignment of codes in categories P05, Disorders of newborn related to slow fetal growth and fetal malnutrition, and P07, Disorders of newborn related to short gestation and low birth weight, not elsewhere classified, should be based on the recorded birth weight and estimated gestational age. Codes from category P05 should not be assigned with codes from category P07.

When both birth weight and gestational age are available, two codes from category P07 should be assigned, with the code for birth weight sequenced before the code for gestational age.

e. Low birth weight and immaturity status
Codes from category P07, Disorders of newborn related to short gestation and low birth weight, not elsewhere classified, are for use for a child or adult who was premature or had a low birth weight as a newborn and this is affecting the patient's current health status.

See Section I.C.21. Factors influencing health status and contact with health services, Status.

f. Bacterial Sepsis of Newborn
Category P36, Bacterial sepsis of newborn, includes congenital sepsis. If a perinate is documented as having sepsis without documentation of congenital or community acquired, the default is congenital and a code from category P36 should be assigned. If the P36 code includes the causal organism, an additional code from category B95, Streptococcus, Staphylococcus, and Enterococcus as the cause of diseases classified elsewhere, or B96, Other bacterial agents as the cause of diseases classified elsewhere, should not be assigned. If the P36 code does not include the causal organism, assign an additional code from category B96. If applicable, use additional codes to identify severe sepsis (R65.2-) and any associated acute organ dysfunction.

g. Stillbirth
Code P95, Stillbirth, is only for use in institutions that maintain separate records for stillbirths. No other code should be used with P95. Code P95 should not be used on the mother's record.

Newborn affected by maternal factors and by complications of pregnancy, labor, and delivery (P00-P04)

Note: These codes are for use when the listed maternal conditions are specified as the cause of confirmed morbidity or potential morbidity which have their origin in the perinatal period (before birth through the first 28 days after birth).

P00- **Newborn affected by <u>maternal conditions</u> that may be <u>unrelated</u> to present pregnancy**

Code first any current condition in newborn

Excludes ❷: encounter for observation of newborn for suspected diseases and conditions ruled out (Z05.-)

newborn affected by maternal complications of pregnancy (P01.-)

newborn affected by maternal endocrine and metabolic disorders (P70-P74)

newborn affected by noxious substances transmitted via placenta or breast milk (P04.-)

P00.0 **Newborn affected by maternal hypertensive disorders**
Newborn affected by maternal conditions classifiable to O10-O11, O13-O16

P00.1 **Newborn affected by maternal renal and urinary tract diseases**
Newborn affected by maternal conditions classifiable to N00-N39

P00.2 **Newborn affected by maternal infectious and parasitic diseases**
AHA 15:3Q:p20 – Suspected sepsis in newborn, ruled out
Newborn affected by maternal infectious disease classifiable to A00-B99, J09 and J10

Excludes 1: infections specific to the perinatal period (P35-P39)
maternal genital tract or other localized infections (P00.8)

P00.3 **Newborn affected by other maternal circulatory and respiratory diseases**
Newborn affected by maternal conditions classifiable to I00-I99, J00-J99, Q20-Q34 and not included in P00.0, P00.2

P00.4 **Newborn affected by maternal nutritional disorders**
Newborn affected by maternal disorders classifiable to E40-E64
Maternal malnutrition NOS

P00.5 **Newborn affected by maternal injury**
Newborn affected by maternal conditions classifiable to O9A.2-

P00.6 **Newborn affected by surgical procedure on mother**
Newborn affected by amniocentesis

Excludes 1: cesarean delivery for present delivery (P03.4)
damage to placenta from amniocentesis, cesarean delivery or surgical induction (P02.1)
previous surgery to uterus or pelvic organs (P03.89)

Excludes ❷: newborn affected by complication of (fetal) intrauterine procedure (P96.5)

P00.7 **Newborn affected by other medical procedures on mother, not elsewhere classified**
Newborn affected by radiation to mother

Excludes 1: damage to placenta from amniocentesis, cesarean delivery or surgical induction (P02.1)
newborn affected by other complications of labor and delivery (P03.-)

P00.8- **Newborn affected by other maternal conditions**

P00.81 **Newborn affected by periodontal disease in mother**

P00.89 **Newborn affected by other maternal conditions**
Newborn affected by conditions classifiable to T80-T88
Newborn affected by maternal genital tract or other localized infections
Newborn affected by maternal systemic lupus erythematosus

P00.9 **Newborn affected by unspecified maternal condition**

P01- **<u>Newborn affected by maternal complications</u> of pregnancy**

Code first any current condition in newborn

Excludes ❷: encounter for observation of newborn for suspected diseases and conditions ruled out (Z05.-)

P01.0 **Newborn affected by incompetent cervix**

P01.1 **Newborn affected by premature rupture of membranes**

P01.2 **Newborn affected by oligohydramnios**

Excludes 1: oligohydramnios due to premature rupture of membranes (P01.1)

P01.3 **Newborn affected by polyhydramnios**
Newborn affected by hydramnios

P01.4 **Newborn affected by ectopic pregnancy**
Newborn affected by abdominal pregnancy

P01.5 **Newborn affected by multiple pregnancy**
Newborn affected by triplet (pregnancy)
Newborn affected by twin (pregnancy)

P01.6 **Newborn affected by maternal death**

P01.7 **Newborn affected by malpresentation before labor**
Newborn affected by breech presentation before labor
Newborn affected by external version before labor
Newborn affected by face presentation before labor
Newborn affected by transverse lie before labor
Newborn affected by unstable lie before labor

P01.8 **Newborn affected by other maternal complications of pregnancy**

P01.9 **Newborn affected by maternal complication of pregnancy, unspecified**

P02- **<u>Newborn affected by complications</u> of placenta, cord and membranes**

Code first any current condition in newborn

Excludes ❷: encounter for observation of newborn for suspected diseases and conditions ruled out (Z05.-)

P02.0 **Newborn affected by placenta previa**

P02.1 **Newborn affected by other forms of placental separation and hemorrhage**
Newborn affected by abruptio placenta
Newborn affected by accidental hemorrhage
Newborn affected by antepartum hemorrhage
Newborn affected by damage to placenta from amniocentesis, cesarean delivery or surgical induction
Newborn affected by maternal blood loss
Newborn affected by premature separation of placenta

P02.2- **Newborn affected by other and unspecified morphological and functional abnormalities of placenta**

P02.20 **Newborn affected by unspecified morphological and functional abnormalities of placenta**

P02.29 **Newborn affected by other morphological and functional abnormalities of placenta**
Newborn affected by placental dysfunction
Newborn affected by placental infarction
Newborn affected by placental insufficiency

P02.3 **Newborn affected by placental transfusion syndromes**
Newborn affected by placental and cord abnormalities resulting in twin-to-twin or other transplacental transfusion

P02.4 **Newborn affected by prolapsed cord**

P02.5 **Newborn affected by other compression of umbilical cord**
Newborn affected by umbilical cord (tightly) around neck
Newborn affected by entanglement of umbilical cord
Newborn affected by knot in umbilical cord

P02.6- **Newborn affected by other and unspecified conditions of umbilical cord**

P02.60 **Newborn affected by unspecified conditions of umbilical cord**

P02.69 **Newborn affected by other conditions of umbilical cord**
Newborn affected by short umbilical cord
Newborn affected by vasa previa

Excludes 1: newborn affected by single umbilical artery (Q27.0)

P02.7 **Newborn affected by chorioamnionitis**
Newborn affected by amnionitis
Newborn affected by membranitis
Newborn affected by placentitis

P02.8 **Newborn affected by other abnormalities of membranes**

P02.9 **Newborn affected by abnormality of membranes, unspecified**

P03- <u>Newborn affected by other complications</u> of labor and delivery
Code first any current condition in newborn
Excludes ❷: encounter for observation of newborn for suspected diseases and conditions ruled out (Z05.-)

P03.0   Newborn affected by breech delivery and extraction

P03.1   Newborn affected by other malpresentation, malposition and disproportion during labor and delivery
Newborn affected by contracted pelvis
Newborn affected by conditions classifiable to O64-O66
Newborn affected by persistent occipitoposterior
Newborn affected by transverse lie

P03.2   Newborn affected by forceps delivery

P03.3   Newborn affected by delivery by vacuum extractor [ventouse]

P03.4   Newborn affected by cesarean delivery

P03.5   Newborn affected by precipitate delivery
Newborn affected by rapid second stage

P03.6   Newborn affected by abnormal uterine contractions
Newborn affected by conditions classifiable to O62.-, except O62.3
Newborn affected by hypertonic labor
Newborn affected by uterine inertia

P03.8-   Newborn affected by other specified complications of labor and delivery

P03.81-   Newborn affected by abnormality in fetal (intrauterine) heart rate or rhythm
Excludes 1:   neonatal cardiac dysrhythmia (P29.1-)

P03.810   Newborn affected by abnormality in fetal (intrauterine) heart rate or rhythm before the onset of labor

P03.811   Newborn affected by abnormality in fetal (intrauterine) heart rate or rhythm during labor

P03.819   Newborn affected by abnormality in fetal (intrauterine) heart rate or rhythm, unspecified as to time of onset

P03.82   Meconium passage during delivery — The presence of meconium at delivery without the presence of the distinctive mixing of meconium staining that is indicative of a stress on the fetus.
*Excludes 1:   meconium aspiration (P24.00, P24.01)
meconium staining (P96.83)*

P03.89   Newborn affected by other specified complications of labor and delivery
Newborn affected by abnormality of maternal soft tissues
Newborn affected by conditions classifiable to O60-O75 and by procedures used in labor and delivery not included in P02.- and P03.0-P03.6
Newborn affected by induction of labor

P03.9   Newborn affected by complication of labor and delivery, unspecified

P04- <u>Newborn affected by noxious substances transmitted via placenta or breast milk</u>
Includes: Nonteratogenic effects of substances transmitted via placenta
*Excludes ❷: congenital malformations (Q00-Q99)
encounter for observation of newborn for suspected diseases and conditions ruled out (Z05.-)
neonatal jaundice from excessive hemolysis due to drugs or toxins transmitted from mother (P58.4)
newborn in contact with and (suspected) exposures hazardous to health not transmitted via placenta or breast milk (Z77.-)*

P04.0   Newborn affected by maternal anesthesia and analgesia in pregnancy, labor and delivery
Newborn affected by reactions and intoxications from maternal opiates and tranquilizers administered during labor and delivery

P04.1   Newborn affected by other maternal medication
Newborn affected by cancer chemotherapy
Newborn affected by cytotoxic drugs
*Excludes 1:   dysmorphism due to warfarin (Q86.2)
fetal hydantoin syndrome (Q86.1)
maternal use of drugs of addiction (P04.4-)*

P04.2   Newborn affected by maternal use of tobacco
Newborn affected by exposure in utero to tobacco smoke
Excludes ❷: newborn exposure to environmental tobacco smoke (P96.81)

P04.3   Newborn affected by maternal use of alcohol
Excludes 1:   fetal alcohol syndrome (Q86.0)

P04.4-   Newborn affected by maternal use of drugs of addiction

P04.41   Newborn affected by maternal use of cocaine
"Crack baby"

P04.49   Newborn affected by maternal use of other drugs of addiction
*Excludes ❷: newborn affected by maternal anesthesia and analgesia (P04.0)
withdrawal symptoms from maternal use of drugs of addiction (P96.1)*

P04.5   Newborn affected by maternal use of nutritional chemical substances

P04.6   Newborn affected by maternal exposure to environmental chemical substances

P04.8   Newborn affected by other maternal noxious substances

P04.9   Newborn affected by maternal noxious substance, unspecified

Disorders of newborn related to length of gestation and fetal growth (P05-P08)

P05-   Disorders of newborn <u>related to slow fetal growth and fetal malnutrition</u>

P05.0-   <u>Newborn light</u> for gestational age
Newborn light-for-dates
Weight below but length above 10th percentile for gestational age

P05.00   Newborn light for gestational age, unspecified weight

P05.01   Newborn light for gestational age, less than 500 grams

P05.02   Newborn light for gestational age, 500-749 grams

P05.03   Newborn light for gestational age, 750-999 grams

P05.04   Newborn light for gestational age, 1000-1249 grams

P05.05   Newborn light for gestational age, 1250-1499 grams

P05.06   Newborn light for gestational age, 1500-1749 grams

P05.07   Newborn light for gestational age, 1750-1999 grams

P05.08   Newborn light for gestational age, 2000-2499 grams

P05.09   Newborn light for gestational age, 2500 grams and over
Newborn light for gestational age, other

P05.1-   <u>Newborn small</u> for gestational age
Newborn small-and-light-for-dates
Newborn small-for-dates
Weight and length below 10th percentile for gestational age

P05.10   Newborn small for gestational age, unspecified weight

P05.11   Newborn small for gestational age, less than 500 grams

P05.12   Newborn small for gestational age, 500-749 grams

P05.13   Newborn small for gestational age, 750-999 grams

P05.14   Newborn small for gestational age, 1000-1249 grams

P05.15   Newborn small for gestational age, 1250-1499 grams

P05.16   Newborn small for gestational age, 1500-1749 grams

P05.17   Newborn small for gestational age, 1750-1999 grams

P05.18   Newborn small for gestational age, 2000-2499 grams

P05.19   Newborn small for gestational age, other
Newborn small for gestational age, 2500 grams and over

P05.2   Newborn affected by fetal (intrauterine) malnutrition <u>not light or small for gestational age</u>
Infant, not light or small for gestational age, showing signs of fetal malnutrition, such as dry, peeling skin and loss of subcutaneous tissue
*Excludes 1:   newborn affected by fetal malnutrition with light for gestational age (P05.0-)
newborn affected by fetal malnutrition with small for gestational age (P05.1-)*

P05.9   Newborn affected by slow intrauterine growth, unspecified
Newborn affected by fetal growth retardation NOS

P03 | P05

P07- **Disorders of newborn related to short gestation and low birth weight,** not elsewhere classified

Note: When both birth weight and gestational age of the newborn are available, both should be coded with birth weight sequenced before gestational age

Includes: The listed conditions, without further specification, as the cause of morbidity or additional care, in newborn

P07.0- **Extremely low birth weight** newborn

Newborn birth weight 999 g. or less

Excludes 1: *low birth weight due to slow fetal growth and fetal malnutrition (P05.-)*

P07.00 Extremely low birth weight newborn, unspecified weight

P07.01 Extremely low birth weight newborn, less than 500 grams

P07.02 Extremely low birth weight newborn, 500-749 grams

P07.03 Extremely low birth weight newborn, 750-999 grams

P07.1- **Other low birth weight** newborn

Newborn birth weight 1000-2499 g.

Excludes 1: *low birth weight due to slow fetal growth and fetal malnutrition (P05.-)*

P07.10 Other low birth weight newborn, unspecified weight

P07.14 Other low birth weight newborn, 1000-1249 grams

P07.15 Other low birth weight newborn, 1250-1499 grams

P07.16 Other low birth weight newborn, 1500-1749 grams

P07.17 Other low birth weight newborn, 1750-1999 grams

P07.18 Other low birth weight newborn, 2000-2499 grams

P07.2- **Extreme immaturity** of newborn

Less than 28 completed weeks (less than 196 completed days) of gestation

P07.20 Extreme immaturity of newborn, unspecified weeks of gestation

Gestational age less than 28 completed weeks NOS

P07.21 Extreme immaturity of newborn, gestational age less than 23 completed weeks

Extreme immaturity of newborn, gestational age less than 23 weeks, 0 days

P07.22 Extreme immaturity of newborn, gestational age 23 completed weeks

Extreme immaturity of newborn, gestational age 23 weeks, 0 days through 23 weeks, 6 days

P07.23 Extreme immaturity of newborn, gestational age 24 completed weeks

Extreme immaturity of newborn, gestational age 24 weeks, 0 days through 24 weeks, 6 days

P07.24 Extreme immaturity of newborn, gestational age 25 completed weeks

Extreme immaturity of newborn, gestational age 25 weeks, 0 days through 25 weeks, 6 days

P07.25 Extreme immaturity of newborn, gestational age 26 completed weeks

Extreme immaturity of newborn, gestational age 26 weeks, 0 days through 26 weeks, 6 days

P07.26 Extreme immaturity of newborn, gestational age 27 completed weeks

Extreme immaturity of newborn, gestational age 27 weeks, 0 days through 27 weeks, 6 days

P07.3- **Preterm** [premature] newborn [other]

28 completed weeks or more but less than 37 completed weeks (196 completed days but less than 259 completed days) of gestation.

Prematurity NOS

P07.30 Preterm newborn, unspecified weeks of gestation

P07.31 Preterm newborn, gestational age 28 completed weeks

Preterm newborn, gestational age 28 weeks, 0 days through 28 weeks, 6 days

P07.32 Preterm newborn, gestational age 29 completed weeks

Preterm newborn, gestational age 29 weeks, 0 days through 29 weeks, 6 days

P07.33 Preterm newborn, gestational age 30 completed weeks

Preterm newborn, gestational age 30 weeks, 0 days through 30 weeks, 6 days

P07.34 Preterm newborn, gestational age 31 completed weeks

Preterm newborn, gestational age 31 weeks, 0 days through 31 weeks, 6 days

P07.35 Preterm newborn, gestational age 32 completed weeks

Preterm newborn, gestational age 32 weeks, 0 days through 32 weeks, 6 days

P07.36 Preterm newborn, gestational age 33 completed weeks

Preterm newborn, gestational age 33 weeks, 0 days through 33 weeks, 6 days

P07.37 Preterm newborn, gestational age 34 completed weeks

Preterm newborn, gestational age 34 weeks, 0 days through 34 weeks, 6 days

P07.38 Preterm newborn, gestational age 35 completed weeks

Preterm newborn, gestational age 35 weeks, 0 days through 35 weeks, 6 days

P07.39 Preterm newborn, gestational age 36 completed weeks

Preterm newborn, gestational age 36 weeks, 0 days through 36 weeks, 6 days

P08- **Disorders of newborn related to** long gestation and high birth weight

Note: When both birth weight and gestational age of the newborn are available, priority of assignment should be given to birth weight

Includes: The listed conditions, without further specification, as causes of morbidity or additional care, in newborn

P08.0 **Exceptionally large newborn baby**

Usually implies a birth weight of 4500 g. or more

Excludes 1: *syndrome of infant of diabetic mother (P70.1)*
syndrome of infant of mother with gestational diabetes (P70.0)

P08.1 **Other heavy for gestational age newborn**

Other newborn heavy- or large-for-dates regardless of period of gestation

Usually implies a birth weight of 4000 g. to 4499 g.

Excludes 1: *newborn with a birth weight of 4500 or more (P08.0)*
syndrome of infant of diabetic mother (P70.1)
syndrome of infant of mother with gestational diabetes (P70.0)

P08.2- **Late newborn, not heavy for gestational age**

AHA 14:1Q:p14 – Post-term newborn

P08.21 **Post-term newborn**

Newborn with gestation period over 40 completed weeks to 42 completed weeks

P08.22 **Prolonged gestation of newborn**

Newborn with gestation period over 42 completed weeks (294 days or more), not heavy- or large-for-dates

Postmaturity NOS

Abnormal findings on neonatal screening (P09)

P09 **Abnormal findings on neonatal screening**

Use additional code to identify signs, symptoms and conditions associated with the screening

Excludes ❷: *nonspecific serologic evidence of human immunodeficiency virus [HIV] (R75)*

Excludes 1: = NOT CODED HERE! (Do not code both)

Excludes ❷: = Not Included Here

P07-P09

Birth trauma (P10-P15)

P10-   <u>Intracranial laceration and hemorrhage due to birth injury</u>
Excludes 1:   intracranial hemorrhage of newborn NOS (P52.9)
    intracranial hemorrhage of newborn due to anoxia or hypoxia
    (P52.-)
    nontraumatic intracranial hemorrhage of newborn (P52.-)

MCC **P10.0**   **Subdural hemorrhage due to birth injury** — The escape of blood below the dura of the infant.
    Subdural hematoma (localized) due to birth injury
    Excludes 1:   subdural hemorrhage accompanying tentorial tear (P10.4)

MCC **P10.1**   **Cerebral hemorrhage due to birth injury** — The escape of blood within the cerebrum of the infant.

CC **P10.2**   **Intraventricular hemorrhage due to birth injury** — The escape of blood within the cerebral ventricles of the infant.

MCC **P10.3**   **Subarachnoid hemorrhage due to birth injury** — The escape of blood below the subarachnoid layer of the meninges of the infant.

MCC **P10.4**   **Tentorial tear due to birth injury** — The disruption of the dura that covers the cerebellum and supports the occipital lobes.

MCC **P10.8**   **Other intracranial lacerations and hemorrhages due to birth injury**

MCC **P10.9**   **Unspecified intracranial laceration and hemorrhage due to birth injury**

P11-   <u>Other</u> birth injuries to <u>central nervous system</u>
MCC **P11.0**   **Cerebral edema due to birth injury** — The accumulation of fluid on the brain.

P11.1   **Other specified brain damage due to birth injury**

MCC **P11.2**   **Unspecified brain damage due to birth injury**

P11.3   **Birth injury to facial nerve** — Traumatic damage to a facial nerve during, or due to, birth.
    Facial palsy due to birth injury

P11.4   **Birth injury to other cranial nerves**

P11.5   **Birth injury to spine and spinal cord** — Traumatic damage to the spine and spinal cord during, or due to, birth.
    Fracture of spine due to birth injury

MCC **P11.9**   **Birth injury to central nervous system, unspecified**

P12-   **Birth injury to <u>scalp</u>** — The traumatic damage to the infant's scalp during, or due to, birth.
P12.0   **Cephalhematoma due to birth injury** — The subcutaneous swelling of the head with blood, often from the application of forceps during delivery.

P12.1   **Chignon (from vacuum extraction) due to birth injury** — The temporary swelling of the scalp due to the suction from the vacuum cap.

CC **P12.2**   **Epicranial subaponeurotic hemorrhage due to birth injury** — The accumulation of blood due to the rupture of blood vessels in the dense connective tissue of the scalp.
    Subgaleal hemorrhage

P12.3   **Bruising of scalp due to birth injury**

P12.4   **Injury of scalp of newborn due to monitoring equipment**
    Sampling incision of scalp of newborn
    Scalp clip (electrode) injury of newborn

P12.8-   **Other birth injuries to scalp**
    P12.81   **Caput succedaneum** — The swelling edema of the scalp produced during labor.
    P12.89   **Other birth injuries to scalp**

P12.9   **Birth injury to scalp, unspecified**

P13-   **Birth injury to <u>skeleton</u>**
Excludes ❷: birth injury to spine (P11.5)

P13.0   **Fracture of skull due to birth injury**

P13.1   **Other birth injuries to skull**
    Excludes 1:   cephalhematoma (P12.0)

P13.2   **Birth injury to femur**

P13.3   **Birth injury to other long bones**

P13.4   **Fracture of clavicle due to birth injury**

P13.8   **Birth injuries to other parts of skeleton**

P13.9   **Birth injury to skeleton, unspecified**

P14-   **Birth injury to <u>peripheral nervous system</u>**
P14.0   **Erb's paralysis due to birth injury** — The loss of the function of small muscles in the hand, due to injury to the fifth and sixth cervical roots.

P14.1   **Klumpke's paralysis due to birth injury** — The loss of muscular control of the arm due to injury of the eighth cervical and first dorsal nerve roots.

P14.2   **Phrenic nerve paralysis due to birth injury** — The loss or impairment of function of the nerve that innervates the pleura, pericardium, diaphragm, peritoneum, and sympathetic plexuses.

P14.3   **Other brachial plexus birth injuries**

P14.8   **Birth injuries to other parts of peripheral nervous system**

P14.9   **Birth injury to peripheral nervous system, unspecified**

P15-   <u>Other birth injuries</u>
P15.0   **Birth injury to liver**
    Rupture of liver due to birth injury

P15.1   **Birth injury to spleen**
    Rupture of spleen due to birth injury

P15.2   **Sternomastoid injury due to birth injury**

P15.3   **Birth injury to eye**
    Subconjunctival hemorrhage due to birth injury
    Traumatic glaucoma due to birth injury

P15.4   **Birth injury to face**
    Facial congestion due to birth injury

P15.5   **Birth injury to external genitalia**

P15.6   **Subcutaneous fat necrosis due to birth injury**

P15.8   **Other specified birth injuries**

P15.9   **Birth injury, unspecified**

Respiratory and cardiovascular disorders specific to the perinatal period (P19-P29)

P19-   **Metabolic acidemia in newborn** — The metabolic disturbance of the normal acid-base balance of the fetus or infant.
    Includes: Metabolic acidemia in newborn

P19.0   **Metabolic acidemia in newborn first noted before onset of labor**

P19.1   **Metabolic acidemia in newborn first noted during labor**

P19.2   **Metabolic acidemia noted at birth**

P19.9   **Metabolic acidemia, unspecified**

P22-   <u>Respiratory distress of newborn</u>
Excludes 1:   respiratory arrest of newborn (P28.81)
    respiratory failure of newborn NOS (P28.5)

MCC **P22.0**   **Respiratory distress syndrome of newborn** — The acute lung underdevelopment condition of the newborn that is characterized by airless alveoli, inelastic lungs, cyanosis, and rapid respirations.
    Cardiorespiratory distress syndrome of newborn
    Hyaline membrane disease
    Idiopathic respiratory distress syndrome [IRDS or RDS] of newborn
    Pulmonary hypoperfusion syndrome
    Respiratory distress syndrome, type I

P22.1   **Transient tachypnea of newborn** — The nonsustained excessive rapidity of respiration.
    Idiopathic tachypnea of newborn
    Respiratory distress syndrome, type II
    Wet lung syndrome — The condition of pulmonary impairment due to excessive and delayed absorption of fluid in the lungs.

P22.8   **Other respiratory distress of newborn**

P22.9   **Respiratory distress of newborn, unspecified**

P10 - P22

P23- <u>Congenital pneumonia</u> — The inflammation of the lungs with exudate-filled air spaces that is present at birth.
    Includes: Infective pneumonia acquired in utero or during birth
    Excludes 1: *neonatal pneumonia resulting from aspiration (P24.-)*

MCC **P23.0** **Congenital pneumonia due to viral agent**
    Use additional code (B97) to identify organism
    Excludes 1: *congenital rubella pneumonitis (P35.0)*

MCC **P23.1** **Congenital pneumonia due to Chlamydia**

MCC **P23.2** **Congenital pneumonia due to staphylococcus**

MCC **P23.3** **Congenital pneumonia due to streptococcus, group B**

MCC **P23.4** **Congenital pneumonia due to Escherichia coli**

MCC **P23.5** **Congenital pneumonia due to Pseudomonas**

MCC **P23.6** **Congenital pneumonia due to other bacterial agents**
    Congenital pneumonia due to Hemophilus influenzae
    Congenital pneumonia due to Klebsiella pneumoniae
    Congenital pneumonia due to Mycoplasma
    Congenital pneumonia due to Streptococcus, except group B
    Use additional code (B95-B96) to identify organism

MCC **P23.8** **Congenital pneumonia due to other organisms**

MCC **P23.9** **Congenital pneumonia, unspecified**

P24- <u>Neonatal aspiration</u> — The inhalation of fluid into the lungs that may result in a significant respiratory compromise.
    Includes: Aspiration in utero and during delivery

    P24.0- <u>Meconium aspiration</u> — The inhalation of fetal intestinal meconium.
        Excludes 1: *meconium passage (without aspiration) during delivery (P03.82)*
        meconium staining (P96.83)

      P24.00 **Meconium aspiration <u>without</u> respiratory symptoms**
        Meconium aspiration NOS

   MCC **P24.01** **Meconium aspiration <u>with respiratory symptoms</u>**
        Meconium aspiration pneumonia
        Meconium aspiration pneumonitis
        Meconium aspiration syndrome NOS
        Use additional code to identify any secondary pulmonary hypertension, if applicable (I27.2)

    P24.1- **Neonatal aspiration of (clear) <u>amniotic fluid</u> and mucus** — The inhalation of the non-meconium stained amniotic fluid.
        Neonatal aspiration of liquor (amnii)

      P24.10 **Neonatal aspiration of (clear) amniotic fluid and mucus <u>without</u> respiratory symptoms**
        Neonatal aspiration of amniotic fluid and mucus NOS

   MCC **P24.11** **Neonatal aspiration of (clear) amniotic fluid and mucus <u>with respiratory symptoms</u>**
        Neonatal aspiration of amniotic fluid and mucus with pneumonia
        Neonatal aspiration of amniotic fluid and mucus with pneumonitis
        Use additional code to identify any secondary pulmonary hypertension, if applicable (I27.2)

    P24.2- **Neonatal aspiration of <u>blood</u>** — The inhalation of blood.

      P24.20 **Neonatal aspiration of blood <u>without</u> respiratory symptoms**
        Neonatal aspiration of blood NOS

   MCC **P24.21** **Neonatal aspiration of blood <u>with respiratory symptoms</u>**
        Neonatal aspiration of blood with pneumonia
        Neonatal aspiration of blood with pneumonitis
        Use additional code to identify any secondary pulmonary hypertension, if applicable (I27.2)

    P24.3- **Neonatal aspiration of <u>milk and regurgitated food</u>**
        Neonatal aspiration of stomach contents

      P24.30 **Neonatal aspiration of milk and regurgitated food <u>without</u> respiratory symptoms**
        Neonatal aspiration of milk and regurgitated food NOS

   MCC **P24.31** **Neonatal aspiration of milk and regurgitated food <u>with respiratory symptoms</u>**
        Neonatal aspiration of milk and regurgitated food with pneumonia
        Neonatal aspiration of milk and regurgitated food with pneumonitis
        Use additional code to identify any secondary pulmonary hypertension, if applicable (I27.2)

    P24.8- **<u>Other</u> neonatal aspiration**

      P24.80 **Other neonatal aspiration <u>without</u> respiratory symptoms**
        Neonatal aspiration NEC

   MCC **P24.81** **Other neonatal aspiration <u>with respiratory symptoms</u>**
        Neonatal aspiration pneumonia NEC
        Neonatal aspiration with pneumonitis NEC
        Neonatal aspiration with pneumonia NOS
        Neonatal aspiration with pneumonitis NOS
        Use additional code to identify any secondary pulmonary hypertension, if applicable (I27.2)

    P24.9 **Neonatal aspiration, <u>unspecified</u>**

P25- <u>Interstitial emphysema</u> and related conditions originating in the perinatal period

MCC **P25.0** **Interstitial emphysema originating in the perinatal period** — The presence of air in the peribronchial and interstitial tissues of the lungs.

MCC **P25.1** **Pneumothorax originating in the perinatal period** — The accumulation of air or gas in the pleural space.

MCC **P25.2** **Pneumomediastinum originating in the perinatal period** — The presence of air or gas in the mediastinum.

MCC **P25.3** **Pneumopericardium originating in the perinatal period** — The presence of air or gas in the pericardium.

MCC **P25.8** **Other conditions related to interstitial emphysema originating in the perinatal period**

P26- <u>Pulmonary hemorrhage</u> originating in the perinatal period — The escape of blood from the lungs.
    Excludes 1: *acute idiopathic hemorrhage in infants over 28 days old (R04.81)*

MCC **P26.0** **Tracheobronchial hemorrhage originating in the perinatal period**

MCC **P26.1** **Massive pulmonary hemorrhage originating in the perinatal period**

MCC **P26.8** **Other pulmonary hemorrhages originating in the perinatal period**

MCC **P26.9** **Unspecified pulmonary hemorrhage originating in the perinatal period**

P27- <u>Chronic respiratory disease</u> originating in the perinatal period
    Excludes 1: *respiratory distress of newborn (P22.0-P22.9)*

MCC **P27.0** **Wilson-Mikity syndrome** — Pulmonary insufficiency caused by the presence of multiple cyst-like areas of hyperaeration with thickening of the interstitial tissues.
    Pulmonary dysmaturity

MCC **P27.1** **Bronchopulmonary dysplasia originating in the perinatal period**

MCC **P27.8** **Other chronic respiratory diseases originating in the perinatal period**
    Congenital pulmonary fibrosis — The formation of fibrous tissue around the pulmonary alveolar walls.
    Ventilator lung in newborn

MCC **P27.9** **Unspecified chronic respiratory disease originating in the perinatal period**

P28-   <u>Other respiratory conditions</u> originating in the perinatal period
Excludes 1:   *congenital malformations of the respiratory system (Q30-Q34)*

CC **P28.0**   **Primary atelectasis of newborn** — The imperfect expansion of the lungs immediately after birth.
     Primary failure to expand terminal respiratory units
     Pulmonary hypoplasia associated with short gestation
     Pulmonary immaturity NOS

P28.1-   **Other and unspecified atelectasis of newborn**

CC **P28.10**   **Unspecified atelectasis of newborn**
     Atelectasis of newborn NOS

CC **P28.11**   **Resorption atelectasis without respiratory distress syndrome**
Excludes 1:   *resorption atelectasis with respiratory distress syndrome (P22.0)*

CC **P28.19**   **Other atelectasis of newborn**
     Partial atelectasis of newborn
     Secondary atelectasis of newborn

CC **P28.2**   **Cyanotic attacks of newborn** — The sudden, severe condition of reduced hemoglobin concentration in the blood characterized by bluish or purple skin discoloration.
Excludes 1:   *apnea of newborn (P28.3-P28.4)*

CC **P28.3**   **Primary sleep apnea of newborn** — The abnormal, periodic cessation of breathing due to a lack of sufficient neural impulses to the respiratory system.
     Central sleep apnea of newborn
     Obstructive sleep apnea of newborn
     Sleep apnea of newborn NOS

CC **P28.4**   **Other apnea of newborn**
     Apnea of prematurity
     Obstructive apnea of newborn
Excludes 1:   *obstructive sleep apnea of newborn (P28.3)*

MCC **P28.5**   **Respiratory failure of newborn** — The sudden onset of severely decreased pulmonary function.
Excludes 1:   *respiratory arrest of newborn (P28.81)*
             respiratory distress of newborn (P22.0-)

P28.8-   **Other specified respiratory conditions of newborn**

MCC **P28.81**   **Respiratory arrest of newborn** — The cessation of breathing.

P28.89   **Other specified respiratory conditions of newborn**
     Congenital laryngeal stridor
     Sniffles in newborn
     Snuffles in newborn
Excludes 1:   *early congenital syphilitic rhinitis (A50.05)*

P28.9   **Respiratory condition of newborn, unspecified**
     Respiratory depression in newborn

P29-   <u>Cardiovascular disorders</u> originating in the perinatal period
Excludes 1:   *congenital malformations of the circulatory system (Q20-Q28)*

P29.0   **Neonatal cardiac failure** — The decreased ability of the heart to pump enough blood to meet the needs of the body's tissues.

P29.1-   **Neonatal cardiac dysrhythmia**

P29.11   **Neonatal tachycardia** — An abnormal, persistent rapid fetal heart rate.

P29.12   **Neonatal bradycardia** — An abnormal, persistent slow fetal heart rate.

P29.2   **Neonatal hypertension** — Abnormally elevated blood pressure.

MCC **P29.3**   **Persistent fetal circulation** — The progressive, severe decrease in the oxygenation of the blood due to the failure of the newborn's circulation to change from the fetal circulation to the normal air-breathing circulation.
     Delayed closure of ductus arteriosus
     (Persistent) pulmonary hypertension of newborn

P29.4   **Transient myocardial ischemia in newborn**

P29.8-   **Other cardiovascular disorders originating in the perinatal period**

MCC **P29.81**   **Cardiac arrest of newborn** — The cessation of cardiac function.

P29.89   **Other cardiovascular disorders originating in the perinatal period**
     AHA 14:4Q:p23 – Possible systolic ejection murmur

P29.9   **Cardiovascular disorder originating in the perinatal period, unspecified**

Infections specific to the perinatal period (P35-P39)

Infections acquired in utero, during birth via the umbilicus, or during the first 28 days after birth
Excludes ❷: *asymptomatic human immunodeficiency virus [HIV] infection status (Z21)*
          congenital gonococcal infection (A54.-)
          congenital pneumonia (P23.-)
          congenital syphilis (A50.-)
          human immunodeficiency virus [HIV] disease (B20)
          infant botulism (A48.51)
          infectious diseases not specific to the perinatal period (A00-B99, J09, J10.-)
          intestinal infectious disease (A00-A09)
          laboratory evidence of human immunodeficiency virus [HIV] (R75)
          tetanus neonatorum (A33)

P35-   <u>Congenital viral diseases</u>
Includes: Infections acquired in utero or during birth

CC **P35.0**   **Congenital rubella syndrome**
     Congenital rubella pneumonitis

MCC **P35.1**   **Congenital cytomegalovirus infection**

MCC **P35.2**   **Congenital herpesviral [herpes simplex] infection**

MCC **P35.3**   **Congenital viral hepatitis**

MCC **P35.8**   **Other congenital viral diseases**
     Congenital varicella [chickenpox]

MCC **P35.9**   **Congenital viral disease, unspecified**

P36-   <u>Bacterial sepsis</u> of newborn — The infectious disease of the newborn that is due to the accumulation and persistence of bacteria and/or their toxins in the blood.
Includes: Congenital sepsis
Use additional code(s), if applicable, to identify severe sepsis (R65.2-) and associated acute organ dysfunction(s)

MCC **P36.0**   **Sepsis of newborn due to streptococcus, group B**

P36.1-   **Sepsis of newborn due to other and unspecified streptococci**

MCC **P36.10**   **Sepsis of newborn due to unspecified streptococci**

MCC **P36.19**   **Sepsis of newborn due to other streptococci**

MCC **P36.2**   **Sepsis of newborn due to Staphylococcus aureus**

P36.3-   **Sepsis of newborn due to other and unspecified staphylococci**

MCC **P36.30**   **Sepsis of newborn due to unspecified staphylococci**

MCC **P36.39**   **Sepsis of newborn due to other staphylococci**

MCC **P36.4**   **Sepsis of newborn due to Escherichia coli**

MCC **P36.5**   **Sepsis of newborn due to anaerobes**

MCC **P36.8**   **Other bacterial sepsis of newborn**
     Use additional code from category B96 to identify organism

MCC **P36.9**   **Bacterial sepsis of newborn, unspecified**

P37-   <u>Other congenital</u> infectious and parasitic diseases
Excludes ❷: *congenital syphilis (A50.-)*
          infectious neonatal diarrhea (A00-A09)
          necrotizing enterocolitis in newborn (P77.-)
          noninfectious neonatal diarrhea (P78.3)
          ophthalmia neonatorum due to gonococcus (A54.31)
          tetanus neonatorum (A33)

MCC **P37.0**   **Congenital tuberculosis**

MCC **P37.1**   **Congenital toxoplasmosis**
     Hydrocephalus due to congenital toxoplasmosis

MCC **P37.2**   **Neonatal (disseminated) listeriosis**

MCC **P37.3**   **Congenital falciparum malaria**

MCC **P37.4**   **Other congenital malaria**

P37.5   **Neonatal candidiasis**

MCC **P37.8**   **Other specified congenital infectious and parasitic diseases**

MCC **P37.9**   **Congenital infectious or parasitic disease, unspecified**

P28 | P37

P38- **Omphalitis** of newborn — Inflamation of the umbilicus.
  Excludes 1:   omphalitis not of newborn (L08.82)
             tetanus omphalitis (A33)
             umbilical hemorrhage of newborn (P51.-)

CC **P38.1** **Omphalitis with mild hemorrhage**

CC **P38.9** **Omphalitis without hemorrhage**
      Omphalitis of newborn NOS

P39- **Other infections** specific to the perinatal period
     Use additional code to identify organism or specific infection

CC **P39.0** **Neonatal infective mastitis** — Inflammation of the newborn breast.
      Excludes 1:   breast engorgement of newborn (P83.4)
                  noninfective mastitis of newborn (P83.4)

P39.1 **Neonatal conjunctivitis and dacryocystitis** — Inflammation of the
     conjunctiva and/or lacrimal sac.
      Neonatal chlamydial conjunctivitis
      Ophthalmia neonatorum NOS
      Excludes 1:   gonococcal conjunctivitis (A54.31)

CC **P39.2** **Intra-amniotic infection affecting newborn, not elsewhere classified**

CC **P39.3** **Neonatal urinary tract infection**

CC **P39.4** **Neonatal skin infection**
      Neonatal pyoderma
      Excludes 1:   pemphigus neonatorum (L00)
                  staphylococcal scalded skin syndrome (L00)

CC **P39.8** **Other specified infections specific to the perinatal period**

CC **P39.9** **Infection specific to the perinatal period, unspecified**

Hemorrhagic and hematological disorders of newborn (P50-P61)

Excludes 1:   congenital stenosis and stricture of bile ducts (Q44.3)
          Crigler-Najjar syndrome (E80.5)
          Dubin-Johnson syndrome (E80.6)
          Gilbert syndrome (E80.4)
          hereditary hemolytic anemias (D55-D58)

P50- **Newborn affected by** **intrauterine (fetal) blood loss** — The diminished
     blood volume of the fetus that affects the fetus and newborn.
      Excludes 1:   congenital anemia from intrauterine (fetal) blood loss (P61.3)

P50.0 **Newborn affected by intrauterine (fetal) blood loss from vasa previa**

P50.1 **Newborn affected by intrauterine (fetal) blood loss from ruptured cord**

P50.2 **Newborn affected by intrauterine (fetal) blood loss from placenta**

P50.3 **Newborn affected by hemorrhage into co-twin**

P50.4 **Newborn affected by hemorrhage into maternal circulation**

P50.5 **Newborn affected by intrauterine (fetal) blood loss from cut end of co-twin's cord**

P50.8 **Newborn affected by other intrauterine (fetal) blood loss**

P50.9 **Newborn affected by intrauterine (fetal) blood loss, unspecified**
      Newborn affected by fetal hemorrhage NOS

P51- **Umbilical hemorrhage** of newborn — The escape of blood from the umbilicus.
  Excludes 1:   omphalitis with mild hemorrhage (P38.1)
             umbilical hemorrhage from cut end of co-twins cord (P50.5)

P51.0 **Massive umbilical hemorrhage of newborn**

P51.8 **Other umbilical hemorrhages of newborn**
      Slipped umbilical ligature NOS

P51.9 **Umbilical hemorrhage of newborn, unspecified**

P52- **Intracranial nontraumatic hemorrhage** of newborn — The escape of blood
     within the skull.
      Includes: Intracranial hemorrhage due to anoxia or hypoxia
      Excludes 1:   intracranial hemorrhage due to birth injury (P10.-)
                  intracranial hemorrhage due to other injury (S06.-)

CC **P52.0** **Intraventricular (nontraumatic) hemorrhage, grade 1, of newborn**
      Subependymal hemorrhage (without intraventricular extension)
      Bleeding into germinal matrix

CC **P52.1** **Intraventricular (nontraumatic) hemorrhage, grade 2, of newborn** — The escape of blood into the ventricles of the brain.
      Subependymal hemorrhage with intraventricular extension
      Bleeding into ventricle

P52.2- **Intraventricular (nontraumatic) hemorrhage, grade 3 and grade 4, of newborn**

MCC **P52.21** **Intraventricular (nontraumatic) hemorrhage, grade 3, of newborn**
      Subependymal hemorrhage with intraventricular extension with enlargement of ventricle

MCC **P52.22** **Intraventricular (nontraumatic) hemorrhage, grade 4, of newborn**
      Bleeding into cerebral cortex
      Subependymal hemorrhage with intracerebral extension

CC **P52.3** **Unspecified intraventricular (nontraumatic) hemorrhage of newborn**

MCC **P52.4** **Intracerebral (nontraumatic) hemorrhage of newborn** — The escape of blood within the brain.

MCC **P52.5** **Subarachnoid (nontraumatic) hemorrhage of newborn** — The escape of blood into the subarachnoid space.

MCC **P52.6** **Cerebellar (nontraumatic) and posterior fossa hemorrhage of newborn**

MCC **P52.8** **Other intracranial (nontraumatic) hemorrhages of newborn**

MCC **P52.9** **Intracranial (nontraumatic) hemorrhage of newborn, unspecified**

P53 **Hemorrhagic disease of newborn** — A bleeding disorder of the
CC   newborn that is caused by a transient vitamin K deficiency.
      Vitamin K deficiency of newborn

P54- **Other neonatal hemorrhages**
  Excludes 1:   newborn affected by (intrauterine) blood loss (P50.-)
             pulmonary hemorrhage originating in the perinatal period (P26.-)

P54.0 **Neonatal hematemesis** — The presence of blood in the vomitus.
      Excludes 1:   neonatal hematemesis due to swallowed maternal blood (P78.2)

MCC **P54.1** **Neonatal melena** — The presence of black, tarry stools due to blood in the feces.
      Excludes 1:   neonatal melena due to swallowed maternal blood (P78.2)

MCC **P54.2** **Neonatal rectal hemorrhage** — The escape of blood from the rectum.

MCC **P54.3** **Other neonatal gastrointestinal hemorrhage** — The escape of blood from the gastrointestinal tract.

CC **P54.4** **Neonatal adrenal hemorrhage** — The escape of blood from the adrenals.

P54.5 **Neonatal cutaneous hemorrhage** — The escape of blood from the skin.
      Neonatal bruising
      Neonatal ecchymoses
      Neonatal petechiae
      Neonatal superficial hematoma
      Excludes ❷: bruising of scalp due to birth injury (P12.3)
                  cephalhematoma due to birth injury (P12.0)

P54.6 **Neonatal vaginal hemorrhage** — [♀] — The escape of blood from the vagina.
      Neonatal pseudomenses

P54.8 **Other specified neonatal hemorrhages**

P54.9 **Neonatal hemorrhage, unspecified**

P
3
8
–
P
5
4

P55-   Hemolytic disease of newborn — The premature destruction of red blood cells of the fetus or newborn.

P55.0   **Rh isoimmunization of newborn** — The premature destruction of red blood cells of the fetus or newborn that is caused by an antigen-antibody reaction of fetal/maternal blood group incompatibility.

P55.1   **ABO isoimmunization of newborn** — The premature destruction of mature red blood cells due to an ABO fetal/maternal blood group incompatibility.
AHA 15:3Q:p20 – ABO incompatibility and Coombs test

P55.8   **Other hemolytic diseases of newborn**

P55.9   **Hemolytic disease of newborn, unspecified**

P56-   Hydrops fetalis due to hemolytic disease
Excludes 1:   hydrops fetalis NOS (P83.2)

MCC **P56.0**   **Hydrops fetalis due to isoimmunization** — The accumulation of massive edema of the newborn that is usually associated with erythroblastosis.

P56.9-   **Hydrops fetalis due to other and unspecified hemolytic disease**

MCC **P56.90**   **Hydrops fetalis due to unspecified hemolytic disease**

MCC **P56.99**   **Hydrops fetalis due to other hemolytic disease**

P57-   Kernicterus

MCC **P57.0**   **Kernicterus due to isoimmunization** — The toxic accumulation of bilirubin in the brain that is due to isoimmunization.

MCC **P57.8**   **Other specified kernicterus**
Excludes 1:   Crigler-Najjar syndrome (E80.5)

MCC **P57.9**   **Kernicterus, unspecified**

P58-   Neonatal jaundice due to other excessive hemolysis — The deposition of yellow bile pigment in the skin due to the premature destruction of blood cells.
Excludes 1:   jaundice due to isoimmunization (P55-P57)

P58.0   **Neonatal jaundice due to bruising**

P58.1   **Neonatal jaundice due to bleeding**

P58.2   **Neonatal jaundice due to infection**

P58.3   **Neonatal jaundice due to polycythemia**

P58.4-   **Neonatal jaundice due to drugs or toxins transmitted from mother or given to newborn**
Code first poisoning due to drug or toxin, if applicable (T36-T65 with fifth or sixth character 1-4 or 6)
Use additional code for adverse effect, if applicable, to identify drug (T36-T50 with fifth or sixth character 5)

P58.41   **Neonatal jaundice due to drugs or toxins transmitted from mother**

P58.42   **Neonatal jaundice due to drugs or toxins given to newborn**

P58.5   **Neonatal jaundice due to swallowed maternal blood**

P58.8   **Neonatal jaundice due to other specified excessive hemolysis**

P58.9   **Neonatal jaundice due to excessive hemolysis, unspecified**

P59-   Neonatal jaundice from other and unspecified causes
AHA 15:3Q:p20 – Hyperbilirubinemia documentation
Excludes 1:   jaundice due to inborn errors of metabolism (E70-E88)
                  kernicterus (P57.-)

P59.0   **Neonatal jaundice associated with preterm delivery** — The deposition of yellow bile pigment in the skin that occurs in preterm infants.
Hyperbilirubinemia of prematurity
Jaundice due to delayed conjugation associated with preterm delivery

MCC **P59.1**   **Inspissated bile syndrome** — The deposition of yellow bile pigment in the skin due to an obstruction of the biliary system.

P59.2-   **Neonatal jaundice from other and unspecified hepatocellular damage** — The deposition of yellow bile pigment in the skin due to an injury to the liver tissue.
Excludes 1:   congenital viral hepatitis (P35.3)

MCC **P59.20**   **Neonatal jaundice from unspecified hepatocellular damage**

MCC **P59.29**   **Neonatal jaundice from other hepatocellular damage**
Neonatal giant cell hepatitis
Neonatal (idiopathic) hepatitis

P59.3   **Neonatal jaundice from breast milk inhibitor**

P59.8   **Neonatal jaundice from other specified causes**

P59.9   **Neonatal jaundice, unspecified**
Neonatal physiological jaundice (intense) (prolonged) NOS

P60   Disseminated intravascular coagulation of newborn — A blood
MCC coagulation disorder in the newborn that is associated with fibrinolysis.
Defibrination syndrome of newborn

P61-   Other perinatal hematological disorders
Excludes 1:   transient hypogammaglobulinemia of infancy (D80.7)

MCC **P61.0**   **Transient neonatal thrombocytopenia** — The temporary decrease in the number of blood platelets in the newborn.
Neonatal thrombocytopenia due to exchange transfusion
Neonatal thrombocytopenia due to idiopathic maternal thrombocytopenia
Neonatal thrombocytopenia due to isoimmunization

P61.1   **Polycythemia neonatorum** — An abnormally increased red blood cell mass in the newborn.

CC **P61.2**   **Anemia of prematurity** — An abnormal reduction of red blood cells in a premature infant.

CC **P61.3**   **Congenital anemia from fetal blood loss** — An abnormal reduction of red blood cells in the newborn due to hemorrhage or other loss of fetal blood.

CC **P61.4**   **Other congenital anemias, not elsewhere classified**
Congenital anemia NOS

MCC **P61.5**   **Transient neonatal neutropenia** — A temporary reduction in the number of neutrophilic leukocytes in the newborn.
Excludes 1:   congenital neutropenia (nontransient) (D70.0)

CC **P61.6**   **Other transient neonatal disorders of coagulation**

P61.8   **Other specified perinatal hematological disorders**

P61.9   **Perinatal hematological disorder, unspecified**

Transitory endocrine and metabolic disorders specific to newborn (P70-P74)

Includes: Transitory endocrine and metabolic disturbances caused by the infant's response to maternal endocrine and metabolic factors, or its adjustment to extrauterine environment

P70-   Transitory disorders of carbohydrate metabolism specific to newborn

P70.0   **Syndrome of infant of mother with gestational diabetes**
Newborn (with hypoglycemia) affected by maternal gestational diabetes
Excludes 1:   newborn (with hypoglycemia) affected by maternal (pre-existing) diabetes mellitus (P70.1)
                  syndrome of infant of a diabetic mother (P70.1)

P70.1   **Syndrome of infant of a diabetic mother**
Newborn (with hypoglycemia) affected by maternal (pre-existing) diabetes mellitus
Excludes 1:   newborn (with hypoglycemia) affected by maternal gestational diabetes (P70.0)
                  syndrome of infant of mother with gestational diabetes (P70.0)

CC **P70.2**   **Neonatal diabetes mellitus** — The metabolic syndrome of faulty pancreatic activity of the newborn.

P70.3   **Iatrogenic neonatal hypoglycemia**

P70.4   **Other neonatal hypoglycemia**
Transitory neonatal hypoglycemia — The abnormally low glucose level of the newborn.

CC **P70.8**   **Other transitory disorders of carbohydrate metabolism of newborn**

P70.9   **Transitory disorder of carbohydrate metabolism of newborn, unspecified**

P71-   Transitory neonatal disorders of calcium and magnesium metabolism

CC **P71.0**   **Cow's milk hypocalcemia in newborn** — The abnormally low levels of calcium in the newborn due the excessive amount of phosphates in cow's milk.

CC **P71.1**   **Other neonatal hypocalcemia**
Excludes 1:   neonatal hypoparathyroidism (P71.4)

CC **P71.2**   **Neonatal hypomagnesemia** — The abnormally low levels of magnesium in the newborn.

CC **P71.3**   **Neonatal tetany without calcium or magnesium deficiency**
Neonatal tetany NOS

CC **P71.4**   **Transitory neonatal hypoparathyroidism**

CC **P71.8**   **Other transitory neonatal disorders of calcium and magnesium metabolism**

CC **P71.9**   **Transitory neonatal disorder of calcium and magnesium metabolism, unspecified**

P 5 5 - P 7 1

P72- Other transitory neonatal endocrine disorders
  Excludes 1: *congenital hypothyroidism with or without goiter (E03.0-E03.1)*
    dyshormogenetic goiter (E07.1)
    Pendred's syndrome (E07.1)

cc **P72.0 Neonatal goiter, not elsewhere classified**
    Transitory congenital goiter with normal functioning

cc **P72.1 Transitory neonatal hyperthyroidism** — The disorder of excessive circulating thyroid hormones of the newborn.
    Neonatal thyrotoxicosis

cc **P72.2 Other transitory neonatal disorders of thyroid function, not elsewhere classified**
    Transitory neonatal hypothyroidism

cc **P72.8 Other specified transitory neonatal endocrine disorders**

P72.9 Transitory neonatal endocrine disorder, unspecified

P74- Other transitory neonatal electrolyte and metabolic disturbances

MCC **P74.0 Late metabolic acidosis of newborn** — The disturbance of the acid-base status of the newborn.
    Excludes 1: *(fetal) metabolic acidosis of newborn (P19)*

P74.1 Dehydration of newborn

P74.2 Disturbances of sodium balance of newborn

P74.3 Disturbances of potassium balance of newborn

P74.4 Other transitory electrolyte disturbances of newborn

cc **P74.5 Transitory tyrosinemia of newborn**

cc **P74.6 Transitory hyperammonemia of newborn**

cc **P74.8 Other transitory metabolic disturbances of newborn**
    Amino-acid metabolic disorders described as transitory

P74.9 Transitory metabolic disturbance of newborn, unspecified

Digestive system disorders of newborn (P76-P78)

P76- Other intestinal obstruction of newborn

P76.0 Meconium plug syndrome — The blocking of the intestine that is due to unusually thick or hard meconium.
    Meconium ileus NOS
    Excludes 1: *meconium ileus in cystic fibrosis (E84.11)*

cc **P76.1 Transitory ileus of newborn** — The temporary obstruction of the newborn's intestine.
    Excludes 1: *Hirschsprung's disease (Q43.1)*

P76.2 Intestinal obstruction due to inspissated milk — The blocking of the intestine that is due to unusual thickening of the milk in the intestine.

P76.8 Other specified intestinal obstruction of newborn
    Excludes 1: *intestinal obstruction classifiable to K56.-*

P76.9 Intestinal obstruction of newborn, unspecified

P77- Necrotizing enterocolitis of newborn — A gastrointestinal disorder involving infection and inflammation that mostly affects premature infants and results in weakening and destruction of the intestinal tissues.

MCC **P77.1 Stage 1 necrotizing enterocolitis in newborn**
    Necrotizing enterocolitis without pneumatosis, without perforation

MCC **P77.2 Stage 2 necrotizing enterocolitis in newborn**
    Necrotizing enterocolitis with pneumatosis, without perforation

MCC **P77.3 Stage 3 necrotizing enterocolitis in newborn**
    Necrotizing enterocolitis with perforation
    Necrotizing enterocolitis with pneumatosis and perforation

MCC **P77.9 Necrotizing enterocolitis in newborn, unspecified**
    Necrotizing enterocolitis in newborn, NOS

P78- Other perinatal digestive system disorders
  Excludes 1: *cystic fibrosis (E84.0-E84.9)*
    neonatal gastrointestinal hemorrhages (P54.0-P54.3)

MCC **P78.0 Perinatal intestinal perforation** — The tearing through the wall of the intestine.
    Meconium peritonitis — Inflammation of the peritoneum in the newborn due to escaped meconium.

P78.1 Other neonatal peritonitis
    Neonatal peritonitis NOS

P78.2 Neonatal hematemesis and melena due to swallowed maternal blood

P78.3 Noninfective neonatal diarrhea
    Neonatal diarrhea NOS

P78.8- Other specified perinatal digestive system disorders

P78.81 Congenital cirrhosis (of liver)

P78.82 Peptic ulcer of newborn

P78.83 Newborn esophageal reflux
    Neonatal esophageal reflux

P78.89 Other specified perinatal digestive system disorders

P78.9 Perinatal digestive system disorder, unspecified

Conditions involving the integument and temperature regulation of newborn (P80-P83)

P80- Hypothermia of newborn

P80.0 Cold injury syndrome
    Severe and usually chronic hypothermia associated with a pink flushed appearance, edema and neurological and biochemical abnormalities
    Excludes 1: *mild hypothermia of newborn (P80.8)*

P80.8 Other hypothermia of newborn
    Mild hypothermia of newborn

P80.9 Hypothermia of newborn, unspecified

P81- Other disturbances of temperature regulation of newborn

P81.0 Environmental hyperthermia of newborn

P81.8 Other specified disturbances of temperature regulation of newborn

P81.9 Disturbance of temperature regulation of newborn, unspecified
    Fever of newborn NOS

P83- Other conditions of integument specific to newborn
  Excludes 1: *congenital malformations of skin and integument (Q80-Q84)*
    hydrops fetalis due to hemolytic disease (P56.-)
    neonatal skin infection (P39.4)
    staphylococcal scalded skin syndrome (L00)
  Excludes ❷: *cradle cap (L21.0)*
    diaper [napkin] dermatitis (L22)

cc **P83.0 Sclerema neonatorum** — The abnormal hardening of the subcutaneous fat that occurs in infants with other neonatal diseases.

P83.1 Neonatal erythema toxicum — The skin condition of small erythematous patches that develop in different locations.

MCC **P83.2 Hydrops fetalis not due to hemolytic disease** — The presence of whole body edema of the newborn that is not due to isoimmunization.
    Hydrops fetalis NOS

P83.3- Other and unspecified edema specific to newborn — The presence of increased amounts of intercellular fluid in the newborn.

cc **P83.30 Unspecified edema specific to newborn**

cc **P83.39 Other edema specific to newborn**

P83.4 Breast engorgement of newborn — The excessive fullness of the breast tissues with a fluid.
    Noninfective mastitis of newborn

P83.5 Congenital hydrocele — [♂] — The accumulation of fluid within the unclosed vaginal process.

P83.6 Umbilical polyp of newborn — The presence of a polypoid nodule of the umbilicus.

P83.8 Other specified conditions of integument specific to newborn
    Bronze baby syndrome
    Neonatal scleroderma
    Urticaria neonatorum

P83.9 Condition of the integument specific to newborn, unspecified

P
7
2
-
P
8
3

Other problems with newborn (P84)

P84 Other problems with newborn
  Acidemia of newborn
  Acidosis of newborn
  Anoxia of newborn NOS
  Asphyxia of newborn NOS
  Hypercapnia of newborn
  Hypoxemia of newborn
  Hypoxia of newborn NOS
  Mixed metabolic and respiratory acidosis of newborn
  Excludes 1:   intracranial hemorrhage due to anoxia or hypoxia (P52.-)
  hypoxic ischemic encephalopathy [HIE] (P91.6-)
  late metabolic acidosis of newborn (P74.0)

Other disorders originating in the perinatal period (P90-P96)

P90 Convulsions of newborn — The involuntary contraction, or series of
MCC   contractions, of the voluntary muscles.
  Excludes 1:   benign myoclonic epilepsy in infancy (G40.3-)
  benign neonatal convulsions (familial) (G40.3-)

P91- Other disturbances of cerebral status of newborn
MCC P91.0   Neonatal cerebral ischemia
MCC P91.1   Acquired periventricular cysts of newborn
MCC P91.2   Neonatal cerebral leukomalacia
    Periventricular leukomalacia
MCC P91.3   Neonatal cerebral irritability
MCC P91.4   Neonatal cerebral depression
MCC P91.5   Neonatal coma
  P91.6- Hypoxic ischemic encephalopathy [HIE] — The condition of cellular
    brain damage due to the insufficient supply of oxygenated blood to the cerebral
    tissues.
    cc P91.60   Hypoxic ischemic encephalopathy [HIE], unspecified
    cc P91.61   Mild hypoxic ischemic encephalopathy [HIE]
    cc P91.62   Moderate hypoxic ischemic encephalopathy [HIE]
    MCC P91.63   Severe hypoxic ischemic encephalopathy [HIE]
  P91.8   Other specified disturbances of cerebral status of newborn
  P91.9   Disturbance of cerebral status of newborn, unspecified

P92- Feeding problems of newborn
  Excludes 1:   feeding problems in child over 28 days old (R63.3)
  P92.0- Vomiting of newborn
    Excludes 1:   vomiting of child over 28 days old (R11.-)
    MCC P92.01   Bilious vomiting of newborn
      Excludes 1:   bilious vomiting in child over 28 days old (R11.14)
    P92.09   Other vomiting of newborn
      Excludes 1:   regurgitation of food in newborn (P92.1)
  P92.1   Regurgitation and rumination of newborn
  P92.2   Slow feeding of newborn
  P92.3   Underfeeding of newborn
  P92.4   Overfeeding of newborn
  P92.5   Neonatal difficulty in feeding at breast
  P92.6   Failure to thrive in newborn
    Excludes 1:   failure to thrive in child over 28 days old (R62.51)
  P92.8   Other feeding problems of newborn
  P92.9   Feeding problem of newborn, unspecified

P93- Reactions and intoxications due to drugs administered to newborn
  **Includes: Reactions and intoxications due to drugs administered to fetus
      affecting newborn**
  *Excludes 1:   jaundice due to drugs or toxins transmitted from mother or
        given to newborn (P58.4-)*
  *reactions and intoxications from maternal opiates,
        tranquilizers and other medication (P04.0-P04.1,P04.4)*
  *withdrawal symptoms from maternal use of drugs of addiction
        (P96.1)*
  *withdrawal symptoms from therapeutic use of drugs in
        newborn (P96.2)*
  cc P93.0   Grey baby syndrome
    Grey syndrome from chloramphenicol administration in newborn
  **cc P93.8   Other reactions and intoxications due to drugs administered
    to newborn**
    Use additional code for adverse effect, if applicable, to identify drug
      (T36-T50 with fifth or sixth character 5)

P94- Disorders of muscle tone of newborn
  cc P94.0   Transient neonatal myasthenia gravis — The autoimmune disorder of
    progressive muscular weakness of the newborn.
    Excludes 1:   myasthenia gravis (G70.0)
  P94.1   Congenital hypertonia
  P94.2   Congenital hypotonia
    Floppy baby syndrome, unspecified
  P94.8   Other disorders of muscle tone of newborn
  P94.9   Disorder of muscle tone of newborn, unspecified

P95 Stillbirth
  Deadborn fetus NOS
  Fetal death of unspecified cause
  Stillbirth NOS
  Excludes 1:   maternal care for intrauterine death (O36.4)
  missed abortion (O02.1)
  outcome of delivery, stillbirth (Z37.1, Z37.3, Z37.4, Z37.7)

P96- Other conditions originating in the perinatal period
  P96.0   Congenital renal failure — The complete, or significantly decreased,
    kidney function.
    Uremia of newborn
  **cc P96.1   Neonatal withdrawal symptoms from maternal use of drugs of
    addiction**
    Drug withdrawal syndrome in infant of dependent mother
    Neonatal abstinence syndrome
    *Excludes 1:   reactions and intoxications from maternal opiates and
          tranquilizers administered during labor and
          delivery (P04.0)*
  **cc P96.2   Withdrawal symptoms from therapeutic use of drugs in
    newborn**
  P96.3   Wide cranial sutures of newborn — The larger than expected soft spots
    between the bony plates of the skull.
    Neonatal craniotabes
  P96.5   Complication to newborn due to (fetal) intrauterine procedure
    Excludes ❷: newborn affected by amniocentesis (P00.6)
  P96.8- Other specified conditions originating in the perinatal period
    **P96.81   Exposure to (parental) (environmental) tobacco smoke in
      the perinatal period**
      *Excludes ❷: newborn affected by in utero exposure to tobacco
          (P04.2)*
      *exposure to environmental tobacco smoke after the
          perinatal period (Z77.22)*
    P96.82   Delayed separation of umbilical cord
    P96.83   Meconium staining — The presence of the distinctive mixing of the
      amniotic fluid and the passed fetal meconium that has occurred prior to
      delivery.
      Excludes 1:   meconium aspiration (P24.00, P24.01)
      meconium passage during delivery (P03.82)
    **P96.89   Other specified conditions originating in the perinatal
      period**
      Use additional code to specify condition
  P96.9   Condition originating in the perinatal period, unspecified
    Congenital debility NOS

P84 - P96

Chapter 17 – Congenital malformations, deformations and chromosomal abnormalities (Q00-Q99)

Note: Codes from this chapter are not for use on maternal or fetal records
Excludes ❷: inborn errors of metabolism (E70-E88)

This chapter contains the following blocks:

Q00-Q07	**Congenital malformations of the nervous system**
Q10-Q18	**Congenital malformations of eye, ear, face and neck**
Q20-Q28	**Congenital malformations of the circulatory system**
Q30-Q34	**Congenital malformations of the respiratory system**
Q35-Q37	**Cleft lip and cleft palate**
Q38-Q45	**Other congenital malformations of the digestive system**
Q50-Q56	**Congenital malformations of genital organs**
Q60-Q64	**Congenital malformations of the urinary system**
Q65-Q79	**Congenital malformations and deformations of the musculoskeletal system**
Q80-Q89	**Other congenital malformations**
Q90-Q99	**Chromosomal abnormalities, not elsewhere classified**

Chapter-Specific Coding Guidelines

C. Chapter-Specific Coding Guidelines

In addition to general coding guidelines, there are guidelines for specific diagnoses and/or conditions in the classification. Unless otherwise indicated, these guidelines apply to all health care settings. Please refer to Section II for guidelines on the selection of principal diagnosis.

17. Chapter 17: Congenital Malformations, Deformations, and Chromosomal Abnormalities (Q00-Q99)

Assign an appropriate code(s) from categories Q00-Q99, Congenital malformations, deformations, and chromosomal abnormalities when a malformation/deformation or chromosomal abnormality is documented. A malformation/deformation/or chromosomal abnormality may be the principal/first-listed diagnosis on a record or a secondary diagnosis.

When a malformation/deformation/or chromosomal abnormality does not have a unique code assignment, assign additional code(s) for any manifestations that may be present.

When the code assignment specifically identifies the malformation/deformation/or chromosomal abnormality, manifestations that are an inherent component of the anomaly should not be coded separately. Additional codes should be assigned for manifestations that are not an inherent component.

Codes from Chapter 17 may be used throughout the life of the patient. If a congenital malformation or deformity has been corrected, a personal history code should be used to identify the history of the malformation or deformity. Although present at birth, malformation/deformation/or chromosomal abnormality may not be identified until later in life. Whenever the condition is diagnosed by the physician, it is appropriate to assign a code from codes Q00-Q99.

For the birth admission, the appropriate code from category Z38, Liveborn infants, according to place of birth and type of delivery, should be sequenced as the principal diagnosis, followed by any congenital anomaly codes, Q00-Q99.

Congenital malformations of the nervous system (Q00-Q07)

Q00- Anencephaly and similar malformations

MCC **Q00.0 Anencephaly** — The congenital absence of part of the skull, brain, and spinal cord.
> **Acephaly** — The congenital absence of the head.
> **Acrania** — The congenital absence of part of the skull.
> **Amyelencephaly** — The congenital absence of part of the brain and spinal cord.
> **Hemianencephaly** — The congenital absence of one half of the brain.
> **Hemicephaly** — The congenital absence of a portion of the cerebrum.

MCC **Q00.1 Craniorachischisis** — The congenital fissure of the skull and spinal column.

MCC **Q00.2 Iniencephaly** — The congenital enlargement of the foramen magnum of the base of the skull with the anomalous formation of the vertebrae.

Q01- Encephalocele — The protrusion of the brain substance through a defect in the skull.
> **Includes: Arnold-Chiari syndrome, type III** — The protrusion of the brain substance and spinal cord through a foramen magnum defect.
> **Encephalocystocele** — The protrusion of the brain substance through a skull defect with an accumulation of fluid.
> **Encephalomyelocele** — The protrusion of the brain substance and spinal cord through a foramen magnum defect.
> **Hydroencephalocele** — The protrusion of the brain substance through a skull defect with an accumulation of fluid.
> **Hydromeningocele, cranial** — The protrusion of a cerebrospinal fluid-filled meningeal sac through a skull defect.
> **Meningocele, cerebral** — The protrusion of the cerebral meninges through a skull defect.
> **Meningoencephalocele** — The protrusion of the brain substance and cerebral meninges through a skull defect.

Excludes 1:   Meckel-Gruber syndrome (Q61.9)

CC **Q01.0 Frontal encephalocele** — A form with a frontal bone defect.

CC **Q01.1 Nasofrontal encephalocele** — A form with a frontal/nasal bone defect.

CC **Q01.2 Occipital encephalocele** — A form with an occipital bone defect.

CC **Q01.8 Encephalocele of other sites**

CC **Q01.9 Encephalocele, unspecified**

Q02 Microcephaly — The congenital smallness of the head.
> **Includes: Hydromicrocephaly** — A form of microcephalus with an abnormally large amount of cerebrospinal fluid.
> **Micrencephalon**

Excludes 1:   Meckel-Gruber syndrome (Q61.9)

Q03- Congenital hydrocephalus — The congenital abnormal accumulation of fluid within the head.
> **Includes: Hydrocephalus in newborn**

Excludes 1:   Arnold-Chiari syndrome, type II (Q07.0-)
acquired hydrocephalus (G91.-)
hydrocephalus due to congenital toxoplasmosis (P37.1)
hydrocephalus with spina bifida (Q05.0-Q05.4)

Q03.0 Malformations of aqueduct of Sylvius — The developmental deviation of the aqueduct of Sylvius.
> **Anomaly of aqueduct of Sylvius**
> **Obstruction of aqueduct of Sylvius, congenital**
> **Stenosis of aqueduct of Sylvius**

Q03.1 Atresia of foramina of Magendie and Luschka — The absence or closure of the foramina of Magendie and Luschka.
> **Dandy-Walker syndrome**

Q03.8 Other congenital hydrocephalus

Q03.9 Congenital hydrocephalus, unspecified

Q04- Other congenital malformations of brain

Excludes 1:   cyclopia (Q87.0)
macrocephaly (Q75.3)

MCC **Q04.0 Congenital malformations of corpus callosum**
> **Agenesis of corpus callosum** — The failure of embryonic development of a portion of the corpus callosum.

MCC **Q04.1 Arhinencephaly** — The absence of the rhinencephalon.

MCC **Q04.2 Holoprosencephaly** — The malformation of the prosencephalon.

Q 0 0 - Q 0 4

MCC **Q04.3** **Other reduction deformities of brain**
    Absence of part of brain — The nonexistence of a portion of the brain.
    Agenesis of part of brain — The failure of embryonic development of a portion of the brain.
    Agyria — A brain malformation that is marked by abnormally developed convolutions of the cerebral cortex that leads to a small brain.
    Aplasia of part of brain — The lack of development of a portion of the brain.
    Hydranencephaly — The lack of development of a portion of the cerebrum and the intracranial cavity is filled with fluid.
    Hypoplasia of part of brain — The incomplete development of a portion of the brain.
    Lissencephaly — The lack of development of folds of the cerebrum.
    Microgyria — The malformation of the brain that is characterized by the development of small convolutions in the cerebrum.
    Pachygyria — The malformation of the brain that is characterized by the development of thick convolutions of the brain.
    Excludes 1:   *congenital malformations of corpus callosum (Q04.0)*

CC **Q04.4** **Septo-optic dysplasia of brain** — The underdevelopment of the optic nerve, pituitary gland, and a midline portion of the brain.

CC **Q04.5** **Megalencephaly** — The excessive size of the head.

CC **Q04.6** **Congenital cerebral cysts** — An encapsulated, fluid-filled sac of the cerebrum.
    Porencephaly — The presence of cysts or cavities in the brain substance.
    Schizencephaly — The presence of cysts or cavities in the clefts of the brain.
    Excludes 1:   *acquired porencephalic cyst (G93.0)*

CC **Q04.8** **Other specified congenital malformations of brain**
    Arnold-Chiari syndrome, type IV — The lack of development of the cerebellum.
    Macrogyria — The excessive size of the convolutions of the brain.

    Q04.9 **Congenital malformation of brain, unspecified**
    Congenital anomaly NOS of brain
    Congenital deformity NOS of brain
    Congenital disease or lesion NOS of brain
    Multiple anomalies NOS of brain, congenital

Q05- **Spina bifida** — The congenital defective closure of the bony portion of the spinal column with protrusion of the spinal cord and meninges.
    Includes: **Hydromeningocele (spinal)** — The protrusion of the cerebrospinal fluid-filled meninges through a vertebral column defect.
        Meningocele (spinal) — The protrusion of the meninges through a vertebral column defect.
        Meningomyelocele — The protrusion of the meninges and part of the spinal cord substance through a vertebral column defect.
        Myelocele — The protrusion of the spinal cord substance through a vertebral column defect.
        Myelomeningocele — The protrusion of the meninges and part of the spinal cord substance through a vertebral column defect.
        Rachischisis — The congenital fissure of the vertebral column.
        Spina bifida (aperta) (cystica) — The protrusion of spinal tissue through a vertebral column defect.
        Syringomyelocele — The protrusion of the spinal cord through a vertebral column defect while remaining connected to the central canal.
    Use additional code for any associated paraplegia (paraparesis) (G82.2-)
    Excludes 1:   *Arnold-Chiari syndrome, type II (Q07.0-)*
                  spina bifida occulta (Q76.0)

CC **Q05.0** <u>Cervical</u> **spina bifida** <u>with hydrocephalus</u> — A form affecting the cervical spinal cord with accumulation of fluid within the cranial meninges.

CC **Q05.1** <u>Thoracic</u> **spina bifida** <u>with hydrocephalus</u> — A form affecting the thoracic spinal cord with accumulation of fluid within the cranial meninges.
    Dorsal spina bifida with hydrocephalus
    Thoracolumbar spina bifida with hydrocephalus

CC **Q05.2** <u>Lumbar</u> **spina bifida** <u>with hydrocephalus</u> — A form affecting the lumbar spinal cord with accumulation of fluid within the cranial meninges.
    Lumbosacral spina bifida with hydrocephalus

CC **Q05.3** <u>Sacral</u> **spina bifida** <u>with hydrocephalus</u> — A form affecting the sacral spinal cord with accumulation of fluid within the cranial meninges.

CC **Q05.4** <u>Unspecified</u> **spina bifida** <u>with hydrocephalus</u>

    Q05.5 <u>Cervical</u> **spina bifida** <u>without</u> hydrocephalus

    Q05.6 <u>Thoracic</u> **spina bifida** <u>without</u> hydrocephalus
    Dorsal spina bifida NOS
    Thoracolumbar spina bifida NOS

    Q05.7 **Lumbar spina bifida** <u>without</u> hydrocephalus
    Lumbosacral spina bifida NOS

    Q05.8 <u>Sacral</u> **spina bifida** <u>without</u> hydrocephalus

    Q05.9 **Spina bifida, <u>unspecified</u>**

Q06- **Other congenital malformations of spinal cord**
    Q06.0 **Amyelia** — The absence of the spinal cord.

    Q06.1 **Hypoplasia and dysplasia of spinal cord**
    Atelomyelia — The incomplete development of the spinal cord.
    Myelatelia — The imperfect development of the spinal cord.
    Myelodysplasia of spinal cord — The deviation of normal development of the spinal cord.

    Q06.2 **Diastematomyelia** — The congenital splitting of the spinal cord by a bony projection.

    Q06.3 **Other congenital cauda equina malformations**

    Q06.4 **Hydromyelia** — The congenital accumulation of fluid in the central portion of the spinal cord.
    Hydrorachis — The accumulation of water in the spinal column.

    Q06.8 **Other specified congenital malformations of spinal cord**

    Q06.9 **Congenital malformation of spinal cord, unspecified**
    Congenital anomaly NOS of spinal cord
    Congenital deformity NOS of spinal cord
    Congenital disease or lesion NOS of spinal cord

Q07- **Other congenital malformations of nervous system**
    Excludes ❷: *congenital central alveolar hypoventilation syndrome (G47.35)*
                familial dysautonomia [Riley-Day] (G90.1)
                neurofibromatosis (nonmalignant) (Q85.0-)

    Q07.0- <u>Arnold-Chiari syndrome</u> — The protrusion of the cerebellum down into the spinal canal.
    Arnold-Chiari syndrome, type II — The protrusion of the cerebellum and medulla oblongata down into the spinal canal.
    Excludes 1:   *Arnold-Chiari syndrome, type III (Q01.-)*
                Arnold-Chiari syndrome, type IV (Q04.8)

        Q07.00 **Arnold-Chiari syndrome** <u>without</u> **spina bifida or hydrocephalus**

        Q07.01 **Arnold-Chiari syndrome** <u>with spina bifida</u>

    CC **Q07.02** **Arnold-Chiari syndrome** <u>with hydrocephalus</u> — A form with accumulation of fluid within the cranial meninges.

    CC **Q07.03** **Arnold-Chiari syndrome** <u>with spina bifida and hydrocephalus</u>

    Q07.8 **Other specified congenital malformations of nervous system**
    Agenesis of nerve — The failure of embryonic development of a nerve.
    Displacement of brachial plexus — The developmental dislocation of the brachial plexus.
    Jaw-winking syndrome — A congenital unilateral ptosis of the eyelid that is of nervous system origin and is momentarily improved by movement of the jaw.
    Marcus Gunn's syndrome

    Q07.9 **Congenital malformation of nervous system, unspecified**
    Congenital anomaly NOS of nervous system
    Congenital deformity NOS of nervous system
    Congenital disease or lesion NOS of nervous system

Q04
-
Q07

Congenital malformations of eye, ear, face and neck (Q10-Q18)

Excludes ❷: cleft lip and cleft palate (Q35-Q37)
   congenital malformation of cervical spine (Q05.0, Q05.5, Q67.5, Q76.0-Q76.4)
   congenital malformation of larynx (Q31.-)
   congenital malformation of lip NEC (Q38.0)
   congenital malformation of nose (Q30.-)
   congenital malformation of parathyroid gland (Q89.2)
   congenital malformation of thyroid gland (Q89.2)

Q10- Congenital malformations of eyelid, lacrimal apparatus and orbit

Excludes 1: cryptophthalmos NOS (Q11.2)
   cryptophthalmos syndrome (Q87.0)

Q10.0 **Congenital ptosis** — The congenital drooping of the upper eyelid.

Q10.1 **Congenital ectropion** — The congenital turning outward of the eyelid margin.

Q10.2 **Congenital entropion** — The congenital turning inward of the eyelid margin.

Q10.3 **Other congenital malformations of eyelid**
   Ablepharon — The partial or complete absence of the eyelids.
   Blepharophimosis, congenital — The reduced size of the eyelids.
   Coloboma of eyelid — A full-thickness defect in the eyelid.
   Congenital absence or agenesis of cilia — The failure of embryonic development of the cilia.
   Congenital absence or agenesis of eyelid — The failure of embryonic development of the eyelid.
   Congenital accessory eyelid — The presence of a supplementary eyelid.
   Congenital accessory eye muscle — The development of supplementary eye muscles.
   Congenital malformation of eyelid NOS

Q10.4 **Absence and agenesis of lacrimal apparatus** — The failure of embryonic development of the lacrimal apparatus.
   Congenital absence of punctum lacrimale

Q10.5 **Congenital stenosis and stricture of lacrimal duct** — The congenital narrowing of the lacrimal ducts.

Q10.6 **Other congenital malformations of lacrimal apparatus**
   Congenital malformation of lacrimal apparatus NOS

Q10.7 **Congenital malformation of orbit**

Q11- Anophthalmos, microphthalmos and macrophthalmos

Q11.0 **Cystic eyeball** — The congenital cystic malformation of the eyeball.

Q11.1 **Other anophthalmos** — The failure of embryonic development of the eye.
   Anophthalmos NOS
   Agenesis of eye
   Aplasia of eye

Q11.2 **Microphthalmos** — The congenital smallness of the eye without associated developmental defects.
   Cryptophthalmos NOS
   Dysplasia of eye
   Hypoplasia of eye
   Rudimentary eye
   Excludes 1: cryptophthalmos syndrome (Q87.0)

Q11.3 **Macrophthalmos** — The larger than normal eyeball.
   Excludes 1: macrophthalmos in congenital glaucoma (Q15.0)

Q12- Congenital lens malformations

Q12.0 **Congenital cataract** — The congenital opacity of the crystalline lens.

Q12.1 **Congenital displaced lens** — The congenital improper position of the lens.

Q12.2 **Coloboma of lens** — A defect in the lens.

Q12.3 **Congenital aphakia** — The congenital absence of the lens.

Q12.4 **Spherophakia** — The abnormal roundness of the lens.

Q12.8 **Other congenital lens malformations**
   Microphakia — The abnormal smallness of the lens.

Q12.9 **Congenital lens malformation, unspecified**

Q13- Congenital malformations of anterior segment of eye

Q13.0 **Coloboma of iris** — The fissure of the iris.
   Coloboma NOS

Q13.1 **Absence of iris** — The congenital absence of the iris.
   Aniridia
   Use additional code for associated glaucoma (H42)

Q13.2 **Other congenital malformations of iris**
   Anisocoria, congenital — The inequality of the pupillary diameters.
   Atresia of pupil — The absence or closure of the pupil.
   Congenital malformation of iris NOS
   Corectopia — The abnormal placement of the pupil.

Q13.3 **Congenital corneal opacity** — The congenital nontransparency of the cornea.

Q13.4 **Other congenital corneal malformations**
   Congenital malformation of cornea NOS
   Microcornea — The abnormal smallness of the cornea.
   Peter's anomaly

Q13.5 **Blue sclera**

Q13.8- **Other congenital malformations of anterior segment of eye**

   Q13.81 **Rieger's anomaly**
      Use additional code for associated glaucoma (H42)

   Q13.89 **Other congenital malformations of anterior segment of eye**

Q13.9 **Congenital malformation of anterior segment of eye, unspecified**

Q14- Congenital malformations of posterior segment of eye

Excludes ❷: optic nerve hypoplasia (H47.03-)

Q14.0 **Congenital malformation of vitreous humor**
   Congenital vitreous opacity — The nontransparency of the vitreous.

Q14.1 **Congenital malformation of retina**
   Congenital retinal aneurysm — The sac-like dilatation of a retinal artery.

Q14.2 **Congenital malformation of optic disc**
   Coloboma of optic disc — The optic disc defect that is due to the incomplete closure of the fetal optic stalk.

Q14.3 **Congenital malformation of choroid**

Q14.8 **Other congenital malformations of posterior segment of eye**
   Coloboma of the fundus — The congenital defect of the fundus.

Q14.9 **Congenital malformation of posterior segment of eye, unspecified**

Q15- Other congenital malformations of eye

Excludes 1: congenital nystagmus (H55.01)
   ocular albinism (E70.31-)
   optic nerve hypoplasia (H47.03-)
   retinitis pigmentosa (H35.52)

Q15.0 **Congenital glaucoma** — The increased intraocular pressure resulting in thickening of the cornea.
   Axenfeld's anomaly — The inherited developmental deviation of the iris and angular structures in the anterior chamber.
   Buphthalmos — The congenital thickening and enlargement of the fibrous coats of the eye.
   Glaucoma of childhood
   Glaucoma of newborn
   Hydrophthalmos
   Keratoglobus, congenital, with glaucoma — The bilateral enlargement of the corneas with a globular shape.
   Macrocornea with glaucoma
   Macrophthalmos in congenital glaucoma
   Megalocornea with glaucoma — The increase in thickness of the cornea.

Q15.8 **Other specified congenital malformations of eye**

Q15.9 **Congenital malformation of eye, unspecified**
   Congenital anomaly of eye
   Congenital deformity of eye

Q16- Congenital malformations of ear causing impairment of hearing

Excludes 1: congenital deafness (H90.-)

Q16.0 **Congenital absence of (ear) auricle**

Q16.1 **Congenital absence, atresia and stricture of auditory canal (external)**
   Congenital atresia or stricture of osseous meatus — The absence or closure of the osseous meatus.

Q16.2 **Absence of eustachian tube**

Q16.3 **Congenital malformation of ear ossicles**
   Congenital fusion of ear ossicles — The immobilizing malformation of the ear ossicles.

Q16.4 **Other congenital malformations of middle ear**
   Congenital malformation of middle ear NOS

Q16.5 **Congenital malformation of inner ear**
   Congenital anomaly of membranous labyrinth — The developmental deviation of the membranous labyrinth.
   Congenital anomaly of organ of Corti — The developmental deviation of the organ of Corti.

Q16.9 **Congenital malformation of ear causing impairment of hearing, unspecified**
   Congenital absence of ear NOS

Q10-Q16

Q17- Other congenital malformations of ear

Excludes 1: congenital malformations of ear with impairment of hearing (Q16.0-Q16.9)
preauricular sinus (Q18.1)

Q17.0 Accessory auricle — The congenital supplementary auricle.
   Accessory tragus — The supplementary cartilaginous projection of the external opening of the ear.
   Polyotia — The development of more than two ears.
   Preauricular appendage or tag — The development of a supplementary preauricular appendage.
   Supernumerary ear — The congenital supplementary auricle.
   Supernumerary lobule — The development of a supplementary ear lobe.

Q17.1 Macrotia — The congenital enlargement of the external ear.

Q17.2 Microtia — The congenital incomplete development of the external ear.

Q17.3 Other misshapen ear
   Pointed ear — A developmental deviation of the external ear in which the ear is pointed.

Q17.4 Misplaced ear — The abnormal location of the ear.
   Low-set ears — The lower than usual location of the ear.
   Excludes 1: cervical auricle (Q18.2)

Q17.5 Prominent ear — A developmental deviation of the external ear in which it protrudes away from the head abnormally.
   Bat ear — A developmental deviation of the external ear in which it grows at a right angle to the head.

Q17.8 Other specified congenital malformations of ear
   Congenital absence of lobe of ear

Q17.9 Congenital malformation of ear, unspecified
   Congenital anomaly of ear NOS

Q18- Other congenital malformations of face and neck

Excludes 1: cleft lip and cleft palate (Q35-Q37)
conditions classified to Q67.0-Q67.4
congenital malformations of skull and face bones (Q75.-)
cyclopia (Q87.0)
dentofacial anomalies [including malocclusion] (M26.-)
malformation syndromes affecting facial appearance (Q87.0)
persistent thyroglossal duct (Q89.2)

Q18.0 Sinus, fistula and cyst of branchial cleft — The congenital failure of the fetal branchial cleft passage to close.
   Branchial vestige

Q18.1 Preauricular sinus and cyst — PREAURICULAR SINUS OR FISTULA – The congenital passage of the pit-like depression of the external ear. PREAURICULAR CYST – The congenital fluid-filled sac resulting from the imperfect fusion of the first and second branchial arches.
   Fistula of auricle, congenital
   Cervicoaural fistula

Q18.2 Other branchial cleft malformations
   Branchial cleft malformation NOS
   Cervical auricle — The congenital flap of skin and yellow cartilage sometimes seen on the side of the neck at the external opening of a persistent branchial cleft.
   Otocephaly — The lack of development of the lower jaw.

Q18.3 Webbing of neck — The congenital web-like tissue that spans the neck to the shoulder.
   Pterygium colli — The thick fold of skin on the side of the neck.

Q18.4 Macrostomia — The congenital exaggeration of the width of the mouth.

Q18.5 Microstomia — The congenital smallness of the width of the mouth.

Q18.6 Macrocheilia — The congenital excessive size of the lips.
   Hypertrophy of lip, congenital

Q18.7 Microcheilia — The congenital smallness of the lips.

Q18.8 Other specified congenital malformations of face and neck
   Medial cyst of face and neck
   Medial fistula of face and neck
   Medial sinus of face and neck

Q18.9 Congenital malformation of face and neck, unspecified
   Congenital anomaly NOS of face and neck

Congenital malformations of the circulatory system (Q20-Q28)

Q20- Congenital malformations of cardiac chambers and connections
Excludes 1: dextrocardia with situs inversus (Q89.3)
mirror-image atrial arrangement with situs inversus (Q89.3)

MCC Q20.0 Common arterial trunk — The congenital absence of a separating septum between the aorta and pulmonary artery.
   Persistent truncus arteriosus
   Excludes 1: aortic septal defect (Q21.4)

MCC Q20.1 Double outlet right ventricle — The congenital malformation of the great vessels in which both the aorta and the pulmonary artery arise from the right ventricle; almost always associated with a ventricular septal defect.
   Taussig-Bing syndrome

MCC Q20.2 Double outlet left ventricle — The congenital malformation of the great vessels in which both the aorta and the pulmonary artery arise from the left ventricle.

MCC Q20.3 Discordant ventriculoarterial connection — The congenital malformation in which the aorta arises from the right ventricle and the pulmonary artery arises from the left ventricle; opposite of normal.
   Dextrotransposition of aorta — The abnormal formation of the aorta in which it arises from the right ventricle.
   Transposition of great vessels (complete)

MCC Q20.4 Double inlet ventricle — The congenital malformation of a three-chambered heart consisting of two atria and one ventricle.
   Common ventricle
   Cor triloculare biatriatum
   Single ventricle

CC Q20.5 Discordant atrioventricular connection — The transposition of the great vessels with inversion of the ventricles.
   Corrected transposition
   Levotransposition
   Ventricular inversion

Q20.6 Isomerism of atrial appendages
   Isomerism of atrial appendages with asplenia or polysplenia

Q20.8 Other congenital malformations of cardiac chambers and connections
   Cor binoculare — The congenital malformation of the heart in which there is a single atrium and a single ventricle.

Q20.9 Congenital malformation of cardiac chambers and connections, unspecified

Q21- Congenital malformations of cardiac septa
Excludes 1: acquired cardiac septal defect (I51.0)

CC Q21.0 Ventricular septal defect — The congenital malformation of the ventricular septum in which there is persistent patency between the ventricles.
   Roger's disease

CC Q21.1 Atrial septal defect — The congenital malformation of the atrial septum in which there is a patency between the two atria with a rim of septum completely around the defect.
   Coronary sinus defect
   Patent or persistent foramen ovale
   Patent or persistent ostium secundum defect (type II)
   Patent or persistent sinus venosus defect

CC Q21.2 Atrioventricular septal defect — The persistent fetal opening between the atrium and ventricle.
   Common atrioventricular canal
   Endocardial cushion defect
   Ostium primum atrial septal defect (type I)

MCC Q21.3 Tetralogy of Fallot
   AHA 14:3Q:p16 – Tetralogy of Fallot
   Ventricular septal defect with pulmonary stenosis or atresia, dextroposition of aorta and hypertrophy of right ventricle

Q21.4 Aortopulmonary septal defect — The developmental deviation of the atrial septum that allows communication between the aorta and the pulmonary artery.
   Aortic septal defect
   Aortopulmonary window

Q21.8 Other congenital malformations of cardiac septa
   Eisenmenger's defect — A form with severe pulmonary hypertension and hypertrophy of the right ventricle.
   Pentalogy of Fallot
   Excludes 1: Eisenmenger's complex (I27.8)
   Eisenmenger's syndrome (I27.8)

Q21.9 Congenital malformation of cardiac septum, unspecified
   Septal (heart) defect NOS

Q17-Q21

Q22- Congenital malformations of pulmonary and tricuspid valves

MCC **Q22.0 Pulmonary valve atresia** — The absence or closure of the pulmonary valve.

CC **Q22.1 Congenital pulmonary valve stenosis** — The reduction in the size of the pulmonary valve orifice.

CC **Q22.2 Congenital pulmonary valve insufficiency** — The developmental deviation in which the pulmonary valve does not completely close.
  Congenital pulmonary valve regurgitation

CC **Q22.3 Other congenital malformations of pulmonary valve**
  Congenital malformation of pulmonary valve NOS
  Supernumerary cusps of pulmonary valve

MCC **Q22.4 Congenital tricuspid stenosis** — The congenital incomplete development of the tricuspid valve.
  Congenital tricuspid atresia

MCC **Q22.5 Ebstein's anomaly** — The congenital malformation of the tricuspid valve attachments.

MCC **Q22.6 Hypoplastic right heart syndrome** — The incomplete development of the right ventricle.

MCC **Q22.8 Other congenital malformations of tricuspid valve**

MCC **Q22.9 Congenital malformation of tricuspid valve, unspecified**

Q23- Congenital malformations of aortic and mitral valves

CC **Q23.0 Congenital stenosis of aortic valve** — The congenital reduction in the size of the aortic valve orifice.
  Congenital aortic atresia
  Congenital aortic stenosis NOS
  Excludes 1:   congenital stenosis of aortic valve in hypoplastic left heart syndrome (Q23.4)
        congenital subaortic stenosis (Q24.4)
        supravalvular aortic stenosis (congenital) (Q25.3)

CC **Q23.1 Congenital insufficiency of aortic valve** — The congenital failure of the aortic valve to close completely.
  Bicuspid aortic valve — The presence of two leaflets instead of three.
  Congenital aortic insufficiency

CC **Q23.2 Congenital mitral stenosis** — The congenital reduction in the size of the mitral valve orifice.
  Congenital mitral atresia

CC **Q23.3 Congenital mitral insufficiency** — The congenital failure of the mitral valve to close completely.

MCC **Q23.4 Hypoplastic left heart syndrome** — The incomplete development of the left ventricle.

Q23.8 Other congenital malformations of aortic and mitral valves

Q23.9 Congenital malformation of aortic and mitral valves, unspecified

Q24- Other congenital malformations of heart
  Excludes 1:   endocardial fibroelastosis (I42.4)

CC **Q24.0 Dextrocardia** — The malforming displacement of the heart with the heart displaced into the abdomen.
  Excludes 1:   dextrocardia with situs inversus (Q89.3)
        isomerism of atrial appendages (with asplenia or polysplenia) (Q20.6)
        mirror-image atrial arrangement with situs inversus (Q89.3)

CC **Q24.1 Levocardia** — The malforming displacement of the heart with the heart in its normal position while the other viscera are transposed.

MCC **Q24.2 Cor triatriatum** — The congenital formation of an accessory atrium into which the pulmonary veins empty.

CC **Q24.3 Pulmonary infundibular stenosis** — The congenital formation of a defective infundibulum of the right ventricle which causes a reduction in pulmonic valve capacity.
  Subvalvular pulmonic stenosis

MCC **Q24.4 Congenital subaortic stenosis** — The congenital formation of a left ventricle obstructive lesion which causes a pressure gradient in the ventricle.

CC **Q24.5 Malformation of coronary vessels** — The developmental deviation of a coronary artery.
  Congenital coronary (artery) aneurysm

MCC **Q24.6 Congenital heart block** — The congenital impairment of heart conduction.

Q24.8 Other specified congenital malformations of heart
  Congenital diverticulum of left ventricle — The sac-like dilatation of the left ventricle.
  Congenital malformation of myocardium — The developmental deviation of the myocardium.
  Congenital malformation of pericardium — The developmental deviation of the pericardium.
  Malposition of heart — The malforming displacement of the heart.
  Uhl's disease — The development of a paper-thin right ventricular wall that dilates easily.

Q24.9 Congenital malformation of heart, unspecified
  Congenital anomaly of heart
  Congenital disease of heart

Q25- Congenital malformations of great arteries

CC **Q25.0 Patent ductus arteriosus** — The congenital persistence of the vessel in the fetus that connects the pulmonary artery and the aorta.
  Patent ductus Botallo
  Persistent ductus arteriosus

PATENT DUCTUS ARTERIOSUS

COARCTATION OF AORTA

CC **Q25.1 Coarctation of aorta** — The congenital discrete narrowing of the aortic arch.
  Coarctation of aorta (preductal) (postductal)
  Stenosis of aorta

Q25.2- Atresia of aorta — The congenital abnormality in size of the aorta.

CC **Q25.21 Interruption of aortic arch** — The congenital discontinuation of a portion of the aortic arch.
  Atresia of aortic arch

CC **Q25.29 Other atresia of aorta**
  Atresia of aorta — The congenital reduction in size of the aorta.

CC **Q25.3 Supravalvular aortic stenosis** — The reduction in size of that portion of the aorta just above the mitral valve.
  Excludes 1:   congenital aortic stenosis NOS (Q23.0)
        congenital stenosis of aortic valve (Q23.0)

Q25.4- Other congenital malformations of aorta
  Excludes 1:   hypoplasia of aorta in hypoplastic left heart syndrome (Q23.4)

CC **Q25.40 Congenital malformation of aorta, unspecified**

CC **Q25.41 Absence and aplasia of aorta** — The nonexistence or lack of development of the aorta.

CC **Q25.42 Hypoplasia of aorta** — The incomplete development of the aorta.

CC **Q25.43 Congenital aneurysm of aorta** — The arterial wall dilatation of the aorta.
  Congenital aneurysm of aortic root
  Congenital aneurysm of aortic sinus

CC **Q25.44 Congenital dilation of aorta** — The widening of the aorta.

CC **Q25.45 Double aortic arch** — The malformation of the aorta consisting of two aortic arches.
  Vascular ring of aorta

Q22-Q25

CC **Q25.46 Tortuous aortic arch** — An anomalous aortic arch.
Persistent convolutions of aortic arch — An anomalous aortic arch which infolds upon itself.

CC **Q25.47 Right aortic arch** — An anomalous aortic arch which passes over the right, rather than the left, bronchus.
Persistent right aortic arch

CC **Q25.48 Anomalous origin of subclavian artery**

CC **Q25.49 Other congenital malformations of aorta**

MCC **Q25.5 Atresia of pulmonary artery** — The absence or closure of the pulmonary artery.

MCC **Q25.6 Stenosis of pulmonary artery** — The reduction in the size of the pulmonary artery lumen.
Supravalvular pulmonary stenosis

Q25.7- Other congenital malformations of pulmonary artery

MCC **Q25.71 Coarctation of pulmonary artery** — The discrete narrowing of the pulmonary artery.

MCC **Q25.72 Congenital pulmonary arteriovenous malformation**
Congenital pulmonary arteriovenous aneurysm — The arteriovenous dilatation of the pulmonary artery.

MCC **Q25.79 Other congenital malformations of pulmonary artery**
Aberrant pulmonary artery — The developmental deviation of the pulmonary artery.
Agenesis of pulmonary artery — The failure of embryonic development of the pulmonary artery.
Congenital aneurysm of pulmonary artery — The dilatation of the pulmonary artery.
Congenital anomaly of pulmonary artery — The congenital developmental deviation of the pulmonary artery.
Hypoplasia of pulmonary artery — The incomplete development of the pulmonary artery.

CC **Q25.8 Other congenital malformations of other great arteries**

CC **Q25.9 Congenital malformation of great arteries, unspecified**

Q26- Congenital malformations of great veins

CC **Q26.0 Congenital stenosis of vena cava** — The reduction in the size of the vena cava lumen.
Congenital stenosis of vena cava (inferior) (superior)

CC **Q26.1 Persistent left superior vena cava** — The failure of the fetal left superior vena cava to close.

CC **Q26.2 Total anomalous pulmonary venous connection** — The congenital malformation of all of the pulmonary veins in which the pulmonary veins empty into the right atrium, or a systemic vein, instead of the left atrium.
Total anomalous pulmonary venous return [TAPVR], subdiaphragmatic — A form contained within the thoracic cavity.
Total anomalous pulmonary venous return [TAPVR], supradiaphragmatic — A form connecting to systemic veins in the abdominal cavity.

CC **Q26.3 Partial anomalous pulmonary venous connection** — The congenital malformation in which some, but not all, of the pulmonary veins empty into the right atrium instead of the left atrium.
Partial anomalous pulmonary venous return

CC **Q26.4 Anomalous pulmonary venous connection, unspecified**

Q26.5 Anomalous portal venous connection

Q26.6 Portal vein-hepatic artery fistula

CC **Q26.8 Other congenital malformations of great veins**
Absence of vena cava (inferior) (superior) — The nonexistence of the vena cava.
Azygos continuation of inferior vena cava
Persistent left posterior cardinal vein — The failure of the fetal left posterior cardinal vein to close.
Scimitar syndrome — The complete or partial venous drainage of the right lung into the inferior vena cava.

CC **Q26.9 Congenital malformation of great vein, unspecified**
Congenital anomaly of vena cava (inferior) (superior) NOS

Q27- Other congenital malformations of peripheral vascular system
Excludes ❷: *anomalies of cerebral and precerebral vessels (Q28.0-Q28.3)*
anomalies of coronary vessels (Q24.5)
anomalies of pulmonary artery (Q25.5-Q25.7)
congenital retinal aneurysm (Q14.1)
hemangioma and lymphangioma (D18.-)

Q27.0 Congenital absence and hypoplasia of umbilical artery — The congenital nonexistence or incomplete development of the umbilical artery.
Single umbilical artery — The presence of one umbilical artery instead of the normal two.

Q27.1 Congenital renal artery stenosis — The reduction in the size of the renal artery lumen.

Q27.2 Other congenital malformations of renal artery
Congenital malformation of renal artery NOS
Multiple renal arteries

Q27.3- Arteriovenous malformation (peripheral) — The abnormally developed arteries and veins of the peripheral vascular system.
Arteriovenous aneurysm — The presence of an abnormal arteriovenous connection of peripheral blood vessels.
Excludes 1: *acquired arteriovenous aneurysm (I77.0)*
Excludes ❷: *arteriovenous malformation of cerebral vessels (Q28.2)*
arteriovenous malformation of precerebral vessels (Q28.0)

CC **Q27.30 Arteriovenous malformation, site unspecified**

Q27.31 Arteriovenous malformation of vessel of upper limb

Q27.32 Arteriovenous malformation of vessel of lower limb

Q27.33 Arteriovenous malformation of digestive system vessel

Q27.34 Arteriovenous malformation of renal vessel

Q27.39 Arteriovenous malformation, other site

CC **Q27.4 Congenital phlebectasia** — The presence of a dilatated vein.

Q27.8 Other specified congenital malformations of peripheral vascular system
Absence of peripheral vascular system
Atresia of peripheral vascular system
Congenital aneurysm (peripheral)
Congenital stricture, artery
Congenital varix
Excludes 1: *arteriovenous malformation (Q27.3-)*

Q27.9 Congenital malformation of peripheral vascular system, unspecified
Anomaly of artery or vein NOS

Q28- Other congenital malformations of circulatory system
Excludes 1: *congenital aneurysm NOS (Q27.8)*
congenital coronary aneurysm (Q24.5)
ruptured cerebral arteriovenous malformation (I60.8)
ruptured malformation of precerebral vessels (I72.0)
Excludes ❷: *congenital peripheral aneurysm (Q27.8)*
congenital pulmonary aneurysm (Q25.79)
congenital retinal aneurysm (Q14.1)

CC **Q28.0 Arteriovenous malformation of precerebral vessels** — The presence of an abnormal precerebral arteriovenous connection.
Congenital arteriovenous precerebral aneurysm (nonruptured)

CC **Q28.1 Other malformations of precerebral vessels** — The abnormally developed precerebral arteries and veins.
Congenital malformation of precerebral vessels NOS
Congenital precerebral aneurysm (nonruptured)

MCC **Q28.2 Arteriovenous malformation of cerebral vessels** — The presence of an abnormal cerebral arteriovenous connection.
Arteriovenous malformation of brain NOS
Congenital arteriovenous cerebral aneurysm (nonruptured)

MCC **Q28.3 Other malformations of cerebral vessels** — The abnormally developed arteries and veins of the brain.
Congenital cerebral aneurysm (nonruptured)
Congenital malformation of cerebral vessels NOS
Developmental venous anomaly

CC **Q28.8 Other specified congenital malformations of circulatory system**
Congenital aneurysm, specified site NEC
Spinal vessel anomaly — The abnormally developed arteries and veins of the spinal vessels.

CC **Q28.9 Congenital malformation of circulatory system, unspecified**

Congenital malformations of the respiratory system (Q30-Q34)

Q30- Congenital malformations of nose
Excludes 1: *congenital deviation of nasal septum (Q67.4)*

Q30.0 Choanal atresia — The congenital occlusion of the nasal choanae that is due to the failure of the embryonic bucconasal membrane to rupture.
Atresia of nares (anterior) (posterior)
Congenital stenosis of nares (anterior) (posterior)

Q30.1 Agenesis and underdevelopment of nose — The failure of embryonic development of the nose.
Congenital absent of nose — The nonexistence of the nose.

Q30.2 Fissured, notched and cleft nose — The developmental deviation of the nose resulting from the incomplete union of the paired nasal primordia.

Q25-Q30

Q30.3   **Congenital perforated nasal septum** — The developmental deviation of the nose marked by turning away from the midline.

Q30.8   **Other congenital malformations of nose**
     Accessory nose — The condition of a supplementary nose.
     Congenital anomaly of nasal sinus wall — The malformation of the wall of a nasal sinus.

Q30.9   **Congenital malformation of nose, unspecified**

Q31-   **Congenital malformations of larynx**
     Excludes 1:   *congenital laryngeal stridor NOS (P28.89)*

Q31.0   **Web of larynx** — The congenital formation of a membrane between the vocal cords.
     Glottic web of larynx
     Subglottic web of larynx
     Web of larynx NOS

cc **Q31.1**   **Congenital subglottic stenosis** — The narrowing of the larynx just below the vocal cords.

cc **Q31.2**   **Laryngeal hypoplasia** — The incomplete development of the larynx.

cc **Q31.3**   **Laryngocele** — The air-sac herniation of the larynx.

cc **Q31.5**   **Congenital laryngomalacia** — The congenital softening of the larynx.

cc **Q31.8**   **Other congenital malformations of larynx**
     Absence of larynx — The failure of embryonic development of the larynx.
     Agenesis of larynx — The failure of embryonic development of the larynx.
     Atresia of larynx — The absence or closure of the larynx.
     Congenital cleft thyroid cartilage — The fissure of the thyroid cartilage resulting from the failure of the parts to fuse during embryonic development.
     Congenital fissure of epiglottis — An abnormal groove in the epiglottis.
     Congenital stenosis of larynx NEC
     Posterior cleft of cricoid cartilage — The fissure of the posterior portion of the cricoid cartilage.

cc **Q31.9**   **Congenital malformation of larynx, unspecified**

Q32-   **Congenital malformations of trachea and bronchus**
     Excludes 1:   *congenital bronchiectasis (Q33.4)*

cc **Q32.0**   **Congenital tracheomalacia** — The congenital softening of the trachea.

cc **Q32.1**   **Other congenital malformations of trachea**
     Atresia of trachea — The absence or closure of the trachea.
     Congenital anomaly of tracheal cartilage — The developmental deviation of the tracheal cartilage.
     Congenital dilatation of trachea — The increased width of the trachea
     Congenital malformation of trachea — The developmental deviation of the trachea.
     Congenital stenosis of trachea — The narrowing of the trachea.
     Congenital tracheocele — The protrusion of the tracheal mucous membrane through the tracheal wall.

cc **Q32.2**   **Congenital bronchomalacia** — The congenital softening of the bronchus.

cc **Q32.3**   **Congenital stenosis of bronchus** — The narrowing of the bronchus.

cc **Q32.4**   **Other congenital malformations of bronchus**
     Absence of bronchus — The failure of embryonic development of the bronchus.
     Agenesis of bronchus — The failure of embryonic development of the bronchus.
     Atresia of bronchus — The absence or closure of the bronchus.
     Congenital diverticulum of bronchus — The mucous membrane herniation of the bronchus.
     Congenital malformation of bronchus NOS

Q33-   **Congenital malformations of lung**

cc **Q33.0**   **Congenital cystic lung** — The congenital development of multiple, small cysts in the lungs.
     Congenital cystic lung disease
     Congenital honeycomb lung — A form marked by the appearance of honeycomb-like, radiolucent shadows on x-ray.
     Congenital polycystic lung disease
     Excludes 1:   *cystic fibrosis (E84.0)*
              cystic lung disease, acquired or unspecified (J98.4)

Q33.1   **Accessory lobe of lung** — The condition of a supplementary lobe.
     Azygos lobe (fissured), lung

MCC **Q33.2**   **Sequestration of lung** — The separation of a lung segment from the bronchial airways.

MCC **Q33.3**   **Agenesis of lung** — The failure of embryonic development of the lung.
     Congenital absence of lung (lobe) — The nonexistence of a portion of a lung.

cc **Q33.4**   **Congenital bronchiectasis** — The congenital dilatation of the bronchi.

Q33.5   **Ectopic tissue in lung**

MCC **Q33.6**   **Congenital hypoplasia and dysplasia of lung**
     Excludes 1:   *pulmonary hypoplasia associated with short gestation (P28.0)*

Q33.8   **Other congenital malformations of lung**

Q33.9   **Congenital malformation of lung, unspecified**

Q34-   **Other congenital malformations of respiratory system**
     Excludes ❷: *congenital central alveolar hypoventilation syndrome (G47.35)*

Q34.0   **Anomaly of pleura** — The developmental deviation of the pleura.

Q34.1   **Congenital cyst of mediastinum** — The fluid-filled sac of the mediastinum.

Q34.8   **Other specified congenital malformations of respiratory system**
     Atresia of nasopharynx — The absence or closure of the nasopharynx.

Q34.9   **Congenital malformation of respiratory system, unspecified**
     Congenital absence of respiratory system
     Congenital anomaly of respiratory system NOS

Cleft lip and cleft palate (Q35-Q37)

Use additional code to identify associated malformation of the nose (Q30.2)
     Excludes 1:   *Robin's syndrome (Q87.0)*

Q35-   **Cleft palate** — The congenital failure of the palate to fuse properly, forming a grooved or fissured depression in the roof of the mouth.
     Includes: **Fissure of palate**
                Palatoschisis
     Excludes 1:   *cleft palate with cleft lip (Q37-)*

Q35.1   **Cleft hard palate**

Q35.3   **Cleft soft palate**

Q35.5   **Cleft hard palate with cleft soft palate**

Q35.7   **Cleft uvula**

Q35.9   **Cleft palate, unspecified**
     Cleft palate NOS

Q36-   **Cleft lip** — The congenital failure of the maxillary and median nasal processes to fuse, forming a groove or fissure in the lip.
     Includes: **Cheiloschisis**
                Congenital fissure of lip
                Harelip
                Labium leporinum
     Excludes 1:   *cleft lip with cleft palate (Q37.-)*

Q36.0   **Cleft lip, bilateral**

Q36.1   **Cleft lip, median**

Q36.9   **Cleft lip, unilateral**
     Cleft lip NOS

Q37-   **Cleft palate with cleft lip** — The congenital failure of the palate and lip to fuse properly, forming a grooved or fissured palate and lip.
     Includes: **Cheilopalatoschisis**

Q37.0   **Cleft hard palate with bilateral cleft lip**

Q37.1   **Cleft hard palate with unilateral cleft lip**
     Cleft hard palate with cleft lip NOS

Q37.2   **Cleft soft palate with bilateral cleft lip**

Q37.3   **Cleft soft palate with unilateral cleft lip**
     Cleft soft palate with cleft lip NOS

Q37.4   **Cleft hard and soft palate with bilateral cleft lip**

Q37.5   **Cleft hard and soft palate with unilateral cleft lip**
     Cleft hard and soft palate with cleft lip NOS

Q37.8   **Unspecified cleft palate with bilateral cleft lip**

Q37.9   **Unspecified cleft palate with unilateral cleft lip**
     Cleft palate with cleft lip NOS

Other congenital malformations of the digestive system (Q38-Q45)

Q38-   **Other congenital malformations of tongue, mouth and pharynx**
     Excludes 1:   *dentofacial anomalies (M26.-)*
                macrostomia (Q18.4)
                microstomia (Q18.5)

Q38.0   **Congenital malformations of lips, not elsewhere classified**
     Congenital fistula of lip
     Congenital malformation of lip NOS
     Van der Woude's syndrome
     Excludes 1:   *cleft lip (Q36.-)*
                cleft lip with cleft palate (Q37.-)
                macrocheilia (Q18.6)
                microcheilia (Q18.7)

Q30 | Q38

Q38.1   Ankyloglossia — The congenital shortness of the tongue frenulum.
   Tongue tie

Q38.2   Macroglossia — The congenital largeness of the tongue.
   Congenital hypertrophy of tongue

Q38.3   Other congenital malformations of tongue
   Aglossia — The congenital absence of the tongue.
   Bifid tongue — The anterior division of the tongue.
   Congenital adhesion of tongue — The congenital restricting fibrous tissue bands of the tongue.
   Congenital fissure of tongue — The congenital groove of the tongue.
   Congenital malformation of tongue NOS
   Double tongue — The anterior division of the tongue.
   Hypoglossia — The incomplete development of the tongue.
   Hypoplasia of tongue — The incomplete development of the tongue.
   Microglossia — The congenital smallness of the tongue.

Q38.4   Congenital malformations of salivary glands and ducts
   Atresia of salivary glands and ducts — The absence or closure of a salivary duct.
   Congenital absence of salivary glands and ducts — The congenital nonexistence of a salivary gland.
   Congenital accessory salivary glands and ducts — The congenital presence of a supplementary salivary gland.
   Congenital fistula of salivary gland — The congenital abnormal passage of a salivary duct.

Q38.5   Congenital malformations of palate, not elsewhere classified
   Congenital absence of uvula — The congenital nonexistence of the uvula.
   Congenital malformation of palate NOS
   Congenital high arched palate
   Excludes 1:   cleft palate (Q35.-)
   *   cleft palate with cleft lip (Q37.-)*

Q38.6   Other congenital malformations of mouth
   Congenital malformation of mouth NOS

Q38.7   Congenital pharyngeal pouch — The congenital sac-like pouch of pharyngeal mucous membrane tissue.
   Congenital diverticulum of pharynx
   Excludes 1:   pharyngeal pouch syndrome (D82.1)

Q38.8   Other congenital malformations of pharynx
   Congenital malformation of pharynx NOS
   Imperforate pharynx — The abnormally closed pharygeal opening.

Q39-   Congenital malformations of esophagus

MCC **Q39.0   Atresia of esophagus without fistula** — The absence or closure of the esophagus.
   Atresia of esophagus NOS

MCC **Q39.1   Atresia of esophagus with tracheo-esophageal fistula** — The absence or closure of the esophagus with the abnormal passage between the esophagus and the trachea.
   Atresia of esophagus with broncho-esophageal fistula

MCC **Q39.2   Congenital tracheo-esophageal fistula without atresia** — The abnormal passage between the esophagus and the trachea.
   Congenital tracheo-esophageal fistula NOS

MCC **Q39.3   Congenital stenosis and stricture of esophagus** — The reduction in the size of the esophageal orifice or the decrease in caliber of the esophageal lumen.

MCC **Q39.4   Esophageal web** — The presence of a web-like structure in the lower esophagus.

CC **Q39.5   Congenital dilatation of esophagus** — The increased size of the esophageal lumen.
   Congenital cardiospasm

CC **Q39.6   Congenital diverticulum of esophagus** — The sac-like pouch of esophageal mucous membrane tissue.
   Congenital esophageal pouch

CC **Q39.8   Other congenital malformations of esophagus**
   Congenital absence of esophagus — The absence or closure of the esophagus.
   Congenital displacement of esophagus — The abnormal anatomical location of the esophagus.
   Congenital duplication of esophagus — The presence of a supplementary esophagus.

CC **Q39.9   Congenital malformation of esophagus, unspecified**

Q40-   Other congenital malformations of upper alimentary tract

Q40.0   Congenital hypertrophic pyloric stenosis — The congenital obstruction of the pyloric orifice.
   Congenital or infantile constriction — The narrowing of the pyloric orifice.
   Congenital or infantile hypertrophy — The enlargement of the pylorus, resulting in the narrowing of the pyloric orifice.
   Congenital or infantile spasm — The involuntary contraction of the muscle surrounding the pyloric orifice.
   Congenital or infantile stenosis — The failure of the pylorus to open completely.
   Congenital or infantile stricture — The decrease in caliber of the pyloric orifice.

Q40.1   Congenital hiatus hernia — The congenital displacement of an organ through the esophageal hiatus in the diaphragm.
   Congenital displacement of cardia through esophageal hiatus
   Excludes 1:   congenital diaphragmatic hernia (Q79.0)

Q40.2   Other specified congenital malformations of stomach
   Congenital displacement of stomach — The abnormal anatomical location of the stomach.
   Congenital diverticulum of stomach — The sac-like pouch of stomach mucous membrane tissue.
   Congenital hourglass stomach — The constriction of the smooth muscle of the stomach, forming an hourglass-shaped appearance.
   Congenital duplication of stomach — The presence of a supplementary stomach.
   Megalogastria — The excessive largeness of the stomach.
   Microgastria — The smallness of the stomach.

Q40.3   Congenital malformation of stomach, unspecified

Q40.8   Other specified congenital malformations of upper alimentary tract

Q40.9   Congenital malformation of upper alimentary tract, unspecified
   Congenital anomaly of upper alimentary tract
   Congenital deformity of upper alimentary tract

Q41-   Congenital absence, atresia and stenosis of small intestine
   Includes: Congenital obstruction, occlusion or stricture of small intestine or intestine NOS
   Excludes 1:   cystic fibrosis with intestinal manifestation (E84.11)
   *   meconium ileus NOS (without cystic fibrosis) (P76.0)*

CC **Q41.0   Congenital absence, atresia and stenosis of duodenum**

CC **Q41.1   Congenital absence, atresia and stenosis of jejunum**
   Apple peel syndrome — The abnormal development of the small bowel marked by the jejunum ending in a blind pouch and the small intestine wrapping itself around.
   Imperforate jejunum — The abnormally closed jejunal lumen.

CC **Q41.2   Congenital absence, atresia and stenosis of ileum**

CC **Q41.8   Congenital absence, atresia and stenosis of other specified parts of small intestine**

CC **Q41.9   Congenital absence, atresia and stenosis of small intestine, part unspecified**
   Congenital absence, atresia and stenosis of intestine NOS

Q42-   Congenital absence, atresia and stenosis of large intestine
   Includes: Congenital obstruction, occlusion and stricture of large intestine

CC **Q42.0   Congenital absence, atresia and stenosis of rectum with fistula** — A form with an abnormal passage.

CC **Q42.1   Congenital absence, atresia and stenosis of rectum without fistula**
   Imperforate rectum — The abnormally closed rectum.

CC **Q42.2   Congenital absence, atresia and stenosis of anus with fistula** — A form with an abnormal passage.

CC **Q42.3   Congenital absence, atresia and stenosis of anus without fistula**
   Imperforate anus — The abnormally closed anus.

CC **Q42.8   Congenital absence, atresia and stenosis of other parts of large intestine**

CC **Q42.9   Congenital absence, atresia and stenosis of large intestine, part unspecified**

Q43-   Other congenital malformations of intestine

Q43.0   Meckel's diverticulum (displaced) (hypertrophic) — The congenital sacculation of the ileum.
   Persistent omphalomesenteric duct
   Persistent vitelline duct

Excludes 1: = NOT CODED HERE! (Do not code both)   *Excludes ➋:* = Not Included Here

CC **Q43.1** **Hirschsprung's disease** — The congenital largeness or dilatation of the colon that is due to absence of ganglion nerve cells of the large intestine.
  Aganglionosis
  Congenital (aganglionic) megacolon

CC **Q43.2** **Other congenital functional disorders of colon**
  Congenital dilatation of colon — The increase in the lumenal width of the colon.

CC **Q43.3** **Congenital malformations of intestinal fixation**
  Congenital omental, anomalous adhesions [bands] — The fibrous tissue abnormally adhering to the omentum.
  Congenital peritoneal adhesions [bands] — The fibrous tissue abnormally adhering to the peritoneum.
  Incomplete rotation of cecum and colon
  Insufficient rotation of cecum and colon
  Jackson's membrane — The fibrous web-like tissue layer that may obstruct the bowel.
  Malrotation of colon — The abnormal rotational displacement of the colon.
  Rotation failure of cecum and colon
  Universal mesentery

CC **Q43.4** **Duplication of intestine** — The presence of an additional intestine.

CC **Q43.5** **Ectopic anus** — The malposition of the anus.

CC **Q43.6** **Congenital fistula of rectum and anus** — The presence of an abnormal passage.
  Excludes 1:   *congenital fistula of anus with absence, atresia and stenosis (Q42.2)*
      congenital fistula of rectum with absence, atresia and stenosis (Q42.0)
      congenital rectovaginal fistula (Q52.2)
      congenital urethrorectal fistula (Q64.73)
      pilonidal fistula or sinus (L05.-)

CC **Q43.7** **Persistent cloaca** — The persistence of the fetal cavity into which the intestinal, urinary, and reproductive ducts open.
  Cloaca NOS

CC **Q43.8** **Other specified congenital malformations of intestine**
  AHA 13:2Q:p31 – Epiploic appendagitis
  Congenital blind loop syndrome
  Congenital diverticulitis, colon
  Congenital diverticulum, intestine — The sac-like pouch of mucous membrane tissue of the colon.
  Dolichocolon — An abnormally long colon.
  Megaloappendix — The abnormal largeness of the appendix.
  Megaloduodenum — The abnormal largeness of the duodenum.
  Microcolon — The abnormal smallness of the colon.
  Transposition of appendix — The malposition of the appendix.
  Transposition of colon — The malposition of the colon.
  Transposition of intestine — The malposition of the intestine.

CC **Q43.9** **Congenital malformation of intestine, unspecified**

Q44- **Congenital malformations of gallbladder, bile ducts and liver**

CC **Q44.0** **Agenesis, aplasia and hypoplasia of gallbladder** — The failure of embryonic development of the gallbladder.
  Congenital absence of gallbladder — The nonexistence of the gallbladder.

CC **Q44.1** **Other congenital malformations of gallbladder**
  Congenital malformation of gallbladder NOS
  Intrahepatic gallbladder — The malposition of the gallbladder within the liver.

MCC **Q44.2** **Atresia of bile ducts** — The congenital absence or closure of a biliary duct.

MCC **Q44.3** **Congenital stenosis and stricture of bile ducts** — The decrease in caliber of a bile duct or passage.

CC **Q44.4** **Choledochal cyst** — The congenital cystic dilatation of the common bile duct.

CC **Q44.5** **Other congenital malformations of bile ducts**
  Accessory hepatic duct — The formation of additional hepatic ducts.
  Biliary duct duplication — The formation of an additional biliary duct.
  Congenital malformation of bile duct NOS
  Cystic duct duplication — The formation of an additional cystic duct.

CC **Q44.6** **Cystic disease of liver** — The congenital formation of multiple cysts in the liver.
  Fibrocystic disease of liver

CC **Q44.7** **Other congenital malformations of liver**
  Accessory liver — The formation of additional liver tissue.
  Alagille's syndrome
  Congenital absence of liver — The nonexistence of part, or all, of the liver.
  Congenital hepatomegaly — The enlargement of the liver.
  Congenital malformation of liver NOS

Q45- **Other congenital malformations of digestive system**
  Excludes ❷: *congenital diaphragmatic hernia (Q79.0)*
      congenital hiatus hernia (Q40.1)

CC **Q45.0** **Agenesis, aplasia and hypoplasia of pancreas** — The failure of embryonic development of the pancreas.
  Congenital absence of pancreas — The nonexistence of the pancreas.

CC **Q45.1** **Annular pancreas** — The developmental deviation in which the pancreas forms a complete ring around the duodenum.

CC **Q45.2** **Congenital pancreatic cyst**

CC **Q45.3** **Other congenital malformations of pancreas and pancreatic duct**
  Accessory pancreas — The inconstant separate part of the head of the pancreas.
  Congenital malformation of pancreas or pancreatic duct NOS
  Excludes 1:   *congenital diabetes mellitus (E10.-)*
      cystic fibrosis (E84.0-E84.9)
      fibrocystic disease of pancreas (E84.-)
      neonatal diabetes mellitus (P70.2)

Q45.8 **Other specified congenital malformations of digestive system**
  Absence (complete) (partial) of alimentary tract NOS
  Duplication of digestive system
  Malposition, congenital of digestive system

Q45.9 **Congenital malformation of digestive system, unspecified**
  Congenital anomaly of digestive system
  Congenital deformity of digestive system

Congenital malformations of genital organs (Q50-Q56)

  Excludes 1:   *androgen insensitivity syndrome (E34.5-)*
      syndromes associated with anomalies in the number and form of chromosomes (Q90-Q99)

Q50- **Congenital malformations of ovaries, fallopian tubes and broad ligaments**

Q50.0- **Congenital absence of ovary** — The nonexistence of an ovary.
  Excludes 1:   *Turner's syndrome (Q96.-)*

  Q50.01 **Congenital absence of ovary, unilateral** — [♀]

  Q50.02 **Congenital absence of ovary, bilateral** — [♀]

Q50.1 **Developmental ovarian cyst** — [♀] – The fluid-filled sac formed by the vestigial structure associated with an ovary.

Q50.2 **Congenital torsion of ovary** — [♀] – The abnormal twisting of an ovary.

Q50.3- **Other congenital malformations of ovary**

  Q50.31 **Accessory ovary** — [♀] – The formation of an additional ovary.

  Q50.32 **Ovarian streak** — [♀]
    46, XX with streak gonads

  Q50.39 **Other congenital malformation of ovary** — [♀]
    Congenital malformation of ovary NOS

Q50.4 **Embryonic cyst of fallopian tube** — [♀] – The congenital development of a fluid-filled sac of embryonic tissue of the fallopian tubes or broad ligaments.
  Fimbrial cyst

Q50.5 **Embryonic cyst of broad ligament** — [♀]
  Epoophoron cyst — The fluid-filled sac formed by the vestigial structure associated with an ovary.
  Parovarian cyst

Q50.6 **Other congenital malformations of fallopian tube and broad ligament** — [♀]
  Absence of fallopian tube and broad ligament — The nonexistence of a fallopian tube or broad ligament.
  Accessory fallopian tube and broad ligament — The formation of an additional fallopian tube or broad ligament.
  Atresia of fallopian tube and broad ligament — The absence or closure of a fallopian tube or broad ligament.
  Congenital malformation of fallopian tube or broad ligament NOS

Q51- **Congenital malformations of uterus and cervix**

Q51.0 **Agenesis and aplasia of uterus** — [♀] – The failure of embryonic development of the uterus.
  Congenital absence of uterus — The nonexistence of the uterus.

Q51.1- **Doubling of uterus with doubling of cervix and vagina** — The congenital malformation of the uterus forming two uterine cavities, cervices, and vaginas.

  Q51.10 **Doubling of uterus with doubling of cervix and vagina without obstruction** — [♀]
    Doubling of uterus with doubling of cervix and vagina NOS

  Q51.11 **Doubling of uterus with doubling of cervix and vagina with obstruction** — [♀]

Q43 - Q51

Q51.2 **Other doubling of uterus** — [♀] – The congenital malformation of the uterus forming two uterine cavities.
  Doubling of uterus NOS
  Septate uterus, complete or partial — The presence of a muscular or fibrous uterine fundus tissue septum that is caused by the failure of the embryonic tissue to be resorbed between the two uterine horns during development.

Q51.3 **Bicornate uterus** — [♀] – The malformation of the two uterine horns.
  Bicornate uterus, complete or partial

Q51.4 **Unicornate uterus** — [♀] – The malformation in which the uterus has one horn.
  Unicornate uterus with or without a separate uterine horn
  Uterus with only one functioning horn

Q51.5 **Agenesis and aplasia of cervix** — [♀] – The failure of embryonic development of the cervix.
  Congenital absence of cervix

Q51.6 **Embryonic cyst of cervix** — [♀] – The congenital fluid-filled sac of embryonic tissue of the cervix.

Q51.7 **Congenital fistulae between uterus and digestive and urinary tracts** — [♀] – The abnormal passage between the uterus and/or the digestive and urinary tracts.

Q51.8- **Other congenital malformations of uterus and cervix**
  Q51.81- **Other congenital malformations of uterus**
    Q51.810 **Arcuate uterus** — [♀] – The presence of a malformed uterine fundus marked by a slightly convex uterine fundus.
      Arcuatus uterus
    Q51.811 **Hypoplasia of uterus** — [♀] – The incomplete embryonic development of the uterus.
    Q51.818 **Other congenital malformations of uterus** — [♀]
      Müllerian anomaly of uterus NEC
  Q51.82- **Other congenital malformations of cervix**
    Q51.820 **Cervical duplication** — [♀] – The congenital presence of two cervices often associated with a didelphys uterus.
    Q51.821 **Hypoplasia of cervix** — [♀] – The incomplete embryonic development of the cervix.
    Q51.828 **Other congenital malformations of cervix** — [♀]

Q51.9 **Congenital malformation of uterus and cervix, unspecified** — [♀]

Q52- **Other congenital malformations of female genitalia**
  Q52.0 **Congenital absence of vagina** — [♀] – The nonexistence of the vagina.
    Vaginal agenesis, total or partial
  Q52.1- **Doubling of vagina** – The congenital malformation of the vagina forming two vaginal canals.
    Excludes 1: *doubling of vagina with doubling of uterus and cervix (Q51.1-)*
    Q52.10 **Doubling of vagina, unspecified** — [♀]
      Septate vagina NOS
    Q52.11 **Transverse vaginal septum** — [♀] – The congenital presence of a fibrous horizontal tissue wall in the vaginal cavity that results in a partial or complete blockage of the vagina.
    Q52.12- **Longitudinal vaginal septum** — The congenital presence of a fibrous vertical tissue wall in the vaginal cavity that essentially creates two vaginal cavities.
      Q52.120 **Longitudinal vaginal septum, nonobstructing** — [♀]
      Q52.121 **Longitudinal vaginal septum, obstructing, right side** — [♀]
      Q52.122 **Longitudinal vaginal septum, obstructing, left side** — [♀]
      Q52.123 **Longitudinal vaginal septum, microperforate, right side** — [♀]
      Q52.124 **Longitudinal vaginal septum, microperforate, left side** — [♀]
      Q52.129 **Other and unspecified longitudinal vaginal septum** — [♀]
  Q52.2 **Congenital rectovaginal fistula** — [♀] – The presence of an abnormal passage between the vagina and rectum.
    Excludes 1: *cloaca (Q43.7)*
  Q52.3 **Imperforate hymen** — [♀] – The abnormally closed vaginal opening.

Q52.4 **Other congenital malformations of vagina** — [♀]
  Canal of Nuck cyst, congenital — The fluid-filled sac formed from the fetal peritoneal membrane that extends down into the inguinal canal.
  Congenital malformation of vagina NOS
  Embryonic vaginal cyst — The fluid-filled sac of embryonal vaginal tissue.
  Gartner's duct cyst — The fluid-filled sac formed in the embryonic remnant of the mesonephric ducts in female development.

Q52.5 **Fusion of labia** — [♀] – The abnormal anatomical connection of the vulvar folds.

Q52.6 **Congenital malformation of clitoris** — [♀] – The incomplete embryonic development of the clitoris.

Q52.7- **Other and unspecified congenital malformations of vulva**
  Q52.70 **Unspecified congenital malformations of vulva** — [♀]
    Congenital malformation of vulva NOS
  Q52.71 **Congenital absence of vulva** — [♀]
  Q52.79 **Other congenital malformations of vulva** — [♀]
    Congenital cyst of vulva — The fluid-filled sac of the vulva.

Q52.8 **Other specified congenital malformations of female genitalia** — [♀]

Q52.9 **Congenital malformation of female genitalia, unspecified** — [♀]

Q53- **Undescended and ectopic testicle**
  Q53.0- **Ectopic testis** — The malposition of a testis.
    Q53.00 **Ectopic testis, unspecified** — [♂]
    Q53.01 **Ectopic testis, unilateral** — [♂]
    Q53.02 **Ectopic testes, bilateral** — [♂]
  Q53.1- **Undescended testicle, unilateral** — The congenital failure of the testis to descend into the scrotum.
    Q53.10 **Unspecified undescended testicle, unilateral** — [♂]
    Q53.11 **Abdominal testis, unilateral** — [♂]
    Q53.12 **Ectopic perineal testis, unilateral** — [♂]
  Q53.2- **Undescended testicle, bilateral**
    Q53.20 **Undescended testicle, unspecified, bilateral** — [♂]
    Q53.21 **Abdominal testis, bilateral** — [♂]
    Q53.22 **Ectopic perineal testis, bilateral** — [♂]
  Q53.9 **Undescended testicle, unspecified** — [♂]
    Cryptorchism NOS

Q54- **Hypospadias** — The congenital opening of the urethra on the under side of the penis.
  Excludes 1: *epispadias (Q64.0)*
  Q54.0 **Hypospadias, balanic** — [♂] – A form opening from the glans of the penis.
    Hypospadias, coronal
    Hypospadias, glandular
  Q54.1 **Hypospadias, penile** — [♂] – A form opening from the under side of the shaft of the penis.
  Q54.2 **Hypospadias, penoscrotal** — [♂] – A form opening from where the penis and scrotum meet.
  Q54.3 **Hypospadias, perineal** — [♂] – A form opening from the perineum.
  Q54.4 **Congenital chordee** — [♂] – The downward bowing of the penis that is usually due to hypospadias.
    Chordee without hypospadias
  Q54.8 **Other hypospadias** — [♂]
    Hypospadias with intersex state
  Q54.9 **Hypospadias, unspecified** — [♂]

Q55- **Other congenital malformations of male genital organs**
  Excludes 1: *congenital hydrocele (P83.5)*
    hypospadias (Q54.-)
  Q55.0 **Absence and aplasia of testis** — [♂] – The nonexistence, or failure of embryonic development of the testis.
    Monorchism — The development of only one testicle.
  Q55.1 **Hypoplasia of testis and scrotum** — [♂] – The incomplete embryonic development of the testis and/or scrotum.
    Fusion of testes — The abnormal anatomical connection of the testes.
  Q55.2- **Other and unspecified congenital malformations of testis and scrotum**
    Q55.20 **Unspecified congenital malformation of testis and scrotum** — [♂]
      Congenital malformation of testis or scrotum NOS
    Q55.21 **Polyorchism** — [♂] – The presence of more than two testicles.

Q51 - Q55

Q55.22 Retractile testis — [♂] — The condition characterized by the testis periodically disappearing from the scrotum.

Q55.23 Scrotal transposition — [♂] — The condition characterized by the scrotum (and testes) being located above the penis.

Q55.29 Other congenital malformations of testis and scrotum — [♂]

Q55.3 Atresia of vas deferens — [♂] — The absence or closure of the vas deferens.
   Code first any associated cystic fibrosis (E84.-)

Q55.4 Other congenital malformations of vas deferens, epididymis, seminal vesicles and prostate — [♂]
   Absence or aplasia of prostate — The nonexistence, or failure of embryonic development of the prostate.
   Absence or aplasia of spermatic cord — The incomplete embryonic development of the spermatic cord.
   Congenital malformation of vas deferens, epididymis, seminal vesicles or prostate NOS

Q55.5 Congenital absence and aplasia of penis — [♂] — The nonexistence, or failure of embryonic development of the penis.

Q55.6- Other congenital malformations of penis

Q55.61 Curvature of penis (lateral) — [♂] — The developmental deviation of the penis.

Q55.62 Hypoplasia of penis — [♂] — The incomplete embryonic development of the penis.
   Micropenis — An abnormally small penis.

Q55.63 Congenital torsion of penis — [♂]
   Excludes 1:   acquired torsion of penis (N48.82)

Q55.64 Hidden penis — [♂] — The developmental deviation of the penis marked by being beneath the skin.
   Buried penis
   Concealed penis
   Excludes 1:   acquired buried penis (N48.83)

Q55.69 Other congenital malformation of penis — [♂]
   Congenital malformation of penis NOS

Q55.7 Congenital vasocutaneous fistula — [♂] — An abnormal passage between the vas deferens and the skin.

Q55.8 Other specified congenital malformations of male genital organs — [♂]

Q55.9 Congenital malformation of male genital organ, unspecified — [♂]
   Congenital anomaly of male genital organ
   Congenital deformity of male genital organ

Q56- Indeterminate sex and pseudohermaphroditism
   Excludes 1:   46,XX true hermaphrodite (Q99.1)
   androgen insensitivity syndrome (E34.5-)
   chimera 46,XX/46,XY true hermaphrodite (Q99.0)
   female pseudohermaphroditism with adrenocortical disorder (E25.-)
   pseudohermaphroditism with specified chromosomal anomaly (Q96-Q99)
   pure gonadal dysgenesis (Q99.1)

Q56.0 Hermaphroditism, not elsewhere classified — The anomaly in which there is both ovarian and testicular tissue.
   Ovotestis — A gonad containing both ovarian and testicular tissue.

Q56.1 Male pseudohermaphroditism, not elsewhere classified — [♂] — A form when testicular tissue is present.
   46, XY with streak gonads
   Male pseudohermaphroditism NOS

Q56.2 Female pseudohermaphroditism, not elsewhere classified — [♀] — A form when ovarian tissue is present.
   Female pseudohermaphroditism NOS

Q56.3 Pseudohermaphroditism, unspecified

Q56.4 Indeterminate sex, unspecified
   Ambiguous genitalia

Congenital malformations of the urinary system (Q60-Q64)

Q60- Renal agenesis and other reduction defects of kidney — The failure, or deviation, of embryonic development of the kidney.
   Includes: Congenital absence of kidney — The nonexistence of the kidney.
   Congenital atrophy of kidney — The wasting of the kidney.
   Infantile atrophy of kidney — A protein-calorie malnutrition of the kidney.

cc **Q60.0 Renal agenesis, unilateral**
cc **Q60.1 Renal agenesis, bilateral**
cc **Q60.2 Renal agenesis, unspecified**
cc **Q60.3 Renal hypoplasia, unilateral**
cc **Q60.4 Renal hypoplasia, bilateral**
cc **Q60.5 Renal hypoplasia, unspecified**
cc **Q60.6 Potter's syndrome** — The failure of embryonic development of the kidney that leads to oligohydramnios.

Q61- Cystic kidney disease — The presence of congenital cysts of the kidneys.
   Excludes 1:   acquired cyst of kidney (N28.1)
   Potter's syndrome (Q60.6)

Q61.0- Congenital renal cyst — The presence of a renal cyst, that is not diagnostic of a specified cystic kidney disease.

cc **Q61.00 Congenital renal cyst, unspecified**
   Cyst of kidney NOS (congenital)

cc **Q61.01 Congenital single renal cyst**
cc **Q61.02 Congenital multiple renal cysts**

Q61.1- Polycystic kidney, infantile type — A disease characterized by the formation of multiple cysts throughout both kidneys, and carried by both members of a pair of homologous chromosomes.
   Polycystic kidney, autosomal recessive

cc **Q61.11 Cystic dilatation of collecting ducts**
cc **Q61.19 Other polycystic kidney, infantile type**

cc **Q61.2 Polycystic kidney, adult type** — A disease characterized by the formation of multiple cysts throughout both kidneys, and carried by only one of a pair of homologous chromosomes.
   Polycystic kidney, autosomal dominant

cc **Q61.3 Polycystic kidney, unspecified**

cc **Q61.4 Renal dysplasia** — A form characterized by the abnormal development of kidney tissue.
   Multicystic dysplastic kidney
   Multicystic kidney (development)
   Multicystic kidney disease — The presence of multiple renal cysts, that is not diagnostic of a specified cystic kidney disease.
   Multicystic renal dysplasia
   Excludes 1:   polycystic kidney disease (Q61.11-Q61.3)

cc **Q61.5 Medullary cystic kidney** — A form characterized by the deteriorization of the medullary tissues of the kidney in which the kidney has a spongy, or porous appearance and feeling.
   Nephronopthisis
   Sponge kidney NOS

cc **Q61.8 Other cystic kidney diseases**
   Fibrocystic kidney
   Fibrocystic renal degeneration or disease

cc **Q61.9 Cystic kidney disease, unspecified**
   Meckel-Gruber syndrome

Q62- Congenital obstructive defects of renal pelvis and congenital malformations of ureter

cc **Q62.0 Congenital hydronephrosis** — The congenital accumulation of urine in the kidney pelvis.

Q62.1- Congenital occlusion of ureter — The congenital blocking of the renal pelvis or ureter.
   Atresia and stenosis of ureter — The decrease in caliber of a ureter.

cc **Q62.10 Congenital occlusion of ureter, unspecified**
cc **Q62.11 Congenital occlusion of ureteropelvic junction** — The congenital blocking of the ureteropelvic junction.
cc **Q62.12 Congenital occlusion of ureterovesical orifice** — The congenital blocking of the ureterovesical junction.

cc **Q62.2 Congenital megaureter** — The developmental dilatation of the ureteral lumen diameter.
   Congenital dilatation of ureter

Q55 - Q62

Q62.3- Other obstructive defects of renal pelvis and ureter

cc **Q62.31 Congenital ureterocele, orthotopic**

cc **Q62.32 Cecoureterocele**
　　　　Ectopic ureterocele

cc **Q62.39 Other obstructive defects of renal pelvis and ureter**
　　　　Ureteropelvic junction obstruction NOS

Q62.4 Agenesis of ureter — The failure of embryonic development of the ureter.
　　　Congenital absence ureter

Q62.5 Duplication of ureter — The developmental deviation in which there are two ureters on the same side.
　　　Accessory ureter — The supplemental formation of an ureter.
　　　Double ureter

Q62.6- Malposition of ureter — The developmental malposition of the ureter.

Q62.60 Malposition of ureter, unspecified

Q62.61 Deviation of ureter

Q62.62 Displacement of ureter

Q62.63 Anomalous implantation of ureter
　　　Ectopia of ureter
　　　Ectopic ureter

Q62.69 Other malposition of ureter

Q62.7 Congenital vesico-uretero-renal reflux

Q62.8 Other congenital malformations of ureter
　　　Anomaly of ureter NOS

Q63- Other congenital malformations of kidney
　　Excludes 1:　congenital nephrotic syndrome (N04.-)

Q63.0 Accessory kidney — The supplemental formation of kidney tissue.

Q63.1 Lobulated, fused and horseshoe kidney — LOBULATED – The developmental deviation in which the kidney forms several lobules. FUSED – The developmental deviation in which both kidneys are connected anatomically. HORSESHOE KIDNEY – The developmental deviation in which the kidneys fuse together and have a horseshoe appearance.

Q63.2 Ectopic kidney — The developmental malposition of the kidney.
　　　Congenital displaced kidney
　　　Malrotation of kidney

Q63.3 Hyperplastic and giant kidney — The excessive development of normal cells of the kidney.
　　　Compensatory hypertrophy of kidney

Q63.8 Other specified congenital malformations of kidney
　　　Congenital renal calculi — The formation of a concretion in the kidney.

Q63.9 Congenital malformation of kidney, unspecified

Q64- Other congenital malformations of urinary system

Q64.0 Epispadias — [♂] – The congenital opening of the urethra on the upper side of the penis.
　　Excludes 1:　hypospadias (Q54.-)

Q64.1- Exstrophy of urinary bladder — The congenital malformation of the bladder and abdominal wall in which the bladder appears to be turned inside out.

cc **Q64.10 Exstrophy of urinary bladder, unspecified**
　　　Ectopia vesicae

cc **Q64.11 Supravesical fissure of urinary bladder**

cc **Q64.12 Cloacal extrophy of urinary bladder**

cc **Q64.19 Other exstrophy of urinary bladder**
　　　Extroversion of bladder

cc **Q64.2 Congenital posterior urethral valves** — The developmental formation of an obstructing urethral tissue valve.

Q64.3- Other atresia and stenosis of urethra and bladder neck

cc **Q64.31 Congenital bladder neck obstruction** — The blocking of the bladder neck.
　　　Congenital obstruction of vesicourethral orifice

cc **Q64.32 Congenital stricture of urethra** — The narrowing of the urethral lumen.

cc **Q64.33 Congenital stricture of urinary meatus** — The narrowing of the urethral opening.

cc **Q64.39 Other atresia and stenosis of urethra and bladder neck**
　　　Atresia and stenosis of urethra and bladder neck NOS

Q64.4 Malformation of urachus — The developmental deviation of the urachus.
　　　Cyst of urachus
　　　Patent urachus
　　　Prolapse of urachus

Q64.5 Congenital absence of bladder and urethra — The nonexistence of the bladder or urethra.

Q64.6 Congenital diverticulum of bladder — The sac-like pouch of bladder tissue.

Q64.7- Other and unspecified congenital malformations of bladder and urethra
　　Excludes 1:　congenital prolapse of bladder (mucosa) (Q79.4)

Q64.70 Unspecified congenital malformation of bladder and urethra
　　　Malformation of bladder or urethra NOS

Q64.71 Congenital prolapse of urethra — The downward displacement of the urethra.

Q64.72 Congenital prolapse of urinary meatus — The downward displacement of the urethral orifice.

Q64.73 Congenital urethrorectal fistula — The abnormal passage between the urethra and the rectum.

Q64.74 Double urethra — The malformation of the urethra in which two normal passages exist.

Q64.75 Double urinary meatus — The malformation of the urinary meatus in which two normal openings exist.

Q64.79 Other congenital malformations of bladder and urethra

Q64.8 Other specified congenital malformations of urinary system

Q64.9 Congenital malformation of urinary system, unspecified
　　　Congenital anomaly NOS of urinary system
　　　Congenital deformity NOS of urinary system

Congenital malformations and deformations of the musculoskeletal system (Q65-Q79)

Q65- Congenital deformities of hip
　　Excludes 1:　clicking hip (R29.4)

Q65.0- Congenital dislocation of hip, unilateral — The congenital displacement of the hip joint (slipping out of the normal socket position).

Q65.00 Congenital dislocation of unspecified hip, unilateral

Q65.01 Congenital dislocation of right hip, unilateral

Q65.02 Congenital dislocation of left hip, unilateral

Q65.1 Congenital dislocation of hip, bilateral

Q65.2 Congenital dislocation of hip, unspecified

Q65.3- Congenital partial dislocation of hip, unilateral — The congenital partial displacement of the hip joint from its normal position.

Q65.30 Congenital partial dislocation of unspecified hip, unilateral

Q65.31 Congenital partial dislocation of right hip, unilateral

Q65.32 Congenital partial dislocation of left hip, unilateral

Q65.4 Congenital partial dislocation of hip, bilateral

Q65.5 Congenital partial dislocation of hip, unspecified

Q65.6 Congenital unstable hip
　　　Congenital dislocatable hip

Q65.8- Other congenital deformities of hip

Q65.81 Congenital coxa valga — The congenital increase in the angle formed by the head of the femur and the shaft of the femur.

Q65.82 Congenital coxa vara — The congenital decrease in the angle formed by the head of the femur and the shaft of the femur.

Q65.89 Other specified congenital deformities of hip
　　　Anteversion of femoral neck — The forward displacement of the head of the femur.
　　　Congenital acetabular dysplasia — The impairment of embryonic development of the acetabulum.

Q65.9 Congenital deformity of hip, unspecified

Q66- Congenital deformities of feet
　　Excludes 1:　reduction defects of feet (Q72.-)
　　　　　　　valgus deformities (acquired) (M21.0-)
　　　　　　　varus deformities (acquired) (M21.1-)

Q66.0 Congenital talipes equinovarus — The congenital turning inward of the heel with turning upward of the inner edge of the foot.

Q66.1 Congenital talipes calcaneovarus — The turning inward of the heel with the turning upward of the toes and forefoot.

Q66.2- Congenital metatarsus (primus) varus — The congenital turning inward of the metatarsals.

Q66.21 Congenital metatarsus primus varus — The congenital turning inward of the first metatarsal.

Q66.22 Congenital metatarsus adductus — The congenital turning inward of all the metatarsals.
  Congenital metatarsus varus

Q66.3 Other congenital varus deformities of feet
  Hallux varus, congenital

Q66.4 Congenital talipes calcaneovalgus — The congenital turning outward of the foot with the turning upward of the toes and forefoot.

Q66.5- Congenital pes planus — The congenital malformation of the bones of the foot causing the arch to flatten (also known as flatfoot).
  Congenital flat foot
  Congenital rigid flat foot
  Congenital spastic (everted) flat foot
  Excludes 1:   *pes planus, acquired (M21.4)*

Q66.50 Congenital pes planus, unspecified foot
Q66.51 Congenital pes planus, right foot
Q66.52 Congenital pes planus, left foot

Q66.6 Other congenital valgus deformities of feet
  Congenital metatarsus valgus

Q66.7 Congenital pes cavus

Q66.8- Other congenital deformities of feet

Q66.80 Congenital vertical talus deformity, unspecified foot
Q66.81 Congenital vertical talus deformity, right foot
Q66.82 Congenital vertical talus deformity, left foot

Q66.89 Other congenital deformities of feet
  Congenital asymmetric talipes
  Congenital clubfoot NOS
  Congenital talipes NOS
  Congenital tarsal coalition
  Hammer toe, congenital

Q66.9 Congenital deformity of feet, unspecified

Q67- Congenital musculoskeletal deformities of head, face, spine and chest
  Excludes 1:   *congenital malformation syndromes classified to Q87.-*
    Potter's syndrome (Q60.6)

Q67.0 Congenital facial asymmetry — The dissimilarity of the facial bones.

Q67.1 Congenital compression facies

Q67.2 Dolichocephaly — The elongation of the head.

Q67.3 Plagiocephaly — The unsymmetrical formation of the head.

Q67.4 Other congenital deformities of skull, face and jaw
  Congenital depressions in skull — The inward displacement of an area of the skull.
  Congenital hemifacial atrophy or hypertrophy
  Deviation of nasal septum, congenital — The displacement of the nasal septum towards one side.
  Squashed or bent nose, congenital
  Excludes 1:   *dentofacial anomalies [including malocclusion] (M26.-)*
    syphilitic saddle nose (A50.5)

cc **Q67.5 Congenital deformity of spine**
  AHA 14:4Q:p26 – Congenital scoliosis
  Congenital postural scoliosis
  Congenital scoliosis NOS
  Excludes 1:   *infantile idiopathic scoliosis (M41.0)*
    scoliosis due to congenital bony malformation (Q76.3)

Q67.6 Pectus excavatum — The congenital depression of the sternum.
  Congenital funnel chest

Q67.7 Pectus carinatum — The congenital prominence of the sternum.
  Congenital pigeon chest

cc **Q67.8 Other congenital deformities of chest**
  Congenital deformity of chest wall NOS

Q68- Other congenital musculoskeletal deformities
  Excludes 1:   *reduction defects of limb(s) (Q71-Q73)*
  Excludes ❷: *congenital myotonic chondrodystrophy (G71.13)*

Q68.0 Congenital deformity of sternocleidomastoid muscle — The congenital malformation of the sternocleidomastoid muscle.
  Congenital contracture of sternocleidomastoid (muscle)
  Congenital (sternomastoid) torticollis — The twisting condition of the neck that is due to malformation of the sternocleidomastoid muscle.
  Sternomastoid tumor (congenital) — The abnormal growth of the sternomastoid region.

cc **Q68.1 Congenital deformity of finger(s) and hand**
  Congenital clubfinger — The turning inward of a finger.
  Spade-like hand (congenital) — The thickened, square-shaped appearance of the hand.

Q68.2 Congenital deformity of knee — The congenital malformation of the knee joint.
  Congenital dislocation of knee — The congenital displacement of the knee joint from its normal position.
  Congenital genu recurvatum — The congenital hyperextension of the knee.

Q68.3 Congenital bowing of femur — The congenital bending of the femur.
  Excludes 1:   *anteversion of femur (neck) (Q65.89)*

Q68.4 Congenital bowing of tibia and fibula — The congenital bending of the tibia or fibula.

Q68.5 Congenital bowing of long bones of leg, unspecified

Q68.6 Discoid meniscus — A thickened, oval (instead of crescent shaped) mass of the meniscus.

Q68.8 Other specified congenital musculoskeletal deformities
  Congenital deformity of clavicle
  Congenital deformity of elbow
  Congenital deformity of forearm
  Congenital deformity of scapula
  Congenital deformity of wrist
  Congenital dislocation of elbow
  Congenital dislocation of shoulder
  Congenital dislocation of wrist

Q69- Polydactyly — The congenital developmental deviation in which there are supernumerary digits.

Q69.0 Accessory finger(s) — The congenital formation of supernumerary fingers of the hand.

Q69.1 Accessory thumb(s) — The congenital formation of the supernumerary thumb of the hand.

Q69.2 Accessory toe(s) — The congenital formation of supernumerary digits of the foot.
  Accessory hallux

Q69.9 Polydactyly, unspecified
  Supernumerary digit(s) NOS

Q70- Syndactyly — The congenital formation of a tissue web between digits.

Q70.0- Fused fingers — The complete fusion of the bones of one digit to another.
  Complex syndactyly of fingers with synostosis

Q70.00 Fused fingers, unspecified hand
Q70.01 Fused fingers, right hand
Q70.02 Fused fingers, left hand
Q70.03 Fused fingers, bilateral

Q70.1- Webbed fingers — The congenital formation of a tissue web between digits.
  Simple syndactyly of fingers without synostosis

Q70.10 Webbed fingers, unspecified hand
Q70.11 Webbed fingers, right hand
Q70.12 Webbed fingers, left hand
Q70.13 Webbed fingers, bilateral

Q70.2- Fused toes — The complete fusion of the bones of one digit to another.
  Complex syndactyly of toes with synostosis

Q70.20 Fused toes, unspecified foot
Q70.21 Fused toes, right foot
Q70.22 Fused toes, left foot
Q70.23 Fused toes, bilateral

Q70.3- Webbed toes — The congenital formation of a tissue web between digits.
  Simple syndactyly of toes without synostosis

Q70.30 Webbed toes, unspecified foot
Q70.31 Webbed toes, right foot
Q70.32 Webbed toes, left foot
Q70.33 Webbed toes, bilateral

Q70.4 Polysyndactyly, unspecified
  Excludes 1:   *specified syndactyly of hand and feet* — code to specified conditions (Q70.0-Q70.3-)

Q70.9 Syndactyly, unspecified
  Symphalangy NOS

Q71- Reduction defects of upper limb — The congenital absence of a portion of the upper limb.

Q71.0- Congenital complete absence of upper limb

Q71.00 Congenital complete absence of unspecified upper limb
Q71.01 Congenital complete absence of right upper limb
Q71.02 Congenital complete absence of left upper limb
Q71.03 Congenital complete absence of upper limb, bilateral

Q66-Q71

Q71.1- Congenital <u>absence of upper arm and forearm with hand present</u>
- **Q71.10** Congenital absence of <u>unspecified</u> upper arm and forearm with hand present
- **Q71.11** Congenital absence of <u>right</u> upper arm and forearm with hand present
- **Q71.12** Congenital absence of <u>left</u> upper arm and forearm with hand present
- **Q71.13** Congenital absence of upper arm and forearm with hand present, <u>bilateral</u>

Q71.2- Congenital <u>absence of both forearm and hand</u>
- **Q71.20** Congenital absence of both forearm and hand, <u>unspecified</u> upper limb
- **Q71.21** Congenital absence of both forearm and hand, <u>right</u> upper limb
- **Q71.22** Congenital absence of both forearm and hand, <u>left</u> upper limb
- **Q71.23** Congenital absence of both forearm and hand, <u>bilateral</u>

Q71.3- Congenital <u>absence of hand and finger</u>
- **Q71.30** Congenital absence of <u>unspecified</u> hand and finger
- **Q71.31** Congenital absence of <u>right</u> hand and finger
- **Q71.32** Congenital absence of <u>left</u> hand and finger
- **Q71.33** Congenital absence of hand and finger, <u>bilateral</u>

Q71.4- <u>Longitudinal reduction</u> defect of <u>radius</u> — The congenital decreased length, or absence, of the radius.
    Clubhand (congenital)
    Radial clubhand
- **Q71.40** Longitudinal reduction defect of <u>unspecified</u> radius
- **Q71.41** Longitudinal reduction defect of <u>right</u> radius
- **Q71.42** Longitudinal reduction defect of <u>left</u> radius
- **Q71.43** Longitudinal reduction defect of radius, <u>bilateral</u>

Q71.5- <u>Longitudinal reduction</u> defect of <u>ulna</u> — The congenital decreased length, or absence, of the ulna.
- **Q71.50** Longitudinal reduction defect of <u>unspecified</u> ulna
- **Q71.51** Longitudinal reduction defect of <u>right</u> ulna
- **Q71.52** Longitudinal reduction defect of <u>left</u> ulna
- **Q71.53** Longitudinal reduction defect of ulna, <u>bilateral</u>

Q71.6- <u>Lobster-claw hand</u> — The absence of one or more of the middle digits of the hand.
- **Q71.60** Lobster-claw hand, <u>unspecified</u> hand
- **Q71.61** Lobster-claw <u>right</u> hand
- **Q71.62** Lobster-claw <u>left</u> hand
- **Q71.63** Lobster-claw hand, <u>bilateral</u>

Q71.8- Other reduction defects of upper limb
- **Q71.81-** Congenital <u>shortening</u> of <u>upper</u> limb — The decreased length of the arm.
  - **Q71.811** Congenital shortening of <u>right</u> upper limb
  - **Q71.812** Congenital shortening of <u>left</u> upper limb
  - **Q71.813** Congenital shortening of upper limb, <u>bilateral</u>
  - **Q71.819** Congenital shortening of <u>unspecified</u> upper limb
- **Q71.89-** <u>Other reduction</u> defects of <u>upper</u> limb
  - **Q71.891** Other reduction defects of <u>right</u> upper limb
  - **Q71.892** Other reduction defects of <u>left</u> upper limb
  - **Q71.893** Other reduction defects of upper limb, <u>bilateral</u>
  - **Q71.899** Other reduction defects of <u>unspecified</u> upper limb

Q71.9- <u>Unspecified reduction</u> defect of upper limb
- **Q71.90** Unspecified reduction defect of <u>unspecified</u> upper limb
- **Q71.91** Unspecified reduction defect of <u>right</u> upper limb
- **Q71.92** Unspecified reduction defect of <u>left</u> upper limb
- **Q71.93** Unspecified reduction defect of upper limb, <u>bilateral</u>

Q72- Reduction defects of lower limb — The congenital absence of a portion of the lower limb.

Q72.0- Congenital <u>complete absence</u> of <u>lower</u> limb
- **Q72.00** Congenital complete absence of <u>unspecified</u> lower limb
- **Q72.01** Congenital complete absence of <u>right</u> lower limb

Q72.02 Congenital complete absence of <u>left</u> lower limb
Q72.03 Congenital complete absence of lower limb, <u>bilateral</u>

Q72.1- Congenital <u>absence of thigh and lower leg with foot present</u>
- **Q72.10** Congenital absence of <u>unspecified</u> thigh and lower leg with foot present
- **Q72.11** Congenital absence of <u>right</u> thigh and lower leg with foot present
- **Q72.12** Congenital absence of <u>left</u> thigh and lower leg with foot present
- **Q72.13** Congenital absence of thigh and lower leg with foot present, <u>bilateral</u>

Q72.2- Congenital <u>absence of both lower leg and foot</u>
- **Q72.20** Congenital absence of both lower leg and foot, <u>unspecified</u> lower limb
- **Q72.21** Congenital absence of both lower leg and foot, <u>right</u> lower limb
- **Q72.22** Congenital absence of both lower leg and foot, <u>left</u> lower limb
- **Q72.23** Congenital absence of both lower leg and foot, <u>bilateral</u>

Q72.3- Congenital <u>absence of foot and toe(s)</u>
- **Q72.30** Congenital absence of unspecified foot and toe(s)
- **Q72.31** Congenital absence of <u>right</u> foot and toe(s)
- **Q72.32** Congenital absence of <u>left</u> foot and toe(s)
- **Q72.33** Congenital absence of foot and toe(s), <u>bilateral</u>

Q72.4- <u>Longitudinal reduction</u> defect of <u>femur</u> — The congenital decreased length, or absence, of the femur.
    Proximal femoral focal deficiency
- **Q72.40** Longitudinal reduction defect of <u>unspecified</u> femur
- **Q72.41** Longitudinal reduction defect of <u>right</u> femur
- **Q72.42** Longitudinal reduction defect of <u>left</u> femur
- **Q72.43** Longitudinal reduction defect of femur, <u>bilateral</u>

Q72.5- <u>Longitudinal reduction</u> defect of <u>tibia</u> — The congenital decreased length, or absence, of the tibia.
- **Q72.50** Longitudinal reduction defect of <u>unspecified</u> tibia
- **Q72.51** Longitudinal reduction defect of <u>right</u> tibia
- **Q72.52** Longitudinal reduction defect of <u>left</u> tibia
- **Q72.53** Longitudinal reduction defect of tibia, <u>bilateral</u>

Q72.6- <u>Longitudinal reduction</u> defect of <u>fibula</u> — The congenital decreased length, or absence, of the fibula.
- **Q72.60** Longitudinal reduction defect of <u>unspecified</u> fibula
- **Q72.61** Longitudinal reduction defect of <u>right</u> fibula
- **Q72.62** Longitudinal reduction defect of <u>left</u> fibula
- **Q72.63** Longitudinal reduction defect of fibula, <u>bilateral</u>

Q72.7- <u>Split foot</u> — The absence of one or more of the middle digits of the hand.
- **Q72.70** Split foot, <u>unspecified</u> lower limb
- **Q72.71** Split foot, <u>right</u> lower limb
- **Q72.72** Split foot, <u>left</u> lower limb
- **Q72.73** Split foot, <u>bilateral</u>

Q72.8- <u>Other reduction</u> defects of <u>lower</u> limb
- **Q72.81-** Congenital <u>shortening</u> of <u>lower</u> limb
  - **Q72.811** Congenital shortening of <u>right</u> lower limb
  - **Q72.812** Congenital shortening of <u>left</u> lower limb
  - **Q72.813** Congenital shortening of lower limb, <u>bilateral</u>
  - **Q72.819** Congenital shortening of <u>unspecified</u> lower limb
- **Q72.89-** <u>Other reduction</u> defects of <u>lower</u> limb
  - **Q72.891** Other reduction defects of <u>right</u> lower limb
  - **Q72.892** Other reduction defects of <u>left</u> lower limb
  - **Q72.893** Other reduction defects of lower limb, <u>bilateral</u>
  - **Q72.899** Other reduction defects of <u>unspecified</u> lower limb

Q72.9- <u>Unspecified reduction</u> defect of lower limb
- **Q72.90** Unspecified reduction defect of <u>unspecified</u> lower limb
- **Q72.91** Unspecified reduction defect of <u>right</u> lower limb
- **Q72.92** Unspecified reduction defect of <u>left</u> lower limb
- **Q72.93** Unspecified reduction defect of lower limb, <u>bilateral</u>

Q71-Q72

Q73- Reduction defects of unspecified limb

Q73.0   Congenital absence of unspecified limb(s)
Amelia NOS

Q73.1   Phocomelia, unspecified limb(s)
Phocomelia NOS

Q73.8   Other reduction defects of unspecified limb(s)
Longitudinal reduction deformity of unspecified limb(s)
Ectromelia of limb NOS
Hemimelia of limb NOS
Reduction defect of limb NOS

Q74- Other congenital malformations of limb(s)
Excludes 1:   polydactyly (Q69.-)
reduction defect of limb (Q71-Q73)
syndactyly (Q70.-)

Q74.0   Other congenital malformations of upper limb(s), including shoulder girdle
Accessory carpal bones — The congenital formation of supplementary carpal bones of the hand.
Cleidocranial dysostosis — The failure of bony development of the cranial bones with absence of part, or all, of the clavicles.
Congenital pseudarthrosis of clavicle — The congenital malformation of the clavicle.
Macrodactylia (fingers) — The congenital largeness of the fingers.
Madelung's deformity — The congenital overgrowth of the distal ulna resulting in deviation of the hand.
Radioulnar synostosis — The congenital fusion of the proximal ends of the radius and ulna.
Sprengel's deformity — The congenital malposition of the scapula above its normal position.
Triphalangeal thumb — The formation of three phalanges of the thumb versus the usual two.

Q74.1   Congenital malformation of knee
Congenital absence of patella — The nonexistence of the patella.
Congenital dislocation of patella — The displacement of the patella.
Congenital genu valgum — The deformity in which the knees are close together.
Congenital genu varum — The deformity in which the knees are more separated.
Rudimentary patella — An imperfectly developed patella.
Excludes 1:   congenital dislocation of knee (Q68.2)
congenital genu recurvatum (Q68.2)
nail patella syndrome (Q87.2)

Q74.2   Other congenital malformations of lower limb(s), including pelvic girdle
Congenital fusion of sacroiliac joint
Congenital malformation of ankle joint
Congenital malformation of sacroiliac joint
Excludes 1:   anteversion of femur (neck) (Q65.89)

CC **Q74.3   Arthrogryposis multiplex congenita**

Q74.8   Other specified congenital malformations of limb(s)

Q74.9   Unspecified congenital malformation of limb(s)
Congenital anomaly of limb(s) NOS

Q75- Other congenital malformations of skull and face bones
Excludes 1:   congenital malformation of face NOS (Q18-)
congenital malformation syndromes classified to Q87-
dentofacial anomalies [including malocclusion] (M26-)
musculoskeletal deformities of head and face (Q67.0-Q67.4)
skull defects associated with congenital anomalies of brain
such as:
anencephaly (Q00.0)
encephalocele (Q01-)
hydrocephalus (Q03-)
microcephaly (Q02)

Q75.0   Craniosynostosis — The premature closure of the skull sutures.
Acrocephaly — The malformation of the skull in which the top of the head is pointed.
Imperfect fusion of skull — The abnormal coherence of the skull bones.
Oxycephaly — The malformation of the skull in which the top of the head is pointed.
Trigonocephaly — The malformation of the skull at the suture of the frontal bones.

Q75.1   Craniofacial dysostosis — The craniofacial malformation consisting of widely-spaced eyes, exophthalmos, optic atrophy, strabismus, acrocephaly, and a beak-shaped nose.
Crouzon's disease

Q75.2   Hypertelorism — The malformation in which the eyes are widely spaced.

Q75.3   Macrocephaly — An overly large head.

Q75.4   Mandibulofacial dysostosis — The craniofacial malformation marked by absent cheek bones, an undersized jaw, and/or an undersized zygoma bone.
Franceschetti syndrome
Treacher Collins syndrome

Q75.5   Oculomandibular dysostosis

Q75.8   Other specified congenital malformations of skull and face bones
Absence of skull bone, congenital — The nonexistence of skull bone(s).
Congenital deformity of forehead — The malformation of the forehead.
Platybasia — The malformation of the occipital and upper vertebral bones in which the base of the skull appears pushed up into the head.

Q75.9   Congenital malformation of skull and face bones, unspecified
Congenital anomaly of face bones NOS
Congenital anomaly of skull NOS

Q76- Congenital malformations of spine and bony thorax
Excludes 1:   congenital musculoskeletal deformities of spine and chest (Q67.5-Q67.8)

Q76.0   Spina bifida occulta — The congenital malformation of the bony spinal canal without impingement upon the spinal cord.
Excludes 1:   meningocele (spinal) (Q05.-)
spina bifida (aperta) (cystica) (Q05.-)

Q76.1   Klippel-Feil syndrome — The congenital reduction in the neck height resulting from absence or incomplete development of cervical vertebrae.
Cervical fusion syndrome

Q76.2   Congenital spondylolisthesis — The congenital forward displacement of a vertebra.
Congenital spondylolysis
Excludes 1:   spondylolisthesis (acquired) (M43.1-)
spondylolysis (acquired) (M43.0-)

CC **Q76.3   Congenital scoliosis due to congenital bony malformation**
Hemivertebra fusion or failure of segmentation with scoliosis

Q76.4- Other congenital malformations of spine, not associated with scoliosis

Q76.41- Congenital kyphosis — The congenital increased convexity of the spinal position.

Q76.411   Congenital kyphosis, occipito-atlanto-axial region

Q76.412   Congenital kyphosis, cervical region

Q76.413   Congenital kyphosis, cervicothoracic region

Q76.414   Congenital kyphosis, thoracic region

Q76.415   Congenital kyphosis, thoracolumbar region

Q76.419   Congenital kyphosis, unspecified region

Q76.42- Congenital lordosis — The congenital increased concavity of the spinal position.

CC **Q76.425   Congenital lordosis, thoracolumbar region**

CC **Q76.426   Congenital lordosis, lumbar region**

CC **Q76.427   Congenital lordosis, lumbosacral region**

CC **Q76.428   Congenital lordosis, sacral and sacrococcygeal region**

CC **Q76.429   Congenital lordosis, unspecified region**

Q76.49   Other congenital malformations of spine, not associated with scoliosis
Congenital absence of vertebra NOS
Congenital fusion of spine NOS
Congenital malformation of lumbosacral (joint) (region) NOS
Congenital malformation of spine NOS
Hemivertebra NOS
Malformation of spine NOS
Platyspondylisis NOS
Supernumerary vertebra NOS

Q76.5   Cervical rib — The congenital formation of an additional rib bone arising from a cervical vertebra.
Supernumerary rib in cervical region

CC **Q76.6   Other congenital malformations of ribs**
Accessory rib — The formation of a supplementary rib.
Congenital absence of rib — The nonexistence of a rib.
Congenital fusion of ribs — The abnormal anatomical connection of the ribs.
Congenital malformation of ribs NOS
Excludes 1:   short rib syndrome (Q77.2)

CC **Q76.7   Congenital malformation of sternum**
Congenital absence of sternum — The nonexistence of the sternum.
Sternum bifidum — The malforming separation of the sternum into 2 parts.

CC **Q76.8   Other congenital malformations of bony thorax**

CC **Q76.9   Congenital malformation of bony thorax, unspecified**

Q73-Q76

Q77- **Osteochondrodysplasia with defects of growth of tubular bones and spine**
  Excludes 1:   mucopolysaccharidosis (E76.0-E76.3)
  Excludes ❷: congenital myotonic chondrodystrophy (G71.13)

Q77.0 **Achondrogenesis** — The lack of embryonic development of the bony cartilage.
    Hypochondrogenesis

Q77.1 **Thanatophoric short stature** — The skeletal deformity marked by extremely short limbs, narrow chest, and underdeveloped lungs.

CC **Q77.2** **Short rib syndrome** — The impairment of embryonic development of the rib cage.
    Asphyxiating thoracic dysplasia [Jeune]

Q77.3 **Chondrodysplasia punctata**
    Excludes 1:   Rhizomelic chondrodysplasia punctata (E71.43)

Q77.4 **Achondroplasia** — The impairment of embryonic development of the bony cartilage.
    Hypochondroplasia
    Osteosclerosis congenita

Q77.5 **Diastrophic dysplasia**

Q77.6 **Chondroectodermal dysplasia** — The congenital malformation of the bony cartilage that is associated with defective development of the skin, hair, and teeth.
    Ellis-van Creveld syndrome

Q77.7 **Spondyloepiphyseal dysplasia**

Q77.8 **Other osteochondrodysplasia with defects of growth of tubular bones and spine**

Q77.9 **Osteochondrodysplasia with defects of growth of tubular bones and spine, unspecified**

Q78- **Other osteochondrodysplasias**
  Excludes ❷: congenital myotonic chondrodystrophy (G71.13)

CC **Q78.0** **Osteogenesis imperfecta** — The congenital brittleness of the bones.
    Fragilitas ossium
    Osteopsathyrosis

Q78.1 **Polyostotic fibrous dysplasia** — The congenital fibrous displacement of bony tissue.
    Albright(-McCune)(-Sternberg) syndrome — The fibrous dysplasia of the bone in association with melanotic pigmentation of the skin.

CC **Q78.2** **Osteopetrosis** — The congenital excessive calcification of the bones.
    Albers-Schönberg syndrome
    Osteosclerosis NOS

Q78.3 **Progressive diaphyseal dysplasia** — The congenital excessive thickness of the bones, especially the long bones.
    Camurati-Engelmann syndrome

Q78.4 **Enchondromatosis** — The overgrowth of cartilage resulting in a thinned cortex of the affected bone.
    Maffucci's syndrome
    Ollier's disease

Q78.5 **Metaphyseal dysplasia** — The congenital thinning of the long bones.
    Pyle's syndrome

Q78.6 **Multiple congenital exostoses** — The congenital development of multiple bony spurs.
    Diaphyseal aclasis

Q78.8 **Other specified osteochondrodysplasias**
    Osteopoikilosis — The congenital excessive calcification of spots of bones.

Q78.9 **Osteochondrodysplasia, unspecified**
    Chondrodystrophy NOS
    Osteodystrophy NOS

Q79- **Congenital malformations of musculoskeletal system, not elsewhere classified**
  Excludes ❷: congenital (sternomastoid) torticollis (Q68.0)

MCC **Q79.0** **Congenital diaphragmatic hernia** — The protrusion of an organ through a defect in the diaphragm.
    Excludes 1:   congenital hiatus hernia (Q40.1)

MCC **Q79.1** **Other congenital malformations of diaphragm**
    Absence of diaphragm — The nonexistence of the diaphragm.
    Congenital malformation of diaphragm NOS
    Eventration of diaphragm — The elevation of the diaphragm from abdominal organ pressure.

MCC **Q79.2** **Exomphalos** — The protrusion of an abdominal organ into the umbilicus.
    Omphalocele — The congenital protrusion of the intestine at the umbilicus.
    Excludes 1:   umbilical hernia (K42.-)

MCC **Q79.3** **Gastroschisis** — A congenital fissure of the abdominal wall with protrusion of the intestine.

MCC **Q79.4** **Prune belly syndrome** — The absence of the lower abdominal rectus and oblique muscles.
    Congenital prolapse of bladder mucosa
    Eagle-Barrett syndrome

Q79.5- **Other congenital malformations of abdominal wall**
    Excludes 1:   umbilical hernia (K42.-)

MCC **Q79.51** **Congenital hernia of bladder** — The protrusion of the bladder through a defect in the abdominal wall.

MCC **Q79.59** **Other congenital malformations of abdominal wall**

CC **Q79.6** **Ehlers-Danlos syndrome** — The congenital syndrome characterized by fragile and hyperelastic tissue, hyperextensibility of joints, visceral malformations, and calcified subcutaneous cysts.

Q79.8 **Other congenital malformations of musculoskeletal system**
    Absence of muscle — The congenital nonexistence of a muscle.
    Absence of tendon — The congenital nonexistence of a tendon.
    Accessory muscle — The congenital formation of an additional muscle.
    Amyotrophia congenita — The incomplete development of a muscle.
    Congenital constricting bands
    Congenital shortening of tendon
    Poland syndrome

Q79.9 **Congenital malformation of musculoskeletal system, unspecified**
    Congenital anomaly of musculoskeletal system NOS
    Congenital deformity of musculoskeletal system NOS

Other congenital malformations (Q80-Q89)

Q80- **Congenital ichthyosis** — The congenital development of rough, dry, and scaly skin.
    Excludes 1:   Refsum's disease (G60.1)

Q80.0 **Ichthyosis vulgaris**

Q80.1 **X-linked ichthyosis**

Q80.2 **Lamellar ichthyosis**
    Collodion baby

Q80.3 **Congenital bullous ichthyosiform erythroderma**

Q80.4 **Harlequin fetus** — The severe form that is marked by thick, horny scales covering the fetus.

Q80.8 **Other congenital ichthyosis**

Q80.9 **Congenital ichthyosis, unspecified**

Q81- **Epidermolysis bullosa** — The hereditary disease marked by the development of bullae and vesicles on the skin.

Q81.0 **Epidermolysis bullosa simplex**
    Excludes 1:   Cockayne's syndrome (Q87.1)

Q81.1 **Epidermolysis bullosa letalis**
    Herlitz' syndrome

Q81.2 **Epidermolysis bullosa dystrophica**

Q81.8 **Other epidermolysis bullosa**

Q81.9 **Epidermolysis bullosa, unspecified**

Q82- **Other congenital malformations of skin**
    Excludes 1:   acrodermatitis enteropathica (E83.2)
              congenital erythropoietic porphyria (E80.0)
              pilonidal cyst or sinus (L05.-)
              Sturge-Weber (-Dimitri) syndrome (Q85.8)

Q82.0 **Hereditary lymphedema** — Edema of the legs resulting from obstruction of the lymphatic system.

Q82.1 **Xeroderma pigmentosum** — The extreme sensitivity of the skin and eyes to light.

Q82.2 **Mastocytosis** — The presence of pink to brown areas on the skin that are caused by abnormal masses of mast cells.
    Urticaria pigmentosa
    Excludes 1:   malignant mastocytosis (C96.2)

Q82.3 **Incontinentia pigmenti** — The congenital developmental deviation of the skin pigment.

Q82.4 **Ectodermal dysplasia (anhidrotic)** — The congenital malformation in which the skin is smooth and glossy, absence of sweat glands, and defective development of the hair.
    Excludes 1:   Ellis-van Creveld syndrome (Q77.6)

Q
7
7
-
Q
8
2

Q82.5 **Congenital non-neoplastic nevus**
  Birthmark NOS
  Flammeus nevus — A congenital malformation of capillary blood vessels within the skin.
  Portwine nevus — A diffuse area of overgrowth of new blood vessels within the skin.
  Sanguineous nevus
  Strawberry nevus — An excessive overgrowth of blood vessels and connective tissue within the skin.
  Vascular nevus NOS
  Verrucous nevus
  Excludes ❷: *café au lait spots (L81.3)*
    lentigo (L81.4)
    nevus NOS (D22.-)
    araneus nevus (I78.1)
    melanocytic nevus (D22.-)
    pigmented nevus (D22.-)
    spider nevus (I78.1)
    stellar nevus (I78.1)

Q82.6 **Congenital sacral dimple** — A congenital indentation of the skin in the lower back just above the crease between the buttocks.
  Parasacaral dimple
  Excludes ❷: *pilonidal cyst with abscess (L05.01)*
    pilonidal cyst without abscess (L05.91)

Q82.8 **Other specified congenital malformations of skin**
  AHA 16:1Q:p17 – Sacral dimple
  Abnormal palmar creases
  Accessory skin tags
  Benign familial pemphigus [Hailey-Hailey]
  Congenital poikiloderma
  Cutis laxa (hyperelastica)
  Dermatoglyphic anomalies
  Inherited keratosis palmaris et plantaris
  Keratosis follicularis [Darier-White]
  Excludes 1: *Ehlers-Danlos syndrome (Q79.6)*

Q82.9 **Congenital malformation of skin, unspecified**

Q83- Congenital malformations of breast
  Excludes ❷: *absence of pectoral muscle (Q79.8)*
    hypoplasia of breast (N64.82)
    micromastia (N64.82)

Q83.0 **Congenital absence of breast with absent nipple** — The congenital nonexistence of a breast and nipple.

Q83.1 **Accessory breast** — The formation of an additional breast.
  Supernumerary breast

Q83.2 **Absent nipple** — The congenital nonexistence of a nipple.

Q83.3 **Accessory nipple** — The formation of an additional nipple.
  Supernumerary nipple

Q83.8 **Other congenital malformations of breast**

Q83.9 **Congenital malformation of breast, unspecified**

Q84- Other congenital malformations of integument

Q84.0 **Congenital alopecia** — The absence of hair, most commonly of the scalp.
  Congenital atrichosis

Q84.1 **Congenital morphological disturbances of hair, not elsewhere classified**
  Beaded hair — The swelling and constrictions in the hair shafts.
  Monilethrix — An inherited disease marked by brittle, beaded hair.
  Pili annulati — The banded appearance discoloration of the hair.
  Excludes 1: *Menkes' kinky hair syndrome (E83.0)*

Q84.2 **Other congenital malformations of hair**
  Congenital hypertrichosis — The excessive growth of hair.
  Congenital malformation of hair NOS
  Persistent lanugo — The continued presence of the fine hair of the fetus.

Q84.3 **Anonychia** — The absence of a nail or nails.
  Excludes 1: *nail patella syndrome (Q87.2)*

Q84.4 **Congenital leukonychia** — The whitish discoloration of the nails.

Q84.5 **Enlarged and hypertrophic nails**
  Congenital onychauxis — The overgrowth of the nails.
  Pachyonychia — The thickening of the nails.

Q84.6 **Other congenital malformations of nails**
  Congenital clubnail — The clubbed appearance of the nails.
  Congenital koilonychia — The formation of thin, concave nails.
  Congenital malformation of nail NOS

Q84.8 **Other specified congenital malformations of integument**
  Aplasia cutis congenita — The congenital absence of a portion of the epidermis.

Q84.9 **Congenital malformation of integument, unspecified**
  Congenital anomaly of integument NOS
  Congenital deformity of integument NOS

Q85- Phakomatoses, not elsewhere classified
  Excludes 1: *ataxia telangiectasia [Louis-Bar] (G11.3)*
    familial dysautonomia [Riley-Day] (G90.1)

Q85.0- Neurofibromatosis (nonmalignant)

  Q85.00 Neurofibromatosis, unspecified

  Q85.01 Neurofibromatosis, type 1
    Von Recklinghausen disease

  Q85.02 Neurofibromatosis, type 2
    Acoustic neurofibromatosis

  Q85.03 Schwannomatosis

  Q85.09 Other neurofibromatosis

cc **Q85.1** **Tuberous sclerosis** — A syndrome characterized by sclerotic patches on the brain and tumors on the lateral ventricles with resultant mental deterioration and epileptic convulsions.
  Bourneville's disease
  Epiloia

cc **Q85.8** **Other phakomatoses, not elsewhere classified**
  Peutz-Jeghers Syndrome
  Sturge-Weber(-Dimitri) syndrome
  von Hippel-Lindau syndrome
  Excludes 1: *Meckel-Gruber syndrome (Q61.9)*

cc **Q85.9** **Phakomatosis, unspecified**
  Hamartosis NOS

Q86- Congenital malformation syndromes due to known exogenous causes, not elsewhere classified
  Excludes ❷: *iodine-deficiency-related hypothyroidism (E00-E02)*
    nonteratogenic effects of substances transmitted via placenta or breast milk (P04.-)

Q86.0 **Fetal alcohol syndrome (dysmorphic)**

Q86.1 **Fetal hydantoin syndrome**
  Meadow's syndrome

Q86.2 **Dysmorphism due to warfarin**

Q86.8 **Other congenital malformation syndromes due to known exogenous causes**

Q87- Other specified congenital malformation syndromes affecting multiple systems
  Use additional code(s) to identify all associated manifestations

Q87.0 **Congenital malformation syndromes predominantly affecting facial appearance**
  Acrocephalopolysyndactyly
  Acrocephalosyndactyly [Apert]
  Cryptophthalmos syndrome
  Cyclopia
  Goldenhar syndrome
  Moebius syndrome
  Oro-facial-digital syndrome
  Robin syndrome
  Whistling face

cc **Q87.1** **Congenital malformation syndromes predominantly associated with short stature**
  Aarskog syndrome
  Cockayne syndrome
  De Lange syndrome
  Dubowitz syndrome
  Noonan syndrome
  Prader-Willi syndrome
  Robinow-Silverman-Smith syndrome
  Russell-Silver syndrome
  Seckel syndrome
  Excludes 1: *Ellis-van Creveld syndrome (Q77.6)*
    Smith-Lemli-Opitz syndrome (E78.72)

cc **Q87.2** **Congenital malformation syndromes predominantly involving limbs**
  Holt-Oram syndrome
  Klippel-Trenaunay-Weber syndrome
  Nail patella syndrome
  Rubinstein-Taybi syndrome
  Sirenomelia syndrome
  Thrombocytopenia with absent radius [TAR] syndrome
  VATER syndrome

Q82 - Q87

cc **Q87.3 Congenital malformation syndromes involving early overgrowth**
Beckwith-Wiedemann syndrome
Sotos syndrome
Weaver syndrome

Q87.4- Marfan's syndrome — A hereditary syndrome characterized by long extremities, dislocation of the optic lens, and dilatation of the ascending aorta.

cc **Q87.40 Marfan's syndrome, unspecified**

Q87.41- Marfan's syndrome with cardiovascular manifestations

cc **Q87.410 Marfan's syndrome with aortic dilation**

cc **Q87.418 Marfan's syndrome with other cardiovascular manifestations**

cc **Q87.42 Marfan's syndrome with ocular manifestations**

cc **Q87.43 Marfan's syndrome with skeletal manifestation**

cc **Q87.5 Other congenital malformation syndromes with other skeletal changes**

Q87.8- Other specified congenital malformation syndromes, not elsewhere classified
Excludes 1:   Zellweger syndrome (E71.510)

cc **Q87.81 Alport syndrome** — A hereditary syndrome characterized by damaged small blood vessels in the kidneys that can lead to kidney disease and failure. **Use additional code to identify stage of chronic kidney disease (N18.1-N18.6)**

cc **Q87.82 Arterial tortuosity syndrome** — A congenital malformation syndrome characterized by elongation and deformation of the pulmonary and systemic arteries.

cc **Q87.89 Other specified congenital malformation syndromes, not elsewhere classified**
Laurence-Moon (-Bardet)-Biedl syndrome

Q89- Other congenital malformations, not elsewhere classified

Q89.0- Congenital absence and malformations of spleen
Excludes 1:   isomerism of atrial appendages (with asplenia or polysplenia) (Q20.6)

cc **Q89.01 Asplenia (congenital)** — The nonexistence of the spleen.

cc **Q89.09 Congenital malformations of spleen** — The congenital developmental deviation of the spleen.
Congenital splenomegaly — The abnormal largeness of the spleen.

Q89.1 Congenital malformations of adrenal gland — The congenital developmental deviation of the adrenal glands.
Excludes 1:   adrenogenital disorders (E25.-)
congenital adrenal hyperplasia (E25.0)

Q89.2 Congenital malformations of other endocrine glands
Congenital malformation of parathyroid or thyroid gland — The congenital developmental deviation of the parathyroid or thyroid gland.
Persistent thyroglossal duct — The abnormal continued patency of the thyroglossal or thyrolingual ducts.
Thyroglossal cyst — The formation of a fluid-filled sac in the thyroglossal duct.
Excludes 1:   congenital goiter (E03.0)
congenital hypothyroidism (E03.1)

cc **Q89.3 Situs inversus** — The lateral transposition of the thoracic or abdominal viscera.
Dextrocardia with situs inversus
Mirror-image atrial arrangement with situs inversus
Situs inversus or transversus abdominalis
Situs inversus or transversus thoracis
Transposition of abdominal viscera
Transposition of thoracic viscera
Excludes 1:   dextrocardia NOS (Q24.0)

MCC **Q89.4 Conjoined twins** — Congenital physically joined twins.
Craniopagus — A form united at the heads.
Dicephaly — A form with two heads and the body of one.
Pygopagus — A form united at the sacrum.
Thoracopagus — A form united at the sternum.

cc **Q89.7 Multiple congenital malformations, not elsewhere classified**
Multiple congenital anomalies NOS
Multiple congenital deformities NOS
Excludes 1:   congenital malformation syndromes affecting multiple systems (Q87.-)

cc **Q89.8 Other specified congenital malformations**
Use additional code(s) to identify all associated manifestations

Q89.9 Congenital malformation, unspecified
Congenital anomaly NOS
Congenital deformity NOS

Chromosomal abnormalities, not elsewhere classified (Q90-Q99)

Excludes ❷: mitochondrial metabolic disorders (E88.4-)

Q90- Down syndrome — The chromosomal abnormality that is characterized by moderate-to-severe mental retardation, sloping forehead, small ear canals, flat-bridged nose, and short phalanges.
Use additional code(s) to identify any associated physical conditions and degree of intellectual disabilities (F70-F79)

Q90.0 Trisomy 21, nonmosaicism (meiotic nondisjunction)

Q90.1 Trisomy 21, mosaicism (mitotic nondisjunction)

Q90.2 Trisomy 21, translocation

Q90.9 Down syndrome, unspecified
Trisomy 21 NOS

Q91- Trisomy 18 and Trisomy 13

cc **Q91.0 Trisomy 18, nonmosaicism (meiotic nondisjunction)**

cc **Q91.1 Trisomy 18, mosaicism (mitotic nondisjunction)**

cc **Q91.2 Trisomy 18, translocation**

cc **Q91.3 Trisomy 18, unspecified** — The chromosomal abnormality that is characterized by mental retardation, neonatal hepatitis, low-set ears, skull malformation, and short digits.

cc **Q91.4 Trisomy 13, nonmosaicism (meiotic nondisjunction)**

cc **Q91.5 Trisomy 13, mosaicism (mitotic nondisjunction)**

cc **Q91.6 Trisomy 13, translocation**

cc **Q91.7 Trisomy 13, unspecified** — The chromosomal abnormality that is characterized by impaired midline facial development, cleft lip and palate, polydactyly, and mental retardation.

Q92- Other trisomies and partial trisomies of the autosomes, not elsewhere classified
Includes: Unbalanced translocations and insertions
Excludes 1:   trisomies of chromosomes 13, 18, 21 (Q90-Q91)

Q92.0 Whole chromosome trisomy, nonmosaicism (meiotic nondisjunction)

Q92.1 Whole chromosome trisomy, mosaicism (mitotic nondisjunction)

Q92.2 Partial trisomy
Less than whole arm duplicated
Whole arm or more duplicated
Excludes 1:   partial trisomy due to unbalanced translocation (Q92.5)

Q92.5 Duplications with other complex rearrangements
Partial trisomy due to unbalanced translocations
Code also any associated deletions due to unbalanced translocations, inversions and insertions (Q93.7)

Q92.6- Marker chromosomes
Trisomies due to dicentrics
Trisomies due to extra rings
Trisomies due to isochromosomes
Individual with marker heterochromatin

Q92.61 Marker chromosomes in normal individual

Q92.62 Marker chromosomes in abnormal individual

Q92.7 Triploidy and polyploidy

Q92.8 Other specified trisomies and partial trisomies of autosomes
Duplications identified by fluorescence in situ hybridization (FISH)
Duplications identified by in situ hybridization (ISH)
Duplications seen only at prometaphase

Q92.9 Trisomy and partial trisomy of autosomes, unspecified

Q93- Monosomies and deletions from the autosomes, not elsewhere classified

Q93.0 Whole chromosome monosomy, nonmosaicism (meiotic nondisjunction)

Q93.1 Whole chromosome monosomy, mosaicism (mitotic nondisjunction)

Q93.2 Chromosome replaced with ring, dicentric or isochromosome

cc **Q93.3 Deletion of short arm of chromosome 4**
Wolff-Hirschorn syndrome

cc **Q93.4 Deletion of short arm of chromosome 5** — The chromosomal abnormality that is characterized by a cat-like cry, widely-spaced eyes, microcephaly, mental retardation, and laryngeal defects.
Cri-du-chat syndrome

cc **Q93.5 Other deletions of part of a chromosome**
Angelman syndrome

Side tab: **Q 8 7 - Q 9 3**

CC **Q93.7** **Deletions with other complex rearrangements**
Deletions due to unbalanced translocations, inversions and insertions
Code also any associated duplications due to unbalanced translocations, inversions and insertions (Q92.5)

Q93.8- **Other deletions from the autosomes**

MCC **Q93.81** **Velo-cardio-facial syndrome** — A condition caused by the deletion of a small segment of the long arm of chromosome 22 that is associated with over thirty different features; most common are cleft palate, heart defects, and characteristic facial appearance.
Deletion 22q11.2

CC **Q93.88** **Other microdeletions**
Miller-Dieker syndrome — A neurodevelopmental disorder caused by the mutation in the LIS1 gene that is characterized by seizures, mental retardation, and early death.
Smith-Magenis syndrome — A condition caused by the deletion of a small segment of chromosome 17 that is characterized by a variety of features including some degree of self injury, sleep disturbances, short stature, and flat facial features.

CC **Q93.89** **Other deletions from the autosomes**
Deletions identified by fluorescence in situ hybridization (FISH)
Deletions identified by in situ hybridization (ISH)
Deletions seen only at prometaphase

CC **Q93.9** **Deletion from autosomes, unspecified**

Q95- **Balanced rearrangements and structural markers, not elsewhere classified**
Includes: Robertsonian and balanced reciprocal translocations and insertions

Q95.0 **Balanced translocation and insertion in normal individual**

Q95.1 **Chromosome inversion in normal individual**

Q95.2 **Balanced autosomal rearrangement in abnormal individual**

Q95.3 **Balanced sex/autosomal rearrangement in abnormal individual**

Q95.5 **Individual with autosomal fragile site**

Q95.8 **Other balanced rearrangements and structural markers**

Q95.9 **Balanced rearrangement and structural marker, unspecified**

Q96- **Turner's syndrome** — The condition of a defective or absent second X chromosome resulting in short stature and undifferentiated gonads with a female phenotype.
Excludes 1:   *Noonan syndrome (Q87.1)*

Q96.0 **Karyotype 45, X** — [♀]

Q96.1 **Karyotype 46, X iso (Xq)** — [♀]
Karyotype 46, isochromosome Xq

Q96.2 **Karyotype 46, X with abnormal sex chromosome, except iso (Xq)** — [♀]
Karyotype 46, X with abnormal sex chromosome, except isochromosome Xq

Q96.3 **Mosaicism, 45, X/46, XX or XY** — [♀]

Q96.4 **Mosaicism, 45, X/other cell line(s) with abnormal sex chromosome** — [♀]

Q96.8 **Other variants of Turner's syndrome** — [♀]

Q96.9 **Turner's syndrome, unspecified** — [♀]

Q97- **Other sex chromosome abnormalities, female phenotype, not elsewhere classified**
Excludes 1:   *Turner's syndrome (Q96.-)*

Q97.0 **Karyotype 47, XXX** — [♀]

Q97.1 **Female with more than three X chromosomes** — [♀]

Q97.2 **Mosaicism, lines with various numbers of X chromosomes** — [♀]

Q97.3 **Female with 46, XY karyotype** — [♀]

Q97.8 **Other specified sex chromosome abnormalities, female phenotype** — [♀]

Q97.9 **Sex chromosome abnormality, female phenotype, unspecified** — [♀]

Q98- **Other sex chromosome abnormalities, male phenotype, not elsewhere classified**

Q98.0 **Klinefelter syndrome karyotype 47, XXY** — [♂] — The condition of an extra X chromosome resulting in the presence of small testes, abnormal Leydig cells, long legs, and a slightly subnormal intelligence.

Q98.1 **Klinefelter syndrome, male with more than two X chromosomes** — [♂]

Q98.3 **Other male with 46, XX karyotype** — [♂]

Q98.4 **Klinefelter syndrome, unspecified** — [♂]

Q98.5 **Karyotype 47, XYY**

Q98.6 **Male with structurally abnormal sex chromosome** — [♂]

Q98.7 **Male with sex chromosome mosaicism** — [♂]

Q98.8 **Other specified sex chromosome abnormalities, male phenotype** — [♂]

Q98.9 **Sex chromosome abnormality, male phenotype, unspecified** — [♂]

Q99- **Other chromosome abnormalities, not elsewhere classified**

Q99.0 **Chimera 46, XX/46, XY**
Chimera 46, XX/46, XY true hermaphrodite

Q99.1 **46, XX true hermaphrodite**
46, XX with streak gonads
46, XY with streak gonads
Pure gonadal dysgenesis

Q99.2 **Fragile X chromosome**
Fragile X syndrome

Q99.8 **Other specified chromosome abnormalities**

Q99.9 **Chromosomal abnormality, unspecified**

Q99 – Q99

Chapter 18 – Symptoms, signs and abnormal clinical and laboratory findings, not elsewhere classified (R00-R99)

Note: This chapter includes symptoms, signs, abnormal results of clinical or other investigative procedures, and ill-defined conditions regarding which no diagnosis classifiable elsewhere is recorded. Signs and symptoms that point rather definitely to a given diagnosis have been assigned to a category in other chapters of the classification. In general, categories in this chapter include the less well-defined conditions and symptoms that, without the necessary study of the case to establish a final diagnosis, point perhaps equally to two or more diseases or to two or more systems of the body. Practically all categories in the chapter could be designated "not otherwise specified", "unknown etiology" or "transient". The Alphabetical Index should be consulted to determine which symptoms and signs are to be allocated here and which to other chapters. The residual subcategories, numbered .8, are generally provided for other relevant symptoms that cannot be allocated elsewhere in the classification. The conditions and signs or symptoms included in categories R00-R94 consist of:

(a) cases for which no more specific diagnosis can be made even after all the facts bearing on the case have been investigated;

(b) signs or symptoms existing at the time of initial encounter that proved to be transient and whose causes could not be determined;

(c) provisional diagnosis in a patient who failed to return for further investigation or care;

(d) cases referred elsewhere for investigation or treatment before the diagnosis was made;

(e) cases in which a more precise diagnosis was not available for any other reason;

(f) certain symptoms, for which supplementary information is provided, that represent important problems in medical care in their own right.

Excludes 2: *abnormal findings on antenatal screening of mother (O28-)*
certain conditions originating in the perinatal period (P04-P96)
signs and symptoms classified in the body system chapters
signs and symptoms of breast (N63, N64.5)

This chapter contains the following blocks:

R00-R09	Symptoms and signs involving the circulatory and respiratory systems
R10-R19	Symptoms and signs involving the digestive system and abdomen
R20-R23	Symptoms and signs involving the skin and subcutaneous tissue
R25-R29	Symptoms and signs involving the nervous and musculoskeletal systems
R30-R39	Symptoms and signs involving the genitourinary system
R40-R46	Symptoms and signs involving cognition, perception, emotional state and behavior
R47-R49	Symptoms and signs involving speech and voice
R50-R69	General symptoms and signs
R70-R79	Abnormal findings on examination of blood, without diagnosis
R80-R82	Abnormal findings on examination of urine, without diagnosis
R83-R89	Abnormal findings on examination of other body fluids, substances and tissues, without diagnosis
R90-R94	Abnormal findings on diagnostic imaging and in function studies, without diagnosis
R97	Abnormal tumor markers
R99	Ill-defined and unknown cause of mortality

Chapter-Specific Coding Guidelines

C. Chapter-Specific Coding Guidelines
In addition to general coding guidelines, there are guidelines for specific diagnoses and/or conditions in the classification. Unless otherwise indicated, these guidelines apply to all health care settings. Please refer to Section II for guidelines on the selection of principal diagnosis.

18. Chapter 18: Symptoms, Signs, and Abnormal Clinical and Laboratory Findings, Not Elsewhere Classified (R00-R99)

Chapter 18 includes symptoms, signs, abnormal results of clinical or other investigative procedures, and ill-defined conditions regarding which no diagnosis classifiable elsewhere is recorded. Signs and symptoms that point to a specific diagnosis have been assigned to a category in other chapters of the classification.

a. Use of symptom codes
Codes that describe symptoms and signs are acceptable for reporting purposes when a related definitive diagnosis has not been established (confirmed) by the provider.

b. Use of a symptom code with a definitive diagnosis code
Codes for signs and symptoms may be reported in addition to a related definitive diagnosis when the sign or symptom is not routinely associated with that diagnosis, such as the various signs and symptoms associated with complex syndromes. The definitive diagnosis code should be sequenced before the symptom code.

Signs or symptoms that are associated routinely with a disease process should not be assigned as additional codes, unless otherwise instructed by the classification.

c. Combination codes that include symptoms
ICD-10-CM contains a number of combination codes that identify both the definitive diagnosis and common symptoms of that diagnosis. When using one of these combination codes, an additional code should not be assigned for the symptom.

d. Repeated falls
Code R29.6, Repeated falls, is for use for encounters when a patient has recently fallen and the reason for the fall is being investigated.

Code Z91.81, History of falling, is for use when a patient has fallen in the past and is at risk for future falls. When appropriate, both codes R29.6 and Z91.81 may be assigned together.

e. Coma scale
The coma scale codes (R40.2-) can be used in conjunction with traumatic brain injury codes, acute cerebrovascular disease or sequelae of cerebrovascular disease codes. These codes are primarily for use by trauma registries, but they may be used in any setting where this information is collected. The coma scale may also be used to assess the status of the central nervous system for other non-trauma conditions, such as monitoring patients in the intensive care unit regardless of medical condition. The coma scale codes should be sequenced after the diagnosis code(s).

These codes, one from each subcategory, are needed to complete the scale. The 7th character indicates when the scale was recorded. The 7th character should match for all three codes.

At a minimum, report the initial score documented on presentation at your facility. This may be a score from the emergency medicine technician (EMT) or in the emergency department. If desired, a facility may choose to capture multiple coma scale scores.

Assign code R40.24, Glasgow coma scale, total score, when only the total score is documented in the medical record and not the individual score(s).

f. Functional quadriplegia
Functional quadriplegia (code R53.2) is the lack of ability to use one's limbs or to ambulate due to extreme debility. It is not associated with neurologic deficit or injury, and code R53.2 should not be used for cases of neurologic quadriplegia. It should only be assigned if functional quadriplegia is specifically documented in the medical record.

g. SIRS due to Non-Infectious Process
The systemic inflammatory response syndrome (SIRS) can develop as a result of certain non-infectious disease processes, such as trauma, malignant neoplasm, or pancreatitis. When SIRS is documented with a noninfectious condition, and no subsequent infection is documented, the code for the underlying condition, such as an injury, should be assigned, followed by code R65.10, Systemic inflammatory response syndrome (SIRS) of non-infectious origin without acute organ dysfunction, or code R65.11, Systemic inflammatory response syndrome (SIRS) of non-infectious origin with acute organ dysfunction. If an associated acute organ dysfunction is documented, the appropriate code(s) for the specific type of organ dysfunction(s) should be assigned in addition to code R65.11. If acute organ dysfunction is documented, but it cannot be determined if the acute organ dysfunction is associated with SIRS or due to another condition (e.g., directly due to the trauma), the provider should be queried.

h. Death NOS
Code R99, Ill-defined and unknown cause of mortality, is only for use in the very limited circumstance when a patient who has already died is brought into an emergency department or other healthcare facility and is pronounced dead upon arrival. It does not represent the discharge disposition of death.

i. NIHSS Stroke Scale
The NIH stroke scale (NIHSS) codes (R29.7- -) can be used in conjunction with acute stroke codes (I63) to identify the patient's neurological status and the severity of the stroke. The stroke scale codes should be sequenced after the acute stroke diagnosis code(s).

At a minimum, report the initial score documented. If desired, a facility may choose to capture multiple stroke scale scores.

See Section I.B.14. for information concerning the medical record documentation that may be used for assignment of the NIHSS codes.

Symptoms and signs involving the circulatory and respiratory systems (R00-R09)

R00- Abnormalities of heart beat
Excludes 1:   *abnormalities originating in the perinatal period (P29.1-)*
Excludes ❷: *specified arrhythmias (I47-I49)*

R00.0 Tachycardia, unspecified
Rapid heart beat
Sinoauricular tachycardia NOS
Sinus [sinusal] tachycardia NOS
Excludes 1:   *neonatal tachycardia (P29.11)*
         paroxysmal tachycardia (I47.-)

R00.1 Bradycardia, unspecified
Sinoatrial bradycardia
Sinus bradycardia
Slow heart beat
Vagal bradycardia
Use additional code for adverse effect, if applicable, to identify drug (T36-T50 with fifth or sixth character 5)
Excludes 1:   *neonatal bradycardia (P29.12)*

R00.2 Palpitations — The rapid, throbbing pulsation of the heart.
Awareness of heart beat

R00.8 Other abnormalities of heart beat

R00.9 Unspecified abnormalities of heart beat

R01- Cardiac murmurs and other cardiac sounds
Excludes 1:   *cardiac murmurs and sounds originating in the perinatal period (P29.8)*

R01.0 Benign and innocent cardiac murmurs — The extra or unusal sound of blood moving through the heart and heart valves.
Functional cardiac murmur

R01.1 Cardiac murmur, unspecified
Cardiac bruit NOS
Heart murmur NOS
Systolic murmur NOS

R01.2 Other cardiac sounds
Cardiac dullness, increased or decreased — The diminished resonance of the heart sounds.
Precordial friction — The rubbing sound of the lower part of the heart.

R03- Abnormal blood-pressure reading, without diagnosis

R03.0 Elevated blood-pressure reading, without diagnosis of hypertension — [Questionable Admission]
Note: This category is to be used to record an episode of elevated blood pressure in a patient in whom no formal diagnosis of hypertension has been made, or as an isolated incidental finding.

R03.1 Nonspecific low blood-pressure reading
Excludes 1:   *hypotension (I95-)*
         maternal hypotension syndrome (O26.5-)
         neurogenic orthostatic hypotension (G90.3)

R04- Hemorrhage from respiratory passages

R04.0 Epistaxis — Bleeding from the nostrils.
Hemorrhage from nose
Nosebleed

R04.1 Hemorrhage from throat — Bleeding from the throat.
Excludes ❷: *hemoptysis (R04.2)*

cc R04.2 Hemoptysis — The coughing-up of blood or bloodstained sputum.
AHA 13:4Q:p118 – Hemoptysis with pneumonia
Blood-stained sputum
Cough with hemorrhage

R04.8- Hemorrhage from other sites in respiratory passages

cc R04.81 Acute idiopathic pulmonary hemorrhage in infants — [Age/0-17] – The presence of blood in the airway of infants without an identifiable cause, and in severe cases with sudden onset of overt bleeding and acute respiratory distress or failure.
AIPHI
Acute idiopathic hemorrhage in infants over 28 days old
Excludes 1:   *perinatal pulmonary hemorrhage (P26.-)*
         von Willebrand's disease (D68.0)

cc R04.89 Hemorrhage from other sites in respiratory passages
Pulmonary hemorrhage NOS

cc R04.9 Hemorrhage from respiratory passages, unspecified

R05 Cough
Excludes 1:   *cough with hemorrhage (R04.2)*
         smoker's cough (J41.0)

R06- Abnormalities of breathing
Excludes 1:   *acute respiratory distress syndrome (J80)*
         respiratory arrest (R09.2)
         respiratory arrest of newborn (P28.81)
         respiratory distress syndrome of newborn (P22.-)
         respiratory failure (J96.-)
         respiratory failure of newborn (P28.5)

R06.0- Dyspnea — Difficult or labored breathing, breathlessness.
Excludes 1:   *tachypnea NOS (R06.82)*
         transient tachypnea of newborn (P22.1)

R06.00 Dyspnea, unspecified

R06.01 Orthopnea — The condition of difficult breathing except when in an upright position.

R06.02 Shortness of breath — The inability to adequately inspirate the lungs.

R06.09 Other forms of dyspnea

R06.1 Stridor — The high-pitched inspiratory sound from the larynx.
Excludes 1:   *congenital laryngeal stridor (P28.89)*
         laryngismus (stridulus) (J38.5)

R06.2 Wheezing — The whistling sound made during breathing.
AHA 16:2Q:p33 – Wheezing due to exposure to electronic cigarette vapors
Excludes 1:   *asthma (J45-)*

cc R06.3 Periodic breathing — The condition marked by increasing and decreasing rates of respiration with periods of apnea.
Cheyne-Stokes breathing

R06.4 Hyperventilation — The abnormally increased breathing resulting in too much oxygen and not enough carbon dioxide in the blood.
Excludes 1:   *psychogenic hyperventilation (F45.8)*

R06.5 Mouth breathing — Breathing predominantly through the mouth instead of the through the nose, often during sleep.
Excludes ❷: *dry mouth NOS (R68.2)*

R06.6 Hiccough — The involuntary, rapid spasm of the diaphragm and lungs with closure of the glottis.
Excludes 1:   *psychogenic hiccough (F45.8)*

R06.7 Sneezing — The extremely rapid expulsion of air from the lungs caused by the irritation of the mucous membrane of the tract.

R06.8- Other abnormalities of breathing

R06.81 Apnea, not elsewhere classified — The abnormal, periodic cessation of breathing.
Apnea NOS
Excludes 1:   *apnea (of) newborn (P28.4)*
         sleep apnea (G47.3-)
         sleep apnea of newborn (primary) (P28.3)

R06.82 Tachypnea, not elsewhere classified — The condition of quick, shallow breathing.
Tachypnea NOS
Excludes 1:   *transitory tachypnea of newborn (P22.1)*

R06.83 Snoring

R06.89 Other abnormalities of breathing
Breath-holding (spells)
Sighing

R06.9 Unspecified abnormalities of breathing

R07- Pain in throat and chest
Excludes 1:   *epidemic myalgia (B33.0)*
Excludes ❷: *jaw pain R68.84*
         pain in breast (N64.4)

R07.0 Pain in throat
Excludes 1:   *chronic sore throat (J31.2)*
         sore throat (acute) NOS (J02.9)
Excludes ❷: *dysphagia (R13.1-)*
         pain in neck (M54.2)

R07.1 Chest pain on breathing
Painful respiration

R07.2 Precordial pain — Chest pain in the area that overlies the heart and lower thorax.

R07.8-   Other chest pain

R07.81   Pleurodynia — Paroxysmal pain in the intercostal muscles.
Pleurodynia NOS
Excludes 1:   epidemic pleurodynia (B33.0)

R07.82   Intercostal pain

R07.89   Other chest pain
Anterior chest-wall pain NOS

R07.9   Chest pain, unspecified

R09-   Other symptoms and signs involving the circulatory and respiratory system
Excludes 1:   acute respiratory distress syndrome (J80)
respiratory arrest of newborn (P28.81)
respiratory distress syndrome of newborn (P22.0)
respiratory failure (J96.-)
respiratory failure of newborn (P28.5)

R09.0-   Asphyxia and hypoxemia
Excludes 1:   asphyxia due to carbon monoxide (T58.-)
asphyxia due to foreign body in respiratory tract (T17.-)
birth (intrauterine) asphyxia (P84)
hypercapnia (R06.4)
hyperventilation (R06.4)
traumatic asphyxia (T71.-)

CC **R09.01   Asphyxia** — The life threatening, severely deficient supply of oxygenated blood to the body's tissues (also refers to stopping of the pulse).

R09.02   Hypoxemia — The abnormal condition of deficient oxygenation of the blood.

R09.1   Pleurisy — Inflammation of the pleura.
Excludes 1:   pleurisy with effusion (J90)

MCC **R09.2   Respiratory arrest** — The cessation of breathing.
Cardiorespiratory failure — The inability of the heart and lungs to perform adequately.
Excludes 1:   cardiac arrest (I46.-)
respiratory arrest of newborn (P28.81)
respiratory distress of newborn (P22.0)
respiratory failure (J96.-)
respiratory failure of newborn (P28.5)
respiratory insufficiency (R06.89)
respiratory insufficiency of newborn (P28.5)

R09.3   Abnormal sputum
Abnormal amount of sputum
Abnormal color of sputum
Abnormal odor of sputum
Excessive sputum
Excludes 1:   blood-stained sputum (R04.2)

R09.8-   Other specified symptoms and signs involving the circulatory and respiratory systems

R09.81   Nasal congestion

R09.82   Postnasal drip

R09.89   Other specified symptoms and signs involving the circulatory and respiratory systems
Bruit (arterial)
Abnormal chest percussion
Feeling of foreign body in throat
Friction sounds in chest
Chest tympany
Choking sensation
Rales
Weak pulse
Excludes ❷: foreign body in throat (T17.2-)
wheezing (R06.2)

Symptoms and signs involving the digestive system and abdomen (R10-R19)

Excludes ❷: congenital or infantile pylorospasm (Q40.0)
gastrointestinal hemorrhage (K92.0-K92.2)
intestinal obstruction (K56.-)
newborn gastrointestinal hemorrhage (P54.0-P54.3)
newborn intestinal obstruction (P76.-)
pylorospasm (K31.3)
signs and symptoms involving the urinary system (R30-R39)
symptoms referable to female genital organs (N94.-)
symptoms referable to male genital organs male (N48-N50)

R10-   Abdominal and pelvic pain
Excludes 1:   renal colic (N23)
Excludes ❷: dorsalgia (M54.-)
flatulence and related conditions (R14.-)

R10.0   Acute abdomen
Severe abdominal pain (generalized) (with abdominal rigidity)
Excludes 1:   abdominal rigidity NOS (R19.3)
generalized abdominal pain NOS (R10.84)
localized abdominal pain (R10.1-R10.3-)

R10.1-   Pain localized to upper abdomen

R10.10   Upper abdominal pain, unspecified

R10.11   Right upper quadrant pain

R10.12   Left upper quadrant pain

R10.13   Epigastric pain
Dyspepsia
Excludes 1:   functional dyspepsia (K30)

R10.2   Pelvic and perineal pain
Excludes 1:   vulvodynia (N94.81)

R10.3-   Pain localized to other parts of lower abdomen

R10.30   Lower abdominal pain, unspecified

R10.31   Right lower quadrant pain

R10.32   Left lower quadrant pain

R10.33   Periumbilical pain

R10.8-   Other abdominal pain

R10.81-   Abdominal tenderness
Abdominal tenderness NOS

R10.811   Right upper quadrant abdominal tenderness

R10.812   Left upper quadrant abdominal tenderness

R10.813   Right lower quadrant abdominal tenderness

R10.814   Left lower quadrant abdominal tenderness

R10.815   Periumbilic abdominal tenderness

R10.816   Epigastric abdominal tenderness

R10.817   Generalized abdominal tenderness

R10.819   Abdominal tenderness, unspecified site

R10.82-   Rebound abdominal tenderness — A form felt upon the release of applied pressure.

R10.821   Right upper quadrant rebound abdominal tenderness

R10.822   Left upper quadrant rebound abdominal tenderness

R10.823   Right lower quadrant rebound abdominal tenderness

R10.824   Left lower quadrant rebound abdominal tenderness

R10.825   Periumbilic rebound abdominal tenderness

R10.826   Epigastric rebound abdominal tenderness

R10.827   Generalized rebound abdominal tenderness

R10.829   Rebound abdominal tenderness, unspecified site

R10.83   Colic — [Age/0-17] — The greater frequency and duration of crying and apparent discomfort.
Colic NOS
Infantile colic
Excludes 1:   colic in adult and child over 12 months old (R10.84)

R10.84   Generalized abdominal pain
Excludes 1:   generalized abdominal pain associated with acute abdomen (R10.0)

R10.9   Unspecified abdominal pain

R0 7 | R10

R11- Nausea and vomiting
  Excludes 1:   *cyclical vomiting associated with migraine (G43.A-)*
                excessive vomiting in pregnancy (O21-)
                hematemesis (K92.0)
                neonatal hematemesis (P54.0)
                newborn vomiting (P92.0-)
                psychogenic vomiting (F50.89)
                vomiting associated with bulimia nervosa (F50.2)
                vomiting following gastrointestinal surgery (K91.0)

  R11.0   Nausea
         Nausea NOS
         Nausea without vomiting
  R11.1- Vomiting
     R11.10   Vomiting, unspecified
            Vomiting NOS
     R11.11   Vomiting without nausea
     R11.12   Projectile vomiting — Vomiting with great force.
     R11.13   Vomiting of fecal matter
     R11.14   Bilious vomiting — Vomitus with bile.
            Bilious emesis
  R11.2   Nausea with vomiting, unspecified
         Persistent nausea with vomiting NOS

R12   Heartburn — The burning sensation in the esophagus.
  Excludes 1:   *dyspepsia NOS (R10.13)*
                functional dyspepsia (K30)

R13- Aphagia and dysphagia
  R13.0   Aphagia
         Inability to swallow
         Excludes 1:   *psychogenic aphagia (F50.9)*
  R13.1- Dysphagia — Difficulty in swallowing.
         Code first, if applicable, dysphagia following cerebrovascular disease (I69. with final characters -91)
         Excludes 1:   *psychogenic dysphagia (F45.8)*
     R13.10   Dysphagia, unspecified
            Difficulty in swallowing NOS
     R13.11   Dysphagia, oral phase — A form involving the cheeks, lips, palate, and tongue in which the food/liquid is chewed in preparation for swallowing.
     R13.12   Dysphagia, oropharyngeal phase — A form involving the tongue base and pharyngeal walls in which the tongue pushes the food or liquid to the back of the mouth, beginning the swallowing process.
     R13.13   Dysphagia, pharyngeal phase — A form involving the pharynx and larynx in which the food or liquid quickly passes through the pharynx.
     R13.14   Dysphagia, pharyngoesophageal phase — A form involving the upper esophageal sphincter in which the food or liquid moves through the esophagus and into the stomach.
     R13.19   Other dysphagia
            Cervical dysphagia
            Neurogenic dysphagia — A form caused by disease or impairment of the nervous system.

R14- Flatulence and related conditions
  Excludes 1:   *psychogenic aerophagy (F45.8)*
  R14.0   Abdominal distension (gaseous)
         Bloating
         Tympanites (abdominal) (intestinal)
  R14.1   Gas pain
  R14.2   Eructation
  R14.3   Flatulence

R15- Fecal incontinence — The inability to control the excretion of feces.
  Includes: Encopresis NOS
  Excludes 1:   *fecal incontinence of nonorganic origin (F98.1)*
  R15.0   Incomplete defecation
         Excludes 1:   *constipation (K59.0-)*
                       fecal impaction (K56.41)
  R15.1   Fecal smearing
         Fecal soiling
  R15.2   Fecal urgency
  R15.9   Full incontinence of feces
         Fecal incontinence NOS

R16- Hepatomegaly and splenomegaly, <u>not elsewhere classified</u>
  R16.0   Hepatomegaly, not elsewhere classified — The abnormal enlargement of the liver.
         Hepatomegaly NOS
  R16.1   Splenomegaly, not elsewhere classified — The abnormal enlargement of the spleen.
         Splenomegaly NOS
  R16.2   Hepatomegaly with splenomegaly, not elsewhere classified — The abnormal enlargement of the liver and spleen.
         Hepatosplenomegaly NOS

R17 **Unspecified jaundice** — The abnormal deposition of bilirubin in the skin resulting in
CC   the yellowish skin discoloration.
  Excludes 1:   *neonatal jaundice (P55, P57-P59)*

R18- Ascites — The abnormal accumulation of serous fluid in the abdominal cavity.
  Includes: Fluid in peritoneal cavity
  Excludes 1:   *ascites in alcoholic cirrhosis (K70.31)*
                ascites in alcoholic hepatitis (K70.11)
                ascites in toxic liver disease with chronic active hepatitis (K71.51)

CC **R18.0   Malignant ascites** — [Unacceptable PDX] – A form due to a malignant neoplasm.
         Code first malignancy, such as:
            Malignant neoplasm of ovary (C56.-)
            Secondary malignant neoplasm of retroperitoneum and peritoneum (C78.6)
CC **R18.8   Other ascites**
         Ascites NOS
         Peritoneal effusion (chronic)

R19- Other symptoms and signs involving the digestive system and abdomen
  Excludes 1:   *acute abdomen (R10.0)*
  R19.0- Intra-abdominal and pelvic swelling, mass and lump
         Excludes 1:   *abdominal distension (gaseous) (R14.-)*
                       ascites (R18.-)
     R19.00   Intra-abdominal and pelvic swelling, mass and lump, <u>unspecified</u> site
     R19.01   <u>Right</u> <u>upper</u> quadrant abdominal swelling, mass and lump
     R19.02   <u>Left</u> <u>upper</u> quadrant abdominal swelling, mass and lump
     R19.03   <u>Right</u> <u>lower</u> quadrant abdominal swelling, mass and lump
     R19.04   <u>Left</u> <u>lower</u> quadrant abdominal swelling, mass and lump
     R19.05   Periumbilic swelling, mass or lump
            Diffuse or generalized umbilical swelling or mass
     R19.06   Epigastric swelling, mass or lump
     R19.07   Generalized intra-abdominal and pelvic swelling, mass and lump
            Diffuse or generalized intra-abdominal swelling or mass NOS
            Diffuse or generalized pelvic swelling or mass NOS
     R19.09   Other intra-abdominal and pelvic swelling, mass and lump
  R19.1- Abnormal bowel sounds
     R19.11   Absent bowel sounds
     R19.12   Hyperactive bowel sounds
     R19.15   Other abnormal bowel sounds
            Abnormal bowel sounds NOS
  R19.2   Visible peristalsis
         Hyperperistalsis — An abnormal increase in the wave-like motion of the intestines.
  R19.3- Abdominal rigidity — The abnormal stiffness of the abdomen.
         Excludes 1:   *abdominal rigidity with severe abdominal pain (R10.0)*
     R19.30   Abdominal rigidity, unspecified site
     R19.31   <u>Right</u> <u>upper</u> quadrant abdominal rigidity
     R19.32   <u>Left</u> <u>upper</u> quadrant abdominal rigidity
     R19.33   <u>Right</u> <u>lower</u> quadrant abdominal rigidity
     R19.34   <u>Left</u> <u>lower</u> quadrant abdominal rigidity
     R19.35   Periumbilic abdominal rigidity
     R19.36   Epigastric abdominal rigidity
     R19.37   Generalized abdominal rigidity

R
1
1
-
R
1
9

R19.4   Change in bowel habit
 Excludes 1:   *constipation (K59.0-)*
                  functional diarrhea (K59.1)

R19.5   Other fecal abnormalities
          Abnormal stool color
          Bulky stools
          Mucus in stools
          Occult blood in feces
          Occult blood in stools
 Excludes 1:   *melena (K92.1)*
                  neonatal melena (P54.1)

R19.6   Halitosis — The condition of offensive or bad breath.

R19.7   Diarrhea, unspecified
          Diarrhea NOS
 Excludes 1:   *functional diarrhea (K59.1)*
                  neonatal diarrhea (P78.3)
                  psychogenic diarrhea (F45.8)

R19.8   Other specified symptoms and signs involving the digestive system and abdomen

Symptoms and signs involving the skin and subcutaneous tissue (R20-R23)

 Excludes ❷: *symptoms relating to breast (N64.4-N64.5)*

R20-   Disturbances of skin sensation
 Excludes 1:   *dissociative anesthesia and sensory loss (F44.6)*
                  psychogenic disturbances (F45.8)

R20.0   Anesthesia of skin — The loss of sensation of the skin.

R20.1   Hypoesthesia of skin — The abnormally decreased sensitivity of the skin.

R20.2   Paresthesia of skin — The abnormal or perverted sensation of the skin.
          Formication
          Pins and needles
          Tingling skin
 Excludes 1:   *acroparesthesia (I73.8)*

R20.3   Hyperesthesia — The abnormally increased sensitivity of the skin.

R20.8   Other disturbances of skin sensation

R20.9   Unspecified disturbances of skin sensation

R21   Rash and other nonspecific skin eruption
          Includes: Rash NOS
 Excludes 1:   *specified type of rash — code to condition*
                  vesicular eruption (R23.8)

R22-   Localized swelling, mass and lump of skin and subcutaneous tissue
          Includes: Subcutaneous nodules (localized) (superficial)
 Excludes 1:   *abnormal findings on diagnostic imaging (R90-R93)*
                  edema (R60-)
                  enlarged lymph nodes (R59-)
                  localized adiposity (E65)
                  swelling of joint (M25.4-)

R22.0   Localized swelling, mass and lump, head

R22.1   Localized swelling, mass and lump, neck

R22.2   Localized swelling, mass and lump, trunk
 Excludes 1:   *intra-abdominal or pelvic mass and lump (R19.0-)*
                  intra-abdominal or pelvic swelling (R19.0-)
 Excludes ❷: *breast mass and lump (N63)*

R22.3- Localized swelling, mass and lump, upper limb
  R22.30   Localized swelling, mass and lump, unspecified upper limb
  R22.31   Localized swelling, mass and lump, right upper limb
  R22.32   Localized swelling, mass and lump, left upper limb
  R22.33   Localized swelling, mass and lump, upper limb, bilateral

R22.4- Localized swelling, mass and lump, lower limb
  R22.40   Localized swelling, mass and lump, unspecified lower limb
  R22.41   Localized swelling, mass and lump, right lower limb
  R22.42   Localized swelling, mass and lump, left lower limb
  R22.43   Localized swelling, mass and lump, lower limb, bilateral

R22.9   Localized swelling, mass and lump, unspecified

R23-   Other skin changes

R23.0   Cyanosis — The condition of reduced hemoglobin concentration in the blood resulting in the bluish or purple skin discoloration.
 Excludes 1:   *acrocyanosis (I73.8)*
                  cyanotic attacks of newborn (P28.2)

R23.1   Pallor — Paleness of the skin.
          Clammy skin

R23.2   Flushing — The sudden redness of the skin.
          Excessive blushing
          Code first, if applicable, menopausal and female climacteric states (N95.1)

R23.3   Spontaneous ecchymoses — Small, hemorrhagic spots on the skin.
          Petechiae
 Excludes 1:   *ecchymoses of newborn (P54.5)*
                  purpura (D69.-)

R23.4   Changes in skin texture
          Desquamation of skin
          Induration of skin
          Scaling of skin
 Excludes 1:   *epidermal thickening NOS (L85.9)*

R23.8   Other skin changes

R23.9   Unspecified skin changes

Symptoms and signs involving the nervous and musculoskeletal systems (R25-R29)

R25-   Abnormal involuntary movements — The condition of bodily movements that are not voluntarily controlled.
 Excludes 1:   *specific movement disorders (G20-G26)*
                  stereotyped movement disorders (F98.4)
                  tic disorders (F95.-)

R25.0   Abnormal head movements

R25.1   Tremor, unspecified — The condition of muscles contracting involuntarily in a rhythmic, oscillating-like pattern in one or more body parts.
 Excludes 1:   *chorea NOS (G25.5)*
                  essential tremor (G25.0)
                  hysterical tremor (F44.4)
                  intention tremor (G25.2)

R25.2   Cramp and spasm
 Excludes ❷: *carpopedal spasm (R29.0)*
                  charley-horse (M62.831)
                  infantile spasms (G40.4-)
                  muscle spasm of back (M62.830)
                  muscle spasm of calf (M62.831)

R25.3   Fasciculation — The condition of small, local muscles contracting involuntarily.
          Twitching NOS

R25.8   Other abnormal involuntary movements

R25.9   Unspecified abnormal involuntary movements

R26-   Abnormalities of gait and mobility — The abnormal deviation of the manner or style of walking.
 Excludes 1:   *ataxia NOS (R27.0)*
                  hereditary ataxia (G11.-)
                  locomotor (syphilitic) ataxia (A52.11)
                  immobility syndrome (paraplegic) (M62.3)

R26.0   Ataxic gait — A form marked by unsteadiness and uncoordinated walk.
          Staggering gait — A form marked by swaying and apparent loss (with recovery) of balance.

R26.1   Paralytic gait — A form marked by loss of motor ability while walking.
          Spastic gait — A form marked by the legs being held together and moving in a stiff manner.

R26.2   Difficulty in walking, not elsewhere classified
 Excludes 1:   *falling (R29.6)*
                  unsteadiness on feet (R26.81)

R26.8- Other abnormalities of gait and mobility
  R26.81   Unsteadiness on feet
  R26.89   Other abnormalities of gait and mobility

R26.9   Unspecified abnormalities of gait and mobility

R
1
9
–
R
2
6

R27- **Other lack of coordination** — The lack of harmonious functioning of the body parts.

 Excludes 1: *ataxic gait (R26.0)*
 hereditary ataxia (G11.-)
 vertigo NOS (R42)

R27.0 **Ataxia, unspecified**
 Excludes 1: *ataxia following cerebrovascular disease (I69. with final characters -93)*

R27.8 **Other lack of coordination**

R27.9 **Unspecified lack of coordination**

R29- **Other symptoms and signs involving the nervous and musculoskeletal systems**

cc **R29.0** **Tetany** — The condition of intermittent tonic spasms involving the extremities.
 Carpopedal spasm — The spasm of the hand or foot, or of the thumbs and great toes.
 Excludes 1: *hysterical tetany (F44.5)*
 neonatal tetany (P71.3)
 parathyroid tetany (E20.9)
 post-thyroidectomy tetany (E89.2)

cc **R29.1** **Meningismus** — The irritation of the brain and spinal cord with symptoms simulating meningitis, but without actual inflammation.

R29.2 **Abnormal reflex**
 Excludes ❷: *abnormal pupillary reflex (H57.0)*
 hyperactive gag reflex (J39.2)
 vasovagal reaction or syncope (R55)

R29.3 **Abnormal posture**

R29.4 **Clicking hip**
 Excludes 1: *congenital deformities of hip (Q65.-)*

cc **R29.5** **Transient paralysis** — The temporary loss of motor function.
 Code first any associated spinal cord injury (S14.0, S14.1-, S24.0, S24.1-, S34.0-, S34.1-)
 Excludes 1: *transient ischemic attack (G45.9)*

R29.6 **Repeated falls**
 Falling
 Tendency to fall
 Excludes ❷: *at risk for falling (Z91.81)*
 history of falling (Z91.81)

R29.7- **National Institutes of Health Stroke Scale (NIHSS) score**
 Code first the type of cerebral infarction (I63.-)

R29.70- NIHSS score 0-9
 R29.700 **NIHSS score 0** — [Unacceptable PDX]
 R29.701 **NIHSS score 1** — [Unacceptable PDX]
 R29.702 **NIHSS score 2** — [Unacceptable PDX]
 R29.703 **NIHSS score 3** — [Unacceptable PDX]
 R29.704 **NIHSS score 4** — [Unacceptable PDX]
 R29.705 **NIHSS score 5** — [Unacceptable PDX]
 R29.706 **NIHSS score 6** — [Unacceptable PDX]
 R29.707 **NIHSS score 7** — [Unacceptable PDX]
 R29.708 **NIHSS score 8** — [Unacceptable PDX]
 R29.709 **NIHSS score 9** — [Unacceptable PDX]

R29.71- NIHSS score 10-19
 R29.710 **NIHSS score 10** — [Unacceptable PDX]
 R29.711 **NIHSS score 11** — [Unacceptable PDX]
 R29.712 **NIHSS score 12** — [Unacceptable PDX]
 R29.713 **NIHSS score 13** — [Unacceptable PDX]
 R29.714 **NIHSS score 14** — [Unacceptable PDX]
 R29.715 **NIHSS score 15** — [Unacceptable PDX]
 R29.716 **NIHSS score 16** — [Unacceptable PDX]
 R29.717 **NIHSS score 17** — [Unacceptable PDX]
 R29.718 **NIHSS score 18** — [Unacceptable PDX]
 R29.719 **NIHSS score 19** — [Unacceptable PDX]

R29.72- NIHSS score 20-29
 R29.720 **NIHSS score 20** — [Unacceptable PDX]
 R29.721 **NIHSS score 21** — [Unacceptable PDX]
 R29.722 **NIHSS score 22** — [Unacceptable PDX]
 R29.723 **NIHSS score 23** — [Unacceptable PDX]
 R29.724 **NIHSS score 24** — [Unacceptable PDX]
 R29.725 **NIHSS score 25** — [Unacceptable PDX]
 R29.726 **NIHSS score 26** — [Unacceptable PDX]
 R29.727 **NIHSS score 27** — [Unacceptable PDX]
 R29.728 **NIHSS score 28** — [Unacceptable PDX]
 R29.729 **NIHSS score 29** — [Unacceptable PDX]

R29.73- NIHSS score 30-39
 R29.730 **NIHSS score 30** — [Unacceptable PDX]
 R29.731 **NIHSS score 31** — [Unacceptable PDX]
 R29.732 **NIHSS score 32** — [Unacceptable PDX]
 R29.733 **NIHSS score 33** — [Unacceptable PDX]
 R29.734 **NIHSS score 34** — [Unacceptable PDX]
 R29.735 **NIHSS score 35** — [Unacceptable PDX]
 R29.736 **NIHSS score 36** — [Unacceptable PDX]
 R29.737 **NIHSS score 37** — [Unacceptable PDX]
 R29.738 **NIHSS score 38** — [Unacceptable PDX]
 R29.739 **NIHSS score 39** — [Unacceptable PDX]

R29.74- NIHSS score 40-42
 R29.740 **NIHSS score 40** — [Unacceptable PDX]
 R29.741 **NIHSS score 41** — [Unacceptable PDX]
 R29.742 **NIHSS score 42** — [Unacceptable PDX]

R29.8- **Other symptoms and signs involving the nervous and musculoskeletal systems**

R29.81- Other symptoms and signs involving the nervous system
 R29.810 **Facial weakness** — The loss or impairment of normal facial muscle control.
 Facial droop
 Excludes 1: *Bell's palsy (G51.0)*
 facial weakness following cerebrovascular disease (I69. with final characters-92)

 R29.818 **Other symptoms and signs involving the nervous system**

R29.89- Other symptoms and signs involving the musculoskeletal system
 Excludes ❷: *pain in limb (M79.6-)*

 R29.890 **Loss of height** — The relatively recent loss of a patient's normal height.
 Excludes 1: *osteoporosis (M80-M81)*

 R29.891 **Ocular torticollis** — The abnormal tilting of the head caused by vision problems.
 Excludes 1: *congenital (sternomastoid) torticollis Q68.0*
 psychogenic torticollis (F45.8)
 spasmodic torticollis (G24.3)
 torticollis due to birth injury (P15.8)
 torticollis NOS M43.6

 R29.898 **Other symptoms and signs involving the musculoskeletal system**

R29.9- **Unspecified symptoms and signs involving the nervous and musculoskeletal systems**

R29.90 **Unspecified symptoms and signs involving the nervous system**

R29.91 **Unspecified symptoms and signs involving the musculoskeletal system**

Excludes 1: = NOT CODED HERE! (Do not code both)

Excludes ❷: = Not Included Here

Symptoms and signs involving the genitourinary system (R30-R39)

R30- Pain associated with micturition
Excludes 1: *psychogenic pain associated with micturition (F45.8)*

R30.0 Dysuria — The condition of painful urination.
Strangury

R30.1 Vesical tenesmus — The sensation of bladder fullness after voiding.

R30.9 Painful micturition, unspecified
Painful urination NOS

R31- Hematuria — The abnormal presence of blood in the urine.
Excludes 1: *hematuria included with underlying conditions, such as:*
acute cystitis with hematuria (N30.01)
recurrent and persistent hematuria in glomerular diseases (N02.-)

R31.0 Gross hematuria — A form that is visible in the urine.

R31.1 Benign essential microscopic hematuria

R31.2- Other microscopic hematuria

R31.21 Asymptomatic microscopic hematuria
AMH

R31.29 Other microscopic hematuria

R31.9 Hematuria, unspecified

R32 Unspecified urinary incontinence
Enuresis NOS
Excludes 1: *functional urinary incontinence (R39.81)*
nonorganic enuresis (F98.0)
stress incontinence and other specified urinary incontinence (N39.3-N39.4-)
urinary incontinence associated with cognitive impairment (R39.81)

R33- Retention of urine — The abnormal accumulation of urine in the bladder due to the inability to urinate.
Excludes 1: *psychogenic retention of urine (F45.8)*

R33.0 Drug-induced retention of urine
Use additional code for adverse effect, if applicable, to identify drug (T36-T50 with fifth or sixth character 5)

R33.8 Other retention of urine
Code first, if applicable, any causal condition, such as:
Enlarged prostate (N40.1)

R33.9 Retention of urine, unspecified

R34 Anuria and oliguria — The lack, or significantly decreased normal amount, of urine.
Excludes 1: *anuria and oliguria complicating abortion or ectopic or molar pregnancy (O00-O07, O08.4)*
anuria and oliguria complicating pregnancy (O26.83-)
anuria and oliguria complicating the puerperium (O90.4)

R35- Polyuria — The condition of passing a large volume of urine in a given period.
Code first, if applicable, any causal condition, such as:
Enlarged prostate (N40.1)
Excludes 1: *psychogenic polyuria (F45.8)*

R35.0 Frequency of micturition — The condition of urination at short intervals without increase in daily volume of urinary output.

R35.1 Nocturia — The condition of excessive urination at night.

R35.8 Other polyuria
Polyuria NOS

R36- Urethral discharge

R36.0 Urethral discharge without blood

R36.1 Hematospermia — [♂] — The abnormal presence of blood in the ejaculate.

R36.9 Urethral discharge, unspecified
Penile discharge NOS
Urethrorrhea

R37 Sexual dysfunction, unspecified

R39- Other and unspecified symptoms and signs involving the genitourinary system

CC R39.0 Extravasation of urine — The escape of urine into the tissues.

R39.1- Other difficulties with micturition
Code first, if applicable, any causal condition, such as:
Enlarged prostate (N40.1)

R39.11 Hesitancy of micturition

R39.12 Poor urinary stream
Weak urinary steam

R39.13 Splitting of urinary stream

R39.14 Feeling of incomplete bladder emptying

R39.15 Urgency of urination
Excludes 1: *urge incontinence (N39.41, N39.46)*

R39.16 Straining to void

R39.19- Other difficulties with micturition

R39.191 Need to immediately re-void

R39.192 Position dependent micturition

R39.198 Other difficulties with micturition

R39.2 Extrarenal uremia — The retention of by-products normally excreted in the urine that is due to non-kidney disorders.
Prerenal uremia
Excludes 1: *uremia NOS (N19)*

R39.8- Other symptoms and signs involving the genitourinary system

R39.81 Functional urinary incontinence
Urinary incontinence due to cognitive impairment, or severe physical disability or immobility
Excludes 1: *stress incontinence and other specified urinary incontinence (N39.3-N39.4-)*
urinary incontinence NOS (R32)

R39.82 Chronic bladder pain

R39.89 Other symptoms and signs involving the genitourinary system

R39.9 Unspecified symptoms and signs involving the genitourinary system

Symptoms and signs involving cognition, perception, emotional state and behavior (R40-R46)

Excludes ②: *symptoms and signs constituting part of a pattern of mental disorder (F01-F99)*

R40- Somnolence, stupor and coma
Excludes 1: *neonatal coma (P91.5)*
somnolence, stupor and coma in diabetes (E08-E13)
somnolence, stupor and coma in hepatic failure (K72-)
somnolence, stupor and coma in hypoglycemia (nondiabetic) (E15)

R40.0 Somnolence
Drowsiness
Excludes 1: *coma (R40.2-)*

R40.1 Stupor — The partial or nearly complete state of unconsciousness.
Catatonic stupor
Semicoma
Excludes 1: *catatonic schizophrenia (F20.2)*
coma (R40.2-)
depressive stupor (F31-F33)
dissociative stupor (F44.2)
manic stupor (F30.2)

R40.2- Coma — A state of profound unconsciousness that is characterized by the inability to be aroused, absence of spontaneous eye movements, response to painful stimuli, and vocalization.
AHA 14:1Q:p19 – Glasgow coma scale (GCS) score
Code first any associated:
Fracture of skull (S02.-)
Intracranial injury (S06.-)
Note: One code from each subcategory, R40.21-R40.23, is required to complete the coma scale

MCC R40.20 Unspecified coma
Coma NOS
Unconsciousness NOS

R40.21- Coma scale, eyes open
The following appropriate 7th character is to be added to subcategory R40.21-:
0 - Unspecified time
1 - In the field [EMT or ambulance]
2 - At arrival to emergency department
3 - At hospital admission
4 - 24 hours or more after hospital admission

MCC-0-4 R40.211- Coma scale, eyes open, never

MCC-0-4 R40.212- Coma scale, eyes open, to pain

R40.213- Coma scale, eyes open, to sound

R40.214- Coma scale, eyes open, spontaneous

R
3
0
–
R
4
0

R40.22- **Coma scale, best verbal response**
The following appropriate 7th character is to be added to subcategory R40.22-:
0 - Unspecified time
1 - In the field [EMT or ambulance]
2 - At arrival to emergency department
3 - At hospital admission
4 - 24 hours or more after hospital admission

MCC-0-4 **R40.221-** **Coma scale, best verbal response, none**

MCC-0-4 **R40.222-** **Coma scale, best verbal response, incomprehensible words**

R40.223- **Coma scale, best verbal response, inappropriate words**

R40.224- **Coma scale, best verbal response, confused conversation**

R40.225- **Coma scale, best verbal response, oriented**

R40.23- **Coma scale, best motor response**
The following appropriate 7th character is to be added to subcategory R40.23-:
0 - Unspecified time
1 - In the field [EMT or ambulance]
2 - At arrival to emergency department
3 - At hospital admission
4 - 24 hours or more after hospital admission

MCC-0-4 **R40.231-** **Coma scale, best motor response, none**

MCC-0-4 **R40.232-** **Coma scale, best motor response, extension**

R40.233- **Coma scale, best motor response, abnormal**

MCC-0-4 **R40.234-** **Coma scale, best motor response, flexion withdrawal**

R40.235- **Coma scale, best motor response, localizes pain**

R40.236- **Coma scale, best motor response, obeys commands**

R40.24- **Glasgow coma scale, total score**
AHA 15:2Q:p17 – Glasgow coma numeric scores
Note: Assign a code from subcategory R40.24, when only the total coma score is documented
The following appropriate 7th character is to be added to subcategory R40.24-:
0 - Unspecified time
1 - In the field [EMT or ambulance]
2 - At arrival to emergency department
3 - At hospital admission
4 - 24 hours or more after hospital admission

R40.241 **Glasgow coma scale score 13-15**

R40.242 **Glasgow coma scale score 9-12**

R40.243 **Glasgow coma scale score 3-8**

R40.244 **Other coma, without documented Glasgow coma scale score, or with partial score reported**

cc **R40.3** **Persistent vegetative state** — A condition characterized by a permanent state of wakefulness without awareness (an eyes-open unconsciousness).

R40.4 **Transient alteration of awareness** — A condition characterized by staring spells or temporary loss of awareness.

R41- **Other symptoms and signs involving cognitive functions and awareness**
Excludes 1: dissociative [conversion] disorders (F44-)
mild cognitive impairment, so stated (G31.84)

R41.0 **Disorientation, unspecified**
Confusion NOS
Delirium NOS

R41.1 **Anterograde amnesia** — The lack of memory for recent events after an amnesia episode.

R41.2 **Retrograde amnesia** — The lack of memory for events preceding the trauma or condition.

R41.3 **Other amnesia**
Amnesia NOS
Memory loss NOS
Excludes 1: amnestic disorder due to known physiologic condition (F04)
amnestic syndrome due to psychoactive substance use (F10-F19 with 5th character .6)
mild memory disturbance due to known physiological condition (F06.8)
transient global amnesia (G45.4)

cc **R41.4** **Neurologic neglect syndrome** — The condition of neurologically originating behavioral abnormalities that are usually the result of dysfunctional sensory stimuli recognition.
Asomatognosia
Hemi-akinesia
Hemi-inattention
Hemispatial neglect
Left-sided neglect
Sensory neglect
Visuospatial neglect
Excludes 1: visuospatial deficit (R41.842)

R41.8- **Other symptoms and signs involving cognitive functions and awareness**

R41.81 **Age-related cognitive decline** — [Age/15-124] — The condition of mental deterioration associated with old age, without mention of psychosis.
Senility NOS

R41.82 **Altered mental status, unspecified**
Change in mental status NOS
Excludes 1: altered level of consciousness (R40.-)
altered mental status due to known condition — code to condition
delirium NOS (R41.0)

R41.83 **Borderline intellectual functioning** — [Unacceptable PDX]
IQ level 71 to 84
Excludes 1: intellectual disabilities (F70-F79)

R41.84- **Other specified cognitive deficit**
Excludes 1: cognitive deficits as sequelae of cerebrovascular disease (I69.01-, I69.11-, I69.21-, I69.31-, I69.81-, I69.91-)

R41.840 **Attention and concentration deficit**
Excludes 1: attention-deficit hyperactivity disorders (F90.-)

R41.841 **Cognitive communication deficit**

R41.842 **Visuospatial deficit**

R41.843 **Psychomotor deficit**

R41.844 **Frontal lobe and executive function deficit**

R41.89 **Other symptoms and signs involving cognitive functions and awareness**
Anosognosia

R41.9 **Unspecified symptoms and signs involving cognitive functions and awareness**

R42 **Dizziness and giddiness** — The disturbed sense of balance and steadiness.
Light-headedness
Vertigo NOS
Excludes 1: vertiginous syndromes (H81.-)
vertigo from infrasound (T75.23)

R43- **Disturbances of smell and taste**

R43.0 **Anosmia** — The loss of the sense of smell.

R43.1 **Parosmia** — The abnormal deviation of the sense of smell.

R43.2 **Parageusia** — The abnormal deviation of the sense of taste, or a bad taste in the mouth.

R43.8 **Other disturbances of smell and taste**
Mixed disturbance of smell and taste

R43.9 **Unspecified disturbances of smell and taste**

R44- **Other symptoms and signs involving general sensations and perceptions**
Excludes 1: alcoholic hallucinations (F1.5)
hallucinations in drug psychosis (F11-F19 with .5)
hallucinations in mood disorders with psychotic symptoms (F30.2, F31.5, F32.3, F33.3)
hallucinations in schizophrenia, schizotypal and delusional disorders (F20-F29)
Excludes ❷: disturbances of skin sensation (R20.-)

cc **R44.0** **Auditory hallucinations** — A sensory perception disorder of sensing external sounds that does not result from an external stimulus.

R44.1 **Visual hallucinations** — A sensory perception disorder of sensing visual images that does not result from an external stimulus.

cc **R44.2** **Other hallucinations**

cc **R44.3** **Hallucinations, unspecified**

R44.8 **Other symptoms and signs involving general sensations and perceptions**

R44.9 **Unspecified symptoms and signs involving general sensations and perceptions**

R 40 - R 44

R45- Symptoms and signs involving emotional state

R45.0 Nervousness
Nervous tension

R45.1 Restlessness and agitation

R45.2 Unhappiness

R45.3 Demoralization and apathy
Excludes 1: anhedonia (R45.84)

R45.4 Irritability and anger

R45.5 Hostility

R45.6 Violent behavior

R45.7 State of emotional shock and stress, unspecified

R45.8- Other symptoms and signs involving emotional state

R45.81 Low self-esteem

R45.82 Worries

R45.83 Excessive crying of child, adolescent or adult
Excludes 1: excessive crying of infant (baby) R68.11

R45.84 Anhedonia

R45.85- Homicidal and suicidal ideations
Excludes 1: suicide attempt (T14.91)

R45.850 Homicidal ideations — [Unacceptable PDX]

CC **R45.851** Suicidal ideations

R45.86 Emotional lability

R45.87 Impulsiveness

R45.89 Other symptoms and signs involving emotional state

R46- Symptoms and signs involving appearance and behavior
Excludes 1: appearance and behavior in schizophrenia, schizotypal and
delusional disorders (F20-F29)
mental and behavioral disorders (F01-F99)

R46.0 Very low level of personal hygiene

R46.1 Bizarre personal appearance

R46.2 Strange and inexplicable behavior

R46.3 Overactivity

R46.4 Slowness and poor responsiveness
Excludes 1: stupor (R40.1)

R46.5 Suspiciousness and marked evasiveness

R46.6 Undue concern and preoccupation with stressful events

R46.7 Verbosity and circumstantial detail obscuring reason for
contact

R46.8- Other symptoms and signs involving appearance and
behavior

R46.81 Obsessive-compulsive behavior — [Unacceptable PDX]
Excludes 1: obsessive-compulsive disorder (F42.-)

R46.89 Other symptoms and signs involving appearance and
behavior — [Unacceptable PDX]

Symptoms and signs involving speech and voice (R47-R49)

R47- Speech disturbances, not elsewhere classified
Excludes 1: autism (F84.0)
cluttering (F80.81)
specific developmental disorders of speech and language
(F80.-)
stuttering (F80.81)

R47.0- Dysphasia and aphasia

CC **R47.01** Aphasia — The absence or impairment of the ability to communicate
through speech, writing, or signs.
Excludes 1: aphasia following cerebrovascular disease
(I69. with final characters -20)
progressive isolated aphasia (G31.01)

R47.02 Dysphasia — The lack of coordination to arrange words in their proper
order.
Excludes 1: dysphasia following cerebrovascular disease
(I69. with final characters -21)

R47.1 Dysarthria and anarthria — Difficulty articulating words of speech.
Excludes 1: dysarthria following cerebrovascular disease
(I69. with final characters -22)

R47.8- Other speech disturbances
Excludes 1: dysarthria following cerebrovascular disease
(I69. with final characters -28)

R47.81 Slurred speech — Slow and distorted speech.

R47.82 Fluency disorder in conditions classified elsewhere —
[Not Allowed as PDX]
Stuttering in conditions classified elsewhere
Code first underlying disease or condition, such as:
Parkinson's disease (G20)
Excludes 1: adult onset fluency disorder (F98.5)
childhood onset fluency disorder (F80.81)
fluency disorder (stuttering) following
cerebrovascular disease (I69. with final
characters-23)

R47.89 Other speech disturbances

R47.9 Unspecified speech disturbances

R48- Dyslexia and other symbolic dysfunctions, not elsewhere classified
Excludes 1: specific developmental disorders of scholastic skills (F81-)

R48.0 Dyslexia and alexia — The inability to read that is due to an organic
disorder.

R48.1 Agnosia — The loss of comprehension of sensory stimuli.
Astereognosia (astereognosis)
Autotopagnosia
Excludes 1: visual object agnosia (R48.3)

R48.2 Apraxia — The inability to perform voluntary movements without any organic
cause.
Excludes 1: apraxia following cerebrovascular disease (I69. with
final characters -90)

R48.3 Visual agnosia — The inability to interpret images that are seen.
Prosopagnosia — The impairment of the ability to recognize familiar faces.
Simultanagnosia (asimultagnosia) — The inability to recognize two or
more objects at the same time.

R48.8 Other symbolic dysfunctions
Acalculia — The inability to perform simple arithmetical calculations.
Agraphia — The difficulty with writing.

R48.9 Unspecified symbolic dysfunctions

R49- Voice and resonance disorders
Excludes 1: psychogenic voice and resonance disorders (F44.4)

R49.0 Dysphonia — The impairment of speaking.
Hoarseness — The rougher than usual quality of the voice.

R49.1 Aphonia — The loss of the ability to produce sounds.
Loss of voice

R49.2- Hypernasality and hyponasality

R49.21 Hypernasality — The increased nasal resonance of the voice.

R49.22 Hyponasality — The decreased nasal resonance of the voice.

R49.8 Other voice and resonance disorders

R49.9 Unspecified voice and resonance disorder
Change in voice NOS
Resonance disorder NOS

General symptoms and signs (R50-R69)

R50- Fever of other and unknown origin — The abnormal elevation of the body's
temperature.
Excludes 1: chills without fever (R68.83)
febrile convulsions (R56.0-)
fever of unknown origin during labor (O75.2)
fever of unknown origin in newborn (P81.9)
hypothermia due to illness (R68.0)
malignant hyperthermia due to anesthesia (T88.3)
puerperal pyrexia NOS (O86.4)

R50.2 Drug-induced fever
Use additional code for adverse effect, if applicable, to identify drug
(T36-T50 with fifth or sixth character 5)
Excludes 1: postvaccination (postimmunization) fever (R50.83)

R50.8- Other specified fever

R50.81 Fever presenting with conditions classified elsewhere —
[Not Allowed as PDX]
Code first underlying condition when associated fever is present,
such as with:
Leukemia (C91-C95)
Neutropenia (D70-)
Sickle-cell disease (D57-)

R50.82 Postprocedural fever — A form that is associated/due to a procedure.
Excludes 1: postprocedural infection (T81.4-)
posttransfusion fever (R50.84)
postvaccination (postimmunization) fever (R50.83)

R
4
5
–
R
5
0

R50.83 Postvaccination fever — A form that is associated/due to a vaccination.
    Postimmunization fever

R50.84 Febrile nonhemolytic transfusion reaction — A form that is associated/due to a transfusion, but not due to hemolysis.
    FNHTR
    Posttransfusion fever

R50.9 Fever, unspecified
    Fever NOS
    Fever of unknown origin [FUO]
    Fever with chills
    Fever with rigors
    Hyperpyrexia NOS
    Persistent fever
    Pyrexia NOS

R51 Headache
    Facial pain NOS
    Excludes 1:   *atypical face pain (G50.1)*
                migraine and other headache syndromes (G43-G44)
                trigeminal neuralgia (G50.0)

R52 Pain, unspecified
    Acute pain NOS
    Generalized pain NOS
    Pain NOS
    Excludes 1:   *acute and chronic pain, not elsewhere classified (G89-)*
                localized pain, unspecified type — *code to pain by site, such*
                  as:
                      abdomen pain (R10-)
                      back pain (M54.9)
                      breast pain (N64.4)
                      chest pain (R07.1-R07.9)
                      ear pain (H92.0-)
                      eye pain (H57.1)
                      headache (R51)
                      joint pain (M25.5-)
                      limb pain (M79.6-)
                      lumbar region pain (M54.5)
                      pelvic and perineal pain (R10.2)
                      shoulder pain (M25.51-)
                      spine pain (M54-)
                      throat pain (R07.0)
                      tongue pain (K14.6)
                      tooth pain (K08.8)
                  pain disorders exclusively related to psychological factors
                      (F45.41)
                  renal colic (N23)

R53- Malaise and fatigue — MALAISE – The vague feeling of bodily discomfort. FATIGUE – The state of decreased bodily efficiency usually resulting from prolonged or excessive exertion.

R53.0 Neoplastic (malignant) related fatigue
    Code first associated neoplasm

R53.1 Weakness
    Asthenia NOS
    Excludes 1:   *age-related weakness (R54)*
                      muscle weakness (M62.8-)
                      sarcopenia (M62.84)
                      senile asthenia (R54)

MCC **R53.2 Functional quadriplegia** — The condition of loss or impairment of function of the limbs that is not due to a neurological or psychological condition.
    Complete immobility due to severe physical disability or frailty
    Excludes 1:   *frailty NOS (R54)*
                      hysterical paralysis (F44.4)
                      immobility syndrome (M62.3)
                      neurologic quadriplegia (G82.5-)
                      quadriplegia (G82.50)

R53.8- Other malaise and fatigue
    Excludes 1:   *combat exhaustion and fatigue (F43.0)*
                      congenital debility (P96.9)
                      exhaustion and fatigue due to depressive episode
                        (F32.-)
                      exhaustion and fatigue due to excessive exertion
                        (T73.3)
                      exhaustion and fatigue due to exposure (T73.2)
                      exhaustion and fatigue due to heat (T67.-)
                      exhaustion and fatigue due to pregnancy (O26.8-)
                      exhaustion and fatigue due to recurrent depressive
                        episode (F33)
                      exhaustion and fatigue due to senile debility (R54)

    R53.81 Other malaise
        Chronic debility
        Debility NOS
        General physical deterioration
        Malaise NOS
        Nervous debility
        Excludes 1:   *age-related physical debility (R54)*

    R53.82 Chronic fatigue, unspecified
        Chronic fatigue syndrome NOS — The abnormal condition of persistent, debilitating fatigue characterized by decreased physical activity, muscle weakness, headaches and depression.
        Excludes 1:   *postviral fatigue syndrome (G93.3)*

    R53.83 Other fatigue
        Fatigue NOS
        Lack of energy
        Lethargy
        Tiredness

R54 Age-related physical debility — [Age/15-124]
    Frailty
    Old age
    Senescence
    Senile asthenia
    Senile debility
    Excludes 1:   *age-related cognitive decline (R41.81)*
                      sarcopenia (M62.84)
                      senile psychosis (F03)
                      senility NOS (R41.81)

R55 Syncope and collapse — SYNCOPE – A brief lapse of consciousness caused by a temporary lack of arterial oxygen to the brain. COLLAPSE – The state of prostration and weakness due to decreased circulation.
    Blackout — A form of syncope that is accompanied by failure of vision.
    Fainting
    Vasovagal attack — A form of syncope associated with abrupt emotional stress.
    Excludes 1:   *cardiogenic shock (R57.0)*
                      carotid sinus syncope (G90.01)
                      heat syncope (T67.1)
                      neurocirculatory asthenia (F45.8)
                      neurogenic orthostatic hypotension (G90.3)
                      orthostatic hypotension (I95.1)
                      postprocedural shock (T81.1-)
                      psychogenic syncope (F48.8)
                      shock NOS (R57.9)
                      shock complicating or following abortion or ectopic or molar
                        pregnancy (O00-O07, O08.3)
                      shock complicating or following labor and delivery (O75.1)
                      Stokes-Adams attack (I45.9)
                      unconsciousness NOS (R40.2-)

R56- Convulsions, not elsewhere classified — A sudden, violent contraction of the voluntary muscle groups.
    Excludes 1:   *dissociative convulsions and seizures (F44.5)*
                      epileptic convulsions and seizures (G40.-)
                      newborn convulsions and seizures (P90)

    R56.0- Febrile convulsions

    CC **R56.00 Simple febrile convulsions** — A form brought on by a high body temperature.
        Febrile convulsion NOS
        Febrile seizure NOS

    CC **R56.01 Complex febrile convulsions** — Fever-associated seizures that are prolonged (usually more than 15 minutes) or reoccur with 24 hours, and usually focus on one part of the body.
        Atypical febrile seizure
        Complex febrile seizure
        Complicated febrile seizure
        Excludes 1:   *status epilepticus (G40.901)*

    CC **R56.1 Post traumatic seizures**
        Excludes 1:   *post traumatic epilepsy (G40.-)*

R
5
0
|
R
5
6

R56.9   Unspecified convulsions
Convulsion disorder
Fit NOS
Recurrent convulsions
Seizure(s) (convulsive) NOS

R57-   Shock, not elsewhere classified
Excludes 1:   *anaphylactic reaction or shock due to adverse food reaction (T78.0-)*
anaphylactic shock due to adverse effect of correct drug or medicament properly administered (T88.6)
anaphylactic shock due to serum (T80.5-)
anaphylactic shock NOS (T78.2)
anesthetic shock (T88.3)
electric shock (T75.4)
obstetric shock (O75.1)
postprocedural shock (T81.1-)
psychic shock (F43.0)
septic shock (R65.21)
shock complicating or following ectopic or molar pregnancy (O00-O07, O08.3)
shock due to lightning (T75.01)
traumatic shock (T79.4)
toxic shock syndrome (A48.3)

MCC **R57.0   Cardiogenic shock** — The failure of peripheral circulation that is due to a decreased cardiac output.

MCC **R57.1   Hypovolemic shock** — The failure of peripheral circulation that is due to a decreased blood volume.

MCC **R57.8   Other shock**

CC **R57.9   Shock, unspecified**
Failure of peripheral circulation NOS

R58   Hemorrhage, not elsewhere classified
Hemorrhage NOS
Excludes 1:   *hemorrhage included with underlying conditions, such as:*
acute duodenal ulcer with hemorrhage (K26.0)
acute gastritis with bleeding (K29.01)
ulcerative enterocolitis with rectal bleeding (K51.01)

R59-   Enlarged lymph nodes
Includes: swollen glands
Excludes 1:   *lymphadenitis NOS (I88.9)*
acute lymphadenitis (L04.-)
chronic lymphadenitis (I88.1)
mesenteric (acute) (chronic) lymphadenitis (I88.0)

R59.0   Localized enlarged lymph nodes

R59.1   Generalized enlarged lymph nodes
Lymphadenopathy NOS

R59.9   Enlarged lymph nodes, unspecified

R60-   Edema, not elsewhere classified — The accumulation of fluid in the intercellular spaces.
Excludes 1:   *angioneurotic edema (T78.3)*
ascites (R18-)
cerebral edema (G93.6)
cerebral edema due to birth injury (P11.0)
edema of larynx (J38.4)
edema of nasopharynx (J39.2)
edema of pharynx (J39.2)
gestational edema (O12.0-)
hereditary edema (Q82.0)
hydrops fetalis NOS (P83.2)
hydrothorax (J94.8)
newborn edema (P83.3)
nutritional edema (E40-E46)
pulmonary edema (J81-)

R60.0   Localized edema

R60.1   Generalized edema

R60.9   Edema, unspecified
Fluid retention NOS

R61   Generalized hyperhidrosis — Excessive sweating occurring over the entire body.
Excessive sweating
Night sweats
Secondary hyperhidrosis
Code first, if applicable, menopausal and female climacteric states (N95.1)
Excludes 1:   *focal (primary) (secondary) hyperhidrosis (L74.5-)*
Frey's syndrome (L74.52)
localized (primary) (secondary) hyperhidrosis (L74.5-)

R62-   Lack of expected normal physiological development in childhood and adults
Excludes 1:   *delayed puberty (E30.0)*
gonadal dysgenesis (Q99.1)
hypopituitarism (E23.0)

R62.0   Delayed milestone in childhood — [Age/0-17]
Delayed attainment of expected physiological developmental stage
Late talker
Late walker

R62.5-   Other and unspecified lack of expected normal physiological development in childhood — The abnormal condition in children that fail to meet the standardized growth and developmental chart progress.
Excludes 1:   *HIV disease resulting in failure to thrive (B20)*
physical retardation due to malnutrition (E45)

R62.50   Unspecified lack of expected normal physiological development in childhood
Infantilism NOS

R62.51   Failure to thrive (child) — [Age/0-17] — A form in which a child loses weight or fails to gain weight.
Failure to gain weight
Excludes 1:   *failure to thrive in child under 28 days old (P92.6)*

R62.52   Short stature (child) — A form in which a child has a slower than normal rate maturation of bone/height for his/her age.
Lack of growth
Physical retardation
Short stature NOS
Excludes 1:   *short stature due to endocrine disorder (E34.3)*

R62.59   Other lack of expected normal physiological development in childhood

R62.7   Adult failure to thrive — [Age/15-124] — The abnormal condition of an adult patient whose health status is deteriorating or not improving.

R63-   Symptoms and signs concerning food and fluid intake
Excludes 1:   *bulimia NOS (F50.2)*
eating disorders of nonorganic origin (F50.-)
malnutrition (E40-E46)

R63.0   Anorexia — The lack or loss of appetite for food.
Loss of appetite
Excludes 1:   *anorexia nervosa (F50.0-)*
loss of appetite of nonorganic origin (F50.89)

R63.1   Polydipsia
Excessive thirst

R63.2   Polyphagia
Excessive eating
Hyperalimentation NOS

R63.3   Feeding difficulties
Feeding problem (elderly) (infant) NOS
Excludes 1:   *feeding problems of newborn (P92.-)*
infant feeding disorder of nonorganic origin (F98.2-)

R63.4   Abnormal weight loss — The relatively recent loss of a patient's usual weight.

R63.5   Abnormal weight gain — The relatively recent increase in a patient's usual weight.
Excludes 1:   *excessive weight gain in pregnancy (O26.0-)*
obesity (E66.-)

R63.6   Underweight — The condition of weighing less than a person's standard weight for his/her height.
Use additional code to identify body mass index (BMI), if known (Z68.-)
Excludes 1:   *abnormal weight loss (R63.4)*
anorexia nervosa (F50.0-)
malnutrition (E40-E46)

R63.8   Other symptoms and signs concerning food and fluid intake

R64   Cachexia — The state of general ill health and malnutrition.
CC   Wasting syndrome
Code first underlying condition, if known
Excludes 1:   *abnormal weight loss (R63.4)*
nutritional marasmus (E41)

R 5 6 ‑ R 6 4

R65- Symptoms and signs specifically associated with systemic inflammation and infection
AHA 14:3Q:p4 – SIRS secondary to pneumonia

R65.1- Systemic inflammatory response syndrome (SIRS) of non-infectious origin
Code first underlying condition, such as:
Heatstroke (T67.0)
Injury and trauma (S00-T88)
Excludes 1: sepsis — code to infection
severe sepsis (R65.2)

CC **R65.10 Systemic inflammatory response syndrome (SIRS) of non-infectious origin without acute organ dysfunction**
Systemic inflammatory response syndrome (SIRS) NOS

MCC **R65.11 Systemic inflammatory response syndrome (SIRS) of non-infectious origin with acute organ dysfunction**
Use additional code to identify specific acute organ dysfunction, such as:
Acute kidney failure (N17.-)
Acute respiratory failure (J96.0-)
Critical illness myopathy (G72.81)
Critical illness polyneuropathy (G62.81)
Disseminated intravascular coagulopathy [DIC] (D65)
Encephalopathy (metabolic) (septic) (G93.41)
Hepatic failure (K72.0-)

R65.2- Severe sepsis
Infection with associated acute organ dysfunction
Sepsis with acute organ dysfunction
Sepsis with multiple organ dysfunction
Systemic inflammatory response syndrome due to infectious process with acute organ dysfunction
Code first underlying infection, such as:
Infection following a procedure (T81.4-)
Infections following infusion, transfusion and therapeutic injection (T80.2-)
Puerperal sepsis (O85)
Sepsis following complete or unspecified spontaneous abortion (O03.87)
Sepsis following ectopic and molar pregnancy (O08.82)
Sepsis following incomplete spontaneous abortion (O03.37)
Sepsis following (induced) termination of pregnancy (O04.87)
Sepsis NOS (A41.9)
Use additional code to identify specific acute organ dysfunction, such as:
Acute kidney failure (N17.-)
Acute respiratory failure (J96.0-)
Critical illness myopathy (G72.81)
Critical illness polyneuropathy (G62.81)
Disseminated intravascular coagulopathy [DIC] (D65)
Encephalopathy (metabolic) (septic) (G93.41)
Hepatic failure (K72.0-)

MCC **R65.20 Severe sepsis without septic shock**
Severe sepsis NOS

MCC **R65.21 Severe sepsis with septic shock** — Sepsis with sepsis-induced hypotension despite fluid resuscitation and inadequate tissue perfusion (failure of peripheral circulation). Septic shock is the final stage in the SIRS-sepsis-severe sepsis-septic shock continuum.

R68- Other general symptoms and signs
R68.0 Hypothermia, not associated with low environmental temperature
Excludes 1: hypothermia NOS (accidental) (T68)
hypothermia due to anesthesia (T88.51)
hypothermia due to low environmental temperature (T68)
newborn hypothermia (P80.-)

R68.1- Nonspecific symptoms peculiar to infancy
Excludes 1: colic, infantile (R10.83)
neonatal cerebral irritability (P91.3)
teething syndrome (K00.7)

R68.11 Excessive crying of infant (baby) — [Age/0-17]
Excludes 1: excessive crying of child, adolescent, or adult (R45.83)

R68.12 Fussy infant (baby) — [Age/0-17]
Irritable infant

R68.13 Apparent life threatening event in infant (ALTE) — [Age/0-17] – A condition that is frightening to the observer that is characterized by various symptoms including cyanosis, apnea, color change, muscle tone change, limb jerking, and choking that is not due to an identifiable diagnosis.
Apparent life threatening event in newborn
Code first confirmed diagnosis, if known
Use additional code(s) for associated signs and symptoms if no confirmed diagnosis established, or if signs and symptoms are not associated routinely with confirmed diagnosis, or provide additional information for cause of ALTE

R68.19 Other nonspecific symptoms peculiar to infancy — [Age/0-17]

R68.2 Dry mouth, unspecified
Excludes 1: dry mouth due to dehydration (E86.0)
dry mouth due to sicca syndrome [Sjögren] (M35.0-)
salivary gland hyposecretion (K11.7)

R68.3 Clubbing of fingers — The distortional enlargement of the fingers.
Clubbing of nails
Excludes 1: congenital clubfinger (Q68.1)

R68.8- Other general symptoms and signs
R68.81 Early satiety
R68.82 Decreased libido — [Age/15-124]
Decreased sexual desire
R68.83 Chills (without fever)
Chills NOS
Excludes 1: chills with fever (R50.9)

R68.84 Jaw pain
Mandibular pain
Maxilla pain
Excludes 1: temporomandibular joint arthralgia (M26.62-)

R68.89 Other general symptoms and signs

R69 Illness, unspecified
Unknown and unspecified cases of morbidity

Abnormal findings on examination of blood, without diagnosis (R70-R79)

Excludes ❷: abnormal findings on antenatal screening of mother (O28.-)
abnormalities of lipids (E78.-)
abnormalities of platelets and thrombocytes (D69.-)
abnormalities of white blood cells classified elsewhere (D70-D72)
coagulation hemorrhagic disorders (D65-D68)
diagnostic abnormal findings classified elsewhere — see Alphabetical Index
hemorrhagic and hematological disorders of newborn (P50-P61)

R70- Elevated erythrocyte sedimentation rate and abnormality of plasma viscosity
R70.0 Elevated erythrocyte sedimentation rate
R70.1 Abnormal plasma viscosity

R71- Abnormality of red blood cells
Excludes 1: anemias (D50-D64)
anemia of premature infant (P61.2)
benign (familial) polycythemia (D75.0)
congenital anemias (P61.2-P61.4)
newborn anemia due to isoimmunization (P55.-)
polycythemia neonatorum (P61.1)
polycythemia NOS (D75.1)
polycythemia vera (D45)
secondary polycythemia (D75.1)

CC **R71.0 Precipitous drop in hematocrit** — A relatively recent, significant, comparative lowering of a patient's hematocrit.
Drop (precipitous) in hemoglobin
Drop in hematocrit

R71.8 Other abnormality of red blood cells
Abnormal red-cell morphology NOS
Abnormal red-cell volume NOS
Anisocytosis — The condition of an excessive variation in the size of erythrocytes in the blood.
Poikilocytosis — The condition of a variation in size of red corpuscles in the blood.

R73- Elevated blood glucose level
Excludes 1:   diabetes mellitus (E08-E13)
diabetes mellitus in pregnancy, childbirth and the puerperium
(O24.-)
neonatal disorders (P70.0-P70.2)
postsurgical hypoinsulinemia (E89.1)

R73.0- Abnormal glucose
Excludes 1:   abnormal glucose in pregnancy (O99.81-)
diabetes mellitus (E08-E13)
dysmetabolic syndrome X (E88.81)
gestational diabetes (O24.4-)
glycosuria (R81)
hypoglycemia (E16.2)

R73.01 Impaired fasting glucose
Elevated fasting glucose

R73.02 Impaired glucose tolerance (oral)
Elevated glucose tolerance

R73.03 Prediabetes
Latent diabetes

R73.09 Other abnormal glucose
Abnormal glucose NOS
Abnormal non-fasting glucose tolerance

R73.9 Hyperglycemia, unspecified

R74- Abnormal serum enzyme levels

R74.0 Nonspecific elevation of levels of transaminase and lactic acid dehydrogenase [LDH]

R74.8 Abnormal levels of other serum enzymes
Abnormal level of acid phosphatase
Abnormal level of alkaline phosphatase
Abnormal level of amylase
Abnormal level of lipase [triacylglycerol lipase]

R74.9 Abnormal serum enzyme level, unspecified

R75 Inconclusive laboratory evidence of human immunodeficiency virus [HIV]
Nonconclusive HIV-test finding in infants
Excludes 1:   asymptomatic human immunodeficiency virus [HIV] infection
status (Z21)
human immunodeficiency virus [HIV] disease (B20)

R76- Other abnormal immunological findings in serum

R76.0 Raised antibody titer
Excludes 1:   isoimmunization in pregnancy (O36.0-O36.1)
isoimmunization affecting newborn (P55-)

R76.1- Nonspecific reaction to test for tuberculosis

R76.11 Nonspecific reaction to tuberculin skin test without active tuberculosis
Abnormal result of Mantoux test
PPD positive
Tuberculin (skin test) positive
Tuberculin (skin test) reactor
Excludes 1:   nonspecific reaction to cell mediated immunity
measurement of gamma interferon antigen
response without active tuberculosis (R76.12)

R76.12 Nonspecific reaction to cell mediated immunity measurement of gamma interferon antigen response without active tuberculosis
Nonspecific reaction to QuantiFERON-TB test (QFT) without
active tuberculosis
Excludes 1:   nonspecific reaction to tuberculin skin test without
active tuberculosis (R76.11)
positive tuberculin skin test (R76.11)

R76.8 Other specified abnormal immunological findings in serum
Raised level of immunoglobulins NOS

R76.9 Abnormal immunological finding in serum, unspecified

R77- Other abnormalities of plasma proteins
Excludes 1:   disorders of plasma-protein metabolism (E88.0)

R77.0 Abnormality of albumin

R77.1 Abnormality of globulin
Hyperglobulinemia NOS

R77.2 Abnormality of alphafetoprotein

R77.8 Other specified abnormalities of plasma proteins

R77.9 Abnormality of plasma protein, unspecified

R78- Findings of drugs and other substances, not normally found in blood
Use additional code to identify the any retained foreign body, if applicable
(Z18.-)
Excludes 1:   mental or behavioral disorders due to psychoactive substance
use (F10-F19)

R78.0 Finding of alcohol in blood
Use additional external cause code (Y90.-), for detail regarding
alcohol level

R78.1 Finding of opiate drug in blood

R78.2 Finding of cocaine in blood

R78.3 Finding of hallucinogen in blood

R78.4 Finding of other drugs of addictive potential in blood

R78.5 Finding of other psychotropic drug in blood

R78.6 Finding of steroid agent in blood

R78.7- Finding of abnormal level of heavy metals in blood

R78.71 Abnormal lead level in blood
Excludes 1:   lead poisoning (T56.0-)

R78.79 Finding of abnormal level of heavy metals in blood

R78.8- Finding of other specified substances, not normally found in blood

cc **R78.81 Bacteremia**
Excludes 1:   sepsis-code to specified infection

R78.89 Finding of other specified substances, not normally found in blood
Finding of abnormal level of lithium in blood

R78.9 Finding of unspecified substance, not normally found in blood

R79- Other abnormal findings of blood chemistry
Use additional code to identify any retained foreign body, if applicable (Z18.-)
Excludes 1:   abnormality of fluid, electrolyte or acid-base balance
(E86-E87)
asymptomatic hyperuricemia (E79.0)
hyperglycemia NOS (R73.9)
hypoglycemia NOS (E16.2)
neonatal hypoglycemia (P70.3-P70.4)
specific findings indicating disorder of amino-acid metabolism
(E70-E72)
specific findings indicating disorder of carbohydrate
metabolism (E73-E74)
specific findings indicating disorder of lipid metabolism (E75.-)

R79.0 Abnormal level of blood mineral
Abnormal blood level of cobalt
Abnormal blood level of copper
Abnormal blood level of iron
Abnormal blood level of magnesium
Abnormal blood level of mineral NEC
Abnormal blood level of zinc
Excludes 1:   abnormal level of lithium (R78.89)
disorders of mineral metabolism (E83.-)
neonatal hypomagnesemia (P71.2)
nutritional mineral deficiency (E58-E61)

R79.1 Abnormal coagulation profile
Abnormal or prolonged bleeding time
Abnormal or prolonged coagulation time
Abnormal or prolonged partial thromboplastin time [PTT]
Abnormal or prolonged prothrombin time [PT]
Excludes 1:   coagulation defects (D68.-)

R79.8- Other specified abnormal findings of blood chemistry

R79.81 Abnormal blood-gas level

R79.82 Elevated C-reactive protein (CRP)

R79.89 Other specified abnormal findings of blood chemistry

R79.9 Abnormal finding of blood chemistry, unspecified

R73-R79

Abnormal findings on examination of urine, without diagnosis (R80-R82)

> **Excludes 1:** abnormal findings on antenatal screening of mother (O28.-)
> diagnostic abnormal findings classified elsewhere — see Alphabetical Index
> specific findings indicating disorder of amino-acid metabolism (E70-E72)
> specific findings indicating disorder of carbohydrate metabolism (E73-E74)

R80- Proteinuria — The presence of excess serum proteins in the urine.
> **Excludes 1:** gestational proteinuria (O12.1-)

   R80.0 Isolated proteinuria
      Idiopathic proteinuria
>   **Excludes 1:** isolated proteinuria with specific morphological lesion (N06.-)

   R80.1 Persistent proteinuria, unspecified

   R80.2 Orthostatic proteinuria, unspecified
      Postural proteinuria

   R80.3 Bence Jones proteinuria — The presence of Bence-Jones protein in the urine.

   R80.8 Other proteinuria

   R80.9 Proteinuria, unspecified
      Albuminuria NOS

R81 Glycosuria — The presence of glucose in the urine.
> **Excludes 1:** renal glycosuria (E74.8)

R82- Other and unspecified abnormal findings in urine
   Includes: Chromoabnormalities in urine
   Use additional code to identify any retained foreign body, if applicable (Z18.-)
> **Excludes 2:** hematuria (R31.-)

cc **R82.0 Chyluria** — The presence of chyle in the urine.
>   **Excludes 1:** filarial chyluria (B74.-)

cc **R82.1 Myoglobinuria** — The presence of myoglobin in the urine.

   R82.2 Biliuria — The presence of bile in the urine.

   R82.3 Hemoglobinuria — The presence of hemoglobin in the urine.
>   **Excludes 1:** hemoglobinuria due to hemolysis from external causes NEC (D59.6)
> hemoglobinuria due to paroxysmal nocturnal [Marchiafava-Micheli] (D59.5)

   R82.4 Acetonuria — The presence of acetone in the urine.
      Ketonuria — The presence of ketone bodies in the urine.

   R82.5 Elevated urine levels of drugs, medicaments and biological substances
      Elevated urine levels of catecholamines
      Elevated urine levels of indoleacetic acid
      Elevated urine levels of 17-ketosteroids
      Elevated urine levels of steroids

   R82.6 Abnormal urine levels of substances chiefly nonmedicinal as to source
      Abnormal urine level of heavy metals

   R82.7- Abnormal findings on microbiological examination of urine
>   **Excludes 1:** colonization status (Z22.-)

     R82.71 Bacteriuria

     R82.79 Other abnormal findings on microbiological examination of urine
        Positive culture findings of urine

   R82.8 Abnormal findings on cytological and histological examination of urine

   R82.9- Other and unspecified abnormal findings in urine

     R82.90 Unspecified abnormal findings in urine

     R82.91 Other chromoabnormalities of urine
        Chromoconversion (dipstick)
        Idiopathic dipstick converts positive for blood with no cellular forms in sediment
>   **Excludes 1:** hemoglobinuria (R82.3)
> myoglobinuria (R82.1)

     R82.99 Other abnormal findings in urine
        Cells and casts in urine
        Crystalluria
        Melanuria

Abnormal findings on examination of other body fluids, substances and tissues, without diagnosis (R83-R89)

> **Excludes 1:** abnormal findings on antenatal screening of mother (O28.-)
> diagnostic abnormal findings classified elsewhere — see Alphabetical Index
>
> **Excludes 2:** abnormal findings on examination of blood, without diagnosis (R70-R79)
> abnormal findings on examination of urine, without diagnosis (R80-R82)
> abnormal tumor markers (R97.-)

R83- Abnormal findings in cerebrospinal fluid

   R83.0 Abnormal level of enzymes in cerebrospinal fluid

   R83.1 Abnormal level of hormones in cerebrospinal fluid

   R83.2 Abnormal level of other drugs, medicaments and biological substances in cerebrospinal fluid

   R83.3 Abnormal level of substances chiefly nonmedicinal as to source in cerebrospinal fluid

   R83.4 Abnormal immunological findings in cerebrospinal fluid

   R83.5 Abnormal microbiological findings in cerebrospinal fluid
      Positive culture findings in cerebrospinal fluid
>   **Excludes 1:** colonization status (Z22.-)

   R83.6 Abnormal cytological findings in cerebrospinal fluid

   R83.8 Other abnormal findings in cerebrospinal fluid
      Abnormal chromosomal findings in cerebrospinal fluid

   R83.9 Unspecified abnormal finding in cerebrospinal fluid

R84- Abnormal findings in specimens from respiratory organs and thorax
   Includes: Abnormal findings in bronchial washings
             Abnormal findings in nasal secretions
             Abnormal findings in pleural fluid
             Abnormal findings in sputum
             Abnormal findings in throat scrapings
> **Excludes 1:** blood-stained sputum (R04.2)

   R84.0 Abnormal level of enzymes in specimens from respiratory organs and thorax

   R84.1 Abnormal level of hormones in specimens from respiratory organs and thorax

   R84.2 Abnormal level of other drugs, medicaments and biological substances in specimens from respiratory organs and thorax

   R84.3 Abnormal level of substances chiefly nonmedicinal as to source in specimens from respiratory organs and thorax

   R84.4 Abnormal immunological findings in specimens from respiratory organs and thorax

   R84.5 Abnormal microbiological findings in specimens from respiratory organs and thorax
      Positive culture findings in specimens from respiratory organs and thorax
>   **Excludes 1:** colonization status (Z22.-)

   R84.6 Abnormal cytological findings in specimens from respiratory organs and thorax

   R84.7 Abnormal histological findings in specimens from respiratory organs and thorax

   R84.8 Other abnormal findings in specimens from respiratory organs and thorax
      Abnormal chromosomal findings in specimens from respiratory organs and thorax

   R84.9 Unspecified abnormal finding in specimens from respiratory organs and thorax

R85- Abnormal findings in specimens from digestive organs and abdominal cavity
   Includes: Abnormal findings in peritoneal fluid
             Abnormal findings in saliva
> **Excludes 1:** cloudy peritoneal dialysis effluent (R88.0)
> fecal abnormalities (R19.5)

   R85.0 Abnormal level of enzymes in specimens from digestive organs and abdominal cavity

   R85.1 Abnormal level of hormones in specimens from digestive organs and abdominal cavity

   R85.2 Abnormal level of other drugs, medicaments and biological substances in specimens from digestive organs and abdominal cavity

R80 – R85

R85.3 Abnormal level of substances chiefly nonmedicinal as to source in specimens from digestive organs and abdominal cavity

R85.4 Abnormal immunological findings in specimens from digestive organs and abdominal cavity

R85.5 Abnormal microbiological findings in specimens from digestive organs and abdominal cavity
   Positive culture findings in specimens from digestive organs and abdominal cavity
   Excludes 1: *colonization status (Z22.-)*

R85.6- Abnormal cytological findings in specimens from digestive organs and abdominal cavity

  R85.61- Abnormal cytologic smear of anus
   Excludes 1: *abnormal cytological findings in specimens from other digestive organs and abdominal cavity (R85.69)*
   anal intraepithelial neoplasia I [AIN I] (K62.82)
   anal intraepithelial neoplasia II [AIN II] (K62.82)
   anal intraepithelial neoplasia III [AIN III] (D01.3)
   carcinoma in situ of anus (histologically confirmed) (D01.3)
   dysplasia (mild) (moderate) of anus (histologically confirmed) (K62.82)
   severe dysplasia of anus (histologically confirmed) (D01.3)
   Excludes ❷: *anal high risk human papillomavirus (HPV) DNA test positive (R85.81)*
   anal low risk human papillomavirus (HPV) DNA test positive (R85.82)

    R85.610 Atypical squamous cells of undetermined significance on cytologic smear of anus (ASC-US)

    R85.611 Atypical squamous cells cannot exclude high grade squamous intraepithelial lesion on cytologic smear of anus (ASC-H)

    R85.612 Low grade squamous intraepithelial lesion on cytologic smear of anus (LGSIL)

    R85.613 High grade squamous intraepithelial lesion on cytologic smear of anus (HGSIL)

    R85.614 Cytologic evidence of malignancy on smear of anus

    R85.615 Unsatisfactory cytologic smear of anus
   Inadequate sample of cytologic smear of anus

    R85.616 Satisfactory anal smear but lacking transformation zone

    R85.618 Other abnormal cytological findings on specimens from anus

    R85.619 Unspecified abnormal cytological findings in specimens from anus
   Abnormal anal cytology NOS
   Atypical glandular cells of anus NOS

  R85.69 Abnormal cytological findings in specimens from other digestive organs and abdominal cavity

R85.7 Abnormal histological findings in specimens from digestive organs and abdominal cavity

R85.8- Other abnormal findings in specimens from digestive organs and abdominal cavity

  R85.81 Anal high risk human papillomavirus (HPV) DNA test positive
   Excludes 1: *anogenital warts due to human papillomavirus (HPV) (A63.0)*
   condyloma acuminatum (A63.0)

  R85.82 Anal low risk human papillomavirus (HPV) DNA test positive
   Use additional code for associated human papillomavirus (B97.7)

  R85.89 Other abnormal findings in specimens from digestive organs and abdominal cavity
   Abnormal chromosomal findings in specimens from digestive organs and abdominal cavity

R85.9 Unspecified abnormal finding in specimens from digestive organs and abdominal cavity

R86- Abnormal findings in specimens from male genital organs
   Includes: Abnormal findings in prostatic secretions
   Abnormal findings in semen, seminal fluid
   Abnormal spermatozoa
   Excludes 1: *azoospermia (N46.0-)*
   oligospermia (N46.1-)

R86.0 Abnormal level of enzymes in specimens from male genital organs — [♂]

R86.1 Abnormal level of hormones in specimens from male genital organs — [♂]

R86.2 Abnormal level of other drugs, medicaments and biological substances in specimens from male genital organs — [♂]

R86.3 Abnormal level of substances chiefly nonmedicinal as to source in specimens from male genital organs — [♂]

R86.4 Abnormal immunological findings in specimens from male genital organs — [♂]

R86.5 Abnormal microbiological findings in specimens from male genital organs — [♂]
   Positive culture findings in specimens from male genital organs
   Excludes 1: *colonization status (Z22.-)*

R86.6 Abnormal cytological findings in specimens from male genital organs — [♂]

R86.7 Abnormal histological findings in specimens from male genital organs — [♂]

R86.8 Other abnormal findings in specimens from male genital organs — [♂]
   Abnormal chromosomal findings in specimens from male genital organs

R86.9 Unspecified abnormal finding in specimens from male genital organs — [♂]

R87- Abnormal findings in specimens from female genital organs
   Includes: Abnormal findings in secretion and smears from cervix uteri
   Abnormal findings in secretion and smears from vagina
   Abnormal findings in secretion and smears from vulva

R87.0 Abnormal level of enzymes in specimens from female genital organs — [♀]

R87.1 Abnormal level of hormones in specimens from female genital organs — [♀]

R87.2 Abnormal level of other drugs, medicaments and biological substances in specimens from female genital organs — [♀]

R87.3 Abnormal level of substances chiefly nonmedicinal as to source in specimens from female genital organs — [♀]

R87.4 Abnormal immunological findings in specimens from female genital organs — [♀]

R87.5 Abnormal microbiological findings in specimens from female genital organs — [♀]
   Positive culture findings in specimens from female genital organs
   Excludes 1: *colonization status (Z22.-)*

R87.6- Abnormal cytological findings in specimens from female genital organs

  R87.61- Abnormal cytological findings in specimens from cervix uteri
   Excludes 1: *abnormal cytological findings in specimens from other female genital organs (R87.69)*
   abnormal cytological findings in specimens from vagina (R87.62-)
   carcinoma in situ of cervix uteri (histologically confirmed) (D06.-)
   cervical intraepithelial neoplasia I [CIN I] (N87.0)
   cervical intraepithelial neoplasia II [CIN II] (N87.1)
   cervical intraepithelial neoplasia III [CIN III] (D06.-)
   dysplasia (mild) (moderate) of cervix uteri (histologically confirmed) (N87.-)
   severe dysplasia of cervix uteri (histologically confirmed) (D06.-)
   Excludes ❷: *cervical high risk human papillomavirus (HPV) DNA test positive (R87.810)*
   cervical low risk human papillomavirus (HPV) DNA test positive (R87.820)

    R87.610 Atypical squamous cells of undetermined significance on cytologic smear of cervix (ASC-US) — [♀]

R 8 5 - R 8 7

R87.611 **Atypical squamous cells cannot exclude high grade squamous intraepithelial lesion** on cytologic smear of cervix (ASC-H) — [♀]

R87.612 **Low grade squamous intraepithelial** lesion on cytologic smear of cervix (LGSIL) — [♀]

R87.613 **High grade squamous intraepithelial** lesion on cytologic smear of cervix (HGSIL) — [♀]

R87.614 **Cytologic evidence of malignancy** on smear of cervix — [♀]

R87.615 **Unsatisfactory** cytologic smear of cervix — [♀]
    Inadequate sample of cytologic smear of cervix

R87.616 **Satisfactory** cervical smear **but lacking transformation zone** — [♀]

R87.618 **Other** abnormal cytological findings on specimens from cervix uteri — [♀]

R87.619 **Unspecified** abnormal cytological findings in specimens from cervix uteri — [♀]
    Abnormal cervical cytology NOS
    Abnormal Papanicolaou smear of cervix NOS
    Abnormal thin preparation smear of cervix NOS
    Atypical endocervical cells of cervix NOS
    Atypical endometrial cells of cervix NOS
    Atypical glandular cells of cervix NOS

R87.62- **Abnormal cytological findings in specimens from vagina**
Use additional code to identify acquired absence of uterus and cervix, if applicable (Z90.71-)
Excludes 1: *abnormal cytological findings in specimens from cervix uteri (R87.61-)*
    abnormal cytological findings in specimens from other female genital organs (R87.69)
    carcinoma in situ of vagina (histologically confirmed) (D07.2)
    dysplasia (mild) (moderate) of vagina (histologically confirmed) (N89.-)
    severe dysplasia of vagina (histologically confirmed) (D07.2)
    vaginal intraepithelial neoplasia I [VAIN I] (N89.0)
    vaginal intraepithelial neoplasia II [VAIN II] (N89.1)
    vaginal intraepithelial neoplasia III [VAIN III] (D07.2)
Excludes ❷: *vaginal high risk human papillomavirus (HPV) DNA test positive (R87.811)*
    vaginal low risk human papillomavirus (HPV) DNA test positive (R87.821)

R87.620 **Atypical squamous cells** of **undetermined significance** on cytologic smear of vagina (ASC-US) — [♀]

R87.621 **Atypical squamous cells cannot exclude high grade squamous intraepithelial lesion** on cytologic smear of vagina (ASC-H) — [♀]

R87.622 **Low grade squamous intraepithelial** lesion on cytologic smear of vagina (LGSIL) — [♀]

R87.623 **High grade squamous intraepithelial** lesion on cytologic smear of vagina (HGSIL) — [♀]

R87.624 **Cytologic evidence of malignancy** on smear of vagina — [♀]

R87.625 **Unsatisfactory** cytologic smear of vagina — [♀]
    Inadequate sample of cytologic smear of vagina

R87.628 **Other** abnormal cytological findings on specimens from vagina — [♀]

R87.629 **Unspecified** abnormal cytological findings in specimens from vagina — [♀]
    Abnormal Papanicolaou smear of vagina NOS
    Abnormal thin preparation smear of vagina NOS
    Abnormal vaginal cytology NOS
    Atypical endocervical cells of vagina NOS
    Atypical endometrial cells of vagina NOS
    Atypical glandular cells of vagina NOS

R87.69 Abnormal cytological findings in specimens from other female genital organs — [♀]
    Abnormal cytological findings in specimens from female genital organs NOS
Excludes 1: *dysplasia of vulva (histologically confirmed) (N90.0-N90.3)*

R87.7 **Abnormal histological findings in specimens from female genital organs** — [♀]
Excludes 1: *carcinoma in situ (histologically confirmed) of female genital organs (D06-D07.3)*
    cervical intraepithelial neoplasia I [CIN I] (N87.0)
    cervical intraepithelial neoplasia II [CIN II] (N87.1)
    cervical intraepithelial neoplasia III [CIN III] (D06.-)
    dysplasia (mild) (moderate) of cervix uteri (histologically confirmed) (N87.-)
    dysplasia (mild) (moderate) of vagina (histologically confirmed) (N89.-)
    severe dysplasia of cervix uteri (histologically confirmed) (D06.-)
    severe dysplasia of vagina (histologically confirmed) (D07.2)
    vaginal intraepithelial neoplasia I [VAIN I] (N89.0)
    vaginal intraepithelial neoplasia II [VAIN II] (N89.1)
    vaginal intraepithelial neoplasia III [VAIN III] (D07.2)

R87.8- **Other abnormal findings in specimens from female genital organs**

R87.81- **High risk human papillomavirus (HPV) DNA test positive from female genital organs**
Excludes 1: *anogenital warts due to human papillomavirus (HPV) (A63.0)*
    condyloma acuminatum (A63.0)

R87.810 **Cervical high risk** human papillomavirus (HPV) DNA test positive — [♀]

R87.811 **Vaginal high risk** human papillomavirus (HPV) DNA test positive — [♀]

R87.82- **Low risk human papillomavirus (HPV) DNA test positive from female genital organs**
Use additional code for associated human papillomavirus (B97.7)

R87.820 **Cervical low risk** human papillomavirus (HPV) DNA test positive — [♀]

R87.821 **Vaginal low risk** human papillomavirus (HPV) DNA test positive — [♀]

R87.89 **Other abnormal findings in specimens from female genital organs** — [♀]
    Abnormal chromosomal findings in specimens from female genital organs

R87.9 **Unspecified abnormal finding in specimens from female genital organs** — [♀]

R88- **Abnormal findings in other body fluids and substances**

R88.0 **Cloudy (hemodialysis) (peritoneal) dialysis effluent**

R88.8 **Abnormal findings in other body fluids and substances**

R89- **Abnormal findings in specimens from other organs, systems and tissues**
Includes: Abnormal findings in nipple discharge
    Abnormal findings in synovial fluid
    Abnormal findings in wound secretions

R89.0 **Abnormal level of enzymes in specimens from other organs, systems and tissues**

R89.1 **Abnormal level of hormones in specimens from other organs, systems and tissues**

R89.2 **Abnormal level of other drugs, medicaments and biological substances in specimens from other organs, systems and tissues**

R89.3 **Abnormal level of substances chiefly nonmedicinal as to source in specimens from other organs, systems and tissues**

R89.4 **Abnormal immunological findings in specimens from other organs, systems and tissues**

R89.5 **Abnormal microbiological findings in specimens from other organs, systems and tissues**
    Positive culture findings in specimens from other organs, systems and tissues
Excludes 1: *colonization status (Z22.-)*

R89.6 **Abnormal cytological findings in specimens from other organs, systems and tissues**

R89.7 **Abnormal histological findings in specimens from other organs, systems and tissues**

R
8
7
-
R
8
9

R89.8 Other abnormal findings in specimens from other organs, systems and tissues
> Abnormal chromosomal findings in specimens from other organs, systems and tissues

R89.9 Unspecified abnormal finding in specimens from other organs, systems and tissues

Abnormal findings on diagnostic imaging and in function studies, without diagnosis (R90-R94)

Includes: Nonspecific abnormal findings on diagnostic imaging by computerized axial tomography [CAT scan]
Nonspecific abnormal findings on diagnostic imaging by magnetic resonance imaging [MRI] [NMR]
Nonspecific abnormal findings on diagnostic imaging by positron emission tomography [PET scan]
Nonspecific abnormal findings on diagnostic imaging by thermography
Nonspecific abnormal findings on diagnostic imaging by ultrasound [echogram]
Nonspecific abnormal findings on diagnostic imaging by X-ray examination

Excludes 1:   *abnormal findings on antenatal screening of mother (O28.-)*
diagnostic abnormal findings classified elsewhere — see Alphabetical Index

R90- Abnormal findings on diagnostic imaging of central nervous system

R90.0 Intracranial space-occupying lesion found on diagnostic imaging of central nervous system

R90.8- Other abnormal findings on diagnostic imaging of central nervous system

R90.81 Abnormal echoencephalogram

R90.82 White matter disease, unspecified

R90.89 Other abnormal findings on diagnostic imaging of central nervous system
> Other cerebrovascular abnormality found on diagnostic imaging of central nervous system

R91- Abnormal findings on diagnostic imaging of lung

R91.1 Solitary pulmonary nodule
> Coin lesion lung
> Solitary pulmonary nodule, subsegmental branch of the bronchial tree

R91.8 Other nonspecific abnormal finding of lung field
> Lung mass NOS found on diagnostic imaging of lung
> Pulmonary infiltrate NOS
> Shadow, lung

R92- Abnormal and inconclusive findings on diagnostic imaging of breast

R92.0 Mammographic microcalcification found on diagnostic imaging of breast — The presence of tiny granule-like deposits of calcium within the breast tissue that is identified by mammography.
Excludes 2:   *mammographic calcification (calculus) found on diagnostic imaging of breast (R92.1)*

R92.1 Mammographic calcification found on diagnostic imaging of breast — The presence of multiple calcium deposits within the breast tissue that is identified by mammography.
> Mammographic calculus found on diagnostic imaging of breast

R92.2 Inconclusive mammogram — A mammogram that has not found an abnormal condition, but requires further testing to rule out abnormal conditions.
AHA 15:1Q:p24 – Dense breasts on mammogram
> Dense breasts NOS
> Inconclusive mammogram NEC
> Inconclusive mammography due to dense breasts
> Inconclusive mammography NEC

R92.8 Other abnormal and inconclusive findings on diagnostic imaging of breast

R93- Abnormal findings on diagnostic imaging of other body structures

R93.0 Abnormal findings on diagnostic imaging of skull and head, not elsewhere classified
Excludes 1:   *intracranial space-occupying lesion found on diagnostic imaging (R90.0)*

R93.1 Abnormal findings on diagnostic imaging of heart and coronary circulation
> Abnormal echocardiogram NOS
> Abnormal heart shadow

R93.2 Abnormal findings on diagnostic imaging of liver and biliary tract
> Nonvisualization of gallbladder

R93.3 Abnormal findings on diagnostic imaging of other parts of digestive tract

R93.4- Abnormal findings on diagnostic imaging of urinary organs
Excludes 2:   *hypertrophy of kidney (N28.81)*

R93.41 Abnormal radiologic findings on diagnostic imaging of renal pelvis, ureter, or bladder
> Filling defect of bladder found on diagnostic imaging
> Filling defect of renal pelvis found on diagnostic imaging
> Filling defect of ureter found on diagnostic imaging

R93.42- Abnormal radiologic findings on diagnostic imaging of kidney

R93.421 Abnormal radiologic findings on diagnostic imaging of right kidney

R93.422 Abnormal radiologic findings on diagnostic imaging of left kidney

R93.429 Abnormal radiologic findings on diagnostic imaging of unspecified kidney

R93.49 Abnormal radiologic findings on diagnostic imaging of other urinary organs

R93.5 Abnormal findings on diagnostic imaging of other abdominal regions, including retroperitoneum

R93.6 Abnormal findings on diagnostic imaging of limbs
Excludes 2:   *abnormal finding in skin and subcutaneous tissue (R93.8)*

R93.7 Abnormal findings on diagnostic imaging of other parts of musculoskeletal system
Excludes 2:   *abnormal findings on diagnostic imaging of skull (R93.0)*

R93.8 Abnormal findings on diagnostic imaging of other specified body structures
> Abnormal finding by radioisotope localization of placenta
> Abnormal radiological finding in skin and subcutaneous tissue
> Mediastinal shift

R93.9 Diagnostic imaging inconclusive due to excess body fat of patient

R94- Abnormal results of function studies
Includes: Abnormal results of radionuclide [radioisotope] uptake studies
Abnormal results of scintigraphy

R94.0- Abnormal results of function studies of central nervous system

R94.01 Abnormal electroencephalogram [EEG]

R94.02 Abnormal brain scan

R94.09 Abnormal results of other function studies of central nervous system

R94.1- Abnormal results of function studies of peripheral nervous system and special senses

R94.11- Abnormal results of function studies of eye

R94.110 Abnormal electro-oculogram [EOG]

R94.111 Abnormal electroretinogram [ERG]
> Abnormal retinal function study

R94.112 Abnormal visually evoked potential [VEP]

R94.113 Abnormal oculomotor study

R94.118 Abnormal results of other function studies of eye

R94.12- Abnormal results of function studies of ear and other special senses

R94.120 Abnormal auditory function study

R94.121 Abnormal vestibular function study

R94.128 Abnormal results of other function studies of ear and other special senses

R94.13- Abnormal results of function studies of peripheral nervous system

R94.130 Abnormal response to nerve stimulation, unspecified

R94.131 Abnormal electromyogram [EMG]
Excludes 1:   *electromyogram of eye (R94.113)*

R94.138 Abnormal results of other function studies of peripheral nervous system

R 8 9 – R 9 4

R94.2   Abnormal results of pulmonary function studies
Reduced ventilatory capacity
Reduced vital capacity

R94.3-   Abnormal results of cardiovascular function studies

R94.30   Abnormal result of cardiovascular function study, unspecified

R94.31   Abnormal electrocardiogram [ECG] [EKG]
Excludes 1:   long QT syndrome (I45.81)

R94.39   Abnormal result of other cardiovascular function study
Abnormal electrophysiological intracardiac studies
Abnormal phonocardiogram
Abnormal vectorcardiogram

R94.4   Abnormal results of kidney function studies
Abnormal renal function test

R94.5   Abnormal results of liver function studies

R94.6   Abnormal results of thyroid function studies

R94.7   Abnormal results of other endocrine function studies
Excludes ❷: abnormal glucose (R73.0-)

R94.8   Abnormal results of function studies of other organs and systems
Abnormal basal metabolic rate [BMR]
Abnormal bladder function test
Abnormal splenic function test

Abnormal tumor markers (R97)

R97-   Abnormal tumor markers — The presence of substances that are produced by tumor cells, or by other cells, in response to neoplastic conditions.
Elevated tumor associated antigens [TAA] — The increased presence of antigens that are relatively restricted to tumor cells.
Elevated tumor specific antigens [TSA] — The increased presence of antigens that are unique to tumor cells.

R97.0   Elevated carcinoembryonic antigen [CEA]

R97.1   Elevated cancer antigen 125 [CA 125] — [♀]

R97.2-   Elevated prostate specific antigen [PSA]

R97.20   Elevated prostate specific antigen [PSA] — [♂, Age/15-124] [Questionable Admission]

R97.21   Rising PSA following treatment for malignant neoplasm of prostate — [♂, Age/15-124] [Questionable Admission]

R97.8   Other abnormal tumor markers

Ill-defined and unknown cause of mortality (R99)

R99   Ill-defined and unknown cause of mortality
Death (unexplained) NOS
Unspecified cause of mortality

R
9
4
-
R
9
9

Chapter 19 – Injury, poisoning and certain other consequences of external causes (S00-T88)
EDUCATIONAL ANNOTATIONS — ILLUSTRATIONS AND DEFINITIONS

Frontal
Parietal
Temporal
Maxilla
Zygomatic
Mandible
6th Cervical Vertebra
Clavicle
1st Rib
Scapula
Sternum
Humerus
12th Thoracic Vertebra
1st Lumbar Vertebra
Radius
5th Lumbar Vertebra
Ulna
Ilium
Pubis
Ischium
Carpals
Metacarpals
Phalanges
Femur
Patella
Tibia
Fibula
Tarsals
Metatarsals
Phalanges

ANTERIOR VIEW OF HUMAN SKELETON

Chapter 19 – Injury, poisoning and certain other consequences of external causes (S00-T88)
EDUCATIONAL ANNOTATIONS — ILLUSTRATIONS AND DEFINITIONS

ARTERIES OF HUMAN BODY

Chapter 19 – Injury, poisoning and certain other consequences of external causes (S00-T88)
EDUCATIONAL ANNOTATIONS — ILLUSTRATIONS AND DEFINITIONS

External Jugular

Internal Jugular

Superior Vena Cava

Pulmonary Arteries

Intercostal

Portal

Renal

Azygos

Superior Mesenteric

Ileo-colic

Ulnar

Radial

Digital

Subclavian

Axillary

Internal Mammary

Brachial

Cephalic

Splenic

Inferior Mesenteric

Inferior Vena Cava

Ovarian/Testicular

Uterine

Iliac

Hypogastric (Internal Iliac)

Common Femoral

Superficial Femoral

Saphenous

Popliteal

Anterior Tibial

Posterior Tibial

Plantar

VEINS OF HUMAN BODY

S00 I S00

Chapter 19 – Injury, poisoning and certain other consequences of external causes (S00-T88)
EDUCATIONAL ANNOTATIONS — ILLUSTRATIONS AND DEFINITIONS

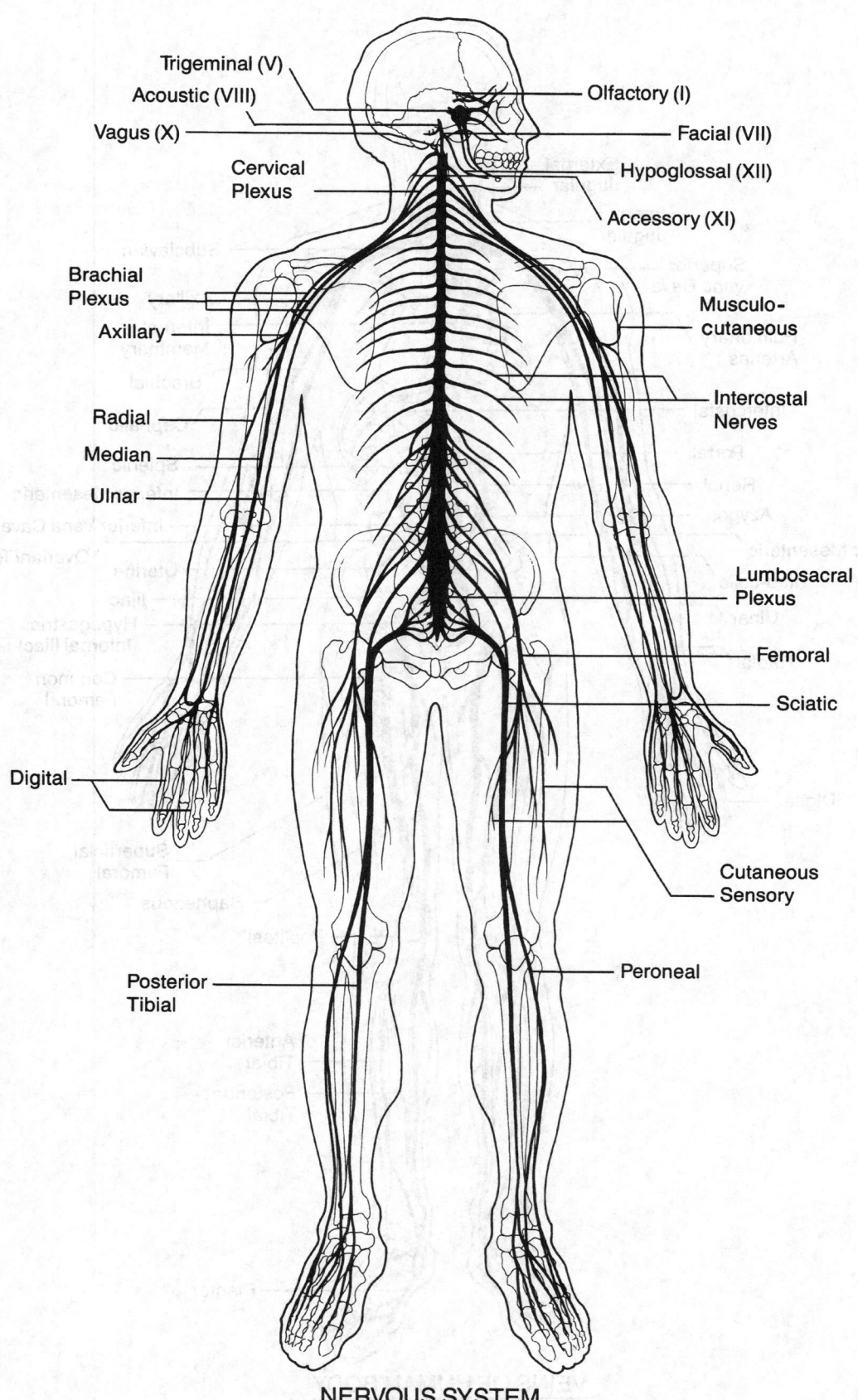

Trigeminal (V)
Acoustic (VIII)
Vagus (X)
Cervical Plexus
Brachial Plexus
Axillary
Radial
Median
Ulnar
Digital
Posterior Tibial

Olfactory (I)
Facial (VII)
Hypoglossal (XII)
Accessory (XI)
Musculo-cutaneous
Intercostal Nerves
Lumbosacral Plexus
Femoral
Sciatic
Cutaneous Sensory
Peroneal

NERVOUS SYSTEM

S00 - S00

Chapter 19 – Injury, poisoning and certain other consequences of external causes (S00-T88)
EDUCATIONAL ANNOTATIONS — ILLUSTRATIONS AND DEFINITIONS

CRANIAL NERVES

1st
2nd
3rd
4th
5th
6th
7th
8th
9th
10th
11th
12th

First Degree Burn

Second Degree Burn

Third Degree Burn

Epidermis

Dermis

Subcutaneous Tissue

EXTENT OF SKIN BURN

9%
18%
9%
9%
1%
18%
18%

BODY SURFACE RULE OF NINES

Occipital
Parietal
Temporal
Sphenoid
Palatine
Vomer
Zygoma
Maxilla

ORBITAL FLOOR AND MALAR BONES

S00 - S00

Chapter 19 – Injury, poisoning and certain other consequences of external causes (S00-T88)
EDUCATIONAL ANNOTATIONS — ILLUSTRATIONS AND DEFINITIONS

Parietal Bone

Frontal Bone

VAULT OF SKULL

Temporal Bone

Occipital Bone

Sphenoid Bone

BASE OF SKULL

Nasal Bones

NASAL BONES

Condylar Process

Coronoid Process

Subcondylar

Alveolar Border

Body

Ramus

Angle of Jaw

MANDIBLE

Dorsal Spine

Transverse Process

Rib Facet

Pedicle

Body

TYPICAL VERTEBRA — SUPERIOR VIEW

Cervical

Dorsal (Thoracic)

Lumbar

Sacrum and Coccyx

VERTEBRAL COLUMN

S00 – S00

Chapter 19 – Injury, poisoning and certain other consequences of external causes (S00-T88)
EDUCATIONAL ANNOTATIONS — ILLUSTRATIONS AND DEFINITIONS

SACRUM AND COCCYX

SCAPULA

RIBS, STERNUM AND LARYNX

CLAVICLE

HUMERUS — ANTERIOR VIEW

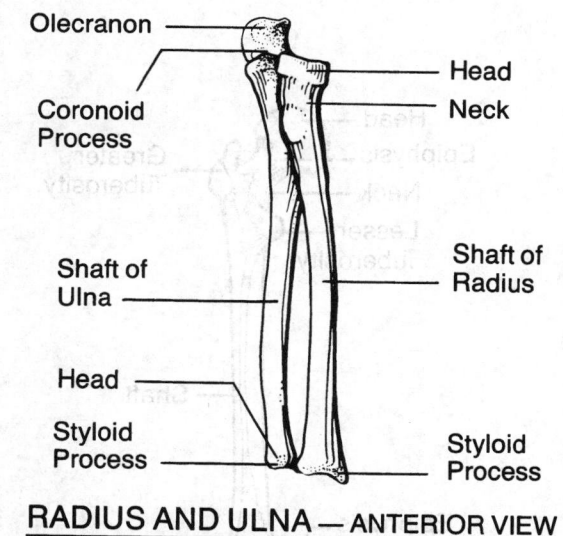

RADIUS AND ULNA — ANTERIOR VIEW

S00 - S00

Chapter 19 – Injury, poisoning and certain other consequences of external causes (S00-T88)
EDUCATIONAL ANNOTATIONS — ILLUSTRATIONS AND DEFINITIONS

Distal Phalanx

Middle Phalanx

Proximal Phalanx

Metacarpals

PHALANGES OF HAND

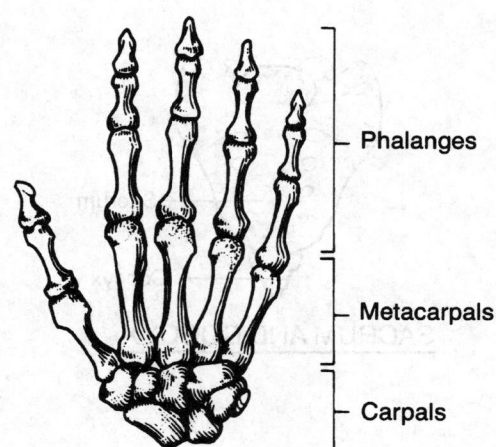

Phalanges

Metacarpals

Carpals

RIGHT HAND — DORSAL VIEW

Neck

Shaft

Base

Base of Thumb

METACARPAL BONES

Trapezium

Trapezoid

Navicular

Capitate

Hamate

Triquetral

Pisiform

Lunate

CARPAL BONES — DORSAL VIEW

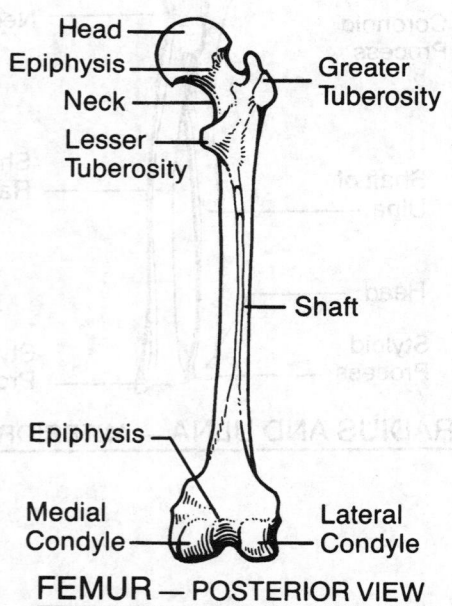

Head

Epiphysis

Neck

Lesser Tuberosity

Greater Tuberosity

Shaft

Epiphysis

Medial Condyle

Lateral Condyle

FEMUR — POSTERIOR VIEW

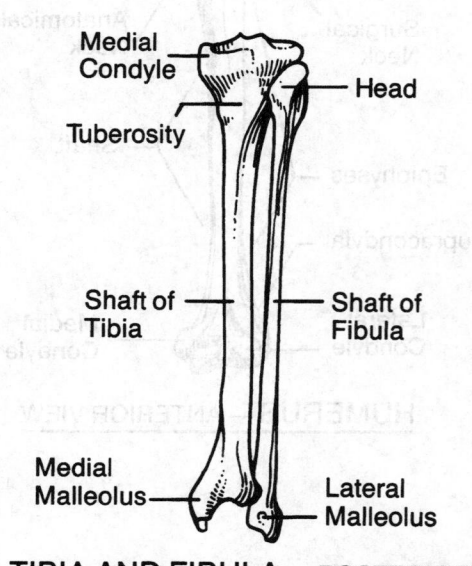

Medial Condyle

Tuberosity

Head

Shaft of Tibia

Shaft of Fibula

Medial Malleolus

Lateral Malleolus

TIBIA AND FIBULA — POSTERIOR VIEW

S00 - S00

Chapter 19 – Injury, poisoning and certain other consequences of external causes (S00-T88)
EDUCATIONAL ANNOTATIONS — ILLUSTRATIONS AND DEFINITIONS

PELVIC BONES

Ilium
Sacrum
Ischium
Pubis

PATELLA — ANTERIOR VIEW

CALCANEUS — MEDIAL VIEW

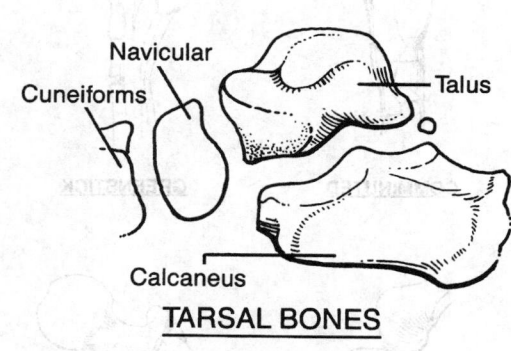

Navicular
Cuneiforms
Talus
Calcaneus

TARSAL BONES

Phalanges
Metatarsals
Tarsals
Talus
Calcaneus

RIGHT FOOT — PLANTAR VIEW

S00-S00

Chapter 19 – Injury, poisoning and certain other consequences of external causes (S00-T88)
EDUCATIONAL ANNOTATIONS — ILLUSTRATIONS AND DEFINITIONS

COLLES'

COMPOUND

COMMINUTED

GREENSTICK

IMPACTED

INTERCONDYLAR

MONTEGGIA

PERTROCHANTERIC

SPIRAL

STELLATE

TRANSCERVICAL

TRANSVERSE

FRACTURE TYPES

Chapter 19 – Injury, poisoning and certain other consequences of external causes (S00-T88)
EDUCATIONAL ANNOTATIONS — ILLUSTRATIONS AND DEFINITIONS

Acetabulum – The round, concave depression in the pelvic bone that articulates with the femoral head forming the hip joint.

Aorta, Abdominal – The abdominal aorta is continuous from the thoracic aorta artery and ends by branching into the right and left common iliac arteries. Many abdominal arteries branch off from the abdominal aorta.

Aorta, Thoracic – The upper most portion of the aorta that lies within the thoracic cavity.

Azygos Vein – The azygos vein drains to the superior vena cava and drains blood from the right side of the posterior thorax.

Carpal – The 8 compact bones of the wrist, forming 2 rows of 4 bones each. The proximal row contains the scaphoid, lunate, pisiform, and triquetrum. The distal row contains the trapezium, trapezoid, capitate, and hamate.

Celiac Artery – The celiac artery (also known as the celiac trunk) branches from the abdominal aorta and then almost immediately (1-2cm) branches into the common hepatic artery, the splenic artery, and left gastric artery.

Clavicle – The paired, straightened S-shaped bones (also known as the collarbones) that connect the sternum with the scapula.

Coccyx – The small wedge-shaped bone (also known as the tailbone) at the end of the spinal column.

Conchae Bone – The 2 small paired bones of the nasal cavity that are attached to the maxilla.

Ethmoid Bone – The single bone located between the orbits that forms the roof of the nasal cavity, part of the floor of the cranial cavity, and part of the orbit.

Facial Bone – Any one of the 14 bones of the facial area below the cranium (2 nasal bones, vomer, 2 conchae, 2 maxilla, mandible, 2 palatine bones, 2 zygomatic bones, 2 lacrimal bones).

Femoral Artery – The femoral artery branches from the external iliac artery and serves the legs.

Femoral Shaft – The middle long portion of the femur.

Femur – The paired long bones (also known as the thigh bone) that articulate at the hip and the knee. It is the longest bone in the body.

Fibula – The paired long slender bones of the lower leg located toward the outside of the lower leg that articulate at the knee and the ankle.

Frontal Bone – The single bone in the front of the skull that also forms part of the roof of the nasal cavity and part of the orbit.

Glenoid Cavity – The shallow, round depression of the scapula that articulates with the humeral head.

Humeral Head – The upper end of the humerus that is part of the shoulder joint.

Humeral Shaft – The middle, long portion of the humerus.

Humerus – The paired, long bones of the upper arm that articulate at the shoulder and the elbow. The capitulum of the humerus articulates with the head of the radius, and the trochlea of the humerus articulates with the trochlear notch of the ulna.

Hyoid Bone – The single horseshoe-shaped bone that lies in the front of the neck and just under the chin and aids in tongue movement and swallowing. It is not directly articulated with any other bone and not considered part of the skull.

Iliac Artery, Common – The common iliac artery branches from the aortic bifurcation of the abdominal aorta and branches almost immediately (4 cm in length) into the internal and external iliac arteries.

Iliac Artery, External – The external iliac artery branches from the common iliac artery and serves the legs.

Inferior Mesenteric Artery – The inferior mesenteric artery branches from the abdominal aorta and serves the descending colon, part of the transverse colon, sigmoid colon, and the upper part of the rectum.

Inferior Vena Cava – The inferior vena cava drains to the right atrium of the heart and drains blood from the common iliac veins.

Innominate Artery – The innominate artery (also known as the brachiocephalic artery) branches from the aortic arch and branches to the right common carotid artery, the internal mammary artery, and the subclavian artery.

Lacrimal Bone – The 2 small paired bones that form the medial side of the orbit and the nasolacrimal canal.

Lower Femur – The distal end of the femur that articulates with the knee joint.

Mandible – The single horseshoe-shaped bone forming the lower jaw.

Maxilla – The 2 fused irregularly-shaped bones that form the upper jaw, the roof of the mouth, and a part of the orbit.

Metacarpal – One of the 5 cylindrical bones of the palm of the hand connecting the carpals to the phalanges of the hand.

Metatarsal – One of the 5 cylindrical bones connecting the tarsals and the phalanges of the foot.

Nasal Bone – The 2 small paired bones that form the bridge of the nose.

S00 - S00

Chapter 19 – Injury, poisoning and certain other consequences of external causes (S00-T88)
EDUCATIONAL ANNOTATIONS — ILLUSTRATIONS AND DEFINITIONS

Occipital Bone – The single bone of the base and back of the skull.

Orbit – The bones (7) which form the orbit (eye socket): Zygomatic, sphenoid, ethmoid, maxilla, lacrimal, palatine, and frontal.

Palatine Bone – The 2 small paired bones at the back of the nasal cavity that form the floor and lateral wall of the nasal cavity, part of the roof of the mouth, and part of the floor of the orbit.

Parietal Bone – The 2 paired bones that form the top and sides of the skull.

Patella – The paired triangular-shaped bones situated at the front of the knee.

Pelvic Bone – Any of the three bones (ilium, ischium, pubis) that connect with the sacrum to form the pelvic girdle.

Phalanx, Finger – The digital bones of the fingers. Each finger contains three bones: Proximal phalanx, intermediate (middle) phalanx, and distal phalanx.

Phalanx, Thumb – The digital bones of the thumb. The thumb contains two bones: Proximal phalanx and distal phalanx.

Phalanx, Toe – The digital bones of the toes. Each toe contains three bones: Proximal phalanx, intermediate (middle) phalanx, and distal phalanx, except the great toe which only has proximal and distal phalanx bones.

Pneumothorax, Traumatic – The traumatic entry of air, blood, or fluid into the pleural space.

Portal Vein – The portal vein drains to the hepatic vein and drains blood from the gastrointestinal tract and liver.

Renal Vein – The renal vein drains to the inferior vena cava and drains blood from the kidney.

Rib – The 12 paired arched bones of the rib cage that partially enclose and protect the chest cavity.

Sacrum – The large wedge-shaped vertebra at the lower end of the spine that connects with S5.

Scapula – The paired flat, triangular bones located in the upper back behind the shoulder (also called the shoulder blade).

Skull – The skull consists of all (22) of the cranial and facial bones. Eight of these bones form the cranium (occipital bone, frontal bone, 2 temporal bones, 2 parietal bones, sphenoid bone, ethmoid bone), and 14 of these bones form the skull below the cranium (2 nasal bones, vomer, 2 conchae, 2 maxilla, mandible, 2 palatine bones, 2 zygomatic bones, 2 lacrimal bones).

Sphenoid Bone – The single winged-shaped bone of the skull floor that forms part of the base of the cranial cavity, sides of the skull, and part of the orbital floor and side.

Splenic Vein – The splenic vein drains to the portal vein and drains blood from the spleen and pancreas.

Sternum – The long flat bone (also known as the breast bone) of the chest that connects to the clavicles and most of the ribs.

Subclavian Artery – The left subclavian artery branches from the aortic arch and serves the thorax, head, and left upper limb. The right subclavian artery branches from the innominate artery (also known as the brachiocephalic artery) and serves the thorax, head, and right upper limb.

Subclavian Vein – The subclavian vein drains to the innominate vein and drains blood from the axillary vein and external jugular vein.

Superior Mesenteric Artery – The superior mesenteric artery branches from the abdominal aorta and serves the duodenum, ascending colon, part of the transverse colon, and pancreas.

Superior Mesenteric Vein – The superior mesenteric vein drains to the portal vein and drains blood from the small intestine.

Superior Vena Cava – The major vein transporting de-oxygenated blood from the upper body and head that empties into the right atrium.

Tarsal – The seven bones of the foot (calcaneus, talus, cuboid, navicular, and the medial, intermediate, and lateral cuneiform bones) distal to the tibia and fibula and proximal to the metatarsal bones.

Temporal Bone – The 2 paired bones that form the lower sides and base of the skull and contain the internal organs and structures of hearing.

Tibia – The paired long bones of the lower leg (also known as the shin bone) that is the innermost bone of the lower leg supporting and articulating with the knee and with the ankle.

Ulna – The paired long bones of the forearms that are closer to the side of the body than the radii.

Vertebra, Cervical – The cervical section of the spinal vertebral column comprised of 7 vertebra, C1-C7.

Vertebra, Lumbar – The lumbar section of the spinal vertebral column comprised of 5 vertebra, S1-S5.

Vertebra, Thoracic – The thoracic section of the spinal vertebral column comprised of 12 vertebra, T1-T12.

Vomer Bone – The single bone of the inferior nasal septum.

Zygomatic Bone – The 2 paired quadrangular bones of the cheeks (also known as the malar bones) that form the cheek prominence and lower-outer part of the orbit.

S00-S00

Chapter 19 – Injury, poisoning and certain other consequences of external causes (S00-T88)

Use additional code to identify any retained foreign body, if applicable (Z18-)

Excludes 1:   *birth trauma (P10-P15)*
              obstetric trauma (O70-O71)

This chapter contains the following blocks:

S00-S09	Injuries to the head
S10-S19	Injuries to the neck
S20-S29	Injuries to the thorax
S30-S39	Injuries to the abdomen, lower back, lumbar spine, pelvis and external genitals
S40-S49	Injuries to the shoulder and upper arm
S50-S59	Injuries to the elbow and forearm
S60-S69	Injuries to the wrist, hand and fingers
S70-S79	Injuries to the hip and thigh
S80-S89	Injuries to the knee and lower leg
S90-S99	Injuries to the ankle and foot
T07	Injuries involving multiple body regions
T14	Injury of unspecified body region
T15-T19	Effects of foreign body entering through natural orifice
T20-T25	Burns and corrosions of external body surface, specified by site
T26-T28	Burns and corrosions confined to eye and internal organs
T30-T32	Burns and corrosions of multiple and unspecified body regions
T33-T34	Frostbite
T36-T50	Poisoning by, adverse effects of and underdosing of drugs, medicaments and biological substances
T51-T65	Toxic effects of substances chiefly nonmedicinal as to source
T66-T78	Other and unspecified effects of external causes
T79	Certain early complications of trauma
T80-T88	Complications of surgical and medical care, not elsewhere classified

Note: Use secondary code(s) from Chapter 20, External causes of morbidity, to indicate cause of injury. Codes within the T section that include the external cause do not require an additional external cause code
The chapter uses the S-section for coding different types of injuries related to single body regions and the T-section to cover injuries to unspecified body regions as well as poisoning and certain other consequences of external causes.

Chapter-Specific Coding Guidelines

C.   Chapter-Specific Coding Guidelines
In addition to general coding guidelines, there are guidelines for specific diagnoses and/or conditions in the classification. Unless otherwise indicated, these guidelines apply to all health care settings. Please refer to Section II for guidelines on the selection of principal diagnosis.

19. Chapter 19: Injury, Poisoning, and Certain Other Consequences of External Causes (S00-T88)

a.   Application of 7th Characters in Chapter 19
Most categories in chapter 19 have a 7th character requirement for each applicable code. Most categories in this chapter have three 7th character values (with the exception of fractures): A, initial encounter, D, subsequent encounter and S, sequela. Categories for traumatic fractures have additional 7th character values. While the patient may be seen by a new or different provider over the course of treatment for an injury, assignment of the 7th character is based on whether the patient is undergoing active treatment and not whether the provider is seeing the patient for the first time.

For complication codes, active treatment refers to treatment for the condition described by the code, even though it may be related to an earlier precipitating problem. For example, code T84.50xA, Infection and inflammatory reaction due to unspecified internal joint prosthesis, initial encounter, is used when active treatment is provided for the infection, even though the condition relates to the prosthetic device, implant or graft that was placed at a previous encounter.

7th character "A" initial encounter is used ~~while~~ for each encounter where the patient is receiving active treatment for the condition. ~~Examples of active treatment are: surgical treatment, emergency department encounter, and evaluation and continuing treatment by the same or a different physician.~~

7th character "D" subsequent encounter is used for encounters after the patient has ~~received~~ completed active treatment of the condition and is receiving routine care for the condition during the healing or recovery phase. ~~Examples of subsequent care are: cast change or removal, an x-ray to check healing status of fracture, removal of external or internal fixation device, medication adjustment, other aftercare and follow up visits following treatment of the injury or condition.~~

The aftercare Z codes should not be used for aftercare for conditions such as injuries or poisonings, where 7th characters are provided to identify subsequent care. For example, for aftercare of an injury, assign the acute injury code with the 7th character "D" (subsequent encounter).

7th character "S", sequela, is for use for complications or conditions that arise as a direct result of an condition, such as scar formation after a burn. The scars are sequelae of the burn. When using 7th character "S", it is necessary to use both the injury code that precipitated the sequela and the code for the sequela itself. The "S" is added only to the injury code, not the sequela code. The 7th character "S" identifies the injury responsible for the sequela. The specific type of sequela (e.g., scar) is sequenced first, followed by the injury code.

See Section I.B.10 Sequela (Late Effects).

b.   Coding of Injuries
When coding injuries, assign separate codes for each injury unless a combination code is provided, in which case the combination code is assigned. Code T07, Unspecified multiple injuries should not be assigned in the inpatient setting unless information for a more specific code is not available. Traumatic injury codes (S00-T14.9) are not to be used for normal, healing surgical wounds or to identify complications of surgical wounds.

The code for the most serious injury, as determined by the provider and the focus of treatment, is sequenced first.

1)   Superficial injuries
Superficial injuries such as abrasions or contusions are not coded when associated with more severe injuries of the same site.

2)   Primary injury with damage to nerves/blood vessels
When a primary injury results in minor damage to peripheral nerves or blood vessels, the primary injury is sequenced first with additional code(s) for injuries to nerves and spinal cord (such as category S04), and/or injury to blood vessels (such as category S15). When the primary injury is to the blood vessels or nerves, that injury should be sequenced first.

c.   Coding of Traumatic Fractures
The principles of multiple coding of injuries should be followed in coding fractures. Fractures of specified sites are coded individually by site in accordance with both the provisions within categories S02, S12, S22, S32, S42, S49, S52, S59, S62, S72, S79, S82, S89, S92 and the level of detail furnished by medical record content.

A fracture not indicated as open or closed should be coded to closed. A fracture not indicated whether displaced or not displaced should be coded to displaced.

More specific guidelines are as follows:

1)   Initial vs. Subsequent Encounter for Fractures
Traumatic fractures are coded using the appropriate 7th character for initial encounter (A, B, C) ~~while~~ for each encounter where the patient is receiving active treatment for the fracture. ~~Examples of active treatment are: surgical treatment, emergency department encounter, and evaluation and continuing (ongoing) treatment by the same or different physician.~~ The appropriate 7th character for initial encounter should also be assigned for a patient who delayed seeking treatment for the fracture or nonunion.

Fractures are coded using the appropriate 7th character for subsequent care for encounters after the patient has completed active treatment of the fracture and is receiving routine care for the fracture during the healing or recovery phase. ~~Examples of fracture aftercare are: cast change or removal, an x ray to check healing status of fracture, removal of external or internal fixation device, medication adjustment, and follow up visits following fracture treatment.~~

Care for complications of surgical treatment for fracture repairs during the healing or recovery phase should be coded with the appropriate complication codes.

Care of complications of fractures, such as malunion and nonunion, should be reported with the appropriate 7th character for subsequent care with nonunion (K, M, N,) or subsequent care with malunion (P, Q, R).

Malunion/nonunion: The appropriate 7th character for initial encounter should also be assigned for a patient who delayed seeking treatment for the fracture or nonunion.

The open fracture designations in the assignment of the 7th character for fractures of the forearm, femur and lower leg, including ankle are based on the Gustilo open fracture classification. When the Gustilo classification type is not specified for an open fracture, the 7th character for open fracture type I or II should be assigned (B, E, H, M, Q).

A code from category M80, not a traumatic fracture code, should be used for any patient with known osteoporosis who suffers a fracture, even if the patient had a minor fall or trauma, if that fall or trauma would not usually break a normal, healthy bone.

See Section I.C.13. Osteoporosis.
The aftercare Z codes should not be used for aftercare for traumatic fractures. For aftercare of a traumatic fracture, assign the acute fracture code with the appropriate 7th character.

S00 I S00

2) Multiple fractures sequencing

Multiple fractures are sequenced in accordance with the severity of the fracture.

d. Coding of Burns and Corrosions

The ICD-10-CM makes a distinction between burns and corrosions. The burn codes are for thermal burns, except sunburns, that come from a heat source, such as a fire or hot appliance. The burn codes are also for burns resulting from electricity and radiation. Corrosions are burns due to chemicals. The guidelines are the same for burns and corrosions.

Current burns (T20-T25) are classified by depth, extent and by agent (X code). Burns are classified by depth as first degree (erythema), second degree (blistering), and third degree (full-thickness involvement). Burns of the eye and internal organs (T26-T28) are classified by site, but not by degree.

1) Sequencing of burn and related condition codes

Sequence first the code that reflects the highest degree of burn when more than one burn is present.

a. When the reason for the admission or encounter is for treatment of external multiple burns, sequence first the code that reflects the burn of the highest degree.

b. When a patient has both internal and external burns, the circumstances of admission govern the selection of the principal diagnosis or first-listed diagnosis.

c. When a patient is admitted for burn injuries and other related conditions such as smoke inhalation and/or respiratory failure, the circumstances of admission govern the selection of the principal or first-listed diagnosis.

2) Burns of the same local site

Classify burns of the same local site (three-character category level, T20-T28) but of different degrees to the subcategory identifying the highest degree recorded in the diagnosis.

3) Non-healing burns

Non-healing burns are coded as acute burns.

Necrosis of burned skin should be coded as a non-healed burn.

4) Infected Burn

For any documented infected burn site, use an additional code for the infection.

5) Assign separate codes for each burn site

When coding burns, assign separate codes for each burn site. Category T30, Burn and corrosion, body region unspecified is extremely vague and should rarely be used.

6) Burns and Corrosions Classified According to Extent of Body Surface Involved

Assign codes from category T31, Burns classified according to extent of body surface involved, or T32, Corrosions classified according to extent of body surface involved, when the site of the burn is not specified or when there is a need for additional data. It is advisable to use category T31 as additional coding when needed to provide data for evaluating burn mortality, such as that needed by burn units. It is also advisable to use category T31 as an additional code for reporting purposes when there is mention of a third-degree burn involving 20 percent or more of the body surface.

Categories T31 and T32 are based on the classic "rule of nines" in estimating body surface involved: head and neck are assigned nine percent, each arm nine percent, each leg 18 percent, the anterior trunk 18 percent, posterior trunk 18 percent, and genitalia one percent. Providers may change these percentage assignments where necessary to accommodate infants and children who have proportionately larger heads than adults, and patients who have large buttocks, thighs, or abdomen that involve burns.

7) Encounters for treatment of sequela of burns

Encounters for the treatment of the late effects of burns or corrosions (i.e., scars or joint contractures) should be coded with a burn or corrosion code with the 7th character "S" for sequela.

8) Sequelae with a late effect code and current burn

When appropriate, both a code for a current burn or corrosion with 7th character "A" or "D" and a burn or corrosion code with 7th character "S" may be assigned on the same record (when both a current burn and sequelae of an old burn exist). Burns and corrosions do not heal at the same rate and a current healing wound may still exist with sequela of a healed burn or corrosion.

See Section I.B.10 Sequela (Late Effects).

9) Use of an external cause code with burns and corrosions

An external cause code should be used with burns and corrosions to identify the source and intent of the burn, as well as the place where it occurred.

e. Adverse Effects, Poisoning, Underdosing and Toxic Effects

Codes in categories T36-T65 are combination codes that include the substance that was taken as well as the intent. No additional external cause code is required for poisonings, toxic effects, adverse effects and underdosing codes.

1) Do not code directly from the Table of Drugs

Do not code directly from the Table of Drugs and Chemicals. Always refer back to the Tabular List.

2) Use as many codes as necessary to describe

Use as many codes as necessary to describe completely all drugs, medicinal or biological substances.

3) If the same code would describe the causative agent

If the same code would describe the causative agent for more than one adverse reaction, poisoning, toxic effect or underdosing, assign the code only once.

4) If two or more drugs, medicinal or biological substances

If two or more drugs, medicinal or biological substances are reported, code each individually unless a combination code is listed in the Table of Drugs and Chemicals.

5) The occurrence of drug toxicity is classified in ICD-10-CM as follows:

(a) Adverse Effect

When coding an adverse effect of a drug that has been correctly prescribed and properly administered, assign the appropriate code for the nature of the adverse effect followed by the appropriate code for the adverse effect of the drug (T36-T50). The code for the drug should have a 5th or 6th character "5" (for example T36.0X5-). Examples of the nature of an adverse effect are tachycardia, delirium, gastrointestinal hemorrhaging, vomiting, hypokalemia, hepatitis, renal failure, or respiratory failure.

(b) Poisoning

When coding a poisoning or reaction to the improper use of a medication (e.g., overdose, wrong substance given or taken in error, wrong route of administration), first assign the appropriate code from categories T36-T50. The poisoning codes have an associated intent as their 5th or 6th character accidental, intentional self-harm, assault and undetermined. If the intent of the poisoning is unknown or unspecified, code the intent as accidental intent. The undetermined intent is only for use if the documentation in the record specifies that the intent cannot be determined. Use additional code(s) for all manifestations of poisonings.

If there is also a diagnosis of abuse or dependence of the substance, the abuse or dependence is assigned as an additional code.

Examples of poisoning include:

(i) Error was made in drug prescription

Errors made in drug prescription or in the administration of the drug by provider, nurse, patient, or other person.

(ii) Overdose of a drug intentionally taken

If an overdose of a drug was intentionally taken or administered and resulted in drug toxicity, it would be coded as a poisoning.

(iii) Nonprescribed drug taken with correctly prescribed and properly administered drug

If a nonprescribed drug or medicinal agent was taken in combination with a correctly prescribed and properly administered drug, any drug toxicity or other reaction resulting from the interaction of the two drugs would be classified as a poisoning.

(iv) Interaction of drug(s) and alcohol

When a reaction results from the interaction of a drug(s) and alcohol, this would be classified as poisoning.

See Section I.C.4. if poisoning is the result of insulin pump malfunctions.

(c) Underdosing

Underdosing refers to taking less of a medication than is prescribed by a provider or a manufacturer's instruction. For underdosing, assign the code from categories T36-T50 (fifth or sixth character "6").

Codes for underdosing should never be assigned as principal or first-listed codes. If a patient has a relapse or exacerbation of the medical condition for which the drug is prescribed because of the reduction in dose, then the medical condition itself should be coded.

Noncompliance (Z91.12-, Z91.13-) or complication of care (Y63.61, Y63.6-Y63.9) codes are to be used with an underdosing code to indicate intent, if known.

S00 - S00

(d) Toxic Effects

When a harmful substance is ingested or comes in contact with a person, this is classified as a toxic effect. The toxic effect codes are in categories T51-T65.

Toxic effect codes have an associated intent: accidental, intentional self-harm, assault and undetermined.

f. Adult and child abuse, neglect and other maltreatment

Sequence first the appropriate code from categories T74.- (Adult and child abuse, neglect and other maltreatment, confirmed) or T76.- (Adult and child abuse, neglect and other maltreatment, suspected) for abuse, neglect and other maltreatment, followed by any accompanying mental health or injury code(s).

If the documentation in the medical record states abuse or neglect it is coded as confirmed (T74.-). It is coded as suspected if it is documented as suspected (T76.-).

For cases of confirmed abuse or neglect an external cause code from the assault section (X92-Y09) should be added to identify the cause of any physical injuries. A perpetrator code (Y07) should be added when the perpetrator of the abuse is known. For suspected cases of abuse or neglect, do not report external cause or perpetrator code.

If a suspected case of abuse, neglect or mistreatment is ruled out during an encounter code Z04.71, Encounter for examination and observation following alleged physical adult abuse, ruled out, or code Z04.72, Encounter for examination and observation following alleged physical child abuse, ruled out, should be used, not a code from T76.

If a suspected case of alleged rape or sexual abuse is ruled out during an encounter code Z04.41, Encounter for examination and observation following alleged ~~physical~~ adult rape ~~abuse, ruled out~~, or code Z04.42, Encounter for examination and observation following alleged child rape ~~or sexual abuse, ruled out~~, should be used, not a code from T76.

See Section I.C.15. Abuse in a pregnant patient.

g. Complications of care

1) General guidelines for complications of care

(a) Documentation of complications of care

See section I.B.16. for information on documentation of complications of care.

2) Pain due to medical devices

Pain associated with devices, implants or grafts left in a surgical site (for example painful hip prosthesis) is assigned to the appropriate code(s) found in Chapter 19, Injury, poisoning, and certain other consequences of external causes. Specific codes for pain due to medical devices are found in the T code section of the ICD-10-CM. Use additional code(s) from category G89 to identify acute or chronic pain due to presence of the device, implant or graft (G89.18 or G89.28).

3) Transplant complications

(a) Transplant complications other than kidney

Codes under category T86, Complications of transplanted organs and tissues, are for use for both complications and rejection of transplanted organs. A transplant complication code is only assigned if the complication affects the function of the transplanted organ. Two codes are required to fully describe a transplant complication: the appropriate code from category T86 and a secondary code that identifies the complication.

Pre-existing conditions or conditions that develop after the transplant are not coded as complications unless they affect the function of the transplanted organs.

See I.C.21. for transplant organ removal status.
See I.C.2. for malignant neoplasm associated with transplanted organ.

(b) Kidney transplant complications

Patients who have undergone kidney transplant may still have some form of chronic kidney disease (CKD) because the kidney transplant may not fully restore kidney function. Code T86.1- should be assigned for documented complications of a kidney transplant, such as transplant failure or rejection or other transplant complication. Code T86.1- should not be assigned for post kidney transplant patients who have chronic kidney (CKD) unless a transplant complication such as transplant failure or rejection is documented. If the documentation is unclear as to whether the patient has a complication of the transplant, query the provider.

Conditions that affect the function of the transplanted kidney, other than CKD, should be assigned a code from subcategory T86.1, Complications of transplanted organ, kidney, and a secondary code that identifies the complication.

For patients with CKD following a kidney transplant, but who do not have a complication such as failure or rejection, *see section I.C.14. Chronic kidney disease and kidney transplant status.*

4) Complication codes that include the external cause

As with certain other T codes, some of the complications of care codes have the external cause included in the code. The code includes the nature of the complication as well as the type of procedure that caused the complication. No external cause code indicating the type of procedure is necessary for these codes.

5) Complications of care codes within the body system chapters

Intraoperative and postprocedural complication codes are found within the body system chapters with codes specific to the organs and structures of that body system. These codes should be sequenced first, followed by a code(s) for the specific complication, if applicable.

Injuries to the head (S00-S09)

Includes: Injuries of ear
Injuries of eye
Injuries of face [any part]
Injuries of gum
Injuries of jaw
Injuries of oral cavity
Injuries of palate
Injuries of periocular area
Injuries of scalp
Injuries of temporomandibular joint area
Injuries of tongue
Injuries of tooth

Code also for any associated infection

*Excludes ❷: burns and corrosions (T20-T32)
effects of foreign body in ear (T16)
effects of foreign body in larynx (T17.3)
effects of foreign body in mouth NOS (T18.0)
effects of foreign body in nose (T17.0-T17.1)
effects of foreign body in pharynx (T17.2)
effects of foreign body on external eye (T15.-)
frostbite (T33-T34)
insect bite or sting, venomous (T63.4)*

S00-   Superficial injury of head

*Excludes 1:   diffuse cerebral contusion (S06.2-)
focal cerebral contusion (S06.3-)
injury of eye and orbit (S05.-)
open wound of head (S01.-)*

The appropriate 7th character is to be added to each code from category S00:
A   Initial encounter
D   Subsequent encounter
S   Sequela

S00.0-   Superficial injury of scalp

S00.00x-   Unspecified superficial injury of scalp

S00.01x-   Abrasion of scalp

S00.02x-   Blister (nonthermal) of scalp

S00.03x-   Contusion of scalp
Bruise of scalp
Hematoma of scalp

S00.04x-   External constriction of part of scalp

S00.05x-   Superficial foreign body of scalp
Splinter in the scalp

S00.06x-   Insect bite (nonvenomous) of scalp

S00.07x-   Other superficial bite of scalp
Excludes 1:   open bite of scalp (S01.05)

S00.1-   Contusion of eyelid and periocular area
Black eye
Excludes ❷: contusion of eyeball and orbital tissues (S05.1)

S00.10x-   Contusion of unspecified eyelid and periocular area

S00.11x-   Contusion of right eyelid and periocular area

S00.12x-   Contusion of left eyelid and periocular area

S00.2-   Other and unspecified superficial injuries of eyelid and periocular area
Excludes ❷: superficial injury of conjunctiva and cornea (S05.0-)

S00.20-   Unspecified superficial injury of eyelid and periocular area

S00.201-   Unspecified superficial injury of right eyelid and periocular area

S00.202-   Unspecified superficial injury of left eyelid and periocular area

S00-S00

S00.209- Unspecified superficial injury of <u>unspecified</u> eyelid and periocular area

S00.21- <u>Abrasion</u> of eyelid and periocular area

S00.211- Abrasion of <u>right</u> eyelid and periocular area

S00.212- Abrasion of <u>left</u> eyelid and periocular area

S00.219- Abrasion of <u>unspecified</u> eyelid and periocular area

S00.22- <u>Blister</u> (nonthermal) of eyelid and periocular area

S00.221- Blister (nonthermal) of <u>right</u> eyelid and periocular area

S00.222- Blister (nonthermal) of <u>left</u> eyelid and periocular area

S00.229- Blister (nonthermal) of <u>unspecified</u> eyelid and periocular area

S00.24- <u>External constriction</u> of eyelid and periocular area

S00.241- External constriction of <u>right</u> eyelid and periocular area

S00.242- External constriction of <u>left</u> eyelid and periocular area

S00.249- External constriction of <u>unspecified</u> eyelid and periocular area

S00.25- <u>Superficial foreign body</u> of eyelid and periocular area
Splinter of eyelid and periocular area
Excludes ❷: retained foreign body in eyelid (H02.81-)

S00.251- Superficial foreign body of <u>right</u> eyelid and periocular area

S00.252- Superficial foreign body of <u>left</u> eyelid and periocular area

S00.259- Superficial foreign body of <u>unspecified</u> eyelid and periocular area

S00.26- <u>Insect bite (nonvenomous)</u> of eyelid and periocular area

S00.261- Insect bite (nonvenomous) of <u>right</u> eyelid and periocular area

S00.262- Insect bite (nonvenomous) of <u>left</u> eyelid and periocular area

S00.269- Insect bite (nonvenomous) of <u>unspecified</u> eyelid and periocular area

S00.27- <u>Other superficial bite</u> of eyelid and periocular area
Excludes 1:   open bite of eyelid and periocular area (S01.15)

S00.271- Other superficial bite of <u>right</u> eyelid and periocular area

S00.272- Other superficial bite of <u>left</u> eyelid and periocular area

S00.279- Other superficial bite of <u>unspecified</u> eyelid and periocular area

S00.3- Superficial injury of <u>nose</u>

S00.30x- Unspecified superficial injury of nose

S00.31x- Abrasion of nose

S00.32x- Blister (nonthermal) of nose

S00.33x- Contusion of nose
Bruise of nose
Hematoma of nose

S00.34x- External constriction of nose

S00.35x- Superficial foreign body of nose
Splinter in the nose

S00.36x- Insect bite (nonvenomous) of nose

S00.37x- Other superficial bite of nose
Excludes 1:   open bite of nose (S01.25)

S00.4- Superficial injury of <u>ear</u>

S00.40- <u>Unspecified</u> superficial injury of ear

S00.401- Unspecified superficial injury of <u>right</u> ear

S00.402- Unspecified superficial injury of <u>left</u> ear

S00.409- Unspecified superficial injury of <u>unspecified</u> ear

S00.41- <u>Abrasion</u> of ear

S00.411- Abrasion of <u>right</u> ear

S00.412- Abrasion of <u>left</u> ear

S00.419- Abrasion of <u>unspecified</u> ear

S00.42- <u>Blister</u> (nonthermal) of ear

S00.421- Blister (nonthermal) of <u>right</u> ear

S00.422- Blister (nonthermal) of <u>left</u> ear

S00.429- Blister (nonthermal) of <u>unspecified</u> ear

S00.43- <u>Contusion</u> of ear
Bruise of ear
Hematoma of ear

S00.431- Contusion of <u>right</u> ear

S00.432- Contusion of <u>left</u> ear

S00.439- Contusion of <u>unspecified</u> ear

S00.44- <u>External constriction</u> of ear

S00.441- External constriction of <u>right</u> ear

S00.442- External constriction of <u>left</u> ear

S00.449- External constriction of <u>unspecified</u> ear

S00.45- <u>Superficial foreign body</u> of ear
Splinter in the ear

S00.451- Superficial foreign body of <u>right</u> ear

S00.452- Superficial foreign body of <u>left</u> ear

S00.459- Superficial foreign body of <u>unspecified</u> ear

S00.46- <u>Insect bite (nonvenomous)</u> of ear

S00.461- Insect bite (nonvenomous) of <u>right</u> ear

S00.462- Insect bite (nonvenomous) of <u>left</u> ear

S00.469- Insect bite (nonvenomous) of <u>unspecified</u> ear

S00.47- <u>Other superficial bite</u> of ear
Excludes 1:   open bite of ear (S01.35)

S00.471- Other superficial bite of <u>right</u> ear

S00.472- Other superficial bite of <u>left</u> ear

S00.479- Other superficial bite of <u>unspecified</u> ear

S00.5- Superficial injury of <u>lip and oral cavity</u>

S00.50- <u>Unspecified</u> superficial injury of lip and oral cavity

S00.501- Unspecified superficial injury of <u>lip</u>

S00.502- Unspecified superficial injury of <u>oral cavity</u>

S00.51- <u>Abrasion</u> of lip and oral cavity

S00.511- Abrasion of lip

S00.512- Abrasion of oral <u>cavity</u>

S00.52- <u>Blister</u> (nonthermal) of lip and oral cavity

S00.521- Blister (nonthermal) of <u>lip</u>

S00.522- Blister (nonthermal) of <u>oral cavity</u>

S00.53- <u>Contusion</u> of lip and oral cavity

S00.531- Contusion of <u>lip</u>
Bruise of lip
Hematoma of oral cavity

S00.532- Contusion of <u>oral cavity</u>
Bruise of lip
Hematoma of oral cavity

S00.54- <u>External constriction</u> of lip and oral cavity

S00.541- External constriction of <u>lip</u>

S00.542- External constriction of <u>oral cavity</u>

S00.55- <u>Superficial foreign body</u> of lip and oral cavity

S00.551- Superficial foreign body of <u>lip</u>
Splinter of lip and oral cavity

S00.552- Superficial foreign body of <u>oral cavity</u>
Splinter of lip and oral cavity

S00.56- <u>Insect bite (nonvenomous)</u> of lip and oral cavity

S00.561- Insect bite (nonvenomous) of <u>lip</u>

S00.562- Insect bite (nonvenomous) of <u>oral cavity</u>

S00.57- <u>Other superficial bite</u> of lip and oral cavity

S00.571- Other superficial bite of <u>lip</u>
Excludes 1:   open bite of lip (S01.551)

S00.572- Other superficial bite of <u>oral cavity</u>
Excludes 1:   open bite of oral cavity (S01.552)

S00.8- <u>Superficial injury of other parts of head</u>
Superficial injuries of face [any part]

S00.80x- Unspecified superficial injury of other part of head

S00.81x- Abrasion of other part of head

S00.82x- Blister (nonthermal) of other part of head

S 0 0 - S 0 0

S00.83x- Contusion of other part of head
Bruise of other part of head
Hematoma of other part of head

S00.84x- External constriction of other part of head

S00.85x- Superficial foreign body of other part of head
Splinter in other part of head

S00.86x- Insect bite (nonvenomous) of other part of head

S00.87x- Other superficial bite of other part of head
Excludes 1:   open bite of other part of head (S01.85)

S00.9- Superficial injury of unspecified part of head

S00.90x- Unspecified superficial injury of unspecified part of head

S00.91x- Abrasion of unspecified part of head

S00.92x- Blister (nonthermal) of unspecified part of head

S00.93x- Contusion of unspecified part of head
Bruise of head
Hematoma of head

S00.94x- External constriction of unspecified part of head

S00.95x- Superficial foreign body of unspecified part of head
Splinter of head

S00.96x- Insect bite (nonvenomous) of unspecified part of head

S00.97x- Other superficial bite of unspecified part of head
Excludes 1:   open bite of head (S01.95)

S01- Open wound of head
Code also any associated:
Injury of cranial nerve (S04.-)
Injury of muscle and tendon of head (S09.1-)
Intracranial injury (S06.-)
Wound infection
Excludes 1:   open skull fracture (S02.- with 7th character B)
Excludes ❷: injury of eye and orbit (S05.-)
traumatic amputation of part of head (S08.-)

The appropriate 7th character is to be added to each code from category S01:
A   Initial encounter
D   Subsequent encounter
S   Sequela

S01.0- Open wound of scalp
Excludes 1:   avulsion of scalp (S08.0)

S01.00x- Unspecified open wound of scalp

S01.01x- Laceration without foreign body of scalp

S01.02x- Laceration with foreign body of scalp
AHA 15:1Q:p5 – Laceration with foreign body of scalp

S01.03x- Puncture wound without foreign body of scalp

S01.04x- Puncture wound with foreign body of scalp

S01.05x- Open bite of scalp
Bite of scalp NOS
Excludes 1:   superficial bite of scalp (S00.06, S00.07-)

S01.1- Open wound of eyelid and periocular area
Open wound of eyelid and periocular area with or without involvement of lacrimal passages

S01.10- Unspecified open wound of eyelid and periocular area

CC-A **S01.101-** Unspecified open wound of right eyelid and periocular area

CC-A **S01.102-** Unspecified open wound of left eyelid and periocular area

CC-A **S01.109-** Unspecified open wound of unspecified eyelid and periocular area

S01.11- Laceration without foreign body of eyelid and periocular area

S01.111- Laceration without foreign body of right eyelid and periocular area

S01.112- Laceration without foreign body of left eyelid and periocular area

S01.119- Laceration without foreign body of unspecified eyelid and periocular area

S01.12- Laceration with foreign body of eyelid and periocular area

S01.121- Laceration with foreign body of right eyelid and periocular area

S01.122- Laceration with foreign body of left eyelid and periocular area

S01.129- Laceration with foreign body of unspecified eyelid and periocular area

S01.13- Puncture wound without foreign body of eyelid and periocular area

S01.131- Puncture wound without foreign body of right eyelid and periocular area

S01.132- Puncture wound without foreign body of left eyelid and periocular area

S01.139- Puncture wound without foreign body of unspecified eyelid and periocular area

S01.14- Puncture wound with foreign body of eyelid and periocular area

S01.141- Puncture wound with foreign body of right eyelid and periocular area

S01.142- Puncture wound with foreign body of left eyelid and periocular area

S01.149- Puncture wound with foreign body of unspecified eyelid and periocular area

S01.15- Open bite of eyelid and periocular area
Bite of eyelid and periocular area NOS
Excludes 1:   superficial bite of eyelid and periocular area (S00.26, S00.27)

S01.151- Open bite of right eyelid and periocular area

S01.152- Open bite of left eyelid and periocular area

S01.159- Open bite of unspecified eyelid and periocular area

S01.2- Open wound of nose

S01.20x- Unspecified open wound of nose

S01.21x- Laceration without foreign body of nose
AHA 15:1Q:p5 – Laceration body of nose

S01.22x- Laceration with foreign body of nose

S01.23x- Puncture wound without foreign body of nose

S01.24x- Puncture wound with foreign body of nose

S01.25x- Open bite of nose
Bite of nose NOS
Excludes 1:   superficial bite of nose (S00.36, S00.37)

S01.3- Open wound of ear

S01.30- Unspecified open wound of ear

S01.301- Unspecified open wound of right ear

S01.302- Unspecified open wound of left ear

S01.309- Unspecified open wound of unspecified ear

S01.31- Laceration without foreign body of ear

S01.311- Laceration without foreign body of right ear

S01.312- Laceration without foreign body of left ear

S01.319- Laceration without foreign body of unspecified ear

S01.32- Laceration with foreign body of ear

S01.321- Laceration with foreign body of right ear

S01.322- Laceration with foreign body of left ear

S01.329- Laceration with foreign body of unspecified ear

S01.33- Puncture wound without foreign body of ear

S01.331- Puncture wound without foreign body of right ear

S01.332- Puncture wound without foreign body of left ear

S01.339- Puncture wound without foreign body of unspecified ear

S01.34- Puncture wound with foreign body of ear

S01.341- Puncture wound with foreign body of right ear

S01.342- Puncture wound with foreign body of left ear

S01.349- Puncture wound with foreign body of unspecified ear

S01.35- Open bite of ear
Bite of ear NOS
Excludes 1:   superficial bite of ear (S00.46, S00.47)

S01.351- Open bite of right ear

S01.352- Open bite of left ear

S01.359- Open bite of unspecified ear

S00 - S01

S01.4- Open wound of <u>cheek and temporomandibular area</u>

S01.40- <u>Unspecified</u> open wound of cheek and temporomandibular area

S01.401- Unspecified open wound of <u>right</u> cheek and temporomandibular area

S01.402- Unspecified open wound of <u>left</u> cheek and temporomandibular area

S01.409- Unspecified open wound of <u>unspecified</u> cheek and temporomandibular area

S01.41- <u>Laceration without</u> foreign body of cheek and temporomandibular area

S01.411- Laceration <u>without</u> foreign body of <u>right</u> cheek and temporomandibular area
AHA 15:1Q:p5 – Laceration of cheek

S01.412- Laceration <u>without</u> foreign body of <u>left</u> cheek and temporomandibular area

S01.419- Laceration <u>without</u> foreign body of <u>unspecified</u> cheek and temporomandibular area

S01.42- <u>Laceration with foreign body</u> of cheek and temporomandibular area

S01.421- Laceration <u>with foreign body</u> of <u>right</u> cheek and temporomandibular area

S01.422- Laceration <u>with foreign body</u> of <u>left</u> cheek and temporomandibular area

S01.429- Laceration <u>with foreign body</u> of <u>unspecified</u> cheek and temporomandibular area

S01.43- <u>Puncture</u> wound <u>without</u> foreign body of cheek and temporomandibular area

S01.431- Puncture wound <u>without</u> foreign body of <u>right</u> cheek and temporomandibular area

S01.432- Puncture wound <u>without</u> foreign body of <u>left</u> cheek and temporomandibular area

S01.439- Puncture wound <u>without</u> foreign body of <u>unspecified</u> cheek and temporomandibular area

S01.44- <u>Puncture</u> wound <u>with foreign body</u> of cheek and temporomandibular area

S01.441- Puncture wound <u>with foreign body</u> of <u>right</u> cheek and temporomandibular area

S01.442- Puncture wound <u>with foreign body</u> of <u>left</u> cheek and temporomandibular area

S01.449- Puncture wound <u>with foreign body</u> of <u>unspecified</u> cheek and temporomandibular area

S01.45- <u>Open bite</u> of cheek and temporomandibular area
Bite of cheek and temporomandibular area NOS
Excludes ❷: superficial bite of cheek and temporomandibular area (S00.86, S00.87)

S01.451- Open bite of <u>right</u> cheek and temporomandibular area

S01.452- Open bite of <u>left</u> cheek and temporomandibular area

S01.459- Open bite of <u>unspecified</u> cheek and temporomandibular area

S01.5- Open wound of <u>lip and oral cavity</u>
Excludes ❷: tooth dislocation (S03.2)
tooth fracture (S02.5)

S01.50- <u>Unspecified</u> open wound of lip and oral cavity

S01.501- Unspecified open wound of <u>lip</u>

S01.502- Unspecified open wound of <u>oral cavity</u>

S01.51- <u>Laceration</u> of lip and oral cavity <u>without</u> foreign body

S01.511- Laceration <u>without</u> foreign body of <u>lip</u>

S01.512- Laceration <u>without</u> foreign body of <u>oral cavity</u>

S01.52- <u>Laceration</u> of lip and oral cavity <u>with foreign body</u>

S01.521- Laceration <u>with foreign body</u> of <u>lip</u>

S01.522- Laceration <u>with foreign body</u> of <u>oral cavity</u>

S01.53- <u>Puncture</u> wound of lip and oral cavity <u>without</u> foreign body

S01.531- Puncture wound <u>without</u> foreign body of <u>lip</u>

S01.532- Puncture wound <u>without</u> foreign body of <u>oral cavity</u>

S01.54- <u>Puncture</u> wound of lip and oral cavity <u>with foreign body</u>

S01.541- Puncture wound <u>with foreign body</u> of <u>lip</u>

S01.542- Puncture wound <u>with foreign body</u> of <u>oral cavity</u>

S01.55- <u>Open bite</u> of lip and oral cavity

S01.551- Open bite of <u>lip</u>
Bite of lip NOS
Excludes 1: superficial bite of lip (S00.571)

S01.552- Open bite of <u>oral cavity</u>
Bite of oral cavity NOS
Excludes 1: superficial bite of oral cavity (S00.572)

S01.8- Open wound of <u>other parts of head</u>

S01.80x- Unspecified open wound of other part of head

S01.81x- Laceration <u>without</u> foreign body of other part of head

S01.82x- Laceration <u>with foreign body</u> of other part of head

S01.83x- Puncture wound <u>without</u> foreign body of other part of head

S01.84x- Puncture wound <u>with foreign body</u> of other part of head

S01.85x- Open bite of other part of head
Bite of other part of head NOS
Excludes 1: superficial bite of other part of head (S00.85)

S01.9- Open wound of <u>unspecified part of head</u>

S01.90x- Unspecified open wound of unspecified part of head

S01.91x- Laceration <u>without</u> foreign body of unspecified part of head

S01.92x- Laceration <u>with foreign body</u> of unspecified part of head

S01.93x- Puncture wound <u>without</u> foreign body of unspecified part of head

S01.94x- Puncture wound <u>with foreign body</u> of unspecified part of head

S01.95x- Open bite of unspecified part of head
Bite of head NOS
Excludes 1: superficial bite of head NOS (S00.97)

S02- <u>Fracture</u> of <u>skull and facial bones</u>
Note: A fracture not indicated as open or closed should be coded to closed
Code also any associated intracranial injury (S06.-)
The appropriate 7th character is to be added to each code from category S02:
A <u>Initial</u> encounter for <u>closed</u> fracture
B <u>Initial</u> encounter for <u>open</u> fracture
D <u>Subsequent</u> encounter for fracture <u>with routine healing</u>
G <u>Subsequent</u> encounter for fracture <u>with delayed healing</u>
K <u>Subsequent</u> encounter for fracture <u>with nonunion</u>
S <u>Sequela</u>

S02.0xx- Fracture of <u>vault</u> of skull
CC-A,K MCC-B Fracture of frontal bone
Fracture of parietal bone

S02.1- Fracture of <u>base</u> of skull
Excludes 1: orbit NOS (S02.8)
Excludes ❷: orbital floor (S02.3-)

S02.10- <u>Unspecified</u> fracture of base of skull
CC-A,K MCC-B **S02.101-** Fracture of base of skull, <u>right</u> side
CC-A,K MCC-B **S02.102-** Fracture of base of skull, <u>left</u> side
CC-A,K MCC-B **S02.109-** Fracture of base of skull, <u>unspecified</u> side

S02.11- Fracture of <u>occiput</u>
CC-A,K MCC-B **S02.110-** Type I occipital condyle fracture, <u>unspecified</u> side
CC-A,K MCC-B **S02.111-** Type II occipital condyle fracture, <u>unspecified</u> side
CC-A,K MCC-B **S02.112-** Type III occipital condyle fracture, <u>unspecified</u> side
CC-A,K MCC-B **S02.113-** Unspecified occipital condyle fracture
CC-A,K MCC-B **S02.118-** Other fracture of occiput, <u>unspecified</u> side
CC-A,K MCC-B **S02.119-** Unspecified fracture of occiput
CC-A,K MCC-B **S02.11A-** Type I occipital condyle fracture, <u>right</u> side
CC-A,K MCC-B **S02.11B-** Type I occipital condyle fracture, <u>left</u> side
CC-A,K MCC-B **S02.11C-** Type II occipital condyle fracture, <u>right</u> side
CC-A,K MCC-B **S02.11D-** Type II occipital condyle fracture, <u>left</u> side
CC-A,K MCC-B **S02.11E-** Type III occipital condyle fracture, <u>right</u> side
CC-A,K MCC-B **S02.11F-** Type III occipital condyle fracture, <u>left</u> side
CC-A,K MCC-B **S02.11G-** Other fracture of occiput, <u>right</u> side

S01 - S02

CC-A,K MCC-B **S02.11H-** Other fracture of occiput, <u>left</u> side

S02.19x- <u>Other</u> fracture of <u>base</u> of skull
CC-A,K MCC-B Fracture of anterior fossa of base of skull
Fracture of ethmoid sinus
Fracture of frontal sinus
Fracture of middle fossa of base of skull
Fracture of orbital roof
Fracture of posterior fossa of base of skull
Fracture of sphenoid
Fracture of temporal bone

S02.2xx- Fracture of <u>nasal bones</u>
CC-B,K

S02.3- Fracture of <u>orbital floor</u>
Excludes 1: *orbit NOS (S02.8)*
Excludes ❷: *orbital roof (S02.1-)*

CC-A,B,K **S02.30x-** Fracture of orbital floor, <u>unspecified</u> side
CC-A,B,K **S02.31x-** Fracture of orbital floor, <u>right</u> side
CC-A,B,K **S02.32x-** Fracture of orbital floor, <u>left</u> side

S02.4- Fracture of <u>malar, maxillary and zygoma bones</u>
Fracture of superior maxilla
Fracture of upper jaw (bone)
Fracture of zygomatic process of temporal bone

S02.40- Fracture of malar, maxillary and zygoma bones, <u>unspecified</u>

CC-A,B,K **S02.400-** Malar fracture, <u>unspecified</u> side
CC-A,B,K **S02.401-** Maxillary fracture, <u>unspecified</u> side
CC-A,B,K **S02.402-** Zygomatic fracture, <u>unspecified</u> side
CC-A,B,K **S02.40A-** Malar fracture, <u>right</u> side
CC-A,B,K **S02.40B-** Malar fracture, <u>left</u> side
CC-A,B,K **S02.40C-** Maxillary fracture, <u>right</u> side
CC-A,B,K **S02.40D-** Maxillary fracture, <u>left</u> side
CC-A,B,K **S02.40E-** Zygomatic fracture, <u>right</u> side
CC-A,B,K **S02.40F-** Zygomatic fracture, <u>left</u> side

S02.41- <u>LeFort</u> fracture
CC-A,B,K **S02.411-** LeFort I fracture
CC-A,B,K **S02.412-** LeFort II fracture
CC-A,B,K **S02.413-** LeFort III fracture

CC-A,B,K **S02.42x-** Fracture of <u>alveolus of maxilla</u>

S02.5xx- Fracture of <u>tooth (traumatic)</u>
CC-K Broken tooth
Excludes 1: *cracked tooth (nontraumatic) (K03.81)*

S02.6- Fracture of <u>mandible</u>
Fracture of lower jaw (bone)

S02.60- Fracture of mandible, unspecified

CC-A,B,K **S02.600-** Fracture of <u>unspecified part of body</u> of mandible, <u>unspecified</u> side
CC-A,B,K **S02.601-** Fracture of <u>unspecified part of body</u> of <u>right</u> mandible
CC-A,B,K **S02.602-** Fracture of <u>unspecified part of body</u> of <u>left</u> mandible
CC-A,B,K **S02.609-** Fracture of mandible, <u>unspecified</u>

S02.61- Fracture of <u>condylar process</u> of mandible
CC-A,B,K **S02.610-** Fracture of condylar process of mandible, <u>unspecified</u> side
CC-A,B,K **S02.611-** Fracture of condylar process of <u>right</u> mandible
CC-A,B,K **S02.612-** Fracture of condylar process of <u>left</u> mandible

S02.62- Fracture of <u>subcondylar process</u> of mandible
CC-A,B,K **S02.620-** Fracture of subcondylar process of mandible, <u>unspecified</u> side
CC-A,B,K **S02.621-** Fracture of subcondylar process of <u>right</u> mandible
CC-A,B,K **S02.622-** Fracture of subcondylar process of <u>left</u> mandible

S02.63- Fracture of <u>coronoid process</u> of mandible
CC-A,B,K **S02.630-** Fracture of coronoid process of mandible, <u>unspecified</u> side
CC-A,B,K **S02.631-** Fracture of coronoid process of <u>right</u> mandible
CC-A,B,K **S02.632-** Fracture of coronoid process of <u>left</u> mandible

S02.64- Fracture of <u>ramus</u> of mandible
CC-A,B,K **S02.640-** Fracture of ramus of mandible, <u>unspecified</u> side
CC-A,B,K **S02.641-** Fracture of ramus of <u>right</u> mandible
CC-A,B,K **S02.642-** Fracture of ramus of <u>left</u> mandible

S02.65- Fracture of <u>angle</u> of mandible
CC-A,B,K **S02.650-** Fracture of angle of mandible, <u>unspecified</u> side
CC-A,B,K **S02.651-** Fracture of angle of <u>right</u> mandible
CC-A,B,K **S02.652-** Fracture of angle of <u>left</u> mandible
CC-A,B,K **S02.66x-** Fracture of <u>symphysis</u> of mandible

S02.67- Fracture of <u>alveolus</u> of mandible
CC-A,B,K **S02.670-** Fracture of alveolus of mandible, <u>unspecified</u> side
CC-A,B,K **S02.671-** Fracture of alveolus of <u>right</u> mandible
CC-A,B,K **S02.672-** Fracture of alveolus of <u>left</u> mandible
CC-A,B,K **S02.69x-** Fracture of mandible of other specified site

S02.8- Fractures of <u>other specified skull and facial bones</u>
Fracture of orbit NOS
Fracture of palate
Excludes 1: *fracture of orbital floor (S02.3-)*
fracture of orbital roof (S02.1-)

CC-A,B,K **S02.80x-** Fracture of other specified skull and facial bones, <u>unspecified</u> side
CC-A,B,K **S02.81x-** Fracture of other specified skull and facial bones, <u>right</u> side
CC-A,B,K **S02.82x-** Fracture of other specified skull and facial bones, <u>left</u> side

S02.9- Fracture of <u>unspecified</u> skull and facial bones

S02.91x- Unspecified fracture of <u>skull</u>
CC-A,K MCC-B

S02.92x- Unspecified fracture of <u>facial bones</u>
CC-A,B,K

S03- <u>Dislocation and sprain</u> of joints and ligaments of <u>head</u>
Includes: Avulsion of joint (capsule) or ligament of head
Laceration of cartilage, joint (capsule) or ligament of head
Sprain of cartilage, joint (capsule) or ligament of head
Traumatic hemarthrosis of joint or ligament of head
Traumatic rupture of joint or ligament of head
Traumatic subluxation of joint or ligament of head
Traumatic tear of joint or ligament of head
Code also any associated open wound
Excludes ❷: *Strain of muscle or tendon of head (S09.1)*

The appropriate 7th character is to be added to each code from category S03:
A <u>Initial</u> encounter
D <u>Subsequent</u> encounter
S <u>Sequela</u>

S03.0- <u>Dislocation</u> of <u>jaw</u>
Dislocation of jaw (cartilage) (meniscus)
Dislocation of mandible
Dislocation of temporomandibular (joint)
S03.00x- Dislocation of jaw, <u>unspecified</u> side
S03.01x- Dislocation of jaw, <u>right</u> side
S03.02x- Dislocation of jaw, <u>left</u> side
S03.03x- Dislocation of jaw, <u>bilateral</u>

S03.1xx- Dislocation of septal cartilage of nose
S03.2xx- Dislocation of tooth

S03.4- <u>Sprain</u> of <u>jaw</u>
Sprain of temporomandibular (joint) (ligament)
S03.40x- Sprain of jaw, <u>unspecified</u> side
S03.41x- Sprain of jaw, <u>right</u> side
S03.42x- Sprain of jaw, <u>left</u> side
S03.43x- Sprain of jaw, <u>bilateral</u>

S03.8xx- Sprain of joints and ligaments of <u>other</u> parts of head
S03.9xx- Sprain of joints and ligaments of <u>unspecified</u> parts of head

S 0 2 ‖ S 0 3

S04- Injury of cranial nerve
The selection of side should be based on the side of the body being affected
Code first any associated intracranial injury (S06.-)
Code also any associated:
  Open wound of head (S01.-)
  Skull fracture (S02.-)
The appropriate 7th character is to be added to each code from category S04:
  A Initial encounter
  D Subsequent encounter
  S Sequela

S04.0- Injury of optic nerve and pathways
Use additional code to identify any visual field defect or blindness (H53.4-, H54)

S04.01- Injury of optic nerve
Injury of 2nd cranial nerve

CC-A **S04.011-** Injury of optic nerve, right eye

CC-A **S04.012-** Injury of optic nerve, left eye

CC-A **S04.019-** Injury of optic nerve, unspecified eye
Injury of optic nerve NOS

CC-A **S04.02x-** Injury of optic chiasm

S04.03- Injury of optic tract and pathways
Injury of optic radiation

CC-A **S04.031-** Injury of optic tract and pathways, right eye

CC-A **S04.032-** Injury of optic tract and pathways, left eye

CC-A **S04.039-** Injury of optic tract and pathways, unspecified eye
Injury of optic tract and pathways NOS

S04.04- Injury of visual cortex

CC-A **S04.041-** Injury of visual cortex, right eye

CC-A **S04.042-** Injury of visual cortex, left eye

CC-A **S04.049-** Injury of visual cortex, unspecified eye
Injury of visual cortex NOS

S04.1- Injury of oculomotor nerve
Injury of 3rd cranial nerve

CC-A **S04.10x-** Injury of oculomotor nerve, unspecified side

CC-A **S04.11x-** Injury of oculomotor nerve, right side

CC-A **S04.12x-** Injury of oculomotor nerve, left side

S04.2- Injury of trochlear nerve
Injury of 4th cranial nerve

CC-A **S04.20x-** Injury of trochlear nerve, unspecified side

CC-A **S04.21x-** Injury of trochlear nerve, right side

CC-A **S04.22x-** Injury of trochlear nerve, left side

S04.3- Injury of trigeminal nerve
Injury of 5th cranial nerve

CC-A **S04.30x-** Injury of trigeminal nerve, unspecified side

CC-A **S04.31x-** Injury of trigeminal nerve, right side

CC-A **S04.32x-** Injury of trigeminal nerve, left side

S04.4- Injury of abducent nerve
Injury of 6th cranial nerve

CC-A **S04.40x-** Injury of abducent nerve, unspecified side

CC-A **S04.41x-** Injury of abducent nerve, right side

CC-A **S04.42x-** Injury of abducent nerve, left side

S04.5- Injury of facial nerve
Injury of 7th cranial nerve

CC-A **S04.50x-** Injury of facial nerve, unspecified side

CC-A **S04.51x-** Injury of facial nerve, right side

CC-A **S04.52x-** Injury of facial nerve, left side

S04.6- Injury of acoustic nerve
Injury of auditory nerve
Injury of 8th cranial nerve

CC-A **S04.60x-** Injury of acoustic nerve, unspecified side

CC-A **S04.61x-** Injury of acoustic nerve, right side

CC-A **S04.62x-** Injury of acoustic nerve, left side

S04.7- Injury of accessory nerve
Injury of 11th cranial nerve

CC-A **S04.70x-** Injury of accessory nerve, unspecified side

CC-A **S04.71x-** Injury of accessory nerve, right side

CC-A **S04.72x-** Injury of accessory nerve, left side

S04.8- Injury of other cranial nerves

S04.81- Injury of olfactory [1st] nerve

CC-A **S04.811-** Injury of olfactory [1st] nerve, right side

CC-A **S04.812-** Injury of olfactory [1st] nerve, left side

CC-A **S04.819-** Injury of olfactory [1st] nerve, unspecified side

S04.89- Injury of other cranial nerves
Injury of vagus [10th] nerve

CC-A **S04.891-** Injury of other cranial nerves, right side

CC-A **S04.892-** Injury of other cranial nerves, left side

CC-A **S04.899-** Injury of other cranial nerves, unspecified side

S04.9xx- Injury of unspecified cranial nerve
CC-A

S05- Injury of eye and orbit
Includes: Open wound of eye and orbit
Excludes ❷: 2nd cranial [optic] nerve injury (S04.0-)
3rd cranial [oculomotor] nerve injury (S04.1-)
open wound of eyelid and periocular area (S01.1-)
orbital bone fracture (S02.1-, S02.3-, S02.8-)
superficial injury of eyelid (S00.1-S00.2)
The appropriate 7th character is to be added to each code from category S05:
  A Initial encounter
  D Subsequent encounter
  S Sequela

S05.0- Injury of conjunctiva and corneal abrasion without foreign body
Excludes 1:   foreign body in conjunctival sac (T15.1)
foreign body in cornea (T15.0)

S05.00x- Injury of conjunctiva and corneal abrasion without foreign body, unspecified eye

S05.01x- Injury of conjunctiva and corneal abrasion without foreign body, right eye

S05.02x- Injury of conjunctiva and corneal abrasion without foreign body, left eye

S05.1- Contusion of eyeball and orbital tissues
Traumatic hyphema
Excludes ❷: black eye NOS (S00.1)
contusion of eyelid and periocular area (S00.1)

S05.10x- Contusion of eyeball and orbital tissues, unspecified eye

S05.11x- Contusion of eyeball and orbital tissues, right eye

S05.12x- Contusion of eyeball and orbital tissues, left eye

S05.2- Ocular laceration and rupture with prolapse or loss of intraocular tissue

CC-A **S05.20x-** Ocular laceration and rupture with prolapse or loss of intraocular tissue, unspecified eye

CC-A **S05.21x-** Ocular laceration and rupture with prolapse or loss of intraocular tissue, right eye

CC-A **S05.22x-** Ocular laceration and rupture with prolapse or loss of intraocular tissue, left eye

S05.3- Ocular laceration without prolapse or loss of intraocular tissue
Laceration of eye NOS

CC-A **S05.30x-** Ocular laceration without prolapse or loss of intraocular tissue, unspecified eye

CC-A **S05.31x-** Ocular laceration without prolapse or loss of intraocular tissue, right eye

CC-A **S05.32x-** Ocular laceration without prolapse or loss of intraocular tissue, left eye

S05.4- Penetrating wound of orbit with or without foreign body
Excludes ❷: retained (old) foreign body following penetrating wound in orbit (H05.5-)

CC-A **S05.40x-** Penetrating wound of orbit with or without foreign body, unspecified eye

CC-A **S05.41x-** Penetrating wound of orbit with or without foreign body, right eye

CC-A **S05.42x-** Penetrating wound of orbit with or without foreign body, left eye

S05.5- <u>Penetrating wound</u> <u>with foreign body</u> of eyeball
    Excludes ❷: retained (old) intraocular foreign body (H44.6-, H44.7)

CC-A **S05.50x-** Penetrating wound <u>with foreign body</u> of <u>unspecified</u> eyeball

CC-A **S05.51x-** Penetrating wound <u>with foreign body</u> of <u>right</u> eyeball

CC-A **S05.52x-** Penetrating wound <u>with foreign body</u> of <u>left</u> eyeball

S05.6- <u>Penetrating wound</u> <u>without</u> foreign body of eyeball
    Ocular penetration NOS

  S05.60x- Penetrating wound <u>without</u> foreign body of <u>unspecified</u> eyeball

  S05.61x- Penetrating wound <u>without</u> foreign body of <u>right</u> eyeball

  S05.62x- Penetrating wound <u>without</u> foreign body of <u>left</u> eyeball

S05.7- <u>Avulsion</u> of eye
    Traumatic enucleation

CC-A **S05.70x-** Avulsion of <u>unspecified</u> eye

CC-A **S05.71x-** Avulsion of <u>right</u> eye

CC-A **S05.72x-** Avulsion of <u>left</u> eye

S05.8- <u>Other injuries</u> of eye and orbit
    Lacrimal duct injury

  S05.8x- <u>Other</u> injuries of eye and orbit

CC-A **S05.8x1-** Other injuries of <u>right</u> eye and orbit

CC-A **S05.8x2-** Other injuries of <u>left</u> eye and orbit

CC-A **S05.8x9-** Other injuries of <u>unspecified</u> eye and orbit

S05.9- <u>Unspecified</u> injury of eye and orbit
    Injury of eye NOS

  S05.90x- Unspecified injury of <u>unspecified</u> eye and orbit

CC-A **S05.91x-** Unspecified injury of <u>right</u> eye and orbit

CC-A **S05.92x-** Unspecified injury of <u>left</u> eye and orbit

S06- <u>Intracranial injury</u>
  Includes: Traumatic brain injury
  Code also any associated:
    Open wound of head (S01.-)
    Skull fracture (S02.-)
  Excludes 1: head injury NOS (S09.90)

> **The appropriate 7th character is to be added to each code from category S06:**
> **A**   <u>Initial</u> encounter
> **D**   <u>Subsequent</u> encounter
> **S**   <u>Sequela</u>

S06.0- <u>Concussion</u>
    Commotio cerebri
    Excludes 1: concussion with other intracranial injuries classified in subcategories S06.1- to S06.6-, S06.81- and S06.82- code to specified intracranial injury

  S06.0x- Concussion

    S06.0x0- Concussion <u>without</u> loss of consciousness

CC-A **S06.0x1-** Concussion <u>with</u> loss of consciousness of <u>30 minutes or less</u>

CC-A **S06.0x9-** Concussion <u>with</u> loss of consciousness of <u>unspecified</u> duration
      Concussion NOS

S06.1- Traumatic cerebral edema
    Diffuse traumatic cerebral edema
    Focal traumatic cerebral edema

  S06.1x- <u>Traumatic cerebral edema</u>
    AHA 15:1Q:p12 – Traumatic cerebral edema

MCC-A **S06.1x0-** Traumatic cerebral edema <u>without</u> loss of consciousness

MCC-A **S06.1x1-** Traumatic cerebral edema <u>with</u> loss of consciousness of <u>30 minutes or less</u>

MCC-A **S06.1x2-** Traumatic cerebral edema <u>with</u> loss of consciousness of <u>31 minutes to 59 minutes</u>

MCC-A **S06.1x3-** Traumatic cerebral edema <u>with</u> loss of consciousness of <u>1 hour to 5 hours 59 minutes</u>

MCC-A **S06.1x4-** Traumatic cerebral edema <u>with</u> loss of consciousness of <u>6 hours to 24 hours</u>

MCC-A **S06.1x5-** Traumatic cerebral edema <u>with</u> loss of consciousness <u>greater than 24</u> hours <u>with return</u> to pre-existing conscious level

MCC-A **S06.1x6-** Traumatic cerebral edema <u>with</u> loss of consciousness <u>greater than 24</u> hours <u>without</u> return to pre-existing conscious level <u>with patient surviving</u>

MCC-A **S06.1x7-** Traumatic cerebral edema <u>with</u> loss of consciousness of <u>any duration with death</u> due to <u>brain injury</u> prior to regaining consciousness

MCC-A **S06.1x8-** Traumatic cerebral edema <u>with</u> loss of consciousness of <u>any duration with death</u> due to <u>other cause</u> prior to regaining consciousness

MCC-A **S06.1x9-** Traumatic cerebral edema with loss of consciousness of <u>unspecified</u> duration
      Traumatic cerebral edema NOS

S06.2- Diffuse traumatic brain injury
    Diffuse axonal brain injury
    Excludes 1: traumatic diffuse cerebral edema (S06.1x-)

  S06.2x- <u>Diffuse traumatic brain injury</u>

    S06.2x0- Diffuse traumatic brain injury <u>without</u> loss of consciousness

CC-A **S06.2x1-** Diffuse traumatic brain injury <u>with</u> loss of consciousness of <u>30 minutes or less</u>

CC-A **S06.2x2-** Diffuse traumatic brain injury <u>with</u> loss of consciousness of <u>31 minutes to 59 minutes</u>

CC-A **S06.2x3-** Diffuse traumatic brain injury <u>with</u> loss of consciousness of <u>1 hour to 5 hours 59 minutes</u>

CC-A **S06.2x4-** Diffuse traumatic brain injury <u>with</u> loss of consciousness of <u>6 hours to 24 hours</u>

CC-A **S06.2x5-** Diffuse traumatic brain injury <u>with</u> loss of consciousness <u>greater than 24</u> hours <u>with return</u> to pre-existing conscious levels

MCC-A **S06.2x6-** Diffuse traumatic brain injury <u>with</u> loss of consciousness <u>greater than 24</u> hours <u>without return</u> to pre-existing conscious level <u>with patient surviving</u>

MCC-A **S06.2x7-** Diffuse traumatic brain injury <u>with</u> loss of consciousness of <u>any duration with death</u> due to <u>brain injury</u> prior to regaining consciousness

MCC-A **S06.2x8-** Diffuse traumatic brain injury <u>with</u> loss of consciousness of <u>any duration with death</u> due to <u>other cause</u> prior to regaining consciousness

CC-A **S06.2x9-** Diffuse traumatic brain injury <u>with</u> loss of consciousness of <u>unspecified</u> duration
      Diffuse traumatic brain injury NOS

S06.3- <u>Focal traumatic brain injury</u>
    Excludes 1: any condition classifiable to S06.4-S06.6 focal cerebral edema (S06.1)

  S06.30- <u>Unspecified</u> focal traumatic brain injury

    S06.300- Unspecified focal traumatic brain injury <u>without</u> loss of consciousness

CC-A **S06.301-** Unspecified focal traumatic brain injury <u>with</u> loss of consciousness of <u>30 minutes or less</u>

CC-A **S06.302-** Unspecified focal traumatic brain injury <u>with</u> loss of consciousness of <u>31 minutes to 59 minutes</u>

CC-A **S06.303-** Unspecified focal traumatic brain injury <u>with</u> loss of consciousness of <u>1 hour to 5 hours 59 minutes</u>

CC-A **S06.304-** Unspecified focal traumatic brain injury <u>with</u> loss of consciousness of <u>6 hours to 24 hours</u>

CC-A **S06.305-** Unspecified focal traumatic brain injury <u>with</u> loss of consciousness <u>greater than 24 hours</u> <u>with return</u> to pre-existing conscious level

MCC-A **S06.306-** Unspecified focal traumatic brain injury <u>with</u> loss of consciousness <u>greater than 24</u> hours <u>without return</u> to pre-existing conscious level <u>with patient surviving</u>

MCC-A **S06.307-** Unspecified focal traumatic brain injury <u>with</u> loss of consciousness of <u>any duration with death</u> due to <u>brain injury</u> prior to regaining consciousness

MCC-A **S06.308-** Unspecified focal traumatic brain injury <u>with</u> loss of consciousness of <u>any duration with death</u> due to <u>other cause</u> prior to regaining consciousness

CC-A **S06.309-** Unspecified focal traumatic brain injury **with** loss of consciousness of **unspecified** duration
Unspecified focal traumatic brain injury NOS

S06.31- Contusion and laceration of right cerebrum

MCC-A **S06.310-** Contusion and laceration of **right** cerebrum **without** loss of consciousness

MCC-A **S06.311-** Contusion and laceration of **right** cerebrum **with** loss of consciousness of **30 minutes or less**

MCC-A **S06.312-** Contusion and laceration of **right** cerebrum **with** loss of consciousness of **31minutes to 59 minutes**

MCC-A **S06.313-** Contusion and laceration of **right** cerebrum **with** loss of consciousness of **1 hour to 5 hours 59 minutes**

MCC-A **S06.314-** Contusion and laceration of **right** cerebrum **with** loss of consciousness of **6 hours to 24 hours**

MCC-A **S06.315-** Contusion and laceration of **right** cerebrum **with** loss of consciousness **greater than 24** hours **with return** to pre-existing conscious level

MCC-A **S06.316-** Contusion and laceration of **right** cerebrum **with** loss of consciousness **greater than 24** hours **without return** to pre-existing conscious level **with patient surviving**

MCC-A **S06.317-** Contusion and laceration of **right** cerebrum **with** loss of consciousness of **any duration with death** due to **brain injury** prior to regaining consciousness

MCC-A **S06.318-** Contusion and laceration of **right** cerebrum **with** loss of consciousness of **any duration with death** due to **other cause** prior to regaining consciousness

MCC-A **S06.319-** Contusion and laceration of **right** cerebrum **with** loss of consciousness of **unspecified** duration
Contusion and laceration of right cerebrum NOS

S06.32- Contusion and laceration of left cerebrum

MCC-A **S06.320-** Contusion and laceration of **left** cerebrum **without** loss of consciousness

MCC-A **S06.321-** Contusion and laceration of **left** cerebrum **with** loss of consciousness of **30 minutes or less**

MCC-A **S06.322-** Contusion and laceration of **left** cerebrum **with** loss of consciousness of **31 minutes to 59 minutes**

MCC-A **S06.323-** Contusion and laceration of **left** cerebrum **with** loss of consciousness of **1 hour to 5 hours 59 minutes**

MCC-A **S06.324-** Contusion and laceration of **left** cerebrum **with** loss of consciousness of **6 hours to 24 hours**

MCC-A **S06.325-** Contusion and laceration of **left** cerebrum **with** loss of consciousness **greater than 24** hours **with return** to pre-existing conscious level

MCC-A **S06.326-** Contusion and laceration of **left** cerebrum **with** loss of consciousness **greater than 24** hours **without return** to pre-existing conscious level **with patient surviving**

MCC-A **S06.327-** Contusion and laceration of **left** cerebrum **with** loss of consciousness of **any duration with death** due to **brain injury** prior to regaining consciousness

MCC-A **S06.328-** Contusion and laceration of **left** cerebrum **with** loss of consciousness of **any duration with death** due to **other cause** prior to regaining consciousness

MCC-A **S06.329-** Contusion and laceration of **left** cerebrum **with** loss of consciousness of **unspecified** duration
Contusion and laceration of left cerebrum NOS

S06.33- Contusion and laceration of cerebrum, unspecified

MCC-A **S06.330-** Contusion and laceration of cerebrum, **unspecified**, **without** loss of consciousness

MCC-A **S06.331-** Contusion and laceration of cerebrum, **unspecified**, **with** loss of consciousness of **30 minutes or less**

MCC-A **S06.332-** Contusion and laceration of cerebrum, **unspecified**, **with** loss of consciousness of **31 minutes to 59 minutes**

MCC-A **S06.333-** Contusion and laceration of cerebrum, **unspecified**, **with** loss of consciousness of **1 hour to 5 hours 59 minutes**

MCC-A **S06.334-** Contusion and laceration of cerebrum, **unspecified**, **with** loss of consciousness of **6 hours to 24 hours**

MCC-A **S06.335-** Contusion and laceration of cerebrum, **unspecified**, **with** loss of consciousness **greater than 24** hours **with return** to pre-existing conscious level

MCC-A **S06.336-** Contusion and laceration of cerebrum, **unspecified**, **with** loss of consciousness **greater than 24** hours **without return** to pre-existing conscious level **with patient surviving**

MCC-A **S06.337-** Contusion and laceration of cerebrum, **unspecified**, **with** loss of consciousness of **any duration with death** due to **brain injury** prior to regaining consciousness

MCC-A **S06.338-** Contusion and laceration of cerebrum, **unspecified**, **with** loss of consciousness of **any duration with death** due to **other cause** prior to regaining consciousness

MCC-A **S06.339-** Contusion and laceration of cerebrum, **unspecified**, **with** loss of consciousness of **unspecified** duration
Contusion and laceration of cerebrum NOS

S06.34- Traumatic hemorrhage of right cerebrum
AHA 15:1Q:p12 – Right frontal intracranial hemorrhage
Traumatic intracerebral hemorrhage and hematoma of right cerebrum

MCC-A **S06.340-** Traumatic hemorrhage of **right** cerebrum **without** loss of consciousness

MCC-A **S06.341-** Traumatic hemorrhage of **right** cerebrum **with** loss of consciousness of **30 minutes or less**

MCC-A **S06.342-** Traumatic hemorrhage of **right** cerebrum **with** loss of consciousness of **31 minutes to 59 minutes**

MCC-A **S06.343-** Traumatic hemorrhage of **right** cerebrum **with** loss of consciousness of **1 hours to 5 hours 59 minutes**

MCC-A **S06.344-** Traumatic hemorrhage of **right** cerebrum **with** loss of consciousness of **6 hours to 24 hours**

MCC-A **S06.345-** Traumatic hemorrhage of **right** cerebrum **with** loss of consciousness greater than 24 hours **with return** to pre-existing conscious level

MCC-A **S06.346-** Traumatic hemorrhage of **right** cerebrum **with** loss of consciousness **greater than 24** hours **without return** to pre-existing conscious level **with patient surviving**

MCC-A **S06.347-** Traumatic hemorrhage of **right** cerebrum **with** loss of consciousness of **any duration with death** due to **brain injury** prior to regaining consciousness

MCC-A **S06.348-** Traumatic hemorrhage of **right** cerebrum **with** loss of consciousness of **any duration with death** due to **other cause** prior to regaining consciousness

MCC-A **S06.349-** Traumatic hemorrhage of **right** cerebrum **with** loss of consciousness of **unspecified** duration
Traumatic hemorrhage of right cerebrum NOS

S06.35- Traumatic hemorrhage of left cerebrum
Traumatic intracerebral hemorrhage and hematoma of left cerebrum

MCC-A **S06.350-** Traumatic hemorrhage of **left** cerebrum **without** loss of consciousness

MCC-A **S06.351-** Traumatic hemorrhage of **left** cerebrum **with** loss of consciousness of **30 minutes or less**

MCC-A **S06.352-** Traumatic hemorrhage of **left** cerebrum **with** loss of consciousness of **31 minutes to 59 minutes**

MCC-A **S06.353-** Traumatic hemorrhage of **left** cerebrum **with** loss of consciousness of **1 hours to 5 hours 59 minutes**

MCC-A **S06.354-** Traumatic hemorrhage of **left** cerebrum **with** loss of consciousness of **6 hours to 24 hours**

MCC-A **S06.355-** Traumatic hemorrhage of **left** cerebrum **with** loss of consciousness **greater than 24** hours **with return** to pre-existing conscious level

MCC-A **S06.356-** Traumatic hemorrhage of **left** cerebrum **with** loss of consciousness greater than 24 hours **without** return to pre-existing conscious level **with patient surviving**

S06
S06
S06

MCC-A **S06.357-** Traumatic hemorrhage of <u>left</u> cerebrum <u>with</u> loss of consciousness of <u>any duration with death</u> due to <u>brain injury</u> prior to regaining consciousness

MCC-A **S06.358-** Traumatic hemorrhage of <u>left</u> cerebrum <u>with</u> loss of <u>any duration with death</u> due to <u>other cause</u> prior to regaining consciousness

MCC-A **S06.359-** Traumatic hemorrhage of <u>left</u> cerebrum <u>with</u> loss of consciousness of <u>unspecified</u> duration
Traumatic hemorrhage of left cerebrum NOS

S06.36- <u>Traumatic hemorrhage</u> of cerebrum, <u>unspecified</u>
Traumatic intracerebral hemorrhage and hematoma, unspecified

MCC-A **S06.360-** Traumatic hemorrhage of cerebrum, <u>unspecified</u>, <u>without</u> loss of consciousness

MCC-A **S06.361-** Traumatic hemorrhage of cerebrum, <u>unspecified</u>, <u>with</u> loss of consciousness of <u>30 minutes or less</u>

MCC-A **S06.362-** Traumatic hemorrhage of cerebrum, <u>unspecified</u>, <u>with</u> loss of consciousness of <u>31 minutes to 59 minutes</u>

MCC-A **S06.363-** Traumatic hemorrhage of cerebrum, <u>unspecified</u>, <u>with</u> loss of consciousness of <u>1 hours to 5 hours 59 minutes</u>

MCC-A **S06.364-** Traumatic hemorrhage of cerebrum, <u>unspecified</u>, <u>with</u> loss of consciousness of <u>6 hours to 24 hours</u>

MCC-A **S06.365-** Traumatic hemorrhage of cerebrum, <u>unspecified</u>, <u>with</u> loss of consciousness <u>greater than 24</u> hours <u>with return</u> to pre-existing conscious level

MCC-A **S06.366-** Traumatic hemorrhage of cerebrum, <u>unspecified</u>, <u>with</u> loss of consciousness <u>greater than 24</u> hours <u>without return</u> to pre-existing conscious level <u>with patient surviving</u>

MCC-A **S06.367-** Traumatic hemorrhage of cerebrum, <u>unspecified</u>, <u>with</u> loss of consciousness of <u>any duration with death</u> due to <u>brain injury</u> prior to regaining consciousness

MCC-A **S06.368-** Traumatic hemorrhage of cerebrum, <u>unspecified</u>, <u>with</u> loss of consciousness of <u>any duration with death</u> due to <u>other cause</u> prior to regaining consciousness

MCC-A **S06.369-** Traumatic hemorrhage of cerebrum, <u>unspecified</u>, <u>with</u> loss of consciousness of <u>unspecified</u> duration
Traumatic hemorrhage of cerebrum NOS

S06.37- <u>Contusion, laceration, and hemorrhage</u> of <u>cerebellum</u>

MCC-A **S06.370-** Contusion, laceration, and hemorrhage of cerebellum <u>without</u> loss of consciousness

CC-A **S06.371-** Contusion, laceration, and hemorrhage of cerebellum <u>with</u> loss of consciousness of <u>30 minutes or less</u>

CC-A **S06.372-** Contusion, laceration, and hemorrhage of cerebellum <u>with</u> loss of consciousness of <u>31 minutes to 59 minutes</u>

CC-A **S06.373-** Contusion, laceration, and hemorrhage of cerebellum <u>with</u> loss of consciousness of <u>1 hour to 5 hours 59</u> minutes

CC-A **S06.374-** Contusion, laceration, and hemorrhage of cerebellum <u>with</u> loss of consciousness of <u>6 hours to 24 hours</u>

CC-A **S06.375-** Contusion, laceration, and hemorrhage of cerebellum <u>with</u> loss of consciousness <u>greater than 24</u> hours <u>with return</u> to pre-existing conscious level

MCC-A **S06.376-** Contusion, laceration, and hemorrhage of cerebellum <u>with</u> loss of consciousness <u>greater than 24</u> hours <u>without return</u> to pre-existing conscious level <u>with patient surviving</u>

MCC-A **S06.377-** Contusion, laceration, and hemorrhage of cerebellum <u>with</u> loss of consciousness of <u>any duration with death</u> due to <u>brain injury</u> prior to regaining consciousness

MCC-A **S06.378-** Contusion, laceration, and hemorrhage of cerebellum <u>with</u> loss of consciousness of <u>any duration with death</u> due to <u>other cause</u> prior to regaining consciousness

CC-A **S06.379-** Contusion, laceration, and hemorrhage of cerebellum <u>with</u> loss of consciousness of <u>unspecified</u> duration
Contusion, laceration, and hemorrhage of cerebellum NOS

S06.38- <u>Contusion, laceration, and hemorrhage</u> of <u>brainstem</u>

MCC-A **S06.380-** Contusion, laceration, and hemorrhage of brainstem <u>without</u> loss of consciousness

CC-A **S06.381-** Contusion, laceration, and hemorrhage of brainstem <u>with</u> loss of consciousness of <u>30 minutes or less</u>

CC-A **S06.382-** Contusion, laceration, and hemorrhage of brainstem <u>with</u> loss of consciousness of <u>31 minutes to 59 minutes</u>

CC-A **S06.383-** Contusion, laceration, and hemorrhage of brainstem <u>with</u> loss of consciousness of <u>1 hour to 5 hours 59</u> minutes

CC-A **S06.384-** Contusion, laceration, and hemorrhage of brainstem <u>with</u> loss of consciousness of <u>6 hours to 24 hours</u>

CC-A **S06.385-** Contusion, laceration, and hemorrhage of brainstem <u>with</u> loss of consciousness <u>greater than 24</u> hours <u>with return</u> to pre-existing conscious level

MCC-A **S06.386-** Contusion, laceration, and hemorrhage of brainstem <u>with</u> loss of consciousness <u>greater than 24</u> hours <u>without return</u> to pre-existing conscious level <u>with patient surviving</u>

MCC-A **S06.387-** Contusion, laceration, and hemorrhage of brainstem <u>with</u> loss of consciousness of <u>any duration with death</u> due to <u>brain injury</u> prior to regaining consciousness

MCC-A **S06.388-** Contusion, laceration, and hemorrhage of brainstem <u>with</u> loss of consciousness of <u>any duration with death</u> due to <u>other cause</u> prior to regaining consciousness

CC-A **S06.389-** Contusion, laceration, and hemorrhage of brainstem <u>with</u> loss of consciousness of <u>unspecified</u> duration
Contusion, laceration, and hemorrhage of brainstem NOS

S06.4- Epidural hemorrhage
Extradural hemorrhage NOS
Extradural hemorrhage (traumatic)

S06.4x- <u>Epidural hemorrhage</u>

MCC-A **S06.4x0-** Epidural hemorrhage <u>without</u> loss of consciousness

MCC-A **S06.4x1-** Epidural hemorrhage <u>with</u> loss of consciousness of <u>30 minutes or less</u>

MCC-A **S06.4x2-** Epidural hemorrhage <u>with</u> loss of consciousness of <u>31 minutes to 59 minutes</u>

MCC-A **S06.4x3-** Epidural hemorrhage <u>with</u> loss of consciousness of <u>1 hour to 5 hours 59 minutes</u>

MCC-A **S06.4x4-** Epidural hemorrhage <u>with</u> loss of consciousness of <u>6 hours to 24 hours</u>

MCC-A **S06.4x5-** Epidural hemorrhage <u>with</u> loss of consciousness <u>greater than 24</u> hours <u>with return</u> to pre-existing conscious level

MCC-A **S06.4x6-** Epidural hemorrhage <u>with</u> loss of consciousness <u>greater than 24</u> hours <u>without return</u> to pre-existing conscious level <u>with patient surviving</u>

MCC-A **S06.4x7-** Epidural hemorrhage <u>with</u> loss of consciousness of <u>any duration with death</u> due to <u>brain injury</u> prior to regaining consciousness

MCC-A **S06.4x8-** Epidural hemorrhage <u>with</u> loss of consciousness of <u>any duration with death</u> due to <u>other causes</u> prior to regaining consciousness

MCC-A **S06.4x9-** Epidural hemorrhage <u>with</u> loss of consciousness of <u>unspecified</u> duration
Epidural hemorrhage NOS

S06
|
S06
|
S06

S06.5- Traumatic subdural hemorrhage

S06.5x- Traumatic subdural hemorrhage

MCC-A **S06.5x0- Traumatic subdural hemorrhage without loss of consciousness**

MCC-A **S06.5x1- Traumatic subdural hemorrhage with loss of consciousness of 30 minutes or less**

MCC-A **S06.5x2- Traumatic subdural hemorrhage with loss of consciousness of 31 minutes to 59 minutes**

MCC-A **S06.5x3- Traumatic subdural hemorrhage with loss of consciousness of 1 hour to 5 hours 59 minutes**

MCC-A **S06.5x4- Traumatic subdural hemorrhage with loss of consciousness of 6 hours to 24 hours**

MCC-A **S06.5x5- Traumatic subdural hemorrhage with loss of consciousness greater than 24 hours with return to pre-existing conscious level**

MCC-A **S06.5x6- Traumatic subdural hemorrhage with loss of consciousness greater than 24 hours without return to pre-existing conscious level with patient surviving**

MCC-A **S06.5x7- Traumatic subdural hemorrhage with loss of consciousness of any duration with death due to brain injury before regaining consciousness**

MCC-A **S06.5x8- Traumatic subdural hemorrhage with loss of consciousness of any duration with death due to other cause before regaining consciousness**

MCC-A **S06.5x9- Traumatic subdural hemorrhage with loss of consciousness of unspecified duration**
Traumatic subdural hemorrhage NOS

S06.6- Traumatic subarachnoid hemorrhage

S06.6x- Traumatic subarachnoid hemorrhage

MCC-A **S06.6x0- Traumatic subarachnoid hemorrhage without loss of consciousness**

MCC-A **S06.6x1- Traumatic subarachnoid hemorrhage with loss of consciousness of 30 minutes or less**

MCC-A **S06.6x2- Traumatic subarachnoid hemorrhage with loss of consciousness of 31 minutes to 59 minutes**

MCC-A **S06.6x3- Traumatic subarachnoid hemorrhage with loss of consciousness of 1 hour to 5 hours 59 minutes**

MCC-A **S06.6x4- Traumatic subarachnoid hemorrhage with loss of consciousness of 6 hours to 24 hours**

MCC-A **S06.6x5- Traumatic subarachnoid hemorrhage with loss of consciousness greater than 24 hours with return to pre-existing conscious level**

MCC-A **S06.6x6- Traumatic subarachnoid hemorrhage with loss of consciousness greater than 24 hours without return to pre-existing conscious level with patient surviving**

MCC-A **S06.6x7- Traumatic subarachnoid hemorrhage with loss of consciousness of any duration with death due to brain injury prior to regaining consciousness**

MCC-A **S06.6x8- Traumatic subarachnoid hemorrhage with loss of consciousness of any duration with death due to other cause prior to regaining consciousness**

MCC-A **S06.6x9- Traumatic subarachnoid hemorrhage with loss of consciousness of unspecified duration**
Traumatic subarachnoid hemorrhage NOS

S06.8- Other specified intracranial injuries

S06.81- Injury of right internal carotid artery, intracranial portion, not elsewhere classified

S06.810- Injury of right internal carotid artery, intracranial portion, not elsewhere classified without loss of consciousness

CC-A **S06.811- Injury of right internal carotid artery, intracranial portion, not elsewhere classified with loss of consciousness of 30 minutes or less**

CC-A **S06.812- Injury of right internal carotid artery, intracranial portion, not elsewhere classified with loss of consciousness of 31 minutes to 59 minutes**

CC-A **S06.813- Injury of right internal carotid artery, intracranial portion, not elsewhere classified with loss of consciousness of 1 hour to 5 hours 59 minutes**

CC-A **S06.814- Injury of right internal carotid artery, intracranial portion, not elsewhere classified with loss of consciousness of 6 hours to 24 hours**

CC-A **S06.815- Injury of right internal carotid artery, intracranial portion, not elsewhere classified with loss of consciousness greater than 24 hours with return to pre-existing conscious level**

MCC-A **S06.816- Injury of right internal carotid artery, intracranial portion, not elsewhere classified with loss of consciousness greater than 24 hours without return to pre-existing conscious level with patient surviving**

MCC-A **S06.817- Injury of right internal carotid artery, intracranial portion, not elsewhere classified with loss of consciousness of any duration with death due to brain injury prior to regaining consciousness**

MCC-A **S06.818- Injury of right internal carotid artery, intracranial portion, not elsewhere classified with loss of consciousness of any duration with death due to other cause prior to regaining consciousness**

CC-A **S06.819- Injury of right internal carotid artery, intracranial portion, not elsewhere classified with loss of consciousness of unspecified duration**
Injury of right internal carotid artery, intracranial portion, not elsewhere classified NOS

S06.82- Injury of left internal carotid artery, intracranial portion, not elsewhere classified

S06.820- Injury of left internal carotid artery, intracranial portion, not elsewhere classified without loss of consciousness

CC-A **S06.821- Injury of left internal carotid artery, intracranial portion, not elsewhere classified with loss of consciousness of 30 minutes or less**

CC-A **S06.822- Injury of left internal carotid artery, intracranial portion, not elsewhere classified with loss of consciousness of 31 minutes to 59 minutes**

CC-A **S06.823- Injury of left internal carotid artery, intracranial portion, not elsewhere classified with loss of consciousness of 1 hour to 5 hours 59 minutes**

CC-A **S06.824- Injury of left internal carotid artery, intracranial portion, not elsewhere classified with loss of consciousness of 6 hours to 24 hours**

CC-A **S06.825- Injury of left internal carotid artery, intracranial portion, not elsewhere classified with loss of consciousness greater than 24 hours with return to pre-existing conscious level**

MCC-A **S06.826- Injury of left internal carotid artery, intracranial portion, not elsewhere classified with loss of consciousness greater than 24 hours without return to pre-existing conscious level with patient surviving**

MCC-A **S06.827- Injury of left internal carotid artery, intracranial portion, not elsewhere classified with loss of consciousness of any duration with death due to brain injury prior to regaining consciousness**

MCC-A **S06.828- Injury of left internal carotid artery, intracranial portion, not elsewhere classified with loss of consciousness of any duration with death due to other cause prior to regaining consciousness**

CC-A **S06.829- Injury of left internal carotid artery, intracranial portion, not elsewhere classified with loss of consciousness of unspecified duration**
Injury of left internal carotid artery, intracranial portion, not elsewhere classified NOS

S06.89- Other specified intracranial injury
Excludes 1:   concussion (S06.0x-)

S06.890- Other specified intracranial injury without loss of consciousness

S06.5 | S06

CC-A **S06.891-** Other specified intracranial injury <u>with</u> loss of consciousness of <u>30 minutes or less</u>

CC-A **S06.892-** Other specified intracranial injury <u>with</u> loss of consciousness of <u>31 minutes to 59 minutes</u>

CC-A **S06.893-** Other specified intracranial injury <u>with</u> loss of consciousness of <u>1 hour to 5 hours 59 minutes</u>

CC-A **S06.894-** Other specified intracranial injury <u>with</u> loss of consciousness of <u>6 hours to 24 hours</u>

CC-A **S06.895-** Other specified intracranial injury <u>with</u> loss of consciousness <u>greater than 24</u> hours <u>with return</u> to pre-existing conscious level

MCC-A **S06.896-** Other specified intracranial injury <u>with</u> loss of consciousness <u>greater than 24</u> hours <u>without return</u> to pre-existing conscious level <u>with patient surviving</u>

MCC-A **S06.897-** Other specified intracranial injury <u>with</u> loss of consciousness of <u>any duration with death</u> due to <u>brain injury</u> prior to regaining consciousness

MCC-A **S06.898-** Other specified intracranial injury <u>with</u> loss of consciousness of <u>any duration with death</u> due to <u>other cause</u> prior to regaining consciousness

CC-A **S06.899-** Other specified intracranial injury <u>with</u> loss of consciousness of <u>unspecified</u> duration

S06.9- **Unspecified intracranial injury**
    Brain injury NOS
    Head injury NOS with loss of consciousness
    Traumatic brain injury NOS
    Excludes 1:   *conditions classifiable to S06.0- to S06.8- code to specified intracranial injury*
                   head injury NOS (S09.90)

S06.9x- <u>Unspecified intracranial injury</u>

    S06.9x0- Unspecified intracranial injury <u>without</u> loss of consciousness

CC-A **S06.9x1-** Unspecified intracranial injury <u>with</u> loss of consciousness of <u>30 minutes or less</u>

CC-A **S06.9x2-** Unspecified intracranial injury <u>with</u> loss of consciousness of <u>31 minutes to 59 minutes</u>

CC-A **S06.9x3-** Unspecified intracranial injury <u>with</u> loss of consciousness of <u>1 hour to 5 hours 59 minutes</u>

CC-A **S06.9x4-** Unspecified intracranial injury <u>with</u> loss of consciousness of <u>6 hours to 24 hours</u>

CC-A **S06.9x5-** Unspecified intracranial injury <u>with</u> loss of consciousness <u>greater than 24</u> hours <u>with return</u> to pre-existing conscious level

MCC-A **S06.9x6-** Unspecified intracranial injury <u>with</u> loss of consciousness <u>greater than 24</u> hours <u>without return</u> to pre-existing conscious level <u>with patient surviving</u>

MCC-A **S06.9x7-** Unspecified intracranial injury <u>with</u> loss of consciousness of <u>any duration with death</u> due to <u>brain injury</u> prior to regaining consciousness

MCC-A **S06.9x8-** Unspecified intracranial injury <u>with</u> loss of consciousness of <u>any duration with death</u> due to <u>other cause</u> prior to regaining consciousness

CC-A **S06.9x9-** Unspecified intracranial injury <u>with</u> loss of consciousness of <u>unspecified</u> duration

S07- **<u>Crushing injury</u> of <u>head</u>**
Use additional code for all associated injuries, such as:
    Intracranial injuries (S06.-)
    Skull fractures (S02.-)

The appropriate 7th character is to be added to each code from category S07:
    A   <u>Initial</u> encounter
    D   <u>Subsequent</u> encounter
    S   <u>Sequela</u>

S07.0xx- Crushing injury of face
CC-A

S07.1xx- Crushing injury of skull
CC-A

S07.8xx- Crushing injury of other parts of head
CC-A

S07.9xx- Crushing injury of head, part <u>unspecified</u>
CC-A

S08- **<u>Avulsion and traumatic amputation</u> of part of head**
Note: An amputation not identified as partial or complete should be coded to complete

The appropriate 7th character is to be added to each code from category S08:
    A   <u>Initial</u> encounter
    D   <u>Subsequent</u> encounter
    S   <u>Sequela</u>

S08.0xx- Avulsion of scalp

S08.1- **<u>Traumatic amputation</u> of <u>ear</u>**
    S08.11- <u>Complete</u> traumatic amputation of ear
        S08.111- Complete traumatic amputation of <u>right</u> ear
        S08.112- Complete traumatic amputation of <u>left</u> ear
        S08.119- Complete traumatic amputation of <u>unspecified</u> ear
    S08.12- <u>Partial</u> traumatic amputation of ear
        S08.121- Partial traumatic amputation of <u>right</u> ear
        S08.122- Partial traumatic amputation of <u>left</u> ear
        S08.129- Partial traumatic amputation of <u>unspecified</u> ear

S08.8- Traumatic amputation of other parts of head
    S08.81- Traumatic amputation of <u>nose</u>
        S08.811- Complete traumatic amputation of nose
        S08.812- Partial traumatic amputation of nose
    S08.89x- Traumatic amputation of other parts of head

S09- **<u>Other and unspecified</u> injuries of head**

The appropriate 7th character is to be added to each code from category S09:
    A   <u>Initial</u> encounter
    D   <u>Subsequent</u> encounter
    S   <u>Sequela</u>

S09.0xx- Injury of blood vessels of head, <u>not elsewhere classified</u>
CC-A   *Excludes 1:*   *injury of cerebral blood vessels (S06.-)*
                          injury of precerebral blood vessels (S15.-)

S09.1- **<u>Injury of muscle and tendon</u> of <u>head</u>**
    Code also any associated open wound (S01.-)
    Excludes ❷: *sprain to joints and ligament of head (S03.9)*
    S09.10x- Unspecified injury of muscle and tendon of head
              Injury of muscle and tendon of head NOS
    S09.11x- Strain of muscle and tendon of head
    S09.12x- Laceration of muscle and tendon of head
    S09.19x- Other specified injury of muscle and tendon of head

S09.2- **<u>Traumatic rupture</u> of <u>ear drum</u>**
    Excludes 1:   *traumatic rupture of ear drum due to blast injury (S09.31-)*
CC-A **S09.20x-** Traumatic rupture of <u>unspecified</u> ear drum
CC-A **S09.21x-** Traumatic rupture of <u>right</u> ear drum
CC-A **S09.22x-** Traumatic rupture of <u>left</u> ear drum

S09.3- Other specified and unspecified injury of <u>middle and inner ear</u>
    Excludes 1:   *injury to ear NOS (S09.91-)*
    Excludes ❷: *injury to external ear (S00.4-, S01.3-, S08.1-)*
    S09.30- <u>Unspecified</u> injury of middle and inner ear
CC-A   **S09.301-** Unspecified injury of <u>right</u> middle and inner ear
CC-A   **S09.302-** Unspecified injury of <u>left</u> middle and inner ear
CC-A   **S09.309-** Unspecified injury of <u>unspecified</u> middle and inner ear
    S09.31- <u>Primary blast</u> injury of ear
              Blast injury of ear NOS
CC-A   **S09.311-** Primary blast injury of <u>right</u> ear
CC-A   **S09.312-** Primary blast injury of <u>left</u> ear
CC-A   **S09.313-** Primary blast injury of ear, <u>bilateral</u>
CC-A   **S09.319-** Primary blast injury of <u>unspecified</u> ear
    S09.39- <u>Other specified injury</u> of middle and inner ear
              Secondary blast injury to ear
CC-A   **S09.391-** Other specified injury of <u>right</u> middle and inner ear
CC-A   **S09.392-** Other specified injury of <u>left</u> middle and inner ear

S06 - S09

CC-A **S09.399-** Other specified injury of <u>unspecified</u> middle and inner ear

S09.8xx- <u>Other</u> specified injuries of head

S09.9- <u>Unspecified</u> injury of face and head

 S09.90x- Unspecified injury of <u>head</u>
  Head injury NOS
  Excludes 1:   brain injury NOS (S06.9-)
  head injury NOS with loss of consciousness (S06.9-)
  intracranial injury NOS (S06.9-)

 S09.91x- Unspecified injury of <u>ear</u>
  Injury of ear NOS

 S09.92x- Unspecified injury of <u>nose</u>
  Injury of nose NOS

 S09.93x- Unspecified injury of <u>face</u>
  Injury of face NOS

Injuries to the neck (S10-S19)

Includes: Injuries of nape
   Injuries of supraclavicular region
   Injuries of throat
Excludes ❷: burns and corrosions (T20-T32)
   effects of foreign body in esophagus (T18.1)
   effects of foreign body in larynx (T17.3)
   effects of foreign body in pharynx (T17.2)
   effects of foreign body in trachea (T17.4)
   frostbite (T33-T34)
   insect bite or sting, venomous (T63.4)

S10- <u>Superficial injury</u> of <u>neck</u>
The appropriate 7th character is to be added to each code from category S10:
 A <u>Initial</u> encounter
 D <u>Subsequent</u> encounter
 S <u>Sequela</u>

 S10.0xx- <u>Contusion</u> of throat
  Contusion of cervical esophagus
  Contusion of larynx
  Contusion of pharynx
  Contusion of trachea

S10.1- <u>Other and unspecified</u> superficial injuries of throat
 S10.10x- Unspecified superficial injuries of throat
 S10.11x- Abrasion of throat
 S10.12x- Blister (nonthermal) of throat
 S10.14x- External constriction of part of throat
 S10.15x- Superficial foreign body of throat
  Splinter in the throat
 S10.16x- Insect bite (nonvenomous) of throat
 S10.17x- Other superficial bite of throat
  Excludes 1:   open bite of throat (S11.85)

S10.8- Superficial injury of <u>other specified parts</u> of neck
 S10.80x- Unspecified superficial injury of other specified part of neck
 S10.81x- Abrasion of other specified part of neck
 S10.82x- Blister (nonthermal) of other specified part of neck
 S10.83x- Contusion of other specified part of neck
 S10.84x- External constriction of other specified part of neck
 S10.85x- Superficial foreign body of other specified part of neck
  Splinter in other specified part of neck
 S10.86x- Insect bite of other specified part of neck
 S10.87x- Other superficial bite of other specified part of neck
  Excludes 1:   open bite of other specified parts of neck (S11.85)

S10.9- Superficial injury of <u>unspecified</u> part of neck
 S10.90x- Unspecified superficial injury of unspecified part of neck
 S10.91x- Abrasion of unspecified part of neck
 S10.92x- Blister (nonthermal) of unspecified part of neck
 S10.93x- Contusion of unspecified part of neck
 S10.94x- External constriction of unspecified part of neck
 S10.95x- Superficial foreign body of unspecified part of neck
 S10.96x- Insect bite of unspecified part of neck

 S10.97x- Other superficial bite of unspecified part of neck

S11- <u>Open wound</u> of <u>neck</u>
Code also any associated:
 Spinal cord injury (S14.0, S14.1-)
 Wound infection
Excludes ❷: open fracture of vertebra (S12.- with 7th character B)
The appropriate 7th character is to be added to each code from category S11:
 A <u>Initial</u> encounter
 D <u>Subsequent</u> encounter
 S <u>Sequela</u>

S11.0- Open wound of larynx and trachea
 S11.01- Open wound of <u>larynx</u>
  Excludes ❷: open wound of vocal cord (S11.03)
 MCC-A **S11.011-** Laceration <u>without</u> foreign body of larynx
 MCC-A **S11.012-** Laceration <u>with foreign body</u> of larynx
 MCC-A **S11.013-** <u>Puncture</u> wound <u>without</u> foreign body of larynx
 MCC-A **S11.014-** <u>Puncture</u> wound <u>with foreign body</u> of larynx
 MCC-A **S11.015-** Open bite of larynx
  Bite of larynx NOS
 MCC-A **S11.019-** Unspecified open wound of larynx
 S11.02- Open wound of <u>trachea</u>
  Open wound of cervical trachea
  Open wound of trachea NOS
  Excludes ❷: open wound of thoracic trachea (S27.5-)
 MCC-A **S11.021-** <u>Laceration</u> <u>without</u> foreign body of trachea
 MCC-A **S11.022-** <u>Laceration</u> <u>with foreign body</u> of trachea
 MCC-A **S11.023-** <u>Puncture</u> wound <u>without</u> foreign body of trachea
 MCC-A **S11.024-** <u>Puncture</u> wound <u>with foreign body</u> of trachea
 MCC-A **S11.025-** Open bite of trachea
  Bite of trachea NOS
 MCC-A **S11.029-** Unspecified open wound of trachea
 S11.03- Open wound of <u>vocal cord</u>
 MCC-A **S11.031-** <u>Laceration</u> <u>without</u> foreign body of vocal cord
 MCC-A **S11.032-** <u>Laceration</u> <u>with foreign body</u> of vocal cord
 MCC-A **S11.033-** <u>Puncture</u> wound <u>without</u> foreign body of vocal cord
 MCC-A **S11.034-** <u>Puncture</u> wound <u>with foreign body</u> of vocal cord
 MCC-A **S11.035-** Open bite of vocal cord
  Bite of vocal cord NOS
 MCC-A **S11.039-** Unspecified open wound of vocal cord

S11.1- Open wound of <u>thyroid gland</u>
 CC-A **S11.10x-** Unspecified open wound of thyroid gland
 CC-A **S11.11x-** Laceration <u>without</u> foreign body of thyroid gland
 CC-A **S11.12x-** Laceration <u>with foreign body</u> of thyroid gland
 CC-A **S11.13x-** <u>Puncture</u> wound <u>without</u> foreign body of thyroid gland
 CC-A **S11.14x-** <u>Puncture</u> wound <u>with foreign body</u> of thyroid gland
 CC-A **S11.15x-** Open bite of thyroid gland
  Bite of thyroid gland NOS

S11.2- Open wound of <u>pharynx and cervical esophagus</u>
  Excludes 1:   open wound of esophagus NOS (S27.8-)
 CC-A **S11.20x-** Unspecified open wound of pharynx and cervical esophagus
 CC-A **S11.21x-** <u>Laceration</u> <u>without</u> foreign body of pharynx and cervical esophagus
 CC-A **S11.22x-** <u>Laceration</u> <u>with foreign body</u> of pharynx and cervical esophagus
 CC-A **S11.23x-** <u>Puncture</u> wound <u>without</u> foreign body of pharynx and cervical esophagus
 CC-A **S11.24x-** <u>Puncture</u> wound <u>with foreign body</u> of pharynx and cervical esophagus
 CC-A **S11.25x-** Open bite of pharynx and cervical esophagus
  Bite of pharynx and cervical esophagus NOS

S11.8- Open wound of <u>other specified parts</u> of neck
 S11.80x- Unspecified open wound of other specified part of neck
 S11.81x- <u>Laceration</u> <u>without</u> foreign body of other specified part of neck
 S11.82x- <u>Laceration</u> <u>with foreign body</u> of other specified part of neck

Excludes 1: = NOT CODED HERE! (Do not code both)

Excludes ❷: = Not Included Here

S11.83x- **Puncture** wound **without** foreign body of other specified part of neck

S11.84x- **Puncture** wound **with foreign body** of other specified part of neck

S11.85x- Open bite of other specified part of neck
Bite of other specified part of neck NOS
Excludes 1: *superficial bite of other specified part of neck (S10.87)*

S11.89x- Other open wound of other specified part of neck

S11.9- Open wound of **unspecified** part of neck

S11.90x- Unspecified open wound of unspecified part of neck

S11.91x- **Laceration without** foreign body of unspecified part of neck

S11.92x- **Laceration with foreign body** of unspecified part of neck

S11.93x- **Puncture** wound **without** foreign body of unspecified part of neck

S11.94x- **Puncture** wound **with foreign body** of unspecified part of neck

S11.95x- Open bite of unspecified part of neck
Bite of neck NOS
Excludes 1: *superficial bite of neck (S10.97)*

S12- **Fracture** of **cervical vertebra** and other parts of neck
Note: A fracture not indicated as nondisplaced or displaced should be classified as displaced
Note: A fracture not indicated as open or closed should be coded to closed
Includes: Fracture of cervical neural arch
Fracture of cervical spine
Fracture of cervical spinous process
Fracture of cervical transverse process
Fracture of cervical vertebral arch
Fracture of neck
Code first any associated cervical spinal cord injury (S14.0, S14.1-)
The appropriate 7th character is to be added to all codes from subcategories S12.0-S12.6:
A **Initial** encounter for **closed** fracture
B **Initial** encounter for **open** fracture
D **Subsequent** encounter for fracture **with routine healing**
G **Subsequent** encounter for fracture **with delayed healing**
K **Subsequent** encounter for fracture **with nonunion**
S **Sequela**

S12.0- Fracture of **first** cervical vertebra
Atlas

S12.00- **Unspecified fracture** of first cervical vertebra

CC-A,K MCC-B S12.000- Unspecified **displaced** fracture of first cervical vertebra

CC-A,K MCC-B S12.001- Unspecified **nondisplaced** fracture of first cervical vertebra

S12.01x- **Stable burst** fracture of first cervical vertebra
CC-A,K MCC-B

S12.02x- **Unstable burst** fracture of first cervical vertebra
CC-A,K MCC-B

S12.03- **Posterior arch** fracture of first cervical vertebra

CC-A,K MCC-B S12.030- **Displaced** posterior arch fracture of first cervical vertebra

CC-A,K MCC-B S12.031- **Nondisplaced** posterior arch fracture of first cervical vertebra

S12.04- **Lateral mass** fracture of first cervical vertebra

CC-A,K MCC-B S12.040- **Displaced** lateral mass fracture of first cervical vertebra

CC-A,K MCC-B S12.041- **Nondisplaced** lateral mass fracture of first cervical vertebra

S12.09- **Other** fracture of first cervical vertebra

CC-A,K MCC-B S12.090- Other **displaced** fracture of first cervical vertebra

CC-A,K MCC-B S12.091- Other **nondisplaced** fracture of first cervical vertebra

S12.1- Fracture of **second** cervical vertebra
Axis

S12.10- **Unspecified fracture** of second cervical vertebra

CC-A,K MCC-B S12.100- Unspecified **displaced** fracture of second cervical vertebra

CC-A,K MCC-B S12.101- Unspecified **nondisplaced** fracture of second cervical vertebra

S12.11- Type II dens fracture

CC-A,K MCC-B S12.110- **Anterior displaced** Type II dens fracture

CC-A,K MCC-B S12.111- **Posterior displaced** Type II dens fracture

CC-A,K MCC-B S12.112- **Nondisplaced** Type II dens fracture

S12.12- **Other dens** fracture

CC-A,K MCC-B S12.120- Other **displaced** dens fracture

CC-A,K MCC-B S12.121- Other **nondisplaced** dens fracture

S12.13- **Unspecified traumatic spondylolisthesis** of second cervical vertebra

CC-A,K MCC-B S12.130- Unspecified traumatic **displaced** spondylolisthesis of second cervical vertebra

CC-A,K MCC-B S12.131- Unspecified traumatic **nondisplaced** spondylolisthesis of second cervical vertebra

S12.14x- **Type III traumatic spondylolisthesis** of second cervical
CC-A,K MCC-B vertebra

S12.15- **Other traumatic spondylolisthesis** of second cervical vertebra

CC-A,K MCC-B S12.150- Other traumatic **displaced** spondylolisthesis of second cervical vertebra

CC-A,K MCC-B S12.151- Other traumatic **nondisplaced** spondylolisthesis of second cervical vertebra

S12.19- **Other fracture** of second cervical vertebra

CC-A,K MCC-B S12.190- Other **displaced** fracture of second cervical vertebra

CC-A,K MCC-B S12.191- Other **nondisplaced** fracture of second cervical vertebra

S12.2- Fracture of **third** cervical vertebra

S12.20- **Unspecified fracture** of third cervical vertebra

CC-A,K MCC-B S12.200- Unspecified **displaced** fracture of third cervical vertebra

CC-A,K MCC-B S12.201- Unspecified **nondisplaced** fracture of third cervical vertebra

S12.23- **Unspecified traumatic spondylolisthesis** of third cervical vertebra

CC-A,K MCC-B S12.230- Unspecified traumatic **displaced** spondylolisthesis of third cervical vertebra

CC-A,K MCC-B S12.231- Unspecified traumatic **nondisplaced** spondylolisthesis of third cervical vertebra

S12.24x- **Type III traumatic spondylolisthesis** of third cervical
CC-A,K MCC-B vertebra

S12.25- **Other traumatic spondylolisthesis** of third cervical vertebra

CC-A,K MCC-B S12.250- Other traumatic **displaced** spondylolisthesis of third cervical vertebra

CC-A,K MCC-B S12.251- Other traumatic **nondisplaced** spondylolisthesis of third cervical vertebra

S12.29- **Other fracture** of third cervical vertebra

CC-A,K MCC-B S12.290- Other **displaced** fracture of third cervical vertebra

CC-A,K MCC-B S12.291- Other **nondisplaced** fracture of third cervical vertebra

S12.3- **Fracture** of **fourth** cervical vertebra

S12.30- **Unspecified fracture** of fourth cervical vertebra

CC-A,K MCC-B S12.300- Unspecified **displaced** fracture of fourth cervical vertebra

CC-A,K MCC-B S12.301- Unspecified **nondisplaced** fracture of fourth cervical vertebra

S12.33- **Unspecified traumatic spondylolisthesis** of fourth cervical vertebra

CC-A,K MCC-B S12.330- Unspecified traumatic **displaced** spondylolisthesis of fourth cervical vertebra

CC-A,K MCC-B S12.331- Unspecified traumatic **nondisplaced** spondylolisthesis of fourth cervical vertebra

S12.34x- **Type III traumatic spondylolisthesis** of fourth cervical
CC-A,K MCC-B vertebra

S12.35- **Other traumatic spondylolisthesis** of fourth cervical vertebra

S11-S12

CC-A,K MCC-B **S12.350-** Other traumatic <u>displaced</u> spondylolisthesis of fourth cervical vertebra

CC-A,K MCC-B **S12.351-** Other traumatic <u>nondisplaced</u> spondylolisthesis of fourth cervical vertebra

S12.39- <u>Other fracture</u> of fourth cervical vertebra

CC-A,K MCC-B **S12.390-** Other <u>displaced</u> fracture of fourth cervical vertebra

CC-A,K MCC-B **S12.391-** Other <u>nondisplaced</u> fracture of fourth cervical vertebra

S12.4- <u>Fracture</u> of <u>fifth</u> cervical vertebra

S12.40- <u>Unspecified fracture</u> of fifth cervical vertebra

CC-A,K MCC-B **S12.400-** Unspecified <u>displaced</u> fracture of fifth cervical vertebra

CC-A,K MCC-B **S12.401-** Unspecified <u>nondisplaced</u> fracture of fifth cervical vertebra

S12.43- <u>Unspecified traumatic spondylolisthesis</u> of fifth cervical vertebra

CC-A,K MCC-B **S12.430-** Unspecified traumatic <u>displaced</u> spondylolisthesis of fifth cervical vertebra

CC-A,K MCC-B **S12.431-** Unspecified traumatic <u>nondisplaced</u> spondylolisthesis of fifth cervical vertebra

S12.44x- <u>Type III traumatic spondylolisthesis</u> of fifth cervical
CC-A,K MCC-B vertebra

S12.45- <u>Other traumatic spondylolisthesis</u> of fifth cervical vertebra

CC-A,K MCC-B **S12.450-** Other traumatic <u>displaced</u> spondylolisthesis of fifth cervical vertebra

CC-A,K MCC-B **S12.451-** Other traumatic <u>nondisplaced</u> spondylolisthesis of fifth cervical vertebra

S12.49- <u>Other fracture</u> of fifth cervical vertebra

CC-A,K MCC-B **S12.490-** Other <u>displaced</u> fracture of fifth cervical vertebra

CC-A,K MCC-B **S12.491-** Other <u>nondisplaced</u> fracture of fifth cervical vertebra

S12.5- <u>Fracture</u> of <u>sixth</u> cervical vertebra

S12.50- <u>Unspecified fracture</u> of sixth cervical vertebra

CC-A,K MCC-B **S12.500-** Unspecified <u>displaced</u> fracture of sixth cervical vertebra

CC-A,K MCC-B **S12.501-** Unspecified <u>nondisplaced</u> fracture of sixth cervical vertebra

S12.53- <u>Unspecified traumatic spondylolisthesis</u> of sixth cervical vertebra

CC-A,K MCC-B **S12.530-** Unspecified traumatic <u>displaced</u> spondylolisthesis of sixth cervical vertebra

CC-A,K MCC-B **S12.531-** Unspecified traumatic <u>nondisplaced</u> spondylolisthesis of sixth cervical vertebra

S12.54x- <u>Type III traumatic spondylolisthesis</u> of sixth cervical
CC-A,K MCC-B vertebra

S12.55- <u>Other traumatic spondylolisthesis</u> of sixth cervical vertebra

CC-A,K MCC-B **S12.550-** Other traumatic <u>displaced</u> spondylolisthesis of sixth cervical vertebra

CC-A,K MCC-B **S12.551-** Other traumatic <u>nondisplaced</u> spondylolisthesis of sixth cervical vertebra

S12.59- <u>Other fracture</u> of sixth cervical vertebra

CC-A,K MCC-B **S12.590-** Other <u>displaced</u> fracture of sixth cervical vertebra

CC-A,K MCC-B **S12.591-** Other <u>nondisplaced</u> fracture of sixth cervical vertebra

S12.6- <u>Fracture</u> of <u>seventh</u> cervical vertebra

S12.60- <u>Unspecified fracture</u> of seventh cervical vertebra

CC-A,K MCC-B **S12.600-** Unspecified <u>displaced</u> fracture of seventh cervical vertebra

CC-A,K MCC-B **S12.601-** Unspecified <u>nondisplaced</u> fracture of seventh cervical vertebra

S12.63- <u>Unspecified traumatic spondylolisthesis</u> of seventh cervical vertebra

CC-A,K MCC-B **S12.630-** Unspecified traumatic <u>displaced</u> spondylolisthesis of seventh cervical vertebra

CC-A,K MCC-B **S12.631-** Unspecified traumatic <u>nondisplaced</u> spondylolisthesis of seventh cervical vertebra

S12.64x- <u>Type III traumatic spondylolisthesis</u> of seventh cervical
CC-A,K MCC-B vertebra

S12.65- <u>Other traumatic spondylolisthesis</u> of seventh cervical vertebra

CC-A,K MCC-B **S12.650-** Other traumatic <u>displaced</u> spondylolisthesis of seventh cervical vertebra

CC-A,K MCC-B **S12.651-** Other traumatic <u>nondisplaced</u> spondylolisthesis of seventh cervical vertebra

S12.69- <u>Other fracture</u> of seventh cervical vertebra

CC-A,K MCC-B **S12.690-** Other <u>displaced</u> fracture of seventh cervical vertebra

CC-A,K MCC-B **S12.691-** Other <u>nondisplaced</u> fracture of seventh cervical vertebra

S12.8xx- <u>Fracture</u> of <u>other parts of neck</u>
MCC-A   Hyoid bone
   Larynx
   Thyroid cartilage
   Trachea

The appropriate 7th character is to be added to code S12.8:
  A <u>Initial</u> encounter
  D <u>Subsequent</u> encounter
  S <u>Sequela</u>

S12.9xx- <u>Fracture</u> of <u>neck, unspecified</u>
CC-A   Fracture of neck NOS
   Fracture of cervical spine NOS
   Fracture of cervical vertebra NOS

The appropriate 7th character is to be added to code S12.9:
  A <u>Initial</u> encounter
  D <u>Subsequent</u> encounter
  S <u>Sequela</u>

S13- <u>Dislocation and sprain</u> of joints and ligaments at <u>neck</u> level
Includes: Avulsion of joint or ligament at neck level
   Laceration of cartilage, joint or ligament at neck level
   Sprain of cartilage, joint or ligament at neck level
   Traumatic hemarthrosis of joint or ligament at neck level
   Traumatic rupture of joint or ligament at neck level
   Traumatic subluxation of joint or ligament at neck level
   Traumatic tear of joint or ligament at neck level
Code also any associated open wound
Excludes ❷: strain of muscle or tendon at neck level (S16.1)

The appropriate 7th character is to be added to each code from category S13:
  A <u>Initial</u> encounter
  D <u>Subsequent</u> encounter
  S <u>Sequela</u>

S13.0xx- <u>Traumatic rupture</u> of <u>cervical intervertebral disc</u>
CC-A   *Excludes 1: rupture or displacement (nontraumatic) of cervical intervertebral disc NOS (M50.-)*

S13.1- <u>Subluxation and dislocation</u> of <u>cervical vertebrae</u>
   Code also any associated:
    Open wound of neck (S11.-)
    Spinal cord injury (S14.1-)
   Excludes ❷: fracture of cervical vertebrae (S12.0-S12.3-)

S13.10- Subluxation and dislocation of <u>unspecified</u> cervical vertebrae

CC-A **S13.100-** <u>Subluxation</u> of unspecified cervical vertebrae

CC-A **S13.101-** <u>Dislocation</u> of unspecified cervical vertebrae

S13.11- Subluxation and dislocation of <u>C0/C1</u> cervical vertebrae
   Subluxation and dislocation of atlantooccipital joint
   Subluxation and dislocation of atloidooccipital joint
   Subluxation and dislocation of occipitoatloid joint

CC-A **S13.110-** <u>Subluxation</u> of C0/C1 cervical vertebrae

CC-A **S13.111-** <u>Dislocation</u> of C0/C1 cervical vertebrae

S13.12- Subluxation and dislocation of <u>C1/C2</u> cervical vertebrae
   Subluxation and dislocation of atlantoaxial joint

CC-A **S13.120-** <u>Subluxation</u> of C1/C2 cervical vertebrae

CC-A **S13.121-** <u>Dislocation</u> of C1/C2 cervical vertebrae

S13.13- Subluxation and dislocation of <u>C2/C3</u> cervical vertebrae

CC-A **S13.130-** <u>Subluxation</u> of C2/C3 cervical vertebrae

CC-A **S13.131-** <u>Dislocation</u> of C2/C3 cervical vertebrae

S13.14- Subluxation and dislocation of <u>C3/C4</u> cervical vertebrae

CC-A **S13.140-** <u>Subluxation</u> of C3/C4 cervical vertebrae

CC-A **S13.141-** <u>Dislocation</u> of C3/C4 cervical vertebrae

S12 - S13

S13.15- Subluxation and dislocation of <u>C4/C5</u> cervical vertebrae
CC-A **S13.150-** <u>Subluxation</u> of C4/C5 cervical vertebrae
CC-A **S13.151-** <u>Dislocation</u> of C4/C5 cervical vertebrae
S13.16- Subluxation and dislocation of <u>C5/C6</u> cervical vertebrae
CC-A **S13.160-** <u>Subluxation</u> of C5/C6 cervical vertebrae
CC-A **S13.161-** <u>Dislocation</u> of C5/C6 cervical vertebrae
S13.17- Subluxation and dislocation of <u>C6/C7</u> cervical vertebrae
CC-A **S13.170-** <u>Subluxation</u> of C6/C7 cervical vertebrae
CC-A **S13.171-** <u>Dislocation</u> of C6/C7 cervical vertebrae
S13.18- Subluxation and dislocation of <u>C7/T1</u> cervical vertebrae
CC-A **S13.180-** <u>Subluxation</u> of C7/T1 cervical vertebrae
CC-A **S13.181-** <u>Dislocation</u> of C7/T1 cervical vertebrae
S13.2- Dislocation of other and <u>unspecified</u> parts of neck
CC-A **S13.20x-** Dislocation of <u>unspecified</u> parts of neck
CC-A **S13.29x-** Dislocation of <u>other</u> parts of neck
S13.4xx- <u>Sprain of ligaments</u> of cervical spine
  Sprain of anterior longitudinal (ligament), cervical
  Sprain of atlanto-axial (joints)
  Sprain of atlanto-occipital (joints)
  Whiplash injury of cervical spine
S13.5xx- Sprain of thyroid region
  Sprain of cricoarytenoid (joint) (ligament)
  Sprain of cricothyroid (joint) (ligament)
  Sprain of thyroid cartilage
S13.8xx- Sprain of joints and ligaments of <u>other</u> parts of neck
S13.9xx- Sprain of joints and ligaments of <u>unspecified</u> parts of neck

S14- <u>Injury of nerves and spinal cord</u> at <u>neck</u> level
  Note: Code to highest level of cervical cord injury
  Code also any associated:
    Fracture of cervical vertebra (S12.0- -S12.6.-)
    Open wound of neck (S11.-)
    Transient paralysis (R29.5)

The appropriate 7th character is to be added to each code from
  category S14:
  A   <u>Initial</u> encounter
  D   <u>Subsequent</u> encounter
  S   <u>Sequela</u>

S14.0xx- <u>Concussion and edema</u> of cervical spinal cord
MCC-A
S14.1- Other and unspecified injuries of cervical spinal cord
  S14.10- <u>Unspecified injury</u> of cervical spinal cord
  MCC-A **S14.101-** Unspecified injury at <u>C1</u> level of cervical spinal
          cord
  MCC-A **S14.102-** Unspecified injury at <u>C2</u> level of cervical spinal
          cord
  MCC-A **S14.103-** Unspecified injury at <u>C3</u> level of cervical spinal
          cord
  MCC-A **S14.104-** Unspecified injury at <u>C4</u> level of cervical spinal
          cord
  MCC-A **S14.105-** Unspecified injury at <u>C5</u> level of cervical spinal
          cord
  MCC-A **S14.106-** Unspecified injury at <u>C6</u> level of cervical spinal
          cord
  MCC-A **S14.107-** Unspecified injury at <u>C7</u> level of cervical spinal
          cord
  MCC-A **S14.108-** Unspecified injury at <u>C8</u> level of cervical spinal
          cord
        S14.109- Unspecified injury at <u>unspecified</u> level of cervical
          spinal cord
          Injury of cervical spinal cord NOS
  S14.11- <u>Complete lesion</u> of cervical spinal cord
  MCC-A **S14.111-** Complete lesion at <u>C1</u> level of cervical spinal cord
  MCC-A **S14.112-** Complete lesion at <u>C2</u> level of cervical spinal cord
  MCC-A **S14.113-** Complete lesion at <u>C3</u> level of cervical spinal cord
  MCC-A **S14.114-** Complete lesion at <u>C4</u> level of cervical spinal cord
  MCC-A **S14.115-** Complete lesion at <u>C5</u> level of cervical spinal cord
  MCC-A **S14.116-** Complete lesion at <u>C6</u> level of cervical spinal cord
  MCC-A **S14.117-** Complete lesion at <u>C7</u> level of cervical spinal cord
  MCC-A **S14.118-** Complete lesion at <u>C8</u> level of cervical spinal cord

S14.119- Complete lesion at <u>unspecified</u> level of cervical
          spinal cord
S14.12- <u>Central cord syndrome</u> of cervical spinal cord
MCC-A **S14.121-** Central cord syndrome at <u>C1</u> level of cervical spinal
          cord
MCC-A **S14.122-** Central cord syndrome at <u>C2</u> level of cervical spinal
          cord
MCC-A **S14.123-** Central cord syndrome at <u>C3</u> level of cervical spinal
          cord
MCC-A **S14.124-** Central cord syndrome at <u>C4</u> level of cervical spinal
          cord
MCC-A **S14.125-** Central cord syndrome at <u>C5</u> level of cervical spinal
          cord
MCC-A **S14.126-** Central cord syndrome at <u>C6</u> level of cervical spinal
          cord
MCC-A **S14.127-** Central cord syndrome at <u>C7</u> level of cervical spinal
          cord
MCC-A **S14.128-** Central cord syndrome at <u>C8</u> level of cervical spinal
          cord
       S14.129- Central cord syndrome at <u>unspecified</u> level of
          cervical spinal cord
S14.13- <u>Anterior cord syndrome</u> of cervical spinal cord
MCC-A **S14.131-** Anterior cord syndrome at <u>C1</u> level of cervical
          spinal cord
MCC-A **S14.132-** Anterior cord syndrome at <u>C2</u> level of cervical
          spinal cord
MCC-A **S14.133-** Anterior cord syndrome at <u>C3</u> level of cervical
          spinal cord
MCC-A **S14.134-** Anterior cord syndrome at <u>C4</u> level of cervical
          spinal cord
MCC-A **S14.135-** Anterior cord syndrome at <u>C5</u> level of cervical
          spinal cord
MCC-A **S14.136-** Anterior cord syndrome at <u>C6</u> level of cervical
          spinal cord
MCC-A **S14.137-** Anterior cord syndrome at <u>C7</u> level of cervical
          spinal cord
MCC-A **S14.138-** Anterior cord syndrome at <u>C8</u> level of cervical
          spinal cord
       S14.139- Anterior cord syndrome at <u>unspecified</u> level of
          cervical spinal cord
S14.14- <u>Brown-Séquard syndrome</u> of cervical spinal cord
MCC-A **S14.141-** Brown-Séquard syndrome at <u>C1</u> level of cervical
          spinal cord
MCC-A **S14.142-** Brown-Séquard syndrome at <u>C2</u> level of cervical
          spinal cord
MCC-A **S14.143-** Brown-Séquard syndrome at <u>C3</u> level of cervical
          spinal cord
MCC-A **S14.144-** Brown-Séquard syndrome at <u>C4</u> level of cervical
          spinal cord
MCC-A **S14.145-** Brown-Séquard syndrome at <u>C5</u> level of cervical
          spinal cord
MCC-A **S14.146-** Brown-Séquard syndrome at <u>C6</u> level of cervical
          spinal cord
MCC-A **S14.147-** Brown-Séquard syndrome at <u>C7</u> level of cervical
          spinal cord
MCC-A **S14.148-** Brown-Séquard syndrome at <u>C8</u> level of cervical
          spinal cord
       S14.149- Brown-Séquard syndrome at <u>unspecified</u> level of
          cervical spinal cord
S14.15- <u>Other incomplete lesions</u> of cervical spinal cord
          Incomplete lesion of cervical spinal cord NOS
          Posterior cord syndrome of cervical spinal cord
MCC-A **S14.151-** Other incomplete lesion at <u>C1</u> level of cervical
          spinal cord
MCC-A **S14.152-** Other incomplete lesion at <u>C2</u> level of cervical
          spinal cord
MCC-A **S14.153-** Other incomplete lesion at <u>C3</u> level of cervical
          spinal cord

S13 - S14

MCC-A **S14.154-** Other incomplete lesion at <u>C4</u> level of cervical spinal cord

MCC-A **S14.155-** Other incomplete lesion at <u>C5</u> level of cervical spinal cord

MCC-A **S14.156-** Other incomplete lesion at <u>C6</u> level of cervical spinal cord

MCC-A **S14.157-** Other incomplete lesion at <u>C7</u> level of cervical spinal cord

MCC-A **S14.158-** Other incomplete lesion at <u>C8</u> level of cervical spinal cord

S14.159- Other incomplete lesion at <u>unspecified</u> level of cervical spinal cord

S14.2xx- Injury of nerve root of cervical spine

S14.3xx- Injury of brachial plexus

S14.4xx- Injury of peripheral nerves of neck

S14.5xx- Injury of cervical sympathetic nerves

S14.8xx- Injury of <u>other</u> specified nerves of neck

S14.9xx- Injury of <u>unspecified</u> nerves of neck

S15- <u>Injury of blood vessels</u> at <u>neck</u> level
Code also any associated open wound (S11.-)

The appropriate 7th character is to be added to each code from category S15:
A <u>Initial</u> encounter
D <u>Subsequent</u> encounter
S <u>Sequela</u>

S15.0- Injury of <u>carotid artery</u> of neck
Injury of carotid artery (common) (external) (internal, extracranial portion)
Injury of carotid artery NOS
Excludes 1: injury of internal carotid artery, intracranial portion (S06.8)

S15.00- <u>Unspecified</u> injury of carotid artery

CC-A **S15.001-** Unspecified injury of <u>right</u> carotid artery

CC-A **S15.002-** Unspecified injury of <u>left</u> carotid artery

CC-A **S15.009-** Unspecified injury of <u>unspecified</u> carotid artery

S15.01- <u>Minor laceration</u> of carotid artery
Incomplete transection of carotid artery
Laceration of carotid artery NOS
Superficial laceration of carotid artery

CC-A **S15.011-** Minor laceration of <u>right</u> carotid artery

CC-A **S15.012-** Minor laceration of <u>left</u> carotid artery

CC-A **S15.019-** Minor laceration of <u>unspecified</u> carotid artery

S15.02- <u>Major laceration</u> of carotid artery
Complete transection of carotid artery
Traumatic rupture of carotid artery

CC-A **S15.021-** Major laceration of <u>right</u> carotid artery

CC-A **S15.022-** Major laceration of <u>left</u> carotid artery

CC-A **S15.029-** Major laceration of <u>unspecified</u> carotid artery

S15.09- <u>Other specified</u> injury of carotid artery

CC-A **S15.091-** Other specified injury of <u>right</u> carotid artery

CC-A **S15.092-** Other specified injury of <u>left</u> carotid artery

CC-A **S15.099-** Other specified injury of <u>unspecified</u> carotid artery

S15.1- Injury of <u>vertebral artery</u>

S15.10- <u>Unspecified</u> injury of vertebral artery

CC-A **S15.101-** Unspecified injury of <u>right</u> vertebral artery

CC-A **S15.102-** Unspecified injury of <u>left</u> vertebral artery

CC-A **S15.109-** Unspecified injury of <u>unspecified</u> vertebral artery

S15.11- <u>Minor laceration</u> of vertebral artery
Incomplete transection of vertebral artery
Laceration of vertebral artery NOS
Superficial laceration of vertebral artery

CC-A **S15.111-** Minor laceration of <u>right</u> vertebral artery

CC-A **S15.112-** Minor laceration of <u>left</u> vertebral artery

CC-A **S15.119-** Minor laceration of <u>unspecified</u> vertebral artery

S15.12- <u>Major laceration</u> of vertebral artery
Complete transection of vertebral artery
Traumatic rupture of vertebral artery

CC-A **S15.121-** Major laceration of <u>right</u> vertebral artery

CC-A **S15.122-** Major laceration of <u>left</u> vertebral artery

CC-A **S15.129-** Major laceration of <u>unspecified</u> vertebral artery

S15.19- <u>Other specified</u> injury of vertebral artery

CC-A **S15.191-** Other specified injury of <u>right</u> vertebral artery

CC-A **S15.192-** Other specified injury of <u>left</u> vertebral artery

CC-A **S15.199-** Other specified injury of <u>unspecified</u> vertebral artery

S15.2- Injury of <u>external jugular vein</u>

S15.20- <u>Unspecified</u> injury of external jugular vein

CC-A **S15.201-** Unspecified injury of <u>right</u> external jugular vein

CC-A **S15.202-** Unspecified injury of <u>left</u> external jugular vein

CC-A **S15.209-** Unspecified injury of <u>unspecified</u> external jugular vein

S15.21- <u>Minor laceration</u> of external jugular vein
Incomplete transection of external jugular vein
Laceration of external jugular vein NOS
Superficial laceration of external jugular vein

CC-A **S15.211-** Minor laceration of <u>right</u> external jugular vein

CC-A **S15.212-** Minor laceration of <u>left</u> external jugular vein

CC-A **S15.219-** Minor laceration of <u>unspecified</u> external jugular vein

S15.22- <u>Major laceration</u> of external jugular vein
Complete transection of external jugular vein
Traumatic rupture of external jugular vein

CC-A **S15.221-** Major laceration of <u>right</u> external jugular vein

CC-A **S15.222-** Major laceration of <u>left</u> external jugular vein

CC-A **S15.229-** Major laceration of <u>unspecified</u> external jugular vein

S15.29- <u>Other specified</u> injury of external jugular vein

CC-A **S15.291-** Other specified injury of <u>right</u> external jugular vein

CC-A **S15.292-** Other specified injury of <u>left</u> external jugular vein

CC-A **S15.299-** Other specified injury of <u>unspecified</u> external jugular vein

S15.3- Injury of <u>internal jugular vein</u>

S15.30- <u>Unspecified</u> injury of internal jugular vein

CC-A **S15.301-** Unspecified injury of <u>right</u> internal jugular vein

CC-A **S15.302-** Unspecified injury of <u>left</u> internal jugular vein

CC-A **S15.309-** Unspecified injury of <u>unspecified</u> internal jugular vein

S15.31- <u>Minor laceration</u> of internal jugular vein
Incomplete transection of internal jugular vein
Laceration of internal jugular vein NOS
Superficial laceration of internal jugular vein

CC-A **S15.311-** Minor laceration of <u>right</u> internal jugular vein

CC-A **S15.312-** Minor laceration of <u>left</u> internal jugular vein

CC-A **S15.319-** Minor laceration of <u>unspecified</u> internal jugular vein

S15.32- <u>Major laceration</u> of internal jugular vein
Complete transection of internal jugular vein
Traumatic rupture of internal jugular vein

CC-A **S15.321-** Major laceration of <u>right</u> internal jugular vein

CC-A **S15.322-** Major laceration of <u>left</u> internal jugular vein

CC-A **S15.329-** Major laceration of <u>unspecified</u> internal jugular vein

S15.39- <u>Other specified</u> injury of internal jugular vein

CC-A **S15.391-** Other specified injury of <u>right</u> internal jugular vein

CC-A **S15.392-** Other specified injury of <u>left</u> internal jugular vein

CC-A **S15.399-** Other specified injury of <u>unspecified</u> internal jugular vein

S15.8xx- Injury of <u>other</u> specified blood vessels at neck level
CC-A

S15.9xx- Injury of <u>unspecified</u> blood vessel at neck level
CC-A

S16- <u>Injury of muscle, fascia and tendon</u> at <u>neck</u> level
Code also any associated open wound (S11.-)
Excludes ❷: sprain of joint or ligament at neck level (S13.9)

The appropriate 7th character is to be added to each code from category S16:
A <u>Initial</u> encounter
D <u>Subsequent</u> encounter
S <u>Sequela</u>

S16.1xx- <u>Strain</u> of muscle, fascia and tendon at neck level

S14-S16

S16.2xx- <u>Laceration</u> of muscle, fascia and tendon at neck level

S16.8xx- <u>Other</u> specified injury of muscle, fascia and tendon at neck level

S16.9xx- <u>Unspecified</u> injury of muscle, fascia and tendon at neck level

S17- <u>Crushing</u> injury of neck
Use additional code for all associated injuries, such as:
   Injury of blood vessels (S15.-)
   Open wound of neck (S11.-)
   Spinal cord injury (S14.0, S14.1-)
   Vertebral fracture (S12.0--S12.3-)

The appropriate 7th character is to be added to each code from category S17:
  A <u>Initial</u> encounter
  D <u>Subsequent</u> encounter
  S <u>Sequela</u>

S17.0xx- Crushing injury of <u>larynx and trachea</u>
CC-A

S17.8xx- Crushing injury of <u>other</u> specified parts of neck
CC-A

S17.9xx- Crushing injury of neck, part <u>unspecified</u>
CC-A

S19- Other specified and unspecified injuries of neck
The appropriate 7th character is to be added to each code from category S19:
  A <u>Initial</u> encounter
  D <u>Subsequent</u> encounter
  S <u>Sequela</u>

S19.8- <u>Other specified</u> injuries of neck

   S19.80x- Other specified injuries of <u>unspecified</u> part of neck

   S19.81x- Other specified injuries of <u>larynx</u>

   S19.82x- Other specified injuries of <u>cervical trachea</u>
      Excludes ❷: other specified injury of thoracic trachea (S27.5-)

   S19.83x- Other specified injuries of <u>vocal cord</u>

   S19.84x- Other specified injuries of <u>thyroid gland</u>

   S19.85x- Other specified injuries of <u>pharynx and cervical esophagus</u>

   S19.89x- Other specified injuries of <u>other specified</u> part of neck

S19.9xx- <u>Unspecified</u> injury of neck

Injuries to the thorax (S20-S29)

Includes: Injuries of breast
           Injuries of chest (wall)
           Injuries of interscapular area
Excludes ❷: burns and corrosions (T20-T32)
       effects of foreign body in bronchus (T17.5)
       effects of foreign body in esophagus (T18.1)
       effects of foreign body in lung (T17.8)
       effects of foreign body in trachea (T17.4)
       frostbite (T33-T34)
       injuries of axilla
       injuries of clavicle
       injuries of scapular region
       injuries of shoulder
       insect bite or sting, venomous (T63.4)

S20- <u>Superficial injury</u> of <u>thorax</u>
The appropriate 7th character is to be added to each code from category S20:
  A <u>Initial</u> encounter
  D <u>Subsequent</u> encounter
  S <u>Sequela</u>

S20.0- <u>Contusion</u> of <u>breast</u>

   S20.00x- Contusion of breast, <u>unspecified</u> breast

   S20.01x- Contusion of <u>right</u> breast

   S20.02x- Contusion of <u>left</u> breast

S20.1- Other and unspecified superficial injuries of <u>breast</u>

  S20.10- <u>Unspecified</u> superficial injuries of breast

     S20.101- Unspecified superficial injuries of breast, <u>right</u> breast

     S20.102- Unspecified superficial injuries of breast, <u>left</u> breast

     S20.109- Unspecified superficial injuries of breast, <u>unspecified</u> breast

  S20.11- <u>Abrasion</u> of breast

     S20.111- Abrasion of breast, <u>right</u> breast

     S20.112- Abrasion of breast, <u>left</u> breast

     S20.119- Abrasion of breast, <u>unspecified</u> breast

  S20.12- <u>Blister</u> (nonthermal) of breast

     S20.121- Blister (nonthermal) of breast, <u>right</u> breast

     S20.122- Blister (nonthermal) of breast, <u>left</u> breast

     S20.129- Blister (nonthermal) of breast, <u>unspecified</u> breast

  S20.14- <u>External constriction</u> of part of breast

     S20.141- External constriction of part of breast, <u>right</u> breast

     S20.142- External constriction of part of breast, <u>left</u> breast

     S20.149- External constriction of part of breast, <u>unspecified</u> breast

  S20.15- <u>Superficial foreign body</u> of breast
     Splinter in the breast

     S20.151- Superficial foreign body of breast, <u>right</u> breast

     S20.152- Superficial foreign body of breast, <u>left</u> breast

     S20.159- Superficial foreign body of breast, <u>unspecified</u> breast

  S20.16- <u>Insect bite (nonvenomous)</u> of breast

     S20.161- Insect bite (nonvenomous) of breast, <u>right</u> breast

     S20.162- Insect bite (nonvenomous) of breast, <u>left</u> breast

     S20.169- Insect bite (nonvenomous) of breast, <u>unspecified</u> breast

  S20.17- <u>Other superficial bite</u> of breast
     Excludes 1: open bite of breast (S21.05-)

     S20.171- Other superficial bite of breast, <u>right</u> breast

     S20.172- Other superficial bite of breast, <u>left</u> breast

     S20.179- Other superficial bite of breast, <u>unspecified</u> breast

S20.2- <u>Contusion</u> of <u>thorax</u>

  S20.20x- Contusion of thorax, <u>unspecified</u>

  S20.21- Contusion of <u>front wall</u> of thorax

     S20.211- Contusion of <u>right</u> front wall of thorax

     S20.212- Contusion of <u>left</u> front wall of thorax

     S20.219- Contusion of <u>unspecified</u> front wall of thorax

  S20.22- Contusion of <u>back wall</u> of thorax

     S20.221- Contusion of <u>right</u> back wall of thorax

     S20.222- Contusion of <u>left</u> back wall of thorax

     S20.229- Contusion of <u>unspecified</u> back wall of thorax

S20.3- Other and unspecified superficial injuries of <u>front wall</u> of thorax

  S20.30- <u>Unspecified</u> superficial injuries of <u>front wall</u> of thorax

     S20.301- Unspecified superficial injuries of <u>right</u> front wall of thorax

     S20.302- Unspecified superficial injuries of <u>left</u> front wall of thorax

     S20.309- Unspecified superficial injuries of <u>unspecified</u> front wall of thorax

  S20.31- <u>Abrasion</u> of <u>front wall</u> of thorax

     S20.311- Abrasion of <u>right</u> front wall of thorax

     S20.312- Abrasion of <u>left</u> front wall of thorax

     S20.319- Abrasion of <u>unspecified</u> front wall of thorax

  S20.32- <u>Blister</u> (nonthermal) of <u>front wall</u> of thorax

     S20.321- Blister (nonthermal) of <u>right</u> front wall of thorax

     S20.322- Blister (nonthermal) of <u>left</u> front wall of thorax

     S20.329- Blister (nonthermal) of <u>unspecified</u> front wall of thorax

  S20.34- <u>External constriction</u> of <u>front wall</u> of thorax

     S20.341- External constriction of <u>right</u> front wall of thorax

     S20.342- External constriction of <u>left</u> front wall of thorax

     S20.349- External constriction of <u>unspecified</u> front wall of thorax

S16 - S20

S20.35- <u>Superficial foreign body</u> of <u>front wall</u> of thorax
Splinter in front wall of thorax
- **S20.351-** Superficial foreign body of <u>right</u> front wall of thorax
- **S20.352-** Superficial foreign body of <u>left</u> front wall of thorax
- **S20.359-** Superficial foreign body of <u>unspecified</u> front wall of thorax

S20.36- <u>Insect bite (nonvenomous)</u> of <u>front wall</u> of thorax
- **S20.361-** Insect bite (nonvenomous) of <u>right</u> front wall of thorax
- **S20.362-** Insect bite (nonvenomous) of <u>left</u> front wall of thorax
- **S20.369-** Insect bite (nonvenomous) of <u>unspecified</u> front wall of thorax

S20.37- <u>Other superficial bite</u> of <u>front wall</u> of thorax
Excludes 1:   open bite of front wall of thorax (S21.14)
- **S20.371-** Other superficial bite of <u>right</u> front wall of thorax
- **S20.372-** Other superficial bite of <u>left</u> front wall of thorax
- **S20.379-** Other superficial bite of <u>unspecified</u> front wall of thorax

S20.4- Other and unspecified superficial injuries of back wall of <u>thorax</u>

S20.40- <u>Unspecified</u> superficial injuries of <u>back wall</u> of thorax
- **S20.401-** Unspecified superficial injuries of <u>right</u> back wall of thorax
- **S20.402-** Unspecified superficial injuries of <u>left</u> back wall of thorax
- **S20.409-** Unspecified superficial injuries of <u>unspecified</u> back wall of thorax

S20.41- <u>Abrasion</u> of <u>back wall</u> of thorax
- **S20.411-** Abrasion of <u>right</u> back wall of thorax
- **S20.412-** Abrasion of <u>left</u> back wall of thorax
- **S20.419-** Abrasion of <u>unspecified</u> back wall of thorax

S20.42- <u>Blister</u> (nonthermal) of <u>back wall</u> of thorax
- **S20.421-** Blister (nonthermal) of <u>right</u> back wall of thorax
- **S20.422-** Blister (nonthermal) of <u>left</u> back wall of thorax
- **S20.429-** Blister (nonthermal) of <u>unspecified</u> back wall of thorax

S20.44- <u>External constriction</u> of <u>back wall</u> of thorax
- **S20.441-** External constriction of <u>right</u> back wall of thorax
- **S20.442-** External constriction of <u>left</u> back wall of thorax
- **S20.449-** External constriction of <u>unspecified</u> back wall of thorax

S20.45- <u>Superficial foreign body</u> of back wall of thorax
Splinter of back wall of thorax
- **S20.451-** Superficial foreign body of <u>right</u> back wall of thorax
- **S20.452-** Superficial foreign body of <u>left</u> back wall of thorax
- **S20.459-** Superficial foreign body of <u>unspecified</u> back wall of thorax

S20.46- <u>Insect bite (nonvenomous)</u> of <u>back wall</u> of thorax
- **S20.461-** Insect bite (nonvenomous) of <u>right</u> back wall of thorax
- **S20.462-** Insect bite (nonvenomous) of <u>left</u> back wall of thorax
- **S20.469-** Insect bite (nonvenomous) of <u>unspecified</u> back wall of thorax

S20.47- <u>Other superficial bite</u> of <u>back wall</u> of thorax
Excludes 1:   open bite of back wall of thorax (S21.24)
- **S20.471-** Other superficial bite of <u>right</u> back wall of thorax
- **S20.472-** Other superficial bite of <u>left</u> back wall of thorax
- **S20.479-** Other superficial bite of <u>unspecified</u> back wall of thorax

S20.9- Superficial injury of <u>unspecified</u> parts of thorax
Excludes 1:   contusion of thorax NOS (S20.20)
- **S20.90x-** Unspecified superficial injury of <u>unspecified</u> parts of thorax
  Superficial injury of thoracic wall NOS
- **S20.91x-** Abrasion of <u>unspecified</u> parts of thorax
- **S20.92x-** Blister (nonthermal) of <u>unspecified</u> parts of thorax
- **S20.94x-** External constriction of <u>unspecified</u> parts of thorax
- **S20.95x-** Superficial foreign body of <u>unspecified</u> parts of thorax
  Splinter in thorax NOS
- **S20.96x-** Insect bite (nonvenomous) of <u>unspecified</u> parts of thorax
- **S20.97x-** Other superficial bite of <u>unspecified</u> parts of thorax
  Excludes 1:   open bite of thorax NOS (S21.95)

S21- <u>Open wound</u> of thorax
Code also any associated injury, such as :
  Injury of heart (S26.-)
  Injury of intrathoracic organs (S27.-)
  Rib fracture (S22.3-, S22.4-)
  Spinal cord injury (S24.0-, S24.1-)
  Traumatic hemothorax (S27.1)
  Traumatic hemopneumothorax (S27.3)
  Traumatic pneumothorax (S27.0)
  Wound infection
Excludes 1:   traumatic amputation (partial) of thorax (S28.1)

The appropriate 7th character is to be added to each code from category S21:
  A <u>Initial</u> encounter
  D <u>Subsequent</u> encounter
  S <u>Sequela</u>

S21.0- Open wound of <u>breast</u>
S21.00- <u>Unspecified</u> open wound of breast
- **S21.001-** Unspecified open wound of <u>right</u> breast
- **S21.002-** Unspecified open wound of <u>left</u> breast
- **S21.009-** Unspecified open wound of <u>unspecified</u> breast

S21.01- <u>Laceration</u> <u>without</u> foreign body of breast
- **S21.011-** Laceration <u>without</u> foreign body of <u>right</u> breast
- **S21.012-** Laceration <u>without</u> foreign body of <u>left</u> breast
- **S21.019-** Laceration <u>without</u> foreign body of <u>unspecified</u> breast

S21.02- <u>Laceration</u> <u>with foreign body</u> of breast
- **S21.021-** Laceration <u>with foreign body</u> of <u>right</u> breast
- **S21.022-** Laceration <u>with foreign body</u> of <u>left</u> breast
- **S21.029-** Laceration <u>with foreign body</u> of <u>unspecified</u> breast

S21.03- <u>Puncture</u> wound <u>without</u> foreign body of breast
- **S21.031-** Puncture wound <u>without</u> foreign body of <u>right</u> breast
- **S21.032-** Puncture wound <u>without</u> foreign body of <u>left</u> breast
- **S21.039-** Puncture wound <u>without</u> foreign body of <u>unspecified</u> breast

S21.04- <u>Puncture</u> wound <u>with foreign body</u> of breast
- **S21.041-** Puncture wound <u>with foreign body</u> of <u>right</u> breast
- **S21.042-** Puncture wound <u>with foreign body</u> of <u>left</u> breast
- **S21.049-** Puncture wound <u>with foreign body</u> of <u>unspecified</u> breast

S21.05- <u>Open bite</u> of breast
  Bite of breast NOS
  Excludes 1:   superficial bite of breast (S20.17)
- **S21.051-** Open bite of <u>right</u> breast
- **S21.052-** Open bite of <u>left</u> breast
- **S21.059-** Open bite of <u>unspecified</u> breast

S21.1- <u>Open wound</u> of <u>front wall</u> of <u>thorax</u> <u>without</u> penetration into thoracic cavity
  Open wound of chest without penetration into thoracic cavity
S21.10- <u>Unspecified</u> open wound of <u>front wall</u> of thorax <u>without</u> penetration into thoracic cavity
CC-A **S21.101-** Unspecified open wound of <u>right</u> front wall of thorax <u>without</u> penetration into thoracic cavity

CC-A **S21.102-** Unspecified open wound of <u>left</u> front wall of thorax <u>without</u> penetration into thoracic cavity

CC-A **S21.109-** Unspecified open wound of <u>unspecified</u> front wall of thorax <u>without</u> penetration into thoracic cavity

S21.11- <u>Laceration without</u> foreign body of front wall of thorax <u>without</u> penetration into thoracic cavity

CC-A **S21.111-** Laceration <u>without</u> foreign body of <u>right</u> front wall of thorax <u>without</u> penetration into thoracic cavity

CC-A **S21.112-** Laceration <u>without</u> foreign body of <u>left</u> front wall of thorax <u>without</u> penetration into thoracic cavity

CC-A **S21.119-** Laceration <u>without</u> foreign body of <u>unspecified</u> front wall of thorax <u>without</u> penetration into thoracic cavity

S21.12- Laceration <u>with foreign body</u> of front wall of thorax <u>without</u> penetration into thoracic cavity

CC-A **S21.121-** Laceration <u>with foreign body</u> of <u>right</u> front wall of thorax <u>without</u> penetration into thoracic cavity

CC-A **S21.122-** Laceration <u>with foreign body</u> of <u>left</u> front wall of thorax <u>without</u> penetration into thoracic cavity

CC-A **S21.129-** Laceration <u>with foreign body</u> of <u>unspecified</u> front wall of thorax <u>without</u> penetration into thoracic cavity

S21.13- <u>Puncture</u> wound <u>without</u> foreign body of front wall of thorax <u>without</u> penetration into thoracic cavity

CC-A **S21.131-** Puncture wound <u>without</u> foreign body of <u>right</u> front wall of thorax <u>without</u> penetration into thoracic cavity

CC-A **S21.132-** Puncture wound <u>without</u> foreign body of <u>left</u> front wall of thorax <u>without</u> penetration into thoracic cavity

CC-A **S21.139-** Puncture wound <u>without</u> foreign body of <u>unspecified</u> front wall of thorax <u>without</u> penetration into thoracic cavity

S21.14- <u>Puncture</u> wound <u>with foreign body</u> of front wall of thorax <u>without</u> penetration into thoracic cavity

CC-A **S21.141-** Puncture wound <u>with foreign body</u> of <u>right</u> front wall of thorax <u>without</u> penetration into thoracic cavity

CC-A **S21.142-** Puncture wound <u>with foreign body</u> of <u>left</u> front wall of thorax <u>without</u> penetration into thoracic cavity

CC-A **S21.149-** Puncture wound <u>with foreign body</u> of <u>unspecified</u> front wall of thorax <u>without</u> penetration into thoracic cavity

S21.15- <u>Open bite</u> of front wall of thorax <u>without</u> penetration into thoracic cavity

Bite of front wall of thorax NOS

Excludes 1:   superficial bite of front wall of thorax (S20.37)

CC-A **S21.151-** Open bite of <u>right</u> front wall of thorax <u>without</u> penetration into thoracic cavity

CC-A **S21.152-** Open bite of <u>left</u> front wall of thorax <u>without</u> penetration into thoracic cavity

CC-A **S21.159-** Open bite of <u>unspecified</u> front wall of thorax <u>without</u> penetration into thoracic cavity

S21.2- <u>Open wound</u> of <u>back wall</u> of <u>thorax without</u> penetration into thoracic cavity

S21.20- <u>Unspecified</u> open wound of <u>back wall</u> of thorax <u>without</u> penetration into thoracic cavity

S21.201- Unspecified open wound of <u>right</u> back wall of thorax <u>without</u> penetration into thoracic cavity

S21.202- Unspecified open wound of <u>left</u> back wall of thorax <u>without</u> penetration into thoracic cavity

S21.209- Unspecified open wound of <u>unspecified</u> back wall of thorax <u>without</u> penetration into thoracic cavity

S21.21- <u>Laceration without</u> foreign body of <u>back wall</u> of thorax <u>without</u> penetration into thoracic cavity

S21.211- Laceration <u>without</u> foreign body of <u>right</u> back wall of thorax <u>without</u> penetration into thoracic cavity

S21.212- Laceration <u>without</u> foreign body of <u>left</u> back wall of thorax <u>without</u> penetration into thoracic cavity

S21.219- Laceration <u>without</u> foreign body of <u>unspecified</u> back wall of thorax <u>without</u> penetration into thoracic cavity

S21.22- <u>Laceration with foreign body</u> of <u>back wall</u> of thorax <u>without</u> penetration into thoracic cavity

S21.221- Laceration <u>with foreign body</u> of <u>right</u> back wall of thorax <u>without</u> penetration into thoracic cavity

S21.222- Laceration <u>with foreign body</u> of <u>left</u> back wall of thorax <u>without</u> penetration into thoracic cavity

S21.229- Laceration <u>with foreign body</u> of <u>unspecified</u> back wall of thorax <u>without</u> penetration into thoracic cavity

S21.23- <u>Puncture</u> wound <u>without</u> foreign body of <u>back wall</u> of thorax <u>without</u> penetration into thoracic cavity

S21.231- Puncture wound <u>without</u> foreign body of <u>right</u> back wall of thorax <u>without</u> penetration into thoracic cavity

S21.232- Puncture wound <u>without</u> foreign body of <u>left</u> back wall of thorax <u>without</u> penetration into thoracic cavity

S21.239- Puncture wound <u>without</u> foreign body of <u>unspecified</u> back wall of thorax <u>without</u> penetration into thoracic cavity

S21.24- <u>Puncture</u> wound <u>with foreign body</u> of <u>back wall</u> of thorax <u>without</u> penetration into thoracic cavity

S21.241- Puncture wound <u>with foreign body</u> of <u>right</u> back wall of thorax <u>without</u> penetration into thoracic cavity

S21.242- Puncture wound <u>with foreign body</u> of <u>left</u> back wall of thorax <u>without</u> penetration into thoracic cavity

S21.249- Puncture wound <u>with foreign body</u> of <u>unspecified</u> back wall of thorax <u>without</u> penetration into thoracic cavity

S21.25- <u>Open bite</u> of <u>back wall</u> of thorax <u>without</u> penetration into thoracic cavity

Bite of back wall of thorax NOS

Excludes 1:   superficial bite of back wall of thorax (S20.47)

S21.251- Open bite of <u>right</u> back wall of thorax <u>without</u> penetration into thoracic cavity

S21.252- Open bite of <u>left</u> back wall of thorax <u>without</u> penetration into thoracic cavity

S21.259- Open bite of <u>unspecified</u> back wall of thorax <u>without</u> penetration into thoracic cavity

S21.3- <u>Open wound</u> of <u>front wall</u> of <u>thorax</u> <u>with penetration into thoracic cavity</u>

Open wound of chest with penetration into thoracic cavity

S21.30- <u>Unspecified</u> open wound of <u>front wall</u> of thorax <u>with penetration into thoracic cavity</u>

MCC-A **S21.301-** Unspecified open wound of <u>right</u> front wall of thorax <u>with penetration</u> into thoracic cavity

MCC-A **S21.302-** Unspecified open wound of <u>left</u> front wall of thorax <u>with penetration</u> into thoracic cavity

MCC-A **S21.309-** Unspecified open wound of <u>unspecified</u> front wall of thorax <u>with penetration</u> into thoracic cavity

S21.31- <u>Laceration without</u> foreign body of <u>front wall</u> of thorax <u>with penetration into thoracic cavity</u>

MCC-A **S21.311-** Laceration <u>without</u> foreign body of <u>right</u> front wall of thorax <u>with penetration</u> into thoracic cavity

MCC-A **S21.312-** Laceration <u>without</u> foreign body of <u>left</u> front wall of thorax <u>with penetration</u> into thoracic cavity

MCC-A **S21.319-** Laceration <u>without</u> foreign body of <u>unspecified</u> front wall of thorax <u>with penetration</u> into thoracic cavity

S21.32- <u>Laceration with foreign body</u> of <u>front wall</u> of thorax <u>with penetration into thoracic cavity</u>

MCC-A **S21.321-** Laceration <u>with foreign body</u> of <u>right</u> front wall of thorax <u>with penetration</u> into thoracic cavity

MCC-A **S21.322-** Laceration <u>with foreign body</u> of <u>left</u> front wall of thorax <u>with penetration</u> into thoracic cavity

S 2 1 - S 2 1

MCC-A **S21.329-** Laceration <u>with foreign body</u> of <u>unspecified</u> front wall of thorax <u>with penetration</u> into thoracic cavity

S21.33- <u>Puncture</u> wound <u>without</u> foreign body of front wall of thorax <u>with penetration into thoracic cavity</u>

MCC-A **S21.331-** Puncture wound <u>without</u> foreign body of <u>right</u> front wall of thorax <u>with penetration</u> into thoracic cavity

MCC-A **S21.332-** Puncture wound <u>without</u> foreign body of <u>left</u> front wall of thorax <u>with penetration</u> into thoracic cavity

MCC-A **S21.339-** Puncture wound <u>without</u> foreign body of <u>unspecified</u> front wall of thorax <u>with penetration</u> into thoracic cavity

S21.34- <u>Puncture</u> wound <u>with foreign body</u> of <u>front wall</u> of thorax <u>with penetration into thoracic cavity</u>

MCC-A **S21.341-** Puncture wound <u>with foreign body</u> of <u>right</u> front wall of thorax <u>with penetration</u> into thoracic cavity

MCC-A **S21.342-** Puncture wound <u>with foreign body</u> of <u>left</u> front wall of thorax <u>with penetration</u> into thoracic cavity

MCC-A **S21.349-** Puncture wound <u>with foreign body</u> of <u>unspecified</u> front wall of thorax <u>with penetration</u> into thoracic cavity

S21.35- <u>Open bite</u> of <u>front wall</u> of thorax <u>with penetration into thoracic cavity</u>
    Excludes 1:   *superficial bite of front wall of thorax (S20.37)*

MCC-A **S21.351-** Open bite of <u>right</u> front wall of thorax <u>with penetration</u> into thoracic cavity

MCC-A **S21.352-** Open bite of <u>left</u> front wall of thorax <u>with penetration</u> into thoracic cavity

MCC-A **S21.359-** Open bite of <u>unspecified</u> front wall of thorax <u>with penetration</u> into thoracic cavity

S21.4- <u>Open wound</u> of <u>back wall</u> of thorax <u>with penetration into thoracic cavity</u>

S21.40- <u>Unspecified</u> open wound of <u>back wall</u> of thorax <u>with penetration into thoracic cavity</u>

MCC-A **S21.401-** Unspecified open wound of <u>right</u> back wall of thorax <u>with penetration</u> into thoracic cavity

MCC-A **S21.402-** Unspecified open wound of <u>left</u> back wall of thorax <u>with penetration</u> into thoracic cavity

MCC-A **S21.409-** Unspecified open wound of <u>unspecified</u> back wall of thorax <u>with penetration</u> into thoracic cavity

S21.41- <u>Laceration</u> <u>without</u> foreign body of <u>back wall</u> of thorax <u>with penetration into thoracic cavity</u>

MCC-A **S21.411-** Laceration <u>without</u> foreign body of <u>right</u> back wall of thorax <u>with penetration</u> into thoracic cavity

MCC-A **S21.412-** Laceration <u>without</u> foreign body of <u>left</u> back wall of thorax <u>with penetration</u> into thoracic cavity

MCC-A **S21.419-** Laceration <u>without</u> foreign body of <u>unspecified</u> back wall of thorax <u>with penetration</u> into thoracic cavity

S21.42- <u>Laceration with foreign body</u> of <u>back wall</u> of thorax <u>with penetration into thoracic cavity</u>

MCC-A **S21.421-** Laceration <u>with foreign body</u> of <u>right</u> back wall of thorax <u>with penetration</u> into thoracic cavity

MCC-A **S21.422-** Laceration <u>with foreign body</u> of <u>left</u> back wall of thorax <u>with penetration</u> into thoracic cavity

MCC-A **S21.429-** Laceration <u>with foreign body</u> of <u>unspecified</u> back wall of thorax <u>with penetration</u> into thoracic cavity

S21.43- <u>Puncture</u> wound <u>without</u> foreign body of <u>back wall</u> of thorax <u>with penetration into thoracic cavity</u>

MCC-A **S21.431-** Puncture wound <u>without</u> foreign body of <u>right</u> back wall of thorax <u>with penetration</u> into thoracic cavity

MCC-A **S21.432-** Puncture wound <u>without</u> foreign body of <u>left</u> back wall of thorax <u>with penetration</u> into thoracic cavity

MCC-A **S21.439-** Puncture wound <u>without</u> foreign body of <u>unspecified</u> back wall of thorax <u>with penetration</u> into thoracic cavity

S21.44- <u>Puncture</u> wound <u>with foreign body</u> of <u>back wall</u> of thorax <u>with penetration into thoracic cavity</u>

MCC-A **S21.441-** Puncture wound <u>with foreign body</u> of <u>right</u> back wall of thorax <u>with penetration</u> into thoracic cavity

MCC-A **S21.442-** Puncture wound <u>with foreign body</u> of <u>left</u> back wall of thorax <u>with penetration</u> into thoracic cavity

MCC-A **S21.449-** Puncture wound <u>with foreign body</u> of <u>unspecified</u> back wall of thorax <u>with penetration</u> into thoracic cavity

S21.45- <u>Open bite</u> of <u>back wall</u> of thorax <u>with penetration into thoracic cavity</u>
    Bite of back wall of thorax NOS
    Excludes 1:   *superficial bite of back wall of thorax (S20.47)*

MCC-A **S21.451-** Open bite of <u>right</u> back wall of thorax <u>with penetration</u> into thoracic cavity

MCC-A **S21.452-** Open bite of <u>left</u> back wall of thorax <u>with penetration</u> into thoracic cavity

MCC-A **S21.459-** Open bite of <u>unspecified</u> back wall of thorax <u>with penetration</u> into thoracic cavity

S21.9- <u>Open wound</u> of <u>unspecified</u> part of thorax
    Open wound of thoracic wall NOS

CC-A **S21.90x-** <u>Unspecified</u> open wound of <u>unspecified</u> part of thorax

CC-A **S21.91x-** <u>Laceration</u> <u>without</u> foreign body of <u>unspecified</u> part of thorax

CC-A **S21.92x-** <u>Laceration</u> <u>with foreign body</u> of <u>unspecified</u> part of thorax

CC-A **S21.93x-** <u>Puncture</u> wound <u>without</u> foreign body of <u>unspecified</u> part of thorax

CC-A **S21.94x-** <u>Puncture</u> wound <u>with foreign body</u> of <u>unspecified</u> part of thorax

CC-A **S21.95x-** <u>Open bite</u> of <u>unspecified</u> part of thorax
    Excludes 1:   *superficial bite of thorax (S20.97)*

S22- <u>Fracture</u> of <u>rib(s), sternum and thoracic spine</u>
    Note: A fracture not indicated as nondisplaced or displaced should be classified to displaced
    Note: A fracture not indicated as open or closed should be coded to closed
    Includes: Fracture of thoracic neural arch
              Fracture of thoracic spinous process
              Fracture of thoracic transverse process
              Fracture of thoracic vertebra
              Fracture of thoracic vertebral arch
    Code first any associated:
      Injury of intrathoracic organ (S27.-)
      Spinal cord injury (S24.0-, S24.1-)
    Excludes 1:   *transection of thorax (S28.1)*
    Excludes ❷: *fracture of clavicle (S42.0-)*
              fracture of scapula (S42.1-)

The appropriate 7th character is to be added to each code from category S22:
  A   <u>Initial</u> encounter for <u>closed</u> fracture
  B   <u>Initial</u> encounter for <u>open</u> fracture
  D   <u>Subsequent</u> encounter for fracture <u>with routine healing</u>
  G   <u>Subsequent</u> encounter for fracture <u>with delayed healing</u>
  K   <u>Subsequent</u> encounter for fracture <u>with nonunion</u>
  S   <u>Sequela</u>

S22.0- <u>Fracture</u> of <u>thoracic vertebra</u>

S22.00- Fracture of <u>unspecified</u> thoracic vertebra

CC-A,K MCC-B **S22.000-** <u>Wedge</u> compression fracture of unspecified thoracic vertebra

CC-A,K MCC-B **S22.001-** <u>Stable burst</u> fracture of unspecified thoracic vertebra

CC-A,K MCC-B **S22.002-** <u>Unstable burst</u> fracture of unspecified thoracic vertebra

CC-A,K MCC-B **S22.008-** <u>Other</u> fracture of unspecified thoracic vertebra

CC-A,K MCC-B **S22.009-** <u>Unspecified</u> fracture of unspecified thoracic vertebra

S22.01- Fracture of <u>first</u> thoracic vertebra

CC-A,K MCC-B **S22.010-** <u>Wedge</u> compression fracture of first thoracic vertebra

CC-A,K MCC-B **S22.011-** <u>Stable burst</u> fracture of first thoracic vertebra

CC-A,K MCC-B **S22.012-** <u>Unstable burst</u> fracture of first thoracic vertebra

CC-A,K MCC-B **S22.018-** <u>Other</u> fracture of first thoracic vertebra

CC-A,K MCC-B **S22.019-** <u>Unspecified</u> fracture of first thoracic vertebra

**S2
1
-
S2
2**

S22.02- Fracture of <u>second</u> thoracic vertebra

CC-A,K MCC-B **S22.020-** <u>Wedge</u> compression fracture of second thoracic vertebra

CC-A,K MCC-B **S22.021-** <u>Stable burst</u> fracture of second thoracic vertebra

CC-A,K MCC-B **S22.022-** <u>Unstable burst</u> fracture of second thoracic vertebra

CC-A,K MCC-B **S22.028-** <u>Other</u> fracture of second thoracic vertebra

CC-A,K MCC-B **S22.029-** <u>Unspecified</u> fracture of second thoracic vertebra

S22.03- Fracture of <u>third</u> thoracic vertebra

CC-A,K MCC-B **S22.030-** <u>Wedge</u> compression fracture of third thoracic vertebra

CC-A,K MCC-B **S22.031-** <u>Stable burst</u> fracture of third thoracic vertebra

CC-A,K MCC-B **S22.032-** <u>Unstable burst</u> fracture of third thoracic vertebra

CC-A,K MCC-B **S22.038-** <u>Other</u> fracture of third thoracic vertebra

CC-A,K MCC-B **S22.039-** <u>Unspecified</u> fracture of third thoracic vertebra

S22.04- Fracture of <u>fourth</u> thoracic vertebra

CC-A,K MCC-B **S22.040-** <u>Wedge</u> compression fracture of fourth thoracic vertebra

CC-A,K MCC-B **S22.041-** <u>Stable burst</u> fracture of fourth thoracic vertebra

CC-A,K MCC-B **S22.042-** <u>Unstable burst</u> fracture of fourth thoracic vertebra

CC-A,K MCC-B **S22.048-** <u>Other</u> fracture of fourth thoracic vertebra

CC-A,K MCC-B **S22.049-** <u>Unspecified</u> fracture of fourth thoracic vertebra

S22.05- Fracture of <u>T5-T6</u> vertebra

CC-A,K MCC-B **S22.050-** <u>Wedge</u> compression fracture of T5-T6 vertebra

CC-A,K MCC-B **S22.051-** <u>Stable burst</u> fracture of T5-T6 vertebra

CC-A,K MCC-B **S22.052-** <u>Unstable burst</u> fracture of T5-T6 vertebra

CC-A,K MCC-B **S22.058-** <u>Other</u> fracture of T5-T6 vertebra

CC-A,K MCC-B **S22.059-** <u>Unspecified</u> fracture of T5-T6 vertebra

S22.06- Fracture of <u>T7-T8</u> vertebra

CC-A,K MCC-B **S22.060-** <u>Wedge</u> compression fracture of T7-T8 vertebra

CC-A,K MCC-B **S22.061-** <u>Stable burst</u> fracture of T7-T8 vertebra

CC-A,K MCC-B **S22.062-** <u>Unstable burst</u> fracture of T7-T8 vertebra

CC-A,K MCC-B **S22.068-** <u>Other</u> fracture of T7-T8 thoracic vertebra

CC-A,K MCC-B **S22.069-** <u>Unspecified</u> fracture of T7-T8 vertebra

S22.07- Fracture of <u>T9-T10</u> vertebra

CC-A,K MCC-B **S22.070-** <u>Wedge</u> compression fracture of T9-T10 vertebra

CC-A,K MCC-B **S22.071-** Stable burst fracture of T9-T10 vertebra

CC-A,K MCC-B **S22.072-** <u>Unstable burst</u> fracture of T9-T10 vertebra

CC-A,K MCC-B **S22.078-** Other fracture of T9-T10 vertebra

CC-A,K MCC-B **S22.079-** <u>Unspecified</u> fracture of T9-T10 vertebra

S22.08- Fracture of <u>T11-T12</u> vertebra

CC-A,K MCC-B **S22.080-** <u>Wedge</u> compression fracture of T11-T12 vertebra

CC-A,K MCC-B **S22.081-** <u>Stable burst</u> fracture of T11-T12 vertebra

CC-A,K MCC-B **S22.082-** <u>Unstable burst</u> fracture of T11-T12 vertebra

CC-A,K MCC-B **S22.088-** <u>Other</u> fracture of T11-T12 vertebra

CC-A,K MCC-B **S22.089-** <u>Unspecified</u> fracture of T11-T12 vertebra

S22.2- Fracture of <u>sternum</u>

S22.20x- <u>Unspecified</u> fracture of sternum
CC-A,K MCC-B

S22.21x- Fracture of <u>manubrium</u>
CC-A,K MCC-B

S22.22x- Fracture of <u>body</u> of sternum
CC-A,K MCC-B

S22.23x- Sternal <u>manubrial dissociation</u>
CC-A,K MCC-B

S22.24x- Fracture of <u>xiphoid process</u>
CC-A,K MCC-B

S22.3- Fracture of <u>one rib</u>

S22.31x- Fracture of one rib, <u>right</u> side
CC-A,K MCC-B

S22.32x- Fracture of one rib, <u>left</u> side
CC-A,K MCC-B

S22.39x- Fracture of one rib, <u>unspecified</u> side
CC-A,K MCC-B

S22.4- <u>Multiple</u> fractures of <u>ribs</u>
Fractures of two or more ribs
Excludes 1:   flail chest (S22.5-)

S22.41x- Multiple fractures of ribs, <u>right</u> side
CC-A,K MCC-B

S22.42x- Multiple fractures of ribs, <u>left</u> side
CC-A,K MCC-B

S22.43x- Multiple fractures of ribs, <u>bilateral</u>
CC-A,K MCC-B

S22.49x- Multiple fractures of ribs, <u>unspecified</u> side
CC-A,K MCC-B

S22.5xx- <u>Flail chest</u>
CC-K MCC-A,B

S22.9xx- Fracture of <u>bony</u> <u>thorax</u>, part <u>unspecified</u>
CC-A,K MCC-B

S23- <u>Dislocation and sprain</u> of joints and ligaments of <u>thorax</u>
Includes: Avulsion of joint or ligament of thorax
Laceration of cartilage, joint or ligament of thorax
Sprain of cartilage, joint or ligament of thorax
Traumatic hemarthrosis of joint or ligament of thorax
Traumatic rupture of joint or ligament of thorax
Traumatic subluxation of joint or ligament of thorax
Traumatic tear of joint or ligament of thorax
Code also any associated open wound
*Excludes ❷: dislocation, sprain of sternoclavicular joint (S43.2, S43.6)
                        strain of muscle or tendon of thorax (S29.01-)*

> **The appropriate 7th character is to be added to each code from category S23:**
> **A**   <u>Initial</u> encounter
> **D**   <u>Subsequent</u> encounter
> **S**   <u>Sequela</u>

S23.0xx- <u>Traumatic rupture</u> of <u>thoracic intervertebral disc</u>
Excludes 1:   rupture or displacement (nontraumatic) of thoracic intervertebral disc NOS (M51.- with fifth character 4)

S23.1- <u>Subluxation and dislocation</u> of <u>thoracic vertebra</u>
Code also any associated:
Open wound of thorax (S21.-)
Spinal cord injury (S24.0-, S24.1-)
Excludes ❷: fracture of thoracic vertebrae (S22.0-)

S23.10- Subluxation and dislocation of <u>unspecified</u> thoracic vertebra

S23.100- <u>Subluxation</u> of unspecified thoracic vertebra

S23.101- <u>Dislocation</u> of unspecified thoracic vertebra

S23.11- Subluxation and dislocation of <u>T1/T2</u> thoracic vertebra

S23.110- <u>Subluxation</u> of T1/T2 thoracic vertebra

S23.111- <u>Dislocation</u> of T1/T2 thoracic vertebra

S23.12- Subluxation and dislocation of <u>T2/T3-T3/T4</u> thoracic vertebra

S23.120- <u>Subluxation</u> of <u>T2/T3</u> thoracic vertebra

S23.121- <u>Dislocation</u> of <u>T2/T3</u> thoracic vertebra

S23.122- <u>Subluxation</u> of <u>T3/T4</u> thoracic vertebra

S23.123- <u>Dislocation</u> of <u>T3/T4</u> thoracic vertebra

S23.13- Subluxation and dislocation of <u>T4/T5-T5/T6</u> thoracic vertebra

S23.130- <u>Subluxation</u> of <u>T4/T5</u> thoracic vertebra

S23.131- <u>Dislocation</u> of <u>T4/T5</u> thoracic vertebra

S23.132- <u>Subluxation</u> of <u>T5/T6</u> thoracic vertebra

S23.133- <u>Dislocation</u> of <u>T5/T6</u> thoracic vertebra

S23.14- Subluxation and dislocation of <u>T6/T7-T7/T8</u> thoracic vertebra

S23.140- <u>Subluxation</u> of <u>T6/T7</u> thoracic vertebra

S23.141- <u>Dislocation</u> of <u>T6/T7</u> thoracic vertebra

S23.142- <u>Subluxation</u> of <u>T7/T8</u> thoracic vertebra

S23.143- <u>Dislocation</u> of <u>T7/T8</u> thoracic vertebra

S23.15- Subluxation and dislocation of <u>T8/T9-T9/T10</u> thoracic vertebra

S23.150- <u>Subluxation</u> of <u>T8/T9</u> thoracic vertebra

S23.151- <u>Dislocation</u> of <u>T8/T9</u> thoracic vertebra

S23.152- <u>Subluxation</u> of <u>T9/T10</u> thoracic vertebra

S23.153- <u>Dislocation</u> of <u>T9/T10</u> thoracic vertebra

S23.16- Subluxation and dislocation of <u>T10/T11-T11/T12</u> thoracic vertebra

S23.160- <u>Subluxation</u> of <u>T10/T11</u> thoracic vertebra

S23.161- <u>Dislocation</u> of <u>T10/T11</u> thoracic vertebra

S23.162- <u>Subluxation</u> of <u>T11/T12</u> thoracic vertebra

S 2 2 - S 2 3

S23.163- <u>Dislocation</u> of <u>T11/T12</u> thoracic vertebra

S23.17- Subluxation and dislocation of T12/L1 thoracic vertebra

S23.170- <u>Subluxation</u> of <u>T12/L1</u> thoracic vertebra

S23.171- <u>Dislocation</u> of <u>T12/L1</u> thoracic vertebra

S23.2- Dislocation of other and <u>unspecified</u> parts of thorax

S23.20x- <u>Dislocation</u> of <u>unspecified</u> part of thorax

S23.29x- <u>Dislocation</u> of <u>other</u> parts of thorax

S23.3xx- <u>Sprain</u> of ligaments of <u>thoracic spine</u>

S23.4- <u>Sprain</u> of ribs and sternum

S23.41x- Sprain of <u>ribs</u>

S23.42- Sprain of <u>sternum</u>

S23.420- Sprain of sternoclavicular (joint) (ligament)

S23.421- Sprain of chondrosternal joint

S23.428- Other sprain of sternum

S23.429- Unspecified sprain of sternum

S23.8xx- Sprain of <u>other</u> specified parts of thorax

S23.9xx- Sprain of <u>unspecified</u> parts of thorax

S24- <u>Injury of nerves and spinal cord</u> at <u>thorax</u> level
   Note: Code to highest level of thoracic spinal cord injury
   Injuries to the spinal cord (S24.0 and S24.1) refer to the cord level
   and not bone level injury, and can affect nerve roots at and below the
   level given.
   Code also any associated:
      Fracture of thoracic vertebra (S22.0-)
      Open wound of thorax (S21.-)
      Transient paralysis (R29.5)
   Excludes ❷: injury of brachial plexus (S14.3)

The appropriate 7th character is to be added to each code from
   category S24:
   A   <u>Initial</u> encounter
   D   <u>Subsequent</u> encounter
   S   <u>Sequela</u>

S24.0xx- <u>Concussion and edema</u> of <u>thoracic</u> spinal cord
MCC-A

S24.1- Other and unspecified injuries of <u>thoracic</u> spinal cord

S24.10- <u>Unspecified</u> injury of <u>thoracic spinal cord</u>

MCC-A S24.101- Unspecified injury at <u>T1</u> level of thoracic spinal cord

MCC-A S24.102- Unspecified injury at <u>T2-T6</u> level of thoracic spinal cord

MCC-A S24.103- Unspecified injury at <u>T7-T10</u> level of thoracic spinal cord

MCC-A S24.104- Unspecified injury at <u>T11-T12</u> level of thoracic spinal cord

S24.109- Unspecified injury at <u>unspecified</u> level of thoracic spinal cord
   Injury of thoracic spinal cord NOS

S24.11- <u>Complete lesion</u> of thoracic spinal cord

MCC-A S24.111- Complete lesion at <u>T1</u> level of thoracic spinal cord

MCC-A S24.112- Complete lesion at <u>T2-T6</u> level of thoracic spinal cord

MCC-A S24.113- Complete lesion at <u>T7-T10</u> level of thoracic spinal cord

MCC-A S24.114- Complete lesion at <u>T11-T12</u> level of thoracic spinal cord

S24.119- Complete lesion at <u>unspecified</u> level of thoracic spinal cord

S24.13- <u>Anterior cord syndrome</u> of thoracic spinal cord

MCC-A S24.131- Anterior cord syndrome at <u>T1</u> level of thoracic spinal cord

MCC-A S24.132- Anterior cord syndrome at <u>T2-T6</u> level of thoracic spinal cord

MCC-A S24.133- Anterior cord syndrome at <u>T7-T10</u> level of thoracic spinal cord

MCC-A S24.134- Anterior cord syndrome at <u>T11-T12</u> level of thoracic spinal cord

S24.139- Anterior cord syndrome at <u>unspecified</u> level of thoracic spinal cord

S24.14- <u>Brown-Séquard syndrome</u> of thoracic spinal cord

MCC-A S24.141- Brown-Séquard syndrome at <u>T1</u> level of thoracic spinal cord

MCC-A S24.142- Brown-Séquard syndrome at <u>T2-T6</u> level of thoracic spinal cord

MCC-A S24.143- Brown-Séquard syndrome at <u>T7-T10</u> level of thoracic spinal cord

MCC-A S24.144- Brown-Séquard syndrome at <u>T11-T12</u> level of thoracic spinal cord

S24.149- Brown-Séquard syndrome at <u>unspecified</u> level of thoracic spinal cord

S24.15- <u>Other incomplete lesions</u> of thoracic spinal cord
   Incomplete lesion of thoracic spinal cord NOS
   Posterior cord syndrome of thoracic spinal cord

MCC-A S24.151- Other incomplete lesion at <u>T1</u> level of thoracic spinal cord

MCC-A S24.152- Other incomplete lesion at <u>T2-T6</u> level of thoracic spinal cord

MCC-A S24.153- Other incomplete lesion at <u>T7-T10</u> level of thoracic spinal cord

MCC-A S24.154- Other incomplete lesion at <u>T11-T12</u> level of thoracic spinal cord

S24.159- Other incomplete lesion at <u>unspecified</u> level of thoracic spinal cord

S24.2xx- Injury of <u>nerve root</u> of thoracic spine

S24.3xx- Injury of <u>peripheral nerves</u> of thorax

S24.4xx- Injury of thoracic <u>sympathetic nervous system</u>
   Injury of cardiac plexus
   Injury of esophageal plexus
   Injury of pulmonary plexus
   Injury of stellate ganglion
   Injury of thoracic sympathetic ganglion

S24.8xx- Injury of <u>other</u> specified nerves of thorax

S24.9xx- Injury of <u>unspecified</u> nerve of thorax

S25- <u>Injury of blood vessels</u> of <u>thorax</u>
   Code also any associated open wound (S21.-)

The appropriate 7th character is to be added to each code from
   category S25:
   A   <u>Initial</u> encounter
   D   <u>Subsequent</u> encounter
   S   <u>Sequela</u>

S25.0- Injury of <u>thoracic aorta</u>
   Injury of aorta NOS

MCC-A S25.00x- <u>Unspecified</u> injury of thoracic aorta

MCC-A S25.01x- <u>Minor</u> laceration of thoracic aorta
   Incomplete transection of thoracic aorta
   Laceration of thoracic aorta NOS
   Superficial laceration of thoracic aorta

MCC-A S25.02x- <u>Major</u> laceration of thoracic aorta
   Complete transection of thoracic aorta
   Traumatic rupture of thoracic aorta

MCC-A S25.09x- <u>Other</u> specified injury of thoracic aorta

S25.1- Injury of <u>innominate or subclavian artery</u>

S25.10- <u>Unspecified</u> injury of <u>innominate or subclavian artery</u>

MCC-A S25.101- Unspecified injury of <u>right</u> innominate or subclavian <u>artery</u>

MCC-A S25.102- Unspecified injury of <u>left</u> innominate or subclavian <u>artery</u>

MCC-A S25.109- Unspecified injury of <u>unspecified</u> innominate or subclavian <u>artery</u>

S25.11- <u>Minor laceration</u> of <u>innominate or subclavian</u> <u>artery</u>
   Incomplete transection of innominate or subclavian artery
   Laceration of innominate or subclavian artery NOS
   Superficial laceration of innominate or subclavian artery

MCC-A S25.111- Minor laceration of <u>right</u> innominate or subclavian <u>artery</u>

MCC-A S25.112- Minor laceration of <u>left</u> innominate or subclavian <u>artery</u>

MCC-A S25.119- Minor laceration of <u>unspecified</u> innominate or subclavian <u>artery</u>

S 2 3 - S 2 5

S25.12- Major laceration of innominate or subclavian artery
　　　Complete transection of innominate or subclavian artery
　　　Traumatic rupture of innominate or subclavian artery

MCC-A S25.121- Major laceration of right innominate or subclavian artery

MCC-A S25.122- Major laceration of left innominate or subclavian artery

MCC-A S25.129- Major laceration of unspecified innominate or subclavian artery

S25.19- Other specified injury of innominate or subclavian artery

MCC-A S25.191- Other specified injury of right innominate or subclavian artery

MCC-A S25.192- Other specified injury of left innominate or subclavian artery

MCC-A S25.199- Other specified injury of unspecified innominate or subclavian artery

S25.2- Injury of superior vena cava
　　　Injury of vena cava NOS

MCC-A S25.20x- Unspecified injury of superior vena cava

MCC-A S25.21x- Minor laceration of superior vena cava
　　　Incomplete transection of superior vena cava
　　　Laceration of superior vena cava NOS
　　　Superficial laceration of superior vena cava

MCC-A S25.22x- Major laceration of superior vena cava
　　　Complete transection of superior vena cava
　　　Traumatic rupture of superior vena cava

MCC-A S25.29x- Other specified injury of superior vena cava

S25.3- Injury of innominate or subclavian vein

S25.30- Unspecified injury of innominate or subclavian vein

MCC-A S25.301- Unspecified injury of right innominate or subclavian vein

MCC-A S25.302- Unspecified injury of left innominate or subclavian vein

MCC-A S25.309- Unspecified injury of unspecified innominate or subclavian vein

S25.31- Minor laceration of innominate or subclavian vein
　　　Incomplete transection of innominate or subclavian vein
　　　Laceration of innominate or subclavian vein NOS
　　　Superficial laceration of innominate or subclavian vein

MCC-A S25.311- Minor laceration of right innominate or subclavian vein

MCC-A S25.312- Minor laceration of left innominate or subclavian vein

MCC-A S25.319- Minor laceration of unspecified innominate or subclavian vein

S25.32- Major laceration of innominate or subclavian vein
　　　Complete transection of innominate or subclavian vein
　　　Traumatic rupture of innominate or subclavian vein

MCC-A S25.321- Major laceration of right innominate or subclavian vein

MCC-A S25.322- Major laceration of left innominate or subclavian vein

MCC-A S25.329- Major laceration of unspecified innominate or subclavian vein

S25.39- Other specified injury of innominate or subclavian vein

MCC-A S25.391- Other specified injury of right innominate or subclavian vein

MCC-A S25.392- Other specified injury of left innominate or subclavian vein

MCC-A S25.399- Other specified injury of unspecified innominate or subclavian vein

S25.4- Injury of pulmonary blood vessels

S25.40- Unspecified injury of pulmonary blood vessels

MCC-A S25.401- Unspecified injury of right pulmonary blood vessels

MCC-A S25.402- Unspecified injury of left pulmonary blood vessels

MCC-A S25.409- Unspecified injury of unspecified pulmonary blood vessels

S25.41- Minor laceration of pulmonary blood vessels
　　　Incomplete transection of pulmonary blood vessels
　　　Laceration of pulmonary blood vessels NOS
　　　Superficial laceration of pulmonary blood vessels

MCC-A S25.411- Minor laceration of right pulmonary blood vessels

MCC-A S25.412- Minor laceration of left pulmonary blood vessels

MCC-A S25.419- Minor laceration of unspecified pulmonary blood vessels

S25.42- Major laceration of pulmonary blood vessels
　　　Complete transection of pulmonary blood vessels
　　　Traumatic rupture of pulmonary blood vessels

MCC-A S25.421- Major laceration of right pulmonary blood vessels

MCC-A S25.422- Major laceration of left pulmonary blood vessels

MCC-A S25.429- Major laceration of unspecified pulmonary blood vessels

S25.49- Other specified injury of pulmonary blood vessels

MCC-A S25.491- Other specified injury of right pulmonary blood vessels

MCC-A S25.492- Other specified injury of left pulmonary blood vessels

MCC-A S25.499- Other specified injury of unspecified pulmonary blood vessels

S25.5- Injury of intercostal blood vessels

S25.50- Unspecified injury of intercostal blood vessels

CC-A S25.501- Unspecified injury of intercostal blood vessels, right side

CC-A S25.502- Unspecified injury of intercostal blood vessels, left side

CC-A S25.509- Unspecified injury of intercostal blood vessels, unspecified side

S25.51- Laceration of intercostal blood vessels

CC-A S25.511- Laceration of intercostal blood vessels, right side

CC-A S25.512- Laceration of intercostal blood vessels, left side

CC-A S25.519- Laceration of intercostal blood vessels, unspecified side

S25.59- Other specified injury of intercostal blood vessels

CC-A S25.591- Other specified injury of intercostal blood vessels, right side

CC-A S25.592- Other specified injury of intercostal blood vessels, left side

CC-A S25.599- Other specified injury of intercostal blood vessels, unspecified side

S25.8- Injury of other blood vessels of thorax
　　　Injury of azygos vein
　　　Injury of mammary artery or vein

S25.80- Unspecified injury of other blood vessels of thorax

CC-A S25.801- Unspecified injury of other blood vessels of thorax, right side

CC-A S25.802- Unspecified injury of other blood vessels of thorax, left side

CC-A S25.809- Unspecified injury of other blood vessels of thorax, unspecified side

S25.81- Laceration of other blood vessels of thorax

CC-A S25.811- Laceration of other blood vessels of thorax, right side

CC-A S25.812- Laceration of other blood vessels of thorax, left side

CC-A S25.819- Laceration of other blood vessels of thorax, unspecified side

S25.89- Other specified injury of other blood vessels of thorax

CC-A S25.891- Other specified injury of other blood vessels of thorax, right side

CC-A S25.892- Other specified injury of other blood vessels of thorax, left side

CC-A S25.899- Other specified injury of other blood vessels of thorax, unspecified side

S25.9- Injury of unspecified blood vessel of thorax

CC-A S25.90x- Unspecified injury of unspecified blood vessel of thorax

CC-A S25.91x- Laceration of unspecified blood vessel of thorax

S25 | S25

CC-A **S25.99x-** <u>Other</u> specified injury of <u>unspecified</u> <u>blood vessel of</u> <u>thorax</u>

S26- Injury of <u>heart</u>
Code also any associated:
Open wound of thorax (S21.-)
Traumatic hemopneumothorax (S27.2)
Traumatic hemothorax (S27.1)
Traumatic pneumothorax (S27.0)

The appropriate 7th character is to be added to each code from category S26:
A <u>Initial</u> encounter
D <u>Subsequent</u> encounter
S <u>Sequela</u>

S26.0- Injury of <u>heart with hemopericardium</u>
CC-A **S26.00x-** <u>Unspecified</u> injury of heart with hemopericardium
CC-A **S26.01x-** <u>Contusion</u> of heart with hemopericardium
S26.02- <u>Laceration</u> of heart <u>with hemopericardium</u>
MCC-A **S26.020-** <u>Mild</u> laceration of heart <u>with hemopericardium</u>
Laceration of heart without penetration of heart chamber
MCC-A **S26.021-** <u>Moderate</u> laceration of heart <u>with hemopericardium</u>
Laceration of heart with penetration of heart chamber
MCC-A **S26.022-** <u>Major</u> laceration of heart <u>with hemopericardium</u>
Laceration of heart with penetration of multiple heart chambers
CC-A **S26.09x-** <u>Other</u> injury of heart <u>with hemopericardium</u>
S26.1- Injury of <u>heart</u> <u>without</u> hemopericardium
CC-A **S26.10x-** <u>Unspecified</u> injury of heart <u>without</u> hemopericardium
CC-A **S26.11x-** <u>Contusion</u> of heart <u>without</u> hemopericardium
MCC-A **S26.12x-** <u>Laceration</u> of heart <u>without</u> hemopericardium
CC-A **S26.19x-** <u>Other</u> injury of heart <u>without</u> hemopericardium
S26.9- Injury of heart, <u>unspecified with or without</u> hemopericardium
CC-A **S26.90x-** <u>Unspecified</u> injury of heart, <u>unspecified with or without</u> hemopericardium
CC-A **S26.91x-** <u>Contusion</u> of heart, <u>unspecified with or without</u> hemopericardium
MCC-A **S26.92x-** <u>Laceration</u> of heart, <u>unspecified with or without</u> hemopericardium
Laceration of heart NOS
CC-A **S26.99x-** <u>Other</u> injury of heart, <u>unspecified with or without</u> hemopericardium

S27- Injury of <u>other and unspecified</u> <u>intrathoracic organs</u>
Code also any associated open wound of thorax (S21.-)
Excludes ❷: injury of cervical esophagus (S10-S19)
injury of trachea (cervical) (S10-S19)

The appropriate 7th character is to be added to each code from category S27:
A <u>Initial</u> encounter
D <u>Subsequent</u> encounter
S <u>Sequela</u>

S27.0xx- Traumatic <u>pneumothorax</u>
CC-A *Excludes 1: spontaneous pneumothorax (J93.-)*
S27.1xx- Traumatic <u>hemothorax</u>
MCC-A
S27.2xx- Traumatic <u>hemopneumothorax</u>
MCC-A
S27.3- Other and unspecified injuries of <u>lung</u>
S27.30- <u>Unspecified</u> injury of lung
CC-A **S27.301-** Unspecified injury of lung, <u>unilateral</u>
CC-A **S27.302-** Unspecified injury of lung, <u>bilateral</u>
CC-A **S27.309-** Unspecified injury of lung, <u>unspecified</u>
S27.31- <u>Primary blast</u> injury of lung
Blast injury of lung NOS
CC-A **S27.311-** Primary blast injury of lung, <u>unilateral</u>
CC-A **S27.312-** Primary blast injury of lung, <u>bilateral</u>
CC-A **S27.319-** Primary blast injury of lung, <u>unspecified</u>
S27.32- <u>Contusion</u> of lung
CC-A **S27.321-** Contusion of lung, <u>unilateral</u>
CC-A **S27.322-** Contusion of lung, <u>bilateral</u>

CC-A **S27.329-** Contusion of lung, <u>unspecified</u>
S27.33- <u>Laceration</u> of lung
MCC-A **S27.331-** Laceration of lung, <u>unilateral</u>
MCC-A **S27.332-** Laceration of lung, <u>bilateral</u>
MCC-A **S27.339-** Laceration of lung, <u>unspecified</u>
S27.39- <u>Other</u> injuries of lung
Secondary blast injury of lung
CC-A **S27.391-** Other injuries of lung, <u>unilateral</u>
CC-A **S27.392-** Other injuries of lung, <u>bilateral</u>
CC-A **S27.399-** Other injuries of lung, <u>unspecified</u>
S27.4- Injury of <u>bronchus</u>
S27.40- <u>Unspecified</u> injury of bronchus
MCC-A **S27.401-** Unspecified injury of bronchus, <u>unilateral</u>
MCC-A **S27.402-** Unspecified injury of bronchus, <u>bilateral</u>
MCC-A **S27.409-** Unspecified injury of bronchus, <u>unspecified</u>
S27.41- <u>Primary blast</u> injury of bronchus
Blast injury of bronchus NOS
MCC-A **S27.411-** Primary blast injury of bronchus, <u>unilateral</u>
MCC-A **S27.412-** Primary blast injury of bronchus, <u>bilateral</u>
MCC-A **S27.419-** Primary blast injury of bronchus, <u>unspecified</u>
S27.42- <u>Contusion</u> of bronchus
MCC-A **S27.421-** Contusion of bronchus, <u>unilateral</u>
MCC-A **S27.422-** Contusion of bronchus, <u>bilateral</u>
MCC-A **S27.429-** Contusion of bronchus, <u>unspecified</u>
S27.43- <u>Laceration</u> of bronchus
MCC-A **S27.431-** Laceration of bronchus, <u>unilateral</u>
MCC-A **S27.432-** Laceration of bronchus, <u>bilateral</u>
MCC-A **S27.439-** Laceration of bronchus, <u>unspecified</u>
S27.49- <u>Other</u> injury of bronchus
Secondary blast injury of bronchus
MCC-A **S27.491-** Other injury of bronchus, <u>unilateral</u>
MCC-A **S27.492-** Other injury of bronchus, <u>bilateral</u>
MCC-A **S27.499-** Other injury of bronchus, <u>unspecified</u>
S27.5- Injury of <u>thoracic</u> <u>trachea</u>
CC-A **S27.50x-** <u>Unspecified</u> injury of thoracic trachea
CC-A **S27.51x-** <u>Primary blast</u> injury of thoracic trachea
Blast injury of thoracic trachea NOS
CC-A **S27.52x-** <u>Contusion</u> of thoracic trachea
CC-A **S27.53x-** <u>Laceration</u> of thoracic trachea
CC-A **S27.59x-** <u>Other</u> injury of thoracic trachea
Secondary blast injury of thoracic trachea
S27.6- Injury of <u>pleura</u>
CC-A **S27.60x-** <u>Unspecified</u> injury of pleura
CC-A **S27.63x-** <u>Laceration</u> of pleura
CC-A **S27.69x-** <u>Other</u> injury of pleura
S27.8- Injury of <u>other specified</u> intrathoracic organs
S27.80- Injury of <u>diaphragm</u>
CC-A **S27.802-** <u>Contusion</u> of diaphragm
CC-A **S27.803-** <u>Laceration</u> of diaphragm
CC-A **S27.808-** <u>Other</u> injury of diaphragm
CC-A **S27.809-** <u>Unspecified</u> injury of diaphragm
S27.81- Injury of <u>esophagus (thoracic part)</u>
MCC-A **S27.812-** <u>Contusion</u> of esophagus (thoracic part)
MCC-A **S27.813-** <u>Laceration</u> of esophagus (thoracic part)
MCC-A **S27.818-** <u>Other</u> injury of esophagus (thoracic part)
MCC-A **S27.819-** <u>Unspecified</u> injury of esophagus (thoracic part)
S27.89- Injury of <u>other specified</u> intrathoracic organs
Injury of lymphatic thoracic duct
Injury of thymus gland
CC-A **S27.892-** <u>Contusion</u> of other specified intrathoracic organs
CC-A **S27.893-** <u>Laceration</u> of other specified intrathoracic organs
CC-A **S27.898-** <u>Other</u> injury of other specified intrathoracic organs
CC-A **S27.899-** <u>Unspecified</u> injury of other specified intrathoracic organs
S27.9xx- Injury of <u>unspecified</u> intrathoracic organ
CC-A

S25
-
S27

S28- Crushing injury of <u>thorax</u>, and traumatic amputation of part of thorax

> The appropriate 7th character is to be added to each code from category S28:
> **A** <u>Initial</u> encounter
> **D** <u>Subsequent</u> encounter
> **S** <u>Sequela</u>

S28.0xx- <u>Crushed</u> chest

> Use additional code for all associated injuries
> *Excludes 1:* flail chest (S22.5)

S28.1xx- <u>Traumatic amputation</u> (partial) of <u>part of thorax</u>, except
CC-A   breast

S28.2- <u>Traumatic amputation</u> of <u>breast</u>

> **S28.21-** <u>Complete</u> traumatic amputation of <u>breast</u>
> > Traumatic amputation of breast NOS
> >
> > **S28.211-** Complete traumatic amputation of <u>right</u> breast
> > **S28.212-** Complete traumatic amputation of <u>left</u> breast
> > **S28.219-** Complete traumatic amputation of <u>unspecified</u> breast
>
> **S28.22-** <u>Partial</u> traumatic amputation of <u>breast</u>
> > **S28.221-** Partial traumatic amputation of <u>right</u> breast
> > **S28.222-** Partial traumatic amputation of <u>left</u> breast
> > **S28.229-** Partial traumatic amputation of <u>unspecified</u> breast

S29- Other and <u>unspecified</u> injuries of thorax

> Code also any associated open wound (S21.-)
> The appropriate 7th character is to be added to each code from category S29:
> **A** <u>Initial</u> encounter
> **D** <u>Subsequent</u> encounter
> **S** <u>Sequela</u>

S29.0- Injury of <u>muscle and tendon</u> at <u>thorax</u> level

> **S29.00-** <u>Unspecified</u> injury of muscle and tendon of thorax
> > **S29.001-** Unspecified injury of muscle and tendon of <u>front wall</u> of thorax
> > **S29.002-** Unspecified injury of muscle and tendon of <u>back wall</u> of thorax
> > **S29.009-** Unspecified injury of muscle and tendon of <u>unspecified</u> wall of thorax
>
> **S29.01-** <u>Strain</u> of muscle and tendon of thorax
> > **S29.011-** Strain of muscle and tendon of <u>front wall</u> of thorax
> > **S29.012-** Strain of muscle and tendon of <u>back wall</u> of thorax
> > **S29.019-** Strain of muscle and tendon of <u>unspecified</u> wall of thorax
>
> **S29.02-** <u>Laceration</u> of muscle and tendon of thorax
> > CC-A **S29.021-** Laceration of muscle and tendon of <u>front wall</u> of thorax
> > **S29.022-** Laceration of muscle and tendon of <u>back wall</u> of thorax
> > CC-A **S29.029-** Laceration of muscle and tendon of <u>unspecified</u> wall of thorax
>
> **S29.09-** <u>Other</u> injury of muscle and tendon of thorax
> > **S29.091-** Other injury of muscle and tendon of <u>front wall</u> of thorax
> > **S29.092-** Other injury of muscle and tendon of <u>back wall</u> of thorax
> > **S29.099-** Other injury of muscle and tendon of <u>unspecified</u> wall of thorax

S29.8xx- <u>Other</u> specified injuries of thorax

S29.9xx- <u>Unspecified</u> injury of thorax

Injuries to the abdomen, lower back, lumbar spine, pelvis and external genitals (S30-S39)

> Includes: Injuries to the abdominal wall
> Injuries to the anus
> Injuries to the buttock
> Injuries to the external genitalia
> Injuries to the flank
> Injuries to the groin
>
> Excludes ❷: burns and corrosions (T20-T32)
> effects of foreign body in anus and rectum (T18.5)
> effects of foreign body in genitourinary tract (T19.-)
> effects of foreign body in stomach, small intestine and colon (T18.2-T18.4)
> frostbite (T33-T34)
> insect bite or sting, venomous (T63.4)

S30- <u>Superficial</u> injury of <u>abdomen, lower back, pelvis and external genitals</u>

> *Excludes ❷:* superficial injury of hip (S70.-)
> The appropriate 7th character is to be added to each code from category S30:
> **A** <u>Initial</u> encounter
> **D** <u>Subsequent</u> encounter
> **S** <u>Sequela</u>

S30.0xx- <u>Contusion</u> of <u>lower back and pelvis</u>

> Contusion of buttock

S30.1xx- <u>Contusion</u> of <u>abdominal wall</u>

> Contusion of flank
> Contusion of groin

S30.2- <u>Contusion</u> of <u>external genital organs</u>

> **S30.20-** Contusion of <u>unspecified</u> external genital organ
> > **S30.201-** Contusion of unspecified external genital organ, <u>male</u> — [♂]
> > **S30.202-** Contusion of unspecified external genital organ, <u>female</u> — [♀]
> **S30.21x-** Contusion of penis — [♂]
> **S30.22x-** Contusion of scrotum and testes — [♂]
> **S30.23x-** Contusion of vagina and vulva — [♀]

S30.3xx- Contusion of anus

S30.8- <u>Other</u> superficial injuries of abdomen, lower back, pelvis and external genitals

> **S30.81-** <u>Abrasion</u> of abdomen, lower back, pelvis and external genitals
> > **S30.810-** Abrasion of lower back and pelvis
> > **S30.811-** Abrasion of abdominal wall
> > **S30.812-** Abrasion of penis — [♂]
> > **S30.813-** Abrasion of scrotum and testes — [♂]
> > **S30.814-** Abrasion of vagina and vulva — [♀]
> > **S30.815-** Abrasion of <u>unspecified</u> external genital organs, <u>male</u> — [♂]
> > **S30.816-** Abrasion of <u>unspecified</u> external genital organs, <u>female</u> — [♀]
> > **S30.817-** Abrasion of anus
>
> **S30.82-** <u>Blister</u> (nonthermal) of abdomen, lower back, pelvis and external genitals
> > **S30.820-** Blister (nonthermal) of lower back and pelvis
> > **S30.821-** Blister (nonthermal) of abdominal wall
> > **S30.822-** Blister (nonthermal) of penis — [♂]
> > **S30.823-** Blister (nonthermal) of scrotum and testes — [♂]
> > **S30.824-** Blister (nonthermal) of vagina and vulva — [♀]
> > **S30.825-** Blister (nonthermal) of <u>unspecified</u> external genital organs, <u>male</u> — [♂]
> > **S30.826-** Blister (nonthermal) of <u>unspecified</u> external genital organs, <u>female</u> — [♀]
> > **S30.827-** Blister (nonthermal) of anus
>
> **S30.84-** <u>External constriction</u> of abdomen, lower back, pelvis and external genitals
> > **S30.840-** External constriction of lower back and pelvis
> > **S30.841-** External constriction of abdominal wall

S 2 8 ‖ S 3 0

S30.842- External constriction of penis — [♂]
  Hair tourniquet syndrome of penis
  Use additional cause code to identify the constricting
    item (W49.0-)

S30.843- External constriction of scrotum and testes — [♂]

S30.844- External constriction of vagina and vulva — [♀]

S30.845- External constriction of unspecified external genital
  organs, male — [♂]

S30.846- External constriction of unspecified external genital
  organs, female — [♀]

S30.85- Superficial foreign body of abdomen, lower back, pelvis
  and external genitals
    Splinter in the abdomen, lower back, pelvis and external
      genitals

S30.850- Superficial foreign body of lower back and pelvis

S30.851- Superficial foreign body of abdominal wall

S30.852- Superficial foreign body of penis — [♂]

S30.853- Superficial foreign body of scrotum and testes —
  [♂]

S30.854- Superficial foreign body of vagina and vulva — [♀]

S30.855- Superficial foreign body of unspecified external
  genital organs, male — [♂]

S30.856- Superficial foreign body of unspecified external
  genital organs, female — [♀]

S30.857- Superficial foreign body of anus

S30.86- Insect bite (nonvenomous) of abdomen, lower back,
  pelvis and external genitals

S30.860- Insect bite (nonvenomous) of lower back and pelvis

S30.861- Insect bite (nonvenomous) of abdominal wall

S30.862- Insect bite (nonvenomous) of penis — [♂]

S30.863- Insect bite (nonvenomous) of scrotum and testes —
  [♂]

S30.864- Insect bite (nonvenomous) of vagina and vulva —
  [♀]

S30.865- Insect bite (nonvenomous) of unspecified external
  genital organs, male — [♂]

S30.866- Insect bite (nonvenomous) of unspecified external
  genital organs, female — [♀]

S30.867- Insect bite (nonvenomous) of anus

S30.87- Other superficial bite of abdomen, lower back, pelvis and
  external genitals
    *Excludes 1:   open bite of abdomen, lower back, pelvis and
      external genitals (S31.05, S31.15, S31.25,
      S31.35, S31.45, S31.55)*

S30.870- Other superficial bite of lower back and pelvis

S30.871- Other superficial bite of abdominal wall

S30.872- Other superficial bite of penis — [♂]

S30.873- Other superficial bite of scrotum and testes — [♂]

S30.874- Other superficial bite of vagina and vulva — [♀]

S30.875- Other superficial bite of unspecified external
  genital organs, male — [♂]

S30.876- Other superficial bite of unspecified external
  genital organs, female — [♀]

S30.877- Other superficial bite of anus

S30.9- Unspecified superficial injury of abdomen, lower back, pelvis
  and external genitals

S30.91x- Unspecified superficial injury of lower back and pelvis

S30.92x- Unspecified superficial injury of abdominal wall

S30.93x- Unspecified superficial injury of penis — [♂]

S30.94x- Unspecified superficial injury of scrotum and testes —
  [♂]

S30.95x- Unspecified superficial injury of vagina and vulva —
  [♀]

S30.96x- Unspecified superficial injury of unspecified external
  genital organs, male — [♂]

S30.97x- Unspecified superficial injury of unspecified external
  genital organs, female — [♀]

S30.98x- Unspecified superficial injury of anus

S31- Open wound of abdomen, lower back, pelvis and external genitals
  Code also any associated:
    Spinal cord injury (S24.0, S24.1-, S34.0-, S34.1-)
    Wound infection
  *Excludes 1:   traumatic amputation of part of abdomen, lower back and
    pelvis (S38.2-, S38.3)*
  *Excludes ❷: open wound of hip (S71.00-S71.02)
    open fracture of pelvis (S32.1- -S32.9 with 7th character B)*

The appropriate 7th character is to be added to each code from
  category S31:
  A   **Initial** encounter
  D   **Subsequent** encounter
  S   **Sequela**

S31.0- Open wound of lower back and pelvis

S31.00- Unspecified open wound of lower back and pelvis

S31.000- Unspecified open wound of lower back and pelvis
  without penetration into retroperitoneum
    Unspecified open wound of lower back and pelvis NOS

MCC-A **S31.001-** Unspecified open wound of lower back and pelvis
  with penetration into retroperitoneum

S31.01- Laceration without foreign body of lower back and pelvis

S31.010- Laceration without foreign body of lower back and
  pelvis without penetration into retroperitoneum
    Laceration without foreign body of lower back and
      pelvis NOS

MCC-A **S31.011-** Laceration without foreign body of lower back and
  pelvis with penetration into retroperitoneum

S31.02- Laceration with foreign body of lower back and pelvis

S31.020- Laceration with foreign body of lower back and
  pelvis without penetration into retroperitoneum
    Laceration with foreign body of lower back and pelvis
      NOS

MCC-A **S31.021-** Laceration with foreign body of lower back and
  pelvis with penetration into retroperitoneum

S31.03- Puncture wound without foreign body of lower back and
  pelvis

S31.030- Puncture wound without foreign body of lower back
  and pelvis without penetration into
  retroperitoneum
    Puncture wound without foreign body of lower back
      and pelvis NOS

MCC-A **S31.031-** Puncture wound without foreign body of lower back
  and pelvis with penetration into retroperitoneum

S31.04- Puncture wound with foreign body of lower back and
  pelvis

S31.040- Puncture wound with foreign body of lower back
  and pelvis without penetration into
  retroperitoneum
    Puncture wound with foreign body of lower back and
      pelvis NOS

MCC-A **S31.041-** Puncture wound with foreign body of lower back
  and pelvis with penetration into retroperitoneum

S31.05- Open bite of lower back and pelvis
  Bite of lower back and pelvis NOS
    *Excludes 1:   superficial bite of lower back and pelvis (S30.860,
      S30.870)*

S31.050- Open bite of lower back and pelvis without
  penetration into retroperitoneum
    Open bite of lower back and pelvis NOS

MCC-A **S31.051-** Open bite of lower back and pelvis with
  penetration into retroperitoneum

S31.1- Open wound of abdominal wall without penetration into
  peritoneal cavity
    Open wound of abdominal wall NOS
    *Excludes ❷: open wound of abdominal wall with penetration into
      peritoneal cavity (S31.6-)*

S31.10- Unspecified open wound of abdominal wall without
  penetration into peritoneal cavity

S31.100- Unspecified open wound of abdominal wall, right
  upper quadrant without penetration into
  peritoneal cavity

S 3 0 - S 3 1

S31.101- Unspecified open wound of abdominal wall, <u>left upper</u> quadrant <u>without</u> penetration into peritoneal cavity

S31.102- Unspecified open wound of abdominal wall, <u>epigastric region</u> <u>without</u> penetration into peritoneal cavity

S31.103- Unspecified open wound of abdominal wall, <u>right lower</u> quadrant <u>without</u> penetration into peritoneal cavity

S31.104- Unspecified open wound of abdominal wall, <u>left lower</u> quadrant <u>without</u> penetration into peritoneal cavity

S31.105- Unspecified open wound of abdominal wall, <u>periumbilic region</u> <u>without</u> penetration into peritoneal cavity

S31.109- Unspecified open wound of abdominal wall, <u>unspecified quadrant</u> <u>without</u> penetration into peritoneal cavity
  Unspecified open wound of abdominal wall NOS

S31.11- <u>Laceration</u> <u>without</u> foreign body of abdominal wall <u>without</u> penetration into peritoneal cavity

S31.110- Laceration <u>without</u> foreign body of abdominal wall, <u>right upper</u> quadrant <u>without</u> penetration into peritoneal cavity

S31.111- Laceration <u>without</u> foreign body of abdominal wall, <u>left upper</u> quadrant <u>without</u> penetration into peritoneal cavity

S31.112- Laceration <u>without</u> foreign body of abdominal wall, <u>epigastric region</u> <u>without</u> penetration into peritoneal cavity

S31.113- Laceration <u>without</u> foreign body of abdominal wall, <u>right lower</u> quadrant <u>without</u> penetration into peritoneal cavity

S31.114- Laceration <u>without</u> foreign body of abdominal wall, <u>left lower</u> quadrant <u>without</u> penetration into peritoneal cavity

S31.115- Laceration <u>without</u> foreign body of abdominal wall, <u>periumbilic region</u> <u>without</u> penetration into peritoneal cavity

S31.119- Laceration <u>without</u> foreign body of abdominal wall, <u>unspecified quadrant</u> <u>without</u> penetration into peritoneal cavity

S31.12- <u>Laceration</u> <u>with foreign body</u> of abdominal wall <u>without</u> penetration into peritoneal cavity

S31.120- Laceration of abdominal wall <u>with foreign body</u>, <u>right upper</u> quadrant <u>without</u> penetration into peritoneal cavity

S31.121- Laceration of abdominal wall <u>with foreign body</u>, <u>left upper</u> quadrant <u>without</u> penetration into peritoneal cavity

S31.122- Laceration of abdominal wall <u>with foreign body</u>, <u>epigastric region</u> <u>without</u> penetration into peritoneal cavity

S31.123- Laceration of abdominal wall <u>with foreign body</u>, <u>right lower</u> quadrant <u>without</u> penetration into peritoneal cavity

S31.124- Laceration of abdominal wall <u>with foreign body</u>, <u>left lower</u> quadrant <u>without</u> penetration into peritoneal cavity

S31.125- Laceration of abdominal wall <u>with foreign body</u>, <u>periumbilic</u> region <u>without</u> penetration into peritoneal cavity

S31.129- Laceration of abdominal wall <u>with foreign body</u>, <u>unspecified quadrant</u> <u>without</u> penetration into peritoneal cavity

S31.13- <u>Puncture</u> wound of abdominal wall <u>without</u> foreign body <u>without</u> penetration into peritoneal cavity

S31.130- Puncture wound of abdominal wall <u>without</u> foreign body, <u>right upper</u> quadrant <u>without</u> penetration into peritoneal cavity

S31.131- Puncture wound of abdominal wall <u>without</u> foreign body, <u>left upper</u> quadrant <u>without</u> penetration into peritoneal cavity

S31.132- Puncture wound of abdominal wall <u>without</u> foreign body, <u>epigastric region</u> <u>without</u> penetration into peritoneal cavity

S31.133- Puncture wound of abdominal wall <u>without</u> foreign body, <u>right lower</u> quadrant <u>without</u> penetration into peritoneal cavity

S31.134- Puncture wound of abdominal wall <u>without</u> foreign body, <u>left lower</u> quadrant <u>without</u> penetration into peritoneal cavity

S31.135- Puncture wound of abdominal wall <u>without</u> foreign body, periumbilic region <u>without</u> penetration into peritoneal cavity

S31.139- Puncture wound of abdominal wall <u>without</u> foreign body, <u>unspecified quadrant</u> <u>without</u> penetration into peritoneal cavity

S31.14- <u>Puncture</u> wound of abdominal wall <u>with foreign body</u> <u>without</u> penetration into peritoneal cavity

S31.140- Puncture wound of abdominal wall <u>with foreign body</u>, <u>right upper</u> quadrant <u>without</u> penetration into peritoneal cavity

S31.141- Puncture wound of abdominal wall <u>with foreign body</u>, <u>left upper</u> quadrant <u>without</u> penetration into peritoneal cavity

S31.142- Puncture wound of abdominal wall <u>with foreign body</u>, <u>epigastric region</u> <u>without</u> penetration into peritoneal cavity

S31.143- Puncture wound of abdominal wall <u>with foreign body</u>, <u>right lower</u> quadrant <u>without</u> penetration into peritoneal cavity

S31.144- Puncture wound of abdominal wall <u>with foreign body</u>, <u>left lower</u> quadrant <u>without</u> penetration into peritoneal cavity

S31.145- Puncture wound of abdominal wall <u>with foreign body</u>, <u>periumbilic region</u> <u>without</u> penetration into peritoneal cavity

S31.149- Puncture wound of abdominal wall <u>with foreign body</u>, <u>unspecified quadrant</u> <u>without</u> penetration into peritoneal cavity

S31.15- <u>Open bite</u> of abdominal wall <u>without</u> penetration into peritoneal cavity
  Bite of abdominal wall NOS
  Excludes 1: *superficial bite of abdominal wall (S30.871)*

S31.150- Open bite of abdominal wall, <u>right upper</u> quadrant <u>without</u> penetration into peritoneal cavity

S31.151- Open bite of abdominal wall, <u>left upper</u> quadrant <u>without</u> penetration into peritoneal cavity

S31.152- Open bite of abdominal wall, <u>epigastric region</u> <u>without</u> penetration into peritoneal cavity

S31.153- Open bite of abdominal wall, <u>right lower</u> quadrant <u>without</u> penetration into peritoneal cavity

S31.154- Open bite of abdominal wall, <u>left lower</u> quadrant <u>without</u> penetration into peritoneal cavity

S31.155- Open bite of abdominal wall, <u>periumbilic region</u> <u>without</u> penetration into peritoneal cavity

S31.159- Open bite of abdominal wall, <u>unspecified quadrant</u> <u>without</u> penetration into peritoneal cavity

S31.2- Open wound of <u>penis</u>
S31.20x- Unspecified open wound of penis —[♂]
S31.21x- Laceration <u>without</u> foreign body of penis —[♂]
S31.22x- Laceration <u>with foreign body</u> of penis —[♂]
S31.23x- Puncture wound <u>without</u> foreign body of penis —[♂]
S31.24x- Puncture wound <u>with foreign body</u> of penis —[♂]
S31.25x- Open bite of penis —[♂]
  Bite of penis NOS
  Excludes 1: *superficial bite of penis (S30.862, S30.872)*

S31.3- Open wound of <u>scrotum and testes</u>

S31.30x- Unspecified open wound of scrotum and testes — [♂]

S31.31x- Laceration <u>without</u> foreign body of scrotum and testes — [♂]

S31.32x- Laceration <u>with foreign body</u> of scrotum and testes — [♂]

S31.33x- Puncture wound <u>without</u> foreign body of scrotum and testes — [♂]

S31.34x- Puncture wound <u>with foreign body</u> of scrotum and testes — [♂]

S31.35x- Open bite of scrotum and testes — [♂]
Bite of scrotum and testes NOS
Excludes 1:   superficial bite of scrotum and testes (S30.863, S30.873)

S31.4- Open wound of <u>vagina and vulva</u>
Excludes 1:   injury to vagina and vulva during delivery (O70.-, O71.4)

S31.40x- Unspecified open wound of vagina and vulva — [♀]

S31.41x- Laceration <u>without</u> foreign body of vagina and vulva — [♀]

S31.42x- Laceration <u>with foreign body</u> of vagina and vulva — [♀]

S31.43x- Puncture wound <u>without</u> foreign body of vagina and vulva — [♀]

S31.44x- Puncture wound <u>with foreign body</u> of vagina and vulva — [♀]

S31.45x- Open bite of vagina and vulva — [♀]
Bite of vagina and vulva NOS
Excludes 1:   superficial bite of vagina and vulva (S30.864, S30.874)

S31.5- Open wound of <u>unspecified external genital organs</u>
Excludes 1:   traumatic amputation of external genital organs (S38.21, S38.22)

S31.50- <u>Unspecified</u> open wound of <u>unspecified</u> external genital organs

S31.501- Unspecified open wound of <u>unspecified</u> external genital organs, <u>male</u> — [♂]

S31.502- Unspecified open wound of <u>unspecified</u> external genital organs, <u>female</u> — [♀]

S31.51- <u>Laceration without</u> foreign body of <u>unspecified</u> external genital organs

S31.511- Laceration <u>without</u> foreign body of <u>unspecified</u> external genital organs, <u>male</u> — [♂]

S31.512- Laceration <u>without</u> foreign body of <u>unspecified</u> external genital organs, <u>female</u> — [♀]

S31.52- <u>Laceration with foreign body</u> of <u>unspecified</u> external genital organs

S31.521- Laceration <u>with foreign body</u> of <u>unspecified</u> external genital organs, <u>male</u> — [♂]

S31.522- Laceration <u>with foreign body</u> of <u>unspecified</u> external genital organs, <u>female</u> — [♀]

S31.53- <u>Puncture</u> wound <u>without</u> foreign body of <u>unspecified</u> external genital organs

S31.531- Puncture wound <u>without</u> foreign body of <u>unspecified</u> external genital organs, <u>male</u> — [♂]

S31.532- Puncture wound <u>without</u> foreign body of <u>unspecified</u> external genital organs, <u>female</u> — [♀]

S31.54- <u>Puncture</u> wound <u>with foreign body</u> of <u>unspecified</u> external genital organs

S31.541- Puncture wound <u>with foreign body</u> of <u>unspecified</u> external genital organs, <u>male</u> — [♂]

S31.542- Puncture wound <u>with foreign body</u> of <u>unspecified</u> external genital organs, <u>female</u> — [♀]

S31.55- <u>Open bite</u> of <u>unspecified external genital organs</u>
Bite of unspecified external genital organs NOS
Excludes 1:   superficial bite of unspecified external genital organs (S30.865, S30.866, S30.875, S30.876)

S31.551- Open bite of <u>unspecified</u> external genital organs, <u>male</u> — [♂]

S31.552- Open bite of <u>unspecified</u> external genital organs, <u>female</u> — [♀]

S31.6- <u>Open wound</u> of <u>abdominal wall</u> <u>with penetration</u> into peritoneal cavity

S31.60- <u>Unspecified</u> open wound of <u>abdominal wall with penetration</u> into peritoneal cavity

MCC-A **S31.600- Unspecified open wound of abdominal wall, <u>right upper</u> quadrant <u>with penetration</u> into peritoneal cavity**

MCC-A **S31.601- Unspecified open wound of abdominal wall, <u>left upper</u> quadrant <u>with penetration</u> into peritoneal cavity**

MCC-A **S31.602- Unspecified open wound of abdominal wall, <u>epigastric region</u> <u>with penetration</u> into peritoneal cavity**

MCC-A **S31.603- Unspecified open wound of abdominal wall, <u>right lower</u> quadrant <u>with penetration</u> into peritoneal cavity**

MCC-A **S31.604- Unspecified open wound of abdominal wall, <u>left lower</u> quadrant <u>with penetration</u> into peritoneal cavity**

MCC-A **S31.605- Unspecified open wound of abdominal wall, <u>periumbilic region</u> <u>with penetration</u> into peritoneal cavity**

MCC-A **S31.609- Unspecified open wound of abdominal wall, <u>unspecified quadrant</u> <u>with penetration</u> into peritoneal cavity**

S31.61- <u>Laceration without</u> foreign body of abdominal wall <u>with penetration</u> into peritoneal cavity

MCC-A **S31.610- Laceration <u>without</u> foreign body of abdominal wall, <u>right upper</u> quadrant <u>with penetration</u> into peritoneal cavity**

MCC-A **S31.611- Laceration <u>without</u> foreign body of abdominal wall, <u>left upper</u> quadrant <u>with penetration</u> into peritoneal cavity**

MCC-A **S31.612- Laceration <u>without</u> foreign body of abdominal wall, <u>epigastric region</u> <u>with penetration</u> into peritoneal cavity**

MCC-A **S31.613- Laceration <u>without</u> foreign body of abdominal wall, <u>right lower</u> quadrant <u>with penetration</u> into peritoneal cavity**

MCC-A **S31.614- Laceration <u>without</u> foreign body of abdominal wall, <u>left lower</u> quadrant <u>with penetration</u> into peritoneal cavity**

MCC-A **S31.615- Laceration <u>without</u> foreign body of abdominal wall, <u>periumbilic region</u> <u>with penetration</u> into peritoneal cavity**

MCC-A **S31.619- Laceration <u>without</u> foreign body of abdominal wall, <u>unspecified quadrant</u> <u>with penetration</u> into peritoneal cavity**

S31.62- <u>Laceration with foreign body</u> of abdominal wall <u>with penetration</u> into peritoneal cavity

MCC-A **S31.620- Laceration <u>with foreign body</u> of abdominal wall, <u>right upper</u> quadrant <u>with penetration</u> into peritoneal cavity**

MCC-A **S31.621- Laceration <u>with foreign body</u> of abdominal wall, <u>left upper</u> quadrant <u>with penetration</u> into peritoneal cavity**

MCC-A **S31.622- Laceration <u>with foreign body</u> of abdominal wall, <u>epigastric region</u> <u>with penetration</u> into peritoneal cavity**

MCC-A **S31.623- Laceration <u>with foreign body</u> of abdominal wall, <u>right lower</u> quadrant <u>with penetration</u> into peritoneal cavity**

MCC-A **S31.624- Laceration <u>with foreign body</u> of abdominal wall, <u>left lower</u> quadrant <u>with penetration</u> into peritoneal cavity**

MCC-A **S31.625- Laceration <u>with foreign body</u> of abdominal wall, <u>periumbilic region</u> <u>with penetration</u> into peritoneal cavity**

S31
S31 - S31

MCC-A **S31.629-** Laceration <u>with foreign body</u> of abdominal wall, <u>unspecified quadrant with penetration</u> into peritoneal cavity

S31.63- <u>Puncture</u> wound <u>without</u> foreign body of abdominal wall <u>with penetration</u> into peritoneal cavity

MCC-A **S31.630-** Puncture wound <u>without</u> foreign body of abdominal wall, <u>right upper</u> quadrant <u>with penetration</u> into peritoneal cavity

MCC-A **S31.631-** Puncture wound <u>without</u> foreign body of abdominal wall, <u>left upper</u> quadrant <u>with penetration</u> into peritoneal cavity

MCC-A **S31.632-** Puncture wound <u>without</u> foreign body of abdominal wall, <u>epigastric region with penetration</u> into peritoneal cavity

MCC-A **S31.633-** Puncture wound <u>without</u> foreign body of abdominal wall, <u>right lower</u> quadrant <u>with penetration</u> into peritoneal cavity

MCC-A **S31.634-** Puncture wound <u>without</u> foreign body of abdominal wall, <u>left lower</u> quadrant <u>with penetration</u> into peritoneal cavity

MCC-A **S31.635-** Puncture wound <u>without</u> foreign body of abdominal wall, <u>periumbilic region with penetration</u> into peritoneal cavity

MCC-A **S31.639-** Puncture wound <u>without</u> foreign body of abdominal wall, <u>unspecified quadrant with penetration</u> into peritoneal cavity

S31.64- <u>Puncture</u> wound <u>with foreign body</u> of abdominal wall <u>with penetration</u> into peritoneal cavity

MCC-A **S31.640-** Puncture wound <u>with foreign body</u> of abdominal wall, <u>right upper</u> quadrant <u>with penetration</u> into peritoneal cavity

MCC-A **S31.641-** Puncture wound <u>with foreign body</u> of abdominal wall, <u>left upper</u> quadrant <u>with penetration</u> into peritoneal cavity

MCC-A **S31.642-** Puncture wound <u>with foreign body</u> of abdominal wall, <u>epigastric region with penetration</u> into peritoneal cavity

MCC-A **S31.643-** Puncture wound <u>with foreign body</u> of abdominal wall, <u>right lower</u> quadrant <u>with penetration</u> into peritoneal cavity

MCC-A **S31.644-** Puncture wound <u>with foreign body</u> of abdominal wall, <u>left lower</u> quadrant <u>with penetration</u> into peritoneal cavity

MCC-A **S31.645-** Puncture wound <u>with foreign body</u> of abdominal wall, <u>periumbilic region with penetration</u> into peritoneal cavity

MCC-A **S31.649-** Puncture wound <u>with foreign body</u> of abdominal wall, <u>unspecified quadrant with penetration</u> into peritoneal cavity

S31.65- <u>Open bite</u> of abdominal wall <u>with penetration</u> into peritoneal cavity
Excludes 1:   superficial bite of abdominal wall (S30.861, S30.871)

MCC-A **S31.650-** Open bite of abdominal wall, <u>right upper</u> quadrant <u>with penetration</u> into peritoneal cavity

MCC-A **S31.651-** Open bite of abdominal wall, <u>left upper</u> quadrant <u>with penetration</u> into peritoneal cavity

MCC-A **S31.652-** Open bite of abdominal wall, <u>epigastric region with penetration</u> into peritoneal cavity

MCC-A **S31.653-** Open bite of abdominal wall, <u>right lower</u> quadrant <u>with penetration</u> into peritoneal cavity

MCC-A **S31.654-** Open bite of abdominal wall, <u>left lower</u> quadrant <u>with penetration</u> into peritoneal cavity

MCC-A **S31.655-** Open bite of abdominal wall, <u>periumbilic region with penetration</u> into peritoneal cavity

MCC-A **S31.659-** Open bite of abdominal wall, <u>unspecified quadrant with penetration</u> into peritoneal cavity

S31.8- <u>Open wound</u> of <u>other parts of abdomen, lower back and pelvis</u>

S31.80- Open wound of <u>unspecified buttock</u>

S31.801- <u>Laceration without</u> foreign body of <u>unspecified</u> buttock

S31.802- <u>Laceration with foreign body</u> of unspecified buttock

S31.803- <u>Puncture</u> wound <u>without</u> foreign body of <u>unspecified</u> buttock

S31.804- <u>Puncture</u> wound <u>with foreign body</u> of <u>unspecified</u> buttock

S31.805- <u>Open bite</u> of <u>unspecified</u> buttock
Bite of buttock NOS
Excludes 1:   superficial bite of buttock (S30.870)

S31.809- <u>Unspecified</u> open wound of <u>unspecified</u> buttock

S31.81- Open wound of <u>right buttock</u>

S31.811- <u>Laceration without</u> foreign body of <u>right</u> buttock

S31.812- <u>Laceration with foreign body</u> of <u>right</u> buttock

S31.813- <u>Puncture</u> wound <u>without</u> foreign body of <u>right</u> buttock

S31.814- <u>Puncture</u> wound <u>with foreign body</u> of <u>right</u> buttock

S31.815- <u>Open bite</u> of <u>right</u> buttock
Bite of right buttock NOS
Excludes 1:   superficial bite of buttock (S30.870)

S31.819- <u>Unspecified</u> open wound of <u>right</u> buttock

S31.82- Open wound of <u>left buttock</u>

S31.821- <u>Laceration without</u> foreign body of <u>left</u> buttock

S31.822- <u>Laceration with foreign body</u> of <u>left</u> buttock

S31.823- <u>Puncture</u> wound <u>without</u> foreign body of <u>left</u> buttock

S31.824- <u>Puncture</u> wound <u>with foreign body</u> of <u>left</u> buttock

S31.825- <u>Open bite</u> of <u>left</u> buttock
Bite of left buttock NOS
Excludes 1:   superficial bite of buttock (S30.870)

S31.829- <u>Unspecified</u> open wound of <u>left</u> buttock

S31.83- Open wound of <u>anus</u>

S31.831- <u>Laceration without</u> foreign body of anus

S31.832- <u>Laceration with foreign body</u> of anus

S31.833- <u>Puncture</u> wound <u>without</u> foreign body of anus

S31.834- <u>Puncture</u> wound <u>with foreign body</u> of anus

S31.835- <u>Open bite</u> of anus
Bite of anus NOS
Excludes 1:   superficial bite of anus (S30.877)

S31.839- <u>Unspecified</u> open wound of anus

S32- Fracture of <u>lumbar</u> spine and pelvis
Note: A fracture not indicated as displaced or nondisplaced should be coded to displaced
Note: A fracture not indicated as opened or closed should be coded to closed
Includes: Fracture of lumbosacral neural arch
Fracture of lumbosacral spinous process
Fracture of lumbosacral transverse process
Fracture of lumbosacral vertebra
Fracture of lumbosacral vertebral arch
Code first any associated spinal cord and spinal nerve injury (S34.-)
Excludes 1:   transection of abdomen (S38.3)
Excludes ❷: fracture of hip NOS (S72.0-)

The appropriate 7th character is to be added to each code from category S32:
  A   <u>Initial</u> encounter for <u>closed</u> fracture
  B   <u>Initial</u> encounter for <u>open</u> fracture
  D   <u>Subsequent</u> encounter for fracture <u>with routine healing</u>
  G   <u>Subsequent</u> encounter for fracture <u>with delayed healing</u>
  K   <u>Subsequent</u> encounter for fracture <u>with nonunion</u>
  S   Sequela

S32.0- <u>Fracture</u> of <u>lumbar vertebra</u>
Fracture of lumbar spine NOS

S32.00- Fracture of <u>unspecified lumbar</u> vertebra

CC-A,K MCC-B **S32.000-** <u>Wedge</u> compression fracture of <u>unspecified</u> lumbar vertebra

S31
-
S32

CC-A,K MCC-B **S32.001-** <u>Stable burst</u> fracture of <u>unspecified</u> lumbar vertebra

CC-A,K MCC-B **S32.002-** <u>Unstable burst</u> fracture of <u>unspecified</u> lumbar vertebra

CC-A,K MCC-B **S32.008-** <u>Other</u> fracture of <u>unspecified</u> lumbar vertebra

CC-A,K MCC-B **S32.009-** <u>Unspecified</u> fracture of <u>unspecified</u> lumbar vertebra

S32.01- Fracture of <u>first</u> lumbar vertebra

CC-A,K MCC-B **S32.010-** <u>Wedge</u> compression fracture of first lumbar vertebra

CC-A,K MCC-B **S32.011-** <u>Stable burst</u> fracture of first lumbar vertebra

CC-A,K MCC-B **S32.012-** <u>Unstable burst</u> fracture of first lumbar vertebra

CC-A,K MCC-B **S32.018-** <u>Other</u> fracture of first lumbar vertebra

CC-A,K MCC-B **S32.019-** <u>Unspecified</u> fracture of first lumbar vertebra

S32.02- Fracture of <u>second</u> lumbar vertebra

CC-A,K MCC-B **S32.020-** <u>Wedge</u> compression fracture of second lumbar vertebra

CC-A,K MCC-B **S32.021-** <u>Stable burst</u> fracture of second lumbar vertebra

CC-A,K MCC-B **S32.022-** <u>Unstable burst</u> fracture of second lumbar vertebra

CC-A,K MCC-B **S32.028-** <u>Other</u> fracture of second lumbar vertebra

CC-A,K MCC-B **S32.029-** <u>Unspecified</u> fracture of second lumbar vertebra

S32.03- Fracture of <u>third</u> lumbar vertebra

CC-A,K MCC-B **S32.030-** <u>Wedge</u> compression fracture of third lumbar vertebra

CC-A,K MCC-B **S32.031-** <u>Stable burst</u> fracture of third lumbar vertebra

CC-A,K MCC-B **S32.032-** <u>Unstable burst</u> fracture of third lumbar vertebra

CC-A,K MCC-B **S32.038-** <u>Other</u> fracture of third lumbar vertebra

CC-A,K MCC-B **S32.039-** <u>Unspecified</u> fracture of third lumbar vertebra

S32.04- Fracture of <u>fourth</u> lumbar vertebra

CC-A,K MCC-B **S32.040-** <u>Wedge</u> compression fracture of fourth lumbar vertebra

CC-A,K MCC-B **S32.041-** <u>Stable burst</u> fracture of fourth lumbar vertebra

CC-A,K MCC-B **S32.042-** <u>Unstable burst</u> fracture of fourth lumbar vertebra

CC-A,K MCC-B **S32.048-** <u>Other</u> fracture of fourth lumbar vertebra

CC-A,K MCC-B **S32.049-** <u>Unspecified</u> fracture of fourth lumbar vertebra

S32.05- Fracture of <u>fifth</u> lumbar vertebra

CC-A,K MCC-B **S32.050-** <u>Wedge</u> compression fracture of fifth lumbar vertebra

CC-A,K MCC-B **S32.051-** <u>Stable burst</u> fracture of fifth lumbar vertebra

CC-A,K MCC-B **S32.052-** <u>Unstable burst</u> fracture of fifth lumbar vertebra

CC-A,K MCC-B **S32.058-** <u>Other</u> fracture of fifth lumbar vertebra

CC-A,K MCC-B **S32.059-** <u>Unspecified</u> fracture of fifth lumbar vertebra

S32.1- Fracture of <u>sacrum</u>
  Note: For vertical fractures, code to most medial fracture extension
  Note: Use two codes if both a vertical and transverse fracture are present
  Code also any associated fracture of pelvic ring (S32.8-)

S32.10x- <u>Unspecified</u> fracture of sacrum
CC-A,K MCC-B

S32.11- Zone I fracture of sacrum
    Vertical sacral ala fracture of sacrum

CC-A,K MCC-B **S32.110-** <u>Nondisplaced</u> Zone I fracture of sacrum

CC-A,K MCC-B **S32.111-** <u>Minimally displaced</u> Zone I fracture of sacrum

CC-A,K MCC-B **S32.112-** <u>Severely displaced</u> Zone I fracture of sacrum

CC-A,K MCC-B **S32.119-** <u>Unspecified</u> Zone I fracture of sacrum

S32.12- Zone II fracture of sacrum
    Vertical foraminal region fracture of sacrum

CC-A,K MCC-B **S32.120-** <u>Nondisplaced</u> Zone II fracture of sacrum

CC-A,K MCC-B **S32.121-** <u>Minimally displaced</u> Zone II fracture of sacrum

CC-A,K MCC-B **S32.122-** <u>Severely displaced</u> Zone II fracture of sacrum

CC-A,K MCC-B **S32.129-** <u>Unspecified</u> Zone II fracture of sacrum

S32.13- Zone III fracture of sacrum
    Vertical fracture into spinal canal region of sacrum

CC-A,K MCC-B **S32.130-** <u>Nondisplaced</u> Zone III fracture of sacrum

CC-A,K MCC-B **S32.131-** <u>Minimally displaced</u> Zone III fracture of sacrum

CC-A,K MCC-B **S32.132-** <u>Severely displaced</u> Zone III fracture of sacrum

CC-A,K MCC-B **S32.139-** <u>Unspecified</u> Zone III fracture of sacrum

S32.14x- Type 1 fracture of sacrum
CC-A,K MCC-B Transverse flexion fracture of sacrum without displacement

S32.15x- Type 2 fracture of sacrum
CC-A,K MCC-B Transverse flexion fracture of sacrum with posterior displacement

S32.16x- Type 3 fracture of sacrum
CC-A,K MCC-B Transverse extension fracture of sacrum with anterior displacement

S32.17x- Type 4 fracture of sacrum
CC-A,K MCC-B Transverse segmental comminution of upper sacrum

S32.19x- <u>Other</u> fracture of sacrum
CC-A,K MCC-B

S32.2xx- Fracture of coccyx
CC-A,K MCC-B

S32.3- Fracture of <u>ilium</u>
    Excludes 1:   fracture of ilium with associated disruption of pelvic ring (S32.8-)

S32.30- <u>Unspecified</u> fracture of ilium

CC-A,K MCC-B **S32.301-** Unspecified fracture of <u>right</u> ilium

CC-A,K MCC-B **S32.302-** Unspecified fracture of <u>left</u> ilium

CC-A,K MCC-B **S32.309-** Unspecified fracture of <u>unspecified</u> ilium

S32.31- <u>Avulsion</u> fracture of ilium

CC-A,K MCC-B **S32.311-** <u>Displaced</u> avulsion fracture of <u>right</u> ilium

CC-A,K MCC-B **S32.312-** <u>Displaced</u> avulsion fracture of <u>left</u> ilium

CC-A,K MCC-B **S32.313-** <u>Displaced</u> avulsion fracture of <u>unspecified</u> ilium

CC-A,K MCC-B **S32.314-** <u>Nondisplaced</u> avulsion fracture of <u>right</u> ilium

CC-A,K MCC-B **S32.315-** <u>Nondisplaced</u> avulsion fracture of <u>left</u> ilium

CC-A,K MCC-B **S32.316-** <u>Nondisplaced</u> avulsion fracture of <u>unspecified</u> ilium

S32.39- <u>Other</u> fracture of ilium

CC-A,K MCC-B **S32.391-** Other fracture of <u>right</u> ilium

CC-A,K MCC-B **S32.392-** Other fracture of <u>left</u> ilium

CC-A,K MCC-B **S32.399-** Other fracture of <u>unspecified</u> ilium

S32.4- Fracture of <u>acetabulum</u>
    Code also any associated fracture of pelvic ring (S32.8-)

S32.40- <u>Unspecified</u> fracture of acetabulum

CC-K MCC-A,B **S32.401-** Unspecified fracture of <u>right</u> acetabulum

CC-K MCC-A,B **S32.402-** Unspecified fracture of <u>left</u> acetabulum

CC-K MCC-A,B **S32.409-** Unspecified fracture of <u>unspecified</u> acetabulum

S32.41- Fracture of <u>anterior wall</u> of acetabulum

CC-K MCC-A,B **S32.411-** <u>Displaced</u> fracture of anterior wall of <u>right</u> acetabulum

CC-K MCC-A,B **S32.412-** <u>Displaced</u> fracture of anterior wall of <u>left</u> acetabulum

CC-K MCC-A,B **S32.413-** <u>Displaced</u> fracture of anterior wall of <u>unspecified</u> acetabulum

CC-K MCC-A,B **S32.414-** <u>Nondisplaced</u> fracture of anterior wall of <u>right</u> acetabulum

CC-K MCC-A,B **S32.415-** <u>Nondisplaced</u> fracture of anterior wall of <u>left</u> acetabulum

CC-K MCC-A,B **S32.416-** <u>Nondisplaced</u> fracture of anterior wall of <u>unspecified</u> acetabulum

S32.42- Fracture of <u>posterior wall</u> of acetabulum

CC-K MCC-A,B **S32.421-** <u>Displaced</u> fracture of posterior wall of <u>right</u> acetabulum

CC-K MCC-A,B **S32.422-** <u>Displaced</u> fracture of posterior wall of <u>left</u> acetabulum

CC-K MCC-A,B **S32.423-** <u>Displaced</u> fracture of posterior wall of <u>unspecified</u> acetabulum

CC-K MCC-A,B **S32.424-** <u>Nondisplaced</u> fracture of posterior wall of <u>right</u> acetabulum

CC-K MCC-A,B **S32.425-** <u>Nondisplaced</u> fracture of posterior wall of <u>left</u> acetabulum

CC-K MCC-A,B **S32.426-** <u>Nondisplaced</u> fracture of posterior wall of <u>unspecified</u> acetabulum

S32.43- Fracture of <u>anterior column [iliopubic]</u> of acetabulum

CC-K MCC-A,B **S32.431-** <u>Displaced</u> fracture of anterior column [iliopubic] of <u>right</u> acetabulum

CC-K MCC-A,B **S32.432-** <u>Displaced</u> fracture of anterior column [iliopubic] of <u>left</u> acetabulum

S 3 2 - S 3 2

CC-K MCC-A,B **S32.433-** <u>Displaced</u> fracture of anterior column [iliopubic] of <u>unspecified</u> acetabulum

CC-K MCC-A,B **S32.434-** <u>Nondisplaced</u> fracture of anterior column [iliopubic] of <u>right</u> acetabulum

CC-K MCC-A,B **S32.435-** <u>Nondisplaced</u> fracture of anterior column [iliopubic] of <u>left</u> acetabulum

CC-K MCC-A,B **S32.436-** <u>Nondisplaced</u> fracture of anterior column [iliopubic] of <u>unspecified</u> acetabulum

S32.44- Fracture of <u>posterior column [ilioischial]</u> of acetabulum

CC-K MCC-A,B **S32.441-** <u>Displaced</u> fracture of posterior column [ilioischial] of <u>right</u> acetabulum

CC-K MCC-A,B **S32.442-** <u>Displaced</u> fracture of posterior column [ilioischial] of <u>left</u> acetabulum

CC-K MCC-A,B **S32.443-** <u>Displaced</u> fracture of posterior column [ilioischial] of <u>unspecified</u> acetabulum

CC-K MCC-A,B **S32.444-** <u>Nondisplaced</u> fracture of posterior column [ilioischial] of <u>right</u> acetabulum

CC-K MCC-A,B **S32.445-** <u>Nondisplaced</u> fracture of posterior column [ilioischial] of <u>left</u> acetabulum

CC-K MCC-A,B **S32.446-** <u>Nondisplaced</u> fracture of posterior column [ilioischial] of <u>unspecified</u> acetabulum

S32.45- <u>Transverse</u> fracture of acetabulum

CC-K MCC-A,B **S32.451-** <u>Displaced</u> transverse fracture of <u>right</u> acetabulum

CC-K MCC-A,B **S32.452-** <u>Displaced</u> transverse fracture of <u>left</u> acetabulum

CC-K MCC-A,B **S32.453-** <u>Displaced</u> transverse fracture of <u>unspecified</u> acetabulum

CC-K MCC-A,B **S32.454-** <u>Nondisplaced</u> transverse fracture of <u>right</u> acetabulum

CC-K MCC-A,B **S32.455-** <u>Nondisplaced</u> transverse fracture of <u>left</u> acetabulum

CC-K MCC-A,B **S32.456-** <u>Nondisplaced</u> transverse fracture of <u>unspecified</u> acetabulum

S32.46- <u>Associated transverse-posterior</u> fracture of acetabulum

CC-K MCC-A,B **S32.461-** <u>Displaced</u> associated transverse-posterior fracture of <u>right</u> acetabulum

CC-K MCC-A,B **S32.462-** <u>Displaced</u> associated transverse-posterior fracture of <u>left</u> acetabulum

CC-K MCC-A,B **S32.463-** <u>Displaced</u> associated transverse-posterior fracture of <u>unspecified</u> acetabulum

CC-K MCC-A,B **S32.464-** <u>Nondisplaced</u> associated transverse-posterior fracture of <u>right</u> acetabulum

CC-K MCC-A,B **S32.465-** <u>Nondisplaced</u> associated transverse-posterior fracture of <u>left</u> acetabulum

CC-K MCC-A,B **S32.466-** <u>Nondisplaced</u> associated transverse-posterior fracture of <u>unspecified</u> acetabulum

S32.47- Fracture of <u>medial wall</u> of acetabulum

CC-K MCC-A,B **S32.471-** <u>Displaced</u> fracture of medial wall of <u>right</u> acetabulum

CC-K MCC-A,B **S32.472-** <u>Displaced</u> fracture of medial wall of <u>left</u> acetabulum

CC-K MCC-A,B **S32.473-** <u>Displaced</u> fracture of medial wall of <u>unspecified</u> acetabulum

CC-K MCC-A,B **S32.474-** <u>Nondisplaced</u> fracture of medial wall of <u>right</u> acetabulum

CC-K MCC-A,B **S32.475-** <u>Nondisplaced</u> fracture of medial wall of <u>left</u> acetabulum

CC-K MCC-A,B **S32.476-** <u>Nondisplaced</u> fracture of medial wall of <u>unspecified</u> acetabulum

S32.48- <u>Dome</u> fracture of acetabulum

CC-K MCC-A,B **S32.481-** <u>Displaced</u> dome fracture of <u>right</u> acetabulum

CC-K MCC-A,B **S32.482-** <u>Displaced</u> dome fracture of <u>left</u> acetabulum

CC-K MCC-A,B **S32.483-** <u>Displaced</u> dome fracture of <u>unspecified</u> acetabulum

CC-K MCC-A,B **S32.484-** <u>Nondisplaced</u> dome fracture of <u>right</u> acetabulum

CC-K MCC-A,B **S32.485-** <u>Nondisplaced</u> dome fracture of <u>left</u> acetabulum

CC-K MCC-A,B **S32.486-** <u>Nondisplaced</u> dome fracture of <u>unspecified</u> acetabulum

S32.49- <u>Other specified</u> fracture of acetabulum

CC-K MCC-A,B **S32.491-** Other specified fracture of <u>right</u> acetabulum

CC-K MCC-A,B **S32.492-** Other specified fracture of <u>left</u> acetabulum

CC-K MCC-A,B **S32.499-** Other specified fracture of <u>unspecified</u> acetabulum

S32.5- Fracture of <u>pubis</u>
> Excludes 1:   fracture of pubis with associated disruption of pelvic ring (S32.8-)

S32.50- <u>Unspecified</u> fracture of pubis

CC-A,K MCC-B **S32.501-** Unspecified fracture of <u>right</u> pubis

CC-A,K MCC-B **S32.502-** Unspecified fracture of <u>left</u> pubis

CC-A,K MCC-B **S32.509-** Unspecified fracture of <u>unspecified</u> pubis

S32.51- Fracture of <u>superior rim</u> of pubis

CC-A,K MCC-B **S32.511-** Fracture of superior rim of <u>right</u> pubis

CC-A,K MCC-B **S32.512-** Fracture of superior rim of <u>left</u> pubis

CC-A,K MCC-B **S32.519-** Fracture of superior rim of <u>unspecified</u> pubis

S32.59- <u>Other specified</u> fracture of pubis

CC-A,K MCC-B **S32.591-** Other specified fracture of <u>right</u> pubis

CC-A,K MCC-B **S32.592-** Other specified fracture of <u>left</u> pubis

CC-A,K MCC-B **S32.599-** Other specified fracture of <u>unspecified</u> pubis

S32.6- Fracture of <u>ischium</u>
> Excludes 1:   fracture of ischium with associated disruption of pelvic ring (S32.8-)

S32.60- <u>Unspecified</u> fracture of ischium

CC-A,K MCC-B **S32.601-** Unspecified fracture of <u>right</u> ischium

CC-A,K MCC-B **S32.602-** Unspecified fracture of <u>left</u> ischium

CC-A,K MCC-B **S32.609-** Unspecified fracture of <u>unspecified</u> ischium

S32.61- <u>Avulsion</u> fracture of ischium

CC-A,K MCC-B **S32.611-** <u>Displaced</u> avulsion fracture of <u>right</u> ischium

CC-A,K MCC-B **S32.612-** <u>Displaced</u> avulsion fracture of <u>left</u> ischium

CC-A,K MCC-B **S32.613-** <u>Displaced</u> avulsion fracture of <u>unspecified</u> ischium

CC-A,K MCC-B **S32.614-** <u>Nondisplaced</u> avulsion fracture of <u>right</u> ischium

CC-A,K MCC-B **S32.615-** <u>Nondisplaced</u> avulsion fracture of <u>left</u> ischium

CC-A,K MCC-B **S32.616-** <u>Nondisplaced</u> avulsion fracture of <u>unspecified</u> ischium

S32.69- <u>Other specified</u> fracture of ischium

CC-A,K MCC-B **S32.691-** Other specified fracture of <u>right</u> ischium

CC-A,K MCC-B **S32.692-** Other specified fracture of <u>left</u> ischium

CC-A,K MCC-B **S32.699-** Other specified fracture of <u>unspecified</u> ischium

S32.8- Fracture of <u>other parts of pelvis</u>
> Code also any associated:
> Fracture of acetabulum (S32.4-)
> Sacral fracture (S32.1-)

S32.81- <u>Multiple</u> fractures of pelvis <u>with disruption of pelvic ring</u>
> Multiple pelvic fractures with disruption of pelvic circle

CC-A,K MCC-B **S32.810-** Multiple fractures of pelvis with <u>stable</u> disruption of pelvic ring

CC-A,K MCC-B **S32.811-** Multiple fractures of pelvis with <u>unstable</u> disruption of pelvic ring

S32.82x- <u>Multiple</u> fractures of pelvis <u>without</u> disruption of pelvic
CC-A,K MCC-B ring
> Multiple pelvic fractures without disruption of pelvic circle

S32.89x- Fracture of <u>other</u> parts of pelvis
CC-A,K MCC-B

S32.9xx- Fracture of <u>unspecified</u> parts of lumbosacral spine and
CC-A,K MCC-B pelvis
> Fracture of lumbosacral spine NOS
> Fracture of pelvis NOS

S32 – S32

S33   Dislocation and sprain of joints and ligaments of lumbar spine and pelvis
   Includes: Avulsion of joint or ligament of lumbar spine and pelvis
               Laceration of cartilage, joint or ligament of lumbar spine and pelvis
               Sprain of cartilage, joint or ligament of lumbar spine and pelvis
               Traumatic hemarthrosis of joint or ligament of lumbar spine and pelvis
               Traumatic rupture of joint or ligament of lumbar spine and pelvis
               Traumatic subluxation of joint or ligament of lumbar spine and pelvis
               Traumatic tear of joint or ligament of lumbar spine and pelvis
   Code also any associated open wound
   Excludes 1:   nontraumatic rupture or displacement of lumbar intervertebral disc NOS (M51.-)
                 obstetric damage to pelvic joints and ligaments (O71.6)
   Excludes ❷: dislocation and sprain of joints and ligaments of hip (S73.-)
                 strain of muscle of lower back and pelvis (S39.01-)

The appropriate 7th character is to be added to each code from category S33:
   A   Initial encounter
   D   Subsequent encounter
   S   Sequela

S33.0xx-   Traumatic rupture of lumbar intervertebral disc
   Excludes 1:   rupture or displacement (nontraumatic) of lumbar intervertebral disc NOS (M51.- with fifth character 6)

S33.1-   Subluxation and dislocation of lumbar vertebra
   Code also any associated:
      Open wound of abdomen, lower back and pelvis (S31)
      Spinal cord injury (S24.0, S24.1-, S34.0-, S34.1-)
   Excludes ❷: fracture of lumbar vertebrae (S32.0-)

   S33.10-   Subluxation and dislocation of unspecified lumbar vertebra
      S33.100-   Subluxation of unspecified lumbar vertebra
      S33.101-   Dislocation of unspecified lumbar vertebra
   S33.11-   Subluxation and dislocation of L1/L2 lumbar vertebra
      S33.110-   Subluxation of L1/L2 lumbar vertebra
      S33.111-   Dislocation of L1/L2 lumbar vertebra
   S33.12-   Subluxation and dislocation of L2/L3 lumbar vertebra
      S33.120-   Subluxation of L2/L3 lumbar vertebra
      S33.121-   Dislocation of L2/L3 lumbar vertebra
   S33.13-   Subluxation and dislocation of L3/L4 lumbar vertebra
      S33.130-   Subluxation of L3/L4 lumbar vertebra
      S33.131-   Dislocation of L3/L4 lumbar vertebra
   S33.14-   Subluxation and dislocation of L4/L5 lumbar vertebra
      S33.140-   Subluxation of L4/L5 lumbar vertebra
      S33.141-   Dislocation of L4/L5 lumbar vertebra
S33.2xx-   Dislocation of sacroiliac and sacrococcygeal joint
S33.3-   Dislocation of other and unspecified parts of lumbar spine and pelvis
   S33.30x-   Dislocation of unspecified parts of lumbar spine and pelvis
   S33.39x-   Dislocation of other parts of lumbar spine and pelvis
S33.4xx-   Traumatic rupture of symphysis pubis
S33.5xx-   Sprain of ligaments of lumbar spine
S33.6xx-   Sprain of sacroiliac joint
S33.8xx-   Sprain of other parts of lumbar spine and pelvis
S33.9xx-   Sprain of unspecified parts of lumbar spine and pelvis

S34-   Injury of lumbar and sacral spinal cord and nerves at abdomen, lower back and pelvis level
   Note: Code to highest level of lumbar cord injury
           Injuries to the spinal cord (S34.0 and S34.1) refer to the cord level and not bone level injury, and can affect nerve roots at and below the level given.
   Code also any associated:
      Fracture of vertebra (S22.0-, S32.0-)
      Open wound of abdomen, lower back and pelvis (S31.-)
      Transient paralysis (R29.5)

The appropriate 7th character is to be added to each code from category S34:
   A   Initial encounter
   D   Subsequent encounter
   S   Sequela

S34.0-   Concussion and edema of lumbar and sacral spinal cord
MCC-A   **S34.01x-**   Concussion and edema of lumbar spinal cord
MCC-A   **S34.02x-**   Concussion and edema of sacral spinal cord
                       Concussion and edema of conus medullaris
S34.1-   Other and unspecified injury of lumbar and sacral spinal cord
   S34.10-   Unspecified injury to lumbar spinal cord
MCC-A   **S34.101-**   Unspecified injury to L1 level of lumbar spinal cord
                       Unspecified injury to lumbar spinal cord level 1
MCC-A   **S34.102-**   Unspecified injury to L2 level of lumbar spinal cord
                       Unspecified injury to lumbar spinal cord level 2
MCC-A   **S34.103-**   Unspecified injury to L3 level of lumbar spinal cord
                       Unspecified injury to lumbar spinal cord level 3
MCC-A   **S34.104-**   Unspecified injury to L4 level of lumbar spinal cord
                       Unspecified injury to lumbar spinal cord level 4
MCC-A   **S34.105-**   Unspecified injury to L5 level of lumbar spinal cord
                       Unspecified injury to lumbar spinal cord level 5
MCC-A   **S34.109-**   Unspecified injury to unspecified level of lumbar spinal cord
   S34.11-   Complete lesion of lumbar spinal cord
MCC-A   **S34.111-**   Complete lesion of L1 level of lumbar spinal cord
                       Complete lesion of lumbar spinal cord level 1
MCC-A   **S34.112-**   Complete lesion of L2 level of lumbar spinal cord
                       Complete lesion of lumbar spinal cord level 2
MCC-A   **S34.113-**   Complete lesion of L3 level of lumbar spinal cord
                       Complete lesion of lumbar spinal cord level 3
MCC-A   **S34.114-**   Complete lesion of L4 level of lumbar spinal cord
                       Complete lesion of lumbar spinal cord level 4
MCC-A   **S34.115-**   Complete lesion of L5 level of lumbar spinal cord
                       Complete lesion of lumbar spinal cord level 5
MCC-A   **S34.119-**   Complete lesion of unspecified level of lumbar spinal cord
   S34.12-   Incomplete lesion of lumbar spinal cord
MCC-A   **S34.121-**   Incomplete lesion of L1 level of lumbar spinal cord
                       Incomplete lesion of lumbar spinal cord level 1
MCC-A   **S34.122-**   Incomplete lesion of L2 level of lumbar spinal cord
                       Incomplete lesion of lumbar spinal cord level 2
MCC-A   **S34.123-**   Incomplete lesion of L3 level of lumbar spinal cord
                       Incomplete lesion of lumbar spinal cord level 3
MCC-A   **S34.124-**   Incomplete lesion of L4 level of lumbar spinal cord
                       Incomplete lesion of lumbar spinal cord level 4
MCC-A   **S34.125-**   Incomplete lesion of L5 level of lumbar spinal cord
                       Incomplete lesion of lumbar spinal cord level 5
MCC-A   **S34.129-**   Incomplete lesion of unspecified level of lumbar spinal cord
   S34.13-   Other and unspecified injury to sacral spinal cord
                 Other injury to conus medullaris
MCC-A   **S34.131-**   Complete lesion of sacral spinal cord
                       Complete lesion of conus medullaris
MCC-A   **S34.132-**   Incomplete lesion of sacral spinal cord
                       Incomplete lesion of conus medullaris
MCC-A   **S34.139-**   Unspecified injury to sacral spinal cord
                       Unspecified injury of conus medullaris
S34.2-   Injury of nerve root of lumbar and sacral spine
   S34.21x-   Injury of nerve root of lumbar spine
   S34.22x-   Injury of nerve root of sacral spine

S33 - S34

S34.3xx- Injury of cauda equina
MCC-A

S34.4xx- Injury of lumbosacral plexus

S34.5xx- Injury of lumbar, sacral and pelvic sympathetic nerves
    Injury of celiac ganglion or plexus
    Injury of hypogastric plexus
    Injury of mesenteric plexus (inferior) (superior)
    Injury of splanchnic nerve

S34.6xx- Injury of peripheral nerve(s) at abdomen, lower back and pelvis level

S34.8xx- Injury of other nerves at abdomen, lower back and pelvis level

S34.9xx- Injury of unspecified nerves at abdomen, lower back and pelvis level

S35- Injury of blood vessels at abdomen, lower back and pelvis level
    Code also any associated open wound (S31.-)
    The appropriate 7th character is to be added to each code from category S35:
      A Initial encounter
      D Subsequent encounter
      S Sequela

S35.0- Injury of abdominal aorta
    Excludes 1: injury of aorta NOS (S25.0)

MCC-A **S35.00x-** Unspecified injury of abdominal aorta

MCC-A **S35.01x-** Minor laceration of abdominal aorta
    Incomplete transection of abdominal aorta
    Laceration of abdominal aorta NOS
    Superficial laceration of abdominal aorta

MCC-A **S35.02x-** Major laceration of abdominal aorta
    Complete transection of abdominal aorta
    Traumatic rupture of abdominal aorta

MCC-A **S35.09x-** Other injury of abdominal aorta

S35.1- Injury of inferior vena cava
    Injury of hepatic vein
    Excludes 1: injury of vena cava NOS (S25.2)

MCC-A **S35.10x-** Unspecified injury of inferior vena cava

MCC-A **S35.11x-** Minor laceration of inferior vena cava
    Incomplete transection of inferior vena cava
    Laceration of inferior vena cava NOS
    Superficial laceration of inferior vena cava

MCC-A **S35.12x-** Major laceration of inferior vena cava
    Complete transection of inferior vena cava
    Traumatic rupture of inferior vena cava

MCC-A **S35.19x-** Other injury of inferior vena cava

S35.2- Injury of celiac or mesenteric artery and branches

  S35.21- Injury of celiac artery

MCC-A **S35.211-** Minor laceration of celiac artery
    Incomplete transection of celiac artery
    Laceration of celiac artery NOS
    Superficial laceration of celiac artery

MCC-A **S35.212-** Major laceration of celiac artery
    Complete transection of celiac artery
    Traumatic rupture of celiac artery

MCC-A **S35.218-** Other injury of celiac artery

MCC-A **S35.219-** Unspecified injury of celiac artery

  S35.22- Injury of superior mesenteric artery

MCC-A **S35.221-** Minor laceration of superior mesenteric artery
    Incomplete transection of superior mesenteric artery
    Laceration of superior mesenteric artery NOS
    Superficial laceration of superior mesenteric artery

MCC-A **S35.222-** Major laceration of superior mesenteric artery
    Complete transection of superior mesenteric artery
    Traumatic rupture of superior mesenteric artery

MCC-A **S35.228-** Other injury of superior mesenteric artery

MCC-A **S35.229-** Unspecified injury of superior mesenteric artery

  S35.23- Injury of inferior mesenteric artery

MCC-A **S35.231-** Minor laceration of inferior mesenteric artery
    Incomplete transection of inferior mesenteric artery
    Laceration of inferior mesenteric artery NOS
    Superficial laceration of inferior mesenteric artery

MCC-A **S35.232-** Major laceration of inferior mesenteric artery
    Complete transection of inferior mesenteric artery
    Traumatic rupture of inferior mesenteric artery

MCC-A **S35.238-** Other injury of inferior mesenteric artery

MCC-A **S35.239-** Unspecified injury of inferior mesenteric artery

  S35.29- Injury of branches of celiac and mesenteric artery
    Injury of gastric artery
    Injury of gastroduodenal artery
    Injury of hepatic artery
    Injury of splenic artery

MCC-A **S35.291-** Minor laceration of branches of celiac and mesenteric artery
    Incomplete transection of branches of celiac and mesenteric artery
    Laceration of branches of celiac and mesenteric artery NOS
    Superficial laceration of branches of celiac and mesenteric artery

MCC-A **S35.292-** Major laceration of branches of celiac and mesenteric artery
    Complete transection of branches of celiac and mesenteric artery
    Traumatic rupture of branches of celiac and mesenteric artery

MCC-A **S35.298-** Other injury of branches of celiac and mesenteric artery

MCC-A **S35.299-** Unspecified injury of branches of celiac and mesenteric artery

S35.3- Injury of portal or splenic vein and branches

  S35.31- Injury of portal vein

MCC-A **S35.311-** Laceration of portal vein

MCC-A **S35.318-** Other specified injury of portal vein

MCC-A **S35.319-** Unspecified injury of portal vein

  S35.32- Injury of splenic vein

MCC-A **S35.321-** Laceration of splenic vein

MCC-A **S35.328-** Other specified injury of splenic vein

MCC-A **S35.329-** Unspecified injury of splenic vein

  S35.33- Injury of superior mesenteric vein

MCC-A **S35.331-** Laceration of superior mesenteric vein

MCC-A **S35.338-** Other specified injury of superior mesenteric vein

MCC-A **S35.339-** Unspecified injury of superior mesenteric vein

  S35.34- Injury of inferior mesenteric vein

MCC-A **S35.341-** Laceration of inferior mesenteric vein

MCC-A **S35.348-** Other specified injury of inferior mesenteric vein

MCC-A **S35.349-** Unspecified injury of inferior mesenteric vein

S35.4- Injury of renal blood vessels

  S35.40- Unspecified injury of renal blood vessel

MCC-A **S35.401-** Unspecified injury of right renal artery

MCC-A **S35.402-** Unspecified injury of left renal artery

MCC-A **S35.403-** Unspecified injury of unspecified renal artery

MCC-A **S35.404-** Unspecified injury of right renal vein

MCC-A **S35.405-** Unspecified injury of left renal vein

MCC-A **S35.406-** Unspecified injury of unspecified renal vein

  S35.41- Laceration of renal blood vessel

MCC-A **S35.411-** Laceration of right renal artery

MCC-A **S35.412-** Laceration of left renal artery

MCC-A **S35.413-** Laceration of unspecified renal artery

MCC-A **S35.414-** Laceration of right renal vein

MCC-A **S35.415-** Laceration of left renal vein

MCC-A **S35.416-** Laceration of unspecified renal vein

  S35.49- Other specified injury of renal blood vessel

MCC-A **S35.491-** Other specified injury of right renal artery

MCC-A **S35.492-** Other specified injury of left renal artery

MCC-A **S35.493-** Other specified injury of unspecified renal artery

MCC-A **S35.494-** Other specified injury of right renal vein

MCC-A **S35.495-** Other specified injury of left renal vein

MCC-A **S35.496-** Other specified injury of unspecified renal vein

S35.5- Injury of iliac blood vessels

MCC-A **S35.50x-** Injury of unspecified iliac blood vessel(s)

  S35.51- Injury of iliac artery or vein
    Injury of hypogastric artery or vein

MCC-A **S35.511-** Injury of right iliac artery

MCC-A **S35.512-** Injury of <u>left</u> iliac <u>artery</u>

MCC-A **S35.513-** Injury of <u>unspecified</u> iliac <u>artery</u>

MCC-A **S35.514-** Injury of <u>right</u> iliac <u>vein</u>

MCC-A **S35.515-** Injury of <u>left</u> iliac <u>vein</u>

MCC-A **S35.516-** Injury of <u>unspecified</u> iliac <u>vein</u>

S35.53- Injury of <u>uterine</u> artery or vein

CC-A **S35.531-** Injury of <u>right</u> uterine <u>artery</u> — [♀]

CC-A **S35.532-** Injury of <u>left</u> uterine <u>artery</u> — [♀]

CC-A **S35.533-** Injury of <u>unspecified</u> uterine <u>artery</u> — [♀]

CC-A **S35.534-** Injury of <u>right</u> uterine <u>vein</u> — [♀]

CC-A **S35.535-** Injury of <u>left</u> uterine <u>vein</u> — [♀]

CC-A **S35.536-** Injury of <u>unspecified</u> uterine <u>vein</u> — [♀]

MCC-A **S35.59x-** Injury of <u>other iliac blood vessels</u>

S35.8- Injury of <u>other blood vessels</u> at <u>abdomen, lower back and pelvis level</u>

  Injury of ovarian artery or vein

S35.8x- Injury of <u>other blood vessels</u> at abdomen, lower back and pelvis level

CC-A **S35.8x1-** <u>Laceration</u> of <u>other</u> blood vessels at abdomen, lower back and pelvis level

CC-A **S35.8x8-** <u>Other</u> specified injury of <u>other</u> blood vessels at abdomen, lower back and pelvis level

CC-A **S35.8x9-** <u>Unspecified</u> injury of <u>other</u> blood vessels at abdomen, lower back and pelvis level

S35.9- Injury of <u>unspecified blood vessel</u> at <u>abdomen, lower back and pelvis level</u>

CC-A **S35.90x-** <u>Unspecified</u> injury of <u>unspecified</u> blood vessel at abdomen, lower back and pelvis level

CC-A **S35.91x-** <u>Laceration</u> of <u>unspecified</u> blood vessel at abdomen, lower back and pelvis level

CC-A **S35.99x-** <u>Other</u> specified injury of <u>unspecified</u> blood vessel at abdomen, lower back and pelvis level

S36- Injury of <u>intra-abdominal organs</u>

  Code also any associated open wound (S31.-)

  The appropriate 7th character is to be added to each code from category S36:
  A <u>Initial</u> encounter
  D <u>Subsequent</u> encounter
  S <u>Sequela</u>

S36.0- Injury of <u>spleen</u>

CC-A **S36.00x-** <u>Unspecified</u> injury of spleen

S36.02- <u>Contusion</u> of spleen
  AHA 15:1Q:p10 – Perisplenic hematoma
  AHA 15:2Q:p36 – Official Correction of 15:1Q:p10

CC-A **S36.020-** <u>Minor</u> contusion of spleen
  Contusion of spleen less than 2 cm

CC-A **S36.021-** <u>Major</u> contusion of spleen
  Contusion of spleen greater than 2 cm

CC-A **S36.029-** <u>Unspecified</u> contusion of spleen

S36.03- <u>Laceration</u> of spleen
  AHA 15:1Q:p10 – Delayed splenic rupture, grade 3 splenic laceration
  AHA 15:2Q:p36 – Official Correction of 15:1Q:p10

CC-A **S36.030-** <u>Superficial</u> (capsular) laceration of spleen
  Laceration of spleen less than 1 cm
  Minor laceration of spleen

MCC-A **S36.031-** <u>Moderate</u> laceration of spleen
  Laceration of spleen 1 to 3 cm

MCC-A **S36.032-** <u>Major</u> laceration of spleen
  Avulsion of spleen
  Laceration of spleen greater than 3 cm
  Massive laceration of spleen
  Multiple moderate lacerations of spleen
  Stellate laceration of spleen

CC-A **S36.039-** <u>Unspecified</u> laceration of spleen

CC-A **S36.09x-** <u>Other</u> injury of spleen

S36.1- Injury of <u>liver and gallbladder and bile duct</u>

S36.11- Injury of <u>liver</u>

CC-A **S36.112-** <u>Contusion</u> of liver

CC-A **S36.113-** <u>Laceration</u> of liver, <u>unspecified</u> degree

CC-A **S36.114-** <u>Minor</u> laceration of liver
  Laceration involving capsule only, or, without significant involvement of hepatic parenchyma [i.e., less than 1 cm deep]

MCC-A **S36.115-** <u>Moderate</u> laceration of liver
  Laceration involving parenchyma but without major disruption of parenchyma [i.e., less than 10 cm long and less than 3 cm deep]

MCC-A **S36.116-** <u>Major</u> laceration of liver
  Laceration with significant disruption of hepatic parenchyma [i.e., greater than 10 cm long and 3 cm deep]
  Multiple moderate lacerations, with or without hematoma
  Stellate laceration of liver

CC-A **S36.118-** <u>Other</u> injury of liver

CC-A **S36.119-** <u>Unspecified</u> injury of liver

S36.12- Injury of <u>gallbladder</u>

CC-A **S36.122-** <u>Contusion</u> of gallbladder

CC-A **S36.123-** <u>Laceration</u> of gallbladder

CC-A **S36.128-** <u>Other</u> injury of gallbladder

CC-A **S36.129-** <u>Unspecified</u> injury of gallbladder

CC-A **S36.13x-** Injury of <u>bile duct</u>

S36.2- Injury of <u>pancreas</u>

S36.20- <u>Unspecified</u> injury of pancreas

CC-A **S36.200-** Unspecified injury of <u>head</u> of pancreas

CC-A **S36.201-** Unspecified injury of <u>body</u> of pancreas

CC-A **S36.202-** Unspecified injury of <u>tail</u> of pancreas

CC-A **S36.209-** Unspecified injury of <u>unspecified</u> part of pancreas

S36.22- <u>Contusion</u> of pancreas

CC-A **S36.220-** Contusion of <u>head</u> of pancreas

CC-A **S36.221-** Contusion of <u>body</u> of pancreas

CC-A **S36.222-** Contusion of <u>tail</u> of pancreas

CC-A **S36.229-** Contusion of <u>unspecified</u> part of pancreas

S36.23- <u>Laceration</u> of pancreas, <u>unspecified</u> degree

CC-A **S36.230-** Laceration of <u>head</u> of pancreas, <u>unspecified</u> degree

CC-A **S36.231-** Laceration of <u>body</u> of pancreas, <u>unspecified</u> degree

CC-A **S36.232-** Laceration of <u>tail</u> of pancreas, <u>unspecified</u> degree

CC-A **S36.239-** Laceration of <u>unspecified</u> part of pancreas, <u>unspecified</u> degree

S36.24- <u>Minor</u> laceration of pancreas

CC-A **S36.240-** Minor laceration of <u>head</u> of pancreas

CC-A **S36.241-** Minor laceration of <u>body</u> of pancreas

CC-A **S36.242-** Minor laceration of <u>tail</u> of pancreas

CC-A **S36.249-** Minor laceration of <u>unspecified</u> part of pancreas

S36.25- <u>Moderate</u> laceration of pancreas

CC-A **S36.250-** Moderate laceration of <u>head</u> of pancreas

CC-A **S36.251-** Moderate laceration of <u>body</u> of pancreas

CC-A **S36.252-** Moderate laceration of <u>tail</u> of pancreas

CC-A **S36.259-** Moderate laceration of <u>unspecified</u> part of pancreas

S36.26- <u>Major</u> laceration of pancreas

CC-A **S36.260-** Major laceration of <u>head</u> of pancreas

CC-A **S36.261-** Major laceration of <u>body</u> of pancreas

CC-A **S36.262-** Major laceration of <u>tail</u> of pancreas

CC-A **S36.269-** Major laceration of <u>unspecified</u> part of pancreas

S36.29- <u>Other</u> injury of pancreas

CC-A **S36.290-** Other injury of <u>head</u> of pancreas

CC-A **S36.291-** Other injury of <u>body</u> of pancreas

CC-A **S36.292-** Other injury of <u>tail</u> of pancreas

CC-A **S36.299-** Other injury of <u>unspecified</u> part of pancreas

S36.3- Injury of <u>stomach</u>

CC-A **S36.30x-** <u>Unspecified</u> injury of stomach

CC-A **S36.32x-** <u>Contusion</u> of stomach

CC-A **S36.33x-** <u>Laceration</u> of stomach

CC-A **S36.39x-** <u>Other</u> injury of stomach

S 3 5 - S 3 6

S36.4-   Injury of <u>small intestine</u>
    S36.40- <u>Unspecified</u> injury of small intestine
    CC-A **S36.400- Unspecified injury of <u>duodenum</u>**
    CC-A **S36.408- Unspecified injury of <u>other</u> part of small intestine**
    CC-A **S36.409- Unspecified injury of <u>unspecified</u> part of small intestine**
    S36.41- <u>Primary blast</u> injury of small intestine
      Blast injury of small intestine NOS
    CC-A **S36.410- Primary blast injury of <u>duodenum</u>**
    CC-A **S36.418- Primary blast injury of <u>other</u> part of small intestine**
    CC-A **S36.419- Primary blast injury of <u>unspecified</u> part of small intestine**
    S36.42- <u>Contusion</u> of small intestine
    CC-A **S36.420- Contusion of <u>duodenum</u>**
    CC-A **S36.428- Contusion of <u>other</u> part of small intestine**
    CC-A **S36.429- Contusion of <u>unspecified</u> part of small intestine**
    S36.43- <u>Laceration</u> of small intestine
    CC-A **S36.430- Laceration of <u>duodenum</u>**
    CC-A **S36.438- Laceration of <u>other</u> part of small intestine**
    CC-A **S36.439- Laceration of <u>unspecified</u> part of small intestine**
    S36.49- <u>Other</u> injury of small intestine
    CC-A **S36.490- Other injury of <u>duodenum</u>**
    CC-A **S36.498- Other injury of <u>other</u> part of small intestine**
    CC-A **S36.499- Other injury of <u>unspecified</u> part of small intestine**
S36.5-   Injury of <u>colon</u>
    Excludes ❷: injury of rectum (S36.6-)
    S36.50- <u>Unspecified</u> injury of colon
    CC-A **S36.500- Unspecified injury of <u>ascending</u> [right] colon**
    CC-A **S36.501- Unspecified injury of <u>transverse</u> colon**
    CC-A **S36.502- Unspecified injury of <u>descending</u> [left] colon**
    CC-A **S36.503- Unspecified injury of <u>sigmoid</u> colon**
    CC-A **S36.508- Unspecified injury of <u>other</u> part of colon**
    CC-A **S36.509- Unspecified injury of <u>unspecified</u> part of colon**
    S36.51- <u>Primary blast</u> injury of colon
      Blast injury of colon NOS
    CC-A **S36.510- Primary blast injury of <u>ascending</u> [right] colon**
    CC-A **S36.511- Primary blast injury of <u>transverse</u> colon**
    CC-A **S36.512- Primary blast injury of <u>descending</u> [left] colon**
    CC-A **S36.513- Primary blast injury of <u>sigmoid</u> colon**
    CC-A **S36.518- Primary blast injury of <u>other</u> part of colon**
    CC-A **S36.519- Primary blast injury of <u>unspecified</u> part of colon**
    S36.52- <u>Contusion</u> of colon
    CC-A **S36.520- Contusion of <u>ascending</u> [right] colon**
    CC-A **S36.521- Contusion of <u>transverse</u> colon**
    CC-A **S36.522- Contusion of <u>descending</u> [left] colon**
    CC-A **S36.523- Contusion of <u>sigmoid</u> colon**
    CC-A **S36.528- Contusion of <u>other</u> part of colon**
    CC-A **S36.529- Contusion of <u>unspecified</u> part of colon**
    S36.53- <u>Laceration</u> of colon
    CC-A **S36.530- Laceration of <u>ascending</u> [right] colon**
    CC-A **S36.531- Laceration of <u>transverse</u> colon**
    CC-A **S36.532- Laceration of <u>descending</u> [left] colon**
    CC-A **S36.533- Laceration of <u>sigmoid</u> colon**
    CC-A **S36.538- Laceration of <u>other</u> part of colon**
    CC-A **S36.539- Laceration of <u>unspecified</u> part of colon**
    S36.59- <u>Other</u> injury of colon
      Secondary blast injury of colon
    CC-A **S36.590- Other injury of <u>ascending</u> [right] colon**
    CC-A **S36.591- Other injury of <u>transverse</u> colon**
    CC-A **S36.592- Other injury of <u>descending</u> [left] colon**
    CC-A **S36.593- Other injury of <u>sigmoid</u> colon**
    CC-A **S36.598- Other injury of <u>other</u> part of colon**
    CC-A **S36.599- Other injury of <u>unspecified</u> part of colon**
S36.6-   Injury of <u>rectum</u>
    CC-A **S36.60x- <u>Unspecified</u> injury of rectum**

CC-A **S36.61x- <u>Primary blast</u> injury of rectum**
      Blast injury of rectum NOS
CC-A **S36.62x- <u>Contusion</u> of rectum**
CC-A **S36.63x- <u>Laceration</u> of rectum**
CC-A **S36.69x- <u>Other</u> injury of rectum**
      Secondary blast injury of rectum
S36.8-   Injury of <u>other intra-abdominal organs</u>
CC-A **S36.81x- Injury of <u>peritoneum</u>**
    S36.89- Injury of <u>other intra-abdominal organs</u>
      Injury of retroperitoneum
    CC-A **S36.892- <u>Contusion</u> of other intra-abdominal organs**
    CC-A **S36.893- <u>Laceration</u> of other intra-abdominal organs**
    CC-A **S36.898- <u>Other</u> injury of other intra-abdominal organs**
    CC-A **S36.899- <u>Unspecified</u> injury of other intra-abdominal organs**
S36.9-   Injury of <u>unspecified</u> intra-abdominal organ
CC-A **S36.90x- <u>Unspecified</u> injury of unspecified intra-abdominal organ**
CC-A **S36.92x- <u>Contusion</u> of unspecified intra-abdominal organ**
CC-A **S36.93x- <u>Laceration</u> of unspecified intra-abdominal organ**
CC-A **S36.99x- <u>Other</u> injury of unspecified intra-abdominal organ**

S37- Injury of <u>urinary and pelvic organs</u>
    Code also any associated open wound (S31.-)
    Excludes 1: obstetric trauma to pelvic organs (O71.-)
    Excludes ❷: injury of peritoneum (S36.81)
               injury of retroperitoneum (S36.89-)
    The appropriate 7th character is to be added to each code from category S37:
    A   <u>Initial</u> encounter
    D   <u>Subsequent</u> encounter
    S   <u>Sequela</u>
    S37.0- Injury of <u>kidney</u>
      Excludes ❷: acute kidney injury (nontraumatic) (N17.9)
    S37.00- <u>Unspecified</u> injury of kidney
    CC-A **S37.001- Unspecified injury of <u>right</u> kidney**
    CC-A **S37.002- Unspecified injury of <u>left</u> kidney**
    CC-A **S37.009- Unspecified injury of <u>unspecified</u> kidney**
    S37.01- <u>Minor contusion</u> of kidney
      Contusion of kidney less than 2 cm
      Contusion of kidney NOS
    CC-A **S37.011- Minor contusion of <u>right</u> kidney**
    CC-A **S37.012- Minor contusion of <u>left</u> kidney**
    CC-A **S37.019- Minor contusion of <u>unspecified</u> kidney**
    S37.02- <u>Major contusion</u> of kidney
      Contusion of kidney greater than 2 cm
    CC-A **S37.021- Major contusion of <u>right</u> kidney**
    CC-A **S37.022- Major contusion of <u>left</u> kidney**
    CC-A **S37.029- Major contusion of <u>unspecified</u> kidney**
    S37.03- <u>Laceration</u> of kidney, unspecified degree
    CC-A **S37.031- Laceration of <u>right</u> kidney, unspecified degree**
    CC-A **S37.032- Laceration of <u>left</u> kidney, unspecified degree**
    CC-A **S37.039- Laceration of <u>unspecified</u> kidney, unspecified degree**
    S37.04- <u>Minor laceration</u> of kidney
      Laceration of kidney less than 1 cm
    CC-A **S37.041- Minor laceration of <u>right</u> kidney**
    CC-A **S37.042- Minor laceration of <u>left</u> kidney**
    CC-A **S37.049- Minor laceration of <u>unspecified</u> kidney**
    S37.05- <u>Moderate laceration</u> of kidney
      Laceration of kidney 1 to 3 cm
    CC-A **S37.051- Moderate laceration of <u>right</u> kidney**
    CC-A **S37.052- Moderate laceration of <u>left</u> kidney**
    CC-A **S37.059- Moderate laceration of <u>unspecified</u> kidney**
    S37.06- <u>Major laceration</u> of kidney
      Avulsion of kidney
      Laceration of kidney greater than 3 cm
      Massive laceration of kidney
      Multiple moderate lacerations of kidney
      Stellate laceration of kidney
    MCC-A **S37.061- Major laceration of <u>right</u> kidney**

S36 - S37

MCC-A **S37.062-** Major laceration of <u>left</u> kidney
MCC-A **S37.069-** Major laceration of <u>unspecified</u> kidney
S37.09- <u>Other</u> injury of kidney
MCC-A **S37.091-** Other injury of <u>right</u> kidney
MCC-A **S37.092-** Other injury of <u>left</u> kidney
MCC-A **S37.099-** Other injury of <u>unspecified</u> kidney
S37.1- Injury of <u>ureter</u>
CC-A **S37.10x-** <u>Unspecified</u> injury of ureter
CC-A **S37.12x-** <u>Contusion</u> of ureter
CC-A **S37.13x-** <u>Laceration</u> of ureter
CC-A **S37.19x-** Other injury of ureter
S37.2- Injury of <u>bladder</u>
CC-A **S37.20x-** <u>Unspecified</u> injury of bladder
CC-A **S37.22x-** <u>Contusion</u> of bladder
CC-A **S37.23x-** <u>Laceration</u> of bladder
CC-A **S37.29x-** <u>Other</u> injury of bladder
S37.3- Injury of <u>urethra</u>
CC-A **S37.30x-** <u>Unspecified</u> injury of urethra
CC-A **S37.32x-** <u>Contusion</u> of urethra
CC-A **S37.33x-** <u>Laceration</u> of urethra
CC-A **S37.39x-** <u>Other</u> injury of urethra
S37.4- Injury of <u>ovary</u>
S37.40- <u>Unspecified</u> injury of ovary
S37.401- Unspecified injury of ovary, <u>unilateral</u> — [♀]
S37.402- Unspecified injury of ovary, <u>bilateral</u> — [♀]
S37.409- Unspecified injury of ovary, <u>unspecified</u> — [♀]
S37.42- <u>Contusion</u> of ovary
S37.421- Contusion of ovary, <u>unilateral</u> — [♀]
S37.422- Contusion of ovary, <u>bilateral</u> — [♀]
S37.429- Contusion of ovary, <u>unspecified</u> — [♀]
S37.43- <u>Laceration</u> of ovary
S37.431- Laceration of ovary, <u>unilateral</u> — [♀]
S37.432- Laceration of ovary, <u>bilateral</u> — [♀]
S37.439- Laceration of ovary, <u>unspecified</u> — [♀]
S37.49- <u>Other</u> injury of ovary
S37.491- Other injury of ovary, <u>unilateral</u> — [♀]
S37.492- Other injury of ovary, <u>bilateral</u> — [♀]
S37.499- Other injury of ovary, <u>unspecified</u> — [♀]
S37.5- Injury of <u>fallopian tube</u>
S37.50- <u>Unspecified</u> injury of fallopian tube
S37.501- Unspecified injury of fallopian tube, <u>unilateral</u> — [♀]
S37.502- Unspecified injury of fallopian tube, <u>bilateral</u> — [♀]
S37.509- Unspecified injury of fallopian tube, <u>unspecified</u> — [♀]
S37.51- <u>Primary blast</u> injury of fallopian tube
Blast injury of fallopian tube NOS
S37.511- Primary blast injury of fallopian tube, <u>unilateral</u> — [♀]
S37.512- Primary blast injury of fallopian tube, <u>bilateral</u> — [♀]
S37.519- Primary blast injury of fallopian tube, <u>unspecified</u> — [♀]
S37.52- <u>Contusion</u> of fallopian tube
S37.521- Contusion of fallopian tube, <u>unilateral</u> — [♀]
S37.522- Contusion of fallopian tube, <u>bilateral</u> — [♀]
S37.529- Contusion of fallopian tube, <u>unspecified</u> — [♀]
S37.53- <u>Laceration</u> of fallopian tube
S37.531- Laceration of fallopian tube, <u>unilateral</u> — [♀]
S37.532- Laceration of fallopian tube, <u>bilateral</u> — [♀]
S37.539- Laceration of fallopian tube, <u>unspecified</u> — [♀]
S37.59- <u>Other</u> injury of fallopian tube
Secondary blast injury of fallopian tube
S37.591- Other injury of fallopian tube, <u>unilateral</u> — [♀]

S37.592- Other injury of fallopian tube, <u>bilateral</u> — [♀]
S37.599- Other injury of fallopian tube, <u>unspecified</u> — [♀]
S37.6- Injury of <u>uterus</u>
Excludes 1: *injury to gravid uterus (O9A.2-)*
injury to uterus during delivery (O71.-)
CC-A **S37.60x-** <u>Unspecified</u> injury of uterus — [♀]
CC-A **S37.62x-** <u>Contusion</u> of uterus — [♀]
CC-A **S37.63x-** <u>Laceration</u> of uterus — [♀]
CC-A **S37.69x-** <u>Other</u> injury of uterus — [♀]
S37.8- Injury of <u>other urinary and pelvic organs</u>
S37.81- Injury of <u>adrenal gland</u>
CC-A **S37.812-** <u>Contusion</u> of adrenal gland
CC-A **S37.813-** <u>Laceration</u> of adrenal gland
CC-A **S37.818-** <u>Other</u> injury of adrenal gland
CC-A **S37.819-** <u>Unspecified</u> injury of adrenal gland
S37.82- Injury of <u>prostate</u>
S37.822- <u>Contusion</u> of prostate — [♂]
S37.823- <u>Laceration</u> of prostate — [♂]
S37.828- <u>Other</u> injury of prostate — [♂]
S37.829- <u>Unspecified</u> injury of prostate — [♂]
S37.89- Injury of other urinary and pelvic organ
CC-A **S37.892-** <u>Contusion</u> of other urinary and pelvic organ
CC-A **S37.893-** <u>Laceration</u> of other urinary and pelvic organ
CC-A **S37.898-** <u>Other</u> injury of other urinary and pelvic organ
CC-A **S37.899-** <u>Unspecified</u> injury of other urinary and pelvic organ
S37.9- Injury of <u>unspecified</u> urinary and pelvic organ
CC-A **S37.90x-** <u>Unspecified</u> injury of unspecified urinary and pelvic organ
CC-A **S37.92x-** <u>Contusion</u> of unspecified urinary and pelvic organ
CC-A **S37.93x-** <u>Laceration</u> of unspecified urinary and pelvic organ
CC-A **S37.99x-** <u>Other</u> injury of unspecified urinary and pelvic organ
S38- <u>Crushing injury</u> and <u>traumatic amputation</u> of <u>abdomen, lower back, pelvis and external genitals</u>
Note: An amputation not identified as partial or complete should be coded to complete
The appropriate 7th character is to be added to each code from category S38:
A <u>Initial</u> encounter
D <u>Subsequent</u> encounter
S <u>Sequela</u>
S38.0- <u>Crushing</u> injury of <u>external genital organs</u>
Use additional code for any associated injuries
S38.00- Crushing injury of <u>unspecified external genital organs</u>
S38.001- Crushing injury of <u>unspecified</u> external genital organs, <u>male</u> — [♂]
S38.002- Crushing injury of <u>unspecified</u> external genital organs, <u>female</u> — [♀]
S38.01x- Crushing injury of <u>penis</u> — [♂]
S38.02x- Crushing injury of <u>scrotum and testis</u> — [♂]
S38.03x- Crushing injury of <u>vulva</u> — [♀]
S38.1xx- Crushing injury of <u>abdomen, lower back, and pelvis</u>
Use additional code for all associated injuries, such as:
Fracture of thoracic or lumbar spine and pelvis (S22.0-, S32.-)
Injury to intra-abdominal organs (S36.-)
Injury to urinary and pelvic organs (S37.-)
Open wound of abdominal wall (S31.-)
Spinal cord injury (S34.0, S34.1-)
Excludes ❷: *crushing injury of external genital organs (S38.0-)*
S38.2- <u>Traumatic amputation</u> of <u>external genital organs</u>
S38.21- Traumatic amputation of <u>female external genital organs</u>
Traumatic amputation of clitoris
Traumatic amputation of labium (majus) (minus)
Traumatic amputation of vulva
S38.211- <u>Complete</u> traumatic amputation of female external genital organs — [♀]
S38.212- <u>Partial</u> traumatic amputation of female external genital organs — [♀]

S37 - S38

S38.22- Traumatic amputation of <u>penis</u>
    S38.221- <u>Complete</u> traumatic amputation of penis —[♂]
    S38.222- <u>Partial</u> traumatic amputation of penis —[♂]
S38.23- Traumatic amputation of <u>scrotum and testis</u>
    S38.231- <u>Complete</u> traumatic amputation of scrotum and
        testis — [♂]
    S38.232- <u>Partial</u> traumatic amputation of scrotum and
        testis — [♂]
S38.3xx-   Transection (partial) of <u>abdomen</u>

S39- <u>Other and unspecified</u> injuries of <u>abdomen, lower back, pelvis and external genitals</u>
    Code also any associated open wound (S31.-)
    Excludes ❷: sprain of joints and ligaments of lumbar spine and pelvis (S33.-)

The appropriate 7th character is to be added to each code from category S39:
  A   <u>Initial</u> encounter
  D   <u>Subsequent</u> encounter
  S   <u>Sequela</u>

S39.0- Injury of <u>muscle, fascia and tendon</u> of <u>abdomen, lower back and pelvis</u>
  S39.00- <u>Unspecified</u> injury of muscle, fascia and tendon of abdomen, lower back and pelvis
    S39.001- Unspecified injury of muscle, fascia and tendon of <u>abdomen</u>
    S39.002- Unspecified injury of muscle, fascia and tendon of <u>lower back</u>
    S39.003- Unspecified injury of muscle, fascia and tendon of <u>pelvis</u>
  S39.01- <u>Strain</u> of muscle, fascia and tendon of abdomen, lower back and pelvis
    S39.011- Strain of muscle, fascia and tendon of <u>abdomen</u>
    S39.012- Strain of muscle, fascia and tendon of <u>lower back</u>
    S39.013- Strain of muscle, fascia and tendon of <u>pelvis</u>
  S39.02- <u>Laceration</u> of muscle, fascia and tendon of abdomen, lower back and pelvis
    S39.021- Laceration of muscle, fascia and tendon of <u>abdomen</u>
    S39.022- Laceration of muscle, fascia and tendon of <u>lower back</u>
    S39.023- Laceration of muscle, fascia and tendon of <u>pelvis</u>
  S39.09- <u>Other injury</u> of muscle, fascia and tendon of abdomen, lower back and pelvis
    S39.091- Other injury of muscle, fascia and tendon of <u>abdomen</u>
    S39.092- Other injury of muscle, fascia and tendon of <u>lower back</u>
    S39.093- Other injury of muscle, fascia and tendon of <u>pelvis</u>
S39.8- <u>Other specified</u> injuries of abdomen, lower back, pelvis and external genitals
  S39.81x- Other specified injuries of <u>abdomen</u>
  S39.82x- Other specified injuries of <u>lower back</u>
  S39.83x- Other specified injuries of <u>pelvis</u>
  S39.84- Other specified injuries of <u>external genitals</u>
    S39.840- <u>Fracture</u> of <u>corpus cavernosum penis</u> — [♂]
    S39.848- <u>Other</u> specified injuries of external genitals
S39.9- <u>Unspecified</u> injury of abdomen, lower back, pelvis and external genitals
  S39.91x- Unspecified injury of <u>abdomen</u>
  S39.92x- Unspecified injury of <u>lower back</u>
  S39.93x- Unspecified injury of <u>pelvis</u>
  S39.94x- Unspecified injury of <u>external genitals</u>

Injuries to the shoulder and upper arm (S40-S49)

Includes: Injuries of axilla
          Injuries of scapular region
Excludes ❷: burns and corrosions (T20-T32)
          frostbite (T33-T34)
          injuries of elbow (S50-S59)
          insect bite or sting, venomous (T63.4)

S40- <u>Superficial injury</u> of <u>shoulder and upper arm</u>
The appropriate 7th character is to be added to each code from category S40:
  A   <u>Initial</u> encounter
  D   <u>Subsequent</u> encounter
  S   <u>Sequela</u>
S40.0- <u>Contusion</u> of shoulder and upper arm
  S40.01- <u>Contusion</u> of <u>shoulder</u>
    S40.011- Contusion of <u>right</u> shoulder
    S40.012- Contusion of <u>left</u> shoulder
    S40.019- Contusion of <u>unspecified</u> shoulder
  S40.02- Contusion of <u>upper arm</u>
    S40.021- Contusion of <u>right</u> upper arm
    S40.022- Contusion of <u>left</u> upper arm
    S40.029- Contusion of <u>unspecified</u> upper arm
S40.2- Other superficial injuries of shoulder
  S40.21- <u>Abrasion</u> of <u>shoulder</u>
    S40.211- Abrasion of <u>right</u> shoulder
    S40.212- Abrasion of <u>left</u> shoulder
    S40.219- Abrasion of <u>unspecified</u> shoulder
  S40.22- <u>Blister</u> (nonthermal) of <u>shoulder</u>
    S40.221- Blister (nonthermal) of <u>right</u> shoulder
    S40.222- Blister (nonthermal) of <u>left</u> shoulder
    S40.229- Blister (nonthermal) of <u>unspecified</u> shoulder
  S40.24- <u>External constriction</u> of <u>shoulder</u>
    S40.241- External constriction of <u>right</u> shoulder
    S40.242- External constriction of <u>left</u> shoulder
    S40.249- External constriction of <u>unspecified</u> shoulder
  S40.25- <u>Superficial foreign body</u> of <u>shoulder</u>
      Splinter in the shoulder
    S40.251- Superficial foreign body of <u>right</u> shoulder
    S40.252- Superficial foreign body of <u>left</u> shoulder
    S40.259- Superficial foreign body of <u>unspecified</u> shoulder
  S40.26- <u>Insect bite (nonvenomous)</u> of <u>shoulder</u>
    S40.261- Insect bite (nonvenomous) of <u>right</u> shoulder
    S40.262- Insect bite (nonvenomous) of <u>left</u> shoulder
    S40.269- Insect bite (nonvenomous) of <u>unspecified</u> shoulder
  S40.27- <u>Other superficial bite</u> of <u>shoulder</u>
    Excludes 1:   open bite of shoulder (S41.05)
    S40.271- Other superficial bite of <u>right</u> shoulder
    S40.272- Other superficial bite of <u>left</u> shoulder
    S40.279- Other superficial bite of <u>unspecified</u> shoulder
S40.8- Other superficial injuries of <u>upper arm</u>
  S40.81- <u>Abrasion</u> of <u>upper arm</u>
    S40.811- Abrasion of <u>right</u> upper arm
    S40.812- Abrasion of <u>left</u> upper arm
    S40.819- Abrasion of <u>unspecified</u> upper arm
  S40.82- <u>Blister</u> (nonthermal) of <u>upper arm</u>
    S40.821- Blister (nonthermal) of <u>right</u> upper arm
    S40.822- Blister (nonthermal) of <u>left</u> upper arm
    S40.829- Blister (nonthermal) of <u>unspecified</u> upper arm
  S40.84- <u>External constriction</u> of <u>upper arm</u>
    S40.841- External constriction of <u>right</u> upper arm
    S40.842- External constriction of <u>left</u> upper arm
    S40.849- External constriction of <u>unspecified</u> upper arm
  S40.85- <u>Superficial foreign body</u> of <u>upper arm</u>
      Splinter in the upper arm
    S40.851- Superficial foreign body of <u>right</u> upper arm
    S40.852- Superficial foreign body of <u>left</u> upper arm

S38 - S40

S40.859- Superficial foreign body of <u>unspecified</u> upper arm

S40.86- <u>Insect bite (nonvenomous)</u> of <u>upper arm</u>

    S40.861- Insect bite (nonvenomous) of <u>right</u> upper arm

    S40.862- Insect bite (nonvenomous) of <u>left</u> upper arm

    S40.869- Insect bite (nonvenomous) of <u>unspecified</u> upper arm

S40.87- <u>Other superficial bite</u> of <u>upper arm</u>
    Excludes 1:   open bite of upper arm (S41.14)
    Excludes ❷: other superficial bite of shoulder (S40.27-)

    S40.871- Other superficial bite of <u>right</u> upper arm

    S40.872- Other superficial bite of <u>left</u> upper arm

    S40.879- Other superficial bite of <u>unspecified</u> upper arm

S40.9- Unspecified superficial injury of shoulder and upper arm

    S40.91- <u>Unspecified superficial injury</u> of <u>shoulder</u>

        S40.911- Unspecified superficial injury of <u>right</u> shoulder

        S40.912- Unspecified superficial injury of <u>left</u> shoulder

        S40.919- Unspecified superficial injury of <u>unspecified</u> shoulder

    S40.92- <u>Unspecified superficial injury</u> of <u>upper arm</u>

        S40.921- Unspecified superficial injury of <u>right</u> upper arm

        S40.922- Unspecified superficial injury of <u>left</u> upper arm

        S40.929- Unspecified superficial injury of <u>unspecified</u> upper arm

S41- Open wound of <u>shoulder and upper arm</u>
    Code also any associated wound infection
    Excludes 1:   traumatic amputation of shoulder and upper arm (S48.-)
    Excludes ❷: open fracture of shoulder and upper arm (S42.- with 7th character B or C)

> **The appropriate 7th character is to be added to each code from category S41:**
> **A**   <u>Initial</u> encounter
> **D**   <u>Subsequent</u> encounter
> **S**   <u>Sequela</u>

S41.0- <u>Open wound</u> of <u>shoulder</u>

    S41.00- <u>Unspecified</u> open wound of <u>shoulder</u>

        S41.001- Unspecified open wound of <u>right</u> shoulder

        S41.002- Unspecified open wound of <u>left</u> shoulder

        S41.009- Unspecified open wound of <u>unspecified</u> shoulder

    S41.01- <u>Laceration without</u> foreign body of <u>shoulder</u>

        S41.011- Laceration <u>without</u> foreign body of <u>right</u> shoulder

        S41.012- Laceration <u>without</u> foreign body of <u>left</u> shoulder

        S41.019- Laceration <u>without</u> foreign body of <u>unspecified</u> shoulder

    S41.02- <u>Laceration with foreign body</u> of <u>shoulder</u>

        S41.021- Laceration <u>with foreign body</u> of <u>right</u> shoulder

        S41.022- Laceration <u>with foreign body</u> of <u>left</u> shoulder

        S41.029- Laceration <u>with foreign body</u> of <u>unspecified</u> shoulder

    S41.03- <u>Puncture</u> wound <u>without</u> foreign body of <u>shoulder</u>

        S41.031- Puncture wound <u>without</u> foreign body of <u>right</u> shoulder

        S41.032- Puncture wound <u>without</u> foreign body of <u>left</u> shoulder

        S41.039- Puncture wound <u>without</u> foreign body of <u>unspecified</u> shoulder

    S41.04- <u>Puncture</u> wound <u>with foreign body</u> of shoulder

        S41.041- Puncture wound <u>with foreign body</u> of <u>right</u> shoulder

        S41.042- Puncture wound <u>with foreign body</u> of <u>left</u> shoulder

        S41.049- Puncture wound <u>with foreign body</u> of <u>unspecified</u> shoulder

    S41.05- Open bite of <u>shoulder</u>
        Bite of shoulder NOS
        Excludes 1:   superficial bite of shoulder (S40.27)

        S41.051- Open bite of <u>right</u> shoulder

        S41.052- Open bite of <u>left</u> shoulder

        S41.059- Open bite of <u>unspecified</u> shoulder

S41.1- <u>Open wound</u> of <u>upper arm</u>

    S41.10- <u>Unspecified</u> open wound of <u>upper arm</u>

        S41.101- Unspecified open wound of <u>right</u> upper arm

        S41.102- Unspecified open wound of <u>left</u> upper arm

        S41.109- Unspecified open wound of <u>unspecified</u> upper arm

    S41.11- <u>Laceration without</u> foreign body of <u>upper arm</u>

        S41.111- Laceration <u>without</u> foreign body of <u>right</u> upper arm

        S41.112- Laceration <u>without</u> foreign body of <u>left</u> upper arm

        S41.119- Laceration <u>without</u> foreign body of <u>unspecified</u> upper arm

    S41.12- <u>Laceration with foreign body</u> of <u>upper arm</u>

        S41.121- Laceration <u>with foreign body</u> of <u>right</u> upper arm

        S41.122- Laceration <u>with foreign body</u> of <u>left</u> upper arm

        S41.129- Laceration <u>with foreign body</u> of <u>unspecified</u> upper arm

    S41.13- <u>Puncture</u> wound <u>without</u> foreign body of <u>upper arm</u>

        S41.131- Puncture wound <u>without</u> foreign body of <u>right</u> upper arm

        S41.132- Puncture wound <u>without</u> foreign body of <u>left</u> upper arm

        S41.139- Puncture wound <u>without</u> foreign body of <u>unspecified</u> upper arm

    S41.14- <u>Puncture</u> wound <u>with foreign body</u> of <u>upper arm</u>

        S41.141- Puncture wound <u>with foreign body</u> of <u>right</u> upper arm

        S41.142- Puncture wound <u>with foreign body</u> of <u>left</u> upper arm

        S41.149- Puncture wound <u>with foreign body</u> of <u>unspecified</u> upper arm

    S41.15- <u>Open bite</u> of <u>upper arm</u>
        Bite of upper arm NOS
        Excludes 1:   superficial bite of upper arm (S40.87)

        S41.151- Open bite of <u>right</u> upper arm

        S41.152- Open bite of <u>left</u> upper arm

        S41.159- Open bite of <u>unspecified</u> upper arm

S42- <u>Fracture</u> of <u>shoulder and upper arm</u>
    Note: A fracture not indicated as displaced or nondisplaced should be coded to displaced
    Note: A fracture not indicated as open or closed should be coded to closed
    Excludes 1:   traumatic amputation of shoulder and upper arm (S48.-)

> **The appropriate 7th character is to be added to all codes from category S42:**
> **A**   <u>Initial</u> encounter for <u>closed</u> fracture
> **B**   <u>Initial</u> encounter for <u>open</u> fracture
> **D**   <u>Subsequent</u> encounter for fracture <u>with routine healing</u>
> **G**   <u>Subsequent</u> encounter for fracture <u>with delayed healing</u>
> **K**   <u>Subsequent</u> encounter for fracture <u>with nonunion</u>
> **P**   <u>Subsequent</u> encounter for fracture <u>with malunion</u>
> **S**   <u>Sequela</u>

S42.0- <u>Fracture</u> of <u>clavicle</u>

    S42.00- <u>Fracture</u> of <u>unspecified</u> part of <u>clavicle</u>

    CC-B,K,P **S42.001-** Fracture of <u>unspecified</u> part of <u>right</u> clavicle

    CC-B,K,P **S42.002-** Fracture of <u>unspecified</u> part of <u>left</u> clavicle

    CC-B,K,P **S42.009-** Fracture of <u>unspecified</u> part of <u>unspecified</u> clavicle

    S42.01- Fracture of <u>sternal end</u> of <u>clavicle</u>

    CC-B,K,P **S42.011-** <u>Anterior displaced</u> fracture of sternal end of <u>right</u> clavicle

    CC-B,K,P **S42.012-** <u>Anterior displaced</u> fracture of sternal end of <u>left</u> clavicle

    CC-B,K,P **S42.013-** <u>Anterior displaced</u> fracture of sternal end of <u>unspecified</u> clavicle
        Displaced fracture of sternal end of clavicle NOS

    CC-B,K,P **S42.014-** <u>Posterior displaced</u> fracture of sternal end of <u>right</u> clavicle

    CC-B,K,P **S42.015-** <u>Posterior displaced</u> fracture of sternal end of <u>left</u> clavicle

    CC-B,K,P **S42.016-** <u>Posterior displaced</u> fracture of sternal end of <u>unspecified</u> clavicle

S40 – S42

CC-B,K,P **S42.017-** <u>Nondisplaced</u> fracture of sternal end of <u>right</u> clavicle

CC-B,K,P **S42.018-** <u>Nondisplaced</u> fracture of sternal end of <u>left</u> clavicle

CC-B,K,P **S42.019-** <u>Nondisplaced</u> fracture of sternal end of <u>unspecified</u> clavicle

S42.02- Fracture of <u>shaft</u> of <u>clavicle</u>

CC-B,K,P **S42.021-** <u>Displaced</u> fracture of shaft of <u>right</u> clavicle

CC-B,K,P **S42.022-** <u>Displaced</u> fracture of shaft of <u>left</u> clavicle

CC-B,K,P **S42.023-** <u>Displaced</u> fracture of shaft of <u>unspecified</u> clavicle

CC-B,K,P **S42.024-** <u>Nondisplaced</u> fracture of shaft of <u>right</u> clavicle

CC-B,K,P **S42.025-** <u>Nondisplaced</u> fracture of shaft of <u>left</u> clavicle

CC-B,K,P **S42.026-** <u>Nondisplaced</u> fracture of shaft of <u>unspecified</u> clavicle

S42.03- Fracture of <u>lateral end</u> of <u>clavicle</u>
    Fracture of acromial end of clavicle

CC-B,K,P **S42.031-** <u>Displaced</u> fracture of lateral end of <u>right</u> clavicle

CC-B,K,P **S42.032-** <u>Displaced</u> fracture of lateral end of <u>left</u> clavicle

CC-B,K,P **S42.033-** <u>Displaced</u> fracture of lateral end of <u>unspecified</u> clavicle

CC-B,K,P **S42.034-** <u>Nondisplaced</u> fracture of lateral end of <u>right</u> clavicle

CC-B,K,P **S42.035-** <u>Nondisplaced</u> fracture of lateral end of <u>left</u> clavicle

CC-B,K,P **S42.036-** <u>Nondisplaced</u> fracture of lateral end of <u>unspecified</u> clavicle

S42.1- Fracture of <u>scapula</u>

S42.10- Fracture of <u>unspecified</u> part of <u>scapula</u>

CC-B,K,P **S42.101-** Fracture of <u>unspecified</u> part of scapula, <u>right</u> shoulder

CC-B,K,P **S42.102-** Fracture of <u>unspecified</u> part of scapula, <u>left</u> shoulder

CC-B,K,P **S42.109-** Fracture of <u>unspecified</u> part of scapula, <u>unspecified</u> shoulder

S42.11- Fracture of <u>body</u> of <u>scapula</u>

CC-B,K,P **S42.111-** <u>Displaced</u> fracture of body of scapula, <u>right</u> shoulder

CC-B,K,P **S42.112-** <u>Displaced</u> fracture of body of scapula, <u>left</u> shoulder

CC-B,K,P **S42.113-** <u>Displaced</u> fracture of body of scapula, <u>unspecified</u> shoulder

CC-B,K,P **S42.114-** <u>Nondisplaced</u> fracture of body of scapula, <u>right</u> shoulder

CC-B,K,P **S42.115-** <u>Nondisplaced</u> fracture of body of scapula, <u>left</u> shoulder

CC-B,K,P **S42.116-** <u>Nondisplaced</u> fracture of body of scapula, <u>unspecified</u> shoulder

S42.12- Fracture of <u>acromial process</u>

CC-B,K,P **S42.121-** <u>Displaced</u> fracture of acromial process, <u>right</u> shoulder

CC-B,K,P **S42.122-** <u>Displaced</u> fracture of acromial process, <u>left</u> shoulder

CC-B,K,P **S42.123-** <u>Displaced</u> fracture of acromial process, <u>unspecified</u> shoulder

CC-B,K,P **S42.124-** <u>Nondisplaced</u> fracture of acromial process, <u>right</u> shoulder

CC-B,K,P **S42.125-** <u>Nondisplaced</u> fracture of acromial process, <u>left</u> shoulder

CC-B,K,P **S42.126-** <u>Nondisplaced</u> fracture of acromial process, <u>unspecified</u> shoulder

S42.13- Fracture of <u>coracoid process</u>

CC-B,K,P **S42.131-** <u>Displaced</u> fracture of coracoid process, <u>right</u> shoulder

CC-B,K,P **S42.132-** <u>Displaced</u> fracture of coracoid process, <u>left</u> shoulder

CC-B,K,P **S42.133-** <u>Displaced</u> fracture of coracoid process, <u>unspecified</u> shoulder

CC-B,K,P **S42.134-** <u>Nondisplaced</u> fracture of coracoid process, <u>right</u> shoulder

CC-B,K,P **S42.135-** <u>Nondisplaced</u> fracture of coracoid process, <u>left</u> shoulder

CC-B,K,P **S42.136-** <u>Nondisplaced</u> fracture of coracoid process, <u>unspecified</u> shoulder

S42.14- Fracture of <u>glenoid cavity</u> of <u>scapula</u>

CC-B,K,P **S42.141-** <u>Displaced</u> fracture of glenoid cavity of scapula, <u>right</u> shoulder

CC-B,K,P **S42.142-** <u>Displaced</u> fracture of glenoid cavity of scapula, <u>left</u> shoulder

CC-B,K,P **S42.143-** <u>Displaced</u> fracture of glenoid cavity of scapula, <u>unspecified</u> shoulder

CC-B,K,P **S42.144-** <u>Nondisplaced</u> fracture of glenoid cavity of scapula, <u>right</u> shoulder

CC-B,K,P **S42.145-** <u>Nondisplaced</u> fracture of glenoid cavity of scapula, <u>left</u> shoulder

CC-B,K,P **S42.146-** <u>Nondisplaced</u> fracture of glenoid cavity of scapula, <u>unspecified</u> shoulder

S42.15- Fracture of <u>neck</u> of <u>scapula</u>

CC-B,K,P **S42.151-** <u>Displaced</u> fracture of neck of scapula, <u>right</u> shoulder

CC-B,K,P **S42.152-** <u>Displaced</u> fracture of neck of scapula, <u>left</u> shoulder

CC-B,K,P **S42.153-** <u>Displaced</u> fracture of neck of scapula, <u>unspecified</u> shoulder

CC-B,K,P **S42.154-** <u>Nondisplaced</u> fracture of neck of scapula, <u>right</u> shoulder

CC-B,K,P **S42.155-** <u>Nondisplaced</u> fracture of neck of scapula, <u>left</u> shoulder

CC-B,K,P **S42.156-** <u>Nondisplaced</u> fracture of neck of scapula, <u>unspecified</u> shoulder

S42.19- Fracture of other part of <u>scapula</u>

CC-B,K,P **S42.191-** Fracture of other part of scapula, <u>right</u> shoulder

CC-B,K,P **S42.192-** Fracture of other part of scapula, <u>left</u> shoulder

CC-B,K,P **S42.199-** Fracture of other part of scapula, <u>unspecified</u> shoulder

S42.2- <u>Fracture</u> of <u>upper end</u> of <u>humerus</u>
    Fracture of proximal end of humerus
    *Excludes ❷: fracture of shaft of humerus (S42.3-)
                    physeal fracture of upper end of humerus (S49.0-)*

S42.20- <u>Unspecified</u> fracture of <u>upper end</u> of <u>humerus</u>

S42.201- Unspecified fracture of upper end of <u>right</u> humerus
CC-A,K,P MCC-B

S42.202- Unspecified fracture of upper end of <u>left</u> humerus
CC-A,K,P MCC-B

S42.209- Unspecified fracture of upper end of <u>unspecified</u> humerus
CC-A,K,P MCC-B

S42.21- <u>Unspecified</u> fracture of <u>surgical neck</u> of <u>humerus</u>
    Fracture of neck of humerus NOS

S42.211- Unspecified <u>displaced</u> fracture of surgical neck of <u>right</u> humerus
CC-A,K,P MCC-B

S42.212- Unspecified <u>displaced</u> fracture of surgical neck of <u>left</u> humerus
CC-A,K,P MCC-B

S42.213- Unspecified <u>displaced</u> fracture of surgical neck of <u>unspecified</u> humerus
CC-A,K,P MCC-B

S42.214- Unspecified <u>nondisplaced</u> fracture of surgical neck of <u>right</u> humerus
CC-A,K,P MCC-B

S42.215- Unspecified <u>nondisplaced</u> fracture of surgical neck of <u>left</u> humerus
CC-A,K,P MCC-B

S42.216- Unspecified <u>nondisplaced</u> fracture of surgical neck of <u>unspecified</u> humerus
CC-A,K,P MCC-B

S42.22- <u>2-part</u> fracture of <u>surgical neck</u> of <u>humerus</u>

S42.221- 2-part <u>displaced</u> fracture of surgical neck of <u>right</u> humerus
CC-A,K,P MCC-B

S42.222- 2-part <u>displaced</u> fracture of surgical neck of <u>left</u> humerus
CC-A,K,P MCC-B

S42.223- 2-part <u>displaced</u> fracture of surgical neck of <u>unspecified</u> humerus
CC-A,K,P MCC-B

S42.224- 2-part <u>nondisplaced</u> fracture of surgical neck of <u>right</u> humerus
CC-A,K,P MCC-B

S42.225- 2-part <u>nondisplaced</u> fracture of surgical neck of <u>left</u> humerus
CC-A,K,P MCC-B

S42 - S42

S42.226- 2-part **nondisplaced** fracture of surgical neck of
CC-A,K,P MCC-B **unspecified** humerus

S42.23- **3-part** fracture of **surgical neck** of **humerus**

S42.231- 3-part fracture of surgical neck of **right** humerus
CC-A,K,P MCC-B

S42.232- 3-part fracture of surgical neck of **left** humerus
CC-A,K,P MCC-B

S42.239- 3-part fracture of surgical neck of **unspecified**
CC-A,K,P MCC-B humerus

S42.24- **4-part** fracture of **surgical neck** of **humerus**

S42.241- 4-part fracture of surgical neck of **right** humerus
CC-A,K,P MCC-B

S42.242- 4-part fracture of surgical neck of **left** humerus
CC-A,K,P MCC-B

S42.249- 4-part fracture of surgical neck of **unspecified**
CC-A,K,P MCC-B humerus

S42.25- Fracture of **greater tuberosity** of **humerus**

S42.251- **Displaced** fracture of greater tuberosity of **right**
CC-A,K,P MCC-B humerus

S42.252- **Displaced** fracture of greater tuberosity of **left**
CC-A,K,P MCC-B humerus

S42.253- **Displaced** fracture of greater tuberosity of
CC-A,K,P MCC-B **unspecified** humerus

S42.254- **Nondisplaced** fracture of greater tuberosity of **right**
CC-A,K,P MCC-B humerus

S42.255- **Nondisplaced** fracture of greater tuberosity of **left**
CC-A,K,P MCC-B humerus

S42.256- **Nondisplaced** fracture of greater tuberosity of
CC-A,K,P MCC-B **unspecified** humerus

S42.26- Fracture of **lesser tuberosity** of **humerus**

S42.261- **Displaced** fracture of lesser tuberosity of **right**
CC-A,K,P MCC-B humerus

S42.262- **Displaced** fracture of lesser tuberosity of **left**
CC-A,K,P MCC-B humerus

S42.263- **Displaced** fracture of lesser tuberosity of
CC-A,K,P MCC-B **unspecified** humerus

S42.264- **Nondisplaced** fracture of lesser tuberosity of **right**
CC-A,K,P MCC-B humerus

S42.265- **Nondisplaced** fracture of lesser tuberosity of **left**
CC-A,K,P MCC-B humerus

S42.266- **Nondisplaced** fracture of lesser tuberosity of
CC-A,K,P MCC-B **unspecified** humerus

S42.27- **Torus fracture** of **upper end** of **humerus**

> The appropriate 7th character is to be added to all codes
> in subcategory S42.27:
> **A** **Initial** encounter for **closed** fracture
> **D** **Subsequent** encounter for fracture **with routine healing**
> **G** **Subsequent** encounter for fracture **with delayed healing**
> **K** **Subsequent** encounter for fracture **with nonunion**
> **P** **Subsequent** encounter for fracture **with malunion**
> **S** Sequela

S42.271- Torus fracture of upper end of **right** humerus
CC-A,K,P

S42.272- Torus fracture of upper end of **left** humerus
CC-A,K,P

S42.279- Torus fracture of upper end of **unspecified** humerus
CC-A,K,P

S42.29- **Other fracture** of **upper end** of **humerus**
Fracture of anatomical neck of humerus
Fracture of articular head of humerus

S42.291- Other **displaced** fracture of upper end of **right**
CC-A,K,P MCC-B humerus

S42.292- Other **displaced** fracture of upper end of **left**
CC-A,K,P MCC-B humerus

S42.293- Other **displaced** fracture of upper end of
CC-A,K,P MCC-B **unspecified** humerus

S42.294- Other **nondisplaced** fracture of upper end of **right**
CC-A,K,P MCC-B humerus

S42.295- Other **nondisplaced** fracture of upper end of **left**
CC-A,K,P MCC-B humerus

S42.296- Other **nondisplaced** fracture of upper end of
CC-A,K,P MCC-B **unspecified** humerus

S42.3- Fracture of **shaft** of **humerus**
Fracture of humerus NOS
Fracture of upper arm NOS
Excludes ❷: *physeal fractures of upper end of humerus (S49.0-)*
physeal fractures of lower end of humerus (S49.1-)

S42.30- **Unspecified** fracture of **shaft** of **humerus**

S42.301- Unspecified fracture of shaft of humerus, **right** arm
CC-A,K,P MCC-B

S42.302- Unspecified fracture of shaft of humerus, **left** arm
CC-A,K,P MCC-B

S42.309- Unspecified fracture of shaft of humerus,
CC-A,K,P MCC-B **unspecified** arm

S42.31- **Greenstick** fracture of **shaft** of **humerus**

> The appropriate 7th character is to be added to all codes
> in subcategory S42.31:
> **A** **Initial** encounter for **closed** fracture
> **D** **Subsequent** encounter for fracture **with routine healing**
> **G** **Subsequent** encounter for fracture **with delayed healing**
> **K** **Subsequent** encounter for fracture **with nonunion**
> **P** **Subsequent** encounter for fracture **with malunion**
> **S** Sequela

S42.311- Greenstick fracture of shaft of humerus, **right** arm
CC-A,K,P

S42.312- Greenstick fracture of shaft of humerus, **left** arm
CC-A,K,P

S42.319- Greenstick fracture of shaft of humerus,
CC-A,K,P **unspecified** arm

S42.32- **Transverse** fracture of **shaft** of **humerus**

S42.321- **Displaced** transverse fracture of shaft of humerus,
CC-A,K,P MCC-B **right** arm

S42.322- **Displaced** transverse fracture of shaft of humerus,
CC-A,K,P MCC-B **left** arm

S42.323- **Displaced** transverse fracture of shaft of humerus,
CC-A,K,P MCC-B **unspecified** arm

S42.324- **Nondisplaced** transverse fracture of shaft of
CC-A,K,P MCC-B humerus, **right** arm

S42.325- **Nondisplaced** transverse fracture of shaft of
CC-A,K,P MCC-B humerus, **left** arm

S42.326- **Nondisplaced** transverse fracture of shaft of
CC-A,K,P MCC-B humerus, **unspecified** arm

S42.33- **Oblique** fracture of **shaft** of **humerus**

S42.331- **Displaced** oblique fracture of shaft of humerus,
CC-A,K,P MCC-B **right** arm

S42.332- **Displaced** oblique fracture of shaft of humerus, **left**
CC-A,K,P MCC-B arm

S42.333- **Displaced** oblique fracture of shaft of humerus,
CC-A,K,P MCC-B **unspecified** arm

S42.334- **Nondisplaced** oblique fracture of shaft of humerus,
CC-A,K,P MCC-B **right** arm

S42.335- **Nondisplaced** oblique fracture of shaft of humerus,
CC-A,K,P MCC-B **left** arm

S42.336- **Nondisplaced** oblique fracture of shaft of humerus,
CC-A,K,P MCC-B **unspecified** arm

S42.34- **Spiral** fracture of **shaft** of **humerus**

S42.341- **Displaced** spiral fracture of shaft of humerus, **right**
CC-A,K,P MCC-B arm

S42.342- **Displaced** spiral fracture of shaft of humerus, **left**
CC-A,K,P MCC-B arm

S42.343- **Displaced** spiral fracture of shaft of humerus,
CC-A,K,P MCC-B **unspecified** arm

S42.344- **Nondisplaced** spiral fracture of shaft of humerus,
CC-A,K,P MCC-B **right** arm

S42.345- **Nondisplaced** spiral fracture of shaft of humerus,
CC-A,K,P MCC-B **left** arm

S42 - S42

S42.346- **Nondisplaced** spiral fracture of shaft of humerus,
CC-A,K,P MCC-B **unspecified** arm

S42.35- **Comminuted** fracture of **shaft** of **humerus**

S42.351- **Displaced** comminuted fracture of shaft of
CC-A,K,P MCC-B humerus, **right arm**

S42.352- **Displaced** comminuted fracture of shaft of
CC-A,K,P MCC-B humerus, **left** arm

S42.353- **Displaced** comminuted fracture of shaft of
CC-A,K,P MCC-B humerus, **unspecified** arm

S42.354- **Nondisplaced** comminuted fracture of shaft of
CC-A,K,P MCC-B humerus, **right** arm

S42.355- **Nondisplaced** comminuted fracture of shaft of
CC-A,K,P MCC-B humerus, **left** arm

S42.356- **Nondisplaced** comminuted fracture of shaft of
CC-A,K,P MCC-B humerus, **unspecified** arm

S42.36- **Segmental** fracture of **shaft** of **humerus**

S42.361- **Displaced** segmental fracture of shaft of humerus,
CC-A,K,P MCC-B **right** arm

S42.362- **Displaced** segmental fracture of shaft of humerus,
CC-A,K,P MCC-B **left** arm

S42.363- **Displaced** segmental fracture of shaft of humerus,
CC-A,K,P MCC-B **unspecified** arm

S42.364- **Nondisplaced** segmental fracture of shaft of
CC-A,K,P MCC-B humerus, **right** arm

S42.365- **Nondisplaced** segmental fracture of shaft of
CC-A,K,P MCC-B humerus, **left** arm

S42.366- **Nondisplaced** segmental fracture of shaft of
CC-A,K,P MCC-B humerus, **unspecified** arm

S42.39- **Other** fracture of **shaft** of **humerus**

S42.391- Other fracture of shaft of **right** humerus
CC-A,K,P MCC-B

S42.392- Other fracture of shaft of **left** humerus
CC-A,K,P MCC-B

S42.399- Other fracture of shaft of **unspecified** humerus
CC-A,K,P MCC-B

S42.4- Fracture of **lower end** of **humerus**
Fracture of distal end of humerus
Excludes ❷: fracture of shaft of humerus (S42.3-)
physeal fracture of lower end of humerus (S49.1-)

S42.40- **Unspecified** fracture of **lower end** of **humerus**
Fracture of elbow NOS

S42.401- Unspecified fracture of lower end of **right** humerus
CC-A,K,P MCC-B

S42.402- Unspecified fracture of lower end of **left** humerus
CC-A,K,P MCC-B

S42.409- Unspecified fracture of lower end of **unspecified**
CC-A,K,P MCC-B humerus

S42.41- **Simple supracondylar** fracture **without** intercondylar
fracture of humerus

S42.411- **Displaced** simple supracondylar fracture **without**
CC-A,K,P MCC-B intercondylar fracture of **right** humerus

S42.412- **Displaced** simple supracondylar fracture **without**
CC-A,K,P MCC-B intercondylar fracture of **left** humerus

S42.413- **Displaced** simple supracondylar fracture **without**
CC-A,K,P MCC-B intercondylar fracture of **unspecified** humerus

S42.414- **Nondisplaced** simple supracondylar fracture
CC-A,K,P MCC-B **without** intercondylar fracture of **right** humerus

S42.415- **Nondisplaced** simple supracondylar fracture
CC-A,K,P MCC-B **without** intercondylar fracture of **left** humerus

S42.416- **Nondisplaced** simple supracondylar fracture
CC-A,K,P MCC-B **without** intercondylar fracture of **unspecified**
humerus

S42.42- **Comminuted supracondylar** fracture **without** intercondylar
fracture of humerus

S42.421- **Displaced** comminuted supracondylar fracture
CC-A,K,P MCC-B **without** intercondylar fracture of **right** humerus

S42.422- **Displaced** comminuted supracondylar fracture
CC-A,K,P MCC-B **without** intercondylar fracture of **left** humerus

S42.423- **Displaced** comminuted supracondylar fracture
CC-A,K,P MCC-B **without** intercondylar fracture of **unspecified**
humerus

S42.424- **Nondisplaced** comminuted supracondylar fracture
CC-A,K,P MCC-B **without** intercondylar fracture of **right** humerus

S42.425- **Nondisplaced** comminuted supracondylar fracture
CC-A,K,P MCC-B **without** intercondylar fracture of **left** humerus

S42.426- **Nondisplaced** comminuted supracondylar fracture
CC-A,K,P MCC-B **without** intercondylar fracture of **unspecified**
humerus

S42.43- Fracture (avulsion) of **lateral epicondyle** of **humerus**

S42.431- **Displaced** fracture (avulsion) of lateral epicondyle
CC-A,K,P MCC-B of **right** humerus

S42.432- **Displaced** fracture (avulsion) of lateral epicondyle
CC-A,K,P MCC-B of **left** humerus

S42.433- **Displaced** fracture (avulsion) of lateral epicondyle
CC-A,K,P MCC-B of **unspecified** humerus

S42.434- **Nondisplaced** fracture (avulsion) of lateral
CC-A,K,P MCC-B epicondyle of **right** humerus

S42.435- **Nondisplaced** fracture (avulsion) of lateral
CC-A,K,P MCC-B epicondyle of **left** humerus

S42.436- **Nondisplaced** fracture (avulsion) of lateral
CC-A,K,P MCC-B epicondyle of **unspecified** humerus

S42.44- Fracture (avulsion) of **medial epicondyle** of humerus

S42.441- **Displaced** fracture (avulsion) of medial epicondyle
CC-A,K,P MCC-B of **right** humerus

S42.442- **Displaced** fracture (avulsion) of medial epicondyle
CC-A,K,P MCC-B of **left** humerus

S42.443- **Displaced** fracture (avulsion) of medial epicondyle
CC-A,K,P MCC-B of **unspecified** humerus

S42.444- **Nondisplaced** fracture (avulsion) of medial
CC-A,K,P MCC-B epicondyle of **right** humerus

S42.445- **Nondisplaced** fracture (avulsion) of medial
CC-A,K,P MCC-B epicondyle of **left** humerus

S42.446- **Nondisplaced** fracture (avulsion) of medial
CC-A,K,P MCC-B epicondyle of **unspecified** humerus

S42.447- **Incarcerated** fracture (avulsion) of medial
CC-A,K,P MCC-B epicondyle of **right** humerus

S42.448- **Incarcerated** fracture (avulsion) of medial
CC-A,K,P MCC-B epicondyle of **left** humerus

S42.449- **Incarcerated** fracture (avulsion) of medial
CC-A,K,P MCC-B epicondyle of **unspecified** humerus

S42.45- Fracture of **lateral condyle** of **humerus**
Fracture of capitellum of humerus

S42.451- **Displaced** fracture of lateral condyle of **right**
CC-A,K,P MCC-B humerus

S42.452- **Displaced** fracture of lateral condyle of **left**
CC-A,K,P MCC-B humerus

S42.453- **Displaced** fracture of lateral condyle of **unspecified**
CC-A,K,P MCC-B humerus

S42.454- **Nondisplaced** fracture of lateral condyle of **right**
CC-A,K,P MCC-B humerus

S42.455- **Nondisplaced** fracture of lateral condyle of **left**
CC-A,K,P MCC-B humerus

S42.456- **Nondisplaced** fracture of lateral condyle of
CC-A,K,P MCC-B **unspecified** humerus

S42.46- Fracture of **medial condyle** of **humerus**
Trochlea fracture of humerus

S42.461- **Displaced** fracture of medial condyle of **right**
CC-A,K,P MCC-B humerus

S42.462- **Displaced** fracture of medial condyle of **left**
CC-A,K,P MCC-B humerus

S42.463- **Displaced** fracture of medial condyle of **unspecified**
CC-A,K,P MCC-B humerus

S42.464- **Nondisplaced** fracture of medial condyle of **right**
CC-A,K,P MCC-B humerus

S42.465- **Nondisplaced** fracture of medial condyle of **left**
CC-A,K,P MCC-B humerus

S42 - S42

S42.466- Nondisplaced fracture of medial condyle of unspecified humerus
CC-A,K,P MCC-B

S42.47- Transcondylar fracture of humerus

S42.471- Displaced transcondylar fracture of right humerus
CC-A,K,P MCC-B

S42.472- Displaced transcondylar fracture of left humerus
CC-A,K,P MCC-B

S42.473- Displaced transcondylar fracture of unspecified humerus
CC-A,K,P MCC-B

S42.474- Nondisplaced transcondylar fracture of right humerus
CC-A,K,P MCC-B

S42.475- Nondisplaced transcondylar fracture of left humerus
CC-A,K,P MCC-B

S42.476- Nondisplaced transcondylar fracture of unspecified humerus
CC-A,K,P MCC-B

S42.48- Torus fracture of lower end of humerus

> The appropriate 7th character is to be added to all codes in subcategory S42.48:
> **A** Initial encounter for closed fracture
> **D** Subsequent encounter for fracture with routine healing
> **G** Subsequent encounter for fracture with delayed healing
> **K** Subsequent encounter for fracture with nonunion
> **P** Subsequent encounter for fracture with malunion
> **S** Sequela

S42.481- Torus fracture of lower end of right humerus
CC-A,K,P

S42.482- Torus fracture of lower end of left humerus
CC-A,K,P

S42.489- Torus fracture of lower end of unspecified humerus
CC-A,K,P

S42.49- Other fracture of lower end of humerus

S42.491- Other displaced fracture of lower end of right humerus
CC-A,K,P MCC-B

S42.492- Other displaced fracture of lower end of left humerus
CC-A,K,P MCC-B

S42.493- Other displaced fracture of lower end of unspecified humerus
CC-A,K,P MCC-B

S42.494- Other nondisplaced fracture of lower end of right humerus
CC-A,K,P MCC-B

S42.495- Other nondisplaced fracture of lower end of left humerus
CC-A,K,P MCC-B

S42.496- Other nondisplaced fracture of lower end of unspecified humerus
CC-A,K,P MCC-B

S42.9- Fracture of shoulder girdle, part unspecified
Fracture of shoulder NOS

S42.90x- Fracture of unspecified shoulder girdle, part unspecified
CC-A,K,P MCC-B

S42.91x- Fracture of right shoulder girdle, part unspecified
CC-A,K,P MCC-B

S42.92x- Fracture of left shoulder girdle, part unspecified
CC-A,K,P MCC-B

S43- Dislocation and sprain of joints and ligaments of shoulder girdle
Includes: Avulsion of joint or ligament of shoulder girdle
Laceration of cartilage, joint or ligament of shoulder girdle
Sprain of cartilage, joint or ligament of shoulder girdle
Traumatic hemarthrosis of joint or ligament of shoulder girdle
Traumatic rupture of joint or ligament of shoulder girdle
Traumatic subluxation of joint or ligament of shoulder girdle
Traumatic tear of joint or ligament of shoulder girdle
Code also any associated open wound
Excludes ❷: *strain of muscle, fascia and tendon of shoulder and upper arm (S46.-)*

> The appropriate 7th character is to be added to each code from category S43:
> **A** Initial encounter
> **D** Subsequent encounter
> **S** Sequela

S43.0- Subluxation and dislocation of shoulder joint
Dislocation of glenohumeral joint
Subluxation of glenohumeral joint

S43.00- Unspecified subluxation and dislocation of shoulder joint
Dislocation of humerus NOS
Subluxation of humerus NOS

S43.001- Unspecified subluxation of right shoulder joint

S43.002- Unspecified subluxation of left shoulder joint

S43.003- Unspecified subluxation of unspecified shoulder joint

S43.004- Unspecified dislocation of right shoulder joint

S43.005- Unspecified dislocation of left shoulder joint

S43.006- Unspecified dislocation of unspecified shoulder joint

S43.01- Anterior subluxation and dislocation of humerus

S43.011- Anterior subluxation of right humerus

S43.012- Anterior subluxation of left humerus

S43.013- Anterior subluxation of unspecified humerus

S43.014- Anterior dislocation of right humerus

S43.015- Anterior dislocation of left humerus

S43.016- Anterior dislocation of unspecified humerus

S43.02- Posterior subluxation and dislocation of humerus

S43.021- Posterior subluxation of right humerus

S43.022- Posterior subluxation of left humerus

S43.023- Posterior subluxation of unspecified humerus

S43.024- Posterior dislocation of right humerus

S43.025- Posterior dislocation of left humerus

S43.026- Posterior dislocation of unspecified humerus

S43.03- Inferior subluxation and dislocation of humerus

S43.031- Inferior subluxation of right humerus

S43.032- Inferior subluxation of left humerus

S43.033- Inferior subluxation of unspecified humerus

S43.034- Inferior dislocation of right humerus

S43.035- Inferior dislocation of left humerus

S43.036- Inferior dislocation of unspecified humerus

S43.08- Other subluxation and dislocation of shoulder joint

S43.081- Other subluxation of right shoulder joint

S43.082- Other subluxation of left shoulder joint

S43.083- Other subluxation of unspecified shoulder joint

S43.084- Other dislocation of right shoulder joint

S43.085- Other dislocation of left shoulder joint

S43.086- Other dislocation of unspecified shoulder joint

S43.1- Subluxation and dislocation of acromioclavicular joint

S43.10- Unspecified dislocation of acromioclavicular joint

S43.101- Unspecified dislocation of right acromioclavicular joint

S43.102- Unspecified dislocation of left acromioclavicular joint

S43.109- Unspecified dislocation of unspecified acromioclavicular joint

S43.11- Subluxation of acromioclavicular joint

S43.111- Subluxation of right acromioclavicular joint

S43.112- Subluxation of left acromioclavicular joint

S43.119- Subluxation of unspecified acromioclavicular joint

S43.12- Dislocation of acromioclavicular joint, 100%-200% displacement

S43.121- Dislocation of right acromioclavicular joint, 100%-200% displacement

S43.122- Dislocation of left acromioclavicular joint, 100%-200% displacement

S43.129- Dislocation of unspecified acromioclavicular joint, 100%-200% displacement

S43.13- Dislocation of acromioclavicular joint, greater than 200% displacement

S43.131- Dislocation of right acromioclavicular joint, greater than 200% displacement

S43.132- Dislocation of left acromioclavicular joint, greater than 200% displacement

S43.139- Dislocation of unspecified acromioclavicular joint, greater than 200% displacement

S43.14- Inferior dislocation of acromioclavicular joint

S43.141- Inferior dislocation of right acromioclavicular joint

S43.142- Inferior dislocation of left acromioclavicular joint

S 4 2 - S 4 3

S43.149- Inferior dislocation of <u>unspecified</u> acromioclavicular joint

S43.15- <u>Posterior</u> dislocation of <u>acromioclavicular joint</u>

S43.151- Posterior dislocation of <u>right</u> acromioclavicular joint

S43.152- Posterior dislocation of <u>left</u> acromioclavicular joint

S43.159- Posterior dislocation of <u>unspecified</u> acromioclavicular joint

S43.2- <u>Subluxation and dislocation</u> of sternoclavicular joint

S43.20- <u>Unspecified subluxation and dislocation</u> of <u>sternoclavicular joint</u>

CC-A **S43.201-** Unspecified <u>subluxation</u> of <u>right</u> sternoclavicular joint

CC-A **S43.202-** Unspecified <u>subluxation</u> of <u>left</u> sternoclavicular joint

CC-A **S43.203-** Unspecified <u>subluxation</u> of <u>unspecified</u> sternoclavicular joint

CC-A **S43.204-** Unspecified <u>dislocation</u> of <u>right</u> sternoclavicular joint

CC-A **S43.205-** Unspecified <u>dislocation</u> of <u>left</u> sternoclavicular joint

CC-A **S43.206-** Unspecified <u>dislocation</u> of <u>unspecified</u> sternoclavicular joint

S43.21- <u>Anterior</u> subluxation and dislocation of <u>sternoclavicular joint</u>

CC-A **S43.211-** Anterior <u>subluxation</u> of <u>right</u> sternoclavicular joint

CC-A **S43.212-** Anterior <u>subluxation</u> of <u>left</u> sternoclavicular joint

CC-A **S43.213-** Anterior <u>subluxation</u> of <u>unspecified</u> sternoclavicular joint

CC-A **S43.214-** Anterior <u>dislocation</u> of <u>right</u> sternoclavicular joint

CC-A **S43.215-** Anterior <u>dislocation</u> of <u>left</u> sternoclavicular joint

CC-A **S43.216-** Anterior <u>dislocation</u> of <u>unspecified</u> sternoclavicular joint

S43.22- <u>Posterior</u> subluxation and dislocation of sternoclavicular joint

CC-A **S43.221-** Posterior <u>subluxation</u> of <u>right</u> sternoclavicular joint

CC-A **S43.222-** Posterior <u>subluxation</u> of <u>left</u> sternoclavicular joint

CC-A **S43.223-** Posterior <u>subluxation</u> of <u>unspecified</u> sternoclavicular joint

CC-A **S43.224-** Posterior <u>dislocation</u> of <u>right</u> sternoclavicular joint

CC-A **S43.225-** Posterior <u>dislocation</u> of <u>left</u> sternoclavicular joint

CC-A **S43.226-** Posterior <u>dislocation</u> of <u>unspecified</u> sternoclavicular joint

S43.3- <u>Subluxation and dislocation</u> of <u>other and unspecified</u> parts of <u>shoulder girdle</u>

S43.30- <u>Subluxation and dislocation</u> of <u>unspecified</u> parts of <u>shoulder girdle</u>
Dislocation of shoulder girdle NOS
Subluxation of shoulder girdle NOS

S43.301- <u>Subluxation</u> of <u>unspecified</u> parts of <u>right</u> shoulder girdle

S43.302- <u>Subluxation</u> of <u>unspecified</u> parts of <u>left</u> shoulder girdle

S43.303- <u>Subluxation</u> of <u>unspecified</u> parts of <u>unspecified</u> shoulder girdle

S43.304- <u>Dislocation</u> of <u>unspecified</u> parts of <u>right</u> shoulder girdle

S43.305- <u>Dislocation</u> of <u>unspecified</u> parts of <u>left</u> shoulder girdle

S43.306- <u>Dislocation</u> of <u>unspecified</u> parts of <u>unspecified</u> shoulder girdle

S43.31- Subluxation and dislocation of <u>scapula</u>

S43.311- <u>Subluxation</u> of <u>right</u> scapula

S43.312- <u>Subluxation</u> of <u>left</u> scapula

S43.313- <u>Subluxation</u> of <u>unspecified</u> scapula

S43.314- <u>Dislocation</u> of <u>right</u> scapula

S43.315- <u>Dislocation</u> of <u>left</u> scapula

S43.316- <u>Dislocation</u> of <u>unspecified</u> scapula

S43.39- Subluxation and dislocation of <u>other parts</u> of <u>shoulder girdle</u>

S43.391- <u>Subluxation</u> of other parts of <u>right</u> shoulder girdle

S43.392- <u>Subluxation</u> of other parts of <u>left</u> shoulder girdle

S43.393- <u>Subluxation</u> of other parts of <u>unspecified</u> shoulder girdle

S43.394- <u>Dislocation</u> of other parts of <u>right</u> shoulder girdle

S43.395- <u>Dislocation</u> of other parts of <u>left</u> shoulder girdle

S43.396- <u>Dislocation</u> of other parts of <u>unspecified</u> shoulder girdle

S43.4- <u>Sprain</u> of shoulder joint

S43.40- <u>Unspecified</u> sprain of <u>shoulder joint</u>

S43.401- Unspecified sprain of <u>right</u> shoulder joint

S43.402- Unspecified sprain of <u>left</u> shoulder joint

S43.409- Unspecified sprain of <u>unspecified</u> shoulder joint

S43.41- <u>Sprain</u> of <u>coracohumeral (ligament)</u>

S43.411- Sprain of <u>right</u> coracohumeral (ligament)

S43.412- Sprain of <u>left</u> coracohumeral (ligament)

S43.419- Sprain of <u>unspecified</u> coracohumeral (ligament)

S43.42- <u>Sprain</u> of <u>rotator cuff capsule</u>
Excludes 1: rotator cuff syndrome (complete) (incomplete), not specified as traumatic (M75.1-)
Excludes ❷: injury of tendon of rotator cuff (S46.0-)

S43.421- Sprain of <u>right</u> rotator cuff capsule

S43.422- Sprain of <u>left</u> rotator cuff capsule

S43.429- Sprain of <u>unspecified</u> rotator cuff capsule

S43.43- <u>Superior glenoid labrum lesion</u>
SLAP lesion

S43.431- Superior glenoid labrum lesion of <u>right</u> shoulder

S43.432- Superior glenoid labrum lesion of <u>left</u> shoulder

S43.439- Superior glenoid labrum lesion of <u>unspecified</u> shoulder

S43.49- <u>Other sprain</u> of <u>shoulder joint</u>

S43.491- Other sprain of <u>right</u> shoulder joint

S43.492- Other sprain of <u>left</u> shoulder joint

S43.499- Other sprain of <u>unspecified</u> shoulder joint

S43.5- <u>Sprain</u> of <u>acromioclavicular joint</u>
Sprain of acromioclavicular ligament

S43.50x- Sprain of <u>unspecified</u> acromioclavicular joint

S43.51x- Sprain of <u>right</u> acromioclavicular joint

S43.52x- Sprain of <u>left</u> acromioclavicular joint

S43.6- <u>Sprain</u> of <u>sternoclavicular joint</u>

S43.60x- Sprain of <u>unspecified</u> sternoclavicular joint

S43.61x- Sprain of <u>right</u> sternoclavicular joint

S43.62x- Sprain of <u>left</u> sternoclavicular joint

S43.8- <u>Sprain</u> of <u>other specified parts</u> of <u>shoulder girdle</u>

S43.80x- Sprain of other specified parts of <u>unspecified</u> shoulder girdle

S43.81x- Sprain of other specified parts of <u>right</u> shoulder girdle

S43.82x- Sprain of other specified parts of <u>left</u> shoulder girdle

S43.9- <u>Sprain</u> of <u>unspecified parts</u> of <u>shoulder girdle</u>

S43.90x- Sprain of <u>unspecified</u> parts of <u>unspecified</u> shoulder girdle
Sprain of shoulder girdle NOS

S43.91x- Sprain of <u>unspecified</u> parts of <u>right</u> shoulder girdle

S43.92x- Sprain of <u>unspecified</u> parts of <u>left</u> shoulder girdle

S43 – S43

S44-   Injury of nerves at shoulder and upper arm level
Code also any associated open wound (S41.-)
Excludes ❷: injury of brachial plexus (S14.3-)

The appropriate 7th character is to be added to each code from category S44:
- **A   Initial encounter**
- **D   Subsequent encounter**
- **S   Sequela**

S44.0-   Injury of ulnar nerve at upper arm level
        Excludes 1:   ulnar nerve NOS (S54.0)
- **S44.00x-   Injury of ulnar nerve at upper arm level, unspecified arm**
- **S44.01x-   Injury of ulnar nerve at upper arm level, right arm**
- **S44.02x-   Injury of ulnar nerve at upper arm level, left arm**

S44.1-   Injury of median nerve at upper arm level
        Excludes 1:   median nerve NOS (S54.1)
- **S44.10x-   Injury of median nerve at upper arm level, unspecified arm**
- **S44.11x-   Injury of median nerve at upper arm level, right arm**
- **S44.12x-   Injury of median nerve at upper arm level, left arm**

S44.2-   Injury of radial nerve at upper arm level
        Excludes 1:   radial nerve NOS (S54.2)
- **S44.20x-   Injury of radial nerve at upper arm level, unspecified arm**
- **S44.21x-   Injury of radial nerve at upper arm level, right arm**
- **S44.22x-   Injury of radial nerve at upper arm level, left arm**

S44.3-   Injury of axillary nerve
- **S44.30x-   Injury of axillary nerve, unspecified arm**
- **S44.31x-   Injury of axillary nerve, right arm**
- **S44.32x-   Injury of axillary nerve, left arm**

S44.4-   Injury of musculocutaneous nerve
- **S44.40x-   Injury of musculocutaneous nerve, unspecified arm**
- **S44.41x-   Injury of musculocutaneous nerve, right arm**
- **S44.42x-   Injury of musculocutaneous nerve, left arm**

S44.5-   Injury of cutaneous sensory nerve at shoulder and upper arm level
- **S44.50x-   Injury of cutaneous sensory nerve at shoulder and upper arm level, unspecified arm**
- **S44.51x-   Injury of cutaneous sensory nerve at shoulder and upper arm level, right arm**
- **S44.52x-   Injury of cutaneous sensory nerve at shoulder and upper arm level, left arm**

S44.8-   Injury of other nerves at shoulder and upper arm level
- **S44.8x-   Injury of other nerves at shoulder and upper arm level**
  - **S44.8x1-   Injury of other nerves at shoulder and upper arm level, right arm**
  - **S44.8x2-   Injury of other nerves at shoulder and upper arm level, left arm**
  - **S44.8x9-   Injury of other nerves at shoulder and upper arm level, unspecified arm**

S44.9-   Injury of unspecified nerve at shoulder and upper arm level
- **S44.90x-   Injury of unspecified nerve at shoulder and upper arm level, unspecified arm**
- **S44.91x-   Injury of unspecified nerve at shoulder and upper arm level, right arm**
- **S44.92x-   Injury of unspecified nerve at shoulder and upper arm level, left arm**

S45-   Injury of blood vessels at shoulder and upper arm level
Code also any associated open wound (S41.-)
Excludes ❷: injury of subclavian artery (S25.1)
*   injury of subclavian vein (S25.3)*

The appropriate 7th character is to be added to each code from category S45:
- **A   Initial encounter**
- **D   Subsequent encounter**
- **S   Sequela**

S45.0-   Injury of axillary artery
- **S45.00-   Unspecified injury of axillary artery**
  - MCC-A **S45.001-   Unspecified injury of axillary artery, right side**
  - MCC-A **S45.002-   Unspecified injury of axillary artery, left side**
  - MCC-A **S45.009-   Unspecified injury of axillary artery, unspecified side**
- **S45.01-   Laceration of axillary artery**
  - MCC-A **S45.011-   Laceration of axillary artery, right side**
  - MCC-A **S45.012-   Laceration of axillary artery, left side**
  - MCC-A **S45.019-   Laceration of axillary artery, unspecified side**
- **S45.09-   Other specified injury of axillary artery**
  - MCC-A **S45.091-   Other specified injury of axillary artery, right side**
  - MCC-A **S45.092-   Other specified injury of axillary artery, left side**
  - MCC-A **S45.099-   Other specified injury of axillary artery, unspecified side**

S45.1-   Injury of brachial artery
- **S45.10-   Unspecified injury of brachial artery**
  - CC-A **S45.101-   Unspecified injury of brachial artery, right side**
  - CC-A **S45.102-   Unspecified injury of brachial artery, left side**
  - CC-A **S45.109-   Unspecified injury of brachial artery, unspecified side**
- **S45.11-   Laceration of brachial artery**
  - CC-A **S45.111-   Laceration of brachial artery, right side**
  - CC-A **S45.112-   Laceration of brachial artery, left side**
  - CC-A **S45.119-   Laceration of brachial artery, unspecified side**
- **S45.19-   Other specified injury of brachial artery**
  - CC-A **S45.191-   Other specified injury of brachial artery, right side**
  - CC-A **S45.192-   Other specified injury of brachial artery, left side**
  - CC-A **S45.199-   Other specified injury of brachial artery, unspecified side**

S45.2-   Injury of axillary or brachial vein
- **S45.20-   Unspecified injury of axillary or brachial vein**
  - CC-A **S45.201-   Unspecified injury of axillary or brachial vein, right side**
  - CC-A **S45.202-   Unspecified injury of axillary or brachial vein, left side**
  - CC-A **S45.209-   Unspecified injury of axillary or brachial vein, unspecified side**
- **S45.21-   Laceration of axillary or brachial vein**
  - CC-A **S45.211-   Laceration of axillary or brachial vein, right side**
  - CC-A **S45.212-   Laceration of axillary or brachial vein, left side**
  - CC-A **S45.219-   Laceration of axillary or brachial vein, unspecified side**
- **S45.29-   Other specified injury of axillary or brachial vein**
  - CC-A **S45.291-   Other specified injury of axillary or brachial vein, right side**
  - CC-A **S45.292-   Other specified injury of axillary or brachial vein, left side**
  - CC-A **S45.299-   Other specified injury of axillary or brachial vein, unspecified side**

S45.3-   Injury of superficial vein at shoulder and upper arm level
- **S45.30-   Unspecified injury of superficial vein at shoulder and upper arm level**
  - CC-A **S45.301-   Unspecified injury of superficial vein at shoulder and upper arm level, right arm**
  - CC-A **S45.302-   Unspecified injury of superficial vein at shoulder and upper arm level, left arm**

S 4 4 - S 4 5

CC-A **S45.309-** Unspecified injury of superficial vein at shoulder and upper arm level, <u>unspecified</u> arm

S45.31- <u>Laceration</u> of <u>superficial vein</u> at <u>shoulder and upper arm level</u>

CC-A **S45.311-** Laceration of superficial vein at shoulder and upper arm level, <u>right</u> arm

CC-A **S45.312-** Laceration of superficial vein at shoulder and upper arm level, <u>left</u> arm

CC-A **S45.319-** Laceration of superficial vein at shoulder and upper arm level, <u>unspecified</u> arm

S45.39- <u>Other specified</u> injury of <u>superficial vein</u> at shoulder and <u>upper arm level</u>

CC-A **S45.391-** Other specified injury of superficial vein at shoulder and upper arm level, <u>right</u> arm

CC-A **S45.392-** Other specified injury of superficial vein at shoulder and upper arm level, <u>left</u> arm

CC-A **S45.399-** Other specified injury of superficial vein at shoulder and upper arm level, <u>unspecified</u> arm

S45.8- Injury of <u>other specified blood vessels</u> at shoulder and upper arm level

S45.80- <u>Unspecified</u> injury of <u>other specified blood vessels</u> <u>at shoulder and upper arm level</u>

CC-A **S45.801-** Unspecified injury of other specified blood vessels at shoulder and upper arm level, <u>right</u> arm

CC-A **S45.802-** Unspecified injury of other specified blood vessels at shoulder and upper arm level, <u>left</u> arm

CC-A **S45.809-** Unspecified injury of other specified blood vessels at shoulder and upper arm level, <u>unspecified</u> arm

S45.81- <u>Laceration</u> of <u>other specified blood vessels</u> at <u>shoulder and upper arm level</u>

CC-A **S45.811-** Laceration of other specified blood vessels at shoulder and upper arm level, <u>right</u> arm

CC-A **S45.812-** Laceration of other specified blood vessels at shoulder and upper arm level, <u>left</u> arm

CC-A **S45.819-** Laceration of other specified blood vessels at shoulder and upper arm level, <u>unspecified</u> arm

S45.89- <u>Other specified injury</u> of <u>other specified blood vessels</u> <u>at shoulder and upper arm level</u>

CC-A **S45.891-** Other specified injury of other specified blood vessels at shoulder and upper arm level, <u>right</u> arm

CC-A **S45.892-** Other specified injury of other specified blood vessels at shoulder and upper arm level, <u>left</u> arm

CC-A **S45.899-** Other specified injury of other specified blood vessels at shoulder and upper arm level, <u>unspecified</u> arm

S45.9- Injury of <u>unspecified blood vessel</u> at shoulder and upper arm level

S45.90- <u>Unspecified</u> injury of <u>unspecified blood vessel</u> at shoulder and upper arm level

CC-A **S45.901-** Unspecified injury of unspecified blood vessel at shoulder and upper arm level, <u>right</u> arm

CC-A **S45.902-** Unspecified injury of unspecified blood vessel at shoulder and upper arm level, <u>left</u> arm

CC-A **S45.909-** Unspecified injury of unspecified blood vessel at shoulder and upper arm level, <u>unspecified</u> arm

S45.91- <u>Laceration</u> of <u>unspecified blood vessel</u> at shoulder and <u>upper arm level</u>

CC-A **S45.911-** Laceration of unspecified blood vessel at shoulder and upper arm level, <u>right</u> arm

CC-A **S45.912-** Laceration of unspecified blood vessel at shoulder and upper arm level, <u>left</u> arm

CC-A **S45.919-** Laceration of unspecified blood vessel at shoulder and upper arm level, <u>unspecified</u> arm

S45.99- <u>Other specified injury</u> of <u>unspecified blood vessel</u> at <u>shoulder and upper arm level</u>

CC-A **S45.991-** Other specified injury of unspecified blood vessel at shoulder and upper arm level, <u>right</u> arm

CC-A **S45.992-** Other specified injury of unspecified blood vessel at shoulder and upper arm level, <u>left</u> arm

---

CC-A **S45.999-** Other specified injury of unspecified blood vessel at shoulder and upper arm level, <u>unspecified</u> arm

S46- Injury of <u>muscle, fascia and tendon</u> at <u>shoulder and upper arm level</u>
Code also any associated open wound (S41.-)
Excludes ❷: *injury of muscle, fascia and tendon at elbow (S56.-)*
sprain of joints and ligaments of shoulder girdle (S43.9)

The appropriate 7th character is to be added to each code from category S46:
A <u>Initial</u> encounter
D <u>Subsequent</u> encounter
S <u>Sequela</u>

S46.0- Injury of <u>muscle(s) and tendon(s)</u> of the <u>rotator cuff of shoulder</u>

S46.00- <u>Unspecified</u> injury of <u>muscle(s) and tendon(s)</u> of the <u>rotator cuff of shoulder</u>

S46.001- Unspecified injury of muscle(s) and tendon(s) of the rotator cuff of <u>right</u> shoulder

S46.002- Unspecified injury of muscle(s) and tendon(s) of the rotator cuff of <u>left</u> shoulder

S46.009- Unspecified injury of muscle(s) and tendon(s) of the rotator cuff of <u>unspecified</u> shoulder

S46.01- <u>Strain</u> of <u>muscle(s) and tendon(s)</u> of the <u>rotator cuff of shoulder</u>

S46.011- Strain of muscle(s) and tendon(s) of the rotator cuff of <u>right</u> shoulder

S46.012- Strain of muscle(s) and tendon(s) of the rotator cuff of <u>left</u> shoulder

S46.019- Strain of muscle(s) and tendon(s) of the rotator cuff of <u>unspecified</u> shoulder

S46.02- <u>Laceration</u> of <u>muscle(s) and tendon(s)</u> of the <u>rotator cuff of shoulder</u>

CC-A **S46.021-** Laceration of muscle(s) and tendon(s) of the rotator cuff of <u>right</u> shoulder

CC-A **S46.022-** Laceration of muscle(s) and tendon(s) of the rotator cuff of <u>left</u> shoulder

CC-A **S46.029-** Laceration of muscle(s) and tendon(s) of the rotator cuff of <u>unspecified</u> shoulder

S46.09- <u>Other injury</u> of <u>muscle(s) and tendon(s)</u> of the <u>rotator cuff of shoulder</u>

S46.091- Other injury of muscle(s) and tendon(s) of the rotator cuff of <u>right</u> shoulder

S46.092- Other injury of muscle(s) and tendon(s) of the rotator cuff of <u>left</u> shoulder

S46.099- Other injury of muscle(s) and tendon(s) of the rotator cuff of <u>unspecified</u> shoulder

S46.1- Injury of <u>muscle, fascia and tendon</u> of <u>long head of biceps</u>

S46.10- <u>Unspecified</u> injury of <u>muscle, fascia and tendon</u> of <u>long head of biceps</u>

S46.101- Unspecified injury of muscle, fascia and tendon of long head of biceps, <u>right</u> arm

S46.102- Unspecified injury of muscle, fascia and tendon of long head of biceps, <u>left</u> arm

S46.109- Unspecified injury of muscle, fascia and tendon of long head of biceps, <u>unspecified</u> arm

S46.11- <u>Strain</u> of <u>muscle, fascia and tendon</u> of <u>long head of biceps</u>

S46.111- Strain of muscle, fascia and tendon of long head of biceps, <u>right</u> arm

S46.112- Strain of muscle, fascia and tendon of long head of biceps, <u>left</u> arm

S46.119- Strain of muscle, fascia and tendon of long head of biceps, <u>unspecified</u> arm

S46.12- <u>Laceration</u> of <u>muscle, fascia and tendon</u> of <u>long head of biceps</u>

CC-A **S46.121-** Laceration of muscle, fascia and tendon of long head of biceps, <u>right</u> arm

CC-A **S46.122-** Laceration of muscle, fascia and tendon of long head of biceps, <u>left</u> arm

S 4 5 – S 4 6

CC-A **S46.129-** Laceration of muscle, fascia and tendon of long head of biceps, <u>unspecified</u> arm

S46.19- <u>Other</u> injury of <u>muscle, fascia and tendon</u> of <u>long head of biceps</u>
- **S46.191-** Other injury of muscle, fascia and tendon of long head of biceps, <u>right</u> arm
- **S46.192-** Other injury of muscle, fascia and tendon of long head of biceps, <u>left</u> arm
- **S46.199-** Other injury of muscle, fascia and tendon of long head of biceps, <u>unspecified</u> arm

S46.2- Injury of <u>muscle, fascia and tendon</u> of <u>other parts of biceps</u>

S46.20- <u>Unspecified</u> injury of <u>muscle, fascia and tendon</u> of <u>other parts of biceps</u>
- **S46.201-** Unspecified injury of muscle, fascia and tendon of other parts of biceps, <u>right</u> arm
- **S46.202-** Unspecified injury of muscle, fascia and tendon of other parts of biceps, <u>left</u> arm
- **S46.209-** Unspecified injury of muscle, fascia and tendon of other parts of biceps, <u>unspecified</u> arm

S46.21- <u>Strain</u> of <u>muscle, fascia and tendon</u> of <u>other parts of biceps</u>
- **S46.211-** Strain of muscle, fascia and tendon of other parts of biceps, <u>right</u> arm
- **S46.212-** Strain of muscle, fascia and tendon of other parts of biceps, <u>left</u> arm
- **S46.219-** Strain of muscle, fascia and tendon of other parts of biceps, <u>unspecified</u> arm

S46.22- <u>Laceration</u> of <u>muscle, fascia and tendon</u> of <u>other parts of biceps</u>
- CC-A **S46.221-** Laceration of muscle, fascia and tendon of other parts of biceps, <u>right</u> arm
- CC-A **S46.222-** Laceration of muscle, fascia and tendon of other parts of biceps, <u>left</u> arm
- CC-A **S46.229-** Laceration of muscle, fascia and tendon of other parts of biceps, <u>unspecified</u> arm

S46.29- <u>Other</u> injury of <u>muscle, fascia and tendon</u> of <u>other parts of biceps</u>
- **S46.291-** Other injury of muscle, fascia and tendon of other parts of biceps, <u>right</u> arm
- **S46.292-** Other injury of muscle, fascia and tendon of other parts of biceps, <u>left</u> arm
- **S46.299-** Other injury of muscle, fascia and tendon of other parts of biceps, <u>unspecified</u> arm

S46.3- Injury of <u>muscle, fascia and tendon</u> of <u>triceps</u>

S46.30- <u>Unspecified</u> injury of <u>muscle, fascia and tendon</u> of <u>triceps</u>
- **S46.301-** Unspecified injury of muscle, fascia and tendon of triceps, <u>right</u> arm
- **S46.302-** Unspecified injury of muscle, fascia and tendon of triceps, <u>left</u> arm
- **S46.309-** Unspecified injury of muscle, fascia and tendon of triceps, <u>unspecified</u> arm

S46.31- <u>Strain</u> of <u>muscle, fascia and tendon</u> of <u>triceps</u>
- **S46.311-** Strain of muscle, fascia and tendon of triceps, <u>right</u> arm
- **S46.312-** Strain of muscle, fascia and tendon of triceps, <u>left</u> arm
- **S46.319-** Strain of muscle, fascia and tendon of triceps, <u>unspecified</u> arm

S46.32- <u>Laceration</u> of <u>muscle, fascia and tendon</u> of <u>triceps</u>
- CC-A **S46.321-** Laceration of muscle, fascia and tendon of triceps, <u>right</u> arm
- CC-A **S46.322-** Laceration of muscle, fascia and tendon of triceps, <u>left</u> arm
- CC-A **S46.329-** Laceration of muscle, fascia and tendon of triceps, <u>unspecified</u> arm

S46.39- <u>Other injury</u> of muscle, fascia and tendon of <u>triceps</u>
- **S46.391-** Other injury of muscle, fascia and tendon of triceps, <u>right</u> arm

S46.392- Other injury of muscle, fascia and tendon of triceps, <u>left</u> arm

S46.399- Other injury of muscle, fascia and tendon of triceps, <u>unspecified</u> arm

S46.8- <u>Injury</u> of <u>other muscles, fascia and tendons</u> at <u>shoulder and upper arm level</u>

S46.80- <u>Unspecified</u> injury of <u>other muscles, fascia and tendons</u> at <u>shoulder and upper arm level</u>
- **S46.801-** Unspecified injury of other muscles, fascia and tendons at shoulder and upper arm level, <u>right</u> arm
- **S46.802-** Unspecified injury of other muscles, fascia and tendons at shoulder and upper arm level, <u>left</u> arm
- **S46.809-** Unspecified injury of other muscles, fascia and tendons at shoulder and upper arm level, <u>unspecified</u> arm

S46.81- <u>Strain</u> of <u>other muscles, fascia and tendons</u> at <u>shoulder and upper arm level</u>
- **S46.811-** Strain of other muscles, fascia and tendons at shoulder and upper arm level, <u>right</u> arm
- **S46.812-** Strain of other muscles, fascia and tendons at shoulder and upper arm level, <u>left</u> arm
- **S46.819-** Strain of other muscles, fascia and tendons at shoulder and upper arm level, <u>unspecified</u> arm

S46.82- <u>Laceration</u> of <u>other muscles, fascia and tendons</u> at <u>shoulder and upper arm level</u>
- CC-A **S46.821-** Laceration of other muscles, fascia and tendons at shoulder and upper arm level, <u>right</u> arm
- CC-A **S46.822-** Laceration of other muscles, fascia and tendons at shoulder and upper arm level, <u>left</u> arm
- CC-A **S46.829-** Laceration of other muscles, fascia and tendons at shoulder and upper arm level, <u>unspecified</u> arm

S46.89- <u>Other injury</u> of <u>other muscles, fascia and tendons</u> at <u>shoulder and upper arm level</u>
- **S46.891-** Other injury of other muscles, fascia and tendons at shoulder and upper arm level, <u>right</u> arm
- **S46.892-** Other injury of other muscles, fascia and tendons at shoulder and upper arm level, <u>left</u> arm
- **S46.899-** Other injury of other muscles, fascia and tendons at shoulder and upper arm level, <u>unspecified</u> arm

S46.9- Injury of <u>unspecified</u> muscle, fascia and tendon at <u>shoulder and upper arm level</u>

S46.90- <u>Unspecified</u> injury of <u>unspecified</u> muscle, fascia and tendon at shoulder and upper arm level
- **S46.901-** Unspecified injury of unspecified muscle, fascia and tendon at shoulder and upper arm level, <u>right</u> arm
- **S46.902-** Unspecified injury of unspecified muscle, fascia and tendon at shoulder and upper arm level, <u>left</u> arm
- **S46.909-** Unspecified injury of <u>unspecified</u> muscle, fascia and tendon at shoulder and upper arm level, <u>unspecified</u> arm

S46.91- <u>Strain</u> of <u>unspecified</u> muscle, fascia and tendon at shoulder and upper arm level
- **S46.911-** Strain of unspecified muscle, fascia and tendon at shoulder and upper arm level, <u>right</u> arm
- **S46.912-** Strain of unspecified muscle, fascia and tendon at shoulder and upper arm level, <u>left</u> arm
- **S46.919-** Strain of unspecified muscle, fascia and tendon at shoulder and upper arm level, <u>unspecified</u> arm

S46.92- <u>Laceration</u> of <u>unspecified</u> muscle, fascia and tendon at <u>shoulder and upper arm level</u>
- CC-A **S46.921-** Laceration of unspecified muscle, fascia and tendon at shoulder and upper arm level, <u>right</u> arm
- CC-A **S46.922-** Laceration of unspecified muscle, fascia and tendon at shoulder and upper arm level, <u>left</u> arm
- CC-A **S46.929-** Laceration of unspecified muscle, fascia and tendon at shoulder and upper arm level, <u>unspecified</u> arm

S4 4 - S4 6

S46.99-   Other injury of unspecified muscle, fascia and tendon at shoulder and upper arm level

     S46.991-   Other injury of unspecified muscle, fascia and tendon at shoulder and upper arm level, right arm

     S46.992-   Other injury of unspecified muscle, fascia and tendon at shoulder and upper arm level, left arm

     S46.999-   Other injury of unspecified muscle, fascia and tendon at shoulder and upper arm level, unspecified arm

S47-   Crushing injury of shoulder and upper arm

Use additional code for all associated injuries

Excludes ❷: *crushing injury of elbow (S57.0-)*

The appropriate 7th character is to be added to each code from category S47:

A   Initial encounter
D   Subsequent encounter
S   Sequela

S47.1xx-   Crushing injury of right shoulder and upper arm

S47.2xx-   Crushing injury of left shoulder and upper arm

S47.9xx-   Crushing injury of shoulder and upper arm, unspecified arm

S48-   Traumatic amputation of shoulder and upper arm

Note: An amputation not identified as partial or complete should be coded to complete

Excludes 1:   *traumatic amputation at elbow level (S58.0)*

The appropriate 7th character is to be added to each code from category S48:

A   Initial encounter
D   Subsequent encounter
S   Sequela

S48.0-   Traumatic amputation at shoulder joint

     S48.01-   Complete traumatic amputation at shoulder joint

     CC-A **S48.011-**   Complete traumatic amputation at right shoulder joint

     CC-A **S48.012-**   Complete traumatic amputation at left shoulder joint

     CC-A **S48.019-**   Complete traumatic amputation at unspecified shoulder joint

     S48.02-   Partial traumatic amputation at shoulder joint

     CC-A **S48.021-**   Partial traumatic amputation at right shoulder joint

     CC-A **S48.022-**   Partial traumatic amputation at left shoulder joint

     CC-A **S48.029-**   Partial traumatic amputation at unspecified shoulder joint

S48.1-   Traumatic amputation at level between shoulder and elbow

     S48.11-   Complete traumatic amputation at level between shoulder and elbow

     CC-A **S48.111-**   Complete traumatic amputation at level between right shoulder and elbow

     CC-A **S48.112-**   Complete traumatic amputation at level between left shoulder and elbow

     CC-A **S48.119-**   Complete traumatic amputation at level between unspecified shoulder and elbow

     S48.12-   Partial traumatic amputation at level between shoulder and elbow

     CC-A **S48.121-**   Partial traumatic amputation at level between right shoulder and elbow

     CC-A **S48.122-**   Partial traumatic amputation at level between left shoulder and elbow

     CC-A **S48.129-**   Partial traumatic amputation at level between unspecified shoulder and elbow

S48.9-   Traumatic amputation of shoulder and upper arm, level unspecified

     S48.91-   Complete traumatic amputation of shoulder and upper arm, level unspecified

     CC-A **S48.911-**   Complete traumatic amputation of right shoulder and upper arm, level unspecified

     CC-A **S48.912-**   Complete traumatic amputation of left shoulder and upper arm, level unspecified

     CC-A **S48.919-**   Complete traumatic amputation of unspecified shoulder and upper arm, level unspecified

     S48.92-   Partial traumatic amputation of shoulder and upper arm, level unspecified

     CC-A **S48.921-**   Partial traumatic amputation of right shoulder and upper arm, level unspecified

     CC-A **S48.922-**   Partial traumatic amputation of left shoulder and upper arm, level unspecified

     CC-A **S48.929-**   Partial traumatic amputation of unspecified shoulder and upper arm, level unspecified

S49-   Other and unspecified injuries of shoulder and upper arm

The appropriate 7th character is to be added to each code from subcategories S49.0 and S49.1:

A   Initial encounter for closed fracture
D   Subsequent encounter for fracture with routine healing
G   Subsequent encounter for fracture with delayed healing
K   Subsequent encounter for fracture with nonunion
P   Subsequent encounter for fracture with malunion
S   Sequela

S49.0-   Physeal fracture of upper end of humerus

     S49.00-   Unspecified physeal fracture of upper end of humerus

     CC-A,K,P **S49.001-**   Unspecified physeal fracture of upper end of humerus, right arm

     CC-A,K,P **S49.002-**   Unspecified physeal fracture of upper end of humerus, left arm

     CC-A,K,P **S49.009-**   Unspecified physeal fracture of upper end of humerus, unspecified arm

     S49.01-   Salter-Harris Type I physeal fracture of upper end of humerus

     CC-A,K,P **S49.011-**   Salter-Harris Type I physeal fracture of upper end of humerus, right arm

     CC-A,K,P **S49.012-**   Salter-Harris Type I physeal fracture of upper end of humerus, left arm

     CC-A,K,P **S49.019-**   Salter-Harris Type I physeal fracture of upper end of humerus, unspecified arm

     S49.02-   Salter-Harris Type II physeal fracture of upper end of humerus

     CC-A,K,P **S49.021-**   Salter-Harris Type II physeal fracture of upper end of humerus, right arm

     CC-A,K,P **S49.022-**   Salter-Harris Type II physeal fracture of upper end of humerus, left arm

     CC-A,K,P **S49.029-**   Salter-Harris Type II physeal fracture of upper end of humerus, unspecified arm

     S49.03-   Salter-Harris Type III physeal fracture of upper end of humerus

     CC-A,K,P **S49.031-**   Salter-Harris Type III physeal fracture of upper end of humerus, right arm

     CC-A,K,P **S49.032-**   Salter-Harris Type III physeal fracture of upper end of humerus, left arm

     CC-A,K,P **S49.039-**   Salter-Harris Type III physeal fracture of upper end of humerus, unspecified arm

     S49.04-   Salter-Harris Type IV physeal fracture of upper end of humerus

     CC-A,K,P **S49.041-**   Salter-Harris Type IV physeal fracture of upper end of humerus, right arm

     CC-A,K,P **S49.042-**   Salter-Harris Type IV physeal fracture of upper end of humerus, left arm

     CC-A,K,P **S49.049-**   Salter-Harris Type IV physeal fracture of upper end of humerus, unspecified arm

     S49.09-   Other physeal fracture of upper end of humerus

     CC-A,K,P **S49.091-**   Other physeal fracture of upper end of humerus, right arm

     CC-A,K,P **S49.092-**   Other physeal fracture of upper end of humerus, left arm

     CC-A,K,P **S49.099-**   Other physeal fracture of upper end of humerus, unspecified arm

S46 | S49

S49.1- <u>Physeal fracture</u> of <u>lower end of humerus</u>

S49.10- <u>Unspecified</u> physeal fracture of <u>lower end</u> of <u>humerus</u>

CC-A,K,P **S49.101-** Unspecified physeal fracture of lower end of humerus, <u>right</u> arm

CC-A,K,P **S49.102-** Unspecified physeal fracture of lower end of humerus, <u>left</u> arm

CC-A,K,P **S49.109-** Unspecified physeal fracture of lower end of humerus, <u>unspecified</u> arm

S49.11- <u>Salter-Harris Type I</u> physeal fracture of <u>lower end</u> of <u>humerus</u>

CC-A,K,P **S49.111-** Salter-Harris Type I physeal fracture of lower end of humerus, <u>right</u> arm

CC-A,K,P **S49.112-** Salter-Harris Type I physeal fracture of lower end of humerus, <u>left</u> arm

CC-A,K,P **S49.119-** Salter-Harris Type I physeal fracture of lower end of humerus, <u>unspecified</u> arm

S49.12- <u>Salter-Harris Type II</u> physeal fracture of <u>lower end</u> of <u>humerus</u>

CC-A,K,P **S49.121-** Salter-Harris Type II physeal fracture of lower end of humerus, <u>right</u> arm

CC-A,K,P **S49.122-** Salter-Harris Type II physeal fracture of lower end of humerus, <u>left</u> arm

CC-A,K,P **S49.129-** Salter-Harris Type II physeal fracture of lower end of humerus, <u>unspecified</u> arm

S49.13- <u>Salter-Harris Type III</u> physeal fracture of <u>lower end</u> of <u>humerus</u>

CC-A,K,P **S49.131-** Salter-Harris Type III physeal fracture of lower end of humerus, <u>right</u> arm

CC-A,K,P **S49.132-** Salter-Harris Type III physeal fracture of lower end of humerus, <u>left</u> arm

CC-A,K,P **S49.139-** Salter-Harris Type III physeal fracture of lower end of humerus, <u>unspecified</u> arm

S49.14- <u>Salter-Harris Type IV</u> physeal fracture of <u>lower end</u> of <u>humerus</u>

CC-A,K,P **S49.141-** Salter-Harris Type IV physeal fracture of lower end of humerus, <u>right</u> arm

CC-A,K,P **S49.142-** Salter-Harris Type IV physeal fracture of lower end of humerus, <u>left</u> arm

CC-A,K,P **S49.149-** Salter-Harris Type IV physeal fracture of lower end of humerus, <u>unspecified</u> arm

S49.19- <u>Other physeal</u> fracture of <u>lower end</u> of <u>humerus</u>

CC-A,K,P **S49.191-** Other physeal fracture of lower end of humerus, <u>right</u> arm

CC-A,K,P **S49.192-** Other physeal fracture of lower end of humerus, <u>left</u> arm

CC-A,K,P **S49.199-** Other physeal fracture of lower end of humerus, <u>unspecified</u> arm

S49.8- <u>Other specified injuries</u> of <u>shoulder and upper arm</u>

The appropriate 7th character is to be added to each code in subcategory S49.8:

  A <u>Initial</u> encounter
  D <u>Subsequent</u> encounter
  S <u>Sequela</u>

S49.80x- Other specified injuries of shoulder and upper arm, <u>unspecified</u> arm

S49.81x- Other specified injuries of <u>right</u> shoulder and upper arm

S49.82x- Other specified injuries of <u>left</u> shoulder and upper arm

S49.9- <u>Unspecified</u> injury of <u>shoulder and upper arm</u>

The appropriate 7th character is to be added to each code in subcategory S49.9:

  A <u>Initial</u> encounter
  D <u>Subsequent</u> encounter
  S <u>Sequela</u>

S49.90x- Unspecified injury of shoulder and upper arm, <u>unspecified</u> arm

S49.91x- Unspecified injury of <u>right</u> shoulder and upper arm

S49.92x- Unspecified injury of <u>left</u> shoulder and upper arm

Injuries to the elbow and forearm (S50-S59)

Excludes ❷: *burns and corrosions (T20-T32)*
       frostbite (T33-T34)
       injuries of wrist and hand (S60-S69)
       insect bite or sting, venomous (T63.4)

S50- <u>Superficial injury</u> of <u>elbow and forearm</u>

Excludes ❷: *superficial injury of wrist and hand (S60.-)*

The appropriate 7th character is to be added to each code from category S50:

  A <u>Initial</u> encounter
  D <u>Subsequent</u> encounter
  S <u>Sequela</u>

S50.0- <u>Contusion</u> of <u>elbow</u>

S50.00x- Contusion of <u>unspecified</u> elbow

S50.01x- Contusion of <u>right</u> elbow

S50.02x- Contusion of <u>left</u> elbow

S50.1- <u>Contusion</u> of <u>forearm</u>

S50.10x- Contusion of <u>unspecified</u> forearm

S50.11x- Contusion of <u>right</u> forearm

S50.12x- Contusion of <u>left</u> forearm

S50.3- <u>Other</u> superficial injuries of <u>elbow</u>

S50.31- <u>Abrasion</u> of <u>elbow</u>

S50.311- Abrasion of <u>right</u> elbow

S50.312- Abrasion of <u>left</u> elbow

S50.319- Abrasion of <u>unspecified</u> elbow

S50.32- <u>Blister</u> (nonthermal) of <u>elbow</u>

S50.321- Blister (nonthermal) of <u>right</u> elbow

S50.322- Blister (nonthermal) of <u>left</u> elbow

S50.329- Blister (nonthermal) of <u>unspecified</u> elbow

S50.34- <u>External constriction</u> of <u>elbow</u>

S50.341- External constriction of <u>right</u> elbow

S50.342- External constriction of <u>left</u> elbow

S50.349- External constriction of <u>unspecified</u> elbow

S50.35- <u>Superficial foreign body</u> of <u>elbow</u>
    Splinter in the elbow

S50.351- Superficial foreign body of <u>right</u> elbow

S50.352- Superficial foreign body of <u>left</u> elbow

S50.359- Superficial foreign body of <u>unspecified</u> elbow

S50.36- <u>Insect bite</u> (nonvenomous) of <u>elbow</u>

S50.361- Insect bite (nonvenomous) of <u>right</u> elbow

S50.362- Insect bite (nonvenomous) of <u>left</u> elbow

S50.369- Insect bite (nonvenomous) of <u>unspecified</u> elbow

S50.37- <u>Other superficial bite</u> of <u>elbow</u>

Excludes 1:   open bite of elbow (S51.04)

S50.371- Other superficial bite of <u>right</u> elbow

S50.372- Other superficial bite of <u>left</u> elbow

S50.379- Other superficial bite of <u>unspecified</u> elbow

S50.8- <u>Other</u> superficial injuries of <u>forearm</u>

S50.81- <u>Abrasion</u> of <u>forearm</u>

S50.811- Abrasion of <u>right</u> forearm

S50.812- Abrasion of <u>left</u> forearm

S50.819- Abrasion of <u>unspecified</u> forearm

S50.82- <u>Blister</u> (nonthermal) of <u>forearm</u>

S50.821- Blister (nonthermal) of <u>right</u> forearm

S50.822- Blister (nonthermal) of <u>left</u> forearm

S50.829- Blister (nonthermal) of <u>unspecified</u> forearm

S50.84- <u>External constriction</u> of <u>forearm</u>

S50.841- External constriction of <u>right</u> forearm

S50.842- External constriction of <u>left</u> forearm

S50.849- External constriction of <u>unspecified</u> forearm

S50.85- <u>Superficial foreign body</u> of <u>forearm</u>
    Splinter in the forearm

S50.851- Superficial foreign body of <u>right</u> forearm

S50.852- Superficial foreign body of <u>left</u> forearm

S50.859- Superficial foreign body of <u>unspecified</u> forearm

S49 - S50 (side tab)

S50.86- <u>Insect bite (nonvenomous)</u> of <u>forearm</u>
- **S50.861-** Insect bite (nonvenomous) of <u>right</u> forearm
- **S50.862-** Insect bite (nonvenomous) of <u>left</u> forearm
- **S50.869-** Insect bite (nonvenomous) of <u>unspecified</u> forearm

S50.87- <u>Other superficial bite</u> of <u>forearm</u>
    Excludes 1:   *open bite of forearm (S51.84)*
- **S50.871-** Other superficial bite of <u>right</u> forearm
- **S50.872-** Other superficial bite of <u>left</u> forearm
- **S50.879-** Other superficial bite of <u>unspecified</u> forearm

S50.9- Unspecified superficial injury of elbow and forearm

S50.90- <u>Unspecified</u> superficial injury of <u>elbow</u>
- **S50.901-** Unspecified superficial injury of <u>right</u> elbow
- **S50.902-** Unspecified superficial injury of <u>left</u> elbow
- **S50.909-** Unspecified superficial injury of <u>unspecified</u> elbow

S50.91- <u>Unspecified</u> superficial injury of <u>forearm</u>
- **S50.911-** Unspecified superficial injury of <u>right</u> forearm
- **S50.912-** Unspecified superficial injury of <u>left</u> forearm
- **S50.919-** Unspecified superficial injury of <u>unspecified</u> forearm

S51- <u>Open wound</u> of <u>elbow and forearm</u>
    AHA 12:4Q:p108 – Open anterior dislocation of the right elbow
    Code also any associated wound infection
    Excludes 1:   *open fracture of elbow and forearm (S52.- with open fracture 7th character)*
                traumatic amputation of elbow and forearm (S58.-)
    Excludes 2:   *open wound of wrist and hand (S61.-)*

> **The appropriate 7th character is to be added to each code from category S51:**
> **A**   <u>Initial</u> encounter
> **D**   <u>Subsequent</u> encounter
> **S**   <u>Sequela</u>

S51.0- <u>Open wound</u> of <u>elbow</u>

S51.00- <u>Unspecified</u> open wound of <u>elbow</u>
- **S51.001-** Unspecified open wound of <u>right</u> elbow
- **S51.002-** Unspecified open wound of <u>left</u> elbow
- **S51.009-** Unspecified open wound of <u>unspecified</u> elbow
      Open wound of elbow NOS

S51.01- <u>Laceration</u> <u>without</u> foreign body of elbow
- **S51.011-** Laceration <u>without</u> foreign body of <u>right</u> elbow
- **S51.012-** Laceration <u>without</u> foreign body of <u>left</u> elbow
- **S51.019-** Laceration <u>without</u> foreign body of <u>unspecified</u> elbow

S51.02- <u>Laceration</u> <u>with foreign body</u> of <u>elbow</u>
- **S51.021-** Laceration <u>with foreign body</u> of <u>right</u> elbow
- **S51.022-** Laceration <u>with foreign body</u> of <u>left</u> elbow
- **S51.029-** Laceration <u>with foreign body</u> of <u>unspecified</u> elbow

S51.03- <u>Puncture</u> wound <u>without</u> foreign body of <u>elbow</u>
- **S51.031-** Puncture wound <u>without</u> foreign body of <u>right</u> elbow
- **S51.032-** Puncture wound <u>without</u> foreign body of <u>left</u> elbow
- **S51.039-** Puncture wound <u>without</u> foreign body of <u>unspecified</u> elbow

S51.04- <u>Puncture</u> wound <u>with foreign body</u> of <u>elbow</u>
- **S51.041-** Puncture wound <u>with foreign body</u> of <u>right</u> elbow
- **S51.042-** Puncture wound <u>with foreign body</u> of <u>left</u> elbow
- **S51.049-** Puncture wound <u>with foreign body</u> of <u>unspecified</u> elbow

S51.05- <u>Open bite</u> of <u>elbow</u>
    Bite of elbow NOS
    Excludes 1:   *superficial bite of elbow (S50.36, S50.37)*
- **S51.051-** Open bite, <u>right</u> elbow
- **S51.052-** Open bite, <u>left</u> elbow
- **S51.059-** Open bite, <u>unspecified</u> elbow

S51.8- <u>Open wound</u> of <u>forearm</u>
    Excludes 2:   *open wound of elbow (S51.0-)*

S51.80- <u>Unspecified</u> open wound of <u>forearm</u>
- **S51.801-** Unspecified open wound of <u>right</u> forearm
- **S51.802-** Unspecified open wound of <u>left</u> forearm
- **S51.809-** Unspecified open wound of <u>unspecified</u> forearm
      Open wound of forearm NOS

S51.81- <u>Laceration</u> <u>without</u> foreign body of <u>forearm</u>
- **S51.811-** Laceration <u>without</u> foreign body of <u>right</u> forearm
- **S51.812-** Laceration <u>without</u> foreign body of <u>left</u> forearm
- **S51.819-** Laceration <u>without</u> foreign body of <u>unspecified</u> forearm

S51.82- <u>Laceration</u> <u>with foreign body</u> of <u>forearm</u>
- **S51.821-** Laceration <u>with foreign body</u> of <u>right</u> forearm
- **S51.822-** Laceration <u>with foreign body</u> of <u>left</u> forearm
- **S51.829-** Laceration <u>with foreign body</u> of <u>unspecified</u> forearm

S51.83- <u>Puncture</u> wound <u>without</u> foreign body of <u>forearm</u>
- **S51.831-** Puncture wound <u>without</u> foreign body of <u>right</u> forearm
- **S51.832-** Puncture wound <u>without</u> foreign body of <u>left</u> forearm
- **S51.839-** Puncture wound <u>without</u> foreign body of <u>unspecified</u> forearm

S51.84- <u>Puncture</u> wound <u>with foreign body</u> of <u>forearm</u>
- **S51.841-** Puncture wound <u>with foreign body</u> of <u>right</u> forearm
- **S51.842-** Puncture wound <u>with foreign body</u> of <u>left</u> forearm
- **S51.849-** Puncture wound <u>with foreign body</u> of <u>unspecified</u> forearm

S51.85- <u>Open bite</u> of <u>forearm</u>
    Bite of forearm NOS
    Excludes 1:   *superficial bite of forearm (S50.86, S50.87)*
- **S51.851-** Open bite of <u>right</u> forearm
- **S51.852-** Open bite of <u>left</u> forearm
- **S51.859-** Open bite of <u>unspecified</u> forearm

S50 – S51

S52- **Fracture** of **forearm**
Note: A fracture not indicated as displaced or nondisplaced should be coded to displaced
Note: A fracture not indicated as open or closed should be coded to closed
Note: The open fracture designations are based on the Gustilo open fracture classification
Excludes 1: traumatic amputation of forearm (S58.-)
Excludes ❷: fracture at wrist and hand level (S62.-)

The appropriate 7th character is to be added to all codes from category S52:
A **Initial** encounter for **closed** fracture
B **Initial** encounter for **open** fracture **type I or II**
     Initial encounter for **open** fracture **NOS**
C **Initial** encounter for **open** fracture **type IIIA, IIIB, or IIIC**
D **Subsequent** encounter for **closed** fracture **with routine healing**
E **Subsequent** encounter for **open** fracture **type I or II with routine healing**
F **Subsequent** encounter for **open** fracture **type IIIA, IIIB, or IIIC with routine healing**
G **Subsequent** encounter for **closed** fracture **with delayed healing**
H **Subsequent** encounter for **open** fracture **type I or II with delayed healing**
J **Subsequent** encounter for **open** fracture **type IIIA, IIIB, or IIIC with delayed healing**
K **Subsequent** encounter for **closed** fracture **with nonunion**
M **Subsequent** encounter for **open** fracture **type I or II with nonunion**
N **Subsequent** encounter for **open** fracture **type IIIA, IIIB, or IIIC with nonunion**
P **Subsequent** encounter for **closed** fracture **with malunion**
Q **Subsequent** encounter for **open** fracture **type I or II with malunion**
R **Subsequent** encounter for **open** fracture **type IIIA, IIIB, or IIIC with malunion**
S **Sequela**

S52.0- Fracture of **upper end** of **ulna**
     Fracture of proximal end of ulna
     Excludes ❷: fracture of elbow NOS (S42.40-)
               fractures of shaft of ulna (S52.2-)

S52.00- **Unspecified** fracture of **upper end** of **ulna**
S52.001- Unspecified fracture of upper end of **right** ulna
CC-K,M,N,P,Q,R MCC-B,C
S52.002- Unspecified fracture of upper end of **left** ulna
CC-K,M,N,P,Q,R MCC-B,C
S52.009- Unspecified fracture of upper end of **unspecified** ulna
CC-K,M,N,P,Q,R MCC-B,C

S52.01- **Torus** fracture of **upper end** of **ulna**
          The appropriate 7th character is to be added to all codes in subcategory S52.01:
          A **Initial** encounter for **closed** fracture
          D **Subsequent** encounter for fracture **with routine healing**
          G **Subsequent** encounter for fracture **with delayed healing**
          K **Subsequent** encounter for fracture **with nonunion**
          P **Subsequent** encounter for fracture **with malunion**
          S **Sequela**
CC-A,K,P **S52.011-** Torus fracture of upper end of **right** ulna
CC-A,K,P **S52.012-** Torus fracture of upper end of **left** ulna
CC-A,K,P **S52.019-** Torus fracture of upper end of **unspecified** ulna
S52.02- Fracture of **olecranon process** **without** intraarticular extension of **ulna**
S52.021- **Displaced** fracture of olecranon process **without** intraarticular extension of **right** ulna
CC-K,M,N,P,Q,R MCC-B,C
S52.022- **Displaced** fracture of olecranon process **without** intraarticular extension of **left** ulna
CC-K,M,N,P,Q,R MCC-B,C
S52.023- **Displaced** fracture of olecranon process **without** intraarticular extension of **unspecified** ulna
CC-K,M,N,P,Q,R MCC-B,C

S52.024- **Nondisplaced** fracture of olecranon process **without** intraarticular extension of **right** ulna
CC-K,M,N,P,Q,R MCC-B,C
S52.025- **Nondisplaced** fracture of olecranon process **without** intraarticular extension of **left** ulna
CC-K,M,N,P,Q,R MCC-B,C
S52.026- **Nondisplaced** fracture of olecranon process **without** intraarticular extension of **unspecified** ulna
CC-K,M,N,P,Q,R MCC-B,C
S52.03- Fracture of **olecranon process with intraarticular extension** of **ulna**
S52.031- **Displaced** fracture of olecranon process with intraarticular extension of **right** ulna
CC-K,M,N,P,Q,R MCC-B,C
S52.032- **Displaced** fracture of olecranon process with intraarticular extension of **left** ulna
CC-K,M,N,P,Q,R MCC-B,C
S52.033- **Displaced** fracture of olecranon process with intraarticular extension of **unspecified** ulna
CC-K,M,N,P,Q,R MCC-B,C
S52.034- **Nondisplaced** fracture of olecranon process with intraarticular extension of **right** ulna
CC-K,M,N,P,Q,R MCC-B,C
S52.035- **Nondisplaced** fracture of olecranon process with intraarticular extension of **left** ulna
CC-K,M,N,P,Q,R MCC-B,C
S52.036- **Nondisplaced** fracture of olecranon process with intraarticular extension of **unspecified** ulna
CC-K,M,N,P,Q,R MCC-B,C
S52.04- Fracture of **coronoid process** of **ulna**
S52.041- **Displaced** fracture of coronoid process of **right** ulna
CC-K,M,N,P,Q,R MCC-B,C
S52.042- **Displaced** fracture of coronoid process of **left** ulna
CC-K,M,N,P,Q,R MCC-B,C
S52.043- **Displaced** fracture of coronoid process of **unspecified** ulna
CC-K,M,N,P,Q,R MCC-B,C
S52.044- **Nondisplaced** fracture of coronoid process of **right** ulna
CC-K,M,N,P,Q,R MCC-B,C
S52.045- **Nondisplaced** fracture of coronoid process of **left** ulna
CC-K,M,N,P,Q,R MCC-B,C
S52.046- **Nondisplaced** fracture of coronoid process of **unspecified** ulna
CC-K,M,N,P,Q,R MCC-B,C
S52.09- **Other** fracture of **upper end** of **ulna**
S52.091- Other fracture of upper end of **right** ulna
CC-K,M,N,P,Q,R MCC-B,C
S52.092- Other fracture of upper end of **left** ulna
CC-K,M,N,P,Q,R MCC-B,C
S52.099- Other fracture of upper end of **unspecified** ulna
CC-K,M,N,P,Q,R MCC-B,C
S52.1- Fracture of **upper end** of **radius**
     Fracture of proximal end of radius
     Excludes ❷: physeal fractures of upper end of radius (S59.2-)
               fracture of shaft of radius (S52.3-)

S52.10- **Unspecified** fracture of **upper end** of **radius**
S52.101- Unspecified fracture of upper end of **right** radius
CC-K,M,N,P,Q,R MCC-B,C
S52.102- Unspecified fracture of upper end of **left** radius
CC-K,M,N,P,Q,R MCC-B,C
S52.109- Unspecified fracture of upper end of **unspecified** radius
CC-K,M,N,P,Q,R MCC-B,C

S52 - S52

S52.11- Torus fracture of upper end of radius

> The appropriate 7th character is to be added to all codes in subcategory S52.11:
> A   Initial encounter for closed fracture
> D   Subsequent encounter for fracture with routine healing
> G   Subsequent encounter for fracture with delayed healing
> K   Subsequent encounter for fracture with nonunion
> P   Subsequent encounter for fracture with malunion
> S   Sequela

CC-A,K,P **S52.111-** Torus fracture of upper end of right radius
CC-A,K,P **S52.112-** Torus fracture of upper end of left radius
CC-A,K,P **S52.119-** Torus fracture of upper end of unspecified radius

S52.12- Fracture of head of radius

S52.121- Displaced fracture of head of right radius
CC-K,M,N,P,Q,R MCC-B,C

S52.122- Displaced fracture of head of left radius
CC-K,M,N,P,Q,R MCC-B,C

S52.123- Displaced fracture of head of unspecified radius
CC-K,M,N,P,Q,R MCC-B,C

S52.124- Nondisplaced fracture of head of right radius
CC-K,M,N,P,Q,R MCC-B,C

S52.125- Nondisplaced fracture of head of left radius
CC-K,M,N,P,Q,R MCC-B,C

S52.126- Nondisplaced fracture of head of unspecified radius
CC-K,M,N,P,Q,R MCC-B,C

S52.13- Fracture of neck of radius

S52.131- Displaced fracture of neck of right radius
CC-K,M,N,P,Q,R MCC-B,C

S52.132- Displaced fracture of neck of left radius
CC-K,M,N,P,Q,R MCC-B,C

S52.133- Displaced fracture of neck of unspecified radius
CC-K,M,N,P,Q,R MCC-B,C

S52.134- Nondisplaced fracture of neck of right radius
CC-K,M,N,P,Q,R MCC-B,C

S52.135- Nondisplaced fracture of neck of left radius
CC-K,M,N,P,Q,R MCC-B,C

S52.136- Nondisplaced fracture of neck of unspecified radius
CC-K,M,N,P,Q,R MCC-B,C

S52.18- Other fracture of upper end of radius

S52.181- Other fracture of upper end of right radius
CC-K,M,N,P,Q,R MCC-B,C

S52.182- Other fracture of upper end of left radius
CC-K,M,N,P,Q,R MCC-B,C

S52.189- Other fracture of upper end of unspecified radius
CC-K,M,N,P,Q,R MCC-B,C

S52.2- Fracture of shaft of ulna

S52.20- Unspecified fracture of shaft of ulna
> Fracture of ulna NOS

S52.201- Unspecified fracture of shaft of right ulna
CC-A,K,M,N,P,Q,R MCC-B,C

S52.202- Unspecified fracture of shaft of left ulna
CC-A,K,M,N,P,Q,R MCC-B,C

S52.209- Unspecified fracture of shaft of unspecified ulna
CC-A,K,M,N,P,Q,R MCC-B,C

S52.21- Greenstick fracture of shaft of ulna

> The appropriate 7th character is to be added to all codes in subcategory S52.21:
> A   Initial encounter for closed fracture
> D   Subsequent encounter for fracture with routine healing
> G   Subsequent encounter for fracture with delayed healing
> K   Subsequent encounter for fracture with nonunion
> P   Subsequent encounter for fracture with malunion
> S   Sequela

CC-A,K,P **S52.211-** Greenstick fracture of shaft of right ulna
CC-A,K,P **S52.212-** Greenstick fracture of shaft of left ulna
CC-A,K,P **S52.219-** Greenstick fracture of shaft of unspecified ulna

S52.22- Transverse fracture of shaft of ulna

S52.221- Displaced transverse fracture of shaft of right ulna
CC-A,K,M,N,P,Q,R MCC-B,C

S52.222- Displaced transverse fracture of shaft of left ulna
CC-A,K,M,N,P,Q,R MCC-B,C

S52.223- Displaced transverse fracture of shaft of unspecified ulna

S52.224- Nondisplaced transverse fracture of shaft of right ulna
CC-A,K,M,N,P,Q,R MCC-B,C

S52.225- Nondisplaced transverse fracture of shaft of left ulna

S52.226- Nondisplaced transverse fracture of shaft of unspecified ulna
CC-A,K,M,N,P,Q,R MCC-B,C

S52.23- Oblique fracture of shaft of ulna

S52.231- Displaced oblique fracture of shaft of right ulna
CC-A,K,M,N,P,Q,R MCC-B,C

S52.232- Displaced oblique fracture of shaft of left ulna
CC-A,K,M,N,P,Q,R MCC-B,C

S52.233- Displaced oblique fracture of shaft of unspecified ulna
CC-A,K,M,N,P,Q,R MCC-B,C

S52.234- Nondisplaced oblique fracture of shaft of right ulna
CC-A,K,M,N,P,Q,R MCC-B,C

S52.235- Nondisplaced oblique fracture of shaft of left ulna
CC-A,K,M,N,P,Q,R MCC-B,C

S52.236- Nondisplaced oblique fracture of shaft of unspecified ulna
CC-A,K,M,N,P,Q,R MCC-B,C

S52.24- Spiral fracture of shaft of ulna

S52.241- Displaced spiral fracture of shaft of ulna, right arm
CC-A,K,M,N,P,Q,R MCC-B,C

S52.242- Displaced spiral fracture of shaft of ulna, left arm
CC-A,K,M,N,P,Q,R MCC-B,C

S52.243- Displaced spiral fracture of shaft of ulna, unspecified arm
CC-A,K,M,N,P,Q,R MCC-B,C

S52.244- Nondisplaced spiral fracture of shaft of ulna, right arm
CC-A,K,M,N,P,Q,R MCC-B,C

S52.245- Nondisplaced spiral fracture of shaft of ulna, left arm
CC-A,K,M,N,P,Q,R MCC-B,C

S52.246- Nondisplaced spiral fracture of shaft of ulna, unspecified arm
CC-A,K,M,N,P,Q,R MCC-B,C

S52.25- Comminuted fracture of shaft of ulna

S52.251- Displaced comminuted fracture of shaft of ulna, right arm
CC-A,K,M,N,P,Q,R MCC-B,C

S52.252- Displaced comminuted fracture of shaft of ulna, left arm
CC-A,K,M,N,P,Q,R MCC-B,C

S52.253- Displaced comminuted fracture of shaft of ulna, unspecified arm
CC-A,K,M,N,P,Q,R MCC-B,C

S52.254- Nondisplaced comminuted fracture of shaft of ulna, right arm
CC-A,K,M,N,P,Q,R MCC-B,C

S52.255- Nondisplaced comminuted fracture of shaft of ulna, left arm
CC-A,K,M,N,P,Q,R MCC-B,C

S52.256- Nondisplaced comminuted fracture of shaft of ulna, unspecified arm
CC-A,K,M,N,P,Q,R MCC-B,C

S52 • S52

S52.26- Segmental fracture of shaft of ulna

S52.261- Displaced segmental fracture of shaft of ulna, **right arm**
CC-A,K,M,N,P,Q,R MCC-B,C

S52.262- Displaced segmental fracture of shaft of ulna, **left arm**
CC-A,K,M,N,P,Q,R MCC-B,C

S52.263- Displaced segmental fracture of shaft of ulna, **unspecified** arm
CC-A,K,M,N,P,Q,R MCC-B,C

S52.264- Nondisplaced segmental fracture of shaft of ulna, **right arm**
CC-A,K,M,N,P,Q,R MCC-B,C

S52.265- Nondisplaced segmental fracture of shaft of ulna, **left arm**
CC-A,K,M,N,P,Q,R MCC-B,C

S52.266- Nondisplaced segmental fracture of shaft of ulna, **unspecified** arm
CC-A,K,M,N,P,Q,R MCC-B,C

S52.27- Monteggia's fracture of ulna
Fracture of upper shaft of ulna with dislocation of radial head

S52.271- Monteggia's fracture of right ulna
CC-K,M,N,P,Q,R MCC-B,C

S52.272- Monteggia's fracture of left ulna
CC-K,M,N,P,Q,R MCC-B,C

S52.279- Monteggia's fracture of unspecified ulna
CC-K,M,N,P,Q,R MCC-B,C

S52.28- Bent bone of ulna

S52.281- Bent bone of right ulna
CC-A,K,M,N,P,Q,R MCC-B,C

S52.282- Bent bone of left ulna
CC-A,K,M,N,P,Q,R MCC-B,C

S52.283- Bent bone of unspecified ulna
CC-A,K,M,N,P,Q,R MCC-B,C

S52.29- Other fracture of shaft of ulna

S52.291- Other fracture of shaft of right ulna
CC-A,K,M,N,P,Q,R MCC-B,C

S52.292- Other fracture of shaft of left ulna
CC-A,K,M,N,P,Q,R MCC-B,C

S52.299- Other fracture of shaft of unspecified ulna
CC-A,K,M,N,P,Q,R MCC-B,C

S52.3- Fracture of shaft of radius

S52.30- Unspecified fracture of shaft of radius

S52.301- Unspecified fracture of shaft of right radius
CC-A,K,M,N,P,Q,R MCC-B,C

S52.302- Unspecified fracture of shaft of left radius
CC-A,K,M,N,P,Q,R MCC-B,C

S52.309- Unspecified fracture of shaft of unspecified radius
CC-A,K,M,N,P,Q,R MCC-B,C

S52.31- Greenstick fracture of shaft of radius

The appropriate 7th character is to be added to all codes in subcategory S52.31:
A   **Initial** encounter for **closed** fracture
D   **Subsequent** encounter for fracture **with routine healing**
G   **Subsequent** encounter for fracture **with delayed healing**
K   **Subsequent** encounter for fracture **with nonunion**
P   **Subsequent** encounter for fracture **with malunion**
S   **Sequela**

CC-A,K,P **S52.311- Greenstick fracture of shaft of radius, right arm**

CC-A,K,P **S52.312- Greenstick fracture of shaft of radius, left arm**

CC-A,K,P **S52.319- Greenstick fracture of shaft of radius, unspecified arm**

S52.32- Transverse fracture of shaft of radius

S52.321- Displaced transverse fracture of shaft of **right radius**
CC-A,K,M,N,P,Q,R MCC-B,C

S52.322- Displaced transverse fracture of shaft of **left** radius
CC-A,K,M,N,P,Q,R MCC-B,C

S52.323- Displaced transverse fracture of shaft of **unspecified** radius
CC-A,K,M,N,P,Q,R MCC-B,C

S52.324- Nondisplaced transverse fracture of shaft of **right** radius
CC-A,K,M,N,P,Q,R MCC-B,C

S52.325- Nondisplaced transverse fracture of shaft of **left** radius
CC-A,K,M,N,P,Q,R MCC-B,C

S52.326- Nondisplaced transverse fracture of shaft of **unspecified** radius
CC-A,K,M,N,P,Q,R MCC-B,C

S52.33- Oblique fracture of shaft of radius

S52.331- Displaced oblique fracture of shaft of **right** radius
CC-A,K,M,N,P,Q,R MCC-B,C

S52.332- Displaced oblique fracture of shaft of **left** radius
CC-A,K,M,N,P,Q,R MCC-B,C

S52.333- Displaced oblique fracture of shaft of **unspecified** radius
CC-A,K,M,N,P,Q,R MCC-B,C

S52.334- Nondisplaced oblique fracture of shaft of **right** radius
CC-A,K,M,N,P,Q,R MCC-B,C

S52.335- Nondisplaced oblique fracture of shaft of **left** radius
CC-A,K,M,N,P,Q,R MCC-B,C

S52.336- Nondisplaced oblique fracture of shaft of **unspecified** radius
CC-A,K,M,N,P,Q,R MCC-B,C

S52.34- Spiral fracture of shaft of radius

S52.341- Displaced spiral fracture of shaft of radius, **right arm**
CC-A,K,M,N,P,Q,R MCC-B,C

S52.342- Displaced spiral fracture of shaft of radius, **left arm**
CC-A,K,M,N,P,Q,R MCC-B,C

S52.343- Displaced spiral fracture of shaft of radius, **unspecified** arm
CC-A,K,M,N,P,Q,R MCC-B,C

S52.344- Nondisplaced spiral fracture of shaft of radius, **right arm**
CC-A,K,M,N,P,Q,R MCC-B,C

S52.345- Nondisplaced spiral fracture of shaft of radius, **left arm**
CC-A,K,M,N,P,Q,R MCC-B,C

S52.346- Nondisplaced spiral fracture of shaft of radius, **unspecified** arm
CC-A,K,M,N,P,Q,R MCC-B,C

S52.35- Comminuted fracture of shaft of radius

S52.351- Displaced comminuted fracture of shaft of radius, **right arm**
CC-A,K,M,N,P,Q,R MCC-B,C

S52.352- Displaced comminuted fracture of shaft of radius, **left arm**
CC-A,K,M,N,P,Q,R MCC-B,C

S52.353- Displaced comminuted fracture of shaft of radius, **unspecified** arm
CC-A,K,M,N,P,Q,R MCC-B,C

S52.354- Nondisplaced comminuted fracture of shaft of radius, **right arm**
CC-A,K,M,N,P,Q,R MCC-B,C

S52.355- Nondisplaced comminuted fracture of shaft of radius, **left arm**
CC-A,K,M,N,P,Q,R MCC-B,C

S52.356- Nondisplaced comminuted fracture of shaft of radius, **unspecified** arm
CC-A,K,M,N,P,Q,R MCC-B,C

S52.36- Segmental fracture of shaft of radius

S52.361- Displaced segmental fracture of shaft of radius, **right arm**
CC-A,K,M,N,P,Q,R MCC-B,C

S52.362- Displaced segmental fracture of shaft of radius, **left arm**
CC-A,K,M,N,P,Q,R MCC-B,C

S52.363- Displaced segmental fracture of shaft of radius, **unspecified** arm
CC-A,K,M,N,P,Q,R MCC-B,C

S52.364- Nondisplaced segmental fracture of shaft of radius, **right arm**
CC-A,K,M,N,P,Q,R MCC-B,C

S 5 2 – S 5 2

S52.365- **Nondisplaced** segmental fracture of shaft of radius, **left arm**
CC-A,K,M,N,P,Q,R MCC-B,C

S52.366- **Nondisplaced** segmental fracture of shaft of radius, **unspecified arm**
CC-A,K,M,N,P,Q,R MCC-B,C

S52.37- **Galeazzi's** fracture
Fracture of lower shaft of radius with radioulnar joint dislocation

S52.371- Galeazzi's fracture of **right** radius
CC-A,K,M,N,P,Q,R MCC-B,C

S52.372- Galeazzi's fracture of **left** radius
CC-A,K,M,N,P,Q,R MCC-B,C

S52.379- Galeazzi's fracture of **unspecified** radius
CC-A,K,M,N,P,Q,R MCC-B,C

S52.38- **Bent bone** of radius

S52.381- Bent bone of **right** radius
CC-A,K,M,N,P,Q,R MCC-B,C

S52.382- Bent bone of **left** radius
CC-A,K,M,N,P,Q,R MCC-B,C

S52.389- Bent bone of **unspecified** radius
CC-A,K,M,N,P,Q,R MCC-B,C

S52.39- **Other** fracture of **shaft** of **radius**

S52.391- Other fracture of shaft of radius, **right arm**
CC-A,K,M,N,P,Q,R MCC-B,C

S52.392- Other fracture of shaft of radius, **left arm**
CC-A,K,M,N,P,Q,R MCC-B,C

S52.399- Other fracture of shaft of radius, **unspecified** arm
CC-A,K,M,N,P,Q,R MCC-B,C

S52.5- Fracture of **lower end** of **radius**
Fracture of distal end of radius
Excludes ❷: physeal fractures of lower end of radius (S59.2-)

S52.50- **Unspecified** fracture of the **lower end** of **radius**

S52.501- Unspecified fracture of the lower end of **right** radius
CC-A,K,M,N,P,Q,R MCC-B,C

S52.502- Unspecified fracture of the lower end of **left** radius
CC-A,K,M,N,P,Q,R MCC-B,C

S52.509- Unspecified fracture of the lower end of **unspecified** radius
CC-A,K,M,N,P,Q,R MCC-B,C

S52.51- **Fracture** of **radial styloid process**

S52.511- **Displaced** fracture of **right** radial styloid process
CC-A,K,M,N,P,Q,R MCC-B,C

S52.512- **Displaced** fracture of **left** radial styloid process
CC-A,K,M,N,P,Q,R MCC-B,C

S52.513- **Displaced** fracture of **unspecified** radial styloid process
CC-A,K,M,N,P,Q,R MCC-B,C

S52.514- **Nondisplaced** fracture of **right** radial styloid process
CC-A,K,M,N,P,Q,R MCC-B,C

S52.515- **Nondisplaced** fracture of **left** radial styloid process
CC-A,K,M,N,P,Q,R MCC-B,C

S52.516- **Nondisplaced** fracture of **unspecified** radial styloid process
CC-A,K,M,N,P,Q,R MCC-B,C

S52.52- **Torus** fracture of **lower end** of **radius**
The appropriate 7th character is to be added to all codes in subcategory S52.52:
A **Initial** encounter for **closed** fracture
D **Subsequent** encounter for fracture **with routine healing**
G **Subsequent** encounter for fracture **with delayed healing**
K **Subsequent** encounter for fracture **with nonunion**
P **Subsequent** encounter for fracture **with malunion**
S **Sequela**

CC-A,K,P S52.521- Torus fracture of lower end of **right** radius
CC-A,K,P S52.522- Torus fracture of lower end of **left** radius
CC-A,K,P S52.529- Torus fracture of lower end of **unspecified** radius

S52.53- **Colles'** fracture

S52.531- Colles' fracture of **right** radius
CC-A,K,M,N,P,Q,R MCC-B,C

S52.532- Colles' fracture of **left** radius
CC-A,K,M,N,P,Q,R MCC-B,C

S52.539- Colles' fracture of **unspecified** radius
CC-A,K,M,N,P,Q,R MCC-B,C

S52.54- **Smith's** fracture

S52.541- Smith's fracture of **right** radius
CC-A,K,M,N,P,Q,R MCC-B,C

S52.542- Smith's fracture of **left** radius
CC-A,K,M,N,P,Q,R MCC-B,C

S52.549- Smith's fracture of **unspecified** radius
CC-A,K,M,N,P,Q,R MCC-B,C

S52.55- **Other extraarticular** fracture of **lower end** of **radius**

S52.551- Other extraarticular fracture of lower end of **right** radius
CC-A,K,M,N,P,Q,R MCC-B,C

S52.552- Other extraarticular fracture of lower end of **left** radius
CC-A,K,M,N,P,Q,R MCC-B,C

S52.559- Other extraarticular fracture of lower end of **unspecified** radius
CC-A,K,M,N,P,Q,R MCC-B,C

S52.56- **Barton's** fracture

S52.561- Barton's fracture of **right** radius
CC-A,K,M,N,P,Q,R MCC-B,C

S52.562- Barton's fracture of **left** radius
CC-A,K,M,N,P,Q,R MCC-B,C

S52.569- Barton's fracture of **unspecified** radius
CC-A,K,M,N,P,Q,R MCC-B,C

S52.57- **Other intraarticular** fracture of **lower end** of **radius**

S52.571- Other intraarticular fracture of lower end of **right** radius
CC-A,K,M,N,P,Q,R MCC-B,C

S52.572- Other intraarticular fracture of lower end of **left** radius
CC-A,K,M,N,P,Q,R MCC-B,C

S52.579- Other intraarticular fracture of lower end of **unspecified** radius
CC-A,K,M,N,P,Q,R MCC-B,C

S52.59- **Other** fractures of **lower end** of **radius**

S52.591- Other fractures of lower end of **right** radius
CC-A,K,M,N,P,Q,R MCC-B,C

S52.592- Other fractures of lower end of **left** radius
CC-A,K,M,N,P,Q,R MCC-B,C

S52.599- Other fractures of lower end of **unspecified** radius
CC-A,K,M,N,P,Q,R MCC-B,C

S52.6- Fracture of **lower end** of **ulna**

S52.60- **Unspecified** fracture of **lower end** of **ulna**

S52.601- Unspecified fracture of lower end of **right** ulna
CC-A,K,M,N,P,Q,R MCC-B,C

S52.602- Unspecified fracture of lower end of **left** ulna
CC-A,K,M,N,P,Q,R MCC-B,C

S52.609- Unspecified fracture of lower end of **unspecified** ulna
CC-A,K,M,N,P,Q,R MCC-B,C

S52.61- Fracture of **ulna styloid process**

S52.611- **Displaced** fracture of **right** ulna styloid process
CC-A,K,M,N,P,Q,R MCC-B,C

S52.612- **Displaced** fracture of **left** ulna styloid process
CC-A,K,M,N,P,Q,R MCC-B,C

S52.613- **Displaced** fracture of **unspecified** ulna styloid process
CC-A,K,M,N,P,Q,R MCC-B,C

S52.614- **Nondisplaced** fracture of **right** ulna styloid process
CC-A,K,M,N,P,Q,R MCC-B,C

S52.615- **Nondisplaced** fracture of **left** ulna styloid process
CC-A,K,M,N,P,Q,R MCC-B,C

S52.616- **Nondisplaced** fracture of **unspecified** ulna styloid process
CC-A,K,M,N,P,Q,R MCC-B,C

S52 - S52 - S52

S52.62- Torus fracture of lower end of ulna

The appropriate 7th character is to be added to all codes in subcategory S52.62:
- **A** Initial encounter for closed fracture
- **D** Subsequent encounter for fracture with routine healing
- **G** Subsequent encounter for fracture with delayed healing
- **K** Subsequent encounter for fracture with nonunion
- **P** Subsequent encounter for fracture with malunion
- **S** Sequela

CC-A,K,P **S52.621-** Torus fracture of lower end of right ulna
CC-A,K,P **S52.622-** Torus fracture of lower end of left ulna
CC-A,K,P **S52.629-** Torus fracture of lower end of unspecified ulna

S52.69- Other fracture of lower end of ulna

S52.691- Other fracture of lower end of right ulna
CC-A,K,M,N,P,Q,R MCC-B,C

S52.692- Other fracture of lower end of left ulna
CC-A,K,M,N,P,Q,R MCC-B,C

S52.699- Other fracture of lower end of unspecified ulna
CC-A,K,M,N,P,Q,R MCC-B,C

S52.9- Unspecified fracture of forearm

S52.90x- Unspecified fracture of unspecified forearm
CC-A,K,M,N,P,Q,R MCC-B,C

S52.91x- Unspecified fracture of right forearm
CC-A,K,M,N,P,Q,R MCC-B,C

S52.92x- Unspecified fracture of left forearm
CC-A,K,M,N,P,Q,R MCC-B,C

S53- Dislocation and sprain of joints and ligaments of elbow

AHA 12:4Q:p108 – Open anterior dislocation of the right elbow

Includes: Avulsion of joint or ligament of elbow
Laceration of cartilage, joint or ligament of elbow
Sprain of cartilage, joint or ligament of elbow
Traumatic hemarthrosis of joint or ligament of elbow
Traumatic rupture of joint or ligament of elbow
Traumatic subluxation of joint or ligament of elbow
Traumatic tear of joint or ligament of elbow

Code also any associated open wound

Excludes 2: strain of muscle, fascia and tendon at forearm level (S56.-)

The appropriate 7th character is to be added to each code from category S53:
- **A** Initial encounter
- **D** Subsequent encounter
- **S** Sequela

S53.0- Subluxation and dislocation of radial head
Dislocation of radiohumeral joint
Subluxation of radiohumeral joint

Excludes 1: Monteggia's fracture-dislocation (S52.27-)

S53.00- Unspecified subluxation and dislocation of radial head
S53.001- Unspecified subluxation of right radial head
S53.002- Unspecified subluxation of left radial head
S53.003- Unspecified subluxation of unspecified radial head
S53.004- Unspecified dislocation of right radial head
S53.005- Unspecified dislocation of left radial head
S53.006- Unspecified dislocation of unspecified radial head

S53.01- Anterior subluxation and dislocation of radial head
Anteriomedial subluxation and dislocation of radial head
S53.011- Anterior subluxation of right radial head
S53.012- Anterior subluxation of left radial head
S53.013- Anterior subluxation of unspecified radial head
S53.014- Anterior dislocation of right radial head
S53.015- Anterior dislocation of left radial head
S53.016- Anterior dislocation of unspecified radial head

S53.02- Posterior subluxation and dislocation of radial head
Posteriolateral subluxation and dislocation of radial head
S53.021- Posterior subluxation of right radial head
S53.022- Posterior subluxation of left radial head
S53.023- Posterior subluxation of unspecified radial head
S53.024- Posterior dislocation of right radial head
S53.025- Posterior dislocation of left radial head
S53.026- Posterior dislocation of unspecified radial head

S53.03- Nursemaid's elbow
AHA 15:1Q:p7 – Right radial head subluxation
S53.031- Nursemaid's elbow, right elbow
S53.032- Nursemaid's elbow, left elbow
S53.033- Nursemaid's elbow, unspecified elbow

S53.09- Other subluxation and dislocation of radial head
S53.091- Other subluxation of right radial head
S53.092- Other subluxation of left radial head
S53.093- Other subluxation of unspecified radial head
S53.094- Other dislocation of right radial head
S53.095- Other dislocation of left radial head
S53.096- Other dislocation of unspecified radial head

S53.1- Subluxation and dislocation of ulnohumeral joint
Subluxation and dislocation of elbow NOS
Excludes 1: dislocation of radial head alone (S53.0-)

S53.10- Unspecified subluxation and dislocation of ulnohumeral joint
S53.101- Unspecified subluxation of right ulnohumeral joint
S53.102- Unspecified subluxation of left ulnohumeral joint
S53.103- Unspecified subluxation of unspecified ulnohumeral joint
S53.104- Unspecified dislocation of right ulnohumeral joint
S53.105- Unspecified dislocation of left ulnohumeral joint
S53.106- Unspecified dislocation of unspecified ulnohumeral joint

S53.11- Anterior subluxation and dislocation of ulnohumeral joint
S53.111- Anterior subluxation of right ulnohumeral joint
S53.112- Anterior subluxation of left ulnohumeral joint
S53.113- Anterior subluxation of unspecified ulnohumeral joint
S53.114- Anterior dislocation of right ulnohumeral joint
S53.115- Anterior dislocation of left ulnohumeral joint
S53.116- Anterior dislocation of unspecified ulnohumeral joint

S53.12- Posterior subluxation and dislocation of ulnohumeral joint
S53.121- Posterior subluxation of right ulnohumeral joint
S53.122- Posterior subluxation of left ulnohumeral joint
S53.123- Posterior subluxation of unspecified ulnohumeral joint
S53.124- Posterior dislocation of right ulnohumeral joint
S53.125- Posterior dislocation of left ulnohumeral joint
S53.126- Posterior dislocation of unspecified ulnohumeral joint

S53.13- Medial subluxation and dislocation of ulnohumeral joint
S53.131- Medial subluxation of right ulnohumeral joint
S53.132- Medial subluxation of left ulnohumeral joint
S53.133- Medial subluxation of unspecified ulnohumeral joint
S53.134- Medial dislocation of right ulnohumeral joint
S53.135- Medial dislocation of left ulnohumeral joint
S53.136- Medial dislocation of unspecified ulnohumeral joint

S53.14- Lateral subluxation and dislocation of ulnohumeral joint
S53.141- Lateral subluxation of right ulnohumeral joint
S53.142- Lateral subluxation of left ulnohumeral joint
S53.143- Lateral subluxation of unspecified ulnohumeral joint
S53.144- Lateral dislocation of right ulnohumeral joint
S53.145- Lateral dislocation of left ulnohumeral joint
S53.146- Lateral dislocation of unspecified ulnohumeral joint

S53.19- Other subluxation and dislocation of ulnohumeral joint
S53.191- Other subluxation of right ulnohumeral joint
S53.192- Other subluxation of left ulnohumeral joint
S53.193- Other subluxation of unspecified ulnohumeral joint

S52 - S53

S53.194- Other <u>dislocation</u> of <u>right</u> ulnohumeral joint
S53.195- Other <u>dislocation</u> of <u>left</u> ulnohumeral joint
S53.196- Other <u>dislocation</u> of <u>unspecified</u> ulnohumeral joint

S53.2- <u>Traumatic rupture</u> of <u>radial collateral ligament</u>
Excludes 1:   sprain of radial collateral ligament NOS (S53.43-)

S53.20x- Traumatic rupture of <u>unspecified</u> radial collateral ligament
S53.21x- Traumatic rupture of <u>right</u> radial collateral ligament
S53.22x- Traumatic rupture of <u>left</u> radial collateral ligament

S53.3- <u>Traumatic rupture</u> of <u>ulnar collateral ligament</u>
Excludes 1:   sprain of ulnar collateral ligament (S53.44-)

S53.30x- Traumatic rupture of <u>unspecified</u> ulnar collateral ligament
S53.31x- Traumatic rupture of <u>right</u> ulnar collateral ligament
S53.32x- Traumatic rupture of <u>left</u> ulnar collateral ligament

S53.4- <u>Sprain</u> of <u>elbow</u>
Excludes ❷: traumatic rupture of radial collateral ligament (S53.2-)
traumatic rupture of ulnar collateral ligament (S53.3-)

S53.40- <u>Unspecified</u> sprain of <u>elbow</u>
S53.401- Unspecified sprain of <u>right</u> elbow
S53.402- Unspecified sprain of <u>left</u> elbow
S53.409- Unspecified sprain of <u>unspecified</u> elbow
Sprain of elbow NOS

S53.41- <u>Radiohumeral</u> (joint) <u>sprain</u>
S53.411- Radiohumeral (joint) sprain of <u>right</u> elbow
S53.412- Radiohumeral (joint) sprain of <u>left</u> elbow
S53.419- Radiohumeral (joint) sprain of <u>unspecified</u> elbow

S53.42- <u>Ulnohumeral</u> (joint) <u>sprain</u>
S53.421- Ulnohumeral (joint) sprain of <u>right</u> elbow
S53.422- Ulnohumeral (joint) sprain of <u>left</u> elbow
S53.429- Ulnohumeral (joint) sprain of <u>unspecified</u> elbow

S53.43- <u>Radial collateral ligament</u> <u>sprain</u>
S53.431- Radial collateral ligament sprain of <u>right</u> elbow
S53.432- Radial collateral ligament sprain of <u>left</u> elbow
S53.439- Radial collateral ligament sprain of <u>unspecified</u> elbow

S53.44- <u>Ulnar collateral ligament</u> <u>sprain</u>
S53.441- Ulnar collateral ligament sprain of <u>right</u> elbow
S53.442- Ulnar collateral ligament sprain of <u>left</u> elbow
S53.449- Ulnar collateral ligament sprain of <u>unspecified</u> elbow

S53.49- <u>Other</u> sprain of <u>elbow</u>
S53.491- Other sprain of <u>right</u> elbow
S53.492- Other sprain of <u>left</u> elbow
S53.499- Other sprain of <u>unspecified</u> elbow

S54- Injury of <u>nerves</u> at <u>forearm level</u>
Code also any associated open wound (S51.-)
Excludes ❷: injury of nerves at wrist and hand level (S64.-)

The appropriate 7th character is to be added to each code from category S54:
A   <u>Initial</u> encounter
D   <u>Subsequent</u> encounter
S   <u>Sequela</u>

S54.0- Injury of <u>ulnar</u> nerve at <u>forearm level</u>
Injury of ulnar nerve NOS
S54.00x- Injury of ulnar nerve at forearm level, <u>unspecified</u> arm
S54.01x- Injury of ulnar nerve at forearm level, <u>right</u> arm
S54.02x- Injury of ulnar nerve at forearm level, <u>left</u> arm

S54.1- Injury of <u>median</u> nerve at <u>forearm level</u>
Injury of median nerve NOS
S54.10x- Injury of median nerve at forearm level, <u>unspecified</u> arm
S54.11x- Injury of median nerve at forearm level, <u>right</u> arm
S54.12x- Injury of median nerve at forearm level, <u>left</u> arm

S54.2- Injury of <u>radial</u> nerve at <u>forearm level</u>
Injury of radial nerve NOS
S54.20x- Injury of radial nerve at forearm level, <u>unspecified</u> arm

S54.21x- Injury of radial nerve at forearm level, <u>right</u> arm
S54.22x- Injury of radial nerve at forearm level, <u>left</u> arm

S54.3- Injury of <u>cutaneous sensory</u> nerve at <u>forearm level</u>
S54.30x- Injury of cutaneous sensory nerve at forearm level, <u>unspecified</u> arm
S54.31x- Injury of cutaneous sensory nerve at forearm level, <u>right</u> arm
S54.32x- Injury of cutaneous sensory nerve at forearm level, <u>left</u> arm

S54.8- Injury of <u>other nerves</u> at <u>forearm level</u>
S54.8x- Injury of other nerves at forearm level
S54.8x1- Injury of other nerves at forearm level, <u>right</u> arm
S54.8x2- Injury of other nerves at forearm level, <u>left</u> arm
S54.8x9- Injury of other nerves at forearm level, <u>unspecified</u> arm

S54.9- Injury of <u>unspecified nerve</u> at <u>forearm level</u>
S54.90x- Injury of unspecified nerve at forearm level, <u>unspecified</u> arm
S54.91x- Injury of unspecified nerve at forearm level, <u>right</u> arm
S54.92x- Injury of unspecified nerve at forearm level, <u>left</u> arm

S55- <u>Injury of blood vessels</u> at <u>forearm level</u>
Code also any associated open wound (S51.-)
Excludes ❷: injury of blood vessels at wrist and hand level (S65.-)
injury of brachial vessels (S45.1-S45.2)

The appropriate 7th character is to be added to each code from category S55:
A   <u>Initial</u> encounter
D   <u>Subsequent</u> encounter
S   <u>Sequela</u>

S55.0- Injury of <u>ulnar artery</u> at <u>forearm level</u>
S55.00- <u>Unspecified</u> injury of <u>ulnar artery</u> at <u>forearm level</u>
CC-A **S55.001-** Unspecified injury of ulnar artery at forearm level, <u>right</u> arm
CC-A **S55.002-** Unspecified injury of ulnar artery at forearm level, <u>left</u> arm
CC-A **S55.009-** Unspecified injury of ulnar artery at forearm level, <u>unspecified</u> arm

S55.01- <u>Laceration</u> of <u>ulnar artery</u> at <u>forearm level</u>
CC-A **S55.011-** Laceration of ulnar artery at forearm level, <u>right</u> arm
CC-A **S55.012-** Laceration of ulnar artery at forearm level, <u>left</u> arm
CC-A **S55.019-** Laceration of ulnar artery at forearm level, <u>unspecified</u> arm

S55.09- <u>Other</u> specified injury of <u>ulnar artery</u> at <u>forearm level</u>
CC-A **S55.091-** Other specified injury of ulnar artery at forearm level, <u>right</u> arm
CC-A **S55.092-** Other specified injury of ulnar artery at forearm level, <u>left</u> arm
CC-A **S55.099-** Other specified injury of ulnar artery at forearm level, <u>unspecified</u> arm

S55.1- Injury of <u>radial artery</u> at <u>forearm level</u>
S55.10- Unspecified injury of radial artery at forearm level
CC-A **S55.101-** Unspecified injury of radial artery at forearm level, <u>right</u> arm
CC-A **S55.102-** Unspecified injury of radial artery at forearm level, <u>left</u> arm
CC-A **S55.109-** Unspecified injury of radial artery at forearm level, <u>unspecified</u> arm

S55.11- <u>Laceration</u> of <u>radial artery</u> at <u>forearm level</u>
CC-A **S55.111-** Laceration of radial artery at forearm level, <u>right</u> arm
CC-A **S55.112-** Laceration of radial artery at forearm level, <u>left</u> arm
CC-A **S55.119-** Laceration of radial artery at forearm level, <u>unspecified</u> arm

S55.19- <u>Other</u> specified injury of <u>radial artery</u> at <u>forearm level</u>
CC-A **S55.191-** Other specified injury of radial artery at forearm level, <u>right</u> arm

CC-A **S55.192-** Other specified injury of radial artery at forearm level, **left** arm

CC-A **S55.199-** Other specified injury of radial artery at forearm level, **unspecified** arm

S55.2- Injury of **vein** at **forearm level**

S55.20- **Unspecified** injury of **vein** at **forearm level**

CC-A **S55.201-** Unspecified injury of vein at forearm level, **right** arm

CC-A **S55.202-** Unspecified injury of vein at forearm level, **left** arm

CC-A **S55.209-** Unspecified injury of vein at forearm level, **unspecified** arm

S55.21- **Laceration** of **vein** at **forearm level**

CC-A **S55.211-** Laceration of vein at forearm level, **right** arm

CC-A **S55.212-** Laceration of vein at forearm level, **left** arm

CC-A **S55.219-** Laceration of vein at forearm level, **unspecified** arm

S55.29- **Other specified injury** of **vein** at **forearm level**

CC-A **S55.291-** Other specified injury of vein at forearm level, **right** arm

CC-A **S55.292-** Other specified injury of vein at forearm level, **left** arm

CC-A **S55.299-** Other specified injury of vein at forearm level, **unspecified** arm

S55.8- Injury of **other blood vessels** at **forearm level**

S55.80- **Unspecified** injury of **other blood vessels** at **forearm level**

CC-A **S55.801-** Unspecified injury of other blood vessels at forearm level, **right** arm

CC-A **S55.802-** Unspecified injury of other blood vessels at forearm level, **left** arm

CC-A **S55.809-** Unspecified injury of other blood vessels at forearm level, **unspecified** arm

S55.81- **Laceration** of **other blood vessels** at **forearm level**

CC-A **S55.811-** Laceration of other blood vessels at forearm level, **right** arm

CC-A **S55.812-** Laceration of other blood vessels at forearm level, **left** arm

CC-A **S55.819-** Laceration of other blood vessels at forearm level, **unspecified** arm

S55.89- **Other specified injury** of **other blood vessels** at **forearm level**

CC-A **S55.891-** Other specified injury of other blood vessels at forearm level, **right** arm

CC-A **S55.892-** Other specified injury of other blood vessels at forearm level, **left** arm

CC-A **S55.899-** Other specified injury of other blood vessels at forearm level, **unspecified** arm

S55.9- Injury of **unspecified blood vessel** at **forearm level**

S55.90- **Unspecified** injury of **unspecified blood vessel** at **forearm level**

CC-A **S55.901-** Unspecified injury of unspecified blood vessel at forearm level, **right** arm

CC-A **S55.902-** Unspecified injury of unspecified blood vessel at forearm level, **left** arm

CC-A **S55.909-** Unspecified injury of unspecified blood vessel at forearm level, **unspecified** arm

S55.91- **Laceration** of **unspecified blood vessel** at **forearm level**

CC-A **S55.911-** Laceration of unspecified blood vessel at forearm level, **right** arm

CC-A **S55.912-** Laceration of unspecified blood vessel at forearm level, **left** arm

CC-A **S55.919-** Laceration of unspecified blood vessel at forearm level, **unspecified** arm

S55.99- **Other specified injury** of **unspecified blood vessel** at **forearm level**

CC-A **S55.991-** Other specified injury of **unspecified** blood vessel at forearm level, **right** arm

CC-A **S55.992-** Other specified injury of **unspecified** blood vessel at forearm level, **left** arm

CC-A **S55.999-** Other specified injury of **unspecified** blood vessel at forearm level, **unspecified** arm

S56- **Injury of muscle, fascia and tendon at forearm level**

Code also any associated open wound (S51.-)

Excludes ❷: injury of muscle, fascia and tendon at or below wrist (S66.-)
sprain of joints and ligaments of elbow (S53.4-)

The appropriate 7th character is to be added to each code from category S56:
A **Initial** encounter
D **Subsequent** encounter
S **Sequela**

S56.0- Injury of **flexor** muscle, fascia and tendon of **thumb** at **forearm level**

S56.00- **Unspecified** injury of **flexor** muscle, fascia and tendon of **thumb** at **forearm level**

S56.001- Unspecified injury of flexor muscle, fascia and tendon of **right** thumb at forearm level

S56.002- Unspecified injury of flexor muscle, fascia and tendon of **left** thumb at forearm level

S56.009- Unspecified injury of flexor muscle, fascia and tendon of **unspecified** thumb at forearm level

S56.01- **Strain** of **flexor** muscle, fascia and tendon of **thumb** at **forearm level**

S56.011- Strain of flexor muscle, fascia and tendon of **right** thumb at forearm level

S56.012- Strain of flexor muscle, fascia and tendon of **left** thumb at forearm level

S56.019- Strain of flexor muscle, fascia and tendon of **unspecified** thumb at forearm level

S56.02- **Laceration** of **flexor** muscle, fascia and tendon of **thumb** at **forearm level**

CC-A **S56.021-** Laceration of flexor muscle, fascia and tendon of **right** thumb at forearm level

CC-A **S56.022-** Laceration of flexor muscle, fascia and tendon of **left** thumb at forearm level

CC-A **S56.029-** Laceration of flexor muscle, fascia and tendon of **unspecified** thumb at forearm level

S56.09- **Other injury** of **flexor** muscle, fascia and tendon of **thumb** at **forearm level**

S56.091- Other injury of flexor muscle, fascia and tendon of **right** thumb at forearm level

S56.092- Other injury of flexor muscle, fascia and tendon of **left** thumb at forearm level

S56.099- Other injury of flexor muscle, fascia and tendon of **unspecified** thumb at forearm level

S56.1- Injury of **flexor** muscle, fascia and tendon **of other and unspecified finger** at **forearm level**

S56.10- **Unspecified** injury of **flexor** muscle, fascia and tendon of other and unspecified **finger** at **forearm level**

S56.101- Unspecified injury of flexor muscle, fascia and tendon of **right index** finger at forearm level

S56.102- Unspecified injury of flexor muscle, fascia and tendon of **left index** finger at forearm level

S56.103- Unspecified injury of flexor muscle, fascia and tendon of **right middle** finger at forearm level

S56.104- Unspecified injury of flexor muscle, fascia and tendon of **left middle** finger at forearm level

S56.105- Unspecified injury of flexor muscle, fascia and tendon of **right ring** finger at forearm level

S56.106- Unspecified injury of flexor muscle, fascia and tendon of **left ring** finger at forearm level

S56.107- Unspecified injury of flexor muscle, fascia and tendon of **right little** finger at forearm level

S56.108- Unspecified injury of flexor muscle, fascia and tendon of **left little** finger at forearm level

S56.109- Unspecified injury of flexor muscle, fascia and tendon of **unspecified finger** at forearm level

S55 - S56

S56.11- **Strain** of flexor muscle, fascia and tendon of other and unspecified finger at forearm level

S56.111- Strain of flexor muscle, fascia and tendon of right index finger at forearm level

S56.112- Strain of flexor muscle, fascia and tendon of left index finger at forearm level

S56.113- Strain of flexor muscle, fascia and tendon of right middle finger at forearm level

S56.114- Strain of flexor muscle, fascia and tendon of left middle finger at forearm level

S56.115- Strain of flexor muscle, fascia and tendon of right ring finger at forearm level

S56.116- Strain of flexor muscle, fascia and tendon of left ring finger at forearm level

S56.117- Strain of flexor muscle, fascia and tendon of right little finger at forearm level

S56.118- Strain of flexor muscle, fascia and tendon of left little finger at forearm level

S56.119- Strain of flexor muscle, fascia and tendon of finger of unspecified finger at forearm level

S56.12- **Laceration** of flexor muscle, fascia and tendon of other and unspecified finger at forearm level

CC-A **S56.121-** Laceration of flexor muscle, fascia and tendon of right index finger at forearm level

CC-A **S56.122-** Laceration of flexor muscle, fascia and tendon of left index finger at forearm level

CC-A **S56.123-** Laceration of flexor muscle, fascia and tendon of right middle finger at forearm level

CC-A **S56.124-** Laceration of flexor muscle, fascia and tendon of left middle finger at forearm level

CC-A **S56.125-** Laceration of flexor muscle, fascia and tendon of right ring finger at forearm level

CC-A **S56.126-** Laceration of flexor muscle, fascia and tendon of left ring finger at forearm level

CC-A **S56.127-** Laceration of flexor muscle, fascia and tendon of right little finger at forearm level

CC-A **S56.128-** Laceration of flexor muscle, fascia and tendon of left little finger at forearm level

CC-A **S56.129-** Laceration of flexor muscle, fascia and tendon of unspecified finger at forearm level

S56.19- **Other injury** of flexor muscle, fascia and tendon of other and unspecified finger at forearm level

S56.191- Other injury of flexor muscle, fascia and tendon of right index finger at forearm level

S56.192- Other injury of flexor muscle, fascia and tendon of left index finger at forearm level

S56.193- Other injury of flexor muscle, fascia and tendon of right middle finger at forearm level

S56.194- Other injury of flexor muscle, fascia and tendon of left middle finger at forearm level

S56.195- Other injury of flexor muscle, fascia and tendon of right ring finger at forearm level

S56.196- Other injury of flexor muscle, fascia and tendon of left ring finger at forearm level

S56.197- Other injury of flexor muscle, fascia and tendon of right little finger at forearm level

S56.198- Other injury of flexor muscle, fascia and tendon of left little finger at forearm level

S56.199- Other injury of flexor muscle, fascia and tendon of unspecified finger at forearm level

S56.2- **Injury** of other flexor muscle, fascia and tendon at forearm level

S56.20- **Unspecified** injury of other flexor muscle, fascia and tendon at forearm level

S56.201- Unspecified injury of other flexor muscle, fascia and tendon at forearm level, right arm

S56.202- Unspecified injury of other flexor muscle, fascia and tendon at forearm level, left arm

S56.209- Unspecified injury of other flexor muscle, fascia and tendon at forearm level, unspecified arm

S56.21- **Strain** of other flexor muscle, fascia and tendon at forearm level

S56.211- Strain of other flexor muscle, fascia and tendon at forearm level, right arm

S56.212- Strain of other flexor muscle, fascia and tendon at forearm level, left arm

S56.219- Strain of other flexor muscle, fascia and tendon at forearm level, unspecified arm

S56.22- **Laceration** of other flexor muscle, fascia and tendon at forearm level

CC-A **S56.221-** Laceration of other flexor muscle, fascia and tendon at forearm level, right arm

CC-A **S56.222-** Laceration of other flexor muscle, fascia and tendon at forearm level, left arm

CC-A **S56.229-** Laceration of other flexor muscle, fascia and tendon at forearm level, unspecified arm

S56.29- **Other injury** of other flexor muscle, fascia and tendon at forearm level

S56.291- Other injury of other flexor muscle, fascia and tendon at forearm level, right arm

S56.292- Other injury of other flexor muscle, fascia and tendon at forearm level, left arm

S56.299- Other injury of other flexor muscle, fascia and tendon at forearm level, unspecified arm

S56.3- **Injury** of extensor or abductor muscles, fascia and tendons of thumb at forearm level

S56.30- **Unspecified** injury of extensor or abductor muscles, fascia and tendons of thumb at forearm level

S56.301- Unspecified injury of extensor or abductor muscles, fascia and tendons of right thumb at forearm level

S56.302- Unspecified injury of extensor or abductor muscles, fascia and tendons of left thumb at forearm level

S56.309- Unspecified injury of extensor or abductor muscles, fascia and tendons of unspecified thumb at forearm level

S56.31- **Strain** of extensor or abductor muscles, fascia and tendons of thumb at forearm level

S56.311- Strain of extensor or abductor muscles, fascia and tendons of right thumb at forearm level

S56.312- Strain of extensor or abductor muscles, fascia and tendons of left thumb at forearm level

S56.319- Strain of extensor or abductor muscles, fascia and tendons of unspecified thumb at forearm level

S56.32- **Laceration** of extensor or abductor muscles, fascia and tendons of thumb at forearm level

CC-A **S56.321-** Laceration of extensor or abductor muscles, fascia and tendons of right thumb at forearm level

CC-A **S56.322-** Laceration of extensor or abductor muscles, fascia and tendons of left thumb at forearm level

CC-A **S56.329-** Laceration of extensor or abductor muscles, fascia and tendons of unspecified thumb at forearm level

S56.39- **Other injury** of extensor or abductor muscles, fascia and tendons of thumb at forearm level

S56.391- Other injury of extensor or abductor muscles, fascia and tendons of right thumb at forearm level

S56.392- Other injury of extensor or abductor muscles, fascia and tendons of left thumb at forearm level

S56.399- Other injury of extensor or abductor muscles, fascia and tendons of unspecified thumb at forearm level

S56.4- **Injury** of extensor muscle, fascia and tendon of other and unspecified finger at forearm level

S56.40- **Unspecified** injury of extensor muscle, fascia and tendon of other and unspecified finger at forearm level

S56.401- Unspecified injury of extensor muscle, fascia and tendon of right index finger at forearm level

S56.402- Unspecified injury of extensor muscle, fascia and tendon of left index finger at forearm level

S56 - S56

S56.403- Unspecified injury of extensor muscle, fascia and tendon of <u>right</u> <u>middle</u> finger at forearm level

S56.404- Unspecified injury of extensor muscle, fascia and tendon of <u>left</u> <u>middle</u> finger at forearm level

S56.405- Unspecified injury of extensor muscle, fascia and tendon of <u>right</u> <u>ring</u> finger at forearm level

S56.406- Unspecified injury of extensor muscle, fascia and tendon of <u>left</u> <u>ring</u> finger at forearm level

S56.407- Unspecified injury of extensor muscle, fascia and tendon of <u>right</u> <u>little</u> finger at forearm level

S56.408- Unspecified injury of extensor muscle, fascia and tendon of <u>left</u> <u>little</u> finger at forearm level

S56.409- Unspecified injury of extensor muscle, fascia and tendon of <u>unspecified</u> <u>finger</u> at forearm level

S56.41- <u>Strain</u> of <u>extensor</u> muscle, fascia and tendon of other and unspecified <u>finger</u> at <u>forearm level</u>

S56.411- Strain of extensor muscle, fascia and tendon of <u>right</u> <u>index</u> finger at forearm level

S56.412- Strain of extensor muscle, fascia and tendon of <u>left</u> <u>index</u> finger at forearm level

S56.413- Strain of extensor muscle, fascia and tendon of <u>right</u> <u>middle</u> finger at forearm level

S56.414- Strain of extensor muscle, fascia and tendon of <u>left</u> <u>middle</u> finger at forearm level

S56.415- Strain of extensor muscle, fascia and tendon of <u>right</u> <u>ring</u> finger at forearm level

S56.416- Strain of extensor muscle, fascia and tendon of <u>left</u> <u>ring</u> finger at forearm level

S56.417- Strain of extensor muscle, fascia and tendon of <u>right</u> <u>little</u> finger at forearm level

S56.418- Strain of extensor muscle, fascia and tendon of <u>left</u> <u>little</u> finger at forearm level

S56.419- Strain of extensor muscle, fascia and tendon of finger, <u>unspecified</u> <u>finger</u> at forearm level

S56.42- <u>Laceration</u> of <u>extensor</u> muscle, fascia and tendon of other and unspecified <u>finger</u> at forearm level

CC-A S56.421- Laceration of extensor muscle, fascia and tendon of <u>right</u> <u>index</u> finger at forearm level

CC-A S56.422- Laceration of extensor muscle, fascia and tendon of <u>left</u> <u>index</u> finger at forearm level

CC-A S56.423- Laceration of extensor muscle, fascia and tendon of <u>right</u> <u>middle</u> finger at forearm level

CC-A S56.424- Laceration of extensor muscle, fascia and tendon of <u>left</u> <u>middle</u> finger at forearm level

CC-A S56.425- Laceration of extensor muscle, fascia and tendon of <u>right</u> <u>ring</u> finger at forearm level

CC-A S56.426- Laceration of extensor muscle, fascia and tendon of <u>left</u> <u>ring</u> finger at forearm level

CC-A S56.427- Laceration of extensor muscle, fascia and tendon of <u>right</u> <u>little</u> finger at forearm level

CC-A S56.428- Laceration of extensor muscle, fascia and tendon of <u>left</u> <u>little</u> finger at forearm level

CC-A S56.429- Laceration of extensor muscle, fascia and tendon of <u>unspecified</u> <u>finger</u> at forearm level

S56.49- <u>Other injury</u> of <u>extensor</u> muscle, fascia and tendon of other and unspecified <u>finger</u> at <u>forearm level</u>

S56.491- Other injury of extensor muscle, fascia and tendon of <u>right</u> <u>index</u> finger at forearm level

S56.492- Other injury of extensor muscle, fascia and tendon of <u>left</u> <u>index</u> finger at forearm level

S56.493- Other injury of extensor muscle, fascia and tendon of <u>right</u> <u>middle</u> finger at forearm level

S56.494- Other injury of extensor muscle, fascia and tendon of <u>left</u> <u>middle</u> finger at forearm level

S56.495- Other injury of extensor muscle, fascia and tendon of <u>right</u> <u>ring</u> finger at forearm level

S56.496- Other injury of extensor muscle, fascia and tendon of <u>left</u> <u>ring</u> finger at forearm level

S56.497- Other injury of extensor muscle, fascia and tendon of <u>right</u> <u>little</u> finger at forearm level

S56.498- Other injury of extensor muscle, fascia and tendon of <u>left</u> <u>little</u> finger at forearm level

S56.499- Other injury of extensor muscle, fascia and tendon of <u>unspecified</u> <u>finger</u> at forearm level

S56.5- <u>Injury</u> of <u>other extensor</u> muscle, fascia and tendon at forearm level

S56.50- <u>Unspecified</u> injury of <u>other extensor</u> muscle, fascia and tendon at <u>forearm level</u>

S56.501- Unspecified injury of other extensor muscle, fascia and tendon at forearm level, <u>right</u> arm

S56.502- Unspecified injury of other extensor muscle, fascia and tendon at forearm level, <u>left</u> arm

S56.509- Unspecified injury of other extensor muscle, fascia and tendon at forearm level, <u>unspecified</u> arm

S56.51- <u>Strain</u> of <u>other extensor</u> muscle, fascia and tendon at <u>forearm level</u>

S56.511- Strain of other extensor muscle, fascia and tendon at forearm level, <u>right</u> arm

S56.512- Strain of other extensor muscle, fascia and tendon at forearm level, <u>left</u> arm

S56.519- Strain of other extensor muscle, fascia and tendon at forearm level, <u>unspecified</u> arm

S56.52- <u>Laceration</u> of <u>other extensor</u> muscle, fascia and tendon at <u>forearm level</u>

CC-A S56.521- Laceration of other extensor muscle, fascia and tendon at forearm level, <u>right</u> arm

CC-A S56.522- Laceration of other extensor muscle, fascia and tendon at forearm level, <u>left</u> arm

CC-A S56.529- Laceration of other extensor muscle, fascia and tendon at forearm level, <u>unspecified</u> arm

S56.59- <u>Other injury</u> of <u>other extensor</u> muscle, fascia and tendon at <u>forearm level</u>

S56.591- Other injury of other extensor muscle, fascia and tendon at forearm level, <u>right</u> arm

S56.592- Other injury of other extensor muscle, fascia and tendon at forearm level, <u>left</u> arm

S56.599- Other injury of other extensor muscle, fascia and tendon at forearm level, <u>unspecified</u> arm

S56.8- <u>Injury</u> of <u>other</u> muscles, fascia and tendons at <u>forearm level</u>

S56.80- <u>Unspecified</u> injury of <u>other</u> muscles, fascia and tendons at <u>forearm level</u>

S56.801- Unspecified injury of other muscles, fascia and tendons at forearm level, <u>right</u> arm

S56.802- Unspecified injury of other muscles, fascia and tendons at forearm level, <u>left</u> arm

S56.809- Unspecified injury of other muscles, fascia and tendons at forearm level, <u>unspecified</u> arm

S56.81- <u>Strain</u> of <u>other</u> muscles, fascia and tendons at <u>forearm level</u>

S56.811- Strain of other muscles, fascia and tendons at forearm level, <u>right</u> arm

S56.812- Strain of other muscles, fascia and tendons at forearm level, <u>left</u> arm

S56.819- Strain of other muscles, fascia and tendons at forearm level, <u>unspecified</u> arm

S56.82- <u>Laceration</u> of <u>other</u> muscles, fascia and tendons at <u>forearm level</u>

CC-A S56.821- Laceration of other muscles, fascia and tendons at forearm level, <u>right</u> arm

CC-A S56.822- Laceration of other muscles, fascia and tendons at forearm level, <u>left</u> arm

CC-A S56.829- Laceration of other muscles, fascia and tendons at forearm level, <u>unspecified</u> arm

S56.89- <u>Other injury</u> of <u>other</u> muscles, fascia and tendons at <u>forearm level</u>

S56.891- Other injury of other muscles, fascia and tendons at forearm level, <u>right</u> arm

S56.892-   Other injury of other muscles, fascia and tendons at forearm level, <u>left</u> arm

S56.899-   Other injury of other muscles, fascia and tendons at forearm level, <u>unspecified</u> arm

S56.9-   <u>Injury</u> of <u>unspecified</u> muscles, fascia and tendons at <u>forearm level</u>

  S56.90-   <u>Unspecified</u> injury of <u>unspecified</u> muscles, fascia and tendons at <u>forearm level</u>

    S56.901-   Unspecified injury of unspecified muscles, fascia and tendons at forearm level, <u>right</u> arm

    S56.902-   Unspecified injury of unspecified muscles, fascia and tendons at forearm level, <u>left</u> arm

    S56.909-   Unspecified injury of unspecified muscles, fascia and tendons at forearm level, <u>unspecified</u> arm

  S56.91-   <u>Strain</u> of <u>unspecified</u> muscles, fascia and tendons at <u>forearm level</u>

    S56.911-   Strain of unspecified muscles, fascia and tendons at forearm level, <u>right</u> arm

    S56.912-   Strain of unspecified muscles, fascia and tendons at forearm level, <u>left</u> arm

    S56.919-   Strain of unspecified muscles, fascia and tendons at forearm level, <u>unspecified</u> arm

  S56.92-   <u>Laceration</u> of <u>unspecified</u> muscles, fascia and tendons at <u>forearm level</u>

CC-A S56.921-   Laceration of unspecified muscles, fascia and tendons at forearm level, <u>right</u> arm

CC-A S56.922-   Laceration of unspecified muscles, fascia and tendons at forearm level, <u>left</u> arm

CC-A S56.929-   Laceration of unspecified muscles, fascia and tendons at forearm level, <u>unspecified</u> arm

  S56.99-   <u>Other injury</u> of <u>unspecified</u> muscles, fascia and tendons at <u>forearm level</u>

    S56.991-   Other injury of unspecified muscles, fascia and tendons at forearm level, <u>right</u> arm

    S56.992-   Other injury of unspecified muscles, fascia and tendons at forearm level, <u>left</u> arm

    S56.999-   Other injury of unspecified muscles, fascia and tendons at forearm level, <u>unspecified</u> arm

S57-   <u>Crushing</u> injury of <u>elbow and forearm</u>
Use additional code(s) for all associated injuries
Excludes ❷: crushing injury of wrist and hand (S67.-)

The appropriate 7th character is to be added to each code from category S57:
A   <u>Initial</u> encounter
D   <u>Subsequent</u> encounter
S   <u>Sequela</u>

  S57.0-   <u>Crushing</u> injury of <u>elbow</u>
    S57.00x-   Crushing injury of <u>unspecified</u> elbow
    S57.01x-   Crushing injury of <u>right</u> elbow
    S57.02x-   Crushing injury of <u>left</u> elbow

  S57.8-   <u>Crushing</u> injury of <u>forearm</u>
    S57.80x-   Crushing injury of <u>unspecified</u> forearm
    S57.81x-   Crushing injury of <u>right</u> forearm
    S57.82x-   Crushing injury of <u>left</u> forearm

S58-   <u>Traumatic amputation</u> of <u>elbow and forearm</u>
Note: An amputation not identified as partial or complete should be coded to complete
Excludes 1:   traumatic amputation of wrist and hand (S68.-)

The appropriate 7th character is to be added to each code from category S58:
A   <u>Initial</u> encounter
D   <u>Subsequent</u> encounter
S   <u>Sequela</u>

  S58.0-   <u>Traumatic amputation</u> at <u>elbow level</u>
    S58.01-   <u>Complete</u> traumatic amputation at <u>elbow level</u>
CC-A S58.011-   Complete traumatic amputation at elbow level, <u>right</u> arm
CC-A S58.012-   Complete traumatic amputation at elbow level, <u>left</u> arm

CC-A S58.019-   Complete traumatic amputation at elbow level, <u>unspecified</u> arm

    S58.02-   <u>Partial</u> traumatic amputation at <u>elbow level</u>
CC-A S58.021-   Partial traumatic amputation at elbow level, <u>right</u> arm
CC-A S58.022-   Partial traumatic amputation at elbow level, <u>left</u> arm
CC-A S58.029-   Partial traumatic amputation at elbow level, <u>unspecified</u> arm

  S58.1-   <u>Traumatic amputation</u> at <u>level between elbow and wrist</u>
    S58.11-   <u>Complete</u> traumatic amputation at <u>level between elbow and wrist</u>
CC-A S58.111-   Complete traumatic amputation at level between elbow and wrist, <u>right</u> arm
CC-A S58.112-   Complete traumatic amputation at level between elbow and wrist, <u>left</u> arm
CC-A S58.119-   Complete traumatic amputation at level between elbow and wrist, <u>unspecified</u> arm

    S58.12-   <u>Partial</u> traumatic amputation at <u>level between elbow and wrist</u>
CC-A S58.121-   Partial traumatic amputation at level between elbow and wrist, <u>right</u> arm
CC-A S58.122-   Partial traumatic amputation at level between elbow and wrist, <u>left</u> arm
CC-A S58.129-   Partial traumatic amputation at level between elbow and wrist, <u>unspecified</u> arm

  S58.9-   <u>Traumatic amputation</u> of forearm, <u>level unspecified</u>
Excludes 1:   traumatic amputation of wrist (S68.-)
    S58.91-   <u>Complete</u> traumatic amputation of forearm, <u>level unspecified</u>
CC-A S58.911-   Complete traumatic amputation of <u>right</u> forearm, level unspecified
CC-A S58.912-   Complete traumatic amputation of <u>left</u> forearm, level unspecified
CC-A S58.919-   Complete traumatic amputation of <u>unspecified</u> forearm, level unspecified

    S58.92-   <u>Partial</u> traumatic amputation of forearm, <u>level unspecified</u>
CC-A S58.921-   Partial traumatic amputation of <u>right</u> forearm, level unspecified
CC-A S58.922-   Partial traumatic amputation of <u>left</u> forearm, level unspecified
CC-A S58.929-   Partial traumatic amputation of <u>unspecified</u> forearm, level unspecified

S59-   <u>Other and unspecified injuries</u> of <u>elbow and forearm</u>
Excludes ❷: other and unspecified injuries of wrist and hand (S69.-)

The appropriate 7th character is to be added to each code from subcategories S59.0, S59.1, and S59.2:
A   <u>Initial</u> encounter for <u>closed</u> fracture
D   <u>Subsequent</u> encounter for fracture <u>with routine healing</u>
G   <u>Subsequent</u> encounter for fracture <u>with delayed healing</u>
K   <u>Subsequent</u> encounter for fracture <u>with nonunion</u>
P   <u>Subsequent</u> encounter for fracture <u>with malunion</u>
S   <u>Sequela</u>

  S59.0-   <u>Physeal</u> fracture of <u>lower end</u> of <u>ulna</u>
    S59.00-   <u>Unspecified physeal</u> fracture of <u>lower end</u> of <u>ulna</u>
CC-A,K,P S59.001-   Unspecified physeal fracture of lower end of ulna, <u>right</u> arm
CC-A,K,P S59.002-   Unspecified physeal fracture of lower end of ulna, <u>left</u> arm
CC-A,K,P S59.009-   Unspecified physeal fracture of lower end of ulna, <u>unspecified</u> arm

    S59.01-   <u>Salter-Harris Type I</u> physeal fracture of <u>lower end</u> of <u>ulna</u>
CC-A,K,P S59.011-   Salter-Harris Type I physeal fracture of lower end of ulna, <u>right</u> arm
CC-A,K,P S59.012-   Salter-Harris Type I physeal fracture of lower end of ulna, <u>left</u> arm
CC-A,K,P S59.019-   Salter-Harris Type I physeal fracture of lower end of ulna, <u>unspecified</u> arm

S56 | S59

S59.02- Salter-Harris Type II physeal fracture of lower end of ulna

CC-A,K,P **S59.021-** Salter-Harris Type II physeal fracture of lower end of ulna, right arm

CC-A,K,P **S59.022-** Salter-Harris Type II physeal fracture of lower end of ulna, left arm

CC-A,K,P **S59.029-** Salter-Harris Type II physeal fracture of lower end of ulna, unspecified arm

S59.03- Salter-Harris Type III physeal fracture of lower end of ulna

CC-A,K,P **S59.031-** Salter-Harris Type III physeal fracture of lower end of ulna, right arm

CC-A,K,P **S59.032-** Salter-Harris Type III physeal fracture of lower end of ulna, left arm

CC-A,K,P **S59.039-** Salter-Harris Type III physeal fracture of lower end of ulna, unspecified arm

S59.04- Salter-Harris Type IV physeal fracture of lower end of ulna

CC-A,K,P **S59.041-** Salter-Harris Type IV physeal fracture of lower end of ulna, right arm

CC-A,K,P **S59.042-** Salter-Harris Type IV physeal fracture of lower end of ulna, left arm

CC-A,K,P **S59.049-** Salter-Harris Type IV physeal fracture of lower end of ulna, unspecified arm

S59.09- Other physeal fracture of lower end of ulna

CC-A,K,P **S59.091-** Other physeal fracture of lower end of ulna, right arm

CC-A,K,P **S59.092-** Other physeal fracture of lower end of ulna, left arm

CC-A,K,P **S59.099-** Other physeal fracture of lower end of ulna, unspecified arm

S59.1- Physeal fracture of upper end of radius

S59.10- Unspecified physeal fracture of upper end of radius

CC-K,P **S59.101-** Unspecified physeal fracture of upper end of radius, right arm

CC-K,P **S59.102-** Unspecified physeal fracture of upper end of radius, left arm

CC-K,P **S59.109-** Unspecified physeal fracture of upper end of radius, unspecified arm

S59.11- Salter-Harris Type I physeal fracture of upper end of radius

CC-K,P **S59.111-** Salter-Harris Type I physeal fracture of upper end of radius, right arm

CC-K,P **S59.112-** Salter-Harris Type I physeal fracture of upper end of radius, left arm

CC-K,P **S59.119-** Salter-Harris Type I physeal fracture of upper end of radius, unspecified arm

S59.12- Salter-Harris Type II physeal fracture of upper end of radius

CC-K,P **S59.121-** Salter-Harris Type II physeal fracture of upper end of radius, right arm

CC-K,P **S59.122-** Salter-Harris Type II physeal fracture of upper end of radius, left arm

CC-K,P **S59.129-** Salter-Harris Type II physeal fracture of upper end of radius, unspecified arm

S59.13- Salter-Harris Type III physeal fracture of upper end of radius

CC-K,P **S59.131-** Salter-Harris Type III physeal fracture of upper end of radius, right arm

CC-K,P **S59.132-** Salter-Harris Type III physeal fracture of upper end of radius, left arm

CC-K,P **S59.139-** Salter-Harris Type III physeal fracture of upper end of radius, unspecified arm

S59.14- Salter-Harris Type IV physeal fracture of upper end of radius

CC-K,P **S59.141-** Salter-Harris Type IV physeal fracture of upper end of radius, right arm

CC-K,P **S59.142-** Salter-Harris Type IV physeal fracture of upper end of radius, left arm

CC-K,P **S59.149-** Salter-Harris Type IV physeal fracture of upper end of radius, unspecified arm

S59.19- Other physeal fracture of upper end of radius

CC-K,P **S59.191-** Other physeal fracture of upper end of radius, right arm

CC-K,P **S59.192-** Other physeal fracture of upper end of radius, left arm

CC-K,P **S59.199-** Other physeal fracture of upper end of radius, unspecified arm

S59.2- Physeal fracture of lower end of radius

S59.20- Unspecified physeal fracture of lower end of radius

CC-A,K,P **S59.201-** Unspecified physeal fracture of lower end of radius, right arm

CC-A,K,P **S59.202-** Unspecified physeal fracture of lower end of radius, left arm

CC-A,K,P **S59.209-** Unspecified physeal fracture of lower end of radius, unspecified arm

S59.21- Salter-Harris Type I physeal fracture of lower end of radius

CC-A,K,P **S59.211-** Salter-Harris Type I physeal fracture of lower end of radius, right arm

CC-A,K,P **S59.212-** Salter-Harris Type I physeal fracture of lower end of radius, left arm

CC-A,K,P **S59.219-** Salter-Harris Type I physeal fracture of lower end of radius, unspecified arm

S59.22- Salter-Harris Type II physeal fracture of lower end of radius

CC-A,K,P **S59.221-** Salter-Harris Type II physeal fracture of lower end of radius, right arm

CC-A,K,P **S59.222-** Salter-Harris Type II physeal fracture of lower end of radius, left arm

CC-A,K,P **S59.229-** Salter-Harris Type II physeal fracture of lower end of radius, unspecified arm

S59.23- Salter-Harris Type III physeal fracture of lower end of radius

CC-A,K,P **S59.231-** Salter-Harris Type III physeal fracture of lower end of radius, right arm

CC-A,K,P **S59.232-** Salter-Harris Type III physeal fracture of lower end of radius, left arm

CC-A,K,P **S59.239-** Salter-Harris Type III physeal fracture of lower end of radius, unspecified arm

S59.24- Salter-Harris Type IV physeal fracture of lower end of radius

CC-A,K,P **S59.241-** Salter-Harris Type IV physeal fracture of lower end of radius, right arm

CC-A,K,P **S59.242-** Salter-Harris Type IV physeal fracture of lower end of radius, left arm

CC-A,K,P **S59.249-** Salter-Harris Type IV physeal fracture of lower end of radius, unspecified arm

S59.29- Other physeal fracture of lower end of radius

CC-A,K,P **S59.291-** Other physeal fracture of lower end of radius, right arm

CC-A,K,P **S59.292-** Other physeal fracture of lower end of radius, left arm

CC-A,K,P **S59.299-** Other physeal fracture of lower end of radius, unspecified arm

S59.8- Other specified injuries of elbow and forearm

The appropriate 7th character is to be added to each code in subcategory S59.8:
A   Initial encounter
D   Subsequent encounter
S   Sequela

S59.80- Other specified injuries of elbow

S59.801- Other specified injuries of right elbow

S59.802- Other specified injuries of left elbow

S59.809- Other specified injuries of unspecified elbow

S59.81- Other specified injuries of forearm

S59.811- Other specified injuries right forearm

S59 - S59

S59.812- Other specified injuries <u>left</u> forearm
S59.819- Other specified injuries <u>unspecified</u> forearm
S59.9- <u>Unspecified injury</u> of <u>elbow and forearm</u>
The appropriate 7th character is to be added to each code in subcategory S59.9:
A <u>Initial</u> encounter
D <u>Subsequent</u> encounter
S <u>Sequela</u>
S59.90- <u>Unspecified injury</u> of <u>elbow</u>
S59.901- Unspecified injury of <u>right</u> elbow
S59.902- Unspecified injury of <u>left</u> elbow
S59.909- Unspecified injury of <u>unspecified</u> elbow
S59.91- <u>Unspecified injury</u> of <u>forearm</u>
S59.911- Unspecified injury of <u>right</u> forearm
S59.912- Unspecified injury of <u>left</u> forearm
S59.919- Unspecified injury of <u>unspecified</u> forearm

Injuries to the wrist, hand and fingers (S60-S69)

Excludes ❷: burns and corrosions (T20-T32)
frostbite (T33-T34)
insect bite or sting, venomous (T63.4)

S60- <u>Superficial injury</u> of <u>wrist, hand and fingers</u>
The appropriate 7th character is to be added to each code from category S60:
A <u>Initial</u> encounter
D <u>Subsequent</u> encounter
S <u>Sequela</u>
S60.0- <u>Contusion</u> of <u>finger</u> <u>without</u> damage to nail
Excludes 1: contusion involving nail (matrix) (S60.1)
S60.00x- <u>Contusion</u> of <u>unspecified</u> finger <u>without</u> damage to nail
Contusion of finger(s) NOS
S60.01- <u>Contusion</u> of <u>thumb</u> <u>without</u> damage to nail
S60.011- Contusion of <u>right</u> thumb without damage to nail
S60.012- Contusion of <u>left</u> thumb without damage to nail
S60.019- Contusion of <u>unspecified</u> thumb without damage to nail
S60.02- <u>Contusion</u> of <u>index</u> finger <u>without</u> damage to nail
S60.021- Contusion of <u>right</u> index finger without damage to nail
S60.022- Contusion of <u>left</u> index finger without damage to nail
S60.029- Contusion of <u>unspecified</u> index finger without damage to nail
S60.03- <u>Contusion</u> of <u>middle</u> finger <u>without</u> damage to nail
S60.031- Contusion of <u>right</u> middle finger without damage to nail
S60.032- Contusion of <u>left</u> middle finger without damage to nail
S60.039- Contusion of <u>unspecified</u> middle finger without damage to nail
S60.04- <u>Contusion</u> of <u>ring</u> finger <u>without</u> damage to nail
S60.041- Contusion of <u>right</u> ring finger without damage to nail
S60.042- Contusion of <u>left</u> ring finger without damage to nail
S60.049- Contusion of <u>unspecified</u> ring finger without damage to nail
S60.05- <u>Contusion</u> of <u>little</u> finger <u>without</u> damage to nail
S60.051- Contusion of <u>right</u> little finger without damage to nail
S60.052- Contusion of <u>left</u> little finger without damage to nail
S60.059- Contusion of <u>unspecified</u> little finger without damage to nail
S60.1- <u>Contusion</u> of <u>finger</u> <u>with damage to nail</u>
S60.10x- <u>Contusion</u> of <u>unspecified</u> finger <u>with damage to nail</u>
S60.11- <u>Contusion</u> of <u>thumb</u> <u>with damage to nail</u>
S60.111- Contusion of <u>right</u> thumb with damage to nail

S60.112- Contusion of <u>left</u> thumb with damage to nail
S60.119- Contusion of <u>unspecified</u> thumb with damage to nail
S60.12- <u>Contusion</u> of <u>index</u> finger <u>with damage to nail</u>
S60.121- Contusion of <u>right</u> index finger with damage to nail
S60.122- Contusion of <u>left</u> index finger with damage to nail
S60.129- Contusion of <u>unspecified</u> index finger with damage to nail
S60.13- <u>Contusion</u> of <u>middle</u> finger <u>with damage to nail</u>
S60.131- Contusion of <u>right</u> middle finger with damage to nail
S60.132- Contusion of <u>left</u> middle finger with damage to nail
S60.139- Contusion of <u>unspecified</u> middle finger with damage to nail
S60.14- <u>Contusion</u> of <u>ring</u> finger <u>with damage to nail</u>
S60.141- Contusion of <u>right</u> ring finger with damage to nail
S60.142- Contusion of <u>left</u> ring finger with damage to nail
S60.149- Contusion of <u>unspecified</u> ring finger with damage to nail
S60.15- <u>Contusion</u> of <u>little</u> finger <u>with damage to nail</u>
S60.151- Contusion of <u>right</u> little finger with damage to nail
S60.152- Contusion of <u>left</u> little finger with damage to nail
S60.159- Contusion of <u>unspecified</u> little finger with damage to nail
S60.2- <u>Contusion</u> of <u>wrist and hand</u>
Excludes ❷: contusion of fingers (S60.0-, S60.1-)
S60.21- <u>Contusion</u> of <u>wrist</u>
S60.211- Contusion of <u>right</u> wrist
S60.212- Contusion of <u>left</u> wrist
S60.219- Contusion of <u>unspecified</u> wrist
S60.22- <u>Contusion</u> of <u>hand</u>
S60.221- Contusion of <u>right</u> hand
S60.222- Contusion of <u>left</u> hand
S60.229- Contusion of <u>unspecified</u> hand
S60.3- <u>Other superficial injuries</u> of <u>thumb</u>
S60.31- <u>Abrasion</u> of <u>thumb</u>
S60.311- Abrasion of <u>right</u> thumb
S60.312- Abrasion of <u>left</u> thumb
S60.319- Abrasion of <u>unspecified</u> thumb
S60.32- <u>Blister</u> (nonthermal) of <u>thumb</u>
S60.321- Blister (nonthermal) of <u>right</u> thumb
S60.322- Blister (nonthermal) of <u>left</u> thumb
S60.329- Blister (nonthermal) of <u>unspecified</u> thumb
S60.34- <u>External constriction</u> of <u>thumb</u>
Hair tourniquet syndrome of thumb
Use additional cause code to identify the constricting item (W49.0-)
S60.341- External constriction of <u>right</u> thumb
S60.342- External constriction of <u>left</u> thumb
S60.349- External constriction of <u>unspecified</u> thumb
S60.35- <u>Superficial foreign body</u> of <u>thumb</u>
Splinter in the thumb
S60.351- Superficial foreign body of <u>right</u> thumb
S60.352- Superficial foreign body of <u>left</u> thumb
S60.359- Superficial foreign body of <u>unspecified</u> thumb
S60.36- <u>Insect bite (nonvenomous)</u> of <u>thumb</u>
S60.361- Insect bite (nonvenomous) of <u>right</u> thumb
S60.362- Insect bite (nonvenomous) of <u>left</u> thumb
S60.369- Insect bite (nonvenomous) of <u>unspecified</u> thumb
S60.37- <u>Other superficial bite</u> of <u>thumb</u>
Excludes 1: open bite of thumb (S61.05-, S61.15-)
S60.371- Other superficial bite of <u>right</u> thumb
S60.372- Other superficial bite of <u>left</u> thumb
S60.379- Other superficial bite of <u>unspecified</u> thumb

S59 | S60

S60.39- Other superficial injuries of thumb
    S60.391- Other superficial injuries of right thumb
    S60.392- Other superficial injuries of left thumb
    S60.399- Other superficial injuries of unspecified thumb
S60.4- Other superficial injuries of other fingers
    S60.41- Abrasion of fingers
        S60.410- Abrasion of right index finger
        S60.411- Abrasion of left index finger
        S60.412- Abrasion of right middle finger
        S60.413- Abrasion of left middle finger
        S60.414- Abrasion of right ring finger
        S60.415- Abrasion of left ring finger
        S60.416- Abrasion of right little finger
        S60.417- Abrasion of left little finger
        S60.418- Abrasion of other finger
            Abrasion of specified finger with unspecified laterality
        S60.419- Abrasion of unspecified finger
    S60.42- Blister (nonthermal) of fingers
        S60.420- Blister (nonthermal) of right index finger
        S60.421- Blister (nonthermal) of left index finger
        S60.422- Blister (nonthermal) of right middle finger
        S60.423- Blister (nonthermal) of left middle finger
        S60.424- Blister (nonthermal) of right ring finger
        S60.425- Blister (nonthermal) of left ring finger
        S60.426- Blister (nonthermal) of right little finger
        S60.427- Blister (nonthermal) of left little finger
        S60.428- Blister (nonthermal) of other finger
            Blister (nonthermal) of specified finger with unspecified laterality
        S60.429- Blister (nonthermal) of unspecified finger
    S60.44- External constriction of fingers
        Hair tourniquet syndrome of finger
        Use additional cause code to identify the constricting item (W49.0-)
        S60.440- External constriction of right index finger
        S60.441- External constriction of left index finger
        S60.442- External constriction of right middle finger
        S60.443- External constriction of left middle finger
        S60.444- External constriction of right ring finger
        S60.445- External constriction of left ring finger
        S60.446- External constriction of right little finger
        S60.447- External constriction of left little finger
        S60.448- External constriction of other finger
            External constriction of specified finger with unspecified laterality
        S60.449- External constriction of unspecified finger
    S60.45- Superficial foreign body of fingers
        Splinter in the finger(s)
        S60.450- Superficial foreign body of right index finger
        S60.451- Superficial foreign body of left index finger
        S60.452- Superficial foreign body of right middle finger
        S60.453- Superficial foreign body of left middle finger
        S60.454- Superficial foreign body of right ring finger
        S60.455- Superficial foreign body of left ring finger
        S60.456- Superficial foreign body of right little finger
        S60.457- Superficial foreign body of left little finger
        S60.458- Superficial foreign body of other finger
            Superficial foreign body of specified finger with unspecified laterality
        S60.459- Superficial foreign body of unspecified finger
    S60.46- Insect bite (nonvenomous) of fingers
        S60.460- Insect bite (nonvenomous) of right index finger
        S60.461- Insect bite (nonvenomous) of left index finger
        S60.462- Insect bite (nonvenomous) of right middle finger
        S60.463- Insect bite (nonvenomous) of left middle finger
        S60.464- Insect bite (nonvenomous) of right ring finger
        S60.465- Insect bite (nonvenomous) of left ring finger

S60.466- Insect bite (nonvenomous) of right little finger
S60.467- Insect bite (nonvenomous) of left little finger
S60.468- Insect bite (nonvenomous) of other finger
    Insect bite (nonvenomous) of specified finger with unspecified laterality
S60.469- Insect bite (nonvenomous) of unspecified finger
S60.47- Other superficial bite of fingers
    Excludes 1:   open bite of fingers (S61.25-, S61.35-)
    S60.470- Other superficial bite of right index finger
    S60.471- Other superficial bite of left index finger
    S60.472- Other superficial bite of right middle finger
    S60.473- Other superficial bite of left middle finger
    S60.474- Other superficial bite of right ring finger
    S60.475- Other superficial bite of left ring finger
    S60.476- Other superficial bite of right little finger
    S60.477- Other superficial bite of left little finger
    S60.478- Other superficial bite of other finger
        Other superficial bite of specified finger with unspecified laterality
    S60.479- Other superficial bite of unspecified finger
S60.5- Other superficial injuries of hand
    Excludes ❷: superficial injuries of fingers (S60.3-, S60.4-)
    S60.51- Abrasion of hand
        S60.511- Abrasion of right hand
        S60.512- Abrasion of left hand
        S60.519- Abrasion of unspecified hand
    S60.52- Blister (nonthermal) of hand
        S60.521- Blister (nonthermal) of right hand
        S60.522- Blister (nonthermal) of left hand
        S60.529- Blister (nonthermal) of unspecified hand
    S60.54- External constriction of hand
        S60.541- External constriction of right hand
        S60.542- External constriction of left hand
        S60.549- External constriction of unspecified hand
    S60.55- Superficial foreign body of hand
        Splinter in the hand
        S60.551- Superficial foreign body of right hand
        S60.552- Superficial foreign body of left hand
        S60.559- Superficial foreign body of unspecified hand
    S60.56- Insect bite (nonvenomous) of hand
        S60.561- Insect bite (nonvenomous) of right hand
        S60.562- Insect bite (nonvenomous) of left hand
        S60.569- Insect bite (nonvenomous) of unspecified hand
    S60.57- Other superficial bite of hand
        Excludes 1:   open bite of hand (S61.45-)
        S60.571- Other superficial bite of hand of right hand
        S60.572- Other superficial bite of hand of left hand
        S60.579- Other superficial bite of hand of unspecified hand
S60.8- Other superficial injuries of wrist
    S60.81- Abrasion of wrist
        S60.811- Abrasion of right wrist
        S60.812- Abrasion of left wrist
        S60.819- Abrasion of unspecified wrist
    S60.82- Blister (nonthermal) of wrist
        S60.821- Blister (nonthermal) of right wrist
        S60.822- Blister (nonthermal) of left wrist
        S60.829- Blister (nonthermal) of unspecified wrist
    S60.84- External constriction of wrist
        S60.841- External constriction of right wrist
        S60.842- External constriction of left wrist
        S60.849- External constriction of unspecified wrist
    S60.85- Superficial foreign body of wrist
        Splinter in the wrist
        S60.851- Superficial foreign body of right wrist
        S60.852- Superficial foreign body of left wrist
        S60.859- Superficial foreign body of unspecified wrist

S60 – S60

S60.86- **Insect bite (nonvenomous)** of **wrist**
- **S60.861-** Insect bite (nonvenomous) of **right** wrist
- **S60.862-** Insect bite (nonvenomous) of **left** wrist
- **S60.869-** Insect bite (nonvenomous) of **unspecified** wrist

S60.87- **Other superficial bite** of **wrist**
> Excludes 1: *open bite of wrist (S61.55)*
- **S60.871-** Other superficial bite of **right** wrist
- **S60.872-** Other superficial bite of **left** wrist
- **S60.879-** Other superficial bite of **unspecified** wrist

S60.9- Unspecified superficial injury of wrist, hand and fingers

S60.91- **Unspecified superficial injury** of **wrist**
- **S60.911-** Unspecified superficial injury of **right** wrist
- **S60.912-** Unspecified superficial injury of **left** wrist
- **S60.919-** Unspecified superficial injury of **unspecified** wrist

S60.92- **Unspecified superficial injury** of **hand**
- **S60.921-** Unspecified superficial injury of **right** hand
- **S60.922-** Unspecified superficial injury of **left** hand
- **S60.929-** Unspecified superficial injury of **unspecified** hand

S60.93- **Unspecified superficial injury** of **thumb**
- **S60.931-** Unspecified superficial injury of **right** thumb
- **S60.932-** Unspecified superficial injury of **left** thumb
- **S60.939-** Unspecified superficial injury of **unspecified** thumb

S60.94- **Unspecified superficial injury** of other **fingers**
- **S60.940-** Unspecified superficial injury of **right** **index** finger
- **S60.941-** Unspecified superficial injury of **left** **index** finger
- **S60.942-** Unspecified superficial injury of **right** **middle** finger
- **S60.943-** Unspecified superficial injury of **left** **middle** finger
- **S60.944-** Unspecified superficial injury of **right** **ring** finger
- **S60.945-** Unspecified superficial injury of **left** **ring** finger
- **S60.946-** Unspecified superficial injury of **right** **little** finger
- **S60.947-** Unspecified superficial injury of **left** **little** finger
- **S60.948-** Unspecified superficial injury of **other** finger
  Unspecified superficial injury of specified finger with unspecified laterality
- **S60.949-** Unspecified superficial injury of **unspecified** finger

S61- **Open wound** of **wrist, hand and fingers**
Code also any associated wound infection
> Excludes 1: *open fracture of wrist, hand and finger (S62.- with 7th character B)*
> *traumatic amputation of wrist and hand (S68.-)*

The appropriate 7th character is to be added to each code from category S61:
- **A** **Initial** encounter
- **D** **Subsequent** encounter
- **S** **Sequela**

S61.0- **Open wound** of **thumb** **without** damage to nail
> Excludes 1: *open wound of thumb with damage to nail (S61.1-)*

S61.00- **Unspecified** open wound of **thumb** **without** damage to nail
- **S61.001-** Unspecified open wound of **right** thumb **without** damage to nail
- **S61.002-** Unspecified open wound of **left** thumb **without** damage to nail
- **S61.009-** Unspecified open wound of **unspecified** thumb **without** damage to nail

S61.01- **Laceration** **without** foreign body of **thumb** **without** damage to nail
- **S61.011-** Laceration **without** foreign body of **right** thumb **without** damage to nail
- **S61.012-** Laceration **without** foreign body of **left** thumb **without** damage to nail
- **S61.019-** Laceration **without** foreign body of **unspecified** thumb **without** damage to nail

S61.02- **Laceration** **with foreign body** of **thumb** **without** damage to nail
- **S61.021-** Laceration **with foreign body** of **right** thumb **without** damage to nail

S61.022- Laceration **with foreign body** of **left** thumb **without** damage to nail
S61.029- Laceration **with foreign body** of **unspecified** thumb **without** damage to nail

S61.03- **Puncture** wound **without** foreign body of **thumb** **without** damage to nail
- **S61.031-** Puncture wound **without** foreign body of **right** thumb **without** damage to nail
- **S61.032-** Puncture wound **without** foreign body of **left** thumb **without** damage to nail
- **S61.039-** Puncture wound **without** foreign body of **unspecified** thumb **without** damage to nail

S61.04- **Puncture** wound **with foreign body** of **thumb** **without** damage to nail
- **S61.041-** Puncture wound **with foreign body** of **right** thumb **without** damage to nail
- **S61.042-** Puncture wound **with foreign body** of **left** thumb **without** damage to nail
- **S61.049-** Puncture wound **with foreign body** of **unspecified** thumb **without** damage to nail

S61.05- **Open bite** of **thumb** **without** damage to nail
Bite of thumb NOS
> Excludes 1: *superficial bite of thumb (S60.36-, S60.37-)*
- **S61.051-** Open bite of **right** thumb **without** damage to nail
- **S61.052-** Open bite of **left** thumb **without** damage to nail
- **S61.059-** Open bite of **unspecified** thumb **without** damage to nail

S61.1- Open wound of thumb **with** damage to nail

S61.10- **Unspecified** **open wound** of **thumb** **with damage to nail**
- **S61.101-** Unspecified open wound of **right** thumb **with damage to nail**
- **S61.102-** Unspecified open wound of **left** thumb **with damage to nail**
- **S61.109-** Unspecified open wound of **unspecified** thumb **with damage to nail**

S61.11- **Laceration** **without** foreign body of **thumb** **with damage to nail**
- **S61.111-** Laceration **without** foreign body of **right** thumb **with damage to nail**
- **S61.112-** Laceration **without** foreign body of **left** thumb **with damage to nail**
- **S61.119-** Laceration **without** foreign body of **unspecified** thumb **with damage to nail**

S61.12- **Laceration** **with foreign body** of **thumb** **with damage to nail**
- **S61.121-** Laceration **with foreign body** of **right** thumb **with damage to nail**
- **S61.122-** Laceration **with foreign body** of **left** thumb **with damage to nail**
- **S61.129-** Laceration **with foreign body** of **unspecified** thumb **with damage to nail**

S61.13- **Puncture** wound **without** foreign body of **thumb** **with damage to nail**
- **S61.131-** Puncture wound **without** foreign body of **right** thumb **with damage to nail**
- **S61.132-** Puncture wound **without** foreign body of **left** thumb **with damage to nail**
- **S61.139-** Puncture wound **without** foreign body of **unspecified** thumb **with damage to nail**

S61.14- **Puncture** wound **with foreign body** of **thumb** **with damage to nail**
- **S61.141-** Puncture wound **with foreign body** of **right** thumb **with damage to nail**
- **S61.142-** Puncture wound **with foreign body** of **left** thumb **with damage to nail**
- **S61.149-** Puncture wound **with foreign body** of **unspecified** thumb **with damage to nail**

S61.15- <u>Open bite</u> of <u>thumb</u> <u>with damage to nail</u>
  Bite of thumb with damage to nail NOS
  Excludes 1: superficial bite of thumb (S60.36-, S60.37-)

  S61.151- Open bite of <u>right</u> thumb <u>with damage to nail</u>

  S61.152- Open bite of <u>left</u> thumb <u>with damage to nail</u>

  S61.159- Open bite of <u>unspecified</u> thumb <u>with damage to nail</u>

S61.2- <u>Open wound</u> of <u>other finger</u> <u>without</u> damage to nail
  Excludes 1: open wound of finger involving nail (matrix) (S61.3-)
  Excludes ❷: open wound of thumb without damage to nail (S61.0-)

  S61.20- <u>Unspecified</u> open wound of <u>other finger</u> <u>without</u> damage to nail

  S61.200- Unspecified open wound of <u>right</u> <u>index</u> finger <u>without</u> damage to nail

  S61.201- Unspecified open wound of <u>left</u> <u>index</u> finger <u>without</u> damage to nail

  S61.202- Unspecified open wound of <u>right</u> <u>middle</u> finger <u>without</u> damage to nail

  S61.203- Unspecified open wound of <u>left</u> <u>middle</u> finger <u>without</u> damage to nail

  S61.204- Unspecified open wound of <u>right</u> <u>ring</u> finger <u>without</u> damage to nail

  S61.205- Unspecified open wound of <u>left</u> <u>ring</u> finger <u>without</u> damage to nail

  S61.206- Unspecified open wound of <u>right</u> <u>little</u> finger <u>without</u> damage to nail

  S61.207- Unspecified open wound of <u>left</u> <u>little</u> finger <u>without</u> damage to nail

  S61.208- Unspecified open wound of <u>other</u> finger <u>without</u> damage to nail
    Unspecified open wound of specified finger with unspecified laterality without damage to nail

  S61.209- Unspecified open wound of <u>unspecified</u> finger <u>without</u> damage to nail

  S61.21- <u>Laceration</u> <u>without</u> foreign body of <u>finger</u> <u>without</u> damage to nail

  S61.210- Laceration <u>without</u> foreign body of <u>right</u> <u>index</u> finger <u>without</u> damage to nail

  S61.211- Laceration <u>without</u> foreign body of <u>left</u> <u>index</u> finger <u>without</u> damage to nail

  S61.212- Laceration <u>without</u> foreign body of <u>right</u> <u>middle</u> finger <u>without</u> damage to nail

  S61.213- Laceration <u>without</u> foreign body of <u>left</u> <u>middle</u> finger <u>without</u> damage to nail

  S61.214- Laceration <u>without</u> foreign body of <u>right</u> <u>ring</u> finger <u>without</u> damage to nail

  S61.215- Laceration <u>without</u> foreign body of <u>left</u> <u>ring</u> finger <u>without</u> damage to nail

  S61.216- Laceration <u>without</u> foreign body of <u>right</u> <u>little</u> finger <u>without</u> damage to nail

  S61.217- Laceration <u>without</u> foreign body of <u>left</u> <u>little</u> finger <u>without</u> damage to nail

  S61.218- Laceration <u>without</u> foreign body of <u>other</u> finger <u>without</u> damage to nail
    Laceration without foreign body of specified finger with unspecified laterality without damage to nail

  S61.219- Laceration <u>without</u> foreign body of <u>unspecified</u> finger <u>without</u> damage to nail

  S61.22- <u>Laceration</u> <u>with foreign body</u> of <u>finger</u> <u>without</u> damage to nail

  S61.220- Laceration <u>with foreign body</u> of <u>right</u> <u>index</u> finger <u>without</u> damage to nail

  S61.221- Laceration <u>with foreign body</u> of <u>left</u> <u>index</u> finger <u>without</u> damage to nail

  S61.222- Laceration <u>with foreign body</u> of <u>right</u> <u>middle</u> finger <u>without</u> damage to nail

  S61.223- Laceration <u>with foreign body</u> of <u>left</u> <u>middle</u> finger <u>without</u> damage to nail

  S61.224- Laceration <u>with foreign body</u> of <u>right</u> <u>ring</u> finger <u>without</u> damage to nail

  S61.225- Laceration <u>with foreign body</u> of <u>left</u> <u>ring</u> finger <u>without</u> damage to nail

  S61.226- Laceration <u>with foreign body</u> of <u>right</u> <u>little</u> finger <u>without</u> damage to nail

  S61.227- Laceration <u>with foreign body</u> of <u>left</u> <u>little</u> finger <u>without</u> damage to nail

  S61.228- Laceration <u>with foreign body</u> of <u>other</u> finger <u>without</u> damage to nail
    Laceration with foreign body of specified finger with unspecified laterality without damage to nail

  S61.229- Laceration <u>with foreign body</u> of <u>unspecified</u> finger <u>without</u> damage to nail

  S61.23- <u>Puncture</u> wound <u>without</u> foreign body of finger <u>without</u> damage to nail

  S61.230- Puncture wound <u>without</u> foreign body of <u>right</u> <u>index</u> finger <u>without</u> damage to nail

  S61.231- Puncture wound <u>without</u> foreign body of <u>left</u> <u>index</u> finger <u>without</u> damage to nail

  S61.232- Puncture wound <u>without</u> foreign body of <u>right</u> <u>middle</u> finger <u>without</u> damage to nail

  S61.233- Puncture wound <u>without</u> foreign body of <u>left</u> <u>middle</u> finger <u>without</u> damage to nail

  S61.234- Puncture wound <u>without</u> foreign body of <u>right</u> <u>ring</u> finger <u>without</u> damage to nail

  S61.235- Puncture wound <u>without</u> foreign body of <u>left</u> <u>ring</u> finger <u>without</u> damage to nail

  S61.236- Puncture wound <u>without</u> foreign body of <u>right</u> <u>little</u> finger <u>without</u> damage to nail

  S61.237- Puncture wound <u>without</u> foreign body of <u>left</u> <u>little</u> finger <u>without</u> damage to nail

  S61.238- Puncture wound <u>without</u> foreign body of other <u>finger</u> <u>without</u> damage to nail
    Puncture wound without foreign body of specified finger with unspecified laterality without damage to nail

  S61.239- Puncture wound <u>without</u> foreign body of <u>unspecified</u> finger <u>without</u> damage to nail

  S61.24- <u>Puncture</u> wound <u>with foreign body</u> of finger <u>without</u> damage to nail

  S61.240- Puncture wound <u>with foreign body</u> of <u>right</u> <u>index</u> finger <u>without</u> damage to nail

  S61.241- Puncture wound <u>with foreign body</u> of <u>left</u> <u>index</u> finger <u>without</u> damage to nail

  S61.242- Puncture wound <u>with foreign body</u> of <u>right</u> <u>middle</u> finger <u>without</u> damage to nail

  S61.243- Puncture wound <u>with foreign body</u> of <u>left</u> <u>middle</u> finger <u>without</u> damage to nail

  S61.244- Puncture wound <u>with foreign body</u> of <u>right</u> <u>ring</u> finger <u>without</u> damage to nail

  S61.245- Puncture wound <u>with foreign body</u> of <u>left</u> <u>ring</u> finger <u>without</u> damage to nail

  S61.246- Puncture wound <u>with foreign body</u> of <u>right</u> <u>little</u> finger <u>without</u> damage to nail

  S61.247- Puncture wound <u>with foreign body</u> of <u>left</u> <u>little</u> finger <u>without</u> damage to nail

  S61.248- Puncture wound <u>with foreign body</u> of <u>other</u> finger <u>without</u> damage to nail
    Puncture wound with foreign body of specified finger with unspecified laterality without damage to nail

  S61.249- Puncture wound <u>with foreign body</u> of <u>unspecified</u> finger <u>without</u> damage to nail

S61.25- <u>Open bite</u> of finger <u>without</u> damage to nail
  Bite of finger without damage to nail NOS
  Excludes 1: superficial bite of finger (S60.46-, S60.47-)

  S61.250- Open bite of <u>right</u> <u>index</u> finger <u>without</u> damage to nail

  S61.251- Open bite of <u>left</u> <u>index</u> finger <u>without</u> damage to nail

  S61.252- Open bite of <u>right</u> <u>middle</u> finger <u>without</u> damage to nail

---

Excludes 1: = NOT CODED HERE! (Do not code both)   **1082**   *Excludes ❷:* = Not Included Here

S61.253- Open bite of <u>left</u> <u>middle</u> finger <u>without</u> damage to nail

S61.254- Open bite of <u>right</u> <u>ring</u> finger <u>without</u> damage to nail

S61.255- Open bite of <u>left</u> <u>ring</u> finger <u>without</u> damage to nail

S61.256- Open bite of <u>right</u> <u>little</u> finger <u>without</u> damage to nail

S61.257- Open bite of <u>left</u> <u>little</u> finger <u>without</u> damage to nail

S61.258- Open bite of other <u>finger</u> <u>without</u> damage to nail
    Open bite of specified finger with unspecified laterality
    without damage to nail

S61.259- Open bite of <u>unspecified</u> finger <u>without</u> damage to nail

S61.3- <u>Open wound of</u> other finger <u>with damage to nail</u>

S61.30- <u>Unspecified open wound</u> of <u>finger</u> <u>with damage to nail</u>

S61.300- Unspecified open wound of <u>right</u> <u>index</u> finger <u>with damage to nail</u>

S61.301- Unspecified open wound of <u>left</u> <u>index</u> finger <u>with damage to nail</u>

S61.302- Unspecified open wound of <u>right</u> <u>middle</u> finger <u>with damage to nail</u>

S61.303- Unspecified open wound of <u>left</u> <u>middle</u> finger <u>with damage to nail</u>

S61.304- Unspecified open wound of <u>right</u> <u>ring</u> finger <u>with damage to nail</u>

S61.305- Unspecified open wound of <u>left</u> <u>ring</u> finger <u>with damage to nail</u>

S61.306- Unspecified open wound of <u>right</u> <u>little</u> finger <u>with damage to nail</u>

S61.307- Unspecified open wound of <u>left</u> <u>little</u> finger <u>with damage to nail</u>

S61.308- Unspecified open wound of <u>other</u> finger <u>with damage to nail</u>
    Unspecified open wound of specified finger with
    unspecified laterality with damage to nail

S61.309- Unspecified open wound of <u>unspecified</u> finger <u>with damage to nail</u>

S61.31- <u>Laceration</u> <u>without</u> foreign body of <u>finger</u> <u>with damage to nail</u>

S61.310- Laceration <u>without</u> foreign body of <u>right</u> <u>index</u> finger <u>with damage to nail</u>

S61.311- Laceration <u>without</u> foreign body of <u>left</u> <u>index</u> finger <u>with damage to nail</u>

S61.312- Laceration <u>without</u> foreign body of <u>right</u> <u>middle</u> finger <u>with damage to nail</u>

S61.313- Laceration <u>without</u> foreign body of <u>left</u> <u>middle</u> finger <u>with damage to nail</u>

S61.314- Laceration <u>without</u> foreign body of <u>right</u> <u>ring</u> finger <u>with damage to nail</u>

S61.315- Laceration <u>without</u> foreign body of <u>left</u> <u>ring</u> finger <u>with damage to nail</u>

S61.316- Laceration <u>without</u> foreign body of <u>right</u> <u>little</u> finger <u>with damage to nail</u>

S61.317- Laceration <u>without</u> foreign body of <u>left</u> <u>little</u> finger <u>with damage to nail</u>

S61.318- Laceration <u>without</u> foreign body of <u>other</u> finger <u>with damage to nail</u>
    Laceration without foreign body of specified finger
    with unspecified laterality with damage to nail

S61.319- Laceration <u>without</u> foreign body of <u>unspecified</u> finger <u>with damage to nail</u>

S61.32- <u>Laceration</u> <u>with foreign body</u> of <u>finger</u> <u>with damage to nail</u>

S61.320- Laceration <u>with foreign body</u> of <u>right</u> <u>index</u> finger <u>with damage to nail</u>

S61.321- Laceration <u>with foreign body</u> of <u>left</u> <u>index</u> finger <u>with damage to nail</u>

S61.322- Laceration <u>with foreign body</u> of <u>right</u> <u>middle</u> finger <u>with damage to nail</u>

S61.323- Laceration <u>with foreign body</u> of <u>left</u> <u>middle</u> finger <u>with damage to nail</u>

S61.324- Laceration <u>with foreign body</u> of <u>right</u> <u>ring</u> finger <u>with damage to nail</u>

S61.325- Laceration <u>with foreign body</u> of <u>left</u> <u>ring</u> finger <u>with damage to nail</u>

S61.326- Laceration <u>with foreign body</u> of <u>right</u> <u>little</u> finger <u>with damage to nail</u>

S61.327- Laceration <u>with foreign body</u> of <u>left</u> <u>little</u> finger <u>with damage to nail</u>

S61.328- Laceration <u>with foreign body</u> of <u>other</u> finger <u>with damage to nail</u>
    Laceration with foreign body of specified finger with
    unspecified laterality with damage to nail

S61.329- Laceration <u>with foreign body</u> of <u>unspecified</u> finger <u>with damage to nail</u>

S61.33- <u>Puncture</u> wound <u>without</u> foreign body of <u>finger</u> with <u>damage to nail</u>

S61.330- Puncture wound <u>without</u> foreign body of <u>right</u> <u>index</u> finger <u>with damage to nail</u>

S61.331- Puncture wound <u>without</u> foreign body of <u>left</u> <u>index</u> finger <u>with damage to nail</u>

S61.332- Puncture wound <u>without</u> foreign body of <u>right</u> <u>middle</u> finger <u>with damage to nail</u>

S61.333- Puncture wound <u>without</u> foreign body of <u>left</u> <u>middle</u> finger <u>with damage to nail</u>

S61.334- Puncture wound <u>without</u> foreign body of <u>right</u> <u>ring</u> finger <u>with damage to nail</u>

S61.335- Puncture wound <u>without</u> foreign body of <u>left</u> <u>ring</u> finger <u>with damage to nail</u>

S61.336- Puncture wound <u>without</u> foreign body of <u>right</u> <u>little</u> finger <u>with damage to nail</u>

S61.337- Puncture wound <u>without</u> foreign body of <u>left</u> <u>little</u> finger <u>with damage to nail</u>

S61.338- Puncture wound <u>without</u> foreign body of <u>other</u> finger <u>with damage to nail</u>
    Puncture wound without foreign body of specified
    finger with unspecified laterality with damage to
    nail

S61.339- Puncture wound <u>without</u> foreign body of <u>unspecified</u> finger <u>with damage to nail</u>

S61.34- <u>Puncture</u> wound <u>with foreign body</u> of <u>finger</u> <u>with damage to nail</u>

S61.340- Puncture wound <u>with foreign body</u> of <u>right</u> <u>index</u> finger <u>with damage to nail</u>

S61.341- Puncture wound <u>with foreign body</u> of <u>left</u> <u>index</u> finger <u>with damage to nail</u>

S61.342- Puncture wound <u>with foreign body</u> of <u>right</u> <u>middle</u> finger <u>with damage to nail</u>

S61.343- Puncture wound <u>with foreign body</u> of <u>left</u> <u>middle</u> finger <u>with damage to nail</u>

S61.344- Puncture wound <u>with foreign body</u> of <u>right</u> <u>ring</u> finger <u>with damage to nail</u>

S61.345- Puncture wound <u>with foreign body</u> of <u>left</u> <u>ring</u> finger <u>with damage to nail</u>

S61.346- Puncture wound <u>with foreign body</u> of <u>right</u> <u>little</u> finger <u>with damage to nail</u>

S61.347- Puncture wound <u>with foreign body</u> of <u>left</u> <u>little</u> finger <u>with damage to nail</u>

S61.348- Puncture wound <u>with foreign body</u> of <u>other</u> finger <u>with damage to nail</u>
    Puncture wound with foreign body of specified finger
    with unspecified laterality with damage to nail

S61.349- Puncture wound <u>with foreign body</u> of <u>unspecified</u> finger <u>with damage to nail</u>

S 6 1 - S 6 1

S61.35- Open bite of finger with damage to nail
Bite of finger with damage to nail NOS
Excludes 1: superficial bite of finger (S60.46-, S60.47-)

S61.350- Open bite of right index finger with damage to nail
S61.351- Open bite of left index finger with damage to nail
S61.352- Open bite of right middle finger with damage to nail
S61.353- Open bite of left middle finger with damage to nail
S61.354- Open bite of right ring finger with damage to nail
S61.355- Open bite of left ring finger with damage to nail
S61.356- Open bite of right little finger with damage to nail
S61.357- Open bite of left little finger with damage to nail
S61.358- Open bite of other finger with damage to nail
Open bite of specified finger with unspecified laterality with damage to nail
S61.359- Open bite of unspecified finger with damage to nail

S61.4- Open wound of hand
S61.40- Unspecified open wound of hand
S61.401- Unspecified open wound of right hand
S61.402- Unspecified open wound of left hand
S61.409- Unspecified open wound of unspecified hand
S61.41- Laceration without foreign body of hand
S61.411- Laceration without foreign body of right hand
S61.412- Laceration without foreign body of left hand
S61.419- Laceration without foreign body of unspecified hand
S61.42- Laceration with foreign body of hand
S61.421- Laceration with foreign body of right hand
S61.422- Laceration with foreign body of left hand
S61.429- Laceration with foreign body of unspecified hand
S61.43- Puncture wound without foreign body of hand
S61.431- Puncture wound without foreign body of right hand
S61.432- Puncture wound without foreign body of left hand
S61.439- Puncture wound without foreign body of unspecified hand
S61.44- Puncture wound with foreign body of hand
S61.441- Puncture wound with foreign body of right hand
S61.442- Puncture wound with foreign body of left hand
S61.449- Puncture wound with foreign body of unspecified hand
S61.45- Open bite of hand
Bite of hand NOS
Excludes 1: superficial bite of hand (S60.56-, S60.57-)
S61.451- Open bite of right hand
S61.452- Open bite of left hand
S61.459- Open bite of unspecified hand

S61.5- Open wound of wrist
S61.50- Unspecified open wound of wrist
S61.501- Unspecified open wound of right wrist
S61.502- Unspecified open wound of left wrist
S61.509- Unspecified open wound of unspecified wrist
S61.51- Laceration without foreign body of wrist
S61.511- Laceration without foreign body of right wrist
S61.512- Laceration without foreign body of left wrist
S61.519- Laceration without foreign body of unspecified wrist
S61.52- Laceration with foreign body of wrist
S61.521- Laceration with foreign body of right wrist
S61.522- Laceration with foreign body of left wrist
S61.529- Laceration with foreign body of unspecified wrist
S61.53- Puncture wound without foreign body of wrist
S61.531- Puncture wound without foreign body of right wrist
S61.532- Puncture wound without foreign body of left wrist
S61.539- Puncture wound without foreign body of unspecified wrist

S61.54- Puncture wound with foreign body of wrist
S61.541- Puncture wound with foreign body of right wrist
S61.542- Puncture wound with foreign body of left wrist
S61.549- Puncture wound with foreign body of unspecified wrist
S61.55- Open bite of wrist
Bite of wrist NOS
Excludes 1: superficial bite of wrist (S60.86-, S60.87-)
S61.551- Open bite of right wrist
S61.552- Open bite of left wrist
S61.559- Open bite of unspecified wrist

S62- Fracture at wrist and hand level
Note: A fracture not indicated as displaced or nondisplaced should be coded to displaced
Note: A fracture not indicated as open or closed should be coded to closed
Excludes 1: traumatic amputation of wrist and hand (S68.-)
Excludes ❷: fracture of distal parts of ulna and radius (S52.-)

The appropriate 7th character is to be added to each code from category S62:
A   Initial encounter for closed fracture
B   Initial encounter for open fracture
D   Subsequent encounter for fracture with routine healing
G   Subsequent encounter for fracture with delayed healing
K   Subsequent encounter for fracture with nonunion
P   Subsequent encounter for fracture with malunion
S   Sequela

S62.0- Fracture of navicular [scaphoid] bone of wrist
S62.00- Unspecified fracture of navicular [scaphoid] bone of wrist
CC-B,K,P **S62.001-** Unspecified fracture of navicular [scaphoid] bone of right wrist
CC-B,K,P **S62.002-** Unspecified fracture of navicular [scaphoid] bone of left wrist
CC-B,K,P **S62.009-** Unspecified fracture of navicular [scaphoid] bone of unspecified wrist
S62.01- Fracture of distal pole of navicular [scaphoid] bone of wrist
Fracture of volar tuberosity of navicular [scaphoid] bone of wrist
CC-B,K,P **S62.011-** Displaced fracture of distal pole of navicular [scaphoid] bone of right wrist
CC-B,K,P **S62.012-** Displaced fracture of distal pole of navicular [scaphoid] bone of left wrist
CC-B,K,P **S62.013-** Displaced fracture of distal pole of navicular [scaphoid] bone of unspecified wrist
CC-B,K,P **S62.014-** Nondisplaced fracture of distal pole of navicular [scaphoid] bone of right wrist
CC-B,K,P **S62.015-** Nondisplaced fracture of distal pole of navicular [scaphoid] bone of left wrist
CC-B,K,P **S62.016-** Nondisplaced fracture of distal pole of navicular [scaphoid] bone of unspecified wrist
S62.02- Fracture of middle third of navicular [scaphoid] bone of wrist
CC-B,K,P **S62.021-** Displaced fracture of middle third of navicular [scaphoid] bone of right wrist
CC-B,K,P **S62.022-** Displaced fracture of middle third of navicular [scaphoid] bone of left wrist
CC-B,K,P **S62.023-** Displaced fracture of middle third of navicular [scaphoid] bone of unspecified wrist
CC-B,K,P **S62.024-** Nondisplaced fracture of middle third of navicular [scaphoid] bone of right wrist
CC-B,K,P **S62.025-** Nondisplaced fracture of middle third of navicular [scaphoid] bone of left wrist
CC-B,K,P **S62.026-** Nondisplaced fracture of middle third of navicular [scaphoid] bone of unspecified wrist
S62.03- Fracture of proximal third of navicular [scaphoid] bone of wrist
CC-B,K,P **S62.031-** Displaced fracture of proximal third of navicular [scaphoid] bone of right wrist
CC-B,K,P **S62.032-** Displaced fracture of proximal third of navicular [scaphoid] bone of left wrist

S 6 1 - S 6 2

CC-B,K,P **S62.033-** <u>Displaced</u> fracture of proximal third of navicular [scaphoid] bone of <u>unspecified</u> wrist

CC-B,K,P **S62.034-** <u>Nondisplaced</u> fracture of proximal third of navicular [scaphoid] bone of <u>right</u> wrist

CC-B,K,P **S62.035-** <u>Nondisplaced</u> fracture of proximal third of navicular [scaphoid] bone of <u>left</u> wrist

CC-B,K,P **S62.036-** <u>Nondisplaced</u> fracture of proximal third of navicular [scaphoid] bone of <u>unspecified</u> wrist

S62.1- Fracture of <u>other and unspecified</u> carpal bone(s)

Excludes ❷: *fracture of scaphoid of wrist (S62.0-)*

S62.10- Fracture of <u>unspecified</u> carpal bone
Fracture of wrist NOS

CC-B,K,P **S62.101-** Fracture of <u>unspecified</u> carpal bone, <u>right</u> wrist

CC-B,K,P **S62.102-** Fracture of <u>unspecified</u> carpal bone, <u>left</u> wrist

CC-B,K,P **S62.109-** Fracture of <u>unspecified</u> carpal bone, <u>unspecified</u> wrist

S62.11- Fracture of <u>triquetrum [cuneiform]</u> bone of <u>wrist</u>

CC-B,K,P **S62.111-** <u>Displaced</u> fracture of triquetrum [cuneiform] bone, <u>right</u> wrist

CC-B,K,P **S62.112-** <u>Displaced</u> fracture of triquetrum [cuneiform] bone, <u>left</u> wrist

CC-B,K,P **S62.113-** <u>Displaced</u> fracture of triquetrum [cuneiform] bone, <u>unspecified</u> wrist

CC-B,K,P **S62.114-** <u>Nondisplaced</u> fracture of triquetrum [cuneiform] bone, <u>right</u> wrist

CC-B,K,P **S62.115-** <u>Nondisplaced</u> fracture of triquetrum [cuneiform] bone, <u>left</u> wrist

CC-B,K,P **S62.116-** <u>Nondisplaced</u> fracture of triquetrum [cuneiform] bone, <u>unspecified</u> wrist

S62.12- Fracture of <u>lunate [semilunar]</u>

CC-B,K,P **S62.121-** <u>Displaced</u> fracture of lunate [semilunar], <u>right</u> wrist

CC-B,K,P **S62.122-** <u>Displaced</u> fracture of lunate [semilunar], <u>left</u> wrist

CC-B,K,P **S62.123-** <u>Displaced</u> fracture of lunate [semilunar], <u>unspecified</u> wrist

CC-B,K,P **S62.124-** <u>Nondisplaced</u> fracture of lunate [semilunar], <u>right</u> wrist

CC-B,K,P **S62.125-** <u>Nondisplaced</u> fracture of lunate [semilunar], <u>left</u> wrist

CC-B,K,P **S62.126-** <u>Nondisplaced</u> fracture of lunate [semilunar], <u>unspecified</u> wrist

S62.13- Fracture of <u>capitate [os magnum]</u> bone

CC-B,K,P **S62.131-** <u>Displaced</u> fracture of capitate [os magnum] bone, <u>right</u> wrist

CC-B,K,P **S62.132-** <u>Displaced</u> fracture of capitate [os magnum] bone, <u>left</u> wrist

CC-B,K,P **S62.133-** <u>Displaced</u> fracture of capitate [os magnum] bone, <u>unspecified</u> wrist

CC-B,K,P **S62.134-** <u>Nondisplaced</u> fracture of capitate [os magnum] bone, <u>right</u> wrist

CC-B,K,P **S62.135-** <u>Nondisplaced</u> fracture of capitate [os magnum] bone, <u>left</u> wrist

CC-B,K,P **S62.136-** <u>Nondisplaced</u> fracture of capitate [os magnum] bone, <u>unspecified</u> wrist

S62.14- Fracture of body of <u>hamate [unciform]</u> bone
Fracture of hamate [unciform] bone NOS

CC-B,K,P **S62.141-** <u>Displaced</u> fracture of body of hamate [unciform] bone, <u>right</u> wrist

CC-B,K,P **S62.142-** <u>Displaced</u> fracture of body of hamate [unciform] bone, <u>left</u> wrist

CC-B,K,P **S62.143-** <u>Displaced</u> fracture of body of hamate [unciform] bone, <u>unspecified</u> wrist

CC-B,K,P **S62.144-** <u>Nondisplaced</u> fracture of body of hamate [unciform] bone, <u>right</u> wrist

CC-B,K,P **S62.145-** <u>Nondisplaced</u> fracture of body of hamate [unciform] bone, <u>left</u> wrist

CC-B,K,P **S62.146-** <u>Nondisplaced</u> fracture of body of hamate [unciform] bone, <u>unspecified</u> wrist

S62.15- Fracture of <u>hook process</u> of <u>hamate [unciform]</u> bone
Fracture of unciform process of hamate [unciform] bone

CC-B,K,P **S62.151-** <u>Displaced</u> fracture of hook process of hamate [unciform] bone, <u>right</u> wrist

CC-B,K,P **S62.152-** <u>Displaced</u> fracture of hook process of hamate [unciform] bone, <u>left</u> wrist

CC-B,K,P **S62.153-** <u>Displaced</u> fracture of hook process of hamate [unciform] bone, <u>unspecified</u> wrist

CC-B,K,P **S62.154-** <u>Nondisplaced</u> fracture of hook process of hamate [unciform] bone, <u>right</u> wrist

CC-B,K,P **S62.155-** <u>Nondisplaced</u> fracture of hook process of hamate [unciform] bone, <u>left</u> wrist

CC-B,K,P **S62.156-** <u>Nondisplaced</u> fracture of hook process of hamate [unciform] bone, <u>unspecified</u> wrist

S62.16- Fracture of <u>pisiform</u>

CC-B,K,P **S62.161-** <u>Displaced</u> fracture of pisiform, <u>right</u> wrist

CC-B,K,P **S62.162-** <u>Displaced</u> fracture of pisiform, <u>left</u> wrist

CC-B,K,P **S62.163-** <u>Displaced</u> fracture of pisiform, <u>unspecified</u> wrist

CC-B,K,P **S62.164-** <u>Nondisplaced</u> fracture of pisiform, <u>right</u> wrist

CC-B,K,P **S62.165-** <u>Nondisplaced</u> fracture of pisiform, <u>left</u> wrist

CC-B,K,P **S62.166-** <u>Nondisplaced</u> fracture of pisiform, <u>unspecified</u> wrist

S62.17- Fracture of <u>trapezium [larger multangular]</u>

CC-B,K,P **S62.171-** <u>Displaced</u> fracture of trapezium [larger multangular], <u>right</u> wrist

CC-B,K,P **S62.172-** <u>Displaced</u> fracture of trapezium [larger multangular], <u>left</u> wrist

CC-B,K,P **S62.173-** <u>Displaced</u> fracture of trapezium [larger multangular], <u>unspecified</u> wrist

CC-B,K,P **S62.174-** <u>Nondisplaced</u> fracture of trapezium [larger multangular], <u>right</u> wrist

CC-B,K,P **S62.175-** <u>Nondisplaced</u> fracture of trapezium [larger multangular], <u>left</u> wrist

CC-B,K,P **S62.176-** <u>Nondisplaced</u> fracture of trapezium [larger multangular], <u>unspecified</u> wrist

S62.18- Fracture of <u>trapezoid [smaller multangular]</u>

CC-B,K,P **S62.181-** <u>Displaced</u> fracture of trapezoid [smaller multangular], <u>right</u> wrist

CC-B,K,P **S62.182-** <u>Displaced</u> fracture of trapezoid [smaller multangular], <u>left</u> wrist

CC-B,K,P **S62.183-** <u>Displaced</u> fracture of trapezoid [smaller multangular], <u>unspecified</u> wrist

CC-B,K,P **S62.184-** <u>Nondisplaced</u> fracture of trapezoid [smaller multangular], <u>right</u> wrist

CC-B,K,P **S62.185-** <u>Nondisplaced</u> fracture of trapezoid [smaller multangular], <u>left</u> wrist

CC-B,K,P **S62.186-** <u>Nondisplaced</u> fracture of trapezoid [smaller multangular], <u>unspecified</u> wrist

S62.2- Fracture of <u>first metacarpal</u> bone

S62.20- <u>Unspecified</u> fracture of <u>first metacarpal</u> bone

CC-B,K,P **S62.201-** Unspecified fracture of first metacarpal bone, <u>right</u> hand

CC-B,K,P **S62.202-** Unspecified fracture of first metacarpal bone, <u>left</u> hand

CC-B,K,P **S62.209-** Unspecified fracture of first metacarpal bone, <u>unspecified</u> hand

S62.21- <u>Bennett's</u> fracture

CC-B,K,P **S62.211-** Bennett's fracture, <u>right</u> hand

CC-B,K,P **S62.212-** Bennett's fracture, <u>left</u> hand

CC-B,K,P **S62.213-** Bennett's fracture, <u>unspecified</u> hand

S62.22- <u>Rolando's</u> fracture

CC-B,K,P **S62.221-** <u>Displaced</u> Rolando's fracture, <u>right</u> hand

CC-B,K,P **S62.222-** <u>Displaced</u> Rolando's fracture, <u>left</u> hand

CC-B,K,P **S62.223-** <u>Displaced</u> Rolando's fracture, <u>unspecified</u> hand

CC-B,K,P **S62.224-** <u>Nondisplaced</u> Rolando's fracture, <u>right</u> hand

CC-B,K,P **S62.225-** <u>Nondisplaced</u> Rolando's fracture, <u>left</u> hand

CC-B,K,P **S62.226-** <u>Nondisplaced</u> Rolando's fracture, <u>unspecified</u> hand

S 6 2 – S 6 2

S62.23- <u>Other</u> fracture of <u>base</u> of <u>first</u> <u>metacarpal</u> bone

CC-B,K,P **S62.231-** Other <u>displaced</u> fracture of base of first metacarpal bone, <u>right</u> hand

CC-B,K,P **S62.232-** Other <u>displaced</u> fracture of base of first metacarpal bone, <u>left</u> hand

CC-B,K,P **S62.233-** Other <u>displaced</u> fracture of base of first metacarpal bone, <u>unspecified</u> hand

CC-B,K,P **S62.234-** Other <u>nondisplaced</u> fracture of base of first metacarpal bone, <u>right</u> hand

CC-B,K,P **S62.235-** Other <u>nondisplaced</u> fracture of base of first metacarpal bone, <u>left</u> hand

CC-B,K,P **S62.236-** Other <u>nondisplaced</u> fracture of base of first metacarpal bone, <u>unspecified</u> hand

S62.24- Fracture of <u>shaft</u> of <u>first</u> <u>metacarpal</u> bone

CC-B,K,P **S62.241-** <u>Displaced</u> fracture of shaft of first metacarpal bone, <u>right</u> hand

CC-B,K,P **S62.242-** <u>Displaced</u> fracture of shaft of first metacarpal bone, <u>left</u> hand

CC-B,K,P **S62.243-** <u>Displaced</u> fracture of shaft of first metacarpal bone, <u>unspecified</u> hand

CC-B,K,P **S62.244-** <u>Nondisplaced</u> fracture of shaft of first metacarpal bone, <u>right</u> hand

CC-B,K,P **S62.245-** <u>Nondisplaced</u> fracture of shaft of first metacarpal bone, <u>left</u> hand

CC-B,K,P **S62.246-** <u>Nondisplaced</u> fracture of shaft of first metacarpal bone, <u>unspecified</u> hand

S62.25- Fracture of <u>neck</u> of <u>first</u> <u>metacarpal</u> bone

CC-B,K,P **S62.251-** <u>Displaced</u> fracture of neck of first metacarpal bone, <u>right</u> hand

CC-B,K,P **S62.252-** <u>Displaced</u> fracture of neck of first metacarpal bone, <u>left</u> hand

CC-B,K,P **S62.253-** <u>Displaced</u> fracture of neck of first metacarpal bone, <u>unspecified</u> hand

CC-B,K,P **S62.254-** <u>Nondisplaced</u> fracture of neck of first metacarpal bone, <u>right</u> hand

CC-B,K,P **S62.255-** <u>Nondisplaced</u> fracture of neck of first metacarpal bone, <u>left</u> hand

CC-B,K,P **S62.256-** <u>Nondisplaced</u> fracture of neck of first metacarpal bone, <u>unspecified</u> hand

S62.29- <u>Other</u> fracture of <u>first</u> <u>metacarpal</u> bone

CC-B,K,P **S62.291-** Other fracture of first metacarpal bone, <u>right</u> hand

CC-B,K,P **S62.292-** Other fracture of first metacarpal bone, <u>left</u> hand

CC-B,K,P **S62.299-** Other fracture of first metacarpal bone, <u>unspecified</u> hand

S62.3- Fracture of <u>other and unspecified</u> <u>metacarpal</u> bone

Excludes ❷: fracture of first metacarpal bone (S62.2-)

S62.30- <u>Unspecified</u> fracture of <u>other</u> <u>metacarpal</u> bone

CC-B,K,P **S62.300-** Unspecified fracture of <u>second</u> metacarpal bone, <u>right</u> hand

CC-B,K,P **S62.301-** Unspecified fracture of <u>second</u> metacarpal bone, <u>left</u> hand

CC-B,K,P **S62.302-** Unspecified fracture of <u>third</u> metacarpal bone, <u>right</u> hand

CC-B,K,P **S62.303-** Unspecified fracture of <u>third</u> metacarpal bone, <u>left</u> hand

CC-B,K,P **S62.304-** Unspecified fracture of <u>fourth</u> metacarpal bone, <u>right</u> hand

CC-B,K,P **S62.305-** Unspecified fracture of <u>fourth</u> metacarpal bone, <u>left</u> hand

CC-B,K,P **S62.306-** Unspecified fracture of <u>fifth</u> metacarpal bone, <u>right</u> hand

CC-B,K,P **S62.307-** Unspecified fracture of <u>fifth</u> metacarpal bone, <u>left</u> hand

CC-B,K,P **S62.308-** Unspecified fracture of <u>other</u> metacarpal bone
Unspecified fracture of specified metacarpal bone with unspecified laterality

CC-B,K,P **S62.309-** Unspecified fracture of <u>unspecified</u> metacarpal bone

S62.31- <u>Displaced</u> fracture of <u>base</u> of <u>other</u> <u>metacarpal</u> bone

CC-B,K,P **S62.310-** <u>Displaced</u> fracture of <u>base</u> of <u>second</u> metacarpal bone, <u>right</u> hand

CC-B,K,P **S62.311-** <u>Displaced</u> fracture of <u>base</u> of <u>second</u> metacarpal bone. <u>left</u> hand

CC-B,K,P **S62.312-** <u>Displaced</u> fracture of <u>base</u> of <u>third</u> metacarpal bone, <u>right</u> hand

CC-B,K,P **S62.313-** <u>Displaced</u> fracture of <u>base</u> of <u>third</u> metacarpal bone, <u>left</u> hand

CC-B,K,P **S62.314-** <u>Displaced</u> fracture of <u>base</u> of <u>fourth</u> metacarpal bone, <u>right</u> hand

CC-B,K,P **S62.315-** <u>Displaced</u> fracture of <u>base</u> of <u>fourth</u> metacarpal bone, <u>left</u> hand

CC-B,K,P **S62.316-** <u>Displaced</u> fracture of <u>base</u> of <u>fifth</u> metacarpal bone, <u>right</u> hand

CC-B,K,P **S62.317-** <u>Displaced</u> fracture of <u>base</u> of <u>fifth</u> metacarpal bone. <u>left</u> hand

CC-B,K,P **S62.318-** <u>Displaced</u> fracture of <u>base</u> of <u>other</u> metacarpal bone
Displaced fracture of base of specified metacarpal bone with unspecified laterality

CC-B,K,P **S62.319-** <u>Displaced</u> fracture of <u>base</u> of <u>unspecified</u> metacarpal bone

S62.32- <u>Displaced</u> fracture of <u>shaft</u> of <u>other</u> <u>metacarpal</u> bone

CC-B,K,P **S62.320-** <u>Displaced</u> fracture of <u>shaft</u> of <u>second</u> metacarpal bone, <u>right</u> hand

CC-B,K,P **S62.321-** <u>Displaced</u> fracture of <u>shaft</u> of <u>second</u> metacarpal bone, <u>left</u> hand

CC-B,K,P **S62.322-** <u>Displaced</u> fracture of <u>shaft</u> of <u>third</u> metacarpal bone, <u>right</u> hand

CC-B,K,P **S62.323-** <u>Displaced</u> fracture of <u>shaft</u> of <u>third</u> metacarpal bone, <u>left</u> hand

CC-B,K,P **S62.324-** <u>Displaced</u> fracture of <u>shaft</u> of <u>fourth</u> metacarpal bone, <u>right</u> hand

CC-B,K,P **S62.325-** <u>Displaced</u> fracture of <u>shaft</u> of <u>fourth</u> metacarpal bone, <u>left</u> hand

CC-B,K,P **S62.326-** <u>Displaced</u> fracture of <u>shaft</u> of <u>fifth</u> metacarpal bone, <u>right</u> hand

CC-B,K,P **S62.327-** <u>Displaced</u> fracture of <u>shaft</u> of <u>fifth</u> metacarpal bone, <u>left</u> hand

CC-B,K,P **S62.328-** <u>Displaced</u> fracture of <u>shaft</u> of <u>other</u> metacarpal bone
Displaced fracture of shaft of specified metacarpal bone with unspecified laterality

CC-B,K,P **S62.329-** <u>Displaced</u> fracture of <u>shaft</u> of <u>unspecified</u> metacarpal bone

S62.33- <u>Displaced</u> fracture of <u>neck</u> of <u>other</u> <u>metacarpal</u> bone

CC-B,K,P **S62.330-** <u>Displaced</u> fracture of <u>neck</u> of <u>second</u> metacarpal bone, <u>right</u> hand

CC-B,K,P **S62.331-** <u>Displaced</u> fracture of <u>neck</u> of <u>second</u> metacarpal bone, <u>left</u> hand

CC-B,K,P **S62.332-** <u>Displaced</u> fracture of <u>neck</u> of <u>third</u> metacarpal bone, <u>right</u> hand

CC-B,K,P **S62.333-** <u>Displaced</u> fracture of <u>neck</u> of <u>third</u> metacarpal bone, <u>left</u> hand

CC-B,K,P **S62.334-** <u>Displaced</u> fracture of <u>neck</u> of <u>fourth</u> metacarpal bone, <u>right</u> hand

CC-B,K,P **S62.335-** <u>Displaced</u> fracture of <u>neck</u> of <u>fourth</u> metacarpal bone, <u>left</u> hand

CC-B,K,P **S62.336-** <u>Displaced</u> fracture of <u>neck</u> of <u>fifth</u> metacarpal bone, <u>right</u> hand

CC-B,K,P **S62.337-** <u>Displaced</u> fracture of <u>neck</u> of <u>fifth</u> metacarpal bone, <u>left</u> hand

CC-B,K,P **S62.338-** <u>Displaced</u> fracture of <u>neck</u> of <u>other</u> metacarpal bone
Displaced fracture of neck of specified metacarpal bone with unspecified laterality

CC-B,K,P **S62.339-** <u>Displaced</u> fracture of <u>neck</u> of <u>unspecified</u> metacarpal bone

S 6 2 - S 6 2

S62.34- Nondisplaced fracture of base of other metacarpal bone

CC-B,K,P **S62.340-** Nondisplaced fracture of base of second metacarpal bone, right hand

CC-B,K,P **S62.341-** Nondisplaced fracture of base of second metacarpal bone, left hand

CC-B,K,P **S62.342-** Nondisplaced fracture of base of third metacarpal bone, right hand

CC-B,K,P **S62.343-** Nondisplaced fracture of base of third metacarpal bone, left hand

CC-B,K,P **S62.344-** Nondisplaced fracture of base of fourth metacarpal bone, right hand

CC-B,K,P **S62.345-** Nondisplaced fracture of base of fourth metacarpal bone, left hand

CC-B,K,P **S62.346-** Nondisplaced fracture of base of fifth metacarpal bone, right hand

CC-B,K,P **S62.347-** Nondisplaced fracture of base of fifth metacarpal bone. left hand

CC-B,K,P **S62.348-** Nondisplaced fracture of base of other metacarpal bone
Nondisplaced fracture of base of specified metacarpal bone with unspecified laterality

CC-B,K,P **S62.349-** Nondisplaced fracture of base of unspecified metacarpal bone

S62.35- Nondisplaced fracture of shaft of other metacarpal bone

CC-B,K,P **S62.350-** Nondisplaced fracture of shaft of second metacarpal bone, right hand

CC-B,K,P **S62.351-** Nondisplaced fracture of shaft of second metacarpal bone, left hand

CC-B,K,P **S62.352-** Nondisplaced fracture of shaft of third metacarpal bone, right hand

CC-B,K,P **S62.353-** Nondisplaced fracture of shaft of third metacarpal bone, left hand

CC-B,K,P **S62.354-** Nondisplaced fracture of shaft of fourth metacarpal bone, right hand

CC-B,K,P **S62.355-** Nondisplaced fracture of shaft of fourth metacarpal bone, left hand

CC-B,K,P **S62.356-** Nondisplaced fracture of shaft of fifth metacarpal bone, right hand

CC-B,K,P **S62.357-** Nondisplaced fracture of shaft of fifth metacarpal bone, left hand

CC-B,K,P **S62.358-** Nondisplaced fracture of shaft of other metacarpal bone
Nondisplaced fracture of shaft of specified metacarpal bone with unspecified laterality

CC-B,K,P **S62.359-** Nondisplaced fracture of shaft of unspecified metacarpal bone

S62.36- Nondisplaced fracture of neck of other metacarpal bone

CC-B,K,P **S62.360-** Nondisplaced fracture of neck of second metacarpal bone, right hand

CC-B,K,P **S62.361-** Nondisplaced fracture of neck of second metacarpal bone, left hand

CC-B,K,P **S62.362-** Nondisplaced fracture of neck of third metacarpal bone, right hand

CC-B,K,P **S62.363-** Nondisplaced fracture of neck of third metacarpal bone, left hand

CC-B,K,P **S62.364-** Nondisplaced fracture of neck of fourth metacarpal bone, right hand

CC-B,K,P **S62.365-** Nondisplaced fracture of neck of fourth metacarpal bone, left hand

CC-B,K,P **S62.366-** Nondisplaced fracture of neck of fifth metacarpal bone, right hand

CC-B,K,P **S62.367-** Nondisplaced fracture of neck of fifth metacarpal bone, left hand

CC-B,K,P **S62.368-** Nondisplaced fracture of neck of other metacarpal bone
Nondisplaced fracture of neck of specified metacarpal bone with unspecified laterality

CC-B,K,P **S62.369-** Nondisplaced fracture of neck of unspecified metacarpal bone

S62.39- Other fracture of other metacarpal bone

CC-B,K,P **S62.390-** Other fracture of second metacarpal bone, right hand

CC-B,K,P **S62.391-** Other fracture of second metacarpal bone, left hand

CC-B,K,P **S62.392-** Other fracture of third metacarpal bone, right hand

CC-B,K,P **S62.393-** Other fracture of third metacarpal bone, left hand

CC-B,K,P **S62.394-** Other fracture of fourth metacarpal bone, right hand

CC-B,K,P **S62.395-** Other fracture of fourth metacarpal bone, left hand

CC-B,K,P **S62.396-** Other fracture of fifth metacarpal bone, right hand

CC-B,K,P **S62.397-** Other fracture of fifth metacarpal bone, left hand

CC-B,K,P **S62.398-** Other fracture of other metacarpal bone
Other fracture of specified metacarpal bone with unspecified laterality

CC-B,K,P **S62.399-** Other fracture of unspecified metacarpal bone

S62.5- Fracture of thumb

S62.50- Fracture of unspecified phalanx of thumb

CC-B,K,P **S62.501-** Fracture of unspecified phalanx of right thumb

CC-B,K,P **S62.502-** Fracture of unspecified phalanx of left thumb

CC-B,K,P **S62.509-** Fracture of unspecified phalanx of unspecified thumb

S62.51- Fracture of proximal phalanx of thumb

CC-B,K,P **S62.511-** Displaced fracture of proximal phalanx of right thumb

CC-B,K,P **S62.512-** Displaced fracture of proximal phalanx of left thumb

CC-B,K,P **S62.513-** Displaced fracture of proximal phalanx of unspecified thumb

CC-B,K,P **S62.514-** Nondisplaced fracture of proximal phalanx of right thumb

CC-B,K,P **S62.515-** Nondisplaced fracture of proximal phalanx of left thumb

CC-B,K,P **S62.516-** Nondisplaced fracture of proximal phalanx of unspecified thumb

S62.52- Fracture of distal phalanx of thumb

CC-B,K,P **S62.521-** Displaced fracture of distal phalanx of right thumb

CC-B,K,P **S62.522-** Displaced fracture of distal phalanx of left thumb

CC-B,K,P **S62.523-** Displaced fracture of distal phalanx of unspecified thumb

CC-B,K,P **S62.524-** Nondisplaced fracture of distal phalanx of right thumb

CC-B,K,P **S62.525-** Nondisplaced fracture of distal phalanx of left thumb

CC-B,K,P **S62.526-** Nondisplaced fracture of distal phalanx of unspecified thumb

S62.6- Fracture of other and unspecified finger(s)
Excludes 2: fracture of thumb (S62.5-)

S62.60- Fracture of unspecified phalanx of finger

CC-B,K,P **S62.600-** Fracture of unspecified phalanx of right index finger

CC-B,K,P **S62.601-** Fracture of unspecified phalanx of left index finger

CC-B,K,P **S62.602-** Fracture of unspecified phalanx of right middle finger

CC-B,K,P **S62.603-** Fracture of unspecified phalanx of left middle finger

CC-B,K,P **S62.604-** Fracture of unspecified phalanx of right ring finger

CC-B,K,P **S62.605-** Fracture of unspecified phalanx of left ring finger

CC-B,K,P **S62.606-** Fracture of unspecified phalanx of right little finger

CC-B,K,P **S62.607-** Fracture of unspecified phalanx of left little finger

CC-B,K,P **S62.608-** Fracture of unspecified phalanx of other finger
Fracture of unspecified phalanx of specified finger with unspecified laterality

CC-B,K,P **S62.609-** Fracture of unspecified phalanx of unspecified finger

S62.61- Displaced fracture of proximal phalanx of finger

CC-B,K,P **S62.610-** Displaced fracture of proximal phalanx of right index finger

S62-S62

CC-B,K,P **S62.611-** <u>Displaced</u> fracture of <u>proximal</u> phalanx of <u>left</u> <u>index</u> finger

CC-B,K,P **S62.612-** <u>Displaced</u> fracture of <u>proximal</u> phalanx of <u>right</u> <u>middle</u> finger

CC-B,K,P **S62.613-** <u>Displaced</u> fracture of <u>proximal</u> phalanx of <u>left</u> <u>middle</u> finger

CC-B,K,P **S62.614-** <u>Displaced</u> fracture of <u>proximal</u> phalanx of <u>right</u> <u>ring</u> finger

CC-B,K,P **S62.615-** <u>Displaced</u> fracture of <u>proximal</u> phalanx of <u>left ring</u> finger

CC-B,K,P **S62.616-** <u>Displaced</u> fracture of <u>proximal</u> phalanx of <u>right</u> <u>little</u> finger

CC-B,K,P **S62.617-** <u>Displaced</u> fracture of <u>proximal</u> phalanx of <u>left little</u> finger

CC-B,K,P **S62.618-** <u>Displaced</u> fracture of <u>proximal</u> phalanx of <u>other</u> finger
Displaced fracture of proximal phalanx of specified finger with unspecified laterality

CC-B,K,P **S62.619-** <u>Displaced</u> fracture of proximal phalanx of <u>unspecified</u> finger

S62.62- <u>Displaced</u> fracture of <u>medial</u> <u>phalanx</u> of <u>finger</u>

CC-B,K,P **S62.620-** <u>Displaced</u> fracture of <u>medial</u> phalanx of <u>right index</u> finger

CC-B,K,P **S62.621-** <u>Displaced</u> fracture of <u>medial</u> phalanx of <u>left index</u> finger

CC-B,K,P **S62.622-** <u>Displaced</u> fracture of <u>medial</u> phalanx of <u>right</u> <u>middle</u> finger

CC-B,K,P **S62.623-** <u>Displaced</u> fracture of <u>medial</u> phalanx of <u>left middle</u> finger

CC-B,K,P **S62.624-** <u>Displaced</u> fracture of <u>medial</u> phalanx of <u>right ring</u> finger

CC-B,K,P **S62.625-** <u>Displaced</u> fracture of <u>medial</u> phalanx of <u>left ring</u> finger

CC-B,K,P **S62.626-** <u>Displaced</u> fracture of <u>medial</u> phalanx of <u>right little</u> finger

CC-B,K,P **S62.627-** <u>Displaced</u> fracture of <u>medial</u> phalanx of <u>left little</u> finger

CC-B,K,P **S62.628-** <u>Displaced</u> fracture of <u>medial</u> phalanx of <u>other</u> finger
Displaced fracture of medial phalanx of specified finger with unspecified laterality

CC-B,K,P **S62.629-** <u>Displaced</u> fracture of <u>medial</u> phalanx of <u>unspecified</u> finger

S62.63- <u>Displaced</u> fracture of <u>distal</u> <u>phalanx</u> of <u>finger</u>

CC-B,K,P **S62.630-** <u>Displaced</u> fracture of <u>distal</u> phalanx of <u>right index</u> finger

CC-B,K,P **S62.631-** <u>Displaced</u> fracture of <u>distal</u> phalanx of <u>left index</u> finger

CC-B,K,P **S62.632-** <u>Displaced</u> fracture of <u>distal</u> phalanx of <u>right middle</u> finger

CC-B,K,P **S62.633-** <u>Displaced</u> fracture of <u>distal</u> phalanx of <u>left middle</u> finger

CC-B,K,P **S62.634-** <u>Displaced</u> fracture of <u>distal</u> phalanx of <u>right ring</u> finger

CC-B,K,P **S62.635-** <u>Displaced</u> fracture of <u>distal</u> phalanx of <u>left ring</u> finger

CC-B,K,P **S62.636-** <u>Displaced</u> fracture of <u>distal</u> phalanx of <u>right little</u> finger

CC-B,K,P **S62.637-** <u>Displaced</u> fracture of <u>distal</u> phalanx of <u>left little</u> finger

CC-B,K,P **S62.638-** <u>Displaced</u> fracture of <u>distal</u> phalanx of <u>other</u> finger
Displaced fracture of distal phalanx of specified finger with unspecified laterality

CC-B,K,P **S62.639-** <u>Displaced</u> fracture of <u>distal</u> phalanx of <u>unspecified</u> finger

S62.64- <u>Nondisplaced</u> fracture of <u>proximal</u> <u>phalanx</u> of <u>finger</u>

CC-B,K,P **S62.640-** <u>Nondisplaced</u> fracture of <u>proximal</u> phalanx of <u>right</u> <u>index</u> finger

CC-B,K,P **S62.641-** <u>Nondisplaced</u> fracture of <u>proximal</u> phalanx of <u>left</u> <u>index</u> finger

CC-B,K,P **S62.642-** <u>Nondisplaced</u> fracture of <u>proximal</u> phalanx of <u>right</u> <u>middle</u> finger

CC-B,K,P **S62.643-** <u>Nondisplaced</u> fracture of <u>proximal</u> phalanx of <u>left</u> <u>middle</u> finger

CC-B,K,P **S62.644-** <u>Nondisplaced</u> fracture of <u>proximal</u> phalanx of <u>right</u> <u>ring</u> finger

CC-B,K,P **S62.645-** <u>Nondisplaced</u> fracture of <u>proximal</u> phalanx of <u>left</u> <u>ring</u> finger

CC-B,K,P **S62.646-** <u>Nondisplaced</u> fracture of <u>proximal</u> phalanx of <u>right</u> <u>little</u> finger

CC-B,K,P **S62.647-** <u>Nondisplaced</u> fracture of <u>proximal</u> phalanx of <u>left</u> <u>little</u> finger

CC-B,K,P **S62.648-** <u>Nondisplaced</u> fracture of <u>proximal</u> phalanx of <u>other</u> finger
Nondisplaced fracture of proximal phalanx of specified finger with unspecified laterality

CC-B,K,P **S62.649-** <u>Nondisplaced</u> fracture of <u>proximal</u> phalanx of <u>unspecified</u> finger

S62.65- <u>Nondisplaced</u> fracture of <u>medial</u> <u>phalanx</u> of <u>finger</u>

CC-B,K,P **S62.650-** <u>Nondisplaced</u> fracture of <u>medial</u> phalanx of <u>right</u> <u>index</u> finger

CC-B,K,P **S62.651-** <u>Nondisplaced</u> fracture of <u>medial</u> phalanx of <u>left</u> <u>index</u> finger

CC-B,K,P **S62.652-** <u>Nondisplaced</u> fracture of <u>medial</u> phalanx of <u>right</u> <u>middle</u> finger

CC-B,K,P **S62.653-** <u>Nondisplaced</u> fracture of <u>medial</u> phalanx of <u>left</u> <u>middle</u> finger

CC-B,K,P **S62.654-** <u>Nondisplaced</u> fracture of <u>medial</u> phalanx of <u>right</u> <u>ring</u> finger

CC-B,K,P **S62.655-** <u>Nondisplaced</u> fracture of <u>medial</u> phalanx of <u>left</u> <u>ring</u> finger

CC-B,K,P **S62.656-** <u>Nondisplaced</u> fracture of <u>medial</u> phalanx of <u>right</u> <u>little</u> finger

CC-B,K,P **S62.657-** <u>Nondisplaced</u> fracture of <u>medial</u> phalanx of <u>left</u> <u>little</u> finger

CC-B,K,P **S62.658-** <u>Nondisplaced</u> fracture of <u>medial</u> phalanx of <u>other</u> finger
Nondisplaced fracture of medial phalanx of specified finger with unspecified laterality

CC-B,K,P **S62.659-** <u>Nondisplaced</u> fracture of <u>medial</u> phalanx of <u>unspecified</u> finger

S62.66- <u>Nondisplaced</u> fracture of <u>distal</u> <u>phalanx</u> of <u>finger</u>

CC-B,K,P **S62.660-** <u>Nondisplaced</u> fracture of <u>distal</u> phalanx of <u>right</u> <u>index</u> finger

CC-B,K,P **S62.661-** <u>Nondisplaced</u> fracture of <u>distal</u> phalanx of <u>left</u> <u>index</u> finger

CC-B,K,P **S62.662-** <u>Nondisplaced</u> fracture of <u>distal</u> phalanx of <u>right</u> <u>middle</u> finger

CC-B,K,P **S62.663-** <u>Nondisplaced</u> fracture of <u>distal</u> phalanx of <u>left</u> <u>middle</u> finger

CC-B,K,P **S62.664-** <u>Nondisplaced</u> fracture of <u>distal</u> phalanx of <u>right</u> <u>ring</u> finger

CC-B,K,P **S62.665-** <u>Nondisplaced</u> fracture of <u>distal</u> phalanx of <u>left ring</u> finger

CC-B,K,P **S62.666-** <u>Nondisplaced</u> fracture of <u>distal</u> phalanx of <u>right</u> <u>little</u> finger

CC-B,K,P **S62.667-** <u>Nondisplaced</u> fracture of <u>distal</u> phalanx of <u>left</u> <u>little</u> finger

CC-B,K,P **S62.668-** <u>Nondisplaced</u> fracture of <u>distal</u> phalanx of <u>other</u> finger
Nondisplaced fracture of distal phalanx of specified finger with unspecified laterality

CC-B,K,P **S62.669-** <u>Nondisplaced</u> fracture of <u>distal</u> phalanx of <u>unspecified</u> finger

S62.9- <u>Unspecified</u> <u>fracture</u> of <u>wrist and hand</u>

CC-B,K,P **S62.90x-** Unspecified fracture of <u>unspecified</u> wrist and hand

CC-B,K,P **S62.91x-** Unspecified fracture of <u>right</u> wrist and hand

CC-B,K,P **S62.92x-** Unspecified fracture of <u>left</u> wrist and hand

S63- **Dislocation and sprain** of joints and ligaments at <u>wrist and hand</u> <u>level</u>

Includes: Avulsion of joint or ligament at wrist and hand level
Laceration of cartilage, joint or ligament at wrist and hand level
Sprain of cartilage, joint or ligament at wrist and hand level
Traumatic hemarthrosis of joint or ligament at wrist and hand level
Traumatic rupture of joint or ligament at wrist and hand level
Traumatic subluxation of joint or ligament at wrist and hand level
Traumatic tear of joint or ligament at wrist and hand level

Code also any associated open wound

Excludes ❷: *strain of muscle, fascia and tendon of wrist and hand (S66.-)*

The appropriate 7th character is to be added to each code from category S63:

A **Initial** encounter
D **Subsequent** encounter
S **Sequela**

S63.0- **Subluxation and dislocation** of <u>wrist and hand joints</u>

S63.00- **Unspecified** subluxation and dislocation of <u>wrist and hand</u>
Dislocation of carpal bone NOS
Dislocation of distal end of radius NOS
Subluxation of carpal bone NOS
Subluxation of distal end of radius NOS

S63.001- Unspecified <u>subluxation</u> of <u>right</u> wrist and hand
S63.002- Unspecified <u>subluxation</u> of <u>left</u> wrist and hand
S63.003- Unspecified <u>subluxation</u> of <u>unspecified</u> wrist and hand
S63.004- Unspecified <u>dislocation</u> of <u>right</u> wrist and hand
S63.005- Unspecified <u>dislocation</u> of <u>left</u> wrist and hand
S63.006- Unspecified <u>dislocation</u> of <u>unspecified</u> wrist and hand

S63.01- Subluxation and dislocation of <u>distal radioulnar joint</u>
S63.011- <u>Subluxation</u> of distal radioulnar joint of <u>right</u> wrist
S63.012- <u>Subluxation</u> of distal radioulnar joint of left wrist
S63.013- <u>Subluxation</u> of distal radioulnar joint of <u>unspecified</u> wrist
S63.014- <u>Dislocation</u> of distal radioulnar joint of <u>right</u> wrist
S63.015- <u>Dislocation</u> of distal radioulnar joint of <u>left</u> wrist
S63.016- <u>Dislocation</u> of distal radioulnar joint of <u>unspecified</u> wrist

S63.02- Subluxation and dislocation of <u>radiocarpal joint</u>
S63.021- <u>Subluxation</u> of radiocarpal joint of <u>right</u> wrist
S63.022- <u>Subluxation</u> of radiocarpal joint of <u>left</u> wrist
S63.023- <u>Subluxation</u> of radiocarpal joint of <u>unspecified</u> wrist
S63.024- <u>Dislocation</u> of radiocarpal joint of <u>right</u> wrist
S63.025- <u>Dislocation</u> of radiocarpal joint of <u>left</u> wrist
S63.026- <u>Dislocation</u> of radiocarpal joint of <u>unspecified</u> wrist

S63.03- Subluxation and dislocation of <u>midcarpal joint</u>
S63.031- <u>Subluxation</u> of midcarpal joint of <u>right</u> wrist
S63.032- <u>Subluxation</u> of midcarpal joint of <u>left</u> wrist
S63.033- <u>Subluxation</u> of midcarpal joint of <u>unspecified</u> wrist
S63.034- <u>Dislocation</u> of midcarpal joint of <u>right</u> wrist
S63.035- <u>Dislocation</u> of midcarpal joint of <u>left</u> wrist
S63.036- <u>Dislocation</u> of midcarpal joint of <u>unspecified</u> wrist

S63.04- Subluxation and dislocation of <u>carpometacarpal joint</u> of thumb
Excludes ❷: *interphalangeal subluxation and dislocation of thumb (S63.1-)*
S63.041- <u>Subluxation</u> of carpometacarpal joint of <u>right</u> thumb
S63.042- <u>Subluxation</u> of carpometacarpal joint of <u>left</u> thumb
S63.043- <u>Subluxation</u> of carpometacarpal joint of <u>unspecified</u> thumb
S63.044- <u>Dislocation</u> of carpometacarpal joint of <u>right</u> thumb
S63.045- <u>Dislocation</u> of carpometacarpal joint of <u>left</u> thumb
S63.046- <u>Dislocation</u> of carpometacarpal joint of <u>unspecified</u> thumb

S63.05- Subluxation and dislocation of <u>other carpometacarpal joint</u>
Excludes ❷: *subluxation and dislocation of carpometacarpal joint of thumb (S63.04-)*
S63.051- <u>Subluxation</u> of other carpometacarpal joint of <u>right</u> hand
S63.052- <u>Subluxation</u> of other carpometacarpal joint of <u>left</u> hand
S63.053- <u>Subluxation</u> of other carpometacarpal joint of <u>unspecified</u> hand
S63.054- <u>Dislocation</u> of other carpometacarpal joint of <u>right</u> hand
S63.055- <u>Dislocation</u> of other carpometacarpal joint of <u>left</u> hand
S63.056- <u>Dislocation</u> of other carpometacarpal joint of <u>unspecified</u> hand

S63.06- Subluxation and dislocation of <u>metacarpal (bone), proximal end</u>
S63.061- <u>Subluxation</u> of metacarpal (bone), proximal end of <u>right</u> hand
S63.062- <u>Subluxation</u> of metacarpal (bone), proximal end of <u>left</u> hand
S63.063- <u>Subluxation</u> of metacarpal (bone), proximal end of <u>unspecified</u> hand
S63.064- <u>Dislocation</u> of metacarpal (bone), proximal end of <u>right</u> hand
S63.065- <u>Dislocation</u> of metacarpal (bone), proximal end of <u>left</u> hand
S63.066- <u>Dislocation</u> of metacarpal (bone), proximal end of <u>unspecified</u> hand

S63.07- Subluxation and dislocation of <u>distal end of ulna</u>
S63.071- <u>Subluxation</u> of distal end of <u>right</u> ulna
S63.072- <u>Subluxation</u> of distal end of <u>left</u> ulna
S63.073- <u>Subluxation</u> of distal end of <u>unspecified</u> ulna
S63.074- <u>Dislocation</u> of distal end of <u>right</u> ulna
S63.075- <u>Dislocation</u> of distal end of <u>left</u> ulna
S63.076- <u>Dislocation</u> of distal end of <u>unspecified</u> ulna

S63.09- <u>Other</u> subluxation and dislocation of <u>wrist and hand</u>
S63.091- Other <u>subluxation</u> of <u>right</u> wrist and hand
S63.092- Other <u>subluxation</u> of <u>left</u> wrist and hand
S63.093- Other <u>subluxation</u> of <u>unspecified</u> wrist and hand
S63.094- Other <u>dislocation</u> of <u>right</u> wrist and hand
S63.095- Other <u>dislocation</u> of <u>left</u> wrist and hand
S63.096- Other <u>dislocation</u> of <u>unspecified</u> wrist and hand

S63.1- Subluxation and dislocation of <u>thumb</u>
S63.10- <u>Unspecified</u> subluxation and dislocation of <u>thumb</u>
S63.101- Unspecified <u>subluxation</u> of <u>right</u> thumb
S63.102- Unspecified <u>subluxation</u> of <u>left</u> thumb
S63.103- Unspecified <u>subluxation</u> of <u>unspecified</u> thumb
S63.104- Unspecified <u>dislocation</u> of <u>right</u> thumb
S63.105- Unspecified <u>dislocation</u> of <u>left</u> thumb
S63.106- Unspecified <u>dislocation</u> of <u>unspecified</u> thumb

S63.11- Subluxation and dislocation of <u>metacarpophalangeal joint</u> of thumb
S63.111- <u>Subluxation</u> of metacarpophalangeal joint of <u>right</u> thumb
S63.112- <u>Subluxation</u> of metacarpophalangeal joint of <u>left</u> thumb
S63.113- <u>Subluxation</u> of metacarpophalangeal joint of <u>unspecified</u> thumb
S63.114- <u>Dislocation</u> of metacarpophalangeal joint of <u>right</u> thumb
S63.115- <u>Dislocation</u> of metacarpophalangeal joint of <u>left</u> thumb
S63.116- <u>Dislocation</u> of metacarpophalangeal joint of <u>unspecified</u> thumb

S 6 3 – S 6 3

S63.12- Subluxation and dislocation of <u>unspecified interphalangeal joint</u> of <u>thumb</u>

   S63.121- <u>Subluxation</u> of unspecified interphalangeal joint of <u>right</u> thumb

   S63.122- <u>Subluxation</u> of unspecified interphalangeal joint of <u>left</u> thumb

   S63.123- <u>Subluxation</u> of unspecified interphalangeal joint of <u>unspecified</u> thumb

   S63.124- <u>Dislocation</u> of unspecified interphalangeal joint of <u>right</u> thumb

   S63.125- <u>Dislocation</u> of unspecified interphalangeal joint of <u>left</u> thumb

   S63.126- <u>Dislocation</u> of unspecified interphalangeal joint of <u>unspecified</u> thumb

S63.13- Subluxation and dislocation of <u>proximal interphalangeal joint</u> of <u>thumb</u>

   S63.131- <u>Subluxation</u> of proximal interphalangeal joint of <u>right</u> thumb

   S63.132- <u>Subluxation</u> of proximal interphalangeal joint of <u>left</u> thumb

   S63.133- <u>Subluxation</u> of proximal interphalangeal joint of <u>unspecified</u> thumb

   S63.134- <u>Dislocation</u> of proximal interphalangeal joint of <u>right</u> thumb

   S63.135- <u>Dislocation</u> of proximal interphalangeal joint of <u>left</u> thumb

   S63.136- <u>Dislocation</u> of proximal interphalangeal joint of <u>unspecified</u> thumb

S63.14- Subluxation and dislocation of <u>distal interphalangeal joint</u> of <u>thumb</u>

   S63.141- <u>Subluxation</u> of distal interphalangeal joint of <u>right</u> thumb

   S63.142- <u>Subluxation</u> of distal interphalangeal joint of <u>left</u> thumb

   S63.143- <u>Subluxation</u> of distal interphalangeal joint of <u>unspecified</u> thumb

   S63.144- <u>Dislocation</u> of distal interphalangeal joint of <u>right</u> thumb

   S63.145- <u>Dislocation</u> of distal interphalangeal joint of <u>left</u> thumb

   S63.146- <u>Dislocation</u> of distal interphalangeal joint of <u>unspecified</u> thumb

S63.2- Subluxation and dislocation of <u>other finger(s)</u>
   Excludes ❷: subluxation and dislocation of thumb (S63.1-)

S63.20- <u>Unspecified subluxation</u> of other <u>finger</u>

   S63.200- Unspecified subluxation of <u>right index</u> finger

   S63.201- Unspecified subluxation of <u>left index</u> finger

   S63.202- Unspecified subluxation of <u>right middle</u> finger

   S63.203- Unspecified subluxation of <u>left middle</u> finger

   S63.204- Unspecified subluxation of <u>right ring</u> finger

   S63.205- Unspecified subluxation of <u>left ring</u> finger

   S63.206- Unspecified subluxation of <u>right little</u> finger

   S63.207- Unspecified subluxation of <u>left little</u> finger

   S63.208- Unspecified subluxation of <u>other</u> finger
      Unspecified subluxation of specified finger with unspecified laterality

   S63.209- Unspecified subluxation of <u>unspecified</u> finger

S63.21- <u>Subluxation</u> of <u>metacarpophalangeal joint</u> of <u>finger</u>

   S63.210- Subluxation of metacarpophalangeal joint of <u>right index</u> finger

   S63.211- Subluxation of metacarpophalangeal joint of <u>left index</u> finger

   S63.212- Subluxation of metacarpophalangeal joint of <u>right middle</u> finger

   S63.213- Subluxation of metacarpophalangeal joint of <u>left middle</u> finger

   S63.214- Subluxation of metacarpophalangeal joint of <u>right ring</u> finger

   S63.215- Subluxation of metacarpophalangeal joint of <u>left ring</u> finger

   S63.216- Subluxation of metacarpophalangeal joint of <u>right little</u> finger

   S63.217- Subluxation of metacarpophalangeal joint of <u>left little</u> finger

   S63.218- Subluxation of metacarpophalangeal joint of <u>other</u> finger
      Subluxation of metacarpophalangeal joint of specified finger with unspecified laterality

   S63.219- Subluxation of metacarpophalangeal joint of <u>unspecified</u> finger

S63.22- <u>Subluxation</u> of <u>unspecified interphalangeal joint</u> of <u>finger</u>

   S63.220- Subluxation of unspecified interphalangeal joint of <u>right index</u> finger

   S63.221- Subluxation of unspecified interphalangeal joint of <u>left index</u> finger

   S63.222- Subluxation of unspecified interphalangeal joint of <u>right middle</u> finger

   S63.223- Subluxation of unspecified interphalangeal joint of <u>left middle</u> finger

   S63.224- Subluxation of unspecified interphalangeal joint of <u>right ring</u> finger

   S63.225- Subluxation of unspecified interphalangeal joint of <u>left ring</u> finger

   S63.226- Subluxation of unspecified interphalangeal joint of <u>right little</u> finger

   S63.227- Subluxation of unspecified interphalangeal joint of <u>left little</u> finger

   S63.228- Subluxation of unspecified interphalangeal joint of <u>other</u> finger
      Subluxation of unspecified interphalangeal joint of specified finger with unspecified laterality

   S63.229- Subluxation of unspecified interphalangeal joint of <u>unspecified</u> finger

S63.23- <u>Subluxation</u> of <u>proximal interphalangeal joint</u> of <u>finger</u>

   S63.230- Subluxation of proximal interphalangeal joint of <u>right index</u> finger

   S63.231- Subluxation of proximal interphalangeal joint of <u>left index</u> finger

   S63.232- Subluxation of proximal interphalangeal joint of <u>right middle</u> finger

   S63.233- Subluxation of proximal interphalangeal joint of <u>left middle</u> finger

   S63.234- Subluxation of proximal interphalangeal joint of <u>right ring</u> finger

   S63.235- Subluxation of proximal interphalangeal joint of <u>left ring</u> finger

   S63.236- Subluxation of proximal interphalangeal joint of <u>right little</u> finger

   S63.237- Subluxation of proximal interphalangeal joint of <u>left little</u> finger

   S63.238- Subluxation of proximal interphalangeal joint of <u>other</u> finger
      Subluxation of proximal interphalangeal joint of specified finger with unspecified laterality

   S63.239- Subluxation of proximal interphalangeal joint of <u>unspecified</u> finger

S63.24- <u>Subluxation</u> of <u>distal interphalangeal joint</u> of <u>finger</u>

   S63.240- Subluxation of distal interphalangeal joint of <u>right index</u> finger

   S63.241- Subluxation of distal interphalangeal joint of <u>left index</u> finger

   S63.242- Subluxation of distal interphalangeal joint of <u>right middle</u> finger

   S63.243- Subluxation of distal interphalangeal joint of <u>left middle</u> finger

   S63.244- Subluxation of distal interphalangeal joint of <u>right ring</u> finger

S63.245- Subluxation of distal interphalangeal joint of <u>left ring</u> finger

S63.246- Subluxation of distal interphalangeal joint of <u>right little</u> finger

S63.247- Subluxation of distal interphalangeal joint of <u>left little</u> finger

S63.248- Subluxation of distal interphalangeal joint of <u>other</u> finger
  Subluxation of distal interphalangeal joint of specified finger with unspecified laterality

S63.249- Subluxation of distal interphalangeal joint of <u>unspecified</u> finger

S63.25- <u>Unspecified</u> <u>dislocation</u> of <u>other</u> <u>finger</u>

S63.250- Unspecified dislocation of <u>right index</u> finger

S63.251- Unspecified dislocation of <u>left index</u> finger

S63.252- Unspecified dislocation of <u>right middle</u> finger

S63.253- Unspecified dislocation of <u>left middle</u> finger

S63.254- Unspecified dislocation of <u>right ring</u> finger

S63.255- Unspecified dislocation of <u>left ring</u> finger

S63.256- Unspecified dislocation of <u>right little</u> finger

S63.257- Unspecified dislocation of <u>left little</u> finger

S63.258- Unspecified dislocation of <u>other</u> finger
  Unspecified dislocation of specified finger with unspecified laterality

S63.259- Unspecified dislocation of <u>unspecified</u> finger
  Unspecified dislocation of specified finger with unspecified laterality

S63.26- <u>Dislocation</u> of <u>metacarpophalangeal joint</u> of <u>finger</u>

S63.260- Dislocation of metacarpophalangeal joint of <u>right index</u> finger

S63.261- Dislocation of metacarpophalangeal joint of <u>left index</u> finger

S63.262- Dislocation of metacarpophalangeal joint of <u>right middle</u> finger

S63.263- Dislocation of metacarpophalangeal joint of <u>left middle</u> finger

S63.264- Dislocation of metacarpophalangeal joint of <u>right ring</u> finger

S63.265- Dislocation of metacarpophalangeal joint of <u>left ring</u> finger

S63.266- Dislocation of metacarpophalangeal joint of <u>right little</u> finger

S63.267- Dislocation of metacarpophalangeal joint of <u>left little</u> finger

S63.268- Dislocation of metacarpophalangeal joint of <u>other</u> finger
  Dislocation of metacarpophalangeal joint of specified finger with unspecified laterality

S63.269- Dislocation of metacarpophalangeal joint of <u>unspecified</u> finger

S63.27- <u>Dislocation</u> of <u>unspecified interphalangeal joint</u> of <u>finger</u>

S63.270- Dislocation of unspecified interphalangeal joint of <u>right index</u> finger

S63.271- Dislocation of unspecified interphalangeal joint of <u>left index</u> finger

S63.272- Dislocation of unspecified interphalangeal joint of <u>right middle</u> finger

S63.273- Dislocation of unspecified interphalangeal joint of <u>left middle</u> finger

S63.274- Dislocation of unspecified interphalangeal joint of <u>right ring</u> finger

S63.275- Dislocation of unspecified interphalangeal joint of <u>left ring</u> finger

S63.276- Dislocation of unspecified interphalangeal joint of <u>right little</u> finger

S63.277- Dislocation of unspecified interphalangeal joint of <u>left little</u> finger

S63.278- Dislocation of unspecified interphalangeal joint of <u>other</u> finger
  Dislocation of unspecified interphalangeal joint of specified finger with unspecified laterality

S63.279- Dislocation of unspecified interphalangeal joint of <u>unspecified</u> finger
  Dislocation of unspecified interphalangeal joint of specified finger without specified laterality

S63.28- Dislocation of <u>proximal interphalangeal joint</u> of <u>finger</u>

S63.280- Dislocation of proximal interphalangeal joint of <u>right index</u> finger

S63.281- Dislocation of proximal interphalangeal joint of <u>left index</u> finger

S63.282- Dislocation of proximal interphalangeal joint of <u>right middle</u> finger

S63.283- Dislocation of proximal interphalangeal joint of <u>left middle</u> finger

S63.284- Dislocation of proximal interphalangeal joint of <u>right ring</u> finger

S63.285- Dislocation of proximal interphalangeal joint of <u>left ring</u> finger

S63.286- Dislocation of proximal interphalangeal joint of <u>right little</u> finger

S63.287- Dislocation of proximal interphalangeal joint of <u>left little</u> finger

S63.288- Dislocation of proximal interphalangeal joint of <u>other</u> finger
  Dislocation of proximal interphalangeal joint of specified finger with unspecified laterality

S63.289- Dislocation of proximal interphalangeal joint of <u>unspecified</u> finger

S63.29- <u>Dislocation</u> of <u>distal interphalangeal joint</u> of <u>finger</u>

S63.290- Dislocation of distal interphalangeal joint of <u>right index</u> finger

S63.291- Dislocation of distal interphalangeal joint of <u>left index</u> finger

S63.292- Dislocation of distal interphalangeal joint of <u>right middle</u> finger

S63.293- Dislocation of distal interphalangeal joint of <u>left middle</u> finger

S63.294- Dislocation of distal interphalangeal joint of <u>right ring</u> finger

S63.295- Dislocation of distal interphalangeal joint of <u>left ring</u> finger

S63.296- Dislocation of distal interphalangeal joint of <u>right little</u> finger

S63.297- Dislocation of distal interphalangeal joint of <u>left little</u> finger

S63.298- Dislocation of distal interphalangeal joint of <u>other</u> finger
  Dislocation of distal interphalangeal joint of specified finger with unspecified laterality

S63.299- Dislocation of distal interphalangeal joint of <u>unspecified</u> finger

S63.3- <u>Traumatic rupture</u> of <u>ligament</u> of <u>wrist</u>

S63.30- <u>Traumatic rupture</u> of <u>unspecified ligament</u> of <u>wrist</u>

S63.301- Traumatic rupture of unspecified ligament of <u>right</u> wrist

S63.302- Traumatic rupture of unspecified ligament of <u>left</u> wrist

S63.309- Traumatic rupture of unspecified ligament of <u>unspecified</u> wrist

S63.31- <u>Traumatic rupture</u> of <u>collateral</u> ligament of <u>wrist</u>

S63.311- Traumatic rupture of collateral ligament of <u>right</u> wrist

S63.312- Traumatic rupture of collateral ligament of <u>left</u> wrist

S63.319- Traumatic rupture of collateral ligament of <u>unspecified</u> wrist

S63.32- <u>Traumatic rupture</u> of <u>radiocarpal</u> ligament

    S63.321- Traumatic rupture of <u>right</u> radiocarpal ligament

    S63.322- Traumatic rupture of <u>left</u> radiocarpal ligament

    S63.329- Traumatic rupture of <u>unspecified</u> radiocarpal ligament

S63.33- <u>Traumatic rupture</u> of <u>ulnocarpal (palmar)</u> ligament

    S63.331- Traumatic rupture of <u>right</u> ulnocarpal (palmar) ligament

    S63.332- Traumatic rupture of <u>left</u> ulnocarpal (palmar) ligament

    S63.339- Traumatic rupture of <u>unspecified</u> ulnocarpal (palmar) ligament

S63.39- <u>Traumatic rupture</u> of <u>other ligament</u> of <u>wrist</u>

    S63.391- Traumatic rupture of other ligament of <u>right</u> wrist

    S63.392- Traumatic rupture of other ligament of <u>left</u> wrist

    S63.399- Traumatic rupture of other ligament of <u>unspecified</u> wrist

S63.4- <u>Traumatic rupture</u> of <u>ligament</u> of <u>finger</u> at <u>metacarpophalangeal and interphalangeal joint(s)</u>

    S63.40- <u>Traumatic rupture</u> of <u>unspecified ligament</u> of <u>finger</u> at <u>metacarpophalangeal and interphalangeal joint</u>

    S63.400- Traumatic rupture of unspecified ligament of <u>right</u> <u>index</u> finger at metacarpophalangeal and interphalangeal joint

    S63.401- Traumatic rupture of unspecified ligament of <u>left</u> <u>index</u> finger at metacarpophalangeal and interphalangeal joint

    S63.402- Traumatic rupture of unspecified ligament of <u>right</u> <u>middle</u> finger at metacarpophalangeal and interphalangeal joint

    S63.403- Traumatic rupture of unspecified ligament of <u>left</u> <u>middle</u> finger at metacarpophalangeal and interphalangeal joint

    S63.404- Traumatic rupture of unspecified ligament of <u>right</u> ring finger at metacarpophalangeal and interphalangeal joint

    S63.405- Traumatic rupture of unspecified ligament of <u>left</u> ring finger at metacarpophalangeal and interphalangeal joint

    S63.406- Traumatic rupture of unspecified ligament of <u>right</u> little finger at metacarpophalangeal and interphalangeal joint

    S63.407- Traumatic rupture of unspecified ligament of <u>left</u> little finger at metacarpophalangeal and interphalangeal joint

    S63.408- Traumatic rupture of unspecified ligament of <u>other</u> finger at metacarpophalangeal and interphalangeal joint

        Traumatic rupture of unspecified ligament of specified finger with unspecified laterality at metacarpophalangeal and interphalangeal joint

    S63.409- Traumatic rupture of unspecified ligament of <u>unspecified</u> finger at metacarpophalangeal and interphalangeal joint

    S63.41- <u>Traumatic rupture</u> of <u>collateral</u> ligament of <u>finger</u> at <u>metacarpophalangeal and interphalangeal joint</u>

    S63.410- Traumatic rupture of collateral ligament of <u>right</u> <u>index</u> finger at metacarpophalangeal and interphalangeal joint

    S63.411- Traumatic rupture of collateral ligament of <u>left</u> <u>index</u> finger at metacarpophalangeal and interphalangeal joint

    S63.412- Traumatic rupture of collateral ligament of <u>right</u> <u>middle</u> finger at metacarpophalangeal and interphalangeal joint

    S63.413- Traumatic rupture of collateral ligament of <u>left</u> <u>middle</u> finger at metacarpophalangeal and interphalangeal joint

S63.414- Traumatic rupture of collateral ligament of <u>right</u> <u>ring</u> finger at metacarpophalangeal and interphalangeal joint

S63.415- Traumatic rupture of collateral ligament of <u>left</u> <u>ring</u> finger at metacarpophalangeal and interphalangeal joint

S63.416- Traumatic rupture of collateral ligament of <u>right</u> <u>little</u> finger at metacarpophalangeal and interphalangeal joint

S63.417- Traumatic rupture of collateral ligament of <u>left</u> <u>little</u> finger at metacarpophalangeal and interphalangeal joint

S63.418- Traumatic rupture of collateral ligament of <u>other</u> finger at metacarpophalangeal and interphalangeal joint

        Traumatic rupture of collateral ligament of specified finger with unspecified laterality at metacarpophalangeal and interphalangeal joint

S63.419- Traumatic rupture of collateral ligament of <u>unspecified</u> finger at metacarpophalangeal and interphalangeal joint

S63.42- <u>Traumatic rupture</u> of <u>palmar ligament</u> of <u>finger</u> at <u>metacarpophalangeal and interphalangeal joint</u>

S63.420- Traumatic rupture of palmar ligament of <u>right</u> <u>index</u> finger at metacarpophalangeal and interphalangeal joint

S63.421- Traumatic rupture of palmar ligament of <u>left</u> <u>index</u> finger at metacarpophalangeal and interphalangeal joint

S63.422- Traumatic rupture of palmar ligament of <u>right</u> <u>middle</u> finger at metacarpophalangeal and interphalangeal joint

S63.423- Traumatic rupture of palmar ligament of <u>left</u> <u>middle</u> finger at metacarpophalangeal and interphalangeal joint

S63.424- Traumatic rupture of palmar ligament of <u>right</u> <u>ring</u> finger at metacarpophalangeal and interphalangeal joint

S63.425- Traumatic rupture of palmar ligament of <u>left</u> <u>ring</u> finger at metacarpophalangeal and interphalangeal joint

S63.426- Traumatic rupture of palmar ligament of <u>right</u> <u>little</u> finger at metacarpophalangeal and interphalangeal joint

S63.427- Traumatic rupture of palmar ligament of <u>left</u> <u>little</u> finger at metacarpophalangeal and interphalangeal joint

S63.428- Traumatic rupture of palmar ligament of <u>other</u> finger at metacarpophalangeal and interphalangeal joint

        Traumatic rupture of palmar ligament of specified finger with unspecified laterality at metacarpophalangeal and interphalangeal joint

S63.429- Traumatic rupture of palmar ligament of <u>unspecified</u> finger at metacarpophalangeal and interphalangeal joint

S63.43- <u>Traumatic rupture</u> of <u>volar plate</u> of <u>finger</u> at <u>metacarpophalangeal and interphalangeal joint</u>

S63.430- Traumatic rupture of volar plate of <u>right</u> <u>index</u> finger at metacarpophalangeal and interphalangeal joint

S63.431- Traumatic rupture of volar plate of <u>left</u> <u>index</u> finger at metacarpophalangeal and interphalangeal joint

S63.432- Traumatic rupture of volar plate of <u>right</u> <u>middle</u> finger at metacarpophalangeal and interphalangeal joint

S63.433- Traumatic rupture of volar plate of <u>left</u> <u>middle</u> finger at metacarpophalangeal and interphalangeal joint

S63
I
S63

S63.434- Traumatic rupture of volar plate of <u>right</u> <u>ring</u> finger at metacarpophalangeal and interphalangeal joint

S63.435- Traumatic rupture of volar plate of <u>left</u> <u>ring</u> finger at metacarpophalangeal and interphalangeal joint

S63.436- Traumatic rupture of volar plate of <u>right</u> <u>little</u> finger at metacarpophalangeal and interphalangeal joint

S63.437- Traumatic rupture of volar plate of <u>left</u> <u>little</u> finger at metacarpophalangeal and interphalangeal joint

S63.438- Traumatic rupture of volar plate of <u>other</u> finger at metacarpophalangeal and interphalangeal joint
Traumatic rupture of volar plate of specified finger with unspecified laterality at metacarpophalangeal and interphalangeal joint

S63.439- Traumatic rupture of volar plate of <u>unspecified</u> finger at metacarpophalangeal and interphalangeal joint

S63.49- <u>Traumatic rupture</u> of <u>other ligament</u> of <u>finger</u> at <u>metacarpophalangeal and interphalangeal joint</u>

S63.490- Traumatic rupture of other ligament of <u>right</u> <u>index</u> finger at metacarpophalangeal and interphalangeal joint

S63.491- Traumatic rupture of other ligament of <u>left</u> <u>index</u> finger at metacarpophalangeal and interphalangeal joint

S63.492- Traumatic rupture of other ligament of <u>right</u> <u>middle</u> finger at metacarpophalangeal and interphalangeal joint

S63.493- Traumatic rupture of other ligament of <u>left</u> <u>middle</u> finger at metacarpophalangeal and interphalangeal joint

S63.494- Traumatic rupture of other ligament of <u>right</u> <u>ring</u> finger at metacarpophalangeal and interphalangeal joint

S63.495- Traumatic rupture of other ligament of <u>left</u> <u>ring</u> finger at metacarpophalangeal and interphalangeal joint

S63.496- Traumatic rupture of other ligament of <u>right</u> <u>little</u> finger at metacarpophalangeal and interphalangeal joint

S63.497- Traumatic rupture of other ligament of <u>left</u> <u>little</u> finger at metacarpophalangeal and interphalangeal joint

S63.498- Traumatic rupture of other ligament of <u>other</u> finger at metacarpophalangeal and interphalangeal joint
Traumatic rupture of ligament of specified finger with unspecified laterality at metacarpophalangeal and interphalangeal joint

S63.499- Traumatic rupture of other ligament of <u>unspecified</u> finger at metacarpophalangeal and interphalangeal joint

S63.5- <u>Other and unspecified</u> <u>sprain</u> of <u>wrist</u>

S63.50- <u>Unspecified</u> sprain of <u>wrist</u>

S63.501- Unspecified sprain of <u>right</u> wrist

S63.502- Unspecified sprain of <u>left</u> wrist

S63.509- Unspecified sprain of <u>unspecified</u> wrist

S63.51- <u>Sprain</u> of <u>carpal (joint)</u>

S63.511- Sprain of carpal joint of <u>right</u> wrist

S63.512- Sprain of carpal joint of <u>left</u> wrist

S63.519- Sprain of carpal joint of <u>unspecified</u> wrist

S63.52- <u>Sprain</u> of <u>radiocarpal joint</u>
Excludes 1:   traumatic rupture of radiocarpal ligament (S63.32-)

S63.521- Sprain of radiocarpal joint of <u>right</u> wrist

S63.522- Sprain of radiocarpal joint of <u>left</u> wrist

S63.529- Sprain of radiocarpal joint of <u>unspecified</u> wrist

S63.59- <u>Other specified sprain</u> of <u>wrist</u>

S63.591- Other specified sprain of <u>right</u> wrist

S63.592- Other specified sprain of <u>left</u> wrist

S63.599- Other specified sprain of <u>unspecified</u> wrist

S63.6- <u>Other and unspecified</u> <u>sprain</u> of <u>finger(s)</u>
Excludes 1:   traumatic rupture of ligament of finger at metacarpophalangeal and interphalangeal joint(s) (S63.4-)

S63.60- <u>Unspecified</u> <u>sprain</u> of <u>thumb</u>

S63.601- Unspecified sprain of <u>right</u> thumb

S63.602- Unspecified sprain of <u>left</u> thumb

S63.609- Unspecified sprain of <u>unspecified</u> thumb

S63.61- <u>Unspecified</u> <u>sprain</u> of other and <u>unspecified</u> <u>finger(s)</u>

S63.610- Unspecified sprain of <u>right</u> <u>index</u> finger

S63.611- Unspecified sprain of <u>left</u> <u>index</u> finger

S63.612- Unspecified sprain of <u>right</u> <u>middle</u> finger

S63.613- Unspecified sprain of <u>left</u> <u>middle</u> finger

S63.614- Unspecified sprain of <u>right</u> <u>ring</u> finger

S63.615- Unspecified sprain of <u>left</u> <u>ring</u> finger

S63.616- Unspecified sprain of <u>right</u> <u>little</u> finger

S63.617- Unspecified sprain of <u>left</u> <u>little</u> finger

S63.618- Unspecified sprain of other <u>finger</u>
Unspecified sprain of specified finger with unspecified laterality

S63.619- Unspecified sprain of <u>unspecified</u> finger

S63.62- <u>Sprain</u> of <u>interphalangeal joint</u> of <u>thumb</u>

S63.621- Sprain of interphalangeal joint of <u>right</u> thumb

S63.622- Sprain of interphalangeal joint of <u>left</u> thumb

S63.629- Sprain of interphalangeal joint of <u>unspecified</u> thumb

S63.63- <u>Sprain</u> of <u>interphalangeal joint</u> of <u>other and unspecified finger(s)</u>

S63.630- Sprain of interphalangeal joint of <u>right</u> <u>index</u> finger

S63.631- Sprain of interphalangeal joint of <u>left</u> <u>index</u> finger

S63.632- Sprain of interphalangeal joint of <u>right</u> <u>middle</u> finger

S63.633- Sprain of interphalangeal joint of <u>left</u> <u>middle</u> finger

S63.634- Sprain of interphalangeal joint of <u>right</u> <u>ring</u> finger

S63.635- Sprain of interphalangeal joint of <u>left</u> <u>ring</u> finger

S63.636- Sprain of interphalangeal joint of <u>right</u> <u>little</u> finger

S63.637- Sprain of interphalangeal joint of <u>left</u> <u>little</u> finger

S63.638- Sprain of interphalangeal joint of <u>other</u> finger

S63.639- Sprain of interphalangeal joint of <u>unspecified</u> finger

S63.64- <u>Sprain</u> of <u>metacarpophalangeal joint</u> of <u>thumb</u>

S63.641- Sprain of metacarpophalangeal joint of <u>right</u> thumb

S63.642- Sprain of metacarpophalangeal joint of <u>left</u> thumb

S63.649- Sprain of metacarpophalangeal joint of <u>unspecified</u> thumb

S63.65- <u>Sprain</u> of <u>metacarpophalangeal joint</u> of <u>other and unspecified finger(s)</u>

S63.650- Sprain of metacarpophalangeal joint of <u>right</u> <u>index</u> finger

S63.651- Sprain of metacarpophalangeal joint of <u>left</u> <u>index</u> finger

S63.652- Sprain of metacarpophalangeal joint of <u>right</u> <u>middle</u> finger

S63.653- Sprain of metacarpophalangeal joint of <u>left</u> <u>middle</u> finger

S63.654- Sprain of metacarpophalangeal joint of <u>right</u> <u>ring</u> finger

S63.655- Sprain of metacarpophalangeal joint of <u>left</u> <u>ring</u> finger

S63.656- Sprain of metacarpophalangeal joint of <u>right</u> <u>little</u> finger

S63.657- Sprain of metacarpophalangeal joint of <u>left</u> <u>little</u> finger

S63 - S63

S63.658- Sprain of metacarpophalangeal joint of <u>other</u> finger
Sprain of metacarpophalangeal joint of specified finger with unspecified laterality

S63.659- Sprain of metacarpophalangeal joint of <u>unspecified</u> finger

S63.68- <u>Other sprain</u> of <u>thumb</u>

S63.681- Other sprain of <u>right</u> thumb

S63.682- Other sprain of <u>left</u> thumb

S63.689- Other sprain of <u>unspecified</u> thumb

S63.69- <u>Other sprain</u> of <u>other and unspecified</u> <u>finger(s)</u>

S63.690- Other sprain of <u>right</u> <u>index</u> finger

S63.691- Other sprain of <u>left</u> <u>index</u> finger

S63.692- Other sprain of <u>right</u> <u>middle</u> finger

S63.693- Other sprain of <u>left</u> <u>middle</u> finger

S63.694- Other sprain of <u>right</u> <u>ring</u> finger

S63.695- Other sprain of <u>left</u> <u>ring</u> finger

S63.696- Other sprain of <u>right</u> <u>little</u> finger

S63.697- Other sprain of <u>left</u> <u>little</u> finger

S63.698- Other sprain of <u>other</u> finger
Other sprain of specified finger with unspecified laterality

S63.699- Other sprain of <u>unspecified</u> finger

S63.8- <u>Sprain</u> of other part of <u>wrist and hand</u>

S63.8x- <u>Sprain</u> of <u>other part</u> of <u>wrist and hand</u>

S63.8x1- Sprain of other part of <u>right</u> wrist and hand

S63.8x2- Sprain of other part of <u>left</u> wrist and hand

S63.8x9- Sprain of other part of <u>unspecified</u> wrist and hand

S63.9- <u>Sprain</u> of <u>unspecified part</u> of <u>wrist and hand</u>

S63.90x- Sprain of unspecified part of <u>unspecified</u> wrist and hand

S63.91x- Sprain of unspecified part of <u>right</u> wrist and hand

S63.92x- Sprain of unspecified part of <u>left</u> wrist and hand

S64- <u>Injury of nerves</u> at <u>wrist and hand level</u>
Code also any associated open wound (S61.-)

The appropriate 7th character is to be added to each code from category S64:
A <u>Initial</u> encounter
D <u>Subsequent</u> encounter
S <u>Sequela</u>

S64.0- Injury of <u>ulnar</u> nerve at <u>wrist and hand level</u>

S64.00x- Injury of ulnar nerve at wrist and hand level of <u>unspecified</u> arm

S64.01x- Injury of ulnar nerve at wrist and hand level of <u>right</u> arm

S64.02x- Injury of ulnar nerve at wrist and hand level of <u>left</u> arm

S64.1- Injury of <u>median</u> nerve at <u>wrist and hand level</u>

S64.10x- Injury of median nerve at wrist and hand level of <u>unspecified</u> arm

S64.11x- Injury of median nerve at wrist and hand level of <u>right</u> arm

S64.12x- Injury of median nerve at wrist and hand level of <u>left</u> arm

S64.2- Injury of <u>radial</u> nerve at <u>wrist and hand level</u>

S64.20x- Injury of radial nerve at wrist and hand level of <u>unspecified</u> arm

S64.21x- Injury of radial nerve at wrist and hand level of <u>right</u> arm

S64.22x- Injury of radial nerve at wrist and hand level of <u>left</u> arm

S64.3- Injury of <u>digital</u> nerve of <u>thumb</u>

S64.30x- Injury of digital nerve of <u>unspecified</u> thumb

S64.31x- Injury of digital nerve of <u>right</u> thumb

S64.32x- Injury of digital nerve of <u>left</u> thumb

S64.4- Injury of <u>digital</u> nerve of <u>other and unspecified</u> finger

S64.40x- Injury of digital nerve of <u>unspecified</u> finger

S64.49- Injury of <u>digital</u> nerve of <u>other</u> finger

S64.490- Injury of digital nerve of <u>right</u> <u>index</u> finger

S64.491- Injury of digital nerve of <u>left</u> <u>index</u> finger

S64.492- Injury of digital nerve of <u>right</u> <u>middle</u> finger

S64.493- Injury of digital nerve of <u>left</u> <u>middle</u> finger

S64.494- Injury of digital nerve of <u>right</u> <u>ring</u> finger

S64.495- Injury of digital nerve of <u>left</u> <u>ring</u> finger

S64.496- Injury of digital nerve of <u>right</u> <u>little</u> finger

S64.497- Injury of digital nerve of <u>left</u> <u>little</u> finger

S64.498- Injury of digital nerve of <u>other</u> finger
Injury of digital nerve of specified finger with unspecified laterality

S64.8- Injury of <u>other nerves</u> at <u>wrist and hand level</u>

S64.8x- Injury of <u>other nerves</u> at <u>wrist and hand level</u>

S64.8x1- Injury of other nerves at wrist and hand level of <u>right</u> arm

S64.8x2- Injury of other nerves at wrist and hand level of <u>left</u> arm

S64.8x9- Injury of other nerves at wrist and hand level of <u>unspecified</u> arm

S64.9- Injury of <u>unspecified nerve</u> at <u>wrist and hand level</u>

S64.90x- Injury of <u>unspecified</u> nerve at wrist and hand level of <u>unspecified</u> arm

S64.91x- Injury of <u>unspecified</u> nerve at wrist and hand level of <u>right</u> arm

S64.92x- Injury of <u>unspecified</u> nerve at wrist and hand level of <u>left</u> arm

S65- <u>Injury of blood vessels</u> at <u>wrist and hand level</u>
Code also any associated open wound (S61.-)

The appropriate 7th character is to be added to each code from category S65:
A <u>Initial</u> encounter
D <u>Subsequent</u> encounter
S <u>Sequela</u>

S65.0- Injury of <u>ulnar artery</u> at <u>wrist and hand level</u>

S65.00- <u>Unspecified</u> injury of <u>ulnar artery</u> at <u>wrist and hand level</u>

CC-A **S65.001-** Unspecified injury of ulnar artery at wrist and hand level of <u>right</u> arm

CC-A **S65.002-** Unspecified injury of ulnar artery at wrist and hand level of <u>left</u> arm

CC-A **S65.009-** Unspecified injury of ulnar artery at wrist and hand level of <u>unspecified</u> arm

S65.01- <u>Laceration</u> of <u>ulnar artery</u> at <u>wrist and hand level</u>

CC-A **S65.011-** Laceration of ulnar artery at wrist and hand level of <u>right</u> arm

CC-A **S65.012-** Laceration of ulnar artery at wrist and hand level of <u>left</u> arm

CC-A **S65.019-** Laceration of ulnar artery at wrist and hand level of <u>unspecified</u> arm

S65.09- <u>Other specified injury</u> of <u>ulnar artery</u> at <u>wrist and hand level</u>

CC-A **S65.091-** Other specified injury of ulnar artery at wrist and hand level of <u>right</u> arm

CC-A **S65.092-** Other specified injury of ulnar artery at wrist and hand level of <u>left</u> arm

CC-A **S65.099-** Other specified injury of ulnar artery at wrist and hand level of <u>unspecified</u> arm

S65.1- Injury of <u>radial artery</u> at <u>wrist and hand level</u>

S65.10- <u>Unspecified</u> injury of <u>radial artery</u> at <u>wrist and hand level</u>

CC-A **S65.101-** Unspecified injury of radial artery at wrist and hand level of <u>right</u> arm

CC-A **S65.102-** Unspecified injury of radial artery at wrist and hand level of <u>left</u> arm

CC-A **S65.109-** Unspecified injury of radial artery at wrist and hand level of <u>unspecified</u> arm

S65.11- <u>Laceration</u> of <u>radial artery</u> at <u>wrist and hand level</u>

CC-A **S65.111-** Laceration of radial artery at wrist and hand level of <u>right</u> arm

S 63 - S 65

CC-A **S65.112-** Laceration of radial artery at wrist and hand level of <u>left</u> arm

CC-A **S65.119-** Laceration of radial artery at wrist and hand level of <u>unspecified</u> arm

S65.19- <u>Other specified injury</u> of <u>radial artery</u> at <u>wrist and hand level</u>

CC-A **S65.191-** Other specified injury of radial artery at wrist and hand level of <u>right</u> arm

CC-A **S65.192-** Other specified injury of radial artery at wrist and hand level of <u>left</u> arm

CC-A **S65.199-** Other specified injury of radial artery at wrist and hand level of <u>unspecified</u> arm

S65.2- <u>Injury of superficial palmar arch</u>

S65.20- <u>Unspecified</u> injury of <u>superficial palmar arch</u>

CC-A **S65.201-** Unspecified injury of superficial palmar arch of <u>right</u> hand

CC-A **S65.202-** Unspecified injury of superficial palmar arch of <u>left</u> hand

CC-A **S65.209-** Unspecified injury of superficial palmar arch of <u>unspecified</u> hand

S65.21- <u>Laceration</u> of <u>superficial palmar arch</u>

CC-A **S65.211-** Laceration of superficial palmar arch of <u>right</u> hand

CC-A **S65.212-** Laceration of superficial palmar arch of <u>left</u> hand

CC-A **S65.219-** Laceration of superficial palmar arch of <u>unspecified</u> hand

S65.29- <u>Other specified injury</u> of <u>superficial palmar arch</u>

CC-A **S65.291-** Other specified injury of superficial palmar arch of <u>right</u> hand

CC-A **S65.292-** Other specified injury of superficial palmar arch of <u>left</u> hand

CC-A **S65.299-** Other specified injury of superficial palmar arch of <u>unspecified</u> hand

S65.3- <u>Injury of deep palmar arch</u>

S65.30- <u>Unspecified</u> injury of <u>deep palmar arch</u>

CC-A **S65.301-** Unspecified injury of deep palmar arch of <u>right</u> hand

CC-A **S65.302-** Unspecified injury of deep palmar arch of <u>left</u> hand

CC-A **S65.309-** Unspecified injury of deep palmar arch of <u>unspecified</u> hand

S65.31- <u>Laceration</u> of <u>deep palmar arch</u>

CC-A **S65.311-** Laceration of deep palmar arch of <u>right</u> hand

CC-A **S65.312-** Laceration of deep palmar arch of <u>left</u> hand

CC-A **S65.319-** Laceration of deep palmar arch of <u>unspecified</u> hand

S65.39- <u>Other specified injury</u> of <u>deep palmar arch</u>

CC-A **S65.391-** Other specified injury of deep palmar arch of <u>right</u> hand

CC-A **S65.392-** Other specified injury of deep palmar arch of <u>left</u> hand

CC-A **S65.399-** Other specified injury of deep palmar arch of <u>unspecified</u> hand

S65.4- <u>Injury of blood vessel</u> of <u>thumb</u>

S65.40- <u>Unspecified</u> injury of <u>blood vessel</u> of <u>thumb</u>

CC-A **S65.401-** Unspecified injury of blood vessel of <u>right</u> thumb

CC-A **S65.402-** Unspecified injury of blood vessel of <u>left</u> thumb

CC-A **S65.409-** Unspecified injury of blood vessel of <u>unspecified</u> thumb

S65.41- <u>Laceration</u> of <u>blood vessel</u> of <u>thumb</u>

CC-A **S65.411-** Laceration of blood vessel of <u>right</u> thumb

CC-A **S65.412-** Laceration of blood vessel of <u>left</u> thumb

CC-A **S65.419-** Laceration of blood vessel of <u>unspecified</u> thumb

S65.49- <u>Other specified injury</u> of <u>blood vessel</u> of <u>thumb</u>

CC-A **S65.491-** Other specified injury of blood vessel of <u>right</u> thumb

CC-A **S65.492-** Other specified injury of blood vessel of <u>left</u> thumb

CC-A **S65.499-** Other specified injury of blood vessel of <u>unspecified</u> thumb

S65.5- <u>Injury of blood vessel</u> of <u>other and unspecified finger</u>

S65.50- <u>Unspecified</u> injury of <u>blood vessel</u> of <u>other and unspecified finger</u>

CC-A **S65.500-** Unspecified injury of blood vessel of <u>right</u> <u>index</u> finger

CC-A **S65.501-** Unspecified injury of blood vessel of <u>left</u> <u>index</u> finger

CC-A **S65.502-** Unspecified injury of blood vessel of <u>right</u> <u>middle</u> finger

CC-A **S65.503-** Unspecified injury of blood vessel of <u>left</u> <u>middle</u> finger

CC-A **S65.504-** Unspecified injury of blood vessel of <u>right</u> <u>ring</u> finger

CC-A **S65.505-** Unspecified injury of blood vessel of <u>left</u> <u>ring</u> finger

CC-A **S65.506-** Unspecified injury of blood vessel of <u>right</u> <u>little</u> finger

CC-A **S65.507-** Unspecified injury of blood vessel of <u>left</u> <u>little</u> finger

CC-A **S65.508-** Unspecified injury of blood vessel of <u>other</u> finger
Unspecified injury of blood vessel of specified finger with unspecified laterality

CC-A **S65.509-** Unspecified injury of blood vessel of <u>unspecified</u> finger

S65.51- <u>Laceration</u> of <u>blood vessel</u> of <u>other and unspecified finger</u>

CC-A **S65.510-** Laceration of blood vessel of <u>right</u> <u>index</u> finger

CC-A **S65.511-** Laceration of blood vessel of <u>left</u> <u>index</u> finger

CC-A **S65.512-** Laceration of blood vessel of <u>right</u> <u>middle</u> finger

CC-A **S65.513-** Laceration of blood vessel of <u>left</u> <u>middle</u> finger

CC-A **S65.514-** Laceration of blood vessel of <u>right</u> <u>ring</u> finger

CC-A **S65.515-** Laceration of blood vessel of <u>left</u> <u>ring</u> finger

CC-A **S65.516-** Laceration of blood vessel of <u>right</u> <u>little</u> finger

CC-A **S65.517-** Laceration of blood vessel of <u>left</u> <u>little</u> finger

CC-A **S65.518-** Laceration of blood vessel of <u>other</u> finger
Laceration of blood vessel of specified finger with unspecified laterality

CC-A **S65.519-** Laceration of blood vessel of <u>unspecified</u> finger

S65.59- <u>Other specified injury</u> of <u>blood vessel</u> of <u>other and unspecified finger</u>

CC-A **S65.590-** Other specified injury of blood vessel of <u>right</u> <u>index</u> finger

CC-A **S65.591-** Other specified injury of blood vessel of <u>left</u> <u>index</u> finger

CC-A **S65.592-** Other specified injury of blood vessel of <u>right</u> <u>middle</u> finger

CC-A **S65.593-** Other specified injury of blood vessel of <u>left</u> <u>middle</u> finger

CC-A **S65.594-** Other specified injury of blood vessel of <u>right</u> <u>ring</u> finger

CC-A **S65.595-** Other specified injury of blood vessel of <u>left</u> <u>ring</u> finger

CC-A **S65.596-** Other specified injury of blood vessel of <u>right</u> <u>little</u> finger

CC-A **S65.597-** Other specified injury of blood vessel of <u>left</u> <u>little</u> finger

CC-A **S65.598-** Other specified injury of blood vessel of <u>other</u> finger
Other specified injury of blood vessel of specified finger with unspecified laterality

CC-A **S65.599-** Other specified injury of blood vessel of <u>unspecified</u> finger

S65.8- <u>Injury of other blood vessels</u> at <u>wrist and hand level</u>

S65.80- <u>Unspecified</u> injury of <u>other blood vessels</u> at <u>wrist and hand level</u>

CC-A **S65.801-** Unspecified injury of other blood vessels at wrist and hand level of <u>right</u> arm

CC-A **S65.802-** Unspecified injury of other blood vessels at wrist and hand level of <u>left</u> arm

S65 – S65

CC-A **S65.809-** Unspecified injury of other blood vessels at wrist and hand level of <u>unspecified</u> arm

S65.81- <u>Laceration</u> of <u>other blood vessels</u> at <u>wrist and hand level</u>

CC-A **S65.811-** Laceration of other blood vessels at wrist and hand level of <u>right</u> arm

CC-A **S65.812-** Laceration of other blood vessels at wrist and hand level of <u>left</u> arm

CC-A **S65.819-** Laceration of other blood vessels at wrist and hand level of <u>unspecified</u> arm

S65.89- <u>Other specified injury</u> of <u>other blood vessels</u> at <u>wrist and hand level</u>

CC-A **S65.891-** Other specified injury of other blood vessels at wrist and hand level of <u>right</u> arm

CC-A **S65.892-** Other specified injury of other blood vessels at wrist and hand level of <u>left</u> arm

CC-A **S65.899-** Other specified injury of other blood vessels at wrist and hand level of <u>unspecified</u> arm

S65.9- Injury of <u>unspecified blood vessel</u> at <u>wrist and hand level</u>

S65.90- <u>Unspecified</u> injury of unspecified blood vessel at wrist and hand level

CC-A **S65.901-** Unspecified injury of unspecified blood vessel at wrist and hand level of <u>right</u> arm

CC-A **S65.902-** Unspecified injury of unspecified blood vessel at wrist and hand level of <u>left</u> arm

CC-A **S65.909-** Unspecified injury of unspecified blood vessel at wrist and hand level of <u>unspecified</u> arm

S65.91- <u>Laceration</u> of <u>unspecified blood vessel</u> at <u>wrist and hand level</u>

CC-A **S65.911-** Laceration of unspecified blood vessel at wrist and hand level of <u>right</u> arm

CC-A **S65.912-** Laceration of unspecified blood vessel at wrist and hand level of <u>left</u> arm

CC-A **S65.919-** Laceration of unspecified blood vessel at wrist and hand level of <u>unspecified</u> arm

S65.99- <u>Other specified injury</u> of <u>unspecified blood vessel</u> at <u>wrist and hand level</u>

CC-A **S65.991-** Other specified injury of unspecified blood vessel at wrist and hand of <u>right</u> arm

CC-A **S65.992-** Other specified injury of unspecified blood vessel at wrist and hand of <u>left</u> arm

CC-A **S65.999-** Other specified injury of unspecified blood vessel at wrist and hand of <u>unspecified</u> arm

S66- <u>Injury of muscle, fascia and tendon</u> at <u>wrist and hand level</u>
Code also any associated open wound (S61.-)

Excludes ❷: sprain of joints and ligaments of wrist and hand (S63.-)

The appropriate 7th character is to be added to each code from category S66:
A <u>Initial</u> encounter
D <u>Subsequent</u> encounter
S <u>Sequela</u>

S66.0- Injury of <u>long flexor muscle, fascia and tendon</u> of <u>thumb</u> at <u>wrist and hand level</u>

S66.00- <u>Unspecified</u> injury of <u>long flexor</u> muscle, fascia and tendon of <u>thumb</u> at <u>wrist and hand level</u>

S66.001- Unspecified injury of long flexor muscle, fascia and tendon of <u>right</u> thumb at wrist and hand level

S66.002- Unspecified injury of long flexor muscle, fascia and tendon of <u>left</u> thumb at wrist and hand level

S66.009- Unspecified injury of long flexor muscle, fascia and tendon of <u>unspecified</u> thumb at wrist and hand level

S66.01- <u>Strain</u> of <u>long flexor</u> muscle, fascia and tendon of <u>thumb</u> at <u>wrist and hand level</u>

S66.011- Strain of long flexor muscle, fascia and tendon of <u>right</u> thumb at wrist and hand level

S66.012- Strain of long flexor muscle, fascia and tendon of <u>left</u> thumb at wrist and hand level

S66.019- Strain of long flexor muscle, fascia and tendon of <u>unspecified</u> thumb at wrist and hand level

S66.02- <u>Laceration</u> of <u>long flexor</u> muscle, fascia and tendon of <u>thumb</u> at <u>wrist and hand level</u>

CC-A **S66.021-** Laceration of long flexor muscle, fascia and tendon of <u>right</u> thumb at wrist and hand level

CC-A **S66.022-** Laceration of long flexor muscle, fascia and tendon of <u>left</u> thumb at wrist and hand level

CC-A **S66.029-** Laceration of long flexor muscle, fascia and tendon of <u>unspecified</u> thumb at wrist and hand level

S66.09- <u>Other specified injury</u> of <u>long flexor</u> muscle, fascia and tendon of <u>thumb</u> at <u>wrist and hand level</u>

S66.091- Other specified injury of long flexor muscle, fascia and tendon of <u>right</u> thumb at wrist and hand level

S66.092- Other specified injury of long flexor muscle, fascia and tendon of <u>left</u> thumb at wrist and hand level

S66.099- Other specified injury of long flexor muscle, fascia and tendon of <u>unspecified</u> thumb at wrist and hand level

S66.1- <u>Injury of flexor muscle, fascia and tendon</u> of <u>other and unspecified finger</u> at <u>wrist and hand level</u>
Excludes ❷: Injury of long flexor muscle, fascia and tendon of thumb at wrist and hand level (S66.0-)

S66.10- <u>Unspecified</u> injury of <u>flexor muscle, fascia and tendon</u> of <u>other and unspecified finger</u> at <u>wrist and hand level</u>

S66.100- Unspecified injury of flexor muscle, fascia and tendon of <u>right index</u> finger at wrist and hand level

S66.101- Unspecified injury of flexor muscle, fascia and tendon of <u>left index</u> finger at wrist and hand level

S66.102- Unspecified injury of flexor muscle, fascia and tendon of <u>right middle</u> finger at wrist and hand level

S66.103- Unspecified injury of flexor muscle, fascia and tendon of <u>left middle</u> finger at wrist and hand level

S66.104- Unspecified injury of flexor muscle, fascia and tendon of <u>right ring</u> finger at wrist and hand level

S66.105- Unspecified injury of flexor muscle, fascia and tendon of <u>left ring</u> finger at wrist and hand level

S66.106- Unspecified injury of flexor muscle, fascia and tendon of <u>right little</u> finger at wristand hand level

S66.107- Unspecified injury of flexor muscle, fascia and tendon of <u>left little</u> finger at wristand hand level

S66.108- Unspecified injury of flexor muscle, fascia and tendon of <u>other</u> finger at wrist and hand level
Unspecified injury of flexor muscle, fascia and tendon of specified finger with unspecified laterality at wrist and hand level

S66.109- Unspecified injury of flexor muscle, fascia and tendon of <u>unspecified</u> finger at wrist and hand level

S66.11- <u>Strain</u> of <u>flexor</u> muscle, fascia and tendon of <u>other and unspecified finger</u> at <u>wrist and hand level</u>

S66.110- Strain of flexor muscle, fascia and tendon of <u>right index</u> finger at wrist and hand level

S66.111- Strain of flexor muscle, fascia and tendon of <u>left index</u> finger at wrist and hand level

S66.112- Strain of flexor muscle, fascia and tendon of <u>right middle</u> finger at wrist and hand level

S66.113- Strain of flexor muscle, fascia and tendon of <u>left middle</u> finger at wrist and hand level

S66.114- Strain of flexor muscle, fascia and tendon of <u>right ring</u> finger at wrist and hand level

S66.115- Strain of flexor muscle, fascia and tendon of <u>left ring</u> finger at wrist and hand level

S66.116- Strain of flexor muscle, fascia and tendon of <u>right little</u> finger at wrist and hand level

S66.117- Strain of flexor muscle, fascia and tendon of <u>left little</u> finger at wrist and hand level

S66.118- Strain of flexor muscle, fascia and tendon of <u>other</u> finger at wrist and hand level
Strain of flexor muscle, fascia and tendon of specified finger with unspecified laterality at wrist and hand level

S66.119- Strain of flexor muscle, fascia and tendon of <u>unspecified</u> finger at <u>wrist and hand level</u>

S66.12- <u>Laceration</u> of <u>flexor</u> muscle, fascia and tendon of <u>other and unspecified finger</u> at <u>wrist and hand level</u>

CC-A **S66.120-** Laceration of flexor muscle, fascia and tendon of <u>right index</u> finger at wrist and hand level

CC-A **S66.121-** Laceration of flexor muscle, fascia and tendon of <u>left index</u> finger at wrist and hand level

CC-A **S66.122-** Laceration of flexor muscle, fascia and tendon of <u>right middle</u> finger at wrist and hand level

CC-A **S66.123-** Laceration of flexor muscle, fascia and tendon of <u>left middle</u> finger at wrist and hand level

CC-A **S66.124-** Laceration of flexor muscle, fascia and tendon of <u>right ring</u> finger at wrist and hand level

CC-A **S66.125-** Laceration of flexor muscle, fascia and tendon of <u>left ring</u> finger at wrist and hand level

CC-A **S66.126-** Laceration of flexor muscle, fascia and tendon of <u>right little</u> finger at wrist and hand level

CC-A **S66.127-** Laceration of flexor muscle, fascia and tendon of <u>left little</u> finger at wrist and hand level

CC-A **S66.128-** Laceration of flexor muscle, fascia and tendon of <u>other</u> finger at wrist and hand level
Laceration of flexor muscle, fascia and tendon of specified finger with unspecified laterality at wrist and hand level

CC-A **S66.129-** Laceration of flexor muscle, fascia and tendon of <u>unspecified</u> finger at wrist and hand level

S66.19- <u>Other injury</u> of <u>flexor</u> muscle, fascia and tendon of <u>other and unspecified finger</u> at <u>wrist and hand level</u>

S66.190- Other injury of flexor muscle, fascia and tendon of <u>right index</u> finger at wrist and hand level

S66.191- Other injury of flexor muscle, fascia and tendon of <u>left index</u> finger at wrist and hand level

S66.192- Other injury of flexor muscle, fascia and tendon of <u>right middle</u> finger at wrist and hand level

S66.193- Other injury of flexor muscle, fascia and tendon of <u>left middle</u> finger at wrist and hand level

S66.194- Other injury of flexor muscle, fascia and tendon of <u>right ring</u> finger at wrist and hand level

S66.195- Other injury of flexor muscle, fascia and tendon of <u>left ring</u> finger at wrist and hand level

S66.196- Other injury of flexor muscle, fascia and tendon of <u>right little</u> finger at wrist and hand level

S66.197- Other injury of flexor muscle, fascia and tendon of <u>left little</u> finger at wrist and hand level

S66.198- Other injury of flexor muscle, fascia and tendon of <u>other</u> finger at wrist and hand level
Other injury of flexor muscle, fascia and tendon of specified finger with unspecified laterality at wrist and hand level

S66.199- Other injury of flexor muscle, fascia and tendon of <u>unspecified</u> finger at wrist and hand level

S66.2- <u>Injury</u> of <u>extensor</u> muscle, fascia and tendon of <u>thumb</u> at <u>wrist and hand level</u>

S66.20- <u>Unspecified</u> injury of <u>extensor</u> muscle, fascia and tendon of <u>thumb</u> at <u>wrist and hand level</u>

S66.201- Unspecified injury of extensor muscle, fascia and tendon of <u>right</u> thumb at wrist and hand level

S66.202- Unspecified injury of extensor muscle, fascia and tendon of <u>left</u> thumb at wrist and hand level

S66.209- Unspecified injury of extensor muscle, fascia and tendon of <u>unspecified</u> thumb at wrist and hand level

S66.21- Strain of <u>extensor</u> muscle, fascia and tendon of <u>thumb</u> at <u>wrist and hand level</u>

S66.211- Strain of extensor muscle, fascia and tendon of <u>right</u> thumb at wrist and hand level

S66.212- Strain of extensor muscle, fascia and tendon of <u>left</u> thumb at wrist and hand level

S66.219- Strain of extensor muscle, fascia and tendon of <u>unspecified</u> thumb at wrist and hand level

S66.22- <u>Laceration</u> of <u>extensor</u> muscle, fascia and tendon of <u>thumb</u> at <u>wrist and hand level</u>

CC-A **S66.221-** Laceration of extensor muscle, fascia and tendon of <u>right</u> thumb at wrist and hand level

CC-A **S66.222-** Laceration of extensor muscle, fascia and tendon of <u>left</u> thumb at wrist and hand level

CC-A **S66.229-** Laceration of extensor muscle, fascia and tendon of <u>unspecified</u> thumb at wrist and hand level

S66.29- <u>Other specified injury</u> of <u>extensor</u> muscle, fascia and tendon of <u>thumb</u> at <u>wrist and hand level</u>

S66.291- Other specified injury of extensor muscle, fascia and tendon of <u>right</u> thumb at wrist and hand level

S66.292- Other specified injury of extensor muscle, fascia and tendon of <u>left</u> thumb at wrist and hand level

S66.299- Other specified injury of extensor muscle, fascia and tendon of <u>unspecified</u> thumb at wrist and hand level

S66.3- <u>Injury</u> of <u>extensor</u> muscle, fascia and tendon of <u>other and unspecified finger</u> at <u>wrist and hand level</u>
Excludes ❷: *Injury of extensor muscle, fascia and tendon of thumb at wrist and hand level (S66.2-)*

S66.30- <u>Unspecified</u> injury of <u>extensor</u> muscle, fascia and tendon of <u>other and unspecified finger</u> at <u>wrist and hand level</u>

S66.300- Unspecified injury of extensor muscle, fascia and tendon of <u>right index</u> finger at wrist and hand level

S66.301- Unspecified injury of extensor muscle, fascia and tendon of <u>left index</u> finger at wrist and hand level

S66.302- Unspecified injury of extensor muscle, fascia and tendon of <u>right middle</u> finger at wrist and hand level

S66.303- Unspecified injury of extensor muscle, fascia and tendon of <u>left middle</u> finger at wrist and hand level

S66.304- Unspecified injury of extensor muscle, fascia and tendon of <u>right ring</u> finger at wrist and hand level

S66.305- Unspecified injury of extensor muscle, fascia and tendon of <u>left ring</u> finger at wrist and hand level

S66.306- Unspecified injury of extensor muscle, fascia and tendon of <u>right little</u> finger at wrist and hand level

S66.307- Unspecified injury of extensor muscle, fascia and tendon of <u>left little</u> finger at wrist and hand level

S66.308- Unspecified injury of extensor muscle, fascia and tendon of <u>other</u> finger at wrist and hand level
Unspecified injury of extensor muscle, fascia and tendon of specified finger with unspecified laterality at wrist and hand level

S66.309- Unspecified injury of extensor muscle, fascia and tendon of <u>unspecified</u> finger at wrist and hand level

S66.31- <u>Strain</u> of <u>extensor</u> muscle, fascia and tendon of <u>other and unspecified finger</u> at <u>wrist and hand level</u>

S66.310- Strain of extensor muscle, fascia and tendon of <u>right index</u> finger at wrist and hand level

S66.311- Strain of extensor muscle, fascia and tendon of <u>left index</u> finger at wrist and hand level

S66.312- Strain of extensor muscle, fascia and tendon of <u>right middle</u> finger at wrist and hand level

S66.313- Strain of extensor muscle, fascia and tendon of <u>left middle</u> finger at wrist and hand level

S66.314- Strain of extensor muscle, fascia and tendon of <u>right ring</u> finger at wrist and hand level

S66.315- Strain of extensor muscle, fascia and tendon of <u>left ring</u> finger at wrist and hand level

S66.316- Strain of extensor muscle, fascia and tendon of <u>right little</u> finger at wrist and hand level

S66.317- Strain of extensor muscle, fascia and tendon of <u>left little</u> finger at wrist and hand level

S66

I

S66

S66.318- Strain of extensor muscle, fascia and tendon of <u>other</u> finger at wrist and hand level

> Strain of extensor muscle, fascia and tendon of specified finger with unspecified laterality at wrist and hand level

S66.319- Strain of extensor muscle, fascia and tendon of <u>unspecified</u> finger at wrist and hand level

S66.32- <u>Laceration</u> of <u>extensor</u> muscle, fascia and tendon of <u>other and unspecified finger</u> at <u>wrist and hand level</u>

CC-A **S66.320-** Laceration of extensor muscle, fascia and tendon of <u>right</u> <u>index</u> finger at wrist and hand level

CC-A **S66.321-** Laceration of extensor muscle, fascia and tendon of <u>left</u> <u>index</u> finger at wrist and hand level

CC-A **S66.322-** Laceration of extensor muscle, fascia and tendon of <u>right</u> middle finger at wrist and hand level

CC-A **S66.323-** Laceration of extensor muscle, fascia and tendon of <u>left</u> <u>middle</u> finger at wrist and hand level

CC-A **S66.324-** Laceration of extensor muscle, fascia and tendon of <u>right</u> <u>ring</u> finger at wrist and hand level

CC-A **S66.325-** Laceration of extensor muscle, fascia and tendon of <u>left</u> <u>ring</u> finger at wrist and hand level

CC-A **S66.326-** Laceration of extensor muscle, fascia and tendon of <u>right</u> <u>little</u> finger at wrist and hand level

CC-A **S66.327-** Laceration of extensor muscle, fascia and tendon of <u>left</u> <u>little</u> finger at wrist and hand level

CC-A **S66.328-** Laceration of extensor muscle, fascia and tendon of <u>other</u> finger at wrist and hand level

> Laceration of extensor muscle, fascia and tendon of specified finger with unspecified laterality at wrist and hand level

CC-A **S66.329-** Laceration of extensor muscle, fascia and tendon of <u>unspecified</u> finger at wrist and hand level

S66.39- <u>Other injury</u> of <u>extensor</u> muscle, fascia and tendon of <u>other and unspecified finger</u> at <u>wrist and hand level</u>

S66.390- Other injury of extensor muscle, fascia and tendon of <u>right</u> <u>index</u> finger at wrist and hand level

S66.391- Other injury of extensor muscle, fascia and tendon of <u>left</u> <u>index</u> finger at wrist and hand level

S66.392- Other injury of extensor muscle, fascia and tendon of <u>right</u> <u>middle</u> finger at wrist and hand level

S66.393- Other injury of extensor muscle, fascia and tendon of <u>left</u> <u>middle</u> finger at wrist and hand level

S66.394- Other injury of extensor muscle, fascia and tendon of <u>right</u> <u>ring</u> finger at wrist and hand level

S66.395- Other injury of extensor muscle, fascia and tendon of <u>left</u> <u>ring</u> finger at wrist and hand level

S66.396- Other injury of extensor muscle, fascia and tendon of <u>right</u> <u>little</u> finger at wrist and hand level

S66.397- Other injury of extensor muscle, fascia and tendon of <u>left</u> <u>little</u> finger at wrist and hand level

S66.398- Other injury of extensor muscle, fascia and tendon of <u>other</u> finger at wrist and hand level

> Other injury of extensor muscle, fascia and tendon of specified finger with unspecified laterality at wrist and hand level

S66.399- Other injury of extensor muscle, fascia and tendon of <u>unspecified</u> finger at wrist and hand level

S66.4- <u>Injury</u> of <u>intrinsic</u> muscle, fascia and tendon of <u>thumb</u> at wrist and hand level

S66.40- <u>Unspecified</u> injury of <u>intrinsic</u> muscle, fascia and tendon of <u>thumb</u> at <u>wrist and hand level</u>

S66.401- Unspecified injury of intrinsic muscle, fascia and tendon of <u>right</u> thumb at wrist and hand level

S66.402- Unspecified injury of intrinsic muscle, fascia and tendon of <u>left</u> thumb at wrist and hand level

S66.409- Unspecified injury of intrinsic muscle, fascia and tendon of <u>unspecified</u> thumb at wrist and hand level

S66.41- <u>Strain</u> of <u>intrinsic</u> muscle, fascia and tendon of <u>thumb</u> at <u>wrist and hand level</u>

S66.411- Strain of intrinsic muscle, fascia and tendon of <u>right</u> thumb at wrist and hand level

S66.412- Strain of intrinsic muscle, fascia and tendon of <u>left</u> thumb at wrist and hand level

S66.419- Strain of intrinsic muscle, fascia and tendon of <u>unspecified</u> thumb at wrist and hand level

S66.42- <u>Laceration</u> of <u>intrinsic</u> muscle, fascia and tendon of <u>thumb</u> at <u>wrist and hand level</u>

CC-A **S66.421-** Laceration of intrinsic muscle, fascia and tendon of <u>right</u> thumb at wrist and hand level

CC-A **S66.422-** Laceration of intrinsic muscle, fascia and tendon of <u>left</u> thumb at wrist and hand level

CC-A **S66.429-** Laceration of intrinsic muscle, fascia and tendon of <u>unspecified</u> thumb at wrist and hand level

S66.49- <u>Other specified injury</u> of <u>intrinsic</u> muscle, fascia and tendon of <u>thumb</u> at <u>wrist and hand level</u>

S66.491- Other specified injury of intrinsic muscle, fascia and tendon of <u>right</u> thumb at wrist and hand level

S66.492- Other specified injury of intrinsic muscle, fascia and tendon of <u>left</u> thumb at wrist and hand level

S66.499- Other specified injury of intrinsic muscle, fascia and tendon of <u>unspecified</u> thumb at wrist and hand level

S66.5- <u>Injury</u> of <u>intrinsic</u> muscle, fascia and tendon of <u>other and unspecified finger</u> at <u>wrist and hand level</u>

Excludes ❷: injury of intrinsic muscle, fascia and tendon of thumb at wrist and hand level (S66.4-)

S66.50- <u>Unspecified</u> injury of <u>intrinsic</u> muscle, fascia and tendon of <u>other and unspecified finger</u> at <u>wrist and hand level</u>

S66.500- Unspecified injury of intrinsic muscle, fascia and tendon of <u>right</u> <u>index</u> finger at wrist and hand level

S66.501- Unspecified injury of intrinsic muscle, fascia and tendon of <u>left</u> <u>index</u> finger at wrist and hand level

S66.502- Unspecified injury of intrinsic muscle, fascia and tendon of <u>right</u> <u>middle</u> finger at wrist and hand level

S66.503- Unspecified injury of intrinsic muscle, fascia and tendon of <u>left</u> <u>middle</u> finger at wrist and hand level

S66.504- Unspecified injury of intrinsic muscle, fascia and tendon of <u>right</u> <u>ring</u> finger at wrist and hand level

S66.505- Unspecified injury of intrinsic muscle, fascia and tendon of <u>left</u> <u>ring</u> finger at wrist and hand level

S66.506- Unspecified injury of intrinsic muscle, fascia and tendon of <u>right</u> <u>little</u> finger at wrist and hand level

S66.507- Unspecified injury of intrinsic muscle, fascia and tendon of <u>left</u> <u>little</u> finger at wrist and hand level

S66.508- Unspecified injury of intrinsic muscle, fascia and tendon of <u>other</u> finger at wrist and hand level

> Unspecified injury of intrinsic muscle, fascia and tendon of specified finger with unspecified laterality at wrist and hand level

S66.509- Unspecified injury of intrinsic muscle, fascia and tendon of <u>unspecified</u> finger at wrist and hand level

S66.51- <u>Strain</u> of <u>intrinsic</u> muscle, fascia and tendon of <u>other and unspecified finger</u> at <u>wrist and hand level</u>

S66.510- Strain of intrinsic muscle, fascia and tendon of <u>right</u> <u>index</u> finger at wrist and hand level

S66.511- Strain of intrinsic muscle, fascia and tendon of <u>left</u> <u>index</u> finger at wrist and hand level

S66.512- Strain of intrinsic muscle, fascia and tendon of <u>right</u> <u>middle</u> finger at wrist and hand level

S66.513- Strain of intrinsic muscle, fascia and tendon of <u>left</u> <u>middle</u> finger at wrist and hand level

S66.514- Strain of intrinsic muscle, fascia and tendon of <u>right</u> <u>ring</u> finger at wrist and hand level

S66.515- Strain of intrinsic muscle, fascia and tendon of <u>left</u> <u>ring</u> finger at wrist and hand level

S66 – S66

S66.516- Strain of intrinsic muscle, fascia and tendon of <u>right</u> <u>little</u> finger at wrist and hand level

S66.517- Strain of intrinsic muscle, fascia and tendon of <u>left</u> <u>little</u> finger at wrist and hand level

S66.518- Strain of intrinsic muscle, fascia and tendon of <u>other</u> finger at wrist and hand level
Strain of intrinsic muscle, fascia and tendon of specified finger with unspecified laterality at wrist and hand level

S66.519- Strain of intrinsic muscle, fascia and tendon of <u>unspecified</u> finger at wrist and hand level

S66.52- <u>Laceration</u> of <u>intrinsic</u> muscle, fascia and tendon of <u>other and unspecified</u> <u>finger</u> at <u>wrist and hand level</u>

CC-A **S66.520-** Laceration of intrinsic muscle, fascia and tendon of <u>right</u> <u>index</u> finger at wrist and hand level

CC-A **S66.521-** Laceration of intrinsic muscle, fascia and tendon of <u>left</u> <u>index</u> finger at wrist and hand level

CC-A **S66.522-** Laceration of intrinsic muscle, fascia and tendon of <u>right</u> middle finger at wrist and hand level

CC-A **S66.523-** Laceration of intrinsic muscle, fascia and tendon of <u>left</u> <u>middle</u> finger at wrist and hand level

CC-A **S66.524-** Laceration of intrinsic muscle, fascia and tendon of <u>right</u> ring finger at wrist and hand level

CC-A **S66.525-** Laceration of intrinsic muscle, fascia and tendon of <u>left</u> <u>ring</u> finger at wrist and hand level

CC-A **S66.526-** Laceration of intrinsic muscle, fascia and tendon of <u>right</u> <u>little</u> finger at wrist and hand level

CC-A **S66.527-** Laceration of intrinsic muscle, fascia and tendon of <u>left</u> little finger at wrist and hand level

CC-A **S66.528-** Laceration of intrinsic muscle, fascia and tendon of <u>other</u> finger at wrist and hand level
Laceration of intrinsic muscle, fascia and tendon of specified finger with unspecified laterality at wrist and hand level

CC-A **S66.529-** Laceration of intrinsic muscle, fascia and tendon of <u>unspecified</u> finger at wrist and hand level

S66.59- <u>Other injury</u> of <u>intrinsic</u> muscle, fascia and tendon of <u>other and unspecified</u> <u>finger</u> at <u>wrist and hand level</u>

S66.590- Other injury of intrinsic muscle, fascia and tendon of <u>right</u> <u>index</u> finger at wrist andhand level

S66.591- Other injury of intrinsic muscle, fascia and tendon of <u>left</u> <u>index</u> finger at wrist and hand level

S66.592- Other injury of intrinsic muscle, fascia and tendon of <u>right</u> <u>middle</u> finger at wrist and hand level

S66.593- Other injury of intrinsic muscle, fascia and tendon of <u>left</u> <u>middle</u> finger at wrist and hand level

S66.594- Other injury of intrinsic muscle, fascia and tendon of <u>right</u> <u>ring</u> finger at wrist and hand level

S66.595- Other injury of intrinsic muscle, fascia and tendon of <u>left</u> <u>ring</u> finger at wrist and hand level

S66.596- Other injury of intrinsic muscle, fascia and tendon of <u>right</u> <u>little</u> finger at wrist and hand level

S66.597- Other injury of intrinsic muscle, fascia and tendon of <u>left</u> <u>little</u> finger at wrist and hand level

S66.598- Other injury of intrinsic muscle, fascia and tendon of <u>other</u> finger at wrist and hand level
Other injury of intrinsic muscle, fascia and tendon of specified finger with unspecified laterality at wrist and hand level

S66.599- Other injury of intrinsic muscle, fascia and tendon of <u>unspecified</u> finger at wrist and hand level

S66.8- <u>Injury</u> of <u>other specified</u> <u>muscles, fascia and tendons</u> at <u>wrist and hand level</u>

S66.80- <u>Unspecified</u> injury of <u>other specified</u> muscles, fascia and tendons at <u>wrist and hand level</u>

S66.801- Unspecified injury of other specified muscles, fascia and tendons at wrist and hand level, <u>right</u> hand

S66.802- Unspecified injury of other specified muscles, fascia and tendons at wrist and hand level, <u>left</u> hand

S66.809- Unspecified injury of other specified muscles, fascia and tendons at wrist and hand level, <u>unspecified</u> hand

S66.81- <u>Strain</u> of <u>other specified</u> muscles, fascia and tendons at <u>wrist and hand level</u>

S66.811- Strain of other specified muscles, fascia and tendons at wrist and hand level, <u>right</u> hand

S66.812- Strain of other specified muscles, fascia and tendons at wrist and hand level, <u>left</u> hand

S66.819- Strain of other specified muscles, fascia and tendons at wrist and hand level, <u>unspecified</u> hand

S66.82- <u>Laceration</u> of <u>other specified</u> muscles, fascia and tendons at <u>wrist and hand level</u>

CC-A **S66.821-** Laceration of other specified muscles, fascia and tendons at wrist and hand level, <u>right</u> hand

CC-A **S66.822-** Laceration of other specified muscles, fascia and tendons at wrist and hand level, <u>left</u> hand

CC-A **S66.829-** Laceration of other specified muscles, fascia and tendons at wrist and hand level, <u>unspecified</u> hand

S66.89- <u>Other injury</u> of <u>other specified</u> muscles, fascia and tendons at <u>wrist and hand level</u>

S66.891- Other injury of other specified muscles, fascia and tendons at wrist and hand level, <u>right</u> hand

S66.892- Other injury of other specified muscles, fascia and tendons at wrist and hand level, <u>left</u> hand

S66.899- Other injury of other specified muscles, fascia and tendons at wrist and hand level, <u>unspecified</u> hand

S66.9- Injury of <u>unspecified</u> muscle, fascia and tendon at <u>wrist and hand level</u>

S66.90- <u>Unspecified</u> injury of <u>unspecified</u> muscle, fascia and tendon at <u>wrist and hand level</u>

S66.901- Unspecified injury of unspecified muscle, fascia and tendon at wrist and hand level, <u>right</u> hand

S66.902- Unspecified injury of unspecified muscle, fascia and tendon at wrist and hand level, <u>left</u> hand

S66.909- Unspecified injury of unspecified muscle, fascia and tendon at wrist and hand level, <u>unspecified</u> hand

S66.91- <u>Strain</u> of <u>unspecified</u> muscle, fascia and tendon at <u>wrist and hand level</u>

S66.911- Strain of unspecified muscle, fascia and tendon at wrist and hand level, <u>right</u> hand

S66.912- Strain of unspecified muscle, fascia and tendon at wrist and hand level, <u>left</u> hand

S66.919- Strain of unspecified muscle, fascia and tendon at wrist and hand level, <u>unspecified</u> hand

S66.92- <u>Laceration</u> of <u>unspecified</u> muscle, fascia and tendon at <u>wrist and hand level</u>

CC-A **S66.921-** Laceration of unspecified muscle, fascia and tendon at wrist and hand level, <u>right</u> hand

CC-A **S66.922-** Laceration of unspecified muscle, fascia and tendon at wrist and hand level, <u>left</u> hand

CC-A **S66.929-** Laceration of unspecified muscle, fascia and tendon at wrist and hand level, <u>unspecified</u> hand

S66.99- <u>Other injury</u> of <u>unspecified</u> muscle, fascia and tendon at <u>wrist and hand level</u>

S66.991- Other injury of unspecified muscle, fascia and tendon at wrist and hand level, <u>right</u> hand

S66.992- Other injury of unspecified muscle, fascia and tendon at wrist and hand level, <u>left</u> hand

S66.999- Other injury of unspecified muscle, fascia and tendon at wrist and hand level, <u>unspecified</u> hand

S66 | S66

S67- **Crushing injury** of **wrist, hand and fingers**
Use additional code for all associated injuries, such as:
Fracture of wrist and hand (S62.-)
Open wound of wrist and hand (S61.-)

The appropriate 7th character is to be added to each code from category S67:
A   **Initial** encounter
D   **Subsequent** encounter
S   **Sequela**

S67.0- **Crushing** injury of **thumb**
S67.00x- Crushing injury of **unspecified** thumb
S67.01x- Crushing injury of **right** thumb
S67.02x- Crushing injury of **left** thumb

S67.1- **Crushing** injury of **other and unspecified finger(s)**
Excludes ❷: crushing injury of thumb (S67.0-)
S67.10x- Crushing injury of **unspecified** finger(s)
S67.19- Crushing injury of **other finger(s)**
S67.190- Crushing injury of **right index** finger
S67.191- Crushing injury of **left index** finger
S67.192- Crushing injury of **right middle** finger
S67.193- Crushing injury of **left middle** finger
S67.194- Crushing injury of **right ring** finger
S67.195- Crushing injury of **left ring** finger
S67.196- Crushing injury of **right little** finger
S67.197- Crushing injury of **left little** finger
S67.198- Crushing injury of **other** finger
Crushing injury of specified finger with unspecified laterality

S67.2- **Crushing** injury of **hand**
Excludes ❷: crushing injury of fingers (S67.1-)
crushing injury of thumb (S67.0-)
S67.20x- Crushing injury of **unspecified** hand
S67.21x- Crushing injury of **right** hand
S67.22x- Crushing injury of **left** hand

S67.3- **Crushing** injury of **wrist**
S67.30x- Crushing injury of **unspecified** wrist
S67.31x- Crushing injury of **right** wrist
S67.32x- Crushing injury of **left** wrist

S67.4- **Crushing** injury of **wrist and hand**
Excludes 1: crushing injury of hand alone (S67.2-)
crushing injury of wrist alone (S67.3-)
Excludes ❷: crushing injury of fingers (S67.1-)
crushing injury of thumb (S67.0-)
S67.40x- Crushing injury of **unspecified** wrist and hand
S67.41x- Crushing injury of **right** wrist and hand
S67.42x- Crushing injury of **left** wrist and hand

S67.9- **Crushing** injury of **unspecified part(s)** of **wrist, hand and fingers**
S67.90x- Crushing injury of unspecified part(s) of **unspecified** wrist, hand and fingers
S67.91x- Crushing injury of unspecified part(s) of **right** wrist, hand and fingers
S67.92x- Crushing injury of unspecified part(s) of **left** wrist, hand and fingers

S68- **Traumatic amputation** of **wrist, hand and fingers**
Note: An amputation not identified as partial or complete should be coded to complete

The appropriate 7th character is to be added to each code from category S68:
A   **Initial** encounter
D   **Subsequent** encounter
S   **Sequela**

S68.0- Traumatic **metacarpophalangeal amputation** of **thumb**
Traumatic amputation of thumb NOS
S68.01- **Complete** traumatic **metacarpophalangeal amputation** of **thumb**
S68.011- Complete traumatic metacarpophalangeal amputation of **right** thumb

S68.012- Complete traumatic metacarpophalangeal amputation of **left** thumb
S68.019- Complete traumatic metacarpophalangeal amputation of **unspecified** thumb
S68.02- **Partial** traumatic **metacarpophalangeal amputation** of **thumb**
S68.021- Partial traumatic metacarpophalangeal amputation of **right** thumb
S68.022- Partial traumatic metacarpophalangeal amputation of **left** thumb
S68.029- Partial traumatic metacarpophalangeal amputation of **unspecified** thumb

S68.1- Traumatic **metacarpophalangeal amputation** of **other and unspecified finger**
Traumatic amputation of finger NOS
Excludes ❷: traumatic metacarpophalangeal amputation of thumb (S68.0-)

S68.11- **Complete** traumatic **metacarpophalangeal** amputation of **other and unspecified finger**
S68.110- Complete traumatic metacarpophalangeal amputation of **right index** finger
S68.111- Complete traumatic metacarpophalangeal amputation of **left index** finger
S68.112- Complete traumatic metacarpophalangeal amputation of **right middle** finger
S68.113- Complete traumatic metacarpophalangeal amputation of **left middle** finger
S68.114- Complete traumatic metacarpophalangeal amputation of **right ring** finger
S68.115- Complete traumatic metacarpophalangeal amputation of **left ring** finger
S68.116- Complete traumatic metacarpophalangeal amputation of **right little** finger
S68.117- Complete traumatic metacarpophalangeal amputation of **left little** finger
S68.118- Complete traumatic metacarpophalangeal amputation of **other** finger
Complete traumatic metacarpophalangeal amputation of specified finger with unspecified laterality
S68.119- Complete traumatic metacarpophalangeal amputation of **unspecified** finger

S68.12- **Partial** traumatic **metacarpophalangeal amputation** of **other and unspecified finger**
S68.120- Partial traumatic metacarpophalangeal amputation of **right index** finger
S68.121- Partial traumatic metacarpophalangeal amputation of **left index** finger
S68.122- Partial traumatic metacarpophalangeal amputation of **right middle** finger
S68.123- Partial traumatic metacarpophalangeal amputation of **left middle** finger
S68.124- Partial traumatic metacarpophalangeal amputation of **right ring** finger
S68.125- Partial traumatic metacarpophalangeal amputation of **left ring** finger
S68.126- Partial traumatic metacarpophalangeal amputation of **right little** finger
S68.127- Partial traumatic metacarpophalangeal amputation of **left little** finger
S68.128- Partial traumatic metacarpophalangeal amputation of **other** finger
Partial traumatic metacarpophalangeal amputation of specified finger with unspecified laterality
S68.129- Partial traumatic metacarpophalangeal amputation of **unspecified** finger

S68.4- Traumatic <u>amputation</u> of <u>hand</u> at <u>wrist level</u>
Traumatic amputation of hand NOS
Traumatic amputation of wrist

S68.41- <u>Complete</u> traumatic <u>amputation</u> of <u>hand</u> at <u>wrist level</u>

CC-A **S68.411-** Complete traumatic amputation of <u>right</u> hand at wrist level

CC-A **S68.412-** Complete traumatic amputation of <u>left</u> hand at wrist level

CC-A **S68.419-** Complete traumatic amputation of <u>unspecified</u> hand at wrist level

S68.42- <u>Partial</u> traumatic <u>amputation</u> of <u>hand</u> at <u>wrist level</u>

CC-A **S68.421-** Partial traumatic amputation of <u>right</u> hand at wrist level

CC-A **S68.422-** Partial traumatic amputation of <u>left</u> hand at wrist level

CC-A **S68.429-** Partial traumatic amputation of <u>unspecified</u> hand at wrist level

S68.5- Traumatic <u>transphalangeal</u> <u>amputation</u> of <u>thumb</u>
Traumatic interphalangeal joint amputation of thumb

S68.51- <u>Complete</u> traumatic <u>transphalangeal</u> <u>amputation</u> of <u>thumb</u>

S68.511- Complete traumatic transphalangeal amputation of <u>right</u> thumb

S68.512- Complete traumatic transphalangeal amputation of <u>left</u> thumb

S68.519- Complete traumatic transphalangeal amputation of <u>unspecified</u> thumb

S68.52- <u>Partial</u> traumatic <u>transphalangeal</u> <u>amputation</u> of <u>thumb</u>

S68.521- Partial traumatic transphalangeal amputation of <u>right</u> thumb

S68.522- Partial traumatic transphalangeal amputation of <u>left</u> thumb

S68.529- Partial traumatic transphalangeal amputation of <u>unspecified</u> thumb

S68.6- Traumatic <u>transphalangeal</u> <u>amputation</u> of <u>other and unspecified finger</u>

S68.61- <u>Complete</u> traumatic <u>transphalangeal</u> <u>amputation</u> of <u>other and unspecified finger(s)</u>

S68.610- Complete traumatic transphalangeal amputation of <u>right index</u> finger

S68.611- Complete traumatic transphalangeal amputation of <u>left index</u> finger

S68.612- Complete traumatic transphalangeal amputation of <u>right middle</u> finger

S68.613- Complete traumatic transphalangeal amputation of <u>left middle</u> finger

S68.614- Complete traumatic transphalangeal amputation of <u>right ring</u> finger

S68.615- Complete traumatic transphalangeal amputation of <u>left ring</u> finger

S68.616- Complete traumatic transphalangeal amputation of <u>right little</u> finger

S68.617- Complete traumatic transphalangeal amputation of <u>left little</u> finger

S68.618- Complete traumatic transphalangeal amputation of <u>other</u> finger
Complete traumatic transphalangeal amputation of specified finger with unspecified laterality

S68.619- Complete traumatic transphalangeal amputation of <u>unspecified</u> finger

S68.62- <u>Partial</u> traumatic <u>transphalangeal</u> <u>amputation</u> of <u>other and unspecified finger</u>

S68.620- Partial traumatic transphalangeal amputation of <u>right index</u> finger

S68.621- Partial traumatic transphalangeal amputation of <u>left index</u> finger

S68.622- Partial traumatic transphalangeal amputation of <u>right middle</u> finger

S68.623- Partial traumatic transphalangeal amputation of <u>left middle</u> finger

S68.624- Partial traumatic transphalangeal amputation of <u>right ring</u> finger

S68.625- Partial traumatic transphalangeal amputation of <u>left ring</u> finger

S68.626- Partial traumatic transphalangeal amputation of <u>right little</u> finger

S68.627- Partial traumatic transphalangeal amputation of <u>left little</u> finger

S68.628- Partial traumatic transphalangeal amputation of <u>other</u> finger
Partial traumatic transphalangeal amputation of specified finger with unspecified laterality

S68.629- Partial traumatic transphalangeal amputation of <u>unspecified</u> finger

S68.7- Traumatic <u>transmetacarpal</u> <u>amputation</u> of <u>hand</u>

S68.71- <u>Complete</u> traumatic <u>transmetacarpal</u> <u>amputation</u> of <u>hand</u>

CC-A **S68.711-** Complete traumatic transmetacarpal amputation of <u>right</u> hand

CC-A **S68.712-** Complete traumatic transmetacarpal amputation of <u>left</u> hand

CC-A **S68.719-** Complete traumatic transmetacarpal amputation of <u>unspecified</u> hand

S68.72- <u>Partial</u> traumatic <u>transmetacarpal</u> <u>amputation</u> of <u>hand</u>

CC-A **S68.721-** Partial traumatic transmetacarpal amputation of <u>right</u> hand

CC-A **S68.722-** Partial traumatic transmetacarpal amputation of <u>left</u> hand

CC-A **S68.729-** Partial traumatic transmetacarpal amputation of <u>unspecified</u> hand

S69- <u>Other and unspecified injuries</u> of <u>wrist, hand and finger(s)</u>
The appropriate 7th character is to be added to each code from category S69:
A <u>Initial</u> encounter
D <u>Subsequent</u> encounter
S <u>Sequela</u>

S69.8- <u>Other specified injuries</u> of <u>wrist, hand and finger(s)</u>

S69.80x- Other specified injuries of <u>unspecified</u> wrist, hand and finger(s)

S69.81x- Other specified injuries of <u>right</u> wrist, hand and finger(s)

S69.82x- Other specified injuries of <u>left</u> wrist, hand and finger(s)

S69.9- <u>Unspecified injury</u> of <u>wrist, hand and finger(s)</u>

S69.90x- Unspecified injury of <u>unspecified</u> wrist, hand and finger(s)

S69.91x- Unspecified injury of <u>right</u> wrist, hand and finger(s)

S69.92x- Unspecified injury of <u>left</u> wrist, hand and finger(s)

Injuries to the hip and thigh (S70-S79)

Excludes ②: burns and corrosions (T20-T32)
frostbite (T33-T34)
snake bite (T63.0-)
venomous insect bite or sting (T63.4-)

S70- <u>Superficial injury</u> of <u>hip and thigh</u>
The appropriate 7th character is to be added to each code from category S70:
A <u>Initial</u> encounter
D <u>Subsequent</u> encounter
S <u>Sequela</u>

S70.0- <u>Contusion</u> of <u>hip</u>

S70.00x- Contusion of <u>unspecified</u> hip

S70.01x- Contusion of <u>right</u> hip

S70.02x- Contusion of <u>left</u> hip

S70.1- <u>Contusion</u> of <u>thigh</u>

S70.10x- Contusion of <u>unspecified</u> thigh

S70.11x- Contusion of <u>right</u> thigh

S70.12x- Contusion of <u>left</u> thigh

S68 – S70

S70.2- **Other superficial injuries** of <u>hip</u>
　S70.21- **Abrasion** of <u>hip</u>
　　S70.211- Abrasion, <u>right</u> hip
　　S70.212- Abrasion, <u>left</u> hip
　　S70.219- Abrasion, <u>unspecified</u> hip
　S70.22- **Blister** (nonthermal) of <u>hip</u>
　　S70.221- Blister (nonthermal), <u>right</u> hip
　　S70.222- Blister (nonthermal), <u>left</u> hip
　　S70.229- Blister (nonthermal), <u>unspecified</u> hip
　S70.24- **External constriction** of <u>hip</u>
　　S70.241- External constriction, <u>right</u> hip
　　S70.242- External constriction, <u>left</u> hip
　　S70.249- External constriction, <u>unspecified</u> hip
　S70.25- **Superficial foreign body** of <u>hip</u>
　　　Splinter in the hip
　　S70.251- Superficial foreign body, <u>right</u> hip
　　S70.252- Superficial foreign body, <u>left</u> hip
　　S70.259- Superficial foreign body, <u>unspecified</u> hip
　S70.26- **Insect bite (nonvenomous)** of <u>hip</u>
　　S70.261- Insect bite (nonvenomous), <u>right</u> hip
　　S70.262- Insect bite (nonvenomous), <u>left</u> hip
　　S70.269- Insect bite (nonvenomous), <u>unspecified</u> hip
　S70.27- **Other superficial bite** of <u>hip</u>
　　　Excludes 1:　open bite of hip (S71.05-)
　　S70.271- Other superficial bite of hip, <u>right</u> hip
　　S70.272- Other superficial bite of hip, <u>left</u> hip
　　S70.279- Other superficial bite of hip, <u>unspecified</u> hip
S70.3- **Other superficial injuries** of <u>thigh</u>
　S70.31- **Abrasion** of <u>thigh</u>
　　S70.311- Abrasion, <u>right</u> thigh
　　S70.312- Abrasion, <u>left</u> thigh
　　S70.319- Abrasion, <u>unspecified</u> thigh
　S70.32- **Blister** (nonthermal) of <u>thigh</u>
　　S70.321- Blister (nonthermal), <u>right</u> thigh
　　S70.322- Blister (nonthermal), <u>left</u> thigh
　　S70.329- Blister (nonthermal), <u>unspecified</u> thigh
　S70.34- **External constriction** of <u>thigh</u>
　　S70.341- External constriction, <u>right</u> thigh
　　S70.342- External constriction, <u>left</u> thigh
　　S70.349- External constriction, <u>unspecified</u> thigh
　S70.35- **Superficial foreign body** of <u>thigh</u>
　　　Splinter in the thigh
　　S70.351- Superficial foreign body, <u>right</u> thigh
　　S70.352- Superficial foreign body, <u>left</u> thigh
　　S70.359- Superficial foreign body, <u>unspecified</u> thigh
　S70.36- **Insect bite (nonvenomous)** of <u>thigh</u>
　　S70.361- Insect bite (nonvenomous), <u>right</u> thigh
　　S70.362- Insect bite (nonvenomous), <u>left</u> thigh
　　S70.369- Insect bite (nonvenomous), <u>unspecified</u> thigh
　S70.37- **Other superficial bite** of <u>thigh</u>
　　　Excludes 1:　open bite of thigh (S71.15)
　　S70.371- Other superficial bite of <u>right</u> thigh
　　S70.372- Other superficial bite of <u>left</u> thigh
　　S70.379- Other superficial bite of <u>unspecified</u> thigh
S70.9- **Unspecified superficial injury** of <u>hip and thigh</u>
　S70.91- **Unspecified** superficial injury of <u>hip</u>
　　S70.911- Unspecified superficial injury of <u>right</u> hip
　　S70.912- Unspecified superficial injury of <u>left</u> hip
　　S70.919- Unspecified superficial injury of <u>unspecified</u> hip
　S70.92- **Unspecified** superficial injury of <u>thigh</u>
　　S70.921- Unspecified superficial injury of <u>right</u> thigh
　　S70.922- Unspecified superficial injury of <u>left</u> thigh
　　S70.929- Unspecified superficial injury of <u>unspecified</u> thigh

S71- **Open wound** of <u>hip and thigh</u>
　Code also any associated wound infection
　Excludes 1:　open fracture of hip and thigh (S72.-)
　　　　　　traumatic amputation of hip and thigh (S78.-)
　Excludes ❷:　bite of venomous animal (T63.-)
　　　　　　open wound of ankle, foot and toes (S91.-)
　　　　　　open wound of knee and lower leg (S81.-)

The appropriate 7th character is to be added to each code from category S71:
　A　<u>Initial</u> encounter
　D　<u>Subsequent</u> encounter
　S　<u>Sequela</u>

S71.0- **Open wound** of <u>hip</u>
　S71.00- **Unspecified** open wound of hip
　　S71.001- Unspecified open wound, <u>right</u> hip
　　S71.002- Unspecified open wound, <u>left</u> hip
　　S71.009- Unspecified open wound, <u>unspecified</u> hip
　S71.01- **Laceration** <u>without</u> foreign body of hip
　　S71.011- Laceration <u>without</u> foreign body, <u>right</u> hip
　　S71.012- Laceration <u>without</u> foreign body, <u>left</u> hip
　　S71.019- Laceration <u>without</u> foreign body, <u>unspecified</u> hip
　S71.02- **Laceration** <u>with foreign body</u> of hip
　　S71.021- Laceration <u>with foreign body</u>, <u>right</u> hip
　　S71.022- Laceration <u>with foreign body</u>, <u>left</u> hip
　　S71.029- Laceration <u>with foreign body</u>, <u>unspecified</u> hip
　S71.03- **Puncture** wound <u>without</u> foreign body of hip
　　S71.031- Puncture wound <u>without</u> foreign body, <u>right</u> hip
　　S71.032- Puncture wound <u>without</u> foreign body, <u>left</u> hip
　　S71.039- Puncture wound <u>without</u> foreign body, <u>unspecified</u> hip
　S71.04- **Puncture** wound <u>with foreign body</u> of hip
　　S71.041- Puncture wound <u>with foreign body</u>, <u>right</u> hip
　　S71.042- Puncture wound <u>with foreign body</u>, <u>left</u> hip
　　S71.049- Puncture wound <u>with foreign body</u>, <u>unspecified</u> hip
　S71.05- **Open bite** of hip
　　　Bite of hip NOS
　　　Excludes 1:　superficial bite of hip (S70.26, S70.27)
　　S71.051- Open bite, <u>right</u> hip
　　S71.052- Open bite, <u>left</u> hip
　　S71.059- Open bite, <u>unspecified</u> hip
S71.1- **Open wound** of <u>thigh</u>
　S71.10- **Unspecified** open wound of thigh
　　S71.101- Unspecified open wound, <u>right</u> thigh
　　S71.102- Unspecified open wound, <u>left</u> thigh
　　S71.109- Unspecified open wound, <u>unspecified</u> thigh
　S71.11- **Laceration** <u>without</u> foreign body of thigh
　　S71.111- Laceration <u>without</u> foreign body, <u>right</u> thigh
　　S71.112- Laceration <u>without</u> foreign body, <u>left</u> thigh
　　S71.119- Laceration <u>without</u> foreign body, <u>unspecified</u> thigh
　S71.12- **Laceration** <u>with foreign body</u> of thigh
　　S71.121- Laceration <u>with foreign body</u>, <u>right</u> thigh
　　S71.122- Laceration <u>with foreign body</u>, <u>left</u> thigh
　　S71.129- Laceration <u>with foreign body</u>, <u>unspecified</u> thigh
　S71.13- **Puncture** wound <u>without</u> foreign body of thigh
　　S71.131- Puncture wound <u>without</u> foreign body, <u>right</u> thigh
　　S71.132- Puncture wound <u>without</u> foreign body, <u>left</u> thigh
　　S71.139- Puncture wound <u>without</u> foreign body, <u>unspecified</u> thigh
　S71.14- **Puncture** wound <u>with foreign body</u> of thigh
　　S71.141- Puncture wound <u>with foreign body</u>, <u>right</u> thigh
　　S71.142- Puncture wound <u>with foreign body</u>, <u>left</u> thigh
　　S71.149- Puncture wound <u>with foreign body</u>, <u>unspecified</u> thigh
　S71.15- **Open bite** of thigh
　　　Bite of thigh NOS
　　　Excludes 1:　superficial bite of thigh (S70.37-)
　　S71.151- Open bite, <u>right</u> thigh

S70-S71

S71.152- Open bite, <u>left</u> thigh

S71.159- Open bite, <u>unspecified</u> thigh

S72- <u>Fracture</u> of <u>femur</u>
Note: A fracture not indicated as displaced or nondisplaced should be coded to displaced
Note: A fracture not indicated as open or closed should be coded to closed
Note: The open fracture designations are based on the Gustilo open fracture classification
Excludes 1:   traumatic amputation of hip and thigh (S78.-)
Excludes ❷: fracture of lower leg and ankle (S82.-)
fracture of foot (S92.-)
periprosthetic fracture of prosthetic implant of hip (T84.040, T84.041)

The appropriate 7th character is to be added to all codes from category S72:
A   <u>Initial</u> encounter for <u>closed</u> fracture
B   <u>Initial</u> encounter for <u>open</u> fracture <u>type I or II</u>
<u>Initial</u> encounter for open fracture NOS
C   <u>Initial</u> encounter for <u>open</u> fracture <u>type IIIA, IIIB, or IIIC</u>
D   <u>Subsequent</u> encounter for <u>closed</u> fracture <u>with routine healing</u>
E   <u>Subsequent</u> encounter for <u>open</u> fracture <u>type I or II</u> <u>with routine healing</u>
F   <u>Subsequent</u> encounter for <u>open</u> fracture <u>type IIIA, IIIB, or IIIC with routine healing</u>
G   <u>Subsequent</u> encounter for <u>closed</u> fracture <u>with delayed healing</u>
H   <u>Subsequent</u> encounter for <u>open</u> fracture <u>type I or II</u> <u>with delayed healing</u>
J   <u>Subsequent</u> encounter for <u>open</u> fracture <u>type IIIA, IIIB, or IIIC with delayed healing</u>
K   <u>Subsequent</u> encounter for <u>closed</u> fracture <u>with nonunion</u>
M   <u>Subsequent</u> encounter for <u>open</u> fracture <u>type I or II</u> <u>with nonunion</u>
N   <u>Subsequent</u> encounter for <u>open</u> fracture <u>type IIIA, IIIB, or IIIC with nonunion</u>
P   <u>Subsequent</u> encounter for <u>closed</u> fracture <u>with malunion</u>
Q   <u>Subsequent</u> encounter for <u>open</u> fracture <u>type I or II</u> <u>with malunion</u>
R   <u>Subsequent</u> encounter for <u>open</u> fracture <u>type IIIA, IIIB, or IIIC with malunion</u>
S   <u>Sequela</u>

S72.0- <u>Fracture</u> of <u>head</u> and <u>neck</u> of <u>femur</u>
Excludes ❷: physeal fracture of upper end of femur (S79.0-)

S72.00- Fracture of <u>unspecified part</u> of <u>neck</u> of femur
Fracture of hip NOS
Fracture of neck of femur NOS

S72.001-   Fracture of unspecified part of neck of <u>right</u> femur
CC-K,M,N,P,Q,R MCC-A,B,C

S72.002-   Fracture of unspecified part of neck of <u>left</u> femur
CC-K,M,N,P,Q,R MCC-A,B,C

S72.009-   Fracture of unspecified part of neck of <u>unspecified</u> femur
CC-K,M,N,P,Q,R MCC-A,B,C

S72.01- <u>Unspecified</u> <u>intracapsular</u> fracture of femur
Subcapital fracture of femur

S72.011-   Unspecified intracapsular fracture of <u>right</u> femur
CC-K,M,N,P,Q,R MCC-A,B,C

S72.012-   Unspecified intracapsular fracture of <u>left</u> femur
CC-K,M,N,P,Q,R MCC-A,B,C

S72.019-   Unspecified intracapsular fracture of <u>unspecified</u> femur
CC-K,M,N,P,Q,R MCC-A,B,C

S72.02- Fracture of <u>epiphysis</u> (separation) (upper) of femur
Transepiphyseal fracture of femur
Excludes 1:   capital femoral epiphyseal fracture (pediatric) of femur (S79.01-)
Salter-Harris Type I physeal fracture of upper end of femur (S79.01-)

S72.021-   <u>Displaced</u> fracture of epiphysis (separation) (upper) of <u>right</u> femur
CC-K,M,N,P,Q,R MCC-A,B,C

S72.022-   <u>Displaced</u> fracture of epiphysis (separation) (upper) of <u>left</u> femur
CC-K,M,N,P,Q,R MCC-A,B,C

S72.023-   <u>Displaced</u> fracture of epiphysis (separation) (upper) of <u>unspecified</u> femur
CC-K,M,N,P,Q,R MCC-A,B,C

S72.024-   <u>Nondisplaced</u> fracture of epiphysis (separation) (upper) of <u>right</u> femur
CC-K,M,N,P,Q,R MCC-A,B,C

S72.025-   <u>Nondisplaced</u> fracture of epiphysis (separation) (upper) of <u>left</u> femur
CC-K,M,N,P,Q,R MCC-A,B,C

S72.026-   <u>Nondisplaced</u> fracture of epiphysis (separation) (upper) of <u>unspecified</u> femur
CC-K,M,N,P,Q,R MCC-A,B,C

S72.03- <u>Midcervical</u> fracture of femur
Transcervical fracture of femur NOS

S72.031-   <u>Displaced</u> midcervical fracture of <u>right</u> femur
CC-K,M,N,P,Q,R MCC-A,B,C

S72.032-   <u>Displaced</u> midcervical fracture of <u>left</u> femur
CC-K,M,N,P,Q,R MCC-A,B,C

S72.033-   <u>Displaced</u> midcervical fracture of <u>unspecified</u> femur
CC-K,M,N,P,Q,R MCC-A,B,C

S72.034-   <u>Nondisplaced</u> midcervical fracture of <u>right</u> femur
CC-K,M,N,P,Q,R MCC-A,B,C

S72.035-   <u>Nondisplaced</u> midcervical fracture of <u>left</u> femur
CC-K,M,N,P,Q,R MCC-A,B,C

S72.036-   <u>Nondisplaced</u> midcervical fracture of <u>unspecified</u> femur
CC-K,M,N,P,Q,R MCC-A,B,C

S72.04- Fracture of <u>base of neck</u> of femur
Cervicotrochanteric fracture of femur

S72.041-   <u>Displaced</u> fracture of base of neck of <u>right</u> femur
CC-K,M,N,P,Q,R MCC-A,B,C

S72.042-   <u>Displaced</u> fracture of base of neck of <u>left</u> femur
CC-K,M,N,P,Q,R MCC-A,B,C

S72.043-   <u>Displaced</u> fracture of base of neck of <u>unspecified</u> femur
CC-K,M,N,P,Q,R MCC-A,B,C

S72.044-   <u>Nondisplaced</u> fracture of base of neck of <u>right</u> femur
CC-K,M,N,P,Q,R MCC-A,B,C

S72.045-   <u>Nondisplaced</u> fracture of base of neck of <u>left</u> femur
CC-K,M,N,P,Q,R MCC-A,B,C

S72.046-   <u>Nondisplaced</u> fracture of base of neck of <u>unspecified</u> femur
CC-K,M,N,P,Q,R MCC-A,B,C

S72.05- <u>Unspecified</u> fracture of <u>head</u> of femur
Fracture of head of femur NOS

S72.051-   <u>Unspecified</u> fracture of head of <u>right</u> femur
CC-K,M,N,P,Q,R MCC-A,B,C

S72.052-   <u>Unspecified</u> fracture of head of <u>left</u> femur
CC-K,M,N,P,Q,R MCC-A,B,C

S72.059-   <u>Unspecified</u> fracture of head of <u>unspecified</u> femur
CC-K,M,N,P,Q,R MCC-A,B,C

S72.06- <u>Articular</u> fracture of <u>head</u> of femur

S72.061-   <u>Displaced</u> articular fracture of head of <u>right</u> femur
CC-K,M,N,P,Q,R MCC-A,B,C

S72.062-   <u>Displaced</u> articular fracture of head of <u>left</u> femur
CC-K,M,N,P,Q,R MCC-A,B,C

S72.063-   <u>Displaced</u> articular fracture of head of <u>unspecified</u> femur
CC-K,M,N,P,Q,R MCC-A,B,C

S72.064-   <u>Nondisplaced</u> articular fracture of head of <u>right</u> femur
CC-K,M,N,P,Q,R MCC-A,B,C

S72.065-   <u>Nondisplaced</u> articular fracture of head of <u>left</u> femur
CC-K,M,N,P,Q,R MCC-A,B,C

S72.066-   <u>Nondisplaced</u> articular fracture of head of <u>unspecified</u> femur
CC-K,M,N,P,Q,R MCC-A,B,C

S72.09- <u>Other fracture</u> of <u>head and neck</u> of femur

S72.091-   Other fracture of head and neck of <u>right</u> femur
CC-K,M,N,P,Q,R MCC-A,B,C

S72.092-   Other fracture of head and neck of <u>left</u> femur
CC-K,M,N,P,Q,R MCC-A,B,C

S71 - S72

S72.099- Other fracture of head and neck of <u>unspecified</u> femur
CC-K,M,N,P,Q,R MCC-A,B,C

S72.1- <u>Pertrochanteric</u> fracture
S72.10- <u>Unspecified</u> trochanteric fracture of femur
Fracture of trochanter NOS
S72.101- Unspecified trochanteric fracture of <u>right</u> femur
CC-K,M,N,P,Q,R MCC-A,B,C
S72.102- Unspecified trochanteric fracture of <u>left</u> femur
CC-K,M,N,P,Q,R MCC-A,B,C
S72.109- Unspecified trochanteric fracture of <u>unspecified</u> femur
CC-K,M,N,P,Q,R MCC-A,B,C

S72.11- Fracture of <u>greater trochanter</u> of femur
S72.111- <u>Displaced</u> fracture of greater trochanter of <u>right</u> femur
CC-K,M,N,P,Q,R MCC-A,B,C
S72.112- <u>Displaced</u> fracture of greater trochanter of <u>left</u> femur
CC-K,M,N,P,Q,R MCC-A,B,C
S72.113- <u>Displaced</u> fracture of greater trochanter of <u>unspecified</u> femur
CC-K,M,N,P,Q,R MCC-A,B,C
S72.114- <u>Nondisplaced</u> fracture of greater trochanter of <u>right</u> femur
CC-K,M,N,P,Q,R MCC-A,B,C
S72.115- <u>Nondisplaced</u> fracture of greater trochanter of <u>left</u> femur
CC-K,M,N,P,Q,R MCC-A,B,C
S72.116- <u>Nondisplaced</u> fracture of greater trochanter of <u>unspecified</u> femur
CC-K,M,N,P,Q,R MCC-A,B,C

S72.12- Fracture of <u>lesser trochanter</u> of femur
S72.121- <u>Displaced</u> fracture of lesser trochanter of <u>right</u> femur
CC-K,M,N,P,Q,R MCC-A,B,C
S72.122- <u>Displaced</u> fracture of lesser trochanter of <u>left</u> femur
CC-K,M,N,P,Q,R MCC-A,B,C
S72.123- <u>Displaced</u> fracture of lesser trochanter of <u>unspecified</u> femur
CC-K,M,N,P,Q,R MCC-A,B,C
S72.124- <u>Nondisplaced</u> fracture of lesser trochanter of <u>right</u> femur
CC-K,M,N,P,Q,R MCC-A,B,C
S72.125- <u>Nondisplaced</u> fracture of lesser trochanter of <u>left</u> femur
CC-K,M,N,P,Q,R MCC-A,B,C
S72.126- <u>Nondisplaced</u> fracture of lesser trochanter of <u>unspecified</u> femur
CC-K,M,N,P,Q,R MCC-A,B,C

S72.13- <u>Apophyseal</u> fracture of femur
Excludes 1: chronic (nontraumatic) slipped upper femoral epiphysis (M93.0-)
S72.131- <u>Displaced</u> apophyseal fracture of <u>right</u> femur
CC-K,M,N,P,Q,R MCC-A,B,C
S72.132- <u>Displaced</u> apophyseal fracture of <u>left</u> femur
CC-K,M,N,P,Q,R MCC-A,B,C
S72.133- <u>Displaced</u> apophyseal fracture of <u>unspecified</u> femur
CC-K,M,N,P,Q,R MCC-A,B,C
S72.134- <u>Nondisplaced</u> apophyseal fracture of <u>right</u> femur
CC-K,M,N,P,Q,R MCC-A,B,C
S72.135- <u>Nondisplaced</u> apophyseal fracture of <u>left</u> femur
CC-K,M,N,P,Q,R MCC-A,B,C
S72.136- <u>Nondisplaced</u> apophyseal fracture of <u>unspecified</u> femur
CC-K,M,N,P,Q,R MCC-A,B,C

S72.14- <u>Intertrochanteric</u> fracture of femur
S72.141- <u>Displaced</u> intertrochanteric fracture of <u>right</u> femur
CC-K,M,N,P,Q,R MCC-A,B,C
S72.142- <u>Displaced</u> intertrochanteric fracture of <u>left</u> femur
CC-K,M,N,P,Q,R MCC-A,B,C
S72.143- <u>Displaced</u> intertrochanteric fracture of <u>unspecified</u> femur
CC-K,M,N,P,Q,R MCC-A,B,C
S72.144- <u>Nondisplaced</u> intertrochanteric fracture of <u>right</u> femur
CC-K,M,N,P,Q,R MCC-A,B,C

S72.145- <u>Nondisplaced</u> intertrochanteric fracture of <u>left</u> femur
CC-K,M,N,P,Q,R MCC-A,B,C
S72.146- <u>Nondisplaced</u> intertrochanteric fracture of <u>unspecified</u> femur
CC-K,M,N,P,Q,R MCC-A,B,C

S72.2- <u>Subtrochanteric</u> fracture of femur
S72.21x- <u>Displaced</u> subtrochanteric fracture of <u>right</u> femur
CC-K,M,N,P,Q,R MCC-A,B,C
S72.22x- <u>Displaced</u> subtrochanteric fracture of <u>left</u> femur
CC-K,M,N,P,Q,R MCC-A,B,C
S72.23x- <u>Displaced</u> subtrochanteric fracture of <u>unspecified</u> femur
CC-K,M,N,P,Q,R MCC-A,B,C
S72.24x- <u>Nondisplaced</u> subtrochanteric fracture of <u>right</u> femur
CC-K,M,N,P,Q,R MCC-A,B,C
S72.25x- <u>Nondisplaced</u> subtrochanteric fracture of <u>left</u> femur
CC-K,M,N,P,Q,R MCC-A,B,C
S72.26x- <u>Nondisplaced</u> subtrochanteric fracture of <u>unspecified</u> femur
CC-K,M,N,P,Q,R MCC-A,B,C

S72.3- Fracture of <u>shaft</u> of femur
S72.30- <u>Unspecified</u> fracture of <u>shaft</u> of femur
S72.301- Unspecified fracture of shaft of <u>right</u> femur
CC-K,M,N,P,Q,R MCC-A,B,C
S72.302- Unspecified fracture of shaft of <u>left</u> femur
CC-K,M,N,P,Q,R MCC-A,B,C
S72.309- Unspecified fracture of shaft of <u>unspecified</u> femur
CC-K,M,N,P,Q,R MCC-A,B,C

S72.32- <u>Transverse</u> fracture of <u>shaft</u> of femur
S72.321- <u>Displaced</u> transverse fracture of shaft of <u>right</u> femur
CC-K,M,N,P,Q,R MCC-A,B,C
S72.322- <u>Displaced</u> transverse fracture of shaft of <u>left</u> femur
CC-K,M,N,P,Q,R MCC-A,B,C
S72.323- <u>Displaced</u> transverse fracture of shaft of <u>unspecified</u> femur
CC-K,M,N,P,Q,R MCC-A,B,C
S72.324- <u>Nondisplaced</u> transverse fracture of shaft of <u>right</u> femur
CC-K,M,N,P,Q,R MCC-A,B,C
S72.325- <u>Nondisplaced</u> transverse fracture of shaft of <u>left</u> femur
CC-K,M,N,P,Q,R MCC-A,B,C
S72.326- <u>Nondisplaced</u> transverse fracture of shaft of <u>unspecified</u> femur
CC-K,M,N,P,Q,R MCC-A,B,C

S72.33- <u>Oblique</u> fracture of <u>shaft</u> of femur
S72.331- <u>Displaced</u> oblique fracture of shaft of <u>right</u> femur
CC-K,M,N,P,Q,R MCC-A,B,C
S72.332- <u>Displaced</u> oblique fracture of shaft of <u>left</u> femur
CC-K,M,N,P,Q,R MCC-A,B,C
S72.333- <u>Displaced</u> oblique fracture of shaft of <u>unspecified</u> femur
CC-K,M,N,P,Q,R MCC-A,B,C
S72.334- <u>Nondisplaced</u> oblique fracture of shaft of <u>right</u> femur
CC-K,M,N,P,Q,R MCC-A,B,C
S72.335- <u>Nondisplaced</u> oblique fracture of shaft of <u>left</u> femur
CC-K,M,N,P,Q,R MCC-A,B,C
S72.336- <u>Nondisplaced</u> oblique fracture of shaft of <u>unspecified</u> femur
CC-K,M,N,P,Q,R MCC-A,B,C

S72.34- <u>Spiral</u> fracture of <u>shaft</u> of femur
S72.341- <u>Displaced</u> spiral fracture of shaft of <u>right</u> femur
CC-K,M,N,P,Q,R MCC-A,B,C
S72.342- <u>Displaced</u> spiral fracture of shaft of <u>left</u> femur
CC-K,M,N,P,Q,R MCC-A,B,C
S72.343- <u>Displaced</u> spiral fracture of shaft of <u>unspecified</u> femur
CC-K,M,N,P,Q,R MCC-A,B,C
S72.344- <u>Nondisplaced</u> spiral fracture of shaft of <u>right</u> femur
CC-K,M,N,P,Q,R MCC-A,B,C
S72.345- <u>Nondisplaced</u> spiral fracture of shaft of <u>left</u> femur
CC-K,M,N,P,Q,R MCC-A,B,C

S72.346- **Nondisplaced** spiral fracture of shaft of **unspecified** femur
CC-K,M,N,P,Q,R MCC-A,B,C

S72.35- **Comminuted** fracture of **shaft** of femur

S72.351- **Displaced** comminuted fracture of shaft of **right** femur
CC-K,M,N,P,Q,R MCC-A,B,C

S72.352- **Displaced** comminuted fracture of shaft of **left** femur
CC-K,M,N,P,Q,R MCC-A,B,C

S72.353- **Displaced** comminuted fracture of shaft of **unspecified** femur
CC-K,M,N,P,Q,R MCC-A,B,C

S72.354- **Nondisplaced** comminuted fracture of shaft of **right** femur
CC-K,M,N,P,Q,R MCC-A,B,C

S72.355- **Nondisplaced** comminuted fracture of shaft of **left** femur
CC-K,M,N,P,Q,R MCC-A,B,C

S72.356- **Nondisplaced** comminuted fracture of shaft of **unspecified** femur
CC-K,M,N,P,Q,R MCC-A,B,C

S72.36- **Segmental** fracture of **shaft** of femur

S72.361- **Displaced** segmental fracture of shaft of **right** femur
CC-K,M,N,P,Q,R MCC-A,B,C

S72.362- **Displaced** segmental fracture of shaft of **left** femur
CC-K,M,N,P,Q,R MCC-A,B,C

S72.363- **Displaced** segmental fracture of shaft of **unspecified** femur
CC-K,M,N,P,Q,R MCC-A,B,C

S72.364- **Nondisplaced** segmental fracture of shaft of **right** femur
CC-K,M,N,P,Q,R MCC-A,B,C

S72.365- **Nondisplaced** segmental fracture of shaft of **left** femur
CC-K,M,N,P,Q,R MCC-A,B,C

S72.366- **Nondisplaced** segmental fracture of shaft of **unspecified** femur
CC-K,M,N,P,Q,R MCC-A,B,C

S72.39- **Other fracture** of **shaft** of femur

S72.391- Other fracture of shaft of **right** femur
CC-K,M,N,P,Q,R MCC-A,B,C

S72.392- Other fracture of shaft of **left** femur
CC-K,M,N,P,Q,R MCC-A,B,C

S72.399- Other fracture of shaft of **unspecified** femur
CC-K,M,N,P,Q,R MCC-A,B,C

S72.4- Fracture of **lower end** of femur
Fracture of distal end of femur
Excludes ❷: *fracture of shaft of femur (S72.3-)*
physeal fracture of lower end of femur (S79.1-)

S72.40- **Unspecified** fracture of **lower end** of femur

S72.401- Unspecified fracture of lower end of **right** femur
CC-A,K,M,N,P,Q,R MCC-B,C

S72.402- Unspecified fracture of lower end of **left** femur
CC-A,K,M,N,P,Q,R MCC-B,C

S72.409- Unspecified fracture of lower end of **unspecified** femur
CC-A,K,M,N,P,Q,R MCC-B,C

S72.41- **Unspecified** **condyle** fracture of **lower end** of femur
Condyle fracture of femur NOS

S72.411- **Displaced** unspecified condyle fracture of lower end of **right** femur
CC-A,K,M,N,P,Q,R MCC-B,C

S72.412- **Displaced** unspecified condyle fracture of lower end of **left** femur
CC-A,K,M,N,P,Q,R MCC-B,C

S72.413- **Displaced** unspecified condyle fracture of lower end of **unspecified** femur
CC-A,K,M,N,P,Q,R MCC-B,C

S72.414- **Nondisplaced** unspecified condyle fracture of lower end of **right** femur
CC-A,K,M,N,P,Q,R MCC-B,C

S72.415- **Nondisplaced** unspecified condyle fracture of lower end of **left** femur
CC-A,K,M,N,P,Q,R MCC-B,C

S72.416- **Nondisplaced** unspecified condyle fracture of lower end of **unspecified** femur
CC-A,K,M,N,P,Q,R MCC-B,C

S72.42- Fracture of **lateral condyle** of femur

S72.421- **Displaced** fracture of lateral condyle of **right** femur
CC-A,K,M,N,P,Q,R MCC-B,C

S72.422- **Displaced** fracture of lateral condyle of **left** femur
CC-A,K,M,N,P,Q,R MCC-B,C

S72.423- **Displaced** fracture of lateral condyle of **unspecified** femur
CC-A,K,M,N,P,Q,R MCC-B,C

S72.424- **Nondisplaced** fracture of lateral condyle of **right** femur
CC-A,K,M,N,P,Q,R MCC-B,C

S72.425- **Nondisplaced** fracture of lateral condyle of **left** femur
CC-A,K,M,N,P,Q,R MCC-B,C

S72.426- **Nondisplaced** fracture of lateral condyle of **unspecified** femur
CC-A,K,M,N,P,Q,R MCC-B,C

S72.43- Fracture of **medial condyle** of femur

S72.431- **Displaced** fracture of medial condyle of **right** femur
CC-A,K,M,N,P,Q,R MCC-B,C

S72.432- **Displaced** fracture of medial condyle of **left** femur
CC-A,K,M,N,P,Q,R MCC-B,C

S72.433- **Displaced** fracture of medial condyle of **unspecified** femur
CC-A,K,M,N,P,Q,R MCC-B,C

S72.434- **Nondisplaced** fracture of medial condyle of **right** femur
CC-A,K,M,N,P,Q,R MCC-B,C

S72.435- **Nondisplaced** fracture of medial condyle of **left** femur
CC-A,K,M,N,P,Q,R MCC-B,C

S72.436- **Nondisplaced** fracture of medial condyle of **unspecified** femur
CC-A,K,M,N,P,Q,R MCC-B,C

S72.44- Fracture of **lower epiphysis** (separation) of femur
Excludes 1: *Salter-Harris Type I physeal fracture of lower end of femur (S79.11-)*

S72.441- **Displaced** fracture of lower epiphysis (separation) of **right** femur
CC-A,K,M,N,P,Q,R MCC-B,C

S72.442- **Displaced** fracture of lower epiphysis (separation) of **left** femur
CC-A,K,M,N,P,Q,R MCC-B,C

S72.443- **Displaced** fracture of lower epiphysis (separation) of **unspecified** femur
CC-A,K,M,N,P,Q,R MCC-B,C

S72.444- **Nondisplaced** fracture of lower epiphysis (separation) of **right** femur
CC-A,K,M,N,P,Q,R MCC-B,C

S72.445- **Nondisplaced** fracture of lower epiphysis (separation) of **left** femur
CC-A,K,M,N,P,Q,R MCC-B,C

S72.446- **Nondisplaced** fracture of lower epiphysis (separation) of **unspecified** femur
CC-A,K,M,N,P,Q,R MCC-B,C

S72.45- **Supracondylar** fracture **without** intracondylar extension of lower end of femur
Supracondylar fracture of lower end of femur NOS
Excludes 1: *supracondylar fracture with intracondylar extension of lower end of femur (S72.46-)*

S72.451- **Displaced** supracondylar fracture **without** intracondylar extension of lower end of **right** femur
CC-A,K,M,N,P,Q,R MCC-B,C

S72.452- **Displaced** supracondylar fracture **without** intracondylar extension of lower end of **left** femur
CC-A,K,M,N,P,Q,R MCC-B,C

S72.453- **Displaced** supracondylar fracture **without** intracondylar extension of lower end of **unspecified** femur
CC-A,K,M,N,P,Q,R MCC-B,C

S72.454- **Nondisplaced** supracondylar fracture **without** intracondylar extension of lower end of **right** femur
CC-A,K,M,N,P,Q,R MCC-B,C

S72 - S72

S72.455- **Nondisplaced** supracondylar fracture **without** intracondylar extension of lower end of **left** femur
CC-A,K,M,N,P,Q,R

S72.456- **Nondisplaced** supracondylar fracture **without** intracondylar extension of lower end of **unspecified** femur
CC-A,K,M,N,P,Q,R MCC-B,C

S72.46- **Supracondylar** fracture **with intracondylar extension** of lower end of femur
Excludes 1: supracondylar fracture without intracondylar extension of lower end of femur (S72.45-)

S72.461- **Displaced** supracondylar fracture **with intracondylar extension** of lower end of **right** femur
CC-A,K,M,N,P,Q,R MCC-B,C

S72.462- **Displaced** supracondylar fracture **with intracondylar extension** of lower end of **left** femur
CC-A,K,M,N,P,Q,R MCC-B,C

S72.463- **Displaced** supracondylar fracture **with intracondylar extension** of lower end of **unspecified** femur
CC-A,K,M,N,P,Q,R MCC-B,C

S72.464- **Nondisplaced** supracondylar fracture **with intracondylar extension** of lower end of **right** femur
CC-A,K,M,N,P,Q,R MCC-B,C

S72.465- **Nondisplaced** supracondylar fracture **with intracondylar extension** of lower end of **left** femur
CC-A,K,M,N,P,Q,R MCC-B,C

S72.466- **Nondisplaced** supracondylar fracture **with intracondylar extension** of lower end of **unspecified** femur
CC-A,K,M,N,P,Q,R MCC-B,C

S72.47- **Torus** fracture of **lower end** of femur

> The appropriate 7th character is to be added to all codes in subcategory S72.47:
> A **Initial** encounter for **closed** fracture
> D **Subsequent** encounter for fracture **with routine healing**
> G **Subsequent** encounter for fracture **with delayed healing**
> K Subsequent encounter for fracture **with nonunion**
> P **Subsequent** encounter for fracture **with malunion**
> S **Sequela**

CC-A,K,P **S72.471-** **Torus** fracture of lower end of **right** femur
CC-A,K,P **S72.472-** **Torus** fracture of lower end of **left** femur
CC-A,K,P **S72.479-** **Torus** fracture of lower end of **unspecified** femur

S72.49- **Other fracture** of **lower end** of femur

S72.491- **Other fracture** of lower end of **right** femur
CC-A,K,M,N,P,Q,R MCC-B,C

S72.492- **Other fracture** of lower end of **left** femur
CC-A,K,M,N,P,Q,R MCC-B,C

S72.499- **Other fracture** of lower end of **unspecified** femur
CC-A,K,M,N,P,Q,R MCC-B,C

S72.8- **Other fracture** of femur

S72.8x- **Other fracture** of femur

S72.8x1- **Other fracture** of **right** femur
CC-K,M,N,P,Q,R MCC-A,B,C

S72.8x2- **Other fracture** of **left** femur
CC-K,M,N,P,Q,R MCC-A,B,C

S72.8x9- **Other fracture** of **unspecified** femur
CC-K,M,N,P,Q,R MCC-A,B,C

S72.9- **Unspecified** fracture of femur
Fracture of thigh NOS
Fracture of upper leg NOS
Excludes 1: fracture of hip NOS (S72.00-, S72.01-)

S72.90x- **Unspecified** fracture of **unspecified** femur
CC-K,M,N,P,Q,R MCC-A,B,C

S72.91x- **Unspecified** fracture of **right** femur
CC-K,M,N,P,Q,R MCC-A,B,C

S72.92x- **Unspecified** fracture of **left** femur
CC-K,M,N,P,Q,R MCC-A,B,C

S73- **Dislocation and sprain** of joint and ligaments of **hip**
Includes: Avulsion of joint or ligament of hip
Laceration of cartilage, joint or ligament of hip
Sprain of cartilage, joint or ligament of hip
Traumatic hemarthrosis of joint or ligament of hip
Traumatic rupture of joint or ligament of hip
Traumatic subluxation of joint or ligament of hip
Traumatic tear of joint or ligament of hip
Code also any associated open wound
Excludes 2: strain of muscle, fascia and tendon of hip and thigh (S76.-)

> The appropriate 7th character is to be added to each code from category S73:
> A **Initial** encounter
> D **Subsequent** encounter
> S **Sequela**

S73.0- **Subluxation and dislocation** of **hip**
Excludes 2: dislocation and subluxation of hip prosthesis (T84.020, T84.021)

S73.00- **Unspecified** subluxation and dislocation of hip
Dislocation of hip NOS
Subluxation of hip NOS

CC-A **S73.001-** Unspecified **subluxation** of **right** hip
CC-A **S73.002-** Unspecified **subluxation** of **left** hip
CC-A **S73.003-** Unspecified **subluxation** of **unspecified** hip
CC-A **S73.004-** Unspecified **dislocation** of **right** hip
CC-A **S73.005-** Unspecified **dislocation** of **left** hip
CC-A **S73.006-** Unspecified **dislocation** of **unspecified** hip

S73.01- **Posterior** subluxation and dislocation of hip
CC-A **S73.011-** Posterior **subluxation** of **right** hip
CC-A **S73.012-** Posterior **subluxation** of **left** hip
CC-A **S73.013-** Posterior **subluxation** of **unspecified** hip
CC-A **S73.014-** Posterior **dislocation** of **right** hip
CC-A **S73.015-** Posterior **dislocation** of **left** hip
CC-A **S73.016-** Posterior **dislocation** of **unspecified** hip

S73.02- **Obturator** subluxation and dislocation of hip
CC-A **S73.021-** Obturator **subluxation** of **right** hip
CC-A **S73.022-** Obturator **subluxation** of **left** hip
CC-A **S73.023-** Obturator **subluxation** of **unspecified** hip
CC-A **S73.024-** Obturator **dislocation** of **right** hip
CC-A **S73.025-** Obturator **dislocation** of **left** hip
CC-A **S73.026-** Obturator **dislocation** of **unspecified** hip

S73.03- **Other anterior** dislocation of hip
CC-A **S73.031-** Other anterior **subluxation** of **right** hip
CC-A **S73.032-** Other anterior **subluxation** of **left** hip
CC-A **S73.033-** Other anterior **subluxation** of **unspecified** hip
CC-A **S73.034-** Other anterior **dislocation** of **right** hip
CC-A **S73.035-** Other anterior **dislocation** of **left** hip
CC-A **S73.036-** Other anterior **dislocation** of **unspecified** hip

S73.04- **Central** dislocation of hip
CC-A **S73.041-** Central **subluxation** of **right** hip
CC-A **S73.042-** Central **subluxation** of **left** hip
CC-A **S73.043-** Central **subluxation** of **unspecified** hip
CC-A **S73.044-** Central **dislocation** of **right** hip
CC-A **S73.045-** Central **dislocation** of **left** hip
CC-A **S73.046-** Central **dislocation** of **unspecified** hip

S73.1- **Sprain** of **hip**
AHA 14:4Q:p25 – Left hip labral tear (sprain)

S73.10- **Unspecified** **sprain** of hip
S73.101- Unspecified sprain of **right** hip
S73.102- Unspecified sprain of **left** hip
S73.109- Unspecified sprain of **unspecified** hip

S73.11- **Iliofemoral ligament** **sprain** of hip
S73.111- Iliofemoral ligament sprain of **right** hip
S73.112- Iliofemoral ligament sprain of **left** hip
S73.119- Iliofemoral ligament sprain of **unspecified** hip

S73.12- **Ischiocapsular (ligament)** **sprain** of hip
S73.121- Ischiocapsular ligament sprain of **right** hip
S73.122- Ischiocapsular ligament sprain of **left** hip

S
7
2
-
S
7
3

Excludes 1: = NOT CODED HERE! (Do not code both)   **1106**   Excludes 2: = Not Included Here

S73.129- Ischiocapsular ligament sprain of <u>unspecified</u> hip
S73.19- <u>Other sprain</u> of hip
S73.191- Other sprain of <u>right</u> hip
S73.192- Other sprain of <u>left</u> hip
S73.199- Other sprain of <u>unspecified</u> hip

S74- <u>Injury of nerves</u> at <u>hip and thigh level</u>
Code also any associated open wound (S71.-)
Excludes ❷: injury of nerves at ankle and foot level (S94.-)
injury of nerves at lower leg level (S84.-)

The appropriate 7th character is to be added to each code from
category S74:
A <u>Initial</u> encounter
D <u>Subsequent</u> encounter
S <u>Sequela</u>

S74.0- Injury of <u>sciatic</u> nerve at <u>hip and thigh level</u>
S74.00x- Injury of sciatic nerve at hip and thigh level,
<u>unspecified</u> leg
S74.01x- Injury of sciatic nerve at hip and thigh level, <u>right</u> leg
S74.02x- Injury of sciatic nerve at hip and thigh level, <u>left</u> leg

S74.1- Injury of <u>femoral</u> nerve at <u>hip and thigh level</u>
S74.10x- Injury of femoral nerve at hip and thigh level,
<u>unspecified</u> leg
S74.11x- Injury of femoral nerve at hip and thigh level, <u>right</u> leg
S74.12x- Injury of femoral nerve at hip and thigh level, <u>left</u> leg

S74.2- Injury of <u>cutaneous sensory</u> nerve at <u>hip and thigh level</u>
S74.20x- Injury of cutaneous sensory nerve at hip and thigh
level, <u>unspecified</u> leg
S74.21x- Injury of cutaneous sensory nerve at hip and high level,
<u>right</u> leg
S74.22x- Injury of cutaneous sensory nerve at hip and thigh
level, <u>left</u> leg

S74.8- Injury of <u>other nerves</u> at <u>hip and thigh level</u>
S74.8x- Injury of <u>other nerves</u> at <u>hip and thigh level</u>
S74.8x1- Injury of other nerves at hip and thigh level, <u>right</u>
leg
S74.8x2- Injury of other nerves at hip and thigh level, <u>left</u>
leg
S74.8x9- Injury of other nerves at hip and thigh level,
<u>unspecified</u> leg

S74.9- Injury of <u>unspecified</u> nerve at <u>hip and thigh level</u>
S74.90x- Injury of unspecified nerve at hip and thigh level,
<u>unspecified</u> leg
S74.91x- Injury of unspecified nerve at hip and thigh level, <u>right</u>
leg
S74.92x- Injury of unspecified nerve at hip and thigh level, <u>left</u>
leg

S75- <u>Injury of blood vessels</u> at <u>hip and thigh level</u>
Code also any associated open wound (S71.-)
Excludes ❷: injury of blood vessels at lower leg level (S85.-)
injury of popliteal artery (S85.0)

The appropriate 7th character is to be added to each code from
category S75:
A <u>Initial</u> encounter
D <u>Subsequent</u> encounter
S <u>Sequela</u>

S75.0- Injury of <u>femoral artery</u>
S75.00- <u>Unspecified</u> injury of <u>femoral artery</u>
MCC-A S75.001- Unspecified injury of femoral artery, <u>right</u> leg
MCC-A S75.002- Unspecified injury of femoral artery, <u>left</u> leg
MCC-A S75.009- Unspecified injury of femoral artery, <u>unspecified</u>
leg
S75.01- <u>Minor laceration</u> of <u>femoral artery</u>
Incomplete transection of femoral artery
Laceration of femoral artery NOS
Superficial laceration of femoral artery
MCC-A S75.011- Minor laceration of femoral artery, <u>right</u> leg
MCC-A S75.012- Minor laceration of femoral artery, <u>left</u> leg
MCC-A S75.019- Minor laceration of femoral artery, <u>unspecified</u> leg

S75.02- <u>Major laceration</u> of <u>femoral artery</u>
Complete transection of femoral artery
Traumatic rupture of femoral artery
MCC-A S75.021- Major laceration of femoral artery, <u>right</u> leg
MCC-A S75.022- Major laceration of femoral artery, <u>left</u> leg
MCC-A S75.029- Major laceration of femoral artery, <u>unspecified</u> leg
S75.09- <u>Other specified injury</u> of <u>femoral artery</u>
MCC-A S75.091- Other specified injury of femoral artery, <u>right</u> leg
MCC-A S75.092- Other specified injury of femoral artery, <u>left</u> leg
MCC-A S75.099- Other specified injury of femoral artery,
<u>unspecified</u> leg

S75.1- Injury of <u>femoral vein</u> at <u>hip and thigh level</u>
S75.10- <u>Unspecified</u> injury of <u>femoral vein</u> at <u>hip and thigh level</u>
MCC-A S75.101- Unspecified injury of femoral vein at hip and thigh
level, <u>right</u> leg
MCC-A S75.102- Unspecified injury of femoral vein at hip and thigh
level, <u>left</u> leg
MCC-A S75.109- Unspecified injury of femoral vein at hip and thigh
level, <u>unspecified</u> leg
S75.11- <u>Minor laceration</u> of <u>femoral vein</u> at <u>hip and thigh level</u>
Incomplete transection of femoral vein at hip and thigh level
Laceration of femoral vein at hip and thigh level NOS
Superficial laceration of femoral vein at hip and thigh level
MCC-A S75.111- Minor laceration of femoral vein at hip and thigh
level, <u>right</u> leg
MCC-A S75.112- Minor laceration of femoral vein at hip and thigh
level, <u>left</u> leg
MCC-A S75.119- Minor laceration of femoral vein at hip and thigh
level, <u>unspecified</u> leg
S75.12- <u>Major laceration</u> of <u>femoral vein</u> at <u>hip and thigh level</u>
Complete transection of femoral vein at hip and thigh level
Traumatic rupture of femoral vein at hip and thigh level
MCC-A S75.121- Major laceration of femoral vein at hip and thigh
level, <u>right</u> leg
MCC-A S75.122- Major laceration of femoral vein at hip and thigh
level, <u>left</u> leg
MCC-A S75.129- Major laceration of femoral vein at hip and thigh
level, <u>unspecified</u> leg
S75.19- <u>Other specified injury</u> of <u>femoral vein</u> at <u>hip and thigh</u>
<u>level</u>
MCC-A S75.191- Other specified injury of femoral vein at hip and
thigh level, <u>right</u> leg
MCC-A S75.192- Other specified injury of femoral vein at hip and
thigh level, <u>left</u> leg
MCC-A S75.199- Other specified injury of femoral vein at hip and
thigh level, <u>unspecified</u> leg

S75.2- Injury of <u>greater saphenous vein</u> at <u>hip and thigh level</u>
Excludes 1: greater saphenous vein NOS (S85.3)
S75.20- <u>Unspecified</u> injury of <u>greater saphenous vein</u> at <u>hip and</u>
<u>thigh level</u>
CC-A S75.201- Unspecified injury of greater saphenous vein at hip
and thigh level, <u>right</u> leg
CC-A S75.202- Unspecified injury of greater saphenous vein at hip
and thigh level, <u>left</u> leg
CC-A S75.209- Unspecified injury of greater saphenous vein at hip
and thigh level, <u>unspecified</u> leg
S75.21- <u>Minor laceration</u> of <u>greater saphenous vein</u> at <u>hip and</u>
<u>thigh level</u>
Incomplete transection of greater saphenous vein at hip and
thigh level
Laceration of greater saphenous vein at hip and thigh level
NOS
Superficial laceration of greater saphenous vein at hip and
thigh level
CC-A S75.211- Minor laceration of greater saphenous vein at hip
and thigh level, <u>right</u> leg
CC-A S75.212- Minor laceration of greater saphenous vein at hip
and thigh level, <u>left</u> leg
CC-A S75.219- Minor laceration of greater saphenous vein at hip
and thigh level, <u>unspecified</u> leg

S73
-
S75

S75.22- <u>Major laceration</u> of <u>greater saphenous</u> <u>vein</u> at <u>hip and</u> <u>thigh level</u>

    Complete transection of greater saphenous vein at hip and thigh level

    Traumatic rupture of greater saphenous vein at hip and thigh level

CC-A **S75.221-** Major laceration of greater saphenous vein at hip and thigh level, <u>right</u> leg

CC-A **S75.222-** Major laceration of greater saphenous vein at hip and thigh level, <u>left</u> leg

CC-A **S75.229-** Major laceration of greater saphenous vein at hip and thigh level, <u>unspecified</u> leg

S75.29- <u>Other specified injury</u> of <u>greater saphenous</u> <u>vein</u> at <u>hip</u> <u>and thigh level</u>

CC-A **S75.291-** Other specified injury of greater saphenous vein at hip and thigh level, <u>right</u> leg

CC-A **S75.292-** Other specified injury of greater saphenous vein at hip and thigh level, <u>left</u> leg

CC-A **S75.299-** Other specified injury of greater saphenous vein at hip and thigh level, <u>unspecified</u> leg

S75.8- Injury of <u>other blood vessels</u> at <u>hip and thigh level</u>

S75.80- <u>Unspecified</u> injury of <u>other blood vessels</u> at <u>hip and thigh</u> <u>level</u>

CC-A **S75.801-** Unspecified injury of other blood vessels at hip and thigh level, <u>right</u> leg

CC-A **S75.802-** Unspecified injury of other blood vessels at hip and thigh level, <u>left</u> leg

CC-A **S75.809-** Unspecified injury of other blood vessels at hip and thigh level, <u>unspecified</u> leg

S75.81- <u>Laceration</u> of <u>other blood vessels</u> at <u>hip and thigh level</u>

CC-A **S75.811-** Laceration of other blood vessels at hip and thigh level, <u>right</u> leg

CC-A **S75.812-** Laceration of other blood vessels at hip and thigh level, <u>left</u> leg

CC-A **S75.819-** Laceration of other blood vessels at hip and thigh level, <u>unspecified</u> leg

S75.89- <u>Other specified injury</u> of <u>other blood vessels</u> at <u>hip and</u> <u>thigh level</u>

CC-A **S75.891-** Other specified injury of other blood vessels at hip and thigh level, <u>right</u> leg

CC-A **S75.892-** Other specified injury of other blood vessels at hip and thigh level, <u>left</u> leg

CC-A **S75.899-** Other specified injury of other blood vessels at hip and thigh level, <u>unspecified</u> leg

S75.9- Injury of <u>unspecified blood vessel</u> at <u>hip and thigh level</u>

S75.90- <u>Unspecified</u> injury of <u>unspecified blood vessel</u> at <u>hip and</u> <u>thigh level</u>

CC-A **S75.901-** Unspecified injury of unspecified blood vessel at hip and thigh level, <u>right</u> leg

CC-A **S75.902-** Unspecified injury of unspecified blood vessel at hip and thigh level, <u>left</u> leg

CC-A **S75.909-** Unspecified injury of unspecified blood vessel at hip and thigh level, <u>unspecified</u> leg

S75.91- <u>Laceration</u> of <u>unspecified blood vessel</u> at <u>hip and thigh</u> <u>level</u>

CC-A **S75.911-** Laceration of unspecified blood vessel at hip and thigh level, <u>right</u> leg

CC-A **S75.912-** Laceration of unspecified blood vessel at hip and thigh level, <u>left</u> leg

CC-A **S75.919-** Laceration of unspecified blood vessel at hip and thigh level, <u>unspecified</u> leg

S75.99- <u>Other specified injury</u> of <u>unspecified blood vessel</u> at <u>hip</u> <u>and thigh level</u>

CC-A **S75.991-** Other specified injury of <u>unspecified</u> blood vessel at hip and thigh level, <u>right</u> leg

CC-A **S75.992-** Other specified injury of <u>unspecified</u> blood vessel at hip and thigh level, <u>left</u> leg

CC-A **S75.999-** Other specified injury of <u>unspecified</u> blood vessel at hip and thigh level, <u>unspecified</u> leg

S76- <u>Injury</u> of <u>muscle, fascia and tendon</u> at <u>hip and thigh level</u>

    Code also any associated open wound (S71.-)

Excludes ❷: *injury of muscle, fascia and tendon at lower leg level (S86)*

         sprain of joint and ligament of hip (S73.1)

The appropriate 7th character is to be added to each code from category S76:

A   <u>Initial</u> encounter

D   <u>Subsequent</u> encounter

S   <u>Sequela</u>

S76.0- Injury of <u>muscle, fascia and tendon</u> of <u>hip</u>

S76.00- <u>Unspecified</u> injury of <u>muscle, fascia and tendon</u> of <u>hip</u>

S76.001- Unspecified injury of muscle, fascia and tendon of <u>right</u> hip

S76.002- Unspecified injury of muscle, fascia and tendon of <u>left</u> hip

S76.009- Unspecified injury of muscle, fascia and tendon of <u>unspecified</u> hip

S76.01- <u>Strain</u> of <u>muscle, fascia and tendon</u> of <u>hip</u>

S76.011- Strain of muscle, fascia and tendon of <u>right</u> hip

S76.012- Strain of muscle, fascia and tendon of <u>left</u> hip

S76.019- Strain of muscle, fascia and tendon of <u>unspecified</u> hip

S76.02- <u>Laceration</u> of <u>muscle, fascia and tendon</u> of <u>hip</u>

CC-A **S76.021-** Laceration of muscle, fascia and tendon of <u>right</u> hip

CC-A **S76.022-** Laceration of muscle, fascia and tendon of <u>left</u> hip

CC-A **S76.029-** Laceration of muscle, fascia and tendon of <u>unspecified</u> hip

S76.09- <u>Other specified injury</u> of <u>muscle, fascia and tendon</u> of <u>hip</u>

S76.091- Other specified injury of muscle, fascia and tendon of <u>right</u> hip

S76.092- Other specified injury of muscle, fascia and tendon of <u>left</u> hip

S76.099- Other specified injury of muscle, fascia and tendon of <u>unspecified</u> hip

S76.1- Injury of <u>quadriceps</u> <u>muscle, fascia and tendon</u>

    Injury of patellar ligament (tendon)

S76.10- <u>Unspecified</u> injury of <u>quadriceps</u> muscle, fascia and tendon

S76.101- Unspecified injury of <u>right</u> quadriceps muscle, fascia and tendon

S76.102- Unspecified injury of <u>left</u> quadriceps muscle, fascia and tendon

S76.109- Unspecified injury of <u>unspecified</u> quadriceps muscle, fascia and tendon

S76.11- <u>Strain</u> of <u>quadriceps</u> muscle, fascia and tendon

S76.111- Strain of <u>right</u> quadriceps muscle, fascia and tendon

S76.112- Strain of <u>left</u> quadriceps muscle, fascia and tendon

S76.119- Strain of <u>unspecified</u> quadriceps muscle, fascia and tendon

S76.12- <u>Laceration</u> of <u>quadriceps</u> muscle, fascia and tendon

CC-A **S76.121-** Laceration of <u>right</u> quadriceps muscle, fascia and tendon

CC-A **S76.122-** Laceration of <u>left</u> quadriceps muscle, fascia and tendon

CC-A **S76.129-** Laceration of <u>unspecified</u> quadriceps muscle, fascia and tendon

S76.19- <u>Other specified injury</u> of <u>quadriceps</u> muscle, fascia and tendon

S76.191- Other specified injury of <u>right</u> quadriceps muscle, fascia and tendon

S76.192- Other specified injury of <u>left</u> quadriceps muscle, fascia and tendon

S76.199- Other specified injury of <u>unspecified</u> quadriceps muscle, fascia and tendon

S 7 5 - S 7 6

S76.2- Injry of <u>adductor muscle, fascia and tendon</u> of <u>thigh</u>

S76.20- <u>Unspecified</u> injury of <u>adductor</u> muscle, fascia and tendon of thigh

S76.201- Unspecified injury of adductor muscle, fascia and tendon of <u>right</u> thigh

S76.202- Unspecified injury of adductor muscle, fascia and tendon of <u>left</u> thigh

S76.209- Unspecified injury of adductor muscle, fascia and tendon of <u>unspecified</u> thigh

S76.21- <u>Strain</u> of <u>adductor</u> muscle, fascia and tendon of <u>thigh</u>

S76.211- Strain of adductor muscle, fascia and tendon of <u>right</u> thigh

S76.212- Strain of adductor muscle, fascia and tendon of <u>left</u> thigh

S76.219- Strain of adductor muscle, fascia and tendon of <u>unspecified</u> thigh

S76.22- <u>Laceration</u> of <u>adductor</u> muscle, fascia and tendon of <u>thigh</u>

CC-A S76.221- Laceration of adductor muscle, fascia and tendon of <u>right</u> thigh

CC-A S76.222- Laceration of adductor muscle, fascia and tendon of <u>left</u> thigh

CC-A S76.229- Laceration of adductor muscle, fascia and tendon of <u>unspecified</u> thigh

S76.29- <u>Other injury</u> of <u>adductor</u> muscle, fascia and tendon of <u>thigh</u>

S76.291- Other injury of adductor muscle, fascia and tendon of <u>right</u> thigh

S76.292- Other injury of adductor muscle, fascia and tendon of <u>left</u> thigh

S76.299- Other injury of adductor muscle, fascia and tendon of <u>unspecified</u> thigh

S76.3- Injury of <u>muscle, fascia and tendon</u> of the <u>posterior muscle group</u> at <u>thigh</u> level

S76.30- <u>Unspecified</u> injury of muscle, fascia and tendon of the <u>posterior muscle group</u> at <u>thigh</u> level

S76.301- Unspecified injury of muscle, fascia and tendon of the posterior muscle group at thigh level, <u>right</u> thigh

S76.302- Unspecified injury of muscle, fascia and tendon of the posterior muscle group at thigh level, <u>left</u> thigh

S76.309- Unspecified injury of muscle, fascia and tendon of the posterior muscle group at thigh level, <u>unspecified</u> thigh

S76.31- <u>Strain</u> of muscle, fascia and tendon of the <u>posterior muscle group</u> at <u>thigh</u> level

S76.311- Strain of muscle, fascia and tendon of the posterior muscle group at thigh level, <u>right</u> thigh

S76.312- Strain of muscle, fascia and tendon of the posterior muscle group at thigh level, <u>left</u> thigh

S76.319- Strain of muscle, fascia and tendon of the posterior muscle group at thigh level, <u>unspecified</u> thigh

S76.32- <u>Laceration</u> of muscle, fascia and tendon of the <u>posterior muscle group</u> at <u>thigh</u> level

CC-A S76.321- Laceration of muscle, fascia and tendon of the posterior muscle group at thigh level, <u>right</u> thigh

CC-A S76.322- Laceration of muscle, fascia and tendon of the posterior muscle group at thigh level, <u>left</u> thigh

CC-A S76.329- Laceration of muscle, fascia and tendon of the posterior muscle group at thigh level, <u>unspecified</u> thigh

S76.39- <u>Other specified injury</u> of muscle, fascia and tendon of the <u>posterior muscle group</u> at <u>thigh</u> level

S76.391- Other specified injury of muscle, fascia and tendon of the posterior muscle group at thigh level, <u>right</u> thigh

S76.392- Other specified injury of muscle, fascia and tendon of the posterior muscle group at thigh level, <u>left</u> thigh

S76.399- Other specified injury of muscle, fascia and tendon of the posterior muscle group at thigh level, <u>unspecified</u> thigh

S76.8- Injury of <u>other specified muscles, fascia and tendons</u> at <u>thigh</u> level

S76.80- <u>Unspecified</u> injury of <u>other specified muscles, fascia and tendons</u> at <u>thigh</u> level

S76.801- Unspecified injury of other specified muscles, fascia and tendons at thigh level, <u>right</u> thigh

S76.802- Unspecified injury of other specified muscles, fascia and tendons at thigh level, <u>left</u> thigh

S76.809- Unspecified injury of other specified muscles, fascia and tendons at thigh level, <u>unspecified</u> thigh

S76.81- <u>Strain</u> of <u>other specified muscles, fascia and tendons</u> at <u>thigh</u> level

S76.811- Strain of other specified muscles, fascia and tendons at thigh level, <u>right</u> thigh

S76.812- Strain of other specified muscles, fascia and tendons at thigh level, <u>left</u> thigh

S76.819- Strain of other specified muscles, fascia and tendons at thigh level, <u>unspecified</u> thigh

S76.82- <u>Laceration</u> of <u>other specified muscles, fascia and tendons</u> at <u>thigh</u> level

CC-A S76.821- Laceration of other specified muscles, fascia and tendons at thigh level, <u>right</u> thigh

CC-A S76.822- Laceration of other specified muscles, fascia and tendons at thigh level, <u>left</u> thigh

CC-A S76.829- Laceration of other specified muscles, fascia and tendons at thigh level, <u>unspecified</u> thigh

S76.89- Other injury of <u>other specified muscles, fascia and tendons</u> at <u>thigh</u> level

S76.891- Other injury of other specified muscles, fascia and tendons at thigh level, <u>right</u> thigh

S76.892- Other injury of other specified muscles, fascia and tendons at thigh level, <u>left</u> thigh

S76.899- Other injury of other specified muscles, fascia and tendons at thigh level, <u>unspecified</u> thigh

S76.9- Injury of <u>unspecified muscles, fascia and tendons</u> at <u>thigh</u> level

S76.90- Unspecified injury of <u>unspecified muscles, fascia and tendons</u> at <u>thigh</u> level

S76.901- Unspecified injury of unspecified muscles, fascia and tendons at thigh level, <u>right</u> thigh

S76.902- Unspecified injury of unspecified muscles, fascia and tendons at thigh level, <u>left</u> thigh

S76.909- Unspecified injury of unspecified muscles, fascia and tendons at thigh level, <u>unspecified</u> thigh

S76.91- <u>Strain</u> of <u>unspecified muscles, fascia and tendons</u> at <u>thigh</u> level

S76.911- Strain of unspecified muscles, fascia and tendons at thigh level, <u>right</u> thigh

S76.912- Strain of unspecified muscles, fascia and tendons at thigh level, <u>left</u> thigh

S76.919- Strain of unspecified muscles, fascia and tendons at thigh level, <u>unspecified</u> thigh

S76.92- <u>Laceration</u> of <u>unspecified muscles, fascia and tendons</u> at <u>thigh</u> level

CC-A S76.921- Laceration of unspecified muscles, fascia and tendons at thigh level, <u>right</u> thigh

CC-A S76.922- Laceration of unspecified muscles, fascia and tendons at thigh level, <u>left</u> thigh

CC-A S76.929- Laceration of unspecified muscles, fascia and tendons at thigh level, <u>unspecified</u> thigh

S76.99- <u>Other specified injury</u> of <u>unspecified muscles, fascia and tendons</u> at <u>thigh</u> level

S76.991- Other specified injury of unspecified muscles, fascia and tendons at thigh level, <u>right</u> thigh

S76.992- Other specified injury of unspecified muscles, fascia and tendons at thigh level, <u>left</u> thigh

S
7
6
|
S
7
6

S76.999- Other specified injury of unspecified muscles, fascia and tendons at thigh level, unspecified thigh

S77- Crushing injury of hip and thigh
Use additional code(s) for all associated injuries
Excludes ❷: crushing injury of ankle and foot (S97.-)
crushing injury of lower leg (S87.-)

The appropriate 7th character is to be added to each code from category S77:
A Initial encounter
D Subsequent encounter
S Sequela

S77.0- Crushing injury of hip
CC-A S77.00x- Crushing injury of unspecified hip
CC-A S77.01x- Crushing injury of right hip
CC-A S77.02x- Crushing injury of left hip

S77.1- Crushing injury of thigh
CC-A S77.10x- Crushing injury of unspecified thigh
CC-A S77.11x- Crushing injury of right thigh
CC-A S77.12x- Crushing injury of left thigh

S77.2- Crushing injury of hip with thigh
S77.20x- Crushing injury of unspecified hip with thigh
S77.21x- Crushing injury of right hip with thigh
S77.22x- Crushing injury of left hip with thigh

S78- Traumatic amputation of hip and thigh
Note: An amputation not identified as partial or complete should be coded to complete
Excludes 1: traumatic amputation of knee (S88.0-)

The appropriate 7th character is to be added to each code from category S78:
A Initial encounter
D Subsequent encounter
S Sequela

S78.0- Traumatic amputation at hip joint
S78.01- Complete traumatic amputation at hip joint
CC-A S78.011- Complete traumatic amputation at right hip joint
CC-A S78.012- Complete traumatic amputation at left hip joint
CC-A S78.019- Complete traumatic amputation at unspecified hip joint
S78.02- Partial traumatic amputation at hip joint
CC-A S78.021- Partial traumatic amputation at right hip joint
CC-A S78.022- Partial traumatic amputation at left hip joint
CC-A S78.029- Partial traumatic amputation at unspecified hip joint

S78.1- Traumatic amputation at level between hip and knee
Excludes 1: traumatic amputation of knee (S88.0-)
S78.11- Complete traumatic amputation at level between hip and knee
CC-A S78.111- Complete traumatic amputation at level between right hip and knee
CC-A S78.112- Complete traumatic amputation at level between left hip and knee
CC-A S78.119- Complete traumatic amputation at level between unspecified hip and knee
S78.12- Partial traumatic amputation at level between hip and knee
CC-A S78.121- Partial traumatic amputation at level between right hip and knee
CC-A S78.122- Partial traumatic amputation at level between left hip and knee
CC-A S78.129- Partial traumatic amputation at level between unspecified hip and knee
S78.9- Traumatic amputation of hip and thigh, level unspecified
S78.91- Complete traumatic amputation of hip and thigh, level unspecified
CC-A S78.911- Complete traumatic amputation of right hip and thigh, level unspecified
CC-A S78.912- Complete traumatic amputation of left hip and thigh, level unspecified

CC-A S78.919- Complete traumatic amputation of unspecified hip and thigh, level unspecified
S78.92- Partial traumatic amputation of hip and thigh, level unspecified
CC-A S78.921- Partial traumatic amputation of right hip and thigh, level unspecified
CC-A S78.922- Partial traumatic amputation of left hip and thigh, level unspecified
CC-A S78.929- Partial traumatic amputation of unspecified hip and thigh, level unspecified

S79- Other and unspecified injuries of hip and thigh
Note: A fracture not indicated as open or closed should be coded to closed
The appropriate 7th character is to be added to each code from subcategories S79.0 and S79.1:
A Initial encounter for closed fracture
D Subsequent encounter for fracture with routine healing
G Subsequent encounter for fracture with delayed healing
K Subsequent encounter for fracture with nonunion
P Subsequent encounter for fracture with malunion
S Sequela

S79.0- Physeal fracture of upper end of femur
Excludes 1: apophyseal fracture of upper end of femur (S72.13-)
nontraumatic slipped upper femoral epiphysis (M93.0-)
S79.00- Unspecified physeal fracture of upper end of femur
CC-K,P MCC-A S79.001- Unspecified physeal fracture of upper end of right femur
CC-K,P MCC-A S79.002- Unspecified physeal fracture of upper end of left femur
CC-K,P MCC-A S79.009- Unspecified physeal fracture of upper end of unspecified femur
S79.01- Salter-Harris Type I physeal fracture of upper end of femur
Acute on chronic slipped capital femoral epiphysis (traumatic)
Acute slipped capital femoral epiphysis (traumatic)
Capital femoral epiphyseal fracture
Excludes 1: chronic slipped upper femoral epiphysis (nontraumatic) (M93.02-)
CC-K,P MCC-A S79.011- Salter-Harris Type I physeal fracture of upper end of right femur
CC-K,P MCC-A S79.012- Salter-Harris Type I physeal fracture of upper end of left femur
CC-K,P MCC-A S79.019- Salter-Harris Type I physeal fracture of upper end of unspecified femur
S79.09- Other physeal fracture of upper end of femur
CC-K,P MCC-A S79.091- Other physeal fracture of upper end of right femur
CC-K,P MCC-A S79.092- Other physeal fracture of upper end of left femur
CC-K,P MCC-A S79.099- Other physeal fracture of upper end of unspecified femur
S79.1- Physeal fracture of lower end of femur
S79.10- Unspecified physeal fracture of lower end of femur
CC-A,K,P S79.101- Unspecified physeal fracture of lower end of right femur
CC-A,K,P S79.102- Unspecified physeal fracture of lower end of left femur
CC-A,K,P S79.109- Unspecified physeal fracture of lower end of unspecified femur
S79.11- Salter-Harris Type I physeal fracture of lower end of femur
CC-A,K,P S79.111- Salter-Harris Type I physeal fracture of lower end of right femur
CC-A,K,P S79.112- Salter-Harris Type I physeal fracture of lower end of left femur
CC-A,K,P S79.119- Salter-Harris Type I physeal fracture of lower end of unspecified femur
S79.12- Salter-Harris Type II physeal fracture of lower end of femur
CC-A,K,P S79.121- Salter-Harris Type II physeal fracture of lower end of right femur
CC-A,K,P S79.122- Salter-Harris Type II physeal fracture of lower end of left femur

CC-A,K,P **S79.129-** Salter-Harris Type II physeal fracture of lower end of <u>unspecified</u> femur

S79.13- <u>Salter-Harris Type III</u> physeal fracture of <u>lower end</u> of <u>femur</u>

CC-A,K,P **S79.131-** Salter-Harris Type III physeal fracture of lower end of <u>right</u> femur

CC-A,K,P **S79.132-** Salter-Harris Type III physeal fracture of lower end of <u>left</u> femur

CC-A,K,P **S79.139-** Salter-Harris Type III physeal fracture of lower end of <u>unspecified</u> femur

S79.14- <u>Salter-Harris Type IV</u> physeal fracture of <u>lower end</u> of <u>femur</u>

CC-A,K,P **S79.141-** Salter-Harris Type IV physeal fracture of lower end of <u>right</u> femur

CC-A,K,P **S79.142-** Salter-Harris Type IV physeal fracture of lower end of <u>left</u> femur

CC-A,K,P **S79.149-** Salter-Harris Type IV physeal fracture of lower end of <u>unspecified</u> femur

S79.19- <u>Other physeal</u> fracture of <u>lower end</u> of <u>femur</u>

CC-A,K,P **S79.191-** Other physeal fracture of lower end of <u>right</u> femur

CC-A,K,P **S79.192-** Other physeal fracture of lower end of <u>left</u> femur

CC-A,K,P **S79.199-** Other physeal fracture of lower end of <u>unspecified</u> femur

S79.8- <u>Other specified injuries</u> of <u>hip</u> and <u>thigh</u>

The appropriate 7th character is to be added to each code in subcategory S79.8:
- A <u>Initial</u> encounter
- D <u>Subsequent</u> encounter
- S <u>Sequela</u>

S79.81- <u>Other specified injuries</u> of <u>hip</u>

S79.811- Other specified injuries of <u>right</u> hip

S79.812- Other specified injuries of <u>left</u> hip

S79.819- Other specified injuries of <u>unspecified</u> hip

S79.82- <u>Other specified injuries</u> of <u>thigh</u>

S79.821- Other specified injuries of <u>right</u> thigh

S79.822- Other specified injuries of <u>left</u> thigh

S79.829- Other specified injuries of <u>unspecified</u> thigh

S79.9- <u>Unspecified injury</u> of <u>hip</u> and <u>thigh</u>

The appropriate 7th character is to be added to each code in subcategory S79.9:
- A <u>Initial</u> encounter
- D <u>Subsequent</u> encounter
- S <u>Sequela</u>

S79.91- <u>Unspecified</u> injury of <u>hip</u>

S79.911- Unspecified injury of <u>right</u> hip

S79.912- Unspecified injury of <u>left</u> hip

S79.919- Unspecified injury of <u>unspecified</u> hip

S79.92- <u>Unspecified</u> injury of <u>thigh</u>

S79.921- Unspecified injury of <u>right</u> thigh

S79.922- Unspecified injury of <u>left</u> thigh

S79.929- Unspecified injury of <u>unspecified</u> thigh

Injuries to the knee and lower leg (S80-S89)

Excludes ❷: *burns and corrosions (T20-T32)*
frostbite (T33-T34)
injuries of ankle and foot, except fracture of ankle and malleolus (S90-S99)
insect bite or sting, venomous (T63.4)

S80- <u>Superficial injury</u> of <u>knee</u> and <u>lower leg</u>
Excludes ❷: *superficial injury of ankle and foot (S90.-)*

The appropriate 7th character is to be added to each code from category S80:
- A <u>Initial</u> encounter
- D <u>Subsequent</u> encounter
- S <u>Sequela</u>

S80.0- <u>Contusion</u> of <u>knee</u>

S80.00x- Contusion of <u>unspecified</u> knee

S80.01x- Contusion of <u>right</u> knee

S80.02x- Contusion of <u>left</u> knee

S80.1- <u>Contusion</u> of <u>lower leg</u>

S80.10x- Contusion of <u>unspecified</u> lower leg

S80.11x- Contusion of <u>right</u> lower leg

S80.12x- Contusion of <u>left</u> lower leg

S80.2- <u>Other superficial injuries</u> of <u>knee</u>

S80.21- <u>Abrasion</u> of knee

S80.211- Abrasion, <u>right</u> knee

S80.212- Abrasion, <u>left</u> knee

S80.219- Abrasion, <u>unspecified</u> knee

S80.22- <u>Blister</u> (nonthermal) of knee

S80.221- Blister (nonthermal), <u>right</u> knee

S80.222- Blister (nonthermal), <u>left</u> knee

S80.229- Blister (nonthermal), <u>unspecified</u> knee

S80.24- <u>External constriction</u> of knee

S80.241- External constriction, <u>right</u> knee

S80.242- External constriction, <u>left</u> knee

S80.249- External constriction, <u>unspecified</u> knee

S80.25- <u>Superficial foreign body</u> of knee
Splinter in the knee

S80.251- Superficial foreign body, <u>right</u> knee

S80.252- Superficial foreign body, <u>left</u> knee

S80.259- Superficial foreign body, <u>unspecified</u> knee

S80.26- <u>Insect bite (nonvenomous)</u> of knee

S80.261- Insect bite (nonvenomous), <u>right</u> knee

S80.262- Insect bite (nonvenomous), <u>left</u> knee

S80.269- Insect bite (nonvenomous), <u>unspecified</u> knee

S80.27- <u>Other superficial bite</u> of knee
Excludes 1:   open bite of knee (S81.05-)

S80.271- Other superficial bite of <u>right</u> knee

S80.272- Other superficial bite of <u>left</u> knee

S80.279- Other superficial bite of <u>unspecified</u> knee

S80.8- <u>Other superficial injuries</u> of <u>lower leg</u>

S80.81- <u>Abrasion</u> of lower leg

S80.811- Abrasion, <u>right</u> lower leg

S80.812- Abrasion, <u>left</u> lower leg

S80.819- Abrasion, <u>unspecified</u> lower leg

S80.82- <u>Blister</u> (nonthermal) of lower leg

S80.821- Blister (nonthermal), <u>right</u> lower leg

S80.822- Blister (nonthermal), <u>left</u> lower leg

S80.829- Blister (nonthermal), <u>unspecified</u> lower leg

S80.84- <u>External constriction</u> of lower leg

S80.841- External constriction, <u>right</u> lower leg

S80.842- External constriction, <u>left</u> lower leg

S80.849- External constriction, <u>unspecified</u> lower leg

S80.85- <u>Superficial foreign body</u> of lower leg
Splinter in the lower leg

S80.851- Superficial foreign body, <u>right</u> lower leg

S80.852- Superficial foreign body, <u>left</u> lower leg

S80.859- Superficial foreign body, <u>unspecified</u> lower leg

S80.86- <u>Insect bite (nonvenomous)</u> of lower leg

S80.861- Insect bite (nonvenomous), <u>right</u> lower leg

S80.862- Insect bite (nonvenomous), <u>left</u> lower leg

S80.869- Insect bite (nonvenomous), <u>unspecified</u> lower leg

S80.87- <u>Other superficial bite</u> of lower leg
Excludes 1:   open bite of lower leg (S81.85-)

S80.871- Other superficial bite, <u>right</u> lower leg

S80.872- Other superficial bite, <u>left</u> lower leg

S80.879- Other superficial bite, <u>unspecified</u> lower leg

S80.9- <u>Unspecified superficial injury</u> of <u>knee</u> and <u>lower leg</u>

S80.91- <u>Unspecified superficial injury</u> of <u>knee</u>

S80.911- Unspecified superficial injury of <u>right</u> knee

S80.912- Unspecified superficial injury of <u>left</u> knee

S80.919- Unspecified superficial injury of <u>unspecified</u> knee

S79 - S80

S80.92- Unspecified superficial injury of lower leg
- **S80.921-** Unspecified superficial injury of right lower leg
- **S80.922-** Unspecified superficial injury of left lower leg
- **S80.929-** Unspecified superficial injury of unspecified lower leg

S81- Open wound of knee and lower leg
Code also any associated wound infection
Excludes 1: open fracture of knee and lower leg (S82.-)
traumatic amputation of lower leg (S88.-)
Excludes ❷: open wound of ankle and foot (S91.-)

The appropriate 7th character is to be added to each code from category S81:
- A Initial encounter
- D Subsequent encounter
- S Sequela

S81.0- Open wound of knee
- **S81.00-** Unspecified open wound of knee
  - **S81.001-** Unspecified open wound, right knee
  - **S81.002-** Unspecified open wound, left knee
  - **S81.009-** Unspecified open wound, unspecified knee
- **S81.01-** Laceration without foreign body of knee
  - **S81.011-** Laceration without foreign body, right knee
  - **S81.012-** Laceration without foreign body, left knee
  - **S81.019-** Laceration without foreign body, unspecified knee
- **S81.02-** Laceration with foreign body of knee
  - **S81.021-** Laceration with foreign body, right knee
  - **S81.022-** Laceration with foreign body, left knee
  - **S81.029-** Laceration with foreign body, unspecified knee
- **S81.03-** Puncture wound without foreign body of knee
  - **S81.031-** Puncture wound without foreign body, right knee
  - **S81.032-** Puncture wound without foreign body, left knee
  - **S81.039-** Puncture wound without foreign body, unspecified knee
- **S81.04-** Puncture wound with foreign body of knee
  - **S81.041-** Puncture wound with foreign body, right knee
  - **S81.042-** Puncture wound with foreign body, left knee
  - **S81.049-** Puncture wound with foreign body, unspecified knee
- **S81.05-** Open bite of knee
  Bite of knee NOS
  Excludes 1: superficial bite of knee (S80.27-)
  - **S81.051-** Open bite, right knee
  - **S81.052-** Open bite, left knee
  - **S81.059-** Open bite, unspecified knee

S81.8- Open wound of lower leg
- **S81.80-** Unspecified open wound of lower leg
  - **S81.801-** Unspecified open wound, right lower leg
  - **S81.802-** Unspecified open wound, left lower leg
  - **S81.809-** Unspecified open wound, unspecified lower leg
- **S81.81-** Laceration without foreign body of lower leg
  - **S81.811-** Laceration without foreign body, right lower leg
  - **S81.812-** Laceration without foreign body, left lower leg
  - **S81.819-** Laceration without foreign body, unspecified lower leg
- **S81.82-** Laceration with foreign body of lower leg
  - **S81.821-** Laceration with foreign body, right lower leg
  - **S81.822-** Laceration with foreign body, left lower leg
  - **S81.829-** Laceration with foreign body, unspecified lower leg
- **S81.83-** Puncture wound without foreign body of lower leg
  - **S81.831-** Puncture wound without foreign body, right lower leg
  - **S81.832-** Puncture wound without foreign body, left lower leg
  - **S81.839-** Puncture wound without foreign body, unspecified lower leg

S81.84- Puncture wound with foreign body of lower leg
  - **S81.841-** Puncture wound with foreign body, right lower leg
  - **S81.842-** Puncture wound with foreign body, left lower leg
  - **S81.849-** Puncture wound with foreign body, unspecified lower leg
S81.85- Open bite of lower leg
  Bite of lower leg NOS
  Excludes 1: superficial bite of lower leg (S80.86-, S80.87-)
  - **S81.851-** Open bite, right lower leg
  - **S81.852-** Open bite, left lower leg
  - **S81.859-** Open bite, unspecified lower leg

S82- Fracture of lower leg, including ankle
AHA 15:1Q:p25 – Comminuted fracture of left distal tibia and fibula
Note: A fracture not indicated as displaced or nondisplaced should be coded to displaced
Note: A fracture not indicated as open or closed should be coded to closed
Note: The open fracture designations are based on the Gustilo open fracture classification
Includes: Fracture of malleolus
Excludes 1: traumatic amputation of lower leg (S88.-)
Excludes ❷: fracture of foot, except ankle (S92.-)
periprosthetic fracture of prosthetic implant of knee (T84.042, T84.043)

The appropriate 7th character is to be added to all codes from category S82:
- A Initial encounter for closed fracture
- B Initial encounter for open fracture type I or II
  Initial encounter for open fracture NOS
- C Initial encounter for open fracture type IIIA, IIIB, or IIIC
- D Subsequent encounter for closed fracture with routine healing
- E Subsequent encounter for open fracture type I or II with routine healing
- F Subsequent encounter for open fracture type IIIA, IIIB, or IIIC with routine healing
- G Subsequent encounter for closed fracture with delayed healing
- H Subsequent encounter for open fracture type I or II with delayed healing
- J Subsequent encounter for open fracture type IIIA, IIIB, or IIIC with delayed healing
- K Subsequent encounter for closed fracture with nonunion
- M Subsequent encounter for open fracture type I or II with nonunion
- N Subsequent encounter for open fracture type IIIA, IIIB, or IIIC with nonunion
- P Subsequent encounter for closed fracture with malunion
- Q Subsequent encounter for open fracture type I or II with malunion
- R Subsequent encounter for open fracture type IIIA, IIIB, or IIIC with malunion
- S Sequela

S82.0- Fracture of patella
  Knee cap
- **S82.00-** Unspecified fracture of patella
  - **S82.001-** Unspecified fracture of right patella
    CC-A,B,C,K,M,N,P,Q,R
  - **S82.002-** Unspecified fracture of left patella
    CC-A,B,C,K,M,N,P,Q,R
  - **S82.009-** Unspecified fracture of unspecified patella
    CC-A,B,C,K,M,N,P,Q,R
- **S82.01-** Osteochondral fracture of patella
  - **S82.011-** Displaced osteochondral fracture of right patella
    CC-A,B,C,K,M,N,P,Q,R
  - **S82.012-** Displaced osteochondral fracture of left patella
    CC-A,B,C,K,M,N,P,Q,R
  - **S82.013-** Displaced osteochondral fracture of unspecified patella
    CC-A,B,C,K,M,N,P,Q,R
  - **S82.014-** Nondisplaced osteochondral fracture of right patella
    CC-A,B,C,K,M,N,P,Q,R
  - **S82.015-** Nondisplaced osteochondral fracture of left patella
    CC-A,B,C,K,M,N,P,Q,R

S82.016- **Nondisplaced** osteochondral fracture of **unspecified** patella
CC-A,B,C,K,M,N,P,Q,R

S82.02- **Longitudinal** fracture of **patella**

S82.021- **Displaced** longitudinal fracture of **right** patella
CC-A,B,C,K,M,N,P,Q,R

S82.022- **Displaced** longitudinal fracture of **left** patella
CC-A,B,C,K,M,N,P,Q,R

S82.023- **Displaced** longitudinal fracture of **unspecified** patella
CC-A,B,C,K,M,N,P,Q,R

S82.024- **Nondisplaced** longitudinal fracture of **right** patella
CC-A,B,C,K,M,N,P,Q,R

S82.025- **Nondisplaced** longitudinal fracture of **left** patella
CC-A,B,C,K,M,N,P,Q,R

S82.026- **Nondisplaced** longitudinal fracture of **unspecified** patella
CC-A,B,C,K,M,N,P,Q,R

S82.03- **Transverse** fracture of **patella**

S82.031- **Displaced** transverse fracture of **right** patella
CC-A,B,C,K,M,N,P,Q,R

S82.032- **Displaced** transverse fracture of **left** patella
CC-A,B,C,K,M,N,P,Q,R

S82.033- **Displaced** transverse fracture of **unspecified** patella
CC-A,B,C,K,M,N,P,Q,R

S82.034- **Nondisplaced** transverse fracture of **right** patella
CC-A,B,C,K,M,N,P,Q,R

S82.035- **Nondisplaced** transverse fracture of **left** patella
CC-A,B,C,K,M,N,P,Q,R

S82.036- **Nondisplaced** transverse fracture of **unspecified** patella
CC-A,B,C,K,M,N,P,Q,R

S82.04- **Comminuted** fracture of **patella**

S82.041- **Displaced** comminuted fracture of **right** patella
CC-A,B,C,K,M,N,P,Q,R

S82.042- **Displaced** comminuted fracture of **left** patella
CC-A,B,C,K,M,N,P,Q,R

S82.043- **Displaced** comminuted fracture of **unspecified** patella
CC-A,B,C,K,M,N,P,Q,R

S82.044- **Nondisplaced** comminuted fracture of **right** patella
CC-A,B,C,K,M,N,P,Q,R

S82.045- **Nondisplaced** comminuted fracture of **left** patella
CC-A,B,C,K,M,N,P,Q,R

S82.046- **Nondisplaced** comminuted fracture of **unspecified** patella
CC-A,B,C,K,M,N,P,Q,R

S82.09- **Other fracture** of **patella**

S82.091- **Other** fracture of **right** patella
CC-A,B,C,K,M,N,P,Q,R

S82.092- **Other** fracture of **left** patella
CC-A,B,C,K,M,N,P,Q,R

S82.099- **Other** fracture of **unspecified** patella
CC-A,B,C,K,M,N,P,Q,R

S82.1- **Fracture** of **upper end** of **tibia**
Fracture of proximal end of tibia
Excludes ❷: *fracture of shaft of tibia (S82.2-)*
physeal fracture of upper end of tibia (S89.0-)

S82.10- **Unspecified** fracture of **upper end** of **tibia**

S82.101- **Unspecified** fracture of upper end of **right** tibia
CC-A,K,M,N,P,Q,R MCC-B,C

S82.102- **Unspecified** fracture of upper end of **left** tibia
CC-A,K,M,N,P,Q,R MCC-B,C

S82.109- **Unspecified** fracture of upper end of **unspecified** tibia
CC-A,K,M,N,P,Q,R MCC-B,C

S82.11- **Fracture** of **tibial spine**

S82.111- **Displaced** fracture of **right** tibial spine
CC-A,K,M,N,P,Q,R MCC-B,C

S82.112- **Displaced** fracture of **left** tibial spine
CC-A,K,M,N,P,Q,R MCC-B,C

S82.113- **Displaced** fracture of **unspecified** tibial spine
CC-A,K,M,N,P,Q,R MCC-B,C

S82.114- **Nondisplaced** fracture of **right** tibial spine
CC-A,K,M,N,P,Q,R MCC-B,C

S82.115- **Nondisplaced** fracture of **left** tibial spine
CC-A,K,M,N,P,Q,R MCC-B,C

S82.116- **Nondisplaced** fracture of **unspecified** tibial spine

S82.12- Fracture of **lateral condyle** of **tibia**

S82.121- **Displaced** fracture of lateral condyle of **right** tibia
CC-A,K,M,N,P,Q,R MCC-B,C

S82.122- **Displaced** fracture of lateral condyle of **left** tibia
CC-A,K,M,N,P,Q,R MCC-B,C

S82.123- **Displaced** fracture of lateral condyle of **unspecified** tibia
CC-A,K,M,N,P,Q,R MCC-B,C

S82.124- **Nondisplaced** fracture of lateral condyle of **right** tibia
CC-A,K,M,N,P,Q,R MCC-B,C

S82.125- **Nondisplaced** fracture of lateral condyle of **left** tibia
CC-A,K,M,N,P,Q,R MCC-B,C

S82.126- **Nondisplaced** fracture of lateral condyle of **unspecified** tibia
CC-A,K,M,N,P,Q,R MCC-B,C

S82.13- Fracture of **medial condyle** of **tibia**

S82.131- **Displaced** fracture of medial condyle of **right** tibia
CC-A,K,M,N,P,Q,R MCC-B,C

S82.132- **Displaced** fracture of medial condyle of **left** tibia
CC-A,K,M,N,P,Q,R MCC-B,C

S82.133- **Displaced** fracture of medial condyle of **unspecified** tibia
CC-A,K,M,N,P,Q,R MCC-B,C

S82.134- **Nondisplaced** fracture of medial condyle of **right** tibia
CC-A,K,M,N,P,Q,R MCC-B,C

S82.135- **Nondisplaced** fracture of medial condyle of **left** tibia
CC-A,K,M,N,P,Q,R MCC-B,C

S82.136- **Nondisplaced** fracture of medial condyle of **unspecified** tibia
CC-A,K,M,N,P,Q,R MCC-B,C

S82.14- **Bicondylar** fracture of **tibia**
Fracture of tibial plateau NOS

S82.141- **Displaced** bicondylar fracture of **right** tibia
CC-A,K,M,N,P,Q,R MCC-B,C

S82.142- **Displaced** bicondylar fracture of **left** tibia
CC-A,K,M,N,P,Q,R MCC-B,C

S82.143- **Displaced** bicondylar fracture of **unspecified** tibia
CC-A,K,M,N,P,Q,R MCC-B,C

S82.144- **Nondisplaced** bicondylar fracture of **right** tibia
CC-A,K,M,N,P,Q,R MCC-B,C

S82.145- **Nondisplaced** bicondylar fracture of **left** tibia
CC-A,K,M,N,P,Q,R MCC-B,C

S82.146- **Nondisplaced** bicondylar fracture of **unspecified** tibia
CC-A,K,M,N,P,Q,R MCC-B,C

S82.15- Fracture of **tibial tuberosity**

S82.151- **Displaced** fracture of **right** tibial tuberosity
CC-A,K,M,N,P,Q,R MCC-B,C

S82.152- **Displaced** fracture of **left** tibial tuberosity
CC-A,K,M,N,P,Q,R MCC-B,C

S82.153- **Displaced** fracture of **unspecified** tibial tuberosity
CC-A,K,M,N,P,Q,R MCC-B,C

S82.154- **Nondisplaced** fracture of **right** tibial tuberosity
CC-A,K,M,N,P,Q,R MCC-B,C

S82.155- **Nondisplaced** fracture of **left** tibial tuberosity
CC-A,K,M,N,P,Q,R MCC-B,C

S82.156- **Nondisplaced** fracture of **unspecified** tibial tuberosity
CC-A,K,M,N,P,Q,R MCC-B,C

S82 – S82

S82.16- Torus fracture of upper end of tibia

The appropriate 7th character is to be added to all codes in subcategory S82.16:

- **A** Initial encounter for closed fracture
- **D** Subsequent encounter for fracture with routine healing
- **G** Subsequent encounter for fracture with delayed healing
- **K** Subsequent encounter for fracture with nonunion
- **P** Subsequent encounter for fracture with malunion
- **S** Sequela

CC-A,K,P **S82.161-** Torus fracture of upper end of right tibia

CC-A,K,P **S82.162-** Torus fracture of upper end of left tibia

CC-A,K,P **S82.169-** Torus fracture of upper end of unspecified tibia

S82.19- Other fracture of upper end of tibia

S82.191- Other fracture of upper end of right tibia
CC-A,K,M,N,P,Q,R MCC-B,C

S82.192- Other fracture of upper end of left tibia
CC-A,K,M,N,P,Q,R MCC-B,C

S82.199- Other fracture of upper end of unspecified tibia
CC-A,K,M,N,P,Q,R MCC-B,C

S82.2- Fracture of shaft of tibia

S82.20- Unspecified fracture of shaft of tibia
Fracture of tibia NOS

S82.201- Unspecified fracture of shaft of right tibia
CC-A,K,M,N,P,Q,R MCC-B,C

S82.202- Unspecified fracture of shaft of left tibia
CC-A,K,M,N,P,Q,R MCC-B,C

S82.209- Unspecified fracture of shaft of unspecified tibia
CC-A,K,M,N,P,Q,R MCC-B,C

S82.22- Transverse fracture of shaft of tibia

S82.221- Displaced transverse fracture of shaft of right tibia
CC-A,K,M,N,P,Q,R MCC-B,C

S82.222- Displaced transverse fracture of shaft of left tibia
CC-A,K,M,N,P,Q,R MCC-B,C

S82.223- Displaced transverse fracture of shaft of unspecified tibia
CC-A,K,M,N,P,Q,R MCC-B,C

S82.224- Nondisplaced transverse fracture of shaft of right tibia
CC-A,K,M,N,P,Q,R MCC-B,C

S82.225- Nondisplaced transverse fracture of shaft of left tibia
CC-A,K,M,N,P,Q,R MCC-B,C

S82.226- Nondisplaced transverse fracture of shaft of unspecified tibia
CC-A,K,M,N,P,Q,R MCC-B,C

S82.23- Oblique fracture of shaft of tibia
AHA 15:1Q:p8 – Nondisplaced oblique fracture of right tibia

S82.231- Displaced oblique fracture of shaft of right tibia
CC-A,K,M,N,P,Q,R MCC-B,C

S82.232- Displaced oblique fracture of shaft of left tibia
CC-A,K,M,N,P,Q,R MCC-B,C

S82.233- Displaced oblique fracture of shaft of unspecified tibia
CC-A,K,M,N,P,Q,R MCC-B,C

S82.234- Nondisplaced oblique fracture of shaft of right tibia
CC-A,K,M,N,P,Q,R MCC-B,C

S82.235- Nondisplaced oblique fracture of shaft of left tibia
CC-A,K,M,N,P,Q,R MCC-B,C

S82.236- Nondisplaced oblique fracture of shaft of unspecified tibia
CC-A,K,M,N,P,Q,R MCC-B,C

S82.24- Spiral fracture of shaft of tibia
Toddler fracture

S82.241- Displaced spiral fracture of shaft of right tibia
CC-A,K,M,N,P,Q,R MCC-B,C

S82.242- Displaced spiral fracture of shaft of left tibia
CC-A,K,M,N,P,Q,R MCC-B,C

S82.243- Displaced spiral fracture of shaft of unspecified tibia
CC-A,K,M,N,P,Q,R MCC-B,C

S82.244- Nondisplaced spiral fracture of shaft of right tibia
CC-A,K,M,N,P,Q,R MCC-B,C

S82.245- Nondisplaced spiral fracture of shaft of left tibia
CC-A,K,M,N,P,Q,R MCC-B,C

S82.246- Nondisplaced spiral fracture of shaft of unspecified tibia
CC-A,K,M,N,P,Q,R MCC-B,C

S82.25- Comminuted fracture of shaft of tibia

S82.251- Displaced comminuted fracture of shaft of right tibia
CC-A,K,M,N,P,Q,R MCC-B,C

S82.252- Displaced comminuted fracture of shaft of left tibia
CC-A,K,M,N,P,Q,R MCC-B,C

S82.253- Displaced comminuted fracture of shaft of unspecified tibia
CC-A,K,M,N,P,Q,R MCC-B,C

S82.254- Nondisplaced comminuted fracture of shaft of right tibia
CC-A,K,M,N,P,Q,R MCC-B,C

S82.255- Nondisplaced comminuted fracture of shaft of left tibia
CC-A,K,M,N,P,Q,R MCC-B,C

S82.256- Nondisplaced comminuted fracture of shaft of unspecified tibia
CC-A,K,M,N,P,Q,R MCC-B,C

S82.26- Segmental fracture of shaft of tibia

S82.261- Displaced segmental fracture of shaft of right tibia
CC-A,K,M,N,P,Q,R MCC-B,C

S82.262- Displaced segmental fracture of shaft of left tibia
CC-A,K,M,N,P,Q,R MCC-B,C

S82.263- Displaced segmental fracture of shaft of unspecified tibia
CC-A,K,M,N,P,Q,R MCC-B,C

S82.264- Nondisplaced segmental fracture of shaft of right tibia
CC-A,K,M,N,P,Q,R MCC-B,C

S82.265- Nondisplaced segmental fracture of shaft of left tibia
CC-A,K,M,N,P,Q,R MCC-B,C

S82.266- Nondisplaced segmental fracture of shaft of unspecified tibia
CC-A,K,M,N,P,Q,R MCC-B,C

S82.29- Other fracture of shaft of tibia

S82.291- Other fracture of shaft of right tibia
CC-A,K,M,N,P,Q,R

S82.292- Other fracture of shaft of left tibia
CC-A,K,M,N,P,Q,R

S82.299- Other fracture of shaft of unspecified tibia

S82.3- Fracture of lower end of tibia
Excludes 1: bimalleolar fracture of lower leg (S82.84-)
fracture of medial malleolus alone (S82.5-)
Maisonneuve's fracture (S82.86-)
pilon fracture of distal tibia (S82.87-)
trimalleolar fractures of lower leg (S82.85-)

S82.30- Unspecified fracture of lower end of tibia

S82.301- Unspecified fracture of lower end of right tibia
CC-B,C,K,M,N,P,Q,R

S82.302- Unspecified fracture of lower end of left tibia
CC-B,C,K,M,N,P,Q,R

S82.309- Unspecified fracture of lower end of unspecified tibia
CC-B,C,K,M,N,P,Q,R

S82.31- Torus fracture of lower end of tibia

The appropriate 7th character is to be added to all codes in subcategory S82.31:

- **A** Initial encounter for closed fracture
- **D** Subsequent encounter for fracture with routine healing
- **G** Subsequent encounter for fracture with delayed healing
- **K** Subsequent encounter for fracture with nonunion
- **P** Subsequent encounter for fracture with malunion
- **S** Sequela

CC-A,K,P **S82.311-** Torus fracture of lower end of right tibia

CC-A,K,P **S82.312-** Torus fracture of lower end of left tibia

CC-A,K,P **S82.319-** Torus fracture of lower end of unspecified tibia

S82.39- Other fracture of lower end of tibia

S82.391- Other fracture of lower end of right tibia
CC-B,C,K,M,N,P,Q,R

S82.392- Other fracture of lower end of left tibia
CC-B,C,K,M,N,P,Q,R

S82.399- Other fracture of lower end of unspecified tibia
CC-B,C,K,M,N,P,Q,R

S82.4- Fracture of shaft of fibula
Excludes ❷: fracture of lateral malleolus alone (S82.6-)

S82.40- Unspecified fracture of shaft of fibula

S82.401- Unspecified fracture of shaft of right fibula
CC-K,M,N,P,Q,R

S82.402- Unspecified fracture of shaft of left fibula
CC-K,M,N,P,Q,R   MCC-B,C

S82.409- Unspecified fracture of shaft of unspecified fibula
CC-K,M,N,P,Q,R   MCC-B,C

S82.42- Transverse fracture of shaft of fibula

S82.421- Displaced transverse fracture of shaft of right fibula
CC-K,M,N,P,Q,R   MCC-B,C

S82.422- Displaced transverse fracture of shaft of left fibula
CC-K,M,N,P,Q,R   MCC-B,C

S82.423- Displaced transverse fracture of shaft of unspecified fibula
CC-K,M,N,P,Q,R   MCC-B,C

S82.424- Nondisplaced transverse fracture of shaft of right fibula
CC-K,M,N,P,Q,R   MCC-B,C

S82.425- Nondisplaced transverse fracture of shaft of left fibula
CC-K,M,N,P,Q,R   MCC-B,C

S82.426- Nondisplaced transverse fracture of shaft of unspecified fibula
CC-K,M,N,P,Q,R   MCC-B,C

S82.43- Oblique fracture of shaft of fibula

S82.431- Displaced oblique fracture of shaft of right fibula
CC-K,M,N,P,Q,R   MCC-B,C

S82.432- Displaced oblique fracture of shaft of left fibula
CC-K,M,N,P,Q,R   MCC-B,C

S82.433- Displaced oblique fracture of shaft of unspecified fibula
CC-K,M,N,P,Q,R   MCC-B,C

S82.434- Nondisplaced oblique fracture of shaft of right fibula
CC-K,M,N,P,Q,R   MCC-B,C

S82.435- Nondisplaced oblique fracture of shaft of left fibula
CC-K,M,N,P,Q,R   MCC-B,C

S82.436- Nondisplaced oblique fracture of shaft of unspecified fibula
CC-K,M,N,P,Q,R   MCC-B,C

S82.44- Spiral fracture of shaft of fibula

S82.441- Displaced spiral fracture of shaft of right fibula
CC-K,M,N,P,Q,R   MCC-B,C

S82.442- Displaced spiral fracture of shaft of left fibula
CC-K,M,N,P,Q,R   MCC-B,C

S82.443- Displaced spiral fracture of shaft of unspecified fibula
CC-K,M,N,P,Q,R   MCC-B,C

S82.444- Nondisplaced spiral fracture of shaft of right fibula
CC-K,M,N,P,Q,R   MCC-B,C

S82.445- Nondisplaced spiral fracture of shaft of left fibula
CC-K,M,N,P,Q,R   MCC-B,C

S82.446- Nondisplaced spiral fracture of shaft of unspecified fibula
CC-K,M,N,P,Q,R   MCC-B,C

S82.45- Comminuted fracture of shaft of fibula

S82.451- Displaced comminuted fracture of shaft of right fibula
CC-K,M,N,P,Q,R   MCC-B,C

S82.452- Displaced comminuted fracture of shaft of left fibula
CC-K,M,N,P,Q,R   MCC-B,C

S82.453- Displaced comminuted fracture of shaft of unspecified fibula
CC-K,M,N,P,Q,R   MCC-B,C

S82.454- Nondisplaced comminuted fracture of shaft of right fibula
CC-K,M,N,P,Q,R   MCC-B,C

S82.455- Nondisplaced comminuted fracture of shaft of left fibula
CC-K,M,N,P,Q,R   MCC-B,C

S82.456- Nondisplaced comminuted fracture of shaft of unspecified fibula
CC-K,M,N,P,Q,R   MCC-B,C

S82.46- Segmental fracture of shaft of fibula

S82.461- Displaced segmental fracture of shaft of right fibula
CC-K,M,N,P,Q,R   MCC-B,C

S82.462- Displaced segmental fracture of shaft of left fibula
CC-K,M,N,P,Q,R   MCC-B,C

S82.463- Displaced segmental fracture of shaft of unspecified fibula
CC-K,M,N,P,Q,R   MCC-B,C

S82.464- Nondisplaced segmental fracture of shaft of right fibula
CC-K,M,N,P,Q,R   MCC-B,C

S82.465- Nondisplaced segmental fracture of shaft of left fibula
CC-K,M,N,P,Q,R   MCC-B,C

S82.466- Nondisplaced segmental fracture of shaft of unspecified fibula
CC-K,M,N,P,Q,R   MCC-B,C

S82.49- Other fracture of shaft of fibula

S82.491- Other fracture of shaft of right fibula
CC-K,M,N,P,Q,R   MCC-B,C

S82.492- Other fracture of shaft of left fibula
CC-K,M,N,P,Q,R   MCC-B,C

S82.499- Other fracture of shaft of unspecified fibula
CC-K,M,N,P,Q,R   MCC-B,C

S82.5- Fracture of medial malleolus
Excludes 1: pilon fracture of distal tibia (S82.87-)
Salter-Harris type III of lower end of tibia (S89.13-)
Salter-Harris type IV of lower end of tibia (S89.14-)

S82.51x- Displaced fracture of medial malleolus of right tibia
CC-B,C,K,M,N,P,Q,R

S82.52x- Displaced fracture of medial malleolus of left tibia
CC-B,C,K,M,N,P,Q,R

S82.53x- Displaced fracture of medial malleolus of unspecified tibia
CC-B,C,K,M,N,P,Q,R

S82.54x- Nondisplaced fracture of medial malleolus of right tibia
CC-B,C,K,M,N,P,Q,R

S82.55x- Nondisplaced fracture of medial malleolus of left tibia
CC-B,C,K,M,N,P,Q,R

S82.56x- Nondisplaced fracture of medial malleolus of unspecified tibia
CC-B,C,K,M,N,P,Q,R

S82.6- Fracture of lateral malleolus
Excludes 1: pilon fracture of distal tibia (S82.87-)

S82.61x- Displaced fracture of lateral malleolus of right fibula
CC-B,C,K,M,N,P,Q,R

S82.62x- Displaced fracture of lateral malleolus of left fibula
CC-B,C,K,M,N,P,Q,R

S82.63x- Displaced fracture of lateral malleolus of unspecified fibula
CC-B,C,K,M,N,P,Q,R

S82.64x- Nondisplaced fracture of lateral malleolus of right fibula
CC-B,C,K,M,N,P,Q,R

S82.65x- Nondisplaced fracture of lateral malleolus of left fibula
CC-B,C,K,M,N,P,Q,R

S82.66x- Nondisplaced fracture of lateral malleolus of unspecified fibula
CC-B,C,K,M,N,P,Q,R

S82 I S82 I S82

S82.8- Other fractures of lower leg

S82.81- Torus fracture of upper end of fibula

The appropriate 7th character is to be added to all codes in subcategory S82.81:
- **A** Initial encounter for closed fracture
- **D** Subsequent encounter for fracture with routine healing
- **G** Subsequent encounter for fracture with delayed healing
- **K** Subsequent encounter for fracture with nonunion
- **P** Subsequent encounter for fracture with malunion
- **S** Sequela

CC-K,P **S82.811-** Torus fracture of upper end of right fibula

CC-K,P **S82.812-** Torus fracture of upper end of left fibula

CC-K,P **S82.819-** Torus fracture of upper end of unspecified fibula

S82.82- Torus fracture of lower end of fibula

The appropriate 7th character is to be added to all codes in subcategory S82.82:
- **A** Initial encounter for closed fracture
- **D** Subsequent encounter for fracture with routine healing
- **G** Subsequent encounter for fracture with delayed healing
- **K** Subsequent encounter for fracture with nonunion
- **P** Subsequent encounter for fracture with malunion
- **S** Sequela

CC-K,P **S82.821-** Torus fracture of lower end of right fibula

CC-K,P **S82.822-** Torus fracture of lower end of left fibula

CC-K,P **S82.829-** Torus fracture of lower end of unspecified fibula

S82.83- Other fracture of upper and lower end of fibula

S82.831- Other fracture of upper and lower end of right fibula
CC-K,M,N,P,Q,R MCC-B,C

S82.832- Other fracture of upper and lower end of left fibula
CC-K,M,N,P,Q,R MCC-B,C

S82.839- Other fracture of upper and lower end of unspecified fibula
CC-K,M,N,P,Q,R MCC-B,C

S82.84- Bimalleolar fracture of lower leg

S82.841- Displaced bimalleolar fracture of right lower leg
CC-B,C,K,M,N,P,Q,R

S82.842- Displaced bimalleolar fracture of left lower leg
CC-B,C,K,M,N,P,Q,R

S82.843- Displaced bimalleolar fracture of unspecified lower leg
CC-B,C,K,M,N,P,Q,R

S82.844- Nondisplaced bimalleolar fracture of right lower leg
CC-B,C,K,M,N,P,Q,R

S82.845- Nondisplaced bimalleolar fracture of left lower leg
CC-B,C,K,M,N,P,Q,R

S82.846- Nondisplaced bimalleolar fracture of unspecified lower leg
CC-B,C,K,M,N,P,Q,R

S82.85- Trimalleolar fracture of lower leg

S82.851- Displaced trimalleolar fracture of right lower leg
CC-B,C,K,M,N,P,Q,R

S82.852- Displaced trimalleolar fracture of left lower leg
CC-B,C,K,M,N,P,Q,R

S82.853- Displaced trimalleolar fracture of unspecified lower leg
CC-B,C,K,M,N,P,Q,R

S82.854- Nondisplaced trimalleolar fracture of right lower leg
CC-B,C,K,M,N,P,Q,R

S82.855- Nondisplaced trimalleolar fracture of left lower leg
CC-B,C,K,M,N,P,Q,R

S82.856- Nondisplaced trimalleolar fracture of unspecified lower leg
CC-B,C,K,M,N,P,Q,R

S82.86- Maisonneuve's fracture

S82.861- Displaced Maisonneuve's fracture of right leg
CC-K,M,N,P,Q,R MCC-B,C

S82.862- Displaced Maisonneuve's fracture of left leg
CC-K,M,N,P,Q,R MCC-B,C

S82.863- Displaced Maisonneuve's fracture of unspecified leg
CC-K,M,N,P,Q,R MCC-B,C

S82.864- Nondisplaced Maisonneuve's fracture of right leg
CC-K,M,N,P,Q,R MCC-B,C

S82.865- Nondisplaced Maisonneuve's fracture of left leg
CC-K,M,N,P,Q,R MCC-B,C

S82.866- Nondisplaced Maisonneuve's fracture of unspecified leg
CC-K,M,N,P,Q,R MCC-B,C

S82.87- Pilon fracture of tibia

S82.871- Displaced pilon fracture of right tibia
CC-B,C,K,M,N,P,Q,R

S82.872- Displaced pilon fracture of left tibia
CC-B,C,K,M,N,P,Q,R

S82.873- Displaced pilon fracture of unspecified tibia
CC-B,C,K,M,N,P,Q,R

S82.874- Nondisplaced pilon fracture of right tibia
CC-B,C,K,M,N,P,Q,R

S82.875- Nondisplaced pilon fracture of left tibia
CC-B,C,K,M,N,P,Q,R

S82.876- Nondisplaced pilon fracture of unspecified tibia
CC-B,C,K,M,N,P,Q,R

S82.89- Other fractures of lower leg

Fracture of ankle NOS

S82.891- Other fracture of right lower leg
CC-B,C,K,M,N,P,Q,R

S82.892- Other fracture of left lower leg
CC-B,C,K,M,N,P,Q,R

S82.899- Other fracture of unspecified lower leg
CC-B,C,K,M,N,P,Q,R

S82.9- Unspecified fracture of lower leg

S82.90x- Unspecified fracture of unspecified lower leg
CC-B,C,K,M,N,P,Q,R

S82.91x- Unspecified fracture of right lower leg
CC-B,C,K,M,N,P,Q,R

S82.92x- Unspecified fracture of left lower leg
CC-B,C,K,M,N,P,Q,R

S83- Dislocation and sprain of joints and ligaments of knee

Includes:
- Avulsion of joint or ligament of knee
- Laceration of cartilage, joint or ligament of knee
- Sprain of cartilage, joint or ligament of knee
- Traumatic hemarthrosis of joint or ligament of knee
- Traumatic rupture of joint or ligament of knee
- Traumatic subluxation of joint or ligament of knee
- Traumatic tear of joint or ligament of knee

Code also any associated open wound

Excludes 1:
- derangement of patella (M22.0-M22.3)
- injury of patellar ligament (tendon) (S76.1-)
- internal derangement of knee (M23.-)
- old dislocation of knee (M24.36)
- pathological dislocation of knee (M24.36)
- recurrent dislocation of knee (M22.0)

Excludes 2: strain of muscle, fascia and tendon of lower leg (S86.-)

The appropriate 7th character is to be added to each code from category S83:
- **A** Initial encounter
- **D** Subsequent encounter
- **S** Sequela

S83.0- Subluxation and dislocation of patella

S83.00- Unspecified subluxation and dislocation of patella

S83.001- Unspecified subluxation of right patella

S83.002- Unspecified subluxation of left patella

S83.003- Unspecified subluxation of unspecified patella

S83.004- Unspecified dislocation of right patella

S83.005- Unspecified dislocation of left patella

S83.006- Unspecified dislocation of unspecified patella

S83.01- Lateral subluxation and dislocation of patella

S83.011- Lateral subluxation of right patella

S83.012- Lateral subluxation of left patella

S83.013- Lateral subluxation of unspecified patella

S83.014- Lateral dislocation of right patella

S83.015- Lateral dislocation of left patella

S 8 2 - S 8 3

S83.016- Lateral dislocation of unspecified patella
S83.09- Other subluxation and dislocation of patella
S83.091- Other subluxation of right patella
S83.092- Other subluxation of left patella
S83.093- Other subluxation of unspecified patella
S83.094- Other dislocation of right patella
S83.095- Other dislocation of left patella
S83.096- Other dislocation of unspecified patella
S83.1- Subluxation and dislocation of knee
Excludes 2: instability of knee prosthesis (T84.022, T84.023)
S83.10- Unspecified subluxation and dislocation of knee
S83.101- Unspecified subluxation of right knee
S83.102- Unspecified subluxation of left knee
S83.103- Unspecified subluxation of unspecified knee
S83.104- Unspecified dislocation of right knee
S83.105- Unspecified dislocation of left knee
S83.106- Unspecified dislocation of unspecified knee
S83.11- Anterior subluxation and dislocation of proximal end of tibia
Posterior subluxation and dislocation of distal end of femur
S83.111- Anterior subluxation of proximal end of tibia, right knee
S83.112- Anterior subluxation of proximal end of tibia, left knee
S83.113- Anterior subluxation of proximal end of tibia, unspecified knee
S83.114- Anterior dislocation of proximal end of tibia, right knee
S83.115- Anterior dislocation of proximal end of tibia, left knee
S83.116- Anterior dislocation of proximal end of tibia, unspecified knee
S83.12- Posterior subluxation and dislocation of proximal end of tibia
Anterior dislocation of distal end of femur
S83.121- Posterior subluxation of proximal end of tibia, right knee
S83.122- Posterior subluxation of proximal end of tibia, left knee
S83.123- Posterior subluxation of proximal end of tibia, unspecified knee
S83.124- Posterior dislocation of proximal end of tibia, right knee
S83.125- Posterior dislocation of proximal end of tibia, left knee
S83.126- Posterior dislocation of proximal end of tibia, unspecified knee
S83.13- Medial subluxation and dislocation of proximal end of tibia
S83.131- Medial subluxation of proximal end of tibia, right knee
S83.132- Medial subluxation of proximal end of tibia, left knee
S83.133- Medial subluxation of proximal end of tibia, unspecified knee
S83.134- Medial dislocation of proximal end of tibia, right knee
S83.135- Medial dislocation of proximal end of tibia, left knee
S83.136- Medial dislocation of proximal end of tibia, unspecified knee
S83.14- Lateral subluxation and dislocation of proximal end of tibia
S83.141- Lateral subluxation of proximal end of tibia, right knee
S83.142- Lateral subluxation of proximal end of tibia, left knee

S83.143- Lateral subluxation of proximal end of tibia, unspecified knee
S83.144- Lateral dislocation of proximal end of tibia, right knee
S83.145- Lateral dislocation of proximal end of tibia, left knee
S83.146- Lateral dislocation of proximal end of tibia, unspecified knee
S83.19- Other subluxation and dislocation of knee
S83.191- Other subluxation of right knee
S83.192- Other subluxation of left knee
S83.193- Other subluxation of unspecified knee
S83.194- Other dislocation of right knee
S83.195- Other dislocation of left knee
S83.196- Other dislocation of unspecified knee
S83.2- Tear of meniscus, current injury
Excludes 1: old bucket-handle tear (M23.2)
S83.20- Tear of unspecified meniscus, current injury
Tear of meniscus of knee NOS
S83.200- Bucket-handle tear of unspecified meniscus, current injury, right knee
S83.201- Bucket-handle tear of unspecified meniscus, current injury, left knee
S83.202- Bucket-handle tear of unspecified meniscus, current injury, unspecified knee
S83.203- Other tear of unspecified meniscus, current injury, right knee
S83.204- Other tear of unspecified meniscus, current injury, left knee
S83.205- Other tear of unspecified meniscus, current injury, unspecified knee
S83.206- Unspecified tear of unspecified meniscus, current injury, right knee
S83.207- Unspecified tear of unspecified meniscus, current injury, left knee
S83.209- Unspecified tear of unspecified meniscus, current injury, unspecified knee
S83.21- Bucket-handle tear of medial meniscus, current injury
S83.211- Bucket-handle tear of medial meniscus, current injury, right knee
S83.212- Bucket-handle tear of medial meniscus, current injury, left knee
S83.219- Bucket-handle tear of medial meniscus, current injury, unspecified knee
S83.22- Peripheral tear of medial meniscus, current injury
S83.221- Peripheral tear of medial meniscus, current injury, right knee
S83.222- Peripheral tear of medial meniscus, current injury, left knee
S83.229- Peripheral tear of medial meniscus, current injury, unspecified knee
S83.23- Complex tear of medial meniscus, current injury
S83.231- Complex tear of medial meniscus, current injury, right knee
S83.232- Complex tear of medial meniscus, current injury, left knee
S83.239- Complex tear of medial meniscus, current injury, unspecified knee
S83.24- Other tear of medial meniscus, current injury
S83.241- Other tear of medial meniscus, current injury, right knee
S83.242- Other tear of medial meniscus, current injury, left knee
S83.249- Other tear of medial meniscus, current injury, unspecified knee
S83.25- Bucket-handle tear of lateral meniscus, current injury
S83.251- Bucket-handle tear of lateral meniscus, current injury, right knee

S83 - S83

S83.252- Bucket-handle tear of lateral meniscus, current injury, <u>left</u> knee

S83.259- Bucket-handle tear of lateral meniscus, current injury, <u>unspecified</u> knee

S83.26- <u>Peripheral tear</u> of <u>lateral meniscus</u>, <u>current injury</u>

S83.261- Peripheral tear of lateral meniscus, current injury, <u>right</u> knee

S83.262- Peripheral tear of lateral meniscus, current injury, <u>left</u> knee

S83.269- Peripheral tear of lateral meniscus, current injury, <u>unspecified</u> knee

S83.27- <u>Complex tear</u> of <u>lateral meniscus</u>, <u>current injury</u>

S83.271- Complex tear of lateral meniscus, current injury, <u>right</u> knee

S83.272- Complex tear of lateral meniscus, current injury, <u>left</u> knee

S83.279- Complex tear of lateral meniscus, current injury, <u>unspecified</u> knee

S83.28- <u>Other tear</u> of <u>lateral meniscus</u>, <u>current injury</u>

S83.281- Other tear of lateral meniscus, current injury, <u>right</u> knee

S83.282- Other tear of lateral meniscus, current injury, <u>left</u> knee

S83.289- Other tear of lateral meniscus, current injury, <u>unspecified</u> knee

S83.3- <u>Tear of articular cartilage</u> of <u>knee</u>, <u>current</u>

S83.30x- Tear of articular cartilage of <u>unspecified</u> knee, current

S83.31x- Tear of articular cartilage of <u>right</u> knee, current

S83.32x- Tear of articular cartilage of <u>left</u> knee, current

S83.4- <u>Sprain</u> of <u>collateral</u> ligament of <u>knee</u>

S83.40- Sprain of <u>unspecified</u> <u>collateral</u> ligament of <u>knee</u>

S83.401- Sprain of unspecified collateral ligament of <u>right</u> knee

S83.402- Sprain of unspecified collateral ligament of <u>left</u> knee

S83.409- Sprain of unspecified collateral ligament of <u>unspecified</u> knee

S83.41- <u>Sprain</u> of <u>medial</u> <u>collateral</u> ligament of <u>knee</u>
    Sprain of tibial collateral ligament

S83.411- Sprain of medial collateral ligament of <u>right</u> knee

S83.412- Sprain of medial collateral ligament of <u>left</u> knee

S83.419- Sprain of medial collateral ligament of <u>unspecified</u> knee

S83.42- <u>Sprain</u> of <u>lateral</u> <u>collateral</u> ligament of <u>knee</u>
    Sprain of fibular collateral ligament

S83.421- Sprain of lateral collateral ligament of <u>right</u> knee

S83.422- Sprain of lateral collateral ligament of <u>left</u> knee

S83.429- Sprain of lateral collateral ligament of <u>unspecified</u> knee

S83.5- <u>Sprain</u> of <u>cruciate</u> ligament of <u>knee</u>

S83.50- <u>Sprain</u> of <u>unspecified</u> <u>cruciate</u> ligament of <u>knee</u>

S83.501- Sprain of unspecified cruciate ligament of <u>right</u> knee

S83.502- Sprain of unspecified cruciate ligament of <u>left</u> knee

S83.509- Sprain of unspecified cruciate ligament of <u>unspecified</u> knee

S83.51- <u>Sprain</u> of <u>anterior</u> <u>cruciate</u> ligament of <u>knee</u>

S83.511- Sprain of anterior cruciate ligament of <u>right</u> knee

S83.512- Sprain of anterior cruciate ligament of <u>left</u> knee

S83.519- Sprain of anterior cruciate ligament of <u>unspecified</u> knee

S83.52- <u>Sprain</u> of <u>posterior</u> <u>cruciate</u> ligament of <u>knee</u>

S83.521- Sprain of posterior cruciate ligament of <u>right</u> knee

S83.522- Sprain of posterior cruciate ligament of <u>left</u> knee

S83.529- Sprain of posterior cruciate ligament of <u>unspecified</u> knee

S83.6- <u>Sprain</u> of the <u>superior tibiofibular joint and ligament</u>

S83.60x- Sprain of the superior tibiofibular joint and ligament, <u>unspecified</u> knee

S83.61x- Sprain of the superior tibiofibular joint and ligament, <u>right</u> knee

S83.62x- Sprain of the superior tibiofibular joint and ligament, <u>left</u> knee

S83.8- <u>Sprain</u> of <u>other specified parts</u> of <u>knee</u>

S83.8x- <u>Sprain</u> of <u>other specified parts</u> of <u>knee</u>

S83.8x1- Sprain of other specified parts of <u>right</u> knee

S83.8x2- Sprain of other specified parts of <u>left</u> knee

S83.8x9- Sprain of other specified parts of <u>unspecified</u> knee

S83.9- <u>Sprain</u> of <u>unspecified site</u> of <u>knee</u>

S83.90x- Sprain of unspecified site of <u>unspecified</u> knee

S83.91x- Sprain of unspecified site of <u>right</u> knee

S83.92x- Sprain of unspecified site of <u>left</u> knee

S84- <u>Injury of nerves</u> at <u>lower leg</u> level
    Code also any associated open wound (S81-)
    Excludes ❷: injury of nerves at ankle and foot level (S94-)
    The appropriate 7th character is to be added to each code from category S84:
    A <u>Initial</u> encounter
    D <u>Subsequent</u> encounter
    S <u>Sequela</u>

S84.0- Injury of <u>tibial</u> nerve at <u>lower leg</u> level

S84.00x- Injury of tibial nerve at lower leg level, <u>unspecified</u> leg

S84.01x- Injury of tibial nerve at lower leg level, <u>right</u> leg

S84.02x- Injury of tibial nerve at lower leg level, <u>left</u> leg

S84.1- Injury of <u>peroneal</u> nerve at <u>lower leg</u> level

S84.10x- Injury of peroneal nerve at lower leg level, <u>unspecified</u> leg

S84.11x- Injury of peroneal nerve at lower leg level, <u>right</u> leg

S84.12x- Injury of peroneal nerve at lower leg level, <u>left</u> leg

S84.2- Injury of <u>cutaneous sensory</u> nerve at <u>lower leg</u> level

S84.20x- Injury of cutaneous sensory nerve at lower leg level, <u>unspecified</u> leg

S84.21x- Injury of cutaneous sensory nerve at lower leg level, <u>right</u> leg

S84.22x- Injury of cutaneous sensory nerve at lower leg level, <u>left</u> leg

S84.8- Injury of other nerves at lower leg level

S84.80- Injury of <u>other nerves</u> at <u>lower leg</u> level

S84.801- Injury of other nerves at lower leg level, <u>right</u> leg

S84.802- Injury of other nerves at lower leg level, <u>left</u> leg

S84.809- Injury of other nerves at lower leg level, <u>unspecified</u> leg

S84.9- Injury of <u>unspecified nerve</u> at <u>lower leg</u> level

S84.90x- Injury of unspecified nerve at lower leg level, <u>unspecified</u> leg

S84.91x- Injury of unspecified nerve at lower leg level, <u>right</u> leg

S84.92x- Injury of unspecified nerve at lower leg level, <u>left</u> leg

S85- <u>Injury of blood vessels</u> at <u>lower leg</u> level
    Code also any associated open wound (S81.-)
    Excludes ❷: injury of blood vessels at ankle and foot level (S95.-)
    The appropriate 7th character is to be added to each code from category S85:
    A <u>Initial</u> encounter
    D <u>Subsequent</u> encounter
    S <u>Sequela</u>

S85.0- Injury of <u>popliteal artery</u>

S85.00- <u>Unspecified</u> injury of <u>popliteal artery</u>

MCC-A S85.001- Unspecified injury of popliteal artery, <u>right</u> leg

MCC-A S85.002- Unspecified injury of popliteal artery, <u>left</u> leg

MCC-A S85.009- Unspecified injury of popliteal artery, <u>unspecified</u> leg

S85.01- <u>Laceration</u> of <u>popliteal artery</u>

MCC-A S85.011- Laceration of popliteal artery, <u>right</u> leg

S 8 3 – S 8 5

MCC-A **S85.012-** Laceration of popliteal artery, <u>left</u> leg
MCC-A **S85.019-** Laceration of popliteal artery, <u>unspecified</u> leg
S85.09- <u>Other specified injury</u> of <u>popliteal artery</u>
MCC-A **S85.091-** Other specified injury of popliteal artery, <u>right</u> leg
MCC-A **S85.092-** Other specified injury of popliteal artery, <u>left</u> leg
MCC-A **S85.099-** Other specified injury of popliteal artery, <u>unspecified</u> leg
S85.1- Injury of <u>tibial artery</u>
S85.10- <u>Unspecified</u> injury of <u>unspecified tibial artery</u>
    Injury of tibial artery NOS
CC-A **S85.101-** Unspecified injury of unspecified tibial artery, <u>right</u> leg
CC-A **S85.102-** Unspecified injury of unspecified tibial artery, <u>left</u> leg
CC-A **S85.109-** Unspecified injury of unspecified tibial artery, <u>unspecified</u> leg
S85.11- <u>Laceration</u> of <u>unspecified tibial artery</u>
CC-A **S85.111-** Laceration of unspecified tibial artery, <u>right</u> leg
CC-A **S85.112-** Laceration of unspecified tibial artery, <u>left</u> leg
CC-A **S85.119-** Laceration of unspecified tibial artery, <u>unspecified</u> leg
S85.12- <u>Other specified injury</u> of <u>unspecified tibial artery</u>
CC-A **S85.121-** Other specified injury of unspecified tibial artery, <u>right</u> leg
CC-A **S85.122-** Other specified injury of unspecified tibial artery, <u>left</u> leg
CC-A **S85.129-** Other specified injury of unspecified tibial artery, <u>unspecified</u> leg
S85.13- <u>Unspecified</u> injury of <u>anterior tibial artery</u>
CC-A **S85.131-** Unspecified injury of anterior tibial artery, <u>right</u> leg
CC-A **S85.132-** Unspecified injury of anterior tibial artery, <u>left</u> leg
CC-A **S85.139-** Unspecified injury of anterior tibial artery, <u>unspecified</u> leg
S85.14- <u>Laceration</u> of <u>anterior tibial artery</u>
CC-A **S85.141-** Laceration of anterior tibial artery, <u>right</u> leg
CC-A **S85.142-** Laceration of anterior tibial artery, <u>left</u> leg
CC-A **S85.149-** Laceration of anterior tibial artery, <u>unspecified</u> leg
S85.15- <u>Other specified injury</u> of <u>anterior tibial artery</u>
CC-A **S85.151-** Other specified injury of anterior tibial artery, <u>right</u> leg
CC-A **S85.152-** Other specified injury of anterior tibial artery, <u>left</u> leg
CC-A **S85.159-** Other specified injury of anterior tibial artery, <u>unspecified</u> leg
S85.16- <u>Unspecified</u> injury of <u>posterior tibial artery</u>
CC-A **S85.161-** Unspecified injury of posterior tibial artery, <u>right</u> leg
CC-A **S85.162-** Unspecified injury of posterior tibial artery, <u>left</u> leg
CC-A **S85.169-** Unspecified injury of posterior tibial artery, <u>unspecified</u> leg
S85.17- <u>Laceration</u> of <u>posterior tibial artery</u>
CC-A **S85.171-** Laceration of posterior tibial artery, <u>right</u> leg
CC-A **S85.172-** Laceration of posterior tibial artery, <u>left</u> leg
CC-A **S85.179** Laceration of posterior tibial artery, <u>unspecified</u> leg
S85.18- <u>Other specified injury</u> of <u>posterior tibial artery</u>
CC-A **S85.181-** Other specified injury of posterior tibial artery, <u>right</u> leg
CC-A **S85.182-** Other specified injury of posterior tibial artery, <u>left</u> leg
CC-A **S85.189** Other specified injury of posterior tibial artery, <u>unspecified</u> leg
S85.2- <u>Injury</u> of <u>peroneal artery</u>
S85.20- <u>Unspecified</u> injury of <u>peroneal artery</u>
CC-A **S85.201-** Unspecified injury of peroneal artery, <u>right</u> leg
CC-A **S85.202-** Unspecified injury of peroneal artery, <u>left</u> leg

CC-A **S85.209** Unspecified injury of peroneal artery, <u>unspecified</u> leg
S85.21- <u>Laceration</u> of <u>peroneal artery</u>
CC-A **S85.211-** Laceration of peroneal artery, <u>right</u> leg
CC-A **S85.212-** Laceration of peroneal artery, <u>left</u> leg
CC-A **S85.219-** Laceration of peroneal artery, <u>unspecified</u> leg
S85.29- <u>Other specified injury</u> of <u>peroneal artery</u>
CC-A **S85.291-** Other specified injury of peroneal artery, <u>right</u> leg
CC-A **S85.292-** Other specified injury of peroneal artery, <u>left</u> leg
CC-A **S85.299-** Other specified injury of peroneal artery, <u>unspecified</u> leg
S85.3- <u>Injury</u> of <u>greater saphenous vein</u> at <u>lower leg</u> level
    Injury of greater saphenous vein NOS
    Injury of saphenous vein NOS
S85.30- <u>Unspecified</u> injury of <u>greater saphenous vein</u> at <u>lower leg</u> level
CC-A **S85.301-** Unspecified injury of greater saphenous vein at lower leg level, <u>right</u> leg
CC-A **S85.302-** Unspecified injury of greater saphenous vein at lower leg level, <u>left</u> leg
CC-A **S85.309-** Unspecified injury of greater saphenous vein at lower leg level, <u>unspecified</u> leg
S85.31- <u>Laceration</u> of <u>greater saphenous vein</u> at <u>lower leg</u> level
CC-A **S85.311-** Laceration of greater saphenous vein at lower leg level, <u>right</u> leg
CC-A **S85.312-** Laceration of greater saphenous vein at lower leg level, <u>left</u> leg
CC-A **S85.319-** Laceration of greater saphenous vein at lower leg level, <u>unspecified</u> leg
S85.39- <u>Other specified injury</u> of <u>greater saphenous vein</u> at <u>lower leg</u> level
CC-A **S85.391-** Other specified injury of greater saphenous vein at lower leg level, <u>right</u> leg
CC-A **S85.392-** Other specified injury of greater saphenous vein at lower leg level, <u>left</u> leg
CC-A **S85.399-** Other specified injury of greater saphenous vein at lower leg level, <u>unspecified</u> leg
S85.4- <u>Injury</u> of <u>lesser saphenous vein</u> at <u>lower leg</u> level
S85.40- <u>Unspecified</u> injury of <u>lesser saphenous vein</u> at <u>lower leg</u> level
CC-A **S85.401-** Unspecified injury of lesser saphenous vein at lower leg level, <u>right</u> leg
CC-A **S85.402-** Unspecified injury of lesser saphenous vein at lower leg level, <u>left</u> leg
CC-A **S85.409-** Unspecified injury of lesser saphenous vein at lower leg level, <u>unspecified</u> leg
S85.41- <u>Laceration</u> of <u>lesser saphenous vein</u> at <u>lower leg</u> level
CC-A **S85.411-** Laceration of lesser saphenous vein at lower leg level, <u>right</u> leg
CC-A **S85.412-** Laceration of lesser saphenous vein at lower leg level, <u>left</u> leg
CC-A **S85.419-** Laceration of lesser saphenous vein at lower leg level, <u>unspecified</u> leg
S85.49- <u>Other specified injury</u> of <u>lesser saphenous vein</u> at <u>lower leg</u> level
CC-A **S85.491-** Other specified injury of lesser saphenous vein at lower leg level, <u>right</u> leg
CC-A **S85.492-** Other specified injury of lesser saphenous vein at lower leg level, <u>left</u> leg
CC-A **S85.499-** Other specified injury of lesser saphenous vein at lower leg level, <u>unspecified</u> leg
S85.5- <u>Injury</u> of <u>popliteal vein</u>
S85.50- <u>Unspecified</u> injury of <u>popliteal vein</u>
MCC-A **S85.501-** Unspecified injury of popliteal vein, <u>right</u> leg
MCC-A **S85.502-** Unspecified injury of popliteal vein, <u>left</u> leg
MCC-A **S85.509-** Unspecified injury of popliteal vein, <u>unspecified</u> leg
S85.51- <u>Laceration</u> of <u>popliteal vein</u>

S 8 5 - S 8 5

MCC-A S85.511- Laceration of popliteal vein, <u>right</u> leg

MCC-A S85.512- Laceration of popliteal vein, <u>left</u> leg

MCC-A S85.519- Laceration of popliteal vein, <u>unspecified</u> leg

S85.59- <u>Other specified injury</u> of <u>popliteal</u> <u>vein</u>

MCC-A S85.591- Other specified injury of popliteal vein, <u>right</u> leg

MCC-A S85.592- Other specified injury of popliteal vein, <u>left</u> leg

MCC-A S85.599- Other specified injury of popliteal vein, <u>unspecified</u> leg

S85.8- <u>Injury</u> of <u>other blood vessels</u> at <u>lower leg</u> level

S85.80- <u>Unspecified</u> injury of other blood vessels at <u>lower leg</u> level

CC-A S85.801- Unspecified injury of other blood vessels at lower leg level, <u>right</u> leg

CC-A S85.802- Unspecified injury of other blood vessels at lower leg level, <u>left</u> leg

CC-A S85.809- Unspecified injury of other blood vessels at lower leg level, <u>unspecified</u> leg

S85.81- <u>Laceration</u> of other blood vessels at <u>lower leg</u> level

CC-A S85.811- Laceration of other blood vessels at lower leg level, <u>right</u> leg

CC-A S85.812- Laceration of other blood vessels at lower leg level, <u>left</u> leg

CC-A S85.819- Laceration of other blood vessels at lower leg level, <u>unspecified</u> leg

S85.89- <u>Other specified injury</u> of <u>other blood vessels</u> at <u>lower leg</u> level

CC-A S85.891- Other specified injury of other blood vessels at lower leg level, <u>right</u> leg

CC-A S85.892- Other specified injury of other blood vessels at lower leg level, <u>left</u> leg

CC-A S85.899- Other specified injury of other blood vessels at lower leg level, <u>unspecified</u> leg

S85.9- <u>Injury</u> of <u>unspecified blood vessel</u> at <u>lower leg</u> level

S85.90- <u>Unspecified</u> injury of <u>unspecified blood vessel</u> at <u>lower leg</u> level

CC-A S85.901- Unspecified injury of unspecified blood vessel at lower leg level, <u>right</u> leg

CC-A S85.902- Unspecified injury of unspecified blood vessel at lower leg level, <u>left</u> leg

CC-A S85.909- Unspecified injury of unspecified blood vessel at lower leg level, <u>unspecified</u> leg

S85.91- <u>Laceration</u> of <u>unspecified blood vessel</u> at <u>lower leg</u> level

CC-A S85.911- Laceration of unspecified blood vessel at lower leg level, <u>right</u> leg

CC-A S85.912- Laceration of unspecified blood vessel at lower leg level, <u>left</u> leg

CC-A S85.919- Laceration of unspecified blood vessel at lower leg level, <u>unspecified</u> leg

S85.99- <u>Other specified injury</u> of <u>unspecified blood vessel</u> at <u>lower leg</u> level

CC-A S85.991- Other specified injury of unspecified blood vessel at lower leg level, <u>right</u> leg

CC-A S85.992- Other specified injury of unspecified blood vessel at lower leg level, <u>left</u> leg

CC-A S85.999- Other specified injury of unspecified blood vessel at lower leg level, <u>unspecified</u> leg

S86- <u>Injury</u> of <u>muscle, fascia and tendon</u> at <u>lower leg</u> level

Code also any associated open wound (S81.-)

Excludes 2: injury of muscle, fascia and tendon at ankle (S96.-)
injury of patellar ligament (tendon) (S76.1-)
sprain of joints and ligaments of knee (S83.-)

The appropriate 7th character is to be added to each code from category S86:
A <u>Initial</u> encounter
D <u>Subsequent</u> encounter
S <u>Sequela</u>

S86.0- <u>Injury</u> of <u>Achilles</u> tendon

S86.00- <u>Unspecified</u> injury of <u>Achilles</u> tendon

S86.001- Unspecified injury of <u>right</u> Achilles tendon

S86.002- Unspecified injury of <u>left</u> Achilles tendon

S86.009- Unspecified injury of <u>unspecified</u> Achilles tendon

S86.01- <u>Strain</u> of <u>Achilles</u> tendon

S86.011- Strain of <u>right</u> Achilles tendon

S86.012- Strain of <u>left</u> Achilles tendon

S86.019- Strain of <u>unspecified</u> Achilles tendon

S86.02- <u>Laceration</u> of <u>Achilles</u> tendon

CC-A S86.021- Laceration of <u>right</u> Achilles tendon

CC-A S86.022- Laceration of <u>left</u> Achilles tendon

CC-A S86.029- Laceration of <u>unspecified</u> Achilles tendon

S86.09- <u>Other specified injury</u> of <u>Achilles</u> tendon

S86.091- Other specified injury of <u>right</u> Achilles tendon

S86.092- Other specified injury of <u>left</u> Achilles tendon

S86.099- Other specified injury of <u>unspecified</u> Achilles tendon

S86.1- <u>Injury</u> of <u>other muscle(s) and tendon(s)</u> of <u>posterior muscle group</u> at <u>lower leg</u> level

S86.10- <u>Unspecified</u> injury of other muscle(s) and tendon(s) of <u>posterior</u> muscle group at <u>lower leg</u> level

S86.101- Unspecified injury of other muscle(s) and tendon(s) of posterior muscle group at lower leg level, <u>right</u> leg

S86.102- Unspecified injury of other muscle(s) and tendon(s) of posterior muscle group at lower leg level, <u>left</u> leg

S86.109- Unspecified injury of other muscle(s) and tendon(s) of posterior muscle group at lower leg level, <u>unspecified</u> leg

S86.11- <u>Strain</u> of other muscle(s) and tendon(s) of <u>posterior</u> muscle group at <u>lower leg</u> level

S86.111- Strain of other muscle(s) and tendon(s) of posterior muscle group at lower leg level, <u>right</u> leg

S86.112- Strain of other muscle(s) and tendon(s) of posterior muscle group at lower leg level, <u>left</u> leg

S86.119- Strain of other muscle(s) and tendon(s) of posterior muscle group at lower leg level, <u>unspecified</u> leg

S86.12- <u>Laceration</u> of other muscle(s) and tendon(s) of <u>posterior</u> muscle group at <u>lower leg</u> level

CC-A S86.121- Laceration of other muscle(s) and tendon(s) of posterior muscle group at lower leg level, <u>right</u> leg

CC-A S86.122- Laceration of other muscle(s) and tendon(s) of posterior muscle group at lower leg level, <u>left</u> leg

CC-A S86.129- Laceration of other muscle(s) and tendon(s) of posterior muscle group at lower leg level, <u>unspecified</u> leg

S86.19- <u>Other injury</u> of other muscle(s) and tendon(s) of <u>posterior</u> muscle group at <u>lower leg</u> level

S86.191- Other injury of other muscle(s) and tendon(s) of posterior muscle group at lower leg level, <u>right</u> leg

S86.192- Other injury of other muscle(s) and tendon(s) of posterior muscle group at lower leg level, <u>left</u> leg

S86.199- Other injury of other muscle(s) and tendon(s) of posterior muscle group at lower leg level, <u>unspecified</u> leg

S85 - S86

S86.2- Injury of muscle(s) and tendon(s) of anterior muscle group at lower leg level

  S86.20- Unspecified injury of muscle(s) and tendon(s) of anterior muscle group at lower leg level

    S86.201- Unspecified injury of muscle(s) and tendon(s) of anterior muscle group at lower leg level, right leg

    S86.202- Unspecified injury of muscle(s) and tendon(s) of anterior muscle group at lower leg level, left leg

    S86.209- Unspecified injury of muscle(s) and tendon(s) of anterior muscle group at lower leg level, unspecified leg

  S86.21- Strain of muscle(s) and tendon(s) of anterior muscle group at lower leg level

    S86.211- Strain of muscle(s) and tendon(s) of anterior muscle group at lower leg level, right leg

    S86.212- Strain of muscle(s) and tendon(s) of anterior muscle group at lower leg level, left leg

    S86.219- Strain of muscle(s) and tendon(s) of anterior muscle group at lower leg level, unspecified leg

  S86.22- Laceration of muscle(s) and tendon(s) of anterior muscle group at lower leg level

    CC-A **S86.221-** Laceration of muscle(s) and tendon(s) of anterior muscle group at lower leg level, right leg

    CC-A **S86.222-** Laceration of muscle(s) and tendon(s) of anterior muscle group at lower leg level, left leg

    CC-A **S86.229-** Laceration of muscle(s) and tendon(s) of anterior muscle group at lower leg level, unspecified leg

  S86.29- Other injury of muscle(s) and tendon(s) of anterior muscle group at lower leg level

    S86.291- Other injury of muscle(s) and tendon(s) of anterior muscle group at lower leg level, right leg

    S86.292- Other injury of muscle(s) and tendon(s) of anterior muscle group at lower leg level, left leg

    S86.299- Other injury of muscle(s) and tendon(s) of anterior muscle group at lower leg level, unspecified leg

S86.3- Injury of muscle(s) and tendon(s) of peroneal muscle group at lower leg level

  S86.30- Unspecified injury of muscle(s) and tendon(s) of peroneal muscle group at lower leg level

    S86.301- Unspecified injury of muscle(s) and tendon(s) of peroneal muscle group at lower leg level, right leg

    S86.302- Unspecified injury of muscle(s) and tendon(s) of peroneal muscle group at lower leg level, left leg

    S86.309- Unspecified injury of muscle(s) and tendon(s) of peroneal muscle group at lower leg level, unspecified leg

  S86.31- Strain of muscle(s) and tendon(s) of peroneal muscle group at lower leg level

    S86.311- Strain of muscle(s) and tendon(s) of peroneal muscle group at lower leg level, right leg

    S86.312- Strain of muscle(s) and tendon(s) of peroneal muscle group at lower leg level, left leg

    S86.319- Strain of muscle(s) and tendon(s) of peroneal muscle group at lower leg level, unspecified leg

  S86.32- Laceration of muscle(s) and tendon(s) of peroneal muscle group at lower leg level

    CC-A **S86.321-** Laceration of muscle(s) and tendon(s) of peroneal muscle group at lower leg level, right leg

    CC-A **S86.322-** Laceration of muscle(s) and tendon(s) of peroneal muscle group at lower leg level, left leg

    CC-A **S86.329-** Laceration of muscle(s) and tendon(s) of peroneal muscle group at lower leg level, unspecified leg

  S86.39- Other injury of muscle(s) and tendon(s) of peroneal muscle group at lower leg level

    S86.391- Other injury of muscle(s) and tendon(s) of peroneal muscle group at lower leg level, right leg

    S86.392- Other injury of muscle(s) and tendon(s) of peroneal muscle group at lower leg level, left leg

    S86.399- Other injury of muscle(s) and tendon(s) of peroneal muscle group at lower leg level, unspecified leg

S86.8- Injury of other muscles and tendons at lower leg level

  S86.80- Unspecified injury of other muscles and tendons at lower leg level

    S86.801- Unspecified injury of other muscle(s) and tendon(s) at lower leg level, right leg

    S86.802- Unspecified injury of other muscle(s) and tendon(s) at lower leg level, left leg

    S86.809- Unspecified injury of other muscle(s) and tendon(s) at lower leg level, unspecified leg

  S86.81- Strain of other muscles and tendons at lower leg level

    S86.811- Strain of other muscle(s) and tendon(s) at lower leg level, right leg

    S86.812- Strain of other muscle(s) and tendon(s) at lower leg level, left leg

    S86.819- Strain of other muscle(s) and tendon(s) at lower leg level, unspecified leg

  S86.82- Laceration of other muscles and tendons at lower leg level

    CC-A **S86.821-** Laceration of other muscle(s) and tendon(s) at lower leg level, right leg

    CC-A **S86.822-** Laceration of other muscle(s) and tendon(s) at lower leg level, left leg

    CC-A **S86.829-** Laceration of other muscle(s) and tendon(s) at lower leg level, unspecified leg

  S86.89- Other injury of other muscles and tendons at lower leg level

    S86.891- Other injury of other muscle(s) and tendon(s) at lower leg level, right leg

    S86.892- Other injury of other muscle(s) and tendon(s) at lower leg level, left leg

    S86.899- Other injury of other muscle(s) and tendon(s) at lower leg level, unspecified leg

S86.9- Injury of unspecified muscle and tendon at lower leg level

  S86.90- Unspecified injury of unspecified muscle and tendon at lower leg level

    S86.901- Unspecified injury of unspecified muscle(s) and tendon(s) at lower leg level, right leg

    S86.902- Unspecified injury of unspecified muscle(s) and tendon(s) at lower leg level, left leg

    S86.909- Unspecified injury of unspecified muscle(s) and tendon(s) at lower leg level, unspecified leg

  S86.91- Strain of unspecified muscle and tendon at lower leg level

    S86.911- Strain of unspecified muscle(s) and tendon(s) at lower leg level, right leg

    S86.912- Strain of unspecified muscle(s) and tendon(s) at lower leg level, left leg

    S86.919- Strain of unspecified muscle(s) and tendon(s) at lower leg level, unspecified leg

  S86.92- Laceration of unspecified muscle and tendon at lower leg level

    CC-A **S86.921-** Laceration of unspecified muscle(s) and tendon(s) at lower leg level, right leg

    CC-A **S86.922-** Laceration of unspecified muscle(s) and tendon(s) at lower leg level, left leg

    CC-A **S86.929-** Laceration of unspecified muscle(s) and tendon(s) at lower leg level, unspecified leg

  S86.99- Other injury of unspecified muscle and tendon at lower leg level

    S86.991- Other injury of unspecified muscle(s) and tendon(s) at lower leg level, right leg

    S86.992- Other injury of unspecified muscle(s) and tendon(s) at lower leg level, left leg

    S86.999- Other injury of unspecified muscle(s) and tendon(s) at lower leg level, unspecified leg

S86 I S86

S87- <u>Crushing injury</u> of <u>lower leg</u>
Use additional code(s) for all associated injuries

Excludes ❷: *crushing injury of ankle and foot (S97.-)*

The appropriate 7th character is to be added to each code from category S87:
- A <u>Initial</u> encounter
- D <u>Subsequent</u> encounter
- S <u>Sequela</u>

S87.0- <u>Crushing</u> injury of <u>knee</u>
- **S87.00x-** Crushing injury of <u>unspecified</u> knee
- **S87.01x-** Crushing injury of <u>right</u> knee
- **S87.02x-** Crushing injury of <u>left</u> knee

S87.8- <u>Crushing</u> injury of <u>lower leg</u>
- **S87.80x-** Crushing injury of <u>unspecified</u> lower leg
- **S87.81x-** Crushing injury of <u>right</u> lower leg
- **S87.82x-** Crushing injury of <u>left</u> lower leg

S88- <u>Traumatic amputation</u> of <u>lower leg</u>
Note: An amputation not identified as partial or complete should be coded to complete

Excludes 1: *traumatic amputation of ankle and foot (S98.-)*

The appropriate 7th character is to be added to each code from category S88:
- A <u>Initial</u> encounter
- D <u>Subsequent</u> encounter
- S <u>Sequela</u>

S88.0- <u>Traumatic amputation</u> at <u>knee</u> level
- **S88.01-** <u>Complete</u> traumatic amputation at knee level
  - CC-A **S88.011-** Complete traumatic amputation at knee level, <u>right</u> lower leg
  - CC-A **S88.012-** Complete traumatic amputation at knee level, <u>left</u> lower leg
  - CC-A **S88.019-** Complete traumatic amputation at knee level, <u>unspecified</u> lower leg
- **S88.02-** <u>Partial</u> traumatic amputation at knee level
  - CC-A **S88.021-** Partial traumatic amputation at knee level, <u>right</u> lower leg
  - CC-A **S88.022-** Partial traumatic amputation at knee level, <u>left</u> lower leg
  - CC-A **S88.029-** Partial traumatic amputation at knee level, <u>unspecified</u> lower leg

S88.1- <u>Traumatic amputation</u> at level <u>between knee and ankle</u>
- **S88.11-** <u>Complete</u> traumatic amputation at level between knee and ankle
  - CC-A **S88.111-** Complete traumatic amputation at level between knee and ankle, <u>right</u> lower leg
  - CC-A **S88.112-** Complete traumatic amputation at level between knee and ankle, <u>left</u> lower leg
  - CC-A **S88.119-** Complete traumatic amputation at level between knee and ankle, <u>unspecified</u> lower leg
- **S88.12-** <u>Partial</u> traumatic amputation at level between knee and ankle
  - CC-A **S88.121-** Partial traumatic amputation at level between knee and ankle, <u>right</u> lower leg
  - CC-A **S88.122-** Partial traumatic amputation at level between knee and ankle, <u>left</u> lower leg
  - CC-A **S88.129-** Partial traumatic amputation at level between knee and ankle, <u>unspecified</u> lower leg

S88.9- <u>Traumatic amputation</u> of <u>lower leg, level unspecified</u>
- **S88.91-** <u>Complete</u> traumatic amputation of lower leg, level unspecified
  - CC-A **S88.911-** Complete traumatic amputation of <u>right</u> lower leg, level unspecified
  - CC-A **S88.912-** Complete traumatic amputation of <u>left</u> lower leg, level unspecified
  - CC-A **S88.919-** Complete traumatic amputation of <u>unspecified</u> lower leg, level unspecified
- **S88.92-** <u>Partial</u> traumatic amputation of lower leg, level unspecified

- CC-A **S88.921-** Partial traumatic amputation of <u>right</u> lower leg, level unspecified
- CC-A **S88.922-** Partial traumatic amputation of <u>left</u> lower leg, level unspecified
- CC-A **S88.929-** Partial traumatic amputation of <u>unspecified</u> lower leg, level unspecified

S89- <u>Other and unspecified injuries</u> of <u>lower leg</u>
Note: A fracture not indicated as open or closed should be coded to closed

Excludes ❷: *other and unspecified injuries of ankle and foot (S99.-)*

The appropriate 7th character is to be added to each code from subcategories S89.0, S89.1, S89.2, and S89.3:
- A <u>Initial</u> encounter for <u>closed</u> fracture
- D <u>Subsequent</u> encounter for fracture <u>with routine healing</u>
- G <u>Subsequent</u> encounter for fracture <u>with delayed healing</u>
- K <u>Subsequent</u> encounter for fracture <u>with nonunion</u>
- P <u>Subsequent</u> encounter for fracture <u>with malunion</u>
- S <u>Sequela</u>

S89.0- <u>Physeal fracture</u> of <u>upper end</u> of <u>tibia</u>
- **S89.00-** <u>Unspecified physeal</u> fracture of <u>upper end</u> of <u>tibia</u>
  - CC-A,K,P **S89.001-** Unspecified physeal fracture of upper end of <u>right</u> tibia
  - CC-A,K,P **S89.002-** Unspecified physeal fracture of upper end of <u>left</u> tibia
  - CC-A,K,P **S89.009-** Unspecified physeal fracture of upper end of <u>unspecified</u> tibia
- **S89.01-** <u>Salter-Harris Type I</u> physeal fracture of <u>upper end</u> of <u>tibia</u>
  - CC-A,K,P **S89.011-** Salter-Harris Type I physeal fracture of upper end of <u>right</u> tibia
  - CC-A,K,P **S89.012-** Salter-Harris Type I physeal fracture of upper end of <u>left</u> tibia
  - CC-A,K,P **S89.019-** Salter-Harris Type I physeal fracture of upper end of <u>unspecified</u> tibia
- **S89.02-** <u>Salter-Harris Type II</u> physeal fracture of <u>upper end</u> of <u>tibia</u>
  - CC-A,K,P **S89.021-** Salter-Harris Type II physeal fracture of upper end of <u>right</u> tibia
  - CC-A,K,P **S89.022-** Salter-Harris Type II physeal fracture of upper end of <u>left</u> tibia
  - CC-A,K,P **S89.029-** Salter-Harris Type II physeal fracture of upper end of <u>unspecified</u> tibia
- **S89.03-** <u>Salter-Harris Type III</u> physeal fracture of <u>upper end</u> of <u>tibia</u>
  - CC-A,K,P **S89.031-** Salter-Harris Type III physeal fracture of upper end of <u>right</u> tibia
  - CC-A,K,P **S89.032-** Salter-Harris Type III physeal fracture of upper end of <u>left</u> tibia
  - CC-A,K,P **S89.039-** Salter-Harris Type III physeal fracture of upper end of <u>unspecified</u> tibia
- **S89.04-** <u>Salter-Harris Type IV</u> physeal fracture of <u>upper end</u> of <u>tibia</u>
  - CC-A,K,P **S89.041-** Salter-Harris Type IV physeal fracture of upper end of <u>right</u> tibia
  - CC-A,K,P **S89.042-** Salter-Harris Type IV physeal fracture of upper end of <u>left</u> tibia
  - CC-A,K,P **S89.049-** Salter-Harris Type IV physeal fracture of upper end of <u>unspecified</u> tibia
- **S89.09-** <u>Other physeal</u> fracture of <u>upper end</u> of <u>tibia</u>
  - CC-A,K,P **S89.091-** Other physeal fracture of upper end of <u>right</u> tibia
  - CC-A,K,P **S89.092-** Other physeal fracture of upper end of <u>left</u> tibia
  - CC-A,K,P **S89.099-** Other physeal fracture of upper end of <u>unspecified</u> tibia
- **S89.1-** <u>Physeal fracture</u> of <u>lower end</u> of <u>tibia</u>
  - **S89.10-** <u>Unspecified physeal</u> fracture of <u>lower end</u> of <u>tibia</u>
    - CC-K,P **S89.101-** Unspecified physeal fracture of lower end of <u>right</u> tibia
    - CC-K,P **S89.102-** Unspecified physeal fracture of lower end of <u>left</u> tibia
    - CC-K,P **S89.109-** Unspecified physeal fracture of lower end of <u>unspecified</u> tibia

S 8 7 - S 8 9

S89.11- <u>Salter-Harris Type I</u> physeal fracture of <u>lower end</u> of <u>tibia</u>

CC-K,P **S89.111-** Salter-Harris Type I physeal fracture of lower end of <u>right</u> tibia

CC-K,P **S89.112-** Salter-Harris Type I physeal fracture of lower end of <u>left</u> tibia

CC-K,P **S89.119-** Salter-Harris Type I physeal fracture of lower end of <u>unspecified</u> tibia

S89.12- <u>Salter-Harris Type II</u> physeal fracture of <u>lower end</u> of <u>tibia</u>

CC-K,P **S89.121-** Salter-Harris Type II physeal fracture of lower end of <u>right</u> tibia

CC-K,P **S89.122-** Salter-Harris Type II physeal fracture of lower end of <u>left</u> tibia

CC-K,P **S89.129-** Salter-Harris Type II physeal fracture of lower end of <u>unspecified</u> tibia

S89.13- <u>Salter-Harris Type III</u> physeal fracture of <u>lower end</u> of <u>tibia</u>

    Excludes 1:   fracture of medial malleolus (adult) (S82.5-)

CC-K,P **S89.131-** Salter-Harris Type III physeal fracture of lower end of <u>right</u> tibia

CC-K,P **S89.132-** Salter-Harris Type III physeal fracture of lower end of <u>left</u> tibia

CC-K,P **S89.139-** Salter-Harris Type III physeal fracture of lower end of <u>unspecified</u> tibia

S89.14- <u>Salter-Harris Type IV</u> physeal fracture of <u>lower end</u> of <u>tibia</u>

    Excludes 1:   fracture of medial malleolus (adult) (S82.5-)

CC-K,P **S89.141-** Salter-Harris Type IV physeal fracture of lower end of <u>right</u> tibia

CC-K,P **S89.142-** Salter-Harris Type IV physeal fracture of lower end of <u>left</u> tibia

CC-K,P **S89.149-** Salter-Harris Type IV physeal fracture of lower end of <u>unspecified</u> tibia

S89.19- <u>Other physeal</u> fracture of <u>lower end</u> of <u>tibia</u>

CC-K,P **S89.191-** Other physeal fracture of lower end of <u>right</u> tibia

CC-K,P **S89.192-** Other physeal fracture of lower end of <u>left</u> tibia

CC-K,P **S89.199-** Other physeal fracture of lower end of <u>unspecified</u> tibia

S89.2- **Physeal fracture** of <u>upper end</u> of <u>fibula</u>

S89.20- <u>Unspecified physeal</u> fracture of <u>upper end</u> of <u>fibula</u>

CC-K,P **S89.201-** Unspecified physeal fracture of upper end of <u>right</u> fibula

CC-K,P **S89.202-** Unspecified physeal fracture of upper end of <u>left</u> fibula

CC-K,P **S89.209-** Unspecified physeal fracture of upper end of <u>unspecified</u> fibula

S89.21- <u>Salter-Harris Type I</u> physeal fracture of <u>upper end</u> of <u>fibula</u>

CC-K,P **S89.211-** Salter-Harris Type I physeal fracture of upper end of <u>right</u> fibula

CC-K,P **S89.212-** Salter-Harris Type I physeal fracture of upper end of <u>left</u> fibula

CC-K,P **S89.219-** Salter-Harris Type I physeal fracture of upper end of <u>unspecified</u> fibula

S89.22- <u>Salter-Harris Type II</u> physeal fracture of <u>upper end</u> of <u>fibula</u>

CC-K,P **S89.221-** Salter-Harris Type II physeal fracture of upper end of <u>right</u> fibula

CC-K,P **S89.222-** Salter-Harris Type II physeal fracture of upper end of <u>left</u> fibula

CC-K,P **S89.229-** Salter-Harris Type II physeal fracture of upper end of <u>unspecified</u> fibula

S89.29- <u>Other physeal</u> fracture of <u>upper end</u> of <u>fibula</u>

CC-K,P **S89.291-** Other physeal fracture of upper end of <u>right</u> fibula

CC-K,P **S89.292-** Other physeal fracture of upper end of <u>left</u> fibula

CC-K,P **S89.299-** Other physeal fracture of upper end of <u>unspecified</u> fibula

S89.3- **Physeal** fracture of <u>lower end</u> of <u>fibula</u>

S89.30- Unspecified physeal fracture of lower end of fibula

CC-K,P **S89.301-** Unspecified physeal fracture of lower end of <u>right</u> fibula

CC-K,P **S89.302-** Unspecified physeal fracture of lower end of <u>left</u> fibula

CC-K,P **S89.309-** Unspecified physeal fracture of lower end of <u>unspecified</u> fibula

S89.31- <u>Salter-Harris Type I</u> physeal fracture of <u>lower end</u> of <u>fibula</u>

CC-K,P **S89.311-** Salter-Harris Type I physeal fracture of lower end of <u>right</u> fibula

CC-K,P **S89.312-** Salter-Harris Type I physeal fracture of lower end of <u>left</u> fibula

CC-K,P **S89.319-** Salter-Harris Type I physeal fracture of lower end of <u>unspecified</u> fibula

S89.32- <u>Salter-Harris Type II</u> physeal fracture of <u>lower end</u> of <u>fibula</u>

CC-K,P **S89.321-** Salter-Harris Type II physeal fracture of lower end of <u>right</u> fibula

CC-K,P **S89.322-** Salter-Harris Type II physeal fracture of lower end of <u>left</u> fibula

CC-K,P **S89.329-** Salter-Harris Type II physeal fracture of lower end of <u>unspecified</u> fibula

S89.39- <u>Other physeal</u> fracture of <u>lower end</u> of <u>fibula</u>

CC-K,P **S89.391-** Other physeal fracture of lower end of <u>right</u> fibula

CC-K,P **S89.392-** Other physeal fracture of lower end of <u>left</u> fibula

CC-K,P **S89.399-** Other physeal fracture of lower end of <u>unspecified</u> fibula

S89.8- <u>Other specified injuries</u> of <u>lower leg</u>

The appropriate 7th character is to be added to each code in subcategory S89.8:

  A <u>Initial</u> encounter
  D <u>Subsequent</u> encounter
  S <u>Sequela</u>

S89.80x- Other specified injuries of <u>unspecified</u> lower leg

S89.81x- Other specified injuries of <u>right</u> lower leg

S89.82x- Other specified injuries of <u>left</u> lower leg

S89.9- <u>Unspecified injury</u> of <u>lower leg</u>

The appropriate 7th character is to be added to each code in subcategory S89.9:

  A <u>Initial</u> encounter
  D <u>Subsequent</u> encounter
  S <u>Sequela</u>

S89.90x- Unspecified injury of <u>unspecified</u> lower leg

S89.91x- Unspecified injury of <u>right</u> lower leg

S89.92x- Unspecified injury of <u>left</u> lower leg

Injuries to the ankle and foot (S90-S99)

Excludes ❷: burns and corrosions (T20-T32)
             fracture of ankle and malleolus (S82.-)
             frostbite (T33-T34)
             insect bite or sting, venomous (T63.4)

S90- **Superficial injury** of <u>ankle, foot and toes</u>

The appropriate 7th character is to be added to each code from category S90:

  A <u>Initial</u> encounter
  D <u>Subsequent</u> encounter
  S <u>Sequela</u>

S90.0- **Contusion** of <u>ankle</u>

S90.00x- Contusion of <u>unspecified</u> ankle

S90.01x- Contusion of <u>right</u> ankle

S90.02x- Contusion of <u>left</u> ankle

S90.1- **Contusion** of <u>toe</u> <u>without</u> damage to nail

S90.11- **Contusion** of <u>great toe</u> <u>without</u> damage to nail

S90.111- Contusion of <u>right</u> great toe <u>without</u> damage to nail

S90.112- Contusion of <u>left</u> great toe <u>without</u> damage to nail

S90.119- Contusion of <u>unspecified</u> great toe <u>without</u> damage to nail

S90.12- <u>Contusion</u> of <u>lesser toe</u> <u>without</u> damage to nail

    S90.121- Contusion of <u>right</u> lesser toe(s) <u>without</u> damage to nail

    S90.122- Contusion of <u>left</u> lesser toe(s) <u>without</u> damage to nail

    S90.129- Contusion of <u>unspecified</u> lesser toe(s) <u>without</u> damage to nail

      Contusion of toe NOS

S90.2- <u>Contusion</u> of <u>toe</u> <u>with damage to nail</u>

  S90.21- Contusion of <u>great toe</u> <u>with</u> damage to nail

    S90.211- Contusion of <u>right</u> great toe with damage to nail

    S90.212- Contusion of <u>left</u> great toe with damage to nail

    S90.219- Contusion of <u>unspecified</u> great toe with damage to nail

  S90.22- <u>Contusion</u> of <u>lesser toe</u> <u>with damage to nail</u>

    S90.221- Contusion of <u>right</u> lesser toe(s) with damage to nail

    S90.222- Contusion of <u>left</u> lesser toe(s) with damage to nail

    S90.229- Contusion of <u>unspecified</u> lesser toe(s) with damage to nail

S90.3- <u>Contusion</u> of <u>foot</u>

    Excludes ❷: contusion of toes (S90.1-, S90.2-)

  S90.30x- Contusion of <u>unspecified</u> foot

      Contusion of foot NOS

  S90.31x- Contusion of <u>right</u> foot

  S90.32x- Contusion of <u>left</u> foot

S90.4- <u>Other superficial injuries</u> of <u>toe</u>

  S90.41- <u>Abrasion</u> of <u>toe</u>

    S90.411- Abrasion, <u>right</u> <u>great</u> toe

    S90.412- Abrasion, <u>left</u> <u>great</u> toe

    S90.413- Abrasion, <u>unspecified</u> <u>great</u> toe

    S90.414- Abrasion, <u>right</u> <u>lesser</u> toe(s)

    S90.415- Abrasion, <u>left</u> <u>lesser</u> toe(s)

    S90.416- Abrasion, <u>unspecified</u> <u>lesser</u> toe(s)

  S90.42- <u>Blister</u> (nonthermal) of <u>toe</u>

    S90.421- Blister (nonthermal), <u>right</u> <u>great</u> toe

    S90.422- Blister (nonthermal), <u>left</u> <u>great</u> toe

    S90.423- Blister (nonthermal), <u>unspecified</u> <u>great</u> toe

    S90.424- Blister (nonthermal), <u>right</u> <u>lesser</u> toe(s)

    S90.425- Blister (nonthermal), <u>left</u> <u>lesser</u> toe(s)

    S90.426- Blister (nonthermal), <u>unspecified</u> <u>lesser</u> toe(s)

  S90.44- <u>External constriction</u> of <u>toe</u>

      Hair tourniquet syndrome of toe

    S90.441- External constriction, <u>right</u> <u>great</u> toe

    S90.442- External constriction, <u>left</u> <u>great</u> toe

    S90.443- External constriction, <u>unspecified</u> <u>great</u> toe

    S90.444- External constriction, <u>right</u> <u>lesser</u> toe(s)

    S90.445- External constriction, <u>left</u> <u>lesser</u> toe(s)

    S90.446- External constriction, <u>unspecified</u> <u>lesser</u> toe(s)

  S90.45- <u>Superficial foreign body</u> of <u>toe</u>

      Splinter in the toe

    S90.451- Superficial foreign body, <u>right</u> <u>great</u> toe

    S90.452- Superficial foreign body, <u>left</u> <u>great</u> toe

    S90.453- Superficial foreign body, <u>unspecified</u> <u>great</u> toe

    S90.454- Superficial foreign body, <u>right</u> <u>lesser</u> toe(s)

    S90.455- Superficial foreign body, <u>left</u> <u>lesser</u> toe(s)

    S90.456- Superficial foreign body, <u>unspecified</u> <u>lesser</u> toe(s)

  S90.46- <u>Insect bite (nonvenomous)</u> of toe

    S90.461- Insect bite (nonvenomous), <u>right</u> <u>great</u> toe

    S90.462- Insect bite (nonvenomous), <u>left</u> <u>great</u> toe

    S90.463- Insect bite (nonvenomous), <u>unspecified</u> <u>great</u> toe

    S90.464- Insect bite (nonvenomous), <u>right</u> <u>lesser</u> toe(s)

    S90.465- Insect bite (nonvenomous), <u>left</u> <u>lesser</u> toe(s)

    S90.466- Insect bite (nonvenomous), <u>unspecified</u> <u>lesser</u> toe(s)

  S90.47- <u>Other superficial bite</u> of toe

    Excludes 1:   open bite of toe (S91.15-, S91.25-)

    S90.471- Other superficial bite of <u>right great</u> toe

    S90.472- Other superficial bite of <u>left great</u> toe

    S90.473- Other superficial bite of <u>unspecified great</u> toe

    S90.474- Other superficial bite of <u>right lesser</u> toe(s)

    S90.475- Other superficial bite of <u>left lesser</u> toe(s)

    S90.476- Other superficial bite of <u>unspecified lesser</u> toe(s)

S90.5- <u>Other superficial injuries</u> of <u>ankle</u>

  S90.51- <u>Abrasion</u> of <u>ankle</u>

    S90.511- Abrasion, <u>right</u> ankle

    S90.512- Abrasion, <u>left</u> ankle

    S90.519- Abrasion, <u>unspecified</u> ankle

  S90.52- <u>Blister</u> (nonthermal) of <u>ankle</u>

    S90.521- Blister (nonthermal), <u>right</u> ankle

    S90.522- Blister (nonthermal), <u>left</u> ankle

    S90.529- Blister (nonthermal), <u>unspecified</u> ankle

  S90.54- <u>External constriction</u> of <u>ankle</u>

    S90.541- External constriction, <u>right</u> ankle

    S90.542- External constriction, <u>left</u> ankle

    S90.549- External constriction, <u>unspecified</u> ankle

  S90.55- <u>Superficial foreign body</u> of <u>ankle</u>

      Splinter in the ankle

    S90.551- Superficial foreign body, <u>right</u> ankle

    S90.552- Superficial foreign body, <u>left</u> ankle

    S90.559- Superficial foreign body, <u>unspecified</u> ankle

  S90.56- <u>Insect bite (nonvenomous)</u> of <u>ankle</u>

    S90.561- Insect bite (nonvenomous), <u>right</u> ankle

    S90.562- Insect bite (nonvenomous), <u>left</u> ankle

    S90.569- Insect bite (nonvenomous), <u>unspecified</u> ankle

  S90.57- <u>Other superficial bite</u> of <u>ankle</u>

    Excludes 1:   open bite of ankle (S91.05-)

    S90.571- Other superficial bite of ankle, <u>right</u> ankle

    S90.572- Other superficial bite of ankle, <u>left</u> ankle

    S90.579- Other superficial bite of ankle, <u>unspecified</u> ankle

S90.8- <u>Other superficial injuries</u> of <u>foot</u>

  S90.81- <u>Abrasion</u> of <u>foot</u>

    S90.811- Abrasion, <u>right</u> foot

    S90.812- Abrasion, <u>left</u> foot

    S90.819- Abrasion, <u>unspecified</u> foot

  S90.82- <u>Blister</u> (nonthermal) of <u>foot</u>

    S90.821- Blister (nonthermal), <u>right</u> foot

    S90.822- Blister (nonthermal), <u>left</u> foot

    S90.829- Blister (nonthermal), <u>unspecified</u> foot

  S90.84- <u>External constriction</u> of <u>foot</u>

    S90.841- External constriction, <u>right</u> foot

    S90.842- External constriction, <u>left</u> foot

    S90.849- External constriction, <u>unspecified</u> foot

  S90.85- <u>Superficial foreign body</u> of <u>foot</u>

      Splinter in the foot

    S90.851- Superficial foreign body, <u>right</u> foot

    S90.852- Superficial foreign body, <u>left</u> foot

    S90.859- Superficial foreign body, <u>unspecified</u> foot

  S90.86- <u>Insect bite (nonvenomous)</u> of <u>foot</u>

    S90.861- Insect bite (nonvenomous), <u>right</u> foot

    S90.862- Insect bite (nonvenomous), <u>left</u> foot

    S90.869- Insect bite (nonvenomous), <u>unspecified</u> foot

  S90.87- <u>Other superficial bite</u> of <u>foot</u>

    Excludes 1:   open bite of foot (S91.35-)

    S90.871- Other superficial bite of <u>right</u> foot

    S90.872- Other superficial bite of <u>left</u> foot

    S90.879- Other superficial bite of <u>unspecified</u> foot

S90
-
S90

S90.9- Unspecified superficial injury of ankle, foot and toe

S90.91- Unspecified superficial injury of ankle

S90.911- Unspecified superficial injury of right ankle

S90.912- Unspecified superficial injury of left ankle

S90.919- Unspecified superficial injury of unspecified ankle

S90.92- Unspecified superficial injury of foot

S90.921- Unspecified superficial injury of right foot

S90.922- Unspecified superficial injury of left foot

S90.929- Unspecified superficial injury of unspecified foot

S90.93- Unspecified superficial injury of toes

S90.931- Unspecified superficial injury of right great toe

S90.932- Unspecified superficial injury of left great toe

S90.933- Unspecified superficial injury of unspecified great toe

S90.934- Unspecified superficial injury of right lesser toe(s)

S90.935- Unspecified superficial injury of left lesser toe(s)

S90.936- Unspecified superficial injury of unspecified lesser toe(s)

S91- Open wound of ankle, foot and toes

Code also any associated wound infection

Excludes 1: open fracture of ankle, foot and toes (S92.-with 7th character B)

traumatic amputation of ankle and foot (S98.-)

The appropriate 7th character is to be added to each code from category S91:

A Initial encounter

D Subsequent encounter

S Sequela

S91.0- Open wound of ankle

S91.00- Unspecified open wound of ankle

S91.001- Unspecified open wound, right ankle

S91.002- Unspecified open wound, left ankle

S91.009- Unspecified open wound, unspecified ankle

S91.01- Laceration without foreign body of ankle

S91.011- Laceration without foreign body, right ankle

S91.012- Laceration without foreign body, left ankle

S91.019- Laceration without foreign body, unspecified ankle

S91.02- Laceration with foreign body of ankle

S91.021- Laceration with foreign body, right ankle

S91.022- Laceration with foreign body, left ankle

S91.029- Laceration with foreign body, unspecified ankle

S91.03- Puncture wound without foreign body of ankle

S91.031- Puncture wound without foreign body, right ankle

S91.032- Puncture wound without foreign body, left ankle

S91.039- Puncture wound without foreign body, unspecified ankle

S91.04- Puncture wound with foreign body of ankle

S91.041- Puncture wound with foreign body, right ankle

S91.042- Puncture wound with foreign body, left ankle

S91.049- Puncture wound with foreign body, unspecified ankle

S91.05- Open bite of ankle

Excludes 1: superficial bite of ankle (S90.56-, S90.57-)

S91.051- Open bite, right ankle

S91.052- Open bite, left ankle

S91.059- Open bite, unspecified ankle

S91.1- Open wound of toe without damage to nail

S91.10- Unspecified open wound of toe without damage to nail

S91.101- Unspecified open wound of right great toe without damage to nail

S91.102- Unspecified open wound of left great toe without damage to nail

S91.103- Unspecified open wound of unspecified great toe without damage to nail

S91.104- Unspecified open wound of right lesser toe(s) without damage to nail

S91.105- Unspecified open wound of left lesser toe(s) without damage to nail

S91.106- Unspecified open wound of unspecified lesser toe(s) without damage to nail

S91.109- Unspecified open wound of unspecified toe(s) without damage to nail

S91.11- Laceration without foreign body of toe without damage to nail

S91.111- Laceration without foreign body of right great toe without damage to nail

S91.112- Laceration without foreign body of left great toe without damage to nail

S91.113- Laceration without foreign body of unspecified great toe without damage to nail

S91.114- Laceration without foreign body of right lesser toe(s) without damage to nail

S91.115- Laceration without foreign body of left lesser toe(s) without damage to nail

S91.116- Laceration without foreign body of unspecified lesser toe(s) without damage to nail

S91.119- Laceration without foreign body of unspecified toe without damage to nail

S91.12- Laceration with foreign body of toe without damage to nail

S91.121- Laceration with foreign body of right great toe without damage to nail

S91.122- Laceration with foreign body of left great toe without damage to nail

S91.123- Laceration with foreign body of unspecified great toe without damage to nail

S91.124- Laceration with foreign body of right lesser toe(s) without damage to nail

S91.125- Laceration with foreign body of left lesser toe(s) without damage to nail

S91.126- Laceration with foreign body of unspecified lesser toe(s) without damage to nail

S91.129- Laceration with foreign body of unspecified toe(s) without damage to nail

S91.13- Puncture wound without foreign body of toe without damage to nail

S91.131- Puncture wound without foreign body of right great toe without damage to nail

S91.132- Puncture wound without foreign body of left great toe without damage to nail

S91.133- Puncture wound without foreign body of unspecified great toe without damage to nail

S91.134- Puncture wound without foreign body of right lesser toe(s) without damage to nail

S91.135- Puncture wound without foreign body of left lesser toe(s) without damage to nail

S91.136- Puncture wound without foreign body of unspecified lesser toe(s) without damage to nail

S91.139- Puncture wound without foreign body of unspecified toe(s) without damage to nail

S91.14- Puncture wound with foreign body of toe without damage to nail

S91.141- Puncture wound with foreign body of right great toe without damage to nail

S91.142- Puncture wound with foreign body of left great toe without damage to nail

S91.143- Puncture wound with foreign body of unspecified great toe without damage to nail

S91.144- Puncture wound with foreign body of right lesser toe(s) without damage to nail

S91.145- Puncture wound with foreign body of left lesser toe(s) without damage to nail

S91.146- Puncture wound with foreign body of unspecified lesser toe(s) without damage to nail

S90 – S91

S91.149- Puncture wound <u>with foreign body</u> of <u>unspecified</u> toe(s) <u>without</u> damage to nail

S91.15- <u>Open bite</u> of <u>toe</u> <u>without</u> damage to nail
> Bite of toe NOS
> *Excludes 1:* superficial bite of toe (S90.46-, S90.47-)

S91.151- Open bite of <u>right great</u> toe <u>without</u> damage to nail

S91.152- Open bite of <u>left great</u> toe <u>without</u> damage to nail

S91.153- Open bite of <u>unspecified great</u> toe <u>without</u> damage to nail

S91.154- Open bite of <u>right lesser</u> toe(s) <u>without</u> damage to nail

S91.155- Open bite of <u>left lesser</u> toe(s) <u>without</u> damage to nail

S91.156- Open bite of <u>unspecified lesser</u> toe(s) <u>without</u> damage to nail

S91.159- Open bite of <u>unspecified</u> toe(s) <u>without</u> damage to nail

S91.2- <u>Open wound</u> of <u>toe</u> <u>with damage to nail</u>

S91.20- <u>Unspecified open wound</u> of <u>toe</u> <u>with damage to nail</u>

S91.201- Unspecified open wound of <u>right great</u> toe <u>with damage to nail</u>

S91.202- Unspecified open wound of <u>left great</u> toe <u>with damage to nail</u>

S91.203- Unspecified open wound of <u>unspecified great</u> toe <u>with damage to nail</u>

S91.204- Unspecified open wound of <u>right lesser</u> toe(s) <u>with damage to nail</u>

S91.205- Unspecified open wound of <u>left lesser</u> toe(s) <u>with damage to nail</u>

S91.206- Unspecified open wound of <u>unspecified lesser</u> toe(s) <u>with damage to nail</u>

S91.209- Unspecified open wound of <u>unspecified</u> toe(s) <u>with damage to nail</u>

S91.21- <u>Laceration without</u> foreign body of toe <u>with damage to nail</u>

S91.211- Laceration <u>without</u> foreign body of <u>right great</u> toe <u>with damage to nail</u>

S91.212- Laceration <u>without</u> foreign body of <u>left great</u> toe <u>with damage to nail</u>

S91.213- Laceration <u>without</u> foreign body of <u>unspecified great</u> toe <u>with damage to nail</u>

S91.214- Laceration <u>without</u> foreign body of <u>right lesser</u> toe(s) <u>with damage to nail</u>

S91.215- Laceration <u>without</u> foreign body of <u>left lesser</u> toe(s) <u>with damage to nail</u>

S91.216- Laceration <u>without</u> foreign body of <u>unspecified lesser</u> toe(s) <u>with damage to nail</u>

S91.219- Laceration <u>without</u> foreign body of <u>unspecified</u> toe(s) <u>with damage to nail</u>

S91.22- <u>Laceration with foreign body</u> of <u>toe</u> <u>with damage to nail</u>

S91.221- Laceration <u>with foreign body</u> of <u>right great</u> toe <u>with damage to nail</u>

S91.222- Laceration <u>with foreign body</u> of <u>left great</u> toe <u>with damage to nail</u>

S91.223- Laceration <u>with foreign body</u> of <u>unspecified great</u> toe <u>with damage to nail</u>

S91.224- Laceration <u>with foreign body</u> of <u>right lesser</u> toe(s) <u>with damage to nail</u>

S91.225- Laceration <u>with foreign body</u> of <u>left lesser</u> toe(s) <u>with damage to nail</u>

S91.226- Laceration <u>with foreign body</u> of <u>unspecified lesser</u> toe(s) <u>with damage to nail</u>

S91.229- Laceration <u>with foreign body</u> of <u>unspecified</u> toe(s) <u>with damage to nail</u>

S91.23- <u>Puncture</u> wound <u>without</u> foreign body of <u>toe</u> <u>with damage to nail</u>

S91.231- Puncture wound <u>without</u> foreign body of <u>right great</u> toe <u>with damage to nail</u>

S91.232- Puncture wound <u>without</u> foreign body of <u>left great</u> toe <u>with damage to nail</u>

S91.233- Puncture wound <u>without</u> foreign body of <u>unspecified great</u> toe <u>with damage to nail</u>

S91.234- Puncture wound <u>without</u> foreign body of <u>right lesser</u> toe(s) <u>with damage to nail</u>

S91.235- Puncture wound <u>without</u> foreign body of <u>left lesser</u> toe(s) <u>with damage to nail</u>

S91.236- Puncture wound <u>without</u> foreign body of <u>unspecified lesser</u> toe(s) <u>with damage to nail</u>

S91.239- Puncture wound <u>without</u> foreign body of <u>unspecified</u> toe(s) <u>with damage to nail</u>

S91.24- <u>Puncture</u> wound <u>with foreign body</u> of <u>toe</u> <u>with damage to nail</u>

S91.241- Puncture wound <u>with foreign body</u> of <u>right great</u> toe <u>with damage to nail</u>

S91.242- Puncture wound <u>with foreign body</u> of <u>left great</u> toe <u>with damage to nail</u>

S91.243- Puncture wound <u>with foreign body</u> of <u>unspecified great</u> toe <u>with damage to nail</u>

S91.244- Puncture wound <u>with foreign body</u> of <u>right lesser</u> toe(s) <u>with damage to nail</u>

S91.245- Puncture wound <u>with foreign body</u> of <u>left lesser</u> toe(s) <u>with damage to nail</u>

S91.246- Puncture wound <u>with foreign body</u> of <u>unspecified lesser</u> toe(s) <u>with damage to nail</u>

S91.249- Puncture wound <u>with foreign body</u> of <u>unspecified</u> toe(s) <u>with damage to nail</u>

S91.25- <u>Open bite</u> of <u>toe</u> <u>with damage to nail</u>
> Bite of toe with damage to nail NOS
> *Excludes 1:* superficial bite of toe (S90.46-, S90.47-)

S91.251- Open bite of <u>right great</u> toe <u>with damage to nail</u>

S91.252- Open bite of <u>left great</u> toe <u>with damage to nail</u>

S91.253- Open bite of <u>unspecified great</u> toe <u>with damage to nail</u>

S91.254- Open bite of <u>right lesser</u> toe(s) <u>with damage to nail</u>

S91.255- Open bite of <u>left lesser</u> toe(s) <u>with damage to nail</u>

S91.256- Open bite of <u>unspecified lesser</u> toe(s) <u>with damage to nail</u>

S91.259- Open bite of <u>unspecified</u> toe(s) <u>with damage to nail</u>

S91.3- <u>Open wound</u> of <u>foot</u>

S91.30- <u>Unspecified</u> open wound of <u>foot</u>

S91.301- Unspecified open wound, <u>right</u> foot

S91.302- Unspecified open wound, <u>left</u> foot

S91.309- Unspecified open wound, <u>unspecified</u> foot

S91.31- <u>Laceration without</u> foreign body of <u>foot</u>

S91.311- Laceration <u>without</u> foreign body, <u>right</u> foot

S91.312- Laceration <u>without</u> foreign body, <u>left</u> foot

S91.319- Laceration <u>without</u> foreign body, <u>unspecified</u> foot

S91.32- <u>Laceration with foreign body</u> of <u>foot</u>

S91.321- Laceration <u>with foreign body</u>, <u>right</u> foot

S91.322- Laceration <u>with foreign body</u>, <u>left</u> foot

S91.329- Laceration <u>with foreign body</u>, <u>unspecified</u> foot

S91.33- <u>Puncture</u> wound <u>without</u> foreign body of <u>foot</u>

S91.331- Puncture wound <u>without</u> foreign body, <u>right</u> foot

S91.332- Puncture wound <u>without</u> foreign body, <u>left</u> foot

S91.339- Puncture wound <u>without</u> foreign body, <u>unspecified</u> foot

S91.34- <u>Puncture</u> wound <u>with foreign body</u> of <u>foot</u>

S91.341- Puncture wound <u>with foreign body</u>, <u>right</u> foot

S91.342- Puncture wound <u>with foreign body</u>, <u>left</u> foot

S91.349- Puncture wound with foreign body, unspecified foot

S91.35- Open bite of foot
Excludes 1: superficial bite of foot (S90.86-, S90.87-)

S91.351- Open bite, right foot

S91.352- Open bite, left foot

S91.359- Open bite, unspecified foot

S92- Fracture of foot and toe, except ankle
Note: A fracture not indicated as displaced or nondisplaced should be coded to displaced
Note: A fracture not indicated as open or closed should be coded to closed
Excludes 1: traumatic amputation of ankle and foot (S98.-)
Excludes ❷: fracture of ankle (S82.-)
fracture of malleolus (S82.-)

The appropriate 7th character is to be added to each code from category S92:
A   Initial encounter for closed fracture
B   Initial encounter for open fracture
D   Subsequent encounter for fracture with routine healing
G   Subsequent encounter for fracture with delayed healing
K   Subsequent encounter for fracture with nonunion
P   Subsequent encounter for fracture with malunion
S   Sequela

S92.0- Fracture of calcaneus
Heel bone
Os calcis
Excludes ❷: physeal fracture of calcaneus (S99.0-)

S92.00- Unspecified fracture of calcaneus
CC-B,K,P S92.001- Unspecified fracture of right calcaneus
CC-B,K,P S92.002- Unspecified fracture of left calcaneus
CC-B,K,P S92.009- Unspecified fracture of unspecified calcaneus

S92.01- Fracture of body of calcaneus
CC-B,K,P S92.011- Displaced fracture of body of right calcaneus
CC-B,K,P S92.012- Displaced fracture of body of left calcaneus
CC-B,K,P S92.013- Displaced fracture of body of unspecified calcaneus
CC-B,K,P S92.014- Nondisplaced fracture of body of right calcaneus
CC-B,K,P S92.015- Nondisplaced fracture of body of left calcaneus
CC-B,K,P S92.016- Nondisplaced fracture of body of unspecified calcaneus

S92.02- Fracture of anterior process of calcaneus
CC-B,K,P S92.021- Displaced fracture of anterior process of right calcaneus
CC-B,K,P S92.022- Displaced fracture of anterior process of left calcaneus
CC-B,K,P S92.023- Displaced fracture of anterior process of unspecified calcaneus
CC-B,K,P S92.024- Nondisplaced fracture of anterior process of right calcaneus
CC-B,K,P S92.025- Nondisplaced fracture of anterior process of left calcaneus
CC-B,K,P S92.026- Nondisplaced fracture of anterior process of unspecified calcaneus

S92.03- Avulsion fracture of tuberosity of calcaneus
CC-B,K,P S92.031- Displaced avulsion fracture of tuberosity of right calcaneus
CC-B,K,P S92.032- Displaced avulsion fracture of tuberosity of left calcaneus
CC-B,K,P S92.033- Displaced avulsion fracture of tuberosity of unspecified calcaneus
CC-B,K,P S92.034- Nondisplaced avulsion fracture of tuberosity of right calcaneus
CC-B,K,P S92.035- Nondisplaced avulsion fracture of tuberosity of left calcaneus
CC-B,K,P S92.036- Nondisplaced avulsion fracture of tuberosity of unspecified calcaneus

S92.04- Other fracture of tuberosity of calcaneus
CC-B,K,P S92.041- Displaced other fracture of tuberosity of right calcaneus
CC-B,K,P S92.042- Displaced other fracture of tuberosity of left calcaneus

CC-B,K,P S92.043- Displaced other fracture of tuberosity of unspecified calcaneus
CC-B,K,P S92.044- Nondisplaced other fracture of tuberosity of right calcaneus
CC-B,K,P S92.045- Nondisplaced other fracture of tuberosity of left calcaneus
CC-B,K,P S92.046- Nondisplaced other fracture of tuberosity of unspecified calcaneus

S92.05- Other extraarticular fracture of calcaneus
CC-B,K,P S92.051- Displaced other extraarticular fracture of right calcaneus
CC-B,K,P S92.052- Displaced other extraarticular fracture of left calcaneus
CC-B,K,P S92.053- Displaced other extraarticular fracture of unspecified calcaneus
CC-B,K,P S92.054- Nondisplaced other extraarticular fracture of right calcaneus
CC-B,K,P S92.055- Nondisplaced other extraarticular fracture of left calcaneus
CC-B,K,P S92.056- Nondisplaced other extraarticular fracture of unspecified calcaneus

S92.06- Intraarticular fracture of calcaneus
CC-B,K,P S92.061- Displaced intraarticular fracture of right calcaneus
CC-B,K,P S92.062- Displaced intraarticular fracture of left calcaneus
CC-B,K,P S92.063- Displaced intraarticular fracture of unspecified calcaneus
CC-B,K,P S92.064- Nondisplaced intraarticular fracture of right calcaneus
CC-B,K,P S92.065- Nondisplaced intraarticular fracture of left calcaneus
CC-B,K,P S92.066- Nondisplaced intraarticular fracture of unspecified calcaneus

S92.1- Fracture of talus
Astragalus

S92.10- Unspecified fracture of talus
CC-B,K,P S92.101- Unspecified fracture of right talus
CC-B,K,P S92.102- Unspecified fracture of left talus
CC-B,K,P S92.109- Unspecified fracture of unspecified talus

S92.11- Fracture of neck of talus
CC-B,K,P S92.111- Displaced fracture of neck of right talus
CC-B,K,P S92.112- Displaced fracture of neck of left talus
CC-B,K,P S92.113- Displaced fracture of neck of unspecified talus
CC-B,K,P S92.114- Nondisplaced fracture of neck of right talus
CC-B,K,P S92.115- Nondisplaced fracture of neck of left talus
CC-B,K,P S92.116- Nondisplaced fracture of neck of unspecified talus

S92.12- Fracture of body of talus
CC-B,K,P S92.121- Displaced fracture of body of right talus
CC-B,K,P S92.122- Displaced fracture of body of left talus
CC-B,K,P S92.123- Displaced fracture of body of unspecified talus
CC-B,K,P S92.124- Nondisplaced fracture of body of right talus
CC-B,K,P S92.125- Nondisplaced fracture of body of left talus
CC-B,K,P S92.126- Nondisplaced fracture of body of unspecified talus

S92.13- Fracture of posterior process of talus
CC-B,K,P S92.131- Displaced fracture of posterior process of right talus
CC-B,K,P S92.132- Displaced fracture of posterior process of left talus
CC-B,K,P S92.133- Displaced fracture of posterior process of unspecified talus
CC-B,K,P S92.134- Nondisplaced fracture of posterior process of right talus
CC-B,K,P S92.135- Nondisplaced fracture of posterior process of left talus
CC-B,K,P S92.136- Nondisplaced fracture of posterior process of unspecified talus

S92.14- Dome fracture of talus
Excludes 1: osteochondritis dissecans (M93.2)

S9 1 – S9 2

CC-B,K,P **S92.141-** <u>Displaced</u> dome fracture of <u>right</u> talus

CC-B,K,P **S92.142-** <u>Displaced</u> dome fracture of <u>left</u> talus

CC-B,K,P **S92.143-** <u>Displaced</u> dome fracture of <u>unspecified</u> talus

CC-B,K,P **S92.144-** <u>Nondisplaced</u> dome fracture of <u>right</u> talus

CC-B,K,P **S92.145-** <u>Nondisplaced</u> dome fracture of <u>left</u> talus

CC-B,K,P **S92.146-** <u>Nondisplaced</u> dome fracture of <u>unspecified</u> talus

S92.15- <u>Avulsion</u> fracture (chip fracture) of <u>talus</u>

CC-B,K,P **S92.151-** <u>Displaced</u> avulsion fracture (chip fracture) of <u>right</u> talus

CC-B,K,P **S92.152-** <u>Displaced</u> avulsion fracture (chip fracture) of <u>left</u> talus

CC-B,K,P **S92.153-** <u>Displaced</u> avulsion fracture (chip fracture) of <u>unspecified</u> talus

CC-B,K,P **S92.154-** <u>Nondisplaced</u> avulsion fracture (chip fracture) of <u>right</u> talus

CC-B,K,P **S92.155-** <u>Nondisplaced</u> avulsion fracture (chip fracture) of <u>left</u> talus

CC-B,K,P **S92.156-** <u>Nondisplaced</u> avulsion fracture (chip fracture) of <u>unspecified</u> talus

S92.19- <u>Other fracture</u> of <u>talus</u>

CC-B,K,P **S92.191-** Other fracture of <u>right</u> talus

CC-B,K,P **S92.192-** Other fracture of <u>left</u> talus

CC-B,K,P **S92.199-** Other fracture of <u>unspecified</u> talus

S92.2- Fracture of <u>other and unspecified</u> <u>tarsal</u> bone(s)

S92.20- Fracture of <u>unspecified</u> tarsal bone(s)

CC-B,K,P **S92.201-** Fracture of <u>unspecified</u> tarsal bone(s) of <u>right</u> foot

CC-B,K,P **S92.202-** Fracture of <u>unspecified</u> tarsal bone(s) of <u>left</u> foot

CC-B,K,P **S92.209-** Fracture of <u>unspecified</u> tarsal bone(s) of <u>unspecified</u> foot

S92.21- Fracture of <u>cuboid</u> bone

CC-B,K,P **S92.211-** <u>Displaced</u> fracture of cuboid bone of <u>right</u> foot

CC-B,K,P **S92.212-** <u>Displaced</u> fracture of cuboid bone of <u>left</u> foot

CC-B,K,P **S92.213-** <u>Displaced</u> fracture of cuboid bone of <u>unspecified</u> foot

CC-B,K,P **S92.214-** <u>Nondisplaced</u> fracture of cuboid bone of <u>right</u> foot

CC-B,K,P **S92.215-** <u>Nondisplaced</u> fracture of cuboid bone of <u>left</u> foot

CC-B,K,P **S92.216-** <u>Nondisplaced</u> fracture of cuboid bone of <u>unspecified</u> foot

S92.22- Fracture of <u>lateral cuneiform</u>

CC-B,K,P **S92.221-** <u>Displaced</u> fracture of lateral cuneiform of <u>right</u> foot

CC-B,K,P **S92.222-** <u>Displaced</u> fracture of lateral cuneiform of <u>left</u> foot

CC-B,K,P **S92.223-** <u>Displaced</u> fracture of lateral cuneiform of <u>unspecified</u> foot

CC-B,K,P **S92.224-** <u>Nondisplaced</u> fracture of lateral cuneiform of <u>right</u> foot

CC-B,K,P **S92.225-** <u>Nondisplaced</u> fracture of lateral cuneiform of <u>left</u> foot

CC-B,K,P **S92.226-** <u>Nondisplaced</u> fracture of lateral cuneiform of <u>unspecified</u> foot

S92.23- Fracture of <u>intermediate cuneiform</u>

CC-B,K,P **S92.231-** <u>Displaced</u> fracture of intermediate cuneiform of <u>right</u> foot

CC-B,K,P **S92.232-** <u>Displaced</u> fracture of intermediate cuneiform of <u>left</u> foot

CC-B,K,P **S92.233-** <u>Displaced</u> fracture of intermediate cuneiform of <u>unspecified</u> foot

CC-B,K,P **S92.234-** <u>Nondisplaced</u> fracture of intermediate cuneiform of <u>right</u> foot

CC-B,K,P **S92.235-** <u>Nondisplaced</u> fracture of intermediate cuneiform of <u>left</u> foot

CC-B,K,P **S92.236-** <u>Nondisplaced</u> fracture of intermediate cuneiform of <u>unspecified</u> foot

S92.24- Fracture of <u>medial cuneiform</u>

CC-B,K,P **S92.241-** <u>Displaced</u> fracture of medial cuneiform of <u>right</u> foot

CC-B,K,P **S92.242-** <u>Displaced</u> fracture of medial cuneiform of <u>left</u> foot

CC-B,K,P **S92.243-** <u>Displaced</u> fracture of medial cuneiform of <u>unspecified</u> foot

CC-B,K,P **S92.244-** <u>Nondisplaced</u> fracture of medial cuneiform of <u>right</u> foot

CC-B,K,P **S92.245-** <u>Nondisplaced</u> fracture of medial cuneiform of <u>left</u> foot

CC-B,K,P **S92.246-** <u>Nondisplaced</u> fracture of medial cuneiform of <u>unspecified</u> foot

S92.25- Fracture of <u>navicular [scaphoid]</u> of <u>foot</u>

CC-B,K,P **S92.251-** <u>Displaced</u> fracture of navicular [scaphoid] of <u>right</u> foot

CC-B,K,P **S92.252-** <u>Displaced</u> fracture of navicular [scaphoid] of <u>left</u> foot

CC-B,K,P **S92.253-** <u>Displaced</u> fracture of navicular [scaphoid] of <u>unspecified</u> foot

CC-B,K,P **S92.254-** <u>Nondisplaced</u> fracture of navicular [scaphoid] of <u>right</u> foot

CC-B,K,P **S92.255-** <u>Nondisplaced</u> fracture of navicular [scaphoid] of <u>left</u> foot

CC-B,K,P **S92.256-** <u>Nondisplaced</u> fracture of navicular [scaphoid] of <u>unspecified</u> foot

S92.3- <u>Fracture</u> of <u>metatarsal</u> bone(s)

Excludes ❷: physeal fracture of metatarsal (S99.1-)

S92.30- Fracture of <u>unspecified</u> <u>metatarsal</u> bone(s)

CC-B,K,P **S92.301-** Fracture of <u>unspecified</u> metatarsal bone(s), <u>right</u> foot

CC-B,K,P **S92.302-** Fracture of <u>unspecified</u> metatarsal bone(s), <u>left</u> foot

CC-B,K,P **S92.309-** Fracture of <u>unspecified</u> metatarsal bone(s), <u>unspecified</u> foot

S92.31- Fracture of first metatarsal bone

CC-B,K,P **S92.311-** <u>Displaced</u> fracture of first metatarsal bone, <u>right</u> foot

CC-B,K,P **S92.312-** <u>Displaced</u> fracture of first metatarsal bone, <u>left</u> foot

CC-B,K,P **S92.313-** <u>Displaced</u> fracture of first metatarsal bone, <u>unspecified</u> foot

CC-B,K,P **S92.314-** <u>Nondisplaced</u> fracture of first metatarsal bone, <u>right</u> foot

CC-B,K,P **S92.315-** <u>Nondisplaced</u> fracture of first metatarsal bone, <u>left</u> foot

CC-B,K,P **S92.316-** <u>Nondisplaced</u> fracture of first metatarsal bone, <u>unspecified</u> foot

S92.32- Fracture of <u>second</u> metatarsal bone

CC-B,K,P **S92.321-** <u>Displaced</u> fracture of second metatarsal bone, <u>right</u> foot

CC-B,K,P **S92.322-** <u>Displaced</u> fracture of second metatarsal bone, <u>left</u> foot

CC-B,K,P **S92.323-** <u>Displaced</u> fracture of second metatarsal bone, <u>unspecified</u> foot

CC-B,K,P **S92.324-** <u>Nondisplaced</u> fracture of second metatarsal bone, <u>right</u> foot

CC-B,K,P **S92.325-** <u>Nondisplaced</u> fracture of second metatarsal bone, <u>left</u> foot

CC-B,K,P **S92.326-** <u>Nondisplaced</u> fracture of second metatarsal bone, <u>unspecified</u> foot

S92.33- Fracture of <u>third</u> metatarsal bone

CC-B,K,P **S92.331-** <u>Displaced</u> fracture of third metatarsal bone, <u>right</u> foot

CC-B,K,P **S92.332-** <u>Displaced</u> fracture of third metatarsal bone, <u>left</u> foot

CC-B,K,P **S92.333-** <u>Displaced</u> fracture of third metatarsal bone, <u>unspecified</u> foot

CC-B,K,P **S92.334-** <u>Nondisplaced</u> fracture of third metatarsal bone, <u>right</u> foot

CC-B,K,P **S92.335-** <u>Nondisplaced</u> fracture of third metatarsal bone, <u>left</u> foot

S92 - S92 *(vertical side tab)*

CC-B,K,P **S92.336-** <u>Nondisplaced</u> fracture of third metatarsal bone, <u>unspecified</u> foot

S92.34- Fracture of <u>fourth</u> metatarsal bone

CC-B,K,P **S92.341-** <u>Displaced</u> fracture of fourth metatarsal bone, <u>right</u> foot

CC-B,K,P **S92.342-** <u>Displaced</u> fracture of fourth metatarsal bone, <u>left</u> foot

CC-B,K,P **S92.343-** <u>Displaced</u> fracture of fourth metatarsal bone, <u>unspecified</u> foot

CC-B,K,P **S92.344-** <u>Nondisplaced</u> fracture of fourth metatarsal bone, <u>right</u> foot

CC-B,K,P **S92.345-** <u>Nondisplaced</u> fracture of fourth metatarsal bone, <u>left</u> foot

CC-B,K,P **S92.346-** <u>Nondisplaced</u> fracture of fourth metatarsal bone, <u>unspecified</u> foot

S92.35- Fracture of <u>fifth</u> metatarsal bone

CC-B,K,P **S92.351-** <u>Displaced</u> fracture of fifth metatarsal bone, <u>right</u> foot

CC-B,K,P **S92.352-** <u>Displaced</u> fracture of fifth metatarsal bone, <u>left</u> foot

CC-B,K,P **S92.353-** <u>Displaced</u> fracture of fifth metatarsal bone, <u>unspecified</u> foot

CC-B,K,P **S92.354-** <u>Nondisplaced</u> fracture of fifth metatarsal bone, <u>right</u> foot

CC-B,K,P **S92.355-** <u>Nondisplaced</u> fracture of fifth metatarsal bone, <u>left</u> foot

CC-B,K,P **S92.356-** <u>Nondisplaced</u> fracture of fifth metatarsal bone, <u>unspecified</u> foot

S92.4- <u>Fracture</u> of <u>great</u> <u>toe</u>
  Excludes ❷: physeal fracture of phalanx of toe (S99.2-)

S92.40- <u>Unspecified</u> fracture of <u>great</u> <u>toe</u>

CC-K,P **S92.401-** <u>Displaced</u> unspecified fracture of <u>right</u> great toe

CC-K,P **S92.402-** <u>Displaced</u> unspecified fracture of <u>left</u> great toe

CC-K,P **S92.403-** <u>Displaced</u> unspecified fracture of <u>unspecified</u> great toe

CC-K,P **S92.404-** <u>Nondisplaced</u> unspecified fracture of <u>right</u> great toe

CC-K,P **S92.405-** <u>Nondisplaced</u> unspecified fracture of <u>left</u> great toe

CC-K,P **S92.406-** <u>Nondisplaced</u> unspecified fracture of <u>unspecified</u> great toe

S92.41- Fracture of <u>proximal phalanx</u> of <u>great</u> <u>toe</u>

CC-K,P **S92.411-** <u>Displaced</u> fracture of proximal phalanx of <u>right</u> great toe

CC-K,P **S92.412-** <u>Displaced</u> fracture of proximal phalanx of <u>left</u> great toe

CC-K,P **S92.413-** <u>Displaced</u> fracture of proximal phalanx of <u>unspecified</u> great toe

CC-K,P **S92.414-** <u>Nondisplaced</u> fracture of proximal phalanx of <u>right</u> great toe

CC-K,P **S92.415-** <u>Nondisplaced</u> fracture of proximal phalanx of <u>left</u> great toe

CC-K,P **S92.416-** <u>Nondisplaced</u> fracture of proximal phalanx of <u>unspecified</u> great toe

S92.42- Fracture of <u>distal phalanx</u> of <u>great</u> <u>toe</u>

CC-K,P **S92.421-** <u>Displaced</u> fracture of distal phalanx of <u>right</u> great toe

CC-K,P **S92.422-** <u>Displaced</u> fracture of distal phalanx of <u>left</u> great toe

CC-K,P **S92.423-** <u>Displaced</u> fracture of distal phalanx of <u>unspecified</u> great toe

CC-K,P **S92.424-** <u>Nondisplaced</u> fracture of distal phalanx of <u>right</u> great toe

CC-K,P **S92.425-** <u>Nondisplaced</u> fracture of distal phalanx of <u>left</u> great toe

CC-K,P **S92.426-** <u>Nondisplaced</u> fracture of distal phalanx of <u>unspecified</u> great toe

S92.49- <u>Other fracture</u> of <u>great</u> <u>toe</u>

CC-K,P **S92.491-** Other fracture of <u>right</u> great toe

CC-K,P **S92.492-** Other fracture of <u>left</u> great toe

CC-K,P **S92.499-** Other fracture of <u>unspecified</u> great toe

S92.5- <u>Fracture</u> of <u>lesser toe(s)</u>
  Excludes ❷: physeal fracture of phalanx of toe (S99.2-)

S92.50- <u>Unspecified</u> fracture of <u>lesser toe(s)</u>

CC-K,P **S92.501-** <u>Displaced</u> unspecified fracture of <u>right</u> lesser toe(s)

CC-K,P **S92.502-** <u>Displaced</u> unspecified fracture of <u>left</u> lesser toe(s)

CC-K,P **S92.503-** <u>Displaced</u> unspecified fracture of <u>unspecified</u> lesser toe(s)

CC-K,P **S92.504-** <u>Nondisplaced</u> unspecified fracture of <u>right</u> lesser toe(s)

CC-K,P **S92.505-** <u>Nondisplaced</u> unspecified fracture of <u>left</u> lesser toe(s)

CC-K,P **S92.506-** <u>Nondisplaced</u> unspecified fracture of <u>unspecified</u> lesser toe(s)

S92.51- Fracture of <u>proximal phalanx</u> of <u>lesser toe(s)</u>

CC-K,P **S92.511-** <u>Displaced</u> fracture of proximal phalanx of <u>right</u> lesser toe(s)

CC-K,P **S92.512-** <u>Displaced</u> fracture of proximal phalanx of <u>left</u> lesser toe(s)

CC-K,P **S92.513-** <u>Displaced</u> fracture of proximal phalanx of <u>unspecified</u> lesser toe(s)

CC-K,P **S92.514-** <u>Nondisplaced</u> fracture of proximal phalanx of <u>right</u> lesser toe(s)

CC-K,P **S92.515-** <u>Nondisplaced</u> fracture of proximal phalanx of <u>left</u> lesser toe(s)

CC-K,P **S92.516-** <u>Nondisplaced</u> fracture of proximal phalanx of <u>unspecified</u> lesser toe(s)

S92.52- Fracture of <u>medial phalanx</u> of <u>lesser toe(s)</u>

CC-K,P **S92.521-** <u>Displaced</u> fracture of medial phalanx of <u>right</u> lesser toe(s)

CC-K,P **S92.522-** <u>Displaced</u> fracture of medial phalanx of <u>left</u> lesser toe(s)

CC-K,P **S92.523-** <u>Displaced</u> fracture of medial phalanx of <u>unspecified</u> lesser toe(s)

CC-K,P **S92.524-** <u>Nondisplaced</u> fracture of medial phalanx of <u>right</u> lesser toe(s)

CC-K,P **S92.525-** <u>Nondisplaced</u> fracture of medial phalanx of <u>left</u> lesser toe(s)

CC-K,P **S92.526-** <u>Nondisplaced</u> fracture of medial phalanx of <u>unspecified</u> lesser toe(s)

S92.53- Fracture of <u>distal phalanx</u> of <u>lesser toe(s)</u>

CC-K,P **S92.531-** <u>Displaced</u> fracture of distal phalanx of <u>right</u> lesser toe(s)

CC-K,P **S92.532-** <u>Displaced</u> fracture of distal phalanx of <u>left</u> lesser toe(s)

CC-K,P **S92.533-** <u>Displaced</u> fracture of distal phalanx of <u>unspecified</u> lesser toe(s)

CC-K,P **S92.534-** <u>Nondisplaced</u> fracture of distal phalanx of <u>right</u> lesser toe(s)

CC-K,P **S92.535-** <u>Nondisplaced</u> fracture of distal phalanx of <u>left</u> lesser toe(s)

CC-K,P **S92.536-** <u>Nondisplaced</u> fracture of distal phalanx of <u>unspecified</u> lesser toe(s)

S92.59- <u>Other fracture</u> of <u>lesser toe(s)</u>

CC-K,P **S92.591-** Other fracture of <u>right</u> lesser toe(s)

CC-K,P **S92.592-** Other fracture of <u>left</u> lesser toe(s)

CC-K,P **S92.599-** Other fracture of <u>unspecified</u> lesser toe(s)

S92.8- <u>Other fracture</u> of <u>foot</u>, except ankle

S92.81- <u>Other</u> fracture of <u>foot</u>
  Sesamoid fracture of foot

CC-B,K,P **S92.811-** Other fracture of <u>right</u> foot

CC-B,K,P **S92.812-** Other fracture of <u>left</u> foot

CC-B,K,P **S92.819-** Other fracture of <u>unspecified</u> foot

S92.9- Unspecified fracture of foot and toe

S92.90- <u>Unspecified</u> fracture of <u>foot</u>

CC-B,K,P **S92.901-** Unspecified fracture of <u>right</u> foot

S92 - S92

CC-B,K,P **S92.902-** Unspecified fracture of <u>left</u> foot

CC-B,K,P **S92.909-** Unspecified fracture of <u>unspecified</u> foot

S92.91- <u>Unspecified</u> fracture of <u>toe</u>

CC-K,P **S92.911-** Unspecified fracture of <u>right</u> toe(s)

CC-K,P **S92.912-** Unspecified fracture of <u>left</u> toe(s)

CC-K,P **S92.919-** Unspecified fracture of <u>unspecified</u> toe(s)

S93- <u>Dislocation and sprain</u> of joints and ligaments at <u>ankle, foot and toe level</u>

Includes: Avulsion of joint or ligament of ankle, foot and toe
Laceration of cartilage, joint or ligament of ankle, foot and toe
Sprain of cartilage, joint or ligament of ankle, foot and toe
Traumatic hemarthrosis of joint or ligament of ankle, foot and toe
Traumatic rupture of joint or ligament of ankle, foot and toe
Traumatic subluxation of joint or ligament of ankle, foot and toe
Traumatic tear of joint or ligament of ankle, foot and toe

Code also any associated open wound

Excludes ❷: *strain of muscle and tendon of ankle and foot (S96.-)*

The appropriate 7th character is to be added to each code from category S93:

A   <u>Initial</u> encounter

D   <u>Subsequent</u> encounter

S   <u>Sequela</u>

S93.0- Subluxation and dislocation of <u>ankle joint</u>

    Subluxation and dislocation of astragalus
    Subluxation and dislocation of fibula, lower end
    Subluxation and dislocation of talus
    Subluxation and dislocation of tibia, lower end

S93.01x- <u>Subluxation</u> of <u>right</u> ankle joint

S93.02x- <u>Subluxation</u> of <u>left</u> ankle joint

S93.03x- <u>Subluxation</u> of <u>unspecified</u> ankle joint

S93.04x- <u>Dislocation</u> of <u>right</u> ankle joint

S93.05x- <u>Dislocation</u> of <u>left</u> ankle joint

S93.06x- <u>Dislocation</u> of <u>unspecified</u> ankle joint

S93.1- Subluxation and dislocation of toe

S93.10- <u>Unspecified</u> subluxation and dislocation of <u>toe</u>

    Dislocation of toe NOS
    Subluxation of toe NOS

S93.101- Unspecified <u>subluxation</u> of <u>right</u> toe(s)

S93.102- Unspecified <u>subluxation</u> of <u>left</u> toe(s)

S93.103- Unspecified <u>subluxation</u> of <u>unspecified</u> toe(s)

S93.104- Unspecified <u>dislocation</u> of <u>right</u> toe(s)

S93.105- Unspecified <u>dislocation</u> of <u>left</u> toe(s)

S93.106- Unspecified <u>dislocation</u> of <u>unspecified</u> toe(s)

S93.11- <u>Dislocation</u> of <u>interphalangeal joint</u>

S93.111- Dislocation of interphalangeal joint of <u>right great</u> toe

S93.112- Dislocation of interphalangeal joint of <u>left great</u> toe

S93.113- Dislocation of interphalangeal joint of <u>unspecified great</u> toe

S93.114- Dislocation of interphalangeal joint of <u>right lesser</u> toe(s)

S93.115- Dislocation of interphalangeal joint of <u>left lesser</u> toe(s)

S93.116- Dislocation of interphalangeal joint of <u>unspecified lesser</u> toe(s)

S93.119- Dislocation of interphalangeal joint of <u>unspecified</u> toe(s)

S93.12- <u>Dislocation</u> of <u>metatarsophalangeal joint</u>

S93.121- Dislocation of metatarsophalangeal joint of <u>right great</u> toe

S93.122- Dislocation of metatarsophalangeal joint of <u>left great</u> toe

S93.123- Dislocation of metatarsophalangeal joint of <u>unspecified great</u> toe

S93.124- Dislocation of metatarsophalangeal joint of <u>right lesser</u> toe(s)

S93.125- Dislocation of metatarsophalangeal joint of <u>left lesser</u> toe(s)

S93.126- Dislocation of metatarsophalangeal joint of <u>unspecified</u> lesser toe(s)

S93.129- Dislocation of metatarsophalangeal joint of <u>unspecified</u> toe(s)

S93.13- <u>Subluxation</u> of <u>interphalangeal joint</u>

S93.131- Subluxation of interphalangeal joint of <u>right great</u> toe

S93.132- Subluxation of interphalangeal joint of <u>left great</u> toe

S93.133- Subluxation of interphalangeal joint of <u>unspecified great</u> toe

S93.134- Subluxation of interphalangeal joint of <u>right lesser</u> toe(s)

S93.135- Subluxation of interphalangeal joint of <u>left lesser</u> toe(s)

S93.136- Subluxation of interphalangeal joint of <u>unspecified lesser</u> toe(s)

S93.139- Subluxation of interphalangeal joint of <u>unspecified</u> toe(s)

S93.14- <u>Subluxation</u> of <u>metatarsophalangeal joint</u>

S93.141- Subluxation of metatarsophalangeal joint of <u>right great</u> toe

S93.142- Subluxation of metatarsophalangeal joint of <u>left great</u> toe

S93.143- Subluxation of metatarsophalangeal joint of <u>unspecified great</u> toe

S93.144- Subluxation of metatarsophalangeal joint of <u>right lesser</u> toe(s)

S93.145- Subluxation of metatarsophalangeal joint of <u>left lesser</u> toe(s)

S93.146- Subluxation of metatarsophalangeal joint of <u>unspecified lesser</u> toe(s)

S93.149- Subluxation of metatarsophalangeal joint of <u>unspecified</u> toe(s)

S93.3- Subluxation and dislocation of <u>foot</u>

Excludes ❷: *dislocation of toe (S93.1-)*

S93.30- <u>Unspecified</u> subluxation and dislocation of <u>foot</u>

    Dislocation of foot NOS
    Subluxation of foot NOS

S93.301- Unspecified <u>subluxation</u> of <u>right</u> foot

S93.302- Unspecified <u>subluxation</u> of <u>left</u> foot

S93.303- Unspecified <u>subluxation</u> of <u>unspecified</u> foot

S93.304- Unspecified <u>dislocation</u> of <u>right</u> foot

S93.305- Unspecified <u>dislocation</u> of <u>left</u> foot

S93.306- Unspecified <u>dislocation</u> of <u>unspecified</u> foot

S93.31- Subluxation and dislocation of <u>tarsal joint</u>

S93.311- <u>Subluxation</u> of tarsal joint of <u>right</u> foot

S93.312- <u>Subluxation</u> of tarsal joint of <u>left</u> foot

S93.313- <u>Subluxation</u> of tarsal joint of <u>unspecified</u> foot

S93.314- <u>Dislocation</u> of tarsal joint of <u>right</u> foot

S93.315- <u>Dislocation</u> of tarsal joint of <u>left</u> foot

S93.316- <u>Dislocation</u> of tarsal joint of <u>unspecified</u> foot

S93.32- Subluxation and dislocation of <u>tarsometatarsal joint</u>

S93.321- <u>Subluxation</u> of tarsometatarsal joint of <u>right</u> foot

S93.322- <u>Subluxation</u> of tarsometatarsal joint of <u>left</u> foot

S93.323- <u>Subluxation</u> of tarsometatarsal joint of <u>unspecified</u> foot

S93.324- <u>Dislocation</u> of tarsometatarsal joint of <u>right</u> foot

S93.325- <u>Dislocation</u> of tarsometatarsal joint of <u>left</u> foot

S93.326- <u>Dislocation</u> of tarsometatarsal joint of <u>unspecified</u> foot

S93.33- <u>Other</u> subluxation and dislocation of <u>foot</u>

S93.331- Other <u>subluxation</u> of <u>right</u> foot

S93.332- Other <u>subluxation</u> of <u>left</u> foot

S93.333- Other <u>subluxation</u> of <u>unspecified</u> foot

S93.334- Other <u>dislocation</u> of <u>right</u> foot

S93.335- Other <u>dislocation</u> of <u>left</u> foot

S 9 2 - S 9 3

S93.336-   Other <u>dislocation</u> of <u>unspecified</u> foot

S93.4-   <u>Sprain</u> of <u>ankle</u>

Excludes ❷: injury of Achilles tendon (S86.0-)

S93.40- <u>Sprain</u> of <u>unspecified ligament</u> of <u>ankle</u>
Sprain of ankle NOS
Sprained ankle NOS

S93.401-   Sprain of unspecified ligament of <u>right</u> ankle

S93.402-   Sprain of unspecified ligament of <u>left</u> ankle

S93.409-   Sprain of unspecified ligament of <u>unspecified</u> ankle

S93.41- <u>Sprain</u> of <u>calcaneofibular</u> ligament

S93.411-   Sprain of calcaneofibular ligament of <u>right</u> ankle

S93.412-   Sprain of calcaneofibular ligament of <u>left</u> ankle

S93.419-   Sprain of calcaneofibular ligament of <u>unspecified</u> ankle

S93.42- <u>Sprain</u> of <u>deltoid</u> ligament

S93.421-   Sprain of deltoid ligament of <u>right</u> ankle

S93.422-   Sprain of deltoid ligament of <u>left</u> ankle

S93.429-   Sprain of deltoid ligament of <u>unspecified</u> ankle

S93.43- <u>Sprain</u> of <u>tibiofibular</u> ligament

S93.431-   Sprain of tibiofibular ligament of <u>right</u> ankle

S93.432-   Sprain of tibiofibular ligament of <u>left</u> ankle

S93.439-   Sprain of tibiofibular ligament of <u>unspecified</u> ankle

S93.49- <u>Sprain</u> of <u>other ligament</u> of <u>ankle</u>
Sprain of internal collateral ligament
Sprain of talofibular ligament

S93.491-   Sprain of other ligament of <u>right</u> ankle

S93.492-   Sprain of other ligament of <u>left</u> ankle

S93.499-   Sprain of other ligament of <u>unspecified</u> ankle

S93.5-   <u>Sprain</u> of <u>toe</u>

S93.50- <u>Unspecified sprain</u> of <u>toe</u>

S93.501-   Unspecified sprain of <u>right</u> <u>great</u> toe

S93.502-   Unspecified sprain of <u>left</u> <u>great</u> toe

S93.503-   Unspecified sprain of <u>unspecified</u> <u>great</u> toe

S93.504-   Unspecified sprain of <u>right</u> <u>lesser</u> toe(s)

S93.505-   Unspecified sprain of <u>left</u> <u>lesser</u> toe(s)

S93.506-   Unspecified sprain of <u>unspecified</u> <u>lesser</u> toe(s)

S93.509-   Unspecified sprain of <u>unspecified</u> toe(s)

S93.51- <u>Sprain</u> of <u>interphalangeal joint</u> of <u>toe</u>

S93.511-   Sprain of interphalangeal joint of <u>right</u> <u>great</u> toe

S93.512-   Sprain of interphalangeal joint of <u>left</u> <u>great</u> toe

S93.513-   Sprain of interphalangeal joint of <u>unspecified</u> <u>great</u> toe

S93.514-   Sprain of interphalangeal joint of <u>right</u> <u>lesser</u> toe(s)

S93.515-   Sprain of interphalangeal joint of <u>left</u> <u>lesser</u> toe(s)

S93.516-   Sprain of interphalangeal joint of <u>unspecified</u> <u>lesser</u> toe(s)

S93.519-   Sprain of interphalangeal joint of <u>unspecified</u> toe(s)

S93.52- <u>Sprain</u> of <u>metatarsophalangeal joint</u> of <u>toe</u>

S93.521-   Sprain of metatarsophalangeal joint of <u>right</u> <u>great</u> toe

S93.522-   Sprain of metatarsophalangeal joint of <u>left</u> <u>great</u> toe

S93.523-   Sprain of metatarsophalangeal joint of <u>unspecified</u> <u>great</u> toe

S93.524-   Sprain of metatarsophalangeal joint of <u>right</u> <u>lesser</u> toe(s)

S93.525-   Sprain of metatarsophalangeal joint of <u>left</u> <u>lesser</u> toe(s)

S93.526-   Sprain of metatarsophalangeal joint of <u>unspecified</u> <u>lesser</u> toe(s)

S93.529-   Sprain of metatarsophalangeal joint of <u>unspecified</u> toe(s)

S93.6-   <u>Sprain</u> of <u>foot</u>

Excludes ❷: sprain of metatarsophalangeal joint of toe (S93.52-)
sprain of toe (S93.5-)

S93.60- <u>Unspecified sprain</u> of <u>foot</u>

S93.601-   Unspecified sprain of <u>right</u> foot

S93.602-   Unspecified sprain of <u>left</u> foot

S93.609-   Unspecified sprain of <u>unspecified</u> foot

S93.61- <u>Sprain</u> of <u>tarsal ligament</u> of <u>foot</u>

S93.611-   Sprain of tarsal ligament of <u>right</u> foot

S93.612-   Sprain of tarsal ligament of <u>left</u> foot

S93.619-   Sprain of tarsal ligament of <u>unspecified</u> foot

S93.62- <u>Sprain</u> of <u>tarsometatarsal ligament</u> of <u>foot</u>

S93.621-   Sprain of tarsometatarsal ligament of <u>right</u> foot

S93.622-   Sprain of tarsometatarsal ligament of <u>left</u> foot

S93.629-   Sprain of tarsometatarsal ligament of <u>unspecified</u> foot

S93.69- <u>Other sprain</u> of <u>foot</u>

S93.691-   Other sprain of <u>right</u> foot

S93.692-   Other sprain of <u>left</u> foot

S93.699-   Other sprain of <u>unspecified</u> foot

S94-   <u>Injury of nerves</u> at <u>ankle and foot level</u>

Code also any associated open wound (S91.-)

The appropriate 7th character is to be added to each code from category S94:
A   <u>Initial</u> encounter
D   <u>Subsequent</u> encounter
S   <u>Sequela</u>

S94.0-   Injury of <u>lateral plantar nerve</u>

S94.00x-   Injury of lateral plantar nerve, <u>unspecified</u> leg

S94.01x-   Injury of lateral plantar nerve, <u>right</u> leg

S94.02x-   Injury of lateral plantar nerve, <u>left</u> leg

S94.1-   Injury of <u>medial plantar nerve</u>

S94.10x-   Injury of medial plantar nerve, <u>unspecified</u> leg

S94.11x-   Injury of medial plantar nerve, <u>right</u> leg

S94.12x-   Injury of medial plantar nerve, <u>left</u> leg

S94.2-   Injury of <u>deep peroneal nerve</u> at <u>ankle and foot level</u>
Injury of terminal, lateral branch of deep peroneal nerve

S94.20x-   Injury of deep peroneal nerve at ankle and foot level, <u>unspecified</u> leg

S94.21x-   Injury of deep peroneal nerve at ankle and foot level, <u>right</u> leg

S94.22x-   Injury of deep peroneal nerve at ankle and foot level, <u>left</u> leg

S94.3-   Injury of <u>cutaneous sensory nerve</u> at <u>ankle and foot level</u>

S94.30x-   Injury of cutaneous sensory nerve at ankle and foot level, <u>unspecified</u> leg

S94.31x-   Injury of cutaneous sensory nerve at ankle and foot level, <u>right</u> leg

S94.32x-   Injury of cutaneous sensory nerve at ankle and foot level, <u>left</u> leg

S94.8-   Injury of other nerves at ankle and foot level

S94.8x- Injury of <u>other nerves</u> at <u>ankle and foot level</u>

S94.8x1-   Injury of other nerves at ankle and foot level, <u>right</u> leg

S94.8x2-   Injury of other nerves at ankle and foot level, <u>left</u> leg

S94.8x9-   Injury of other nerves at ankle and foot level, <u>unspecified</u> leg

S94.9-   Injury of <u>unspecified nerve</u> at <u>ankle and foot level</u>

S94.90x-   Injury of unspecified nerve at ankle and foot level, <u>unspecified</u> leg

S94.91x-   Injury of unspecified nerve at ankle and foot level, <u>right</u> leg

S94.92x-   Injury of unspecified nerve at ankle and foot level, <u>left</u> leg

S93 - S94

S95- Injury of blood vessels at ankle and foot level
Code also any associated open wound (S91.-)
Excludes ❷: injury of posterior tibial artery and vein (S85.1-, S85.8-)

The appropriate 7th character is to be added to each code from category S95:
A Initial encounter
D Subsequent encounter
S Sequela

S95.0- Injury of dorsal artery of foot

S95.00- Unspecified injury of dorsal artery of foot

CC-A **S95.001-** Unspecified injury of dorsal artery of right foot

CC-A **S95.002-** Unspecified injury of dorsal artery of left foot

CC-A **S95.009-** Unspecified injury of dorsal artery of unspecified foot

S95.01- Laceration of dorsal artery of foot

CC-A **S95.011-** Laceration of dorsal artery of right foot

CC-A **S95.012-** Laceration of dorsal artery of left foot

CC-A **S95.019-** Laceration of dorsal artery of unspecified foot

S95.09- Other specified injury of dorsal artery of foot

CC-A **S95.091-** Other specified injury of dorsal artery of right foot

CC-A **S95.092-** Other specified injury of dorsal artery of left foot

CC-A **S95.099-** Other specified injury of dorsal artery of unspecified foot

S95.1- Injury of plantar artery of foot

S95.10- Unspecified injury of plantar artery of foot

CC-A **S95.101-** Unspecified injury of plantar artery of right foot

CC-A **S95.102-** Unspecified injury of plantar artery of left foot

CC-A **S95.109-** Unspecified injury of plantar artery of unspecified foot

S95.11- Laceration of plantar artery of foot

CC-A **S95.111-** Laceration of plantar artery of right foot

CC-A **S95.112-** Laceration of plantar artery of left foot

CC-A **S95.119-** Laceration of plantar artery of unspecified foot

S95.19- Other specified injury of plantar artery of foot

CC-A **S95.191-** Other specified injury of plantar artery of right foot

CC-A **S95.192-** Other specified injury of plantar artery of left foot

CC-A **S95.199-** Other specified injury of plantar artery of unspecified foot

S95.2- Injury of dorsal vein of foot

S95.20- Unspecified injury of dorsal vein of foot

CC-A **S95.201-** Unspecified injury of dorsal vein of right foot

CC-A **S95.202-** Unspecified injury of dorsal vein of left foot

CC-A **S95.209-** Unspecified injury of dorsal vein of unspecified foot

S95.21- Laceration of dorsal vein of foot

CC-A **S95.211-** Laceration of dorsal vein of right foot

CC-A **S95.212-** Laceration of dorsal vein of left foot

CC-A **S95.219-** Laceration of dorsal vein of unspecified foot

S95.29- Other specified injury of dorsal vein of foot

CC-A **S95.291-** Other specified injury of dorsal vein of right foot

CC-A **S95.292-** Other specified injury of dorsal vein of left foot

CC-A **S95.299-** Other specified injury of dorsal vein of unspecified foot

S95.8- Injury of other blood vessels at ankle and foot level

S95.80- Unspecified injury of other blood vessels at ankle and foot level

CC-A **S95.801-** Unspecified injury of other blood vessels at ankle and foot level, right leg

CC-A **S95.802-** Unspecified injury of other blood vessels at ankle and foot level, left leg

CC-A **S95.809-** Unspecified injury of other blood vessels at ankle and foot level, unspecified leg

S95.81- Laceration of other blood vessels at ankle and foot level

CC-A **S95.811-** Laceration of other blood vessels at ankle and foot level, right leg

CC-A **S95.812-** Laceration of other blood vessels at ankle and foot level, left leg

CC-A **S95.819-** Laceration of other blood vessels at ankle and foot level, unspecified leg

S95.89- Other specified injury of other blood vessels at ankle and foot level

CC-A **S95.891-** Other specified injury of other blood vessels at ankle and foot level, right leg

CC-A **S95.892-** Other specified injury of other blood vessels at ankle and foot level, left leg

CC-A **S95.899-** Other specified injury of other blood vessels at ankle and foot level, unspecified leg

S95.9- Injury of unspecified blood vessel at ankle and foot level

S95.90- Unspecified injury of unspecified blood vessel at ankle and foot level

CC-A **S95.901-** Unspecified injury of unspecified blood vessel at ankle and foot level, right leg

CC-A **S95.902-** Unspecified injury of unspecified blood vessel at ankle and foot level, left leg

CC-A **S95.909-** Unspecified injury of unspecified blood vessel at ankle and foot level, unspecified leg

S95.91- Laceration of unspecified blood vessel at ankle and foot level

CC-A **S95.911-** Laceration of unspecified blood vessel at ankle and foot level, right leg

CC-A **S95.912-** Laceration of unspecified blood vessel at ankle and foot level, left leg

CC-A **S95.919-** Laceration of unspecified blood vessel at ankle and foot level, unspecified leg

S95.99- Other specified injury of unspecified blood vessel at ankle and foot level

CC-A **S95.991-** Other specified injury of unspecified blood vessel at ankle and foot level, right leg

CC-A **S95.992-** Other specified injury of unspecified blood vessel at ankle and foot level, left leg

CC-A **S95.999-** Other specified injury of unspecified blood vessel at ankle and foot level, unspecified leg

S96- Injury of muscle and tendon at ankle and foot level
Code also any associated open wound (S91.-)
Excludes ❷: injury of Achilles tendon (S86.0-)
sprain of joints and ligaments of ankle and foot (S93.-)

The appropriate 7th character is to be added to each code from category S96:
A Initial encounter
D Subsequent encounter
S Sequela

S96.0- Injury of muscle and tendon of long flexor muscle of toe at ankle and foot level

S96.00- Unspecified injury of muscle and tendon of long flexor muscle of toe at ankle and foot level

S96.001- Unspecified injury of muscle and tendon of long flexor muscle of toe at ankle and foot level, right foot

S96.002- Unspecified injury of muscle and tendon of long flexor muscle of toe at ankle and foot level, left foot

S96.009- Unspecified injury of muscle and tendon of long flexor muscle of toe at ankle and foot level, unspecified foot

S96.01- Strain of muscle and tendon of long flexor muscle of toe at ankle and foot level

S96.011- Strain of muscle and tendon of long flexor muscle of toe at ankle and foot level, right foot

S96.012- Strain of muscle and tendon of long flexor muscle of toe at ankle and foot level, left foot

S96.019- Strain of muscle and tendon of long flexor muscle of toe at ankle and foot level, unspecified foot

S96.02- Laceration of muscle and tendon of long flexor muscle of toe at ankle and foot level

CC-A **S96.021-** Laceration of muscle and tendon of long flexor muscle of toe at ankle and foot level, right foot

CC-A **S96.022-** Laceration of muscle and tendon of long flexor muscle of toe at ankle and foot level, <u>left</u> foot

CC-A **S96.029-** Laceration of muscle and tendon of long flexor muscle of toe at ankle and foot level, <u>unspecified</u> foot

S96.09- <u>Other injury</u> of muscle and tendon of <u>long flexor muscle</u> of <u>toe</u> at <u>ankle and foot level</u>

　　S96.091- Other injury of muscle and tendon of long flexor muscle of toe at ankle and foot level, <u>right</u> foot

　　S96.092- Other injury of muscle and tendon of long flexor muscle of toe at ankle and foot level, <u>left</u> foot

　　S96.099- Other injury of muscle and tendon of long flexor muscle of toe at ankle and foot level, <u>unspecified</u> foot

S96.1- <u>Injury</u> of muscle and tendon of <u>long extensor muscle</u> of <u>toe</u> at <u>ankle and foot level</u>

S96.10- <u>Unspecified</u> injury of muscle and tendon of <u>long extensor muscle</u> of <u>toe</u> at <u>ankle and foot level</u>

　　S96.101- Unspecified injury of muscle and tendon of long extensor muscle of toe at ankle and foot level, <u>right</u> foot

　　S96.102- Unspecified injury of muscle and tendon of long extensor muscle of toe at ankle and foot level, <u>left</u> foot

　　S96.109- Unspecified injury of muscle and tendon of long extensor muscle of toe at ankle and foot level, <u>unspecified</u> foot

S96.11- <u>Strain</u> of muscle and tendon of <u>long extensor muscle</u> of <u>toe</u> at <u>ankle and foot level</u>

　　S96.111- Strain of muscle and tendon of long extensor muscle of toe at ankle and foot level, <u>right</u> foot

　　S96.112- Strain of muscle and tendon of long extensor muscle of toe at ankle and foot level, <u>left</u> foot

　　S96.119- Strain of muscle and tendon of long extensor muscle of toe at ankle and foot level, <u>unspecified</u> foot

S96.12- <u>Laceration</u> of muscle and tendon of <u>long extensor muscle</u> of <u>toe</u> at <u>ankle and foot level</u>

CC-A **S96.121-** Laceration of muscle and tendon of long extensor muscle of toe at ankle and foot level, <u>right</u> foot

CC-A **S96.122-** Laceration of muscle and tendon of long extensor muscle of toe at ankle and foot level, <u>left</u> foot

CC-A **S96.129-** Laceration of muscle and tendon of long extensor muscle of toe at ankle and foot level, <u>unspecified</u> foot

S96.19- <u>Other specified injury</u> of muscle and tendon of <u>long extensor muscle</u> of <u>toe</u> at <u>ankle and foot level</u>

　　S96.191- Other specified injury of muscle and tendon of long extensor muscle of toe at ankle and foot level, <u>right</u> foot

　　S96.192- Other specified injury of muscle and tendon of long extensor muscle of toe at ankle and foot level, <u>left</u> foot

　　S96.199- Other specified injury of muscle and tendon of long extensor muscle of toe at ankle and foot level, <u>unspecified</u> foot

S96.2- <u>Injury</u> of <u>intrinsic muscle and tendon</u> at <u>ankle and foot level</u>

S96.20- <u>Unspecified</u> injury of <u>intrinsic muscle and tendon</u> at <u>ankle and foot level</u>

　　S96.201- Unspecified injury of intrinsic muscle and tendon at ankle and foot level, <u>right</u> foot

　　S96.202- Unspecified injury of intrinsic muscle and tendon at ankle and foot level, <u>left</u> foot

　　S96.209- Unspecified injury of intrinsic muscle and tendon at ankle and foot level, <u>unspecified</u> foot

S96.21- <u>Strain</u> of <u>intrinsic muscle and tendon</u> at <u>ankle and foot level</u>

　　S96.211- Strain of intrinsic muscle and tendon at ankle and foot level, <u>right</u> foot

S96.212- Strain of intrinsic muscle and tendon at ankle and foot level, <u>left</u> foot

S96.219- Strain of intrinsic muscle and tendon at ankle and foot level, <u>unspecified</u> foot

S96.22- <u>Laceration</u> of <u>intrinsic muscle and tendon</u> at <u>ankle and foot level</u>

CC-A **S96.221-** Laceration of intrinsic muscle and tendon at ankle and foot level, <u>right</u> foot

CC-A **S96.222-** Laceration of intrinsic muscle and tendon at ankle and foot level, <u>left</u> foot

CC-A **S96.229-** Laceration of intrinsic muscle and tendon at ankle and foot level, <u>unspecified</u> foot

S96.29- <u>Other specified injury</u> of <u>intrinsic muscle and tendon</u> at <u>ankle and foot level</u>

　　S96.291- Other specified injury of intrinsic muscle and tendon at ankle and foot level, <u>right</u> foot

　　S96.292- Other specified injury of intrinsic muscle and tendon at ankle and foot level, <u>left</u> foot

　　S96.299- Other specified injury of intrinsic muscle and tendon at ankle and foot level, <u>unspecified</u> foot

S96.8- <u>Injury</u> of <u>other specified muscles and tendons</u> at <u>ankle and foot level</u>

S96.80- <u>Unspecified</u> injury of <u>other specified muscles and tendons</u> at <u>ankle and foot level</u>

　　S96.801- Unspecified injury of other specified muscles and tendons at ankle and foot level, <u>right</u> foot

　　S96.802- Unspecified injury of other specified muscles and tendons at ankle and foot level, <u>left</u> foot

　　S96.809- Unspecified injury of other specified muscles and tendons at ankle and foot level, <u>unspecified</u> foot

S96.81- <u>Strain</u> of <u>other specified muscles and tendons</u> at <u>ankle and foot level</u>

　　S96.811- Strain of other specified muscles and tendons at ankle and foot level, <u>right</u> foot

　　S96.812- Strain of other specified muscles and tendons at ankle and foot level, <u>left</u> foot

　　S96.819- Strain of other specified muscles and tendons at ankle and foot level, <u>unspecified</u> foot

S96.82- <u>Laceration</u> of <u>other specified muscles and tendons</u> at <u>ankle and foot level</u>

CC-A **S96.821-** Laceration of other specified muscles and tendons at ankle and foot level, <u>right</u> foot

CC-A **S96.822-** Laceration of other specified muscles and tendons at ankle and foot level, <u>left</u> foot

CC-A **S96.829-** Laceration of other specified muscles and tendons at ankle and foot level, <u>unspecified</u> foot

S96.89- <u>Other specified injury</u> of <u>other specified muscles and tendons</u> at <u>ankle and foot level</u>

　　S96.891- Other specified injury of other specified muscles and tendons at ankle and foot level, <u>right</u> foot

　　S96.892- Other specified injury of other specified muscles and tendons at ankle and foot level, <u>left</u> foot

　　S96.899- Other specified injury of other specified muscles and tendons at ankle and foot level, <u>unspecified</u> foot

S96.9- <u>Injury</u> of <u>unspecified muscle and tendon</u> at <u>ankle and foot level</u>

S96.90- <u>Unspecified</u> injury of <u>unspecified muscle and tendon</u> at <u>ankle and foot level</u>

　　S96.901- Unspecified injury of unspecified muscle and tendon at ankle and foot level, <u>right</u> foot

　　S96.902- Unspecified injury of unspecified muscle and tendon at ankle and foot level, <u>left</u> foot

　　S96.909- Unspecified injury of unspecified muscle and tendon at ankle and foot level, <u>unspecified</u> foot

S96.91- <u>Strain</u> of <u>unspecified muscle and tendon</u> at <u>ankle and foot level</u>

　　S96.911- Strain of unspecified muscle and tendon at ankle and foot level, <u>right</u> foot

S96 – S96

S96.912- Strain of unspecified muscle and tendon at ankle and foot level, **left** foot

S96.919- Strain of unspecified muscle and tendon at ankle and foot level, **unspecified** foot

S96.92- **Laceration** of **unspecified muscle and tendon** at **ankle and foot level**

CC-A S96.921- Laceration of unspecified muscle and tendon at ankle and foot level, **right** foot

CC-A S96.922- Laceration of unspecified muscle and tendon at ankle and foot level, **left** foot

CC-A S96.929- Laceration of unspecified muscle and tendon at ankle and foot level, **unspecified** foot

S96.99- **Other specified injury** of **unspecified muscle and tendon** at **ankle and foot level**

S96.991- Other specified injury of unspecified muscle and tendon at ankle and foot level, **right** foot

S96.992- Other specified injury of unspecified muscle and tendon at ankle and foot level, **left** foot

S96.999- Other specified injury of unspecified muscle and tendon at ankle and foot level, **unspecified** foot

S97- **Crushing injury** of **ankle and foot**
Use additional code(s) for all associated injuries

The appropriate 7th character is to be added to each code from category S97:
A **Initial** encounter
D **Subsequent** encounter
S **Sequela**

S97.0- **Crushing** injury of **ankle**

S97.00x- Crushing injury of **unspecified** ankle

S97.01x- Crushing injury of **right** ankle

S97.02x- Crushing injury of **left** ankle

S97.1- **Crushing** injury of **toe**

S97.10- **Crushing** injury of **unspecified toe(s)**

S97.101- Crushing injury of unspecified **right** toe(s)

S97.102- Crushing injury of unspecified **left** toe(s)

S97.109- Crushing injury of unspecified toe(s)
Crushing injury of toe NOS

S97.11- **Crushing** injury of **great toe**

S97.111- Crushing injury of **right** great toe

S97.112- Crushing injury of **left** great toe

S97.119- Crushing injury of **unspecified** great toe

S97.12- **Crushing** injury of **lesser toe(s)**

S97.121- Crushing injury of **right** lesser toe(s)

S97.122- Crushing injury of **left** lesser toe(s)

S97.129- Crushing injury of **unspecified** lesser toe(s)

S97.8- **Crushing** injury of **foot**

S97.80x- Crushing injury of **unspecified** foot
Crushing injury of foot NOS

S97.81x- Crushing injury of **right** foot

S97.82x- Crushing injury of **left** foot

S98- **Traumatic amputation** of **ankle and foot**
Note: An amputation not identified as partial or complete should be coded to complete

The appropriate 7th character is to be added to each code from category S98:
A **Initial** encounter
D **Subsequent** encounter
S **Sequela**

S98.0- **Traumatic** **amputation** of **foot** at **ankle level**

S98.01- **Complete** traumatic amputation of foot at ankle level

CC-A S98.011- Complete traumatic amputation of **right** foot at ankle level

CC-A S98.012- Complete traumatic amputation of **left** foot at ankle level

CC-A S98.019- Complete traumatic amputation of **unspecified** foot at ankle level

S98.02- **Partial** traumatic amputation of foot at ankle level

CC-A S98.021- Partial traumatic amputation of **right** foot at ankle level

CC-A S98.022- Partial traumatic amputation of **left** foot at ankle level

CC-A S98.029- Partial traumatic amputation of **unspecified** foot at ankle level

S98.1- **Traumatic** **amputation** of **one toe**

S98.11- **Complete** traumatic amputation of **great** toe

S98.111- Complete traumatic amputation of **right** great toe

S98.112- Complete traumatic amputation of **left** great toe

S98.119- Complete traumatic amputation of **unspecified** great toe

S98.12- **Partial** traumatic amputation of **great** toe

S98.121- Partial traumatic amputation of **right** great toe

S98.122- Partial traumatic amputation of **left** great toe

S98.129- Partial traumatic amputation of **unspecified** great toe

S98.13- **Complete** traumatic amputation of **one lesser toe**
Traumatic amputation of toe NOS

S98.131- Complete traumatic amputation of one **right** lesser toe

S98.132- Complete traumatic amputation of one **left** lesser toe

S98.139- Complete traumatic amputation of one **unspecified** lesser toe

S98.14- **Partial** traumatic amputation of **one lesser toe**

S98.141- Partial traumatic amputation of one **right** lesser toe

S98.142- Partial traumatic amputation of one **left** lesser toe

S98.149- Partial traumatic amputation of one **unspecified** lesser toe

S98.2- **Traumatic** **amputation** of **two or more lesser toes**

S98.21- **Complete** traumatic amputation of two or more lesser toes

S98.211- Complete traumatic amputation of two or more **right** lesser toes

S98.212- Complete traumatic amputation of two or more **left** lesser toes

S98.219- Complete traumatic amputation of two or more **unspecified** lesser toes

S98.22- **Partial** traumatic amputation of two or more lesser toes

S98.221- Partial traumatic amputation of two or more **right** lesser toes

S98.222- Partial traumatic amputation of two or more **left** lesser toes

S98.229- Partial traumatic amputation of two or more **unspecified** lesser toes

S98.3- **Traumatic** **amputation** of **midfoot**

S98.31- **Complete** traumatic amputation of midfoot

CC-A S98.311- Complete traumatic amputation of **right** midfoot

CC-A S98.312- Complete traumatic amputation of **left** midfoot

CC-A S98.319- Complete traumatic amputation of **unspecified** midfoot

S98.32- **Partial** traumatic amputation of midfoot

CC-A S98.321- Partial traumatic amputation of **right** midfoot

CC-A S98.322- Partial traumatic amputation of **left** midfoot

CC-A S98.329- Partial traumatic amputation of **unspecified** midfoot

S98.9- **Traumatic** **amputation** of foot, **level unspecified**

S98.91- **Complete** traumatic amputation of foot, **level unspecified**

CC-A S98.911- Complete traumatic amputation of **right** foot, level unspecified

CC-A S98.912- Complete traumatic amputation of **left** foot, level unspecified

CC-A S98.919- Complete traumatic amputation of **unspecified** foot, level unspecified

S 9 6 - S 9 8

S98.92- **Partial** traumatic amputation of foot, **level unspecified**
CC-A S98.921- Partial traumatic amputation of **right** foot, level unspecified
CC-A S98.922- Partial traumatic amputation of **left** foot, level unspecified
CC-A S98.929- Partial traumatic amputation of **unspecified** foot, level unspecified

S99- **Other and unspecified injuries** of **ankle and foot**
  S99.0- **Physeal fracture** of **calcaneus**
  The appropriate 7th character is to be added to each code from subcategory S99.0:
  A **Initial** encounter for **closed** fracture
  B **Initial** encounter for **open** fracture
  D **Subsequent** encounter for fracture **with routine healing**
  G **Subsequent** encounter for fracture **with delayed healing**
  K **Subsequent** encounter for fracture **with nonunion**
  P **Subsequent** encounter for fracture **with malunion**
  S **Sequela**

    S99.00- **Unspecified** physeal fracture of calcaneus
      S99.001- Unspecified physeal fracture of **right** calcaneus
      S99.002- Unspecified physeal fracture of **left** calcaneus
      S99.009- Unspecified physeal fracture of **unspecified** calcaneus
    S99.01- **Salter-Harris Type I** physeal fracture of calcaneus
      S99.011- Salter-Harris **Type I** physeal fracture of **right** calcaneus
      S99.012- Salter-Harris **Type I** physeal fracture of **left** calcaneus
      S99.019- Salter-Harris **Type I** physeal fracture of **unspecified** calcaneus
    S99.02- **Salter-Harris Type II** physeal fracture of calcaneus
      S99.021- Salter-Harris **Type II** physeal fracture of **right** calcaneus
      S99.022- Salter-Harris **Type II** physeal fracture of **left** calcaneus
      S99.029- Salter-Harris **Type II** physeal fracture of **unspecified** calcaneus
    S99.03- **Salter-Harris Type III** physeal fracture of calcaneus
      S99.031- Salter-Harris **Type III** physeal fracture of **right** calcaneus
      S99.032- Salter-Harris **Type III** physeal fracture of **left** calcaneus
      S99.039- Salter-Harris **Type III** physeal fracture of **unspecified** calcaneus
    S99.04- **Salter-Harris Type IV** physeal fracture of calcaneus
      S99.041- Salter-Harris **Type IV** physeal fracture of **right** calcaneus
      S99.042- Salter-Harris **Type IV** physeal fracture of **left** calcaneus
      S99.049- Salter-Harris **Type IV** physeal fracture of **unspecified** calcaneus
    S99.09- **Other** physeal fracture of calcaneus
      S99.091- Other physeal fracture of **right** calcaneus
      S99.092- Other physeal fracture of **left** calcaneus
      S99.099- Other physeal fracture of **unspecified** calcaneus

  S99.1- **Physeal fracture** of **metatarsal**
  The appropriate 7th character is to be added to each code from subcategory S99.1:
  A **Initial** encounter for **closed** fracture
  B **Initial** encounter for **open** fracture
  D **Subsequent** encounter for fracture **with routine healing**
  G **Subsequent** encounter for fracture **with delayed healing**
  K **Subsequent** encounter for fracture **with nonunion**
  P **Subsequent** encounter for fracture **with malunion**
  S **Sequela**

    S99.10- **Unspecified** physeal fracture of metatarsal
      S99.101- Unspecified physeal fracture of **right** metatarsal
      S99.102- Unspecified physeal fracture of **left** metatarsal
      S99.109- Unspecified physeal fracture of **unspecified** metatarsal
    S99.11- **Salter-Harris Type I** physeal fracture of metatarsal
      S99.111- Salter-Harris **Type I** physeal fracture of **right** metatarsal
      S99.112- Salter-Harris **Type I** physeal fracture of **left** metatarsal
      S99.119- Salter-Harris **Type I** physeal fracture of **unspecified** metatarsal
    S99.12- **Salter-Harris Type II** physeal fracture of metatarsal
      S99.121- Salter-Harris **Type II** physeal fracture of **right** metatarsal
      S99.122- Salter-Harris **Type II** physeal fracture of **left** metatarsal
      S99.129- Salter-Harris **Type II** physeal fracture of **unspecified** metatarsal
    S99.13- **Salter-Harris Type III** physeal fracture of metatarsal
      S99.131- Salter-Harris **Type III** physeal fracture of **right** metatarsal
      S99.132- Salter-Harris **Type III** physeal fracture of **left** metatarsal
      S99.139- Salter-Harris **Type III** physeal fracture of **unspecified** metatarsal
    S99.14- **Salter-Harris Type IV** physeal fracture of metatarsal
      S99.141- Salter-Harris **Type IV** physeal fracture of **right** metatarsal
      S99.142- Salter-Harris **Type IV** physeal fracture of **left** metatarsal
      S99.149- Salter-Harris **Type IV** physeal fracture of **unspecified** metatarsal
    S99.19- **Other** physeal fracture of metatarsal
      S99.191- Other physeal fracture of **right** metatarsal
      S99.192- Other physeal fracture of **left** metatarsal
      S99.199- Other physeal fracture of **unspecified** metatarsal

  S99.2- **Physeal fracture** of **phalanx of toe**
  The appropriate 7th character is to be added to each code from subcategory S99.2:
  A **Initial** encounter for **closed** fracture
  B **Initial** encounter for **open** fracture
  D **Subsequent** encounter for fracture **with routine healing**
  G **Subsequent** encounter for fracture **with delayed healing**
  K **Subsequent** encounter for fracture **with nonunion**
  P **Subsequent** encounter for fracture **with malunion**
  S **Sequela**

    S99.20- **Unspecified** physeal fracture of phalanx of toe
      S99.201- Unspecified physeal fracture of phalanx of **right** toe
      S99.202- Unspecified physeal fracture of phalanx of **left** toe
      S99.209- Unspecified physeal fracture of phalanx of **unspecified** toe
    S99.21- **Salter-Harris Type I** physeal fracture of phalanx of toe
      S99.211- Salter-Harris **Type I** physeal fracture of phalanx of **right** toe
      S99.212- Salter-Harris **Type I** physeal fracture of phalanx of **left** toe

S98
–
S99

S99.219- Salter-Harris <u>Type I</u> physeal fracture of phalanx of <u>unspecified</u> toe
S99.22- <u>Salter-Harris Type II physeal fracture of phalanx of toe</u>
    S99.221- Salter-Harris <u>Type II</u> physeal fracture of phalanx of <u>right</u> toe
    S99.222- Salter-Harris <u>Type II</u> physeal fracture of phalanx of <u>left</u> toe
    S99.229- Salter-Harris <u>Type II</u> physeal fracture of phalanx of <u>unspecified</u> toe
S99.23- <u>Salter-Harris Type III physeal fracture of phalanx of toe</u>
    S99.231- Salter-Harris <u>Type III</u> physeal fracture of phalanx of <u>right</u> toe
    S99.232- Salter-Harris <u>Type III</u> physeal fracture of phalanx of <u>left</u> toe
    S99.239- Salter-Harris <u>Type III</u> physeal fracture of phalanx of <u>unspecified</u> toe
S99.24- <u>Salter-Harris Type IV physeal fracture of phalanx of toe</u>
    S99.241- Salter-Harris <u>Type IV</u> physeal fracture of phalanx of <u>right</u> toe
    S99.242- Salter-Harris <u>Type IV</u> physeal fracture of phalanx of <u>left</u> toe
    S99.249- Salter-Harris <u>Type IV</u> physeal fracture of phalanx of <u>unspecified</u> toe
S99.29- <u>Other</u> physeal fracture of phalanx of toe
    S99.291- Other physeal fracture of phalanx of <u>right</u> toe
    S99.292- Other physeal fracture of phalanx of <u>left</u> toe
    S99.299- Other physeal fracture of phalanx of <u>unspecified</u> toe
S99.8- <u>Other specified injuries</u> of ankle and foot

The appropriate 7th character is to be added to each code from subcategory S99.8:
A <u>Initial</u> encounter
D <u>Subsequent</u> encounter
S <u>Sequela</u>

  S99.81- <u>Other specified injuries</u> of <u>ankle</u>
    S99.811- Other specified injuries of <u>right</u> ankle
    S99.812- Other specified injuries of <u>left</u> ankle
    S99.819- Other specified injuries of <u>unspecified</u> ankle
  S99.82- <u>Other specified injuries</u> of <u>foot</u>
    S99.821- Other specified injuries of <u>right</u> foot
    S99.822- Other specified injuries of <u>left</u> foot
    S99.829- Other specified injuries of <u>unspecified</u> foot
S99.9- <u>Unspecified injury</u> of ankle and foot

The appropriate 7th character is to be added to each code from subcategory S99.9:
A <u>Initial</u> encounter
D <u>Subsequent</u> encounter
S <u>Sequela</u>

  S99.91- <u>Unspecified</u> injury of <u>ankle</u>
    S99.911- Unspecified injury of <u>right</u> ankle
    S99.912- Unspecified injury of <u>left</u> ankle
    S99.919- Unspecified injury of <u>unspecified</u> ankle
  S99.92- <u>Unspecified</u> injury of <u>foot</u>
    S99.921- Unspecified injury of <u>right</u> foot
    S99.922- Unspecified injury of <u>left</u> foot
    S99.929- Unspecified injury of <u>unspecified</u> foot

S99

S99 - S99

Injury, poisoning and certain other consequences of external causes (T07-T88)

Injuries involving multiple body regions (T07)

> **Excludes 1:** burns and corrosions (T20-T32)
> frostbite (T33-T34)
> insect bite or sting, venomous (T63.4)
> sunburn (L55-)

T07   Unspecified multiple injuries
> **Excludes 1:** injury NOS (T14-)

Injury of unspecified body region (T14)

T14-   Injury of unspecified body region
> **Excludes 1:** multiple unspecified injuries (T07)

T14.8   Other injury of unspecified body region
Abrasion NOS
Contusion NOS
Crush injury NOS
Fracture NOS
Skin injury NOS
Vascular injury NOS

T14.9-   Unspecified injury

T14.90   Injury, unspecified
Injury NOS

T14.91   Suicide attempt
Attempted suicide NOS

Effects of foreign body entering through natural orifice (T15-T19)

> **Excludes ❷:** foreign body accidentally left in operation wound (T81.5-)
> foreign body in penetrating wound — see open wound by body region
> residual foreign body in soft tissue (M79.5)
> splinter, without open wound — see superficial injury by body region

T15-   Foreign body on external eye
> **Excludes ❷:** foreign body in penetrating wound of orbit and eye ball (S05.4-, S05.5-)
> open wound of eyelid and periocular area (S01.1-)
> retained foreign body in eyelid (H02.8-)
> retained (old) foreign body in penetrating wound of orbit and eye ball (H05.5-, H44.6-, H44.7-)
> superficial foreign body of eyelid and periocular area (S00.25-)

The appropriate 7th character is to be added to each code from category T15:
A   Initial encounter
D   Subsequent encounter
S   Sequela

T15.0-   Foreign body in cornea
T15.00x-   Foreign body in cornea, unspecified eye
T15.01x-   Foreign body in cornea, right eye
T15.02x-   Foreign body in cornea, left eye

T15.1-   Foreign body in conjunctival sac
T15.10x-   Foreign body in conjunctival sac, unspecified eye
T15.11x-   Foreign body in conjunctival sac, right eye
T15.12x-   Foreign body in conjunctival sac, left eye

T15.8-   Foreign body in other and multiple parts of external eye
Foreign body in lacrimal punctum
T15.80x-   Foreign body in other and multiple parts of external eye, unspecified eye
T15.81x-   Foreign body in other and multiple parts of external eye, right eye
T15.82x-   Foreign body in other and multiple parts of external eye, left eye

T15.9-   Foreign body on external eye, part unspecified
T15.90x-   Foreign body on external eye, part unspecified, unspecified eye
T15.91x-   Foreign body on external eye, part unspecified, right eye
T15.92x-   Foreign body on external eye, part unspecified, left eye

T16-   Foreign body in ear
Includes: Foreign body in auditory canal
The appropriate 7th character is to be added to each code from category T16:
A   Initial encounter
D   Subsequent encounter
S   Sequela

T16.1xx-   Foreign body in right ear
T16.2xx-   Foreign body in left ear
T16.9xx-   Foreign body in ear, unspecified ear

T17-   Foreign body in respiratory tract
The appropriate 7th character is to be added to each code from category T17:
A   Initial encounter
D   Subsequent encounter
S   Sequela

T17.0xx-   Foreign body in nasal sinus
T17.1xx-   Foreign body in nostril
Foreign body in nose NOS

T17.2-   Foreign body in pharynx
Foreign body in nasopharynx
Foreign body in throat NOS
T17.20-   Unspecified foreign body in pharynx
T17.200-   Unspecified foreign body in pharynx causing asphyxiation
T17.208-   Unspecified foreign body in pharynx causing other injury
T17.21-   Gastric contents in pharynx
Aspiration of gastric contents into pharynx
Vomitus in pharynx
T17.210-   Gastric contents in pharynx causing asphyxiation
T17.218-   Gastric contents in pharynx causing other injury
T17.22-   Food in pharynx
Bones in pharynx
Seeds in pharynx
T17.220-   Food in pharynx causing asphyxiation
T17.228-   Food in pharynx causing other injury
T17.29-   Other foreign object in pharynx
T17.290-   Other foreign object in pharynx causing asphyxiation
T17.298-   Other foreign object in pharynx causing other injury

T17.3-   Foreign body in larynx
T17.30-   Unspecified foreign body in larynx
T17.300-   Unspecified foreign body in larynx causing asphyxiation
T17.308-   Unspecified foreign body in larynx causing other injury
T17.31-   Gastric contents in larynx
Aspiration of gastric contents into larynx
Vomitus in larynx
T17.310-   Gastric contents in larynx causing asphyxiation
T17.318-   Gastric contents in larynx causing other injury
T17.32-   Food in larynx
Bones in larynx
Seeds in larynx
T17.320-   Food in larynx causing asphyxiation
T17.328-   Food in larynx causing other injury
T17.39-   Other foreign object in larynx
T17.390-   Other foreign object in larynx causing asphyxiation
T17.398-   Other foreign object in larynx causing other injury

T07 - T17

T17.4-   Foreign body in <u>trachea</u>
   T17.40- <u>Unspecified</u> foreign body in trachea
   CC-A **T17.400-**   Unspecified foreign body in trachea <u>causing asphyxiation</u>
   CC-A **T17.408-**   Unspecified foreign body in trachea <u>causing other injury</u>
   T17.41- Gastric contents in <u>trachea</u>
      Aspiration of gastric contents into trachea
      Vomitus in trachea
   CC-A **T17.410-**   Gastric contents in trachea <u>causing asphyxiation</u>
   CC-A **T17.418-**   Gastric contents in trachea <u>causing other injury</u>
   T17.42- Food in <u>trachea</u>
      Bones in trachea
      Seeds in trachea
   CC-A **T17.420-**   Food in trachea <u>causing asphyxiation</u>
   CC-A **T17.428-**   Food in trachea <u>causing other injury</u>
   T17.49- <u>Other foreign object</u> in <u>trachea</u>
   CC-A **T17.490-**   Other foreign object in trachea <u>causing asphyxiation</u>
   CC-A **T17.498-**   Other foreign object in trachea <u>causing other injury</u>
T17.5-   Foreign body in <u>bronchus</u>
   T17.50- <u>Unspecified</u> foreign body in <u>bronchus</u>
   CC-A **T17.500-**   Unspecified foreign body in bronchus <u>causing asphyxiation</u>
   CC-A **T17.508-**   Unspecified foreign body in bronchus <u>causing other injury</u>
   T17.51- <u>Gastric contents</u> in <u>bronchus</u>
      Aspiration of gastric contents into bronchus
      Vomitus in bronchus
   CC-A **T17.510-**   Gastric contents in bronchus <u>causing asphyxiation</u>
   CC-A **T17.518-**   Gastric contents in bronchus <u>causing other injury</u>
   T17.52- <u>Food</u> in <u>bronchus</u>
      Bones in bronchus
      Seeds in bronchus
   CC-A **T17.520-**   Food in bronchus <u>causing asphyxiation</u>
   CC-A **T17.528-**   Food in bronchus <u>causing other injury</u>
   T17.59- <u>Other foreign object</u> in <u>bronchus</u>
   CC-A **T17.590-**   Other foreign object in bronchus <u>causing asphyxiation</u>
   CC-A **T17.598-**   Other foreign object in bronchus <u>causing other injury</u>
T17.8-   Foreign body <u>in other parts of respiratory tract</u>
      Foreign body in bronchioles
      Foreign body in lung
   T17.80- <u>Unspecified</u> foreign body <u>in other parts of respiratory tract</u>
   CC-A **T17.800-**   Unspecified foreign body in other parts of respiratory tract <u>causing asphyxiation</u>
   CC-A **T17.808-**   Unspecified foreign body in other parts of respiratory tract <u>causing other injury</u>
   T17.81- <u>Gastric contents</u> in other parts of respiratory tract
      Aspiration of gastric contents into other parts of respiratory tract
      Vomitus in other parts of respiratory tract
   CC-A **T17.810-**   Gastric contents in other parts of respiratory tract <u>causing asphyxiation</u>
   CC-A **T17.818-**   Gastric contents in other parts of respiratory tract <u>causing other injury</u>
   T17.82- <u>Food</u> in other parts of respiratory tract
      Bones in other parts of respiratory tract
      Seeds in other parts of respiratory tract
   CC-A **T17.820-**   Food in other parts of respiratory tract <u>causing asphyxiation</u>
   CC-A **T17.828-**   Food in other parts of respiratory tract <u>causing other injury</u>
   T17.89- <u>Other foreign object</u> <u>in other parts of respiratory tract</u>
   CC-A **T17.890-**   Other foreign object in other parts of respiratory tract <u>causing asphyxiation</u>
   CC-A **T17.898-**   Other foreign object in other parts of respiratory tract <u>causing other injury</u>

T17.9-   Foreign body <u>in respiratory tract</u>, <u>part unspecified</u>
   T17.90- <u>Unspecified</u> foreign body in respiratory tract, part unspecified
      T17.900-   Unspecified foreign body in respiratory tract, part unspecified <u>causing asphyxiation</u>
      T17.908-   Unspecified foreign body in respiratory tract, part unspecified <u>causing other injury</u>
   T17.91- <u>Gastric contents in respiratory tract</u>, <u>part unspecified</u>
      Aspiration of gastric contents into respiratory tract, part unspecified
      Vomitus in trachea respiratory tract, part unspecified
      T17.910-   Gastric contents in respiratory tract, part unspecified <u>causing asphyxiation</u>
      T17.918-   Gastric contents in respiratory tract, part unspecified <u>causing other injury</u>
   T17.92- <u>Food</u> <u>in respiratory tract</u>, <u>part unspecified</u>
      Bones in respiratory tract, part unspecified
      Seeds in respiratory tract, part unspecified
      T17.920-   Food in respiratory tract, part unspecified <u>causing asphyxiation</u>
      T17.928-   Food in respiratory tract, part unspecified <u>causing other injury</u>
   T17.99- <u>Other foreign object</u> <u>in respiratory tract</u>, <u>part unspecified</u>
      T17.990-   Other foreign object in respiratory tract, part unspecified in <u>causing asphyxiation</u>
      T17.998-   Other foreign object in respiratory tract, part unspecified <u>causing other injury</u>

T18-   <u>Foreign body in alimentary tract</u>
   Excludes ➋: foreign body in pharynx (T17.2-)
   The appropriate 7th character is to be added to each code from category T18:
   A   <u>Initial</u> encounter
   D   <u>Subsequent</u> encounter
   S   <u>Sequela</u>
   T18.0xx-   Foreign body in <u>mouth</u>
   T18.1-   Foreign body in <u>esophagus</u>
      Excludes ➋: foreign body in respiratory tract (T17.-)
      T18.10- <u>Unspecified</u> foreign body in <u>esophagus</u>
         T18.100-   Unspecified foreign body in esophagus <u>causing compression of trachea</u>
            Unspecified foreign body in esophagus causing obstruction of respiration
         T18.108-   Unspecified foreign body in esophagus <u>causing other injury</u>
      T18.11- <u>Gastric contents</u> in <u>esophagus</u>
         Vomitus in esophagus
         T18.110-   Gastric contents in esophagus <u>causing compression of trachea</u>
            Gastric contents in esophagus causing obstruction of respiration
         T18.118-   Gastric contents in esophagus <u>causing other injury</u>
      T18.12- <u>Food</u> in <u>esophagus</u>
         Bones in esophagus
         Seeds in esophagus
         T18.120-   Food in esophagus <u>causing compression of trachea</u>
            Food in esophagus causing obstruction of respiration
         T18.128-   Food in esophagus <u>causing other injury</u>
      T18.19- <u>Other foreign object</u> in <u>esophagus</u>
         T18.190-   Other foreign object in esophagus <u>causing compression of trachea</u>
            Other foreign body in esophagus causing obstruction of respiration
         T18.198-   Other foreign object in esophagus <u>causing other injury</u>
   T18.2xx-   Foreign body in stomach
   T18.3xx-   Foreign body in small intestine
   T18.4xx-   Foreign body in colon
   T18.5xx-   Foreign body in anus and rectum
      Foreign body in rectosigmoid (junction)
   T18.8xx-   Foreign body in other parts of alimentary tract

T17-T18 (side tab)

T18.9xx-   Foreign body of alimentary tract, part unspecified
    Foreign body in digestive system NOS
    Swallowed foreign body NOS

T19-   **Foreign body in genitourinary tract**
Excludes ❷: *complications due to implanted mesh (T83.7-)*
    mechanical complications of contraceptive device (intrauterine) (vaginal) (T83.3-)
    presence of contraceptive device (intrauterine) (vaginal) (Z97.5)

The appropriate 7th character is to be added to each code from category T19:
A   Initial encounter
D   Subsequent encounter
S   Sequela

T19.0xx-   Foreign body in urethra
T19.1xx-   Foreign body in bladder
T19.2xx-   Foreign body in vulva and vagina —[♀]
T19.3xx-   Foreign body in uterus —[♀]
T19.4xx-   Foreign body in penis —[♂]
T19.8xx-   Foreign body in other parts of genitourinary tract
T19.9xx-   Foreign body in genitourinary tract, part unspecified

Burns and corrosions (T20-T32)

Includes: Burns (thermal) from electrical heating appliances
    Burns (thermal) from electricity
    Burns (thermal) from flame
    Burns (thermal) from friction
    Burns (thermal) from hot air and hot gases
    Burns (thermal) from hot objects
    Burns (thermal) from lightning
    Burns (thermal) from radiation
    Chemical burn [corrosion] (external) (internal)
    Scalds
Excludes ❷: *erythema [dermatitis] ab igne (L59.0)*
    radiation-related disorders of the skin and subcutaneous tissue (L55-L59)
    sunburn (L55.-)

Burns and corrosions of external body surface, specified by site (T20-T25)

Includes: Burns and corrosions of first degree [erythema]
    Burns and corrosions of second degree [blisters][epidermal loss]
    Burns and corrosions of third degree [deep necrosis of underlying tissue] [full- thickness skin loss]
Use additional code from category T31 or T32 to identify extent of body surface involved

T20-   **Burn and corrosion of head, face, and neck**
Excludes ❷: *burn and corrosion of ear drum (T28.41, T28.91)*
    burn and corrosion of eye and adnexa (T26.-)
    burn and corrosion of mouth and pharynx (T28.0)

The appropriate 7th character is to be added to each code from category T20:
A   Initial encounter
D   Subsequent encounter
S   Sequela

T20.0-   Burn of unspecified degree of head, face, and neck
    Use additional external cause code to identify the source, place and intent of the burn (X00-X19, X75-X77, X96-X98, Y92)

    T20.00x-   Burn of unspecified degree of head, face, and neck, unspecified site

    T20.01-   Burn of unspecified degree of ear [any part, except ear drum]
        Excludes ❷: *burn of ear drum (T28.41-)*

        T20.011-   Burn of unspecified degree of right ear [any part, except ear drum]

        T20.012-   Burn of unspecified degree of left ear [any part, except ear drum]

        T20.019-   Burn of unspecified degree of unspecified ear [any part, except ear drum]

    T20.02x-   Burn of unspecified degree of lip(s)
    T20.03x-   Burn of unspecified degree of chin
    T20.04x-   Burn of unspecified degree of nose (septum)
    T20.05x-   Burn of unspecified degree of scalp [any part]

T20.06x-   Burn of unspecified degree of forehead and cheek
T20.07x-   Burn of unspecified degree of neck
T20.09x-   Burn of unspecified degree of multiple sites of head, face, and neck

T20.1-   Burn of first degree of head, face, and neck
    Use additional external cause code to identify the source, place and intent of the burn (X00-X19, X75-X77, X96-X98, Y92)

    T20.10x-   Burn of first degree of head, face, and neck, unspecified site

    T20.11-   Burn of first degree of ear [any part, except ear drum]
        Excludes ❷: *burn of ear drum (T28.41-)*

        T20.111-   Burn of first degree of right ear [any part, except ear drum]

        T20.112-   Burn of first degree of left ear [any part, except ear drum]

        T20.119-   Burn of first degree of unspecified ear [any part, except ear drum]

    T20.12x-   Burn of first degree of lip(s)
    T20.13x-   Burn of first degree of chin
    T20.14x-   Burn of first degree of nose (septum)
    T20.15x-   Burn of first degree of scalp [any part]
    T20.16x-   Burn of first degree of forehead and cheek
    T20.17x-   Burn of first degree of neck
    T20.19x-   Burn of first degree of multiple sites of head, face, and neck

T20.2-   Burn of second degree of head, face, and neck
    Use additional external cause code to identify the source, place and intent of the burn (X00-X19, X75-X77, X96-X98, Y92)

    T20.20x-   Burn of second degree of head, face, and neck, unspecified site

    T20.21-   Burn of second degree of ear [any part, except ear drum]
        Excludes ❷: *burn of ear drum (T28.41-)*

        T20.211-   Burn of second degree of right ear [any part, except ear drum]

        T20.212-   Burn of second degree of left ear [any part, except ear drum]

        T20.219-   Burn of second degree of unspecified ear [any part, except ear drum]

    T20.22x-   Burn of second degree of lip(s)
    T20.23x-   Burn of second degree of chin
    T20.24x-   Burn of second degree of nose (septum)
    T20.25x-   Burn of second degree of scalp [any part]
    T20.26x-   Burn of second degree of forehead and cheek
    T20.27x-   Burn of second degree of neck
    T20.29x-   Burn of second degree of multiple sites of head, face, and neck

T20.3-   Burn of third degree of head, face, and neck
    Use additional external cause code to identify the source, place and intent of the burn (X00-X19, X75-X77, X96-X98, Y92)

CC-A T20.30x-   Burn of third degree of head, face, and neck, unspecified site

    T20.31-   Burn of third degree of ear [any part, except ear drum]
        AHA 15:1Q:p18 – Status post third degree burn of left external ear
        Excludes ❷: *burn of ear drum (T28.41-)*

CC-A   T20.311-   Burn of third degree of right ear [any part, except ear drum]

CC-A   T20.312-   Burn of third degree of left ear [any part, except ear drum]

CC-A   T20.319-   Burn of third degree of unspecified ear [any part, except ear drum]

CC-A T20.32x-   Burn of third degree of lip(s)
CC-A T20.33x-   Burn of third degree of chin
CC-A T20.34x-   Burn of third degree of nose (septum)
CC-A T20.35x-   Burn of third degree of scalp [any part]
CC-A T20.36x-   Burn of third degree of forehead and cheek
CC-A T20.37x-   Burn of third degree of neck

T18 - T20

CC-A **T20.39x-**   Burn of <u>third</u> degree of multiple sites of head, face, and neck

T20.4-   <u>Corrosion</u> of <u>unspecified degree</u> of <u>head, face, and neck</u>
Code first (T51-T65) to identify chemical and intent
Use additional external cause code to identify place (Y92)

   T20.40x-   <u>Corrosion</u> of <u>unspecified degree</u> of <u>head, face, and neck, unspecified</u> site

   T20.41-   <u>Corrosion</u> of <u>unspecified degree</u> of <u>ear</u> [any part, except ear drum]
Excludes ❷: corrosion of ear drum (T28.91-)

     T20.411-   Corrosion of unspecified degree of <u>right</u> ear [any part, except ear drum]

     T20.412-   Corrosion of unspecified degree of <u>left</u> ear [any part, except ear drum]

     T20.419-   Corrosion of unspecified degree of <u>unspecified</u> ear [any part, except ear drum]

   T20.42x-   <u>Corrosion</u> of <u>unspecified degree</u> of lip(s)

   T20.43x-   <u>Corrosion</u> of <u>unspecified degree</u> of chin

   T20.44x-   <u>Corrosion</u> of <u>unspecified degree</u> of nose (septum)

   T20.45x-   <u>Corrosion</u> of <u>unspecified degree</u> of scalp [any part]

   T20.46x-   <u>Corrosion</u> of <u>unspecified degree</u> of forehead and cheek

   T20.47x-   <u>Corrosion</u> of <u>unspecified degree</u> of neck

   T20.49x-   <u>Corrosion</u> of <u>unspecified degree</u> of multiple sites of head, face, and neck

T20.5-   <u>Corrosion</u> of <u>first</u> degree of <u>head, face, and neck</u>
Code first (T51-T65) to identify chemical and intent
Use additional external cause code to identify place (Y92)

   T20.50x-   <u>Corrosion</u> of <u>first</u> degree of <u>head, face, and neck, unspecified</u> site

   T20.51-   <u>Corrosion</u> of <u>first</u> degree of <u>ear</u> [any part, except ear drum]
Excludes ❷: corrosion of ear drum (T28.91-)

     T20.511-   Corrosion of first degree of <u>right</u> ear [any part, except ear drum]

     T20.512-   Corrosion of first degree of <u>left</u> ear [any part, except ear drum]

     T20.519-   Corrosion of first degree of <u>unspecified</u> ear [any part, except ear drum]

   T20.52x-   <u>Corrosion</u> of <u>first</u> degree of lip(s)

   T20.53x-   <u>Corrosion</u> of <u>first</u> degree of chin

   T20.54x-   <u>Corrosion</u> of <u>first</u> degree of nose (septum)

   T20.55x-   <u>Corrosion</u> of <u>first</u> degree of scalp [any part]

   T20.56x-   <u>Corrosion</u> of <u>first</u> degree of forehead and cheek

   T20.57x-   <u>Corrosion</u> of <u>first</u> degree of neck

   T20.59x-   <u>Corrosion</u> of <u>first</u> degree of multiple sites of head, face, and neck

T20.6-   <u>Corrosion</u> of <u>second</u> degree of <u>head, face, and neck</u>
Code first (T51-T65) to identify chemical and intent
Use additional external cause code to identify place (Y92)

   T20.60x-   <u>Corrosion</u> of <u>second</u> degree of <u>head, face, and neck, unspecified</u> site

   T20.61-   <u>Corrosion</u> of <u>second</u> degree of <u>ear</u> [any part, except ear drum]
Excludes ❷: corrosion of ear drum (T28.91-)

     T20.611-   Corrosion of second degree of <u>right</u> ear [any part, except ear drum]

     T20.612-   Corrosion of second degree of <u>left</u> ear [any part, except ear drum]

     T20.619-   Corrosion of second degree of <u>unspecified</u> ear [any part, except ear drum]

   T20.62x-   <u>Corrosion</u> of <u>second</u> degree of lip(s)

   T20.63x-   <u>Corrosion</u> of <u>second</u> degree of chin

   T20.64x-   <u>Corrosion</u> of <u>second</u> degree of nose (septum)

   T20.65x-   <u>Corrosion</u> of <u>second</u> degree of scalp [any part]

   T20.66x-   <u>Corrosion</u> of <u>second</u> degree of forehead and cheek

   T20.67x-   <u>Corrosion</u> of <u>second</u> degree of neck

   T20.69x-   <u>Corrosion</u> of <u>second</u> degree of multiple sites of head, face, and neck

---

T20.7-   <u>Corrosion</u> of <u>third</u> degree of <u>head, face, and neck</u>
Code first (T51-T65) to identify chemical and intent
Use additional external cause code to identify place (Y92)

CC-A **T20.70x-**   <u>Corrosion</u> of <u>third</u> degree of <u>head, face, and neck, unspecified</u> site

   T20.71-   <u>Corrosion</u> of <u>third</u> degree of <u>ear</u> [any part, except ear drum]
Excludes ❷: corrosion of ear drum (T28.91-)

CC-A **T20.711-**   Corrosion of third degree of <u>right</u> ear [any part, except ear drum]

CC-A **T20.712-**   Corrosion of third degree of <u>left</u> ear [any part, except ear drum]

CC-A **T20.719-**   Corrosion of third degree of <u>unspecified</u> ear [any part, except ear drum]

CC-A **T20.72x-**   <u>Corrosion</u> of <u>third</u> degree of lip(s)

CC-A **T20.73x-**   <u>Corrosion</u> of <u>third</u> degree of chin

CC-A **T20.74x-**   <u>Corrosion</u> of <u>third</u> degree of nose (septum)

CC-A **T20.75x-**   <u>Corrosion</u> of <u>third</u> degree of scalp [any part]

CC-A **T20.76x-**   <u>Corrosion</u> of <u>third</u> degree of forehead and cheek

CC-A **T20.77x-**   <u>Corrosion</u> of <u>third</u> degree of neck

CC-A **T20.79x-**   <u>Corrosion</u> of <u>third</u> degree of multiple sites of head, face, and neck

T21-   <u>Burn and corrosion</u> of <u>trunk</u>
Includes: Burns and corrosion of hip region
Excludes ❷: burns and corrosion of axilla (T22.- with fifth character 4)
burns and corrosion of scapular region (T22.- with fifth character 6)
burns and corrosion of shoulder (T22. with fifth character 5)

The appropriate 7th character is to be added to each code from category T21:
A   <u>Initial</u> encounter
D   <u>Subsequent</u> encounter
S   <u>Sequela</u>

T21.0-   Burn of <u>unspecified degree</u> of <u>trunk</u>
Use additional external cause code to identify the source, place and intent of the burn (X00-X19, X75-X77, X96-X98, Y92)

   T21.00x-   Burn of <u>unspecified degree</u> of trunk, <u>unspecified</u> site

   T21.01x-   Burn of <u>unspecified degree</u> of <u>chest wall</u>
Burn of of unspecified degree of breast

   T21.02x-   Burn of <u>unspecified degree</u> of <u>abdominal wall</u>
Burn of unspecified degree of flank
Burn of unspecified degree of groin

   T21.03x-   Burn of <u>unspecified degree</u> of <u>upper back</u>
Burn of unspecified degree of interscapular region

   T21.04x-   Burn of <u>unspecified degree</u> of <u>lower back</u>

   T21.05x-   Burn of <u>unspecified degree</u> of <u>buttock</u>
Burn of unspecified degree of anus

   T21.06x-   Burn of <u>unspecified degree</u> of <u>male genital region</u> — [♂]
Burn of unspecified degree of penis
Burn of unspecified degree of scrotum
Burn of unspecified degree of testis

   T21.07x-   Burn of <u>unspecified degree</u> of <u>female genital region</u> — [♀]
Burn of unspecified degree of labium (majus) (minus)
Burn of unspecified degree of perineum
Burn of unspecified degree of vulva
Excludes ❷: burn of vagina (T28.3)

   T21.09x-   Burn of <u>unspecified degree</u> of <u>other</u> site of trunk

T21.1-   Burn of <u>first</u> degree of <u>trunk</u>
Use additional external cause code to identify the source, place and intent of the burn (X00-X19, X75-X77, X96-X98, Y92)

   T21.10x-   Burn of <u>first</u> degree of trunk, <u>unspecified</u> site

   T21.11x-   Burn of <u>first</u> degree of <u>chest wall</u>
Burn of first degree of breast

   T21.12x-   Burn of <u>first</u> degree of <u>abdominal wall</u>
Burn of first degree of flank
Burn of first degree of groin

   T21.13x-   Burn of <u>first</u> degree of <u>upper back</u>
Burn of first degree of interscapular region

   T21.14x-   Burn of <u>first</u> degree of <u>lower back</u>

T21.15x- Burn of <u>first</u> degree of <u>buttock</u>
Burn of first degree of anus

T21.16x- Burn of <u>first</u> degree of <u>male genital region</u> — [♂]
Burn of first degree of penis
Burn of first degree of scrotum
Burn of first degree of testis

T21.17x- Burn of <u>first</u> degree of <u>female genital region</u> — [♀]
Burn of first degree of labium (majus) (minus)
Burn of first degree of perineum
Burn of first degree of vulva

Excludes ❷: burn of vagina (T28.3)

T21.19x- Burn of <u>first</u> degree of <u>other</u> site of trunk

T21.2- Burn of <u>second</u> degree of <u>trunk</u>
Use additional external cause code to identify the source, place and intent of the burn (X00-X19, X75-X77, X96-X98, Y92)

T21.20x- Burn of <u>second</u> degree of trunk, <u>unspecified</u> site

T21.21x- Burn of <u>second</u> degree of <u>chest wall</u>
Burn of second degree of breast

T21.22x- Burn of <u>second</u> degree of <u>abdominal wall</u>
Burn of second degree of flank
Burn of second degree of groin

T21.23x- Burn of <u>second</u> degree of <u>upper back</u>
Burn of second degree of interscapular region

T21.24x- Burn of <u>second</u> degree of <u>lower back</u>

T21.25x- Burn of <u>second</u> degree of <u>buttock</u>
Burn of second degree of anus

T21.26x- Burn of <u>second</u> degree of <u>male genital region</u> — [♂]
Burn of second degree of penis
Burn of second degree of scrotum
Burn of second degree of testis

T21.27x- Burn of <u>second</u> degree of <u>female genital region</u> — [♀]
Burn of second degree of labium (majus) (minus)
Burn of second degree of perineum
Burn of second degree of vulva

Excludes ❷: burn of vagina (T28.3)

T21.29x- Burn of <u>second</u> degree of <u>other</u> site of trunk

T21.3- Burn of <u>third</u> degree of <u>trunk</u>
Use additional external cause code to identify the source, place and intent of the burn (X00-X19, X75-X77, X96-X98, Y92)

CC-A **T21.30x-** Burn of <u>third</u> degree of trunk, <u>unspecified</u> site

CC-A **T21.31x-** Burn of <u>third</u> degree of <u>chest wall</u>
Burn of third degree of breast

CC-A **T21.32x-** Burn of <u>third</u> degree of <u>abdominal wall</u>
Burn of third degree of flank
Burn of third degree of groin

CC-A **T21.33x-** Burn of <u>third</u> degree of <u>upper back</u>
Burn of third degree of interscapular region

CC-A **T21.34x-** Burn of <u>third</u> degree of <u>lower back</u>

CC-A **T21.35x-** Burn of <u>third</u> degree of <u>buttock</u>
Burn of third degree of anus

CC-A **T21.36x-** Burn of <u>third</u> degree of <u>male genital region</u> — [♂]
Burn of third degree of penis
Burn of third degree of scrotum
Burn of third degree of testis

CC-A **T21.37x-** Burn of <u>third</u> degree of <u>female genital region</u> — [♀]
Burn of third degree of labium (majus) (minus)
Burn of third degree of perineum
Burn of third degree of vulva

Excludes ❷: burn of vagina (T28.3)

CC-A **T21.39x-** Burn of <u>third</u> degree of <u>other</u> site of trunk

T21.4- <u>Corrosion</u> of <u>unspecified degree</u> of <u>trunk</u>
Code first (T51-T65) to identify chemical and intent
Use additional external cause code to identify place (Y92)

T21.40x- <u>Corrosion</u> of <u>unspecified degree</u> of trunk, <u>unspecified</u> site

T21.41x- <u>Corrosion</u> of <u>unspecified degree</u> of <u>chest wall</u>
Corrosion of unspecified degree of breast

T21.42x- <u>Corrosion</u> of <u>unspecified degree</u> of <u>abdominal wall</u>
Corrosion of unspecified degree of flank
Corrosion of unspecified degree of groin

T21.43x- <u>Corrosion</u> of <u>unspecified degree</u> of <u>upper back</u>
Corrosion of unspecified degree of interscapular region

T21.44x- <u>Corrosion</u> of <u>unspecified degree</u> of <u>lower back</u>

T21.45x- <u>Corrosion</u> of <u>unspecified degree</u> of <u>buttock</u>
Corrosion of unspecified degree of anus

T21.46x- <u>Corrosion</u> of <u>unspecified degree</u> of <u>male genital region</u> — [♂]
Corrosion of unspecified degree of penis
Corrosion of unspecified degree of scrotum
Corrosion of unspecified degree of testis

T21.47x- <u>Corrosion</u> of <u>unspecified degree</u> of <u>female genital region</u> — [♀]
Corrosion of unspecified degree of labium (majus) (minus)
Corrosion of unspecified degree of perineum
Corrosion of unspecified degree of vulva

Excludes ❷: corrosion of vagina (T28.8)

T21.49x- <u>Corrosion</u> of <u>unspecified degree</u> of <u>other</u> site of trunk

T21.5- <u>Corrosion</u> of <u>first</u> degree of <u>trunk</u>
Code first (T51-T65) to identify chemical and intent
Use additional external cause code to identify place (Y92)

T21.50x- <u>Corrosion</u> of <u>first</u> degree of trunk, <u>unspecified</u> site

T21.51x- <u>Corrosion</u> of <u>first</u> degree of <u>chest wall</u>
Corrosion of first degree of breast

T21.52x- <u>Corrosion</u> of <u>first</u> degree of <u>abdominal wall</u>
Corrosion of first degree of flank
Corrosion of first degree of groin

T21.53x- <u>Corrosion</u> of <u>first</u> degree of <u>upper back</u>
Corrosion of first degree of interscapular region

T21.54x- <u>Corrosion</u> of <u>first</u> degree of <u>lower back</u>

T21.55x- <u>Corrosion</u> of <u>first</u> degree of <u>buttock</u>
Corrosion of first degree of anus

T21.56x- <u>Corrosion</u> of <u>first</u> degree of <u>male genital region</u> — [♂]
Corrosion of first degree of penis
Corrosion of first degree of scrotum
Corrosion of first degree of testis

T21.57x- <u>Corrosion</u> of <u>first</u> degree of <u>female genital region</u> — [♀]
Corrosion of first degree of labium (majus) (minus)
Corrosion of first degree of perineum
Corrosion of first degree of vulva

Excludes ❷: corrosion of vagina (T28.8)

T21.59x- <u>Corrosion</u> of <u>first</u> degree of <u>other</u> site of trunk

T21.6- <u>Corrosion</u> of <u>second</u> degree of <u>trunk</u>
Code first (T51-T65) to identify chemical and intent
Use additional external cause code to identify place (Y92)

T21.60x- <u>Corrosion</u> of <u>second</u> degree of trunk, <u>unspecified</u> site

T21.61x- <u>Corrosion</u> of <u>second</u> degree of <u>chest wall</u>
Corrosion of second degree of breast

T21.62x- <u>Corrosion</u> of <u>second</u> degree of <u>abdominal wall</u>
Corrosion of second degree of flank
Corrosion of second degree of groin

T21.63x- <u>Corrosion</u> of <u>second</u> degree of <u>upper back</u>
Corrosion of second degree of interscapular region

T21.64x- <u>Corrosion</u> of <u>second</u> degree of <u>lower back</u>

T21.65x- <u>Corrosion</u> of <u>second</u> degree of <u>buttock</u>
Corrosion of second degree of anus

T21.66x- <u>Corrosion</u> of <u>second</u> degree of <u>male genital region</u> — [♂]
Corrosion of second degree of penis
Corrosion of second degree of scrotum
Corrosion of second degree of testis

T21.67x- <u>Corrosion</u> of <u>second</u> degree of <u>female genital region</u> — [♀]
Corrosion of second degree of labium (majus) (minus)
Corrosion of second degree of perineum
Corrosion of second degree of vulva

Excludes ❷: corrosion of vagina (T28.8)

T21.69x- <u>Corrosion</u> of <u>second</u> degree of <u>other</u> site of trunk

T21.7- <u>Corrosion</u> of <u>third</u> degree of <u>trunk</u>
Code first (T51-T65) to identify chemical and intent
Use additional external cause code to identify place (Y92)

CC-A **T21.70x-** <u>Corrosion</u> of <u>third</u> degree of trunk, <u>unspecified</u> site

CC-A **T21.71x-** <u>Corrosion</u> of <u>third</u> degree of <u>chest wall</u>
Corrosion of third degree of breast

CC-A **T21.72x-** <u>Corrosion</u> of <u>third</u> degree of <u>abdominal wall</u>
Corrosion of third degree of flank
Corrosion of third degree of groin

T 2 1 - T 2 1

CC-A **T21.73x-** <u>Corrosion</u> of <u>third</u> degree of <u>upper back</u>
Corrosion of third degree of interscapular region

CC-A **T21.74x-** <u>Corrosion</u> of <u>third</u> degree of <u>lower back</u>

CC-A **T21.75x-** <u>Corrosion</u> of <u>third</u> degree of <u>buttock</u>
Corrosion of third degree of anus

CC-A **T21.76x-** <u>Corrosion</u> of <u>third</u> degree of <u>male genital region</u> — [♂]
Corrosion of third degree of penis
Corrosion of third degree of scrotum
Corrosion of third degree of testis

CC-A **T21.77x-** <u>Corrosion</u> of <u>third</u> degree of <u>female genital region</u> — [♀]
Corrosion of third degree of labium (majus) (minus)
Corrosion of third degree of perineum
Corrosion of third degree of vulva

Excludes ❷: corrosion of vagina (T28.8)

CC-A **T21.79x-** <u>Corrosion</u> of <u>third</u> degree of <u>other</u> site of trunk

T22- <u>Burn and corrosion</u> of <u>shoulder and upper limb</u>, <u>except wrist and hand</u>

Excludes ❷: burn and corrosion of interscapular region (T21.-)
burn and corrosion of wrist and hand (T23.-)

The appropriate 7th character is to be added to each code from category T22:
A <u>Initial</u> encounter
D <u>Subsequent</u> encounter
S <u>Sequela</u>

T22.0- Burn of <u>unspecified degree</u> of <u>shoulder and upper limb</u>, <u>except wrist and hand</u>
Use additional external cause code to identify the source, place and intent of the burn (X00-X19, X75-X77, X96-X98, Y92)

T22.00x- Burn of <u>unspecified degree</u> of <u>shoulder and upper limb</u>, except wrist and hand, <u>unspecified</u> site

T22.01- Burn of <u>unspecified degree</u> of <u>forearm</u>
T22.011- Burn of unspecified degree of <u>right</u> forearm
T22.012- Burn of unspecified degree of <u>left</u> forearm
T22.019- Burn of unspecified degree of <u>unspecified</u> forearm

T22.02- Burn of <u>unspecified degree</u> of <u>elbow</u>
T22.021- Burn of unspecified degree of <u>right</u> elbow
T22.022- Burn of unspecified degree of <u>left</u> elbow
T22.029- Burn of unspecified degree of <u>unspecified</u> elbow

T22.03- Burn of <u>unspecified degree</u> of <u>upper arm</u>
T22.031- Burn of unspecified degree of <u>right</u> upper arm
T22.032- Burn of unspecified degree of <u>left</u> upper arm
T22.039- Burn of unspecified degree of <u>unspecified</u> upper arm

T22.04- Burn of <u>unspecified degree</u> of <u>axilla</u>
T22.041- Burn of unspecified degree of <u>right</u> axilla
T22.042- Burn of unspecified degree of <u>left</u> axilla
T22.049- Burn of unspecified degree of <u>unspecified</u> axilla

T22.05- Burn of <u>unspecified degree</u> of <u>shoulder</u>
T22.051- Burn of unspecified degree of <u>right</u> shoulder
T22.052- Burn of unspecified degree of <u>left</u> shoulder
T22.059- Burn of unspecified degree of <u>unspecified</u> shoulder

T22.06- Burn of <u>unspecified degree</u> of <u>scapular region</u>
T22.061- Burn of unspecified degree of <u>right</u> scapular region
T22.062- Burn of unspecified degree of <u>left</u> scapular region
T22.069- Burn of unspecified degree of <u>unspecified</u> scapular region

T22.09- Burn of <u>unspecified degree</u> of <u>multiple</u> sites of shoulder and upper limb, except wrist and hand
T22.091- Burn of unspecified degree of multiple sites of <u>right</u> shoulder and upper limb, except wrist and hand
T22.092- Burn of unspecified degree of multiple sites of <u>left</u> shoulder and upper limb, except wrist and hand
T22.099- Burn of unspecified degree of multiple sites of <u>unspecified</u> shoulder and upper limb, except wrist and hand

T22.1- Burn of <u>first</u> degree of <u>shoulder and upper limb</u>, <u>except wrist and hand</u>
Use additional external cause code to identify the source, place and intent of the burn (X00-X19, X75-X77, X96-X98, Y92)

T22.10x- Burn of <u>first</u> degree of <u>shoulder and upper limb</u>, except wrist and hand, <u>unspecified</u> site

T22.11- Burn of <u>first</u> degree of <u>forearm</u>
T22.111- Burn of first degree of <u>right</u> forearm
T22.112- Burn of first degree of <u>left</u> forearm
T22.119- Burn of first degree of <u>unspecified</u> forearm

T22.12- Burn of <u>first</u> degree of <u>elbow</u>
T22.121- Burn of first degree of <u>right</u> elbow
T22.122- Burn of first degree of <u>left</u> elbow
T22.129- Burn of first degree of <u>unspecified</u> elbow

T22.13- Burn of <u>first</u> degree of <u>upper arm</u>
T22.131- Burn of first degree of <u>right</u> upper arm
T22.132- Burn of first degree of <u>left</u> upper arm
T22.139- Burn of first degree of <u>unspecified</u> upper arm

T22.14- Burn of <u>first</u> degree of <u>axilla</u>
T22.141- Burn of first degree of <u>right</u> axilla
T22.142- Burn of first degree of <u>left</u> axilla
T22.149- Burn of first degree of <u>unspecified</u> axilla

T22.15- Burn of <u>first</u> degree of <u>shoulder</u>
T22.151- Burn of first degree of <u>right</u> shoulder
T22.152- Burn of first degree of <u>left</u> shoulder
T22.159- Burn of first degree of <u>unspecified</u> shoulder

T22.16- Burn of <u>first</u> degree of <u>scapular region</u>
T22.161- Burn of first degree of <u>right</u> scapular region
T22.162- Burn of first degree of <u>left</u> scapular region
T22.169- Burn of first degree of <u>unspecified</u> scapular region

T22.19- Burn of <u>first</u> degree of <u>multiple</u> sites of shoulder and upper limb, except wrist and hand
T22.191- Burn of first degree of multiple sites of <u>right</u> shoulder and upper limb, except wrist and hand
T22.192- Burn of first degree of multiple sites of <u>left</u> shoulder and upper limb, except wrist and hand
T22.199- Burn of first degree of multiple sites of <u>unspecified</u> shoulder and upper limb, except wrist and hand

T22.2- Burn of <u>second</u> degree of <u>shoulder and upper limb</u>, <u>except wrist and hand</u>
Use additional external cause code to identify the source, place and intent of the burn (X00-X19, X75-X77, X96-X98, Y92)

T22.20x- Burn of <u>second</u> degree of <u>shoulder and upper limb</u>, except wrist and hand, <u>unspecified</u> site

T22.21- Burn of <u>second</u> degree of <u>forearm</u>
T22.211- Burn of second degree of <u>right</u> forearm
T22.212- Burn of second degree of <u>left</u> forearm
T22.219- Burn of second degree of <u>unspecified</u> forearm

T22.22- Burn of <u>second</u> degree of <u>elbow</u>
T22.221- Burn of second degree of <u>right</u> elbow
T22.222- Burn of second degree of <u>left</u> elbow
T22.229- Burn of second degree of <u>unspecified</u> elbow

T22.23- Burn of <u>second</u> degree of <u>upper arm</u>
T22.231- Burn of second degree of <u>right</u> upper arm
T22.232- Burn of second degree of <u>left</u> upper arm
T22.239- Burn of second degree of <u>unspecified</u> upper arm

T22.24- Burn of <u>second</u> degree of <u>axilla</u>
T22.241- Burn of second degree of <u>right</u> axilla
T22.242- Burn of second degree of <u>left</u> axilla
T22.249- Burn of second degree of <u>unspecified</u> axilla

T22.25- Burn of <u>second</u> degree of <u>shoulder</u>
T22.251- Burn of second degree of <u>right</u> shoulder
T22.252- Burn of second degree of <u>left</u> shoulder
T22.259- Burn of second degree of <u>unspecified</u> shoulder

T22.26- Burn of <u>second</u> degree of <u>scapular region</u>
T22.261- Burn of second degree of <u>right</u> scapular region

T21-T22

T22.262-   Burn of second degree of <u>left</u> scapular region
T22.269-   Burn of second degree of <u>unspecified</u> scapular region

T22.29- Burn of <u>second</u> degree of <u>multiple</u> sites of shoulder and upper limb, except wrist and hand

T22.291-   Burn of second degree of multiple sites of <u>right</u> shoulder and upper limb, except wrist and hand
T22.292-   Burn of second degree of multiple sites of <u>left</u> shoulder and upper limb, except wrist and hand
T22.299-   Burn of second degree of multiple sites of <u>unspecified</u> shoulder and upper limb, except wrist and hand

T22.3- Burn of <u>third</u> degree of <u>shoulder and upper limb, except wrist and hand</u>
Use additional external cause code to identify the source, place and intent of the burn (X00-X19, X75-X77, X96-X98, Y92)

CC-A **T22.30x-** Burn of <u>third</u> degree of shoulder and upper limb, except wrist and hand, <u>unspecified</u> site

T22.31- Burn of <u>third</u> degree of <u>forearm</u>
CC-A T22.311-   Burn of third degree of <u>right</u> forearm
CC-A T22.312-   Burn of third degree of <u>left</u> forearm
CC-A T22.319-   Burn of third degree of <u>unspecified</u> forearm

T22.32- Burn of <u>third</u> degree of <u>elbow</u>
CC-A T22.321-   Burn of third degree of <u>right</u> elbow
CC-A T22.322-   Burn of third degree of <u>left</u> elbow
CC-A T22.329-   Burn of third degree of <u>unspecified</u> elbow

T22.33- Burn of <u>third</u> degree of <u>upper arm</u>
CC-A T22.331-   Burn of third degree of <u>right</u> upper arm
CC-A T22.332-   Burn of third degree of <u>left</u> upper arm
CC-A T22.339-   Burn of third degree of <u>unspecified</u> upper arm

T22.34- Burn of <u>third</u> degree of <u>axilla</u>
CC-A T22.341-   Burn of third degree of <u>right</u> axilla
CC-A T22.342-   Burn of third degree of <u>left</u> axilla
CC-A T22.349-   Burn of third degree of <u>unspecified</u> axilla

T22.35- Burn of <u>third</u> degree of <u>shoulder</u>
CC-A T22.351-   Burn of third degree of <u>right</u> shoulder
CC-A T22.352-   Burn of third degree of <u>left</u> shoulder
CC-A T22.359-   Burn of third degree of <u>unspecified</u> shoulder

T22.36- Burn of <u>third</u> degree of <u>scapular region</u>
CC-A T22.361-   Burn of third degree of <u>right</u> scapular region
CC-A T22.362-   Burn of third degree of <u>left</u> scapular region
CC-A T22.369-   Burn of third degree of <u>unspecified</u> scapular region

T22.39 Burn of <u>third</u> degree of <u>multiple</u> sites of shoulder and upper limb, except wrist and hand
CC-A T22.391-   Burn of third degree of multiple sites of <u>right</u> shoulder and upper limb, except wrist and hand
CC-A T22.392-   Burn of third degree of multiple sites of <u>left</u> shoulder and upper limb, except wrist and hand
CC-A T22.399-   Burn of third degree of multiple sites of <u>unspecified</u> shoulder and upper limb, except wrist and hand

T22.4- <u>Corrosion</u> of <u>unspecified degree</u> of <u>shoulder and upper limb, except wrist and hand</u>
Code first (T51-T65) to identify chemical and intent
Use additional external cause code to identify place (Y92)

T22.40x- <u>Corrosion</u> of <u>unspecified degree</u> of <u>shoulder and upper limb, except wrist and hand, unspecified</u> site

T22.41- <u>Corrosion</u> of <u>unspecified degree</u> of <u>forearm</u>
T22.411-   Corrosion of unspecified degree of <u>right</u> forearm
T22.412-   Corrosion of unspecified degree of <u>left</u> forearm
T22.419-   Corrosion of unspecified degree of <u>unspecified</u> forearm

T22.42- <u>Corrosion</u> of <u>unspecified degree</u> of <u>elbow</u>
T22.421-   Corrosion of unspecified degree of <u>right</u> elbow
T22.422-   Corrosion of unspecified degree of <u>left</u> elbow
T22.429-   Corrosion of unspecified degree of <u>unspecified</u> elbow

T22.43- <u>Corrosion</u> of <u>unspecified degree</u> of <u>upper arm</u>
T22.431-   Corrosion of unspecified degree of <u>right</u> upper arm
T22.432-   Corrosion of unspecified degree of <u>left</u> upper arm
T22.439-   Corrosion of unspecified degree of <u>unspecified</u> upper arm

T22.44- <u>Corrosion</u> of <u>unspecified degree</u> of <u>axilla</u>
T22.441-   Corrosion of unspecified degree of <u>right</u> axilla
T22.442-   Corrosion of unspecified degree of <u>left</u> axilla
T22.449-   Corrosion of unspecified degree of <u>unspecified</u> axilla

T22.45- <u>Corrosion</u> of <u>unspecified degree</u> of <u>shoulder</u>
T22.451-   Corrosion of unspecified degree of <u>right</u> shoulder
T22.452-   Corrosion of unspecified degree of <u>left</u> shoulder
T22.459-   Corrosion of unspecified degree of <u>unspecified</u> shoulder

T22.46- <u>Corrosion</u> of <u>unspecified degree</u> of <u>scapular region</u>
T22.461-   Corrosion of unspecified degree of <u>right</u> scapular region
T22.462-   Corrosion of unspecified degree of <u>left</u> scapular region
T22.469-   Corrosion of unspecified degree of <u>unspecified</u> scapular region

T22.49- <u>Corrosion</u> of <u>unspecified degree</u> of <u>multiple</u> sites of shoulder and upper limb, except wrist and hand
T22.491-   Corrosion of unspecified degree of multiple sites of <u>right</u> shoulder and upper limb, except wrist and hand
T22.492-   Corrosion of unspecified degree of multiple sites of <u>left</u> shoulder and upper limb, except wrist and hand
T22.499-   Corrosion of unspecified degree of multiple sites of <u>unspecified</u> shoulder and upper limb, except wrist and hand

T22.5- <u>Corrosion</u> of <u>first</u> degree of <u>shoulder and upper limb, except wrist and hand</u>
Code first (T51-T65) to identify chemical and intent
Use additional external cause code to identify place (Y92)

T22.50x- <u>Corrosion</u> of <u>first</u> degree of <u>shoulder and upper limb</u>, except wrist and hand <u>unspecified</u> site

T22.51- <u>Corrosion</u> of <u>first</u> degree of <u>forearm</u>
T22.511-   Corrosion of first degree of <u>right</u> forearm
T22.512-   Corrosion of first degree of <u>left</u> forearm
T22.519-   Corrosion of first degree of <u>unspecified</u> forearm

T22.52- <u>Corrosion</u> of <u>first</u> degree of <u>elbow</u>
T22.521-   Corrosion of first degree of <u>right</u> elbow
T22.522-   Corrosion of first degree of <u>left</u> elbow
T22.529-   Corrosion of first degree of <u>unspecified</u> elbow

T22.53- <u>Corrosion</u> of <u>first</u> degree of <u>upper arm</u>
T22.531-   Corrosion of first degree of <u>right</u> upper arm
T22.532-   Corrosion of first degree of <u>left</u> upper arm
T22.539-   Corrosion of first degree of <u>unspecified</u> upper arm

T22.54- <u>Corrosion</u> of <u>first</u> degree of <u>axilla</u>
T22.541-   Corrosion of first degree of <u>right</u> axilla
T22.542-   Corrosion of first degree of <u>left</u> axilla
T22.549-   Corrosion of first degree of <u>unspecified</u> axilla

T22.55- <u>Corrosion</u> of <u>first</u> degree of <u>shoulder</u>
T22.551-   Corrosion of first degree of <u>right</u> shoulder
T22.552-   Corrosion of first degree of <u>left</u> shoulder
T22.559-   Corrosion of first degree of <u>unspecified</u> shoulder

T22.56- <u>Corrosion</u> of <u>first</u> degree of <u>scapular region</u>
T22.561-   Corrosion of first degree of <u>right</u> scapular region
T22.562-   Corrosion of first degree of <u>left</u> scapular region
T22.569-   Corrosion of first degree of <u>unspecified</u> scapular region

T22.59- Corrosion of first degree of multiple sites of shoulder and upper limb, except wrist and hand

    T22.591- Corrosion of first degree of multiple sites of right shoulder and upper limb, except wrist and hand

    T22.592- Corrosion of first degree of multiple sites of left shoulder and upper limb, except wrist and hand

    T22.599- Corrosion of first degree of multiple sites of unspecified shoulder and upper limb, except wrist and hand

T22.6- Corrosion of second degree of shoulder and upper limb, except wrist and hand
Code first (T51-T65) to identify chemical and intent
Use additional external cause code to identify place (Y92)

    T22.60x- Corrosion of second degree of shoulder and upper limb, except wrist and hand, unspecified site

    T22.61- Corrosion of second degree of forearm

    T22.611- Corrosion of second degree of right forearm

    T22.612- Corrosion of second degree of left forearm

    T22.619- Corrosion of second degree of unspecified forearm

    T22.62- Corrosion of second degree of elbow

    T22.621- Corrosion of second degree of right elbow

    T22.622- Corrosion of second degree of left elbow

    T22.629- Corrosion of second degree of unspecified elbow

    T22.63- Corrosion of second degree of upper arm

    T22.631- Corrosion of second degree of right upper arm

    T22.632- Corrosion of second degree of left upper arm

    T22.639- Corrosion of second degree of unspecified upper arm

    T22.64- Corrosion of second degree of axilla

    T22.641- Corrosion of second degree of right axilla

    T22.642- Corrosion of second degree of left axilla

    T22.649- Corrosion of second degree of unspecified axilla

    T22.65- Corrosion of second degree of shoulder

    T22.651- Corrosion of second degree of right shoulder

    T22.652- Corrosion of second degree of left shoulder

    T22.659- Corrosion of second degree of unspecified shoulder

    T22.66- Corrosion of second degree of scapular region

    T22.661- Corrosion of second degree of right scapular region

    T22.662- Corrosion of second degree of left scapular region

    T22.669- Corrosion of second degree of unspecified scapular region

    T22.69- Corrosion of second degree of multiple sites of shoulder and upper limb, except wrist and hand

    T22.691- Corrosion of second degree of multiple sites of right shoulder and upper limb, except wrist and hand

    T22.692- Corrosion of second degree of multiple sites of left shoulder and upper limb, except wrist and hand

    T22.699- Corrosion of second degree of multiple sites of unspecified shoulder and upper limb, except wrist and hand

T22.7- Corrosion of third degree of shoulder and upper limb, except wrist and hand
Code first (T51-T65) to identify chemical and intent
Use additional external cause code to identify place (Y92)

CC-A T22.70x- Corrosion of third degree of shoulder and upper limb, except wrist and hand, unspecified site

    T22.71- Corrosion of third degree of forearm

CC-A T22.711- Corrosion of third degree of right forearm

CC-A T22.712- Corrosion of third degree of left forearm

CC-A T22.719- Corrosion of third degree of unspecified forearm

    T22.72- Corrosion of third degree of elbow

CC-A T22.721- Corrosion of third degree of right elbow

CC-A T22.722- Corrosion of third degree of left elbow

CC-A T22.729- Corrosion of third degree of unspecified elbow

    T22.73- Corrosion of third degree of upper arm

CC-A T22.731- Corrosion of third degree of right upper arm

CC-A T22.732- Corrosion of third degree of left upper arm

CC-A T22.739- Corrosion of third degree of unspecified upper arm

    T22.74- Corrosion of third degree of axilla

CC-A T22.741- Corrosion of third degree of right axilla

CC-A T22.742- Corrosion of third degree of left axilla

CC-A T22.749- Corrosion of third degree of unspecified axilla

    T22.75- Corrosion of third degree of shoulder

CC-A T22.751- Corrosion of third degree of right shoulder

CC-A T22.752- Corrosion of third degree of left shoulder

CC-A T22.759- Corrosion of third degree of unspecified shoulder

    T22.76- Corrosion of third degree of scapular region

CC-A T22.761- Corrosion of third degree of right scapular region

CC-A T22.762- Corrosion of third degree of left scapular region

CC-A T22.769- Corrosion of third degree of unspecified scapular region

    T22.79- Corrosion of third degree of multiple sites of shoulder and upper limb, except wrist and hand

CC-A T22.791- Corrosion of third degree of multiple sites of right shoulder and upper limb, except wrist and hand

CC-A T22.792- Corrosion of third degree of multiple sites of left shoulder and upper limb, except wrist and hand

CC-A T22.799- Corrosion of third degree of multiple sites of unspecified shoulder and upper limb, except wrist and hand

T23- Burn and corrosion of wrist and hand

The appropriate 7th character is to be added to each code from category T23:
  A Initial encounter
  D Subsequent encounter
  S Sequela

T23.0- Burn of unspecified degree of wrist and hand
Use additional external cause code to identify the source, place and intent of the burn (X00-X19, X75-X77, X96-X98, Y92)

    T23.00- Burn of unspecified degree of hand, unspecified site

    T23.001- Burn of unspecified degree of right hand, unspecified site

    T23.002- Burn of unspecified degree of left hand, unspecified site

    T23.009- Burn of unspecified degree of unspecified hand, unspecified site

    T23.01- Burn of unspecified degree of thumb (nail)

    T23.011- Burn of unspecified degree of right thumb (nail)

    T23.012- Burn of unspecified degree of left thumb (nail)

    T23.019- Burn of unspecified degree of unspecified thumb (nail)

    T23.02- Burn of unspecified degree of single finger (nail) except thumb

    T23.021- Burn of unspecified degree of single right finger (nail) except thumb

    T23.022- Burn of unspecified degree of single left finger (nail) except thumb

    T23.029- Burn of unspecified degree of unspecified single finger (nail) except thumb

    T23.03- Burn of unspecified degree of multiple fingers (nail), not including thumb

    T23.031- Burn of unspecified degree of multiple right fingers (nail), not including thumb

    T23.032- Burn of unspecified degree of multiple left fingers (nail), not including thumb

    T23.039- Burn of unspecified degree of unspecified multiple fingers (nail), not including thumb

    T23.04- Burn of unspecified degree of multiple fingers (nail), including thumb

    T23.041- Burn of unspecified degree of multiple right fingers (nail), including thumb

    T23.042- Burn of unspecified degree of multiple left fingers (nail), including thumb

T22 - T23

T23.049- Burn of unspecified degree of <u>unspecified</u> multiple fingers (nail), including thumb

T23.05- Burn of <u>unspecified degree</u> of <u>palm</u>

T23.051- Burn of unspecified degree of <u>right</u> palm

T23.052- Burn of unspecified degree of <u>left</u> palm

T23.059- Burn of unspecified degree of <u>unspecified</u> palm

T23.06- Burn of <u>unspecified degree</u> of <u>back of hand</u>

T23.061- Burn of unspecified degree of back of <u>right</u> hand

T23.062- Burn of unspecified degree of back of <u>left</u> hand

T23.069- Burn of unspecified degree of back of <u>unspecified</u> hand

T23.07- Burn of <u>unspecified degree</u> of <u>wrist</u>

T23.071- Burn of unspecified degree of <u>right</u> wrist

T23.072- Burn of unspecified degree of <u>left</u> wrist

T23.079- Burn of unspecified degree of <u>unspecified</u> wrist

T23.09- Burn of <u>unspecified degree</u> of <u>multiple</u> sites of <u>wrist and hand</u>

T23.091- Burn of unspecified degree of multiple sites of <u>right</u> wrist and hand

T23.092- Burn of unspecified degree of multiple sites of <u>left</u> wrist and hand

T23.099- Burn of unspecified degree of multiple sites of <u>unspecified</u> wrist and hand

T23.1- Burn of <u>first</u> degree of <u>wrist and hand</u>
Use additional external cause code to identify the source, place and intent of the burn (X00-X19, X75-X77, X96-X98, Y92)

T23.10- Burn of <u>first</u> degree of hand, <u>unspecified</u> site

T23.101- Burn of first degree of <u>right</u> hand, unspecified site

T23.102- Burn of first degree of <u>left</u> hand, unspecified site

T23.109- Burn of first degree of <u>unspecified</u> hand, unspecified site

T23.11- Burn of <u>first</u> degree of <u>thumb</u> (nail)

T23.111- Burn of first degree of <u>right</u> thumb (nail)

T23.112- Burn of first degree of <u>left</u> thumb (nail)

T23.119- Burn of first degree of <u>unspecified</u> thumb (nail)

T23.12- Burn of <u>first</u> degree of <u>single finger</u> (nail) <u>except thumb</u>

T23.121- Burn of first degree of single <u>right</u> finger (nail) except thumb

T23.122- Burn of first degree of single <u>left</u> finger (nail) except thumb

T23.129- Burn of first degree of <u>unspecified</u> single finger (nail) except thumb

T23.13- Burn of <u>first</u> degree of <u>multiple fingers</u> (nail), <u>not including thumb</u>

T23.131- Burn of first degree of multiple <u>right</u> fingers (nail), not including thumb

T23.132- Burn of first degree of multiple <u>left</u> fingers (nail), not including thumb

T23.139- Burn of first degree of <u>unspecified</u> multiple fingers (nail), not including thumb

T23.14- Burn of <u>first</u> degree of <u>multiple fingers</u> (nail), <u>including thumb</u>

T23.141- Burn of first degree of multiple <u>right</u> fingers (nail), including thumb

T23.142- Burn of first degree of multiple <u>left</u> fingers (nail), including thumb

T23.149- Burn of first degree of <u>unspecified</u> multiple fingers (nail), including thumb

T23.15- Burn of <u>first</u> degree of <u>palm</u>

T23.151- Burn of first degree of <u>right</u> palm

T23.152- Burn of first degree of <u>left</u> palm

T23.159- Burn of first degree of <u>unspecified</u> palm

T23.16- Burn of <u>first</u> degree of <u>back of hand</u>

T23.161- Burn of first degree of back of <u>right</u> hand

T23.162- Burn of first degree of back of <u>left</u> hand

T23.169- Burn of first degree of back of <u>unspecified</u> hand

T23.17- Burn of <u>first</u> degree of <u>wrist</u>

T23.171- Burn of first degree of <u>right</u> wrist

T23.172- Burn of first degree of <u>left</u> wrist

T23.179- Burn of first degree of <u>unspecified</u> wrist

T23.19- Burn of <u>first</u> degree of <u>multiple</u> sites of <u>wrist and hand</u>

T23.191- Burn of first degree of multiple sites of <u>right</u> wrist and hand

T23.192- Burn of first degree of multiple sites of <u>left</u> wrist and hand

T23.199- Burn of first degree of multiple sites of <u>unspecified</u> wrist and hand

T23.2- Burn of <u>second</u> degree of <u>wrist and hand</u>
Use additional external cause code to identify the source, place and intent of the burn (X00-X19, X75-X77, X96-X98, Y92)

T23.20- Burn of <u>second</u> degree of hand, <u>unspecified</u> site

T23.201- Burn of second degree of <u>right</u> hand, unspecified site

T23.202- Burn of second degree of <u>left</u> hand, unspecified site

T23.209- Burn of second degree of unspecified hand, <u>unspecified</u> site

T23.21- Burn of <u>second</u> degree of <u>thumb</u> (nail)

T23.211- Burn of second degree of <u>right</u> thumb (nail)

T23.212- Burn of second degree of <u>left</u> thumb (nail)

T23.219- Burn of second degree of <u>unspecified</u> thumb (nail)

T23.22- Burn of <u>second</u> degree of <u>single finger</u> (nail) <u>except thumb</u>

T23.221- Burn of second degree of single <u>right</u> finger (nail) except thumb

T23.222- Burn of second degree of single <u>left</u> finger (nail) except thumb

T23.229- Burn of second degree of <u>unspecified</u> single finger (nail) except thumb

T23.23- Burn of <u>second</u> degree of <u>multiple fingers</u> (nail), <u>not including thumb</u>

T23.231- Burn of second degree of multiple <u>right</u> fingers (nail), not including thumb

T23.232- Burn of second degree of multiple <u>left</u> fingers (nail), not including thumb

T23.239- Burn of second degree of <u>unspecified</u> multiple fingers (nail), not including thumb

T23.24- Burn of <u>second</u> degree of <u>multiple fingers</u> (nail), <u>including thumb</u>

T23.241- Burn of second degree of multiple <u>right</u> fingers (nail), including thumb

T23.242- Burn of second degree of multiple <u>left</u> fingers (nail), including thumb

T23.249- Burn of second degree of <u>unspecified</u> multiple fingers (nail), including thumb

T23.25- Burn of <u>second</u> degree of <u>palm</u>

T23.251- Burn of second degree of <u>right</u> palm

T23.252- Burn of second degree of <u>left</u> palm

T23.259- Burn of second degree of <u>unspecified</u> palm

T23.26- Burn of <u>second</u> degree of <u>back of hand</u>

T23.261- Burn of second degree of back of <u>right</u> hand

T23.262- Burn of second degree of back of <u>left</u> hand

T23.269- Burn of second degree of back of <u>unspecified</u> hand

T23.27- Burn of <u>second</u> degree of <u>wrist</u>

T23.271- Burn of second degree of <u>right</u> wrist

T23.272- Burn of second degree of <u>left</u> wrist

T23.279- Burn of second degree of <u>unspecified</u> wrist

T23.29- Burn of <u>second</u> degree of <u>multiple</u> sites of <u>wrist and hand</u>

T23.291- Burn of second degree of multiple sites of <u>right</u> wrist and hand

T23.292- Burn of second degree of multiple sites of <u>left</u> wrist and hand

T23.299- Burn of second degree of multiple sites of <u>unspecified</u> wrist and hand

T23.3- Burn of <u>third</u> degree of <u>wrist and hand</u>
Use additional external cause code to identify the source, place and intent of the burn (X00-X19, X75-X77, X96-X98, Y92)

T23.30- Burn of <u>third</u> degree of hand, <u>unspecified</u> site

CC-A **T23.301-** Burn of third degree of <u>right</u> hand, unspecified site

CC-A **T23.302-** Burn of third degree of <u>left</u> hand, unspecified site

CC-A **T23.309-** Burn of third degree of <u>unspecified</u> hand, unspecified site

T23.31- Burn of <u>third</u> degree of <u>thumb</u> (nail)

CC-A **T23.311-** Burn of third degree of <u>right</u> thumb (nail)

CC-A **T23.312-** Burn of third degree of <u>left</u> thumb (nail)

CC-A **T23.319-** Burn of third degree of <u>unspecified</u> thumb (nail)

T23.32- Burn of <u>third</u> degree of <u>single finger</u> (nail) <u>except thumb</u>

CC-A **T23.321-** Burn of third degree of single <u>right</u> finger (nail) except thumb

CC-A **T23.322-** Burn of third degree of single <u>left</u> finger (nail) except thumb

CC-A **T23.329-** Burn of third degree of <u>unspecified</u> single finger (nail) except thumb

T23.33- Burn of <u>third</u> degree of <u>multiple</u> fingers (nail), <u>not including thumb</u>

CC-A **T23.331-** Burn of third degree of multiple <u>right</u> fingers (nail), not including thumb

CC-A **T23.332-** Burn of third degree of multiple <u>left</u> fingers (nail), not including thumb

CC-A **T23.339-** Burn of third degree of <u>unspecified</u> multiple fingers (nail), not including thumb

T23.34- Burn of <u>third</u> degree of <u>multiple</u> fingers (nail), <u>including thumb</u>

CC-A **T23.341-** Burn of third degree of multiple <u>right</u> fingers (nail), including thumb

CC-A **T23.342-** Burn of third degree of multiple <u>left</u> fingers (nail), including thumb

CC-A **T23.349-** Burn of third degree of <u>unspecified</u> multiple fingers (nail), including thumb

T23.35- Burn of <u>third</u> degree of <u>palm</u>

CC-A **T23.351-** Burn of third degree of <u>right</u> palm

CC-A **T23.352-** Burn of third degree of <u>left</u> palm

CC-A **T23.359-** Burn of third degree of <u>unspecified</u> palm

T23.36- Burn of <u>third</u> degree of <u>back of hand</u>

CC-A **T23.361-** Burn of third degree of back of <u>right</u> hand

CC-A **T23.362-** Burn of third degree of back of <u>left</u> hand

CC-A **T23.369-** Burn of third degree of back of <u>unspecified</u> hand

T23.37- Burn of <u>third</u> degree of <u>wrist</u>

CC-A **T23.371-** Burn of third degree of <u>right</u> wrist

CC-A **T23.372-** Burn of third degree of <u>left</u> wrist

CC-A **T23.379-** Burn of third degree of <u>unspecified</u> wrist

T23.39- Burn of <u>third</u> degree of <u>multiple</u> sites of <u>wrist and hand</u>

CC-A **T23.391-** Burn of third degree of multiple sites of <u>right</u> wrist and hand

CC-A **T23.392-** Burn of third degree of multiple sites of <u>left</u> wrist and hand

CC-A **T23.399-** Burn of third degree of multiple sites of <u>unspecified</u> wrist and hand

T23.4- <u>Corrosion</u> of <u>unspecified degree</u> of <u>wrist and hand</u>
Code first (T51-T65) to identify chemical and intent
Use additional external cause code to identify place (Y92)

T23.40- <u>Corrosion</u> of <u>unspecified degree</u> of hand, <u>unspecified</u> site

T23.401- Corrosion of unspecified degree of <u>right</u> hand, unspecified site

T23.402- Corrosion of unspecified degree of <u>left</u> hand, unspecified site

T23.409- Corrosion of unspecified degree of <u>unspecified</u> hand, unspecified site

T23.41- <u>Corrosion</u> of <u>unspecified degree</u> of <u>thumb</u> (nail)

T23.411- Corrosion of unspecified degree of <u>right</u> thumb (nail)

T23.412- Corrosion of unspecified degree of <u>left</u> thumb (nail)

T23.419- Corrosion of unspecified degree of <u>unspecified</u> thumb (nail)

T23.42- <u>Corrosion</u> of <u>unspecified degree</u> of <u>single finger</u> (nail) <u>except thumb</u>

T23.421- Corrosion of unspecified degree of single <u>right</u> finger (nail) except thumb

T23.422- Corrosion of unspecified degree of single <u>left</u> finger (nail) except thumb

T23.429- Corrosion of unspecified degree of <u>unspecified</u> single finger (nail) except thumb

T23.43- <u>Corrosion</u> of <u>unspecified degree</u> of <u>multiple</u> fingers (nail), <u>not including thumb</u>

T23.431- Corrosion of unspecified degree of multiple <u>right</u> fingers (nail), not including thumb

T23.432- Corrosion of unspecified degree of multiple <u>left</u> fingers (nail), not including thumb

T23.439- Corrosion of unspecified degree of <u>unspecified</u> multiple fingers (nail), not including thumb

T23.44- <u>Corrosion</u> of <u>unspecified degree</u> of <u>multiple</u> fingers (nail), <u>including thumb</u>

T23.441- Corrosion of unspecified degree of multiple <u>right</u> fingers (nail), including thumb

T23.442- Corrosion of unspecified degree of multiple <u>left</u> fingers (nail), including thumb

T23.449- Corrosion of unspecified degree of <u>unspecified</u> multiple fingers (nail), including thumb

T23.45- <u>Corrosion</u> of <u>unspecified degree</u> of <u>palm</u>

T23.451- Corrosion of unspecified degree of <u>right</u> palm

T23.452- Corrosion of unspecified degree of <u>left</u> palm

T23.459- Corrosion of unspecified degree of <u>unspecified</u> palm

T23.46- <u>Corrosion</u> of <u>unspecified degree</u> of <u>back of hand</u>

T23.461- Corrosion of unspecified degree of back of <u>right</u> hand

T23.462- Corrosion of unspecified degree of back of <u>left</u> hand

T23.469- Corrosion of unspecified degree of back of <u>unspecified</u> hand

T23.47- <u>Corrosion</u> of <u>unspecified degree</u> of <u>wrist</u>

T23.471- Corrosion of unspecified degree of <u>right</u> wrist

T23.472- Corrosion of unspecified degree of <u>left</u> wrist

T23.479- Corrosion of unspecified degree of <u>unspecified</u> wrist

T23.49- <u>Corrosion</u> of <u>unspecified degree</u> of <u>multiple</u> sites of <u>wrist and hand</u>

T23.491- Corrosion of unspecified degree of multiple sites of <u>right</u> wrist and hand

T23.492- Corrosion of unspecified degree of multiple sites of <u>left</u> wrist and hand

T23.499- Corrosion of unspecified degree of multiple sites of <u>unspecified</u> wrist and hand

T23.5- <u>Corrosion</u> of <u>first</u> degree of <u>wrist and hand</u>
Code first (T51-T65) to identify chemical and intent
Use additional external cause code to identify place (Y92)

T23.50- <u>Corrosion</u> of <u>first</u> degree of hand, <u>unspecified</u> site

T23.501- Corrosion of first degree of <u>right</u> hand, unspecified site

T23.502- Corrosion of first degree of <u>left</u> hand, unspecified site

T23.509- Corrosion of first degree of <u>unspecified</u> hand, unspecified site

T23.51- <u>Corrosion</u> of <u>first</u> degree of <u>thumb</u> (nail)

T23.511- Corrosion of first degree of <u>right</u> thumb (nail)

T23-T23

T23.512- Corrosion of first degree of <u>left</u> thumb (nail)

T23.519- Corrosion of first degree of <u>unspecified</u> thumb (nail)

T23.52- <u>Corrosion</u> of <u>first</u> degree of <u>single finger</u> (nail) <u>except thumb</u>

T23.521- Corrosion of first degree of single <u>right</u> finger (nail) except thumb

T23.522- Corrosion of first degree of single <u>left</u> finger (nail) except thumb

T23.529- Corrosion of first degree of <u>unspecified</u> single finger (nail) except thumb

T23.53- <u>Corrosion</u> of <u>first</u> degree of <u>multiple fingers</u> (nail), <u>not including thumb</u>

T23.531- Corrosion of first degree of multiple <u>right</u> fingers (nail), not including thumb

T23.532- Corrosion of first degree of multiple <u>left</u> fingers (nail), not including thumb

T23.539- Corrosion of first degree of <u>unspecified</u> multiple fingers (nail), not including thumb

T23.54- <u>Corrosion</u> of <u>first</u> degree of <u>multiple fingers</u> (nail), <u>including thumb</u>

T23.541- Corrosion of first degree of multiple <u>right</u> fingers (nail), including thumb

T23.542- Corrosion of first degree of multiple <u>left</u> fingers (nail), including thumb

T23.549- Corrosion of first degree of <u>unspecified</u> multiple fingers (nail), including thumb

T23.55- <u>Corrosion</u> of <u>first</u> degree of <u>palm</u>

T23.551- Corrosion of first degree of <u>right</u> palm

T23.552- Corrosion of first degree of <u>left</u> palm

T23.559- Corrosion of first degree of <u>unspecified</u> palm

T23.56- <u>Corrosion</u> of <u>first</u> degree of <u>back of hand</u>

T23.561- Corrosion of first degree of back of <u>right</u> hand

T23.562- Corrosion of first degree of back of <u>left</u> hand

T23.569- Corrosion of first degree of back of <u>unspecified</u> hand

T23.57- <u>Corrosion</u> of <u>first</u> degree of <u>wrist</u>

T23.571- Corrosion of first degree of <u>right</u> wrist

T23.572- Corrosion of first degree of <u>left</u> wrist

T23.579- Corrosion of first degree of <u>unspecified</u> wrist

T23.59- <u>Corrosion</u> of <u>first</u> degree of <u>multiple</u> sites of <u>wrist and hand</u>

T23.591- Corrosion of first degree of multiple sites of <u>right</u> wrist and hand

T23.592- Corrosion of first degree of multiple sites of <u>left</u> wrist and hand

T23.599- Corrosion of first degree of multiple sites of <u>unspecified</u> wrist and hand

T23.6- <u>Corrosion</u> of <u>second</u> degree of <u>wrist and hand</u>
Code first (T51-T65) to identify chemical and intent
Use additional external cause code to identify place (Y92)

T23.60- <u>Corrosion</u> of <u>second</u> degree of hand, <u>unspecified</u> site

T23.601- Corrosion of second degree of <u>right</u> hand, unspecified site

T23.602- Corrosion of second degree of <u>left</u> hand, unspecified site

T23.609- Corrosion of second degree of <u>unspecified</u> hand, unspecified site

T23.61- <u>Corrosion</u> of <u>second</u> degree of <u>thumb</u> (nail)

T23.611- Corrosion of second degree of <u>right</u> thumb (nail)

T23.612- Corrosion of second degree of <u>left</u> thumb (nail)

T23.619- Corrosion of second degree of <u>unspecified</u> thumb (nail)

T23.62- <u>Corrosion</u> of <u>second</u> degree of <u>single finger</u> (nail) <u>except thumb</u>

T23.621- Corrosion of second degree of single <u>right</u> finger (nail) except thumb

T23.622- Corrosion of second degree of single <u>left</u> finger (nail) except thumb

T23.629- Corrosion of second degree of <u>unspecified</u> single finger (nail) except thumb

T23.63- <u>Corrosion</u> of <u>second</u> degree of <u>multiple fingers</u> (nail), <u>not including thumb</u>

T23.631- Corrosion of second degree of multiple <u>right</u> fingers (nail), not including thumb

T23.632- Corrosion of second degree of multiple <u>left</u> fingers (nail), not including thumb

T23.639- Corrosion of second degree of <u>unspecified</u> multiple fingers (nail), not including thumb

T23.64- <u>Corrosion</u> of <u>second</u> degree of <u>multiple fingers</u> (nail), <u>including thumb</u>

T23.641- Corrosion of second degree of multiple <u>right</u> fingers (nail), including thumb

T23.642- Corrosion of second degree of multiple <u>left</u> fingers (nail), including thumb

T23.649- Corrosion of second degree of <u>unspecified</u> multiple fingers (nail), including thumb

T23.65- <u>Corrosion</u> of <u>second</u> degree of <u>palm</u>

T23.651- Corrosion of second degree of <u>right</u> palm

T23.652- Corrosion of second degree of <u>left</u> palm

T23.659- Corrosion of second degree of <u>unspecified</u> palm

T23.66- <u>Corrosion</u> of <u>second</u> degree of <u>back of hand</u>

T23.661- Corrosion of second degree back of <u>right</u> hand

T23.662- Corrosion of second degree back of <u>left</u> hand

T23.669- Corrosion of second degree back of <u>unspecified</u> hand

T23.67- <u>Corrosion</u> of <u>second</u> degree of <u>wrist</u>

T23.671- Corrosion of second degree of <u>right</u> wrist

T23.672- Corrosion of second degree of <u>left</u> wrist

T23.679- Corrosion of second degree of <u>unspecified</u> wrist

T23.69- <u>Corrosion</u> of <u>second</u> degree of <u>multiple</u> sites of <u>wrist and hand</u>

T23.691- Corrosion of second degree of multiple sites of <u>right</u> wrist and hand

T23.692- Corrosion of second degree of multiple sites of <u>left</u> wrist and hand

T23.699- Corrosion of second degree of multiple sites of <u>unspecified</u> wrist and hand

T23.7- <u>Corrosion</u> of <u>third</u> degree of <u>wrist and hand</u>
Code first (T51-T65) to identify chemical and intent
Use additional external cause code to identify place (Y92)

T23.70- <u>Corrosion</u> of <u>third</u> degree of hand, <u>unspecified</u> site

CC-A **T23.701-** Corrosion of third degree of <u>right</u> hand, unspecified site

CC-A **T23.702-** Corrosion of third degree of <u>left</u> hand, unspecified site

CC-A **T23.709-** Corrosion of third degree of <u>unspecified</u> hand, unspecified site

T23.71- <u>Corrosion</u> of <u>third</u> degree of <u>thumb</u> (nail)

CC-A **T23.711-** Corrosion of third degree of <u>right</u> thumb (nail)

CC-A **T23.712-** Corrosion of third degree of <u>left</u> thumb (nail)

CC-A **T23.719-** Corrosion of third degree of <u>unspecified</u> thumb (nail)

T23.72- <u>Corrosion</u> of <u>third</u> degree of <u>single finger</u> (nail) <u>except thumb</u>

CC-A **T23.721-** Corrosion of third degree of single <u>right</u> finger (nail) except thumb

CC-A **T23.722-** Corrosion of third degree of single <u>left</u> finger (nail) except thumb

CC-A **T23.729-** Corrosion of third degree of <u>unspecified</u> single finger (nail) except thumb

T23.73- <u>Corrosion</u> of <u>third</u> degree of <u>multiple fingers</u> (nail), <u>not including thumb</u>

CC-A **T23.731-** Corrosion of third degree of multiple <u>right</u> fingers (nail), not including thumb

T23 - T23

CC-A **T23.732-** Corrosion of third degree of multiple <u>left</u> fingers (nail), not including thumb

CC-A **T23.739-** Corrosion of third degree of <u>unspecified</u> multiple fingers (nail), not including thumb

T23.74- <u>Corrosion</u> of <u>third</u> degree of <u>multiple fingers</u> (nail), <u>including thumb</u>

CC-A **T23.741-** Corrosion of third degree of multiple <u>right</u> fingers (nail), including thumb

CC-A **T23.742-** Corrosion of third degree of multiple <u>left</u> fingers (nail), including thumb

CC-A **T23.749-** Corrosion of third degree of <u>unspecified</u> multiple fingers (nail), including thumb

T23.75- <u>Corrosion</u> of <u>third</u> degree of <u>palm</u>

CC-A **T23.751-** Corrosion of third degree of <u>right</u> palm

CC-A **T23.752-** Corrosion of third degree of <u>left</u> palm

CC-A **T23.759-** Corrosion of third degree of <u>unspecified</u> palm

T23.76- <u>Corrosion</u> of <u>third</u> degree of <u>back of hand</u>

CC-A **T23.761-** Corrosion of third degree of back of <u>right</u> hand

CC-A **T23.762-** Corrosion of third degree of back of <u>left</u> hand

CC-A **T23.769-** Corrosion of third degree back of <u>unspecified</u> hand

T23.77- <u>Corrosion</u> of <u>third</u> degree of <u>wrist</u>

CC-A **T23.771-** Corrosion of third degree of <u>right</u> wrist

CC-A **T23.772-** Corrosion of third degree of <u>left</u> wrist

CC-A **T23.779-** Corrosion of third degree of <u>unspecified</u> wrist

T23.79- <u>Corrosion</u> of <u>third</u> degree of <u>multiple</u> sites of <u>wrist and hand</u>

CC-A **T23.791-** Corrosion of third degree of multiple sites of <u>right</u> wrist and hand

CC-A **T23.792-** Corrosion of third degree of multiple sites of <u>left</u> wrist and hand

CC-A **T23.799-** Corrosion of third degree of multiple sites of <u>unspecified</u> wrist and hand

T24- <u>Burn and corrosion</u> of <u>lower limb</u>, <u>except ankle and foot</u>
Excludes ❷: burn and corrosion of ankle and foot (T25.-)
burn and corrosion of hip region (T21.-)

The appropriate 7th character is to be added to each code from category T24:
A <u>Initial</u> encounter
D <u>Subsequent</u> encounter
S <u>Sequela</u>

T24.0- Burn of <u>unspecified degree</u> of <u>lower limb</u>, <u>except ankle and foot</u>
Use additional external cause code to identify the source, place and intent of the burn (X00-X19, X75-X77, X96-X98, Y92)

T24.00- Burn of <u>unspecified degree</u> of <u>unspecified</u> site of <u>lower limb</u>, <u>except ankle and foot</u>

T24.001- Burn of unspecified degree of unspecified site of <u>right</u> lower limb, except ankle and foot

T24.002- Burn of unspecified degree of unspecified site of <u>left</u> lower limb, except ankle and foot

T24.009- Burn of unspecified degree of unspecified site of <u>unspecified</u> lower limb, except ankle and foot

T24.01- Burn of <u>unspecified degree</u> of <u>thigh</u>

T24.011- Burn of unspecified degree of <u>right</u> thigh

T24.012- Burn of unspecified degree of <u>left</u> thigh

T24.019- Burn of unspecified degree of <u>unspecified</u> thigh

T24.02- Burn of <u>unspecified degree</u> of <u>knee</u>

T24.021- Burn of unspecified degree of <u>right</u> knee

T24.022- Burn of unspecified degree of <u>left</u> knee

T24.029- Burn of unspecified degree of <u>unspecified</u> knee

T24.03- Burn of <u>unspecified degree</u> of <u>lower leg</u>

T24.031- Burn of unspecified degree of <u>right</u> lower leg

T24.032- Burn of unspecified degree of <u>left</u> lower leg

T24.039- Burn of unspecified degree of <u>unspecified</u> lower leg

T24.09- Burn of <u>unspecified degree</u> of <u>multiple</u> sites of <u>lower limb</u>, <u>except ankle and foot</u>

T24.091- Burn of unspecified degree of multiple sites of <u>right</u> lower limb, except ankle and foot

T24.092- Burn of unspecified degree of multiple sites of <u>left</u> lower limb, except ankle and foot

T24.099- Burn of unspecified degree of multiple sites of <u>unspecified</u> lower limb, except ankle and foot

T24.1- Burn of <u>first</u> degree of <u>lower limb</u>, <u>except ankle and foot</u>
Use additional external cause code to identify the source, place and intent of the burn (X00-X19, X75-X77, X96-X98, Y92)

T24.10- Burn of <u>first</u> degree of <u>unspecified</u> site of <u>lower limb</u>, <u>except ankle and foot</u>

T24.101- Burn of first degree of unspecified site of <u>right</u> lower limb, except ankle and foot

T24.102- Burn of first degree of unspecified site of <u>left</u> lower limb, except ankle and foot

T24.109- Burn of first degree of unspecified site of <u>unspecified</u> lower limb, except ankle and foot

T24.11- Burn of <u>first</u> degree of <u>thigh</u>

T24.111- Burn of first degree of <u>right</u> thigh

T24.112- Burn of first degree of <u>left</u> thigh

T24.119- Burn of first degree of <u>unspecified</u> thigh

T24.12- Burn of <u>first</u> degree of <u>knee</u>

T24.121- Burn of first degree of <u>right</u> knee

T24.122- Burn of first degree of <u>left</u> knee

T24.129- Burn of first degree of <u>unspecified</u> knee

T24.13- Burn of <u>first</u> degree of <u>lower leg</u>

T24.131- Burn of first degree of <u>right</u> lower leg

T24.132- Burn of first degree of <u>left</u> lower leg

T24.139- Burn of first degree of <u>unspecified</u> lower leg

T24.19- Burn of <u>first</u> degree of <u>multiple</u> sites of <u>lower limb</u>, <u>except ankle and foot</u>

T24.191- Burn of first degree of multiple sites of <u>right</u> lower limb, except ankle and foot

T24.192- Burn of first degree of multiple sites of <u>left</u> lower limb, except ankle and foot

T24.199- Burn of first degree of multiple sites of <u>unspecified</u> lower limb, except ankle and foot

T24.2- Burn of <u>second</u> degree of <u>lower limb</u>, <u>except ankle and foot</u>
Use additional external cause code to identify the source, place and intent of the burn (X00-X19, X75-X77, X96-X98, Y92)

T24.20- Burn of <u>second</u> degree of <u>unspecified</u> site of <u>lower limb</u>, <u>except ankle and foot</u>

T24.201- Burn of second degree of unspecified site of <u>right</u> lower limb, except ankle and foot

T24.202- Burn of second degree of unspecified site of <u>left</u> lower limb, except ankle and foot

T24.209- Burn of second degree of unspecified site of <u>unspecified</u> lower limb, except ankle and foot

T24.21- Burn of <u>second</u> degree of <u>thigh</u>

T24.211- Burn of second degree of <u>right</u> thigh

T24.212- Burn of second degree of <u>left</u> thigh

T24.219- Burn of second degree of <u>unspecified</u> thigh

T24.22- Burn of <u>second</u> degree of <u>knee</u>

T24.221- Burn of second degree of <u>right</u> knee

T24.222- Burn of second degree of <u>left</u> knee

T24.229- Burn of second degree of <u>unspecified</u> knee

T24.23- Burn of <u>second</u> degree of <u>lower leg</u>

T24.231- Burn of second degree of <u>right</u> lower leg

T24.232- Burn of second degree of <u>left</u> lower leg

T24.239- Burn of second degree of <u>unspecified</u> lower leg

T24.29- Burn of <u>second</u> degree of <u>multiple</u> sites of <u>lower limb</u>, <u>except ankle and foot</u>

T24.291- Burn of second degree of multiple sites of <u>right</u> lower limb, except ankle and foot

T24.292- Burn of second degree of multiple sites of <u>left</u> lower limb, except ankle and foot

T24.299- Burn of second degree of multiple sites of <u>unspecified</u> lower limb, except ankle and foot

T24.3- Burn of <u>third</u> degree of <u>lower limb</u>, <u>except ankle and foot</u>
Use additional external cause code to identify the source, place and intent of the burn (X00-X19, X75-X77, X96-X98, Y92)

T24.30- Burn of <u>third</u> degree of <u>unspecified</u> site of <u>lower limb</u>, <u>except ankle and foot</u>

CC-A **T24.301-** Burn of third degree of <u>unspecified</u> site of <u>right</u> lower limb, except ankle and foot

CC-A **T24.302-** Burn of third degree of <u>unspecified</u> site of <u>left</u> lower limb, except ankle and foot

CC-A **T24.309-** Burn of third degree of <u>unspecified</u> site of <u>unspecified</u> lower limb, except ankle and foot

T24.31- Burn of <u>third</u> degree of <u>thigh</u>

CC-A **T24.311-** Burn of third degree of <u>right</u> thigh

CC-A **T24.312-** Burn of third degree of <u>left</u> thigh

CC-A **T24.319-** Burn of third degree of <u>unspecified</u> thigh

T24.32- Burn of <u>third</u> degree of <u>knee</u>

CC-A **T24.321-** Burn of third degree of <u>right</u> knee

CC-A **T24.322-** Burn of third degree of <u>left</u> knee

CC-A **T24.329-** Burn of third degree of <u>unspecified</u> knee

T24.33- Burn of <u>third</u> degree of <u>lower leg</u>

CC-A **T24.331-** Burn of third degree of <u>right</u> lower leg

CC-A **T24.332-** Burn of third degree of <u>left</u> lower leg

CC-A **T24.339-** Burn of third degree of <u>unspecified</u> lower leg

T24.39- Burn of <u>third</u> degree of <u>multiple</u> sites of <u>lower limb</u>, <u>except ankle and foot</u>

CC-A **T24.391-** Burn of third degree of multiple sites of <u>right</u> lower limb, except ankle and foot

CC-A **T24.392-** Burn of third degree of multiple sites of <u>left</u> lower limb, except ankle and foot

CC-A **T24.399-** Burn of third degree of multiple sites of <u>unspecified</u> lower limb, except ankle and foot

T24.4- <u>Corrosion</u> of <u>unspecified degree</u> of <u>lower limb</u>, <u>except ankle and foot</u>
Code first (T51-T65) to identify chemical and intent
Use additional external cause code to identify place (Y92)

T24.40- <u>Corrosion</u> of <u>unspecified degree</u> of <u>unspecified</u> site of <u>lower limb</u>, <u>except ankle and foot</u>

T24.401- Corrosion of unspecified degree of <u>unspecified</u> site of <u>right</u> lower limb, except ankle and foot

T24.402- Corrosion of unspecified degree of <u>unspecified</u> site of <u>left</u> lower limb, except ankle and foot

T24.409- Corrosion of unspecified degree of <u>unspecified</u> site of <u>unspecified</u> lower limb, except ankle and foot

T24.41- <u>Corrosion</u> of <u>unspecified degree</u> of <u>thigh</u>

T24.411- Corrosion of unspecified degree of <u>right</u> thigh

T24.412- Corrosion of unspecified degree of <u>left</u> thigh

T24.419- Corrosion of unspecified degree of <u>unspecified</u> thigh

T24.42- <u>Corrosion</u> of <u>unspecified degree</u> of <u>knee</u>

T24.421- Corrosion of unspecified degree of <u>right</u> knee

T24.422- Corrosion of unspecified degree of <u>left</u> knee

T24.429- Corrosion of unspecified degree of <u>unspecified</u> knee

T24.43- <u>Corrosion</u> of <u>unspecified degree</u> of <u>lower leg</u>

T24.431- Corrosion of unspecified degree of <u>right</u> lower leg

T24.432- Corrosion of unspecified degree of <u>left</u> lower leg

T24.439- Corrosion of unspecified degree of <u>unspecified</u> lower leg

T24.49- <u>Corrosion</u> of <u>unspecified degree</u> of <u>multiple</u> sites of <u>lower limb</u>, <u>except ankle and foot</u>

T24.491- Corrosion of unspecified degree of multiple sites of <u>right</u> lower limb, except ankle and foot

T24.492- Corrosion of unspecified degree of multiple sites of <u>left</u> lower limb, except ankle and foot

T24.499- Corrosion of unspecified degree of multiple sites of <u>unspecified</u> lower limb, except ankle and foot

T24.5- <u>Corrosion</u> of <u>first</u> degree of <u>lower limb</u>, <u>except ankle and foot</u>
Code first (T51-T65) to identify chemical and intent
Use additional external cause code to identify place (Y92)

T24.50- <u>Corrosion</u> of <u>first</u> degree of <u>unspecified</u> site of <u>lower limb</u>, <u>except ankle and foot</u>

T24.501- Corrosion of first degree of unspecified site of <u>right</u> lower limb, except ankle and foot

T24.502- Corrosion of first degree of unspecified site of <u>left</u> lower limb, except ankle and foot

T24.509- Corrosion of first degree of unspecified site of <u>unspecified</u> lower limb, except ankle and foot

T24.51- <u>Corrosion</u> of <u>first</u> degree of <u>thigh</u>

T24.511- Corrosion of first degree of <u>right</u> thigh

T24.512- Corrosion of first degree of <u>left</u> thigh

T24.519- Corrosion of first degree of <u>unspecified</u> thigh

T24.52- <u>Corrosion</u> of <u>first</u> degree of <u>knee</u>

T24.521- Corrosion of first degree of <u>right</u> knee

T24.522- Corrosion of first degree of <u>left</u> knee

T24.529- Corrosion of first degree of <u>unspecified</u> knee

T24.53- <u>Corrosion</u> of <u>first</u> degree of <u>lower leg</u>

T24.531- Corrosion of first degree of <u>right</u> lower leg

T24.532- Corrosion of first degree of <u>left</u> lower leg

T24.539- Corrosion of first degree of <u>unspecified</u> lower leg

T24.59- <u>Corrosion</u> of <u>first</u> degree of <u>multiple</u> sites of <u>lower limb</u>, <u>except ankle and foot</u>

T24.591- Corrosion of first degree of multiple sites of <u>right</u> lower limb, except ankle and foot

T24.592- Corrosion of first degree of multiple sites of <u>left</u> lower limb, except ankle and foot

T24.599- Corrosion of first degree of multiple sites of <u>unspecified</u> lower limb, except ankle and foot

T24.6- <u>Corrosion</u> of <u>second</u> degree of <u>lower limb</u>, <u>except ankle and foot</u>
Code first (T51-T65) to identify chemical and intent
Use additional external cause code to identify place (Y92)

T24.60- <u>Corrosion</u> of <u>second</u> degree of <u>unspecified</u> site of <u>lower limb</u>, <u>except ankle and foot</u>

T24.601- Corrosion of second degree of unspecified site of <u>right</u> lower limb, except ankle and foot

T24.602- Corrosion of second degree of unspecified site of <u>left</u> lower limb, except ankle and foot

T24.609- Corrosion of second degree of unspecified site of <u>unspecified</u> lower limb, except ankle and foot

T24.61- <u>Corrosion</u> of <u>second</u> degree of <u>thigh</u>

T24.611- Corrosion of second degree of <u>right</u> thigh

T24.612- Corrosion of second degree of <u>left</u> thigh

T24.619- Corrosion of second degree of <u>unspecified</u> thigh

T24.62- <u>Corrosion</u> of <u>second</u> degree of <u>knee</u>

T24.621- Corrosion of second degree of <u>right</u> knee

T24.622- Corrosion of second degree of <u>left</u> knee

T24.629- Corrosion of second degree of <u>unspecified</u> knee

T24.63- <u>Corrosion</u> of <u>second</u> degree of <u>lower leg</u>

T24.631- Corrosion of second degree of <u>right</u> lower leg

T24.632- Corrosion of second degree of <u>left</u> lower leg

T24.639- Corrosion of second degree of <u>unspecified</u> lower leg

T24.69- <u>Corrosion</u> of <u>second</u> degree of <u>multiple</u> sites of <u>lower limb</u>, <u>except ankle and foot</u>

T24.691- Corrosion of second degree of multiple sites of <u>right</u> lower limb, except ankle and foot

T24.692- Corrosion of second degree of multiple sites of <u>left</u> lower limb, except ankle and foot

T24.699- Corrosion of second degree of multiple sites of <u>unspecified</u> lower limb, except ankle and foot

T24.7- Corrosion of third degree of lower limb, except ankle and foot
Code first (T51-T65) to identify chemical and intent
Use additional external cause code to identify place (Y92)

T24.70- Corrosion of third degree of unspecified site of lower limb, except ankle and foot

CC-A **T24.701-** Corrosion of third degree of unspecified site of right lower limb, except ankle and foot

CC-A **T24.702-** Corrosion of third degree of unspecified site of left lower limb, except ankle and foot

CC-A **T24.709-** Corrosion of third degree of unspecified site of unspecified lower limb, except ankle and foot

T24.71- Corrosion of third degree of thigh

CC-A **T24.711-** Corrosion of third degree of right thigh

CC-A **T24.712-** Corrosion of third degree of left thigh

CC-A **T24.719-** Corrosion of third degree of unspecified thigh

T24.72- Corrosion of third degree of knee

CC-A **T24.721-** Corrosion of third degree of right knee

CC-A **T24.722-** Corrosion of third degree of left knee

CC-A **T24.729-** Corrosion of third degree of unspecified knee

T24.73- Corrosion of third degree of lower leg

CC-A **T24.731-** Corrosion of third degree of right lower leg

CC-A **T24.732-** Corrosion of third degree of left lower leg

CC-A **T24.739-** Corrosion of third degree of unspecified lower leg

T24.79- Corrosion of third degree of multiple sites of lower limb, except ankle and foot

CC-A **T24.791-** Corrosion of third degree of multiple sites of right lower limb, except ankle and foot

CC-A **T24.792-** Corrosion of third degree of multiple sites of left lower limb, except ankle and foot

CC-A **T24.799-** Corrosion of third degree of multiple sites of unspecified lower limb, except ankle and foot

T25- Burn and corrosion of ankle and foot
The appropriate 7th character is to be added to each code from category T25:
A Initial encounter
D Subsequent encounter
S Sequela

T25.0- Burn of unspecified degree of ankle and foot
Use additional external cause code to identify the source, place and intent of the burn (X00-X19, X75-X77, X96-X98, Y92)

T25.01- Burn of unspecified degree of ankle

T25.011- Burn of unspecified degree of right ankle

T25.012- Burn of unspecified degree of left ankle

T25.019- Burn of unspecified degree of unspecified ankle

T25.02- Burn of unspecified degree of foot
Excludes ❷: burn of unspecified degree of toe(s) (nail) (T25.03-)

T25.021- Burn of unspecified degree of right foot

T25.022- Burn of unspecified degree of left foot

T25.029- Burn of unspecified degree of unspecified foot

T25.03- Burn of unspecified degree of toe(s) (nail)

T25.031- Burn of unspecified degree of right toe(s) (nail)

T25.032- Burn of unspecified degree of left toe(s) (nail)

T25.039- Burn of unspecified degree of unspecified toe(s) (nail)

T25.09- Burn of unspecified degree of multiple sites of ankle and foot

T25.091- Burn of unspecified degree of multiple sites of right ankle and foot

T25.092- Burn of unspecified degree of multiple sites of left ankle and foot

T25.099- Burn of unspecified degree of multiple sites of unspecified ankle and foot

T25.1- Burn of first degree of ankle and foot
Use additional external cause code to identify the source, place and intent of the burn (X00-X19, X75-X77, X96-X98, Y92)

T25.11- Burn of first degree of ankle

T25.111- Burn of first degree of right ankle

T25.112- Burn of first degree of left ankle

T25.119- Burn of first degree of unspecified ankle

T25.12- Burn of first degree of foot
Excludes ❷: burn of first degree of toe(s) (nail) (T25.13-)

T25.121- Burn of first degree of right foot

T25.122- Burn of first degree of left foot

T25.129- Burn of first degree of unspecified foot

T25.13- Burn of first degree of toe(s) (nail)

T25.131- Burn of first degree of right toe(s) (nail)

T25.132- Burn of first degree of left toe(s) (nail)

T25.139- Burn of first degree of unspecified toe(s) (nail)

T25.19- Burn of first degree of multiple sites of ankle and foot

T25.191- Burn of first degree of multiple sites of right ankle and foot

T25.192- Burn of first degree of multiple sites of left ankle and foot

T25.199- Burn of first degree of multiple sites of unspecified ankle and foot

T25.2- Burn of second degree of ankle and foot
Use additional external cause code to identify the source, place and intent of the burn (X00-X19, X75-X77, X96-X98, Y92)

T25.21- Burn of second degree of ankle

T25.211- Burn of second degree of right ankle

T25.212- Burn of second degree of left ankle

T25.219- Burn of second degree of unspecified ankle

T25.22- Burn of second degree of foot
Excludes ❷: burn of second degree of toe(s) (nail) (T25.23-)

T25.221- Burn of second degree of right foot

T25.222- Burn of second degree of left foot

T25.229- Burn of second degree of unspecified foot

T25.23- Burn of second degree of toe(s) (nail)

T25.231- Burn of second degree of right toe(s) (nail)

T25.232- Burn of second degree of left toe(s) (nail)

T25.239- Burn of second degree of unspecified toe(s) (nail)

T25.29- Burn of second degree of multiple sites of ankle and foot

T25.291- Burn of second degree of multiple sites of right ankle and foot

T25.292- Burn of second degree of multiple sites of left ankle and foot

T25.299- Burn of second degree of multiple sites of unspecified ankle and foot

T25.3- Burn of third degree of ankle and foot
Use additional external cause code to identify the source, place and intent of the burn (X00-X19, X75-X77, X96-X98, Y92)

T25.31- Burn of third degree of ankle

CC-A **T25.311-** Burn of third degree of right ankle

CC-A **T25.312-** Burn of third degree of left ankle

CC-A **T25.319-** Burn of third degree of unspecified ankle

T25.32- Burn of third degree of foot
Excludes ❷: burn of third degree of toe(s) (nail) (T25.33-)

CC-A **T25.321-** Burn of third degree of right foot

CC-A **T25.322-** Burn of third degree of left foot

CC-A **T25.329-** Burn of third degree of unspecified foot

T25.33- Burn of third degree of toe(s) (nail)

CC-A **T25.331-** Burn of third degree of right toe(s) (nail)

CC-A **T25.332-** Burn of third degree of left toe(s) (nail)

CC-A **T25.339-** Burn of third degree of unspecified toe(s) (nail)

T25.39- Burn of third degree of multiple sites of ankle and foot

CC-A **T25.391-** Burn of third degree of multiple sites of right ankle and foot

CC-A **T25.392-** Burn of third degree of multiple sites of left ankle and foot

CC-A **T25.399-** Burn of third degree of multiple sites of unspecified ankle and foot

T24-T25

T25.4-　Corrosion of unspecified degree of ankle and foot
Code first (T51-T65) to identify chemical and intent
Use additional external cause code to identify place (Y92)

T25.41-　Corrosion of unspecified degree of ankle

T25.411-　Corrosion of unspecified degree of right ankle

T25.412-　Corrosion of unspecified degree of left ankle

T25.419-　Corrosion of unspecified degree of unspecified ankle

T25.42-　Corrosion of unspecified degree of foot
Excludes ❷:　corrosion of unspecified degree of toe(s) (nail) (T25.43-)

T25.421-　Corrosion of unspecified degree of right foot

T25.422-　Corrosion of unspecified degree of left foot

T25.429-　Corrosion of unspecified degree of unspecified foot

T25.43-　Corrosion of unspecified degree of toe(s) (nail)

T25.431-　Corrosion of unspecified degree of right toe(s) (nail)

T25.432-　Corrosion of unspecified degree of left toe(s) (nail)

T25.439-　Corrosion of unspecified degree of unspecified toe(s) (nail)

T25.49-　Corrosion of unspecified degree of multiple sites of ankle and foot

T25.491-　Corrosion of unspecified degree of multiple sites of right ankle and foot

T25.492-　Corrosion of unspecified degree of multiple sites of left ankle and foot

T25.499-　Corrosion of unspecified degree of multiple sites of unspecified ankle and foot

T25.5-　Corrosion of first degree of ankle and foot
Code first (T51-T65) to identify chemical and intent
Use additional external cause code to identify place (Y92)

T25.51-　Corrosion of first degree of ankle

T25.511-　Corrosion of first degree of right ankle

T25.512-　Corrosion of first degree of left ankle

T25.519-　Corrosion of first degree of unspecified ankle

T25.52-　Corrosion of first degree of foot
Excludes ❷:　corrosion of first degree of toe(s) (nail) (T25.53-)

T25.521-　Corrosion of first degree of right foot

T25.522-　Corrosion of first degree of left foot

T25.529-　Corrosion of first degree of unspecified foot

T25.53-　Corrosion of first degree of toe(s) (nail)

T25.531-　Corrosion of first degree of right toe(s) (nail)

T25.532-　Corrosion of first degree of left toe(s) (nail)

T25.539-　Corrosion of first degree of unspecified toe(s) (nail)

T25.59-　Corrosion of first degree of multiple sites of ankle and foot

T25.591-　Corrosion of first degree of multiple sites of right ankle and foot

T25.592-　Corrosion of first degree of multiple sites of left ankle and foot

T25.599-　Corrosion of first degree of multiple sites of unspecified ankle and foot

T25.6-　Corrosion of second degree of ankle and foot
Code first (T51-T65) to identify chemical and intent
Use additional external cause code to identify place (Y92)

T25.61-　Corrosion of second degree of ankle

T25.611-　Corrosion of second degree of right ankle

T25.612-　Corrosion of second degree of left ankle

T25.619-　Corrosion of second degree of unspecified ankle

T25.62-　Corrosion of second degree of foot
Excludes ❷:　corrosion of second degree of toe(s) (nail) (T25.63-)

T25.621-　Corrosion of second degree of right foot

T25.622-　Corrosion of second degree of left foot

T25.629-　Corrosion of second degree of unspecified foot

T25.63-　Corrosion of second degree of toe(s) (nail)

T25.631-　Corrosion of second degree of right toe(s) (nail)

T25.632-　Corrosion of second degree of left toe(s) (nail)

T25.639-　Corrosion of second degree of unspecified toe(s) (nail)

T25.69　Corrosion of second degree of multiple sites of ankle and foot

T25.691-　Corrosion of second degree of right ankle and foot

T25.692-　Corrosion of second degree of left ankle and foot

T25.699-　Corrosion of second degree of unspecified ankle and foot

T25.7-　Corrosion of third degree of ankle and foot
Code first (T51-T65) to identify chemical and intent
Use additional external cause code to identify place (Y92)

T25.71-　Corrosion of third degree of ankle

CC-A T25.711-　Corrosion of third degree of right ankle

CC-A T25.712-　Corrosion of third degree of left ankle

CC-A T25.719-　Corrosion of third degree of unspecified ankle

T25.72-　Corrosion of third degree of foot
Excludes ❷: corrosion of third degree of toe(s) (nail) (T25.73-)

CC-A T25.721-　Corrosion of third degree of right foot

CC-A T25.722-　Corrosion of third degree of left foot

CC-A T25.729-　Corrosion of third degree of unspecified foot

T25.73-　Corrosion of third degree of toe(s) (nail)

CC-A T25.731-　Corrosion of third degree of right toe(s) (nail)

CC-A T25.732-　Corrosion of third degree of left toe(s) (nail)

CC-A T25.739-　Corrosion of third degree of unspecified toe(s) (nail)

T25.79-　Corrosion of third degree of multiple sites of ankle and foot

CC-A T25.791-　Corrosion of third degree of multiple sites of right ankle and foot

CC-A T25.792-　Corrosion of third degree of multiple sites of left ankle and foot

CC-A T25.799-　Corrosion of third degree of multiple sites of unspecified ankle and foot

Burns and corrosions confined to eye and internal organs (T26-T28)

T26-　Burn and corrosion confined to eye and adnexa
The appropriate 7th character is to be added to each code from category T26:
A　Initial encounter
D　Subsequent encounter
S　Sequela

T26.0-　Burn of eyelid and periocular area
Use additional external cause code to identify the source, place and intent of the burn (X00-X19, X75-X77, X96-X98, Y92)

T26.00x-　Burn of unspecified eyelid and periocular area

T26.01x-　Burn of right eyelid and periocular area

T26.02x-　Burn of left eyelid and periocular area

T26.1-　Burn of cornea and conjunctival sac
Use additional external cause code to identify the source, place and intent of the burn (X00-X19, X75-X77, X96-X98, Y92)

T26.10x-　Burn of cornea and conjunctival sac, unspecified eye

T26.11x-　Burn of cornea and conjunctival sac, right eye

T26.12x-　Burn of cornea and conjunctival sac, left eye

T26.2-　Burn with resulting rupture and destruction of eyeball
Use additional external cause code to identify the source, place and intent of the burn (X00-X19, X75-X77, X96-X98, Y92)

CC-A T26.20x-　Burn with resulting rupture and destruction of unspecified eyeball

CC-A T26.21x-　Burn with resulting rupture and destruction of right eyeball

CC-A T26.22x-　Burn with resulting rupture and destruction of left eyeball

T26.3-　Burns of other specified parts of eye and adnexa
Use additional external cause code to identify the source, place and intent of the burn (X00-X19, X75-X77, X96-X98, Y92)

T26.30x-　Burns of other specified parts of unspecified eye and adnexa

T25 - T26

T26.31x-   Burns of other specified parts of <u>right</u> eye and adnexa

T26.32x-   Burns of other specified parts of <u>left</u> eye and adnexa

T26.4-   Burn of eye and adnexa, part <u>unspecified</u>
Use additional external cause code to identify the source, place and intent of the burn (X00-X19, X75-X77, X96-X98, Y92)

T26.40x-   Burn of <u>unspecified</u> eye and adnexa, part <u>unspecified</u>

T26.41x-   Burn of <u>right</u> eye and adnexa, part <u>unspecified</u>

T26.42x-   Burn of <u>left</u> eye and adnexa, part <u>unspecified</u>

T26.5-   <u>Corrosion</u> of <u>eyelid and periocular area</u>
Code first (T51-T65) to identify chemical and intent
Use additional external cause code to identify place (Y92)

T26.50x-   Corrosion of <u>unspecified</u> eyelid and periocular area

T26.51x-   Corrosion of <u>right</u> eyelid and periocular area

T26.52x-   Corrosion of <u>left</u> eyelid and periocular area

T26.6-   <u>Corrosion</u> of <u>cornea and conjunctival sac</u>
Code first (T51-T65) to identify chemical and intent
Use additional external cause code to identify place (Y92)

T26.60x-   Corrosion of cornea and conjunctival sac, <u>unspecified</u> eye

T26.61x-   Corrosion of cornea and conjunctival sac, <u>right</u> eye

T26.62x-   Corrosion of cornea and conjunctival sac, <u>left</u> eye

T26.7-   <u>Corrosion with resulting rupture and destruction of eyeball</u>
Code first (T51-T65) to identify chemical and intent
Use additional external cause code to identify place (Y92)

CC-A T26.70x-   Corrosion with resulting rupture and destruction of <u>unspecified</u> eyeball

CC-A T26.71x-   Corrosion with resulting rupture and destruction of <u>right</u> eyeball

CC-A T26.72x-   Corrosion with resulting rupture and destruction of <u>left</u> eyeball

T26.8-   <u>Corrosions</u> of <u>other specified parts</u> of <u>eye and adnexa</u>
Code first (T51-T65) to identify chemical and intent
Use additional external cause code to identify place (Y92)

T26.80x-   Corrosions of other specified parts of <u>unspecified</u> eye and adnexa

T26.81x-   Corrosions of other specified parts of <u>right</u> eye and adnexa

T26.82x-   Corrosions of other specified parts of <u>left</u> eye and adnexa

T26.9-   <u>Corrosion</u> of eye and adnexa, part <u>unspecified</u>
Code first (T51-T65) to identify chemical and intent
Use additional external cause code to identify place (Y92)

T26.90x-   Corrosion of <u>unspecified</u> eye and adnexa, part <u>unspecified</u>

T26.91x-   Corrosion of <u>right</u> eye and adnexa, part <u>unspecified</u>

T26.92x-   Corrosion of <u>left</u> eye and adnexa, part <u>unspecified</u>

T27-   <u>Burn and corrosion</u> of <u>respiratory tract</u>
Use additional external cause code to identify the source and intent of the burn (X00-X19, X75-X77, X96-X98)
Use additional external cause code to identify place (Y92)

The appropriate 7th character is to be added to each code from category T27:
A   <u>Initial</u> encounter
D   <u>Subsequent</u> encounter
S   <u>Sequela</u>

T27.0xx-   Burn of larynx and trachea
CC-A

T27.1xx-   Burn involving larynx and trachea with lung
CC-A

T27.2xx-   Burn of other parts of respiratory tract
CC-A   Burn of thoracic cavity

T27.3xx-   Burn of respiratory tract, part <u>unspecified</u>
CC-A   Code first (T51-T65) to identify chemical and intent for codes T27.4-T27.7

T27.4xx-   <u>Corrosion</u> of larynx and trachea
CC-A

T27.5xx-   <u>Corrosion</u> involving larynx and trachea with lung
CC-A

T27.6xx-   <u>Corrosion</u> of other parts of respiratory tract
CC-A

T27.7xx-   <u>Corrosion</u> of respiratory tract, part <u>unspecified</u>
CC-A

T28-   <u>Burn and corrosion</u> of <u>other internal organs</u>
Use additional external cause code to identify the source and intent of the burn (X00-X19, X75-X77, X96-X98)
Use additional external cause code to identify place (Y92)

The appropriate 7th character is to be added to each code from category T28:
A   <u>Initial</u> encounter
D   <u>Subsequent</u> encounter
S   <u>Sequela</u>

T28.0xx-   Burn of mouth and pharynx

T28.1xx-   Burn of esophagus
CC-A

T28.2xx-   Burn of other parts of alimentary tract
CC-A

T28.3xx-   Burn of internal genitourinary organs

T28.4xx-   Burns of other and unspecified internal organs

T28.40x-   Burn of <u>unspecified</u> internal organ

T28.41-   Burn of <u>ear drum</u>

T28.411-   Burn of <u>right</u> ear drum

T28.412-   Burn of <u>left</u> ear drum

T28.419-   Burn of <u>unspecified</u> ear drum

T28.49x-   Burn of <u>other</u> internal organ
Code first (T51-T65) to identify chemical and intent for T28.5-T28.9-

T28.5xx-   <u>Corrosion</u> of mouth and pharynx

T28.6xx-   <u>Corrosion</u> of esophagus
CC-A

T28.7xx-   <u>Corrosion</u> of other parts of alimentary tract
CC-A

T28.8xx-   <u>Corrosion</u> of internal genitourinary organs

T28.9xx-   <u>Corrosions</u> of other and unspecified internal organs

T28.90x-   Corrosions of <u>unspecified</u> internal organs

T28.91-   Corrosions of <u>ear drum</u>

T28.911-   Corrosions of <u>right</u> ear drum

T28.912-   Corrosions of <u>left</u> ear drum

T28.919-   Corrosions of <u>unspecified</u> ear drum

T28.99x-   Corrosions of <u>other</u> internal organs

T26-T28

Burns and corrosions of multiple and unspecified body regions (T30-T32)

T30-   Burn and corrosion, body region unspecified

T30.0   Burn of unspecified body region, unspecified degree
> Note: This code is not for inpatient use. Code to specified site and degree of burns
> Burn NOS
> Multiple burns NOS

T30.4   Corrosion of unspecified body region, unspecified degree
> Note: This code is not for inpatient use. Code to specified site and degree of corrosion
> Corrosion NOS
> Multiple corrosion NOS

T31-   Burns classified according to extent of body surface involved
> Note: This category is to be used as the primary code only when the site of the burn is unspecified. It should be used as a supplementary code with categories T20-T25 when the site is specified.

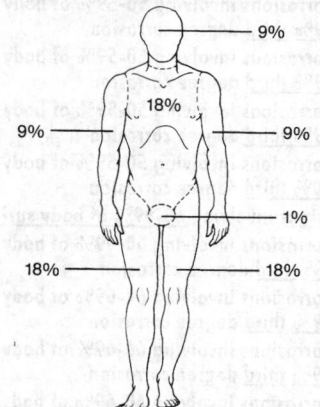

9%
18%
9%   9%
1%
18%   18%

BODY SURFACE RULE OF NINES

First Degree Burn — Epidermis
Second Degree Burn — Dermis
Third Degree Burn — Subcutaneous Tissue

EXTENT OF SKIN BURN

T31.0   Burns involving less than 10% of body surface

T31.1-   Burns involving 10-19% of body surface
- cc **T31.10**   Burns involving 10-19% of body surface with 0% to 9% third degree burns
  Burns involving 10-19% of body surface NOS
- cc **T31.11**   Burns involving 10-19% of body surface with 10-19% third degree burns

T31.2-   Burns involving 20-29% of body surface
- cc **T31.20**   Burns involving 20-29% of body surface with 0% to 9% third degree burns
  Burns involving 20-29% of body surface NOS
- MCC **T31.21**   Burns involving 20-29% of body surface with 10-19% third degree burns
- MCC **T31.22**   Burns involving 20-29% of body surface with 20-29% third degree burns

T31.3-   Burns involving 30-39% of body surface
- cc **T31.30**   Burns involving 30-39% of body surface with 0% to 9% third degree burns
  Burns involving 30-39% of body surface NOS
- MCC **T31.31**   Burns involving 30-39% of body surface with 10-19% third degree burns
- MCC **T31.32**   Burns involving 30-39% of body surface with 20-29% third degree burns

- MCC **T31.33**   Burns involving 30-39% of body surface with 30-39% third degree burns

T31.4-   Burns involving 40-49% of body surface
- cc **T31.40**   Burns involving 40-49% of body surface with 0% to 9% third degree burns
  Burns involving 40-49% of body surface NOS
- MCC **T31.41**   Burns involving 40-49% of body surface with 10-19% third degree burns
- MCC **T31.42**   Burns involving 40-49% of body surface with 20-29% third degree burns
- MCC **T31.43**   Burns involving 40-49% of body surface with 30-39% third degree burns
- MCC **T31.44**   Burns involving 40-49% of body surface with 40-49% third degree burns

T31.5-   Burns involving 50-59% of body surface
- cc **T31.50**   Burns involving 50-59% of body surface with 0% to 9% third degree burns
  Burns involving 50-59% of body surface NOS
- MCC **T31.51**   Burns involving 50-59% of body surface with 10-19% third degree burns
- MCC **T31.52**   Burns involving 50-59% of body surface with 20-29% third degree burns
- MCC **T31.53**   Burns involving 50-59% of body surface with 30-39% third degree burns
- MCC **T31.54**   Burns involving 50-59% of body surface with 40-49% third degree burns
- MCC **T31.55**   Burns involving 50-59% of body surface with 50-59% third degree burns

T31.6-   Burns involving 60-69% of body surface
- cc **T31.60**   Burns involving 60-69% of body surface with 0% to 9% third degree burns
  Burns involving 60-69% of body surface NOS
- MCC **T31.61**   Burns involving 60-69% of body surface with 10-19% third degree burns
- MCC **T31.62**   Burns involving 60-69% of body surface with 20-29% third degree burns
- MCC **T31.63**   Burns involving 60-69% of body surface with 30-39% third degree burns
- MCC **T31.64**   Burns involving 60-69% of body surface with 40-49% third degree burns
- MCC **T31.65**   Burns involving 60-69% of body surface with 50-59% third degree burns
- MCC **T31.66**   Burns involving 60-69% of body surface with 60-69% third degree burns

T31.7-   Burns involving 70-79% of body surface
- cc **T31.70**   Burns involving 70-79% of body surface with 0% to 9% third degree burns
  Burns involving 70-79% of body surface NOS
- MCC **T31.71**   Burns involving 70-79% of body surface with 10-19% third degree burns
- MCC **T31.72**   Burns involving 70-79% of body surface with 20-29% third degree burns
- MCC **T31.73**   Burns involving 70-79% of body surface with 30-39% third degree burns
- MCC **T31.74**   Burns involving 70-79% of body surface with 40-49% third degree burns
- MCC **T31.75**   Burns involving 70-79% of body surface with 50-59% third degree burns
- MCC **T31.76**   Burns involving 70-79% of body surface with 60-69% third degree burns
- MCC **T31.77**   Burns involving 70-79% of body surface with 70-79% third degree burns

T30 - T31

T31.8-   Burns involving 80-89% of body surface
- cc **T31.80**   Burns involving 80-89% of body surface with 0% to 9% third degree burns
   - Burns involving 80-89% of body surface NOS
- mcc **T31.81**   Burns involving 80-89% of body surface with 10-19% third degree burns
- mcc **T31.82**   Burns involving 80-89% of body surface with 20-29% third degree burns
- mcc **T31.83**   Burns involving 80-89% of body surface with 30-39% third degree burns
- mcc **T31.84**   Burns involving 80-89% of body surface with 40-49% third degree burns
- mcc **T31.85**   Burns involving 80-89% of body surface with 50-59% third degree burns
- mcc **T31.86**   Burns involving 80-89% of body surface with 60-69% third degree burns
- mcc **T31.87**   Burns involving 80-89% of body surface with 70-79% third degree burns
- mcc **T31.88**   Burns involving 80-89% of body surface with 80-89% third degree burns

T31.9-   Burns involving 90% or more of body surface
- cc **T31.90**   Burns involving 90% or more of body surface with 0% to 9% third degree burns
   - Burns involving 90% or more of body surface NOS
- mcc **T31.91**   Burns involving 90% or more of body surface with 10-19% third degree burns
- mcc **T31.92**   Burns involving 90% or more of body surface with 20-29% third degree burns
- mcc **T31.93**   Burns involving 90% or more of body surface with 30-39% third degree burns
- mcc **T31.94**   Burns involving 90% or more of body surface with 40-49% third degree burns
- mcc **T31.95**   Burns involving 90% or more of body surface with 50-59% third degree burns
- mcc **T31.96**   Burns involving 90% or more of body surface with 60-69% third degree burns
- mcc **T31.97**   Burns involving 90% or more of body surface with 70-79% third degree burns
- mcc **T31.98**   Burns involving 90% or more of body surface with 80-89% third degree burns
- mcc **T31.99**   Burns involving 90% or more of body surface with 90% or more third degree burns

T32-   Corrosions classified according to extent of body surface involved
   Note: This category is to be used as the primary code only when the site of the corrosion is unspecified. It may be used as a supplementary code with categories T20-T25 when the site is specified.

T32.0   Corrosions involving less than 10% of body surface

T32.1-   Corrosions involving 10-19% of body surface
- cc **T32.10**   Corrosions involving 10-19% of body surface with 0% to 9% third degree corrosion
   - Corrosions involving 10-19% of body surface NOS
- cc **T32.11**   Corrosions involving 10-19% of body surface with 10-19% third degree corrosion

T32.2-   Corrosions involving 20-29% of body surface
- cc **T32.20**   Corrosions involving 20-29% of body surface with 0% to 9% third degree corrosion
- mcc **T32.21**   Corrosions involving 20-29% of body surface with 10-19% third degree corrosion
- mcc **T32.22**   Corrosions involving 20-29% of body surface with 20-29% third degree corrosion

T32.3-   Corrosions involving 30-39% of body surface
- cc **T32.30**   Corrosions involving 30-39% of body surface with 0% to 9% third degree corrosion
- mcc **T32.31**   Corrosions involving 30-39% of body surface with 10-19% third degree corrosion
- mcc **T32.32**   Corrosions involving 30-39% of body surface with 20-29% third degree corrosion
- mcc **T32.33**   Corrosions involving 30-39% of body surface with 30-39% third degree corrosion

T32.4-   Corrosions involving 40-49% of body surface
- cc **T32.40**   Corrosions involving 40-49% of body surface with 0% to 9% third degree corrosion
- mcc **T32.41**   Corrosions involving 40-49% of body surface with 10-19% third degree corrosion
- mcc **T32.42**   Corrosions involving 40-49% of body surface with 20-29% third degree corrosion
- mcc **T32.43**   Corrosions involving 40-49% of body surface with 30-39% third degree corrosion
- mcc **T32.44**   Corrosions involving 40-49% of body surface with 40-49% third degree corrosion

T32.5-   Corrosions involving 50-59% of body surface
- cc **T32.50**   Corrosions involving 50-59% of body surface with 0% to 9% third degree corrosion
- mcc **T32.51**   Corrosions involving 50-59% of body surface with 10-19% third degree corrosion
- mcc **T32.52**   Corrosions involving 50-59% of body surface with 20-29% third degree corrosion
- mcc **T32.53**   Corrosions involving 50-59% of body surface with 30-39% third degree corrosion
- mcc **T32.54**   Corrosions involving 50-59% of body surface with 40-49% third degree corrosion
- mcc **T32.55**   Corrosions involving 50-59% of body surface with 50-59% third degree corrosion

T32.6-   Corrosions involving 60-69% of body surface
- cc **T32.60**   Corrosions involving 60-69% of body surface with 0% to 9% third degree corrosion
- mcc **T32.61**   Corrosions involving 60-69% of body surface with 10-19% third degree corrosion
- mcc **T32.62**   Corrosions involving 60-69% of body surface with 20-29% third degree corrosion
- mcc **T32.63**   Corrosions involving 60-69% of body surface with 30-39% third degree corrosion
- mcc **T32.64**   Corrosions involving 60-69% of body surface with 40-49% third degree corrosion
- mcc **T32.65**   Corrosions involving 60-69% of body surface with 50-59% third degree corrosion
- mcc **T32.66**   Corrosions involving 60-69% of body surface with 60-69% third degree corrosion

T32.7-   Corrosions involving 70-79% of body surface
- cc **T32.70**   Corrosions involving 70-79% of body surface with 0% to 9% third degree corrosion
- mcc **T32.71**   Corrosions involving 70-79% of body surface with 10-19% third degree corrosion
- mcc **T32.72**   Corrosions involving 70-79% of body surface with 20-29% third degree corrosion
- mcc **T32.73**   Corrosions involving 70-79% of body surface with 30-39% third degree corrosion
- mcc **T32.74**   Corrosions involving 70-79% of body surface with 40-49% third degree corrosion
- mcc **T32.75**   Corrosions involving 70-79% of body surface with 50-59% third degree corrosion
- mcc **T32.76**   Corrosions involving 70-79% of body surface with 60-69% third degree corrosion
- mcc **T32.77**   Corrosions involving 70-79% of body surface with 70-79% third degree corrosion

T32.8-   Corrosions involving 80-89% of body surface
- cc **T32.80**   Corrosions involving 80-89% of body surface with 0% to 9% third degree corrosion
- mcc **T32.81**   Corrosions involving 80-89% of body surface with 10-19% third degree corrosion
- mcc **T32.82**   Corrosions involving 80-89% of body surface with 20-29% third degree corrosion
- mcc **T32.83**   Corrosions involving 80-89% of body surface with 30-39% third degree corrosion
- mcc **T32.84**   Corrosions involving 80-89% of body surface with 40-49% third degree corrosion

T
3
1
-
T
3
2

MCC **T32.85** Corrosions involving 80-89% of body surface <u>with 50-59% third</u> degree corrosion

MCC **T32.86** Corrosions involving 80-89% of body surface <u>with 60-69% third</u> degree corrosion

MCC **T32.87** Corrosions involving 80-89% of body surface <u>with 70-79% third</u> degree corrosion

MCC **T32.88** Corrosions involving 80-89% of body surface <u>with 80-89% third</u> degree corrosion

T32.9- <u>Corrosions</u> involving <u>90% or more of body surface</u>

CC **T32.90** Corrosions involving 90% or more of body surface <u>with 0% to 9% third</u> degree corrosion

MCC **T32.91** Corrosions involving 90% or more of body surface <u>with 10-19% third</u> degree corrosion

MCC **T32.92** Corrosions involving 90% or more of body surface <u>with 20-29% third</u> degree corrosion

MCC **T32.93** Corrosions involving 90% or more of body surface <u>with 30-39% third</u> degree corrosion

MCC **T32.94** Corrosions involving 90% or more of body surface <u>with 40-49% third</u> degree corrosion

MCC **T32.95** Corrosions involving 90% or more of body surface <u>with 50-59% third</u> degree corrosion

MCC **T32.96** Corrosions involving 90% or more of body surface <u>with 60-69% third</u> degree corrosion

MCC **T32.97** Corrosions involving 90% or more of body surface <u>with 70-79% third</u> degree corrosion

MCC **T32.98** Corrosions involving 90% or more of body surface <u>with 80-89% third</u> degree corrosion

MCC **T32.99** Corrosions involving 90% or more of body surface <u>with 90% or more third</u> degree corrosion

Frostbite (T33-T34)

Excludes ❷: hypothermia and other effects of reduced temperature (T68, T69.-)

T33- <u>Superficial</u> frostbite
Includes: Frostbite with partial thickness skin loss
The appropriate 7th character is to be added to each code from category T33:
  A <u>Initial</u> encounter
  D <u>Subsequent</u> encounter
  S <u>Sequela</u>

T33.0- Superficial frostbite of head

 T33.01- Superficial frostbite of <u>ear</u>

 CC-A **T33.011-** Superficial frostbite of <u>right</u> ear

 CC-A **T33.012-** Superficial frostbite of <u>left</u> ear

 CC-A **T33.019-** Superficial frostbite of <u>unspecified</u> ear

CC-A **T33.02x-** Superficial frostbite of nose

CC-A **T33.09x-** Superficial frostbite of other part of head

T33.1xx- Superficial frostbite of neck
CC-A

T33.2xx- Superficial frostbite of thorax
CC-A

T33.3xx- Superficial frostbite of abdominal wall, lower back and pelvis
CC-A

T33.4- Superficial frostbite of <u>arm</u>
  Excludes ❷: superficial frostbite of wrist and hand (T33.5-)

CC-A **T33.40x-** Superficial frostbite of <u>unspecified</u> arm

CC-A **T33.41x-** Superficial frostbite of <u>right</u> arm

CC-A **T33.42x-** Superficial frostbite of <u>left</u> arm

T33.5- Superficial frostbite of wrist, hand, and fingers

 T33.51- Superficial frostbite of <u>wrist</u>

 CC-A **T33.511-** Superficial frostbite of <u>right</u> wrist

 CC-A **T33.512-** Superficial frostbite of <u>left</u> wrist

 CC-A **T33.519-** Superficial frostbite of <u>unspecified</u> wrist

 T33.52- Superficial frostbite of <u>hand</u>
   Excludes ❷: superficial frostbite of fingers (T33.53-)

 CC-A **T33.521-** Superficial frostbite of <u>right</u> hand

 CC-A **T33.522-** Superficial frostbite of <u>left</u> hand

 CC-A **T33.529-** Superficial frostbite of <u>unspecified</u> hand

 T33.53- Superficial frostbite of <u>finger(s)</u>

 CC-A **T33.531-** Superficial frostbite of <u>right</u> finger(s)

 CC-A **T33.532-** Superficial frostbite of <u>left</u> finger(s)

 CC-A **T33.539-** Superficial frostbite of <u>unspecified</u> finger(s)

T33.6- Superficial frostbite of <u>hip and thigh</u>

CC-A **T33.60x-** Superficial frostbite of <u>unspecified</u> hip and thigh

CC-A **T33.61x-** Superficial frostbite of <u>right</u> hip and thigh

CC-A **T33.62x-** Superficial frostbite of <u>left</u> hip and thigh

T33.7- Superficial frostbite of <u>knee and lower leg</u>
  Excludes ❷: superficial frostbite of ankle and foot (T33.8-)

CC-A **T33.70x-** Superficial frostbite of <u>unspecified</u> knee and lower leg

CC-A **T33.71x-** Superficial frostbite of <u>right</u> knee and lower leg

CC-A **T33.72x-** Superficial frostbite of <u>left</u> knee and lower leg

T33.8- Superficial frostbite of ankle, foot, and toe(s)

 T33.81- Superficial frostbite of <u>ankle</u>

 CC-A **T33.811-** Superficial frostbite of <u>right</u> ankle

 CC-A **T33.812-** Superficial frostbite of <u>left</u> ankle

 CC-A **T33.819-** Superficial frostbite of <u>unspecified</u> ankle

 T33.82- Superficial frostbite of <u>foot</u>

 CC-A **T33.821-** Superficial frostbite of <u>right</u> foot

 CC-A **T33.822-** Superficial frostbite of <u>left</u> foot

 CC-A **T33.829-** Superficial frostbite of <u>unspecified</u> foot

 T33.83- Superficial frostbite of <u>toe(s)</u>

 CC-A **T33.831-** Superficial frostbite of <u>right</u> toe(s)

 CC-A **T33.832-** Superficial frostbite of <u>left</u> toe(s)

 CC-A **T33.839-** Superficial frostbite of <u>unspecified</u> toe(s)

T33.9- Superficial frostbite of other and unspecified sites

CC-A **T33.90x-** Superficial frostbite of <u>unspecified</u> sites
  Superficial frostbite NOS

CC-A **T33.99x-** Superficial frostbite of <u>other</u> sites
  Superficial frostbite of leg NOS
  Superficial frostbite of trunk NOS

T34- <u>Frostbite with tissue necrosis</u>
The appropriate 7th character is to be added to each code from category T34:
  A <u>Initial</u> encounter
  D <u>Subsequent</u> encounter
  S <u>Sequela</u>

T34.0- Frostbite <u>with tissue necrosis</u> of head

 T34.01- Frostbite <u>with tissue necrosis</u> of <u>ear</u>

 CC-A **T34.011-** Frostbite with tissue necrosis of <u>right</u> ear

 CC-A **T34.012-** Frostbite with tissue necrosis of <u>left</u> ear

 CC-A **T34.019-** Frostbite with tissue necrosis of <u>unspecified</u> ear

CC-A **T34.02x-** Frostbite <u>with tissue necrosis</u> of nose

CC-A **T34.09x-** Frostbite <u>with tissue necrosis</u> of other part of head

T34.1xx- Frostbite <u>with tissue necrosis</u> of neck
CC-A

T34.2xx- Frostbite <u>with tissue necrosis</u> of thorax
CC-A

T34.3xx- Frostbite <u>with tissue necrosis</u> of abdominal wall, lower back and pelvis
CC-A

T34.4- Frostbite <u>with tissue necrosis</u> of <u>arm</u>
  Excludes ❷: frostbite with tissue necrosis of wrist and hand (T34.5-)

CC-A **T34.40x-** Frostbite with tissue necrosis of <u>unspecified</u> arm

CC-A **T34.41x-** Frostbite with tissue necrosis of <u>right</u> arm

CC-A **T34.42x-** Frostbite with tissue necrosis of <u>left</u> arm

T34.5- Frostbite <u>with tissue necrosis</u> of wrist, hand, and finger(s)

 T34.51- Frostbite <u>with tissue necrosis</u> of <u>wrist</u>

 CC-A **T34.511-** Frostbite with tissue necrosis of <u>right</u> wrist

 CC-A **T34.512-** Frostbite with tissue necrosis of <u>left</u> wrist

 CC-A **T34.519-** Frostbite with tissue necrosis of <u>unspecified</u> wrist

 T34.52- Frostbite <u>with tissue necrosis</u> of <u>hand</u>
   Excludes ❷: frostbite with tissue necrosis of finger(s) (T34.53-)

 CC-A **T34.521-** Frostbite with tissue necrosis of <u>right</u> hand

 CC-A **T34.522-** Frostbite with tissue necrosis of <u>left</u> hand

 CC-A **T34.529-** Frostbite with tissue necrosis of <u>unspecified</u> hand

T
3
2
-
T
3
4

T34.53- Frostbite <u>with tissue necrosis</u> of <u>finger(s)</u>

CC-A **T34.531- Frostbite with tissue necrosis of <u>right</u> finger(s)**

CC-A **T34.532- Frostbite with tissue necrosis of <u>left</u> finger(s)**

CC-A **T34.539- Frostbite with tissue necrosis of <u>unspecified</u> finger(s)**

T34.6- Frostbite <u>with tissue necrosis</u> of <u>hip and thigh</u>

CC-A **T34.60x- Frostbite with tissue necrosis of <u>unspecified</u> hip and thigh**

CC-A **T34.61x- Frostbite with tissue necrosis of <u>right</u> hip and thigh**

CC-A **T34.62x- Frostbite with tissue necrosis of <u>left</u> hip and thigh**

T34.7- Frostbite <u>with tissue necrosis</u> of <u>knee and lower leg</u>

  Excludes ❷: frostbite with tissue necrosis of ankle and foot (T34.8-)

CC-A **T34.70x- Frostbite with tissue necrosis of <u>unspecified</u> knee and lower leg**

CC-A **T34.71x- Frostbite with tissue necrosis of <u>right</u> knee and lower leg**

CC-A **T34.72x- Frostbite with tissue necrosis of <u>left</u> knee and lower leg**

T34.8- Frostbite <u>with tissue necrosis</u> of ankle, foot, and toe(s)

  T34.81- Frostbite <u>with tissue necrosis</u> of <u>ankle</u>

CC-A **T34.811- Frostbite with tissue necrosis of <u>right</u> ankle**

CC-A **T34.812- Frostbite with tissue necrosis of <u>left</u> ankle**

CC-A **T34.819- Frostbite with tissue necrosis of <u>unspecified</u> ankle**

  T34.82- Frostbite <u>with tissue necrosis</u> of <u>foot</u>

CC-A **T34.821- Frostbite with tissue necrosis of <u>right</u> foot**

CC-A **T34.822- Frostbite with tissue necrosis of <u>left</u> foot**

CC-A **T34.829- Frostbite with tissue necrosis of <u>unspecified</u> foot**

  T34.83- Frostbite <u>with tissue necrosis</u> of <u>toe(s)</u>

CC-A **T34.831- Frostbite with tissue necrosis of <u>right</u> toe(s)**

CC-A **T34.832- Frostbite with tissue necrosis of <u>left</u> toe(s)**

CC-A **T34.839- Frostbite with tissue necrosis of <u>unspecified</u> toe(s)**

T34.9- Frostbite <u>with tissue necrosis</u> of other and unspecified sites

CC-A **T34.90x- Frostbite with tissue necrosis of <u>unspecified</u> sites**
      Frostbite with tissue necrosis NOS

CC-A **T34.99x- Frostbite with tissue necrosis of <u>other</u> sites**
      Frostbite with tissue necrosis of leg NOS
      Frostbite with tissue necrosis of trunk NOS

Poisoning by, adverse effects of and underdosing of drugs, medicaments and biological substances (T36-T50)

Includes: Adverse effect of correct substance properly administered
             Poisoning by overdose of substance
             Poisoning by wrong substance given or taken in error
             Underdosing by (inadvertantly) (deliberately) taking less substance than prescribed or instructed

Code first, for adverse effects, the nature of the adverse effect, such as:
  Adverse effect NOS (T88.7)
  Aspirin gastritis (K29-)
  Blood disorders (D56-D76)
  Contact dermatitis (L23-L25)
  Dermatitis due to substances taken internally (L27-)
  Nephropathy (N14.0-N14.2)

Note: The drug giving rise to the adverse effect should be identified by use of codes from categories T36-T50 with fifth or sixth character 5.

Use additional code(s) to specifiy:
  Manifestations of poisoning
  Underdosing of medication regime (Z91.12-, Z91.13-)
  Underdosing or failure in dosage during medical and surgical care (Y63.6, Y63.8-Y63.9)

Excludes 1:   toxic reaction to local anesthesia in pregnancy (O29.3-)

Excludes ❷: abuse and dependence of psychoactive substances (F10-F19)
            abuse of non-dependence-producing substances (F55-)
            drug reaction and poisoning affecting newborn (P00-P96)
            pathological drug intoxication (inebriation) (F10-F19)

* Indicates the complete list of specific drugs and chemicals included in each drug and chemical category for codes T36-T65, taken directly from the Official Table of Drugs & Chemicals.

T36- Poisoning by, adverse effect of and underdosing of <u>systemic antibiotics</u>

  Excludes 1:   antineoplastic antibiotics (T45.1-)
            locally applied antibiotic NEC (T49.0)
            topically used antibiotic for ear, nose and throat (T49.6)
            topically used antibiotic for eye (T49.5)

The appropriate 7th character is to be added to each code from category T36:

  A   <u>Initial</u> encounter
  D   <u>Subsequent</u> encounter
  S   <u>Sequela</u>

T36.0-   Poisoning by, adverse effect of and underdosing of <u>penicillins</u>

T36.0 - DRUGS/CHEMS*		
Adicillin	Ciclacillin	Penethamate
Amdinocilline	Clemizole penicillin	Penicillin (any)
Amoxicillin	Clometocillin	Phenbenicillin
Ampicillin	Cloxacillin	Pheneticillin
Ancillin	Cyclacillin	Phenoxymethyl penicillin
Apalcillin	Dicloxacillin	Phenthicillin
Aspoxicillin	Flucloxacillin	Piperacillin
Azidocillin	Hetacillin	Pivampicillin
Azlocillin	Hydrabamine penicillin	Pivmecillinam
Bacampicillin	Imipenem	Procaine, benzylpenicillin
Benethamine penicillin	Isoxazolyl penicillin	Procaine, penicillin G
Benzathine benzylpenicillin	Mecillinam	Propicillin
Benzathine penicillin	Metampicillin	Sodium nafcillin
Benzyl penicillin	Methicillin	Sulbactam
Benzylpenicillin	Methoxybenzyl penicillin	Sulbenicillin
Carbenicillin	Meticillin	Sultamicillin
Carfecillin	Mezlocillin	Talampicillin
Carindacillin	Nafcillin	Temocillin
Cephalosporins, N	Oxacillin	Ticarcillin
(adicillin)	Penamecillin	Xantocillin

T36.0x- Poisoning by, adverse effect of and underdosing of penicillins

  T36.0x1- Poisoning by penicillins, <u>accidental</u> (unintentional)
         Poisoning by penicillins NOS

  T36.0x2- Poisoning by penicillins, <u>intentional</u> self-harm

  T36.0x3- Poisoning by penicillins, <u>assault</u>

  T36.0x4- Poisoning by penicillins, <u>undetermined</u>

  T36.0x5- <u>Adverse effect</u> of penicillins

  T36.0x6- <u>Underdosing</u> of penicillins

T3 4 - T3 6

T36.1-   Poisoning by, adverse effect of and underdosing of cephalosporins and other beta-lactam antibiotics

T36.1 - DRUGS/CHEMS*		
Antibiotic, cephalosporin (group)	Cefbuperazone	Cefteram
Antibiotic, b-lactam NEC	Cefetamet	Ceftezole
Aztreonam	Cefixime	Ceftizoxime
Cefacetrile	Cefmenoxime	Ceftriaxone
Cefaclor	Cefmetazole	Cefuroxime
Cefadroxil	Cefminox	Cefuzonam
Cefalexin	Cefonicid	Cephalexin
Cefaloglycin	Cefoperazone	Cephaloglycin
Cefaloridine	Ceforanide	Cephaloridine
Cefalosporins	Cefotaxime	Cephalosporins
Cefalotin	Cefotetan	Cephalothin
Cefamandole	Cefotiam	Cephalotin
Cefamycin antibiotic	Cefoxitin	Cephradine
Cefapirin	Cefpimizole	Clavulanic acid
Cefatrizine	Cefpiramide	Flomoxef
Cefazedone	Cefradine	Latamoxef
Cefazolin	Cefroxadine	
	Cefsulodin	
	Ceftazidime	

T36.1x-   Poisoning by, adverse effect of and underdosing of cephalosporins and other beta-lactam antibiotics

T36.1x1-   Poisoning by cephalosporins and other beta-lactam antibiotics, accidental (unintentional)
     Poisoning by cephalosporins and other beta-lactam antibiotics NOS

T36.1x2-   Poisoning by cephalosporins and other beta-lactam antibiotics, intentional self-harm

T36.1x3-   Poisoning by cephalosporins and other beta-lactam antibiotics, assault

T36.1x4-   Poisoning by cephalosporins and other beta-lactam antibiotics, undetermined

T36.1x5-   Adverse effect of cephalosporins and other beta-lactam antibiotics

T36.1x6-   Underdosing of cephalosporins and other beta-lactam antibiotics

T36.2-   Poisoning by, adverse effect of and underdosing of chloramphenicol group

T36.2 - DRUGS/CHEMS*		
Antibiotic, chloramphenicol (group)	Chloramphenicol	Cloramfenicol
	Chloromycetin	Thiamphenicol
	Cloponone	

T36.2x-   Poisoning by, adverse effect of and underdosing of chloramphenicol group

T36.2x1-   Poisoning by chloramphenicol group, accidental (unintentional)
     Poisoning by chloramphenicol group NOS

T36.2x2-   Poisoning by chloramphenicol group, intentional self-harm

T36.2x3-   Poisoning by chloramphenicol group, assault

T36.2x4-   Poisoning by chloramphenicol group, undetermined

T36.2x5-   Adverse effect of chloramphenicol group

T36.2x6-   Underdosing of chloramphenicol group

T36.3-   Poisoning by, adverse effect of and underdosing of macrolides

T36.3 - DRUGS/CHEMS*		
Antibiotic, macrolides	Kitasamycin	Rokitamycin
Azithromycin	Macrolide, antibiotic	Roxithromycin
Erythromycin (salts)	Midecamycin	Spiramycin
Ilotycin	Miokamycin	TAO
Josamycin	Oleandomycin	Triacetyloleandomycin
	Pristinamycin	Troleandomycin

T36.3x-   Poisoning by, adverse effect of and underdosing of macrolides

T36.3x1-   Poisoning by macrolides, accidental (unintentional)
     Poisoning by macrolides NOS

T36.3x2-   Poisoning by macrolides, intentional self-harm

T36.3x3-   Poisoning by macrolides, assault

T36.3x4-   Poisoning by macrolides, undetermined

T36.3x5-   Adverse effect of macrolides

T36.3x6-   Underdosing of macrolides

T36.4-   Poisoning by, adverse effect of and underdosing of tetracyclines

T36.4 - DRUGS/CHEMS*		
Achromycin	Demeclocycline	Methacycline
Antibiotic, tetracycline (group)	Demethylchlortetracycline	Minocycline
Aureomycin	Demethyltetracycline	Oxytetracycline
Chlormethylenecycline	DMCT	Penimepicycline
Chlortetracycline	Doxycycline	Polycycline
Clomocycline	Guamecycline	Rolitetracycline
Declomycin	Lymecycline	Terramycin
	Meclocycline	Tetracycline
	Metacycline	

T36.4x-   Poisoning by, adverse effect of and underdosing of tetracyclines

T36.4x1-   Poisoning by tetracyclines, accidental (unintentional)
     Poisoning by tetracyclines NOS

T36.4x2-   Poisoning by tetracyclines, intentional self-harm

T36.4x3-   Poisoning by tetracyclines, assault

T36.4x4-   Poisoning by tetracyclines, undetermined

T36.4x5-   Adverse effect of tetracyclines

T36.4x6-   Underdosing of tetracyclines

T36.5-   Poisoning by, adverse effect of and underdosing of aminoglycosides
     Poisoning by, adverse effect of and underdosing of streptomycin

T36.5 - DRUGS/CHEMS*		
Amikacin	Bekanamycin	Netilmicin
Antibiotic, aminoglycoside	Dibekacin	Novobiocin
Antibiotic, antimycobacterial	Dihydrostreptomycin	Paromomycin
Anti-infective, antimycobacterial, antibiotics	Framycetin	Ribostamycin
	Garamycin	Sisomicin
Antimycobacterial drug, antibiotics	Gentamicin	Spectinomycin
	Isepamicin	Streptoduocin
	Kanamycin	Streptomycin (derivative)
Antituberculars, antibiotics	Kantrex	Streptonivicin
Astromicin	Micronomicin	Streptovarycin
	Mycifradin	Tobramycin
	Neomycin (derivatives)	

T36.5x-   Poisoning by, adverse effect of and underdosing of aminoglycosides

T36.5x1-   Poisoning by aminoglycosides, accidental (unintentional)
     Poisoning by aminoglycosides NOS

T36.5x2-   Poisoning by aminoglycosides, intentional self-harm

T36.5x3-   Poisoning by aminoglycosides, assault

T36.5x4-   Poisoning by aminoglycosides, undetermined

T36.5x5-   Adverse effect of aminoglycosides

T36.5x6-   Underdosing of aminoglycosides

T36.6-   Poisoning by, adverse effect of and underdosing of rifampicins

T36.6 - DRUGS/CHEMS*		
Ansamycin	Rifamide	Rifaximin
Isoniazid with rifampicin	Rifampicin	
Rifabutin	Rifampin	
	Rifamycin	

T36.6x-   Poisoning by, adverse effect of and underdosing of rifampicins

T36.6x1-   Poisoning by rifampicins, accidental (unintentional)
     Poisoning by rifampicins NOS

T36.6x2-   Poisoning by rifampicins, intentional self-harm

T36.6x3-   Poisoning by rifampicins, assault

T36.6x4-   Poisoning by rifampicins, undetermined

T36.6x5-   Adverse effect of rifampicins

T36.6x6-   Underdosing of rifampicins

T
3
6
-
T
3
6

T36.7- Poisoning by, adverse effect of and underdosing of antifungal antibiotics, systemically used

T36.7 - DRUGS/CHEMS*	Fungizone	Nilstat
Amphotericin B	Grifulvin	Nystatin
Antibiotic, antifungal	Griseofulvin	Pimaricin
Antifungal, antibiotic (systemic)	Hachimycin	Trichomycin
	Mepartricin	
Fulvicin	Mycostatin	

T36.7x- Poisoning by, adverse effect of and underdosing of <u>antifungal antibiotics, systemically used</u>

    T36.7x1- Poisoning by antifungal antibiotics, systemically used, <u>accidental</u> (unintentional)
        Poisoning by antifungal antibiotics, systemically used NOS

    T36.7x2- Poisoning by antifungal antibiotics, systemically used, <u>intentional</u> self-harm

    T36.7x3- Poisoning by antifungal antibiotics, systemically used, <u>assault</u>

    T36.7x4- Poisoning by antifungal antibiotics, systemically used, <u>undetermined</u>

    T36.7x5- <u>Adverse effect</u> of antifungal antibiotics, systemically used

    T36.7x6- <u>Underdosing</u> of antifungal antibiotics, systemically used

T36.8- Poisoning by, adverse effect of and underdosing of other systemic antibiotics

T36.8 - DRUGS/CHEMS*	Colistimethate	Neosporin
Aerosporin	Colistin	Norfloxacin
Albamycin	Co-trimoxazole	Ofloxacin
Amfomycin	Enoxacin	Polymyxin
Amphomycin	Enviomycin	Polymyxin B
Antibiotic, intestinal	Fleroxacin	Ristocetin
Antibiotic, polypeptide	Fosfomycin	Sodium fusidate
Antibiotic, specified NEC	Fugillin	Sulfamethoxazole with trimethoprim
Anti-infective, antibiotics, specified NEC	Fumadil	Sulfomyxin
Betamicin	Fumagillin	Teicoplanin
Capreomycin	Fusafungine	Trimethoprim with sulfamethoxazole
Carbomycin	Fusidate (ethanolamine) (sodium)	Vancomycin
Cathomycin	Fusidic acid	Viomycin
Ciprofloxacin	Lincomycin	Virginiamycin
Clindamycin	Magnamycin	
Colimycin	Mycitracin	

T36.8x- Poisoning by, adverse effect of and underdosing of <u>other systemic antibiotics</u>

    T36.8x1- Poisoning by other systemic antibiotics, <u>accidental</u> (unintentional)
        Poisoning by other systemic antibiotics NOS

    T36.8x2- Poisoning by other systemic antibiotics, <u>intentional</u> self-harm

    T36.8x3- Poisoning by other systemic antibiotics, <u>assault</u>

    T36.8x4- Poisoning by other systemic antibiotics, <u>undetermined</u>

    T36.8x5- <u>Adverse effect</u> of other systemic antibiotics

    T36.8x6- <u>Underdosing</u> of other systemic antibiotics

T36.9- Poisoning by, adverse effect of and underdosing of <u>unspecified systemic antibiotic</u>

T36.9 - DRUGS/CHEMS*
Antibiotic NEC
Anti-infective, antibiotics

T36.91x- Poisoning by unspecified systemic antibiotic, <u>accidental</u> (unintentional)
    Poisoning by systemic antibiotic NOS

T36.92x- Poisoning by unspecified systemic antibiotic, <u>intentional</u> self-harm

T36.93x- Poisoning by unspecified systemic antibiotic, <u>assault</u>

T36.94x- Poisoning by unspecified systemic antibiotic, <u>undetermined</u>

T36.95x- <u>Adverse effect</u> of unspecified systemic antibiotic

T36.96x- <u>Underdosing</u> of unspecified systemic antibiotic

T37- Poisoning by, adverse effect of and underdosing of <u>other systemic anti-infectives and antiparasitics</u>

Excludes 1:   *anti-infectives topically used for ear, nose and throat (T49.6-)*
      anti-infectives topically used for eye (T49.5-)
      locally applied anti-infectives NEC (T49.0-)

The appropriate 7th character is to be added to each code from category T37:
  A   <u>Initial</u> encounter
  D   <u>Subsequent</u> encounter
  S   <u>Sequela</u>

T37.0- Poisoning by, adverse effect of and underdosing of sulfonamides

T37.0 - DRUGS/CHEMS*	Sulfaethidole	Sulfaproxyline
Acedapsone	Sulfafurazole	Sulfapyridine
Acesulfamethoxypyridazine	Sulfaguanidine	Sulfapyrimidine
Acetylsulfamethoxypyrida zine	Sulfalene	Sulfasalazine
	Sulfaloxate	Sulfasuxidine
Azosulfamide	Sulfaloxic acid	Sulfasymazine
Azulfidine	Sulfamerazine	Sulfathiazole
Diaphenylsulfone	Sulfameter	Sulfisomidine
Disulfanilamide	Sulfamethazine	Sulfisoxazole
Neoprontosil	Sulfamethizole	Sulfonamide NEC
Phthalylsulfathiazole	Sulfamethoxazole	Sulphadiazine
Prontosil	Sulfamethoxydiazine	Sulphadimethoxine
Salazosulfapyridine	Sulfamethoxypyridazine	Sulphadimidine
Salicylazosulfapyridine	Sulfamethylthiazole	Sulphafurazole
Succinylsulfathiazole	Sulfametoxydiazine	Sulphamethizole
Sulfachlorpyridazine	Sulfamonomethoxine	Sulphamethoxazole
Sulfacitine	Sulfamoxole	Sulphaphenazole
Sulfadiasulfone sodium	Sulfanilamide	Sulphapyridine
Sulfadiazine	Sulfanilylguanidine	Sulphasalazine
Sulfadimethoxine	Sulfaperin	Trisulfapyrimidines
Sulfadimidine	Sulfaphenazole	
Sulfadoxine	Sulfaphenylthiazole	

T37.0x- Poisoning by, adverse effect of and underdosing of <u>sulfonamides</u>

    T37.0x1- Poisoning by sulfonamides, <u>accidental</u> (unintentional)
        Poisoning by sulfonamides NOS

    T37.0x2- Poisoning by sulfonamides, <u>intentional</u> self-harm

    T37.0x3- Poisoning by sulfonamides, <u>assault</u>

    T37.0x4- Poisoning by sulfonamides, <u>undetermined</u>

    T37.0x5- <u>Adverse effect</u> of sulfonamides

    T37.0x6- <u>Underdosing</u> of sulfonamides

T37.1- Poisoning by, adverse effect of and underdosing of antimycobacterial drugs
  Excludes 1:   rifampicins (T36.6-)
                 streptomycin (T36.5-)

T37.1 - DRUGS/CHEMS*		
Acetosulfone (sodium)	Diaminodiphenylsulfone	Potassium aminosalicylate
Aldesulfone sodium	Diasone (sodium)	Promacetin
Aminosalicylic acid	Etambutol	Promin
Aminosalylum	Ethambutol	Prothionamide
Anti-infective,	Ethionamide	Protionamide
antimycobacterial NEC	Ethioniamide	Pyrazinamide
Antimycobacterial drug	Ethyl chaulmoograte	Pyrazinoic acid (amide)
NEC	Fenamisal	Rifampicin with isoniazid
Antimycobacterial drug,	Glucosulfone sodium	Rimifon
combination	Glyconiazide	Salinazid
Antituberculars	INH	Sodium acetosulfone
Avlosulfon	Isoniazid	Sodium glucosulfone
Benzamidosalicylate	Isoniazid with	Sodium sulfoxone
(calcium)	thioacetazone	Solapsone
Benzoylpas calcium	Isonicotinic acid hydrazide	Solasulfone
Bromosalicylhydroxamic	Izoniazid	Sulfonazide
acid	Izoniazid with	Sulfones
Calcium	thioacetazone	Sulfoxone
benzamidosalicylate	Methaniazide	Sulphadione
Chaulmosulfone	Morinamide	Terizidone
Clofazimine	Morphazinamide	Thiambutosine
Cyanacetyl hydrazide	Nydrazid	Thioacetazone
Cycloserine	Para-aminosalicylic acid	Thioacetazone, with
DADPS	PAS	isoniazid
Dapsone	Pasiniazid	Thiocarlide
DDS	Pentylsalicylamide	Tiocarlide
	Pirazinamide	Trecator

T37.1x- Poisoning by, adverse effect of and underdosing of antimycobacterial drugs

  T37.1x1- Poisoning by antimycobacterial drugs, accidental (unintentional)
            Poisoning by antimycobacterial drugs NOS
  T37.1x2- Poisoning by antimycobacterial drugs, intentional self-harm
  T37.1x3- Poisoning by antimycobacterial drugs, assault
  T37.1x4- Poisoning by antimycobacterial drugs, undetermined
  T37.1x5- Adverse effect of antimycobacterial drugs
  T37.1x6- Underdosing of antimycobacterial drugs

T37.2- Poisoning by, adverse effect of and underdosing of antimalarials and drugs acting on other blood protozoa
  Excludes 1:   hydroxyquinoline derivatives (T37.8-)

T37.2 - DRUGS/CHEMS*		
8-Aminoquinoline drugs	Chloroguanide	Pentaquine
Amodiaquine	Chloroquine	Primaquine
Amopyroquin(e)	Chlorproguanil	Proguanil
Anti-infective, antimalarial	Cinchona	Pyrimethamine
Anti-infective,	Cinchonine alkaloids	Pyrimethamine with
antiprotozoal, blood	Cycloguanil embonate	sulfadoxine
Antimalarial	Daraprim	Quinacrine
Antimalarial, prophylactic	Eflornithine	Quinine
NEC	Guanatol	Quinocide
Antimalarial, pyrimidine	Halofantrine	Schizontozide (blood)
derivative	Isopentaquine	(tissue)
Antiprotozoal drug, blood	Mefloquine	Sulfadoxine with
Aralen	Mepacrine	pyrimethamine
Camoquin	Paludrine	
	Pamaquine (naphthoute)	

T37.2x- Poisoning by, adverse effect of and underdosing of antimalarials and drugs acting on other blood protozoa
  T37.2x1- Poisoning by antimalarials and drugs acting on other blood protozoa, accidental (unintentional)
            Poisoning by antimalarials and drugs acting on other blood protozoa NOS
  T37.2x2- Poisoning by antimalarials and drugs acting on other blood protozoa, intentional self-harm
  T37.2x3- Poisoning by antimalarials and drugs acting on other blood protozoa, assault
  T37.2x4- Poisoning by antimalarials and drugs acting on other blood protozoa, undetermined
  T37.2x5- Adverse effect of antimalarials and drugs acting on other blood protozoa
  T37.2x6- Underdosing of antimalarials and drugs acting on other blood protozoa

T37.3- Poisoning by, adverse effect of and underdosing of other antiprotozoal drugs

T37.3 - DRUGS/CHEMS*		
Acetarsol	Clefamide	Ornidazole
Acterol	Dehydroemetine	Oxophenarsine
Aminitrozole	DHE	Pentamidine
Anti-infective,	Difetarsone	Phanquinone
antiprotozoal NEC	Diloxanide	Phanquone
Antimony,	Emetine	Secnidazole
dimercaptosuccinate	Etofamide	Sodium antimony
Antimony, sodium	Flagyl	gluconate
dimercaptosuccinate	Glaucarubin	Sodium stibogluconate
Antiprotozoal drug NEC	Glycobiarsol	Stibogluconate
Antitrichomonal drug	Hydroxystilbamidine	Stilbamidine (isetionate)
Arsthinol	Melarsonyl potassium	Teclozan
Azanidazole	Melarsoprol	Tenonitrozole
Benznidazole	Misonidazole	Tinidazole
Bialamicol	Nifurtimox	Trichomonacides NEC
Carbarsone	Nimorazole	Tryparsamide
	Nitrimidazine	

T37.3x- Poisoning by, adverse effect of and underdosing of other antiprotozoal drugs
  T37.3x1- Poisoning by other antiprotozoal drugs, accidental (unintentional)
            Poisoning by other antiprotozoal drugs NOS
  T37.3x2- Poisoning by other antiprotozoal drugs, intentional self-harm
  T37.3x3- Poisoning by other antiprotozoal drugs, assault
  T37.3x4- Poisoning by other antiprotozoal drugs, undetermined
  T37.3x5- Adverse effect of other antiprotozoal drugs
  T37.3x6- Underdosing of other antiprotozoal drugs

T37-T37-T37

T37.4- Poisoning by, adverse effect of and underdosing of anthelminthics

T37.4 - DRUGS/CHEMS*		
Alantolactone	Dichlorophen	Piperazine
Albendazole	Diethyl carbamazine	Praziquantel
Amphotalide	Diethylcarbamazine	Pumpkin seed extract
Anthelmintic NEC	Dithiazanine iodide	Pyrantel
Antihiolimine	Fenbendazole	Pyrvinium chloride
Antifilarial drug	Filix mas	Santonin
Antihelmintics	Flubendazole	Spigelia (root)
Antihookworm drug	Helenin	Stibophen
Anti-infective, anthelmintic	Ivermectin	Suramin (sodium)
Antinematode drug	Levamisole	Teroxalene
Antiplatyhelmintic drug	Lucanthone	Tetrachloroethylene,
Antischistosomal drug	Male fern extract	medicinal
Antitapeworm drug	Mebendazole	Tetramisole
Antiwhipworm drug	Niclosamide	Thiabendazole
Ascaridole	Niridazole	Tiabendazole
Aspidium (oleoresin)	Nitrothiazol	Urea stibamine
Bephenium	Oxamniquine	Veroxil
hydroxynaphthoate	Oxantel	Viprynium
Bithionol, anthelminthic	Pelletierine tannate	Wormseed, American
Bitoscanate	Perchloroethylene,	
Chenopodium	medicinal	
	Pinkroot	

T37.4x- Poisoning by, adverse effect of and underdosing of anthelminthics

T37.4x1- Poisoning by anthelminthics, <u>accidental</u> (unintentional)
    Poisoning by anthelminthics NOS

T37.4x2- Poisoning by anthelminthics, <u>intentional</u> self-harm

T37.4x3- Poisoning by anthelminthics, <u>assault</u>

T37.4x4- Poisoning by anthelminthics, <u>undetermined</u>

T37.4x5- <u>Adverse effect</u> of anthelminthics

T37.4x6- <u>Underdosing</u> of anthelminthics

T37.5- Poisoning by, adverse effect of and underdosing of antiviral drugs

> Excludes 1:   amantadine (T42.8-)
>   cytarabine (T45.1-)

T37.5 - DRUGS/CHEMS*		
ABOB	Dideoxyinosine	Metisazone
Aciclovir	Flumidin	Moroxydine
Acyclovir	Foscarnet sodium	Ribavirin
Adenine, arabinoside	Fosfonet sodium	Rimantadine
Anti-infective, antiviral	Ganciclovir (sodium)	Thymopentin
Antiviral drug NEC	Ibacitabine	Trifluridine
Ara-A	Inosine pranobex	Tromantadine
Azidothymidine	Interferon (alpha) (beta)	Vidarabine
AZT	(gamma)	Virugon
Dideoxycytidine	Methisazone	Zalcitabine
	Methisoprinol	Zidovudine

T37.5x- Poisoning by, adverse effect of and underdosing of antiviral drugs

T37.5x1- Poisoning by antiviral drugs, <u>accidental</u> (unintentional)
    Poisoning by antiviral drugs NOS

T37.5x2- Poisoning by antiviral drugs, <u>intentional</u> self-harm

T37.5x3- Poisoning by antiviral drugs, <u>assault</u>

T37.5x4- Poisoning by antiviral drugs, <u>undetermined</u>

T37.5x5- <u>Adverse effect</u> of antiviral drugs

T37.5x6- <u>Underdosing</u> of antiviral drugs

T37.8- Poisoning by, adverse effect of and underdosing of other specified systemic anti-infectives and antiparasitics
    Poisoning by, adverse effect of and underdosing of hydroxyquinoline derivatives
> Excludes 1:   antimalarial drugs (T37.2-)

T37.8 - DRUGS/CHEMS*		
Akritoin	Fluconazole	Nifurtoinol
Anti-infective, arsenical	Flucytosine	Nitrofurantoin
Anti-infective, heavy metals	Flumequine	Nitroxoline
NEC	Flunidazole	Oxolinic acid
Antimony, anti-infectives	Fluorocytosine	Oxyquinoline (derivatives)
Antimony, potassium	Furazolidone	Pefloxacin
(sodium) tartrate	Hexamine (mandelate)	Pipemidic acid
Antimony, tartrated	Hexetidine	Piromidic acid
Antiparasitic drug, specified	Hydroxychloroquine	Potassium antimony
NEC	Hydroxyquinoline	'tartrate'
Arsenic anti-infectives	(derivatives) NEC	Quiniobine
Arsphenamine (silver)	Iodobismitol	Quinoline (derivatives) NEC
Bismarsen	Iodochlorhydroxyquin	Rosoxacin
Bismuth salts, anti-	Iodochlorhydroxyquinoline	Salvarsan 606 (neosilver)
infectives	Iodoquinol	(silver)
Bismuth salts, subsalicylate	Itraconazole	Silver arsphenamine
Bismuth salts,	Lead, anti-infectives	Silver salvarsan
sulfarsphenamine	Mandelic acid	Sodium cacodylate, anti-
Bithionol	Mapharsen	infective
Broxyquinoline	Meglumine antimoniate	Stovarsal
Chiniofon	Mercury, anti-infective,	Sulfarsphenamine
Cinoxacin	systemic	Tartar emetic
Clioquinol	Methenamine (mandelate)	Tartrated antimony (anti-
Croconazole	Methyl glucamine	infective)
Dichlorhydroxyquinoline	antimonate	Thiobismol
Diiodohydroxyquin	Metronidazol	Thiocarbarsone
Diiodohydroxyquinoline	Nalidixic acid	Tin, anti-infectives
Diodoquin	Neoarsphenamine	Trimethoprim
Disinfectant, intestinal	Neosalvarsan	Urinary anti-infective
Floraquin	Neosilversalvarsan	Vioform
	Nifuratel	Xibornol

T37.8x- Poisoning by, adverse effect of and underdosing of <u>other specified systemic anti-infectives and antiparasitics</u>

T37.8x1- Poisoning by other specified systemic anti-infectives and antiparasitics, <u>accidental</u> (unintentional)
    Poisoning by other specified systemic anti-infectives and antiparasitics NOS

T37.8x2- Poisoning by other specified systemic anti-infectives and antiparasitics, <u>intentional</u> self-harm

T37.8x3- Poisoning by other specified systemic anti-infectives and antiparasitics, <u>assault</u>

T37.8x4- Poisoning by other specified systemic anti-infectives and antiparasitics, <u>undetermined</u>

T37.8x5- <u>Adverse effect</u> of other specified systemic anti-infectives and antiparasitics

T37.8x6- <u>Underdosing</u> of other specified systemic anti-infectives and antiparasitics

T37.9- Poisoning by, adverse effect of and underdosing of <u>unspecified systemic anti-infective and antiparasitics</u>

T37.9 - DRUGS/CHEMS*		
Acriflavine	Anti-infective NEC	Ethoxazene
Ammonium mandelate	Anti-infective, mixed	Furadantin
Antifungal, anti-infective	Antiparasitic drug	Furoxone
NEC	(systemic)	Nifuraldezone
	Calcium mandelate	Serenium (hydrochloride)

T37.91x- Poisoning by unspecified systemic anti-infective and antiparasitics, <u>accidental</u> (unintentional)
    Poisoning by, adverse effect of and underdosing of systemic anti-infective and antiparasitics NOS

T37.92x- Poisoning by unspecified systemic anti-infective and antiparasitics, <u>intentional</u> self-harm

T37.93x- Poisoning by unspecified systemic anti-infective and antiparasitics, <u>assault</u>

T37.94x- Poisoning by unspecified systemic anti-infective and antiparasitics, <u>undetermined</u>

T37.95x- <u>Adverse effect</u> of unspecified systemic anti-infective and antiparasitic

T37.96x- <u>Underdosing</u> of unspecified systemic anti-infectives and antiparasitics

T3 7 – T37

T38- Poisoning by, adverse effect of and underdosing of <u>hormones and their synthetic substitutes and antagonists</u>, <u>not elsewhere classified</u>

Excludes 1:　mineralocorticoids and their antagonists (T50.0-)
　　　　　　oxytocic hormones (T48.0-)
　　　　　　parathyroid hormones and derivatives (T50.9-)

The appropriate 7th character is to be added to each code from category T38:
A　<u>Initial</u> encounter
D　<u>Subsequent</u> encounter
S　<u>Sequela</u>

T38.0- Poisoning by, adverse effect of and underdosing of glucocorticoids and synthetic analogues

Excludes 1:　glucocorticoids, topically used (T49.-)

T38.0 - DRUGS/CHEMS*		
Adrenal (extract, cortex or medulla) (glucocorticoids) (hormones) (mineralocorticoids)	Corticosteroid	Glucocorticoids
Aristocort	Cortisone (acetate)	Glucocorticosteroid
Celestone	Cortivazol	Hormone, adrenal cortical steroids
Clocortolone	Cortogen	Hydeltra
Cloprednol	Cortone	Hydrocortone
Compound E (cortisone)	Cortril	Kenacort
Compound F (hydrocortisone)	Decadron	Meprednisone
Cortate	Deflazacort	Methyl prednisolone
Cort-Dome	Deltasone	Paramethasone
Cortef	Deltra	Percorten
	Dexamethasone	Prednisolone
	DOCA	Prednisone
	Florinef	Prednylidene
	Fluohydrocortisone	Steroid
	Fluorinated corticosteroids	
	Fluprednisolone	

T38.0x- Poisoning by, adverse effect of and underdosing of <u>glucocorticoids and synthetic analogues</u>

T38.0x1- Poisoning by glucocorticoids and synthetic analogues, <u>accidental</u> (unintentional)
Poisoning by glucocorticoids and synthetic analogues NOS

T38.0x2- Poisoning by glucocorticoids and synthetic analogues, <u>intentional</u> self-harm

T38.0x3- Poisoning by glucocorticoids and synthetic analogues, <u>assault</u>

T38.0x4- Poisoning by glucocorticoids and synthetic analogues, <u>undetermined</u>

T38.0x5- <u>Adverse effect</u> of glucocorticoids and synthetic analogues

T38.0x6- <u>Underdosing</u> of glucocorticoids and synthetic analogues

T38.1- Poisoning by, adverse effect of and underdosing of thyroid hormones and substitutes

T38.1 - DRUGS/CHEMS*		
Cytomel	Levoid	Synthroid
Detrothyronine	Levothyroxine	Thyroglobulin
Dextrothyroxin	Levothyroxine sodium	Thyroid (hormone)
Dextrothyroxine sodium	Liothyronine	Thyrolar
Euthroid	Liotrix	Thyroxine
Hormone, thyroid	Proloid	Tiratricol
I-thyroxine sodium	Sodium l-triiodothyronine	Titroid
Letter	Sodium (L)-triiodothyronine	Triiodothyronine

T38.1x- Poisoning by, adverse effect of and underdosing of <u>thyroid hormones and substitutes</u>

T38.1x1- Poisoning by thyroid hormones and substitutes, <u>accidental</u> (unintentional)
Poisoning by thyroid hormones and substitutes NOS

T38.1x2- Poisoning by thyroid hormones and substitutes, <u>intentional</u> self-harm

T38.1x3- Poisoning by thyroid hormones and substitutes, <u>assault</u>

T38.1x4- Poisoning by thyroid hormones and substitutes, <u>undetermined</u>

T38.1x5- <u>Adverse effect</u> of thyroid hormones and substitutes

T38.1x6- <u>Underdosing</u> of thyroid hormones and substitutes

T38.2- Poisoning by, adverse effect of and underdosing of antithyroid drugs

T38.2 - DRUGS/CHEMS*		
Antithyroid drug NEC	Methimazole	Sodium iodide I-131, therapeutic
Benzylthiouracil	Methyl thiouracil	Tapazole
Carbimazole	Methylthiouracil	Thiamazole
Diiodotyrosine	Potassium perchlorate, antithyroid	Thiocarbamide
Iodine 131, therapeutic	Potassium perchlorate, medicinal	Thiouracil (benzyl) (methyl) (propyl)
Iodine for thyroid conditions (antithyroid)	Propyl thiouracil	Thiourea
Iothiouracil	Propylthiouracil	
Methiacil		

T38.2x- Poisoning by, adverse effect of and underdosing of <u>antithyroid drugs</u>

T38.2x1- Poisoning by antithyroid drugs, <u>accidental</u> (unintentional)
Poisoning by antithyroid drugs NOS

T38.2x2- Poisoning by antithyroid drugs, <u>intentional</u> self-harm

T38.2x3- Poisoning by antithyroid drugs, <u>assault</u>

T38.2x4- Poisoning by antithyroid drugs, <u>undetermined</u>

T38.2x5- <u>Adverse effect</u> of antithyroid drugs

T38.2x6- <u>Underdosing</u> of antithyroid drugs

T38.3- Poisoning by, adverse effect of and underdosing of insulin and oral hypoglycemic [antidiabetic] drugs

T38.3 - DRUGS/CHEMS*		
Acetohexamide	Glisolamide	Insulin, slow acting
Antidiabetic NEC	Glisoxepide	Insulin, zinc, protamine injection
Antidiabetic, biguanide	Globin zinc insulin	Insulin, zinc, suspension (amorphous) (crystalline)
Antidiabetic, biguanide and sulfonyl combined	Glucagon	Isophane insulin
Antidiabetic, combined	Glyburide	Lente lietin (insulin)
Antidiabetic, sulfonylurea	Glyclopyramide	Metformin
Biguanide derivatives, oral	Glycyclamide	Neutral insulin injection
Buformin	Glymidine sodium	NPH Iletin (insulin)
Carbutamide	Hormone, antidiabetic agents	Orinase
Chlorpropamide	Iletin	Phenformin
DBI	Insular tissue extract	Phenylethylbiguanide
Diabinese	Insulin (amorphous) (globin) (isophane) (Lente) (NPH) (Semilente) (Ultralente) (zinc)	Protamine sulfate, zinc insulin
Dimethyl diguanide		PZI
Dymelor		Sodium tolbutamide
Extended insulin zinc suspension	Insulin, defalan	Sulfonylurea derivatives, oral
Glibenclamide	Insulin, human	Tolazamide
Glibornuride	Insulin, injection, soluble	Tolbutamide (sodium)
Gliclazide	Insulin, injection, soluble, biphasic	
Glimidine	Insulin, intermediate acting	
Glipizide	Insulin, protamine zinc	
Gliquidone		

T38.3x- Poisoning by, adverse effect of and underdosing of <u>insulin and oral hypoglycemic [antidiabetic] drugs</u>

T38.3x1- Poisoning by insulin and oral hypoglycemic [antidiabetic] drugs, <u>accidental</u> (unintentional)
Poisoning by insulin and oral hypoglycemic [antidiabetic] drugs NOS

T38.3x2- Poisoning by insulin and oral hypoglycemic [antidiabetic] drugs, <u>intentional</u> self-harm

T38.3x3- Poisoning by insulin and oral hypoglycemic [antidiabetic] drugs, <u>assault</u>

T38.3x4- Poisoning by insulin and oral hypoglycemic [antidiabetic] drugs, <u>undetermined</u>

T38.3x5- <u>Adverse effect</u> of insulin and oral hypoglycemic [antidiabetic] drugs

T38.3x6- <u>Underdosing</u> of insulin and oral hypoglycemic [antidiabetic] drugs

T38 | T38 | T38

T38.4- Poisoning by, adverse effect of and underdosing of oral contraceptives
    Poisoning by, adverse effect of and underdosing of multiple- and single-ingredient oral contraceptive preparations

T38.4 - DRUGS/CHEMS*		
Antifertility pill	Ethynodiol with mestranol diacetate	Norlestrin
Contraceptive (oral)	Etinodiol	Norlutin
Demulen	Etynodiol	Oracon
Enovid	Levonorgestrel	Oral contraceptives
Ethinylestradiol, with levonorgestrel	Lynestrenol	Ortho-Novum
	Norethindrone	Ovral
Ethinylestradiol, with norethisterone	Norethisterone (acetate) (enantate)	Ovulen
		Progestin, oral contraceptive
Ethynodiol	Norgestrel	Quingestanol
	Norgestrienone	

T38.4x- Poisoning by, adverse effect of and underdosing of <u>oral contraceptives</u>

  T38.4x1- Poisoning by oral contraceptives, <u>accidental</u> (unintentional)
      Poisoning by oral contraceptives NOS

  T38.4x2- Poisoning by oral contraceptives, <u>intentional</u> self-harm

  T38.4x3- Poisoning by oral contraceptives, <u>assault</u>

  T38.4x4- Poisoning by oral contraceptives, <u>undetermined</u>

  T38.4x5- <u>Adverse effect</u> of oral contraceptives

  T38.4x6- <u>Underdosing</u> of oral contraceptives

T38.5- Poisoning by, adverse effect of and underdosing of other estrogens and progestogens
    Poisoning by, adverse effect of and underdosing of estrogens and progestogens mixtures and substitutes

T38.5 - DRUGS/CHEMS*		
Allylestrenol	Estrogen, conjugated	Norethisterone with ethynylestradiol
Anhydrohydroxy-progesterone	Estrone	
	Estropipate	Noretynodrel
Antineoplastic combination, estrogen	Ethinylestradiol, ethinyloestradiol	Normethandrone
		Oestradiol
Chlormadinone	Ethisterone	Oestriol
Chlorotrianisene	Fosfestrol	Oestrogen
Chlortrianisene	Gestonorone caproate	Oestrone
Clomifene	Gonadal tissue extract, female	Ovarian hormone
Clomiphene		Ovarian stimulant
Conjugated estrogenic substances	Hexestrol	Oxendolone
	Hexoestrol	Piperazine estrone sulfate
	Hormone, ovarian	Polyestradiol phosphate
Delalutin	Hydroxyestrone	Polyoestradiol phosphate
Demegestone	Hydroxyprogesterone	Pregnandiol
Desogestrel	Hydroxyprogesterone caproate	Pregneninolone
Diaethylstilboestrolum		Premarin
Dienestrol	Isopregnenone	Progesterone
Dienoestrol	Levonorgestrel with ethinylestradiol	Progestin
Diethyl stilbestrol		Progestogen NEC
Diethylstilbestrol	Lipo-Lutin	Progestone
Diethylstilboestrol	Lutocylol	Proluton
Dimestrol	Lutromone	Promegestone
Dimethisterone	Medrogestone	Provera
Dydrogesterone	Medroxyprogesterone acetate (depot)	Quinestradiol
Epiestriol		Quinestradol
Epimestrol	Megestrol	Quinestrol
Estradiol	Mestranol	Steroid, antineoplastic, hormone, estrogen
Estradiol benzoate	Methallenestril	
Estriol	Methallenoestril	Stilbestrol
Estrogen	Methylestrenolone	Stilboestrol
Estrogen, with progesterone	Nomegestrol	Tace

T38.5x- Poisoning by, adverse effect of and underdosing of <u>other estrogens and progestogens</u>

  T38.5x1- Poisoning by other estrogens and progestogens, <u>accidental</u> (unintentional)
      Poisoning by other estrogens and progestogens NOS

  T38.5x2- Poisoning by other estrogens and progestogens, <u>intentional</u> self-harm

  T38.5x3- Poisoning by other estrogens and progestogens, <u>assault</u>

  T38.5x4- Poisoning by other estrogens and progestogens, <u>undetermined</u>

T38.5x5- <u>Adverse effect</u> of other estrogens and progestogens

T38.5x6- <u>Underdosing</u> of other estrogens and progestogens

T38.6- Poisoning by, adverse effect of and underdosing of antigonadotrophins, antiestrogens, antiandrogens, not elsewhere classified
    Poisoning by, adverse effect of and underdosing of tamoxifen

T38.6 - DRUGS/CHEMS*		
Antiandrogen NEC	Danazol	Ormeloxifene
Antiestrogen NEC	Flutamide	Taleranol
Antigonadotrophin NEC	Mifepristone	Tamoxifen
Cyproterone	Nafoxidine	Toremifene
	Nilutamide	

T38.6x- Poisoning by, adverse effect of and underdosing of <u>antigonadotrophins, antiestrogens, antiandrogens, not elsewhere classified</u>

  T38.6x1- Poisoning by antigonadotrophins, antiestrogens, antiandrogens, not elsewhere classified, <u>accidental</u> (unintentional)
      Poisoning by antigonadotrophins, antiestrogens, antiandrogens, not elsewhere classified NOS

  T38.6x2- Poisoning by antigonadotrophins, antiestrogens, antiandrogens, not elsewhere classified, <u>intentional</u> self-harm

  T38.6x3- Poisoning by antigonadotrophins, antiestrogens, antiandrogens, not elsewhere classified, <u>assault</u>

  T38.6x4- Poisoning by antigonadotrophins, antiestrogens, antiandrogens, not elsewhere classified, <u>undetermined</u>

  T38.6x5- <u>Adverse effect</u> of antigonadotrophins, antiestrogens, antiandrogens, not elsewhere classified

  T38.6x6- <u>Underdosing</u> of antigonadotrophins, antiestrogens, antiandrogens, not elsewhere classified

T38.7- Poisoning by, adverse effect of and underdosing of androgens and anabolic congeners

T38.7 - DRUGS/CHEMS*		
Anabolic steroid	Ethylestrenol	Nandrolone
Androgen	Fluoxymesterone	Norethandrolone
Androgen-estrogen mixture	Gonadal tissue extract, male	Nortestosterone (furanpropionate)
Androstalone	Hormone, androgenic	Oxandrolone
Androstanolone	Macrolide, anabolic drug	Oxymesterone
Androsterone	Mepitiostane	Oxymetholone
Antineoplastic steroid	Mestanolone	Prasterone
Calusterone	Mesterolone	Stanolone
Chlorodehydromethyl-testosterone	Metandienone	Stanozolol
	Metandrostenolone	Steroid, anabolic
Congener, anabolic	Metenolone	Steroid, androgenic
Dromostanolone	Methandienone	Steroid, antineoplastic, hormone
Drostanolone	Methandiol	
Durabolin	Methandrostenolone	Testolactone
Epitiostanol	Methenolone	Testosterone
Estanozolol	Methyl androstanolone	Zeranol
Estradiol with testosterone	Methyl testosterone	
Ethyl estranol	Methyltestosterone	

T38.7x- Poisoning by, adverse effect of and underdosing of <u>androgens and anabolic congeners</u>

  T38.7x1- Poisoning by androgens and anabolic congeners, <u>accidental</u> (unintentional)
      Poisoning by androgens and anabolic congeners NOS

  T38.7x2- Poisoning by androgens and anabolic congeners, <u>intentional</u> self-harm

  T38.7x3- Poisoning by androgens and anabolic congeners, <u>assault</u>

  T38.7x4- Poisoning by androgens and anabolic congeners, <u>undetermined</u>

  T38.7x5- <u>Adverse effect</u> of androgens and anabolic congeners

  T38.7x6- <u>Underdosing</u> of androgens and anabolic congeners

T38.8- Poisoning by, adverse effect of and underdosing of other and unspecified hormones and synthetic substitutes

T38.80- Poisoning by, adverse effect of and underdosing of unspecified hormones and synthetic substitutes

T38.80 - DRUGS/CHEMS*
Hormone

T38.801- Poisoning by unspecified hormones and synthetic substitutes, <u>accidental</u> (unintentional)
Poisoning by unspecified hormones and synthetic substitutes NOS

T38.802- Poisoning by unspecified hormones and synthetic substitutes, <u>intentional</u> self-harm

T38.803- Poisoning by unspecified hormones and synthetic substitutes, <u>assault</u>

T38.804- Poisoning by unspecified hormones and synthetic substitutes, <u>undetermined</u>

T38.805- <u>Adverse effect</u> of unspecified hormones and synthetic substitutes

T38.806- <u>Underdosing</u> of unspecified hormones and synthetic substitutes

T38.81- Poisoning by, adverse effect of and underdosing of <u>anterior pituitary [adenohypophyseal] hormones</u>

T38.81 - DRUGS/CHEMS*		
ACTH	HGH (human growth hormone)	Menotropins
Adrenocorticotrophic hormone	Hormone, anterior pituitary NEC	Pergonal
Adrenocorticotrophin	Hormone, follicle stimulating	Pituitary extracts, anterior
Alsactide		Prolactin
Anterior pituitary hormone NEC	Hormone, gonadotropic, pituitary	Seractide
Corticotropin	Hormone, growth	Somatotropin
Cosyntropin	Hormone, luteinizing	Somatrem
Follicle-stimulating hormone, human	Hormone, pituitary, anterior	Somatropin
FSH	Human growth hormone (HGH)	Tetracosactide
Gonadotropin, pituitary	Luteinizing hormone	Tetracosactrin
Growth hormone		Thyreotrophic hormone
		Thyrotrophin
		Thyrotropic hormone
		TSH
		Urofollitropin

T38.811- Poisoning by anterior pituitary [adenohypophyseal] hormones, <u>accidental</u> (unintentional)
Poisoning by anterior pituitary [adenohypophyseal] hormones NOS

T38.812- Poisoning by anterior pituitary [adenohypophyseal] hormones, <u>intentional</u> self-harm

T38.813- Poisoning by anterior pituitary [adenohypophyseal] hormones, <u>assault</u>

T38.814- Poisoning by anterior pituitary [adenohypophyseal] hormones, <u>undetermined</u>

T38.815- <u>Adverse effect</u> of anterior pituitary [adenohypophyseal] hormones

T38.816- <u>Underdosing</u> of anterior pituitary [adenohypophyseal] hormones

T38.89- Poisoning by, adverse effect of and underdosing of <u>other hormones and synthetic substitutes</u>

T38.89 - DRUGS/CHEMS*	Hormone, antidiuretic	Pituitrin
ADH	Hormone, gonadotropic	Placental hormone
Antidiuretic hormone	Hormone, pituitary (posterior) NEC	Posterior pituitary hormone NEC
Buserelin		
Chorionic gonadotropin	Hormone, specified, NEC	Protirelin
DDAVP	Hypophysis, posterior	Sermorelin
Deamino-D-arginine vasopressin	Leuprolide	Somatorelin
	Lypressin	Terlipressin
Desmopressin	Lysine vasopressin	Thymus extract
Enterogastrone	Melanocyte-stimulating hormone	Vasopressin
Felypressin		Vasopressor drugs
Gonadorelin	Pitressin (tannate)	
Gonadotropin	Pituitary extracts (posterior)	
Gonadotropin, chorionic		

T38.891- Poisoning by other hormones and synthetic substitutes, <u>accidental</u> (unintentional)
Poisoning by other hormones and synthetic substitutes NOS

T38.892- Poisoning by other hormones and synthetic substitutes, <u>intentional</u> self-harm

T38.893- Poisoning by other hormones and synthetic substitutes, <u>assault</u>

T38.894- Poisoning by other hormones and synthetic substitutes, <u>undetermined</u>

T38.895- <u>Adverse effect</u> of other hormones and synthetic substitutes

T38.896- <u>Underdosing</u> of other hormones and synthetic substitutes

T38.9- Poisoning by, adverse effect of and underdosing of other and unspecified hormone antagonists

T38.90- Poisoning by, adverse effect of and underdosing of <u>unspecified hormone antagonists</u>

T38.90 - DRUGS/CHEMS*
Gonadal tissue extract

T38.901- Poisoning by unspecified hormone antagonists, <u>accidental</u> (unintentional)
Poisoning by unspecified hormone antagonists NOS

T38.902- Poisoning by unspecified hormone antagonists, <u>intentional</u> self-harm

T38.903- Poisoning by unspecified hormone antagonists, <u>assault</u>

T38.904- Poisoning by unspecified hormone antagonists, <u>undetermined</u>

T38.905- <u>Adverse effect</u> of unspecified hormone antagonists

T38.906- <u>Underdosing</u> of unspecified hormone antagonists

T38.99- Poisoning by, adverse effect of and underdosing of <u>other hormone antagonists</u>

T38.99 - DRUGS/CHEMS*	Somatostatin
Octreotide	Trilostane

T38.991- Poisoning by other hormone antagonists, <u>accidental</u> (unintentional)
Poisoning by other hormone antagonists NOS

T38.992- Poisoning by other hormone antagonists, <u>intentional</u> self-harm

T38.993- Poisoning by other hormone antagonists, <u>assault</u>

T38.994- Poisoning by other hormone antagonists, <u>undetermined</u>

T38.995- <u>Adverse effect</u> of other hormone antagonists

T38.996- <u>Underdosing</u> of other hormone antagonists

T
3
8
–
T
3
8

T39- **Poisoning by, adverse effect of and underdosing of <u>nonopioid analgesics, antipyretics and antirheumatics</u>**

The appropriate 7th character is to be added to each code from category T39:
- A   <u>Initial</u> encounter
- D   <u>Subsequent</u> encounter
- S   <u>Sequela</u>

T39.0-   **Poisoning by, adverse effect of and underdosing of <u>salicylates</u>**

T39.01-   **Poisoning by, adverse effect of and underdosing of <u>aspirin</u>**
   Poisoning by, adverse effect of and underdosing of acetylsalicylic acid

T39.01 - DRUGS/CHEMS*		
Acetylsalicylic acid (enteric coated) (salts)	Aluminium bis (acetylsalicylate)	Calcium actylsalicylate
Alka-seltzer	Aspirin (aluminum) (soluble)	Calcium carbaspirin
Aluminium aspirin	Bufferin	Carbaspirin
		Fiorinal
		Rhodine

T39.011-   Poisoning by aspirin, <u>accidental</u> (unintentional)

T39.012-   Poisoning by aspirin, <u>intentional</u> self-harm

T39.013-   Poisoning by aspirin, <u>assault</u>

T39.014-   Poisoning by aspirin, <u>undetermined</u>

T39.015-   <u>Adverse effect</u> of aspirin

T39.016-   <u>Underdosing</u> of aspirin

T39.09-   **Poisoning by, adverse effect of and underdosing of <u>other salicylates</u>**

T39.09 - DRUGS/CHEMS*		
Aluminium salicylate	Diflunisal	Salicylic acid, derivative
Calcium salicylate	Magnesium salicylate	Salicylic acid, salts
Carbethyl salicylate	Salicylamide	Salsalate
Choline salicylate	Salicylate NEC	Sodium salicylate
	Salicylic acid, congeners	Sodium thiosalicylate

T39.091-   Poisoning by salicylates, <u>accidental</u> (unintentional)
   Poisoning by salicylates NOS

T39.092-   Poisoning by salicylates, <u>intentional</u> self-harm

T39.093-   Poisoning by salicylates, <u>assault</u>

T39.094-   Poisoning by salicylates, <u>undetermined</u>

T39.095-   <u>Adverse effect</u> of salicylates

T39.096-   <u>Underdosing</u> of salicylates

T39.1-   **Poisoning by, adverse effect of and underdosing of <u>4-Aminophenol derivatives</u>**

T39.1 - DRUGS/CHEMS*		
P-Acetamidophenol	Analgesic, aromatic NEC	Para-acetamidophenol
Acetaminophen	Aniline analgesic	Para-aminophenol derivatives
Acetaminosalol	Aniline derivatives, therapeutic NEC	Paracetamol
Acetanilide	Bromo-seltzer	Phenacetin
Acetophenetedin	Exalgin	
4-Aminophenol derivatives	Panadol	

T39.1x-   **Poisoning by, adverse effect of and underdosing of 4-Aminophenol derivatives**

T39.1x1-   Poisoning by 4-Aminophenol derivatives, <u>accidental</u> (unintentional)
   Poisoning by 4-Aminophenol derivatives NOS

T39.1x2-   Poisoning by 4-Aminophenol derivatives, <u>intentional</u> self-harm

T39.1x3-   Poisoning by 4-Aminophenol derivatives, <u>assault</u>

T39.1x4-   Poisoning by 4-Aminophenol derivatives, <u>undetermined</u>

T39.1x5-   <u>Adverse effect</u> of 4-Aminophenol derivatives

T39.1x6-   <u>Underdosing</u> of 4-Aminophenol derivatives

T39.2-   **Poisoning by, adverse effect of and underdosing of pyrazolone derivatives**

T39.2 - DRUGS/CHEMS*		
Amidopyrine	Feprazone	Phenazone
Aminofenazone	Hydroxyphenylbutazone	Phenyl butazone
Aminophenazone	Indocin	Phenylbutazone
Aminopyrine	Isopropylaminophenazone	Propyphenazone
Analgesic, pyrazole	Kebuzone	Pyramidon
Analgin	Ketazon	Pyrazole (derivatives)
Antipyrine	Metamizole sodium	Pyrazolone analgesic NEC
Azapropazone	Methampyrone	Ramifenazone
Butazolidin	Mofebutazone	Sulfamazone
Clofezone	Monophenylbutazone	Sulfamidopyrine
Coal tar, medicinal, analgesics NEC	Myochrysin(e)	Sulpyrine
Diphenylbutazone	Nifenazone	Suxibuzone
Dipyrone	Noramidopyrine	Tandearil, tanderil
Fenazone	Noramidopyrine methanesulfonate sodium	
Fenylbutazone	Oxyphenbutazone	

T39.2x-   **Poisoning by, adverse effect of and underdosing of <u>pyrazolone derivatives</u>**

T39.2x1-   Poisoning by pyrazolone derivatives, <u>accidental</u> (unintentional)
   Poisoning by pyrazolone derivatives NOS

T39.2x2-   Poisoning by pyrazolone derivatives, <u>intentional</u> self-harm

T39.2x3-   Poisoning by pyrazolone derivatives, <u>assault</u>

T39.2x4-   Poisoning by pyrazolone derivatives, <u>undetermined</u>

T39.2x5-   <u>Adverse effect</u> of pyrazolone derivatives

T39.2x6-   <u>Underdosing</u> of pyrazolone derivatives

T39.3-   **Poisoning by, adverse effect of and underdosing of <u>other nonsteroidal anti-inflammatory drugs [NSAID]</u>**

T39.31-   **Poisoning by, adverse effect of and underdosing of <u>propionic acid derivatives</u>**
   Poisoning by, adverse effect of and underdosing of fenoprofen
   Poisoning by, adverse effect of and underdosing of flurbiprofen
   Poisoning by, adverse effect of and underdosing of ibuprofen
   Poisoning by, adverse effect of and underdosing of ketoprofen
   Poisoning by, adverse effect of and underdosing of naproxen
   Poisoning by, adverse effect of and underdosing of oxaprozin

T39.31 - DRUGS/CHEMS*		
Aleve	Carprofen	Naproxen
Analgesic, anti-inflammatory NEC, propionic acid derivative	Esflurbiprofen	Oxaprozin
	Fenoprofen	Suprofen
	Flurbiprofen	Tiaprofenic acid
Anti-inflammatory drug, nonsteroidal, propionic acid derivative	Ibufenac	
	Ibuprofen	
	Ibuproxam	
	Ketoprofen	

T39.311-   Poisoning by propionic acid derivatives, <u>accidental</u> (unintentional)

T39.312-   Poisoning by propionic acid derivatives, <u>intentional</u> self-harm

T39.313-   Poisoning by propionic acid derivatives, <u>assault</u>

T39.314-   Poisoning by propionic acid derivatives, <u>undetermined</u>

T39.315-   <u>Adverse effect</u> of propionic acid derivatives

T39.316-   <u>Underdosing</u> of propionic acid derivatives

T39.39-   **Poisoning by, adverse effect of and underdosing of <u>other nonsteroidal anti-inflammatory drugs [NSAID]</u>**

T39.39 - DRUGS/CHEMS*		
Anti-inflammatory drug NEC	Fenflumizole	Nimesulide
	Flufenamic acid	Piroxicam
Anti-inflammatory drug, nonsteroidal NEC	Indometacin	Proquazone
	Indomethacin	Sulindac
Anti-inflammatory drug, specified NEC	Isoxicam	Tenoxicam
	Meclofenamate	Tolmetin
Diclofenac	Meclofenamic acid	Ufenamate
Etodolac	Mefenamic acid	Zomepirac
	Nabumetone	

T39.391-   Poisoning by other nonsteroidal anti-inflammatory drugs [NSAID], <u>accidental</u> (unintentional)
   Poisoning by other nonsteroidal anti-inflammatory drugs NOS

T39.392- **Poisoning** by other nonsteroidal anti-inflammatory drugs [NSAID], <u>intentional</u> self-harm

T39.393- **Poisoning** by other nonsteroidal anti-inflammatory drugs [NSAID], <u>assault</u>

T39.394- **Poisoning** by other nonsteroidal anti-inflammatory drugs [NSAID], <u>undetermined</u>

T39.395- <u>Adverse effect</u> of other nonsteroidal anti-inflammatory drugs [NSAID]

T39.396- <u>Underdosing</u> of other nonsteroidal anti-inflammatory drugs [NSAID]

T39.4- **Poisoning by, adverse effect of and underdosing of antirheumatics, not elsewhere classified**

Excludes 1:   poisoning by, adverse effect of and underdosing of glucocorticoids (T38.0-)
poisoning by, adverse effect of and underdosing of salicylates (T39.0-)

T39.4 - DRUGS/CHEMS*	Auranofin	Glucosamine sulfate
Analgesic, antirheumatic NEC	Aurothioglucose	Gold salts
Antiphlogistic NEC	Aurothioglycanide	Indomethacin farnesil
Antirheumatic NEC	Aurothiomalate sodium	Sodium aurothiomalate
	Aurotioprol	Sodium aurothiosulfate

T39.4x- **Poisoning by, adverse effect of and underdosing of <u>antirheumatics</u>, <u>not elsewhere classified</u>**

T39.4x1- **Poisoning by antirheumatics, not elsewhere classified, <u>accidental</u> (unintentional)**
Poisoning by antirheumatics, not elsewhere classified NOS

T39.4x2- **Poisoning by antirheumatics, not elsewhere classified, <u>intentional</u> self-harm**

T39.4x3- **Poisoning by antirheumatics, not elsewhere classified, <u>assault</u>**

T39.4x4- **Poisoning by antirheumatics, not elsewhere classified, <u>undetermined</u>**

T39.4x5- <u>Adverse effect</u> of antirheumatics, not elsewhere classified

T39.4x6- <u>Underdosing</u> of antirheumatics, not elsewhere classified

T39.8- **Poisoning by, adverse effect of and underdosing of other nonopioid analgesics and antipyretics, not elsewhere classified**

T39.8 - DRUGS/CHEMS*	Fluradoline	Phenyramidol,
Acetylphenylhydrazine	Glafenine	phenyramidon
Analgesic, specified NEC	Jamaica dogwood (bark)	Piroxicam, beta-
Antipyretic, specified NEC	Ketorolac	cyclodextrin complex
Carbiphene	Lefetamine	Piscidia (bark) (erythrina)
Clonixin	Meptazinol	Pyrabital
Cropropamide	Methopholine	Pyridium
Crotethamide	Metofoline	Rimazolium metilsulfate
Cryogenine	Nefopam	Sumatriptan
Cyclopyrabital	Oxetorone	Tiaramide
Darvon	Pentosan polysulfate	Tinoridine
Diclonixine	(sodium)	Versidyne
Doloxene	Perisoxal	Viminol
Emorfazone	Phenazopyridine	Zactane
Etomide	Phenicarbazide	
Floctafenine		

T39.8x- **Poisoning by, adverse effect of and underdosing of <u>other nonopioid analgesics and antipyretics</u>, <u>not elsewhere classified</u>**

T39.8x1- **Poisoning by other nonopioid analgesics and antipyretics, not elsewhere classified, <u>accidental</u> (unintentional)**
Poisoning by other nonopioid analgesics and antipyretics, not elsewhere classified NOS

T39.8x2- **Poisoning by other nonopioid analgesics and antipyretics, not elsewhere classified, <u>intentional</u> self-harm**

T39.8x3- **Poisoning by other nonopioid analgesics and antipyretics, not elsewhere classified, <u>assault</u>**

T39.8x4- **Poisoning by other nonopioid analgesics and antipyretics, not elsewhere classified, <u>undetermined</u>**

T39.8x5- <u>Adverse effect</u> of other nonopioid analgesics and antipyretics, not elsewhere classified

T39.8x6- <u>Underdosing</u> of other nonopioid analgesics and antipyretics, not elsewhere classified

T39.9- **Poisoning by, adverse effect of and underdosing of <u>unspecified nonopioid analgesic, antipyretic and antirheumatic</u>**

T39.9 - DRUGS/CHEMS*	Analgesic, non-narcotic	Antipyretic
Analgesic	NEC	
Analgesic, anti-inflammatory NEC	Analgesic, non-narcotic NEC, combination	

T39.91x- **Poisoning by unspecified nonopioid analgesic, antipyretic and antirheumatic, <u>accidental</u> (unintentional)**
Poisoning by nonopioid analgesic, antipyretic and antirheumatic NOS

T39.92x- **Poisoning by unspecified nonopioid analgesic, antipyretic and antirheumatic, <u>intentional</u> self-harm**

T39.93x- **Poisoning by unspecified nonopioid analgesic, antipyretic and antirheumatic, <u>assault</u>**

T39.94x- **Poisoning by unspecified nonopioid analgesic, antipyretic and antirheumatic, <u>undetermined</u>**

T39.95x- <u>Adverse effect</u> of unspecified nonopioid analgesic, antipyretic and antirheumatic

T39.96x- <u>Underdosing</u> of unspecified nonopioid analgesic, antipyretic and antirheumatic

T40- **Poisoning by, adverse effect of and underdosing of <u>narcotics and psychodysleptics [hallucinogens]</u>**

Excludes ❷: *drug dependence and related mental and behavioral disorders due to psychoactive substance use (F10.-F19.-)*

The appropriate 7th character is to be added to each code from category T40:
A   <u>Initial</u> encounter
D   <u>Subsequent</u> encounter
S   <u>Sequela</u>

T40.0- **Poisoning by, adverse effect of and underdosing of opium**

T40.0 - DRUGS/CHEMS*	Opium alkaloids,	Pantopon
Laudanum	standardized powdered	Papaveretum
Opium alkaloids (total)	Opium alkaloids, tincture (camphorated)	Paregoric

T40.0x- **Poisoning by, adverse effect of and underdosing of <u>opium</u>**

T40.0x1- **Poisoning by opium, <u>accidental</u> (unintentional)**
Poisoning by opium NOS

T40.0x2- **Poisoning by opium, <u>intentional</u> self-harm**

T40.0x3- **Poisoning by opium, <u>assault</u>**

T40.0x4- **Poisoning by opium, <u>undetermined</u>**

T40.0x5- <u>Adverse effect</u> of opium

T40.0x6- <u>Underdosing</u> of opium

T40.1- **Poisoning by and adverse effect of heroin**

T40.1 - DRUGS/CHEMS*	Diacetylmorphine	Heroin
Acetomorphine	Diamorphine	

T40.1x- **Poisoning by and adverse effect of <u>heroin</u>**

T40.1x1- **Poisoning by heroin, <u>accidental</u> (unintentional)**
Poisoning by heroin NOS

T40.1x2- **Poisoning by heroin, <u>intentional</u> self-harm**

T40.1x3- **Poisoning by heroin, <u>assault</u>**

T40.1x4- **Poisoning by heroin, <u>undetermined</u>**

T40.2- Poisoning by, adverse effect of and underdosing of other opioids

T40.2 - DRUGS/CHEMS*	Dihydrohydroxy-	Metopon
14-hydroxydihydro	morphinone	Morfin
morphinone	Dihydroisocodeine	Morphine
Acemorphan	Dihydromorphine	Morpholinylethylmorphine
Acetorphine	Dihydromorphinone	Nicomorphine
Acetyldihydrocodeine	Dihydroxycodeinone	Nisentil
Acetyldihydrocodeinone	Dilaudid	Normorphine
Alvodine	Dimethyl meperidine	Numorphan
Antitussive, codeine	Dionin	Opioid NEC
mixture	Drocode	Oxycodone
Antitussive, opiate	Dromoran	Oxymorphone
Benzomorphan	Ethyl morphine	Palfium
Benzyl morphine	Ethylmorphine	Paracodin
Blue velvet	Etorphine	Parzone
Cliradon	Eucodal	Percodan
Codeine	Heptalgin	Peronine
Cough mixture, containing	Hycodan	Phenadoxone
opiates	Hydrocodone	Phenomorphan
Demerol	Hydromorphinol	Piminodine
Desocodeine	Hydromorphinone	Pipadone
Desomorphine	Hydromorphone	Prinadol
Dextrorphan	Hydroxydihydrocodeinone	Promedol
Difencloxazine	Leritine	Racemoramide
Dihydrocodeine	Levo-dromoran	Racemorphan
Dihydrocodein-one	Methyl dihydromorphinone	Thebaine
Dihydrohydroxycodein-one	Methyl morphine NEC	
	Methylmorphine	

T40.2x- Poisoning by, adverse effect of and underdosing of other opioids

T40.2x1- Poisoning by other opioids, accidental (unintentional)
  Poisoning by other opioids NOS

T40.2x2- Poisoning by other opioids, intentional self-harm

T40.2x3- Poisoning by other opioids, assault

T40.2x4- Poisoning by other opioids, undetermined

T40.2x5- Adverse effect of other opioids

T40.2x6- Underdosing of other opioids

T40.3- Poisoning by, adverse effect of and underdosing of methadone

T40.3 - DRUGS/CHEMS*	Dolophine	Methadone
Amidone	Levo-iso-methadone	Physeptone

T40.3x- Poisoning by, adverse effect of and underdosing of methadone

T40.3x1- Poisoning by methadone, accidental (unintentional)
  Poisoning by methadone NOS

T40.3x2- Poisoning by methadone, intentional self-harm

T40.3x3- Poisoning by methadone, assault

T40.3x4- Poisoning by methadone, undetermined

T40.3x5- Adverse effect of methadone

T40.3x6- Underdosing of methadone

T40.4- Poisoning by, adverse effect of and underdosing of other synthetic narcotics

T40.4 - DRUGS/CHEMS*	Eptazocine	Pentazocine
Alfentanil	Ethoheptazine	Pethidine
Alphaprodine	Fentanyl	Phenazocine
Anileridine	Isonipecaine	Phenoperidine
Bezitramide	Ketobemidone	Piritramide
Buprenorphine	Levopropoxyphene	Profadol
Butorphanol	Levorphanol	Propoxyphene
Dextromoramide	Meperidine	Sufentanil
Dextropropoxyphene	Nalbuphine	Tilidine
Dipipanone	Narcotic, synthetic	Tramadol

T40.4x- Poisoning by, adverse effect of and underdosing of other synthetic narcotics

T40.4x1- Poisoning by other synthetic narcotics, accidental (unintentional)
  Poisoning by other synthetic narcotics NOS

T40.4x2- Poisoning by other synthetic narcotics, intentional self-harm

T40.4x3- Poisoning by other synthetic narcotics, assault

T40.4x4- Poisoning by other synthetic narcotics, undetermined

T40.4x5- Adverse effect of other synthetic narcotics

T40.4x6- Underdosing of other synthetic narcotics

T40.5- Poisoning by, adverse effect of and underdosing of cocaine

T40.5 - DRUGS/CHEMS*	Cocaine
Coca (leaf)	Crack

T40.5x- Poisoning by, adverse effect of and underdosing of cocaine
  AHA 16:2Q:p8 – Overdose of crack cocaine, intent

T40.5x1- Poisoning by cocaine, accidental (unintentional)
  Poisoning by cocaine NOS

T40.5x2- Poisoning by cocaine, intentional self-harm

T40.5x3- Poisoning by cocaine, assault

T40.5x4- Poisoning by cocaine, undetermined

T40.5x5- Adverse effect of cocaine

T40.5x6- Underdosing of cocaine

T40.6- Poisoning by, adverse effect of and underdosing of other and unspecified narcotics

T40.60- Poisoning by, adverse effect of and underdosing of unspecified narcotics

T40.60 - DRUGS/CHEMS*	Analgesic, narcotic NEC,	Opiate NEC
Analgesic, narcotic NEC	obstetric	
Analgesic, narcotic NEC,	Narcotic (drug)	
combination	Narcotic analgesic NEC	

T40.601- Poisoning by unspecified narcotics, accidental (unintentional)
  Poisoning by narcotics NOS

T40.602- Poisoning by unspecified narcotics, intentional self-harm

T40.603- Poisoning by unspecified narcotics, assault

T40.604- Poisoning by unspecified narcotics, undetermined

T40.605- Adverse effect of unspecified narcotics

T40.606- Underdosing of unspecified narcotics

T40.69- Poisoning by, adverse effect of and underdosing of other narcotics

T40.69 - DRUGS/CHEMS*
Narcotic, specified NEC

T40.691- Poisoning by other narcotics, accidental (unintentional)
  Poisoning by other narcotics NOS

T40.692- Poisoning by other narcotics, intentional self-harm

T40.693- Poisoning by other narcotics, assault

T40.694- Poisoning by other narcotics, undetermined

T40.695- Adverse effect of other narcotics

T40.696- Underdosing of other narcotics

T40.7-   Poisoning by, adverse effect of and underdosing of cannabis (derivatives)

T40.7 - DRUGS/CHEMS*		
Afghanistan black	Central nervous system depressants, cannabis sativa	Lebanese red
Bhang		Marihuana
Cannabinol	Dronabinol	Marijuana
Cannabis (derivatives)	Ganja	Nabilone
	Hashish	Pot
	Indian hemp	Tetrahydrocannabinol
		THC

T40.7x- Poisoning by, adverse effect of and underdosing of cannabis (derivatives)

   T40.7x1- Poisoning by cannabis (derivatives), <u>accidental</u> (unintentional)
         Poisoning by cannabis NOS

   T40.7x2- Poisoning by cannabis (derivatives), <u>intentional</u> self-harm

   T40.7x3- Poisoning by cannabis (derivatives), <u>assault</u>

   T40.7x4- Poisoning by cannabis (derivatives), <u>undetermined</u>

   T40.7x5- <u>Adverse effect</u> of cannabis (derivatives)

   T40.7x6- <u>Underdosing</u> of cannabis (derivatives)

T40.8-   Poisoning by and adverse effect of lysergide [LSD]

T40.8 - DRUGS/CHEMS*	
D-lysergic acid diethylamide	LSD
	Lysergic acid diethylamide
	Lysergide

T40.8x- Poisoning by and adverse effect of lysergide [LSD]

   T40.8x1- Poisoning by lysergide [LSD], <u>accidental</u> (unintentional)
         Poisoning by lysergide [LSD] NOS

   T40.8x2- Poisoning by lysergide [LSD], <u>intentional</u> self-harm

   T40.8x3- Poisoning by lysergide [LSD], <u>assault</u>

   T40.8x4- Poisoning by lysergide [LSD], <u>undetermined</u>

T40.9-   Poisoning by, adverse effect of and underdosing of other and unspecified psychodysleptics [hallucinogens]

T40.90- Poisoning by, adverse effect of and underdosing of <u>unspecified psychodysleptics [hallucinogens]</u>

T40.90 - DRUGS/CHEMS*	
Central nervous system depressants, hallucinogenics	Hallucinogen NEC
	Megahallucinogen
	Psychodysleptic drug NEC
	Psychotomimetic agents

   T40.901- Poisoning by unspecified psychodysleptics [hallucinogens], <u>accidental</u> (unintentional)

   T40.902- Poisoning by unspecified psychodysleptics [hallucinogens], <u>intentional</u> self-harm

   T40.903- Poisoning by unspecified psychodysleptics [hallucinogens], <u>assault</u>

   T40.904- Poisoning by unspecified psychodysleptics [hallucinogens], <u>undetermined</u>

   T40.905- <u>Adverse effect</u> of unspecified psychodysleptics [hallucinogens]

   T40.906- <u>Underdosing</u> of unspecified psychodysleptics

T40.99- Poisoning by, adverse effect of and underdosing of <u>other psychodysleptics [hallucinogens]</u>

T40.99 - DRUGS/CHEMS*		
Bufotenine	Magic mushroom	Peyote
Diethyltryptamine (DET)	Mescal buttons	Phencyclidine
Dimethyl tryptamine	Mescaline	Psilocin
Hawaiian Woodrose seeds	Morning glory seeds	Psilocybin
Heavenly Blue (morning glory)	PCP, meaning phencyclidine	Psilocybine
	Pearly Gates (morning glory seeds)	Yohimbic acid

   T40.991- Poisoning by other psychodysleptics [hallucinogens], <u>accidental</u> (unintentional)
         Poisoning by other psychodysleptics [hallucinogens] NOS

   T40.992- Poisoning by other psychodysleptics [hallucinogens], <u>intentional</u> self-harm

   T40.993- Poisoning by other psychodysleptics [hallucinogens], <u>assault</u>

   T40.994- Poisoning by other psychodysleptics [hallucinogens], <u>undetermined</u>

   T40.995- <u>Adverse effect</u> of other psychodysleptics [hallucinogens]

   T40.996- <u>Underdosing</u> of other psychodysleptics

T41-   Poisoning by, adverse effect of and underdosing of <u>anesthetics and therapeutic gases</u>
   Excludes 1:   benzodiazepines (T42.4-)
            cocaine (T40.5-)
            complications of anesthesia during pregnancy (O29.-)
            complications of anesthesia during labor and delivery (O74.-)
            complications of anesthesia during the puerperium (O89.-)
            opioids (T40.0-T40.2-)

   The appropriate 7th character is to be added to each code from category T41:
   A   <u>Initial</u> encounter
   D   <u>Subsequent</u> encounter
   S   <u>Sequela</u>

T41.0-   Poisoning by, adverse effect of and underdosing of inhaled anesthetics
   Excludes 1:   oxygen (T41.5-)

T41.0 - DRUGS/CHEMS*		
Anesthesia, endotracheal	Diethyl ether (vapor) — see also Ether	Fluothane
Anesthesia, inhalation	Divinyl ether	Fluroxene
Anesthetic, gaseous NEC	Enflurane	Gas, anesthetic
Anesthetic, halogenated hydrocarbon derivatives NEC	Ether (vapor)	Halothane
	Ether, anesthetic	Isoflurane
	Ether, divinyl	Laughing gas
Central nervous system depressants, anesthetic, gases NEC	Ether, ethyl (medicinal)	Methoxyflurane
	Ethyl bromide (anesthetic)	Nitrous oxide
	Ethyl chloride (anesthetic)	Trichloroethylene, anesthetic (gas)
Chloroform, anesthetic	Ethyl chloride, anesthetic, inhaled	Trifluoroethyl vinyl ether
Chloroform, water, concentrated	Ethylene, anesthetic (general)	Trilene
		Vinesthene, vinethene
		Vinyl ether

T41.0x- Poisoning by, adverse effect of and underdosing of <u>inhaled anesthetics</u>

   T41.0x1- Poisoning by inhaled anesthetics, <u>accidental</u> (unintentional)
         Poisoning by inhaled anesthetics NOS

   T41.0x2- Poisoning by inhaled anesthetics, <u>intentional</u> self-harm

   T41.0x3- Poisoning by inhaled anesthetics, <u>assault</u>

   T41.0x4- Poisoning by inhaled anesthetics, <u>undetermined</u>

   T41.0x5- <u>Adverse effect</u> of inhaled anesthetics

   T41.0x6- <u>Underdosing</u> of inhaled anesthetics

T41.1-   Poisoning by, adverse effect of and underdosing of intravenous anesthetics
      Poisoning by, adverse effect of and underdosing of thiobarbiturates

T41.1 - DRUGS/CHEMS*		
Alfadolone	Butyl thiobarbital sodium	Pentothal
Alfaxalone	Central nervous system depressants, anesthetic, intravenous	Sernyl
Alphadolone		Sodium thiopental
Alphaxalone	Etomidate	Surital
Anesthetic, intravenous NEC	Evipal sodium	Thialbarbital
	Evipan sodium	Thiamylal
Anesthetic, thiobarbiturate	Hexobarbital, sodium	Thiamylal sodium
Barbiturate anesthetic (intravenous)	Intranarcon	Thiobarbital sodium
	Kemithal	Thiobarbiturate anesthetic
Brevital (sodium)	Methohexital	Thiobutabarbital sodium
Buthalitone (sodium)	Methohexitone	Thiopental (sodium)
		Thiopentone (sodium)

T41.1x- Poisoning by, adverse effect of and underdosing of <u>intravenous anesthetics</u>

   T41.1x1- Poisoning by intravenous anesthetics, <u>accidental</u> (unintentional)
         Poisoning by intravenous anesthetics NOS

   T41.1x2- Poisoning by intravenous anesthetics, <u>intentional</u> self-harm

   T41.1x3- Poisoning by intravenous anesthetics, <u>assault</u>

   T41.1x4- Poisoning by intravenous anesthetics, <u>undetermined</u>

   T41.1x5- <u>Adverse effect</u> of intravenous anesthetics

   T41.1x6- <u>Underdosing</u> of intravenous anesthetics

T40 - T41

T41.2- **Poisoning by, adverse effect of and underdosing of other and unspecified general anesthetics**

T41.20- **Poisoning by, adverse effect of and underdosing of unspecified general anesthetics**

T41.20 - DRUGS/CHEMS*		
Anesthesia, potentiated	Anesthetic, with muscle relaxant, general	Central nervous system depressants, anesthetic (general) NEC
Anesthesia, rectal	Anesthetic, general NEC	
Anesthesia, rectal, general	Anesthetic, rectal	Depressant, central nervous system, general anesthetic
Anesthetic, with muscle relaxant	Anesthetic, rectal, general	
		Premedication anesthetic

T41.201- **Poisoning by unspecified general anesthetics, accidental (unintentional)**
 Poisoning by general anesthetics NOS

T41.202- **Poisoning by unspecified general anesthetics, intentional self-harm**

T41.203- **Poisoning by unspecified general anesthetics, assault**

T41.204- **Poisoning by unspecified general anesthetics, undetermined**

T41.205- **Adverse effect of unspecified general anesthetics**

T41.206- **Underdosing of unspecified general anesthetics**

T41.29- **Poisoning by, adverse effect of and underdosing of other general anesthetics**

T41.29 - DRUGS/CHEMS*		
Cyclopropane	Ketamine	Propofol
Disoprofol	Minaxolone	Sodium oxybate
Hexobarbital, rectal	Oxybate sodium	Tiletamine
	Propanidid	Tribromoethanol, rectal

T41.291- **Poisoning by other general anesthetics, accidental (unintentional)**
 Poisoning by other general anesthetics NOS

T41.292- **Poisoning by other general anesthetics, intentional self-harm**

T41.293- **Poisoning by other general anesthetics, assault**

T41.294- **Poisoning by other general anesthetics, undetermined**

T41.295- **Adverse effect of other general anesthetics**

T41.296- **Underdosing of other general anesthetics**

T41.3- **Poisoning by, adverse effect of and underdosing of local anesthetics**
 Cocaine (topical)

 Excludes 2: *poisoning by cocaine used as a central nervous system stimulant (T40.5x1-T40.5x4)*

T41.3 - DRUGS/CHEMS*		
Amethocaine (regional) (spinal)	Blockain, infiltration (subcutaneous)	Cinchocaine, topical (surface)
Amyleine, regional	Blockain, nerve block (peripheral) (plexus)	Citanest
Amylocaine (regional) (infiltration) (nerve block) (spinal) (topical)	Blockain, topical (surface)	Citanest, infiltration (subcutaneous)
	Bupivacaine	Citanest, nerve block (peripheral) (plexus)
Anesthesia, caudal	Bupivacaine, infiltration (subcutaneous)	Cocaine, topical anesthetic
Anesthesia, epidural	Bupivacaine, nerve block (peripheral) (plexus)	Cyclaine
Anesthesia, local		Cyclomethycaine
Anesthesia, mucosal	Bupivacaine, spinal	Dibucaine
Anesthesia, nerve blocking	Butacaine	Dibucaine, topical (surface)
Anesthesia, plexus blocking	Butamben	Dimethocaine
Anesthesia, rectal, local	Butanilicaine	Diperodon
Anesthesia, regional	Butyl aminobenzoate	Dorsacaine
Anesthesia, surface	Butyn	Dyclone
Anesthetic, with muscle relaxant, local	Carbocaine	Dyclonine
	Carbocaine, infiltration (subcutaneous)	Endocaine
Anesthetic, infiltration NEC		EPAB
Anesthetic, local NEC	Carbocaine, nerve block (peripheral) (plexus)	Ethocaine (infiltration) (topical)
Anesthetic, rectal, local	Carbocaine, topical	Ethocaine, nerve block (peripheral) (plexus)
Anesthetic, regional NEC	(surface)	
Anesthetic, spinal NEC	Chloroprocaine	Ethocaine, spinal
Anesthetic, topical	Chloroprocaine, infiltration (subcutaneous)	Ethyl aminobenzoate
Aptocaine		Ethyl chloride, anesthetic (local)
Articaine	Chloroprocaine, nerve block (peripheral) (plexus)	Etidocaine
Benoxinate		Etidocaine, infiltration (subcutaneous)
Benzamine	Chloroprocaine, spinal	
Benzocaine	Cinchocaine	
Betoxycaine		
Blockain		

T41.3 - DRUGS/CHEMS* — Continued		
Etidocaine, nerve (peripheral) (plexus)	Novocain, spinal	Procaine, spinal
	Nupercaine (spinal anesthetic)	Proparacaine
Eucaine	Nupercaine, topical (surface)	Propitocaine
Hexylcaine		Propitocaine, infiltration (subcutaneous)
Leucinocaine	Ophthaine	
Lidocaine	Ophthetic	Propitocaine, nerve block (peripheral) (plexus)
Lidocaine, regional	Orthocaine	
Lidocaine, spinal	Oxetacaine	Propoxycaine
Lignocaine	Oxethazine	Propoxycaine, infiltration (subcutaneous)
Lignocaine, regional	Oxybuprocaine	
Lignocaine, spinal	Percaine (spinal)	Propoxycaine, nerve block (peripheral) (plexus)
Marcaine	Percaine, topical (surface)	
Marcaine, infiltration (subcutaneous)	Phenacaine	Propoxycaine, topical (surface)
	Piperocaine	
Marcaine, nerve block (peripheral) (plexus)	Piperocaine, infiltration (subcutaneous)	Proxymetacaine
		Quotane
Mepivacaine	Piperocaine, nerve block (peripheral) (plexus)	Stovaine
Mepivacaine epidural		Stovaine, infiltration (subcutaneous)
Meprylcaine	Piperocaine, topical (surface)	
Metabutethamine		Stovaine, nerve block (peripheral) (plexus)
Metycaine	Pitkin's solution	
Metycaine, infiltration (subcutaneous)	Pontocaine (hydrochloride) (infiltration) (topical)	Stovaine, spinal
		Stovaine, topical (surface)
Metycaine, nerve block (peripheral) (plexus)	Pontocaine, nerve block (peripheral) (plexus)	Surfacaine
		Tetracaine
Metycaine, topical (surface)	Pontocaine, spinal	Tetracaine, nerve block (peripheral) (plexus)
Nesacaine	Prilocaine	
Nesacaine, infiltration (subcutaneous)	Prilocaine, infiltration (subcutaneous)	Tetracaine, regional
		Tetracaine, spinal
Nesacaine, nerve block (peripheral) (plexus)	Prilocaine, nerve block (peripheral) (plexus)	Trimecaine
		Tronothane
Novocain (infiltration) (topical)	Prilocaine, regional	Xylocaine (infiltration) (topical)
	Procaine	
Novocain, nerve block (peripheral) (plexus)	Procaine, nerve block (peripheral) (plexus)	Xylocaine, nerve block (peripheral) (plexus)
	Procaine, regional	Xylocaine, spinal

T41.3x- **Poisoning by, adverse effect of and underdosing of local anesthetics**

T41.3x1- **Poisoning by local anesthetics, accidental (unintentional)**
 Poisoning by local anesthetics NOS

T41.3x2- **Poisoning by local anesthetics, intentional self-harm**

T41.3x3- **Poisoning by local anesthetics, assault**

T41.3x4- **Poisoning by local anesthetics, undetermined**

T41.3x5- **Adverse effect of local anesthetics**

T41.3x6- **Underdosing of local anesthetics**

T41.4- **Poisoning by, adverse effect of and underdosing of unspecified anesthetic**

T41.4 - DRUGS/CHEMS*
Anesthetic NEC — see also Anesthesia

T41.41x- **Poisoning by unspecified anesthetic, accidental (unintentional)**
 Poisoning by anesthetic NOS

T41.42x- **Poisoning by unspecified anesthetic, intentional self-harm**

T41.43x- **Poisoning by unspecified anesthetic, assault**

T41.44x- **Poisoning by unspecified anesthetic, undetermined**

T41.45x- **Adverse effect of unspecified anesthetic**

T41.46x- **Underdosing of unspecified anesthetics**

T41.5- **Poisoning by, adverse effect of and underdosing of therapeutic gases**

T41.5 - DRUGS/CHEMS*	
Carbon dioxide, medicinal	Gas, therapeutic
	Oxygen

T41.5x- **Poisoning by, adverse effect of and underdosing of therapeutic gases**

T41.5x1- **Poisoning by therapeutic gases, accidental (unintentional)**
 Poisoning by therapeutic gases NOS

T41.5x2- Poisoning by therapeutic gases, <u>intentional</u> self-harm

T41.5x3- Poisoning by therapeutic gases, <u>assault</u>

T41.5x4- Poisoning by therapeutic gases, <u>undetermined</u>

T41.5x5- <u>Adverse effect</u> of therapeutic gases

T41.5x6- <u>Underdosing</u> of therapeutic gases

T42- Poisoning by, adverse effect of and underdosing of <u>antiepileptic, sedative-hypnotic and antiparkinsonism drugs</u>

Excludes ❷: *drug dependence and related mental and behavioral disorders due to psychoactive substance use (F10.-F19.-)*

The appropriate 7th character is to be added to each code from category T42:
A   <u>Initial</u> encounter
D   <u>Subsequent</u> encounter
S   <u>Sequela</u>

T42.0- Poisoning by, adverse effect of and underdosing of hydantoin derivatives

T42.0 - DRUGS/CHEMS*	Epanutin	Methetoin
Albutoin	Ethotoin	Methoin
Anticonvulsant, hydantoin	Hydantoin derivative NEC	Phenantoin
Dilantin	Mephenytoin	Phenytoin
Diphenylhydantoin	Metetoin	

T42.0x- Poisoning by, adverse effect of and underdosing of <u>hydantoin derivatives</u>

T42.0x1- Poisoning by hydantoin derivatives, <u>accidental</u> (unintentional)
Poisoning by hydantoin derivatives NOS

T42.0x2- Poisoning by hydantoin derivatives, <u>intentional</u> self-harm

T42.0x3- Poisoning by hydantoin derivatives, <u>assault</u>

T42.0x4- Poisoning by hydantoin derivatives, <u>undetermined</u>

T42.0x5- <u>Adverse effect</u> of hydantoin derivatives

T42.0x6- <u>Underdosing</u> of hydantoin derivatives

T42.1- Poisoning by, adverse effect of and underdosing of iminostilbenes
Poisoning by, adverse effect of and underdosing of carbamazepine

T42.1 - DRUGS/CHEMS*	Iminostilbene	Tegretol
Carbamazepine	Oxcarbazepine	

T42.1x- Poisoning by, adverse effect of and underdosing of <u>iminostilbenes</u>

T42.1x1- Poisoning by iminostilbenes, <u>accidental</u> (unintentional)
Poisoning by iminostilbenes NOS

T42.1x2- Poisoning by iminostilbenes, <u>intentional</u> self-harm

T42.1x3- Poisoning by iminostilbenes, <u>assault</u>

T42.1x4- Poisoning by iminostilbenes, <u>undetermined</u>

T42.1x5- <u>Adverse effect</u> of iminostilbenes

T42.1x6- <u>Underdosing</u> of iminostilbenes

T42.2- Poisoning by, adverse effect of and underdosing of succinimides and oxazolidinediones

T42.2 - DRUGS/CHEMS*	Mesuximide	Phensuximide
Aloxidone	Methsuximide	Succinimide, antiepileptic
Anticonvulsant, oxazolidinedione	Morsuximide	or anticonvulsant
	Oxazolidine derivatives	Tridione
Anticonvulsant, succinimide	Oxazolidinedione	Trimethadione
Ethadione	(derivative)	Troxidone
Ethosuximide	Paradione	
Isoethadione	Paramethadione	

T42.2x- Poisoning by, adverse effect of and underdosing of <u>succinimides and oxazolidinediones</u>

T42.2x1- Poisoning by succinimides and oxazolidinediones, <u>accidental</u> (unintentional)
Poisoning by succinimides and oxazolidinediones NOS

T42.2x2- Poisoning by succinimides and oxazolidinediones, <u>intentional</u> self-harm

T42.2x3- Poisoning by succinimides and oxazolidinediones, <u>assault</u>

T42.2x4- Poisoning by succinimides and oxazolidinediones, <u>undetermined</u>

T42.2x5- <u>Adverse effect</u> of succinimides and oxazolidinediones

T42.2x6- <u>Underdosing</u> of succinimides and oxazolidinediones

T42.3- Poisoning by, adverse effect of and underdosing of barbiturates

Excludes 1: *poisoning by, adverse effect of and underdosing of thiobarbiturates (T41.1-)*

T42.3 - DRUGS/CHEMS*	Dormiral	Noptil
Agrypnal	Enhexymal	Nunol
Allobarbital	Eskabarb	Ortal (sodium)
Allylisopropylmalonylurea	Ethobral	Pentobarbital
Allypropymal	Etilfen	Pentobarbital, sodium
Alurate	Etoval	Pentobarbitone
Amobarbital (sodium)	Euneryl	Pentymal
Amylobarbitone	Evipal	Pernocton
Amytal (sodium)	Evipan	Pernoston
Anticonvulsant, barbiturate	Febarbamate	Phanodorm, phanodorn
Anticonvulsant, combination (with barbiturate)	Fenobarbital	Phemitone
	Gardenal	Phenemal
	Gardepanyl	Phenobal
Aprobarbital	Gemonil	Phenobarbital
Barbenyl	Heptabarb	Phenobarbital with mephenytoin
Barbital	Heptabarbital	
Barbital, sodium	Heptabarbitone	Phenobarbital with phenytoin
Barbitone	Hexemal	
Barbiturate NEC	Hexethal (sodium)	Phenobarbital, sodium
Barbiturate with tranquilizer	Hexobarbital	Phenobarbitone
	Ipral	Phenonyl
Brallobarbital	Lotusate	Phenylmethylbarbitone
Butabarbital (sodium)	Luminal	Phenytoin with phenobarbital
Butabarbitone	Meballymal	
Butabarpal	Mebaral	Probarbital
Butalbital	Mebumal	Propallylonal
Butallylonal	Medinal	Proxibarbal
Butethal	Medomin	Quinalbarbital
Butisol (sodium)	Mephebarbital	Quinalbarbitone sodium
Butobarbital	Mephenytoin with phenobarbital	Secbutabarbital
Butobarbital sodium		Secbutabarbitone
Butobarbitone	Mephobarbital	Secobarbital
Carbrital	Metharbital	Seconal
Central nervous system depressants, barbiturates	Methitural	Sodium amytal
	Methobarbital, methobarbitone	Sodium barbiturate
		Somonal
Cyclobarbital	Methylhexabital	Soneryl
Cyclobarbitone	Methylphenobarbital	Talbutal
Delvinal	Mysoline	Veramon
Dial, sedative	Nealbarbital	Veronal
Diallylbarbituric acid	Nembutal	Vinbarbital, vinbarbitone
Diallymal	Neonal	Vinyl bital
Diemal	Neraval	Vinylbital
Diethyl barbituric acid	Neravan	
Difebarbamate	Neurobarb	

T42.3x- Poisoning by, adverse effect of and underdosing of <u>barbiturates</u>

T42.3x1- Poisoning by barbiturates, <u>accidental</u> (unintentional)
Poisoning by barbiturates NOS

T42.3x2- Poisoning by barbiturates, <u>intentional</u> self-harm

T42.3x3- Poisoning by barbiturates, <u>assault</u>

T42.3x4- Poisoning by barbiturates, <u>undetermined</u>

T42.3x5- <u>Adverse effect</u> of barbiturates

T42.3x6- <u>Underdosing</u> of barbiturates

T41 - T42

T42.4- Poisoning by, adverse effect of and underdosing of benzodiazepines

T42.4 - DRUGS/CHEMS*	Delorazepam	Nimetazepam
Alprazolam	Diazepam	Nitrazepam
Bentazepam	Estazolam	Nordazepam
Benzodiapin	Ethyl loflazepate	Oxazepam
Benzodiazepine NEC	Etizolam	Oxazolam
Bromazepam	Fludiazepam	Perlapine
Brotizolam	Flunitrazepam	Pinazepam
Camazepam	Flurazepam	Prazepam
Carpipramine	Flutazolam	Quazepam
Central nervous system	Flutoprazepam	Rohypnol
depressants,	Halazepam	Serax
benzodiazepines	Haloxazolam	Temazepam
Chlordiazepoxide	Ketazolam	Tetrazepam
Clobazam	Librium	Tofisopam
Clonazepam	Loprazolam	Tranquilizer,
Clorazepate (dipotassium)	Lorazepam	benzodiazepine NEC
Clotiazepam	Lormetazepam	Tranxene
Cloxazolam	Medazepam	Triazolam
Clozapine	Mexazolam	Valium
Dalmane	Midazolam	

T42.4x- Poisoning by, adverse effect of and underdosing of benzodiazepines

T42.4x1- Poisoning by benzodiazepines, accidental (unintentional)
Poisoning by benzodiazepines NOS

T42.4x2- Poisoning by benzodiazepines, intentional self-harm

T42.4x3- Poisoning by benzodiazepines, assault

T42.4x4- Poisoning by benzodiazepines, undetermined

T42.4x5- Adverse effect of benzodiazepines

T42.4x6- Underdosing of benzodiazepines

T42.5- Poisoning by, adverse effect of and underdosing of mixed antiepileptics

T42.5 - DRUGS/CHEMS*	Antiepilepsy agent, mixed
Antiepilepsy agent, combination	

T42.5x- Poisoning by, adverse effect of and underdosing of antiepileptics

T42.5x1- Poisoning by mixed antiepileptics, accidental (unintentional)
Poisoning by mixed antiepileptics NOS

T42.5x2- Poisoning by mixed antiepileptics, intentional self-harm

T42.5x3- Poisoning by mixed antiepileptics, assault

T42.5x4- Poisoning by mixed antiepileptics, undetermined

T42.5x5- Adverse effect of mixed antiepileptics

T42.5x6- Underdosing of mixed antiepileptics

T42.6- Poisoning by, adverse effect of and underdosing of other antiepileptic and sedative-hypnotic drugs
Poisoning by, adverse effect of and underdosing of methaqualone
Poisoning by, adverse effect of and underdosing of valproic acid
Excludes 1: poisoning by, adverse effect of and underdosing of carbamazepine (T42.1-)

T42.6 - DRUGS/CHEMS*	Central nervous system	Petrichloral
Acecarbromal	depressants, sedatives	Phenacemide
Acetylcarbromal	sedative-hypnotics,	Phenergan
Acetylpheneturide	specified NEC	Pheneturide
Allylisopropylacetylurea	Chloral	Phthalimidoglutarimide
Allyltribromide	Chloral derivative	Placidyl
Ammonium bromide	Chloralhydrate	Potassium bromide
Anticonvulsant, hypnotic	Chloralamide	Primidone
NEC	Chloralodol	Progabide
Anticonvulsant,	Chlorbutol	Propionaidehyde
pyrimidinedione	Chlorethiazol	(medicinal)
Anticonvulsant, specified	Chloretone	Pyrithyldione
NEC	Chlorhexadol	Quaalude
Antiepilepsy agent,	Chlormethiazole	Sedative, mixed NEC
specified, NEC	Chlormezanone	Sedormid
Apronalide	Clomethiazole	Serenesil
Avomine	Cloral betaine	Sodium bromide
Barbexaclone	Croton, chloral	Sodium valproate
Beclamide	Dichloralphenozone	Somnos
Beta-Chlor	Diethylsulfone-	Sopor
Bromal (hydrate)	diethylmethane	Soporific drug, specified
Bromide salts	Divalproex	type NEC
Bromine compounds	Doriden	Sulfonal
(medicinal)	Dormison	Sulfonethylmethane
Bromine sedative	Ectylurea	Sulfonmethane
Bromisoval	Ethchlorvynol	Sulthiame
Bromisovalum	Ethinamate	Sultiame
Bromoform	Etifoxine	Tetronal
Bromural	Glutethimide	Toloxatone
Bromvaletone	Hexapropymate	Tranquilizer with hypnotic
Butyl chloral (hydrate)	Hypnotic, specified NEC	or sedative
Butylchloral hydrate	Lactuca (virosa) (extract)	Tribromacetaldehyde
Calcium bromide	Lactucarium	Tribromomethane
Calcium bromolactobionate	Lettuce opium	Trichloroethanol
Carbamate (sedative)	Levanil	Trichloroethyl phosphate
Carbromal	Levoprome	Triclofos
Central nervous system	Meparfynol	Trional
depressants, bromides	Methaqualone (compound)	Triple bromides
Central nervous system	Methyl parafynol	Valerian root
depressants, chloral	Methyl sulfonal	Valerian tincture
hydrate	Methylparafynol	Valmid
Central nervous system	Methylpentynol,	Valnoctamide
depressants, hypnotics,	methylpenthynol	Valproate (sodium)
specified NEC	Methyprylon	Valproic acid
Central nervous system	Niaprazine	Valpromide
depressants,	Noctec	Vigabatrin
paraldehyde	Noludar	Welldorm
Central nervous system	Paracetaldehyde	Zolpidem
depressants, sedatives	Paraldehyde	Zopiclone
sedative-hypnotics,	Pentaerythritol, chloral	
mixed NEC	Periclor	

T42.6x- Poisoning by, adverse effect of and underdosing of other antiepileptic and sedative-hypnotic drugs

T42.6x1- Poisoning by other antiepileptic and sedative-hypnotic drugs, accidental (unintentional)
Poisoning by other antiepileptic and sedative-hypnotic drugs NOS

T42.6x2- Poisoning by other antiepileptic and sedative-hypnotic drugs, intentional self-harm

T42.6x3- Poisoning by other antiepileptic and sedative-hypnotic drugs, assault

T42.6x4- Poisoning by other antiepileptic and sedative-hypnotic drugs, undetermined

T42.6x5- Adverse effect of other antiepileptic and sedative-hypnotic drugs

T42.6x6- Underdosing of other antiepileptic and sedative-hypnotic drugs

T42.7- Poisoning by, adverse effect of and underdosing of <u>unspecified antiepileptic and sedative-hypnotic drugs</u>

T42.7 - DRUGS/CHEMS*	Central nervous system	Hypnotic
Anticonvulsant	depressants, sedatives	Hypnotic, anticonvulsant
Antiepilepsy agent	sedative-hypnotics	Sedative NEC
Central nervous system	Depressant, central nervous	Sleeping draught, pill
depressants	system (anesthetic) —	Soporific
Central nervous system	see also Central nervous	Soporific drug
depressants, hypnotics	system, depressants	

T42.71x- Poisoning by unspecified antiepileptic and sedative-hypnotic drugs, <u>accidental</u> (unintentional)
  Poisoning by antiepileptic and sedative-hypnotic drugs NOS

T42.72x- Poisoning by unspecified antiepileptic and sedative-hypnotic drugs, <u>intentional</u> self-harm

T42.73x- Poisoning by unspecified antiepileptic and sedative-hypnotic drugs, <u>assault</u>

T42.74x- Poisoning by unspecified antiepileptic and sedative-hypnotic drugs, <u>undetermined</u>

T42.75x- <u>Adverse effect</u> of unspecified antiepileptic and sedative-hypnotic drugs

T42.76x- <u>Underdosing</u> of unspecified antiepileptic and sedative-hypnotic drugs

T42.8- Poisoning by, adverse effect of and underdosing of antiparkinsonism drugs and other central muscle-tone depressants
  Poisoning by, adverse effect of and underdosing of amantadine

T42.8 - DRUGS/CHEMS*	Deprenyl	Muscle affecting agents,
Afloqualone	Depressant, central nervous	relaxants, central
Amantadine	system, muscle tone	nervous system
Antiparkinsonism drug NEC	Depressant, muscle tone,	Muscle-tone depressant,
Antirigidity drug NEC	central	central NEC
Baclofen	Diethazine	Muscle-tone depressant,
Benserazide	Difluoromethyldopa	central, specified NEC
Benzatropine	Disipal	Orphenadrine
Benztropine, antiparkinson	Dopa	(hydrochloride)
Bromocriptine	Idrocilamide	Pergolide
Cabergoline	L-dopa	Phenprobamate
Carbidopa (with levodopa)	Levodopa	Piribedil
Carisoprodol	Levodopa with carbidopa	Rela
Central nervous system	Lisuride	Relaxant, muscle, central
depressants, muscle	Mephenamin(e)	nervous system
relaxants	Mephenesin	Selegiline
Central nervous system	Mephenoxalone	Soma
muscle-tone depressants	Mesulergine	Styramate
Chlorphenesin	Metaxalone	Tizanidine
Chlorzoxazone	Metergoline	Tolserol
Dantrolene	Methocarbamol	Zoxazolamine
Deprenalin		

T42.8x- Poisoning by, adverse effect of and underdosing of <u>antiparkinsonism drugs and other central muscle-tone depressants</u>

T42.8x1- Poisoning by antiparkinsonism drugs and other central muscle-tone depressants, <u>accidental</u> (unintentional)
  Poisoning by antiparkinsonism drugs and other central muscle-tone depressants NOS

T42.8x2- Poisoning by antiparkinsonism drugs and other central muscle-tone depressants, <u>intentional</u> self-harm

T42.8x3- Poisoning by antiparkinsonism drugs and other central muscle-tone depressants, <u>assault</u>

T42.8x4- Poisoning by antiparkinsonism drugs and other central muscle-tone depressants, <u>undetermined</u>

T42.8x5- <u>Adverse effect</u> of antiparkinsonism drugs and other central muscle-tone depressants

T42.8x6- <u>Underdosing</u> of antiparkinsonism drugs and other central muscle-tone depressants

T43- Poisoning by, adverse effect of and underdosing of <u>psychotropic drugs</u>, <u>not elsewhere classified</u>

Excludes 1: appetite depressants (T50.5-)
  barbiturates (T42.3-)
  benzodiazepines (T42.4-)
  methaqualone (T42.6-)
  psychodysleptics [hallucinogens] (T40.7-T40.9-)

Excludes ❷: drug dependence and related mental and behavioral disorders due to psychoactive substance use (F10.- -F19.-)

The appropriate 7th character is to be added to each code from category T43:
A <u>Initial</u> encounter
D <u>Subsequent</u> encounter
S <u>Sequela</u>

T43.0- Poisoning by, adverse effect of and underdosing of tricyclic and tetracyclic antidepressants

T43.01- Poisoning by, adverse effect of and underdosing of <u>tricyclic antidepressants</u>

T43.01 - DRUGS/CHEMS*	Desmethylimipramine	Noxiptiline
Allegron	Dibenzepin	Opipramol
Amineptine	Dosulepin	Pertofrane
Amitriptyline	Dothiepin	Protriptyline
Amitriptylinoxide	Doxepin	Quinupramine
Amoxapine	Imipramine	Saroten
Antidepressant, tricyclic	Iprindole	Sinequan
Butriptyline	Laroxyl	Tofranil
Chlorimipramine	Lofepramine	Trimipramine
Cianopramine	Melitracen	Tryptizol
Clomipramine	Metapramine	
Desipramine	Nortriptyline	

T43.011- Poisoning by tricyclic antidepressants, <u>accidental</u> (unintentional)
  Poisoning by tricyclic antidepressants NOS

T43.012- Poisoning by tricyclic antidepressants, <u>intentional</u> self-harm

T43.013- Poisoning by tricyclic antidepressants, <u>assault</u>

T43.014- Poisoning by tricyclic antidepressants, <u>undetermined</u>

T43.015- <u>Adverse effect</u> of tricyclic antidepressants

T43.016- <u>Underdosing</u> of tricyclic antidepressants

T43.02- Poisoning by, adverse effect of and underdosing of <u>tetracyclic antidepressants</u>

T43.02 - DRUGS/CHEMS*	Maprotiline	Mirtazapine
Antidepressant, tetracyclic	Mianserin	Oxaprotiline

T43.021- Poisoning by tetracyclic antidepressants, <u>accidental</u> (unintentional)
  Poisoning by tetracyclic antidepressants NOS

T43.022- Poisoning by tetracyclic antidepressants, <u>intentional</u> self-harm

T43.023- Poisoning by tetracyclic antidepressants, <u>assault</u>

T43.024- Poisoning by tetracyclic antidepressants, <u>undetermined</u>

T43.025- <u>Adverse effect</u> of tetracyclic antidepressants

T43.026- <u>Underdosing</u> of tetracyclic antidepressants

T43.1- Poisoning by, adverse effect of and underdosing of monoamine-oxidase-inhibitor antidepressants

T43.1x- Poisoning by, adverse effect of and underdosing of <u>monoamine-oxidase-inhibitor antidepressants</u>

T43.1 - DRUGS/CHEMS*	Inhibitor, monoamine	Monoamine oxidase
Amiflamine	oxidase, hydrazine	inhibitor NEC
Antidepressant,	Iproclozide	Monoamine oxidase
monoamine oxidase	Iproniazid	inhibitor, hydrazine
inhibitor	Isocarboxazid	Nardil
Clorgiline	MAO inhibitors	Nialamide
Hydrazine monoamine	Marplan	Parnate
oxidase inhibitors	Marsilid	Phenelzine
Inhibitor, monoamine	Mebanazine	Pheniprazine
oxidase NEC	Moclobemide	Safrazine
		Tranylcypromine

T 4 2 - T 4 3

T43.1x1- Poisoning by monoamine-oxidase-inhibitor antidepressants, <u>accidental</u> (unintentional)
Poisoning by monoamine-oxidase-inhibitor antidepressants NOS

T43.1x2- Poisoning by monoamine-oxidase-inhibitor antidepressants, <u>intentional</u> self-harm

T43.1x3- Poisoning by monoamine-oxidase-inhibitor antidepressants, <u>assault</u>

T43.1x4- Poisoning by monoamine-oxidase-inhibitor antidepressants, <u>undetermined</u>

T43.1x5- <u>Adverse effect</u> of monoamine-oxidase-inhibitor antidepressants

T43.1x6- <u>Underdosing</u> of monoamine-oxidase-inhibitor antidepressants

T43.2- Poisoning by, adverse effect of and underdosing of other and unspecified antidepressants

T43.20- Poisoning by, adverse effect of and underdosing of <u>unspecified antidepressants</u>

T43.20 - DRUGS/CHEMS*	
Antidepressant	Psychotherapeutic drug, antidepressants — see also Antidepressant
Central nervous system stimulants, antidepressants	

T43.201- Poisoning by unspecified antidepressants, <u>accidental</u> (unintentional)
Poisoning by antidepressants NOS

T43.202- Poisoning by unspecified antidepressants, <u>intentional</u> self-harm

T43.203- Poisoning by unspecified antidepressants, <u>assault</u>

T43.204- Poisoning by unspecified antidepressants, <u>undetermined</u>

T43.205- <u>Adverse effect</u> of unspecified antidepressants

T43.206- <u>Underdosing</u> of unspecified antidepressants

T43.21- Poisoning by, adverse effect of and underdosing of <u>selective serotonin and norepinephrinere uptake inhibitors</u>
Poisoning by, adverse effect of and underdosing of SSNRI antidepressants

T43.21 - DRUGS/CHEMS*	
Antidepressant, selective serotonin norepinephrine reuptake inhibitor	Antidepressant, triazolopyridine
	Trazodone
	Venlafaxine

T43.211- Poisoning by selective serotonin and norepinephrine reuptake inhibitors, <u>accidental</u> (unintentional)

T43.212- Poisoning by selective serotonin and norepinephrine reuptake inhibitors, <u>intentional</u> self-harm

T43.213- Poisoning by selective serotonin and norepinephrine reuptake inhibitors, <u>assault</u>

T43.214- Poisoning by selective serotonin and norepinephrine reuptake inhibitors, <u>undetermined</u>

T43.215- <u>Adverse effect</u> of selective serotonin and norepinephrine reuptake inhibitors

T43.216- <u>Underdosing</u> of selective serotonin and norepinephrine reuptake inhibitors

T43.22- Poisoning by, adverse effect of and underdosing of <u>selective serotonin reuptake inhibitors</u>
Poisoning by, adverse effect of and underdosing of SSRI antidepressants

T43.22 - DRUGS/CHEMS*		
Antidepressant, selective serotonin reuptake inhibitor	Citalopram	Indalpine
	Femoxetine	Prozac
	Fluoxetine	Zimeldine
	Fluvoxamine	

T43.221- Poisoning by selective serotonin reuptake inhibitors, <u>accidental</u> (unintentional)

T43.222- Poisoning by selective serotonin reuptake inhibitors, <u>intentional</u> self-harm

T43.223- Poisoning by selective serotonin reuptake inhibitors, <u>assault</u>

T43.224- Poisoning by selective serotonin reuptake inhibitors, <u>undetermined</u>

T43.225- <u>Adverse effect</u> of selective serotonin reuptake inhibitors

T43.226- <u>Underdosing</u> of selective serotonin reuptake inhibitors

T43.29- Poisoning by, adverse effect of and underdosing of <u>other antidepressants</u>

T43.29 - DRUGS/CHEMS*		
Amfebutamone	Bupropion	Prazitone
Antidepressant, specified NEC	Diclofensine	Thiazesim
	Minaprine	Tianeptine
	Nomifensine	Viloxazine
Bifemelane	Oxitriptan	

T43.291- Poisoning by other antidepressants, <u>accidental</u> (unintentional)
Poisoning by other antidepressants NOS

T43.292- Poisoning by other antidepressants, <u>intentional</u> self-harm

T43.293- Poisoning by other antidepressants, <u>assault</u>

T43.294- Poisoning by other antidepressants, <u>undetermined</u>

T43.295- <u>Adverse effect</u> of other antidepressants

T43.296- <u>Underdosing</u> of other antidepressants

T43.3- Poisoning by, adverse effect of and underdosing of phenothiazine antipsychotics and neuroleptics

T43.3 - DRUGS/CHEMS*		
Acepromazine	Mequitazine	Stemetil
Acetophenazine	Mesoridazine	Sulforidazine
Alimemazine	Methdilazine	Thiazinamium metilsulfate
Butaperazine	Methopromazine	Thiethylperazine
Carfenazine	Methotrimeprazine	Thiopropazate
Carphenazine	Methoxypromazine	Thioproperazine
Chlorpromazine	Metofenazate	Thioridazine
Compazine	Oxomemazine	Thorazine
Cyamemazine	Pecazine	Tindal
Dimetotiazine	Perazine	Tranquilizer, dimethylamine
Dioxopromethazine	Periciazine	Tranquilizer, ethylamine
Dixyrazine	Perphenazine	Tranquilizer, penothiazine NEC
Ethyl aminophenothiazine	Phenothiazine (psychotropic) NEC	
Fentazin	Piperacetazine	Tranquilizer, phenothiazine-based
Fluopromazine	Pipotiazine	Tranquilizer, piperazine NEC
Fluphenazine	Plegicil	
Isopromethazine	Prochlorperazine	Tranquilizer, piperidine
Largactil	Promazine	Tranquilizer, propylamine
Levomepromazine	Promethazine (teoclate)	Trifluoperazine
Levopromazine	Propylaminophenothiazine	Triflupromazine
Mellaril	Sparine	
Mepazine	Stelazine	

T43.3x- Poisoning by, adverse effect of and underdosing of <u>phenothiazine antipsychotics and neuroleptics</u>

T43.3x1- Poisoning by phenothiazine antipsychotics and neuroleptics, <u>accidental</u> (unintentional)
Poisoning by phenothiazine antipsychotics and neuroleptics NOS

T43.3x2- Poisoning by phenothiazine antipsychotics and neuroleptics, <u>intentional</u> self-harm

T43.3x3- Poisoning by phenothiazine antipsychotics and neuroleptics, <u>assault</u>

T43.3x4- Poisoning by phenothiazine antipsychotics and neuroleptics, <u>undetermined</u>

T43.3x5- <u>Adverse effect</u> of phenothiazine antipsychotics and neuroleptics

T43.3x6- <u>Underdosing</u> of phenothiazine antipsychotics and neuroleptics

T43 - T43

T43.4- **Poisoning by, adverse effect of and underdosing of butyrophenone and thiothixene neuroleptics**

T43.4 - DRUGS/CHEMS*		
Benperidol	Flupentixol	Thiothixene
Bromperidol	Haloperidol	Timiperone
Butyrophenone (-based	Lenperone	Tiotixene
tranquilizers)	Melperone	Tranquilizer,
Chlorprothixene	Methyl peridol	butyrophenone NEC
Clopenthixol	Moperone	Trifluperidol
Fluanisone	Pipamperone	Triperidol
Flupentixol	Spiperone	Zuclopenthixol
	Spiroperidol	

T43.4x- **Poisoning by, adverse effect of and underdosing of butyrophenone and thiothixene neuroleptics**

T43.4x1- **Poisoning by butyrophenone and thiothixene neuroleptics, accidental (unintentional)**
Poisoning by butyrophenone and thiothixene neuroleptics NOS

T43.4x2- **Poisoning by butyrophenone and thiothixene neuroleptics, intentional self-harm**

T43.4x3- **Poisoning by butyrophenone and thiothixene neuroleptics, assault**

T43.4x4- **Poisoning by butyrophenone and thiothixene neuroleptics, undetermined**

T43.4x5- **Adverse effect of butyrophenone and thiothixene neuroleptics**

T43.4x6- **Underdosing of butyrophenone and thiothixene neuroleptics**

T43.5- **Poisoning by, adverse effect of and underdosing of other and unspecified antipsychotics and neuroleptics**
Excludes 1:   poisoning by, adverse effect of and underdosing of rauwolfia (T46.5-)

T43.50- **Poisoning by, adverse effect of and underdosing of unspecified antipsychotics and neuroleptics**

T43.50 - DRUGS/CHEMS*		
Antianxiety drug NEC	Depressant,	Tranquilizer NEC
Antihallucinogen	psychotherapeutic	Tranquilizer, major NEC
Antipsychotic drug	Neuroleptic drug NEC	
Ataractic drug NEC	Psychotherapeutic drug,	
	tranquilizers NEC	

T43.501- **Poisoning by unspecified antipsychotics and neuroleptics, accidental (unintentional)**
Poisoning by antipsychotics and neuroleptics NOS

T43.502- **Poisoning by unspecified antipsychotics and neuroleptics, intentional self-harm**

T43.503- **Poisoning by unspecified antipsychotics and neuroleptics, assault**

T43.504- **Poisoning by unspecified antipsychotics and neuroleptics, undetermined**

T43.505- **Adverse effect of unspecified antipsychotics and neuroleptics**

T43.506- **Underdosing of unspecified antipsychotics and neuroleptics**

T43.59- **Poisoning by, adverse effect of and underdosing of other antipsychotics and neuroleptics**

T43.59 - DRUGS/CHEMS*		
Aminophenylpyridone	Hydroxyzine	Raclopride
Amisulpride	Lithium gluconate	Remoxipride
Amperozide	Lithium salts (carbonate)	Setoperone
Amphenidone	Loxapine	Spirilene
Antipsychotic drug,	Mebutamate	Sulpiride
specified NEC	Meprobam	Sultopride
Azacyclonol	Meprobamate	Taractan
Benzperidin	Miltown	Tetrabenazine
Benzperidol	Molindone	Tiapride
Buspirone	Mosapramine	Tranquilizer, carbamate
Captodiame, captodiamine	Nemonapride	Tranquilizer, hydroxyzine
Clotiapine	Olanzapine	Tranquilizer, specified NEC
Droperidol	Oxanamide	Tranquilizer, thioxanthene
Emylcamate	Oxypertine	NEC
Enpiprazole	Penfluridol	Tybamate
Equanil	Phenaglycodol	Zotepine
Fluspirilene	Pimozide	Zyprexa
Hydroxyphenamate	Procalmidol	
	Prothipendyl	

T43.591- **Poisoning by other antipsychotics and neuroleptics, accidental (unintentional)**
Poisoning by other antipsychotics and neuroleptics NOS

T43.592- **Poisoning by other antipsychotics and neuroleptics, intentional self-harm**

T43.593- **Poisoning by other antipsychotics and neuroleptics, assault**

T43.594- **Poisoning by other antipsychotics and neuroleptics, undetermined**

T43.595- **Adverse effect of other antipsychotics and neuroleptics**

T43.596- **Underdosing of other antipsychotics and neuroleptics**

T43.6- **Poisoning by, adverse effect of and underdosing of psychostimulants**
Excludes 1:   poisoning by, adverse effect of and underdosing of cocaine (T40.5-)

T43.60- **Poisoning by, adverse effect of and underdosing of unspecified psychostimulant**

T43.60 - DRUGS/CHEMS*		
Central nervous system	Psychostimulant	Stimulant, central nervous
stimulants	Stimulant, central nervous	system,
Cerebral stimulants	system — see also	psychotherapeutic NEC —
Cerebral stimulants,	Psychostimulant	see also
psychotherapeutic		Psychotherapeutic drug

T43.601- **Poisoning by unspecified psychostimulants, accidental (unintentional)**
Poisoning by psychostimulants NOS

T43.602- **Poisoning by unspecified psychostimulants, intentional self-harm**

T43.603- **Poisoning by unspecified psychostimulants, assault**

T43.604- **Poisoning by unspecified psychostimulants, undetermined**

T43.605- **Adverse effect of unspecified psychostimulants**

T43.606- **Underdosing of unspecified psychostimulants**

T43.61- **Poisoning by, adverse effect of and underdosing of caffeine**

T43.61 - DRUGS/CHEMS*	Psychostimulant, caffeine
Caffeine	

T43.611- **Poisoning by caffeine, accidental (unintentional)**
Poisoning by caffeine NOS

T43.612- **Poisoning by caffeine, intentional self-harm**

T43.613- **Poisoning by caffeine, assault**

T43.614- **Poisoning by caffeine, undetermined**

T43.615- **Adverse effect of caffeine**

T43.616- **Underdosing of caffeine**

T43 - T43

T43.62- Poisoning by, adverse effect of and underdosing of <u>amphetamines</u>
Poisoning by, adverse effect of and underdosing of methamphetamines

T43.62 - DRUGS/CHEMS*	Dexamphetamine	Methylenedioxyamphetamine
Amfetamine	Dexedrine	
Amfetaminil	Dextroamphetamine	Methylenedioxymethamphetamine
Amphetamine NEC	Ecstasy	
Benzedrine (amphetamine)	MDMA	Psychostimulant, amphetamine
Central nervous system stimulants, amphetamines	Metamfetamine	
	Methamphetamine	Speed
	Methedrine	Tenamfetamine
Desoxyephedrine	Methyl amphetamine	
Dexamfetamine	Methylamphetamine	

T43.621- Poisoning by amphetamines, <u>accidental</u> (unintentional)
Poisoning by amphetamines NOS

T43.622- Poisoning by amphetamines, <u>intentional</u> self-harm

T43.623- Poisoning by amphetamines, <u>assault</u>

T43.624- Poisoning by amphetamines, <u>undetermined</u>

T43.625- <u>Adverse effect</u> of amphetamines

T43.626- <u>Underdosing</u> of amphetamines

T43.63- Poisoning by, adverse effect of and underdosing of <u>methylphenidate</u>

T43.63 - DRUGS/CHEMS*	Psychostimulant,
Methyl phenidate	methylphenidate
Methylphenidate	Ritalin

T43.631- Poisoning by methylphenidate, <u>accidental</u> (unintentional)
Poisoning by methylphenidate NOS

T43.632- Poisoning by methylphenidate, <u>intentional</u> self-harm

T43.633- Poisoning by methylphenidate, <u>assault</u>

T43.634- Poisoning by methylphenidate, <u>undetermined</u>

T43.635- <u>Adverse effect</u> of methylphenidate

T43.636- <u>Underdosing</u> of methylphenidate

T43.69- Poisoning by, adverse effect of and underdosing of <u>other psychostimulants</u>

T43.69 - DRUGS/CHEMS*	Etryptamine	Preludin
Catha (edulis) (tea)	Fencamfamine	Prolintane
Central nervous system stimulants, specified NEC	Fenetylline	Psychostimulant, specified NEC
	Khat	
Cerebral stimulants, specified NEC	Meclofenoxate	Stimulant, central nervous system, specified NEC
	Pipradrol	

T43.691- Poisoning by other psychostimulants, <u>accidental</u> (unintentional)
Poisoning by other psychostimulants NOS

T43.692- Poisoning by other psychostimulants, <u>intentional</u> self-harm

T43.693- Poisoning by other psychostimulants, <u>assault</u>

T43.694- Poisoning by other psychostimulants, <u>undetermined</u>

T43.695- <u>Adverse effect</u> of other psychostimulants

T43.696- <u>Underdosing</u> of other psychostimulants

T43.8- Poisoning by, adverse effect of and underdosing of other psychotropic drugs

T43.8 - DRUGS/CHEMS*	Inhibitor, postsynaptic	Nizofenone
4-Aminobutyric acid	Lithane	Psychotherapeutic drug, specified NEC
Eskalith	Lithonate	
GABA	Memantine	Psychotropic drug, specified NEC
Gamma-aminobutyric acid	Namenda	

T43.8x- Poisoning by, adverse effect of and underdosing of <u>other psychotropic drugs</u>

T43.8x1- Poisoning by other psychotropic drugs, <u>accidental</u> (unintentional)
Poisoning by other psychotropic drugs NOS

T43.8x2- Poisoning by other psychotropic drugs, <u>intentional</u> self-harm

T43.8x3- Poisoning by other psychotropic drugs, <u>assault</u>

T43.8x4- Poisoning by other psychotropic drugs, <u>undetermined</u>

T43.8x5- <u>Adverse effect</u> of other psychotropic drugs

T43.8x6- <u>Underdosing</u> of other psychotropic drugs

T43.9- Poisoning by, adverse effect of and underdosing of <u>unspecified psychotropic drug</u>

T43.9 - DRUGS/CHEMS*	Psychotherapeutic drug NEC	Psychotropic drug NEC

T43.91x- Poisoning by unspecified psychotropic drug, <u>accidental</u> (unintentional)
Poisoning by psychotropic drug NOS

T43.92x- Poisoning by unspecified psychotropic drug, <u>intentional</u> self-harm

T43.93x- Poisoning by unspecified psychotropic drug, <u>assault</u>

T43.94x- Poisoning by unspecified psychotropic drug, <u>undetermined</u>

T43.95x- <u>Adverse effect</u> of unspecified psychotropic drug

T43.96x- <u>Underdosing</u> of unspecified psychotropic drug

T44- Poisoning by, adverse effect of and underdosing of <u>drugs primarily affecting the autonomic nervous system</u>

The appropriate 7th character is to be added to each code from category T44:
A   <u>Initial</u> encounter
D   <u>Subsequent</u> encounter
S   <u>Sequela</u>

T44.0- Poisoning by, adverse effect of and underdosing of anticholinesterase agents

T44.0 - DRUGS/CHEMS*	DFP	Galantamine
Ambenonium (chloride)	Diflos	Isoflurophate
Anticholinesterase	Difluorophate	Neomycin with neostigmine
Anticholinesterase, organophosphorus	Diisopropylfluorophosphonate	Neostigmine bromide
Anticholinesterase, reversible	Distigmine (bromide)	Prostigmin
	Dyflos	Pyridostigmine bromide
Cholinergic organophosphorus	Edrophonium	Tacrine
	Edrophonium chloride	Tetrahydroaminoacridine

T44.0x- Poisoning by, adverse effect of and underdosing of <u>anticholinesterase agents</u>

T44.0x1- Poisoning by anticholinesterase agents, <u>accidental</u> (unintentional)
Poisoning by anticholinesterase agents NOS

T44.0x2- Poisoning by anticholinesterase agents, <u>intentional</u> self-harm

T44.0x3- Poisoning by anticholinesterase agents, <u>assault</u>

T44.0x4- Poisoning by anticholinesterase agents, <u>undetermined</u>

T44.0x5- <u>Adverse effect</u> of anticholinesterase agents

T44.0x6- <u>Underdosing</u> of anticholinesterase agents

T44.1- Poisoning by, adverse effect of and underdosing of other parasympathomimetics [cholinergics]

T44.1 - DRUGS/CHEMS*	Carbachol	Parasympathomimetic drug NEC
Aceclidine	Carbamylcholine chloride	
Acetylcholine (chloride) (derivative)	Cholinergic (drug) NEC	Pilocarpine
	Cholinergic muscle tone enhancer	Pilocarpus (jaborandi) extract
Arecoline		
Benzpyrinium bromide	Cholinergic trimethyl ammonium propanediol	
Bethanechol		
Bethanechol chloride	Methacholine	

T44.1x- Poisoning by, adverse effect of and underdosing of <u>other parasympathomimetics [cholinergics]</u>

T44.1x1- Poisoning by other parasympathomimetics [cholinergics], <u>accidental</u> (unintentional)
Poisoning by other parasympathomimetics [cholinergics] NOS

T44.1x2- Poisoning by other parasympathomimetics [cholinergics], <u>intentional</u> self-harm

T43 – T44

T44.1x3- Poisoning by other parasympathomimetics [cholinergics], <u>assault</u>

T44.1x4- Poisoning by other parasympathomimetics [cholinergics], <u>undetermined</u>

T44.1x5- <u>Adverse effect</u> of other parasympathomimetics [cholinergics]

T44.1x6- <u>Underdosing</u> of other parasympathomimetics

T44.2- Poisoning by, adverse effect of and underdosing of ganglionic blocking drugs

T44.2 - DRUGS/CHEMS*		
Ganglionic blocking drug NEC	Pempidine	Tetraethylammonium chloride
Ganglionic blocking drug, specified NEC	Pentamethonium bromide	Tetrylammonium chloride
Hexamethonium bromide	Pentapyrrolinium (bitartrate)	Trimetaphan camsilate
Mecamylamine	Pentolonium tartrate	Trimethaphan
	Quarternary ammonium, ganglion blocking	Trimethidinium

T44.2x- Poisoning by, adverse effect of and underdosing of <u>ganglionic blocking drugs</u>

T44.2x1- Poisoning by ganglionic blocking drugs, <u>accidental</u> (unintentional)
　　Poisoning by ganglionic blocking drugs NOS

T44.2x2- Poisoning by ganglionic blocking drugs, <u>intentional</u> self-harm

T44.2x3- Poisoning by ganglionic blocking drugs, <u>assault</u>

T44.2x4- Poisoning by ganglionic blocking drugs, <u>undetermined</u>

T44.2x5- <u>Adverse effect</u> of ganglionic blocking drugs

T44.2x6- <u>Underdosing</u> of ganglionic blocking drugs

T44.3- Poisoning by, adverse effect of and underdosing of other parasympatholytics [anticholinergics and antimuscarinics] and spasmolytics
　　Poisoning by, adverse effect of and underdosing of papaverine

T44.3 - DRUGS/CHEMS*		
Adiphenine	Dibutoline sulfate	Methantheline
Alverine	Dicyclomine	Methanthelinium bromide
Ambutonium bromide	Dicycloverine	Methixene
Aminopentamide	Diisopromine	Methscopolamine bromide
Amprotropine	Diphemanil	Methyl atropine
Aniscoropine	Diphemanil metilsulfate	Methylatropine nitrate
Anisotropine methylbromide	Drotaverine	Methylbenactyzium bromide
Antagonist, extrapyramidal NEC	Duboisine	Metixene
	Dyphylline	Milverine
	Emepronium (salts)	Moxaverine
Anticholinergic NEC	Emepronium bromide	Muscle affecting agents, relaxants, smooth
Antimuscarinic NEC	Ethaverine	
Artane	Ethopropazine	
Atropine	Etomidoline	Mydriacyl
Atropine derivative	Etybenzatropine	Octatropine methyl bromide
Atropine methonitrate	Euphthalmine	
Belladonna alkaloids	Extrapyramidal antagonist NEC	Otilonium bromide
Belladonna extract	Fenoverine	Oxapium iodide
Belladonna herb	Flavoxate	Oxybutynin
Benactyzine	Flopropione	Oxyphencyclimine
Benaprizine	Gefarnate	Oxyphenonium bromide
Benzhexol	Glycopyrrolate	Papaverine
Benzilonium bromide	Glycopyrronium	Parasympatholytic NEC
Benztropine, anticholinergic	Glycopyrronium bromide	Penthienate bromide
	Hexasonium iodide	Phenglutarimide
Bevonium metilsulfate	Hexocyclium	Pinaverium bromide
Biperiden	Hexocyclium metilsulfate	Pipenzolate bromide
Bornaprine	Homatropine	Piperidolate
Butethamate	Homatropine methylbromide	Pipethanate
Butropium bromide		Poldine metilsulfate
Butyl scopolamine bromide	Hyoscine	Pramiverine
Camylofin	Hyoscyamine	Pridinol
Caramiphen	Hyoscyamus	Prifinium bromide
Carpronium chloride	Hyoscyamus, dry extract	Pro-Banthine
Chlorbenzoxamine	Isometheptene	Procyclidine
Cimetropium bromide	Isopropamide	Profenamine
Clidinium bromide	Isopropamide iodide	Profenil
Clorotepine	Levsin	Propantheline
Cogentin	Mebeverine	Propantheline bromide
Cyclodrine	Meladrazine	Quarternary ammonium, parasympatholytic
Cyclopentolate	Mepenzolate	
Cycrimine	Mepenzolate bromide	Relaxant, muscle, smooth NEC
Dexetimide	Mepiperphenidol	Rociverine

T44.3 - DRUGS/CHEMS* — Continued		
Scopolamine	Tiemonium	Trimebutine
Scopolia extract	Tiemonium, iodide	Trimeprazine (tartrate)
Smooth muscle relaxant	Tifenamil	Triperiden
Spacoline	Tigloidine	Trithiozine
Spasmolytic, anticholinergics	Timepidium bromide	Tritiozine
	Tiquizium bromide	Tropacine
Spasmolytic, autonomic	Tolperisone	Tropatepine
Spasmolytic, quaternary ammonium	Toquizine	Tropicamide
	Trasentine	Trospium chloride
Sulmetozine	Triampyzine	Valethamate bromide
Thiphenamil	Tricyclamol chloride	
	Tridihexethyl iodide	
	Trihexyphenidyl	

T44.3x- Poisoning by, adverse effect of and underdosing of <u>other parasympatholytics [anticholinergics and antimuscarinics] and spasmolytics</u>

T44.3x1- Poisoning by other parasympatholytics [anticholinergics and antimuscarinics] and spasmolytics, <u>accidental</u> (unintentional)
　　Poisoning by other parasympatholytics [anticholinergics and antimuscarinics] and spasmolytics NOS

T44.3x2- Poisoning by other parasympatholytics [anticholinergics and antimuscarinics] and spasmolytics, <u>intentional</u> self-harm

T44.3x3- Poisoning by other parasympatholytics [anticholinergics and antimuscarinics] and spasmolytics, <u>assault</u>

T44.3x4- Poisoning by other parasympatholytics [anticholinergics and antimuscarinics] and spasmolytics, <u>undetermined</u>

T44.3x5- <u>Adverse effect</u> of other parasympatholytics [anticholinergics and antimuscarinics] and spasmolytics

T44.3x6- <u>Underdosing</u> of other parasympatholytics [anticholinergics and antimuscarinics] and spasmolytics

T44.4- Poisoning by, adverse effect of and underdosing of predominantly alpha-adrenoreceptor agonists
　　Poisoning by, adverse effect of and underdosing of metaraminol

T44.4 - DRUGS/CHEMS*		
Agonist, predominantly alpha-adrenoreceptor	Etilefrine	Norfenefrine
	Gepefrine	Oxedrine
Aplonidine	Levarterenol	Paredrine
Apraclonidine (hydrochloride)	Metaraminol	Phenylephrine
	Methoxamine	Privine
Cyclopentamine	Noradrenaline	Propyl hexadrine
	Norepinephrine	

T44.4x- Poisoning by, adverse effect of and underdosing of <u>predominantly alpha-adrenoreceptor agonists</u>

T44.4x1- Poisoning by predominantly alpha-adrenoreceptor agonists, <u>accidental</u> (unintentional)
　　Poisoning by predominantly alpha-adrenoreceptor agonists NOS

T44.4x2- Poisoning by predominantly alpha-adrenoreceptor agonists, <u>intentional</u> self-harm

T44.4x3- Poisoning by predominantly alpha-adrenoreceptor agonists, <u>assault</u>

T44.4x4- Poisoning by predominantly alpha-adrenoreceptor agonists, <u>undetermined</u>

T44.4x5- <u>Adverse effect</u> of predominantly alpha-adrenoreceptor agonists

T44.4x6- <u>Underdosing</u> of predominantly alpha-adrenoreceptor agonists

T44 - T44

T44.5- Poisoning by, adverse effect of and underdosing of predominantly beta-adrenoreceptor agonists

> Excludes 1: poisoning by, adverse effect of and underdosing of beta-adrenoreceptor agonists used in asthmatherapy (T48.6-)

T44.5 - DRUGS/CHEMS*		
Adrenalin	Beclomethasone	Procaterol
Adrenaline	Budesonide	Racepinefrin
Agonist, predominantly	Dobutamine	Ritodrine
beta-adrenoreceptor	Epinephrine	Xamoterol
Angiotensin	Isoetharine	
	Prenalterol	

T44.5x- Poisoning by, adverse effect of and underdosing of predominantly beta-adrenoreceptor agonists

T44.5x1- Poisoning by predominantly beta-adrenoreceptor agonists, accidental (unintentional)
>   Poisoning by predominantly beta-adrenoreceptor agonists NOS

T44.5x2- Poisoning by predominantly beta-adrenoreceptor agonists, intentional self-harm

T44.5x3- Poisoning by predominantly beta-adrenoreceptor agonists, assault

T44.5x4- Poisoning by predominantly beta-adrenoreceptor agonists, undetermined

T44.5x5- Adverse effect of predominantly beta-adrenoreceptor agonists

T44.5x6- Underdosing of predominantly beta-adrenoreceptor agonists

T44.6- Poisoning by, adverse effect of and underdosing of alpha-adrenoreceptor antagonists

> Excludes 1: poisoning by, adverse effect of and underdosing of ergot alkaloids (T48.0)

T44.6 - DRUGS/CHEMS*		
Alpha adrenergic blocking	Dibenamine	Prazosin
drug	Dibenzyline	Priscol, Priscoline
Antagonist, alpha-	Doxazosin	Tamsulosin
adrenoreceptor	Flomax	Terazosin
Bunazosin	Hydergine	
	Indoramin	

T44.6x- Poisoning by, adverse effect of and underdosing of alpha-adrenoreceptor antagonists

T44.6x1- Poisoning by alpha-adrenoreceptor antagonists, accidental (unintentional)
>   Poisoning by alpha-adrenoreceptor antagonists NOS

T44.6x2- Poisoning by alpha-adrenoreceptor antagonists, intentional self-harm

T44.6x3- Poisoning by alpha-adrenoreceptor antagonists, assault

T44.6x4- Poisoning by alpha-adrenoreceptor antagonists, undetermined

T44.6x5- Adverse effect of alpha-adrenoreceptor antagonists

T44.6x6- Underdosing of alpha-adrenoreceptor antagonists

T44.7- Poisoning by, adverse effect of and underdosing of beta-adrenoreceptor antagonists

T44.7 - DRUGS/CHEMS*		
Acebutolol	Bisoprolol	Nadolol
Adrenergic, blocking agent	Bopindolol	Oxprenolol
NEC, beta, heart	Bunitrolol	Penbutolol
Alprenolol	Bupranolol	Pindolol
Antagonist, beta-	Carazolol	Practolol
adrenoreceptor	Carteolol	Pronetalol
Atenolol	Celiprolol	Propranolol
Beta adrenergic blocking	Esmolol	Sotalol
agent, heart	Indenolol	Tertatolol
Betaxolol	Inderal	Timolol
Bevantolol	Mepindolol	Tolamolol
	Metoprolol	

T44.7x- Poisoning by, adverse effect of and underdosing of beta-adrenoreceptor antagonists

T44.7x1- Poisoning by beta-adrenoreceptor antagonists, accidental (unintentional)
>   Poisoning by beta-adrenoreceptor antagonists NOS

T44.7x2- Poisoning by beta-adrenoreceptor antagonists, intentional self-harm

T44.7x3- Poisoning by beta-adrenoreceptor antagonists, assault

T44.7x4- Poisoning by beta-adrenoreceptor antagonists, undetermined

T44.7x5- Adverse effect of beta-adrenoreceptor antagonists

T44.7x6- Underdosing of beta-adrenoreceptor antagonists

T44.8- Poisoning by, adverse effect of and underdosing of centrally-acting and adrenergic-neuron-blocking agents

> Excludes 1: poisoning by, adverse effect of and underdosing of clonidine (T46.5)
>   poisoning by, adverse effect of and underdosing of guanethidine (T46.5)

T44.8 - DRUGS/CHEMS*		
Adrenergic, blocking agent	Antiadrenergic NEC	Sympatholytic,
NEC	Labetalol	haloalkylamine
Alfuzosin (hydrochloride)	Medroxalol	
	Sympatholytic NEC	

T44.8x- Poisoning by, adverse effect of and underdosing of centrally-acting and adrenergic-neuron-blocking agents

T44.8x1- Poisoning by centrally-acting and adrenergic-neuron-blocking agents, accidental (unintentional)
>   Poisoning by centrally-acting and adrenergic-neuron-blocking agents NOS

T44.8x2- Poisoning by centrally-acting and adrenergic-neuron-blocking agents, intentional self-harm

T44.8x3- Poisoning by centrally-acting and adrenergic-neuron-blocking agents, assault

T44.8x4- Poisoning by centrally-acting and adrenergic-neuron-blocking agents, undetermined

T44.8x5- Adverse effect of centrally-acting and adrenergic-neuron-blocking agents

T44.8x6- Underdosing of centrally-acting and adrenergic-neuron-blocking agents

T44.9- Poisoning by, adverse effect of and underdosing of other and unspecified drugs primarily affecting the autonomic nervous system
>   Poisoning by, adverse effect of and underdosing of drug stimulating both alpha and beta-adrenoreceptors

T44.90- Poisoning by, adverse effect of and underdosing of unspecified drugs primarily affecting the autonomic nervous system

T44.90 - DRUGS/CHEMS*		
Adrenergic NEC	Autonomic nervous system	Sympathomimetic NEC
	agent NEC	

T44.901- Poisoning by unspecified drugs primarily affecting the autonomic nervous system, accidental (unintentional)
>   Poisoning by unspecified drugs primarily affecting the autonomic nervous system NOS

T44.902- Poisoning by unspecified drugs primarily affecting the autonomic nervous system, intentional self-harm

T44.903- Poisoning by unspecified drugs primarily affecting the autonomic nervous system, assault

T44.904- Poisoning by unspecified drugs primarily affecting the autonomic nervous system, undetermined

T44.905- Adverse effect of unspecified drugs primarily affecting the autonomic nervous system

T44.906- Underdosing of unspecified drugs primarily affecting the autonomic nervous system

T44.99- Poisoning by, adverse effect of and underdosing of other drugs primarily affecting the autonomic nervous system

T44.99 - DRUGS/CHEMS*		
Adrenergic, specified NEC	Dopamine	Mephentermine
Amezinium metilsulfate	Ephedra	Phenylpropanolamine
Angiotensinamide	Ephedrine	Pseudoephedrine
Benzedrex	Ibopamine	Sympathomimetic, specified
	Isoephedrine	NEC

T44.991- Poisoning by other drug primarily affecting the autonomic nervous system, accidental (unintentional)
>   Poisoning by other drugs primarily affecting the autonomic nervous system NOS

T4 4 - T4 4

T44.992- Poisoning by other drug primarily affecting the autonomic nervous system, _intentional_ self-harm

T44.993- Poisoning by other drug primarily affecting the autonomic nervous system, _assault_

T44.994- Poisoning by other drug primarily affecting the autonomic nervous system, _undetermined_

T44.995- _Adverse effect_ of other drug primarily affecting the autonomic nervous system

T44.996- _Underdosing_ of other drug primarily affecting the autonomic nervous system

T45- Poisoning by, adverse effect of and underdosing of _primarily systemic and hematological agents_, _not elsewhere classified_

The appropriate 7th character is to be added to each code from category T45:
- **A** _Initial_ encounter
- **D** _Subsequent_ encounter
- **S** _Sequela_

T45.0- Poisoning by, adverse effect of and underdosing of antiallergic and antiemetic drugs

Excludes 1: _poisoning by, adverse effect of and underdosing of phenothiazine-based neuroleptics (T43.3)_

T45.0 - DRUGS/CHEMS*		
Acrivastine	Cinnarizine	Methaphenilene
Alizapride	Clemastine	Methapyrilene
Antazolin(e)	Clemizole	Metoclopramide
Antiallergic NEC	Clorfenamine	Moxastine
Antiemetic drug	Cyclizine	Nytol
Antihistamine	Cyproheptadine	Ondansetron
Antinausea drug	Deptropine	Oxatomide
Antistine	Dexbrompheniramine	Percogesic – see also
Antivertigo drug	Dexchlorpheniramine	Acetaminophen
Astemizole	Dibenzheptropine	Periactin
Azatadine	Difenidol	Phenindamine
Azelastine	Dimenhydrinate	Pheniramine
Bamipine	Dimetane	Phenyltoloxamine
Benadryl	Dimethindene	Pimethixene
Benzhydramine (chloride)	Dimetindene	Pipamazine
Benzquinamide	Diphenhydramine	Pipoxizine
Bisulepin (hydrochloride)	Diphenidol	Piprinhydrinate
Bonine	Diphenylpyraline	Propiomazine
Bromazine	Domperidone	Pyrathiazine
Bromodiphenhydramine	Doxylamine	Pyribenzamine
Brompheniramine	Dramamine	Pyrilamine
Buclizine	Embramine	Pyrrobutamine
Carbinoxamine	Granisetron	Rotoxamine
Cerium oxalate	Homochlorcyclizine	Setastine
Cerous oxalate	Isothipendyl	Sleep-eze
Cetirizine	Ketotifen	Sominex
Cetoxime	Levocabastine	Terfenadine
Chlorcyclizine	(hydrochloride)	Thenyldiamine
Chloropyramine	Loratidine	Thonzylamine (systemic)
Chloropyrilene	Magnesium thiosulfate	Tigan
Chlorothen	Marezine	Tranilast
Chlorphenamine	Mebhydrolin	Trimethobenzamide
Chlorpheniramine	Meclizine (hydrochloride)	Trimeton
Chlorphenoxamine	Meclozine	Tripelennamine
Chlor-Trimeton	Mephenhydramine	Triprolidine
	Mepyramine	Tritoqualine

T45.0x- Poisoning by, adverse effect of and underdosing of _antiallergic and antiemetic drugs_

T45.0x1- Poisoning by antiallergic and antiemetic drugs, _accidental_ (unintentional)
　　Poisoning by antiallergic and antiemetic drugs NOS

T45.0x2- Poisoning by antiallergic and antiemetic drugs, _intentional_ self-harm

T45.0x3- Poisoning by antiallergic and antiemetic drugs, _assault_

T45.0x4- Poisoning by antiallergic and antiemetic drugs, _undetermined_

T45.0x5- _Adverse effect_ of antiallergic and antiemetic drugs

T45.0x6- _Underdosing_ of antiallergic and antiemetic drugs

T45.1- Poisoning by, adverse effect of and underdosing of antineoplastic and immunosuppressive drugs

Excludes 1: _poisoning by, adverse effect of and underdosing of tamoxifen (T38.6)_

T45.1 - DRUGS/CHEMS*		
Aclarubicin	2-Deoxy-5-fluorouridine	Myleran
Actinomycin C	5-Deoxy-5-fluorouridine	Nimustine
Actinomycin D	Dibromodulcitol	Nitrogen mustard
Adriamycin	Dibromomannitol	Olivomycin
Alkylating drug NEC	Doxifluridine	Oncovin
(antimyeloproliferative)	Doxorubicin	Paroxypropione
(lymphatic)	DTIC	Pentostatin
Altretamine	Elliptinium acetate	Peplomycin
Amethopterin	Enocitabine	Phenyl hydrazine,
Aminoglutethimide	Epirubicin	antineoplastic
Aminopterin sodium	Estramustine	Phenylalanine mustard
Amsacrine	Ethyl carbamate	Pipobroman
Antagonist, folic acid	Etoglucid	Pirarubicin
Antagonist, pyrimidine	Etoposide	Plicamycin
Anthramycin	FAC (fluorouracil +	Porfiromycin
Antibiotic, anticancer	doxorubicin	Prednimustine
Antibiotic, antineoplastic	+ cyclophosphamide)	Procarbazine
Anticancer agents NEC	Floxuridine	Pteroyltriglutamate
Antimetabolite	Fluorodeoxyuridine	Purine analogue
Antimitotic agent	Fluorouracil	(antineoplastic)
Antineoplastic NEC	Folic acid, antagonist	Purinethol
Antineoplastic antibiotics	Ftorafur	Pyrimidine antagonist
Antineoplastic alkaloidal	Gold, colloidal (I98Au)	Razoxane
Antineoplastic combination	Goserelin	Rubidomycin
Ara-C	Hexamethylmelamine	Rufocromomycin
Asparaginase	Hormone, cancer therapy	Sarcolysin
Azacitidine	Hydroxycarbamide	Sarkomycin
Azaribine	Hydroxyurea	Semustine
Azaserine	Idarubicin	Sodium aminopterin
Azatepa	Ifosfamide	Streptozocin
Azathioprine	Imidazole-4-carboxamide	Streptozotocin
BCNU	Immunosuppressive drug	Tauromustine
Benzcarbimine	Inproquone	Tegafur
Bleomycin	Iproplatin	TEM
Broxuridine	Isophosphamide	Teniposide
Busulfan, busulphan	Leukeran	TEPA
Cactinomycin	Lomustine	Thalidomide
Cancer chemotherapy drug	Lonidamine	Thioguanine
regimen	M-AMSA	Thiotepa
Carboplatin	Mannomustine	Tioguanine
Carboquone	Matulane	Treosulfan
Carmofur	Mechlorethamine	Tretamine
Carmustine	Melphalan	Triaziquone
Chlorambucil	Mercaptopurine	Trichlormethine
Chlorhexamide	Methotrexate	Trichlorotriethylamine
Chlormethine	Methyl CCNU	Triethanomelamine
Chloropurine	Metoprine	Triethylenemelamine
Chromic phosphate 32P	Mithramycin	Triethylenephosphoramide
Chromomycin A3	Mitobronitol	Triethylenethio-
Ciclosporin	Mitoguazone	phosphoramide
Cisplatin	Mitolactol	Trimetrexate
Colaspase	Mitomycin	Trimustine
Corynebacterium parvum	Mitopodozide	Trofosfamide
Cycloleucin	Mitotane	Uracil mustard
Cyclophosphamide	Mitoxantrone	Uramustine
Cyclosporin	Mopidamol	Urethane
Cytarabine	MOPP (mechlorethamine	Vinblastine
Cytosine arabinoside	+ vincristine +	Vincamine
Cytoxan	prednisone +	Vincristine
Dacarbazine	procarbazine)	Vindesine
Dactinomycin	Muromonab-CD3	Vinorelbine tartrate
Daunomycin	Mustard, nitrogen	Zinostatin
Daunorubicin	Mustine	Zorubicin
Demecolcine	M-vac	
	Myelobromal	

T45.1x- Poisoning by, adverse effect of and underdosing of _antineoplastic and immunosuppressive drugs_

T45.1x1- Poisoning by antineoplastic and immunosuppressive drugs, _accidental_ (unintentional)
　　Poisoning by antineoplastic and immunosuppressive drugs NOS

T45.1x2- Poisoning by antineoplastic and immunosuppressive drugs, _intentional_ self-harm

T45.1x3- Poisoning by antineoplastic and immunosuppressive drugs, _assault_

T 4 4 - T 4 5

T45.1x4-   Poisoning by antineoplastic and immunosuppressive drugs, <u>undetermined</u>

T45.1x5-   <u>Adverse effect</u> of antineoplastic and immunosuppressive drugs
> AHA 14:4Q:p22 – Adverse effect of antineoplastic drug

T45.1x6-   <u>Underdosing</u> of antineoplastic and immunosuppressive drugs

T45.2-   Poisoning by, adverse effect of and underdosing of vitamins
> Excludes ❷: poisoning by, adverse effect of and underdosing of
> nicotinic acid (derivatives) (T46.7)
> poisoning by, adverse effect of and underdosing of iron
> (T45.4)
> poisoning by, adverse effect of and underdosing of
> vitamin K (T45.7)

T45.2 - DRUGS/CHEMS*	Dexpanthenol	Retinol
Acetiamine	Dextro calcium	Riboflavin
Adenine	pantothenate	Thiamine
Alfacalcidol	Dextro pantothenyl alcohol	Tocoferol
Alpha tocoferol (acetate)	Dihydrotachysterol	Tocopherol
Aneurine	Ergocalciferol	Tocopherol acetate
Ascorbic acid	Esculin	Viosterol
Axerophthol	Esculoside	Vitamin NEC
Benfotiamine	Flavine adenine	Vitamin A
Betacarotene	dinucleotide	Vitamin B NEC
Biotin	Folic acid with ferrous salt	Vitamin B1
Bisbentiamine	Fursultiamine	Vitamin B2
Bisbutiamine	Ilopan	Vitamin B6
Calcifediol	Lactoflavin	Vitamin B12
Calciferol	Niacinamide	Vitamin B15
Calcitriol	Nicotinamide	Vitamin C
Calcium pantothenate	Octotiamine	Vitamin D
Carotene	Oleovitamin A	Vitamin D2
Cetotiamine	Pangamic acid	Vitamin D3
Cevitamic acid	Panthenol	Vitamin E
Cholecalciferol	Pantothenic acid	Vitamin E acetate
Cobalamine	Prosultiamine	Vitamin PP
Cod-liver oil	Provitamin A	Yeast
Colecalciferol	Pyridoxal phosphate	Yeast, dried
Cozyme	Pyridoxine	

T45.2x-   Poisoning by, adverse effect of and underdosing of <u>vitamins</u>

   T45.2x1-   Poisoning by vitamins, <u>accidental</u> (unintentional)
>   Poisoning by vitamins NOS

   T45.2x2-   Poisoning by vitamins, <u>intentional</u> self-harm

   T45.2x3-   Poisoning by vitamins, <u>assault</u>

   T45.2x4-   Poisoning by vitamins, <u>undetermined</u>

   T45.2x5-   <u>Adverse effect</u> of vitamins

   T45.2x6-   <u>Underdosing</u> of vitamins
>   Excludes 1:   vitamin deficiencies (E50-E56)

T45.3-   Poisoning by, adverse effect of and underdosing of enzymes

T45.3 - DRUGS/CHEMS*	Chymotrypsin	Hyaluronidase
Alglucerase	Cocarboxylase	Hyazyme
Alidase	Deoxyribonuclease	Pancreatic dornase
Alpha amylase	(pancreatic)	Penicillinase
Brinase	Diffusin	Pronase
Bromelains	Enzodase	Serrapeptase
Catalase	Enzyme NEC	Streptodornase
Chymar	Enzyme, fibrolytic	Sutilains
Chymopapain	Enzyme, thrombolytic	Trypsin

T45.3x-   Poisoning by, adverse effect of and underdosing of <u>enzymes</u>

   T45.3x1-   Poisoning by enzymes, <u>accidental</u> (unintentional)
>   Poisoning by enzymes NOS

   T45.3x2-   Poisoning by enzymes, <u>intentional</u> self-harm

   T45.3x3-   Poisoning by enzymes, <u>assault</u>

   T45.3x4-   Poisoning by enzymes, <u>undetermined</u>

   T45.3x5-   <u>Adverse effect</u> of enzymes

   T45.3x6-   <u>Underdosing</u> of enzymes

T45.4-   Poisoning by, adverse effect of and underdosing of iron and its compounds

T45.4 - DRUGS/CHEMS*	Ferrodextrane	Iron, dextran injection
Calcium ferrous citrate	Ferropolimaler	Iron, salts
Dextriferron	Ferrous phosphate	Iron, sorbitex
Ferric chloride	Ferrous salt	Iron, sorbitol citric acid
Ferric citrate	Ferrous salt with folic acid	complex
Ferric hydroxide, colloidal	Ferrous fumarate,	Isomaltose, ferric complex
Ferric hydroxide,	gluconate, lactate, salt	Jectofer
polymaltose	NEC, sulfate (medicinal)	Polyferose
Ferric pyrophosphate	Iron (compounds)	Sodium iron edetate
Ferritin	(medicinal) NEC	
Ferrocholinate	Iron, ammonium	

T45.4x-   Poisoning by, adverse effect of and underdosing of <u>iron and its compounds</u>

   T45.4x1-   Poisoning by iron and its compounds, <u>accidental</u> (unintentional)
>   Poisoning by iron and its compounds NOS

   T45.4x2-   Poisoning by iron and its compounds, <u>intentional</u> self-harm

   T45.4x3-   Poisoning by iron and its compounds, <u>assault</u>

   T45.4x4-   Poisoning by iron and its compounds, <u>undetermined</u>

   T45.4x5-   <u>Adverse effect</u> of iron and its compounds

   T45.4x6-   <u>Underdosing</u> of iron and its compounds
>   Excludes 1:   iron deficiency (E61.1)

T45.5-   Poisoning by, adverse effect of and underdosing of anticoagulants and antithrombotic drugs

  T45.51-   Poisoning by, adverse effect of and underdosing of <u>anticoagulants</u>
> AHA 16:1Q:p14 – Duodenal ulcer with hemorrhage due to
> Coumadin therapy

T45.51 - DRUGS/CHEMS*	Diphenadione	Nicoumalone
Acenocoumarin	Drotrecogin alfa	Panwarfin
Acenocoumarol	Enoxaparin (sodium)	Phenindione
Anisindione	Ethyl biscoumacetate	Phenprocoumon
Anticoagulant NEC	Ethylidene dicoumarin	Prothrombin synthesis
Bishydroxycoumarin	Ethylidene dicoumarol	inhibitor
Bromindione	Fluindione	Sintrom
Coumadin	Heparin (sodium)	Tioclomarol
Coumarin	Heparin-fraction	Warfarin
Coumetarol	Heparinoid (systemic)	Xigris
Cumetharol	Indandione (derivatives)	Zovant
Danilone	Indendione (derivatives)	
Dicoumarol, dicoumarin,	Inhibitor, prothrombin	
dicumarol	synthesis	

   T45.511-   Poisoning by anticoagulants, <u>accidental</u> (unintentional)
>   Poisoning by anticoagulants NOS

   T45.512-   Poisoning by anticoagulants, <u>intentional</u> self-harm

   T45.513-   Poisoning by anticoagulants, <u>assault</u>

   T45.514-   Poisoning by anticoagulants, <u>undetermined</u>

   T45.515-   <u>Adverse effect</u> of anticoagulants
> AHA 13:2Q:p34 – Warfarin induced skin necrosis

   T45.516-   <u>Underdosing</u> of anticoagulants

  T45.52-   Poisoning by, adverse effect of and underdosing of <u>antithrombotic drugs</u>
> AHA 16:1Q:p15 – Hemorrhage due to Prasugrel (Effient®)
> Poisoning by, adverse effect of and underdosing of
> antiplatelet drugs
> Excludes ❷: poisoning by, adverse effect of and underdosing of
> aspirin (T39.01-)
> poisoning by, adverse effect of and underdosing of
> acetylsalicylic acid (T39.01-)

T45.52 - DRUGS/CHEMS*	Prostacyclin	Triflusal
Epoprostenol	Prostaglandin (I2)	
Indobufen	Ticlopidine	

   T45.521-   Poisoning by antithrombotic drugs, <u>accidental</u> (unintentional)
>   Poisoning by antithrombotic drug NOS

   T45.522-   Poisoning by antithrombotic drugs, <u>intentional</u> self-harm

T45.523- **Poisoning** by antithrombotic drugs, <u>assault</u>
T45.524- **Poisoning** by antithrombotic drugs, <u>undetermined</u>
T45.525- <u>Adverse effect</u> of antithrombotic drugs
T45.526- <u>Underdosing</u> of antithrombotic drugs

T45.6- **Poisoning** by, adverse effect of and underdosing of fibrinolysis-affecting drugs

T45.60- **Poisoning** by, adverse effect of and underdosing of <u>unspecified fibrinolysis-affecting drugs</u>

T45.60 - DRUGS/CHEMS*
Fibrinolysis, affecting drug

T45.601- **Poisoning** by unspecified fibrinolysis-affecting drugs, <u>accidental</u> (unintentional)
    Poisoning by fibrinolysis-affecting drug NOS
T45.602- **Poisoning** by unspecified fibrinolysis-affecting drugs, <u>intentional</u> self-harm
T45.603- **Poisoning** by unspecified fibrinolysis-affecting drugs, <u>assault</u>
T45.604- **Poisoning** by unspecified fibrinolysis-affecting drugs, <u>undetermined</u>
T45.605- <u>Adverse effect</u> of unspecified fibrinolysis-affecting drugs
T45.606- <u>Underdosing</u> of unspecified fibrinolysis-affecting drugs

T45.61- **Poisoning** by, adverse effect of and underdosing of <u>thrombolytic drugs</u>

T45.61 - DRUGS/CHEMS*	Plasminogen (tissue)	Thrombolysin
Alteplase	activator	Urokinase
Anistreplase	Rt-PA	
Fibrinolytic drug	Streptokinase	

T45.611- **Poisoning** by thrombolytic drug, <u>accidental</u> (unintentional)
    Poisoning by thrombolytic drug NOS
T45.612- **Poisoning** by thrombolytic drug, <u>intentional</u> self-harm
T45.613- **Poisoning** by thrombolytic drug, <u>assault</u>
T45.614- **Poisoning** by thrombolytic drug, <u>undetermined</u>
T45.615- <u>Adverse effect</u> of thrombolytic drugs
T45.616- <u>Underdosing</u> of thrombolytic drugs

T45.62- **Poisoning** by, adverse effect of and underdosing of <u>hemostatic drugs</u>

T45.62 - DRUGS/CHEMS*	Epsilon amino-caproic acid	Inhibitor, fibrinolysis
Aminocaproic acid	Fibrinolysis, inhibitor NEC	Tranexamic acid
Antifibrinolytic drug	Hemostatic	
Aprotinin	Hemostatic, drug, systemic	

T45.621- **Poisoning** by hemostatic drug, <u>accidental</u> (unintentional)
    Poisoning by hemostatic drug NOS
T45.622- **Poisoning** by hemostatic drug, <u>intentional</u> self-harm
T45.623- **Poisoning** by hemostatic drug, <u>assault</u>
T45.624- **Poisoning** by hemostatic drug, <u>undetermined</u>
T45.625- <u>Adverse effect</u> of hemostatic drug
T45.626- <u>Underdosing</u> of hemostatic drugs

T45.69- **Poisoning** by, adverse effect of and underdosing of <u>other fibrinolysis-affecting drugs</u>

T45.69 - DRUGS/CHEMS*	Ancrod
Aminomethylbenzoic acid	Fibrinolysin (human)

T45.691- **Poisoning** by other fibrinolysis-affecting drugs, <u>accidental</u> (unintentional)
    Poisoning by other fibrinolysis-affecting drug NOS
T45.692- **Poisoning** by other fibrinolysis-affecting drugs, <u>intentional</u> self-harm
T45.693- **Poisoning** by other fibrinolysis-affecting drugs, <u>assault</u>
T45.694- **Poisoning** by other fibrinolysis-affecting drugs, <u>undetermined</u>

T45.695- <u>Adverse effect</u> of other fibrinolysis-affecting drugs
T45.696- <u>Underdosing</u> of other fibrinolysis-affecting drugs

T45.7- **Poisoning** by, adverse effect of and underdosing of anticoagulant antagonists, vitamin K and other coagulants

T45.7 - DRUGS/CHEMS*	Factor IX complex	Phytomenadione
Acetomenaphthone	Gelatin, absorbable	Phytonadione
Antagonist, anticoagulant	(sponge)	Protamine sulfate
Anticoagulant, antagonist	Gelfoam	Prothrombin activator
Antihemophilic globulin	Heparin, action reverser	Russel's viper venin
concentrate	Hexadimethrine (bromide)	Snake venom or bite,
Antihemophilic plasma,	Menadiol	hemocoagulase
dried	Menadiol sodium sulfate	Sponge, absorbable
Antiheparin drug	Menadione	(gelatin)
Coagulant NEC	Menadione sodium bisulfite	Thrombin
Cotarnine	Menaphthone	Thromboplastin
Cytozyme	Menaquinone	Vitamin K NEC
Etamsylate	Menatetrenone	Vitamin K1
Ethamsylate	Phylloquinone	Vitamin K2

T45.7x- **Poisoning** by, adverse effect of and underdosing of <u>anticoagulant antagonists, vitamin K and other coagulants</u>

T45.7x1- **Poisoning** by anticoagulant antagonists, vitamin K and other coagulants, <u>accidental</u> (unintentional)
    Poisoning by anticoagulant antagonists, vitamin K and other coagulants NOS
T45.7x2- **Poisoning** by anticoagulant antagonists, vitamin K and other coagulants, <u>intentional</u> self-harm
T45.7x3- **Poisoning** by anticoagulant antagonists, vitamin K and other coagulants, <u>assault</u>
T45.7x4- **Poisoning** by anticoagulant antagonists, vitamin K and other coagulants, <u>undetermined</u>
T45.7x5- <u>Adverse effect</u> of anticoagulant antagonists, vitamin K and other coagulants
T45.7x6- <u>Underdosing</u> of anticoagulant antagonist, vitamin K and other coagulants
    Excludes 1:   vitamin K deficiency (E56.1)

T45.8- **Poisoning** by, adverse effect of and underdosing of other primarily systemic and hematological agents
    Poisoning by, adverse effect of and underdosing of liver preparations and other antianemic agents
    Poisoning by, adverse effect of and underdosing of natural blood and blood products
    Poisoning by, adverse effect of and underdosing of plasma substitute
    Excludes ❷: poisoning by, adverse effect of and underdosing of immunoglobulin (T50.Z1)
       poisoning by, adverse effect of and underdosing of iron (T45.4)
       transfusion reactions (T80-)

T45.8x- **Poisoning** by, adverse effect of and underdosing of <u>other primarily systemic and hematological agents</u>

T45.8 - DRUGS/CHEMS*	Calcium EDTA	Fibrinogen (human)
Albumin (bovine) (human	Calcium folinate	Folacin
serum (salt-poor))	Calcium leucovorin	Folic acid
(normal human serum)	Citrovorum (factor)	Folinic acid
Aminoethylisothiourium	Cobalt, medicinal (trace)	Gelatin (intravenous)
Antagonist, heavy metal	(chloride)	Haptendextran
Anti-anemic (drug)	Copper, medicinal (trace)	Heavy metal antidote
(preparation)	Cyanocobalamin	Hematin
Antidote, heavy metal	Deferoxamine	Hematinic preparation
Antihemophilic factor	Desferrioxamine	Hematological agent,
Antihemophilic fraction	Dextran (40) (70) (150)	specified NEC
Antihemophilic human	Dimercaprol (British anti-	HES
plasma	lewisite)	Hetastarch
BAL	Dimercaptopropanol	Human albumin
Blood (derivatives)	Edathamil disodium	Hydroxocobalamin
(natural) (plasma)	Edetate, disodium	Hydroxyethyl starch
(whole)	(calcium)	Leucovorin (factor)
Blood, dried	EPO	Liver extract
Blood, expander NEC	Epoetin alpha	Liver extract for parenteral
Blood, fraction NEC	Erythropoietin	use
Blood, substitute	Erythropoietin, human	Liver fraction 1
(macromolecular)	Factor I (fibrinogen)	Liver hydrolysate
British antilewisite	Factor III (thromboplastin)	LMD
Calcium disodium	Factor VIII (antihemophilic	Mecobalamin
edathamil	Factor) (concentrate)	
Calcium disodium edetate	Factor IX complex, human	

T45 – T45 – T45

---

x

T45.8 - DRUGS/CHEMS* – Continued	Polyvinylpyrrolidone	Sodium edetate
Natural blood (product)	Potassium aminobenzoate	Sodium feredetate
Normal serum albumin (human), salt-poor	Povidone	Sodium glutamate
	Pteroylglutamic acid	Sodium lactate (compound solution)
Oxypolygelatin	PVP	
Packed red cells	Red blood cells, packed	Sodium phosphate, cellulose
Plasma	Saccharated iron oxide	
Plasma expander NEC	Serum, complement (inhibitor)	Systemic drug, specified NEC
Plasma protein fraction (human)	Serum, hemolytic complement	Trace element NEC
Plasmanate	Sodium calcium edetate	Trientine
Polygeline	Sodium dehydrocholate	Vitamin hematopoietic
Polyvidone	Sodium dipantoyl ferrate	Whole blood (human)

T45.8x1- **Poisoning by other primarily systemic and hematological agents, accidental (unintentional)**
Poisoning by other primarily systemic and hematological agents NOS

T45.8x2- **Poisoning by other primarily systemic and hematological agents, intentional self-harm**

T45.8x3- **Poisoning by other primarily systemic and hematological agents, assault**

T45.8x4- **Poisoning by other primarily systemic and hematological agents, undetermined**

T45.8x5- **Adverse effect of other primarily systemic and hematological agents**

T45.8x6- **Underdosing of other primarily systemic and hematological agents**

T45.9- **Poisoning by, adverse effect of and underdosing of unspecified primarily systemic and hematological agent**

T45.9 - DRUGS/CHEMS*	
Blood, drug affecting NEC	Hematological agent
	Systemic drug

T45.91x- **Poisoning by unspecified primarily systemic and hematological agent, accidental (unintentional)**
Poisoning by primarily systemic and hematological agent NOS

T45.92x- **Poisoning by unspecified primarily systemic and hematological agent, intentional self-harm**

T45.93x- **Poisoning by unspecified primarily systemic and hematological agent, assault**

T45.94x- **Poisoning by unspecified primarily systemic and hematological agent, undetermined**

T45.95x- **Adverse effect of unspecified primarily systemic and hematological agent**

T45.96x- **Underdosing of unspecified primarily systemic and hematological agent**

T46- **Poisoning by, adverse effect of and underdosing of agents primarily affecting the cardiovascular system**

Excludes 1: poisoning by, adverse effect of and underdosing of metaraminol (T44.4)

The appropriate 7th character is to be added to each code from category T46:
A **Initial** encounter
D **Subsequent** encounter
S **Sequela**

T46.0- **Poisoning by, adverse effect of and underdosing of cardiac-stimulant glycosides and drugs of similar action**

T46.0 - DRUGS/CHEMS*	Digitalis lanata	Metildigoxin
Acetyldigitoxin	Digitalis purpurea	Oleandrin
Acetyldigoxin	Digitoxin	Ouabain(e)
Alpha acetyldigoxin	Digitoxose	Pengitoxin
b-acetyldigoxin	Digoxin	Peruvoside
Cardiotonic (glycoside) NEC	Digoxine	Proscillaridin
Cerberin	Gitalin	Squill
Ch'an su	Gitalin, amorphous	Strofantina
Convallaria glycosides	Gitaloxin	Strophanthin (g) (k)
Crataegus extract	Gitoxin	Strophanthus
Cymarin	Glycoside, cardiac (stimulant)	Strophantin
Deslanoside	Lanatosides	Strophantin-g
Digitalin(e)	Meproscillarin	
Digitalis (leaf) (glycoside)		

T46.0x- **Poisoning by, adverse effect of and underdosing of cardiac-stimulant glycosides and drugs of similar action**

T46.0x1- **Poisoning by cardiac-stimulant glycosides and drugs of similar action, accidental (unintentional)**
Poisoning by cardiac-stimulant glycosides and drugs of similar action NOS

T46.0x2- **Poisoning by cardiac-stimulant glycosides and drugs of similar action, intentional self-harm**

T46.0x3- **Poisoning by cardiac-stimulant glycosides and drugs of similar action, assault**

T46.0x4- **Poisoning by cardiac-stimulant glycosides and drugs of similar action, undetermined**

T46.0x5- **Adverse effect of cardiac-stimulant glycosides and drugs of similar action**

T46.0x6- **Underdosing of cardiac-stimulant glycosides and drugs of similar action**

T46.1- **Poisoning by, adverse effect of and underdosing of calcium-channel blockers**

T46.1 - DRUGS/CHEMS*	Iproveratril	Nisoldipine
Bepridil	Isradipine	Nitrendipine
Blockers, calcium channel	Lidoflazine	Oxodipine
Diltiazem	Monoxidine hydrochloride	Tiapamil
Felodipine	Nicardipine	Verapamil
Fendiline	Nifedipine	
Gallopamil	Nimodipine	

T46.1x- **Poisoning by, adverse effect of and underdosing of calcium-channel blockers**

T46.1x1- **Poisoning by calcium-channel blockers, accidental (unintentional)**
Poisoning by calcium-channel blockers NOS

T46.1x2- **Poisoning by calcium-channel blockers, intentional self-harm**

T46.1x3- **Poisoning by calcium-channel blockers, assault**

T46.1x4- **Poisoning by calcium-channel blockers, undetermined**

T46.1x5- **Adverse effect of calcium-channel blockers**

T46.1x6- **Underdosing of calcium-channel blockers**

T46.2- **Poisoning by, adverse effect of and underdosing of other antidysrhythmic drugs, not elsewhere classified**
    Excludes 1:   *poisoning by, adverse effect of and underdosing of beta-adrenoreceptor antagonists (T44.7-)*

T46.2 - DRUGS/CHEMS*	Cardiac rhythm regulator,	Mexiletine
Adenosine (phosphate)	specified NEC	Pilsicainide (hydrochloride)
Ajmaline	Chinidin(e)	Prajmalium bitartrate
Amiodarone	Cibenzoline	Procainamide
Antidysrhythmic NEC	Depressant, cardiac	Pronestyl (hydrochloride)
Aprindine	Encainide	Propafenone
Bretylium tosilate	Flecainide	Quinaglute
Bunaftine	Hydroquinidine	Quinidine
Cardiac depressants	Lorajmine	Tocainide
Cardiac rhythm regulator	Lorcainide	

T46.2x- **Poisoning by, adverse effect of and underdosing of <u>other antidysrhythmic drugs</u>**
    T46.2x1- **Poisoning by other antidysrhythmic drugs, <u>accidental</u> (unintentional)**
         Poisoning by other antidysrhythmic drugs NOS
    T46.2x2- **Poisoning by other antidysrhythmic drugs, <u>intentional</u> self-harm**
    T46.2x3- **Poisoning by other antidysrhythmic drugs, <u>assault</u>**
    T46.2x4- **Poisoning by other antidysrhythmic drugs, <u>undetermined</u>**
    T46.2x5- **<u>Adverse effect</u> of other antidysrhythmic drugs**
    T46.2x6- **<u>Underdosing</u> of other antidysrhythmic drugs**

T46.3- **Poisoning by, adverse effect of and underdosing of coronary vasodilators**
     Poisoning by, adverse effect of and underdosing of dipyridamole
    Excludes 1:   *poisoning by, adverse effect of and underdosing of calcium-channel blockers (T46.1)*

T46.3 - DRUGS/CHEMS*	Heptaminol	Pentaerythritol, tetranitrate
Amikhelline	Hexadiline	NEC
Amyl nitrite	Hexadylamine	Pentaerythrityl tetranitrate
Bendazol	Hexobendine	Pentrinat
Benziodarone	Ipriflavone	Perhexilene
Carbocromen	Isoamyl nitrite	Perhexiline (maleate)
Chromonar	Isosorbide dinitrate	Peritrate
Coronary vasodilator NEC	Itramin tosilate	Piridoxilate
Cromonar	Khellin	Prenylamine
Diisopropylamine	Khelloside	Propatylnitrate
Dilazep	Mannitol hexanitrate	Sorbide nitrate
Dimoxyline	Molsidomine	Sweet niter spirit
Dioxyline	Nicorandil	Tenitramine
Dipyridamole	Nitrate, organic	Terodiline
Efloxate	Nitrite, amyl (medicinal)	Trapidil
Eritrityl tetranitrate	(vapor)	Triethanolamine, trinitrate
Erythrityl tetranitrate	Nitroglycerin, nitro-glycerol	(biphosphate)
Erythrol tetranitrate	(medicinal)	Trinitrine
Etafenone	Nitrous ether spirit	Trolnitrate (phosphate)
Fenalcomine	Octyl nitrite	Vasodilator, coronary NEC
Fluorosol	Organonitrate NEC	Visnadine
Glyceryl nitrate	Oxyfedrine	
Glyceryl trinitrate	Pentaerythritol	

T46.3x- **Poisoning by, adverse effect of and underdosing of <u>coronary vasodilators</u>**
    T46.3x1- **Poisoning by coronary vasodilators, <u>accidental</u> (unintentional)**
         Poisoning by coronary vasodilators NOS
    T46.3x2- **Poisoning by coronary vasodilators, <u>intentional</u> self-harm**
    T46.3x3- **Poisoning by coronary vasodilators, <u>assault</u>**
    T46.3x4- **Poisoning by coronary vasodilators, <u>undetermined</u>**
    T46.3x5- **<u>Adverse effect</u> of coronary vasodilators**
    T46.3x6- **<u>Underdosing</u> of coronary vasodilators**

T46.4- **Poisoning by, adverse effect of and underdosing of angiotensin-converting-enzyme inhibitors**

T46.4 - DRUGS/CHEMS*	Enalaprilat	Perindopril
Alacepril	Fosinopril	Quinapril
Benazepril	Fosinopril, sodium	Ramipril
Captopril	Inhibitor, angiotensin-	Spirapril
Cilazapril	converting enzyme	Zofenopril
Enalapril	Lisinopril	

T46.4x- **Poisoning by, adverse effect of and underdosing of <u>angiotensin-converting-enzyme inhibitors</u>**
    T46.4x1- **Poisoning by angiotensin-converting-enzyme inhibitors, <u>accidental</u> (unintentional)**
         Poisoning by angiotensin-converting-enzyme inhibitors NOS
    T46.4x2- **Poisoning by angiotensin-converting-enzyme inhibitors, <u>intentional</u> self-harm**
    T46.4x3- **Poisoning by angiotensin-converting-enzyme inhibitors, <u>assault</u>**
    T46.4x4- **Poisoning by angiotensin-converting-enzyme inhibitors, <u>undetermined</u>**
    T46.4x5- **<u>Adverse effect</u> of angiotensin-converting-enzyme inhibitors**
    T46.4x6- **<u>Underdosing</u> of angiotensin-converting-enzyme inhibitors**

T46.5- **Poisoning by, adverse effect of and underdosing of other antihypertensive drugs**
    Excludes 2:   *poisoning by, adverse effect of and underdosing of beta-adrenoreceptor antagonists (T44.7)*
         poisoning by, adverse effect of and underdosing of calcium-channel blockers (T46.1)
         poisoning by, adverse effect of and underdosing of diuretics (T50.0-T50.2)

T46.5 - DRUGS/CHEMS*	Guanabenz	Protoveratrine(s) (A) (B)
Aldomet	Guanacline	Raudixin
Alkavervir	Guanadrel	Rautensin
Alseroxylon	Guanethidine	Rautina
Amiquinsin	Guanfacine	Rautotal
Antagonist, serotonin	Guanochlor	Rauwiloid
Antihypertensive drug NEC	Guanoclor	Rauwoldin
Apresoline	Guanoctine	Rauwolfia (alkaloids)
Benzapril hydrochloride	Guanoxabenz	Rescinnamine
Betanidine	Guanoxan	Reserpin(e)
Bethanidine	Harmonyl	Sandril
Budralazine	Hydralazine	Saralasin
Cadralazine	Hypotensive NEC	Serpasil
Clonidine	Indapamide	Singoserp
Cryptenamine (tannates)	Lacidipine	Sodium nitroferricyanide
Debrisoquine	Methoserpidine	Sodium nitroprusside
Deserpidine	Methyldopa	Syrosingopine
DHE 45	Methyldopate	Teprotide
Diazoxide	Methysergide	Todralazine
Dihydralazine	Metirosine	Tolonidine
Dihydrazine	Moderil	Urapidil
Dihydroergotamine	Nitroprusside	Veratrine
Endralazine	Pargyline	Veratrum, alkaloids
Ergotamine	Pinacidil	

T46.5x- **Poisoning by, adverse effect of and underdosing of <u>other antihypertensive drugs</u>**
    T46.5x1- **Poisoning by other antihypertensive drugs, <u>accidental</u> (unintentional)**
         Poisoning by other antihypertensive drugs NOS
    T46.5x2- **Poisoning by other antihypertensive drugs, <u>intentional</u> self-harm**
    T46.5x3- **Poisoning by other antihypertensive drugs, <u>assault</u>**
    T46.5x4- **Poisoning by other antihypertensive drugs, <u>undetermined</u>**
    T46.5x5- **<u>Adverse effect</u> of other antihypertensive drugs**
    T46.5x6- **<u>Underdosing</u> of other antihypertensive drugs**

T 4 6 - T 4 6

T46.6- Poisoning by, adverse effect of and underdosing of antihyperlipidemic and antiarteriosclerotic drugs

T46.6 - DRUGS/CHEMS*		
Acipimox	Clinofibrate	Linolenic acid
Allyl disulfide	Clofibrate	Lovastatin
Aluminium clofibrate	Clofibride	Mesoglycan
Antiarteriosclerotic drug	Clotibric acid	Oleic acid
Anticholesterolemic drug	Colestipol	Pirozadil
NEC	Colestyramine	Polidexide (sulfate)
Antihyperlipidemic drug	Cyamopsis tetragono-loba	Pravastatin
Antilipemic drug NEC	Detaxtran	Probucol
b-benzalbutyramide	Ethylparachloro-	Ronifibrate
Benfluorex	phenoxyisobutyrate	Safflower oil
Benzalbutyramide	Etiroxate	Simfibrate
Benzyl nicotinate	Etofibrate	Simvastatin
Bezafibrate	Etofylline clofibrate	Sitosterols
Binifibrate	Fenofibrate	Soysterol
b-sitosterol(s)	Gemfibrozil	Sunflower seed oil
Cholesterol-lowering	Guar gum (medicinal)	Triparanol
agents	Halofenate	Unsaturated fatty acid
Cholestyramine (resin)	Ion exchange resin,	
Ciprofibrate	cholestyramine	
	Linoleic acid	

T46.6x- Poisoning by, adverse effect of and underdosing of antihyperlipidemic and antiarteriosclerotic drugs

   T46.6x1- Poisoning by antihyperlipidemic and antiarteriosclerotic drugs, accidental (unintentional)
      Poisoning by antihyperlipidemic and antiarteriosclerotic drugs NOS

   T46.6x2- Poisoning by antihyperlipidemic and antiarteriosclerotic drugs, intentional self-harm

   T46.6x3- Poisoning by antihyperlipidemic and antiarteriosclerotic drugs, assault

   T46.6x4- Poisoning by antihyperlipidemic and antiarteriosclerotic drugs, undetermined

   T46.6x5- Adverse effect of antihyperlipidemic and antiarteriosclerotic drugs

   T46.6x6- Underdosing of antihyperlipidemic and antiarteriosclerotic drugs

T46.7- Poisoning by, adverse effect of and underdosing of peripheral vasodilators
   Poisoning by, adverse effect of and underdosing of nicotinic acid (derivatives)
   Excludes 1:   poisoning by, adverse effect of and underdosing of papaverine (T44.3)

T46.7 - DRUGS/CHEMS*		
Alprostadil	Etofylline	Pentoxifylline
Aluminium nicotinate	Flunarizine	Phenoxybenzamine
Azapetine	Hepronicate	Phentolamine
Bamethan (sulfate)	Hydromethylpyridine	Prostaglandin E1
Bencyclane	Ifenprodil	Raubasine
Betahistine	Iloprost	Sildenafil
Brovincamine	Inositol nicotinate	Suloctidil
Buflomedil	Isoxsuprine	Tadalafil
Buphenine	Kallidinogenase	Tetranicotinoyl fructose
Butalamine	Kallikrein	Thurfyl nicotinate
Cetiedil	Lipo-alprostadil	Thymoxamine
Ciclonicate	Minoxidil	Tolazoline
Cinepazide	Moxisylyte	Trimetazidine
Cyclandelate	Naftidrofuryl (oxalate)	Vardenafil
Dihydroergocornine	Niacin	Vasodilan
Dihydroergocristine	Nicametate	Vasodilator, peripheral NEC
(mesilate)	Nicergoline	Vinburnine
Dihydroergokryptine	Nicofuranose	Vinpocetine
Dihydroergotoxine	Nicotinic acid	Viquidil
Dihydroergotoxine mesilate	Nicotinyl alcohol	Vitamin B, nicotinic acid
Ergoloid mesylates	Nylidrin	Xanthinol nicotinate
	Pentifylline	Xanthinol nicotinate

T46.7x- Poisoning by, adverse effect of and underdosing of peripheral vasodilators

   T46.7x1- Poisoning by peripheral vasodilators, accidental (unintentional)
      Poisoning by peripheral vasodilators NOS

   T46.7x2- Poisoning by peripheral vasodilators, intentional self-harm

   T46.7x3- Poisoning by peripheral vasodilators, assault

   T46.7x4- Poisoning by peripheral vasodilators, undetermined

   T46.7x5- Adverse effect of peripheral vasodilators

   T46.7x6- Underdosing of peripheral vasodilators

T46.8- Poisoning by, adverse effect of and underdosing of antivaricose drugs, including sclerosing agents

T46.8 - DRUGS/CHEMS*		
Antivaricose drug	Monoethanolamine oleate	Sodium tetradecyl sulfate
Dextrose, concentrated	Phenol, in oil injection	Sotradecol
solution, intravenous	Polidocanol	Varicose reduction drug
Ethanolamine oleate	Sclerosing agent	Venous sclerosing drug NEC
Monoethanolamine	Sodium morrhuate	Zinc, antivaricose
	Sodium psylliate	

T46.8x- Poisoning by, adverse effect of and underdosing of antivaricose drugs, including sclerosing agents

   T46.8x1- Poisoning by antivaricose drugs, including sclerosing agents, accidental (unintentional)
      Poisoning by antivaricose drugs, including sclerosing agents NOS

   T46.8x2- Poisoning by antivaricose drugs, including sclerosing agents, intentional self-harm

   T46.8x3- Poisoning by antivaricose drugs, including sclerosing agents, assault

   T46.8x4- Poisoning by antivaricose drugs, including sclerosing agents, undetermined

   T46.8x5- Adverse effect of antivaricose drugs, including sclerosing agents

   T46.8x6- Underdosing of antivaricose drugs, including sclerosing agents

T46.9- Poisoning by, adverse effect of and underdosing of other and unspecified agents primarily affecting the cardiovascular system

T46.90- Poisoning by, adverse effect of and underdosing of unspecified agents primarily affecting the cardiovascular system

T46.90 - DRUGS/CHEMS*	Cardiovascular drug NEC
Capillary-active drug NEC	

   T46.901- Poisoning by unspecified agents primarily affecting the cardiovascular system, accidental (unintentional)

   T46.902- Poisoning by unspecified agents primarily affecting the cardiovascular system, intentional self-harm

   T46.903- Poisoning by unspecified agents primarily affecting the cardiovascular system, assault

   T46.904- Poisoning by unspecified agents primarily affecting the cardiovascular system, undetermined

   T46.905- Adverse effect of unspecified agents primarily affecting the cardiovascular system

   T46.906- Underdosing of unspecified agents primarily affecting the cardiovascular system

T46.99- Poisoning by, adverse effect of and underdosing of other agents primarily affecting the cardiovascular system

T46.99 - DRUGS/CHEMS*		
Aconite (wild)	Calcium dobesilate	Naftazone
Aconitine	Chlorisondamine chloride	Phenopyrazone
Aconitum ferox	Diosmin	Pholedrine
Adrenochrome (derivative)	Escin	Rutinum
((mono) semicarbazone)	Ethoxazorutoside	Rutoside
Aurantiin	Flavodic acid	Tribenoside
Benzopyrone	Hesperidin	Troxerutin
Bioflavonoid(s)	Leucocianidol	
	Metescufylline	

   T46.991- Poisoning by other agents primarily affecting the cardiovascular system, accidental (unintentional)

   T46.992- Poisoning by other agents primarily affecting the cardiovascular system, intentional self-harm

   T46.993- Poisoning by other agents primarily affecting the cardiovascular system, assault

   T46.994- Poisoning by other agents primarily affecting the cardiovascular system, undetermined

T46 - T46

T46.995-   Adverse effect of other agents primarily affecting the cardiovascular system

T46.996-   Underdosing of other agents primarily affecting the cardiovascular system

T47-   Poisoning by, adverse effect of and underdosing of <u>agents primarily affecting the gastrointestinal system</u>

The appropriate 7th character is to be added to each code from category T47:
- **A**   <u>Initial</u> encounter
- **D**   <u>Subsequent</u> encounter
- **S**   <u>Sequela</u>

T47.0-   Poisoning by, adverse effect of and underdosing of histamine H2-receptor blockers

T47.0 - DRUGS/CHEMS*		
Antagonist, H2 receptor	Famotidine	Roxatidine
Cimetidine	Nizatidine	
	Ranitidine	

T47.0x-   Poisoning by, adverse effect of and underdosing of <u>histamine H2-receptor blockers</u>

T47.0x1-   Poisoning by histamine H2-receptor blockers, <u>accidental</u> (unintentional)
        Poisoning by histamine H2-receptor blockers NOS

T47.0x2-   Poisoning by histamine H2-receptor blockers, <u>intentional</u> self-harm

T47.0x3-   Poisoning by histamine H2-receptor blockers, <u>assault</u>

T47.0x4-   Poisoning by histamine H2-receptor blockers, <u>undetermined</u>

T47.0x5-   <u>Adverse effect</u> of histamine H2-receptor blockers

T47.0x6-   <u>Underdosing</u> of histamine H2-receptor blockers

T47.1-   Poisoning by, adverse effect of and underdosing of other antacids and anti-gastric-secretion drugs

T47.1 - DRUGS/CHEMS*		
Alexitol sodium	Bismuth salts, aluminate	Misoprostol
Algeldrate	Burimamide	Omeprazole
Almagate	Calcium carbonate	Ornoprostil
Almasilate	Carbenoxolone	Pepstatin
Aloglutamol	Cetraxate	Pirenzepine
Aluminium carbonate (gel, basic)	Chalk, precipitated	Potassium glucaldrate
	Dihydroxyaluminum aminoacetate	Proglumide
Aluminium chlorhydroxide-complex		Rolaids
	Dihydroxyaluminum sodium carbonate	Rosaprostol
Aluminium glycinate		Simaldrate
Aluminium hydroxide (gel)	Dimethicone	Simethicone
Aluminium hydroxide-magnesium carb. gel	Dimeticone	Soda, bicarb
	Enprostil	Sodium bicarbonate
Aluminium magnesium silicate	Hydrotalcite	Sodium glucaldrate
	Magaldrate	Sodium polyhydroxyaluminium monocarbonate
Aluminium phosphate	Magnesia magma	
Aluminium silicate	Magnesium carbonate	
Aluminium sodium silicate	Magnesium hydroxide	Sucralfate
Antacid NEC	Magnesium oxide	Sulglicotide
Anti-gastric-secretion drug NEC	Magnesium trisilicate	Triple carbonate
	Methylpolysiloxane	Vitamin ulceroprotectant
Benexate	Metiamide	
	Milk of magnesia	

T47.1x-   Poisoning by, adverse effect of and underdosing of <u>other antacids and anti-gastric-secretion drugs</u>

T47.1x1-   Poisoning by other antacids and anti-gastric-secretion drugs, <u>accidental</u> (unintentional)
        Poisoning by other antacids and anti-gastric-secretion drugs NOS

T47.1x2-   Poisoning by other antacids and anti-gastric-secretion drugs, <u>intentional</u> self-harm

T47.1x3-   Poisoning by other antacids and anti-gastric-secretion drugs, <u>assault</u>

T47.1x4-   Poisoning by other antacids and anti-gastric-secretion drugs, <u>undetermined</u>

T47.1x5-   <u>Adverse effect</u> of other antacids and anti-gastric-secretion drugs

T47.1x6-   <u>Underdosing</u> of other antacids and anti-gastric-secretion drugs

T47.2-   Poisoning by, adverse effect of and underdosing of stimulant laxatives

T47.2 - DRUGS/CHEMS*		
Aloes	Danthron	Phenolphthalein
Aloin	Dantron	Picosulfate (sodium)
Bisacodyl	Dianthone	Potassium sulfate
Bisoxatin	Dihydroxyanthraquinone	Rhubarb, dry extract
Bryonia	Dulcolax	Rhubarb, tincture, compound
Carter's Little Pills	Elaterium	
Cascara (sagrada)	Ex-Lax (phenolphthalein)	Scammony
Castor oil	Frangula	Senna
Cathartic, anthacene derivative	Frangula, extract	Sennoside A+B
	Gamboge	Sodium phosphate, dibasic
Cathartic, contact	Hinkle's pills	Sodium phosphate, monobasic
Cathartic, irritant NEC	Jalap	
Cathartic, vegetable	Laxative, stimulant	Sodium picosulfate
Chrysazin	Mineral oil, emulsion	Squirting cucumber (cathartic)
Colocynth	Oleum ricini	
Croton (oil)	Oxyphenisatine	Sulisatin
	Phenisatin	Yellow phenolphthalein

T47.2x-   Poisoning by, adverse effect of and underdosing of <u>stimulant laxatives</u>

T47.2x1-   Poisoning by stimulant laxatives, <u>accidental</u> (unintentional)
        Poisoning by stimulant laxatives NOS

T47.2x2-   Poisoning by stimulant laxatives, <u>intentional</u> self-harm

T47.2x3-   Poisoning by stimulant laxatives, <u>assault</u>

T47.2x4-   Poisoning by stimulant laxatives, <u>undetermined</u>

T47.2x5-   <u>Adverse effect</u> of stimulant laxatives

T47.2x6-   <u>Underdosing</u> of stimulant laxatives

T47.3-   Poisoning by, adverse effect of and underdosing of saline and osmotic laxatives

T47.3 - DRUGS/CHEMS*		
Carbamide	Lactulose	Potassium bisulfate
Cathartic, saline	Laxative, osmotic	Urea
Epsom salt	Laxative, saline	
	Mannitol	

T47.3x-   Poisoning by and adverse effect of <u>saline and osmotic laxatives</u>

T47.3x1-   Poisoning by saline and osmotic laxatives, <u>accidental</u> (unintentional)
        Poisoning by saline and osmotic laxatives NOS

T47.3x2-   Poisoning by saline and osmotic laxatives, <u>intentional</u> self-harm

T47.3x3-   Poisoning by saline and osmotic laxatives, <u>assault</u>

T47.3x4-   Poisoning by saline and osmotic laxatives, <u>undetermined</u>

T47.3x5-   <u>Adverse effect</u> of saline and osmotic laxatives

T47.3x6-   <u>Underdosing</u> of saline and osmotic laxatives

T46 - T47

T47.4- **Poisoning by, adverse effect of and underdosing of other laxatives**

T47.4 - DRUGS/CHEMS*		
Agar	Fiber, dietary	Paraffin(s), liquid
Arachis oil, cathartic	Glycerin	(medicinal)
Atonia drug, intestinal	Glycerol	Peach kernel oil (emulsion)
Bran (wheat)	Ispagula	Peanut oil (emulsion) NEC
Bulk filler, cathartic	Ispagula, husk	Petrolatum, liquid
Calcium dioctyl	Karaya (gum)	Phosphate, laxative
sulfosuccinate	Konsyl	Poloxalkol
Carboxymethyl-cellulose	Laxative NEC	Poloxamer
Carmellose	Linseed	Polycarbophil
Cathartic NEC	Liquid paraffin	Psyllium hydrophilic
Cathartic, bulk	Liquid petrolatum	mucilloid
Cathartic, emollient NEC	Magnesium citrate	Purgative NEC – see also
Cathartic, mucilage	Magnesium sulfate	Cathartic
Cellulose, cathartic	Metamucil	Soap, enema
Cellulose, hydroxyethyl	Methyl cellulose	Sodium basic phosphate
Colace	Methylcellulose	Sodium dioctyl
Dioctyl sulfosuccinate	Methylcellulose, laxative	sulfosuccinate
(calcium) (sodium)	Mineral oil (laxative)	Sodium sulfate
Docusate sodium	(medicinal)	Sorbitol
Ethylhydroxycellulose	Mucilage, plant	Sterculia
Fecal softener	Olive oil (medicinal) NEC	Tartrate, laxative

T47.4x- **Poisoning by, adverse effect of and underdosing of other laxatives**

   T47.4x1- **Poisoning by other laxatives, accidental (unintentional)**
       Poisoning by other laxatives NOS

   T47.4x2- **Poisoning by other laxatives, intentional self-harm**

   T47.4x3- **Poisoning by other laxatives, assault**

   T47.4x4- **Poisoning by other laxatives, undetermined**

   T47.4x5- **Adverse effect of other laxatives**

   T47.4x6- **Underdosing of other laxatives**

T47.5- **Poisoning by, adverse effect of and underdosing of digestants**

T47.5 - DRUGS/CHEMS*		
Amylase	Decholin	Hydrochloric acid,
Anise oil	Dehydrocholic acid	medicinal (digestant)
Antiflatulent	Diastase	Lipancreatin
Betaine	Digestant NEC	Ox bile extract
b-galactosidase	Dill	Pancreatin
Bile salts	Elastase	Pancrelipase
Carminative	Enzyme, gastric	Papain
Chenodeoxycholic acid	Enzyme, intestinal	Papain, digestant
Chenodiol	Florantyrone	Peppermint (oil)
Cholagogues	b-Galactosidase	Pepsin
Choleretic	Gastric enzymes	Pepsin, digestant
Cholic acid	Gentian	Phenylpropanol
Citric acid	Ginger	Protease
Cytochrome C	Glutamic acid	Tilactase

T47.5x- **Poisoning by, adverse effect of and underdosing of digestants**

   T47.5x1- **Poisoning by digestants, accidental (unintentional)**
       Poisoning by digestants NOS

   T47.5x2- **Poisoning by digestants, intentional self-harm**

   T47.5x3- **Poisoning by digestants, assault**

   T47.5x4- **Poisoning by digestants, undetermined**

   T47.5x5- **Adverse effect of digestants**

   T47.5x6- **Underdosing of digestants**

T47.6- **Poisoning by, adverse effect of and underdosing of antidiarrheal drugs**
   Excludes ❷: *poisoning by, adverse effect of and underdosing of systemic antibiotics and other anti-infectives (T36-T37)*

T47.6 - DRUGS/CHEMS*		
Activated charcoal – see	Charcoal	Lactobacillus acidophilus
also Charcoal, medicinal	Charcoal, activated – see	Lactobacillus acidophilus,
Aluminium tannate	also Charcoal, medicinal	compound
Amylopectin	Charcoal, medicinal	Lactobacillus bifidus,
Antidiarrheal drug NEC	(activated)	lyophilized
Antidiarrheal drug,	Charcoal, medicinal,	Lactobacillus bulgaricus
absorbent	antidiarrheal	Lactobacillus sporogenes
Attapulgite	Difenoxin	Lignin hemicellulose
Bacillus, subtilis	Diphenoxylate	Lomotil
Bismuth salts	Fetoxilate	Loperamide
Bismuth salts,	Intestinal motility control	Miyari bacteria
subcarbonate	drug	Pectin
Carbo medicinalis	Kaolin	Saccharomyces boulardii
	Kaolin, light	

T47.6x- **Poisoning by, adverse effect of and underdosing of antidiarrheal drugs**

   T47.6x1- **Poisoning by antidiarrheal drugs, accidental (unintentional)**
       Poisoning by antidiarrheal drugs NOS

   T47.6x2- **Poisoning by antidiarrheal drugs, intentional self-harm**

   T47.6x3- **Poisoning by antidiarrheal drugs, assault**

   T47.6x4- **Poisoning by antidiarrheal drugs, undetermined**

   T47.6x5- **Adverse effect of antidiarrheal drugs**

   T47.6x6- **Underdosing of antidiarrheal drugs**

T47.7- **Poisoning by, adverse effect of and underdosing of emetics**

T47.7 - DRUGS/CHEMS*		
Apomorphine	Copper sulfate, cupric,	Emetic NEC
Copper, emetic	medicinal, emetic	Ipecac
	Copper sulfate, medicinal,	Mustard (emetic)
	emetic	Mustard, black

T47.7x- **Poisoning by, adverse effect of and underdosing of emetics**

   T47.7x1- **Poisoning by emetics, accidental (unintentional)**
       Poisoning by emetics NOS

   T47.7x2- **Poisoning by emetics, intentional self-harm**

   T47.7x3- **Poisoning by emetics, assault**

   T47.7x4- **Poisoning by emetics, undetermined**

   T47.7x5- **Adverse effect of emetics**

   T47.7x6- **Underdosing of emetics**

T47.8- **Poisoning by, adverse effect of and underdosing of other agents primarily affecting gastrointestinal system**

T47.8 - DRUGS/CHEMS*		
Algin	Clebopride	Ion exchange resin,
Ammonium sulfonate resin	Dimethyl polysiloxane	intestinal
Bacillus, lactobacillus	Gastrointestinal drug,	Liquorice, extract
Bromopride	biological	Mesalazine
Carrageenan	Gastrointestinal drug,	Olsalazine
Charcoal, medicinal, poison	specified NEC	Pancreatic digestive
control	Glucurolactone	secretion stimulant
Charcoal, medicinal,	Hepatic secretion stimulant	Polysilane
specified use other than	Intestinal motility control	Sodium alginate
for diarrhea	drug, biological	Sodium amylosulfate
Cisapride	Ion exchange resin, anion	Sulfated amylopectin

T47.8x- **Poisoning by, adverse effect of and underdosing of other agents primarily affecting gastrointestinal system**

   T47.8x1- **Poisoning by other agents primarily affecting gastrointestinal system, accidental (unintentional)**
       Poisoning by other agents primarily affecting gastrointestinal system NOS

   T47.8x2- **Poisoning by other agents primarily affecting gastrointestinal system, intentional self-harm**

   T47.8x3- **Poisoning by other agents primarily affecting gastrointestinal system, assault**

   T47.8x4- **Poisoning by other agents primarily affecting gastrointestinal system, undetermined**

T47 - T47

T47.8x5- <u>Adverse effect</u> of other agents primarily affecting gastrointestinal system

T47.8x6- <u>Underdosing</u> of other agents primarily affecting gastrointestinal system

T47.9- Poisoning by, adverse effect of and underdosing of <u>unspecified agents primarily affecting the gastrointestinal system</u>

T47.9 - DRUGS/CHEMS*
Gastrointestinal drug

T47.91x- Poisoning by unspecified agents primarily affecting the gastrointestinal system, <u>accidental</u> (unintentional)
Poisoning by agents primarily affecting the gastrointestinal system NOS

T47.92x- Poisoning by unspecified agents primarily affecting the gastrointestinal system, <u>intentional</u> self-harm

T47.93x- Poisoning by unspecified agents primarily affecting the gastrointestinal system, <u>assault</u>

T47.94x- Poisoning by unspecified agents primarily affecting the gastrointestinal system, <u>undetermined</u>

T47.95x- <u>Adverse effect</u> of unspecified agents primarily affecting the gastrointestinal system

T47.96x- <u>Underdosing</u> of unspecified agents primarily affecting the gastrointestinal system

T48- Poisoning by, adverse effect of and underdosing of <u>agents primarily acting on smooth and skeletal muscles and the respiratory system</u>

The appropriate 7th character is to be added to each code from category T48:
A <u>Initial</u> encounter
D <u>Subsequent</u> encounter
S <u>Sequela</u>

T48.0- Poisoning by, adverse effect of and underdosing of oxytocic drugs
Excludes 1:   *poisoning by, adverse effect of and underdosing of estrogens, progestogens and antagonists (T38.4-T38.6)*

T48.0 - DRUGS/CHEMS*		
Carboprost	Ergotrate	Oxytocin (synthetic)
Dinoprost	Gemeprost	Pitocin
Dinoprostone	Hormone, oxytocic	Prostaglandin E2
Ergobasine	Methergine	Prostaglandin F2 alpha
Ergometrine	Methyl ergometrine	Sparteine
Ergonovine	Methyl ergonovine	Sulprostone
Ergot, derivative	Methylergometrine	Syntocinon
Ergot, medicinal (alkaloids)	Methylergonovine	Tocosamine
Ergot, prepared	Muscle affecting agents, oxytocic	Vetrabutine
Ergotocine	Oxytocic drug NEC	

T48.0x- Poisoning by, adverse effect of and underdosing of <u>oxytocic drugs</u>

T48.0x1- Poisoning by oxytocic drugs, <u>accidental</u> (unintentional)
Poisoning by oxytocic drugs NOS

T48.0x2- Poisoning by oxytocic drugs, <u>intentional</u> self-harm

T48.0x3- Poisoning by oxytocic drugs, <u>assault</u>

T48.0x4- Poisoning by oxytocic drugs, <u>undetermined</u>

T48.0x5- <u>Adverse effect</u> of oxytocic drugs

T48.0x6- <u>Underdosing</u> of oxytocic drugs

T48.1- Poisoning by, adverse effect of and underdosing of skeletal muscle relaxants [neuromuscular blocking agents]

T48.1 - DRUGS/CHEMS*		
Aclatonium napadisilate	Gallamine (triethiodide)	Relaxant, muscle, anesthetic
Alcuronium (chloride)	Hexafluorenium bromide	Relaxant, muscle, skeletal NEC
Anesthesia, muscle relaxation	Hexafluronium (bromide)	
	Hexanuorenium	
Atracurium besilate	Hexcarbacholine bromide	Skeletal muscle relaxants
Carbolonium (bromide)	Laudexium	Spasmolytic, skeletal muscle NEC
Curare, curarine	Methocarbamol, skeletal muscle relaxant	
Cyclobenzaprine	Mivacurium chloride	Succinylcholine
Decamethonium (bromide)	Muscle affecting agents, relaxants, skeletal	Suxamethonium (chloride)
Dimethyl tubocurarine		Suxethonium (chloride)
Dimethyltubocurarinium chloride	Myoneural blocking agents	Tubocurare
	Neuromuscular blocking drug	Tubocurarine (chloride)
Fazadinium bromide		Urari
	Pancuronium (bromide)	Vecuronium bromide
Flaxedil		Woorali

T48.1x- Poisoning by, adverse effect of and underdosing of <u>skeletal muscle relaxants [neuromuscular blocking agents]</u>

T48.1x1- Poisoning by skeletal muscle relaxants [neuromuscular blocking agents], <u>accidental</u> (unintentional)
Poisoning by skeletal muscle relaxants [neuromuscular blocking agents] NOS

T48.1x2- Poisoning by skeletal muscle relaxants [neuromuscular blocking agents], <u>intentional</u> self-harm

T48.1x3- Poisoning by skeletal muscle relaxants [neuromuscular blocking agents], <u>assault</u>

T48.1x4- Poisoning by skeletal muscle relaxants [neuromuscular blocking agents], <u>undetermined</u>

T48.1x5- <u>Adverse effect</u> of skeletal muscle relaxants [neuromuscular blocking agents]

T48.1x6- <u>Underdosing</u> of skeletal muscle relaxants [neuromuscular blocking agents]

T48.2- Poisoning by, adverse effect of and underdosing of other and unspecified drugs acting on muscles

T48.20- Poisoning by, adverse effect of and underdosing of <u>unspecified drugs acting on muscles</u>

T48.20 - DRUGS/CHEMS*	Muscle affecting agents,	Muscle-action drug NEC
Muscle affecting agents NEC	relaxants	

T48.201- Poisoning by unspecified drugs acting on muscles, <u>accidental</u> (unintentional)
Poisoning by unspecified drugs acting on muscles NOS

T48.202- Poisoning by unspecified drugs acting on muscles, <u>intentional</u> self-harm

T48.203- Poisoning by unspecified drugs acting on muscles, <u>assault</u>

T48.204- Poisoning by unspecified drugs acting on muscles, <u>undetermined</u>

T48.205- <u>Adverse effect</u> of unspecified drugs acting on muscles

T48.206- <u>Underdosing</u> of unspecified drugs acting on muscles

T48.29- Poisoning by, adverse effect of and underdosing of <u>other drugs acting on muscles</u>

T48.29 - DRUGS/CHEMS*	Dipropyline	Metaproterenol
Botox	Hydrastine	Orciprenaline
Bruceine	Lututrin	Strychnine, medicinal

T48.291- Poisoning by other drugs acting on muscles, <u>accidental</u> (unintentional)
Poisoning by other drugs acting on muscles NOS

T48.292- Poisoning by other drugs acting on muscles, <u>intentional</u> self-harm

T48.293- Poisoning by other drugs acting on muscles, <u>assault</u>

T48.294- Poisoning by other drugs acting on muscles, <u>undetermined</u>

T48.295- <u>Adverse effect</u> of other drugs acting on muscles

T48.296- <u>Underdosing</u> of other drugs acting on muscles

T47 - T48

T48.3- **Poisoning by, adverse effect of and underdosing of antitussives**

T48.3 - DRUGS/CHEMS*	Dibunate sodium	Oxeladin (citrate)
Antitussive NEC	Dimemorfan	Oxolamine
Benproperine	Dimethoxanate	Pentoxyverine
Benzonatate	Dropropizine	Pholcodine
Bibenzonium bromide	Ethyl dibunate	Picoperine
Butamirate	Fedrilate	Pipazetate
Carbetapentane	Fominoben	Piperidione
Chlophedianol	Isoaminile (citrate)	Prenoxdiazine
Clobutinol	Levdropropizine	Romilar
Clofedanol	Methorate	Tessalon
Cloperastine	Narcotine	Thebacon
Clophedianol	Nectadon	Tipepidine
Dextromethorphan	Noscapine	Zipeprol

T48.3x- **Poisoning by, adverse effect of and underdosing of antitussives**

T48.3x1- **Poisoning by antitussives, accidental (unintentional)**
Poisoning by antitussives NOS

T48.3x2- **Poisoning by antitussives, intentional self-harm**

T48.3x3- **Poisoning by antitussives, assault**

T48.3x4- **Poisoning by antitussives, undetermined**

T48.3x5- **Adverse effect of antitussives**

T48.3x6- **Underdosing of antitussives**

T48.4- **Poisoning by, adverse effect of and underdosing of expectorants**

T48.4 - DRUGS/CHEMS*	Expectorant NEC	Mucomyst
Acetylcysteine	Glycerol, iodinated	Organidin
Ambroxol	Glyceryl gualacolate	Potassium iodide
Ammonium chloride, expectorant	Glycyrrhiza extract	Quillaja extract
	Glycyrrhizic acid	Respaire
Bromhexine	Glycyrrhizinate potassium	Respiratory drug,
Calcium iodide	Guaiacol derivatives	expectorant NEC
Carbocisteine	Guaifenesin	Senega syrup
S-Carboxymethyl-cysteine	Guaimesal	Sobrerol
Cough mixture (syrup)	Guaiphenesin	Sodium dibunate
Cough mixture, expectorants	Hydriodic acid	Sputum viscosity-lowering drug
	Iodide, potassium (expectorant) NEC	
Creosote, medicinal (expectorant)	Iodinated glycerol	Stepronin
Creosote, syrup	Ipecacuanha	Sulfogaiacol
Deglycyrrhizinized extract of licorice	Letosteine	Superinone
	Liquorice	Tenoglicin
Domiodol	Mecysteine	Terpin (cis) hydrate
Dornase	Mesna	Tyloxapol
Eprazinone	Mucolytic drug	

T48.4x- **Poisoning by, adverse effect of and underdosing of expectorants**

T48.4x1- **Poisoning by expectorants, accidental (unintentional)**
Poisoning by expectorants NOS

T48.4x2- **Poisoning by expectorants, intentional self-harm**

T48.4x3- **Poisoning by expectorants, assault**

T48.4x4- **Poisoning by expectorants, undetermined**

T48.4x5- **Adverse effect of expectorants**

T48.4x6- **Underdosing of expectorants**

T48.5- **Poisoning by, adverse effect of and underdosing of other anti-common-cold drugs**
Poisoning by, adverse effect of and underdosing of decongestants
Excludes ❷: poisoning by, adverse effect of and underdosing of antipyretics, NEC (T39.9-)
poisoning by, adverse effect of and underdosing of non-steroidal antiinflammatory drugs (T39.3-)
poisoning by, adverse effect of and underdosing of salicylates (T39.0-)

T48.5 - DRUGS/CHEMS*	Decongestant, nasal, combination	Sympathomimetic, anti-common-cold
Amidefrine mesilate		
Anti-common-cold drug NEC	Fenoxazoline	Thonzylamine, mucosal decongestant
APC	Indanazoline	
Benzoin (tincture)	Menthol	Tramazoline
Cinnamedrine	Metizoline	Tuaminoheptane
Contac	Naphazoline	Tymazoline
Decongestant, nasal (mucosa)	Oxymetazoline	Xylometazoline
	Propylhexedrine	
	Respiratory drug, anti-common-cold NEC	

T48.5x- **Poisoning by, adverse effect of and underdosing of other anti-common-cold drugs**

T48.5x1- **Poisoning by other anti-common-cold drugs, accidental (unintentional)**
Poisoning by other anti-common-cold drugs NOS

T48.5x2- **Poisoning by other anti-common-cold drugs, intentional self-harm**

T48.5x3- **Poisoning by other anti-common-cold drugs, assault**

T48.5x4- **Poisoning by other anti-common-cold drugs, undetermined**

T48.5x5- **Adverse effect of other anti-common-cold drugs**

T48.5x6- **Underdosing of other anti-common-cold drugs**

T48.6- **Poisoning by, adverse effect of and underdosing of antiasthmatics, not elsewhere classified**
Poisoning by, adverse effect of and underdosing of beta-adrenoreceptor agonists used in asthma therapy
Excludes 1: poisoning by, adverse effect of and underdosing of beta-adrenoreceptor agonists not used in asthma therapy (T44.5)
poisoning by, adverse effect of and underdosing of anterior pituitary [adenohypophyseal] hormones (T38.8)

T48.6 - DRUGS/CHEMS*	Ethyl noradrenaline	Respiratory drug, antiasthmatic NEC
Acefylline piperazine	Ethylenediamine theophylline	
Acepifylline		Rimiterol
Albuterol	Ethylnorepinephrine	Salbutamol
Ambuphylline	Fenoterol	Salmeterol
Aminophylline	Flunisolide	Sodium cromoglicate
Amlexanox	Flutropium bromide	Spasmolytic, bronchial NEC
Antiasthmatic drug NEC	Folium stramoniae	Stramonium
Bambuterol	Glyphylline	Sympathomimetic, bronchodilator
Bamifylline	Hexoprenaline	
Bitolterol	Ibuterol	Terbutaline
Bronchodilator NEC	Ipratropium (bromide)	Theobromine (calcium salicylate)
Broxaterol	Isoetarine	
Bufrolin	Isoprenaline	Theobromine, sodium salicylate
Bufylline	Isoproterenol	
Butetamate	Levalbuterol	Theophylline
Carbuterol	Levoproxyphylline	Theophylline
Choline	Methoxyphenamine	Theophylline, aminobenzoic acid
Choline theophyllinate	Nedocromil	
Clenbuterol	Oxitropium bromide	Theophylline, ethylenediamine
Clorprenaline	Oxtriphylline	
Cromoglicic acid	Pemirolast (potassium)	Theophylline, piperazine p-amino-benzoate
Cromolyn	Pirbuterol	
Doxantrazole	Protokylol	Tretoquinol
Enprofylline	Proxyphylline	Tulobuterol
Etafedrine	Reproterol	
Etamiphyllin		

T48.6x- **Poisoning by, adverse effect of and underdosing of antiasthmatics**

T48.6x1- **Poisoning by antiasthmatics, accidental (unintentional)**
Poisoning by antiasthmatics NOS

T 4 8 – T 4 8

T48.6x2- Poisoning by antiasthmatics, <u>intentional</u> self-harm
T48.6x3- Poisoning by antiasthmatics, <u>assault</u>
T48.6x4- Poisoning by antiasthmatics, <u>undetermined</u>
T48.6x5- <u>Adverse effect</u> of antiasthmatics
T48.6x6- <u>Underdosing</u> of antiasthmatics

T48.9- Poisoning by, adverse effect of and underdosing of other and unspecified agents primarily acting on the respiratory system

 T48.90- Poisoning by, adverse effect of and underdosing of <u>unspecified agents primarily acting on the respiratory system</u>

T48.90 - DRUGS/CHEMS* Stimulant, respiratory
Respiratory drug NEC
Respiratory drug, stimulant

  T48.901- Poisoning by unspecified agents primarily acting on the respiratory system, <u>accidental</u> (unintentional)
  T48.902- Poisoning by unspecified agents primarily acting on the respiratory system, <u>intentional</u> self-harm
  T48.903- Poisoning by unspecified agents primarily acting on the respiratory system, <u>assault</u>
  T48.904- Poisoning by unspecified agents primarily acting on the respiratory system, <u>undetermined</u>
  T48.905- <u>Adverse effect</u> of unspecified agents primarily acting on the respiratory system
  T48.906- <u>Underdosing</u> of unspecified agents primarily acting on the respiratory system

 T48.99- Poisoning by, adverse effect of and underdosing of <u>other agents primarily acting on the respiratory system</u>

T48.99 - DRUGS/CHEMS* Helium, medicinal
Ammonia, aromatic spirit

  T48.991- Poisoning by other agents primarily acting on the respiratory system, <u>accidental</u> (unintentional)
  T48.992- Poisoning by other agents primarily acting on the respiratory system, <u>intentional</u> self-harm
  T48.993- Poisoning by other agents primarily acting on the respiratory system, <u>assault</u>
  T48.994- Poisoning by other agents primarily acting on the respiratory system, <u>undetermined</u>
  T48.995- <u>Adverse effect</u> of other agents primarily acting on the respiratory system
  T48.996- <u>Underdosing</u> of other agents primarily acting on the respiratory system

T49- Poisoning by, adverse effect of and underdosing of <u>topical agents primarily affecting skin and mucous membrane and by ophthalmological, otorhinolaryngological and dental drugs</u>
Includes: Poisoning by, adverse effect of and underdosing of glucocorticoids, topically used

The appropriate 7th character is to be added to each code from category T49:
A <u>Initial</u> encounter
D <u>Subsequent</u> encounter
S <u>Sequela</u>

T49.0- Poisoning by, adverse effect of and underdosing of local antifungal, anti-infective and anti-inflammatory drugs

T49.0 - DRUGS/CHEMS*		
Achromycin, topical NEC	Buclosamide	Desonide
Acriflavinium chloride	Butoconazole (nitrate)	Desoximetasone
Acrinol	Cadexomer iodine	Dettol (external
Acrisorcin	Calomel	medication)
Adrenal, topical NEC	Camomile	Dexamethasone, topical
Aerosporin, topical NEC	Candeptin	NEC
Akrinol	Candicidin	Diamthazole
Alclometasone	Carbamide, peroxide	Dibromopropamidine
Alkonium (bromide)	Carbol fuchsin	isethionate
Allethrin	Carfusin	Dibrompropamidine
Aluminium acetate solution	Castellani's paint	Dicophane
Aluminium sulfate	Ceepryn	Diethyltoluamide
Amcinonide	Celestone, topical	Diflorasone
Aminacrine	Cetalkonium (chloride)	Diflucortolone
Aminoacridine	Cethexonium chloride	Diiodohydroxyquin, topical
Ammoniated mercury	Cetrimide	Dimazole
Amphotericin B, topical	Cetrimonium (bromide)	Dixanthogen
Antibiotic, fungicidal (local)	Cetylpyridinium chloride	Dodicin
Antibiotic, local	Chamomile	Dofamium chloride
Antifungal, disinfectant,	Chloramine T	Domiphen (bromide)
local	Chloramine, topical	Dye, antiseptic
Antifungal, topical	Chloramphenicol, topical	Econazole
Anti-infective, bismuth,	NEC	Erythromycin, topical NEC
local	Chlordantoin	Ethacridine
Anti-infective, local NEC	Chlorhexidine	Ethylene oxide, medicinal
Anti-infective, local,	Chlorhydroxyquinolin	Eurax
specified NEC	Chlorinated lime, and boric	Exalamide
Anti-infective, topical NEC	acid solution	Fenticlor
Anti-inflammatory drug,	Chlorinated soda solution	Florinef, topical NEC
local	Chlorobutanol	Fluclorolone acetonide
Antiparasitic drug, local	Chlorocresol	Fludrocortisone, topical
Antiprotozoal drug, local	Chloromycetin, topical NEC	NEC
Antiseptics (external)	Chloroxylenol	Fludroxycortide
(medicinal)	Chlorphenesin, topical	Flumethasone
Argyrol	(antifungal)	Fluocinolone (acetonide)
Aristocort, topical NEC	Chlorquinaldol	Fluocinonide
Asiaticoside	Chlorquinol	Fluocortin (butyl)
Aureomycin, topical NEC	Ciclopirox (olamine)	Fluocortolone
Azelaic acid	Clobetasol	Fluohydrocortisone, topical
Bacimycin	Clobetasone	NEC
Bacitracin zinc	Clodantoin	Fluonid
Bacitracin zinc with	Clofenotane	Fluormetholone
neomycin	Clotrimazole	Fluorometholone
Bacitracin zinc, topical NEC	Cloxiquine	Fluprednidene
Basic fuchsin	Copper gluconate	Flurandrenolide
Benisone	Copper oleate	Flurandrenolone
Benzalkonium (chloride)	Cordran	Flurobate
Benzethonium (chloride)	Cort-Dome, topical NEC	Fungizone, topical
Benzoic acid	Cortef, topical NEC	Furacin
Benzoic acid with salicylic	Corticosteroid, topical NEC	Furazolium chloride
acid	Cortisol	Gamma-benzene
Benzoxonium chloride	Cortisol, topical NEC	hexachloride
Benzoyl peroxide	Cortisone, topical NEC	(medicinal)
Benzydamine	Cortril, topical NEC	Gamma-BHC (medicinal) –
Benzyl alcohol	Creosol (compound)	see also Gamma-
Benzyl benzoate	Creosote (coal tar)	benzene hexachloride
Benzyl Benzoic acid	(beechwood)	Garamycin, topical NEC
Betamethasone	Cresol(s)	Gentamicin, topical NEC
Betamethasone, topical	Cresol(s) and soap solution	Gentian, violet
BHC (medicinal)	Cresyl acetate	Gexane
Bismuth salts, formic iodide	Cresylic acid	Glutaral (medicinal)
Bismuth salts,	Crotamiton	Glutaraldehyde, medicinal
glycolylarsenate	Crystal violet	Glyceryl triacetate (topical)
Boracic acid	Cupric gluconate	Gramicidin
Boric acid	Cupric oleate	Halcinolone
Bromochlorosalicylanilide	Dakin's solution	Halcinonide
Bromosalicylchloranitide	Decadron, topical NEC	Halethazole
	Dequalinium (chloride)	

T48 - T49

T49.0 - DRUGS/CHEMS*
– Continued

Halometasone	Methyl paraben	Pyrogallol
Haloprogin	Methyl prednisolone, topical NEC	Quarternary ammonium, anti-infective
Halotex	Methyl rosaniline NEC	Retinoic acid
Halquinols	Methylbenzethonium chloride	Salicylhydroxamic acid
HCH, medicinal	Methylrosaniline	Silvadene
Hedaquinium	Methylrosanilinium chloride	Silver
Hexachlorophene	Micatin	Silver, anti-infectives
Hexamidine	Miconazole	Silver, colloidal
Hydrargaphen	Mometasone	Silver nitrate
Hydrargyri amino-chloridum	Monistat	Sodium hypochlorite, medicinal (anti-infective) (external)
Hydrocortisone (derivatives)	Monosulfiram	
Hydrocortisone, aceponate	Mupirocin	Sodium hyposulfite
Hydrocortisone, topical NEC	Mycifradin, topical	Sodium perborate, medicinal
Hydrocortone, topical NEC	Mycostatin, topical	Sodium propionate
Hydrogen peroxide	Myralact	Sporostacin
Hydroxytoluene, medicinal	Naftifine	Staphisagria or stavesacre (pediculicide)
Hypochlorite	Natamycin	
Ichthammol	Neomycin with bacitracin	Steroid, topical NEC
Ilotycin, topical NEC	Neomycin, topical NEC	Sulbentine
Iodide NEC — see also Iodine	Neosporin, topical NEC	Sulfacetamide
	Nilstat, topical	Sulfadiazine, silver (topical)
Iodide, mercury (ointment)	Nitrofural	
Iodide, methylate	Nitrofurazone	Sulfamylon
Iodine (antiseptic, external) (tincture) NEC	Nitromersol	Sulfiram
	Nitrozone	Sulfur, ointment
Iodine solution	Noxytiolin	Synalar
Iodochlorhydroxyquin, topical	Nystatin, topical	Terconazole
	Orthoboric acid	Tetracycline, topical NEC
Iodoform	Oxiconazole	Tetramethylthiuram, medicinal
Isoconazole	Oxychlorosene	
Ketoconazole	Oxylone	Thimerosal
Kwell, anti-infective (topical)	Parachlorophenol (camphorated)	Thiomersal
	Paramethasone acetate	Thymol
Laurolinium	Peruvian balsam	Ticlatone
Lidex	Phenoctide	Tioconazole
Lindane, medicinal	Phenol	Tolciclate
Locorten	Phenothrin	Tolnaftate
Lysozyme	Phenoxyethanol	Tretinoin
Mafenide	Phenylmercuric acetate	Triacetin
Magnesium peroxide	Phenylmercuric borate	Triamcinolone
Malathion (medicinal)	Phenylmercuric nitrate	Triamcinolone, hexacetonide
Maphenide	Piketoprofen	
Medrysone	Polymyxin B, topical NEC	Triamcinolone, topical NEC
Melaleuca alternifolia oil	Polynoxylin	Triclobisonium chloride
Merbromin	Polyoxymethyleneurea	Triclocarban
Mercaptobenzothiazole salts	Potassium iodate	Triclosan
	Potassium permanganate, medicinal	Tridesilon
Mercurochrome		Undecenoic acid
Mercury, ammoniated	Povidone, iodine	Undecoylium
Mercury, anti-infective, local	Prednicarbate	Undecylenic acid (derivatives)
	Prednisolone, steaglate	
Mercury, anti-infective, topical	Prednisolone, topical NEC	Urea peroxide
	Proflavine	Valisone
Mercury, chloride (ammoniated)	Propamidine	Vioform, topical
	Propiolactone	Zephiran (topical)
Mercury, oxide, yellow	Propion gel	Zinc, anti-infectives
Merthiolate	Propionate (calcium) (sodium)	Zinc bacitracin
Mesulfen		Zinc peroxide
Metactesylacetate	Pyrethrum extract	Zinc sulfate, topical NEC
Metaphen	Pyrogallic acid	Zinc undecylenate

T49.0x- Poisoning by, adverse effect of and underdosing of <u>local antifungal, anti-infective and anti-inflammatory drugs</u>

T49.0x1- Poisoning by local antifungal, anti-infective and anti-inflammatory drugs, <u>accidental</u> (unintentional)
Poisoning by local antifungal, anti-infective and anti-inflammatory drugs NOS

T49.0x2- Poisoning by local antifungal, anti-infective and anti-inflammatory drugs, <u>intentional</u> self-harm

T49.0x3- Poisoning by local antifungal, anti-infective and anti-inflammatory drugs, <u>assault</u>

T49.0x4- Poisoning by local antifungal, anti-infective and anti-inflammatory drugs, <u>undetermined</u>

T49.0x5- <u>Adverse effect</u> of local antifungal, anti-infective and anti-inflammatory drugs

T49.0x6- <u>Underdosing</u> of local antifungal, anti-infective and anti-inflammatory drugs

T49.1- Poisoning by, adverse effect of and underdosing of antipruritics

T49.1 - DRUGS/CHEMS*

Antipruritic drug NEC	ESDT (ether-soluble tar distillate)	Pramocaine
Benzamine, lactate		Pramoxine
b-eucaine	Fluticasone propionate	Quinisocaine
Coal tar	Juniper tar	Tar, distillate
Dimethisoquin	Phenol, medicinal	Tar, medicinal
	Phenolic preparation	Tar, ointment

T49.1x- Poisoning by, adverse effect of and underdosing of <u>antipruritics</u>

T49.1x1- Poisoning by antipruritics, <u>accidental</u> (unintentional)
Poisoning by antipruritics NOS

T49.1x2- Poisoning by antipruritics, <u>intentional</u> self-harm

T49.1x3- Poisoning by antipruritics, <u>assault</u>

T49.1x4- Poisoning by antipruritics, <u>undetermined</u>

T49.1x5- <u>Adverse effect</u> of antipruritics

T49.1x6- <u>Underdosing</u> of antipruritics

T49.2- Poisoning by, adverse effect of and underdosing of local astringents and local detergents

T49.2 - DRUGS/CHEMS*

Acetic acid medicinal (lotion)	Detergent, local	Septisol
	Detergent, medicinal	Soap, medicinal, soft
Aluminium acetate	Dial (soap)	Soap, superfatted
Aluminium chloride	Duponol (C) (EP)	Sodium lauryl (sulfate)
Aluminium diacetate	Green soap	Sulfatostearate
Aluminium subacetate	Hamamelis	Tannic acid
Antihemorrhoidal preparation	Hexa-germ	Tannic acid, medicinal (astringent)
	Iproheptine	
Antiperspirant NEC	Lauryl sulfoacetate	Thiram, medicinal
Astringent (local)	Lead acetate	Vegetable extract, astringent
Astringent, specified NEC	Lowila	
Detergent	Methyl salicylate	Witch hazel
Detergent, external medication	pHisoHex	
	Polyethanolamine alkyl sulfate	

T49.2x- Poisoning by, adverse effect of and underdosing of <u>local astringents and local detergents</u>

T49.2x1- Poisoning by local astringents and local detergents, <u>accidental</u> (unintentional)
Poisoning by local astringents and local detergents NOS

T49.2x2- Poisoning by local astringents and local detergents, <u>intentional</u> self-harm

T49.2x3- Poisoning by local astringents and local detergents, <u>assault</u>

T49.2x4- Poisoning by local astringents and local detergents, <u>undetermined</u>

T49.2x5- <u>Adverse effect</u> of local astringents and local detergents

T49.2x6- <u>Underdosing</u> of local astringents and local detergents

T49 - T49

T49.3- Poisoning by, adverse effect of and underdosing of emollients, demulcents and protectants

T49.3 - DRUGS/CHEMS*		
Acetic acid with sodium acetate (ointment)	Filtering cream	Plaster dressing
Acrylic resin	Flaxseed (medicinal)	Plastic dressing
Allylthiourea	Homosalate	Polyethylene adhesive
Aluminium ointment (surgical) (topical)	Hydrophilic lotion	Protectant, skin NEC
Aluminium topical NEC	Hydrous wool fat	Pyroxylin
Aminobenzoic acid (-p)	Lanolin	Rose water ointment
Arachis oil	Liquid petrolatum, topical	Salicylate, methyl
Barrier cream	Mecrilate	Salol
Bentonite	Meladinin	Silicone, medicinal
Benzophenones	Melanizing agents	Solar lotion
Betula oil	Meloxine	Sulisobenzone
Calamine (lotion)	Methoxa-Dome	Sweet oil (birch)
Carbowax	Mexenone	Talc powder
Cellulose, nitrates (topical)	Mineral oil, topical	Talcum
Chlordiethyl benzamide	Nutmeg oil (liniment)	Thiosinamine
Cold cream	Octafonium (chloride)	Titanium dioxide
Collodion	Oil, wintergreen (bitter) NEC	Titanium ointment
Colophony adhesive	Oily preparation (for skin)	Titanium oxide
Corn starch	Ointment NEC	Trimethylpsoralen
Cornhusker's lotion	Oxsoralen	Trisoralen
Cottonseed oil	PABA	Ultraviolet light protectant
Cyanoacrylate adhesive	Padimate	Unna's boot
Demulcent (external)	Para-aminobenzoic acid	Vaseline
Demulcent, specified NEC	Peanut oil, topical	Wintergreen (oil)
Diethyl toluamide, medicinal	Petrolatum	Wool fat (hydrous)
Dimethyl phthlate	Petrolatum, hydrophilic	Xanthotoxin
Emollient NEC	Petrolatum, liquid, topical	Zinc, gelatin
	Petrolatum, red veterinary	Zinc oxide
	Petrolatum, white	Zinc oxide, plaster
	Phenyl salicylate	Zinc stearate

T49.3x- Poisoning by, adverse effect of and underdosing of <u>emollients, demulcents and protectants</u>

T49.3x1- Poisoning by emollients, demulcents and protectants, <u>accidental</u> (unintentional)
Poisoning by emollients, demulcents and protectants NOS

T49.3x2- Poisoning by emollients, demulcents and protectants, <u>intentional</u> self-harm

T49.3x3- Poisoning by emollients, demulcents and protectants, <u>assault</u>

T49.3x4- Poisoning by emollients, demulcents and protectants, <u>undetermined</u>

T49.3x5- <u>Adverse effect</u> of emollients, demulcents and protectants

T49.3x6- <u>Underdosing</u> of emollients, demulcents and protectants

---

T49.4- Poisoning by, adverse effect of and underdosing of keratolytics, keratoplastics, and other hair treatment drugs and preparations

T49.4 - DRUGS/CHEMS*		
Allantoin	Dimethylamine sulfate	Salicylic acid with benzoic acid
Alum (medicinal)	Dithranol	Savin (oil)
Ammonium ichthyosulronate	Enzyme, local action	Selenium disulfide or sulfide
Anthralin	Enzyme, proteolytic	Selenium sulfide
Antiseborrheics	Ethyl chloride, local	Selsun
Bleaching agent (medicinal)	Ethyl fumarate	Silver nitrate, toughened (keratolytic)
Butantrone	Euresol	Silver sulfadiazine
Cade oil	Flowers of sulfur	Sulfur, sulfurated, sulfuric, sulfurous, sulfuryl (compounds NEC) (medicinal)
Cadmium sulfide (medicinal) NEC	Fumaric acid	
Capsicum	Hair dye	
Carbazochrome (salicylate) (sodium sulfonate)	Hair preparation NEC	Sulfur, medicinal (keratolytic) (ointment) NEC
Carbon dioxide, snow	Hemostyptic	
Cellulose, oxidized	Ichthyol	Thioglycolate
Chlorothymol	Isopropyl alcohol, medicinal	Tioxolone
Chloroxine	Keratolytic drug NEC	Triacetoxyanthracene
Chrysarobin	Keratolytic drug, anthracene	Trichloroacetic acid, medicinal
Coal tar, medicinal (ointment)	Keratoplastic NEC	Trioxysalen
Collagenase	Lassar's paste	Vleminckx's solution
Corn cures	Methyl nicotinate	White lotion (keratolytic)
Depilatory	Monobenzone	Xenysalate
Desloughing agent	Podophyllum (resin)	Zinc pyrithionate
Diachylon plaster	Preparation, local	
Dimethyl sulfoxide, medicinal	Pyrithione zinc	
	Resorcin, resorcinol, medicinal	
	Rubefacient	
	Salicylic acid	

T49.4x- Poisoning by, adverse effect of and underdosing of <u>keratolytics, keratoplastics, and other hair treatment drugs and preparations</u>

T49.4x1- Poisoning by keratolytics, keratoplastics, and other hair treatment drugs and preparations, <u>accidental</u> (unintentional)
Poisoning by keratolytics, keratoplastics, and other hair treatment drugs and preparations NOS

T49.4x2- Poisoning by keratolytics, keratoplastics, and other hair treatment drugs and preparations, <u>intentional</u> self-harm

T49.4x3- Poisoning by keratolytics, keratoplastics, and other hair treatment drugs and preparations, <u>assault</u>

T49.4x4- Poisoning by keratolytics, keratoplastics, and other hair treatment drugs and preparations, <u>undetermined</u>

T49.4x5- <u>Adverse effect</u> of keratolytics, keratoplastics, and other hair treatment drugs and preparations

T49.4x6- <u>Underdosing</u> of keratolytics, keratoplastics, and other hair treatment drugs and preparations

T49.5- Poisoning by, adverse effect of and underdosing of ophthalmological drugs and preparations

T49.5 - DRUGS/CHEMS*		
Achromycin, ophthalmic preparation	Bacimycin, ophthalmic preparation	Colistin sulfate (eye preparation)
Adrenal, ophthalmic preparation	Bacitracin zinc, ophthalmic preparation	Contact lens solution
Aerosporin, ophthalmic preparation	Befunolol	Copper sulfate, cupric, medicinal, eye
Ammonium acid tartrate	Benzalkonium, ophthalmic preparation	Copper sulfate, medicinal, eye
Antibiotic, eye	Bibrocathol	Cort-Dome, ophthalmic preparation
Anticholinesterase, reversible, ophthalmological	Boracic acid, ophthalmic preparation	Cortef, ophthalmic preparation
Anti-infective, eye NEC	Boric acid, ophthalmic preparation	Corticosteroid, ophthalmic
Anti-infective, ophthalmic preparation	Chloramphenicol, ophthalmic preparation	Cortisol, ophthalmic preparation
Antiviral drug, eye	Chloromycetin, ophthalmic preparation	Cortisone, ophthalmic preparation
Argyrol, ophthalmic preparation	Chloroptic	Cortogen, ophthalmic preparation
Aristocort, ophthalmic preparation	Chymar, ophthalmic preparation	Cortone, ophthalmic preparation
Aureomycin, ophthalmic preparation	Chymotrypsin, ophthalmic preparation	Cortril, ophthalmic preparation

T49.5 - DRUGS/CHEMS* – Continued		
Cycloplegic drug	Hydrocortisone, ophthalmic preparation	Prednisolone, ophthalmic preparation
Decadron, ophthalmic preparation	Hydrocortone, ophthalmic preparation	Propylparaben (ophthalmic)
Demecarium (bromide)	Hydroxyamphetamine	Silver nitrate, ophthalmic preparation
Dendrid	Hypromellose	
Dexamethasone, ophthalmic preparation	Ilotycin, ophthalmic preparation	Silver, protein
Dipivefrine	Irrigating fluid, eye	Sodium borate, cleanser, eye
Echothiophate, echothiopate, ecothiopate	Lachesine	Steroid, ophthalmic preparation
	Levobunolol	Stoxil
Ecothiopate iodide	Lubricant, eye	Sulfacetamide, ophthalmic preparation
Edoxudine	Merthiolate, ophthalmic preparation	
Erythromycin, ophthalmic preparation	Methyl prednisolone, ophthalmic preparation	Sulfisoxazole, ophthalmic preparation
Eserine	Methylparaben (ophthalmic)	Sulfonamide, eye
Eucatropine	Metipranolol	Tear solution
External medications, ophthalmic preparation	Miotic drug	Tetracycline, ophthalmic preparation
Eye agents (anti-infective)	Mycitracin, ophthalmic preparation	Tetrahydrozoline
Eye drug NEC	Mydriatic drug	Tetryzoline
Florinef, ophthalmic preparation	Neomycin, ophthalmic preparation	Thimerosal, ophthalmic preparation
Fludrocortisone, ophthalmic preparation	Neosporin, ophthalmic preparation	Topical action drug, eye
Fluohydrocortisone, ophthalmic preparation	Orthoboric acid, ophthalmic preparation	Triamcinolone, ophthalmic preparation
Fluorometholone, ophthalmic preparation	Oxylone, ophthalmic preparation	Tyrothricin, ophthalmic preparation
Fluorphenylalanine	Phospholine	Visine
Garamycin, ophthalmic preparation	Physostigmine	Zephiran, ophthalmic preparation
Gentamicin, ophthalmic preparation	Polymyxin B, ophthalmic preparation	Zinc sulfate
	Polymyxin E sulfate (eye preparation)	Zinc sulfate, ophthalmic solution
Herplex		

T49.5x- Poisoning by, adverse effect of and underdosing of ophthalmological drugs and preparations

T49.5x1- Poisoning by ophthalmological drugs and preparations, accidental (unintentional)
Poisoning by ophthalmological drugs and preparations NOS

T49.5x2- Poisoning by ophthalmological drugs and preparations, intentional self-harm

T49.5x3- Poisoning by ophthalmological drugs and preparations, assault

T49.5x4- Poisoning by ophthalmological drugs and preparations, undetermined

T49.5x5- Adverse effect of ophthalmological drugs and preparations

T49.5x6- Underdosing of ophthalmological drugs and preparations

T49.6- Poisoning by, adverse effect of and underdosing of otorhinolaryngological drugs and preparations

T49.6 - DRUGS/CHEMS*		
Adrenal, ENT agent	Cetylpyridinium chloride, lozenges	Ear drug NEC
Aerosporin, ENT agent	Chloramphenicol, ENT agent	Ear preparations
Alkaline antiseptic solution (aromatic)		ENT preparations (anti-infectives)
Ambazone	Chloromycetin, ENT agent	External medications, ENT agent
Amylmetacresol	Chloromycetin, otic solution	
Antibiotic, ENT	Copper sulfate, cupric, medicinal, ear	Florinef, ENT agent
Antibiotic, throat		Fludrocortisone, ENT agent
Anti-infective, ENT	Copper sulfate, medicinal, ear	Fluohydrocortisone, ENT agent
Argyrol, ENT agent	Corbadrine	
Aristocort, ENT agent	Cort-Dome, ENT agent	Glycerol, borax
Bacitracin zinc, ENT agent	Cortef, ENT agent	Hydrocortisone, ENT agent
Biclotymol	Corticosteroid, ENT agent	Hydrocortone, ENT agent
Bisdequalinium (salts) (diacetate)	Cortisol, ENT agent	Levonordefrin
	Cortisone, ENT agent	Lozenges (throat)
Boracic acid, ENT agent	Cortogen, ENT agent	Methyl prednisolone, ENT agent
Boric acid, ENT agent	Cortone, ENT agent	
Ceepryn, ENT agent	Cortril, ENT agent	Mouthwash (antiseptic) (zinc chloride)
Ceepryn, lozenges	Decadron, ENT agent	
Cetylpyridinium chloride, ENT agent	Dexamethasone, ENT agent	Nasal drug NEC
	Dichlorobenzyl alcohol	Neomycin, ENT agent

T49.6 - DRUGS/CHEMS* – Continued		
Neosporin, ENT agent	Polymyxin B, ENT agent	Triamcinolone, ENT agent
Nose preparations	Prednisolone, ENT agent	Tyrothricin
Orthoboric acid, ENT agent	Steroid, ENT agent	Tyrothricin, ENT agent
Otorhinolaryngological drug NEC	Thenoic acid	Zinc chloride (mouthwash)
	Throat drug NEC	Zinc sulfate, ENT agent
	Topical action drug, ear, nose or throat	

T49.6x- Poisoning by, adverse effect of and underdosing of otorhinolaryngological drugs and preparations

T49.6x1- Poisoning by otorhinolaryngological drugs and preparations, accidental (unintentional)
Poisoning by otorhinolaryngological drugs and preparations NOS

T49.6x2- Poisoning by otorhinolaryngological drugs and preparations, intentional self-harm

T49.6x3- Poisoning by otorhinolaryngological drugs and preparations, assault

T49.6x4- Poisoning by otorhinolaryngological drugs and preparations, undetermined

T49.6x5- Adverse effect of otorhinolaryngological drugs and preparations

T49.6x6- Underdosing of otorhinolaryngological drugs and preparations

T49.7- Poisoning by, adverse effect of and underdosing of dental drugs, topically applied

T49.7 - DRUGS/CHEMS*		
Dental drug, topical application NEC	External medications, dental agent	Oil, cloves
Dentifrice	Fluoride, medicinal, dental use	Pulp, devitalizing paste
Dressing, live pulp	Fluoride, stannous	Pulp, dressing
Eucalyptus oil	Fluoristan	Stannous fluoride

T49.7x- Poisoning by, adverse effect of and underdosing of dental drugs, topically applied

T49.7x1- Poisoning by dental drugs, topically applied, accidental (unintentional)
Poisoning by dental drugs, topically applied NOS

T49.7x2- Poisoning by dental drugs, topically applied, intentional self-harm

T49.7x3- Poisoning by dental drugs, topically applied, assault

T49.7x4- Poisoning by dental drugs, topically applied, undetermined

T49.7x5- Adverse effect of dental drugs, topically applied

T49.7x6- Underdosing of dental drugs, topically applied

T49.8- Poisoning by, adverse effect of and underdosing of other topical agents
Poisoning by, adverse effect of and underdosing of spermicides

T49.8 - DRUGS/CHEMS*		
Benoquin	Dextromoramide, topical	Octoxinol (9)
Camphor, medicinal	Elase	Panthenol, topical
Cantharides, cantharidin, cantharis	Enzyme, depolymerizing	Podophyllotoxin
	External medications, specified NEC	Preparation H
Carbamide, topical	Gelfilm	Santyl
Cell stimulants and proliferants	Heet	Scarlet red
	Irrigating fluid (vaginal)	Skin agents, specified NEC
Charcoal, medicinal, topical	Lactic acid	Sodium borate, therapeutic
Chloresium	Local action drug NEC	Spanish fly
Contraceptive, vaginal	Lytta (vitatta)	Spermicide
Cosmetic preparation	Mucous membrane agents, specified NEC	Topical action drug, specified NEC
Cosmetics		Tosylchloramide sodium
Demelanizing agents	Nonoxinol	Urea, topical
Deodorant spray (feminine hygiene)	Nonylphenoxy (polyethoxy-ethanol)	Vaginal contraceptives

T49.8x- Poisoning by, adverse effect of and underdosing of other topical agents

T49.8x1- Poisoning by other topical agents, accidental (unintentional)
Poisoning by other topical agents NOS

T49.8x2- Poisoning by other topical agents, intentional self-harm

T49.8x3- Poisoning by other topical agents, assault

T49.8x4- Poisoning by other topical agents, undetermined

T49 - T49

T49.8x5- __Adverse effect__ of other topical agents

T49.8x6- __Underdosing__ of other topical agents

T49.9- Poisoning by, adverse effect of and underdosing of __unspecified topical agent__

T49.9 - DRUGS/CHEMS*	Lotions NEC	Topical action drug NEC
External medications (skin) (mucous membrane)	Mucous membrane agents (external)	Topical action drug, skin
Liniments NEC	Skin agents (external)	

T49.91x- Poisoning by unspecified topical agent, __accidental__ (unintentional)

T49.92x- Poisoning by unspecified topical agent, __intentional__ self-harm

T49.93x- Poisoning by unspecified topical agent, __assault__

T49.94x- Poisoning by unspecified topical agent, __undetermined__

T49.95x- __Adverse effect__ of unspecified topical agent

T49.96x- __Underdosing__ of unspecified topical agent

T50- Poisoning by, adverse effect of and underdosing of __diuretics and other and unspecified drugs, medicaments and biological substances__

The appropriate 7th character is to be added to each code from category T50:
A __Initial__ encounter
D __Subsequent__ encounter
S __Sequela__

T50.0- Poisoning by, adverse effect of and underdosing of mineralocorticoids and their antagonists

T50.0 - DRUGS/CHEMS*	Corticosteroid, mineral	Mineralocorticosteroid
Aldactone	Deoxycortone	Potassium canrenoate
Aldosterone	Desoxycorticosteroid	Salt-retaining
Antagonist, aldosterone	Desoxycortone	mineralocorticoid
Canrenoic acid	Fludrocortisone	Spironolactone
Canrenone	Fluorhydrocortisone	

T50.0x- Poisoning by, adverse effect of and underdosing of __mineralocorticoids and their antagonists__

T50.0x1- Poisoning by mineralocorticoids and their antagonists, __accidental__ (unintentional)
    Poisoning by mineralocorticoids and their antagonists NOS

T50.0x2- Poisoning by mineralocorticoids and their antagonists, __intentional__ self-harm

T50.0x3- Poisoning by mineralocorticoids and their antagonists, __assault__

T50.0x4- Poisoning by mineralocorticoids and their antagonists, __undetermined__

T50.0x5- __Adverse effect__ of mineralocorticoids and their antagonists

T50.0x6- __Underdosing__ of mineralocorticoids and their antagonists

T50.1- Poisoning by, adverse effect of and underdosing of loop [high-ceiling] diuretics

T50.1 - DRUGS/CHEMS*	Ethacrynic acid	Piretanide
Bumetanide	Etozolin	Sodium ethacrynate
Diuretic, loop (high-ceiling)	Frusemide	Ticrynafen
Edecrin	Furosemide	Tienilic acid
Etacrynate sodium	Lasix	
Etacrynic acid	Lyovac Sodium Edecrin	

T50.1x- Poisoning by, adverse effect of and underdosing of __loop [high-ceiling] diuretics__

T50.1x1- Poisoning by loop [high-ceiling] diuretics, __accidental__ (unintentional)
    Poisoning by loop [high-ceiling] diuretics NOS

T50.1x2- Poisoning by loop [high-ceiling] diuretics, __intentional__ self-harm

T50.1x3- Poisoning by loop [high-ceiling] diuretics, __assault__

T50.1x4- Poisoning by loop [high-ceiling] diuretics, __undetermined__

T50.1x5- __Adverse effect__ of loop [high-ceiling] diuretics

T50.1x6- __Underdosing__ of loop [high-ceiling] diuretics

T50.2- Poisoning by, adverse effect of and underdosing of carbonic-anhydrase inhibitors, benzothiadiazides and other diuretics
    Poisoning by, adverse effect of and underdosing of acetazolamide

T50.2 - DRUGS/CHEMS*	Diucardin	Mercurophylline
Acetazolamide	Diupres	Mercury, diuretic NEC
Altizide	Diuretic NEC	Mersalyl
Amiloride	Diuretic, benzothiadiazine	Methazolamide
Aminometradine	Diuretic, carbonic acid	Methyclothiazide
Amisometradine	anhydrase inhibitors	Meticrane
Anhydron	Diuretic, furfuryl NEC	Metolazone
Bendrofluazide	Diuretic, mercurial NEC	Osmotic diuretics
Bendroflumethiazide	Diuretic, osmotic	Penflutizide
Benzothiadiazides	Diuretic, purine NEC	Polythiazide
Benzthiazide	Diuretic, saluretic NEC	Purine diuretics
Benzylhydrochlorthiazide	Diuretic, sulfonamide	Quinethazone
Butizide	Diuretic, thiazide NEC	Regroton
Carbonic acid gas,	Diuretic, xanthine	Renese
anhydrase inhibitor NEC	Diurgin	Salicylate, theobromine
Cardrase	Diuril	calcium
Chlorazanil	Epitizide	Saluretic NEC
Chlormerodrin	Equisetum, diuretic	Saluron
Chlorothiazide	Ethamide	Sodium mersalate
Chlortalidone	Ethiazide	Teclothiazide
Chlorthalidone	Ethoxzolamide	Tetrachlormethiazide
Clofenamide	Fenquizone	Thiazides (diuretics)
Clopamide	Flumethiazide	Thiomercaptomerin
Clorexolone	Hydrochlorothiazide	Thiomerin
Cyclopenthiazide	Hydroflumethiazide	Tiamizide
Cyclothiazide	Hydromox	Triamterene
Diamox	Inhibitor, carbonic	Trichlormethiazide
Dichlorphenamide	anhydrase	Tripamide
Diclofenamide	Mefruside	Trometamol
Dihydroxypropyl	Meralluride	Tromethamine
theophylline	Merbaphen	Xanthine diuretics
Diphylline	Mercaptomerin	Xipamide
Diprophylline	Mercumatilin	Zaroxolyn
Disulfamide	Mercuramide	

T50.2x- Poisoning by, adverse effect of and underdosing of __carbonic-anhydrase inhibitors, benzothiadiazides and other diuretics__

T50.2x1- Poisoning by carbonic-anhydrase inhibitors, benzothiadiazides and other diuretics, __accidental__ (unintentional)
    Poisoning by carbonic-anhydrase inhibitors, benzothiadiazides and other diuretics NOS

T50.2x2- Poisoning by carbonic-anhydrase inhibitors, benzothiadiazides and other diuretics, __intentional__ self-harm

T50.2x3- Poisoning by carbonic-anhydrase inhibitors, benzothiadiazides and other diuretics, __assault__

T50.2x4- Poisoning by carbonic-anhydrase inhibitors, benzothiadiazides and other diuretics, __undetermined__

T50.2x5- __Adverse effect__ of carbonic-anhydrase inhibitors, benzothiadiazides and other diuretics

T50.2x6- __Underdosing__ of carbonic-anhydrase inhibitors, benzothiadiazides and other diuretics

T50.3- Poisoning by, adverse effect of and underdosing of electrolytic, caloric and water-balance agents
    Poisoning by, adverse effect of and underdosing of oral rehydration salts

T50.3 - DRUGS/CHEMS*	Caloric agent	Hartmann's solution
Acetic acid irrigating	Carbacrylamine (resin)	Invert sugar
solution	Cation exchange resin	Ion exchange resin, cation
Amino acids	Dextrose	Lactated potassic saline
Aminoacetic acid	Dialysis solution	Levulose
(derivatives)	(intraperitoneal)	Magnesium silicofluoride
Antikaluretic	Electrolyte balance drug	Mineral salt NEC
Calcium	Electrolytes NEC	Oral rehydration salts
Calcium glubionate	Electrolytic agent NEC	Peritoneal dialysis solution
Calcium gluconate	Fructose	Polyaminostyrene resins
Calcium	Galactose	Potassic saline injection
gluconogalactogluc-	Glucose	(lactated)
onate	Glucose with sodium	Potassium (salts) NEC
Calcium lactate	chloride	Potassium chloride
Calcium phosphate	Glycerol, intravenous	Potassium-removing resin
Calcium salts	Glycine	Potassium-retaining drug

T
4
9
-
T
5
0

T50.3 - DRUGS/CHEMS* – Continued		
Rehydration salts (oral)	Sodium chloride with glucose	Sodium removing resins
Replacement solution	Sodium cyclamate	Sodium salt NEC
Ringer (lactate) solution	Sodium, free salt	Sodium-removing resin
Sodium acid phosphate	Sodium hydrogen carbonate	Sucrose
Sodium biphosphate	Sodium polystyrene sulfonate	Travert
Sodium chloride		Water balance drug
		Water, distilled
		Water, purified

T50.3x- Poisoning by, adverse effect of and underdosing of <u>electrolytic, caloric and water-balance agents</u>

T50.3x1- Poisoning by electrolytic, caloric and water-balance agents, <u>accidental</u> (unintentional)
　Poisoning by electrolytic, caloric and water-balance agents NOS

T50.3x2- Poisoning by electrolytic, caloric and water-balance agents, <u>intentional</u> self-harm

T50.3x3- Poisoning by electrolytic, caloric and water-balance agents, <u>assault</u>

T50.3x4- Poisoning by electrolytic, caloric and water-balance agents, <u>undetermined</u>

T50.3x5- <u>Adverse effect</u> of electrolytic, caloric and water-balance agents

T50.3x6- <u>Underdosing</u> of electrolytic, caloric and water-balance agents

T50.4- Poisoning by, adverse effect of and underdosing of drugs affecting uric acid metabolism

T50.4 - DRUGS/CHEMS*		
Allopurinol	Etebenecid	Sulfinpyrazone
Atophan	Ethebenecid	Sulphinpyrazone
Benemid	Neocinchophen	Tisopurine
Benzbromarone	Oxipurinol	Urate oxidase
Cinchophen	Phenoquin	Uric acid metabolism drug NEC
Colchicine	Probenecid	
	Spindle inactivator	Uricosuric agent

T50.4x- Poisoning by, adverse effect of and underdosing of <u>drugs affecting uric acid metabolism</u>

T50.4x1- Poisoning by drugs affecting uric acid metabolism, <u>accidental</u> (unintentional)
　Poisoning by drugs affecting uric acid metabolism NOS

T50.4x2- Poisoning by drugs affecting uric acid metabolism, <u>intentional</u> self-harm

T50.4x3- Poisoning by drugs affecting uric acid metabolism, <u>assault</u>

T50.4x4- Poisoning by drugs affecting uric acid metabolism, <u>undetermined</u>

T50.4x5- <u>Adverse effect</u> of drugs affecting uric acid metabolism

T50.4x6- <u>Underdosing</u> of drugs affecting uric acid metabolism

T50.5- Poisoning by, adverse effect of and underdosing of appetite depressants

T50.5 - DRUGS/CHEMS*		
Amfepramone	Chlorphentermine	Fenproporex
Aminorex	Clobenzorex	Levopropylhexedrine
Anorexiant (central)	Cloforex	Mazindol
Anorexic agents	Clortermine	Mefenorex
Appetite depressants, central	Depressant, appetite	Norpseudoephedrine
Benzamphetamine	Depressant, appetite, central	Oxazimedrine
Benzfetamine	Dexfenfluramine	Phenbutrazate
Benzphetamine	Diethyl propion	Phendimetrazine
Bulk filler	Diethylpropion	Phenmetrazine
Cathine	Fenbutrazate	Phentermine
	Fenfluramine	

T50.5x- Poisoning by, adverse effect of and underdosing of <u>appetite depressants</u>

T50.5x1- Poisoning by appetite depressants, <u>accidental</u> (unintentional)
　Poisoning by appetite depressants NOS

T50.5x2- Poisoning by appetite depressants, <u>intentional</u> self-harm

T50.5x3- Poisoning by appetite depressants, <u>assault</u>

T50.5x4- Poisoning by appetite depressants, <u>undetermined</u>

T50.5x5- <u>Adverse effect</u> of appetite depressants

T50.5x6- <u>Underdosing</u> of appetite depressants

T50.6- Poisoning by, adverse effect of and underdosing of antidotes and chelating agents
　Poisoning by, adverse effect of and underdosing of alcohol deterrents

T50.6 - DRUGS/CHEMS*		
Alcohol, deterrent NEC	Ethylenedinitrilotetra-acetate	Pralidoxime, chloride
Antabuse	Fytic acid, nonasodium	Protopam
Antidote NEC	Glutathione	Prussian blue, therapeutic
Calcium carbimide	Methylene blue	Pyridine, aldoxime methiodide
Chelating agent NEC	Methylthionine chloride	Pyridine, aldoxime methyl chloride
Cholinesterase reactivator	Methylthioninium chloride	Sodium nitrite
Cysteamine	Nitrefazole	Sodium phytate
Deterrent, alcohol	Obidoxime chloride	Sodium thiosulfate
Detoxifying agent	PAM (pralidoxime)	Sodium versenate
Disodium edetate	Penicillamine	Tetraethylthiuram disulfide
Disulfiram	Potassium ferric hexacyanoferrate (medicinal)	Trisodium hydrogen edetate
EDTA		Versenate
Ethylenediaminetetra-acetic acid	Pralidoxime (iodide)	

T50.6x- Poisoning by, adverse effect of and underdosing of <u>antidotes and chelating agents</u>

T50.6x1- Poisoning by antidotes and chelating agents, <u>accidental</u> (unintentional)
　Poisoning by antidotes and chelating agents NOS

T50.6x2- Poisoning by antidotes and chelating agents, <u>intentional</u> self-harm

T50.6x3- Poisoning by antidotes and chelating agents, <u>assault</u>

T50.6x4- Poisoning by antidotes and chelating agents, <u>undetermined</u>

T50.6x5- <u>Adverse effect</u> of antidotes and chelating agents

T50.6x6- <u>Underdosing</u> of antidotes and chelating agents

T50.7- Poisoning by, adverse effect of and underdosing of analeptics and opioid receptor antagonists

T50.7 - DRUGS/CHEMS*		
Almitrine	Crotethamide with cropropamide	Nikethamide
Amiphenazole	Cyclazocine	Opiate, antagonists
Analeptic NEC	Dimefline	Pemoline
Antagonist, narcotic analgesic	Dimorpholamine	Pentetrazole
Antagonist, opiate	Doxapram	Pentylenetetrazole
Bemegride	Etamivan	Picrotoxin
Bicuculline	Ethamivan	Pimeclone
Central nervous system stimulants, analeptics	Leptazol	Prethcamide
	Levallorphan	Stimulant, central nervous system, analeptics
Central nervous system stimulants, opiate antagonists	Lobeline	
	Morphine, antagonist	Stimulant, central nervous system, opiate antagonist
	Nalorphine	
Cropropamide with crotethamide	Naloxone	
	Naltrexone	
	Narcotic antagonist	

T50.7x- Poisoning by, adverse effect of and underdosing of <u>analeptics and opioid receptor antagonists</u>

T50.7x1- Poisoning by analeptics and opioid receptor antagonists, <u>accidental</u> (unintentional)
　Poisoning by analeptics and opioid receptor antagonists NOS

T50.7x2- Poisoning by analeptics and opioid receptor antagonists, <u>intentional</u> self-harm

T50.7x3- Poisoning by analeptics and opioid receptor antagonists, <u>assault</u>

T50.7x4- Poisoning by analeptics and opioid receptor antagonists, <u>undetermined</u>

T50.7x5- <u>Adverse effect</u> of analeptics and opioid receptor antagonists

T50.7x6- <u>Underdosing</u> of analeptics and opioid receptor antagonists

T50 - T50

T50.8- Poisoning by, adverse effect of and underdosing of diagnostic agents

T50.8 - DRUGS/CHEMS*		
Acetrizoate (sodium)	Iodinated human serum albumin (131I)	Pentagastrin
Acetrizoic acid	Iodine 125 — see also	Peptavlon
Adipiodone	Radiation sickness, and	Phenobutiodil
Alcohol, diagnostic (gastric function)	Exposure to radioactivce isotopes	Phenol, red
Ametazole	Iodine 131 — see also	Phenolsulfonphthalein
Amidotrizoate	Radiation sickness, and	Propyl iodone
Aminohippuric acid	Exposure to radioactivce isotopes	Propyliodone
Angio-Conray	Iodine, diagnostic	PSP (phenolsulfon-phthalein)
Azuresin	Iodipamide	Radioactive drug NEC
Barium, diagnostic agent	Iodized (poppy seed) oil	Radio-opaque (drugs) (materials)
Barium, sulfate (medicinal)	Iodocholesterol (131I)	Renografin
Bentiromide	Iodohippuric acid	Rose bengal sodium (131I)
Betazole	Iodopanoic acid	Rubidium chloride Rb82
Biligrafin	Iodophthalein (sodium)	Secretin
Bilopaque	Iodopyracet	Selenomethionine (75Se)
Bromsulfophthalein	Iodoxamic acid	Sincalide
Bunamiodyl	Iofendylate	Skin test antigen
Calcium ipodate	Ioglycamic acid	Sodium acetrizoate
Cardiografin	Iohexol	Sodium amidotrizoate
Cardio-green	Iopamidol	Sodium cacodylate (nonmedicinal) NEC
Ceruletide	Iopanoic acid	Sodium diatrizoate
Cholebrine	Iophenoic acid	Sodium indigotin disulfonate
Cholecystokinin	Iopodate, sodium	Sodium iodide I-131
Cholografin	Iopodic acid	Sodium iodohippurate (131I)
Chromium sesquioxide	Iopromide	Sodium iopodate
Coccidioidin	Iopydol	Sodium iothalamate
Congo red	Iotalamic acid	Sodium metrizoate
Contrast medium, radiography	Iothalamate	Sodium para-aminohippurate
Diagnostic agent NEC	Iotrol	Sodium pertechnetate Tc99m
Diatrizoate	Iotrolan	Sodium tyropanoate
Diodone	Iotroxate	Sulfan blue (diagnostic dye)
Dye, diagnostic agents	Iotroxic acid	Sulfobromophthalein (sodium)
Ethiodized oil (131 I)	Ioversol	Sulfobromphthalein
Evans blue	Ioxaglate	Sulfonphthal, sulfonphthol
Fludeoxyglucose (18F)	Ioxaglic acid	Sulkowitch's reagent
Fluorescein	Ioxitalamic acid	Sulphan blue
Frei antigen	Ipodate, calcium	Telepaque
Gadopentetic acid	Iprofenin	Thorium dioxide suspension
Gastrografin	Lidofenin	Toxin, diphtheria (Schick Test)
Histalog	Lygranum (skin test)	Tuberculin, purified protein derivative (PPD)
Histamine (phosphate)	Lymphogranuloma venereum antigen	Tyropanoate
Histoplasmin	Meglumine diatrizoate	Urokon
Hypaque	Meglumine iodipamide	Xenon (127Xe) (133Xe)
Indigo carmine	Meglumine iotroxate	
Indocyanine green	Methiodal sodium	
Inulin	Metrizamide	
Iobenzamic acid	Metrizoic acid	
Iocarmic acid	Metyrapone	
Iocetamic acid	Mumps skin test antigen	
Iodamide	Oragrafin	
Iodinated contrast medium	Penicilloyl polylysine	

T50.8x- Poisoning by, adverse effect of and underdosing of diagnostic agents

T50.8x1- Poisoning by diagnostic agents, accidental (unintentional)
   Poisoning by diagnostic agents NOS

T50.8x2- Poisoning by diagnostic agents, intentional self-harm

T50.8x3- Poisoning by diagnostic agents, assault

T50.8x4- Poisoning by diagnostic agents, undetermined

T50.8x5- Adverse effect of diagnostic agents

T50.8x6- Underdosing of diagnostic agents

T50.A- Poisoning by, adverse effect of and underdosing of bacterial vaccines

T50.A1- Poisoning by, adverse effect of and underdosing of pertussis vaccine, including combinations with a pertussis component

T50.A1 - DRUGS/CHEMS*		
Diphtheria, toxoid, with tetanus toxoid, with pertussis component	Tetanus toxoid or vaccine, toxoid, with diphtheria toxoid, with pertussis	Vaccine, pertussis, with diphtheria
Diphtheria, vaccine, combination, including pertussis	Triple vaccine, DPT	Vaccine, pertussis, with diphtheria, and tetanus
Pertussis immune serum vaccine (with diphtheria toxoid) (with tetanus toxoid)	Triple vaccine, including pertussis	Vaccine, pertussis, with other component
	Vaccine, bacterial with, pertussis component	
	Vaccine, diphtheria, with pertussis component	
	Vaccine, diphtheria, with tetanus, and pertussis	
	Vaccine, pertussis	

T50.A11- Poisoning by pertussis vaccine, including combinations with a pertussis component, accidental (unintentional)

T50.A12- Poisoning by pertussis vaccine, including combinations with a pertussis component, intentional self-harm

T50.A13- Poisoning by pertussis vaccine, including combinations with a pertussis component, assault

T50.A14- Poisoning by pertussis vaccine, including combinations with a pertussis component, undetermined

T50.A15- Adverse effect of pertussis vaccine, including combinations with a pertussis component

T50.A16- Underdosing of pertussis vaccine, including combinations with a pertussis component

T50.A2- Poisoning by, adverse effect of and underdosing of mixed bacterial vaccines without a pertussis component

T50.A2 - DRUGS/CHEMS*		
Diphtheria, toxoid, with tetanus toxoid	Toxoid, combined	Vaccine, diphtheria, with tetanus
Diphtheria, vaccine, combination, without pertussis	Vaccine, bacterial with, other bacterial component	Vaccine, rickettsial, with bacterial component
Tetanus toxoid or vaccine, toxoid with diphtheria toxoid	Vaccine, bacterial with, viral-rickettsial component	
	Vaccine, bacterial, mixed NEC	

T50.A21- Poisoning by mixed bacterial vaccines without a pertussis component, accidental (unintentional)

T50.A22- Poisoning by mixed bacterial vaccines without a pertussis component, intentional self-harm

T50.A23- Poisoning by mixed bacterial vaccines without a pertussis component, assault

T50.A24- Poisoning by mixed bacterial vaccines without a pertussis component, undetermined

T50.A25- Adverse effect of mixed bacterial vaccines without a pertussis component

T50.A26- Underdosing of mixed bacterial vaccines without a pertussis component

T50.A9- Poisoning by, adverse effect of and underdosing of other bacterial vaccines

T50.A9 - DRUGS/CHEMS*		
BCG (vaccine)	Tetanus toxoid or vaccine	Vaccine, meningococcal
Cholera vaccine	Tetanus toxoid or vaccine, toxoid	Vaccine, paratyphoid
Diphtheria, toxoid	Toxoid, diphtheria	Vaccine, plague
Diphtheria, vaccine	Toxoid, tetanus	Vaccine, rickettsial NEC
Meningococcal vaccine	Typhoid-paratyphoid vaccine	Vaccine, Rocky Mountain spotted fever
Menningovax (-AC) (-C)	Typhus vaccine	Vaccine, TAB
Paratyphoid vaccine	Vaccine, bacterial NEC	Vaccine, tetanus
Plague vaccine	Vaccine, BCG	Vaccine, typhoid
Rickettsial vaccine NEC	Vaccine, cholera	Vaccine, typhus
Rocky Mountain spotted fever vaccine	Vaccine, diphtheria	

T50.A91- Poisoning by other bacterial vaccines, accidental (unintentional)

T50.A92- Poisoning by other bacterial vaccines, intentional self-harm

T50 / T5A

T50.A93- Poisoning by other bacterial vaccines, <u>assault</u>

T50.A94- Poisoning by other bacterial vaccines, <u>undetermined</u>

T50.A95- <u>Adverse effect</u> of other bacterial vaccines

T50.A96- <u>Underdosing</u> of other bacterial vaccines

T50.B- Poisoning by, adverse effect of and underdosing of viral vaccines

T50.B1- Poisoning by, adverse effect of and underdosing of <u>smallpox vaccines</u>

T50.B1 - DRUGS/CHEMS*	Vaccine, smallpox
Smallpox vaccine	

T50.B11- Poisoning by smallpox vaccines, <u>accidental</u> (unintentional)

T50.B12- Poisoning by smallpox vaccines, <u>intentional</u> self-harm

T50.B13- Poisoning by smallpox vaccines, <u>assault</u>

T50.B14- Poisoning by smallpox vaccines, <u>undetermined</u>

T50.B15- <u>Adverse effect</u> of smallpox vaccines

T50.B16- <u>Underdosing</u> of smallpox vaccines

T50.B9- Poisoning by, adverse effect of and underdosing of <u>other viral vaccines</u>

T50.B9 - DRUGS/CHEMS*	Rabies vaccine	Vaccine, poliovirus
Diplovax	Rubella vaccine	Vaccine, rabies
Hepatitis B vaccine	Rubeola vaccine	Vaccine, respiratory
Influenza vaccine	Synagis	syncytial virus
Measles virus vaccine	Triple vaccine, MMR	Vaccine, rubella
(attenuated)	Vaccine, influenza	Vaccine, sabin oral
Meruvax	Vaccine, measles	Vaccine, viral NEC
Mumps vaccine	Vaccine, measles, with	Vaccine, yellow fever
Mumpsvax	mumps and rubella	Viral vaccine NEC
Orimune	Vaccine, mumps	Yellow fever vaccine
Poliomyelitis vaccine	Vaccine, poliomyelitis	

T50.B91- Poisoning by other viral vaccines, <u>accidental</u> (unintentional)

T50.B92- Poisoning by other viral vaccines, <u>intentional</u> self-harm

T50.B93- Poisoning by other viral vaccines, <u>assault</u>

T50.B94- Poisoning by other viral vaccines, <u>undetermined</u>

T50.B95- <u>Adverse effect</u> of other viral vaccines

T50.B96- <u>Underdosing</u> of other viral vaccines

T50.Z- Poisoning by, adverse effect of and underdosing of other vaccines and biological substances

T50.Z1- Poisoning by, adverse effect of and underdosing of <u>immunoglobulin</u>

T50.Z1 - DRUGS/CHEMS*	Gamma globulin	Rabies immune globulin
AHLG	Gamulin	(human)
Anti-D immunoglobulin	Globulin, antilymphocytic	Rh (D) immune globulin
(human)	Globulin, antirhesus	(human)
Antidiphtheria serum	Globulin, antivenin	RhoGAM
Anti-human lymphocytic	Globulin, antiviral	Serum, antibotulinus
globulin	Hepatitis B immune	Serum, anticytotoxic
Antirabies hyperimmune	globulin	Serum, antidiphtheria
serum	Homo-tet	Serum, antimeningococcus
Antiscorpion sera	Horse anti-human	Serum, anti-Rh
Antitetanus	lymphocytic serum	Serum, anti-snake-bite
immunoglobulin	Human immune serum	Serum, antitetanic
Antitoxin	Hypertussis	Serum, antitoxic
Antitoxin, diphtheria	Immu-G	Serum, convalescent
Antitoxin, gas gangrene	Immuglobin	Serum, immune (human)
Antitoxin, tetanus	Immune globulin	Serum, protective NEC
Antivenin, antivenom	Immune serum globulin	Spider, antivenin
(sera)	Immunoglobin human	Tetanus toxoid or vaccine,
Antivenin, crotaline	(intravenous) (normal)	antitoxin
Antivenin, spider bite	Immunoglobin human,	Tetanus toxoid or vaccine,
Black widow spider	unmodified	immune globulin
antivenin	Immu-tetanus	(human)
Botulinus anti-toxin (type	Mumps immune globulin	Vaccinia immune globulin
A, B)	(human)	
Diphtheria, antitoxin	Pertussis immune serum	
Gamimune	(human)	

T50.Z11- Poisoning by immunoglobulin, <u>accidental</u> (unintentional)

T50.Z12- Poisoning by immunoglobulin, <u>intentional</u> self-harm

T50.Z13- Poisoning by immunoglobulin, <u>assault</u>

T50.Z14- Poisoning by immunoglobulin, <u>undetermined</u>

T50.Z15- <u>Adverse effect</u> of immunoglobulin

T50.Z16- <u>Underdosing</u> of immunoglobulin

T50.Z9- Poisoning by, adverse effect of and underdosing of <u>other vaccines and biological substances</u>

T50.Z9 - DRUGS/CHEMS*	Pegademase, bovine
Glandular extract	Vaccine NEC
(medicinal) NEC	Vaccine, antineoplastic

T50.Z91- Poisoning by other vaccines and biological substances, <u>accidental</u> (unintentional)

T50.Z92- Poisoning by other vaccines and biological substances, <u>intentional</u> self-harm

T50.Z93- Poisoning by other vaccines and biological substances, <u>assault</u>

T50.Z94- Poisoning by other vaccines and biological substances, <u>undetermined</u>

T50.Z95- <u>Adverse effect</u> of other vaccines and biological substances

T50.Z96- <u>Underdosing</u> of other vaccines and biological substances

T50.9- Poisoning by, adverse effect of and underdosing of other and unspecified drugs, medicaments and biological substances

T50.90- Poisoning by, adverse effect of and underdosing of <u>unspecified drugs, medicaments and biological substances</u>

T50.90 - DRUGS/CHEMS*	Lactose (as excipient)	Salt-replacing drug
Acidifying agent NEC	Lipotropic drug NEC	Sodium-free salt
Adjunct, pharmaceutical	Medicament NEC	Soothing syrup
Alkalinizing agents	Nutritional supplement	Spray, medicinal NEC
(medicinal)	Pharmaceutical, adjunct	Starch
Alkalizing agent NEC	NEC	Stone-dissolving drug
Biological substance NEC	Pharmaceutical, excipient	Sweetener
Dietetic drug NEC	NEC	Tablets — see also specified
Drug NEC	Pharmaceutical, sweetener	substance
Dye, pharmaceutical NEC	Pharmaceutical, viscous	Tonic NEC
Elemental diet	agent	Viscous agent
Excipients, pharmaceutical	Preservative, medicinal	
Headache cures, drugs,	Saccharin	
powders NEC	Salt substitute	

T50.901- Poisoning by unspecified drugs, medicaments and biological substances, <u>accidental</u> (unintentional)

T50.902- Poisoning by unspecified drugs, medicaments and biological substances, <u>intentional</u> self-harm

T50.903- Poisoning by unspecified drugs, medicaments and biological substances, <u>assault</u>

T50.904- Poisoning by unspecified drugs, medicaments and biological substances, <u>undetermined</u>

T50.905- <u>Adverse effect</u> of unspecified drugs, medicaments and biological substances

T50.906- <u>Underdosing</u> of unspecified drugs, medicaments and biological substances

T5A-T50

T50.99- Poisoning by, adverse effect of and underdosing of <u>other drugs, medicaments and biological substances</u>

<u>T50.99 - DRUGS/CHEMS*</u>		
Acetohydroxamic acid	Diacetyl monoxime	Methylethyl cellulose
Acitretin	Drug, specified NEC	Monooctanoin
Ammonium chloride	Elcatonin	Octanoin
Arginine	Epomediol	Orazamide
Arginine glutamate	Etidronate	Ornithine aspartate
Baking soda	Etidronic acid (disodium	Oxalic acid, ammonium salt
Bergapten	salt)	Palm kernel oil
BHA	Etretinate	Parathormone
Borate(s) buffer	Fat suspension, intravenous	Parathyroid extract
Bromophenol blue reagent	Fluoride, medicinal NEC	Phenaphthazine reagent
Butylated hydroxy-anisole	Gallium citrate	Potassium citrate
Calcitonin	Gelsemine	Protein hydrolysate
Calcium chloride	Gluconic acid	Psoralens (medicinal)
Calcium chloride,	Glycerophosphate	Serotonin
anhydrous	Guaiac reagent	Silibinin
Calculus-dissolving drug	Hormone, parathyroid	Silymarin
Canthaxanthin	(derivatives)	Sodium citrate
Cetomacrogol	Inositol	Sodium iodide
Chlorophyll	Intravenous, amino acids	Sodium magnesium citrate
Choline chloride	Intravenous, fat suspension	Sodium propyl
Choline dihydrogen citrate	Iodine 125, therapeutic	hydroxybenzoate
Cianidanol	Isotretinoin	Teriparatide (acetate)
Clodronic acid	Levocarnitine	Thioctamide
Cochineal, medicinal	Levoglutamide	Thioctic acid
products	Macrogol	Tidiacic
Coenzyme A	Manganese, medicinal	Tiopronin
Cogalactoiso-merase	Methionine	Tragacanth
Collagen	Methoxsalen	Ursodeoxycholic acid
Colorant – see also Dye	5-Methoxypsoralen (5-	Ursodiol
Cyclamate	MOP)	Vienna red, pharmaceutical
Deanol (aceglumate)	8-Methoxypsoralen (8-	dye
	MOP)	

T50.991- Poisoning by other drugs, medicaments and biological substances, <u>accidental</u> (unintentional)

T50.992- Poisoning by other drugs, medicaments and biological substances, <u>intentional</u> self-harm

T50.993- Poisoning by other drugs, medicaments and biological substances, <u>assault</u>

T50.994- Poisoning by other drugs, medicaments and biological substances, <u>undetermined</u>

T50.995- <u>Adverse effect</u> of other drugs, medicaments and biological substances

T50.996- <u>Underdosing</u> of other drugs, medicaments and biological substances

Toxic effects of substances chiefly nonmedicinal as to source (T51-T65)

Note: When no intent is indicated code to accidental. Undetermined intent is only for use when there is specific documentation in the record that the intent of the toxic effect cannot be determined.

Use additional code(s):
For all associated manifestations of toxic effect, such as: respiratory conditions due to external agents (J60-J70)
Personal history of foreign body fully removed (Z87.821)
To identify any retained foreign body, if applicable (Z18.-)

Excludes 1: contact with and (suspected) exposure to toxic substances (Z77.-)

T51-   Toxic effect of <u>alcohol</u>

> **The appropriate 7th character is to be added to each code from category T51:**
> **A   <u>Initial</u> encounter**
> **D   <u>Subsequent</u> encounter**
> **S   <u>Sequela</u>**

T51.0-   Toxic effect of ethanol
  Toxic effect of ethyl alcohol
  Excludes ❷: acute alcohol intoxication or "hangover" effects (F10.129, F10.229, F10.929)
      drunkenness (F10.129, F10.229, F10.929)
      pathological alcohol intoxication (F10.129, F10.229, F10.929)

<u>T51.0 - DRUGS/CHEMS*</u>	Alcohol, industrial	Ethyl alcohol, beverage
Absinthe (beverage)	Alcohol, preparation for	Grain alcohol
Alcohol, absolute	consumption	Industrial alcohol
(beverage)	Alcohol, surgical	Neutral spirits
Alcohol, beverage	Central nervous system	Neutral spirits, beverage
Alcohol, dehydrated	depressants, ethanol	Spirit(s) (neutral) NEC
(beverage)	Denatured alcohol	Spirit(s), beverage
Alcohol, denatured	Ethanol	Spirit(s), industrial
Alcohol, ethyl (beverage)	Ethanol, beverage	Spirit(s), surgical
Alcohol, grain (beverage)	Ethyl alcohol	

T51.0x- Toxic effect of <u>ethanol</u>

T51.0x1- Toxic effect of ethanol, <u>accidental</u> (unintentional)
      Toxic effect of ethanol NOS

T51.0x2- Toxic effect of ethanol, <u>intentional</u> self-harm

T51.0x3- Toxic effect of ethanol, <u>assault</u>

T51.0x4- Toxic effect of ethanol, <u>undetermined</u>

T51.1-   Toxic effect of methanol
  Toxic effect of methyl alcohol

<u>T51.1 - DRUGS/CHEMS*</u>	Antifreeze, alcohol	Methyl carbinol
Alcohol, antifreeze	Canned heat	Methylated spirit
Alcohol, methyl	Carbinol	Radiator alcohol
Alcohol, radiator	Methanol (vapor)	Wood alcohol or spirit
Alcohol, wood	Methyl alcohol	Zerone

T51.1x- Toxic effect of <u>methanol</u>

T51.1x1- Toxic effect of methanol, <u>accidental</u> (unintentional)
      Toxic effect of methanol NOS

T51.1x2- Toxic effect of methanol, <u>intentional</u> self-harm

T51.1x3- Toxic effect of methanol, <u>assault</u>

T51.1x4- Toxic effect of methanol, <u>undetermined</u>

T51.2-   Toxic effect of 2-Propanol
  Toxic effect of isopropyl alcohol

<u>T51.2 - DRUGS/CHEMS*</u>	Alcohol, rubbing	2-Propanol
2-propanol	Dimethyl carbinol	Rubbing alcohol
Alcohol, isopropyl	Isopropanol	
Alcohol, propyl, secondary	Isopropyl alcohol	

T51.2x- Toxic effect of <u>2-Propanol</u>

T51.2x1- Toxic effect of 2-Propanol, <u>accidental</u> (unintentional)
      Toxic effect of 2-Propanol NOS

T51.2x2- Toxic effect of 2-Propanol, <u>intentional</u> self-harm

T51.2x3- Toxic effect of 2-Propanol, <u>assault</u>

T51.2x4- Toxic effect of 2-Propanol, <u>undetermined</u>

T50 - T51

T51.3- Toxic effect of fusel oil
 Toxic effect of amyl alcohol
 Toxic effect of butyl [1-butanol] alcohol
 Toxic effect of propyl [1-propanol] alcohol

T51.3 - DRUGS/CHEMS*	Butanol	Methyl butanol
1-propanol	Butyl alcohol	Methyl propylcarbinol
Alcohol, amyl	Butyl carbinol	Pentanol
Alcohol, butyl	Diethyl carbinol	1-Propanol
Alcohol, propyl	Ethyl carbinol	Propyl alcohol
Amyl alcohol	Fusel oil (any) (amyl)	Propyl carbinol
Amylene hydrate	(butyl) (propyl), vapor	Trimethylcarbinol

T51.3x- Toxic effect of fusel oil

T51.3x1- Toxic effect of fusel oil, accidental (unintentional)
 Toxic effect of fusel oil NOS

T51.3x2- Toxic effect of fusel oil, intentional self-harm

T51.3x3- Toxic effect of fusel oil, assault

T51.3x4- Toxic effect of fusel oil, undetermined

T51.8- Toxic effect of other alcohols

T51.8 - DRUGS/CHEMS*	Antifreeze, ethylene glycol	Hexahydrocresol(s)
Alcohol, allyl	Bay rum	Hexahydrophenol
Alcohol, specified type NEC	Cyclohexanol	Hexalen
Allyl alcohol	Ethyl methylcarbinol	Methyl cyclohexanol

T51.8x- Toxic effect of other alcohols

T51.8x1- Toxic effect of other alcohols, accidental (unintentional)
 Toxic effect of other alcohols NOS

T51.8x2- Toxic effect of other alcohols, intentional self-harm

T51.8x3- Toxic effect of other alcohols, assault

T51.8x4- Toxic effect of other alcohols, undetermined

T51.9- Toxic effect of unspecified alcohol

T51.9 - DRUGS/CHEMS*
Alcohol

T51.91x- Toxic effect of unspecified alcohol, accidental (unintentional)

T51.92x- Toxic effect of unspecified alcohol, intentional self-harm

T51.93x- Toxic effect of unspecified alcohol, assault

T51.94x- Toxic effect of unspecified alcohol, undetermined

T52- Toxic effect of organic solvents
 Excludes 1: halogen derivatives of aliphatic and aromatic hydrocarbons
     (T53.-)

The appropriate 7th character is to be added to each code from category T52:
 A Initial encounter
 D Subsequent encounter
 S Sequela

T52.0- Toxic effects of petroleum products
 Toxic effects of gasoline [petrol]
 Toxic effects of kerosene [paraffin oil]
 Toxic effects of paraffin wax
 Toxic effects of ether petroleum
 Toxic effects of naphtha petroleum
 Toxic effects of spirit petroleum

T52.0 - DRUGS/CHEMS*	Kerosene, kerosine,	Petrol
Automobile fuel	insecticide	Petrol, vapor
Benzol vapor	Kerosene, kerosine, vapor	Petrolatum, nonmedicinal
Brasso	Lighter fluid	Petroleum (products) NEC
Cigarette lighter fluid	Ligroin(e) (solvent)	Petroleum, solids
Coal tar, naphtha (solvent)	Lubricating oil NEC	Petroleum, solvents
Crude oil	Mineral oil, nonmedicinal	Petroleum, vapor
Ethyl formate NEC (solvent)	Mineral spirits	Solvent, industrial,
Ethylidene diethyl ether	Naphtha (painters')	naphtha
Fuel, automobile	(petroleum)	Solvent, industrial,
Fuel, automobile, vapor	Naphtha, solvent	petroleum
NEC	Naphtha, vapor	Spirit(s), mineral
Gas, oil	Oil, lubricating	Tar NEC
Gasoline	Paraffin(s) (wax)	Tractor fuel NEC
Gasoline, vapor	Paraffin(s), liquid,	Wax (paraffin) (petroleum)
Kerosene, kerosine (fuel)	nonmedicinal	Wax, floor
(solvent) NEC	Pesticide, kerosene	White spirit

T52.0x- Toxic effects of petroleum products

T52.0x1- Toxic effect of petroleum products, accidental (unintentional)
 Toxic effects of petroleum products NOS

T52.0x2- Toxic effect of petroleum products, intentional self-harm

T52.0x3- Toxic effect of petroleum products, assault

T52.0x4- Toxic effect of petroleum products, undetermined

T52.1- Toxic effects of benzene
 Excludes 1: homologues of benzene (T52.2)
     nitroderivatives and aminoderivatives of benzene and
      its homologues (T65.3)

T52.1 - DRUGS/CHEMS*	Diphenylmethane dye)
Benzene	
Benzol (benzene)	

T52.1x- Toxic effects of benzene

T52.1x1- Toxic effect of benzene, accidental (unintentional)
 Toxic effects of benzene NOS

T52.1x2- Toxic effect of benzene, intentional self-harm

T52.1x3- Toxic effect of benzene, assault

T52.1x4- Toxic effect of benzene, undetermined

T52.2- Toxic effects of homologues of benzene
 Toxic effects of toluene [methylbenzene]
 Toxic effects of xylene [dimethylbenzene]

T52.2 - DRUGS/CHEMS*	Hexylresorcinol	Toluol (liquid)
Benzene, homologues	Hydroquinone	Toluol, vapor
(acetyl) (dimethyl)	Methyl benzene	Xylene (vapor)
(methyl) (solvent)	Methyl benzol	Xylol (vapor)
Butyltoluene	Toluene (liquid)	

T52.2x- Toxic effects of homologues of benzene

T52.2x1- Toxic effect of homologues of benzene, accidental (unintentional)
 Toxic effects of homologues of benzene NOS

T52.2x2- Toxic effect of homologues of benzene, intentional self-harm

T52.2x3- Toxic effect of homologues of benzene, assault

T52.2x4- Toxic effect of homologues of benzene, undetermined

T52.3- Toxic effects of glycols

T52.3 - DRUGS/CHEMS*	Diethylene glycol	Ethylene glycol(s), dinitrate
Butyl carbitol	(monoacetate)	Ethylene glycol(s),
Butyl cellosolve	(monobutyl ether)	monobutyl ether
Carbitol	(monoethyl ether)	Glycols (ether)
	2-Ethoxyethanol	2-Methoxyethanol
	Ethylene dinitrate	Nitroglycol

T52.3x- Toxic effects of glycols

T52.3x1- Toxic effect of glycols, accidental (unintentional)
 Toxic effects of glycols NOS

T52.3x2- Toxic effect of glycols, intentional self-harm

T52.3x3- Toxic effect of glycols, assault

T52.3x4- Toxic effect of glycols, undetermined

T52.4- Toxic effects of ketones

T52.4 - DRUGS/CHEMS*	Dimethyl ketone	MEK (methyl ethyl ketone)
Acetone (chlorinated) (oils)	Dimethyl ketone, vapor	Methyl acetate
(vapor)	Hexanone, 2-hexanone	Methyl acetone
Acetophenone	Hexone	Methyl ethyl ketone
Butanone, 2-butanone	Hydroxymethylpenta-none	Methyl isobutyl ketone
Cyclohexanone	Ketols	
Diacetone alcohol	Ketone oils	

T52.4x- Toxic effects of ketones

T52.4x1- Toxic effect of ketones, accidental (unintentional)
 Toxic effects of ketones NOS

T52.4x2- Toxic effect of ketones, intentional self-harm

T52.4x3- Toxic effect of ketones, assault

T52.4x4- Toxic effect of ketones, undetermined

T51 - T52

T52.8-   Toxic effects of other organic solvents

T52.8 - DRUGS/CHEMS*		
Acetal	Diethylene dioxide	Hexahydrobenzol
Acetaldehyde (vapor)	Dimethyl carbonate	Hexamethylene
Acetic acid ester (solvent)	Dimethyl sulfoxide	Isobutyl acetate
(vapor)	(nonmedicinal)	Isopropyl acetate
Acetic ether (vapor)	Dimethylformamide	Isopropyl ether
Acetonitrile	Dioxane	Limonene
Amyl acetate	Dipentene	Methyl benzoate
Amyl formate	Epichlorhydrin,	Methyl carbonate
Benzyl acetate	epichlorohydrin	Methyl cyclohexane
Butyl acetate (secondary)	Ether, ethyl, nonmedicinal	Methyl cyclohexanone
Butyl butyrate	Ether, solvent	Methyl cyclohexyl acetate
Butyl formate	Ethyl acetate	Methyl sulfate, liquid
Butyl lactate	Ethyl aldehyde, liquid	Nitropropane
Butyl propionate	Ethyl benzoate	Oil, Niobe
Cyclohexane	Ethyl carbonate	Paint solvent NEC
Cyclohexyl acetate	ether – see also Ether	Paint stripper
Decahydronaphthalene	Ethyl hydroxyisobutyrate	Pimelic ketone
Decalin	NEC (solvent)	Pyridine
Dekalin	Ethyl lactate NEC (solvent)	Solvent, industrial,
Dichlorhydrin	Ethyl oxybutyrate NEC	specified NEC
Dichloroethane	(solvent)	Stripper (paint) (solvent)
Dichlorohydrin, alpha-	Ethylene chlorohydrin	Tetrahydrofuran
dichlorohydrin	Ethylene dichloride	Tetrahydronaphthalene
Diethyl carbonate	Ethylene glycol(s)	Tetralin
Diethyl oxide	Furfural	Turpentine (spirits of)
	Glue NEC	Turpentine, vapor

T52.8x- Toxic effects of other organic solvents

T52.8x1- Toxic effect of other organic solvents, accidental (unintentional)
      Toxic effects of other organic solvents NOS

T52.8x2- Toxic effect of other organic solvents, intentional self-harm

T52.8x3- Toxic effect of other organic solvents, assault

T52.8x4- Toxic effect of other organic solvents, undetermined

T52.9-   Toxic effects of unspecified organic solvent

T52.9 - DRUGS/CHEMS*		
Cellosolve	Methyl cellosolve	Tricresyl phosphate, solvent
Cleaner, of paint or varnish	Nail polish remover	Varnish, cleaner
Dialkyl carbonate	Paint cleaner	
Industrial solvents (fumes)	Phosphate, solvent	
(vapors)	Polyester resin hardener	
	Solvent, industrial NEC	

T52.91x- Toxic effect of unspecified organic solvent, accidental (unintentional)

T52.92x- Toxic effect of unspecified organic solvent, intentional self-harm

T52.93x- Toxic effect of unspecified organic solvent, assault

T52.94x- Toxic effect of unspecified organic solvent, undetermined

T53-   Toxic effect of halogen derivatives of aliphatic and aromatic hydrocarbons

The appropriate 7th character is to be added to each code from category T53:
A   Initial encounter
D   Subsequent encounter
S   Sequela

T53.0-   Toxic effects of carbon tetrachloride
      Toxic effects of tetrachloromethane

T53.0 - DRUGS/CHEMS*		
Carbon tetrachloride	Carbon tetrachloride, liquid	Carbon tetrachloride,
(vapor) NEC	(cleansing agent) NEC	solvent

T53.0x- Toxic effects of carbon tetrachloride

T53.0x1- Toxic effect of carbon tetrachloride, accidental (unintentional)
      Toxic effects of carbon tetrachloride NOS

T53.0x2- Toxic effect of carbon tetrachloride, intentional self-harm

T53.0x3- Toxic effect of carbon tetrachloride, assault

T53.0x4- Toxic effect of carbon tetrachloride, undetermined

T53.1-   Toxic effects of chloroform
      Toxic effects of trichloromethane

T53.1 - DRUGS/CHEMS*	Chloroform, solvent
Chloroform (fumes)	
(vapor)	

T53.1x- Toxic effects of chloroform

T53.1x1- Toxic effect of chloroform, accidental (unintentional)
      Toxic effects of chloroform NOS

T53.1x2- Toxic effect of chloroform, intentional self-harm

T53.1x3- Toxic effect of chloroform, assault

T53.1x4- Toxic effect of chloroform, undetermined

T53.2-   Toxic effects of trichloroethylene
      Toxic effects of trichloroethene

T53.2 - DRUGS/CHEMS*	Trichloroethylene (liquid)
Trichlorethane	(vapor)
Trichlorethylene	Trichloroethylene, vapor
Trichloroethane	NEC

T53.2x- Toxic effects of trichloroethylene

T53.2x1- Toxic effect of trichloroethylene, accidental (unintentional)
      Toxic effects of trichloroethylene NOS

T53.2x2- Toxic effect of trichloroethylene, intentional self-harm

T53.2x3- Toxic effect of trichloroethylene, assault

T53.2x4- Toxic effect of trichloroethylene, undetermined

T53.3-   Toxic effects of tetrachloroethylene
      Toxic effects of perchloroethylene
      Toxic effect of tetrachloroethene

T53.3 - DRUGS/CHEMS*	Tetrachloroethylene
Perchloroethylene	(liquid)
Perchloroethylene, vapor	Tetrachloroethylene, vapor

T53.3x- Toxic effects of tetrachloroethylene

T53.3x1- Toxic effect of tetrachloroethylene, accidental (unintentional)
      Toxic effects of tetrachloroethylene NOS

T53.3x2- Toxic effect of tetrachloroethylene, intentional self-harm

T53.3x3- Toxic effect of tetrachloroethylene, assault

T53.3x4- Toxic effect of tetrachloroethylene, undetermined

T53.4-   Toxic effects of dichloromethane
      Toxic effects of methylene chloride

T53.4 - DRUGS/CHEMS*	Dichloromethane, vapor	Methylene chloride or
Dichloromethane (solvent)		dichloride (solvent) NEC

T53.4x- Toxic effects of dichloromethane

T53.4x1- Toxic effect of dichloromethane, accidental (unintentional)
      Toxic effects of dichloromethane NOS

T53.4x2- Toxic effect of dichloromethane, intentional self-harm

T53.4x3- Toxic effect of dichloromethane, assault

T53.4x4- Toxic effect of dichloromethane, undetermined

T53.5-   Toxic effects of chlorofluorocarbons

T53.5 - DRUGS/CHEMS*	Fumes, freons	Refrigerant gas
Chlorofluorocarbons	Gas, refrigerant	(chlorofluoro-carbon)
Dichlorodifluoromethane	(chlorofluorocarbon)	Trichlorofluoromethane
Freon		NEC

T53.5x- Toxic effects of chlorofluorocarbons

T53.5x1- Toxic effect of chlorofluorocarbons, accidental (unintentional)
      Toxic effects of chlorofluorocarbons NOS

T53.5x2- Toxic effect of chlorofluorocarbons, intentional self-harm

T53.5x3- Toxic effect of chlorofluorocarbons, assault

T53.5x4- Toxic effect of chlorofluorocarbons, undetermined

T 5 2 - T 5 3

T53.6- Toxic effects of other halogen derivatives of aliphatic hydrocarbons

T53.6 - DRUGS/CHEMS*	Chloropicrin (fumes)	HCH
Acetyl (bromide) (chloride)	Dibromoethane	Hexachlorocyclohexane
Acetylene dichloride	Sym-Dichloroethyl ether	Lindane (insecticide)
Acetylene tetrachloride	Dichloroethylene	(nonmedicinal) (vapor)
(vapor)	Ethyl chloride, solvent	Pentachloroethane
Amyl chloride	Ethylene chlorohydrin,	Pentalin
Amylene dichloride	vapor	Sym-dichloroethyl ether
BHC, nonmedicinal (vapor)	Ethylene dichloride, vapor	Tetrachloroethane
Chlorex	Ethylidene chloride NEC	Tetrachloroethane, vapor
Chlorinated camphene	Fluorocarbon monomer	Tetrachloroethane, vapor,
Chlorobromomethane (fire	Gamma-benzene	paint or varnish
extinguisher)	hexachloride,	Trichloropropane
Chloroethylene	nonmedicinal, vapor	

T53.6x- Toxic effects of <u>other halogen derivatives of aliphatic hydrocarbons</u>

T53.6x1- Toxic effects of other halogen derivatives of aliphatic hydrocarbons, <u>accidental</u> (unintentional)
Toxic effects of other halogen derivatives of aliphatic hydrocarbons NOS

T53.6x2- Toxic effect of other halogen derivatives of aliphatic hydrocarbons, <u>intentional</u> self-harm

T53.6x3- Toxic effect of other halogen derivatives of aliphatic hydrocarbons, <u>assault</u>

T53.6x4- Toxic effect of other halogen derivatives of aliphatic hydrocarbons, <u>undetermined</u>

T53.7- Toxic effects of other halogen derivatives of aromatic hydrocarbons

T53.7 - DRUGS/CHEMS*	Chlorodinitrobenzene	Dioxin
Chlorbenzene, chlorbenzol	Chlorodinitrobenzene, dust	Methoxychlor
Chlorinated diphenyl	or vapor	Methoxy-DDT
Chlorinated naphthalene,	Chlorodiphenyl	Monochlorobenzene
industrial (non-	Chloronitrobenzene	Orthodichlorobenzene
pesticide)	Chloronitrobenzene, dust	Pentachloronaphthalene
Chloroaniline	or vapor	TCDD
Chlorobenzene,	Chlorophenol	2,3,7,8-Tetrachlorodibenzo-
chlorbenzol	Dichlorobenzene	p-dioxin

T53.7x- Toxic effects of <u>other halogen derivatives of aromatic hydrocarbons</u>

T53.7x1- Toxic effect of other halogen derivatives of aromatic hydrocarbons, <u>accidental</u> (unintentional)
Toxic effects of other halogen derivatives of aromatic hydrocarbons NOS

T53.7x2- Toxic effect of other halogen derivatives of aromatic hydrocarbons, <u>intentional</u> self-harm

T53.7x3- Toxic effect of other halogen derivatives of aromatic hydrocarbons, <u>assault</u>

T53.7x4- Toxic effect of other halogen derivatives of aromatic hydrocarbons, <u>undetermined</u>

T53.9- Toxic effects of <u>unspecified halogen derivatives of aliphatic and aromatic hydrocarbons</u>

T53.9 - DRUGS/CHEMS*	Chlorinated hydrocarbons,
Chlorinated hydrocarbons	solvents
NEC	

T53.91x- Toxic effect of unspecified halogen derivatives of aliphatic and aromatic hydrocarbons, <u>accidental</u> (unintentional)

T53.92x- Toxic effect of unspecified halogen derivatives of aliphatic and aromatic hydrocarbons, <u>intentional</u> self-harm

T53.93x- Toxic effect of unspecified halogen derivatives of aliphatic and aromatic hydrocarbons, <u>assault</u>

T53.94x- Toxic effect of unspecified halogen derivatives of aliphatic and aromatic hydrocarbons, <u>undetermined</u>

T54- Toxic effect of <u>corrosive substances</u>
The appropriate 7th character is to be added to each code from category T54:
A <u>Initial</u> encounter
D <u>Subsequent</u> encounter
S <u>Sequela</u>

T54.0- Toxic effects of phenol and phenol homologues

T54.0 - DRUGS/CHEMS*	Hydroxytoluene	Phenol, nonmedicinal NEC
Aminophenol	(nonmedicinal)	
Carbolic acid — see also	Nitrophenol	
Phenol	Phenol, disinfectant	

T54.0x- Toxic effects of <u>phenol and phenol homologues</u>

T54.0x1- Toxic effect of phenol and phenol homologues, <u>accidental</u> (unintentional)
Toxic effects of phenol and phenol homologues NOS

T54.0x2- Toxic effect of phenol and phenol homologues, <u>intentional</u> self-harm

T54.0x3- Toxic effect of phenol and phenol homologues, <u>assault</u>

T54.0x4- Toxic effect of phenol and phenol homologues, <u>undetermined</u>

T54.1- Toxic effects of other corrosive organic compounds

T54.1 - DRUGS/CHEMS*	Aziridine (chelating)	Creolin, disinfectant
Acrolein, liquid	Corrosive aromatics	Disinfectant, aromatic
Aromatics, corrosive	Corrosive aromatics,	Ethylene imine
Aromatics, corrosive,	disinfectant	Hydrazine
disinfectants	Creolin	Lysol

T54.1x- Toxic effects of <u>other corrosive organic compounds</u>

T54.1x1- Toxic effect of other corrosive organic compounds, <u>accidental</u> (unintentional)
Toxic effects of other corrosive organic compounds NOS

T54.1x2- Toxic effect of other corrosive organic compounds, <u>intentional</u> self-harm

T54.1x3- Toxic effect of other corrosive organic compounds, <u>assault</u>

T54.1x4- Toxic effect of other corrosive organic compounds, <u>undetermined</u>

T54.2- Toxic effects of corrosive acids and acid-like substances
Toxic effects of hydrochloric acid
Toxic effects of sulfuric acid

T54.2 - DRUGS/CHEMS*	Mineral acids	Phosphoric acid
Acetic acid	Nitric acid (liquid)	Picric acid
Acid (corrosive) NEC	Nitrohydrochloric acid	Saniflush (cleaner)
Aqua fortis	Nitrous acid (liquid)	Storage battery (cells)
Battery acid or fluid	Oil, vitriol (liquid)	(acid)
Corrosive acid NEC	Oil, vitriol, fumes	Sulfur, acid
Formic acid	Orthotolidine (reagent)	Sulfuric acid
Hydrazoic acid, azides	Osmic acid (liquid)	Trichloroacetic acid,
Hydrochloric acid (liquid)	Osmic acid, fumes	trichloracetic acid
Hydrofluoric acid (liquid)	Oxalic acid	

T54.2x- Toxic effects of <u>corrosive acids and acid-like substances</u>

T54.2x1- Toxic effect of corrosive acids and acid-like substances, <u>accidental</u> (unintentional)
Toxic effects of corrosive acids and acid-like substances NOS

T54.2x2- Toxic effect of corrosive acids and acid-like substances, <u>intentional</u> self-harm

T54.2x3- Toxic effect of corrosive acids and acid-like substances, <u>assault</u>

T54.2x4- Toxic effect of corrosive acids and acid-like substances, <u>undetermined</u>

T53 - T54

T54.3- **Toxic effects of corrosive alkalis and alkali-like substances**
Toxic effects of potassium hydroxide
Toxic effects of sodium hydroxide

T54.3 - DRUGS/CHEMS*	Caustic(s) hydroxide	Potassium hydroxide
Alkali (caustic)	Caustic(s) potash	Quicklime
Ammonia, liquid (household)	Caustic(s) soda	Soda (caustic)
	Chloride of lime (bleach)	Sodium carbonate NEC
Ammonium carbonate	Chlorinated lime (bleach)	Sodium hydroxide
Ammonium compounds (household) NEC	Chlorine bleach	Sodium hypochlorite (bleach) NEC
	Disinfectant, alkaline	
Ammonium compounds, industrial	Drano (drain cleaner)	Sodium hypochlorite, disinfectant
	Hydroxide, caustic	
Calcium hydrate, hydroxide	Lime (chloride)	Sodium hypochlorite, vapor
Calcium hypochlorite	Lye (concentrated)	Triethanolamine NEC
Calcium oxide	Potash (caustic)	Triethanolamine, detergent
Caustic(s) alkali	Potassium carbonate	

T54.3x- **Toxic effects of corrosive alkalis and alkali-like substances**
- **T54.3x1-** Toxic effect of corrosive alkalis and alkali-like substances, **accidental** (unintentional)
  Toxic effects of corrosive alkalis and alkali-like substances NOS
- **T54.3x2-** Toxic effect of corrosive alkalis and alkali-like substances, **intentional** self-harm
- **T54.3x3-** Toxic effect of corrosive alkalis and alkali-like substances, **assault**
- **T54.3x4-** Toxic effect of corrosive alkalis and alkali-like substances, **undetermined**

T54.9- **Toxic effects of unspecified corrosive substance**

T54.9 - DRUGS/CHEMS*	Clorox (bleach)	Oxidizing agent NEC
Bleach	Corrosive NEC	Purex (bleach)
Borate(s) cleanser	Corrosive fumes NEC	Sodium chlorate, herbicide
Borax (cleanser)	Corrosive, specified NEC	
Caustic(s) NEC	Fluoride, not pesticide NEC	
Caustic(s) specified NEC	Fumes, corrosive NEC	

T54.91x- Toxic effect of unspecified corrosive substance, **accidental** (unintentional)
T54.92x- Toxic effect of unspecified corrosive substance, **intentional** self-harm
T54.93x- Toxic effect of unspecified corrosive substance, **assault**
T54.94x- Toxic effect of unspecified corrosive substance, **undetermined**

T55- Toxic effect of **soaps and detergents**

The appropriate 7th character is to be added to each code from category T55:
- **A** **Initial** encounter
- **D** **Subsequent** encounter
- **S** **Sequela**

T55.0- **Toxic effect of soaps**

T55.0 - DRUGS/CHEMS*	Soap (powder) (product)	Soft soap
Shampoo	Sodium perborate, soap	

T55.0x- **Toxic effect of soaps**
- **T55.0x1-** Toxic effect of soaps, **accidental** (unintentional)
  Toxic effect of soaps NOS
- **T55.0x2-** Toxic effect of soaps, **intentional** self-harm
- **T55.0x3-** Toxic effect of soaps, **assault**
- **T55.0x4-** Toxic effect of soaps, **undetermined**

T55.1- **Toxic effect of detergents**

T55.1 - DRUGS/CHEMS*	Detergent, specified NEC
Detergent, nonmedicinal	

T55.1x- **Toxic effect of detergents**
- **T55.1x1-** Toxic effect of detergents, **accidental** (unintentional)
  Toxic effect of detergents NOS
- **T55.1x2-** Toxic effect of detergents, **intentional** self-harm
- **T55.1x3-** Toxic effect of detergents, **assault**
- **T55.1x4-** Toxic effect of detergents, **undetermined**

T56- **Toxic effect of metals**
Includes: Toxic effects of fumes and vapors of metals
Toxic effects of metals from all sources, except medicinal substances
Use additional code to identify any retained metal foreign body, if applicable (Z18.0-, T18.1-)
Excludes 1:   arsenic and its compounds (T57.0)
manganese and its compounds (T57.2)

The appropriate 7th character is to be added to each code from category T56:
- **A** **Initial** encounter
- **D** **Subsequent** encounter
- **S** **Sequela**

T56.0- **Toxic effects of lead and its compounds**

T56.0 - DRUGS/CHEMS*	Lead carbonate, paint	Lead oxide
Antiknock (tetraethyl lead)	Lead chromate	Lead oxide, paint
Chromate, lead — see also Lead	Lead chromate, paint	Lead paint
	Lead dioxide	Lead salts
Chromate, lead paint	Lead, inorganic	Lead, specified compound NEC
Lead (dust) (fumes) (vapor) NEC	Lead iodide	
	Lead iodide, pigment (paint)	Lead, tetra-ethyl
Lead alkyl (fuel additive)		Paint, lead (fumes)
Lead, antiknock compound (tetraethyl)	Lead monoxide (dust)	Tetraethyl, lead
	Lead monoxide, paint	
Lead carbonate	Lead, organic	

T56.0x- **Toxic effects of lead and its compounds**
- **T56.0x1-** Toxic effect of lead and its compounds, **accidental** (unintentional)
  Toxic effects of lead and its compounds NOS
- **T56.0x2-** Toxic effect of lead and its compounds, **intentional** self-harm
- **T56.0x3-** Toxic effect of lead and its compounds, **assault**
- **T56.0x4-** Toxic effect of lead and its compounds, **undetermined**

T56.1- **Toxic effects of mercury and its compounds**

T56.1 - DRUGS/CHEMS*	Mercury, mercurial, mercuric, mercurous (compounds) (cyanide) (fumes) (nonmedicinal) (vapor) NEC	Mercury, chloride, fungicide
Corrosive sublimate		Mercury, fungicide
Ethyl mercuric chloride		Mercury, organic (fungicide)
Fulminate of mercury		

T56.1x- **Toxic effects of mercury and its compounds**
- **T56.1x1-** Toxic effect of mercury and its compounds, **accidental** (unintentional)
  Toxic effects of mercury and its compounds NOS
- **T56.1x2-** Toxic effect of mercury and its compounds, **intentional** self-harm
- **T56.1x3-** Toxic effect of mercury and its compounds, **assault**
- **T56.1x4-** Toxic effect of mercury and its compounds, **undetermined**

T56.2- **Toxic effects of chromium and its compounds**

T56.2 - DRUGS/CHEMS*	Chromate, dust or mist	Chromium
Bichromates, fumes	Chromic acid	Chromyl chloride
Chromate	Chromic acid, dust or mist	Potassium bichromate

T56.2x- **Toxic effects of chromium and its compounds**
- **T56.2x1-** Toxic effect of chromium and its compounds, **accidental** (unintentional)
  Toxic effect of chromium and its compounds NOS
- **T56.2x2-** Toxic effect of chromium and its compounds, **intentional** self-harm
- **T56.2x3-** Toxic effect of chromium and its compounds, **assault**
- **T56.2x4-** Toxic effect of chromium and its compounds, **undetermined**

T54
–
T56

T56.3- Toxic effects of cadmium and its compounds

> **T56.3** - DRUGS/CHEMS*
> Cadmium (chloride)
> (fumes) (oxide)

T56.3x- Toxic effects of cadmium and its compounds

T56.3x1- Toxic effect of cadmium and its compounds, accidental (unintentional)
    Toxic effects of cadmium and its compounds NOS

T56.3x2- Toxic effect of cadmium and its compounds, intentional self-harm

T56.3x3- Toxic effect of cadmium and its compounds, assault

T56.3x4- Toxic effect of cadmium and its compounds, undetermined

T56.4- Toxic effects of copper and its compounds

> **T56.4** - DRUGS/CHEMS*   Copper sulfate, cupric   Cuprous sulfate – see also
> Copper (dust) (fumes)   Copper sulfate, cuprous   Copper sulfate
> (nonmedicinal) NEC   Cupric sulfate
> Copper sulfate

T56.4x- Toxic effects of copper and its compounds

T56.4x1- Toxic effect of copper and its compounds, accidental (unintentional)
    Toxic effects of copper and its compounds NOS

T56.4x2- Toxic effect of copper and its compounds, intentional self-harm

T56.4x3- Toxic effect of copper and its compounds, assault

T56.4x4- Toxic effect of copper and its compounds, undetermined

T56.5- Toxic effects of zinc and its compounds

> **T56.5** - DRUGS/CHEMS*   Zinc chromate
> Zinc (compounds) (fumes)   Zinc, pesticides
> (vapor) NEC

T56.5x- Toxic effects of zinc and its compounds

T56.5x1- Toxic effect of zinc and its compounds, accidental (unintentional)
    Toxic effects of zinc and its compounds NOS

T56.5x2- Toxic effect of zinc and its compounds, intentional self-harm

T56.5x3- Toxic effect of zinc and its compounds, assault

T56.5x4- Toxic effect of zinc and its compounds, undetermined

T56.6- Toxic effects of tin and its compounds

> **T56.6** - DRUGS/CHEMS*
> Tin (chloride) (dust)
> (oxide) NEC

T56.6x- Toxic effects of tin and its compounds

T56.6x1- Toxic effect of tin and its compounds, accidental (unintentional)
    Toxic effects of tin and its compounds NOS

T56.6x2- Toxic effect of tin and its compounds, intentional self-harm

T56.6x3- Toxic effect of tin and its compounds, assault

T56.6x4- Toxic effect of tin and its compounds, undetermined

T56.7- Toxic effects of beryllium and its compounds

> **T56.7** - DRUGS/CHEMS*
> Beryllium (compounds)

T56.7x- Toxic effects of beryllium and its compounds

T56.7x1- Toxic effect of beryllium and its compounds, accidental (unintentional)
    Toxic effects of beryllium and its compounds NOS

T56.7x2- Toxic effect of beryllium and its compounds, intentional self-harm

T56.7x3- Toxic effect of beryllium and its compounds, assault

T56.7x4- Toxic effect of beryllium and its compounds, undetermined

T56.8- Toxic effects of other metals

T56.81- Toxic effect of thallium

> **T56.81** - DRUGS/CHEMS*   Thallium (compounds)
> Metals, thallium   (dust) NEC

T56.811- Toxic effect of thallium, accidental (unintentional)
    Toxic effect of thallium NOS

T56.812- Toxic effect of thallium, intentional self-harm

T56.813- Toxic effect of thallium, assault

T56.814- Toxic effect of thallium, undetermined

T56.89- Toxic effects of other metals

> **T56.89** - DRUGS/CHEMS*   Golden sulfide of antimony   Silver, nonmedicinal (dust)
> Alum, nonmedicinal   Iron, nonmedicinal   Stibine
>   (ammonium)   Lithium   Tellurium
>   (potassium)   Magnesium NEC   Tellurium, fumes
> Antimony (compounds)   Metals, specified NEC   Titanium (compounds)
>   (vapor) NEC   Nickel (carbonyl) (tetra-   (vapor)
> Antimony, hydride   carbonyl) (fumes)   Titanium tetrachloride
> Brass (fumes)   (vapor)   Titanocene
> Cobalt (nonmedicinal)   Nickelocene   Vanadium
>   (fumes) (industrial)   Selenium NEC

T56.891- Toxic effect of other metals, accidental (unintentional)
    Toxic effects of other metals NOS

T56.892- Toxic effect of other metals, intentional self-harm

T56.893- Toxic effect of other metals, assault

T56.894- Toxic effect of other metals, undetermined

T56.9- Toxic effects of unspecified metal

> **T56.9** - DRUGS/CHEMS*   Metals, dust, fumes, or   Metals, light, dust, fumes,
> Metals (heavy)   vapor NEC   or vapor NEC
> (nonmedicinal)   Metals, light NEC   Smelter fumes NEC

T56.91x- Toxic effect of unspecified metal, accidental (unintentional)

T56.92x- Toxic effect of unspecified metal, intentional self-harm

T56.93x- Toxic effect of unspecified metal, assault

T56.94x- Toxic effect of unspecified metal, undetermined

T57- Toxic effect of other inorganic substances

The appropriate 7th character is to be added to each code from category T57:
A   Initial encounter
D   Subsequent encounter
S   Sequela

T57.0- Toxic effect of arsenic and its compounds

> **T57.0** - DRUGS/CHEMS*   Diphenylchloroarsine, not   Lewisite (gas), not in war
> Arsenate of lead   in war   Paris green
> Arsenate of lead, herbicide   Ethyl dichloroarsine   Paris green, insecticide
> Arsenic, arsenicals   (vapor)   Pesticide, arsenic
>   (compounds) (dust)   Fowler's solution   Potassium arsenite
>   (vapor) NEC   Hexahydrocresol(s)   (solution)
> Arsenic pesticide (dust)   arsenide   Realgar
>   (fumes)   Hexahydrocresol(s)   Scheele's green
> Arsine (gas)   arseniurated   Scheele's green, insecticide
> Cacodyl, cacodylic acid   Hexahydrocresol(s) sulfide,   Schweinfurth green
> Chlorovinyldichloro-arsine,   arseniurated   Schweinfurth green,
>   not in war   Hydrogen arsenide   insecticide
> Copper arsenate, arsenite   Hydrogen, arseniureted   Sodium arsenate
> Cupric acetoarsenite   Hydrogen sulfide,   Trioxide of arsenic
> Cupric arsenate   arseniureted   Vienna green
> Dimethyl arsine, arsinic   Lead arsenate, arsenite   Vienna red
>   acid   (dust) (herbicide)   White arsenic
>   (insecticide) (vapor)

T57.0x- Toxic effect of arsenic and its compounds

T57.0x1- Toxic effect of arsenic and its compounds, accidental (unintentional)
    Toxic effect of arsenic and its compounds NOS

T57.0x2- Toxic effect of arsenic and its compounds, intentional self-harm

T57.0x3- Toxic effect of arsenic and its compounds, assault

T57.0x4- Toxic effect of arsenic and its compounds, undetermined

T57.1-   Toxic effect of phosphorus and its compounds
　　Excludes 1:   organophosphate insecticides (T60.0)

T57.1 - DRUGS/CHEMS*	Phosphine, fumigant
Hydrogen phosphureted	Phosphorus (compound)
Phosphine	NEC

T57.1x-   Toxic effect of phosphorus and its compounds

T57.1x1-   Toxic effect of phosphorus and its compounds, accidental (unintentional)
　　　Toxic effect of phosphorus and its compounds NOS

T57.1x2-   Toxic effect of phosphorus and its compounds, intentional self-harm

T57.1x3-   Toxic effect of phosphorus and its compounds, assault

T57.1x4-   Toxic effect of phosphorus and its compounds, undetermined

T57.2-   Toxic effect of manganese and its compounds

T57.2 - DRUGS/CHEMS*
Manganese (dioxide)
(salts)

T57.2x-   Toxic effect of manganese and its compounds

T57.2x1-   Toxic effect of manganese and its compounds, accidental (unintentional)
　　　Toxic effect of manganese and its compounds NOS

T57.2x2-   Toxic effect of manganese and its compounds, intentional self-harm

T57.2x3-   Toxic effect of manganese and its compounds, assault

T57.2x4-   Toxic effect of manganese and its compounds, undetermined

T57.3-   Toxic effect of hydrogen cyanide

T57.3 - DRUGS/CHEMS*	Gas, cyanide	Hydrogen cyanide (salts)
Cyanide(s), dust or gas	HCN	Hydrogen cyanide, gas
(inhalation) NEC	Hexahydrocresol(s) cyanide	Prussic acid, vapor
Cyanide(s), hydrogen	Hydrocyanic acid (liquid)	

T57.3x-   Toxic effect of hydrogen cyanide

T57.3x1-   Toxic effect of hydrogen cyanide, accidental (unintentional)
　　　Toxic effect of hydrogen cyanide NOS

T57.3x2-   Toxic effect of hydrogen cyanide, intentional self-harm

T57.3x3-   Toxic effect of hydrogen cyanide, assault

T57.3x4-   Toxic effect of hydrogen cyanide, undetermined

T57.8-   Toxic effect of other specified inorganic substances

T57.8 - DRUGS/CHEMS*	Boron	Hexahydrocresol(s)
Asbestos	Boron hydride NEC	sulfurated
Barium (carbonate)	Boron hydride, fumes or	Hydrogen chloride
(chloride) (sulfite)	gas	Potassium fluoride
Bichromates (calcium)	Calcium cyanide	Potassium nitrate
(potassium) (sodium)	Chloramine	Sodium bichromate
(crystals)	Decaborane	Sodium borate, cleanser
Borane complex	Hexahydrocresol(s)	
Borate(s)	Fluoride (liquid)	
Borate(s) sodium	Hexahydrocresol(s) sulfate	

T57.8x-   Toxic effect of other specified inorganic substances

T57.8x1-   Toxic effect of other specified inorganic substances, accidental (unintentional)
　　　Toxic effect of other specified inorganic substances NOS

T57.8x2-   Toxic effect of other specified inorganic substances, intentional self-harm

T57.8x3-   Toxic effect of other specified inorganic substances, assault

T57.8x4-   Toxic effect of other specified inorganic substances, undetermined

T57.9-   Toxic effect of unspecified inorganic substance

T57.9 - DRUGS/CHEMS*
Inorganic substance

T57.91x-   Toxic effect of unspecified inorganic substance, accidental (unintentional)

T57.92x-   Toxic effect of unspecified inorganic substance, intentional self-harm

T57.93x-   Toxic effect of unspecified inorganic substance, assault

T57.94x-   Toxic effect of unspecified inorganic substance, undetermined

T58-   Toxic effect of carbon monoxide
　Includes:　Asphyxiation from carbon monoxide
　　　　Toxic effect of carbon monoxide from all sources

The appropriate 7th character is to be added to each code from category T58:
　A　**Initial** encounter
　D　**Subsequent** encounter
　S　**Sequela**

T58.0-   Toxic effect of carbon monoxide from motor vehicle exhaust
　　Toxic effect of exhaust gas from gas engine
　　Toxic effect of exhaust gas from motor pump

T58.0 - DRUGS/CHEMS*	Carbon monoxide, exhaust	Exhaust gas (engine)
Carbon monoxide, exhaust	gas, gas engine	(motor vehicle)
gas (motor) not in	Carbon monoxide, exhaust	Fuel, automobile, exhaust
transit	gas, motor pump	gas, not in transit
Carbon monoxide, exhaust	Carbon monoxide, exhaust	Gas, exhaust
gas, combustion engine,	gas, motor vehicle, not	Gas, garage
any not in watercraft	in transit	Gas, motor exhaust, not in
Carbon monoxide, exhaust	Carbon monoxide, motor	transit
gas, farm tractor, not in	exhaust gas, not in	Motor exhaust gas
transit	transit	

T58.01x-   Toxic effect of carbon monoxide from motor vehicle exhaust, accidental (unintentional)

T58.02x-   Toxic effect of carbon monoxide from motor vehicle exhaust, intentional self-harm

T58.03x-   Toxic effect of carbon monoxide from motor vehicle exhaust, assault

T58.04x-   Toxic effect of carbon monoxide from motor vehicle exhaust, undetermined

T58.1-   Toxic effect of carbon monoxide from utility gas
　　Toxic effect of acetylene
　　Toxic effect of gas NOS used for lighting, heating, cooking
　　Toxic effect of water gas

T58.1 - DRUGS/CHEMS*	Carbon monoxide, fuel,	Carbon monoxide, utility
Acetylene, incomplete	utility, in mobile	gas
combustion of	container	Carbon monoxide, utility
Butane, incomplete	Carbon monoxide, fuel,	gas, piped
combustion	piped (natural)	Carbon monoxide, water
Carbon monoxide, butane	Carbon monoxide,	gas
(distributed in mobile	illuminating gas	Gas, acetylene, incomplete
container)	Carbon monoxide, piped	combustion of
Carbon monoxide, butane,	gas (manufactured)	Gas, illuminating (after
distributed through	(natural)	combustion)
pipes	Carbon monoxide, propane	Gas, stove (after
Carbon monoxide, coal, gas	(distributed in mobile	combustion)
(piped)	container)	Gas, water
Carbon monoxide, fuel, gas	Carbon monoxide,	Illuminating gas (after
(piped)	propane, distributed	combustion)
Carbon monoxide, fuel,	through pipes	Natural gas, incomplete
gas, in mobile container	Carbon monoxide, stove	combustion
Carbon monoxide, fuel,	gas	Propane, incomplete
utility	Carbon monoxide, stove	combustion
	gas, piped	

T58.11x-   Toxic effect of carbon monoxide from utility gas, accidental (unintentional)

T58.12x-   Toxic effect of carbon monoxide from utility gas, intentional self-harm

T58.13x-   Toxic effect of carbon monoxide from utility gas, assault

T58.14x-   Toxic effect of carbon monoxide from utility gas, undetermined

T57 - T58

T58.2- **Toxic effect of carbon monoxide from incomplete combustion of other domestic fuels**
Toxic effect of carbon monoxide from incomplete combustion of coal, coke, kerosene, wood

T58.2 - DRUGS/CHEMS*	Carbon monoxide, kerosene (in domestic stoves, fireplaces)	Coke fumes or gas (carbon monoxide)
Carbon monoxide, charcoal fumes	Carbon monoxide, wood (in domestic stoves, fireplaces)	Furnace (coal burning) (domestic), gas from
Carbon monoxide, coal		Gas, coal
Carbon monoxide, coal, solid (in domestic stoves, fireplaces)	Charcoal, fumes (carbon monoxide)	Gas, from wood- or coal-burning stove or fireplace
Carbon monoxide, coke (in domestic stoves, fireplaces)	Coal (carbon monoxide from) — see also Carbon, monoxide, coal	
Carbon monoxide, fuel (in domestic use)		

T58.2x- **Toxic effect of carbon monoxide from incomplete combustion of other domestic fuels**

T58.2x1- Toxic effect of carbon monoxide from incomplete combustion of other domestic fuels, **accidental** (unintentional)

T58.2x2- Toxic effect of carbon monoxide from incomplete combustion of other domestic fuels, **intentional** self-harm

T58.2x3- Toxic effect of carbon monoxide from incomplete combustion of other domestic fuels, **assault**

T58.2x4- Toxic effect of carbon monoxide from incomplete combustion of other domestic fuels, **undetermined**

T58.8- **Toxic effect of carbon monoxide from other source**
Toxic effect of carbon monoxide from blast furnace gas
Toxic effect of carbon monoxide from fuels in industrial use
Toxic effect of carbon monoxide from kiln vapor

T58.8 - DRUGS/CHEMS*	Carbon monoxide, producer gas	Gas, blast furnace
Blast furnace gas (carbon monoxide from)	Carbon monoxide, specified source NEC	Gas, fuel, industrial use
Carbon monoxide, blast furnace gas	Charcoal, fumes, industrial	Gas, kiln
Carbon monoxide, industrial fuels or gases, any	Coke fumes or gas, industrial	Gas, producer
	Fuel, industrial, incomplete combustion	Kiln gas or vapor (carbon monoxide)
Carbon monoxide, kiln gas or vapor	Furnace, gas from, industrial	Producer gas
		Vapor, kiln (carbon monoxide)

T58.8x- **Toxic effect of carbon monoxide from other source**

T58.8x1- Toxic effect of carbon monoxide from other source, **accidental** (unintentional)

T58.8x2- Toxic effect of carbon monoxide from other source, **intentional** self-harm

T58.8x3- Toxic effect of carbon monoxide from other source, **assault**

T58.8x4- Toxic effect of carbon monoxide from other source, **undetermined**

T58.9- **Toxic effect of carbon monoxide from unspecified source**

T58.9 - DRUGS/CHEMS*
Carbon monoxide (from incomplete combustion)

T58.91x- Toxic effect of carbon monoxide from unspecified source, **accidental** (unintentional)

T58.92x- Toxic effect of carbon monoxide from unspecified source, **intentional** self-harm

T58.93x- Toxic effect of carbon monoxide from unspecified source, **assault**

T58.94x- Toxic effect of carbon monoxide from unspecified source, **undetermined**

T59- **Toxic effect of other gases, fumes and vapors**
Includes: Aerosol propellants
Excludes 1:   chlorofluorocarbons (T53.5)

The appropriate 7th character is to be added to each code from category T59:
A   Initial encounter
D   Subsequent encounter
S   Sequela

T59.0- **Toxic effect of nitrogen oxides**

T59.0 - DRUGS/CHEMS*	Nitric oxide (gas)
Fumes, nitrogen dioxide	Nitrogen

T59.0x- **Toxic effect of nitrogen oxides**

T59.0x1- Toxic effect of nitrogen oxides, **accidental** (unintentional)
Toxic effect of nitrogen oxides NOS

T59.0x2- Toxic effect of nitrogen oxides, **intentional** self-harm

T59.0x3- Toxic effect of nitrogen oxides, **assault**

T59.0x4- Toxic effect of nitrogen oxides, **undetermined**

T59.1- **Toxic effect of sulfur dioxide**

T59.1 - DRUGS/CHEMS*	Smog
Fumes, sulfur dioxide	Sulfur, dioxide (gas)

T59.1x- **Toxic effect of sulfur dioxide**

T59.1x1- Toxic effect of sulfur dioxide, **accidental** (unintentional)
Toxic effect of sulfur dioxide NOS

T59.1x2- Toxic effect of sulfur dioxide, **intentional** self-harm

T59.1x3- Toxic effect of sulfur dioxide, **assault**

T59.1x4- Toxic effect of sulfur dioxide, **undetermined**

T59.2- **Toxic effect of formaldehyde**

T59.2 - DRUGS/CHEMS*	Formalin
Formaldehyde (solution), gas or vapor	Formalin, vapor

T59.2x- **Toxic effect of formaldehyde**

T59.2x1- Toxic effect of formaldehyde, **accidental** (unintentional)
Toxic effect of formaldehyde NOS

T59.2x2- Toxic effect of formaldehyde, **intentional** self-harm

T59.2x3- Toxic effect of formaldehyde, **assault**

T59.2x4- Toxic effect of formaldehyde, **undetermined**

T59.3- **Toxic effect of lacrimogenic gas**
Toxic effect of tear gas

T59.3 - DRUGS/CHEMS*	Chloroacetophenone	Lacrimogenic gas
Brombenzylcyanide	Ethyl iodoacetate	Mace
Bromobenzylcyanide	Gas, lacrimogenic	Methyl chloroformate
Chloroacetone	Gas, tear	Tear gas

T59.3x- **Toxic effect of lacrimogenic gas**

T59.3x1- Toxic effect of lacrimogenic gas, **accidental** (unintentional)
Toxic effect of lacrimogenic gas NOS

T59.3x2- Toxic effect of lacrimogenic gas, **intentional** self-harm

T59.3x3- Toxic effect of lacrimogenic gas, **assault**

T59.3x4- Toxic effect of lacrimogenic gas, **undetermined**

T59.4- **Toxic effect of chlorine gas**

T59.4 - DRUGS/CHEMS*	Chlorine disinfectant
Chlorine (fumes) (gas)	Chlorine releasing agents
Chlorine compound gas NEC	NEC
	Gas, chlorine

T59.4x- **Toxic effect of chlorine gas**

T59.4x1- Toxic effect of chlorine gas, **accidental** (unintentional)
Toxic effect of chlorine gas NOS

T59.4x2- Toxic effect of chlorine gas, **intentional** self-harm

T59.4x3- Toxic effect of chlorine gas, **assault**

T59.4x4- Toxic effect of chlorine gas, **undetermined**

T
5
8
|
T
5
9

T59.5-   Toxic effect of fluorine gas and hydrogen fluoride

T59.5 - DRUGS/CHEMS*	
Fluorine (gas)	Hydrogen fluoride Hydrogen fluoride, vapor

T59.5x-   Toxic effect of <u>fluorine gas and hydrogen fluoride</u>

    T59.5x1-   Toxic effect of fluorine gas and hydrogen fluoride, <u>accidental</u> (unintentional)
        Toxic effect of fluorine gas and hydrogen fluoride NOS

    T59.5x2-   Toxic effect of fluorine gas and hydrogen fluoride, <u>intentional</u> self-harm

    T59.5x3-   Toxic effect of fluorine gas and hydrogen fluoride, <u>assault</u>

    T59.5x4-   Toxic effect of fluorine gas and hydrogen fluoride, <u>undetermined</u>

T59.6-   Toxic effect of hydrogen sulfide

T59.6 - DRUGS/CHEMS*		
Hexahydrocresol(s) sulfide (gas)	Hydrogen sulfide Hydrogen, sulfureted Hydrosulfuric acid (gas)	Sulfur, hydrogen

T59.6x-   Toxic effect of <u>hydrogen sulfide</u>

    T59.6x1-   Toxic effect of hydrogen sulfide, <u>accidental</u> (unintentional)
        Toxic effect of hydrogen sulfide NOS

    T59.6x2-   Toxic effect of hydrogen sulfide, <u>intentional</u> self-harm

    T59.6x3-   Toxic effect of hydrogen sulfide, <u>assault</u>

    T59.6x4-   Toxic effect of hydrogen sulfide, <u>undetermined</u>

T59.7-   Toxic effect of carbon dioxide

T59.7 - DRUGS/CHEMS*		
Carbon dioxide (gas)	Carbon dioxide, nonmedicinal Carbonic acid gas	Choke damp

T59.7x-   Toxic effect of <u>carbon dioxide</u>

    T59.7x1-   Toxic effect of carbon dioxide, <u>accidental</u> (unintentional)
        Toxic effect of carbon dioxide NOS

    T59.7x2-   Toxic effect of carbon dioxide, <u>intentional</u> self-harm

    T59.7x3-   Toxic effect of carbon dioxide, <u>assault</u>

    T59.7x4-   Toxic effect of carbon dioxide, <u>undetermined</u>

T59.8-   Toxic effect of other specified gases, fumes and vapors

    T59.81-   Toxic effect of <u>smoke</u>
        AHA 13:4Q:p121 – Acute respiratory failure due to smoke inhalation
        Smoke inhalation
        Excludes ❷: toxic effect of cigarette (tobacco) smoke (T65.22-)

T59.81 - DRUGS/CHEMS*
Smoke NEC

        T59.811-   Toxic effect of smoke, <u>accidental</u> (unintentional)
            Toxic effect of smoke NOS

        T59.812-   Toxic effect of smoke, <u>intentional</u> self-harm

        T59.813-   Toxic effect of smoke, <u>assault</u>

        T59.814-   Toxic effect of smoke, <u>undetermined</u>

    T59.89-   Toxic effect of <u>other specified gases, fumes and vapors</u>

T59.89 - DRUGS/CHEMS*		
Acetylene (gas) Acetylene, industrial Acridine, vapor Acrolein (gas) Alcohol, vapor (from any type of alcohol) Ammonia (fumes) (gas) (vapor) Ammonium compounds, fumes (any usage) Amyl acetate, vapor Anticholinesterase, organophosphorus, nerve gas Boron trifluoride Brake fluid vapor Bromine vapor	Butane (distributed in mobile container) Butane, distributed through pipes Cholinergic organophosphorus, nerve gas Coal tar, fumes Combustion gas, prior to combustion Cordite vapor Cyanic acid (gas) Cyanogen (chloride) (gas) NEC Decaborane, fumes Diazomethane (gas) Diborane (gas) Dichloroethyl sulfide, not in war	Dichloroformoxine, not in war Dimethyl sulfate (fumes) Dinitrobenzene, vapor Dinitrobenzol, vapor Domestic gas, prior to combustion Dynamite, fumes Ethidium chloride (vapor) Ethyl aldehyde (vapor) Ethylene (gas) Ethylene oxide (fumigant) (nonmedicinal) Ferrovanadium (fumes) Firedamp Formic acid, vapor

T59.89 - DRUGS/CHEMS* – Continued		
Fuel, gas (domestic use) – see also Carbon, monoxide, fuel, utility Fuel, gas, utility Fuel, gas, utility, in mobile container Fuel, gas, utility, piped (natural) Fumes, hydrocarbons Fumes, hydrocarbons, petroleum (liquefied) Fumes, hydrocarbons, petroleum, distributed through pipes (pure or mixed with air) Fumes, petroleum (liquefied) Fumes, petroleum, distributed through pipes (pure or mixed with air) Fumes, polyester Fumes, specified source NEC – see also substance, specified Gas, acetylene Gas, from utility, prior to combustion Gas, fuel, prior to combustion Gas, fuel, utility Gas, fuel, utility, in mobile container Gas, fuel, utility, piped (natural) Gas, hydrocarbon NEC Gas, hydrocarbon, liquefied, piped	Gas, illuminating, prior to combustion Gas, marsh Gas, mustard, not in war Gas, natural Gas, petroleum (liquefied) (distributed in mobile containers) Gas, petroleum, piped (pure or mixed with air) Gas, piped (manufactured) (natural) NEC Gas, refrigerant, not chlorofluoro-carbon Gas, stove, prior to combustion Gas, utility (for cooking, heating, or lighting) (piped) NEC Gas, utility, in mobile container Gas, utility, piped (natural) Helium (nonmedicinal) NEC Hexahydrocresol(s) cyanide, gas Hexahydrocresol(s) Fluoride, vapor Hydrocarbon gas Hydrocarbon gas, liquefied (mobile container) Hydrocarbon gas, liquefied, piped (natural) Hydrochloric acid, vapor Hydrofluoric acid, vapor Hydrogen Hydroquinone, vapor Illuminating gas, prior to combustion Industrial fumes Iodine vapor	Ligroin(e), vapor Liquefied petroleum gases Liquefied petroleum gases, piped (pure or mixed with air) Marsh gas Methane Methanethiol Methyl bromide (gas) Methyl chloride (gas) Methyl mercaptan Methyl sulfate (fumes) Natural gas (piped) Nitric acid, vapor Nitroaniline, vapor Nitrous acid, fumes Oil, fumes Ozone Paint fumes NEC Phosgene (gas) Polyester fumes Polyester resin hardener, fumes Polytetrafluoroethylene (inhaled) Propane (distributed in mobile container) Propane, distributed through pipes Propylene Pyridine, vapor Refrigerant gas, not chlorofluoro-carbon Selenium, fumes Sternutator gas Sulfur, vapor NEC Tar, fumes Toluidine, vapor Vapor, specified source NEC Vinyl chloride

        T59.891-   Toxic effect of other specified gases, fumes and vapors, <u>accidental</u> (unintentional)

        T59.892-   Toxic effect of other specified gases, fumes and vapors, <u>intentional</u> self-harm

        T59.893-   Toxic effect of other specified gases, fumes and vapors, <u>assault</u>

        T59.894-   Toxic effect of other specified gases, fumes and vapors, <u>undetermined</u>

T59.9-   Toxic effect of <u>unspecified gases, fumes and vapors</u>

T59.9 - DRUGS/CHEMS*		
Fumes (from) Gas Gas, air contaminants, source or type not specified	Gas, nerve, not in war Gas, sewer Gas, specified source NEC Lung irritant (gas) NEC Mustard gas, not in war Nerve gas, not in war	Sewer gas Vapor – see also Gas

    T59.91x-   Toxic effect of unspecified gases, fumes and vapors, <u>accidental</u> (unintentional)

    T59.92x-   Toxic effect of unspecified gases, fumes and vapors, <u>intentional</u> self-harm

    T59.93x-   Toxic effect of unspecified gases, fumes and vapors, <u>assault</u>

    T59.94x-   Toxic effect of unspecified gases, fumes and vapors, <u>undetermined</u>

T59 - T59

T60- **Toxic effect of pesticides**

Includes: Toxic effect of wood preservatives

The appropriate 7th character is to be added to each code from category T60:

A   Initial encounter
D   Subsequent encounter
S   Sequela

T60.0- **Toxic effect of organophosphate and carbamate insecticides**

T60.0 - DRUGS/CHEMS*		
Aldicarb	Demephion -O and -S	Mevinphos
Anticholinesterase,	Demeton -O and -S	Mipafox
organophosphorus,	Diazinon	Naled
insecticide	Dicapthon	Octamethyl
Azinphos (ethyl) (methyl)	Dichlorvos	pyrophosphoramide
Benomyl	Dicrotophos	OMPA
Carbamate (insecticide)	Dimefox	Organophosphates
Carbamate, herbicide	Dimethoate	Paraoxon
Carbamate, insecticide	Dimethyl parathion	Parathion
Carbaril	Dimetilan	Phenylsulfthion
Carbaryl	Dioxathion	Phorate
Carbophenothion	Disulfoton	Phosdrin
Chlorfenvinphos	Dithiocarbamate	Phosfolan
Chlormephos	EPN	Phosphamidon
Chloropyrifos	Ethion	Phosphate, organic
Chlorthion	Fenthion	Phosphorus, pesticide
Chlorthiophos	Fluorophosphate insecticide	Propoxur
Cholinergic	HETP	Prothoate
organophosphorus,	Hexaethyl tetraphos-phate	Quinalphos
insecticide	Hexahydrocresol(s)	Schradan
Compound 3422	phophorated	TEPP
(parathion)	Insecticide, carbamate	Terbufos
Compound 3911 (phorate)	Insecticide,	Tetraethyl pyrophosphate
Compound 4049	corganophosphorus	Thiocarbamate (insecticide)
(malathion)	Leptophos	Thiofos
Compound 4069	Malathion, insecticide	Thionazin
(malathion)	Mephosfolan	Trichlorfon
Compound 4124	Metaphos	Trichloronate
(dicapthon)	Methyl demeton	Zineb
Coumaphos	Methyl parathion	
	Metrifonate	

T60.0x- **Toxic effect of organophosphate and carbamate insecticides**

T60.0x1- **Toxic effect of organophosphate and carbamate insecticides, accidental (unintentional)**
Toxic effect of organophosphate and carbamate insecticides NOS

T60.0x2- **Toxic effect of organophosphate and carbamate insecticides, intentional self-harm**

T60.0x3- **Toxic effect of organophosphate and carbamate insecticides, assault**

T60.0x4- **Toxic effect of organophosphate and carbamate insecticides, undetermined**

T60.1- **Toxic effect of halogenated insecticides**

Excludes 1:   chlorinated hydrocarbon (T53.-)

T60.1 - DRUGS/CHEMS*		
2,4,5-T (trichloropheno	Diflubenzuron	PCP, meaning
xyacetic acid)	Endrin	pentachlorophenol
Aldrin (dust)	Heptachlor	PCP, meaning
Chlordan(e) (dust)	Insecticide, cchlorinated	pentachlorophenol,
Chlorex, insecticide	Insecticide, corganochlorine	insecticide
Chlorinated naphthalene	Isobenzan	Pentachlorophenol
(insecticide)	Kelevan	(pesticide)
Chlorophenothane	Kwell (insecticide)	Pentachlorophenol,
Compound 269 (endrin)	Mirex	insecticide
Compound 497 (dieldrin)	Moth balls,	Permethrin
Compound 3956 (toxaphene)	paradichlorobenzene	Pesticide, chlorinated
Cryolite (vapor)	Naphthalene, chlorinated	Pesticide, organochlorine
Cryolite, insecticide	Naphthalene, chlorinated,	(compounds)
Cyhalothrin	vapor	Sodium monofluoroacetate
Cypermethrin	Naphthalene, insecticide or	(pesticide)
DDT (dust)	moth repellent,	Strobane
Deltamethrin	chlorinated	Tar, camphor
Dieldrin (vapor)	Naphthalene, vapor,	Toxaphene (dust) (spray)
	chlorinated	

T60.1x- **Toxic effect of halogenated insecticides**

T60.1x1- **Toxic effect of halogenated insecticides, accidental (unintentional)**
Toxic effect of halogenated insecticides NOS

T60.1x2- **Toxic effect of halogenated insecticides, intentional self-harm**

T60.1x3- **Toxic effect of halogenated insecticides, assault**

T60.1x4- **Toxic effect of halogenated insecticides, undetermined**

T60.2- **Toxic effect of other insecticides**

T60.2 - DRUGS/CHEMS*		
Azadirachta	Endosulfan	Pesticide, naphthalene
Camphor, insecticide	Moth balls — see also	Phenothiazine, insecticide
Copper arsenate, arsenite,	Pesticides	Pyrethrin, pyrethrum
insecticide	Moth balls, naphthalene	(nonmedicinal)
Copper, insecticide	Naphthalene (non-	Rotenone
Cyphenothrin	chlorinated)	Sabadilla, pesticide
D-Con, insecticide	Naphthalene, insecticide or	Sodium selenate
DDE (bis(chlorophenyl)-	moth repellent	Tetramethrin
dichloroethylene)	Naphthalene, vapor	Vienna green, insecticide
Derris root	Nicotine (insecticide)	
	(spray) (sulfate) NEC	

T60.2x- **Toxic effect of other insecticides**

T60.2x1- **Toxic effect of other insecticides, accidental (unintentional)**
Toxic effect of other insecticides NOS

T60.2x2- **Toxic effect of other insecticides, intentional self-harm**

T60.2x3- **Toxic effect of other insecticides, assault**

T60.2x4- **Toxic effect of other insecticides, undetermined**

T60.3- **Toxic effect of herbicides and fungicides**

T60.3 - DRUGS/CHEMS*		
2,4-D	Dichloronaphthoquinone	Paraquat
(dichlorophenoxyacetic	2,4-Dichlorophenoxyacetic	PCP, meaning
acid)	acid	pentachlorophenol,
Ammonium sulfamate	Dichloropropene	fungicide
Antifungal, nonmedicinal	Dichloropropionic acid	PCP, meaning
(spray)	Dinoseb	pentachlorophenol,
Auramine fungicide	Diquat (dibromide)	herbicide
Benzimidazole	Diuron	Pentachlorophenol,
Bordeaux mixture	DNBP	fungicide
Bromoxynil	Endothall	Pentachlorophenol,
Captafol	Ethylidene diacetate	herbicide
Captan	Fertilizers with herbicide	Plant food or fertilizer,
Chlorate (potassium)	mixture	containing herbicide
(sodium) NEC	Folpet	Propachlor
Chlorate, herbicide	Formaldehyde, fungicide	Propanil
Chloroacetic acid	Formalin, fungicide	Simazine
Chloropicrin, fungicide	Fungicide NEC	Sodium cacodylate,
Chlorothalonil	(nonmedicinal)	herbicide
Copper, fungicide	Glyphosate	2,4,5-T
Copper sulfate, cupric,	HCB	Tetramethylthiuram
fungicide	Herbicide NEC	(disulfide) NEC
Copper sulfate, fungicide	Hexachlorobenzene (vapor)	Thiram
Cupric acetate	MCPA	TMTD
Cycloheximide	Mecoprop	Triazine (herbicide)
2,4-D	Methyl isothiocyanate	Triazole (herbicide)
Dalapon (sodium)	Methylchlorophenoxy-acetic	2,4,5-
Dicamba	acid	Trichlorophenoxyacetic
Dichlobenil	Monochloroacetic acid	acid
Dichlone	Monuron	Verdigris
	Paraformaldehyde	Weed killers NEC

T60.3x- **Toxic effect of herbicides and fungicides**

T60.3x1- **Toxic effect of herbicides and fungicides, accidental (unintentional)**
Toxic effect of herbicides and fungicides NOS

T60.3x2- **Toxic effect of herbicides and fungicides, intentional self-harm**

T60.3x3- **Toxic effect of herbicides and fungicides, assault**

T60.3x4- **Toxic effect of herbicides and fungicides, undetermined**

T60 - T60

T60.4- Toxic effect of rodenticides

> *Excludes 1:*   strychnine and its salts (T65.1)
> thallium (T56.81-)

T60.4 - DRUGS/CHEMS*	Crimidine	Rough-on-rats
ANTU (alpha naphthylthiourea)	D-Con, rodenticide	Scilla, rat poison
Barium, pesticide	Diphacinone	Scillaren
Barium, rodenticide	Diphenadione, rodenticide	Sodium fluoroacetate (dust) (pesticide)
Brodifacoum	Naphthylthiourea (ANTU)	Squill, rat poison
Bromethalin	Norbormide	Thallium, pesticide
Chloralose	Pesticide, thallium	Warfarin, rodenticide
Chlorophacinone	Pindone	Warfarin, sodium
Compound 1080 (sodium fluoroacetate)	Pyriminil	Zinc phosphide
	Rat poison NEC	
	Red squill (scilliroside)	
Coumadin, rodenticide	Rodenticide NEC	

T60.4x- Toxic effect of rodenticides

T60.4x1- Toxic effect of rodenticides, accidental (unintentional)
> Toxic effect of rodenticides NOS

T60.4x2- Toxic effect of rodenticides, intentional self-harm

T60.4x3- Toxic effect of rodenticides, assault

T60.4x4- Toxic effect of rodenticides, undetermined

T60.8- Toxic effect of other pesticides

T60.8 - DRUGS/CHEMS*	Fluoracetate	Petroleum, pesticide
Acaricide	Fluoride (nonmedicinal) (pesticide) (sodium) NEC	Phenol, pesticide
Antimony, pesticide (vapor)		Piperonyl butoxide
Azobenzene smoke, acaricide	Fluoroacetate	Seed disinfectant or dressing
	Metaldehyde (snail killer)	
Chlorinated pesticide NEC	NEC	Snail killer NEC
Chloropicrin, fumigant	Methyl bromide, fumigant	Tetradifon
Chloropicrin, pesticide	Pesticide, petroleum (distillate) (products)	
Deet	NEC	
Dibromochloropropane		
Diethyl toluamide (nonmedicinal)	Pesticide, specified ingredient NEC	

T60.8x- Toxic effect of other pesticides

T60.8x1- Toxic effect of other pesticides, accidental (unintentional)
> Toxic effect of other pesticides NOS

T60.8x2- Toxic effect of other pesticides, intentional self-harm

T60.8x3- Toxic effect of other pesticides, assault

T60.8x4- Toxic effect of other pesticides, undetermined

T60.9- Toxic effect of unspecified pesticide

T60.9 - DRUGS/CHEMS*	Black leaf (40)	Pesticide, mixture (of compounds)
Pesticide (dust) (fumes) (vapor) NEC	D-Con	
	Fumigant NEC	Preservative, wood
Antrol — see also by specific chemical substance	Horticulture agent with pesticide	Sulfur, pesticide (vapor)
Antrol, fungicide	Insecticide NEC	
Black flag	Insecticide, cmixed	

T60.91x- Toxic effect of unspecified pesticide, accidental (unintentional)

T60.92x- Toxic effect of unspecified pesticide, intentional self-harm

T60.93x- Toxic effect of unspecified pesticide, assault

T60.94x- Toxic effect of unspecified pesticide, undetermined

T61- Toxic effect of noxious substances eaten as seafood

> *Excludes 1:*   allergic reaction to food, such as:
> anaphylactic reaction or shock due to adverse food reaction (T78.0-)
> bacterial foodborne intoxications (A05.-)
> dermatitis (L23.6, L25.4, L27.2)
> food protein-induced enterocolitis syndrome (K52.21)
> food protein-induced enteropathy (K52.22)
> gastroenteritis (noninfective) (K52.29)
> toxic effect of aflatoxin and other mycotoxins (T64)
> toxic effect of cyanides (T65.0-)
> toxic effect of harmful algae bloom (T65.82-)
> toxic effect of hydrogen cyanide (T57.3-)
> toxic effect of mercury (T56.1-)
> toxic effect of red tide (T65.82-)

The appropriate 7th character is to be added to each code from category T61:
A   **Initial** encounter
D   **Subsequent** encounter
S   **Sequela**

T61.0- Ciguatera fish poisoning

T61.0 - DRUGS/CHEMS*	Fish, ciguatera
Ciguatoxin	

T61.01x- Ciguatera fish poisoning, accidental (unintentional)

T61.02x- Ciguatera fish poisoning, intentional self-harm

T61.03x- Ciguatera fish poisoning, assault

T61.04x- Ciguatera fish poisoning, undetermined

T61.1- Scombroid fish poisoning
> Histamine-like syndrome

T61.1 - DRUGS/CHEMS*	Scombrotoxin
Fish, scombroid	

T61.11x- Scombroid fish poisoning, accidental (unintentional)

T61.12x- Scombroid fish poisoning, intentional self-harm

T61.13x- Scombroid fish poisoning, assault

T61.14x- Scombroid fish poisoning, undetermined

T61.7- Other fish and shellfish poisoning

T61.77- Other fish poisoning

T61.77 - DRUGS/CHEMS*	Tetradotoxin
Fish, specified NEC	

T61.771- Other fish poisoning, accidental (unintentional)

T61.772- Other fish poisoning, intentional self-harm

T61.773- Other fish poisoning, assault

T61.774- Other fish poisoning, undetermined

T61.78- Other shellfish poisoning

T61.78 - DRUGS/CHEMS*	Food, shellfish	Shellfish, noxious, nonbacterial
Fish, shell	Mussel, noxious	

T61.781- Other shellfish poisoning, accidental (unintentional)

T61.782- Other shellfish poisoning, intentional self-harm

T61.783- Other shellfish poisoning, assault

T61.784- Other shellfish poisoning, undetermined

T61.8- Toxic effect of other seafood

T61.8 - DRUGS/CHEMS*	Food, seafood, specified NEC	Seafood, specified NEC

T61.8x- Toxic effect of other seafood

T61.8x1- Toxic effect of other seafood, accidental (unintentional)

T61.8x2- Toxic effect of other seafood, intentional self-harm

T61.8x3- Toxic effect of other seafood, assault

T61.8x4- Toxic effect of other seafood, undetermined

T61.9- Toxic effect of unspecified seafood

T61.9 - DRUGS/CHEMS*	Food, fish — see also Fish	Seafood
Fish, noxious, nonbacterial	Food, seafood	

T61.91x- Toxic effect of unspecified seafood, accidental (unintentional)

T61.92x- Toxic effect of unspecified seafood, intentional self-harm

T61.93x- Toxic effect of unspecified seafood, assault

T61.94x- Toxic effect of unspecified seafood, undetermined

T60 - T61

T62-   Toxic effect of <u>other noxious substances eaten as food</u>

Excludes 1:   allergic reaction to food, such as:
         anaphylactic shock (reaction) due to adverse food reaction
              (T78.0-)
         bacterial food borne intoxications (A05.-)
         dermatitis (L23.6, L25.4, L27.2)
         food protein-induced enterocolitis syndrome (K52.21)
         food protein-induced enteropathy (K52.22)
         gastroenteritis (noninfective) (K52.29)
      toxic effect of aflatoxin and other mycotoxins (T64)
      toxic effect of cyanides (T65.0-)
      toxic effect of hydrogen cyanide (T57.3-)
      toxic effect of mercury (T56.1-)

The appropriate 7th character is to be added to each code from
category T62:
  A   <u>Initial</u> encounter
  D   <u>Subsequent</u> encounter
  S   <u>Sequela</u>

T62.0-   Toxic effect of ingested mushrooms

T62.0 - DRUGS/CHEMS*	Food, mushrooms	Mushroom, noxious
Amanita phalloides	Fungi, noxious, used as	Toadstool
Amanitine	food	

T62.0x-   Toxic effect of <u>ingested mushrooms</u>

> **T62.0x1-   Toxic effect of ingested mushrooms, <u>accidental</u> (unintentional)**
>   Toxic effect of ingested mushrooms NOS

> **T62.0x2-   Toxic effect of ingested mushrooms, <u>intentional</u> self-harm**

> **T62.0x3-   Toxic effect of ingested mushrooms, <u>assault</u>**

> **T62.0x4-   Toxic effect of ingested mushrooms, <u>undetermined</u>**

T62.1-   Toxic effect of ingested berries

T62.1 - DRUGS/CHEMS*	Deadly nightshade, berry	Plant, noxious, used as
Actaea spicata, berry	Elder berry, (unripe)	food, berries
Akee	Food, berries	Poisonous berries
Anamirta cocculus	Mezereon berries	Privet berries
Berries, poisonous	Nightshade, deadly, berry	Sambucus canadensis berry
Cocculus indicus	Phytolacca decandra	Solanine berries
Convallaria majalis, berry	berries	Solanum dulcamara berries
Daphne, berry		

T62.1x-   Toxic effect of <u>ingested berries</u>

> **T62.1x1-   Toxic effect of ingested berries, <u>accidental</u> (unintentional)**
>   Toxic effect of ingested berries NOS

> **T62.1x2-   Toxic effect of ingested berries, <u>intentional</u> self-harm**

> **T62.1x3-   Toxic effect of ingested berries, <u>assault</u>**

> **T62.1x4-   Toxic effect of ingested berries, <u>undetermined</u>**

T62.2-   Toxic effect of other ingested (parts of) plant(s)

T62.2 - DRUGS/CHEMS*	Cuckoopint	Jamaica ginger, root
Abrine	Cyclamen europaeum	Jatropha
Abrus (seed)	Cytisus laburnum	Jatropha curcas
Actaea spicata	Cytisus scoparius	Jequirity (bean)
Aethusa cynapium	Daphne (gnidium)	Jimson weed (stramonium)
African boxwood	(mezereum)	Jimson weed, seeds
Amygdaline	Darnel	Kosam seed
Anemone pulsatilla	Deadly nightshade – see	Laburnum (seeds)
Bearsfoot	also Belladonna	Laburnum, leaves
Bittersweet	Delphinium	Larkspur
Black henbane	Elder	Lathyrus (seed)
Brucia	Equisetum	Laurel, black or cherry
Buttercups	Food, plants	Ligustrum vulgare
Calabar bean	Food, seeds	Lily of the valley
Caladium seguinum	Fool's parsley	Lobelia
Cassava	Foxglove	Lolium temulentum
Castor bean	Gaultheria procumbens	Meadow saffron
Cerbera (odallam)	Gelsemium (sempervirens)	Melia azedarach
Chelidonium majus	Goldylocks	Mezereon
Cherry laurel	Gratiola officinalis	Monkshood
Cicuta maculata or virosa	Green hellebore	Myristica fragrans
Cicutoxin	Hedge hyssop	Nerium oleander
Claviceps purpurea	Hellebore (black) (green)	Nicotiana (plant)
Clematis vitalba	(white)	Nightshade, deadly
Colchicum	Hemlock	(solanum) – see also
Coniine, conine	Henbane	Belladonna
Conium (maculatum)	Holly berries	Oleander
Convallaria majalis	Ilex	
Cowbane	Indian tobacco	

T62.2 - DRUGS/CHEMS*	Prunus virginiana	Tansy
— Contiued	Pulsatilla	Thornapple
Physostigma venenosum	Ranunculus	Tobacco, Indian
Phytolacca decandra	Ricin	Urtica
Piper cubeba	Ricinus communis	Veratrum, album
Plant, noxious, used as	Rue	Veratrum, viride
food	Ruta (graveolens)	Water, hemlock
Plant, noxious, used as	Sabadilla (plant)	White hellebore
food, seeds	Sambucus canadensis	Wild black cherry
Plant, noxious, used as	Sanguinaria canadensis	Wild poisonous plants NEC
food, specified type NEC	Seeds (poisonous)	Wisterine
Pokeweed (any part)	Solanine	Yellow jasmine
Pride of China	Solanum dulcamara	Yew
Primula (veris)	Spurge flax	Zygadenus (venenosus)
Privet	Spurges	
Prunus laurocerasus	Stramonium, natural state	

T62.2x-   Toxic effect of <u>other ingested (parts of) plant(s)</u>

> **T62.2x1-   Toxic effect of other ingested (parts of) plant(s), <u>accidental</u> (unintentional)**
>   Toxic effect of other ingested (parts of) plant(s) NOS

> **T62.2x2-   Toxic effect of other ingested (parts of) plant(s), <u>intentional</u> self-harm**

> **T62.2x3-   Toxic effect of other ingested (parts of) plant(s), <u>assault</u>**

> **T62.2x4-   Toxic effect of other ingested (parts of) plant(s), <u>undetermined</u>**

T62.8-   Toxic effect of other specified noxious substances eaten as food

T62.8 - DRUGS/CHEMS*	Food, specified NEC	Oil, bitter almond
Bitter almond oil	Meat, noxious	Pyrrolizidine alkaloids
Bone meal	Noxious foodstuff, specified	
Coffee	NEC	

T62.8x-   Toxic effect of <u>other specified noxious substances eaten as food</u>

> **T62.8x1-   Toxic effect of other specified noxious substances eaten as food, <u>accidental</u> (unintentional)**
>   Toxic effect of other specified noxious substances eaten as food NOS

> **T62.8x2-   Toxic effect of other specified noxious substances eaten as food, <u>intentional</u> self-harm**

> **T62.8x3-   Toxic effect of other specified noxious substances eaten as food, <u>assault</u>**

> **T62.8x4-   Toxic effect of other specified noxious substances eaten as food, <u>undetermined</u>**

T62.9-   Toxic effect of <u>unspecified noxious substance eaten as food</u>

T62.9 - DRUGS/CHEMS*	Food, foodstuffs, noxious,	Noxious foodstuff
	nonbacterial, NEC	

T62.91x-   Toxic effect of unspecified noxious substance eaten as food, <u>accidental</u> (unintentional)
   Toxic effect of unspecified noxious substance eaten as food NOS

T62.92x-   Toxic effect of unspecified noxious substance eaten as food, <u>intentional</u> self-harm

T62.93x-   Toxic effect of unspecified noxious substance eaten as food, <u>assault</u>

T62.94x-   Toxic effect of unspecified noxious substance eaten as food, <u>undetermined</u>

T6 2 - T6 2

T63- Toxic effect of <u>contact with venomous animals and plants</u>
  Includes: Bite or touch of venomous animal
              Pricked or stuck by thorn or leaf
  Excludes ❷: ingestion of toxic animal or plant (T61.-, T62.-)

The appropriate 7th character is to be added to each code from category T63:
  A <u>Initial</u> encounter
  D <u>Subsequent</u> encounter
  S <u>Sequela</u>

T63.0- Toxic effect of snake venom

T63.00- Toxic effect of <u>unspecified snake venom</u>

> **T63.00** - DRUGS/CHEMS*   Venom, snake
> Snake venom or bite

T63.001- Toxic effect of unspecified snake venom, <u>accidental</u> (unintentional)
  Toxic effect of unspecified snake venom NOS

T63.002- Toxic effect of unspecified snake venom, <u>intentional</u> self-harm

T63.003- Toxic effect of unspecified snake venom, <u>assault</u>

T63.004- Toxic effect of unspecified snake venom, <u>undetermined</u>

T63.01- Toxic effect of <u>rattlesnake venom</u>

> **T63.01** - DRUGS/CHEMS*   Venom, snake, rattlesnake
> Rattlesnake (venom)

T63.011- Toxic effect of rattlesnake venom, <u>accidental</u> (unintentional)
  Toxic effect of rattlesnake venom NOS

T63.012- Toxic effect of rattlesnake venom, <u>intentional</u> self-harm

T63.013- Toxic effect of rattlesnake venom, <u>assault</u>

T63.014- Toxic effect of rattlesnake venom, <u>undetermined</u>

T63.02- Toxic effect of <u>coral snake venom</u>

> **T63.02** - DRUGS/CHEMS*   Venom, snake, coral snake
> Coral snake (bite) (venom)

T63.021- Toxic effect of coral snake venom, <u>accidental</u> (unintentional)
  Toxic effect of coral snake venom NOS

T63.022- Toxic effect of coral snake venom, <u>intentional</u> self-harm

T63.023- Toxic effect of coral snake venom, <u>assault</u>

T63.024- Toxic effect of coral snake venom, <u>undetermined</u>

T63.03- Toxic effect of <u>taipan venom</u>

> **T63.03** - DRUGS/CHEMS*
> Venom, snake, taipan

T63.031- Toxic effect of taipan venom, <u>accidental</u> (unintentional)
  Toxic effect of taipan venom NOS

T63.032- Toxic effect of taipan venom, <u>intentional</u> self-harm

T63.033- Toxic effect of taipan venom, <u>assault</u>

T63.034- Toxic effect of taipan venom, <u>undetermined</u>

T63.04- Toxic effect of <u>cobra venom</u>

> **T63.04** - DRUGS/CHEMS*   Venom, snake, cobra
> Cobra (venom)

T63.041- Toxic effect of cobra venom, <u>accidental</u> (unintentional)
  Toxic effect of cobra venom NOS

T63.042- Toxic effect of cobra venom, <u>intentional</u> self-harm

T63.043- Toxic effect of cobra venom, <u>assault</u>

T63.044- Toxic effect of cobra venom, <u>undetermined</u>

T63.06- Toxic effect of venom of <u>other North and South American snake</u>

> **T63.06** - DRUGS/CHEMS*   Fer de lance (bite) (venom)   Water moccasin (venom)
> Copperhead snake (bite)   Venom, snake, American
> (venom)   (North) (South) NEC

T63.061- Toxic effect of venom of other North and South American snake, <u>accidental</u> (unintentional)
  Toxic effect of venom of other North and South American snake NOS

T63.062- Toxic effect of venom of other North and South American snake, <u>intentional</u> self-harm

T63.063- Toxic effect of venom of other North and South American snake, <u>assault</u>

T63.064- Toxic effect of venom of other North and South American snake, <u>undetermined</u>

T63.07- Toxic effect of venom of <u>other Australian snake</u>

> **T63.07** - DRUGS/CHEMS*
> Venom, snake, Australian

T63.071- Toxic effect of venom of other Australian snake, <u>accidental</u> (unintentional)
  Toxic effect of venom of other Australian snake NOS

T63.072- Toxic effect of venom of other Australian snake, <u>intentional</u> self-harm

T63.073- Toxic effect of venom of other Australian snake, <u>assault</u>

T63.074- Toxic effect of venom of other Australian snake, <u>undetermined</u>

T63.08- Toxic effect of venom of <u>other African and Asian snake</u>

> **T63.08** - DRUGS/CHEMS*   Venom, snake, Asian
> Venom, snake, African NEC

T63.081- Toxic effect of venom of other African and Asian snake, <u>accidental</u> (unintentional)
  Toxic effect of venom of other African and Asian snake NOS

T63.082- Toxic effect of venom of other African and Asian snake, <u>intentional</u> self-harm

T63.083- Toxic effect of venom of other African and Asian snake, <u>assault</u>

T63.084- Toxic effect of venom of other African and Asian snake, <u>undetermined</u>

T63.09- Toxic effect of <u>venom of other snake</u>

> **T63.09** - DRUGS/CHEMS*   Venom, snake, specified
> Krait (venom)   NEC
> Sea snake (bite) (venom)   Viper (venom)

T63.091- Toxic effect of venom of other snake, <u>accidental</u> (unintentional)
  Toxic effect of venom of other snake NOS

T63.092- Toxic effect of venom of other snake, <u>intentional</u> self-harm

T63.093- Toxic effect of venom of other snake, <u>assault</u>

T63.094- Toxic effect of venom of other snake, <u>undetermined</u>

T63.1- Toxic effect of <u>venom of other reptiles</u>

T63.11- Toxic effect of <u>venom of gila monster</u>

> **T63.11** - DRUGS/CHEMS*   Venom, reptile, gila
> Gila monster (venom)   monster

T63.111- Toxic effect of venom of gila monster, <u>accidental</u> (unintentional)
  Toxic effect of venom of gila monster NOS

T63.112- Toxic effect of venom of gila monster, <u>intentional</u> self-harm

T63.113- Toxic effect of venom of gila monster, <u>assault</u>

T63.114- Toxic effect of venom of gila monster, <u>undetermined</u>

T63.12- Toxic effect of <u>venom of other venomous lizard</u>

> **T63.12** - DRUGS/CHEMS*   Venom, lizard
> Lizard (bite) (venom)   Venom, reptile, lizard NEC

T63.121- Toxic effect of venom of other venomous lizard, <u>accidental</u> (unintentional)
  Toxic effect of venom of other venomous lizard NOS

T63.122- Toxic effect of venom of other venomous lizard, <u>intentional</u> self-harm

T63.123- Toxic effect of venom of other venomous lizard, <u>assault</u>

T63.124- Toxic effect of venom of other venomous lizard, <u>undetermined</u>

T63 - T63

T63.19- Toxic effect of <u>venom of other reptiles</u>

T63.19 - DRUGS/CHEMS*	
Venom, reptile	

T63.191- Toxic effect of venom of other reptiles, <u>accidental</u> (unintentional)

Toxic effect of venom of other reptiles NOS

T63.192- Toxic effect of venom of other reptiles, <u>intentional</u> self-harm

T63.193- Toxic effect of venom of other reptiles, <u>assault</u>

T63.194- Toxic effect of venom of other reptiles, <u>undetermined</u>

T63.2- Toxic effect of venom of scorpion

T63.2 - DRUGS/CHEMS*	
Venom, scorpion	

T63.2x- Toxic effect of <u>venom of scorpion</u>

T63.2x1- Toxic effect of venom of scorpion, <u>accidental</u> (unintentional)

Toxic effect of venom of scorpion NOS

T63.2x2- Toxic effect of venom of scorpion, <u>intentional</u> self-harm

T63.2x3- Toxic effect of venom of scorpion, <u>assault</u>

T63.2x4- Toxic effect of venom of scorpion, <u>undetermined</u>

T63.3- Toxic effect of venom of spider

T63.30- Toxic effect of <u>unspecified spider venom</u>

T63.30 - DRUGS/CHEMS*	
Venom, spider	

T63.301- Toxic effect of unspecified spider venom, <u>accidental</u> (unintentional)

T63.302- Toxic effect of unspecified spider venom, <u>intentional</u> self-harm

T63.303- Toxic effect of unspecified spider venom, <u>assault</u>

T63.304- Toxic effect of unspecified spider venom, <u>undetermined</u>

T63.31- Toxic effect of <u>venom of black widow spider</u>

T63.31 - DRUGS/CHEMS*	Venom, spider, black widow
Black widow spider (bite)	

T63.311- Toxic effect of venom of black widow spider, <u>accidental</u> (unintentional)

T63.312- Toxic effect of venom of black widow spider, <u>intentional</u> self-harm

T63.313- Toxic effect of venom of black widow spider, <u>assault</u>

T63.314- Toxic effect of venom of black widow spider, <u>undetermined</u>

T63.32- Toxic effect of <u>venom of tarantula</u>

T63.32 - DRUGS/CHEMS*	Venom, spider, tarantula
Tarantula (venomous)	

T63.321- Toxic effect of venom of tarantula, <u>accidental</u> (unintentional)

T63.322- Toxic effect of venom of tarantula, <u>intentional</u> self-harm

T63.323- Toxic effect of venom of tarantula, <u>assault</u>

T63.324- Toxic effect of venom of tarantula, <u>undetermined</u>

T63.33- Toxic effect of <u>venom of brown recluse spider</u>

T63.33 - DRUGS/CHEMS*	Venom, spider, brown
Brown recluse spider (bite) (venom)	recluse

T63.331- Toxic effect of venom of brown recluse spider, <u>accidental</u> (unintentional)

T63.332- Toxic effect of venom of brown recluse spider, <u>intentional</u> self-harm

T63.333- Toxic effect of venom of brown recluse spider, <u>assault</u>

T63.334- Toxic effect of venom of brown recluse spider, <u>undetermined</u>

T63.39- Toxic effect of <u>venom of other spider</u>

T63.39 - DRUGS/CHEMS*	Spider (bite) (venom)
Brown spider (bite) (venom)	Venom, spider, specified NEC

T63.391- Toxic effect of venom of other spider, <u>accidental</u> (unintentional)

T63.392- Toxic effect of venom of other spider, <u>intentional</u> self-harm

T63.393- Toxic effect of venom of other spider, <u>assault</u>

T63.394- Toxic effect of venom of other spider, <u>undetermined</u>

T63.4- Toxic effect of venom of other arthropods

T63.41- Toxic effect of <u>venom of centipedes and venomous millipedes</u>

T63.41 - DRUGS/CHEMS*	Millipede (tropical) (venomous)	Venom, millipede (tropical)
Centipede (bite)	Venom, centipede	

T63.411- Toxic effect of venom of centipedes and venomous millipedes, <u>accidental</u> (unintentional)

T63.412- Toxic effect of venom of centipedes and venomous millipedes, <u>intentional</u> self-harm

T63.413- Toxic effect of venom of centipedes and venomous millipedes, <u>assault</u>

T63.414- Toxic effect of venom of centipedes and venomous millipedes, <u>undetermined</u>

T63.42- Toxic effect of <u>venom of ants</u>

T63.42 - DRUGS/CHEMS*	Insect (sting), venomous, ant	Venom, ant
Ant (bite) (sting)		

T63.421- Toxic effect of venom of ants, <u>accidental</u> (unintentional)

T63.422- Toxic effect of venom of ants, <u>intentional</u> self-harm

T63.423- Toxic effect of venom of ants, <u>assault</u>

T63.424- Toxic effect of venom of ants, <u>undetermined</u>

T63.43- Toxic effect of <u>venom of caterpillars</u>

T63.43 - DRUGS/CHEMS*	Insect (sting), venomous, caterpillar
Caterpillar (sting)	

T63.431- Toxic effect of venom of caterpillars, <u>accidental</u> (unintentional)

T63.432- Toxic effect of venom of caterpillars, <u>intentional</u> self-harm

T63.433- Toxic effect of venom of caterpillars, <u>assault</u>

T63.434- Toxic effect of venom of caterpillars, <u>undetermined</u>

T63.44- Toxic effect of <u>venom of bees</u>

T63.44 - DRUGS/CHEMS*	Insect (sting), venomous, bee	Venom, bee
Bee (sting) (venom)		

T63.441- Toxic effect of venom of bees, <u>accidental</u> (unintentional)

T63.442- Toxic effect of venom of bees, <u>intentional</u> self-harm

T63.443- Toxic effect of venom of bees, <u>assault</u>

T63.444- Toxic effect of venom of bees, <u>undetermined</u>

T63.45- Toxic effect of <u>venom of hornets</u>

T63.45 - DRUGS/CHEMS*	Insect (sting), venomous, hornet	Venom, hornet
Hornet (sting)		

T63.451- Toxic effect of venom of hornets, <u>accidental</u> (unintentional)

T63.452- Toxic effect of venom of hornets, <u>intentional</u> self-harm

T63.453- Toxic effect of venom of hornets, <u>assault</u>

T63.454- Toxic effect of venom of hornets, <u>undetermined</u>

T63.46- Toxic effect of <u>venom of wasps</u>

Toxic effect of yellow jacket

T63.46 - DRUGS/CHEMS*	Venom, wasp
Insect (sting), venomous, wasp	Wasp (sting)

T63.461- Toxic effect of venom of wasps, <u>accidental</u> (unintentional)

T63 - T63

T63.462- Toxic effect of venom of wasps, <u>intentional</u> self-harm

T63.463- Toxic effect of venom of wasps, <u>assault</u>

T63.464- Toxic effect of venom of wasps, <u>undetermined</u>

T63.48- Toxic effect of <u>venom of other arthropod</u>

T63.48 - DRUGS/CHEMS*	Insect (sting), venomous	Venom, insect NEC
Arthropod (venomous) NEC	Venom, arthropod NEC	

T63.481- Toxic effect of venom of other arthropod, <u>accidental</u> (unintentional)

T63.482- Toxic effect of venom of other arthropod, <u>intentional</u> self-harm

T63.483- Toxic effect of venom of other arthropod, <u>assault</u>

T63.484- Toxic effect of venom of other arthropod, <u>undetermined</u>

T63.5- Toxic effect of <u>contact with venomous fish</u>

    Excludes ❷: poisoning by ingestion of fish (T61.-)

T63.51- Toxic effect of <u>contact with stingray</u>

T63.51 - DRUGS/CHEMS*	Venom, sting ray
Venom, marine, sting ray	

T63.511- Toxic effect of contact with stingray, <u>accidental</u> (unintentional)

T63.512- Toxic effect of contact with stingray, <u>intentional</u> self-harm

T63.513- Toxic effect of contact with stingray, <u>assault</u>

T63.514- Toxic effect of contact with stingray, <u>undetermined</u>

T63.59- Toxic effect of <u>contact with other venomous fish</u>

T63.59 - DRUGS/CHEMS*	Venom, marine, fish
Venom, fish	

T63.591- Toxic effect of contact with other venomous fish, <u>accidental</u> (unintentional)

T63.592- Toxic effect of contact with other venomous fish, <u>intentional</u> self-harm

T63.593- Toxic effect of contact with other venomous fish, <u>assault</u>

T63.594- Toxic effect of contact with other venomous fish, <u>undetermined</u>

T63.6- Toxic effect of <u>contact with other venomous marine animals</u>

    Excludes 1: sea-snake venom (T63.09)

    Excludes ❷: poisoning by ingestion of shellfish (T61.78-)

T63.61- Toxic effect of <u>contact with Portugese Man-o-war</u>

    Toxic effect of contact with bluebottle

T63.61 - DRUGS/CHEMS*	Venom, marine, animals,
Venom, marine, animals,	Portugese Man-o-war
bluebottle	

T63.611- Toxic effect of contact with Portugese Man-o-war, <u>accidental</u> (unintentional)

T63.612- Toxic effect of contact with Portugese Man-o-war, <u>intentional</u> self-harm

T63.613- Toxic effect of contact with Portugese Man-o-war, <u>assault</u>

T63.614- Toxic effect of contact with Portugese Man-o-war, <u>undetermined</u>

T63.62- Toxic effect of <u>contact with other jellyfish</u>

T63.62 - DRUGS/CHEMS*	Venom, marine, animals,
Jellyfish (sting)	jellyfish NEC

T63.621- Toxic effect of contact with other jellyfish, <u>accidental</u> (unintentional)

T63.622- Toxic effect of contact with other jellyfish, <u>intentional</u> self-harm

T63.623- Toxic effect of contact with other jellyfish, <u>assault</u>

T63.624- Toxic effect of contact with other jellyfish, <u>undetermined</u>

T63.63- Toxic effect of <u>contact with sea anemone</u>

T63.63 - DRUGS/CHEMS*	Venom, marine, animals,
Sea anemone (sting)	sea anemone

T63.631- Toxic effect of contact with sea anemone, <u>accidental</u> (unintentional)

T63.632- Toxic effect of contact with sea anemone, <u>intentional</u> self-harm

T63.633- Toxic effect of contact with sea anemone, <u>assault</u>

T63.634- Toxic effect of contact with sea anemone, <u>undetermined</u>

T63.69- Toxic effect of <u>contact with other venomous marine animals</u>

T63.69 - DRUGS/CHEMS*	Nematocyst (sting)	Venom, marine, animals,
Coral (sting)	Sea cucumber (sting)	specified NEC
Marine (sting)	Sea urchin spine (puncture)	
Marine, animals (sting)	Venom, marine, animals	

T63.691- Toxic effect of contact with other venomous marine animals, <u>accidental</u> (unintentional)

T63.692- Toxic effect of contact with other venomous marine animals, <u>intentional</u> self-harm

T63.693- Toxic effect of contact with other venomous marine animals, <u>assault</u>

T63.694- Toxic effect of contact with other venomous marine animals, <u>undetermined</u>

T63.7- Toxic effect of contact with venomous plant

T63.71- Toxic effect of <u>contact with venomous marine plant</u>

T63.71 - DRUGS/CHEMS*	Venom, marine, plants
Marine, plants (sting)	Venom, plant, marine

T63.711- Toxic effect of contact with venomous marine plant, <u>accidental</u> (unintentional)

T63.712- Toxic effect of contact with venomous marine plant, <u>intentional</u> self-harm

T63.713- Toxic effect of contact with venomous marine plant, <u>assault</u>

T63.714- Toxic effect of contact with venomous marine plant, <u>undetermined</u>

T63.79- Toxic effect of <u>contact with other venomous plant</u>

T63.79 - DRUGS/CHEMS*
Venom, plant NEC

T63.791- Toxic effect of contact with other venomous plant, <u>accidental</u> (unintentional)

T63.792- Toxic effect of contact with other venomous plant, <u>intentional</u> self-harm

T63.793- Toxic effect of contact with other venomous plant, <u>assault</u>

T63.794- Toxic effect of contact with other venomous plant, <u>undetermined</u>

T63.8- Toxic effect of contact with other venomous animals

T63.81- Toxic effect of <u>contact with venomous frog</u>

    Excludes 1: contact with nonvenomous frog (W62.0)

T63.81 - DRUGS/CHEMS*
Venom, frog

T63.811- Toxic effect of contact with venomous frog, <u>accidental</u> (unintentional)

T63.812- Toxic effect of contact with venomous frog, <u>intentional</u> self-harm

T63.813- Toxic effect of contact with venomous frog, <u>assault</u>

T63.814- Toxic effect of contact with venomous frog, <u>undetermined</u>

T63.82- Toxic effect of contact <u>with venomous toad</u>

    Excludes 1: contact with nonvenomous toad (W62.1)

T63.82 - DRUGS/CHEMS*
Venom, toad

T63.821- Toxic effect of contact with venomous toad, <u>accidental</u> (unintentional)

T63.822- Toxic effect of contact with venomous toad, <u>intentional</u> self-harm

T63.823- Toxic effect of contact with venomous toad, <u>assault</u>

T63.824- Toxic effect of contact with venomous toad, <u>undetermined</u>

T
6
3
-
T
6
3

T63.83- Toxic effect of contact <u>with other venomous amphibian</u>
  Excludes 1:   contact with nonvenomous amphibian (W62.9)

T63.83 - DRUGS/CHEMS*
Venom, amphibian NEC

    T63.831- Toxic effect of contact with other venomous amphibian, <u>accidental</u> (unintentional)
    T63.832- Toxic effect of contact with other venomous amphibian, <u>intentional</u> self-harm
    T63.833- Toxic effect of contact with other venomous amphibian, <u>assault</u>
    T63.834- Toxic effect of contact with other venomous amphibian, <u>undetermined</u>

T63.89- Toxic effect of contact <u>with other venomous animals</u>

T63.89 - DRUGS/CHEMS*
Venom, animal NEC

    T63.891- Toxic effect of contact with other venomous animals, <u>accidental</u> (unintentional)
    T63.892- Toxic effect of contact with other venomous animals, <u>intentional</u> self-harm
    T63.893- Toxic effect of contact with other venomous animals, <u>assault</u>
    T63.894- Toxic effect of contact with other venomous animals, <u>undetermined</u>

T63.9- Toxic effect of contact with <u>unspecified venomous animal</u>

T63.9 - DRUGS/CHEMS*
Venom, venomous (bite) (sting)

    T63.91x- Toxic effect of contact with unspecified venomous animal, <u>accidental</u> (unintentional)
    T63.92x- Toxic effect of contact with unspecified venomous animal, <u>intentional</u> self-harm
    T63.93x- Toxic effect of contact with unspecified venomous animal, <u>assault</u>
    T63.94x- Toxic effect of contact with unspecified venomous animal, <u>undetermined</u>

T64- Toxic effect of <u>aflatoxin and other mycotoxin food contaminants</u>
The appropriate 7th character is to be added to each code from category T64:
  A   <u>Initial</u> encounter
  D   <u>Subsequent</u> encounter
  S   <u>Sequela</u>

T64.0- Toxic effect of <u>aflatoxin</u>

T64.0 - DRUGS/CHEMS*	Mycotoxins, aflatoxin
Aflatoxin	

    T64.01x- Toxic effect of aflatoxin, <u>accidental</u> (unintentional)
    T64.02x- Toxic effect of aflatoxin, <u>intentional</u> self-harm
    T64.03x- Toxic effect of aflatoxin, <u>assault</u>
    T64.04x- Toxic effect of aflatoxin, <u>undetermined</u>

T64.8- Toxic effect of <u>other mycotoxin food contaminants</u>

T64.8 - DRUGS/CHEMS*	Mycotoxins
Ergot NEC	Mycotoxins, specified NEC

    T64.81x- Toxic effect of other mycotoxin food contaminants, <u>accidental</u> (unintentional)
    T64.82x- Toxic effect of other mycotoxin food contaminants, <u>intentional</u> self-harm
    T64.83x- Toxic effect of other mycotoxin food contaminants, <u>assault</u>
    T64.84x- Toxic effect of other mycotoxin food contaminants, <u>undetermined</u>

T65- Toxic effect of <u>other and unspecified substances</u>
The appropriate 7th character is to be added to each code from category T65:
  A   <u>Initial</u> encounter
  D   <u>Subsequent</u> encounter
  S   <u>Sequela</u>

T65.0- Toxic effect of cyanides
  Excludes 1:   hydrogen cyanide (T57.3-)

T65.0 - DRUGS/CHEMS*	Cyanide(s), pesticide (dust)	Potassium cyanide
2,4-toluene diisocyanate	(fumes)	Prussic acid
Aliphatic thiocyanates	Dicyanogen (gas)	Sodium cyanide
Alkylisocyanate	Gas, dicyanogen	TDI (vapor)
Cyanide(s) (compounds)	Gas, hydrocyanic acid	Toluene diisocyanate
(potassium) (sodium)	Hydrocyanic acid, gas	Tolylene-2,4-diisocyanate
NEC	Isocyanate	
Cyanide(s), fumigant	Pesticide, cyanide	

  T65.0x- Toxic effect of <u>cyanides</u>
    T65.0x1- Toxic effect of cyanides, <u>accidental</u> (unintentional)
      Toxic effect of cyanides NOS
    T65.0x2- Toxic effect of cyanides, <u>intentional</u> self-harm
    T65.0x3- Toxic effect of cyanides, <u>assault</u>
    T65.0x4- Toxic effect of cyanides, <u>undetermined</u>

T65.1- Toxic effect of <u>strychnine and its salts</u>

T65.1 - DRUGS/CHEMS*	Nux vomica	Strychnine (nonmedicinal)
Brucine	Pesticide, strychnine	(pesticide) (salts)

  T65.1x- Toxic effect of <u>strychnine and its salts</u>
    T65.1x1- Toxic effect of strychnine and its salts, <u>accidental</u> (unintentional)
      Toxic effect of strychnine and its salts NOS
    T65.1x2- Toxic effect of strychnine and its salts, <u>intentional</u> self-harm
    T65.1x3- Toxic effect of strychnine and its salts, <u>assault</u>
    T65.1x4- Toxic effect of strychnine and its salts, <u>undetermined</u>

T65.2- Toxic effect of tobacco and nicotine
  Excludes 2:   nicotine dependence (F17.-)

T65.21- Toxic effect of <u>chewing tobacco</u>

T65.21 - DRUGS/CHEMS*
Snuff

    T65.211- Toxic effect of chewing tobacco, <u>accidental</u> (unintentional)
      Toxic effect of chewing tobacco NOS
    T65.212- Toxic effect of chewing tobacco, <u>intentional</u> self-harm
    T65.213- Toxic effect of chewing tobacco, <u>assault</u>
    T65.214- Toxic effect of chewing tobacco, <u>undetermined</u>

T65.22- Toxic effect of <u>tobacco cigarettes</u>
    Toxic effect of tobacco smoke
    Use additional code for exposure to second hand tobacco smoke (Z57.31, Z77.22)

T65.22 - DRUGS/CHEMS*	Nicotine from tobacco,	Tobacco smoke, second-
Cigarettes (tobacco)	cigarettes	hand
	Tobacco, cigarettes	

    T65.221- Toxic effect of tobacco cigarettes, <u>accidental</u> (unintentional)
      Toxic effect of tobacco cigarettes NOS
    T65.222- Toxic effect of tobacco cigarettes, <u>intentional</u> self-harm
    T65.223- Toxic effect of tobacco cigarettes, <u>assault</u>
    T65.224- Toxic effect of tobacco cigarettes, <u>undetermined</u>

T65.29- Toxic effect of <u>other tobacco and nicotine</u>

T65.29 - DRUGS/CHEMS*	Nicotine, not insecticide
Nicotine from tobacco	Tobacco NEC

    T65.291- Toxic effect of other tobacco and nicotine, <u>accidental</u> (unintentional)
      Toxic effect of other tobacco and nicotine NOS
    T65.292- Toxic effect of other tobacco and nicotine, <u>intentional</u> self-harm

T63 - T65

T65.293- Toxic effect of other tobacco and nicotine, <u>assault</u>

T65.294- Toxic effect of other tobacco and nicotine, <u>undetermined</u>

T65.3- Toxic effect of nitroderivatives and aminoderivatives of benzene and its homologues
Toxic effect of anilin [benzenamine]
Toxic effect of nitrobenzene
Toxic effect of trinitrotoluene

<u>T65.3</u> - DRUGS/CHEMS*	Dinitrophenol	Phenyl enediamine
Aniline (dye) (liquid)	Diphenylamine	Phenyl hydrazine
Aniline vapor	DNOC	Phenylenediamine
Anisidine	Dynamite	Tetryl
Azobenzene smoke	Methoxyaniline	TNT (fumes)
Benzenamine	Methyl aminophenol	Toluylenediamine
Binitrobenzol	Nitramine	Trinitrobenzol
Dichlorbenzidine	Nitroaniline	Trinitrophenol
Dinitro (-ortho-)cresol (pesticide) (spray)	Nitrobenzene, nitrobenzol	Trinitrotoluene (fumes)
	Nitrobenzene, vapor	
Dinitrobenzene	Nitrodiphenyl	
Dinitrobenzol	Nitrosodimethylamine	
Dinitrobutylphenol	Nitrotoluene, nitrotoluol	
Dinitrocyclohexylphenol	Nitrotoluene, vapor	

T65.3x- Toxic effect of <u>nitroderivatives and aminoderivatives of benzene and its homologues</u>

T65.3x1- Toxic effect of nitroderivatives and aminoderivatives of benzene and its homologues, <u>accidental</u> (unintentional)
Toxic effect of nitroderivatives and aminoderivatives of benzene and its homologues NOS

T65.3x2- Toxic effect of nitroderivatives and aminoderivatives of benzene and its homologues, <u>intentional</u> self-harm

T65.3x3- Toxic effect of nitroderivatives and aminoderivatives of benzene and its homologues, <u>assault</u>

T65.3x4- Toxic effect of nitroderivatives and aminoderivatives of benzene and its homologues, <u>undetermined</u>

T65.4- Toxic effect of carbon disulfide

<u>T65.4</u> - DRUGS/CHEMS*	Carbon bisulfide vapor	Carbon disulfide, vapor
Carbon bisulfide (liquid)	Carbon disulfide (liquid)	Varnish

T65.4x- Toxic effect of <u>carbon disulfide</u>

T65.4x1- Toxic effect of carbon disulfide, <u>accidental</u> (unintentional)
Toxic effect of carbon disulfide NOS

T65.4x2- Toxic effect of carbon disulfide, <u>intentional</u> self-harm

T65.4x3- Toxic effect of carbon disulfide, <u>assault</u>

T65.4x4- Toxic effect of carbon disulfide, <u>undetermined</u>

T65.5- Toxic effect of nitroglycerin and other nitric acids and esters
Toxic effect of 1,2,3-Propanetriol trinitrate

<u>T65.5</u> - DRUGS/CHEMS*	Nitroglycerin,
Nitroglycerin, nonmedicinal	nonmedicinal, fumes

T65.5x- Toxic effect of <u>nitroglycerin and other nitric acids and esters</u>

T65.5x1- Toxic effect of nitroglycerin and other nitric acids and esters, <u>accidental</u> (unintentional)
Toxic effect of nitroglycerin and other nitric acids and esters NOS

T65.5x2- Toxic effect of nitroglycerin and other nitric acids and esters, <u>intentional</u> self-harm

T65.5x3- Toxic effect of nitroglycerin and other nitric acids and esters, <u>assault</u>

T65.5x4- Toxic effect of nitroglycerin and other nitric acids and esters, <u>undetermined</u>

T65.6- Toxic effect of paints and dyes, not elsewhere classified

<u>T65.6</u> - DRUGS/CHEMS*	Cochineal	Oil, colors
Acridine	Dye NEC	Paint NEC
Auramine dye	Lacquer	Stains

T65.6x- Toxic effect of <u>paints and dyes</u>, <u>not elsewhere classified</u>

T65.6x1- Toxic effect of paints and dyes, not elsewhere classified, <u>accidental</u> (unintentional)
Toxic effect of paints and dyes NOS

T65.6x2- Toxic effect of paints and dyes, not elsewhere classified, <u>intentional</u> self-harm

T65.6x3- Toxic effect of paints and dyes, not elsewhere classified, <u>assault</u>

T65.6x4- Toxic effect of paints and dyes, not elsewhere classified, <u>undetermined</u>

T65.8- Toxic effect of other specified substances

T65.81- Toxic effect of <u>latex</u>

<u>T65.81</u> - DRUGS/CHEMS*
Latex

T65.811- Toxic effect of latex, <u>accidental</u> (unintentional)
Toxic effect of latex NOS

T65.812- Toxic effect of latex, <u>intentional</u> self-harm

T65.813- Toxic effect of latex, <u>assault</u>

T65.814- Toxic effect of latex, <u>undetermined</u>

T65.82- Toxic effect of <u>harmful algae and algae toxins</u>
Toxic effect of (harmful) algae bloom NOS
Toxic effect of blue-green algae bloom
Toxic effect of brown tide
Toxic effect of cyanobacteria bloom
Toxic effect of Florida red tide
Toxic effect of pfiesteria piscicida
Toxic effect of red tide

<u>T65.82</u> - DRUGS/CHEMS*
Algae (harmful) (toxin)

T65.821- Toxic effect of harmful algae and algae toxins, <u>accidental</u> (unintentional)
Toxic effect of harmful algae and algae toxins NOS

T65.822- Toxic effect of harmful algae and algae toxins, <u>intentional</u> self-harm

T65.823- Toxic effect of harmful algae and algae toxins, <u>assault</u>

T65.824- Toxic effect of harmful algae and algae toxins, <u>undetermined</u>

T65.83- Toxic effect of <u>fiberglass</u>

<u>T65.83</u> - DRUGS/CHEMS*
Fiberglass

T65.831- Toxic effect of fiberglass, <u>accidental</u> (unintentional)
Toxic effect of fiberglass NOS

T65.832- Toxic effect of fiberglass, <u>intentional</u> self-harm

T65.833- Toxic effect of fiberglass, <u>assault</u>

T65.834- Toxic effect of fiberglass, <u>undetermined</u>

T65 - T65

T65.89- Toxic effect of <u>other specified substances</u>

<u>T65.89 - DRUGS/CHEMS*</u>	Naphthol	Reducing agent, industrial
Acetaldehyde liquid	Naphthylamine	NEC
Acetic anhydride	Nitrocellulose	Resorcin, resorcinol
Acrylamide	Nitrocellulose, lacquer	(nonmedicinal)
Acrylonitrile	Nitronaphthalene	Scouring powder
Adhesive NEC	Oil (of)	Silicone NEC
Amyl propionate	PBB (polybrominated	Sodium bisulfate
Antiaris toxicaria	biphenyls)	Sodium chlorate NEC
Auramine	PCB	Sodium chromate
Benzidine	Permanganate	Sodium metasilicate
Bergamot oil	Phosphate	Sodium nitrate (oxidizing
Cleaner, cleansing agent,	Phosphate, tricresyl	agent)
type not specified	Phthalates	Sodium oxalate
Cleaner, specified type NEC	Phthalic anhydride	Sodium oxide/peroxide
Cordite	Pine oil (disinfectant)	Sodium perborate
Diethylhexylphthalate	Pitch	(nonmedicinal) NEC
Dimethyl sulfate, liquid	Plant food or fertilizer NEC	Soldering fluid
Disinfectant	Polish (car) (floor)	Solid substance, specified
Epoxy resin	(furniture) (metal)	NEC
Fertilizers NEC	(porcelain) (silver)	Spray, cosmetic
Furniture polish	Polish, abrasive	Styrene
Glutaral, nonmedicinal	Polish, porcelain	Tartaric acid
Glutaraldehyde	Polychlorinated biphenyl	Thioglycolic acid
(nonmedicinal)	Potassium chlorate NEC	Toilet deodorizer
Grease	Potassium ferric	Toluidine
Guano	hexacyanoferrate,	Tricresyl phosphate
Ink	nonmedicinal	Triorthocresyl phosphate
Isophorone	Potassium oxalate	Triphenylphosphate
Jamaica ginger	Potassium perchlorate	Vinyl acetate
Liquid, specified NEC	(nonmedicinal) NEC	Vinyl bromide
Liquor creosolis compositus	Potassium permanganate	Vinylidene chloride
Methyl acrylate	(nonmedicinal)	Wax, automobile
Methyl hydrazine	Preservative	Whitewash
Methyl iodide	(nonmedicinal)	Window cleaning fluid
Monosodium glutamate	Prussian blue, commercial	
Myristicin	Psoralene (nonmedicinal)	

T65.891- Toxic effect of other specified substances, <u>accidental</u> (unintentional)
Toxic effect of other specified substances NOS

T65.892- Toxic effect of other specified substances, <u>intentional</u> self-harm

T65.893- Toxic effect of other specified substances, <u>assault</u>

T65.894- Toxic effect of other specified substances, <u>undetermined</u>

T65.9- Toxic effect of <u>unspecified substance</u>

<u>T65.9 - DRUGS/CHEMS*</u>	Bismuth salts,	Liquid substance
Agricultural agent NEC	nonmedicinal	Poison NEC
Aerosol spray NEC	(compounds) NEC	Solid substance
Air contaminant (s),	Chemical substance NEC	Spray (aerosol)
source/type NOS	Horticulture agent NEC	
Antifreeze	Ingested substance NEC	

T65.91x- Toxic effect of unspecified substance, <u>accidental</u> (unintentional)
Poisoning NOS

T65.92x- Toxic effect of unspecified substance, <u>intentional</u> self-harm

T65.93x- Toxic effect of unspecified substance, <u>assault</u>

T65.94x- Toxic effect of unspecified substance, <u>undetermined</u>

Other and unspecified effects of external causes (T66-T78)

T66.xxx- Radiation sickness, <u>unspecified</u>
Excludes 1: radiation gastroenteritis and colitis (K52.0)
radiation pneumonitis (J70.0)
radiation related disorders of the skin and subcutaneous tissue (L55-L59)
specified adverse effects of radiation, such as:
burns (T20-T31)
leukemia (C91-C95)
sunburn (L55.-)

The appropriate 7th character is to be added to code T66:
A <u>Initial</u> encounter
D <u>Subsequent</u> encounter
S <u>Sequela</u>

T67- Effects of heat and light
Excludes 1: erythema [dermatitis] ab igne (L59.0)
malignant hyperpyrexia due to anesthesia (T88.3)
radiation-related disorders of the skin and subcutaneous tissue (L55-L59)
Excludes 2: burns (T20-T31)
sunburn (L55.-)
sweat disorder due to heat (L74-L75)

The appropriate 7th character is to be added to each code from category T67:
A <u>Initial</u> encounter
D <u>Subsequent</u> encounter
S <u>Sequela</u>

T67.0xx- Heatstroke and sunstroke
CC-A
Heat apoplexy
Heat pyrexia
Siriasis
Thermoplegia
Use additional code(s) to identify any associated complications of heatstroke, such as:
Coma and stupor (R40.-)
Systemic inflammatory response syndrome (R65.1-)

T67.1xx- Heat syncope
Heat collapse

T67.2xx- Heat cramp

T67.3xx- Heat exhaustion, anhydrotic
Heat prostration due to water depletion
Excludes 1: heat exhaustion due to salt depletion (T67.4)

T67.4xx- Heat exhaustion due to salt depletion
Heat prostration due to salt (and water) depletion

T67.5xx- Heat exhaustion, <u>unspecified</u>
Heat prostration NOS

T67.6xx- Heat fatigue, transient

T67.7xx- Heat edema

T67.8xx- Other effects of heat and light

T67.9xx- Effect of heat and light, <u>unspecified</u>

T68xxx- Hypothermia
Accidental hypothermia
Hypothermia NOS
Use additional code to identify source of exposure:
Exposure to excessive cold of man-made origin (W93)
Exposure to excessive cold of natural origin (X31)
Excludes 1: hypothermia following anesthesia (T88.51)
hypothermia not associated with low environmental temperature (R68.0)
hypothermia of newborn (P80.-)
Excludes 2: frostbite (T33-T34)

The appropriate 7th character is to be added to code T68:
A <u>Initial</u> encounter
D <u>Subsequent</u> encounter
S <u>Sequela</u>

T65 - T68

T69-   Other effects of reduced temperature
Use additional code to identify source of exposure:
Exposure to excessive cold of man-made origin (W93)
Exposure to excessive cold of natural origin (X31)
Excludes ❷: *frostbite (T33-T34)*
The appropriate 7th character is to be added to each code from category T69:
A   Initial encounter
D   Subsequent encounter
S   Sequela

T69.0-   Immersion hand and foot
    T69.01-   Immersion hand
       T69.011-   Immersion hand, right hand
       T69.012-   Immersion hand, left hand
       T69.019-   Immersion hand, unspecified hand
    T69.02-   Immersion foot
          Trench foot
   CC-A **T69.021-**   Immersion foot, right foot
   CC-A **T69.022-**   Immersion foot, left foot
   CC-A **T69.029-**   Immersion foot, unspecified foot
T69.1xx-   Chilblains
T69.8xx-   Other specified effects of reduced temperature
T69.9xx-   Effect of reduced temperature, unspecified

T70-   Effects of air pressure and water pressure
The appropriate 7th character is to be added to each code from category T70:
A   Initial encounter
D   Subsequent encounter
S   Sequela

T70.0xx-   Otitic barotrauma
          Aero-otitis media
          Effects of change in ambient atmospheric pressure or water pressure on ears
T70.1xx-   Sinus barotrauma
          Aerosinusitis
          Effects of change in ambient atmospheric pressure on sinuses
T70.2-   Other and unspecified effects of high altitude
       Excludes ❷: *polycythemia due to high altitude (D75.1)*
    T70.20x-   Unspecified effects of high altitude
    T70.29x-   Other effects of high altitude
          Alpine sickness
          Anoxia due to high altitude
          Barotrauma NOS
          Hypobaropathy
          Mountain sickness
T70.3xx-   Caisson disease [decompression sickness]
  CC-A
          Compressed-air disease
          Diver's palsy or paralysis
T70.4xx-   Effects of high-pressure fluids
          Hydraulic jet injection (industrial)
          Pneumatic jet injection (industrial)
          Traumatic jet injection (industrial)
T70.8xx-   Other effects of air pressure and water pressure
T70.9xx-   Effect of air pressure and water pressure, unspecified

T71-   Asphyxiation
Mechanical suffocation
Traumatic suffocation
Excludes 1:   *acute respiratory distress (syndrome) (J80)*
           anoxia due to high altitude (T70.2)
           asphyxia NOS (R09.01)
           asphyxia from carbon monoxide (T58-)
           asphyxia from inhalation of food or foreign body (T17-)
           asphyxia from other gases, fumes and vapors (T59-)
           respiratory distress (syndrome) in newborn (P22-)
The appropriate 7th character is to be added to each code from category T71:
A   Initial encounter
D   Subsequent encounter
S   Sequela

T71.1-   Asphyxiation due to mechanical threat to breathing
          Suffocation due to mechanical threat to breathing
    T71.11-   Asphyxiation due to smothering under pillow
   CC-A **T71.111-**   Asphyxiation due to smothering under pillow, accidental
          Asphyxiation due to smothering under pillow NOS
   CC-A **T71.112-**   Asphyxiation due to smothering under pillow, intentional self-harm
   CC-A **T71.113-**   Asphyxiation due to smothering under pillow, assault
   CC-A **T71.114-**   Asphyxiation due to smothering under pillow, undetermined
    T71.12-   Asphyxiation due to plastic bag
   CC-A **T71.121-**   Asphyxiation due to plastic bag, accidental
          Asphyxiation due to plastic bag NOS
   CC-A **T71.122-**   Asphyxiation due to plastic bag, intentional self-harm
   CC-A **T71.123-**   Asphyxiation due to plastic bag, assault
   CC-A **T71.124-**   Asphyxiation due to plastic bag, undetermined
    T71.13-   Asphyxiation due to being trapped in bed linens
   CC-A **T71.131-**   Asphyxiation due to being trapped in bed linens, accidental
          Asphyxiation due to being trapped in bed linens NOS
   CC-A **T71.132-**   Asphyxiation due to being trapped in bed linens, intentional self-harm
   CC-A **T71.133-**   Asphyxiation due to being trapped in bed linens, assault
   CC-A **T71.134-**   Asphyxiation due to being trapped in bed linens, undetermined
    T71.14-   Asphyxiation due to smothering under another person's body (in bed)
   CC-A **T71.141-**   Asphyxiation due to smothering under another person's body (in bed), accidental
          Asphyxiation due to smothering under another person's body (in bed) NOS
   CC-A **T71.143-**   Asphyxiation due to smothering under another person's body (in bed), assault
   CC-A **T71.144-**   Asphyxiation due to smothering under another person's body (in bed), undetermined
    T71.15-   Asphyxiation due to smothering in furniture
   CC-A **T71.151-**   Asphyxiation due to smothering in furniture, accidental
          Asphyxiation due to smothering in furniture NOS
   CC-A **T71.152-**   Asphyxiation due to smothering in furniture, intentional self-harm
   CC-A **T71.153-**   Asphyxiation due to smothering in furniture, assault
   CC-A **T71.154-**   Asphyxiation due to smothering in furniture, undetermined

T69 - T71

T71.16- Asphyxiation due to <u>hanging</u>
Hanging by window shade cord
Use additional code for any associated injuries, such as:
Crushing injury of neck (S17.-)
Fracture of cervical vertebrae (S12.0-S12.2-)
Open wound of neck (S11.-)

CC-A **T71.161-** Asphyxiation due to hanging, <u>accidental</u>
Asphyxiation due to hanging NOS
Hanging NOS

CC-A **T71.162-** Asphyxiation due to hanging, <u>intentional</u> self-harm

CC-A **T71.163-** Asphyxiation due to hanging, <u>assault</u>

CC-A **T71.164-** Asphyxiation due to hanging, <u>undetermined</u>

T71.19- Asphyxiation due to <u>mechanical threat to breathing due to other causes</u>

CC-A **T71.191-** Asphyxiation due to mechanical threat to breathing due to other causes, <u>accidental</u>
Asphyxiation due to other causes NOS

CC-A **T71.192-** Asphyxiation due to mechanical threat to breathing due to other causes, <u>intentional</u> self-harm

CC-A **T71.193-** Asphyxiation due to mechanical threat to breathing due to other causes, <u>assault</u>

CC-A **T71.194-** Asphyxiation due to mechanical threat to breathing due to other causes, <u>undetermined</u>

T71.2- Asphyxiation due to <u>systemic oxygen deficiency due to low oxygen content in ambient air</u>
Suffocation due to systemic oxygen deficiency due to low oxygen content in ambient air

CC-A **T71.20x-** Asphyxiation due to systemic oxygen deficiency due to low oxygen content in ambient air due to <u>unspecified cause</u>

CC-A **T71.21x-** Asphyxiation due to <u>cave-in or falling earth</u>
Use additional code for any associated cataclysm (X34-X38)

T71.22- Asphyxiation due to <u>being trapped in a car trunk</u>

CC-A **T71.221-** Asphyxiation due to being trapped in a car trunk, <u>accidental</u>

CC-A **T71.222-** Asphyxiation due to being trapped in a car trunk, <u>intentional</u> self-harm

CC-A **T71.223-** Asphyxiation due to being trapped in a car trunk, <u>assault</u>

CC-A **T71.224-** Asphyxiation due to being trapped in a car trunk, <u>undetermined</u>

T71.23- Asphyxiation due to <u>being trapped in a (discarded) refrigerator</u>

CC-A **T71.231-** Asphyxiation due to being trapped in a (discarded) refrigerator, <u>accidental</u>

CC-A **T71.232-** Asphyxiation due to being trapped in a (discarded) refrigerator, <u>intentional</u> self-harm

CC-A **T71.233-** Asphyxiation due to being trapped in a (discarded) refrigerator, <u>assault</u>

CC-A **T71.234-** Asphyxiation due to being trapped in a (discarded) refrigerator, <u>undetermined</u>

CC-A **T71.29x-** Asphyxiation due to <u>being trapped in other low oxygen environment</u>

T71.9xx- Asphyxiation due to <u>unspecified cause</u>
CC-A Suffocation (by strangulation) due to unspecified cause
Suffocation NOS
Systemic oxygen deficiency due to low oxygen content in ambient air due to unspecified cause
Systemic oxygen deficiency due to mechanical threat to breathing due to unspecified cause
Traumatic asphyxia NOS

T73- Effects of other deprivation
The appropriate 7th character is to be added to each code from category T73:
A <u>Initial</u> encounter
D <u>Subsequent</u> encounter
S <u>Sequela</u>

T73.0xx- Starvation
Deprivation of food

T73.1xx- Deprivation of water

T73.2xx- Exhaustion due to exposure

T73.3xx- Exhaustion due to excessive exertion
Exhaustion due to overexertion

T73.8xx- Other effects of deprivation

T73.9xx- Effect of deprivation, unspecified

T74- Adult and child abuse, neglect and other maltreatment, <u>confirmed</u>
Use additional code, if applicable, to identify any associated current injury
Use additional external cause code to identify perpetrator, if known (Y07-)
Excludes 1:   *abuse and maltreatment in pregnancy (O9A.3-, O9A.4-, O9A.5-)*
adult and child maltreatment, suspected (T76-)
The appropriate 7th character is to be added to each code from category T74:
A <u>Initial</u> encounter
D <u>Subsequent</u> encounter
S <u>Sequela</u>

T74.0- <u>Neglect or abandonment</u>, <u>confirmed</u>

CC-A **T74.01x-** <u>Adult</u> neglect or abandonment, <u>confirmed</u> — [Age/15-124]

CC-A **T74.02x-** <u>Child</u> neglect or abandonment, <u>confirmed</u> — [Age/0-17]

T74.1- <u>Physical abuse</u>, <u>confirmed</u>
Excludes ❷: *sexual abuse (T74.2-)*

CC-A **T74.11x-** <u>Adult</u> physical abuse, <u>confirmed</u> — [Age/15-124]

CC-A **T74.12x-** <u>Child</u> physical abuse, <u>confirmed</u> — [Age/0-17]
Excludes ❷: *shaken infant syndrome (T74.4)*

T74.2- <u>Sexual abuse</u>, <u>confirmed</u>
Rape, confirmed
Sexual assault, confirmed

CC-A **T74.21x-** <u>Adult</u> sexual abuse, <u>confirmed</u> — [Age/15-124]

CC-A **T74.22x-** <u>Child</u> sexual abuse, <u>confirmed</u> — [Age/0-17]

T74.3- <u>Psychological abuse</u>, <u>confirmed</u>

T74.31x- <u>Adult</u> psychological abuse, <u>confirmed</u> — [Age/15-124]

CC-A **T74.32x-** <u>Child</u> psychological abuse, <u>confirmed</u> — [Age/0-17]

T74.4xx- Shaken infant syndrome — [Age/0-17]
CC-A

T74.9- <u>Unspecified maltreatment</u>, <u>confirmed</u>

CC-A **T74.91x-** Unspecified <u>adult</u> maltreatment, <u>confirmed</u> — [Age/15-124]

CC-A **T74.92x-** Unspecified <u>child</u> maltreatment, <u>confirmed</u> — [Age/0-17]

T75- Other and unspecified effects of other external causes
Excludes 1: *adverse effects NEC (T78.-)*
Excludes ❷: *burns (electric) (T20-T31)*
The appropriate 7th character is to be added to each code from category T75:
A <u>Initial</u> encounter
D <u>Subsequent</u> encounter
S <u>Sequela</u>

T75.0- Effects of lightning
Struck by lightning

T75.00x- Unspecified effects of lightning
Struck by lightning NOS

T75.01x- Shock due to being struck by lightning

T75.09x- Other effects of lightning
Use additional code for other effects of lightning

T75.1xx- Unspecified effects of drowning and nonfatal submersion
CC-A Immersion
Excludes 1: *specified effects of drowning — code to effects*

T75.2-   **Effects of vibration**
  T75.20x-   Unspecified effects of vibration
  T75.21x-   Pneumatic hammer syndrome
  T75.22x-   Traumatic vasospastic syndrome
  T75.23x-   Vertigo from infrasound
              Excludes 1:   *vertigo NOS (R42)*
  T75.29-   Other effects of vibration
T75.3xx-   **Motion sickness**
            Airsickness
            Seasickness
            Travel sickness
            Use additional external cause code to identify vehicle or type of
              motion (Y92.81-, Y93.5-)
T75.4xx-   **Electrocution**
            Shock from electric current
            Shock from electroshock gun (taser)
T75.8-   **Other specified effects of external causes**
  T75.81x-   Effects of abnormal gravitation [G] forces
  T75.82x-   Effects of weightlessness
  T75.89x-   Other specified effects of external causes

T76-   **Adult and child abuse, neglect and other maltreatment, _suspected_**
        Use additional code, if applicable, to identify any associated current injury
        Excludes 1:   *adult and child maltreatment, confirmed (T74.-)*
                         suspected abuse and maltreatment in pregnancy (O9A.3-,
                           O9A.4-, O9A.5-)
                         suspected adult physical abuse, ruled out (Z04.71)
                         suspected adult sexual abuse, ruled out (Z04.41)
                         suspected child physical abuse, ruled out (Z04.72)
                         suspected child sexual abuse, ruled out (Z04.42)

The appropriate 7th character is to be added to each code from
  category T76:
  A   Initial encounter
  D   Subsequent encounter
  S   Sequela

T76.0-   **Neglect or abandonment, suspected**
CC-A T76.01x-   **Adult** neglect or abandonment, suspected — [Age/15-124]
CC-A T76.02x-   **Child** neglect or abandonment, suspected — [Age/0-17]
T76.1-   **Physical abuse, suspected**
CC-A T76.11x-   **Adult** physical abuse, suspected — [Age/15-124]
CC-A T76.12x-   **Child** physical abuse, suspected — [Age/0-17]
T76.2-   **Sexual abuse, suspected**
            Rape, suspected
            Sexual abuse, suspected
          Excludes 1:   *alleged abuse, ruled out (Z04.7)*
CC-A T76.21x-   **Adult** sexual abuse, suspected — [Age/15-124]
CC-A T76.22x-   **Child** sexual abuse, suspected — [Age/0-17]
T76.3-   **Psychological abuse, suspected**
  T76.31x-   **Adult** psychological abuse, suspected — [Age/15-124]
CC-A T76.32x-   **Child** psychological abuse, suspected — [Age/0-17]
T76.9-   **Unspecified maltreatment, suspected**
CC-A T76.91x-   Unspecified **adult** maltreatment, suspected —
                  [Age/15-124]
CC-A T76.92x-   Unspecified **child** maltreatment, suspected — [Age/0-17]

T78-   **Adverse effects, _not elsewhere classified_**
        Excludes ❷: *complications of surgical and medical care NEC (T80-T88)*
The appropriate 7th character is to be added to each code from
  category T78:
  A   Initial encounter
  D   Subsequent encounter
  S   Sequela
T78.0-   **Anaphylactic reaction due to food**
            Anaphylactic reaction due to adverse food reaction
            Anaphylactic shock or reaction due to nonpoisonous foods
            Anaphylactoid reaction due to food
CC-A T78.00x-   Anaphylactic reaction due to unspecified food
CC-A T78.01x-   Anaphylactic reaction due to peanuts
CC-A T78.02x-   Anaphylactic reaction due to shellfish (crustaceans)
CC-A T78.03x-   Anaphylactic reaction due to other fish
CC-A T78.04x-   Anaphylactic reaction due to fruits and vegetables
CC-A T78.05x-   Anaphylactic reaction due to tree nuts and seeds
              Excludes ❷: *anaphylactic reaction due to peanuts (T78.01)*

CC-A T78.06x-   Anaphylactic reaction due to food additives
CC-A T78.07x-   Anaphylactic reaction due to milk and dairy products
CC-A T78.08x-   Anaphylactic reaction due to eggs
CC-A T78.09x-   Anaphylactic reaction due to other food products
T78.1xx-   **Other adverse food reactions, _not elsewhere classified_**
            Use additional code to identify the type of reaction, if applicable
            Excludes 1:   *anaphylactic reaction or shock due to adverse food*
                               reaction (T78.0-)
                             anaphylactic reaction due to food (T78.0-)
                             bacterial food borne intoxications (A05-)
            Excludes ❷: *allergic and dietetic gastroenteritis and colitis*
                               (K52.29)
                             allergic rhinitis due to food (J30.5)
                             dermatitis due to food in contact with skin (L23.6,
                               L24.6, L25.4)
                             dermatitis due to ingested food (L27.2)
                             food protein-induced enterocolitis syndrome (K52.21)
                             food protein-induced enteropathy (K52.22)
T78.2xx-   **Anaphylactic shock, _unspecified_**
CC-A   Allergic shock
            Anaphylactic reaction
            Anaphylaxis
            Excludes 1:   *anaphylactic reaction or shock due to adverse effect*
                               of correct medicinal substance properly
                               administered (T88.6)
                             anaphylactic reaction or shock due to adverse food
                               reaction (T78.0-)
                             anaphylactic reaction or shock due to serum (T80.5)
T78.3xx-   **Angioneurotic edema**
            Allergic angioedema
            Giant urticaria
            Quincke's edema
            Excludes 1:   *serum urticaria (T80.6-)*
                             urticaria (L50-)
T78.4-   **Other and unspecified allergy**
          Excludes 1:   *specified types of allergic reaction such as:*
                             allergic diarrhea (K52.29)
                             allergic gastroenteritis and colitis (K52.29)
                             dermatitis (L23-L25, L27.-)
                             food protein-induced enterocolitis syndrome (K52.21)
                             food protein-induced enteropathy (K52.22)
                             hay fever (J30.1)
  T78.40x-   **Allergy, unspecified**
              Allergic reaction NOS
              Hypersensitivity NOS
  T78.41x-   **Arthus phenomenon**
              Arthus reaction
  T78.49x-   **Other allergy**
T78.8xx-   **Other adverse effects, not elsewhere classified**

Certain early complications of trauma (T79)

T79- Certain early complications of trauma, <u>not elsewhere classified</u>
Excludes ❷: acute respiratory distress syndrome (J80)
      complications occurring during or following medical procedures
        (T80-T88)
      complications of surgical and medical care NEC (T80-T88)
      newborn respiratory distress syndrome (P22.0)

The appropriate 7th character is to be added to each code from
    category T79:
    A   <u>Initial</u> encounter
    D   <u>Subsequent</u> encounter
    S   <u>Sequela</u>

T79.0xx-   **Air embolism (traumatic)**
MCC-A   Excludes 1:   air embolism complicating abortion or ectopic or
              molar pregnancy (O00-O07, O08.2)
           air embolism complicating pregnancy, childbirth and
              the puerperium (O88.0)
           air embolism following infusion, transfusion, and
              therapeutic injection (T80.0)
           air embolism following procedure NEC (T81.7-)

T79.1xx-   **Fat embolism (traumatic)**
MCC-A   Excludes 1:   fat embolism complicating:
           abortion or ectopic or molar pregnancy
              (O00-O07, O08.2)
           pregnancy, childbirth and the puerperium (O88.8)

T79.2xx-   **Traumatic secondary and recurrent hemorrhage and seroma**
CC-A

T79.4xx-   **Traumatic shock**
MCC-A   **Shock (immediate) (delayed) following injury**
    Excludes 1:   anaphylactic shock due to adverse food reaction
              (T78.0-)
           anaphylactic shock due to correct medicinal substance
              properly administered (T88.6)
           anaphylactic shock due to serum (T80.5-)
           anaphylactic shock NOS (T78.2)
           anesthetic shock (T88.2)
           electric shock (T75.4)
           nontraumatic shock NEC (R57-)
           obstetric shock (O75.1)
           postprocedural shock (T81.1-)
           septic shock (R65.21)
           shock complicating abortion or ectopic or molar
              pregnancy (O00-O07, O08.3)
           shock due to lightning (T75.01)
           shock NOS (R57.9)

T79.5xx-   **Traumatic anuria**
MCC-A   **Crush syndrome**
    Renal failure following crushing

T79.6xx-   **Traumatic ischemia of muscle**
    Traumatic rhabdomyolysis
    Volkmann's ischemic contracture
    Excludes ❷: anterior tibial syndrome (M76.8)
           compartment syndrome (traumatic) (T79.A-)
           nontraumatic ischemia of muscle (M62.2-)

T79.7xx-   **Traumatic subcutaneous emphysema**
CC-A   Excludes 1:   emphysema NOS (J43)
           emphysema (subcutaneous) resulting from a
              procedure (T81.82)

T79.A-   **Traumatic compartment syndrome**
    Excludes 1:   fibromyalgia (M79.7)
           nontraumatic compartment syndrome (M79.A-)
           traumatic ischemic infarction of muscle (T79.6)

CC-A **T79.A0x-**   **Compartment syndrome, <u>unspecified</u>**
        Compartment syndrome NOS

T79.A1-   Traumatic compartment syndrome of <u>upper extremity</u>
        Traumatic compartment syndrome of shoulder, arm, forearm,
        wrist, hand, and fingers

CC-A **T79.A11-**   **Traumatic compartment syndrome of <u>right</u> upper
           extremity**

CC-A **T79.A12-**   **Traumatic compartment syndrome of <u>left</u> upper
           extremity**

CC-A **T79.A19-**   **Traumatic compartment syndrome of <u>unspecified</u>
           upper extremity**

T79.A2-   Traumatic compartment syndrome of <u>lower extremity</u>
        Traumatic compartment syndrome of hip, buttock, thigh, leg,
        foot, and toes

CC-A **T79.A21-**   **Traumatic compartment syndrome of <u>right</u> lower
           extremity**

CC-A **T79.A22-**   **Traumatic compartment syndrome of <u>left</u> lower
           extremity**

CC-A **T79.A29-**   **Traumatic compartment syndrome of <u>unspecified</u>
           lower extremity**

CC-A **T79.A3x-**   **Traumatic compartment syndrome of <u>abdomen</u>**

CC-A **T79.A9x-**   **Traumatic compartment syndrome of <u>other</u> sites**

T79.8xx-   **Other early complications of trauma**

T79.9xx-   **Unspecified early complication of trauma**

Complications of surgical and medical care, not elsewhere classified (T80-T88)

Use additional code for adverse effect, if applicable, to identify drug (T36-
    T50 with fifth or sixth character 5)
Use additional code(s) to identify the specified condition resulting from the
    complication
Use additional code to identify devices involved and details of circumstances
    (Y62-Y82)
Excludes ❷: any encounters with medical care for postprocedural conditions
           in which no complications are present, such as:
              artificial opening status (Z93-)
              closure of external stoma (Z43-)
              fitting and adjustment of external prosthetic device (Z44-)
           burns and corrosions from local applications and irradiation
              (T20-T32)
           complications of surgical procedures during pregnancy,
              childbirth and the puerperium (O00-O9A)
           mechanical complication of respirator [ventilator] (J95.850)
           poisoning and toxic effects of drugs and chemicals (T36-T65
              with fifth or sixth characters 1-4 or 6)
           postprocedural fever (R50.82)
            specified complications classified elsewhere, such as:
              cerebrospinal fluid leak from spinal puncture (G97.0)
              colostomy malfunction (K94.0-)
               disorders of fluid and electrolyte imbalance (E86-E87)
              functional disturbances following cardiac surgery (I97.0-I97.1)
              intraoperative and postprocedural complications of specified
                 body systems (D78-, E36-, E89-, G97.3-, G97.4, H59.3-,
                 H59-, H95.2-, H95.3, I97.4-, I97.5, J95.6-, J95.7,
                 K91.6-, L76-, M96-, N99-)
              ostomy complications (J95.0-, K94.-, N99.5-)
              postgastric surgery syndromes (K91.1)
              postlaminectomy syndrome NEC (M96.1)
              postmastectomy lymphedema syndrome (I97.2)
              postsurgical blind-loop syndrome (K91.2)
              ventilator associated pneumonia (J95.851)

T80-   **Complications following <u>infusion, transfusion and therapeutic
      injection</u>**
    Includes: Complications following perfusion
    Excludes ❷: bone marrow transplant rejection (T86.01)
           febrile nonhemolytic transfusion reaction (R50.84)
           fluid overload due to transfusion (E87.71)
           posttransfusion purpura (D69.51)
           transfusion associated circulatory overload (TACO) (E87.71)
           transfusion (red blood cell) associated hemochromatosis
              (E83.111)
           transfusion related acute lung injury (TRALI) (J95.84)

The appropriate 7th character is to be added to each code from
    category T80:
    A   <u>Initial</u> encounter
    D   <u>Subsequent</u> encounter
    S   <u>Sequela</u>

T80.0xx-   <u>Air embolism</u> following infusion, transfusion and
MCC-A   therapeutic injection

T80.1xx-   <u>Vascular</u> complications following infusion, transfusion and
CC-A   therapeutic injection
    Use additional code to identify the vascular complication
    Excludes ❷: extravasation of vesicant agent (T80.81-)
           infiltration of vesicant agent (T80.81-)
           postprocedural vascular complications (T81.7-)
           vascular complications specified as due to prosthetic
              devices, implants and grafts (T82.8-, T83.8-,
              T84.8-, T85.8-)

T79 - T80 (side tab)

T80.2- <u>Infections</u> following infusion, transfusion and therapeutic injection
Use additional code to identify the specific infection, such as:
Sepsis (A41.9)
Use additional code (R65.2-) to identify severe sepsis, if applicable
Excludes ❷: *infections specified as due to prosthetic devices, implants and grafts (T82.6-T82.7, T83.5-T83.6, T84.5-T84.7, T85.7)*
postprocedural infections (T81.4-)

T80.21- Infection <u>due to central venous catheter</u>
Infection due to pulmonary artery catheter (Swan-Ganz catheter)

CC-A **T80.211-** <u>Bloodstream</u> infection due to central venous catheter
Bloodstream infection due to Hickman catheter
Bloodstream infection due to peripherally inserted central catheter (PICC)
Bloodstream infection due to portacath (port-a-cath)
Bloodstream infection due to pulmonary artery catheter
Bloodstream infection due to triple lumen catheter
Bloodstream infection due to umbilical venous catheter
Catheter-related bloodstream infection (CRBSI) NOS
Central line-associated bloodstream infection (CLABSI)

CC-A **T80.212-** <u>Local</u> infection due to central venous catheter
Exit or insertion site infection
Local infection due to Hickman catheter
Local infection due to peripherally inserted central catheter (PICC)
Local infection due to portacath (port-a-cath)
Local infection due to pulmonary artery catheter
Local infection due to triple lumen catheter
Local infection due to umbilical venous catheter
Port or reservoir infection
Tunnel infection

CC-A **T80.218-** <u>Other</u> infection due to central venous catheter
Other central line-associated infection
Other infection due to Hickman catheter
Other infection due to peripherally inserted central catheter (PICC)
Other infection due to portacath (port-a-cath)
Other infection due to pulmonary artery catheter
Other infection due to triple lumen catheter
Other infection due to umbilical venous catheter

CC-A **T80.219-** <u>Unspecified</u> infection due to central venous catheter
Central line-associated infection NOS
Unspecified infection due to Hickman catheter
Unspecified infection due to peripherally inserted central catheter (PICC)
Unspecified infection due to portacath (port-a-cath)
Unspecified infection due to pulmonary artery catheter
Unspecified infection due to triple lumen catheter
Unspecified infection due to umbilical venous catheter

CC-A **T80.22x-** <u>Acute infection</u> following transfusion, infusion, or injection of <u>blood and blood products</u>

CC-A **T80.29x-** Infection following <u>other infusion, transfusion and therapeutic injection</u>

T80.3- <u>ABO incompatibility reaction</u> due to transfusion of blood or blood products
Excludes 1: *minor blood group antigens reactions (Duffy) (E) (K(ell)) (Kidd) (Lewis) (M) (N) (P) (S) (T80.A)*

CC-A **T80.30x-** ABO incompatibility reaction due to transfusion of blood or blood products, <u>unspecified</u>
ABO incompatibility blood transfusion NOS
Reaction to ABO incompatibility from transfusion NOS

T80.31- ABO incompatibility <u>with hemolytic transfusion reaction</u>

CC-A **T80.310-** ABO incompatibility with <u>acute</u> hemolytic transfusion reaction
ABO incompatibility with hemolytic transfusion reaction less than 24 hours after transfusion
Acute hemolytic transfusion reaction (AHTR) due to ABO incompatibility

CC-A **T80.311-** ABO incompatibility with <u>delayed</u> hemolytic transfusion reaction
ABO incompatibility with hemolytic transfusion reaction 24 hours or more after transfusion
Delayed hemolytic transfusion reaction (DHTR) due to ABO incompatibility

CC-A **T80.319-** ABO incompatibility with hemolytic transfusion reaction, <u>unspecified</u>
ABO incompatibility with hemolytic transfusion reaction at unspecified time after transfusion
Hemolytic transfusion reaction (HTR) due to ABO incompatibility NOS

CC-A **T80.39x-** <u>Other</u> ABO incompatibility reaction due to transfusion of blood or blood products
Delayed serologic transfusion reaction (DSTR) from ABO incompatibility
Other ABO incompatible blood transfusion
Other reaction to ABO incompatible blood transfusion

T80.4- <u>Rh incompatibility reaction</u> due to transfusion of blood or blood products
Reaction due to incompatibility of Rh antigens (C) (c) (D) (E) (e)

CC-A **T80.40x-** Rh incompatibility reaction due to transfusion of blood or blood products, <u>unspecified</u>
Reaction due to Rh factor in transfusion NOS
Rh incompatible blood transfusion NOS

T80.41- Rh incompatibility <u>with hemolytic transfusion reaction</u>

CC-A **T80.410-** Rh incompatibility with <u>acute</u> hemolytic transfusion reaction
Acute hemolytic transfusion reaction (AHTR) due to Rh incompatibility
Rh incompatibility with hemolytic transfusion reaction less than 24 hours after transfusion

CC-A **T80.411-** Rh incompatibility with <u>delayed</u> hemolytic transfusion reaction
Delayed hemolytic transfusion reaction (DHTR) due to Rh incompatibility
Rh incompatibility with hemolytic transfusion reaction 24 hours or more after transfusion

CC-A **T80.419-** Rh incompatibility with hemolytic transfusion reaction, <u>unspecified</u>
Rh incompatibility with hemolytic transfusion reaction at unspecified time after transfusion
Hemolytic transfusion reaction (HTR) due to Rh incompatibility NOS

CC-A **T80.49x-** <u>Other</u> Rh incompatibility reaction due to transfusion of blood or blood products
Delayed serologic transfusion reaction (DSTR) from Rh incompatibility
Other reaction to Rh incompatible blood transfusion

T80.A- <u>Non-ABO incompatibility reaction</u> due to transfusion of blood or blood products
Reaction due to incompatibility of minor antigens (Duffy) (Kell) (Kidd) (Lewis) (M) (N) (P) (S)

CC-A **T80.A0x-** Non-ABO incompatibility reaction due to transfusion of blood or blood products, <u>unspecified</u>
Non-ABO antigen incompatibility reaction from transfusion NOS

T80.A1- Non-ABO incompatibility <u>with hemolytic transfusion reaction</u>

CC-A **T80.A10-** Non-ABO incompatibility with <u>acute</u> hemolytic transfusion reaction
Acute hemolytic transfusion reaction (AHTR) due to non-ABO incompatibility
Non-ABO incompatibility with hemolytic transfusion reaction less than 24 hours after transfusion

CC-A **T80.A11-** Non-ABO incompatibility with <u>delayed</u> hemolytic transfusion reaction
Delayed hemolytic transfusion reaction (DHTR) due to non-ABO incompatibility
Non-ABO incompatibility with hemolytic transfusion reaction 24 or more hours after transfusion

CC-A **T80.A19-** Non-ABO incompatibility with hemolytic transfusion reaction, <u>unspecified</u>
Hemolytic transfusion reaction (HTR) due to non-ABO incompatibility NOS
Non-ABO incompatibility with hemolytic transfusion reaction at unspecified time after transfusion

CC-A **T80.A9x-** <u>Other</u> non-ABO incompatibility reaction due to transfusion of blood or blood products
Delayed serologic transfusion reaction (DSTR) from non-ABO incompatibility
Other reaction to non-ABO incompatible blood transfusion

T80 – T80

T80.5-   **Anaphylactic reaction due to serum**
Allergic shock due to serum
Anaphylactic shock due to serum
Anaphylactoid reaction due to serum
Anaphylaxis due to serum
> Excludes 1:   ABO incompatibility reaction due to transfusion of blood or blood products (T80.3-)
> allergic reaction or shock NOS (T78.2)
> anaphylactic reaction or shock NOS (T78.2)
> anaphylactic reaction or shock due to adverse effect of correct medicinal substance properly administered (T88.6)
> other serum reaction (T80.6-)

CC-A **T80.51x-**   **Anaphylactic reaction due to administration of blood and blood products**

CC-A **T80.52x-**   **Anaphylactic reaction due to vaccination**

CC-A **T80.59x-**   **Anaphylactic reaction due to other serum**

T80.6-   **Other serum reactions**
Intoxication by serum
Protein sickness
Serum rash
Serum sickness
Serum urticaria
> Excludes ❷: serum hepatitis (B16-B19)

CC-A **T80.61x-**   **Other serum reaction due to administration of blood and blood products**

CC-A **T80.62x-**   **Other serum reaction due to vaccination**

CC-A **T80.69x-**   **Other serum reaction due to other serum**

T80.8-   **Other complications following infusion, transfusion and therapeutic injection**

T80.81-   **Extravasation of vesicant agent**
Infiltration of vesicant agent

CC-A **T80.810-**   **Extravasation of vesicant antineoplastic chemotherapy**
Infiltration of vesicant antineoplastic chemotherapy

CC-A **T80.818-**   **Extravasation of other vesicant agent**
Infiltration of other vesicant agent

T80.89x-   **Other complications following infusion, transfusion and therapeutic injection**
Delayed serologic transfusion reaction (DSTR), unspecified incompatibility
Use additional code to identify graft-versus-host reaction, if applicable, (D89.81-)

T80.9-   **Unspecified complication following infusion, transfusion and therapeutic injection**

T80.90x-   **Unspecified complication following infusion and therapeutic injection**

T80.91-   **Hemolytic transfusion reaction, unspecified incompatibility**
> Excludes 1:   ABO incompatibility with hemolytic transfusion reaction (T80.31-)
> Non-ABO incompatibility with hemolytic transfusion reaction (T80.A1-)
> Rh incompatibility with hemolytic transfusion reaction (T80.41-)

CC-A **T80.910-**   **Acute hemolytic transfusion reaction, unspecified incompatibility**

CC-A **T80.911-**   **Delayed hemolytic transfusion reaction, unspecified incompatibility**

CC-A **T80.919-**   **Hemolytic transfusion reaction, unspecified incompatibility, unspecified as acute or delayed**
Hemolytic transfusion reaction NOS

T80.92x-   **Unspecified transfusion reaction**
Transfusion reaction NOS

T81-   **Complications of procedures, not elsewhere classified**
Use additional code for adverse effect, if applicable, to identify drug (T36-T50 with fifth or sixth character 5)
> Excludes ❷: complications following immunization (T88.0-T88.1)
> complications following infusion, transfusion and therapeutic injection (T80-)
> complications of transplanted organs and tissue (T86-)
> specified complications classified elsewhere, such as:
> complication of prosthetic devices, implants and grafts (T82-T85)
> dermatitis due to drugs and medicaments (L23.3, L24.4, L25.1, L27.0-L27.1)
> endosseous dental implant failure (M27.6-)
> floppy iris syndrome (IFIS) (intraoperative) H21.81
> intraoperative and postprocedural complications of specific body system (D78.-, E36.-, E89.-, G97.3-, G97.4, H59.3-, H59.-, H95.2-, H95.3, I97.4-, I97.5, J95, K91.-, L76.-, M96.-, N99.-)
> ostomy complications (J95.0-, K94.-, N99.5-)
> plateau iris syndrome (post-iridectomy) (postprocedural) H21.82
> poisoning and toxic effects of drugs and chemicals (T36-T65 with fifth or sixth character 1-4 or 6)

> The appropriate 7th character is to be added to each code from category T81:
> **A**   **Initial** encounter
> **D**   **Subsequent** encounter
> **S**   **Sequela**

T81.1-   **Postprocedural shock**
AHA 15:1Q:p23 – Penny lodged in proximal esophagus
Shock during or resulting from a procedure, not elsewhere classified
> Excludes 1:   anaphylactic shock NOS (T78.2)
> anaphylactic shock due to correct substance properly administered (T88.6)
> anaphylactic shock due to serum (T80.5-)
> anesthetic shock (T88.2)
> electric shock (T75.4)
> obstetric shock (O75.1)
> septic shock (R65.21)
> shock following abortion or ectopic or molar pregnancy (O00-O07, O08.3)
> traumatic shock (T79.4)

CC-A **T81.10x-**   **Postprocedural shock, unspecified**
Collapse NOS during or resulting from a procedure, not elsewhere classified
Postprocedural failure of peripheral circulation
Postprocedural shock NOS

MCC-A **T81.11x-**   **Postprocedural cardiogenic shock**

MCC-A **T81.12x-**   **Postprocedural septic shock** — [Unacceptable PDX]
Postprocedural endotoxic shock resulting from a procedure, not elsewhere classified
Postprocedural gram-negative shock resulting from a procedure, not elsewhere classified
Code first underlying infection
Use additional code, to identify any associated acute organ dysfunction, if applicable

MCC-A **T81.19x-**   **Other postprocedural shock**
Postprocedural hypovolemic shock

T80 - T81

T81.3-   Disruption of wound, not elsewhere classified
  AHA 14:1Q:p23 – Nonhealing surgical wound
  Disruption of any suture materials or other closure methods
  Excludes 1:   *breakdown (mechanical) of permanent sutures*
                      (T85.612)
                  displacement of permanent sutures (T85.622)
                  disruption of cesarean delivery wound (O90.0)
                  disruption of perineal obstetric wound (O90.1)
                  mechanical complication of permanent sutures NEC
                      (T85.692)

CC-A **T81.30x-**   Disruption of wound, unspecified
                      Disruption of wound NOS

CC-A **T81.31x-**   Disruption of external operation (surgical) wound, not
                      elsewhere classified
                      Dehiscence of operation wound NOS
                      Disruption of operation wound NOS
                      Disruption or dehiscence of closure of cornea
                      Disruption or dehiscence of closure of mucosa
                      Disruption or dehiscence of closure of skin and
                          subcutaneous tissue
                      Full-thickness skin disruption or dehiscence
                      Superficial disruption or dehiscence of operation wound
                  Excludes 1:   *dehiscence of amputation stump (T87.81)*

CC-A **T81.32x-**   Disruption of internal operation (surgical) wound, not
                      elsewhere classified
                      Deep disruption or dehiscence of operation wound NOS
                      Disruption or dehiscence of closure of internal organ or
                          other internal tissue
                      Disruption or dehiscence of closure of muscle or muscle flap
                      Disruption or dehiscence of closure of ribs or rib cage
                      Disruption or dehiscence of closure of skull or craniotomy
                      Disruption or dehiscence of closure of sternum or
                          sternotomy
                      Disruption or dehiscence of closure of tendon or ligament
                      Disruption or dehiscence of closure of superficial or
                          muscular fascia

CC-A **T81.33x-**   Disruption of traumatic injury wound repair
                      Disruption or dehiscence of closure of traumatic laceration
                          (external) (internal)

T81.4xx-   Infection following a procedure
CC-A
                  AHA 14:1Q:p23 – Nonhealing surgical wound
                  Intra-abdominal abscess following a procedure
                  Postprocedural infection, not elsewhere classified
                  Sepsis following a procedure
                  Stitch abscess following a procedure
                  Subphrenic abscess following a procedure
                  Wound abscess following a procedure
                  Use additional code to identify infection
                  Use additional code (R65.2-) to identify severe sepsis, if applicable
                  Excludes 1:   *obstetric surgical wound infection (O86.0)*
                                  postprocedural fever NOS (R50.82)
                                  postprocedural retroperitoneal abscess (K68.11)
                  Excludes ❷: *bleb associated endophthalmitis (H59.4-)*
                                  infection due to infusion, transfusion and therapeutic
                                      injection (T80.2-)
                                  infection due to prosthetic devices, implants and
                                      grafts (T82.6-T82.7, T83.5-T83.6, T84.5-T84.7,
                                      T85.7)

T81.5-   Complications of foreign body accidentally left in body
                following procedure
                  AHA 14:4Q:p24 – Loose cement fragment in hip joint

T81.50-   Unspecified complication of foreign body accidentally left
                in body following procedure

CC-A **T81.500-**   Unspecified complication of foreign body
                      accidentally left in body following surgical
                      operation

CC-A **T81.501-**   Unspecified complication of foreign body
                      accidentally left in body following infusion or
                      transfusion

CC-A **T81.502-**   Unspecified complication of foreign body
                      accidentally left in body following kidney dialysis

CC-A **T81.503-**   Unspecified complication of foreign body
                      accidentally left in body following injection or
                      immunization

CC-A **T81.504-**   Unspecified complication of foreign body
                      accidentally left in body following endoscopic
                      examination

CC-A **T81.505-**   Unspecified complication of foreign body
                      accidentally left in body following heart
                      catheterization

CC-A **T81.506-**   Unspecified complication of foreign body
                      accidentally left in body following aspiration,
                      puncture or other catheterization

CC-A **T81.507-**   Unspecified complication of foreign body
                      accidentally left in body following removal of
                      catheter or packing

CC-A **T81.508-**   Unspecified complication of foreign body
                      accidentally left in body following other procedure

CC-A **T81.509-**   Unspecified complication of foreign body
                      accidentally left in body following unspecified
                      procedure

T81.51-   Adhesions due to foreign body accidentally left in body
                following procedure

CC-A **T81.510-**   Adhesions due to foreign body accidentally left in
                      body following surgical operation

CC-A **T81.511-**   Adhesions due to foreign body accidentally left in
                      body following infusion or transfusion

CC-A **T81.512-**   Adhesions due to foreign body accidentally left in
                      body following kidney dialysis

CC-A **T81.513-**   Adhesions due to foreign body accidentally left in
                      body following injection or immunization

CC-A **T81.514-**   Adhesions due to foreign body accidentally left in
                      body following endoscopic examination

CC-A **T81.515-**   Adhesions due to foreign body accidentally left in
                      body following heart catheterization

CC-A **T81.516-**   Adhesions due to foreign body accidentally left in
                      body following aspiration, puncture or other
                      catheterization

CC-A **T81.517-**   Adhesions due to foreign body accidentally left in
                      body following removal of catheter or packing

CC-A **T81.518-**   Adhesions due to foreign body accidentally left in
                      body following other procedure

CC-A **T81.519-**   Adhesions due to foreign body accidentally left in
                      body following unspecified procedure

T81.52-   Obstruction due to foreign body accidentally left in body
                following procedure

CC-A **T81.520-**   Obstruction due to foreign body accidentally left in
                      body following surgical operation

CC-A **T81.521-**   Obstruction due to foreign body accidentally left in
                      body following infusion or transfusion

CC-A **T81.522-**   Obstruction due to foreign body accidentally left in
                      body following kidney dialysis

CC-A **T81.523-**   Obstruction due to foreign body accidentally left in
                      body following injection or immunization

CC-A **T81.524-**   Obstruction due to foreign body accidentally left in
                      body following endoscopic examination

CC-A **T81.525-**   Obstruction due to foreign body accidentally left in
                      body following heart catheterization

CC-A **T81.526-**   Obstruction due to foreign body accidentally left in
                      body following aspiration, puncture or other
                      catheterization

CC-A **T81.527-**   Obstruction due to foreign body accidentally left in
                      body following removal of catheter or packing

CC-A **T81.528-**   Obstruction due to foreign body accidentally left in
                      body following other procedure

CC-A **T81.529-**   Obstruction due to foreign body accidentally left in
                      body following unspecified procedure

T81.53-   Perforation due to foreign body accidentally left in body
                following procedure

CC-A **T81.530-**   Perforation due to foreign body accidentally left in
                      body following surgical operation

CC-A **T81.531-**   Perforation due to foreign body accidentally left in
                      body following infusion or transfusion

CC-A **T81.532-**   Perforation due to foreign body accidentally left in
                      body following kidney dialysis

T 8 1 - T 8 1

CC-A **T81.533-** Perforation due to foreign body accidentally left in body following <u>injection or immunization</u>

CC-A **T81.534-** Perforation due to foreign body accidentally <u>left</u> in body following <u>endoscopic examination</u>

CC-A **T81.535-** Perforation due to foreign body accidentally left in body following <u>heart catheterization</u>

CC-A **T81.536-** Perforation due to foreign body accidentally <u>left</u> in body following <u>aspiration, puncture or other catheterization</u>

CC-A **T81.537-** Perforation due to foreign body accidentally left in body following <u>removal of catheter or packing</u>

CC-A **T81.538-** Perforation due to foreign body accidentally left in body following <u>other procedure</u>

CC-A **T81.539-** Perforation due to foreign body accidentally left in body following <u>unspecified procedure</u>

T81.59- <u>Other complications</u> of <u>foreign body accidentally left in body following procedure</u>
   Excludes ❷: obstruction or perforation due to prosthetic devices and implants intentionally left in body (T82.0-T82.5, T83.0-T83.4, T83.7, T84.0-T84.4, T85.0-T85.6)

CC-A **T81.590-** Other complications of foreign body accidentally left in body following <u>surgical operation</u>

CC-A **T81.591-** Other complications of foreign body accidentally left in body following <u>infusion or transfusion</u>

CC-A **T81.592-** Other complications of foreign body accidentally left in body following <u>kidney dialysis</u>

CC-A **T81.593-** Other complications of foreign body accidentally left in body following <u>injection or immunization</u>

CC-A **T81.594-** Other complications of foreign body accidentally left in body following <u>endoscopic examination</u>

CC-A **T81.595-** Other complications of foreign body accidentally left in body following <u>heart catheterization</u>

CC-A **T81.596-** Other complications of foreign body accidentally left in body following <u>aspiration, puncture or other catheterization</u>

CC-A **T81.597-** Other complications of foreign body accidentally left in body following <u>removal of catheter or packing</u>

CC-A **T81.598-** Other complications of foreign body accidentally left in body following <u>other procedure</u>

CC-A **T81.599-** Other complications of foreign body accidentally left in body following <u>unspecified procedure</u>

T81.6- <u>Acute reaction</u> to <u>foreign substance accidentally left during a procedure</u>
   Excludes ❷: complications of foreign body accidentally left in body cavity or operation wound following procedure (T81.5-)

CC-A **T81.60x-** <u>Unspecified</u> acute reaction to foreign substance accidentally left during a procedure

CC-A **T81.61x-** <u>Aseptic peritonitis</u> due to foreign substance accidentally left during a procedure
   Chemical peritonitis

CC-A **T81.69x-** <u>Other acute reaction</u> to foreign substance accidentally left during a procedure

T81.7- <u>Vascular complications following a procedure</u>, <u>not elsewhere classified</u>
   Air embolism following procedure NEC
   Phlebitis or thrombophlebitis resulting from a procedure
   *Excludes 1:   embolism complicating abortion or ectopic or molar pregnancy (O00-O07, O08.2)
      embolism complicating pregnancy, childbirth and the puerperium (O88.-)
      traumatic embolism (T79.0)*
   *Excludes ❷: embolism due to prosthetic devices, implants and grafts (T82.8-, T83.81, T84.-, T85.81-)
      embolism following infusion, transfusion and therapeutic injection (T80.0)*

T81.71- Complication of <u>artery</u> following a procedure, not elsewhere classified

CC-A **T81.710-** Complication of <u>mesenteric</u> artery following a procedure, not elsewhere classified

CC-A **T81.711-** Complication of <u>renal</u> artery following a procedure, not elsewhere classified

CC-A **T81.718-** Complication of <u>other artery</u> following a procedure, not elsewhere classified

CC-A **T81.719-** Complication of <u>unspecified artery</u> following a procedure, not elsewhere classified

CC-A **T81.72x-** Complication of <u>vein</u> following a procedure, not elsewhere classified

T81.8- Other complications of procedures, <u>not elsewhere classified</u>
   *Excludes ❷: hypothermia following anesthesia (T88.51)
      malignant hyperpyrexia due to anesthesia (T88.3)*

T81.81x- Complication of inhalation therapy

T81.82x- Emphysema (subcutaneous) resulting from a procedure

CC-A **T81.83x-** Persistent postprocedural fistula

T81.89x- Other complications of procedures, not elsewhere classified
   AHA 14:1Q:p23 – Nonhealing surgical wound
   Use additional code to specify complication, such as:
      Postprocedural delirium (F05)

T81.9xx- Unspecified complication of procedure

T82- <u>Complications of cardiac and vascular prosthetic devices, implants and grafts</u>
   Excludes ❷: failure and rejection of transplanted organs and tissue (T86.-)
   The appropriate 7th character is to be added to each code from category T82:
   A <u>Initial</u> encounter
   D <u>Subsequent</u> encounter
   S <u>Sequela</u>

T82.0- <u>Mechanical</u> complication of <u>heart valve prosthesis</u>
   Mechanical complication of artificial heart valve
   Excludes 1:   mechanical complication of biological heart valve graft (T82.22-)

CC-A **T82.01x-** Breakdown (mechanical) of heart valve prosthesis

CC-A **T82.02x-** Displacement of heart valve prosthesis
   Malposition of heart valve prosthesis

CC-A **T82.03x-** Leakage of heart valve prosthesis

CC-A **T82.09x-** Other mechanical complication of heart valve prosthesis
   Obstruction (mechanical) of heart valve prosthesis
   Perforation of heart valve prosthesis
   Protrusion of heart valve prosthesis

T82.1- <u>Mechanical</u> complication of <u>cardiac electronic device</u>

T82.11- Breakdown (mechanical) of cardiac electronic device

CC-A **T82.110-** Breakdown (mechanical) of cardiac electrode

CC-A **T82.111-** Breakdown (mechanical) of cardiac pulse generator (battery)

CC-A **T82.118-** Breakdown (mechanical) of other cardiac electronic device

CC-A **T82.119-** Breakdown (mechanical) of unspecified cardiac electronic device

T82.12- <u>Displacement</u> of <u>cardiac electronic device</u>
   Malposition of cardiac electronic device

CC-A **T82.120-** Displacement of cardiac electrode

CC-A **T82.121-** Displacement of cardiac pulse generator (battery)

CC-A **T82.128-** Displacement of other cardiac electronic device

CC-A **T82.129-** Displacement of unspecified cardiac electronic device

T82.19- <u>Other mechanical</u> complication of <u>cardiac electronic device</u>
   Leakage of cardiac electronic device
   Obstruction of cardiac electronic device
   Perforation of cardiac electronic device
   Protrusion of cardiac electronic device

CC-A **T82.190-** Other mechanical complication of cardiac electrode

CC-A **T82.191-** Other mechanical complication of cardiac pulse generator (battery)

CC-A **T82.198-** Other mechanical complication of other cardiac electronic device

CC-A **T82.199-** Other mechanical complication of unspecified cardiac device

T81 - T82 *(side tab)*

T82.2-   **Mechanical** complication of coronary artery bypass graft and biological heart valve graft
     Excludes 1:   *mechanical complication of artificial heart valve prosthesis (T82.0-)*

T82.21-   **Mechanical** complication of <u>coronary artery bypass graft</u>

CC-A **T82.211-**   Breakdown (mechanical) of coronary artery bypass graft

CC-A **T82.212-**   Displacement of coronary artery bypass graft
     Malposition of coronary artery bypass graft

CC-A **T82.213-**   Leakage of coronary artery bypass graft

CC-A **T82.218-**   Other mechanical complication of coronary artery bypass graft
     Obstruction, mechanical of coronary artery bypass graft
     Perforation of coronary artery bypass graft
     Protrusion of coronary artery bypass graft

T82.22-   **Mechanical** complication of <u>biological heart valve graft</u>

CC-A **T82.221-**   Breakdown (mechanical) of biological heart valve graft

CC-A **T82.222-**   Displacement of biological heart valve graft
     Malposition of biological heart valve graft

CC-A **T82.223-**   Leakage of biological heart valve graft

CC-A **T82.228-**   Other mechanical complication of biological heart valve graft
     Obstruction of biological heart valve graft
     Perforation of biological heart valve graft
     Protrusion of biological heart valve graft

T82.3-   **Mechanical** complication of <u>other vascular grafts</u>

T82.31-   **Breakdown** (mechanical) of other vascular grafts

CC-A **T82.310-**   Breakdown (mechanical) of aortic (bifurcation) graft (replacement)

CC-A **T82.311-**   Breakdown (mechanical) of carotid arterial graft (bypass)

CC-A **T82.312-**   Breakdown (mechanical) of femoral arterial graft (bypass)

CC-A **T82.318-**   Breakdown (mechanical) of other vascular grafts

CC-A **T82.319-**   Breakdown (mechanical) of <u>unspecified</u> vascular grafts

T82.32-   **Displacement** of other vascular grafts
     Malposition of other vascular grafts

CC-A **T82.320-**   Displacement of aortic (bifurcation) graft (replacement)

CC-A **T82.321-**   Displacement of carotid arterial graft (bypass)

CC-A **T82.322-**   Displacement of femoral arterial graft (bypass)

CC-A **T82.328-**   Displacement of other vascular grafts

CC-A **T82.329-**   Displacement of <u>unspecified</u> vascular grafts

T82.33-   **Leakage** of other vascular grafts

CC-A **T82.330-**   Leakage of aortic (bifurcation) graft (replacement)

CC-A **T82.331-**   Leakage of carotid arterial graft (bypass)

CC-A **T82.332-**   Leakage of femoral arterial graft (bypass)

CC-A **T82.338-**   Leakage of other vascular grafts

CC-A **T82.339-**   Leakage of <u>unspecified</u> vascular graft

T82.39-   **Other mechanical** complication of other vascular grafts
     Obstruction (mechanical) of other vascular grafts
     Perforation of other vascular grafts
     Protrusion of other vascular grafts

CC-A **T82.390-**   Other mechanical complication of aortic (bifurcation) graft (replacement)

CC-A **T82.391-**   Other mechanical complication of carotid arterial graft (bypass)

CC-A **T82.392-**   Other mechanical complication of femoral arterial graft (bypass)

CC-A **T82.398-**   Other mechanical complication of other vascular grafts

CC-A **T82.399-**   Other mechanical complication of <u>unspecified</u> vascular grafts

T82.4-   **Mechanical** complication of <u>vascular dialysis catheter</u>
     Mechanical complication of hemodialysis catheter
     Excludes 1:   *mechanical complication of intraperitoneal dialysis catheter (T85.62)*

CC-A **T82.41x-**   Breakdown (mechanical) of vascular dialysis catheter

CC-A **T82.42x-**   Displacement of vascular dialysis catheter
     Malposition of vascular dialysis catheter

CC-A **T82.43x-**   Leakage of vascular dialysis catheter

CC-A **T82.49x-**   Other complication of vascular dialysis catheter
     Obstruction (mechanical) of vascular dialysis catheter
     Perforation of vascular dialysis catheter
     Protrusion of vascular dialysis catheter

T82.5-   **Mechanical** complication of <u>other cardiac and vascular devices and implants</u>
     Excludes ❷: *mechanical complication of epidural and subdural infusion catheter (T85.61)*

T82.51-   **Breakdown** (mechanical) of other cardiac and vascular devices and implants

CC-A **T82.510-**   Breakdown (mechanical) of surgically created arteriovenous fistula

CC-A **T82.511-**   Breakdown (mechanical) of surgically created arteriovenous shunt

CC-A **T82.512-**   Breakdown (mechanical) of artificial heart

CC-A **T82.513-**   Breakdown (mechanical) of balloon (counterpulsation) device

CC-A **T82.514-**   Breakdown (mechanical) of infusion catheter

CC-A **T82.515-**   Breakdown (mechanical) of umbrella device

CC-A **T82.518-**   Breakdown (mechanical) of other cardiac and vascular devices and implants

CC-A **T82.519-**   Breakdown (mechanical) of unspecified cardiac and vascular devices and implants

T82.52-   **Displacement** of other cardiac and vascular devices and implants
     Malposition of other cardiac and vascular devices and implants

CC-A **T82.520-**   Displacement of surgically created arteriovenous fistula

CC-A **T82.521-**   Displacement of surgically created arteriovenous shunt

CC-A **T82.522-**   Displacement of artificial heart

CC-A **T82.523-**   Displacement of balloon (counterpulsation) device

CC-A **T82.524-**   Displacement of infusion catheter

CC-A **T82.525-**   Displacement of umbrella device

CC-A **T82.528-**   Displacement of other cardiac and vascular devices and implants

CC-A **T82.529-**   Displacement of unspecified cardiac and vascular devices and implants

T82.53-   **Leakage** of other cardiac and vascular devices and implants

CC-A **T82.530-**   Leakage of surgically created arteriovenous fistula

CC-A **T82.531-**   Leakage of surgically created arteriovenous shunt

CC-A **T82.532-**   Leakage of artificial heart

CC-A **T82.533-**   Leakage of balloon (counterpulsation) device

CC-A **T82.534-**   Leakage of infusion catheter

CC-A **T82.535-**   Leakage of umbrella device

CC-A **T82.538-**   Leakage of other cardiac and vascular devices and implants

CC-A **T82.539-**   Leakage of unspecified cardiac and vascular devices and implants

T82.59-   **Other mechanical** complication of other cardiac and vascular devices and implants
     Obstruction (mechanical) of other cardiac and vascular devices and implants
     Perforation of other cardiac and vascular devices and implants
     Protrusion of other cardiac and vascular devices and implants

CC-A **T82.590-**   Other mechanical complication of surgically created arteriovenous fistula

CC-A **T82.591-**   Other mechanical complication of surgically created arteriovenous shunt

T82 - T82

CC-A **T82.592-** Other mechanical complication of artificial heart

CC-A **T82.593-** Other mechanical complication of balloon (counterpulsation) device

CC-A **T82.594-** Other mechanical complication of infusion catheter

CC-A **T82.595-** Other mechanical complication of umbrella device

CC-A **T82.598-** Other mechanical complication of other cardiac and vascular devices and implants

CC-A **T82.599-** Other mechanical complication of unspecified cardiac and vascular devices andimplants

T82.6xx- <u>Infection and inflammatory reaction</u> due to <u>cardiac valve prosthesis</u>
CC-A
Use additional code to identify infection

T82.7xx- <u>Infection and inflammatory reaction</u> due to <u>other cardiac and vascular devices, implants and grafts</u>
CC-A
Use additional code to identify infection

T82.8- <u>Other specified complications</u> of <u>cardiac and vascular prosthetic devices, implants and grafts</u>

T82.81- <u>Embolism</u> due to cardiac and vascular prosthetic devices, implants and grafts

CC-A **T82.817-** Embolism due to cardiac prosthetic devices, implants and grafts

CC-A **T82.818-** Embolism due to vascular prosthetic devices, implants and grafts

T82.82- <u>Fibrosis</u> due to cardiac and vascular prosthetic devices, implants and grafts

CC-A **T82.827-** Fibrosis due to cardiac prosthetic devices, implants and grafts

CC-A **T82.828-** Fibrosis due to vascular prosthetic devices, implants and grafts

T82.83- <u>Hemorrhage</u> due to cardiac and vascular prosthetic devices, implants and grafts

CC-A **T82.837-** Hemorrhage due to cardiac prosthetic devices, implants and grafts

CC-A **T82.838-** Hemorrhage due to vascular prosthetic devices, implants and grafts

T82.84- <u>Pain</u> due to cardiac and vascular prosthetic devices, implants and grafts

CC-A **T82.847-** Pain due to cardiac prosthetic devices, implants and grafts

CC-A **T82.848-** Pain due to vascular prosthetic devices, implants and grafts

T82.85- <u>Stenosis</u> due to cardiac and vascular prosthetic devices, implants and grafts

CC-A **T82.855-** Stenosis of coronary artery stent
In-stent stenosis (restenosis) of coronary artery stent
Restenosis of coronary artery stent

CC-A **T82.856-** Stenosis of peripheral vascular stent
In-stent stenosis (restenosis) of peripheral vascular stent
Restenosis of peripheral vascular stent

CC-A **T82.857-** Stenosis of other cardiac prosthetic devices, implants and grafts

CC-A **T82.858-** Stenosis of other vascular prosthetic devices, implants and grafts

T82.86- <u>Thrombosis</u> of cardiac and vascular prosthetic devices, implants and grafts

CC-A **T82.867-** Thrombosis due to cardiac prosthetic devices, implants and grafts

CC-A **T82.868-** Thrombosis due to vascular prosthetic devices, implants and grafts

T82.89- <u>Other specified complication</u> of cardiac and vascular prosthetic devices, implants and grafts

CC-A **T82.897-** Other specified complication of cardiac prosthetic devices, implants and grafts

CC-A **T82.898-** Other specified complication of vascular prosthetic devices, implants and grafts

T82.9xx- <u>Unspecified</u> complication of cardiac and vascular prosthetic device, implant and graft
CC-A

T83- <u>Complications of genitourinary prosthetic devices, implants and grafts</u>
Excludes ❷: *failure and rejection of transplanted organs and tissue (T86.-)*

The appropriate 7th character is to be added to each code from category T83:
A <u>Initial</u> encounter
D <u>Subsequent</u> encounter
S <u>Sequela</u>

T83.0- <u>Mechanical</u> complication of <u>urinary catheter</u>
Excludes ❷: *complications of stoma of urinary tract (N99.5-)*

T83.01- <u>Breakdown</u> (mechanical) of urinary catheter

CC-A **T83.010-** Breakdown (mechanical) of <u>cystostomy</u> catheter

T83.011- Breakdown (mechanical) of <u>indwelling urethral</u> catheter

T83.012- Breakdown (mechanical) of <u>nephrostomy</u> catheter

T83.018- Breakdown (mechanical) of <u>other</u> urinary catheter
Breakdown (mechanical) of Hopkins catheter
Breakdown (mechanical) of ileostomy catheter
Breakdown (mechanical) of urostomy catheter

T83.02- <u>Displacement</u> of urinary catheter
Malposition of urinary catheter

CC-A **T83.020-** Displacement of <u>cystostomy</u> catheter

T83.021- Displacement of <u>indwelling urethral</u> catheter

T83.022- Displacement of <u>nephrostomy</u> catheter

T83.028- Displacement of <u>other</u> urinary catheter
Displacement of Hopkins catheter
Displacement of ileostomy catheter
Displacement of urostomy catheter

T83.03- <u>Leakage</u> of urinary catheter

CC-A **T83.030-** Leakage of <u>cystostomy</u> catheter

T83.031- Leakage of <u>indwelling urethral</u> catheter

T83.032- Leakage of <u>nephrostomy</u> catheter

T83.038- Leakage of <u>other</u> urinary catheter
Leakage of Hopkins catheter
Leakage of ileostomy catheter
Leakage of urostomy catheter

T83.09- <u>Other mechanical</u> complication of urinary catheter
Obstruction (mechanical) of urinary catheter
Perforation of urinary catheter
Protrusion of urinary catheter

CC-A **T83.090-** Other mechanical complication of <u>cystostomy</u> catheter

T83.091- Other mechanical complication of <u>indwelling urethral</u> catheter

T83.092- Other mechanical complication of <u>nephrostomy</u> catheter

T83.098- Other mechanical complication of <u>other</u> urinary catheter
Other mechanical complication of Hopkins catheter
Other mechanical complication of ileostomy catheter
Other mechanical complication of urostomy catheter

T83.1- <u>Mechanical</u> complication of <u>other urinary devices and implants</u>

T83.11- <u>Breakdown</u> (mechanical) of other urinary devices and implants

CC-A **T83.110-** Breakdown (mechanical) of <u>urinary electronic stimulator device</u>
Excludes ❷: *breakdown (mechanical) of electrode (lead) for sacral nerve neurostimulator (T85.111)*
breakdown (mechanical) of implanted electronic sacral neurostimulator, pulse generator or receiver (T85.113)

CC-A **T83.111-** Breakdown (mechanical) of <u>implanted urinary sphincter</u>

CC-A **T83.112-** Breakdown (mechanical) of <u>indwelling ureteral stent</u>

CC-A **T83.113-** Breakdown (mechanical) of <u>other</u> urinary <u>stents</u>
Breakdown (mechanical) of ileal conduit stent
Breakdown (mechanical) of nephroureteral stent

CC-A **T83.118-** Breakdown (mechanical) of <u>other</u> urinary <u>devices</u> and implants

T82 - T83

T83.12- <u>Displacement</u> of other urinary devices and implants
Malposition of other urinary devices and implants

CC-A **T83.120-** Displacement of <u>urinary electronic stimulator device</u>
Excludes ❷: *displacement of electrode (lead) for sacral nerve neurostimulator (T85.121)*
displacement of implanted electronic sacral neurostimulator, pulse generator or receiver (T85.123)

CC-A **T83.121-** Displacement of <u>implanted urinary sphincter</u>

CC-A **T83.122-** Displacement of <u>indwelling ureteral stent</u>

CC-A **T83.123-** Displacement of <u>other</u> urinary <u>stents</u>
Displacement of ileal conduit stent
Displacement of nephroureteral stent

CC-A **T83.128-** Displacement of <u>other</u> urinary <u>devices</u> and implants

T83.19- <u>Other mechanical complication</u> of other urinary devices and implants
Leakage of other urinary devices and implants
Obstruction (mechanical) of other urinary devices and implants
Perforation of other urinary devices and implants
Protrusion of other urinary devices and implants

CC-A **T83.190-** Other mechanical complication of <u>urinary electronic stimulator device</u>
Excludes ❷: *other mechanical complication of electrode (lead) for sacral nerve neurostimulator (T85.191)*
other mechanical complication of implanted electronic sacral neurostimulator, pulse generator or receiver (T85.193)

CC-A **T83.191-** Other mechanical complication of <u>implanted urinary sphincter</u>

CC-A **T83.192-** Other mechanical complication of <u>indwelling ureteral stent</u>

CC-A **T83.193-** Other mechanical complication of <u>other</u> urinary stent
Other mechanical complication of ileal conduit stent
Other mechanical complication of nephroureteral stent

CC-A **T83.198-** Other mechanical complication of <u>other</u> urinary <u>devices</u> and implants

T83.2- <u>Mechanical</u> complication of <u>graft of urinary organ</u>

CC-A **T83.21x-** <u>Breakdown</u> (mechanical) of graft of urinary organ

CC-A **T83.22x-** <u>Displacement</u> of graft of urinary organ
Malposition of graft of urinary organ

CC-A **T83.23x-** <u>Leakage</u> of graft of urinary organ

CC-A **T83.24x-** <u>Erosion</u> of graft of urinary organ

CC-A **T83.25x-** <u>Exposure</u> of graft of urinary organ

CC-A **T83.29x-** <u>Other</u> mechanical complication of graft of urinary organ
Obstruction (mechanical) of graft of urinary organ
Perforation of graft of urinary organ
Protrusion of graft of urinary organ

T83.3- <u>Mechanical</u> complication of <u>intrauterine contraceptive device</u>

T83.31x- <u>Breakdown</u> (mechanical) of intrauterine contraceptive device — [♀]

T83.32x- <u>Displacement</u> of intrauterine contraceptive device — [♀]
Malposition of intrauterine contraceptive device
Missing string of intrauterine contraceptive device

T83.39x- <u>Other</u> mechanical complication of intrauterine contraceptive device — [♀]
Leakage of intrauterine contraceptive device
Obstruction (mechanical) of intrauterine contraceptive device
Perforation of intrauterine contraceptive device
Protrusion of intrauterine contraceptive device

T83.4- <u>Mechanical</u> complication of <u>other prosthetic devices, implants and grafts of genital tract</u>

T83.41- <u>Breakdown</u> (mechanical) of other prosthetic devices, implants and grafts of genital tract

CC-A **T83.410-** Breakdown (mechanical) of <u>implanted penile prosthesis</u> — [♂]
Breakdown (mechanical) of penile prosthesis cylinder
Breakdown (mechanical) of penile prosthesis pump
Breakdown (mechanical) of penile prosthesis reservoir

CC-A **T83.411-** Breakdown (mechanical) of <u>implanted testicular prosthesis</u> — [♂]

CC-A **T83.418-** Breakdown (mechanical) of <u>other</u> prosthetic devices, implants and grafts of genital tract

T83.42- <u>Displacement</u> of other prosthetic devices, implants and grafts of genital tract
Malposition of other prosthetic devices, implants and grafts of genital tract

CC-A **T83.420-** Displacement of <u>implanted penile prosthesis</u> — [♂]
Displacement of penile prosthesis cylinder
Displacement of penile prosthesis pump
Displacement of penile prosthesis reservoir

CC-A **T83.421-** Displacement of <u>implanted testicular prosthesis</u> — [♂]

CC-A **T83.428-** Displacement of <u>other</u> prosthetic devices, implants and grafts of genital tract

T83.49- <u>Other mechanical complication</u> of other prosthetic devices, implants and grafts of genital tract
Leakage of other prosthetic devices, implants and grafts of genital tract
Obstruction, mechanical of other prosthetic devices, implants and grafts of genital tract
Perforation of other prosthetic devices, implants and grafts of genital tract
Protrusion of other prosthetic devices, implants and grafts of genital tract

CC-A **T83.490-** Other mechanical complication of <u>implanted penile prosthesis</u> — [♂]
Other mechanical complication of penile prosthesis cylinder
Other mechanical complication of penile prosthesis pump
Other mechanical complication of penile prosthesis reservoir

CC-A **T83.491-** Other mechanical complication of <u>implanted testicular prosthesis</u> — [♂]

CC-A **T83.498-** Other mechanical complication of <u>other</u> prosthetic devices, implants and grafts of genital tract

T83.5- <u>Infection and inflammatory reaction</u> due to <u>prosthetic device, implant and graft in urinary system</u>
Use additional code to identify infection

T83.51- Infection and inflammatory reaction due to urinary catheter
Excludes ❷: *complications of stoma of urinary tract (N99.5-)*

CC-A **T83.510-** Infection and inflammatory reaction due to <u>cystostomy</u> catheter

CC-A **T83.511-** Infection and inflammatory reaction due to <u>indwelling urethral</u> catheter

CC-A **T83.512-** Infection and inflammatory reaction due to <u>nephrostomy</u> catheter

CC-A **T83.518-** Infection and inflammatory reaction due to <u>other</u> urinary catheter
Infection and inflammatory reaction due to Hopkins catheter
Infection and inflammatory reaction due to ileostomy catheter
Infection and inflammatory reaction due to urostomy catheter

T83 – T83

T83.59-   Infection and inflammatory reaction due to prosthetic device, implant and graft in urinary system

CC-A **T83.590-**   Infection and inflammatory reaction due to implanted urinary neurostimulation device

     Excludes ❷: *infection and inflammatory reaction due to electrode lead of sacral nerve neurostimulator (T85.732)*

           infection and inflammatory reaction due to pulse generator or receiver of sacral nerve neurostimulator (T85.734)

CC-A **T83.591-**   Infection and inflammatory reaction due to implanted urinary sphincter

CC-A **T83.592-**   Infection and inflammatory reaction due to indwelling ureteral stent

CC-A **T83.593-**   Infection and inflammatory reaction due to other urinary stents
     Infection and inflammatory reaction due to ileal conduit stents
     Infection and inflammatory reaction due to nephroureteral stent

CC-A **T83.598-**   Infection and inflammatory reaction due to other prosthetic device, implant and graft in urinary system

T83.6-   Infection and inflammatory reaction due to prosthetic device, implant and graft in genital tract
     Use additional code to identify infection

CC-A **T83.61x-**   Infection and inflammatory reaction due to implanted penile prosthesis
     Infection and inflammatory reaction due to penile prosthesis cylinder
     Infection and inflammatory reaction due to penile prosthesis pump
     Infection and inflammatory reaction due to penile prosthesis reservoir

CC-A **T83.62x-**   Infection and inflammatory reaction due to implanted testicular prosthesis

CC-A **T83.69x-**   Infection and inflammatory reaction due to other prosthetic device, implant and graft in genital tract

T83.7-   Complications due to implanted mesh and other prosthetic materials

   T83.71-   Erosion of implanted mesh and other prosthetic materials to surrounding organ or tissue

     T83.711-   Erosion of implanted vaginal mesh to surrounding organ or tissue — [♀]
       Erosion of implanted vaginal mesh into pelvic floor muscles

    CC-A **T83.712-**   Erosion of implanted urethral mesh to surrounding organ or tissue
       Erosion of implanted female urethral sling
       Erosion of implanted male urethral sling
       Erosion of implanted urethral mesh into pelvic floor muscles

    CC-A **T83.713-**   Erosion of implanted urethral bulking agent to surrounding organ or tissue

    CC-A **T83.714-**   Erosion of implanted ureteral bulking agent to surrounding organ or tissue

    CC-A **T83.718-**   Erosion of other implanted mesh to organ or tissue

    CC-A **T83.719-**   Erosion of other prosthetic materials to surrounding organ or tissue

   T83.72-   Exposure of implanted mesh and other prosthetic materials to surrounding organ or tissue
     Extrusion of implanted mesh

     T83.721-   Exposure of implanted vaginal mesh into vagina — [♀]
       Exposure of implanted vaginal mesh through vaginal wall

    CC-A **T83.722-**   Exposure of implanted urethral mesh into urethra
       Exposure of implanted female urethral sling
       Exposure of implanted male urethral sling
       Exposure of implanted urethral mesh through urethral wall

    CC-A **T83.723-**   Exposure of implanted urethral bulking agent into urethra

CC-A **T83.724-**   Exposure of implanted ureteral bulking agent into ureter

CC-A **T83.728-**   Exposure of other implanted mesh into organ or tissue

CC-A **T83.729-**   Exposure of other prosthetic materials into organ or tissue

CC-A **T83.79x-**   Other specified complications due to other genitourinary prosthetic materials

T83.8-   Other specified complications of genitourinary prosthetic devices, implants and grafts

CC-A **T83.81x-**   Embolism due to genitourinary prosthetic devices, implants and grafts

CC-A **T83.82x-**   Fibrosis due to genitourinary prosthetic devices, implants and grafts

CC-A **T83.83x-**   Hemorrhage due to genitourinary prosthetic devices, implants and grafts

CC-A **T83.84x-**   Pain due to genitourinary prosthetic devices, implants and grafts

CC-A **T83.85x-**   Stenosis due to genitourinary prosthetic devices, implants and grafts

CC-A **T83.86x-**   Thrombosis due to genitourinary prosthetic devices, implants and grafts

CC-A **T83.89x-**   Other specified complication of genitourinary prosthetic devices, implants and grafts

T83.9xx-   Unspecified complication of genitourinary prosthetic device, implant and graft
CC-A

T84-   Complications of internal orthopedic prosthetic devices, implants and grafts
     Excludes ❷: *failure and rejection of transplanted organs and tissues (T86.-)*
           fracture of bone following insertion of orthopedic implant, joint prosthesis or bone plate (M96.6)

> **The appropriate 7th character is to be added to each code from category T84:**
> **A**   Initial encounter
> **D**   Subsequent encounter
> **S**   Sequela

T84.0-   Mechanical complication of internal joint prosthesis

   T84.01-   Broken internal joint prosthesis
     Breakage (fracture) of prosthetic joint
     Broken prosthetic joint implant
     Excludes 1:   *periprosthetic joint implant fracture (T84.04)*

    CC-A **T84.010-**   Broken internal right hip prosthesis

    CC-A **T84.011-**   Broken internal left hip prosthesis

    CC-A **T84.012-**   Broken internal right knee prosthesis

    CC-A **T84.013-**   Broken internal left knee prosthesis

    CC-A **T84.018-**   Broken internal joint prosthesis, other site
       Use additional code to identify the joint (Z96.6-)

    CC-A **T84.019-**   Broken internal joint prosthesis, unspecified site

   T84.02-   Dislocation of internal joint prosthesis
     Instability of internal joint prosthesis
     Subluxation of internal joint prosthesis

    CC-A **T84.020-**   Dislocation of internal right hip prosthesis

    CC-A **T84.021-**   Dislocation of internal left hip prosthesis

    CC-A **T84.022-**   Instability of internal right knee prosthesis

    CC-A **T84.023-**   Instability of internal left knee prosthesis

    CC-A **T84.028-**   Dislocation of other internal joint prosthesis
       Use additional code to identify the joint (Z96.6-)

    CC-A **T84.029-**   Dislocation of unspecified internal joint prosthesis

   T84.03-   Mechanical loosening of internal prosthetic joint
     Aseptic loosening of prosthetic joint

    CC-A **T84.030-**   Mechanical loosening of internal right hip prosthetic joint

    CC-A **T84.031-**   Mechanical loosening of internal left hip prosthetic joint

    CC-A **T84.032-**   Mechanical loosening of internal right knee prosthetic joint

    CC-A **T84.033-**   Mechanical loosening of internal left knee prosthetic joint

T83 - T84 *(side tab)*

CC-A **T84.038-** Mechanical loosening of <u>other</u> internal prosthetic joint
  Use additional code to identify the joint (Z96.6-)

CC-A **T84.039-** Mechanical loosening of <u>unspecified</u> internal prosthetic joint

T84.05- <u>Periprosthetic osteolysis</u> of internal prosthetic joint
  Use additional code to identify major osseous defect, if applicable (M89.7-)

CC-A **T84.050-** Periprosthetic osteolysis of internal prosthetic <u>right hip</u> joint

CC-A **T84.051-** Periprosthetic osteolysis of internal prosthetic <u>left hip</u> joint

CC-A **T84.052-** Periprosthetic osteolysis of internal prosthetic <u>right knee</u> joint

CC-A **T84.053-** Periprosthetic osteolysis of internal prosthetic <u>left knee</u> joint

CC-A **T84.058-** Periprosthetic osteolysis of <u>other</u> internal prosthetic joint
  Use additional code to identify the joint (Z96.6-)

CC-A **T84.059-** Periprosthetic osteolysis of <u>unspecified</u> internal prosthetic joint

T84.06- <u>Wear of articular bearing surface</u> of internal prosthetic joint

CC-A **T84.060-** Wear of articular bearing surface of internal prosthetic <u>right hip</u> joint

CC-A **T84.061-** Wear of articular bearing surface of internal prosthetic <u>left hip</u> joint

CC-A **T84.062-** Wear of articular bearing surface of internal prosthetic <u>right knee</u> joint

CC-A **T84.063-** Wear of articular bearing surface of internal prosthetic <u>left knee</u> joint

CC-A **T84.068-** Wear of articular bearing surface of <u>other</u> internal prosthetic joint
  Use additional code to identify the joint (Z96.6-)

CC-A **T84.069-** Wear of articular bearing surface of <u>unspecified</u> internal prosthetic joint

T84.09- <u>Other mechanical complication</u> of internal joint prosthesis
  Prosthetic joint implant failure NOS

CC-A **T84.090-** Other mechanical complication of internal <u>right hip</u> prosthesis

CC-A **T84.091-** Other mechanical complication of internal <u>left hip</u> prosthesis

CC-A **T84.092-** Other mechanical complication of internal <u>right knee</u> prosthesis

CC-A **T84.093-** Other mechanical complication of internal <u>left knee</u> prosthesis

CC-A **T84.098-** Other mechanical complication of <u>other</u> internal joint prosthesis
  Use additional code to identify the joint (Z96.6-)

CC-A **T84.099-** Other mechanical complication of <u>unspecified</u> internal joint prosthesis

T84.1- <u>Mechanical complication of internal fixation device of bones of limb</u>
  Excludes ❷: mechanical complication of internal fixation device of bones of feet (T84.2-)
   mechanical complication of internal fixation device of bones of fingers (T84.2-)
   mechanical complication of internal fixation device of bones of hands (T84.2-)
   mechanical complication of internal fixation device of bones of toes (T84.2-)

T84.11- <u>Breakdown</u> (mechanical) of internal fixation device of bones of limb

CC-A **T84.110-** Breakdown (mechanical) of internal fixation device of <u>right humerus</u>

CC-A **T84.111-** Breakdown (mechanical) of internal fixation device of <u>left humerus</u>

CC-A **T84.112-** Breakdown (mechanical) of internal fixation device of bone of <u>right forearm</u>

CC-A **T84.113-** Breakdown (mechanical) of internal fixation device of bone of <u>left forearm</u>

CC-A **T84.114-** Breakdown (mechanical) of internal fixation device of <u>right femur</u>

CC-A **T84.115-** Breakdown (mechanical) of internal fixation device of <u>left femur</u>

CC-A **T84.116-** Breakdown (mechanical) of internal fixation device of bone of <u>right lower leg</u>

CC-A **T84.117-** Breakdown (mechanical) of internal fixation device of bone of <u>left lower leg</u>

CC-A **T84.119-** Breakdown (mechanical) of internal fixation device of <u>unspecified</u> bone of limb

T84.12- <u>Displacement</u> of internal fixation device of bones of limb
  Malposition of internal fixation device of bones of limb

CC-A **T84.120-** Displacement of internal fixation device of <u>right humerus</u>

CC-A **T84.121-** Displacement of internal fixation device of <u>left humerus</u>

CC-A **T84.122-** Displacement of internal fixation device of bone of <u>right forearm</u>

CC-A **T84.123-** Displacement of internal fixation device of bone of <u>left forearm</u>

CC-A **T84.124-** Displacement of internal fixation device of <u>right femur</u>

CC-A **T84.125-** Displacement of internal fixation device of <u>left femur</u>

CC-A **T84.126-** Displacement of internal fixation device of bone of <u>right lower leg</u>

CC-A **T84.127-** Displacement of internal fixation device of bone of <u>left lower leg</u>

CC-A **T84.129-** Displacement of internal fixation device of <u>unspecified</u> bone of limb

T84.19- <u>Other mechanical complication</u> of internal fixation device of bones of limb
  Obstruction (mechanical) of internal fixation device of bones of limb
  Perforation of internal fixation device of bones of limb
  Protrusion of internal fixation device of bones of limb

CC-A **T84.190-** Other mechanical complication of internal fixation device of <u>right humerus</u>

CC-A **T84.191-** Other mechanical complication of internal fixation device of <u>left humerus</u>

CC-A **T84.192-** Other mechanical complication of internal fixation device of bone of <u>right forearm</u>

CC-A **T84.193-** Other mechanical complication of internal fixation device of bone of <u>left forearm</u>

CC-A **T84.194-** Other mechanical complication of internal fixation device of <u>right femur</u>

CC-A **T84.195-** Other mechanical complication of internal fixation device of <u>left femur</u>

CC-A **T84.196-** Other mechanical complication of internal fixation device of bone of <u>right lower leg</u>

CC-A **T84.197-** Other mechanical complication of internal fixation device of bone of <u>left lower leg</u>

CC-A **T84.199-** Other mechanical complication of internal fixation device of <u>unspecified</u> bone of limb

T84.2- <u>Mechanical complication of internal fixation device of other bones</u>

T84.21- <u>Breakdown</u> (mechanical) of internal fixation device of other bones

CC-A **T84.210-** Breakdown (mechanical) of internal fixation device of bones of <u>hand and fingers</u>

CC-A **T84.213-** Breakdown (mechanical) of internal fixation device of bones of <u>foot and toes</u>

CC-A **T84.216-** Breakdown (mechanical) of internal fixation device of <u>vertebrae</u>

CC-A **T84.218-** Breakdown (mechanical) of internal fixation device of <u>other bones</u>

T84 - T84

T84.22- <u>Displacement</u> of internal fixation device of other bones
  Malposition of internal fixation device of other bones

CC-A **T84.220-** Displacement of internal fixation device of bones of <u>hand and fingers</u>

CC-A **T84.223-** Displacement of internal fixation device of bones of <u>foot and toes</u>

CC-A **T84.226-** Displacement of internal fixation device of <u>vertebrae</u>

CC-A **T84.228-** Displacement of internal fixation device of <u>other bones</u>

T84.29- <u>Other mechanical complication</u> of internal fixation device of other bones
  Obstruction (mechanical) of internal fixation device of other bones
  Perforation of internal fixation device of other bones
  Protrusion of internal fixation device of other bones

CC-A **T84.290-** Other mechanical complication of internal fixation device of bones of <u>hand and fingers</u>

CC-A **T84.293-** Other mechanical complication of internal fixation device of bones of <u>foot and toes</u>

CC-A **T84.296-** Other mechanical complication of internal fixation device of <u>vertebrae</u>

CC-A **T84.298-** Other mechanical complication of internal fixation device of <u>other bones</u>

T84.3- <u>Mechanical complication</u> of <u>other bone devices, implants and grafts</u>
  Excludes ❷: *other complications of bone graft (T86.83-)*

T84.31- <u>Breakdown</u> (mechanical) of other bone devices, implants and grafts

CC-A **T84.310-** Breakdown (mechanical) of electronic bone stimulator

CC-A **T84.318-** Breakdown (mechanical) of other bone devices, implants and grafts

T84.32- <u>Displacement</u> of other bone devices, implants and grafts
  Malposition of other bone devices, implants and grafts

CC-A **T84.320-** Displacement of electronic bone stimulator

CC-A **T84.328-** Displacement of other bone devices, implants and grafts
  AHA 14:4Q:p28 – Dislodged proximal hooks and growing rods

T84.39- <u>Other mechanical complication</u> of other bone devices, implants and grafts
  Obstruction (mechanical) of other bone devices, implants and grafts
  Perforation of other bone devices, implants and grafts
  Protrusion of other bone devices, implants and grafts

CC-A **T84.390-** Other mechanical complication of electronic bone stimulator

CC-A **T84.398-** Other mechanical complication of other bone devices, implants and grafts

T84.4- <u>Mechanical</u> complication of <u>other internal orthopedic devices, implants and grafts</u>

T84.41- <u>Breakdown</u> (mechanical) of other internal orthopedic devices, implants and grafts

CC-A **T84.410-** Breakdown (mechanical) of muscle and tendon graft

CC-A **T84.418-** Breakdown (mechanical) of other internal orthopedic devices, implants and grafts

T84.42- <u>Displacement</u> of other internal orthopedic devices, implants and grafts
  Malposition of other internal orthopedic devices, implants and grafts

CC-A **T84.420-** Displacement of muscle and tendon graft

CC-A **T84.428-** Displacement of other internal orthopedic devices, implants and grafts

T84.49- <u>Other mechanical complication</u> of other internal orthopedic devices, implants and grafts
  Mechanical complication of other internal orthopedic devices, implants and grafts NOS
  Obstruction (mechanical) of other internal orthopedic devices, implants and grafts
  Perforation of other internal orthopedic devices, implants and grafts
  Protrusion of other internal orthopedic devices, implants and grafts

CC-A **T84.490-** Other mechanical complication of muscle and tendon graft

CC-A **T84.498-** Other mechanical complication of other internal orthopedic devices, implants and grafts

T84.5- <u>Infection and inflammatory reaction</u> due to <u>internal joint prosthesis</u>
  AHA 15:1Q:p16 – Infection after a primary left total hip replacement
  Use additional code to identify infection

CC-A **T84.50x-** Infection and inflammatory reaction due to <u>unspecified</u> internal joint prosthesis

CC-A **T84.51x-** Infection and inflammatory reaction due to internal <u>right hip</u> prosthesis

CC-A **T84.52x-** Infection and inflammatory reaction due to internal <u>left hip</u> prosthesis

CC-A **T84.53x-** Infection and inflammatory reaction due to internal <u>right knee</u> prosthesis

CC-A **T84.54x-** Infection and inflammatory reaction due to internal <u>left knee</u> prosthesis

CC-A **T84.59x-** Infection and inflammatory reaction due to <u>other</u> internal joint prosthesis

T84.6- <u>Infection and inflammatory reaction</u> due to <u>internal fixation device</u>
  Use additional code to identify infection

CC-A **T84.60x-** Infection and inflammatory reaction due to internal fixation device of <u>unspecified</u> site

T84.61- Infection and inflammatory reaction due to internal fixation device of <u>arm</u>

CC-A **T84.610-** Infection and inflammatory reaction due to internal fixation device of <u>right humerus</u>

CC-A **T84.611-** Infection and inflammatory reaction due to internal fixation device of <u>left humerus</u>

CC-A **T84.612-** Infection and inflammatory reaction due to internal fixation device of <u>right radius</u>

CC-A **T84.613-** Infection and inflammatory reaction due to internal fixation device of <u>left radius</u>

CC-A **T84.614-** Infection and inflammatory reaction due to internal fixation device of <u>right ulna</u>

CC-A **T84.615-** Infection and inflammatory reaction due to internal fixation device of <u>left ulna</u>

CC-A **T84.619-** Infection and inflammatory reaction due to internal fixation device of <u>unspecified</u> bone of arm

T84.62- Infection and inflammatory reaction due to internal fixation device of <u>leg</u>

CC-A **T84.620-** Infection and inflammatory reaction due to internal fixation device of <u>right femur</u>

CC-A **T84.621-** Infection and inflammatory reaction due to internal fixation device of <u>left femur</u>

CC-A **T84.622-** Infection and inflammatory reaction due to internal fixation device of <u>right tibia</u>

CC-A **T84.623-** Infection and inflammatory reaction due to internal fixation device of <u>left tibia</u>

CC-A **T84.624-** Infection and inflammatory reaction due to internal fixation device of <u>right fibula</u>

CC-A **T84.625-** Infection and inflammatory reaction due to internal fixation device of <u>left fibula</u>

CC-A **T84.629-** Infection and inflammatory reaction due to internal fixation device of <u>unspecified</u> bone of leg

CC-A **T84.63x-** Infection and inflammatory reaction due to internal fixation device of <u>spine</u>

CC-A **T84.69x-** Infection and inflammatory reaction due to internal fixation device of <u>other site</u>

T84
-
T84

T84.7xx-   Infection and inflammatory reaction due to other internal
CC-A   orthopedic prosthetic devices, implants and grafts
Use additional code to identify infection

T84.8-   Other specified complications of internal orthopedic
prosthetic devices, implants and grafts

CC-A **T84.81x-**   Embolism due to internal orthopedic prosthetic devices,
implants and grafts

CC-A **T84.82x-**   Fibrosis due to internal orthopedic prosthetic devices,
implants and grafts

CC-A **T84.83x-**   Hemorrhage due to internal orthopedic prosthetic
devices, implants and grafts

CC-A **T84.84x-**   Pain due to internal orthopedic prosthetic devices,
implants and grafts

CC-A **T84.85x-**   Stenosis due to internal orthopedic prosthetic devices,
implants and grafts

CC-A **T84.86x-**   Thrombosis due to internal orthopedic prosthetic
devices, implants and grafts

CC-A **T84.89x-**   Other specified complication of internal orthopedic
prosthetic devices, implants and grafts

T84.9xx-   Unspecified complication of internal orthopedic prosthetic
CC-A   device, implant and graft

T85-   Complications of other internal prosthetic devices, implants and
grafts
AHA 15:1Q:p15 – Graft prolapse
Excludes ❷: failure and rejection of transplanted organs and tissue (T86-)

The appropriate 7th character is to be added to each code from
category T85:
   A   Initial encounter
   D   Subsequent encounter
   S   Sequela

T85.0-   Mechanical complication of ventricular intracranial
(communicating) shunt

CC-A **T85.01x-**   Breakdown (mechanical) of ventricular intracranial
(communicating) shunt

CC-A **T85.02x-**   Displacement of ventricular intracranial
(communicating) shunt
Malposition of ventricular intracranial (communicating)
shunt

CC-A **T85.03x-**   Leakage of ventricular intracranial (communicating)
shunt

CC-A **T85.09x-**   Other mechanical complication of ventricular
intracranial (communicating) shunt
Obstruction (mechanical) of ventricular intracranial
(communicating) shunt
Perforation of ventricular intracranial (communicating)
shunt
Protrusion of ventricular intracranial (communicating) shunt

T85.1-   Mechanical complication of implanted electronic stimulator of
nervous system

T85.11-   Breakdown (mechanical) of implanted electronic
stimulator of nervous system

CC-A **T85.110-**   Breakdown (mechanical) of implanted electronic
neurostimulator of brain electrode (lead)

CC-A **T85.111-**   Breakdown (mechanical) of implanted electronic
neurostimulator of peripheral nerve electrode
(lead)
Breakdown of electrode (lead) for cranial nerve
neurostimulators
Breakdown of electrode (lead) for gastric
neurostimulator
Breakdown of electrode (lead) for sacral nerve
neurostimulator
Breakdown of electrode (lead) for vagal nerve
neurostimulators

CC-A **T85.112-**   Breakdown (mechanical) of implanted electronic
neurostimulator of spinal cord electrode (lead)

CC-A **T85.113-**   Breakdown (mechanical) of implanted electronic
neurostimulator, generator
Breakdown (mechanical) of implanted electronic
neurostimulator generator, brain, peripheral,
gastric, spinal
Breakdown (mechanical) of implanted electronic sacral
neurostimulator, pulse generator or receiver

CC-A **T85.118-**   Breakdown (mechanical) of other implanted
electronic stimulator of nervous system

T85.12-   Displacement of implanted electronic stimulator of
nervous system
Malposition of implanted electronic stimulator of nervous
system

CC-A **T85.120-**   Displacement of implanted electronic
neurostimulator of brain electrode (lead)

CC-A **T85.121-**   Displacement of implanted electronic
neurostimulator of peripheral nerve electrode
(lead)
Displacement of electrode (lead) for cranial nerve
neurostimulators
Displacement of electrode (lead) for gastric
neurostimulator
Displacement of electrode (lead) for sacral nerve
neurostimulator
Displacement of electrode (lead) for vagal nerve
neurostimulators

CC-A **T85.122-**   Displacement of implanted electronic
neurostimulator of spinal cord electrode (lead)

CC-A **T85.123-**   Displacement of implanted electronic
neurostimulator, generator
Displacement of implanted electronic neurostimulator
generator, brain, peripheral, gastric, spinal
Displacement of implanted electronic sacral
neurostimulator, pulse generator or receiver

CC-A **T85.128-**   Displacement of other implanted electronic
stimulator of nervous system

T85.19-   Other mechanical complication of implanted electronic
stimulator of nervous system
Leakage of implanted electronic stimulator of nervous system
Obstruction (mechanical) of implanted electronic stimulator of
nervous system
Perforation of implanted electronic stimulator of nervous
system
Protrusion of implanted electronic stimulator of nervous
system

CC-A **T85.190-**   Other mechanical complication of implanted
electronic neurostimulator of brain electrode (lead)

CC-A **T85.191-**   Other mechanical complication of implanted
electronic neurostimulator of peripheral nerve
electrode (lead)
Other mechanical complication of electrode (lead) for
cranial nerve neurostimulators
Other mechanical complication of electrode (lead) for
gastric neurostimulator
Other mechanical complication of electrode (lead) for
sacral nerve neurostimulator
Other mechanical complication of electrode (lead) for
vagal nerve neurostimulators

CC-A **T85.192-**   Other mechanical complication of implanted
electronic neurostimulator of spinal cord electrode
(lead)

CC-A **T85.193-**   Other mechanical complication of implanted
electronic neurostimulator, generator
Other mechanical complication of implanted electronic
neurostimulator generator, brain, peripheral,
gastric, spinal
Other mechanical complication of implanted electronic
sacral neurostimulator, pulse generator or receiver

CC-A **T85.199-**   Other mechanical complication of other implanted
electronic stimulator of nervous system

T85.2-   Mechanical complication of intraocular lens

CC-A **T85.21x-**   Breakdown (mechanical) of intraocular lens

CC-A **T85.22x-**   Displacement of intraocular lens
Malposition of intraocular lens

CC-A **T85.29x-**   Other mechanical complication of intraocular lens
Obstruction (mechanical) of intraocular lens
Perforation of intraocular lens
Protrusion of intraocular lens

T84
-
T85

T85.3-　**Mechanical** complication of <u>other ocular prosthetic devices, implants and grafts</u>

　　Excludes ❷:　other complications of corneal graft (T86.84-)

T85.31-　**Breakdown** (mechanical) of other ocular prosthetic devices, implants and grafts

CC-A **T85.310-**　Breakdown (mechanical) of prosthetic orbit of <u>right</u> eye

CC-A **T85.311-**　Breakdown (mechanical) of prosthetic orbit of <u>left</u> eye

T85.318-　Breakdown (mechanical) of <u>other</u> ocular prosthetic devices, implants and grafts

T85.32-　**Displacement** of other ocular prosthetic devices, implants and grafts

　　Malposition of other ocular prosthetic devices, implants and grafts

CC-A **T85.320-**　Displacement of prosthetic orbit of <u>right</u> eye

CC-A **T85.321-**　Displacement of prosthetic orbit of <u>left</u> eye

T85.328-　Displacement of <u>other</u> ocular prosthetic devices, implants and grafts

T85.39-　**Other mechanical** complication of other ocular prosthetic devices, implants and grafts

　　Obstruction (mechanical) of other ocular prosthetic devices, implants and grafts
　　Perforation of other ocular prosthetic devices, implants and grafts
　　Protrusion of other ocular prosthetic devices, implants and grafts

CC-A **T85.390-**　Other mechanical complication of prosthetic orbit of <u>right</u> eye

CC-A **T85.391-**　Other mechanical complication of prosthetic orbit of <u>left</u> eye

T85.398-　Other mechanical complication of <u>other</u> ocular prosthetic devices, implants and grafts

T85.4-　**Mechanical** complication of <u>breast prosthesis and implant</u>

CC-A **T85.41x-**　**Breakdown** (mechanical) of breast prosthesis and implant

CC-A **T85.42x-**　**Displacement** of breast prosthesis and implant
　　Malposition of breast prosthesis and implant

CC-A **T85.43x-**　**Leakage** of breast prosthesis and implant

CC-A **T85.44x-**　**Capsular contracture** of breast implant

CC-A **T85.49x-**　**Other mechanicalm** complication of breast prosthesis and implant
　　Obstruction (mechanical) of breast prosthesis and implant
　　Perforation of breast prosthesis and implant
　　Protrusion of breast prosthesis and implant

T85.5-　**Mechanical** complication of <u>gastrointestinal prosthetic devices, implants and grafts</u>

T85.51-　**Breakdown** (mechanical) of gastrointestinal prosthetic devices, implants and grafts

CC-A **T85.510-**　Breakdown (mechanical) of <u>bile duct prosthesis</u>

CC-A **T85.511-**　Breakdown (mechanical) of <u>esophageal anti-reflux device</u>

CC-A **T85.518-**　Breakdown (mechanical) of <u>other</u> gastrointestinal prosthetic devices, implants and grafts

T85.52-　**Displacement** of gastrointestinal prosthetic devices, implants and grafts
　　Malposition of gastrointestinal prosthetic devices, implants and grafts

CC-A **T85.520-**　Displacement of <u>bile duct prosthesis</u>

CC-A **T85.521-**　Displacement of <u>esophageal anti-reflux device</u>

CC-A **T85.528-**　Displacement of <u>other</u> gastrointestinal prosthetic devices, implants and grafts

T85.59-　**Other mechanical** complication of gastrointestinal prosthetic devices, implants and
　　Obstruction, mechanical of gastrointestinal prosthetic devices, implants and grafts
　　Perforation of gastrointestinal prosthetic devices, implants and grafts
　　Protrusion of gastrointestinal prosthetic devices, implants and grafts

CC-A **T85.590-**　Other mechanical complication of <u>bile duct prosthesis</u>

CC-A **T85.591-**　Other mechanical complication of <u>esophageal anti-reflux device</u>

CC-A **T85.598-**　Other mechanical complication of <u>other</u> gastrointestinal prosthetic devices, implants and grafts

T85.6-　**Mechanical** complication of <u>other specified internal and external prosthetic devices, implants and grafts</u>

T85.61-　**Breakdown** (mechanical) of other specified internal prosthetic devices, implants and grafts

CC-A **T85.610-**　Breakdown (mechanical) of <u>cranial or spinal infusion catheter</u>
　　Breakdown (mechanical) of epidural infusion catheter
　　Breakdown (mechanical) of intrathecal infusion catheter
　　Breakdown (mechanical) of subarachnoid infusion catheter
　　Breakdown (mechanical) of subdural infusion catheter

CC-A **T85.611-**　Breakdown (mechanical) of <u>intraperitoneal dialysis catheter</u>
　　Excludes 1:　mechanical complication of vascular dialysis catheter (T82.4-)

CC-A **T85.612-**　Breakdown (mechanical) of <u>permanent sutures</u>
　　Excludes 1:　mechanical complication of permanent (wire) suture used in bone repair (T84.1-T84.2)

CC-A **T85.613-**　Breakdown (mechanical) of <u>artificial skin graft and decellularized allodermis</u>
　　Failure of artificial skin graft and decellularized allodermis
　　Non-adherence of artificial skin graft and decellularized allodermis
　　Poor incorporation of artificial skin graft and decellularized allodermis
　　Shearing of artificial skin graft and decellularized allodermis

CC-A **T85.614-**　Breakdown (mechanical) of <u>insulin pump</u>

CC-A **T85.615-**　Breakdown (mechanical) of other nervous system device, implant or graft
　　Breakdown (mechanical) of intrathecal infusion pump

CC-A **T85.618-**　Breakdown (mechanical) of <u>other</u> specified internal prosthetic devices, implants and grafts

T85.62-　**Displacement** of other specified internal prosthetic devices, implants and grafts
　　Malposition of other specified internal prosthetic devices, implants and grafts

CC-A **T85.620-**　Displacement of <u>cranial or spinal infusion catheter</u>
　　Displacement of epidural infusion catheter
　　Displacement of intrathecal infusion catheter
　　Displacement of subarachnoid infusion catheter
　　Displacement of subdural infusion catheter

CC-A **T85.621-**　Displacement of <u>intraperitoneal dialysis catheter</u>
　　Excludes 1:　mechanical complication of vascular dialysis catheter (T82.4-)

CC-A **T85.622-**　Displacement of <u>permanent sutures</u>
　　Excludes 1:　mechanical complication of permanent (wire) suture used in bone repair (T84.1-T84.2)

CC-A **T85.623-**　Displacement of <u>artificial skin graft and decellularized allodermis</u>
　　Dislodgement of artificial skin graft and decellularized allodermis
　　Displacement of artificial skin graft and decellularized allodermis

CC-A **T85.624-**　Displacement of <u>insulin pump</u>

CC-A **T85.625-**　Displacement of other nervous system device, implant or graft
　　Displacement of intrathecal infusion pump

CC-A **T85.628-**　Displacement of <u>other</u> specified internal prosthetic devices, implants and grafts

T85.63-　**Leakage** of other specified internal prosthetic devices, implants and grafts

CC-A **T85.630-**　Leakage of <u>cranial or spinal infusion catheter</u>
　　Leakage of epidural infusion catheter
　　Leakage of intrathecal infusion catheter
　　Leakage of subarachnoid infusion catheter
　　Leakage of subdural infusion catheter

CC-A **T85.631-** Leakage of <u>intraperitoneal dialysis catheter</u>
  Excludes 1:   *mechanical complication of vascular dialysis catheter (T82.4)*

CC-A **T85.633-** Leakage of <u>insulin pump</u>

CC-A **T85.635-** Leakage of other nervous system device, implant or graft
  Leakage of intrathecal infusion pump

CC-A **T85.638-** Leakage of <u>other</u> specified internal prosthetic devices, implants and grafts

T85.69- <u>Other mechanical</u> complication of other specified internal prosthetic devices, implants and grafts
  Obstruction, mechanical of other specified internal prosthetic devices, implants and grafts
  Perforation of other specified internal prosthetic devices, implants and grafts
  Protrusion of other specified internal prosthetic devices, implants and grafts

CC-A **T85.690-** Other mechanical complication of <u>cranial or spinal infusion catheter</u>
  Other mechanical complication of epidural infusion catheter
  Other mechanical complication of intrathecal infusion catheter
  Other mechanical complication of subarachnoid infusion catheter
  Other mechanical complication of subdural infusion catheter

CC-A **T85.691-** Other mechanical complication of <u>intraperitoneal dialysis catheter</u>
  Excludes 1:   *mechanical complication of vascular dialysis catheter (T82.4)*

CC-A **T85.692-** Other mechanical complication of <u>permanent sutures</u>
  Excludes 1:   *mechanical complication of permanent (wire) suture used in bone repair (T84.1-T84.2)*

CC-A **T85.693-** Other mechanical complication of <u>artificial skin graft and decellularized allodermis</u>

CC-A **T85.694-** Other mechanical complication of <u>insulin pump</u>

CC-A **T85.695-** Other mechanical complication of other nervous system device, implant or graft
  Other mechanical complication of intrathecal infusion pump

CC-A **T85.698-** Other mechanical complication of <u>other</u> specified internal prosthetic devices, implants and grafts
  Mechanical complication of nonabsorbable surgical material NOS

T85.7- <u>Infection and inflammatory reaction</u> due to <u>other internal prosthetic devices, implants and grafts</u>
  Use additional code to identify infection

CC-A **T85.71x-** Infection and inflammatory reaction due to <u>peritoneal dialysis catheter</u>

CC-A **T85.72x-** Infection and inflammatory reaction due to <u>insulin pump</u>

T85.73- <u>Infection and inflammatory reaction</u> due to <u>nervous system devices, implants and graft</u>

CC-A **T85.730-** Infection and inflammatory reaction due to <u>ventricular intracranial (communicating) shunt</u>

CC-A **T85.731-** Infection and inflammatory reaction due to implanted electronic <u>neurostimulator of brain</u>, electrode (lead)

CC-A **T85.732-** Infection and inflammatory reaction due to implanted electronic <u>neurostimulator of peripheral nerve</u>, electrode (lead)
  Infection and inflammatory reaction due to electrode (lead) for cranial nerve neurostimulators
  Infection and inflammatory reaction due to electrode (lead) for gastric neurostimulator
  Infection and inflammatory reaction due to electrode (lead) for sacral nerve neurostimulator
  Infection and inflammatory reaction due to electrode (lead) for vagal nerve neurostimulators

CC-A **T85.733-** Infection and inflammatory reaction due to implanted electronic <u>neurostimulator of spinal cord</u>, electrode (lead)

CC-A **T85.734-** Infection and inflammatory reaction due to implanted electronic <u>neurostimulator, generator</u>
  Generator pocket infection

CC-A **T85.735-** Infection and inflammatory reaction due to cranial or spinal <u>infusion catheter</u>
  Infection and inflammatory reaction due to epidural catheter
  Infection and inflammatory reaction due to intrathecal infusion catheter
  Infection and inflammatory reaction due to subarachnoid catheter
  Infection and inflammatory reaction due to subdural catheter

CC-A **T85.738-** Infection and inflammatory reaction due to <u>other</u> nervous system device, implant or graft
  Infection and inflammatory reaction due to intrathecal infusion pump

CC-A **T85.79x-** Infection and inflammatory reaction due to <u>other</u> internal prosthetic devices, implants and grafts

T85.8- <u>Other specified complications</u> of internal prosthetic devices, implants and grafts, not elsewhere classified

T85.81- <u>Embolism</u> due to internal prosthetic devices, implants and grafts, not elsewhere classified

CC-A,D **T85.810-** Embolism due to <u>nervous system</u> prosthetic devices, implants and grafts

T85.818- Embolism due to <u>other</u> internal prosthetic devices, implants and grafts

T85.82- <u>Fibrosis</u> due to internal prosthetic devices, implants and grafts, not elsewhere classified

CC-A,D **T85.820-** Fibrosis due to <u>nervous system</u> prosthetic devices, implants and grafts

T85.828- Fibrosis due to <u>other</u> internal prosthetic devices, implants and grafts

T85.83- <u>Hemorrhage</u> due to internal prosthetic devices, implants and grafts, not elsewhere classified

CC-A,D **T85.830-** Hemorrhage due to <u>nervous system</u> prosthetic devices, implants and grafts

T85.838- Hemorrhage due to <u>other</u> internal prosthetic devices, implants and grafts

T85.84- <u>Pain</u> due to internal prosthetic devices, implants and grafts, not elsewhere classified

CC-A,D **T85.840-** Pain due to <u>nervous system</u> prosthetic devices, implants and grafts

T85.848- Pain due to <u>other</u> internal prosthetic devices, implants and grafts

T85.85- <u>Stenosis</u> due to internal prosthetic devices, implants and grafts, not elsewhere classified

CC-A,D **T85.850-** Stenosis due to <u>nervous system</u> prosthetic devices, implants and grafts

T85.858- Stenosis due to <u>other</u> internal prosthetic devices, implants and grafts

T85.86- <u>Thrombosis</u> due to internal prosthetic devices, implants and grafts, not elsewhere classified

CC-A,D **T85.860-** Thrombosis due to <u>nervous system</u> prosthetic devices, implants and grafts

T85.868- Thrombosis due to <u>other</u> internal prosthetic devices, implants and grafts

T85.89- <u>Other specified complication</u> of internal prosthetic devices, implants and grafts, not elsewhere classified
  Erosion or breakdown of subcutaneous device pocket

CC-A,D **T85.890-** Other specified complication of nervous system prosthetic devices, implants and grafts

T85.898- Other specified complication of other internal prosthetic devices, implants and grafts

T85.9xx- <u>Unspecified</u> complication of internal prosthetic device, implant and graft
  Complication of internal prosthetic device, implant and graft NOS

T85 - T85 - T85

T86- <u>Complications of transplanted organs and tissue</u>
Use additional code to identify other transplant complications, such as:
Graft-versus-host disease (D89.81-)
Malignancy associated with organ transplant (C80.2)
Post-transplant lymphoproliferative disorders (PTLD) (D47.Z1)

T86.0- Complications of <u>bone marrow transplant</u>
CC **T86.00** <u>Unspecified</u> complication of bone marrow transplant
CC **T86.01** Bone marrow transplant <u>rejection</u>
CC **T86.02** Bone marrow transplant <u>failure</u>
CC **T86.03** Bone marrow transplant <u>infection</u>
CC **T86.09** <u>Other</u> complications of bone marrow transplant

T86.1- Complications of <u>kidney transplant</u>
CC **T86.10** <u>Unspecified</u> complication of kidney transplant
CC **T86.11** Kidney transplant <u>rejection</u>
CC **T86.12** Kidney transplant <u>failure</u>
AHA 13:1Q:p24 – Kidney transplant failure with stage IV chronic kidney disease
CC **T86.13** Kidney transplant <u>infection</u>
Use additional code to specify infection
CC **T86.19** <u>Other</u> complication of kidney transplant

T86.2- Complications of <u>heart transplant</u>
Excludes 1: complication of:
artificial heart device (T82.5)
heart-lung transplant (T86.3)
CC **T86.20** <u>Unspecified</u> complication of heart transplant
CC **T86.21** Heart transplant <u>rejection</u>
CC **T86.22** Heart transplant <u>failure</u>
CC **T86.23** Heart transplant <u>infection</u>
Use additional code to specify infection
T86.29- <u>Other</u> complications of heart transplant
CC **T86.290** <u>Cardiac allograft vasculopathy</u>
Excludes 1: atherosclerosis of coronary arteries
(I25.75-, I25.76-, I25.81-)
CC **T86.298** <u>Other</u> complications of heart transplant

T86.3- Complications of <u>heart-lung transplant</u>
CC **T86.30** <u>Unspecified</u> complication of heart-lung transplant
CC **T86.31** Heart-lung transplant <u>rejection</u>
CC **T86.32** Heart-lung transplant <u>failure</u>
CC **T86.33** Heart-lung transplant <u>infection</u>
Use additional code to specify infection
CC **T86.39** <u>Other</u> complications of heart-lung transplant

T86.4- Complications of <u>liver transplant</u>
CC **T86.40** <u>Unspecified</u> complication of liver transplant
CC **T86.41** Liver transplant <u>rejection</u>
CC **T86.42** Liver transplant <u>failure</u>
CC **T86.43** Liver transplant <u>infection</u>
Use additional code to identify infection, such as:
Cytomegalovirus (CMV) infection (B25.-)
CC **T86.49** <u>Other</u> complications of liver transplant

CC **T86.5** Complications of <u>stem cell transplant</u>
Complications from stem cells from peripheral blood
Complications from stem cells from umbilical cord

T86.8- Complications of other transplanted organs and tissues
T86.81- Complications of <u>lung transplant</u>
Excludes 1: complication of heart-lung transplant (T86.3-)
CC **T86.810** Lung transplant <u>rejection</u>
CC **T86.811** Lung transplant <u>failure</u>
CC **T86.812** Lung transplant <u>infection</u>
Use additional code to specify infection
CC **T86.818** <u>Other</u> complications of lung transplant
CC **T86.819** <u>Unspecified</u> complication of lung transplant

T86.82- Complications of <u>skin graft (allograft) (autograft)</u>
Excludes ❷: complication of artificial skin graft (T85.693)
CC **T86.820** Skin graft (allograft) <u>rejection</u>
CC **T86.821** Skin graft (allograft) (autograft) <u>failure</u>
CC **T86.822** Skin graft (allograft) (autograft) <u>infection</u>
Use additional code to specify infection
CC **T86.828** <u>Other</u> complications of skin graft (allograft) (autograft)
CC **T86.829** <u>Unspecified</u> complication of skin graft (allograft) (autograft)

T86.83- Complications of <u>bone graft</u>
Excludes ❷: mechanical complications of bone graft (T84.3-)
CC **T86.830** Bone graft <u>rejection</u>
CC **T86.831** Bone graft <u>failure</u>
CC **T86.832** Bone graft <u>infection</u>
Use additional code to specify infection
CC **T86.838** <u>Other</u> complications of bone graft
CC **T86.839** <u>Unspecified</u> complication of bone graft

T86.84- Complications of <u>corneal transplant</u>
Excludes ❷: mechanical complications of corneal graft (T85.3-)
CC **T86.840** Corneal transplant <u>rejection</u>
CC **T86.841** Corneal transplant <u>failure</u>
CC **T86.842** Corneal transplant <u>infection</u>
Use additional code to specify infection
CC **T86.848** <u>Other</u> complications of corneal transplant
CC **T86.849** <u>Unspecified</u> complication of corneal transplant

T86.85- Complication of <u>intestine transplant</u>
CC **T86.850** Intestine transplant <u>rejection</u>
CC **T86.851** Intestine transplant <u>failure</u>
CC **T86.852** Intestine transplant <u>infection</u>
Use additional code to specify infection
CC **T86.858** <u>Other</u> complications of intestine transplant
CC **T86.859** <u>Unspecified</u> complication of intestine transplant

T86.89- Complications of <u>other transplanted tissue</u>
Transplant failure or rejection of pancreas
CC **T86.890** Other transplanted tissue <u>rejection</u>
CC **T86.891** Other transplanted tissue <u>failure</u>
CC **T86.892** Other transplanted tissue <u>infection</u>
Use additional code to specify infection
CC **T86.898** <u>Other</u> complications of other transplanted tissue
CC **T86.899** <u>Unspecified</u> complication of other transplanted tissue

T86.9- Complication of <u>unspecified transplanted organ and tissue</u>
CC **T86.90** <u>Unspecified</u> complication of unspecified transplanted organ and tissue
CC **T86.91** Unspecified transplanted organ and tissue <u>rejection</u>
CC **T86.92** Unspecified transplanted organ and tissue <u>failure</u>
CC **T86.93** Unspecified transplanted organ and tissue <u>infection</u>
Use additional code to specify infection
CC **T86.99** <u>Other</u> complications of unspecified transplanted organ and tissue

T86 - T86

T87-   Complications peculiar to reattachment and amputation

  T87.0-   Complications of reattached (part of) upper extremity

    T87.0x-   Complications of reattached (part of) upper extremity

    cc **T87.0x1**   Complications of reattached (part of) right upper extremity

    cc **T87.0x2**   Complications of reattached (part of) left upper extremity

    cc **T87.0x9**   Complications of reattached (part of) unspecified upper extremity

  T87.1-   Complications of reattached (part of) lower extremity

    T87.1x-   Complications of reattached (part of) lower extremity

    cc **T87.1x1**   Complications of reattached (part of) right lower extremity

    cc **T87.1x2**   Complications of reattached (part of) left lower extremity

    cc **T87.1x9**   Complications of reattached (part of) unspecified lower extremity

  cc **T87.2**   Complications of other reattached body part

  T87.3-   Neuroma of amputation stump

    T87.30   Neuroma of amputation stump, unspecified extremity

    T87.31   Neuroma of amputation stump, right upper extremity

    T87.32   Neuroma of amputation stump, left upper extremity

    T87.33   Neuroma of amputation stump, right lower extremity

    T87.34   Neuroma of amputation stump, left lower extremity

  T87.4-   Infection of amputation stump

    cc **T87.40**   Infection of amputation stump, unspecified extremity

    cc **T87.41**   Infection of amputation stump, right upper extremity

    cc **T87.42**   Infection of amputation stump, left upper extremity

    cc **T87.43**   Infection of amputation stump, right lower extremity

    cc **T87.44**   Infection of amputation stump, left lower extremity

  T87.5-   Necrosis of amputation stump

    T87.50   Necrosis of amputation stump, unspecified extremity

    T87.51   Necrosis of amputation stump, right upper extremity

    T87.52   Necrosis of amputation stump, left upper extremity

    T87.53   Necrosis of amputation stump, right lower extremity

    T87.54   Necrosis of amputation stump, left lower extremity

  T87.8-   Other complications of amputation stump

    T87.81   Dehiscence of amputation stump

    T87.89   Other complications of amputation stump

        Amputation stump contracture
        Amputation stump contracture of next proximal joint
        Amputation stump edema
        Amputation stump flexion
        Amputation stump hematoma

        Excludes ❷: *phantom limb syndrome (G54.6-G54.7)*

  T87.9   Unspecified complications of amputation stump

T88-   Other complications of surgical and medical care, not elsewhere classified

  Excludes ❷: *complication following infusion, transfusion and therapeutic injection (T80.-)*
    complication following procedure NEC (T81.-)
    complications of anesthesia in labor and delivery (O74.-)
    complications of anesthesia in pregnancy (O29.-)
    complications of anesthesia in puerperium (O89.-)
    complications of devices, implants and grafts (T82-T85)
    complications of obstetric surgery and procedure (O75.4)
    dermatitis due to drugs and medicaments (L23.3, L24.4, L25.1, L27.0-L27.1)
    poisoning and toxic effects of drugs and chemicals (T36-T65 with fifth or sixth character 1-4 or 6)
    specified complications classified elsewhere

> **The appropriate 7th character is to be added to each code from category T88:**
> **A**   Initial encounter
> **D**   Subsequent encounter
> **S**   Sequela

T88.0xx-   Infection following immunization

CC-A   Sepsis following immunization

T88.1xx-   Other complications following immunization, not elsewhere classified

CC-A   Generalized vaccinia
    Rash following immunization

  Excludes 1:   *vaccinia not from vaccine (B08.011)*
  Excludes ❷: *anaphylactic shock due to serum (T80.5-)*
    other serum reactions (T80.6-)
    postimmunization arthropathy (M02.2)
    postimmunization encephalitis (G04.02)
    postimmunization fever (R50.83)

T88.2xx-   Shock due to anesthesia

CC-A   Use additional code for adverse effect, if applicable, to identify drug (T41- with fifth or sixth character 5)

  Excludes 1:   *complications of anesthesia (in):*
    labor and delivery (O74-)
    pregnancy (O29-)
    puerperium (O89-)
    postprocedural shock NOS (T81.1-)

T88.3xx-   Malignant hyperthermia due to anesthesia

CC-A   Use additional code for adverse effect, if applicable, to identify drug (T41- with fifth or sixth character 5)

T88.4xx-   Failed or difficult intubation

T88.5-   Other complications of anesthesia

  Use additional code for adverse effect, if applicable, to identify drug (T41- with fifth or sixth character 5)

  T88.51x-   Hypothermia following anesthesia

  T88.52x-   Failed moderate sedation during procedure

    Failed conscious sedation during procedure

    Excludes ❷: *personal history of failed moderate sedation (Z92.83)*

  T88.53x-   Unintended awareness under general anesthesia during procedure

    Excludes ❷: *personal history of unintended awareness under general anesthesia (Z92.84)*

  T88.59x-   Other complications of anesthesia

T88.6xx-   Anaphylactic reaction due to adverse effect of correct drug or medicament properly administered

CC-A   Anaphylactic shock due to adverse effect of correct drug or medicament properly administered
    Anaphylactoid reaction NOS
    Use additional code for adverse effect, if applicable, to identify drug (T36-T50 with fifth or sixth character 5)

  Excludes 1:   *anaphylactic reaction due to serum (T80.5)*

T88.7xx-   Unspecified adverse effect of drug or medicament

    Drug hypersensitivity NOS
    Drug reaction NOS
    Use additional code for adverse effect, if applicable, to identify drug (T36-T50 with fifth or sixth character 5)

  Excludes 1:   *specified adverse effects of drugs and medicaments (A00-R94 and T80-T88.6, T88.8)*

T88.8xx-   Other specified complications of surgical and medical care, not elsewhere classified

    Use additional code to identify the complication

T88.9xx-   Complication of surgical and medical care, unspecified

T87 - T88

Chapter 20 – External causes of morbidity (V00-Y99)

Note: This chapter permits the classification of environmental events and circumstances as the cause of injury, and other adverse effects. Where a code from this section is applicable, it is intended that it shall be used secondary to a code from another chapter of the Classification indicating the nature of the condition. Most often, the condition will be classifiable to Chapter 19, Injury, poisoning and certain other consequences of external causes (S00-T88). Other conditions that may be stated to be due to external causes are classified in Chapters I to XVIII. For these conditions, codes from Chapter 20 should be used to provide additional information as to the cause of the condition.

This chapter contains the following blocks:

V00-X58	Accidents
V00-V99	Transport accidents
V00-V09	Pedestrian injured in transport accident
V10-V19	Pedal cycle rider injured in transport accident
V20-V29	Motorcycle rider injured in transport accident
V30-V39	Occupant of three-wheeled motor vehicle injured in transport accident
V40-V49	Car occupant injured in transport accident
V50-V59	Occupant of pick-up truck or van injured in transport accident
V60-V69	Occupant of heavy transport vehicle injured in transport accident
V70-V79	Bus occupant injured in transport accident
V80-V89	Other land transport accidents
V90-V94	Water transport accidents
V95-V97	Air and space transport accidents
V98-V99	Other and unspecified transport accidents
W00-W19	Slipping, tripping, stumbling and falls
W20-W49	Exposure to inanimate mechanical forces
W50-W64	Exposure to animate mechanical forces
W65-W74	Accidental non-transport drowning and submersion
W85-W99	Exposure to electric current, radiation and extreme ambient air temperature and pressure
X00-X08	Exposure to smoke, fire and flames
X10-X19	Contact with heat and hot substances
X30-X39	Exposure to forces of nature
X50	Overexertion and strenuous or repetitive movements
X52-X58	Accidental exposure to other specified factors
X71-X83	Intentional self-harm
X92-Y09	Assault
Y21-Y33	Event of undetermined intent
Y35-Y38	Legal intervention, operations of war, military operations, and terrorism
Y62-Y69	Misadventures to patients during surgical and medical care
Y70-Y82	Medical devices associated with adverse incidents in diagnostic and therapeutic use
Y83-Y84	Surgical and other medical procedures as the cause of abnormal reaction of the patient, or of later complication, without mention of misadventure at the time of the procedure
Y90-Y99	Supplementary factors related to causes of morbidity classified elsewhere

Accidents (V00-X58)

Transport accidents (V00-V99)

Note: This section is structured in 12 groups. Those relating to land transport accidents (V00-V89) reflect the victim's mode of transport and are subdivided to identify the victim's "counterpart" or the type of event. The vehicle of which the injured person is an occupant is identified in the first two characters since it is seen as the most important factor to identify for prevention purposes. A transport accident is one in which the vehicle involved must be moving or running or in use for transport purposes at the time of the accident.

Use additional code to identify:
Airbag injury (W22.1)
Type of street or road (Y92.4-)
Use of cellular telephone and other electronic equipment at the time of the transport accident (Y93.C-)

Excludes 1:   agricultural vehicles in stationary use or maintenance (W31-)
assault by crashing of motor vehicle (Y03-)
automobile or motor cycle in stationary use or maintenance — code to type of accident
crashing of motor vehicle, undetermined intent (Y32)
intentional self-harm by crashing of motor vehicle (X82)

Excludes ❷: transport accidents due to cataclysm (X34-X38)

Definitions related to transport accidents:

(a) A transport accident (V00-V99) is any accident involving a device designed primarily for, or used at the time primarily for, conveying persons or goods from one place to another.

(b) A public highway [trafficway] or street is the entire width between property lines (or other boundary lines) of land open to the public as a matter of right or custom for purposes of moving persons or property from one place to another. A roadway is that part of the public highway designed, improved and customarily used for vehicular traffic.

(c) A traffic accident is any vehicle accident occurring on the public highway [i.e. originating on, terminating on, or involving a vehicle partially on the highway]. A vehicle accident is assumed to have occurred on the public highway unless another place is specified, except in the case of accidents involving only off-road motor vehicles, which are classified as nontraffic accidents unless the contrary is stated.

(d) A nontraffic accident is any vehicle accident that occurs entirely in any place other than a public highway.

(e) A pedestrian is any person involved in an accident who was not at the time of the accident riding in or on a motor vehicle, railway train, streetcar or animal-drawn or other vehicle, or on a pedal cycle or animal. This includes, a person changing a tire, working on a parked car, or a person on foot. It also includes the user of a pedestrian conveyance such as a babystroller, ice-skates, skis, sled, roller skates, a skateboard, nonmotorized or motorized wheelchair, motorized mobility scooter, or nonmotorized scooter.

(f) A driver is an occupant of a transport vehicle who is operating or intending to operate it.

(g) A passenger is any occupant of a transport vehicle other than the driver, except a person traveling on the outside of the vehicle.

(h) A person on the outside of a vehicle is any person being transported by a vehicle but not occupying the space normally reserved for the driver or passengers, or the space intended for the transport of property. This includes a person traveling on the bodywork, bumper, fender, roof, running board or step of a vehicle, as well as, hanging on the outside of the vehicle.

(i) A pedal cycle is any land transport vehicle operated solely by nonmotorized pedals including a bicycle or tricycle.

(j) A pedal cyclist is any person riding a pedal cycle or in a sidecar or trailer attached to a pedal cycle.

(k) A motorcycle is a two-wheeled motor vehicle with one or two riding saddles and sometimes with a third wheel for the support of a sidecar. The sidecar is considered part of the motorcycle. This includes a moped, motor scooter, or motorized bicycle.

(l) A motorcycle rider is any person riding a motorcycle or in a sidecar or trailer attached to the motorcycle.

(m) A three-wheeled motor vehicle is a motorized tricycle designed primarily for on-road use. This includes a motor-driven tricycle, a motorized rickshaw, or a three-wheeled motor car.

(n) A car [automobile] is a four-wheeled motor vehicle designed primarily for carrying up to 7 persons. A trailer being towed by the car is considered part of the car. It does not include a van or minivan – see definition (o).

(o) A pick-up truck or van is a four or six-wheeled motor vehicle designed for carrying passengers as well as property or cargo weighing less than the local limit for classification as a heavy goods vehicle, and not requiring a special driver's license. This includes a minivan and a sport-utility vehicle (SUV).

(p) A heavy transport vehicle is a motor vehicle designed primarily for carrying property, meeting local criteria for classification as a heavy goods vehicle in terms of weight and requiring a special driver's license.

(q) A bus (coach) is a motor vehicle designed or adapted primarily for carrying more than 10 passengers, and requiring a special driver's license.

(r) A railway train or railway vehicle is any device, with or without freight or passenger cars coupled to it, designed for traffic on a railway track. This includes subterranean (subways) or elevated trains.

(s) A streetcar is a device designed and used primarily for transporting passengers within a municipality, running on rails, usually subject to normal traffic control signals, and operated principally on a right-of-way that forms part of the roadway. This includes a tram or trolley that runs on rails. A trailer being towed by a streetcar is considered part of the streetcar.

(t) A special vehicle mainly used on industrial premises is a motor vehicle designed primarily for use within the buildings and premises of industrial or commercial establishments. This includes battery-powered airport passenger vehicles or baggage/mail trucks, forklifts, coal-cars in a coal mine, logging cars and trucks used in mines or quarries.

(u) A special vehicle mainly used in agriculture is a motor vehicle designed specifically for use in farming and agriculture (horticulture), to work the land, tend and harvest crops and transport materials on the farm. This includes harvesters, farm machinery and tractor and trailers.

(v) A special construction vehicle is a motor vehicle designed specifically for use on construction and demolition sites. This includes bulldozers, diggers, earth levellers, dump trucks, backhoes, front-end loaders, pavers, and mechanical shovels.

(w) **A special all-terrain vehicle** is a motor vehicle of special design to enable it to negotiate over rough or soft terrain, snow or sand. Examples of special design are high construction, special wheels and tires, tracks, and support on a cushion of air. This includes snow mobiles, all-terrain vehicles (ATV), and dune buggies. It does not include passenger vehicle designated as Sport Utility Vehicles (SUV).

(x) **A watercraft** is any device designed for transporting passengers or goods on water. This includes motor or sail boats, ships, and hovercraft.

(y) **An aircraft** is any device for transporting passengers or goods in the air. This includes hot-air balloons, gliders, helicopters and airplanes.

(z) **A military vehicle** is any motorized vehicle operating on a public roadway owned by the military and being operated by a member of the military.

Chapter-Specific Coding Guidelines

C. Chapter-Specific Coding Guidelines
In addition to general coding guidelines, there are guidelines for specific diagnoses and/or conditions in the classification. Unless otherwise indicated, these guidelines apply to all health care settings. Please refer to Section II for guidelines on the selection of principal diagnosis.

20. Chapter 20: External Causes of Morbidity (V00-Y99)

The external causes of morbidity codes should never be sequenced as the first-listed or principal diagnosis.

External cause codes are intended to provide data for injury research and evaluation of injury prevention strategies. These codes capture how the injury or health condition happened (cause), the intent (unintentional or accidental; or intentional, such as suicide or assault), the place where the event occurred the activity of the patient at the time of the event, and the person's status (e.g., civilian, military).

There is no national requirement for mandatory ICD-10-CM external cause code reporting. Unless a provider is subject to a state-based external cause code reporting mandate or these codes are required by a particular payer, reporting of ICD-10-CM codes in Chapter 20, External Causes of Morbidity, is not required. In the absence of a mandatory reporting requirement, providers are encouraged to voluntarily report external cause codes, as they provide valuable data for injury research and evaluation of injury prevention strategies.

a. General External Cause Coding Guidelines

1) Used with any code in the range of A00.0-T88.9, Z00-Z99
An external cause code may be used with any code in the range of A00.0-T88.9, Z00-Z99, classification that is a health condition due to an external cause. Though they are most applicable to injuries, they are also valid for use with such things as infections or diseases due to an external source, and other health conditions, such as a heart attack that occurs during strenuous physical activity.

2) External cause code used for length of treatment
Assign the external cause code, with the appropriate 7th character (initial encounter, subsequent encounter or sequela) for each encounter for which the injury or condition is being treated.
Most categories in chapter 20 have a 7th character requirement for each applicable code. Most categories in this chapter have three 7th character values: A, initial encounter, D, subsequent encounter and S, sequela. While the patient may be seen by a new or different provider over the course of treatment for an injury or condition, assignment of the 7th character for external cause should match the 7th character of the code assigned for the associated injury or condition for the encounter.

3) Use the full range of external cause codes
Use the full range of external cause codes to completely describe the cause, the intent, the place of occurrence, and if applicable, the activity of the patient at the time of the event, and the patient's status, for all injuries, and other health conditions due to an external cause.

4) Assign as many external cause codes as necessary
Assign as many external cause codes as necessary to fully explain each cause. If only one external code can be recorded, assign the code most related to the principal diagnosis.

5) The selection of the appropriate external cause code
The selection of the appropriate external cause code is guided by the Alphabetic Index of External Causes and by Inclusion and Exclusion notes in the Tabular List.

6) External cause code can never be a principal diagnosis
An external cause code can never be a principal (first-listed) diagnosis.

7) Combination external cause codes
Certain of the external cause codes are combination codes that identify sequential events that result in an injury, such as a fall which results in striking against an object. The injury may be due to either event or both. The combination external cause code used should correspond to the sequence of events regardless of which caused the most serious injury.

8) No external cause code needed in certain circumstances
No external cause code from Chapter 20 is needed if the external cause and intent are included in a code from another chapter (e.g. T36.0x1- Poisoning by penicillins, accidental (unintentional)).

b. Place of Occurrence Guideline
Codes from category Y92, Place of occurrence of the external cause, are secondary codes for use after other external cause codes to identify the location of the patient at the time of injury or other condition.

Generally, a place of occurrence code is assigned only once, at the initial encounter for treatment. However, in the rare instance that a new injury occurs during hospitalization, an additional place of occurrence code may be assigned. No 7th characters are used for Y92.

Do not use place of occurrence code Y92.9 if the place is not stated or is not applicable.

c. Activity Code
Assign a code from category Y93, Activity code, to describe the activity of the patient at the time the injury or other health condition occurred.

An activity code is used only once, at the initial encounter for treatment. Only one code from Y93 should be recorded on a medical record.

The activity codes are not applicable to poisonings, adverse effects, misadventures or sequela.

Do not assign Y93.9, Unspecified activity, if the activity is not stated.

A code from category Y93 is appropriate for use with external cause and intent codes if identifying the activity provides additional information about the event.

d. Place of Occurrence, Activity, and Status Codes Used with other External Cause Code
When applicable, place of occurrence, activity, and external cause status codes are sequenced after the main external cause code(s). Regardless of the number of external cause codes assigned, there should be only one place of occurrence code, one activity code, and one external cause status code assigned to an encounter.

e. If the Reporting Format Limits the Number of External Cause Codes
If the reporting format limits the number of external cause codes that can be used in reporting clinical data, report the code for the cause/intent most related to the principal diagnosis. If the format permits capture of additional external cause codes, the cause/intent, including medical misadventures, of the additional events should be reported rather than the codes for place, activity, or external status.

f. Multiple External Cause Coding Guidelines
More than one external cause code is required to fully describe the external cause of an illness or injury. The assignment of external cause codes should be sequenced in the following priority:
If two or more events cause separate injuries, an external cause code should be assigned for each cause. The first-listed external cause code will be selected in the following order:

External codes for child and adult abuse take priority over all other external cause codes.
See Section I.C.19. Child and Adult abuse guidelines.

External cause codes for terrorism events take priority over all other external cause codes except child and adult abuse.

External cause codes for cataclysmic events take priority over all other external cause codes except child and adult abuse and terrorism.

External cause codes for transport accidents take priority over all other external cause codes except cataclysmic events, child and adult abuse and terrorism.

Activity and external cause status codes are assigned following all causal (intent) external cause codes.

The first-listed external cause code should correspond to the cause of the most serious diagnosis due to an assault, accident, or self-harm, following the order of hierarchy listed above.

g. Child and Adult Abuse Guideline
Adult and child abuse, neglect and maltreatment are classified as assault. Any of the assault codes may be used to indicate the external cause of any injury resulting from the confirmed abuse.

For confirmed cases of abuse, neglect and maltreatment, when the perpetrator is known, a code from Y07, Perpetrator of maltreatment and neglect, should accompany any other assault codes.

See Section I.C.19. Adult and child abuse, neglect and other maltreatment.

h. Unknown or Undetermined Intent Guideline
If the intent (accident, self-harm, assault) of the cause of an injury or other condition is unknown or unspecified, code the intent as accidental intent. All transport accident categories assume accidental intent.

1) Use of undetermined intent
External cause codes for events of undetermined intent are only for use if the documentation in the record specifies that the intent cannot be determined.

i. Sequelae (Late Effects) of External Cause Guidelines

1) Sequelae external cause codes
Sequela are reported using the external cause code with the 7th character "S" for sequela. These codes should be used with any report of a late effect or sequela resulting from a previous injury.

See Section I.B.10 Sequela (Late Effects).

2) Sequela external cause code with a related current injury
A sequela external cause code should never be used with a related current nature of injury code.

3) Use of sequela external cause codes for subsequent visits
Use a late effect external cause code for subsequent visits when a late effect of the initial injury is being treated. Do not use a late effect external cause code for subsequent visits for follow-up care (e.g., to assess healing, to receive rehabilitative therapy) of the injury when no late effect of the injury has been documented.

j. Terrorism Guidelines

1) Cause of injury identified by the Federal Government (FBI) as terrorism
When the cause of an injury is identified by the Federal Government (FBI) as terrorism, the first-listed external cause code should be a code from category Y38, Terrorism. The definition of terrorism employed by the FBI is found at the inclusion note at the beginning of category Y38. Use additional code for place of occurrence (Y92.-). More than one Y38 code may be assigned if the injury is the result of more than one mechanism of terrorism.

2) Cause of an injury is suspected to be the result of terrorism
When the cause of an injury is suspected to be the result of terrorism a code from category Y38 should not be assigned. Suspected cases should be classified as assault.

3) Code Y38.9, Terrorism, secondary effects
Assign code Y38.9, Terrorism, secondary effects, for conditions occurring subsequent to the terrorist event. This code should not be assigned for conditions that are due to the initial terrorist act.

It is acceptable to assign code Y38.9 with another code from Y38 if there is an injury due to the initial terrorist event and an injury that is a subsequent result of the terrorist event.

k. External cause status
A code from category Y99, External cause status, should be assigned whenever any other external cause code is assigned for an encounter, including an Activity code, except for the events noted below. Assign a code from category Y99, External cause status, to indicate the work status of the person at the time the event occurred. The status code indicates whether the event occurred during military activity, whether a non-military person was at work, whether an individual including a student or volunteer was involved in a non-work activity at the time of the causal event.

A code from Y99, External cause status, should be assigned, when applicable, with other external cause codes, such as transport accidents and falls. The external cause status codes are not applicable to poisonings, adverse effects, misadventures or late effects.

Do not assign a code from category Y99 if no other external cause codes (cause, activity) are applicable for the encounter.

An external cause status code is used only once, at the initial encounter for treatment. Only one code from Y99 should be recorded on a medical record.

Do not assign code Y99.9, Unspecified external cause status, if the status is not stated.

Pedestrian injured in transport accident (V00-V09)

Includes: Person changing tire on transport vehicle
Person examining engine of vehicle broken down in (on side of) road
Excludes 1: *fall due to non-transport collision with other person (W03)*
pedestrian on foot falling (slipping) on ice and snow (W00-)
struck or bumped by another person (W51)

V00- Pedestrian conveyance accident
Use additional place of occurrence and activity external cause codes, if known (Y92-, Y93-)
Excludes 1: *collision with another person without fall (W51)*
fall due to person on foot colliding with another person on foot (W03)
fall from non-moving wheelchair, nonmotorized scooter and motorized mobility scooter without collision (W05-)
pedestrian (conveyance) collision with other land transport vehicle (V01-V09)
pedestrian on foot falling (slipping) on ice and snow (W00-)

The appropriate 7th character is to be added to each code from category V00:
A   Initial encounter
D   Subsequent encounter
S   Sequela

V00.0- Pedestrian on foot injured in collision with pedestrian conveyance
V00.01x- Pedestrian on foot injured in collision with roller-skater
V00.02x- Pedestrian on foot injured in collision with skateboarder
V00.09x- Pedestrian on foot injured in collision with other pedestrian conveyance

V00.1- Rolling-type pedestrian conveyance accident
Excludes 1: *accident with babystroller (V00.82-)*
accident with wheelchair (powered) (V00.81-)
accident with motorized mobility scooter (V00.83-)

V00.11- In-line roller-skate accident
V00.111- Fall from in-line roller-skates
V00.112- In-line roller-skater colliding with stationary object
V00.118- Other in-line roller-skate accident
Excludes 1: *roller-skater collision with other land transport vehicle (V01-V09 with 5th character 1)*

V00.12- Non-in- line roller-skate accident
V00.121- Fall from non-in-line roller-skates
V00.122- Non-in-line roller-skater colliding with stationary object
V00.128- Other non-in-line roller-skating accident
Excludes 1: *roller-skater collision with other land transport vehicle (V01-V09 with 5th character 1)*

V00.13- Skateboard accident
V00.131- Fall from skateboard
V00.132- Skateboarder colliding with stationary object
V00.138- Other skateboard accident
Excludes 1: *skateboarder collision with other land transport vehicle (V01-V09 with 5th character 2)*

V00.14- Scooter (nonmotorized) accident
Excludes 1: *motorscooter accident (V20-V29)*
V00.141- Fall from scooter (nonmotorized)
V00.142- Scooter (nonmotorized) colliding with stationary object
V00.148- Other scooter (nonmotorized) accident
Excludes 1: *scooter (nonmotorized) collision with other land transport vehicle (V01-V09 with fifth character 9)*

V00.15- Heelies accident
Rolling shoe
Wheeled shoe
Wheelies accident
V00.151- Fall from heelies
V00.152- Heelies colliding with stationary object

V00 - V09

V00.158- Other heelies accident

V00.18- Accident on other rolling-type pedestrian conveyance

V00.181- Fall from other rolling-type pedestrian conveyance

V00.182- Pedestrian on other rolling-type pedestrian conveyance colliding with stationary object

V00.188- Other accident on other rolling-type pedestrian conveyance

V00.2- <u>Gliding-type pedestrian</u> conveyance accident

V00.21- Ice-skates accident

V00.211- Fall from ice-skates

V00.212- Ice-skater colliding with stationary object

V00.218- Other ice-skates accident
Excludes 1:   *ice-skater collision with other land transport vehicle (V01-V09 with 5th digit 9)*

V00.22- Sled accident

V00.221- Fall from sled

V00.222- Sledder colliding with stationary object

V00.228- Other sled accident
Excludes 1:   *sled collision with other land transport vehicle (V01-V09 with 5th digit 9)*

V00.28- Other gliding-type pedestrian conveyance accident

V00.281- Fall from other gliding-type pedestrian conveyance

V00.282- Pedestrian on other gliding-type pedestrian conveyance colliding with stationary object

V00.288- Other accident on other gliding-type pedestrian conveyance
Excludes 1:   *gliding-type pedestrian conveyance collision with other land transport vehicle (V01-V09 with 5th digit 9)*

V00.3- Flat-bottomed pedestrian conveyance accident

V00.31- <u>Snowboard accident</u>

V00.311- Fall from snowboard

V00.312- Snowboarder colliding with stationary object

V00.318- Other snowboard accident
Excludes 1:   *snowboarder collision with other land transport vehicle (V01-V09 with 5th digit 9)*

V00.32- <u>Snow-ski accident</u>

V00.321- Fall from snow-skis
AHA 15:1Q:p12 – Fell down while cross country skiing

V00.322- Snow-skier colliding with stationary object

V00.328- Other snow-ski accident
Excludes 1:   *snow-skier collision with other land transport vehicle (V01-V09 with 5th digit 9)*

V00.38- Other flat-bottomed pedestrian conveyance accident

V00.381- Fall from other flat-bottomed pedestrian conveyance

V00.382- Pedestrian on other flat-bottomed pedestrian conveyance colliding with stationary object

V00.388- Other accident on other flat-bottomed pedestrian conveyance

V00.8- Accident on other pedestrian conveyance

V00.81- Accident with <u>wheelchair</u> (powered)

V00.811- Fall from moving wheelchair (powered)
Excludes 1:   *fall from non-moving wheelchair (W05.0)*

V00.812- Wheelchair (powered) colliding with stationary object

V00.818- Other accident with wheelchair (powered)

V00.82- Accident with <u>babystroller</u>

V00.821- Fall from babystroller

V00.822- Babystroller colliding with stationary object

V00.828- Other accident with babystroller

V00.83- Accident with <u>motorized mobility scooter</u>

V00.831- Fall from motorized mobility scooter
Excludes 1:   *fall from non-moving motorized mobility scooter (W05.2)*

V00.832- Motorized mobility scooter colliding with stationary object

V00.838- Other accident with motorized mobility scooter

V00.89- Accident on other pedestrian conveyance

V00.891- Fall from other pedestrian conveyance

V00.892- Pedestrian on other pedestrian conveyance colliding with stationary object

V00.898- Other accident on other pedestrian conveyance
Excludes 1:   *other pedestrian (conveyance) collision with other land transport vehicle (V01-V09 with 5th digit 9)*

V01- <u>Pedestrian injured in collision</u> with <u>pedal cycle</u>
The appropriate 7th character is to be added to each code from category V01:
A   <u>Initial</u> encounter
D   <u>Subsequent</u> encounter
S   <u>Sequela</u>

V01.0- <u>Pedestrian injured in collision</u> with <u>pedal cycle</u> in <u>nontraffic</u> accident

V01.00x- Pedestrian on foot injured in collision with pedal cycle in nontraffic accident
Pedestrian NOS injured in collision with pedal cycle in nontraffic accident

V01.01x- Pedestrian on roller-skates injured in collision with pedal cycle in nontraffic accident

V01.02x- Pedestrian on skateboard injured in collision with pedal cycle in nontraffic accident

V01.09x- Pedestrian with other conveyance injured in collision with pedal cycle in nontraffic accident
Pedestrian with babystroller injured in collision with pedal cycle in nontraffic accident
Pedestrian on ice-skates injured in collision with pedal cycle in nontraffic accident
Pedestrian on nonmotorized scooter injured in collision with pedal cycle in nontraffic accident
Pedestrian on sled injured in collision with pedal cycle in nontraffic accident
Pedestrian on snowboard injured in collision with pedal cycle in nontraffic accident
Pedestrian on snow-skis injured in collision with pedal cycle in nontraffic accident
Pedestrian in wheelchair (powered) injured in collision with pedal cycle in nontraffic accident
Pedestrian in motorized mobility scooter injured in collision with pedal cycle in nontraffic accident

V01.1- <u>Pedestrian injured in collision</u> with <u>pedal cycle</u> in <u>traffic</u> accident

V01.10x- Pedestrian on foot injured in collision with pedal cycle in traffic accident
Pedestrian NOS injured in collision with pedal cycle in traffic accident

V01.11x- Pedestrian on roller-skates injured in collision with pedal cycle in traffic accident

V01.12x- Pedestrian on skateboard injured in collision with pedal cycle in traffic accident

V01.19x- Pedestrian with other conveyance injured in collision with pedal cycle in traffic accident
Pedestrian with babystroller injured in collision with pedal cycle in traffic accident
Pedestrian on ice-skates injured in collision with pedal cycle in traffic accident
Pedestrian on nonmotorized scooter injured in collision with pedal cycle in traffic accident
Pedestrian on sled injured in collision with pedal cycle in traffic accident
Pedestrian on snowboard injured in collision with pedal cycle in traffic accident
Pedestrian on snow-skis injured in collision with pedal cycle in traffic accident
Pedestrian in wheelchair (powered) injured in collision with pedal cycle in traffic accident
Pedestrian in motorized mobility scooter injured in collision with pedal cycle in traffic accident

V01.9- **Pedestrian injured in collision** with **pedal cycle**, **unspecified** whether traffic or nontraffic accident

V01.90x- Pedestrian on foot injured in collision with pedal cycle, unspecified whether traffic or nontraffic accident
> Pedestrian NOS injured in collision with pedal cycle, unspecified whether traffic or nontraffic accident

V01.91x- Pedestrian on roller-skates injured in collision with pedal cycle, unspecified whether traffic or nontraffic accident

V01.92x- Pedestrian on skateboard injured in collision with pedal cycle, unspecified whether traffic or nontraffic accident

V01.99x- Pedestrian with other conveyance injured in collision with pedal cycle, unspecified whether traffic or nontraffic accident
> Pedestrian with babystroller injured in collision with pedal cycle, unspecified whether traffic or nontraffic accident
> Pedestrian on ice-skates injured in collision with pedal cycle unspecified, whether traffic or nontraffic accident
> Pedestrian on nonmotorized scooter injured in collision with pedal cycle, unspecified whether traffic or nontraffic accident
> Pedestrian on sled injured in collision with pedal cycle unspecified, whether traffic or nontraffic accident
> Pedestrian on snowboard injured in collision with pedal cycle, unspecified whether traffic or nontraffic accident
> Pedestrian on snow-skis injured in collision with pedal cycle, unspecified whether traffic or nontraffic accident
> Pedestrian in wheelchair (powered) injured in collision with pedal cycle, unspecified whether traffic or nontraffic accident
> Pedestrian in motorized mobility scooter injured in collision with pedal cycle, unspecified whether traffic or nontraffic accident

V02- **Pedestrian injured in collision** with **two- or three-wheeled motor vehicle**

The appropriate 7th character is to be added to each code from category V02:

A   **Initial** encounter
D   **Subsequent** encounter
S   **Sequela**

V02.0- **Pedestrian injured in collision** with **two- or three-wheeled motor vehicle** in **nontraffic** accident

V02.00x- Pedestrian on foot injured in collision with two- or three-wheeled motor vehicle in nontraffic accident
> Pedestrian NOS injured in collision with two- or three-wheeled motor vehicle in nontraffic accident

V02.01x- Pedestrian on roller-skates injured in collision with two- or three-wheeled motor vehicle in nontraffic accident

V02.02x- Pedestrian on skateboard injured in collision with two- or three-wheeled motor vehicle in nontraffic accident

V02.09x- Pedestrian with other conveyance injured in collision with two- or three-wheeled motorvehicle in nontraffic accident
> Pedestrian with babystroller injured in collision with two- or three-wheeled motor vehicle in nontraffic accident
> Pedestrian on ice-skates injured in collision with two- or three-wheeled motor vehicle in nontraffic accident
> Pedestrian on nonmotorized scooter injured in collision with two- or three-wheeled motor vehicle in nontraffic accident
> Pedestrian on sled injured in collision with two- or three-wheeled motor vehicle in nontraffic accident
> Pedestrian on snowboard injured in collision with two- or three-wheeled motor vehicle in nontraffic accident
> Pedestrian on snow-skis injured in collision with two- or three-wheeled motor vehicle in nontraffic accident
> Pedestrian in wheelchair (powered) injured in collision with two- or three-wheeled motor vehicle in nontraffic accident
> Pedestrian in motorized mobility scooter injured in collision with two- or three-wheeled motor vehicle in nontraffic accident

V02.1- **Pedestrian injured in collision** with **two- or three-wheeled motor vehicle** in **traffic** accident

V02.10x- Pedestrian on foot injured in collision with two- or three-wheeled motor vehicle in traffic accident
> Pedestrian NOS injured in collision with two- or three-wheeled motor vehicle in traffic accident

V02.11x- Pedestrian on roller-skates injured in collision with two- or three-wheeled motor vehicle intraffic accident

V02.12x- Pedestrian on skateboard injured in collision with two- or three-wheeled motor vehicle intraffic accident

V02.19x- Pedestrian with other conveyance injured in collision with two- or three-wheeled motorvehicle in traffic accident
> Pedestrian with babystroller injured in collision with two- or three-wheeled motor vehicle in traffic accident
> Pedestrian on ice-skates injured in collision with two- or three-wheeled motor vehicle in traffic accident
> Pedestrian on nonmotorized scooter injured in collision with two- or three-wheeled motor vehicle in traffic accident
> Pedestrian on sled injured in collision with two- or three-wheeled motor vehicle in traffic accident
> Pedestrian on snowboard injured in collision with two- or three-wheeled motor vehicle in traffic accident
> Pedestrian on snow-skis injured in collision with two- or three-wheeled motor vehicle in traffic accident
> Pedestrian in wheelchair (powered) injured in collision with two- or three-wheeled motor vehicle in traffic accident
> Pedestrian in motorized mobility scooter injured in collision with two- or three-wheeled motor vehicle in traffic accident

V02.9- **Pedestrian injured in collision** with **two- or three-wheeled motor vehicle**, **unspecified** whether traffic or nontraffic accident

V02.90x- Pedestrian on foot injured in collision with two- or three-wheeled motor vehicle, unspecified whether traffic or nontraffic accident
> Pedestrian NOS injured in collision with two- or three-wheeled motor vehicle, unspecified whether traffic or nontraffic accident

V02.91x- Pedestrian on roller-skates injured in collision with two- or three-wheeled motor vehicle, unspecified whether traffic or nontraffic accident

V02.92x- Pedestrian on skateboard injured in collision with two- or three-wheeled motor vehicle, unspecified whether traffic or nontraffic accident

V02.99x- Pedestrian with other conveyance injured in collision with two- or three-wheeled motor vehicle, unspecified whether traffic or nontraffic accident
> Pedestrian with babystroller injured in collision with two- or three-wheeled motor vehicle, unspecified whether traffic or nontraffic accident
> Pedestrian on ice-skates injured in collision with two- or three-wheeled motor vehicle, unspecified whether traffic or nontraffic accident
> Pedestrian on nonmotorized scooter injured in collision with two- or three-wheeled motor vehicle, unspecified whether traffic or nontraffic accident
> Pedestrian on sled injured in collision with two- or three-wheeled motor vehicle, unspecified whether traffic or nontraffic accident
> Pedestrian on snowboard injured in collision with two- or three-wheeled motor vehicle, unspecified whether traffic or nontraffic accident
> Pedestrian on snow-skis injured in collision with two- or three-wheeled motor vehicle, unspecified whether traffic or nontraffic accident
> Pedestrian in wheelchair (powered) injured in collision with two- or three-wheeled motor vehicle, unspecified whether traffic or nontraffic accident
> Pedestrian in motorized mobility scooter injured in collision with two- or three-wheeled motor vehicle, unspecified whether traffic or nontraffic accident

V01 – V02

V03- **Pedestrian injured in collision** with **car, pick-up truck or van**

The appropriate 7th character is to be added to each code from category V03:
A   **Initial** encounter
D   **Subsequent** encounter
S   **Sequela**

V03.0- **Pedestrian injured in collision** with **car, pick-up truck or van** in **nontraffic** accident

  V03.00x- Pedestrian on foot injured in collision with car, pick-up truck or van in nontraffic accident
    Pedestrian NOS injured in collision with car, pick-up truck or van in nontraffic accident

  V03.01x- Pedestrian on roller-skates injured in collision with car, pick-up truck or van in nontraffic accident

  V03.02x- Pedestrian on skateboard injured in collision with car, pick-up truck or van in nontraffic accident

  V03.09x- Pedestrian with other conveyance injured in collision with **car, pick-up truck or van** in **nontraffic** accident
    Pedestrian with babystroller injured in collision with car, pick-up truck or van in nontraffic accident
    Pedestrian on ice-skates injured in collision with car, pick-up truck or van in nontraffic accident
    Pedestrian on nonmotorized scooter injured in collision with car, pick-up truck or van in nontraffic accident
    Pedestrian on sled injured in collision with car, pick-up truck or van in nontraffic accident
    Pedestrian on snowboard injured in collision with car, pick-up truck or van in nontraffic accident
    Pedestrian on snow-skis injured in collision with car, pick-up truck or van in nontraffic accident
    Pedestrian in wheelchair (powered) injured in collision with car, pick-up truck or van in nontraffic accident
    Pedestrian in motorized mobility scooter injured in collision with car, pick-up truck or van in nontraffic accident

V03.1- **Pedestrian injured in collision** with **car, pick-up truck or van in traffic** accident

  V03.10x- Pedestrian on foot injured in collision with car, pick-up truck or van in traffic accident
    Pedestrian NOS injured in collision with car, pick-up truck or van in traffic accident

  V03.11x- Pedestrian on roller-skates injured in collision with car, pick-up truck or van in traffic accident

  V03.12x- Pedestrian on skateboard injured in collision with car, pick-up truck or van in traffic accident

  V03.19x- Pedestrian with other conveyance injured in collision with car, pick-up truck or van in traffic accident
    Pedestrian with babystroller injured in collision with car, pick-up truck or van in traffic accident
    Pedestrian on ice-skates injured in collision with car, pick-up truck or van in traffic accident
    Pedestrian on nonmotorized scooter injured in collision with car, pick-up truck or van in traffic accident
    Pedestrian on sled injured in collision with car, pick-up truck or van in traffic accident
    Pedestrian on snowboard injured in collision with car, pick-up truck or van in traffic accident
    Pedestrian on snow-skis injured in collision with car, pick-up truck or van in traffic accident
    Pedestrian in wheelchair (powered) injured in collision with car, pick-up truck or van in traffic accident
    Pedestrian in motorized mobility scooter injured in collision with car, pick-up truck or van in traffic accident

V03.9- **Pedestrian injured in collision** with **car, pick-up truck or van, unspecified** whether traffic or nontraffic accident

  V03.90x- Pedestrian on foot injured in collision with car, pick-up truck or van, unspecified whether traffic or nontraffic accident
    Pedestrian NOS injured in collision with car, pick-up truck or van, unspecified whether traffic or nontraffic accident

  V03.91x- Pedestrian on roller-skates injured in collision with car, pick-up truck or van, unspecified whether traffic or nontraffic accident

  V03.92x- Pedestrian on skateboard injured in collision with car, pick-up truck or van, unspecified whether traffic or nontraffic accident

  V03.99x- Pedestrian with other conveyance injured in collision with car, pick-up truck or van, unspecified whether traffic or nontraffic accident
    Pedestrian with babystroller injured in collision with car, pick-up truck or van, unspecified whether traffic or nontraffic accident
    Pedestrian on ice-skates injured in collision with car, pick-up truck or van, unspecified whether traffic or nontraffic accident
    Pedestrian on nonmotorized scooter injured in collision with car, pick-up truck or van, unspecified whether traffic or nontraffic accident
    Pedestrian on sled injured in collision with car, pick-up truck or van in nontraffic accident
    Pedestrian on snowboard injured in collision with car, pick-up truck or van, unspecified whether traffic or nontraffic accident
    Pedestrian on snow-skis injured in collision with car, pick-up truck or van, unspecified whether traffic or nontraffic accident
    Pedestrian in wheelchair (powered) injured in collision with car, pick-up truck or van, unspecified whether traffic or nontraffic accident
    Pedestrian in motorized mobility scooter injured in collision with car, pick-up truck or van, unspecified whether traffic or nontraffic accident

V04- **Pedestrian injured in collision** with **heavy transport vehicle or bus**

Excludes 1:   *pedestrian injured in collision with military vehicle (V09.01, V09.21)*

The appropriate 7th character is to be added to each code from category V04:
A   **Initial** encounter
D   **Subsequent** encounter
S   **Sequela**

V04.0- **Pedestrian injured in collision** with **heavy transport vehicle or bus** in **nontraffic** accident

  V04.00x- Pedestrian on foot injured in collision with heavy transport vehicle or bus in nontraffic accident
    Pedestrian NOS injured in collision with heavy transport vehicle or bus in nontraffic accident

  V04.01x- Pedestrian on roller-skates injured in collision with heavy transport vehicle or bus in nontraffic accident

  V04.02x- Pedestrian on skateboard injured in collision with heavy transport vehicle or bus in nontraffic accident

  V04.09x- Pedestrian with other conveyance injured in collision with heavy transport vehicle or bus in nontraffic accident
    Pedestrian with babystroller injured in collision with heavy transport vehicle or bus in nontraffic accident
    Pedestrian on ice-skates injured in collision with heavy transport vehicle or bus in nontraffic accident
    Pedestrian on nonmotorized scooter injured in collision with heavy transport vehicle or bus in nontraffic accident
    Pedestrian on sled injured in collision with heavy transport vehicle or bus in nontraffic accident
    Pedestrian on snowboard injured in collision with heavy transport vehicle or bus in nontraffic accident
    Pedestrian on snow-skis injured in collision with heavy transport vehicle or bus in nontraffic accident
    Pedestrian in wheelchair (powered) injured in collision with heavy transport vehicle or bus in nontraffic accident
    Pedestrian in motorized mobility scooter injured in collision with heavy transport vehicle or bus in nontraffic accident

V04.1- **Pedestrian injured in collision** with **heavy transport vehicle or bus** in **traffic** accident

  V04.10x- Pedestrian on foot injured in collision with heavy transport vehicle or bus in traffic accident
    Pedestrian NOS injured in collision with heavy transport vehicle or bus in traffic accident

  V04.11x- Pedestrian on roller-skates injured in collision with heavy transport vehicle or bus in traffic accident

  V04.12x- Pedestrian on skateboard injured in collision with heavy transport vehicle or bus in traffic accident

V03-V04 (side tab)

V04.19x- Pedestrian with other conveyance injured in collision with heavy transport vehicle or bus in traffic accident
> Pedestrian with babystroller injured in collision with heavy transport vehicle or bus in traffic accident
> Pedestrian on ice-skates injured in collision with heavy transport vehicle or bus in traffic accident
> Pedestrian on nonmotorized scooter injured in collision with heavy transport vehicle or bus in traffic accident
> Pedestrian on sled injured in collision with heavy transport vehicle or bus in traffic accident
> Pedestrian on snowboard injured in collision with heavy transport vehicle or bus in traffic accident
> Pedestrian on snow-skis injured in collision with heavy transport vehicle or bus in traffic accident
> Pedestrian in wheelchair (powered) injured in collision with heavy transport vehicle or bus in traffic accident
> Pedestrian in motorized mobility scooter injured in collision with heavy transport vehicle or bus in traffic accident

V04.9- Pedestrian injured in collision with heavy transport vehicle or bus, unspecified whether traffic or nontraffic accident

V04.90x- Pedestrian on foot injured in collision with heavy transport vehicle or bus, unspecified whether traffic or nontraffic accident
> Pedestrian NOS injured in collision with heavy transport vehicle or bus, unspecified whether traffic or nontraffic accident

V04.91x- Pedestrian on roller-skates injured in collision with heavy transport vehicle or bus, unspecified whether traffic or nontraffic accident

V04.92x- Pedestrian on skateboard injured in collision with heavy transport vehicle or bus, unspecified whether traffic or nontraffic accident

V04.99x- Pedestrian with other conveyance injured in collision with heavy transport vehicle or bus, unspecified whether traffic or nontraffic accident
> Pedestrian with babystroller injured in collision with heavy transport vehicle or bus, unspecified whether traffic or nontraffic accident
> Pedestrian on ice-skates injured in collision with heavy transport vehicle or bus, unspecified whether traffic or nontraffic accident
> Pedestrian on nonmotorized scooter injured in collision with heavy transport vehicle or bus, unspecified whether traffic or nontraffic accident
> Pedestrian on sled injured in collision with heavy transport vehicle or bus, unspecified whether traffic or nontraffic accident
> Pedestrian on snowboard injured in collision with heavy transport vehicle or bus, unspecified whether traffic or nontraffic accident
> Pedestrian on snow-skis injured in collision with heavy transport vehicle or bus, unspecified whether traffic or nontraffic accident
> Pedestrian in wheelchair (powered) injured in collision with heavy transport vehicle or bus, unspecified whether traffic or nontraffic accident
> Pedestrian in motorized mobility scooter injured in collision with heavy transport vehicle or bus, unspecified whether traffic or nontraffic accident

V05- Pedestrian injured in collision with railway train or railway vehicle

The appropriate 7th character is to be added to each code from category V05:
A   Initial encounter
D   Subsequent encounter
S   Sequela

V05.0- Pedestrian injured in collision with railway train or railway vehicle in nontraffic accident

V05.00x- Pedestrian on foot injured in collision with railway train or railway vehicle in nontraffic accident
> Pedestrian NOS injured in collision with railway train or railway vehicle in nontraffic accident

V05.01x- Pedestrian on roller-skates injured in collision with railway train or railway vehicle in nontraffic accident

V05.02x- Pedestrian on skateboard injured in collision with railway train or railway vehicle in nontraffic accident

V05.09x- Pedestrian with other conveyance injured in collision with railway train or railway vehicle in nontraffic accident
> Pedestrian with babystroller injured in collision with railway train or railway vehicle in nontraffic accident
> Pedestrian on ice-skates injured in collision with railway train or railway vehicle in nontraffic accident
> Pedestrian on nonmotorized scooter injured in collision with railway train or railway vehicle in nontraffic accident
> Pedestrian on sled injured in collision with railway train or railway vehicle in nontraffic accident
> Pedestrian on snowboard injured in collision with railway train or railway vehicle in nontraffic accident
> Pedestrian on snow-skis injured in collision with railway train or railway vehicle in nontraffic accident
> Pedestrian in wheelchair (powered) injured in collision with railway train or railway vehicle in nontraffic accident
> Pedestrian in motorized mobility scooter injured in collision with railway train or railway vehicle in nontraffic accident

V05.1- Pedestrian injured in collision with railway train or railway vehicle in traffic accident

V05.10x- Pedestrian on foot injured in collision with railway train or railway vehicle in traffic accident
> Pedestrian NOS injured in collision with railway train or railway vehicle in traffic accident

V05.11x- Pedestrian on roller-skates injured in collision with railway train or railway vehicle in traffic accident

V05.12x- Pedestrian on skateboard injured in collision with railway train or railway vehicle in traffic accident

V05.19x- Pedestrian with other conveyance injured in collision with railway train or railway vehicle in traffic accident
> Pedestrian with babystroller injured in collision with railway train or railway vehicle in traffic accident
> Pedestrian on ice-skates injured in collision with railway train or railway vehicle in traffic accident
> Pedestrian on nonmotorized scooter injured in collision with railway train or railway vehicle in traffic accident
> Pedestrian on sled injured in collision with railway train or railway vehicle in traffic accident
> Pedestrian on snowboard injured in collision with railway train or railway vehicle in traffic accident
> Pedestrian on snow-skis injured in collision with railway train or railway vehicle in traffic accident
> Pedestrian in wheelchair (powered) injured in collision with railway train or railway vehicle in traffic accident
> Pedestrian in motorized mobility scooter injured in collision with railway train or railway vehicle in traffic accident

V05.9- Pedestrian injured in collision with railway train or railway vehicle, unspecified whether traffic or nontraffic accident

V05.90x- Pedestrian on foot injured in collision with railway train or railway vehicle, unspecified whether traffic or nontraffic accident
> Pedestrian NOS injured in collision with railway train or railway vehicle, unspecified whether traffic or nontraffic accident

V05.91x- Pedestrian on roller-skates injured in collision with railway train or railway vehicle, unspecified whether traffic or nontraffic accident

V05.92x- Pedestrian on skateboard injured in collision with railway train or railway vehicle, unspecified whether traffic or nontraffic accident

V04-V05

V05.99x- Pedestrian with other conveyance injured in collision with railway train or railway vehicle, unspecified whether traffic or nontraffic accident

Pedestrian with babystroller injured in collision with railway train or railway vehicle, unspecified whether traffic or nontraffic

Pedestrian on ice-skates injured in collision with railway train or railway vehicle, unspecified whether traffic or nontraffic

Pedestrian on nonmotorized scooter injured in collision with railway train or railway vehicle, unspecified whether traffic or nontraffic

Pedestrian on sled injured in collision with railway train or railway vehicle, unspecified whether traffic or nontraffic

Pedestrian on snowboard injured in collision with railway train or railway vehicle, unspecified whether traffic or nontraffic

Pedestrian on snow-skis injured in collision with railway train or railway vehicle, unspecified whether traffic or nontraffic

Pedestrian in wheelchair (powered) injured in collision with railway train or railway vehicle, unspecified whether traffic or nontraffic

Pedestrian in motorized mobility scooter injured in collision with railway train or railway vehicle, unspecified whether traffic or nontraffic

V06- Pedestrian injured in collision with other nonmotor vehicle
Includes: Collision with animal-drawn vehicle, animal being ridden, nonpowered streetcar
Excludes 1: pedestrian injured in collision with pedestrian conveyance (V00.0-)

The appropriate 7th character is to be added to each code from category V06:
A Initial encounter
D Subsequent encounter
S Sequela

V06.0- Pedestrian injured in collision with other nonmotor vehicle in nontraffic accident

V06.00x- Pedestrian on foot injured in collision with other nonmotor vehicle in nontraffic accident
Pedestrian NOS injured in collision with other nonmotor vehicle in nontraffic accident

V06.01x- Pedestrian on roller-skates injured in collision with other nonmotor vehicle in nontraffic accident

V06.02x- Pedestrian on skateboard injured in collision with other nonmotor vehicle in nontraffic accident

V06.09x- Pedestrian with other conveyance injured in collision with other nonmotor vehicle in nontraffic accident
Pedestrian with babystroller injured in collision with other nonmotor vehicle in nontraffic accident
Pedestrian on ice-skates injured in collision with other nonmotor vehicle in nontraffic accident
Pedestrian on nonmotorized scooter injured in collision with other nonmotor vehicle in nontraffic accident
Pedestrian on sled injured in collision with other nonmotor vehicle in nontraffic accident
Pedestrian on snowboard injured in collision with other nonmotor vehicle in nontraffic accident
Pedestrian on snow-skis injured in collision with other nonmotor vehicle in nontraffic accident
Pedestrian in wheelchair (powered) injured in collision with other nonmotor vehicle in nontraffic accident
Pedestrian in motorized mobility scooter injured in collision with other nonmotor vehicle in nontraffic accident

V06.1- Pedestrian injured in collision with other nonmotor vehicle in traffic accident

V06.10x- Pedestrian on foot injured in collision with other nonmotor vehicle in traffic accident
Pedestrian NOS injured in collision with other nonmotor vehicle in traffic accident

V06.11x- Pedestrian on roller-skates injured in collision with other nonmotor vehicle in traffic accident

V06.12x- Pedestrian on skateboard injured in collision with other nonmotor vehicle in traffic accident

V06.19x- Pedestrian with other conveyance injured in collision with other nonmotor vehicle in traffic accident
Pedestrian with babystroller injured in collision with other nonmotor vehicle in nontraffic accident
Pedestrian on ice-skates injured in collision with other nonmotor vehicle in nontraffic accident
Pedestrian on nonmotorized scooter injured in collision with other nonmotor vehicle in traffic accident
Pedestrian on sled injured in collision with other nonmotor vehicle in traffic accident
Pedestrian on snowboard injured in collision with other nonmotor vehicle in traffic accident
Pedestrian on snow-skis injured in collision with other nonmotor vehicle in traffic accident
Pedestrian in wheelchair (powered) injured in collision with other nonmotor vehicle in traffic accident
Pedestrian in motorized mobility scooter injured in collision with other nonmotor vehicle in traffic accident

V06.9- Pedestrian injured in collision with other nonmotor vehicle, unspecified whether traffic or nontraffic accident

V06.90x- Pedestrian on foot injured in collision with other nonmotor vehicle, unspecified whether traffic or nontraffic accident
Pedestrian NOS injured in collision with other nonmotor vehicle, unspecified whether traffic or nontraffic accident

V06.91x- Pedestrian on roller-skates injured in collision with other nonmotor vehicle, unspecified whether traffic or nontraffic accident

V06.92x- Pedestrian on skateboard injured in collision with other nonmotor vehicle, unspecified whether traffic or nontraffic accident

V06.99x- Pedestrian with other conveyance injured in collision with other nonmotor vehicle, unspecified whether traffic or nontraffic accident
Pedestrian with babystroller injured in collision with other nonmotor vehicle, unspecified whether traffic or nontraffic accident
Pedestrian on ice-skates injured in collision with other nonmotor vehicle, unspecified whether traffic or nontraffic accident
Pedestrian on nonmotorized scooter injured in collision with other nonmotor vehicle, unspecified whether traffic or nontraffic accident
Pedestrian on sled injured in collision with other nonmotor vehicle, unspecified whether traffic or nontraffic accident
Pedestrian on snowboard injured in collision with other nonmotor vehicle, unspecified whether traffic or nontraffic accident
Pedestrian on snow-skis injured in collision with other nonmotor vehicle, unspecified whether traffic or nontraffic accident
Pedestrian in wheelchair (powered) injured in collision with other nonmotor vehicle, unspecified whether traffic or nontraffic accident
Pedestrian in motorized mobility scooter injured in collision with other nonmotor vehicle, unspecified whether traffic or nontraffic accident

V09- Pedestrian injured in other and unspecified transport accidents
The appropriate 7th character is to be added to each code from category V09:
A Initial encounter
D Subsequent encounter
S Sequela

V09.0- Pedestrian injured in nontraffic accident involving other and unspecified motor vehicles

V09.00x- Pedestrian injured in nontraffic accident involving unspecified motor vehicles

V09.01x- Pedestrian injured in nontraffic accident involving military vehicle

V09.09x- Pedestrian injured in nontraffic accident involving other motor vehicles
Pedestrian injured in nontraffic accident by special vehicle

V09.1xx- Pedestrian injured in unspecified nontraffic accident

V09.2- 　Pedestrian injured in traffic accident involving other and unspecified motor vehicles

V09.20x- 　Pedestrian injured in traffic accident involving unspecified motor vehicles

V09.21x- 　Pedestrian injured in traffic accident involving military vehicle

V09.29x- 　Pedestrian injured in traffic accident involving other motor vehicles

V09.3xx- 　Pedestrian injured in unspecified traffic accident

V09.9xx- 　Pedestrian injured in unspecified transport accident

Pedal cycle rider injured in transport accident (V10-V19)

Includes: 　Any non-motorized vehicle, excluding an animal-drawn vehicle, or a sidecar or trailer attached to the pedal cycle

Excludes ❷: 　*rupture of pedal cycle tire (W37.0)*

V10- 　<u>Pedal cycle rider injured in collision</u> with <u>pedestrian or animal</u>

Excludes 1: 　*pedal cycle rider collision with animal-drawn vehicle or animal being ridden (V16.-)*

The appropriate 7th character is to be added to each code from category
V10:
A 　<u>Initial</u> encounter
D 　<u>Subsequent</u> encounter
S 　<u>Sequela</u>

V10.0xx- 　Pedal cycle driver injured in collision with pedestrian or animal in nontraffic accident

V10.1xx- 　Pedal cycle passenger injured in collision with pedestrian or animal in nontraffic accident

V10.2xx- 　Unspecified pedal cyclist injured in collision with pedestrian or animal in nontraffic accident

V10.3xx- 　Person boarding or alighting a pedal cycle injured in collision with pedestrian or animal

V10.4xx- 　Pedal cycle driver injured in collision with pedestrian or animal in traffic accident

V10.5xx- 　Pedal cycle passenger injured in collision with pedestrian or animal in traffic accident

V10.9xx- 　Unspecified pedal cyclist injured in collision with pedestrian or animal in traffic accident

V11- 　<u>Pedal cycle rider injured in collision</u> with <u>other pedal cycle</u>

The appropriate 7th character is to be added to each code from category
V11:
A 　<u>Initial</u> encounter
D 　<u>Subsequent</u> encounter
S 　<u>Sequela</u>

V11.0xx- 　Pedal cycle driver injured in collision with other pedal cycle in nontraffic accident

V11.1xx- 　Pedal cycle passenger injured in collision with other pedal cycle in nontraffic accident

V11.2xx- 　Unspecified pedal cyclist injured in collision with other pedal cycle in nontraffic accident

V11.3xx- 　Person boarding or alighting a pedal cycle injured in collision with other pedal cycle

V11.4xx- 　Pedal cycle driver injured in collision with other pedal cycle in traffic accident

V11.5xx- 　Pedal cycle passenger injured in collision with other pedal cycle in traffic accident

V11.9xx- 　Unspecified pedal cyclist injured in collision with other pedal cycle in traffic accident

V12- 　<u>Pedal cycle rider injured in collision</u> with <u>two- or three-wheeled motor vehicle</u>

The appropriate 7th character is to be added to each code from category
V12:
A 　<u>Initial</u> encounter
D 　<u>Subsequent</u> encounter
S 　<u>Sequela</u>

V12.0xx- 　Pedal cycle driver injured in collision with two- or three-wheeled motor vehicle in nontraffic accident

V12.1xx- 　Pedal cycle passenger injured in collision with two- or three-wheeled motor vehicle in nontraffic accident

V12.2xx- 　Unspecified pedal cyclist injured in collision with two- or three-wheeled motor vehicle in nontraffic accident

V12.3xx- 　Person boarding or alighting a pedal cycle injured in collision with two- or three-wheeled motor vehicle

V12.4xx- 　Pedal cycle driver injured in collision with two- or three-wheeled motor vehicle in traffic accident

V12.5xx- 　Pedal cycle passenger injured in collision with two- or three-wheeled motor vehicle in traffic accident

V12.9xx- 　Unspecified pedal cyclist injured in collision with two- or three-wheeled motor vehicle in traffic accident

V13- 　<u>Pedal cycle rider injured in collision</u> with <u>car, pick-up truck or van</u>

The appropriate 7th character is to be added to each code from category
V13:
A 　<u>Initial</u> encounter
D 　<u>Subsequent</u> encounter
S 　<u>Sequela</u>

V13.0xx- 　Pedal cycle driver injured in collision with car, pick-up truck or van in nontraffic accident

V13.1xx- 　Pedal cycle passenger injured in collision with car, pick-up truck or van in nontraffic accident

V13.2xx- 　Unspecified pedal cyclist injured in collision with car, pick-up truck or van in nontraffic accident

V13.3xx- 　Person boarding or alighting a pedal cycle injured in collision with car, pick-up truck or van

V13.4xx- 　Pedal cycle driver injured in collision with car, pick-up truck or van in traffic accident

V13.5xx- 　Pedal cycle passenger injured in collision with car, pick-up truck or van in traffic accident

V13.9xx- 　Unspecified pedal cyclist injured in collision with car, pick-up truck or van in traffic accident

V14- 　<u>Pedal cycle rider injured in collision</u> with <u>heavy transport vehicle or bus</u>

Excludes 1: 　*pedal cycle rider injured in collision with military vehicle (V19.81)*

The appropriate 7th character is to be added to each code from category
V14:
A 　<u>Initial</u> encounter
D 　<u>Subsequent</u> encounter
S 　<u>Sequela</u>

V14.0xx- 　Pedal cycle driver injured in collision with heavy transport vehicle or bus in nontraffic accident

V14.1xx- 　Pedal cycle passenger injured in collision with heavy transport vehicle or bus in nontraffic accident

V14.2xx- 　Unspecified pedal cyclist injured in collision with heavy transport vehicle or bus in nontraffic accident

V14.3xx- 　Person boarding or alighting a pedal cycle injured in collision with heavy transport vehicle or bus

V14.4xx- 　Pedal cycle driver injured in collision with heavy transport vehicle or bus in traffic accident

V14.5xx- 　Pedal cycle passenger injured in collision with heavy transport vehicle or bus in traffic accident

V14.9xx- 　Unspecified pedal cyclist injured in collision with heavy transport vehicle or bus in traffic accident

V15- 　<u>Pedal cycle rider injured in collision</u> with <u>railway train or railway vehicle</u>

The appropriate 7th character is to be added to each code from category
V15:
A 　<u>Initial</u> encounter
D 　<u>Subsequent</u> encounter
S 　<u>Sequela</u>

V15.0xx- 　Pedal cycle driver injured in collision with railway train or railway vehicle in nontraffic accident

V15.1xx- 　Pedal cycle passenger injured in collision with railway train or railway vehicle in nontraffic accident

V15.2xx- 　Unspecified pedal cyclist injured in collision with railway train or railway vehicle in nontraffic accident

V15.3xx- 　Person boarding or alighting a pedal cycle injured in collision with railway train or railway vehicle

V15.4xx- 　Pedal cycle driver injured in collision with railway train or railway vehicle in traffic accident

V15.5xx- 　Pedal cycle passenger injured in collision with railway train or railway vehicle in traffic accident

V15.9xx- Unspecified pedal cyclist injured in collision with railway train or railway vehicle in traffic accident

V16- Pedal cycle rider injured in collision with other nonmotor vehicle
Includes: Collision with animal-drawn vehicle, animal being ridden, streetcar

The appropriate 7th character is to be added to each code from category V16:
A **Initial** encounter
D **Subsequent** encounter
S **Sequela**

V16.0xx- Pedal cycle driver injured in collision with other nonmotor vehicle in nontraffic accident

V16.1xx- Pedal cycle passenger injured in collision with other nonmotor vehicle in nontraffic accident

V16.2xx- Unspecified pedal cyclist injured in collision with other nonmotor vehicle in nontraffic accident

V16.3xx- Person boarding or alighting a pedal cycle injured in collision with other nonmotor vehicle in nontraffic accident

V16.4xx- Pedal cycle driver injured in collision with other nonmotor vehicle in traffic accident

V16.5xx- Pedal cycle passenger injured in collision with other nonmotor vehicle in traffic accident

V16.9xx- Unspecified pedal cyclist injured in collision with other nonmotor vehicle in traffic accident

V17- Pedal cycle rider injured in collision with fixed or stationary object

The appropriate 7th character is to be added to each code from category V17:
A **Initial** encounter
D **Subsequent** encounter
S **Sequela**

V17.0xx- Pedal cycle driver injured in collision with fixed or stationary object in nontraffic accident

V17.1xx- Pedal cycle passenger injured in collision with fixed or stationary object in nontraffic accident

V17.2xx- Unspecified pedal cyclist injured in collision with fixed or stationary object in nontraffic accident

V17.3xx- Person boarding or alighting a pedal cycle injured in collision with fixed or stationary object

V17.4xx- Pedal cycle driver injured in collision with fixed or stationary object in traffic accident

V17.5xx- Pedal cycle passenger injured in collision with fixed or stationary object in traffic accident

V17.9xx- Unspecified pedal cyclist injured in collision with fixed or stationary object in traffic accident

V18- Pedal cycle rider injured in noncollision transport accident
Includes: Fall or thrown from pedal cycle (without antecedent collision)
Overturning pedal cycle NOS
Overturning pedal cycle without collision

The appropriate 7th character is to be added to each code from category V18:
A **Initial** encounter
D **Subsequent** encounter
S **Sequela**

V18.0xx- Pedal cycle driver injured in noncollision transport accident in nontraffic accident

V18.1xx- Pedal cycle passenger injured in noncollision transport accident in nontraffic accident

V18.2xx- Unspecified pedal cyclist injured in noncollision transport accident in nontraffic accident

V18.3xx- Person boarding or alighting a pedal cycle injured in noncollision transport accident

V18.4xx- Pedal cycle driver injured in noncollision transport accident in traffic accident

V18.5xx- Pedal cycle passenger injured in noncollision transport accident in traffic accident

V18.9xx- Unspecified pedal cyclist injured in noncollision transport accident in traffic accident

V19- Pedal cycle rider injured in other and unspecified transport accidents

The appropriate 7th character is to be added to each code from category V19:
A **Initial** encounter
D **Subsequent** encounter
S **Sequela**

V19.0- Pedal cycle driver injured in collision with other and unspecified motor vehicles in nontraffic accident

V19.00x- Pedal cycle driver injured in collision with unspecified motor vehicles in nontraffic accident

V19.09x- Pedal cycle driver injured in collision with other motor vehicles in nontraffic accident

V19.1- Pedal cycle passenger injured in collision with other and unspecified motor vehicles in nontraffic accident

V19.10x- Pedal cycle passenger injured in collision with unspecified motor vehicles in nontraffic accident

V19.19x- Pedal cycle passenger injured in collision with other motor vehicles in nontraffic accident

V19.2- Unspecified pedal cyclist injured in collision with other and unspecified motor vehicles in nontraffic accident

V19.20x- Unspecified pedal cyclist injured in collision with unspecified motor vehicles in nontraffic accident
Pedal cycle collision NOS, nontraffic

V19.29x- Unspecified pedal cyclist injured in collision with other motor vehicles in nontraffic accident

V19.3xx- Pedal cyclist (driver) (passenger) injured in unspecified nontraffic accident
Pedal cycle accident NOS, nontraffic
Pedal cyclist injured in nontraffic accident NOS

V19.4- Pedal cycle driver injured in collision with other and unspecified motor vehicles in traffic accident

V19.40x- Pedal cycle driver injured in collision with unspecified motor vehicles in traffic accident

V19.49x- Pedal cycle driver injured in collision with other motor vehicles in traffic accident

V19.5- Pedal cycle passenger injured in collision with other and unspecified motor vehicles in traffic accident

V19.50x- Pedal cycle passenger injured in collision with unspecified motor vehicles in traffic accident

V19.59x- Pedal cycle passenger injured in collision with other motor vehicles in traffic accident

V19.6- Unspecified pedal cyclist injured in collision with other and unspecified motor vehicles in traffic accident

V19.60x- Unspecified pedal cyclist injured in collision with unspecified motor vehicles in traffic accident
Pedal cycle collision NOS (traffic)

V19.69x- Unspecified pedal cyclist injured in collision with other motor vehicles in traffic accident

V19.8- Pedal cyclist (driver) (passenger) injured in other specified transport accidents

V19.81x- Pedal cyclist (driver) (passenger) injured in transport accident with military vehicle

V19.88x- Pedal cyclist (driver) (passenger) injured in other specified transport accidents

V19.9xx- Pedal cyclist (driver) (passenger) injured in unspecified traffic accident
Pedal cycle accident NOS

V
1
5
-
V
1
9

Motorcycle rider injured in transport accident (V20-V29)

Includes: Moped
            Motorcycle with sidecar
            Motorized bicycle
            Motor scooter
Excludes 1:   three-wheeled motor vehicle (V30-V39)

V20-   Motorcycle rider injured in collision with pedestrian or animal
Excludes 1:   motorcycle rider collision with animal-drawn vehicle or animal
              being ridden (V26.-)

The appropriate 7th character is to be added to each code from category
V20:
A   **Initial** encounter
D   **Subsequent** encounter
S   **Sequela**

V20.0xx-   Motorcycle driver injured in collision with pedestrian or animal in nontraffic accident
V20.1xx-   Motorcycle passenger injured in collision with pedestrian or animal in nontraffic accident
V20.2xx-   Unspecified motorcycle rider injured in collision with pedestrian or animal in nontraffic accident
V20.3xx-   Person boarding or alighting a motorcycle injured in collision with pedestrian or animal
V20.4xx-   Motorcycle driver injured in collision with pedestrian or animal in traffic accident
V20.5xx-   Motorcycle passenger injured in collision with pedestrian or animal in traffic accident
V20.9xx-   Unspecified motorcycle rider injured in collision with pedestrian or animal in traffic accident

V21-   Motorcycle rider injured in collision with pedal cycle
The appropriate 7th character is to be added to each code from category
V21:
A   **Initial** encounter
D   **Subsequent** encounter
S   **Sequela**

V21.0xx-   Motorcycle driver injured in collision with pedal cycle in nontraffic accident
V21.1xx-   Motorcycle passenger injured in collision with pedal cycle in nontraffic accident
V21.2xx-   Unspecified motorcycle rider injured in collision with pedal cycle in nontraffic accident
V21.3xx-   Person boarding or alighting a motorcycle injured in collision with pedal cycle
V21.4xx-   Motorcycle driver injured in collision with pedal cycle in traffic accident
V21.5xx-   Motorcycle passenger injured in collision with pedal cycle in traffic accident
V21.9xx-   Unspecified motorcycle rider injured in collision with pedal cycle in traffic accident

V22-   Motorcycle rider injured in collision with two- or three-wheeled motor vehicle
The appropriate 7th character is to be added to each code from category
V22:
A   **Initial** encounter
D   **Subsequent** encounter
S   **Sequela**

V22.0xx-   Motorcycle driver injured in collision with two- or three-wheeled motor vehicle in nontraffic accident
V22.1xx-   Motorcycle passenger injured in collision with two- or three-wheeled motor vehicle in nontraffic accident
V22.2xx-   Unspecified motorcycle rider injured in collision with two- or three-wheeled motor vehicle in nontraffic accident
V22.3xx-   Person boarding or alighting a motorcycle injured in collision with two- or three-wheeled motor vehicle
V22.4xx-   Motorcycle driver injured in collision with two- or three-wheeled motor vehicle in traffic accident
V22.5xx-   Motorcycle passenger injured in collision with two- or three-wheeled motor vehicle in traffic accident
V22.9xx-   Unspecified motorcycle rider injured in collision with two- or three-wheeled motor vehicle in traffic accident

V23-   Motorcycle rider injured in collision with car, pick-up truck or van
The appropriate 7th character is to be added to each code from category
V23:
A   **Initial** encounter
D   **Subsequent** encounter
S   **Sequela**

V23.0xx-   Motorcycle driver injured in collision with car, pick-up truck or van in nontraffic accident
V23.1xx-   Motorcycle passenger injured in collision with car, pick-up truck or van in nontraffic accident
V23.2xx-   Unspecified motorcycle rider injured in collision with car, pick-up truck or van in nontraffic accident
V23.3xx-   Person boarding or alighting a motorcycle injured in collision with car, pick-up truck or van
V23.4xx-   Motorcycle driver injured in collision with car, pick-up truck or van in traffic accident
V23.5xx-   Motorcycle passenger injured in collision with car, pick-up truck or van in traffic accident
V23.9xx-   Unspecified motorcycle rider injured in collision with car, pick-up truck or van in traffic accident

V24-   Motorcycle rider injured in collision with heavy transport vehicle or bus
Excludes 1:   motorcycle rider injured in collision with military vehicle
              (V29.81)

The appropriate 7th character is to be added to each code from category
V24:
A   **Initial** encounter
D   **Subsequent** encounter
S   **Sequela**

V24.0xx-   Motorcycle driver injured in collision with heavy transport vehicle or bus in nontraffic accident
V24.1xx-   Motorcycle passenger injured in collision with heavy transport vehicle or bus in nontraffic accident
V24.2xx-   Unspecified motorcycle rider injured in collision with heavy transport vehicle or bus in nontraffic accident
V24.3xx-   Person boarding or alighting a motorcycle injured in collision with heavy transport vehicle or bus
V24.4xx-   Motorcycle driver injured in collision with heavy transport vehicle or bus in traffic accident
V24.5xx-   Motorcycle passenger injured in collision with heavy transport vehicle or bus in traffic accident
V24.9xx-   Unspecified motorcycle rider injured in collision with heavy transport vehicle or bus in traffic accident

V25-   Motorcycle rider injured in collision with railway train or railway vehicle
The appropriate 7th character is to be added to each code from category
V25:
A   **Initial** encounter
D   **Subsequent** encounter
S   **Sequela**

V25.0xx-   Motorcycle driver injured in collision with railway train or railway vehicle in nontraffic accident
V25.1xx-   Motorcycle passenger injured in collision with railway train or railway vehicle in nontraffic accident
V25.2xx-   Unspecified motorcycle rider injured in collision with railway train or railway vehicle in nontraffic accident
V25.3xx-   Person boarding or alighting a motorcycle injured in collision with railway train or railway vehicle
V25.4xx-   Motorcycle driver injured in collision with railway train or railway vehicle in traffic accident
V25.5xx-   Motorcycle passenger injured in collision with railway train or railway vehicle in traffic accident
V25.9xx-   Unspecified motorcycle rider injured in collision with railway train or railway vehicle in traffic accident

V20-V25

V26- <u>Motorcycle rider injured in collision</u> with <u>other nonmotor vehicle</u>

Includes: Collision with animal-drawn vehicle, animal being ridden, streetcar

The appropriate 7th character is to be added to each code from category V26:

A <u>Initial</u> encounter
D <u>Subsequent</u> encounter
S <u>Sequela</u>

V26.0xx- Motorcycle driver injured in collision with other nonmotor vehicle in nontraffic accident

V26.1xx- Motorcycle passenger injured in collision with other nonmotor vehicle in nontraffic accident

V26.2xx- Unspecified motorcycle rider injured in collision with other nonmotor vehicle in nontraffic accident

V26.3xx- Person boarding or alighting a motorcycle injured in collision with other nonmotor vehicle

V26.4xx- Motorcycle driver injured in collision with other nonmotor vehicle in traffic accident

V26.5xx- Motorcycle passenger injured in collision with other nonmotor vehicle in traffic accident

V26.9xx- Unspecified motorcycle rider injured in collision with other nonmotor vehicle in traffic accident

V27- <u>Motorcycle rider injured in collision</u> with <u>fixed or stationary object</u>

The appropriate 7th character is to be added to each code from category V27:

A <u>Initial</u> encounter
D <u>Subsequent</u> encounter
S <u>Sequela</u>

V27.0xx- Motorcycle driver injured in collision with fixed or stationary object in nontraffic accident

V27.1xx- Motorcycle passenger injured in collision with fixed or stationary object in nontraffic accident

V27.2xx- Unspecified motorcycle rider injured in collision with fixed or stationary object in nontraffic accident

V27.3xx- Person boarding or alighting a motorcycle injured in collision with fixed or stationary object

V27.4xx- Motorcycle driver injured in collision with fixed or stationary object in traffic accident

V27.5xx- Motorcycle passenger injured in collision with fixed or stationary object in traffic accident

V27.9xx- Unspecified motorcycle rider injured in collision with fixed or stationary object in traffic accident

V28- <u>Motorcycle rider injured</u> in <u>noncollision</u> transport accident

Includes: Fall or thrown from motorcycle (without antecedent collision)
Overturning motorcycle NOS
Overturning motorcycle without collision

The appropriate 7th character is to be added to each code from category V28:

A <u>Initial</u> encounter
D <u>Subsequent</u> encounter
S <u>Sequela</u>

V28.0xx- Motorcycle driver injured in noncollision transport accident in nontraffic accident

V28.1xx- Motorcycle passenger injured in noncollision transport accident in nontraffic accident

V28.2xx- Unspecified motorcycle rider injured in noncollision transport accident in nontraffic accident

V28.3xx- Person boarding or alighting a motorcycle injured in noncollision transport accident

V28.4xx- Motorcycle driver injured in noncollision transport accident in traffic accident

V28.5xx- Motorcycle passenger injured in noncollision transport accident in traffic accident

V28.9xx- Unspecified motorcycle rider injured in noncollision transport accident in traffic accident

V29- <u>Motorcycle rider injured</u> in <u>other and unspecified transport accidents</u>

The appropriate 7th character is to be added to each code from category V29:

A <u>Initial</u> encounter
D <u>Subsequent</u> encounter
S <u>Sequela</u>

V29.0- Motorcycle driver injured in collision with other and unspecified motor vehicles in nontraffic accident

V29.00x- Motorcycle driver injured in collision with unspecified motor vehicles in nontraffic accident

V29.09x- Motorcycle driver injured in collision with other motor vehicles in nontraffic accident

V29.1- Motorcycle passenger injured in collision with other and unspecified motor vehicles in nontraffic accident

V29.10x- Motorcycle passenger injured in collision with unspecified motor vehicles in nontraffic accident

V29.19x- Motorcycle passenger injured in collision with other motor vehicles in nontraffic accident

V29.2- Unspecified motorcycle rider injured in collision with other and unspecified motor vehicles in nontraffic accident

V29.20x- Unspecified motorcycle rider injured in collision with unspecified motor vehicles in nontraffic accident
Motorcycle collision NOS, nontraffic

V29.29x- Unspecified motorcycle rider injured in collision with other motor vehicles in nontraffic accident

V29.3xx- Motorcycle rider (driver) (passenger) injured in unspecified nontraffic accident
Motorcycle accident NOS, nontraffic
Motorcycle rider injured in nontraffic accident NOS

V29.4- Motorcycle driver injured in collision with other and unspecified motor vehicles in traffic accident

V29.40x- Motorcycle driver injured in collision with unspecified motor vehicles in traffic accident

V29.49x- Motorcycle driver injured in collision with other motor vehicles in traffic accident

V29.5- Motorcycle passenger injured in collision with other and unspecified motor vehicles in traffic accident

V29.50x- Motorcycle passenger injured in collision with unspecified motor vehicles in traffic accident

V29.59x- Motorcycle passenger injured in collision with other motor vehicles in traffic accident

V29.6- Unspecified motorcycle rider injured in collision with other and unspecified motor vehicles in traffic accident

V29.60x- Unspecified motorcycle rider injured in collision with unspecified motor vehicles in traffic accident
Motorcycle collision NOS (traffic)

V29.69x- Unspecified motorcycle rider injured in collision with other motor vehicles in traffic accident

V29.8- Motorcycle rider (driver) (passenger) injured in other specified transport accidents

V29.81x- Motorcycle rider (driver) (passenger) injured in transport accident with military vehicle

V29.88x- Motorcycle rider (driver) (passenger) injured in other specified transport accidents

V29.9xx- Motorcycle rider (driver) (passenger) injured in unspecified traffic accident
Motorcycle accident NOS

Occupant of three-wheeled motor vehicle injured in transport accident (V30-V39)

Includes: Motorized tricycle
Motorized rickshaw
Three-wheeled motor car

Excludes 1: all-terrain vehicles (V86.-)
motorcycle with sidecar (V20-V29)
vehicle designed primarily for off-road use (V86.-)

V30- **Occupant of three-wheeled motor vehicle injured in collision with pedestrian or animal**

Excludes 1: three-wheeled motor vehicle collision with animal-drawn vehicle or animal being ridden (V36.-)

The appropriate 7th character is to be added to each code from category V30:
A   Initial encounter
D   Subsequent encounter
S   Sequela

V30.0xx-   Driver of three-wheeled motor vehicle injured in collision with pedestrian or animal in nontraffic accident

V30.1xx-   Passenger in three-wheeled motor vehicle injured in collision with pedestrian or animal in nontraffic accident

V30.2xx-   Person on outside of three-wheeled motor vehicle injured in collision with pedestrian or animal in nontraffic accident

V30.3xx-   Unspecified occupant of three-wheeled motor vehicle injured in collision with pedestrian or animal in nontraffic accident

V30.4xx-   Person boarding or alighting a three-wheeled motor vehicle injured in collision with pedestrian or animal

V30.5xx-   Driver of three-wheeled motor vehicle injured in collision with pedestrian or animal in traffic accident

V30.6xx-   Passenger in three-wheeled motor vehicle injured in collision with pedestrian or animal in traffic accident

V30.7xx-   Person on outside of three-wheeled motor vehicle injured in collision with pedestrian or animal in traffic accident

V30.9xx-   Unspecified occupant of three-wheeled motor vehicle injured in collision with pedestrian or animal in traffic accident

V31- **Occupant of three-wheeled motor vehicle injured in collision with pedal cycle**

The appropriate 7th character is to be added to each code from category V31:
A   Initial encounter
D   Subsequent encounter
S   Sequela

V31.0xx-   Driver of three-wheeled motor vehicle injured in collision with pedal cycle in nontraffic accident

V31.1xx-   Passenger in three-wheeled motor vehicle injured in collision with pedal cycle in nontraffic accident

V31.2xx-   Person on outside of three-wheeled motor vehicle injured in collision with pedal cycle in nontraffic accident

V31.3xx-   Unspecified occupant of three-wheeled motor vehicle injured in collision with pedal cycle in nontraffic accident

V31.4xx-   Person boarding or alighting a three-wheeled motor vehicle injured in collision with pedal cycle

V31.5xx-   Driver of three-wheeled motor vehicle injured in collision with pedal cycle in traffic accident

V31.6xx-   Passenger in three-wheeled motor vehicle injured in collision with pedal cycle in traffic accident

V31.7xx-   Person on outside of three-wheeled motor vehicle injured in collision with pedal cycle in traffic accident

V31.9xx-   Unspecified occupant of three-wheeled motor vehicle injured in collision with pedal cycle in traffic accident

V32- **Occupant of three-wheeled motor vehicle injured in collision with two- or three-wheeled motor vehicle**

The appropriate 7th character is to be added to each code from category V32:
A   Initial encounter
D   Subsequent encounter
S   Sequela

V32.0xx-   Driver of three-wheeled motor vehicle injured in collision with two- or three-wheeled motor vehicle in nontraffic accident

V32.1xx-   Passenger in three-wheeled motor vehicle injured in collision with two- or three-wheeled motor vehicle in nontraffic accident

V32.2xx-   Person on outside of three-wheeled motor vehicle injured in collision with two- or three-wheeled motor vehicle in nontraffic accident

V32.3xx-   Unspecified occupant of three-wheeled motor vehicle injured in collision with two- or three-wheeled motor vehicle in nontraffic accident

V32.4xx-   Person boarding or alighting a three-wheeled motor vehicle injured in collision with two- or three-wheeled motor vehicle

V32.5xx-   Driver of three-wheeled motor vehicle injured in collision with two- or three-wheeled motor vehicle in traffic accident

V32.6xx-   Passenger in three-wheeled motor vehicle injured in collision with two- or three-wheeled motor vehicle in traffic accident

V32.7xx-   Person on outside of three-wheeled motor vehicle injured in collision with two- or three-wheeled motor vehicle in traffic accident

V32.9xx-   Unspecified occupant of three-wheeled motor vehicle injured in collision with two- or three-wheeled motor vehicle in traffic accident

V33- **Occupant of three-wheeled motor vehicle injured in collision with car, pick-up truck or van**

The appropriate 7th character is to be added to each code from category V33:
A   Initial encounter
D   Subsequent encounter
S   Sequela

V33.0xx-   Driver of three-wheeled motor vehicle injured in collision with car, pick-up truck or van in nontraffic accident

V33.1xx-   Passenger in three-wheeled motor vehicle injured in collision with car, pick-up truck or van in nontraffic accident

V33.2xx-   Person on outside of three-wheeled motor vehicle injured in collision with car, pick-up truck or van in nontraffic accident

V33.3xx-   Unspecified occupant of three-wheeled motor vehicle injured in collision with car, pick-up truck or van in nontraffic accident

V33.4xx-   Person boarding or alighting a three-wheeled motor vehicle injured in collision with car, pick-up truck or van

V33.5xx-   Driver of three-wheeled motor vehicle injured in collision with car, pick-up truck or van in traffic accident

V33.6xx-   Passenger in three-wheeled motor vehicle injured in collision with car, pick-up truck or van in traffic accident

V33.7xx-   Person on outside of three-wheeled motor vehicle injured in collision with car, pick-up truck or van in traffic accident

V33.9xx-   Unspecified occupant of three-wheeled motor vehicle injured in collision with car, pick-up truck or van in traffic accident

V30 - V33

V34- Occupant of three-wheeled motor vehicle injured in collision with heavy transport vehicle or bus

Excludes 1:   occupant of three-wheeled motor vehicle injured in collision with military vehicle (V39.81)

The appropriate 7th character is to be added to each code from category V34:
A   Initial encounter
D   Subsequent encounter
S   Sequela

V34.0xx- Driver of three-wheeled motor vehicle injured in collision with heavy transport vehicle or bus in nontraffic accident

V34.1xx- Passenger in three-wheeled motor vehicle injured in collision with heavy transport vehicle or bus in nontraffic accident

V34.2xx- Person on outside of three-wheeled motor vehicle injured in collision with heavy transport vehicle or bus in nontraffic accident

V34.3xx- Unspecified occupant of three-wheeled motor vehicle injured in collision with heavy transport vehicle or bus in nontraffic accident

V34.4xx- Person boarding or alighting a three-wheeled motor vehicle injured in collision with heavy transport vehicle or bus

V34.5xx- Driver of three-wheeled motor vehicle injured in collision with heavy transport vehicle or bus in traffic accident

V34.6xx- Passenger in three-wheeled motor vehicle injured in collision with heavy transport vehicle or bus in traffic accident

V34.7xx- Person on outside of three-wheeled motor vehicle injured in collision with heavy transport vehicle or bus in traffic accident

V34.9xx- Unspecified occupant of three-wheeled motor vehicle injured in collision with heavy transport vehicle or bus in traffic accident

V35- Occupant of three-wheeled motor vehicle injured in collision with railway train or railway vehicle

The appropriate 7th character is to be added to each code from category V35:
A   Initial encounter
D   Subsequent encounter
S   Sequela

V35.0xx- Driver of three-wheeled motor vehicle injured in collision with railway train or railway vehicle in nontraffic accident

V35.1xx- Passenger in three-wheeled motor vehicle injured in collision with railway train or railway vehicle in nontraffic accident

V35.2xx- Person on outside of three-wheeled motor vehicle injured in collision with railway train or railway vehicle in nontraffic accident

V35.3xx- Unspecified occupant of three-wheeled motor vehicle injured in collision with railway train or railway vehicle in nontraffic accident

V35.4xx- Person boarding or alighting a three-wheeled motor vehicle injured in collision with railway train or railway vehicle

V35.5xx- Driver of three-wheeled motor vehicle injured in collision with railway train or railway vehicle in traffic accident

V35.6xx- Passenger in three-wheeled motor vehicle injured in collision with railway train or railway vehicle in traffic accident

V35.7xx- Person on outside of three-wheeled motor vehicle injured in collision with railway train or railway vehicle in traffic accident

V35.9xx- Unspecified occupant of three-wheeled motor vehicle injured in collision with railway train or railway vehicle in traffic accident

V36- Occupant of three-wheeled motor vehicle injured in collision with other nonmotor vehicle

Includes: Collision with animal-drawn vehicle, animal being ridden, streetcar

The appropriate 7th character is to be added to each code from category V36:
A   Initial encounter
D   Subsequent encounter
S   Sequela

V36.0xx- Driver of three-wheeled motor vehicle injured in collision with other nonmotor vehicle in nontraffic accident

V36.1xx- Passenger in three-wheeled motor vehicle injured in collision with other nonmotor vehicle in nontraffic accident

V36.2xx- Person on outside of three-wheeled motor vehicle injured in collision with other nonmotor vehicle in nontraffic accident

V36.3xx- Unspecified occupant of three-wheeled motor vehicle injured in collision with other nonmotor vehicle in nontraffic accident

V36.4xx- Person boarding or alighting a three-wheeled motor vehicle injured in collision with other nonmotor vehicle

V36.5xx- Driver of three-wheeled motor vehicle injured in collision with other nonmotor vehicle in traffic accident

V36.6xx- Passenger in three-wheeled motor vehicle injured in collision with other nonmotor vehicle in traffic accident

V36.7xx- Person on outside of three-wheeled motor vehicle injured in collision with other nonmotor vehicle in traffic accident

V36.9xx- Unspecified occupant of three-wheeled motor vehicle injured in collision with other nonmotor vehicle in traffic accident

V37- Occupant of three-wheeled motor vehicle injured in collision with fixed or stationary object

The appropriate 7th character is to be added to each code from category V37:
A   Initial encounter
D   Subsequent encounter
S   Sequela

V37.0xx- Driver of three-wheeled motor vehicle injured in collision with fixed or stationary object in nontraffic accident

V37.1xx- Passenger in three-wheeled motor vehicle injured in collision with fixed or stationary object in nontraffic accident

V37.2xx- Person on outside of three-wheeled motor vehicle injured in collision with fixed or stationary object in nontraffic accident

V37.3xx- Unspecified occupant of three-wheeled motor vehicle injured in collision with fixed or stationary object in nontraffic accident

V37.4xx- Person boarding or alighting a three-wheeled motor vehicle injured in collision with fixed or stationary object

V37.5xx- Driver of three-wheeled motor vehicle injured in collision with fixed or stationary object in traffic accident

V37.6xx- Passenger in three-wheeled motor vehicle injured in collision with fixed or stationary object in traffic accident

V37.7xx- Person on outside of three-wheeled motor vehicle injured in collision with fixed or stationary object in traffic accident

V37.9xx- Unspecified occupant of three-wheeled motor vehicle injured in collision with fixed or stationary object in traffic accident

V34 - V37

V38- Occupant of three-wheeled motor vehicle injured in noncollision transport accident

Includes: Fall or thrown from three-wheeled motor vehicle
Overturning of three-wheeled motor vehicle NOS
Overturning of three-wheeled motor vehicle without collision

The appropriate 7th character is to be added to each code from category V38:
   A   Initial encounter
   D   Subsequent encounter
   S   Sequela

V38.0xx- Driver of three-wheeled motor vehicle injured in noncollision transport accident in nontraffic accident

V38.1xx- Passenger in three-wheeled motor vehicle injured in noncollision transport accident in nontraffic accident

V38.2xx- Person on outside of three-wheeled motor vehicle injured in noncollision transport accident in nontraffic accident

V38.3xx- Unspecified occupant of three-wheeled motor vehicle injured in noncollision transport accident in nontraffic accident

V38.4xx- Person boarding or alighting a three-wheeled motor vehicle injured in noncollision transport accident

V38.5xx- Driver of three-wheeled motor vehicle injured in noncollision transport accident in traffic accident

V38.6xx- Passenger in three-wheeled motor vehicle injured in noncollision transport accident in traffic accident

V38.7xx- Person on outside of three-wheeled motor vehicle injured in noncollision transport accident in traffic accident

V38.9xx- Unspecified occupant of three-wheeled motor vehicle injured in noncollision transport accident in traffic accident

V39- Occupant of three-wheeled motor vehicle injured in other and unspecified transport accidents

The appropriate 7th character is to be added to each code from category V39:
   A   Initial encounter
   D   Subsequent encounter
   S   Sequela

V39.0- Driver of three-wheeled motor vehicle injured in collision with other and unspecified motor vehicles in nontraffic accident

V39.00x- Driver of three-wheeled motor vehicle injured in collision with unspecified motor vehicles in nontraffic accident

V39.09x- Driver of three-wheeled motor vehicle injured in collision with other motor vehicles in nontraffic accident

V39.1- Passenger in three-wheeled motor vehicle injured in collision with other and unspecified motor vehicles in nontraffic accident

V39.10x- Passenger in three-wheeled motor vehicle injured in collision with unspecified motor vehicles in nontraffic accident

V39.19x- Passenger in three-wheeled motor vehicle injured in collision with other motor vehicles in nontraffic accident

V39.2- Unspecified occupant of three-wheeled motor vehicle injured in collision with other and unspecified motor vehicles in nontraffic accident

V39.20x- Unspecified occupant of three-wheeled motor vehicle injured in collision with unspecified motor vehicles in nontraffic accident
   Collision NOS involving three-wheeled motor vehicle, nontraffic

V39.29x- Unspecified occupant of three-wheeled motor vehicle injured in collision with other motor vehicles in nontraffic accident

V39.3xx- Occupant (driver) (passenger) of three-wheeled motor vehicle injured in unspecified nontraffic accident
   Accident NOS involving three-wheeled motor vehicle, nontraffic
   Occupant of three-wheeled motor vehicle injured in nontraffic accident NOS

V39.4- Driver of three-wheeled motor vehicle injured in collision with other and unspecified motor vehicles in traffic accident

V39.40x- Driver of three-wheeled motor vehicle injured in collision with unspecified motor vehicles in traffic accident

V39.49x- Driver of three-wheeled motor vehicle injured in collision with other motor vehicles in traffic accident

V39.5- Passenger in three-wheeled motor vehicle injured in collision with other and unspecified motor vehicles in traffic accident

V39.50x- Passenger in three-wheeled motor vehicle injured in collision with unspecified motor vehicles in traffic accident

V39.59x- Passenger in three-wheeled motor vehicle injured in collision with other motor vehicles in traffic accident

V39.6- Unspecified occupant of three-wheeled motor vehicle injured in collision with other and unspecified motor vehicles in traffic accident

V39.60x- Unspecified occupant of three-wheeled motor vehicle injured in collision with unspecified motor vehicles in traffic accident
   Collision NOS involving three-wheeled motor vehicle (traffic)

V39.69x- Unspecified occupant of three-wheeled motor vehicle injured in collision with other motor vehicles in traffic accident

V39.8- Occupant (driver) (passenger) of three-wheeled motor vehicle injured in other specified transport accidents

V39.81x- Occupant (driver) (passenger) of three-wheeled motor vehicle injured in transport accident with military vehicle

V39.89x- Occupant (driver) (passenger) of three-wheeled motor vehicle injured in other specified transport accidents

V39.9xx- Occupant (driver) (passenger) of three-wheeled motor vehicle injured in unspecified traffic accident
   Accident NOS involving three-wheeled motor vehicle

Car occupant injured in transport accident (V40-V49)

Includes: A four-wheeled motor vehicle designed primarily for carrying passengers
Automobile (pulling a trailer or camper)

Excludes 1:   bus (V50-V59)
minibus (V50-V59)
minivan (V50-V59)
motorcoach (V70-V79)
pick-up truck (V50-V59)
sport utility vehicle (SUV) (V50-V59)

V40- Car occupant injured in collision with pedestrian or animal

Excludes 1:   car collision with animal-drawn vehicle or animal being ridden (V46.-)

The appropriate 7th character is to be added to each code from category V40:
   A   Initial encounter
   D   Subsequent encounter
   S   Sequela

V40.0xx- Car driver injured in collision with pedestrian or animal in nontraffic accident

V40.1xx- Car passenger injured in collision with pedestrian or animal in nontraffic accident

V40.2xx- Person on outside of car injured in collision with pedestrian or animal in nontraffic accident

V40.3xx- Unspecified car occupant injured in collision with pedestrian or animal in nontraffic accident

V40.4xx- Person boarding or alighting a car injured in collision with pedestrian or animal

V40.5xx- Car driver injured in collision with pedestrian or animal in traffic accident

V40.6xx- Car passenger injured in collision with pedestrian or animal in traffic accident

V40.7xx- Person on outside of car injured in collision with pedestrian or animal in traffic accident

V38
–
V40

V40.9xx- Unspecified car occupant injured in collision with pedestrian or animal in traffic accident

V41- <u>Car occupant injured in collision</u> with <u>pedal cycle</u>

The appropriate 7th character is to be added to each code from category V41:
- **A** <u>Initial</u> encounter
- **D** <u>Subsequent</u> encounter
- **S** <u>Sequela</u>

V41.0xx- Car driver injured in collision with pedal cycle in nontraffic accident

V41.1xx- Car passenger injured in collision with pedal cycle in nontraffic accident

V41.2xx- Person on outside of car injured in collision with pedal cycle in nontraffic accident

V41.3xx- Unspecified car occupant injured in collision with pedal cycle in nontraffic accident

V41.4xx- Person boarding or alighting a car injured in collision with pedal cycle

V41.5xx- Car driver injured in collision with pedal cycle in traffic accident

V41.6xx- Car passenger injured in collision with pedal cycle in traffic accident

V41.7xx- Person on outside of car injured in collision with pedal cycle in traffic accident

V41.9xx- Unspecified car occupant injured in collision with pedal cycle in traffic accident

V42- <u>Car occupant injured in collision</u> with <u>two- or three-wheeled motor vehicle</u>

The appropriate 7th character is to be added to each code from category V42:
- **A** <u>Initial</u> encounter
- **D** <u>Subsequent</u> encounter
- **S** <u>Sequela</u>

V42.0xx- Car driver injured in collision with two- or three-wheeled motor vehicle in nontraffic accident

V42.1xx- Car passenger injured in collision with two- or three-wheeled motor vehicle in nontraffic accident

V42.2xx- Person on outside of car injured in collision with two- or three-wheeled motor vehicle in nontraffic accident

V42.3xx- Unspecified car occupant injured in collision with two- or three-wheeled motor vehicle in nontraffic accident

V42.4xx- Person boarding or alighting a car injured in collision with two- or three-wheeled motor vehicle

V42.5xx- Car driver injured in collision with two- or three-wheeled motor vehicle in traffic accident

V42.6xx- Car passenger injured in collision with two- or three-wheeled motor vehicle in traffic accident

V42.7xx- Person on outside of car injured in collision with two- or three-wheeled motor vehicle in traffic accident

V42.9xx- Unspecified car occupant injured in collision with two- or three-wheeled motor vehicle in traffic accident

V43- <u>Car occupant injured in collision</u> with <u>car, pick-up truck or van</u>

The appropriate 7th character is to be added to each code from category V43:
- **A** <u>Initial</u> encounter
- **D** <u>Subsequent</u> encounter
- **S** <u>Sequela</u>

V43.0- Car driver injured in collision with car, pick-up truck or van in nontraffic accident

V43.01x- Car driver injured in collision with sport utility vehicle in nontraffic accident

V43.02x- Car driver injured in collision with other type car in nontraffic accident

V43.03x- Car driver injured in collision with pick-up truck in nontraffic accident

V43.04x- Car driver injured in collision with van in nontraffic accident

V43.1- Car passenger injured in collision with car, pick-up truck or van in nontraffic accident

V43.11x- Car passenger injured in collision with sport utility vehicle in nontraffic accident

V43.12x- Car passenger injured in collision with other type car in nontraffic accident

V43.13x- Car passenger injured in collision with pick-up in nontraffic accident

V43.14x- Car passenger injured in collision with van in nontraffic accident

V43.2- Person on outside of car injured in collision with car, pick-up truck or van in nontraffic accident

V43.21x- Person on outside of car injured in collision with sport utility vehicle in nontraffic accident

V43.22x- Person on outside of car injured in collision with other type car in nontraffic accident

V43.23x- Person on outside of car injured in collision with pick-up truck in nontraffic accident

V43.24x- Person on outside of car injured in collision with van in nontraffic accident

V43.3- Unspecified car occupant injured in collision with car, pick-up truck or van in nontraffic accident

V43.31x- Unspecified car occupant injured in collision with sport utility vehicle in nontraffic accident

V43.32x- Unspecified car occupant injured in collision with other type car in nontraffic accident

V43.33x- Unspecified car occupant injured in collision with pick-up truck in nontraffic accident

V43.34x- Unspecified car occupant injured in collision with van in nontraffic accident

V43.4- Person boarding or alighting a car injured in collision with car, pick-up truck or van

V43.41x- Person boarding or alighting a car injured in collision with sport utility vehicle

V43.42x- Person boarding or alighting a car injured in collision with other type car

V43.43x- Person boarding or alighting a car injured in collision with pick-up truck

V43.44x- Person boarding or alighting a car injured in collision with van

V43.5- Car driver injured in collision with car, pick-up truck or van in traffic accident

V43.51x- Car driver injured in collision with sport utility vehicle in traffic accident

V43.52x- Car driver injured in collision with other type car in traffic accident

V43.53x- Car driver injured in collision with pick-up truck in traffic accident

V43.54x- Car driver injured in collision with van in traffic accident

V43.6- Car passenger injured in collision with car, pick-up truck or van in traffic accident

V43.61x- Car passenger injured in collision with sport utility vehicle in traffic accident

AHA 15:1Q:p5 – Car passenger injured in collision with sport utility vehicle in traffic accident

V43.62x- Car passenger injured in collision with other type car in traffic accident

V43.63x- Car passenger injured in collision with pick-up truck in traffic accident

V43.64x- Car passenger injured in collision with van in traffic accident

V43.7- Person on outside of car injured in collision with car, pick-up truck or van in traffic accident

V43.71x- Person on outside of car injured in collision with sport utility vehicle in traffic accident

V43.72x- Person on outside of car injured in collision with other type car in traffic accident

V43.73x- Person on outside of car injured in collision with pick-up truck in traffic accident

V43.74x- Person on outside of car injured in collision with van in traffic accident

V43.9- Unspecified car occupant injured in collision with car, pick-up truck or van in traffic accident

V43.91x- Unspecified car occupant injured in collision with sport utility vehicle in traffic accident

V43.92x- Unspecified car occupant injured in collision with other type car in traffic accident

V43.93x- Unspecified car occupant injured in collision with pick-up truck in traffic accident

V43.94x- Unspecified car occupant injured in collision with van in traffic accident

V44- Car occupant injured in collision with heavy transport vehicle or bus

Excludes 1: car occupant injured in collision with military vehicle (V49.81)

The appropriate 7th character is to be added to each code from category V44:
- **A** Initial encounter
- **D** Subsequent encounter
- **S** Sequela

V44.0xx- Car driver injured in collision with heavy transport vehicle or bus in nontraffic accident

V44.1xx- Car passenger injured in collision with heavy transport vehicle or bus in nontraffic accident

V44.2xx- Person on outside of car injured in collision with heavy transport vehicle or bus in nontraffic accident

V44.3xx- Unspecified car occupant injured in collision with heavy transport vehicle or bus in nontraffic accident

V44.4xx- Person boarding or alighting a car injured in collision with heavy transport vehicle or bus

V44.5xx- Car driver injured in collision with heavy transport vehicle or bus in traffic accident

V44.6xx- Car passenger injured in collision with heavy transport vehicle or bus in traffic accident

V44.7xx- Person on outside of car injured in collision with heavy transport vehicle or bus in traffic accident

V44.9xx- Unspecified car occupant injured in collision with heavy transport vehicle or bus in traffic accident

V45- Car occupant injured in collision with railway train or railway vehicle

The appropriate 7th character is to be added to each code from category V45:
- **A** Initial encounter
- **D** Subsequent encounter
- **S** Sequela

V45.0xx- Car driver injured in collision with railway train or railway vehicle in nontraffic accident

V45.1xx- Car passenger injured in collision with railway train or railway vehicle in nontraffic accident

V45.2xx- Person on outside of car injured in collision with railway train or railway vehicle in nontraffic accident

V45.3xx- Unspecified car occupant injured in collision with railway train or railway vehicle in nontraffic accident

V45.4xx- Person boarding or alighting a car injured in collision with railway train or railway vehicle

V45.5xx- Car driver injured in collision with railway train or railway vehicle in traffic accident

V45.6xx- Car passenger injured in collision with railway train or railway vehicle in traffic accident

V45.7xx- Person on outside of car injured in collision with railway train or railway vehicle in traffic accident

V45.9xx- Unspecified car occupant injured in collision with railway train or railway vehicle in traffic accident

V46- Car occupant injured in collision with other nonmotor vehicle

Includes: Collision with animal-drawn vehicle, animal being ridden, streetcar

The appropriate 7th character is to be added to each code from category V46:
- **A** Initial encounter
- **D** Subsequent encounter
- **S** Sequela

V46.0xx- Car driver injured in collision with other nonmotor vehicle in nontraffic accident

V46.1xx- Car passenger injured in collision with other nonmotor vehicle in nontraffic accident

V46.2xx- Person on outside of car injured in collision with other nonmotor vehicle in nontraffic accident

V46.3xx- Unspecified car occupant injured in collision with other nonmotor vehicle in nontraffic accident

V46.4xx- Person boarding or alighting a car injured in collision with other nonmotor vehicle

V46.5xx- Car driver injured in collision with other nonmotor vehicle in traffic accident

V46.6xx- Car passenger injured in collision with other nonmotor vehicle in traffic accident

V46.7xx- Person on outside of car injured in collision with other nonmotor vehicle in traffic accident

V46.9xx- Unspecified car occupant injured in collision with other nonmotor vehicle in traffic accident

V47- Car occupant injured in collision with fixed or stationary object

The appropriate 7th character is to be added to each code from category V47:
- **A** Initial encounter
- **D** Subsequent encounter
- **S** Sequela

V47.0xx- Car driver injured in collision with fixed or stationary object in nontraffic accident

V47.1xx- Car passenger injured in collision with fixed or stationary object in nontraffic accident

V47.2xx- Person on outside of car injured in collision with fixed or stationary object in nontraffic accident

V47.3xx- Unspecified car occupant injured in collision with fixed or stationary object in nontraffic accident

V47.4xx- Person boarding or alighting a car injured in collision with fixed or stationary object

V47.5xx- Car driver injured in collision with fixed or stationary object in traffic accident

V47.6xx- Car passenger injured in collision with fixed or stationary object in traffic accident

V47.7xx- Person on outside of car injured in collision with fixed or stationary object in traffic accident

V47.9xx- Unspecified car occupant injured in collision with fixed or stationary object in traffic accident

V48- Car occupant injured in noncollision transport accident

Includes: Overturning car NOS
Overturning car without collision

The appropriate 7th character is to be added to each code from category V48:
- **A** Initial encounter
- **D** Subsequent encounter
- **S** Sequela

V48.0xx- Car driver injured in noncollision transport accident in nontraffic accident

V48.1xx- Car passenger injured in noncollision transport accident in nontraffic accident

V48.2xx- Person on outside of car injured in noncollision transport accident in nontraffic accident

V48.3xx- Unspecified car occupant injured in noncollision transport accident in nontraffic accident

V48.4xx- Person boarding or alighting a car injured in noncollision transport accident

V48.5xx- Car driver injured in noncollision transport accident in traffic accident

V43 – V48

V48.6xx- Car passenger injured in noncollision transport accident in traffic accident

V48.7xx- Person on outside of car injured in noncollision transport accident in traffic accident

V48.9xx- Unspecified car occupant injured in noncollision transport accident in traffic accident

V49- Car occupant injured in other and unspecified transport accidents

The appropriate 7th character is to be added to each code from category V49:

A   Initial encounter
D   Subsequent encounter
S   Sequela

V49.0- Driver injured in collision with other and unspecified motor vehicles in nontraffic accident

V49.00x- Driver injured in collision with unspecified motor vehicles in nontraffic accident

V49.09x- Driver injured in collision with other motor vehicles in nontraffic accident

V49.1- Passenger injured in collision with other and unspecified motor vehicles in nontraffic accident

V49.10x- Passenger injured in collision with unspecified motor vehicles in nontraffic accident

V49.19x- Passenger injured in collision with other motor vehicles in nontraffic accident

V49.2- Unspecified car occupant injured in collision with other and unspecified motor vehicles in nontraffic accident

V49.20x- Unspecified car occupant injured in collision with unspecified motor vehicles in nontraffic accident
          Car collision NOS, nontraffic

V49.29x- Unspecified car occupant injured in collision with other motor vehicles in nontraffic accident

V49.3xx- Car occupant (driver) (passenger) injured in unspecified nontraffic accident
          Car accident NOS, nontraffic
          Car occupant injured in nontraffic accident NOS

V49.4- Driver injured in collision with other and unspecified motor vehicles in traffic accident

V49.40x- Driver injured in collision with unspecified motor vehicles in traffic accident

V49.49x- Driver injured in collision with other motor vehicles in traffic accident

V49.5- Passenger injured in collision with other and unspecified motor vehicles in traffic accident

V49.50x- Passenger injured in collision with unspecified motor vehicles in traffic accident

V49.59x- Passenger injured in collision with other motor vehicles in traffic accident

V49.6- Unspecified car occupant injured in collision with other and unspecified motor vehicles in traffic accident

V49.60x- Unspecified car occupant injured in collision with unspecified motor vehicles in traffic accident
          Car collision NOS (traffic)

V49.69x- Unspecified car occupant injured in collision with other motor vehicles in traffic accident

V49.8- Car occupant (driver) (passenger) injured in other specified transport accidents

V49.81x- Car occupant (driver) (passenger) injured in transport accident with military vehicle

V49.88x- Car occupant (driver) (passenger) injured in other specified transport accidents

V49.9xx- Car occupant (driver) (passenger) injured in unspecified traffic accident
          Car accident NOS

Occupant of pick-up truck or van injured in transport accident (V50-V59)

Includes: A four or six wheel motor vehicle designed primarily for carrying passengers and property but weighing less than the local limit for classification as a heavy goods vehicle
            Minibus
            Minivan
            Sport utility vehicle (SUV)
            Truck
            Van

Excludes 1:   heavy transport vehicle (V60-V69)

V50- Occupant of pick-up truck or van injured in collision with pedestrian or animal

Excludes 1:   pick-up truck or van collision with animal-drawn vehicle or animal being ridden (V56.-)

The appropriate 7th character is to be added to each code from category V50:

A   Initial encounter
D   Subsequent encounter
S   Sequela

V50.0xx- Driver of pick-up truck or van injured in collision with pedestrian or animal in nontraffic accident

V50.1xx- Passenger in pick-up truck or van injured in collision with pedestrian or animal in nontraffic accident

V50.2xx- Person on outside of pick-up truck or van injured in collision with pedestrian or animal in nontraffic accident

V50.3xx- Unspecified occupant of pick-up truck or van injured in collision with pedestrian or animal in nontraffic accident

V50.4xx- Person boarding or alighting a pick-up truck or van injured in collision with pedestrian or animal

V50.5xx- Driver of pick-up truck or van injured in collision with pedestrian or animal in traffic accident

V50.6xx- Passenger in pick-up truck or van injured in collision with pedestrian or animal in traffic accident

V50.7xx- Person on outside of pick-up truck or van injured in collision with pedestrian or animal in traffic accident

V50.9xx- Unspecified occupant of pick-up truck or van injured in collision with pedestrian or animal in traffic accident

V51- Occupant of pick-up truck or van injured in collision with pedal cycle

The appropriate 7th character is to be added to each code from category V51:

A   Initial encounter
D   Subsequent encounter
S   Sequela

V51.0xx- Driver of pick-up truck or van injured in collision with pedal cycle in nontraffic accident

V51.1xx- Passenger in pick-up truck or van injured in collision with pedal cycle in nontraffic accident

V51.2xx- Person on outside of pick-up truck or van injured in collision with pedal cycle in nontraffic accident

V51.3xx- Unspecified occupant of pick-up truck or van injured in collision with pedal cycle in nontraffic accident

V51.4xx- Person boarding or alighting a pick-up truck or van injured in collision with pedal cycle

V51.5xx- Driver of pick-up truck or van injured in collision with pedal cycle in traffic accident

V51.6xx- Passenger in pick-up truck or van injured in collision with pedal cycle in traffic accident

V51.7xx- Person on outside of pick-up truck or van injured in collision with pedal cycle in traffic accident

V51.9xx- Unspecified occupant of pick-up truck or van injured in collision with pedal cycle in traffic accident

V52- **Occupant of pick-up truck or van injured in collision** with <u>two- or three-wheeled motor vehicle</u>

The appropriate 7th character is to be added to each code from category V52:
A **Initial** encounter
D **Subsequent** encounter
S **Sequela**

V52.0xx- Driver of pick-up truck or van injured in collision with two- or three-wheeled motor vehicle in nontraffic accident

V52.1xx- Passenger in pick-up truck or van injured in collision with two- or three-wheeled motor vehicle in nontraffic accident

V52.2xx- Person on outside of pick-up truck or van injured in collision with two- or three-wheeled motor vehicle in nontraffic accident

V52.3xx- Unspecified occupant of pick-up truck or van injured in collision with two- or three-wheeled motor vehicle in nontraffic accident

V52.4xx- Person boarding or alighting a pick-up truck or van injured in collision with two- or three-wheeled motor vehicle

V52.5xx- Driver of pick-up truck or van injured in collision with two- or three-wheeled motor vehicle in traffic accident

V52.6xx- Passenger in pick-up truck or van injured in collision with two- or three-wheeled motor vehicle in traffic accident

V52.7xx- Person on outside of pick-up truck or van injured in collision with two- or three-wheeled motor vehicle in traffic accident

V52.9xx- Unspecified occupant of pick-up truck or van injured in collision with two- or three-wheeled motor vehicle in traffic accident

V53- **Occupant of pick-up truck or van injured in collision** with <u>car, pick-up truck or van</u>

The appropriate 7th character is to be added to each code from category V53:
A **Initial** encounter
D **Subsequent** encounter
S **Sequela**

V53.0xx- Driver of pick-up truck or van injured in collision with car, pick-up truck or van in nontraffic accident

V53.1xx- Passenger in pick-up truck or van injured in collision with car, pick-up truck or van in nontraffic accident

V53.2xx- Person on outside of pick-up truck or van injured in collision with car, pick-up truck or van in nontraffic accident

V53.3xx- Unspecified occupant of pick-up truck or van injured in collision with car, pick-up truck or van in nontraffic accident

V53.4xx- Person boarding or alighting a pick-up truck or van injured in collision with car, pick-up truck or van

V53.5xx- Driver of pick-up truck or van injured in collision with car, pick-up truck or van in traffic accident

V53.6xx- Passenger in pick-up truck or van injured in collision with car, pick-up truck or van in traffic accident

V53.7xx- Person on outside of pick-up truck or van injured in collision with car, pick-up truck or van in traffic accident

V53.9xx- Unspecified occupant of pick-up truck or van injured in collision with car, pick-up truck or van in traffic accident

V54- **Occupant of pick-up truck or van injured in collision** with <u>heavy transport vehicle or bus</u>

Excludes 1:   *occupant of pick-up truck or van injured in collision with military vehicle (V59.81)*

The appropriate 7th character is to be added to each code from category V54:
A **Initial** encounter
D **Subsequent** encounter
S **Sequela**

V54.0xx- Driver of pick-up truck or van injured in collision with heavy transport vehicle or bus in nontraffic accident

V54.1xx- Passenger in pick-up truck or van injured in collision with heavy transport vehicle or bus in nontraffic accident

V54.2xx- Person on outside of pick-up truck or van injured in collision with heavy transport vehicle or bus in nontraffic accident

V54.3xx- Unspecified occupant of pick-up truck or van injured in collision with heavy transport vehicle or bus in nontraffic accident

V54.4xx- Person boarding or alighting a pick-up truck or van injured in collision with heavy transport vehicle or bus

V54.5xx- Driver of pick-up truck or van injured in collision with heavy transport vehicle or bus in traffic accident

V54.6xx- Passenger in pick-up truck or van injured in collision with heavy transport vehicle or bus in traffic accident

V54.7xx- Person on outside of pick-up truck or van injured in collision with heavy transport vehicle or bus in traffic accident

V54.9xx- Unspecified occupant of pick-up truck or van injured in collision with heavy transport vehicle or bus in traffic accident

V55- **Occupant of pick-up truck or van injured in collision** with <u>railway train or railway vehicle</u>

The appropriate 7th character is to be added to each code from category V55:
A **Initial** encounter
D **Subsequent** encounter
S **Sequela**

V55.0xx- Driver of pick-up truck or van injured in collision with railway train or railway vehicle in nontraffic accident

V55.1xx- Passenger in pick-up truck or van injured in collision with railway train or railway vehicle in nontraffic accident

V55.2xx- Person on outside of pick-up truck or van injured in collision with railway train or railway vehicle in nontraffic accident

V55.3xx- Unspecified occupant of pick-up truck or van injured in collision with railway train or railway vehicle in nontraffic accident

V55.4xx- Person boarding or alighting a pick-up truck or van injured in collision with railway train or railway vehicle

V55.5xx- Driver of pick-up truck or van injured in collision with railway train or railway vehicle in traffic accident

V55.6xx- Passenger in pick-up truck or van injured in collision with railway train or railway vehicle in traffic accident

V55.7xx- Person on outside of pick-up truck or van injured in collision with railway train or railway vehicle in traffic accident

V55.9xx- Unspecified occupant of pick-up truck or van injured in collision with railway train or railway vehicle in traffic accident

V56- **Occupant of pick-up truck or van injured in collision** with <u>other nonmotor vehicle</u>

Includes: Collision with animal-drawn vehicle, animal being ridden, streetcar

The appropriate 7th character is to be added to each code from category V56:
A **Initial** encounter
D **Subsequent** encounter
S **Sequela**

V56.0xx- Driver of pick-up truck or van injured in collision with other nonmotor vehicle in nontraffic accident

V56.1xx- Passenger in pick-up truck or van injured in collision with other nonmotor vehicle in nontraffic accident

V56.2xx- Person on outside of pick-up truck or van injured in collision with other nonmotor vehicle in nontraffic accident

V56.3xx- Unspecified occupant of pick-up truck or van injured in collision with other nonmotor vehicle in nontraffic accident

V56.4xx- Person boarding or alighting a pick-up truck or van injured in collision with other nonmotor vehicle

V56.5xx- Driver of pick-up truck or van injured in collision with other nonmotor vehicle in traffic accident

V56.6xx- Passenger in pick-up truck or van injured in collision with other nonmotor vehicle in traffic accident

V56.7xx- Person on outside of pick-up truck or van injured in collision with other nonmotor vehicle in traffic accident

V52 - V56

V56.9xx-   Unspecified occupant of pick-up truck or van injured in collision with other nonmotor vehicle in traffic accident

V57-   Occupant of pick-up truck or van injured in collision with fixed or stationary object

The appropriate 7th character is to be added to each code from category V57:

   A   Initial encounter
   D   Subsequent encounter
   S   Sequela

V57.0xx-   Driver of pick-up truck or van injured in collision with fixed or stationary object in nontraffic accident

V57.1xx-   Passenger in pick-up truck or van injured in collision with fixed or stationary object in nontraffic accident

V57.2xx-   Person on outside of pick-up truck or van injured in collision with fixed or stationary object in nontraffic accident

V57.3xx-   Unspecified occupant of pick-up truck or van injured in collision with fixed or stationary object in nontraffic accident

V57.4xx-   Person boarding or alighting a pick-up truck or van injured in collision with fixed or stationary object

V57.5xx-   Driver of pick-up truck or van injured in collision with fixed or stationary object in traffic accident

V57.6xx-   Passenger in pick-up truck or van injured in collision with fixed or stationary object in traffic accident

V57.7xx-   Person on outside of pick-up truck or van injured in collision with fixed or stationary object in traffic accident

V57.9xx-   Unspecified occupant of pick-up truck or van injured in collision with fixed or stationary object in traffic accident

V58-   Occupant of pick-up truck or van injured in noncollision transport accident

Includes: Overturning pick-up truck or van NOS
          Overturning pick-up truck or van without collision

The appropriate 7th character is to be added to each code from category V58:

   A   Initial encounter
   D   Subsequent encounter
   S   Sequela

V58.0xx-   Driver of pick-up truck or van injured in noncollision transport accident in nontraffic accident

V58.1xx-   Passenger in pick-up truck or van injured in noncollision transport accident in nontraffic accident

V58.2xx-   Person on outside of pick-up truck or van injured in noncollision transport accident in nontraffic accident

V58.3xx-   Unspecified occupant of pick-up truck or van injured in noncollision transport accident in nontraffic accident

V58.4xx-   Person boarding or alighting a pick-up truck or van injured in noncollision transport accident

V58.5xx-   Driver of pick-up truck or van injured in noncollision transport accident in traffic accident

V58.6xx-   Passenger in pick-up truck or van injured in noncollision transport accident in traffic accident

V58.7xx-   Person on outside of pick-up truck or van injured in noncollision transport accident in traffic accident

V58.9xx-   Unspecified occupant of pick-up truck or van injured in noncollision transport accident in traffic accident

V59-   Occupant of pick-up truck or van injured in other and unspecified transport accidents

The appropriate 7th character is to be added to each code from category V59:

   A   Initial encounter
   D   Subsequent encounter
   S   Sequela

V59.0-   Driver of pick-up truck or van injured in collision with other and unspecified motor vehicles in nontraffic accident

V59.00x-   Driver of pick-up truck or van injured in collision with unspecified motor vehicles in nontraffic accident

V59.09x-   Driver of pick-up truck or van injured in collision with other motor vehicles in nontraffic accident

V59.1-   Passenger in pick-up truck or van injured in collision with other and unspecified motor vehicles in nontraffic accident

V59.10x-   Passenger in pick-up truck or van injured in collision with unspecified motor vehicles in nontraffic accident

V59.19x-   Passenger in pick-up truck or van injured in collision with other motor vehicles in nontraffic accident

V59.2-   Unspecified occupant of pick-up truck or van injured in collision with other and unspecified motor vehicles in nontraffic accident

V59.20x-   Unspecified occupant of pick-up truck or van injured in collision with unspecified motor vehicles in nontraffic accident

       Collision NOS involving pick-up truck or van, nontraffic

V59.29x-   Unspecified occupant of pick-up truck or van injured in collision with other motor vehicles in nontraffic accident

V59.3xx-   Occupant (driver) (passenger) of pick-up truck or van injured in unspecified nontraffic accident

       Accident NOS involving pick-up truck or van, nontraffic
       Occupant of pick-up truck or van injured in nontraffic accident NOS

V59.4-   Driver of pick-up truck or van injured in collision with other and unspecified motor vehicles in traffic accident

V59.40x-   Driver of pick-up truck or van injured in collision with unspecified motor vehicles in traffic accident

V59.49x-   Driver of pick-up truck or van injured in collision with other motor vehicles in traffic accident

V59.5-   Passenger in pick-up truck or van injured in collision with other and unspecified motor vehicles in traffic accident

V59.50x-   Passenger in pick-up truck or van injured in collision with unspecified motor vehicles in traffic accident

V59.59x-   Passenger in pick-up truck or van injured in collision with other motor vehicles in traffic accident

V59.6-   Unspecified occupant of pick-up truck or van injured in collision with other and unspecified motor vehicles in traffic accident

V59.60x-   Unspecified occupant of pick-up truck or van injured in collision with unspecified motor vehicles in traffic accident

       Collision NOS involving pick-up truck or van (traffic)

V59.69x-   Unspecified occupant of pick-up truck or van injured in collision with other motor vehicles in traffic accident

V59.8-   Occupant (driver) (passenger) of pick-up truck or van injured in other specified transport accidents

V59.81x-   Occupant (driver) (passenger) of pick-up truck or van injured in transport accident with military vehicle

V59.88x-   Occupant (driver) (passenger) of pick-up truck or van injured in other specified transport accidents

V59.9xx-   Occupant (driver) (passenger) of pick-up truck or van injured in unspecified traffic accident

       Accident NOS involving pick-up truck or van

Occupant of heavy transport vehicle injured in transport accident (V60-V69)

Includes: 18 wheeler
 Armored car
 Panel truck
Excludes 1: *bus*
 motorcoach

V60- **Occupant of heavy transport vehicle injured in collision** with **pedestrian or animal**
Excludes 1: *heavy transport vehicle collision with animal-drawn vehicle or animal being ridden (V66.-)*

The appropriate 7th character is to be added to each code from category V60:
A **Initial** encounter
D **Subsequent** encounter
S **Sequela**

V60.0xx- Driver of heavy transport vehicle injured in collision with pedestrian or animal in nontraffic accident
V60.1xx- Passenger in heavy transport vehicle injured in collision with pedestrian or animal in nontraffic accident
V60.2xx- Person on outside of heavy transport vehicle injured in collision with pedestrian or animal in nontraffic accident
V60.3xx- Unspecified occupant of heavy transport vehicle injured in collision with pedestrian or animal in nontraffic accident
V60.4xx- Person boarding or alighting a heavy transport vehicle injured in collision with pedestrian or animal
V60.5xx- Driver of heavy transport vehicle injured in collision with pedestrian or animal in traffic accident
V60.6xx- Passenger in heavy transport vehicle injured in collision with pedestrian or animal in traffic accident
V60.7xx- Person on outside of heavy transport vehicle injured in collision with pedestrian or animal in traffic accident
V60.9xx- Unspecified occupant of heavy transport vehicle injured in collision with pedestrian or animal in traffic accident

V61- **Occupant of heavy transport vehicle injured in collision** with **pedal cycle**

The appropriate 7th character is to be added to each code from category V61:
A **Initial** encounter
D **Subsequent** encounter
S **Sequela**

V61.0xx- Driver of heavy transport vehicle injured in collision with pedal cycle in nontraffic accident
V61.1xx- Passenger in heavy transport vehicle injured in collision with pedal cycle in nontraffic accident
V61.2xx- Person on outside of heavy transport vehicle injured in collision with pedal cycle in nontraffic accident
V61.3xx- Unspecified occupant of heavy transport vehicle injured in collision with pedal cycle in nontraffic accident
V61.4xx- Person boarding or alighting a heavy transport vehicle injured in collision with pedal cycle while boarding or alighting
V61.5xx- Driver of heavy transport vehicle injured in collision with pedal cycle in traffic accident
V61.6xx- Passenger in heavy transport vehicle injured in collision with pedal cycle in traffic accident
V61.7xx- Person on outside of heavy transport vehicle injured in collision with pedal cycle in traffic accident
V61.9xx- Unspecified occupant of heavy transport vehicle injured in collision with pedal cycle in traffic accident

V62- **Occupant of heavy transport vehicle injured in collision** with **two- or three-wheeled motor vehicle**

The appropriate 7th character is to be added to each code from category V62:
A **Initial** encounter
D **Subsequent** encounter
S **Sequela**

V62.0xx- Driver of heavy transport vehicle injured in collision with two- or three-wheeled motor vehicle in nontraffic accident
V62.1xx- Passenger in heavy transport vehicle injured in collision with two- or three-wheeled motor vehicle in nontraffic accident
V62.2xx- Person on outside of heavy transport vehicle injured in collision with two- or three-wheeled motor vehicle in nontraffic accident
V62.3xx- Unspecified occupant of heavy transport vehicle injured in collision with two- or three-wheeled motor vehicle in nontraffic accident
V62.4xx- Person boarding or alighting a heavy transport vehicle injured in collision with two- or three-wheeled motor vehicle
V62.5xx- Driver of heavy transport vehicle injured in collision with two- or three-wheeled motor vehicle in traffic accident
V62.6xx- Passenger in heavy transport vehicle injured in collision with two- or three-wheeled motor vehicle in traffic accident
V62.7xx- Person on outside of heavy transport vehicle injured in collision with two- or three-wheeled motor vehicle in traffic accident
V62.9xx- Unspecified occupant of heavy transport vehicle injured in collision with two- or three-wheeled motor vehicle in traffic accident

V63- **Occupant of heavy transport vehicle injured in collision** with **car, pick-up truck or van**

The appropriate 7th character is to be added to each code from category V63:
A **Initial** encounter
D **Subsequent** encounter
S **Sequela**

V63.0xx- Driver of heavy transport vehicle injured in collision with car, pick-up truck or van in nontraffic accident
V63.1xx- Passenger in heavy transport vehicle injured in collision with car, pick-up truck or van in nontraffic accident
V63.2xx- Person on outside of heavy transport vehicle injured in collision with car, pick-up truck or van in nontraffic accident
V63.3xx- Unspecified occupant of heavy transport vehicle injured in collision with car, pick-up truck or van in nontraffic accident
V63.4xx- Person boarding or alighting a heavy transport vehicle injured in collision with car, pick-up truck or van
V63.5xx- Driver of heavy transport vehicle injured in collision with car, pick-up truck or van in traffic accident
V63.6xx- Passenger in heavy transport vehicle injured in collision with car, pick-up truck or van in traffic accident
V63.7xx- Person on outside of heavy transport vehicle injured in collision with car, pick-up truck or van in traffic accident
V63.9xx- Unspecified occupant of heavy transport vehicle injured in collision with car, pick-up truck or van in traffic accident

V64- **Occupant of heavy transport vehicle injured in collision** with **heavy transport vehicle or bus**
Excludes 1: *occupant of heavy transport vehicle injured in collision with military vehicle (V69.81)*

The appropriate 7th character is to be added to each code from category V64:
A **Initial** encounter
D **Subsequent** encounter
S **Sequela**

V64.0xx- Driver of heavy transport vehicle injured in collision with heavy transport vehicle or bus in nontraffic accident
V64.1xx- Passenger in heavy transport vehicle injured in collision with heavy transport vehicle or bus in nontraffic accident
V64.2xx- Person on outside of heavy transport vehicle injured in collision with heavy transport vehicle or bus in nontraffic accident
V64.3xx- Unspecified occupant of heavy transport vehicle injured in collision with heavy transport vehicle or bus in nontraffic accident
V64.4xx- Person boarding or alighting a heavy transport vehicle injured in collision with heavy transport vehicle or bus while boarding or alighting

V60 - V64

V64.5xx- Driver of heavy transport vehicle injured in collision with heavy transport vehicle or bus in traffic accident

V64.6xx- Passenger in heavy transport vehicle injured in collision with heavy transport vehicle or bus in traffic accident

V64.7xx- Person on outside of heavy transport vehicle injured in collision with heavy transport vehicle or bus in traffic accident

V64.9xx- Unspecified occupant of heavy transport vehicle injured in collision with heavy transport vehicle or bus in traffic accident

V65- Occupant of heavy transport vehicle injured in collision with railway train or railway vehicle

The appropriate 7th character is to be added to each code from category V65:
A Initial encounter
D Subsequent encounter
S Sequela

V65.0xx- Driver of heavy transport vehicle injured in collision with railway train or railway vehicle in nontraffic accident

V65.1xx- Passenger in heavy transport vehicle injured in collision with railway train or railway vehicle in nontraffic accident

V65.2xx- Person on outside of heavy transport vehicle injured in collision with railway train or railway vehicle in nontraffic accident

V65.3xx- Unspecified occupant of heavy transport vehicle injured in collision with railway train or railway vehicle in nontraffic accident

V65.4xx- Person boarding or alighting a heavy transport vehicle injured in collision with railway train or railway vehicle

V65.5xx- Driver of heavy transport vehicle injured in collision with railway train or railway vehicle in traffic accident

V65.6xx- Passenger in heavy transport vehicle injured in collision with railway train or railway vehicle in traffic accident

V65.7xx- Person on outside of heavy transport vehicle injured in collision with railway train or railway vehicle in traffic accident

V65.9xx- Unspecified occupant of heavy transport vehicle injured in collision with railway train or railway vehicle in traffic accident

V66- Occupant of heavy transport vehicle injured in collision with other nonmotor vehicle

Includes: Collision with animal-drawn vehicle, animal being ridden, streetcar

The appropriate 7th character is to be added to each code from category V66:
A Initial encounter
D Subsequent encounter
S Sequela

V66.0xx- Driver of heavy transport vehicle injured in collision with other nonmotor vehicle in nontraffic accident

V66.1xx- Passenger in heavy transport vehicle injured in collision with other nonmotor vehicle in nontraffic accident

V66.2xx- Person on outside of heavy transport vehicle injured in collision with other nonmotor vehicle in nontraffic accident

V66.3xx- Unspecified occupant of heavy transport vehicle injured in collision with other nonmotor vehicle in nontraffic accident

V66.4xx- Person boarding or alighting a heavy transport vehicle injured in collision with other nonmotor vehicle

V66.5xx- Driver of heavy transport vehicle injured in collision with other nonmotor vehicle in traffic accident

V66.6xx- Passenger in heavy transport vehicle injured in collision with other nonmotor vehicle in traffic accident

V66.7xx- Person on outside of heavy transport vehicle injured in collision with other nonmotor vehicle in traffic accident

V66.9xx- Unspecified occupant of heavy transport vehicle injured in collision with other nonmotor vehicle in traffic accident

V67- Occupant of heavy transport vehicle injured in collision with fixed or stationary object

The appropriate 7th character is to be added to each code from category V67:
A Initial encounter
D Subsequent encounter
S Sequela

V67.0xx- Driver of heavy transport vehicle injured in collision with fixed or stationary object in nontraffic accident

V67.1xx- Passenger in heavy transport vehicle injured in collision with fixed or stationary object in nontraffic accident

V67.2xx- Person on outside of heavy transport vehicle injured in collision with fixed or stationary object in nontraffic accident

V67.3xx- Unspecified occupant of heavy transport vehicle injured in collision with fixed or stationary object in nontraffic accident

V67.4xx- Person boarding or alighting a heavy transport vehicle injured in collision with fixed or stationary object

V67.5xx- Driver of heavy transport vehicle injured in collision with fixed or stationary object in traffic accident

V67.6xx- Passenger in heavy transport vehicle injured in collision with fixed or stationary object in traffic accident

V67.7xx- Person on outside of heavy transport vehicle injured in collision with fixed or stationary object in traffic accident

V67.9xx- Unspecified occupant of heavy transport vehicle injured in collision with fixed or stationary object in traffic accident

V68- Occupant of heavy transport vehicle injured in noncollision transport accident

Includes: Overturning heavy transport vehicle NOS
           Overturning heavy transport vehicle without collision

The appropriate 7th character is to be added to each code from category V68:
A Initial encounter
D Subsequent encounter
S Sequela

V68.0xx- Driver of heavy transport vehicle injured in noncollision transport accident in nontraffic accident

V68.1xx- Passenger in heavy transport vehicle injured in noncollision transport accident in nontraffic accident

V68.2xx- Person on outside of heavy transport vehicle injured in noncollision transport accident in nontraffic accident

V68.3xx- Unspecified occupant of heavy transport vehicle injured in noncollision transport accident in nontraffic accident

V68.4xx- Person boarding or alighting a heavy transport vehicle injured in noncollision transport accident

V68.5xx- Driver of heavy transport vehicle injured in noncollision transport accident in traffic accident

V68.6xx- Passenger in heavy transport vehicle injured in noncollision transport accident in traffic accident

V68.7xx- Person on outside of heavy transport vehicle injured in noncollision transport accident in traffic accident

V68.9xx- Unspecified occupant of heavy transport vehicle injured in noncollision transport accident in traffic accident

V69- Occupant of heavy transport vehicle injured in other and unspecified transport accidents

The appropriate 7th character is to be added to each code from category V69:
A Initial encounter
D Subsequent encounter
S Sequela

V69.0- Driver of heavy transport vehicle injured in collision with other and unspecified motor vehicles in nontraffic accident

V69.00x- Driver of heavy transport vehicle injured in collision with unspecified motor vehicles in nontraffic accident

V69.09x- Driver of heavy transport vehicle injured in collision with other motor vehicles in nontraffic accident

V69.1- Passenger in heavy transport vehicle injured in collision with other and unspecified motor vehicles in nontraffic accident

V69.10x- Passenger in heavy transport vehicle injured in collision with unspecified motor vehicles in nontraffic accident

V69.19x- Passenger in heavy transport vehicle injured in collision with other motor vehicles in nontraffic accident

V69.2- Unspecified occupant of heavy transport vehicle injured in collision with other and unspecified motor vehicles in nontraffic accident

V69.20x- Unspecified occupant of heavy transport vehicle injured in collision with unspecified motor vehicles in nontraffic accident

  Collision NOS involving heavy transport vehicle, nontraffic

V69.29x- Unspecified occupant of heavy transport vehicle injured in collision with other motor vehicles in nontraffic accident

V69.3xx- Occupant (driver) (passenger) of heavy transport vehicle injured in unspecified nontraffic accident

  Accident NOS involving heavy transport vehicle, nontraffic
  Occupant of heavy transport vehicle injured in nontraffic accident NOS

V69.4- Driver of heavy transport vehicle injured in collision with other and unspecified motor vehicles intraffic accident

V69.40x- Driver of heavy transport vehicle injured in collision with unspecified motor vehicles in traffic accident

V69.49x- Driver of heavy transport vehicle injured in collision with other motor vehicles in traffic accident

V69.5- Passenger in heavy transport vehicle injured in collision with other and unspecified motor vehicles in traffic accident

V69.50x- Passenger in heavy transport vehicle injured in collision with unspecified motor vehicles in traffic accident

V69.59x- Passenger in heavy transport vehicle injured in collision with other motor vehicles in traffic accident

V69.6- Unspecified occupant of heavy transport vehicle injured in collision with other and unspecified motor vehicles in traffic accident

V69.60x- Unspecified occupant of heavy transport vehicle injured in collision with unspecified motor vehicles in traffic accident

  Collision NOS involving heavy transport vehicle (traffic)

V69.69x- Unspecified occupant of heavy transport vehicle injured in collision with other motor vehicles in traffic accident

V69.8- Occupant (driver) (passenger) of heavy transport vehicle injured in other specified transport accidents

V69.81x- Occupant (driver) (passenger) of heavy transport vehicle injured in transport accidents with military vehicle

V69.88x- Occupant (driver) (passenger) of heavy transport vehicle injured in other specified transport accidents

V69.9xx- Occupant (driver) (passenger) of heavy transport vehicle injured in unspecified traffic accident

  Accident NOS involving heavy transport vehicle

Bus occupant injured in transport accident (V70-V79)

Includes: Motorcoach
Excludes 1:   minibus (V50-V59)

V70- Bus occupant injured in collision with pedestrian or animal
Excludes 1:   bus collision with animal-drawn vehicle or animal being ridden (V76.-)

The appropriate 7th character is to be added to each code from category V70:
 A   Initial encounter
 D   Subsequent encounter
 S   Sequela

V70.0xx- Driver of bus injured in collision with pedestrian or animal in nontraffic accident

V70.1xx- Passenger on bus injured in collision with pedestrian or animal in nontraffic accident

V70.2xx- Person on outside of bus injured in collision with pedestrian or animal in nontraffic accident

V70.3xx- Unspecified occupant of bus injured in collision with pedestrian or animal in nontraffic accident

V70.4xx- Person boarding or alighting from bus injured in collision with pedestrian or animal

V70.5xx- Driver of bus injured in collision with pedestrian or animal in traffic accident

V70.6xx- Passenger on bus injured in collision with pedestrian or animal in traffic accident

V70.7xx- Person on outside of bus injured in collision with pedestrian or animal in traffic accident

V70.9xx- Unspecified occupant of bus injured in collision with pedestrian or animal in traffic accident

V71- Bus occupant injured in collision with pedal cycle
The appropriate 7th character is to be added to each code from category V71:
 A   Initial encounter
 D   Subsequent encounter
 S   Sequela

V71.0xx- Driver of bus injured in collision with pedal cycle in nontraffic accident

V71.1xx- Passenger on bus injured in collision with pedal cycle in nontraffic accident

V71.2xx- Person on outside of bus injured in collision with pedal cycle in nontraffic accident

V71.3xx- Unspecified occupant of bus injured in collision with pedal cycle in nontraffic accident

V71.4xx- Person boarding or alighting from bus injured in collision with pedal cycle

V71.5xx- Driver of bus injured in collision with pedal cycle in traffic accident

V71.6xx- Passenger on bus injured in collision with pedal cycle in traffic accident

V71.7xx- Person on outside of bus injured in collision with pedal cycle in traffic accident

V71.9xx- Unspecified occupant of bus injured in collision with pedal cycle in traffic accident

V72- Bus occupant injured in collision with two- or three-wheeled motor vehicle
The appropriate 7th character is to be added to each code from category V72:
 A   Initial encounter
 D   Subsequent encounter
 S   Sequela

V72.0xx- Driver of bus injured in collision with two- or three-wheeled motor vehicle in nontraffic accident

V72.1xx- Passenger on bus injured in collision with two- or three-wheeled motor vehicle in nontraffic accident

V72.2xx- Person on outside of bus injured in collision with two- or three-wheeled motor vehicle in nontraffic accident

V72.3xx- Unspecified occupant of bus injured in collision with two- or three-wheeled motor vehicle in nontraffic accident

V72.4xx- Person boarding or alighting from bus injured in collision with two- or three-wheeled motor vehicle

V72.5xx- Driver of bus injured in collision with two- or three-wheeled motor vehicle in traffic accident

V72.6xx- Passenger on bus injured in collision with two- or three-wheeled motor vehicle in traffic accident

V72.7xx- Person on outside of bus injured in collision with two- or three-wheeled motor vehicle in traffic accident

V72.9xx- Unspecified occupant of bus injured in collision with two- or three-wheeled motor vehicle in traffic accident

V73- Bus occupant injured in collision with car, pick-up truck or van

The appropriate 7th character is to be added to each code from category V73:
- A   Initial encounter
- D   Subsequent encounter
- S   Sequela

V73.0xx- Driver of bus injured in collision with car, pick-up truck or van in nontraffic accident

V73.1xx- Passenger on bus injured in collision with car, pick-up truck or van in nontraffic accident

V73.2xx- Person on outside of bus injured in collision with car, pick-up truck or van in nontraffic accident

V73.3xx- Unspecified occupant of bus injured in collision with car, pick-up truck or van in nontraffic accident

V73.4xx- Person boarding or alighting from bus injured in collision with car, pick-up truck or van

V73.5xx- Driver of bus injured in collision with car, pick-up truck or van in traffic accident

V73.6xx- Passenger on bus injured in collision with car, pick-up truck or van in traffic accident

V73.7xx- Person on outside of bus injured in collision with car, pick-up truck or van in traffic accident

V73.9xx- Unspecified occupant of bus injured in collision with car, pick-up truck or van in traffic accident

V74- Bus occupant injured in collision with heavy transport vehicle or bus

Excludes 1:   bus occupant injured in collision with military vehicle (V79.81)

The appropriate 7th character is to be added to each code from category V74:
- A   Initial encounter
- D   Subsequent encounter
- S   Sequela

V74.0xx- Driver of bus injured in collision with heavy transport vehicle or bus in nontraffic accident

V74.1xx- Passenger on bus injured in collision with heavy transport vehicle or bus in nontraffic accident

V74.2xx- Person on outside of bus injured in collision with heavy transport vehicle or bus in nontraffic accident

V74.3xx- Unspecified occupant of bus injured in collision with heavy transport vehicle or bus in nontraffic accident

V74.4xx- Person boarding or alighting from bus injured in collision with heavy transport vehicle or bus

V74.5xx- Driver of bus injured in collision with heavy transport vehicle or bus in traffic accident

V74.6xx- Passenger on bus injured in collision with heavy transport vehicle or bus in traffic accident

V74.7xx- Person on outside of bus injured in collision with heavy transport vehicle or bus in traffic accident

V74.9xx- Unspecified occupant of bus injured in collision with heavy transport vehicle or bus in traffic accident

V75- Bus occupant injured in collision with railway train or railway vehicle

The appropriate 7th character is to be added to each code from category V75:
- A   Initial encounter
- D   Subsequent encounter
- S   Sequela

V75.0xx- Driver of bus injured in collision with railway train or railway vehicle in nontraffic accident

V75.1xx- Passenger on bus injured in collision with railway train or railway vehicle in nontraffic accident

V75.2xx- Person on outside of bus injured in collision with railway train or railway vehicle in nontraffic accident

V75.3xx- Unspecified occupant of bus injured in collision with railway train or railway vehicle in nontraffic accident

V75.4xx- Person boarding or alighting from bus injured in collision with railway train or railway vehicle

V75.5xx- Driver of bus injured in collision with railway train or railway vehicle in traffic accident

V75.6xx- Passenger on bus injured in collision with railway train or railway vehicle in traffic accident

V75.7xx- Person on outside of bus injured in collision with railway train or railway vehicle in traffic accident

V75.9xx- Unspecified occupant of bus injured in collision with railway train or railway vehicle in traffic accident

V76- Bus occupant injured in collision with other nonmotor vehicle

Includes: Collision with animal-drawn vehicle, animal being ridden, streetcar

The appropriate 7th character is to be added to each code from category V76:
- A   Initial encounter
- D   Subsequent encounter
- S   Sequela

V76.0xx- Driver of bus injured in collision with other nonmotor vehicle in nontraffic accident

V76.1xx- Passenger on bus injured in collision with other nonmotor vehicle in nontraffic accident

V76.2xx- Person on outside of bus injured in collision with other nonmotor vehicle in nontraffic accident

V76.3xx- Unspecified occupant of bus injured in collision with other nonmotor vehicle in nontraffic accident

V76.4xx- Person boarding or alighting from bus injured in collision with other nonmotor vehicle

V76.5xx- Driver of bus injured in collision with other nonmotor vehicle in traffic accident

V76.6xx- Passenger on bus injured in collision with other nonmotor vehicle in traffic accident

V76.7xx- Person on outside of bus injured in collision with other nonmotor vehicle in traffic accident

V76.9xx- Unspecified occupant of bus injured in collision with other nonmotor vehicle in traffic accident

V77- Bus occupant injured in collision with fixed or stationary object

The appropriate 7th character is to be added to each code from category V77:
- A   Initial encounter
- D   Subsequent encounter
- S   Sequela

V77.0xx- Driver of bus injured in collision with fixed or stationary object in nontraffic accident

V77.1xx- Passenger on bus injured in collision with fixed or stationary object in nontraffic accident

V77.2xx- Person on outside of bus injured in collision with fixed or stationary object in nontraffic accident

V77.3xx- Unspecified occupant of bus injured in collision with fixed or stationary object in nontraffic accident

V77.4xx- Person boarding or alighting from bus injured in collision with fixed or stationary object

V77.5xx- Driver of bus injured in collision with fixed or stationary object in traffic accident

V77.6xx- Passenger on bus injured in collision with fixed or stationary object in traffic accident

V77.7xx- Person on outside of bus injured in collision with fixed or stationary object in traffic accident

V77.9xx- Unspecified occupant of bus injured in collision with fixed or stationary object in traffic accident

V78- **Bus occupant injured** in **noncollision** **transport accident**
Includes: Overturning bus NOS
            Overturning bus without collision

The appropriate 7th character is to be added to each code from category
V78:
A   **Initial** encounter
D   **Subsequent** encounter
S   **Sequela**

V78.0xx- Driver of bus injured in noncollision transport accident in nontraffic accident

V78.1xx- Passenger on bus injured in noncollision transport accident in nontraffic accident

V78.2xx- Person on outside of bus injured in noncollision transport accident in nontraffic accident

V78.3xx- Unspecified occupant of bus injured in noncollision transport accident in nontraffic accident

V78.4xx- Person boarding or alighting from bus injured in noncollision transport accident

V78.5xx- Driver of bus injured in noncollision transport accident in traffic accident

V78.6xx- Passenger on bus injured in noncollision transport accident in traffic accident

V78.7xx- Person on outside of bus injured in noncollision transport accident in traffic accident

V78.9xx- Unspecified occupant of bus injured in noncollision transport accident in traffic accident

V79- **Bus occupant injured** in **other and unspecified transport accidents**

The appropriate 7th character is to be added to each code from category
V79:
A   **Initial** encounter
D   **Subsequent** encounter
S   **Sequela**

V79.0- Driver of bus injured in collision with other and unspecified motor vehicles in nontraffic accident

V79.00x- Driver of bus injured in collision with unspecified motor vehicles in nontraffic accident

V79.09x- Driver of bus injured in collision with other motor vehicles in nontraffic accident

V79.1- Passenger on bus injured in collision with other and unspecified motor vehicles in nontraffic accident

V79.10x- Passenger on bus injured in collision with unspecified motor vehicles in nontraffic accident

V79.19x- Passenger on bus injured in collision with other motor vehicles in nontraffic accident

V79.2- Unspecified bus occupant injured in collision with other and unspecified motor vehicles in nontraffic accident

V79.20x- Unspecified bus occupant injured in collision with unspecified motor vehicles in nontraffic accident
            Bus collision NOS, nontraffic

V79.29x- Unspecified bus occupant injured in collision with other motor vehicles in nontraffic accident

V79.3xx- Bus occupant (driver) (passenger) injured in unspecified nontraffic accident
            Bus accident NOS, nontraffic
            Bus occupant injured in nontraffic accident NOS

V79.4- Driver of bus injured in collision with other and unspecified motor vehicles in traffic accident

V79.40x- Driver of bus injured in collision with unspecified motor vehicles in traffic accident

V79.49x- Driver of bus injured in collision with other motor vehicles in traffic accident

V79.5- Passenger on bus injured in collision with other and unspecified motor vehicles in traffic accident

V79.50x- Passenger on bus injured in collision with unspecified motor vehicles in traffic accident

V79.59x- Passenger on bus injured in collision with other motor vehicles in traffic accident

V79.6- Unspecified bus occupant injured in collision with other and unspecified motor vehicles in traffic accident

V79.60x- Unspecified bus occupant injured in collision with unspecified motor vehicles in traffic accident
            Bus collision NOS (traffic)

V79.69x- Unspecified bus occupant injured in collision with other motor vehicles in traffic accident

V79.8- Bus occupant (driver) (passenger) injured in other specified transport accidents

V79.81x- Bus occupant (driver) (passenger) injured in transport accidents with military vehicle

V79.88x- Bus occupant (driver) (passenger) injured in other specified transport accidents

V79.9xx- Bus occupant (driver) (passenger) injured in unspecified traffic accident
            Bus accident NOS

Other land transport accidents (V80-V89)

V80- **Animal-rider or occupant of animal-drawn vehicle injured in transport accident**

The appropriate 7th character is to be added to each code from category
V80:
A   **Initial** encounter
D   **Subsequent** encounter
S   **Sequela**

V80.0- Animal-rider or occupant of animal drawn vehicle injured **by fall from or being thrown from animal or animal-drawn vehicle in noncollision accident**

V80.01- Animal-rider injured by fall from or being thrown from animal in noncollision accident

V80.010- Animal-rider injured by fall from or being thrown from horse in noncollision accident

V80.018- Animal-rider injured by fall from or being thrown from other animal in noncollision accident

V80.02x- Occupant of animal-drawn vehicle injured by fall from or being thrown from animal-drawn vehicle in noncollision accident
            Overturning animal-drawn vehicle NOS
            Overturning animal-drawn vehicle without collision

V80.1- Animal-rider or occupant of animal-drawn vehicle injured in **collision with pedestrian or animal**
   Excludes 1: *animal-rider or animal-drawn vehicle collision with animal-drawn vehicle or animal being ridden (V80.7)*

V80.11x- Animal-rider injured in collision with pedestrian or animal

V80.12x- Occupant of animal-drawn vehicle injured in collision with pedestrian or animal

V80.2- Animal-rider or occupant of animal-drawn vehicle injured in **collision with pedal cycle**

V80.21x- Animal-rider injured in collision with pedal cycle

V80.22x- Occupant of animal-drawn vehicle injured in collision with pedal cycle

V80.3- Animal-rider or occupant of animal-drawn vehicle injured in **collision with two- or three-wheeled motor vehicle**

V80.31x- Animal-rider injured in collision with two- or three-wheeled motor vehicle

V80.32x- Occupant of animal-drawn vehicle injured in collision with two- or three-wheeled motor vehicle

V80.4- Animal-rider or occupant of animal-drawn vehicle injured in **collision with car, pick-up truck, van, heavy transport vehicle or bus**
   Excludes 1: *animal-rider injured in collision with military vehicle (V80.910)*
               occupant of animal-drawn vehicle injured in collision with military vehicle (V80.920)

V80.41x- Animal-rider injured in collision with car, pick-up truck, van, heavy transport vehicle or bus

V
7
8
I
V
8
0

V80.42x- Occupant of animal-drawn vehicle injured in collision with car, pick-up truck, van, heavy transport vehicle or bus

V80.5- Animal-rider or occupant of animal-drawn vehicle injured in <u>collision with other specified motor vehicle</u>

> **V80.51x-** Animal-rider injured in collision with other specified motor vehicle
>
> **V80.52x-** Occupant of animal-drawn vehicle injured in collision with other specified motor vehicle

V80.6- Animal-rider or occupant of animal-drawn vehicle injured in <u>collision with railway train or railway vehicle</u>

> **V80.61x-** Animal-rider injured in collision with railway train or railway vehicle
>
> **V80.62x-** Occupant of animal-drawn vehicle injured in collision with railway train or railway vehicle

V80.7- Animal-rider or occupant of animal-drawn vehicle injured in <u>collision with other nonmotor vehicles</u>

> **V80.71-** Animal-rider or occupant of animal-drawn vehicle injured in collision with animal being ridden
>
> > **V80.710-** Animal-rider injured in collision with other animal being ridden
> >
> > **V80.711-** Occupant of animal-drawn vehicle injured in collision with animal being ridden
>
> **V80.72-** Animal-rider or occupant of animal-drawn vehicle injured in collision with other animal-drawn vehicle
>
> > **V80.720-** Animal-rider injured in collision with animal-drawn vehicle
> >
> > **V80.721-** Occupant of animal-drawn vehicle injured in collision with other animal-drawn vehicle
>
> **V80.73-** Animal-rider or occupant of animal-drawn vehicle injured in collision with streetcar
>
> > **V80.730-** Animal-rider injured in collision with streetcar
> >
> > **V80.731-** Occupant of animal-drawn vehicle injured in collision with streetcar
>
> **V80.79-** Animal-rider or occupant of animal-drawn vehicle injured in collision with other nonmotor vehicles
>
> > **V80.790-** Animal-rider injured in collision with other nonmotor vehicles
> >
> > **V80.791-** Occupant of animal-drawn vehicle injured in collision with other nonmotor vehicles

V80.8- Animal-rider or occupant of animal-drawn vehicle injured in <u>collision with fixed or stationary object</u>

> **V80.81x-** Animal-rider injured in collision with fixed or stationary object
>
> **V80.82x-** Occupant of animal-drawn vehicle injured in collision with fixed or stationary object

V80.9- Animal-rider or occupant of animal-drawn vehicle injured in <u>other and unspecified transport accidents</u>

> **V80.91-** Animal-rider injured in other and unspecified transport accidents
>
> > **V80.910-** Animal-rider injured in transport accident with military vehicle
> >
> > **V80.918-** Animal-rider injured in other transport accident
> >
> > **V80.919-** Animal-rider injured in unspecified transport accident
> >
> > Animal rider accident NOS
>
> **V80.92-** Occupant of animal-drawn vehicle injured in other and unspecified transport accidents
>
> > **V80.920-** Occupant of animal-drawn vehicle injured in transport accident with military vehicle
> >
> > **V80.928-** Occupant of animal-drawn vehicle injured in other transport accident
> >
> > **V80.929-** Occupant of animal-drawn vehicle injured in unspecified transport accident
> >
> > Animal-drawn vehicle accident NOS

V81- <u>Occupant of railway train or railway vehicle injured</u> in <u>transport accident</u>

Includes: Derailment of railway train or railway vehicle
Person on outside of train

Excludes 1: streetcar (V82.-)

The appropriate 7th character is to be added to each code from category V81:

- **A** <u>Initial</u> encounter
- **D** <u>Subsequent</u> encounter
- **S** <u>Sequela</u>

V81.0xx- Occupant of railway train or railway vehicle injured in <u>collision with motor vehicle in nontraffic accident</u>

Excludes 1: occupant of railway train or railway vehicle injured due to collision with military vehicle (V81.83)

V81.1xx- Occupant of railway train or railway vehicle injured in <u>collision with motor vehicle in traffic accident</u>

Excludes 1: occupant of railway train or railway vehicle injured due to collision with military vehicle (V81.83)

V81.2xx- Occupant of railway train or railway vehicle injured in <u>collision with or hit by rolling stock</u>

V81.3xx- Occupant of railway train or railway vehicle injured in <u>collision with other object</u>

Railway collision NOS

V81.4xx- Person injured while boarding or alighting from railway train or railway vehicle

V81.5xx- Occupant of railway train or railway vehicle injured by fall in railway train or railway vehicle

V81.6xx- Occupant of railway train or railway vehicle injured by fall from railway train or railway vehicle

V81.7xx- Occupant of railway train or railway vehicle injured in derailment without antecedent collision

V81.8- Occupant of railway train or railway vehicle injured in other specified railway accidents

> **V81.81x-** Occupant of railway train or railway vehicle injured due to explosion or fire on train
>
> **V81.82x-** Occupant of railway train or railway vehicle injured due to object falling onto train
>
> > Occupant of railway train or railway vehicle injured due to falling earth onto train
> > Occupant of railway train or railway vehicle injured due to falling rocks onto train
> > Occupant of railway train or railway vehicle injured due to falling snow onto train
> > Occupant of railway train or railway vehicle injured due to falling trees onto train
>
> **V81.83x-** Occupant of railway train or railway vehicle injured due to collision with military vehicle
>
> **V81.89x-** Occupant of railway train or railway vehicle injured due to other specified railway accident

V81.9xx- Occupant of railway train or railway vehicle injured in unspecified railway accident

Railway accident NOS

V82- <u>Occupant of powered streetcar injured</u> in <u>transport accident</u>

Includes: Interurban electric car
Person on outside of streetcar
Tram (car)
Trolley (car)

Excludes 1: bus (V70-V79)
motorcoach (V70-V79)
nonpowered streetcar (V76.-)
train (V81.-)

The appropriate 7th character is to be added to each code from category V82:

- **A** <u>Initial</u> encounter
- **D** <u>Subsequent</u> encounter
- **S** <u>Sequela</u>

V82.0xx- Occupant of streetcar injured in collision with motor vehicle in nontraffic accident

V82.1xx- Occupant of streetcar injured in collision with motor vehicle in traffic accident

V82.2xx- Occupant of streetcar injured in collision with or hit by rolling stock

V80 - V82

V82.3xx- Occupant of streetcar injured in collision with other object
> *Excludes 1:*   *collision with animal-drawn vehicle or animal being ridden (V82.8)*

V82.4xx- Person injured while boarding or alighting from streetcar

V82.5xx- Occupant of streetcar injured by fall in streetcar
> *Excludes 1:*   *fall in streetcar:*
> *while boarding or alighting (V82.4)*
> *with antecedent collision (V82.0-V82.3)*

V82.6xx- Occupant of streetcar injured by fall from streetcar
> *Excludes 1:*   *fall from streetcar:*
> *while boarding or alighting (V82.4)*
> *with antecedent collision (V82.0-V82.3)*

V82.7xx- Occupant of streetcar injured in derailment without antecedent collision
> *Excludes 1:*   *occupant of streetcar injured in derailment with antecedent collision (V82.0-V82.3)*

V82.8xx- Occupant of streetcar injured in other specified transport accidents
> Streetcar collision with military vehicle
> Streetcar collision with train or nonmotor vehicles

V82.9xx- Occupant of streetcar injured in unspecified traffic accident
> Streetcar accident NOS

V83- <u>Occupant of special vehicle mainly used on industrial premises injured</u> in <u>transport accident</u>
> Includes: Battery-powered airport passenger vehicle
> Battery-powered truck (baggage) (mail)
> Voal-car in mine
> Forklift (truck)
> Logging car
> Self-propelled industrial truck
> Station baggage truck (powered)
> Tram, truck, or tub (powered) in mine or quarry
> *Excludes 1:*   *special construction vehicles (V85.-)*
> *special industrial vehicle in stationary use or maintenance (W31.-)*

The appropriate 7th character is to be added to each code from category V83:
A	**Initial** encounter
D	**Subsequent** encounter
S	**Sequela**

V83.0xx- Driver of special industrial vehicle injured in traffic accident

V83.1xx- Passenger of special industrial vehicle injured in traffic accident

V83.2xx- Person on outside of special industrial vehicle injured in traffic accident

V83.3xx- Unspecified occupant of special industrial vehicle injured in traffic accident

V83.4xx- Person injured while boarding or alighting from special industrial vehicle

V83.5xx- Driver of special industrial vehicle injured in nontraffic accident

V83.6xx- Passenger of special industrial vehicle injured in nontraffic accident

V83.7xx- Person on outside of special industrial vehicle injured in nontraffic accident

V83.9xx- Unspecified occupant of special industrial vehicle injured in nontraffic accident
> Special-industrial-vehicle accident NOS

V84- <u>Occupant of special vehicle mainly used in agriculture injured</u> in <u>transport accident</u>
> Includes: Self-propelled farm machinery
> Tractor (and trailer)
> *Excludes 1:*   *animal-powered farm machinery accident (W30.8-)*
> *contact with combine harvester (W30.0)*
> *special agricultural vehicle in stationary use or maintenance (W30.-)*

The appropriate 7th character is to be added to each code from category V84:
A	**Initial** encounter
D	**Subsequent** encounter
S	**Sequela**

V84.0xx- Driver of special agricultural vehicle injured in traffic accident

V84.1xx- Passenger of special agricultural vehicle injured in traffic accident

V84.2xx- Person on outside of special agricultural vehicle injured in traffic accident

V84.3xx- Unspecified occupant of special agricultural vehicle injured in traffic accident

V84.4xx- Person injured while boarding or alighting from special agricultural vehicle

V84.5xx- Driver of special agricultural vehicle injured in nontraffic accident

V84.6xx- Passenger of special agricultural vehicle injured in nontraffic accident

V84.7xx- Person on outside of special agricultural vehicle injured in nontraffic accident

V84.9xx- Unspecified occupant of special agricultural vehicle injured in nontraffic accident
> Special-agricultural vehicle accident NOS

V85- <u>Occupant of special construction vehicle injured</u> in <u>transport accident</u>
> Includes: Bulldozer
> Digger
> Dump truck
> Earth-leveller
> Mechanical shovel
> Road-roller
> *Excludes 1:*   *special industrial vehicle (V83.-)*
> *special construction vehicle in stationary use or maintenance (W31.-)*

The appropriate 7th character is to be added to each code from category V85:
A	**Initial** encounter
D	**Subsequent** encounter
S	**Sequela**

V85.0xx- Driver of special construction vehicle injured in traffic accident

V85.1xx- Passenger of special construction vehicle injured in traffic accident

V85.2xx- Person on outside of special construction vehicle injured in traffic accident

V85.3xx- Unspecified occupant of special construction vehicle injured in traffic accident

V85.4xx- Person injured while boarding or alighting from special construction vehicle

V85.5xx- Driver of special construction vehicle injured in nontraffic accident

V85.6xx- Passenger of special construction vehicle injured in nontraffic accident

V85.7xx- Person on outside of special construction vehicle injured in nontraffic accident

V85.9xx- Unspecified occupant of special construction vehicle injured in nontraffic accident
> Special-construction-vehicle accident NOS

V86- <u>Occupant of special all-terrain or other off-road motor vehicle, injured</u> in <u>transport accident</u>
> *Excludes 1:*   *special all-terrain vehicle in stationary use or maintenance (W31.-)*
> *sport-utility vehicle (V50-V59)*
> *three-wheeled motor vehicle designed for on-road use (V30-V39)*

The appropriate 7th character is to be added to each code from category V86:
A	**Initial** encounter
D	**Subsequent** encounter
S	**Sequela**

V86.0- Driver of special all-terrain or other off-road motor vehicle injured in traffic accident

V86.01x- Driver of ambulance or fire engine injured in traffic accident

V86.02x- Driver of snowmobile injured in traffic accident

V86.03x- Driver of dune buggy injured in traffic accident

V86.04x- Driver of military vehicle injured in traffic accident

V82 - V86

V86.09x- Driver of other special all-terrain or other off-road motor vehicle injured in traffic accident
    Driver of dirt bike injured in traffic accident
    Driver of go cart injured in traffic accident
    Driver of golf cart injured in traffic accident

V86.1- Passenger of special all-terrain or other off-road motor vehicle injured in traffic accident

V86.11x- Passenger of ambulance or fire engine injured in traffic accident

V86.12x- Passenger of snowmobile injured in traffic accident

V86.13x- Passenger of dune buggy injured in traffic accident

V86.14x- Passenger of military vehicle injured in traffic accident

V86.19x- Passenger of other special all-terrain or other off-road motor vehicle injured in traffic accident
    Passenger of dirt bike injured in traffic accident
    Passenger of go cart injured in traffic accident
    Passenger of golf cart injured in traffic accident

V86.2- Person on outside of special all-terrain or other off-road motor vehicle injured in traffic accident

V86.21x- Person on outside of ambulance or fire engine injured in traffic accident

V86.22x- Person on outside of snowmobile injured in traffic accident

V86.23x- Person on outside of dune buggy injured in traffic accident

V86.24x- Person on outside of military vehicle injured in traffic accident

V86.29x- Person on outside of other special all-terrain or other off-road motor vehicle injured in traffic accident
    Person on outside of dirt bike injured in traffic accident
    Person on outside of go cart injured in traffic accident
    Person on outside of golf cart injured in traffic accident

V86.3- Unspecified occupant of special all-terrain or other off-road motor vehicle injured in traffic accident

V86.31x- Unspecified occupant of ambulance or fire engine injured in traffic accident

V86.32x- Unspecified occupant of snowmobile injured in traffic accident

V86.33x- Unspecified occupant of dune buggy injured in traffic accident

V86.34x- Unspecified occupant of military vehicle injured in traffic accident

V86.39x- Unspecified occupant of other special all-terrain or other off-road motor vehicle injured in traffic accident
    Unspecified occupant of dirt bike injured in traffic accident
    Unspecified occupant of go cart injured in traffic accident
    Unspecified occupant of golf cart injured in traffic accident

V86.4- Person injured while boarding or alighting from special all-terrain or other off-road motor vehicle

V86.41x- Person injured while boarding or alighting from ambulance or fire engine

V86.42x- Person injured while boarding or alighting from snowmobile

V86.43x- Person injured while boarding or alighting from dune buggy

V86.44x- Person injured while boarding or alighting from military vehicle

V86.49x- Person injured while boarding or alighting from other special all-terrain or other off-road motor vehicle
    Person injured while boarding or alighting from dirt bike
    Person injured while boarding or alighting from go cart
    Person injured while boarding or alighting from golf cart

V86.5- Driver of special all-terrain or other off-road motor vehicle injured in nontraffic accident

V86.51x- Driver of ambulance or fire engine injured in nontraffic accident

V86.52x- Driver of snowmobile injured in nontraffic accident

V86.53x- Driver of dune buggy injured in nontraffic accident

V86.54x- Driver of military vehicle injured in nontraffic accident

V86.59x- Driver of other special all-terrain or other off-road motor vehicle injured in nontraffic accident
    Driver of dirt bike injured in nontraffic accident
    Driver of go cart injured in nontraffic accident
    Driver of golf cart injured in nontraffic accident

V86.6- Passenger of special all-terrain or other off-road motor vehicle injured in nontraffic accident

V86.61x- Passenger of ambulance or fire engine injured in nontraffic accident

V86.62x- Passenger of snowmobile injured in nontraffic accident

V86.63x- Passenger of dune buggy injured in nontraffic accident

V86.64x- Passenger of military vehicle injured in nontraffic accident

V86.69x- Passenger of other special all-terrain or other off-road motor vehicle injured in nontraffic accident
    Passenger of dirt bike injured in nontraffic accident
    Passenger of go cart injured in nontraffic accident
    Passenger of golf cart injured in nontraffic accident

V86.7- Person on outside of special all-terrain or other off-road motor vehicle injured in nontraffic accident

V86.71x- Person on outside of ambulance or fire engine injured in nontraffic accident

V86.72x- Person on outside of snowmobile injured in nontraffic accident

V86.73x- Person on outside of dune buggy injured in nontraffic accident

V86.74x- Person on outside of military vehicle injured in nontraffic accident

V86.79x- Person on outside of other special all-terrain or other off-road motor vehicles injured in nontraffic accident
    Person on outside of dirt bike injured in nontraffic accident
    Person on outside of go cart injured in nontraffic accident
    Person on outside of golf cart injured in nontraffic accident

V86.9- Unspecified occupant of special all-terrain or other off-road motor vehicle injured in nontraffic accident

V86.91x- Unspecified occupant of ambulance or fire engine injured in nontraffic accident

V86.92x- Unspecified occupant of snowmobile injured in nontraffic accident

V86.93x- Unspecified occupant of dune buggy injured in nontraffic accident

V86.94x- Unspecified occupant of military vehicle injured in nontraffic accident

V86.99x- Unspecified occupant of other special all-terrain or other off-road motor vehicle injured in nontraffic accident
    All-terrain motor-vehicle accident NOS
    Off-road motor-vehicle accident NOS
    Other motor-vehicle accident NOS
    Unspecified occupant of dirt bike injured in nontraffic accident
    Unspecified occupant of go cart injured in nontraffic accident
    Unspecified occupant of golf cart injured in nontraffic accident

V87- <u>Traffic accident of specified type but victim's mode of transport unknown</u>
Excludes 1:   *collision involving:*
      pedal cycle (V10-V19)
      pedestrian (V01-V09)

The appropriate 7th character is to be added to each code from category **V87:**

A   <u>Initial</u> encounter
D   <u>Subsequent</u> encounter
S   <u>Sequela</u>

V87.0xx- Person injured in collision between car and two- or three-wheeled powered vehicle (traffic)

V87.1xx- Person injured in collision between other motor vehicle and two- or three-wheeled motor vehicle (traffic)

V87.2xx- Person injured in collision between car and pick-up truck or van (traffic)

V87.3xx- Person injured in collision between car and bus (traffic)

V87.4xx-　Person injured in collision between car and heavy transport vehicle (traffic)

V87.5xx-　Person injured in collision between heavy transport vehicle and bus (traffic)

V87.6xx-　Person injured in collision between railway train or railway vehicle and car (traffic)

V87.7xx-　Person injured in collision between other specified motor vehicles (traffic)

V87.8xx-　Person injured in other specified noncollision transport accidents involving motor vehicle (traffic)

V87.9xx-　Person injured in other specified (collision) (noncollision) transport accidents involving nonmotor vehicle (traffic)

V88-　**Nontraffic accident of specified type but victim's mode of transport unknown**

　　Excludes 1:　collision involving:
　　　　pedal cycle (V10-V19)
　　　　pedestrian (V01-V09)

　　The appropriate 7th character is to be added to each code from category V88:
　　A　**Initial** encounter
　　D　**Subsequent** encounter
　　S　**Sequela**

V88.0xx-　Person injured in collision between car and two- or three-wheeled motor vehicle, nontraffic

V88.1xx-　Person injured in collision between other motor vehicle and two- or three-wheeled motor vehicle, nontraffic

V88.2xx-　Person injured in collision between car and pick-up truck or van, nontraffic

V88.3xx-　Person injured in collision between car and bus, nontraffic

V88.4xx-　Person injured in collision between car and heavy transport vehicle, nontraffic

V88.5xx-　Person injured in collision between heavy transport vehicle and bus, nontraffic

V88.6xx-　Person injured in collision between railway train or railway vehicle and car, nontraffic

V88.7xx-　Person injured in collision between other specified motor vehicle, nontraffic

V88.8xx-　Person injured in other specified noncollision transport accidents involving motor vehicle, nontraffic

V88.9xx-　Person injured in other specified (collision)(noncollision) transport accidents involving nonmotor vehicle, nontraffic

V89-　**Motor- or nonmotor-vehicle accident, type of vehicle unspecified**

　　The appropriate 7th character is to be added to each code from category V89:
　　A　**Initial** encounter
　　D　**Subsequent** encounter
　　S　**Sequela**

V89.0xx-　Person injured in unspecified motor-vehicle accident, nontraffic
　　　　Motor-vehicle accident NOS, nontraffic

V89.1xx-　Person injured in unspecified nonmotor-vehicle accident, nontraffic
　　　　Nonmotor-vehicle accident NOS (nontraffic)

V89.2xx-　Person injured in unspecified motor-vehicle accident, traffic
　　　　Motor-vehicle accident [MVA] NOS
　　　　Road (traffic) accident [RTA] NOS

V89.3xx-　Person injured in unspecified nonmotor-vehicle accident, traffic
　　　　Nonmotor-vehicle traffic accident NOS

V89.9xx-　Person injured in unspecified vehicle accident
　　　　Collision NOS

Water transport accidents (V90-V94)

V90-　**Drowning and submersion due to accident to watercraft**

　　Excludes 1:　civilian water transport accident involving military watercraft (V94.81-)
　　　　fall into water not from watercraft (W16.-)
　　　　military watercraft accident in military or war operations (Y36.0-, Y37.0-)
　　　　water-transport-related drowning or submersion without accident to watercraft (V92.-)

　　The appropriate 7th character is to be added to each code from category V90:
　　A　**Initial** encounter
　　D　**Subsequent** encounter
　　S　**Sequela**

V90.0-　Drowning and submersion **due to watercraft overturning**

V90.00x-　Drowning and submersion due to merchant ship overturning

V90.01x-　Drowning and submersion due to passenger ship overturning
　　　　Drowning and submersion due to Ferry-boat overturning
　　　　Drowning and submersion due to Liner overturning

V90.02x-　Drowning and submersion due to fishing boat overturning

V90.03x-　Drowning and submersion due to other powered watercraft overturning
　　　　Drowning and submersion due to Hovercraft (on open water) overturning
　　　　Drowning and submersion due to Jet ski overturning

V90.04x-　Drowning and submersion due to sailboat overturning

V90.05x-　Drowning and submersion due to canoe or kayak overturning

V90.06x-　Drowning and submersion due to (nonpowered) inflatable craft overturning

V90.08x-　Drowning and submersion due to other unpowered watercraft overturning
　　　　Drowning and submersion due to windsurfer overturning

V90.09x-　Drowning and submersion due to unspecified watercraft overturning
　　　　Drowning and submersion due to boat NOS overturning
　　　　Drowning and submersion due to ship NOS overturning
　　　　Drowning and submersion due to watercraft NOS overturning

V90.1-　Drowning and submersion **due to watercraft sinking**

V90.10x-　Drowning and submersion due to merchant ship sinking

V90.11x-　Drowning and submersion due to passenger ship sinking
　　　　Drowning and submersion due to Ferry-boat sinking
　　　　Drowning and submersion due to Liner sinking

V90.12x-　Drowning and submersion due to fishing boat sinking

V90.13x-　Drowning and submersion due to other powered watercraft sinking
　　　　Drowning and submersion due to Hovercraft (on open water) sinking
　　　　Drowning and submersion due to Jet ski sinking

V90.14x-　Drowning and submersion due to sailboat sinking

V90.15x-　Drowning and submersion due to canoe or kayak sinking

V90.16x-　Drowning and submersion due to (nonpowered) inflatable craft sinking

V90.18x-　Drowning and submersion due to other unpowered watercraft sinking

V90.19x-　Drowning and submersion due to unspecified watercraft sinking
　　　　Drowning and submersion due to boat NOS sinking
　　　　Drowning and submersion due to ship NOS sinking
　　　　Drowning and submersion due to watercraft NOS sinking

V90.2-　Drowning and submersion **due to falling or jumping from burning watercraft**

V90.20x-　Drowning and submersion due to falling or jumping from burning merchant ship

V
8
7
-
V
9
0

V90.21x- **Drowning and submersion due to falling or jumping from burning passenger ship**
Drowning and submersion due to falling or jumping from burning Ferry-boat
Drowning and submersion due to falling or jumping from burning Liner

V90.22x- **Drowning and submersion due to falling or jumping from burning fishing boat**

V90.23x- **Drowning and submersion due to falling or jumping from other burning powered watercraft**
Drowning and submersion due to falling and jumping from burning Hovercraft (on open water)
Drowning and submersion due to falling and jumping from burning Jet ski

V90.24x- **Drowning and submersion due to falling or jumping from burning sailboat**

V90.25x- **Drowning and submersion due to falling or jumping from burning canoe or kayak**

V90.26x- **Drowning and submersion due to falling or jumping from burning (nonpowered) inflatable craft**

V90.27x- **Drowning and submersion due to falling or jumping from burning water-skis**

V90.28x- **Drowning and submersion due to falling or jumping from other burning unpowered watercraft**
Drowning and submersion due to falling and jumping from burning surf-board
Drowning and submersion due to falling and jumping from burning windsurfer

V90.29x- **Drowning and submersion due to falling or jumping from unspecified burning watercraft**
Drowning and submersion due to falling or jumping from burning boat NOS
Drowning and submersion due to falling or jumping from burning ship NOS
Drowning and submersion due to falling or jumping from burning watercraft NOS

V90.3- **Drowning and submersion due to falling or jumping from crushed watercraft**

V90.30x- **Drowning and submersion due to falling or jumping from crushed merchant ship**

V90.31x- **Drowning and submersion due to falling or jumping from crushed passenger ship**
Drowning and submersion due to falling and jumping from crushed Ferry boat
Drowning and submersion due to falling and jumping from crushed Liner

V90.32x- **Drowning and submersion due to falling or jumping from crushed fishing boat**

V90.33x- **Drowning and submersion due to falling or jumping from other crushed powered watercraft**
Drowning and submersion due to falling and jumping from crushed Hovercraft
Drowning and submersion due to falling and jumping from crushed Jet ski

V90.34x- **Drowning and submersion due to falling or jumping from crushed sailboat**

V90.35x- **Drowning and submersion due to falling or jumping from crushed canoe or kayak**

V90.36x- **Drowning and submersion due to falling or jumping from crushed (nonpowered) inflatable craft**

V90.37x- **Drowning and submersion due to falling or jumping from crushed water-skis**

V90.38x- **Drowning and submersion due to falling or jumping from other crushed unpowered watercraft**
Drowning and submersion due to falling and jumping from crushed surf-board
Drowning and submersion due to falling and jumping from crushed windsurfer

V90.39x- **Drowning and submersion due to falling or jumping from crushed unspecified watercraft**
Drowning and submersion due to falling and jumping from crushed boat NOS
Drowning and submersion due to falling and jumping from crushed ship NOS
Drowning and submersion due to falling and jumping from crushed watercraft NOS

V90.8- **Drowning and submersion due to other accident to watercraft**

V90.80x- **Drowning and submersion due to other accident to merchant ship**

V90.81x- **Drowning and submersion due to other accident to passenger ship**
Drowning and submersion due to other accident to Ferry-boat
Drowning and submersion due to other accident to Liner

V90.82x- **Drowning and submersion due to other accident to fishing boat**

V90.83x- **Drowning and submersion due to other accident to other powered watercraft**
Drowning and submersion due to other accident to Hovercraft (on open water)
Drowning and submersion due to other accident to Jet ski

V90.84x- **Drowning and submersion due to other accident to sailboat**

V90.85x- **Drowning and submersion due to other accident to canoe or kayak**

V90.86x- **Drowning and submersion due to other accident to (nonpowered) inflatable craft**

V90.87x- **Drowning and submersion due to other accident to water-skis**

V90.88x- **Drowning and submersion due to other accident to other unpowered watercraft**
Drowning and submersion due to other accident to surf-board
Drowning and submersion due to other accident to windsurfer

V90.89x- **Drowning and submersion due to other accident to unspecified watercraft**
Drowning and submersion due to other accident to boat NOS
Drowning and submersion due to other accident to ship NOS
Drowning and submersion due to other accident to watercraft NOS

V91- **Other injury due to accident to watercraft**
Includes: Any injury except drowning and submersion as a result of an accident to watercraft
Excludes 1: *civilian water transport accident involving military watercraft (V94.81-)*
military watercraft accident in military or war operations (Y36, Y37.-)
Excludes ❷: *drowning and submersion due to accident to watercraft (V90.-)*

The appropriate 7th character is to be added to each code from category V91:
A Initial encounter
D Subsequent encounter
S Sequela

V91.0- **Burn due to watercraft on fire**
Excludes 1: *burn from localized fire or explosion on board ship without accident to watercraft (V93.-)*

V91.00x- **Burn due to merchant ship on fire**

V91.01x- **Burn due to passenger ship on fire**
Burn due to Ferry-boat on fire
Burn due to Liner on fire

V91.02x- **Burn due to fishing boat on fire**

V91.03x- **Burn due to other powered watercraft on fire**
Burn due to Hovercraft (on open water) on fire
Burn due to Jet ski on fire

V91.04x- **Burn due to sailboat on fire**

V91.05x- **Burn due to canoe or kayak on fire**

V91.06x- **Burn due to (nonpowered) inflatable craft on fire**

V91.07x- **Burn due to water-skis on fire**

V91.08x- **Burn due to other unpowered watercraft on fire**

V91.09x- **Burn due to unspecified watercraft on fire**
Burn due to boat NOS on fire
Burn due to ship NOS on fire
Burn due to watercraft NOS on fire

V90-V91

V91.1- **Crushed** between watercraft and other watercraft or other object due to collision
    Crushed by lifeboat after abandoning ship in a collision
    NOTE: Select the specified type of watercraft that the victim was on at the time of the collision

V91.10x- Crushed between merchant ship and other watercraft or other object due to collision

V91.11x- Crushed between passenger ship and other watercraft or other object due to collision
    Crushed between Ferry-boat and other watercraft or other object due to collision
    Crushed between Liner and other watercraft or other object due to collision

V91.12x- Crushed between fishing boat and other watercraft or other object due to collision

V91.13x- Crushed between other powered watercraft and other watercraft or other object due to collision
    Crushed between Hovercraft (on open water) and other watercraft or other object due to collision
    Crushed between Jet ski and other watercraft or other object due to collision

V91.14x- Crushed between sailboat and other watercraft or other object due to collision

V91.15x- Crushed between canoe or kayak and other watercraft or other object due to collision

V91.16x- Crushed between (nonpowered) inflatable craft and other watercraft or other object due to collision

V91.18x- Crushed between other unpowered watercraft and other watercraft or other object due to collision
    Crushed between surfboard and other watercraft or other object due to collision
    Crushed between windsurfer and other watercraft or other object due to collision

V91.19x- Crushed between unspecified watercraft and other watercraft or other object due to collision
    Crushed between boat NOS and other watercraft or other object due to collision
    Crushed between ship NOS and other watercraft or other object due to collision
    Crushed between watercraft NOS and other watercraft or other object due to collision

V91.2- **Fall** due to collision between watercraft and other watercraft or other object
    Fall while remaining on watercraft after collision
    Note: Select the specified type of watercraft that the victim was on at the time of the collision
    Excludes 1:   *crushed between watercraft and other watercraft and other object due to collision (V91.1-)*
        drowning and submersion due to falling from crushed watercraft (V90.3-)

V91.20x- Fall due to collision between merchant ship and other watercraft or other object

V91.21x- Fall due to collision between passenger ship and other watercraft or other object
    Fall due to collision between Ferry-boat and other watercraft or other object
    Fall due to collision between Liner and other watercraft or other object

V91.22x- Fall due to collision between fishing boat and other watercraft or other object

V91.23x- Fall due to collision between other powered watercraft and other watercraft or other object
    Fall due to collision between Hovercraft (on open water) and other watercraft or other object
    Fall due to collision between Jet ski and other watercraft or other object

V91.24x- Fall due to collision between sailboat and other watercraft or other object

V91.25x- Fall due to collision between canoe or kayak and other watercraft or other object

V91.26x- Fall due to collision between (nonpowered) inflatable craft and other watercraft or other object

V91.29x- Fall due to collision between unspecified watercraft and other watercraft or other object
    Fall due to collision between boat NOS and other watercraft or other object
    Fall due to collision between ship NOS and other watercraft or other object
    Fall due to collision between watercraft NOS and other watercraft or other object

V91.3- **Hit or struck by falling object** due to accident to watercraft
    Hit or struck by falling object (part of damaged watercraft or other object) after falling or jumping from damaged watercraft
    Excludes ❷: *drowning or submersion due to fall or jumping from damaged watercraft (V90.2-, V90.3-)*

V91.30x- Hit or struck by falling object due to accident to merchant ship

V91.31x- Hit or struck by falling object due to accident to passenger ship
    Hit or struck by falling object due to accident to Ferry-boat
    Hit or struck by falling object due to accident to Liner

V91.32x- Hit or struck by falling object due to accident to fishing boat

V91.33x- Hit or struck by falling object due to accident to other powered watercraft
    Hit or struck by falling object due to accident to Hovercraft (on open water)
    Hit or struck by falling object due to accident to Jet ski

V91.34x- Hit or struck by falling object due to accident to sailboat

V91.35x- Hit or struck by falling object due to accident to canoe or kayak

V91.36x- Hit or struck by falling object due to accident to (nonpowered) inflatable craft

V91.37x- Hit or struck by falling object due to accident to water-skis
    Hit by water-skis after jumping off of waterskis

V91.38x- Hit or struck by falling object due to accident to other unpowered watercraft
    Hit or struck by surf-board after falling off damaged surf-board
    Hit or struck by object after falling off damaged windsurfer

V91.39x- Hit or struck by falling object due to accident to unspecified watercraft
    Hit or struck by falling object due to accident to boat NOS
    Hit or struck by falling object due to accident to ship NOS
    Hit or struck by falling object due to accident to watercraft NOS

V91.8- **Other injury** due to other accident to watercraft

V91.80x- Other injury due to other accident to merchant ship

V91.81x- Other injury due to other accident to passenger ship
    Other injury due to other accident to Ferry-boat
    Other injury due to other accident to Liner

V91.82x- Other injury due to other accident to fishing boat

V91.83x- Other injury due to other accident to other powered watercraft
    Other injury due to other accident to Hovercraft (on open water)
    Other injury due to other accident to Jet ski

V91.84x- Other injury due to other accident to sailboat

V91.85x- Other injury due to other accident to canoe or kayak

V91.86x- Other injury due to other accident to (nonpowered) inflatable craft

V91.87x- Other injury due to other accident to water-skis

V91.88x- Other injury due to other accident to other unpowered watercraft
    Other injury due to other accident to surf-board
    Other injury due to other accident to windsurfer

V91.89x- Other injury due to other accident to unspecified watercraft
    Other injury due to other accident to boat NOS
    Other injury due to other accident to ship NOS
    Other injury due to other accident to watercraft NOS

V91 - V91

V92- **Drowning and submersion** **due to accident on board watercraft,**
without accident to watercraft
  Excludes 1:   civilian water transport accident involving military watercraft
                    (V94.81-)
              drowning or submersion due to accident to watercraft (V90-
                    V91)
              drowning or submersion of diver who voluntarily jumps from
                    boat not involved in an accident (W16.711, W16.721)
              fall into water without watercraft (W16.-)
              military watercraft accident in military or war operations (Y36,
                    Y37)

  The appropriate 7th character is to be added to each code from category
  V92:
  A   Initial encounter
  D   Subsequent encounter
  S   Sequela

V92.0- **Drowning and submersion** **due to fall off watercraft**
          Drowning and submersion due to fall from gangplank of watercraft
          Drowning and submersion due to fall overboard watercraft
  Excludes ②: hitting head on object or bottom of body of water due
                    to fall from watercraft (V94.0-)

V92.00x- **Drowning and submersion due to fall off merchant ship**

V92.01x- **Drowning and submersion due to fall off passenger**
          ship
          Drowning and submersion due to fall off Ferry-boat
          Drowning and submersion due to fall off Liner

V92.02x- **Drowning and submersion due to fall off fishing boat**

V92.03x- **Drowning and submersion due to fall off other powered**
          watercraft
          Drowning and submersion due to fall off Hovercraft (on
               open water)
          Drowning and submersion due to fall off Jet ski

V92.04x- **Drowning and submersion due to fall off sailboat**

V92.05x- **Drowning and submersion due to fall off canoe or**
          kayak

V92.06x- **Drowning and submersion due to fall off (nonpowered)**
          inflatable craft

V92.07x- **Drowning and submersion due to fall off water-skis**
  Excludes 1:   drowning and submersion due to falling off
                    burning water-skis (V90.27)
              drowning and submersion due to falling off
                    crushed water-skis (V90.37)
              hit by boat while water-skiing NOS (V94.-)

V92.08x- **Drowning and submersion due to fall off other**
          unpowered watercraft
          Drowning and submersion due to fall off surf-board
          Drowning and submersion due to fall off windsurfer
  Excludes 1:   drowning and submersion due to fall off burning
                    unpowered watercraft (V90.28)
              drowning and submersion due to fall off crushed
                    unpowered watercraft (V90.38)
              drowning and submersion due to fall off
                    damaged unpowered watercraft (V90.88)
              drowning and submersion due to rider of
                    nonpowered watercraft being hit by other
                    watercraft (V94.-)
              other injury due to rider of nonpowered
                    watercraft being hit by other watercraft
                    (V94.-)

V92.09x- **Drowning and submersion due to fall off unspecified**
          watercraft
          Drowning and submersion due to fall off boat NOS
          Drowning and submersion due to fall off ship
          Drowning and submersion due to fall off watercraft NOS

V92.1- **Drowning and submersion** **due to being thrown overboard by**
          motion of watercraft
  Excludes 1:   drowning and submersion due to fall off surf-board
                    (V92.08)
              drowning and submersion due to fall off water-skis
                    (V92.07)
              drowning and submersion due to fall off windsurfer
                    (V92.08)

V92.10x- **Drowning and submersion due to being thrown**
          overboard by motion of merchant ship

V92.11x- **Drowning and submersion due to being thrown**
          overboard by motion of passenger ship
          Drowning and submersion due to being thrown overboard
               by motion of Ferry-boat
          Drowning and submersion due to being thrown overboard
               by motion of Liner

V92.12x- **Drowning and submersion due to being thrown**
          overboard by motion of fishing boat

V92.13x- **Drowning and submersion due to being thrown**
          overboard by motion of other powered watercraft
          Drowning and submersion due to being thrown overboard
               by motion of Hovercraft

V92.14x- **Drowning and submersion due to being thrown**
          overboard by motion of sailboat

V92.15x- **Drowning and submersion due to being thrown**
          overboard by motion of canoe or kayak

V92.16x- **Drowning and submersion due to being thrown**
          overboard by motion of (nonpowered) inflatable craft

V92.19x- **Drowning and submersion due to being thrown**
          overboard by motion of unspecified watercraft
          Drowning and submersion due to being thrown overboard
               by motion of boat NOS
          Drowning and submersion due to being thrown overboard
               by motion of ship NOS
          Drowning and submersion due to being thrown overboard
               by motion of watercraft NOS

V92.2- **Drowning and submersion** **due to being washed overboard**
          from watercraft
          Code first any associated cataclysm (X37.0-)

V92.20x- **Drowning and submersion due to being washed**
          overboard from merchant ship

V92.21x- **Drowning and submersion due to being washed**
          overboard from passenger ship
          Drowning and submersion due to being washed overboard
               from Ferry-boat
          Drowning and submersion due to being washed overboard
               from Liner

V92.22x- **Drowning and submersion due to being washed**
          overboard from fishing boat

V92.23x- **Drowning and submersion due to being washed**
          overboard from other powered watercraft
          Drowning and submersion due to being washed overboard
               from Hovercraft (on open water)
          Drowning and submersion due to being washed overboard
               from Jet ski

V92.24x- **Drowning and submersion due to being washed**
          overboard from sailboat

V92.25x- **Drowning and submersion due to being washed**
          overboard from canoe or kayak

V92.26x- **Drowning and submersion due to being washed**
          overboard from (nonpowered) inflatable craft

V92.27x- **Drowning and submersion due to being washed**
          overboard from water-skis
  Excludes 1:   drowning and submersion due to fall off water-
                    skis (V92.07)

V92.28x- **Drowning and submersion due to being washed**
          overboard from other unpowered watercraft
          Drowning and submersion due to being washed overboard
               from surf-board
          Drowning and submersion due to being washed overboard
               from windsurfer

V92.29x- **Drowning and submersion due to being washed**
          overboard from unspecified watercraft
          Drowning and submersion due to being washed overboard
               from boat NOS
          Drowning and submersion due to being washed overboard
               from ship NOS
          Drowning and submersion due to being washed overboard
               from watercraft NOS

V93-   **Other injury due to accident on board watercraft,** without accident to watercraft

Excludes 1:   *civilian water transport accident involving military watercraft (V94.81-)*

other injury due to accident to watercraft (V91.-)

military watercraft accident in military or war operations (Y36, Y37.-)

Excludes ❷: *drowning and submersion due to accident on board watercraft, without accident to watercraft (V92.-)*

The appropriate 7th character is to be added to each code from category V93:

A   **Initial** encounter

D   **Subsequent** encounter

S   **Sequela**

V93.0-   **Burn** due to localized fire on board watercraft

Excludes 1:   *burn due to watercraft on fire (V91.0-)*

V93.00x-   **Burn due to localized fire on board merchant vessel**

V93.01x-   **Burn due to localized fire on board passenger vessel**
Burn due to localized fire on board Ferry-boat
Burn due to localized fire on board Liner

V93.02x-   **Burn due to localized fire on board fishing boat**

V93.03x-   **Burn due to localized fire on board other powered watercraft**
Burn due to localized fire on board Hovercraft
Burn due to localized fire on board Jet ski

V93.04x-   **Burn due to localized fire on board sailboat**

V93.09x-   **Burn due to localized fire on board unspecified watercraft**
Burn due to localized fire on board boat NOS
Burn due to localized fire on board ship NOS
Burn due to localized fire on board watercraft NOS

V93.1-   **Other burn** on board watercraft
Burn due to source other than fire on board watercraft

Excludes 1:   *burn due to watercraft on fire (V91.0-)*

V93.10x-   **Other burn on board merchant vessel**

V93.11x-   **Other burn on board passenger vessel**
Other burn on board Ferry-boat
Other burn on board Liner

V93.12x-   **Other burn on board fishing boat**

V93.13x-   **Other burn on board other powered watercraft**
Other burn on board Hovercraft
Other burn on board Jet ski

V93.14x-   **Other burn on board sailboat**

V93.19x-   **Other burn on board unspecified watercraft**
Other burn on board boat NOS
Other burn on board ship NOS
Other burn on board watercraft NOS

V93.2-   **Heat exposure** on board watercraft

Excludes 1:   *exposure to man-made heat not aboard watercraft (W92)*

exposure to natural heat while on board watercraft (X30)

exposure to sunlight while on board watercraft (X32)

Excludes ❷: *burn due to fire on board watercraft (V93.0-)*

V93.20x-   **Heat exposure on board merchant ship**

V93.21x-   **Heat exposure on board passenger ship**
Heat exposure on board Ferry-boat
Heat exposure on board Liner

V93.22x-   **Heat exposure on board fishing boat**

V93.23x-   **Heat exposure on board other powered watercraft**
Heat exposure on board hovercraft

V93.24x-   **Heat exposure on board sailboat**

V93.29x-   **Heat exposure on board unspecified watercraft**
Heat exposure on board boat NOS
Heat exposure on board ship NOS
Heat exposure on board watercraft NOS

V93.3-   **Fall** on board watercraft

Excludes 1:   *fall due to collision of watercraft (V91.2-)*

V93.30x-   **Fall on board merchant ship**

V93.31x-   **Fall on board passenger ship**
Fall on board Ferry-boat
Fall on board Liner

V93.32x-   **Fall on board fishing boat**

V93.33x-   **Fall on board other powered watercraft**
Fall on board Hovercraft (on open water)
Fall on board Jet ski

V93.34x-   **Fall on board sailboat**

V93.35x-   **Fall on board canoe or kayak**

V93.36x-   **Fall on board (nonpowered) inflatable craft**

V93.38x-   **Fall on board other unpowered watercraft**

V93.39x-   **Fall on board unspecified watercraft**
Fall on board boat NOS
Fall on board ship NOS
Fall on board watercraft NOS

V93.4-   **Struck by falling object** on board watercraft
Hit by falling object on board watercraft

Excludes 1:   *struck by falling object due to accident to watercraft (V91.3)*

V93.40x-   **Struck by falling object on merchant ship**

V93.41x-   **Struck by falling object on passenger ship**
Struck by falling object on Ferry-boat
Struck by falling object on Liner

V93.42x-   **Struck by falling object on fishing boat**

V93.43x-   **Struck by falling object on other powered watercraft**
Struck by falling object on Hovercraft

V93.44x-   **Struck by falling object on sailboat**

V93.48x-   **Struck by falling object on other unpowered watercraft**

V93.49x-   **Struck by falling object on unspecified watercraft**

V93.5-   **Explosion** on board watercraft
Boiler explosion on steamship

Excludes ❷: *fire on board watercraft (V93.0-)*

V93.50x-   **Explosion on board merchant ship**

V93.51x-   **Explosion on board passenger ship**
Explosion on board Ferry-boat
Explosion on board Liner

V93.52x-   **Explosion on board fishing boat**

V93.53x-   **Explosion on board other powered watercraft**
Explosion on board Hovercraft
Explosion on board Jet ski

V93.54x-   **Explosion on board sailboat**

V93.59x-   **Explosion on board unspecified watercraft**
Explosion on board boat NOS
Explosion on board ship NOS
Explosion on board watercraft NOS

V93.6-   **Machinery accident** on board watercraft

Excludes 1:   *machinery explosion on board watercraft (V93.4-)*

machinery fire on board watercraft (V93.0-)

V93.60x-   **Machinery accident on board merchant ship**

V93.61x-   **Machinery accident on board passenger ship**
Machinery accident on board Ferry-boat
Machinery accident on board Liner

V93.62x-   **Machinery accident on board fishing boat**

V93.63x-   **Machinery accident on board other powered watercraft**
Machinery accident on board Hovercraft

V93.64x-   **Machinery accident on board sailboat**

V93.69x-   **Machinery accident on board unspecified watercraft**
Machinery accident on board boat NOS
Machinery accident on board ship NOS
Machinery accident on board watercraft NOS

V93.8-   **Other injury** due to other accident on board watercraft
Accidental poisoning by gases or fumes on watercraft

V93.80x-   **Other injury due to other accident on board merchant ship**

V93.81x-   **Other injury due to other accident on board passenger ship**
Other injury due to other accident on board Ferry-boat
Other injury due to other accident on board Liner

V93.82x-   **Other injury due to other accident on board fishing boat**

V93.83x-   **Other injury due to other accident on board other powered watercraft**
Other injury due to other accident on board Hovercraft
Other injury due to other accident on board Jet ski

V93.84x-   **Other injury due to other accident on board sailboat**

V93.85x-   **Other injury due to other accident on board canoe or kayak**

V
9
3
-
V
9
3

V93.86x- Other injury due to other accident on board (nonpowered) inflatable craft

V93.87x- Other injury due to other accident on board water-skis
Hit or struck by object while waterskiing

V93.88x- Other injury due to other accident on board other unpowered watercraft
Hit or struck by object while surfing
Hit or struck by object while on board windsurfer

V93.89x- Other injury due to other accident on board unspecified watercraft
Other injury due to other accident on board boat NOS
Other injury due to other accident on board ship NOS
Other injury due to other accident on board watercraft NOS

V94- <u>Other and unspecified water transport accidents</u>
Excludes 1: military watercraft accidents in military or war operations (Y36, Y37)

The appropriate 7th character is to be added to each code from category V94:
A <u>Initial</u> encounter
D <u>Subsequent</u> encounter
S <u>Sequela</u>

V94.0xx- Hitting object or bottom of body of water due to fall from watercraft
Excludes ❷: drowning and submersion due to fall from watercraft (V92.0-)

V94.1- Bather struck by watercraft
Swimmer hit by watercraft

V94.11x- Bather struck by powered watercraft

V94.12x- Bather struck by nonpowered watercraft

V94.2- Rider of nonpowered watercraft struck by other watercraft

V94.21x- Rider of nonpowered watercraft struck by other nonpowered watercraft
Canoer hit by other nonpowered watercraft
Surfer hit by other nonpowered watercraft
Windsurfer hit by other nonpowered watercraft

V94.22x- Rider of nonpowered watercraft struck by powered watercraft
Canoer hit by motorboat
Surfer hit by motorboat
Windsurfer hit by motorboat

V94.3- Injury to rider of (inflatable) watercraft being pulled behind other watercraft

V94.31x- Injury to rider of (inflatable) recreational watercraft being pulled behind other watercraft
Injury to rider of inner-tube pulled behind motor boat

V94.32x- Injury to rider of non-recreational watercraft being pulled behind other watercraft
Injury to occupant of dingy being pulled behind boat or ship
Injury to occupant of life-raft being pulled behind boat or ship

V94.4xx- Injury to barefoot water-skier
Injury to person being pulled behind boat or ship

V94.8- Other water transport accident

V94.81- Water transport accident involving military watercraft

V94.810- Civilian watercraft involved in water transport accident with military watercraft
Passenger on civilian watercraft injured due to accident with military watercraft

V94.811- Civilian in water injured by military watercraft

V94.818- Other water transport accident involving military watercraft

V94.89x- Other water transport accident

V94.9xx- Unspecified water transport accident
Water transport accident NOS

Air and space transport accidents (V95-V97)
Excludes 1: military aircraft accidents in military or war operations (Y36, Y37)

V95- <u>Accident to powered aircraft causing injury to occupant</u>
The appropriate 7th character is to be added to each code from category V95:
A <u>Initial</u> encounter
D <u>Subsequent</u> encounter
S <u>Sequela</u>

V95.0- <u>Helicopter</u> accident injuring occupant

V95.00x- Unspecified helicopter accident injuring occupant

V95.01x- Helicopter crash injuring occupant

V95.02x- Forced landing of helicopter injuring occupant

V95.03x- Helicopter collision injuring occupant
Helicopter collision with any object, fixed, movable or moving

V95.04x- Helicopter fire injuring occupant

V95.05x- Helicopter explosion injuring occupant

V95.09x- Other helicopter accident injuring occupant

V95.1- <u>Ultralight, microlight or powered-glider</u> accident injuring occupant

V95.10x- Unspecified ultralight, microlight or powered-glider accident injuring occupant

V95.11x- Ultralight, microlight or powered-glider crash injuring occupant

V95.12x- Forced landing of ultralight, microlight or powered-glider injuring occupant

V95.13x- Ultralight, microlight or powered-glider collision injuring occupant
Ultralight, microlight or powered-glider collision with any object, fixed, movable or moving

V95.14x- Ultralight, microlight or powered-glider fire injuring occupant

V95.15x- Ultralight, microlight or powered-glider explosion injuring occupant

V95.19x- Other ultralight, microlight or powered-glider accident injuring occupant

V95.2- <u>Other private fixed-wing aircraft</u> accident injuring occupant

V95.20x- Unspecified accident to other private fixed-wing aircraft, injuring occupant

V95.21x- Other private fixed-wing aircraft crash injuring occupant

V95.22x- Forced landing of other private fixed-wing aircraft injuring occupant

V95.23x- Other private fixed-wing aircraft collision injuring occupant
Other private fixed-wing aircraft collision with any object, fixed, movable or moving

V95.24x- Other private fixed-wing aircraft fire injuring occupant

V95.25x- Other private fixed-wing aircraft explosion injuring occupant

V95.29x- Other accident to other private fixed-wing aircraft injuring occupant

V95.3- <u>Commercial fixed-wing aircraft accident</u> injuring occupant

V95.30x- Unspecified accident to commercial fixed-wing aircraft injuring occupant

V95.31x- Commercial fixed-wing aircraft crash injuring occupant

V95.32x- Forced landing of commercial fixed-wing aircraft injuring occupant

V95.33x- Commercial fixed-wing aircraft collision injuring occupant
Commercial fixed-wing aircraft collision with any object, fixed, movable or moving

V95.34x- Commercial fixed-wing aircraft fire injuring occupant

V95.35x- Commercial fixed-wing aircraft explosion injuring occupant

V95.39x- Other accident to commercial fixed-wing aircraft injuring occupant

V93 – V95

V95.4- Spacecraft accident injuring occupant
V95.40x- Unspecified spacecraft accident injuring occupant
V95.41x- Spacecraft crash injuring occupant
V95.42x- Forced landing of spacecraft injuring occupant
V95.43x- Spacecraft collision injuring occupant
Spacecraft collision with any object, fixed, moveable or moving
V95.44x- Spacecraft fire injuring occupant
V95.45x- Spacecraft explosion injuring occupant
V95.49x- Other spacecraft accident injuring occupant
V95.8xx- Other powered aircraft accidents injuring occupant
V95.9xx- Unspecified aircraft accident injuring occupant
Aircraft accident NOS
Air transport accident NOS

V96- Accident to nonpowered aircraft causing injury to occupant
The appropriate 7th character is to be added to each code from category V96:
A Initial encounter
D Subsequent encounter
S Sequela
V96.0- Balloon accident injuring occupant
V96.00x- Unspecified balloon accident injuring occupant
V96.01x- Balloon crash injuring occupant
V96.02x- Forced landing of balloon injuring occupant
V96.03x- Balloon collision injuring occupant
Balloon collision with any object, fixed, moveable or moving
V96.04x- Balloon fire injuring occupant
V96.05x- Balloon explosion injuring occupant
V96.09x- Other balloon accident injuring occupant
V96.1- Hang-glider accident injuring occupant
V96.10x- Unspecified hang-glider accident injuring occupant
V96.11x- Hang-glider crash injuring occupant
V96.12x- Forced landing of hang-glider injuring occupant
V96.13x- Hang-glider collision injuring occupant
Hang-glider collision with any object, fixed, moveable or moving
V96.14x- Hang-glider fire injuring occupant
V96.15x- Hang-glider explosion injuring occupant
V96.19x- Other hang-glider accident injuring occupant
V96.2- Glider (nonpowered) accident injuring occupant
V96.20x- Unspecified glider (nonpowered) accident injuring occupant
V96.21x- Glider (nonpowered) crash injuring occupant
V96.22x- Forced landing of glider (nonpowered) injuring occupant
V96.23x- Glider (nonpowered) collision injuring occupant
Glider (nonpowered) collision with any object, fixed, moveable or moving
V96.24x- Glider (nonpowered) fire injuring occupant
V96.25x- Glider (nonpowered) explosion injuring occupant
V96.29x- Other glider (nonpowered) accident injuring occupant
V96.8xx- Other nonpowered-aircraft accidents injuring occupant
Kite carrying a person accident injuring occupant
V96.9xx- Unspecified nonpowered-aircraft accident injuring occupant
Nonpowered-aircraft accident NOS

V97- Other specified air transport accidents
The appropriate 7th character is to be added to each code from category V97:
A Initial encounter
D Subsequent encounter
S Sequela
V97.0xx- Occupant of aircraft injured in other specified air transport accidents
Fall in, on or from aircraft in air transport accident
Excludes 1: accident while boarding or alighting aircraft (V97.1)
V97.1xx- Person injured while boarding or alighting from aircraft

V97.2- Parachutist accident
V97.21x- Parachutist entangled in object
Parachutist landing in tree
V97.22x- Parachutist injured on landing
V97.29x- Other parachutist accident
V97.3- Person on ground injured in air transport accident
V97.31x- Hit by object falling from aircraft
Hit by crashing aircraft
Injured by aircraft hitting house
Injured by aircraft hitting car
V97.32x- Injured by rotating propeller
V97.33x- Sucked into jet engine
V97.39x- Other injury to person on ground due to air transport accident
V97.8- Other air transport accidents, not elsewhere classified
Excludes 1: aircraft accident NOS (V95.9)
exposure to changes in air pressure during ascent or descent (W94.-)
V97.81- Air transport accident involving military aircraft
V97.810- Civilian aircraft involved in air transport accident with military aircraft
Passenger in civilian aircraft injured due to accident with military aircraft
V97.811- Civilian injured by military aircraft
V97.818- Other air transport accident involving military aircraft
V97.89x- Other air transport accidents, not elsewhere classified
Injury from machinery on aircraft

Other and unspecified transport accidents (V98-V99)

Excludes 1: vehicle accident, type of vehicle unspecified (V89.-)
V98- Other specified transport accidents
The appropriate 7th character is to be added to each code from category V98:
A Initial encounter
D Subsequent encounter
S Sequela
V98.0xx- Accident to, on or involving cable-car, not on rails
Caught or dragged by cable-car, not on rails
Fall or jump from cable-car, not on rails
Object thrown from or in cable-car, not on rails
V98.1xx- Accident to, on or involving land-yacht
V98.2xx- Accident to, on or involving ice yacht
V98.3xx- Accident to, on or involving ski lift
Accident to, on or involving ski chair-lift
Accident to, on or involving ski-lift with gondola
V98.8xx- Other specified transport accidents
V99.xxx- Unspecified transport accident
The appropriate 7th character is to be added to code V99
A Initial encounter
D Subsequent encounter
S Sequela

Other external causes of accidental injury (W00-X58)

Slipping, tripping, stumbling and falls (W00-W19)

Excludes 1:   *assault involving a fall (Y01-Y02)*
                  fall from animal (V80.-)
                  fall (in) (from) machinery (in operation) (W28-W31)
                  fall (in) (from) transport vehicle (V01-V99)
                  intentional self-harm involving a fall (X80-X81)

Excludes ❷: *at risk for fall (history of fall) Z91.81*
                  fall (in) (from) burning building (X00.-)
                  fall into fire (X00-X04, X08-X09)

W00- <u>Fall due to <u>ice and snow</u></u>
          Includes: Pedestrian on foot falling (slipping) on ice and snow
          Excludes 1:   *fall on (from) ice and snow involving pedestrian conveyance*
                          (V00.-)
                          fall from stairs and steps not due to ice and snow (W10.-)

The appropriate 7th character is to be added to each code from category
W00:
A   <u>Initial</u> encounter
D   <u>Subsequent</u> encounter
S   <u>Sequela</u>

W00.0xx- Fall on same level due to ice and snow

W00.1xx- Fall from stairs and steps due to ice and snow

W00.2xx- Other fall from one level to another due to ice and snow

W00.9xx- Unspecified fall due to ice and snow

W01- <u>Fall on same level from slipping, tripping and stumbling</u>
          Includes: Fall on moving sidewalk
          Excludes 1:   *fall due to bumping (striking) against object (W18.0-)*
                          fall in shower or bathtub (W18.2-)
                          fall on same level NOS (W18.30)
                          fall on same level from slipping, tripping and stumbling due to
                          ice or snow (W00.0)
                          fall off or from toilet (W18.1-)
                          slipping, tripping and stumbling NOS (W18.40)
                          slipping, tripping and stumbling without falling (W18.4-)

The appropriate 7th character is to be added to each code from category
W01:
A   <u>Initial</u> encounter
D   <u>Subsequent</u> encounter
S   <u>Sequela</u>

W01.0xx- Fall on same level from slipping, tripping and stumbling
              <u>without</u> subsequent striking against object
              Falling over animal

W01.1- Fall on same level from slipping, tripping and stumbling <u>with</u>
            <u>subsequent striking against object</u>

    W01.10x- Fall on same level from slipping, tripping and
                   stumbling with subsequent striking against unspecified
                   object

    W01.11- Fall on same level from slipping, tripping and
                   stumbling with subsequent striking against <u>sharp</u>
                   object

        W01.110- Fall on same level from slipping, tripping and
                          stumbling with subsequent striking against sharp
                          <u>glass</u>

        W01.111- Fall on same level from slipping, tripping and
                          stumbling with subsequent striking against <u>power</u>
                          <u>tool or machine</u>

        W01.118- Fall on same level from slipping, tripping and
                          stumbling with subsequent striking against <u>other</u>
                          sharp object

        W01.119- Fall on same level from slipping, tripping and
                          stumbling with subsequent striking against
                          <u>unspecified</u> sharp object

    W01.19-Fall on same level from slipping, tripping and stumbling
                   <u>with subsequent striking against other object</u>

        W01.190- Fall on same level from slipping, tripping and
                          stumbling with subsequent striking against
                          <u>furniture</u>

        W01.198- Fall on same level from slipping, tripping and
                          stumbling with subsequent striking against <u>other</u>
                          object

W03.xxx- <u>Other fall</u> on <u>same level</u> due to <u>collision with another person</u>
              AHA 15:1Q:p8 – Tripped over another player
              Fall due to non-transport collision with other person
          Excludes 1:   *collision with another person without fall (W51)*
                          crushed or pushed by a crowd or human stampede
                          (W52)
                          fall involving pedestrian conveyance (V00-V09)
                          fall due to ice or snow (W00)
                          fall on same level NOS (W18.30)

The appropriate 7th character is to be added to code W03:
A   <u>Initial</u> encounter
D   <u>Subsequent</u> encounter
S   <u>Sequela</u>

W04.xxx- <u>Fall while being carried or supported by other persons</u>
              Accidentally dropped while being carried

The appropriate 7th character is to be added to code W04:
A   <u>Initial</u> encounter
D   <u>Subsequent</u> encounter
S   <u>Sequela</u>

W05- <u>Fall</u> from <u>non-moving</u> wheelchair, nonmotorized scooter and
          motorized mobility scooter
          Excludes 1:   *fall from moving wheelchair (powered) (V00.811)*
                          fall from moving motorized mobility scooter (V00.831)
                          fall from nonmotorized scooter (V00.141)

The appropriate 7th character is to be added to each code from category
W05:
A   <u>Initial</u> encounter
D   <u>Subsequent</u> encounter
S   <u>Sequela</u>

W05.0xx- Fall from non-moving <u>wheelchair</u>

W05.1xx- Fall from non-moving <u>nonmotorized scooter</u>

W05.2xx- Fall from non-moving <u>motorized mobility scooter</u>

W06.xxx- <u>Fall</u> from <u>bed</u>
              The appropriate 7th character is to be added to code W06:
              A   <u>Initial</u> encounter
              D   <u>Subsequent</u> encounter
              S   <u>Sequela</u>

W07.xxx- <u>Fall</u> from <u>chair</u>
              The appropriate 7th character is to be added to code W07:
              A   <u>Initial</u> encounter
              D   <u>Subsequent</u> encounter
              S   <u>Sequela</u>

W08.xxx- <u>Fall</u> from <u>other furniture</u>
              The appropriate 7th character is to be added to code W08:
              A   <u>Initial</u> encounter
              D   <u>Subsequent</u> encounter
              S   <u>Sequela</u>

W09- <u>Fall</u> on and from <u>playground equipment</u>
          Excludes 1:   *fall involving recreational machinery (W31)*

The appropriate 7th character is to be added to each code from category
W09:
A   <u>Initial</u> encounter
D   <u>Subsequent</u> encounter
S   <u>Sequela</u>

W09.0xx- Fall on or from playground slide

W09.1xx- Fall from playground swing

W09.2xx- Fall on or from jungle gym

W09.8xx- Fall on or from other playground equipment

W10- <u>Fall</u> on and from <u>stairs and steps</u>
          Excludes 1:   *Fall from stairs and steps due to ice and snow (W00.1)*

The appropriate 7th character is to be added to each code from category
W10:
A   <u>Initial</u> encounter
D   <u>Subsequent</u> encounter
S   <u>Sequela</u>

W10.0xx- Fall (on) (from) escalator

W10.1xx- Fall (on) (from) sidewalk curb

W10.2xx- Fall (on) (from) incline
              Fall (on) (from) ramp

W10.8xx- Fall (on) (from) other stairs and steps

W10.9xx- Fall (on) (from) unspecified stairs and steps

W00-W10

W11.xxx- Fall on and from ladder
The appropriate 7th character is to be added to code W11:
A   Initial encounter
D   Subsequent encounter
S   Sequela

W12.xxx- Fall on and from scaffolding
The appropriate 7th character is to be added to code W12:
A   Initial encounter
D   Subsequent encounter
S   Sequela

W13- Fall from, out of or through building or structure
The appropriate 7th character is to be added to each code from category W13:
A   Initial encounter
D   Subsequent encounter
S   Sequela

W13.0xx- Fall from, out of or through balcony
Fall from, out of or through railing

W13.1xx- Fall from, out of or through bridge

W13.2xx- Fall from, out of or through roof

W13.3xx- Fall through floor

W13.4xx- Fall from, out of or through window
Excludes ❷: fall with subsequent striking against sharp glass (W01.110)

W13.8xx- Fall from, out of or through other building or structure
Fall from, out of or through viaduct
Fall from, out of or through wall
Fall from, out of or through flag-pole

W13.9xx- Fall from, out of or through building, not otherwise specified
Excludes 1: collapse of a building or structure (W20.-)
fall or jump from burning building or structure (X00.-)

W14.xxx- Fall from tree
The appropriate 7th character is to be added to code W14:
A   Initial encounter
D   Subsequent encounter
S   Sequela

W15.xxx- Fall from cliff
The appropriate 7th character is to be added to code W15:
A   Initial encounter
D   Subsequent encounter
S   Sequela

W16- Fall, jump or diving into water
Excludes 1: accidental non-watercraft drowning and submersion not involving fall (W65-W74)
effects of air pressure from diving (W94.-)
fall into water from watercraft (V90-V94)
hitting an object or against bottom when falling from watercraft (V94.0)
Excludes ❷: striking or hitting diving board (W21.4)

The appropriate 7th character is to be added to each code from category W16:
A   Initial encounter
D   Subsequent encounter
S   Sequela

W16.0- Fall into swimming pool
Fall into swimming pool NOS
Excludes 1: fall into empty swimming pool (W17.3)

W16.01-Fall into swimming pool striking water surface
W16.011- Fall into swimming pool striking water surface causing drowning and submersion
Excludes 1: drowning and submersion while in swimming pool without fall (W67)

W16.012- Fall into swimming pool striking water surface causing other injury

W16.02-Fall into swimming pool striking bottom
W16.021- Fall into swimming pool striking bottom causing drowning and submersion
Excludes 1: drowning and submersion while in swimming pool without fall (W67)

W16.022- Fall into swimming pool striking bottom causing other injury

W16.03-Fall into swimming pool striking wall
W16.031- Fall into swimming pool striking wall causing drowning and submersion
Excludes 1: drowning and submersion while in swimming pool without fall (W67)

W16.032- Fall into swimming pool striking wall causing other injury

W16.1- Fall into natural body of water
Fall into lake
Fall into open sea
Fall into river
Fall into stream

W16.11-Fall into natural body of water striking water surface
W16.111- Fall into natural body of water striking water surface causing drowning and submersion
Excludes 1: drowning and submersion while in natural body of water without fall (W69)

W16.112- Fall into natural body of water striking water surface causing other injury

W16.12-Fall into natural body of water striking bottom
W16.121- Fall into natural body of water striking bottom causing drowning and submersion
Excludes 1: drowning and submersion while in natural body of water without fall (W69)

W16.122- Fall into natural body of water striking bottom causing other injury

W16.13-Fall into natural body of water striking side
W16.131- Fall into natural body of water striking side causing drowning and submersion
Excludes 1: drowning and submersion while in natural body of water without fall (W69)

W16.132- Fall into natural body of water striking side causing other injury

W16.2- Fall in (into) filled bathtub or bucket of water
W16.21-Fall in (into) filled bathtub
Excludes 1: fall into empty bathtub (W18.2)

W16.211- Fall in (into) filled bathtub causing drowning and submersion
Excludes 1: drowning and submersion while in filled bathtub without fall (W65)

W16.212- Fall in (into) filled bathtub causing other injury

W16.22-Fall in (into) bucket of water
W16.221- Fall in (into) bucket of water causing drowning and submersion

W16.222- Fall in (into) bucket of water causing other injury

W16.3- Fall into other water
Fall into fountain
Fall into reservoir

W16.31-Fall into other water striking water surface
W16.311- Fall into other water striking water surface causing drowning and submersion
Excludes 1: drowning and submersion while in other water without fall (W73)

W16.312- Fall into other water striking water surface causing other injury

W16.32-Fall into other water striking bottom
W16.321- Fall into other water striking bottom causing drowning and submersion
Excludes 1: drowning and submersion while in other water without fall (W73)

W16.322- Fall into other water striking bottom causing other injury

W16.33-Fall into other water striking wall
W16.331- Fall into other water striking wall causing drowning and submersion
Excludes 1: drowning and submersion while in other water without fall (W73)

W16.332 Fall into other water striking wall causing other injury

W11-W16

W16.4- <u>Fall</u> into <u>unspecified water</u>

    W16.41x- Fall into unspecified water <u>causing drowning and submersion</u>

    W16.42x- Fall into unspecified water <u>causing other injury</u>

W16.5- <u>Jumping or diving</u> into <u>swimming pool</u>

    W16.51- Jumping or diving into swimming pool <u>striking water surface</u>

        W16.511- Jumping or diving into swimming pool striking water surface causing drowning and submersion

            Excludes 1:   *drowning and submersion while in swimming pool without jumping or diving (W67)*

        W16.512- Jumping or diving into swimming pool striking water surface <u>causing other injury</u>

    W16.52- Jumping or diving into swimming pool <u>striking bottom</u>

        W16.521- Jumping or diving into swimming pool striking bottom <u>causing drowning and submersion</u>

            Excludes 1:   *drowning and submersion while in swimming pool without jumping or diving (W67)*

        W16.522- Jumping or diving into swimming pool striking bottom <u>causing other injury</u>

    W16.53- Jumping or diving into swimming pool <u>striking wall</u>

        W16.531- Jumping or diving into swimming pool striking wall <u>causing drowning and submersion</u>

            Excludes 1:   *drowning and submersion while in swimming pool without jumping or diving (W67)*

        W16.532- Jumping or diving into swimming pool striking wall <u>causing other injury</u>

W16.6- <u>Jumping or diving</u> into <u>natural body of water</u>

    Jumping or diving into lake

    Jumping or diving into open sea

    Jumping or diving into river

    Jumping or diving into stream

    W16.61- Jumping or diving into natural body of water <u>striking water surface</u>

        W16.611- Jumping or diving into natural body of water striking water surface <u>causing drowning and submersion</u>

            Excludes 1:   *drowning and submersion while in natural body of water without jumping or diving (W69)*

        W16.612- Jumping or diving into natural body of water striking water surface <u>causing other injury</u>

    W16.62- Jumping or diving into natural body of water <u>striking bottom</u>

        W16.621- Jumping or diving into natural body of water striking bottom <u>causing drowning and submersion</u>

            Excludes 1:   *drowning and submersion while in natural body of water without jumping ordiving (W69)*

        W16.622- Jumping or diving into natural body of water striking bottom <u>causing other injury</u>

W16.7- Jumping or diving from <u>boat</u>

    Excludes 1:   *fall from boat into water — see watercraft accident (V90-V94)*

    W16.71- Jumping or diving from boat <u>striking water surface</u>

        W16.711- Jumping or diving from boat striking water surface <u>causing drowning and submersion</u>

        W16.712- Jumping or diving from boat striking water surface <u>causing other injury</u>

    W16.72- Jumping or diving from boat <u>striking bottom</u>

        W16.721- Jumping or diving from boat striking bottom <u>causing drowning and submersion</u>

        W16.722- Jumping or diving from boat striking bottom <u>causing other injury</u>

W16.8- Jumping or diving into <u>other</u> water

    Jumping or diving into fountain

    Jumping or diving into reservoir

    W16.81- Jumping or diving into other water <u>striking water surface</u>

        W16.811- Jumping or diving into other water striking water surface <u>causing drowning and submersion</u>

            Excludes 1:   *drowning and submersion while in other water without jumping or diving (W73)*

        W16.812- Jumping or diving into other water striking water surface <u>causing other injury</u>

    W16.82- Jumping or diving into other water <u>striking bottom</u>

        W16.821- Jumping or diving into other water striking bottom <u>causing drowning and submersion</u>

            Excludes 1:   *drowning and submersion while in other water without jumping or diving (W73)*

        W16.822- Jumping or diving into other water striking bottom <u>causing other injury</u>

    W16.83- Jumping or diving into other water <u>striking wall</u>

        W16.831- Jumping or diving into other water striking wall <u>causing drowning and submersion</u>

            Excludes 1:   *drowning and submersion while in other water without jumping or diving (W73)*

        W16.832- Jumping or diving into other water striking wall <u>causing other injury</u>

W16.9- Jumping or diving into <u>unspecified water</u>

    W16.91x- Jumping or diving into unspecified water <u>causing drowning and submersion</u>

    W16.92x- Jumping or diving into unspecified water <u>causing other injury</u>

W17- <u>Other fall</u> <u>from one level to another</u>

    The appropriate 7th character is to be added to each code from category W17:

    A   <u>Initial</u> encounter

    D   <u>Subsequent</u> encounter

    S   <u>Sequela</u>

W17.0xx- Fall into well

W17.1xx- Fall into storm drain or manhole

W17.2xx- Fall into hole

    Fall into pit

W17.3xx- Fall into empty swimming pool

    Excludes 1:   *fall into filled swimming pool (W16.0-)*

W17.4xx- Fall from dock

W17.8- Other fall from one level to another

    W17.81x- Fall down embankment (hill)

    W17.82x- Fall from (out of) grocery cart

        Fall due to grocery cart tipping over

    W17.89x- Other fall from one level to another

        Fall from cherry picker

        Fall from lifting device

        Fall from mobile elevated work platform [MEWP]

        Fall from sky lift

W18- Other <u>slipping, tripping and stumbling and falls</u>

    The appropriate 7th character is to be added to each code from category W18:

    A   <u>Initial</u> encounter

    D   <u>Subsequent</u> encounter

    S   <u>Sequela</u>

W18.0- Fall due to <u>bumping against object</u>

    Striking against object with subsequent fall

    Excludes 1:   *fall on same level due to slipping, tripping, or stumbling with subsequent striking against object (W01.1-)*

    W18.00x- Striking against unspecified object with subsequent fall

    W18.01x- Striking against sports equipment with subsequent fall

    W18.02x- Striking against glass with subsequent fall

    W18.09x- Striking against other object with subsequent fall

W18.1- Fall from or off <u>toilet</u>

    W18.11x- Fall from or off toilet without subsequent striking against object

        Fall from (off) toilet NOS

W16-W18

W18.12x- Fall from or off toilet with subsequent striking against object

W18.2xx- Fall in (into) <u>shower or empty bathtub</u>
    Excludes 1:   *fall in full bathtub causing drowning or submersion (W16.21-)*

W18.3- Other and unspecified fall on same level

W18.30x- Fall on same level, unspecified

W18.31x- Fall on same level due to stepping on an object
    Fall on same level due to stepping on an animal
    Excludes 1:   *slipping, tripping and stumbling without fall due to stepping on animal (W18.41)*

W18.39x- Other fall on same level

W18.4- Slipping, tripping and stumbling <u>without falling</u>
    Excludes 1:   *collision with another person without fall (W51)*

W18.40x- Slipping, tripping and stumbling without falling, unspecified

W18.41x- Slipping, tripping and stumbling without falling due to stepping on object
    Slipping, tripping and stumbling without falling due to stepping on animal
    Excludes 1:   *slipping, tripping and stumbling with fall due to stepping on animal (W18.31)*

W18.42x- Slipping, tripping and stumbling without falling due to stepping into hole or opening

W18.43x- Slipping, tripping and stumbling without falling due to stepping from one level to another

W18.49x- Other slipping, tripping and stumbling without falling

W19.xxx- <u>Unspecified fall</u>
    Accidental fall NOS
    The appropriate 7th character is to be added to code W19:
    A <u>Initial</u> encounter
    D <u>Subsequent</u> encounter
    S <u>Sequela</u>

Exposure to inanimate mechanical forces (W20-W49)

    Excludes 1:   *assault (X92-Y09)*
            contact or collision with animals or persons (W50-W64)
            exposure to inanimate mechanical forces involving military or war operations (Y36-, Y37-)
            intentional self-harm (X71-X83)

W20- <u>Struck by thrown, projected or falling object</u>
    Code first any associated:
    Cataclysm (X34-X39)
    Lightning strike (T75.00)
    Excludes 1:   *falling object in machinery accident (W24, W28-W31)*
            falling object in transport accident (V01-V99)
            object set in motion by explosion (W35-W40)
            object set in motion by firearm (W32-W34)
            struck by thrown sports equipment (W21.-)

    The appropriate 7th character is to be added to each code from category W20:
    A <u>Initial</u> encounter
    D <u>Subsequent</u> encounter
    S <u>Sequela</u>

W20.0xx- Struck by falling object in cave-in
    Excludes ❷: *asphyxiation due to cave-in (T71.21)*

W20.1xx- Struck by object due to collapse of building
    Excludes 1:   *struck by object due to collapse of burning building (X00.2, X02.2)*

W20.8xx- Other cause of strike by thrown, projected or falling object
    Excludes 1:   *struck by thrown sports equipment (W21.-)*

W21- <u>Striking against or struck</u> by <u>sports equipment</u>
    Excludes 1:   *assault with sports equipment (Y08.0-)*
            striking against or struck by sports equipment with subsequent fall (W18.01)

    The appropriate 7th character is to be added to each code from category W21:
    A <u>Initial</u> encounter
    D <u>Subsequent</u> encounter
    S <u>Sequela</u>

W21.0- Struck by <u>hit or thrown ball</u>

W21.00x- Struck by hit or thrown ball, unspecified type

W21.01x- Struck by football

W21.02x- Struck by soccer ball

W21.03x- Struck by baseball

W21.04x- Struck by golf ball

W21.05x- Struck by basketball

W21.06x- Struck by volleyball

W21.07x- Struck by softball

W21.09x- Struck by other hit or thrown ball

W21.1- Struck by <u>bat, racquet or club</u>

W21.11x- Struck by baseball bat

W21.12x- Struck by tennis racquet

W21.13x- Struck by golf club

W21.19x- Struck by other bat, racquet or club

W21.2- Struck by <u>hockey stick or puck</u>

W21.21- Struck by hockey <u>stick</u>

W21.210- Struck by ice hockey stick

W21.211- Struck by field hockey stick

W21.22- Struck by hockey <u>puck</u>

W21.220- Struck by ice hockey puck

W21.221- Struck by field hockey puck

W21.3- Struck by <u>sports foot wear</u>

W21.31x- Struck by shoe cleats
    Stepped on by shoe cleats

W21.32x- Struck by skate blades
    Skated over by skate blades

W21.39x- Struck by other sports foot wear

W21.4xx- Striking against <u>diving board</u>
    Use additional code for subsequent falling into water, if applicable (W16.-)

W21.8- Striking against or struck by <u>other</u> sports equipment

W21.81x- Striking against or struck by football helmet

W21.89x- Striking against or struck by other sports equipment

W21.9xx- Striking against or struck by <u>unspecified</u> sports equipment

W22- <u>Striking</u> against or struck by <u>other objects</u>
    Excludes 1:   *striking against or struck by object with subsequent fall (W18.09)*

    The appropriate 7th character is to be added to each code from category W22:
    A <u>Initial</u> encounter
    D <u>Subsequent</u> encounter
    S <u>Sequela</u>

W22.0- Striking against <u>stationary object</u>
    Excludes 1:   *striking against stationary sports equipment (W21.8)*

W22.01x- Walked into wall

W22.02x- Walked into lamppost

W22.03x- Walked into furniture

W22.04- Striking against wall of swimming pool

W22.041- Striking against wall of swimming pool causing drowning and submersion
    Excludes 1:   *drowning and submersion while swimming without striking against wall (W67)*

W22.042- Striking against wall of swimming pool causing other injury

W22.09x- Striking against other stationary object

W22.1- Striking against or struck by <u>automobile airbag</u>

W22.10x- Striking against or struck by unspecified automobile airbag

W22.11x- Striking against or struck by driver side automobile airbag

W22.12x- Striking against or struck by front passenger side automobile airbag

W22.19x- Striking against or struck by other automobile airbag

W22.8xx- Striking against or struck by other objects
    Striking against or struck by object NOS
    Excludes 1:   *struck by thrown, projected or falling object (W20.-)*

W23- **Caught, crushed, jammed or pinched** **in or between objects**

Excludes 1:   *injury caused by cutting or piercing instruments (W25-W27)*
injury caused by firearms malfunction (W32.1, W33.1-, W34.1-)
injury caused by lifting and transmission devices (W24.-)
injury caused by machinery (W28-W31)
injury caused by nonpowered hand tools (W27.-)
injury caused by transport vehicle being used as a means of
transportation (V01-V99)
injury caused by struck by thrown, projected or falling object
(W20.-)

The appropriate 7th character is to be added to each code from category
W23:
A **Initial** encounter
D **Subsequent** encounter
S **Sequela**

W23.0xx- Caught, crushed, jammed, or pinched between moving
objects

W23.1xx- Caught, crushed, jammed, or pinched between stationary
objects

W24- Contact with **lifting and transmission devices**, not elsewhere
classified
Excludes 1:   *transport accidents (V01-V99)*

The appropriate 7th character is to be added to each code from category
W24:
A **Initial** encounter
D **Subsequent** encounter
S **Sequela**

W24.0xx- Contact with lifting devices, not elsewhere classified
Contact with chain hoist
Contact with drive belt
Contact with pulley (block)

W24.1xx- Contact with transmission devices, not elsewhere classified
Contact with transmission belt or cable

W25.xxx- **Contact with sharp glass**
Code first any associated:
Injury due to flying glass from explosion or firearm discharge
(W32-W40)
Transport accident (V00-V99)
Excludes 1:   *fall on same level due to slipping, tripping and*
stumbling with subsequent striking against sharp
glass (W01.10)
striking against sharp glass with subsequent fall
(W18.02)
Excludes ❷: *glass embedded in skin (W45.-)*

The appropriate 7th character is to be added to code W25:
A **Initial** encounter
D **Subsequent** encounter
S **Sequela**

W26- Contact with **other sharp objects**
Excludes ❷: *sharp object(s) embedded in skin (W45.-)*

The appropriate 7th character is to be added to each code from category
W26:
A **Initial** encounter
D **Subsequent** encounter
S **Sequela**

W26.0xx- Contact with knife
Excludes 1:   *contact with electric knife (W29.1)*

W26.1xx- Contact with sword or dagger

W26.2xx- Contact with edge of stiff paper
Paper cut

W26.8xx- Contact with other sharp object(s), not elsewhere classified
Contact with tin can lid

W26.9xx- Contact with unspecified sharp object(s)

W27- Contact with **nonpowered hand tool**

The appropriate 7th character is to be added to each code from category
W27:
A **Initial** encounter
D **Subsequent** encounter
S **Sequela**

W27.0xx- Contact with **workbench tool**
Contact with auger
Contact with axe
Contact with chisel
Contact with handsaw
Contact with screwdriver

W27.1xx- Contact with **garden tool**
Contact with hoe
Contact with nonpowered lawn mower
Contact with pitchfork
Contact with rake

W27.2xx- Contact with **scissors**

W27.3xx- Contact with **needle (sewing)**
Excludes 1:   *contact with hypodermic needle (W46.-)*

W27.4xx- Contact with **kitchen utensil**
Contact with fork
Contact with ice-pick
Contact with can-opener NOS

W27.5xx- Contact with **paper-cutter**

W27.8xx- Contact with **other nonpowered hand tool**
Contact with nonpowered sewing machine
Contact with shovel

W28.xxx- Contact with **powered lawn mower**
Powered lawn mower (commercial) (residential)
Excludes 1:   *contact with nonpowered lawn mower (W27.1)*
Excludes ❷: *exposure to electric current (W86.-)*

The appropriate 7th character is to be added to code W28:
A **Initial** encounter
D **Subsequent** encounter
S **Sequela**

W29- Contact with **other powered hand tools and household machinery**
Excludes 1:   *contact with commercial machinery (W31.82)*
contact with hot household appliance (X15)
contact with nonpowered hand tool (W27.-)
exposure to electric current (W86)

The appropriate 7th character is to be added to each code from category
W29:
A **Initial** encounter
D **Subsequent** encounter
S **Sequela**

W29.0xx- Contact with powered **kitchen** appliance
Contact with blender
Contact with can-opener
Contact with garbage disposal
Contact with mixer

W29.1xx- Contact with electric knife

W29.2xx- Contact with other powered **household** machinery
Contact with electric fan
Contact with powered dryer (clothes) (powered) (spin)
Contact with washing-machine
Contact with sewing machine

W29.3xx- Contact with powered **garden** and **outdoor** hand tools and
machinery
Contact with chainsaw
Contact with edger
Contact with garden cultivator (tiller)
Contact with hedge trimmer
Contact with other powered garden tool
Excludes 1:   *contact with powered lawn mower (W28)*

W29.4xx- Contact with **nail gun**

W29.8xx- Contact with **other** powered powered hand tools and
household machinery
Contact with do-it-yourself tool NOS

W30- Contact with **agricultural** machinery
Includes: Animal-powered farm machine
Excludes 1:   *agricultural transport vehicle accident (V01-V99)*
explosion of grain store (W40.8)
exposure to electric current (W86.-)

The appropriate 7th character is to be added to each code from category
W30:
A **Initial** encounter
D **Subsequent** encounter
S **Sequela**

W30.0xx- Contact with combine harvester
Contact with reaper
Contact with thresher

W30.1xx- Contact with power take-off devices (PTO)

W30.2xx- Contact with hay derrick

W30.3xx- Contact with grain storage elevator
Excludes 1:   *explosion of grain store (W40.8)*

W30.8-   Contact with other specified agricultural machinery

     W30.81x-   Contact with agricultural transport vehicle in stationary use

         Contact with agricultural transport vehicle under repair, not on public roadway

         Excludes 1:   *agricultural transport vehicle accident (V01-V99)*

     W30.89x-   Contact with other specified agricultural machinery

W30.9xx-   Contact with unspecified agricultural machinery

     Contact with farm machinery NOS

W31-   Contact with <u>other and unspecified</u> machinery

     Excludes 1:   *contact with agricultural machinery (W30.-)*

         contact with machinery in transport under own power or being towed by a vehicle (V01-V99)

         exposure to electric current (W86)

The appropriate 7th character is to be added to each code from category W31:

A   <u>Initial</u> encounter

D   <u>Subsequent</u> encounter

S   <u>Sequela</u>

W31.0xx-   Contact with mining and earth-drilling machinery

     Contact with bore or drill (land) (seabed)

     Contact with shaft hoist

     Contact with shaft lift

     Contact with undercutter

W31.1xx-   Contact with metalworking machines

     Contact with abrasive wheel

     Contact with forging machine

     Contact with lathe

     Contact with mechanical shears

     Contact with metal drilling machine

     Contact with milling machine

     Contact with power press

     Contact with rolling-mill

     Contact with metal sawing machine

W31.2xx-   Contact with powered woodworking and forming machines

     Contact with band saw

     Contact with bench saw

     Contact with circular saw

     Contact with molding machine

     Contact with overhead plane

     Contact with powered saw

     Contact with radial saw

     Contact with sander

     Excludes 1:   *nonpowered woodworking tools (W27.0)*

W31.3xx-   Contact with prime movers

     Contact with gas turbine

     Contact with internal combustion engine

     Contact with steam engine

     Contact with water driven turbine

W31.8-   Contact with other specified machinery

     W31.81x-   Contact with recreational machinery

         Contact with roller coaster

     W31.82x-   Contact with other commercial machinery

         Contact with commercial electric fan

         Contact with commercial kitchen appliances

         Contact with commercial powered dryer (clothes) (powered) (spin)

         Contact with commercial washing-machine

         Contact with commercial sewing machine

         Excludes 1:   *contact with household machinery (W29.-)*

             contact with powered lawn mower (W28)

     W31.83x-   Contact with special construction vehicle in stationary use

         Contact with special construction vehicle under repair, not on public roadway

         Excludes 1:   *special construction vehicle accident (V01-V99)*

     W31.89x-   Contact with other specified machinery

W31.9xx-   Contact with unspecified machinery

     Contact with machinery NOS

W32-   <u>Accidental handgun discharge and malfunction</u>

     Includes: Accidental discharge and malfunction of gun for single hand use

         Accidental discharge and malfunction of pistol

         Accidental discharge and malfunction of revolver

     Handgun discharge and malfunction NOS

     Excludes 1:   *accidental airgun discharge and malfunction (W34.010, W34.110)*

         accidental BB gun discharge and malfunction (W34.010, W34.110)

         accidental pellet gun discharge and malfunction (W34.010, W34.110)

         accidental shotgun discharge and malfunction (W33.01, W33.11)

         assault by handgun discharge (X93)

         handgun discharge involving legal intervention (Y35.0-)

         handgun discharge involving military or war operations (Y36.4-)

         intentional self-harm by handgun discharge (X72)

         Very pistol discharge and malfunction (W34.09, W34.19)

The appropriate 7th character is to be added to each code from category W32:

A   <u>Initial</u> encounter

D   <u>Subsequent</u> encounter

S   <u>Sequela</u>

W32.0xx-   Accidental <u>handgun discharge</u>

W32.1xx-   Accidental <u>handgun malfunction</u>

     Injury due to explosion of handgun (parts)

     Injury due to malfunction of mechanism or component of handgun

     Injury due to recoil of handgun

     Powder burn from handgun

W33-   <u>Accidental rifle, shotgun and larger firearm discharge and malfunction</u>

     Includes: Rifle, shotgun and larger firearm discharge and malfunction NOS

     Excludes 1:   *accidental airgun discharge and malfunction (W34.010, W34.110)*

         accidental BB gun discharge and malfunction (W34.010, W34.110)

         accidental handgun discharge and malfunction (W32.-)

         accidental pellet gun discharge and malfunction (W34.010, W34.110)

         assault by rifle, shotgun and larger firearm discharge (X94)

         firearm discharge involving legal intervention (Y35.0-)

         firearm discharge involving military or war operations (Y36.4-)

         intentional self-harm by rifle, shotgun and larger firearm discharge (X73)

The appropriate 7th character is to be added to each code from category W33:

A   <u>Initial</u> encounter

D   <u>Subsequent</u> encounter

S   <u>Sequela</u>

W33.0-   Accidental rifle, shotgun and larger firearm <u>discharge</u>

     W33.00x-   Accidental discharge of unspecified larger firearm

         Discharge of unspecified larger firearm NOS

     W33.01x-   Accidental discharge of shotgun

         Discharge of shotgun NOS

     W33.02x-   Accidental discharge of hunting rifle

         Discharge of hunting rifle NOS

     W33.03x-   Accidental discharge of machine gun

         Discharge of machine gun NOS

     W33.09x-   Accidental discharge of other larger firearm

         Discharge of other larger firearm NOS

W33.1-   Accidental rifle, shotgun and larger firearm <u>malfunction</u>

     Injury due to explosion of rifle, shotgun and larger firearm (parts)

     Injury due to malfunction of mechanism or component of rifle, shotgun and larger firearm

     Injury due to piercing, cutting, crushing or pinching due to (by) slide trigger mechanism, scope or other gunpart

     Injury due to recoil of rifle, shotgun and larger firearm

     Powder burn from rifle, shotgun and larger firearm

     W33.10x-   Accidental malfunction of unspecified larger firearm

         Malfunction of unspecified larger firearm NOS

     W33.11x-   Accidental malfunction of shotgun

         Malfunction of shotgun NOS

W30 – W33

W33.12x- Accidental malfunction of hunting rifle
　　　　Malfunction of hunting rifle NOS

W33.13x- Accidental malfunction of machine gun
　　　　Malfunction of machine gun NOS

W33.19x- Accidental malfunction of other larger firearm
　　　　Malfunction of other larger firearm NOS

W34- Accidental discharge and malfunction from other and unspecified firearms and guns

The appropriate 7th character is to be added to each code from category W34:
A **Initial** encounter
D **Subsequent** encounter
S **Sequela**

W34.0- Accidental discharge from other and unspecified firearms and guns
　　　　AHA 15:1Q:p17 – Accidental gunshot wound

W34.00x- Accidental discharge from unspecified firearms or gun
　　　　Discharge from firearm NOS
　　　　Gunshot wound NOS
　　　　Shot NOS

W34.01- Accidental discharge of gas, air or spring-operated guns

W34.010- Accidental discharge of airgun
　　　　Accidental discharge of BB gun
　　　　Accidental discharge of pellet gun

W34.011- Accidental discharge of paintball gun
　　　　Accidental injury due to paintball discharge

W34.018- Accidental discharge of other gas, air or spring-operated gun

W34.09x- Accidental discharge from other specified firearms
　　　　Accidental discharge from Very pistol [flare]

W34.1- Accidental malfunction from other and unspecified firearms and guns

W34.10x- Accidental malfunction from unspecified firearms or gun
　　　　Firearm malfunction NOS

W34.11- Accidental malfunction of gas, air or spring-operated guns

W34.110- Accidental malfunction of airgun
　　　　Accidental malfunction of BB gun
　　　　Accidental malfunction of pellet gun

W34.111- Accidental malfunction of paintball gun
　　　　Accidental injury due to paintball gun malfunction

W34.118- Accidental malfunction of other gas, air or spring-operated gun

W34.19x- Accidental malfunction from other specified firearms
　　　　Accidental malfunction from Very pistol [flare]

W35.xxx- **Explosion and rupture of boiler**
　Excludes 1: explosion and rupture of boiler on watercraft (V93.4)

The appropriate 7th character is to be added to code W35:
A **Initial** encounter
D **Subsequent** encounter
S **Sequela**

W36- Explosion and rupture of gas cylinder

The appropriate 7th character is to be added to each code from category W36:
A **Initial** encounter
D **Subsequent** encounter
S **Sequela**

W36.1xx- Explosion and rupture of aerosol can
W36.2xx- Explosion and rupture of air tank
W36.3xx- Explosion and rupture of pressurized-gas tank
W36.8xx- Explosion and rupture of other gas cylinder
W36.9xx- Explosion and rupture of unspecified gas cylinder

W37- Explosion and rupture of pressurized tire, pipe or hose

The appropriate 7th character is to be added to each code from category W37:
A **Initial** encounter
D **Subsequent** encounter
S **Sequela**

W37.0xx- Explosion of bicycle tire
W37.8xx- Explosion and rupture of other pressurized tire, pipe or hose

W38.xxx- **Explosion and rupture of other specified pressurized devices**

The appropriate 7th character is to be added to code W38
A **Initial** encounter
D **Subsequent** encounter
S **Sequela**

W39.xxx- **Discharge of firework**

The appropriate 7th character is to be added to code W39
A **Initial** encounter
D **Subsequent** encounter
S **Sequela**

W40- Explosion of other materials
　Excludes 1: assault by explosive material (X96)
　　　　explosion involving legal intervention (Y35.1-)
　　　　explosion involving military or war operations (Y36.0-, Y36.2-)
　　　　intentional self-harm by explosive material (X75)

The appropriate 7th character is to be added to each code from category W40:
A **Initial** encounter
D **Subsequent** encounter
S **Sequela**

W40.0xx- Explosion of blasting material
　　　　Explosion of blasting cap
　　　　Explosion of detonator
　　　　Explosion of dynamite
　　　　Explosion of explosive (any) used in blasting operations

W40.1xx- Explosion of explosive gases
　　　　Explosion of acetylene
　　　　Explosion of butane
　　　　Explosion of coal gas
　　　　Explosion in mine NOS
　　　　Explosion of explosive gas
　　　　Explosion of fire damp
　　　　Explosion of gasoline fumes
　　　　Explosion of methane
　　　　Explosion of propane

W40.8xx- Explosion of other specified explosive materials
　　　　Explosion in dump NOS
　　　　Explosion in factory NOS
　　　　Explosion in grain store
　　　　Explosion in munitions
　Excludes 1: explosion involving legal intervention (Y35.1-)
　　　　explosion involving military or war operations (Y36.0-, Y36.2-)

W40.9xx- Explosion of unspecified explosive materials
　　　　Explosion NOS

W42- Exposure to noise

The appropriate 7th character is to be added to each code from category W42:
A **Initial** encounter
D **Subsequent** encounter
S **Sequela**

W42.0xx- Exposure to supersonic waves
W42.9xx- Exposure to other noise
　　　　Exposure to sound waves NOS

W33 - W42

W45- Foreign body or object entering through skin
Includes: Foreign body or object embedded in skin
Nail embedded in skin
Excludes ❷: *contact with hand tools (nonpowered) (powered) (W27-W29)*
contact with other sharp object(s) (W26.-)
contact with sharp glass (W25.-)
struck by objects (W20-W22)
The appropriate 7th character is to be added to each code from category W45:
A   Initial encounter
D   Subsequent encounter
S   Sequela

W45.0xx- Nail entering through skin

W45.8xx- Other foreign body or object entering through skin
Splinter in skin NOS

W46- Contact with hypodermic needle
The appropriate 7th character is to be added to each code from category W46:
A   Initial encounter
D   Subsequent encounter
S   Sequela

W46.0xx- Contact with hypodermic needle
Hypodermic needle stick NOS

W46.1xx- Contact with contaminated hypodermic needle

W49- Exposure to other inanimate mechanical forces
Includes: Exposure to abnormal gravitational [G] forces
Exposure to inanimate mechanical forces NEC
Excludes 1:   exposure to inanimate mechanical forces involving military or war operations (Y36.-, Y37.-)
The appropriate 7th character is to be added to each code from category W49:
A   Initial encounter
D   Subsequent encounter
S   Sequela

W49.0- Item causing external constriction
W49.01x- Hair causing external constriction
W49.02x- String or thread causing external constriction
W49.03x- Rubber band causing external constriction
W49.04x- Ring or other jewelry causing external constriction
W49.09x- Other specified item causing external constriction

W49.9xx- Exposure to other inanimate mechanical forces

Exposure to animate mechanical forces (W50-W64)

Excludes 1:   toxic effect of contact with venomous animals and plants (T63.-)

W50- Accidental hit, strike, kick, twist, bite or scratch by another person
Includes: Hit, strike, kick, twist, bite, or scratch by another person NOS
Excludes 1:   assault by bodily force (Y04)
struck by objects (W20-W22)
The appropriate 7th character is to be added to each code from category W50:
A   Initial encounter
D   Subsequent encounter
S   Sequela

W50.0xx- Accidental hit or strike by another person
Hit or strike by another person NOS

W50.1xx- Accidental kick by another person
Kick by another person NOS

W50.2xx- Accidental twist by another person
AHA 15:1Q:p7 – Brother twisted his right elbow
Twist by another person NOS

W50.3xx- Accidental bite by another person
Human bite
Bite by another person NOS

W50.4xx- Accidental scratch by another person
Scratch by another person NOS

W51.xxx- Accidental striking against or bumped into by another person
Excludes 1:   assault by striking against or bumping into by another person (Y04.2)
fall due to collision with another person (W03)
The appropriate 7th character is to be added to code W51:
A   Initial encounter
D   Subsequent encounter
S   Sequela

W52.xxx- Crushed, pushed or stepped on by crowd or human stampede
Crushed, pushed or stepped on by crowd or human stampede with or without fall
The appropriate 7th character is to be added to code W52:
A   Initial encounter
D   Subsequent encounter
S   Sequela

W53- Contact with rodent
Includes: Contact with saliva, feces or urine of rodent
The appropriate 7th character is to be added to each code from category W53:
A   Initial encounter
D   Subsequent encounter
S   Sequela

W53.0- Contact with mouse
W53.01x- Bitten by mouse
W53.09x- Other contact with mouse

W53.1- Contact with rat
W53.11x- Bitten by rat
W53.19x- Other contact with rat

W53.2- Contact with squirrel
W53.21x- Bitten by squirrel
W53.29x- Other contact with squirrel

W53.8- Contact with other rodent
W53.81x- Bitten by other rodent
W53.89x- Other contact with other rodent

W54- Contact with dog
Includes: Contact with saliva, feces or urine of dog
The appropriate 7th character is to be added to each code from category W54:
A   Initial encounter
D   Subsequent encounter
S   Sequela

W54.0xx- Bitten by dog
W54.1xx- Struck by dog
Knocked over by dog
W54.8xx- Other contact with dog

W55- Contact with other mammals
Includes: Contact with saliva, feces or urine of mammal
Excludes 1:   animal being ridden- see transport accidents
bitten or struck by dog (W54)
bitten or struck by rodent (W53.-)
contact with marine mammals (W56.-)
The appropriate 7th character is to be added to each code from category W55:
A   Initial encounter
D   Subsequent encounter
S   Sequela

W55.0- Contact with cat
W55.01x- Bitten by cat
W55.03x- Scratched by cat
W55.09x- Other contact with cat

W55.1- Contact with horse
W55.11x- Bitten by horse
W55.12x- Struck by horse
W55.19x- Other contact with horse

W55.2- Contact with cow
Contact with bull
W55.21x- Bitten by cow
W55.22x- Struck by cow
Gored by bull
W55.29x- Other contact with cow

W55.3-   **Contact with** <u>other hoof stock</u>
     Contact with goats
     Contact with sheep
   W55.31x-   **Bitten by other hoof stock**
   W55.32x-   **Struck by other hoof stock**
      Gored by goat
      Gored by ram
   W55.39x-   **Other contact with other hoof stock**

W55.4-   **Contact with** <u>pig</u>
   W55.41x-   **Bitten by pig**
   W55.42x-   **Struck by pig**
   W55.49x-   **Other contact with pig**

W55.5-   **Contact with** <u>raccoon</u>
   W55.51x-   **Bitten by raccoon**
   W55.52x-   **Struck by raccoon**
   W55.59x-   **Other contact with raccoon**

W55.8-   **Contact with** <u>other mammals</u>
   W55.81x-   **Bitten by other mammals**
   W55.82x-   **Struck by other mammals**
   W55.89x-   **Other contact with other mammals**

W56-   **Contact with** <u>nonvenomous marine animal</u>
   Excludes 1:   contact with venomous marine animal (T63.-)
   The appropriate 7th character is to be added to each code from category
     W56:
     A   <u>Initial</u> encounter
     D   <u>Subsequent</u> encounter
     S   <u>Sequela</u>

W56.0-   **Contact with** <u>dolphin</u>
   W56.01x-   **Bitten by dolphin**
   W56.02x-   **Struck by dolphin**
   W56.09x-   **Other contact with dolphin**

W56.1-   **Contact with** <u>sea lion</u>
   W56.11x-   **Bitten by sea lion**
   W56.12x-   **Struck by sea lion**
   W56.19x-   **Other contact with sea lion**

W56.2-   **Contact with** <u>orca</u>
     Contact with killer whale
   W56.21x-   **Bitten by orca**
   W56.22x-   **Struck by orca**
   W56.29x-   **Other contact with orca**

W56.3-   **Contact with** <u>other marine mammals</u>
   W56.31x-   **Bitten by other marine mammals**
   W56.32x-   **Struck by other marine mammals**
   W56.39x-   **Other contact with other marine mammals**

W56.4-   **Contact with** <u>shark</u>
   W56.41x-   **Bitten by shark**
   W56.42x-   **Struck by shark**
   W56.49x-   **Other contact with shark**

W56.5-   **Contact with** <u>other fish</u>
   W56.51x-   **Bitten by other fish**
   W56.52x-   **Struck by other fish**
   W56.59x-   **Other contact with other fish**

W56.8-   **Contact with** <u>other nonvenomous marine animals</u>
   W56.81x-   **Bitten by other nonvenomous marine animals**
   W56.82x-   **Struck by other nonvenomous marine animals**
   W56.89x-   **Other contact with other nonvenomous marine animals**

W57.xxx-   **Bitten or stung by** <u>nonvenomous insect and other</u>
<u>nonvenomous arthropods</u>
   Excludes 1:   contact with venomous insects and arthropods (T63.2-,
           T63.3-, T63.4-)
   The appropriate 7th character is to be added to code W57:
     A   <u>Initial</u> encounter
     D   <u>Subsequent</u> encounter
     S   <u>Sequela</u>

W58-   **Contact with** <u>crocodile or alligator</u>
   The appropriate 7th character is to be added to each code from category
     W58:
     A   <u>Initial</u> encounter
     D   <u>Subsequent</u> encounter
     S   <u>Sequela</u>

W58.0-   **Contact with** <u>alligator</u>
   W58.01x-   **Bitten by alligator**
   W58.02x-   **Struck by alligator**
   W58.03x-   **Crushed by alligator**
   W58.09x-   **Other contact with alligator**

W58.1-   **Contact with** <u>crocodile</u>
   W58.11x-   **Bitten by crocodile**
   W58.12x-   **Struck by crocodile**
   W58.13x-   **Crushed by crocodile**
   W58.19x-   **Other contact with crocodile**

W59-   **Contact with** <u>other nonvenomous reptiles</u>
   Excludes 1:   contact with venomous reptile (T63.0-, T63.1-)
   The appropriate 7th character is to be added to each code from category
     W59:
     A   <u>Initial</u> encounter
     D   <u>Subsequent</u> encounter
     S   <u>Sequela</u>

W59.0-   **Contact with** <u>nonvenomous lizards</u>
   W59.01x-   **Bitten by nonvenomous lizards**
   W59.02x-   **Struck by nonvenomous lizards**
   W59.09x-   **Other contact with nonvenomous lizards**
      Exposure to nonvenomous lizards

W59.1-   **Contact with** <u>nonvenomous snakes</u>
   W59.11x-   **Bitten by nonvenomous snake**
   W59.12x-   **Struck by nonvenomous snake**
   W59.13x-   **Crushed by nonvenomous snake**
   W59.19x-   **Other contact with nonvenomous snake**

W59.2-   **Contact with** <u>turtles</u>
     Excludes 1:   contact with tortoises (W59.8-)
   W59.21x-   **Bitten by turtle**
   W59.22x-   **Struck by turtle**
   W59.29x-   **Other contact with turtle**
      Exposure to turtles

W59.8-   **Contact with** <u>other nonvenomous reptiles</u>
   W59.81x-   **Bitten by other nonvenomous reptiles**
   W59.82x-   **Struck by other nonvenomous reptiles**
   W59.83x-   **Crushed by other nonvenomous reptiles**
   W59.89x-   **Other contact with other nonvenomous reptiles**

W60.xxx-   **Contact with** <u>nonvenomous plant thorns and spines and sharp</u>
<u>leaves</u>
   Excludes 1:   contact with venomous plants (T63.7-)
   The appropriate 7th character is to be added to code W60
     A   <u>Initial</u> encounter
     D   <u>Subsequent</u> encounter
     S   <u>Sequela</u>

W61-   **Contact with** <u>birds (domestic) (wild)</u>
   Includes: Contact with excreta of birds
   The appropriate 7th character is to be added to each code from category
     W61:
     A   <u>Initial</u> encounter
     D   <u>Subsequent</u> encounter
     S   <u>Sequela</u>

W61.0-   **Contact with** <u>parrot</u>
   W61.01x-   **Bitten by parrot**
   W61.02x-   **Struck by parrot**
   W61.09x-   **Other contact with parrot**
      Exposure to parrots

W 5 5 - W 6 1

W61.1- Contact with <u>macaw</u>
  W61.11x- Bitten by macaw
  W61.12x- Struck by macaw
  W61.19x- Other contact with macaw
      Exposure to macaws
W61.2- Contact with <u>other psittacines</u>
  W61.21x- Bitten by other psittacines
  W61.22x- Struck by other psittacines
  W61.29x- Other contact with other psittacines
      Exposure to other psittacines
W61.3- Contact with <u>chicken</u>
  W61.32x- Struck by chicken
  W61.33x- Pecked by chicken
  W61.39x- Other contact with chicken
      Exposure to chickens
W61.4- Contact with <u>turkey</u>
  W61.42x- Struck by turkey
  W61.43x- Pecked by turkey
  W61.49x- Other contact with turkey
W61.5- Contact with <u>goose</u>
  W61.51x- Bitten by goose
  W61.52x- Struck by goose
  W61.59x- Other contact with goose
W61.6- Contact with <u>duck</u>
  W61.61x- Bitten by duck
  W61.62x- Struck by duck
  W61.69x- Other contact with duck
W61.9- Contact with <u>other birds</u>
  W61.91x- Bitten by other birds
  W61.92x- Struck by other birds
  W61.99x- Other contact with other birds
      Contact with bird NOS

W62- Contact with <u>nonvenomous amphibians</u>
  Excludes 1:   contact with venomous amphibians (T63.81-R63.83)
  The appropriate 7th character is to be added to each code from category W62:
      A   <u>Initial</u> encounter
      D   <u>Subsequent</u> encounter
      S   <u>Sequela</u>
  W62.0xx- Contact with nonvenomous frogs
  W62.1xx- Contact with nonvenomous toads
  W62.9xx- Contact with other nonvenomous amphibians

W64.xxx- <u>Exposure to other animate mechanical forces</u>
  Includes: Exposure to nonvenomous animal NOS
  Excludes 1:   contact with venomous animal (T63.-)
  The appropriate 7th character is to be added to code W64:
      A   <u>Initial</u> encounter
      D   <u>Subsequent</u> encounter
      S   <u>Sequela</u>

Accidental non-transport drowning and submersion (W65-W74)

Excludes 1:   accidental drowning and submersion due to fall into water (W16.-)
            accidental drowning and submersion due to water transport accident (V90.-, V92.-)
Excludes ❷: accidental drowning and submersion due to cataclysm (X34-X39)

W65.xxx- <u>Accidental drowning and submersion while in bath-tub</u>
  Excludes 1:   accidental drowning and submersion due to fall in (into) bathtub (W16.211)
  The appropriate 7th character is to be added to code W65:
      A   <u>Initial</u> encounter
      D   <u>Subsequent</u> encounter
      S   <u>Sequela</u>

W67.xxx- <u>Accidental drowning and submersion while in swimming-pool</u>
  Excludes 1:   accidental drowning and submersion due to fall into swimming pool (W16.011, W16.021, W16.031)
            accidental drowning and submersion due to striking into wall of swimming pool (W22.041)
  The appropriate 7th character is to be added to code W67:
      A   <u>Initial</u> encounter
      D   <u>Subsequent</u> encounter
      S   <u>Sequela</u>

W69.xxx- <u>Accidental drowning and submersion while in natural water</u>
      Accidental drowning and submersion while in lake
      Accidental drowning and submersion while in open sea
      Accidental drowning and submersion while in river
      Accidental drowning and submersion while in stream
  Excludes 1:   accidental drowning and submersion due to fall into natural body of water (W16.111, W16.121, W16.131)
  The appropriate 7th character is to be added to code W69:
      A   <u>Initial</u> encounter
      D   <u>Subsequent</u> encounter
      S   <u>Sequela</u>

W73.xxx- <u>Other specified cause of accidental non-transport drowning and submersion</u>
      Accidental drowning and submersion while in quenching tank
      Accidental drowning and submersion while in reservoir
  Excludes 1:   accidental drowning and submersion due to fall into other water (W16.311, W16.321, W16.331)
  The appropriate 7th character is to be added to code W73:
      A   <u>Initial</u> encounter
      D   <u>Subsequent</u> encounter
      S   <u>Sequela</u>

W74.xxx- <u>Unspecified cause of accidental drowning and submersion</u>
      Drowning NOS
  The appropriate 7th character is to be added to code W74:
      A   <u>Initial</u> encounter
      D   <u>Subsequent</u> encounter
      S   <u>Sequela</u>

Exposure to electric current, radiation and extreme ambient air temperature and pressure (W85-W99)

Excludes 1:   exposure to:
            lightning (T75.0-)
            natural cold (X31)
            natural heat (X30)
            natural radiation NOS (X39)
            radiological procedure and radiotherapy (Y84.2)
            sunlight (X32)
            failure in dosage of radiation or temperature during surgical and medical care (Y63.2-Y63.5)

W85.xxx- <u>Exposure to electric transmission lines</u>
      Broken power line
  The appropriate 7th character is to be added to code W85:
      A   <u>Initial</u> encounter
      D   <u>Subsequent</u> encounter
      S   <u>Sequela</u>

W61 - W85

W86- Exposure to other specified electric current

The appropriate 7th character is to be added to each code from category W86:

- **A** Initial encounter
- **D** Subsequent encounter
- **S** Sequela

W86.0xx- Exposure to domestic wiring and appliances

W86.1xx- Exposure to industrial wiring, appliances and electrical machinery
Exposure to conductors
Exposure to control apparatus
Exposure to electrical equipment and machinery
Exposure to transformers

W86.8xx- Exposure to other electric current
Exposure to wiring and appliances in or on farm (not farmhouse)
Exposure to wiring and appliances outdoors
Exposure to wiring and appliances in or on public building
Exposure to wiring and appliances in or on residential institutions
Exposure to wiring and appliances in or on schools

W88- Exposure to ionizing radiation

Excludes 1:   exposure to sunlight (X32)

The appropriate 7th character is to be added to each code from category W88:

- **A** Initial encounter
- **D** Subsequent encounter
- **S** Sequela

W88.0xx- Exposure to X-rays

W88.1xx- Exposure to radioactive isotopes

W88.8xx- Exposure to other ionizing radiation

W89- Exposure to man-made visible and ultraviolet light

Includes: Exposure to welding light (arc)

Excludes 1:   exposure to sunlight (X32)

The appropriate 7th character is to be added to each code from category W89:

- **A** Initial encounter
- **D** Subsequent encounter
- **S** Sequela

W89.0xx- Exposure to welding light (arc)

W89.1xx- Exposure to tanning bed

W89.8xx- Exposure to other man-made visible and ultraviolet light

W89.9xx- Exposure to unspecified man-made visible and ultraviolet light

W90- Exposure to other nonionizing radiation

Excludes 1:   exposure to sunlight (X32)

The appropriate 7th character is to be added to each code from category W90:

- **A** Initial encounter
- **D** Subsequent encounter
- **S** Sequela

W90.0xx- Exposure to radiofrequency

W90.1xx- Exposure to infrared radiation

W90.2xx- Exposure to laser radiation

W90.8xx- Exposure to other nonionizing radiation

W92.xxx- Exposure to excessive heat of man-made origin

The appropriate 7th character is to be added to code W92:

- **A** Initial encounter
- **D** Subsequent encounter
- **S** Sequela

W93- Exposure to excessive cold of man-made origin

The appropriate 7th character is to be added to each code from category W93:

- **A** Initial encounter
- **D** Subsequent encounter
- **S** Sequela

W93.0- Contact with or inhalation of dry ice

W93.01x- Contact with dry ice

W93.02x- Inhalation of dry ice

W93.1- Contact with or inhalation of liquid air

W93.11x- Contact with liquid air
Contact with liquid hydrogen
Contact with liquid nitrogen

W93.12x- Inhalation of liquid air
Inhalation of liquid hydrogen
Inhalation of liquid nitrogen

W93.2xx- Prolonged exposure in deep freeze unit or refrigerator

W93.8xx- Exposure to other excessive cold of man-made origin

W94- Exposure to high and low air pressure and changes in air pressure

The appropriate 7th character is to be added to each code from category W94:

- **A** Initial encounter
- **D** Subsequent encounter
- **S** Sequela

W94.0xx- Exposure to prolonged high air pressure

W94.1- Exposure to prolonged low air pressure

W94.11x- Exposure to residence or prolonged visit at high altitude

W94.12x- Exposure to other prolonged low air pressure

W94.2- Exposure to rapid changes in air pressure during ascent

W94.21x- Exposure to reduction in atmospheric pressure while surfacing from deep-water diving

W94.22x- Exposure to reduction in atmospheric pressure while surfacing from underground

W94.23x- Exposure to sudden change in air pressure in aircraft during ascent

W94.29x- Exposure to other rapid changes in air pressure during ascent

W94.3- Exposure to rapid changes in air pressure during descent

W94.31x- Exposure to sudden change in air pressure in aircraft during descent

W94.32x- Exposure to high air pressure from rapid descent in water

W94.39x- Exposure to other rapid changes in air pressure during descent

W99.xxx- Exposure to other man-made environmental factors

The appropriate 7th character is to be added to code W99:

- **A** Initial encounter
- **D** Subsequent encounter
- **S** Sequela

Exposure to smoke, fire and flames (X00-X08)

Excludes 1:   arson (X97)
Excludes 2:   explosions (W35-W40)
lightning (T75.0-)
transport accident (V01-V99)

X00- Exposure to uncontrolled fire in building or structure

Includes: Conflagration in building or structure

Code first any associated cataclysm

Excludes 2:   exposure to ignition or melting of nightwear (X05)
exposure to ignition or melting of other clothing and apparel (X06.-)
exposure to other specified smoke, fire and flames (X08.-)

The appropriate 7th character is to be added to each code from category X00:

- **A** Initial encounter
- **D** Subsequent encounter
- **S** Sequela

X00.0xx- Exposure to flames in uncontrolled fire in building or structure

X00.1xx- Exposure to smoke in uncontrolled fire in building or structure

X00.2xx- Injury due to collapse of burning building or structure in uncontrolled fire

Excludes 1:   injury due to collapse of building not on fire (W20.1)

X00.3xx- Fall from burning building or structure in uncontrolled fire

X00.4xx- Hit by object from burning building or structure in uncontrolled fire

X00.5xx- Jump from burning building or structure in uncontrolled fire

X00.8xx- Other exposure to uncontrolled fire in building or structure

W 8 6 I X 0 0

X01- Exposure to <u>uncontrolled fire, not in</u> building or structure
Includes: Exposure to forest fire

The appropriate 7th character is to be added to each code from category X01:
- **A** <u>Initial</u> encounter
- **D** <u>Subsequent</u> encounter
- **S** <u>Sequela</u>

X01.0xx- Exposure to <u>flames</u> in uncontrolled fire, not in building or structure

X01.1xx- Exposure to <u>smoke</u> in uncontrolled fire, not in building or structure

X01.3xx- <u>Fall</u> due to uncontrolled fire, not in building or structure

X01.4xx- <u>Hit</u> by object due to uncontrolled fire, not in building or structure

X01.8xx- <u>Other</u> exposure to uncontrolled fire, not in building or structure

X02- Exposure to <u>controlled fire</u> in <u>building or structure</u>
Includes: Exposure to fire in fireplace
Exposure to fire in stove

The appropriate 7th character is to be added to each code from category X02:
- **A** <u>Initial</u> encounter
- **D** <u>Subsequent</u> encounter
- **S** <u>Sequela</u>

X02.0xx- Exposure to <u>flames</u> in controlled fire in building or structure

X02.1xx- Exposure to <u>smoke</u> in controlled fire in building or structure

X02.2xx- Injury due to <u>collapse</u> of burning building or structure in controlled fire
Excludes 1: injury due to collapse of building not on fire (W20.1)

X02.3xx- <u>Fall</u> from burning building or structure in controlled fire

X02.4xx- <u>Hit by object</u> from burning building or structure in controlled fire

X02.5xx- <u>Jump</u> from burning building or structure in controlled fire

X02.8xx- <u>Other</u> exposure to controlled fire in building or structure

X03- Exposure to <u>controlled fire, not in</u> building or structure
Includes: Exposure to bon fire
Exposure to camp-fire
Exposure to trash fire

The appropriate 7th character is to be added to each code from category X03:
- **A** <u>Initial</u> encounter
- **D** <u>Subsequent</u> encounter
- **S** <u>Sequela</u>

X03.0xx- Exposure to <u>flames</u> in controlled fire, not in building or structure

X03.1xx- Exposure to <u>smoke</u> in controlled fire, not in building or structure

X03.3xx- <u>Fall</u> due to controlled fire, not in building or structure

X03.4xx- <u>Hit by object</u> due to controlled fire, not in building or structure

X03.8xx- <u>Other</u> exposure to controlled fire, not in building or structure

X04.xxx- Exposure to ignition of highly flammable material
Includes: Exposure to ignition of gasoline
Exposure to ignition of kerosene
Exposure to ignition of petrol
Excludes ❷: exposure to ignition or melting of nightwear (X05)
exposure to ignition or melting of other clothing and apparel (X06)

The appropriate 7th character is to be added to code X04:
- **A** <u>Initial</u> encounter
- **D** <u>Subsequent</u> encounter
- **S** <u>Sequela</u>

X05.xxx- Exposure to <u>ignition or melting of nightwear</u>
Excludes ❷: exposure to <u>uncontrolled</u> fire in building or structure (X00.-)
exposure to <u>uncontrolled</u> fire, not in building or structure (X01.-)
exposure to <u>controlled</u> fire in building or structure (X02.-)
exposure to controlled fire, not in building or structure (X03.-)
exposure to ignition of highly flammable materials (X04.-)

The appropriate 7th character is to be added to code X05:
- **A** <u>Initial</u> encounter
- **D** <u>Subsequent</u> encounter
- **S** <u>Sequela</u>

X06- Exposure to <u>ignition or melting of other clothing and apparel</u>
Excludes ❷: exposure to uncontrolled fire in building or structure (X00.-)
exposure to uncontrolled fire, not in building or structure (X01.-)
exposure to controlled fire in building or structure (X02.-)
exposure to controlled fire, not in building or structure (X03.-)
exposure to ignition of highly flammable materials (X04.-)

The appropriate 7th character is to be added to each code from category X06:
- **A** <u>Initial</u> encounter
- **D** <u>Subsequent</u> encounter
- **S** <u>Sequela</u>

X06.0xx- Exposure to ignition of plastic jewelry

X06.1xx- Exposure to melting of plastic jewelry

X06.2xx- Exposure to ignition of other clothing and apparel

X06.3xx- Exposure to melting of other clothing and apparel

X08- Exposure to <u>other specified smoke, fire and flames</u>
The appropriate 7th character is to be added to each code from category X08:
- **A** <u>Initial</u> encounter
- **D** <u>Subsequent</u> encounter
- **S** <u>Sequela</u>

X08.0- Exposure to <u>bed fire</u>
Exposure to mattress fire

X08.00x- Exposure to bed fire due to unspecified burning material

X08.01x- Exposure to bed fire due to burning cigarette

X08.09x- Exposure to bed fire due to other burning material

X08.1- Exposure to <u>sofa fire</u>

X08.10x- Exposure to sofa fire due to unspecified burning material

X08.11x- Exposure to sofa fire due to burning cigarette

X08.19x- Exposure to sofa fire due to other burning material

X08.2- Exposure to <u>other furniture fire</u>

X08.20x- Exposure to other furniture fire due to unspecified burning material

X08.21x- Exposure to other furniture fire due to burning cigarette

X08.29x- Exposure to other furniture fire due to other burning material

X08.8xx- Exposure to <u>other specified smoke, fire and flames</u>

Contact with heat and hot substances (X10-X19)

Excludes 1: exposure to excessive natural heat (X30)
exposure to fire and flames (X00-X09)

X10- Contact with <u>hot drinks, food, fats and cooking oils</u>
The appropriate 7th character is to be added to each code from category X10:
- **A** <u>Initial</u> encounter
- **D** <u>Subsequent</u> encounter
- **S** <u>Sequela</u>

X10.0xx- Contact with hot drinks

X10.1xx- Contact with hot food

X10.2xx- Contact with fats and cooking oils

X01 - X10

X11- Contact with <u>hot tap-water</u>
Includes: Contact with boiling tap-water
            Contact with boiling water NOS
Excludes 1:   contact with water heated on stove (X12)
The appropriate 7th character is to be added to each code from category
X11:
A   <u>Initial</u> encounter
D   <u>Subsequent</u> encounter
S   <u>Sequela</u>

X11.0xx- Contact with hot water in bath or tub
Excludes 1:   contact with running hot water in bath or tub (X11.1)

X11.1xx- Contact with running hot water
Contact with hot water running out of hose
Contact with hot water running out of tap

X11.8xx- Contact with other hot tap-water
Contact with hot water in bucket
Contact with hot tap-water NOS

X12.xxx- Contact with <u>other hot fluids</u>
Contact with water heated on stove
Excludes 1:   hot (liquid) metals (X18)
The appropriate 7th character is to be added to code X12:
A   <u>Initial</u> encounter
D   <u>Subsequent</u> encounter
S   <u>Sequela</u>

X13- Contact with <u>steam and other hot vapors</u>
The appropriate 7th character is to be added to each code from category
X13:
A   <u>Initial</u> encounter
D   <u>Subsequent</u> encounter
S   <u>Sequela</u>

X13.0xx- Inhalation of steam and other hot vapors

X13.1xx- Other contact with steam and other hot vapors

X14- Contact with <u>hot air and other hot gases</u>
The appropriate 7th character is to be added to each code from category
X14:
A   <u>Initial</u> encounter
D   <u>Subsequent</u> encounter
S   <u>Sequela</u>

X14.0xx- Inhalation of hot air and gases

X14.1xx- Other contact with hot air and other hot gases

X15- Contact with <u>hot household appliances</u>
Excludes 1:   contact with heating appliances (X16)
*   contact with powered household appliances (W29.-)*
*   exposure to controlled fire in building or structure due to*
*   household appliance (X02.8)*
*   exposure to household appliances electrical current (W86.0)*
The appropriate 7th character is to be added to each code from category
X15:
A   <u>Initial</u> encounter
D   <u>Subsequent</u> encounter
S   <u>Sequela</u>

X15.0xx- Contact with hot stove (kitchen)

X15.1xx- Contact with hot toaster

X15.2xx- Contact with hotplate

X15.3xx- Contact with hot saucepan or skillet

X15.8xx- Contact with other hot household appliances
Contact with cooker
Contact with kettle
Contact with light bulbs

X16.xxx- Contact with <u>hot heating appliances, radiators and pipes</u>
Excludes 1:   contact with powered appliances (W29.-)
*   exposure to controlled fire in building or structure due*
*   to appliance (X02.8)*
*   exposure to industrial appliances electrical current*
*   (W86.1)*
The appropriate 7th character is to be added to code X16:
A   <u>Initial</u> encounter
D   <u>Subsequent</u> encounter
S   <u>Sequela</u>

X17.xxx- Contact with <u>hot engines, machinery and tools</u>
Excludes 1:   contact with hot heating appliances, radiators and pipes
*   (X16)*
*   contact with hot household appliances (X15)*
The appropriate 7th character is to be added to code X17:
A   <u>Initial</u> encounter
D   <u>Subsequent</u> encounter
S   <u>Sequela</u>

X18.xxx- Contact with <u>other hot metals</u>
Contact with liquid metal
The appropriate 7th character is to be added to code X18:
A   <u>Initial</u> encounter
D   <u>Subsequent</u> encounter
S   <u>Sequela</u>

X19.xxx- Contact with <u>other heat and hot substances</u>
Excludes 1:   objects that are not normally hot, e.g., an object made
*   hot by a house fire (X00-X09)*
The appropriate 7th character is to be added to code X19:
A   <u>Initial</u> encounter
D   <u>Subsequent</u> encounter
S   <u>Sequela</u>

Exposure to forces of nature (X30-X39)

X30.xxx- Exposure to <u>excessive natural heat</u>
Exposure to excessive heat as the cause of sunstroke
Exposure to heat NOS
Excludes 1:   excessive heat of man-made origin (W92)
*   exposure to man-made radiation (W89)*
*   exposure to sunlight (X32)*
*   exposure to tanning bed (W89)*
The appropriate 7th character is to be added to code X30:
A   <u>Initial</u> encounter
D   <u>Subsequent</u> encounter
S   <u>Sequela</u>

X31.xxx- Exposure to <u>excessive natural cold</u>
Excessive cold as the cause of chilblains NOS
Excessive cold as the cause of immersion foot or hand
Exposure to cold NOS
Exposure to weather conditions
Excludes 1:   cold of man-made origin (W93.-)
*   contact with or inhalation of dry ice (W93.-)*
*   contact with or inhalation of liquefied gas (W93.-)*
The appropriate 7th character is to be added to code X31:
A   <u>Initial</u> encounter
D   <u>Subsequent</u> encounter
S   <u>Sequela</u>

X32.xxx- Exposure to <u>sunlight</u>
Excludes 1:   man-made radiation (tanning bed) (W89)
The appropriate 7th character is to be added to code X32:
A   <u>Initial</u> encounter
D   <u>Subsequent</u> encounter
S   <u>Sequela</u>

X34.xxx- Earthquake
Excludes ❷: tidal wave (tsunami) due to earthquake (X37.41)
The appropriate 7th character is to be added to code X34:
A   <u>Initial</u> encounter
D   <u>Subsequent</u> encounter
S   <u>Sequela</u>

X35.xxx- Volcanic eruption
Excludes ❷: tidal wave (tsunami) due to volcanic eruption (X37.41)
The appropriate 7th character is to be added to code X35:
A   <u>Initial</u> encounter
D   <u>Subsequent</u> encounter
S   <u>Sequela</u>

X11-X35

X36-   Avalanche, landslide and other earth movements

Includes: Victim of mudslide of cataclysmic nature

Excludes 1:   *earthquake (X34)*

Excludes ❷: *transport accident involving collision with avalanche or landslide not in motion (V01-V99)*

The appropriate 7th character is to be added to each code from category X36:

     A   <u>Initial</u> encounter

     D   <u>Subsequent</u> encounter

     S   <u>Sequela</u>

X36.0xx-   Collapse of dam or man-made structure causing earth movement

X36.1xx-   Avalanche, landslide, or mudslide

X37-   <u>Cataclysmic storm</u>

The appropriate 7th character is to be added to each code from category X37:

     A   <u>Initial</u> encounter

     D   <u>Subsequent</u> encounter

     S   <u>Sequela</u>

X37.0xx-   Hurricane

     Storm surge

     Typhoon

X37.1xx-   Tornado

     Cyclone

     Twister

X37.2xx-   Blizzard (snow) (ice)

X37.3xx-   Dust storm

X37.4-   Tidalwave

     X37.41x-   Tidal wave due to earthquake or volcanic eruption

         Tidal wave NOS

         Tsunami

     X37.42x-   Tidal wave due to storm

     X37.43x-   Tidal wave due to landslide

X37.8xx-   Other cataclysmic storms

     Cloudburst

     Torrential rain

     Excludes ❷: *flood (X38)*

X37.9xx-   Unspecified cataclysmic storm

     Storm NOS

     Excludes 1:   *collapse of dam or man-made structure causing earth movement (X39.0)*

X38.xxx-   Flood

     Flood arising from remote storm

     Flood of cataclysmic nature arising from melting snow

     Flood resulting directly from storm

     Excludes 1:   *collapse of dam or man-made structure causing earth movement (X39.0)*

                 tidal wave NOS (X37.41)

                 tidal wave caused by storm (X37.2)

The appropriate 7th character is to be added to code X38:

     A   <u>Initial</u> encounter

     D   <u>Subsequent</u> encounter

     S   <u>Sequela</u>

X39-   Exposure to <u>other forces of nature</u>

The appropriate 7th character is to be added to each code from category X39:

     A   <u>Initial</u> encounter

     D   <u>Subsequent</u> encounter

     S   <u>Sequela</u>

X39.0-   Exposure to natural radiation

     Excludes 1:   *contact with and (suspected) exposure to radon and other naturally occuring radiation (Z77.123)*

                 exposure to man-made radiation (W88-W90)

                 exposure to sunlight (X32)

     X39.01x-   Exposure to radon

     X39.08x-   Exposure to other natural radiation

X39.8xx-   Other exposure to forces of nature

Overexertion and strenuous or repetitive movements (X50)

X50-   Overexertion and strenuous or repetitive movement or load

The appropriate 7th character is to be added to each code from category X50:

     A   <u>Initial</u> encounter

     D   <u>Subsequent</u> encounter

     S   <u>Sequela</u>

X50.0xx-   Overexertion from strenuous movements

     Lifting heavy objects

     Lifting weights

X50.1xx-   Overexertion from prolonged static or awkward postures

     Prolonged bending

     Prolonged kneeling

     Prolonged reaching

     Prolonged sitting

     Prolonged standing

     Prolonged twisting

     Static bending

     Static kneeling

     Static reaching

     Static sitting

     Static standing

     Static twisting

X50.3xx-   Overexertion from repetitive movements

     Use of hand as hammer

     Excludes ❷: *overuse from prolonged static or awkward postures (X50.1)*

X50.9xx-   Other and unspecified overexertion or strenuous movements or postures

     Contact pressure

     Contact stress

Accidental exposure to other specified factors (X52-X58)

X52.xxx-   Prolonged stay in weightless environment

     Weightlessness in spacecraft (simulator)

The appropriate 7th character is to be added to code X52:

     A   <u>Initial</u> encounter

     D   <u>Subsequent</u> encounter

     S   <u>Sequela</u>

X58.xxx-   Exposure to other specified factors

     Accident NOS

     Exposure NOS

The appropriate 7th character is to be added to code X58:

     A   <u>Initial</u> encounter

     D   <u>Subsequent</u> encounter

     S   <u>Sequela</u>

Intentional self-harm (X71-X83)

Purposely self-inflicted injury

Suicide (attempted)

X71-   <u>Intentional self-harm</u> by <u>drowning and submersion</u>

The appropriate 7th character is to be added to each code from category X71:

     A   <u>Initial</u> encounter

     D   <u>Subsequent</u> encounter

     S   <u>Sequela</u>

X71.0xx-   Intentional self-harm by drowning and submersion while in <u>bathtub</u>

X71.1xx-   Intentional self-harm by drowning and submersion <u>while in swimming pool</u>

X71.2xx-   Intentional self-harm by drowning and submersion after <u>jump into swimming pool</u>

X71.3xx-   Intentional self-harm by drowning and submersion in <u>natural water</u>

X71.8xx-   <u>Other</u> intentional self-harm by drowning and submersion

X71.9xx-   Intentional self-harm by drowning and submersion, <u>unspecified</u>

X
3
6
–
X
7
1

X72.xxx- <u>Intentional self-harm</u> by <u>handgun discharge</u>
Intentional self-harm by gun for single hand use
Intentional self-harm by pistol
Intentional self-harm by revolver
Excludes 1: Very pistol (X74.8)
The appropriate 7th character is to be added to code X72:
  A <u>Initial</u> encounter
  D <u>Subsequent</u> encounter
  S <u>Sequela</u>

X73- <u>Intentional self-harm</u> by <u>rifle, shotgun and larger firearm discharge</u>
Excludes 1: airgun (X74.01)
The appropriate 7th character is to be added to each code from category X73:
  A <u>Initial</u> encounter
  D <u>Subsequent</u> encounter
  S <u>Sequela</u>

X73.0xx- Intentional self-harm by shotgun discharge
X73.1xx- Intentional self-harm by hunting rifle discharge
X73.2xx- Intentional self-harm by machine gun discharge
X73.8xx- Intentional self-harm by other larger firearm discharge
X73.9xx- Intentional self-harm by unspecified larger firearm discharge

X74- <u>Intentional self-harm</u> by <u>other and unspecified firearm and gun discharge</u>
The appropriate 7th character is to be added to each code from category X74:
  A <u>Initial</u> encounter
  D <u>Subsequent</u> encounter
  S <u>Sequela</u>

X74.0- Intentional self-harm by gas, air or spring-operated guns
  X74.01x- Intentional self-harm by airgun
    Intentional self-harm by BB gun discharge
    Intentional self-harm by pellet gun discharge
  X74.02x- Intentional self-harm by paintball gun
  X74.09x- Intentional self-harm by other gas, air or spring-operated gun
X74.8xx- Intentional self-harm by other firearm discharge
    Intentional self-harm by Very pistol [flare] discharge
X74.9xx- Intentional self-harm by unspecified firearm discharge

X75.xxx- <u>Intentional self-harm</u> by <u>explosive material</u>
The appropriate 7th character is to be added to code X75:
  A <u>Initial</u> encounter
  D <u>Subsequent</u> encounter
  S <u>Sequela</u>

X76.xxx- <u>Intentional self-harm</u> by <u>smoke, fire and flames</u>
The appropriate 7th character is to be added to code X76:
  A <u>Initial</u> encounter
  D <u>Subsequent</u> encounter
  S <u>Sequela</u>

X77- <u>Intentional self-harm</u> by <u>steam, hot vapors and hot objects</u>
The appropriate 7th character is to be added to each code from category X77:
  A <u>Initial</u> encounter
  D <u>Subsequent</u> encounter
  S <u>Sequela</u>

X77.0xx- Intentional self-harm by steam or hot vapors
X77.1xx- Intentional self-harm by hot tap water
X77.2xx- Intentional self-harm by other hot fluids
X77.3xx- Intentional self-harm by hot household appliances
X77.8xx- Intentional self-harm by other hot objects
X77.9xx- Intentional self-harm by unspecified hot objects

X78- <u>Intentional self-harm</u> by <u>sharp object</u>
The appropriate 7th character is to be added to each code from category X78:
  A <u>Initial</u> encounter
  D <u>Subsequent</u> encounter
  S <u>Sequela</u>

X78.0xx- Intentional self-harm by sharp glass
X78.1xx- Intentional self-harm by knife
X78.2xx- Intentional self-harm by sword or dagger

X78.8xx- Intentional self-harm by other sharp object
X78.9xx- Intentional self-harm by unspecified sharp object

X79.xxx- <u>Intentional self-harm</u> by <u>blunt object</u>
The appropriate 7th character is to be added to code X79:
  A <u>Initial</u> encounter
  D <u>Subsequent</u> encounter
  S <u>Sequela</u>

X80.xxx- <u>Intentional self-harm</u> by <u>jumping from a high place</u>
Intentional fall from one level to another
The appropriate 7th character is to be added to code X80:
  A <u>Initial</u> encounter
  D <u>Subsequent</u> encounter
  S <u>Sequela</u>

X81- <u>Intentional self-harm</u> by <u>jumping or lying in front of moving object</u>
The appropriate 7th character is to be added to each code from category X81:
  A <u>Initial</u> encounter
  D <u>Subsequent</u> encounter
  S <u>Sequela</u>

X81.0xx- Intentional self-harm by jumping or lying in front of motor vehicle
X81.1xx- Intentional self-harm by jumping or lying in front of (subway) train
X81.8xx- Intentional self-harm by jumping or lying in front of other moving object

X82- <u>Intentional self-harm</u> by <u>crashing of motor vehicle</u>
The appropriate 7th character is to be added to each code from category X82:
  A <u>Initial</u> encounter
  D <u>Subsequent</u> encounter
  S <u>Sequela</u>

X82.0xx- Intentional collision of motor vehicle with other motor vehicle
X82.1xx- Intentional collision of motor vehicle with train
X82.2xx- Intentional collision of motor vehicle with tree
X82.8xx- Other intentional self-harm by crashing of motor vehicle

X83- <u>Intentional self-harm</u> by <u>other specified means</u>
Excludes 1: intentional self-harm by poisoning or contact with toxic substance — see Table of Drugs and Chemicals
The appropriate 7th character is to be added to each code from category X83:
  A <u>Initial</u> encounter
  D <u>Subsequent</u> encounter
  S <u>Sequela</u>

X83.0xx- Intentional self-harm by crashing of aircraft
X83.1xx- Intentional self-harm by electrocution
X83.2xx- Intentional self-harm by exposure to extremes of cold
X83.8xx- Intentional self-harm by other specified means

Assault (X92-Y09)

Includes: Homicide
    Injuries inflicted by another person with intent to injure or kill, by any means
Excludes 1: injuries due to legal intervention (Y35.-)
    injuries due to operations of war (Y36.-)
    injuries due to terrorism (Y38.-)

X92- <u>Assault</u> by <u>drowning and submersion</u>
The appropriate 7th character is to be added to each code from category X92:
  A <u>Initial</u> encounter
  D <u>Subsequent</u> encounter
  S <u>Sequela</u>

X92.0xx- Assault by drowning and submersion while in bathtub
X92.1xx- Assault by drowning and submersion while in swimming pool
X92.2xx- Assault by drowning and submersion after push into swimming pool
X92.3xx- Assault by drowning and submersion in natural water
X92.8xx- Other assault by drowning and submersion
X92.9xx- Assault by drowning and submersion, unspecified

X 7 2 - X 9 2

X93.xxx-   Assault by handgun discharge
Assault by discharge of gun for single hand use
Assault by discharge of pistol
Assault by discharge of revolver
Excludes 1:   Very pistol (X95.8)
The appropriate 7th character is to be added to code X93:
- **A   Initial** encounter
- **D   Subsequent** encounter
- **S   Sequela**

X94-   Assault by rifle, shotgun and larger firearm discharge
Excludes 1:   airgun (X95.01)
The appropriate 7th character is to be added to each code from category X94:
- **A   Initial** encounter
- **D   Subsequent** encounter
- **S   Sequela**

X94.0xx-   Assault by shotgun
X94.1xx-   Assault by hunting rifle
X94.2xx-   Assault by machine gun
X94.8xx-   Assault by other larger firearm discharge
X94.9xx-   Assault by unspecified larger firearm discharge

X95-   Assault by other and unspecified firearm and gun discharge
The appropriate 7th character is to be added to each code from category X95:
- **A   Initial** encounter
- **D   Subsequent** encounter
- **S   Sequela**

X95.0-   Assault by gas, air or spring-operated guns
X95.01x-   Assault by airgun discharge
Assault by BB gun discharge
Assault by pellet gun discharge
X95.02x-   Assault by paintball gun discharge
X95.09x-   Assault by other gas, air or spring-operated gun
X95.8xx-   Assault by other firearm discharge
Assault by Very pistol [flare] discharge
X95.9xx-   Assault by unspecified firearm discharge

X96-   Assault by explosive material
Excludes 1:   incendiary device (X97)
terrorism involving explosive material (Y38.2-)
The appropriate 7th character is to be added to each code from category X96:
- **A   Initial** encounter
- **D   Subsequent** encounter
- **S   Sequela**

X96.0xx-   Assault by antipersonnel bomb
Excludes 1:   antipersonnel bomb use in military or war (Y36.2-)
X96.1xx-   Assault by gasoline bomb
X96.2xx-   Assault by letter bomb
X96.3xx-   Assault by fertilizer bomb
X96.4xx-   Assault by pipe bomb
X96.8xx-   Assault by other specified explosive
X96.9xx-   Assault by unspecified explosive

X97.xxx-   Assault by smoke, fire and flames
Assault by arson
Assault by cigarettes
Assault by incendiary device
The appropriate 7th character is to be added to code X97:
- **A   Initial** encounter
- **D   Subsequent** encounter
- **S   Sequela**

X98-   Assault by steam, hot vapors and hot objects
The appropriate 7th character is to be added to each code from category X98:
- **A   Initial** encounter
- **D   Subsequent** encounter
- **S   Sequela**

X98.0xx-   Assault by steam or hot vapors
X98.1xx-   Assault by hot tap water
X98.2xx-   Assault by hot fluids
X98.3xx-   Assault by hot household appliances

X98.8xx-   Assault by other hot objects
X98.9xx-   Assault by unspecified hot objects

X99-   Assault by sharp object
Excludes 1:   assault by strike by sports equipment (Y08.0-)
The appropriate 7th character is to be added to each code from category X99:
- **A   Initial** encounter
- **D   Subsequent** encounter
- **S   Sequela**

X99.0xx-   Assault by sharp glass
X99.1xx-   Assault by knife
X99.2xx-   Assault by sword or dagger
X99.8xx-   Assault by other sharp object
X99.9xx-   Assault by unspecified sharp object
Assault by stabbing NOS

Y00.xxx-   Assault by blunt object
Excludes 1:   assault by strike by sports equipment (Y08.0-)
The appropriate 7th character is to be added to code Y00:
- **A   Initial** encounter
- **D   Subsequent** encounter
- **S   Sequela**

Y01.xxx-   Assault by pushing from high place
The appropriate 7th character is to be added to code Y01:
- **A   Initial** encounter
- **D   Subsequent** encounter
- **S   Sequela**

Y02-   Assault by pushing or placing victim in front of moving object
The appropriate 7th character is to be added to each code from category Y02:
- **A   Initial** encounter
- **D   Subsequent** encounter
- **S   Sequela**

Y02.0xx-   Assault by pushing or placing victim in front of motor vehicle
Y02.1xx-   Assault by pushing or placing victim in front of (subway) train
Y02.8xx-   Assault by pushing or placing victim in front of other moving object

Y03-   Assault by crashing of motor vehicle
The appropriate 7th character is to be added to each code from category Y03:
- **A   Initial** encounter
- **D   Subsequent** encounter
- **S   Sequela**

Y03.0xx-   Assault by being hit or run over by motor vehicle
Y03.8xx-   Other assault by crashing of motor vehicle

Y04-   Assault by bodily force
Excludes 1:   assault by:
submersion (X92.-)
use of weapon (X93-X95, X99, Y00)
The appropriate 7th character is to be added to each code from category Y04:
- **A   Initial** encounter
- **D   Subsequent** encounter
- **S   Sequela**

Y04.0xx-   Assault by unarmed brawl or fight
Y04.1xx-   Assault by human bite
Y04.2xx-   Assault by strike against or bumped into by another person
Y04.8xx-   Assault by other bodily force
Assault by bodily force NOS

X93 - Y04

Y07- **Perpetrator** of <u>assault, maltreatment and neglect</u>
Note: Codes from this category are for use only in cases of confirmed abuse (T74-)
Note: Selection of the correct perpetrator code is based on the relationship between the perpetrator and the victim
Includes: Perpetrator of abandonment
Perpetrator of emotional neglect
Perpetrator of mental cruelty
Perpetrator of physical abuse
Perpetrator of physical neglect
Perpetrator of sexual abuse
Perpetrator of torture

Y07.0- **Spouse or partner**, perpetrator of maltreatment and neglect
Spouse or partner, perpetrator of maltreatment and neglect against spouse or partner

Y07.01 Husband, perpetrator of maltreatment and neglect

Y07.02 Wife, perpetrator of maltreatment and neglect

Y07.03 Male partner, perpetrator of maltreatment and neglect

Y07.04 Female partner, perpetrator of maltreatment and neglect

Y07.1- **Parent** (adoptive) (biological), perpetrator of maltreatment and neglect

Y07.11 Biological father, perpetrator of maltreatment and neglect

Y07.12 Biological mother, perpetrator of maltreatment and neglect

Y07.13 Adoptive father, perpetrator of maltreatment and neglect

Y07.14 Adoptive mother, perpetrator of maltreatment and neglect

Y07.4- **Other family member**, perpetrator of maltreatment and neglect

Y07.41- **Sibling**, perpetrator of maltreatment and neglect
Excludes 1: stepsibling, perpetrator of maltreatment and neglect (Y07.435, Y07.436)

Y07.410 Brother, perpetrator of maltreatment and neglect

Y07.411 Sister, perpetrator of maltreatment and neglect

Y07.42- Foster parent, perpetrator of maltreatment and neglect

Y07.420 Foster father, perpetrator of maltreatment and neglect

Y07.421 Foster mother, perpetrator of maltreatment and neglect

Y07.43- **Stepparent or stepsibling**, perpetrator of maltreatment and neglect

Y07.430 Stepfather, perpetrator of maltreatment and neglect

Y07.432 Male friend of parent (co-residing in household), perpetrator of maltreatment and neglect

Y07.433 Stepmother, perpetrator of maltreatment and neglect

Y07.434 Female friend of parent (co-residing in household), perpetrator of maltreatment and neglect

Y07.435 Stepbrother, perpetrator or maltreatment and neglect

Y07.436 Stepsister, perpetrator of maltreatment and neglect

Y07.49- **Other family member**, perpetrator of maltreatment and neglect

Y07.490 Male cousin, perpetrator of maltreatment and neglect

Y07.491 Female cousin, perpetrator of maltreatment and neglect

Y07.499 Other family member, perpetrator of maltreatment and neglect

Y07.5- **Non-family member**, perpetrator of maltreatment and neglect

Y07.50 **Unspecified** non-family member, perpetrator of maltreatment and neglect

Y07.51- **Daycare provider**, perpetrator of maltreatment and neglect

Y07.510 At-home childcare provider, perpetrator of maltreatment and neglect

Y07.511 Daycare center childcare provider, perpetrator of maltreatment and neglect

Y07.512 At-home adultcare provider, perpetrator of maltreatment and neglect

Y07.513 Adultcare center provider, perpetrator of maltreatment and neglect

Y07.519 Unspecified daycare provider, perpetrator of maltreatment and neglect

Y07.52- **Healthcare provider**, perpetrator of maltreatment and neglect

Y07.521 Mental health provider, perpetrator of maltreatment and neglect

Y07.528 Other therapist or healthcare provider, perpetrator of maltreatment and neglect
Nurse perpetrator of maltreatment and neglect
Occupational therapist perpetrator of maltreatment and neglect
Physical therapist perpetrator of maltreatment and neglect
Speech therapist perpetrator of maltreatment and neglect

Y07.529 Unspecified healthcare provider, perpetrator of maltreatment and neglect

Y07.53 **Teacher or instructor**, perpetrator of maltreatment and neglect
Coach, perpetrator of maltreatment and neglect

Y07.59 **Other** <u>non-family</u> member, perpetrator of maltreatment and neglect

Y07.9 Unspecified perpetrator of maltreatment and neglect

Y08- **Assault** by other specified means
The appropriate 7th character is to be added to each code from category Y08:
A   **Initial** encounter
D   **Subsequent** encounter
S   **Sequela**

Y08.0- Assault by strike by sport equipment

Y08.01x- Assault by strike by hockey stick

Y08.02x- Assault by strike by baseball bat

Y08.09x- Assault by strike by other specified type of sport equipment

Y08.8- Assault by other specified means

Y08.81x- Assault by crashing of aircraft

Y08.89x- Assault by other specified means

Y09 Assault by unspecified means
Assassination (attempted) NOS
Homicide (attempted) NOS
Manslaughter (attempted) NOS
Murder (attempted) NOS

Event of undetermined intent (Y21-Y33)

Note: Undetermined intent is only for use when there is specific documentation in the record that the intent of the injury cannot be determined. If no such documentation is present, code to accidental (unintentional).

Y21- **Drowning and submersion, <u>undetermined intent</u>**
The appropriate 7th character is to be added to each code from category Y21:
A   **Initial** encounter
D   **Subsequent** encounter
S   **Sequela**

Y21.0xx- Drowning and submersion while in bathtub, undetermined intent

Y21.1xx- Drowning and submersion after fall into bathtub, undetermined intent

Y21.2xx- Drowning and submersion while in swimming pool, undetermined intent

Y21.3xx- Drowning and submersion after fall into swimming pool, undetermined intent

Y21.4xx- Drowning and submersion in natural water, undetermined intent

Y21.8xx- Other drowning and submersion, undetermined intent

Y21.9xx- Unspecified drowning and submersion, undetermined intent

Y07 – Y21

Excludes 1: = NOT CODED HERE! (Do not code both)   **1284**   *Excludes ❷:* = Not Included Here

Y22.xxx- Handgun discharge, <u>undetermined intent</u>
Discharge of gun for single hand use, undetermined intent
Discharge of pistol, undetermined intent
Discharge of revolver, undetermined intent
Excludes ❷: Very pistol (Y24.8)
The appropriate 7th character is to be added to code Y22:
A   <u>Initial</u> encounter
D   <u>Subsequent</u> encounter
S   <u>Sequela</u>

Y23- Rifle, shotgun and larger firearm discharge, <u>undetermined intent</u>
Excludes ❷: airgun (Y24.0)
The appropriate 7th character is to be added to each code from category Y23:
A   <u>Initial</u> encounter
D   <u>Subsequent</u> encounter
S   <u>Sequela</u>

Y23.0xx- Shotgun discharge, undetermined intent
Y23.1xx- Hunting rifle discharge, undetermined intent
Y23.2xx- Military firearm discharge, undetermined intent
Y23.3xx- Machine gun discharge, undetermined intent
Y23.8xx- Other larger firearm discharge, undetermined intent
Y23.9xx- Unspecified larger firearm discharge, undetermined intent

Y24- Other and unspecified firearm discharge, <u>undetermined intent</u>
The appropriate 7th character is to be added to each code from category Y24:
A   <u>Initial</u> encounter
D   <u>Subsequent</u> encounter
S   <u>Sequela</u>

Y24.0xx- Airgun discharge, undetermined intent
BB gun discharge, undetermined intent
Pellet gun discharge, undetermined intent
Y24.8xx- Other firearm discharge, undetermined intent
Paintball gun discharge, undetermined intent
Very pistol [flare] discharge, undetermined intent
Y24.9xx- Unspecified firearm discharge, undetermined intent

Y25.xxx- Contact with explosive material, <u>undetermined intent</u>
The appropriate 7th character is to be added to code Y25:
A   <u>Initial</u> encounter
D   <u>Subsequent</u> encounter
S   <u>Sequela</u>

Y26.xxx- Exposure to smoke, fire and flames, <u>undetermined intent</u>
The appropriate 7th character is to be added to code Y26:
A   <u>Initial</u> encounter
D   <u>Subsequent</u> encounter
S   <u>Sequela</u>

Y27- Contact with steam, hot vapors and hot objects, <u>undetermined intent</u>
The appropriate 7th character is to be added to each code from category Y27:
A   <u>Initial</u> encounter
D   <u>Subsequent</u> encounter
S   <u>Sequela</u>

Y27.0xx- Contact with steam and hot vapors, undetermined intent
Y27.1xx- Contact with hot tap water, undetermined intent
Y27.2xx- Contact with hot fluids, undetermined intent
Y27.3xx- Contact with hot household appliance, undetermined intent
Y27.8xx- Contact with other hot objects, undetermined intent
Y27.9xx- Contact with unspecified hot objects, undetermined intent

Y28- Contact with sharp object, <u>undetermined intent</u>
The appropriate 7th character is to be added to each code from category Y28:
A   <u>Initial</u> encounter
D   <u>Subsequent</u> encounter
S   <u>Sequela</u>

Y28.0xx- Contact with sharp glass, undetermined intent
Y28.1xx- Contact with knife, undetermined intent
Y28.2xx- Contact with sword or dagger, undetermined intent
Y28.8xx- Contact with other sharp object, undetermined intent
Y28.9xx- Contact with unspecified sharp object, undetermined intent

Y29.xxx- Contact with blunt object, <u>undetermined intent</u>
The appropriate 7th character is to be added to code Y29:
A   <u>Initial</u> encounter
D   <u>Subsequent</u> encounter
S   <u>Sequela</u>

Y30.xxx- Falling, jumping or pushed from a high place, <u>undetermined intent</u>
Victim falling from one level to another, undetermined intent
The appropriate 7th character is to be added to code Y30:
A   <u>Initial</u> encounter
D   <u>Subsequent</u> encounter
S   <u>Sequela</u>

Y31.xxx- Falling, lying or running before or into moving object, <u>undetermined intent</u>
The appropriate 7th character is to be added to code Y31:
A   <u>Initial</u> encounter
D   <u>Subsequent</u> encounter
S   <u>Sequela</u>

Y32.xxx- Crashing of motor vehicle, <u>undetermined intent</u>
The appropriate 7th character is to be added to code Y32:
A   <u>Initial</u> encounter
D   <u>Subsequent</u> encounter
S   <u>Sequela</u>

Y33.xxx- Other specified events, <u>undetermined intent</u>
The appropriate 7th character is to be added to code Y33:
A   <u>Initial</u> encounter
D   <u>Subsequent</u> encounter
S   <u>Sequela</u>

Legal intervention, operations of war, military operations, and terrorism (Y35-Y38)

Y35- <u>Legal intervention</u>
Includes: Any injury sustained as a result of an encounter with any law enforcement official, serving in any capacity at the time of the encounter, whether on-duty or off-duty. Includes: injury to law enforcement official, suspect and bystander
The appropriate 7th character is to be added to code Y35:
A   <u>Initial</u> encounter
D   <u>Subsequent</u> encounter
S   <u>Sequela</u>

Y35.0- Legal intervention involving <u>firearm discharge</u>
Y35.00- Legal intervention involving unspecified firearm discharge
Legal intervention involving gunshot wound
Legal intervention involving shot NOS
Y35.001- Legal intervention involving <u>unspecified firearm</u> discharge, <u>law enforcement official injured</u>
Y35.002- Legal intervention involving unspecified firearm discharge, <u>bystander</u> injured
Y35.003- Legal intervention involving unspecified firearm discharge, <u>suspect</u> injured
Y35.01- Legal intervention involving injury by <u>machine gun</u>
Y35.011- Legal intervention involving injury by machine gun, <u>law enforcement official injured</u>
Y35.012- Legal intervention involving injury by machine gun, <u>bystander</u> injured
Y35.013- Legal intervention involving injury by machine gun, <u>suspect</u> injured
Y35.02- Legal intervention involving injury by <u>handgun</u>
Y35.021- Legal intervention involving injury by handgun, <u>law enforcement official injured</u>
Y35.022- Legal intervention involving injury by handgun, <u>bystander</u> injured
Y35.023- Legal intervention involving injury by handgun, <u>suspect</u> injured
Y35.03- Legal intervention involving injury by <u>rifle pellet</u>
Y35.031- Legal intervention involving injury by rifle pellet, <u>law enforcement official injured</u>
Y35.032- Legal intervention involving injury by rifle pellet, <u>bystander</u> injured

Y22 - Y35

Y35.033- Legal intervention involving injury by rifle pellet, <u>suspect</u> injured

Y35.04- Legal intervention involving injury by <u>rubber bullet</u>

Y35.041- Legal intervention involving injury by rubber bullet, <u>law enforcement official injured</u>

Y35.042- Legal intervention involving injury by rubber bullet, <u>bystander</u> injured

Y35.043- Legal intervention involving injury by rubber bullet, <u>suspect</u> injured

Y35.09- Legal intervention involving <u>other firearm discharge</u>

Y35.091- Legal intervention involving other firearm discharge, <u>law enforcement official injured</u>

Y35.092- Legal intervention involving other firearm discharge, <u>bystander</u> injured

Y35.093- Legal intervention involving other firearm discharge, <u>suspect</u> injured

Y35.1- Legal intervention involving <u>explosives</u>

Y35.10- Legal intervention involving unspecified explosives

Y35.101- Legal intervention involving unspecified explosives, <u>law enforcement official injured</u>

Y35.102- Legal intervention involving unspecified explosives, <u>bystander</u> injured

Y35.103- Legal intervention involving unspecified explosives, <u>suspect</u> injured

Y35.11- Legal intervention involving injury by <u>dynamite</u>

Y35.111- Legal intervention involving injury by dynamite, law <u>enforcement official injured</u>

Y35.112- Legal intervention involving injury by dynamite, <u>bystander</u> injured

Y35.113- Legal intervention involving injury by dynamite, <u>suspect</u> injured

Y35.12- Legal intervention involving injury by <u>explosive shell</u>

Y35.121- Legal intervention involving injury by explosive shell, <u>law enforcement official injured</u>

Y35.122- Legal intervention involving injury by explosive shell, <u>bystander</u> injured

Y35.123- Legal intervention involving injury by explosive shell, <u>suspect</u> injured

Y35.19- Legal intervention involving <u>other explosives</u>
Legal intervention involving injury by grenade
Legal intervention involving injury by mortar bomb

Y35.191- Legal intervention involving other explosives, <u>law enforcement official injured</u>

Y35.192- Legal intervention involving other explosives, <u>bystander</u> injured

Y35.193- Legal intervention involving other explosives, <u>suspect</u> injured

Y35.2- Legal intervention involving <u>gas</u>
Legal intervention involving asphyxiation by gas
Legal intervention involving poisoning by gas

Y35.20- Legal intervention involving <u>unspecified</u> gas

Y35.201- Legal intervention involving unspecified gas, <u>law enforcement official injured</u>

Y35.202- Legal intervention involving unspecified gas, <u>bystander</u> injured

Y35.203- Legal intervention involving unspecified gas, <u>suspect</u> injured

Y35.21- Legal intervention involving injury by <u>tear gas</u>

Y35.211- Legal intervention involving injury by tear gas, <u>law enforcement official injured</u>

Y35.212- Legal intervention involving injury by tear gas, <u>bystander</u> injured

Y35.213- Legal intervention involving injury by tear gas, <u>suspect</u> injured

Y35.29- Legal intervention involving <u>other gas</u>

Y35.291- Legal intervention involving other gas, <u>law enforcement official injured</u>

Y35.292- Legal intervention involving other gas, <u>bystander</u> injured

Y35.293- Legal intervention involving other gas, <u>suspect</u> injured

Y35.3- Legal intervention involving <u>blunt objects</u>
Legal intervention involving being hit or struck by blunt object

Y35.30- Legal intervention involving <u>unspecified</u> blunt objects

Y35.301- Legal intervention involving unspecified blunt objects, <u>law enforcement official injured</u>

Y35.302- Legal intervention involving unspecified blunt objects, <u>bystander</u> injured

Y35.303- Legal intervention involving unspecified blunt objects, <u>suspect</u> injured

Y35.31- Legal intervention involving <u>baton</u>

Y35.311- Legal intervention involving baton, <u>law enforcement official injured</u>

Y35.312- Legal intervention involving baton, <u>bystander</u> injured

Y35.313- Legal intervention involving baton, <u>suspect</u> injured

Y35.39- Legal intervention involving <u>other blunt objects</u>

Y35.391- Legal intervention involving other blunt objects, <u>law enforcement official injured</u>

Y35.392- Legal intervention involving other blunt objects, <u>bystander</u> injured

Y35.393- Legal intervention involving other blunt objects, <u>suspect</u> injured

Y35.4- Legal intervention involving <u>sharp objects</u>
Legal intervention involving being cut by sharp objects
Legal intervention involving being stabbed by sharp objects

Y35.40- Legal intervention involving <u>unspecified</u> sharp objects

Y35.401- Legal intervention involving unspecified sharp objects, <u>law enforcement official injured</u>

Y35.402- Legal intervention involving unspecified sharp objects, <u>bystander</u> injured

Y35.403- Legal intervention involving unspecified sharp objects, <u>suspect</u> injured

Y35.41- Legal intervention involving <u>bayonet</u>

Y35.411- Legal intervention involving bayonet, <u>law enforcement official injured</u>

Y35.412- Legal intervention involving bayonet, <u>bystander</u> injured

Y35.413- Legal intervention involving bayonet, <u>suspect</u> injured

Y35.49- Legal intervention involving <u>other sharp objects</u>

Y35.491- Legal intervention involving other sharp objects, <u>law enforcement official injured</u>

Y35.492- Legal intervention involving other sharp objects, <u>bystander</u> injured

Y35.493- Legal intervention involving other sharp objects, <u>suspect</u> injured

Y35.8- Legal intervention involving <u>other specified means</u>

Y35.81- Legal intervention involving <u>manhandling</u>

Y35.811- Legal intervention involving manhandling, <u>law enforcement official injured</u>

Y35.812- Legal intervention involving manhandling, <u>bystander</u> injured

Y35.813- Legal intervention involving manhandling, <u>suspect</u> injured

Y35.89- Legal intervention involving <u>other specified means</u>

Y35.891- Legal intervention involving other specified means, <u>law enforcement official injured</u>

Y35.892- Legal intervention involving other specified means, <u>bystander</u> injured

Y35.893- Legal intervention involving other specified means, <u>suspect</u> injured

Y35.9- Legal intervention, <u>means unspecified</u>

Y35.91- Legal intervention, means unspecified, <u>law enforcement official injured</u>

Y35.92- Legal intervention, means unspecified, <u>bystander</u> injured

Y35.93- Legal intervention, means unspecified, <u>suspect</u> injured

Y36- Operations of war

AHA 14:3Q:p4 – Encounters for treatment of conditions due to war

Includes: Injuries to military personnel and civilians caused by war, civil insurrection, and peacekeeping missions

Excludes 1: injury to military personnel occurring during peacetime military operations (Y37.-)

military vehicles involved in transport accidents with non-military vehicle during peacetime (V09.01, V09.21, V19.81, V29.81, V39.81, V49.81, V59.81, V69.81, V79.81)

The appropriate 7th character is to be added to each code from category Y36:

A   Initial encounter
D   Subsequent encounter
S   Sequela

Y36.0- War operations involving explosion of marine weapons

Y36.00- War operations involving explosion of unspecified marine weapon

War operations involving underwater blast NOS

Y36.000- War operations involving explosion of unspecified marine weapon, military personnel

Y36.001- War operations involving explosion of unspecified marine weapon, civilian

Y36.01- War operations involving explosion of depth-charge

Y36.010- War operations involving explosion of depth-charge, military personnel

Y36.011- War operations involving explosion of depth-charge, civilian

Y36.02- War operations involving explosion of marine mine

War operations involving explosion of marine mine, at sea or in harbor

Y36.020- War operations involving explosion of marine mine, military personnel

Y36.021- War operations involving explosion of marine mine, civilian

Y36.03- War operations involving explosion of sea-based artillery shell

Y36.030- War operations involving explosion of sea-based artillery shell, military personnel

Y36.031- War operations involving explosion of sea-based artillery shell, civilian

Y36.04- War operations involving explosion of torpedo

Y36.040- War operations involving explosion of torpedo, military personnel

Y36.041- War operations involving explosion of torpedo, civilian

Y36.05- War operations involving accidental detonation of onboard marine weapons

Y36.050- War operations involving accidental detonation of onboard marine weapons, military personnel

Y36.051- War operations involving accidental detonation of onboard marine weapons, civilian

Y36.09- War operations involving explosion of other marine weapons

Y36.090- War operations involving explosion of other marine weapons, military personnel

Y36.091- War operations involving explosion of other marine weapons, civilian

Y36.1- War operations involving destruction of aircraft

Y36.10- War operations involving unspecified destruction of aircraft

Y36.100- War operations involving unspecified destruction of aircraft, military personnel

Y36.101- War operations involving unspecified destruction of aircraft, civilian

Y36.11- War operations involving destruction of aircraft due to enemy fire or explosives

War operations involving destruction of aircraft due to air to air missile

War operations involving destruction of aircraft due to explosive placed on aircraft

War operations involving destruction of aircraft due to rocket propelled grenade [RPG]

War operations involving destruction of aircraft due to small arms fire

War operations involving destruction of aircraft due to surface to air missile

Y36.110- War operations involving destruction of aircraft due to enemy fire or explosives, military personnel

Y36.111- War operations involving destruction of aircraft due to enemy fire or explosives, civilian

Y36.12- War operations involving destruction of aircraft due to collision with other aircraft

Y36.120- War operations involving destruction of aircraft due to collision with other aircraft, military personnel

Y36.121- War operations involving destruction of aircraft due to collision with other aircraft, civilian

Y36.13- War operations involving destruction of aircraft due to onboard fire

Y36.130- War operations involving destruction of aircraft due to onboard fire, military personnel

Y36.131- War operations involving destruction of aircraft due to onboard fire, civilian

Y36.14- War operations involving destruction of aircraft due to accidental detonation of onboard munitions and explosives

Y36.140- War operations involving destruction of aircraft due to accidental detonation of onboard munitions and explosives, military personnel

Y36.141- War operations involving destruction of aircraft due to accidental detonation of onboard munitions and explosives, civilian

Y36.19- War operations involving other destruction of aircraft

Y36.190- War operations involving other destruction of aircraft, military personnel

Y36.191- War operations involving other destruction of aircraft, civilian

Y36.2- War operations involving other explosions and fragments

Excludes 1: war operations involving explosion of aircraft (Y36.1-)

war operations involving explosion of marine weapons (Y36.0-)

war operations involving explosion of nuclear weapons (Y36.5-)

war operations involving explosion occurring after cessation of hostilities (Y36.8-)

Y36.20- War operations involving unspecified explosion and fragments

War operations involving air blast NOS
War operations involving blast NOS
War operations involving blast fragments NOS
War operations involving blast wave NOS
War operations involving blast wind NOS
War operations involving explosion NOS
War operations involving explosion of bomb NOS

Y36.200- War operations involving unspecified explosion and fragments, military personnel

Y36.201- War operations involving unspecified explosion and fragments, civilian

Y36.21- War operations involving explosion of aerial bomb

Y36.210- War operations involving explosion of aerial bomb, military personnel

Y36.211- War operations involving explosion of aerial bomb, civilian

Y36.22- War operations involving explosion of guided missile

Y36.220- War operations involving explosion of guided missile, military personnel

Y36.221- War operations involving explosion of guided missile, civilian

Y36 - Y36

Y36.23- War operations involving explosion of <u>improvised explosive device [IED]</u>

    War operations involving explosion of person-borne improvised explosive device [IED]

    War operations involving explosion of vehicle-borne improvised explosive device [IED]

    War operations involving explosion of roadside improvised explosive device [IED]

    Y36.230- War operations involving explosion of improvised explosive device [IED], <u>military</u> personnel

    Y36.231- War operations involving explosion of improvised explosive device [IED], <u>civilian</u>

Y36.24- War operations involving explosion due to <u>accidental detonation and discharge of own munitions or munitions launch device</u>

    Y36.240- War operations involving explosion due to accidental detonation and discharge of own munitions or munitions launch-device, <u>military</u> personnel

    Y36.241- War operations involving explosion due to accidental detonation and discharge of own munitions or munitions launch device, <u>civilian</u>

Y36.25- War operations involving <u>fragments from munitions</u>

    Y36.250- War operations involving fragments from munitions, <u>military</u> personnel

    Y36.251- War operations involving fragments from munitions, <u>civilian</u>

Y36.26 War operations involving fragments of <u>improvised explosive device [IED]</u>

    War operations involving fragments of person-borne improvised explosive device [IED]

    War operations involving fragments of vehicle-borne improvised explosive device [IED]

    War operations involving fragments of roadside improvised explosive device [IED]

    Y36.260- War operations involving fragments of improvised explosive device [IED], <u>military</u> personnel

    Y36.261- War operations involving fragments of improvised explosive device [IED], <u>civilian</u>

Y36.27- War operations involving <u>fragments from weapons</u>

    Y36.270- War operations involving fragments from weapons, <u>military</u> personnel

    Y36.271- War operations involving fragments from weapons, <u>civilian</u>

Y36.29- War operations involving <u>other explosions and fragments</u>

    War operations involving explosion of grenade

    War operations involving explosions of land mine

    War operations involving shrapnel NOS

    Y36.290- War operations involving other explosions and fragments, <u>military</u> personnel

    Y36.291- War operations involving other explosions and fragments, <u>civilian</u>

Y36.3- War operations involving <u>fires, conflagrations and hot substances</u>

    War operations involving smoke, fumes, and heat from fires, conflagrations and hot substances

    Excludes 1:   *war operations involving fires and conflagrations aboard military aircraft (Y36.1-)*

        war operations involving fires and conflagrations aboard military watercraft (Y36.0-)

        war operations involving fires and conflagrations caused indirectly by conventional weapons (Y36.2-)

        war operations involving fires and thermal effects of nuclear weapons (Y36.53-)

Y36.30- War operations involving <u>unspecified</u> fire, conflagration and hot substance

    Y36.300- War operations involving unspecified fire, conflagration and hot substance, <u>military</u> personnel

    Y36.301- War operations involving unspecified fire, conflagration and hot substance, <u>civilian</u>

Y36.31- War operations involving <u>gasoline bomb</u>

    War operations involving incendiary bomb

    War operations involving petrol bomb

    Y36.310- War operations involving gasoline bomb, <u>military</u> personnel

    Y36.311- War operations involving gasoline bomb, <u>civilian</u>

Y36.32- War operations involving <u>incendiary bullet</u>

    Y36.320- War operations involving incendiary bullet, <u>military</u> personnel

    Y36.321- War operations involving incendiary bullet, <u>civilian</u>

Y36.33- War operations involving <u>flamethrower</u>

    Y36.330- War operations involving flamethrower, <u>military</u> personnel

    Y36.331- War operations involving flamethrower, <u>civilian</u>

Y36.39- War operations involving <u>other</u> fires, conflagrations and hot substances

    Y36.390- War operations involving other fires, conflagrations and hot substances, <u>military</u> personnel

    Y36.391- War operations involving other fires, conflagrations and hot substances, <u>civilian</u>

Y36.4- War operations involving <u>firearm discharge and other forms of conventional warfare</u>

Y36.41- War operations involving <u>rubber bullets</u>

    Y36.410- War operations involving rubber bullets, <u>military</u> personnel

    Y36.411- War operations involving rubber bullets, <u>civilian</u>

Y36.42- War operations involving <u>firearms pellets</u>

    Y36.420- War operations involving firearms pellets, <u>military</u> personnel

    Y36.421- War operations involving firearms pellets, <u>civilian</u>

Y36.43- War operations involving <u>other</u> firearms discharge

    War operations involving bullets NOS

    Excludes 1:   *war operations involving munitions fragments (Y36.25-)*

        war operations involving incendiary bullets (Y36.32-)

    Y36.430- War operations involving other firearms discharge, <u>military</u> personnel

    Y36.431- War operations involving other firearms discharge, <u>civilian</u>

Y36.44- War operations involving <u>unarmed hand to hand combat</u>

    Excludes 1:   *war operations involving combat using blunt or piercing object (Y36.45-)*

        war operations involving intentional restriction of air and airway (Y36.46-)

        war operations involving unintentional restriction of air and airway (Y36.47-)

    Y36.440- War operations involving unarmed hand to hand combat, <u>military</u> personnel

    Y36.441- War operations involving unarmed hand to hand combat, <u>civilian</u>

Y36.45- War operations involving combat <u>using blunt or piercing object</u>

    Y36.450- War operations involving combat using blunt or piercing object, <u>military</u> personnel

    Y36.451- War operations involving combat using blunt or piercing object, <u>civilian</u>

Y36.46- War operations involving <u>intentional restriction of air and airway</u>

    Y36.460- War operations involving intentional restriction of air and airway, <u>military</u> personnel

    Y36.461- War operations involving intentional restriction of air and airway, <u>civilian</u>

Y36.47- War operations involving <u>unintentional restriction of air and airway</u>

    Y36.470- War operations involving unintentional restriction of air and airway, <u>military</u> personnel

    Y36.471- War operations involving unintentional restriction of air and airway, <u>civilian</u>

Y36 - Y36

Y36.49- War operations involving <u>other</u> forms of conventional warfare

    Y36.490- War operations involving other forms of conventional warfare, <u>military</u> personnel

    Y36.491- War operations involving other forms of conventional warfare, <u>civilian</u>

Y36.5- War operations involving <u>nuclear weapons</u>
    War operations involving dirty bomb NOS

    Y36.50- War operations involving <u>unspecified</u> effect of nuclear weapon

        Y36.500- War operations involving unspecified effect of nuclear weapon, <u>military</u> personnel

        Y36.501- War operations involving unspecified effect of nuclear weapon, <u>civilian</u>

    Y36.51- War operations involving <u>direct blast effect</u> of nuclear weapon
        War operations involving blast pressure of nuclear weapon

        Y36.510- War operations involving direct blast effect of nuclear weapon, <u>military</u> personnel

        Y36.511- War operations involving direct blast effect of nuclear weapon, <u>civilian</u>

    Y36.52- War operations involving <u>indirect blast effect</u> of nuclear weapon
        War operations involving being thrown by blast of nuclear weapon
        War operations involving being struck or crushed by blast debris of nuclear weapon

        Y36.520- War operations involving indirect blast effect of nuclear weapon, <u>military</u> personnel

        Y36.521- War operations involving indirect blast effect of nuclear weapon, <u>civilian</u>

    Y36.53- War operations involving <u>thermal radiation effect</u> of nuclear weapon
        War operations involving direct heat from nuclear weapon
        War operation involving fireball effects from nuclear weapon

        Y36.530- War operations involving thermal radiation effect of nuclear weapon, <u>military</u> personnel

        Y36.531- War operations involving thermal radiation effect of nuclear weapon, <u>civilian</u>

    Y36.54- War operation involving <u>nuclear radiation effects</u> of nuclear weapon
        War operation involving acute radiation exposure from nuclear weapon
        War operation involving exposure to immediate ionizing radiation from nuclear weapon
        War operation involving fallout exposure from nuclear weapon
        War operation involving secondary effects of nuclear weapons

        Y36.540- War operation involving nuclear radiation effects of nuclear weapon, <u>military</u> personnel

        Y36.541- War operation involving nuclear radiation effects of nuclear weapon, <u>civilian</u>

    Y36.59- War operation involving <u>other</u> effects of nuclear weapons

        Y36.590- War operation involving other effects of nuclear weapons, <u>military</u> personnel

        Y36.591- War operation involving other effects of nuclear weapons, <u>civilian</u>

Y36.6- War operations involving <u>biological weapons</u>

    Y36.6x- War operations involving biological weapons

        Y36.6x0- War operations involving biological weapons, <u>military</u> personnel

        Y36.6x1- War operations involving biological weapons, <u>civilian</u>

Y36.7- War operations involving <u>chemical weapons and other forms of unconventional warfare</u>
    Excludes 1:   *war operations involving incendiary devices (Y36.3-, Y36.5-)*

    Y36.7x- War operations involving <u>chemical weapons and other forms of unconventional warfare</u>

        Y36.7x0- War operations involving chemical weapons and other forms of unconventional warfare, <u>military</u> personnel

        Y36.7x1- War operations involving chemical weapons and other forms of unconventional warfare, <u>civilian</u>

Y36.8- War operations occurring <u>after cessation of hostilities</u>
    War operations classifiable to categories Y36.0-Y36.8 but occurring after cessation of hostilities

    Y36.81- Explosion of <u>mine</u> placed during <u>war</u> operations but <u>exploding after</u> cessation of hostilities

        Y36.810- Explosion of mine placed during <u>war</u> operations but exploding after cessation of hostilities, <u>military</u> personnel

        Y36.811- Explosion of mine placed during <u>war</u> operations but exploding after cessation of hostilities, <u>civilian</u>

    Y36.82- Explosion of <u>bomb</u> placed during <u>war</u> operations but <u>exploding after</u> cessation of hostilities

        Y36.820- Explosion of bomb placed during <u>war</u> operations but exploding after cessation of hostilities, <u>military</u> personnel

        Y36.821- Explosion of bomb placed during <u>war</u> operations but exploding after cessation of hostilities, <u>civilian</u>

    Y36.88- <u>Other</u> <u>war</u> operations <u>occurring after</u> cessation of hostilities

        Y36.880- Other <u>war</u> operations occurring after cessation of hostilities, <u>military</u> personnel

        Y36.881- Other <u>war</u> operations occurring after cessation of hostilities, <u>civilian</u>

    Y36.89- <u>Unspecified</u> <u>war</u> operations <u>occurring after</u> cessation of hostilities

        Y36.890- Unspecified <u>war</u> operations occurring after cessation of hostilities, <u>military</u> personnel

        Y36.891- Unspecified <u>war</u> operations occurring after cessation of hostilities, <u>civilian</u>

Y36.9- Other and unspecified <u>war</u> operations

    Y36.90- <u>War</u> operations, <u>unspecified</u>

    Y36.91- <u>War</u> operations involving <u>unspecified weapon of mass destruction [WMD]</u>

    Y36.92- <u>War</u> operations involving <u>friendly fire</u>

Y37- <u>Military operations</u>
    Includes: Injuries to military personnel and civilians <u>occurring during peacetime</u> on military property and <u>during routine military exercises and operations</u>
    Excludes 1:   *military aircraft involved in aircraft accident with civilian aircraft (V97.81-)*
        military vehicles involved in transport accident with civilian vehicle (V09.01, V09.21, V19.81, V29.81, V39.81, V49.81, V59.81, V69.81, V79.81)
        military watercraft involved in water transport accident with civilian watercraft (V94.81-)
        war operations (Y36.-)

> The appropriate 7th character is to be added to each code from category Y37:
> A   <u>Initial</u> encounter
> D   <u>Subsequent</u> encounter
> S   <u>Sequela</u>

Y37.0- Military operations involving <u>explosion of marine weapons</u>

    Y37.00- Military operations involving explosion of <u>unspecified</u> marine weapon
        Military operations involving underwater blast NOS

        Y37.000- Military operations involving explosion of unspecified marine weapon, <u>military</u> personnel

        Y37.001- Military operations involving explosion of unspecified marine weapon, <u>civilian</u>

    Y37.01- Military operations involving explosion of <u>depth-charge</u>

        Y37.010- Military operations involving explosion of depth-charge, <u>military</u> personnel

        Y37.011- Military operations involving explosion of depth-charge, <u>civilian</u>

    Y37.02- Military operations involving explosion of <u>marine mine</u>
        Military operations involving explosion of marine mine, at sea or in harbor

        Y37.020- Military operations involving explosion of marine mine, <u>military</u> personnel

Y36 - Y37

Y37.021- Military operations involving explosion of marine mine, <u>civilian</u>

Y37.03- Military operations involving explosion of <u>sea-based artillery shell</u>

Y37.030- Military operations involving explosion of sea-based artillery shell, <u>military</u> personnel

Y37.031- Military operations involving explosion of sea-based artillery shell, <u>civilian</u>

Y37.04- Military operations involving explosion of <u>torpedo</u>

Y37.040- Military operations involving explosion of torpedo, <u>military</u> personnel

Y37.041- Military operations involving explosion of torpedo, <u>civilian</u>

Y37.05- Military operations involving <u>accidental detonation of onboard marine weapons</u>

Y37.050- Military operations involving accidental detonation of onboard marine weapons, <u>military</u> personnel

Y37.051- Military operations involving accidental detonation of onboard marine weapons, <u>civilian</u>

Y37.09- Military operations involving explosion of <u>other marine weapons</u>

Y37.090- Military operations involving explosion of other marine weapons, <u>military</u> personnel

Y37.091- Military operations involving explosion of other marine weapons, <u>civilian</u>

Y37.1- Military operations involving <u>destruction of aircraft</u>

Y37.10- Military operations involving <u>unspecified</u> destruction of aircraft

Y37.100- Military operations involving unspecified destruction of aircraft, <u>military</u> personnel

Y37.101- Military operations involving unspecified destruction of aircraft, <u>civilian</u>

Y37.11- Military operations involving destruction of aircraft <u>due to enemy fire or explosives</u>

Military operations involving destruction of aircraft due to air to air missile

Military operations involving destruction of aircraft due to explosive placed on aircraft

Military operations involving destruction of aircraft due to rocket propelled grenade [RPG]

Military operations involving destruction of aircraft due to small arms fire

Military operations involving destruction of aircraft due to surface to air missile

Y37.110- Military operations involving destruction of aircraft due to enemy fire or explosives, <u>military</u> personnel

Y37.111- Military operations involving destruction of aircraft due to enemy fire or explosives, <u>civilian</u>

Y37.12- Military operations involving destruction of aircraft <u>due to collision with other aircraft</u>

Y37.120- Military operations involving destruction of aircraft due to collision with other aircraft, <u>military</u> personnel

Y37.121- Military operations involving destruction of aircraft due to collision with other aircraft, <u>civilian</u>

Y37.13- Military operations involving destruction of aircraft <u>due to onboard fire</u>

Y37.130- Military operations involving destruction of aircraft due to onboard fire, <u>military</u> personnel

Y37.131- Military operations involving destruction of aircraft due to onboard fire, <u>civilian</u>

Y37.14- Military operations involving destruction of aircraft <u>due to accidental detonation of onboard munitions and explosives</u>

Y37.140- Military operations involving destruction of aircraft due to accidental detonation of onboard munitions and explosives, <u>military</u> personnel

Y37.141- Military operations involving destruction of aircraft due to accidental detonation of onboard munitions and explosives, <u>civilian</u>

Y37.19- Military operations involving <u>other destruction of aircraft</u>

Y37.190- Military operations involving other destruction of aircraft, <u>military</u> personnel

Y37.191- Military operations involving other destruction of aircraft, <u>civilian</u>

Y37.2- Military operations involving <u>other explosions and fragments</u>

Excludes 1: *military operations involving explosion of aircraft (Y37.1-)*
military operations involving explosion of marine weapons (Y37.0-)
military operations involving explosion of nuclear weapons (Y37.5-)

Y37.20- Military operations involving <u>unspecified</u> explosion and fragments

Military operations involving air blast NOS
Military operations involving blast NOS
Military operations involving blast fragments NOS
Military operations involving blast wave NOS
Military operations involving blast wind NOS
Military operations involving explosion NOS
Military operations involving explosion of bomb NOS

Y37.200- Military operations involving unspecified explosion and fragments, <u>military</u> personnel

Y37.201- Military operations involving unspecified explosion and fragments, <u>civilian</u>

Y37.21- Military operations involving explosion of <u>aerial bomb</u>

Y37.210- Military operations involving explosion of aerial bomb, <u>military</u> personnel

Y37.211- Military operations involving explosion of aerial bomb, <u>civilian</u>

Y37.22- Military operations involving explosion of <u>guided missile</u>

Y37.220- Military operations involving explosion of guided missile, <u>military</u> personnel

Y37.221- Military operations involving explosion of guided missile, <u>civilian</u>

Y37.23- Military operations involving explosion of <u>improvised explosive device [IED]</u>

Military operations involving explosion of person-borne improvised explosive device [IED]
Military operations involving explosion of vehicle-borne improvised explosive device [IED]
Military operations involving explosion of roadside improvised explosive device [IED]

Y37.230- Military operations involving explosion of improvised explosive device [IED], <u>military</u> personnel

Y37.231- Military operations involving explosion of improvised explosive device [IED], <u>civilian</u>

Y37.24- Military operations involving explosion due to <u>accidental detonation and discharge of own munitions or munitions launch device</u>

Y37.240- Military operations involving explosion due to accidental detonation and discharge of own munitions or munitions launch device, <u>military</u> personnel

Y37.241- Military operations involving explosion due to accidental detonation and discharge of own munitions or munitions launch device, <u>civilian</u>

Y37.25- Military operations involving <u>fragments from munitions</u>

Y37.250- Military operations involving fragments from munitions, <u>military</u> personnel

Y37.251- Military operations involving fragments from munitions, <u>civilian</u>

Y37.26- Military operations involving <u>fragments of improvised explosive device [IED]</u>

Military operations involving fragments of person-borne improvised explosive device [IED]
Military operations involving fragments of vehicle-borne improvised explosive device [IED]
Military operations involving fragments of roadside improvised explosive device [IED]

Y37.260- Military operations involving fragments of improvised explosive device [IED], <u>military</u> personnel

Y37
–
Y37

Y37.261- Military operations involving fragments of
improvised explosive device [IED], civilian

Y37.27- Military operations involving fragments from weapons

Y37.270- Military operations involving fragments from
weapons, military personnel

Y37.271- Military operations involving fragments from
weapons, civilian

Y37.29- Military operations involving other explosions and
fragments
Military operations involving explosion of grenade
Military operations involving explosions of land mine
Military operations involving shrapnel NOS

Y37.290- Military operations involving other explosions and
fragments, military personnel

Y37.291- Military operations involving other explosions and
fragments, civilian

Y37.3- Military operations involving fires, conflagrations and hot
substances
Military operations involving smoke, fumes, and heat from fires,
conflagrations and hot substances
Excludes 1:   military operations involving fires and conflagrations
aboard military aircraft (Y37.1-)
military operations involving fires and conflagrations
aboard military watercraft (Y37.0-)
military operations involving fires and conflagrations
caused indirectly by conventional weapons
(Y37.2-)
military operations involving fires and thermal effects
of nuclear weapons (Y36.53-)

Y37.30- Military operations involving unspecified fire,
conflagration and hot substance

Y37.300- Military operations involving unspecified fire,
conflagration and hot substance, military
personnel

Y37.301- Military operations involving unspecified fire,
conflagration and hot substance, civilian

Y37.31- Military operations involving gasoline bomb
Military operations involving incendiary bomb
Military operations involving petrol bomb

Y37.310- Military operations involving gasoline bomb,
military personnel

Y37.311- Military operations involving gasoline bomb,
civilian

Y37.32- Military operations involving incendiary bullet

Y37.320- Military operations involving incendiary bullet,
military personnel

Y37.321- Military operations involving incendiary bullet,
civilian

Y37.33- Military operations involving flamethrower

Y37.330- Military operations involving flamethrower,
military personnel

Y37.331- Military operations involving flamethrower, civilian

Y37.39- Military operations involving other fires, conflagrations
and hot substances

Y37.390- Military operations involving other fires,
conflagrations and hot substances, military
personnel

Y37.391- Military operations involving other fires,
conflagrations and hot substances, civilian

Y37.4- Military operations involving firearm discharge and other
forms of conventional warfare

Y37.41- Military operations involving rubber bullets

Y37.410- Military operations involving rubber bullets,
military personnel

Y37.411- Military operations involving rubber bullets,
civilian

Y37.42- Military operations involving firearms pellets

Y37.420- Military operations involving firearms pellets,
military personnel

Y37.421- Military operations involving firearms pellets,
civilian

Y37.43- Military operations involving other firearms discharge
Military operations involving bullets NOS
Excludes 1:   military operations involving munitions fragments
(Y37.25-)
military operations involving incendiary bullets
(Y37.32-)

Y37.430- Military operations involving other firearms
discharge, military personnel

Y37.431- Military operations involving other firearms
discharge, civilian

Y37.44- Military operations involving unarmed hand to hand
combat
Excludes 1:   military operations involving combat using blunt or
piercing object (Y37.45-)
military operations involving intentional restriction
of air and airway (Y37.46-)
military operations involving unintentional
restriction of air and airway (Y37.47-)

Y37.440- Military operations involving unarmed hand to
hand combat, military personnel

Y37.441- Military operations involving unarmed hand to
hand combat, civilian

Y37.45- Military operations involving combat using blunt or
piercing object

Y37.450- Military operations involving combat using blunt or
piercing object, military personnel

Y37.451- Military operations involving combat using blunt or
piercing object, civilian

Y37.46- Military operations involving intentional restriction of air
and airway

Y37.460- Military operations involving intentional restriction
of air and airway, military personnel

Y37.461- Military operations involving intentional restriction
of air and airway, civilian

Y37.47- Military operations involving unintentional restriction of
air and airway

Y37.470- Military operations involving unintentional
restriction of air and airway, military personnel

Y37.471- Military operations involving unintentional
restriction of air and airway, civilian

Y37.49- Military operations involving other forms of conventional
warfare

Y37.490- Military operations involving other forms of
conventional warfare, military personnel

Y37.491- Military operations involving other forms of
conventional warfare, civilian

Y37.5- Military operations involving nuclear weapons
Military operation involving dirty bomb NOS

Y37.50- Military operations involving unspecified effect of nuclear
weapon

Y37.500- Military operations involving unspecified effect of
nuclear weapon, military personnel

Y37.501- Military operations involving unspecified effect of
nuclear weapon, civilian

Y37.51- Military operations involving direct blast effect of nuclear
weapon
Military operations involving blast pressure of nuclear weapon

Y37.510- Military operations involving direct blast effect of
nuclear weapon, military personnel

Y37.511- Military operations involving direct blast effect of
nuclear weapon, civilian

Y37.52- Military operations involving indirect blast effect of
nuclear weapon
Military operations involving being thrown by blast of nuclear
weapon
Military operations involving being struck or crushed by blast
debris of nuclear weapon

Y37.520- Military operations involving indirect blast effect
of nuclear weapon, military personnel

Y37.521- Military operations involving indirect blast effect
of nuclear weapon, civilian

Y37-Y37

Y37.53- Military operations involving <u>thermal radiation effect</u> of nuclear weapon
    Military operations involving direct heat from nuclear weapon
    Military operation involving fireball effects from nuclear weapon

    Y37.530- Military operations involving thermal radiation effect of nuclear weapon, <u>military</u> personnel

    Y37.531- Military operations involving thermal radiation effect of nuclear weapon, <u>civilian</u>

Y37.54- Military operation involving <u>nuclear radiation effects</u> of nuclear weapon
    Military operation involving acute radiation exposure from nuclear weapon
    Military operation involving exposure to immediate ionizing radiation from nuclear weapon
    Military operation involving fallout exposure from nuclear weapon
    Military operation involving secondary effects of nuclear weapons

    Y37.540- Military operation involving nuclear radiation effects of nuclear weapon, <u>military</u> personnel

    Y37.541- Military operation involving nuclear radiation effects of nuclear weapon, <u>civilian</u>

Y37.59- Military operation involving <u>other</u> effects of nuclear weapons

    Y37.590- Military operation involving other effects of nuclear weapons, <u>military</u> personnel

    Y37.591- Military operation involving other effects of nuclear weapons, <u>civilian</u>

Y37.6- Military operations involving <u>biological weapons</u>

    Y37.6x- Military operations involving biological weapons

        Y37.6x0- Military operations involving biological weapons, <u>military</u> personnel

        Y37.6x1- Military operations involving biological weapons, <u>civilian</u>

Y37.7- Military operations involving <u>chemical weapons and other forms of unconventional warfare</u>
    Excludes 1:   *military operations involving incendiary devices (Y36.3-, Y36.5-)*

    Y37.7x- Military operations involving <u>chemical weapons</u> and other forms of unconventional warfare

        Y37.7x0- Military operations involving chemical weapons and other forms of unconventional warfare, <u>military</u> personnel

        Y37.7x1- Military operations involving chemical weapons and other forms of unconventional warfare, <u>civilian</u>

Y37.9- Other and unspecified military operations

    Y37.90x- Military operations, <u>unspecified</u>

    Y37.91x- Military operations involving <u>unspecified weapon of mass destruction [WMD]</u>

    Y37.92x- Military operations involving <u>friendly fire</u>

Y38- **Terrorism**
    Note: These codes are for use to identify injuries resulting from the unlawful use of force or violence against persons or property to intimidate or coerce a Government, the civilian population, or any segment thereof, in furtherance of political or social objective
    Use additional code for place of occurrence (Y92.-)
    The appropriate 7th character is to be added to each code from category Y38:
    A   <u>Initial</u> encounter
    D   <u>Subsequent</u> encounter
    S   <u>Sequela</u>

Y38.0- Terrorism involving <u>explosion of marine weapons</u>
    Terrorism involving depth-charge
    Terrorism involving marine mine
    Terrorism involving mine NOS, at sea or in harbor
    Terrorism involving sea-based artillery shell
    Terrorism involving torpedo
    Terrorism involving underwater blast

    Y38.0x- Terrorism involving explosion of <u>marine weapons</u>

        Y38.0x1- Terrorism involving explosion of marine weapons, <u>public safety official</u> injured

        Y38.0x2- Terrorism involving explosion of marine weapons, <u>civilian</u> injured

        Y38.0x3- Terrorism involving explosion of marine weapons, <u>terrorist</u> injured

Y38.1- Terrorism involving <u>destruction of aircraft</u>
    Terrorism involving aircraft burned
    Terrorism involving aircraft exploded
    Terrorism involving aircraft being shot down
    Terrorism involving aircraft used as a weapon

    Y38.1x- Terrorism involving destruction of aircraft

        Y38.1x1- Terrorism involving destruction of aircraft, <u>public safety official</u> injured

        Y38.1x2- Terrorism involving destruction of aircraft, <u>civilian</u> injured

        Y38.1x3- Terrorism involving destruction of aircraft, <u>terrorist</u> injured

Y38.2- Terrorism involving <u>other explosions and fragments</u>
    Terrorism involving antipersonnel (fragments) bomb
    Terrorism involving blast NOS
    Terrorism involving explosion NOS
    Terrorism involving explosion of breech block
    Terrorism involving explosion of cannon block
    Terrorism involving explosion (fragments) of artillery shell
    Terrorism involving explosion (fragments) of bomb
    Terrorism involving explosion (fragments) of grenade
    Terrorism involving explosion (fragments) of guided missile
    Terrorism involving explosion (fragments) of land mine
    Terrorism involving explosion of mortar bomb
    Terrorism involving explosion of munitions
    Terrorism involving explosion (fragments) of rocket
    Terrorism involving explosion (fragments) of shell
    Terrorism involving shrapnel
    Terrorism involving mine NOS, on land
    Excludes 1:   *terrorism involving explosion of nuclear weapon (Y38.5)*
        terrorism involving suicide bomber (Y38.81)

    Y38.2x- Terrorism involving other explosions and fragments

        Y38.2x1- Terrorism involving other explosions and fragments, <u>public safety official</u> injured

        Y38.2x2- Terrorism involving other explosions and fragments, <u>civilian</u> injured

        Y38.2x3- Terrorism involving other explosions and fragments, <u>terrorist</u> injured

Y38.3- Terrorism involving <u>fires, conflagration and hot substances</u>
    Terrorism involving conflagration NOS
    Terrorism involving fire NOS
    Terrorism involving petrol bomb
    Excludes 1:   *terrorism involving fire or heat of nuclear weapon (Y38.5)*

    Y38.3x- Terrorism involving fires, conflagration and hot substances

        Y38.3x1- Terrorism involving fires, conflagration and hot substances, <u>public safety official</u> injured

        Y38.3x2- Terrorism involving fires, conflagration and hot substances, <u>civilian</u> injured

        Y38.3x3- Terrorism involving fires, conflagration and hot substances, <u>terrorist</u> injured

Y38.4- Terrorism involving <u>firearms</u>
    Terrorism involving carbine bullet
    Terrorism involving machine gun bullet
    Terrorism involving pellets (shotgun)
    Terrorism involving pistol bullet
    Terrorism involving rifle bullet
    Terrorism involving rubber (rifle) bullet

    Y38.4x- Terrorism involving firearms

        Y38.4x1- Terrorism involving firearms, <u>public safety official</u> injured

        Y38.4x2- Terrorism involving firearms, <u>civilian</u> injured

        Y38.4x3- Terrorism involving firearms, <u>terrorist</u> injured

Y38.5- Terrorism involving <u>nuclear weapons</u>
    Terrorism involving blast effects of nuclear weapon
    Terrorism involving exposure to ionizing radiation from nuclear weapon
    Terrorism involving fireball effect of nuclear weapon
    Terrorism involving heat from nuclear weapon

    Y38.5x- Terrorism involving nuclear weapons

        Y38.5x1- Terrorism involving nuclear weapons, <u>public safety official</u> injured

Side tab: Y37 – Y38

Y38.5x2- Terrorism involving nuclear weapons, <u>civilian</u> injured

Y38.5x3- Terrorism involving nuclear weapons, <u>terrorist</u> injured

Y38.6- Terrorism involving <u>biological weapons</u>
Terrorism involving anthrax
Terrorism involving cholera
Terrorism involving smallpox

Y38.6x- Terrorism involving biological weapons

Y38.6x1- Terrorism involving biological weapons, <u>public safety official</u> injured

Y38.6x2- Terrorism involving biological weapons, <u>civilian</u> injured

Y38.6x3- Terrorism involving biological weapons, <u>terrorist</u> injured

Y38.7- Terrorism involving <u>chemical weapons</u>
Terrorism involving gases, fumes, chemicals
Terrorism involving hydrogen cyanide
Terrorism involving phosgene
Terrorism involving sarin

Y38.7x- Terrorism involving chemical weapons

Y38.7x1- Terrorism involving chemical weapons, <u>public safety official</u> injured

Y38.7x2- Terrorism involving chemical weapons, <u>civilian</u> injured

Y38.7x3- Terrorism involving chemical weapons, <u>terrorist</u> injured

Y38.8- Terrorism involving <u>other and unspecified means</u>

Y38.80x- Terrorism involving <u>unspecified</u> means
Terrorism NOS

Y38.81- Terrorism involving <u>suicide bomber</u>

Y38.811- Terrorism involving suicide bomber, <u>public safety official</u> injured

Y38.812- Terrorism involving suicide bomber, <u>civilian</u> injured

Y38.89- Terrorism involving <u>other means</u>
Terrorism involving drowning and submersion
Terrorism involving lasers
Terrorism involving piercing or stabbing instruments

Y38.891- Terrorism involving other means, <u>public safety official</u> injured

Y38.892- Terrorism involving other means, <u>civilian</u> injured

Y38.893- Terrorism involving other means, <u>terrorist</u> injured

Y38.9- Terrorism, <u>secondary effects</u>
Note: This code is for use to identify conditions occurring subsequent to a terrorist attack not those that are due to the initial terrorist attack.

Y38.9x- Terrorism, secondary effects

Y38.9x1- Terrorism, secondary effects, <u>public safety official</u> injured

Y38.9x2- Terrorism, secondary effects, <u>civilian</u> injured

Complications of medical and surgical care (Y62-Y84)

Includes: Complications of medical devices
Surgical and medical procedures as the cause of abnormal reaction of the patient, or of later complication, without mention of misadventure at the time of the procedure

Misadventures to patients during surgical and medical care (Y62-Y69)

Excludes 1: surgical and medical procedures as the cause of abnormal reaction of the patient, without mention of misadventure at the time of the procedure (Y83-Y84)

Excludes ❷: breakdown or malfunctioning of medical device (during procedure) (after implantation) (ongoing use) (Y70-Y82)

Y62- <u>Failure of sterile precautions</u> during surgical and medical care

Y62.0 Failure of sterile precautions during <u>surgical operation</u>

Y62.1 Failure of sterile precautions during <u>infusion or transfusion</u>

Y62.2 Failure of sterile precautions during <u>kidney dialysis and other perfusion</u>

Y62.3 Failure of sterile precautions during <u>injection or immunization</u>

Y62.4 Failure of sterile precautions during <u>endoscopic examination</u>

Y62.5 Failure of sterile precautions during <u>heart catheterization</u>

Y62.6 Failure of sterile precautions during <u>aspiration, puncture and other catheterization</u>

Y62.8 Failure of sterile precautions during <u>other</u> surgical and medical care

Y62.9 Failure of sterile precautions during <u>unspecified</u> surgical and medical care

Y63- <u>Failure in dosage</u> during surgical and medical care
Excludes ❷: accidental overdose of drug or wrong drug given in error (T36-T50)

Y63.0 <u>Excessive amount</u> of blood or other fluid given during transfusion or infusion

Y63.1 <u>Incorrect dilution</u> of fluid used during infusion

Y63.2 <u>Overdose of radiation</u> given during therapy

Y63.3 <u>Inadvertent exposure</u> of patient to radiation during medical care

Y63.4 Failure in dosage in <u>electroshock or insulin-shock therapy</u>

Y63.5 <u>Inappropriate temperature</u> in local application and packing

Y63.6 <u>Underdosing</u> and <u>nonadministration</u> of necessary drug, medicament or biological substance

Y63.8 Failure in dosage during <u>other</u> surgical and medical care

Y63.9 Failure in dosage during <u>unspecified</u> surgical and medical care

Y64- <u>Contaminated</u> medical or biological substances

Y64.0 Contaminated medical or biological substance, <u>transfused or infused</u>

Y64.1 Contaminated medical or biological substance, <u>injected or used for immunization</u>

Y64.8 Contaminated medical or biological substance <u>administered by other means</u>

Y64.9 Contaminated medical or biological substance administered by <u>unspecified</u> means
Administered contaminated medical or biological substance NOS

Y65- <u>Other misadventures</u> during surgical and medical care

Y65.0 <u>Mismatched</u> blood in transfusion

Y65.1 <u>Wrong</u> fluid used in infusion — [Wrong Procedure Performed]

Y65.2 <u>Failure in suture or ligature</u> during surgical operation — [Wrong Procedure Performed]

Y65.3 <u>Endotracheal tube wrongly placed</u> during anesthetic procedure — [Wrong Procedure Performed]

Y65.4 <u>Failure to introduce or to remove</u> other tube or instrument

Y65.5- Performance of <u>wrong procedure</u> (operation)

Y65.51 Performance of wrong procedure (operation) on correct patient
Wrong device implanted into correct surgical site
Excludes 1: performance of correct procedure (operation) on wrong side or body part (Y65.53)

Y38 - Y65

Y65.52   **Performance of procedure (operation) on patient not scheduled for surgery**
Performance of procedure (operation) intended for another patient
Performance of procedure (operation) on wrong patient

Y65.53   **Performance of correct procedure (operation) on <u>wrong side or body part</u>**
Performance of correct procedure (operation) on wrong side
Performance of correct procedure (operation) on wrong site

Y65.8   <u>Other</u> specified misadventures during surgical and medical care

Y66   <u>Nonadministration</u> of <u>surgical and medical care</u>
Premature cessation of surgical and medical care
Excludes 1:   *DNR status (Z66)*
palliative care (Z51.5)

Y69   <u>Unspecified</u> misadventure during surgical and medical care

Medical devices associated with adverse incidents in diagnostic and therapeutic use (Y70-Y82)

Includes: Breakdown or malfunction of medical devices (during use) (after implantation) (ongoing use)
Excludes ❷: *breakdown or malfunctioning of medical device (after implantation) (during procedure) (ongoing use) (Y70-Y82)*
later complications following use of medical devices without breakdown or malfunctioning of device (Y83-Y84)
misadventure to patients during surgical and medical care, classifiable to (Y62-Y69)
surgical and other medical procedures as the cause of abnormal reaction of the patient, or of later complication, without mention of misadventure at the time of the procedure (Y83-Y84)

Y70-   <u>Anesthesiology devices</u> <u>associated with adverse incidents</u>

Y70.0   **Diagnostic and monitoring anesthesiology devices associated with adverse incidents**

Y70.1   **Therapeutic (nonsurgical) and rehabilitative anesthesiology devices associated with adverse incidents**

Y70.2   **Prosthetic and other implants, materials and accessory anesthesiology devices associated with adverse incidents**

Y70.3   **Surgical instruments, materials and anesthesiology devices (including sutures) associated with adverse incidents**

Y70.8   **Miscellaneous anesthesiology devices associated with adverse incidents, not elsewhere classified**

Y71-   <u>Cardiovascular devices</u> <u>associated with adverse incidents</u>

Y71.0   **Diagnostic and monitoring cardiovascular devices associated with adverse incidents**

Y71.1   **Therapeutic (nonsurgical) and rehabilitative cardiovascular devices associated with adverse incidents**

Y71.2   **Prosthetic and other implants, materials and accessory cardiovascular devices associated with adverse incidents**

Y71.3   **Surgical instruments, materials and cardiovascular devices (including sutures) associated with adverse incidents**

Y71.8   **Miscellaneous cardiovascular devices associated with adverse incidents, not elsewhere classified**

Y72-   <u>Otorhinolaryngological devices</u> <u>associated with adverse incidents</u>

Y72.0   **Diagnostic and monitoring otorhinolaryngological devices associated with adverse incidents**

Y72.1   **Therapeutic (nonsurgical) and rehabilitative otorhinolaryngological devices associated with adverse incidents**

Y72.2   **Prosthetic and other implants, materials and accessory otorhinolaryngological devices associated with adverse incidents**

Y72.3   **Surgical instruments, materials and otorhinolaryngological devices (including sutures) associated with adverse incidents**

Y72.8   **Miscellaneous otorhinolaryngological devices associated with adverse incidents, not elsewhere classified**

Y73-   <u>Gastroenterology and urology devices</u> <u>associated with adverse incidents</u>

Y73.0   **Diagnostic and monitoring gastroenterology and urology devices associated with adverse incidents**

Y73.1   **Therapeutic (nonsurgical) and rehabilitative gastroenterology and urology devices associated with adverse incidents**

Y73.2   **Prosthetic and other implants, materials and accessory gastroenterology and urology devices associated with adverse incidents**

Y73.3   **Surgical instruments, materials and gastroenterology and urology devices (including sutures) associated with adverse incidents**

Y73.8   **Miscellaneous gastroenterology and urology devices associated with adverse incidents, not elsewhere classified**

Y74-   <u>General hospital and personal-use devices</u> <u>associated with adverse incidents</u>

Y74.0   <u>Diagnostic</u> and monitoring general hospital and personal-use devices associated with adverse incidents

Y74.1   <u>Therapeutic</u> (nonsurgical) and rehabilitative general hospital and personal-use devices associated with adverse incidents

Y74.2   <u>Prosthetic</u> and other implants, materials and accessory general hospital and personal-use devices associated with adverse incidents

Y74.3   <u>Surgical</u> instruments, materials and general hospital and personal-use devices (including sutures) associated with adverse incidents

Y74.8   <u>Miscellaneous</u> general hospital and personal-use devices associated with adverse incidents, not elsewhere classified

Y75-   <u>Neurological devices</u> <u>associated with adverse incidents</u>

Y75.0   <u>Diagnostic</u> and monitoring neurological devices associated with adverse incidents

Y75.1   <u>Therapeutic</u> (nonsurgical) and rehabilitative neurological devices associated with adverse incidents

Y75.2   <u>Prosthetic</u> and other implants, materials and neurological devices associated with adverse incidents

Y75.3   <u>Surgical</u> instruments, materials and neurological devices (including sutures) associated with adverse incidents

Y75.8   <u>Miscellaneous</u> neurological devices associated with adverse incidents, not elsewhere classified

Y76-   <u>Obstetric and gynecological devices</u> <u>associated with adverse incidents</u>

Y76.0   <u>Diagnostic</u> and monitoring obstetric and gynecological devices associated with adverse incidents — [♀]

Y76.1   <u>Therapeutic</u> (nonsurgical) and rehabilitative obstetric and gynecological devices associated with adverse incidents — [♀]

Y76.2   <u>Prosthetic</u> and other implants, materials and accessory obstetric and gynecological devices associated with adverse incidents — [♀]

Y76.3   <u>Surgical</u> instruments, materials and obstetric and gynecological devices (including sutures) associated with adverse incidents — [♀]

Y76.8   <u>Miscellaneous</u> obstetric and gynecological devices associated with adverse incidents, not elsewhere classified — [♀]

Y77-   <u>Ophthalmic devices</u> <u>associated with adverse incidents</u>

Y77.0   <u>Diagnostic</u> and monitoring ophthalmic devices associated with adverse incidents

Y77.1   <u>Therapeutic</u> (nonsurgical) and rehabilitative ophthalmic devices associated with adverse incidents

Y77.2   <u>Prosthetic</u> and other implants, materials and accessory ophthalmic devices associated with adverse incidents

Y77.3   <u>Surgical</u> instruments, materials and ophthalmic devices (including sutures) associated with adverse incidents

Y77.8   <u>Miscellaneous</u> ophthalmic devices associated with adverse incidents, not elsewhere classified

Y78-   Radiological devices associated with adverse incidents

Y78.0   Diagnostic and monitoring radiological devices associated with adverse incidents

Y78.1   Therapeutic (nonsurgical) and rehabilitative radiological devices associated with adverse incidents

Y78.2   Prosthetic and other implants, materials and accessory radiological devices associated with adverse incidents

Y78.3   Surgical instruments, materials and radiological devices (including sutures) associated with adverse incidents

Y78.8   Miscellaneous radiological devices associated with adverse incidents, not elsewhere classified

Y79-   Orthopedic devices associated with adverse incidents

Y79.0   Diagnostic and monitoring orthopedic devices associated with adverse incidents

Y79.1   Therapeutic (nonsurgical) and rehabilitative orthopedic devices associated with adverse incidents

Y79.2   Prosthetic and other implants, materials and accessory orthopedic devices associated with adverse incidents

Y79.3   Surgical instruments, materials and orthopedic devices (including sutures) associated with adverse incidents

Y79.8   Miscellaneous orthopedic devices associated with adverse incidents, not elsewhere classified

Y80-   Physical medicine devices associated with adverse incidents

Y80.0   Diagnostic and monitoring physical medicine devices associated with adverse incidents

Y80.1   Therapeutic (nonsurgical) and rehabilitative physical medicine devices associated with adverse incidents

Y80.2   Prosthetic and other implants, materials and accessory physical medicine devices associated with adverse incidents

Y80.3   Surgical instruments, materials and physical medicine devices (including sutures) associated with adverse incidents

Y80.8   Miscellaneous physical medicine devices associated with adverse incidents, not elsewhere classified

Y81-   General- and plastic-surgery devices associated with adverse incidents

Y81.0   Diagnostic and monitoring general- and plastic-surgery devices associated with adverse incidents

Y81.1   Therapeutic (nonsurgical) and rehabilitative general- and plastic-surgery devices associated with adverse incidents

Y81.2   Prosthetic and other implants, materials and accessory general- and plastic-surgery devices associated with adverse incidents

Y81.3   Surgical instruments, materials and general- and plastic-surgery devices (including sutures) associated with adverse incidents

Y81.8   Miscellaneous general- and plastic-surgery devices associated with adverse incidents, not elsewhere classified

Y82-   Other and unspecified medical devices associated with adverse incidents

Y82.8   Other medical devices associated with adverse incidents

Y82.9   Unspecified medical devices associated with adverse incidents

Surgical and other medical procedures as the cause of abnormal reaction of the patient, or of later complication, without mention of misadventure at the time of the procedure (Y83-Y84)

Excludes 1:   misadventures to patients during surgical and medical care, classifiable to (Y62-Y69)

Excludes ❷: breakdown or malfunctioning of medical device (after implantation) (during procedure) (ongoing use) (Y70-Y82)

Y83-   Surgical operation and other surgical procedures as the cause of abnormal reaction of the patient, or of later complication, without mention of misadventure at the time of the procedure

Y83.0   Surgical operation with transplant of whole organ as the cause of abnormal reaction of the patient, or of later complication, without mention of misadventure at the time of the procedure

Y83.1   Surgical operation with implant of artificial internal device as the cause of abnormal reaction of the patient, or of later complication, without mention of misadventure at the time of the procedure

Y83.2   Surgical operation with anastomosis, bypass or graft as the cause of abnormal reaction of the patient, or of later complication, without mention of misadventure at the time of the procedure

Y83.3   Surgical operation with formation of external stoma as the cause of abnormal reaction of the patient, or of later complication, without mention of misadventure at the time of the procedure

Y83.4   Other reconstructive surgery as the cause of abnormal reaction of the patient, or of later complication, without mention of misadventure at the time of the procedure

Y83.5   Amputation of limb(s) as the cause of abnormal reaction of the patient, or of later complication, without mention of misadventure at the time of the procedure

Y83.6   Removal of other organ (partial) (total) as the cause of abnormal reaction of the patient, or of later complication, without mention of misadventure at the time of the procedure

Y83.8   Other surgical procedures as the cause of abnormal reaction of the patient, or of later complication, without mention of misadventure at the time of the procedure

Y83.9   Surgical procedure, unspecified as the cause of abnormal reaction of the patient, or of later complication, without mention of misadventure at the time of the procedure

Y84-   Other medical procedures as the cause of abnormal reaction of the patient, or of later complication, without mention of misadventure at the time of the procedure

Y84.0   Cardiac catheterization as the cause of abnormal reaction of the patient, or of later complication, without mention of misadventure at the time of the procedure

Y84.1   Kidney dialysis as the cause of abnormal reaction of the patient, or of later complication, without mention of misadventure at the time of the procedure

Y84.2   Radiological procedure and radiotherapy as the cause of abnormal reaction of the patient, or of later complication, without mention of misadventure at the time of the procedure

Y84.3   Shock therapy as the cause of abnormal reaction of the patient, or of later complication, without mention of misadventure at the time of the procedure

Y84.4   Aspiration of fluid as the cause of abnormal reaction of the patient, or of later complication, without mention of misadventure at the time of the procedure

Y84.5   Insertion of gastric or duodenal sound as the cause of abnormal reaction of the patient, or of later complication, without mention of misadventure at the time of the procedure

Y84.6   Urinary catheterization as the cause of abnormal reaction of the patient, or of later complication, without mention of misadventure at the time of the procedure

Y78 I Y84

Y84.7 <u>Blood-sampling</u> as the cause of abnormal reaction of the patient, or of later complication, without mention of misadventure at the time of the procedure

Y84.8 <u>Other</u> medical procedures as the cause of abnormal reaction of the patient, or of later complication, without mention of misadventure at the time of the procedure

AHA 14:4Q:p24 – Durotomy secondary to previous epidural injections

Y84.9 Medical procedure, <u>unspecified</u> as the cause of abnormal reaction of the patient, or of later complication, without mention of misadventure at the time of the procedure

Supplementary factors related to causes of morbidity classified elsewhere (Y90-Y99)

Note: These categories may be used to provide supplementary information concerning causes of morbidity. They are not to be used for single-condition coding.

Y90- <u>Evidence of alcohol involvement determined by blood alcohol level</u>
Code first any associated alcohol related disorders (F10)

Y90.0 Blood alcohol level of less than 20 mg/100 ml

Y90.1 Blood alcohol level of 20-39 mg/100 ml

Y90.2 Blood alcohol level of 40-59 mg/100 ml

Y90.3 Blood alcohol level of 60-79 mg/100 ml

Y90.4 Blood alcohol level of 80-99 mg/100 ml

Y90.5 Blood alcohol level of 100-119 mg/100 ml

Y90.6 Blood alcohol level of 120-199 mg/100 ml

Y90.7 Blood alcohol level of 200-239 mg/100 ml

Y90.8 Blood alcohol level of 240 mg/100 ml or more

Y90.9 Presence of alcohol in blood, level not specified

Y92- <u>Place of occurrence</u> of the <u>external cause</u>
Note: The following category is for use, when relevant, to identify the place of occurrence of the external cause. Use in conjunction with an activity code.
Note: Place of occurrence should be recorded only at the initial encounter for treatment.

Y92.0- <u>Non-institutional (private) residence</u> as the place of occurrence of the external cause
Excludes 1: *abandoned or derelict house (Y92.89)*
home under construction but not yet occupied (Y92.6-)
institutional place of residence (Y92.1-)

Y92.00- <u>Unspecified</u> non-institutional (private) residence as the place of occurrence of the external cause

Y92.000 <u>Kitchen</u> of unspecified non-institutional (private) residence as the place of occurrence of the external cause

Y92.001 <u>Dining room</u> of unspecified non-institutional (private) residence as the place of occurrence of the external cause

Y92.002 <u>Bathroom</u> of unspecified non-institutional (private) residence single-family (private) house as the place of occurrence of the external cause

Y92.003 <u>Bedroom</u> of unspecified non-institutional (private) residence as the place of occurrence of the external cause

Y92.007 <u>Garden or yard</u> in unspecified non-institutional (private) residence as the place of occurrence of the external cause

Y92.008 <u>Other</u> place in unspecified non-institutional (private) residence as the place of occurrence of the external cause

Y92.009 <u>Unspecified</u> place in unspecified non-institutional (private) residence as the place of occurrence of the external cause
Home (NOS) as the place of occurrence of the external cause

Y92.01- <u>Single-family</u> non-institutional (private) house as the place of occurrence of the external cause
Farmhouse as the place of occurrence of the external cause
Excludes 1: *barn (Y92.71)*
chicken coop or hen house (Y92.72)
farm field (Y92.73)
orchard (Y92.74)
single family mobile home or trailer (Y92.02-)
slaughter house (Y92.86)

Y92.010 <u>Kitchen</u> of single-family (private) house as the place of occurrence of the external cause

Y92.011 <u>Dining room</u> of single-family (private) house as the place of occurrence of the external cause

Y92.012 <u>Bathroom</u> of single-family (private) house as the place of occurrence of the external cause

Y92.013 <u>Bedroom</u> of single-family (private) house as the place of occurrence of the external cause

Y92.014 <u>Private driveway</u> to single-family (private) house as the place of occurrence of the external cause

Y92.015 <u>Private garage</u> of single-family (private) house as the place of occurrence of the external cause

Y92.016 <u>Swimming-pool</u> in single-family (private) house or garden as the place of occurrence of the external cause

Y92.017 <u>Garden or yard</u> in single-family (private) house as the place of occurrence of the external cause

Y92.018 <u>Other</u> place in single-family (private) house as the place of occurrence of the external cause

Y92.019 <u>Unspecified</u> place in single-family (private) house as the place of occurrence of the external cause

Y92.02- <u>Mobile home</u> as the place of occurrence of the external cause

Y92.020 <u>Kitchen</u> in mobile home as the place of occurrence of the external cause

Y92.021 <u>Dining room</u> in mobile home as the place of occurrence of the external cause

Y92.022 <u>Bathroom</u> in mobile home as the place of occurrence of the external cause

Y92.023 <u>Bedroom</u> in mobile home as the place of occurrence of the external cause

Y92.024 <u>Driveway</u> of mobile home as the place of occurrence of the external cause

Y92.025 <u>Garage</u> of mobile home as the place of occurrence of the external cause

Y92.026 <u>Swimming-pool</u> of mobile home as the place of occurrence of the external cause

Y92.027 <u>Garden or yard</u> of mobile home as the place of occurrence of the external cause

Y92.028 <u>Other</u> place in mobile home as the place of occurrence of the external cause

Y92.029 <u>Unspecified</u> place in mobile home as the place of occurrence of the external cause

Y92.03- <u>Apartment</u> as the place of occurrence of the external cause
Condominium as the place of occurrence of the external cause
Co-op apartment as the place of occurrence of the external cause

Y92.030 <u>Kitchen</u> in apartment as the place of occurrence of the external cause

Y92.031 <u>Bathroom</u> in apartment as the place of occurrence of the external cause

Y92.032 <u>Bedroom</u> in apartment as the place of occurrence of the external cause

Y92.038 <u>Other</u> place in apartment as the place of occurrence of the external cause

Y92.039 <u>Unspecified</u> place in apartment as the place of occurrence of the external cause

Y84-Y92

Y92.04- <u>Boarding-house</u> as the place of occurrence of the external cause

Y92.040 <u>Kitchen</u> in boarding-house as the place of occurrence of the external cause

Y92.041 <u>Bathroom</u> in boarding-house as the place of occurrence of the external cause

Y92.042 <u>Bedroom</u> in boarding-house as the place of occurrence of the external cause

Y92.043 <u>Driveway</u> of boarding-house as the place of occurrence of the external cause

Y92.044 <u>Garage</u> of boarding-house as the place of occurrence of the external cause

Y92.045 <u>Swimming-pool</u> of boarding-house as the place of occurrence of the external cause

Y92.046 <u>Garden or yard</u> of boarding-house as the place of occurrence of the external cause

Y92.048 <u>Other</u> place in boarding-house as the place of occurrence of the external cause

Y92.049 <u>Unspecified</u> place in boarding-house as the place of occurrence of the external cause

Y92.09- <u>Other</u> non-institutional residence as the place of occurrence of the external cause

Y92.090 <u>Kitchen</u> in other non-institutional residence as the place of occurrence of the external cause

Y92.091 <u>Bathroom</u> in other non-institutional residence as the place of occurrence of the external cause

Y92.092 <u>Bedroom</u> in other non-institutional residence as the place of occurrence of the external cause

Y92.093 <u>Driveway</u> of other non-institutional residence as the place of occurrence of the external cause

Y92.094 <u>Garage</u> of other non-institutional residence as the place of occurrence of the external cause

Y92.095 <u>Swimming-pool</u> of other non-institutional residence as the place of occurrence of the external cause

Y92.096 <u>Garden or yard</u> of other non-institutional residence as the place of occurrence of the external cause

Y92.098 <u>Other</u> place in other non-institutional residence as the place of occurrence of the external cause

Y92.099 <u>Unspecified</u> place in other non-institutional residence as the place of occurrence of the external cause

Y92.1- <u>Institutional (nonprivate) residence</u> as the place of occurrence of the external cause

Y92.10 <u>Unspecified</u> residential institution as the place of occurrence of the external cause

Y92.11- <u>Children's home and orphanage</u> as the place of occurrence of the external cause

Y92.110 <u>Kitchen</u> in children's home and orphanage as the place of occurrence of the external cause

Y92.111 <u>Bathroom</u> in children's home and orphanage as the place of occurrence of the external cause

Y92.112 <u>Bedroom</u> in children's home and orphanage as the place of occurrence of the external cause

Y92.113 <u>Driveway</u> of children's home and orphanage as the place of occurrence of the external cause

Y92.114 <u>Garage</u> of children's home and orphanage as the place of occurrence of the external cause

Y92.115 <u>Swimming-pool</u> of children's home and orphanage as the place of occurrence of the external cause

Y92.116 <u>Garden or yard</u> of children's home and orphanage as the place of occurrence of the external cause

Y92.118 <u>Other</u> place in children's home and orphanage as the place of occurrence of the external cause

Y92.119 <u>Unspecified</u> place in children's home and orphanage as the place of occurrence of the external cause

Y92.12- <u>Nursing home</u> as the place of occurrence of the external cause

Home for the sick as the place of occurrence of the external cause

Hospice as the place of occurrence of the external cause

Y92.120 <u>Kitchen</u> in nursing home as the place of occurrence of the external cause

Y92.121 <u>Bathroom</u> in nursing home as the place of occurrence of the external cause

Y92.122 <u>Bedroom</u> in nursing home as the place of occurrence of the external cause

Y92.123 <u>Driveway</u> of nursing home as the place of occurrence of the external cause

Y92.124 <u>Garage</u> of nursing home as the place of occurrence of the external cause

Y92.125 <u>Swimming-pool</u> of nursing home as the place of occurrence of the external cause

Y92.126 <u>Garden or yard</u> of nursing home as the place of occurrence of the external cause

Y92.128 <u>Other</u> place in nursing home as the place of occurrence of the external cause

Y92.129 <u>Unspecified</u> place in nursing home as the place of occurrence of the external cause

Y92.13- <u>Military base</u> as the place of occurrence of the external cause

Excludes 1:   *military training grounds (Y92.83)*

Y92.130 <u>Kitchen</u> on military base as the place of occurrence of the external cause

Y92.131 <u>Mess hall</u> on military base as the place of occurrence of the external cause

Y92.133 <u>Barracks</u> on military base as the place of occurrence of the external cause

Y92.135 <u>Garage</u> on military base as the place of occurrence of the external cause

Y92.136 <u>Swimming-pool</u> on military base as the place of occurrence of the external cause

Y92.137 <u>Garden or yard</u> on military base as the place of occurrence of the external cause

Y92.138 <u>Other</u> place on military base as the place of occurrence of the external cause

Y92.139 <u>Unspecified</u> place military base as the place of occurrence of the external cause

Y92.14- <u>Prison</u> as the place of occurrence of the external cause

Y92.140 <u>Kitchen</u> in prison as the place of occurrence of the external cause

Y92.141 <u>Dining room</u> in prison as the place of occurrence of the external cause

Y92.142 <u>Bathroom</u> in prison as the place of occurrence of the external cause

Y92.143 <u>Cell</u> of prison as the place of occurrence of the external cause

Y92.146 <u>Swimming-pool</u> of prison as the place of occurrence of the external cause

Y92.147 <u>Courtyard</u> of prison as the place of occurrence of the external cause

Y92.148 <u>Other</u> place in prison as the place of occurrence of the external cause

Y92.149 <u>Unspecified</u> place in prison as the place of occurrence of the external cause

Y92.15- <u>Reform school</u> as the place of occurrence of the external cause

Y92.150 <u>Kitchen</u> in reform school as the place of occurrence of the external cause

Y92.151 <u>Dining room</u> in reform school as the place of occurrence of the external cause

Y92.152 <u>Bathroom</u> in reform school as the place of occurrence of the external cause

Y92.153 <u>Bedroom</u> in reform school as the place of occurrence of the external cause

Y92 - Y92

Y92.154 <u>Driveway</u> of reform school as the place of occurrence of the external cause

Y92.155 <u>Garage</u> of reform school as the place of occurrence of the external cause

Y92.156 <u>Swimming-pool</u> of reform school as the place of occurrence of the external cause

Y92.157 <u>Garden or yard</u> of reform school as the place of occurrence of the external cause

Y92.158 <u>Other</u> place in reform school as the place of occurrence of the external cause

Y92.159 <u>Unspecified</u> place in reform school as the place of occurrence of the external cause

Y92.16- <u>School dormitory</u> as the place of occurrence of the external cause

Excludes 1: *reform school as the place of occurrence of the external cause (Y92.15-)*
school buildings and grounds as the place of occurrence of the external cause (Y92.2-)
school sports and athletic areas as the place of occurrence of the external cause (Y92.3-)

Y92.160 <u>Kitchen</u> in school dormitory as the place of occurrence of the external cause

Y92.161 <u>Dining room</u> in school dormitory as the place of occurrence of the external cause

Y92.162 <u>Bathroom</u> in school dormitory as the place of occurrence of the external cause

Y92.163 <u>Bedroom</u> in school dormitory as the place of occurrence of the external cause

Y92.168 <u>Other</u> place in school dormitory as the place of occurrence of the external cause

Y92.169 <u>Unspecified</u> place in school dormitory as the place of occurrence of the external cause

Y92.19- <u>Other specified residential institution</u> as the place of occurrence of the external cause

Y92.190 <u>Kitchen</u> in other specified residential institution as the place of occurrence of the external cause

Y92.191 <u>Dining room</u> in other specified residential institution as the place of occurrence of the external cause

Y92.192 <u>Bathroom</u> in other specified residential institution as the place of occurrence of the external cause

Y92.193 <u>Bedroom</u> in other specified residential institution as the place of occurrence of the external cause

Y92.194 <u>Driveway</u> of other specified residential institution as the place of occurrence of the external cause

Y92.195 <u>Garage</u> of other specified residential institution as the place of occurrence of the external cause

Y92.196 <u>Pool</u> of other specified residential institution as the place of occurrence of the external cause

Y92.197 <u>Garden or yard</u> of other specified residential institution as the place of occurrence of the external cause

Y92.198 <u>Other</u> place in other specified residential institution as the place of occurrence of the external cause

Y92.199 <u>Unspecified</u> place in other specified residential institution as the place of occurrence of the external cause

Y92.2- <u>School, other institution and public administrative area</u> as the place of occurrence of the external cause

Building and adjacent grounds used by the general public or by a particular group of the public

Excludes 1: *building under construction as the place of occurrence of the external cause (Y92.6)*
residential institution as the place of occurrence of the external cause (Y92.1)
school dormitory as the place of occurrence of the external cause (Y92.16-)
sports and athletics area of schools as the place of occurrence of the external cause (Y92.3-)

Y92.21- <u>School (private) (public) (state)</u> as the place of occurrence of the external cause

Y92.210 <u>Daycare center</u> as the place of occurrence of the external cause

Y92.211 <u>Elementary school</u> as the place of occurrence of the external cause

Kindergarten as the place of occurrence of the external cause

Y92.212 <u>Middle school</u> as the place of occurrence of the external cause

Y92.213 <u>High school</u> as the place of occurrence of the external cause

Y92.214 <u>College</u> as the place of occurrence of the external cause

University as the place of occurrence of the external cause

Y92.215 <u>Trade school</u> as the place of occurrence of the external cause

Y92.218 <u>Other</u> school as the place of occurrence of the external cause

Y92.219 <u>Unspecified</u> school as the place of occurrence of the external cause

Y92.22 <u>Religious institution</u> as the place of occurrence of the external cause

Church as the place of occurrence of the external cause
Mosque as the place of occurrence of the external cause
Synagogue as the place of occurrence of the external cause

Y92.23- <u>Hospital</u> as the place of occurrence of the external cause

Excludes 1: *ambulatory (outpatient) health services establishments (Y92.53-)*
home for the sick as the place of occurrence of the external cause (Y92.12-)
hospice as the place of occurrence of the external cause (Y92.12-)
nursing home as the place of occurrence of the external cause (Y92.12-)

Y92.230 <u>Patient room</u> in hospital as the place of occurrence of the external cause

Y92.231 <u>Patient bathroom</u> in hospital as the place of occurrence of the external cause

Y92.232 <u>Corridor</u> of hospital as the place of occurrence of the external cause

Y92.233 <u>Cafeteria</u> of hospital as the place of occurrence of the external cause

Y92.234 <u>Operating room</u> of hospital as the place of occurrence of the external cause

Y92.238 <u>Other</u> place in hospital as the place of occurrence of the external cause

Y92.239 <u>Unspecified</u> place in hospital as the place of occurrence of the external cause

Y92.24- <u>Public administrative building</u> as the place of occurrence of the external cause

Y92.240 <u>Courthouse</u> as the place of occurrence of the external cause

Y92.241 <u>Library</u> as the place of occurrence of the external cause

Y92.242 <u>Post office</u> as the place of occurrence of the external cause

Y92.243 <u>City hall</u> as the place of occurrence of the external cause

Y92.248   **Other** public administrative building as the place of occurrence of the external cause

Y92.25-   **Cultural building** as the place of occurrence of the external cause

Y92.250   **Art Gallery** as the place of occurrence of the external cause

Y92.251   **Museum** as the place of occurrence of the external cause

Y92.252   **Music hall** as the place of occurrence of the external cause

Y92.253   **Opera house** as the place of occurrence of the external cause

Y92.254   **Theater (live)** as the place of occurrence of the external cause

Y92.258   **Other** cultural public building as the place of occurrence of the external cause

Y92.26   **Movie house or cinema** as the place of occurrence of the external cause

Y92.29   **Other** specified public building as the place of occurrence of the external cause
     Assembly hall as the place of occurrence of the external cause
     Clubhouse as the place of occurrence of the external cause

Y92.3-   **Sports and athletics area** as the place of occurrence of the external cause

Y92.31-   **Athletic court** as the place of occurrence of the external cause
     Excludes 1:   *tennis court in private home or garden (Y92.09)*

Y92.310   **Basketball** court as the place of occurrence of the external cause

Y92.311   **Squash** court as the place of occurrence of the external cause

Y92.312   **Tennis** court as the place of occurrence of the external cause

Y92.318   **Other** athletic court as the place of occurrence of the external cause

Y92.32-   **Athletic field** as the place of occurrence of the external cause

Y92.320   **Baseball** field as the place of occurrence of the external cause

Y92.321   **Football** field as the place of occurrence of the external cause

Y92.322   **Soccer** field as the place of occurrence of the external cause

Y92.328   **Other** athletic field as the place of occurrence of the external cause
     Cricket field as the place of occurrence of the external cause
     Hockey field as the place of occurrence of the external cause

Y92.33-   **Skating rink** as the place of occurrence of the external cause

Y92.330   **Ice skating** rink (indoor) (outdoor) as the place of occurrence of the external cause

Y92.331   **Roller skating** rink as the place of occurrence of the external cause

Y92.34   **Swimming pool (public)** as the place of occurrence of the external cause
     Excludes 1:   *swimming pool in private home or garden (Y92.016)*

Y92.39   **Other** specified sports and athletic area as the place of occurrence of the external cause
     Golf-course as the place of occurrence of the external cause
     Gymnasium as the place of occurrence of the external cause
     Riding-school as the place of occurrence of the external cause
     Stadium as the place of occurrence of the external cause

Y92.4-   **Street, highway and other paved roadways** as the place of occurrence of the external cause
     Excludes 1:   *private driveway of residence (Y92.014, Y92.024, Y92.043, Y92.093, Y92.113, Y92.123, Y92.154, Y92.194)*

Y92.41-   **Street and highway** as the place of occurrence of the external cause

Y92.410   **Unspecified** street and highway as the place of occurrence of the external cause
     Road NOS as the place of occurrence of the external cause

Y92.411   **Interstate highway** as the place of occurrence of the external cause
     Freeway as the place of occurrence of the external cause
     Motorway as the place of occurrence of the external cause

Y92.412   **Parkway** as the place of occurrence of the external cause

Y92.413   **State road** as the place of occurrence of the external cause

Y92.414   **Local residential or business street** as the place of occurrence of the external cause

Y92.415   **Exit ramp or entrance ramp** of street or highway as the place of occurrence of the external cause

Y92.48-   **Other paved roadways** as the place of occurrence of the external cause

Y92.480   **Sidewalk** as the place of occurrence of the external cause

Y92.481   **Parking lot** as the place of occurrence of the external cause

Y92.482   **Bike path** as the place of occurrence of the external cause

Y92.488   **Other** paved roadways as the place of occurrence of the external cause

Y92.5-   **Trade and service area** as the place of occurrence of the external cause
     Excludes 1:   *garage in private home (Y92.015)*
                 schools and other public administration buildings (Y92.2-)

Y92.51-   **Private commercial establishments** as the place of occurrence of the external cause

Y92.510   **Bank** as the place of occurrence of the external cause

Y92.511   **Restaurant or café** as the place of occurrence of the external cause

Y92.512   **Supermarket**, store or market as the place of occurrence of the external cause

Y92.513   **Shop** (commercial) as the place of occurrence of the external cause

Y92.52-   **Service areas** as the place of occurrence of the external cause

Y92.520   **Airport** as the place of occurrence of the external cause

Y92.521   **Bus station** as the place of occurrence of the external cause

Y92.522   **Railway station** as the place of occurrence of the external cause

Y92.523   **Highway rest stop** as the place of occurrence of the external cause

Y92.524   **Gas station** as the place of occurrence of the external cause
     Petroleum station as the place of occurrence of the external cause
     Service station as the place of occurrence of the external cause

Y92.53- **Ambulatory health services establishments** as the place of occurrence of the external cause

Y92.530   **Ambulatory surgery center** as the place of occurrence of the external cause

Outpatient surgery center, including that connected with a hospital as the place of occurrence of the external cause

Same day surgery center, including that connected with a hospital as the place of occurrence of the external cause

Y92.531   **Health care provider office** as the place of occurrence of the external cause

Physician office as the place of occurrence of the external cause

Y92.532   **Urgent care center** as the place of occurrence of the external cause

Y92.538   **Other** ambulatory health services establishments as the place of occurrence of the external cause

Y92.59   **Other** trade areas as the place of occurrence of the external cause

Office building as the place of occurrence of the external cause

Casino as the place of occurrence of the external cause

Garage (commercial) as the place of occurrence of the external cause

Hotel as the place of occurrence of the external cause

Radio or television station as the place of occurrence of the external cause

Shopping mall as the place of occurrence of the external cause

Warehouse as the place of occurrence of the external cause

Y92.6-   **Industrial and construction area** as the place of occurrence of the external cause

Y92.61   **Building [any] under construction** as the place of occurrence of the external cause

Y92.62   **Dock or shipyard** as the place of occurrence of the external cause

Dockyard as the place of occurrence of the external cause

Dry dock as the place of occurrence of the external cause

Shipyard as the place of occurrence of the external cause

Y92.63   **Factory** as the place of occurrence of the external cause

Factory building as the place of occurrence of the external cause

Factory premises as the place of occurrence of the external cause

Industrial yard as the place of occurrence of the external cause

Y92.64   **Mine or pit** as the place of occurrence of the external cause

Mine as the place of occurrence of the external cause

Y92.65   **Oil rig** as the place of occurrence of the external cause

Pit (coal) (gravel) (sand) as the place of occurrence of the external cause

Y92.69   **Other** specified industrial and construction area as the place of occurrence of the external cause

Gasworks as the place of occurrence of the external cause

Power-station (coal) (nuclear) (oil) as the place of occurrence of the external cause

Tunnel under construction as the place of occurrence of the external cause

Workshop as the place of occurrence of the external cause

Y92.7-   **Farm** as the place of occurrence of the external cause

Ranch as the place of occurrence of the external cause

Excludes 1:   *farmhouse and home premises of farm (Y92.01-)*

Y92.71   **Barn** as the place of occurrence of the external cause

Y92.72   **Chicken coop** as the place of occurrence of the external cause

Hen house as the place of occurrence of the external cause

Y92.73   **Farm field** as the place of occurrence of the external cause

Y92.74   **Orchard** as the place of occurrence of the external cause

Y92.79   **Other** farm location as the place of occurrence of the external cause

Y92.8-   **Other places** as the place of occurrence of the external cause

Y92.81-   **Transport vehicle** as the place of occurrence of the external cause

Excludes 1:   *transport accidents (V00-V99)*

Y92.810   **Car** as the place of occurrence of the external cause

Y92.811   **Bus** as the place of occurrence of the external cause

Y92.812   **Truck** as the place of occurrence of the external cause

Y92.813   **Airplane** as the place of occurrence of the external cause

Y92.814   **Boat** as the place of occurrence of the external cause

Y92.815   **Train** as the place of occurrence of the external cause

Y92.816   **Subway car** as the place of occurrence of the external cause

Y92.818   **Other** transport vehicle as the place of occurrence of the external cause

Y92.82-   **Wilderness area**

Y92.820   **Desert** as the place of occurrence of the external cause

Y92.821   **Forest** as the place of occurrence of the external cause

Y92.828   **Other** wilderness area as the place of occurrence of the external cause

Swamp as the place of occurrence of the external cause

Mountain as the place of occurrence of the external cause

Marsh as the place of occurrence of the external cause

Prairie as the place of occurrence of the external cause

Y92.83-   **Recreation area** as the place of occurrence of the external cause

Y92.830   **Public park** as the place of occurrence of the external cause

Y92.831   **Amusement park** as the place of occurrence of the external cause

Y92.832   **Beach** as the place of occurrence of the external cause

Seashore as the place of occurrence of the external cause

Y92.833   **Campsite** as the place of occurrence of the external cause

Y92.834   **Zoological garden (Zoo)** as the place of occurrence of the external cause

Y92.838   **Other** recreation area as the place of occurrence of the external cause

Y92.84   **Military training ground** as the place of occurrence of the external cause

Y92.85   **Railroad track** as the place of occurrence of the external cause

Y92.86   **Slaughter house** as the place of occurrence of the external cause

Y92.89   **Other** specified places as the place of occurrence of the external cause

Derelict house as the place of occurrence of the external cause

Y92.9   **Unspecified** place or not applicable

Y93- Activity codes

Note: Category Y93 is provided for use to indicate the activity of the person seeking healthcare for an injury or health condition, such as a heart attack while shoveling snow, which resulted from, or was contributed to, by the activity. These codes are appropriate for use for both acute injuries, such as those from chapter 19, and conditions that are due to the long-term, cumulative effects of an activity, such as those from chapter 13. They are also appropriate for use with external cause codes for cause and intent if identifying the activity providesadditional information on the event. These codes should be used in conjunction with codes for external cause status (Y99) and place of occurrence (Y92).

This section contains the following broad activity categories:

Y93.0	Activities involving walking and running
Y93.1	Activities involving water and water craft
Y93.2	Activities involving ice and snow
Y93.3	Activities involving climbing, rappelling, and jumping off
Y93.4	Activities involving dancing and other rhythmic movement
Y93.5	Activities involving other sports and athletics played individually
Y93.6	Activities involving other sports and athletics played as a team or group
Y93.7	Activities involving other specified sports and athletics
Y93.A	Activities involving other cardiorespiratory exercise
Y93.B	Activities involving other muscle strengthening exercises
Y93.C	Activities involving computer technology and electronic devices
Y93.D	Activities involving arts and handcrafts
Y93.E	Activities involving personal hygiene and interior property and clothing maintenance
Y93.F	Activities involving caregiving
Y93.G	Activities involving food preparation, cooking and grilling
Y93.H	Activities involving exterior property and land maintenance, building and construction
Y93.I	Activities involving roller coasters and other types of external motion
Y93.J	Activities involving playing musical instrument
Y93.K	Activities involving animal care
Y93.8	Activities, other specified
Y93.9	Activity, unspecified

Y93.0- Activities involving walking and running
Excludes 1: activity, walking an animal (Y93.K1)
activity, walking or running on a treadmill (Y93.A1)

Y93.01 Activity, walking, marching and hiking
Activity, walking, marching and hiking on level or elevated terrain
Excludes 1: activity, mountain climbing (Y93.31)

Y93.02 Activity, running

Y93.1- Activities involving water and water craft
Excludes 1: activities involving ice (Y93.2-)

Y93.11 Activity, swimming

Y93.12 Activity, springboard and platform diving

Y93.13 Activity, water polo

Y93.14 Activity, water aerobics and water exercise

Y93.15 Activity, underwater diving and snorkeling
Activity, SCUBA diving

Y93.16 Activity, rowing, canoeing, kayaking, rafting and tubing
Activity, canoeing, kayaking, rafting and tubing in calm and turbulent water

Y93.17 Activity, water skiing and wake boarding

Y93.18 Activity, surfing, windsurfing and boogie boarding
Activity, water sliding

Y93.19 Activity, other involving water and watercraft
Activity involving water NOS
Activity, parasailing
Activity, water survival training and testing

Y93.2- Activities involving ice and snow
Excludes 1: activity, shoveling ice and snow (Y93.H1)

Y93.21 Activity, ice skating
Activity, figure skating (singles) (pairs)
Activity, ice dancing
Excludes 1: activity, ice hockey (Y93.22)

Y93.22 Activity, ice hockey

Y93.23 Activity, snow (alpine) (downhill) skiing, snow boarding, sledding, tobogganing and snowtubing
Excludes 1: activity, cross country skiing (Y93.24)

Y93.24 Activity, cross country skiing
Activity, nordic skiing

Y93.29 Activity, other involving ice and snow
Activity involving ice and snow NOS

Y93.3- Activities involving climbing, rappelling and jumping off
Excludes 1: activity, hiking on level or elevated terrain (Y93.01)
activity, jumping rope (Y93.56)
activity, trampoline jumping (Y93.44)

Y93.31 Activity, mountain climbing, rock climbing and wall climbing

Y93.32 Activity, rappelling

Y93.33 Activity, BASE jumping
Activity, Building, Antenna, Span, Earth jumping

Y93.34 Activity, bungee jumping

Y93.35 Activity, hang gliding

Y93.39 Activity, other involving climbing, rappelling and jumping off

Y93.4- Activities involving dancing and other rhythmic movement
Excludes 1: activity, martial arts (Y93.75)

Y93.41 Activity, dancing

Y93.42 Activity, yoga

Y93.43 Activity, gymnastics
Activity, rhythmic gymnastics
Excludes 1: activity, trampolining (Y93.44)

Y93.44 Activity, trampolining

Y93.45 Activity, cheerleading

Y93.49 Activity, other involving dancing and other rhythmic movements

Y93.5- Activities involving other sports and athletics played individually
Excludes 1: activity, dancing (Y93.41)
activity, gymnastic (Y93.43)
activity, trampolining (Y93.44)
activity, yoga (Y93.42)

Y93.51 Activity, roller skating (inline) and skateboarding

Y93.52 Activity, horseback riding

Y93.53 Activity, golf

Y93.54 Activity, bowling

Y93.55 Activity, bike riding

Y93.56 Activity, jumping rope

Y93.57 Activity, non-running track and field events
Excludes 1: activity, running (any form) (Y93.02)

Y93.59 Activity, other involving other sports and athletics played individually
Excludes 1: activities involving climbing, rappelling, and jumping (Y93.3-)
activities involving ice and snow (Y93.2-)
activities involving walking and running (Y93.0-)
activities involving water and watercraft (Y93.1-)

Y93.6- Activities involving other sports and athletics played as a team or group
Excludes 1: activity, ice hockey (Y93.22)
activity, water polo (Y93.13)

Y93.61 Activity, american tackle football
Activity, football NOS

Y93.62 Activity, american flag or touch football

Y93.63 Activity, rugby

Y93.64 Activity, baseball
Activity, softball

Y93 I Y93

Y93.65   Activity, lacrosse and field hockey
       AHA 15:1Q:p8 – Playing lacrosse

Y93.66   Activity, soccer

Y93.67   Activity, basketball

Y93.68   Activity, volleyball (beach) (court)

Y93.6A   Activity, physical games generally associated with school recess, summer camp and children
       Activity, capture the flag
       Activity, dodge ball
       Activity, four square
       Activity, kickball

Y93.69   Activity, other involving other sports and athletics played as a team or group
       Activity, cricket

Y93.7-   Activities involving <u>other specified sports and athletics</u>

Y93.71   Activity, boxing

Y93.72   Activity, wrestling

Y93.73   Activity, racquet and hand sports
       Activity, handball
       Activity, racquetball
       Activity, squash
       Activity, tennis

Y93.74   Activity, frisbee
       Activity, ultimate frisbee

Y93.75   Activity, martial arts
       Activity, combatives

Y93.79   Activity, other specified sports and athletics
       Excludes 1:   sports and athletics activities specified in categories Y93.0-Y93.6

Y93.A-   Activities involving <u>other cardiorespiratory exercise</u>
       Activities involving physical training

Y93.A1   Activity, exercise machines primarily for cardiorespiratory conditioning
       Activity, elliptical and stepper machines
       Activity, stationary bike
       Activity, treadmill

Y93.A2   Activity, calisthenics
       Activity, jumping jacks
       Activity, warm up and cool down

Y93.A3   Activity, aerobic and step exercise

Y93.A4   Activity, circuit training

Y93.A5   Activity, obstacle course
       Activity, challenge course
       Activity, confidence course

Y93.A6   Activity, grass drills
       Activity, guerilla drills

Y93.A9   Activity, other involving cardiorespiratory exercise
       Excludes 1:   activities involving cardiorespiratory exercise specified in categories Y93.0-Y93.7

Y93.B-   Activities involving other <u>muscle strengthening exercises</u>

Y93.B1   Activity, exercise machines primarily for muscle strengthening

Y93.B2   Activity, push-ups, pull-ups, sit-ups

Y93.B3   Activity, free weights
       Activity, barbells
       Activity, dumbbells

Y93.B4   Activity, pilates

Y93.B9   Activity, other involving muscle strengthening exercises
       Excludes 1:   activities involving muscle strengthening specified in categories Y93.0-Y93.A

Y93.C-   Activities involving <u>computer technology and electronic devices</u>
       Excludes 1:   activity, electronic musical keyboard or instruments (Y93.J-)

Y93.C1   Activity, computer keyboarding
       Activity, electronic game playing using keyboard or other stationary device

Y93.C2   Activity, hand held interactive electronic device
       Activity, cellular telephone and communication device
       Activity, electronic game playing using interactive device
       Excludes 1:   activity, electronic game playing using keyboard or other stationary device (Y93.C1)

Y93.C9   Activity, other involving computer technology and electronic devices

Y93.D-   Activities involving <u>arts and handcrafts</u>
       Excludes 1:   activities involving playing musical instrument (Y93.J-)

Y93.D1   Activity, knitting and crocheting

Y93.D2   Activity, sewing

Y93.D3   Activity, furniture building and finishing
       Activity, furniture repair

Y93.D9   Activity, other involving arts and handcrafts

Y93.E-   Activities involving <u>personal hygiene and interior property and clothing maintenance</u>
       Excludes 1:   activities involving cooking and grilling (Y93.G-)
                 activities involving exterior property and land maintenance, building and construction (Y93.H-)
                 activities involving caregiving (Y93.F-)
                 activity, dishwashing (Y93.G1)
                 activity, food preparation (Y93.G1)
                 activity, gardening (Y93.H2)

Y93.E1   Activity, personal bathing and showering

Y93.E2   Activity, laundry

Y93.E3   Activity, vacuuming

Y93.E4   Activity, ironing

Y93.E5   Activity, floor mopping and cleaning

Y93.E6   Activity, residential relocation
       Activity, packing up and unpacking involved in moving to a new residence

Y93.E8   Activity, other personal hygiene

Y93.E9   Activity, other interior property and clothing maintenance

Y93.F-   Activities involving <u>caregiving</u>
       Activity involving the provider of caregiving

Y93.F1   Activity, caregiving, bathing

Y93.F2   Activity, caregiving, lifting

Y93.F9   Activity, other caregiving

Y93.G-   Activities involving <u>food preparation, cooking and grilling</u>

Y93.G1   Activity, food preparation and clean up
       Activity, dishwashing

Y93.G2   Activity, grilling and smoking food

Y93.G3   Activity, cooking and baking
       Activity, use of stove, oven and microwave oven

Y93.G9   Activity, other involving cooking and grilling

Y93.H-   Activities involving <u>exterior property and land maintenance, building and construction</u>

Y93.H1   Activity, digging, shoveling and raking
       Activity, dirt digging
       Activity, raking leaves
       Activity, snow shoveling

Y93.H2   Activity, gardening and landscaping
       Activity, pruning, trimming shrubs, weeding

Y93.H3   Activity, building and construction

Y93.H9   Activity, other involving exterior property and land maintenance, building and construction

Y93.I-   Activities involving <u>roller coasters and other types of external motion</u>

Y93.I1   Activity, roller coaster riding

Y93.I9   Activity, other involving external motion

Y93.J-   Activities involving <u>playing musical instrument</u>
       Activity involving playing electric musical instrument

Y93.J1   Activity, piano playing
       Activity, musical keyboard (electronic) playing

Y93.J2   Activity, drum and other percussion instrument playing

Y93.J3   Activity, string instrument playing

Y93.J4   Activity, winds and brass instrument playing

Y93.K-   Activities involving <u>animal care</u>
       Excludes 1:   activity, horseback riding (Y93.52)

Y93.K1   Activity, walking an animal

Y93.K2   Activity, milking an animal

Y93.K3   Activity, grooming and shearing an animal

Y93.K9   Activity, other involving animal care

Y
9
3
-
Y
9
3

Y93.8- **Activities, <u>other specified</u>**

    Y93.81 **Activity, refereeing a sports activity**

    Y93.82 **Activity, spectator at an event**

    Y93.83 **Activity, rough housing and horseplay**

        AHA 15:1Q:p7 – Rough housing

    Y93.84 **Activity, sleeping**

    Y93.85 **Activity, choking game**

        Activity, blackout game

        Activity, fainting game

        Activity, pass out game

    Y93.89 **Activity, other specified**

Y93.9 **Activity, <u>unspecified</u>**

Y95 **Nosocomial condition**

    AHA 13:4Q:p119 – Healthcare associated pneumonia

Y99- **<u>External cause status</u>**

    Note: A single code from category Y99 should be used in conjunction with the external cause code(s) assigned to a record to indicate the status of the person at the time the event occurred.

Y99.0 **Civilian activity done for income or pay**

    Civilian activity done for financial or other compensation

    Excludes 1: *military activity (Y99.1)*

              volunteer activity (Y99.2)

Y99.1 **Military activity**

    Excludes 1: *activity of off duty military personnel (Y99.8)*

Y99.2 **Volunteer activity**

    Excludes 1: *activity of child or other family member assisting in compensated work of other family member (Y99.8)*

Y99.8 **Other external cause status**

    Activity NEC

    Activity of child or other family member assisting in compensated work of other family member

    Hobby not done for income

    Leisure activity

    Off-duty activity of military personnel

    Recreation or sport not for income or while a student

    Student activity

    Excludes 1: *civilian activity done for income or compensation (Y99.0)*

              military activity (Y99.1)

Y99.9 **Unspecified external cause status**

Y
9
9
I
Y
9
9

Chapter 21 – Factors influencing health status and contact with health services (Z00-Z99)

Note: Z codes represent reasons for encounters. A corresponding procedure code must accompany a Z code if a procedure is performed. Categories Z00-Z99 are provided for occasions when circumstances other than a disease, injury or external cause classifiable to categories A00-Y89 are recorded as "diagnoses" or "problems". This can arise in two main ways:

(a) When a person who may or may not be sick encounters the health services for some specific purpose, such as to receive limited care or service for a current condition, to donate an organ or tissue, to receive prophylactic vaccination (immunization), or to discuss a problem which is in itself not a disease or injury.

(b) When some circumstance or problem is present which influences the person's health status but is not in itself a current illness or injury.

This chapter contains the following blocks:

Z00-Z13	Persons encountering health services for examinations
Z14-Z15	Genetic carrier and genetic susceptibility to disease
Z16	Resistance to antimicrobial drugs
Z17	Estrogen receptor status
Z18	Retained foreign body fragments
Z19	Hormone sensitivity malignancy status
Z20-Z29	Persons with potential health hazards related to communicable diseases
Z30-Z39	Persons encountering health services in circumstances related to reproduction
Z40-Z53	Encounters for other specific health care
Z55-Z65	Persons with potential health hazards related to socioeconomic and psychosocial circumstances
Z66	Do not resuscitate status
Z67	Blood type
Z68	Body mass index (BMI)
Z69-Z76	Persons encountering health services in other circumstances
Z77-Z99	Persons with potential health hazards related to family and personal history and certain conditions influencing health status

Chapter-Specific Coding Guidelines

C. Chapter-Specific Coding Guidelines

In addition to general coding guidelines, there are guidelines for specific diagnoses and/or conditions in the classification. Unless otherwise indicated, these guidelines apply to all health care settings. Please refer to Section II for guidelines on the selection of principal diagnosis.

21. Chapter 21: Factors Influencing Health Status and Contact with Health Services (Z00-Z99)

Note: The chapter specific guidelines provide additional information about the use of Z codes for specified encounters.

a. Use of Z codes in any healthcare setting

Z codes are for use in any healthcare setting. Z codes may be used as either a first-listed (principal diagnosis code in the inpatient setting) or secondary code, depending on the circumstances of the encounter.
Certain Z codes may only be used as first-listed or principal diagnosis.

b. Z Codes indicate a reason for an encounter

Z codes are not procedure codes. A corresponding procedure code must accompany a Z code to describe any procedure performed.

c. Categories of Z Codes

1) Contact/Exposure

Category Z20 indicates contact with, and suspected exposure to, communicable diseases. These codes are for patients who do not show any sign or symptom of a disease but are suspected to have been exposed to it by close personal contact with an infected individual or are in an area where a disease is epidemic.

Category Z77, Other contact with and (suspected) exposures hazardous to health, indicates contact with and suspected exposures hazardous to health.

Contact/exposure codes may be used as a first-listed code to explain an encounter for testing, or, more commonly, as a secondary code to identify a potential risk.

2) Inoculations and vaccinations

Code Z23 is for encounters for inoculations and vaccinations. It indicates that a patient is being seen to receive a prophylactic inoculation against a disease. Procedure codes are required to identify the actual administration of the injection and the type(s) of immunizations given. Code Z23 may be used as a secondary code if the inoculation is given as a routine part of preventive health care, such as a well-baby visit.

3) Status

Status codes indicate that a patient is either a carrier of a disease or has the sequelae or residual of a past disease or condition. This includes such things as the presence of prosthetic or mechanical devices resulting from past treatment. A status code is informative, because the status may affect the course of treatment and its outcome. A status code is distinct from a history code. The history code indicates that the patient no longer has the condition.

A status code should not be used with a diagnosis code from one of the body system chapters, if the diagnosis code includes the information provided by the status code. For example, code Z94.1, Heart transplant status, should not be used with a code from subcategory T86.2, Complications of heart transplant. The status code does not provide additional information. The complication code indicates that the patient is a heart transplant patient.

For encounters for weaning from a mechanical ventilator, assign a code from subcategory J96.1, Chronic respiratory failure, followed by code Z99.11, Dependence on respirator [ventilator] status.

The status Z codes/categories are:

Z14   Genetic carrier
Genetic carrier status indicates that a person carries a gene, associated with a particular disease, which may be passed to offspring who may develop that disease. The person does not have the disease and is not at risk of developing the disease.

Z15   Genetic susceptibility to disease
Genetic susceptibility indicates that a person has a gene that increases the risk of that person developing the disease.
Codes from category Z15 should not be used as principal or first-listed codes. If the patient has the condition to which he/she is susceptible, and that condition is the reason for the encounter, the code for the current condition should be sequenced first. If the patient is being seen for follow-up after completed treatment for this condition, and the condition no longer exists, a follow-up code should be sequenced first, followed by the appropriate personal history and genetic susceptibility codes. If the purpose of the encounter is genetic counseling associated with procreative management, code Z31.5, Encounter for genetic counseling, should be assigned as the first-listed code, followed by a code from category Z15. Additional codes should be assigned for any applicable family or personal history.

Z16	Resistance to antimicrobial drugs

This code indicates that a patient has a condition that is resistant to antimicrobial drug treatment. Sequence the infection code first.

Z17	Estrogen receptor status
Z18	Retained foreign body fragments
Z19	Hormone sensitivity malignancy status
Z21	Asymptomatic HIV infection status

This code indicates that a patient has tested positive for HIV but has manifested no signs or symptoms of the disease.

Z22	Carrier of infectious disease

Carrier status indicates that a person harbors the specific organisms of a disease without manifest symptoms and is capable of transmitting the infection.

Z28.3	Underimmunization status
Z33.1	Pregnant state, incidental

This code is a secondary code only for use when the pregnancy is in no way complicating the reason for visit. Otherwise, a code from the obstetric chapter is required.

Z66	Do not resuscitate

This code may be used when it is documented by the provider that a patient is on do not resuscitate status at any time during the stay.

Z67	Blood type
Z68	Body mass index (BMI)

As with all other secondary diagnosis codes, the BMI codes should only be assigned when they meet the definition of a reportable diagnosis (see Section III, Reporting Additional Diagnoses).

Z74.01	Bed confinement status
Z76.82	Awaiting organ transplant status
Z78	Other specified health status

Code Z78.1, Physical restraint status, may be used when it is documented by the provider that a patient has been put in restraints during the current encounter. Please note that this code should not be reported when it is documented by the provider that a patient is temporarily restrained during a procedure.

Z00 - Z00

Z79   Long-term (current) drug therapy
Codes from this category indicate a patient's continuous use of a prescribed drug (including such things as aspirin therapy) for the long-term treatment of a condition or for prophylactic use. It is not for use for patients who have addictions to drugs. This subcategory is not for use of medications for detoxification or maintenance programs to prevent withdrawal symptoms in patients with drug dependence (e.g., methadone maintenance for opiate dependence). Assign the appropriate code for the drug dependence instead.

Assign a code from Z79 if the patient is receiving a medication for an extended period as a prophylactic measure (such as for the prevention of deep vein thrombosis) or as treatment of a chronic condition (such as arthritis) or a disease requiring a lengthy course of treatment (such as cancer). Do not assign a code from category Z79 for medication being administered for a brief period of time to treat an acute illness or injury (such as a course of antibiotics to treat acute bronchitis).

Z88   Allergy status to drugs, medicaments and biological substances
Except: Z88.9, Allergy status to unspecified drugs, medicaments and biological substances status

Z89   Acquired absence of limb

Z90   Acquired absence of organs, not elsewhere classified

Z91.0-   Allergy status, other than to drugs and biological substances

Z92.82   Status post administration of tPA (rtPA) in a different facility within the last 24 hours prior to admission to a current facility.
Assign code Z92.82, Status post administration of tPA (rtPA) in a different facility within the last 24 hours prior to admission to current facility, as a secondary diagnosis when a patient is received by transfer into a facility and documentation indicates they were administered tissue plasminogen activator (tPA) within the last 24 hours prior to admission to the current facility.

This guideline applies even if the patient is still receiving the tPA at the time they are received into the current facility.

The appropriate code for the condition for which the tPA was administered (such as cerebrovascular disease or myocardial infarction) should be assigned first.

Code Z92.82 is only applicable to the receiving facility record and not to the transferring facility record.

Z93   Artificial opening status

Z94   Transplanted organ and tissue status

Z95   Presence of cardiac and vascular implants and grafts

Z96   Presence of other functional implants

Z97   Presence of other devices

Z98   Other postprocedural states
Assign code Z98.85, Transplanted organ removal status, to indicate that a transplanted organ has been previously removed. This code should not be assigned for the encounter in which the transplanted organ is removed. The complication necessitating removal of the transplant organ should be assigned for that encounter.

See section I.C19. for information on the coding of organ transplant complications.

Z99   Dependence on enabling machines and devices, not elsewhere classified
Note: Categories Z89-Z90 and Z93-Z99 are for use only if there are no complications or malfunctions of the organ or tissue replaced, the amputation site or the equipment on which the patient is dependent.

4) **History (of)**
There are two types of history Z codes, personal and family. Personal history codes explain a patient's past medical condition that no longer exists and is not receiving any treatment, but that has the potential for recurrence, and therefore may require continued monitoring.

Family history codes are for use when a patient has a family member(s) who has had a particular disease that causes the patient to be at higher risk of also contracting the disease.

Personal history codes may be used in conjunction with follow-up codes and family history codes may be used in conjunction with screening codes to explain the need for a test or procedure. History codes are also acceptable on any medical record regardless of the reason for visit. A history of an illness, even if no longer present, is important information that may alter the type of treatment ordered.

The history Z code categories are:
Z80   Family history of primary malignant neoplasm
Z81   Family history of mental and behavioral disorders
Z82   Family history of certain disabilities and chronic diseases (leading to disablement)
Z83   Family history of other specific disorders
Z84   Family history of other conditions

Z85   Personal history of malignant neoplasm
Z86   Personal history of certain other diseases
Z87   Personal history of other diseases and conditions
Z91.4-   Personal history of psychological trauma, not elsewhere classified
Z91.5   Personal history of self-harm
Z91.8-   Other specified personal risk factors, not elsewhere classified
Exception: Z91.83, Wandering in diseases classified elsewhere
Z92   Personal history of medical treatment
Except: Z92.0, Personal history of contraception
Except: Z92.82, Status post administration of tPA (rtPA) in a different facility within the last 24 hours prior to admission to a current facility

5) **Screening**
Screening is the testing for disease or disease precursors in seemingly well individuals so that early detection and treatment can be provided for those who test positive for the disease (e.g., screening mammogram).

The testing of a person to rule out or confirm a suspected diagnosis because the patient has some sign or symptom is a diagnostic examination, not a screening. In these cases, the sign or symptom is used to explain the reason for the test.

A screening code may be a first-listed code if the reason for the visit is specifically the screening exam. It may also be used as an additional code if the screening is done during an office visit for other health problems. A screening code is not necessary if the screening is inherent to a routine examination, such as a pap smear done during a routine pelvic examination.

Should a condition be discovered during the screening then the code for the condition may be assigned as an additional diagnosis.

The Z code indicates that a screening exam is planned. A procedure code is required to confirm that the screening was performed.

The screening Z codes/categories:
Z11   Encounter for screening for infectious and parasitic diseases
Z12   Encounter for screening for malignant neoplasms
Z13   Encounter for screening for other diseases and disorders
Except: Z13.9, Encounter for screening, unspecified
Z36   Encounter for antenatal screening for mother

6) **Observation**
There are ~~two~~ three observation Z code categories. They are for use in very limited circumstances when a person is being observed for a suspected condition that is ruled out. The observation codes are not for use if an injury or illness or any signs or symptoms related to the suspected condition are present. In such cases the diagnosis/symptom code is used with the corresponding external cause code.

The observation codes are to be used as principal diagnosis only. The only exception to this is when the principal diagnosis is required to be a code from category Z38, Liveborn infants according to place of birth and type of delivery. Then a code from category Z05, Encounter for observation and evaluation of newborn for suspected diseases and conditions ruled out, is sequenced after the Z38 code. Additional codes may be used in addition to the observation code but only if they are unrelated to the suspected condition being observed.

Codes from subcategory Z03.7, Encounter for suspected maternal and fetal conditions ruled out, may either be used as a first-listed or as an additional code assignment depending on the case. They are for use in very limited circumstances on a maternal record when an encounter is for a suspected maternal or fetal condition that is ruled out during that encounter (for example, a maternal or fetal condition may be suspected due to an abnormal test result). These codes should not be used when the condition is confirmed. In those cases, the confirmed condition should be coded. In addition, these codes are not for use if an illness or any signs or symptoms related to the suspected condition or problem are present. In such cases the diagnosis/symptom code is used.

Additional codes may be used in addition to the code from subcategory Z03.7, but only if they are unrelated to the suspected condition being evaluated.

Codes from subcategory Z03.7 may not be used for encounters for antenatal screening of mother. *See Section I.C.21. Screening.*

For encounters for suspected fetal condition that are inconclusive following testing and evaluation, assign the appropriate code from category O35, O36, O40 or O41.

The observation Z code categories:
Z03   Encounter for medical observation for suspected diseases and conditions ruled out
Z04   Encounter for examination and observation for other reasons
Except: Z04.9, Encounter for examination and observation for unspecified reason
Z05   Encounter for observation and evaluation of newborn for suspected diseases and conditions ruled out

Z00-Z99

7) Aftercare

Aftercare visit codes cover situations when the initial treatment of a disease has been performed and the patient requires continued care during the healing or recovery phase, or for the long-term consequences of the disease. The aftercare Z code should not be used if treatment is directed at a current, acute disease. The diagnosis code is to be used in these cases. Exceptions to this rule are codes Z51.0, Encounter for antineoplastic radiation therapy, and codes from subcategory Z51.1, Encounter for antineoplastic chemotherapy and immunotherapy. These codes are to be first-listed, followed by the diagnosis code when a patient's encounter is solely to receive radiation therapy, chemotherapy, or immunotherapy for the treatment of a neoplasm. If the reason for the encounter is more than one type of antineoplastic therapy, code Z51.0 and a code from subcategory Z51.1 may be assigned together, in which case one of these codes would be reported as a secondary diagnosis.

The aftercare Z codes should also not be used for aftercare for injuries. For aftercare of an injury, assign the acute injury code with the appropriate 7th character (for subsequent encounter).

The aftercare codes are generally first-listed to explain the specific reason for the encounter. An aftercare code may be used as an additional code when some type of aftercare is provided in addition to the reason for admission and no diagnosis code is applicable. An example of this would be the closure of a colostomy during an encounter for treatment of another condition.

Aftercare codes should be used in conjunction with other aftercare codes or diagnosis codes to provide better detail on the specifics of an aftercare encounter visit, unless otherwise directed by the classification. Should a patient receive multiple types of antineoplastic therapy during the same encounter, code Z51.0, Encounter for antineoplastic radiation therapy, and codes from subcategory Z51.1, Encounter for antineoplastic chemotherapy and immunotherapy, may be used together on a record. The sequencing of multiple aftercare codes depends on the circumstances of the encounter.

Certain aftercare Z code categories need a secondary diagnosis code to describe the resolving condition or sequelae. For others, the condition is included in the code title.

Additional Z code aftercare category terms include fitting and adjustment, and attention to artificial openings.

Status Z codes may be used with aftercare Z codes to indicate the nature of the aftercare. For example code Z95.1, Presence of aortocoronary bypass graft, may be used with code Z48.812, Encounter for surgical aftercare following surgery on the circulatory system, to indicate the surgery for which the aftercare is being performed. A status code should not be used when the aftercare code indicates the type of status, such as using Z43.0, Encounter for attention to tracheostomy, with Z93.0, Tracheostomy status.

The aftercare Z category/codes:
Z42	Encounter for plastic and reconstructive surgery following medical procedure or healed injury
Z43	Encounter for attention to artificial openings
Z44	Encounter for fitting and adjustment of external prosthetic device
Z45	Encounter for adjustment and management of implanted device
Z46	Encounter for fitting and adjustment of other devices
Z47	Orthopedic aftercare
Z48	Encounter for other postprocedural aftercare
Z49	Encounter for care involving renal dialysis
Z51	Encounter for other aftercare and medical care

8) Follow-up

The follow-up codes are used to explain continuing surveillance following completed treatment of a disease, condition, or injury. They imply that the condition has been fully treated and no longer exists. They should not be confused with aftercare codes, or injury codes with a 7th character for subsequent encounter, that explain ongoing care of a healing condition or its sequelae. Follow-up codes may be used in conjunction with history codes to provide the full picture of the healed condition and its treatment. The follow-up code is sequenced first, followed by the history code.

A follow-up code may be used to explain multiple visits. Should a condition be found to have recurred on the follow-up visit, then the diagnosis code for the condition should be assigned in place of the follow-up code.

The follow-up Z code categories:
Z08	Encounter for follow-up examination after completed treatment for malignant neoplasm
Z09	Encounter for follow-up examination after completed treatment for conditions other than malignant neoplasm
Z39	Encounter for maternal postpartum care and examination

9) Donor

Codes in category Z52, Donors of organs and tissues, are used for living individuals who are donating blood or other body tissue. These codes are only for individuals donating for others, not for self-donations. They are not used to identify cadaveric donations.

10) Counseling

Counseling Z codes are used when a patient or family member receives assistance in the aftermath of an illness or injury, or when support is required in coping with family or social problems. They are not used in conjunction with a diagnosis code when the counseling component of care is considered integral to standard treatment.
The counseling Z codes/categories:
Z30.0-	Encounter for general counseling and advice on contraception
Z31.5	Encounter for genetic counseling
Z31.6-	Encounter for general counseling and advice on procreation
Z32.2	Encounter for childbirth instruction
Z32.3	Encounter for childcare instruction
Z69	Encounter for mental health services for victim and perpetrator of abuse
Z70	Counseling related to sexual attitude, behavior and orientation
Z71	Persons encountering health services for other counseling and medical advice, not elsewhere classified
Z76.81	Expectant mother prebirth pediatrician visit

11) Encounters for Obstetrical and Reproductive Services

See Section I.C.15. Pregnancy, Childbirth, and the Puerperium, for further instruction on the use of these codes.

Z codes for pregnancy are for use in those circumstances when none of the problems or complications included in the codes from the Obstetrics chapter exist (a routine prenatal visit or postpartum care). Codes in category Z34, Encounter for supervision of normal pregnancy, are always first-listed and are not to be used with any other code from the OB chapter.

Codes in category Z3A, Weeks of gestation, may be assigned to provide additional information about the pregnancy. Category Z3A codes should not be assigned for pregnancies with abortive outcomes (categories O00-O08), elective termination of pregnancy (code Z33.32), nor for postpartum conditions, as category Z3A is not applicable to these conditions. The date of the admission should be used to determine weeks of gestation for inpatient admissions that encompass more than one gestational week.

The outcome of delivery, category Z37, should be included on all maternal delivery records. It is always a secondary code. Codes in category Z37 should not be used on the newborn record.

Z codes for family planning (contraceptive) or procreative management and counseling should be included on an obstetric record either during the pregnancy or the postpartum stage, if applicable.

Z codes/categories for obstetrical and reproductive services:
Z30	Encounter for contraceptive management
Z31	Encounter for procreative management
Z32.2	Encounter for childbirth instruction
Z32.3	Encounter for childcare instruction
Z33	Pregnant state
Z34	Encounter for supervision of normal pregnancy
Z36	Encounter for antenatal screening of mother
Z3A	Weeks of gestation
Z37	Outcome of delivery
Z39	Encounter for maternal postpartum care and examination
Z76.81	Expectant mother prebirth pediatrician visit

12) Newborns and Infants

See Section I.C.16. Newborn (Perinatal) Guidelines, for further instruction on the use of these codes.

Newborn Z codes/categories:
Z76.1	Encounter for health supervision and care of foundling
Z00.1-	Encounter for routine child health examination
Z38	Liveborn infants according to place of birth and type of delivery

13) Routine and administrative examinations

The Z codes allow for the description of encounters for routine examinations, such as, a general check-up, or, examinations for administrative purposes, such as, a pre-employment physical. The codes are not to be used if the examination is for diagnosis of a suspected condition or for treatment purposes. In such cases the diagnosis code is used. During a routine exam, should a diagnosis or condition be discovered, it should be coded as an additional code. Pre-existing and chronic conditions and history codes may also be included as additional codes as long as the examination is for administrative purposes and not focused on any particular condition.

Z00 - Z00

Some of the codes for routine health examinations distinguish between "with" and "without" abnormal findings. Code assignment depends on the information that is known at the time the encounter is being coded. For example, if no abnormal findings were found during the examination, but the encounter is being coded before test results are back, it is acceptable to assign the code for "without abnormal findings." When assigning a code for "with abnormal findings," additional code(s) should be assigned to identify the specific abnormal finding(s).

Pre-operative examination and pre-procedural laboratory examination Z codes are for use only in those situations when a patient is being cleared for a procedure or surgery and no treatment is given.

The Z codes/categories for routine and administrative examinations:

Z00	Encounter for general examination without complaint, suspected or reported diagnosis
Z01	Encounter for other special examination without complaint, suspected or reported diagnosis
Z02	Encounter for administrative examination
	Except: Z02.9, Encounter for administrative examinations, unspecified
Z32.0-	Encounter for pregnancy test

14) Miscellaneous Z codes

The miscellaneous Z codes capture a number of other health care encounters that do not fall into one of the other categories. Certain of these codes identify the reason for the encounter; others are for use as additional codes that provide useful information on circumstances that may affect a patient's care and treatment.

Prophylactic Organ Removal

For encounters specifically for prophylactic removal of an organ (such as prophylactic removal of breasts due to a genetic susceptibility to cancer or a family history of cancer), the principal or first-listed code should be a code from category Z40, Encounter for prophylactic surgery, followed by the appropriate codes to identify the associated risk factor (such as genetic susceptibility or family history).

If the patient has a malignancy of one site and is having prophylactic removal at another site to prevent either a new primary malignancy or metastatic disease, a code for the malignancy should also be assigned in addition to a code from subcategory Z40.0, Encounter for prophylactic surgery for risk factors related to malignant neoplasms. A Z40.0 code should not be assigned if the patient is having organ removal for treatment of a malignancy, such as the removal of the testes for the treatment of prostate cancer.

Miscellaneous Z codes/categories:

Z28	Immunization not carried out
	Except: Z28.3, Underimmunization status
Z29	Encounter for other prophylactic measures
Z40	Encounter for prophylactic surgery
Z41	Encounter for procedures for purposes other than remedying health state
	Except: Z41.9, Encounter for procedure for purposes other than remedying health state, unspecified
Z53	Persons encountering health services for specific procedures and treatment, not carried out
Z55	Problems related to education and literacy
Z56	Problems related to employment and unemployment
Z57	Occupational exposure to risk factors
Z58	Problems related to physical environment
Z59	Problems related to housing and economic circumstances
Z60	Problems related to social environment
Z62	Problems related to upbringing
Z63	Other problems related to primary support group, including family circumstances
Z64	Problems related to certain psychosocial circumstances
Z65	Problems related to other psychosocial circumstances
Z72	Problems related to lifestyle
	Note: These codes should be assigned only when the documentation specifies that the patient has an associated problem
Z73	Problems related to life management difficulty
Z74	Problems related to care provider dependency
	Except: Z74.01, Bed confinement status
Z75	Problems related to medical facilities and other health care
Z76.0	Encounter for issue of repeat prescription
Z76.3	Healthy person accompanying sick person
Z76.4	Other boarder to healthcare facility
Z76.5	Malingerer [conscious simulation]
Z91.1-	Patient's noncompliance with medical treatment and regimen
Z91.83	Wandering in diseases classified elsewhere
Z91.89	Other specified personal risk factors, not elsewhere classified

15) Nonspecific Z codes

Certain Z codes are so non-specific, or potentially redundant with other codes in the classification, that there can be little justification for their use in the inpatient setting. Their use in the outpatient setting should be limited to those instances when there is no further documentation to permit more precise coding. Otherwise, any sign or symptom or any other reason for visit that is captured in another code should be used.

Nonspecific Z codes/categories:

Z02.9	Encounter for administrative examinations, unspecified
Z04.9	Encounter for examination and observation for unspecified reason
Z13.9	Encounter for screening, unspecified
Z41.9	Encounter for procedure for purposes other than remedying health state, unspecified
Z52.9	Donor of unspecified organ or tissue
Z86.59	Personal history of other mental and behavioral disorders
Z88.9	Allergy status to unspecified drugs, medicaments and biological substances status
Z92.0	Personal history of contraception

16) Z Codes That May Only be Principal/First-Listed Diagnosis

The following Z codes/categories may only be reported as the principal/first-listed diagnosis, except when there are multiple encounters on the same day and the medical records for the encounters are combined:

Z00	Encounter for general examination without complaint, suspected or reported diagnosis Except: Z00.6
Z01	Encounter for other special examination without complaint, suspected or reported diagnosis
Z02	Encounter for administrative examination
Z03	Encounter for medical observation for suspected diseases and conditions ruled out
Z04	Encounter for examination and observation for other reasons
Z31.81	Encounter for male factor infertility in female patient
~~Z31.82~~	~~Encounter for Rh incompatibility status~~
Z31.83	Encounter for assisted reproductive fertility procedure cycle
Z31.84	Encounter for fertility preservation procedure
Z34	Encounter for supervision of normal pregnancy
Z39	Encounter for maternal postpartum care and examination
Z38	Liveborn infants according to place of birth and type of delivery
Z42	Encounter for plastic and reconstructive surgery following medical procedure or healed injury
Z51.0	Encounter for antineoplastic radiation therapy
Z51.1-	Encounter for antineoplastic chemotherapy and immunotherapy
Z52	Donors of organs and tissues
	Except: Z52.9, Donor of unspecified organ or tissue
Z76.1	Encounter for health supervision and care of foundling
Z76.2	Encounter for health supervision and care of other healthy infant and child
Z99.12	Encounter for respirator [ventilator] dependence during power failure

Persons encountering health services for examinations (Z00-Z13)

Note: Nonspecific abnormal findings disclosed at the time of these examinations are classified to categories R70-R94.
Excludes 1: *examinations related to pregnancy and reproduction (Z30-Z36, Z39.-)*

Z00- **Encounter for <u>general examination</u> <u>without</u> complaint, suspected or reported diagnosis**
Excludes 1: *encounter for examination for administrative purposes (Z02.-)*
Excludes ❷: *encounter for pre-procedural examinations (Z01.81-)*
special screening examinations (Z11-Z13)

Z00.0- **Encounter for general adult medical examination**
Encounter for adult periodic examination (annual) (physical) and any associated laboratory and radiologic examinations
Excludes 1: *encounter for examination of sign or symptom- code to sign or symptom*
general health check-up of infant or child (Z00.12.-)

Z00.00 **Encounter for general adult medical examination <u>without</u> abnormal findings** — [Age/15-124] [Unacceptable PDX]
AHA 16:1Q:p36 – Adult exam with history of COPD and smoking
Encounter for adult health check-up NOS

Z00.01 **Encounter for general adult medical examination <u>with</u> abnormal findings** — [Age/15-124] [Unacceptable PDX]
AHA 16:1Q:p36 – Adult exam with acute exacerbation of COPD
AHA 16:1Q:p35 – Adult exam with elevated blood pressure
Use additional code to identify abnormal findings

Z00.1- **Encounter for newborn, infant and child health examinations**
Z00.11- **<u>Newborn health examination</u>**
Health check for child under 29 days old
Use additional code to identify any abnormal findings
Excludes 1: *health check for child over 28 days old (Z00.12-)*

Z00.110 **Health examination for newborn <u>under 8 days old</u>** — [Age/0] [Unacceptable PDX]
Health check for newborn under 8 days old

Z00.111 **Health examination for newborn <u>8 to 28 days old</u>** — [Age/0] [Unacceptable PDX]
Health check for newborn 8 to 28 days old
Newborn weight check

Z00.12- **Encounter for <u>routine child health examination</u>**
Encounter for development testing of infant or child
Health check (routine) for child over 28 days old
Excludes 1: *health check for child under 29 days old (Z00.11-)*
health supervision of foundling or other healthy infant or child (Z76.1-Z76.2)
newborn health examination (Z00.11-)

Z00.121 **Encounter for routine child health examination <u>with</u> abnormal findings** — [Age/0-17] [Unacceptable PDX]
AHA 16:1Q:p35 – Well-child exam with acute exacerbation of mild persistent asthma
AHA 16:1Q:p34 – Well-infant exam with findings of otitis media
Use additional code to identify abnormal findings

Z00.129 **Encounter for routine child health examination <u>without</u> abnormal findings** — [Age/0-17] [Unacceptable PDX]
AHA 16:1Q:p34 – Well-child exam with previous diagnosis of viral bronchitis
Encounter for routine child health examination NOS

Z00.2 **Encounter for examination for period of rapid growth in childhood** — [Age/0-17] [Unacceptable PDX]

Z00.3 **Encounter for examination for adolescent development state** — [Age/0-17] [Unacceptable PDX]
Encounter for puberty development state

Z00.5 **Encounter for examination of potential donor of organ and tissue** — [Unacceptable PDX]

Z00.6 **Encounter for examination for normal comparison and control in clinical research program**
Examination of participant or control in clinical research program

Z00.7- **Encounter for <u>examination for period of delayed growth in childhood</u>**
Z00.70 **Encounter for examination for period of delayed growth in childhood <u>without</u> abnormal findings** — [Age/0-17] [Unacceptable PDX]

Z00.71 **Encounter for examination for period of delayed growth in childhood <u>with abnormal findings</u>** — [Age/0-17] [Unacceptable PDX]
Use additional code to identify abnormal findings

Z00.8 **Encounter for other general examination** — [Unacceptable PDX]
Encounter for health examination in population surveys

Z01- **Encounter for <u>other special examination</u> <u>without</u> complaint, suspected or reported diagnosis**
Includes: Routine examination of specific system
Note: Codes from category Z01 represent the reason for the encounter. A separate procedure code is required to identify any examinations or procedures performed.
Excludes 1: *encounter for examination for administrative purposes (Z02.-)*
encounter for examination for suspected conditions, proven not to exist (Z03.-)
encounter for laboratory and radiologic examinations as a component of general medical examinations (Z00.0-)
encounter for laboratory, radiologic and imaging examinations for sign(s) and symptom(s) — code to the sign(s) or symptom(s)
Excludes ❷: *screening examinations (Z11-Z13)*

Z01.0- **Encounter for <u>examination of eyes and vision</u>**
Excludes 1: *examination for driving license (Z02.4)*

Z01.00 **Encounter for examination of eyes and vision <u>without</u> abnormal findings**
Encounter for examination of eyes and vision NOS

Z01.01 **Encounter for examination of eyes and vision <u>with</u> abnormal findings**
Use additional code to identify abnormal findings

Z01.1- **Encounter for <u>examination of ears and hearing</u>**
Z01.10 **Encounter for examination of ears and hearing <u>without</u> abnormal findings** — [Unacceptable PDX]
Encounter for examination of ears and hearing NOS

Z01.11- **Encounter for examination of ears and hearing <u>with</u> abnormal findings**
Z01.110 **Encounter for hearing examination following failed hearing screening** — [Unacceptable PDX]

Z01.118 **Encounter for examination of ears and hearing with other abnormal findings** — [Unacceptable PDX]
Use additional code to identify abnormal findings

Z01.12 **Encounter for hearing conservation and treatment** — [Unacceptable PDX]

Z01.2- **Encounter for <u>dental examination and cleaning</u>**
Z01.20 **Encounter for dental examination and cleaning <u>without</u> abnormal findings** — [Unacceptable PDX]
Encounter for dental examination and cleaning NOS

Z01.21 **Encounter for dental examination and cleaning <u>with</u> abnormal findings** — [Unacceptable PDX]
Use additional code to identify abnormal findings

Z01.3- **Encounter for <u>examination of blood pressure</u>**
Z01.30 **Encounter for examination of blood pressure <u>without</u> abnormal findings** — [Unacceptable PDX]
Encounter for examination of blood pressure NOS

Z01.31 **Encounter for examination of blood pressure <u>with</u> abnormal findings** — [Unacceptable PDX]
Use additional code to identify abnormal findings

Z01.4- Encounter for <u>gynecological examination</u>
>   *Excludes ❷:* *pregnancy examination or test (Z32.0-)*
>   *routine examination for contraceptive maintenance (Z30.4-)*

Z01.41- Encounter for <u>routine</u> gynecological examination
>   Encounter for general gynecological examination with or without cervical smear
>   Encounter for gynecological examination (general) (routine) NOS
>   Encounter for pelvic examination (annual) (periodic)
>   Use additional code:
>   For screening for human papillomavirus, if applicable, (Z11.51)
>   For screening vaginal pap smear, if applicable (Z12.72)
>   To identify acquired absence of uterus, if applicable (Z90.71-)
>   *Excludes 1:* *gynecologic examination status-post hysterectomy for malignant condition (Z08)*
>   *screening cervical pap smear not a part of a routine gynecological examination (Z12.4)*

Z01.411 Encounter for gynecological examination (general) (routine) <u>with abnormal findings</u> — [♀]
>   Use additional code to identify abnormal findings

Z01.419 Encounter for gynecological examination (general) (routine) <u>without</u> abnormal findings — [♀]

Z01.42 Encounter for cervical smear to confirm findings of recent normal smear following initial abnormal smear — [♀]

Z01.8- Encounter for other specified special examinations

Z01.81- Encounter for <u>preprocedural examinations</u>
>   Encounter for preoperative examinations
>   Encounter for radiological and imaging examinations as part of preprocedural examination

Z01.810 Encounter for preprocedural <u>cardiovascular</u> examination

Z01.811 Encounter for preprocedural <u>respiratory</u> examination

Z01.812 Encounter for preprocedural <u>laboratory</u> examination — [Unacceptable PDX]
>   Blood and urine tests prior to treatment or procedure

Z01.818 Encounter for <u>other</u> preprocedural examination — [Unacceptable PDX]
>   Encounter for preprocedural examination NOS
>   Encounter for examinations prior to antineoplastic chemotherapy

Z01.82 Encounter for allergy testing — [Unacceptable PDX]
>   *Excludes 1:* *encounter for antibody response examination (Z01.84)*

Z01.83 Encounter for blood typing — [Unacceptable PDX]
>   Encounter for Rh typing

Z01.84 Encounter for antibody response examination — [Unacceptable PDX]
>   Encounter for immunity status testing
>   *Excludes 1:* *encounter for allergy testing (Z01.82)*

Z01.89 Encounter for other specified special examinations — [Unacceptable PDX]

Z02- Encounter for <u>administrative examination</u>

Z02.0 Encounter for examination for admission to educational institution — [Unacceptable PDX]
>   Encounter for examination for admission to preschool (education)
>   Encounter for examination for re-admission to school following illness or medical treatment

Z02.1 Encounter for pre-employment examination

Z02.2 Encounter for examination for admission to residential institution — [Unacceptable PDX]
>   *Excludes 1:* *examination for admission to prison (Z02.89)*

Z02.3 Encounter for examination for recruitment to armed forces

Z02.4 Encounter for examination for driving license — [Unacceptable PDX]

Z02.5 Encounter for examination for participation in sport — [Unacceptable PDX]
>   *Excludes 1:* *blood-alcohol and blood-drug test (Z02.83)*

Z02.6 Encounter for examination for insurance purposes — [Unacceptable PDX]

Z02.7- Encounter for issue of medical certificate
>   *Excludes 1:* *encounter for general medical examination (Z00-Z01, Z02.0-Z02.6, Z02.8-Z02.9)*

Z02.71 Encounter for disability determination — [Unacceptable PDX]
>   Encounter for issue of medical certificate of incapacity
>   Encounter for issue of medical certificate of invalidity

Z02.79 Encounter for issue of other medical certificate — [Unacceptable PDX]

Z02.8- Encounter for other administrative examinations

Z02.81 Encounter for paternity testing

Z02.82 Encounter for adoption services — [Unacceptable PDX]

Z02.83 Encounter for blood-alcohol and blood-drug test
>   Use additional code for findings of alcohol or drugs in blood (R78.-)

Z02.89 Encounter for other administrative examinations — [Unacceptable PDX]
>   Encounter for examination for admission to prison
>   Encounter for examination for admission to summer camp
>   Encounter for immigration examination
>   Encounter for naturalization examination
>   Encounter for premarital examination
>   *Excludes 1:* *health supervision of foundling or other healthy infant or child (Z76.1-Z76.2)*

Z02.9 Encounter for administrative examinations, unspecified — [Unacceptable PDX]

Z03- Encounter for <u>medical observation for suspected diseases and conditions</u> ruled out
>   Note: This category is to be used when a person without a diagnosis is suspected of having an abnormal condition, without signs or symptoms, which requires study, but after examination and observation, is ruled out. This category is also for use for administrative and legal observation status.
>   *Excludes 1:* *contact with and (suspected) exposures hazardous to health (Z77.-)*
>   *newborn observation for suspected condition, ruled out (P00-P04)*
>   *person with feared complaint in whom no diagnosis is made (Z71.1)*
>   *signs or symptoms under study — code to signs or symptoms*

Z03.6 Encounter for observation for suspected toxic effect from ingested substance ruled out
>   Encounter for observation for suspected adverse effect from drug
>   Encounter for observation for suspected poisoning

Z03.7- Encounter for <u>suspected maternal and fetal conditions</u> ruled out
>   Encounter for suspected maternal and fetal conditions not found
>   *Excludes 1:* *known or suspected fetal anomalies affecting management of mother, not ruled out (O26.-, O35.-, O36.-, O40.-, O41.-)*

Z03.71 Encounter for suspected problem <u>with amniotic cavity and membrane</u> ruled out — [♀, Age/12-55] [Unacceptable PDX]
>   Encounter for suspected oligohydramnios ruled out
>   Encounter for suspected polyhydramnios ruled out

Z03.72 Encounter for suspected <u>placental problem</u> ruled out — [♀, Age/12-55] [Unacceptable PDX]

Z03.73 Encounter for suspected <u>fetal anomaly</u> ruled out — [♀, Age/12-55] [Unacceptable PDX]

Z03.74 Encounter for suspected <u>problem with fetal growth</u> ruled out — [♀, Age/12-55] [Unacceptable PDX]

Z03.75 Encounter for suspected <u>cervical shortening</u> ruled out — [♀, Age/12-55] [Unacceptable PDX]

Z03.79 Encounter for <u>other</u> suspected maternal and fetal conditions <u>ruled out</u> — [♀, Age/12-55] [Unacceptable PDX]

Z03.8- Encounter for observation for other suspected diseases and conditions ruled out

Z03.81- Encounter for observation for suspected exposure to biological agents ruled out

Z03.810 Encounter for observation for suspected exposure to anthrax ruled out

Z03.818 Encounter for observation for suspected exposure to other biological agents ruled out

Z03.89 Encounter for observation for other suspected diseases and conditions ruled out

Z01-Z03

Z04- **Encounter for examination and observation for other reasons**
Includes: Encounter for examination for medicolegal reasons
Note: This category is to be used when a person without a diagnosis is suspected of having an abnormal condition, without signs or symptoms, which requires study, but after examination and observation, is ruled out. This category is also for use for administrative and legal observation status.

Z04.1 **Encounter for examination and observation following transport accident**
Excludes 1:   encounter for examination and observation following work accident (Z04.2)

Z04.2 **Encounter for examination and observation following work accident**

Z04.3 **Encounter for examination and observation following other accident**

Z04.4- **Encounter for examination and observation following alleged rape**
Encounter for examination and observation of victim following alleged rape
Encounter for examination and observation of victim following alleged sexual abuse

Z04.41 **Encounter for examination and observation following alleged adult rape** — [Age/15-124]
Suspected adult rape, ruled out
Suspected adult sexual abuse, ruled out

Z04.42 **Encounter for examination and observation following alleged child rape** — [Age/0-17]
Suspected child rape, ruled out
Suspected child sexual abuse, ruled out

Z04.6 **Encounter for general psychiatric examination, requested by authority**

Z04.7- **Encounter for examination and observation following alleged physical abuse**

Z04.71 **Encounter for examination and observation following alleged adult physical abuse** — [Age/15-124]
Suspected adult physical abuse, ruled out
Excludes 1:   confirmed case of adult physical abuse (T74.-)
encounter for examination and observation following alleged adult sexual abuse (Z04.41)
suspected case of adult physical abuse, not ruled out (T76.-)

Z04.72 **Encounter for examination and observation following alleged child physical abuse** — [Age/0-17]
Suspected child physical abuse, ruled out
Excludes 1:   confirmed case of child physical abuse (T74.-)
encounter for examination and observation following alleged child sexual abuse (Z04.42)
suspected case of child physical abuse, not ruled out (T76.-)

Z04.8 **Encounter for examination and observation for other specified reasons** — [Unacceptable PDX]
Encounter for examination and observation for request for expert evidence

Z04.9 **Encounter for examination and observation for unspecified reason** — [Unacceptable PDX]
Encounter for observation NOS

Z05- **Encounter for observation and examination of newborn for suspected diseases and conditions ruled out**
This category is to be used for newborns, within the neonatal period (the first 28 days of life), who are suspected of having an abnormal condition unrelated to exposure from the mother or the birth process, but without signs or symptoms, and which, after examination and observation, is ruled out.
Excludes ❷: newborn observation for suspected condition, related to exposure from the mother or birth process (P00-P04)

Z05.0 **Observation and evaluation of newborn for suspected cardiac condition ruled out** — [Age/0] [Unacceptable PDX]

Z05.1 **Observation and evaluation of newborn for suspected infectious condition ruled out** — [Age/0] [Unacceptable PDX]

Z05.2 **Observation and evaluation of newborn for suspected neurological condition ruled out** — [Age/0] [Unacceptable PDX]

Z05.3 **Observation and evaluation of newborn for suspected respiratory condition ruled out** — [Age/0] [Unacceptable PDX]

Z05.4- **Observation and evaluation of newborn for suspected genetic, metabolic or immunologic condition ruled out**

Z05.41 **Observation and evaluation of newborn for suspected genetic condition ruled out** — [Age/0] [Unacceptable PDX]

Z05.42 **Observation and evaluation of newborn for suspected metabolic condition ruled out** — [Age/0] [Unacceptable PDX]

Z05.43 **Observation and evaluation of newborn for suspected immunologic condition ruled out** — [Age/0] [Unacceptable PDX]

Z05.5 **Observation and evaluation of newborn for suspected gastrointestinal condition ruled out** — [Age/0] [Unacceptable PDX]

Z05.6 **Observation and evaluation of newborn for suspected genitourinary condition ruled out** — [Age/0] [Unacceptable PDX]

Z05.7- **Observation and evaluation of newborn for suspected skin, subcutaneous, musculoskeletal and connective tissue condition ruled out**

Z05.71 **Observation and evaluation of newborn for suspected skin and subcutaneous tissue condition ruled out** — [Age/0] [Unacceptable PDX]

Z05.72 **Observation and evaluation of newborn for suspected musculoskeletal condition ruled out** — [Age/0] [Unacceptable PDX]

Z05.73 **Observation and evaluation of newborn for suspected connective tissue condition ruled out** — [Age/0] [Unacceptable PDX]

Z05.8 **Observation and evaluation of newborn for other specified suspected condition ruled out** — [Age/0] [Unacceptable PDX]

Z05.9 **Observation and evaluation of newborn for unspecified suspected condition ruled out** — [Age/0] [Unacceptable PDX]

Z08 **Encounter for follow-up examination after completed treatment for malignant neoplasm** — [Unacceptable PDX]
Medical surveillance following completed treatment
Use additional code to identify any acquired absence of organs (Z90.-)
Use additional code to identify the personal history of malignant neoplasm (Z85.-)
Excludes 1:   aftercare following medical care (Z43-Z49, Z51)

Z09 **Encounter for follow-up examination after completed treatment for conditions other than malignant neoplasm** — [Unacceptable PDX]
Medical surveillance following completed treatment
Use additional code to identify any applicable history of disease code (Z86.- Z87.-)
Excludes 1:   aftercare following medical care (Z43-Z49, Z51)
surveillance of contraception (Z30.4-)
surveillance of prosthetic and other medical devices (Z44-Z46)

Z11- **Encounter for screening for infectious and parasitic diseases**
Note: Screening is the testing for disease or disease precursors in asymptomatic individuals so that early detection and treatment can be provided for those who test positive for the disease.
Excludes 1:   encounter for diagnostic examination — code to sign or symptom

Z11.0 **Encounter for screening for intestinal infectious diseases** — [Unacceptable PDX]

Z11.1 **Encounter for screening for respiratory tuberculosis** — [Unacceptable PDX]

Z11.2 **Encounter for screening for other bacterial diseases** — [Unacceptable PDX]

Z11.3 **Encounter for screening for infections with a predominantly sexual mode of transmission** — [Unacceptable PDX]
Excludes ❷: encounter for screening for human immunodeficiency virus [HIV] (Z11.4)
encounter for screening for human papillomavirus (Z11.51)

Z11.4 **Encounter for screening for human immunodeficiency virus [HIV]** — [Unacceptable PDX]

Z04-Z11

Z11.5- Encounter for screening for other viral diseases
Excludes ❷: encounter for screening for viral intestinal disease (Z11.0)

Z11.51 Encounter for screening for human papillomavirus (HPV) — [Unacceptable PDX]

Z11.59 Encounter for screening for other viral diseases — [Unacceptable PDX]

Z11.6 Encounter for screening for other protozoal diseases and helminthiases — [Unacceptable PDX]
Excludes ❷: encounter for screening for protozoal intestinal disease (Z11.0)

Z11.8 Encounter for screening for other infectious and parasitic diseases — [Unacceptable PDX]
Encounter for screening for chlamydia
Encounter for screening for rickettsial
Encounter for screening for spirochetal
Encounter for screening for mycoses

Z11.9 Encounter for screening for infectious and parasitic diseases, unspecified — [Unacceptable PDX]

Z12- Encounter for <u>screening for malignant neoplasms</u>
AHA 15:1Q:p24 – Screening mammogram
Note: Screening is the testing for disease or disease precursors in asymptomatic individuals so that early detection and treatment can be provided for those who test positive for the disease.
Use additional code to identify any family history of malignant neoplasm (Z80.-)
Excludes 1:   encounter for diagnostic examination — code to sign or symptom

Z12.0 Encounter for screening for malignant neoplasm of <u>stomach</u> — [Unacceptable PDX]

Z12.1- Encounter for screening for malignant neoplasm of <u>intestinal tract</u>

Z12.10 Encounter for screening for malignant neoplasm of intestinal tract, <u>unspecified</u> — [Unacceptable PDX]

Z12.11 Encounter for screening for malignant neoplasm of <u>colon</u> — [Unacceptable PDX]
Encounter for screening colonoscopy NOS

Z12.12 Encounter for screening for malignant neoplasm of <u>rectum</u> — [Unacceptable PDX]

Z12.13 Encounter for screening for malignant neoplasm of <u>small intestine</u> — [Unacceptable PDX]

Z12.2 Encounter for screening for malignant neoplasm of <u>respiratory organs</u> — [Unacceptable PDX]

Z12.3- Encounter for screening for malignant neoplasm of <u>breast</u>

Z12.31 Encounter for screening <u>mammogram</u> for malignant neoplasm of breast — [Unacceptable PDX]
Excludes 1:   inconclusive mammogram (R92.2)

Z12.39 Encounter for <u>other screening</u> for malignant neoplasm of breast — [Unacceptable PDX]

Z12.4 Encounter for screening for malignant neoplasm of <u>cervix</u> — [♀] [Unacceptable PDX]
Encounter for screening pap smear for malignant neoplasm of cervix
Excludes 1:   when screening is part of general gynecological examination (Z01.4-)
Excludes ❷: encounter for screening for human papillomavirus (Z11.51)

Z12.5 Encounter for screening for malignant neoplasm of <u>prostate</u> — [♂]

Z12.6 Encounter for screening for malignant neoplasm of <u>bladder</u> — [Unacceptable PDX]

Z12.7- Encounter for screening for malignant neoplasm of other genitourinary organs

Z12.71 Encounter for screening for malignant neoplasm of <u>testis</u> — [♂] [Unacceptable PDX]

Z12.72 Encounter for screening for malignant neoplasm of <u>vagina</u> — [♀] [Unacceptable PDX]
Vaginal pap smear status-post hysterectomy for non-malignant condition
Use additional code to identify acquired absence of uterus (Z90.71-)
Excludes 1:   vaginal pap smear status-post hysterectomy for malignant conditions (Z08)

Z12.73 Encounter for screening for malignant neoplasm of <u>ovary</u> — [♀] [Unacceptable PDX]

Z12.79 Encounter for screening for malignant neoplasm of <u>other genitourinary organs</u> — [Unacceptable PDX]

Z12.8- Encounter for screening for malignant neoplasm of other sites

Z12.81 Encounter for screening for malignant neoplasm of <u>oral cavity</u> — [Unacceptable PDX]

Z12.82 Encounter for screening for malignant neoplasm of <u>nervous system</u> — [Unacceptable PDX]

Z12.83 Encounter for screening for malignant neoplasm of <u>skin</u> — [Unacceptable PDX]

Z12.89 Encounter for screening for malignant neoplasm of <u>other sites</u> — [Unacceptable PDX]

Z12.9 Encounter for screening for malignant neoplasm, <u>site unspecified</u> — [Unacceptable PDX]

Z13- Encounter for <u>screening for other diseases and disorders</u>
Note: Screening is the testing for disease or disease precursors in asymptomatic individuals so that early detection and treatment can be provided for those who test positive for the disease.
Excludes 1:   encounter for diagnostic examination — code to sign or symptom

Z13.0 Encounter for screening for diseases of the blood and blood-forming organs and certain disorders involving the immune mechanism — [Unacceptable PDX]

Z13.1 Encounter for screening for diabetes mellitus — [Unacceptable PDX]

Z13.2- Encounter for screening for nutritional, metabolic and other endocrine disorders

Z13.21 Encounter for screening for nutritional disorder — [Unacceptable PDX]

Z13.22- Encounter for screening for metabolic disorder

Z13.220 Encounter for screening for lipoid disorders — [Unacceptable PDX]
Encounter for screening for cholesterol level
Encounter for screening for hypercholesterolemia
Encounter for screening for hyperlipidemia

Z13.228 Encounter for screening for other metabolic disorders — [Unacceptable PDX]

Z13.29 Encounter for screening for other suspected endocrine disorder — [Unacceptable PDX]
Excludes 1:   encounter for screening for diabetes mellitus (Z13.1)

Z13.4 Encounter for screening for certain developmental disorders in childhood — [Age/0-17] [Unacceptable PDX]
Encounter for screening for developmental handicaps in early childhood
Excludes 1:   routine development testing of infant or child (Z00.1-)

Z13.5 Encounter for screening for eye and ear disorders — [Unacceptable PDX]
*Excludes ❷: encounter for general hearing examination (Z01.1-)
encounter for general vision examination (Z01.0-)*

Z13.6 Encounter for screening for cardiovascular disorders — [Unacceptable PDX]

Z13.7- Encounter for screening for genetic and chromosomal anomalies
Excludes 1:   genetic testing for procreative management (Z31.4-)

Z13.71 Encounter for nonprocreative screening for genetic disease carrier status — [Unacceptable PDX]

Z13.79 Encounter for other screening for genetic and chromosomal anomalies — [Unacceptable PDX]

Z13.8- Encounter for screening for other specified diseases and disorders
Excludes ❷: screening for malignant neoplasms (Z12.-)

Z13.81- Encounter for screening for digestive system disorders

Z13.810 Encounter for screening for upper gastrointestinal disorder — [Unacceptable PDX]

Z13.811 Encounter for screening for lower gastrointestinal disorder — [Unacceptable PDX]
Excludes 1:   encounter for screening for intestinal infectious disease (Z11.0)

Z13.818 Encounter for screening for other digestive system disorders — [Unacceptable PDX]

Excludes 1: = NOT CODED HERE! (Do not code both)   **1312**   *Excludes ❷: = Not Included Here*

Z13.82- **Encounter for screening for musculoskeletal disorder**

    Z13.820   **Encounter for screening for osteoporosis** — [Unacceptable PDX]

    Z13.828   **Encounter for screening for other musculoskeletal disorder** — [Unacceptable PDX]

Z13.83   **Encounter for screening for respiratory disorder NEC** — [Unacceptable PDX]

    Excludes 1:   *encounter for screening for respiratory tuberculosis (Z11.1)*

Z13.84   **Encounter for screening for dental disorders** — [Unacceptable PDX]

Z13.85- **Encounter for screening for nervous system disorders**

    Z13.850   **Encounter for screening for traumatic brain injury** — [Unacceptable PDX]

    Z13.858   **Encounter for screening for other nervous system disorders** — [Unacceptable PDX]

Z13.88   **Encounter for screening for disorder due to exposure to contaminants** — [Unacceptable PDX]

    Excludes 1:   *those exposed to contaminants without suspected disorders (Z57.-, Z77.-)*

Z13.89   **Encounter for screening for other disorder** — [Unacceptable PDX]

    Encounter for screening for genitourinary disorders

Z13.9   **Encounter for screening, unspecified** — [Unacceptable PDX]

Genetic carrier and genetic susceptibility to disease (Z14-Z15)

Z14- **Genetic carrier**

Z14.0- **Hemophilia A carrier**

    Z14.01   **Asymptomatic hemophilia A carrier** — [Unacceptable PDX]

    Z14.02   **Symptomatic hemophilia A carrier** — [Unacceptable PDX]

Z14.1   **Cystic fibrosis carrier** — [Unacceptable PDX]

Z14.8   **Genetic carrier of other disease** — [Unacceptable PDX]

Z15- **Genetic susceptibility to disease**

   Includes: Confirmed abnormal gene

   Use additional code, if applicable, for any associated family history of the disease (Z80-Z84)

   Excludes 1:   *chromosomal anomalies (Q90-Q99)*

Z15.0- **Genetic susceptibility to malignant neoplasm**

   Code first, if applicable, any current malignant neoplasm (C00-C75, C81-C96)

   Use additional code, if applicable, for any personal history of malignant neoplasm (Z85-)

    Z15.01   **Genetic susceptibility to malignant neoplasm of breast** — [Unacceptable PDX]

    Z15.02   **Genetic susceptibility to malignant neoplasm of ovary** — [♀] [Unacceptable PDX]

    Z15.03   **Genetic susceptibility to malignant neoplasm of prostate** — [♂] [Unacceptable PDX]

    Z15.04   **Genetic susceptibility to malignant neoplasm of endometrium** — [♀] [Unacceptable PDX]

    Z15.09   **Genetic susceptibility to other malignant neoplasm** — [Unacceptable PDX]

Z15.8- **Genetic susceptibility to other disease**

    Z15.81   **Genetic susceptibility to multiple endocrine neoplasia [MEN]** — [Unacceptable PDX]

    Excludes 1:   *multiple endocrine neoplasia [MEN] syndromes (E31.2-)*

    Z15.89   **Genetic susceptibility to other disease** — [Unacceptable PDX]

Resistance to antimicrobial drugs (Z16)

Z16- <u>**Resistance**</u> **to antimicrobial drugs**

   Note: The codes in this category are provided for use as additional codes to identify the resistance and nonresponsiveness of a condition to antimicrobial drugs.

   Code first the infection

   Excludes 1:   *methicillin resistant Staphylococcus aureus infection (A49.02)*
          methicillin resistant Staphylococcus aureus infection in diseases classified elsewhere (B95.62)
          methicillin resistant Staphylococcus aureus pneumonia (J15.212)
          sepsis due to methicillin resistant Staphylococcus aureus (A41.02)

Z16.1- **Resistance to** <u>beta lactam</u> **antibiotics**

    Z16.10   **Resistance to unspecified beta lactam antibiotics** — [Unacceptable PDX]

    Z16.11   **Resistance to** <u>penicillins</u> — [Unacceptable PDX]
         Resistance to amoxicillin
         Resistance to ampicillin

    Z16.12   **Extended spectrum beta lactamase (ESBL) resistance** — [Unacceptable PDX]

    Z16.19   **Resistance to other specified beta lactam antibiotics** — [Unacceptable PDX]
         Resistance to cephalosporins

Z16.2- **Resistance to** <u>other antibiotics</u>

    Z16.20   **Resistance to unspecified antibiotic** — [Unacceptable PDX]
         Resistance to antibiotics NOS

    Z16.21   **Resistance to vancomycin** — [Unacceptable PDX]

    Z16.22   **Resistance to vancomycin related antibiotics** — [Unacceptable PDX]

    Z16.23   **Resistance to quinolones and fluoroquinolones** — [Unacceptable PDX]

    Z16.24   **Resistance to multiple antibiotics** — [Unacceptable PDX]

    Z16.29   **Resistance to other single specified antibiotic** — [Unacceptable PDX]
         Resistance to aminoglycosides
         Resistance to macrolides
         Resistance to sulfonamides
         Resistance to tetracyclines

Z16.3- **Resistance to other** <u>antimicrobial</u> **drugs**

   Excludes 1:   *resistance to antibiotics (Z16.1-, Z16.2-)*

    Z16.30   **Resistance to unspecified antimicrobial drugs** — [Unacceptable PDX]
         Drug resistance NOS

    Z16.31   **Resistance to antiparasitic drug(s)** — [Unacceptable PDX]
         Resistance to quinine and related compounds

    Z16.32   **Resistance to antifungal drug(s)** — [Unacceptable PDX]

    Z16.33   **Resistance to antiviral drug(s)** — [Unacceptable PDX]

    Z16.34- **Resistance to** <u>antimycobacterial</u> **drug(s)**
         Resistance to tuberculostatics

      Z16.341   **Resistance to single antimycobacterial drug** — [Unacceptable PDX]
            Resistance to antimycobacterial drug NOS

      Z16.342   **Resistance to multiple antimycobacterial drugs** — [Unacceptable PDX]

    Z16.35   **Resistance to multiple antimicrobial drugs** — [Unacceptable PDX]

    Excludes 1:   *resistance to multiple antibiotics only (Z16.24)*

    Z16.39   **Resistance to other specified antimicrobial drug** — [Unacceptable PDX]

Estrogen receptor status (Z17)

Z17- **Estrogen receptor status**

   Code first malignant neoplasm of breast (C50-)

Z17.0   **Estrogen receptor positive status [ER+]** — [Unacceptable PDX]

Z17.1   **Estrogen receptor negative status [ER-]** — [Unacceptable PDX]

Retained foreign body fragments (Z18)

Z18- Retained foreign body fragments
Includes: Embedded fragment (status)
Embedded splinter (status)
Retained foreign body status
Excludes 1: *artificial joint prosthesis status (Z96.6-)*
foreign body accidentally left during a procedure (T81.5-)
foreign body entering through orifice (T15-T19)
in situ cardiac device (Z95.-)
organ or tissue replaced by means other than transplant (Z96.-, Z97.-)
organ or tissue replaced by transplant (Z94.-)
personal history of retained foreign body fully removed Z87.821
superficial foreign body (non-embedded splinter) — code to superficial foreign body, by site

Z18.0- Retained radioactive fragments
Z18.01 Retained depleted uranium fragments — [Unacceptable PDX]
Z18.09 Other retained radioactive fragments — [Unacceptable PDX]
Other retained depleted isotope fragments
Retained nontherapeutic radioactive fragments

Z18.1- Retained metal fragments
Excludes 1: *retained radioactive metal fragments (Z18.01-Z18.09)*
Z18.10 Retained metal fragments, unspecified — [Unacceptable PDX]
Retained metal fragment NOS
Z18.11 Retained <u>magnetic</u> metal fragments — [Unacceptable PDX]
Z18.12 Retained <u>nonmagnetic</u> metal fragments — [Unacceptable PDX]

Z18.2 Retained plastic fragments — [Unacceptable PDX]
Acrylics fragments
Diethylhexylphthalates fragments
Isocyanate fragments

Z18.3- Retained organic fragments
Z18.31 Retained animal quills or spines — [Unacceptable PDX]
Z18.32 Retained tooth — [Unacceptable PDX]
Z18.33 Retained wood fragments — [Unacceptable PDX]
Z18.39 Other retained organic fragments — [Unacceptable PDX]

Z18.8- Other specified retained foreign body
Z18.81 Retained glass fragments — [Unacceptable PDX]
Z18.83 Retained stone or crystalline fragments — [Unacceptable PDX]
Retained concrete or cement fragments
Z18.89 Other specified retained foreign body fragments — [Unacceptable PDX]

Z18.9 Retained foreign body fragments, unspecified material — [Unacceptable PDX]

Hormone sensitivity malignancy status (Z19)

Z19- Hormone sensitivity malignancy status
Code first malignant neoplasm – see Table of Neoplasms, by site, malignant
Z19.1 Hormone sensitive malignancy status — [Unacceptable PDX]
Z19.2 Hormone resistant malignancy status — [Unacceptable PDX]
Castrate resistant prostate malignancy status

Persons with potential health hazards related to communicable diseases (Z20-Z29)

Z20- <u>Contact with and (suspected) exposure to communicable diseases</u>
Excludes 1: *carrier of infectious disease (Z22.-)*
diagnosed current infectious or parasitic disease — see Alphabetic Index
Excludes 2: *personal history of infectious and parasitic diseases (Z86.1-)*
Z20.0- Contact with and (suspected) exposure to intestinal infectious diseases
Z20.01 Contact with and (suspected) exposure to intestinal infectious diseases due to Escherichia coli (E. coli)
Z20.09 Contact with and (suspected) exposure to other intestinal infectious diseases — [Unacceptable PDX]
Z20.1 Contact with and (suspected) exposure to tuberculosis — [Unacceptable PDX]
Z20.2 Contact with and (suspected) exposure to infections with a predominantly sexual mode of transmission — [Unacceptable PDX]

Z20.3 Contact with and (suspected) exposure to rabies — [Unacceptable PDX]
Z20.4 Contact with and (suspected) exposure to rubella — [Unacceptable PDX]
Z20.5 Contact with and (suspected) exposure to viral hepatitis
Z20.6 Contact with and (suspected) exposure to human immunodeficiency virus [HIV]
Excludes 1: *asymptomatic human immunodeficiency virus [HIV] HIV infection status (Z21)*
Z20.7 Contact with and (suspected) exposure to pediculosis, acariasis and other infestations — [Unacceptable PDX]
Z20.8- Contact with and (suspected) exposure to other communicable diseases
Z20.81- Contact with and (suspected) exposure to other bacterial communicable diseases
Z20.810 Contact with and (suspected) exposure to anthrax — [Unacceptable PDX]
Z20.811 Contact with and (suspected) exposure to meningococcus
Z20.818 Contact with and (suspected) exposure to other bacterial communicable diseases — [Unacceptable PDX]
Z20.82- Contact with and (suspected) exposure to other viral communicable diseases
Z20.820 Contact with and (suspected) exposure to varicella
Z20.828 Contact with and (suspected) exposure to other viral communicable diseases
Z20.89 Contact with and (suspected) exposure to other communicable diseases — [Unacceptable PDX]
Z20.9 Contact with and (suspected) exposure to unspecified communicable disease — [Unacceptable PDX]

Z21 Asymptomatic human immunodeficiency virus [HIV] infection status — [Questionable Admission]
HIV positive NOS
Code first human immunodeficiency virus [HIV] disease complicating pregnancy, childbirth and the puerperium, if applicable (O98.7-)
Excludes 1: *acquired immunodeficiency syndrome (B20)*
contact with human immunodeficiency virus [HIV] (Z20.6)
exposure to human immunodeficiency virus [HIV] (Z20.6)
human immunodeficiency virus [HIV] disease (B20)
inconclusive laboratory evidence of human immunodeficiency virus [HIV] (R75)

Z22- <u>Carrier of infectious disease</u>
Includes: Colonization status
Suspected carrier
Excludes 2: *carrier of viral hepatitis (B18.-)*
Z22.0 Carrier of typhoid — [Unacceptable PDX]
Z22.1 Carrier of other intestinal infectious diseases — [Unacceptable PDX]
Z22.2 Carrier of diphtheria — [Unacceptable PDX]
Z22.3- Carrier of other specified bacterial diseases
Z22.31 Carrier of bacterial disease due to meningococci — [Unacceptable PDX]
Z22.32- Carrier of bacterial disease due to staphylococci
Z22.321 Carrier or suspected carrier of methicillin susceptible Staphylococcus aureus — [Unacceptable PDX]
MSSA colonization
Z22.322 Carrier or suspected carrier of methicillin resistant Staphylococcus aureus — [Unacceptable PDX]
MRSA colonization
Z22.33- Carrier of bacterial disease due to streptococci
Z22.330 Carrier of Group B streptococcus — [Unacceptable PDX]
Excludes 1: *carrier of streptococcus group B (GBS) complicating pregnancy, childbirth and the puerperium (O99.-)*
Z22.338 Carrier of other streptococcus — [Unacceptable PDX]
Z22.39 Carrier of other specified bacterial diseases — [Unacceptable PDX]
Z22.4 Carrier of infections with a predominantly sexual mode of transmission — [Unacceptable PDX]

Z22.6 Carrier of human T-lymphotropic virus type-1 [HTLV-1] infection — [Unacceptable PDX]

Z22.8 Carrier of other infectious diseases — [Unacceptable PDX]

Z22.9 Carrier of infectious disease, unspecified — [Unacceptable PDX]

Z23 Encounter for immunization — [Unacceptable PDX]
Code first any routine childhood examination
Note: Procedure codes are required to identify the types of immunizations given.

Z28- Immunization not carried out and underimmunization status
Includes:　Vaccination not carried out

Z28.0- Immunization not carried out because of contraindication

Z28.01 Immunization not carried out because of acute illness of patient — [Unacceptable PDX]

Z28.02 Immunization not carried out because of chronic illness or condition of patient — [Unacceptable PDX]

Z28.03 Immunization not carried out because of immune compromised state of patient — [Unacceptable PDX]

Z28.04 Immunization not carried out because of patient allergy to vaccine or component — [Unacceptable PDX]

Z28.09 Immunization not carried out because of other contraindication — [Unacceptable PDX]

Z28.1 Immunization not carried out because of patient decision for reasons of belief or group pressure — [Unacceptable PDX]
Immunization not carried out because of religious belief

Z28.2- Immunization not carried out because of patient decision for other and unspecified reason

Z28.20 Immunization not carried out because of patient decision for unspecified reason — [Unacceptable PDX]

Z28.21 Immunization not carried out because of patient refusal — [Unacceptable PDX]

Z28.29 Immunization not carried out because of patient decision for other reason — [Unacceptable PDX]

Z28.3 Underimmunization status — [Unacceptable PDX]
Delinquent immunization status
Lapsed immunization schedule status

Z28.8- Immunization not carried out for other reason

Z28.81 Immunization not carried out due to patient having had the disease — [Unacceptable PDX]

Z28.82 Immunization not carried out because of caregiver refusal — [Unacceptable PDX]
Immunization not carried out because of guardian refusal
Immunization not carried out because of parent refusal
Excludes 1:　immunization not carried out because of caregiver refusal because of religious belief (Z28.1)

Z28.89 Immunization not carried out for other reason — [Unacceptable PDX]

Z28.9 Immunization not carried out for unspecified reason — [Unacceptable PDX]

Z29- Encounter for other prophylactic measures
Excludes 1:　desensitization to allergens (Z51.6)
prophylactic surgery (Z40.-)

Z29.1- Encounter for prophylactic immunotherapy
Encounter for administration of immunoglobulin

Z29.11 Encounter for prophylactic immunotherapy for respiratory syncytial virus (RSV) — [Unacceptable PDX]

Z29.12 Encounter for prophylactic antivenin — [Unacceptable PDX]

Z29.13 Encounter for prophylactic Rho(D) immune globulin — [Unacceptable PDX]

Z29.14 Encounter for prophylactic rabies immune globin — [Unacceptable PDX]

Z29.3 Encounter for prophylactic fluoride administration — [Unacceptable PDX]

Z29.8 Encounter for other specified prophylactic measures — [Unacceptable PDX]

Z29.9 Encounter for prophylactic measures, unspecified — [Unacceptable PDX]

Persons encountering health services in circumstances related to reproduction (Z30-Z39)

Z30- Encounter for contraceptive management

Z30.0- Encounter for general counseling and advice on contraception

Z30.01- Encounter for initial prescription of contraceptives
Excludes 1:　encounter for surveillance of contraceptives (Z30.4-)

Z30.011 Encounter for initial prescription of contraceptive pills — [♀] [Unacceptable PDX]

Z30.012 Encounter for prescription of emergency contraception — [♀] [Unacceptable PDX]
Encounter for postcoital contraception

Z30.013 Encounter for initial prescription of injectable contraceptive — [♀] [Unacceptable PDX]

Z30.014 Encounter for initial prescription of intrauterine contraceptive device — [♀] [Unacceptable PDX]
Excludes 1:　encounter for insertion of intrauterine contraceptive device (Z30.430, Z30.432)

Z30.015 Encounter for initial prescription of vaginal ring hormonal contraceptive — [♀] [Unacceptable PDX]

Z30.016 Encounter for initial prescription of transdermal patch hormonal contraceptive device — [♀] [Unacceptable PDX]

Z30.017 Encounter for initial prescription of implantable subdermal contraceptive — [♀] [Unacceptable PDX]

Z30.018 Encounter for initial prescription of other contraceptives — [♀] [Unacceptable PDX]
Encounter for initial prescription of barrier contraception
Encounter for initial prescription of diaphragm

Z30.019 Encounter for initial prescription of contraceptives, unspecified — [♀] [Unacceptable PDX]

Z30.02 Counseling and instruction in natural family planning to avoid pregnancy — [Unacceptable PDX]

Z30.09 Encounter for other general counseling and advice on contraception — [Unacceptable PDX]
Encounter for family planning advice NOS

Z30.2 Encounter for sterilization

Z30.4- Encounter for surveillance of contraceptives

Z30.40 Encounter for surveillance of contraceptives, unspecified — [Unacceptable PDX]

Z30.41 Encounter for surveillance of contraceptive pills — [♀] [Unacceptable PDX]
Encounter for repeat prescription for contraceptive pill

Z30.42 Encounter for surveillance of injectable contraceptive — [♀] [Unacceptable PDX]

Z30.43- Encounter for surveillance of intrauterine contraceptive device

Z30.430 Encounter for insertion of intrauterine contraceptive device — [♀] [Unacceptable PDX]

Z30.431 Encounter for routine checking of intrauterine contraceptive device — [♀] [Unacceptable PDX]

Z30.432 Encounter for removal of intrauterine contraceptive device — [♀] [Unacceptable PDX]

Z30.433 Encounter for removal and reinsertion of intrauterine contraceptive device — [♀] [Unacceptable PDX]
Encounter for replacement of intrauterine contraceptive device

Z30.44 Encounter for surveillance of vaginal ring hormonal contraceptive device — [♀] [Unacceptable PDX]

Z30.45 Encounter for surveillance of transdermal patch hormonal contraceptive device — [♀] [Unacceptable PDX]

Z30.46 Encounter for surveillance of implantable subdermal contraceptive — [♀] [Unacceptable PDX]
Encounter for checking, reinsertion or removal of implantable subdermal contraceptive

Z 2 2 - Z 3 0

Z30.49 **Encounter for surveillance of other contraceptives** — [♀]
[Unacceptable PDX]
Encounter for surveillance of barrier contraception
Encounter for surveillance of diaphragm

Z30.8 **Encounter for other contraceptive management** —
[Unacceptable PDX]
Encounter for postvasectomy sperm count
Encounter for routine examination for contraceptive maintenance
Excludes 1: *sperm count following sterilization reversal (Z31.42)*
sperm count for fertility testing (Z31.41)

Z30.9 **Encounter for contraceptive management, unspecified** —
[Unacceptable PDX]

Z31- **Encounter for** <u>procreative management</u>
Excludes 1: *complications associated with artificial fertilization (N98.-)*
female infertility (N97.-)
male infertility (N46.-)

Z31.0 **Encounter for reversal of previous sterilization**

Z31.4- **Encounter for procreative investigation and testing**
Excludes 1: *postvasectomy sperm count (Z30.8)*

Z31.41 **Encounter for fertility testing** — [Unacceptable PDX]
Encounter for fallopian tube patency testing
Encounter for sperm count for fertility testing

Z31.42 **Aftercare following sterilization reversal** —
[Unacceptable PDX]
Sperm count following sterilization reversal

Z31.43- **Encounter for genetic testing of** <u>female</u> **for procreative management**
Use additional code for recurrent pregnancy loss, if applicable
(N96, O26.2-)
Excludes 1: *nonprocreative genetic testing (Z13.7-)*

Z31.430 **Encounter of female for testing for genetic disease carrier status for procreative management** — [♀]
[Unacceptable PDX]

Z31.438 **Encounter for other genetic testing of female for procreative management** — [♀] [Unacceptable PDX]

Z31.44- **Encounter for genetic testing of** <u>male</u> **for procreative management**
Excludes 1: *nonprocreative genetic testing (Z13.7-)*

Z31.440 **Encounter of male for testing for genetic disease carrier status for procreative management** — [♂]
[Unacceptable PDX]

Z31.441 **Encounter for testing of male partner of patient with recurrent pregnancy loss** — [♂, Age/15-124]
[Unacceptable PDX]

Z31.448 **Encounter for other genetic testing of male for procreative management** — [♂, Age/15-124]
[Unacceptable PDX]

Z31.49 **Encounter for other procreative investigation and testing** — [Unacceptable PDX]

Z31.5 **Encounter for genetic counseling** — [Unacceptable PDX]

Z31.6- **Encounter for general counseling and advice on procreation**

Z31.61 **Procreative counseling and advice using natural family planning** — [Unacceptable PDX]

Z31.62 **Encounter for fertility preservation counseling** —
[Unacceptable PDX]
Encounter for fertility preservation counseling prior to cancer therapy
Encounter for fertility preservation counseling prior to surgical removal of gonads

Z31.69 **Encounter for other general counseling and advice on procreation** — [Unacceptable PDX]

Z31.7 **Encounter for procreative management and counseling for gestational carrier** — [Unacceptable PDX]
Excludes 1: *pregnant state, gestational carrier (Z33.3)*

Z31.8- **Encounter for other procreative management**

Z31.81 **Encounter for male factor infertility in female patient** —
[♀] [Unacceptable PDX]

Z31.82 **Encounter for Rh incompatibility status** — [♀]
[Unacceptable PDX]
AHA 14:4Q:p17 – Prophylactic injection of anti-D antibodies during prenatal visit

Z31.83 **Encounter for assisted reproductive fertility procedure cycle** — [♀] [Unacceptable PDX]
Patient undergoing in vitro fertilization cycle
Use additional code to identify the type of infertility
Excludes 1: *pre-cycle diagnosis and testing — code to reason for encounter*

Z31.84 **Encounter for fertility preservation procedure** —
[Unacceptable PDX]
Encounter for fertility preservation procedure prior to cancer therapy
Encounter for fertility preservation procedure prior to surgical removal of gonads

Z31.89 **Encounter for other procreative management** —
[Unacceptable PDX]

Z31.9 **Encounter for procreative management, unspecified** —
[Unacceptable PDX]

Z32- **Encounter for pregnancy test and childbirth and childcare instruction**

Z32.0- **Encounter for pregnancy test**

Z32.00 **Encounter for pregnancy test, result unknown** — [♀]
Encounter for pregnancy test NOS

Z32.01 **Encounter for pregnancy test, result positive** —
[♀, Age/12-55]

Z32.02 **Encounter for pregnancy test, result negative** — [♀]

Z32.2 **Encounter for childbirth instruction** — [Unacceptable PDX]

Z32.3 **Encounter for childcare instruction** — [Unacceptable PDX]
Encounter for prenatal or postpartum childcare instruction

Z33- **Pregnant state**

Z33.1 **Pregnant state, incidental** — [♀, Age/12-55] [Unacceptable PDX]
Pregnant state NOS
Excludes 1: *complications of pregnancy (O00-O9A)*
pregnant state, gestational carrier (Z33.3)

Z33.2 **Encounter for elective termination of pregnancy** —
[♀, Age/12-55]
Excludes 1: *early fetal death with retention of dead fetus (O02.1)*
late fetal death (O36.4)
spontaneous abortion (O03)

Z33.3 **Pregnant state, gestational carrier** — [♀, Age/12-55]
[Unacceptable PDX]
Excludes 1: *encounter for procreative management and counseling for gestational carrier (Z31.7)*

Z34- **Encounter for** <u>supervision of normal pregnancy</u>
Excludes 1: *any complication of pregnancy (O00-O9A)*
encounter for pregnancy test (Z32.0-)
encounter for supervision of high risk pregnancy (O09-)

Z34.0- **Encounter for supervision of** <u>normal</u> <u>first</u> **pregnancy**

Z34.00 **Encounter for supervision of normal** <u>first</u> **pregnancy,** <u>unspecified trimester</u> — [♀, Age/12-55] [Unacceptable PDX]

Z34.01 **Encounter for supervision of normal** <u>first</u> **pregnancy,** <u>first trimester</u> — [♀, Age/12-55] [Unacceptable PDX]

Z34.02 **Encounter for supervision of normal** <u>first</u> **pregnancy,** <u>second trimester</u> — [♀, Age/12-55] [Unacceptable PDX]

Z34.03 **Encounter for supervision of normal** <u>first</u> **pregnancy,** <u>third trimester</u> — [♀, Age/12-55] [Unacceptable PDX]

Z34.8- **Encounter for supervision of** <u>other normal</u> **pregnancy**
AHA 14:4Q:p17 – Prophylactic injection of anti-D antibodies during prenatal visit

Z34.80 **Encounter for supervision of other normal pregnancy,** <u>unspecified trimester</u> — [♀, Age/12-55] [Unacceptable PDX]

Z34.81 **Encounter for supervision of other normal pregnancy,** <u>first trimester</u> — [♀, Age/12-55] [Unacceptable PDX]

Z34.82 **Encounter for supervision of other normal pregnancy,** <u>second trimester</u> — [♀, Age/12-55] [Unacceptable PDX]

Z34.83 **Encounter for supervision of other normal pregnancy,** <u>third trimester</u> — [♀, Age/12-55] [Unacceptable PDX]

Z34.9- **Encounter for supervision of normal pregnancy,** <u>unspecified</u>

Z34.90 **Encounter for supervision of normal pregnancy, unspecified,** <u>unspecified trimester</u> — [♀, Age/12-55]
[Unacceptable PDX]

Z34.91 **Encounter for supervision of normal pregnancy, unspecified,** <u>first trimester</u> — [♀, Age/12-55] [Unacceptable PDX]

Z30 - Z34

Z34.92 **Encounter for supervision of normal pregnancy, unspecified, <u>second trimester</u>** — [♀, Age/12-55] [Unacceptable PDX]

Z34.93 **Encounter for supervision of normal pregnancy, unspecified, <u>third trimester</u>** — [♀, Age/12-55] [Unacceptable PDX]

Z36 **Encounter for antenatal screening of mother** — [♀, Age/12-55] [Unacceptable PDX]

    Excludes 1:   abnormal findings on antenatal screening of mother (O28.-) diagnostic examination- code to sign or symptom encounter for suspected maternal and fetal conditions ruled out (Z03.7-) suspected fetal condition affecting management of pregnancy — code to condition in Chapter 15

    Excludes ❷: genetic counseling and testing (Z31.43-, Z31.5) routine prenatal care (Z34)

Z3A- <u>Weeks of gestation</u>

    AHA 13:2Q:p33 – Use date of admission for weeks of gestation

    AHA 14:1Q:p14 – Discrepancies in documentation of gestational age

    AHA 14:3Q:p17 – Weeks of gestation not applicable in ectopic pregnancies

    Note: Codes from category Z3A are for use, only on the maternal record, to indicate the weeks of gestation of the pregnancy, if known.

    Code first complications of pregnancy, childbirth and the puerperium (O00-O9A)

Z3A.0- **Weeks of gestation of pregnancy, unspecified or less than 10 weeks**

    Z3A.00 **Weeks of gestation of pregnancy not specified** — [♀, Age/12-55] [Unacceptable PDX]

    Z3A.01 **Less than 8 weeks of gestation of pregnancy** — [♀, Age/12-55] [Unacceptable PDX]

    Z3A.08 **8 weeks of gestation of pregnancy** — [♀, Age/12-55] [Unacceptable PDX]

    Z3A.09 **9 weeks of gestation of pregnancy** — [♀, Age/12-55] [Unacceptable PDX]

Z3A.1- **Weeks of gestation of pregnancy, weeks 10-19**

    Z3A.10 **10 weeks of gestation of pregnancy** — [♀, Age/12-55] [Unacceptable PDX]

    Z3A.11 **11 weeks of gestation of pregnancy** — [♀, Age/12-55] [Unacceptable PDX]

    Z3A.12 **12 weeks of gestation of pregnancy** — [♀, Age/12-55] [Unacceptable PDX]

    Z3A.13 **13 weeks of gestation of pregnancy** — [♀, Age/12-55] [Unacceptable PDX]

    Z3A.14 **14 weeks of gestation of pregnancy** — [♀, Age/12-55] [Unacceptable PDX]

    Z3A.15 **15 weeks of gestation of pregnancy** — [♀, Age/12-55] [Unacceptable PDX]

    Z3A.16 **16 weeks of gestation of pregnancy** — [♀, Age/12-55] [Unacceptable PDX]

    Z3A.17 **17 weeks of gestation of pregnancy** — [♀, Age/12-55] [Unacceptable PDX]

    Z3A.18 **18 weeks of gestation of pregnancy** — [♀, Age/12-55] [Unacceptable PDX]

    Z3A.19 **19 weeks of gestation of pregnancy** — [♀, Age/12-55] [Unacceptable PDX]

Z3A.2- **Weeks of gestation of pregnancy, weeks 20-29**

    Z3A.20 **20 weeks of gestation of pregnancy** — [♀, Age/12-55] [Unacceptable PDX]

    Z3A.21 **21 weeks of gestation of pregnancy** — [♀, Age/12-55] [Unacceptable PDX]

    Z3A.22 **22 weeks of gestation of pregnancy** — [♀, Age/12-55] [Unacceptable PDX]

    Z3A.23 **23 weeks of gestation of pregnancy** — [♀, Age/12-55] [Unacceptable PDX]

    Z3A.24 **24 weeks of gestation of pregnancy** — [♀, Age/12-55] [Unacceptable PDX]

    Z3A.25 **25 weeks of gestation of pregnancy** — [♀, Age/12-55] [Unacceptable PDX]

    Z3A.26 **26 weeks of gestation of pregnancy** — [♀, Age/12-55] [Unacceptable PDX]

    Z3A.27 **27 weeks of gestation of pregnancy** — [♀, Age/12-55] [Unacceptable PDX]

Z3A.28 **28 weeks of gestation of pregnancy** — [♀, Age/12-55] [Unacceptable PDX]

Z3A.29 **29 weeks of gestation of pregnancy** — [♀, Age/12-55] [Unacceptable PDX]

Z3A.3- **Weeks of gestation of pregnancy, weeks 30-39**

    Z3A.30 **30 weeks of gestation of pregnancy** — [♀, Age/12-55] [Unacceptable PDX]

    Z3A.31 **31 weeks of gestation of pregnancy** — [♀, Age/12-55] [Unacceptable PDX]

    Z3A.32 **32 weeks of gestation of pregnancy** — [♀, Age/12-55] [Unacceptable PDX]

    Z3A.33 **33 weeks of gestation of pregnancy** — [♀, Age/12-55] [Unacceptable PDX]

    Z3A.34 **34 weeks of gestation of pregnancy** — [♀, Age/12-55] [Unacceptable PDX]

    Z3A.35 **35 weeks of gestation of pregnancy** — [♀, Age/12-55] [Unacceptable PDX]

    Z3A.36 **36 weeks of gestation of pregnancy** — [♀, Age/12-55] [Unacceptable PDX]

    Z3A.37 **37 weeks of gestation of pregnancy** — [♀, Age/12-55] [Unacceptable PDX]

    Z3A.38 **38 weeks of gestation of pregnancy** — [♀, Age/12-55] [Unacceptable PDX]

    Z3A.39 **39 weeks of gestation of pregnancy** — [♀, Age/12-55] [Unacceptable PDX]

Z3A.4- **Weeks of gestation of pregnancy, weeks 40 or greater**

    Z3A.40 **40 weeks of gestation of pregnancy** — [♀, Age/12-55] [Unacceptable PDX]

    Z3A.41 **41 weeks of gestation of pregnancy** — [♀, Age/12-55] [Unacceptable PDX]

    Z3A.42 **42 weeks of gestation of pregnancy** — [♀, Age/12-55] [Unacceptable PDX]

    Z3A.49 **Greater than 42 weeks of gestation of pregnancy** — [♀, Age/12-55] [Unacceptable PDX]

    AHA 14:4Q:p23 – 42 weeks of gestation or more

Z37- <u>Outcome of delivery</u>

    Note: This category is intended for use as an additional code to identify the outcome of delivery on the mother's record. It is not for use on the newborn record.

    Excludes 1:   stillbirth (P95)

Z37.0 **Single live birth** — [♀, Age/12-55] [Unacceptable PDX]

Z37.1 **Single stillbirth** — [♀, Age/12-55] [Unacceptable PDX]

Z37.2 **Twins, both liveborn** — [♀, Age/12-55] [Unacceptable PDX]

Z37.3 **Twins, one liveborn and one stillborn** — [♀, Age/12-55] [Unacceptable PDX]

Z37.4 **Twins, both stillborn** — [♀, Age/12-55] [Unacceptable PDX]

Z37.5- **Other multiple births, all liveborn**

    Z37.50 **Multiple births, unspecified, all liveborn** — [♀, Age/12-55] [Unacceptable PDX]

    Z37.51 **Triplets, all liveborn** — [♀, Age/12-55] [Unacceptable PDX]

    Z37.52 **Quadruplets, all liveborn** — [♀, Age/12-55] [Unacceptable PDX]

    Z37.53 **Quintuplets, all liveborn** — [♀, Age/12-55] [Unacceptable PDX]

    Z37.54 **Sextuplets, all liveborn** — [♀, Age/12-55] [Unacceptable PDX]

    Z37.59 **Other multiple births, all liveborn** — [♀, Age/12-55] [Unacceptable PDX]

Z37.6- **Other multiple births, some liveborn**

    Z37.60 **Multiple births, unspecified, some liveborn** — [♀, Age/12-55] [Unacceptable PDX]

    Z37.61 **Triplets, some liveborn** — [♀, Age/12-55] [Unacceptable PDX]

    Z37.62 **Quadruplets, some liveborn** — [♀, Age/12-55] [Unacceptable PDX]

    Z37.63 **Quintuplets, some liveborn** — [♀, Age/12-55] [Unacceptable PDX]

    Z37.64 **Sextuplets, some liveborn** — [♀, Age/12-55] [Unacceptable PDX]

    Z37.69 **Other multiple births, some liveborn** — [♀, Age/12-55] [Unacceptable PDX]

Z37.7 **Other multiple births, all stillborn** — [♀, Age/12-55] [Unacceptable PDX]

Z3A-Z37

Z37.9   Outcome of delivery, unspecified — [♀, Age/12-55]
[Unacceptable PDX]
Multiple birth NOS
Single birth NOS

Z38-   Liveborn infants according to place of birth and type of delivery
Note: This category is for use as the principal code on the initial record of a newborn baby. It is to be used for the initial birth record only. It is not to be used on the mother's record.
AHA 15:2Q:p15 – Physician reporting of Z38 category codes

Z38.0-   Single liveborn infant, born in hospital
Single liveborn infant, born in birthing center or other health care facility

Z38.00   Single liveborn infant, delivered vaginally — [Age/0]

Z38.01   Single liveborn infant, delivered by cesarean — [Age/0]

Z38.1   Single liveborn infant, born outside hospital — [Age/0]

Z38.2   Single liveborn infant, unspecified as to place of birth — [Age/0]
Single liveborn infant NOS

Z38.3-   Twin liveborn infant, born in hospital

Z38.30   Twin liveborn infant, delivered vaginally — [Age/0]

Z38.31   Twin liveborn infant, delivered by cesarean — [Age/0]

Z38.4   Twin liveborn infant, born outside hospital — [Age/0]

Z38.5   Twin liveborn infant, unspecified as to place of birth — [Age/0]

Z38.6-   Other multiple liveborn infant, born in hospital

Z38.61   Triplet liveborn infant, delivered vaginally — [Age/0]

Z38.62   Triplet liveborn infant, delivered by cesarean — [Age/0]

Z38.63   Quadruplet liveborn infant, delivered vaginally — [Age/0]

Z38.64   Quadruplet liveborn infant, delivered by cesarean — [Age/0]

Z38.65   Quintuplet liveborn infant, delivered vaginally — [Age/0]

Z38.66   Quintuplet liveborn infant, delivered by cesarean — [Age/0]

Z38.68   Other multiple liveborn infant, delivered vaginally — [Age/0]

Z38.69   Other multiple liveborn infant, delivered by cesarean — [Age/0]

Z38.7   Other multiple liveborn infant, born outside hospital — [Age/0]

Z38.8   Other multiple liveborn infant, unspecified as to place of birth — [Age/0]

Z39-   Encounter for maternal postpartum care and examination

Z39.0   Encounter for care and examination of mother immediately after delivery — [♀, Age/12-55]
Care and observation in uncomplicated cases when the delivery occurs outside a healthcare facility
Excludes 1:   care for postpartum complication — see Alphabetic index

Z39.1   Encounter for care and examination of lactating mother — [♀, Age/12-55] [Unacceptable PDX]
Encounter for supervision of lactation
Excludes 1:   disorders of lactation (O92.-)

Z39.2   Encounter for routine postpartum follow-up — [♀, Age/12-55] [Unacceptable PDX]

Encounters for other specific health care (Z40-Z53)

NOTE: Categories Z40-Z53 are intended for use to indicate a reason for care. They may be used for patients who have already been treated for a disease or injury, but who are receiving aftercare or prophylactic care, or care to consolidate the treatment, or to deal with a residual state.
Excludes ❷: follow-up examination for medical surveillance after treatment (Z08-Z09)

Z40-   Encounter for prophylactic surgery
Excludes 1:   organ donations (Z52.-)
therapeutic organ removal — code to condition

Z40.0-   Encounter for prophylactic surgery for risk factors related to malignant neoplasms
Admission for prophylactic organ removal
Use additional code to identify risk factor

Z40.00   Encounter for prophylactic removal of unspecified organ

Z40.01   Encounter for prophylactic removal of breast

Z40.02   Encounter for prophylactic removal of ovary — [♀]

Z40.09   Encounter for prophylactic removal of other organ

Z40.8   Encounter for other prophylactic surgery — [Unacceptable PDX]

Z40.9   Encounter for prophylactic surgery, unspecified — [Unacceptable PDX]

Z41-   Encounter for procedures for purposes other than remedying health state

Z41.1   Encounter for cosmetic surgery
Encounter for cosmetic breast implant
Encounter for cosmetic procedure
Excludes 1:   encounter for plastic and reconstructive surgery following medical procedure or healed injury (Z42-)
encounter for post-mastectomy breast implantation (Z42.1)

Z41.2   Encounter for routine and ritual male circumcision — [♂]

Z41.3   Encounter for ear piercing — [Unacceptable PDX]

Z41.8   Encounter for other procedures for purposes other than remedying health state

Z41.9   Encounter for procedure for purposes other than remedying health state, unspecified — [Unacceptable PDX]

Z42-   Encounter for plastic and reconstructive surgery following medical procedure or healed injury
Excludes 1:   encounter for cosmetic plastic surgery (Z41.1)
encounter for plastic surgery for treatment of current injury — code to relevent injury

Z42.1   Encounter for breast reconstruction following mastectomy — [Age/15-124]
Excludes 1:   deformity and disproportion of reconstructed breast (N65.1-)

Z42.8   Encounter for other plastic and reconstructive surgery following medical procedure or healed injury

Z43-   Encounter for attention to artificial openings
Includes: Closure of artificial openings
Passage of sounds or bougies through artificial openings
Reforming artificial openings
Removal of catheter from artificial openings
Toilet or cleansing of artificial openings
Excludes 1:   artificial opening status only, without need for care (Z93.-)
complications of external stoma (J95.0-, K94.-, N99.5-)
Excludes ❷: fitting and adjustment of prosthetic and other devices (Z44-Z46)

Z43.0   Encounter for attention to tracheostomy

cc **Z43.1**   Encounter for attention to gastrostomy

Z43.2   Encounter for attention to ileostomy

Z43.3   Encounter for attention to colostomy

Z43.4   Encounter for attention to other artificial openings of digestive tract

Z43.5   Encounter for attention to cystostomy

Z43.6   Encounter for attention to other artificial openings of urinary tract
Encounter for attention to nephrostomy
Encounter for attention to ureterostomy
Encounter for attention to urethrostomy

Z43.7   Encounter for attention to artificial vagina

Z43.8   Encounter for attention to other artificial openings

Z37-Z43

Z43.9   **Encounter for attention to unspecified artificial opening —** [Unacceptable PDX]

Z44-   **Encounter for <u>fitting and adjustment of external prosthetic device</u>**
Includes: Removal or replacement of external prosthetic device
Excludes 1:   malfunction or other complications of device — see Alphabetical Index
           presence of prosthetic device (Z97.-)

Z44.0-   **Encounter for fitting and adjustment of <u>artificial arm</u>**

  Z44.00-   **Encounter for fitting and adjustment of <u>unspecified</u> artificial arm**

    Z44.001   **Encounter for fitting and adjustment of unspecified <u>right</u> artificial arm**

    Z44.002   **Encounter for fitting and adjustment of unspecified <u>left</u> artificial arm**

    Z44.009   **Encounter for fitting and adjustment of unspecified artificial arm, <u>unspecified</u> arm**

  Z44.01-   **Encounter for fitting and adjustment of <u>complete</u> artificial arm**

    Z44.011   **Encounter for fitting and adjustment of complete <u>right</u> artificial arm**

    Z44.012   **Encounter for fitting and adjustment of complete <u>left</u> artificial arm**

    Z44.019   **Encounter for fitting and adjustment of complete artificial arm, <u>unspecified</u> arm**

  Z44.02-   **Encounter for fitting and adjustment of <u>partial</u> artificial arm**

    Z44.021   **Encounter for fitting and adjustment of partial artificial <u>right</u> arm**

    Z44.022   **Encounter for fitting and adjustment of partial artificial <u>left</u> arm**

    Z44.029   **Encounter for fitting and adjustment of partial artificial arm, <u>unspecified</u> arm**

Z44.1-   **Encounter for <u>fitting and adjustment of artificial leg</u>**

  Z44.10-   **Encounter for fitting and adjustment of unspecified artificial leg**

    Z44.101   **Encounter for fitting and adjustment of unspecified <u>right</u> artificial leg**

    Z44.102   **Encounter for fitting and adjustment of unspecified <u>left</u> artificial leg**

    Z44.109   **Encounter for fitting and adjustment of unspecified artificial leg, <u>unspecified</u> leg**

  Z44.11-   **Encounter for fitting and adjustment of <u>complete</u> artificial leg**

    Z44.111   **Encounter for fitting and adjustment of complete <u>right</u> artificial leg**

    Z44.112   **Encounter for fitting and adjustment of complete <u>left</u> artificial leg**

    Z44.119   **Encounter for fitting and adjustment of complete artificial leg, <u>unspecified</u> leg**

  Z44.12-   **Encounter for fitting and adjustment of <u>partial</u> artificial leg**

    Z44.121   **Encounter for fitting and adjustment of partial artificial <u>right</u> leg**

    Z44.122   **Encounter for fitting and adjustment of partial artificial <u>left</u> leg**

    Z44.129   **Encounter for fitting and adjustment of partial artificial leg, unspecified leg**

Z44.2-   **Encounter for <u>fitting and adjustment of artificial eye</u>**
Excludes 1:   mechanical complication of ocular prosthesis (T85.3)

  Z44.20   **Encounter for fitting and adjustment of artificial eye, <u>unspecified</u>**

  Z44.21   **Encounter for fitting and adjustment of artificial <u>right</u> eye**

  Z44.22   **Encounter for fitting and adjustment of artificial <u>left</u> eye**

Z44.3-   **Encounter for <u>fitting and adjustment of external breast prosthesis</u>**
Excludes 1:   complications of breast implant (T85.4-)
           encounter for adjustment or removal of breast implant (Z45.81-)
           encounter for initial breast implant insertion for cosmetic breast augmentation (Z41.1)
           encounter for breast reconstruction following mastectomy (Z42.1)

  Z44.30   **Encounter for fitting and adjustment of external breast prosthesis, <u>unspecified</u> breast**

  Z44.31   **Encounter for fitting and adjustment of external <u>right</u> breast prosthesis**

  Z44.32   **Encounter for fitting and adjustment of external <u>left</u> breast prosthesis**

Z44.8   **Encounter for fitting and adjustment of other external prosthetic devices**

Z44.9   **Encounter for fitting and adjustment of unspecified external prosthetic device — [Unacceptable PDX]**

Z45-   **Encounter for <u>adjustment and management of implanted device</u>**
Includes: Removal or replacement of implanted device
Excludes 1:   malfunction or other complications of device — see Alphabetical Index
           presence of prosthetic and other devices (Z95-Z97)
Excludes ❷: encounter for fitting and adjustment of non-implanted device (Z46-)

Z45.0-   **Encounter for adjustment and management of <u>cardiac device</u>**

  Z45.01-   **Encounter for adjustment and management of cardiac <u>pacemaker</u>**
Encounter for adjustment and management of cardiac resynchronization therapy pacemaker (CRT-P)
Excludes 1:   encounter for adjustment and management of automatic implantable cardiac defibrillator with synchronous cardiac pacemaker (Z45.02)

    Z45.010   **Encounter for checking and testing of cardiac pacemaker <u>pulse generator [battery]</u> —** [Questionable Admission]
Encounter for replacing cardiac pacemaker pulse generator [battery]

    Z45.018   **Encounter for adjustment and management of <u>other part of cardiac pacemaker</u> —** [Questionable Admission]

  Z45.02   **Encounter for adjustment and management of automatic implantable <u>cardiac defibrillator</u> —** [Questionable Admission]
Encounter for adjustment and management of automatic implantable cardiac defibrillator with synchronous cardiac pacemaker
Encounter for adjustment and management of cardiac resynchronization therapy defibrillator (CRT-D)

  Z45.09   **Encounter for adjustment and management of other cardiac device — [Questionable Admission]**

Z45.1   **Encounter for adjustment and management of <u>infusion pump</u>**

Z45.2   **Encounter for adjustment and management of <u>vascular access device</u>**
Encounter for adjustment and management of vascular catheters
Excludes 1:   encounter for adjustment and management of renal dialysis catheter (Z49.01)

Z45.3-   **Encounter for <u>adjustment and management of implanted devices of the special senses</u>**

  Z45.31   **Encounter for adjustment and management of implanted visual substitution device**

  Z45.32-   **Encounter for adjustment and management of <u>implanted hearing device</u>**
Excludes 1:   Encounter for fitting and adjustment of hearing aide (Z46.1)

    Z45.320   **Encounter for adjustment and management of <u>bone conduction device</u>**

    Z45.321   **Encounter for adjustment and management of <u>cochlear device</u>**

    Z45.328   **Encounter for adjustment and management of <u>other</u> implanted hearing device**

Z43 - Z45

Z45.4- Encounter for <u>adjustment and management of implanted nervous system device</u>
AHA 14:3Q:p19 – Replacement of Baclofen pump and catheter

Z45.41 Encounter for adjustment and management of <u>cerebrospinal fluid drainage device</u>
Encounter for adjustment and management of cerebral ventricular (communicating) shunt

Z45.42 Encounter for adjustment and management of <u>neuropacemaker</u> (brain) (peripheral nerve) (spinal cord)

Z45.49 Encounter for adjustment and management of <u>other</u> implanted nervous system device
AHA 14:4Q:p26 – Encounter for adjustment of vertical expandable prosthetic titanium rib (VEPTR)
AHA 14:4Q:p27 – Encounter for open lengthening of growing rods

Z45.8- Encounter for adjustment and management of <u>other implanted devices</u>

Z45.81- Encounter for <u>adjustment or removal of breast implant</u>
Encounter for elective implant exchange (different material) (different size)
Encounter removal of tissue expander without synchronous insertion of permanent implant
Excludes 1:   *complications of breast implant (T85.4-)*
encounter for initial breast implant insertion for cosmetic breast augmentation (Z41.1)
encounter for breast reconstruction following mastectomy (Z42.1)

Z45.811 Encounter for adjustment or removal of <u>right</u> breast implant

Z45.812 Encounter for adjustment or removal of <u>left</u> breast implant

Z45.819 Encounter for adjustment or removal of <u>unspecified</u> breast implant

Z45.82 Encounter for adjustment or removal of myringotomy device (stent) (tube) — [Unacceptable PDX]

Z45.89 Encounter for adjustment and management of other implanted devices — [Unacceptable PDX]

Z45.9 Encounter for adjustment and management of unspecified implanted device — [Unacceptable PDX]

Z46- Encounter for <u>fitting and adjustment of other devices</u>
Includes: Removal or replacement of other device
Excludes 1:   *malfunction or other complications of device — see Alphabetical Index*
Excludes ❷: *encounter for fitting and management of implanted devices (Z45-)*
issue of repeat prescription only (Z76.0)
presence of prosthetic and other devices (Z95-Z97)

Z46.0 Encounter for fitting and adjustment of <u>spectacles and contact lenses</u> — [Unacceptable PDX]

Z46.1 Encounter for fitting and adjustment of <u>hearing aid</u> — [Unacceptable PDX]
Excludes 1:   *encounter for adjustment and management of implanted hearing device (Z45.32-)*

Z46.2 Encounter for fitting and adjustment of other devices related to nervous system and special senses
Excludes ❷: *encounter for adjustment and management of implanted nervous system device (Z45.4-)*
encounter for adjustment and management of implanted visual substitution device (Z45.31)

Z46.3 Encounter for fitting and adjustment of <u>dental prosthetic device</u>
Encounter for fitting and adjustment of dentures

Z46.4 Encounter for fitting and adjustment of <u>orthodontic</u> device — [Unacceptable PDX]

Z46.5- Encounter for fitting and adjustment of <u>other gastrointestinal appliance and device</u>
Excludes 1:   *encounter for attention to artificial openings of digestive tract (Z43.1-Z43.4)*

Z46.51 Encounter for fitting and adjustment of <u>gastric lap band</u> — [Unacceptable PDX]

Z46.59 Encounter for fitting and adjustment of <u>other</u> gastrointestinal appliance and device — [Unacceptable PDX]

Z46.6 Encounter for fitting and adjustment of <u>urinary device</u> — [Unacceptable PDX]
Excludes ❷: *attention to artificial openings of urinary tract (Z43.5, Z43.6)*

Z46.8- Encounter for fitting and adjustment of other specified devices

Z46.81 Encounter for fitting and adjustment of <u>insulin pump</u> — [Unacceptable PDX]
Encounter for insulin pump titration
Encounter for insulin pump instruction and training

Z46.82 Encounter for fitting and adjustment of <u>non-vascular catheter</u>

Z46.89 Encounter for fitting and adjustment of <u>other</u> specified devices — [Unacceptable PDX]
Encounter for fitting and adjustment of wheelchair

Z46.9 Encounter for fitting and adjustment of unspecified device — [Unacceptable PDX]

Z47- <u>Orthopedic aftercare</u>
Excludes 1:   *aftercare for healing fracture — code to fracture with 7th character D*

Z47.1 Aftercare following <u>joint replacement</u> surgery
Use additional code to identify the joint (Z96.6-)

Z47.2 Encounter for <u>removal of internal fixation device</u>
Excludes 1:   *encounter for adjustment of internal fixation device for fracture treatment — code to fracture with appropriate 7th character*
encounter for removal of external fixation device — code to fracture with 7th character D
infection or inflammatory reaction to internal fixation device (T84.6-)
mechanical complication of internal fixation device (T84.1-)

Z47.3- Aftercare following <u>explantation of joint prosthesis</u>
AHA 15:1Q:p16 – Insertion of new hip prosthesis after removal of previous
Aftercare following explantation of joint prosthesis, staged procedure
Encounter for joint prosthesis insertion following prior explantation of joint prosthesis

Z47.31 Aftercare following explantation of <u>shoulder</u> joint prosthesis
Excludes 1:   *acquired absence of shoulder joint following prior explantation of shoulder joint prosthesis (Z89.23-)*
shoulder joint prosthesis explantation status (Z89.23-)

Z47.32 Aftercare following explantation of <u>hip</u> joint prosthesis
Excludes 1:   *acquired absence of hip joint following prior explantation of hip joint prosthesis (Z89.62-)*
hip joint prosthesis explantation status (Z89.62-)

Z47.33 Aftercare following explantation of <u>knee</u> joint prosthesis
Excludes 1:   *acquired absence of knee joint following prior explantation of knee joint prosthesis (Z89.52-)*
knee joint prosthesis explantation status (Z89.52-)

Z47.8- Encounter for <u>other orthopedic aftercare</u>

Z47.81 Encounter for orthopedic aftercare <u>following surgical amputation</u>
Use additional code to identify the limb amputated (Z89.-)

Z47.82 Encounter for orthopedic aftercare <u>following scoliosis surgery</u>

Z47.89 Encounter for <u>other</u> orthopedic aftercare

Z48- Encounter for <u>other postprocedural aftercare</u>
Excludes 1:   *encounter for follow-up examination after completed treatment (Z08-Z09)*
Excludes ❷: *encounter for attention to artificial openings (Z43.-)*
encounter for fitting and adjustment of prosthetic and other devices (Z44-Z46)

Z48.0- Encounter for attention to dressings, sutures and drains
Excludes 1:   *encounter for planned postprocedural wound closure (Z48.1)*

Z48.00 Encounter for change or removal of nonsurgical wound dressing — [Unacceptable PDX]
Encounter for change or removal of wound dressing NOS

Z48.01 Encounter for change or removal of surgical wound dressing — [Unacceptable PDX]

Z48.02 Encounter for removal of sutures — [Unacceptable PDX]
    Encounter for removal of staples

Z48.03 Encounter for change or removal of drains

Z48.1 Encounter for planned postprocedural wound closure
    Excludes 1: encounter for attention to dressings and sutures (Z48.0-)

Z48.2- Encounter for <u>aftercare following organ transplant</u>

cc **Z48.21** Encounter for aftercare following <u>heart</u> transplant

cc **Z48.22** Encounter for aftercare following <u>kidney</u> transplant

cc **Z48.23** Encounter for aftercare following <u>liver</u> transplant

cc **Z48.24** Encounter for aftercare following <u>lung</u> transplant

Z48.28- Encounter for aftercare following <u>multiple</u> organ transplant

  cc **Z48.280** Encounter for aftercare following <u>heart-lung transplant</u>

  Z48.288 Encounter for aftercare following <u>multiple organ transplant</u>

Z48.29- Encounter for aftercare following <u>other</u> organ transplant

  cc **Z48.290** Encounter for aftercare following <u>bone marrow</u> transplant

  Z48.298 Encounter for aftercare following <u>other</u> organ transplant

Z48.3 Aftercare following <u>surgery for neoplasm</u>
    Use additional code to identify the neoplasm

Z48.8- Encounter for other specified postprocedural aftercare

Z48.81- Encounter for surgical aftercare following surgery on specified body systems
    Note: These codes identify the body system requiring aftercare. They are for use in conjunction with other aftercare codes to fully explain the aftercare encounter. The condition treated should also be coded if still present.
    Excludes 1: aftercare for injury — code the injury with 7th character D
        aftercare following surgery for neoplasm (Z48.3)
    Excludes ❷: aftercare following organ transplant (Z48.2-)
        orthopedic aftercare (Z47.-)

Z48.810 Encounter for surgical aftercare following surgery on the sense organs

Z48.811 Encounter for surgical aftercare following surgery on the nervous system
    Excludes ❷: encounter for surgical aftercare following surgery on the sense organs (Z48.810)

Z48.812 Encounter for surgical aftercare following surgery on the circulatory system

Z48.813 Encounter for surgical aftercare following surgery on the respiratory system

Z48.814 Encounter for surgical aftercare following surgery on the teeth or oral cavity

Z48.815 Encounter for surgical aftercare following surgery on the digestive system

Z48.816 Encounter for surgical aftercare following surgery on the genitourinary system
    Excludes 1: encounter for aftercare following sterilization reversal (Z31.42)

Z48.817 Encounter for surgical aftercare following surgery on the skin and subcutaneous tissue

Z48.89 Encounter for other specified surgical aftercare

Z49- Encounter for care involving renal dialysis
    Code also associated end stage renal disease (N18.6)

Z49.0- Preparatory care for renal dialysis
    Encounter for dialysis instruction and training

Z49.01 Encounter for fitting and adjustment of <u>extracorporeal dialysis catheter</u>
    Removal or replacement of renal dialysis catheter
    Toilet or cleansing of renal dialysis catheter

Z49.02 Encounter for fitting and adjustment of <u>peritoneal dialysis catheter</u> — [Unacceptable PDX]

Z49.3- Encounter for adequacy testing for <u>dialysis</u>

Z49.31 Encounter for adequacy testing for <u>hemodialysis</u> — [Unacceptable PDX]

Z49.32 Encounter for adequacy testing for <u>peritoneal dialysis</u> — [Unacceptable PDX]
    Encounter for peritoneal equilibration test

Z51- Encounter for other aftercare and medical care
    Code also condition requiring care
    Excludes 1: follow-up examination after treatment (Z08-Z09)

Z51.0 Encounter for <u>antineoplastic radiation therapy</u>

Z51.1- Encounter for antineoplastic chemotherapy and immunotherapy
    Excludes ❷: encounter for chemotherapy and immunotherapy for nonneoplastic condition — code to condition

Z51.11 Encounter for <u>antineoplastic chemotherapy</u>
    AHA 15:3Q:p19 – Admitted for chemotherapy

Z51.12 Encounter for <u>antineoplastic immunotherapy</u>

Z51.5 Encounter for palliative care — [Unacceptable PDX]

Z51.6 Encounter for desensitization to allergens — [Unacceptable PDX]

Z51.8- Encounter for other specified aftercare
    Excludes 1: holiday relief care (Z75.5)

Z51.81 Encounter for therapeutic drug level monitoring
    Code also any long-term (current) drug therapy (Z79.-)
    Excludes 1: encounter for blood-drug test for administrative or medicolegal reasons (Z02.83)

Z51.89 Encounter for other specified aftercare — [Unacceptable PDX, Requires Secondary DX]

Z52- <u>Donors of organs and tissues</u>
    AHA 12:4Q:p99 – Domino liver transplant
    Includes: Autologous and other living donors
    Excludes 1: cadaveric donor — omit code
        examination of potential donor (Z00.5)

Z52.0- <u>Blood donor</u>

Z52.00- <u>Unspecified</u> blood donor

Z52.000 Unspecified donor, whole blood — [Unacceptable PDX]

Z52.001 Unspecified donor, stem cells — [Unacceptable PDX]

Z52.008 Unspecified donor, other blood — [Unacceptable PDX]

Z52.01- <u>Autologous</u> blood donor

Z52.010 Autologous donor, whole blood — [Unacceptable PDX]

Z52.011 Autologous donor, stem cells — [Unacceptable PDX]

Z52.018 Autologous donor, other blood — [Unacceptable PDX]

Z52.09- <u>Other blood</u> donor
    Volunteer donor

Z52.090 Other blood donor, whole blood — [Unacceptable PDX]

Z52.091 Other blood donor, stem cells — [Unacceptable PDX]

Z52.098 Other blood donor, other blood — [Unacceptable PDX]

Z52.1- <u>Skin</u> donor

Z52.10 Skin donor, unspecified

Z52.11 Skin donor, autologous

Z52.19 Skin donor, other

Z52.2- <u>Bone</u> donor

Z52.20 Bone donor, unspecified

Z52.21 Bone donor, autologous

Z52.29 Bone donor, other

Z52.3 Bone marrow donor

Z52.4 Kidney donor

Z52.5 Cornea donor

Z52.6 Liver donor

Z52.8- Donor of other specified organs or tissues

Z52.81- <u>Egg (Oocyte) donor</u>

Z52.810 Egg (Oocyte) donor <u>under age 35</u>, <u>anonymous recipient</u> — [♀] [Unacceptable PDX]
    Egg donor under age 35 NOS

Z52.811 Egg (Oocyte) donor <u>under age 35</u>, <u>designated recipient</u> — [♀] [Unacceptable PDX]

Z52.812 Egg (Oocyte) donor <u>age 35 and over</u>, <u>anonymous recipient</u> — [♀] [Unacceptable PDX]
    Egg donor age 35 and over NOS

Z52.813 Egg (Oocyte) donor <u>age 35 and over</u>, <u>designated recipient</u> — [♀] [Unacceptable PDX]

Z52.819 Egg (Oocyte) donor, <u>unspecified</u> — [♀] [Unacceptable PDX]

Z52.89 Donor of other specified organs or tissues

Z52.9 Donor of unspecified organ or tissue
Donor NOS

Z53- Persons encountering health services for <u>specific procedures and treatment</u>, <u>not carried out</u>

Z53.0- Procedure and treatment not carried out because of <u>contraindication</u>

Z53.01 Procedure and treatment not carried out <u>due to patient smoking</u> — [Unacceptable PDX]

Z53.09 Procedure and treatment not carried out <u>because of other contraindication</u> — [Unacceptable PDX]

Z53.1 Procedure and treatment not carried out <u>because of patient's decision for reasons of belief and group pressure</u> — [Unacceptable PDX]

Z53.2- Procedure and treatment not carried out <u>because of patient's decision for other and unspecified reasons</u>

Z53.20 Procedure and treatment not carried out because of patient's decision for unspecified reasons — [Unacceptable PDX]

Z53.21 Procedure and treatment not carried out due to patient leaving prior to being seen by healthcare provider — [Unacceptable PDX]

Z53.29 Procedure and treatment not carried out because of patient's decision for other reasons — [Unacceptable PDX]

Z53.3- <u>Procedure converted to open procedure</u>

Z53.31 <u>Laparoscopic</u> surgical procedure converted to open procedure — [Unacceptable PDX]

Z53.32 <u>Thoracoscopic</u> surgical procedure converted to open procedure — [Unacceptable PDX]

Z53.33 <u>Arthroscopic</u> surgical procedure converted to open procedure — [Unacceptable PDX]

Z53.39 <u>Other specified</u> procedure converted to open procedure — [Unacceptable PDX]

Z53.8 Procedure and treatment <u>not carried out for other reasons</u> — [Unacceptable PDX]

Z53.9 Procedure and treatment <u>not carried out</u>, <u>unspecified</u> reason — [Unacceptable PDX]

Persons with potential health hazards related to socioeconomic and psychosocial circumstances (Z55-Z65)

Z55- Problems related to education and literacy
Excludes 1: *disorders of psychological development (F80-F89)*

Z55.0 Illiteracy and low-level literacy — [Unacceptable PDX]

Z55.1 Schooling unavailable and unattainable — [Unacceptable PDX]

Z55.2 Failed school examinations — [Unacceptable PDX]

Z55.3 Underachievement in school — [Unacceptable PDX]

Z55.4 Educational maladjustment and discord with teachers and classmates — [Unacceptable PDX]

Z55.8 Other problems related to education and literacy — [Unacceptable PDX]
Problems related to inadequate teaching

Z55.9 Problems related to education and literacy, unspecified — [Unacceptable PDX]
Academic problems NOS

Z56- Problems related to employment and unemployment
Excludes ❷: *occupational exposure to risk factors (Z57.-)*
problems related to housing and economic circumstances (Z59.-)

Z56.0 Unemployment, unspecified — [Unacceptable PDX]

Z56.1 Change of job — [Age/15-124] [Unacceptable PDX]

Z56.2 Threat of job loss — [Unacceptable PDX]

Z56.3 Stressful work schedule — [Unacceptable PDX]

Z56.4 Discord with boss and workmates — [Unacceptable PDX]

Z56.5 Uncongenial work environment — [Unacceptable PDX]
Difficult conditions at work

Z56.6 Other physical and mental strain related to work — [Unacceptable PDX]

Z56.8- Other problems related to employment

Z56.81 Sexual harassment on the job — [Unacceptable PDX]

Z56.82 Military deployment status — [Unacceptable PDX]
Individual (civilian or military) currently deployed in theater or in support of military war, peacekeeping and humanitarian operations

Z56.89 Other problems related to employment — [Unacceptable PDX]

Z56.9 Unspecified problems related to employment — [Unacceptable PDX]
Occupational problems NOS

Z57- Occupational exposure to risk factors

Z57.0 Occupational exposure to noise — [Unacceptable PDX]

Z57.1 Occupational exposure to radiation — [Unacceptable PDX]

Z57.2 Occupational exposure to dust — [Unacceptable PDX]

Z57.3- Occupational exposure to other air contaminants

Z57.31 Occupational exposure to environmental tobacco smoke — [Unacceptable PDX]
Excludes ❷: *exposure to environmental tobacco smoke (Z77.22)*

Z57.39 Occupational exposure to other air contaminants — [Unacceptable PDX]

Z57.4 Occupational exposure to toxic agents in agriculture — [Unacceptable PDX]
Occupational exposure to solids, liquids, gases or vapors in agriculture

Z57.5 Occupational exposure to toxic agents in other industries — [Unacceptable PDX]
Occupational exposure to solids, liquids, gases or vapors in other industries

Z57.6 Occupational exposure to extreme temperature — [Unacceptable PDX]

Z57.7 Occupational exposure to vibration — [Unacceptable PDX]

Z57.8 Occupational exposure to other risk factors — [Unacceptable PDX]

Z57.9 Occupational exposure to unspecified risk factor — [Unacceptable PDX]

Z59- Problems related to housing and economic circumstances
Excludes ❷: *problems related to upbringing (Z62.-)*

Z59.0 Homelessness — [Unacceptable PDX]

Z59.1 Inadequate housing — [Unacceptable PDX]
Lack of heating
Restriction of space
Technical defects in home preventing adequate care
Unsatisfactory surroundings
Excludes 1: *problems related to the natural and physical environment (Z77.1-)*

Z59.2 Discord with neighbors, lodgers and landlord — [Unacceptable PDX]

Z59.3 Problems related to living in residential institution — [Unacceptable PDX]
Boarding-school resident
Excludes 1: *institutional upbringing (Z62.2)*

Z59.4 Lack of adequate food and safe drinking water — [Unacceptable PDX]
Inadequate drinking water supply
Excludes 1: *effects of hunger (T73.0)*
inappropriate diet or eating habits (Z72.4)
malnutrition (E40-E46)

Z59.5 Extreme poverty — [Unacceptable PDX]

Z59.6 Low income — [Unacceptable PDX]

Z59.7 Insufficient social insurance and welfare support — [Unacceptable PDX]

Z59.8 Other problems related to housing and economic circumstances — [Unacceptable PDX]
Foreclosure on loan
Isolated dwelling
Problems with creditors

Z59.9 Problem related to housing and economic circumstances, unspecified — [Unacceptable PDX]

Z52-Z59

Z60- **Problems related to social environment**

Z60.0 **Problems of adjustment to life-cycle transitions** — [Unacceptable PDX]
    Empty nest syndrome
    Phase of life problem
    Problem with adjustment to retirement [pension]

Z60.2 **Problems related to living alone** — [Unacceptable PDX]

Z60.3 **Acculturation difficulty** — [Unacceptable PDX]
    Problem with migration
    Problem with social transplantation

Z60.4 **Social exclusion and rejection** — [Unacceptable PDX]
    Exclusion and rejection on the basis of personal characteristics, such as unusual physical appearance, illness or behavior.
    Excludes 1: *target of adverse discrimination such as for racial or religious reasons (Z60.5)*

Z60.5 **Target of (perceived) adverse discrimination and persecution** — [Unacceptable PDX]
    Excludes 1: *social exclusion and rejection (Z60.4)*

Z60.8 **Other problems related to social environment** — [Unacceptable PDX]

Z60.9 **Problem related to social environment, unspecified** — [Unacceptable PDX]

Z62- **Problems related to upbringing**
    Includes: Current and past negative life events in childhood
        Current and past problems of a child related to upbringing
    Excludes ❷: *maltreatment syndrome (T74.-)*
        problems related to housing and economic circumstances (Z59.-)

Z62.0 **Inadequate parental supervision and control** — [Unacceptable PDX]

Z62.1 **Parental overprotection** — [Unacceptable PDX]

Z62.2- **Upbringing away from parents**
    Excludes 1: *problems with boarding school (Z59.3)*

Z62.21 **Child in welfare custody** — [Age/0-17] [Unacceptable PDX]
    Child in care of non-parental family member
    Child in foster care
    Excludes ❷: *problem for parent due to child in welfare custody (Z63.5)*

Z62.22 **Institutional upbringing** — [Unacceptable PDX]
    Child living in orphanage or group home

Z62.29 **Other upbringing away from parents** — [Unacceptable PDX]

Z62.3 **Hostility towards and scapegoating of child** — [Age/0-17] [Unacceptable PDX]

Z62.6 **Inappropriate (excessive) parental pressure** — [Unacceptable PDX]

Z62.8- **Other specified problems related to upbringing**

Z62.81- **Personal history of abuse in childhood**

Z62.810 **Personal history of physical and sexual abuse in childhood** — [Unacceptable PDX]
    Excludes 1: *current child physical abuse (T74.12-, T76.12-)*
        current child sexual abuse (T74.22-, T76.22-)

Z62.811 **Personal history of psychological abuse in childhood** — [Unacceptable PDX]
    Excludes 1: *current child psychological abuse (T74.32-, T76.32-)*

Z62.812 **Personal history of neglect in childhood** — [Unacceptable PDX]
    Excludes 1: *current child neglect (T74.02, T76.02-)*

Z62.819 **Personal history of unspecified abuse in childhood** — [Unacceptable PDX]
    Excludes 1: *current child abuse NOS (T74.92, T76.92-)*

Z62.82- **Parent-child conflict**

Z62.820 **Parent-biological child conflict** — [Unacceptable PDX]
    Parent-child problem NOS

Z62.821 **Parent-adopted child conflict** — [Unacceptable PDX]

Z62.822 **Parent-foster child conflict** — [Unacceptable PDX]

Z62.89- **Other specified problems related to upbringing**

Z62.890 **Parent-child estrangement NEC** — [Unacceptable PDX]

Z62.891 **Sibling rivalry** — [Unacceptable PDX]

Z62.898 **Other specified problems related to upbringing** — [Unacceptable PDX]

Z62.9 **Problem related to upbringing, unspecified** — [Unacceptable PDX]

Z63- **Other problems related to primary support group, including family circumstances**
    Excludes ❷: *maltreatment syndrome (T74.-, T76)*
        parent-child problems (Z62.-)
        problems related to negative life events in childhood (Z62.-)
        problems related to upbringing (Z62.-)

Z63.0 **Problems in relationship with spouse or partner** — [Unacceptable PDX]
    Excludes 1: *counseling for spousal or partner abuse problems (Z69.1)*
        counseling related to sexual attitude, behavior, and orientation (Z70.-)

Z63.1 **Problems in relationship with in-laws** — [Unacceptable PDX]

Z63.3- **Absence of family member**
    Excludes 1: *absence of family member due to disappearance and death (Z63.4)*
        absence of family member due to separation and divorce (Z63.5)

Z63.31 **Absence of family member due to military deployment** — [Unacceptable PDX]
    Individual or family affected by other family member being on military deployment
    Excludes 1: *family disruption due to return of family member from military deployment (Z63.71)*

Z63.32 **Other absence of family member** — [Unacceptable PDX]

Z63.4 **Disappearance and death of family member** — [Unacceptable PDX]
    AHA 14:1Q:p25 – Bereavement
    Assumed death of family member
    Bereavement

Z63.5 **Disruption of family by separation and divorce** — [Unacceptable PDX]
    Marital estrangement

Z63.6 **Dependent relative needing care at home** — [Unacceptable PDX]

Z63.7- **Other stressful life events affecting family and household**

Z63.71 **Stress on family due to return of family member from military deployment** — [Unacceptable PDX]
    Individual or family affected by family member having returned from military deployment (current or past conflict)

Z63.72 **Alcoholism and drug addiction in family** — [Unacceptable PDX]

Z63.79 **Other stressful life events affecting family and household** — [Unacceptable PDX]
    Anxiety (normal) about sick person in family
    Health problems within family
    Ill or disturbed family member
    Isolated family

Z63.8 **Other specified problems related to primary support group** — [Unacceptable PDX]
    Family discord NOS
    Family estrangement NOS
    High expressed emotional level within family
    Inadequate family support NOS
    Inadequate or distorted communication within family

Z63.9 **Problem related to primary support group, unspecified** — [Unacceptable PDX]
    Relationship disorder NOS

Z64- **Problems related to certain psychosocial circumstances**

Z64.0 **Problems related to unwanted pregnancy** — [♀] [Unacceptable PDX]

Z64.1 **Problems related to multiparity** — [♀] [Unacceptable PDX]

Z64.4 **Discord with counselors** — [Unacceptable PDX]
    Discord with probation officer
    Discord with social worker

Z65- **Problems related to other psychosocial circumstances**

Z65.0 **Conviction in civil and criminal proceedings without imprisonment** — [Unacceptable PDX]

Z65.1 **Imprisonment and other incarceration** — [Unacceptable PDX]

Z65.2 **Problems related to release from prison** — [Unacceptable PDX]

Z65.3 **Problems related to other legal circumstances** — [Unacceptable PDX]
    Arrest
    Child custody or support proceedings
    Litigation
    Prosecution

Z60
I
Z65

Z65.4   Victim of crime and terrorism — [Unacceptable PDX]
   Victim of torture

Z65.5   Exposure to disaster, war and other hostilities —
   [Unacceptable PDX]
   Excludes 1:   target of perceived discrimination or persecution
   (Z60.5)

**Z65.8   Other specified problems related to psychosocial
   circumstances** — [Unacceptable PDX]

Z65.9   Problem related to unspecified psychosocial circumstances —
   [Unacceptable PDX]

Do not resuscitate status (Z66)

Z66   Do not resuscitate — [Unacceptable PDX]
   DNR status

Blood type (Z67)

Z67-   Blood type

Z67.1-   Type A blood
   Z67.10   Type A blood, Rh positive — [Unacceptable PDX]
   Z67.11   Type A blood, Rh negative — [Unacceptable PDX]

Z67.2-   Type B blood
   Z67.20   Type B blood, Rh positive — [Unacceptable PDX]
   Z67.21   Type B blood, Rh negative — [Unacceptable PDX]

Z67.3-   Type AB blood
   Z67.30   Type AB blood, Rh positive — [Unacceptable PDX]
   Z67.31   Type AB blood, Rh negative — [Unacceptable PDX]

Z67.4-   Type O blood
   Z67.40   Type O blood, Rh positive — [Unacceptable PDX]
   Z67.41   Type O blood, Rh negative — [Unacceptable PDX]

Z67.9-   Unspecified blood type
   Z67.90   Unspecified blood type, Rh positive — [Unacceptable PDX]
   Z67.91   Unspecified blood type, Rh negative — [Unacceptable PDX]

Body mass index [BMI] (Z68)

Z68-   Body mass index [BMI]
   Kilograms per meters squared
   Note: BMI adult codes are for use for persons 21 years of age or older.
   Note: BMI pediatric codes are for use for persons 2-20 years of age. These
     percentiles are based on the growth charts published by the Centers
     for Disease Control and Prevention (CDC).

cc **Z68.1   Body mass index (BMI) 19 or less, adult** — [Age/15-124]
   [Unacceptable PDX]

Z68.2-   Body mass index (BMI) 20-29, adult
   Z68.20   Body mass index (BMI) 20.0-20.9, adult — [Age/15-124]
     [Unacceptable PDX]
   Z68.21   Body mass index (BMI) 21.0-21.9, adult — [Age/15-124]
     [Unacceptable PDX]
   Z68.22   Body mass index (BMI) 22.0-22.9, adult — [Age/15-124]
     [Unacceptable PDX]
   Z68.23   Body mass index (BMI) 23.0-23.9, adult — [Age/15-124]
     [Unacceptable PDX]
   Z68.24   Body mass index (BMI) 24.0-24.9, adult — [Age/15-124]
     [Unacceptable PDX]
   Z68.25   Body mass index (BMI) 25.0-25.9, adult — [Age/15-124]
     [Unacceptable PDX]
   Z68.26   Body mass index (BMI) 26.0-26.9, adult — [Age/15-124]
     [Unacceptable PDX]
   Z68.27   Body mass index (BMI) 27.0-27.9, adult — [Age/15-124]
     [Unacceptable PDX]
   Z68.28   Body mass index (BMI) 28.0-28.9, adult — [Age/15-124]
     [Unacceptable PDX]
   Z68.29   Body mass index (BMI) 29.0-29.9, adult — [Age/15-124]
     [Unacceptable PDX]

Z68.3-   Body mass index (BMI) 30-39, adult
   Z68.30   Body mass index (BMI) 30.0-30.9, adult — [Age/15-124]
     [Unacceptable PDX]
   Z68.31   Body mass index (BMI) 31.0-31.9, adult — [Age/15-124]
     [Unacceptable PDX]
   Z68.32   Body mass index (BMI) 32.0-32.9, adult — [Age/15-124]
     [Unacceptable PDX]
   Z68.33   Body mass index (BMI) 33.0-33.9, adult — [Age/15-124]
     [Unacceptable PDX]
   Z68.34   Body mass index (BMI) 34.0-34.9, adult — [Age/15-124]
     [Unacceptable PDX]
   Z68.35   Body mass index (BMI) 35.0-35.9, adult — [Age/15-124]
     [Unacceptable PDX]
   Z68.36   Body mass index (BMI) 36.0-36.9, adult — [Age/15-124]
     [Unacceptable PDX]
   Z68.37   Body mass index (BMI) 37.0-37.9, adult — [Age/15-124]
     [Unacceptable PDX]
   Z68.38   Body mass index (BMI) 38.0-38.9, adult — [Age/15-124]
     [Unacceptable PDX]
   Z68.39   Body mass index (BMI) 39.0-39.9, adult — [Age/15-124]
     [Unacceptable PDX]

Z68.4-   Body mass index (BMI) 40 or greater, adult
cc **Z68.41   Body mass index (BMI) 40.0-44.9, adult** — [Age/15-124]
     [Unacceptable PDX]
cc **Z68.42   Body mass index (BMI) 45.0-49.9, adult** — [Age/15-124]
     [Unacceptable PDX]
cc **Z68.43   Body mass index (BMI) 50.0-59.9, adult** — [Age/15-124]
     [Unacceptable PDX]
cc **Z68.44   Body mass index (BMI) 60.0-69.9, adult** — [Age/15-124]
     [Unacceptable PDX]
cc **Z68.45   Body mass index (BMI) 70 or greater, adult** — [Age/15-124]
     [Unacceptable PDX]

Z68.5-   Body mass index (BMI) pediatric
   **Z68.51   Body mass index (BMI) pediatric, less than 5th percentile
     for age** — [Unacceptable PDX]
   **Z68.52   Body mass index (BMI) pediatric, 5th percentile to less
     than 85th percentile for age** — [Unacceptable PDX]
   **Z68.53   Body mass index (BMI) pediatric, 85th percentile to less
     than 95th percentile for age** — [Unacceptable PDX]
   **Z68.54   Body mass index (BMI) pediatric, greater than or equal to
     95th percentile for age** — [Unacceptable PDX]

Persons encountering health services in other circumstances (Z69-Z76)

**Z69-   Encounter for mental health services for victim and perpetrator of
   abuse**
   Includes: Counseling for victims and perpetrators of abuse

Z69.0-   Encounter for mental health services for child abuse problems
   **Z69.01-   Encounter for mental health services for parental child
     abuse**
     **Z69.010   Encounter for mental health services for victim of
       parental child abuse** — [Age/0-17]
     **Z69.011   Encounter for mental health services for
       perpetrator of parental child abuse** —
       [Unacceptable PDX]
       Excludes 1:   encounter for mental health services for
         non-parental child abuse (Z69.02-)

   **Z69.02-   Encounter for mental health services for non-parental
     child abuse**
     **Z69.020   Encounter for mental health services for victim of
       non-parental child abuse** — [Age/0-17]
     **Z69.021   Encounter for mental health services for
       perpetrator of non-parental child abuse** —
       [Unacceptable PDX]

**Z69.1-   Encounter for mental health services for spousal or partner
   abuse problems**
   **Z69.11   Encounter for mental health services for victim of spousal
     or partner abuse** — [Unacceptable PDX]

Z65-Z69

Z69.12 Encounter for mental health services for <u>perpetrator</u> of spousal or partner abuse — [Unacceptable PDX]

Z69.8- Encounter for mental health services for victim or perpetrator of <u>other</u> abuse

Z69.81 Encounter for mental health services for <u>victim</u> of other abuse — [Unacceptable PDX]
Encounter for rape victim counseling

Z69.82 Encounter for mental health services for <u>perpetrator</u> of other abuse — [Unacceptable PDX]

Z70- Counseling related to sexual attitude, behavior and orientation
Includes: Encounter for mental health services for sexual attitude, behavior and orientation
Excludes ❷: contraceptive or procreative counseling (Z30-Z31)

Z70.0 Counseling related to sexual attitude — [Unacceptable PDX]

Z70.1 Counseling related to patient's sexual behavior and orientation — [Unacceptable PDX]
Patient concerned regarding impotence
Patient concerned regarding non-responsiveness
Patient concerned regarding promiscuity
Patient concerned regarding sexual orientation

Z70.2 Counseling related to sexual behavior and orientation of third party — [Unacceptable PDX]
Advice sought regarding sexual behavior and orientation of child
Advice sought regarding sexual behavior and orientation of partner
Advice sought regarding sexual behavior and orientation of spouse

Z70.3 Counseling related to combined concerns regarding sexual attitude, behavior and orientation — [Unacceptable PDX]

Z70.8 Other sex counseling — [Unacceptable PDX]
Encounter for sex education

Z70.9 Sex counseling, unspecified — [Unacceptable PDX]

Z71- Persons encountering health services for other counseling and medical advice, not elsewhere classified
Excludes ❷: contraceptive or procreation counseling (Z30-Z31)
*   sex counseling (Z70.-)*

Z71.0 Person encountering health services to consult on behalf of another person — [Unacceptable PDX]
Person encountering health services to seek advice or treatment for non-attending third party
Excludes ❷: anxiety (normal) about sick person in family (Z63.7)
*   expectant (adoptive) parent(s) pre-birth pediatrician visit (Z76.81)*

Z71.1 Person with feared health complaint in whom no diagnosis is made — [Unacceptable PDX]
Person encountering health services with feared condition which was not demonstrated
Person encountering health services in which problem was normal state
"Worried well"
Excludes 1:   medical observation for suspected diseases and conditions proven not to exist (Z03.-)

Z71.2 Person consulting for explanation of examination or test findings — [Unacceptable PDX]

Z71.3 Dietary counseling and surveillance — [Unacceptable PDX]
Use additional code for any associated underlying medical condition
Use additional code to identify body mass index (BMI), if known (Z68.-)

Z71.4- <u>Alcohol abuse counseling and surveillance</u>
Use additional code for alcohol abuse or dependence (F10.-)

Z71.41 Alcohol abuse counseling and surveillance of <u>alcoholic</u> — [Unacceptable PDX]

Z71.42 Counseling for <u>family member of alcoholic</u> — [Unacceptable PDX]
Counseling for significant other, partner, or friend of alcoholic

Z71.5- Drug abuse counseling and surveillance
Use additional code for drug abuse or dependence (F11-F16, F18-F19)

Z71.51 Drug abuse counseling and surveillance of drug abuser — [Unacceptable PDX]

Z71.52 Counseling for <u>family member of drug abuser</u> — [Unacceptable PDX]
Counseling for significant other, partner, or friend of drug abuser

Z71.6 Tobacco abuse counseling — [Unacceptable PDX]
Use additional code for nicotine dependence (F17.-)

Z71.7 Human immunodeficiency virus [HIV] counseling — [Unacceptable PDX]

Z71.8- Other specified counseling
Excludes ❷: counseling for contraception (Z30.0-)
*   counseling for genetics (Z31.5)*
*   counseling for procreative management (Z31.6-)*

Z71.81 Spiritual or religious counseling — [Unacceptable PDX]

Z71.89 Other specified counseling — [Unacceptable PDX]

Z71.9 Counseling, unspecified — [Unacceptable PDX]
Encounter for medical advice NOS

Z72- Problems related to lifestyle
Excludes ❷: problems related to life-management difficulty (Z73.-)
*   problems related to socioeconomic and psychosocial circumstances (Z55-Z65)*

Z72.0 Tobacco use — [Unacceptable PDX]
Tobacco use NOS
Excludes 1:   history of tobacco dependence (Z87.891)
*   nicotine dependence (F17.2-)*
*   tobacco dependence (F17.2-)*
*   tobacco use during pregnancy (O99.33-)*

Z72.3 Lack of physical exercise — [Unacceptable PDX]

Z72.4 Inappropriate diet and eating habits — [Unacceptable PDX]
Excludes 1:   behavioral eating disorders of infancy or childhood (F98.2.-F98.3)
*   eating disorders (F50.-)*
*   lack of adequate food (Z59.4)*
*   malnutrition and other nutritional deficiencies (E40-E64)*

Z72.5- High risk sexual behavior
Promiscuity
Excludes 1:   paraphilias (F65)

Z72.51 High risk heterosexual behavior — [Unacceptable PDX]

Z72.52 High risk homosexual behavior — [Unacceptable PDX]

Z72.53 High risk bisexual behavior — [Unacceptable PDX]

Z72.6 Gambling and betting — [Unacceptable PDX]
Excludes 1:   compulsive or pathological gambling (F63.0)

Z72.8- Other problems related to lifestyle

Z72.81- Antisocial behavior
Excludes 1:   conduct disorders (F91.-)

Z72.810 Child and adolescent antisocial behavior — [Age/0-17]
Antisocial behavior (child) (adolescent) without manifest psychiatric disorder
Delinquency NOS
Group delinquency
Offenses in the context of gang membership
Stealing in company with others
Truancy from school

Z72.811 Adult antisocial behavior — [Age/15-124]
Adult antisocial behavior without manifest psychiatric disorder

Z72.82- Problems related to sleep

Z72.820 Sleep deprivation
Lack of adequate sleep
Excludes 1:   insomnia (G47.0-)

Z72.821 Inadequate sleep hygiene — [Unacceptable PDX]
Bad sleep habits
Irregular sleep habits
Unhealthy sleep wake schedule
Excludes 1:   insomnia (F51.0-, G47.0-)

Z72.89 Other problems related to lifestyle — [Unacceptable PDX]
Self-damaging behavior

Z72.9 Problem related to lifestyle, unspecified — [Unacceptable PDX]

Z73- Problems related to life management difficulty
Excludes ❷: problems related to socioeconomic and psychosocial circumstances (Z55-Z65)

Z73.0 Burn-out — [Unacceptable PDX]

Z73.1 Type A behavior pattern — [Unacceptable PDX]

Z73.2 Lack of relaxation and leisure — [Unacceptable PDX]

Z73.3 Stress, not elsewhere classified — [Unacceptable PDX]
Physical and mental strain NOS
Excludes 1:   stress related to employment or unemployment (Z56.-)

Z69 - Z73

Z73.4 Inadequate social skills, not elsewhere classified — [Unacceptable PDX]

Z73.5 Social role conflict, not elsewhere classified — [Unacceptable PDX]

Z73.6 Limitation of activities due to disability — [Unacceptable PDX]
  Excludes 1: care-provider dependency (Z74.-)

Z73.8- Other problems related to life management difficulty
  Z73.81- Behavioral insomnia of childhood
    Z73.810 Behavioral insomnia of childhood, sleep-onset association type — [Age/0-17] [Unacceptable PDX]
    Z73.811 Behavioral insomnia of childhood, limit setting type — [Age/0-17] [Unacceptable PDX]
    Z73.812 Behavioral insomnia of childhood, combined type — [Age/0-17] [Unacceptable PDX]
    Z73.819 Behavioral insomnia of childhood, unspecified type — [Age/0-17] [Unacceptable PDX]
  Z73.82 Dual sensory impairment — [Unacceptable PDX]
  Z73.89 Other problems related to life management difficulty — [Unacceptable PDX]

Z73.9 Problem related to life management difficulty, unspecified — [Unacceptable PDX]

Z74- Problems related to care provider dependency
  Excludes 2: dependence on enabling machines or devices NEC (Z99.-)

Z74.0- Reduced mobility
  Z74.01 Bed confinement status — [Unacceptable PDX]
    Bedridden
  Z74.09 Other reduced mobility — [Unacceptable PDX]
    Chairridden
    Reduced mobility NOS
    Excludes 2: wheelchair dependence (Z99.3)

Z74.1 Need for assistance with personal care — [Unacceptable PDX]

Z74.2 Need for assistance at home and no other household member able to render care — [Unacceptable PDX]

Z74.3 Need for continuous supervision — [Unacceptable PDX]

Z74.8 Other problems related to care provider dependency — [Unacceptable PDX]

Z74.9 Problem related to care provider dependency, unspecified — [Unacceptable PDX]

Z75- Problems related to medical facilities and other health care
  Z75.0 Medical services not available in home — [Unacceptable PDX]
    Excludes 1: no other household member able to render care (Z74.2)
  Z75.1 Person awaiting admission to adequate facility elsewhere — [Unacceptable PDX]
  Z75.2 Other waiting period for investigation and treatment — [Unacceptable PDX]
  Z75.3 Unavailability and inaccessibility of health-care facilities — [Unacceptable PDX]
    Excludes 1: bed unavailable (Z75.1)
  Z75.4 Unavailability and inaccessibility of other helping agencies — [Unacceptable PDX]
  Z75.5 Holiday relief care — [Unacceptable PDX]
  Z75.8 Other problems related to medical facilities and other health care — [Unacceptable PDX]
  Z75.9 Unspecified problem related to medical facilities and other health care — [Unacceptable PDX]

Z76- Persons encountering health services in other circumstances
  AHA 14:2Q:p10 – Encounter for Neulasta to prevent infection
  Z76.0 Encounter for issue of repeat prescription — [Unacceptable PDX]
    Encounter for issue of repeat prescription for appliance
    Encounter for issue of repeat prescription for medicaments
    Encounter for issue of repeat prescription for spectacles
    Excludes 2: issue of medical certificate (Z02.7)
      repeat prescription for contraceptive (Z30.4-)
  Z76.1 Encounter for health supervision and care of foundling

Z76.2 Encounter for health supervision and care of other healthy infant and child — [Age/0-17] [Unacceptable PDX]
  Encounter for medical or nursing care or supervision of healthy infant under circumstances such as adverse socioeconomic conditions at home
  Encounter for medical or nursing care or supervision of healthy infant under circumstances such as awaiting foster or adoptive placement
  Encounter for medical or nursing care or supervision of healthy infant under circumstances such as maternal illness
  Encounter for medical or nursing care or supervision of healthy infant under circumstances such as number of children at home preventing or interfering with normal care

Z76.3 Healthy person accompanying sick person

Z76.4 Other boarder to healthcare facility
  Excludes 1: homelessness (Z59.0)

Z76.5 Malingerer [conscious simulation]
  Person feigning illness (with obvious motivation)
  Excludes 1: factitious disorder (F68.1-)
    peregrinating patient (F68.1-)

Z76.8- Persons encountering health services in other specified circumstances
  Z76.81 Expectant parent(s) prebirth pediatrician visit — [Unacceptable PDX]
    Pre-adoption pediatrician visit for adoptive parent(s)
  Z76.82 Awaiting organ transplant status — [Unacceptable PDX]
    Patient waiting for organ availability
  Z76.89 Persons encountering health services in other specified circumstances — [Unacceptable PDX]
    Persons encountering health services NOS

Persons with potential health hazards related to family and personal history and certain conditions influencing health status (Z77-Z99)

Code also any follow-up examination (Z08-Z09)

Z77- Other contact with and (suspected) exposures hazardous to health
  Includes: Contact with and (suspected) exposures to potential hazards to health
  Excludes 2: contact with and (suspected) exposure to communicable diseases (Z20.-)
    exposure to (parental) (environmental) tobacco smoke in the perinatal period (P96.81)
    newborn affected by noxious substances transmitted via placenta or breast milk (P04.-)
    occupational exposure to risk factors (Z57.-)
    retained foreign body (Z18.-)
    retained foreign body fully removed (Z87.821)
    toxic effects of substances chiefly nonmedicinal as to source (T51-T65)

Z77.0- Contact with and (suspected) exposure to hazardous, chiefly nonmedicinal, chemicals
  Z77.01- Contact with and (suspected) exposure to hazardous metals
    Z77.010 Contact with and (suspected) exposure to arsenic — [Unacceptable PDX]
    Z77.011 Contact with and (suspected) exposure to lead — [Unacceptable PDX]
    Z77.012 Contact with and (suspected) exposure to uranium — [Unacceptable PDX]
      Excludes 1: retained depleted uranium fragments (Z18.01)
    Z77.018 Contact with and (suspected) exposure to other hazardous metals — [Unacceptable PDX]
      Contact with and (suspected) exposure to chromium compounds
      Contact with and (suspected) exposure to nickel dust
  Z77.02- Contact with and (suspected) exposure to hazardous aromatic compounds
    Z77.020 Contact with and (suspected) exposure to aromatic amines — [Unacceptable PDX]
    Z77.021 Contact with and (suspected) exposure to benzene — [Unacceptable PDX]

Z73-Z77

Z77.028 **Contact with and (suspected) exposure to other hazardous aromatic compounds** — [Unacceptable PDX]
Aromatic dyes NOS
Polycyclic aromatic hydrocarbons

Z77.09- **Contact with and (suspected) exposure to other hazardous, chiefly nonmedicinal, chemicals**

Z77.090 **Contact with and (suspected) exposure to asbestos** — [Unacceptable PDX]

Z77.098 **Contact with and (suspected) exposure to other hazardous, chiefly nonmedicinal, chemicals** — [Unacceptable PDX]
Dyes NOS

Z77.1- **Contact with and (suspected) exposure to environmental pollution and hazards in the physical environment**

Z77.11- **Contact with and (suspected) exposure to environmental pollution**

Z77.110 **Contact with and (suspected) exposure to air pollution** — [Unacceptable PDX]

Z77.111 **Contact with and (suspected) exposure to water pollution** — [Unacceptable PDX]

Z77.112 **Contact with and (suspected) exposure to soil pollution** — [Unacceptable PDX]

Z77.118 **Contact with and (suspected) exposure to other environmental pollution** — [Unacceptable PDX]

Z77.12- **Contact with and (suspected) exposure to hazards in the physical environment**

Z77.120 **Contact with and (suspected) exposure to mold (toxic)** — [Unacceptable PDX]

Z77.121 **Contact with and (suspected) exposure to harmful algae and algae toxins** — [Unacceptable PDX]
Contact with and (suspected) exposure to (harmful) algae bloom NOS
Contact with and (suspected) exposure to blue-green algae bloom
Contact with and (suspected) exposure to brown tide
Contact with and (suspected) exposure to cyanobacteria bloom
Contact with and (suspected) exposure to Florida red tide
Contact with and (suspected) exposure to pfiesteria piscicida
Contact with and (suspected) exposure to red tide

Z77.122 **Contact with and (suspected) exposure to noise** — [Unacceptable PDX]

Z77.123 **Contact with and (suspected) exposure to radon and other naturally occuring radiation** — [Unacceptable PDX]
Excludes ❷: radiation exposure as the cause of a confirmed condition (W88-W90, X39.0-)
radiation sickness NOS (T66)

Z77.128 **Contact with and (suspected) exposure to other hazards in the physical environment** — [Unacceptable PDX]

Z77.2- **Contact with and (suspected) exposure to other hazardous substances**

Z77.21 **Contact with and (suspected) exposure to potentially hazardous body fluids** — [Unacceptable PDX]

Z77.22 **Contact with and (suspected) exposure to environmental tobacco smoke (acute) (chronic)** — [Unacceptable PDX]
Exposure to second hand tobacco smoke (acute) (chronic)
Passive smoking (acute) (chronic)
Excludes 1: nicotine dependence (F17.-)
tobacco use (Z72.0)
Excludes ❷: occupational exposure to environmental tobacco smoke (Z57.31)

Z77.29 **Contact with and (suspected) exposure to other hazardous substances** — [Unacceptable PDX]
AHA 16:2Q:p33 – Wheezing due to exposure to electronic cigarette vapors

Z77.9 **Other contact with and (suspected) exposures hazardous to health** — [Unacceptable PDX]

Z78- **Other specified health status**
Excludes ❷: asymptomatic human immunodeficiency virus [HIV] infection status (Z21)
postprocedural status (Z93-Z99)
sex reassignment status (Z87.890)

Z78.0 **Asymptomatic menopausal state** — [♀, Age/15-124] [Unacceptable PDX]
Menopausal state NOS
Postmenopausal status NOS
Excludes ❷: symptomatic menopausal state (N95.1)

Z78.1 **Physical restraint status** — [Unacceptable PDX]
Excludes 1: physical restraint due to a procedure — omit code

Z78.9 **Other specified health status** — [Unacceptable PDX]

Z79- **Long term (current) drug therapy**
Includes: Long term (current) drug use for prophylactic purposes
Code also any therapeutic drug level monitoring (Z51.81)
Excludes ❷: drug abuse and dependence (F11-F19)
drug use complicating pregnancy, childbirth, and the puerperium (O99.32-)
long term (current) use of oral antidiabetic drugs (Z79.84)
long term (current) use of oral hypoglycemic drugs (Z79.84)

Z79.0- **Long term (current) use of anticoagulants and antithrombotics/antiplatelets**
Excludes ❷: long term (current) use of aspirin (Z79.82)

Z79.01 **Long term (current) use of anticoagulants**

Z79.02 **Long term (current) use of antithrombotics/antiplatelets** — [Unacceptable PDX]

Z79.1 **Long term (current) use of non-steroidal anti-inflammatories (NSAID)** — [Unacceptable PDX]
Excludes ❷: long term (current) use of aspirin (Z79.82)

Z79.2 **Long term (current) use of antibiotics** — [Unacceptable PDX]

Z79.3 **Long term (current) use of hormonal contraceptives**
Long term (current) use of birth control pill or patch

Z79.4 **Long term (current) use of insulin**

Z79.5- **Long term (current) use of steroids**

Z79.51 **Long term (current) use of inhaled steroids** — [Unacceptable PDX]

Z79.52 **Long term (current) use of systemic steroids** — [Unacceptable PDX]

Z79.8- **Other long term (current) drug therapy**

Z79.81- **Long term (current) use of agents affecting estrogen receptors and estrogen levels**
Code first, if applicable:
Malignant neoplasm of breast (C50.-)
Malignant neoplasm of prostate (C61)
Use additional code, if applicable, to identify:
Estrogen receptor positive status (Z17.0)
Family history of breast cancer (Z80.3)
Genetic susceptibility to malignant neoplasm (cancer) (Z15.0-)
Personal history of breast cancer (Z85.3)
Personal history of prostate cancer (Z85.46)
Postmenopausal status (Z78.0)
Excludes 1: hormone replacement therapy (postmenopausal) (Z79.890)

Z79.810 **Long term (current) use of selective estrogen receptor modulators (SERMs)** — [Unacceptable PDX]
Long term (current) use of raloxifene (Evista)
Long term (current) use of tamoxifen (Nolvadex)
Long term (current) use of toremifene (Fareston)

Z79.811 **Long term (current) use of aromatase inhibitors** — [Unacceptable PDX]
Long term (current) use of anastrozole (Arimidex)
Long term (current) use of exemestane (Aromasin)
Long term (current) use of letrozole (Femara)

Z79.818 **Long term (current) use of other agents affecting estrogen receptors and estrogen levels** — [Unacceptable PDX]
Long term (current) use of estrogen receptor downregulators
Long term (current) use of fulvestrant (Faslodex)
Long term (current) use of gonadotropin-releasing hormone (GnRH) agonist
Long term (current) use of goserelin acetate (Zoladex)
Long term (current) use of leuprolide acetate (leuprorelin) (Lupron)
Long term (current) use of megestrol acetate (Megace)

Z77-Z79

Z79.82 Long term (current) use of <u>aspirin</u>

Z79.83 Long term (current) use of <u>bisphosphonates</u> — [Unacceptable PDX]

Z79.84 Long term (current) use of <u>oral hypoglycemic drugs</u> — [Unacceptable PDX]
Long term (current) use of oral antidiabetic drugs
Excludes ❷: long term (current) use of insulin (Z79.4)

Z79.89- Other long term (current) drug therapy

Z79.890 <u>Hormone replacement therapy</u> (postmenopausal) — [Unacceptable PDX]

Z79.891 Long term (current) use of <u>opiate analgesic</u>
Long term (current) use of methadone for pain management
Excludes 1: methadone use NOS (F11.9-)
use of methadone for treatment of heroin addiction (F11.2-)

Z79.899 Other long term (current) drug therapy
AHA 15:3Q:p21 – Immunocompromised state due to immunosuppresant medication

Z80- <u>Family history</u> of <u>primary malignant neoplasm</u>

Z80.0 Family history of malignant neoplasm of digestive organs — [Unacceptable PDX]
Conditions classifiable to C15-C26

Z80.1 Family history of malignant neoplasm of trachea, bronchus and lung — [Unacceptable PDX]
Conditions classifiable to C33-C34

Z80.2 Family history of malignant neoplasm of other respiratory and intrathoracic organs — [Unacceptable PDX]
Conditions classifiable to C30-C32, C37-C39

Z80.3 Family history of malignant neoplasm of breast — [Unacceptable PDX]
Conditions classifiable to C50.-

Z80.4- Family history of malignant neoplasm of genital organs
Conditions classifiable to C51-C63

Z80.41 Family history of malignant neoplasm of ovary — [Unacceptable PDX]

Z80.42 Family history of malignant neoplasm of prostate — [Unacceptable PDX]

Z80.43 Family history of malignant neoplasm of testis — [Unacceptable PDX]

Z80.49 Family history of malignant neoplasm of other genital organs — [Unacceptable PDX]

Z80.5- Family history of malignant neoplasm of urinary tract
Conditions classifiable to C64-C68

Z80.51 Family history of malignant neoplasm of kidney — [Unacceptable PDX]

Z80.52 Family history of malignant neoplasm of bladder — [Unacceptable PDX]

Z80.59 Family history of malignant neoplasm of other urinary tract organ — [Unacceptable PDX]

Z80.6 Family history of leukemia — [Unacceptable PDX]
Conditions classifiable to C91-C95

Z80.7 Family history of other malignant neoplasms of lymphoid, hematopoietic and related tissues — [Unacceptable PDX]
Conditions classifiable to C81-C90, C96.-

Z80.8 Family history of malignant neoplasm of other organs or systems — [Unacceptable PDX]
Conditions classifiable to C00-C14, C40-C49, C69-C79

Z80.9 Family history of malignant neoplasm, unspecified — [Unacceptable PDX]
Conditions classifiable to C80.1

Z81- <u>Family history</u> of <u>mental and behavioral disorders</u>

Z81.0 Family history of intellectual disabilities — [Unacceptable PDX]
Conditions classifiable to F70-F79

Z81.1 Family history of alcohol abuse and dependence — [Unacceptable PDX]
Conditions classifiable to F10.-

Z81.2 Family history of tobacco abuse and dependence — [Unacceptable PDX]
Conditions classifiable to F17.-

Z81.3 Family history of other psychoactive substance abuse and dependence — [Unacceptable PDX]
Conditions classifiable to F11-F16, F18-F19

Z81.4 Family history of other substance abuse and dependence — [Unacceptable PDX]
Conditions classifiable to F55

Z81.8 Family history of other mental and behavioral disorders — [Unacceptable PDX]
Conditions classifiable elsewhere in F01-F99

Z82- <u>Family history</u> of <u>certain disabilities and chronic diseases (leading to disablement)</u>

Z82.0 Family history of epilepsy and other diseases of the nervous system — [Unacceptable PDX]
Conditions classifiable to G00-G99

Z82.1 Family history of blindness and visual loss — [Unacceptable PDX]
Conditions classifiable to H54.-

Z82.2 Family history of deafness and hearing loss — [Unacceptable PDX]
Conditions classifiable to H90-H91

Z82.3 Family history of stroke — [Unacceptable PDX]
Conditions classifiable to I60-I64

Z82.4- Family history of ischemic heart disease and other diseases of the circulatory system
Conditions classifiable to I00-I52, I65-I99

Z82.41 Family history of sudden cardiac death — [Unacceptable PDX]

Z82.49 Family history of ischemic heart disease and other diseases of the circulatory system — [Unacceptable PDX]

Z82.5 Family history of asthma and other chronic lower respiratory diseases — [Unacceptable PDX]
Conditions classifiable to J40-J47
Excludes ❷: family history of other diseases of the respiratory system (Z83.6)

Z82.6- Family history of arthritis and other diseases of the musculoskeletal system and connective tissue
Conditions classifiable to M00-M99

Z82.61 Family history of arthritis — [Unacceptable PDX]

Z82.62 Family history of osteoporosis — [Unacceptable PDX]

Z82.69 Family history of other diseases of the musculoskeletal system and connective tissue — [Unacceptable PDX]

Z82.7- Family history of congenital malformations, deformations and chromosomal abnormalities
Conditions classifiable to Q00-Q99

Z82.71 Family history of polycystic kidney — [Unacceptable PDX]

Z82.79 Family history of other congenital malformations, deformations and chromosomal abnormalities — [Unacceptable PDX]

Z82.8 Family history of other disabilities and chronic diseases leading to disablement, not elsewhere classified — [Unacceptable PDX]

Z83- <u>Family history</u> of <u>other specific disorders</u>
Excludes ❷: contact with and (suspected) exposure to communicable disease in the family (Z20.-)

Z83.0 Family history of human immunodeficiency virus [HIV] disease — [Unacceptable PDX]
Conditions classifiable to B20

Z83.1 Family history of other infectious and parasitic diseases — [Unacceptable PDX]
Conditions classifiable to A00-B19, B25-B94, B99

Z83.2 Family history of diseases of the blood and blood-forming organs and certain disorders involving the immune mechanism — [Unacceptable PDX]
Conditions classifiable to D50-D89

Z83.3 Family history of diabetes mellitus — [Unacceptable PDX]
Conditions classifiable to E08-E13

Z83.4- Family history of other endocrine, nutritional and metabolic diseases
Conditions classifiable to E00-E07, E15-E88

Z83.41 Family history of multiple endocrine neoplasia [MEN] syndrome — [Unacceptable PDX]

Z83.42 Family history of familial hypercholesterolemia — [Unacceptable PDX]

Z79 - Z83

Z83.49 Family history of other endocrine, nutritional and metabolic diseases — [Unacceptable PDX]

Z83.5- Family history of eye and ear disorders

Z83.51- Family history of eye disorders
Conditions classifiable to H00-H53, H55-H59
Excludes ❷: family history of blindness and visual loss (Z82.1)

Z83.511 Family history of glaucoma — [Unacceptable PDX]

Z83.518 Family history of other specified eye disorder — [Unacceptable PDX]

Z83.52 Family history of ear disorders — [Unacceptable PDX]
Conditions classifiable to H60-H83, H92-H95
Excludes ❷: family history of deafness and hearing loss (Z82.2)

Z83.6 Family history of other diseases of the respiratory system — [Unacceptable PDX]
Conditions classifiable to J00-J39, J60-J99
Excludes ❷: family history of asthma and other chronic lower respiratory diseases (Z82.5)

Z83.7- Family history of diseases of the digestive system
Conditions classifiable to K00-K93

Z83.71 Family history of colonic polyps — [Unacceptable PDX]
Excludes 1: family history of malignant neoplasm of digestive organs (Z80.0)

Z83.79 Family history of other diseases of the digestive system — [Unacceptable PDX]

Z84- Family history of other conditions

Z84.0 Family history of diseases of the skin and subcutaneous tissue — [Unacceptable PDX]
Conditions classifiable to L00-L99

Z84.1 Family history of disorders of kidney and ureter — [Unacceptable PDX]
Conditions classifiable to N00-N29

Z84.2 Family history of other diseases of the genitourinary system — [Unacceptable PDX]
Conditions classifiable to N30-N99

Z84.3 Family history of consanguinity — [Unacceptable PDX]

Z84.8- Family history of other specified conditions

Z84.81 Family history of carrier of genetic disease — [Unacceptable PDX]

Z84.82 Family history of sudden infant death syndrome — [Unacceptable PDX]
Family history of SIDS

Z84.89 Family history of other specified conditions — [Unacceptable PDX]

Z85- Personal history of malignant neoplasm
Code first any follow-up examination after treatment of malignant neoplasm (Z08)
Use additional code to identify:
Alcohol use and dependence (F10.-)
Exposure to environmental tobacco smoke (Z77.22)
History of tobacco dependence (Z87.891)
Occupational exposure to environmental tobacco smoke (Z57.31)
Tobacco dependence (F17.-)
Tobacco use (Z72.0)
*Excludes ❷: personal history of benign neoplasm (Z86.01-)
personal history of carcinoma-in-situ (Z86.00-)*

Z85.0- Personal history of malignant neoplasm of digestive organs

Z85.00 Personal history of malignant neoplasm of unspecified digestive organ — [Unacceptable PDX]

Z85.01 Personal history of malignant neoplasm of esophagus — [Unacceptable PDX]
Conditions classifiable to C15

Z85.02- Personal history of malignant neoplasm of stomach

Z85.020 Personal history of malignant carcinoid tumor of stomach — [Unacceptable PDX]
Conditions classifiable to C7A.092

Z85.028 Personal history of other malignant neoplasm of stomach — [Unacceptable PDX]
Conditions classifiable to C16

Z85.03- Personal history of malignant neoplasm of large intestine

Z85.030 Personal history of malignant carcinoid tumor of large intestine — [Unacceptable PDX]
Conditions classifiable to C7A.022-C7A.025, C7A.029

Z85.038 Personal history of other malignant neoplasm of large intestine — [Unacceptable PDX]
Conditions classifiable to C18

Z85.04- Personal history of malignant neoplasm of rectum, rectosigmoid junction, and anus

Z85.040 Personal history of malignant carcinoid tumor of rectum — [Unacceptable PDX]
Conditions classifiable to C7A.026

Z85.048 Personal history of other malignant neoplasm of rectum, rectosigmoid junction, and anus — [Unacceptable PDX]
Conditions classifiable to C19-C21

Z85.05 Personal history of malignant neoplasm of liver — [Unacceptable PDX]
Conditions classifiable to C22

Z85.06- Personal history of malignant neoplasm of small intestine

Z85.060 Personal history of malignant carcinoid tumor of small intestine — [Unacceptable PDX]
Conditions classifiable to C7A.01-

Z85.068 Personal history of other malignant neoplasm of small intestine — [Unacceptable PDX]
Conditions classifiable to C17

Z85.07 Personal history of malignant neoplasm of pancreas — [Unacceptable PDX]
Conditions classifiable to C25

Z85.09 Personal history of malignant neoplasm of other digestive organs — [Unacceptable PDX]

Z85.1- Personal history of malignant neoplasm of trachea, bronchus and lung

Z85.11- Personal history of malignant neoplasm of bronchus and lung

Z85.110 Personal history of malignant carcinoid tumor of bronchus and lung — [Unacceptable PDX]
Conditions classifiable to C7A.090

Z85.118 Personal history of other malignant neoplasm of bronchus and lung — [Unacceptable PDX]
Conditions classifiable to C34

Z85.12 Personal history of malignant neoplasm of trachea — [Unacceptable PDX]
Conditions classifiable to C33

Z85.2- Personal history of malignant neoplasm of other respiratory and intrathoracic organs

Z85.20 Personal history of malignant neoplasm of unspecified respiratory organ — [Unacceptable PDX]

Z85.21 Personal history of malignant neoplasm of larynx — [Unacceptable PDX]
Conditions classifiable to C32

Z85.22 Personal history of malignant neoplasm of nasal cavities, middle ear, and accessory sinuses — [Unacceptable PDX]
Conditions classifiable to C30-C31

Z85.23- Personal history of malignant neoplasm of thymus

Z85.230 Personal history of malignant carcinoid tumor of thymus — [Unacceptable PDX]
Conditions classifiable to C7A.091

Z85.238 Personal history of other malignant neoplasm of thymus — [Unacceptable PDX]
Conditions classifiable to C37

Z85.29 Personal history of malignant neoplasm of other respiratory and intrathoracic organs — [Unacceptable PDX]

Z85.3 Personal history of malignant neoplasm of breast — [Unacceptable PDX]
Conditions classifiable to C50.-

Z85.4- Personal history of malignant neoplasm of genital organs
Conditions classifiable to C51-C63

Z85.40 Personal history of malignant neoplasm of unspecified female genital organ — [♀] [Unacceptable PDX]

Z85.41 Personal history of malignant neoplasm of cervix uteri — [♀] [Unacceptable PDX]

Z85.42 Personal history of malignant neoplasm of other parts of uterus — [♀] [Unacceptable PDX]

Z85.43 Personal history of malignant neoplasm of ovary — [♀] [Unacceptable PDX]

Z85.44 Personal history of malignant neoplasm of other female genital organs — [♀] [Unacceptable PDX]

Z85.45 Personal history of malignant neoplasm of unspecified male genital organ — [♂] [Unacceptable PDX]

Z85.46 Personal history of malignant neoplasm of prostate — [♂] [Unacceptable PDX]

Z85.47 Personal history of malignant neoplasm of testis — [♂] [Unacceptable PDX]

Z85.48 Personal history of malignant neoplasm of epididymis — [♂] [Unacceptable PDX]

Z85.49 Personal history of malignant neoplasm of other male genital organs — [♂] [Unacceptable PDX]

Z85.5- Personal history of malignant neoplasm of urinary tract
Conditions classifiable to C64-C68

Z85.50 Personal history of malignant neoplasm of unspecified urinary tract organ — [Unacceptable PDX]

Z85.51 Personal history of malignant neoplasm of bladder — [Unacceptable PDX]

Z85.52- Personal history of malignant neoplasm of kidney
Excludes 1:   personal history of malignant neoplasm of renal pelvis (Z85.53)

Z85.520 Personal history of malignant carcinoid tumor of kidney — [Unacceptable PDX]
Conditions classifiable to C7A.093

Z85.528 Personal history of other malignant neoplasm of kidney — [Unacceptable PDX]
Conditions classifiable to C64

Z85.53 Personal history of malignant neoplasm of renal pelvis — [Unacceptable PDX]

Z85.54 Personal history of malignant neoplasm of ureter — [Unacceptable PDX]

Z85.59 Personal history of malignant neoplasm of other urinary tract organ — [Unacceptable PDX]

Z85.6 Personal history of leukemia — [Unacceptable PDX]
Conditions classifiable to C91-C95
Excludes 1:   leukemia in remission C91.0-C95.9 with 5th character 1

Z85.7- Personal history of other malignant neoplasms of lymphoid, hematopoietic and related tissues

Z85.71 Personal history of Hodgkin lymphoma — [Unacceptable PDX]
Conditions classifiable to C81

Z85.72 Personal history of non-Hodgkin lymphomas — [Unacceptable PDX]
Conditions classifiable to C82-C85

Z85.79 Personal history of other malignant neoplasms of lymphoid, hematopoietic and related tissues — [Unacceptable PDX]
Conditions classifiable to C88-C90, C96
Excludes 1:   multiple myeloma in remission (C90.01)
plasma cell leukemia in remission (C90.11)
plasmacytoma in remission (C90.21)

Z85.8- Personal history of malignant neoplasms of other organs and systems
Conditions classifiable to C00-C14, C40-C49, C69-C79, C7A.098, C76-C79

Z85.81- Personal history of malignant neoplasm of lip, oral cavity, and pharynx

Z85.810 Personal history of malignant neoplasm of tongue — [Unacceptable PDX]

Z85.818 Personal history of malignant neoplasm of other sites of lip, oral cavity, and pharynx — [Unacceptable PDX]

Z85.819 Personal history of malignant neoplasm of unspecified site of lip, oral cavity, and pharynx — [Unacceptable PDX]

Z85.82- Personal history of malignant neoplasm of skin

Z85.820 Personal history of malignant melanoma of skin — [Unacceptable PDX]
Conditions classifiable to C43

Z85.821 Personal history of Merkel cell carcinoma — [Unacceptable PDX]
Conditions classifiable to C4A

Z85.828 Personal history of other malignant neoplasm of skin — [Unacceptable PDX]
Conditions classifiable to C44

Z85.83- Personal history of malignant neoplasm of bone and soft tissue

Z85.830 Personal history of malignant neoplasm of bone — [Unacceptable PDX]

Z85.831 Personal history of malignant neoplasm of soft tissue — [Unacceptable PDX]
Excludes ❷: personal history of malignant neoplasm of skin (Z85.82-)

Z85.84- Personal history of malignant neoplasm of eye and nervous tissue

Z85.840 Personal history of malignant neoplasm of eye — [Unacceptable PDX]

Z85.841 Personal history of malignant neoplasm of brain — [Unacceptable PDX]

Z85.848 Personal history of malignant neoplasm of other parts of nervous tissue — [Unacceptable PDX]

Z85.85- Personal history of malignant neoplasm of endocrine glands

Z85.850 Personal history of malignant neoplasm of thyroid — [Unacceptable PDX]

Z85.858 Personal history of malignant neoplasm of other endocrine glands — [Unacceptable PDX]

Z85.89 Personal history of malignant neoplasm of other organs and systems — [Unacceptable PDX]

Z85.9 Personal history of malignant neoplasm, unspecified — [Unacceptable PDX]
Conditions classifiable to C7A.00, C80.1

Z86- Personal history of certain other diseases
Code first any follow-up examination after treatment (Z09)

Z86.0- Personal history of in situ and benign neoplasms and neoplasms of uncertain behavior
Excludes ❷: personal history of malignant neoplasms (Z85.-)

Z86.00- Personal history of in situ neoplasm
Conditions classifiable to D00-D09

Z86.000 Personal history of in situ neoplasm of breast — [Unacceptable PDX]

Z86.001 Personal history of in situ neoplasm of cervix uteri — [♀] [Unacceptable PDX]
Personal history of cervical intraepithelial neoplasia III [CIN III]

Z86.008 Personal history of in situ neoplasm of other site — [Unacceptable PDX]
Personal history of vaginal intraepithelial neoplasia III [VAIN III]
Personal history of vulvar intraepithelial neoplasia III [VIN III]

Z86.01- Personal history of benign neoplasm

Z86.010 Personal history of colonic polyps — [Unacceptable PDX]

Z86.011 Personal history of benign neoplasm of the brain — [Unacceptable PDX]

Z86.012 Personal history of benign carcinoid tumor — [Unacceptable PDX]

Z86.018 Personal history of other benign neoplasm — [Unacceptable PDX]

Z85 - Z86

Z86.03   Personal history of neoplasm of uncertain behavior —
[Unacceptable PDX]

Z86.1-   <u>Personal history</u> of <u>infectious and parasitic diseases</u>
Conditions classifiable to A00-B89, B99
Excludes 1:   *personal history of infectious diseases specific to a body system*
         sequelae of infectious and parasitic diseases (B90-B94)

Z86.11   Personal history of tuberculosis — [Unacceptable PDX]

Z86.12   Personal history of poliomyelitis — [Unacceptable PDX]

Z86.13   Personal history of malaria — [Unacceptable PDX]

Z86.14   Personal history of methicillin resistant Staphylococcus aureus infection — [Unacceptable PDX]
     Personal history of MRSA infection

Z86.19   Personal history of other infectious and parasitic diseases — [Unacceptable PDX]

Z86.2   <u>Personal history</u> of <u>diseases of the blood and blood-forming organs and certain disorders involving the immune mechanism</u> — [Unacceptable PDX]
     Conditions classifiable to D50-D89

Z86.3-   <u>Personal history</u> of <u>endocrine, nutritional and metabolic diseases</u>
     Conditions classifiable to E00-E88

Z86.31   Personal history of diabetic foot ulcer — [Unacceptable PDX]
Excludes ❷: *current diabetic foot ulcer (E08.621, E09.621, E10.621, E11.621, E13.621)*

Z86.32   Personal history of gestational diabetes — [♀]
[Unacceptable PDX]
     Pesonal history of conditions classifiable to O24.4-
Excludes 1:   *gestational diabetes mellitus in current pregnancy (O24.4-)*

Z86.39   Personal history of other endocrine, nutritional and metabolic disease — [Unacceptable PDX]

Z86.5-   <u>Personal history</u> of <u>mental and behavioral disorders</u>
     Conditions classifiable to F40-F59

Z86.51   Personal history of combat and operational stress reaction — [Age/15-124] [Unacceptable PDX]

Z86.59   Personal history of other mental and behavioral disorders — [Unacceptable PDX]

Z86.6-   <u>Personal history</u> of <u>diseases of the nervous system and sense organs</u>
     Conditions classifiable to G00-G99, H00-H95

Z86.61   Personal history of infections of the central nervous system — [Unacceptable PDX]
     Personal history of encephalitis
     Personal history of meningitis

Z86.69   Personal history of other diseases of the nervous system and sense organs — [Unacceptable PDX]

Z86.7-   <u>Personal history</u> of <u>diseases of the circulatory system</u>
     Conditions classifiable to I00-I99
Excludes ❷: *old myocardial infarction (I25.2)*
       personal history of anaphylactic shock (Z87.892)
       postmyocardial infarction syndrome (I24.1)

Z86.71-   Personal history of venous thrombosis and embolism

Z86.711   Personal history of pulmonary embolism — [Unacceptable PDX]

Z86.718   Personal history of other venous thrombosis and embolism — [Unacceptable PDX]

Z86.72   Personal history of thrombophlebitis — [Unacceptable PDX]

Z86.73   Personal history of transient ischemic attack (TIA), and cerebral infarction without residual deficits —
[Unacceptable PDX]
     Personal history of prolonged reversible ischemic neurological deficit (PRIND)
     Personal history of stroke NOS without residual deficits
Excludes 1:   *personal history of traumatic brain injury (Z87.820)*
       sequelae of cerebrovascular disease (I69.-)

Z86.74   Personal history of sudden cardiac arrest —
[Unacceptable PDX]
     Personal history of sudden cardiac death successfully resuscitated

Z86.79   Personal history of other diseases of the circulatory system — [Unacceptable PDX]

Z87-   <u>Personal history</u> of <u>other diseases and conditions</u>
Code first any follow-up examination after treatment (Z09)

Z87.0-   Personal history of diseases of the <u>respiratory system</u>
     Conditions classifiable to J00-J99

Z87.01   Personal history of pneumonia (recurrent) —
[Unacceptable PDX]

Z87.09   Personal history of other diseases of the respiratory system — [Unacceptable PDX]

Z87.1-   Personal history of diseases of the <u>digestive system</u>
     Conditions classifiable to K00-K93

Z87.11   Personal history of peptic ulcer disease — [Unacceptable PDX]

Z87.19   Personal history of other diseases of the digestive system — [Unacceptable PDX]

Z87.2   Personal history of diseases of the <u>skin and subcutaneous tissue</u> — [Unacceptable PDX]
     Conditions classifiable to L00-L99
Excludes ❷: *personal history of diabetic foot ulcer (Z86.31)*

Z87.3-   Personal history of diseases of the <u>musculoskeletal system and connective tissue</u>
     Conditions classifiable to M00-M99
Excludes ❷: *personal history of (healed) traumatic fracture (Z87.81)*

Z87.31-   Personal history of (healed) nontraumatic fracture

Z87.310   Personal history of (healed) osteoporosis fracture — [Unacceptable PDX]
     Personal history of (healed) fragility fracture
     Personal history of (healed) collapsed vertebra due to osteoporosis

Z87.311   Personal history of (healed) other pathological fracture — [Unacceptable PDX]
     Personal history of (healed) collapsed vertebra NOS
Excludes ❷: *personal history of osteoporosis fracture (Z87.310)*

Z87.312   Personal history of (healed) stress fracture —
[Unacceptable PDX]
     Personal history of (healed) fatigue fracture

Z87.39   Personal history of other diseases of the musculoskeletal system and connective tissue — [Unacceptable PDX]

Z87.4-   Personal history of diseases of <u>genitourinary system</u>
     Conditions classifiable to N00-N99

Z87.41-   Personal history of <u>dysplasia</u> of the <u>female genital tract</u>
Excludes 1:   *personal history of intraepithelial neoplasia III of female genital tract (Z87.001, Z87.008)*
       personal history of malignant neoplasm of female genital tract (Z85.40-Z85.44)

Z87.410   Personal history of cervical dysplasia — [♀]
[Unacceptable PDX]

Z87.411   Personal history of vaginal dysplasia — [♀]
[Unacceptable PDX]

Z87.412   Personal history of vulvar dysplasia — [♀]
[Unacceptable PDX]

Z87.42   Personal history of <u>other</u> diseases of the <u>female genital tract</u> — [♀] [Unacceptable PDX]

Z87.43-   Personal history of diseases of <u>male genital organs</u>

Z87.430   Personal history of prostatic dysplasia — [♂]
[Unacceptable PDX]
Excludes 1:   *personal history of malignant neoplasm of prostate (Z85.46)*

Z87.438   Personal history of other diseases of male genital organs — [♂] [Unacceptable PDX]

Z87.44-   Personal history of diseases of <u>urinary system</u>
Excludes 1:   *personal history of malignant neoplasm of cervix uteri (Z85.41)*

Z87.440   Personal history of urinary (tract) infections —
[Unacceptable PDX]

Z87.441   Personal history of nephrotic syndrome —
[Unacceptable PDX]

Z87.442   Personal history of urinary calculi — [Unacceptable PDX]
     Personal history of kidney stones

Z87.448   Personal history of other diseases of urinary system — [Unacceptable PDX]

Z 8 6 – Z 8 7

Z87.5- Personal history of complications of pregnancy, childbirth and the puerperium

Conditions classifiable to O00-O9A

Excludes ❷: recurrent pregnancy loss (N96)

Z87.51 Personal history of pre-term labor — [♀] [Unacceptable PDX]

Excludes 1: current pregnancy with history of pre-term labor (O09.21-)

Z87.59 Personal history of other complications of pregnancy, childbirth and the puerperium — [♀] [Unacceptable PDX]

Personal history of trophoblastic disease

Z87.7- Personal history of (corrected) congenital malformations

Conditions classifiable to Q00-Q89 that have been repaired or corrected

Excludes 1: congenital malformations that have been partially corrected or repair but which still require medical treatment — code to condition

Excludes ❷: other postprocedural states (Z98.-)

personal history of medical treatment (Z92.-)

presence of cardiac and vascular implants and grafts (Z95.-)

presence of other devices (Z97.-)

presence of other functional implants (Z96.-)

transplanted organ and tissue status (Z94.-)

Z87.71- Personal history of (corrected) congenital malformations of genitourinary system

Z87.710 Personal history of (corrected) hypospadias — [♂] [Unacceptable PDX]

Z87.718 Personal history of other specified (corrected) congenital malformations of genitourinary system — [Unacceptable PDX]

Z87.72- Personal history of (corrected) congenital malformations of nervous system and senseorgans

Z87.720 Personal history of (corrected) congenital malformations of eye — [Unacceptable PDX]

Z87.721 Personal history of (corrected) congenital malformations of ear — [Unacceptable PDX]

Z87.728 Personal history of other specified (corrected) congenital malformations of nervous system and sense organs — [Unacceptable PDX]

Z87.73- Personal history of (corrected) congenital malformations of digestive system

Z87.730 Personal history of (corrected) cleft lip and palate — [Unacceptable PDX]

Z87.738 Personal history of other specified (corrected) congenital malformations of digestive system — [Unacceptable PDX]

Z87.74 Personal history of (corrected) congenital malformations of heart and circulatory system — [Unacceptable PDX]

Z87.75 Personal history of (corrected) congenital malformations of respiratory system — [Unacceptable PDX]

Z87.76 Personal history of (corrected) congenital malformations of integument, limbs and musculoskeletal system — [Unacceptable PDX]

Z87.79- Personal history of other (corrected) congenital malformations

Z87.790 Personal history of (corrected) congenital malformations of face and neck — [Unacceptable PDX]

Z87.798 Personal history of other (corrected) congenital malformations — [Unacceptable PDX]

Z87.8- Personal history of other specified conditions

Excludes ❷: personal history of self harm (Z91.5)

Z87.81 Personal history of (healed) traumatic fracture — [Unacceptable PDX]

Excludes ❷: personal history of (healed) nontraumatic fracture (Z87.31-)

Z87.82- Personal history of other (healed) physical injury and trauma

Conditions classifiable to S00-T88, except traumatic fractures

Z87.820 Personal history of traumatic brain injury — [Unacceptable PDX]

Excludes 1: personal history of transient ischemic attack (TIA), and cerebral infarction without residual deficits (Z86.73)

Z87.821 Personal history of retained foreign body fully removed — [Unacceptable PDX]

Z87.828 Personal history of other (healed) physical injury and trauma — [Unacceptable PDX]

Z87.89- Personal history of other specified conditions

Z87.890 Personal history of sex reassignment

Z87.891 Personal history of nicotine dependence — [Unacceptable PDX]

Excludes 1: current nicotine dependence (F17.2-)

Z87.892 Personal history of anaphylaxis — [Unacceptable PDX]

Code also allergy status, such as:

Allergy status to drugs, medicaments and biological substances (Z88-)

Allergy status, other than to drugs and biological substances (Z91.0-)

Z87.898 Personal history of other specified conditions — [Unacceptable PDX]

AHA 13:1Q:p21 – Methamphetamine abuse in prolonged remission

Z88- Allergy status to drugs, medicaments and biological substances

Excludes ❷: allergy status, other than to drugs and biological substances (Z91.0-)

Z88.0 Allergy status to penicillin — [Unacceptable PDX]

Z88.1 Allergy status to other antibiotic agents status — [Unacceptable PDX]

Z88.2 Allergy status to sulfonamides status — [Unacceptable PDX]

Z88.3 Allergy status to other anti-infective agents status — [Unacceptable PDX]

Z88.4 Allergy status to anesthetic agent status — [Unacceptable PDX]

Z88.5 Allergy status to narcotic agent status — [Unacceptable PDX]

Z88.6 Allergy status to analgesic agent status — [Unacceptable PDX]

Z88.7 Allergy status to serum and vaccine status — [Unacceptable PDX]

Z88.8 Allergy status to other drugs, medicaments and biological substances status — [Unacceptable PDX]

Z88.9 Allergy status to unspecified drugs, medicaments and biological substances status — [Unacceptable PDX]

Z89- Acquired absence of limb

Includes: Amputation status

Postprocedural loss of limb

Post-traumatic loss of limb

Excludes 1: acquired deformities of limbs (M20-M21)

congenital absence of limbs (Q71-Q73)

Z89.0- Acquired absence of thumb and other finger(s)

Z89.01- Acquired absence of thumb

Z89.011 Acquired absence of right thumb — [Unacceptable PDX]

Z89.012 Acquired absence of left thumb — [Unacceptable PDX]

Z89.019 Acquired absence of unspecified thumb — [Unacceptable PDX]

Z89.02- Acquired absence of other finger(s)

Excludes ❷: acquired absence of thumb (Z89.01-)

Z89.021 Acquired absence of right finger(s) — [Unacceptable PDX]

Z89.022 Acquired absence of left finger(s) — [Unacceptable PDX]

Z89.029 Acquired absence of unspecified finger(s) — [Unacceptable PDX]

Z89.1- Acquired absence of hand and wrist

Z89.11- Acquired absence of hand

Z89.111 Acquired absence of right hand — [Unacceptable PDX]

Z89.112 Acquired absence of left hand — [Unacceptable PDX]

Z89.119 Acquired absence of unspecified hand — [Unacceptable PDX]

Z87 - Z89

Z89.12- Acquired absence of <u>wrist</u>
Disarticulation at wrist

Z89.121 Acquired absence of <u>right</u> wrist — [Unacceptable PDX]

Z89.122 Acquired absence of <u>left</u> wrist — [Unacceptable PDX]

Z89.129 Acquired absence of <u>unspecified</u> wrist —
[Unacceptable PDX]

Z89.2- Acquired absence of upper limb above wrist

Z89.20- Acquired absence of <u>upper limb, unspecified level</u>

Z89.201 Acquired absence of <u>right</u> upper limb, unspecified level — [Unacceptable PDX]

Z89.202 Acquired absence of <u>left</u> upper limb, unspecified level — [Unacceptable PDX]

Z89.209 Acquired absence of <u>unspecified</u> upper limb, unspecified level — [Unacceptable PDX]
Acquired absence of arm NOS

Z89.21- Acquired absence of <u>upper limb below elbow</u>

Z89.211 Acquired absence of <u>right</u> upper limb below elbow — [Unacceptable PDX]

Z89.212 Acquired absence of <u>left</u> upper limb below elbow — [Unacceptable PDX]

Z89.219 Acquired absence of <u>unspecified</u> upper limb below elbow — [Unacceptable PDX]

Z89.22- Acquired absence of <u>upper limb above elbow</u>
Disarticulation at elbow

Z89.221 Acquired absence of <u>right</u> upper limb above elbow — [Unacceptable PDX]

Z89.222 Acquired absence of <u>left</u> upper limb above elbow — [Unacceptable PDX]

Z89.229 Acquired absence of <u>unspecified</u> upper limb above elbow — [Unacceptable PDX]

Z89.23- Acquired absence of <u>shoulder</u>
Acquired absence of shoulder joint following explantation of shoulder joint prosthesis, with or without presence of antibiotic-impregnated cement spacer

Z89.231 Acquired absence of <u>right</u> shoulder —
[Unacceptable PDX]

Z89.232 Acquired absence of <u>left</u> shoulder — [Unacceptable PDX]

Z89.239 Acquired absence of <u>unspecified</u> shoulder —
[Unacceptable PDX]

Z89.4- Acquired absence of toe(s), foot, and ankle

Z89.41- Acquired absence of <u>great toe</u>

Z89.411 Acquired absence of <u>right</u> great toe —
[Unacceptable PDX]

Z89.412 Acquired absence of <u>left</u> great toe —
[Unacceptable PDX]

Z89.419 Acquired absence of <u>unspecified</u> great toe —
[Unacceptable PDX]

Z89.42- Acquired absence of <u>other toe(s)</u>
Excludes ❷: acquired absence of great toe (Z89.41-)

Z89.421 Acquired absence of other <u>right</u> toe(s) —
[Unacceptable PDX]

Z89.422 Acquired absence of other <u>left</u> toe(s) —
[Unacceptable PDX]

Z89.429 Acquired absence of other toe(s), <u>unspecified</u> side — [Unacceptable PDX]

Z89.43- Acquired absence of <u>foot</u>

Z89.431 Acquired absence of <u>right</u> foot — [Unacceptable PDX]

Z89.432 Acquired absence of <u>left</u> foot — [Unacceptable PDX]

Z89.439 Acquired absence of <u>unspecified</u> foot —
[Unacceptable PDX]

Z89.44- Acquired absence of <u>ankle</u>
Disarticulation of ankle

Z89.441 Acquired absence of <u>right</u> ankle — [Unacceptable PDX]

Z89.442 Acquired absence of <u>left</u> ankle — [Unacceptable PDX]

Z89.449 Acquired absence of <u>unspecified</u> ankle —
[Unacceptable PDX]

Z89.5- Acquired absence of <u>leg below knee</u>

Z89.51- Acquired absence of leg below knee

Z89.511 Acquired absence of <u>right</u> leg below knee —
[Unacceptable PDX]

Z89.512 Acquired absence of <u>left</u> leg below knee —
[Unacceptable PDX]

Z89.519 Acquired absence of <u>unspecified</u> leg below knee —
[Unacceptable PDX]

Z89.52- Acquired absence of knee
Acquired absence of knee joint following explantation of knee joint prosthesis, with or without presence of antibiotic-impregnated cement spacer

Z89.521 Acquired absence of <u>right</u> knee — [Unacceptable PDX]

Z89.522 Acquired absence of <u>left</u> knee — [Unacceptable PDX]

Z89.529 Acquired absence of <u>unspecified</u> knee —
[Unacceptable PDX]

Z89.6- Acquired absence of leg above knee

Z89.61- Acquired absence of <u>leg above knee</u>
Acquired absence of leg NOS
Disarticulation at knee

Z89.611 Acquired absence of <u>right</u> leg above knee —
[Unacceptable PDX]

Z89.612 Acquired absence of <u>left</u> leg above knee —
[Unacceptable PDX]

Z89.619 Acquired absence of <u>unspecified</u> leg above knee —
[Unacceptable PDX]

Z89.62- Acquired absence of <u>hip</u>
Acquired absence of hip joint following explantation of hip joint prosthesis, with or without presence of antibiotic-impregnated cement spacer
Disarticulation at hip

Z89.621 Acquired absence of <u>right</u> hip joint —
[Unacceptable PDX]

Z89.622 Acquired absence of <u>left</u> hip joint — [Unacceptable PDX]

Z89.629 Acquired absence of <u>unspecified</u> hip joint —
[Unacceptable PDX]

Z89.9 Acquired absence of limb, <u>unspecified</u> — [Unacceptable PDX]

Z90- <u>Acquired absence</u> of organs, <u>not elsewhere classified</u>
Includes: Postprocedural or post-traumatic loss of body part NEC
Excludes 1:   congenital absence — see Alphabetical Index
Excludes ❷: postprocedural absence of endocrine glands (E89.-)

Z90.0- Acquired absence of part of head and neck

Z90.01 Acquired absence of eye — [Unacceptable PDX]

Z90.02 Acquired absence of larynx — [Unacceptable PDX]

Z90.09 Acquired absence of other part of head and neck —
[Unacceptable PDX]
Acquired absence of nose
Excludes ❷: teeth (K08.1)

Z90.1- Acquired absence of <u>breast and nipple</u>

Z90.10 Acquired absence of <u>unspecified</u> breast and nipple

Z90.11 Acquired absence of <u>right</u> breast and nipple

Z90.12 Acquired absence of <u>left</u> breast and nipple

Z90.13 Acquired absence of <u>bilateral</u> breasts and nipples

Z90.2 Acquired absence of lung [part of] — [Unacceptable PDX]

Z90.3 Acquired absence of stomach [part of] — [Unacceptable PDX]

Z90.4- Acquired absence of other specified parts of digestive tract

Z90.41 Acquired absence of pancreas
Code also exocrine pancreatic insufficiency (K86.81)
Use additional code to identify any associated:
Insulin use (Z79.4)
Diabetes mellitus, postpancreatectomy (E13.-)

Z90.410 Acquired total absence of pancreas —
[Unacceptable PDX]
Acquired absence of pancreas NOS

Z90.411 Acquired partial absence of pancreas —
[Unacceptable PDX]

Z90.49 Acquired absence of other specified parts of digestive tract — [Unacceptable PDX]

Z90.5 Acquired absence of kidney — [Unacceptable PDX]

Z
8
9
–
Z
9
0

Z90.6 Acquired absence of other parts of urinary tract —
[Unacceptable PDX]
Acquired absence of bladder

Z90.7- Acquired absence of genital organ(s)
Excludes 1: *personal history of sex reassignment (Z87.890)*
Excludes ❷: *female genital mutilation status (N90.81-)*

Z90.71- Acquired absence of cervix and uterus

Z90.710 Acquired absence of <u>both cervix and uterus</u> — [♀]
[Unacceptable PDX]
Acquired absence of uterus NOS
Status post total hysterectomy

Z90.711 Acquired absence of <u>uterus with remaining cervical stump</u> — [♀] [Unacceptable PDX]
Status post partial hysterectomy with remaining cervical stump

Z90.712 Acquired absence of <u>cervix with remaining uterus</u> — [♀] [Unacceptable PDX]

Z90.72- Acquired absence of <u>ovaries</u>

Z90.721 Acquired absence of ovaries, <u>unilateral</u> — [♀]
[Unacceptable PDX]

Z90.722 Acquired absence of ovaries, <u>bilateral</u> — [♀]
[Unacceptable PDX]

Z90.79 Acquired absence of other genital organ(s) —
[Unacceptable PDX]

Z90.8- Acquired absence of other organs

Z90.81 Acquired absence of spleen — [Unacceptable PDX]

Z90.89 Acquired absence of other organs — [Unacceptable PDX]

Z91- Personal risk factors, not elsewhere classified
Excludes ❷: *contact with and (suspected) exposures hazardous to health (Z77-)*
exposure to pollution and other problems related to physical environment (Z77.1-)
occupational exposure to risk factors (Z57-)
personal history of physical injury and trauma (Z87.81, Z87.82-)

Z91.0- <u>Allergy status</u>, other than to drugs and biological substances
Excludes ❷: *allergy status to drugs, medicaments, and biological substances (Z88-)*

Z91.01- <u>Food</u> allergy status
Excludes ❷: *food additives allergy status (Z91.02)*

Z91.010 Allergy to peanuts — [Unacceptable PDX]

Z91.011 Allergy to milk products — [Unacceptable PDX]
Excludes 1: *lactose intolerance (E73-)*

Z91.012 Allergy to eggs — [Unacceptable PDX]

Z91.013 Allergy to seafood — [Unacceptable PDX]
Allergy to shellfish
Allergy to octopus or squid ink

Z91.018 Allergy to other foods — [Unacceptable PDX]
Allergy to nuts other than peanuts

Z91.02 <u>Food additives</u> allergy status — [Unacceptable PDX]

Z91.03- <u>Insect</u> allergy status

Z91.030 Bee allergy status — [Unacceptable PDX]

Z91.038 Other insect allergy status — [Unacceptable PDX]

Z91.04- <u>Nonmedicinal substance</u> allergy status

Z91.040 Latex allergy status — [Unacceptable PDX]
Latex sensitivity status

Z91.041 Radiographic dye allergy status — [Unacceptable PDX]
Allergy status to contrast media used for diagnostic X-ray procedure

Z91.048 Other nonmedicinal substance allergy status —
[Unacceptable PDX]

Z91.09 <u>Other</u> allergy status, other than to drugs and biological substances — [Unacceptable PDX]

Z91.1- <u>Patient's noncompliance with medical treatment and regimen</u>

Z91.11 Patient's noncompliance with <u>dietary regimen</u> —
[Unacceptable PDX]

Z91.12- Patient's <u>intentional underdosing</u> of medication regimen
Code first underdosing of medication (T36-T50) with fifth or sixth character 6
Excludes 1: *adverse effect of prescribed drug taken as directed — code to adverse effect*
poisoning (overdose) — code to poisoning

Z91.120 Patient's intentional underdosing of medication regimen <u>due to financial hardship</u> —
[Unacceptable PDX]

Z91.128 Patient's intentional underdosing of medication regimen <u>for other reason</u> — [Unacceptable PDX]

Z91.13- Patient's <u>unintentional underdosing</u> of medication regimen
Code first underdosing of medication (T36-T50) with fifth or sixth character 6
Excludes 1: *adverse effect of prescribed drug taken as directed — code to adverse effect*
poisoning (overdose) — code to poisoning

Z91.130 Patient's unintentional underdosing of medication regimen <u>due to age-related debility</u> —
[Unacceptable PDX]

Z91.138 Patient's unintentional underdosing of medication regimen <u>for other reason</u> — [Unacceptable PDX]

Z91.14 Patient's <u>other noncompliance</u> with <u>medication regimen</u> — [Unacceptable PDX]
Patient's underdosing of medication NOS

Z91.15 Patient's <u>noncompliance</u> with renal dialysis —
[Unacceptable PDX]

Z91.19 Patient's <u>noncompliance</u> with other medical treatment and regimen — [Unacceptable PDX]

Z91.4- Personal history of psychological trauma, not elsewhere classified

Z91.41- Personal history of adult abuse
Excludes ❷: *personal history of abuse in childhood (Z62.81-)*

Z91.410 Personal history of adult physical and sexual abuse — [Age/15-124] [Unacceptable PDX]
Excludes 1: *current adult physical abuse (T74.11, T76.11)*
current adult sexual abuse (T74.21, T76.11)

Z91.411 Personal history of adult psychological abuse —
[Age/15-124] [Unacceptable PDX]

Z91.412 Personal history of adult neglect — [Age/15-124]
[Unacceptable PDX]
Excludes 1: *current adult neglect (T74.01, T76.01)*

Z91.419 Personal history of unspecified adult abuse —
[Age/15-124] [Unacceptable PDX]

Z91.49 Other personal history of psychological trauma, not elsewhere classified — [Unacceptable PDX]

Z91.5 Personal history of self-harm — [Unacceptable PDX]
Personal history of parasuicide
Personal history of self-poisoning
Personal history of suicide attempt

Z91.8- Other specified personal risk factors, not elsewhere classified

Z91.81 <u>History of falling</u> — [Unacceptable PDX]
At risk for falling

Z91.82 Personal history of military deployment — [Age/15-124]
[Unacceptable PDX]
Individual (civilian or military) with past history of military war, peacekeeping and humanitarian deployment (current or past conflict)
Returned from military deployment

Z91.83 Wandering in diseases classified elsewhere —
[Not Allowed as PDX]
Code first underlying disorder, such as:
Alzheimer's disease (G30.-)
Autism or pervasive developmental disorder (F84.-)
Intellectual disabilities (F70-F79)
Unspecified dementia with behavioral disturbance (F03.9-)

Z91.89 Other specified personal risk factors, not elsewhere classified — [Unacceptable PDX]

Z90 - Z91

Z92- **Personal history** of medical treatment
Excludes ❷: *postprocedural states (Z98-)*

Z92.0 **Personal history of <u>contraception</u>** — [Unacceptable PDX]
Excludes 1: *counseling or management of current contraceptive practices (Z30-)*
long term (current) use of contraception (Z79.3)
presence of (intrauterine) contraceptive device (Z97.5)

Z92.2- **Personal history of <u>drug therapy</u>**
Excludes ❷: *long term (current) drug therapy (Z79-)*

Z92.21 **Personal history of antineoplastic chemotherapy** — [Unacceptable PDX]

Z92.22 **Personal history of monoclonal drug therapy** — [Unacceptable PDX]

Z92.23 **Personal history of estrogen therapy** — [Unacceptable PDX]

Z92.24- **Personal history of steroid therapy**

Z92.240 **Personal history of inhaled steroid therapy** — [Unacceptable PDX]

Z92.241 **Personal history of systemic steroid therapy** — [Unacceptable PDX]
Personal history of steroid therapy NOS

Z92.25 **Personal history of <u>immunosupression therapy</u>** — [Unacceptable PDX]
Excludes ❷: *personal history of steroid therapy (Z92.24)*

Z92.29 **Personal history of other drug therapy** — [Unacceptable PDX]

Z92.3 **Personal history of <u>irradiation</u>** — [Unacceptable PDX]
Personal history of exposure to therapeutic radiation
Excludes 1: *exposure to radiation in the physical environment (Z77.12)*
occupational exposure to radiation (Z57.1)

Z92.8- **Personal history of <u>other</u> medical treatment**

Z92.81 **Personal history of extracorporeal membrane oxygenation (ECMO)** — [Unacceptable PDX]

Z92.82 **Status post administration of tPA (rtPA) in a different facility within the last 24 hours prior to admission to current facility** — [Unacceptable PDX]
AHA 13:4Q:p124 – tPA (rtPA) in a different facility within the last 24 hours
Code first condition requiring tPA administration, such as:
Acute cerebral infarction (I63-)
Acute myocardial infarction (I21-, I22-)

Z92.83 **Personal history of failed moderate sedation** — [Unacceptable PDX]
Personal history of failed conscious sedation
Excludes ❷: *failed moderate sedation during procedure (T88.52)*

Z92.84 **Personal history of unintended awareness under general anesthesia** — [Unacceptable PDX]
Excludes ❷: *unintended awareness under general anesthesia during procedure (T88.53)*

Z92.89 **Personal history of other medical treatment** — [Unacceptable PDX]

Z93- **Artificial opening status**
Excludes 1: *artificial openings requiring attention or management (Z43.-)*
complications of external stoma (J95.0-, K94.-, N99.5-)

Z93.0 **Tracheostomy status** — [Unacceptable PDX]

Z93.1 **Gastrostomy status** — [Unacceptable PDX]

Z93.2 **Ileostomy status** — [Unacceptable PDX]

Z93.3 **Colostomy status** — [Unacceptable PDX]

Z93.4 **Other artificial openings of gastrointestinal tract status** — [Unacceptable PDX]

Z93.5- **Cystostomy status**

Z93.50 **Unspecified cystostomy status** — [Unacceptable PDX]

Z93.51 **Cutaneous-vesicostomy status** — [Unacceptable PDX]

Z93.52 **Appendico-vesicostomy status** — [Unacceptable PDX]

Z93.59 **Other cystostomy status** — [Unacceptable PDX]

Z93.6 **Other artificial openings of urinary tract status** — [Unacceptable PDX]
Nephrostomy status
Ureterostomy status
Urethrostomy status

Z93.8 **Other artificial opening status** — [Unacceptable PDX]

Z93.9 **Artificial opening status, unspecified** — [Unacceptable PDX]

Z94- **Transplanted organ and tissue status**
Includes: Organ or tissue replaced by heterogenous or homogenous transplant
Excludes 1: *complications of transplanted organ or tissue — see Alphabetical Index*
Excludes ❷: *presence of vascular grafts (Z95.-)*

cc **Z94.0** **Kidney transplant status** — [Unacceptable PDX]

cc **Z94.1** **Heart transplant status** — [Unacceptable PDX]
Excludes 1: *artificial heart status (Z95.812)*
heart-valve replacement status (Z95.2-Z95.4)

cc **Z94.2** **Lung transplant status** — [Unacceptable PDX]

cc **Z94.3** **Heart and lungs transplant status** — [Unacceptable PDX]

cc **Z94.4** **Liver transplant status** — [Unacceptable PDX]

Z94.5 **Skin transplant status** — [Unacceptable PDX]
Autogenous skin transplant status

Z94.6 **Bone transplant status** — [Unacceptable PDX]

Z94.7 **Corneal transplant status** — [Unacceptable PDX]

Z94.8- **Other transplanted organ and tissue status**

cc **Z94.81** **Bone marrow transplant status** — [Unacceptable PDX]

cc **Z94.82** **Intestine transplant status** — [Unacceptable PDX]

cc **Z94.83** **Pancreas transplant status** — [Unacceptable PDX]

cc **Z94.84** **Stem cells transplant status** — [Unacceptable PDX]

Z94.89 **Other transplanted organ and tissue status** — [Unacceptable PDX]

Z94.9 **Transplanted organ and tissue status, unspecified** — [Unacceptable PDX]

Z95- **Presence of cardiac and vascular implants and grafts**
Excludes 1: *complications of cardiac and vascular devices, implants and grafts (T82.-)*

Z95.0 **Presence of cardiac pacemaker** — [Unacceptable PDX]
Presence of cardiac resynchronization therapy (CRT-P) pacemaker
Excludes 1: *adjustment or management of cardiac device (Z45.0-)*
adjustment or management of cardiac pacemaker (Z45.0)
presence of automatic (implantable) cardiac defibrillator with synchronous cardiac pacemaker (Z95.810)

Z95.1 **Presence of aortocoronary bypass graft** — [Unacceptable PDX]
Presence of coronary artery bypass graft

Z95.2 **Presence of prosthetic heart valve** — [Unacceptable PDX]
Presence of heart valve NOS

Z95.3 **Presence of xenogenic heart valve** — [Unacceptable PDX]

Z95.4 **Presence of other heart-valve replacement** — [Unacceptable PDX]

Z95.5 **Presence of coronary angioplasty implant and graft** — [Unacceptable PDX]
Excludes 1: *coronary angioplasty status without implant and graft (Z98.61)*

Z95.8- **Presence of other cardiac and vascular implants and grafts**

Z95.81- **Presence of other cardiac implants and grafts**

Z95.810 **Presence of automatic (implantable) cardiac defibrillator** — [Unacceptable PDX]
Presence of automatic (implantable) cardiac defibrillator with synchronous cardiac pacemaker
Presence of cardiac resynchronization therapy defibrillator (CRT-D)
Presence of cardioverter-defibrillator (ICD)

cc **Z95.811** **Presence of heart assist device** — [Unacceptable PDX]

cc **Z95.812** **Presence of fully implantable artificial heart** — [Unacceptable PDX]

Z95.818 **Presence of other cardiac implants and grafts** — [Unacceptable PDX]

Z95.82- **Presence of other vascular implants and grafts**

Z95.820 **Peripheral vascular angioplasty status with implants and grafts** — [Unacceptable PDX]
Excludes 1: *peripheral vascular angioplasty without implant and graft (Z98.62)*

Z95.828 **Presence of other vascular implants and grafts** — [Unacceptable PDX]
Presence of intravascular prosthesis NEC

Z92 - Z95

Excludes 1: = NOT CODED HERE! (Do not code both)   **1335**   *Excludes ❷:* = Not Included Here

Z95.9 Presence of cardiac and vascular implant and graft, unspecified — [Unacceptable PDX]

Z96- Presence of other functional implants
Excludes 2: complications of internal prosthetic devices, implants and grafts (T82-T85)
fitting and adjustment of prosthetic and other devices (Z44-Z46)

Z96.0 Presence of urogenital implants — [Unacceptable PDX]

Z96.1 Presence of intraocular lens — [Unacceptable PDX]
Presence of pseudophakia

Z96.2- Presence of otological and audiological implants
Z96.20 Presence of otological and audiological implant, unspecified — [Unacceptable PDX]
Z96.21 Cochlear implant status — [Unacceptable PDX]
Z96.22 Myringotomy tube(s) status — [Unacceptable PDX]
Z96.29 Presence of other otological and audiological implants — [Unacceptable PDX]
Presence of bone-conduction hearing device
Presence of eustachian tube stent
Stapes replacement

Z96.3 Presence of artificial larynx — [Unacceptable PDX]

Z96.4- Presence of endocrine implants
Z96.41 Presence of insulin pump (external) (internal) — [Unacceptable PDX]
Z96.49 Presence of other endocrine implants — [Unacceptable PDX]

Z96.5 Presence of tooth-root and mandibular implants — [Unacceptable PDX]

Z96.6- Presence of orthopedic joint implants
AHA 15:1Q:p16 – Presence of left artificial hip joint
Z96.60 Presence of unspecified orthopedic joint implant — [Unacceptable PDX]
Z96.61- Presence of artificial shoulder joint
Z96.611 Presence of right artificial shoulder joint — [Unacceptable PDX]
Z96.612 Presence of left artificial shoulder joint — [Unacceptable PDX]
Z96.619 Presence of unspecified artificial shoulder joint — [Unacceptable PDX]
Z96.62- Presence of artificial elbow joint
Z96.621 Presence of right artificial elbow joint — [Unacceptable PDX]
Z96.622 Presence of left artificial elbow joint — [Unacceptable PDX]
Z96.629 Presence of unspecified artificial elbow joint — [Unacceptable PDX]
Z96.63- Presence of artificial wrist joint
Z96.631 Presence of right artificial wrist joint — [Unacceptable PDX]
Z96.632 Presence of left artificial wrist joint — [Unacceptable PDX]
Z96.639 Presence of unspecified artificial wrist joint — [Unacceptable PDX]
Z96.64- Presence of artificial hip joint
Hip-joint replacement (partial) (total)
Z96.641 Presence of right artificial hip joint — [Unacceptable PDX]
Z96.642 Presence of left artificial hip joint — [Unacceptable PDX]
Z96.643 Presence of artificial hip joint, bilateral — [Unacceptable PDX]
Z96.649 Presence of unspecified artificial hip joint — [Unacceptable PDX]

Z96.65- Presence of artificial knee joint
Z96.651 Presence of right artificial knee joint — [Unacceptable PDX]
Z96.652 Presence of left artificial knee joint — [Unacceptable PDX]
Z96.653 Presence of artificial knee joint, bilateral — [Unacceptable PDX]
Z96.659 Presence of unspecified artificial knee joint — [Unacceptable PDX]
Z96.66- Presence of artificial ankle joint
Z96.661 Presence of right artificial ankle joint — [Unacceptable PDX]
Z96.662 Presence of left artificial ankle joint — [Unacceptable PDX]
Z96.669 Presence of unspecified artificial ankle joint — [Unacceptable PDX]
Z96.69- Presence of other orthopedic joint implants
Z96.691 Finger-joint replacement of right hand — [Unacceptable PDX]
Z96.692 Finger-joint replacement of left hand — [Unacceptable PDX]
Z96.693 Finger-joint replacement, bilateral — [Unacceptable PDX]
Z96.698 Presence of other orthopedic joint implants — [Unacceptable PDX]

Z96.7 Presence of other bone and tendon implants — [Unacceptable PDX]
Presence of skull plate

Z96.8- Presence of other specified functional implants
Z96.81 Presence of artificial skin — [Unacceptable PDX]
Z96.89 Presence of other specified functional implants — [Unacceptable PDX]

Z96.9 Presence of functional implant, unspecified — [Unacceptable PDX]

Z97- Presence of other devices
Excludes 1: complications of internal prosthetic devices, implants and grafts (T82-T85)
fitting and adjustment of prosthetic and other devices (Z44-Z46)
Excludes 2: presence of cerebrospinal fluid drainage device (Z98.2)

Z97.0 Presence of artificial eye — [Unacceptable PDX]

Z97.1- Presence of artificial limb (complete) (partial)
Z97.10 Presence of artificial limb (complete) (partial), unspecified — [Unacceptable PDX]
Z97.11 Presence of artificial right arm (complete) (partial) — [Unacceptable PDX]
Z97.12 Presence of artificial left arm (complete) (partial) — [Unacceptable PDX]
Z97.13 Presence of artificial right leg (complete) (partial) — [Unacceptable PDX]
Z97.14 Presence of artificial left leg (complete) (partial) — [Unacceptable PDX]
Z97.15 Presence of artificial arms, bilateral (complete) (partial) — [Unacceptable PDX]
Z97.16 Presence of artificial legs, bilateral (complete) (partial) — [Unacceptable PDX]

Z97.2 Presence of dental prosthetic device (complete) (partial) — [Unacceptable PDX]
Presence of dentures (complete) (partial)

Z97.3 Presence of spectacles and contact lenses — [Unacceptable PDX]

Z97.4 Presence of external hearing-aid — [Unacceptable PDX]

Z97.5 Presence of (intrauterine) contraceptive device — [♀] [Unacceptable PDX]
Excludes 1: checking, reinsertion or removal of implantable subdermal contraceptive (Z30.46)
checking, reinsertion or removal of intrauterine contraceptive device (Z30.43-)

Z97.8 Presence of other specified devices — [Unacceptable PDX]

Z95-Z97

Z98- Other postprocedural states
Excludes ❷: aftercare (Z43-Z49, Z51)
follow-up medical care (Z08-Z09)
postprocedural complication — see Alphabetical Index

Z98.0 Intestinal bypass and anastomosis status — [Unacceptable PDX]
Excludes ❷: bariatric surgery status (Z98.84)
gastric bypass status (Z98.84)
obesity surgery status (Z98.84)

Z98.1 Arthrodesis status — [Unacceptable PDX]

Z98.2 Presence of cerebrospinal fluid drainage device — [Unacceptable PDX]
Presence of CSF shunt

Z98.3 Post therapeutic collapse of lung status — [Unacceptable PDX]
Code first underlying disease

Z98.4- Cataract extraction status
Use additional code to identify intraocular lens implant status (Z96.1)
Excludes 1: aphakia (H27.0)

Z98.41 Cataract extraction status, right eye — [Unacceptable PDX]

Z98.42 Cataract extraction status, left eye — [Unacceptable PDX]

Z98.49 Cataract extraction status, unspecified eye — [Unacceptable PDX]

Z98.5- Sterilization status
Excludes 1: female infertility (N97.-)
male infertility (N46.-)

Z98.51 Tubal ligation status — [♀] [Unacceptable PDX]

Z98.52 Vasectomy status — [♂, Age/15-124] [Unacceptable PDX]

Z98.6- Angioplasty status

Z98.61 Coronary angioplasty status — [Unacceptable PDX]
Excludes 1: coronary angioplasty status with implant and graft (Z95.5)

Z98.62 Peripheral vascular angioplasty status — [Unacceptable PDX]
Excludes 1: peripheral vascular angioplasty status with implant and graft (Z95.820)

Z98.8- Other specified postprocedural states

Z98.81- Dental procedure status

Z98.810 Dental sealant status — [Unacceptable PDX]

Z98.811 Dental restoration status — [Unacceptable PDX]
Dental crown status
Dental fillings status

Z98.818 Other dental procedure status — [Unacceptable PDX]

Z98.82 Breast implant status — [Unacceptable PDX]
Excludes 1: breast implant removal status (Z98.86)

Z98.83 Filtering (vitreous) bleb after glaucoma surgery status — [Unacceptable PDX]
Excludes 1: Inflammation (infection) of postprocedural bleb (H59.4-)

Z98.84 Bariatric surgery status — [Unacceptable PDX]
Gastric banding status
Gastric bypass status for obesity
Obesity surgery status
Excludes 1: bariatric surgery status complicating pregnancy, childbirth, or the puerperium (O99.84)
Excludes ❷: intestinal bypass and anastomosis status (Z98.0)

Z98.85 Transplanted organ removal status — [Unacceptable PDX]
Transplanted organ previously removed due to complication, failure, rejection or infection
Excludes 1: encounter for removal of transplanted organ — code to complication of transplanted organ (T86.-)

Z98.86 Personal history of breast implant removal — [Unacceptable PDX]

Z98.87- Personal history of in utero procedure

Z98.870 Personal history of in utero procedure during pregnancy — [♀] [Unacceptable PDX]
Excludes ❷: complications from in utero procedure for current pregnancy (O35.7)
supervision of current pregnancy with history of in utero procedure during previous pregnancy (O09.82-)

Z98.871 Personal history of in utero procedure while a fetus — [Unacceptable PDX]

Z98.89- Other specified postprocedural states

Z98.890 Other specified postprocedural states — [Unacceptable PDX]
Personal history of surgery, not elsewhere classified

Z98.891 History of uterine scar from previous surgery — [Unacceptable PDX]
Excludes 1: maternal care due to uterine scar from previous surgery (O34.2-)

Z99- Dependence on enabling machines and devices, not elsewhere classified
Excludes 1: cardiac pacemaker status (Z95.0)

Z99.0 Dependence on aspirator — [Unacceptable PDX]

Z99.1- Dependence on respirator
Dependence on ventilator

cc **Z99.11** Dependence on respirator [ventilator] status

cc **Z99.12** Encounter for respirator [ventilator] dependence during power failure
Excludes 1: mechanical complication of respirator [ventilator] (J95.850)

Z99.2 Dependence on renal dialysis — [Unacceptable PDX]
Hemodialysis status
Peritoneal dialysis status
Presence of arteriovenous shunt for dialysis
Renal dialysis status NOS
Excludes 1: encounter for fitting and adjustment of dialysis catheter (Z49.0-)
Excludes ❷: noncompliance with renal dialysis (Z91.15)

Z99.3 Dependence on wheelchair — [Unacceptable PDX]
Wheelchair confinement status
Code first cause of dependence, such as:
Muscular dystrophy (G71.0)
Obesity (E66.-)

Z99.8- Dependence on other enabling machines and devices

Z99.81 Dependence on supplemental oxygen — [Unacceptable PDX]
Dependence on long-term oxygen

Z99.89 Dependence on other enabling machines and devices — [Unacceptable PDX]
Dependence on machine or device NOS

Z
9
9
-
Z
9
9

NOTES

NOTES

NOTES

NOTES

NOTES

NOTES

NOTES

NOTES

[   ]

NOTES

NOTES

NOTES

[   ]

NOTES